W9-DBL-663

Textbook of **Pediatric Infectious Diseases**

FIFTH EDITION

Textbook of Pediatric Infectious Diseases

VOLUME 2

Ralph D. Feigin, M.D.

J. S. Abercrombie Professor and Chairman, Department of Pediatrics, and Distinguished Service Professor, Baylor College of Medicine
Physician-in-Chief, Texas Children's Hospital
Physician-in-Chief, Service of Pediatrics, Ben Taub General Hospital
Chief, Pediatric Service, The Methodist Hospital
Houston, Texas

James D. Cherry M.D., M.Sc.

Professor of Pediatrics
David Geffen School of Medicine at UCLA
Member, Division of Infectious Diseases
Mattel Children's Hospital at UCLA
Los Angeles, California

Gail J. Demmler, M.D.

Professor, Department of Pediatrics
Baylor College of Medicine
Director, Diagnostic Virology Laboratory
Texas Children's Hospital
Houston, Texas

Sheldon L. Kaplan, M.D.

Professor and Vice-Chairman of Clinical Affairs, Department of Pediatrics
Baylor College of Medicine
Chief, Infectious Disease Service
Texas Children's Hospital
Houston, Texas

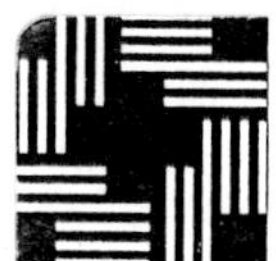

SAUNDERS
An Imprint of Elsevier Science

SAUNDERS
An Imprint of Elsevier Science

The Curtis Center
Independence Square West
Philadelphia, Pennsylvania 19106

Volume 1: Part no. 9997620194
Volume 2: Part no. 9997620208
Two-volume set ISBN 0-7216-9329-6

TEXTBOOK OF PEDIATRIC INFECTIOUS DISEASES

Notice

Pharmacology is an ever-changing field. Standard safety precautions must be followed, but as new research and clinical experience broaden our knowledge, changes in treatment and drug therapy may become necessary or appropriate. Readers are advised to check the most current product information provided by the manufacturer of each drug to be administered to verify the recommended dose, the method and duration of administration, and contraindications. It is the responsibility of the treating physician, relying on experience and knowledge of the patient, to determine dosages and the best treatment for each individual patient. Neither the Publisher nor the editor assumes any liability for any injury and/or damage to persons or property arising from this publication.

The Publisher

Library of Congress Cataloging-in-Publication Data

Textbook of pediatric infectious diseases/[edited by] Ralph D. Feigin... [et al.].-- 5th ed.
p.; cm.
Includes bibliographical references and index.
ISBN 0-7216-9329-6
1. Communicable diseases in children. I. Feigin, Ralph D.
[DNLM: 1. Communicable diseases—Child. 2. Pediatrics—methods. WC 100 T355 2004]
RJ401 .T49 2004
618.92′9—dc21 2002026835

Acquisitions Editor: Judy Fletcher
Developmental Editor: Melissa Dudlick
Project Manager: Lee Ann Draud

Printed in the United States of America

Last digit is the print number: 9 8 7 6 5 4 3 2 1

To our spouses—
Judith Feigin, Jeanne Cherry, Richard Demmler, and Marsha Kaplan.

our children—
Susan Feigin Harris and Jonathan Harris, Michael and Barbara Feigin, Debra Feigin Sukin and Steven Sukin; James Cherry, Jeffrey Cherry and Kass Hogan, Susan Cherry, Kenneth Cherry and Jennifer Carbry; Emily, Matthew, Amy, and Anna Rose Demmler; and Lauren Kaplan, Mindy Kaplan Langland and Lance Langland

and our grandchildren—
Rebecca and Sarah Harris, Matthew and Rachel Feigin, Jacob Sukin, and Ferguson and Dennis Carbry

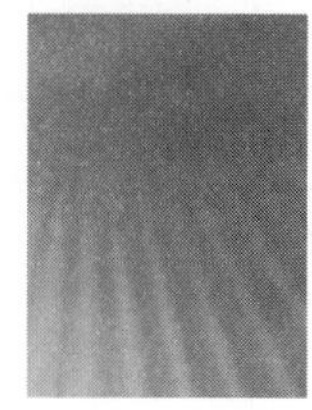

CONTRIBUTORS

John G. Aaskov, Ph.D., F.R.C.Path.
Senior Lecturer, School of Life Sciences, Queensland University of Technology, Brisbane, Australia
Ross River Virus Arthritis; Murray Valley Encephalitis

Susan M. Abdel-Rahman, Pharm.D.
Associate Professor, Department of Pediatrics, University of Missouri—Kansas City, School of Medicine; Director, Developmental Pharmacokinetic and Pharmacodynamic Core Lab, Pediatric Clinical Pharmacology and Medical Toxicology, Children's Mercy Hospital and Clinics, Kansas City, Missouri
The Pharmacokinetic-Pharmacodynamic Interface: Determinants of Anti-infective Drug Action and Efficacy in Pediatrics

Walid Abuhammour, M.D.
Associate Professor of Pediatrics, Department of Pediatric Infectious Diseases, Michigan State University College of Human Medicine; Associate Professor of Pediatrics, Department of Pediatric Infectious Diseases, Hurley Medical Center, East Lansing, Michigan
Antimicrobial Prophylaxis

Cristoph Aebi, M.D.
Head, Pediatric Infectious Diseases Unit, Department of Pediatrics and Institute for Infectious Diseases, University of Bern, Bern, Switzerland
Tick-Borne Encephalitis

Joshua J. Alexander, M.D.
Assistant Professor of Physician Medicine and Rehabilitation and Pediatrics, University of North Carolina at Chapel Hill School of Medicine, Chapel Hill, North Carolina
Otitis Externa

Marvin E. Ament, M.D.
Distinguished Professor of Pediatrics and Chief, Division of Gastroenterology and Nutrition, David Geffen School of Medicine at UCLA, Los Angeles, California
Esophagitis

Donald C. Anderson, M.D.
Adjunct Professor of Pediatrics, Baylor College of Medicine, Houston, Texas; Senior Vice President and Chief Scientific Officer, Adaptive Therapeutics, La Solla, California
Pneumocystis carinii Pneumonia

Marsha S. Anderson, M.D.
Assistant Professor, Department of Pediatrics, University of Colorado School of Medicine; Director of Inpatient Medicine, Children's Hospital, Denver, Colorado
Meningococcal Disease

Stephen S. Arnon, M.D.
Founder and Chief, Infant Botulism Treatment and Prevention Program, California Department of Health Services, Berkeley, California
Infant Botulism

Ann M. Arvin, M.D.
Lucille Packard Professor, Department of Pediatrics and Microbiology and Immunology, Stanford University School of Medicine; Chief, Infectious Disease Service, Lucille Packard Children's Hospital, Stanford, California
Herpes Simplex Viruses 1 and 2

Jane T. Atkins, M.D.
Department of Pediatrics, University of Texas—Houston Medical School, Houston, Texas
Cryptosporidiosis, Cyclospora Infection, Isosporiasis, and Microsporidiosis

Robert L. Atmar, M.D.
Associate Professor, Department of Medicine, Molecular Virology, and Microbiology, Baylor College of Medicine; Chairman, Infection Control, Ben Taub General Hospital, Houston, Texas
Rhinoviruses

Carol J. Baker, M.D.
Professor and Texas Children's Hospital Foundation Chair in Pediatric Infectious Diseases, Department of Pediatrics, Molecular Virology, and Microbiology, Baylor College of Medicine; Attending Physician, Infectious Diseases Section, Texas Children's Hospital; Medical Director of Infection Control, Women's Hospital of Texas, Houston, Texas
Cervical Lymphadenitis; Group B Streptococcal Infections

Stephen J. Barenkamp, M.D.
Professor of Pediatrics and Molecular Microbiology, Department of Pediatrics, St. Louis University School of Medicine; Director, Division of Pediatric Infectious Diseases, Cardinal Glennon Children's Hospital, St. Louis, Missouri
Other *Haemophilus* Species

Elizabeth D. Barnett, M.D.
Associate Professor of Pediatrics, Boston University School of Medicine; Department of Pediatrics, Boston Medical Center, Boston, Massachusetts
Malaria

Robert D. Basow, M.D.
Community Preceptor Attending, Department of Community Pediatrics, University of Massachusetts Medical Center, Worcester, Massachusetts
Streptobacillus moniliformis (Rat-Bite Fever); *Spirillum minus* (Rat-Bite Fever)

William R. Beisel, M.D., F.A.C.P.
Adjunct Professor (retired), W. Harry Feinstone Department of Molecular Mirobiology and Immunology, Johns Hopkins School of Hygiene and Public Health, Baltimore, Maryland
Metabolic Response of the Host to Infections

Beth P. Bell, M.D., M.P.H.
Chief, Epidemiology Branch, Division of Viral Hepatitis, National Center for Infectious Diseases, Centers for Disease Control and Prevention, Atlanta, Georgia
Hepatitis A Virus

Gil Benard, M.D., Ph.D.
Medical Researcher, Clinical and Experimental Allergy and Immunology Laboratory, Medical School of the University of São Paulo, São Paulo, Brazil
Paracoccidioidomycosis

David I. Bernstein, M.D.
Professor, Department of Pediatrics, University of Cincinnati; Director, Division of Infectious Diseases, Cincinnati Children's Hospital, Cincinnati, Ohio
Rotaviruses

Charles D. Bluestone, M.D.
Eberly Professor of Pediatric Otolaryngology, Department of Otolaryngology, University of Pittsburgh School of Medicine; Director, Department of Pediatric Otolaryngology, Children's Hospital of Pittsburgh, Pittsburgh, Pennsylvania
Otitis Media

Michael D. Blum, M.D.
Assistant Vice President, Global Safety Surveillance and Epidemiology, Wyeth Research, Collegeville, Pennsylvania
Aspergillus Infections

Jeffrey L. Blumer, Ph.D., M.D.
Professor, Department of Pediatrics and Pharmacology, Case Western Reserve University; Chief, Department of Pediatric Pharmacology and Critical Care, Rainbow Babies and Children's Hospital, Cleveland, Ohio
Antibiotic Resistance

Robert Bortolussi, M.D., F.R.C.P.C.
Professor of Pediatrics, Department of Pediatrics and Microbiology and Immunology, Dalhousie University Faculty of Medicine; Chief of Research, IWK Health Centre, Halifax, Nova Scotia, Canada
Listeriosis

Thomas G. Boyce, M.D., M.P.H.
Assistant Professor of Pediatrics, Mayo Medical School; Consultant, Pediatric Infectious Diseases, Mayo Clinic, Rochester, Minnesota
Miscellaneous Gram-Positive Cocci; *Erysipelothrix rhusiopathiae;* Miscellaneous Gram-Positive Bacilli; *Citrobacter; Enterobacter; Klebsiella; Morganella morganii; Proteus; Providencia; Serratia;* Miscellaneous Enterobacteria; *Vibrio vulnificus;* Miscellaneous Non-Enterobacteriaceae Fermentative Bacilli; *Achromobacter* (*Alcaligenes*); *Eikenella corrodens; Chryseobacterium (Flavobacterium)*

Kenneth M. Boyer, M.D.
Women's Board Professor of Pediatrics, Rush Medical College of Rush University; Chairman, Department of Pediatrics, Rush Children's Hospital, Chicago, Illinois
Nonbacterial Pneumonia; *Borrelia* (Relapsing Fever); Toxoplasmosis

John S. Bradley, M.D.
Director, Division of Infectious Diseases, Children's Hospital and Health Center, San Diego, California
Peritonitis and Intra-abdominal Abscess; Retroperitoneal Infections; Outpatient Intravenous Antibiotic Therapy for Serious Infections

Michael T. Brady, M.D.
Professor and Vice Chair for Clinical Affairs, Department of Pediatrics, Ohio State University College of Medicine and Public Health; Associate Medical Director, Department of Pediatrics, Children's Hospital, Columbus, Columbus, Ohio
Pseudomonas and Related Genera

Kathryn Brady-McCreery, M.D.
Assistant Professor, Baylor College of Medicine; Staff Pediatric Ophthalmologist, Texas Children's Hospital, Houston, Texas
Ocular Infectious Diseases

William J. Britt, M.D.
Charles A. Alford Professor of Pediatrics, Professor of Pediatrics, Microbiology, and Neurology, University of Alabama School of Medicine; Attending Physician, Children's Hospital of Alabama and University of Alabama Hospitals, Birmingham, Alabama
Transmissible Spongiform Encephalopathies (Creutzfeldt-Jakob Disease, Gertsmann-Sträussler-Scheinker Disease, Kuru, Fatal Familial Insomnia, New Variant Creutzfeldt-Jakob Disease)

Annemarie Broderick, M.B., B.Ch., M.R.C.P.I.
Fellow, Combined Program in Pediatric Gastroenterology and Nutrition, Department of Pediatrics, Harvard Medical School; Fellow, Combined Program in Pediatric Gastroenterology and Nutrition, Department of Pediatric Gastroenterology and Nutrition, Children's Hospital, Boston; Fellow, Combined Program in Pediatric Gastroenterology and Nutrition; Department of Pediatric Gastroenterology, Massachusetts General Hospital, Boston, Massachusetts
Hepatitis B and D Viruses

David A. Bruckner, Sc.D.
Chief, Division of Laboratory Medicine, Department of Pathology and Laboratory Medicine, David Geffen School of Medicine at UCLA; Chief Operating Officer, Clinical Laboratories, UCLA Hospital Systems, Los Angeles, California
Nomenclature for Aerobic and Anaerobic Bacteria

Carrie L. Byington, M.D.
Associate Professor, Department of Pediatrics and Infectious Diseases, University of Utah, Salt Lake City, Utah
Streptobacillus moniliformis (Rat-Bite Fever); *Spirillum minus* (Rat-Bite Fever)

Judith R. Campbell, M.D.
Associate Professor, Pediatrics/Infectious Diseases Section, Baylor College of Medicine; Attending Physician, Texas Children's Hospital, Houston, Texas
Parotitis; Peritonitis and Intra-abdominal Abscess

Thomas S. Carothers, M.D.
Pediatric Ophthalmology and Adult Strabismus, Virginia Eye Institute, Richmond, Virginia
Ocular Infectious Diseases

Mariam R. Chacko, M.D.
Associate Professor, Department of Pediatrics, and Medical Director, Baylor Teen Health Clinics, Baylor College of Medicine; Attending Physician, Texas Children's Hospital, Houston, Texas
Genital Infections in Childhood and Adolescence; *Calymmatobacterium granulomatis; Trichomonas* Infections

Louisa E. Chapman, M.D.
Assistant to the Director for Biological Therapeutics, Division of AIDS, STD, and TB Laboratory Research, National Center for Infectious Diseases, Centers for Disease Control and Prevention, Atlanta, Georgia
Hantaviruses

Rémi N. Charrel, M.D., Ph.D.
Unité des Virus Émergents, Faculté de Médecine, Université de la Mediterranée, Marseilles, France
Arenaviral Hemorrhagic Fevers; Filoviral Hemorrhagic Fever: Marburg and Ebola Virus Fevers

James D. Cherry, M.D., M.Sc.
Professor of Pediatrics, David Geffen School of Medicine at UCLA; Member, Division of Infectious Diseases, Mattel Children's Hospital at UCLA, Los Angeles, California
Epidemiology of Infectious Diseases; The Common Cold; Pharyngitis (Pharyngitis, Tonsillitis, Tonsillopharyngitis, and Nasopharyngitis); Herpangina; Pharyngoconjunctival Fever; Sinusitis; Mastoiditis; Epiglottitis (Supraglottitis); Croup (Laryngitis, Laryngotracheitis, Spasmodic Croup, Laryngotracheobronchitis, Bacterial Tracheitis, and Laryngotracheobronchopneumonitis); Acute Bronchitis; Aseptic Meningitis and Viral Meningitis; Encephalitis and Meningoencephalitis; Cutaneous Manifestations of Systemic Infections; Roseola Infantum (Exanthem Subitum); *Arcanobacterium haemolyticum;* Pertussis and Other *Bordetella* Infections; Tetanus; Human Parvoviruses B19; Adenoviruses; Smallpox (Variola Virus); Other Poxviruses; Enteroviruses and Parechoviruses; Reoviruses; Rubella Virus; Measles Virus; Mumps Virus; Severe Acute Respiratory Syndrome (SARS); *Mycoplasma* and *Ureaplasma* Infections; Use of the Diagnostic Virology Laboratory

P. Joan Chesney, M.D.
Professor of Pediatrics, Division of Infectious Diseases, University of Tennessee, Memphis, College of Medicine; Active Staff, Department of Pediatrics, Le Bonheur Children's Medical Center; Director, Office of Academic Programs, St. Jude Children's Research Hospital, Memphis, Tennessee
Toxic Shock Syndrome

Javier Chinen, M.D., Ph.D.
Staff Clinician, Genetic and Molecular Biology Branch, National Human Genome Research Institute—National Institutes of Health, Bethesda, Maryland
Primary Immunodeficiencies

Natascha Ching, M.D.
Clinical Instructor, Department of Pediatrics, David Geffen School of Medicine at UCLA; Attending Physician, Department of Pediatrics, Division of Pediatric Infectious Diseases, Mattel Children's Hospital at UCLA, Los Angeles, California
Mycoplasma and *Ureaplasma* Infections

H. Fred Clark, D.V.M., Ph.D.
Research Professor, Department of Pediatrics, University of Pennsylvania School of Medicine; Adjunct Professor, Wistar Institute, Philadelphia, Pennsylvania
Rabies Virus

John R. Clark, Jr., M.D.
Resident in Pediatrics, Department of Pediatrics, Baylor College of Medicine; Resident in Pediatrics, Department of Pediatrics, Texas Children's Hospital, Houston, Texas
Parotitis

Thomas G. Cleary, M.D.
Professor of Pediatrics, Department of Pediatrics, Pediatric Infectious Diseases Division, University of Texas—Houston Medical School; Professor of Pediatrics, Department of Pediatric Infectious Diseases, Memorial Hermann Children's Hospital, Houston, Texas
Approach to Patients with Gastrointestinal Tract Infections and Food Poisoning; *Bacillus cereus; Shigella; Salmonella; Vibrio parahaemolyticus; Campylobacter jejuni;* Cryptosporidiosis, *Cyclospora* Infection, Isosporiasis, and Microsporidiosis

David K. Coats, M.D.
Associate Professor of Ophthalmology and Pediatrics, Department of Ophthalmology, Baylor College of Medicine; Chief, Section of Pediatric Ophthalmology, Department of Pediatric Ophthalmology, Texas Children's Hospital, Houston, Texas
Ocular Infectious Diseases

Armando G. Correa, M.D.
Assistant Professor, Department of Pediatrics, Mayo Medical School; Senior Associate Consultant, Department of Pediatric and Adolescent Medicine, Mayo Clinic, Rochester, Minnesota
Coagulase-Positive Staphylococcal Infections *(Staphylococcus aureus); Acinetobacter;* Clostridial Intoxication and Infection

J. Thomas Cross, Jr., M.D., M.P.H.
Vice President, Education, MEDStudy Corporation, Colorado Springs, Colorado
Fungal Meningitis; Other Mycobacteria

Ronald Dagan, M.D.
Professor of Pediatrics and Infectious Diseases, Faculty of Health Sciences, Ben-Gurion University of the Negev; Director, Pediatric Infectious Disease Unit, Soroka University Medical Center, Beer-Sheva, Israel
Pneumococcal Infections

Adnan S. Dajani, M.D.
Professor Emeritus of Pediatrics, Wayne State University School of Medicine; Director Emeritus, Division of Infectious Diseases, Children's Hospital of Michigan, Detroit, Michigan
Antimicrobial Prophylaxis

Toni Darville, M.D.
Associate Professor of Pediatrics and Microbiology/Immunology, Department of Pediatrics, University of Arkansas for Medical Sciences, Little Rock, Arkansas
Nocardia

Jeffrey P. Davis, M.D.
Adjunct Professor, Departments of Pediatrics and Preventative Medicine, University of Wisconsin Medical School; Chief Medical Officer and State Epidemiologist for Communicable Diseases, Bureau of Public Health, Wisconsin Division of Health, Madison, Wisconsin
Toxic Shock Syndrome

Gail J. Demmler, M.D.
Professor, Department of Pediatrics, Baylor College of Medicine; Director, Diagnostic Virology Laboratory, Texas Children's Hospital, Houston, Texas
Hepatitis; Opportunistic Infections in Kidney Transplantation; Human Polyomaviruses and Papillomaviruses; Cytomegalovirus; Antiviral Agents

Penelope H. Dennehy, M.D.
Professor, Department of Pediatrics, Brown University School of Medicine; Associate Director, Department of Pediatric Infectious Diseases, Rhode Island Hospital, Providence, Rhode Island
Active Immunizing Agents

Jaime G. Deville, M.D
Assistant Clinical Professor, Department of Pediatrics, David Geffen School of Medicine at UCLA; Attending Physician, Department of Pediatrics, Mattel Children's Hospital at UCLA, Los Angeles, California
Sinusitis

Jan E. Drutz, M.D.
Professor, Department of Pediatrics, Baylor College of Medicine; Director, Residents' Primary Care Group Clinic, Department of Pediatrics, Texas Children's Hospital, Houston, Texas
Arthropods

Desmond F. Duff, M.B., F.R.C.P.I., F.A.A.P.
Consultant, Paediatric Cardiologist, Our Lady's Hospital for Sick Children, Dublin, Ireland
Myocarditis

Paul H. Edelstein, M.D.
Professor, Department of Pathology and Laboratory Medicine, University of Pennsylvania School of Medicine; Director of Clinical Microbiology, Hospital of the University of Pennsylvania, Philadelphia, Pennsylvania
Legionnaires' Disease, Pontiac Fever, and Related Illnesses

Kathryn M. Edwards, M.D.
Professor of Pediatrics, Department of Pediatrics, and Vice Chair for Clinical Research, Vanderbilt University School of Medicine; Attending Physician, Vanderbilt Children's Hospital, Nashville, Tennessee
Bartonella: Cat Scratch Disease

Morven S. Edwards, M.D.
Professor, Department of Pediatrics, Baylor College of Medicine; Attending Physician, Department of Pediatrics, Texas Children's Hospital and Ben Taub General Hospital, Houston, Texas
Mediastinitis; Anthrax; Rickettisal Diseases; Animal Bites

B. Keith English, M.D.
Professor, Department of Pediatrics, University of Tennessee Health Science Center and Children's Foundation Research Center; Division Chief, Department of Infectious Diseases, Le Bonheur Children's Medical Center, Memphis, Tennessee
Enterococcal and Viridans Streptococcal Infections

Leland L. Fan, M.D.
Professor, Department of Pediatrics, Baylor College of Medicine; Department of Pediatrics, Texas Children's Hospital, Houston, Texas
Chronic Interstitial Pneumonitis and Hypersensitivity Pneumonitis

Ralph D. Feigin, M.D.
J. S. Abercrombie Professor and Chairman, Department of Pediatrics, and Distinguished Service Professor, Baylor College of Medicine; Physician-in-Chief, Texas Children's Hospital; Physician-in-Chief, Service of Pediatrics, Ben Taub General Hospital; Chief, Pediatric Service, The Methodist Hospital, Houston Texas
Interaction of Infection and Nutrition; Otitis Externa; Bacterial Meningitis beyond the Neonatal Period; Fever without Source and Fever of Unknown Origin; Diphtheria; *Aeromonas;* Tularemia; Leptospirosis; Rickettsial Diseases

George D. Ferry, M.D.
Professor of Pediatrics, Department of Pediatrics, Baylor College of Medicine and Texas Children's Hospital; Department of Pediatrics, Ben Taub General Hospital, Houston, Texas
Antibiotic-Associated Colitis

Philip R. Fischer, M.D.
Profesor of Pediatrics and Consultant, Pediatric and Adolescent Medicine, Mayo Medical School and Mayo Clinic, Rochester, Minnesota
Schistosomiasis

Randall G. Fisher, M.D.
Assistant Professor of Pediatrics, Eastern Virginia Medical School; Medical Director, Division of Pediatric Infectious Diseases, and Attending Physician, Children's Hospital of the King's Daughters, Norfolk, Virginia
Miscellaneous Gram-Positive Cocci; *Erysipelothrix rhusiopathiae;* Miscellaneous Gram-Positive Bacilli; *Citrobacter; Enterobacter; Klebsiella; Morganella morganii; Proteus; Providencia; Serratia;* Miscellaneous Enterobacteria; *Vibrio vulnificus;* Miscellaneous Non-Enterobacteriaceae Fermentative Bacilli; *Achromobacter (Alcaligenes); Eikenella corrodens; Chryseobacterium (Flavobacterium)*

Patricia M. Flynn, M.D.
Professor, Departments of Pediatrics and Preventative Medicine, University of Tennessee, Memphis, College of Medicine; Member, Department of Infectious Diseases, St. Jude Children's Research Hospital, Memphis, Tennessee
Candidiasis

Thomas R. Flynn, D.M.D.
Assistant Professor of Oral and Maxillofacial Surgery, Department of Oral and Maxillofacial Surgery, and Director, Predoctoral Oral and Maxillofacial Surgery Education, Harvard School of Dental Medicine; Associate Visiting Surgeon, Department of Oral and Maxiollofacial Surgery, Massachusetts General Hospital; Associate Attending Physician, Department of Dentistry, Brigham and Women's Hospital, Boston, Massachusetts
Infections of the Oral Cavity

David W. Fraser, M.D.
Yardley, Pennsylvania
Public Health Considerations

Lisa M. Frenkel, M.D.
Associate Professor, Department of Pediatrics and Laboratory Medicine, University of Washington School of Medicine; Children's Hospital and Regional Medical Center, Seattle, Washington
Dientamoeba fragilis Infections

Richard A. Friedman, M.D., M.B.A.
Assistant Professor of Pediatrics, Baylor College of Medicine; Chief, Arrhythmia and Pacing Services, and Chief, Cardiology Clinic, Texas Children's Hospital, Houston, Texas
Infectious Pericarditis; Myocarditis

David R. Fulton, M.D.
Associate Professor of Pediatrics, Harvard Medical School; Chief, Cardiology Outpatient Services, and Senior Associate in Cardiology, Department of Cardiology, Children's Hospital, Boston, Boston, Massachusetts
Noninfectious Carditis

Lynne S. Garcia, M.S., M.T., F.A.A.M.
Director, LSG & Associates, Santa Monica, California
Classification and Nomenclature of Human Parasites

Michael A. Gerber, M.D.
Professor, Department of Pediatrics, University of Cincinnati College of Medicine; Attending Physician, Division of Infectious Diseases, Cincinnati Children's Hospital Medical Center, Cincinnati, Ohio
Group A, Group C, and Group G Beta-Hemolytic Streptococcal Infections

Anne A. Gershon, M.D.
Professor, Department of Pediatrics, Columbia University College of Physicians and Surgeons; Director, Division of Pediatric Infectious Diseases, Department of Pediatrics, Columbia University Medical Center, New York, New York
Varicella-Zoster Virus

Mark A. Gilger, M.D.
Associate Professor of Pediatrics, Department of Pediatrics—Gastroenterology, Baylor College of Medicine; Director, Gastrointestinal Procedures Suite, Texas Children's Hospital, Houston, Texas
Whipple Disease; *Helicobacter pylori*

Daniel G. Glaze, M.D.
Associate Professor, Department of Pediatrics and Neurology, and Medical Director, Blue Bird Circle Rett Center, Department of Pediatrics, Baylor College of Medicine; Medical Director, Texas Children's Hospital Sleep Disorders Center, Department of Neurophysiology, Texas Children's Hospital; Medical Director, The Methodist Hospital Sleep Disorders Center, Department of Neurophysiology, The Methodist Hospital, Houston, Texas
Guillain-Barré Syndrome

W. Paul Glezen, M.D.
Professor, Department of Molecular Virology and Microbiology, Department of Pediatrics, Baylor College of Medicine; Adjunct Professor, Department of Epidemiology, School of Public Health, University of Texas Health Science Center; Attending Pediatrician, Department of Pediatrics, Ben Taub General Hospital; Courtesy Staff, Infectious Diseases, Texas Children's Hospital, Houston, Texas
Influenza Viruses

Mary P. Glodé, M.D.
Professor of Pediatrics, University of Colorado Health Sciences Center; Vice-Chair, Department of Pediatrics, and Chief, Section of Pediatric Infectious Diseases, Children's Hospital and University of Colorado Health Sciences Center, Denver, Colorado
Meningococcal Disease

Donald A. Goldmann, M.D.
Professor of Pediatrics, Harvard Medical School; Hospital Epidemiologist, Division of Infectious Diseases, Children's Hospital, Boston, Boston, Massachusetts
Nosocomial Infections; Prevention and Control of Nosocomial Infections in Health Care Facilities That Serve Children

Ellie J. C. Goldstein, M.D.
Clinical Professor, David Geffen School of Medicine at UCLA, Los Angeles; Director, R. M. Alden Research Laboratory, Santa Monica, California
Human Bites

Maria D. Goldstein, M.D.
Associate Clinical Professor, Department of Pediatrics, University of New Mexico Medical School; District Health Officer, Public Health Division, New Mexico Department of Health, Albuquerque, New Mexico
Plague *(Yersinia pestis)*

Nira A. Goldstein, M.D.
Assistant Professor, Division of Pediatric Otolaryngology, State University of New York Downstate Medical Center; Attending Physician, Division of Pediatric Otolaryngology, University Hospital of Brooklyn, Long Island College Hospital, and Kings County Hospital Center, Brooklyn, New York
Peritonsillar, Retropharyngeal, and Parapharyngeal Abscesses

Edmond T. Gonzales, Jr., M.D.
Professor of Urology, Scott Department of Urology, Baylor College of Medicine; Head, Department of Surgery; Chief, Pediatric Urology Service, Texas Children's Hospital, Houston, Texas
Renal Abscess; Prostatitis

Blanca E. Gonzalez, M.D.
Postdoctoral Clinical Fellow, Department of Pediatrics, Section of Infectious Diseases, Baylor College of Medicine, Houston, Texas
Cholera

Howard P. Goodkin, M.D., Ph.D.
Assistant Professor of Neurology and Pediatrics, Department of Neurology, University of Virginia, Charlottesville, Virginia
Parameningeal Infections; Transverse Myelitis or Myelopathy

Simin Goral, M.D.
Associate Professor, Division of Nephrology, University of Pennsylvania Medical Center, Philadelphia, Pennsylvania
Bartonella: Cat-Scratch Disease

Michael Green, M.D., M.P.H.
Professor of Pediatrics and Surgery, Department of Pediatrics, University of Pittsburgh School of Medicine; Professor of Pediatrics and Surgery, Division of Allergy, Immunology, and Infectious Diseases, Children's Hospital of Pittsburgh, Pittsburgh, Pennsylvania
Opportunistic Infections in Liver Transplantation

David Greenberg, M.D.
Lecturer, Faculty of Health Sciences, Ben-Gurion University of the Negev; Senior Physician, Specialist in Pediatrics and Infectious Diseases, Soroka University Medical Center, Beer-Sheva, Israel
Pneumococcal Infections

Andreas H. Groll, M.D.
Head, Infectious Disease Research Program, Department of Pediatric Hematology/Oncology, University Children's Hospital, Muenster, Germany
Antifungal Agents

Charles Grose, M.D.
Professor, Departments of Pediatrics and Microbiology, University of Iowa College of Medicine; Professor and Director of Infectious Diseases, Department of Pediatrics, University of Iowa Hospital, Iowa City, Iowa
Pyomyositis and Bacterial Myositis; Human Herpesviruses 6, 7, and 8

William C. Gruber, M.D.
Vice President, Clinical Research, Wyeth Vaccines Research, Wyeth Research, Pearl River, New York
Miscellaneous Gram-Positive Cocci; *Erysipelothrix rhusiopathiae;* Miscellaneous Gram-Positive Bacilli; *Citrobacter; Enterobacter; Klebsiella; Morganella morganii; Proteus; Providencia; Serratia;* Miscellaneous Enterobacteria; *Vibrio vulnificus;* Miscellaneous Non-Enterobacteriaceae Fermentative Bacilli; *Achromobacter (Alcaligenes); Eikenella corrodens; Chryseobacterium (Flavobacterium)*

Duane J. Gubler, Sc.D.
Director, Division of Vector-Borne Infectious Diseases, Centers for Disease Control and Prevention, Fort Collins, Colorado
Yellow Fever

Roberto A. Guerrero, M.D.
Children's Gastroenterology of South Florida, P.A., West Palm Beach, Florida
Whipple Disease

Laura T. Gutman, M.D.
Duke University Medical Center, Durham, North Carolina
Syphilis

Caroline Breese Hall, M.D.
Professor of Pediatrics and Infectious Diseases in Medicine, Department of Pediatrics, University of Rochester, School of Medicine and Dentistry, Rochester, New York
Parainfluenza Viruses; Respiratory Syncytial Virus

Scott B. Halstead, M.D.
Adjunct Professor, Department of Preventive Medicine and Biometrics, Uniformed Services University of the Health Sciences, Bethesda, Maryland
Chikungunya; Dengue and Dengue Hemorrhagic Fever

Margaret R. Hammerschlag, M.D.
Professor, Department of Pediatrics and Medicine, and Director, Division of Pediatric Infectious Diseases, State University of New York Downstate Medical Center; Attending Physician, University Hospital of Brooklyn and Kings County Hospital Center, Brooklyn, New York
Peritonsillar, Retropharyngeal, and Parapharyngeal Abscesses; *Chlamydia* Infections

I. Celine Hanson, M.D.
Adjunct Professor, Department of Pediatrics, Baylor College of Medicine; Regional Medical Director, Texas Department of Health, Houston, Texas
Chronic Bronchitis; Lentiviruses (Human Immunodeficiency Virus Type I and the Acquired Immunodeficiency Syndrome)

Rick E. Harrison, M.D.
Professor of Clinical Pediatrics, Division of Critical Care, David Geffen School of Medicine at UCLA; Chief of Staff, UCLA Medical Center, Los Angeles, California
Tetanus

C. Mary Healy, M.D., M.R.C.P. (UK)
Clinical Postdoctoral Fellow, Department of Pediatrics, Section of Infectious Diseases, Baylor College of Medicine and Texas Children's Hospital, Houston, Texas
Cervical Lymphadenitis

Ulrich Heininger, M.D.
Professor of Pediatrics, University of Basel Medical School; Chair, Division of Pediatric Infectious Diseases and Vaccines, University Children's Hospital, Basel, Switzerland
Pertussis and Other *Bordetella* Infections

Gloria P. Heresi, M.D.
Associate Professor, Department of Pediatrics, Pediatric Infectious Diseases Division, University of Texas—Houston Medical School; Associate Professor, Department of Pediatrics, Memorial Hermann Children's Hospital, Houston, Texas
Campylobacter jejuni

Paula M. Hertel, M.D.
Postdoctoral Fellow, Department of Pediatric Gastroenterology and Nutrition, Baylor College of Medicine; Postdoctoral Fellow, Department of Pediatric Gastroenterology and Nutrition, Texas Children's Hospital, Houston, Texas
Diphtheria

Peter W. Hiatt, M.D.
Associate Professor, Department of Pediatrics, Baylor College of Medicine; Attending Faculty, Texas Children's Hospital, Houston, Texas
Cystic Fibrosis; Adult Respiratory Distress Syndrome in Children

Harry R. Hill, M.D.
Professor of Pathology, Pediatrics, and Medicine, Department of Pathology, University of Utah Salt Lake City, Salt Lake City, Utah
Immunomodulating Agents

Ellis K. L. Hon, M.B.B.S., F.A.A.P.
Assistant Professor, Department of Paediatrics, Chinese University of Hong Kong; Honorary Medical Officer, Prince of Wales Hospital, Shatin, Hong Kong, China
Severe Acute Respiratory Syndrome (SARS)

Margaret K. Hostetter, M.D.
Chair, Department of Pediatrics, and Professor of Pediatrics and Microbiology, Yale University School of Medicine; Physician-in-Chief, Yale–New Haven Children's Hospital, New Haven, Connecticut
Infectious Disease Problems of International Adoptees and Refugees

Peter J. Hotez, M.D., Ph.D.
Professor and Chair, Department of Microbiology and Tropical Medicine, George Washington University; Senior Fellow, Sabin Vaccine Institute, Washington, DC
Amebiasis; *Blastocystis hominis* Infection; *Entamoeba coli* Infection; *Balantidium coli* Infection; Parasitic Nematode Infections; Drugs for Parasitic Infections

Dexter H. Howard, Ph.D.
Professor Emeritus of Microbiology and Immunology, Department of Microbiology, Immunology, and Molecular Genetics, David Geffen School of Medicine at UCLA; Consultant in Medical Mycology, Department of Microbiology, UCLA Clinical Laboratories, Los Angeles, California
Classification of Fungi

Walter T. Hughes, M.D.
Professor, Department of Pediatrics, University of Tennessee, Memphis, College of Medicine; Emeritus Member, Department of Infectious Diseases, St. Jude Children's Research Hospital, Memphis, Tennessee
Candidiasis; Cryptococcosis; *Pneumocystis carinii* Pneumonia

David A. Hunstad, M.D.
Instructor, Departments of Pediatrics and Molecular Microbiology, Washington University School of Medicine; Attending Physician, Department of Pediatrics, St. Louis Children's Hospital, St. Louis, Missouri
Molecular Determinants of Microbial Pathogenesis

Eugene S. Hurwitz, M.D.
Clinical Assistant Professor, Department of Pediatrics, Emory University School of Medicine; Respiratory Disease Management Associates, LLC, Atlanta, Georgia
Reye Syndrome

W. Charles Huskins, M.D., M.Sc.
Assistant Professor, Department of Pediatrics, Mayo Medical School; Consultant, Department of Pediatric and Adolescent Medicine, Division of Pediatric Infectious Diseases, Mayo Clinic, Rochester, Minnesota
Nosocomial Infections; Prevention and Control of Nosocomial Infections in Health Care Facilities That Serve Children

Mary Anne Jackson, M.D.
Professor of Pediatrics, University of Missouri—Kansas City School of Medicine; Chief, Pediatric Infectious Diseases Section, Children's Mercy Hospitals and Clinics, Kansas City, Missouri
Skin Infections

Michael R. Jacobs, M.B., B.Ch., Ph.D.
Professor of Pathology, Case Western Reserve University; Director of Clinical Microbiology, University Hospitals of Cleveland, Cleveland, Ohio
Pneumococcal Infections

Richard F. Jacobs, M.D.
Horace C. Cabe Professor of Pediatrics, Department of Pediatrics, University of Arkansas for Medical Sciences; Chief, Pediatric Infectious Diseases, Arkansas Children's Hospital, Little Rock, Arkansas
Pleural Effusions and Empyema; Lung Abscess; Fungal Meningitis; Other Mycobacteria; *Nocardia; Actinobacillus actinomycetemcomitans;* Actinomycosis

Ravi Jhaveri, M.D.
Associate, Division of Infectious Diseases, Department of Pediatrics, Duke University Medical Center, Durham, North Carolina
Cutaneous Manifestations of Systemic Infections

Maureen M. Jonas, M.D.
Associate Professor, Department of Pediatrics, Harvard Medical School; Associate in Gastroenterology, Department of Medicine, Children's Hospital Boston, Boston, Massachusetts
Hepatitis B and D Viruses; Hepatitis C Virus

Edward L. Kaplan, M.D.
Professor of Pediatrics, Department of Pediatrics, University of Minnesota Medical School; Attending Physician, Department of Pediatrics, Fairview University Medical Center, Minneapolis, Minnesota
Group A, Group C, and Group G Beta-Hemolytic Streptococcal Infections

Sheldon L. Kaplan, M.D.
Professor and Vice-Chairman of Clinical Affairs, Department of Pediatrics, Baylor College of Medicine; Chief, Infectious Disease Service, Texas Children's Hospital, Houston, Texas
Infectious Pericarditis; Renal Abscess; Prostatitis; Pyogenic Liver Abscess; Bacteremia and Septic Shock; Infection in Pediatric Heart Transplant Recipients; Diarrhea- and Dysentery-Causing *Escherichia coli;* Public Health Considerations; Use of the Bacteriology, Mycology, and Parasitology Laboratories

Saul J. Karpen, M.D., Ph.D.
Associate Professor, Department of Pediatrics, Baylor College of Medicine; Director, Texas Children's Liver Center, Houston, Texas
Cholangitis and Cholecystitis

Michael Katz, M.D.
Reuben S. Carpentier Professor Emeritus of Pediatrics, Department of Pediatrics, Columbia University College of Physicians and Surgeons; Consulant Emeritus, Department of Pediatrics, New York–Presbyterian Hospital, New York; Senior Vice President for Research and Global Programs, March of Dimes Birth Defects Foundation, White Plains, New York
Parasitic Nematode Infections

Gregory L. Kearns, Pharm.D., Ph.D.
Professor, Department of Pediatrics and Pharmacology, University of Missouri—Kansas City, School of Medicine; Division Chief, Pediatric Clinical Pharmacology and Medical Toxicology, Children's Mercy Hospital and Clinics, Kansas City, Missouri
The Pharmacokinetic-Pharmacodynamic Interface: Determinants of Anti-infective Drug Action and Efficacy in Pediatrics

Margaret A. Keller, M.D.
Professor, Department of Pediatrics, University of California, Los Angeles, Harbor-UCLA Medical Center; Director, Program for Pediatric HIV/AIDS, and Attending Physician, Department of Pediatrics, Harbor-UCLA Medical Center; Acting Chief, Pediatric Infectious Diseases, Department of Pediatrics, Harbor-UCLA Medical Center, Torrance, California
Passive Immunization

Gerald T. Keusch, M.D.
Associate Director for International Research and Director, Fogarty International Center, National Institutes of Health, Bethesda, Maryland
Diarrhea- and Dysentery-Causing *Escherichia coli;* Cholera

Martin B. Kleiman, M.D.
Ryan White Professor of Pediatrics, Indiana University School of Medicine; Director, Pediatric Infectious Diseases, Department of Pediatrics, James Whitcomb Riley Hospital for Children, Indianapolis, Indiana
Histoplasmosis

Jerome O. Klein, M.D.
Professor of Pediatrics, Boston University School of Medicine; Vice-Chairman for Academic Affairs, Department of Pediatrics, Boston Medical Center, Boston, Massachusetts
Otitis Media; Bacterial Pneumonias

Mark W. Kline, M.D.
Professor of Pediatrics, Head, Section of Retrovirology, Baylor College of Medicine; Attending Physician, Texas Children's Hospital, Houston, Texas
Primary Immunodeficiences

Heidi M. Kokkinos, M.T. (ASCP), B.S.
Core Technologist, Mycology Laboratory, University of California, Los Angeles; Clinical Laboratory Scientist, Department of Pathology and Laboratory Medicine, UCLA Medical Center, Los Angeles, California
Classification of Fungi

Peter J. Krause, M.D.
Professor, Department of Pediatrics, University of Connecticut School of Medicine, Farmington; Director of Infectious Diseases, Department of Pediatrics, Connecticut Children's Medical Center, Hartford, Connecticut
Babeisosis

Leonard R. Krilov, M.D.
Professor of Pediatrics, Department of Pediatrics, State University of New York at Stony Brook School of Medicine, Stony Brook; Chief, Pediatric Infectious Diseases, Department of Pediatrics, Winthrop University Hospital, Mineola, New York
Chronic Fatigue Syndrome

Paul Krogstad, M.D.
Associate Professor, Departments of Pediatrics and Molecular and Medical Pharmacology, David Geffen School of Medicine at UCLA, Los Angeles, California
Osteomyelitis and Septic Arthritis

Thomas L. Kuhls, M.D.
Chief, Department of Pediatrics, Norman Regional Hospital, Norman, Oklahoma
Appendicitis and Pelvic Abscess; Pancreatitis; *Kingella* Species

Timothy R. La Pine, M.D.
Adjunct Professor of Pathology and Pediatrics, Department of Pathology, University of Utah School of Medicine, Salt Lake City, Utah
Immunomodulating Agents

Ching C. Lau, M.D., Ph.D.
Assistant Professor, Department of Pediatrics, Division of Hematology-Oncology, Baylor College of Medicine; Attending Physician, Texas Children's Cancer Center, Texas Children's Hospital, Houston, Texas
Tularemia

Charles T. Leach, M.D.
Professor, Department of Pediatrics, and Chief, Division of Infectious Diseases, University of Texas Health Science Center at San Antonio; Attending Physician, Department of Pediatrics, Christus Santa Rosa Children's Hospital and University Hospital, San Antonio, Texas
Epstein-Barr Virus

Robert J. Leggiadro, M.D.
Professor, Department of Pediatrics, University of Medicine and Dentistry of New Jersey, Robert Wood Johnson Medical School, Newark; Vice Chairman, Department of Pediatrics, Hackensack University Medical Center, Hackensack, New Jersey
Other *Campylobacter* Species; Bioterrorism

Diana Lennon, M.B., Ch.B., F.R.A.C.P.
Professor of Population Health, Child, and Youth, Department of Paediatrics, University of Auckland; Paediatrician in Infectious Diseases, Department of Paediatrics, Starship Children's Hospital, Auckland, New Zealand
Acute Rheumatic Fever

Chi Wai Leung, M.B.B.S., F.R.C.P.C.H., F.R.C.P. (Edin.)
Consultant Paediatrician, Department of Paediatrics and Adolescent Medicine, Princess Margaret Hospital; Honorary Clinical Associate Professor of Paediatrics, University of Hong Kong, Hong Kong, China
Severe Acute Respiratory Syndrome (SARS)

Karen Lewis, M.D.
Physician Trainer, Office of Bioterrorism, Arizona Department of Health Sciences, Phoenix, Arizona
Mastoiditis

Albert M. Li, M.B.Bch., M.R.C.P. (UK)
Assistant Professor, Department of Paediatrics, Chinese University of Hong Kong, Honorary Medical Officer, Prince of Wales Hospital, Shatin, Hong Kong, China
Severe Acute Respiratory Syndrome (SARS)

Martin I. Lorin, M.D.
Professor, Department of Pediatrics, Baylor College of Medicine; Attending Physician, Texas Children's Hospital, Houston, Texas
Fever: Pathogenesis and Treatment; Fever without Source and Fever of Unknown Origin

Jorge Luján-Zilbermann, M.D.
Assistant Professor, Department of Pediatrics, Division of Infectious Diseases, University of South Florida College of Medicine; Attending Physician, Division of Pediatric Infectious Diseases, Tampa General Hospital, Tampa; Attending Physician, Division of Infectious Diseases, All Children's Hospital, St. Petersburg, Florida
Opportunistic Infections in Hematopoietic Stem Cell Transplantation

Timothy Mailman, M.D., F.R.C.P.C.
Assistant Professor, Department of Pediatrics, Dalhousie University Faculty of Medicine; Director of Microbiology, Department of Pediatrics, IWK Health Centre, Halifax, Nova Scotia, Canada
Listeriosis

Susan A. Maloney, M.D., M.H.Sc.
Chief Epidemiologist and Special Studies, Division of Global Migration and Quarantine, Centers for Disease Control and Prevention, Atlanta, Georgia
International Travel Issues for Children

Harold S. Margolis, M.D.
Director, Division of Viral Hepatitis, Centers for Disease Control and Prevention, Atlanta, Georgia
Hepatitis A Virus

Edward O. Mason, Jr., Ph.D.
Professor, Department of Pediatrics and Department of Virology and Microbiology, Baylor College of Medicine; Director, Infectious Disease Laboratory, Texas Children's Hospital, Houston, Texas
Use of the Bacteriology, Mycology, and Parasitology Laboratories; Use of the Serology Laboratory

David O. Matson, M.D., Ph.D.
Professor, Department of Pediatrics, Eastern Virginia Medical School; Attending Physician, Department of Infectious Diseases, Children's Hospital of The King's Daughters; Head, Department of Infectious Diseases Section, Center for Pediatric Research, Norfolk, Virginia
Caliciviruses and Hepatitis E Virus

Alan N. Mayer, M.D., Ph.D.
Instructor, Department of Pediatrics, Harvard Medical School; Assistant, Division of Gastroenterology, Children's Hospital, Boston, Massachusetts
Hepatitis C Virus

Marc A. Mazade, M.D.
Consultant, Department of Infectious Diseases, PID Associates, Dallas, Texas
Infections Related to Craniofacial Surgical Procedures

George H. McCracken, Jr., M.D.
Professor of Pediatrics, The GlaxoSmithKline Distinguished Professor of Pediatric Infectious Disease, and The Sarah M. and Charles E. Seay Chair in Pediatric Infectious Disease, University of Texas Southwestern Medical Center at Dallas; Attending Physician, Children's Medical Center of Dallas, Dallas, Texas
Perinatal Bacterial Diseases; Antibacterial Therapeutic Agents

Kenneth McIntosh, M.D.
Professor, Department of Pediatrics, Harvard Medical School; Senior Associate in Medicine, Division of Infectious Diseases, Children's Hospital, Boston, Boston, Massachusetts
Coronaviruses and Toroviruses

James E. McJunkin, M.D.
Professor, Department of Pediatrics, Robert C. Byrd Health Sciences Center, Charleston Division; Attending Physician, Charleston Area Medical Center, Charleston, West Virginia
La Crosse Encephalitis and Other California Serogroup Viruses

Kelly T. McKee, Jr., M.D.
Managing Research Physician, Camber Corporation, U.S. Army Medical Research Institute of Infectious Diseases, Fort Detrick, Maryland
Hantaviruses

Rima L. McLeod, M.D.
Jules and Doris Stein RPB Professor, Department of Visual Sciences, Pathology, Committees of Molecular Medicine, Genetics, and Immunology, University of Chicago; Attending Physician, Department of Medicine, University of Chicago Hospitals; Attending Physician, Department of Ophthalmology, Michael Reese Hospital and Medical Center, Chicago, Illinois
Toxoplasmosis

Wayne M. Meyers, M.D., Ph.D., D.Sc. (Hon)
Research Affiliate, Tulane Primate Research Center, Tulane University, Covington, Louisiana; Chief, Mycobacteriology Branch, and Registrar, Leprosy Registry, American Registry of Pathology, Armed Forces Institute of Pathology, Washington, DC
Leprosy and Buruli Ulcer: The Major Cutaneous Mycobacterioses

Ian C. Michelow, M.B.B.Ch., D.T.M.&H., F.C.Paed.(SA)
Instructor, Department of Pediatrics, Harvard Medical School; Assistant in Pediatrics, Department of Infectious Diseases, Massachusetts General Hospital, Boston, Massachusetts
Antibacterial Therapeutic Agents

James N. Miller, Ph.D.
Professor Emeritus on Recall, Department of Microbiology, Immunology, and Molecular Genetics, David Geffen School of Medicine at UCLA, Los Angeles, California
Nonvenereal Treponematoses

Marjorie J. Miller, Dr.P.H.
Senior Specialist, Clinical Laboratories—Microbiology, University of California Medical Center, Los Angeles, Los Angeles, California
Classification and Nomenclature of Viruses; Use of the Diagnostic Virology Laboratory

Linda L. Minnich, M.S.
Adjunct Assistant Professor, Robert C. Byrd Health Sciences Center, Charleston Division; Virologist, Charleston Area Medical Center, Charleston, West Virginia
La Crosse Encephalitis and Other California Serogroup Viruses

Sudipta Misra, M.D.
Assistant Professor, Department of Pediatrics, and Chief, Division of Gastroenterology, University of Illinois College of Medicine at Peoria, Peoria, Illinois
Esophagitis

Lynne M. Mofenson, M.D.
Chief, Pediatric Adolescent and Maternal AIDS Branch, National Institute of Child Health and Human Development, National Institutes of Health, Bethesda, Maryland
Oncoviruses (Human T-Cell Lymphotropic Viruses Types I and II) and Lentiviruses (Human Immunodeficiency Virus Type 2)

Edward A. Mortimer, Jr., M.D.*
University Professor Emeritus, Department of Epidemiology and Biostatistics, Case Western Reserve University, Cleveland, Ohio
Epidemiology of Infectious Diseases
*Deceased

James R. Murphy, Ph.D.
Professor, Department of Pediatrics, Pediatric Infectious Diseases, University of Texas—Houston Medical School, Houston, Texas
Campylobacter jejuni

Edmund A. S. Nelson, M.B.Ch.B., F.R.C.P.C.H., F.R.C.P. (UK)
Associate Professor, Department of Paediatrics, and affiliated member of the School of Public Health, Chinese University of Hong Kong; Honorary Consultant, Prince of Wales Hospital, Shatin, Hong Kong, China
Severe Acute Respiratory Syndrome (SARS)

Karin A. Nielsen, M.D., M.P.H.
Assistant Clinical Professor, Department of Pediatrics—Division of Infectious Diseases, David Geffen School of Medicine at UCLA; Attending Physician, Department of Pediatric Infectious Diseases, Mattel Children's Hospital of UCLA; Attending Physician, Maternal Child Immunology Clinic—HIV Medicine, UCLA Care Clinic, Los Angeles, California
Herpangina; Aseptic Meningitis and Viral Meningitis

Michael D. Nissen, B.Med.Sc, M.B.B.S., F.R.A.C.P., F.R.C.P.A.
Senior Lecturer, Department of Paediatrics and Child Health, University of Queensland School of Medicine; Director, Department of Infectious Diseases, Royal Children's Hospital, Herston, Queensland, Australia
Human Metapneumovirus: *Paramyxoviridae*

Christopher M. Oermann, M.D.
Assistant Professor, Department of Pediatrics, Baylor College of Medicine; Attending Faculty, Pulmonary Medicine Service, Texas Children's Hospital, Houston, Texas
Adult Respiratory Distress Syndrome in Children

Christian C. Patrick, M.D., Ph.D.
Chief of Staff and Senior Vice President for Medical Affairs, Miami Children's Hospital, Miami, Florida
Opportunistic Infections in Hematopoietic Stem Cell Transplantation; Coagulase-Negative Staphylococcal Infections

Evelyn A. Paysse, M.D.
Assistant Professor of Ophthalmology and Pediatrics, Department of Ophthalmology, Baylor College of Medicine; Active Staff, Department of Pediatric Ophthalmology and Strabismus, Texas Children's Hospital, Houston, Texas
Ocular Infectious Diseases

Eric Pearlman, M.D., Ph.D.
Assistant Professor, Department of Pediatrics, Mercer University School of Medicine (Savannah Campus); Staff Physician, Savannah Neurology, Savannah, Georgia
Bacterial Meningitis beyond the Neonatal Period

Georges Peter, M.D.
Professor of Pediatrics and Vice Chair for Faculty Affairs, Department of Pediatrics, Brown University School of Medicine; Director, Division of Pediatric Infectious Diseases, Department of Pediatrics, Rhode Island Hospital and Hasbro Children's Hospital, Providence, Rhode Island
Active Immunizing Agents

C. J. Peters, M.D.
John Sealy Distinguished University Chair in Tropical and Emerging Virology, Department of Microbiology and Immunology/Pathology, University of Texas Medical Branch, Galveston, Texas
Hantaviruses

Larry K. Pickering, M.D., F.A.A.P.
Professor of Pediatrics, Department of Pediatrics, Emory University School of Medicine; Senior Advisor to the Director, National Immunization Program, Centers for Disease Control and Prevention, Atlanta, Georgia
Approach to Patients with Gastrointestinal Tract Infections and Food Poisoning

Joseph F. Piecuch, D.M.D., M.D.
Clinical Professor, Department of Oral and Maxillofacial Surgery, University of Connecticut School of Dental Medicine, Farmington; Director, Oral and Maxillofacial Surgery Section, Hartford Hospital, Hartford, Connecticut
Infections of the Oral Cavity

Francisco P. Pinheiro, M.D., Ph.D.
Department of Arborivus, Instituto Evandro Chagas, Belém, Brazil
Oropouche Fever

Stanley A. Plotkin, M.D.
Emeritus Professor, Department of Pediatrics, University of Pennsylvania School of Medicine, Philadelphia; Medical and Scientific Advisor, Aventis Pasteur, Swiftwater, Pennsylvania
Rabies Virus

Scott L. Pomeroy, M.D., Ph.D.
Associate Professor, Department of Neurology, Harvard Medical School; Senior Associate, Department of Neurology, Children's Hospital, Boston, Massachusetts
Parameningeal Infections; Transverse Myelitis or Myelopathy

Alice Pong, M.D.
Department of Pediatric Infectious Diseases, Children's Hospital and Health Center, San Diego, California
Retroperitoneal Infections

Joan S. Purcell, M.D., F.A.A.P.
Chair, Department of Pediatrics, The Woodlands Memorial Hospital; Vice President, Step Pediatrics, The Woodlands, Texas
Trichomonas Infections

Jack S. Remington, M.D.
Palo Alto Medical Foundation, Palo Alto, California
Toxoplasmosis

Angela Restrepo-Moreno, Ph.D.
Senior Researcher, Medical and Experimental Mycology Group, Corporación para Investigaciones Biológicas (CIB), Medellín, Colombia
Paracoccidioidomycosis

Carina A. Rodriguez, M.D.
Postdoctoral Fellow, University of Tennessee, Memphis, College of Medicine, and Department of Infectious Diseases, St. Jude Children's Research Hospital, Memphis, Tennessee
Coagulase-Negative Staphylococcal Infections

Judith L. Rowen, M.D.
Associate Professor, Department of Pediatrics, University of Texas Medical Branch, Galveston, Texas
Group B Streptococcal Infections; Miscellaneous Mycoses

Xavier Sáez-Llorens, M.D.
Professor of Pediatrics and Infectious Diseases, University of Panama School of Medicine; Vice-Chairman and Head of Infectious Diseases, Hospital del Niño, Panama City, Panama
Perinatal Bacterial Diseases

Lisa Saiman, M.D., M.P.H.
Associate Professor of Clinical Pediatrics, Department of Pediatrics, Columbia University College of Physicians and Surgeons; Associate Attending Pediatrician, Department of Pediatrics, and Hospital Epidemiologist, Department of Pediatrics and Epidemiology, Children's Hospital of New York, New York, New York
Cystic Fibrosis

Joseph W. St. Geme III, M.D.
Professor and Director of Pediatric Infectious Diseases, Department of Pediatrics and Molecular Microbiology, Washington University School of Medicine; Attending Physician, Department of Pediatrics, St. Louis Children's Hospital, St. Louis, Missouri
Molecular Determinants of Microbial Pathogenesis

Pablo J. Sánchez, M.D.
Professor, Department of Pediatrics, Division of Neonatal-Perinatal Medicine and Pediatric Infectious Diseases, University of Texas Southwestern Medical School; Professor of Pediatrics, Division of Neonatal-Perinatal Medicine and Pediatric Infectious Diseases, Parkland Health and Hospital Systems and Children's Medical Center of Dallas, Dallas, Texas
Viral Infections of the Fetus and Neonate; Syphilis

Carlos A. Sattler, M.D.
Associate Director, Biologics Clinical Research, Merck Research Laboratories, West Point, Pennsylvania
Coagulase-Positive Staphylococcal Infections *(Staphylococcus aureus); Stenotrophomonas (Xanthomonas) maltophilia*

Jane G. Schaller, M.D.
Karp Professor of Pediatrics Emerita, Department of Pediatrics, Tufts University School of Medicine; Chief, Division of Pediatric Rheumatology, Tufts–New England Medical Center, Boston, Massachusetts
Noninfectious Carditis

Kenneth O. Schowengerdt, Jr., M.D.
Associate Professor, Department of Pediatrics, University of Florida College of Medicine; Medical Director, Pediatric Heart Transplant Program, University of Florida and Shands Transplant Center, Gainesville, Florida
Myocarditis

Gordon E. Schutze, M.D.
Professor of Pediatrics and Pathology and Pediatric Program Director, Department of Pediatrics, University of Arkansas for Medical Sciences; Attending Physician, Arkansas Children's Hospital, Little Rock, Arkansas
Blastomycosis

James S. Seidel, M.D., Ph.D.*
Professor, Department of Pediatrics, David Geffen School of Medicine at UCLA, Los Angeles; Chief, Division of General and Emergency Pediatrics, Department of Emergency Medicine and Pediatrics, Harbor-UCLA Medical Center, Torrance, California
Giardiasis; *Naegleria, Acanthamoeba,* and *Balamuthia*
*Deceased

Alan M. Shapiro, M.D., Ph.D.
Fellow, Division of Pediatric Infectious Diseases, Department of Pediatrics, David Geffen School of Medicine at UCLA, Los Angeles, California
Arcanobacterium haemolyticum

Craig N. Shapiro, M.D.
Medical Epidemiologist, Division of Viral Hepatitis, National Center for Infectious Diseases, Centers for Disease Control and Prevention, Atlanta, Georgia
Hepatitis A Virus

Eugene D. Shapiro, M.D.
Professor of Pediatrics, Epidemiology, and Investigative Medicine, Departments of Pediatrics, Epidemiology, and Public Health and the Children's Clinical Research Center, Yale University School of Medicine; Attending Pediatrician, Children's Hospital at Yale–New Haven, New Haven, Connecticut
Epidemiology and Biostatistics

Nina L. Shapiro, M.D.
Assistant Professor, Division of Head and Neck Surgery, David Geffen School of Medicine at UCLA; Attending Physician, Division of Head and Neck Surgery, UCLA Medical Center, Los Angeles, California
Sinusitis; Mastoiditis

William T. Shearer, M.D., Ph.D.
Professor of Pediatrics and Immunology, Baylor College of Medicine; Chief, Allergy and Immunology Service, Texas Children's Hospital, Houston, Texas
Chronic Bronchitis; Primary Immunodeficiences; Lentiviruses (Human Immunodeficiency Virus Type I and the Acquired Immunodeficiency Syndrome)

Ziad M. Shehab, M.D.
Professor of Clinical Pediatrics and Pathology, University of Arizona College of Medicine; Section Chief, Pediatric Infectious Diseases, and Clerkship Director, Department of Pediatrics, University of Arizona Health Sciences Center; Department of Pediatrics, University Medical Center and Tucson Medical Center, Tucson; Department of Pediatrics, Maricopa Medical Center, Phoenix, Arizona
Coccidioidomycosis

Jerry L. Shenep, M.D.
Professor of Pediatrics, University of Tennessee Health Science Center; Member, Department of Infectious Diseases, St. Jude Children's Research Hospital, Memphis, Tennessee
Enterococcal and Viridans Streptococcal Infections

W. Donald Shields, M.D.
Chief of Pediatric Neurology, Department of Pediatrics, David Geffen School of Medicine at UCLA, Los Angeles, California
Encephalitis and Meningoencephalitis

Robert E. Shope, M.D.
Professor of Pathology, Center for Tropical Diseases, University of Texas Medical Branch, Galveston, Texas
Rift Valley Fever

Stanford T. Shulman, M.D.
Professor of Pediatrics, Department of Pediatrics, Feinberg School of Medicine, Northwestern University; Chief, Division of Infectious Diseases, Children's Memorial Hospital, Chicago, Illinois
Kawasaki Disease

Constantine Simos, D.M.D.
Visiting Assistant Professor, Department of Oral and Maxillofacial Surgery, Tufts University, Boston, Massachusetts; Active Staff, Department of Oral and Maxillofacial Surgery, Robert Wood Johnson University Hospital; Active Staff, Department of Oral and Maxillofacial Surgery, St. Peter's University Hospital, New Brunswick, New Jersey
Infections of the Oral Cavity

Arnold L. Smith, M.D.
Professor, Department of Pathobiology, University of Washington School of Public Health; Member, Department of Bacterial Pathogens, Seattle Biomedical Research Institute, Seattle, Washington
Meningococcal Disease

Kimberly C. Smith, M.D., M.P.H.
Associate Professor, Department of Pediatrics, University of Texas—Houston Medical School, Houston, Texas
Tuberculosis

Jason S. Soden, M.D.
Department of Pediatrics, Baylor College of Medicine, Houston, Texas
Cholangitis and Cholecystitis

Steven L. Solomon, M.D.
Chief, Healthcare Outcomes Branch, Division of Healthcare Quality Promotion, National Center for Infectious Diseases, Centers for Disease Control and Prevention, Atlanta, Georgia
Public Health Considerations

Mary A. Staat, M.D., M.P.H.
Associate Professor, Department of Pediatrics, University of Cincinnati College of Medicine; Associate Professor, Department of Pediatrics, Division of Infectious Diseases, Cincinnati Children's Hospital Medical Center, Cincinnati, Ohio
Genital Infections in Childhood and Adolescence

Jeffrey R. Starke, M.D.
Professor, Department of Pediatrics, Baylor College of Medicine; Chief, Department of Pediatrics, Ben Taub General Hospital, Houston, Texas
Infective Endocarditis; Tuberculosis

Barbara W. Stechenberg, M.D.
Professor, Department of Pediatrics, Tufts University School of Medicine, Boston; Vice Chair and Director, Pediatric Infectious Diseases, Department of Pediatrics, Baystate Medical Center Children's Hospital, Springfield, Massachusetts
Eosinophilic Meningitis; *Moraxella catarrhalis;* Diphtheria; *Pasteurella multocida;* Bartonellosis; *Borrelia* (Lyme Disease)

Leah A. Stephenson, M.D.
Department of Pediatrics, Baylor College of Medicine, Houston, Texas
Interaction of Infection and Nutrition

E. Richard Stiehm, M.D.
Professor of Pediatrics, Department of Pediatrics, David Geffen School of Medicine at UCLA; Attending Pediatrician, Mattel Children's Hospital at UCLA, Los Angeles, California
Passive Immunization

Alan D. Strickland, M.D.
Clute, Texas
Amebiasis

Ciro V. Sumaya, M.D., M.P.H.T.M.
Dean, School of Rural Public Health, Cox Endowed Chair in Medicine, and Professor, Department of Pediatrics, Texas A & M University System Health Science Center, College Station; Attending Physician, Scott and White Hospital and Clinic, Temple, Texas
Epstein-Barr Virus

Douglas S. Swanson, M.D.
Assistant Professor, Department of Pediatrics, University of Missouri—Kansas City School of Medicine; Pediatrician, Department of Pediatric Infectious Diseases, Children's Mercy Hospital and Clinics, Kansas City, Missouri
Indigenous Flora

Tina Tan, M.D.
Associate Professor, Department of Pediatrics, Feinberg School of Medicine, Northwestern University; Infectious Diseases Attending, Co-Director, Travel Medicine Clinic, and Director, International Adoptee Clinic, Children's Memorial Hospital, Chicago, Illinois
Infections Related to Prosthetic or Artificial Devices

Herbert B. Tanowitz, M.D., F.A.C.P.
Professor of Pathology and Medicine, Department of Pathology, Albert Einstein College of Medicine of Yeshiva University; Attending Physician, Department of Medicine, Weiler Hospital–Montefiore Medical Center; Attending Physician, Department of Medicine and Pathology, Jacobs Medical Center, Bronx, New York
Leishmaniasis; Trypanosomiasis

Robert B. Tesh, M.D.
George Dock Distinguished Professor of Pathology, Department of Pathology, University of Texas Medical Branch; Member, Center for Biodefense and Emerging Infectious Diseases, University of Texas Medical Branch, Galveston, Texas
Crimean-Congo Hemorrhagic Fever; Phlebotomus Fever (Sandfly Fever)

Philip Toltzis, M.D.
Associate Professor, Department of Pediatrics, Case Western Reserve University School of Medicine; Attending Physician, Division of Pediatric Pharmacology and Critical Care, Rainbow Babies and Children's Hospital, Cleveland, Ohio
Antibiotic Resistance

Richard G. Topazian, D.D.S.
Professor Emeritus, Department of Oral and Maxillofacial Surgery, University of Connecticut School of Dental Medicine, Farmington, Connecticut
Infections of the Oral Cavity

Michael F. Tosi, M.D.
Associate Professor of Pediatrics, Sections of Leukocyte Biology and Infectious Diseases, Baylor College of Medicine, Houston, Texas
Immunologic and Phagocytic Responses to Infection

Jeffrey A. Towbin, M.D.
Professor, Department of Pediatrics (Cardiology) and Molecular and Human Genetics, Baylor College of Medicine; Associate Chief, Pediatric Cardiology, Texas Children's Hospital; Medical Director, Pediatrics Heart Failure and Transplant Service, Texas Children's Hospital; Texas Children's Hospital Foundation Chair in Pediatric Cardiac Research, Texas Children's Hospital, Houston, Texas
Myocarditis

Amelia P. A. Travassos da Rosa, B.Sc.
Visiting Scientist, Department of Pathology, University of Texas Medical Branch, Galveston, Texas
Oropouche Fever

Theodore F. Tsai, M.D., M.P.H.
Senior Director of Medical Affairs, Vaccines Division, Wyeth, Collegeville, Pennsylvania
Orbiviruses and Coltiviruses; Eastern Equine Encephalitis; Western Equine Encephalitis; Venezuelan Equine Encephalitis; Other Alphaviral Infections; St. Louis Encephalitis; Japanese Encephalitis; Tick-Borne Encephalitis; Other Flaviviral Infections; La Crosse Encephalitis and Other California Serogroup Viruses

Jerrold A. Turner, M.D., F.A.C.P., D.T.M.&H.
Professor Emeritus of Clinical Medicine and Microbiology, Department of Immunology and Molecular Genetics, David Geffen School of Medicine at UCLA, Los Angeles; Director, Turner Parasitology, Carson, California
Cestodes; Trematodes

Xilla T. Ussery, M.D.
Associate Director, Clinical Development, Infectious Diseases, Pfizer Inc., New London, Connecticut
Other Anaerobic Infections

Jesus G. Vallejo, M.D.
Assistant Professor of Pediatrics and Medicine, Section of Infectious Disease and Winters Center for Heart Failure Research, Baylor College of Medicine; Attending Physician, Infectious Disease Service, Texas Children's Hospital, Houston, Texas
Myocarditis; Cholera

John A. Vanchiere, M.D., Ph.D.
Assistant Professor, Department of Pediatrics, Section of Infectious Diseases, Baylor College of Medicine, Houston, Texas
Human Polyomaviruses and Papillomaviruses

Pedro Fernando da C. Vasconcelos, M.D., Ph.D.
Chief, Department of Arbovirus, Instituto Evandro Chagas, Belém, Brazil
Oropouche Fever

Ellen R. Wald, M.D.
Professor of Pediatrics and Otolaryngology, Department of Pediatrics, University of Pittsburgh School of Medicine; Chief, Division of Allergy, Immunology, and Infectious Diseases, Department of Pediatrics, Children's Hospital, Pittsburgh, Pennsylvania
Uvulitis; Genitourinary Tract Infections; Infections in Daycare Environments

Thomas J. Walsh, M.D.
Senior Investigator and Chief, Immunocompromised Host Section, Pediatric Oncology Branch, National Cancer Institute, Bethesda, Maryland
Antifungal Agents

Joel I. Ward, M.D.
Professor, Department of Pediatrics, David Geffen School of Medicine at UCLA, Los Angeles; Director, UCLA Center for Vaccine Research, and Director, Hospital Infection Control, Department of Pediatrics, Harbor—UCLA Medical Center, Torrance, California
Haemophilus influenzae

Richard L. Ward, Ph.D.
Professor, Department of Infectious Diseases, Children's Hospital Medical Center, Cincinnati, Ohio
Rotaviruses

Michelle Weinberg, M.D., M.P.H.
Medical Epidemiologist, Division of Global Migration and Quarantine, Centers for Disease Control and Prevention, Atlanta, Georgia
International Travel Issues for Children

Robert C. Welliver, M.D.
Professor, Department of Pediatrics, State University of New York at Buffalo; Co-Director, Division of Infectious Diseases, Department of Pediatrics, Women's and Children's Hospital of Buffalo, Buffalo, New York
Bronchiolitis and Infectious Asthma

J. Gary Wheeler, M.D.
Professor of Pediatrics, Department of Pediatric Infectious Diseases, University of Arkansas for Medical Sciences; Attending Physician, Arkansas Children's Hospital, Little Rock, Arkansas
Pleural Effusions and Empyema; Lung Abscess

A. Clinton White, Jr., M.D.
Associate Professor, Infectious Disease Section, Department of Medicine, Baylor College of Medicine; Chief, Section of Infectious Diseases, Department of Medicine, Ben Taub General Hospital, Houston, Texas
Schistosomiasis

Suzanne Whitworth, M.D.
Department of Pediatric Infectious Diseases, Cook Children's Medical Center, Fort Worth, Texas
Actinobacillus actinomycetemcomitans; Actinomycosis

Bernhard L. Wiedermann, M.D.
Associate Professor and Vice Chair for Education, Department of Pediatrics, George Washington University School of Medicine and Health Sciences; Attending in Infectious Diseases and Director, Medical Education and Pediatric Residency Training Program, Children's National Medical Center, Washington, DC
Miscellaneous Causes of Myositis; *Aspergillus* Infections; Sporotrichosis; Zygomycosis

Murray Wittner, M.D.
Professor of Pathology and Parasitology, Department of Pathology, Albert Einstein College of Medicine of Yeshiva University; Attending Physician, Department of Medicine and Pathology, Montefiore Medical Center, Bronx, New York
Leishmaniasis; Trypanosomiasis

Charles R. Woods, Jr., M.D.
Associate Professor of Pediatrics, Wake Forest University School of Medicine; Attending Physician, Brenner Children's Hospital, Winston-Salem, North Carolina
Genital Infections in Childhood and Adolescence; Gonococcal Infections; Other *Yersinia* Species

Ram Yogev, M.D.
Professor, Department of Pediatrics, Feinberg School of Medicine, Northwestern University; Associate Division Head and Director, Section of Pediatric, Adolescent, and Maternal HIV Infection, Department of Infectious Diseases, Children's Memorial Hospital, Chicago, Illinois
Infections Related to Prosthetic or Artificial Devices

Edward J. Young, M.D.
Professor, Department of Medicine and Molecular Virology and Microbiology, Baylor College of Medicine; Staff Physician, Infectious Diseases Section, Veterans Affairs Medical Center, Houston, Texas
Brucellosis

PREFACE

Despite the dramatic reduction in morbidity and mortality rates related to infectious diseases that followed the introduction of antimicrobial therapy, as well as active and passive immunization efforts, infectious diseases remain the leading cause of morbidity in infants and children. Children continue to experience three to nine respiratory infections annually, requiring visits to physicians that outnumber the visits made for the purpose of well-child care. Infectious diseases also are the most common cause of school absenteeism. In more recent years, the emergence of resistance to multiple antibiotics by a large number of bacterial microorganisms as well as the identification of new infectious diseases such as severe acute respiratory syndrome (SARS) also have contributed to the morbidity and mortalities related to infectious disease processes.

The first edition of our text was written because we and many of our colleagues were concerned that no single reference text existed that comprehensively covered infectious diseases in children and adolescents. With each subsequent edition, including this one, our goal has been to provide comprehensive coverage of all subjects pertinent to the study of infectious diseases in these populations. Any attempt to summarize our present understanding of infectious diseases for serious students of the subject is a formidable task. In many areas, new information continues to accrue so rapidly that material becomes dated before it can appear in a text of this magnitude. Nonetheless, we have endeavored with the help of many of our colleagues to provide the most comprehensive and up-to-date discussion of this field.

To provide a text as comprehensive and authoritative as possible, we have enlisted contributions from a large number of individuals whose collective expertise is responsible for whatever success we may have had in meeting our objective. We offer our most profound appreciation to the 245 fellow contributors from 180 universities or institutions in 12 countries for their professional expertise and devoted scholarship. Their cooperation and willingness to work with us leave us deeply in their debt.

We also are pleased to have enlisted for this fifth edition of our text the help of two additional co-editors whose expertise and scholarship have enhanced this endeavor immeasurably.

Dr. Gail J. Demmler is Professor in the Department of Pediatrics at Baylor College of Medicine and Director of the Diagnostic Virology Laboratory at Texas Children's Hospital. Dr. Demmler is a nationally recognized pediatric virologist whose own area of clinical and research expertise has been in the fields of cytomegalovirus infections, influenza virus infections, and pediatric human immunodeficiency virus (HIV) infections. Dr. Demmler has served for many years on the Executive and Program Committees of the Pediatric Academic Societies and currently is President of the Society for Pediatric Research. She also holds fellowship status in the Infectious Disease Society of America.

Dr. Sheldon L. Kaplan currently serves as Professor and Vice Chair for Clinical Affairs in the Department of Pediatrics at Baylor College of Medicine and as Chief of the Infectious Disease Service at Texas Children's Hospital. A Fellow of the Infectious Disease Society of America, Dr. Kaplan also is President of the Pediatric Infectious Diseases Society. Dr. Kaplan has done extensive work in the field of bacterial infections with specific emphasis on treatment of infections caused by antibiotic-resistant microorganisms. He also has served as Editor of *Current Therapy in Pediatric Infectious Diseases*.

Once again, infectious diseases are discussed according to organ systems that may be affected, as well as individually by microorganisms. In all sections in which diseases related to specific agents are discussed, emphasis has been placed, to the greatest extent possible, on the specificity of clinical manifestations that may be related to the organism causing the disease. Detailed information regarding the best means to establish a diagnosis and explicit recommendations for therapy are provided.

The entire text has been revised extensively. This edition continues the format that we initiated in the fourth edition in that infections with specific microorganisms have been reorganized to provide appropriate emphasis on the common features that may relate specific microorganisms to each other. Thus, all gram-positive coccal organisms are presented sequentially and are followed by gram-negative cocci, gram-positive bacilli, enterobacteria, gram-negative coccobacilli, Treponemataceae, anaerobic bacteria, and so forth. In addition, special sections of the text have been devoted to discussions of each of the following: molecular determinants of microbial pathogenesis; immunologic and phagocytic responses to infection; metabolic response of the host to infections; interaction of infection and nutrition; pathogenesis and treatment of fever; indigenous flora; epidemiology of infectious diseases; congenital immune deficiency; acquired immunodeficiency syndrome (AIDS) and other acquired immunodeficiency diseases; Kawasaki disease; chronic fatigue syndrome; international travel issues for children; infectious disease problems of international adoptees and refugees; nosocomial infections; prevention and control of infections in hospitalized children; pharmacology and pharmacokinetics of antibacterial, antiviral, antifungal, and antiparasitic agents; public health considerations; infections in daycare environments; and use of the bacteriology, mycology, parasitology, virology, and serology laboratories. The section on opportunistic infections in the compromised host has been divided into multiple chapters as follows: opportunistic infections in children with bone marrow transplantation; infections in pediatric heart transplant recipients; opportunistic infections in children with liver transplantation; opportunistic infections in children with kidney transplantation; infections related to prosthetics or artificial devices; and infections related to craniofacial surgical procedures. This reorganization has been necessitated by the large number of individuals, particularly post-transplantation recipients, who now serve as the source of many infectious disease problems and constitute a large part of the consulting practice of many pediatric infectious disease physicians.

With some sadness, we have introduced into the text for the first time a section on bioterrorism, which was necessitated by the current state of world affairs. The section on immunomodulating agents and their potential use in the treatment of infectious diseases has been expanded because information on this subject has become more extensive since the publication of the last edition. Specific sections also have been devoted to human and animal bites. The subject of biostatistics as applicable to the subspecialty of infectious diseases also has been included. A section on human metapneumovirus has been added to the chapter on respiratory syncytial virus infection, and a section on SARS has been added to the chapter on coronaviruses.

This book could not have been brought to fruition without the help and assistance of many individuals whose names do not appear in the text. No words are sufficient to adequately convey our gratitude appropriately; we hope that they know they have our heartfelt thanks.

We would like to single out certain individuals for specific mention. We cannot adequately convey our appreciation for the thousands of hours devoted by Dr. Lee Ligon, who edited and also proofread every word of the text that was submitted, as well as the galleys and page proofs. We are equally indebted to Mary Campbell, who spent an equivalent amount of time and who was specifically responsible for the coordination of the editorial effort, correspondence with our contributors and with the publisher, and coordination of the manuscript preparation process. She also typed and retyped many sections of the text. We also appreciate the assistance provided to Mary Campbell and to the editors by Tracey Ramsey and Carrel Briley, as well as the help provided by Brooke Taylor, Anabel Alvarez, Vionna Cabal, and Margarita Santiago.

We also appreciate the help and support of Judith Fletcher, Melissa Dudlick, Jennifer Shreiner, and Lee Ann Draud at Saunders, as well as the continued editorial guidance of Lisette Bralow who has helped us with every edition of this text.

Finally, we would like to thank the Baylor College of Medicine and Texas Children's Hospital in Houston, Texas, and the David Geffen School of Medicine at UCLA and the Mattel UCLA Children's Hospital for providing an environment that is supportive of intellectual pursuits.

Ralph D. Feigin, M.D.
James D. Cherry, M.D.

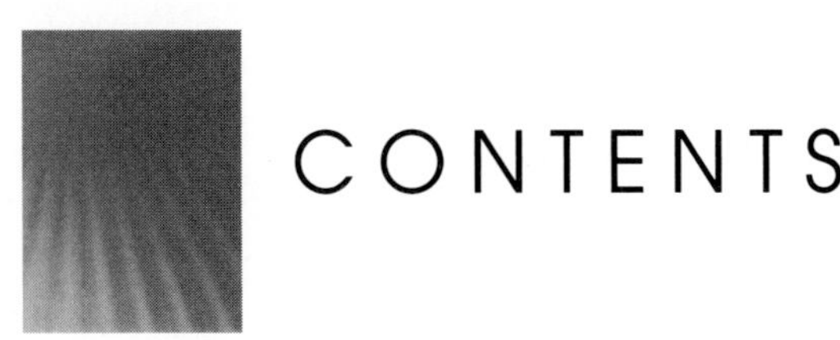

CONTENTS

Color plates appear between pages 762–763, 1976–1977, and 2720–2721.

VOLUME 1

PART I

Host-Parasite Relationships and the Pathogenesis of Infectious Diseases

PART II

Infections of Specific Organ Systems

SECTION I

UPPER RESPIRATORY TRACT INFECTIONS

SECTION II

LOWER RESPIRATORY TRACT INFECTIONS

SECTION III

INFECTIONS OF THE HEART

SECTION IV

CENTRAL NERVOUS SYSTEM INFECTIONS

SECTION V

GENITOURINARY TRACT INFECTIONS

SUBSECTION 5

GRAM-NEGATIVE COCCOBACILLI

VOLUME 2

SECTION XVIII

CHLAMYDIA

SECTION XIX

RICKETTSIAL DISEASES

SECTION XX

MYCOPLASMA

SECTION XXI

FUNGAL DISEASES

SECTION XXII

PARASITIC DISEASES

SUBSECTION 1

PROTOZOA

A AMEBAE

B FLAGELLATES (INTESTINAL)

C CILIATES (INTESTINAL)

D COCCIDIA, INICNOSPORIDIA (INTESTINAL)

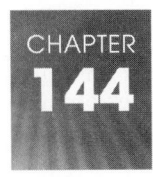

Streptobacillus moniliformis (Rat-Bite Fever)

CARRIE L. BYINGTON ■ ROBERT D. BASOW

Rat-bite fever is an acute febrile illness usually acquired in humans from the bite of a rat or other rodent. It is a zoonosis with worldwide distribution.[97] *Streptobacillus moniliformis* is the leading cause of rat-bite fever in the United States, but in Asia, the illness is caused most often by a spirochete, *Spirillum minus*[40] (see Chapter 149). Infection with *S. moniliformis* is characterized by a relapsing fever, rash, and prominent arthralgia and arthritis. Infection may be acquired after the bite of an animal, by skin or mucous membrane contact with an infected animal, or by ingestion of food or water contaminated by rats. When the organism is acquired by ingestion, the resulting illness is termed *Haverhill fever*, after an outbreak that occurred in Haverhill, Massachusetts, in 1926.[55, 59]

History

The first description of rat-bite fever is found in the 2500-year-old Indian *Compendium of Medicine*, the *Susruta Samhita*.[17] In this text, a description of the illness is given that remains valid today: "The blood of any part of the human body coming in contact with the semen of rats or scratched with their nails or teeth is vitiated and gives rise to the appearance of nodes, swellings, eruptions of circular erythematous patches on skin, pustules, violent and acute erysipelas, breaking pain in the joints, extreme pain in the body, fever, anemia, aversion to food, shivering, and horripilation." The disease also was known in ancient Japan, where treatment consisted of local application of herbs and dynamite to cause an "explosion in the wound."[17]

The first modern accounts of the disease are found in a lecture by professor Eli Ives at Yale University in 1831.[30] The first case report was published in 1839.[95] In 1900, Miyake gave a detailed description of the disease, which he named *sodoku*, from the Japanese *so* (rat) and *doku* (poison).[52] Blake, Schottmüller, and Levaditi were the first to isolate and describe the causative agent of streptobacillary rat-bite fever in 1914, 1916, and 1925, respectively.[11, 45, 80] The organism has been known as *Streptothrix muris ratti* and *Streptobacillus muris minus* but currently is referred to as *S. moniliformis*.[37]

Haverhill fever was reported first in 1926 after an outbreak of epidemic illness that was traced to contaminated milk.[59] The illness originally was called *erythema arthriticum epidemicum*. Shortly thereafter, the causative organism was isolated and named *Haverhillia multiformis* and was shown to be identical to *S. moniliformis*.[55]

Epidemiology

Approximately 200 cases of rat-bite fever have been reported in the United States.* In addition, the disease has been reported worldwide.† *S. moniliformis* is responsible for most of the cases seen in North America, whereas the spirillary form is seen more commonly in Asia. One case of spirillary rat-bite fever has been reported in the American literature since 1969.[18] Two outbreaks of Haverhill fever are reported in the literature.[49, 55]

Rat-bite fever currently is not a reportable illness in the United States; hence, its true incidence is unknown. Although it is considered to be rare, the illness likely is underdiagnosed. More than 2 million animal bites are reported yearly in the United States, and rat bites account for at least 1 percent of them.[26] A review of animal bites in Maryland during a 3-year period found that approximately 4.7 percent were caused by rats or lagomorphs.[21] Among bitten patients, the risk for rat-bite fever is significant, with reported rates between 4 and 11 percent.[67, 94] One half of all reported cases of rat-bite fever in the United States since the 1970s have involved children, usually younger than 12 years of age.[20] Not surprisingly, children living in crowded urban centers or rural impoverished areas seem to be at greatest risk.[21, 38, 64, 92] Most of the other reported cases involve laboratory personnel who handle rats.[3]

Rat-bite fever usually is transmitted through the bite of a rat but also may be transmitted by rat scratches.[6, 20] Rat-bite fever also has been reported after handling of pet rats and in individuals who dwell in rat-infested homes.[29, 76] Rat-bite fever was reported after varicella in a child who handled pet rats frequently while she had open skin lesions, and septic arthritis was reported in a child who kissed pet rats.[36, 61]

Between 10 and 100 percent of rats, both wild and laboratory, carry *S. moniliformis* as normal nasopharyngeal flora and excrete it in their urine.[3, 87] The disease also has been transmitted to humans from mice,[65] squirrels,[51] weasels,[22] gerbils,[96] and such rat-eating carnivores as cats,[32, 53] dogs,[56, 68] and pigs.[93] *S. moniliformis* also can cause disease in turkeys,[54] guinea pigs,[42] koalas,[75] and spinifex hopping mice.[39] These animals could pose a potential source of infection in humans.

Haverhill fever is transmitted by ingestion of food or water contaminated by rats. Previous outbreaks have involved unpasteurized milk, ice cream made from raw milk, and water.[49, 59]

Bacteriology

S. moniliformis is a pleomorphic, microaerophilic, nonmotile, nonencapsulated, non–acid-fast, gram-negative bacillus. It measures 1 to 5 μm in length.[37] The organism is oxidase and catalase negative and will ferment glucose, maltose, fructose, galactose, and salicin.[37]

The organism is fastidious and requires special handling for isolation. Optimal growth is achieved in trypticase soy agar or broth supplemented with 20 percent horse or rabbit serum.[55] Alternatively, brain-heart infusion broth supplemented with *Panmede* (a papain digest of ox liver) also has been shown to support the growth of *S. moniliformis*.[85] Sodium polyanethol sulfonate (SPS), which is added to most aerobic blood culture bottles at a concentration of

*See references 2, 3, 5–7, 13, 18, 20, 25, 38, 61.

†See references 4, 8–10, 14, 24, 35, 43, 44, 49, 77, 81.

0.05 percent, inhibits the growth of *S. moniliformis* at concentrations as low as 0.0125 percent.[84] Blood culture bottles without SPS added should be used for primary isolation of *S. moniliformis* when rat-bite fever is suspected. SPS is not added to anaerobic blood culture bottles, and *S. moniliformis* may be isolated from standard anaerobic culture. Cultures should be incubated at 35° to 37° C in a humid environment with a partial pressure of carbon dioxide between 8 and 10 percent.

The morphologic characteristics of the bacteria are dependent on its environment.[55] In favorable media, the typical appearance is that of short rods that may grow in chains. Under other conditions, the organism tends to grow in long, interwoven filaments that commonly contain beaded and fusiform swellings throughout their length. In broth culture, colonies usually appear in 2 to 10 days.[37] The colonies are white, soft "puffballs" 1 to 2 mm in diameter. On blood agar plates, the colonies are round, gray, and glistening and measure 1 to 2 mm in diameter after 2 to 3 days of incubation.[37]

Stable L-forms of the organism develop spontaneously in vivo or in vitro. These cell wall–deficient forms have a fried egg appearance, with dark centers and lacy edges, when grown on solid media.[37, 57] They are resistant to penicillin and other antibiotics active against the bacterial cell wall. L-Phase variants may deposit in tissues and prolong the symptoms of illness.[24]

Clinical Manifestations

Streptobacillary rat-bite fever typically has an incubation period of fewer than 7 days, with a reported range of 1 to 22 days.[13] Young children have a predilection for shorter incubation times. The illness is characterized by the acute onset of shaking chills, fever, headache, and vomiting. Usually, the bite site is well healed, without evidence of inflammation or regional adenopathy. Within the first week of illness, more than 50 percent of patients develop arthralgia or arthritis with or without joint effusion. The arthritis, usually involving large joints, tends to be migratory, nonsymmetric, and extremely painful.[4, 29, 38, 81] Within 1 to 8 days after the onset of fever, approximately 75 percent of patients develop a pink-red maculopapular rash that frequently involves the palms and soles.[20, 50, 60] The rash, lasting as long as 3 weeks, may be generalized, petechial, purpuric, or pustular, and approximately 20 percent desquamate. With untreated infection, persistent or recurrent episodes of fever and arthritis may occur.[30, 89] The rash generally does not recur. The untreated mortality rate of *S. moniliformis* infection is 10 percent overall.[5, 64, 70] The prognosis generally is excellent in patients treated with antibiotics, and the mortality rate is thought to be less than 1.5 percent. However, infection in infants younger than 3 months of age may be particularly severe or fatal, even with appropriate antibiotic therapy.[47, 50, 82]

Haverhill fever is similar to streptobacillary rat-bite fever, with the abrupt onset of fever and chills (100%), rash (95%), and arthritis (97%).[1, 50] Generally, the incubation period is 1 to 3 days. Upper respiratory and gastrointestinal complaints are common. Multiple recurrences of fever are found rarely, and the rash tends to be small and uniform in size.[49]

Complications of *S. moniliformis* infection include anemia,[70] formation of cutaneous or subcutaneous abscesses,[5, 35, 57, 91] interstitial pneumonia,[50, 82] mastoiditis,[58] meningitis,[8, 82] pericardial effusion,[15] pancreatitis, prostatitis,[97] and septic arthritis.[36, 46, 73, 77] Abscess formation of organs, including the brain,[23] the female genital tract,[57] and the spleen,[16] has been reported. Unusual and potentially devastating complications include chorioamnionitis[28] and periarteritis nodosa.[63] The most frequent serious complication is that of bacterial endocarditis, which was uniformly fatal in the pre-antibiotic era.[48, 66, 74, 86] Six cases of endocarditis occurring in children younger than 18 years of age have been reported since 1934.[50, 62, 71, 82, 86, 88] Five of the six patients died during the acute illness. Four received no antibiotic treatment. Endocarditis caused by *S. moniliformis* has been reported recently in an adult with human immunodeficiency virus infection.[69] The patient recovered with antibiotic therapy.

Iron-deficiency anemia is the only complication that has been reported after Haverhill fever.[49] No reported fatalities due to Haverhill fever have been reported, and the prognosis is excellent.[49]

Pathophysiology and Pathology

The factors influencing the virulence of *S. moniliformis* are not well described. The organism has an affinity for synovial tissue in both animals and humans, but the mechanisms by which *S. moniliformis* produces arthritis are unknown.[33, 34, 38, 41, 46, 79, 90] Studies performed in mice indicate that *S. moniliformis* is only slightly immunogenic, producing mild leukocytosis and minimal homologous antibody production.[78, 79] In addition, the organism is resistant to phagocytic destruction.[78] These factors may allow the development of chronic infection.

The pathologic features of streptobacillary rat-bite fever have been described in a limited number of autopsy reports. Common features include ulcerative endocarditis with secondary septic embolization in the liver and spleen, septic arthritis, and interstitial pneumonia.[11, 82] The pure interstitial pneumonia is atypical of bacterial infections. Mononuclear meningitis and erythrophagocytosis also have been reported.[82] In most reports, little histologic evidence of inflammation at the site of the bite is found.[50]

Diagnosis

The correct diagnosis of rat-bite fever requires a high index of suspicion on the part of the physician. The diagnosis is suggested in a febrile patient with a history of rat exposure, but in most clinical settings, the exposure history is not elucidated until after the diagnosis is made.

Nonspecific signs include an elevation in the white blood cell count, usually in the range of 10,000 to 30,000 cells/mm^3 with a left shift, a mild anemia, and a false-positive serologic test for syphilis, which may occur in 25 percent of patients.[70] Direct visualization of the organism on Giemsa stain of blood or joint fluid may suggest the diagnosis. Serologic assays currently are not available for humans. An enzyme-linked immunosorbent assay has been developed and is being used to monitor infection in rodent colonies.[12] Molecular methods, such as the polymerase chain reaction, may offer hope in the future for detection of *S. moniliformis* from culture-negative specimens.[31]

Currently, diagnosis depends on culturing the organism. The organism has been cultured from blood, joint fluid, abscesses, pericardial fluid, meninges, and tissues obtained at autopsy.[15] *S. moniliformis* possesses strict growth requirements, and choice of culture media and technique is of critical importance for optimal growth of the bacterium (see section "Bacteriology"). In general, routine aerobic blood cultures are not satisfactory for isolation.

If the organism is isolated, it may be identified rapidly using gas-liquid chromatography. *S. moniliformis* has a characteristic fatty acid profile, with major peaks being palmitic, linoleic, oleic, and stearic acid.[57, 72] Electrophoretic protein patterns that can distinguish Haverhill fever strains from rat-bite fever strains also have been described.[19]

The differential diagnosis for streptobacillary rat-bite fever includes illness caused by *S. minus*, which may be indistinguishable (see Chapter 149). It also includes all relapsing fevers, such as *Borrelia recurrentis*, malaria, and typhoid. Rickettsial disease, especially Rocky Mountain spotted fever, must be considered.[60] Other infectious entities include leptospirosis, Lyme disease, disseminated gonococcal infection, meningococcemia, brucellosis, syphilis, and viral infections, especially those caused by enteroviruses or human parvoviruses. Acute rheumatic fever also should be considered. Noninfectious entities include drug reactions, collagen vascular disease, and Pel-Ebstein fever.

Treatment and Prevention

In proven cases of streptobacillary rat-bite fever, the treatment of choice is penicillin G. In adults, the dosage of penicillin should be no less than 400,000 to 600,000 IU/day continued for at least 7 days.[70] If no response is seen within 2 days, the dosage should be increased to 1.2 million IU/day. Children have been treated successfully with 20,000 to 50,000 units/kg/day of intramuscular or intravenous penicillin, up to a maximum of 1.2 million IU/day.[83] In children who do not require hospitalization, oral penicillin V, 1 to 2 g/day in divided doses, may be given.[83] In penicillin-allergic adults, both streptomycin and tetracycline have been effective.[60, 81] In children, streptomycin and erythromycin have been used. However, treatment failures with erythromycin have been reported.[35] Newer antibiotics, including cefuroxime, cefotaxime, gentamicin, and ciprofloxacin, have good activity against *S. moniliformis* in vitro.[27] Several reports document successful treatment with cephalosporins, including cefuroxime and ceftriaxone.[6, 20, 36, 69]

Endocarditis secondary to *S. moniliformis* should be treated with high-dose penicillin G in combination with streptomycin or gentamicin. In children, the dosage is 160,000 to 240,000 IU/kg/day, up to the adult maximum of 20 million IU/day.[74, 83] Treatment should be continued for at least 4 weeks. Antibiotic susceptibility testing of the organism should be performed, and minimum inhibitory and bactericidal concentrations for several antimicrobial agents should be determined. A peak serum minimum bactericidal concentration of at least 1:8 is desirable. Recently, successful treatment of endocarditis with ceftriaxone in combination with gentamicin was reported.[69]

Haverhill fever is treated in much the same way, with penicillin G currently being the drug of choice. Most individuals can be treated as outpatients.

Rat-bite fever can be prevented by controlling rodents in urban areas, properly handling rodents, and avoiding unpasteurized milk products. If a rat bites an individual, prophylactic antibiotics, such as amoxicillin or amoxicillin-clavulanic acid, probably would prevent rat-bite fever, but current data do not support the routine use of antibiotics after all rat bites. Some authors would suggest that, because of the serious nature of rat-bite fever in young infants, infants younger than 3 months of age who are bitten by a rat receive prophylaxis.[47]

REFERENCES

1. Albritten, F., Sheely, R., and Jeffers, W.: *Haverhillia multiformis* septicemia: Etiologic and clinical relationship to rat-bite fever. J. A. M. A. *114:*2360–2363, 1940.
2. Anderson, D., and Marrie, T. J.: Septic arthritis due to *Streptobacillus moniliformis*. Arthritis Rheum. *30:*229–230, 1987.
3. Anderson, L. C., Leary, S. L., and Manning, P. J.: Rat-bite fever in animal research laboratory personnel. Lab. Anim. Sci. *33:*292–294, 1983.
4. Anglada, A., Comas, L., Euras, J. M., et al.: [Arthritis caused by *Streptobacillus moniliformis*: A case of fever induced by a rat bite]. Med. Clin. (Barc.) *94:*535–537, 1990.
5. Anonymous: Rat-bite fever in a college student—California. M. M. W. R. Morb. Mortal. Wkly. Rep. *33:*318–320, 1984.
6. Anonymous: Rat-bite fever—New Mexico, 1996. M. M. W. R. Morb. Mortal. Wkly. Rep. *47:*89–91, 1998.
7. Arkless, H. A.: Rat-bite fever at Albert Einstein Medical Center. Pa. Med. *73:*49, 1970.
8. Atala, A., Correa, C. N., Correa, W. M., et al.: [Meningitis caused by *Streptobacillus moniliformis*]. Rev. Paul. Med. *82:*175–178, 1973.
9. Ban, R., Bajolet-Laudinat, O., Eschard, J. P., et al.: [Acute purulent polyarthritis induced by *Streptobacillus moniliformis*]. Presse Med. *20:*1515–1516, 1991.
10. Bhatt, K. M., and Mirza, N. B.: Rat bite fever: A case report of a Kenyan. East Afr. Med. J. *69:*542–543, 1992.
11. Blake, F.: The etiology of rat-bite fever. J. Exp. Med. *23:*39–60, 1916.
12. Boot, R., Bakker, R. H., Thuis, H., et al.: An enzyme-linked immunosorbent assay (ELISA) for monitoring rodent colonies for *Streptobacillus moniliformis* antibodies. Lab. Anim. *27:*350–357, 1993.
13. Brown, T., and Nunemaker, J.: Rat-bite fever: Review of American cases with reevaluation of its etiology and report of cases. Bull. Johns Hopkins Hosp. *70:*201–202, 1942.
14. Buranakitjaroen, P., Nilganuwong, S., and Gherunpong, V.: Rat-bite fever caused by *Streptobacillus moniliformis*. Southeast Asian J. Trop. Med. Public Health *25:*778–781, 1994.
15. Carbeck, R. B., Murphy, J. F., and Britt, E. M.: Streptobacillary rat-bite fever with massive pericardial effusion. J. A. M. A. *201:*703–704, 1967.
16. Chulay, J. D., and Lankerani, M. R.: Splenic abscess: Report of 10 cases and review of the literature. Am. J. Med. *61:*513–522, 1976.
17. Cohen, H: Rat-bite fever: Contributions to its history and war significance. Bull. Hist. Med. *15:*108–115, 1944.
18. Cole, J. S., Stoll, R. W., and Bulger, R. J.: Rat-bite fever: Report of three cases. Ann. Intern. Med. *71:*979–981, 1969.
19. Costas, M., and Owen, R. J.: Numerical analysis of electrophoretic protein patterns of *Streptobacillus moniliformis* strains from human, murine and avian infections. J. Med. Microbiol. *23:*303–311, 1987.
20. Cunningham, B. B., Paller, A. S., and Katz, B. Z.: Rat bite fever in a pet lover. J. Am. Acad. Dermatol. *38:*330–332, 1998.
21. De Hoff, J. B., and Ross, L.: Animal bites. Md. State Med. J. *30:*35–45, 1981.
22. Dick, G., and Turncliff, R.: Streptothrix isolated from the blood of a patient bitten by a weasel. J. Infect. Dis. *23:*183–187, 1918.
23. Dijkmans, B. A., Thomeer, R. T., Vielvoye, G. J., et al.: Brain abscess due to *Streptobacillus moniliformis* and Actinobacterium meyerii. Infection *12:*262–264, 1984.
24. Dolman, C: Two cases of rat-bite fever due to *Streptobacillus moniliformis*. Can. J. Public Health *42*:228–241, 1951.
25. Dow, G. R., Rankin, R. J., and Saunders, B. W.: Rat-bite fever. N. Z. Med. J *105:*133, 1992.
26. Edwards, M.: Animal bites. *In* Feigin, R., Cherry, J. (eds.): Textbook of Pediatric Infectious Diseases. Vol. 2. Philadelphia, WB Saunders, 1998, pp. 2248–2253.
27. Edwards, R., and Finch, R. G.: Characterisation and antibiotic susceptibilities of *Streptobacillus moniliformis*. J. Med. Microbiol. *21:*39–42, 1986.
28. Faro, S., Walker, C., and Pierson, R. L.: Amnionitis with intact amniotic membranes involving *Streptobacillus moniliformis*. Obstet. Gynecol. *55:*9S–11S, 1980.
29. Fordham, J. N., McKay-Ferguson, E., Davies, A., et al.: Rat bite fever without the bite. Ann. Rheum. Dis. *51:*411–412, 1992.
30. Francis, E.: Rat-bite fever and relapsing fever in the United States. Trans. Assoc. Am. Physicians *47:*143–151, 1932.
31. Fredricks, D. N., and Relman, D. A.: Application of polymerase chain reaction to the diagnosis of infectious diseases. Clin. Infect. Dis. *29:* 475–488, 1999.
32. Gascard, E., Vignoli, R., Moulard, J. C., et al.: [Case of febrile eruption after a cat bite: *Streptobacillus moniliformis* septicemia?]. Mars. Med. *104:*861–864, 1967.
33. Glastonbury, J. R., Morton, J. G., and Matthews, L. M.: *Streptobacillus moniliformis* infection in Swiss white mice. J. Vet. Diagn. Invest. *8:* 202–209, 1996.
34. Glunder, G., Hinz, K. H., and Stiburek, B.: [Joint disease in turkeys caused by *Streptobacillus moniliformis* in Germany]. Dtsch. Tierarztl. Wochenschr. *89:*367–370, 1982.
35. Hagelskjaer, L., Sorensen, I., and Randers, E.: *Streptobacillus moniliformis* infection: 2 cases and a literature review. Scand. J. Infect. Dis. *30:*309–311, 1998.
36. Hockman, D. E., Pence, C. D., Whittler, R. R., et al.: Septic arthritis of the hip secondary to rat bite fever: A case report. Clin. Orthop. *380:*173–176, 2000.

37. Holmes, B., Pickett, M., and Hollis, D.: *Streptobacillus moniliformis. In:* Murray, P. (ed.): Manual of Clinical Microbiology. Washington, DC, ASM Press, 1995, pp. 506–507.
38. Holroyd, K. J., Reiner, A. P., and Dick, J. D.: *Streptobacillus moniliformis* polyarthritis mimicking rheumatoid arthritis: An urban case of rat bite fever. Am. J. Med. *85:*711–714, 1988.
39. Hopkinson, W. I., and Lloyd, J. M.: *Streptobacillus moniliformis* septicaemia in spinifex hopping mice *(Notomys alexis).* Aust. Vet. J. *57:* 533–534, 1981.
40. Ito, A.: [Rat-bite fever]. Ryoikibetsu Shokogun Shirizu *24:*300, 1999.
41. Kaspareit-Rittinghausen, J., Wullenweber, M., Deerberg, F., et al.: [Pathological changes in *Streptobacillus moniliformis* infection of C57bl/6J mice]. Berl. Munch. Tierarztl. Wochenschr. *103:*84–87, 1990.
42. Kirchner, B. K., Lake, S. G., and Wightman, S. R.: Isolation of *Streptobacillus moniliformis* from a guinea pig with granulomatous pneumonia. Lab. Anim. Sci. *42:*519–521, 1992.
43. Konstantopoulos, K., Skarpas, P., Hitjazis, F., et al.: Rat bite fever in a Greek child. Scand. J. Infect. Dis. *24:*531–533, 1992.
44. Latrille, J., Verdaguer, P., Aubertin, J., et al.: [Septicemia caused by *Haverilla moniliformis*]. J. Med. Bord. *143:*677–684, 1966.
45. Levaditi, C., Nicolau, S., and Poindoux, P.: Sur le role etiologique de *Streptobacillus moniliformis* (nov. spec.) dans l'erytheme polymorphe aigu septicemique. Compt. Rend. Acad. Sci. *180:*1188–1190, 1925.
46. Mandel, D. R.: Streptobacillary fever. An unusual cause of infectious arthritis. Cleve. Clin. Q. *52:*203–205, 1985.
47. Mathiasen, T., and Rix, M.: [Rat-bite: An infant bitten by a rat]. Ugeskr. Laeger. *155:*1475–1476, 1993.
48. McCormack, R. C., Kaye, D., and Hook, E. W.: Endocarditis due to *Streptobacillus moniliformis.* J. A. M. A. *200:*77–79, 1967.
49. McEvoy, M. B., Noah, N. D., and Pilsworth, R.: Outbreak of fever caused by *Streptobacillus moniliformis.* Lancet *2:*1361–1363, 1987.
50. McHugh, T, P., Bartlett, R. L., Raymond, J. I.: Rat bite fever: Report of a fatal case. Ann. Emerg. Med. *14:*1116–1118, 1985.
51. McMillan, B., and Boulger, L. R.: Squirrel-bite fever. Trans. R. Soc. Trop. Med. Hyg. *62:*567, 1968.
52. Miyake, H.: Gerber die rattenbiskrankheit. Mitt. Grenzgeb. Med. Chir. *5:*231–262, 1900.
53. Mock, H., and Morrow, A.: Rat-bite fever transmitted from a cat bite. Ill. Med. J. *61:*67–70, 1932.
54. Mohamed, Y. S., Moorhead, P. D., and Bohl, E. H.: Natural *Streptobacillus moniliformis* infection of turkeys, and attempts to infect turkeys, sheep, and pigs. Avian Dis. *13:*379–385, 1969.
55. Parker, F., and Hudson, N.: The etiology of Haverhill fever (erythema arthriticum epidemicum). Am. J. Pathol. *2:*357–379, 1926.
56. Peel, M. M.: Dog-associated bacterial infections in humans: Isolates submitted to an Australian reference laboratory, 1981–1992. Pathology *25:*379–384, 1993.
57. Pins, M. R., Holden, J. M., Yang, J. M., et al.: Isolation of presumptive *Streptobacillus moniliformis* from abscesses associated with the female genital tract. Clin. Infect. Dis. *22:*471–476, 1996.
58. Pirodda, E.: [Atypical otomastoiditis due to Haverhillia multiformis *(Streptobacillus moniliformis)*]. Otorinolaringol. Ital. *34:*23–32, 1965.
59. Place, E., Sutton, H., Willner, O.: Erythema arthriticum epidemicum: Preliminary report. Boston Med. Surg. J. *194:*285–287, 1926.
60. Portnoy, B. L., Satterwhite, T. K., and Dyckman, J. D.: Rat bite fever misdiagnosed as Rocky Mountain spotted fever. South. Med. J. *72:* 607–609, 1979.
61. Prager, L., and Frenck, R. W., Jr.: *Streptobacillus moniliformis* infection in a child with chickenpox. Pediatr. Infect. Dis. J. *13:*417–418, 1994.
62. Priest, W: Penicillin therapy in subacute bacterial endocarditis. Arch. Intern. Med. *79:*333–359, 1947.
63. Prouty, M., and Shater, E.: Periarteritis nodosa associated with rat-bite fever due to *Streptobacillus moniliformis* (erythema arthriticum epidemicum). J. Pediatr. *36:*605–613, 1950.
64. Raffin, B. J., and Freemark, M.: Streptobacillary rat-bite fever: A pediatric problem. Pediatrics *64:*214–217, 1979.
65. Reitzel, R., Haim, A., and Prindle, K.: Rat bite fever from a field mouse. J. A. M. A. *106:*1090, 1936.
66. Rey, J. L., Laurans, G., Pleskof, A., et al.: [*Streptobacillus moniliformis* endocarditis: Apropos of 2 cases]. Ann. Cardiol. Angeiol. (Paris) *36:*297–300, 1987.
67. Richter, C.: Incidence of rat bites and rat-bite fever in Baltimore. J. A. M. A. *128:*324, 1945.
68. Ripley, H., and Van Sant, H.: Rat-bite fever acquired from a dog. J. A. M. A. *102:*1917, 1934.
69. Rordorf, T., Zuger, C., Zbinden, R., et al.: *Streptobacillus moniliformis* endocarditis in an HIV-positive patient. Infection *28:*393–394, 2000.
70. Roughgarden, J.: Antimicrobial therapy of rat-bite fever. Arch. Intern. Med. *116:*39–53, 1965.
71. Roundtree, P., and Rohan, M.: A fatal human infection with *Streptobacillus moniliformis.* Med. J. Aust. *1:*359, 1941.
72. Rowbotham, T. J.: Rapid identification of *Streptobacillus moniliformis.* Lancet *2:*567, 1983.
73. Rumley, R. L., Patrone, N. A., and White, L.: Rat-bite fever as a cause of septic arthritis: A diagnostic dilemma. Ann. Rheum. Dis. *46:*793–795, 1987.
74. Rupp, M. E.: *Streptobacillus moniliformis* endocarditis: Case report and review. Clin. Infect. Dis. *14:*769–772, 1992.
75. Russell, E. G., and Straube, E. F.: Streptobacillary pleuritis in a koala *(Phascolarctos cinereus).* J. Wildl. Dis. *15:*391–394, 1979.
76. Rygg, M., and Bruun, C. F.: Rat bite fever *(Streptobacillus moniliformis)* with septicemia in a child. Scand. J. Infect. Dis. *24:*535–540, 1992.
77. Saez Villaverde, R., Alvarez Lario, B., Alegre Lopez, J., et al.: [*Streptobacillus moniliformis* septic oligoarthritis (fever caused by rat bite)]. Rev. Clin. Esp. *196:*413–415, 1996.
78. Savage, N. L.: Host-parasite relationships in experimental *Streptobacillus moniliformis* arthritis in mice. Infect. Immun. *5:*183–190, 1972.
79. Savage, N. L., Joiner, G. N., and Florey, D. W.: Clinical, microbiological, and histological manifestations of *Streptobacillus moniliformis*–induced arthritis in mice. Infect. Immun. *34:*605–609, 1981.
80. Schottmüller, H.: Zur aetiologie und klinik der bisskrankheit. Dermatol. Wochenschr. *58*(Suppl.):77–103, 1914.
81. Schuurman, B., van Griethuysen, A. J., Marcelis, J. H., et al.: [Rat bite fever after a bite from a tame pet rat]. Ned. Tijdschr. Geneeskd. *142:*2006–2009, 1998.
82. Sens, M. A., Brown, E. W., Wilson, L. R., et al.: Fatal *Streptobacillus moniliformis* infection in a two-month-old infant. Am. J. Clin. Pathol. *91:*612–616, 1989.
83. Shackelford, P.: Rat-bite fever. *In* Kaplan, S. (ed.): Current Therapy in Pediatric Infectious Disease. St. Louis, Mosby–Year Book, 1993, p. 235.
84. Shanson, D. C., Gazzard, B. G., Midgley, J., et al.: *Streptobacillus moniliformis* isolated from blood in four cases of Haverhill fever. Lancet *2:*92–94, 1983.
85. Shanson, D. C., Pratt, J., and Greene, P.: Comparison of media with and without "Panmede" for the isolation of *Streptobacillus moniliformis* from blood cultures and observations on the inhibitory effect of sodium polyanethol sulphonate. J. Med. Microbiol. *19:*181–186, 1985.
86. Simon, M. W., and Wilson, H. D.: *Streptobacillus moniliformis* endocarditis: A case report. Clin. Pediatr. (Phila.) *25:*110–111, 1986.
87. Strangeways, W.: Rats as carriers of *Streptobacillus moniliformis.* J. Pathol. Bacteriol. *37:*45–51, 1933.
88. Stuart-Harris, C., Wells, A., Rosher, H.: Four cases of infective endocarditis due to organisms similar to *Haemophilus parainfluenza* and one case due to pleomorphic *Streptobacillus.* J. Pathol. Bacteriol. *41:*407–421, 1935.
89. Taber, L. H., and Feigin, R. D.: Spirochetal infections. Pediatr. Clin. North Am. *26:*377–413, 1979.
90. Taylor, J. D., Stephens, C. P., Duncan, R. G., et al.: Polyarthritis in wild mice *(Mus musculus)* caused by *Streptobacillus moniliformis.* Aust. Vet. J. *71:*143–145, 1994.
91. Vasseur, E., Joly, P., Nouvellon, M., et al.: Cutaneous abscess: A rare complication of *Streptobacillus moniliformis* infection. Br. J. Dermatol. *129:*95–96, 1993.
92. Vasseur, E., Joly, P., Nouvellon, M., et al.: [*Streptobacillus moniliformis*: A rare anthropozoonosis sometimes observed in urban area]. Ann. Dermatol. Venereol. *120:*813–814, 1993.
93. Washburn, R.: *Streptobacillus moniliformis* (rat-bite fever). *In* Mandell, G., Bennett, J., Dolin, R. (eds.): Principles and Practice of Infectious Diseases. Vol. 2. New York, Churchill Livingstone, 1995, pp. 2084–2086.
94. Watkins, C.: Rat-bite fever. J. Pediatr. *28:*429–488, 1946.
95. Wilcox, W.: Violent symptoms from the bite of a rat. Am. J. Med. Sci. *26:* 245–246, 1839.
96. Wilkins, E. G., Millar, J. G., Cockcroft, P. M., et al.: Rat-bite fever in a gerbil breeder. J. Infect. *16:*177–180, 1988.
97. Wullenweber, M.: *Streptobacillus moniliformis*: A zoonotic pathogen. Taxonomic considerations, host species, diagnosis, therapy, geographical distribution. Lab. Anim. *29:*1–15, 1995.

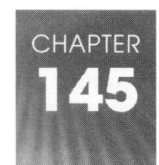

CHAPTER 145

Bartonella: Cat-Scratch Disease

SIMIN GORAL ■ KATHRYN M. EDWARDS

Cat-scratch disease (CSD) usually is an acute, self-limited infection that begins as a papule or nodule at the site of inoculation by a cat, followed by regional lymphadenopathy. *Bartonella henselae* is the causative agent of CSD. In a small number of patients, more serious systemic complications, including involvement of the central nervous system, liver, spleen, bone, eyes, and skin, may occur. Although CSD was recognized as a clinical entity in the 1930s, the first written report, by Debre from France, was not published until 1950.

Etiology

For more than 40 years, numerous attempts were made to isolate the responsible organism from infected nodes in patients with CSD. The first clue was recognized in 1983, when Wear and colleagues used Warthin-Starry silver stain to demonstrate small, pleomorphic, gram-negative bacilli in lymph nodes and skin papules from patients with CSD.[18] Initial attempts to culture the bacillus were unsuccessful. In 1988, an organism was isolated by English and associates from the lymph nodes of patients with CSD and subsequently classified as *Afipia felis*.[7] The discovery of bacillary angiomatosis and its association with *Bartonella* (formerly *Rochalimaea*) *henselae* encouraged further investigation of the role of this newly recognized organism in CSD.[15] In 1992, Regnery and colleagues demonstrated elevated antibodies to *B. henselae* using indirect fluorescent antibody (IFA) test in serum samples from patients with suspected CSD.[14] Researchers also have shown that patients with CSD who were tested by enzyme-linked immunosorbent assay (ELISA) had significant serologic responses to *B. henselae* and *Bartonella quintana* but not to *A. felis,* thus suggesting that the causative agent of CSD was antigenically related to the *Bartonella* genus and not to *Afipia*.[17] In a physician survey to identify cases of CSD occurring during a 13-month period in cat owners in Connecticut, Zangwill and colleagues demonstrated that of 45 patients with clinical CSD, 38 had antibody titers of 1:64 and higher for *B. henselae* as compared with only 4 of 112 samples from controls ($p < .001$).[20] CSD was associated strongly with owning a kitten. Finally, the use of polymerase chain reaction (PCR) for amplification of ribosomal DNA helped confirm the causative agent of CSD as *B. henselae*.[2] Eventually, PCR amplification was used to detect *B. henselae* not only in purulent material aspirated from involved nodes but also in CSD skin test material.[1, 10, 16] Subsequently, *B. henselae* was cultured from lymph nodes obtained from patients with CSD.

B. henselae is a fastidious, gram-negative bacillus requiring an incubation period of up to 5 weeks to culture. It belongs to the genus *Bartonella,* along with other species such as *Bartonella bacilliformis* (the agent of Carrión disease) and *B. quintana* (the agent of trench fever). Colony morphology varies from small, dry, gray-white colonies to smooth, creamy yellow colonies.

Transmission

Domesticated house cats are healthy carriers of *B. henselae,* and cat fleas *(Ctenocephalides felis)* play a major role in cat-to-cat transmission. Approximately 90 percent of patients with CSD have a history of exposure to cats, particularly a kitten with fleas, and a scratch or a bite from a kitten. Although they remain asymptomatic, domestic cats serve as persistent reservoirs for *B. henselae*. Blood samples cultured from pet and impounded cats in the San Francisco Bay region grew *B. henselae* in 41 percent. *B. henselae* also was detected in fleas from infected cats by both direct culture and PCR. Interestingly, Chang and colleagues recently tested adult *Ixodes pacificus* ticks in Santa Clara County, California, and demonstrated that 19.2 percent of ticks were PCR-positive for *Bartonella*.[6] Although they could not demonstrate whether the *Bartonella* strains were alive and transmissible, these results suggest that *I. pacificus* ticks can carry pathogenic *Bartonella* spp. This finding should alert clinicians to consider the possibility of *Bartonella* infection in humans after tick bites.

Epidemiology

CSD occurs worldwide and generally affects children and young adults. The Centers for Disease Control and Prevention estimates that more than 24,000 cases of CSD occur annually in the United States; of those cases, approximately 2000 require hospitalization. Higher rates of disease are reported in the autumn and winter. Zangwill and colleagues suggested that the seasonality of CSD could be explained by the breeding patterns of cats and fleas, as well as increased contact with kittens, which often are kept indoors during the winter months.[20]

Pathology

Pathologic examination of the primary inoculation lesion demonstrates dermal necrosis with variable numbers of histiocytes and occasional multinucleated giant cells accompanied by scattered microabscesses with neutrophils, eosinophils, lymphocytes, and plasma cells. The epidermal changes are nonspecific and consist of parakeratosis, hyperkeratosis, edema, and exocytosis of inflammatory cells. Characteristic findings in the lymph nodes, similar to the primary lesion, are follicular hyperplasia, focal cortical necrosis, and necrotizing granulomata with central microabscesses and palisading histiocytes. A perivascular neutrophilic infiltrate may be present. Subsequently, the lesions progress to small cortical granulomata and "stellate microabscesses" within the granulomata. Warthin-Starry or Steiner silver impregnation stains may reveal pleomorphic bacilli in clusters or short chains within the areas of central necrosis or around small vessels. Bacteria are visualized easily in early lesions. Granulomata with microabscess formation also can be found in other sites such as the liver, spleen, and bone. Because other infections such as tularemia and fungal and mycobacterial infection may have similar histopathologic characteristics, these findings on a biopsy specimen must be correlated with the clinical findings and serologic studies.

Recent observations have identified important new properties of *B. henselae*. By inducing activation of the nuclear factor NFκB and expression of adhesion molecules, *B. henselae* infects and activates endothelial cells, an important step in the pathogenesis of CSD and bacillary angiomatosis.[8] Recently, animal studies have shown that interferon-γ–mediated activation of macrophages is involved in clearing *B. henselae* infection and that microbicidal activity is mediated to a large extent by nitric oxide.[13] The importance of cell-mediated immunity in CSD is suggested by the positive skin reaction and the granulomatous lesions noted in biopsy specimens.

Clinical Manifestations and Course

The most common clinical manifestation of CSD is gradual regional lymph node enlargement that occurs after the patient incurs a distal scratch. An inoculation site can be detected in two thirds of patients. The clinical course may last as long as 2 to 3 months, sometimes longer. Fever, malaise, headache, and muscle aches are seen often. Physical examination usually reveals only lymphadenopathy and skin papules at the inoculation site (Fig. 145–1). Within 2 weeks of a scratch or contact with a cat, the lymph nodes draining the site of inoculation become enlarged and tender. Lymphadenopathy occurs in more than 90 percent of patients with CSD. In approximately 50 percent of cases, regional lymphadenopathy is the only manifestation of the disease and most commonly occurs in the head and neck area, followed by the upper and lower extremities. Suppuration of the involved lymph nodes occurs in approximately 10 percent of patients (Fig. 145–2). Constitutional symptoms of fever, malaise, fatigue, anorexia, emesis, and headache are common but usually mild occurrences. Occasionally (≈10%), patients can have more unusual manifestations such as Parinaud oculoglandular syndrome (Fig. 145–3), neuroretinitis, subacute iritis, optic neuritis, and focal chorioretinitis. Patients with Parinaud oculoglandular syndrome manifest conjunctivitis and preauricular adenopathy. The affected eye usually has pain, is nonpruritic, and shows no evidence of discharge. Most patients recover from Parinaud syndrome spontaneously without residua in 2 to 4 months.

Hepatosplenic CSD is an important cause of prolonged fever in children and should be included in the differential diagnosis of a child with fever of unknown origin. Before diagnosis, these children usually have fever for several weeks (mean, 3 weeks); weight loss and abdominal pain are common.[3] Joint pain, headache, and chills also may be noted. Hepatic or splenic enlargement (or both) are found in half of these children. Ultrasound or computed tomography (CT) usually demonstrates typical lesions in the liver or spleen that are almost diagnostic of this entity (Fig. 145–4).

Neurologic complications are reported in approximately 2 percent of the estimated 24,000 patients in the United States who contract CSD annually. Encephalopathy is the manifestation most commonly reported. Typically, 1 to 6 weeks after the onset of lymphadenopathy, fever and seizures develop, followed by confusion and disorientation. CT of the head generally is normal. Cerebrospinal fluid shows minimal pleocytosis or elevated protein levels. Electroencephalographic findings frequently are abnormal, with diffuse slowing or focal abnormalities found in most patients. Neurologic recovery almost always is complete within a week, but persistent deficits or a need for prolonged anticonvulsant therapy has been reported.

Patients also may have skin lesions, including maculopapular rash, erythema nodosum, and thrombocytopenic purpura. Other systemic manifestations include hepatitis, splenic involvement, hemolytic anemia, atypical pneumonia, pulmonary nodules, endocarditis, bone involvement such as osteolytic bone lesions and osteomyelitis, an infectious mononucleosis–like syndrome, persistent febrile illness, and disseminated bartonellosis. Bacillary angiomatosis, bacillary peliosis (dilated capillaries or multiple blood-filled cavernous

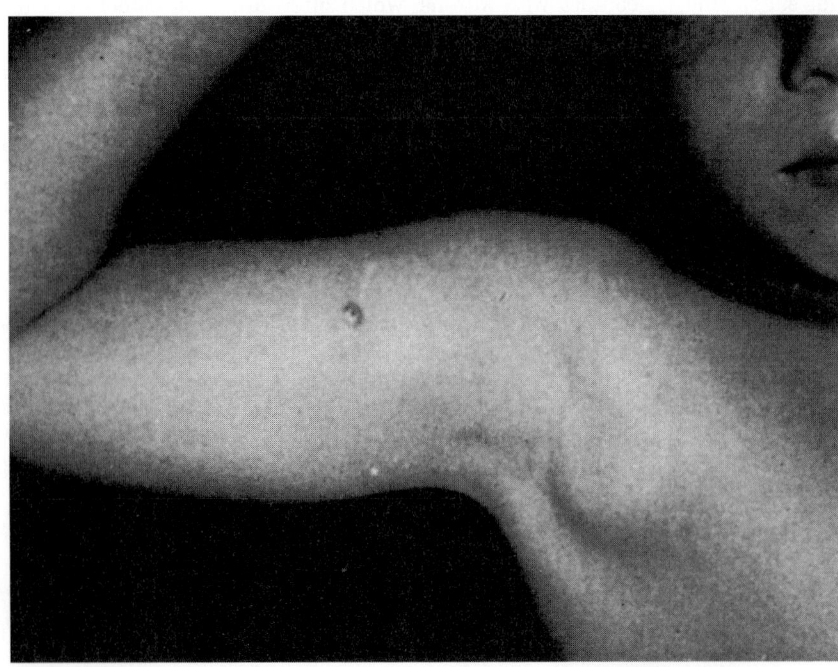

FIGURE 145–1 ■ Cat-scratch disease involving an axillary lymph node with primary granuloma of the upper part of the arm. Note that the primary lesion is within the line of a healed scratch. (Courtesy of Hugh A. Carithers, M.D.)

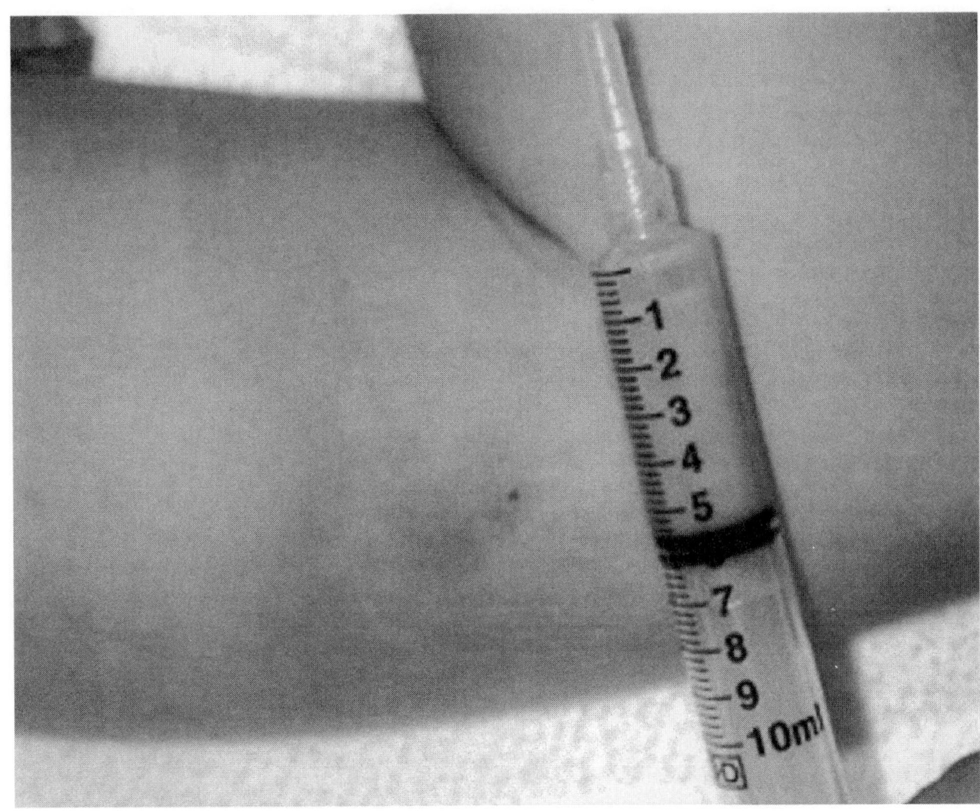

FIGURE 145–2 ■ Purulent material aspirated from an epitrochlear lymph node of a child with cat-scratch disease. The primary lesion was on the index finger.

spaces in biopsy specimens), and relapsing fever with bacteremia can develop in immunocompromised subjects.

Diagnosis

Until recently, the clinical diagnosis of CSD required the presence of at least three of the following: a history of contact with a cat and the presence of a scratch or a primary lesion, a positive skin test, regional lymphadenopathy with negative studies for other potential causes of lymphadenopathy, and characteristic histopathologic findings in a biopsy specimen. The difficulty in isolating organisms in routine culture of lymph node specimens from patients with suspected CSD has created significant problems over the years. An intradermal skin test composed of heated purulent lymph node material from patients with CSD was used for many years to aid in the diagnosis. Although the skin test is 90 to 98 percent sensitive and specific for the diagnosis of CSD, the material is not readily available, is not standardized, and is not licensed for routine use. In addition, the potential for transmission of other infectious agents with this test currently prohibits its use.

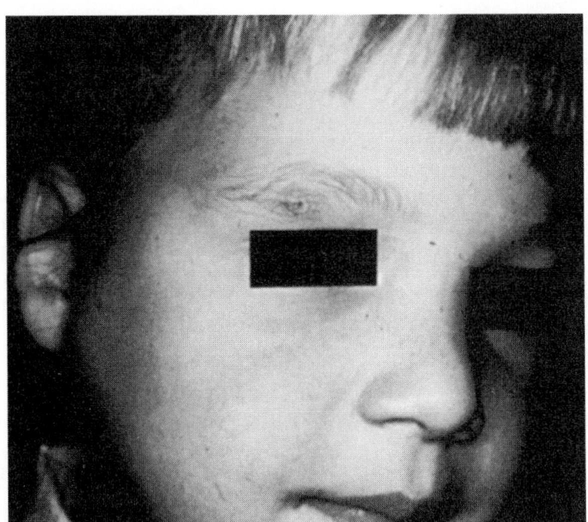

FIGURE 145–3 ■ Child with the oculoglandular syndrome of Parinaud as a manifestation of cat-scratch disease. Note the parotid swelling and the primary site in the right eyebrow. (Courtesy of James D. Cherry, M.D.)

Recently, specific diagnostic tests such as IFA and ELISA to assess serum antibodies against *B. henselae* and PCR amplification to identify *B. henselae* DNA sequences in tissues have reduced the need for performing skin testing and invasive surgical diagnostic procedures. Giladi and colleagues developed a new enzyme immunoassay for IgM and IgG that uses *N*-lauroylsarcosine–insoluble outer membrane antigens from agar-grown *B. henselae* and demonstrated an increased sensitivity of the test.[9] A high antibody titer (>1:64) is suggestive of recent infection. Detection of a significant elevation in titer between acute and convalescent sera may be confirmatory. Currently, with a very sensitive species- and strain-specific assay involving PCR amplification of highly variable regions of the 16S ribosomal RNA gene sequence of *Bartonella,* CSD can be diagnosed in animals also. Different methods of collecting and handling blood can affect isolation of this pathogen. Brenner and colleagues reported that frozen blood specimens from cats infected with *B. henselae* collected in ethylenediaminetetraacetic acid (EDTA) provided the highest colony counts.[5] These authors suggested that host-cell lysis and disruption of cell membranes improved the sensitivity and rapidity of colony formation of *B. henselae.*

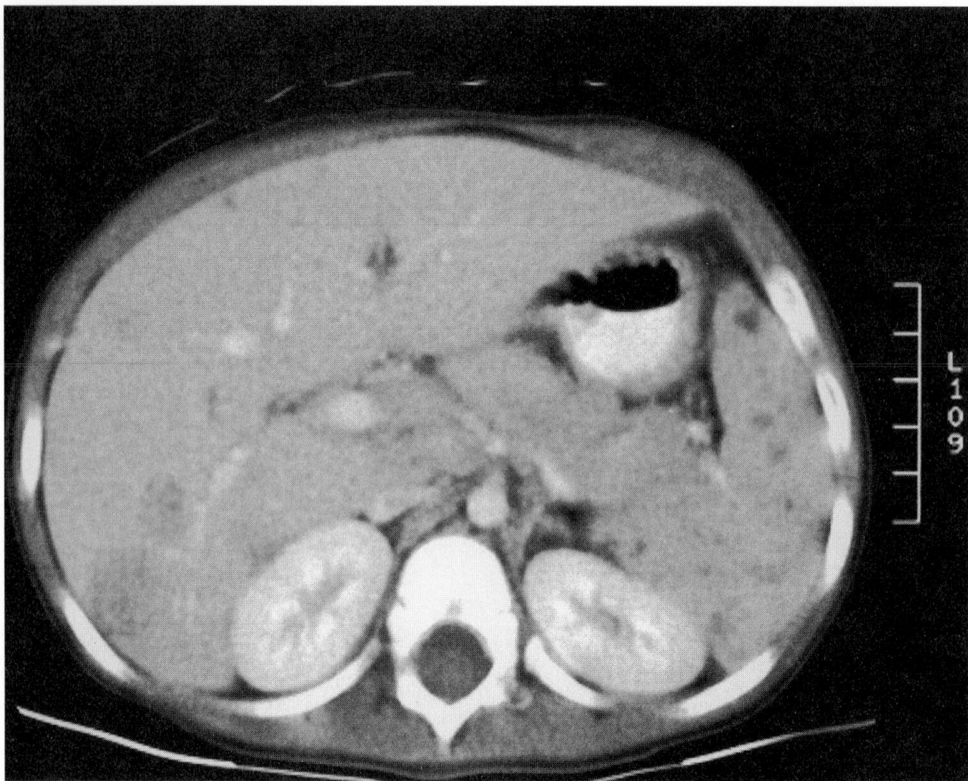

FIGURE 145–4 ■ Multiple hypodense lesions in the liver and spleen on computed tomography seen in a child with prolonged fever, abdominal pain, and positive *Bartonella henselae* serology.

The differential diagnosis of CSD includes various infections such as other forms of bacterial adenitis, typical or atypical mycobacterial infections, lymphogranuloma venereum, infectious mononucleosis, tularemia, plague, sporotrichosis, blastomycosis, histoplasmosis, syphilis, human immunodeficiency virus infection, and other conditions such as benign and malignant tumors, sarcoidosis, and Kawasaki disease.

Treatment

In an immunocompetent host, typical CSD is self-limited and resolves spontaneously in 1 to 2 months without antibiotics. In Margileth's retrospective review of 202 patients with CSD, rifampin was more effective (87%) than were ciprofloxacin, gentamicin, and trimethoprim-sulfamethoxazole.[12] Rifampin (20 mg/kg/day in two doses for 14 days) also may be useful in decreasing the duration of fever in children with hepatosplenic CSD.[3] Penicillins, cephalosporins, tetracycline, and erythromycin had minimal or no clinical efficacy. In a prospective, randomized, double-blind, placebo-controlled study, therapy with oral azithromycin for 5 days was very effective in reducing the lymph node volume measured by three-dimensional ultrasonography within the first month of treatment.[4] Adults and children weighing more than 100 lb were given an initial single dose of 500 mg azithromycin on day 1 of treatment and 250 mg on days 2 to 5 as single daily doses. Patients weighing less received the liquid preparation of 10 mg/kg on day 1 and 5 mg/kg on days 2 to 5. Unfortunately, the only randomized, prospective, controlled study, mentioned earlier, does not address management of the systemic manifestations of CSD. Clarithromycin therapy also has been reported to be effective both in vitro (in Vero cell cultures) and in vivo (in humans for hip osteomyelitis). Recently, the in vitro susceptibility of *Bartonella* and *Rickettsia* to different fluoroquinolones was tested.[11] Levofloxacin exhibited the greatest activity against *B. elizabethae* and *B. quintana*. Reports of the duration of antibiotic therapy have varied from 5 days in immunocompetent patients to 6 weeks in patients with atypical CSD or in immunocompromised patients. High-dose corticosteroid therapy has been used in a few cases of CSD encephalopathy.[19]

The application of moist soaks and local heat, the use of analgesics, limitation of activity of the affected limb, and aspiration of fluctuant material in the nodes may relieve the pain and resolve the inflammation.

Prognosis and Prevention

Typically, the prognosis of CSD is excellent without any sequelae. Although patients with atypical findings and involvement of other organs may have a prolonged course and antibiotics may need to be used, the prognosis is good. Reinfection is extremely rare, and isolation is unnecessary. Currently, preventive measures such as vaccines are not available. Routine veterinary visits, control of flea and tick infestations, and declawing of young kittens are the current practical preventive measures for CSD.

REFERENCES

1. Anderson, B., Kelly, C., Threlkel, R., et al.: Detection of *Rochalimaea henselae* in cat-scratch disease skin test antigens. J. Infect. Dis. *168*:1034–1036, 1993.
2. Anderson, B., Sims, K., Regnery, R., et al.: Detection of *Rochalimaea henselae* DNA in specimens from cat scratch disease patients by PCR. J. Clin. Microbiol. *32*:942–948, 1994.
3. Arisoy, E. S., Correa, A. G., Wagner, M. C., and Kaplan, S. L.: Hepatosplenic cat-scratch disease in children: Selected clinical feature and treatment. Clin. Infect. Dis. *28*:778–784, 1999.

4. Bass, J. W., Freitas, B. C., Freitas, A. D., et al.: Prospective randomized, double blind, placebo-controlled evaluation of azithromycin for treatment of cat-scratch disease. Pediatr. Infect. Dis. *17*:447–452, 1998.
5. Brenner, S. A., Rooney, J. A., Manzewitsch, P., et al.: Isolation of *Bartonella (Rochalimaea) henselae:* Effects of methods of blood collection and handling. J. Clin. Microbiol. *35*:544–547, 1997.
6. Chang, C. C., Chomel, B. B., Kasten, R. W., et al.: Molecular evidence of *Bartonella* spp in questing adult *Ixodes pacificus* ticks in California. J. Clin. Microbiol. *39*:1221–1226, 2001.
7. English, C. K., Wear, D. J., Margileth, A. M., et al.: Cat-scratch disease: Isolation and culture of the bacterial agent. J. A. M. A. *259*:1347–1352, 1988
8. Fuhrmann, O., Arvand, M., Gohler, A., et al.: *Bartonella henselae* induces NF-kappa B–dependent upregulation of adhesion molecules in cultured human endothelial cells: Possible role of outer membrane proteins as pathogenic factors. Infect. Immun. *69*:5088–5097, 2001.
9. Giladi, M., Kletter, Y., Avidor, B., et al.: Enzyme immunoassay for the diagnosis of cat-scratch disease defined by polymerase chain reaction. Clin. Infect. Dis. *33*:1852–1858, 2001.
10. Goral, S., Anderson, B., Hager, C., et al.: Detection of *Rochalimaea henselae* DNA by polymerase chain reaction from suppurative nodes of children with cat scratch disease. Pediatr. Infect. Dis. J. *13*:994–997, 1994.
11. Ives, T. J., Marston, E., Regnery, R. L., et al.: In vitro susceptibilities of *Bartonella* and *Rickettsia* spp. to fluoroquinolone antibiotics as determined by immunofluorescent antibody analysis of infected Vero cell monolayers. Int. J. Antimicrob. Agents *18*:217–222, 2001.
12. Margileth, A. M.: Antibiotic therapy for cat-scratch disease: Clinical study of therapeutic outcome of 268 patients and a review of the literature. Pediatr. Infect. Dis. J. *11*:474, 1992.
13. Musso, T., Badolato, R., Ravarino, D., et al.: Interaction of *Bartonella henselae* with the murine macrophage cell line J774: Infection and proinflammatory response. Infect. Immun. *69*:5974–5980, 2001.
14. Regnery, R. L., Olson, J. G., Perkins, B. A., et al.: Serological response to *"Rochalimaea henselae"* antigen in suspected cat-scratch disease. Lancet *339*:1443–1445, 1992.
15. Relman, D. A., Loutit, J. S., Schmidt, T. M., et al.: The agent of bacillary angiomatosis: An approach to the identification of uncultured pathogens. N. Engl. J. Med. *323*:1573–1580, 1990.
16. Scott, M. A., McCurley, T. L., Vnencak-Jones, C. L., et al.: Cat scratch disease—detection of *Bartonella henselae* DNA in archival biopsies from patients with clinically, serologically and histologically defined disease. Am. J. Pathol. *149*:2161–2167, 1996.
17. Szelc-Kelly, C. M., Goral, S., Perez-Perez, G. I., et al.: Serologic responses to *Bartonella* and *Afipia* in patients with confirmed cat scratch disease. Pediatrics *96*:1137–1142, 1995.
18. Wear, D. J., Margileth, A. M., Hadfield, T. L., et al.: Cat scratch disease: A bacterial infection. Science *221*:1403–1405, 1983.
19. Weston, K. D., Tran, T., Kimmel, K., et al.: Possible role of high-dose corticosteroids in the treatment of cat-scratch disease encephalopathy. J. Child Neurol. *16*:762–763, 2001.
20. Zangwill, K. M., Hamilton, D. H., Perkins, B. A., et al.: Cat scratch disease in Connecticut: Epidemiology, risk factors, and evaluation of a new diagnostic test. N. Engl. J. Med. *329*:8–13, 1993.

SUBSECTION **6**

TREPONEMATACEAE

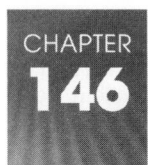

Borrelia (Relapsing Fever)

KENNETH M. BOYER

Relapsing fever is a vector-borne bacterial infection that is characterized by recurring febrile attacks separated by periods of relative well-being. Spirochetes of the genus *Borrelia* cause the disease. It may be transmitted by lice (epidemic relapsing fever) or ticks (endemic relapsing fever).

Relapsing fever first was differentiated from other intermittently febrile conditions in 1868 by Obermeir,[8] who noted the presence of "myriads of living and actively motile spirilla in the blood of relapsing fever patients during the febrile attack." At the turn of the century, Mackie in India and Nicolle in Tunisia elucidated transmission of the epidemic disease by the human body louse. Concurrently, in equatorial Africa, Dutton and Todd discovered that sporadic cases could be transmitted by argasid (soft) ticks.

Massive outbreaks of louse-borne relapsing fever accompanied the social and hygienic disruption in Europe and North Africa that occurred in the wake of both World Wars. At present, louse-borne disease is reported in appreciable numbers only from Ethiopia and Sudan. Tick-borne relapsing fever persists as an uncommon, but widely dispersed, infection in many countries, including the western portion of the United States.[21, 23]

The Organism

The borreliae that cause relapsing fever differ from other pathogenic spirochetes (such as *Leptospira* and *Treponema*) in their loose-coiled morphology and ready staining by Wright or Giemsa stain. These two characteristics permit identification of the organisms in blood smears, a diagnostic finding that is unique among bacterial diseases (Fig. 146–1). *Borrelia burgdorferi,* the cause of Lyme disease, is not seen in peripheral smears, an important point in the differential diagnosis.

Borrelia microorganisms are extremely fastidious in cultivation, and taxonomic classification has depended on the specificity of strain-vector relationships.[14, 26] *Borrelia recurrentis* is transmitted by the human body louse *(Pediculus humanus humanus).* The other species that cause relapsing fever are transmitted by ticks of the genus *Ornithodoros* (Table 146–1).

Propagation of *B. recurrentis, Borrelia crocidurae, Borrelia hispanica, Borrelia hermsii,* and *Borrelia turicatae* in complex artificial media has been accomplished.[34] In common with other pathogenic spirochetes, borreliae

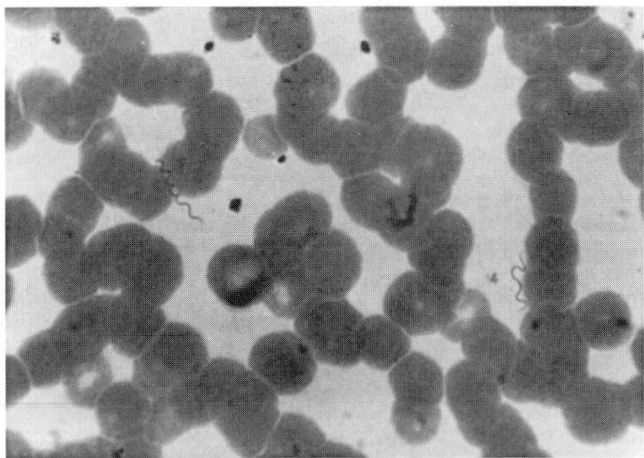

FIGURE 146–1 ■ *Borrelia hermsii* spirochetes in the peripheral blood smear of a 20-year-old patient with tick-borne relapsing fever (Wright stain, ×1000). (From Boyer, K. M., Munford, R. S., Maupin, G. O., et al.: Tick-borne relapsing fever: An interstate outbreak originating at Grand Canyon National Park. Am. J. Epidemiol. *105*:469–479, 1977.)

require long-chain fatty acids for growth. They are microaerophilic and metabolize glucose by glycolysis, with resulting accumulation of lactic acid. Further study of metabolism and DNA homology eventually may simplify their taxonomy. The guanine and cytosine content in the multiple copies of borrelial genomic DNA is an exceptionally low 27 to 32 percent.[3] *B. burgdorferi* has 30 to 44 percent DNA homology with *B. hermsii.*[31] It is clearly a distinct species and perhaps a distinct genus. The 86 percent DNA homology between the two North American relapsing fever spirochetes *B. turicatae* and *B. hermsii,* however, suggests a much closer taxonomic and evolutionary relationship.[3] Analysis of plasmid DNA, protein profiles, and reactivity with specific monoclonal antibodies now permits definitive speciation of isolates that have been recovered in culture.[1]

Transmission

Body lice that transmit relapsing fever become infected by feeding on a spirochetemic patient. Ingested spirochetes enter the hemolymph through the gut epithelium and multiply there. Except for the central ganglion, other tissues such as the salivary glands and genital organs are not invaded. Once infected, lice remain so for their entire life but do not transmit the organism to their progeny. Transmission to humans takes place by contamination of the bite wound with infectious hemolymph when lice are crushed or wounded by scratching. Intermediate hosts for *B. recurrentis* other than humans are not known.[27]

The development of borreliae in *Ornithodoros* ticks differs from that in body lice. After the tick engorges on an infected host, spirochetes invade all tissues, including the salivary glands and, in most instances, the female genital tract. The latter phenomenon results in transovarial infection of progeny, an important survival mechanism. Once infected, ticks remain capable of transmitting infection for years via secretions of infectious saliva or coxal fluid. *Ornithodoros* ticks typically are night feeders and take blood meals lasting an average of 15 minutes, after which they detach themselves. Their bites usually are painless and are noted infrequently. With the exception of *Ornithodoros moubata,* ticks that transmit relapsing fever are maintained in nature by intermediate hosts. Rodents and other small mammals are the major reservoirs of both ticks and tick-borne borreliae.[13, 26, 27, 59]

Epidemiology

The epidemiology of relapsing fever is determined by the habits of its vectors. Acquisition of louse-borne relapsing fever occurs under conditions of crowding, cold weather, and poor hygiene, which favor the spread of lice. Thus, epidemics have occurred in the setting of wars, earthquakes, famines, and floods, often in association with epidemic typhus. In Addis Ababa, Ethiopia, where an estimated 1000 cases of louse-borne relapsing fever occur each year, nomadic tribesmen and seasonal laborers living in conditions of extreme poverty are at risk.[12]

Most foci of tick-borne relapsing fever exist in nature in rather closed environments, such as rodent burrows, nests, or caves. In Africa, Asia, and South America, primitive dwellings with dirt floors, thatched roofs, and rodent nests often harbor endemic species of *Ornithodoros.* In more sophisticated societies, people become part of these ecologic systems only when "roughing it." In the western portion of the United States, for example, where *Ornithodoros hermsi* transmits most cases, a history of sleeping in old summer cabins in forested mountain areas is the rule.[24, 30, 55, 59] In well-studied outbreaks occurring at Browne Mountain, Spokane County, Washington,[56] Big Bear Lake, San

TABLE 146–1 ■ IMPORTANT BORRELIAE CAUSING RELAPSING FEVER, THEIR VECTORS, AND THEIR CURRENT GEOGRAPHIC DISTRIBUTION

Borrelia Species	*Vector*	Geographic Distribution
B. recurrentis	*Pediculus humanus humanus*	Ethiopia, Sudan
B. caucasica	*Ornithodoros verrucosus*	Iraq, southwestern former U.S.S.R.
B. crocidurae	*Ornithodoros erraticus* (small variant)	North Africa, Middle East
B. duttonii	*Ornithodoros moubata*	East and Central Africa
B. hermsii	*Ornithodoros hermsi*	Western United States and Canada
B. hispanica	*Ornithodoros erraticus* (large variant)	Spain, western North Africa
B. latyschewii	*Ornithodoros tartakowskyi*	Iran, central Asia
B. mazzottii	*Ornithodoros talaje*	Mexico, Central America
B. parkeri	*Ornithodoros parkeri*	Western United States
B. persica	*Ornithodoros tholozani*	Middle East, western Asia
B. turicatae	*Ornithodoros turicata*	Southwestern United States, Mexico
B. venezuelensis	*Ornithodoros rudis*	Northern South America

Data from references 5, 13, 14, 26.

Bernardino County, California,[19] and North Rim, Grand Canyon National Park, Arizona,[9, 20] cabins that were the sources of cases were found to contain large rodent nests from which infective ticks were recovered.

Pathogenesis and Pathology

Borreliae undergo spontaneous antigenic variation both in vivo and in vitro.[46, 53] Repeated episodes of dense spirochetemia (10^5 to 10^8 organisms/mL), each involving a different antigenic variant, account for the cyclic nature of relapsing fever in infected humans. Borreliae isolated directly from infectious ticks exhibit much less antigenic diversity.[4, 37, 49] In relapsing fever borreliae, the immunodominant surface protein is called variable major protein (VMP). In serial passage in mice, the progeny of a single organism can give rise to as many as 40 antigenically distinctive VMPs.[2, 33, 46] Different VMPs have some sequence homology but generally differ by considerably more than a single point mutation.[5, 43] The VMP genes of *B. hermsii* are located on multiple copies of linear plasmids. Antigenic variation can be conferred by interplasmidic and intraplasmidic recombination events, as well as by point mutations in the VMP gene. The mechanisms are reminiscent of those used in B cells to generate antibody diversity.[3, 35, 43, 46] With each remission of the disease, the antibodies produced against the variant strain result in immobilization, opsonization, and agglutination.[16, 18, 37] Agglutinated organisms are phagocytosed and cleared from the circulation. Experimental animal studies indicate that during remissions, borreliae persist in the central nervous system, bone marrow, spleen, and liver.[27]

Major pathologic findings in fatal cases include widespread petechial hemorrhaging of visceral surfaces, splenomegaly and hepatomegaly (often with multiple necrotic foci), and diffuse histiocytic interstitial myocarditis.[27, 32] Other features of cases with a fatal outcome include intercurrent infections such as pneumonia, salmonellosis, or reactivated malaria; hemorrhages in the central nervous system; meningitis; disseminated intravascular coagulation; splenic rupture; hepatic coma; and cardiac arrhythmia.[27, 32]

Borreliae cross the placenta, and infection during pregnancy results in abortion or severe infection of full-term neonates.[28, 52]

Clinical Manifestations

After an incubation period of 5 to 11 days, relapsing fever has a sudden onset with high fever (39 to 41° C [102.2 to 105.8° F]), chills, headache, and myalgia.[23] An initial illness of 3 to 6 days' duration will be followed by approximately a week during which the patient is afebrile and feels weak but improved. Relapse occurs with "flulike" symptoms similar to those of the initial episode. As many as 10 febrile attacks have been recorded in untreated tick-borne cases, whereas 4 episodes is the usual maximum in louse-borne disease. Resolution of the febrile attacks, either spontaneously or after antibiotic administration, is by crisis. Relapses become progressively shorter and milder as the afebrile intervals lengthen[10] (Fig. 146–2).

Other clinical features are inconstant and reflect the nature of the infecting organism and the condition of the host. *B. recurrentis* and *B. duttonii* infections are uniformly severe; infections by other species tend to be somewhat milder. Splenomegaly and hepatomegaly, often with associated tenderness, are characteristic. A fleeting macular rash on the trunk, which may become generalized or petechial, is a common finding. Meningeal irritation, iridocyclitis, epistaxis, and myocarditis are more variable in their incidence but may be prominent features.[32, 51] Inflammation at the site of inoculation and regional lymphadenopathy are not seen. Thrombocytopenia, hyperbilirubinemia, and elevated liver enzymes are frequent laboratory abnormalities.

Diagnosis and Differential Diagnosis

Although an appropriate history of exposure is by far the most helpful clue to the diagnosis of relapsing fever,[36] physicians caring for patients who have vacationed in distant endemic areas may not consider the possibility. Often, an alert hematology technician first makes the diagnosis by

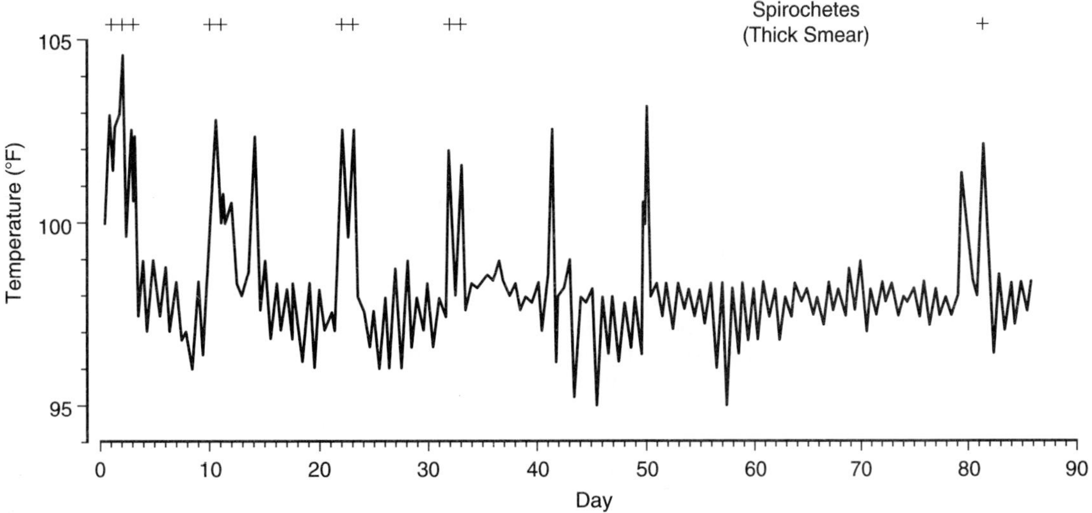

FIGURE 146–2 ■ Febrile course of untreated tick-borne relapsing fever caused by *Borrelia duttonii*. Thick blood smears were examined for spirochetes on each day of illness, with positive results indicated by *plus signs*. (Adapted from Breinl, A., Dutton, J. E., Kinghorn, A., et al.: An experimental study of the parasite of the African tick fever. Memoir XXI of the Liverpool School of Tropical Medicine. London, Williams & Norgate, 1906.)

recognizing loosely coiled spirochetes in a Wright-stained smear of the patient's peripheral blood. Although routine smears usually are positive while the patient has fever, increased sensitivity is obtained by examination of dehemoglobinized thick smears or buffy coat preparations stained with Giemsa[29] or acridine orange.[50] Species-specific fluoresceinated monoclonal antibodies can enhance further the detection of borreliae in blood smears.[48] Immature laboratory mice, in which spirochetemia readily develops after intraperitoneal inoculation with infected blood, provide the most sensitive system for specific diagnosis during late relapses or remission periods.[26] Because of the fastidiousness of *Borrelia,* performing routine blood cultures is helpful only in excluding other causes of bacteremia.

A serologic diagnosis now can be achieved with indirect fluorescent antibody tests and confirmatory immunoblotting,[21] although these tests are limited by antigenic variability. False-positive results can occur in patients with Lyme disease and other spirochetal infections.[33] Conversely, enzyme-linked immunosorbent assays and immunoblot serologic tests for Lyme disease may yield false-positive results in patients with relapsing fever.[21, 45]

Because of its nonspecific initial symptoms and spontaneous remissions, relapsing fever may be misdiagnosed as influenza or enteroviral infection. The "saddleback" fever pattern of Colorado tick fever may resemble relapsing fever, but this condition may be recognized by its characteristic leukopenia. Other tick-transmitted illnesses, such as Lyme borreliosis, tularemia, Rocky Mountain spotted fever, and human ehrlichiosis, may be suggested by a history of tick exposure. In developing countries, malaria, typhoid fever, and rickettsial diseases may show similar clinical findings and are important to differentiate. The microgametocytes of *Plasmodium vivax* may look similar to borreliae in a peripheral blood smear.[22] The periodic fevers, such as familial Mediterranean fever, hyper-IgD syndrome, and the "FAPA" syndrome (fever, aphthous stomatitis, pharyngitis, and adenitis) may resemble relapsing fever but generally have longer intervals between febrile episodes.[38] Empiric treatment with broad-spectrum antibiotics may modify the characteristic fever pattern of relapsing fever or cure it before a diagnosis is made.

Treatment

Because of difficulties in cultivation, no in vitro data are available to compare the efficacy of antimicrobial agents against relapsing fever borreliae. Oral or parenteral tetracycline, erythromycin, and chloramphenicol are clinically effective, whereas intramuscular procaine penicillin G and oral ampicillin result in relapse rates of approximately 5 and 30 percent, respectively. Probably ceftriaxone and amoxicillin also are effective drugs, as indicated by anecdotal experience[33] and by analogy to their efficacy in Lyme disease. The newer macrolides clarithromycin and azithromycin also may have efficacy. Doxycycline (100 mg orally), tetracycline (250 mg intravenously or 500 mg orally), and erythromycin (250 mg intravenously or 500 mg orally) have been used successfully as single-dose regimens for the treatment of adults with louse-borne relapsing fever in Ethiopia.[17, 41, 42] Such regimens have the advantages of low cost and at least partial efficacy against other louse-borne diseases such as typhus.

Erythromycin is considered the drug of choice for children younger than 8 years, whereas tetracycline is considered the drug of choice for older patients. For a febrile patient, however, oral phenoxymethyl penicillin (a single dose of 7.5 mg/kg) or intravenous penicillin G (10,000 U/kg infused over a period of 30 minutes) is recommended as initial therapy. Either should lead to gradual clearance of circulating spirochetes and defervescence. Thereafter, a 10-day course of oral erythromycin or tetracycline (40 mg/kg/day of either drug divided every 6 hours) will eradicate tissue spirochetes and prevent relapse.[42] For an afebrile child between relapses, erythromycin or tetracycline may be given alone without initial penicillin therapy.

Other than the choice of antimicrobial therapy, the major concern in treating relapsing fever is the frequent occurrence of the Jarisch-Herxheimer reaction in the first hours after initiating therapy. This response, an exaggeration of the crisis that normally terminates febrile attacks, is characterized by rigors and hyperthermia followed by drenching sweats, hypotension, and prostration.[11] It may be fatal in louse-borne disease but generally is less severe in tick-borne cases. Rapid clearance of bloodstream spirochetes initiates the process.[11, 17, 54, 58] Release of inflammatory mediators, such as tumor necrosis factor, interleukin-6, and interleukin-8, after bacterial lysis or phagocytosis probably is the major pathophysiologic mechanism.[6, 15, 16, 18, 40, 44] Purified VMPs are potent triggers of production of tumor necrosis factor by human monocytes.[57]

Three approaches to controlling this response have been tried—supportive measures, gradual killing of spirochetes, and pharmacologic blockade. The usual supportive measures involve volume expansion and antipyretics. Penicillins result in slower elimination of circulating borreliae and yield a more prolonged, but less severe reaction than tetracycline or erythromycin does.[47, 58] Steroids (e.g., hydrocortisone) and pure opioid antagonists (e.g., naloxone) do not block the reaction. The opioid antagonist and partial agonist meptazinol (available in Great Britain; not licensed in the United States) effectively blocks the reaction.[54] Fekade and colleagues[25] demonstrated that pretreatment with sheep anti–tumor necrosis factor–α Fab antibody fragments suppresses Jarisch-Herxheimer reactions and reduces the associated increases in plasma concentrations of interleukin-6 and interleukin-8.

At present, the most reasonable approach to limiting Jarisch-Herxheimer reactions is to provide close nursing supervision (either in the hospital or in an office or emergency treatment room) during the first 12 hours after initiation of therapy. During this period, an intravenous line should be in place. The use of oral penicillin as initial therapy is recommended. Positioning, volume expansion, sponging, and antipyretics should be used as necessary to control changes in blood pressure, pulse, and temperature.

Prognosis

With current therapy, case-fatality rates from relapsing fever are less than 5 percent.[44] Without treatment, louse-borne disease, in particular, carries a much higher risk of fatality. Fatal cases of tick-borne disease in North America are rare. Late relapses may occur, particularly in patients with an incompletely treated central nervous system "sanctuary."[39] In untreated cases, immunity persists for several years. In treated cases, the duration of immunity is unknown.

Prevention

Louse-borne relapsing fever is internationally notifiable to the World Health Organization. Tick-borne relapsing fever is reportable to state health authorities in the United States only in California, but its occurrence in national parks and other public recreational settings renders optional reporting desirable.

Prevention of relapsing fever is largely a problem of avoiding its vectors. In outbreaks of louse-borne disease, time-honored measures, such as environmental dusting with insecticide, cutting hair short, laundering at 49° C (120° F), and applying residual insecticides to clothing and bedding, have been effective.[7] In individual cases of louse-borne disease, eradication of pediculosis with 5 percent permethrin or 1 percent lindane is an essential adjunct to specific therapy.

In endemic foci of tick-borne disease, the habits of *Ornithodoros* and humans determine the environmental and personal measures necessary.[9, 19, 20] In the United States, increasing utilization of wilderness recreational areas by the public calls for increased awareness of relapsing fever and its potential transmission. Dwellings in endemic areas should be constructed with "rodent-proof" foundations and soffits. In unsatisfactory buildings, removal of rodent nesting materials and liberal spraying of walls, floors, ceilings, and crawl spaces with 1.1 percent *o*-isopropoxyphenyl *N*-methylcarbamate (Baygon) or a similar residual insecticide are proven preventive measures.[9] The use of insect repellents has been recommended in some instances, but their effectiveness is not established.

REFERENCES

1. Banerjee, S. N., Banerjee, M., Fernando, K., et al.: Tick-borne relapsing fever in British Columbia, Canada: First isolation of *Borrelia hermsii.* J. Clin. Microbiol. *36*:3505–3508, 1998.
2. Barbour, A. G., Barrera, O., and Judd, R. C.: Structural analysis of the variable major proteins of *Borrelia hermsii.* J. Exp. Med. *158*:2127–2140, 1983.
3. Barbour, A. G., Carter, C. J., Burman, N., et al.: Tandem insertion sequence-like elements define the expression site for variable antigen genes of *Borrelia hermsii.* Infect. Immun. *59*:390–397, 1991.
4. Barbour, A. G., Carter, C. J., and Sohaskey, C. D.: Surface protein variation by expression site switching in the relapsing fever agent *Borrelia hermsii.* Infect. Immun. *68*:7114–7121, 2000.
5. Barbour, A. G., and Hayes, S. F.: Biology of *Borrelia* species. Microbiol. Rev. *50*:381–400, 1986.
6. Barbour, A. G., Todd, W. J., and Stoenner, H. G.: Action of penicillin on *Borrelia hermsii.* Antimicrob. Agents Chemother. *21*:823–829, 1982.
7. Benenson, A. S.: Control of Communicable Diseases Manual: An Official Report of the American Public Health Association. Washington, DC, American Public Health Association, 1995, pp. 345–347, 392–395.
8. Birkhaug, K.: Otto H. F. Obermeier. *In* Moulton, F. R. (ed.): A Symposium on Relapsing Fever in the Americas. Washington, DC, American Association for the Advancement of Science, 1942, pp. 7–14.
9. Boyer, K. M., Munford, R. S., Maupin, G. O., et al.: Tick-borne relapsing fever: An interstate outbreak originating at Grand Canyon National Park. Am. J. Epidemiol. *105*:469–479, 1977.
10. Breinl, A., Dutton, J. E., Kinghorn, A., et al.: An experimental study of the parasite of the African tick fever. Memoir XXI of the Liverpool School of Tropical Medicine. London, Williams & Norgate, 1906.
11. Bryceson, A. D. M.: Clinical pathology of the Jarisch-Herxheimer reaction. J. Infect. Dis. *133*:696–704, 1976.
12. Bryceson, A. D. M., Parry, E. H. O., Perine, P. L., et al.: Louse-borne relapsing fever. Q. J. Med. *39*:129–170, 1970.
13. Burgdorfer, W.: Epidemiology of the relapsing fevers. *In* Johnson, R. C. (ed.): The Biology of Parasitic Spirochetes. New York, Academic Press, 1976, pp. 191–200.
14. Burgdorfer, W., Rosa, P. A., and Schwan, T. G.: *Borrelia. In* Murray, P. R., Barou, E. J., Pfaller, M. A., et al. (eds.): Manual of Clinical Microbiology. Washington, DC, American Society for Microbiology, 1995, pp. 626–635.
15. Butler, T.: Relapsing fever: New lessons about antibiotic action. Ann. Intern. Med. *102*:397–399, 1985.
16. Butler, T., Aikawa, M., Habte-Michael, A., et al.: Phagocytosis of *Borrelia recurrentis* by blood polymorphonuclear leukocytes is enhanced by antibiotic treatment. Infect. Immun. *28*:1009–1013, 1980.
17. Butler, T., Jones, P. K., and Wallace, C. K.: *Borrelia recurrentis* infection: Single-dose antibiotic regimens and management of the Jarisch-Herxheimer reaction. J. Infect. Dis. *137*:573–577, 1978.
18. Butler, T., Spagnuolo, P. J., Goldsmith, G. H., et al.: Interaction of *Borrelia* spirochetes with human mononuclear leukocytes causes production of leukocytic pyrogen and thromboplastin. J. Lab. Clin. Med. *99*:709–721, 1982.
19. Centers for Disease Control and Prevention: Common source outbreak of relapsing fever: California. M. M. W. R. Morb. Mortal. Wkly. Rep. *39*(34): 579, 585–586, 1990.
20. Centers for Disease Control and Prevention: Outbreak of relapsing fever—Grand Canyon National Park, Arizona, 1991. M. M. W. R. Morb. Mortal. Wkly. Rep. *40*(18):296–297, 303, 1991.
21. Dworkin, M. S., Anderson, D. E., Jr., Schwan, R. G., et al: Tick-borne relapsing fever in the northwestern United States and southwestern Canada. Clin. Infect. Dis. *26*:122–131, 1998.
22. Dworkin, M. S., Anderson, D. E., Thompson, E., et al.: Photo quiz: Relapse of *Plasmodium vivax* malaria with the presence of microgametes. Clin. Infect. Dis. *24*:447–448, 1997.
23. Dworkin, M. S., Schwan, T. G., and Anderson, D. E., Jr.: Tick-borne relapsing fever in North America. Med. Clin. North Am. *86*:417–433, 2002.
24. Edall, T. A., Emerson, J. K., Maupin, G. O., et al.: Tick-borne relapsing fever in Colorado: Historical review and report of cases. J. A. M. A. *241*: 2279–2282, 1979.
25. Fekade, D., Knox, K., Hussein K., et al.: Prevention of Jarisch-Herxheimer reactions by treatment with antibodies against tumor necrosis factor α. N. Engl. J. Med. *335*:311–315, 1996.
26. Felsenfeld, O.: *Borrelia,* human relapsing fever, and parasite-vector-host relationships. Bacteriol. Rev. *29*:46–74, 1965.
27. Felsenfeld, O.: *Borrelia:* Strains, Vectors, Human and Animal Borreliosis. St. Louis, Warren H. Green, 1971.
28. Fuchs, P. C., and Oyama, A. A.: Neonatal relapsing fever due to transplacental transmission of *Borrelia.* J. A. M. A. *208*:690–692, 1969.
29. Goldsmid, J. M., and Mahomed, K.: The use of the microhematocrit for the recovery of *Borrelia duttonii* from the blood. Am. J. Clin. Pathol. *58*:165–169, 1972.
30. Horton, J. M., and Blaser, M. J.: The spectrum of relapsing fever in the Rocky Mountains. Arch. Intern. Med. *145*:871–875, 1985.
31. Hyde, F. W., and Johnson, R. C.: Genetic relationship of Lyme disease spirochetes to *Borrelia, Treponema,* and *Leptospira* spp. J. Clin. Microbiol. *20*:151–154, 1984.
32. Judge, D. M., Samuel, I., Perine, P. L., et al.: Louse-borne relapsing fever in man. Arch. Pathol. *97*:136–140, 1974.
33. Kehl, K. S.: Relapsing fever: Role of borrelial antigens. Clin. Microbiol. Newsl. *7*:25–27, 1985.
34. Kelly, R. T.: Cultivation of *Borrelia hermsii.* Science *173*:443–444, 1971.
35. Kitten, T., and Barbour, A. G.: Juxtaposition of expressed variable antigen genes with a conserved telomere in the bacterium *Borrelia hermsii.* Proc. Natl. Acad. Sci. U. S. A. *87*:6077–6081, 1990.
36. Le, C. T.: Tick-borne relapsing fever in children. Pediatrics *66*:963–966, 1980.
37. Meleney, H. E.: Relapse phenomena of *Spironema recurrentis.* J. Exp. Med. *48*:65–82, 1928.
38. Miller, L. C., Sisson, B. A., Tucker, L. B., et al.: Prolonged fevers of unknown origin in children: Patterns of presentation and outcome. J. Pediatr. *129*:419–423, 1996.
39. Nassif, X., Dupont, B., Fleury, J., et al.: Ceftriaxone in relapsing fever. Lancet *2*:394, 1988.
40. Negussie, Y., Remick, D. G., DeForge, L. E., et al.: Detection of plasma tumor necrosis factor, interleukins 6 and 8 during the Jarisch-Herxheimer reaction of relapsing fever. J. Exp. Med. *175*:1207–1212, 1992.
41. Perine, P. L., Krause, D. W., Awoke, S., et al.: Single-dose doxycycline treatment of louse-borne relapsing fever and endemic typhus. Lancet *2*:742–744, 1974.
42. Perine, P. L., and Tekly, B.: Antibiotic treatment of louse-borne relapsing fever in Ethiopia: A report of 377 cases. Am. J. Trop. Med. Hyg. *32*: 1096–1100, 1983.
43. Plasterk, R. H. A., Simon, M. I., and Barbour, A. G.: Transposition of structural genes to an expression sequence on a linear plasmid causes antigenic variation in the bacterium *Borrelia hermsii.* Nature *318*:257–263, 1985.
44. Randolph, J. D., Norgard, M. V., Brandt, M. E., et al.: Lipoproteins of *Borrelia burgdorferi* and *Treponema pallidum* activate cachectin/tumor necrosis factor synthesis: Analysis using a CAT reporter construct. J. Immunol. *147*:1968–1974, 1991.
45. Rath, P. U., Ragler, G., Schonberg, A., et al.: Relapsing fever and its serological discrimination from Lyme borreliosis. Infection *20*:283–286, 1992.
46. Restrepo, B. I., and Barbour, A. G.: Antigenic diversity in the bacterium *B. hermsii* through "somatic mutations" in rearranged *vmp* genes. Cell *78*:867–876, 1994.
47. Salih, S. Y., and Mustafa, D.: Louse-borne relapsing fever. II. Combined penicillin and tetracycline therapy in 160 Sudanese patients. Trans. R. Soc. Trop. Med. Hyg. *71*:49–51, 1977.
48. Schwan, T. G., Gage, K. L., Karstens, R. L., et al.: Identification of the tick-borne relapsing fever spirochete *Borrelia hermsii* by using a species-specific monoclonal antibody. J. Clin. Microbiol. *30*:790–795, 1992.

49. Schwan, T. G., and Hinnebusch, B. J.: Bloodstream- versus tick-associated variants of a relapsing fever bacterium. Science *280*:1938–1940, 1998.
50. Sciotto, C. G., Lauer, B. A., White, W. L., et al.: Detection of *Borrelia* in acridine orange–stained blood smears by fluorescence microscopy. Arch. Pathol. Lab. Med. *107*:384–386, 1983.
51. Southern, P. M., and Sanford, J. P.: Relapsing fever: A clinical and microbiological review. Medicine (Baltimore) *48*:129–149, 1969.
52. Steenbarger, J. R.: Congenital tick-borne relapsing fever: Report of a case with first documentation of transplacental transmission. Birth Defects *18*:39–45, 1982.
53. Stoenner, H. G., Dodd, T., and Larsen, C.: Antigenic variation of *Borrelia hermsii*. J. Exp. Med. *156*:1297–1311, 1982.
54. Teklu, B., Habte-Michael, A., Warrell, D. A., et al.: Meptazinol diminishes the Jarisch-Herxheimer reaction of relapsing fever. Lancet *1*:835–839, 1983.
55. Trevejo, R. T., Schreifer, M. E., Gage, K. L., et al.: An interstate outbreak of tick-borne relapsing fever among vacationers at a Rocky Mountain cabin. Am. J. Trop. Med. Hyg. *58*:743–747, 1998.
56. Thompson, R. S., Burgdorfer, W., Russell, R., et al.: Outbreak of tick-borne relapsing fever in Spokane County, Washington. J. A. M. A. *310*: 1045–1050, 1969.
57. Vidal, V., Scragg, I. G., Cutler, S. J., et al: Variable major lipoprotein is a principal TNF-inducing factor of louse-borne relapsing fever. Nat. Med. *4*:1416–1420, 1998.
58. Warrell, D. A., Perine, P. L., Krause, D. W., et al.: Pathophysiology and immunology of the Jarisch-Herxheimer reaction in louse-borne relapsing fever: Comparison of tetracycline and slow release penicillin. J. Infect. Dis. *147*:898–909, 1983.
59. Wynns, H. L.: The epidemiology of relapsing fever. *In* Moulton, F. R. (ed.): A Symposium on Relapsing Fever in the Americas. Washington, DC, American Association for the Advancement of Science, 1942, pp. 100–105.

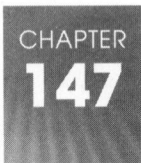

CHAPTER 147 *Borrelia* (Lyme Disease)

BARBARA W. STECHENBERG

Lyme disease, recognized initially in 1975, first was brought to medical attention through the concern of two mothers from Lyme, Connecticut; one contacted the Connecticut State Health Department, and the other contacted physicians at Yale about the unusual illness spreading through their community, a small town approximately 15 km north of Long Island Sound near the mouth of the Connecticut River. Their inquiries sparked an intensive clinical and epidemiologic investigation that has yielded much of the information about this disorder—its wide spectrum of clinical manifestations, etiology, pathogenesis, and treatment.

From these investigations, a distinct pattern of signs and symptoms emerged as a newly described disorder. Actually, the characteristic skin lesions soon were recognized as erythema (chronicum) migrans, a skin lesion that had been associated with a similar, but more limited, illness in Europe since the early 1920s.

The Organism

Because of certain epidemiologic characteristics, particularly the geographic and seasonal clustering of cases, an infectious etiology, particularly associated with an arthropod or other vector, was sought. Early speculation that Lyme disease might be caused by a virus diminished with the report of rapid resolution of erythema migrans and other symptoms with early treatment with penicillin or tetracycline.[103]

In 1982, Burgdorfer and associates[18] isolated a *Treponema*-like spirochete from the midgut of the tick *Ixodes scapularis* (also called *Ixodes dammini*). The spirochete has irregular coils ranging in size from 10 to 30 μm in length and from 0.18 to 0.25 μm in diameter. Electron microscopy demonstrates their close association with the microvillar brush border of intestinal epithelium.

When infected *I. scapularis* ticks were allowed to feed on New Zealand white rabbits, no immediate adverse effect occurred. However, 10 to 12 weeks after tick engorgement, small skin lesions developed that progressed into typical erythema migrans. The sera of all exposed rabbits yielded high titers of antibody to the spirochetes by indirect immunofluorescence. Sera from nine patients with clinically diagnosed Lyme disease also demonstrated positive reactions.[18]

The etiologic role of these spirochetes has been defined further. Steere and associates[101] isolated the spirochete from blood, skin, and cerebrospinal fluid (CSF) of 3 of 56 patients with Lyme disease and from 21 of 110 *I. scapularis* ticks studied. More than 90 percent of the patients had a characteristic immunoglobulin M (IgM) and IgG antibody response; IgM antibody titers reached a peak between the third and sixth weeks after onset, and IgG antibodies rose slowly to reach a peak when arthritis was present. Benach and associates[13] isolated the same spirochete from 2 of 36 patients with Lyme disease in New York. These patients also had a similar rise in antispirochetal antibodies. Berger and his group[16] demonstrated the spirochete in 6 of 14 patients in whom the cutaneous lesions of erythema migrans were studied; four of the six positive specimens were obtained from the peripheries of lesions. Berger was able to demonstrate the organisms in secondary lesions.[16]

Although morphologically similar to known pathogenic *Treponema* organisms, the spirochete found in the *I. scapularis* tick is distinctive because it grows on artificial media. Growth of this fastidious, microaerophilic organism occurs best at 33° C in a complex liquid medium called Barbour-Stoenner-Kelly medium.[8] The organism has an apparent slime layer, an outer membrane that is associated loosely with the underlying structures, flagella (7 to 11), a cell wall, and cytoplasmic constituents.[101] It is coiled more loosely and is longer than are other spirochetes. It resembles borreliae most closely and has been designated *Borrelia burgdorferi*.

B. burgdorferi contains many different proteins. Six outer-membrane proteins that act as surface antigens have been identified: outer-surface protein A (OspA; 30 to 32 kd), outer-surface protein B (OspB; 34 kd), outer-surface protein C (OspC; 22 to 25 kd), outer-surface protein D (OspD; 28 to 30 kd), outer-surface protein E (OspE; 19 kd), and outer-surface protein F (OspF; 26 kd). Other polypeptides include the 41-kd flagellar antigen, several heat shock proteins, and a 93-kd antigen that is part of the protoplasmic cylinder. A 49-kilobase linear plasmid contains genes that encode for the two major outer surface proteins, OspA and OspB.[9] In fact, all isolates of *B. burgdorferi* examined have had four to nine pieces of extrachromosomal plasmid DNA, both supercoiled and linear.[10] The complete genome of *B. burgdorferi* (strain B 31) has been sequenced. The genome consists of approximately 1.5 megabases.[38] The only known virulence factors of *B. burgdorferi* are the surface proteins that allow for attachment to mammalian cells.

Strain differences in DNA and plasmid composition,[60] ultrastructure, and outer-surface proteins among American and European strains have been identified; the European strains generally are more diverse. Three genomic groups of the *B. burgdorferi* sensu lato complex have been identified using several methods. To date, all North American strains have belonged to group *B. burgdorferi* sensu stricto. All three groups have been found in Europe, but group 2, *Borrelia garinii,* and group 3, *Borrelia afzelii,* occur more commonly.[7, 19] These differences may account for variability in clinical expression.

Epidemiology

Evidence for the tick vector had accumulated early in the investigations. During 1977, the incidence of Lyme disease was 30 times greater on the eastern bank of the Connecticut River than on the western shore.[97, 110] Case-control studies of patients, mainly children and young adults and their neighbors, revealed that patients did not participate in more outdoor activities but were more likely to have a cat or farm animal, a pet with ticks, or a tick bite in the year of the study. Ixodid ticks were identified as the likely vector. These ticks have a complex life cycle that spans 2 years, during which they feed once during each of their three stages. In the United States, the white-footed mouse is the preferred host for both the larval and the nymph stages. The larvae feed in late summer, whereas the nymphs feed in spring or early summer. Of importance is that this animal is the host for both of these stages and that it is tolerant to infection. The host-seeking behavior of the nymphs in late May is what initiates the Lyme disease season each year. Although the prevalence of spirochetes in this stage (20–25%) is approximately half that found in the adult, nymphs are responsible for nearly 90 percent of Lyme disease cases,[37] which may be related to their smaller size, their greater abundance, and the coincidence of their peak feeding activity with human outdoor activity. The white-tailed deer is the preferred host for the adult stages and acts as the reservoir during winter months. The adult tick feeds in the fall or winter.

Since the association of the *Ixodes* genus of tick with a large number of cases reported from the Lyme, Connecticut, area, Lyme disease has been reported in at least 46 states and now is the most common vector-borne disease in the United States. More than 15,000 cases are reported each year, representing a 25-fold increase since national surveillance began in 1982. The major geographic areas with clusters of cases include the eastern seaboard (particularly from Massachusetts to Maryland), the upper Midwest (Wisconsin and Minnesota), and the West (California, Nevada, Utah, and Oregon). Massachusetts, Rhode Island, Connecticut, New York, New Jersey, Maryland, Delaware, and Pennsylvania all have incidences of Lyme disease greater than the national rate (6.0 per 100,000). These states account for 92 percent of the nationally reported cases.[64] In the East, the tick associated with disease is the *I. scapularis* or *I. dammini* tick; in the West, it is *Ixodes pacificus*, which prefers to feed on lizards that are not susceptible to infection, thus accounting for the low frequency of disease. In the East and Upper Midwest, these same ticks may be co-infected with *Babesia microti* and *Ehrlichia phagocytophilia.*[109]

In Europe, cases of erythema migrans with and without meningopolyneuritis have occurred within the range of the *Ixodes ricinus* tick, although one case described outside the range of this vector has been ascribed to mosquito bites.[85] The highest frequencies of disease occur in Middle Europe and Scandinavia. The infection has been documented in Russia, China, and Japan. In Asia, the vector is *Ixodes persulcatus.* Isolated cases over a wide distribution, including Australia, where none of the vectors recognized currently are known to exist, suggest that the disease may be more widespread than first realized and may have a broader range of potential vectors. Mosquitoes and deer flies may become infected with the organism but do not appear to be able to transmit the organism to humans.[66]

B. burgdorferi is widespread in the animal kingdom. Virtually any feral or domestic animal can act as an intermediate host. Birds frequently are carriers and may account for the unusual dispersal pattern of Lyme disease.[4] The greatest reservoir continues to be white-footed mice and deer. Wild animals do not develop illness; however, clinical Lyme disease may occur in domestic animals, such as dogs and horses.

As expected with this vector, the disease has a high occurrence in the summer and early fall, with clustering of patients in wooded and sparsely settled areas. The age range of reported cases has been from 2 to 88 years, with a slight male predominance. In 1999, 25 percent of cases were in people younger than 15 years of age.[64]

Pathogenesis

Lyme disease appears to result from direct infection by and the immune response of the host to *B. burgdorferi*. The spirochete is injected into the bloodstream through the saliva of the tick or deposited on the skin in fecal material.[14] After an incubation period of 3 to 32 days, the spirochete may invade or migrate to the skin, causing erythema migrans, or enter the bloodstream, migrating to distant sites. The organism has shown in vitro resistance to elimination by phagocytic cells, thereby increasing infectivity of the spirochete.[40] It has been isolated from CSF of patients with neurologic symptoms up to 10 weeks after the initial tick bite. Success with antibiotic treatment provides evidence that the spirochete still is alive when arthritis is present.[100] The late complications probably are caused by a direct effect of infection with viable organisms and the immunologic response to them. The spirochete can adhere to many different types of mammalian cells and is a potent inducer of tumor necrosis factor and interleukin-1β and interleukin-6.[47] In a rat model, permeability changes in the blood-brain barrier begin within 12 hours of inoculation of the organism, and the spirochete can be cultured from CSF within 24 hours.[39]

Initially, the immune response seems to be suppressed, which may aid dissemination. The specific IgM response peaks between the third and sixth weeks of infection. It often is associated with polyclonal activation of B cells, causing elevated total serum IgM levels, circulating immune complexes, and cryoglobulins.[50] The specific IgG response develops initially during the first 6 to 8 weeks but then matures for months with the development of a wide array of antibodies to both protein and nonprotein antigens. The unusual persistence of the IgM response in patients with severe disease suggests that such patients have a defect in their helper T-cell function needed to switch from IgM to IgG production.[101] Patients with severe and prolonged illness, particularly arthritis or neurologic disease, often have the B-cell alloantigen HLA-DR4.[99]

Histologically, all affected tissues show infiltration of lymphocytes and plasma cells. Some degree of vascular damage may be seen in many sites, suggesting that the organism may have been in or around the vessels. *B. burgdorferi* seems to survive for long periods in certain areas, particularly the skin, nervous system, and joints. With the development of animal models and expansion of knowledge about the immune response to this infection, new information is accumulating about the pathogenesis of this disease, which is well described in a recent excellent review by Steere.[93]

Clinical Manifestations

The clinical findings in Lyme disease can be divided into three stages on the basis of chronologic relationship to the original bite. In the first stage, the presence of the skin lesions is the most prominent symptom; in the second stage, cardiac and neurologic findings predominate; and in the third stage, arthritis is the most common symptom. Any of these findings may occur in isolation or recurrently. Asbrink and Hovmark[5] proposed a clinical classification analogous to that of syphilis, with early infection divided into stage 1 (localized erythema migrans), followed days to weeks later by stage 2 (early disseminated infection), with late or persistent infection as stage 3.

The most common of the clinical manifestations is the skin rash, erythema migrans (Fig. 147–1). This rash usually begins 3 to 30 days after a tick bite, although only approximately one third of patients give a specific history of a bite, which may relate to the small size of the tick. An erythematous macule or papule forms at the site of the bite. It gradually enlarges to form a large, plaquelike, erythematous annular lesion. The median diameter is 16 cm, but it may reach 68 cm.[17] The outer border usually is erythematous and flat, although it may be indurated. The middle area may show clearing, but the center sometimes is indurated or erythematous or may have vesicles. The lesions often are hot to touch and otherwise asymptomatic but may burn, prickle, or itch. They may occur on any area of the body; usual sites include the thigh, buttocks, and axillae; intertriginous areas; or places where underwear may be tight. Mucosal lesions do not occur. Multiple secondary annular lesions occur in 20 to 50 percent of the patients, usually within a few days of the manifestation of the primary lesion. These secondary lesions are evidence of dissemination (stage 2).

The average duration of the initial skin lesion is approximately 3 weeks. It gradually resolves, sometimes with a bluish hue as it fades. Lesions can recur for up to a year or more, often coincident with subsequent attacks of arthritis. Among patients treated with appropriate antibiotics, the lesions usually resolve within several days.

The skin lesions often are associated with systemic symptoms, most commonly malaise, fatigue, headache, stiff neck, and arthralgias; additionally, backache, myalgias, nausea, vomiting, and sore throat may be present. Fever usually is low grade, but the patient's temperature can be as high as 40° C with chills. Fever occurs more commonly in children than adults.[112] Lymphadenopathy, usually regional and associated with erythema migrans but occasionally generalized, may occur. Occasionally, a malar rash, conjunctivitis, or pharyngitis is present. In approximately 10 percent of patients, signs and symptoms consistent with anicteric hepatitis, including hepatomegaly and right upper quadrant tenderness, are present. Most symptoms resolve over the course of a few days, but some patients experience intermittent and fluctuating symptoms for a period of several weeks. Feder and associates[35] described a group of five children who presented with a flulike illness without erythema migrans that was documented serologically as Lyme disease.

Another skin lesion seen in early disseminated disease is *Borrelia* lymphocytoma. Seen in Europe in approximately 1 percent of cases of Lyme disease, it usually presents as a firm, red, red-brown, or red-purple nodule or papule, seen principally on the pinna of the ear in children or on the nipple or areola in adults.[67]

The late skin manifestation is acrodermatitis chronica atrophicans, a progressive dermatologic condition that develops slowly with increasing erythema and pigmentation changes of the skin of an extremity, which spreads over its extensor surface. After initial hyperpigmentation, hypopigmented areas develop, and eventually the skin

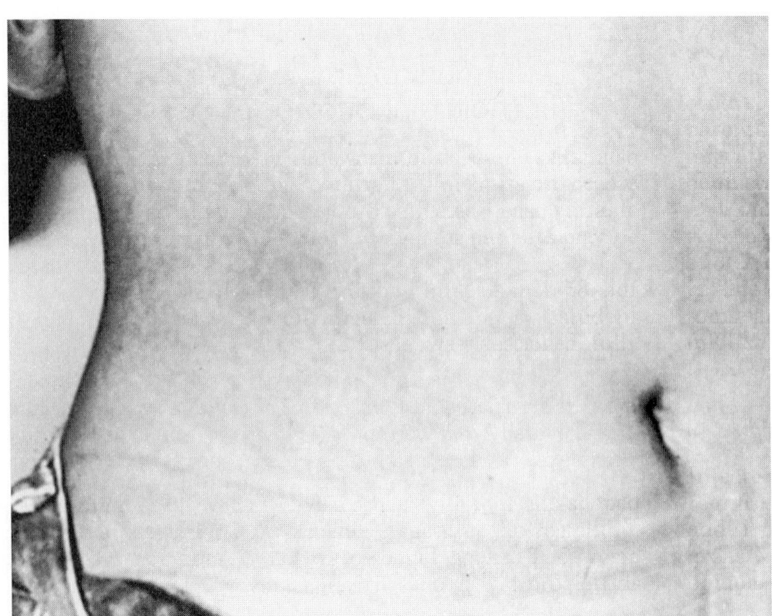

FIGURE 147–1 ■ The typical skin lesion of Lyme disease, erythema (chronicum) migrans. The lesion had progressed from about 3 cm to this size within a week. (Courtesy of Drs. Jane Grant-Kels and Nadine Wenner.)

becomes frail. It is seen primarily in European cases. This condition has been associated with elevated antibodies to *B. burgdorferi* and response to antibiotic therapy.[70] Other associated lesions are fibrotic nodules, other sclerotic and atrophic lesions, and, rarely, eosinophilic fasciitis and progressive facial hemiatrophy.[45, 67]

Although early Lyme disease can cause symptoms of meningeal irritation and headache, they usually are benign and self-limited. Neurologic abnormalities occur roughly within 4 weeks (range, 2 to 11 weeks, but can be up to months) after the tick bite. The spectrum of involvement is wide and includes aseptic meningitis, meningoencephalitis, chorea, cerebellar ataxia, cranial neuritis, radiculopathies, mononeuritis multiplex, and myelitis.[25, 48, 77] The most common occurrence is aseptic meningitis, presenting with headache and stiff neck and often associated with nausea and vomiting, sensory disturbance, photophobia, and irritability. Findings in the CSF are similar to those seen in patients with viral meningitis. The symptoms may occur intermittently for weeks, with mild headache persisting between attacks until spontaneous remission occurs. In a series comparing children with Lyme and those with viral meningitis, Eppes and associates[34] showed that those with Lyme meningitis were more likely to have lower temperature, longer duration of symptoms, associated papilledema or cranial neuropathy, and milder pleocytosis. As many as two thirds of adult patients exhibit subtle findings of parenchymal abnormality or encephalitis[36] with somnolence, emotional lability, memory loss, poor concentration, or behavioral changes. In a series of children with neurologic manifestations, changes in behavior that did not predate the Lyme disease occurred rarely, as did meningoradiculitis and peripheral neuropathy syndromes.[12]

The seventh cranial nerve is involved most frequently in Lyme disease; unilateral or bilateral facial palsies occur in as many as 11 percent of patients.[21] Seventh nerve palsy is seen in approximately 50 percent of patients with meningitis; it also can occur alone. Other cranial nerves, particularly III and IV, are involved less frequently. Several children with pseudotumor cerebri in association with Lyme disease have been reported.[12, 45, 76]

Neurologic involvement can occur in the third stage of illness months to years after the initial infection. These patients present with neuropsychiatric symptoms, focal central nervous system disease, or, rarely, severe incapacitating fatigue.[48, 73] These findings are extremely rare occurrences in children.[12, 88]

Conjunctivitis is an infrequent early ophthalmologic manifestation that usually is transient.[94] A case has been described of iritis progressing to panophthalmitis and unilateral blindness.[98] Spirochetes consistent with *B. burgdorferi* were found in vitreous debris. Other eye manifestations include optic neuritis, iritis, and keratitis.[11] Rothermel and colleagues[81] recently described four cases of optic neuropathy in children with Lyme disease: two children had optic neuritis, one had papilledema, and one had both.

Cardiac abnormalities occur in approximately 10 percent of untreated patients, usually within several weeks (average, 5 weeks; range, 3 to 21 weeks after the bite). Seen most commonly in young adult males, they range from fluctuating degrees of atrioventricular block to myopericarditis and left ventricular dysfunction.[69, 95] Cardiac involvement usually is brief (3 days to 6 weeks). Patients with cardiac involvement usually have other evidence of more severe systemic disease, such as fever, rash, arthritis, or neurologic findings. Although described in children, these cardiac findings are uncommon occurrences among pediatric patients.

The second most common manifestation of Lyme disease after erythema migrans is arthritis, which occurs in approximately one half of the patients without treatment.[26, 104] It begins typically 4 weeks after the skin lesion (5 to 6 weeks after the bite), although the time span can vary from less than 1 week to many months, and a small percentage of patients do not recall having any skin lesions. The arthritis usually is of sudden onset, monoarticular or oligoarticular, and occasionally migratory. Large joints, often those closest to the initial rash, are affected most commonly. The knee is by far the joint involved most frequently, followed by the shoulder, elbow, temporomandibular joint, ankle, wrist, and hip.[30] They become swollen, warm, and painful but rarely red. The usual duration of the first episode is approximately 1 week, but sometimes the episode persists for several months.

Recurrent attacks of arthritis are common occurrences. Among the initial 51 patients studied, 35 (69%) had recurrent attacks.[94, 104] The median number of recurrent attacks was three. During recurrences, usually more joints are involved than in the initial episode. These attacks last approximately 1 week, with intervals of 1 week to 2 years between attacks. Children experience complete remissions between attacks; however, adults often have persistent asymptomatic joint effusions or mild morning stiffness. Approximately 10 percent of all patients with Lyme disease develop a severe chronic erosive arthritis; it occurs approximately 1 year after the initial manifestations and often is associated with HLA-DR4.[99] A rare, unusual complication is rupture of a Baker cyst, which causes a pseudothrombophlebitis.

Other unusual manifestations of Lyme disease include recurrent hepatitis,[44] myositis,[6] eosinophilic lymphadenitis,[75] and adult respiratory distress syndrome.[57] Simultaneous co-infection with the agent of babesiosis or human granulocytic ehrlichiosis may increase the severity of illness or present a more confusing picture.[109]

Maternal-fetal transmission of *B. burgdorferi* has been documented in two infants, one with congenital heart disease,[84] the other with encephalitis.[111] Neither case had evidence of tissue inflammation. A stillbirth that occurred after maternal Lyme disease also has been reported.[65] An analysis of 19 cases of Lyme disease occurring during pregnancy revealed five pregnancies (26%) with adverse outcomes. They occurred in all three trimesters, and no two were the same.[68] In a study of 463 infants, no association between congenital malformations and the presence of antibody to *B. burgdorferi* in cord blood or IgM antibody could be established.[113]

Strobino and associates,[107] in a prospective study of about 2000 pregnant women in an endemic area, found no evidence of fetal wasting, prematurity, or congenital malformations attributable to Lyme disease. In a follow-up study, they found no associated congenital heart disease.[106] Gerber and Zalneraitis[43] surveyed pediatric neurologists in a large endemic area to determine the prevalence of clinically significant nervous system disease that might be attributable to transplacental transmission; they found no cases that met their case definition.

The association of Lyme disease with adverse fetal outcomes appears to be unusual; however, the importance of continued surveillance of pregnant women, as well as prompt diagnosis and treatment, should be emphasized.

Differential Diagnosis

When the characteristic erythema migrans rash is present and recognized, identifying the etiology of subsequent symptoms should pose little problem. However, particularly when the presentation is atypical, the differential diagnosis is broad.

If the rash is not recognized as erythema migrans, it may be confused with streptococcal cellulitis. Erythema multiforme might be a consideration, but the lesions in that disorder often are smaller and urticarial or vesicular, are seen on mucosal surfaces, and often are associated with drug exposure. Erythema marginatum usually is smaller and less annular. If a necrotic or vesicular center is present in the erythema migrans lesion, it may resemble the lesion of tularemia, but the latter is not expansive and not associated with similar complications. Occasionally, a superficial reaction to a tick bite proves confusing, but usually the time course helps. A hiatus of at least 3 days should occur between the bite and development of erythema migrans.

Distinguishing Lyme disease from acute rheumatic fever is particularly important. If the skin lesion is misdiagnosed and migratory arthritis is noted in association with nonspecific electrocardiographic changes, such as prolonged PR interval, one might assume erroneously that the modified Jones criteria have been fulfilled. Fortunately, in Lyme disease, usually no evidence of antecedent streptococcal infection is present, and the specific natures of rheumatologic and cardiac involvement are different.

Other forms of arthritis that may be confused with Lyme disease include (1) pauciarticular juvenile rheumatoid arthritis, (2) psoriatic arthritis, (3) reactive arthritis associated with *Salmonella, Shigella,* or *Yersinia* spp. infections, (4) Reiter syndrome, and (5) postinfectious or infectious arthritis, such as that associated with rubella, hepatitis B, or echoviruses. Several distinctive features usually allow prompt differentiation from Lyme disease.

The major neurologic manifestation of aseptic meningitis may be confused with enteroviral, leptospiral, or early tuberculous meningitis. When it becomes more chronic and relapsing, one must consider sarcoidosis, Mollaret meningitis, Behçet disease, and multiple sclerosis.

Specific Diagnosis

The diagnosis of Lyme disease is made best on clinical and epidemiologic grounds and often can be established early in the course of illness from the gross appearance of erythema migrans.

Routine laboratory testing usually is nonspecific and not helpful. The sedimentation rate often is elevated. Leukocyte counts commonly are normal. Serum glutamic-oxaloacetic transaminase and serum glutamic-pyruvic transaminase levels may be elevated mildly early in the course of the disease. Complement studies may be normal, low, or high. Serum IgG and IgA usually are normal; however, IgM and cryoglobulin IgM often are elevated, particularly in patients with severe disease or in those who later develop neurologic complications or arthritis. Immune complexes as measured by Clq binding (or other methods) may be found in patients with Lyme disease and may be involved in the pathogenesis. They may be present at the time of diagnosis and then clear in those patients without neurologic or cardiac involvement or localize to the synovium in those with arthritis.[50]

Examination of the synovial fluid in patients with arthritis demonstrates elevated leukocyte counts from 500 to 98,000 cells/mm^3, with a predominance of polymorphonuclear leukocytes. Total protein usually is between 3 and 8 g/dL.

Patients with aseptic meningitis often have CSF pleocytosis, with counts ranging from 25 to 450 cells/mm^3, usually with a lymphocytic predominance. Total protein may be elevated mildly, and glucose levels (CSF-to-blood ratio) usually are normal.

Culture of *B. burgdorferi* from specimens permits definitive diagnosis; however, the yield from cultures is too low to render them practical for diagnosis. Therefore, serology currently is the only practical laboratory technique used for diagnosis. Although indirect immunofluorescence first was used to evaluate the immune response to *B. burgdorferi*, the enzyme-linked immunosorbent assay (ELISA) appears to be more sensitive and specific.[23, 82] However, because no standardization of testing has been established, interlaboratory variation in results may be marked.[51, 56] Any serologic results must be interpreted with care. Serologic testing should be undertaken only when the clinical and epidemiologic investigations suggest Lyme disease as the diagnosis.

False-negative results are common occurrences early in the infection.[91] Only 20 to 30 percent of patients have positive responses, usually IgM, in the first few weeks of infection. However, Berardi and associates[15] have developed a sensitive capture IgM ELISA that demonstrates an IgM response in as many as 90 percent of patients with early disease. Some patients treated with antibiotics early in the course of disease may not show an antibody response. In one study, 17 patients with a variety of symptoms were found to be seronegative but to have mononuclear cells with a proliferative response to *B. burgdorferi*.[27] The significance of such responses remains to be seen, but this finding should be considered extremely uncommon.

Techniques to increase sensitivity, specificity, or both include ELISA using flagellar antigen,[49] immunoblotting,[46] and polymerase chain reaction (PCR).[72] Immunoblotting, particularly, may be used to identify false-positive results.[80] The Western blot or immunoblotting separates surface and subsurface proteins of *B. burgdorferi* by polyacrylamide gel electrophoresis, which then are reacted with patients' sera. This technique is more specific than is ELISA or immunofluorescent assay and is particularly useful in identifying false-positive results.[42, 46, 80]

As a result of a national conference on serologic diagnosis of Lyme disease, the Centers for Disease Control and Prevention recommend a two-test approach for active disease and for previous infection using a sensitive enzyme immunoassay or immunofluorescent assay followed by a Western blot if the initial test is positive or equivocal.[20] Negative results need not be validated. For Western blot in the first 4 weeks of disease, both IgM and IgG procedures should be performed. A positive IgM test result alone is not recommended for use for determining active disease in patients with illnesses of greater than 1 month's duration because of a high false-positive rate due to the lower specificity of the IgM immunoblot.[114] If serologic results in a patient with suspected early Lyme disease are negative, paired acute and convalescent specimens should be obtained. Serum samples from patients with disseminated or late-stage disease almost always have a strong IgG response to *B. burgdorferi* antigens. A recommendation is that an IgM immunoblot result be considered positive if two of the following three bands are present: 24 kd (OspC), 39 kd (BmpA), or 41 kd (Fla).[33] An IgG immunoblot result is considered positive if 5 of the following 10 bands are present: 18 kd, 21 kd (OspC), 28 kd, 30 kd, 39 kd (BmpA0), 41 kd (Fla), 45 kd, 58 kd, 66 kd, or 93 kd.[31]

In addition to having false-positive results, 5 to 10 percent of patients in the United States have asymptomatic *B. burgdorferi* infection; these serologic results may interfere with making the diagnosis of another significant illness. In fact, because IgM or IgG antibody responses to the organism may persist for 10 to 20 years after active disease, linking testing to appropriate clinical scenarios is important.[55]

PCR has been used to amplify and detect *B. burgdorferi* DNA in cultured spirochetes, infected animals, and patients with Lyme disease.[72, 78, 86] DNA sequences can be detected in blood, urine, CSF, skin, and synovial fluid. *B. burgdorferi* DNA was detected in 75 of 88 synovial fluid samples from patients with Lyme disease.[72] The usefulness of PCR in clinical situations is an area of active research, but its use may be limited by problems with sensitivity and specificity.[72, 78, 86] The Lyme urine antigen test is unreliable for the diagnosis of suspected Lyme disease.[56, 58]

Diagnosing neurologic manifestations of Lyme disease is particularly difficult. Comparing intrathecal antibody assay results with serum results may be helpful.[96]

Because of the delay in specific antibody response and the possible ablation of this response in patients with localized disease who are treated early, recognition of the clinical picture—erythema migrans, a flulike or meningitis-like illness in the summer, or both—is essential for providing prompt diagnosis and treatment. Laboratory evaluation is unnecessary in early disease and should be used only to support a clinical diagnosis of Lyme disease, in later stages.

Treatment

Even before the spirochete was identified as the causative agent of Lyme disease, antibiotic treatment of adults with penicillin or tetracycline was associated with more rapid resolution of the rash and its associated symptoms.[103] Subsequent studies have confirmed that impression; tetracycline may be more effective in preventing late complications (meningoencephalitis, myocarditis, and arthritis) of the disease.[102] None of 88 patients treated with tetracycline developed such complications, compared with 7.5 percent (3 of 40) of a group of patients treated with penicillin. However, nearly one half of all treated patients still had minor late symptoms, such as headache, musculoskeletal pain, and lethargy. These complications correlated significantly with the initial severity of illness.

Antibiotic sensitivities to *B. burgdorferi* have been determined in vitro and in experimental animals.[52, 54] Although the methods are not standardized, the consensus is that the organism is highly sensitive to tetracycline. It also is susceptible to ampicillin, ceftriaxone, and imipenem. Unlike *Treponema pallidum*, *B. burgdorferi* is only moderately sensitive to penicillin. Aminoglycosides and rifampin have no activity, whereas oxacillin and chloramphenicol are only moderately active. Erythromycin appears active in vitro but may be less so in vivo.

In fact, azithromycin and clarithromycin both are more active, although the clinical efficacy of either is controversial.[29] A trial comparing azithromycin and amoxicillin for the treatment of erythema migrans showed amoxicillin to be significantly more effective.[62] Newer oral cephalosporins, particularly cefixime and cefuroxime axetil, hold promise.[3, 53] Cefuroxime axetil was comparable with doxycycline in a clinical trial in patients with early Lyme disease.[63]

Recommendations for treatment continue to evolve. The Infectious Diseases Society of America recently presented evidence-based guidelines for treatment.[115] For early localized or disseminated Lyme disease, doxycycline, 100 mg twice a day for 14 to 21 days, is effective for adults and children older than 8 years of age. In younger children, amoxicillin, 30 to 50 mg/kg/day in three divided doses, for the same duration appears to be the best choice, with cefuroxime axetil, 30 to 40 mg/kg/day in two divided doses, as an alternative. For penicillin-allergic children who cannot tolerate a cephalosporin, erythromycin, 30 to 50 mg/kg/day in four divided doses, for the same period may be used, although its efficacy is less clear. The duration of treatment is based on clinical response. Multicenter studies of patients with early disease show similar efficacy with doxycycline, amoxicillin, and cefuroxime axetil. Some patients may have subjective symptoms after receiving treatment, but objective evidence of persistent infection or relapse are very uncommon findings.

Patients with isolated seventh nerve palsy should be treated with oral regimens to prevent further complications. If the palsy is associated with other neurologic complications, parenteral therapy should be initiated.

Neurologic complications, particularly Lyme meningitis, have been treated successfully with large doses of penicillin G (20 million IU/day) in adults.[105] No large trials have been reported in children; however, penicillin, 300,000 IU/kg/day, appeared to be beneficial in two cases of pseudotumor cerebri.[76] The exquisite sensitivity of the organism to ceftriaxone renders it an attractive alternative for parenteral therapy, and it has become the drug of choice. The dose of ceftriaxone is 75 to 100 mg/kg/day up to 2 g a day. In a study of 23 patients with late Lyme disease, Dattwyler and associates[26] reported superior efficacy of ceftriaxone over penicillin. Cefotaxime is a reasonable alternative. The duration of parenteral therapy for neurologic or rheumatologic disease is not clear but should be a minimum of 14 days (as long as 4 weeks). The signs and symptoms of acute neuroborreliosis usually resolve within weeks. Even patients with late encephalopathy can be treated successfully with ceftriaxone.[61]

Patients with established Lyme arthritis also have been treated successfully with high-dose penicillin but without universal efficacy.[100] In an uncontrolled study of 33 children with arthritis, 31 were treated with oral therapy alone for 3 to 4 weeks, with elimination of synovitis and recurrent attacks.[24, 32] Oral therapy with either doxycycline or amoxicillin for 4 weeks is a reasonable approach for children without neurologic involvement. Persistent or recurrent arthritis may be treated with a subsequent oral course or parenteral treatment with ceftriaxone.

The self-limited nature of the acute arthritis obviates the need for any analgesics other than acetaminophen or nonsteroidal anti-inflammatory agents. Patients with chronic arthritis usually have been treated with the nonsteroidal anti-inflammatory agents.

Patients with cardiac complications usually do not require specific treatment other than an oral antibiotic regimen if they have first- or second-degree atrioventricular block. Patients with third-degree block should be treated with parenteral therapy such as ceftriaxone, although no clinical data support this approach. Those with heart block may require temporary pacing.[95]

Prognosis and Prevention

Most patients with Lyme disease, particularly those treated promptly with an appropriate antibiotic, have an uncomplicated course. Series in children point to an excellent prognosis in most cases. A review of 65 children treated for erythema migrans and followed for a mean of longer than 3 years found them all to be well and without findings of late Lyme disease.[83] Another prospective study of children with newly diagnosed disease of any stage found that all the children were cured.[88] Rose and associates[79] described 44 children with arthritis who all had an excellent prognosis. A study of cognitive sequelae in children treated for Lyme disease showed no differences between the Lyme disease and control groups.[1] In fact, a study of children with arthritis who initially were untreated for at least 4 years found few children with late or chronic problems.[108] A recent study of 90 children also suggested an excellent prognosis.[41]

After receiving appropriate treatment for Lyme disease, a small percentage of patients continue to have subjective symptoms, mainly musculoskeletal pain, fatigue, and neurocognitive difficulties, sometimes called *chronic Lyme disease*. It is an extremely rare occurrence in children. A large study showed no difference in frequency of pain and fatigue in adult patients who had had Lyme disease compared with age-matched controls.[87] In a recent study of adult patients with post-Lyme syndrome, comparison of treatment with intravenous ceftriaxone followed by doxycycline and treatment with appropriate placebos for a total of 3 months showed no significant differences between the groups.[58]

For the small percentage of patients with chronic arthritis, the course may be variable, although the illness may resolve after 12 to 16 months. With earlier treatment, this group should be held to a minimum.

The prompt recognition of this disease with its diverse manifestations should lead to early treatment and resolution. The best prevention is avoidance of contact with the tick vector.

Even in endemic areas where a large percentage of the ticks are infected, the chance of acquiring disease is not great and depends in part on the duration of attachment of the tick. Attachment for more than 24 hours is required.[74] A recent study using mice and nymphal *I. scapularis* revealed that no transmission occurred in the first 24 hours, with maximum transmission occurring between 48 and 72 hours.[28] A small study of prophylactic antibiotics for tick bites showed a low risk for acquiring disease that was similar to the risk for adverse reaction to penicillin.[22] In a study of prophylaxis after tick bites in a highly endemic area, the risk for development of infection in the placebo-treated group was only 1.2 percent. The authors concluded that, even in an endemic area, the use of routine prophylactic antibiotics is not indicated.[89] A recent trial demonstrated that a single 200-mg dose of doxycycline can effectively prevent Lyme disease if given within 72 hours of the tick bite.[71] One cannot generalize this finding to less endemic areas, other antibiotic regimens, or unidentified, unengorged ticks.[90] However, in certain situations, such as a highly engorged tick on a pregnant woman, prophylaxis might be considered.

Important preventive measures include (1) avoiding high-risk areas, particularly wooded, grassy areas; (2) when walking in such areas, wearing light-colored, long pants tucked into socks, sneakers, and long-sleeved shirts; (3) using insect repellents such as DEET (for skin) and permethrin (for clothing); (4) most important, conducting careful "tick patrols" every day or after every potential exposure to look carefully for the ticks; and (5) removing ticks by pulling them straight out with tweezers or protected fingers.

Active immunization against *B. burgdorferi* consisting of recombinant OspA in adjuvant was available commercially in the United States for appropriate patients at least 15 years of age. In phase III efficacy and safety trials, vaccine efficacy to prevent definite Lyme disease was 49 percent after two injections and 76 percent after three injections.[56] The most important factor in protection was the strength of the antibody response to the OspA epitope. The Advisory Committee on Immunization Practices of the Centers for Disease Control and Prevention advised consideration of vaccination for Lyme disease for people 15 to 70 years old who live or work in high-risk areas and who have frequent or prolonged exposure to the ticks.[2] However, this vaccine no longer is available. A recent trial showed similar safety and higher geometric mean antibody titers compared with adults.[92] Studies of other vaccines are ongoing. Vigilance for tick bites will continue to be the most important preventive measure.

REFERENCES

1. Adams, W. V., Rose, C. D., Eppes, S. C., et al.: Cognitive effects of Lyme disease in children. Pediatrics *94*:185–189, 1994.
2. Advisory Committee on Immunization Practices: Recommendations for the use of Lyme disease vaccine. M. M. W. R. Morb. Mortal. Wkly. Rep. 48(RR-7): 1–24, 1999. (Erratum: M. M. W. R. *48*:833, 1999).
3. Agger, W. A., Callister, S. M., and Jobe, D. A.: In vitro susceptibles of *Borrelia burgdorferi* to five oral cephalosporins and ceftriaxone. Antimicrob. Agents Chemother. *36*:1788–1790, 1995.
4. Anderson, J. F., and Magnarelli, L. A.: Avian and mammalian hosts for spirochete-infected ticks and insects in a Lyme disease focus in Connecticut. Yale J. Biol. Med. *57*:627–641, 1984.
5. Asbrink, E., and Hovmark, A.: Early and late cutaneous manifestations of Ixodes-borne borreliosis (erythema migrans borreliosis, Lyme borreliosis). Ann. N. Y. Acad. Sci. *539*:4–15, 1988.
6. Atlas, E., Novak, S. N., Duray, P. H., et al.: Lyme myositis: Muscle invasion by *Borrelia burgdorferi*. Ann. Intern. Med. *109*:245–246, 1988.
7. Baranton, G, Postic, D. Saint-Girons, I., et al.: Delineation of *Borrelia Burgdorferi* sensu stricto, *Borrelia garinii* sp. nov. and group VS461 associated with Lyme borreliosis. Int. Syst. Bacteriol. *42*:378–383, 1992.
8. Barbour, A. G.: Isolation and cultivation of Lyme disease spirochetes. Yale J. Biol. Med. *57*:521–525, 1984.
9. Barbour, A. G.: The molecular biology of Borrelia. Rev. Infect. Dis. *11*:S1470–S1474, 1989.
10. Barbour, A. G.: Plasmid analysis of *Borrelia burgdorferi*, the Lyme disease agent. J. Clin. Microbiol. *26*:475–478, 1988.
11. Baum, J., Barza, M., Weinstein, P., et al.: Bilateral keratitis as a manifestation of Lyme disease. Am. J. Ophthalmol. *105*:75–77, 1988.
12. Belman, A. L., Iyer, M., Coyle, P. K., et al.: Neurologic manifestations in children with North American Lyme disease. Neurology *43*:2609–2614, 1994.
13. Benach, J. L., Bosler, E. M., Hanrahan, J. P., et al.: Spirochetes isolated from the blood of two patients with Lyme disease. N. Engl. J. Med. *308*:740–742, 1983.
14. Benach, J. L., Coleman, J. L., Skinner, R. A., et al.: Adult *Ixodes dammini* on rabbits: A hypothesis for the development and transmission of *Borrelia burgdorferi*. J. Infect. Dis. *155*:1300–1306, 1987.
15. Berardi, V. P., Weeks, K. E., and Steere, A. C.: Serodiagnosis of early Lyme disease: Analysis of IgM and IgG antibody responses by using an antibody capture enzyme immunoassay. J. Infect. Dis. *158*:754–760, 1988.
16. Berger, B. W., Clemmensen, O. J., and Ackerman, A. B.: Lyme disease is a spirochetosis: A review of the disease and evidence for its cause. Am. J. Dermatopathol. *5*:111–124, 1983.
17. Bruhn, F. W.: Lyme disease. Am. J. Dis. Child. *138*:467–470, 1984.
18. Burgdorfer, W., Barbour, A. G., Hayes, S. F., et al.: Lyme disease: A tick-borne spirochetosis? Science *216*:1317–1319, 1982.
19. Canica, M. M., Nato, F., duMerle, L., et al.: Monoclonal antibodies for identification of *B. burgdorferi*. sp. nov. associated with late cutaneous manifestations of Lyme borreliosis. Scand. J. Infect. Dis. *25*:441–448, 1993.
20. Centers for Disease Control and Prevention: Recommendations for test performance and interpretation from the second national conference on serologic diagnosis of Lyme disease. M. M. W. R. *44*:590–591, 1995.
21. Clark, J. R., Carlson, R. D., Sasaki, C. T., et al.: Facial paralysis in Lyme disease. Laryngoscope *95*:1341–1345, 1985.
22. Costello, C. M., Steere, A. C., Pinkerton, R. E., et al.: Prospective study of tick bites in an endemic area for Lyme disease. J. Infect. Dis. *159*: 136–139, 1989.
23. Craft, J. E., Grodzicki, R. L., and Steere, A. C.: Antibody response in Lyme disease: Evaluation of diagnostic tests. J. Infect. Dis. *149*:789–795, 1984.
24. Culp, R. W., Eichenfield, A. H., Davidson, R. S., et al.: Lyme arthritis in children. J. Bone Joint Surg. [Am.] *69*:96–99, 1987.
25. Darras, B. T., Annunziato, D., and Leggiadro, R. J.: Lyme disease with neurologic abnormalities. Pediatr. Infect. Dis. *2*:47–49, 1982.
26. Dattwyler, R. J., Halperin, J. J., Volkman, D. J., et al.: Treatment of late Lyme borreliosis: Randomized comparison of ceftriaxone and penicillin. Lancet *1*:1191–1194, 1988.
27. Dattwyler, R. J., Volkman, D. J., Luft, B. J., et al.: Seronegative Lyme disease: Dissociation of specific T- and B-lymphocyte responses to *Borrelia burgdorferi*. N. Engl. J. Med. *319*:1441–1446, 1988.
28. des Vignes, F., Piesman, J., Jeffernan, R., and Schulze, T. L.: Effect of tick removal on transmission of *Borrelia burgdorferi* and *Ehrlichia phagocytophila* by *Ixodes scapularis* nymphs. J. Infect. Dis. *183*:773–778, 2001.
29. Dever, L. L., Jogensen, J. H., and Barbour, A. G.: Comparative in vitro activities of clarithromycin, azithromycin, and erythromycin against *Borrelia burgdorferi*. Antimicrob. Agents Chemother. *37*:1700–1706, 1993.
30. Doughty, R. A.: Lyme disease. Pediatr. Rev. *6*:20–25, 1984.
31. Dressler, F., Whalen, J. A., Reinhardt, B. N., et al.: Western blotting in the serodiagnosis of Lyme disease. J. Infect. *167*:392–400, 1993.
32. Eichenfield, A. H., Goldsmith, D. P., Benach, J. L., et al.: Childhood Lyme arthritis: Experience in an endemic area. J. Pediatr. *109*:753–758, 1986.

33. Engstrom, S. M., Snoop, E., and Johnson, R. C.: Immunoblot interpretation criteria for serodiagnosis of early Lyme disease. J. Clin. Microbiol. *33*:419–427, 1995.
34. Eppes, S. C., Nelson D. K., Lewis, L. L. and Klein, J. D.: Characterization of Lyme meningitis and comparison with viral meningitis in children. Pediatrics *103*:957–960, 1999.
35. Feder, H. M., Gerber, M. A., Drause, P. J., et al.: Early Lyme disease: A flu-like illness without erythema migrans. Pediatrics *91*:456–459, 1993.
36. Feder, H. M., Zalneraitis, E. L., and Reik, L.: Lyme disease: Acute focal meningoencephalitis in a child. Pediatrics *82*:931–934, 1988.
37. Fish, D.: Environmental risk and prevention of Lyme disease. Am. J. Med. *98*(Suppl. 4A):2S–7S, 1995.
38. Fraser, C. M., Casjens S., Huang W. M., et al.: Genomic sequence of a Lyme disease spirochete, *Borrelia burgdorferi*. Nature *390*:580–586, 1997.
39. Garcia-Monco, J. C., Villar, B. F., Alen, J. C., et al.: *Borrelia burgdorferi* in the central nervous system: Experimental and clinical evidence of early invasion. J. Infect. Dis. *161*:1187–1193, 1990.
40. Georgilis, K., Steere, A. C., and Klempner, M. S.: Infectivity of *Borrelia burgdorferi* correlates with resistance to elimination by phagocytic cells. J. Infect. Dis. *163*:150–155, 1991.
41. Gerber, M. A., Zemel L. S., and Shapiro, E. D.: Lyme arthritis in children: Clinical epidemiology and long-term outcomes. Pediatrics *102*:905–908, 1998.
42. Gerber, M. D., and Shapiro, E. D.: Diagnosis of Lyme disease in children. J. Pediatr. *121*:157–162, 1992.
43. Gerber, M. D., and Zalneraitis, E. L.: Childhood neurologic disorders and Lyme disease during pregnancy. Pediatr. Neurol. *11*:41–43, 1994.
44. Goellner, M. H., Agger, W. A., Burgess, J. H., et al.: Hepatitis due to recurrent Lyme disease. Ann. Intern. Med. *108*:707–708, 1988.
45. Granter, S. R, Barnhill, R. L., Hewins, M. E., et al.: Identification of *Borrelia burgdorferi* in diffuse fasciitis with peripheral eosinophilia: *Borrelia fasciitis*. J. A. M. A. *272*:1283–1285, 1994.
46. Grodzicki, R. L., and Steere, A. C.: Comparison of immunoblotting and indirect enzyme-linked immunosorbent assay using different antigen preparations for diagnosing early Lyme disease. J. Infect. Dis. *157*: 790–797, 1988.
47. Habicht, G. S., Katona, L. I., and Benach, J. L.: Cytokines and the pathogenesis of neuroborreliosis: *B. burgdorferi* induces glioma cells to secrete interleukin-6. J. Infect. Dis. *164*:568–574, 1991.
48. Halperin, J. J., Luft, B. J., Anand, A. K., et al.: Lyme neuroborreliosis: Central nervous system manifestations. Neurology *39*:753–759, 1989.
49. Hansen, K., and Asbrink, E.: Serodiagnosis of erythema migrans and acrodermatitis chronica atrophicans by the *Borrelia burgdorferi* flagellum enzyme-linked immunosorbent assay. J. Clin. Microbiol. *27*:545–551, 1989.
50. Hardin, J. A., Steere, A. C., and Malawista, S. E.: Immune complexes and the evolution of Lyme arthritis. N. Engl. J. Med. *301*:1358, 1979.
51. Hedberg, C. W., Osterholm, M. T., MacDonald, K. L., et al.: An interlaboratory study of antibody to *Borrelia burgdorferi*. J. Infect. Dis. *6*:1325–1327, 1987.
52. Johnson, R. C., Klein, G. C., Schmid, G. P., et al.: Susceptibility of the Lyme disease spirochete to seven antimicrobial agents. Yale J. Biol. Med. *57*:549–553, 1984.
53. Johnson, R. C., Kodner, C. B., Jurkovich, P. J., et al.: Comparative in vitro and in vivo susceptibilities of the Lyme disease spirochete *Borrelia burgdorferi* to cefuroxime and other antimicrobial agents. Antimicrob. Agents Chemother. *34*:2133–2136, 1990.
54. Johnson, R. C., Kodner, C., and Russel, M.: In vitro and in vivo susceptibility of the Lyme disease spirochete, *Borrelia burgdorferi* to four antimicrobial agents. Antimicrob. Agents Chemother. *31*:164–167, 1987.
55. Kalish, R. A., McHugh G., Granquist J., et al.: Persistence of immunoglobulin M or immunoglobulin G antibody responses after active Lyme disease. Clin. Infect. Dis. *33*:780–785, 2001.
56. Keller, D., Koster, F. T., Marks, D. H., et al.: Safety and immunogenicity of a recombinant outer surface protein A Lyme vaccine. J. A. M. A. *27*: 1764–1768, 1994.
57. Kirsch, M., Ruben, F. L., Steere, A. C., et al.: Fatal adult respiratory distress syndrome in a patient with Lyme disease. J. A. M. A. *259*: 2737–2739, 1988.
58. Klempner, M. S., Hu, L. T., Evans J., et al.: Two controlled trials of antibiotic treatment in patients with persistent symptoms and a history of Lyme disease. N. Engl. J. Med. *345*:85–92, 2001.
59. Klempner, M. S., Schmid C. H., Hu, L., et al.: Intralaboratory reliability of serologic and urine testing for Lyme disease. Am. J. Med. *110*:217–219, 2001.
60. LeFebvre, R. B., Perng, G. C., and Johnson, R. C.: Characterization of *Borrelia burgdorferi* isolates by restriction endonuclease analysis and DNA hybridization. J. Clin. Microbiol. *27*:636–639, 1989.
61. Logigian, E. L., Kaplan, R. F., and Steere, A. C.: Successful treatment of Lyme encephalopathy with intravenous ceftriaxone. J. Infect. Dis. *180*:377–383, 1999.
62. Luft, B. J., Dattwyler, R. J., Johnson, R. C., et al.: Azithromycin compared with amoxicillin in the treatment of erythema migrans: A double-blind, randomized, controlled trial. Ann. Intern. Med. *124*:785–791, 1996.
63. Luger, S. W., Paparone, P., Wormser, G. P., et al.: Comparison of cefuroxime axetil and doxycycline in treatment of patients with early Lyme disease associated with erythema migrans. Antimicrob. Agents Chemother. *39*:661–667, 1995.
64. Lyme disease, United States, 1999: Centers for Disease Control and Prevention. M. M. W. R. Morb. Mortal. Wkly. Rep. *50*:181–185, 2001.
65. MacDonald, A. B., Benach, J. L., and Burgdorfer, W.: Still birth following maternal Lyme disease. N. Y. State J. Med. *87*:615–616, 1987.
66. Magnarelli, L. A., and Anderson, J. F.: Ticks and biting insects infected with the etiologic agent of Lyme disease, *Borrelia burgdorferi*. J. Clin. Microbiol. *26*:1482–1486, 1988.
67. Malane, M. S., Grant-Kels, J. M., Feder, H. M., et al.: Diagnosis of Lyme disease based on dermatologic manifestations. Ann. Intern. Med. *114*: 490–498, 1991.
68. Markowitz, L. E., Steere, A. C., Benach, J. L., et al.: Lyme disease during pregnancy. J. A. M. A. *255*:3394–3396, 1986.
69. McAlister, H. F., Klementowicz, P. T., Andrews, C., et al.: Lyme carditis: An important cause of reversible heart block. Ann. Intern. Med. *110*: 339–345, 1989.
70. Nadal, D., Gundelfinger, R., Flueler, U., et al.: Acrodermatitis chronica atrophicans. Arch. Dis. Child. *63*:72–74, 1988.
71. Nadelman, R. B., Nowakowski J., Fish, D., et al.: Prophylaxis with single-dose doxycycline for the prevention of Lyme disease after an *Ixodes scapularis* tick bite. N. Engl. J. Med. *345*:79–84, 2001.
72. Nocton, J. J., Dressler, F., Rutledge, B. J., et al.: Detection of *Borrelia burgdorferi* DNA by polymerase chain reaction in synovial fluid from patients with Lyme arthritis. N. Engl. J. Med. *330*:329–334, 1994.
73. Pachner, A. R., Duray, P., and Steere, A. C.: Central nervous system manifestations of Lyme disease. Arch. Neurol. *46*:790–795, 1989.
74. Piesman, J., Mather, T. N., Sinsky, R. J., et al.: Duration of tick attachment and *Borrelia burgdorferi* transmission. J. Clin. Microbiol. *25*: 557–558, 1987.
75. Ramakrishnan, T., Gloster, E., Bonagura, V. R., et al.: Eosinophilic lymphadenitis in Lyme disease. Pediatr. Infect. Dis. *8*:180–181, 1989.
76. Raucher, H. S., Kaufman, D. M., Goldfarb, J., et al.: Pseudotumor cerebri and Lyme disease: A new association. J. Pediatr. *107*:931–933, 1985.
77. Reik, L., Steere, A. C., Bartenhagen, N. H., et al.: Neurologic abnormalities of Lyme disease. Medicine *58*:281–294, 1979.
78. Rosa, P. A., and Schwan, T. G.: A specific and sensitive assay for the Lyme disease spirochete *Borrelia burgdorferi* using the polymerase chain reaction. J. Infect. Dis. *160*:1018–1029, 1989.
79. Rose, C. D., Fawcett, P. T., Epps, S. C., et al.: Pediatric Lyme arthritis: Clinical spectrum and outcome. J. Pediatr. Orthop. *14*:238–241, 1994.
80. Rose, C. D., Fawcett, P. T., Singsen, B. H., et al.: Use of Western blot and enzyme-linked immunosorbent assays to assist in the diagnosis of Lyme disease. Pediatrics *88*:465–470, 1991.
81. Rothermel H., Hedges, T. R., III, and Steere, A. C.: Optic neuropathy in children with Lyme disease. Pediatrics *108*:477–481, 2001.
82. Russell, H., Sampson, J. S., Schmid, G. P., et al.: Enzyme-linked immunoabsorbent assay and indirect immunofluorescence assay for Lyme disease. J. Infect. Dis. *149*:465–470, 1984.
83. Salazar, J. C., Gerber, M. A., and Goff, C. W.: Longterm outcome of Lyme disease in children given early treatment. J. Pediatr. *122*:591–593, 1993.
84. Schlesinger, P. A., Duray, P. H., Durk, B. A., et al.: Maternal-fetal transmission of the Lyme disease spirochete, *Borrelia burgdorferi*. Ann. Intern. Med. *103*:67–68, 1985.
85. Schmid, G. P.: The global distribution of Lyme disease. Rev. Infect. Dis. *7*:41–50, 1985.
86. Schwartz, I., Wormser, G. P., Schwartz, J. J., et al.: Diagnosis of early Lyme disease by polymerase chain reaction amplification and culture of skin biopsies from erythema migrans lesions. J. Clin. Microbiol. *30*: 3082–3088, 1992.
87. Seltzer, E. G., Gerber M. A., Cartter, M. L., et.al.: Long-term outcomes in persons with Lyme disease. J. A. M. A. 283:609–616, 2000.
88. Shapiro, E. D.: Lyme disease in children. Am. J. Med. *98*(Suppl. 4A): 69S–73S, 1995.
89. Shapiro, E. D., Gerber, M. A., Holabird, N. B., et al.: A controlled trial of antimicrobial prophylaxis for Lyme disease after deer-tick bites. N. Engl. J. Med. *327*:1769–1773, 1992.
90. Shapiro, E. D.: Doxycycline for tick bites not for everyone. N. Engl. J. Med. *345*:133–134, 2001.
91. Shrestha, M., Grodzicki, R. L., and Steere, A. C.: Diagnosing early Lyme disease. Am. J. Med. *78*:235–240, 1985.
92. Sikand, V. K., Halsey, N., Krause, P. J., et al.: *Borrelia burgdorferi* outer surface protein A vaccine against Lyme disease in healthy children and adolescents: A randomized controlled trial. Pediatrics *108*:123–128, 2001.
93. Steere, A. C.: Lyme disease. N. Engl. J. Med. *345*:115–125, 2001.
94. Steere, A. C., Bartenhagen, N. H., Craft, J. E., et al.: The early clinical manifestations of Lyme disease. Ann. Intern. Med. *99*:22–26, 1983.
95. Steere, A. C., Batsford, W. P., Weinberg, M., et al.: Lyme carditis: Cardiac abnormalities of Lyme disease. Ann. Intern. Med. *93*:8–16, 1980.
96. Steere, A. C., Berardi, V. P., Weeks, K. E., et al.: Evaluation of the intrathecal antibody response to *Borrelia burgdorferi* as a diagnostic test for Lyme neuroborreliosis. J. Infect. Dis. *161*:1203–1209, 1990.

97. Steere, A. C., Broderick, T. F., and Malawista, S. E.: Erythema chronicum migrans and Lyme arthritis: Epidemiologic evidence for a tick vector. Am. J. Epidemiol. *108*:312–321, 1978.
98. Steere, A. C., Duray, P. H., Kauffmann, D. J. H., et al.: Unilateral blindness caused by infection with the Lyme disease spirochete, *Borrelia burgdorferi*. Ann. Intern. Med. *103*:382–384, 1985.
99. Steere, A. C., Dwyer, E., and Winchester, R.: Association of chronic Lyme arthritis with HLA-DR4 and HLA-DR2 alleles. N. Engl. J. Med. *323*:219–223, 1990.
100. Steere, A. C., Green, J., Schoen, R. T., et al.: Successful parenteral penicillin therapy of established Lyme arthritis. N. Engl. J. Med. *312*:869–874, 1985.
101. Steere, A. C., Grodzicki, R. L., Kernblatt, A. N., et al.: The spirochetal etiology of Lyme disease. N. Engl. J. Med. *308*:733–740, 1983.
102. Steere, A. C., Hutchinson, G. J., Rahn, D. W., et al.: Treatment of the early manifestations of Lyme disease. Ann. Intern. Med. *99*:22–26, 1983.
103. Steere, A. C., Malawista, S. E., Newman, J. H., et al.: Antibiotic therapy in Lyme disease. Ann. Intern. Med. *93*:1–8, 1980.
104. Steere, A. C., Malawista, S. E., Snydman, D. R., et al.: Lyme arthritis. Arthritis Rheum. *20*:7–17, 1977.
105. Steere, A. C., Pachner, A. R., and Malawista, S. E.: Neurologic abnormalities of Lyme disease: Successful treatment with high-dose intravenous penicillin. Ann. Intern. Med. *99*:767–772, 1983.
106. Strobino, B. A., Abid, S., Gewitz, M., et al.: Maternal Lyme disease and congenital heart disease: A case control study in an endemic area. Am. J. Obstet. Gynecol. *180*:711–716, 1999.
107. Strobino, B. A., Williams, C. L., Abid, S., et al.: Lyme disease and pregnancy outcome: A prospective study of two thousand prenatal patients. Am. J. Obstet. Gynecol. *169*:367–374, 1993.
108. Szer, I. S., Taylor, E., and Steere, A. C.: The long-term course of Lyme arthritis in children. N. Engl. J. Med. *325*:159–163, 1991.
109. Thompson, C., Spielman A., and Krause P. J.: Coinfecting deer-associated zoonoses: Lyme disease, babesiosis and ehrlichiosis. Clin. Infect. Dis. *33*:676–685, 2001.
110. Wallis, R. C., Brown, S. E., Kloter, K. O., et al.: Erythema chronicum migrans and Lyme arthritis: Field study of ticks. Am. J. Epidemiol. *105*:322–327, 1978.
111. Weber, K., Bratzke, H. J., Neubert, U., et al.: *Borrelia burgdorferi* in a newborn despite oral penicillin for Lyme borreliosis during pregnancy. Pediatr. Infect. Dis. *7*:286–289, 1988.
112. Williams, C. L., Strobino, B., Lee, A., et al.: Lyme disease in childhood: Clinical and epidemiologic features of ninety cases. Pediatr. Infect. Dis. *9*:10–14, 1990.
113. Williams, C. L., Benach, J. L., Curran, A. S., et al.: Lyme disease during pregnancy: A cord blood serosurvey. Ann. N. Y. Acad. Sci. *539*:504–506, 1988.
114. Wormser, G. P., Aguero-Rosenfeld, M. E., and Nadelman, R. B.: Lyme disease serology: Problems and opportunities. J. A. M. A. *282*:79–80, 1999.
115. Wormser, G. P., Nadelman, R. B., Dattwyler, R. J., et al.: Practice guidelines for the treatment of Lyme disease. Clin. Infect. Dis. *31*:S1–S14, 2000.

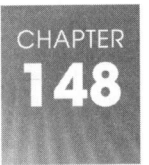

CHAPTER 148 Leptospirosis

RALPH D. FEIGIN

History

Weil[176] is credited with providing the first description of leptospirosis in 1886. Not until 1915, however, was the causal agent, "spirochaeta icterohaemorrhagiae," identified by Inada and associates.[85] Two years earlier, Stimson[148] unknowingly had identified the same organism within sections of kidney obtained from a patient who had been diagnosed incorrectly as having yellow fever.

Noguchi[113] first recovered this organism from a Norway rat in 1917; in 1922, the first case of Weil disease in a person associated with rat exposure was identified.[171] For many years, the rat was considered the only animal host of *Leptospira icterohaemorrhagiae*. In 1944, Randall and Cooper[120] isolated this agent from a naturally infected dog, and *L. icterohaemorrhagiae* subsequently has been associated with many animal hosts, including goats, swine, cattle, and hamsters.

In 1938 and 1939, Meyer and associates[104] popularized the concept that infection with *Leptospira canicola* caused disease in dogs and humans in the United States. "Canicola fever" first was reported in Great Britain in 1946,[14] and in 1951, 40 percent of the dogs in Great Britain were noted to be seropositive.[33] Surveys have confirmed the presence of *L. canicola* infection in species other than dogs.[132, 168]

In 1950, Gochenour and colleagues[72] identified *Leptospira pomona* as the agent responsible for leptospirosis in cows. Widespread *L. pomona* infection among cattle in the United States was recognized quickly, and, in time, this finding stimulated extensive epidemiologic investigations in livestock. Infections of cattle with *Leptospira hebdomidis* and *Leptospira grippotyphosa* were identified, and, concomitantly, infections of swine and horses with *L. pomona* were documented.[80] In Europe, *L. pomona* was identified as the agent responsible for "swineherd disease," and it was recovered from other domestic animals as well. In 1951, the first human cases of *L. pomona* infection were identified.

Many new serotypes of leptospires were recognized after the establishment in the early 1950s of serologic diagnostic services for leptospires by the Centers for Disease Control and Prevention (CDC) and the Walter Reed Army Institute of Research. Along with the identification of additional leptospiral serotypes, the spectrum of clinical disease associated with infection by leptospires was elucidated. Patients with autumnal fever (a disease in Japanese peasants and potters) and Fort Bragg fever (a febrile illness associated with pretibial eruptions described in army recruits) were shown to suffer from leptospirosis caused by *Leptospira autumnalis*.[128] "Mud fever," "pea-pickers disease," and "European swamp fever," terms that were used to describe a disease of undetermined etiology in East Germany, the Far East, and western Poland, were shown to be examples of leptospirosis caused by *L. grippotyphosa*.[38, 71] Seven-day fever in Japan, Wycon fever and Bushy Creek fever in the United States, canefield fever in Australia, and swineherd disease in Europe were identified as examples of infection caused by *L. hebdomidis, L. canicola, L. pomona, Leptospira australis,* and *L. pomona,* respectively.[18, 23, 28, 44, 80]

Leptospirosis is a disease now thought to be caused most likely by a single family of organisms that has multiple serogroups and serotypes[3] and is characterized by a broad spectrum of clinical findings.[117] In the *Leptospira* genus, the species *Leptospira interrogans* is pathogenic for animals and humans.[13] At least 180 strains, called *serovars* (serotypes), which are divided into serogroups on the basis of common antigens, have been identified.

Epidemiology

ANIMAL RESERVOIRS

Among mammals, rodents are the most important reservoir of leptospires, but nearly all mammals may be infected and can transmit the disease. In various parts of the world, rats, field mice, moles, gerbils, coypus, hedgehogs, shrews, dogs, foxes, jackals, mongooses, civets, skunks, raccoons, bandicoots, opossums, and cattle have been implicated as sources of human infection.* Leptospires also have been isolated in reptiles and birds, but the epidemiologic significance of these animals in terms of maintenance of the organism in nature or transmission of disease to humans is not clear. For many species, infectivity rates of 10 to 50 percent have been reported frequently.[80] During epizootics, the circulation of leptospires among many species of animals living within a given biocenosis has been well recognized.[49]

A biologic equilibrium exists between some strains of leptospires and numerous species of animals whereby these organisms remain within the convoluted tubules of the kidneys of the host without producing any pathogenic effect on the tubular epithelium. When this equilibrium is not established, the animal may become ill or may die.[15, 58] Studies performed in skunks suggest that local resistance appears soon after infection occurs. The failure of leptospires to elicit a significant systemic antibody response in certain animal species may be due to development of this local immunity.[153] Some animals fail to develop homologous antibody titers but harbor leptospires in the kidneys for extended periods.[153] Thus, lack of a positive titer to leptospires, as determined during the course of serologic surveys of animal populations, does not indicate absence of infection. For this reason, serologic surveys of animal populations cannot reflect accurately the true incidence of leptospiral infection.

A particular host species may serve as a reservoir for one or more serotypes of leptospires, and a particular serotype may be hosted by many different animal species. Turner[162, 165] stressed that a particular animal species serves commonly as a reservoir for selected serotypes but temporarily may be infected and serve as an incidental host for other serotypes with which it usually is not infected. Two or more animal hosts for the same serotype may be present in the same geographic area. These newer insights have replaced earlier epidemiologic concepts of leptospirosis concerning a "host of election." Although any animal susceptible to infection by leptospires may become a urinary "shedder" of the organisms temporarily, only selected animal species with "biologic sympathy" for a particular strain of leptospires can become a principal or maintenance host of the serotype.[15]

TRANSMISSION OF LEPTOSPIRES TO HUMANS

Transmission of leptospires to humans occurs after either contact with blood, urine, tissues, or organs of infected animals or exposure to an environment that has been contaminated by leptospires. Humans usually represent a dead end in the chain of infection because although person-to-person transmission is possible theoretically, it is rare. Upon direct exposure of humans to infected animals, leptospires may enter breaks in the skin or may penetrate the mucous membranes, including the conjunctiva, nasopharynx, and vagina.[18, 50, 127, 162] Human-to-human transmission has been reported through human milk obtained by a breast-fed infant from a lactating mother who was infected with *L. interrogans*.[27]

*See references 15, 50, 54, 58, 78, 128, 159, 162, 165, 166.

Indirect transmission of leptospires to humans (from soil or water) depends on the presence of an environment that favors the survival of leptospires outside the animal host. A warm climate (25° C [77° F]), the presence of moisture, and pH values of soil or surface water between 6.2 and 8.0 are optimal for survival of leptospires. These conditions prevail in many tropical regions throughout the year and in temperate climates during the late spring, summer, and autumn months. Conversely, survival of leptospires outside the animal host is impeded by chemical pollution, salinity, and various absorptive properties of clay in the soil.[50, 162]

Smith and Self[140] demonstrated survival of leptospires in cultures of infected soil for 43 days. *L. icterohaemorrhagiae* recovered from the soil of lawns in suburban communities has been indicted in an epidemic of leptospirosis in Missouri,[39] and a case of human leptospirosis has been reported in a soil scientist who became infected after handling a soil sample that had been collected in North Queensland, Australia, and transported 1100 miles during a period of 48 hours.[158]

Fresh water, particularly that contaminated by rat urine, has been recognized as an important vehicle for transmission of leptospiral infection.[70, 162] Drinking water from a fountain also has been associated with an outbreak of leptospirosis.[35] The urine of infected cows may contain as many as 100 million leptospires per milliliter. If conditions are favorable, surface water contaminated by the urine of infected cattle may remain infectious for several weeks.[36]

Venereal transmission of leptospirosis is important in rodents and can occur in livestock. Leptospires have been recovered from the semen of bulls and have been transmitted by artificial insemination and by coitus. The possibility of seminal transmission in humans remains speculative.[41] Transplacental infection of the fetus in utero is well documented in livestock and other animals and may occur in humans.[45, 50, 162, 164]

The importance of occupation as related to the risk for leptospirosis was emphasized in 1965.[80] Disease appeared to occur most frequently in people with occupations that required exposure to cattle or swine or to water contaminated by rat urine. During the past several decades, the number of cases acquired during outdoor recreation has increased. In rural areas, the U.S. Department of Agriculture promoted and aided in the development of farm ponds. These ponds, along with streams and rivers, are used widely for recreation and as a water supply for livestock and wild animals.[116] That many outbreaks of human leptospirosis have been attributed to water used for dual purposes is not surprising.[23, 67, 123, 128]

More recently, leptospirosis has become a more frequent occurrence in children, students, and housewives than in adults with occupational exposure; cases from urban and suburban communities have been reported more frequently than have cases from rural areas.[39] The dog has been incriminated increasingly as an important vector and as a reservoir of this disease. Although immunization of dogs against leptospirosis is possible, an important note to remember is that (1) the immunization may not prevent the dog from having renal carriage and excreting the organism, (2) canine immunity after immunization may persist for but 1 year, and (3) immunity, when established, is effective only for those serotypes found in the canine vaccine.[15] The immunized pet dog has been identified as a previously unrecognized threat to people.[15] The exact prevalence in each community of immunized dogs that excrete leptospires is unknown. In one survey of suburban and urban areas, however, between 15 and 40 percent of dogs were found to be infected.[22] These data are consistent with reports from the CDC; dogs were implicated in 58 percent of the 820 known cases of leptospirosis reported between 1962 and 1971.[39]

In a study performed in Detroit, 90 percent of rats carried *L. icterohemorrhagiae.*[53] Strain-specific tests comparing antibody titers in the sera of inner-city and suburban children were performed. Thirty-one percent of inner-city children had antibodies against *L. icterohaemorrhagiae;* 10 percent of suburban children also had antibodies to this organism.

Pathophysiology

After penetration of the skin or mucous membranes, leptospires invade the bloodstream and spread throughout the body to produce the protean manifestation of the disease.[59, 60, 145] Stavitsky[145] has suggested that the speed with which the leptospire revolves in a corkscrew fashion enables it to bore through connective tissue. This suggestion correlates with observations in humans, which show that leptospires regularly invade the anterior chamber of the eye and the subarachnoid space without eliciting a significant inflammatory response.[77] Volland and Brede[170] detected hyaluronidase in fluid filtered from leptospiral cultures and cited it as a reason for the unusual invasive property of leptospires.

Specific factors responsible for the virulence of leptospires remain unknown. The possible role played by animal hosts in determining the virulence of leptospires for humans remains speculative. Faine[59] compared the fate of virulent and nonvirulent strains of *L. icterohaemorrhagiae* in guinea pigs. Both strains behaved similarly after intraperitoneal infection, but virulent organisms survived and multiplied, whereas avirulent strains did not. Both virulent and avirulent strains were taken up by fixed phagocytes in reticuloendothelial tissues in vivo. Phagocytosis or chemotaxis was not noted with either strain in vitro or in vivo. Virulent and avirulent strains appeared to be identical serologically. Faine[60] also showed that the severity of lesions correlated positively with the number of organisms present and that a discrete number of organisms were required to cause death. The logarithm of the dose for strains of a given virulence was related constantly to survival time after ingestion. This relationship was correlated with growth rate in vivo. Faine[59] also suggested that the low proportion of virulent organisms within avirulent strains permitted modification of the disease process by antibodies that have sufficient time to develop before the disease process becomes irreversible. He hypothesized that virulence results from the selective multiplication of virulent leptospires in vivo. This hypothesis was supported by the fact that maximum virulence can be regained after a single animal passage that follows isolation in culture. Virulence may be lost in culture by mutation to nonvirulent forms.

Nonspecific resistance to leptospirosis is not mediated by differences in phagocytosis of leptospires among animals. Specific resistance, however, apparently is mediated by antibody. Antibody increases the efficacy of clearance of leptospires from the bloodstream by enhancing opsonization and, hence, improving phagocytosis.[44] Wang and associates[172] demonstrated that polymorphonuclear leukocytes are not an efficient defense factor for pathogenic leptospires in nonimmune hosts. Virulence of leptospires appears to be related to their ability to resist killing both by serum and by neutrophils.

Clinical and histologic findings in human and animal leptospirosis have suggested that the pathogenicity of leptospirosis may be, in part, the result of enzyme, toxin, or other metabolites that are elaborated by or released from lysed leptospires.[2, 8, 9, 11, 21, 59, 66, 74, 76, 81, 119, 156] Imamura and associates[84] demonstrated the presence of a thermostable dermal necrotizing toxin in extracts of suspension of *L. icterohaemorrhagiae* by noting the necrotizing effects that occurred after intradermal injection into guinea pigs or rabbits. The skin-necrotizing effect was attributed to the presence of insoluble particles of leptospires in the sonification supernatant.[57]

Clinical and histologic findings observed in leptospirosis are similar to those noted in animals given endotoxin, which suggests that the endotoxin may, in part, be responsible for the pathogenic action of leptospires.[155] Arean and associates[11] were unable to demonstrate the presence of endotoxin in extracts of leptospires and concluded that *L. icterohaemorrhagiae* contained either no endotoxin or one that was labile and readily destroyed by chemical agents in the process of infection. Further study by the same investigators, however, suggested the elaboration of some other undefined toxins that may play a role in the pathogenic action of leptospires.[10] The inoculation of rabbits by Gourley and Low[75] intravenously with disintegrated cells or extracts of cells of *L. canicola* and *L. icterohaemorrhagiae* has been followed by fever, leukopenia, thrombocytopenia, and, later, leukocytosis. Their findings suggested the presence of endotoxin in these serotypes. Finco and Low,[63] using preparations *of L. canicola* organisms and several bioassay procedures, showed that *L. canicola* had little ability to elicit biologic responses characteristic of endotoxins. One thousand to 1 million more *L. canicola* organisms (on the basis of dry weight) were required to produce a febrile response in rabbits of a magnitude similar to that elicited by *Escherichia coli.* The results suggest that *L. canicola* contains material with weak endotoxin activity. Massive quantities of *L. canicola* would be required to produce endotoxin-related disease. Finco and Low[63] concluded that (1) other factors related to leptospiral infection may increase the susceptibility of the host to endotoxin during leptospirosis, or (2) endotoxin from the intestinal lumen may gain access to the bloodstream during the course of leptospirosis.

The development of hemolytic anemia and jaundice in patients with leptospirosis has suggested a role for hemolysis in the pathogenesis of this disease. Alexander and associates[5] reported the presence of a heat-labile, oxygen-stable, nondialyzable hemolysin in the supernate of leptospiral cultures; subsequently, Russell[125] noted that this hemolysin could be inhibited by leptospiral antiserum. Hemolysis may persist during leptospirosis, despite the development of serum antibodies, which suggests that circulating hemolysin is adsorbed by erythrocytes early in the course of leptospirosis and that the erythrocytes lyse subsequently,[21, 109] despite the presence of circulating antibody. The hemolysin is thermolabile and can be inactivated by trypsin and precipitated by ammonium sulfates, which suggests that it is, in part, a protein moiety.[5, 8] To date, attempts to isolate hemolysins from strains of *L. icterohaemorrhagiae* have failed. The precise role of hemolysins in human disease remains unclear.

A toxic and pathogenic potential in vivo for lipid products of leptospiral metabolism has been suggested.[2] The cell wall of the leptospire is high in lipid content; component fatty acids vary among leptospiral strains. Lipids are used as a source of energy by the leptospires.[2] Saprophytic leptospires invariably possess lipase activity, whereas pathogenic leptospires may be lipase positive or lipase negative.[2] Kasarov and Addamiano[91] investigated the lipolytic activity of leptospires on serum lipoproteins. On the basis of their ability to attack these lipoproteins, leptospires can be divided into three groups: (1) strains that degrade lecithin and sphingomyelin, (2) strains that degrade neither lecithin nor sphingomyelin, and (3) strains that degrade lecithin but not sphingomyelin. Virulent leptospires behaved as group 1 and 2 strains, whereas saprophytic leptospires behaved as a group 3 strain.

A prominent feature of experimental leptospirosis is hemorrhagic diathesis that increases in severity before death.[9] Many investigators have attributed bleeding to depletion of serum prothrombin, to thrombocytopenia, or to both.[43, 77, 119] Prothrombin activity, however, can be corrected in children and adults with leptospirosis by the administration of vitamin K without otherwise altering the severity of the hemorrhagic diathesis.[9, 69, 148] Moreover, thrombocytopenia is not a consistent concomitant in patients who bleed during the course of leptospirosis. For these reasons, the hemorrhagic diathesis most likely reflects widespread damage to the capillary endothelium.[11, 38, 54, 172] The precise mechanism of capillary injury is uncertain, but the damage has been suggested to be induced by toxin.[9] Generally, hemorrhage is restricted to the skin or mucosal surfaces, but, rarely, death may follow the occurrence of a massive gastrointestinal hemorrhage or bleeding into a vital organ.[77]

In humans, profound derangement in hepatic function has been demonstrated. Liver cell necrosis, however, occurs infrequently, and, thus, the activity of aspartate aminotransferase and alanine aminotransferase generally is elevated only slightly.

The most striking clinical manifestation of hepatic dysfunction is jaundice. Laboratory evidence of hepatic involvement in human leptospirosis includes the following: impaired bromsulfophthalein excretion, positive cephalin flocculation reactions, reduced esterification of cholesterol, abnormal galactose tolerance test, impaired production of the clotting factors dependent on vitamin K, decreased serum albumin, and increased serum globulins. These abnormalities have been noted in icteric and anicteric patients with leptospirosis.

Several theories attempt to explain the jaundice of leptospirosis. Early investigation suggested that hyperbilirubinemia was the result of a hemolytic anemia.[20] Considerable evidence does not support the hemolytic theory; attempts to demonstrate hemolysin elaboration by *L. icterohaemorrhagiae,* a serotype associated frequently with hyperbilirubinemia in humans, have failed repeatedly.[9] Variability in the presence of anemia, the poor temporal association between anemia (when present) and the development of icterus, the absence of hemoglobinuria and reticulocytosis, and generally normal fecal urobilinogen values provide evidence that hemolysis is not the cause of jaundice in many patients with leptospirosis.[119]

On the other hand, a significant hemolytic process can be documented in selected patients.[156] Hemoglobinuria has been documented early in the course of leptospirosis, even before the development of jaundice.[7, 87] Significant anemia is a feature only of icteric cases of leptospirosis. Most likely, hemolysis occurs in selected cases of severe leptospirosis in humans, and it may contribute to the development of jaundice in some cases.[54, 156]

One must conclude that the hepatic manifestations of leptospirosis, including jaundice, most likely are the result of hepatocellular injury because hemolysis is not a consistent finding and neither intrahepatic nor extrahepatic biliary stasis has been observed morphologically or clinically.[9, 119, 171] Although hepatocellular injury occurs, hepatocellular destruction is not significant, as reflected by the complete recovery without residual hepatic dysfunction, even in survivors of severe icteric leptospirosis. Histologic changes that have been observed consistently include disorganization of liver cell plates; variations in the shape and size of parenchymal cells; large numbers of bi-, tri-, and multinucleated cells with bizarre nuclei; proliferation of Kupffer cells with erythrophagocytosis; and cholestasis associated with scant infiltrates of round cells in the periportal spaces.[8, 25, 54] These changes also have been observed in anicteric patients.[25] Electron microscopy has demonstrated alterations in cell membranes, alteration or destruction of mitochondria, and a predominance of smooth over rough endoplasmic reticulum in hepatocytes, reflecting an altered protein turnover.[52]

Additional evidence of hepatocellular damage is provided by the histochemical demonstration of reduced activity of succinic, isocitric, glutamic, and lactate dehydrogenases concomitant with functional alteration,[10] findings suggesting that the fundamental hepatic lesion is subcellular and that critical cellular enzyme systems somehow are affected. Presumably, hepatocellular damage is not caused by the direct action of leptospiral organisms because the most severe pathologic changes are noted at a time when leptospires are difficult to demonstrate in tissue section.[74] Moreover, leptospires rarely have been identified in sections of hepatic tissue. The elaboration of one or more toxins by leptospires or the release of various products after lysis, which may be injurious to hepatocytes, is the most plausible explanation for hepatic injury at this time.

Renal failure is an important cause of death in patients with leptospirosis. In patients who have died during the first week of disease, renal changes included cloudy swelling or isolated tubular epithelial cell necrosis previously involving the distal convoluted tubule and the ascending loop of Henle, isolated foci of acute vasculitis, segmental thickening of the basement membrane, and isolated areas of mild interstitial edema with lymphocytic infiltrates. In patients who have died during the second week of the illness, numerous foci of tubular epithelial necrosis have been apparent. Interstitial edema and infiltrates of lymphocytes, monocytes, plasma cells, and neutrophils are more prominent. When patients die after the 12th day of illness, the inflammatory infiltrate is widespread and involves the medulla as well as the cortex. Foci of tubular necrosis and interstitial inflammation are large, irregular, and packed densely with plasma cells, monocytes, lymphocytes, and neutrophils. Cells lining the lumen of the renal tubules are distended and disorganized and contain hyaline, granular, epithelial, and even bile casts. The glomeruli show mesangial hyperplasia, focal fusion of foot processes, moderate cloudy swelling of the epithelium in the Bowman capsule, and basement membrane thickening.[8, 10, 47, 52, 83, 94, 139, 177] The changes observed in epithelial cells may be responsible for the protein leak observed clinically as proteinuria.[42] Leptospires have been demonstrated in the liver or renal tubules and less frequently in the interstices of the renal cortex.[8, 54, 94]

Hypokalemia may be noted in patients with leptospirosis who develop acute renal failure. The studies of Abdulkader and associates[1] suggest that these findings are a result of renal potassium wasting potentialized by increased secretion of aldosterone and cortisol.

Although some investigators[83] have emphasized that interstitial nephritis is the fundamental lesion of leptospirosis, renal failure primarily is the result of tubular damage. Interstitial nephritis occurs primarily in patients who have survived until inflammation has had an opportunity to develop. Interstitial nephritis frequently is absent in patients with fulminant disease.[8]

Hypoxia may contribute significantly to the pathogenesis of renal dysfunction in leptospirosis. The focal distribution of the lesions suggests a relationship to impaired renal blood flow. Even in relatively mild cases of leptospirosis in which glomerular function remains unaffected, tubular function as measured by the excretion of paraaminohippurate is reduced markedly.[13, 47] In severe cases, the tubular maximum for paraaminohippurate becomes negligible, and glomerular filtration drops precipitously. On the basis of observations of this type, researchers have concluded that impaired renal blood flow is the fundamental alteration of the nephropathy of leptospirosis. Histochemical and enzymatic studies also demonstrate hypoxic damage and suggest renal ischemia.[10] Diminution in renal perfusion in leptospirosis also is suggested by the clinical occurrence of hypovolemia, hypotension, and circulatory collapse.[25, 57, 67, 95] The reversible oliguria frequently observed during the course of leptospirosis has been attributed to reduced renal blood flow resulting from hypotension, a deficit of extracellular fluid, or both.[54] During periods of oliguria, decreased glomerular filtration rates have been noted. Renal function recovers first by restitution of glomerular function; subsequently, and more slowly, renal tubular function improves.[9]

Hypovolemia or hypotension in patients with leptospirosis may reflect dehydration secondary to vomiting, increased insensible water loss, diminished intake of fluid, and, rarely, massive gastrointestinal hemorrhage.[54, 64] A decrease in intravascular volume caused by a shift of fluid from the intravascular to the extracellular spaces as a result of severe endothelial injury also may occur.

Rarely, during human leptospirosis, adrenal insufficiency occurs after hemorrhagic infarction of the adrenal glands.[142] Vascular collapse observed terminally in fatal cases may reflect, in part, adrenal insufficiency secondary to hemorrhage. However, it cannot be the cause of the reversible state of shock that is noted early during the course of leptospirosis.

Cardiac dysfunction also may lead to hypoperfusion in severe leptospirosis. Focal hemorrhagic myocarditis, acute coronary arteritis, pericarditis, aortitis, and cardiac arrhythmias also have been documented well. Rarely, sudden death results from congestive heart failure or arrhythmias.[8, 51, 134, 142, 152] Cardiac malfunction also may develop secondary to hypertension, hypovolemia, electrolyte imbalance, or uremia. Peripheral vascular collapse in leptospirosis most often occurs regardless of any cardiac involvement, obvious dehydration, or massive hemorrhage. Regardless of the etiologic factor, shock is a common occurrence in the course of severe leptospirosis.

Pulmonary lesions in leptospirosis generally are the result of hemorrhage rather than of acute inflammation. In selected cases, acute inflammation is noted but generally reflects a secondary pyogenic infection. Localized or confluent hemorrhagic pneumonitis may be noted, and petechial and ecchymotic hemorrhages are noted throughout the lungs, pleura, and tracheobronchial tree.[136] Acute hemorrhagic lobar pneumonia and massive hemoptysis have been observed in fatal cases.[12] Silverstein[136] suggested that pulmonary capillary damage was the result of a toxin because leptospires have not been demonstrated in the lungs.

Central or peripheral nervous system involvement may be striking. Most investigators agree that signs of meningeal inflammation cannot be attributed to invasion of the meninges by leptospires. Leptospires frequently are isolated from cerebrospinal fluid (CSF) that otherwise is normal; thus, reaction to the presence of leptospires in the meninges appears to be minimal. The leptospires disappear rapidly after onset of meningeal signs, usually during the second week of disease. Because meningeal reaction occurs only after the development of antibody, leptospiral meningitis has been suggested to be a reflection of an antigen-antibody reaction.[15, 77] Meningitis as a result of hypersensitivity may explain the absence of pleocytosis in the early stages of meningeal involvement, the abrupt onset of meningitis at the end of the first week of leptospiral disease, and the good prognosis of patients with leptospirosis who have involvement of the central nervous system.

Pathologic examination of the meninges may reveal nothing[8] or may show thickening of the meninges, a slight increase in the number of arachnoid cells, and a predominance of mononuclear cells in the exudate.[12]

Uncommon features of leptospirosis include encephalitis, myelitis, radiculitis, and peripheral neuritis. When present, they occur during the second week of illness.[54] These neurologic findings also may be the result of hypersensitivity reactions similar to those seen in other postinfectious encephalitis syndromes.[105, 106] Koppisch and Bond,[94] however, demonstrated perivascular infiltration of blood vessels in the spinal cord, basal ganglia, hippocampus, and white matter of the cerebellum and in the subcortical areas of the cerebrum; these changes are not pathologic features of postinfectious viral encephalitis.[8, 73] In certain cases, neurologic manifestations have been attributed to subarachnoid, peripapillary, and subdural hemorrhages.[34, 36]

The aqueous humor provides a protective environment for leptospires; despite the development of high antibody titers in serum, leptospires may remain viable in the anterior chamber of the eye for many months.[4] Persistence of leptospires in the aqueous humor may be responsible for the recurrent, chronic, or latent uveitis syndromes that have been seen in patients with leptospirosis. The acute ocular inflammatory response that occurs during the leptospirotic phase of the disease generally disappears without complications and with little or no opacification of the vitreous. Chronic ocular involvement occurs less commonly but is more significant because anterior uveal inflammation and vitreous opacification may occur. Development of a hypopyon during the course of leptospirosis may be followed by loss of vision. Pathologic descriptions of ocular tissue from patients with leptospirosis are limited, which precludes a better understanding of the pathogenesis of the ocular involvement.

The myalgia reported so frequently in patients with leptospirosis most likely relates to the pathologic process that has been noted.[95] Biopsy specimens obtained early in the course of leptospirosis have vacuoles within the cytoplasm of the myofibril. Subsequent focal cytoplasmic changes include fragmentation and loss of cellular detail, which results in homogeneous or irregular acidophilic masses. Polymorphonuclear infiltrates that may be noted in affected areas are minimal, even in muscle fibers that are affected severely. Infiltration by sarcoblasts, with new myofibril formation, leads ultimately to healing without significant fibrosis.[26, 87] Histologic changes in the muscles of patients with mild infection usually are minimal.[54] Pathologic evidence of myopathy resolves completely and promptly in most cases; pathologic changes usually are absent in the muscles of patients dying in the second week of disease.[156]

The selective involvement of certain muscle groups in some patients with leptospirosis is not explained. Any or all muscles may be affected; generalized myalgia occurs commonly. Myalgia is an early clinical feature concurrent with leptospirosis, and these clinical findings are correlated with the timing of the histologic changes in muscle. Generally, muscle pain subsides promptly as leptospiral agglutinin titers develop and the septicemic stage of leptospirosis ends. These observations are consistent with active invasion of skeletal muscle by leptospires, rather than from a toxin-related effect.[95, 143] Antigens of leptospires have been demonstrated by fluorescent antibody techniques in patients infected with *L. icterohemorrhagiae.*[135]

The epicardium, endocardium, and myocardium all may be involved during leptospirosis. Arean[8] described focal or diffuse epicardial hemorrhages with or without lymphocytic and monocytic infiltrates in 10 fatal cases. In four patients, mesothelial desquamation and fibrin formation in the pericardial cavity also were noted. Myocardial changes included focal or diffuse lesions characterized by interstitial edema with fragmented fibers and infiltrates of monocytes, lymphocytes, and plasma cells. Neutrophilic infiltrates also were observed in most necrotic foci. Aortic insufficiency caused by focal endocarditis involving the aortic valves also was noted.[8] Patchy interstitial edema, cellular infiltrates, necrosis, and focal hemorrhagic lesions have been noted in other patients.[73, 156] In most cases, these findings are not mirrored by clinical findings. Rarely, leptospires have been demonstrated in myocardium.[54]

Except for focal hemorrhages, no characteristic lesions have been noted in adrenal glands, lymph nodes, spleen, gastrointestinal tract, pancreas, ureter, or bladder. Interstitial edema with monocytic and lymphocytic infiltrates has been found in testicular tissue associated with impaired spermatogenesis.[73] Bone involvement in leptospirosis is not a significant feature clinically or pathologically, and no explanation accounts for the apparent failure of leptospires to proliferate in bone.[86]

Clinical Manifestations

Leptospirosis is an acute systemic infection characterized by extensive vasculitis. Serologic surveys in human populations indicate that a large number of subclinical infections also occur. Surveys of veterinarians and packinghouse and abattoir workers reveal positive leptospiral titers in 5 to 16 percent of people tested.[88, 107, 108, 157]

A low index of suspicion of this disorder in physicians, coupled with the diversity and nonspecificity of its presentation, accounts for the significant number of cases that go unrecognized. In one series of 483 proven cases, only 17 percent were diagnosed initially as leptospirosis.[23]

The incubation period generally is 7 to 12 days, but a range of 2 to 20 days has been noted.[130, 145, 166] The incubation period does not vary significantly among serotypes and is not of prognostic significance. Variability in incubation period may be attributed to the dose of virulent organisms to which the host is exposed and to the portal of entry of the organism.[130, 145, 166]

The clinical course of leptospirosis varies, but generally it is predictable: both anicteric and icteric leptospirosis follow a biphasic course (Fig. 148–1).

The first stage (septicemic phase) is characterized by acute systemic infection. The onset of symptoms is abrupt. This phase terminates after 4 to 7 days; symptomatic improvement and defervescence of fever coincide with disappearance of leptospires from the blood, CSF, and all other tissues, with the exception of the aqueous humor and renal parenchyma. Antibody titers to leptospires develop rapidly; this immune response heralds the second or "immune" stage of the illness.

The immune or second stage lasts 4 to 30 days. Leptospiruria is prevalent and continues for 1 week to 1 month; generally, it is unaffected by antibiotic therapy. Meningitis or hepatic or renal manifestations, when present, reach peak intensity during this stage of the disease.

ANICTERIC LEPTOSPIROSIS

Ninety percent or more of all leptospirosis patients are anicteric. They frequently escape definitive diagnosis because jaundice and azotemia are absent. The onset of the septicemic phase of anicteric leptospirosis is abrupt[55] and is heralded by fever, malaise, headache, myalgia, and, occasionally, prostration and circulatory collapse.[100] Chills, remittent fever, headaches, severe myalgia, and abdominal pain are prominent for 4 to 7 days. Fever defervesces by lysis, and other symptoms resolve. Death is an extraordinarily rare occurrence in the first stage of anicteric illness. Some patients with anicteric leptospirosis do not experience a biphasic illness and remain asymptomatic after the first week.[55]

The second phase of anicteric disease may be characterized by fever, uveitis, rash, headache, and meningitis. If present, fever usually is of brief duration and has a lower

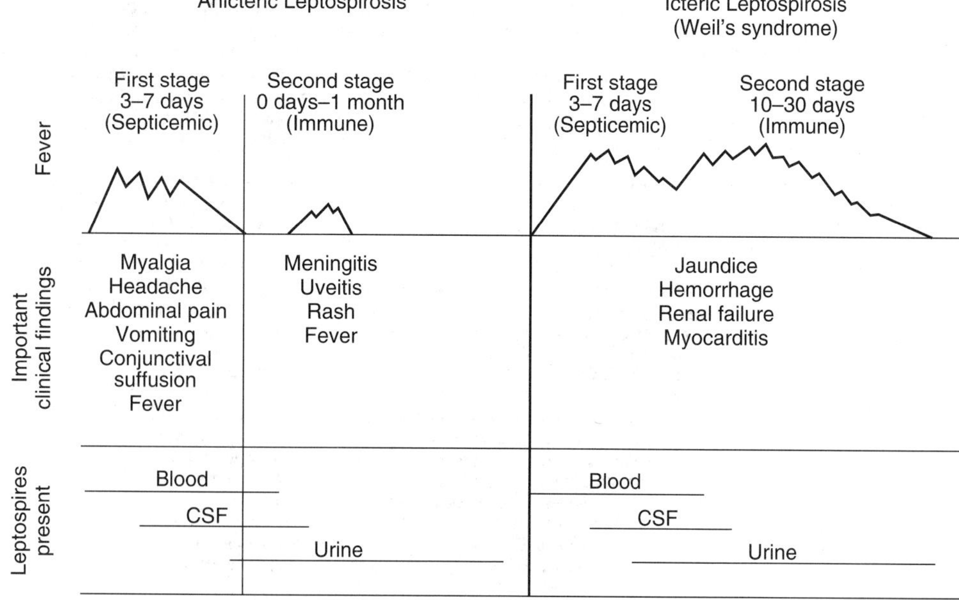

FIGURE 148–1 ■ The clinical course of leptospirosis: anicteric and icteric disease.

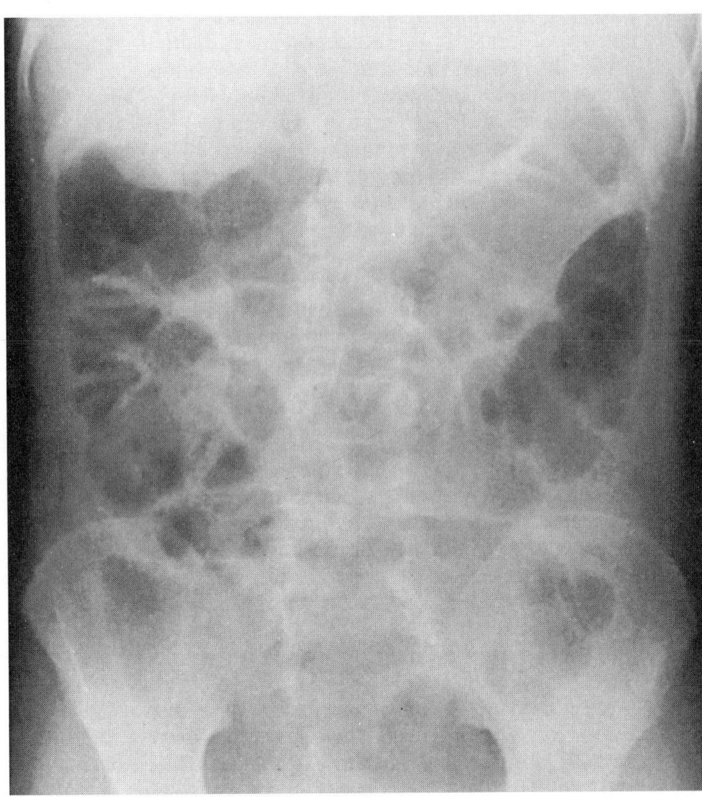

FIGURE 148–2 ■ Radiograph demonstrating a dilated, opaque gallbladder protruding from the inferior margin of the liver, presenting nonobstructed toxic dilation of the gallbladder in a child with leptospirosis.

peak than that of the septicemic phase.[54, 55, 80] Maximum temperatures range from 38.2° to 40.6° C (100° to 105° F), with one or more daily peaks. Recurrence of fever 2 or 3 weeks after leptospirosis resolves is not unusual, but no reports of the isolation of leptospires from blood document relapse on these occasions. Relapse occurs generally when the immune response of the host is peaking and at a time of maximal leptospiruria, which suggests an allergic or immune basis for the febrile episodes.[25] Headache may be intense and generally is not controlled well by analgesics. Generally, it is frontal in distribution and characterized as bitemporal or occipital. It may be associated with retrobulbar pain.[46, 54, 55] Persistence or recurrence of headache after termination of the septicemic phase of disease usually indicates the onset of meningitis. The factors responsible for headache in the septicemic phase of leptospirosis are unknown.

Restlessness, nocturnal confusion, mood disturbances, and mild alterations in consciousness usually occur briefly and commonly in both stages of leptospirosis.[54, 80] Delirium, hallucinations, psychotic behavior, and suicidal tendencies have been reported.[54, 80]

Anorexia, nausea, vomiting, and abdominal pain may be reported in both stages of anicteric disease. Constipation, diarrhea, and gastrointestinal hemorrhage also have been documented.[54, 100, 113] Generally, hemorrhagic complications are associated exclusively with icteric disease.

Physical examination during the septicemic stage may reveal dehydration, muscle tenderness, conjunctival suffusion, generalized lymphadenopathy, hepatosplenomegaly, and skin rashes that may be macular, maculopapular, erythematous, urticarial, petechial, purpuric, hemorrhagic, or desquamating. Skin lesions are most prominent over the trunk, but any area of the body may be affected. Pretibial eruptions have been noted in patients with infection caused by *L. autumnalis,* but other serotypes also may cause disease with pretibial eruptions. Recurrent, transient, urticarial eruptions have appeared for many days after resolution of other manifestations of leptospirosis. Pharyngitis, rales, arthritis, and nonpitting edema occur less commonly.* Tachycardia is a common occurrence, and cardiac arrhythmias occur occasionally.[115, 142] Hypotension rarely occurs in anicteric leptospirosis.[55]

Muscle pain and tenderness may be generalized, but the muscles of the calf, lumbosacral spine, and abdomen are affected most frequently. Tenderness and rigidity of the abdominal wall may suggest the possibility of an acute surgical abdomen. Tenderness of the muscles adjacent to the cervical spine often causes nuchal rigidity in patients without meningeal involvement. Muscle tenderness usually subsides with termination of the septicemic stage of the disease.

Conjunctival suffusion, photophobia, ocular pain, and conjunctival hemorrhage are more specifically helpful diagnostic signs. Chemosis and inflammatory exudates generally are absent, despite marked conjunctival infection. In anicteric disease, conjunctival infection primarily involves the bulbar conjunctiva only. It appears by the third day of illness and disappears 3 days to 3 weeks later.

Abdominal pain and tenderness, when associated with vomiting and hypoactive bowel sounds, clearly suggest the possibility of a surgical abdomen and present a challenging diagnostic problem because acute intraabdominal catastrophes may complicate the natural history of this disease. Nonobstructive, toxic dilation of the gallbladder requiring cholecystotomy has been noted repeatedly in children with leptospirosis (Fig. 148–2). Pain of this type must be differentiated from myositis, subperitoneal or subserosal hemorrhages, abdominal wall causalgia, or pancreatitis, all of which may occur in some children with anicteric or icteric disease.

*See references 6, 8, 24, 46, 55, 80, 87, 100, 126, 161, 166.

Pulmonary involvement may be observed in anicteric patients, generally during the septicemic phase, and usually is manifested by a dry, hacking cough, occasionally productive of blood-stained sputum, or by the finding of infiltrates on a chest radiograph.[24, 118, 136] Hemoptysis, chest pain, respiratory distress, and cyanosis appear rarely during anicteric disease.[118] Hemoptysis, when present, clears in 3 to 5 days. Physical examination of the chest may reveal rales, evidence of consolidation, or pleural or pericardial friction rub.

Chest radiographs may show (1) confluent infiltrates or massive consolidation representing larger areas of pulmonary hemorrhage; (2) small, patchy, snowflake-like lesions in the periphery of the lung fields that are restricted to a few intercostal spaces or disseminated widely; and (3) solitary, patchy lesions with ill-defined margins.[118, 173] Of these radiographic appearances, the second is most common. Small pleural effusions are rare occurrences in anicteric disease,[173] and hilar adenopathy has not been described. Although the chest radiograph may help delineate the extent of pulmonary disease, it does not provide information that could be considered pathognomonic of leptospirosis.

Other signs and symptoms of the septicemic phase of anicteric leptospirosis that have been reported include parotitis,[20] orchitis,[149] epididymitis,[80] prostatitis,[80] otitis media,[24] arthralgia,[24, 54, 80] and monoarticular or polyarticular arthritis.[52]

The hallmark of the immune phase of anicteric leptospirosis is meningitis, and it is reflected by CSF pleocytosis with or without meningeal symptoms or signs. During the leptospirotic phase, leptospires may be found in the subarachnoid space unassociated with the presence of inflammatory cells. As an antibody titer develops, leptospires are cleared rapidly from the CSF, and an inflammatory response develops.[54] If the CSF is examined during the second week of illness in all patients with anicteric leptospirosis, a meningeal reaction can be demonstrated in more than 80 percent, but only 50 percent of these patients have clinical signs and symptoms of meningitis.[37, 54] The severity of meningitis varies and does not correlate with the severity of other clinical manifestations of leptospirosis. Symptoms referable to the nervous system usually subside within 1 or 2 days but rarely persist for 2 or 3 weeks. The CSF pleocytosis may persist for 2 to 3 months but generally disappears within 7 to 21 days.[54] In some cases, patients are asymptomatic during the septicemic phase of leptospirosis but seek medical attention during the immune phase because of headache, vomiting, and nuchal rigidity. Papilledema rarely has been observed in patients with leptospirosis.[34]

Lumbar puncture may reveal CSF pressures varying from normal to 350 mm H_2O. Mean values generally are less than 200 mm H_2O.[82] Cell counts within CSF vary from normal to more than 500 cells/mm^3; generally, fewer than 500 cells have been reported.[54, 80] Polymorphonuclear leukocytes predominate early in the immune phase, but mononuclear cells subsequently predominate. Protein concentrations within the CSF range from normal to 300 mg/dL. In some cases, protein values have been elevated in the absence of pleocytosis. Abnormal values may persist for several weeks after clinical symptoms resolve.[24, 37, 80, 101, 102] Glucose concentrations within the CSF generally are normal.[37, 55, 101]

Encephalitis, focal weakness, spasticity, paralysis, nystagmus, peripheral neuritis, cranial nerve paralysis, seizures, radiculitis, visual disturbances, myelitis, or Guillain-Barré syndrome may appear with or subsequent to the immune stage of anicteric disease.[54, 57, 80, 101, 105, 123, 169] Generally, these symptoms resolve, but complete resolution may require several weeks to months. Neurologic sequelae secondary to central nervous system hemolysis may occur.[34, 36]

The anterior uveal tract may be affected as early as the third week of illness, but symptoms may be found up to 1 year after the onset of leptospirosis. The conjunctival suffusion (characteristic during the septicemic phase) is not found in the immune stage of the disease. Rather, iritis, iridocyclitis, and, occasionally, chorioretinitis are noted.[23, 54, 55, 80] Uveal involvement may be unilateral or bilateral and may occur as a single, self-limited episode, as recurrent episodes, or as a chronic unrelenting process.[30, 54] The severity of the uveitis does not correlate with the severity of other clinical manifestations. When uveitis is transient or self-limited, complete healing is the rule, but, in some cases, blindness and cataract formation are noted.

The precise incidence of involvement of the uveal tract is unclear because symptoms may be minimal or may not appear until after other clinical manifestations have resolved completely. The generally benign course of uveitis may be attributable to the capacity of leptospires to survive in the aqueous humor without eliciting an intense inflammatory response.[55] Despite the presence of high titers of specific antibodies to leptospires in the serum, antibodies to leptospires are absent or found in low titer in the aqueous humor.

Leptospiruria is the rule during the immune stage of anicteric leptospirosis, and it is not associated with impaired renal function. In contrast to many animal species, humans do not serve as a reservoir for leptospires; leptospiruria is transient. In anicteric patients, proteinuria, pyuria, microscopic hematuria, and mild to moderate azotemia may be observed.[24]

The white blood cell count may be low, normal, or elevated. Neutrophilia is the rule, regardless of the total white blood cell count. Leukocytosis generally is associated with hepatic involvement. Anemia is an inconsistent finding; when present, it may be attributable to blood loss, vascular damage, or hemolysis. In the absence of blood loss, significant anemia is not a manifestation of anicteric cases. The sedimentation rate consistently is elevated.

ICTERIC LEPTOSPIROSIS (WEIL SYNDROME)

The term *Weil syndrome* should be applied to define a form of leptospirosis that is distinctive in clinical expression but nonspecific with respect to serotypic etiologic agents. In addition to having the symptoms and signs of anicteric leptospirosis, Weil syndrome is set apart by the presence of impaired hepatic and renal function, vascular collapse, hemorrhage, severe alterations in consciousness, and a high mortality rate.

Weil syndrome may be heterogeneous in presentation, and the course may be dominated by symptoms of renal, hepatic, or vascular dysfunction. Jaundice and azotemia may be so severe that the biphasic course of illness is not observed. Fever may persist without defervescence between the septicemic and immune stages and is more prominent and of longer duration during the immune stage than in anicteric cases. The mortality rate, despite adequate supportive care, is between 5 and 10 percent.

Jaundice remains the hallmark of Weil syndrome. The intensity of jaundice varies; maximum total serum bilirubin concentration in the range of 60 to 80 mg/dL has been reported.[101] Usually, the bilirubin concentration is less than 20 mg/dL. Both direct- and indirect-reacting bilirubin levels increase, but an increase in the direct fraction usually accounts for most of the bilirubin elevation.[146] Jaundice may appear as early as the third day of illness or may not appear until the second week.[12, 55] The concentration of serum bilirubin peaks within the first 7 days after onset of jaundice in 85 percent of cases.[119]

Modest elevations of serum alkaline phosphatase and depressed activity of plasma prothrombin are noted occasionally.[119] Hypoprothrombinemia responds uniformly to parenteral administration of vitamin K. Serum albumin may be depressed; concentrations of 2 to 2.5 g are not unexpected.[146] Aspartate aminotransferase and alanine aminotransferase are elevated minimally; these values rarely exceed 100 and 200 U, respectively. Abnormal cephalothin flocculation and thymic turbidity values generally are noted, and the urine may contain bilirubin and urobilinogen.

Hepatomegaly is found in approximately 24 percent of patients, a frequency that is no greater than that in anicteric cases.[54] Transient biliary obstruction, probably intrahepatic, may occur, but no evidence that obstructive phenomena are the primary mechanism of impaired hepatic function exists. Even in severely icteric cases, acholic stools generally are not observed.[54, 80] Pruritus has been reported rarely in patients with leptospirosis.[54] The presence of abnormal urinary urobilinogen values in the absence of acholic stools suggests the patency of the biliary tract in most cases.[119]

In some reports of children with leptospirosis, acalculous cholecystitis has been seen in 55 percent of cases.[147] In these cases, right upper quadrant pain, tenderness, and a palpable mass were present. Abdominal radiographs confirmed the presence of a mass in the region of the gallbladder. When cholecystotomy was performed, a massively distended gallbladder containing colorless bile was noted. Routine aerobic and anaerobic cultures of bile were negative, but cultures for leptospires were positive.

Hepatic dysfunction is not an important cause of death in patients with leptospirosis. It is present, however, in most patients who die of this disease, and, conversely, a fatal outcome is extremely rare in the absence of hepatic dysfunction.[24] Renal dysfunction, cardiovascular collapse, and hemorrhagic complications occur most often in patients whose icterus is most prominent.

Renal dysfunction may be observed in all forms of leptospirosis, regardless of the severity of disease or of the serotype causing infection.[24, 54, 80] Symptoms attributable to functional renal impairment generally are observed only during icteric leptospirosis.[12, 24, 54, 55, 166] During the leptospirotic phase, abnormal urinalysis results are noted in as many as 80 percent of cases.[24, 54, 147] Proteinuria is the most frequent abnormality and generally is mild. Hyaline or granular casts and cellular elements (red and white blood cells) may be found in the urinary sediment. Microscopic or gross hematuria is noted in many patients and most likely reflects the presence of a hemorrhagic diathesis rather than glomerular injury.[169]

Fatal cases of icteric leptospirosis in which urinalysis results were normal have been reported.[12] Abnormalities of urinary sediment and proteinuria may persist for weeks in patients without significant azotemia.[19]

Oliguria or anuria may be noted as early as the third day of illness but occurs more commonly after the first week. Generally, blood urea nitrogen values remain below 100 mg/dL, but values may exceed 300 mg/dL in some cases.[80, 114] The height of the blood urea nitrogen value is not of prognostic value in individual cases, but in groups of patients, it correlates well with outcome.[156]

Azotemic patients with leptospirosis can be divided into two groups: (1) those with decreased renal perfusion (urine osmolality [Uosm]–to–plasma osmolality [Posm] ratio of about 2:1) and a good response to fluid administration, and (2) those with a Uosm-to-Posm ratio close to 1:1, with impaired resorption of sodium and water from the renal tubules and no response to fluid administration. The manifestations of the second group of patients are those of acute tubular necrosis. The factors responsible for oliguria in the first group of patients (those with prerenal azotemia), including hypotension, shock, and volume depletion, if uncorrected, ultimately may progress to acute tubular necrosis as well.

Anuria is an ominous sign, and diuresis is a good prognostic omen.[12] Impairment in renal function may persist, and fatalities have been recorded after the onset of diuresis.[114] Hyposthenuria can persist for months in some cases.[55] Some evidence of renal disease has been demonstrated by renal function tests and renal biopsies for as long as 6 months after the onset of leptospirosis.[17] Renal failure is the principal cause of death in patients with leptospirosis, but it generally is reversible in time.

Cardiac involvement is a relatively infrequent occurrence, but when it is present, congestive heart failure and cardiovascular collapse may occur.[55, 87] Electrocardiographic changes are seen in all forms of leptospirosis.[115] In one series of patients, electrocardiograms obtained during the first week of illness were abnormal in 90 percent of patients at a time when none had signs or symptoms of congestive failure, pericarditis, or hypotension.[115] The electrocardiographic abnormalities disappeared by 10 days in most cases. The electrocardiographic changes that have been described are nonspecific findings common to many infectious diseases or attributable to fever alone.[115]

Cerebrovascular accidents may be noted in patients with leptospirosis.[97] In one study of 21 cases in which postmortem examination was performed, subarachnoid hemorrhage was described in one case, cerebral hemorrhage in two, and recent cerebral infarction in one.

Hyponatremia is a rather consistent finding in patients with severe icteric leptospirosis. The hyponatremia appears to be the result of (1) failure of the sodium pump, which causes sodium to move intracellularly in exchange for potassium, and (2) a redistribution of fluid such that the extracellular fluid space is expanded at the expense of the intracellular space. Hyponatremia in these patients may be unresponsive to either sodium replacement or fluid restriction. It is treated best by fluid restriction, which can be continued unless systemic blood pressure falls. Clinical improvement in the patient generally follows a spontaneous increase in serum sodium, which may occur before any other evidence of clinical improvement is noted.

Laboratory Diagnosis

Whenever possible, the physician should use laboratory facilities in which cultural and serologic tests for leptospirosis are performed routinely. I recommend that specimens be sent to the standard reference laboratory, the National Leptospirosis Laboratory at the CDC in Atlanta. Despite proper collection and handling of specimens, obtaining laboratory confirmation of cases of leptospirosis may be difficult, even for facilities with skill in this area.

A confirmed case of leptospirosis, as defined by the U.S. Department of Health and Human Services, fulfills one of the following criteria: (1) clinical specimens that are culture positive for leptospires, or (2) clinical symptoms compatible with leptospirosis and either a seroconversion or a fourfold or greater rise in the microscopic agglutination titer between acute and convalescent sera specimens obtained 2 or more weeks apart and studied at the same laboratory.

Presumptive leptospirosis is defined as the presentation of clinical symptoms that are compatible with leptospirosis and a microscopic agglutination titer of 1:100 or greater, a positive macroscopic agglutination slide test reaction on a single serum specimen obtained after the onset of symptoms, or a stable microscopic agglutination titer of 1:100 or greater in two or more serum specimens obtained after the onset of symptoms.

IDENTIFICATION BY CULTURE

Leptospires can be recovered from blood or CSF obtained from patients during the septicemic stage of illness or from urine during the immune stage. Other than these body fluids, only tissue sections obtained by biopsy or at necropsy are sources from which organisms can be recovered. Rarely, organisms are isolated from intraocular fluid during convalescence.[4]

Media for the cultivation of leptospires generally contain a buffered solution, with or without peptone and with or without 0.1 to 0.2 percent agar to which rabbit serum has been added to provide a final concentration in the medium of 5 to 10 percent. In addition, a pH between 7.2 and 7.8 appears to be essential. Clinical materials obtained for culture frequently are contaminated; antimicrobial agents, including neomycin, vancomycin, or bacitracin, added to leptospiral media in low concentration have been found to be effective in reducing contamination and exert little if any effect on leptospires.

For routine use, Fletcher semisolid medium[65] or EMJH semisolid medium[89, 145] is recommended. Stuart medium[150] has been used to prepare and maintain antigens for serologic tests. Tween 80-albumin medium (OAC) was developed not long ago and is available commercially. This medium appears to be superior for primary isolation of leptospires.

Several solid media are available but appear to be most useful for the isolation and purification of leptospires from contaminated natural materials, such as water.[151, 164] The preparation, use, and maintenance of these solid media and other media are described in other works.[103, 151, 164]

Multiple cultures should be obtained from patients with leptospirosis because the concentration of organisms in blood at any point in time is low.[89] Freshly drawn blood is most desirable, but leptospires may remain viable in anticoagulated blood for up to 11 days.[150] Blood should be inoculated into several tubes of semisolid media. The number of drops of blood placed into each tube should be varied (one to four drops). Excessive amounts of blood inhibit the growth of leptospires; hence, a small inoculum yields the best results.[65] Cultures are incubated at 28° to 30° C (82.4° to 86° F) in the dark for 6 weeks or longer.

In semisolid media, leptospires grow in a concentrated ring about 0.5 to 1 cm below the surface. Growth may not be detected in Fletcher semisolid media for several weeks but may occur earlier in polysorbate medium.

Contaminated specimens or suspensions of primary cultures in which contamination is suspected may be inoculated into hamsters. Upon death of any animal, phlebotomy or necropsy is performed, and sections of liver, kidney, and brain then are recultured in appropriate semisolid media.

If collected during the septicemic phase, CSF may be cultured in the same manner as blood is.

Urine serves as the main source from which leptospires can be isolated during the immune and convalescent phases of leptospirosis. A clean-voided urine may be inoculated directly into an appropriate semisolid medium. Urine specimens must be diluted with sterile, buffered saline solution to ensure growth.[156] Best results are obtained by adding 0.1 mL of urine to 0.9 mL of buffered saline before inoculation into 5 mL of semisolid medium. This procedure can be continued with four additional dilutions. Other bacterial contaminants that may be present in undiluted urine cultures generally do not survive in these cultures after dilution.[151]

IDENTIFICATION BY MEANS OTHER THAN CULTURE

The morphologic appearances of all members of the genus *Leptospira* are similar. They are slender, threadlike organisms about 0.1 µm in diameter and 6 to 12 µm in length, tightly coiled on their long axis. Like other spirochetes, they cannot be seen in wet preparations by lightfield microscopy, but on darkfield examination they may be observed readily. For the detection of one leptospire per high-power field by darkfield examination, a concentration of 10,000 to 20,000 leptospires per milliliter of fluid is needed.[164] At best, darkfield examination should be considered an aid that may suggest but not establish a diagnosis of leptospirosis.

Leptospires can be stained by several silver impregnation techniques.[32, 92, 103, 151, 164] The modified method of Van Orden has been used at the CDC for demonstrating organisms in tissue sections of liver, kidney, or other tissues. Infecting serotypes cannot be differentiated by silver impregnation techniques. Leptospiral antigen also has been detected by the use of an immunoperoxidase staining procedure.[62]

Fluorescent-antibody techniques may be applied successfully to the detection of leptospires in urine or tissue.[110, 111, 151, 164] This test is based on specific antigen-antibody reactions using fluorescence-tagged antisera. In theory, the fluorescent-antibody reaction should demonstrate distorted and fragmented, as well as whole, organisms, but caution is required. Control specimens that have been treated with unlabeled antiserum before addition of fluorescein-labeled antiserum should be employed.[103] The control specimen should not fluoresce. The fluorescent-antibody technique may provide the physician with useful information in the course of the disease in some patients. Positive results, however, are considered only as presumptive evidence of infection.

In addition to this technique, DNA hybridization techniques or nucleic acid amplification procedures, including polymerase chain reaction (PCR) protocols using leptospiral-specific cDNA probes or oligonucleotide primers, can be used to detect the presence of leptospires in body fluids or culture supernatants. These techniques are being developed in the laboratories of the Leptospirosis Branch at the CDC, but proof of their superiority in terms of sensitivity or specificity in detecting leptospiral organisms in body fluids or other clinical samples has not been established yet.

SEROLOGIC TESTS

Evaluating serologic findings to supplement clinical and epidemiologic information generally is recommended as a first step in establishing a diagnosis of leptospirosis. One of the most widely used specific serologic tests for leptospirosis has been the microscopic agglutination test (MAT), in which live antigen is used. This test is time consuming and potentially hazardous to the technician but is considered the reference test against which all other tests are evaluated. Formalinized antigens can be used for the MAT, and they are preferred in some laboratories, but the titers obtained are lower than those obtained with live antigens, and more cross-reactions with heterologous serotypes occur. Generally, serum is used for the MAT or other agglutination tests, but CSF, urine, bile, or aqueous humor may be employed.[103]

In the United States, 20 leptospiral strains representative of the serogroups known to be present in this country currently are used to prepare antigens for MATs performed at the CDC. Serotypes representative of serogroups in other countries can be added to the battery, and others may be deleted, if desired. Killed antigens remain stable for at least 12 months and are available commercially either individually or in pools. Sulzer and associates[151] have provided detailed descriptions of the methods for performance of the MAT. Modifications of the MAT have been developed and include the semimicro method and microtiter techniques.[68]

A newer serologic test diffusion in gel, the enzyme-linked immunosorbent assay (ELISA), has been compared with MAT for the serologic diagnosis of leptospirosis.[49] The results suggest that this test is a viable alternative to the MAT because of its sensitivity, potential for standardization, and simplicity. Variations of this test have been developed; rapid serodiagnosis of leptospirosis with the use of an immunoglobulin M (IgM)-specific dot ELISA has proved to be as sensitive and specific as are MATs.[174] The dot ELISAs are inexpensive and simple to perform, and they use minute volumes of leptospiral antigens.

The IgM-PK ELISA, an assay for IgM employing a proteinase K–treated antigen, was compared with the Leptoteste-S macroagglutination test (Centers for Disease Control and Prevention, Atlanta, GA) and with the MAT for the diagnosis of leptospirosis. All three tests were comparable in the ability to detect the presence of leptospirosis infection. Both the IgM-PK ELISA and Leptoteste-S tests differed statistically from the MAT in terms of the positivity of the acute-phase sera. Thirty-eight percent of patients with leptospirosis were identified earlier with either test than when the MAT was used. The IgM-PK ELISA, which had a sensitivity of 89.9 percent and a specificity of 97.4 percent, has been suggested as the test of choice for those laboratories that are equipped to perform ELISA.[122]

A slide agglutination test available commercially has been compared to the ELISA IgM and has yielded equivalent results for the diagnosis of leptospirosis. The slide agglutination test is inexpensive and can be performed more quickly and more easily than can ELISA, rendering it a useful test for laboratories that are less well equipped than those in which IgM ELISA currently is performed.[31]

Lepto Dipstick (Royal Tropical Institute, Amsterdam, The Netherlands), a dipstick assay for detection of *Leptospira*-specific IgM antibodies in sera, has been studied as a method for the diagnosis of leptospirosis in situations in which laboratory facilities may not be available.[141] The dipstick test results correlated well (93.2% observed agreement) with results obtained by the IgM ELISA leptospiral antigen detection method. The dipstick test is a valuable and useful tool for the rapid screening for leptospirosis and may be useful in the field for detecting and monitoring outbreaks of leptospirosis.

Other tests that may be used for the serologic diagnosis of leptospirosis include a complement-fixation assay,[40] a hemolytic test,[40] an indirect immunofluorescent test,[160] an erythrocyte-sensitizing substance test,[40] and countercurrent immunoelectrophoresis.[112] These tests are genus specific and may yield positive results earlier in the course of leptospirosis than do the agglutination tests. Their results also revert to negative earlier; therefore, these tests are of little value for serologic surveys. They may be of value in distinguishing current from past infections when agglutination test results are equivocal.[150, 151] Other works[40, 48, 121, 160, 164] provide specific details concerning the use of these techniques.

An indirect hemagglutination test offers the advantage of detecting antibodies as early as the fourth day after the onset of illness. It is genus specific, is less time consuming, and requires but one antigen in the test system. It has an excellent sensitivity and specificity, and some investigators have suggested that it may replace the MAT as the screening test of choice.[151] Effler and colleagues,[56] however, reported discouraging results when this test was used for the diagnosis of leptospirosis in Hawaii.

Agglutination tests have been considered to be serotype specific. Because of the antigenic complexity of leptospires, however, cross-agglutination reactions occur; serotypes that belong to the same serogroup cross-react at high titers. Early in the course of leptospirosis, heterologous reactions may be stronger than are homologous reactions. Because of these paradoxic cross-reactions, one should not depend on serologic determination alone to define the infecting serotype. When agglutination tests are performed on serial specimens over time, the homologous reaction becomes the dominant one in most cases. Performing agglutination absorption studies may be necessary to define the infecting serotype in some cases. The antigen (serotype) that absorbs out agglutinin to all the serotypes in a serogroup most likely is the infecting serotype.[103, 146, 163]

A passive microcapsule agglutination test that uses chemically stable microcapsules instead of sheep erythrocytes has been developed.[12] Compared with the MAT, the passive microcapsule agglutination test showed a relatively greater degree of genus specificity and 4- to 32-fold higher titers. The sensitized microcapsules were stable for at least 1 year. This test is simple to perform and reproducible and can be employed readily in the routine laboratory. Moreover, the test appears to be more sensitive than is the MAT in the early stages of leptospirosis.[133]

A positive leptospiral agglutination reaction generally is not found until the 6th to 12th day of illness, and maximal levels are reached at between 21 and 28 days. After recovery, low titers may persist for many years. One blood sample should be obtained early in the course of illness, and a second one should be obtained at the end of 1 month. Negative reactions in serial samples do not exclude the possibility of leptospirosis because patients may be infected with a serotype not included in the battery of test antigens or with a previously unrecognized serotype. Moreover, the titer may have peaked before the acute-phase specimen was collected. Antibiotic therapy also may suppress the development of positive titers or delay their appearance.[78, 103] Peak microscopic agglutination titers of 1:3000 to 1:100,000 usually are reached during the third week of illness.[54, 163] An unchanging titer of 1:100 on two successive serum specimens has been defined as sufficient for making a presumptive diagnosis of leptospirosis. A fourfold increase in titers between acute and convalescent sera is indisputable evidence of active leptospirosis.

Leptospira DNA may be detected by PCR. Romero and colleagues[98] reported that PCR was more likely to facilitate the early diagnosis of leptospiral aseptic meningitis than was either the IgM ELISA or MAT test.

Nonradioactive arbitrarily primed PCR assays can be used to discriminate species of *Leptospira*.[98]

Treatment

To be of maximum therapeutic benefit, an antimicrobial agent would have to be administered before invading organisms damage the endothelium of blood vessels and various organs or tissues. One of the problems in evaluating the efficacy of treatment is the fact that, generally, leptospirosis is a self-limited disease with a favorable prognosis. Even patients with severe icteric leptospirosis may recover without specific treatment.

Most claims of the beneficial value of antimicrobial agents in human leptospirosis are based on the response of individual patients rather than on controlled studies. Hall and associates[79] compared the effects of penicillin, chloramphenicol, chlortetracycline (Aureomycin), and oxytetracycline (Terramycin) with placebo in 67 confirmed cases of leptospirosis. No appreciable effect of antibiotics could be demonstrated on the duration or severity of illness or on the prevention or amelioration of central nervous system, hepatic, renal, or hemorrhagic complications of this disease. Moreover, the duration of leptospiremia and the persistence of organisms in CSF were not altered by treatment. Kocen[93] compared the effects of penicillin given on the fourth day of illness in 28 patients with a control group of 33 who were given only supportive care and reported that the duration of fever was shorter and the incidences of jaundice, meningismus, renal involvement, and hemorrhagic manifestations were diminished in the treated group.[93] None of these controlled studies was entirely satisfactory with respect to randomization of patients.

McClain and associates[99] studied the therapeutic efficacy of doxycycline in military recruits contracting leptospirosis while training at the Jungle Operations Training Center in Panama. Twenty-nine patients with anicteric disease were treated in a randomized, double-blinded fashion with doxycycline, 100 mg orally twice a day, or with placebo. Therapy was administered for 7 days in the hospital, after which patients were followed for 3 weeks. The duration of illness before therapy and the severity of illness were similar in both study groups. Doxycycline shortened the duration of illness by 2 days and favorably influenced fever, malaise, headache, and myalgias. Treatment also prevented leptospiruria, and no significant adverse effects of doxycycline administration were observed.

In another randomized, double-blinded, placebo-controlled field trial at the same military training site, Takafuji and associates[154] demonstrated that doxycycline (200-mg oral dose) given weekly or at the completion of jungle training was highly effective in preventing the onset of clinical leptospirosis. Twenty cases of disease were documented in the placebo group (attack rate, 4.2 percent), compared with only one case in the treatment group (attack rate, 0.2 percent), findings supporting the prophylactic utility of doxycycline in this setting.

Watt and associates[175] reported the results of a trial in which a 7-day course of large intravenous doses of penicillin (4 million U/m^2/day) was compared with placebo in a randomized, double-blinded trial involving 42 patients. All of the patients had severe, advanced disease. Every measurable aspect of the disease was affected favorably by penicillin. The duration of fever was shortened significantly ($P < .005$) in the group receiving penicillin. Penicillin therapy decreased the number of days of hospitalization and prevented development of leptospiruria. These investigators concluded that intravenous penicillin should be given to patients with severe leptospirosis, even if therapy can be initiated only late in the course of their disease.

Treatment with penicillin or tetracycline (to be avoided in children younger than 9 years of age) should be initiated if the diagnosis of leptospirosis is suspected early in the course of the disease. Parenteral aqueous penicillin G, 6 to 8 million U/m^2/day in six divided doses, should provide optimal blood and tissue concentration of penicillin. For patients sensitive to penicillin, tetracycline, 10 to 20 mg/kg/day intravenously, or 25 to 50 mg/kg/day orally in four divided doses for 1 week, should be provided.

The management of leptospirosis requires careful attention to supportive care. Fluid and electrolyte balance requires meticulous attention. Dehydration, cardiovascular collapse, and acute renal failure may require prompt and specific treatment. In some cases, acute renal failure may be prevented by ensuring adequate renal perfusion and appropriate fluid administration early in the course of disease, when prerenal azotemia and shock may be seen.[19, 137] If prerenal azotemia is suspected, diuresis should be attempted promptly with administration of a fluid or colloid load designed to expand extracellular volume and replace extracellular fluid deficits.[19] In patients who do not respond to such therapy, acute tubular necrosis may be suspected, and appropriate fluid restriction should be initiated. If azotemia is severe or prolonged, peritoneal dialysis or hemodialysis should be instituted.[61, 167] The use of exchange transfusion has been suggested in patients with marked hyperbilirubinemia.[111, 114, 138]

The use of corticosteroids in the treatment of severe cases has not been evaluated critically, but their use in patients with impending hepatic coma has been suggested.[55] Anecdotal reports also suggest that corticosteroids may be of value in patients with profound hypotension or shock.

Prevention

Benches in rat-infested, fish-gutting sheds and sewers may be decontaminated. Hygienic conditions should be encouraged in slaughterhouses, farmyard buildings, and bathing pools. In addition to hygiene, prevention of leptospirosis primarily depends on immunization of animals. Immunization of workers at high risk for acquiring leptospirosis has been used successfully in mines in Japan and Poland and in rice fields in Italy and Spain.[162]

Leptospire bacterins are available commercially and have been evaluated for safety and efficacy in laboratory animals and in domestic livestock.[29, 90, 129, 144] The degree of protection that is attained depends largely on the antigenic potential of the immunizing agent. Requirements for *L. pomona* vaccine used in cattle are such that not more than one eight-hundredth of the dose recommended for cattle must protect 80 percent of hamsters challenged intraperitoneally 14 to 18 days after vaccination with a dose of 100 hamster LD_{50}s. In contrast, most dogs are immunized with a vaccine that is but one tenth of the potency of that used for cattle. Most dogs so immunized have been protected against disease but not necessarily from carrying and excreting leptospires in their urine. Trends documenting that many cases of leptospirosis in children have been associated with contact with dogs suggest that more stringent requirements for the immunization of pet dogs are needed.

A randomized trial of doxycycline compared with placebo was undertaken to assess the efficacy of doxycycline prophylaxis in the prevention of infection and disease caused by leptospires during outbreaks in North Andaman.[131] Leptospiral infection was not prevented, but the patients who received doxycycline and who subsequently developed disease had lower morbidity and mortality rates.

REFERENCES

1. Abdulkader, R. C. R. M., Seguro, A. C., Malheiro, P. S., et al.: Peculiar electrolytic and hormonal abnormalities in acute renal failure due to leptospirosis. Am. J. Trop. Med. *54*:1–6, 1996.
2. Abdussalam, M., Alexander, A. D., Babudieri, B., et al.: Research needs in leptospirosis. Bull. W. H. O. *47*:113–122, 1971–1972.
3. Addamiano, L.: Classificazione serologica di alcuniceppi di leptospire provenienti dall Indonesia [Serological classification of strains of Leptospira from Indonesia]. Rend. 1st Super. Sanita. *22*:5–12, 1959.
4. Alexander, A., Baer, A., Fair, J. P., et al.: Leptospiral uveitis: Report of bacteriologically verified cases. Arch. Ophthalmol. *48*:292–297, 1952.

5. Alexander, A. D., Smith, O. H., Hiatt, C. W., et al.: Presence of hemolysin in cultures of pathogenic leptospires. Proc. Soc. Exp. Biol. Med. *91*: 205–211, 1956.
6. Allen, G. L., Weber, D. R., and Russell, P. K.: The clinical picture of leptospirosis in American soldiers in Vietnam. Milit. Med. *133*:275–280, 1968.
7. Alston, J. M., and Broom, J. C.: Leptospirosis in Man and Animals. Edinburgh and London, E. & S. Livingston, 1958.
8. Arean, V. M.: The pathologic anatomy and pathogenesis of fatal human leptospirosis (Weil's disease). Am. J. Pathol. *40*:393–414, 1962.
9. Arean, V. M.: Studies on the pathogenesis of leptospirosis. II. A clinicopathologic evaluation of hepatic and renal function in experimental leptospiral infections. Lab. Invest. *11*:273–288, 1962.
10. Arean, V. M., and Henry, J. B.: Studies on the pathogenesis of leptospirosis. IV. The behavior of transaminases and oxidative enzymes in experimental leptospirosis: A histochemical and biochemical assay. Am. J. Trop. Med. Hyg. *13*:430–442, 1964.
11. Arean, V. M., Sarasin, G., and Green, J. H.: The pathogenesis of leptospirosis: Toxin production by *Leptospira icterohemorrhagiae*. Am. J. Vet. Res. *25*:836–842, 1964.
12. Arimitsu, Y., Kobayashi, S., Akama, K., et al.: Development of a simple serological method for diagnosing leptospirosis: A microcapsule agglutination test. J. Clin. Microbiol. *15*:835–841, 1982.
13. Austoni, M., and Cora, D.: Data on the pathogenesis and therapy of acute renal insufficiency in leptospirosis. Clin. Ter. *18*:233–243, 1960.
14. Baber, M. D., and Stuart, R. D.: Leptospirosis canicola: Case treated with penicillin. Lancet *2*:594–596, 1946.
15. Babudieri, B.: Animal reservoirs of leptospires. Ann. N. Y. Acad. Sci. *70*: 393–413, 1958.
16. Babudieri, B.: Laboratory diagnosis of leptospirosis. Bull. W. H. O. *24*: 45–58, 1961.
17. Bain, B. J., Ribush, N. T., Nicoll, P., et al.: Renal failure and transient paraproteinemia due to *Leptospira pomona*. Arch. Intern. Med. *131*: 740–745, 1973.
18. Barciscewski, M., and Domanski, E.: Przypadek zakazenia choroba Weila w pracowni [Case of Weil's disease acquired in a laboratory]. Pol. Typ. Lek. *6*:1550–1551, 1951.
19. Barrett-Connor, E., Child, C. M., and Carter, M. J.: Renal failure in leptospirosis. South. Med. J. *63*:580–583, 1970.
20. Basile, C.: Pathology and pathogenesis of spirochetosis icterohemorrhagiae. J. Pathol. Bacteriol. *24*:277–285, 1921.
21. Bauer, D. C., Eames, L. N., Sleight, S. D., et al.: The significance of leptospiral hemolysin in the pathogenesis of *Leptospira pomona* infections. J. Infect. Dis. *108*:229–236, 1961.
22. Beck, A., and Barbehenn, K. R.: The Status of Leptospirosis in the St. Louis Area: Final Report to the Commissioners of Health. St. Louis City and University City, Missouri, 1974.
23. Beeson, P. B., Hankey, D. D., and Cooper, C. F., Jr.: Leptospiral iridocyclitis: Evidence of human infection with *Leptospira pomona* in the United States. J. A. M. A. *145*:229–230, 1951.
24. Berman, S. J., Tsai, C., Holmes, K., et al.: Sporadic anicteric leptospirosis in South Vietnam: A study in 150 patients. Ann. Intern. Med. *79*:167–173, 1973.
25. Bhamarapravati, N., Boonyapaknavig, V., Viranuvatti, V., et al.: Liver changes in leptospirosis: A study of needle biopsies in twenty-two cases. Am. J. Proctol. *17*:480–487, 1966.
26. Blake, F. G.: Weil's disease in the United States: Report of a case in Connecticut. N. Engl. J. Med. *223*:5561–5565, 1940.
27. Bolin, C. A., and Koellner, P.: Human-to-human transmission of *Leptospira interrogans* by milk. J. Infect. Dis. *158*:246–247, 1988.
28. Bowdoin, C. D.: New disease entity. J. Med. Assoc. Ga. *31*:437, 1942.
29. Bramel, R. G., and Scheidy, S. F.: The effect of revaccination of horses and cattle with *Leptospira pomona* bacterin. J. Am. Vet. Med. Assoc. *128*: 399–400, 1956.
30. Brand, N., and Moshe, H. B.: Human leptospirosis associated with eye complications. Isr. Med. J. *22*:182–184, 1963.
31. Brandão, A. P., Camargo, E. D., Emilson, D., et al.: Macroscopic agglutination test for rapid diagnosis of human leptospirosis. J. Clin. Microbiol. *36*:3138–3142, 1998.
32. Bridges, C. H., and Luna, L.: Kerr's improved Warthin-Starry technic. Lab. Invest. *6*:357–367, 1957.
33. Broom, J. C.: Canicola fever in Great Britain. Monthly Bull. Ministry Health *10*:258–265, 1951.
34. Buzzard, E. M., and Wylie, J. A. H.: Meningitis leptospirosa. Lancet *2*:417–420, 1947.
35. Cacciapuoti, B., Ciceroni, L., Maffei, C., et al.: A waterborne outbreak of leptospirosis. Am. J. Epidemiol. *126*:535–545, 1987.
36. Carayon, A., and Fouin, G.: Encephalite pseudotumorale et leptomeningite hemorragique en "plaques" sousdurales, complication tardive d'une leptospirose icterohemorrhagique en Extreme-Orient. Med. Trop. *13*:698–702, 1953; Bull. Hyg. *29*:1226–1227, 1954.
37. Cargill, W. H., Jr., and Beeson, P. B.: The value of spinal fluid examination as a diagnostic procedure in Weil's disease. Ann. Intern. Med. *27*:396–400, 1947.
38. Carrasco, E. D., and Dunkelberg, W. E.: European swamp fever: Leptospirosis due to leptospiral grippotyphosa: A case report. Milit. Med. *127*:569–570, 1962.
39. Centers for Disease Control: Annual Summary of Leptospirosis for 1972. Atlanta, 1974.
40. Chang, R. S., Smith, O. J. W., McComb, D. C., et al.: The use of erythrocyte-sensitizing substance in the diagnosis of leptospirosis. Am. J. Trop. Med. Hyg. *6*:101–107, 1957.
41. Chung, H. L., Ts'ao, W. C., Mo, P. S., et al.: Transplacental or congenital infection of leptospirosis: Clinical and experimental observations. Chin. Med. J. (Peking) *82*:777–782, 1963.
42. Chung, J.: Electron microscopic aspects of renal pathology. *In* Becker, E. L. (ed.): Structural Basis of Renal Disease. New York, Harper & Row, 1968, pp. 132–196.
43. Clapper, M., and Myers, G. B.: Clinical manifestations of Weil's disease with particular reference to meningitis. Arch. Intern. Med. *72*:18–30, 1943.
44. Cockburn, T. A., Vavra, J. D., Spencer, S. S., et al.: Human leptospirosis associated with a swimming pool, diagnosed after eleven years. Am. J. Hyg. *60*:1–7, 1954.
45. Coghlan, J. D., and Norval, J.: Canicola fever in man from contact with infected pigs: Further observations. Br. Med. J. *1*:1711–1713, 1960.
46. Cohn, A. P., and Howard, A. A.: Common characteristics of leptospirosis: A report of 11 cases. Ann. Intern. Med. *54*:57–65, 1961.
47. Cora, D.: La funzionalita renale nel morbo di Weil. G. Clin. Med. *37*:1295, 1956.
48. Cox, D. C.: Hemolysis of sheep erythrocytes sensitized with leptospiral extracts. Proc. Soc. Exp. Biol. Med. *90*:610–615, 1955.
49. Cursons, R., and Pyke, P.: Diffusion in gel-enzyme-linked immunosorbent assay: A new serological test for leptospirosis. J. Clin. Pathol. *34*: 1128–1131, 1981.
50. Daniels, W. B., and Grennan, H. A.: Pretibial fever, an obscure disease. J. A. M. A. *122*:361–365, 1943.
51. de Brito, T., Morais, C. F., Yasuda, P. H., et al.: Cardiovascular involvement in human and experimental leptospirosis: Pathologic findings and immunohistochemical detection of leptospiral antigen. Ann. Trop. Med. Parasitol. *81*:207–214, 1987.
52. de Brito, T., Penna, D. O., Pereira, V. C., et al.: Kidney biopsies in human leptospirosis: A biochemical and electron microscopy study. Virchows Arch. [A] *343*:124–135, 1967.
53. Demers, R. Y., Thiermann, A., Demers, P., et al.: Exposure to *Leptospira icterohaemorrhagiae* in inner city and suburban children: A serologic comparison. J. Fam. Pract. *17*:1007–1011, 1983.
54. Edwards, G. A., and Domm, B. M.: Human leptospirosis. Medicine (Baltimore) *39*:117–156, 1960.
55. Edwards, G. A., and Domm, B. M.: Leptospirosis. II. Med. Times *94*: 1086–1095, 1966.
56. Effler, P. V., Domen, H. Y., Bragg, S. L., et al.: Evaluation of the indirect hemagglutination assay for diagnosis of acute leptospirosis in Hawaii. J. Clin. Microbiol. *38*:1081–1084, 2000.
57. Elian, M., Tamir, M., and Bornstein, B.: Unusual case of brachial plexitis in relation to leptospires and Coxsackie virus. Confin. Neurol. *26*:1–6, 1965.
58. Emanuel, M. L., Mackerras, I. M., and Smith, D. J.: The epidemiology of leptospirosis in North Queensland. I. General surgery of animal hosts. J. Hyg. (Camb.) *62*:451–484, 1964.
59. Faine, S.: Virulence in *Leptospira*. I. Reactions of guineapigs to experimental infection with *Leptospira icterohemorrhagiae*. Br. J. Exp. Pathol. *38*:1–8, 1957.
60. Faine, S.: Virulence in *Leptospira*. II. The growth in vivo of virulent *Leptospira icterohemorrhagiae*. Br. J. Exp. Pathol. *38*:8–14, 1957.
61. Feigin, R. D., Lobes, L. A., Anderson, D. C., et al.: Human leptospirosis from immunized dogs. Ann. Intern. Med. *79*:777–785, 1973.
62. Ferreira Alvas, V. A., Vianna, M. R., Yasuda, P. H., et al.: Detection of leptospiral antigens in the human liver and kidney using an immunoperoxidase staining procedure. J. Pathol. *115*:125–131, 1987.
63. Finco, D. R., and Low, D. G.: Endotoxin properties of *Leptospira canicola*. Am. J. Vet. Res. *28*:1863–1872, 1967.
64. Finco, D. R., and Low, D. G.: Water, electrolyte, and acid-base alterations in experimental canine leptospirosis. Am. J. Vet. Res. *29*:1799–1807, 1968.
65. Fletcher, W.: Recent work on leptospirosis, tsutsugamushi disease and tropical typhus in the Federated Malay States. Trans. R. Soc. Trop. Med. Hyg. *21*:265–288, 1928.
66. Fukushima, B., and Hosoya, S.: Sci. Rep. Govt. Inst. Infect. Dis., Tokyo Imperial University *5*:151–169, 1926.
67. Galton, M. M., Menges, R. W., Shotts, E. B., Jr., et al.: Leptospirosis. PHS Publication No. 951. Washington, DC, U.S. Government Printing Office, 1962.
68. Galton, M. M., Sulzer, C. R., Santa Rosa, A., et al.: Application of a microtechnique to the agglutination test for leptospiral antibodies. Appl. Microbiol. *13*:81–85, 1965.
69. Geszti, O., Chung, H. L., and Ts'ao, W. C.: Studies on blood coagulation disorders in experimental leptospirosis. Chin. Med. J. *75*:603–615, 1957.

70. Gillespie, R. W., and Ryn, J.: Epidemiology of leptospirosis. Am. J. Public Health *53*:950–955, 1963.
71. Gochenour, W. S., Jr., Smadel, J. E., Jackson, E. B., et al.: Leptospiral etiology of Fort Bragg fever. Public Health Rep. *67*:811–813, 1952.
72. Gochenour, W. S., Jr., Yager, R. H., and Wetmore, P. W.: Antigenic similarity of bovine strains of leptospira (United States) and *Leptospira pomona*. Proc. Soc. Exp. Biol. Med. *74*:199–202, 1950.
73. Goebel, A., and Koburg, E.: Experimentelle untersuchungen zur frage der nierenveranderungen bei respirattorescher insuffizienz [Experimental studies on the problem of kidney changes in respiratory insufficiency]. Beitr. Pathol. Anat. *120*:111–124, 1959.
74. Gourley, I. M.: Studies of Experimental Canine Leptospirosis. Thesis, University of Minnesota Graduate School, Minneapolis, 1962.
75. Gourley, I. M., and Low, D. G.: In vitro aggregation of canine blood platelets and liquefaction of blood clots by leptospires. Am. J. Vet. Res. *23*:1252–1256, 1962.
76. Green, J. H., and Arean, V. M.: Virulence and distribution of *Leptospira icterohemorrhagiae* in experimental guinea pig infections. Am. J. Vet. Res. *25*:264–267, 1964.
77. Gsell, O.: Leptospirosis. Bern, Hans Huber Verlag, 1952.
78. Gsell, O.: Epidemiology of the leptospiroses. *In* Symposium of the Leptospiroses, December 11–12, 1952. Medical Science Publication No. 1. Washington, DC, U.S. Government Printing Office, 1953, pp. 4–23.
79. Hall, H. E., Hightower, J. A., Rivera, R. D., et al.: Evaluation of antibiotic therapy in human leptospirosis. Ann. Intern. Med. *35*:981–998, 1951.
80. Heath, C. W., Jr., Alexander, A. D., and Galton, M. M.: Leptospirosis in the United States. N. Engl. J. Med. *273*:857–922, 1965.
81. Hubbart, W. R.: Immunologic Studies on Leptospirosis. Thesis, University of California Graduate School, Los Angeles, 1964.
82. Hubbert, W. T., and Humphrey, G. L.: Epidemiology of leptospirosis in California: A cause of aseptic meningitis. Calif. Med. *108*:113–116, 1968.
83. Hutchison, J. H., Poppard, J. S., White, M. H. G., et al.: Outbreak of Weil's disease in the British army in Italy; clinical study; post-mortem and histological findings. Br. Med. J. *1*:81–83, 1946.
84. Imamura, S., Kuribayashi, K., and Kameta, M.: Studies on toxins of pathogenic *Leptospira*. Jpn. J. Microbiol. *1*:43–47, 1957.
85. Inada, R., Ido, Y., Hoki, R., et al.: The etiology, mode of infection and specific therapy of Weil's disease (spirochaetosis icterohaemorrhagica). J. Exp. Med. *23*:377–402, 1916.
86. Jacobs, J. H.: Spondylitis following Weil's disease. Ann. Rheum. Dis. *10*:61–63, 1951.
87. Jeghers, H. J., Houghton, J. D., and Foley, J. A.: Weil's disease: Report of case with postmortem observations and review of recent literature. Arch. Pathol. *20*:447–476, 1935.
88. Johnson, D. W.: The Australian leptospiroses. Med. J. Aust. *2*:724–731, 1950.
89. Johnson, R. C., and Harris, V. G.: Differentiation of pathogenic and saprophytic leptospires. I. Growth at low temperatures. J. Bacteriol. *94*:27–31, 1967.
90. Kahrs, R. F., and Baker, J. A.: Combined vaccines for dairy cattle. U.S. Livestock Sanitary Association, Proceedings of 69th Annual Meeting, 1966, p. 177.
91. Kasarov, L. B., and Addamiano, L.: Metabolism of the lipoproteins of serum by leptospires: Degradation of the triglycerides. J. Med. Microbiol. *2*:165–168, 1969.
92. Kerr, D. A.: Improved Warthin-Starry technique of staining spirochetes in tissue section. Am. J. Clin. Pathol. *2*(Tech. Suppl.):63–67, 1938.
93. Kocen, R. S.: Leptospirosis, a comparison of symptomatic and penicillin therapy. Br. Med. J. *1*:1181–1183, 1962.
94. Koppisch, E., and Bond, W. M.: The morbid anatomy of human leptospirosis: A report on thirteen fatal cases. *In* Symposium on the Leptospiroses, December 11–12, 1952. Medical Science Publication No. 1. Washington, DC, U.S. Government Printing Office, 1953, pp. 83–105.
95. Laurain, A. R.: Lesions of skeletal muscle in leptospirosis: Review of reports and an experimental study. Am. J. Pathol. *31*:501–514, 1955.
96. Lawson, J. H.: Leptospirosis in the west of Scotland. Scott. Med. J. *1*:220–224, 1972.
97. Lessa, I., and Cortes, E.: Cerebrovascular accident as a complication of leptospirosis. Lancet *2*:1113, 1981.
98. Letocart, M., Baranton, G., and Perolat, P.: Rapid identification of pathogenic *Leptospira* species (*Leptospira interrogans*, *L. borgpetersenii*, and *L. kirschneri*) with species-specific DNA probes produced by arbitrarily primed PCR. J. Clin. Microbiol. *35*:248–253, 1997.
99. McClain, J. B., Ballou, W. R., Harrison, S. M., et al.: Doxycycline therapy for leptospirosis. Ann. Intern. Med. *100*:696–698, 1984.
100. McCrumb, F. R., Jr., Stockard, J. L., Robinson, C. R., et al.: Leptospirosis in Malaya. I. Sporadic cases among military and civilian personnel. Am. J. Trop. Med. Hyg. *6*:238–256, 1952.
101. McCulloch, W. F., Braun, J. L., and Robinson, R. G.: Leptospiral meningitis. J. Iowa Med. Soc. *52*:728–731, 1962.
102. McNee, J. W.: Spirochaetal jaundice: The morbid anatomy and mechanism of production of the icterus. J. Pathol. Bacteriol. *23*:342–349, 1919.
103. Menges, R. W., Galton, M. M., and Hall, A. D.: Diagnosis of leptospirosis from urine specimens by direct culture following bladder tapping. J. Am. Vet. Med. Assoc. *132*:58–60, 1958.
104. Meyer, K. F., Anderson-Stewart, B., and Eddie, B.: Canine leptospirosis in the United States. J. Am. Vet. Med. Assoc. *95*:710–729, 1939.
105. Middleton, J. E.: Canicola fever with neurological complications. Br. Med. J. *2*:25–26, 1955.
106. Miller, H. G., Stanton, J. B., and Gibbons, J. L.: Parainfectious encephalomyelitis and related syndromes: A critical review of the neurological complication of certain specific fevers. Q. J. Med. *25*:427, 1956.
107. Miller, N. G., and Wilson, R. B.: In vivo and in vitro observations of *Leptospira pomona* by electron microscopy. J. Bacteriol. *84*:569–576, 1962.
108. Morse, E. V., Allen, V., and Worley, G., Jr.: Brucellosis and leptospirosis serological test results on serums of Wisconsin veterinarians. J. Am. Vet. Med. Assoc. *126*:59, 1955.
109. Morse, E. V., Morter, R. L., Langham, R. F., et al.: Experimental bovine leptospirosis, *Leptospira pomona* infection. J. Infect. Dis. *101*:129–136, 1957.
110. Moulton, J. E., and Howarth, J. A.: The demonstration of *Leptospira canicola* in hamster kidneys by means of fluorescent antibody. Cornell Vet. *47*:524–532, 1957.
111. Murphy, K. J.: Exchange transfusion and albumin infusion for severe leptospiral jaundice. Med. J. Aust. *1*:1299–1300, 1969.
112. Myers, D. M.: Serodiagnosis of human leptospirosis by countercurrent immunoelectrophoresis. J. Clin. Microbiol. *25*:897–899, 1987.
113. Noguchi, H.: *Spirochaeta icterohaemorrhagiae* in American wild rats and its relation to the Japanese and European strains. J. Exp. Med. *25*:755–763, 1917.
114. Ooi, B. S., Chen, B. T. M., Tan, K. K., et al.: Human renal leptospirosis. Am. J. Trop. Med. Hyg. *21*:336–341, 1972.
115. Parsons, M.: Electrocardiographic changes in leptospirosis. Br. Med. J. *2*:201–203, 1965.
116. Pertzelan, A., and Pruzanski, W.: *Leptospira canicola* infection: Report of 81 cases and review of the literature. Am. J. Trop. Med. Hyg. *12*:75–81, 1963.
117. Peter, G.: Leptospirosis: A zoonosis of protean manifestations. Pediatr. Infect. Dis. *1*:282–288, 1982.
118. Poh, S. C., and Soh, C. S.: Lung manifestations in leptospirosis. Thorax *25*:751–755, 1970.
119. Ramos-Morales, F., Diaz-Rivera, R. S., Cintron-Rivera, A. A., et al.: The pathogenesis of leptospiral jaundice. Ann. Intern. Med. *51*:861–878, 1959.
120. Randall, R., and Cooper, H. R.: Golden hamster *(Cricetus auratus)* as test animal for diagnosis of leptospirosis. Science *100*:133–134, 1944.
121. Randall, R., Wetmore, P. W., and Warner, A. R.: Sonic-vibrated leptospirae as antigens in complement fixation test for diagnosis of leptospirosis. J. Lab. Clin. Med. *34*:1411–1415, 1949.
122. Ribeiro, M. A., Brando, A. P., and Romero, E. C.: Evaluation of diagnostic tests for human leptospirosis. Braz. J. Med. Biol. Res. *29*:773–777, 1996.
123. Rimpan, W.: Die Leptospirose. Munich, Urban & Schwarzenberg, 1950.
124. Romero, E. C., Billerbeck, A. E. C., Sando, V. S., et al.: Detection of *Leptospira* DNA in patients with aseptic meningitis by PCR. J. Clin. Microbiol. *36*:1453–1455, 1998.
125. Russell, C. M.: A hemolysin associated with leptospirae. J. Immunol. *77*:405–409, 1956.
126. Russell, R. W. R.: Clinical features of tropical leptospirosis. Ann. Trop. Med. Parasitol. *53*:416–420, 1959.
127. Sarasin, G., Tucker, D. N., and Arean, V. M.: Accidental laboratory infection caused by *Leptospira icterohaemorrhagiae:* Report of a case. Am. J. Clin. Pathol. *40*:146–150, 1963.
128. Schaeffer, M.: Leptospiral meningitis: Investigation of a water-borne epidemic due to *L. pomona*. J. Clin. Invest. *30*:670–671, 1951.
129. Scheidy, S. F.: Leptospirosis vaccination studies in cattle, swine, sheep, and horses. J. Am. Vet. Med. Assoc. *131*:366–368, 1957.
130. Schuffner, W.: Recent work on leptospirosis. Trans. R. Soc. Trop. Med. Hyg. *28*:7–37, 1934.
131. Sehgal, S. C., Sugunan, A. P., Murhekar, M. V., et al.: Randomized controlled trial of doxycycline prophylaxis against leptospirosis in an endemic area. Int. J. Antimicrob. Agents *13*:249–255, 2000.
132. Seiler, H. E., Noval, J., and Coghlan, J. D.: Leptospirosis in piggery workers. Nature *177*:1042, 1956.
133. Seki, M., Sato, T., Arimitsu, Y., et al.: One-point method for serological diagnosis of leptospirosis: A microcapsule agglutination test. Epidemiol. Infect. *99*:399–405, 1987.
134. Senekjie, H. A.: The clinical manifestations of leptospirosis in Louisiana. J. A. M. A. *126*:5–10, 1944.
135. Sheldon, W. H.: Lesions of muscle in spirochetal jaundice (Weil's disease; spirochetoses icterohemorrhagica). Arch. Intern. Med. *75*:119–124, 1945.
136. Silverstein, C. M.: Pulmonary manifestations of leptospirosis. Radiology *61*:327–334, 1953.
137. Sitprija, V.: Renal involvement in human leptospirosis. Br. Med. J. *2*:656–658, 1968.

138. Sitprija, V., and Chusilp, S.: Renal failure and hyperbilirubinemia in leptospirosis: Treatment with exchange transfusion. Med. J. Aust. *1*:171–173, 1973.
139. Sitprija, V., and Evans, H.: The kidney in human leptospirosis. Am. J. Med. *49*:780–788, 1970.
140. Smith, D. J. W., and Self, H. R.: Observations on the survival of *Leptospira australis* A in soil and water. J. Hyg. (Lond.) *53*:436–444, 1955.
141. Smits, H. L., Ananyina, Y. V., Chereshsky, A., et al.: International multicenter evaluation of the clinical utility of a dipstick assay for detection of *Leptospira*-specific immunoglobulin M antibodies in human serum specimens. J. Clin. Microbiol. *37*:2904–2909, 1999.
142. Sodeman, W. A., and Kilough, J. H.: Cardiac manifestations of Weil's disease. Am. J. Trop. Med. *31*:479–488, 1951.
143. Solbrig, A. U., Sher, J. H., and Kula, R. W.: Rhabdomyolysis in leptospirosis (Weil's disease). J. Infect. Dis. *156*:692–693, 1987.
144. Stalheim, O. H., and Wilson, J. B.: Antigenicity and immunogenicity of leptospires grown in chemically characterized medium. Am. J. Vet. Res. *25*:1277–1280, 1964.
145. Stavitsky, A. B.: Studies on the pathogenesis of leptospirosis. J. Infect. Dis. *76*:179–192, 1945.
146. Sterling, K.: Hepatic function in Weil's disease. Gastroenterology *15*:52–58, 1950.
147. Stiles, W. W., Goldstein, J. D., and McCann, W. S.: Leptospiral nephritis. J. A. M. A. *131*:1271–1274, 1946.
148. Stimson, A. M.: Note on an organism found in yellow-fever tissue. Public Health Rep. *22*:541, 1907.
149. Stoenner, H. G., and Marlean, D.: Leptospirosis ballum contracted from Swiss albino mice. Arch. Intern. Med. *101*:606–610, 1958.
150. Stuart, R. D.: Transport problems in public health bacteriology: The use of transport media and other devices to maintain the viability of bacteria in specimens. Can. J. Public Health *47*:115–122, 1956.
151. Sulzer, C. R., Glosser, J. W., Rogers, F., et al.: Evaluation of an indirect hemagglutination test for the diagnosis of human leptospirosis. J. Clin. Microbiol. *2*:218–221, 1975.
152. Sutliff, W. D., Shepard, R., and Dunham, W. B.: Acute *Leptospira pomona* arthritis and myocarditis. Ann. Intern. Med. *39*:134–140, 1953.
153. Tabel, H., and Karstad, L.: The renal carrier state of experimental *Leptospira pomona* infections in skunks *(Mephitis mephitis)*. Am. J. Epidemiol. *85*:9–15, 1967.
154. Takafuji, E. T., Kirkpatrick, J. W., Miller, R. N., et al.: An efficacy trial of doxycycline chemoprophylaxis against leptospirosis. N. Engl. J. Med. *310*:497–500, 1984.
155. Thomas, L.: Physiological disturbances produced by endotoxins. Annu. Rev. Physiol. *16*:467–490, 1954.
156. Thomson, J. G.: Fatal Weil's disease with myocarditis in South Africa. S. Afr. Med. J. *38*:696–700, 1964.
157. Tobie, J. E., and McCullough, N. B.: Serologic evidence of *Leptospira pomona* infections in meat inspectors. J. Am. Vet. Med. Assoc. *138*:434–436, 1961.
158. Tonge, J. I., and Smith, D. J.: Leptospirosis acquired from soil. Med. J. Aust. *48*:711–712, 1961.
159. Torten, M., Birnbaum, S., Klingberg, M. A., et al.: Epidemiologic investigation of an outbreak of leptospirosis in the Upper Galilee, Israel. Am. J. Epidemiol. *91*:52–58, 1970.
160. Torten, M., Shenberg, E., and van der Hoeden, J.: The use of immunofluorescence in the diagnosis of human leptospirosis by a genus-specific antigen. J. Infect. Dis. *116*:537–543, 1966.
161. Trimble, A. P.: Clinical aspects of leptospirosis in Malaya. Proc. R. Soc. Med. *50*:125–128, 1957.
162. Turner, L. H.: Leptospirosis. I. Trans. R. Soc. Trop. Med. Hyg. *61*: 842–855, 1967.
163. Turner, L. H.: Leptospirosis. II. Trans. R. Soc. Trop. Med. Hyg. *62*: 880–899, 1968.
164. Turner, L. H.: Leptospirosis. III. Maintenance, isolation and demonstration of leptospires. Trans. R. Soc. Trop. Med. Hyg. *64*:623–646, 1970.
165. Turner, L. H.: Leptospirosis. Br. Med. J. *1*:231–235, 1969.
166. Turner, L. H.: Leptospirosis. Br. Med. J. *1*:537–540, 1973.
167. Valek, K., Neuwirtova, R., and Chytil, M.: Treatment of acute renal failure in the course of Weil's disease by the artificial kidney. Rev. Czech. Med. *5*:32–39, 1959.
168. van der Hoeden, J., Shenberg, E., and Torten, M.: The epidemiological complexity of *Leptospira canicola* infection of man and animals in Israel. Isr. J. Med. Sci. *3*:880–884, 1967.
169. Van Thiele, P. H.: The Leptospiroses. Leiden, Universitaire Pers Leiden, 1948.
170. Volland, W., and Brede, H. D.: Zur frage der hyaluronidasebildung durch Leptospiren: Ein beitrag zum problem der meningitisentstehung und der blut-gehirnschranke [On the production of hyaluronidase by leptospires with reference to meningitis and the hemoencephalic barrier]. Med. Monatsschr. *5*:698, 1951; Bull. Hyg. (Lond.) *27*:251–252, 1952.
171. Wadsworth, A., Langworthy, H. V., Stewart, F. O., et al.: Infectious jaundice occurring in New York State: Preliminary report of an investigation, with report of a case of accidental infection of the human subject with *Leptospira icterohaemorrhagiae* from the rat. J. A. M. A. *78*:1120, 1922.
172. Wang, B., Sullivan, J., Sullivan, G. W., et al.: Interaction of leptospires with human polymorphonuclear neutrophils. Infect. Immun. *44*: 459–464, 1984.
173. Wang, C. P., Chi, C. W., and Lu, F. L.: Studies on anicteric leptospirosis. III. Roentgenologic observations of pulmonary changes. Chin. Med. J. (Peking) *84*:298–306, 1965.
174. Watt, G., Alquiza, L. M., Padre, L. P., et al.: The rapid diagnosis of leptospirosis: A prospective comparison of the DOT enzyme-linked immunosorbent assay and the genus-specific microscopic agglutination test at different stages of illness. J. Infect. Dis. *157*:840–842, 1988.
175. Watt, G., Padre, L. P., Tuazon, M. L., et al.: Placebo-controlled trial of intravenous penicillin for severe and late leptospirosis. Lancet *1*:433–435, 1988.
176. Weil, A.: Ueber eine eigenthumliche, mit milztumor, icterus und nephritis einhergehende, acute infectionskrankheit. Dtsch. Arch. Klin. Med. *39*: 209–232, 1886.
177. Wylie, J. A. H.: Relative importance of renal and hepatic lesions in experimental leptospirosis icterohemorrhagiae. J. Pathol. Bacteriol. *58*:351–358, 1946.

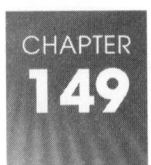

CHAPTER 149 *Spirillum minus* (Rat-Bite Fever)

CARRIE L. BYINGTON ■ ROBERT D. BASOW

Spirillum minus is one of the causative agents of rat-bite fever, or sodoku. Rat-bite fever also may be caused by *Streptobacillus moniliformis* (see Chapter 144). *S. minus* is a spirochete that was isolated first by Futaki and associates in 1917.[5] The original name for the organism was *Spirochaeta morsus muris*. *S. minus* is the most frequent cause of rat-bite fever in Asia.[9] Only one case of spirillary rat-bite fever has been reported in the American literature since 1969.[3]

Bacteriology

S. minus is a short, rigid, aerobic, gram-negative, flagellated spirochete measuring 2 to 5 μm in length. The organism is thicker than *Treponema pallidum* and usually contains two to five regular sharp turns along its length. On darkfield microscopy, the organism moves quickly, using the terminal flagellum.[5] In general, researchers agree that *S. minus*, like other spirochetes, does not grow on artificial media and requires animal inoculation for successful isolation.[15] However, two reports in the literature describe the isolation of *S. minus* in broth.[8, 14] The cases, however, may have represented other infectious illnesses.

Epidemiology and Pathology

The epidemiology of spirillary rat-bite fever is similar to that of the streptobacillary form. Disease appears to be transmitted primarily through rat bites. Approximately 25 percent of rats are carriers of *S. minus* in the nasopharynx, and rats with conjunctivitis have been shown to have *S. minus* in the eye discharges that drain into their mouths.[11] Disease has not been reported after oral ingestion of the organism. Human-to-human transmission has not been reported but conceivably could occur during blood transfusions.

Gunning[6] has given an excellent description of the pathologic changes of *S. minus* infection. The infection provokes edema, mononuclear leukocyte infiltration, and necrosis at the site of inoculation. Regional lymph nodes are hyperplastic. The relapsing symptoms are associated with invasion of the blood by spirilla. Toxic, hemorrhagic, or necrotic changes may occur in the liver and kidney.

Clinical Manifestations

The incubation period of spirillary rat-bite fever typically is longer than that of the streptobacillary form, averaging 14 to 18 days, with a range of 1 to 36 days.[2] The disease is heralded by the appearance of an indurated lesion at the site of the initially healed bite, which coincides with the onset of fever and chills. Chancre formation or ulceration may occur at the site, and regional lymphadenopathy occurs commonly. The temperature may reach 41° C in a stepwise fashion over the course of 2 to 4 days and fall abruptly.[6] Six to eight regularly occurring relapses of fever separated by afebrile periods lasting 3 to 7 days may ensue. During febrile periods, the patient also may experience myalgia, headache, and vomiting. About 50 percent of patients develop a purple to red-brown rash consisting of large macules with occasional indurated erythematous plaques or urticarial lesions.[15] As opposed to streptobacillary rat-bite fever, joint manifestations are rare occurrences. In untreated cases, the illness may persist for 3 to 8 weeks, but relapses have occurred after months or years.[13]

Spontaneous cures are the general rule, but several untreated cases have persisted for longer than 1 year.[15] The untreated mortality rate is reported to be 6.5 percent.[2] In protracted, untreated cases, severe complications include endocarditis,[8] meningitis,[10] myocarditis, hepatitis, and nephritis.[4] Anemia, weight loss, and severe diarrhea are common complications in infants and children. Epididymitis, nuchal rigidity, headache, pleurisy, pleural effusion, and splenomegaly also have been reported.[12]

The differential diagnosis includes streptobacillary rat-bite fever and many other infectious and noninfectious diseases (see Chapter 144 for details).

Diagnosis

Definitive diagnosis requires isolation and identification of the spirochete. Although the organism rarely may be seen on peripheral blood smear[1] or darkfield examination of ulcer exudate,[7] animal inoculation usually is required for isolation. Blood or wound aspirates are injected intraperitoneally into guinea pigs or mice. The spirochetes then may be recovered in 5 to 15 days from the animals' blood, which is examined under darkfield microscopy. This process is time consuming and may not be available in most centers. In addition, the inoculated animals must be screened carefully for prior *Spirillum* spp. carriage.

Nonspecific diagnostic criteria include a false-positive test for syphilis in 50 percent of patients, white blood cell count between 10,000 and 20,000 cells/mm^3, and a moderate anemia.[2, 15] No specific serologic tests exist for *S. minus*. Molecular methods, such as the polymerase chain reaction, may offer hope in the future for detection of *S. minus*.[4]

Treatment

S. minus is considerably more sensitive to penicillin than is *S. moniliformis*. In one study, a dosage as low as 24,000 units/day for 5 days was shown to be effective.[13] However, because distinguishing spirillary disease from streptobacillary disease is difficult and the two may coexist, treating with dosages effective against *S. moniliformis* in the acute stage is important (see Chapter 144 for further details).

REFERENCES

1. Bhatt, K. M., and Mirza, N. B.: Rat bite fever: A case report of a Kenyan. East Afr. Med. J. *69:*542–543, 1992.
2. Brown, T., and Nunemaker, J.: Rat-bite fever: Review of American cases with reevaluation of its etiology and report of cases. Bull. Johns Hopkins Hosp. *70:*201–202, 1942.
3. Cole, J. S., Stoll, R. W., and Bulger, R. J.: Rat-bite fever: Report of three cases. Ann. Intern. Med. *71:*979–981, 1969.
4. Fredricks, D. N., and Relman, D. A.: Application of polymerase chain reaction to the diagnosis of infectious diseases. Clin. Infect. Dis. *29:*475–488, 1999.
5. Futaki, K., Takaki, I., and Taniguchi, T.: *Spirochaeta morsus muris* n. sp.: The cause of rat-bite fever. J. Exp. Med. *25:*33–44, 1917.
6. Gunning, J.: Rat-bite fever. *In:* Hunter, G., Swartzwelder, J., Clyde, D. (eds.): Tropical Medicine. Philadelphia, W. B. Saunders, 1976, pp. 245–247.
7. Hinrichsen, S. L., Ferraz, S., Romeiro, M., et al.: [Sodoku—a case report]. Rev. Soc. Bras. Med. Trop. *25:*135–138, 1992.
8. Hitzig, W., and Liebman, A.: Subacute endocarditis associated with a spirillum: Report of a case with repeated isolation of the organism from the blood. Arch. Intern. Med. *73:*415, 1944.
9. Ito, A.: [Rat-bite fever]. Ryoikibetsu Shokogun Shirizu *24:*300, 1999.
10. Kiefer, H., Froscher, W., and Mohr, H. P.: [Rat bite disease with meningoencephalitic involvement]. Med. Klin. *76:*653–655, 1981.
11. McDermott, E: Rat-bite fever: Study of experimental disease with critical review of the literature. Q. J. Med. *21:*433–458, 1928.
12. Robertson, A.: *Spirillum minus*: Etiological agent of rat-bite fever. Ann. Trop. Med. *24:*367, 1930.
13. Roughgarden, J.: Antimicrobial therapy of rat-bite fever. Arch. Intern. Med. *116:*39–53, 1965.
14. Shwartzman, G., Florman, A., and Bass, M.: Repeated recovery of a spirillum by blood culture from two children with prolonged and recurrent fevers. Pediatrics *8:*227, 1951.
15. Taber, L. H., and Feigin, R. D.: Spirochetal infections. Pediatr. Clin. North Am. *26:*377–413, 1979.

CHAPTER 150

Syphilis

PABLO J. SÁNCHEZ ■ LAURA T. GUTMAN

Syphilis first was recognized in Europe at the end of the 15th century. It appeared initially in the Mediterranean area, from which it spread and rapidly reached epidemic proportions. Although the European origin of the disease is unknown, the possibility that the disease was introduced from the West Indies by Columbus' crew has been considered. Alternatively, endemic African disease may have been imported by travelers. Some people also consider it probable that the endemic yaws and bejel of African people appeared as virulent syphilis in a susceptible European population.

Syphilis initially was called the "Italian disease," the "French disease," and the "great pox" (as distinguished from smallpox). Its venereal transmission was not recognized until the 18th century. Delineation of the characteristics of syphilis was hindered by the confusion of its symptoms with those of gonorrhea. In 1767, John Hunter, a great English experimental biologist and physician, inoculated himself with urethral exudate from a patient with gonorrhea. Unfortunately, the patient also had syphilis, and the subsequent symptoms experienced by Hunter convinced two generations of physicians of the unity of gonorrhea and syphilis. The separate nature of gonorrhea and syphilis was demonstrated in 1838 by Ricord, who reported his observations on more than 2500 human inoculations. Recognition of the stages of syphilis occurred afterward, and in 1905, Schaudinn and Hoffman discovered the causative agent. The following year, Wassermann introduced the diagnostic blood test that bears his name.

The Organism

Morphologic characteristics are the primary features by which members of the family Spirochaetaceae are placed into a single taxon. Spirochetes are helix-shaped, heterotrophic bacteria. These organisms are slender, coiled, and flexible, with one or more complete turns in the helix. Spirochetes are motile, their motility resulting from the action of axial fibrils rather than flagella. Five genera are included in the family Spirochaetaceae, of which only *Treponema, Borrelia,* and *Leptospira* spp. cause major human illness. Differentiation among genera of the family Spirochaetaceae is based primarily on morphology of the organism.

The name *Treponema* is derived from the Greek words meaning "turning thread." Individual organisms are 5 to 20 μm in length and 0.092 to 0.5 μm in diameter and have finely tapered ends. Whole cells appear to have a flat wave with one or more planes per cell that gives the appearance of a helical coil. Each cell has 8 to 14 waves distributed evenly. They exhibit a sluggish mobility, with drifting motion and graceful flexuous movements. These organisms rarely rotate but are motile in liquid and solid media.

The internal structure of *Treponema pallidum* in general is similar to that of other spirochetes. An outermost thin, three-layered membrane surrounds the protoplasmic cylinder of the cell. Intracytoplasmic microtubules have been described, and such structures may be specific for *Treponema*.

The six axial fibrils are long, flagellum-like intracellular organelles that originate at either end of the cell from knoblike structures and extend toward the other end. Axial fibrils are variable in length but overlap one another near the middle of the cell. These fibrils are thought to determine the spiral shape of the cells and are responsible for the characteristic motility exhibited by members of the Spirochaetaceae.

Recently, the complete genome of *T. pallidum* subspecies *pallidum* (Nichols strain) was sequenced by the whole genome rapid sequencing method.[44] The *T. pallidum* genome is a circular chromosome containing 1,138,006 base pairs with 1041 predicted coding sequences. In addition, by a polyacrylamide gel electrophoresis technique, the major constituent proteins of *T. pallidum,* including integral membrane proteins with apparent molecular masses of 47, 34, 17, and 15 kd, have been characterized.[95] These lipoprotein antigens are highly immunogenic in laboratory animals and humans.[8, 63]

Virulent strains of *T. pallidum* are propagated by intratesticular inoculation of rabbits, and the inability to propagate the organisms in vitro has hampered study of these microorganisms. The division time of the organism in rabbits is approximately 30 hours. Velocity sedimentation with discontinuous gradients of Hypaque has been used to purify and concentrate treponemes extracted from infected rabbit testes. These organisms retain the antigens for the fluorescence test, although motility is lost.

Limited cultivation of *T. pallidum* on monolayers of baby hamster kidney cells in 7 percent carbon dioxide has been reported. Research on the in vitro characteristics of these organisms also has resulted in the description of adherence of virulent *T. pallidum* to primary cell cultures of rabbit testicular cells and to an established continuous line of human epithelial cells (HEp-2). To date, however, direct in vitro culture for the diagnosis of *T. pallidum* disease has not been possible.

Transmission

ACQUIRED SYPHILIS

Syphilis is not a highly contagious disease. A person who has had sexual contact with an infected partner has an approximately 30 percent chance of acquiring disease. The median infectious dose (ID_{50}) in humans has been estimated experimentally to be 57 organisms. *T. pallidum* has the capability of invading intact mucous membranes or skin in areas of abrasion. Direct inoculation from contact with an infected person is necessary for infection because survival of the organism outside the host is very limited. Sexual contact is the common method of transmission of acquired disease, and the site of inoculation usually is on the genital organs: the vagina or cervix in females and the penis in males. Other sites include the lips, breast, tongue, and abraded areas of the skin. Examining physicians and pathologists may be infected by contact if appropriate barrier protection is not provided.

CONGENITAL SYPHILIS

Congenital syphilis usually results from transplacental infection of the developing fetus from maternal spirochetemia, but a newborn occasionally may be infected at delivery by contact with an infectious lesion present in the birth canal or perineum. Intrauterine transmission is supported by isolation of the organism from umbilical cord blood and amniotic fluid,[49, 93, 119, 142] detection of spirochetes in the placenta and umbilical cord in association with typical histopathologic changes,[43, 103] and detection of specific IgM antibody to *T. pallidum* in neonatal serum obtained at birth.[75, 85, 117, 119] Isolation of *T. pallidum* from as many as 74 percent of amniotic fluid specimens obtained from women with early syphilis also suggests that the organism is capable of traversing the fetal membranes, gaining access to amniotic fluid, and causing fetal infection.[76] Breast-feeding is not associated with the transmission of syphilis unless the mother has a chancre on her breast.

Transmission of syphilis to the fetus can occur throughout pregnancy. Occasional reports in the literature describing treponemes in fetal tissue or placentas before the fifth month of gestation were disputed for decades.[36] The Langhans cell layer of the cytotrophoblast was thought to form a placental barrier against treponemal invasion of the fetus. However, researchers subsequently demonstrated that the layer of Langhans cells in the placenta persisted throughout pregnancy. In addition, in 1976, Harter and Benirschke[54] visualized spirochetes by Warthin-Starry silver stain and immunofluorescence in tissue from two aborted fetuses at gestational ages of 9 and 10 weeks. The expected inflammatory response was not observed in these two fetuses, but such changes have been found in infected fetuses after the 15th week of pregnancy. These investigators noted that researchers who described syphilitic fetuses or placentas in the older literature worked with products of spontaneous abortion. Such fetal loss caused by syphilis occurred only after 18 weeks of gestation, thus implying that the fetal loss was a reflection of the damage incurred as a result of the host response to the organism. The observation of sequential acquisition by the fetus of the ability to respond to a variety of antigens suggests that inflammation can be present only after the fetus acquires the immunologic ability to recognize the treponeme.[130] The more recent detection of spirochetes in amniotic fluid obtained by amniocentesis from a woman with early syphilis at 14 weeks of pregnancy clearly has shown that the fetus can be infected with *T. pallidum* in early pregnancy.[92] Vertical transmission, however, does increase with advancing gestation.

Vertical transmission is related directly to the maternal stage of syphilis, with early syphilis resulting in significantly higher transmission rates than noted with late latent infection. In general, the greater the time that has elapsed since the woman's primary or secondary infection, the less likely she is to transmit disease to the fetus. Ingraham in 1951 reported that among 251 women with syphilis of up to 4 years' duration, 41 percent of their infants were liveborn and had congenital syphilis, 25 percent were stillborn, 14 percent died in the neonatal period, 21 percent had low birth weight but no evidence of syphilis, and only 18 percent were normal full-term infants.[59] In contrast, only 2 percent of infants born to mothers with late disease had congenital syphilis. In 1952, Fiumara and colleagues[41] reported that untreated primary or secondary syphilis resulted in 50 percent of infants contracting congenital syphilis, whereas the other half either were stillborn or premature or died in the neonatal period. With early latent infection, 40 percent of the infants had congenital syphilis, whereas with late latent disease, syphilis developed in only 10 percent. These data are supported by a recent study of Sheffield and associates,[127] in which mothers with primary, secondary, early latent, and late latent infection had transmission rates of 29, 59, 50, and 13 percent, respectively.

Syphilis is one of the ulcer-causing diseases associated with increased sexual transmission of human immunodeficiency virus (HIV). In this regard, increasing proportions of newborns who are infected with congenital syphilis also are born to mothers with HIV, and vice versa. The contribution of maternal co-infection with *T. pallidum* and HIV to vertical transmission of either syphilis or HIV has not been elucidated fully. Virulent *T. pallidum* can promote the induction of HIV gene expression in macrophages, possibly resulting in increased systemic HIV levels and more rapid progression of the HIV infection.[138] The significance of this finding in relation to maternal-to-infant transmission of HIV is not known. A recent study noted higher rates of congenital syphilis in infants born to co-infected mothers, but the diagnosis of congenital syphilis was based on a surveillance definition used by the Centers for Disease Control and Prevention (CDC) and not on strict diagnostic criteria.[123]

Epidemiology

The introduction of penicillin in 1942 and its subsequent widespread use in the 1950s resulted in a marked decline in the occurrence of syphilis in the United States. After an increase in cases in the early 1960s, syphilis again declined in the 1970s, only to have a dramatic resurgence from 1986 to 1991.[19, 27, 108] The rapid increase in the rate and number of cases of primary and secondary syphilis in adults during these years, specifically in women of child-bearing age, resulted in a significant increase in rates of congenital syphilis. Rates of syphilis were greatest in blacks and Hispanics residing in large urban centers, and the disease was centered in populations in which substance abuse, particularly crack cocaine, was a common occurrence and in which prostitution was practiced. One of the cycles of infection occurs in groups in which sex is exchanged for drugs. Among persons who trade sex for drugs, the identities of sexual partners often are unknown, thus rendering partner notification, a traditional syphilis control measure, virtually impossible.[19] Other factors that may have contributed to the increased rates of syphilis included underfunded and overwhelmed public health resources, the use of spectinomycin for treatment of penicillinase-producing *Neisseria gonorrhoeae* because spectinomycin is not effective against incubating syphilis, and failure to implement safer sexual practices, especially among adolescents and young adults. In general, persons who acquire syphilis characteristically are young and often promiscuous, having had contact with an average of five persons during the incubation period. Because of the high rate of dual infection (8%) with *N. gonorrhoeae,* some persons identified and treated for gonorrhea with ceftriaxone also will be treated for syphilis while in the preprimary stage of disease.

Strenuous attempts were made to control syphilis, and current syphilis rates are the lowest ever reported in the United States.[20] Reasons include (1) wider screening practices because of medical and public awareness of the syphilis epidemic of the late 1980s that led to identification and treatment of infected individuals; (2) increased state and local funding for such syphilis control programs as partner notification, community-based screening and presumptive treatment strategies, and risk reduction counseling; (3) introduction of HIV prevention programs that target prevention of other sexually transmitted diseases; (4) decrease in crack cocaine use and sex-for-drugs behavior; and, possibly, (5) the development of acquired immunity to syphilis in high-risk populations, which has resulted in less reacquisition of infectious syphilis. Currently, syphilis is occurring in fewer geographic areas in the United States, with most new cases reported from less than 1 percent of counties that are disproportionately clustered in the southeastern United States, an area that has less than 20 percent of the total U.S. population. It is occurring in racial and ethnic minorities who live in poverty and whose medical care is poor. In addition, focal clusters of early syphilis continue to arise and have been associated primarily with homosexual activity, but also with the illicit use of drugs. Although the possibility now exists for eventual control and elimination of endemic syphilis and the CDC has funded a National Plan for Elimination of Syphilis from the United States, continued surveillance is mandatory.[133]

In 1987, the reported rate of congenital syphilis was 10.5 cases per 100,000 live births. By 1991, 4398 cases of congenital syphilis (107/100,000 live births) had been reported. These rates reflect a reporting case definition that was changed in 1988[19, 146] and resulted in an almost fourfold increase in cases reported to the CDC.[27] However, a genuine increase also occurred in actual cases and case rates as a result of the increase in early syphilis in women.[66] Case rates of congenital syphilis were greatest in the Northeast (186.2 cases/100,000) and lowest in the Midwest (54.8/100,000).[37] In 1988, researchers recognized that the previous definitions of congenital syphilis that had been used for surveillance and treatment decisions were difficult to apply to the clinical setting because they required a diagnosis that often could be made only over a period of weeks or months. During that period, many children were lost to follow-up and, therefore, were neither treated nor reported.[27] Because of the high incidence of congenital disease in infants born to inadequately treated mothers, current definitions of congenital syphilis for a presumptive case (which should be reported and treated) require only (1) that the infant be born to a mother with untreated or inadequately treated syphilis or (2) that the child have physical or laboratory signs of congenital syphilis. A summary of the surveillance case definition used since 1988 is presented in Table 150–1.

Minor differences exist in the case definitions of congenital syphilis as formulated by several agencies and experts.[113] For example, some experts also would consider a newborn who is well clinically but was born to a mother who had contact within 90 days before delivery with a person who had primary or secondary syphilis and had not been treated or had been treated inadequately as a presumptive case, even if the mother has nonreactive serology. Although recommendations for therapy commonly have assumed that adequate treatment of a mother with primary or secondary syphilis during pregnancy will prevent congenital syphilis with a high degree of reliability, reasons to doubt this premise have emerged.[3, 82, 145] In particular, treatment failures in which syphilis developed in the infant despite maternal therapy have been reported when the mother initially was treated within 30 days of delivery.[12, 14, 81, 83, 112] Therefore, infants born to mothers who were treated within 30 days of delivery are considered to have been treated inadequately, and the baby should receive appropriate therapy. The various circumstances in which maternal therapy may be presumed to be subtherapeutic are presented in Table 150–2. The consequences of inadequate treatment of the mother are shown in Table 150–3. In that experience, 13 percent of the children born to inadequately treated mothers had congenital syphilis, all of which were neurosyphilis.[111]

TABLE 150–1 ■ SURVEILLANCE CASE DEFINITION FOR CONGENITAL SYPHILIS

A *confirmed case* of congenital syphilis is an infant in whom *Treponema pallidum* is identified by darkfield microscopy, fluorescent antibody, or other specific stains in specimens from lesions, placenta, umbilical cord, amniotic fluid, or autopsy material

A *presumptive case* of congenital syphilis is either of the following:
Any infant whose mother had untreated or inadequately treated* syphilis at delivery, regardless of findings in the infant, *or*
Any infant or child who has a reactive treponemal test for syphilis and any one of the following:
1. Any evidence of congenital syphilis on physical examination *or*
2. Any evidence of congenital syphilis on long bone radiograph *or*
3. Reactive cerebrospinal fluid VDRL *or*
4. Elevated cerebrospinal fluid cell count or protein (without other cause) *or*
5. Quantitative nontreponemal serologic titers that are fourfold higher than the mother's (both drawn at birth) *or*
6. Reactive test for FTA-ABS 19S IgM antibody

A *syphilitic stillbirth* is defined as death of a fetus weighing >500 g or having a gestational age >20 wk in which the mother had untreated or inadequately treated syphilis at delivery

*Inadequate treatment consists of any nonpenicillin therapy or penicillin given less than 30 days before delivery.
FTA-ABS, fluorescent treponema/antibody absorption; VDRL, Venereal Disease Research Laboratory.
Adapted from Centers for Disease Control and Prevention: Congenital syphilis—New York City, 1986–1988. M. M. W. R. Morb. Mortal. Wkly. Rep. *38*(48):828, 1989.

Undoubtedly, substantial under-reporting of infected infants did occur previously,[145] but the revised surveillance definition does not represent diagnostic criteria. Rather, it reflects the public health burden of the disease because these infants require medical and public health interventions. Despite this change in reporting guidelines, the number of cases of congenital syphilis has continued to decline since 1991 because of the decreasing number of syphilis cases in the United States.[21] Worldwide, however, syphilis remains a considerable public health problem, particularly in Eastern Europe and the developing countries of Latin America and Africa.

Congenital syphilis is a disease that should be almost fully amenable to eradication if currently available prenatal health measures are implemented completely. Table 150–4 presents two studies of the prenatal care of women who

TABLE 150–2 ■ CIRCUMSTANCES IN WHICH MATERNAL THERAPY FOR SYPHILIS MAY BE SUBTHERAPEUTIC OR INADEQUATE

Treatment with a nonpenicillin regimen
History of material treatment not documented fully or verifiable
Treatment during the month before delivery
Treatment in HIV-infected women
Serial post-therapy assays of maternal nontreponemal antibody titers were not performed
Serial post-therapy assays of maternal nontreponemal antibody titers did not show a fourfold decline in titer after treatment of early syphilis, thus not permitting assessment of the adequacy of therapy and suggesting the possibility of failure to eradicate infection
Serial post-therapy assays of maternal nontreponemal antibody titers show a fourfold increase in titer, suggesting reinfection or relapse

TABLE 150–3 ■ CLINICAL FINDINGS OF 148 INFANTS WHOSE MOTHERS HAD SYPHILIS AND WHOSE TREATMENT WAS ADEQUATE, INADEQUATE, OR NOT PROVIDED

	Maternal Treatment		
Infant Findings	None (n = 72)	Inadequate (n = 31)	Adequate (n = 45)
Clinical disease	3	0	0
Positive CSF VDRL test	7	4	0
Abnormal bone radiograph	6	0	0
Stillbirth	6	0	0
Total (any abnormality)	22 (31%)	4 (13%)	0

CSF, cerebrospinal fluid; VDRL, Venereal Disease Research Laboratory.
From Reyes, M. P., Hunt, N., Ostrea, E. M., et al: Material/congenital syphilis in a large tertiary care urban hospital. Clin. Infect. Dis. *17*: 1041–1046, 1993.

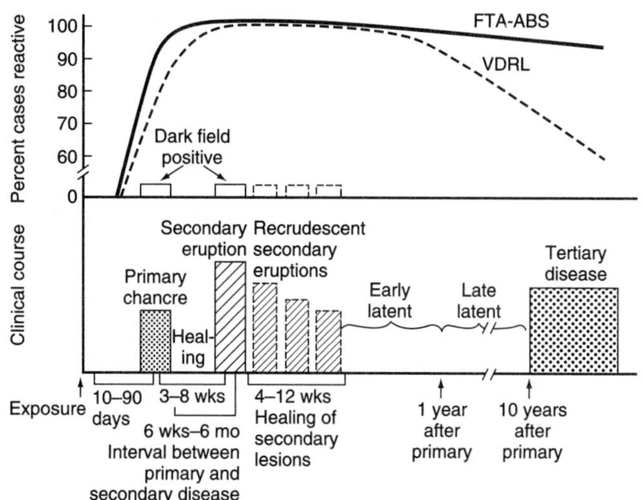

FIGURE 150–1 ■ The course of untreated syphilis.

delivered infants with congenital syphilis and indicates the hurdles that control of the disease will have to overcome.[28, 82] Lack of prenatal care is by far the most important one.

Little doubt exists that penicillin was a major reason for the decline in treponematosis seen in the early 1950s.[38] Other factors must be considered in the attempted eradication of these infections. For example, nonvenereal endemic treponemal infections (endemic syphilis, bejel, yaws, pinta) have continued to flourish, despite the introduction of penicillin, in underdeveloped areas of the world where hygiene is poor. Progress in control of these diseases requires that institution of mass treatment programs be coupled with effort to improve local living conditions. In areas where these measures could be accomplished, a resulting decline in endemic treponematosis has occurred.

Pathology

Syphilis often is a lifelong infection that progresses in three clear characteristic stages (Fig. 150–1). After initial invasion through mucous membranes or the skin, the organism undergoes rapid multiplication and is disseminated widely. Spread through the perivascular lymphatics and then through the systemic circulation probably occurs even before clinical development of the primary lesion. Ten to 90 days later, usually within 3 to 4 weeks, the patient mounts an inflammatory response to the infection at the site of the inoculation. The resulting lesion, a chancre, is characterized by the profuse discharge of spirochetes; an accumulation of mononuclear leukocytes, lymphocytes, and plasma cells; and swelling of capillary endothelia. The regional lymph nodes are enlarged, and the cellular infiltrate resembles that of the primary lesions. Resolution of the primary lesion is by fibrosis.

Secondary lesions develop when tissues of ectodermal origin, such as the skin, mucous membranes, and central nervous system (CNS), participate in an inflammatory response. Mucous patches in the mouth are caused by local vasculitis. The cellular infiltrate resembles that of the primary lesion, with a predominance of plasma cells. Little or no necrosis occurs, and healing is without scarring but may include pigmentary changes.

Tertiary syphilis may involve any organ system and often is asymmetric. Gummata are lesions typified by extensive necrosis, a few giant cells, and a paucity of organisms. They commonly occur in internal organs, bone, and skin. The other major form of tertiary lesions is a diffuse chronic inflammation, with plasma cells and lymphocytes but without caseation, that may result in an aneurysm of the aorta, paralytic dementia, or tabes dorsalis. Chronic swelling of the capillary endothelium and fibrosis are responsible for the characteristic tissue changes.

Congenital syphilis is a result of hematogenous infection and disseminated involvement of almost all viscera. The intense inflammatory response occurs in the perivascular framework and interstitial stroma rather than the parenchyma.[90] Bone, liver, pancreas, intestine, kidney, and spleen are the tissues involved most reproducibly and severely. Other tissues, such as the brain, pituitary gland,[14] lymph nodes, and lungs, may be infected as well. The gastrointestinal tract shows a pattern of mononuclear cell infiltration in the mucosa and submucosa, with subsequent widening of the submucosa by the ensuing fibrosis. This event is most prominent in the small bowel. In the kidney, perivascular inflammation, particularly in the juxtamedullary region, is evident. The basic architecture of the tissue

TABLE 150–4 ■ PRENATAL CARE AND THE OCCURRENCE* OF CONGENITAL SYPHILIS IN INFANTS

	Mascola et al., 1984[82] (*n* = 50)	**Coles et al., 1995[28] (*n* = 318)**
No prenatal care	56	46
First prenatal test negative; testing not repeated in late pregnancy	6	14
Medical mismanagement	6	10
Failure of conventional prenatal syphilis treatment of mother	8	5
Negative maternal syphilis test at delivery	14	—
Infection late in pregnancy or no prenatal care until late in pregnancy	—	20
Mother not tested	8	3
Laboratory error	2	—

*Numbers represent percentages of total cases in the studies.
Adapted from Gutman, L. T.: Congenital syphilis. *In* Mandell, G. L. (ed.): Atlas of Infectious Disease. Vol. 5. Sexually Transmitted Diseases. Philadelphia, Current Medicine, 1996.

influences the ultimate pattern of involvement. For example, the deposition of collagen around arteries of the spleen produces a typical onion-skin appearance. The periosteum and epiphyses are the most affected portions of bone, and syphilitic granulation tissue may interfere with bone formation. Pancreatitis with typical inflammation and fibrosis also is observed. The fetus or newborn shows diffuse extramedullary hematopoiesis in many tissues. The placenta of infants with congenital syphilis often is large, thick, and pale. Three histopathologic features commonly are seen: enlarged and hypercellular villi, proliferative fetal vascular changes, and both acute and chronic inflammation of the villi.[47, 126] Erythroblastosis involving the placenta has been noted more commonly in stillborn infants with congenital syphilis than in liveborn infants with or without syphilis.[126] Spirochetes may be identified in placental tissue by conventional staining, although they may be difficult to visualize. Nucleic acid amplification methods also have been used to identify the *T. pallidum* genome in involved placental specimens.[47] In addition, the umbilical cord may exhibit significant inflammation with abscess-like foci of necrosis located within the Wharton jelly and centered around the umbilical vessels, a condition termed necrotizing funisitis.[43, 126] Macroscopically, the umbilical cord resembles a "barber's pole" in that the edematous portions have a spiral striped zone of red and pale blue discoloration, interspersed with streaks of chalky white. Histochemical staining may demonstrate spirochetes within the wall of the umbilical vessels. Placental and umbilical cord histopathologic studies should be performed in every case of suspected syphilis.[126]

Pathogenesis and Immune Response

The pathogenesis of syphilis will not be understood until we can comprehend why on the one hand a vigorous host immune response to infection occurs but, on the other hand, the infection may persist for life in the presence of this response. In addition, previous infection does not confer resistance to reinfection. Information concerning host and bacterial interactions that may pertain to these questions is described briefly.

TREPONEMAL VIRULENCE-ASSOCIATED FACTORS

Virulent *T. pallidum* organisms attach to host cells during parasitism and are oriented by their proximal hook to the host cell surface. A ligand-receptor adherence mechanism involving the treponemal outer-membrane proteins appears to exist. Virulent strains attach to metabolically active mammalian cells, and treponemes are capable of multiplication only during attachment. Fetal and infant cells appear to support treponemal growth maximally, and capillary cells are the prime target of parasitism. Virulent treponemal strains produce hyaluronidase, which may facilitate the perivascular infiltration that is apparent by histopathologic study. These strains also may invade the ground substance that joins capillary endothelial cells.

Virulent *T. pallidum* is coated with fibronectin of host origin. This coating appears to protect the organism from antibody-mediated phagocytosis, allows the organism to adhere to the surface of host phagocytes with only limited ingestion of the organisms, may block complement-mediated lysis of the coated treponemes, and, finally, may allow the treponemes to additionally acquire physiologically active host proteins, such as ceruloplasmin and transferrin, on which they are dependent.[100]

HOST RESPONSE

Treponemes appear to persist in extracellular loci with little or no inflammatory response elicited. Polymorphonuclear leukocytes are known to ingest virulent treponemes, incorporate them into phagocytic vacuoles, and degranulate and digest *T. pallidum*. In addition, phagocytosis occurs relatively slowly and is facilitated by the presence of immune serum.[2] However, relatively large numbers of treponemes are needed to elicit this response, and small numbers may escape recognition.[87]

Alterations in host-cell–mediated immunity occur during the primary and secondary stages of syphilis. During the early stages of disease, all aspects of cell-mediated immunity, including responses to nonspecific T-cell mitogens, are suppressed. Blastogenesis to treponemal antigens is not demonstrable until late in secondary disease. Natural killer cell activity is increased in early primary syphilis and depressed in secondary and latent syphilis.[62] Some evidence supports the idea that lymphocytes from previously infected animals confer moderate protection to nonimmune animals. However, the extent to which these alterations in cellular function during infection affect the outcome or progression of disease remains uncertain.

During the initial infection with *T. pallidum,* humoral IgG and IgM antibodies are detectable by the time that the chancre appears. In primary syphilis, the main IgG subclass is IgG1, whereas in secondary syphilis, IgG1 and IgG3 predominate.[10] If the patient is treated adequately, IgM antibody declines during the next 1 to 2 years, but IgG antibody usually persists throughout the lifetime of the patient. The stages of syphilis evolve, in spite of the humoral antibody response.

Persons with untreated syphilis have a relative resistance to reinfection; consequently, the development of a chancre with reinfection is unusual and probably depends on the challenge inoculum. After re-exposure, increased humoral antibody levels may develop in untreated persons.

In persons who have been treated for syphilis, especially if treatment was given during the secondary or earlier stages, the protective effect of previous disease is minor, and active disease after reinfection is a common event. This effect applies to persons who maintain a reactive nontreponemal antibody test (Serofast), as well as to those who are sero-nonreactive. Patients who have been treated for congenital syphilis also may acquire symptomatic disease.[40, 98] In summary, although active or previous syphilis modifies the response of the patient to subsequent reinfection, protection is only relative and is unreliable.

Secondary syphilis and congenital infection may be accompanied by nephrotic syndrome. The nephrosis characteristically responds rapidly to penicillin, and light microscopy reveals membranous glomerulonephritis with glomerular mesangial cell proliferation. The subendothelial basement membrane deposits contain IgG and C3 or only globulin. Acute syphilitic glomerulonephritis appears to be an immune complex disease.[15, 45, 64] In infants with congenital syphilis, analysis of circulating immune complexes by immunoblotting methods has demonstrated the presence of an 83-kd *T. pallidum* antigen.[34] Similar findings have been made with secondary syphilis.

Clinical Manifestations

The course of untreated syphilis characteristically progresses through three or four stages over a period of many years. Information on the natural history of untreated syphilis comes primarily from follow-up studies of almost

2000 untreated syphilitic patients who were seen initially between 1891 and 1910 in the clinic of Dr. Boeck. Subsequent studies of these patients by Dr. Bruusgaard and by other epidemiologists later provided the basis for most of our concepts of the consequences of this disease. A summary of some of these studies has been compiled by Clark and Danbolt.[26] Figure 150–1 depicts some of the characteristics of an untreated course of disease.

ACQUIRED SYPHILIS

Most recognized syphilitic disease in children is congenital. Acquired syphilis in prepubertal children seldom is reported and is assumed to resemble the clinical course of acquired syphilis in adulthood. Children with acquired syphilis should be assumed to have been infected through contact during sexual abuse, unless another method of transmission is identified. Although the acquisition of syphilis during sexual abuse seems to be a relatively uncommon event, one of the authors (L.T.G.) has treated two children who acquired syphilis through abuse; one had progressed to general paresis, and the other had concurrent primary and secondary disease. All patients with syphilis should be tested for HIV infection.[22]

The decision to screen for syphilis during the medical evaluation of a child who is suspected of having been abused sexually should be decided on an individual basis because the prevalence of sexually transmitted diseases (STDs) is low in these circumstances. Situations in which screening is recommended include the following: the perpetrator has an STD or is at high risk of having one, such as residing in a community or being in a social setting in which the prevalence of STDs is high; multiple perpetrators are involved; the child has another STD such as HIV infection or has physical signs of sexual abuse; STDs are present in siblings, other children, or adults in the household; the child is a postpubertal patient; and the patient or family requests such screening.[11, 69, 128, 129] A difficult aspect of follow-up is the requirement for repeat serologic assays in 3 to 6 months because the initial test may not detect incubating syphilis.

Primary Disease

The chancre of primary syphilis typically is a single lesion, nontender and firm, with a clean surface, raised border, and reddish color. It may be overlooked by women because it frequently is situated on the cervix or vaginal wall. Systemic signs or symptoms are absent, but the adjacent lymph nodes frequently are enlarged and nontender (see elsewhere[51] for depictions of children with acquired primary syphilis).

Secondary Disease

Two to 10 weeks after the primary lesions appear, the patient may experience secondary disease. Prominent findings include fever, sore throat, generalized lymphadenopathy, headache, and rash. Involvement of the palms and soles occurs commonly, in contradistinction to many other dermatologic conditions. On mucous membranes, the lesions may appear as white mucous patches. Condylomata lata occur around moist areas such as the anus and vagina. All secondary lesions of the skin and mucous membranes are highly infectious. Acquired syphilis in early childhood may have minimal dermal findings.[1]

Latent Disease

After the clinical signs of secondary disease resolve, the patient enters the stage of latent disease. Latent syphilis refers to infection in individuals who have reactive serologic tests for syphilis but no clinical manifestations. The first year after infection is considered early latent infection, and the subsequent period is late latent syphilis. Early latent syphilis originally was classified as being within 4 years of infection based on the time when mucocutaneous lesions may recur. Recent classification of early latent syphilis is based on the period of highest communicability, which is in the first year after infection. If the duration of syphilis infection cannot be determined, the disease is classified as syphilis of unknown duration; clinical management and treatment should be the same as for late latent infection. If therapy for syphilis initially is given during the latent stage, the patient is unlikely to show regression of nontreponemal antibody levels. Approximately 60 percent of untreated patients in the late latent stage continue to have an asymptomatic course, whereas symptoms of late or tertiary disease develop in 30 to 40 percent. Progression of disease from late latent to late symptomatic syphilis usually is prevented if appropriate antimicrobial therapy is given at this stage (see elsewhere[51] for depictions of children with acquired secondary syphilis).

Tertiary Disease

Three to 10 years after the last evidence of secondary disease, nonprogressive, localized lesions of the dermal elements or supporting structures of the body, called *gummata*, may develop. Because these lesions are relatively quiescent, the term benign tertiary syphilis often is used. Spirochetes are extremely sparse or absent. The gummatous reaction primarily is a pronounced immunologic reaction of the host.

Neurosyphilis

During the early stage of syphilis, approximately a third of all patients have involvement of the CNS. If untreated, late neurosyphilis develops in only half of these patients. The interval between primary disease and late neurosyphilis is usually more than 5 years. However, in several of the few children recognized to have acquired (versus congenital) late neurosyphilis, symptomatic disease has developed at a very early age. The disease possibly progresses more rapidly in children than in adults.

Late neurosyphilis may be asymptomatic or, if symptomatic, may occur in a variety of ways. Classic manifestations include paralytic dementia, tabes dorsalis, amyotrophic lateral sclerosis, meningovascular syphilis, seizures, optic atrophy, and gummatous changes of the cord. Neurosyphilis may resemble virtually any other neurologic disease.

Cardiovascular Syphilis

Approximately 10 to 40 years after having primary syphilis, signs of cardiovascular involvement may develop in untreated patients. Most commonly involved are the great vessels of the heart, where syphilitic aortitis and pulmonary arteritis develop. The inflammatory reaction also may cause stenosis, with resulting angina, myocardial insufficiency, and death.

SYPHILIS IN PREGNANCY

Pregnancy has no known effect on the clinical course of syphilis. Untreated syphilis, however, can affect the outcome of pregnancy profoundly and result in spontaneous abortion, stillbirth, nonimmune hydrops fetalis,[9, 16] premature delivery, perinatal death, and two characteristic syndromes of congenital disease, early and late congenital syphilis (see later).[50, 118] The outcome of untreated fetal infection is variable. Intrauterine death occurs in an estimated 25 percent of infections, with abortion usually taking place after the first trimester. Perinatal death may occur in another 25 to 30 percent of untreated infected babies.[90] In a study of the perinatal outcome of congenital syphilis, the infant fatality rate was 464 per 1000 infected births. Of the fatalities, 27 percent were neonatal deaths and 73 percent were stillbirths.[112] Currently, the majority of infected infants, if not hydropic at birth, will survive the neonatal period, most likely because of early identification and treatment of infected infants, as well as improved neonatal care.

The investigations of Taber and Huber[136] illustrate the importance of recognition and appropriate treatment of syphilis in pregnant women. In this study, syphilis was not diagnosed in 22 women with the disease during pregnancy, and therefore, they did not receive prenatal therapy. Eleven infants were monitored without initial therapy. At delivery, all were clinically asymptomatic, four had a reactive Venereal Disease Research Laboratory (VDRL) test, five had a nonreactive VDRL test, and two were not tested. All these infants were readmitted with obvious disease and multisystem involvement, three with proven spirochetal hepatitis, two with nephrotic syndrome, and three with CNS findings. This experience again emphasizes the importance of transmission of infection late in gestation, which leads to the delivery of infants who are well clinically but whose disease emerges in the weeks after delivery if untreated.[35]

CONGENITAL SYPHILIS

At the onset of congenital syphilis, *T. pallidum* is liberated directly into the circulation of the fetus, with subsequent development of spirochetemia and widespread dissemination. The clinical, laboratory, and radiographic abnormalities of congenital syphilis are a consequence of active infection with *T. pallidum* and the resultant inflammatory response induced in various body organs and tissues. The severity of these manifestations is extremely variable and can range from overwhelming involvement of multiple organs and body systems, as seen in fetal hydrops, to only laboratory or radiographic abnormalities. Most infants born to mothers with untreated syphilis appear completely normal at birth and have no clinical or laboratory evidence of infection. Manifestations of disease may develop in these infants several months to years later if left untreated.[25] The signs and symptoms of congenital syphilis are divided arbitrarily into early manifestations, which appear in the first 2 years of life, and late manifestations, which emerge anytime thereafter, usually near puberty.

Early Congenital Syphilis

The abnormal physical and laboratory findings in early congenital syphilis are varied and unpredictable.[105] Table 150–5 lists the major physical and laboratory findings from 310 reported cases of early congenital syphilis. These rates undoubtedly are minimal rates for each finding. The onset is between birth and approximately 3 months of age, with most cases occurring within the first 5 weeks of life.

TABLE 150–5 ■ FINDINGS IN 310 CASES OF EARLY CONGENITAL SYPHILIS

Findings	Number of Patients
Hepatomegaly	100
Skeletal abnormalities	91
Birth weight <2500 g	51
Skin lesions	45
Hyperbilirubinemia	40
Pneumonia	51
Splenomegaly	56
Severe anemia, hydrops, edema	50
Snuffles, nasal discharge	27
Painful limbs	22
Pancreatitis	14
Cerebrospinal fluid abnormalities	21
Nephritis	11
Failure to thrive	10
Testicular mass	1
Chorioretinitis	1
Hypoglobulinemia	1

Data from references 16, 30, 64, 71, 96, 112, 136, 137.

SKELETAL SYSTEM. Bone involvement, the most common manifestation of congenital syphilis, occurs in 60 to 80 percent of infants with clinical signs of syphilis. In addition, it may be the only abnormality seen in infants born to mothers with untreated syphilis. Because of their frequency and early appearance, the roentgenographic changes in the bones, termed osteochondritis and periostitis, are of diagnostic value.[30] The femur and humerus are involved most often. Roentgenographically, accumulating calcified matrix is seen at the epiphyseal margin, which may be smooth or serrated. The serrated appearance is known as the Wegner sign and represents points of calcified cartilage along the nutrient cartilage canal. A zone of rarefaction at the metaphysis may be seen that represents syphilitic granulation tissue containing a few scattered calcified remnants and a mass of connective tissue containing areas of perivascular infiltration of small round cells. Irregular areas of increased density and rarefaction produce the moth-eaten appearance of the roentgenogram. The demineralization and osseous destruction of the upper medial tibial metaphysis is called the Wimberger sign. Previously thought to be specific for syphilis, the Wimberger sign also may occur in osteomyelitis and hyperparathyroidism. Epiphyseal separation may occur as a result of a fracture of the brittle layer of calcified cartilage. Irregular periosteal thickening also is a common occurrence. The changes usually are present at birth but may appear in the first few weeks of life. The bone changes are self-limited and generally heal within the first 6 months, even in the absence of specific therapy. They may be painful lesions, and pain on motion often leads an affected infant to appear to have limb paralysis, termed the "pseudoparalysis of Parrot."

RHINITIS. The development of rhinitis, coryza, or snuffles is likely to mark the onset of congenital syphilis. Usually, they appear in the first week of life and seldom later than the third month. The snuffles are more severe and persist longer than the common cold does, often are bloody, and frequently are associated with laryngitis. Secondary bacterial superinfection may result in a purulent appearance. The nasal discharge is teeming with spirochetes and should be examined by darkfield microscopy to confirm its diagnosis.

RASH. The syphilitic rash usually appears 1 to 2 weeks after the rhinitis. The typical eruption is maculopapular and consists of small spots that are dark red-copper. If the rash is present at birth, it often is disseminated widely and bullous and is called pemphigus syphiliticus. It is most severe on the hands and feet. The bullous fluid contains many spirochetes. The rash forms slowly, taking 1 to 3 weeks, and is followed by desquamation and crusting. As the rash fades, the lesions become coppery or dusky red, and the pigmentation may persist (see elsewhere[51] for depictions of a variety of cutaneous manifestations of early congenital syphilis).

FISSURES AND MUCOUS PATCHES. Fissures and mucous patches are not seen often but are highly characteristic features of congenital syphilis. The fissures develop about the lips, nares, and anus. They bleed readily and heal with scarring. A cluster of scars radiating around the mouth is termed *rhagades* and is a characteristic of late congenital syphilis. Mucous patches may be found on any of the mucous membranes, especially in the mouth and genitalia. Condylomata are raised, moist lesions appearing on areas of the skin where moisture or friction are present. They are highly infectious because they contain many spirochetes.

HEMATOLOGIC FINDINGS. Anemia, thrombocytopenia, hemolytic processes, and both leukopenia and leukocytosis are characteristic of congenital syphilis. The hemolytic process is Coombs test–negative and often accompanied by cryoglobulinemia, immune complex formation, and macroglobulinemia. The hemolysis, like the liver disease, is refractory to therapy and may persist for weeks. Paroxysmal nocturnal hemoglobinuria is a late manifestation of congenital syphilis.

CENTRAL NERVOUS SYSTEM INVOLVEMENT. In the era before penicillin therapy, findings of meningovascular disease developed in approximately 15 percent of infants with congenital syphilis. These findings included meningitis, meningeal irritation, bulging fontanelle, cranial nerve palsies, seizures, and hydrocephalus.[58] In addition, involvement of the pituitary gland in congenital syphilis occurs relatively commonly and is noted in approximately 40 percent of autopsy cases[96]; such involvement consists of interstitial inflammation and fibrosis with gumma formation in the anterior lobe. Clinical disease in affected infants is manifested by persistent hypoglycemia and diabetes insipidus.[31, 94]

Most infants infected with *T. pallidum,* however, are completely asymptomatic, and CNS involvement is inferred from cerebrospinal fluid (CSF) abnormalities such as reactivity on a VDRL test, pleocytosis, and elevated protein content. Because of the wide range of normal values for CSF protein, red blood cells, and white blood cells in the neonatal period, defining the proportion of infants with congenital syphilis who have abnormalities in these laboratory values has been difficult. Current consensus identifies an abnormal CSF white blood cell count in infants being evaluated for possible congenital syphilis as more than 25 cells/mm^3 and protein as greater than 150 mg/dL (>170 mg/dL if infant is premature). A reactive CSF VDRL test is considered to be specific for neurosyphilis in older children and adults. However, in neonates, the significance of a reactive CSF VDRL test is suspect because maternal nontreponemal IgG antibodies can pass from maternal to fetal and neonatal serum and then diffuse into the CSF. Moreover, children may fail to have a reactive VDRL test on initial examination but still be subject to the later signs of neurosyphilis.

With the use of rabbit infectivity testing, which involves inoculation of CSF into rabbits to determine the presence of the spirochete in the CSF specimen, Michelow and coworkers[85] found that CNS invasion with *T. pallidum* occurs in 41 percent of infants who have clinical, laboratory, or radiographic abnormalities consistent with congenital syphilis. None of these infants had clinical signs of neurologic disease. When compared with isolation of spirochetes in CSF by rabbit inoculation, the sensitivity and specificity of a reactive VDRL test, elevated white blood cell count, and elevated protein in CSF were 54 and 90 percent, 38 and 88 percent, and 56 and 78 percent, respectively. These investigators also documented CNS infection in three infants who had normal CSF studies. With current methodologies, the best indicator of CNS infection in neonates is an abnormal evaluation consisting of an abnormal physical examination, anemia, thrombocytopenia, CSF abnormalities, and abnormal bone radiographs. A normal evaluation renders CNS infection extremely uncommon.

PNEUMONIA. Syphilitic pneumonia has been a common finding in congenital syphilis, particularly in developing countries. The classic roentgenographic appearance is one of complete opacification of both lung fields and is termed "pneumonia alba." More commonly today, a fluffy, diffuse infiltrate involving all lung areas is seen on chest radiographs. At autopsy, pneumonia alba consists of a focal obliterative fibrosis with scarring and thickening of the alveolar walls and loss of alveolar spaces. Follow-up evaluation of children who have recovered from congenital syphilis has shown that at least 10 percent may have chronic pulmonary disease, particularly if they were premature and required mechanical ventilation.

HEPATOSPLENOMEGALY. Hepatomegaly is the most common clinical sign in congenital syphilis. Its occurrence in the fetus has been documented by ultrasonography, and it may be a marker of maternal treatment during pregnancy but inadequate treatment of the fetal infection.[55] Hepatosplenomegaly often is caused by extramedullary hematopoiesis. Hepatomegaly may occur in the absence of splenomegaly, but unlike congenital cytomegalovirus infection, the reverse does not occur. Neonatal syphilitic hepatitis is associated with visible spirochetes in biopsy specimens of liver tissue and with jaundice and cholestasis. Aspartate aminotransferase, alkaline phosphatase, and alanine aminotransferase values often are elevated, and direct hyperbilirubinemia is a common finding. The prothrombin time may be delayed. The liver disease often resolves slowly, even after apparently adequate therapy. Liver disease may be exacerbated by penicillin therapy before improving.[124]

ECTODERMAL CHANGES. Ectodermal changes in syphilitic infants include suppuration and exfoliation of the nails, loss of hair and eyebrows, choroiditis, and iritis.

OTHER FINDINGS. Other clinical manifestations of congenital syphilis are nonimmune fetal hydrops, possibly intrauterine growth restriction, generalized lymphadenopathy, fever, failure to thrive, nephrotic syndrome, and myocarditis.[17] Eye involvement has been manifested as chorioretinitis, cataract, glaucoma, and chancre of the eyelid. Gastrointestinal manifestations include rectal bleeding caused by syphilitic ileitis, necrotizing enterocolitis, malabsorption secondary to fibrosis of the gastrointestinal tract, and fetal bowel dilatation as seen on antenatal ultrasonography.[112] Some children with symptomatic congenital syphilis also may have sepsis caused by other bacteria, including *Escherichia coli,* group B streptococci, and *Yersinia* spp.

Neonates and infants with congenital syphilis may resemble babies with other illnesses peculiar to newborns, including toxoplasmosis, rubella, cytomegalovirus infection, herpes simplex virus infection, "sepsis" of the newborn, blood group incompatibilities, battered child syndrome, "periostitis" of prematurity, neonatal hepatitis, and osteomyelitis.

Late Congenital Syphilis

The late manifestations or stigmata of congenital syphilis are the result of scarring from the early systemic disease or reactions to persistent inflammation. Such manifestations include involvement of the teeth, bones, eyes, and eighth nerve; gummata in the viscera, skin, or mucous membranes; and neurosyphilis[42] (Table 150–6). Late manifestations of infection develop in approximately 40 percent of surviving

TABLE 150–6 ■ STIGMATA OF LATE CONGENITAL SYPHILIS*

Stigmata	Percentage of Total Patients
Frontal boss of Parrot	87
Short maxilla	84
High palatal arch	76
Hutchinson triad	75
Hutchinson teeth	63
Interstitial keratitis	9
Eighth nerve deafness	3
Saddle nose	73
Mulberry molars	65
Higouménaki sign	39
Relative protuberance of the mandible	26
Rhagades	7
Saber shin	4
Scaphoid scapulae	0.7
Clutton joint	0.3

*An analysis of 271 patients.
Adapted from Fiumara, N. J., and Lessell, S.: Manifestations of late congenital syphilis. Arch. Dermatol. *102*:78–83, 1970. Copyright 1970, American Medical Association.

and untreated, infected infants, as reported in the early literature. Some of these changes can be prevented by treatment of the mother during pregnancy or treatment of the infant while younger than 3 months. In contrast, treatment of 15 children at 4 months of age or later resulted in 7 with dental changes.[102] Other stigmata (e.g., keratitis, saber shins) may occur or progress despite appropriate therapy in the infant. Nonspecific sequelae of congenital syphilis have not been described well because follow-up studies of children with congenital syphilis are minimal. However, the experience of one of the authors (P.J.S.) has been that in general, infants in whom congenital syphilis is diagnosed and who are treated appropriately in the neonatal period do well, at least through early childhood. We have every reason to be hopeful and optimistic with the families of these children, even if they are symptomatic and have CNS involvement at diagnosis.

DENTITION. Characteristic changes are found in the permanent upper central incisors, which demonstrate a notched appearance of the biting edges; radiographic study leads to the diagnosis, even while deciduous teeth are in place. Such dentition is termed Hutchinson teeth, which are also small and hypoplastic and, therefore, widely spaced with abnormal enamelization. If the first molars have maldeveloped cusps, the finding is called mulberry or moon molars.

INTERSTITIAL KERATITIS. Interstitial keratitis is the most common late lesion. It may develop in a patient at any age between 4 and 30 years or later, but it characteristically appears when the patient is close to puberty. A ground-glass appearance of the cornea may be noted, along with vascularization of the adjacent sclera. These changes become bilateral and usually lead to blindness. It has been seen in adolescent patients despite previous and appropriate administration of penicillin therapy during infancy. At the time of its occurrence, keratitis is not affected by penicillin therapy, but it may respond transiently to corticosteroid treatment.

CENTRAL NERVOUS SYSTEM. The same manifestations of neurosyphilis seen in acquired syphilis may occur in congenital syphilis. Paresis develops more frequently and tabes dorsalis less frequently in the congenital form than in the acquired form of the disease. Cranial nerve palsies and optic atrophy are prominent signs.

EIGHTH NERVE DEAFNESS. Hearing loss usually is sudden and appears when the patient is approximately 8 to 10 years of age. It often accompanies interstitial keratitis. The constellation of eighth nerve deafness, interstitial keratitis, and Hutchinson teeth is called the Hutchinson triad. The hearing loss generally involves the higher frequencies, and normal conversational tones become affected later. It may respond to long-term corticosteroid treatment.

BONE AND JOINT CHANGES. Bone changes include sclerosing lesions, saber shin, and frontal bossing, which are sequelae of periostitis involving the frontal bone and tibia. Periosteal reaction of the sternoclavicular portion of the clavicle may lead to the Higouménaki sign. The gummatous or destructive lesions include saddle nose deformity, which occurs as a sequelae of rhinitis. Perforation of the hard palate is almost pathognomonic of congenital syphilis. Clutton joints are uncommon findings and represent painless arthritis of the knees and, rarely, other joints.

CUTANEOUS LESIONS. Rhagades represent scars resulting from persistent rhinitis during infancy and rarely are seen today.

Diagnosis

Efforts to diagnose infectious syphilis suffer from lack of a method to culture the organism on laboratory media. Methods used in the diagnosis of syphilis include (1) direct visualization of the organism in infected fluids or lesions by darkfield microscopy or fluorescent antibody technique, (2) demonstration of the organism by special stains on histopathologic examination of tissue,[53, 110] (3) animal inoculation (rabbit infectivity test), (4) demonstration of serologic reactions typical of syphilis, and (5) detection of *T. pallidum* DNA in a clinical specimen.[18]

The rabbit infectivity test is the current gold standard for identification of viable *T. pallidum* in clinical specimens and has a sensitivity of less than 10 organisms.[77, 79] It involves intratesticular inoculation of the specimen into a rabbit, demonstration of seroconversion and orchitis, and subsequent visualization of motile spirochetes by darkfield microscopy in testicular tissue. The rabbit infectivity test, however, is performed only in research laboratories and may take several months for identification of the organism. Recently, *T. pallidum* DNA has been detected by polymerase chain reaction (PCR) in such body fluids as amniotic fluid and infant blood, CSF, and endotracheal aspirates.[49, 85] PCR remains a research tool; it is not yet available commercially.

In the clinical setting, the diagnosis of syphilis is made by visualization of the spirochete by darkfield microscopy or special staining and serology. The diagnosis may be made by darkfield microscopy in patients with a primary syphilis lesion (chancre), as well as in those with active secondary lesions. Because this diagnosis depends on direct visualization of motile spirochetes, the organisms must be active and viable. Previous use of many antibiotics rapidly destroys the motility of the organisms, as do many topical disinfectants. Serous fluid from the base of the lesion should be collected for darkfield examination. Syphilitic lesions of the mouth may harbor indigenous treponemes whose morphologic similarity to pathogenic species can confuse the interpretation of findings. Direct darkfield examination is particularly helpful, however, in making a diagnosis early in the disease, before the development of seroreactivity. If a darkfield microscope is unavailable, a direct fluorescent antibody stain for *T. pallidum* may be used.[16] Exudate is collected in capillary tubes or slides and stained with specific antibody.

TABLE 150–7 ■ STANDARD SEROLOGIC TESTS FOR SYPHILIS

			Percent Reactivity during		
		Test	Primary Stage	Secondary Stage	Tertiary Stage
Nontreponemal	Extracts of tissue (cardiolipin-lecithin-cholesterol)	VDRL	78	95	71
		RPR	86	98	73
Treponemal	*Treponema pallidum*	MHA-TP*	76	100	94
		FTA-ABS	84	100	97

*MHA-TP has been replaced with the *T. pallidum* particle agglutination (TP-PA) test.
FTA-ABS, fluorescent treponemal antibody absorption; MHA-TP, microhemagglutination assay—*T. pallidum*; RPR, rapid plasma reagin; VDRL, Venereal Disease Research Laboratory.

Amniotic fluid may be examined for the presence of spirochetes by darkfield microscopy or fluorescent antitreponemal staining; the finding of spirochetes may be a marker for more severe fetal disease.[48, 141] On a practical basis, however, the diagnosis is made by serologic methods.[74, 143]

SEROLOGIC TESTS

The two types of serologic tests for syphilis are nontreponemal antibody tests and treponemal antibody tests (Table 150–7). Although the latter tests indicate the presence of a treponemal infection, they cross-react with the antigen of other treponemal diseases, such as those causing yaws and pinta. Therefore, no test is specific for syphilis, and no test is completely sensitive. Efforts to produce a more sensitive and more specific test are continuing. A promising approach is the use of recombinant clones expressing immunogenic proteins of *T. pallidum* to investigate pathogen-specific antigens.[60] Some of these products are being investigated for use as diagnostic material.[119]

NONTREPONEMAL TESTS. The original test for syphilis, as described by Wassermann, used syphilitic tissue as complement-fixing antigen to detect the presence of antibody (reagin) induced by *T. pallidum*. Extracts of other normal tissue, such as beef heart, had similar properties, and purification and standardization of these materials led to the use of a preparation containing cardiolipin and lecithin in cholesterol as antigen.

Two tests currently using cardiolipin, lecithin, and cholesterol are the VDRL and rapid plasma reagin (RPR) tests. These tests measure mostly IgG but also IgM antibodies nondiscriminatively. The tests provide similar clinical information and have similar advantages. The RPR titer is often one to two dilutions higher than that obtained with the VDRL test, so caution must be exercised when making clinical decisions on the basis of results obtained from these two tests performed on the same patient. Both are inexpensive to perform and demonstrate rising and falling antibody titers that often correlate with the adequacy of therapy and the clinical status of the patient. A fourfold increase in RPR or VDRL titer is indicative of active disease, whereas a fourfold decrease suggests adequate therapy. Disadvantages include a relatively high proportion of biologic acute and chronic false-positive reactions and an increasing proportion of false-negative reactions in the later stages of untreated syphilis. The main technical difficulty is a negative reaction caused by the prozone phenomenon. It occurs in 1 to 2 percent of individuals, usually with secondary syphilis, and is due to the presence of an excess amount of reagin antibody in the patient's undiluted serum that prevents flocculation. Diluting the serum sample before testing overcomes this inhibition and results in a positive reaction. Because the RPR test generally is more sensitive than is the VDRL test, it is preferred for the screening of pregnant women. The VDRL test, however, is recommended for use on CSF.

The RPR test is used commonly to screen pregnant women for possible infection with *T. pallidum*. Transplacental passage of IgG antibodies to the infant means that mothers with positive RPR tests usually will transmit these antibodies to their infants. A review of the relationship of maternal to newborn VDRL tests was included in the study by Taber and Huber[136] of mothers in whom the disease was undiagnosed and untreated. Although 12 of 22 mothers had VDRL test results two to four times that of their babies, 6 of these women and their babies had nonreactive serology at the time of delivery. These and other data have shown that an infant seldom has a VDRL test of greater titer than that of its mother, even if the infant was incubating congenital syphilis.[134] Nonetheless, the finding of a fourfold-higher titer in infant serum than that seen in maternal serum when both sera are obtained at the same time is indicative of active infection in the infant. Even if the infant is asymptomatic, a 10-day course of penicillin therapy should be given.

TREPONEMAL TESTS. The most significant development of the past 3 decades in the serologic study of syphilis was the detection of treponemal antibody by fluorescein-labeled antihuman antibody. These tests are used to confirm the validity of a positive nontreponemal test and to diagnose late stages of syphilis. The tests are both sensitive and reliable.

Fluorescent treponemal antibody absorption (FTA-ABS) tests use lyophilized Nichols strain organisms as antigen and are tests that measure both IgG and IgM antibodies. Antigen is fixed to a slide, and the test serum is applied to allow reaction of antitreponemal antibody with antigen. The slide is layered with fluorescein isothiocyanate–labeled antihuman gamma-globulin, and the presence or absence of antibody is determined by fluorescent microscopy.

Test sera are pre-absorbed with sorbent to eliminate group-reactive antibody. Thus, the test is rendered relatively specific for disease with virulent treponemal species, usually *T. pallidum*. However, the FTA-ABS test is expensive and time consuming. Therefore, it is recommended not for general screening but for confirmation of positive nontreponemal tests and diagnosis of later stages of syphilis in which the results of nontreponemal tests may be negative.

Microhemagglutination tests and, specifically, the *T. pallidum* particle agglutination (TP-PA) test depend on passive hemagglutination of erythrocytes or latex particles that have been sensitized with Nichols strain *T. pallidum*. The test has been automated and is both easy to perform technically and inexpensive. The TP-PA test has largely replaced the FTA-ABS test as the most efficient specific test for detecting antibody to *T. pallidum*. It is as sensitive as is the FTA-ABS test, except for primary syphilis. Like the FTA-ABS test, it is unlikely to revert to a nonreactive state after treatment of the patient, unless treatment is given very early.

IgM TESTS. In the diagnosis of congenital syphilis, a means of differentiating between passive transplacental transfer of maternal antibody to the fetus and production of endogenous antitreponemal antibody by the fetus would be most helpful. Because antibodies of the IgM class do not cross the placenta, detection of IgM antibody in fetal or neonatal serum would indicate antibody production by the fetus because of active fetal infection. Unfortunately, no IgM assay that is commercially available is sufficiently sensitive and specific to recommend for routine use in the evaluation of infants born to mothers with syphilis. The fluorescent treponemal antibody test that measures IgM antitreponemal antibodies, the IgM FTA-ABS test, has been associated with false-positive and false-negative results.[4, 65, 116] When the test was refined further by use of the IgM fraction of neonatal serum only, it had a sensitivity of 73 percent.[134] The test is also insensitive when the onset of disease is delayed. Occasional false-positive IgM FTA-ABS test results occur because of the presence of an IgM anti-IgG antibody, or rheumatoid factor. For these reasons, the CDC has recommended that the IgM FTA-ABS test be suspended for diagnostic testing of newborns, and the test is available only as a provisional test. Efforts to develop a sensitive and specific serologic test for congenital syphilis have led to the identification of antigenic components of *T. pallidum* that are epitopes for the immune response. A 34-kd membrane protein is a lipoprotein[135] and the target of IgM antibody formation in the sera of some congenitally infected infants.[33] The Captia Syphilis M test is an enzyme-linked immunosorbent assay that uses this treponemal protein; it is available commercially but showed a sensitivity of 88 percent in infants with clinical and laboratory findings of congenital syphilis.[72, 134]

Immunoblotting has been used to characterize the specific neonatal IgM antibody responses to *T. pallidum*. Specific IgM antibodies directed against *T. pallidum* antigens with apparent molecular masses of 72, 47, 45, 42, 37, 17, and 15 kd have been detected in the sera of fetuses[55] and infants with clinical findings of congenital syphilis and in 20 to 40 percent of asymptomatic infants born to mothers with untreated syphilis.[33, 75, 85, 117, 119, 122] IgM reactivity against the 47-kd antigen, a membrane lipoprotein of the organism, has been the most consistent finding. Similar reactivities also have been seen in the CSF of infants with congenital syphilis.[75, 121] A recent study demonstrated that a reactive serum IgM immunoblot identified all 17 infants in whom spirochetes were detected in CSF by rabbit infectivity testing.[85] Effort to develop rapid diagnostic tests based on these findings is in progress.[70] In addition, immunoblotting has been used to detect similar IgA reactivities in infants with congenital syphilis.[122]

POLYMERASE CHAIN REACTION. PCR has been used on neonatal blood and CSF for the diagnosis of congenital syphilis.[49, 85, 119] When compared with isolation of the organism by rabbit infectivity testing, the sensitivity and specificity of PCR on CSF was 65 to 71 percent and 97 to 100 percent, respectively.[85, 119] In 17 infants who had spirochetes detected in CSF by rabbit inoculation, a blood PCR test was the best predictor of CNS infection with *T. pallidum*.[85] This finding further supports the concept that spirochetes gain access to the CNS by a hematogenous route.

FALSE-POSITIVE REACTIONS

All the available serologic tests for syphilis produce occasional reactive results in patients for whom no other evidence of syphilitic infection is present. These reactions usually are called biologic false-positive (BFP) and are distinct from positive reactions that occur because of technical error. Most BFP reactions occur with nontreponemal tests, and approximately 1 percent of normal adults will have a BFP reaction by nontreponemal antigen tests. These reactions probably are not more common findings in pregnant women than in the general population. Reaginic antibody is reactive with at least 200 antigens other than those of *T. pallidum*, and although the specific stimulus for this antibody in syphilis and other diseases is unknown, it may represent antibody to cellular lipoidal antigens of the host that are liberated during various diseases. For clinical purposes, BFP reactions may be classified as acute, in which the reactivity resolves within 6 months, or chronic, in which reactivity is persistent.

ACUTE BIOLOGIC FALSE-POSITIVE REACTIONS. Most BFP reactions are detected by nontreponemal tests and occur in patients with other acute illnesses, especially pneumonia, hepatitis, and viral exanthematous disease, or after vaccinations. The prognosis for the patient's health is not affected by the finding. The titer of antibody is usually low, less than 1:8, and in most instances the FTS-ABS test is nonreactive. Approximately two thirds of patients with BFP reactions have acute reactions, and reactivity subsides in 6 months or less.

CHRONIC BIOLOGIC FALSE-POSITIVE REACTIONS. Many patients with chronic BFP reactions have or acquire systemic disease. Drug addiction, chronic hepatitis, old age, leprosy, and collagen vascular disease, especially systemic lupus erythematosus, are associated highly with chronic BFP reactions. There may be a familial predisposition to this finding. The antibody detected by the VDRL test in chronic BFP reactions is predominantly IgM, whereas in syphilis, it is mainly IgG. Patients with chronic BFP reactions and systemic lupus erythematosus frequently also have a reactive FTA-ABS test.[73] The triosephosphate isomerase test may be helpful in the differential diagnosis in these instances. A particularly concerning finding has been that a relative increase in both acute and chronic BFP reactions appears to exist in women infected with HIV.[6]

EVALUATION AND DIAGNOSIS OF EARLY CONGENITAL SYPHILIS

The diagnosis of congenital syphilis is established by the observation of spirochetes in body fluids or tissue and is suggested by the results of serologic tests, physical examination, laboratory tests (including CSF examination), and radiographs of long bones. Pathologic examination of the placenta or umbilical cord by specific fluorescent antitreponemal antibody staining is recommended.[47, 104] The decision to evaluate and ultimately treat an infant for congenital syphilis is based on clinical, serologic, and epidemiologic considerations. The evaluation includes an assessment of the mother for general risk factors for increased rates of syphilis (Table 150–8), followed by an evaluation of the mother's current known serologic status (Table 150–9). If the mother

TABLE 150–8 ■ GENERAL MATERNAL RISK FACTORS ASSOCIATED WITH INCREASED RATES OF EARLY SYPHILIS IN PREGNANCY

Infection with HIV
Adolescent or unmarried status
History of sexually transmitted disease
Substance abuse, especially cocaine
Inadequate or absent prenatal care
Prostitution or promiscuity
Localized populations or geographic areas
Treatment of gonorrhea with ciprofloxacin or spectinomycin
Poor communication among medical personnel regarding maternal/infant status

Data from references 32, 68, 99, 111, 140.

has been treated, the clinician must assess the adequacy of therapy.

If the mother's serologic assays have been positive, the infant must be assessed for clinically apparent disease. Both the nontreponemal (RPR) and treponemal (TP-PA) tests measure IgG antibody and, therefore, do not distinguish disease of the infant from maternally derived antibody. Many infants are born to women who have had syphilis in the past, received therapy, and remained seroreactive. Their infants also will be seroreactive. Ensuring that the infant does not have congenital disease in the immediate newborn period may not be possible.

An approach to the evaluation of infants born to mothers with reactive serologic tests for syphilis is presented in Figure 150–2 and Table 150–10. Testing of all pregnant women with syphilis for co-infection with HIV is recommended strongly, even though infants born to co-infected mothers do not require any different evaluation for syphilis.[22] All infants born to mothers with reactive serologic tests for syphilis should have a serum quantitative nontreponemal test performed and a thorough physical examination that focuses on finding evidence of congenital syphilis. The nontreponemal test that is performed on the infant should be the same test that was performed on the mother to be able to compare serologic titers. Though uncommon, a

TABLE 150–9 ■ COMPONENTS OF THE EPIDEMIOLOGIC EVALUATION OF AN INFANT'S MOTHER FOR POSSIBLE SYPHILIS THAT WILL AID IN EVALUATION AND TREATMENT OF THE INFANT

Evaluate the mother for a previous history of syphilis or major risk factors for syphilis (see Table 150–8)
If the mother received therapy for syphilis, evaluate the course of therapy for adequacy in the treatment of congenital syphilis (see Table 150–2)
Evaluate the current maternal status with a nontreponemal test (e.g., Venereal Disease Research Laboratory, rapid plasma reagin) and, if reactive, a treponemal test (e.g., fluorescent treponemal antibody absorption, *Treponema pallidum* particle agglutination test)
If the mother is identified clinically or through contact tracing as having early syphilis during the 3 mo after delivery, re-evaluate the infant and consider therapy at that time
Note that higher maternal titers to nontreponemal tests are associated with failure of maternal therapy to prevent congenital disease[84]
Note that an unknown duration of maternal syphilis is associated with failure of maternal therapy to prevent congenital disease[84]

serum quantitative nontreponemal titer that is fourfold or greater than the corresponding maternal titer is diagnostic of congenital syphilis; when it has occurred, one of the authors (P.J.S.) has isolated spirochetes from the blood or CSF of all infants. The CDC recommends that the infant's serologic test be performed on serum and not umbilical cord blood because false-positive test results have been reported with the use of umbilical cord blood as a result of contamination of the specimen with maternal blood and Wharton jelly. Some clinicians, however, continue to use umbilical cord blood because it is readily available and easily collected; appropriate care should be exercised during its collection to minimize contamination with maternal blood.[23] In addition, false-negative test results may occur when the maternal titer is of low dilution; this event argues for maternal screening rather than screening of infant serum.

Infants who have an abnormal physical examination that is consistent with congenital syphilis, a serum quantitative nontreponemal serologic titer that is fourfold or greater than the mother's, or a positive darkfield or fluorescent antibody test of body fluid should have a complete blood cell count (CBC) and platelet count performed, as well as CSF examination for cell count, protein content, and VDRL test. Other tests such as bone and chest roentgenograms, liver function tests, cranial ultrasound, ophthalmologic examination, and auditory brain stem response should be performed as clinically indicated. These infants are considered to have *proved or highly probable disease*; spirochetemia with invasion of the CNS occurs in approximately 40 to 50 percent of these infants.[85] Although these infants must receive a full course of penicillin therapy, which will treat possible neurosyphilis, detection of CNS abnormalities at the initial evaluation is beneficial for follow-up purposes. Nonetheless, the diagnosis of congenital neurosyphilis is difficult to establish (see "Clinical Manifestations"). The presence of red blood cells in the CSF as a result of traumatic lumbar puncture can produce a false-positive serologic reaction. Examination of the CSF for *T. pallidum* DNA by PCR may prove more useful for the diagnosis of congenital neurosyphilis.[49, 85, 119]

Infants who have a normal physical examination and a serum quantitative nontreponemal test that is less than fourfold the maternal titer require further evaluation and treatment that depend on the maternal treatment history and stage of infection (see Fig. 150–2 and Table 150–10). Whether a complete evaluation (lumbar puncture, long bone radiographs, and CBC and platelet count) should be performed on the infant depends on the maternal treatment history and planned treatment of the infant (see "Treatment"). If the mother did not receive any previous syphilis treatment or the treatment was inadequate, such evaluation must be performed and be completely normal if a single intramuscular dose of benzathine penicillin G therapy is administered. Though preferred to help establish a diagnosis of congenital syphilis, a complete evaluation is not necessary if a full 10-day course of parenteral penicillin is provided because such therapy would treat for the possibility of congenital infection.[13, 86] The need to perform a lumbar puncture has been questioned because the yield of abnormal findings from examination of CSF has been very low in some experiences and appreciable in others.[12, 39, 111] However, a primary benefit of performing CSF studies in infants who are receiving a 10-day parenteral course of aqueous or procaine penicillin therapy is identification of infants for whom follow-up of abnormal CSF results should be ensured. Likewise, long bone radiographs are abnormal in approximately 65 percent of infants with clinical findings of syphilis but only in a minority of asymptomatic infants. The finding of

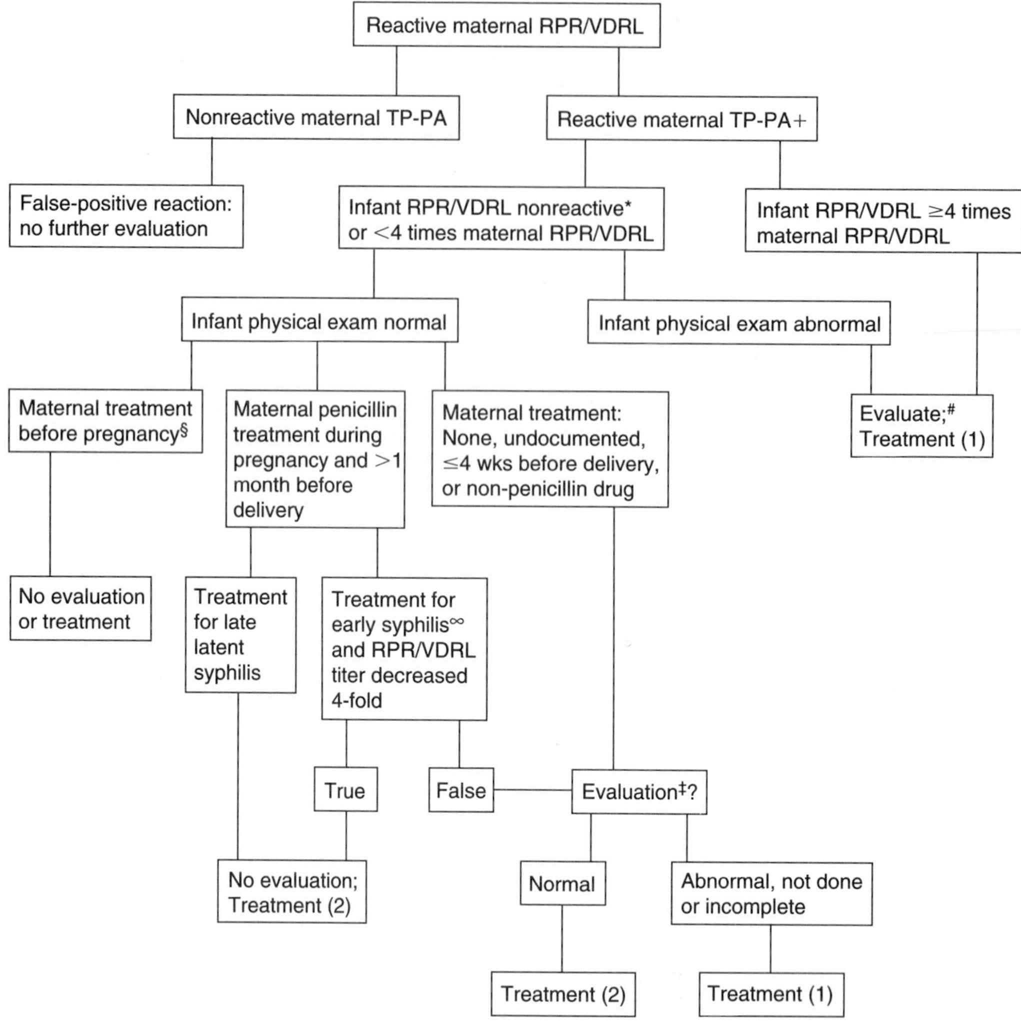

\+ Test for HIV-antibody. Infants of HIV-Ab ⊕ mothers do not require different evaluation or treatment.
* Infant's RPR may be nonreactive due to low maternal RPR titer or recent maternal infection. If the mother has untreated or inadequately treated syphilis and the infant's physical exam is normal, treat infant with a single IM injection of benzathine penicillin (50,000 U/kg). No further evaluation is needed.
\# Evaluation consists of CBC, platelet count; CSF examination for cell count, protein, and quantitative response; eye exam; chest X-ray; liver function tests; urine or meconium toxicology.
§ Women who maintain a VDRL titer ≤1:2 (RPR ≤1:4) beyond 1 year following successful treatment are considered serofast.
∞ Early syphilis: primary, secondary or early latent infection.
‡ CBC, platelet count; CSF examination for cell count, protein, and quantitative VDRL; long bone x-rays.

Treatment:
(1) Aqueous penicillin G 50,000 U/kg IV q 12 hr (≤1 wk of age), q 8 hr (>1 wk), or procaine penicillin G 50,000 U/kg IM single daily dose × 10 days.
(2) Benzathine pencillin G 50,000 U/kg IM × 1 dose.

FIGURE 150–2 ■ Algorithm for evaluation and treatment of infants born to mothers with reactive serologic tests for syphilis.

osteochondritis or periostitis in an infant born to a mother with reactive serologic tests for syphilis is indicative of congenital syphilis, and the infant requires a full course of penicillin therapy for highly probable disease. Such an infant, however, is likely to have CNS infection even if no clinical signs of neurosyphilis are present, and close clinical and serologic follow-up would be indicated.[85]

After the newborn period, children with syphilis should have a lumbar puncture performed for evaluation of CSF to detect asymptomatic neurosyphilis. In addition, birth and maternal records should be reviewed to assess whether such children have acquired or congenital syphilis.[25] Children with acquired syphilis should be evaluated for the possibility of sexual abuse.

Treatment

T. pallidum is extremely sensitive to penicillin, as defined by experimental animal work. The minimal inhibitory

TABLE 150–10 ■ TREATMENT GUIDELINES FOR CONGENITAL SYPHILIS

Scenario	Maternal Stage Treatment	Recommended Evaluation	Regimen
Infant with proven or highly probable disease: a. Abnormal physical examination *or* b. Abnormal evaluation* *or* c. Serum nontreponemal titer ≥4 × maternal titer *or* d. Visualization of spirochete in clinical specimen	Any or none	CSF analysis: VDRL, cell count, protein CBC and differential, platelet count As clinically indicated: long bone radiographs, liver function tests, cranial ultrasound, eye examination, hearing evaluation	**Aqueous penicillin** G, 50,000 U/kg IV q12h (≤1 wk), q8h (>1 wk, ≤4 wk), q6h (>4 wk) × 10 days *or* **Procaine penicillin G,** 50,000 U/kg IM × 10 days (≤4 wk)
Infant with *normal* physical examination and serum nontreponemal titer <4 x maternal titer	Any stage of infection *and* No treatment *or* Inadequate or undocumented treatment *or* Erythromycin or nonpenicillin treatment *or* Therapy ≤4 wk before delivery *or* Adequate therapy >1 mo before delivery, but maternal nontreponemal titers have not decreased fourfold after treatment of early syphilis (primary, secondary, early latent syphilis)	CSF analysis: VDRL, cell count, protein CBC and differential, platelet count Long bone radiographs a. If *all* normal: treatment A b. If *any* abnormal or not done†: Treatment B	Treatment A: Benzathine penicillin G‡, 50,000 U/kg IM Treatment B: Aqueous penicillin G, 50,000 U/Kg IV q12h (≤1 wk), q8h (>1 wk, ≤4 wk), q6h (>4 wk) × 10 days *or* Procaine penicillin G, 50,000 U/kg IM × 10 days (≤4 wk)
	Adequate therapy >1 mo before delivery and appropriate for stage of infection *or* Maternal nontreponemal titer decreased fourfold after treatment of early syphilis *or* Maternal nontreponemal titers remained stable and low for late syphilis *and* No evidence of reinfection or relapse	No evaluation	**Benzathine penicillin G** 50,000 U/kg IM × 1§
	Adequate therapy before pregnancy and stable nontreponemal titers (VDRL ≤1:2 or RPR ≤1:4) throughout pregnancy	No evaluation	No treatment‖
Congenital syphilis in child beyond 28 days of age	Any or none	CSF analysis: VDRL, cell count, protein CBC and differential, platelet count As clinically indicated: long bone radiographs, liver function tests, cranial ultrasound, eye examination, hearing evaluation	**Aqueous penicillin G** 50,000 U/kg IV q4–6h × 10 days *And* ?Benzathine penicillin G¶ 50,000 U/Kg

*CSF examination (VDRL test, cell count, protein), bone radiographs, CBC, platelets, umbilical cord or serum VDRL/RPR (same test as performed on maternal serum).
†If the infant's nontreponemal test is nonreactive, no evaluation is required, but the infant should receive treatment A.
‡Clinical and serologic follow-up must be certain.
§Some experts would not treat but provide close serologic follow-up.
‖Benzathine penicillin G, 50,000 U/kg IM × 1, if follow-up is uncertain.
¶Some experts prefer prolonged therapy by administration of a single dose of benzathine penicillin G after the 10-day course of intravenous aqueous penicillin G.
CBC, complete blood count; CSF, cerebrospinal fluid; RPR, rapid plasma reagin; VDRL, Venereal Disease Research Laboratory.
Adapted from Centers for Disease Control and Prevention: Sexually transmitted diseases treatment guidelines 2002. M.M.W.R. Recomm. Rep. *51*(RR-6):26–28, 2002; American Academy of Pediatrics: Syphilis. *In*, Pickering, L. K. (ed):. 2000 Red Book: Report of the Committee on Infectious Diseases. 25th ed. Elk Grove Village, IL. American Academy of Pediatrics, 2000, pp. 547–559.

concentration of penicillin is approximately 0.004 U (or 0.0025 μg/mL). No evidence exists of increasing resistance to penicillin by the spirochetes, but such confirmation would come only from recognition of therapeutic failures. Effective treatment of syphilis must maintain a minimal inhibitory concentration of 0.03 U/mL of penicillin in serum (or CSF) for 7 to 10 days. Therapy is designed to achieve and maintain several times the necessary inhibiting levels and to avoid penicillin-free intervals during therapy. Penicillin remains the drug of first choice because of its established efficacy and minimal toxicity.

ACQUIRED SYPHILIS

Early syphilis, specifically, primary, secondary, and early latent infection, is treated with benzathine penicillin G, 50,000 U/kg up to the adult dose of 2.4 million U intramuscularly in a single dose.[22] Late latent syphilis requires benzathine penicillin G, 150,000 U/kg up to the adult dose of 7.2 million U administered as 50,000 U/kg up to the adult dose of 2.4 million U weekly for 3 weeks. When the duration of infection is not known, the patient should be treated as those who have late latent disease.

All patients with syphilis should be tested for HIV infection at diagnosis, and if they have early syphilis, they should be retested 3 to 6 months later. Because neurosyphilis may be asymptomatic and can be defined accurately only by examination of CSF, the CDC recommends performance of a lumbar puncture in the following situations: (1) neurologic or ophthalmic signs or symptoms, (2) active tertiary syphilis, (3) treatment failure, and (4) HIV infection with late latent syphilis or syphilis of unknown duration.[22] Benzathine penicillin does not produce inhibitory CSF levels of penicillin reliably.[132] Therefore, shorter-acting penicillins must be used for neurosyphilis. In evaluating a patient for neurosyphilis, a CSF specimen without contamination by peripheral blood is needed.[61] The recommended therapy for neurosyphilis is aqueous crystalline penicillin G, 18 to 24 million U/day administered as 3 to 4 million U intravenously every 4 hours or a continuous infusion for 10 to 14 days. An alternative regimen consists of procaine penicillin, 2.4 million U intramuscularly once daily, plus probenecid, 500 mg orally four times per day, both for 10 to 14 days. Because these regimens are shorter than that used for late latent syphilis, some experts recommend the additional administration of benzathine penicillin G, 2.4 million U intramuscularly once per week for up to 3 weeks, after completion of the 10- to 14-day course. Older children with definite acquired syphilis and a normal neurologic and CSF examination may be treated with benzathine penicillin G, 50,000 U/kg intramuscularly to a maximal dose of 2.4 million U. Children with neurosyphilis should receive aqueous penicillin G, 200,000 to 300,000 U/kg/day intravenously administered as 50,000 U/kg every 4 to 6 hours for 10 to 14 days. Similar to adults, an additional dose of benzathine penicillin G, 50,000 U/kg intramuscularly, may be given after the 10 to 14-day intravenous penicillin treatment. Evaluation and treatment of early syphilis in HIV-infected individuals are the same as for HIV-uninfected persons.[114] HIV-infected individuals who have late latent syphilis or syphilis of unknown duration should have their CSF examined for evidence of neurosyphilis before treatment; further management and treatment are dependent on the CSF findings. Close serologic follow-up of HIV-infected persons is mandatory to detect treatment failure and the need for CSF examination and re-treatment.

Data to support the use of alternatives to penicillin for the treatment of syphilis are limited. Any history of penicillin allergy should be documented clearly, and whenever possible, patients should receive skin testing, desensitization, and therapy with penicillin.[22] Doxycycline (100 mg orally twice daily) and tetracycline (500 mg four times daily) have been administered for 14 days for the treatment of early syphilis and 28 days for late latent infection and syphilis of unknown duration. Close serologic follow-up is mandatory. Neither of these therapies is recommended for children younger than 8 years. Ceftriaxone (100 mg/kg/day, maximum of 1 g daily) given either intravenously or intramuscularly for 8 to 10 days may be effective for the treatment of early syphilis.[56] Preliminary data also suggest that azithromycin as a single dose of 2 g may be effective in adults.[22]

Two to 12 hours after the treatment of syphilis, an acute systemic (Jarisch-Herxheimer) reaction usually consisting of headache, malaise, temperature to 38° C or higher, and resolution within a day develop in a variable proportion of patients. The reaction is observed most commonly in the early stages of syphilis, probably represents a reaction to liberated endotoxin,[46] and does not affect the course of recovery. In the later stages of syphilis, the reaction develops in fewer than one in four patients. Most reactions in late syphilis are clinically insignificant, but an occasional reaction may produce damage to the CNS or cardiovascular system.

SYPHILIS IN PREGNANCY

Pregnant women with reactive serologic tests for syphilis should be considered infected unless an adequate treatment history is documented and sequential nontreponemal antibody titers have declined. They should receive the same penicillin regimen appropriate for the stage of syphilis.[143] For early syphilis, many experts recommend that an additional dose of benzathine penicillin G be provided 1 week after the initial dose. Management and treatment decisions may be guided further by the use of fetal ultrasonography. Evidence of fetal infection may require additional doses of benzathine penicillin G until the resolution of fetal abnormalities. The Jarisch-Herxheimer reaction may complicate treatment and result in preterm labor and fetal decelerations, although concern for its occurrence should not delay treatment.[67, 89] No alternative to penicillin is available; pregnant women who have a history of penicillin allergy should undergo skin testing, desensitization, and treatment with penicillin.[144] Erythromycin is not recommended because infants have been born with congenital syphilis after maternal treatment with erythromycin. Any therapy other than penicillin is considered to be inadequate fetal therapy.[38, 101]

Women infected with syphilis and HIV should receive treatment regimens corresponding to their stage of syphilis. Follow-up on treated HIV-infected women must be thorough and frequent.[52, 88]

Patients who received ceftriaxone therapy for gonorrhea have a high rate of cure of preprimary syphilis, but failures have occurred, and its efficacy in pregnancy is not well studied.[56] This regimen, therefore, cannot be assumed to have provided adequate therapy for syphilis in pregnancy.

CONGENITAL SYPHILIS

INFANTS WITH EITHER PROVEN OR HIGHLY PROBABLE DISEASE. Infants who have findings on physical examination that are consistent with congenital syphilis, a quantitative nontreponemal serologic titer that is at least fourfold greater than the mother's titer, or spirochetes visualized in body fluids should be treated with aqueous crystalline penicillin G, 50,000 U/kg per dose intravenously every 12 hours during the first 7 days of life and every 8 hours thereafter for 10 days, or procaine penicillin G, 50,000 U/kg per dose intramuscularly in a single daily dose for 10 days[22] (see Table 150–10). Although levels of penicillin achieved in the CSF after procaine therapy are lower than those seen with intravenous penicillin treatment, the clinical significance is unclear.[7] No treatment failures have been reported after the administration of procaine penicillin therapy. If more than 1 day of penicillin therapy is missed, the entire course should be restarted. During a recent penicillin shortage in the United States, ampicillin was recommended as an alternative agent, although insufficient data exist for routine administration of ampicillin. When possible, a full 10-day course of penicillin is preferred even if ampicillin was provided initially for possible sepsis. Data also are lacking on the use of ceftriaxone in these infants. Infants born to mothers co-infected with syphilis and HIV do not require more intense or prolonged treatment of syphilis than that recommended for all infants.

INFANTS WITH A NORMAL PHYSICAL EXAMINATION AND A SERUM QUANTITATIVE NONTREPONEMAL SEROLOGIC TITER THAT IS THE SAME OR LESS THAN FOURFOLD THE MATERNAL TITER. Treatment decisions for these "asymptomatic" infants are based on the maternal history of syphilis and past treatment. The following situations are associated with a high likelihood that the infant may be infected with *T. pallidum* and should receive treatment: (1) the mother was not treated, was inadequately treated, or has no documentation of having received treatment[104]; (2) the mother was treated with erythromycin or another nonpenicillin regimen; (3) the mother received treatment 4 weeks or less before delivery[14]; and (4) the mother has early syphilis and a nontreponemal titer that has either not decreased fourfold or has increased fourfold. If the infant's nontreponemal test is reactive, the infant should be evaluated with a CBC and differential, platelet count, long bone radiographs, and CSF analysis for the VDRL test, cell count, and protein content[22] (see Fig. 150–2 and Table 150–10). If the entire evaluation is normal and follow-up is certain, the infant may receive benzathine penicillin G, 50,000 U/kg as a single intramuscular dose. If any part of the evaluation is abnormal or not done or if follow-up is uncertain, treatment should consist of aqueous penicillin G or procaine penicillin G (see earlier) for 10 days. If the infant's nontreponemal serum test is nonreactive, the evaluation may be omitted, but the infant should be treated with a single intramuscular dose of benzathine penicillin for the possibility of incubating syphilis. Some experts prefer that all infants born to mothers with untreated syphilis receive parenteral penicillin therapy for 10 days, even if the evaluation is normal, because many of these infants are likely to be infected with *T. pallidum,* especially if the mother has secondary syphilis at delivery or has seroconverted during the pregnancy.[22]

Recent studies have re-evaluated the efficacy of treatment regimens for asymptomatic infants born to mothers in whom treatment of possible syphilis was suboptimal.[97, 104] Paryani and colleagues[97] randomized 152 infants to receive either one injection of benzathine penicillin or a 10-day course of parenteral procaine penicillin. All study infants were asymptomatic on physical examination and had a normal CSF evaluation, normal radiographic studies of the long bones, and no visceral abnormalities. The results of both forms of therapy were excellent, with no treatment failures. This study indicates that single-dose therapy may have a high rate of success when the infant has negative studies and is asymptomatic. Failure of such therapy in three infants has been reported; however, the frequency appears to be low, but is unknown.[12, 145] None of the three infants in whom clinical signs of congenital syphilis developed several weeks after having received a single intramuscular dose of benzathine penicillin were fully evaluated for congenital syphilis at birth. The concern has been that infected but asymptomatic infants may have infection of the CNS and fail therapy with benzathine penicillin because it does not achieve treponemicidal concentrations in CSF.[132] Recently, using rabbit inoculation, Michelow and colleagues[85] have shown that invasion of the CNS occurs infrequently in infants with normal results on clinical, laboratory, and radiographic evaluation.

Infants do not require any evaluation in the following situations: (1) the mother was treated during the pregnancy, treatment was appropriate for the stage of infection, and treatment was administered longer than 4 weeks before delivery; (2) the mother's nontreponemal titers decreased fourfold after appropriate therapy for early syphilis or remained stable and low for late syphilis; and (3) the mother has no evidence of reinfection or relapse. The CDC, however, recommends that these infants receive a single dose of benzathine penicillin G, 50,000 U/kg intramuscularly. Infection of the fetus may occur despite appropriate maternal therapy during pregnancy; failure rates of maternal treatment for prevention of fetal infection have been reported to be from 2 to 14 percent and are more common with maternal secondary syphilis.[3, 29, 92, 125] Treating the infant at birth may prevent the development of clinical disease if these infants were infected in utero. However, some specialists would not treat the infant but provide close serologic follow-up only.

If the mother's treatment was adequate before pregnancy and the mother's nontreponemal serologic titer remained low and stable during pregnancy and at delivery, no evaluation or treatment is recommended by the CDC. However, some specialists provide a single intramuscular dose of benzathine penicillin if follow-up is uncertain because of the remote possibility of reinfection in the mother. These infants are at very low risk of having congenital syphilis; for the most part, these mothers are serofast.[91]

After the neonatal period, all children in whom congenital syphilis is diagnosed should be evaluated with a CBC and differential, platelet count, and CSF examination. Other tests such as auditory brain stem responses should be performed as clinically indicated. These children, as well as those with late congenital syphilis, should be treated with 200,000 to 300,000 U/kg/day of aqueous crystalline penicillin G given as 50,000 U/kg every 4 to 6 hours for a minimum of 10 to 14 days.

The Jarisch-Herxheimer reaction may complicate the treatment of congenital syphilis. It rarely is seen in newborns, although it occurs more commonly when syphilis is treated later in infancy. It usually is manifested by fever, but cardiovascular collapse and seizures also have been reported.

Follow-up Evaluation

Table 150–11 summarizes recommendations concerning the follow-up of infants after treatment of congenital syphilis, as well as seroreactive infants who were not treated because of the presumed adequacy of management of the mother's serologic status.[57, 58, 106] Infants born to mothers with syphilis should have serial quantitative nontreponemal tests performed until the test results show nonreactivity.[53, 109] Similarly, infants who are seronegative but whose mothers acquired syphilis late in gestation should be monitored via serial testing after penicillin therapy is instituted.

Follow-up for infants who received appropriate penicillin therapy for possible syphilis can be incorporated into routine pediatric care at 2, 4, 6, 12, 15, and 24 months. These infants should demonstrate a fourfold decrease in nontreponemal serologic titer. In infants with congenital syphilis, nontreponemal serologic tests become nonreactive within 6 to 12 months after appropriate treatment. Uninfected infants usually become seronegative by 6 months of age.[24] Infants with persistently low, stable titers of nontreponemal tests beyond 1 year of age may require re-treatment.

Untreated infants may benefit from having a nontreponemal test performed at 1 month of age. Untreated infants who are not seronegative by 6 months of age should be re-evaluated clinically and treated. If the nontreponemal titer increases fourfold in any infant during follow-up, full evaluation and treatment are indicated. All infants and children should be evaluated thoroughly for the extent of disease if they have serologic evidence of failure of treatment or recurrent disease. Such evaluation should, at a minimum, consist of CSF examination, CBC, and platelet count. Other tests such as long bone radiographs, liver function tests, hearing evaluation, and ophthalmologic assessment can be performed as clinically indicated.

A reactive treponemal test beyond 18 months of age when the infant has lost all maternal antibody confirms the diagnosis of congenital syphilis. This event, however, occurs in the minority of infants with congenital syphilis as proved by

TABLE 150–11 ■ RECOMMENDED FOLLOW-UP OF INFANTS BORN TO MOTHERS WITH SYPHILIS

Nontreponemal test (e.g., RPR)

Treated infant: Perform at 2, 4, 6, 12, 15, and 24 mo of age (or post-therapy) until nonreactive. The nontreponemal test titer should decrease fourfold within 6 mo after treatment and be nonreactive by 6 to 12 mo. If the test remains reactive ≥12 mo after treatment, consider re-evaluation and re-treatment. If the nontreponemal test titer increases fourfold, full re-evaluation and re-treatment for proved disease is required.

Untreated infant: Perform at 1, 2, 4, 6, 12, 15, and 24 mo of age (or post-therapy) until nonreactive. The nontreponemal test titer should decrease fourfold within 6 mo after treatment and be nonreactive by 6 mo. If the nontreponemal assay is reactive at 6 mo, re-evaluate the child (including CSF examination) and treat. If the nontreponemal test titer increases fourfold, full evaluation and treatment for proved disease are required.

Treponemal test (e.g., TP-PA): Perform at 12 mo. If reactive, repeat at 18 and 24 mo of age*

Abnormal CSF examination at diagnosis: repeat the CSF examination (Venereal Disease Research Laboratory test, cell count, protein content) at 6 mo of age (or post-therapy). If abnormal and no other explanation is found, re-treat the infant

Monitor yearly for neurologic, hearing, and ophthalmic disorders

Monitor developmental status and assess school function

*Approximately 30% of infected children will maintain a reactive treponemal test beyond 18 months of age. This finding, however, confirms the diagnosis of congenital syphilis. If the child was not treated previously, treatment of proved congenital syphilis is mandatory.

CSF, cerebrospinal fluid; RPR, rapid plasma reagin; TP-PA, *Treponema pallidum* particle agglutination test.

Adapted from Ikeda, M. K., and Jenson, H. B.: Evaluation and treatment of congenital syphilis. J. Pediatr. *117*:843–852, 1990; Rathbun, K. C.: Congenital syphilis: A proposal for improved surveillance, diagnosis and treatment. Sex. Transm. Dis. *10*:102–107, 1983; Ingall, D., Sánchez, P.J.: Syphilis. *In* Remington, J. S., and Klein J. O. (eds.):. Infectious Diseases of the Fetus and Newborn Infant. 5th ed. Philadelphia, W.B. Saunders, 2001, pp. 643–681.

isolation of spirochetes via inoculation of infant blood or CSF into rabbits. If the child did not previously receive treatment, a full evaluation and treatment are indicated.

Infants with abnormal CSF findings should have a repeat lumbar puncture performed 6 months after therapy. A reactive CSF VDRL test result or an abnormal protein content or cell count at that time is an indication for re-treatment.

Adults and older children with primary or secondary syphilis should be examined clinically and serologically at least 6 and 12 months after receiving treatment. Failure of nontreponemal titers to decrease fourfold within 6 months of treatment is indicative of probable treatment failure. These individuals should be re-evaluated for HIV infection and consideration given to performance of a lumbar puncture for detection of unrecognized neurosyphilis and re-treatment.[115] For latent syphilis, subsequent follow-up with quantitative serology at 6, 12, and 24 months is recommended. Failure of a fourfold decrease in initially elevated nontreponemal serologic titers (>1:32) within 12 to 24 months of therapy is an indication for examination of CSF and re-treatment. Re-treatment of syphilis also is recommended when clinical signs or symptoms persist or recur or if a sustained fourfold increase in titer of a nontreponemal serologic test is noted. Patients with neurosyphilis require examination and repeat CSF evaluation every 6 months until the cell count is normal. If the cell count is not decreased after 6 months or the CSF is not normal after 2 years, re-treatment should be considered.

In most patients receiving appropriate therapy during the primary or secondary stages, active disease is arrested totally and permanently. Persistent seroreactivity as measured by the FTA-ABS test may be avoided if treatment is given during the preprimary stage, but very infrequently thereafter. Nonetheless, progression to tertiary disease seldom, if ever, occurs. Similarly, therapy during early or late latent syphilis averts the development of symptomatic tertiary disease. Antimicrobial therapy for symptomatic neurosyphilis, optic neuritis, and cardiovascular syphilis may not be followed by significant clinical improvement, and established damage to vital organs may fail to resolve.

Prevention

Methods to control the spread of syphilis have relied extensively on treatment of case contacts. Persons with active syphilis are interviewed to identify all sexual contacts that may have occurred: (1) 3 months plus the duration of symptoms for primary syphilis, (2) 6 months plus the duration of symptoms for secondary syphilis, and (3) 1 year for early latent syphilis. Contacts are examined, tested serologically, and treated appropriately even if seronegative. Advantage is taken of the long incubation period of syphilis by preventing disease in contacts before they themselves can transmit infection.

Adverse outcomes of pregnancy and congenital infection can be prevented effectively by providing routine prenatal serologic screening and penicillin treatment of infected women and their sexual partners.[131, 139] All pregnant women should have a nontreponemal serologic test for syphilis at the first prenatal visit. For communities and populations in which the prevalence of syphilis is high or for patients at increased risk of contracting the disease, serologic testing should be performed at 28 weeks' gestation and at delivery because some women may acquire syphilis during the pregnancy.[5] In the absence of clinical symptoms or proven exposure to an active case and with a negative treponemal test, treatment may be withheld and studies repeated in 4 weeks because it probably represents a BFP result. When epidemiologic, clinical, or serologic evidence of infection is present or the diagnosis cannot be excluded, treatment should be instituted.

Serologic screening tests should be performed on maternal serum and not on the infant's serum or umbilical cord blood.[107] An infant's serologic titer usually is one to two dilutions less than that of the mother's titer; therefore, an infant may have a nonreactive serologic test for syphilis when the maternal titer is of low dilution. Some of these infants, especially those born to mothers with no previous treatment of syphilis, will require therapy for prevention of late-onset disease. They would have been missed if only infant screening had been performed.

Limitations of the current screening practices also exist. A falsely negative nontreponemal test can result from a prozone phenomenon. In addition, a negative maternal nontreponemal test at delivery will not exclude incubating syphilis or even primary syphilis if nontreponemal and treponemal antibodies have not yet reached detectable concentrations.[35, 120] Infants born to such mothers may be infected and experience clinical disease in the ensuing 3 to 14 weeks. Repeat screening of mothers who reside in areas with a high prevalence of syphilis or who engage in high-risk behavior may be advisable at the first postpartum visit.

A policy statement of the CDC is that no infant should leave the hospital without the serologic status of the infant's mother having been documented at least once during pregnancy and preferably again at delivery.[22, 80] In this era of early and very early discharge from the hospital after deliveries, fulfilling the policy goal may require careful planning and advocacy by the clinician.

All syphilis cases must be reported to the local public health department. This practice allows for contact investigation, appropriate follow-up, and identification of core environments and populations in which the greatest transmission of syphilis is occurring in a particular community. Despite great progress in recent years, the prevention, control, and even elimination of endemic syphilis in the United States remain elusive goals in public health policy.

REFERENCES

1. Ackerman, A. B., Goldfaden, G., and Cosmides, J. C.: Acquired syphilis in early childhood. Arch. Dermatol. *106*:92, 1972.
2. Alder, J. D., Friess, L., Tengowski, M., et al.: Phagocytosis of opsonized *Treponema pallidum* subsp. *pallidum* proceeds slowly. Infect. Immun. *58*:1167–1173, 1990.
3. Alexander, J. M., Sheffield, J. S., Sanchez, P. J., et al.: Efficacy of treatment for syphilis in pregnancy. Obstet. Gynecol. *93*:5–8, 1999.
4. Alford, C. A., Jr., Polt, S. S., Cassady, G. E., et al.: γ-M-fluorescent treponemal antibody in the diagnosis of congenital syphilis. N. Engl. J. Med. *280*:1086–1091, 1969.
5. Al-Salihi, F. L., Curran, J. P., and Shteir, O. A.: Occurrence of fetal syphilis after a nonreactive early gestational serologic test. J. Pediatr. *78*:121–123, 1971.
6. Augenbraun, M. H., DeHovitz, J. A., Feldman, J., et al.: Biological false-positive syphilis test results for women infected with human immunodeficiency virus. Clin. Infect. Dis. *19*:1040–1044, 1994.
7. Azimi, P. H., Janner, D., Berne, P., et al.: Concentrations of procaine and aqueous penicillin in the cerebrospinal fluid of infants treated for congenital syphilis. J. Pediatr. *124*:649, 1994.
8. Baker-Zander, S. A., Hook, E. W., III, Bonin, P., et al.: Antigens of *Treponema pallidum* recognized by IgG and IgM antibodies during syphilis in humans. J. Infect. Dis. *151*:264, 1985.
9. Barton, J. R., Thorpe, E. M., Shaver, D. C., et al.: Nonimmune hydrops fetalis associated with maternal infection with syphilis. Am. J. Obstet. Gynecol. *167*:56, 1992.
10. Baughn, R. E., Jorizzo, J. L., Adams, C. B., et al.: Ig class and IgG subclass responses to *Treponema pallidum* in patients with syphilis. J. Clin. Immunol. *8*:128–139, 1988.
11. Bays, J., and Chadwick, D.: The serologic test for syphilis in sexually abused children and adolescents. Adolesc. Pediatr. Gynecol. *4*:148–151, 1991.
12. Beck-Sague, C., and Alexander, R.: Failure of benzathine penicillin G treatment in early congenital syphilis. Pediatr. Infect. Dis. *6*:1061–1064, 1987.
13. Beeram, M. R., Chopde, N., Dawood, Y., et al.: Lumbar puncture in the evaluation of possible asymptomatic congenital syphilis in neonates. J. Pediatr. *128*:125–129, 1996.
14. Benzick, A. E., Wirthwein, D. P., Weinberg, A., et al.: Pituitary gland gumma in congenital syphilis after failed maternal treatment: A case report: Pediatrics *104*(1):e1–e4, 1999.
15. Braunstein, G. D., Lewis, E. J., Galvanek, E. G., et al.: The nephrotic syndrome associated with secondary syphilis. Am. J. Med. *48*:643–648, 1970.
16. Bromberg, K., Rawstron, S., and Tannis, G.: Diagnosis of congenital syphilis by combining *Treponema pallidum*-specific IgM detection with immunofluorescent antigen detection of *T. pallidum*. J. Infect. Dis. *168*: 238, 1993.
17. Bulova, S. I., Schwartz, E., and Harrer, W. V.: Hydrops fetalis and congenital syphilis. Pediatrics *49*:285–287, 1972.
18. Burstain, J. M., Grimprel, E., Lukehart, S. A., et al.: Sensitive detection of *Treponema pallidum* by using the polymerase chain reaction. J. Clin. Microbiol. *29*:62, 1991.
19. Centers for Disease Control and Prevention: Congenital syphilis—New York City, 1986–1988. M. M. W. R. Morb. Mortal. Wkly. Rep. *38*(48): 825–829, 1989.
20. Centers for Disease Control and Prevention: Primary and secondary syphilis—United States, 1999. M. M. W. R. Morb. Mortal. Wkly. Rep. *50*(7):113–117, 2001.
21. Centers for Disease Control and Prevention: Congenital syphilis—United States, 2000. M. M. W. R. Morb. Mortal. Wkly. Rep. *50*(27):573–577, 2001.
22. Centers for Disease Control and Prevention: Sexually transmitted diseases treatment guidelines 2002. M. M. W. R. Recomm. Rep. *51*(RR-6): 18–30, 2002.
23. Chabra, R. S., Brion, L. P., Castro, M., et al.: Comparison of maternal sera, cord blood and neonatal sera for detecting presumptive congenital syphilis: Relationship with maternal treatment. Pediatrics *91*:88–91, 1993.
24. Chang, S. N., Chung, K.-Y., Lee, M.-G., and Lee, J. B.: Seroreversion of the serological tests for syphilis in the newborns born to treated syphilitic mothers. Genitourin. Med. *71*:68–70, 1995.
25. Christian, C. W., Lavelle, J., and Bell, L. M.: Preschoolers with syphilis. Pediatrics *103*:e4, 1999.
26. Clark, E. G., and Danbolt, N.: The Oslo study of the natural course of untreated syphilis: An epidemiologic investigation based on a re-study of the Boeck-Bruusgaard material. Med. Clin. North Am. *48*:613–623, 1964.
27. Cohen, D. A., Boyd, D., Pabhudas, I., et al.: The effects of case definition, maternal screening, and reporting criteria on rates of congenital syphilis. Am. J. Public Health *80*:316–317, 1990.
28. Coles, F. B., Hipp, S. S., Siberstein, G. S., et al.: Congenital syphilis surveillance in upstate New York, 1989–1992: Implications for prevention and clinical management. J. Infect. Dis. *171*:732–735, 1995.
29. Conover, C. S., Rend, C. A., Miller, G. B., Jr., and Schmid, G. P.: Congenital syphilis after treatment of maternal syphilis with a penicillin regimen exceeding CDC guidelines. Infect. Dis. Obstet. Gynecol. *6*:134–137, 1998.
30. Cremin, B. J., and Fisher, R. M.: The lesions of congenital syphilis. Br. J. Radiol. *43*:333–341, 1970.
31. Daaboul, J. J., Kartchner, W., and Jones, K. L.: Neonatal hypoglycemia caused by hypopituitarism in infants with congenital syphilis. J. Pediatr. *123*:983–985, 1993.
32. Desenclos, J.-C. A., Scaggs, M., and Wroten, J. E.: Characteristics of mothers of live infants with congenital syphilis in Florida, 1987–1989. Am. J. Epidemiol. *136*:657–661, 1992.
33. Dobson, S. R. M., Taber, L. H., and Baughn, R. E.: Recognition of *Treponema pallidum* antigens by IgM and IgG antibodies in congenitally infected newborns and their mothers. J. Infect. Dis. *157*:903–910, 1988.
34. Dobson, S. R. M., Taber, L. H., and Baughn, R. E.: Characterization of the components in circulating immune complexes from infants with congenital syphilis. J. Infect. Dis. *158*:940–947, 1988.
35. Dorfman, D. H., and Glaser, J. H.: Congenital syphilis presenting in infants after the newborn period. N. Engl. J. Med. *323*:1299–1302, 1990.
36. Dorman, H. G., and Sahyun, B. F.: Identification and significance of spirochetes in placenta: Report of 105 cases with positive findings. Am. J. Obstet. Gynecol. *33*:954–967, 1937.
37. Dunn, R. A., Webster, L. A., Nakashima, A. K., and Sylvester, G. C.: Surveillance for geographic and secular trends in congenital syphilis—United States, 1983–1991. Morb. Mortal. Wkly. Rep. CDC Surveill. Summ. *42*(6):59–71, 1993.
38. Fenton, L. J., and Light, I. J.: Congenital syphilis after maternal treatment with erythromycin. Obstet. Gynecol. *47*:492–494, 1976.
39. Finelli, L., Crayne, E. M., and Spitalny, K. C.: Treatment of infants with reactive syphilis serology, New Jersey. Pediatrics *102*:e27, 1998.
40. Fiumara, N. J.: Acquired syphilis in three patients with congenital syphilis. N. Engl. J. Med. *290*:1110–1120, 1974.
41. Fiumara, N. J., Fleming, W. L., Downing, J. G., et al.: The incidence of prenatal syphilis at the Boston City Hospital. N. Engl. J. Med. *247*:48, 1952.
42. Fiumara, N. J., and Lessell, S.: Manifestations of late congenital syphilis. Arch. Dermatol. *102*:78–83, 1970.
43. Fojaca, R. M., Hensely, G. T., and Moskowitz, L.: Congenital syphilis and necrotizing funisitis. J. A. M. A. *12*:1788, 1989.
44. Fraser, C. M., Morris, S. J., Weinstock, G. M., et al.: Complete genome sequence of *Treponema pallidum,* the syphilis spirochete. Science *281*:375, 1998.
45. Gamble, C. N., and Reardan, J. B.: Immunopathogenesis of syphilitic glomerulonephritis. N. Engl. J. Med. *292*:449–454, 1975.
46. Gelfand, J. A., Elin, R. J., Berry, F. W., Jr., et al.: Endotoxemia associated with the Jarisch-Herxheimer reaction. N. Engl. J. Med. *295*:211–213, 1976.
47. Genest, D. R., Choi-Hong, S. R., Tate, J. E., et al.: Diagnosis of congenital syphilis from placental examination: Comparison of histopathology, Steiner stain, and polymerase chain reaction for *Treponema pallidum* DNA. Hum. Pathol. *27*:366–372, 1996.
48. Glover, D. D., Winter, C. A., Charles, D., et al.: Diagnostic considerations in intra-amniotic syphilis. Sex. Transm. Dis. *12*:145–149, 1985.
49. Grimprel, E., Sanchez, P. J., Wendel, G. D., Jr., et al.: Use of polymerase chain reaction and rabbit infectivity testing to detect *Treponema pallidum* in amniotic fluids, fetal and neonatal sera, and cerebrospinal fluid. J. Clin. Microbiol. *29*:171, 1991.
50. Gust, D. A., Levine, W. C., St. Louis, M. E., et al.: Mortality associated with congenital syphilis in the United States, 1992–1998. Pediatrics *109*:e79, 2002.
51. Gutman, L. T.: Congenital syphilis. *In* Mandell, G. L. (ed.): Atlas of Infectious Disease. Vol. 5. Sexually Transmitted Diseases. Philadelphia, Current Medicine, 1996.
52. Haas, J. S., Bolan, G., Larsen, S. A., et al.: Sensitivity of treponemal tests for detecting prior treated syphilis during human immunodeficiency virus infection. J. Infect. Dis. *162*:862–866, 1990.
53. Hardy, J. B., Hardy, P. H., and Oppenheimer, E. H.: Failure of penicillin in a newborn with congenital syphilis. J. A. M. A. *212*:1345, 1970.
54. Harter, C. A., and Benirschke, K.: Fetal syphilis in the first trimester. Am. J. Obstet. Gynecol. *124*:705–711, 1976.

55. Hollier, L. M., Harstad, T. W., Sanchez, P. J., et al.: Fetal syphilis: Clinical and laboratory characteristics. Obstet. Gynecol. *97*:947–953, 2001.
56. Hook, E. W., Roddy, R. E., and Hardsfield, H. H.: Ceftriaxone therapy for incubating and early syphilis. J. Infect. Dis. *158*:881–884, 1988.
57. Ikeda, M. K., and Jenson, H. B.: Evaluation and treatment of congenital syphilis. J. Pediatr. *117*:843–852, 1990.
58. Ingall, D., Sánchez, P. J.: Syphilis. *In* Remington, J. S., and Klein, J. O. (eds.): Infectious Diseases of the Fetus and Newborn Infant. 5th ed. Philadelphia, W. B. Saunders, 2001, pp. 643–681.
59. Ingraham, N. R.: The value of penicillin alone in the prevention and treatment of congenital syphilis. Acta. Derm. Venereol. *31*(Suppl. 24):60, 1951.
60. Isaacs, R. D., and Radolf, J. D.: Molecular approaches to improved syphilis serodiagnosis. Serodiagn. Immunother. Infect. Dis. *3*:299–306, 1989.
61. Izzat, N. N., Bartruff, J. K., Glicksman, J. M., et al.: Validity of the VDRL test on cerebrospinal fluid contaminated by blood. Br. J. Vener. Dis. *47*: 162–164, 1971.
62. Jensen, J. R., Thestrup-Pedersen, K., and From, E.: Fluctuations in natural killer cell activity in early syphilis. Br. J. Vener. Dis. *59*:30–32, 1983.
63. Jones, S. A., Marchitto, K. S., Miller, J. N., et al.: Monoclonal antibody with hemagglutination, immobilization, and neutralization activities defines an immunodominant, 47,000 mol wt, surface-exposed immunogen of *Treponema pallidum* (Nichols). J. Exp. Med. *160*:1404, 1984.
64. Kaplan, B. S., Wiglesworth, F. W., Marks, M. I., et al.: The glomerulopathy of congenital syphilis: An immune deposit disease. J. Pediatr. *81*:1154–1156, 1972.
65. Kaufman, R. E., Olansky, D. C., and Wiesner, P. J.: The FTA-ABS (IgM) test for neonatal congenital syphilis: A critical review. J. Am. Vener. Dis. Assoc. *1*:78–84, 1974.
66. Klass, P. E., Brown, E. R., and Pelton, S. I.: The incidence of prenatal syphilis at the Boston City Hospital: A comparison across four decades. Pediatrics *94*:24–28, 1994.
67. Klein, V. R., Cox, S. M., Mitchell, M. D., and Wendel, G. D., Jr.: The Jarisch-Herxheimer reaction complicating syphilotherapy in pregnancy. Obstet. Gynecol. *92*:375–380, 1990.
68. Knight, J., Richardson, A. C., and White, K. C.: The role of syphilis serology in the evaluation of suspected sexual abuse. Pediatr. Infect. Dis. J. *11*:125–127, 1992.
69. Lande, M. B., Richardson, A. C., and White, K. C.: The role of syphilis in the evaluation of suspected sexual abuse. Pediatr. Infect. Dis. J. *11*: 125–127, 1992.
70. Larsen, S. A., Steiner, B. M., and Rudolph, A. H.: Laboratory diagnosis and interpretation of tests for syphilis. Clin. Microbiol. Rev. *8*:1–21, 1995.
71. Lascari, A. D., Diamond, J., and Nolan, B. E.: Anemia as the only presenting manifestation of congenital syphilis. Clin. Pediatr. *15*:90–91, 1976.
72. Lefevre, J. C., Betrand, M. A., and Bauriaud, R.: Evaluation of the Captia enzyme immunoassays for detection of immunoglobulins G and M to *Treponema pallidum* in syphilis. J. Clin. Microbiol. *28*:1704–1707, 1990.
73. Lesser, R. P., and O'Connell, E. J.: Positive fluorescent treponemal antibody test in systemic lupus erythematosus in childhood: Report of a case. J. Pediatr. *79*:1006–1008, 1971.
74. Lewis, L. L.: Congenital syphilis: Serologic diagnosis in the young infant. Infect. Dis. Clin. North Am. *6*:31, 1992.
75. Lewis, L. L., Taber, L. H., and Baughn, R. E.: Evaluation of immunoglobulin M Western blot analysis in the diagnosis of congenital syphilis. J. Clin. Microbiol. *28*:296, 1990.
76. Lucas, M. J., Theriot, S. K., and Wendel, G. D.: Doppler systolic-diastolic ratios in pregnancies complicated by syphilis. Obstet. Gynecol. *77*:217, 1991.
77. Lukehart, S. A., Hook, E. W., III, Baker-Zander, S. A., et al.: Invasion of the central nervous system by *Treponema pallidum:* Implications for diagnoses and therapy. Ann. Intern. Med. *109*:855, 1988.
78. Macias, E. G., Eller, J. J., Huber, T. W., et al.: Immunofluorescence of tracheal secretions in neonatal syphilis. Pediatrics *53*:947–949, 1974.
79. Magnuson, H. J., Eagle, H., and Fleischman, R.: The minimal infectious inoculum of *Spirochaeta pallida* (Nichols strain), and a consideration of its rate of multiplication in vivo. Am. J. Syphilis Gonorrhea Vener. Dis. *32*:1, 1948.
80. Martin, D., Bertrand, J., McKegney, C., et al.: Congenital syphilis surveillance and newborn evaluation in a low-incidence state. Arch. Pediatr. Adolesc. Med. *155*:140–144, 2001.
81. Mascola, L., Pelosi, R., and Alexander, C. E.: Inadequate treatment of syphilis in pregnancy. Am. J. Obstet. Gynecol. *150*:945–947, 1984.
82. Mascola, L., Pelosi, R., Blount, J. H., et al.: Congenital syphilis: Why is it still occurring? J. A. M. A. *252*:1719–1722, 1984.
83. Mascola, L., Pelosi, R., Blount, J. H., et al.: Congenital syphilis revisited. Am. J. Dis. Child. *139*:575–580, 1985.
84. McFarlin, B. L., Bottoms, S. F., Dock, B. S., et al.: Epidemic syphilis: Maternal factors associated with congenital infection. Am. J. Obstet. Gynecol. *170*:535–540, 1994.
85. Michelow, I. C., Wendel, G. D., Jr., Norgard, M. V., et al.: Central nervous system infection in congenital syphilis. N. Engl. J. Med. *346*:1792–1798, 2002.
86. Moyer, V. A., Schneider, V., Yetman, R., et al.: Contribution of long-bone radiographs to the management of congenital syphilis in the newborn infant. Arch. Pediatr. Adolesc. Med. *152*:353–357, 1998.
87. Musher, D. M., Hague-Park, M., Gyorkey, F., et al.: The interaction between *Treponema pallidum* and human polymorphonuclear leukocytes. J. Infect. Dis. *147*:77–86, 1983.
88. Musher, D. M., Hamill, R. J., and Baughn, R. E.: Effect of human immunodeficiency virus (HIV) infection on the course of syphilis and on the response to treatment. Ann. Intern. Med. *113*:872–881, 1990.
89. Myles, T. D., Elam, G., Park-Hwang, E., and Nguyen, T.: The Jarisch-Herxheimer reaction and fetal monitoring changes in pregnant women treated for syphilis. Obstet. Gynecol. *92*:859–864, 1998.
90. Nabarro, J. N. D.: Congenital Syphilis. Baltimore, Williams & Wilkins, 1954.
91. Nathan, L., Bawdon, R. E., Sidawi, E., et al.: Penicillin levels following administration of benzathine penicillin G in pregnancy. Obstet. Gynecol. *82*:338, 1993.
92. Nathan, L., Bohman, V. R., Sánchez, P. J., et al.: In utero infection with *Treponema pallidum* in early pregnancy. Prenat. Diagn. *17*:119, 1997.
93. Nathan, L., Twickler, D. M., Peters, M. T., et al.: Fetal syphilis: Correlation of sonographic findings and rabbit infectivity testing of amniotic fluid. J. Ultrasound Med. *2*:97, 1993.
94. Nolt, D., Saad, R., Kouatli, A., et al.: Survival with hypopituitarism from congenital syphilis. Pediatrics *109*(4):e1–e4, 2002.
95. Norris, S. J., Alderete, J. E., Axelson, N. H., et al.: Identity of *Treponema pallidum* subsp. *pallidum* polypeptides: Correlation of sodium dodecyl sulfate–polyacrylamide gel electrophoresis results from different laboratories. Electrophoresis *8*:77, 1987.
96. Oppenheimer, E. H., and Hardy, J. B.: Congenital syphilis in the newborn infant: Clinical and pathological observations in recent cases. Johns Hopkins Med. J. *129*:63–82, 1971.
97. Paryani, S. G., Vaugh, A. J., Crosby, M., et al.: Treatment of asymptomatic congenital syphilis benzathine versus procaine penicillin G therapy. J. Pediatr. *125*:471–475, 1994.
98. Pavithran, K.: Acquired syphilis in a patient with late congenital syphilis. Sex. Transm. Dis. *14*:119–121, 1987.
99. Peterman, T. A., Zaidi, A. A., Lieb, S., et al.: Incubating syphilis in patients treated for gonorrhea: A comparison of treatment regimens. J. Infect. Dis. *170*:689–692, 1994.
100. Peterson, K., Baseman, J. B., and Alderete, J. F.: *Treponema pallidum* receptor binding proteins interact with fibronectin. J. Exp. Med. *157*: 1958–1970, 1983.
101. Philipson, A., Sabeth, L. D., and Charles, D.: Transplacental passage of erythromycin and clindamycin. N. Engl. J. Med. *288*:1219–1221, 1973.
102. Putkonen, T.: Does early treatment prevent dental changes in congenital syphilis? Acta Derm. Venerol. *43*:240–249, 1963.
103. Qureshi, F., Jacques, S. M., and Reyes, M. P.: Placental histopathology in syphilis. Hum. Pathol. *24*:779–784, 1993.
104. Radcliffe, M., Meyer, M., Roditi, D., and Malan, A.: Single-dose benzathine penicillin in infants at risk of congenital syphilis—results of a randomised study. S. Afr. Med. J. *87*:62–65, 1997.
105. Rathbun, K. C.: Congenital syphilis. Sex. Transm. Dis. *10*:93–99, 1983.
106. Rathbun, K. C.: Congenital syphilis: A proposal for improved surveillance, diagnosis and treatment. Sex. Transm. Dis. *10*:102–107, 1983.
107. Rawstron, S. A., and Bromberg, K.: Comparison of maternal and newborn serologic tests for syphilis. Am. J. Dis. Child. *145*:1383–1388, 1991.
108. Rawstron, S. A., Jenkins, S., Blanchard, S., et al.: Maternal and congenital syphilis in Brooklyn, NY: Epidemiology, transmission, and diagnosis. Am. J. Dis. Child. *147*:727, 1993.
109. Rawstron, S. A., Mehta, S., Marcellino, L., et al.: Congenital syphilis and fluorescent treponemal antibody test reactivity after the age of 1 year. Sex. Transm. Dis. *28*:412–416, 2001.
110. Rawstron, S. A., Vetrano, J., Tannis, G., and Bromberg, K.: Congenital syphilis: Detection of *Treponema pallidum* in stillborns. Clin. Infect. Dis. *24*:24, 1997.
111. Reyes, M. P., Hunt, N., Ostrea, E. M., et al.: Maternal/congenital syphilis in a large tertiary care urban hospital. Clin. Infect. Dis. *17*:1041–1046, 1993.
112. Ricci, J. M., Fojaco, R. M., and O'Sullivan, M. J.: Congenital syphilis: The University of Miami/Jackson Memorial Medical Center experience, 1986–1988. Obstet. Gynecol. *74*:687–693, 1989.
113. Risser, W. L., and Hwang, L.-Y.: Problems in the current case definitions of congenital syphilis. J. Pediatr. *129*:499–505, 1996.
114. Rolfs, R. T., Joesoef, J. R., Hendershot, E. F., et al.: A randomized trial of enhanced therapy for early syphilis in patients with and without human immunodeficiency virus infection. N. Engl. J. Med. *337*:307, 1997.
115. Romanowski, B., Sutherland, R., and Fick, G. H.: Serologic response to treatment of infectious syphilis. Ann. Intern. Med. *114*:1005–1009, 1991.
116. Rosen, E. U., and Richardson, N. J.: A reappraisal of the value of the IgM fluorescent treponemal antibody absorption test in the diagnosis of congenital syphilis. J. Pediatr. *87*:38–42, 1975.
117. Sánchez, P. J., McCracken, G. H., Wendel, G. D., et al.: Molecular analysis of the fetal IgM response to *Treponema pallidum* antigens: Implications for improved serodiagnosis of congenital syphilis. J. Infect. Dis. *159*:508–517, 1989.

118. Sánchez, P. J., and Wendel, G. D.: Syphilis in pregnancy. Clin. Perinatol. *24*:71–90, 1997.
119. Sánchez, P. J., Wendel, G. D., Grimpel, E., et al.: Evaluation of molecular methodologies and rabbit infectivity testing for the diagnosis of congenital syphilis and central nervous system invasion by *Treponema pallidum*. J. Infect. Dis. *167*:148–157, 1993.
120. Sánchez, P. J., Wendel, G. D., and Norgard, M. V.: Congenital syphilis associated with negative results of maternal serologic tests at delivery. Am. J. Dis. Child. *145*:967, 1991.
121. Sánchez, P. J., Wendel, G. D., Norgard, M. V.: IgM antibody to *Treponema pallidum* in cerebrospinal fluid of infants with congenital syphilis. Am. J. Dis. Child. *146*:1171, 1992.
122. Schmitz, J. L., Gertis, K. S., Mauney, C., et al.: Laboratory diagnosis of congenital syphilis by immunoglobulin M (IgM) and IgA immunoblotting. Clin. Diagn. Lab. Immunol. *1*:32, 1994.
123. Schulte, J. M., Burkham, S., Hamaker, D., et al.: Syphilis among HIV-infected mothers and their infants in Texas from 1988 to 1994. Sex. Transm. Dis. *28*:315–320, 2001.
124. Shah, M. C., and Barton, L. L.: Congenital syphilitic hepatitis. Pediatr. Infect. Dis. *8*:891–892, 1989.
125. Sheffield, J. S., Sánchez, P. J., Morris, G., et al.: Congenital syphilis after maternal treatment for syphilis during pregnancy. Am. J. Obstet. Gynecol. *186*:569–573, 2002.
126. Sheffield, J. S., Sánchez, P. J., Wendel, G. D., Jr., et al.: Placental histopathology of congenital syphilis. Obstet. Gynecol. *100*:20, 2002.
127. Sheffield, J. S., Wendel, G. D., Jr., Zeray, F., et al.: Congenital syphilis: The influence of maternal stage of syphilis on vertical transmission. Abstract. Am. J. Obstet. Gynecol. *180*(Suppl.):85, 1999.
128. Shew, M. L., and Fortenberry, J. D.: Syphilis screening in adolescents. J. Adolesc. Health *13*:303–305, 1992.
129. Silber, T. J., and Milard, M. F.: The clinical spectrum of syphilis in adolescence. Adolesc. Health Care *5*:112–116, 1984.
130. Silverstein, A. M.: Congenital syphilis and the timing of immunogenesis in the human fetus. Nature *194*:196–197, 1962.
131. Southwick, K. L., Guidry, H. M., Weldon, M. M., et al.: An epidemic of congenital syphilis in Jefferson County, Texas, 1994–1995: Inadequate prenatal syphilis testing after an outbreak in adults. Am. J. Public Health. *89*:557, 1999.
132. Speer, M. E., Taber, L. H., Clark, D. B., et al.: Cerebrospinal fluid levels of benzathine penicillin in the neonate. J. Pediatr. *91*:996–997, 1977.
133. St. Louis, M. E., and Wasserheit, J. M.: Elimination of syphilis in the United States. Science *281*:353, 1998.
134. Stoll, B. J., Lee, F. K., Larsen, S., et al.: Clinical and serologic evaluation of neonates for congenital syphilis: A continuing diagnostic dilemma. J. Infect. Dis. *167*:415–422, 1993.
135. Swancott, M. A., Radolf, J. D., and Norgard, M. V.: The 34-kilodalton membrane immunogen of *Treponema pallidum* is a lipoprotein. Infect. Immun. *58*:384–392, 1990.
136. Taber, L. H., and Huber, T. W.: Congenital syphilis. Prog. Clin. Biol. Res. *3*:183–190, 1975.
137. Tan, K. L.: The re-emergence of early congenital syphilis. Acta Pediatr. *62*:601–607, 1973.
138. Theus, S. A., Harrich, D. A., Gaynor, R., et al.: *Treponema pallidum,* lipoproteins, and synthetic lipoprotein analogues induce human immunodeficiency virus type 1 gene expression in monocytes via NF-κB activation. J. Infect. Dis. *177*:941–950, 1998.
139. Warner, L., Rochat, R. W., Fichtner, R. R., et al.: Missed opportunities for congenital syphilis prevention in an urban southeastern hospital. Sex. Transm. Dis. *28*:92–98, 2001.
140. Webber, M. P., Lambert, G., Bateman, D. A., et al.: Maternal risk factors for congenital syphilis: A case-control study. Am. J. Epidemiol. *137*:415–422, 1993.
141. Wendel, G. D., Maberry, M. C., Christmas, J. T., et al.: Examination of amniotic fluid in diagnosing congenital syphilis with fetal death. Obstet. Gynecol. *74*:967–970, 1989.
142. Wendel, G. D., Sánchez, P. J., Peters, M. T., et al.: Identification of *Treponema pallidum* in amniotic fluid and fetal blood from pregnancies complicated by congenital syphilis. Obstet. Gynecol. *78*:890, 1991.
143. Wendel, G. D., Jr., Sheffield, J. S., Hollier, L. M., et al.: Treatment of syphilis in pregnancy and prevention of congenital syphilis. Clin. Infect. Dis. *35*(Suppl. 2):200–209, 2002.
144. Wendel, G. D., Jr., Stark, B. J., Jamison, R. B., et al.: Penicillin allergy and desensitization in serious infections during pregnancy. N. Engl. J. Med. *312*:1229, 1985.
145. Woolf, A., Wilfert, C. M., Kelsey, D. B., et al.: Childhood syphilis in North Carolina. N. C. Med. J. *41*:443–449, 1980.
146. Zenker, P. N., and Berman, S. M.: Congenital syphilis: Reporting and reality. Am. J. Public Health *80*:271–272, 1990.

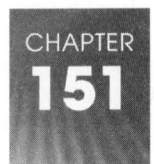

Nonvenereal Treponematoses

JAMES N. MILLER

Pinta, yaws, and endemic syphilis are the three chronic granulomatous diseases that constitute the pathogenic nonvenereal treponematoses of humans. These diseases are caused by morphologically indistinguishable treponemes found almost exclusively in underdeveloped populations of the tropical and bordering arid areas of the world. On the basis of 100 percent DNA sequence homology for the etiologic agents of syphilis and yaws[35] and the consideration by most investigators that the etiologic agent of endemic syphilis is a variant of *Treponema pallidum*,[27] the pathogenic treponemes have been given subspecies designations as follows: syphilis, *T. pallidum* subspecies *pallidum* (*T. pallidum*); yaws, *T. pallidum* subspecies *pertenue* (*Treponema pertenue*); endemic syphilis, *T. pallidum* subspecies *endemicum* (*T. pallidum*). The designation for the causative agent of pinta remains *Treponema carateum* (*Treponema herrejoni*).

Agents responsible for the nonvenereal treponematoses are transmitted from person to person by means of skin or mucous membrane contact. Close contact with children or young adults, traumatized areas of skin, lack of clothing, and poor personal hygiene are important factors in transmission of these diseases. All three nonvenereal treponematoses are potentially debilitating diseases that have enormous social and economic implications within endemic areas. Although their worldwide prevalence in general has been reduced considerably by means of seroepidemiologic and mass treatment campaigns sponsored by the World Health Organization (WHO) and the United Nations International Children's Emergency Fund (UNICEF), they remain a public health problem in several areas of the world where sporadic outbreaks continue to occur.[39, 53]

These diseases have existed for centuries. In theory, they appear to have originated from mutant forms of ancient treponemes, commencing with the human acquisition of pinta from an animal infection in the Euro-Afro-Asian landmass some time before 20,000 BC. Pinta presumably spread throughout the world by 15,000 BC and became isolated in the Americas by shifting continents. By 10,000 BC, climate-induced mutations gave rise to yaws in the tropical areas of Asia and Africa, as the benign pinta-producing treponemes became more invasive and destructive. The emergence of the Bering Strait isolated the Americas. Finally, in the arid lands bordering the tropical zones, yaws-producing treponemes again mutated by 7000 BC. Natural selection within populations more fully clothed gave rise to treponemes that spread not by skin contact but by mucous membrane contact, namely, the etiologic agent of bejel or endemic syphilis.[18]

On morphologic examination, the treponemes are thin, tightly coiled organisms that do not stain or stain poorly with the usual aniline dyes. They contain 4 to 14 spirals and are actively motile by virtue of periplasmic flagella. The organisms are quite fragile and sensitive to drying, atmospheric oxygen, and temperatures above 35°C (95°F). Although limited multiplication of *T. pallidum* subspecies *pallidum* has been achieved in a tissue-culture system,[10] it has not been accomplished as yet with the nonvenereal pathogenic treponemes. Furthermore, none of the human pathogenic treponemes has been cultured in or on artificial media. They can, however, be identified by darkfield microscopy in infected skin or mucous membrane lesions.

Material should be removed aseptically and immediately examined unstained. In tissue from biopsy material, silver impregnation methods can be used to identify organisms,[25] but care must be taken to distinguish them from morphologically similar tissue artifacts. Little can be done to distinguish the various species of pathogenic treponemes. Clinical and epidemiologic features of each disease state from which the treponeme is recovered constitute the primary method of differentiation. Despite differences in methods of transmission, clinical disease, and geographic distribution, all human treponemes remain sensitive to penicillin.[51] Although not practical, further differentiation is based on the response of animal models to experimental infection.[22, 28, 40, 44, 45] Each of the pathogenic treponemes stimulates cross-reactive antibodies assayed in the serologic diagnosis of the human diseases by nontreponemal and treponemal tests. Furthermore, varying degrees of homologous resistance and cross-immunity exist after infection with any of these spirochetes.[22, 23, 31, 33, 44, 49]

Pinta

Pinta (mal del pinto, carate) is a chronic, contagious, nonvenereally transmitted treponemal disease presumed to be the most primitive of the human treponematoses. It can affect children and adults of all age groups, producing dyschromic skin lesions without pathogenic involvement of deeper organ structures. Pinta is not a fatal disease but a disfiguring one, which results in social ostracism and an inability to adjust to an urban society.

BIOLOGY AND IMMUNOLOGY

Pinta is caused by *T. carateum*, which is morphologically indistinguishable from the other pathogenic treponemes. The organism is characterized primarily by its isolation from patients with clinically apparent pinta and by its lack of pathogenicity for small laboratory animals. Only the chimpanzee has been shown to be susceptible to experimental infection.[28, 29] Human studies by Medina[33] suggest that *T. carateum* induces significant protection against homologous reinfection as well as cross-immunity against the treponemes of yaws and syphilis; however, these two subspecies of *T. pallidum* fail to confer cross-protection against *T. carateum*.[33]

EPIDEMIOLOGY

Pinta is found primarily among the primitive, underprivileged Indians of tropical Central and South America. It occurs in major river basins of Mexico, Venezuela, Colombia, Brazil, Peru, and Ecuador. Cases also have been reported in Argentina, Chile, Haiti, Guatemala, Dominican Republic, Honduras, Nicaragua, and Bolivia. Pinta rarely occurs at higher elevations in the mountain regions of these countries. Coastal areas surprisingly are devoid of the disease. In the early 1920s, approximately 500,000 cases occurred throughout Latin America; however, today, as a result of the seroepidemiologic and mass treatment campaigns, few cases have been reported.

The disease is found where poor hygienic and crowded conditions exist. Although endemic areas basically are rural, tribal tradition allows very close contact among its members. These tropical societies, with their absence of shoes and clothes, continually subject exposed skin to trauma and to contact with infectious lesions. Transmission of *T. carateum* occurs primarily by intimate skin-to-skin contact; a break in the skin is required for invasion of the treponeme. Pinta is not acquired congenitally or by blood transfusion. The proposed transmission of the disease by insect vectors has been disproved[33]; insects probably initiate disease by producing the necessary breaks in the skin.[9] Pinta is distributed equally between males and females and among all races in endemic areas. Furthermore, it is acquired primarily by young adults aged 15 to 20 years,[39] frequently spreading to family members because of crowded living conditions.

PATHOGENESIS AND PATHOLOGY

T. carateum penetrates skin through breaks in the epidermis, with resultant damage restricted to the dermal and epidermal tissues. The organisms multiply in these layers, eliciting cellular proliferation as well as a plasma cell, lymphocyte, and macrophage infiltration. The resulting primary lesion may appear on any area of exposed skin but most often occurs on the legs, the dorsum of the foot, the forearms, or the back of the hands.[39] The lesion enlarges as a result of continual progression and direct extension or by coalescing with adjacent primary lesions; occasionally, a regional lymphadenopathy develops. Secondary lesions, known as pintids, result from treponemal dissemination and exhibit a cellular proliferation and infiltration similar to that of the primary lesion. In contrast to venereal syphilis, blood vessels remain intact and do not show proliferation. The dyschromic or multicolored nature of the primary and secondary lesions is more characteristic of older than of younger lesions, in which pigmentary changes usually are minimal. The variously pigmented older lesions may show hyperkeratosis or parakeratosis. Large numbers of treponemes can be found throughout the dermis and epidermis in the highly contagious primary and secondary lesions.

Late pinta is characterized by pigmentary changes, from dyschromic treponeme-containing lesions to achromic treponeme-free lesions.[39] This depigmentation process occurs at different rates even within the same lesion, which gives rise to different degrees of hypochromia and atrophy around dyschromic and achromic lesions.[39] A concomitant lack of hair follicles and sebaceous glands may occur.[7]

CLINICAL MANIFESTATIONS

Pinta is characterized by a continuing production of early infectious lesions from either direct extension or dissemination and by the concomitant presence of lesions in various stages of dyschromia and achromia. The lesions are not well delineated, often merge, and may be accompanied by regional lymphadenopathy. Primary, secondary, and tertiary stages may or may not occur simultaneously.

The early stage of pinta includes the initial lesions, occasional regional lymphadenopathy, and secondary lesions resulting from treponemal dissemination. A primary lesion (not always evident) develops after an incubation period of 3 days to 2 months, usually 2 to 3 weeks. The primary lesion begins as one or more small erythematous papules that may appear scaly and indurated. The papules progressively enlarge during the course of 1 to 3 months, often coalescing, becoming pigmented and more scaly and erythematous, and developing heaped-up margins. Occasionally, an accompanying regional lymphadenopathy is present. The lesion may disappear in several months or may continue to enlarge for several years, forming larger psoriasiform plaques that coalesce further.

The primary lesions of pinta generally overlap development of the secondary lesions or pintids, which appear 3 to 9 months after infection. During this stage, dissemination occurs, and almost any area of the skin can be involved. The lesions occur typically on exposed areas of skin and are variously pigmented. The degree of pigmentation is related to the state of lesion development, the age of the lesion, the degree of sun exposure, and the host's natural pigmentation. Pintids begin as small, scaly papules that gradually enlarge and coalesce. Several colors may exist within the same lesion. Initially, pintids usually are red to violaceous; later, they become slate blue, gray, or black as a result of photosensitization. Lesions on the legs typically are yellowish brown or dark brown.

Serologic surveys suggest that a latent form of pinta exists, although it has not been established clearly.[8]

The late stage of pinta is characterized by the development of depigmented lesions. Achromia usually begins several years after the onset of the disease but may appear as early as 3 months. Areas of depigmentation spread slowly, leaving large achromic lesions as the end result. Early achromia tends to be asymmetric, whereas later depigmented lesions are symmetric. Characteristic of the Cuban form of pinta is the development of hyperkeratosis of the palms and soles.

DIAGNOSIS

A presumptive diagnosis of pinta is based on the typical clinical presentation of a patient from a known endemic area. Laboratory tests are essential in characterizing pinta as a treponemal disease and include darkfield examination of early lesions and serologic tests for syphilis.

Darkfield examination of fluid obtained from the initial lesion or from pintids generally reveals the presence of treponemes. As the lesions become achromic, treponemes are more difficult to find. For all practical purposes, achromic lesions are devoid of organisms. Silver impregnation of biopsy material from skin lesions or lymph nodes may reveal the organisms, but care must be taken in differentiating treponemes from tissue artifact. Both the nontreponemal and treponemal tests, originally designed for use in venereal syphilis, may not become reactive until as late as 4 months after the development of the initial lesion. Reactivity with these assays points to the antigenic cross-reactivity among the pathogenic treponemes and the inability to differentiate among the treponematoses solely on this basis.[39] Furthermore, an important note is that the nontreponemal tests are, at best, screening procedures; false-positive reactions caused by a variety of conditions and nontreponemal diseases can occur.[36] Many chronic dermatologic entities characterized by scaly, psoriasiform lesions or by dyschromia or depigmentation can be confused with pinta in endemic areas. Maculopapulosquamous diseases, including psoriasis, parapsoriasis and lichen planus, as well as such dyschromic dermatologic diseases as vitiligo, ochronosis, and argyria, must be taken into consideration. Combined nontreponemal and treponemal tests will aid greatly in the differentiation.

PROGNOSIS

Pinta is not a fatal disease; it produces changes related only to the skin. Untreated, the patient frequently develops large achromic cutaneous blemishes. The major resulting problem is one of social ostracism from the community. These infected members are removed from the urban society and find refuge in the rural areas. This isolation further separates the patient from the principal sources of medical therapy.

TREATMENT AND PREVENTION

The treatment of choice is benzathine penicillin G; those older than 10 years of age with clinical disease in a period of latency or in the incubatory stage and contacts of cases should receive 1.2 million units of benzathine penicillin G intramuscularly in a single dose; children younger than 10 years of age should receive 600,000 units in a single dose by the same route.[39, 53] Tetracycline is the antibiotic of choice for penicillin-allergic patients older than 8 years of age and not pregnant. The recommended dose is 500 mg by mouth four times daily for 15 days (total dose of 30 g)[39]; children between 8 and 15 years of age may be given one half the dose.[39] Studies to determine the effectiveness of erythromycin have not been reported, although the same dosage and route as recommended for tetracycline probably are effective for those 8 years of age or older[39]; those younger than 8 years of age should be given doses adjusted for their body weight.[39]

The clinical response to therapy is remarkably slow in pinta. Primary and early secondary lesions take 4 to 6 months to disappear, whereas late secondary lesions require 6 to 12 months for complete healing to occur.[41] Hyperchromic lesions heal without residua, and hypochromic lesions often result in depigmented areas. Old achromic lesions usually remain intact without repigmentation. In general, the serologic response to therapy is absent or slow in pinta. Treponemal tests tend to remain reactive for life; nontreponemal tests may take years to decline after adequate therapy.[34]

Early campaigns to eradicate pinta proved that the prevalence of the disease could be reduced significantly by improving personal hygiene, by initiating mass treatment of patients and contacts with penicillin, and by initiating seroepidemiologic campaigns.

Yaws

Yaws (framboesia, pian, buba, bouba) is a communicable, nonvenereally transmitted treponematosis of the tropical zones. The disease is characterized by its early acquisition (usually before puberty) and its chronic, relapsing pattern of early benign lesions separated by periods of latency that terminate with late destructive lesions of skin, bones, and cartilaginous tissues.

Historically, yaws is another ancient treponematosis that, in theory, arose around 10,000 BC in Africa and Asia from a mutant form of pinta more suitable to tropical climates. From here, the disease was brought to the Americas by

African slaves and occurs today almost exclusively among their descendants. The interesting distribution of yaws in South America, for example, corresponds to the distribution of people of African descent.[18] A very prevalent disease in the early part of this century, yaws was estimated to have affected more than 50 million people. Although seroepidemiologic and mass treatment campaigns sponsored by the WHO and UNICEF have reduced its overall prevalence drastically,[16] endemic areas of concern continue to exist.[39, 53]

BIOLOGY AND IMMUNOLOGY

T. pallidum subspecies *pertenue*, the etiologic agent of yaws, is morphologically identical to other pathogenic treponemes. The organisms can be stored in either 15 percent glycerol at −70°C (−94°F) or liquid nitrogen and still retain their virulence for long periods.[25, 48] Rabbits experimentally infected by both the intratesticular and intradermal routes produce visible lesions and regional lymphadenopathy.[22, 48] However, four features commonly observed in experimental yaws infection differentiate it from experimental syphilis in the rabbit: (1) the relative absence of induration in the initial testicular lesions; (2) small focal lesions in or immediately beneath the visceral tunic of the testis, which give rise to a granular periorchitis; (3) the relative absence of induration in initial skin lesions; and (4) the relative scarcity of generalized (metastatic) lesions.[48] Both outbred and inbred hamsters can be infected experimentally with yaws treponeme strains by the intradermal route in the groin, with the production of chronic, ulcerative skin lesions and, in most cases, generalized lymphadenopathy.[22, 44, 48] In contrast, intradermal groin infection of hamsters with *T. pallidum* subspecies *pallidum* rarely produces skin lesions but consistently results in generalized lymphadenopathy with larger numbers of treponemes within the nodes.[22, 45, 48]

On the basis of human and experimental studies, the organism stimulates a significant degree of homologous resistance to reinfection and superinfection as well as cross-immunity to *T. pallidum* subspecies *pallidum* and *endemicum*.[22, 26, 32, 44, 48]

EPIDEMIOLOGY

Yaws is a disease of tropical countries found primarily among the rural populations. It exists in the warm, moist, endemic areas of rural Africa, Southeast Asia, the Caribbean, and central and southern Africa. As indicated, seroepidemiologic and mass treatment campaigns have resulted in a significant reduction in prevalence of the disease in most of these areas. However, the failure of many countries to integrate active control measures into the functions of local health services has led to a gradual build-up and extension of yaws reservoirs, with the emergence of significant numbers of new, active cases since 1974 in Ghana, Togo, Benin, Indonesia, and the Ivory Coast.[53] In a WHO survey in the Central African Republic, Congo, and Gabori, clinical yaws was detected in more than 20 percent of the Pygmy population, and reactive serologic tests were obtained in 80 percent.[53]

Poor hygiene, close crowding among children (especially in sleeping areas), and lack of protective clothing facilitate transmission of the disease by direct skin-to-skin contact, whereby *T. pallidum* subspecies *pertenue* enters traumatized exposed areas from an infected lesion. The usual portals of entry are the lower extremities, head, face, and mouth. The presence of treponemal antibodies and isolation of treponemes (most probably *T. pallidum* subspecies *pertenue* from West African monkeys[2, 11]) suggest the possibility that primates in this area may act as a reservoir for spread of the disease.

Yaws usually is acquired before puberty and, therefore, is most prevalent among children. Because such a large percentage of the population contracts the disease in infancy, young children represent the primary reservoir. Older children and adults generally are not infectious; therefore, congenital and sexual transmission does not occur. Both males and females are affected equally.

PATHOGENESIS AND PATHOLOGY

T. pallidum subspecies *pertenue* enters the host through abraded skin, most frequently below the knees. The organisms multiply locally and in the regional lymph nodes; epithelial hyperplasia and plasma cell, lymphocytic, and macrophage infiltration are elicited. The end result is the formation of a primary lesion and lymphadenopathy containing numerous treponemes. Shortly after their introduction into the host, organisms are carried to skin, bone, and cartilage through the circulation. Disseminated treponemes in these tissues multiply; elicit a chronic inflammatory response similar to that seen in the primary lesion; and produce distant papillomas, lymphadenopathy, hyperkeratosis, and bone involvement that develop uninterruptedly until they are reversed by either immune mechanisms or treatment. In contrast to those associated with venereal syphilis, vascular changes are discrete or do not occur in cutaneous yaws.

The untreated primary and secondary cutaneous lesions generally heal with only minimal scarring unless they are complicated by secondary bacterial infection. The healing process and maintenance of latency appear to involve both humoral and cellular mechanisms of immunity.[43] Relapses may occur during latency and, together with late disease, may be caused by a breakdown in the immune state, the development of antigenic variation by the treponeme, or both.

The late gummatous lesions are thought to be caused by a hypersensitivity-induced mechanism similar to that postulated for the syphilitic gumma. Bone changes in late yaws most often involve the long bones and manifest as hypertrophic periostitis, gummatous periostitis, osteitis, and nodular or generalized osteomyelitis.[19] Juxtaarticular nodules occur near major joints and are characterized as nonspecific granulomata.[6]

CLINICAL MANIFESTATIONS

Yaws is a chronic, debilitating disease characterized by early infectious lesions; periods of latency and relapse; and late destructive lesions of cutaneous, subcutaneous, cartilaginous, and bony tissue. After an incubation period of 9 to 90 days (usually about 3 weeks), the primary lesion forms at the site of inoculation and is accompanied by regional lymphadenopathy. The lesion typically appears as a raised papule that enlarges to become a hyperkeratotic papilloma measuring 2 to 5 cm in diameter, referred to as a *mother yaw*. It undergoes shallow ulceration and persists from a few months to as long as 3 years, at which time healing occurs with a resultant hypopigmented scar.[6]

Before or weeks to months after healing of the mother yaw, crops of secondary, generalized, nondestructive papular lesions appear together with lymphadenopathy and malaise. Some papules fade, whereas others enlarge to become papillomatous lesions referred to as *satellite secondaries* or *daughter yaws*. The multiple papillomas are circular, raised, red-yellow lesions with a granular, lobulated, and verrucous surface. They contain numerous treponemes, usually measure 1 to 3 cm in diameter, and produce a yellow discharge that dries to form a black scab. Hyperkeratotic involvement of the palms and soles occurs commonly. Painful fissuring of the soles may cause the patient to walk on the sides of the feet, thus producing the characteristic gait of crab yaws.[6] Bone pain may be severe, and nondestructive long bone lesions, including periostitis, osteitis, and osteomyelitis, may occur.[6, 17]

Untreated secondary lesions may persist for longer than 6 months, at which time, owing to the development of host immune mechanisms, they usually heal without scars or residual defects unless ulceration caused by secondary bacterial infection occurs. Of note is that during the dry season, early yaws lesions often are atypical, tending to be macular and fewer in number; papillomas, which are small, scanty, dry, flat, and grayish in appearance and of short duration (about 1 month), are confined mainly to the hidden, protected, moist skin folds.[37, 39, 50]

Despite healing, some treponemes evade the immune process and persist in the affected tissues (latency). Latency frequently is interrupted by relapses, which tend to occur several times over a 3- to 5-year period. Fewer lesions are produced with each relapse, and they tend to be localized to the periaxillary, perianal, or circumoral area.[39] After cessation of the relapses and usually after a latent period of 3 to several years, tertiary lesions occur in as many as 10 percent of patients[39]; the latent state persists in the remaining patients for their lifetime.

The tertiary lesions characteristically are solitary and destructive; they involve skin, subcutaneous tissue, bone, or cartilage and most commonly occur after the onset of puberty. Painful hyperkeratosis of the palms and soles similar to that seen in early yaws frequently occurs. Other lesions develop as ulcerating, subcutaneous nodules and may heal spontaneously to form scars or extend widely from their margins. The scarring results in depigmentation and, at times, contractions. Bone deformities of late yaws include chronic hypertrophic periostitis, osteitis, gummatous periostitis, and osteomyelitis, each of which may ulcerate through the skin.[19] Gangosa, or rhinopharyngitis mutilans, the destructive gummatous ulceration of the skin and bones of the central face, as well as juxtaarticular nodules, ganglions of tendon sheaths, and sabre tibiae, also may occur as manifestations of the late disease.[19] Gondou, a hypertrophic osteitis of the frontal processes of the maxillae once commonly seen among western Africans with yaws, is not a proven manifestation of the disease.[6]

DIAGNOSIS

As with the other nonvenereal treponematoses, a presumptive diagnosis is based largely on clinical presentation of the disease in an endemic area. The diagnosis of yaws in nonendemic areas or during periods of latency is difficult to make. Although darkfield examination of early lesions and lymph nodes permits visualization of treponemes, late lesions usually contain few, if any, organisms. Silver impregnation of biopsy material from late lesions or lymph nodes may reveal treponemes, but again, care must be taken in differentiating the organisms from tissue artifact.

Nontreponemal and treponemal tests for syphilis become reactive during the first few weeks of illness, a reflection, again, of the shared antigens of pathogenic treponemes. As previously indicated, care must be taken in the use of only nontreponemal tests in diagnosis because of the possibility of false-positive reactions among patients with nontreponemal diseases or conditions.[36] Furthermore, differentiating the treponematoses from one another solely on the basis of serologic testing is not possible because of shared antigens.[12, 39] The coexistence of yaws and endemic syphilis in certain geographic locations, together with their often identical clinical manifestations, renders both darkfield and serologic assays useless for differentiating these diseases in such areas.[39] Similar limitations are applicable in differentiating venereal syphilis from yaws or endemic syphilis in nonendemic areas.[39] Under these circumstances, the diagnosis can be based only on a careful history and epidemiologic data.[39] In tropical areas, numerous other diseases may be confused with yaws.[21, 39] Impetigo and chronic tropical ulcers are found frequently and usually respond to penicillin therapy. Ecthyma may produce ulcers that occasionally are similar to the ulcerative papillomas of yaws. Other diseases that must be differentiated from yaws skin lesions include vitamin deficiencies, early leprosy, venereal syphilis, tinea versicolor, molluscum contagiosum, scabies, lichen planus, plantar warts, tungiasis, psoriasis, and cutaneous leishmaniasis. Sickle-cell disease, tuberculosis, and bacterial osteomyelitis may produce clinical manifestations that mimic the bone lesions of yaws. Combined nontreponemal and treponemal tests aid greatly in the differentiation.

PROGNOSIS

Yaws is not a benign disease. If left untreated, it can produce destructive, disfiguring lesions of the face, feet, and hands, as well as disabling and painful lesions of the fingers and long bones. Ulcers near joints may result in crippling contractures. Secondary bacterial infection of ulcers and of protruding bone lesions can result in further permanent damage to skin and bone tissues. Fractures generally are not a problem.

TREATMENT AND PREVENTION

As with pinta, the treatment of choice is benzathine penicillin G; those older than 10 years of age with clinical disease, in a period of latency, or in the incubatory stages, as well as contacts of cases, should receive 1.2 million units of benzathine penicillin G intramuscularly in a single dose; children younger than 10 years of age should receive 600,000 units in a single dose by the same route.[39, 53] Tetracycline is the antibiotic of choice for penicillin-allergic patients older than 8 years of age and not pregnant. The recommended dosage is 500 mg by mouth four times daily for 15 days (total dose of 30 g)[39]; children between 8 and 15 years of age may be given one-half the dose.[39] Studies to determine the efficacy of erythromycin have not been reported, although the same dosage and route as recommended for tetracycline probably are effective for those 8 years of age or older[39]; those younger than 8 years of age should be given doses adjusted for their body weight.[39]

Therapy renders early lesions noninfectious in a few days, with complete healing in 7 to 10 days. Recurrences after treatment may occur as a result of reinfection.[20] Late lesions heal more slowly after therapy and may require surgery. Nontreponemal test titers may revert to nonreactive if the patient is treated early in the course of the disease. However, the longer the patient remains untreated, the more slowly conversion to seronegativity occurs.[5] As with each of the treponemal diseases, treponemal tests remain reactive for life after adequate therapy.

Improvement of living conditions and the general hygiene of the community, mass treatment of patients and contacts, and seroepidemiologic campaigns contribute significantly to the prevention of yaws.

Endemic Syphilis

Endemic syphilis (bejel, njovera, siti, dichuchwa) is a chronic, nonvenereally transmitted disease of prepubescent children. It occurs in the warm, dry, arid regions of the world[39]; lesions are confined to the skin, bone, and cartilage. The disease, known to exist for centuries in Africa, has been recorded in epidemic proportions in areas where conditions among children allow transmission. As with yaws, although seroepidemiologic and mass treatment campaigns have reduced its overall prevalence drastically,[16, 39] endemic areas of concern continue to exist.[38, 39, 53]

BIOLOGY AND IMMUNOLOGY

T. pallidum subspecies *endemicum*, the etiologic agent of endemic syphilis, morphologically is identical to the other pathogenic treponemes. Like *T. pallidum* subspecies *pallidum* and *pertenue*, the organisms can be stored in 15 percent glycerol at −70°C (−94°F) or in liquid nitrogen and still retain their virulence for long periods.[25, 48] *T. pallidum* subspecies *endemicum* exhibits further similarity to these treponemes by producing visible lesions and generalized lymphadenopathy in rabbits experimentally infected by the intratesticular and intradermal routes.[22, 48] However, the degree of lesion induration generally is less than that observed in *T. pallidum* subspecies *pallidum* infection, whereas the frequency of granular periorchitis is intermediate between that seen with strains of yaws and venereal syphilis treponemes.[22, 48] As with *T. pallidum* subspecies *pertenue* infection, but in contrast to infection with *T. pallidum* subspecies *pallidum*, generalized (metastatic) lesions have not been observed in the rabbit.[22] Further similarities to the yaws treponeme are evidenced by the response of hamsters to infection. Both outbred and inbred hamsters can be infected experimentally by the intradermal route in the groin, with the production of chronic, ulcerative skin lesions and generalized lymphadenopathy.[22, 45, 48] However, as indicated earlier, infection of hamsters with *T. pallidum* subspecies *pallidum* by the same route rarely produces skin lesions but consistently results in generalized lymphadenopathy with large numbers of treponemes in the nodes.[22, 45, 48]

On the basis of experimental studies in inbred hamsters, *T. pallidum* subspecies *endemicum* stimulates a high degree of homologous resistance to reinfection as well as cross-immunity to *T. pallidum* subspecies *pallidum* and *pertenue*.[45]

EPIDEMIOLOGY

Endemic syphilis continues to persist in the warm, drier desert areas bordering the tropical belt. It is prevalent primarily among the seminomadic rural populations in the Arabian peninsula and along the southern border of the Sahara desert in Africa known as the Sahel region[38, 39]; a significant resurgence occurred in Mali, Mauritania, Niger, and the upper Volta during the 1970s.[39, 53] Although scattered endemic foci did exist in central Asia, Australia, the former Yugoslavia, and India, they now virtually have been eliminated from these areas by mass treatment campaigns.[38, 39]

As with pinta and yaws, endemic syphilis propagates under conditions of poor hygiene, crowding, and little or no clothing. Oral mucous membrane transmission is favored through contaminated objects, such as drinking vessels and kitchen utensils, as well as through contact with saliva-contaminated fingers and mouth-to-mouth contact.[4, 24] Transmission may occur through direct oral lesion–to-skin contact.[39] Occasionally, a previously uninfected nursing mother will develop a primary lesion on or near the nipple after the transfer of treponemes from her infected infant.[14, 52] Congenital transmission does not occur, and the role of insect vectors, such as flies, is uncertain.

Endemic syphilis occurs predominantly among children, with onset usually in those younger than 15 years of age[4] and with equal sex distribution. Spread occurs most commonly within the family, and active disease can be present in more than one family member at any given time.

PATHOGENESIS AND PATHOLOGY

T. pallidum subspecies *endemicum* enters the host most often through the oral mucosa. The relatively small number of treponemes introduced into a susceptible host usually precludes the local multiplication and host inflammatory response required to produce a visible primary buccal lesion.[14] When a primary lesion does occur, it appears as a papule or ulcer resulting from a chronic inflammatory response to the proliferating organisms consisting of plasma cell, lymphocytic, and macrophage infiltration. Endothelial cell swelling of small blood vessels also is evident.

The organisms are carried to the regional lymph nodes within a few hours of entry, commonly into the oral mucosa portal entry. They multiply and elicit epithelial hyperplasia as well as plasma cell, lymphocytic, and macrophage infiltration, with resultant lymphadenopathy. Dissemination occurs through the circulation, and the organisms are carried to the skin, bone, oral mucosa, axillae, and anogenital regions, where they multiply and elicit a chronic inflammatory response characterized by a cellular infiltration, as seen in the lymph nodes. Vascular changes and perivascular cuffing are prominent.

The untreated early lesions heal as a result of mechanisms thought to involve both humoral and cellular immune responses by the host,[42] and the disease enters into a state of latency. Maintenance of latency is thought to involve similar mechanisms. The occurrence of infectious relapses during the latent period still is uncertain.

The late lesions of endemic syphilis are strikingly similar to those of late yaws. Both late disease and relapses (if they occur) may be due to a hypersensitivity-induced mechanism similar to that postulated for the syphilitic gumma.[14, 15] Juxtaarticular nodules may occur and represent a nonspecific granulomatous response occurring near major joints.[6] The rarity of cardiovascular and neurologic manifestations may be due to the slow acquisition of small numbers of organisms over a long period, which results in the immunologic protection of the heart and nervous system.[14, 30]

CLINICAL MANIFESTATIONS

Endemic syphilis is a chronic, often debilitating disease characterized by early infectious secondary lesions, variable periods of latency, and late destructive lesions of cutaneous, subcutaneous, and bone tissues. As indicated, primary lesions are rare findings. They appear usually on the breast or nipple as a papule or shallow ulcer similar to that seen in primary venereal syphilis after an approximate 3-week incubation period[1]; they may persist for years before healing.[24]

Even without the appearance of a primary lesion, generalized infection occurs as a result of early dissemination. The onset begins after an incubation period thought to approximate that of secondary venereal syphilis and is characterized by the presence of highly infectious, relatively painless, ulcerative mucous patches on the oropharyngeal mucosa, including the tongue, lips, palate, tonsils, and larynx, with accompanying regional lymphadenopathy. Involvement of the larynx usually results in hoarseness.[6] Split papules or angular stomatitis occurs at the angles of the mouth. Osteoperiostitis of the long bones of the lower extremities, similar to that seen in yaws, is a common early manifestation causing nocturnal leg pains.[6] Occasionally, axillary and anogenital secondary-type lesions result, which consist of condylomata similar to yaws or dry papilloma annular patches, with accompanying axillary and inguinal lymphadenopathy. Disseminated papules that are indistinguishable from those seen in secondary venereal syphilis may occur. Other forms of cutaneous lesions can occur but are rare.

Untreated secondary lesions may persist for 6 to 9 months, at which time healing occurs because of the development of host immunity. This period of latency is variable and, like yaws, may last for 3 to several years.

Most patients develop tertiary manifestations. Late lesions generally occur during adolescence or adult life and may resemble those seen in either late yaws or late venereal syphilis. Gummata may affect any part of the body but commonly occur in the nasopharynx, skin, and bone, resulting in destructive, disfiguring, chronic ulcerations characteristic of gangosa or gangosa-like lesions. Late gummatous lesions can occur during childhood, possibly as a result of superinfection in an already infected host.[13] Bone involvement also is a common finding and results in painful lesions. This condition involves osteitis with gumma formation and, like yaws, periostitis affecting most frequently the long bones of the lower extremities. Bilateral synovitis, especially of the knees, occasionally may occur with concomitant juxtaarticular nodules.[13] The cardiovascular and neurologic findings common to venereal syphilis rarely occur in endemic syphilis; when clinical manifestations do occur, they usually are atypical and very mild.[3]

Endemic syphilis appears to have become "clinically attenuated" in Saudi Arabia.[38] Once florid, the classic disease seems to have been replaced by a milder form in which the number, severity, and duration of both early and late lesions are reduced and seroreactive latent infection is increased.[38] The most common late manifestation observed in this study was painful osteoperiostitis of the legs affecting mainly the tibia and fibula. Researchers have postulated that attenuation has occurred owing to improvement in hygienic conditions, with resultant less reexposure to potential superinfection.[38]

DIAGNOSIS

Endemic syphilis, like pinta and yaws, is diagnosed presumptively from the typical clinical presentation of patients living in known endemic areas. The diagnosis of the disease as a treponemal infection can be confirmed by the darkfield examination of serous exudate from mucous membrane or cutaneous lesions and by the use of both nontreponemal and treponemal serologic tests. Seroreactivity approaches 100 percent in patients presenting with clinical manifestations characteristic of early secondary endemic syphilis. It bears repeating, however, that the coexistence of yaws and endemic syphilis in certain geographic locations, together with their often indistinguishable clinical manifestations, renders both darkfield and serologic assays useless for differentiating these diseases in such areas.[39] Similarly, in nonendemic areas, venereal syphilis may not be distinguishable from yaws or endemic syphilis by the use of these laboratory procedures. In these circumstances, the diagnosis can be based only on a careful case history and epidemiologic data.[39] The same nontreponemal diseases that can simulate the clinical manifestations of yaws and venereal syphilis also can confuse the diagnosis of endemic syphilis, which again stresses the importance of using both nontreponemal and treponemal serologic tests in the differential diagnosis.

PROGNOSIS

The main complication of endemic syphilis is the destructive gummatous lesions of the face and bones. Severely disfiguring and disabling, these lesions prevent the patient from working effectively in the community. Many of the bone lesions are extremely painful and incapacitating. The prognosis for the rare cardiovascular and neurologic manifestations is unknown.

TREATMENT AND PREVENTION

Like the other pathogenic human treponemes, *T. pallidum* subspecies *endemicum* is highly susceptible to penicillin G. It should be administered to those older than 10 years of age with clinical disease, in a period of latency, or in the incubatory stage and to contacts of cases as the long-acting benzathine penicillin G in a single intramuscular dose of 1.2 million units; children younger than 10 years of age should be given 600,000 units in a single dose by the same route.[39, 53] In the penicillin-allergic patient older than 8 years of age and not pregnant, tetracycline is the antibiotic of choice. The recommended dose is 500 mg by mouth, four times daily for 15 days (total dose of 30 g)[39]; children between 8 and 15 years of age may be given half the dose.[39] Studies to determine the efficacy of erythromycin have not been reported, although the same dosage and route as recommended for tetracycline probably are effective for those 8 years of age or older[39]; those younger than 8 years of age should be given doses adjusted for their body weight.[39]

Infectious lesions rapidly disappear, and relapses usually are prevented after therapy. As in yaws, nontreponemal test titers may revert to nonreactive if the patient is treated early in the course of the disease. However, treatment during the later stages may result in the persistence of relatively high titers.[5] As with each of the treponemal diseases, treponemal tests remain reactive for life after adequate therapy.

Control of the disease in endemic areas requires mass treatment and seroepidemiologic campaigns coupled with an improvement in the hygiene of the community.

REFERENCES

1. Akrawi, F.: Is bejel syphilis? Br. J. Vener. Dis. *25*:115–123, 1949.
2. Baylet, R., Thivolet, J., Sepetjian, M., et al.: La treponematose naturelle ouverte du singe *Papio papio* en Casamance. Bull. Soc. Pathol. Exot. *64*:842–846, 1971.
3. Csonka, G. W.: Clinical aspects of bejel. Br. J. Vener. Dis. *29*:95–103, 1953.
4. Cutler, J. C.: Endemic syphilis, yaws, and pinta. *In* Johnson, R. C. (ed.): The Biology of Parasitic Spirochetes. New York, Academic Press, 1976, pp. 365–373.

5. Demis, D. J.: Nonsyphilitic treponematoses. *In* Hoeprich, P. D. (ed.): Infectious Diseases. New York, Harper & Row, 1977, pp. 823–835.
6. Dooley, J. R., and Binford, C. H.: Treponematoses. *In* Binford, C. H., and Connor, D. H. (eds.): Pathology of Tropical and Extraordinary Diseases. Vol. 1. Washington, DC, Armed Forces Institute of Pathology, 1976, pp. 10–117.
7. Edmundson, W. F.: Pinta. *In* Demis, D. J., Dobson, R. C., and McGuire, J. (eds.): Clinical Dermatology. Vol. 3. New York, Harper & Row, 1976, pp. 1–12.
8. Edmundson, W. F., Demis, D. J., and Bejarino, G.: A clinico-serologic study of pinta in the Alto Beni Region, Bolivia. Dermatol. Int. *6*:64–76, 1967.
9. Edmundson, W. F., Lopez Rico, A., and Olansky, S.: A study of pinta in the Tepalcatepec Basin, Michoacan, Mexico. Am. J. Syph. *37*:201–225, 1953.
10. Fieldsteel, A. H., Cox, D. L., and Moeckli, R. A.: Cultivation of virulent *Treponema pallidum* in tissue culture. Infect. Immun. *32*:908–915, 1981.
11. Fribourg-Blanc, A., Niel, G., and Mollaret, H. H.: Note sur quelques aspects immunologiques du cynocephale african. Bull. Soc. Pathol. Exot. *56*:474–485, 1963.
12. Garner, M. F., Backhouse, J. L., Cook, C. A., et al.: Fluorescent treponemal antibody absorption (FTA-ABS) test in yaws. Br. J. Vener. Dis. *46*: 284–286, 1970.
13. Grin, E. I.: Endemic syphilis (bejel). *In* Demis, D. J., Dobson, R. C., and McGuire, J. (eds.): Clinical Dermatology. Vol. 3. New York, Harper & Row, 1976, pp. 1–7.
14. Grin, E. I.: Epidemiology and control of endemic syphilis. W. H. O. Monogr. Ser. *11*, 1953.
15. Guthe, T., and Luger, A.: Epidemiologic aspects of nonvenereal endemic syphilis. Dermatologica *115*:248–272, 1957.
16. Guthe, T., and Wilcox, R. R.: Changing concepts in the epidemiology and control of the treponematoses. Chron. W. H. O., Special Number *8*:33–69, 1954.
17. Hackett, C. J.: Bone Lesions of Yaws in Uganda. Oxford, Blackwell Scientific Publications, 1951.
18. Hackett, C. J.: On the origin of the human treponematoses. Bull. W. H. O. *29*:7–41, 1963.
19. Hackett, C. J.: Yaws. *In* Demis, D. J., Dobson, R. C., and McGuire, J. (eds.): Clinical Dermatology. Vol. 3. New York, Harper & Row, 1976, pp. 1–19.
20. Hackett, C. J., and Guthe, T.: Some important aspects of yaws eradication. Bull. W. H. O. *15*:869–896, 1956.
21. Hackett, C. J., and Loewenthal, L. J. A.: Differential diagnosis of yaws. W. H. O. Monogr. Ser. *45*:1–88, 1960.
22. Hardy, P. H.: Pathogenic treponemes. *In* Johnson, R. C. (ed.): The Biology of Parasitic Spirochetes. New York, Academic Press, 1976, pp. 107–119.
23. Hill, K. R.: Non-specific factors in the epidemiology of yaws. Bull. W. H. O. *8*:17–47, 1953.
24. Hudson, E. H.: Non-venereal Syphilis. Edinburgh, E. & S. Livingstone, Ltd., 1958.
25. Kelly, R. T.: Treponema. *In* Lennette, E. H., Spaulding, E. H., and Truant, J. P. (eds.): Manual of Clinical Microbiology. Washington, DC, American Society for Microbiology, 1975, pp. 358–360.
26. Knox, J. M., Musher, D., and Guzick, N. D.: The pathogenesis of syphilis and the related treponematoses. *In* Johnson, R. C. (ed.): The Biology of Parasitic Spirochetes. New York, Academic Press, 1976, pp. 249–259.
27. Krieg, N. R., and Holt, J. G. (eds.): Bergey's Manual of Systematic Bacteriology. Vol. 1. Baltimore/London, Williams & Wilkins, 1984, p. 50.
28. Kuhn, U. S. G., III, Medina, R., Cohen, P. G., et al.: Inoculation pinta in chimpanzees. Br. J. Vener. Dis. *46*:311–312, 1970.
29. Kuhn, U. S. G., III, Varela, G., Chandler, Jr., F. W., et al.: Experimental pinta in the chimpanzee. J. A. M. A. *206*:829, 1968.
30. Luger, A., and Schmid, E. E.: Immunity of the central nervous system in endemic syphilis. Dermatol. Wochenschr. *143*:617–637, 1961.
31. Magnuson, H. J., Thomas, E. W., Olansky, M. D., et al.: Inoculation syphilis in human volunteers. Medicine *35*:33–82, 1956.
32. McLeod, C. P., and Magnuson, H. J.: Study of cross-immunity between syphilis and yaws in treated rabbits. J. Vener. Dis. Infect. *32*:305–309, 1951.
33. Medina, R.: Pinta in South America. *In* Fogarty International Center Symposium Documents: Yaws and Other Endemic Treponematoses. April 16–18, 1984.
34. Mesa, J., Restrepo, A., and Cortes, A.: A study of fluorescent treponemal antibody absorption (FTA-ABS) and VDRL tests in pinta. Int. J. Dermatol. *12*:135–138, 1973.
35. Miao, R. M., and Fieldsteel, A. H.: Genetic relationship between *Treponema pallidum* and *Treponema pertenue*, two noncultivable human pathogens. J. Bacteriol. *141*:427–429, 1980.
36. Miller, J. N.: Value and limitations of nontreponemal and treponemal tests in the laboratory diagnosis of syphilis. Clin. Obstet. Gynecol. *18*:191–203, 1975.
37. Niemal, P. L. A., Brunings, E. A., and Menke, H. E.: Attenuated yaws in Surinam. Br. J. Vener. Dis. *55*:99–101, 1979.
38. Pace, J. L., and Csonka, G. W.: Endemic non-venereal syphilis (bejel) in Saudi Arabia. Br. J. Vener. Dis. *60*:293–297, 1984.
39. Perine, P. L., Hopkins, D. R., Niemel, P. L. A., et al.: Handbook of Endemic Treponematoses. Geneva, World Health Organization, 1984.
40. Pierce, C. S., Wicher, K., and Nakeeb, S.: Experimental syphilis: Guinea pig model. Br. J. Vener. Dis. *59*:157–168, 1983.
41. Rein, C. R.: Bacteriologic and serologic aspects of pinta. Am. J. Syph. *38*:336–340, 1954.
42. Schell, R. F., Chan, J. K., and LeFrock, J. L.: Endemic syphilis: Passive transfer of resistance with serum and cells in hamsters. J. Infect. Dis. *140*:378–383, 1979.
43. Schell, R. F., LeFrock, J. L., and Babu, J. P.: Passive transfer of resistance to frambesial infection in hamsters. Infect. Immun. *21*:430–435, 1978.
44. Schell, R. F., LeFrock, J. L., Babu, J. P., et al.: Use of CB hamster in the study of *Treponema pertenue*. Br. J. Vener. Dis. *55*:316–319, 1979.
45. Schell, R. F., LeFrock, J. L., Chan, J. K., et al.: LSH hamster model of syphilitic infection. Infect. Immun. *28*:909–913, 1980.
46. Schöbl, O., and Miyao, I.: Immunologic relation between yaws and syphilis. Philipp. J. Sci. *40*:91–109, 1929.
47. Turner, T. B.: The resistance of yaws and syphilis patients to reinoculation with yaws spirochetes. Am. J. Hyg. *23*:431–448, 1936.
48. Turner, T. B., and Hollander, D. H.: Biology of the Treponematoses. Geneva, World Health Organization, 1957.
49. Turner, T. B., McLeod, C. P., and Updyke, E. L.: Crossimmunity in experimental syphilis, yaws, and venereal spirochetosis of rabbits. Am. J. Hyg. *46*:287–295, 1947.
50. Vorst, F. A.: Attenuating endemic treponematoses. Thesis, University of Amsterdam, 1974.
51. Wilcox, R. R.: Changing patterns of treponemal disease. Br. J. Vener. Dis. *50*:169–178, 1974.
52. Wilcox, R. R.: Endemic syphilis in Africa. S. Afr. Med. J. *25*:501–504, 1951.
53. WHO Technical Report Series No. 674: Treponemal Infections. Geneva, World Health Organization, 1982.

ANAEROBIC BACTERIA

CHAPTER 152 Clostridial Intoxication and Infection

ARMANDO G. CORREA

Clostridia are obligate anaerobic, spore-forming bacilli that usually are positive on Gram stain. Of the more than 80 species of *Clostridium,* at least 14 are potentially pathogenic in humans, mostly by virtue of their biologically active proteins (toxins). These ubiquitous organisms frequently are found in soil, sewage, decaying tissue, and the intestinal tract of humans and other animals.[10] Human disease caused by *Clostridium tetani* is discussed in Chapter 154.

Botulism

Botulism is an acute descending flaccid paralysis that results when the neurotoxin of *Clostridium botulinum* blocks neuromuscular transmission. Five clinical forms of botulism have been identified: infant (the most common), *"classic"* or food-borne, wound, hidden or "unclassified," and inadvertent. The fourth category, hidden or "unclassified," was created by the Centers for Disease Control and Prevention (CDC) for adult patients who lack an apparent food or wound source of botulinum toxin[9] and whose cases hypothetically may have an infant-type pathogenesis.[1] Inadvertent botulism, the form of botulism most recently recognized, is an unintended consequence of the treatment of certain movement disorders (such as dystonia) with botulinum toxin A. Recently, the potential use of botulinum toxin as a bioterrorist agent has become an important concern. Infant botulism is discussed in Chapter 153.

EPIDEMIOLOGY AND ETIOLOGY

Seven antigenically distinct types of botulinum toxin are designated by the letters A through G. Disease in humans is caused by toxin types A, B, E, F (rarely), and possibly G.[4, 12, 16, 17, 26, 27, 31, 35, 37] Types C and D cause botulism in animals.[16, 37] From 1973 to 1996, a median of 24 cases of food-borne botulism, 3 cases of wound botulism, and 71 cases of infant botulism were reported annually to the CDC.[35] In the United States, approximately 50 percent of the food-borne cases are caused by toxin A and another 25 percent each by toxins E and B. Type A occurs primarily in the western states, whereas type B is seen more commonly in the eastern states. Type E outbreaks occur more frequently in Alaska and the Great Lakes region.

Botulinum toxin is considered the most potent and lethal of all naturally occurring compounds. It is heat-labile; 5 minutes of boiling destroys the toxin, and little remains after 30 minutes of exposure at 80° C. Toxin is produced by *C. botulinum* at all temperatures at which growth occurs (3° C to 48 °C). Toxin also is formed at all pH values at which growth occurs (pH 4.8 to 8.5), but the toxin is unstable at pH values greater than 7. The presence of organisms in improperly processed acidic food, however, can allow toxin production to occur.[16, 17, 37] Type E toxin may be produced quickly in small fragments of fish exposed to air and at lower pH values and cooler temperatures than noted with other toxin types.[16]

Most outbreaks of botulism in the United States are traceable to home-processed foods; however, in recent years, the proportion of cases that result from restaurant-associated outbreaks has increased significantly.[35] The most important food vehicles are vegetables, fish, fruits, and condiments. Type E botulism almost always is traceable to fish and fish products, but types A and B also may be involved in outbreaks related to this type of food. Recent outbreaks have been traced to unusual foods, such as potato salad and sautéed onions served by restaurants and commercial frozen pot pies mishandled at home.

Wound botulism results from infection of traumatized tissue by *C. botulinum* type A or B and subsequent production of toxin.[31] In the United States, approximately 80 percent of cases are caused by toxin A and 20 percent by toxin B.[35] Although infrequently reported, wound infection is a disease of pediatric concern: approximately half the cases in the United States that occurred before 1991 were in children and teenagers, most of whom were boys with compound extremity fractures. In recent years, however, most new cases have occurred in users of contaminated injectable black tar heroin.[1, 10, 35]

PATHOPHYSIOLOGY

Botulinum toxin is absorbed from the proximal part of the intestine or an infected wound into the lymphatics and then distributed hematogenously to peripheral cholinergic nerve synapses, most notably the neuromuscular junction. The toxin does not cross the blood-brain barrier. The nerve endings take up the toxin, which then irreversibly blocks release of acetylcholine and clinically results in flaccid paralysis.[16, 17, 37] The cranial nerves are affected earliest and often most severely. Death occurs mainly from respiratory muscle paralysis (asphyxia) or its complications, such as cardiac arrhythmia, aspiration, and pneumonia. Recovery occurs by regeneration of terminal motor neurons and the formation of new motor end-plates.

CLINICAL MANIFESTATIONS

The illness begins as a descending symmetric motor paralysis first affecting muscles supplied by the cranial nerves.[16] No sensory disturbance occurs, although vision may be impaired and hearing distorted because of cranial nerve involvement.

Mental processes remain clear, but anxiety and agitation may be present. Fever is absent unless a secondary bacterial infection occurs. The triad of bulbar palsies (including a sluggish or absent pupillary response to light), lucid sensorium, and absent fever always should bring botulism to mind.

Common symptoms include blurred vision, diplopia, dysarthria, and dysphagia. The degree of ocular involvement is quite variable; in severe cases, the pupils may become fixed and dilated. The mucous membranes of the mouth, tongue, and pharynx may be so dry that pain results, which may lead to the mistaken diagnosis of pharyngitis. Dizziness or vertigo may occur. Urinary retention may be seen, occasionally with stress incontinence.

Two thirds of patients have no gastrointestinal symptoms. In those who do, with type A or type B botulism the gastrointestinal manifestations are primarily abdominal pain, cramps, fullness, and diarrhea. However, after an initial period of diarrhea, constipation or obstipation may be noted and, indeed, is more typical of the disease. In contrast to those with the other types, most patients with type E botulism first have gastrointestinal symptoms. Included are nausea, vomiting, substernal burning or pain, abdominal distention, and decreased bowel sounds. The most common signs encountered in botulism are respiratory impairment; specific muscle weakness or paralysis; eye muscle involvement, including ptosis; dry throat, mouth, or tongue; dilated fixed pupils; and ataxia. Respiratory involvement, even aside from aspiration pneumonia, is a fairly common occurrence. Vital capacity is a more sensitive indicator of respiratory compromise than is measurement of blood gas. Postural hypotension, nystagmus, and somnolence may be noted.

The usual interval between the ingestion of food and the onset of symptoms is 18 to 36 hours, but it may be as short as a few hours or as long as 8 days. In general, patients with shorter incubation periods are affected more severely and have a poorer prognosis. The shortness of the incubation period and the severity of illness correlate with the amount of toxin ingested. Although the syndrome is similar for each toxin type, type A toxin has been associated with more severe disease and a higher mortality rate than has either type B or type E toxin.[44]

The symptoms of wound botulism are similar to those of food botulism, but some important differences may occur.[31] Fever may or may not be present. Constipation occurs, but nausea and vomiting do not. Unilateral sensory changes in association with the trauma or infection may be noted. The wound itself may have grossly purulent drainage, but sometimes the wounds show no evidence of infection. The incubation period of wound botulism is usually 4 to 14 days.

In the event of an intentional food-borne poisoning with botulism toxin, the signs and symptoms probably would resemble those of naturally occurring food-borne botulism.[35] If the aerosolized toxin from a bioterrorist attack were to be inhaled, the incubation period might be slightly longer, and gastrointestinal symptoms might not occur.[35]

DIFFERENTIAL DIAGNOSIS

The differential diagnosis of botulism includes myasthenia gravis, cerebral vascular accidents, Guillain-Barré syndrome (particularly the Miller-Fisher variant), tick paralysis, paralytic shellfish poisoning, chemical intoxication, diphtheritic polyneuritis, psychiatric disease, and the Eaton-Lambert syndrome.[16, 37]

Ordinary bacterial food poisoning usually is not a problem in the differential diagnosis because of the absence of cranial nerve involvement. Chemical food poisoning may cause neurologic manifestations, but the signs almost always appear within minutes or at most hours after the consumption of contaminated food. Atropine poisoning has a very rapid onset and is distinctive because of facial flushing and hallucinations. Shellfish and fish poisonings have a rapid onset and often cause characteristic paresthesias, tremors, and other signs. Mushroom poisoning results in severe abdominal pain, violent vomiting, diarrhea, and coma.

Myasthenia gravis usually spares pupillary oculomotor function. An edrophonium (Tensilon) test should be performed. Guillain-Barré syndrome can mimic botulism but usually shows ascending peripheral paralysis and, later, cranial nerve involvement. Muscle cramps, paresthesias, and an elevated protein content in cerebrospinal fluid in the absence of cells help distinguish this disease. Electromyography may be extremely useful in differentiating botulism from atypical cases of Guillain-Barré syndrome.

The problem of identifying a case is complicated by reports of patients with features not characteristic of either botulism or the action of botulinum toxin, such as paresthesias, asymmetric weakness of the extremities, asymmetric ptosis, slightly elevated cerebrospinal fluid protein, and a "positive" response to edrophonium. Some of these symptoms may be a consequence of the high anxiety that prevails in persons who know that they have eaten a food containing botulinum toxin.

SPECIFIC DIAGNOSIS

Confirmation of the diagnosis of botulism depends primarily on detection of the toxin or the organism in the patient or in the implicated food or wound.[16, 37] Specimens to be examined for botulinum toxin include serum, gastric contents or vomitus, feces (at least 50 g when possible), and exudates from wounds and tissues. These specimens, particularly blood specimens, should be obtained as soon as possible and before antitoxin is given. When feasible, 30 mL of blood should be drawn into a large vacuum tube and sent without separation of the serum to the nearest laboratory capable of performing the mouse neutralization test and other tests for toxin. State health departments or the CDC can provide advice regarding specimen collection and handling and laboratories to which samples can be sent (see later).

Specimens should be refrigerated and examined as quickly as possible after collection. Whenever feasible, suspect food should be kept sealed in the original container. Sterile unbreakable containers should be used for other food samples. Specimens to be shipped to laboratories must be placed in leak-proof containers, packed with ice in a second leak-proof, insulated container, and marked "Danger, hazardous material." Extreme caution should be used in handling materials that may contain botulinum toxin because even minute quantities of toxin acquired by ingestion, inhalation, or absorption through the eye or a break in the skin may cause profound intoxication and death.

Laboratory confirmation of suspected botulism should be attempted, even late in the clinical course. Detection of the organism itself may be achieved by culture (preferably by means of spore selection procedures and a selective medium), by fluorescent antibody technique, and in a presumptive manner, by gas chromatography.

Toxin is detected in serum or stool specimens in approximately 46 percent of clinically diagnosed cases. When stool specimens also are cultured for *C. botulinum,* confirmatory evidence is obtained in approximately 70 percent of botulism cases.[35, 44] Thus, detection of *C. botulinum* toxin or organisms in the stool of a symptomatic person should be considered diagnostic.

TREATMENT

The mainstay of therapy in all forms of botulism is meticulous supportive care, with particular attention paid to the respiratory and nutritional needs of the patient and to anticipation of potential complications for the purpose of preventing them.[16, 17] Symptomatic persons known to have ingested toxin-containing food should be hospitalized, with careful monitoring of respiratory and cardiac function. Measurement of vital capacity has been a useful index of clinical status in adult patients.

In cases of food-borne botulism, if the patient is seen early, emetics and gastric lavage should be used to reduce the amount of unabsorbed toxin; in the absence of ileus, cathartic agents may be helpful. Magnesium-containing cathartic agents should be avoided because they may enhance the action of botulinum toxin. Trivalent antitoxin (types A, B, and E) or bivalent antitoxin (types A and B), both of equine origin, frequently are considered in the management of food-borne botulism in adults, although conclusive evidence of their efficacy is lacking.[16, 40] The antitoxin is used to neutralize circulating botulinum toxin molecules that are not yet bound to nerve endings. The dose currently recommended in adults is 1 vial per patient as a single dose.[35] Hypersensitivity reactions have been reported in approximately 9 percent of persons treated with equine sera, so skin testing should be performed before administration of the antitoxin. Treatment of a single patient with suspected or proven food-borne botulism requires immediate notification of state and federal (CDC) health officials, who also are the antitoxin source, because the food responsible for the index patient's illness still may be available to other persons. The appropriate initial contact is via the state health department. If this agency cannot be reached, the CDC should be contacted immediately (CDC telephone: 404-639-2206, days, or 404-639-2888, nights). Presently, a human-derived botulinum antitoxin is available in the United States exclusively for the treatment of infantile botulism.

In the event of a potential exposure to contaminated food, the following procedures should be implemented. Locate all persons who ate the suspect food and determine whether any have symptoms or signs of botulism.[16] If the patients are seen soon after the suspect meal, the use of gastric lavage, emetics, and cathartics deserves consideration. Arrange to have antitoxin easily available. Collect and refrigerate any samples of the suspect food that may remain. The health authorities should assist the clinician with these tasks. Obtain the fecal and serum specimens needed to establish the diagnosis. If neurologic signs are present, try to identify defective neuromuscular transmission by electromyelography. If neurologic signs are absent, the patient and family should be informed of the early signs of botulinum intoxication and be instructed to return at the first manifestation of ptosis, diplopia, blurred vision, dysphonia, dysarthria, or dysphagia. Because of the serious side effects of equine botulinum antitoxin, prophylactic administration of it to asymptomatic persons who have ingested food known to contain botulinum toxin generally is not recommended.[1]

When wound botulism is suspected, exploration and débridement of the site must be undertaken, ideally after administration of antitoxin has begun. Arrangements should be made to obtain material for anaerobic culture in the operating room and begin antibiotic therapy there. High-dose penicillin (250,000 to 400,000 U/kg/day for 10 to 14 days) is the drug of choice. Guanidine, aminopyridine, steroids, and intravenous immunoglobulin have been used to treat a small number of cases of food-borne and wound botulism, but convincing evidence of their efficacy is lacking.

PROGNOSIS

With the emphasis on mechanical ventilation and intensive supportive care, the mortality rate from botulism has decreased steadily from 60 percent in the 1950s to 5 to 10 percent at the present time. It is lower with type B and type C disease than with type A.[4] The mortality rate is lower in individuals younger than 20 years. An important factor, as noted, is the dose of toxin ingested as reflected by the length of the incubation period. The longer the incubation period, the better the prognosis. If the index case in an outbreak can be detected early, other patients exposed to the same food will have a much better prognosis. Recovery may be prolonged, and some symptoms (e.g., fatigability) may persist for as long as 1 year. Most patients recover entirely.

PREVENTION

Local and state health authorities and the CDC should be notified immediately of all suspected cases of botulism so that appropriate investigations can be undertaken. Although commercial products still are occasionally responsible for botulism, control measures taken by the industry have done a great deal to prevent botulism from this source. Home canners still must be instructed regarding appropriate means for sterilizing containers and food before preserving and for adequate cooking of food before serving.[16, 37] In canning, a pressure cooker must be used to obtain temperatures well above boiling to destroy the spores of *C. botulinum* types A and B. For certain foods, a temperature of 116° C is recommended. Spores of *C. botulinum* are destroyed at 120° C after 30 minutes. Pressure cookers set at 15 lb will achieve this temperature, but correction for higher altitudes must be made. Home-canned foods should be boiled for 10 minutes before serving. Food containers that appear to bulge may contain gas produced by *C. botulinum* and should not be opened. A pentavalent botulinum toxoid vaccine has been used in military personnel to protect them from a biologic warfare assault. It is given in three subcutaneous doses and leads to detectable antibodies in 83 percent of subjects.[10]

Clostridial Infections

Clostridia are encountered less commonly in infections than non–spore-forming anaerobic bacteria are, but these spore formers rarely may produce devastating disease. Overall, clostridia are present in 5 to 10 percent of anaerobic or mixed anaerobic infections.[4, 13, 16, 42] *Clostridium perfringens* is the species encountered most commonly. It may be isolated in pure culture but more commonly is part of a mixed flora involving other anaerobes and nonanaerobes as well at times. Other species that are important clinically or encountered commonly (or both) include *Clostridium novyi, Clostridium septicum, Clostridium bifermentans, Clostridium histolyticum,* and *Clostridium sordellii* (together with *C. perfringens,* these species commonly are referred to as the "gas gangrene group"); *C. tetani* (see Chapter 154); *Clostridium difficile,* a major pathogen in pseudomembranous colitis; and a group of clostridia important in infections other than gas gangrene or myonecrosis (wound infection, abscesses, bacteremia, etc.)—*C. perfringens, Clostridium ramosum, C. bifermentans, Clostridium sphenoides, Clostridium sporogenes,* and others.

Clostridia may be involved in a wide variety of infections throughout the body. Certain of these infections have a distinctive clinical picture; they are discussed in this chapter. Many other infections, including peritonitis, intra-abdominal infection, wound infection, soft tissue infection, and, occasionally, pleuropulmonary infection, central nervous system infection, and urinary tract infection, are not distinctive and will not be discussed specifically here. Emphysematous cholecystitis involving *C. perfringens* has distinctive features, but it is not encountered in the pediatric age group and thus is not discussed. Bacteremia involving *C. perfringens* may or may not have characteristic features. The distinctive intravascular hemolysis that may occur with *C. perfringens* bacteremia is discussed in connection with female genital tract infections caused by this organism.

EPIDEMIOLOGY

The vast majority of clostridial infections are of endogenous origin. Even those secondary to trauma and contamination of a wound with foreign bodies usually involve *C. perfringens* or other clostridia from the host's flora, chiefly the intestinal tract.

PATHOPHYSIOLOGY

The principal sites of normal carriage of *C. perfringens* in humans are the colon and the vagina.[16, 17] Many other clostridial species are found in the bowel. These organisms may gain access to tissues through wounds (surgical or traumatic), by virtue of perforation of abdominal viscera, or because of local disease such as tumor. The organism then may grow in tissues if the oxidation-reduction potential is low or host defense mechanisms are impaired, or both. Factors favoring anaerobic growth include necrotic tissue, a poor blood supply, the presence of foreign bodies, or previous multiplication of other bacteria in the wound leading to a lowered oxidation-reduction potential.

C. perfringens produces at least a dozen different extracellular toxins or other factors that account for its pathogenicity.[16] The most important of the five major lethal toxins is alpha-toxin, a lecithinase and the main toxin responsible for destruction of tissue, hemolysis, and death. Other important factors include collagenase, hyaluronidase, leukocidin, deoxyribonuclease, and fibrinolysin. The enterotoxins produced by some strains of *C. perfringens* and *C. difficile* are important in the pathogenesis of certain gastrointestinal diseases, which are discussed. Gas gangrene, or clostridial myonecrosis, is characterized by profound toxicity, necrosis of muscle, edema, thrombosis of small vessels, gas bubbles in the tissues, and minimal infiltration of leukocytes (probably caused by destruction of leukocytes at the site).

CLINICAL MANIFESTATIONS

Gas Gangrene or Myonecrosis

Although other clostridia also are involved in gas gangrene, *C. perfringens* is the causative species in approximately 90 to 95 percent of cases. Gas gangrene usually results from contamination of open wounds involving muscle. The tissue destruction in gas gangrene is related to the profound attenuation in blood flow as a result of activation of platelet responses by the alpha-toxin of *C. perfringens*.[5] Clostridial myonecrosis may occur in the absence of a traumatic wound. This disease is referred to as spontaneous myonecrosis and is caused by bacteremic seeding of muscle with either *C. perfringens* or *C. septicum*. In spontaneous myonecrosis, the source of the organism typically is the bowel, and the usual predisposing factors are mucosal tumors of the bowel or ulcerations produced by cytotoxic chemotherapy.[17] Only a handful of cases of spontaneous myonecrosis in children have been described.[32]

The typical case of clostridial myonecrosis is manifested by the sudden appearance of pain in the region of a wound.[16] The pain increases in severity but remains localized to the infected area. Subsequently, local swelling and edema occur, and a thin hemorrhagic exudate appears. The pulse is very rapid, out of proportion to the mild temperature elevation. Initially, the skin is tense, white, somewhat colder than normal, and very tender. Bronze discoloration appears and increases with time. The process extends and becomes more severe, and the patient becomes toxemic. The skin becomes dusky or bronzed, and bullae filled with dark-red or purple fluid appear. Crepitus caused by gas may be noted, but the amount of gas produced generally is small. A peculiar sweet smell may be noted in some cases. Occasionally, a fetid odor that probably reflects the presence of a *Clostridium* organism other than *C. perfringens* may be present.[17] Toxic delirium and, later, overwhelming prostration and toxemia may develop. Some patients are alert and apprehensive, whereas others are apathetic. Later in the course of the disease, shock supervenes. At surgery, early changes in muscle consist primarily of edema and pallor, but increased reddening with mottled purple is present. The consistency of the muscle may be pasty or mucoid, and contractility disappears. Eventually, the muscle becomes diffusely gangrenous, dark greenish-purple or black, friable, and even liquefied.

Soft Tissue Infection

C. perfringens and other clostridia also may be involved in less dramatic and less serious infections ranging from minor superficial infections to anaerobic cellulitis and necrotizing fasciitis.[17] The clinical picture in these various infections is no different from that noted with other types of organisms and thus is not discussed further here.

Septic Abortion and Puerperal Sepsis

C. perfringens infections of the uterus usually occur after incomplete abortions are induced under nonsterile conditions.[16] Occasionally, this type of infection will develop after spontaneous abortion, prolonged labor, ruptured membranes, or operative interference with pregnancy. Early symptoms include uterine bleeding, suprapubic and back pain, chills, and fever.[16, 17] The incubation period after the precipitating event usually is several days, but it may be less than 24 hours. In addition to vaginal bleeding, a foul-smelling, brown vaginal discharge containing necrotic tissue often is present. The uterus is tender, and the lower abdominal wall may be tense. Nausea, vomiting, and diarrhea may occur. Generalized peritonitis may complicate the picture. The most striking systemic manifestation of the disease, however, is massive intravascular hemolysis with hemoglobinemia, hemoglobinuria, and jaundice. Shock and acute renal failure may complicate the picture. Intrauterine gas formation may be detected.

Neonatal Sepsis and Meningitis

A small number of cases of sepsis or meningitis (or both) caused by *Clostridium* have been reported in newborns.[18, 20, 25, 33, 39] Although some of these neonatal cases have been associated with invasive procedures or devitalized tissue, others have not had an obvious source.[20, 25, 33] In several of these cases, the systemic infection involved both the mother and infant. The typical clinical picture in neonatal infections is one of fulminant septic shock, intravascular hemolysis, respiratory distress, and rapid death. Pneumatocephalus may occur in the presence of meningitis.

Pseudomembranous Colitis

Pseudomembranous colitis represents the most severe end of a disease spectrum that the toxins of *C. difficile* can produce. It generally is characterized by profuse watery diarrhea, abdominal cramps, fever, and small (2 to 5 mm) raised, yellowish plaques on the colonic mucosa.[17, 21] At the other end of the spectrum are found asymptomatic carriage and mild diarrhea. *C. difficile* diarrhea and colitis almost invariably occur after the administration of antimicrobial drugs, the most common precipitants being ampicillin, clindamycin, and cephalosporins.[17] However, almost any antibacterial agent can set off the illness. Sporadic cases not associated with antibiotics have been recognized. *C. difficile* disease is related to the action of one or both of its toxins, known as A and B. Toxin A is responsible primarily for the enterotoxic activity of *C. difficile,* whereas toxin B is much more potent as a cytotoxin than toxin A is.[24] The spectrum of *C. difficile*–associated diarrhea ranges from a trivial, self-limited disease to that of a severe illness simulating an intra-abdominal catastrophe. Fever to 104° C, leukocytosis to 25,000 cells/mm^3, and hypoalbuminemia occur in approximately 25 percent of patients. Stools range from 3 or 4 to 20 per day and may be loose, watery, or bloody with mucus; associated abdominal cramping is a relatively common event.[17] Occasionally, pseudomembranous colitis may be caused by *Staphylococcus aureus* or by clostridia other than *C. difficile* (e.g., *C. perfringens* type C).

Many determinants of the illness remain to be clarified. Toddlers and especially infants may harbor the bacterium and its toxins asymptomatically within the intestinal flora, whereas in healthy older children and adults, *C. difficile* is found infrequently (approximately 2% intestinal carriage rate).[28, 43] Possibly, receptors for *C. difficile* toxin may be decreased or absent in younger children.[14] Genetic analysis of the pathogenicity locus in *C. difficile* may help distinguish pathogenic from nonpathogenic strains of *C. difficile* in the future.[11] Children's facilities and hospitals have been identified as major reservoirs of *C. difficile.* Important risk factors for the development of disease are situations that would decrease the protective effect of the normal intestinal flora (such as antimicrobial therapy, repeated enemas, or intestinal surgery) and thereby allow the bacteria to proliferate and elaborate toxin. Asymptomatic colonization with *C. difficile* may be seen in a proportion of pediatric oncology patients,[6] as well as in children with prolonged hospital stays.

Other Enteric Infections

A mild and self-limited, but very common, form of food poisoning may be caused by *C. perfringens,* with meat and meat products being the major vehicles for such outbreaks.[16, 17] Food poisoning is caused by a heat-labile enterotoxin produced by *C. perfringens* type A. The incubation period after ingestion of the contaminated food varies from 6 to 24 hours but usually is 8 to 12 hours. The major symptoms are crampy abdominal pain and diarrhea. Stools are liquid but do not contain blood or mucus. Nausea may be noted on occasion, but vomiting and fever seldom are present. The illness usually lasts less than 24 hours.

Rarely, *C. perfringens* also may produce a very severe type of enteritis known as enteritis necroticans. Although food poisoning is produced by *C. perfringens* type A, necrotizing enteritis involves the beta-toxin of *C. perfringens* type C.[29] Consumption of excessive amounts of rich food by people normally on a low protein diet who have decreased levels of digestive proteases seems to be an important background factor. Additionally, proteases may be blocked by ingestion of the trypsin inhibitors found in sweet potatoes. In some cases, consumption of contaminated canned meat is involved. In New Guinea, where this condition is known as "pigbel," enteritis necroticans in children is associated with traditional pig-feasting activities in which large quantities of pork are consumed. The disease is characterized by abdominal cramps, vomiting, shock, diarrhea (sometimes bloody), and acute inflammation of the small intestine with areas of necrosis and gangrene, particularly in the jejunum. A 12-year-old diabetic boy in whom enteritis necroticans developed after the ingestion of pig intestines (chitterlings) was reported recently.[34]

Miscellaneous Infections Caused by Clostridia

Fewer than 40 cases of septic arthritis attributable to *Clostridium* spp., including several pediatric patients, have been reported.[23] Anaerobic osteomyelitis caused by *Clostridium* also is a rare finding.[19] Aggressive surgical débridement and prolonged antibiotic therapy are warranted in the treatment of anaerobic musculoskeletal infections.[36]

The clinical spectrum of clostridial bacteremia ranges from an asymptomatic patient with an incidental positive blood culture to fulminant sepsis syndrome.[8] Bacteremia with *C. septicum* is considered a unique syndrome associated with malignancies, particularly leukemia and colon cancer, and it has a devastating clinical course.[30] Infections with this organism also have been linked to children with cyclic neutropenia.[2] In a recent review of 28 pediatric patients with *C. septicum* bacteremia, Caya noted that all of them had underlying cancer or gastrointestinal disease.[7] The overall mortality rate was 72 percent. Five cases of *C. septicum* infection occurring after *Escherichia coli* O157–induced hemolytic-uremic syndrome have been described.[3]

Panophthalmitis involving *C. perfringens* or, occasionally, other clostridia is secondary to penetrating injury, usually with retention of a foreign body.[16] Pain and loss of vision occur within 12 hours after the injury. By 18 hours, evidence of fulminating panophthalmitis is present and consists of chemosis and brawny swelling of the lids, proptosis, hypopyon, increased intraocular tension, gas bubbles in the anterior chamber, and necrosis of the wound margins. Intracranial infections involving *Clostridium,* usually as a result of penetrating trauma with items such as a lawn dart or an arrow, have been described.

Pneumatosis cystoides intestinalis can be produced in animals by *C. perfringens,* and this organism has been recovered from this process in humans.[16, 17] Pneumatosis cystoides intestinalis may be found in conjunction with toxic megacolon and neonatal necrotizing enterocolitis and as a complication of ileal bypass for obesity.

SPECIFIC DIAGNOSIS

The diagnosis of gas gangrene must be made on clinical grounds. The presence of a gas-forming infection and recovery of *C. perfringens* from the wound do not establish the diagnosis of gas gangrene. The key to this diagnosis is demonstration of myonecrosis. Clostridial myonecrosis must be differentiated from other gas-forming soft tissue infections, which may or may not involve *C. perfringens,* and from other causes of myonecrosis. The sudden onset, extreme toxemia, and severe pain that are noted in clostridial myonecrosis represent important differential features. Entities such as anaerobic cellulitis and streptococcal myonecrosis have a gradual onset, slight toxemia, and less pain than seen with clostridial myonecrosis. Synergistic nonclostridial anaerobic myonecrosis is a severe infection characterized by discrete areas of blue-gray necrosis of skin, along with extensive involvement of the underlying soft tissue and muscle and foul "dish-water" pus. Anaerobic cellulitis typically has much more gas and does not involve muscle.

In streptococcal myonecrosis, edema of the muscle is present initially, and then the muscle has a hemorrhagic appearance.[16] Specimens for Gram staining and culture should be obtained from the involved muscle rather than the surface of the wound. Large gram-positive rods will be demonstrated on Gram stain in clostridial myonecrosis; no white blood cells may be demonstrable, or the white blood cells present may be distorted significantly as a result of the toxin of *C. perfringens* acting on them. Anaerobic cellulitis typically shows a mixture of organisms, which may include *C. perfringens.* Streptococcal myonecrosis reveals anaerobic streptococci, sometimes along with group A streptococci, *S. aureus,* and other organisms.[16] In synergistic nonclostridial anaerobic myonecrosis, *Bacteroides* organisms seem to be key pathogens, together with anaerobic cocci and nonanaerobic gram-negative bacilli.[17] Of importance when obtaining material for culture is to place it under anaerobic conditions promptly for transport to the laboratory. Anaerobic blood cultures also should be performed.

Uterine infection by *C. perfringens* varies in severity from secondary invasion of necrotic material into the uterus or a dead fetus to invasion of intact uterine muscle producing myonecrosis and physometra.[16] Although bacteremia is a relatively uncommon finding in gas gangrene, uterine infection with *C. perfringens* frequently is accompanied by sepsis, which leads to the dramatic picture of intravascular hemolysis described earlier. Demonstration of severe hemolytic anemia in association with uterine infection essentially is diagnostic. Anaerobic blood cultures should be performed.

Clostridia, particularly *C. perfringens,* occasionally are isolated from the blood of a patient with a clinically benign course. The usual scenario is that a hospitalized patient has a single fever spike of unclear etiology, and blood cultures are performed as part of the evaluation; by the time that the culture becomes positive, no evidence of an infectious process is present. This transient and benign bacteremia probably originates from the colonic flora.[6]

C. perfringens food poisoning usually is seen in the setting of a sizable outbreak.[17] The organism grows to high counts in the responsible food and then sets up an infection in the host, with production of enterotoxin in the colon of patients. Demonstration of large numbers of *C. perfringens* ($>10^5$/g) in the implicated food and demonstration of the same serotype of *C. perfringens* in the stool of affected individuals and in the food are important in documenting the nature of the food poisoning. Enterotoxin also may be found in the stool of affected individuals, and the *C. perfringens* recovered from stool or food can be demonstrated to produce enterotoxin in vitro. Necrotizing enteritis caused by *C. perfringens* may be suspected by virtue of the dramatic clinical picture and confirmed by demonstration of *C. perfringens* type C in the stool or suspect food or demonstration of serum antibody to the beta-toxin of the organism.

C. difficile–associated diarrhea should be suspected in children with diarrhea who have received antibiotics within the previous 2 months or whose diarrhea begins 72 hours after hospitalization.[15] Typically, toxin testing of a single stool specimen will establish the diagnosis, but occasionally, repeat testing or endoscopy may be necessary. The finding of exudative plaques (pseudomembranes) and a hyperemic, friable mucosa by direct endoscopic visualization suggests the diagnosis of pseudomembranous colitis. Although *C. difficile* is isolated conveniently by the use of a selective medium, distinction between toxigenic and nonpathogenic strains cannot be made. Its toxin B (cytotoxin) is identified most easily by tissue culture assay, which remains the gold standard for diagnosis of antibiotic-associated diarrhea.[17] A simple latex particle agglutination test for detection of *C. difficile* is available, although it is considered relatively insensitive and nonspecific and, for that reason, no longer is recommended.[41]

In recent years, commercially available enzyme immunoassay (EIA) kits that detect toxin B or both toxin A and B have become the preferred method of diagnosis.[41] The EIAs in general are easy to perform, relatively inexpensive, and specific. Polymerase chain reaction amplification tests for toxins A and B have been designed but are not available commercially.

Interpreting the significance of finding *C. difficile* or its toxins in very young patients with diarrhea is difficult because infants and toddlers have such a high rate of asymptomatic carriage.[28, 43] Quantitation of toxin or organisms has not correlated with the presence or absence of symptoms. Consequently, once the possible presence of other diarrhea-producing pathogens (e.g., rotavirus, *Salmonella)* has been excluded, efforts should be made to stop the presumptive precipitating antibacterial agent. If diarrhea with mucus or blood persists, endoscopy should be considered and specific therapy begun.

TREATMENT

The most important aspect of treating clostridial myonecrosis is immediate surgical intervention consisting of radical débridement and drainage and decompression of the fascial compartments.[16, 17] The wound should not be closed after this surgery. Of crucial importance is that all bits of necrotic muscle and other tissue be removed. Polyvalent gas gangrene antitoxin was never established firmly as being beneficial in the context of modern therapy, and this product is no longer available in the United States. Hyperbaric oxygen is recommended enthusiastically by some physicians, but no definitive evidence that its use reduces mortality rates has been shown. It does facilitate demarcation of a limb with impaired vascular supply, and it appears to slow down or arrest local spread of the gangrenous infection. Clearly, however, hyperbaric oxygen must not be used as a substitute for any of the important principles of surgical management. Antimicrobial therapy also is important as an adjunct, with high-dose penicillin G (250,000 to 400,000 U/kg/day) being the drug of choice.[16, 17] In individuals allergic to penicillin G, clindamycin or metronidazole may be used. In addition, chloramphenicol is routinely active against all clostridia. The combination of penicillin and clindamycin has been used widely on the basis of experimental animal models that have shown enhanced efficacy with such a combination.[38]

Clostridial cellulitis is treated by incision plus drainage and antimicrobial therapy. Radical débridement is not necessary, but it is important to lay the tissues open to effect proper drainage and permit removal of all necrotic tissue.[16, 17]

Uterine curettage should be performed for diagnosis and treatment of postabortal or puerperal clostridial infections.[16] Hysterectomy may be required if the myometrium is involved and if the patient's condition is deteriorating. At times, perforation of the uterus may be present without the typical clinical findings. Exchange transfusion has been recommended for sepsis caused by *C. perfringens* when significant intravascular hemolysis is present.

Food poisoning caused by *C. perfringens* is self-limited and requires no therapy. Antitoxin to the beta-toxin produced by *C. perfringens* type C has been of considerable benefit in the treatment of necrotizing enteritis caused by this organism.

In any serious infection caused by *C. perfringens* or other clostridia, the usual supportive measures for shock, dehydration, anemia, and renal insufficiency are implemented as indicated.

Treatment of *C. difficile*–associated disease involves discontinuation of the offending antibiotic regimen when feasible. Isolates of *C. difficile* are susceptible to metronidazole and vancomycin. Oral or intravenous metronidazole (30 mg/kg/day in four divided doses) is considered the drug of choice. With the recent and rapid increase in the recovery of vancomycin-resistant enterococci, many experts[15] and the CDC have suggested that oral vancomycin (40 mg/kg/day in four divided doses) be used to treat *C. difficile*–induced diarrhea only in patients who are critically ill or those who do not respond to metronidazole. The efficacy of intravenous vancomycin is uncertain. Orally administered bacitracin also may be useful, although some experts suggest that it may be less effective than is metronidazole or vancomycin. Antimicrobial agents typically are administered for 7 to 10 days, but as many as 20 percent of patients may experience a relapse requiring a second course of treatment. The use of cholestyramine or probiotics, such as *Saccharomyces* or *Lactobacillus,* in adult patients with multiple relapses has been advocated by some physicians, but such treatment has not been evaluated in children with disease caused by *C. difficile*.

PROGNOSIS

The mortality rate with gas gangrene varies between 15 and 35 percent and is worse when large muscle groups, such as those of the buttock, thigh, leg, and shoulder, are involved or when areas that are difficult to débride, such as the viscera and pelvis, are involved with disease. Clostridial cellulitis has a much better prognosis, but aggressive therapy still is important to minimize mortality rates. The mortality rate in postabortal clostridial sepsis remains 50 to 85 percent. *C. perfringens* food poisoning has an excellent prognosis, but mortality rates are significant with necrotizing enteritis caused by *C. perfringens* type C.

PREVENTION

Wounds involving areas with large muscle masses are particularly prone to gas gangrene, as are compound fractures, severe crushing injuries, and injuries secondary to high-velocity missiles. Extensive laceration or devitalization of muscle tissue, impairment of the main blood supply to a limb or large muscle group, and contamination by dirt and particularly by bowel contents all predispose to the development of clostridial myonecrosis. The most important aspect of prophylaxis by far is early and adequate surgical management.[16, 17] All devitalized tissue must be débrided; meticulous hemostasis is very important. Primary closure and tight packing of the wound should be avoided. All aspects of the wound must be drained adequately. If a cast must be applied, it should be bivalved from the outset. Hyperbaric oxygen is not indicated prophylactically. Antimicrobial prophylaxis, however, definitely is indicated. Penicillin is the drug of choice and should be given as early as possible after injury. Of emphasis is that antimicrobial prophylaxis is strictly adjunctive and far from adequate by itself. Bathing, particularly showering, and application of a compress wet with an iodophor for 15 minutes have been shown to reduce the skin count of *C. perfringens* significantly and minimize the likelihood of postoperative gas gangrene. This type of decontamination, of course, also may be useful in the management of traumatic wounds.

Prevention of clostridial uterine infection involves ensuring that all products of conception are removed during abortion and that retained portions of the placenta are removed immediately after the third stage of labor. Prolonged labor should be anticipated when possible and analgesics administered judiciously. During labor, particularly with ruptured membranes, pelvic and rectal examinations should be kept to a minimum. During delivery, trauma should be minimized and lacerations repaired according to accepted surgical principles.

Proper sanitation in food-preparing facilities and adequate refrigeration are important safeguards against *C. perfringens* food poisoning. In areas where necrotizing enteritis caused by *C. perfringens* type C is found with some frequency (such as in Papua New Guinea), a *C. perfringens* type C toxoid has been given with encouraging results.

Contact isolation for the duration of the illness is recommended for hospitalized children with *C. difficile*–associated diarrhea. Meticulous handwashing, the use of gloves for handling contaminated objects and fomites, environmental cleaning and disinfection, and limiting the use of antimicrobial agents have been advocated widely to control the transmission of *C. difficile* in health care facilities.[22]

REFERENCES

1. American Academy of Pediatrics: Clostridial infections. *In* Pickering, L. K. (ed.): 2000 Red Book: Report of the Committee on Infectious diseases. 25th ed. Elk Grove Village, IL, American Academy of Pediatrics, 2000, pp. 212–219.
2. Bar-Joseph, G., Halberthal, M., Sweed, Y., et al.: *Clostridium septicum* infection in children with cyclic neutropenia. J. Pediatr. *131*:317–319, 1997.
3. Barnham, M., and Weightman, N.: *Clostridium septicum* infection and hemolytic-uremic syndrome. Emerg. Infect. Dis. *4*:321–324, 1998.
4. Brook, I.: Anaerobic Infections in Childhood. Boston, G. K. Hall, 1983.
5. Bryant, A. E., Chen, R. Y. Z., Nagata, Y., et al.: Clostridial gas gangrene. I. Cellular and molecular mechanisms of microvascular dysfunction induced by exotoxins of *Clostridium perfringens*. J. Infect. Dis. *182*: 799–807, 2000.
6. Burgener, D., Sirakas, S., Eagles G., et al.: A prospective study of *Clostridium difficile* infection and colonization in pediatric oncology patients. Pediatr. Infect. Dis. J. *16*:1131–1134, 1997.
7. Caya, J. G.: *Clostridium septicum* bacteremia in the pediatric population. Arch. Pathol. Lab. Med. *124*:1583, 2000.
8. Caya J. G., and Truant, A. L.: Clostridial bacteremia in the non-infant pediatric population: A report of two cases and review of the literature. Pediatr. Infect. Dis. J. *18*:291–298, 1999.
9. Centers for Disease Control and Prevention: Botulism. M. M. W. R. Recomm. Rep. *46*(RR-10):1–55, 1997.
10. Cherington, M.: Clinical spectrum of botulism. Muscle Nerve *21*:701–710, 1998.
11. Cohen, S. H., Tang, Y. J., and Silva, J.: Analysis of the pathogenicity locus in *Clostridium difficile* strains. J. Infect. Dis. *181*:659–663, 2000.
12. Dowell, V. R., Jr.: Botulism and tetanus: Selected epidemiologic and microbiologic aspects. Rev. Infect. Dis. *6*(Suppl. 1):202–207, 1984.

13. Dunkle, L. M., Brotherton, T. J., and Feigin, R. D.: Anaerobic infections in children: A prospective study. Pediatrics *57*:311–320, 1976.
14. Eglow, R., Pothoukalis, C., and Itzkowitz, S.: Diminished *Clostridium difficile* toxin A sensitivity in newborn rabbit ilium is associated with decreased toxin A receptor. J. Clin. Invest. *90*:822–829, 1992.
15. Fekety, R.: Guidelines for the diagnosis and management of *Clostridium difficile*-associated diarrhea and colitis. Am. J. Gastroenterol. *92*: 739–750, 1997.
16. Finegold, S. M.: Anaerobic Bacteria in Human Disease. New York, Academic Press, 1977.
17. Finegold, S. M., and George, W. L. (eds.): Anaerobic Infections in Humans. San Diego, Academic Press, 1989.
18. Freedman, S., and Hollander, M.: *Clostridium perfringens* septicemia as a postoperative complication of the newborn infant. J. Pediatr. *71*:576–578, 1967.
19. Gaglani, M. J., Murray, J. C., Morad, A. B., and Edwards, M. E.: Chronic osteomyelitis caused by *Clostridium difficile* in an adolescent with sickle cell disease. Pediatr. Infect. Dis. J. *15*:1054–1056, 1996.
20. Gallaher, K. J., and Marks, K. H.: Clostridial infection as a cause of fulminant congenital sepsis neonatorum. Am. J. Perinatol. *8*:370–372, 1991.
21. George, W. L.: Antimicrobial agent–associated colitis and diarrhea: Historical background and clinical aspects. Rev. Infect. Dis. *6*(Suppl. 1):208–213, 1984.
22. Gerding, D. N., Johnson, S., Peterson, L. R., et al.: *Clostridium difficile*-associated diarrhea and colitis. Infect. Control Hosp. Epidemiol. *16*:459–477, 1995.
23. Gredlein, C. M., Silverman, M. L., and Downey, M. S.: Polymicrobial septic arthritis due to *Clostridium* species: Case report and review. Clin. Infect. Dis. *30*:590–594, 2000.
24. Hatheway C. L.: Toxigenic clostridia. Clin. Microbiol. Rev. *3*:66–98, 1990.
25. Heidemann, S. M., Meert, K. L., Perrin, E., and Sarnaik, A. P.: Primary clostridial meningitis in infancy. Pediatr. Infect. Dis. J. *8*:126–128, 1989.
26. Horowitz, M. A., Hughes, J. M., Merson, M. H., et al.: Food-borne botulism in the United States, 1970–1975. J. Infect. Dis. *136*:153–159, 1977.
27. Hughes, L. M., Blumenthal, J. R., Merson, M. H., et al.: Clinical features of types A and B food-borne botulism. Ann. Intern. Med. *95*:442–445, 1981.
28. Jarvis, W. R., and Feldman, R. A.: *Clostridium difficile* and gastroenteritis: How strong is the association in children? Pediatr. Infect. Dis. *3*:4–6, 1984.
29. Lawrence, G., and Walker, P. D.: Pathogenesis of enteritis necroticans in Papua, New Guinea. Lancet *1*:125–126, 1976.
30. Lorber, B.: Gas gangrene and other *Clostridium*-associated diseases. *In* Mandell, G. L., Bennett, J. E., and Dolin, R. (eds.): Mandell, Douglas and Bennett's Principles and Practice of Infectious Diseases. 5th ed. Philadelphia, Churchill Livingstone, 2000, pp. 2549–2561.
31. Merson, M. H., and Dowell, V. R., Jr.: Epidemiologic, clinical and laboratory aspects of wound botulism. N. Engl. J. Med. *289*:1005–1010, 1973.
32. Minutti, C. Z., Immergluck, L. C., and Schmidt, M. L.: Spontaneous gas gangrene due to *Clostridium perfringens*. Clin. Infect. Dis. *28*:159–160, 1999.
33. Motz, R. A., James, A. G., and Dove, B.: *Clostridium perfringens* meningitis in a newborn infant. Pediatr. Infect. Dis. J. *8*:708–710, 1996.
34. Petrillo, T. M., Beck-Sague, C. M., Songer, J. G., et al.: Enteritis necroticans (pigbel) in a diabetic child. N. Engl. J. Med. *342*:1250–1253, 2000.
35. Shapiro R. L., Hatheway C., and Swerdlow D. L.: Botulism in the United States; a clinical and epidemiologic review. Ann. Intern. Med. *129*: 221–228, 1998.
36. Shetty, A. K., Heinrich, S. D., and Steele, R. W.: *Clostridium septicum* osteomyelitis: Case report and review. Pediatr. Infect. Dis. J. *17*:927–928, 1998.
37. Smith, L., and Sugiyama, H.: Botulism: The Organism, Its Toxins, the Disease. 2nd ed. Springfield, IL, Charles C Thomas, 1977.
38. Stevens D. L., Laine B. M., and Mitten J. E.: Comparison of single and combination antimicrobial agents for prevention of experimental gas gangrene caused by *Clostridium perfringens*. Antimicrob. Agents Chemother. *31*:312–316, 1987.
39. Stunden, R. J., Brown, R. A., Rode, H., et al.: Umbilical gangrene in the newborn. J. Pediatr. Surg. *23*:130–134, 1988.
40. Tacket, C. O., Shandera, W. X., Mann, J. M., et al.: Equine antitoxin use and other factors that predict outcome in type A food-borne botulism. Am. J. Med. *76*:794–798, 1984.
41. Thielman, N. M.: Antibiotic-associated colitis. *In* Mandell, G. L., Bennett, J. E., and Dolin, R. (eds.): Mandell, Douglas and Bennett's Principles and Practice of Infectious Diseases. 5th ed. Philadelphia, Churchill Livingstone, 2000, pp. 1111–1126.
42. Thirumoorthia, M. C., Keen, B. M., and Djani, A. S.: Anaerobic infections in children: A prospective study. J. Clin. Microbiol. *3*:318–323, 1976.
43. Welch, D. F., and Marks, M. I.: Is *Clostridium difficile* pathogenic in infants? J. Pediatr. *100*:393–395, 1982.
44. Woodruff, B. A., Griffin P. M., and McCroskey, L. M., et al.: Clinical and laboratory comparison of botulism from toxin types A, B, and E in the United States, 1975–1988. J. Infect. Dis. *166*:1281–1286, 1992.

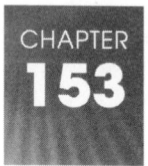

CHAPTER 153 Infant Botulism

STEPHEN S. ARNON

Of the three forms of human botulism (food-borne, wound, and infant), infant botulism is the most recently recognized (1976) and the most common in the United States. Now recognized globally, infant botulism results from a unique pathogenesis. Ingested spores of *Clostridium botulinum* germinate, colonize the infant colon, and produce botulinum neurotoxin. The toxin then is absorbed, binds to peripheral cholinergic synapses, and causes flaccid paralysis. Knowledge of this intestinal pathogenesis resulted in the discovery of novel pathogenic strains of *Clostridium baratii* and *Clostridium butyricum,* each of which can make a botulinum-like neurotoxin and cause the clinical picture of infant botulism. Discovery of these strains enlarged the number of organisms known to cause the "intestinal toxemias of infancy," of which infant botulism is the prototype.[4] Parenthetically, adults and older children rarely may become susceptible to infant-type botulism after broad-spectrum antibiotic treatment, intestinal surgery, or inflammatory bowel disease[6, 22, 29, 49] or in association with Meckel diverticulum or bone marrow transplantation procedures.[74]

History

Infant botulism is not a new disease; rather, it is a recently recognized one. The first laboratory-proven case of human infant botulism occurred in California in 1931, although it was misdiagnosed at the time.[13] Decades later and well before the etiology of the disease was apparent, the characteristic clinical features of infant botulism had become evident to discerning observers. In 1974, Grover and associates[34] described nine patients from Pennsylvania with a neurologic syndrome of undetermined cause that from today's perspective almost certainly was infant botulism. The same idiopathic syndrome was recognized in southern California and was reported by Ramseyer and colleagues[67] in 1976 to have a characteristic electromyographic pattern. In 1977, Clay and associates[23] linked their eight patients to infant botulism.

The first report of frank botulism in infancy was described by Pickett and colleagues[66] in 1976. Although the source of botulinum neurotoxin in their two patients was undetermined, the possibility of in vivo production of it was suggested.[51, 66] The diagnosis of botulism in these and other California patients was established by identification of *C. botulinum* toxin and organisms in the infants' feces.[51] Evidence also was obtained that ingested spores of *C. botulinum* had produced the toxin in the infants' intestinal tract.[9, 51, 94]

In subsequent years, the clinical spectrum of infant botulism was found to include mild, outpatient cases and, in some but not all[18] locations, sudden unexpected death indistinguishable from typical sudden infant death syndrome.[10, 58, 65, 79, 90] In 1985, a *C. baratii* strain that produced a type F–like botulinum neurotoxin was recognized belatedly as the true cause of a case of infant botulism that occurred in New Mexico in 1979,[35, 38] and in 1986, a *C. butyricum* strain that produced a type E–like botulinum neurotoxin was recognized as the cause of two cases of infant botulism in Rome, Italy.[14] These latter two novel clostridia were discovered only because they caused human infant botulism; their existence suggests that others like them await discovery.

Etiologic Agent

C. botulinum is a gram-positive, spore-forming, obligate anaerobe for which the natural habitat worldwide is the soil. Consequently, *C. botulinum* is as ubiquitous as the dust on which it may travel, and, hence, its spores commonly are present on fresh fruits, vegetables, and other agricultural products such as honey. Strains of *C. botulinum* are so diverse in their biochemical capabilities that they would not be grouped as a single species except for the similar neurotoxin molecule that each strain produces[78]; at present, *C. botulinum* is subdivided into six groups based on metabolic characteristics.[62] Almost all cases of infant botulism in the United States have been caused by group I proteolytic type A or type B strains. Unusual strains of *C. baratii* and *C. butyricum* that make botulinum-like toxins E and F also cause infant botulism.[14, 35, 62, 83, 93]

In general, each vegetative cell of *C. botulinum* produces just one of seven serologically distinguishable toxins, which arbitrarily have been assigned the letters A to G. Antitoxin raised against one toxin type does not protect against any of the other six types. The different toxin types serve as convenient epidemiologic and clinical markers. Each toxin molecule is a simple protein consisting of two polypeptide chains of approximately 100,000 d (heavy chain) and 50,000 d (light chain) joined by a disulfide bond. Botulinum toxin is the most poisonous substance known.[31] For this reason and because of the ease with which it may be produced, transported, and disseminated, the Centers for Disease Control and Prevention (CDC) has listed botulinum toxin as one of the six "class A" (most dangerous) potential bioweapon agents.[12] By extrapolation from studies involving adult primates, the lethal dose in the bloodstream of humans is approximately 1 ng/kg body weight.[12, 31] Its potency in infants may be even higher because of the narrowness of their pharyngeal airway.[91]

After centuries of evoking awe and mystery, the basis of the phenomenal potency of the botulinum (and tetanus) toxins was shown to be enzymatic. The light chain of each neurotoxin is a Zn^{2+}-containing protease that hydrolyzes one or more of three intracellular proteins needed for vesicle fusion and acetylcholine release into the synaptic cleft.[55, 60]

Pathogenesis

Infant botulism is not the diminutive form of food-borne botulism and, hence, is not "infantile botulism." Rather, infant botulism results from a unique infectious disease pathway and was so named to emphasize that fact.[2, 4, 51] Ingested spores of *C. botulinum* germinate, colonize the infant colon, and produce botulinum neurotoxin.[9, 36, 53, 54, 63, 94] The toxin subsequently is absorbed and carried by the bloodstream to peripheral cholinergic synapses, to which it binds irreversibly. The light chain then is taken into the cytosol of the neuron, where it blocks the release of acetylcholine by enzymatic cleavage of "fusion complex" proteins.[55,60] Clinically, the most important of the peripheral cholinergic synapses is the neuromuscular junction; the toxin's action results in flaccid paralysis and hypotonia. Preganglionic cholinergic synapses in the autonomic nervous system also may be affected.[48,72]

By use of a mouse model system of intestinal colonization (in which the animals paradoxically remained symptom-free), Sugiyama and colleagues[17, 54, 84] demonstrated that the intestinal microflora of adult animals ordinarily prevents colonization of the gut by *C. botulinum*. Administration of 10^6 type A spores failed to colonize the intestine of normal adult mice, whereas after treatment for 2½ days with a combination of oral erythromycin and kanamycin, half the mice could be colonized by just 2×10^4 spores. When the antibiotic-treated mice were placed in cages with normal mice, they lost their susceptibility to intestinal colonization after 3 days.[17] (Mice normally are coprophagic.) In addition, adult germ-free mice could be colonized intestinally by just 10 *C. botulinum* type A spores. When the germ-free adult animals were placed in a room with conventional mice, in 3 days the formerly germ-free animals became resistant to colonization by 10^5 spores.[54]

In contrast to the experimental work with adult mice, normal infant mice were susceptible to intestinal colonization by *C. botulinum* spores.[84] Like human infants, the normal infant mice were susceptible to colonization for only a limited period (7 to 13 days of age). Susceptibility of the infant mice peaked between days 8 and 11 in a pattern reminiscent of the peaking of susceptibility seen between 2 and 4 months of age in human infant botulism[7, 84] (Fig. 153–1). The infective dose of spores for infant mice was much smaller than that of their antibiotic-treated adult counterparts; the 50 percent infective dose for normal infants was only 700 spores. In one experiment, just 10 spores colonized an infant mouse.[84] The minimal infective dose of *C. botulinum* spores for human infants is not known, but from exposure to spore-containing honey, it has been estimated to be as low as 10 to 100.[11]

Recognition of the central role of the host intestinal microflora in determining susceptibility or resistance to colonization by *C. botulinum* has directed attention to factors that may influence the composition of the normal microflora. Diet may be the most important of these factors. When compared with adult-type flora, infant flora is simpler, with fewer genera and species. The dominant members vary, depending in part on whether the infant is fed only breast milk, only formula milk, or a mixture of the two.[81] In addition, the composition of the intestinal flora is changed if solid foods such as cereal become part of the infant's diet. The normal human infant microflora contains several bacterial species, mainly *Bifidobacterium* and *Bacteroides,* that in vitro can inhibit the multiplication of *C. botulinum.*[86]

The onset of infant botulism occurs at a significantly younger age in formula-fed infants (7.6 weeks) than in breast-fed infants (13.7 weeks),[8] perhaps reflecting the earlier availability in formula-fed infants of suitable ecologic niches[8, 48, 81, 82] and the formula-fed infants' lack of immune factors (e.g., secretory IgA, lactoferrin) contained in human milk.[2, 3, 33] In addition, the introduction of solid foods may

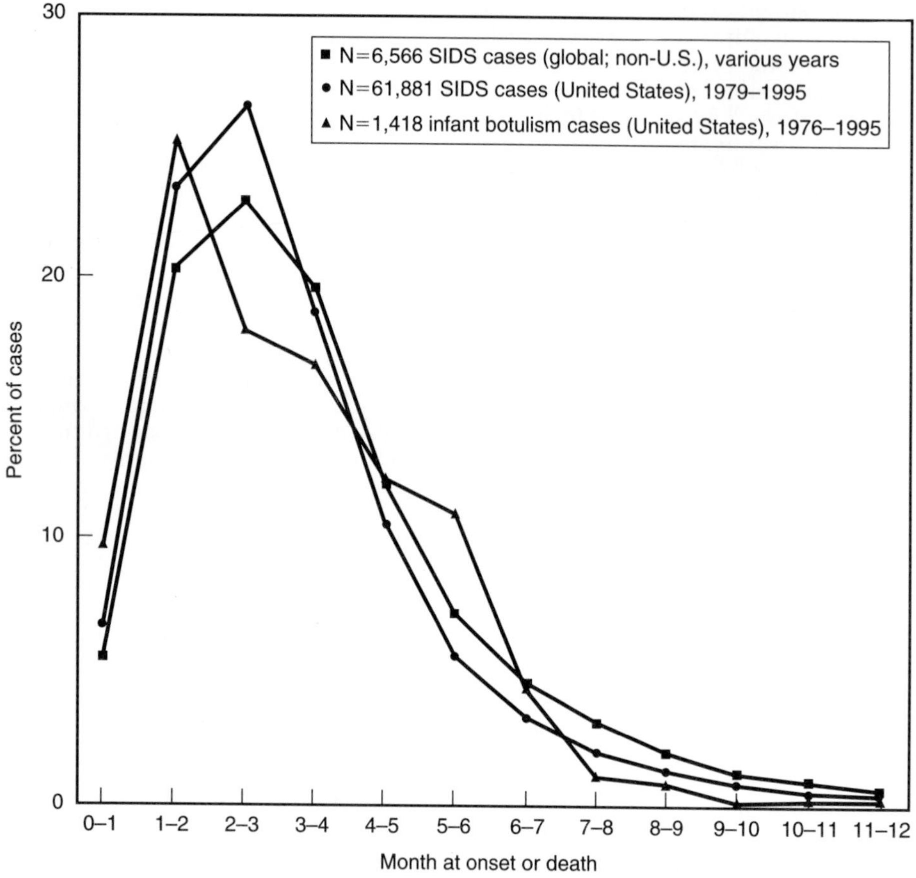

FIGURE 153–1 ■ Age distributions of infant botulism and sudden infant death syndrome (SIDS).

"perturb" the intestinal microflora[81] and thereby aid *C. botulinum* colonization.[2, 7, 48, 80]

An additional physiologic risk factor for infant botulism is slower gut motility, as measured by the frequency of defecation before the onset of illness.[80] Less than one bowel movement per day is a risk factor for both breast-fed and formula-fed infants, but it occurred in just 50 percent of cases.[73] Whether a Meckel diverticulum may predispose to the acquisition of infant botulism caused by *C. botulinum,* as it appears to do for infant botulism caused by *C. butyricum,* is not known.[28, 70]

Epidemiology

Any discussion of the epidemiology of infant botulism should be prefaced by the caveat that almost all information presently available is derived from study of only part of the clinical spectrum, namely, hospitalized patients. Accordingly, current perspectives may need to be modified as the outpatient and sudden-death portions of the clinical spectrum become defined more fully. Furthermore, the perceived incidence remains more a reflection of physician awareness and access to diagnostic testing than of the actual occurrence of disease. Almost half (41.6%) of U.S. cases have been reported from California, which has the largest number of births of any state. However, California does not have the highest incidence of infant botulism once adjustment is made for differences in annual births (Table 153–1). Notably, 8 of the 11 states with the highest incidence are located west of the Rocky Mountains, and 6 of the 8 are contiguous.

A unique epidemiologic feature of infant botulism is its age distribution, which perhaps coincidentally, is virtually identical to the age distribution of sudden infant death syndrome[7, 10, 19, 80] (see Fig. 153–1). All cases of infant botulism reported to date have occurred in children younger than 1 year. Some 95 percent of cases occur in the first 6 months of life; the remaining 5 percent are distributed over the subsequent 6 months. The youngest known patient was 6 days old at onset,[41,89] and the oldest was 351 days.[39] The illness has occurred in all major racial and ethnic groups and in approximately equal proportions in males and females. A national seasonality is not evident.

Infant botulism has been reported from all inhabited continents except Africa. In the United States, with four exceptions, all hospitalized cases known as of December

TABLE 153–1 ■ CASES AND INCIDENCE OF INFANT BOTULISM, TOP 11 STATES IN INCIDENCE, UNITED STATES, 1977–2001

State	Cases	Incidence*
Delaware	32	12.4
Hawaii	43	9.0
Utah	78	7.6
California	799	6.2
Pennsylvania	224	5.5
Oregon	40	3.7
Washington	63	3.4
Idaho	15	3.2
New Jersey	86	3.0
New Mexico	21	3.0
Nevada	21	2.9

*Per 100,000 live births per year. Montana was the state with the 12th highest incidence at 2.5.

2001 were caused by either *C. botulinum* type A or type B (or in one case, by both). Forty-nine of the 50 states, representing all regions of the country, including Alaska and Hawaii, now have reported infant botulism. Only Rhode Island has not. In general, the distribution of cases by toxin type has paralleled the distribution of toxin types in U.S. soils,[77] with type B cases predominating from the great plains eastward and type A cases predominating from the Rocky Mountains westward. Of the four exceptional toxin types, two cases in New Mexico and Oregon resulted from a type F–like toxin produced by *C. baratii* strains,[35, 38, 62] and the other two cases were caused by a *C. botulinum* strain that produced mostly type B and some type F toxin (designated type Bf). One patient with Bf illness lived in New Mexico, and the other patient had traveled there immediately before the onset of illness. A third type Bf case occurred in England.[76]

Geographic clustering has been noted. In Pennsylvania, 43 of 53 cases in the period 1977 to 1983 occurred in four suburban counties that form an arc bordering the city of Philadelphia.[47] In Colorado, three type A cases occurred in separate families in a small town with approximately 300 annual births. Two of the infants had used the same crib sequentially; environmental samples, including the crib, soil, and household dust, yielded *C. botulinum* type A.[42] In California, two type A cases occurred 5 years apart in the children of two families who lived one house apart. In another California family, two infants born successively each acquired type A infant botulism, but the third child born in sequence did not. Soil and dust specimens from the house where all three infants lived contained *C. botulinum* type A.

The role of breast-feeding and formula-feeding as factors possibly predisposing to the development of illness remains unsettled. All studies to date have identified an association between being breast-fed and being hospitalized for infant botulism.[3, 8, 47, 48, 56, 80, 90] This finding has resulted in one perspective that holds that breast-feeding predisposes to the development of illness,[47, 48, 80] whereas the other perspective holds that breast-feeding slows its onset sufficiently to permit hospitalization to occur.[2, 3, 7, 8] However, among hospitalized patients, the mean age at onset of botulism in formula-fed infants (7.6 weeks) was significantly younger and approximately half that of breast-fed infants (13.8 weeks). In addition, the fulminant-onset infant botulism patients who stopped breathing and died at home all were formula-fed.[8] The relative susceptibility of formula-fed and breast-fed infants to the acquisition of infant botulism and the resultant severity of their disease may reflect differences in the availability of suitable ecologic niches in the intestinal flora for *C. botulinum*, differences in the availability of immune factors (such as lactoferrin and secretory IgA) contained in human milk but not in formula milk,[33] or other differences not identified yet.

Honey is the one dietary reservoir of *C. botulinum* spores thus far definitively linked to infant botulism by both laboratory and epidemiologic evidence.* To date, 35 instances worldwide are known in which *C. botulinum* spores have been found in the actual honey fed to an affected infant before the onset of illness. In each instance, the toxin type (A or B) of the spores in the honey matched the toxin type (A or B) of the *C. botulinum* that caused the infant's illness; the probability that such perfect concordance occurred by chance is less than 1 in 10 billion. *C. botulinum* spores have been found in honey from the United States, Argentina, Australia, Canada, China (Taiwan also), Denmark, Finland, Italy, Norway, Spain, Japan, and Central America,* but not in honey from the United Kingdom.[16] For these reasons and because honey is not nutritionally essential, all major pediatric, public health, and honey industry agencies in the United States have joined in the recommendation that honey not be fed to infants. In 2000, several honey brands sold in the United States began to carry a warning to not feed honey to infants; an equivalent label first appeared on British honey in 1996.

Discussion of the possible role of corn syrup in infant botulism is necessitated by two reports. In 1982, the U.S. Food and Drug Administration (FDA) found *C. botulinum* type B spores in approximately 0.5 percent (5 of 961) of previously unopened retail samples of light and dark corn syrup[44]; the manufacturer then made changes in the production process. In 1989, the CDC reported a 2-year epidemiologic study of U.S. cases from all states except California.[80] By subgrouping patients by age and using logistic regression modeling techniques, researchers were able to obtain a statistical association between the triad of corn syrup exposure, breast-feeding, and an age of 2 months or older at onset.[61, 80]

In contrast to these reports, a 1988 Canadian survey found no *C. botulinum* spores in 43 corn syrup samples.[37] A 1991 FDA market survey of 738 syrup samples (354 of which were light corn syrup and 271 were dark corn syrup) concluded that none contained *C. botulinum* spores.[46] A California study (unpublished) of 103 corn syrup samples, 72 of which had been fed to infants who subsequently became ill with infant botulism, did not find *C. botulinum* in any sample. In addition, a 1979 epidemiologic study that simply compared corn syrup exposure rates in 41 cases and 107 control infants identified feeding of corn syrup as a significant protective factor against the acquisition of type A infant botulism.[11] The explanation offered for the latter observation was that if a parent chose corn syrup as a sweetener for the infant, honey was unlikely to have been fed to the child as a second sweetener. Thus, on the basis of evidence presently available, corn syrup does not appear to be a source of *C. botulinum* spores or a risk factor for the acquisition of infant botulism. In addition to corn syrups, honey and hundreds of traditional and nontraditional infant food items, including formula milk, have been examined and found to not contain *C. botulinum.*[43]

Besides honey, potential environmental sources of *C. botulinum* spores have been identified in many locales. Soil in Pennsylvania,[48] soil and cistern water in Australia,[57] and soil and vacuum cleaner dust[7] obtained from case homes in California were found to contain *C. botulinum,* the toxin type of which (A or B) in each instance matched that of the ill infant. However, despite the foregoing findings, it deserves emphasis that for most cases of infant botulism, no source of *C. botulinum* spores is ever identified, even circumstantially. In these cases, the illness probably was acquired by swallowing spores adherent to airborne microscopic (invisible) dust.

Clinical Manifestations

Like other infectious diseases, infant botulism produces a spectrum of clinical severity.[2, 7, 10, 48, 65, 72, 79, 90] To date, almost all recognized infants have been sufficiently hypotonic and weak to need hospitalization. Consequently, the present picture of infant botulism is derived from hospitalized patients. However, botulinism in outpatient infants who displayed only a few days of lethargy, poor feeding, and some decrease in the

*See references 9, 11, 15, 37, 40, 44, 52, 69, 85.

*See references 11, 15, 37, 40, 44, 50, 52, 59, 69, 85.

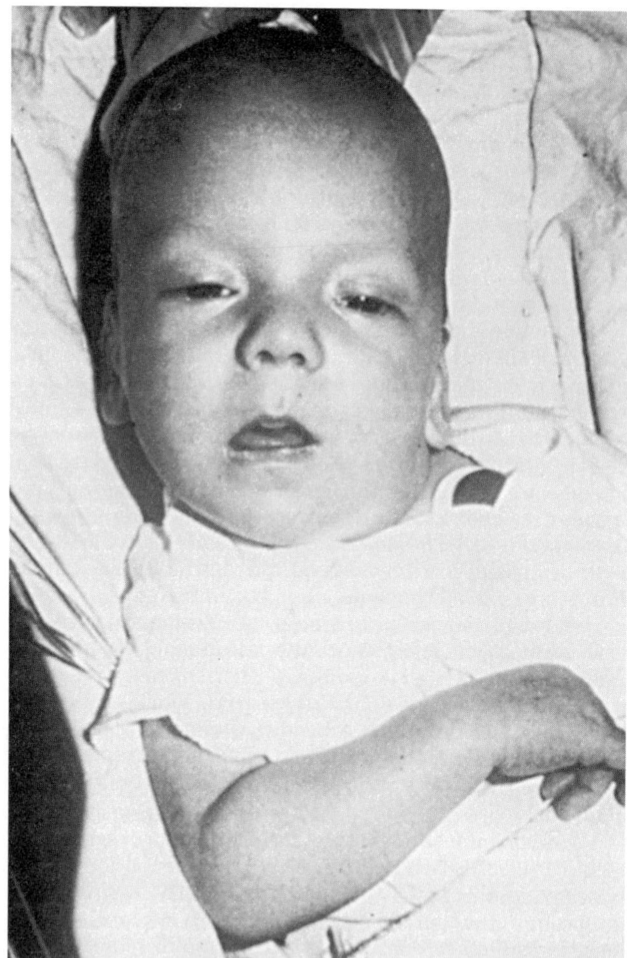

FIGURE 153–2 ■ Mildly affected, 7-week-old infant with botulism. Note the minimal signs, including ptosis, mildly disconjugate gaze, expressionless face, slack jaw, and neck and arm hypotonia.

frequency of bowel movements has been detected by alert physicians familiar with the more "classic" illness. At the opposite end of the clinical spectrum are the few patients with histories and manifestations indistinguishable from those of typical cases of sudden infant death syndrome (crib death),[10, 65, 79, 90] approximately 1 in 20 of which (in California) appears to result from fulminant infant botulism.[7, 10]

The onset of infant botulism ranges from the insidious to the abrupt. At one extreme are patients who were nursing normally 6 hours before becoming so floppy that acute meningitis was the initial diagnosis, and at the other extreme are patients who returned to their physicians four times in a week as the signs of illness gradually became evident.

In the "classic" case, the first sign of illness almost always is constipation (defined as 3 or more days without defecation in a previously regular infant), yet the constipation often is overlooked. A few patients (<5%) will not have a history of constipation. Usually, a mother first notices listlessness, lethargy, and poor feeding, together with breast engorgement if the infant had been nursing. The increasing weakness during the ensuing 1 to 4 days typically brings the baby to medical attention.

Botulism is manifested clinically as a symmetric, descending paralysis. Early in the course, weakness and hypotonia characterize the illness, and the remainder of the physical examination not involving the neuromuscular system is normal. The first signs of illness are found in the cranial nerves; *it is not possible to have infant botulism without having bulbar palsies.* The typical patient has an expressionless face, a feeble cry, ptosis (evident when the eyelids must work against gravity), poor head control, and generalized weakness and hypotonia (Fig. 153–2). Eye muscle paralysis varies, and the pupils often are midposition and initially briskly reactive (Table 153–2). The gag, suck, and swallow reflexes are impaired, as is the corneal reflex if it is tested repetitively. Deep tendon reflexes often are normal at initial evaluation and diminish subsequently as the paralysis extends and increases. The "frog legs" sign frequently is seen. Patients are afebrile unless a secondary infection (e.g., aspiration pneumonia) is present.

The results of most laboratory and clinical studies are normal. At admission, evidence of mild dehydration and fat mobilization may be present because of diminished oral intake. Occasionally at admission, the cerebrospinal fluid (CSF) protein concentration becomes elevated because of the mild dehydration. If infant botulism is suspected soon after admission, electroencephalography, computed tomography, and magnetic resonance imaging seldom are required, but if performed, these examinations yield nonspecific or normal results. Electromyography may offer rapid bedside confirmation of the clinical diagnosis (see "Differential Diagnosis and Diagnosis").[24, 27]

Small amounts (<5 mouse median lethal doses [LD_{50}]/mL) of botulinum toxin occasionally may be identified in serum specimens if they are collected early in the illness.[14, 36, 64, 88, 92] In one report, almost one patient in eight had toxin demonstrable in serum.[36] The definitive diagnostic laboratory study is examination of feces for the presence of *C. botulinum* organisms and toxin, which is the only way to identify the neurotoxin type (A, B, or other) responsible for the illness. Clinically suspected cases that lack an identified toxin type are not included in official tallies of infant botulism.[20, 21]

The usual hospital course of untreated infant botulism has certain general features.[43, 48, 72] After the increasing weakness has necessitated admission, the weakness and hypotonia continue to progress and usually become generalized. The deep tendon reflexes, which may be normal at admission, may diminish or disappear temporarily. The

TABLE 153–2 ■ NEUROLOGIC SIGNS HELPFUL IN THE DIAGNOSIS OF INFANT BOTULISM

Test	Findings
1.	Take the patient to a dark room. Shine a bright light into the eye; note the quickness of pupillary constriction. Remove the light when the constriction is maximal; let the pupil dilate again. Then immediately repeat the light, continuing thus for 1 to 3 minutes. The initially brisk pupillary response may become sluggish and the pupil unable to constrict maximally. (Fatigability with repetitive muscle contraction is the clinical hallmark of botulism.)
2.	Shine a bright light onto the fovea and keep it there for 1 to 3 minutes, even if the infant tries to deviate the eyes. Latent ophthalmoplegia may be elicited, and/or purposeful efforts to avoid the light may diminish.
3.	Place a clean fifth finger in the infant's mouth while taking care to not obstruct the airway. Note the strength and duration of the reflex sucking. The suck is weak and poorly sustained. The gag reflex strength also may be quickly checked (if the infant has not been fed recently).

Adapted from Arnon, S. S.: Infant botulism. Annu. Rev. Med. *31*: 541–560, 1980. Reproduced with permission from Annual Reviews, Inc.

TABLE 153–3 ■ COMPLICATIONS OF INFANT BOTULISM

Adult respiratory distress syndrome
Aspiration
Clostridium difficile colitis
Fracture of the femur (nosocomial)
Inappropriate antidiuretic hormone secretion
Misplaced or plugged endotracheal tube
Necrotizing enterocolitis
Otitis media
Pneumonia
Recurrent atelectasis
Seizures secondary to hyponatremia
Sepsis
Tension pneumothorax
Transfusion reaction
Urinary tract infection
Subglottic stenosis
Tracheal granuloma
Tracheitis
Tracheomalacia

TABLE 153–4 ■ WORKING DIFFERENTIAL DIAGNOSIS OF INFANT BOTULISM

Admission Diagnoses	Subsequent Working Diagnoses
Rule out sepsis	Hypothyroidism
Dehydration	Metabolic encephalopathy
Viral syndrome	Amino acid metabolic disorder
Pneumonia	Heavy metal poisoning (Pb, Mg, As)
Idiopathic hypotonia	Drug ingestion
Failure to thrive	Poliomyelitis
	Medium-chain acyl-CoA dehydrogenase deficiency
	Brain stem encephalitis
	Myasthenia gravis
	Viral polyneuritis
	Guillain-Barré syndrome
	Hirschsprung disease
	Werdnig-Hoffmann disease

nadir of paresis and paralysis in untreated patients usually occurs within 1 to 2 weeks after admission; such patients often remain at their nadir for as long as 1 to 3 weeks before showing signs of improvement. However, once strength and tone begin to return, improvement continues steadily and gradually over the ensuing weeks in the absence of complications (Table 153–3).

In the California experience, infant botulism does not have a biphasic or relapsing course, and perceived "relapses" have been found, in retrospect, to be an indication of either the onset of a complication (see Table 153–3) or premature discharge. However, the clinical experience elsewhere with regard to relapses has been different.[32, 68, 72] The patient is ready for discharge when the gag, suck, and swallow reflexes are sufficiently strong to both protect the airway against accidental aspiration and ensure the adequacy of oral intake. Parents also may be taught to feed by gavage at home. In either situation, discharge may occur safely while head lag and constipation are still present.

Differential Diagnosis and Diagnosis

When initially brought to medical attention, patients with infant botulism often are so mildly weak and hypotonic that the illness is not suspected. Even today, more than 25 years after initial recognition of the disease, suspected sepsis remains the most common admission diagnosis for patients with infant botulism. A careful history (constipation commonly is overlooked) and physical examination (especially cranial nerve function) usually provide sufficient information for correct identification of infant botulism and render most additional testing for the other entities typically suspected unnecessary (Table 153–4).

The diagnosis of infant botulism is established by identification of *C. botulinum* organisms in the feces of an infant with clinical signs consistent with the paralyzing action of botulinum toxin.[20, 43, 45, 51, 63] Extensive studies have demonstrated that *C. botulinum* is not part of the normal resident flora of infants or adults.[7, 36, 81, 82] If the fecal specimen is obtained sufficiently early in the course of the illness, it also will contain botulinum toxin. Because of the patient's constipation, an enema with sterile, nonbacteriostatic water (not saline) commonly is needed to obtain a fecal specimen for diagnostic examination. The mouse neutralization test remains the most sensitive and specific assay for identifying botulinum toxin.[21] Laboratory diagnosis to identify the toxin type responsible for the illness is essential for the case to be registered as infant botulism and is important for prognosis; the mean hospital stay is significantly longer in untreated type A cases (see "Treatment").[2] Physicians are reminded that in most states, botulism or suspected botulism (all types) is an immediately reportable illness.

At the bedside, electromyography sometimes can be helpful in ambiguous situations; when a clinically weak muscle is tested, electromyography often discloses a pattern known by the acronym BSAP (brief, small, abundant motor unit potentials).[9, 24, 27, 30, 72, 75] The edrophonium (Tensilon) test does not need to be performed because congenital myasthenia gravis can be excluded by history, and de novo myasthenia does not occur at this age because of the immaturity of an infant's immune system. Likewise, Guillain-Barré syndrome documented by finding a consistently elevated protein concentration in CSF occurs rarely, if at all, in infancy. In infant botulism, the CSF protein concentration is normal, the occasional exception being that of a specimen collected while the child is dehydrated.

Treatment

Specific therapy for infant botulism is now available. In California, a 5-year, randomized, double-blinded, placebo-controlled treatment trial demonstrated the apparent safety and efficacy of human-derived botulinum antitoxin, known formally as botulism immune globulin intravenous (human) (BIG-IV).[5, 45] The use of BIG-IV reduced the mean hospital stay per case from approximately 5.5 weeks to approximately 2.5 weeks ($p <.001$), as well as the mean hospitalization cost per case by approximately $70,000 ($p <.001$). Treatment with BIG-IV should be started as early in the illness as possible. In the United States, BIG-IV may be obtained from the California Department of Health Services (24-hour telephone: 510-231-7600) under a U.S. FDA–approved Treatment Investigational New Drug (IND) protocol; the license application for BIG-IV is under review at the FDA.

Successful management of infant botulism also depends on meticulous supportive care and anticipation and avoidance of potentially fatal complications (see Table 153–3). Feeding and breathing generally require the most attention. At admission, patients should undergo cardiac, respiratory, and transcutaneous blood gas monitoring (especially carbon dioxide pressure) until it is clear that the paralysis no longer is progressing. An endotracheal tube often is needed to maintain and protect the airway, even in the absence of a need for mechanical ventilation. Particular care should be taken to protect the patient from the acquisition of nosocomially acquired *C. difficile* colitis.[71]

A third cornerstone of management is forbearance. Antibiotics should be reserved to treat the principal secondary infections (pneumonia, urinary tract infection, otitis media) because their use may result in lysis of intraintestinal *C. botulinum* and liberation of intracellular neurotoxin into the gut lumen. This potential problem may be avoided by the use of nalidixic acid or trimethoprim-sulfamethoxazole, antibiotics to which *C. botulinum* is known to be resistant.[87]

Performing a tracheostomy is not necessary.[1, 72] Improved airway management can be accomplished by two simple positioning measures. First, for expansion of the thoracic cage and assistance in diaphragmatic function, patients should be placed in an older-style crib, the rigid bottom mattress of which can be lifted to tilt the entire body to a 30-degree angle. Second, for tipping the head back and to maintain normal curvature of the neck and airway, a soft cloth should be rolled to the thickness of approximately three fingers and placed under just the child's neck. This maneuver allows oral secretions to drain away from the trachea into the true posterior pharynx, where they are swallowed most easily.

The use of intravenous feeding (hyperalimentation) is discouraged because of its potential for causing secondary infection and the success obtained with nasogastric or nasojejunal tube feeding. Mother's milk is the nutritional fluid of choice. Isolation measures or "enteric precautions" are not required, but meticulous handwashing is. Soiled diapers should be autoclaved because they can be expected to contain botulinum neurotoxin, as well as viable spores and vegetative cells of *C. botulinum*. For this reason, staff with open lesions on their hands should not handle the diapers.

The hospital stay of all 508 California patients hospitalized between 1976 and 1991 averaged just over 1 month (4.9 weeks). However, the mean length of stay differed significantly ($p < .0001$) between the 307 type A cases (5.7 weeks) and the 201 type B cases (3.6 weeks), in large part because the major complications and multimonth hospitalizations occurred mainly in type A cases. Thus, untreated illness caused by type A toxin appears to be potentially, but not invariably, more severe than that caused by type B toxin. With the use of BIG-IV, the mean hospital stay has been reduced to approximately 2.5 weeks for patients with either type A or type B infant botulism.

Outcome and Prognosis

Recovery from infant botulism occurs through regeneration of the poisoned terminal unmyelinated nerve endings. The newly synthesized nerve twigs then induce the formation of new motor end-plates that are functionally and morphologically indistinguishable from the original ones.[25, 26] In experimental animals and in humans, completion of this process takes several weeks.[26] Consequently, in the absence of hypoxic cerebral complications, full and complete recovery of strength and tone is the expected outcome of infant botulism. In addition, because botulinum toxin does not cross the blood-brain barrier to any functional degree, the child's intelligence and personality remain as originally endowed. Parents often need reassurance on this latter point. Reinfection with the same or a different type of *C. botulinum* toxin has not occurred. In hospitalized patients in the United States, the case-fatality ratio is less than 1 percent, a reflection of and tribute to the high quality of intensive care given to these critically ill infants. In other countries, the experience has not been so fortunate.

Prevention

At present, the one known way to prevent the acquisition of infant botulism is not to feed honey to infants, and all major pediatric and public health agencies have endorsed this recommendation. Breast-feeding may help moderate the rapidity of onset and the severity of illness. Persuasive evidence that links infant botulism to the ingestion of corn or other syrups is lacking. Mean hospital costs in California (1984 to 1991) exceeded $100,000 per case (2001 dollars; data collection began in 1984), and the patient with the most protracted illness was hospitalized for 10 months in 1988 at a cost of more than $1,000,000 (2001 dollars). These economic facts combine with humanitarian considerations to make a compelling case for the prevention and effective treatment of infant botulism.

SUGGESTED READINGS

Schiavo, G., Matteoli, M., and Montecucco, C.: Neurotoxins affecting Neuroexocytosis. Physiol. Rev. *80*:717–766, 2000. (677 refs)

Smith, L. D. S., and Sugiyama, H.: Botulism: The Organism, Its Toxins, the Disease. 2nd ed. Springfield, IL, Charles C Thomas, 1988.

REFERENCES

1. Anderson, T. D, Shah, U. K., Schreiner, M. D., and Jacobs, I. N.: Airway complications of infant botulism: Ten-year experience with 60 cases. Otolaryngol. Head Neck Surg. *126*:234–239, 2002.
2. Arnon, S. S.: Infant botulism. Annu. Rev. Med. *31*:541–560, 1980.
3. Arnon, S. S.: Breast feeding and toxigenic intestinal infections: Missing links in crib death? Rev. Infect. Dis. *6*(Suppl.):193–201, 1984.
4. Arnon, S. S.: Infant botulism: Anticipating the second decade. J. Infect. Dis. *154*:201–206, 1986.
5. Arnon, S. S.: Clinical trial of human botulism immune globulin. *In* Das Gupta, B. R. (ed.): Botulinum and Tetanus Neurotoxins: Neurotransmission and Biomedical Aspects. New York, Plenum Press, 1993, pp. 477–482.
6. Arnon, S. S.: Botulism as an intestinal toxemia. *In* Blaser, M. J., Smith, P. D., Ravdin, J. I., et al. (eds.): Infections of the Gastrointestinal Tract. New York, Raven Press, 1995, pp. 257–271.
7. Arnon, S. S., Damus, K., and Chin, J.: Infant botulism: Epidemiology and relation to sudden infant death syndrome. Epidemiol. Rev. *3*:45–66, 1981.
8. Arnon, S. S., Damus, K., Thompson, B., et al.: Protective role of human milk against sudden death from infant botulism. J. Pediatr. *100*:568–573, 1982.
9. Arnon, S. S., Midura, T. F., Clay, S. A., et al.: Infant botulism: Epidemiological, clinical, and laboratory aspects. J. A. M. A. *237*:1946–1951, 1977.
10. Arnon, S. S., Midura, T. F., Damus, K., et al.: Intestinal infection and toxin production by *Clostridium botulinum* as one cause of sudden infant death syndrome. Lancet *1*:1273–1277, 1978.
11. Arnon, S. S., Midura, T. F., Damus, K., et al.: Honey and other environmental risk factors for infant botulism. J. Pediatr. *94*:331–336, 1979.
12. Arnon, S. S., Schechter, R., Inglesby, T. V., et al.: Botulinum toxin as a biological weapon: Medical and public health management. J. A. M. A. *285*:1059–1070, 2001.
13. Arnon, S. S., Werner, S. B., Faber, H. K., et al.: Infant botulism in 1931: Discovery of a misclassified case. Am. J. Dis. Child. *133*:580–582, 1979.
14. Aureli, P., Fenicia, L., Pasolini, B., et al.: Two cases of type E infant botulism in Italy caused by neurotoxigenic *Clostridium butyricum*. J. Infect. Dis. *54*:207–211, 1986.
15. Aureli P., Franciosa, G., Fenicia, L.: Infant botulism and honey in Europe: A commentary. Pediatr. Infect. Dis. J. *21*:866–868, 2002.
16. Berry, P. R., Gilbert, R. J., Oliver, R. W. A., et al.: Some preliminary studies on the low incidence of infant botulism in the United Kingdom. Corres. J. Clin. Pathol. *40*:121, 1987.
17. Burr, D. H., Sugiyama, H., and Jarvis, G.: Susceptibility to enteric botulinum colonization of antibiotic-treated adult mice. Infect. Immun. *36*:103–106, 1982.
18. Byard, R. W., Moore, L., Bourne, A. J., et al.: *Clostridium botulinum* and sudden infant death syndrome: A 10 year prospective study. J. Paediatr. Child Health *28*:156–157, 1992.

19. Centers for Disease Control and Prevention: Sudden infant death syndrome: United States, 1983–1994. M. M. W. R. Morb. Mortal. Wkly. Rep. *45*:859–863, 1996.
20. Centers for Disease Control and Prevention: Case definitions for infectious conditions under public health surveillance. M. M. W. R. Recomm. Rep. *46*(RR-10):7–8, 1997.
21. Centers for Disease Control and Prevention: Botulism in the United States, 1899–1996. Handbook for Epidemiologists, Clinicians, and Laboratory Workers. Atlanta, Centers for Disease Control, 1998.
22. Chia, J. K., Clark, J. B., Ryan, C. A., et al.: Botulism in an adult associated with food-borne intestinal infection with *Clostridium botulinum*. N. Engl. J. Med. *315*:239–240, 1986.
23. Clay, S. A., Ramseyer, J. C., Fishman, L. S., et al.: Acute infantile motor unit disorder: Infantile botulism? Arch. Neurol. *345*:236–243, 1977.
24. Cornblath, D. R., Sladky, J. T., and Sumner, A. J.: Clinical electrophysiology of infantile botulism. Muscle Nerve *6*:448–452, 1983.
25. De Pavia, A., Meunier, F. A., Molgo, J., et al.: Functional repair of motor endplates after botulinum neurotoxin type A poisoning: Biphasic switch of synaptic activity between nerve sprouts and their parent terminals. Proc. Natl. Acad. Sci. U. S. A. *96*:3200–3205, 1999.
26. Duchen, L. W.: Motor nerve growth induced by botulinum toxin as a regenerative phenomenon. Proc. R. Soc. Med. *65*:196–197, 1972.
27. Engel, W. K.: Brief, small, abundant motor-unit action potentials: A further critique of electromyographic interpretation. Neurology *25*: 173–176, 1975.
28. Fenicia, L., Franciosa, G., Pourshaban, M., and Aureli, P.: Intestinal toxemia botulism in two young people caused by *Clostridium butyricum* type E (and addendum). Clin. Infect. Dis. *29*:1381–1387, 1999.
29. Freedman, M., Armstrong, R. M., Killian, J. M., et al.: Botulism in a patient with jejunoileal bypass. Ann. Neurol. *20*:641–643, 1986.
30. Graf, W. D., Hays, R. M., Astley, S. J., and Mendelman, P. M.: Electrodiagnostic reliability in the diagnosis of infant botulism. J. Pediatr. *120*: 747–749, 1992.
31. Gill, D. M.: Bacterial toxins: A table of lethal amounts. Microbiol. Rev. *46*: 86–94, 1982.
32. Glauser, T. A., Maguire, H. C., and Sladky, J. T.: Relapse of infant botulism. Ann. Neurol. *28*:187–189, 1990.
33. Goldman, A. S., and Goldblum, R. M.: Immunologic system in human milk: Characteristics and effects. *In* Lebenthal, E. (ed.): Textbook of Gastroenterology and Nutrition in Infancy. 2nd ed. New York, Raven Press, 1989, pp. 135–142.
34. Grover, W. D., Peckham, G. J., and Berman, P. H.: Recovery following cranial nerve dysfunction and muscle weakness in infancy. Dev. Med. Child. Neurol. *16*:163–171, 1974.
35. Hall, J. D., McCroskey, L. M., Pincomb, B. J., et al.: Isolation of an organism resembling *Clostridium barati* which produces type F botulinal toxin from an infant with botulism. J. Clin. Microbiol. *21*:654–655, 1985.
36. Hatheway, C. L., and McCroskey, L. M.: Examination of feces and serum for diagnosis of infant botulism in 336 patients. J. Clin. Microbiol. *25*: 2334–2338, 1987.
37. Hauschild, A. H. W., Hilsheimer, R., Weiss, K. F., et al.: *Clostridium botulinum* in honey, syrups and dry infant cereals. J. Food Protect. *51*: 892–894, 1988.
38. Hoffman, R. E., Pincomb, B. J., Skeels, M. R., et al.: Type F infant botulism. Am. J. Dis. Child. *136*:270–271, 1982.
39. Hubert, P., Roy, C., and Caille, B.: Un cas de botulisme chez un nourrisson de 11 mois. Arch. Fr. Pediatr. *44*:129–130, 1987.
40. Huhtanen, C. N., Knox, D., and Shimanuki, H.: Incidence and origin of *Clostridium botulinum* spores in honey. J. Food Protect. *44*:812–815, 1981.
41. Hurst, D. L., and Marsh, W. W.: Early severe infantile botulism. J. Pediatr. *122*:909–911, 1993.
42. Istre, G. R., Compton, R., Novotny, T., et al.: Infant botulism: Three cases in a small town. Am. J. Dis. Child. *140*:1013–1014, 1986.
43. Johnson, R. O., Clay, S. A., and Arnon, S. S.: Diagnosis and management of infant botulism. Am. J. Dis. Child. *133*:586–593, 1979.
44. Kautter, D. A., Lilly, T., Jr., Solomon, H. M., et al.: *Clostridium botulinum* spores in infant foods: A survey. J. Food Protect. *45*: 1028–1029, 1982.
45. Lewis, G. E., Jr.: Approaches to the prophylaxis, immunotherapy, and chemotherapy of botulism. *In* Lewis, G. E., Jr. (ed.): Biomedical Aspects of Botulism. New York, Academic Press, 1981, pp. 261–270.
46. Lilly, T., Jr., Rhodehamel, E. J., Kautter, D. A., et al.: Incidence of *Clostridium botulinum* spores in corn syrup and other syrups. J. Food Protect. *54*:585–587, 1991.
47. Long, S. S.: Epidemiologic study of infant botulism in Pennsylvania: Report of the infant botulism study group. J. Pediatr. *75*:928–934, 1985.
48. Long, S. S., Gajeweski, J. L., Brown, L. W., et al.: Clinical, laboratory, and environmental features of infant botulism in southeastern Pennsylvania. Pediatrics *75*:935–941, 1985.
49. McCroskey, L. M., and Hatheway, C. L.: Laboratory findings in four cases of adult botulism suggest colonization of the intestinal tract. J. Clin. Microbiol. *26*:1052–1054, 1988.
50. Nakano, H., Okabe, T., Hashimoto, H., and Sakaguchi, G.: Incidence of *Clostridium botulinum* in honey of various origins. Jpn. J. Med. Sci. Biol. *43*:183–195, 1990.
51. Midura, T. F., and Arnon, S. S.: Infant botulism: Identification of *Clostridium botulinum* and its toxins in faeces. Lancet *2*:934–936, 1976.
52. Midura, T. F., Snowden, S., Wood, R. M., et al.: Isolation of *Clostridium botulinum* from honey. J. Clin. Microbiol. *9*:282–283, 1979.
53. Mills, D. C., and Arnon, S. S.: The large intestine as the site of *Clostridium botulinum* colonization in human infant botulism. J. Infect. Dis. *156*: 997–998, 1987.
54. Moberg, L. J., and Sugiyama, H.: Microbial ecologic basis of infant botulism as studied with germfree mice. Infect. Immun. *25*:653–657, 1979.
55. Montecucco, C., and Schiavo, G.: Tetanus and botulism neurotoxins: A new group of zinc proteases. Trends Biochem. Sci. *18*:324–327, 1993.
56. Morris, J. G., Jr., Snyder, J. D., Wilson, R., et al.: Infant botulism in the United States: An epidemiologic study of cases occurring outside of California. Am. J. Public Health *73*:1385–1388, 1983.
57. Murrell, W. G., and Stewart, B. J.: Botulism in New South Wales, 1980–1981. Med. J. Aust. *1*:13–17, 1983.
58. Murrell, W. G., Stewart, B. J., O'Neill, C., et al.: Enterotoxigenic bacteria in sudden infant death syndrome. J. Med. Microbiol. *39*:114–127, 1993.
59. Nevas, M., Hielm, S., Lindstrom, M., et al.: High prevalence of *Clostridium botulinum* types A and B in honey samples detected by polymerase chain reaction. Int. J. Food Microbiol. *72*:45–52, 2002.
60. Niemann, H., Blasi, J., and Jahn, R.: Clostridial neurotoxins: New tools for dissecting exocytosis. Trends Cell. Biol. *4*:179–185, 1994.
61. Olsen, S. J., and Swerdlow, D. L.: Risk of infant botulism from corn syrup. Pediatr. Infect. Dis. J. *19*:584–585, 2000.
62. Paisley, J. W., Lauer, B. A., and Arnon, S. S.: A second case of infant botulism type F caused by *Clostridium baratii*. Pediatr. Infect. Dis. J. *14*: 912–914, 1995.
63. Paton, J. C., Lawrence, A. J., and Manson, J. I.: Quantitation of *Clostridium botulinum* organisms and toxin in the feces of an infant with botulism. J. Clin. Microbiol. *15*:1–4, 1982.
64. Paton, J. C., Lawrence, A. J., and Steven, I. M.: Quantities of *Clostridium botulinum* organisms and toxin in feces and presence of *Clostridium botulinum* toxin in the serum of an infant with botulism. J. Clin. Microbiol. *17*:13–15, 1983.
65. Peterson, D. R., Eklund, M. W., and Chinn, N. M.: The sudden infant death syndrome and infant botulism. Rev. Infect. Dis. *1*(Suppl.):630–634, 1979.
66. Pickett, J., Berg, B., Chaplin, E., et al.: Syndrome of botulism in infancy: Clinical and electrophysiologic study. N. Engl. J. Med. *295*:770–772, 1976.
67. Ramseyer, J. C., Clay, S. A., and Fishman, L. S.: Electromyographic studies in acute infantile polyneuropathy. Neurology *26*:364, 1976.
68. Ravid, S., Maytal, J., and Eviatar, L.: Biphasic course of infant botulism. Pediatr. Neurol. *23*:338–339, 2000.
69. Sakaguchi, G., Sakaguchi, S., Kamata, Y., et al.: Distinct characteristics of *Clostridium botulinum* type A strains and their toxin associated with infant botulism in Japan. Int. J. Food Microbiol. *11*:231–242, 1990.
70. Schechter, R., and Arnon, S. S.: Where Marco Polo meets Meckel: Type E botulism from *Clostridium butyricum*. Clin. Infect. Dis. *29*:1388–1393, 1999.
71. Schechter, R., Peterson, B., McGee, J., et al.: *Clostridium difficile* colitis associated with infant botulism: Near-fatal case analogous to Hirschsprung's enterocolitis. Clin. Infect. Dis. *29*:367–374, 1999.
72. Schreiner, M. S., Field, E., and Ruddy, R.: Infant botulism: A review of 12 years' experience at the Children's Hospital of Philadelphia. Pediatrics *87*:159–165, 1991.
73. Schwarz, P. J., Arnon, J. M., and Arnon, S. S.: Epidemiological aspects of infant botulism in California, 1976–1991. *In* DasGupta, B. R. (ed.): Botulinum and Tetanus Neurotoxins: Neurotransmission and Biomedical Aspects. New York, Plenum Press, 1993.
74. Shen, W. -P. V., Felsing, N., Lang, D., et al.: Development of infant botulism in a 3-year-old female with neuroblastoma following autologous bone marrow transplantation. Bone Marrow Transplant. *13*:345–347, 1994.
75. Sheth, R. D., Lotz, B. P., Hecox, K. E., and Waclawik, A. J.: Infantile botulism: Pitfalls in electrodiagnosis. J. Child Neurol. *14*:156–158, 1999.
76. Smith, G. E., Hinde, F., Westmoreland, D., et al.: Infantile botulism. Arch. Dis. Child. *64*:871–872, 1989.
77. Smith, L. D. S.: The occurrence of *Clostridium botulinum* and *Clostridium tetani* in the soil of the United States. Health Lab. Sci. *15*:74–80, 1978.
78. Smith, L. D. S., and Sugiyama, H.: Botulism: The Organism, Its Toxins, the Disease. 2nd ed. Springfield, IL, Charles C Thomas, 1988.
79. Sonnabend, O. A. R., Sonnabend, W. F. F., Krech, U., et al.: Continuous microbiological and pathological study of 70 sudden and unexpected deaths: Toxigenic intestinal *Clostridium botulinum* infection in 9 cases of sudden infant death syndrome. Lancet *1*:237–240, 1985.
80. Spika, J. S., Shaffer, N., Hargrett-Bean, N., et al.: Risk factors for infant botulism in the United States. Am. J. Dis. Child. *143*:828–832, 1989.
81. Stark, P. L., and Lee, A.: The microbial ecology of the large bowel of breast-fed and formula-fed infants during the first year of life. J. Med. Microbiol. *15*:189–203, 1982.
82. Stark, P. L., and Lee, A.: Clostridia isolated from the feces of infants during the first year of life. J. Pediatr. *100*:362–365, 1982.

83. Suen, J. C., Hatheway, C. L., Steigerwalt, A. G., et al.: Genetic confirmation of identities of neurotoxigenic *Clostridium barati* and *Clostridium butyricum* implicated as agents of infant botulism. J. Clin. Microbiol. *26*:2191–2192, 1988.
84. Sugiyama, H., and Mills, D. C.: Intraintestinal toxin in infant mice challenged intragastrically with *Clostridium botulinum* spores. Infect. Immun. *21*:59–63, 1978.
85. Sugiyama, H., Mills, D. C., and Kuo, L. -J. C.: Number of *Clostridium botulinum* spores in honey. J. Food Protect. *41*:848–850, 1978.
86. Sullivan, N. M., Mills, D. C., Riemann, H. P., and Arnon, S. S.: Inhibition of growth of *Clostridium botulinum* by intestinal microflora isolated from healthy infants. Microbiol. Ecol. Health Dis. *1*:179–192, 1988.
87. Swenson, J. M., Thornsberry, C., McCroskey, L. M., et al.: Susceptibility of *Clostridium botulinum* to thirteen antimicrobial agents. Antimicrob. Agents Chemother. *18*:13–19, 1980.
88. Takahashi, M., Noda, H., Takeshita, S. et al.: Attempts to quantify *Clostridium botulinum* type A toxin and antitoxin in serum of two cases of infant botulism in Japan. Jpn. J. Med. Sci. Biol. *43*:233–237, 1990.
89. Thilo, E. H., and Townsend, S. F.: Infant botulism at 1 week of age: Report of two cases. Pediatrics *92*:151–153, 1993.
90. Thompson, J. A., Glasgow, L. A., Warpinski, J. R., et al.: Infant botulism: Clinical spectrum and epidemiology. Pediatrics *66*:936–942, 1980.
91. Tonkin, S.: Sudden infant death syndrome: Hypothesis of causation. Pediatrics *55*:650–661, 1975.
92. Toyoguchi, S., Tsugu, H., Nariai, A., et al.: Infant botulism with Down syndrome. Acta Pediatr. Jpn. *33*:394–397, 1991.
93. Trethon, A., Budai, J., Herendi, A., et al.: Infant botulism. Orv. Hetil. *28*:1497–1499, 1995.
94. Wilcke, B. W., Jr., Midura, T. F., and Arnon, S. S.: Quantitative evidence of intestinal colonization by *Clostridium botulinum* in four cases of infant botulism. J. Infect. Dis. *141*:419–423, 1980.

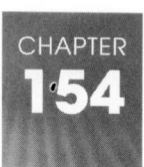

CHAPTER 154 Tetanus

JAMES D. CHERRY ■ RICK E. HARRISON

Tetanus is caused by the anaerobic, spore-forming bacillus *Clostridium tetani*, an organism present in soil and human and animal feces. The clinical symptoms are not caused by infection but result from a specific toxin, tetanospasmin, that is produced at the site of injury and acts primarily on the spinal cord but also on the brain, motor end-plates, and autonomic nerves. The disease may appear as a local form or a more generalized syndrome. It is characterized by tonic spasms of skeletal muscles, little or no fever, and occasional spasms of the glottis and larynx. Bilateral trismus is the most common sign. Active immunization is highly protective. Although tetanus is well controlled today in developed countries throughout the world, it remains a major cause of death in developing countries.[26] In 1993, an estimated 515,000 deaths were caused by neonatal tetanus.

History

The first description of tetanus in recorded medical history probably was written by Hippocrates.[53] A vivid picture of the clinical course of the disease was recorded by Aretaeus the Cappadocian in the second century.[6] Very little of importance was added to this knowledge during the next 18 centuries. The transmissibility of tetanus was demonstrated by Carle and Rattone[23] in 1884. They reported that when the sciatic nerves of rabbits were injected with the contents of a human "pustule," the characteristic disease developed in the animals in 2 to 3 days; inoculation of tissue obtained from their nervous systems into healthy rabbits produced a similar syndrome. The role of soil in the pathogenesis of tetanus was demonstrated by Nicolaier[77] in 1884; although he saw the organism, he was unable to recover it.

The bacterium responsible for the disease was identified first by Rosenbach,[90] who described a bacillus containing a round terminal spore in pus obtained from a human case; tetanus developed when the purulent exudate was injected into animals. *C. tetani* was isolated by Kitasato,[59] who fulfilled Koch's postulates with it in 1889. One year later, von Behring and Kitasato[107] reported the appearance of specific antitoxin in the serum of animals given injections of the tetanus toxin produced by the organism. This finding was followed, in 1926, by the development of toxoid, injections of which produced immunity.

Microbiology

The vegetative form of *C. tetani* is a gram-positive, spore-forming, motile, anaerobic bacillus that measures 0.3 to 0.5 μm in width and 2.0 to 2.5 μm in length; in culture, long filament-like cells develop.[12, 20, 108, 111] *C. tetani* is a strict anaerobe that grows best at 33° C to 37° C; it can be cultured in many different routine media used for anaerobic organisms, such as thioglycolate, casein hydrolysate, and cooked meat. Enhanced growth occurs in medium supplemented with reducing substances and maintained at neutral or alkaline pH. With growth, gas with a fetid odor usually is produced.

The first step in the process of spore formation is the development of a bulge at one end of the organism; this bulge contains the spore and is responsible for the characteristic drumstick or tennis racquet appearance. As sporulation progresses, the organism decreases in length and the spores are extruded. They stain poorly by the Gram method. Sporulation occurs in tissues as well as in vitro and is dependent on the composition of the medium and the temperature of the culture. Enhanced sporulation occurs in the presence of oleic acid, phosphates, 1 to 2 percent sodium chloride, and manganese salts.[12, 20, 108] In vivo, sporulation is enhanced by lactic acid and other substances toxic to cells. Sporulation is inhibited by high and low temperatures (>41° C and <25° C), glucose, fatty acids, and potassium salts. The metabolic activity of *C. tetani* is limited; carbohydrates and proteins are digested poorly, and the vegetative, nonsporulated forms are killed easily by heat and numerous disinfecting agents. In contrast, the spores are resistant to boiling and phenol, cresol, 1:1000 bichloride of mercury, and other disinfectants; however, they are destroyed by heating at 120° C for 15 to 20 minutes. If not exposed to sunlight, the spores may survive in soil for months to years. They also may constitute part of the normal intestinal microflora of some horses, cows, guinea pigs, sheep, dogs, cats, rats, chickens, and humans.

Three nonpathogenic clostridia are present in soil and in human and animal feces: *Clostridium tetanomorphum, Clostridium tertium,* and *Clostridium tetanoides.* Diagnostic confusion may occur because they are morphologically similar to the organism responsible for tetanus. *C. tetani* is recovered much more commonly from cultivated than from virgin or uncultivated soil. Rural dwellers and people engaged in agricultural occupations have a higher rate of intestinal, skin, and oral carriage of the organism than city dwellers have. Dust and dirt from houses, streets, and operating rooms, as well as solutions of heroin, have been found to be contaminated with the organism.

Epidemiology

SOURCE OF EXPOSURE

The predominant reservoir of *C. tetani* is the soil; it is also part of the normal flora of the intestinal tract of animals, both herbivores and omnivores.[108] Intestinal spores and bacilli are shed in the feces of animals and contribute to the soil reservoir.

The worldwide morbidity and mortality attributable to tetanus is related inversely to adequate immunization with tetanus toxoid and directly to suboptimal hygiene and childbirth practices and wound care.[108] Throughout the world, tetanus has a seasonal trend: more cases occur in the summer or in "wet" seasons. Rates of illness are highest in countries that are located near the equator and have fertile soil.

Acute wounds, including relatively minor ones, are the site of most *C. tetani* infections leading to tetanus. In addition, infection may occur after parenteral drug use and surgical procedures. In many cases, the source of exposure is unknown. The source of infection in neonatal tetanus is the umbilical cord or stump as a result of unsterile delivery conditions and unhygienic cultural rituals involving the umbilical stump.[54, 55]

INCIDENCE

The reported incidence of tetanus and tetanus-related deaths in the United States from 1947 to 1997 is presented in Figure 154–1, and the reported cases and their incidence are presented by age group and fatal cases for 1995 to 1997 in Figure 154–2.[25] From 1947 through 1976, the incidence of tetanus fell 10-fold; since 1976, the continued decrease in incidence has been less than twofold. During the same period, mortality rates fell from 91 percent in 1947 to 44 percent in 1976 to 11 percent in 1995 to 1997.

As noted in Figure 154–2, 35 percent of the patients were 60 years or older, 60 percent were 20 to 59 years old, and only 5 percent were younger than 20 years.[25, 27] Of the 124 cases of tetanus reported in 1995 to 1997, the immunization status was known in 58 (46%). Of this group, 47 percent were not immunized and 72 percent had two or fewer doses of vaccine. Sixteen patients had received three or more doses of vaccine. Of these 16 patients, 2 were younger than 20 years of age. One was a 14-year-old boy who had been bitten by a dog and had received his last vaccine dose 2 years previously. He had sought medical care after his injury. The other case occurred in a 15-year-old boy injured in a moped crash. His last vaccine dose had been 11 years previously, and he received tetanus toxoid within 6 hours of his injury. Forty percent of the cases in 1995 to 1997 occurred in females.

Pathogenesis

Tetanus is, by strictest definition, not a true infection. Spores introduced at a site of injury remain harmless until, stimulated by a variety of factors, they are converted to vegetative forms that multiply but do not produce injury to tissue or provoke an inflammatory response. The clinical syndrome is caused entirely by toxin elaborated in the area where the vegetative cells are growing. *C. tetani* produces two exotoxins: tetanolysin and tetanospasmin. Tetanolysin induces hemolysis but plays no role in the disease. The activity of tetanospasmin is responsible for all the clinical features of the disease. Purified tetanospasmin is a protein with a molecular weight of approximately 67,000 Da.[81] One milligram contains 6,400,000 lethal doses for mice; 0.00001 mg may kill a 20-g mouse in 2 hours. With the exception of the toxin produced by *Clostridium botulinum*, tetanospasmin currently is the most potent known poison. Humans are most susceptible to this agent and require only 1/2500 and 1/350,000 of the dose fatal for cats and chickens, respectively.

C. tetani is introduced into an area of injury as the spore, the form usually present in soil and intestinal contents. Disease does not develop until the spores are converted to

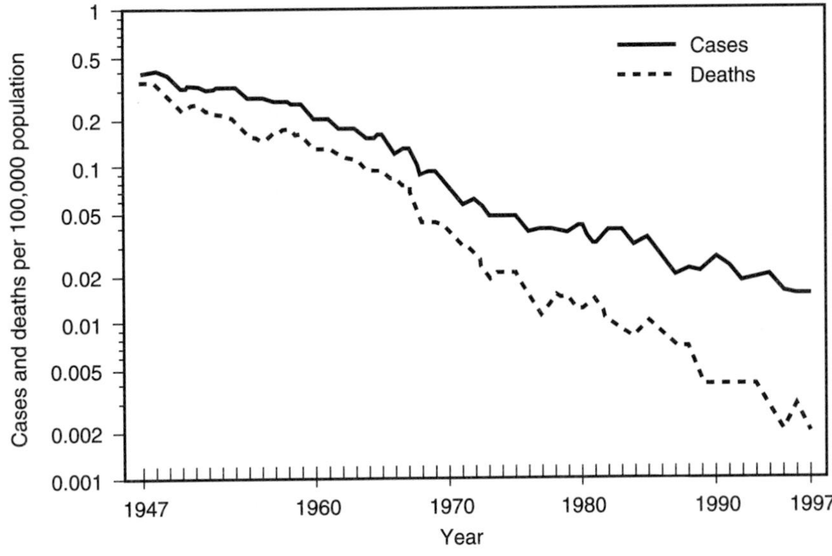

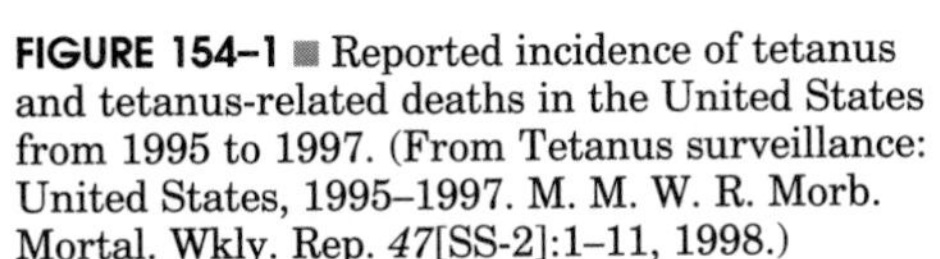
FIGURE 154–1 ■ Reported incidence of tetanus and tetanus-related deaths in the United States from 1995 to 1997. (From Tetanus surveillance: United States, 1995–1997. M. M. W. R. Morb. Mortal. Wkly. Rep. *47*[SS-2]:1–11, 1998.)

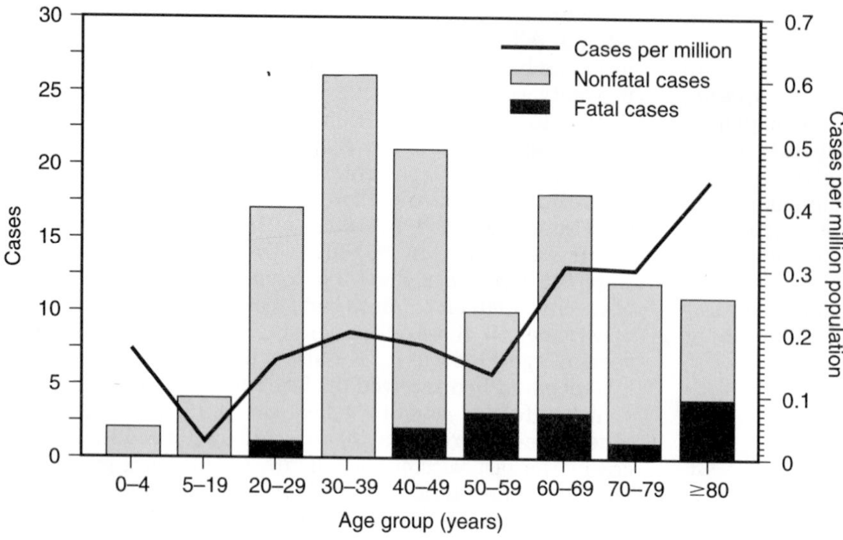

FIGURE 154–2 ■ Reported tetanus cases and incidence rates by age group in the United States in 1995 and 1997. (From Tetanus surveillance: United States, 1995–1997. M. M. W. R. Morb. Mortal. Wkly. Rep. *47*[SS-2]:1–11, 1998.)

the toxin-elaborating bacillus, which does not follow the simple inoculation of spores. When these spores are injected with very sharp needles into animals so that tissue is not injured but merely separated, tetanus does not develop. However, the addition of a small quantity of calcium chloride to a suspension of spores before injection is performed leads to development of the typical disease. This development is not caused by a specific effect of the cation on conversion of the spore to the vegetative form of the organism but is related to the necrosis of tissue produced by it, which leads to a reduction in oxidation-reduction potential and oxygen tension, factors involved in vegetation of the spore; the same effects are produced by the presence of a foreign body, trauma, or a localized suppurative process.

The pathway by which toxin, elaborated at the site at which *C. tetani* is multiplying, reaches the central nervous system (CNS) has been a matter of controversy. Researchers first thought that tetanospasmin was absorbed chiefly by motor nerve endings and then traveled along axis cylinders to the anterior horn cells.[82] Symptoms of the disease were thought to appear only after the toxin had reached the nervous system, with the initial tetanic contractions occurring first in the injured extremity, then in the opposite limb, and finally, as the toxin diffused through the spinal cord, in all the muscles. A small amount of toxin was suggested to be absorbed into the lymph and carried to the bloodstream, from which it was taken up by motor nerve endings in various parts of the body.[71]

Abel and associates[1] postulated that toxin reached the nervous system via the arterial circulation and suggested the following series of events. Some of the toxin diffuses from the local site of injury into adjacent skeletal muscle and acts on the neuromuscular organs to produce a state of maintained contraction: *local tetanus*. Some toxin also enters the lymphatics and bloodstream, from which it is taken up by specifically reactive cells in the spinal cord, medulla, and the motor end-organs of muscle.

Friedemann and colleagues[46] noted that tetanus toxin did not penetrate the blood-brain barrier, and, therefore, they questioned hematogenous transmission. This finding led researchers to focus attention on transport of tetanospasmin in nerves. Wright and coworkers[114] observed that direct injection of toxin into the vagal, facial, or hypoglossal nerves of rabbits led, within 24 hours, to the development of a syndrome characteristic of involvement of the brain stem, as indicated by the appearance of strabismus, immobility of the hairs in the nasal cavity, salivation, bradycardia, and torticollis. Inoculation of the vagus resulted in the successive development of these manifestations; those dependent on innervation from motor nuclei in close proximity to the nerve tended to appear early. This hypothesis is supported by observations indicating that a variety of substances, including India ink and radioactive compounds, migrate along peripheral nerves to the CNS after intraneural injection.[43] This observation, together with the demonstration by numerous investigators that toxin is present in the peripheral nerves closest to the site of inoculation, supports the concept of transport of tetanospasmin in the tissues of the nervous system.

Knowledge of the specific mechanisms involved in the absorption of tetanus toxin and its mechanisms of action on body cells is incomplete. Most of the evidence presently available indicates that some element of the peripheral nerve is involved. Whether transport occurs in the axis cylinder, the perineural space, or the lymphatics remains unsettled. Tetanus toxin is carried to the neurons of the sciatic nerve via the neurofibrillae in axis cylinders at a rate of approximately 3.35 mm/hr.[89]

Pathophysiology

Tetanospasmin exerts its effects in four areas of the nervous system: (1) the motor end-plates in skeletal muscle, (2) the spinal cord, (3) the brain, and (4) (in some cases) the sympathetic nervous system.*

MOTOR END-PLATES IN SKELETAL MUSCLE

Tetanus toxin has been noted to interfere with neuromuscular transmission. Release of acetylcholine from the nerve terminals in muscle is inhibited. The presence of tetanospasmin in the transverse and terminal sacs of the longitudinal elements of the sarcotubular system of the skeletal muscles suggests that it acts by interfering with contraction coupling or with the mechanisms involved in contraction and relaxation. These phenomena probably are involved in the pathogenesis of local tetanus.

*See references 16, 18, 19, 22, 33, 56, 57, 96, 105, 116.

SPINAL CORD

The effects of the toxin on the spinal cord are practically identical to those produced by strychnine. It does not act on reflex arcs that include only sensory and motor neurons (two-neuron or monosynaptic reflexes). However, the toxin profoundly alters the activity of the more complex polysynaptic reflexes involving interneurons, thereby leading to the inhibition of antagonists. Hyperpolarization of the membranes of neurons, a mechanism normally operating when direct inhibitory pathways are stimulated, is suppressed. The depolarization associated with excitation is not affected. Whether tetanospasmin blocks inhibitory synapses by preventing release of the inhibitory transmitter substance or by suppressing the action of this substance on the membrane of motor neurons is unknown. Selective blocking of inhibitory synapses in the CNS appears adequate to account for the primary phenomena of tetanus. Unchecked and uncoordinated excitatory impulses multiply and traverse reflex pathways to produce the characteristic tetanic spasms of muscles.

BRAIN

Researchers have suggested that the action of tetanospasmin on the brain may be responsible for the typical seizures of tetanus.[16] This hypothesis is supported, in part, by the observation that cerebral gangliosides fix the toxin. The antidromic inhibition of evoked cortical activity is decreased. The effects of tetanospasmin on the brain are the same as those on the spinal cord, as well as those that occur after exposure to strychnine.

SYMPATHETIC NERVOUS SYSTEM

Manifestations indicating dysfunction of the sympathetic nervous system have been observed in some patients with tetanus. Signs and symptoms include profuse sweating, peripheral vasoconstriction, labile hypertension, cardiac arrhythmias, tachycardia, increased output of carbon dioxide, elevated urinary concentration of catecholamines, and hypotension late in the course of the disease.

Clinical Manifestations

Although it may be as short as 1 day or as long as several months, the incubation period of tetanus is usually 3 to 21 days. A direct relationship may exist between the distance of the site of invasion by *C. tetani* from the CNS and the length of the interval between injury and the onset of disease; the greater the distance between the local area and the CNS, the longer, in general, the incubation period. Sustained or separate, repeated tonic spasms of isolated or multiple muscles are the characteristic clinical feature of the disease. Tetanus may appear in two forms: local and generalized.

LOCAL TETANUS

The occurrence of local tetanus probably is more common than recognized. Although local tetanus is thought to occur infrequently, it probably is so because it may be uncommon as an isolated syndrome or because by the time that diffuse involvement has occurred, the spasms in the muscles in the area of the site of entry of the organism cannot be separated from the generalized spasms. Local manifestations frequently precede the development of the generalized disorder. The characteristic abnormality in local tetanus is unyielding, persistent, painful rigidity of the group of muscles that lie in close proximity to the site at which *C. tetani* was introduced. Local tetanus often is present when a dose of antitoxin has been given that is adequate to inactivate circulating toxin but insufficient to neutralize what has accumulated at the site of injury. Symptoms may persist for several weeks or months and finally disappear without leaving any residua.[72] Local tetanus may be the only manifestation, usually is mild, and has a fatality rate of approximately 1 percent.

Cephalic tetanus is a variant of local tetanus. It generally occurs after the introduction of *C. tetani* in the course of injuries to the scalp, eye, face, ear, or neck; in conjunction with chronic otitis media; and, rarely, after tonsillectomy.[7] Insect bites on the face or head, especially if secondarily infected by pyogenic organisms, also may serve as portals of entry for the organism. The incubation period of this syndrome is short, frequently no more than 1 to 2 days. The principal distinctive clinical features are palsies of cranial nerves III, IV, VII, IX, X, and XII; they may be involved singly or in any combination. Dysfunction may persist for days or many months. In general, the prognosis for survival is poor. However, if death does not intervene, complete recovery without residual neurologic dysfunction is the rule. In some, but not all instances, generalized tetanus may develop during the course of the cephalic form of the disease.

GENERALIZED TETANUS

Generalized tetanus is the most common manifestation of the disease.[87, 109] Despite the general impression that inoculation of the organism is associated most frequently with deep penetrating injury, the portal of entry in approximately 80 percent of cases is an insignificant wound.[82] Burns, injuries induced by blank cartridges, deep punctures, furunculosis, dental extraction, embedded splinters, decubitus ulcers, hypodermic injections, and compound fractures complicated by chronic active osteomyelitis are typical situations in which tetanus may develop because the environment in the tissues is optimal (decrease in oxidation-reduction potential and tension of oxygen) for conversion of spores to the toxin-producing vegetative organisms. Iatrogenic disease has occurred after the use of smallpox vaccine and surgical sutures contaminated with the spores of *C. tetani*. It also has occurred as a postoperative complication in patients exposed to the organisms present in the dust of operating rooms.[84, 86, 95] Very *minor* injuries, such as penetration by "clean" sewing needles and bites by chiggers, bees, and scorpions, have been recorded as portals of entry. Tetanus also has occurred after induced abortions, usually performed under poor asepsis.

The initial manifestation in more than 50 percent of cases of generalized tetanus is trismus; it may be unilateral early in the disease but becomes bilateral within a short time. In some cases, it may be absent during the entire course of the illness or appear only after other abnormalities have become evident. In some instances, the only symptoms and signs may be irritability, restlessness, stiffness of the neck, difficulty swallowing, and rigidity of the abdominal or thoracic muscles; these symptoms may be present singly or in various combinations. The diagnostic importance of trismus cannot be overemphasized despite the fact that it may be associated with numerous disorders unrelated to tetanus. Among these disorders are postmeasles encephalitis, trichinosis, suppurative and other types of parotitis, tender cervical lymphadenopathy, infected impacted upper molar teeth, and exposure to phenothiazine drugs.

As the activity of tetanospasmin persists, groups of muscles other than the masseters may become involved, including tonic spasms of the jaw, neck, back, and abdomen. Unrelenting trismus leads to the development of a characteristic facial expression, the sardonic smile (risus sardonicus). The abdominal and spinal muscles may become rigid. Intense and sustained contraction of the muscles of the chest and back results in persistent opisthotonos; in young children, this condition may be so severe that the youngster lies on one side with the soles of the feet resting on top of the head.

Generalized seizures, tetanospasms, are unique in their appearance and peculiar to this disease. Characteristically, a sudden burst of tonic contractions of all groups of muscles occurs and leads to the development of opisthotonos, flexion and abduction of the arms, clenching of the fists on the chest, and extension of the legs. Pain in the spastic muscles usually is severe. Glottal and laryngeal spasm with the chest in the position of full inspiration may develop in some patients. During such an episode, the face becomes florid, the neck veins are distended markedly, and cyanosis develops. All the features of this syndrome are consistent with an intense and sustained Valsalva maneuver; unless the tonic contraction of the glottis and larynx subsides or a tracheostomy is performed, death results. Dysphagia and hydrophobia may develop as isolated phenomena in the absence of a generalized tetanospasm. Dysuria or urinary retention also may occur.

Electroencephalographic studies of patients have indicated involvement of the brain. Of 106 patients studied by Luisto,[65] 76 percent were found to have abnormal electroencephalograms. When patients of the same age and sex who had not had tetanus were compared with 40 individuals who had contracted the disease 7 years earlier, the latter were found to have more muscle fatigue and cramps; difficulty in speech, balance, and memory; and more peripheral paresis, muscular atrophy, decreased or absent tendon reflexes, and impaired mental capacity.[58]

The generalized seizures of tetanus often are triggered by very slight external stimuli, such as a light breeze, talking, a bump on the bed, or slight touching of the patient. The intense work generated by sustained or frequently repeated tetanospasms often leads to increases in body temperature of 2° F to 5° F or more.

The intense suffering of patients with the generalized tonic seizures of tetanus and the total frustration of the physician, who in ancient times had to stand by helplessly, unable to alter the course of the disease, were described best by Aretaeus[6] in the second century BC; no better description has ever appeared:

> *An inhuman calamity! An unseemly sight! A spectacle painful even to the beholder, an incurable malady! Owing to the distortion, not to be recognized by the dearest friends; and hence the prayers of the spectators, which formerly would have been reckoned not pious, now becomes good, that the patient may depart from life, or being a deliverance from the pains and unseemly evils attendant on it. But neither can the physician, though present and looking on, furnish any assistance, as regards life, relief from pain or from deformity. For if he should wish to straighten the limbs, he can do so only by cutting and breaking those of a living man. With them, then, who are overpowered by this disease, he can merely sympathize. This is the great misfortune of the physician.*

Heroin Addicts

When generalized tetanus develops in persons addicted to heroin, many of the clinical features differ from those present in people who do not use drugs. Among them are much higher levels of fever; absence of trismus at onset and throughout the course of the disease or its appearance some time after other manifestations have been present; marked stiffness of the neck and back, which in the absence of trismus may be confused with meningitis (the normal cerebrospinal fluid of tetanus excludes this possibility); and early onset of coma. Prophylaxis is less effective in addicted than nonaddicted persons. The fatality rate approaches 100 percent.

Neonatal Tetanus

Although neonatal tetanus is of very minor importance in developed areas of the world, it has been a major cause of death in infants in developing countries.[26, 27, 61, 67, 100, 108] In 1993, an estimated 515,000 deaths worldwide were caused by neonatal tetanus.[26] These deaths occurred predominantly in Southeast Asia (34.2%), Africa (28.2%), the western Pacific, including China (21.4%), and the eastern Mediterranean region (15.7%). The global mortality rate in 1993 was estimated to be 4.1 per 1000 live births. The very high frequency of neonatal tetanus in these areas probably is related to conditions surrounding the birth of infants. Most babies are born in very unhygienic environments; delivery rarely takes place in an adequate hospital. In addition, unclean instruments are used to sever the umbilical cord, rags often contaminated with soil or feces are used as dressings, and mud and manure are applied directly to the umbilical stump. In a study in Senegal that examined risk factors for development of neonatal tetanus, the major source of *C. tetani* was found to be the hands of the birth attendant, and the mode of contamination of the infant was related to the method that the birth attendant and the mother used to dress the umbilical cord stump.[61] In rural Pakistan, the ritual of bundling (wrapping the baby for prolonged periods in a sheepskin cover after the application of cow dung) is a significant risk factor for acquisition of neonatal tetanus.[10]

Neonatal tetanus usually begins 3 to 14 days after birth with poor sucking and excessive crying.[109] Manifestations include trismus, difficulty swallowing, other tetanic spasms, and, frequently, marked opisthotonos.

A study of the causes of death in patients with neonatal tetanus by Salimpour[92] indicated pulmonary disease to be most common. Bronchopneumonia or hemorrhage in the lungs (or both) was the most frequent finding at autopsy. Among the nonpulmonary disorders responsible for a fatal outcome were hepatitis, omphalitis, cerebral hemorrhage, thrombosis, and rupture of the renal vein. As has been noted not only in infants but also in older children and adults with tetanus, any gross or histologic abnormalities are very uncommon findings. The complications described by Salimpour,[92] especially those involving the lungs, probably are related to aspiration associated with the laryngoglottal spasm characteristic of the disease. Newborns who survived tetanus in rural Kenya often had evidence of brain damage.[8] Indicators of a poor prognosis for neonates include age younger than 10 days when admitted to the hospital, symptoms of less than 5 days' duration, the presence of risus sardonicus, and fever.[67]

Diagnosis

DIFFERENTIAL DIAGNOSIS

The differential diagnosis depends on the major clinical manifestations of the illness.[108] Cephalic tetanus may be confused with Bell palsy, trigeminal neuritis, and encephalitis, whereas generalized tetanus can be confused with rabies, strychnine poisoning, and phenothiazine reactions. Trismus can result from dental problems, tonsillitis, peritonsillar abscess, temporomandibular joint dysfunction, and parotitis. Tetany caused by hypocalcemia or hyperventilation should be considered as well.

SPECIFIC DIAGNOSIS

The diagnosis of tetanus is established on the basis of the history of an injury, particularly one in which either soil or fecal material has been introduced. In a small number of cases, especially those in which a relatively long incubation period has occurred, the site of entry of the organism may be healed and undetectable. Laboratory studies are of little help. Peripheral leukocytosis may or may not be present. The characteristic gram-positive rods, some of which may contain subterminal spores, may be seen occasionally in stained material obtained from the wound that has served as the portal of entry. Anaerobic cultures of exudate or necrotic tissue may grow typical sporulated rods and vegetative forms, but the yield of positive findings tends to be low.[29]

Low or undetectable levels of serum antitoxin at the time of onset of the illness is supportive of the diagnosis, but occasionally, serum antitoxin is present.[108] Rises in antitoxin titer occur uncommonly after infection, so the use of paired sera for retrospective diagnosis usually is not helpful; in addition, this form of serologic diagnosis is not possible when therapy included active immunization. In selected cases, electrophysiologic studies of the masseter muscle may be helpful.[9] A characteristic absence or shortening of the silent period occurs as a result of failure of Renshaw cell inhibition; exaggerated f-responses indicating hyperexcitability also may be noted.

Treatment

Management of generalized tetanus is directed to the following goals:

1. Neutralization of toxin still present in the blood before it comes in contact with the nervous system. Neutralization is accomplished by the administration of antitoxin as soon as the possibility of the disease is suspected or confirmed.[12] However, no acceptable evidence has shown that toxin can be inactivated by antitoxin once the toxin is fixed to tissues. In fact, the effectiveness of even large doses of antitoxin in reducing the fatality rate has been questioned.
2. Surgical removal of the site of entry of the organism, when possible, to eliminate the "factory" in which tetanospasmin is being produced. Omphalectomy has been performed with good results in children with neonatal tetanus.[34] Hysterectomy has been recommended when the disease has complicated induced and often septic abortions; however, patients for whom the infected uterus is not removed occasionally may survive. When the surgical procedure may be mutilating, as is the case with lesions on the face, it should not be performed.
3. Constant and meticulous nursing care.
4. Close monitoring of fluid, electrolyte, and caloric balance because it frequently is abnormal, especially in patients with high temperature and repeated seizures, as well as in those unable to take food or liquids because of severe trismus, dysphagia, or hydrophobia.

The slightest external stimulus may precipitate potentially lethal seizures in persons with diffuse disease. For this reason, of extreme importance is that all therapeutic and other manipulations be well coordinated and carefully scheduled so that the risk of producing a tetanospasm is reduced to a minimum. All maneuvers are performed best after patients have received optimal sedation and relaxation. A quiet, darkened room in which the light is subdued and the doors padded, removed as far as possible from the mainstream of hospital traffic, is ideal, but at the same time the patient requires constant monitoring and observation in an intensive care environment.

The antitoxin of choice for the treatment of tetanus is human tetanus immune globulin (TIG) at a dose of 3000 to 6000 U intramuscularly; a second dose does not appear to be necessary. When TIG is not available, equine antitoxin (EA) may be used, but it should be avoided if at all possible. The dose of EA is 100,000 U; one half is injected intramuscularly after appropriate tests to rule out sensitivity to horse serum have been performed. If the EA is well tolerated, the remainder is given intravenously *slowly*. Patients sensitized to horse serum must be desensitized. An intramuscular injection of 80,000 U of EA produces maximal concentrations of antibody in the blood in 48 to 72 hours; very good levels may be maintained for 7 days.[103, 104] Intravenous administration of the same dose yields concentrations of 40 or more U of antitoxin per milliliter of serum after 6 hours; it may persist for approximately 48 hours. Essentially no difference in the circulating quantities of antitoxin exists 7 days after it is given by either route. Local instillation of antitoxin around the known or suspected wound may be of value if excision cannot be performed; it also has been recommended before surgical removal of the injured area.

Penicillin kills the vegetative forms of *C. tetani*. Until recently, parenteral administration of penicillin G, 100,000 U/kg/day intravenously every 6 hours for 10 days has been recommended in all cases of tetanus. Observations have suggested that penicillin may act as an agonist to tetanospasmin by inhibiting the release of gamma-aminobutyric acid (GABA).[108] Because of this possibility and the results of a controlled study in Indonesia, metronidazole has become the antimicrobial treatment of choice in many centers.[4] The metronidazole dosage is 30 mg/kg/day intravenously given every 6 hours after an initial dose of 15 mg/kg. The usual duration of therapy is 7 to 10 days.

The spasticity and seizures of tetanus are caused by exaggerated reflex responses to afferent stimuli as a result of suppression of balancing central inhibition. Several classes of drugs that act at different sites along the reflex pathway are useful for control of these manifestations. Among them are hypnotics and sedatives, which reduce sensory input and generalized excitability; general anesthetics, which produce broad depression of the CNS; centrally acting muscle relaxants or spinal depressants, which lower reflex activity and decrease motor output from the spinal cord; and neuromuscular blocking agents, which inhibit the transmission of excess motor nerve activity to effector muscles.

The ideal drug for the treatment of tetanus must control seizures and decrease spasticity without impairing respiration, voluntary movement, or consciousness. The activity of an agent in inhibiting the convulsions induced by strychnine usually has been a reliable guide for the prediction of effectiveness in the management of tetanus. However, it may not be reliable always. For example, although the phenothiazines act as anticonvulsants in both naturally occurring and experimentally produced tetanus, they fail to control seizures induced by strychnine. Creech and associates[32] point out, "It may be concluded that any type of sedative or hypnotic agent, when properly administered so as to avoid respiratory depression, has the same effect or lack of effect upon the outcome of tetanus."

Historically, many different drugs have been used for patients with tetanus. Secobarbital sodium (Seconal) and pentobarbital (Nembutal) have been favored for their relatively short half-life.[56, 73] Barbiturates, however, may have deleterious effects on both the respiratory and cardiovascular systems. A patient heavily sedated with barbiturates often will have a rise in carbon dioxide pressure and a fall in oxygen pressure, as well as hypotension and a fall in cardiac output. In addition, barbiturates have a lower therapeutic index than do the benzodiazepines.[83] Chlorpromazine (Thorazine) also has been used to control the muscle spasms of tetanus, but it has some drawbacks.[30] Chlorpromazine actually may lower the seizure threshold and should be administered, if at all, only with concomitant anticonvulsant therapy. The acute dystonic reactions occasionally seen with chlorpromazine can confuse markedly the picture in a patient with tetanic spasms and rigidity. Akathisia, the need of the patient to be in constant movement, is another extrapyramidal effect occasionally seen with the phenothiazines and would be undesirable in a patient susceptible to tetanic spasms. Meprobamate historically was used to control the tonic spasms of tetanus.[80] It is relatively ineffective when given orally or intramuscularly (dissolved in propylene glycol).[73]

The barbiturates, phenothiazines, and meprobamate are no longer first-line antispasmodic drugs; benzodiazepines are the preferred drugs for the spasms and rigidity associated with tetanus.[31] They also have the advantage of being potent anticonvulsants, as well as sedative hypnotic agents. Additionally, they are GABA agonists and perhaps partially overcome the effect of tetanospasmin interfering with the normally inhibitory effect of GABA.[105] Diazepam (Valium) and lorazepam (Ativan) have been the benzodiazepines most frequently used for tetanus. Lorazepam has a somewhat longer half-life and may be preferred for this reason. Very large total daily doses of diazepam (500 mg) or lorazepam (200 mg) may be required.[106] Both drugs are formulated in propylene glycol solution for intravenous administration, and the large doses required may result in significant propylene glycol toxicity, including metabolic acidosis. For this reason, an enteral preparation that is free of propylene glycol should be given enterally if at all possible.[13]

Midazolam (Versed) is a short-acting benzodiazepine that is soluble in water and thus does not include propylene glycol in the parenteral formulation. Because of its short half-life, it should be administered as a continuous infusion, and an initial infusion dose of 0.1 to 0.3 mg/kg/hr may be required. The benzodiazepines all induce tachyphylaxis and will require escalation of dosage with time. The dosage should be titrated to prevent tetanic spasms and provide adequate sedation instead of being a specified dose. To avoid causing withdrawal symptoms after long-term use, the benzodiazepines should be tapered during the course of several weeks.

If the benzodiazepines are unable to control the spasms and rigidity associated with tetanus, intrathecal baclofen should be considered. Baclofen is a GABA receptor agonist that directly stimulates the postsynaptic GABA beta receptors on synapses blocked by tetanus toxin, thereby restoring physiologic inhibition of the alpha motor neuron. Numerous centers have described the efficacy of intrathecal baclofen for treating tetanus, although its safety and efficacy have not been established in children younger than 4 years of age.[14, 38, 39]

When the benzodiazepines and intrathecal baclofen are unable to control the spasms and rigidity associated with tetanus, neuromuscular blockade is indicated. Although succinylcholine has been used in the past,[45] newer agents have supplanted it. Additionally, theoretic reasons provide the basis to avoid the use of succinylcholine. With functional denervation of the motor end-plate in neuromuscular junctions directly affected by tetanospasmin, succinylcholine may result in exaggerated potassium release and hyperkalemia. This condition has been associated with cardiac dysrhythmias and death in other denervating conditions. For this reason, nondepolarizing agents should be used. Potential agents would include pancuronium, vecuronium, atracurium, and rocuronium.

Pancuronium can cause tachycardia via blockade of cardiac muscarinic receptors and, therefore, would be relatively contraindicated in patients with autonomic instability. Atracurium has a metabolite, laudanosine, that has been shown in animals to have cerebral excitatory effects, including seizures. In addition, atracurium may cause release of histamine with resultant pruritus and a decrease in blood pressure. Vecuronium and rocuronium only rarely induce the release of histamine and have no effect on either autonomic ganglia or cardiac muscarinic receptors, thus rendering them the preferred neuromuscular-blocking agents for tetanus.[55]

Neuromuscular-blocking drugs should be used only by physicians experienced in their use in a critical care environment, typically anesthesiologists or intensivists.[60] Although neuromuscular blockers formerly were used at low doses to preserve diaphragmatic function and spontaneous respiration, current thought is that they should be administered in conjunction with endotracheal intubation and ventilatory support. Remembering that neuromuscular-blocking drugs have no effect on cortical function and have no sedative effect is critical. The benzodiazepines are good sedatives and have significant amnestic effect. They are not, however, analgesics, and if pain is present (such as from previous muscle spasms), morphine sulfate is an effective analgesic. It also may be helpful in treating sympathetic hyperactivity. If sympathetic overactivity remains problematic, a combined alpha- and beta-receptor blocker such as labetalol should be used. The use of a beta-blocker such as propranolol alone should be avoided because the unopposed alpha-mediated vasoconstriction could lead to significant hypertension. Clonidine and epidural anesthesia are alternative therapies for increased sympathetic discharge. A combination of epidural bupivacaine and sufentanil has been used by some physicians to treat the sympathetic overactivity.[11]

The management approach to a patient with tetanus spasms or rigidity should be one of escalation of therapy based on need. Benzodiazepines should be administered initially, with high doses often being required. If the benzodiazepines are not effective, intrathecal baclofen may be used.[38, 39] If these therapies are inadequate or result in airway compromise or inadequate ventilation, endotracheal intubation should be performed with a nondepolarizing neuromuscular-blocking agent. Intubation also should be performed if spasms result in obstruction of the airway. Some physicians have advocated that heroin addicts with tetanus have an airway established because of the fulminant course of the disease.[80]

Sixty-six percent of 103 children 1 to 12 years of age with severe tetanus studied by Wesley and Pathes[110] required management with total muscle paralysis and intermittent positive-pressure ventilation. The death rate in this group was 14.5 percent.

Although reports[76] have documented that intrathecal administration of antitetanus serum did not improve the rate of survival in neonatal tetanus, the results of a study by Mongi and colleagues[74] led them to recommend this form of therapy. They found that intrathecal serotherapy may be of great value in the management of tetanus. Their experience indicated that the death rate from this disease in patients given intrathecal therapy was 45 percent; in those who did not receive this agent, it was 82 percent. However, the results of a recent meta-analysis led Abrutyn and Berlin[2] to conclude that intrathecal therapy with either EA or TIG is not of proven benefit and, therefore, should be given only during well-designed, controlled therapeutic trials.

Very careful attention must be paid to care of the skin, bladder, mouth, and bowel of patients with tetanus. Adequate fluid and electrolyte balance must be maintained. Feeding by gavage in patients unable to eat because of severe trismus, dysphagia, or hydrophobia has been suggested as a means of ensuring optimal caloric intake. Gastric emptying may be impaired, and a transpyloric feeding tube will facilitate adequate nutritional support with a continuous infusion of age-appropriate enteral formula. Transpyloric placement of the feeding tube also may decrease the risk of aspiration.

The use of dantrolene with conservative treatment has been reported to significantly reduce the fatality rate associated with tetanus.[3] The need to block both the sympathetic and the parasympathetic nervous systems to stabilize hemodynamics has been suggested. Such blockade may be produced by spinal anesthesia.[97] Patients with tetanus treated with metronidazole have been found to have a lower fatality rate, a shorter stay in the hospital, and an improved response to treatment.[4] Intravenous administration of morphine to patients with tetanus has been noted to reduce arterial blood pressure and systemic vascular resistance.[87]

Patients who have survived an episode of tetanus must be immunized actively after recovery because antitoxin usually is not detectable in the serum for as long as 3 months after recovery.[103] Recurrent attacks of the disease rarely occur, however.[21]

Studies in mice have shown that adrenocortical steroids are without effect in altering the course of tetanus. The administration of cortisone after a significant delay between the injection of toxin and antitoxin or after clinical manifestations have appeared was found not only to be without benefit but also to decrease the effectiveness of the antitoxin.[28] Other studies also have indicated a lack of therapeutic effect[50, 104] but have not demonstrated deleterious effects. Critically evaluated clinical experience has confirmed this finding.[63]

Prognosis

The average fatality rate associated with tetanus ranges from 25 to 70 percent, but mortality rates can be reduced to 10 to 30 percent with modern intensive care.[88, 108] The risk of death in patients with tetanus neonatorum is particularly high; it was reported to be 99.5 percent in a group of 5794 infants in 1930.[52] With modern treatment and high-intensity supportive care, the mortality rate associated with neonatal tetanus can be reduced to approximately 25 percent.[108] Heroin addicts are highly susceptible to the development of very severe disease and are likely to die.[58]

A variety of other factors play an important role in determining the outcome of tetanus. Patients in the second and third decades of life have a higher rate of recovery than do those who are elderly. An inverse relationship exists between the length of the incubation period and the risk, first pointed out by Hippocrates. The risk of death is approximately 58 percent when the interval between injury and the onset of tetanus is 2 to 10 days. When the interval is 11 to 22 days or longer, fatality rates have been 35 to 17 percent, respectively. A relationship also appears to exist between the period elapsing from the time of appearance of the first signs of tetanus and development of the first seizure or maximal intensity of the disease; the shorter this interval, the poorer the prognosis.[29]

The clinical form of tetanus also influences the outcome. Cephalic tetanus and tetanus neonatorum are associated with the highest incidence of death. In contrast, local tetanus, unless complicated by development of the generalized syndrome, has an excellent prognosis. The early administration of prophylactic antitoxin markedly increases the frequency of survival, even when tetanus develops.

Cause of Death

Because the clinical course of tetanus may be prolonged and the therapy used is complex and potentially dangerous, the cause of death often is not clear. Animals may die after the injection of toxin without any recognizable signs of the disease appearing.[44] Studies in parabiotic rats have suggested that tetanospasmin exerts a lethal effect on the respiratory center.[94] Involvement of the medulla has been observed in experimental animals and humans in whom episodes of respiratory failure, often in the absence of seizures, have been described.[60, 114] The action of the toxin on brain tissue has been postulated to be the cause of hyperpyrexia, tachycardia, hypotension, bulbar palsy, and cardiac arrest.[75] Myocardial damage also may occur; both histologic and electrocardiographic abnormalities have been described.[79]

Death may occur during a convulsion, but the specific mechanisms involved are not always clear. Laryngospasm and disturbances in electrolyte balance may play important roles. Pneumonia complicating aspiration, induced by an inability to swallow and oversedation, occurs commonly. It may be directly responsible for death or may contribute to a fatal outcome by increasing the degree of anoxia of the respiratory center.

Prevention

As noted in Figure 154–1, tetanus in the United States has decreased dramatically, and this decline can be attributed to routine universal use of tetanus toxoid and improved wound management, including the use of tetanus prophylaxis in emergency departments.

ACTIVE IMMUNIZATION

For complete information regarding tetanus immunization, the reader is referred to the most recent recommendations of the Advisory Committee on Immunization Practices of the U. S. Public Health Service,[24] the recommendations of the Committee on Infectious Diseases of the American Academy of Pediatrics,[5] and product information from vaccine manufacturers.

In the United States, primary immunization against tetanus is performed in conjunction with immunization against diphtheria and pertussis in the form of diphtheria and tetanus toxoids and acellular pertussis vaccine adsorbed (DTaP). The schedule involves an initial series of three doses of vaccine at 2, 4, and 6 months of age, a reinforcing dose at 12 to 18 months of age, and a booster dose at 4 to 6 years of age. After the initial series, additional booster doses of adult-type diphtheria and tetanus toxoids adsorbed (Td) are recommended at 10-year intervals. The minimal serum level of antitoxin needed for protection is 0.01 IU/mL.[36, 66, 68, 98] After the initial three-dose series, the reinforcing dose, and the booster dose in the schedule just described, levels of antitoxin 100- to 1000-fold higher than 0.01 IU/mL are attained, and levels higher than 0.01 IU/mL persist in nearly all vaccinees until the scheduled subsequent dose.

TETANUS PROPHYLAXIS IN WOUND MANAGEMENT

Antimicrobial prophylaxis against tetanus is neither practical nor useful in managing wounds. Wound cleaning, débridement when indicated, and proper immunization are important factors. The need for tetanus toxoid (active immunization), with or without TIG (passive immunization), depends on both the condition of the wound and the patient's vaccination history[24] (Table 154–1). Rarely has tetanus occurred in persons with documentation of having received a primary series of toxoid injections.

A thorough attempt must be made to determine whether a patient has completed primary vaccination. Patients with unknown or uncertain previous vaccination histories should be considered to have had no previous tetanus toxoid doses. Persons who served in the military since 1941 can be considered to have received at least one dose. Although most people in the military since 1941 may have completed a primary series of tetanus toxoid, such protection cannot be assumed for each individual. Patients who have not completed a primary series may require tetanus toxoid and passive immunization at the time of wound cleaning and débridement (see Table 154–1).

The evidence available indicates that complete primary vaccination with tetanus toxoid provides long-lasting protection for 10 or more years in most recipients. Consequently, after complete primary tetanus vaccination, boosters—even for wound management—need be given only every 10 years when wounds are minor and uncontaminated. For other wounds, a booster is appropriate if the patient has not received tetanus toxoid within the preceding 5 years. Antitoxin antibodies rapidly develop in persons who have received at least two doses of tetanus toxoid.

TABLE 154–1 ■ SUMMARY GUIDE TO TETANUS PROPHYLAXIS IN ROUTINE WOUND MANAGEMENT, 1991

History of Adsorbed Tetanus Toxoid (Doses)	Clean, Minor Wounds		All Other Wounds*	
	Td†	TIG	Td†	TIG
Unknown or < three	Yes	No	Yes	Yes
≥Three‡	No§	No	No‖	No

*Such as, but not limited to wounds contaminated with dirt, feces, soil, and saliva; puncture wounds; avulsions; and wounds resulting from missiles, crushing, burns, and frostbite.
†For children younger than 7 years, diphtheria-tetanus-pertussis vaccine (diphtheria-tetanus if pertussis vaccine is contraindicated) is preferred to tetanus toxoid alone. For persons 7 years or older, Td is preferred to tetanus toxoid alone.
‡If only three doses of fluid toxoid have been received, a fourth dose of toxoid, preferably an adsorbed toxoid, should be given.
§Yes, if older than 10 years since the last dose.
‖Yes, if older than 5 years since the last dose (more frequent boosters are not needed and can accentuate side effects).
Td, adult-type diphtheria and tetanus toxoids; TIG, tetanus immune globulin.
From Centers for Disease Control: Diphtheria, tetanus and pertussis: Recommendations for vaccine use and other preventive measures; recommendations of the Immunization Practices Advisory Committee (ACIP). M. M. W. R. *40* (RR-10):2–28, 1991.

Td is the preferred preparation for active tetanus immunization in the wound management of patients 7 years of age or older. Because a large proportion of adults are susceptible, this plan enhances diphtheria protection. Thus, by taking advantage of acute health care visits, such as for wound management, some patients can be protected who otherwise would remain susceptible. For routine wound management in children younger than 7 years of age who are not vaccinated adequately, DTaP should be used instead of single-antigen tetanus toxoid. Td may be used if pertussis vaccine is contraindicated. For patients of all ages who are inadequately vaccinated, completion of primary vaccination at the time of discharge or at follow-up visits should be ensured.

If passive immunization is needed, human TIG is the product of choice. It provides protection longer than antitoxin of animal origin does and causes fewer adverse reactions. The TIG prophylactic dose currently recommended for wounds of average severity is 250 U intramuscularly. When tetanus toxoid and TIG are given concurrently, separate syringes and separate sites should be used. The Advisory Committee on Immunization Practices recommends the use of only adsorbed toxoid in this situation.

NEONATAL TETANUS

Several approaches have been taken to reduce the incidence and fatality rate of neonatal tetanus in developing areas of the world. Among these approaches are (1) educating pregnant women concerning the danger of using contaminated materials for cutting the umbilical cord and covering the stump, (2) training midwives in the application of modern techniques of obstetric asepsis, (3) developing hospitals in which babies are born under strict asepsis, and (4) immunizing all women of child-bearing age or, if such immunization is not possible, all who are pregnant. Clearly, immunizing all individuals in all developing areas may not be feasible. If universal immunization is not possible, emphasis should be placed on immunizing women of child-bearing age. Studies performed by the World Health Organization (WHO) have demonstrated that such immunization is practical and leads to an appreciable reduction in the incidence of neonatal tetanus.[40–42, 100] Babies born to mothers who have been immunized during pregnancy not only have adequate levels of circulating antibody but also are protected against acquiring the disease. The level of protective antibody in newborns and the magnitude of the transfer rate of passive immunity to tetanus directly depend on the level of tetanus antitoxin in maternal serum. Mothers who had tetanus antitoxin levels of 1.28 IU/mL or more could transfer protection to almost all the newborns (97% to 100%), irrespective of the doses of tetanus toxoid administered. However, mothers who had received two doses of tetanus toxoid during pregnancy not only conferred good protection but also transferred high antitoxin levels to their newborns.[93]

In 1989, the WHO adopted a resolution to eliminate neonatal tetanus worldwide,[112] and in 1990, the World Summit for Children issued a declaration for global elimination of neonatal tetanus by the end of 1995.[26, 113] In 1993, the WHO's goal was defined as elimination of neonatal tetanus as a public health problem by reducing its incidence to less than 1 case per 1000 live births for all health districts.[48]

From 1989 to 1993, the rate of vaccination coverage with two or more doses of tetanus toxoid administered to pregnant women in risk areas increased from 27 to 45 percent. To achieve and maintain neonatal tetanus elimination, 80 percent or more of infants need to be protected at birth through vaccination of their mothers with at least two doses of tetanus toxoid or through clean delivery and cord care practices.[48]

REFERENCES

1. Abel, J. J., Firor, W. M., and Chalain, W.: Researches on tetanus. IX. Further evidence to show that tetanus toxin is not carried to central neurons by way of the axis cylinders of motor nerves. Bull. Johns Hopkins Hosp. *63*:373–403, 1938.
2. Abrutyn, E., and Berlin, J. A.: Intrathecal therapy in tetanus: A meta-analysis. J. A. M. A. *266*:2262–2267, 1991.
3. Aguilar Bernal, O. R., Bender, M. A., and Lacy, M. E.: Efficacy of dantrolene sodium in management of tetanus in children. J. R. Soc. Med. *79*:277–281, 1986.
4. Ahmadsyah, I., and Salim, A.: Treatment of tetanus: An open study to compare the efficacy of procaine penicillin with metronidazole in the treatment of moderate tetanus. B. M. J. *29*:640–650, 1985.
5. American Academy of Pediatrics: Active and passive immunization; tetanus. *In* Pickering, L. K. (ed.): 2000 Red Book: Report of the Committee on Infectious Diseases. 25th ed. Elk Grove Village, IL, American Academy of Pediatrics, 2000, pp. 1-79, 563–568.
6. Aretaeus: Tetanus. *In* Major, R. H.: Classic Descriptions of Disease. 2nd ed. Springfield, IL, Charles C Thomas, 1939, pp. 148–149.
7. Bagratuni, L.: Cephalic tetanus. B. M. J. *1*:461–463, 1952.
8. Barlow, J. L., Mung'ala-Odera, V., Gona, J., et al.: Brain damage after neonatal tetanus in a rural Kenyan hospital. Trop. Med. Int. Health *6*:305–308, 2001.
9. Bartlett, J. G.: *Clostridium tetani. In* Gorbac, S. L., Bartlett, J. G., and Blacklow, N. R. (eds.): Infectious Diseases. Philadelphia, W. B. Saunders, 1992, pp. 1580–1583.
10. Bennett, J., Schooley, M., Traverso, H., et al.: Bundling, a newly identified risk factor for neonatal tetanus: Implications for global control. Int. J. Epidemiol. *25*:879–884, 1996.
11. Bhagwanjee, S., Bosenberg, A. T., and Muckart, D. J.: Management of sympathetic overactivity in tetanus with epidural bupivacaine and sufentanil: Experience with 11 patients. Crit. Care Med. *27*:1721–1725, 1999.
12. Bizzini, B.: Tetanus. *In* Germanier, R. (ed.): Bacterial Vaccines. Orlando, FL, Academic, 1984, pp. 38–68.
13. Bleck, T. P.: Tetanus: Pathophysiology, management and prophylaxis. Dis. Mon. *37*:545–603, 1991.
14. Boots, R. J., Lipman, J., O'Callaghan, J., et al.: The treatment of tetanus with intrathecal baclofen. Anesth. Intensive Care *28*:438–442, 2000.
15. Botticelli, J. T., and Waisbren, B. A.: Tetanus in an urban community. Am. J. Med. Sci. *242*:44–50, 1961.
16. Bradley, K., Easton, D. M., and Eccles, J. C.: Investigation of primary or direct inhibition. J. Physiol. *122*:474–478, 1953.
17. Brand, D. A., Acampora, D., Gottlieb, L. D., et al.: Adequacy of antitetanus prophylaxis in six hospital emergency rooms. N. Engl. J. Med. *308*: 630–640, 1983.
18. Brooks, V. B., and Asanuma, H.: Action of tetanus toxin in the cerebral cortex. Science *137*:674–676, 1962.
19. Brooks, V. B., Curtis, D. R., and Eccles, J. C.: Mode of action of tetanus toxin. Nature *175*:120–121, 1955.
20. Bytchenko, B.: Microbiology of tetanus. *In* Veronesi, R. (ed.): Tetanus: Important New Concepts. Amsterdam, Excerpta Medica, 1981, pp. 28–39.
21. Cain, H. O., and Falco, F. G.: Recurrent tetanus. Calif. Med. *97*:31–33, 1962.
22. Carrea, R., and Lanari, A.: Chronic effect of tetanus toxin applied locally to the cerebral cortex of the dog. Science *137*:342–343, 1962.
23. Carle and Rattone: Studio esperimentale sull'eziologia del tetano. G. Acad. Med. Torino *32*:174–180, 1884.
24. Centers for Disease Control: Diphtheria, tetanus and pertussis: Recommendations for vaccine use and other preventive measures; recommendations of the Immunization Practices Advisory Committee (ACIP). M. M. W. R. Recomm. Rep. *40*(RR-10):2–28, 1991.
25. Centers for Disease Control and Prevention: Tetanus surveillance: United States, 1980–1994. M. M. W. R. Morb. Mortal. Wkly. Rep. *47*(SS-2):1–13, 1998.
26. Centers for Disease Control and Prevention: Progress toward the global elimination of neonatal tetanus, 1989–1993. M. M. W. R. Morb. Mortal. Wkly. Rep. *43*(48):885–887, 893–894, 1994.
27. Centers for Disease Control and Prevention: Progress toward elimination of neonatal tetanus: Egypt, 1988–1994. M. M. W. R. Morb. Mortal. Wkly. Rep. *45*(4):89–92, 1996.
28. Chang, T. W., and Weinstein, L.: Effect of cortisone on treatment of tetanus with antitoxin. Proc. Soc. Exp. Biol. Med. *94*:431–433, 1957.
29. Christensen, N. A., and Thurber, D. L.: Clinical experience with tetanus: 91 cases. Staff Meetings Mayo Clin. *32*:146–157, 1957.
30. Cole, A. C. E., and Robertson, D. H. H.: Chlorpromazine in the management of tetanus. Lancet *2*:1063–1064, 1955.
31. Cordova, A. B.: Control of the spasms of tetanus with diazepam (Valium). Clin. Pediatr. (Phila.) *8*:712–716, 1969.
32. Creech, O., Glover, A., and Ochsner, A.: Tetanus: Evaluation of treatment at Charity Hospital, New Orleans, Louisiana. Ann. Surg. *146*:369, 1957.
33. Davies, J. R., Morgan, R. S., Wright, E. A., et al.: The effect of local tetanus intoxication of the hind limb reflexes of the rabbit. Arch. Int. Physiol. *62*:248–263, 1954.
34. Dietrich, H. F.: Tetanus neonatorum. J. A. M. A. *147*:1038–1040, 1951.
35. Edsall, G.: Specific prophylaxis of tetanus. J. A. M. A. *171*:417–427, 1959.
36. Edsall, G.: Problems in the immunology and control of tetanus. Med. J. Aust. *2*:216–220, 1976.
37. Edsall, G., Elliott, M. W., Peebles, T. C., et al.: Excessive use of tetanus boosters. J. A. M. A. *202*:17–19, 1967.
38. Engrand, N., Guerot, E., Rouamba, A., et al.: The efficacy of intrathecal baclofen in severe tetanus. Anesthesiology *90*:1773–1776, 1999.
39. Engrand, N., Vilian, G., Rouamba, A., et al.: Value of intrathecal baclofen in the treatment of severe tetanus in the tropical milieu. Med. Trop. (Mars.) *60*:385–388, 2000.
40. Expanded Programme on Immunization. Reduction of neonatal deaths by immunizing women against tetanus: Wkly. Epidemiol. Rec. *56*:185–186, 1981.
41. Expanded Programme on Immunization. Prevention of neonatal tetanus. Wkly. Epidemiol. Rec. *57*:137–142, 1982.
42. Expanded Programme on Immunization. Global Advisory Group Meeting. Weekly Advisory Group Meeting. Wkly. Epidemiol. Rec. *58*:15–18, 1983.
43. Fedinec, A. A., and Matzke, H. A.: The role of tissue spaces and nerve fibers in the spread of tetanus toxin in the rat. Univ. Kansas Sci. Bull. *38*:1439–1498, 1958.
44. Firor, W. M., Lamont, A., and Shumacker, H. B.: Studies on the cause of death in tetanus. Ann. Surg. *111*:246, 1940.
45. Forrester, A. T. T.: Treatment of tetanus with succinylcholine. B. M. J. *2*:342–344, 1954.
46. Friedemann, U., Zuger, B., and Hollander, A.: Investigations on the pathogenesis of tetanus, I and II. J. Immunol. *36*:473–484, 485–488, 1939.
47. Friedlander, F. C.: Tetanus neonatorum. J. Pediatr. *39*:448–454, 1951.
48. Global Advisory Group: Expanded Program on Immunization. Global Advisory Group—Part II. Achieving the major disease control goals. Wkly. Epidemiol. Rec. *69*(5):29–31, 34–35, 1994.
49. Godfrey, M. P., Parsons, V., and Rawstron, J. R.: Rapid destruction of antitetanus serum in a patient previously sensitized to horse serum. Lancet *2*:1229–1230, 1960.
50. Green, A. E., Ambrus, J. L., and Gershenfeld, L.: Effect of cortisone and desoxycorticosterone on infection with tetanus spores and on toxicity of tetanus toxin. Antibiot. Chemother. *3*:1221, 1953.
51. Gurses, N., and Aydin, M.: Factors affecting prognosis of neonatal tetanus. Scand. J. Infect. Dis. *25*:353–355, 1993.
52. Hines, E. A., Jr.: Tetanus neonatorum: Report of a case with recovery. Am. J. Dis. Child. *39*:560–572, 1930.
53. Hippocrates: Tetanus. *In* Major, H. H. (ed.): Classic Descriptions of Disease. 2nd ed. Springfield, IL, Charles C Thomas, 1939, pp. 148–149.
54. Hlady, W. G., Bennett, J. V., Samadi, A. R., et al.: Neonatal tetanus in rural Bangladesh: Risk factors and toxoid efficacy. Am. J. Public Health *82*:1365–1369, 1992.
55. Howder, C. L.: Cardiopulmonary Pharmacology. Baltimore, Williams & Wilkins, 1996, p. 316.
56. Jenkins, M. T., and Luhn, N. R.: Active management of tetanus. Anesthesiology *23*:690–709, 1962.
57. Kaeser, H. E., and Saner, A.: Tetanus toxin, a neuromuscular blocking agent. Nature *223*:842, 1969.
58. Kerr, J. H., Corbett, J. L., Prys-Roberts, C., et al.: Involvement of the sympathetic nervous system in tetanus. Lancet *2*:236–241, 1968.
59. Kitasato, S.: Über den tetanus Bacillus. Z. Hyg. Infektkr. *7*:225–234, 1889.
60. Laurence, D. R., and Webster, R. A.: Pathologic physiology, pharmacology and therapeutics of tetanus. Clin. Pharmacol. Ther. *4*:36–72, 1963.
61. Leroy, O., and Garenne, M.: Risk factors of neonatal tetanus in Senegal. Int. J. Epidemiol. *20*:521–526, 1991.
62. Levinson, A., Marska, R. L., and Shein, M. K.: Tetanus in heroin addicts. J. A. M. A. *157*:658–660, 1955.
63. Lewis, R. A., Satoskar, R. S., Joag, C. G., et al.: Cortisone and hydrocortisone given parenterally and orally in severe tetanus. J. A. M. A. *156*:479, 1954.
64. Luisto, M.: Outcome and neurological sequelae of patients after tetanus. Acta Neurol. Scand. *80*:504–511, 1989.
65. Luisto, M.: Tetanus in Finland: Diagnostic problems and complications. Ann. Med. *22*:15–19, 1990.
66. MacLennan, R., Schofield, F. D., Pitman, M., et al.: Immunization against neonatal tetanus in New Guinea: Antitoxin response of pregnant women to adjuvant and plain toxoids. Bull. World Health Organ. *32*:683–697, 1965.
67. Malgaard, B., Mutie, D. M., and Kimani, G.: A cluster survey of mortality due to neonatal tetanus in Kenya. Int. J. Epidemiol. *12*:124–127, 1988.
68. McComb, J. A.: The prophylactic dose of homologous tetanus antitoxin. N. Engl. J. Med. *270*:175–178, 1964.
69. McComb, J. A., and Dwyer, R. C.: Passive-active immunization with tetanus immune globulin (human). N. Engl. J. Med. *268*:857–862, 1963.

70. Mellanby, J., Van Heyningen, W. E., and Whitaker, V. P.: Fixation of tetanus toxin by subcellular fractions of brain. J. Neurochem. *12*:77–79, 1965.
71. Meyer, H., and Ransom, F.: Untersuchungen über den Tetanus. Arch. Exp. Pathol. Pharmakol. *49*:369–416, 1903.
72. Millard, A. H.: Local tetanus. Lancet *2*:844–846, 1954.
73. Miller, C. L., and Stoelting, V. K.: Recent evaluation of the treatment of tetanus. J. A. M. A. *168*:393–394, 1958.
74. Mongi, P. S., Moise, R. L., Msengi, A. E., et al.: Tetanus neonatorum experience with intrathecal serotherapy at Muhumbili Medical Center. Am. Trop. Med. *7*:27–31, 1987.
75. Montgomery, R. D.: The cause of death in tetanus. West Indian Med. J. *10*:84, 1961.
76. Nesquay, E., and Nkrumah, F. K.: Failure of intrathecal antitetanus serum to improve survival in neonatal tetanus. Arch. Dis. Child. *58*: 276–278, 1983.
77. Nicolaier, A.: Über infectiosen Tetanus. Dtsch. Med. Wochenschr. *10*:842–884, 1884.
78. Peebles, T. C., Levine, L., Eldred, M. C., et al.: Tetanus-toxoid emergency boosters. N. Engl. J. Med. *280*:575–581, 1969.
79. Perez, L. R.: The electrocardiogram in tetanus. Rev. Clin. Esp. *75*:20, 1959.
80. Perlstein, M. A., Stein, M. D., and Elam, H.: Routine treatment of tetanus. J. A. M. A. *173*:1536–1541, 1960.
81. Pillemer, L., Wittler, R. G., and Grossberg, D. B.: The isolation and crystallization of tetanal toxin. Science *103*:615–616, 1946.
82. Pratt, E. L.: Clinical tetanus: A study of 56 cases, with special reference to methods of prevention and a plan for evaluating treatment. J. A. M. A. *129*:1243–1247, 1945.
83. Rall, T. W.: Hypnotics and sedatives. *In* Goodman and Gilman's The Pharmacologic Basis of Therapeutics. Section III. Drugs Acting on the Central Nervous System. New York, Pergamon, 1990, pp. 345–382.
84. Ramon, G., and Zoeller, C.: L'immunite antitetanique par l'anatoxine chez l'homme. Presse Med. *34*:485, 1926.
85. Risk, W. S., Bosch, E. P., Kimura, J., et al.: Chronic tetanus: Clinical report and histochemistry of muscle. Muscle Nerve *4*:363–366, 1981.
86. Robinson, D. T., McLeod, J. S., and Downie, A. W.: Dust in surgical theatres. Lancet *1*:152–154, 1946.
87. Rock, D. A., Wesley, A. G., Pather, M., et al.: Morphine in tetanus: The management of sympathetic nervous system overactivity. S. Afr. Med. *20*:666–668, 1986.
88. Romitti, M., Romitti, F., Banchini, E.: Tetanus. Physiopathology and intensive care treatment. Minerva Anestesiol. *66*:445–460, 2000.
89. Roofe, P. G.: Role of the axis cylinder in transport of tetanus toxin. Science *105*:180–181, 1947.
90. Rosenbach: Arch. Klin. Chir. *34*:306, 1887.
91. Rubbo, S. D., and Suri, J. C.: Passive immunization against tetanus with human immune globulin. B. M. J. *2*:79–81, 1962.
92. Salimpour, R.: Cause of death in tetanus neonatorum. Arch. Dis. Child. *32*:587–589, 1977.
93. Sangpetchsong, V., Vichaikummart, S., Vichitnant, A., et al.: Transfer of transplacental immunity from unimmunized and immunized mothers. Southeast Asian J. Trop. Med. Public Health *15*:275–280, 1984.
94. Schellenberg, D. B., and Matzke, H. A.: The development of tetanus in parabiotic rats. J. Immunol. *80*:367, 1958.
95. Sevitt, S.: Source of two hospital-infected cases of tetanus. Lancet *2*:1075–1078, 1949.
96. Sherrington, C. S.: The Integrative Action of the Nervous System. New York, Yale University Press, 1906, pp. 303, 112.
97. Shibuya, M., Sugimoto, H., Sugimoto, T., et al.: The use of spinal anesthesia in severe tetanus with autonomic disturbances. J. Trauma *29*:1423–1429, 1989.
98. Smith, J. W. G.: Diphtheria and tetanus toxoids. Br. Med. Bull. *25*:177–182, 1969.
99. Smolens, J., Vogt, A. B., Crawford, M. N., et al.: The persistence in the human circulation of horse and human tetanus antitoxins. J. Pediatr. *59*:899–902, 1961.
100. Stanfield, J. P., and Galazaka, A.: Neonatal tetanus in the world today. Bull. World Health Organ. *62*:647–669, 1984.
101. Tallman, J. F., Gallagher, D. W.: The GABAergic system: A locus of benzodiazepine action. Annu. Rev. Neurosci. *8*:21–44, 1985.
102. Talmage, D. W., Dixon, F. J., Bukantz, S. C., et al.: Antigen elimination from the blood as an early manifestation of the immune response. J. Immunol. *67*:243–255, 1951.
103. Turner, T. B., Stafford, E. S., and Goldman, L.: Studies on the duration of protection afforded by active immunization against tetanus. Bull. Johns Hopkins Hosp. *94*:204–217, 1954.
104. Turner, T. B., Velasco-Joven, E. A., and Prudovsky, S.: Studies on the prophylaxis and treatment of tetanus. Bull. Johns Hopkins Hosp. *102*:71–84, 1958.
105. Van Heyningen, W. E., and Miller, P. A.: The fixation of tetanus toxin by ganglioside. J. Gen. Microbiol. *24*:107–119, 1961.
106. Vassa, T., Yahnik, V. H., Joshi, K. R., et al.: Comparative clinical trial of diazepam with other conventional drugs in tetanus. Postgrad. Med. J. *50*:755–758, 1974.
107. Von Behring, E., and Kitasato, S.: Über des zustandekommen der Diphterie-Immunitat und der Tetanus-Immunitat bei Tieren. Dtsch. Med. Wochenschr. *16*:1113–1114, 1890.
108. Wassilak, S. G. F., Orenstein, W. A., and Sutter, R. W.: Tetanus toxoid. *In* Plotkin, S. A., and Mortimer, E. A. (eds.): Vaccines. 2nd ed. Philadelphia, W. B. Saunders, 1994, pp. 57–90.
109. Weinstein, L.: Tetanus. N. Engl. J. Med. *289*:1293–1296, 1973.
110. Wesley, A. G., and Pathes, M.: Tetanus in children: An 11 year review. Ann. Trop. Med. Paediatr. *7*:32–37, 1987.
111. Willis, A. T.: *Clostridium*: The spore-bearing anaerobes. *In* Wilson, G., Miles, A., and Parker, M. T. (eds.): Topley and Wilson's Principles of Bacteriology, Virology and Immunity. Vol. 2. Baltimore, Williams & Wilkins, 1983, pp. 442–475.
112. World Health Assembly: Expanded Program on Immunization. Geneva, World Health Organization, May 19, 1989 (Resolution WHA42.32).
113. World Health Organization: Revised Plan of Action for Neonatal Tetanus Elimination. Publication No. WHO/EPI/GEN/93.13. Geneva, World Health Organization, Expanded Program on Immunization, 1993.
114. Wright, E. A., Morgan, R. S., and Wright, G. P.: Tetanus intoxication of the brain stem in rabbits. J. Pathol. Bacteriol. *62*:569–583, 1950.
115. Young, L. S., LaForce, F. M., and Bennett, J. V.: An evaluation of serologic and antimicrobial therapy in the treatment of tetanus in the United States. J. Infect. Dis. *120*:153–159, 1969.
116. Zacks, S. I., and Shef, M. F.: Tetanus toxin: Fine structure localization of binding sites in striated muscle. Science *159*:643–644, 1968.

Actinomycosis

SUZANNE WHITWORTH ■ RICHARD F. JACOBS

Human actinomycosis is a clinical illness with a typical histologic presentation that is caused by a variety of pathogens. It often is polymicrobial, and *Actinobacillus actinomycetemcomitans* frequently is a co-pathogen. It is endogenous worldwide, with sporadic cases reported annually. Occurrence of the disease is unrelated to age, sex, season, or occupation, although it is a decidedly uncommon event in the pediatric population. These organisms have the ability to spread locally without regard to fascial planes or other anatomic barriers. Actinomycosis is characterized by localized swelling with suppuration, abscess formation, and draining sinuses. The abscesses have fibrous walls and are filled with pus and characteristic sulfur granules. The three most common types of actinomycosis are oral and cervicofacial, pulmonary, and abdominal. However, involvement of the liver, female reproductive tract, and brain has been described. Definitive diagnosis of the infection rests on isolation of the organism from pus or identification of sulfur granules on histopathologic sections of biopsy material. Adequate treatment generally consists of surgical removal of the lesion or prolonged antibiotic therapy.

Microbiology

The clinical entity of actinomycosis is caused by species of the genera *Actinomyces* and *Propionibacterium*. Human actinomycosis most often is caused by *Actinomyces israelii,* although *Actinomyces naeslundii, Actinomyces viscosus, Actinomyces odontolyticus, and Actinomyces meyeri*, also are causes of human illness. *Arcanobacterium pyogenes* (previously in the *Actinomyces* genus) also causes human actinomycosis. Other species more recently shown to cause human disease include *Arcanobacterium europae, Arcanobacterium turicensis,* and *Arcanobacterium radingae.*[18] *Arcanobacterium bovis, Arcanobacterium denticolens, Arcanobacterium howellii, Arcanobacterium hordeovulneris*, and *Arcanobacterium slackii* are primarily animal pathogens. *Propionibacterium propionica* is the only species in the *Propionibacterium* genus that is a cause of human actinomycosis.

These bacterial organisms are irregular, non–spore-forming, non–acid-fast, nonmotile, gram-positive rods. They grow in most rich culture media and have varying oxygen requirements. For example, *A. israelii* requires anaerobic conditions for growth. *A. viscosus*, however, grows in an aerobic environment with carbon dioxide. These species ferment carbohydrates as their source of energy for growth.[6] These organisms now are firmly classified as prokaryotic bacteria, although they originally were thought to be fungi because of the mycelial appearance of the organisms in sulfur granules and because of their branching morphology. However, neither genus contains chitin or glucans, which are characteristic macromolecules of fungi. In addition, they reproduce by bacillary fusion, are sensitive to antibiotics, and are resistant to antifungal agents. These organisms are members of the endogenous flora of mucous membranes. *A. israelii* always is found in the oral cavity when the appropriate anaerobic culture technique is used. It also has been found in the gastrointestinal tract, bronchi, and female genital tract.[16]

A. actinomycetemcomitans is a fastidious, gram-negative rod that frequently complicates actinomycosis caused by *A. israelii* (see Chapter 131). In addition to being associated with actinomycosis, it has been implicated as a pathogen in periodontal disease and is part of the oral flora. This organism is characterized by slow growth in culture and the need for incubation in an atmosphere enhanced with carbon dioxide.[8] Other bacterial species isolated concomitantly in human actinomycosis are *Eikenella corrodens* and *Fusobacterium, Bacteroides, Capnocytophaga, Staphylococcus,* and *Streptococcus* spp., and Enterobacteriaceae.

Pathogenesis

The organisms that cause actinomycosis normally are found in the oral flora from infancy to adulthood. Actinomyces are primary colonizers that initiate formation of plaque and set the stage for infectious disease development. These bacteria adhere tenaciously to both the hard and soft tissue surfaces of the oral cavity.[27] Disruption of this mucous membrane likely is the initiating event for oral and cervicofacial disease. The organisms then invade locally and spread without regard to fascial planes. The exact mechanism for this spread is unknown but may be related to the ability of these organisms to suppress part of the host immune system. Organisms of the *Actinomyces* genus have been shown to be chemotactic, to activate lymphocyte blastogenesis, and to stimulate the release of lysosomal enzymes from polymorphonuclear leukocytes and macrophages.[6] In addition, the co-pathogens involved in this infection may reduce local oxygen tension. Dental extractions are associated with mucosal breaks and tissue necrosis and may predispose to oral or cervicofacial actinomycosis.[15] Hematogenous dissemination eventually can occur but does so uncommonly. Gastrointestinal disease probably is associated with the disruption of the mucosal barrier, similar to oral and cervicofacial disease.[16] Organisms causing pulmonary actinomycosis likely reach the lungs through aspiration. Thoracic actinomycosis usually is a complication of localized pulmonary parenchymal infection. Actinomycetes produce enzymes and thus spread by extension into lungs, pleura, and chest wall without regard to tissue planes.[22] Numerous reports in the literature associate actinomycosis with intrauterine devices (IUDs), and some question exists regarding the association of foreign bodies with actinomycosis.[3]

Pathology

Actinomycosis most commonly presents as a chronic infection with single or multiple indurated swellings. These lesions eventually soften, become fluctuant, and suppurate. The walls are fibrous and firm and often described as wooden, which frequently results in their confusion with neoplasms. Over the course of time, sinus tracts form and extend through the overlying skin or to adjacent bones or tissues. The overlying skin may have a bluish hue.[16]

Histologically, a typical lesion has a central purulent area containing neutrophils and sulfur granules, surrounded by an outer zone of granulation with collagen fibers and fibroblasts. Sulfur granules are firm, yellowish granules containing the organisms, and are virtually diagnostic of actinomycosis, although they can be seen in nocardiosis and botryomycosis. In addition to neutrophils, lymphocytes and plasma cells frequently are seen in the lesions; eosinophils and multinucleated giant cells occasionally are seen.[16]

Clinical Manifestations

There are three important sites of actinomycotic infection. The order of frequency of occurrence is oral and cervicofacial, abdominal, and pulmonary. Actinomycosis resembles several other chronic inflammatory diseases and must be differentiated from mycotic infections, tuberculosis, appendicitis, *Yersinia enterocolitica* pseudoappendicitis, osteomyelitis, amebiasis, hepatic abscess, and other chronic bacterial infections, including nocardiosis.

Because oral and cervicofacial actinomycosis occurs after disruption of the mucous membranes in the mouth or oropharynx, patients who have this type of actinomycosis may have a history of oral surgery, dental procedures, or trauma to the mouth. They may present clinically with pain, trismus, firm swelling, and fistulas with drainage that contains the characteristic sulfur granules (Figs. 155–1 and 155–2). Patients most commonly have a chronic disease course but may present acutely with cellulitis. Infection may spread through the sinus tracts to the cranial bones, which gives rise to meningitis. Bone is not involved early in the disease, but later a periostitis may develop. A case of thyroiditis presumed to be secondary to an oral source has been reported in a pediatric patient.[26] The marked ability of the organisms in the disease to burrow through tissue planes and even bone differentiates actinomycosis from nocardiosis and is an important characteristic of this infection. The cervicofacial type of actinomycosis, or "lumpy jaw," has the best prognosis. With surgical débridement and excision as an adjunct to proper antibiotic therapy, the disease usually is cured.

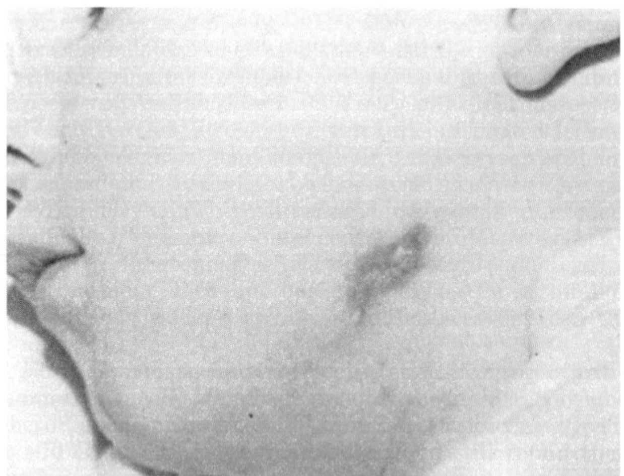

FIGURE 155–1 ■ Actinomycosis. Cervicofacial disease with draining sinus tracts due to *Actinomyces israelii*.

Because abdominal actinomycosis also is the result of disruption of the mucosa of the gastrointestinal tract, patients may present with a history of gastrointestinal surgery, diverticulitis, or appendicitis. The patient also may have a history of trauma to the abdomen. Patients may have chills, fever, night sweats, and weight loss. The course is indolent and similar to that of tuberculous peritonitis. Because appendicitis is the most common predisposing event, on physical examination, the patients may have a hard, irregular mass in the ileocecal area that softens and then drains to the outside. Extension from such foci usually is by direct continuity (or, rarely, is hematogenous) and involves any tissue or organ, including muscle, liver, spleen, kidney, fallopian tubes, ovaries, uterus, testes, bladder, or rectum. A delayed diagnosis of actinomycosis involving the abdomen or pelvis is typical.

The diagnosis of pulmonary actinomycosis depends on a high index of suspicion because neither the clinical nor radiographic presentation is specific. Patients may have a history of, or risk factors for, aspiration. This type of actinomycosis also occurs after introduction of a colonized foreign body. Patients with oral or cervicofacial or abdominal actinomycotic infections are at risk for developing pulmonary infection from direct or hematogenous spread. A history of these preexisting infections should heighten the index of suspicion. Pulmonary actinomycosis may present as an endobronchial infection, a tumor-like lesion, diffuse pneumonia, or a pleural effusion.[1, 10] The presence of chronic pleural effusion, underlying lung changes, and periosteal rib involvement is indicative of actinomycosis but seldom is reported.[25] The principal symptoms include chest pain, fever, productive cough, and weight loss. The infection frequently dissects along tissue planes and may extend through the chest wall or diaphragm, producing multiple sinuses. These characteristic sinus tracts contain small abscesses and purulent drainage. Adults with thoracic actinomycosis usually have abnormal local defenses, such as chronic bronchitis, bronchiectasis, or emphysema. However, pediatric patients have been shown to have predisposing factors less often.[22] The differential diagnosis of pulmonary actinomycosis includes tuberculosis, lung abscess, nocardiosis, fungal infection, and botryomycosis.

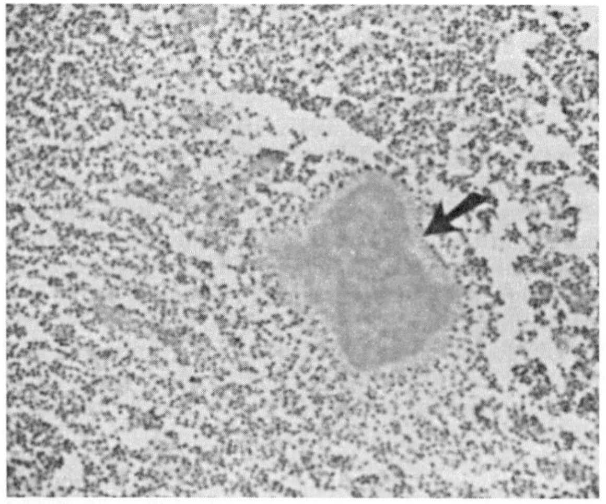

FIGURE 155–2 ■ Abscess containing actinomycotic granule surrounded by purulent exudate. The peripheral clubbing *(arrow)* is stained by eosin. (Hematoxylin and eosin; original magnification ×52.)

Women wearing IUDs are at risk for the development of pelvic actinomycosis. These patients may present with vaginal discharge, pelvic pain, abdominal pain, menorrhagia, fever, pelvic mass, a history of pelvic inflammatory disease, or a history of prolonged IUD use. The risk is more significant if the IUD has been in place for longer than 2 to 3 years. These devices are thought to cause an inflammatory response in the endometrium with focal necrosis. This anaerobic environment encourages the growth of *A. israelii*. In these patients, removal of the IUD and treatment with antibiotics are necessary.[3]

Hepatic involvement occurs in approximately 15 percent of cases of abdominal actinomycosis. Involvement of the liver can occur through direct extension from a subdiaphragmatic or subhepatic abscess. It also is a common finding in disseminated actinomycosis.[16] Occult disruption of the gastrointestinal mucosa with spread of organisms through the portal vein may provide a portal of entry for the organisms in cases of primary or isolated hepatic disease. Presenting symptoms may include fever, abdominal pain, anorexia, weight loss, nausea, vomiting, shoulder pain, back pain, or diarrhea. The presentation usually is indolent, with 1 to 6 months of symptoms. On physical examination, the patient commonly has fever, abdominal tenderness, and hepatomegaly. A palpable abdominal mass, jaundice, or draining sinuses may be present. Disseminated intravascular coagulation has been reported to occur.[24] Hepatic actinomycosis has been reported to occur in children who have undergone appendectomies.[9] Other causes of liver masses included in the differential diagnosis are pyogenic abscess, amebiasis, and malignancy.

Laryngeal actinomycosis rarely has been reported in older teenagers.[12] Colonization of the oropharynx with these organisms may be involved in the development of obstructive tonsillar hypertrophy.[15] Several adult cases of pericardial actinomycosis are reported in the literature.[4] Actinomycetes have been isolated from nearly every organ in the body, including the kidneys, brain, heart, breasts, mastoids, male genitourinary tract, and eyes. *A. pyogenes* has been implicated only rarely as a cause of human infection, but cases of septicemia, endocarditis, meningitis, arthritis, empyema, pneumonia, otitis media, cystitis, mastoiditis, appendicitis, and cutaneous infection have been reported.[2, 5]

Actinomycosis does not seem to be associated commonly with human immunodeficiency virus infection, perhaps because these patients frequently are in the health care system and have close monitoring. They may be treated for other infections with intermittent antibiotic therapy that also treats subclinical actinomycosis. Thoracic and oral cases have been reported, however, and all immunocompromised hosts should be monitored closely for this potential group of pathogens.[14, 23]

A. actinomycetemcomitans is a pathogen in at least 30 percent of actinomycotic infections.[8] Failure to recognize this organism and treat it adequately has resulted in clinical relapse and deterioration in infected patients with actinomycosis.[11, 27] Severe forms of periodontitis, particularly localized juvenile periodontitis, also are associated with this pathogen, and studies have shown that it is related strongly to children in the 10- to 19-year-old age group.[19] Additionally, it is one of the HACEK (HACEK includes *Haemophilus aphrophilus, Cardiobacterium hominis, Eikenella corrodens*, and *Kingella kingae*) organisms that has a propensity for infecting heart valves. Endocarditis caused by this organism usually is insidious, with fever occurring in fewer than 50 percent of cases.[8] This organism also has been reported to cause pericarditis, meningitis, brain abscess, parotitis, synovitis, osteomyelitis, urinary tract infection, pneumonia, and empyema.[8]

Diagnosis

To make a definitive diagnosis of actinomycosis, the clinician must isolate the causative organism from tissue or pus from a normally sterile body site, such as the lungs. Isolation of the organism from the oral cavity or the female genital tract without clinical evidence of disease is, therefore, not diagnostic. Because the organisms that cause actinomycosis are exquisitely sensitive to antibiotics, clinical specimens must be obtained before initiating their use. The specimens should be processed carefully to maintain anaerobic conditions. They should undergo routine Gram stain, which will reveal gram-positive rods that are not acid fast and appear in diphtheroidal arrangements with or without branching.[6] The Gram stain is more sensitive than is culture, particularly if the patient has been given antibiotics. Immunofluorescence is available for confirmation of organisms in biopsy specimens with suggestive Gram stains. Growth on media usually appears within 5 to 7 days but may take 2 to 4 weeks.[16]

True microbiologic identification of these organisms occurs uncommonly, and diagnosis most often rests on the clinical picture, with identification of the characteristic sulfur granules. The sulfur granules may be found by drawing pus from a lesion, on the bandage covering the lesion, or in surgical specimens (see Fig. 155–2). Pus that is poured down the side of a glass will leave sulfur granules adhering to the sides so that the granules will be identified more easily. On hematoxylin and eosin stain, the granules are eosinophilic or variably surrounded by a radiating fringe of eosinophilic clubs. The formation of granules is a hallmark of actinomycosis and is related to a bacterial secretion that cements elements of *Actinomyces* spp. together. However, the formation of granules related to various nonfilamentous bacteria such as *Staphylococcus aureus* or *Pseudomonas* spp. is called botryomycosis or bacterial pseudomycosis, and they can look grossly similar to the typical sulfur granules of actinomycosis.[10] Washed, crushed actinomycotic granules or well-mixed pus in the absence of granules is cultured on a rich medium, such as brain-heart infusion blood agar, and incubated anaerobically and aerobically with added carbon dioxide. Plates can be examined at 24 hours and after 5 to 7 days for the characteristic colonies of *Actinomyces* spp.[6]

Various imaging modalities have been useful in diagnosing and characterizing actinomycosis. Computed tomography has been shown to help differentiate between inflammatory masses and tumors. Additionally, the location, extension, and relation between the mass and surrounding structures can be defined better. Ultrasonography has been shown in one report to reveal a mass with an ill-defined margin that was hypoechoic with intrinsic hyperechoic spots.[17] Currently, no skin tests are available for screening purposes, and no useful serologic tests are available for actinomycosis.[4]

A. actinomycetemcomitans can be cultured on blood and chocolate agar but grows poorly on MacConkey agar. The cultures require incubation in an enhanced carbon dioxide atmosphere. Growth of the organism in a blood culture may take as long as 9 days in patients with endocarditis, and thus the cultures should be held longer. The organism on Gram stain appears coccoid to coccobacillary.[8] Molecular techniques based on nonamplification nucleic acid probes or on polymerase chain reaction can provide rapid and accurate identification of *A. actinomycetemcomitans*.[7] Because of the frequency of co-infection with this organism in cases of actinomycosis, attempts always should be made to isolate this organism in these patients.

Treatment

The mainstays of therapy for actinomycosis remain surgical débridement or removal of the lesion and prolonged antimicrobial therapy. Most experts still recommend drainage of abscesses, fistulotomy, sinus tract excision, and debulking of large masses, although numerous successful outcomes with antimicrobial therapy alone are reported in the literature.[9, 16] The option to treat medically and observe for clinical response seems reasonable in the stable, noncritical patient. The antibiotic of choice is penicillin. The recommended total duration of therapy ranges from 6 to 12 months. For patients who are allergic to penicillin, use of tetracycline or erythromycin is acceptable. Other alternatives are clindamycin, chloramphenicol, and the third-generation cephalosporins. Administration of daily ceftriaxone for 3 weeks followed by prolonged administration of ampicillin was effective treatment in one case.[22] Thoracic actinomycosis has been treated successfully with a total duration of therapy of only 4 months.[20] Failure to respond to adequate treatment has been noted in patients with underlying malignancy. Because the disease is an uncommon occurrence in children and no significant randomized prospective treatment trials have been performed, most authors still recommend 4 to 6 weeks of intravenous therapy followed by oral therapy for a prolonged period. The duration of total therapy is based on clinical and radiographic follow-up. Numerous cases of actinomycosis in various forms that have been treated successfully with therapy having a total duration of 3 to 6 months are reported in the literature. Certainly in cases for which surgical débridement or incision and drainage have occurred, a shorter duration of therapy would be reasonable provided close clinical follow-up can be ensured.

REFERENCES

1. Coodley, E. L., Yoshinaka, R.: Pleural effusion as the major manifestation of actinomycosis. Chest. *106*:1615–1617, 1994.
2. Drancourt, M.: Two cases of *Actinomyces pyogenes* infection in humans. Eur. J. Microbiol. Infect. Dis. *12*:55–57, 1993.
3. Evans, D. P. T.: *Actinomyces israelii* in the female genital tract: A review. Genitourin. Med. *69*:54–59,1993.

4. Fife, T. D., Finegold S. M., and Grennan T.: Pericardial actinomycosis: Case report and review. Rev. Infect. Dis. *13*:120–126, 1991.
5. Gahrn-Hansen, B., and Frederiksen W.: Human infections with *Actinomyces pyogenes (Corynebacterium pyogenes)*. Diag. Microbiol. Infect. Dis. *15*:349–354, 1992.
6. Gerencser, M. A.: *Actinomyces, Arachnia,* and *Streptomyces. In* Baron, S. (ed.): Medical Microbiology. 3rd ed. New York, Churchill Livingstone, 1991, pp. 469–477.
7. Leys, J. E., Griffen, A. L., Strong, S. J., et al.: Detection and strain identification of *Actinobacillus actinomycetemcomitans* by nested PCR. J. Clin. Microbiol. *32*:1288–1294, 1994.
8. McGowan, J. E., and Steinberg, J. P.: Other gram-negative bacilli. *In* Mandell, G. L., Bennett, J. E., and Dolin, R. (eds.): Principles and Practices of Infectious Diseases. New York, Churchill Livingstone, 1995, pp. 2106–2107.
9. Miyamoto, M. I., and Fang, F. C.: Pyogenic liver abscess involving *Actinomyces*: Case report and review. Clin. Infect. Dis. *16*:303–309, 1993.
10. de Montpreville, V., Nashashibi, N., Dulmet, E. M.: Actinomycosis and other bronchopulmonary infections with bacterial granules. Ann. Diagn. Pathol. *3*:67–74, 1999.
11. Morris, J. F., and Sewell, D. L.: Necrotizing pneumonia caused by mixed infection with *Actinobacillus actinomycetemcomitans* and *Actinomyces israelii:* Case report and review. Clin. Infect. Dis. *18*:450–452, 1994.
12. Nelson, E. G., and Tybor, A. G.: Actinomycosis of the larynx. Ear Nose Throat J. *71*:356–358, 1992.
13. Nisengard, R. J., Mikulski, L., McDuffie, D., et al.: Development of a rapid latex agglutination test for periodontal pathogens. J. Periodontol. *63*:611–617, 1992.
14. Ossorio, M. A., Fields, C. L., Byrd, R. P., and Roy, T. M.: Thoracic actinomycosis and human immunodeficiency virus infection. South. Med. J. *90*:1136–1138, 1997.
15. Pransky, M., Feldman, J. I., Kearns, D. B., et al.: Actinomycosis in obstructive tonsillar hypertrophy and recurrent tonsillitis. Arch. Otolaryngol. *117*:883–885, 1991.
16. Russo, T. A.: Agents of actinomycosis. *In* Mandell, G. L., Bennett, J. E., and Dolin, R. (eds.): Principles and Practices of Infectious Diseases. New York, Churchill Livingstone, 1995, pp. 2280–2288.
17. Sa'do, B., Kazunori, Y., Yuasa, K., et al.: Multimodality imaging of cervicofacial actinomycosis. Oral Surg. Oral Med. Oral Pathol. *76*: 772–778, 1993.
18. Sabbe, L. J. M., Van De Merwe, D., Schouls, L., et al.: Clinical spectrum of infections due to the newly described *Actinomyces* species *A. turicensis, A. radingae,* and *A. europaeus*. J. Clin. Microbiol. *37*:8–13, 1999.
19. Savitt, E. D., and Kent, R. L.: Distribution of *Actinobacillus actinomycetemcomitans* and *Porphyromonas gingivalis*. J. Periodontol. *62*: 490–494, 1991.
20. Skoutelis, A., Petrochilow, J., and Bassaris, H.: Successful treatment of thoracic actinomycosis with ceftriaxone. Clin. Infect. Dis. *19*:161–162, 1994.
21. Slots, J.: *Actinobacillus actinomycetemcomitans* and *Porphyromonas gingivalis* in periodontal disease: Introduction. Periodontology 2000 *20*: 7–13, 1999.
22. Snape, P. S.: Thoracic actinomycosis: An unusual childhood infection. South. Med. J. *86*:222–224, 1993.
23. Spadari, F., Tartaglia, G. M., Spadari, E., and Fazio, N.: Oral actinomycosis in acquired immunodeficiency syndrome. Int. J. S. T. D. A. I. D. S. *9*: 424–426, 1998.
24. Sugano, S., Matuda, T., Suzuki, T., et al.: Hepatic actinomycosis: Case report and review of the literature in Jpn. J. Gastroenterol. *32*:672–676, 1997.
25. Sumoza, D., Raad, I., and Douglas, E.: Differentiating thoracic actinomycosis from lung cancer. Infect. Med. *17*:695–698, 2000.
26. Trites, J., and Evans, M.: Actinomycotic thyroiditis in a child. J. Pediatr. Surg. *33*:781–782, 1998.
27. Tyrrell, J., Noone, P., and Prichard, J. S.: Thoracic actinomycosis complicated by *Actinobacillus actinomycetemcomitans:* Case report and review of literature. Respir. Med. *86*:341–343, 1992.
28. Yeung, M. K.: Molecular and genetic analyses of actinomyces spp. Crit. Rev. Oral Biol. Med. *10*(2):120–138, 1999.

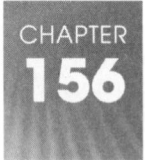

CHAPTER 156 Other Anaerobic Infections

XILLA T. USSERY

During the 17th century, Antonie van Leeuwenhoek observed that certain bacteria required an environment without oxygen to grow and replicate. In 1861, after discovering bacterial fermentation, Pasteur introduced the term *anaérobies*. In 1896, Welch described what now is recognized as the anaerobe *Clostridium perfringens*. During the first half of the 20th century, numerous studies documented the importance of anaerobic bacteria in abdominal and gynecologic infections, but these studies largely were unrecognized. Only after the discovery of relatively simple anaerobic culture techniques was the significance of these bacteria in clinical infections appreciated.

Anaerobic infections have been studied most extensively in adults, but several studies have documented the importance of anaerobic infections in infants and children. Indeed, although anaerobic infections occur less frequently in children than in adults, they should be considered in high-risk situations and in cases of unexplained sepsis.

Bacteriology

The anaerobic bacteria involved in clinical infections are a small portion of the vast taxonomy of existing anaerobes (Table 156–1). Anaerobic bacteria, like aerobic bacteria, are categorized according to their morphologic characteristics and Gram-staining properties. The primary characteristic of anaerobic bacteria that differentiates them from their aerobic counterparts is that they need an environment without oxygen. Unlike aerobic metabolism, anaerobic metabolism does not use oxygen as the final electron acceptor. In fact, oxygen adversely affects the oxidation-reduction (redox) potential of anaerobic bacteria. The redox potential is the ability to accept electrons. Studies have shown that for many anaerobes, the maximal redox potential above which they cannot grow occurs at pH 7.0. The reason is not entirely clear, but it probably is related to the inability of anaerobes in higher redox environments to maintain critical enzymes in a reduced state. Indeed, the limiting factor in the cultivation of anaerobes is oxygen toxicity.[95]

The reasons for oxygen toxicity are related to several chemical processes.[75] Some anaerobes lack the enzyme catalase; when oxygen is present, the bacteria are destroyed by the hydrogen peroxide that is generated. This mechanism appears operative in some species of *Bifidobacterium* and *Clostridium*. However, other species, including *Peptostreptococcus*, *Prevotella,* and *Bacteroides,* are aero-intolerant despite the presence of measurable quantities of catalase. For many species of anaerobes, when oxygen is added to the culture medium, growth is inhibited without a demonstrable

TABLE 156–1 ■ CLINICALLY SIGNIFICANT ANAEROBIC BACTERIA

Gram-positive
Bacilli (spore forming)
Clostridium
Bacilli (non-spore forming)
Proprionibacterium
Actinomyces
Lactobacillus
Eubacterium
Bifidobacterium
Cocci
Peptostreptococcus
Gram-negative
Bacilli
Bacillas fragilis group
Prevotella
Porphyromonas
Fusobacterium
Bilophila wadsworthia
Sutterella wadsworthensis
Cocci
Veillonella

accumulation of hydrogen peroxide. Furthermore, many species do not grow even after catalase is added to this culture medium. Clearly, the absence of catalase does not fully explain why oxygen is toxic to anaerobes. Other anaerobes lack the enzyme superoxide dismutase, which in the presence of oxygen generates a toxic intermediate superoxide anion. However, even strains that produce superoxide dismutase remain strictly anaerobic.

In vivo growth of anaerobic bacteria does not require an oxygen-free environment because reducing substances are the natural by-products of metabolism. However, in vitro growth depends on the creation of an environment in which oxygen is reduced sufficiently or absent. Therefore, specimens for culture should not be exposed to air before laboratory inoculation onto a reduced medium. Ideally, specimens should be placed in an anaerobic transport device as soon as possible. Aspirates and tissue are preferable to swabs. Liquid specimens should be transported to the laboratory in sterile tubes rather than in syringes with capped needles (to prevent needle-stick injuries). All specimens should be transported rapidly (within 30 minutes) to the laboratory so that they can be placed in an oxygen-free environment as soon as possible.[49, 52]

Once the anaerobes are in the laboratory, microbiologic techniques to cultivate them include the supplementation of media with reducing substances such as thioglycolate, dithiothreitol, cysteine, iron shavings, and chopped meat. Although broth media incubated under aerobic conditions and supplemented with reducing substances supports some anaerobic growth, the solid media used for isolation and identification of anaerobes must be processed and incubated in an oxygen-free environment.[80] Furthermore, such media should contain antibiotics to suppress the growth of facultative organisms that might otherwise overgrow the anaerobes.

The traditional method of identifying and classifying anaerobic bacteria is analysis of carbohydrate fermentation reactions. One such method uses the sodium dodecyl sulfate–polyacrylamide gel electrophoresis (SDS-PAGE) technique for analysis of whole-cell proteins. These methods are the standard against which newer techniques are measured. Agar dilution, broth macrodilution and microdilution, and the E test are the techniques used most widely for susceptibility testing of individual isolates. Guidelines for susceptibility testing are found in the National Committee for Clinical Laboratory Standards (NCCLS) manual,[96] and information regarding the cultivation of anaerobic bacteria is available in several standard guides and textbooks.[124]

Epidemiology

Anaerobic infections occur less frequently in children than in adults, probably because children are less likely than are adults to have certain predisposing chronic conditions and types of infections that often involve anaerobes (e.g., lung, liver, and peritoneal abscesses; empyema; obstetric and gynecologic infections).

Most anaerobic infections result from disruption of endogenous flora. However, some infections, such as those caused by certain *Clostridium* spp. (e.g., wound botulism, tetanus), are of exogenous origin. Nosocomially acquired infections and those caused by animal and human bites are other examples of exogenously acquired infections that often involve anaerobic bacteria.

The epidemiology of antimicrobial resistance among anaerobes is evolving rapidly and varies by locale. In recent years, many anaerobic bacteria have demonstrated increased resistance to the antimicrobial agents commonly used, thus complicating empiric therapy for infections with these bacteria. This resistance is especially true among the *Bacillus fragilis* group, for which several studies have shown increasing resistance to β-lactam antibiotics and to clindamycin.[8, 62, 64, 70] In one survey of seven medical centers in the Chicago area, among *B. fragilis* group isolates, 21 to 50 percent were resistant to clindamycin and 14 to 75 percent were resistant to piperacillin. In the same study, resistance was lowest for metronidazole, imipenem, piperacillin-tazobactam, ticarcillin–clavulanic acid, and ampicillin-sulbactam.[70]

For anaerobes such as *Clostridium*, *Peptostreptococcus*, and *Prevotella*, antimicrobial resistance rates are lower, but rates of resistance to clindamycin, trovafloxacin, and penicillin are increasing.[70] These data highlight the importance of conducting periodic hospital surveys of antimicrobial susceptibility patterns so that adequate antimicrobial coverage can be provided for anaerobic infections.

Pathogenesis

The pathogenesis of anaerobic infections reflects a complex interaction among bacterial virulence factors, host defense mechanisms, and synergy with other organisms. The distinguishing characteristics of anaerobic infections include suppuration, abscess formation, tissue destruction, foul odor, and, occasionally, formation of gas. The virulence of anaerobic bacteria is a result of adherence factors, surface constituents (capsular polysaccharide and lipopolysaccharide, or endotoxin), and toxin production.

Bacterial adherence mechanisms are important for establishing colonization and infection. Some strains of *Prevotella melaninogenica* and *Fusobacterium nucleatum* preferentially adhere to the epithelial cells found in crevices within the oral cavity.[76, 88, 101] Pili enable adherence to mucosal membranes,[117] and the capsule resists opsonophagocytosis.[111, 116]

Surface constituents also play a role in the pathogenesis of anaerobic infections. For instance, thrombophlebitis, which is associated with some species of *Bacteroides,* is the result of activation of Hageman factor (clotting factor XII) by lipopolysaccharide.[9] Furthermore, the capsular polysaccharide of *B. fragilis* not only resists phagocytosis but also promotes the formation of abscesses.[41, 83, 102, 103, 115]

Many anaerobic bacteria elaborate proteolytic toxins that enhance cell necrosis. For example, the kappa-toxin produced by *C. perfringens* causes collagen degradation, necrosis, and extravasation of blood.[118] Furthermore, in mixed infections, these toxins may contribute to the virulence of relatively nonpathogenic organisms. Metabolic products such as the ammonia produced by some strains of *P. melaninogenica* may cause further tissue damage.

Clinical Manifestations

Anaerobic infections frequently involve the endogenous flora of adjacent mucosal surfaces and usually are the result of an alteration in these surfaces that compromises tissue. Devitalized tissue provides the necessary oxygen-free environment that enhances the growth of anaerobic bacteria. Introduction of organisms into host tissues can occur through breaks in mucosal surfaces or through invasion of organisms with enhanced adherence mechanisms. Whatever the mechanism for initiation, polymicrobial infection with endogenous flora often occurs.

Predisposing conditions for anaerobic infection in children include immunosuppression, renal insufficiency, malignancy, chronic infection, and tissue compromise after surgery, injury, shock, or vascular embarrassment.

The clinical manifestations of anaerobic infections are similar to those of aerobic infections. Some anaerobic infections, however, such as pleuropulmonary and pelvic infections, occur much less commonly in children than in adults. Serious anaerobic infections are seen more frequently in compromised hosts or in newborn infants than in otherwise healthy children. The outcome in patients with severe anaerobic infections is dependent on the underlying disease and the time elapsed until appropriate therapy is provided; prompt recognition is associated with a better outcome.

BACTEREMIA

When cultures are obtained properly, anaerobes have been found to cause 5 to 10 percent of clinically significant bacteremic episodes in infants and children.[13, 55] In one study, anaerobic bacteremia occurred twice as frequently in newborn infants as in older children and accounted for 12 percent of all cases of neonatal bacteremia.[55] This percentage is not surprising because after delivery, neonates are colonized with maternal vaginal flora that contains both aerobic and anaerobic bacteria. Predisposing factors for anaerobic bacteremia in neonates include perinatal maternal complications (e.g., premature rupture of membranes), prematurity, and necrotizing enterocolitis.[24] In neonates, the mortality rate associated with anaerobic bacteremia ranges from 4 to 38 percent; higher mortality rates are associated with clinically significant disease such as necrotizing enterocolitis.[48, 55, 68]

In children older than 1 month of age, anaerobic bacteremia typically occurs in those with chronic disease or immunosuppression.[55] Often, the bacteremia can be traced to a gastrointestinal source, which includes the oral cavity. Indeed, 66 to 75 percent of clinically significant episodes of anaerobic bacteremia are caused by gram-negative bacilli, predominantly of the *B. fragilis* group. The strains next most commonly involved are *Peptostreptococcus* (10% of isolates) and *Clostridium* (5–10% of isolates).[114] The clinical features of anaerobic bacteremia are indistinguishable from those of aerobic bacteremia.

HEAD AND NECK INFECTION

Chronic otitis media, acute and chronic mastoiditis, chronic sinusitis, peritonsillar abscess, odontogenic infections, and deep neck space infections often involve anaerobes.[14, 44, 45, 100]

In patients with chronic otitis media, the bacteria isolated most frequently from middle ear cultures are *Staphylococcus aureus*, *Pseudomonas aeruginosa,* and anaerobes. Indeed, when appropriate culture techniques are used, 33 to 55 percent of cultures yield anaerobic bacteria, either alone or as part of a mixed infection with aerobic bacteria.[11, 21, 43, 82, 123] The predominant organisms include anaerobic gram-positive cocci and *Bacteroides* and *Clostridium* spp. Additionally, in patients with acute otitis media, anaerobes have been recovered from 5 to 15 percent of middle ear cultures.[42]

Similarly, in patients with acute sinusitis, anaerobic bacteria are recovered from approximately 10 percent of sinus cultures. In contrast, in patients with chronic sinusitis, the predominant pathogens isolated from sinus culture are anaerobic bacteria. In one study, cultures from 37 of 40 children with chronic sinusitis yielded bacteria. Of these 37 cultures, all yielded anaerobic bacteria, either alone (62%) or as part of a mixed infection with aerobic bacteria (38%).[18]

In saliva, the ratio of anaerobic to aerobic bacteria is 10:1.[59] Therefore, one is not surprised to find that anaerobic bacteria are involved in the overwhelming majority of odontogenic infections (periodontitis, periapical and dental abscesses, gingivitis, etc.) and associated infections such as peritonsillar abscesses (quinsy), cervical adenitis, and deep neck space infections.[12, 17, 33, 39, 97] In one study of peritonsillar abscesses in children, anaerobic bacteria were isolated from all 16 patients in whom aspiration was performed. The isolated pathogens included various gram-positive cocci and *Fusobacterium*, *Bacteroides*, and *Clostridium* spp. Two thirds of patients had β-lactamase–producing organisms recovered.[17]

Deep neck space infections are potentially life-threatening and often are preceded by oral, dental, and pharyngeal infections. Retropharyngeal and prevertebral space infections are characterized by dysphagia, hoarseness, bulging of the posterior of the pharynx, and often, stiff neck. Submandibular space infection, or Ludwig angina, has a characteristic clinical picture of rapidly progressive, submental, spreading cellulitis that elevates the tongue from the floor of the mouth and may lead to complete airway compromise. Other clinical features include dysphagia, trismus, drooling, voice change, and dyspnea. Systemic toxicity is severe, and surgical decompression is the mainstay of treatment.[94] Another serious complication of perimandibular infection is Lemierre syndrome, which is associated with *Fusobacterium necrophorum* bacteremia, jugular vein septic thrombophlebitis, metastatic abscess (lung, liver, or elsewhere), and a foul-smelling tonsillar pseudomembrane.

CENTRAL NERVOUS SYSTEM

Anaerobic bacteria can cause a variety of intracranial infections, including brain abscess, subdural empyema, epidural abscess, and meningitis.[7, 15, 20, 77, 105] In children, predisposing conditions for brain abscess include chronic infections of the ears, mastoids, sinuses, or oropharynx; cyanotic congenital heart disease; skull fracture or penetrating head injury; and neurosurgery.[105] Although in adults, pulmonary disease is the most frequent cause of a metastatic focus to the brain, such is not the case for children. In general, the predisposing condition (e.g., chronic sinusitis) determines both the anatomic location of the abscess and the organism or organisms isolated.

In some studies of brain abscess in children, anaerobic bacteria have been causative more than 80 percent of the time, either alone or as part of a mixed infection with aerobes.[15, 26] The predominant anaerobes involved in brain abscess include those found in the sinuses and oropharynx, such as *Bacteroides, Fusobacterium, Prevotella,* and *Actinomyces* spp.[15]

The prognosis for patients with brain abscess is related to the anatomic location of the abscess, the ease with which it can be drained surgically, and the degree to which its mass effect compromises the intracranial contents. A brain abscess of sufficient size generally responds best to drainage, although surgical drainage of multiple or loculated abscesses may be impractical. For abscesses with a diameter greater than 2 cm, the outcome is improved with surgical drainage, and excision remains the management of choice for well-encapsulated lesions. Smaller lesions and those that have not yet encapsulated can improve with prolonged antimicrobial therapy alone.[6, 7, 93] The mortality rate associated with brain abscess is 11 to 14 percent, although lesions located in the cerebral hemispheres have significantly better prognoses than do those in the cerebellum or brain stem structures.[78, 110]

Anaerobic meningitis rarely occurs in children, although when it does, it usually is a complication of a cerebrospinal fluid (CSF) shunt or a respiratory tract infection. Anaerobes involved in CSF shunt infections often are those of cutaneous (e.g., *Propionibacterium acnes*) or enteric (e.g., *B. fragilis*) origin.[28, 40]

INTRA-ABDOMINAL

In children, secondary peritonitis and intra-abdominal abscesses are a consequence of disruption of the integrity of the intestinal wall as a result of perforation, obstruction, infarction, or trauma. Secondary peritonitis usually is associated with appendicitis, but it also occurs with volvulus, intussusception, incarcerated hernia, or rupture of the Meckel diverticulum or as a complication of intestinal mucosal disease.[27]

Anaerobic bacteria are the predominant organisms in the gastrointestinal tract; therefore, after bowel perforation occurs, they frequently are isolated from peritoneal or abscess cultures.[10, 67, 92, 122] Intra-abdominal infections in children frequently involve both aerobic bacteria (e.g., *Escherichia coli, Enterococcus* spp.) and anaerobic bacteria (*B. fragilis, Peptostreptococcus* and *Clostridium* spp.).[27, 67] Several studies have confirmed similar findings for secondary peritonitis and retroperitoneal and liver abscesses.[10, 32, 36, 37, 92, 113] In one study of children with appendicitis, although *B. fragilis* and *Peptostreptococcus micros* were the predominant species (73% and 66% of the isolates, respectively), several other anaerobic bacteria (*Bilophila wadsworthia, F. nucleatum, Eggerthella lenta,* and a previously undescribed bile-resistant, pigment-producing gram-negative rod) also were isolated.[107]

Appropriate management of intra-abdominal infections in children includes surgical drainage and administration of antimicrobial agents effective against both aerobic and anaerobic bacteria. Secondary peritonitis, intra-abdominal abscesses, and abdominal wound infections in otherwise normal hosts are associated with a good prognosis when effective therapy is administered and surgical drainage is performed, which is true also for bacteremia associated with intra-abdominal anaerobic infections. However, when endotoxic shock, disseminated intravascular coagulopathy, or metastatic foci of infection supervene, the prognosis of a favorable outcome decreases.

SKIN AND SOFT TISSUE INFECTIONS

Anaerobic bacteria can be involved in a variety of skin and soft tissue infections, both superficial and deep. Superficial infections with potential anaerobic involvement are paronychia, infected ulcers, gastrostomy or tracheostomy site infections, secondary infections of scabies lesions, and cellulitis.[16, 29, 31, 35, 38] Anaerobic infections of the subcutaneous tissue include bite wounds (both human and animal), cutaneous abscesses, anaerobic cellulitis, bacterial synergistic gangrene, infected pilonidal cysts, and burn wounds. Deeper infections of the muscle and fascia include necrotizing fasciitis, gas gangrene (clostridial myonecrosis), synergistic necrotizing cellulitis, and Fournier gangrene (necrotizing fasciitis of the male genital area).[23, 65, 66, 81, 121, 125, 127]

Anaerobic bacteria recovered from skin and soft tissue infections vary by location and circumstance (e.g., soil contamination, bite wound). The anaerobes encountered most frequently include the *B. fragilis* group, anaerobic gram-positive cocci, and other *Bacteroides, Prevotella, Porphyromonas, Fusobacterium,* and *Clostridium* spp. Aerobic bacteria such as *S. aureus*, group A beta-hemolytic streptococci, alpha-hemolytic and nonhemolytic streptococci, *Enterobacter,* and *E. coli* also are involved often.[35, 38] For bite wound infections, the predominant bacteria include *Pasteurella multocida, S. aureus, Staphylococcus intermedius,* alpha-hemolytic streptococci, *Capnocytophaga canimorsus,* and other oral flora.[23, 65, 66] When cultures from bite wounds are obtained appropriately, anaerobic bacteria (*Fusobacterium, Bacteroides, Porphyromonas,* and *Prevotella*) have been isolated from 75 percent of cultures, either alone or as part of a mixed infection with aerobic bacteria.[23, 125]

Infections involving the muscle and fascia often are associated with severe systemic toxicity, are potentially life-threatening, and require prompt recognition, surgical management, and antimicrobial therapy. In spite of severe toxicity, the early stages of necrotizing fasciitis can be difficult to diagnose because local findings often are subtle and nonspecific (edema, erythema, superficial skin lesions, cellulitis).[63, 112] A definitive diagnosis usually is made at the time of surgery. Mortality rates can exceed 50 percent; mortality is dependent on the time elapsed until surgical débridement. By facilitating early recognition, the use of bedside frozen section biopsies can decrease mortality rates from 73 to 12.5 percent.[121]

OSTEOMYELITIS

Anaerobic osteomyelitis is not a common event in children. When it does occur, it usually is a result of direct extension from a contiguous focus (e.g., mucous membrane) rather than from bacteremia. In one study of children with anaerobic osteomyelitis, predisposing conditions included chronic mastoiditis, chronic sinusitis, decubitus ulcers, periodontal abscesses, bite wounds, paronychia, trauma, and scalp infection after fetal monitoring. Of 26 cases, 15 (57%) had osteomyelitis of the skull and facial bones.[22]

Although the clinical manifestations of anaerobic osteomyelitis do not differ from those of aerobic osteomyelitis, they often are more subtle.[99] Radiographically, anaerobic osteomyelitis can mimic malignant osseous tumors.[99] Thus, specimens should be obtained for anaerobic culture whenever drainage or biopsy procedures are performed, and anaerobic infections should be considered in osteomyelitis of unclear etiology.[99, 106]

The predominant organisms include anaerobic cocci and *Bacteroides, Fusobacterium,* and *Clostridium* spp.[22] Finally, like most infections that involve anaerobic bacteria, anaerobic osteomyelitis often is polymicrobial, so antimicrobial therapy should be directed initially against both aerobic and anaerobic organisms.[22, 106]

PLEUROPULMONARY INFECTIONS

Anaerobic pleuropulmonary infections occur less frequently in children than in adults. However, certain types of pulmonary infection (aspiration pneumonia, lung abscess) often involve anaerobic bacteria.[25] Predisposing conditions for lung abscess include aspiration caused by neurologic impairment, foreign body aspiration, poor oral hygiene, gingivitis, periodontitis, cystic fibrosis, and immunosuppression.[34, 57] Ideally, specimens for culture should be obtained by percutaneous or transtracheal aspiration of the abscess. Under these circumstances, anaerobic bacteria (e.g., *Peptostreptococcus*, *Peptococcus*, and *Bacteroides* spp.) often are found as part of a mixed infection with aerobic bacteria (e.g., alpha-hemolytic streptococci, group A beta-hemolytic streptococci, *E. coli*, and *Klebsiella pneumoniae*).[34] Thus, antimicrobial therapy should be directed against both anaerobes and gram-positive aerobes.

Anaerobic bacteria also have been recovered from cultures of sputum obtained from children with ventilator-associated pneumonia. In one such study, strict anaerobes were recovered from sputum culture specimens that were obtained with protective brush catheters after endotracheal suctioning, followed by rapid transport to the laboratory. Of 10 children with ventilator-associated pneumonia, 9 had anaerobic bacteria recovered from sputum culture (e.g., *Prevotella*, *Porphyromonas*, *Peptostreptococcus*, *Fusobacterium*, and *Bacteroides* spp.), either alone (3 children) or as part of a mixed infection with aerobic bacteria (6 children).[30]

Diagnosis

The diagnosis of anaerobic infections requires a high index of suspicion. A few anaerobic infections are diagnosed clinically (tetanus, botulism, and gas gangrene), and for these infections, culture results can be misleading. However, most anaerobic infections are diagnosed by both clinical and microbiologic methods. Radiographs demonstrating gas in infected tissues may be helpful, although often they are nonspecific. When anaerobic infections are suspected, specimens for culture must be collected properly, without contamination from the endogenous flora of adjacent mucous membranes. For example, expectorated sputum or sinus drainage can be contaminated with mucosal flora and yield unreliable culture results. Ideally, these specimens should be obtained by aspiration that bypasses the oropharyngeal mucosa. In general, acceptable specimens for culture include blood, aspirates of body fluid or deep wounds, and material obtained surgically. Gram-stained smears of aspirated material should be examined and used to complement culture results.

Biochemical tests and gas-liquid chromatography of metabolites may be used to identify anaerobic bacteria. Molecular genetic methods such as DNA hybridization, chromosomal DNA probes, and species-specific polymerase chain reaction also allow identification of anaerobic isolates.[51, 86, 87, 90, 91] Direct immunofluorescence on a variety of organisms has been used for rapid detection of anaerobic bacteria, although nonspecific reactions do occur.[128] Enzyme immunoassay kits for the rapid detection of *Clostridium difficile* toxin in stool have been available commercially for some time, with sensitivities ranging between 93 and 100 percent.[1]

Treatment

Treatment of anaerobic infections often involves surgical drainage or débridement (or both), combined with appropriate antimicrobial therapy. If surgery is required, it must be performed promptly to ensure an adequate therapeutic outcome. Antimicrobial therapy for common site-specific anaerobic infections in children is presented in Table 156–2. Other therapeutic modalities, such as hyperbaric oxygen, have been used in certain instances, but experience in children is limited and clear recommendations cannot be made.

Antimicrobial agents with the most potent activity against anaerobic bacteria include metronidazole, imipenem, chloramphenicol, and the β-lactam/β-lactamase inhibitor combinations. Historically, clindamycin and some of the cephalosporins have been good alternatives, but in recent years, many anaerobic bacteria have become increasingly resistant to these drugs.[71, 119]

Empiric antimicrobial therapy for the management of anaerobic infections should be based on an assessment of the probable pathogens, local susceptibility patterns, and previous antimicrobial use. Furthermore, because anaerobes often are recovered as part of a mixed infection, optimal therapy should provide coverage for both aerobic and anaerobic bacteria. Therapy should be adjusted when the antimicrobial susceptibility of the pathogens isolated is known. Given the nationwide variability in susceptibility patterns, such testing is important to determine optimal therapy.[53, 56, 109] In general, susceptibility testing should be performed for the following groups: seriously ill patients or those who require prolonged therapy, patients who do not respond to initial therapy or have a relapse, and patients with novel or resistant organisms.[60]

The duration of antimicrobial therapy for anaerobic infections does not differ from that for aerobic infections. Minor soft tissue infection usually is treated for 10 to 14 days, septicemia for 10 days to 3 weeks, bone and joint infection for 6 weeks or more, and brain abscess for a minimum of 6 to 8 weeks.

Serious anaerobic infections should be treated with intravenous antimicrobial agents at the maximal approved dosages (after adjusting for individual renal and hepatic function) because these infections frequently involve devitalized tissue and abscess formation, which results in poor tissue penetration of antimicrobial agents.

PENICILLINS

Penicillin G is the drug of choice for most non–β-lactamase–producing organisms, including gram-positive anaerobic bacteria (e.g., anaerobic streptococci, *Clostridium* spp., and non–spore-forming, gram-positive bacilli). However, in most gram-negative anaerobic bacilli (e.g., the *B. fragilis* group and *Prevotella*, *Porphyromonas*, and *Fusobacterium* spp.), a high incidence of β-lactamase production occurs, and, therefore, penicillin G should not be used to treat serious infections with these organisms.[4, 73, 85, 98]

Penicillin therapy for susceptible organisms can be rendered ineffective by other β-lactamase–producing organisms at the site of infection. These organisms release β-lactamase into the environment, which degrades the penicillin. The addition of a β-lactamase inhibitor (e.g., clavulanic acid, sulbactam, or tazobactam) to the β-lactam antibiotic (e.g., amoxicillin, ampicillin, piperacillin, or ticarcillin) can overcome this problem. β-Lactam/β-lactamase inhibitor combinations have the advantage of being well tolerated and having a broad spectrum of antibacterial activity. Of the

TABLE 156–2 ■ ANTIMICROBIAL THERAPY FOR SITE-SPECIFIC ANAEROBIC INFECTIONS

Site	Pathogen	Therapy
Intracranial	*Bacteroides* *Fusobacterium* *Prevotella* *Actinomyces* *Propionibacterium*	Metronidazole Meropenem
Dental	*Bacteroides* *Fusobacterium* *Clostridium* *Porphyromonas* *Peptostreptococcus*	Clindamycin Penicillin Metronidazole Amoxicillin + CA
Upper respiratory tract	*Bacteroides* *Fusobacterium* *Prevotella* *Porphyromonas* *Clostridium* *Peptostreptococcus*	Clindamycin Metronidazole Amoxicillin + CA
Pulmonary	*Bacillus fragilis* group *Fusobacterium* *Prevotella* *Porphyromonas* Anaerobic gram-positive cocci	Clindamycin Ticarcillin + CA Ampicillin + SU Imipenem or meropenem Amoxicillin + CA
Abdominal/pelvic	*B. fragilis* group *Peptostreptococcus* *Clostridium* *Fusobacterium* *Bilophila wadsworthia*	Clindamycin Cefoxitin Metronidazole Piperacillin + TA Imipenem or meropenem Ampicillin + SU Ticarcillin + CA
Skin/soft tissue	*B. fragilis* group Anaerobic gram-positive cocci *Bacteroides* *Prevotella* Porphyromonas *Fusobacterium* *Clostridium*	Clindamycin Cefoxitin Metronidazole Amoxicillin + CA Ampicillin + SU Ticarcillin + CA Clindamycin
Bone/joint	Anaerobic cocci *Bacteroides* *Fusobacterium* *Clostridium*	Imipenem or meropenem Metronidazole Ticarcillin + CA Imipenem or meropenem
Bacteremia	*B. fragilis* group *Peptostreptococcus* *Clostridium* *Fusobacterium* *Propionibacterium*	Metronidazole Cefoxitin Ticarcillin + CA Clindamycin Amoxicillin + CA

*Chloramphenicol may be used for intracranial, pulmonary, and bone/joint infections.
CA, clavulanic acid; SU, sulbactam; TA, tazobactam

combinations available, recent in vitro data suggest that more species of clinically important anaerobic bacteria are more susceptible to ampicillin-sulbactam than to either piperacillin-tazobactam or ticarcillin–clavulanic acid.[61]

METRONIDAZOLE

Metronidazole is a nitroimidazole antibiotic with excellent activity against most anaerobic gram-negative organisms. However, non–spore-forming, anaerobic, gram-positive bacilli (e.g., *Actinomyces* and *Propionibacterium*) and gram-positive cocci (e.g., *Peptostreptococcus*) often are resistant to metronidazole.[5] Metronidazole enters the cell by passive diffusion and undergoes a reductive process that produces a metabolite toxic to cells. This process requires a low redox potential, in part explaining why metronidazole is not active against aerobic bacteria.[126] Thus, metronidazole should not be used as a single agent for polymicrobial infections with aerobic bacteria.

Metronidazole penetrates well into many tissues, including the central nervous system (CNS), and is thus an effective medication for serious anaerobic infections, including brain abscess, skin and soft tissue infection, bone and joint infection, and even endocarditis.[19, 58, 84] It is the drug of choice for the treatment of pseudomembranous colitis caused by *C. difficile*. Although metronidazole is well tolerated generally, when given in large or prolonged doses, CNS side effects, including seizures, encephalopathy, cerebellar dysfunction, and peripheral neuropathy, have been reported.

CLINDAMYCIN

Clindamycin is a derivative of the antibiotic lincomycin and has essentially replaced it because of better absorption and a broader spectrum of activity. Clindamycin is active against most anaerobes, including anaerobic gram-positive cocci, gram-positive non–spore-forming bacilli (e.g., *Actinomyces* and *Propionibacterium*), *C. perfringens*, and anaerobic gram-negative bacilli (e.g., *Bacteroides*, *Prevotella,* and *Porphyromonas*). It also is active against most aerobic gram-positive bacteria, including *Streptococcus pneumoniae*, viridans streptococci, and methicillin-susceptible *S. aureus*. However, clindamycin is not active against *Enterococcus* spp. or aerobic gram-negative bacteria. Furthermore, some anaerobic cocci and *B. fragilis* isolates are resistant to clindamycin. In one study, of 253 anaerobic isolates from pediatric infections, 22 percent of peptostreptococcal isolates and 13 percent of *B. fragilis* isolates were resistant to clindamycin at a concentration of 4 μg/mL.[51] Hospital-acquired infections with members of the *B. fragilis* group also have been shown to be associated with resistance to clindamycin.[54]

Clindamycin penetrates well into most tissues and fluids, with the exception of CSF.[104] Therefore, it should be considered for the treatment of anaerobic infections outside the CNS. Clindamycin, combined with an antimicrobial agent that has aerobic gram-negative activity, is sufficient for treating some polymicrobial infections. Furthermore, clindamycin is a useful alternative in patients allergic to penicillin. Clindamycin generally is well tolerated, although diarrhea is a common side effect.

CHLORAMPHENICOL

Chloramphenicol, a nitrobenzene moiety, penetrates bacterial cells by facilitated diffusion and binds reversibly to the 50S ribosomal subunit. It has a broad spectrum of antimicrobial activity against many gram-positive and gram-negative bacteria, as well as rickettsiae. It penetrates the CNS well and has particularly good activity against anaerobic bacteria, including *B. fragilis*. In addition, resistance to chloramphenicol occurs rarely. Unfortunately, its use is limited because of potential serious side effects, including "gray baby" syndrome, a rare but fatal aplastic anemia, and dose-dependent bone marrow suppression.

CEPHALOSPORINS

The cephalosporins have a six-member hydrothiazine ring connected to the β-lactam ring, which must remain intact for effective antimicrobial activity to occur. The cephalosporins, like the penicillins, kill susceptible bacteria by interfering with cell wall synthesis. The first-generation cephalosporins are similar to penicillin G with respect to activity against anaerobic bacteria. Among the cephalosporins, the second-generation agent cefoxitin has the most potent activity against the *B. fragilis* group. However, at some centers, 6 to 20 percent of *B. fragilis* group isolates and 18 percent of *Clostridium* isolates are resistant to cefoxitin.[8, 70] Third-generation cephalosporins are inferior to cefoxitin with respect to anaerobic activity.

CARBAPENEMS (IMIPENEM, MEROPENEM)

Imipenem-cilastatin is a parenteral carbapenem that consists of imipenem, a crystalline derivative of thienamycin, and cilastatin, a potent inhibitor of renal dehydropeptidase I. Although cilastatin lacks antimicrobial activity, it prevents renal metabolism, and, therefore, the compound is not associated with nephrotoxicity. Imipenem has activity against a wide variety of anaerobic and aerobic, gram-positive and gram-negative bacteria. In general, with respect to *Bacteroides* spp. and other anaerobic bacteria, the activity of imipenem is equal to or superior to that of clindamycin, metronidazole, amoxicillin–clavulanic acid, and cefoxitin.[8, 70, 74, 120]

QUINOLONES

Fluoroquinolones bind to the A subunits of DNA gyrase, thereby preventing DNA supercoiling and unraveling and, consequently, halting DNA replication. They have a rapid bactericidal effect against most susceptible organisms, and, like the macrolides, they penetrate into tissues and mammalian cells extremely well. Although the early fluoroquinolone antibiotics (e.g., ciprofloxacin and ofloxacin) have limited activity against anaerobic bacteria, the newer fluoroquinolones (e.g., trovafloxacin, gatifloxacin, and moxifloxacin) have improved activity against several important pathogens, including anaerobic bacteria.[2, 3, 69, 72] However, resistance to quinolones has emerged in some strains of previously susceptible aerobic (e.g., methicillin-sensitive and -resistant *S. aureus*, *S. pneumoniae*, and *P. aeruginosa*) and anaerobic bacteria (e.g., the *B. fragilis* group and *Prevotella*, *Peptostreptococcus*, and *Clostridium* spp.).[70, 108]

Fluoroquinolones are safe and effective in adult patients with a variety of infections, but arthrotoxicity in juvenile animals has limited their use in children, growing adolescents, and pregnant and lactating women. Nevertheless, over the years, many children have received quinolones for a variety of infections, mostly on a compassionate-use basis. Although cases of quinolone-associated joint effusion and pain have been described in the literature,[46, 47, 79, 89] most cases were associated with pefloxacin and all but one were not associated with long-term sequelae. The one exception was a subject in whom other etiologies could not be excluded.[47]

MACROLIDES (ERYTHROMYCIN, AZITHROMYCIN, CLARITHROMYCIN)

The macrolides inhibit protein synthesis by reversibly binding to the 50S ribosome subunit of sensitive bacteria. In general, the macrolides have fairly good in vitro activity against anaerobic bacteria, with the exception of *B. fragilis* and *Fusobacterium* spp. Clarithromycin is the most active against oral gram-positive anaerobes (e.g., *Actinomyces*, *Propionibacterium*, *Lactobacillus*, and *Bifidobacterium* spp.).[129] Macrolides also are active against *Prevotella* and *Porphyromonas* and certain clostridia, although they have poor or inconsistent activity against other gram-negative anaerobic bacilli.

GLYCOPEPTIDES (VANCOMYCIN, TEICOPLANIN)

Vancomycin is a tricyclic glycopeptide that inhibits cell wall synthesis. Its activity is limited to gram-positive bacteria, both aerobic and anaerobic.

Prevention

Preventing the development of anaerobic infections involves precluding conditions that promote the introduction and proliferation of anaerobes in healthy tissue. Preventive measures include cleaning and débriding wounds properly, removing foreign bodies promptly, maintaining an adequate tissue blood supply, applying good surgical technique, avoiding aspiration of gastric contents, and using antimicrobial agents appropriately for prophylaxis and treatment. Tetanus is the only anaerobic infection that can be prevented by immunization. The use of antitoxin is applicable to both tetanus and botulism.

REFERENCES

1. Altaie, S. S., Meyer, P., and Dryja, D.: Comparison of two commercially available enzyme immunoassays for detection of *Clostridium difficile* in stool specimens. J. Clin. Microbiol. *32*:51–53, 1994.
2. Appelbaum, P. C.: Quinolone activity against anaerobes. Drugs *58*(Suppl. 2):60–64, 1999.
3. Appelbaum, P. C., and Hunter, P. A.: The fluoroquinolone antibacterials: Past, present and future perspectives. Int. J. Antimicrob. Agents *16*:5–15, 2000.
4. Appelbaum, P. C., Spangler, S. K., and Jacobs, M. R.: β-Lactamase production and susceptibilities to amoxicillin, amoxicillin-clavulanate, ticarcillin, ticarcillin/clavulanate, cefoxitin, imipenem, and metronidazole of 320 non-*Bacteroides fragilis Bacteroides* isolates and 129 fusobacteria from 28 US centers. Antimicrob. Agents Chemother. *34*:1546–1550, 1990.
5. Appelbaum, P. C., Spangler, S. K., and Jacobs, M. R.: Susceptibility of 539 gram-positive and gram-negative anaerobes to new agents, including RP59500, biapenem, trospectomycin and piperacillin/tazobactam. J. Antimicrob. Chemother. *32*:223–231, 1993.
6. Barsoum, A. H., Lewis, H. C., and Cannillo, K. L.: Nonoperative treatment of multiple brain abscesses. Surg. Neurol. *16*:283–287, 1981.
7. Berg, B., Franklin, G., Cuneo, R., et al.: Nonsurgical cure of brain abscess: Early diagnosis and follow-up with computerized tomography. Ann. Neurol. *3*:474–478, 1978.
8. Betriu, C., Gomez, M., Rodriguez-Avial, I., et al.: Trends in antimicrobial resistance of the *Bacteroides fragilis* group over an 11-year period (1989–2000). Poster C2-64. Presented at the 41st Interscience Conference on Antimicrobial Agents and Chemotherapy, 2001, Chicago.
9. Bjornson, H. S.: Activation of Hageman factor by lipopolysaccharides of *B. fragilis, B. vulgatus* and *Fusobacterium mortiferum*. Rev. Infect. Dis. *6*(Suppl.):30–33, 1984.
10. Brook, I.: Bacterial studies of peritoneal cavity and postoperative surgical wound drainage following perforated appendix in children. Ann. Surg. *192*:208–212, 1980.
11. Brook, I.: Chronic otitis media in children: Microbiological studies. Am. J. Dis. Child. *134*:564–566, 1980.
12. Brook, I.: Aerobic and anaerobic bacteriology of cervical adenitis in children. Clin. Pediatr. (Phila.) *19*:693–696, 1980.
13. Brook, I.: Anaerobic bacteremia in children. Am. J. Dis. Child. *134*: 1052–1056, 1980.
14. Brook, I.: Aerobic and anaerobic bacteriology of chronic mastoiditis in children. Am. J. Dis. Child. *135*:478–479, 1981.
15. Brook, I.: Bacteriology of intracranial abscess in children. J. Neurosurg. *54*:484–488, 1981.
16. Brook, I.: Bacteriologic study of paronychia in children. Am. J. Surg. *141*:703–705, 1981.
17. Brook, I.: Aerobic and anaerobic bacteriology of peritonsillar abscess in children. Acta Paediatr. Scand. *70*:831–835, 1981.
18. Brook, I.: Bacteriologic features of chronic sinusitis in children. J. A. M. A. *246*:967–969, 1981.
19. Brook, I.: Treatment of anaerobic infections in children with metronidazole. Dev. Pharmacol. Ther. *6*:187–198, 1983.
20. Brook, I.: Anaerobic meningitis in an infant associated with pilonidal cyst abscess. Clin. Neurol. Neurosurg. *87*:131–132, 1985.
21. Brook, I.: Prevalence of β-lactamase producing bacteria in chronic suppurative otitis media. Am. J. Dis. Child. *139*:280–283, 1985.
22. Brook, I.: Anaerobic osteomyelitis in children. Pediatr. Infect. Dis. *5*:550–556, 1986.
23. Brook, I.: Microbiology of human and animal bite wounds in children. Pediatr. Infect. Dis. J. *6*:29–32, 1987.
24. Brook, I.: Bacteremia due to anaerobic bacteria in newborns. J. Perinatol. *10*:351–356, 1990.
25. Brook, I.: Microbiology of empyema in children and adolescents. Pediatrics *85*:722–726, 1990.
26. Brook, I.: Aerobic and anaerobic bacteriology of intracranial abscesses. Pediatr. Neurol. *8*:210–214, 1992.
27. Brook, I.: Intra-abdominal infections in children. Drugs *46*:53–62, 1993.
28. Brook, I.: Infections caused by *Propionibacterium* in children. Clin. Pediatr. (Phila.) *33*:485–490, 1994.
29. Brook, I.: Aerobic and anaerobic microbiology of gastrostomy-site wound infections in children. Clin. Infect. Dis. *20*(Suppl. 2):257–258, 1995.
30. Brook, I.: Pneumonia in mechanically ventilated children. Scand. J. Infect. Dis. *27*:619–622, 1995.
31. Brook, I.: Microbiology of secondary bacterial infection in scabies lesions. J. Clin. Microbiol. *33*:2139–2140, 1995.
32. Brook, I.: Microbiology of retroperitoneal abscesses in children. J. Med. Microbiol. *48*:679–700, 1999.
33. Brook, I.: Anaerobic infections in children. Adv. Pediatr. *47*:395–437, 2000.
34. Brook, I., and Finegold, S. M.: Bacteriology and therapy of lung abscess in children. J. Pediatr. *94*:10–12, 1979.
35. Brook, I., and Finegold, S. M.: Aerobic and anaerobic bacteriology of cutaneous abscesses in children. Pediatrics *67*:891–895, 1981.
36. Brook, I., and Fraizer, E. H.: Role of anaerobic bacteria in liver abscesses in children. Pediatr. Infect. Dis. J. *12*:743–746, 1993.
37. Brook, I., and Frazier, E. H.: Aerobic and anaerobic microbiology of retroperitoneal abscesses. Clin. Infect. Dis. *26*:938–941, 1998.
38. Brook, I., Frazier, E. H., Yeager, J. K.: Microbiology of infected poison ivy dermatitis. Br. J. Dermatol. *142*:943–946, 2000.
39. Brook, I., Grimm, S., and Kielich, R. B.: Bacteriology of acute periapical abscess in children. J. Endodont. *7*:378–380, 1981.
40. Brook, I., Johnson, N., Overturf, G. D., et al.: Mixed bacterial meningitis: A complication of ventriculo- and lumbo-peritoneal shunts. J. Neurosurg. *47*:961–964, 1977.
41. Brook, I., Myhal, L. A., and Dorsey, C. H.: Encapsulation and pilus formation of *Bacteroides* spp. in normal flora, abscesses and blood. J. Infect. *25*:251–257, 1992.
42. Brook, I., and Schwartz, R.: Anaerobic bacteria in acute otitis media. Acta Otolaryngol. *91*:111–114, 1981.
43. Brook, I., and Yocum, P.: Quantitative bacterial cultures and beta-lactamase activity in chronic suppurative otitis media. Ann. Otol. Rhinol. Laryngol. *98*:293–297, 1989.
44. Brook, I., Yocum, P., and Shah, K.: Surface vs. core-tonsillar aerobic and anaerobic flora in recurrent tonsillitis. J. A. M. A. *244*:1696–1698, 1980.
45. Busch, D. F.: Anaerobes in infection of the head and neck and ear, nose and throat. Rev. Infect. Dis. *6*(Suppl.):115-–122, 1984.
46. Chang, H., Chung, M.-H., Kim, J. I. H., and Kim, J.-H.: Pefloxacin-induced arthropathy in an adolescent with brain abscess. Scand. J. Infect. Dis. *28*:641–643, 1996.
47. Chevalier, X., Albengres, E., Voisin, M.-C., et al.: A case of destructive polyarthropathy in a 17-year old youth following pefloxacin treatment. Drug Saf. 7:310–314, 1992.
48. Chow, A. W., Leake, R. D., Yamauchi, T., et al.: The significance of anaerobes in neonatal bacteremia: Analysis of 23 cases and review of the literature. Pediatrics *54*:736–745, 1974.
49. Citron, D. M.: Specimen collection and transport, anaerobic culture techniques and identification of anaerobes. Rev. Infect. Dis. *6*(Suppl.):51–58, 1984.
50. Citron, D. M., Goldstein, E. J. C., Kenner, M. A., et al.: Activity of ampicillin/sulbactam, ticarcillin/clavulanate, clarithromycin and eleven other antimicrobial agents against anaerobic bacteria isolated from infections in children. Clin. Infect. Dis. *20*(Suppl. 2):356–360, 1995.
51. Claros, M. C., Citron, D. M., Gerardo, S. H., et al.: Characterization of indole-negative *Bacteroides fragilis* group species with use of polymerase chain reaction fingerprinting and resistance profiles. Clin. Infect. Dis. *23*(Suppl. 1):66–72, 1996.
52. Collee, J. G.: Factors contributing to loss of anaerobic bacteria in transit from the patient to the laboratory. Infection *8*(Suppl.):145–147, 1980.
53. Cuchural, G., Jacobus, N., Gorbach, S. L., et al.: A survey of *Bacteroides* susceptibility in the United States. J. Antimicrob. Chemother. *8*:27–31, 1981.
54. Dalmau, D., Cayouette, M., Lamothe, F., et al.: Clindamycin resistance in the *Bacteroides fragilis* group: Association with hospital-acquired infections. Clin. Infect. Dis. *24*:874–877, 1997.
55. Dunkle, L. M., Brotherton, T. J., and Feigin, R. D.: Anaerobic infections in children: A prospective survey. Pediatrics *57*:311–320, 1976.
56. Edson, R. S., Rosenblatt, J. E., Lee, D. T., et al.: Recent experience with antimicrobial susceptibility of anaerobic bacteria. Mayo Clin. Proc. *57*:734–741, 1982.
57. Emanuel, B., and Shulman, S. T.: Lung abscess in infants and children. Clin. Pediatr. (Phila.) *34*:2–6, 1995.
58. Feng, J., and Austin, T. W.: Anaerobic vertebral osteomyelitis. Can. Med. Assoc. J. *145*:132–3, 1991.
59. Finegold, S. M.: Anaerobic Bacteria in Human Disease. New York, Academic Press, 1977, p. 29.
60. Finegold, S. M.: Perspective on susceptibility testing of anaerobic bacteria. Clin. Infect. Dis. *25*(Suppl. 2):251–253, 1997.
61. Finegold, S. M.: In vitro efficacy of β-lactam/β-lactamase inhibitor combinations against bacteria involved in mixed infections. Int. J. Antimicrob. Agents *12*(Suppl. 1):9–14, 1999.
62. Finegold, S. M., and Wexler, H. M.: Present status of therapy for anaerobic infections. Clin. Infect. Dis. *23*(Suppl. 1):9–14, 1996.
63. Freeman, H. P., Oluwole, S. F., Ganepola, G. A. P., and Dy, E.: Necrotizing fasciitis. Am. J. Surg. *142*:377–383, 1981.
64. Golan, Y., Jacobus, N. V., McDermott, L. A., et al.: Clindamycin resistance (CR) among *Bacteroides fragilis* group (Bf): Analysis by site of infection. Poster C2–63. Presented at the 41st Interscience Conference on Antimicrobial Agents and Chemotherapy, 2001, Chicago.
65. Goldstein, E. J. C.: Bite wounds and infection. Clin. Infect. Dis. *14*:633–640, 1992.
66. Goldstein, E. J. C., and Richwald, G. A.: Human and animal bite wounds. Am. Fam. Physician *36*:101–109, 1987.
67. Gorenstein, A., Gewurtz, G., Serour, F., and Somekh, E.: Postappendectomy intra-abdominal abscess: A therapeutic approach. Arch. Dis. Child. *70*:400–402, 1994.

68. Harrod, J. R., and Stevens, D. A.: Anaerobic infections in the newborn infant. J. Pediatr. *85*:399–402, 1974.
69. Hecht, D. W., and Osmolski, J. R.: Comparison of activities of trovafloxacin (CP-99,219) and five other agents against 585 anaerobes with use of three media. Clin. Infect. Dis. *23*(Suppl. 1):44–50, 1996.
70. Hecht, D. W., and Osmolski, J. R.: Antibiotic resistance among 547 anaerobes from Chicago area medical centers. Abstract C2-62. Poster C2-62. Presented at the 41st Interscience Conference on Antimicrobial Agents and Chemotherapy, 2001, Chicago.
71. Hecht, D. W., Osmolski, J. R., and O'Keefe, J. P.: Variation in the susceptibility of *Bacteroides fragilis* group isolates from six Chicago hospitals. Clin. Infect. Dis. *16*(Suppl. 4):357–360, 1993.
72. Hecht, D. W., and Wexler, H. M.: In vitro susceptibility of anaerobes to quinolones in the United States. Clin. Infect. Dis. *23*(Suppl. 1):2–8, 1996.
73. Heimdahl, A., Vonkonow, L., and Nord, C. E.: Isolation of beta-lactamase–producing *Bacteroides* strains associated with clinical failures with penicillin treatment of human orofacial infection. Arch. Oral Biol. *25*:689–692, 1980.
74. Hellinger, W. C., and Brewer, N. S.: Carbapenems and monobactams: Imipenem, meropenem, and aztreonam. Mayo Clin. Proc. *74*:420–434, 1999.
75. Hewitt, L. F.: Influence of hydrogen ion concentration and oxidation-reduction conditions on bacterial behavior. Symp. Soc. Gen. Microbiol. *7*:42, 1957.
76. Hofstad, T.: Pathogenicity of anaerobic gram negative rods: Possible mechanisms. Rev. Infect. Dis. *6*:189–199, 1984.
77. Jacobs, J. A., Hendriks, J. J. E., Verschure, P. D. M., et al.: Meningitis due to *Fusobacterium necrophorum* subspecies *necrophorum:* Case report and review of the literature. Infection *21*:57–60, 1993.
78. Jadavji, T., Humphreys, R. P., and Prober, C. G.: Brain abscesses in infants and children. Pediatr. Infect. Dis. *4*:394–398, 1985.
79. Jawad, A. S. M.: Cystic fibrosis and drug-induced arthropathy. Br. J. Rheumatol. *28*:179–180, 1989.
80. Jonsimies-Somer, H. R., and Finegold, S. M.: Problems encountered in clinical anaerobic bacteriology. Rev. Infect. Dis. *6*(Suppl.):45–50, 1984.
81. Kaiser, R. E., and Cerra, F. B.: Progressive necrotizing surgical infections: A unified approach. J. Trauma *21*:349–353, 1981.
82. Karma, P., Jokipii, L., Ojala, K., et al.: Bacteriology of the chronically discharging middle ear. Acta Otolaryngol. *86*:110–114, 1978.
83. Kasper, D. L., Lindberg, A. A., Weintraub, A., et al.: Capsular polysaccharides and lipopolysaccharides from two strains of *Bacteroides fragilis.* Rev. Infect. Dis. *6*(Suppl.):25–29, 1984.
84. Kolander, S. A., Cosgrove, E. M., and Molavi, A.: Clostridial endocarditis: Report of a case caused by *Clostridium bifermentans* and review of the literature. Arch. Intern. Med. *149*:455–456, 1989.
85. Könönen, E., Nyfors, S., Mättö, J., et al.: β-Lactamase production by oral pigmented *Prevotella* species isolated from young children. Clin. Infect. Dis. *25*(Suppl. 2):272–274, 1997.
86. Kuritza, A. P., Getty, C. E., Shaughnessy, P., et al.: DNA probes for identification of clinically important *Bacteroides* species. J. Clin. Microbiol. *23*:343–349, 1986.
87. La Fontaine, S., Egerton, J. R., and Rood, J. I.: Detection of *Dichelobacter nodosus* using species-specific oligonucleotides as PCR primers. Vet. Microbiol. *35*:101–117, 1993.
88. Lee, S. W., Alexander, B., and McGowan, B.: Purification, characterization and serologic characteristics of *Bacteroides nodosus* pili and use of a purified pili vaccine in sheep. Am. J. Vet. Res. *44*:1676–1681, 1983.
89. Le Loet, X., Fessard, C., Noblet, C., et al.: Severe polyarthropathy in an adolescent treated with pefloxacin. Letter. J. Rheumatol. *18*:1941–1942, 1991.
90. Loos, B. G., Mayrand, D., Genco, R. J., and Dickinson, D. P.: Genetic heterogeneity of *Porphyromonas (Bacteroides) gingivalis* by genomic DNA finger-printing. J. Dent. Res. 69:1488–1493, 1990.
91. Love, D. N., and Bailey, G. D.: Chromosomal DNA probes for the identification of *Bacteroides tectum* and *Bacteroides fragilis* from the oral cavity of cats. Vet. Microbiol. *34*:89–95, 1993.
92. Marchildon, M. B., and Dudgeon, D. L.: Perforated appendicitis: Current experience in a children's hospital. Ann. Surg. *185*:84–87, 1977.
93. Mathiesen, G. E., Meyer, R. D., George, W. L., et al.: Brain abscess and cerebritis. Rev. Infect. Dis. *6*(Suppl.):101–106, 1984.
94. Meyers, B. R., Lawson, W., and Hirschman, S. Z.: Ludwig's angina: Case report with review of bacteriology and current therapy. Am. J. Med. *53*:257–260, 1972.
95. Morris, J. G.: Oxygen tolerance/intolerance of anaerobic bacteria. *In* Gottschalk, G., Pennig, N., and Werner, H. (eds.): Anaerobes and Anaerobic Infections. Stuttgart, Germany, Gustav Fischer Verlag, 1980.
96. National Committee for Clinical Laboratory Standards: Methods for Antimicrobial Susceptibility Testing of Anaerobic Bacteria; Approved Standard. 5th ed. NCCLS Document M11-A5 [ISBN 1-56238-429-5]. NCCLS, 940 West Valley Road, Suite 1400, Wayne, PA 19087-1898, 2001.
97. Newman, M. G.: Anaerobic oral and dental infection. Rev. Infect. Dis. *6*(Suppl.):107–114, 1984.
98. Nord, C. E.: Mechanisms of ß-lactam resistance in anaerobic bacteria. Rev. Infect. Dis. *8*(Suppl. 5):543–548, 1986.
99. Ogden, J. A., and Light, T. R.: Pediatric osteomyelitis. III. Anaerobic microorganisms. Clin. Orthop. *145*:230–236, 1979.
100. Ogle, J. W., and Lauer, B. A.: Acute mastoiditis: Diagnosis and complications. Am. J. Dis. Child. 140:1178–1182, 1986.
101. Okuda, K., Slots, J., and Genco, R. J.: *Bacteroides gingivalis, Bacteroides asaccharolyticus,* and *Bacteroides melaninogenicus* subspecies: Cell surface morphology and adherence to erythrocytes and human buccal epithelial cells. Curr. Microbiol. *6*:7–12, 1981.
102. Onderdonk, A. B., Kasper, D. L., Cisneros, R. L., et al.: The capsular polysaccharide of *Bacteroides fragilis* as a virulence factor. J. Infect. Dis. *136*:82–89, 1977.
103. Onderdonk, A. B., Shapiro, M. E., Finberg, R. W., et al.: Use of a model of intra-abdominal sepsis for studies of the pathogenicity of *B. fragilis.* Rev. Infect. Dis. *6*(Suppl.):91–95, 1984.
104. Panzer, J. D., Brown, D. C., Epstein, W. L., et al.: Clindamycin levels in various body tissues and fluids. J. Clin. Pharmacol. New Drugs *12*:259–262, 1972.
105. Patrick, C. C., and Kaplan, S. L.: Current concepts in the pathogenesis and management of brain abscesses in children. Pediatr. Clin. North Am. *35*:625–636, 1988.
106. Raff, M. J., and Melo, J. C.: Anaerobic osteomyelitis. Medicine (Baltimore) *57*:83–103, 1978.
107. Rautio, M., Saxén, H., Siitonen, A., et al.: Bacteriology of histopathologically defined appendicitis in children. Pediatr. Infect. Dis. J. *19*: 1078–1083, 2000.
108. Robson, H. G., and Lavallee, J.: Rapidly increasing resistance of *Streptococcus pneumoniae* to penicillin, macrolides and fluoroquinolones in a Canadian teaching hospital. Poster C2–704. Presented at the 41st Interscience Conference on Antimicrobial Agents and Chemotherapy, 2001, Chicago.
109. Rosenblatt, J. E.: Antimicrobial susceptibility testing of anaerobic bacteria. Rev. Infect. Dis. *6*(Suppl.):242–248, 1984.
110. Rosenblum, M. L., Hoff, J. T., Norman, D., et al.: Decreased mortality from brain abscesses since advent of computerized tomography. J. Neurosurg. *49*:658–663, 1978.
111. Rotstein, O. D.: Interactions between leukocytes and anaerobic bacteria in polymicrobial surgical infections. Clin. Infect. Dis. *16*(Suppl. 4): 190–194, 1993.
112. Rouse, T. M., Malangoni, M. A., and Schulte, W. J.: Necrotizing fasciitis: A preventable disaster. Surgery *92*:765–770, 1982.
113. Sabbaj, J.: Anaerobes in liver abscess. Rev. Infect. Dis. *6*(Suppl.): 152–156, 1984.
114. Salonen, J. H., Eerola, E., and Meurman, O.: Clinical significance and outcome of anaerobic bacteremia. Clin. Infect. Dis. *26*:1413–1417, 1998.
115. Shapiro, M. E., Onderdonk, A. B., Kasper, D. L., et al.: Cellular immunity to *Bacteroides fragilis* capsular polysaccharide. J. Exp. Med. *155*: 1188–1197, 1982.
116. Simon, G. L., Klempner, M. S., Kasper, D. L., et al.: Alterations in opsonophagocytic killing by neutrophils of *Bacteroides fragilis* associated with animal and laboratory passage: Effect of capsular polysaccharide. J. Infect. Dis. *145*:72–77, 1982.
117. Slots, J., and Gibbons, R. J.: Attachment of *Bacteroides melaninogenicus* subsp. *asaccharolyticus* to oral surfaces and its possible role in colonization of the mouth of periodontal pockets. Infect. Immun. *19*:254–264, 1978.
118. Smith, L. D.: Virulence factors of *C. perfringens.* Rev. Infect. Dis. *1*:254–260, 1979.
119. Snydman, D. R., and Cuchural, G. J.: Susceptibility variations in *Bacteroides fragilis*: A national survey. Infect. Dis. Clin. Pract. *3*(Suppl.): 34–43, 1994.
120. Snydman, D. R., McDermott, L., Cuchural, G. J., Jr., et al.: Analysis of trends in antimicrobial resistance patterns among clinical isolates of *Bacteroides fragilis* group species from 1990 to 1994. Clin. Infect. Dis. *23*(Suppl. 1):54–65, 1996.
121. Stamenkovic, I., and Lew, P. D.: Early recognition of potentially fatal necrotizing fasciitis. N. Engl. J. Med. *310*:1689–1693, 1984.
122. Stone, J. H.: Bacterial flora of appendicitis in children. J. Pediatr. Surg. *11*:37–45, 1976.
123. Sugita, R., Kawamura, S., and Ichikawa, G.: Studies on anaerobic bacteria in chronic otitis media. Laryngoscope *91*:816–821, 1981.
124. Summanen, P., Baron, E. J., Citron, D. M., et al.: Wadsworth Anaerobic Bacteriology Manual. 5th ed. Belmont, CA, Star Publishing, 1993.
125. Talan, D. A., Citron, D. M., Abrahamian, F. M., et al.: Bacteriologic analysis of infected dog and cat bites. N. Engl. J. Med. *340*:85–92, 1999.
126. Tally, F. P., and Sullivan, C. E.: Metronidazole: In vitro activity, pharmacology and efficacy in anaerobic bacterial infections. Pharmacotherapy *1*:28–38, 1981.
127. Weinstein, L., and Barza, M. A.: Gas gangrene. N. Engl. J. Med. *289*:1129–1131, 1973.
128. Weissfeld, A. S., and Sonnenwirth, A. C.: Rapid detection and identification of *B. fragilis* and *B. melaninogenicus* by immunofluorescence. J. Clin. Microbiol. *13*:798–800, 1981.
129. Williams, J. D., Maskell, J. P., Shain, H., et al.: Comparative in-vitro activity of azithromycin, macrolides (erythromycin, clarithromycin and spiramycin) and streptogramin RP 59500 against oral organisms. J. Antimicrob. Chemother. *30*:27–37, 1992.

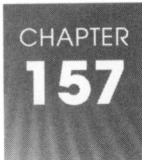

CHAPTER 157 Classification and Nomenclature of Viruses

MARJORIE J. MILLER

Viruses originally were differentiated from other microorganisms by their small size and their filterability. Initial efforts to classify viruses were based on disease, pathogenesis, organ tropisms, and epidemiologic characteristics rather than physicochemical properties of the virus particle. During the 1950s and 1960s, many new viruses were being discovered while evidence of virus structure and composition also was emerging, prompting proposals that viruses be grouped on the basis of shared virion properties. The herpesvirus,[1] myxovirus,[2] and poxvirus[5] groups were among the first taxonomic groups delineated. As more information concerning the physicochemical characteristics of viruses accumulated, the need for a universal system of classification and nomenclature became apparent.

The International Committee on Nomenclature of Viruses (ICNV) was established in 1966 at the International Congress of Microbiology in Moscow, some 20 years after a bacterial taxonomy first was published and 75 years after the discovery of viruses. The ICNV became the International Committee on Taxonomy of Viruses (ICTV), which operates under the auspices of the Virology Division of the International Union of Microbiological Societies, in 1973. The ICTV classifies viruses isolated from vertebrates, invertebrates, plants, fungi, protozoa, bacteria, and mycoplasmas and publishes periodic reports summarizing the most recent developments in viral taxonomy.[6–9, 11, 15, 16] Interim updates were published in *Intervirology* and more recently in *Archives of Virology*. Additional information on virus taxonomy can be accessed through the Internet at www.ncbi.nlm.nih.gov/ICTV/ and through a worldwide universal virus database (ICTVdB) being developed through the cooperation of the Australian National University (ANU, http//life.anu.edu.au/viruses/welcome.htm) in Canberra, the American Type Culture Collection, and the U.S. National Science Foundation (mirror Internet sites are NCBI, Bethesda, MD: www.ncbi.nlm.nih.gov/ICTVdB/welcome.htm and IACR, Rothamsted, UK: www.bbsrc.ac.uk/mirror/auz/welcome.htm).

The hierarchic levels of virus taxonomy consist of order, family, subfamily, genus, and species based on structural, physicochemical, biologic, and replicative properties of viruses.[11] Structural characteristics include size, shape, presence or absence of an envelope, and capsid symmetry. Physicochemical characterization is based on type, strandedness, and the number of segments of nucleic acid as well as the number and size of proteins and their functional activities. Biologic properties include host range, serologic relationships, pathogenicity, and transmission; replicative properties include nucleic acid replication, transcription, and translation.

Virus orders comprise groups of families that share common characteristics (e.g., biochemical composition, virus replication strategy, particle structure, and general genomic organization) distinguishable from other orders and families. Virus orders are designated with the suffix-*virales*. Currently, the ICTV has approved two orders, the order *Mononegavirales* comprising the families *Paramyxoviridae*, *Rhabdoviridae*, and *Filoviridae* and the order *Nidovirales* comprising the families *Coronaviridae* and *Arteriviridae*.

Virus families represent groups of genera that share common characteristics distinct from viruses of other families. Virus families are designated with the suffix *-viridae*. Most families have unique virion morphology, genome structure, or strategies of replication (Fig. 157–1). Virus subfamilies are designated with the suffix *-virinae* and have been introduced in four families: *Poxviridae (Chorodopoxvirinae)*, *Herpesviridae (Alpha-, Beta-, Gammaherpesvirinae)*, *Parvoviridae (Parvovirinae)*, and *Paramyxoviridae (Paramyxovirinae, Pneumovirinae)* (Table 157–1).

Virus genera consist of groups of species that share common characteristics different from those of members of other genera. Common properties within a genus include virus replication strategy, genome size, organization, numbers of segments, sequence homologies, and vector transmission. Virus genera are designated with the suffix *-virus*.

The species taxon is the most fundamental unit in biologic classification, but the viruses have proved to be the most difficult with which to deal, requiring years before a definition of virus species was accepted internationally. In 1991, the ICTV accepted the definition of a virus species proposed by van Regenmortel[12]: "A virus species is defined as a polythetic class of viruses that constitutes a replicating lineage and occupies a particular ecological niche." Members of a polythetic class have several properties in common, although no single common attribute is present in all members, thereby accommodating the inherent variability of viruses. Common species properties include genome rearrangement, sequence homologies, serologic relationships, vector transmission, host range, pathogenicity, tissue tropism, and geographic distribution.[15] Some properties of viruses used in taxonomy are listed in Table 157–2.[11]

The ICTV also has established criteria for formal virus nomenclature[15] and recommended abbreviations for virus names.[4, 15] In formal taxonomic usage, the names of orders, families, subfamilies, genera, and species are printed in italics and the first letter of the name is capitalized. This form applies when using a species name to refer to a taxonomic category (e.g., in the Materials and Methods section of a paper when describing the particular virus used in the study). Some examples of formal taxonomic terminology are *Poliovirus*, genus *Enterovirus*, family *Picornaviridae* or *Human herpesvirus 1* (Herpes simplex virus type 1), genus

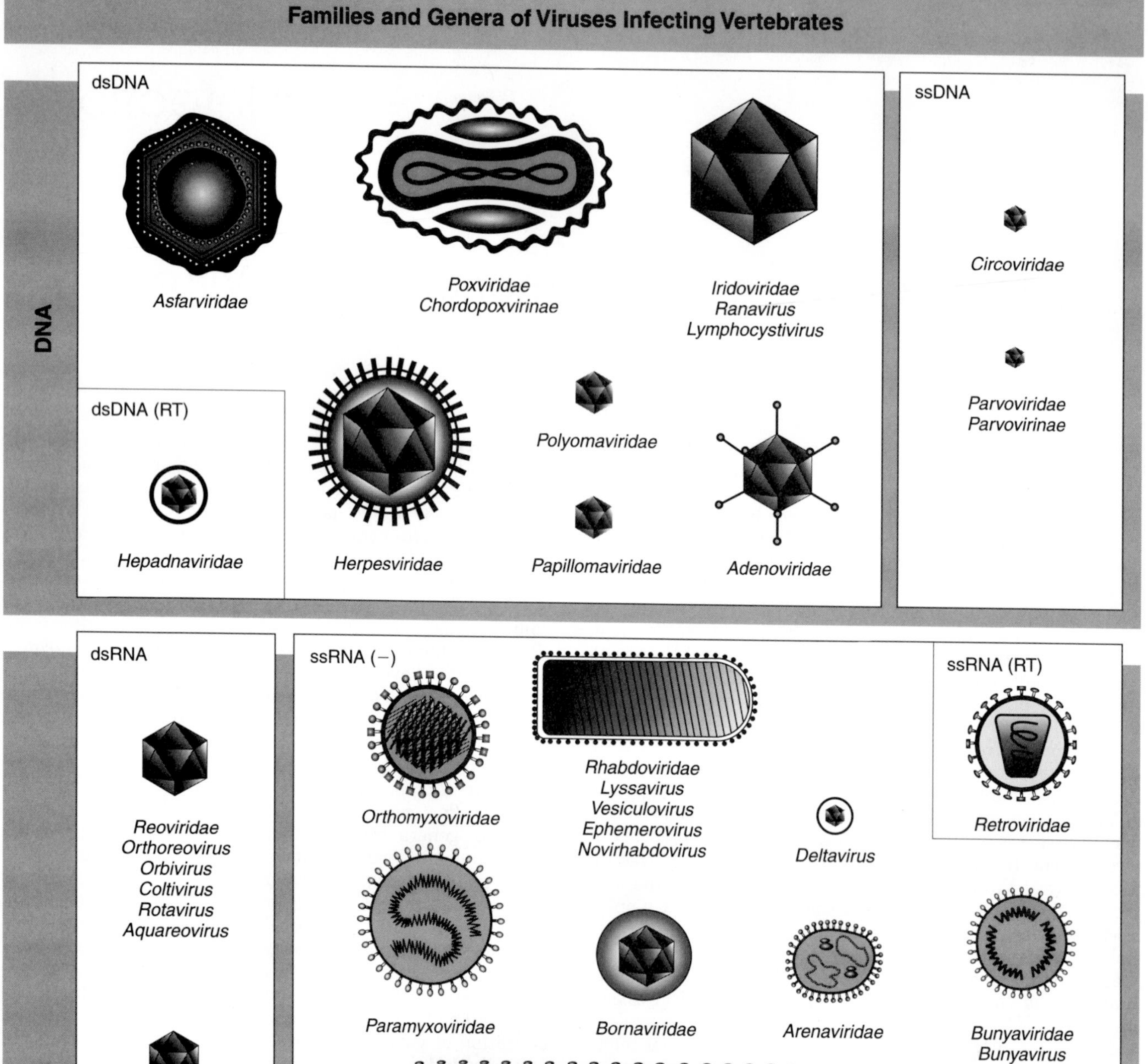

FIGURE 157–1 ■ Diagram illustrating the shapes and relative sizes of animal viruses of the major families. (From Van Regenmortel, M. H. V., Fauquet, C. M., Bishop, D. H. L., et al. [eds.]: Virus Taxonomy: Classification and Nomenclature of Viruses. Seventh Report of the International Committee on Taxonomy of Viruses. Academic Press, 2000, p. 30.)

TABLE 157–1 ■ CLASSIFICATION AND NOMENCLATURE OF REPRESENTATIVE VIRUSES AFFECTING HUMANS

Family	Subfamily	Genus	Representative Species Pathogenic for Humans (abbreviation, disease, synonym, or no. of members)
DNA Viruses			
Poxviridae	*Chordopoxvirinae*	*Orthopoxvirus*	*Vaccinia virus* (VACV) *Variola virus* (VARV)
		Parapoxvirus	*Orf virus* (ORFH, contagious pustular dermatitis) *Pseudocowpox virus* (PCPV, milkers' nodule)
		Molluscipoxvirus	*Molluscum contagiosum virus* (MOCV)
		Yatapoxvirus	*Yaba monkey tumor virus, tanapox virus* (YMTV, TANV)
Herpesviridae	*Alphaherpesvirinae*	*Simplexvirus*	*Human herpesvirus 1* (HHV-1, herpes simplex virus type 1) *Human herpesvirus 2* (HHV-2, herpes simplex virus type 2) *Cercopithecine herpesvirus 1* (CeHV-1, monkey B virus)
		Varicellovirus	*Human herpesvirus 3* (HHV-3, varicella-zoster virus)
	Betaherpesvirinae	*Cytomegalovirus*	*Human herpesvirus 5* (HHV-5, cytomegalovirus)
		Roseolovirus	*Human herpesvirus 6* (HHV-6, human B lymphotropic virus) *Human herpesvirus 7* (HHV-7)
	Gammaherpesvirinae	*Lymphocryptovirus*	*Human herpesvirus 4* (HHV-4, Epstein-Barr virus)
		Rhadinovirus	*Human herpesvirus 8* (HHV-8, Kaposi sarcoma-associated herpesvirus)
Adenoviridae		*Mastadenovirus*	*Human adenovirus A* (HAdV-A; 12, 18, 31) *Human adenovirus B* (HAdV-B; 3, 7, 11, 14, 16, 21, 34, 35, 50) *Human adenovirus C* (HAdV-C; 1, 2, 5, 6) *Human adenovirus D* (HAdV-D; 8–10, 13, 15, 17, 19, 20, 22–30, 32, 33, 36–39, 42–49, 51) *Human adenovirus E* (HAdV-E; 4) *Human adenovirus F* (HAdV-F; 40, 41)
Papillomaviridae		*Papillomavirus*	*Human papillomavirus* (HPV, 80)
Polyomaviridae		*Polyomavirus*	*BK polyomavirus* (BKPyV, polyomavirus hominis 1) *JC polyomavirus* (JCPyV, polyomavirus hominis 2)
Parvoviridae	*Parvovirinae*	*Erythrovirus*	*B19 virus* (B19V, human parvovirus, erythema infectiosum or fifth disease)
Hepadnaviridae		*Orthohepadnavirus*	*Hepatitis B virus* (HBV)
RNA Viruses			
Reoviridae		*Orthoreovirus*	*Mammalian orthoreovirus* (MRV, 3)
		Coltivirus	*Colorado tick fever virus* (CTFV)
		Orbivirus	*Changuinola virus* (CGLV; 12); *Great Island virus* (GIV; 36)
		Rotavirus	*Rotavirus A, B,* and *C* (RV-A, RV-B, RV-C, numerous serotypes)
Paramyxoviridae	*Paramyxovirinae*	*Respirovirus*	*Human parainfluenza virus 1 and 3* (HPIV-1, HPIV-3)
		Morbillivirus	*Measles virus* (MeV)
		Rubulavirus	*Mumps virus* (MUV), *Human parainfluenza virus 2* (HPIV-2) and *4* (HPIV-4 a and b)
	Pneumovirinae	*Pneumovirus*	*Human respiratory syncytial virus* (HRSV)
		Metapneumovirus	*Human metapneumovirus* (HMPV)
Rhabdoviridae		*Vesiculovirus*	*Vesicular stomatitis Indiana virus* (VSIV)
		Lyssavirus	*Rabies virus* (RABV)
Filoviridae		*Marburg-like virus*	*Lake Victoria marburgvirus* (LVMARV)
		Ebola-like virus	*Zaire ebolavirus* (ZEBOV), *Reston ebolavirus* (REBOV)
Orthomyxoviridae		*Influenzavirus A*	*Influenza A virus* (FLUAV)
		Influenzavirus B	*Influenza B virus* (FLUBV)
		Influenzavirus C	*Influenza C virus* (FLUCV)
Bunyaviridae		*Bunyavirus*	*Bunyamwera virus* (BUNV, Bunyamwera serogroup), *California encephalitis virus* (CEV, California serogroup), (mosquito- and culicoid fly-transmitted; ~47 species, >161 serotypes)
		Hantavirus	*Hantaan virus* (HTNV, Korean hemorrhagic fever or hemorrhagic fever with renal syndrome), *Sin Nombre virus* (SNV, Four Corners hantavirus, hantavirus pulmonary syndrome), and others (rodent-associated, ~22 species)
		Nairovirus	*Crimean-Congo hemorrhagic fever virus* (CCHFV); (tick-transmitted, 8 species, >34 strains)
		Phlebovirus	*Sandfly fever Naples virus* (SFNV), *Rift Valley fever virus* (RVFV) (sandfly-borne primarily); *Uukuniemi virus* (UUKV) (phlebotomine-, tick-, and mosquito-transmitted; ~9 species, 35 strains)

(Continued)

TABLE 157–1 ■ CLASSIFICATION AND NOMENCLATURE OF REPRESENTATIVE VIRUSES AFFECTING HUMANS—Cont'd

Family	Subfamily	Genus	Representative Species Pathogenic for Humans (abbreviation, disease, synonym, or no. of members)
Arenaviridae		*Arenavirus*	*Lymphocytic choriomeningitis virus* (LCMV) *Lassa virus* (LASV) *Junin virus* (JUNV, Argentine hemorrhagic fever virus) *Machupo virus* (MAVC, Bolivian hemorrhagic fever virus)
Picornaviridae		*Enterovirus*	*Poliovirus* (PV, Human poliovirus 1–3) *Human enterovirus A* (HEV-A, 10 serotypes; human coxsackie A viruses 2, 3, 5, 7, 8, 10, 12, 14, 16; human enterovirus 71) *Human enterovirus B* (HEV-B, 36 serotypes; human coxsackie B viruses 1–6; human coxsackie virus A9; human echovirus 1–21 and 24–33; human enterovirus 69) *Human enterovirus C* (HEV-C, 11 serotypes; human coxsackie viruses A1, A11, A13, A15, A17–22, A24) *Human enterovirus D* (HEV-D, 2 serotypes; human enteroviruses 68 and 70)
		Parechovirus	*Human parechovirus* (HPeV; human parechovirus 1, formerly echovirus 22; human parechovirus 2, formerly echovirus 23)
		Rhinovirus	*Human rhinovirus A* (HRV-A, 18 serotypes) *Human rhinovirus B* (HRV-B, 13 serotypes) (unassigned serotypes, 82)
		Hepatovirus	*Hepatitis A virus* (HAV, enterovirus 72)
Caliciviridae		*Norovirus*	*Norwalk virus* (NV, 7 strains)
		Sapovirus	*Sapporo virus* (SV, 6 strains)
Astroviridae		*Mamastrovirus*	*Human astrovirus* (HAstV, 8)
Coronaviridae		*Coronavirus*	*Human coronavirus* (HCoV-229E and HCoV-CC43)
Flaviviridae		*Flavivirus*	*St. Louis encephalitis virus* (SLEV), *Yellow fever virus* (YFV), *Dengue virus* (DENV), and *West Nile virus* (WNV) (group B arboviruses, mosquito-borne, ~27) *Kyasanur Forest disease virus* (KFDV), *tick-borne encephalitis virus* (TBEV) (tick-borne, ~15) Vector-unassociated viruses (~17)
		Hepacivirus	*Hepatitis C virus* (HCV, parenterally transmitted non-A, non-B hepatitis) *Hepatitis G virus* (HGV-1)
Togaviridae		*Alphavirus*	*Western, Eastern,* and *Venezuelan equine encephalitis viruses* (WEEV, EEEV, VEEV); *Ross River* and *Sindbis viruses* (RRV, SINV) (group A arboviruses, mosquito-borne, ~27)
		Rubivirus	*Rubella virus* (RUBV)
Retroviridae	*Orthoretrovirinae*	*Deltaretrovirus*	*Primate T-cell lymphotropic virus 1* (PTLV-1, human T-lymphotropic virus 1) *Primate T-cell lymphotrophic virus 2* (PTLV-2, human T-lymphotropic virus 2)
		Lentivirus	*Human immunodeficiency viruses 1 and 2*
Subviral Agents (Satellites, Viroids, and Agents of Spongiform Encephalopathies)			
Prions			Kuru, Creutzfeldt-Jakob disease (CJD), Gerstmann-Sträussler-Scheinker syndrome (GSS), fatal familial insomnia (FFI)
Unclassified Viruses			
		Delta virus	*Hepatitis delta virus* (HDV)
		Heptitis E–like viruses	*Hepatitis E virus* (HEV, enterically transmitted non-A, non-B hepatitis)

TABLE 157–2 ■ REPRESENTATIVE PROPERTIES USED IN VIRUS TAXONOMY

Virion Properties

- Morphology
  - Size
  - Shape
  - Presence, absence of envelope and peplomers
  - Capsid structure, symmetry
- Physical properties
  - Molecular mass
  - Buoyant density
  - Sedimentation coefficient
  - pH stability
  - Thermal stability
  - Solvent, detergent stability
  - Cation (Mg^{++}, Mn^{++}) stability
  - Radiation stability
- Genome
  - Type of nucleic acid, DNA or RNA
  - Strandedness, single- or double-stranded
  - Linear or circular
  - Sense—positive, negative, or ambisense
  - Number of segments
  - Size
  - Presence or absence and type of 5′ terminal cap
  - Nucleotide sequence comparisons
- Protein properties
  - Number
  - Size
  - Functional activities
  - Amino acid sequence comparisons
- Lipids
  - Presence or absence
  - Nature
- Carbohydrates
  - Presence or absence
  - Nature

Genome Organization and Replication

- Organization
- Strategy of replication
- Characteristics of transcription
- Characteristics of translation and post-translational processing
- Site of accumulation of assembly, maturation, and release

Antigenic Properties

- Serologic relationships
- Mapping epitopes

Biologic Properties

- Host range
- Pathogenesis
- Tissue tropisms, pathology
- Mode of transmission
- Vector relationships
- Geographic distribution

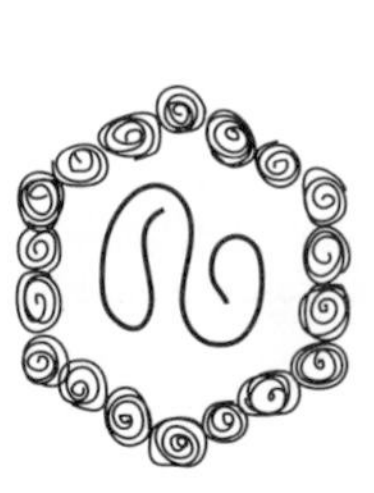

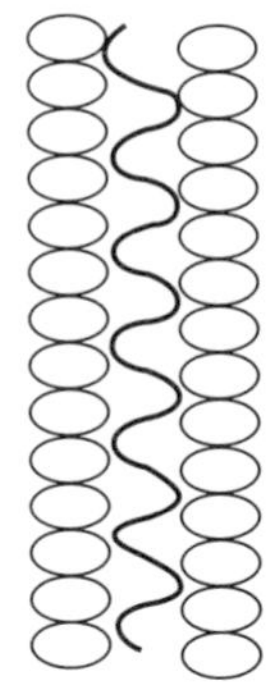
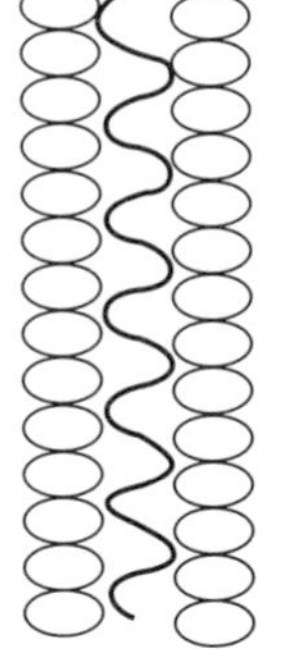
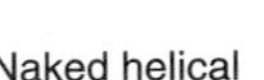

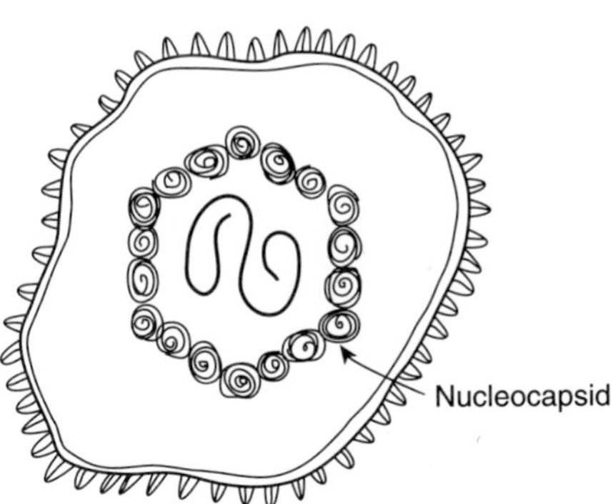

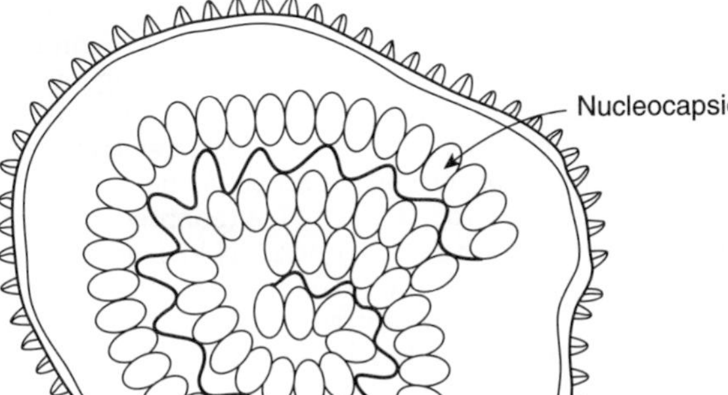

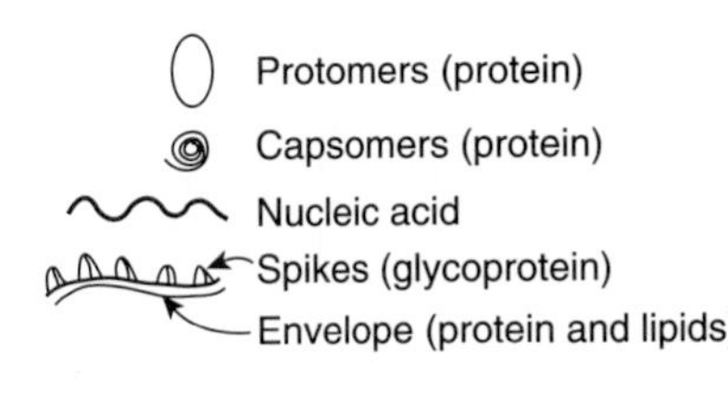

FIGURE 157–2 ■ Schematic diagram of simple forms of virions and their components. The naked icosahedral virions resemble small crystals; the naked helical virions resemble rods with a fine regular helical pattern in their surface. The enveloped icosahedral virions are composed of icosahedral nucleocapsids surrounded by the envelope; the enveloped helical virions are helical nucleocapsids bent to form a coarse, often irregular, coil within the envelope. (From Davis, B. D., Dulbecco, R., Eisen, H. N., et al.: Microbiology. 4th ed. Philadelphia, J. B. Lippincott, 1990, p. 772.)

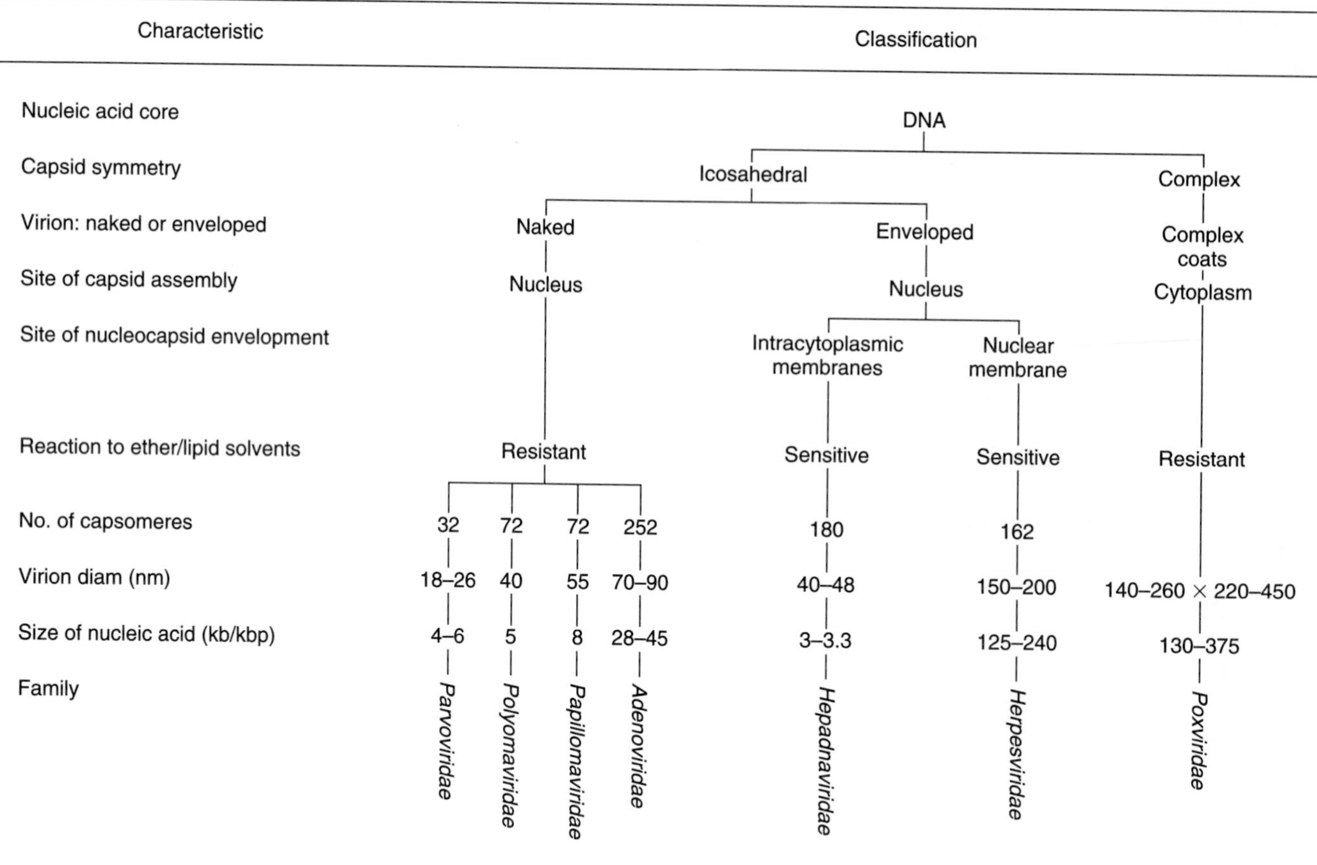

FIGURE 157–3 ■ Classification of major DNA-containing viruses affecting humans. (Adapted from Melnick, J. L. Nomenclature and classification of viruses. *In* Feigin, R. D., and Cherry, J. D. [eds.]: Textbook of Pediatric Infectious Diseases. 4th ed. Philadelphia, WB Saunders, 1998, pp. 1603–1607.)

Simplexvirus, subfamily *Alphaherpesvirinae*, family *Herpesviridae*. Thereafter, vernacular names can be used throughout the publication. In informal vernacular usage when referring to virions or virus particles, or if used as an adjective, italics and capital initial letters are not required and the names are written in lower-case Roman script (e.g., "poliovirus cytopathic effect" or "picornaviruses/polioviruses were inoculated into cell culture").[13, 14] Viruses with uncertain taxonomic status are considered "tentative" species, and names are not italicized although the initial letter is capitalized. Although not part of the formal International Code, abbreviations also have been recommended by the ICTV for every virus name in order to reduce the possibility of duplication when new abbreviations are proposed[4, 15] (see Fig. 157–1).

Figure 157–2 is a schematic diagram showing the basic forms and composition of viruses. The type of nucleic acid, capsid symmetry, presence or absence of an envelope, and peplomers (spikes) all are characteristics used in classification. Figure 157–1 is a more detailed diagram not only illustrating relative shapes and sizes of families and genera of vertebrate viruses but also indicating the type and nature (single-stranded [ss], double-stranded [ds], sense [+/–]) of the nucleic acid, presence of reverse transcriptase (RT), and presence or absence of an envelope.

Figures 157–3 and 157–4 (adapted from ref. 10) show the classification of DNA and RNA virus families, respectively, using some of the taxonomic characteristics listed in Table 157–2. Representative DNA and RNA viruses affecting humans are listed in Table 157–1 using the most recent

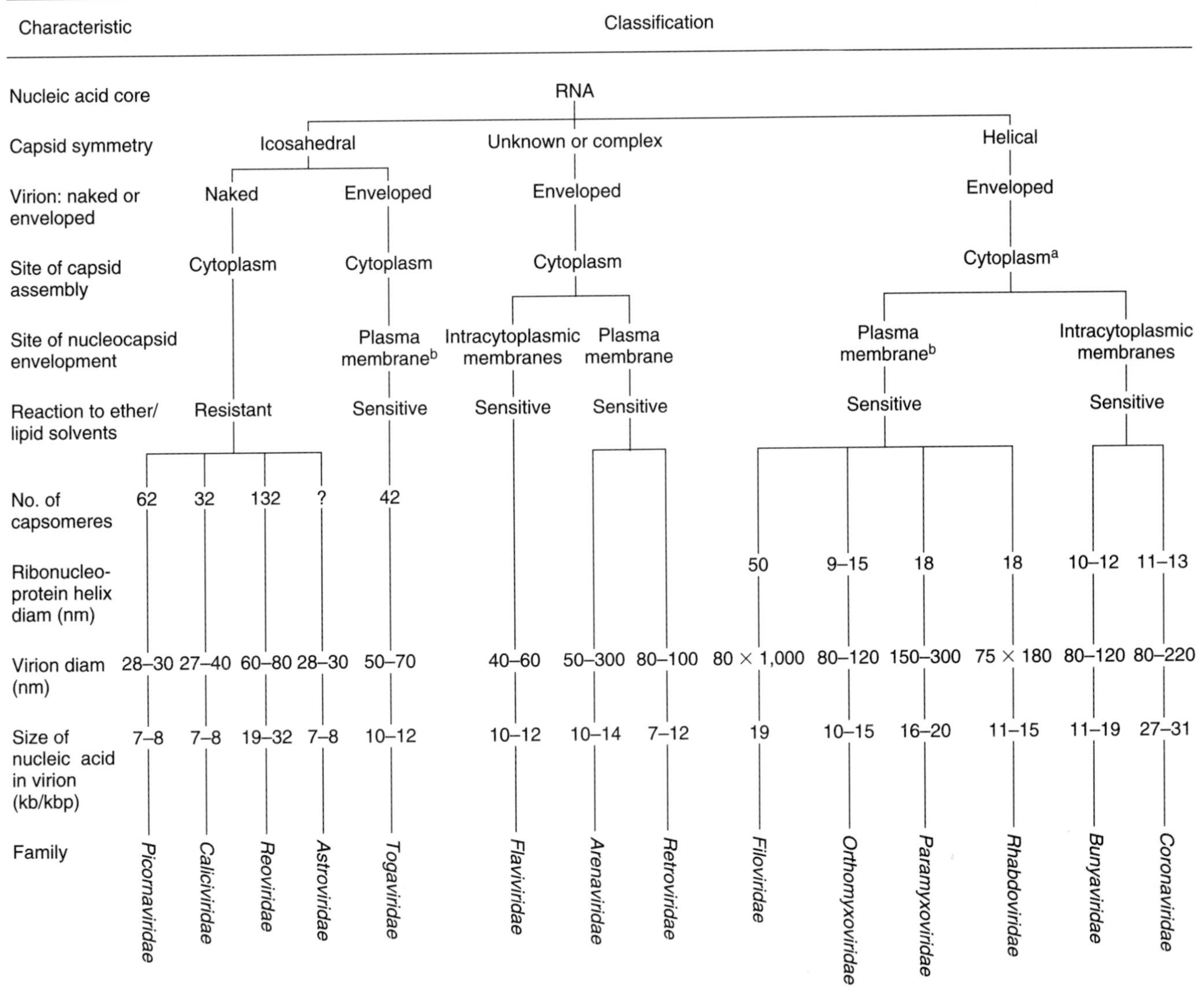

FIGURE 157–4 ■ Classification of major RNA-containing viruses affecting humans. (Adapted from Melnick, J. L. Nomenclature and classification of viruses. *In* Feigin, R. D., and Cherry, J. D. [eds.]: Textbook of Pediatric Infectious Diseases. 4th ed. Philadelphia, WB Saunders, 1998, pp. 1603–1607.)

nomenclature reported by the ICTV (for a complete listing, see reference 15).

REFERENCES

1. Andrewes, C. H.: Nomenclature of viruses. Nature *173*:260–261, 1954.
2. Andrewes, C. H., Bang, F. B., and Burnet, F. M.: A short description of the Myxovirus group (influenza and related viruses). Virology *1*:176–180, 1955.
3. Davis, B. D., Dulbecco, R., and Eisen, H. N., et al.: Microbiology. 4th ed. Philadelphia, J. B. Lippincott, 1990.
4. Fauquet, C. M., and Pringle, C. R.: Abbreviations for vertebrate virus species names. Arch. Virol. *144*:1865–1880, 1999.
5. Fenner, F., and Burnet, F. M.: A short description of the poxvirus group (vaccinia and related viruses). Virology *4*:305–310, 1957.
6. Fenner, F.: Classification and nomenclature of viruses. Second report of the International Committee on Taxonomy of Viruses. Intervirology *7*:1–116, 1976.
7. Francki, R. I. B., Fauquet, C. M., Knudson, D. L., et al. (eds.): Classification and nomenclature of viruses. Fifth Report of the International Committee on Taxonomy of Viruses. Arch. Virol. *2*(Suppl.):1–450, 1991.
8. Matthews, R. E. F.: Classification and nomenclature of viruses. Third report of the International Committee on Taxonomy of Viruses. Intervirology *12*:129–296, 1979.
9. Matthews, R. E. F.: Classification and nomenclature of viruses. Fourth report of the International Committee on Taxonomy of Viruses. Intervirology *17*:1–199, 1982.
10. Melnick, J. L.: Nomenclature and classification of viruses. *In* Feigin, R. D., and Cherry, J. D. (eds.): Textbook of Pediatric Infectious Diseases. 4th ed. Philadelphia, W. B. Saunders, 1998.
11. Murphy, F. A., Fauquet, C. M., Bishop, D. H. L., et al. (eds.): Virus taxonomy. Sixth report of the International Committee on Taxonomy of Viruses. Arch Virol *10*(Suppl.):1–503, 1995.
12. Van Regenmortel, M. H. V.: Virus species, a much overlooked but essential concept in virus classification. Intervirology *31*:241–254, 1990.
13. Van Regenmortel, M. H. V.: How to write the names of virus species. Arch Virol *144*:1041–1042, 1999.
14. Van Regenmortel, M. H. V.: On the relative merits of italics, Latin and binomial nomenclature in virus taxonomy. Arch Virol *145*:433–441, 2000.
15. Van Regenmortel, M. H. V., Fauquet, C. M., Bishop, D. H. L., et al. (eds.): Virus taxonomy. Classification and nomenclature of viruses. Seventh report of the International Committee on Taxonomy of Viruses. San Diego, Academic Press, 2000.
16. Wildy, P.: Classification and nomenclature of viruses: First report of the International Committee on Nomenclature of Viruses. Monographs in Virology. Vol. 5. Basel, S. Karger, 1971.

DNA VIRUSES

SUBSECTION 1

PARVOVIRIDAE

CHAPTER 158 Human Parvovirus B19

JAMES D. CHERRY

The family *Parvoviridae* includes two subfamilies: *Parvovirinae* and *Densovirinae*.[119, 184] The subfamily *Parvovirinae* has three genera: *Erythrovirus, Parvovirus,* and *Dependovirus;* the subfamily *Densovirinae* also has three genera: *Densovirus, Iteravirus,* and *Centravirus.* Densonucleosis viruses (*Densovirus* spp.) infect insect hosts and have not been found in humans or mammals.[23, 202] Human parvovirus B19 is the only member of the recently created genus *Erythrovirus;* originally, it was classified in the genus *Parvovirus.* In spite of this reclassification, the contemporary literature still refers to this *Erythrovirus* as parvovirus B19. This virus is autonomous and does not require the presence of a helper virus.

Erythema infectiosum is the common clinical manifestation of parvovirus B19 infection. Other clinical findings include arthralgia and arthritis, aplastic crisis in patients with red blood cell defects, chronic anemia in immunocompromised patients, fetal hydrops, neurologic disease, and a variety of other significant illnesses.

History

The first parvoviruses to be discovered infecting humans were found in stool specimens by electron microscopy.[203] These fecal parvoviruses have been linked with gastrointestinal symptoms, often in outbreaks associated with the consumption of shellfish.[72, 267] Their precise pathogenic role remains unclear because these viruses also may be found in the feces of asymptomatic individuals.[203]

In 1974, a second type of parvovirus was noted in the serum of asymptomatic blood donors.[63] Discovered by chance as an agent responsible for false-positive results in the counterimmunoelectrophoresis tests then in use for the detection of hepatitis B virus surface antigen, they were revealed by electron microscopy to be uniform icosahedral particles with a mean diameter of 23 nm.

Preliminary studies of the physicochemical nature of this agent suggested its probable identity as a member of the family *Parvoviridae*.[63] In the following years, reports concerning this virus named it variously as human parvovirus-like agent, serum parvovirus-like virus,[58] and B19[244] after one of the original isolates. After elucidation of its chemical properties in 1983,[54, 257] the virus was referred to as human parvovirus—or human serum parvovirus—to denote that it is distinct from the fecal viral particles. Today, the virus most commonly is called human parvovirus B19 or just B19 virus.[5, 59, 124]

For many years after its discovery, B19 virus infection appeared to be either asymptomatic or associated with a nonspecific febrile illness.[244] However, in the early 1980s, the central role of B19 virus in the etiology of aplastic crisis in chronic hemolytic anemia was identified.[52, 71, 123, 216, 239] Soon thereafter came the appreciation that erythema infectiosum (fifth disease) is the common manifestation of B19 virus infection.[12] Approximately 17 years ago, the association between B19 virus infection in pregnancy and fetal death was observed, and during the past 15 years, the clinical spectrum of B19 virus infection has broadened considerably.*

Although human parvovirus B19 was not discovered until 1974, its most common clinical disease (erythema infectiosum) was described 200 years ago.[29]

Tschamer's report in 1889 was considered by most reviewers to be the first description of erythema infectiosum.[264] However, Boysen[29] noted that an English dermatologist, Robert Willan, had reported the illness first in 1799 and then more completely in 1840.

After Tschamer's report came a succession of Austrian and German reports of the illness.[29] Tschamer thought that erythema infectiosum was a manifestation of rubella, but a few years later, Escherich[79] suggested that it was a specific disease. Stricker[256] in 1899 gave the name erythema infectiosum to the clinical entity.

In 1905, Shaw,[243] after having observed cases of erythema infectiosum in Austria, published the first account in the American literature. Herrick[112] was the first to document in detail an outbreak in the United States; however, cases of erythema infectiosum had been observed previously in St. Louis[300] and in Hamburg, New York.[112] During the last 70 years, numerous outbreaks and epidemics have been described in North America.† Erythema infectiosum frequently is referred to as fifth disease and in the past also was called ring rubella, large-spotted disease, and epidemic megaloerythema.

Properties of the Virus

Human parvovirus B19 is a naked icosahedral virus with a mean diameter of 23 nm and a mean buoyant density in

*See references 4, 26, 50, 109, 115, 124, 125, 183, 207, 233, 238, 290.

†See references 3, 14, 17, 18, 21, 31, 43, 48, 53, 56, 60, 73, 84, 87, 92, 96, 128, 149, 150, 154, 172, 185, 208, 209, 218, 246, 277, 278, 286, 288, 303.

cesium chloride of 1.43 g/dL.[63] The capsid is formed from two major structural proteins (VP1 and VP2) discernible by sodium dodecyl sulfate–polyacrylamide gel electrophoresis.[54] VP2 is the major structural protein, with a molecular weight of 58 kd; VP1 has a molecular weight of 84 kd. Ninety-six percent of the capsid is VP2, and 4 percent is VP1. The major nonstructural protein (NS1) has a molecular weight of 77 kd. The genome consists of a single molecule of single-stranded DNA approximately 5.6 kb in length.[67] The DNA in B19 virus occurs as both plus and minus strands in approximately equal numbers.[124] When virions are disrupted with protease, the two complementary strands anneal to form a stable duplex.[257] At each end of the molecule are palindromic sequences forming "hairpin" loops. The hairpin at the 3′ end of the genome serves as a primer for DNA polymerases. The hairpin duplex at the 5′ end of the molecule consists of sequences that are neither complementary to those at the 3′ end, as is found in dependoviruses, nor as highly complementary within this 5′ end as are those at the 3′ end.[64]

Parvovirus infectivity is relatively heat-stable, tolerant of a wide range of pH, and resistant to ether.[13] Successful replication of parvoviruses can be accomplished only in a dividing cell because of the absolute requirement for host-cell function or functions found in late S phase.[106] Human parvovirus B19 can be propagated only in human erythropoietic cells from the bone marrow and in primary fetal liver culture.[36, 202, 252, 253, 260]

The cellular receptor for B19 virus infection is the blood group P antigen.[33] This antigen is found on erythroblasts, megakaryoblasts, and endothelial cells. People who lack the P protein are resistant to infection with B19 virus.[35]

Antigenically, this human parvovirus is distinct from the parvovirus-like particles found in feces,[204] as well as from the human dependoviruses and autonomous animal parvoviruses.[63] However, the nucleotide sequence and hybridization results reported by Turton and associates[267] suggest that the viruses from gastroenteritis cases in 1977 and 1986 are similar to B19. In contrast to animal parvoviruses, no hemagglutinin has been demonstrated.

The degree to which B19 virus is related to other mammalian parvovirus types has been investigated by the technique of DNA:DNA hybridization. Although no relationship is discernible with the human dependoviruses, a distant evolutionary relationship to the genomes of the autonomous parvoviruses of rodents is apparent. Interestingly, this relationship is closer than that between B19 virus and the parvoviruses infecting domestic animals (bovine, feline, and canine parvoviruses).[64]

Many recent studies have examined genetic variability in parvovirus B19 isolates.[26, 77, 88, 111, 122, 126] In general, sequence divergence usually is less than 1 percent. Hemauer and associates[111] suggested that greater genome variability occurs in isolates from patients with persistent infections than in isolates from patients with acute infections. Erdman and colleagues[77] noted that geographically defined genetic lineages of parvovirus B19 existed but that no particular genotype was associated with a specific clinical manifestation.

Parvovirus B19 does not grow in routine tissue cultures. It will grow in erythroid progenitor cells from human bone marrow, fetal liver, erythroid cells from a patient with erythroleukemia, and human umbilical cord and peripheral blood.[124, 201] It grows only in dividing cells, and, therefore, all the aforementioned tissue culture systems require the addition of erythropoietin. Parvovirus B19 also has been propagated in megakaryoblastoid cell lines.

Epidemiology

Outbreaks of erythema infectiosum have been observed throughout the world, but most reports have come from nontropical regions. The epidemic pattern of erythema infectiosum is surprisingly similar to that of rubella. Community epidemics are most prevalent in the winter and spring, and they usually last for 3 to 6 months. In a review of 30 well-described epidemics,* 26 had their onset in the period from December through May, and 23 of the 30 peaked in March, April, or May. When the North American literature for a 50-year period is examined, a cyclic pattern is evident, with peaks in disease activity occurring approximately every 6 years. The peak periods last for an average of 3 years. A longitudinal study of aplastic crisis in persons with sickle-cell anemia in Jamaica suggested peaks in incidence occur every 2 to 3 years in this island population.[239]

The case-to-case interval of erythema infectiosum is reported to be between 4 and 14 days.[3, 12, 73, 96, 212, 277, 288] In an elementary school epidemic, Greenwald and Bashe[96] noted that the mean case-to-case interval was 8.7 days. Ager and associates[3] in their studies noted clustering of intervals between cases of 7 to 11 days. The data of Wilcox and Evans[288] on multiple cases in households suggest that the case-to-case interval usually is closer to 12 to 14 days. In a volunteer study in which adults were inoculated intranasally, the incubation time to onset of the rash was 17 to 18 days.[9] From this study, the case-to-case interval in the community would be expected to be between 6 and 12 days because virus shedding occurs between days 5 and 12 of infection. This prediction accords well with intervals in the studies noted earlier, as well as intervals observed in patients with hematologic diseases and aplastic crisis.[176]

In epidemics, the attack rate is high. Lauer and colleagues[149] noted an overall attack rate of 24.3 percent in schoolchildren in grades kindergarten through eighth grade. Similar attack rates were noted in two other school-related outbreaks.[73, 96] In the community as a whole, the attack rate is highest in children 5 to 14 years of age,[2, 3] but secondary cases occur in preschool children, teachers, and parents. In the home, secondary cases are reported more commonly in mothers than in fathers.[3] In school epidemics, the attack rate is considerably higher in girls than in boys.[3, 73, 149] Prevalence studies of serum IgG antibody to B19 virus have noted that 40 to 60 percent of adults and 2 to 21 percent of children younger than 11 years are seropositive.[5–7, 58] Nosocomial infections do occur; most often, the index case is an unrecognized, chronically infected patient.[2, 144, 211] During community outbreaks, the risk of acquisition in hospital workers is no greater than that in other community residents.

Although erythema infectiosum long had been postulated to be transmitted by droplet via the respiratory tract,[3] proof of this route was not obtained until a group of volunteers were infected successfully with B19 virus after intranasal inoculation. One week after inoculation, virus was excreted from the respiratory tract for 6 days.[9]

Parvovirus B19 infection also can be transmitted by blood transfusion and clotting factor concentrates but not by immunoglobulin preparations.[165, 178, 292]

Pathogenesis and Pathology

The pathogenesis of parvovirus disease involves two quite separate components. The first is caused by the lytic infection

*See references 3, 7, 14, 18, 29, 31, 48, 53, 56, 60, 73, 84, 96, 112, 128, 149, 150, 154, 185, 209, 218, 246, 255, 277, 285, 288, 303.

of susceptible dividing cells and the second by interaction with the products of the immune response.

As stated earlier, parvoviruses replicate only in dividing cells. Thus, infection of an organ or tissue in which a significant proportion of the cells are dividing may give rise to organ-specific disease. This condition is seen clearly in canine and feline parvovirus infections, in which virus replication in the crypt cells of the intestine gives rise to a severe and often fatal enteritis.[102, 158]

Parvovirus B19 is thought not to infect cells of the gastrointestinal tract; virus could not be detected in the feces of volunteers,[9] nor have viruses of this type been found in stool specimens.

Gaining entry via the respiratory tract, the virus sets up a systemic infection with copious viremia (Fig. 158–1) in which 10^{10} or 10^{11} virus particles per milliliter of blood is not an uncommon finding.[9, 213]

Parvovirus infection results in profound reticulocytopenia for some 7 to 10 days, commencing during viremia.[9] In vitro studies on cultured bone marrow and peripheral blood have shown that B19 virus inhibits the formation of blast-forming erythroid colonies, thus suggesting that an early erythrocyte precursor cell is susceptible to virus infection. Granulocytes and megakaryocytes are unaffected by virus in these in vitro systems. However, during B19 virus infection in a normal host, clinically insignificant lymphopenia and neutropenia occur, as does a drop in platelet number.[9, 212] The mechanisms of the loss of these cells from the peripheral blood remain to be determined. Srivastava and associates[252] noted that B19 virus infection of bone marrow cells in culture results in suppression of megakaryocyte colony formation. In this study, tropism of B19 virus for cells other than the erythroid progenitor cell appeared to take place, although viral DNA replication did not occur in the megakaryocyte-enriched fractions. They suggested that the virus might be toxic to cell populations that are nonpermissive for viral DNA replication.

As noted in Figure 158–1, viremia ends at the time of appearance of specific IgM antibody. In addition, researchers have found that the appearance of antibody neutralizes the inhibitory effect of B19 virus on erythrocyte colony formation in vitro.[297] The early IgM response is almost entirely VP2-specific. IgG antibody first appears

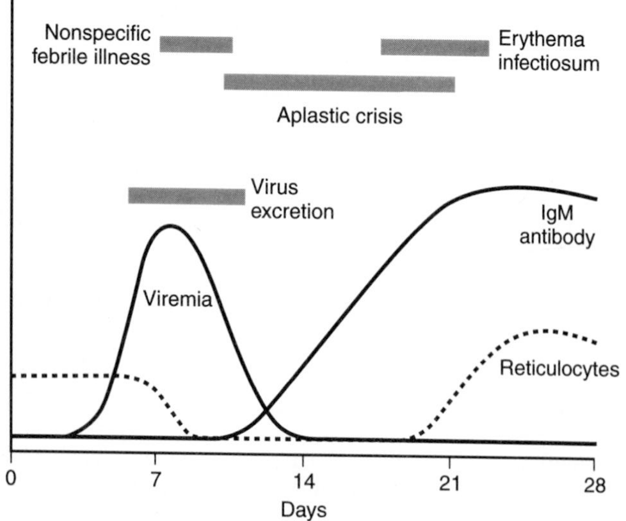

FIGURE 158–1 ■ Selected virologic, immunologic, hematologic, and clinical events in parvovirus B19 virus infection.

approximately 2 weeks after exposure and later becomes the major antibody subclass; in contrast to the initial IgM response, the IgG response is directed at VP1 rather than VP2. The role of cellular immunity in recovery from infection is unclear. Most patients with persistent infection have T-cell as well as other immune defects suggesting a cellular component in the host response.[26] Surprisingly, few studies of cellular immunity have been performed in patients with parvovirus B19 infection.[85, 145, 275] von Poblotzki and associates[275] showed that the T cells of persons with parvovirus B19 antibody had HLA class II–restricted responses against B19 structural proteins. Fraussila and colleagues[85] demonstrated virus-specific helper T-cell proliferation in recently and remotely infected patients. Their data suggested that B cells that recognize the viral capsid (VP1 and VP2) receive class II–restricted help from $CD4^+$ T lymphocytes.

The most common result of infection with B19 virus is erythema infectiosum. Figure 158–1 shows that the symptoms of this disease begin 17 or 18 days after inoculation and that approximately 1 week later, virus can be detected in either throat swabs or blood. Skin biopsy results have been reported in three studies.[21, 97, 116] In three skin biopsy specimens from regions of reticulated eruption, Bard and Perry[21] noted either normal skin or very mild inflammatory changes. Hoffman[116] described edema in the epidermis and perivascular infiltration with mononuclear cells; he also noted swelling of the endothelium of superficial vessels and cleavage spaces between the epidermis and dermis. The histopathology was investigated in 10 cases by Grimmer and Joseph.[97] They reported dilation of blood vessels with lymphocytic and occasional plasma cell perivascular infiltration. However, the clinical manifestations of many of the cases in the epidemic that Grimmer and Joseph[97] studied were quite atypical.

Virus-specific IgM is present at the time of onset of the rash in erythema infectiosum, so although the mechanisms of production of the rash (and arthralgia) of erythema infectiosum remain to be elucidated, postulating an immune-mediated pathogenesis is not unreasonable. The perivascular infiltrations noted by Hoffman[116] would support this suggestion. However, Schwarz and colleagues[237] have found both viral capsid proteins and viral DNA in a skin biopsy specimen of the rash from a patient with erythema infectiosum. They, therefore, suggest that the rash may be a direct effect of the virus rather than being immune complex mediated.

Intrauterine infection results in infection of the fetus and, frequently, abortion.* The main finding in infected fetuses is hydrops fetalis, which results from the anemia caused by infection of the erythrocyte precursor cells. Intranuclear inclusions are seen in nucleated red blood cells, and viral particles are identified in the same cells by electron microscopy.[47]

In immunocompromised patients, persistent infection with B19 virus often occurs[145] as a result of failure to produce effective neutralizing antibodies.

Clinical Manifestations

Infection with human parvovirus B19 results in a spectrum of clinical manifestations; classic cases of erythema infectiosum occupy a central position in this spectrum. Other major manifestations include arthritis and arthralgia, intrauterine infection and hydrops fetalis, transient aplastic crisis in patients with a variety of underlying hemolytic illnesses,

*See references 4, 5, 43, 47, 92, 131, 215, 222, 235, 290, 296.

and persistent infection with chronic anemia in patients with immunodeficiencies. In addition, subclinical, nonexanthematous infection occurs, especially in children.[9, 212]

Other less common illnesses include myocarditis, vasculitis, glomerulonephritis, and neurologic disease. In addition to the established parvovirus B19 disease associations is an ever-expanding list of illness categories in which evidence of parvovirus B19 infection has been found. These illnesses are presented in Table 158–1.

ERYTHEMA INFECTIOSUM

Although a search of the literature relating to erythema infectiosum outbreaks reveals a conspicuous absence of prodromal symptoms in patients, infected volunteers have had febrile episodes with nonspecific symptoms of headache, chills, myalgia, and malaise accompanying the viremic phase of the B19 virus infection[9] (see Fig. 158–1). These symptoms last for 2 to 3 days and coincide with excretion of virus from the pharynx. This phase is followed by a period of 7 days during which individuals are free of symptoms before the onset of the second, or exanthematous, phase of illness. Probably, the relatively long period between symptoms in this biphasic illness has prevented recognition of the link between these nonspecific prodromal symptoms and erythema infectiosum.

The exanthem in classic cases of erythema infectiosum occurs in three stages.[3, 17, 31, 48, 51, 53, 96, 243, 277–279] The first stage begins 18 days after the acquisition of infection and is characterized by a fiery red rash on the cheeks (see Fig. 65–6) (slapped-cheek appearance). The edges of the involved areas may be raised slightly, and a relatively circumoral pallor is present. At this stage, the appearance may be suggestive of scarlet fever, drug sensitivity or other allergic reaction, or collagen vascular disease. The facial exanthem is aggravated by the transition from outdoors to a warm room.

The second stage of the exanthem occurs 1 to 4 days after the onset of facial involvement and consists of the appearance of an erythematous, maculopapular rash on the trunk and limbs. This rash is discrete initially but spreads to involve large areas. Toward the end of this stage, central clearing of the rash from these areas gives the characteristic lacy or reticular pattern (see Fig. 65–7).

The third stage of the exanthem is highly variable in duration, lasting from 1 to 3 or more weeks, and is characterized by marked changes in the intensity of the rash, with periodic complete evanescence and recrudescence. These fluctuations are related to environmental factors such as exposure to sunlight and temperature (a hot bath may result in recrudescence in an apparently recovered child).

The rash often is pruritic, especially in adults, and it generally is more prominent on the extensor surfaces; the palms and soles rarely are affected. Slight desquamation has been noted in a small number of patients in most reviews.

Although classic cases of erythema infectiosum are easy to recognize clinically, especially during outbreaks, wide variation in the form of the exanthem can be noted—from a very faint, fleeting rash to a florid exanthem, confluent over large areas (see Fig. 65–8). In many cases, the illness may be indistinguishable from rubella.

The overwhelming majority of cases of erythema infectiosum have no enanthem. Kerr and Marsh[128] and Condon[60] noted a few children with pharyngitis.

Other symptoms and signs occur uncommonly in erythema infectiosum (Table 158–2). In general, complaints are more frequent in adults than children. Headache is noted in approximately one fifth of childhood cases and approximately one half of afflicted adults. Joint pain and swelling and myalgia are particularly troublesome in adults.

Routine laboratory studies are of little use in erythema infectiosum. The leukocyte count usually is normal, although mild eosinophilia is noted occasionally.[17, 29, 278, 279]

The most common complication of erythema infectiosum is joint involvement; it is relatively rare in children (<10% of cases) but is the norm in adults and occurs in 80 percent or more of cases.* A range of severity from mild arthralgia to frank arthritis is observed. The joints most commonly involved are the knees, ankles, and proximal interphalangeal joints; symptoms usually are bilateral. The joint involvement usually is transient and lasts only a few days. In some individuals, symptoms may persist for some weeks

TABLE 158–1 ■ REPORTED UNUSUAL CLINICAL FINDINGS IN PATIENTS WITH LABORATORY EVIDENCE OF PARVOVIRUS B19 VIRUS INFECTION

Persistent arthritis
- Juvenile rheumatoid arthritis[51, 133]
- Rheumatoid arthritis[193, 254, 261]
- Adult Still disease[155, 214]

Neurologic disease
- Encephalitis[19, 110]
- Meningitis[44, 143, 199, 255, 258]
- Postinfectious neuralgic amyotropy[205]
- Guillain-Barré syndrome[169]
- Facial palsy[162]
- Carpal tunnel syndrome[230]
- Numbness and tingling of fingers[299]

Myocarditis[75, 190, 227]

Cutaneous manifestations
- Papular-purpuric gloves and socks syndrome[16, 25, 100, 200, 247]
- Vesiculopustular exanthema[188]
- Erythema multiforme[90]
- Henoch-Schönlein syndrome[273]
- Petechial and purpuric rashes[1, 61, 70, 153]
- Pruritus without rash[157]

Hematologic manifestations
- Thrombocytopenic purpura[82, 118, 152, 295]
- Pancytopenia[103, 180]
- Hemophagocytic syndrome[28, 180, 266, 270, 283, 298]
- Neutropenia[163]
- Diamond-Blackfan syndrome[107, 262]
- Splenic sequestration[160]

Other manifestations
- Glomerulonephritis[143, 287]
- Kawasaki disease[117, 192]
- Behçet disease[132]
- Polyarteritis nodosa[274]
- Wegener granulomatosis[194]
- Leukocytoclastic vasculitis[62]
- Giant-cell arteritis[89]
- Systemic sclerosis[81]
- Systemic lupus erythematosus[191]
- Hepatitis[70, 148, 251, 293]
- Raynaud phenomenon[104]
- Pseudoappendicitis or mesenteric lymphadenitis[174]
- Cervical lymphadenopathy[265]
- Parotitis[162]
- Pneumonia[175, 282]
- Chronic infection without immunosuppresion but with
  - Chronic hemolytic anemia[126]
  - Persistent arthralgia[126]
  - Chronic fatigue syndrome[120, 126, 130]
  - Recurrent paresthesias[80]
  - Fibromyalgia[22]

*See references 5, 11, 12, 17, 109, 186, 219, 221, 280, 286.

TABLE 158–2 ■ FREQUENCY OF SYMPTOMS AND SIGNS IN ERYTHEMA INFECTIOSUM

Sign or Symptom	Percent Occurrence	
	Children	Adults
Rash	100	100
Pruritus	15	50
Headache	20	50
Fever	15	25
Sore throat	15	15
Coryza	10	15
Cough	8	8
Sore eyes	10	10
Anorexia	15	22
Nausea	7	26
Vomiting	4	7
Diarrhea	4	12
Abdominal pain	10	15
Joint pain	10	70
Joint swelling	5	60
Myalgia	4	50

Data from references 3, 73, 96, 278.

or, rarely, months. When joint involvement occurs after an exanthem, the diagnosis may be inferred, but such is not invariably the case. As with rubella, the frequency of arthralgia and arthritis is higher in women than men.

Other complications of erythema infectiosum include cases of transient hemolytic anemia, encephalitis with recovery but without residua, encephalopathy in a 9-month-old boy resulting in permanent sequelae, thrombocytopenic purpura, Henoch-Schönlein purpura, myocarditis, and pseudoappendicitis.[19, 82, 101, 118, 151, 152, 174, 227, 280]

OTHER EXANTHEMS

Grimmer and Joseph[97] described cases in which the rashes were morbilliform, hemorrhagic, urticarial, vesicular, and erythema multiforme–like. Their studies were conducted during an epidemic of erythema infectiosum in Berlin, Germany, in which an estimated 50,000 persons were affected. The cases with markedly unusual manifestations quite possibly were not of the same etiology as the typical cases. However, other authors also have noted papular, purpuric, vesicular, urticarial, and morbilliform eruptions.[48, 60, 61, 153, 160, 188, 209]

García-Tapia and associates[90] described a 5-year-old girl with erythema multiforme bullosum but without other systemic manifestations; the patient's serum had B19 virus–specific IgM antibody. Several adults with a papular-purpuric or petechial "glove and sock" syndrome have been described.[16, 25, 100, 247] A 13-year-old girl who had a simultaneous infection with human herpesvirus 7 and parvovirus B19 and papular-purpuric gloves and socks syndrome has been described.[200] Henoch-Schönlein syndrome and other vasculitic rashes also have been reported.[1, 62, 70, 204, 233, 273]

Grimmer and Joseph[97] stated that most of their patients in the Berlin epidemic had dark red spots on the pharynx, gums, soft palate, and uvula. These cases, again, must be regarded with some suspicion because the investigators also noted genital lesions and conjunctivitis in a few patients.

APLASTIC CRISIS

In individuals with chronic hemolytic anemia, the profound reticulocytopenia of human parvovirus B19 infection results in depression of hemoglobin concentrations to critical levels.* With resolution of the infection, reticulocytes reappear in the peripheral blood and hemoglobin concentrations return to the normal steady-state values for these patients. This transient arrest in production of erythrocytes is termed *aplastic crisis* and may occur in any individual whose erythrocytes have a short life span. Examples of such conditions include sickle-cell anemia,[94, 239] hereditary spherocytosis,[78, 103, 123, 198] thalassemia,[153, 216] glucose-6-phosphate dehydrogenase deficiency,[93] and pyruvate kinase deficiency.[71]

Serjeant and coworkers[240] studied the epidemiology of B19 virus infection over time in 308 children with homozygous sickle-cell disease and in 239 controls with normal hemoglobin. B19 virus infection accounted for all 91 aplastic crises that occurred. Twenty-three additional patients with sickle-cell disease had B19 virus infections; of these, 10 had mild hematologic changes and 13 had no changes. By 15 years of age, approximately 40 percent of the sickle-cell group and the control group had IgG antibody to B19 virus, thus indicating equal infection rates in the two groups. No patient or control had two infections caused by B19 virus.

Rao and colleagues[217] found that 70 percent of patients with transient aplastic crisis admitted to their hospitals during a 7-year period had B19 viral infections. No patients had chronic or recurrent infections. In a study of 48 patients with aplastic crises, Mallouh and Qudah[161] found B19 virus infection in 91 percent. In addition to the anemia, 21 percent of the patients had leukopenia, 27 percent had neutropenia, and 42 percent had thrombocytopenia. The same investigators noted acute splenic sequestration together with aplastic crisis in three patients with sickle-cell disease and B19 virus infection.[160] Lowenthal and associates[156] noted three young adults with sickle-cell acute chest syndrome associated with B19 virus infection.

Interestingly, reports of exanthematous illness occurring after aplastic crisis are rare. However, patients with aplastic crisis require transfusion with packed cells, and rashes occurring after such treatment possibly would be regarded as transfusion reactions. Joint symptoms occur fairly frequently in conditions such as sickle-cell anemia, so, although they may occur as a result of B19 infection, they may be diagnosed as "painful crises."

As noted earlier, human parvovirus B19 infection does not result invariably in aplastic crisis in a chronic hemolytic anemic patient. Some individuals escape this complication if they have been transfused recently,[8] possibly because of a protective effect of transfused antibody (more than 60% of donors are immune), the substitution of longer-lived, donated erythrocytes for the patients' own fragile ones, or a combination of these two mechanisms. Certainly, among individuals suffering the more severe form of beta-thalassemia, aplastic crisis is a rare complication; in such cases, the anemia is so severe that the patient is maintained by regular, frequent transfusions.

In populations in which aplastic crisis does occur, the severity of the episode varies among individuals, perhaps reflecting the variation in erythrocyte life span among these patients.[8]

OTHER HEMATOLOGIC MANIFESTATIONS

In addition to pure red blood cell aplasia, numerous other hematologic manifestations, including thrombocytopenic

*See references 5, 8, 43, 71, 93, 94, 103, 123, 153, 176, 198, 216, 225, 239, 257, 296, 297.

purpura, pancytopenia, hemophagocytic syndrome, neutropenia, and Diamond-Blackfan syndrome, have been observed in association with B19 virus infection.* Thrombocytopenia has been noted as an isolated event, thus suggesting idiopathic thrombocytopenic purpura or an association with aplastic crisis.[82, 118, 152, 183, 295]

Pancytopenia has been observed in association with aplastic crisis, and hemophagocytosis often is demonstrated.† Yufu and coauthors[298] described a 15-year-old girl with hemophagocytic syndrome and lymphadenopathy resembling histiocytic necrotizing lymphadenitis (Kikuchi disease).

McClain and colleagues[163] studied 19 children with immune-mediated neutropenia and found by polymerase chain reaction (PCR) assay of bone marrow specimens that 15 had evidence of B19 virus infection.

ARTHRITIS AND ARTHRALGIA

As noted earlier, acute arthritis and arthralgia occur commonly in erythema infectiosum. In most instances, the joint symptoms subside within a few weeks, but arthralgia and arthritis persist occasionally. Researchers also have observed that the joint manifestations caused by B19 virus infection can occur without any exanthem or with an exanthem not typical of erythema infectiosum. These findings have led to investigations related to the role of B19 virus in rheumatoid arthritis (RA).‡

Nocton and associates[196] described the clinical characteristics of 22 children seen in their rheumatology clinic with joint complaints and evidence of recent B19 virus infection. Of this group, 16 were girls and 6 were boys. The youngest patient was 2 years old, and the oldest was 19 years of age. Seven of the patients had associated rashes, but none had typical erythema infectiosum. One of these children had a petechial rash on the lower extremities, and another child had a past history of urticaria. Fever, anorexia, malaise, or fatigue occurred in 11 of the patients.

Of the 22 patients, 20 had arthritis and 2 had arthralgias only. The knee joints were involved most commonly. The frequency of specific joint involvement was as follows: knees, 82 percent; ankles and wrist, 41 percent; elbows, 32 percent; neck, small joints of the hands and feet, and hips, 27 percent; shoulders, 23 percent; and sternoclavicular joints, 9 percent. Ten of the patients had involvement of five or more joints, and in 12 patients, the pattern was pauciarticular, with four or fewer joints involved; 2 patients had only a single joint involved, and 2 had migratory illness.

The duration of the arthritis or arthralgia was less than 6 weeks in 50 percent of the children and less than 4 months in 64 percent of the patients. Of the 11 children with illness lasting longer than 2 months, 6 had manifestations that fulfilled the criteria for the diagnosis of juvenile rheumatoid arthritis (JRA). Selected laboratory results were as follows: the erythrocyte sedimentation rate was greater than 25 mm in 32 percent of the children, antinuclear antibody titers were greater than 1:40 in 7 of 21 of the patients, and 3 of 6 children had a low total hemolytic complement (CH_{50}) value.

The relationship between B19 virus infection and JRA, RA, and adult Still disease has been studied extensively during the last 15 years, but the findings are difficult to interpret.* Clearly, B19 virus can cause illnesses that fulfill the criteria for diagnosis of JRA[37, 196, 286] and adult Still disease.[125, 155] However, three possible scenarios need to be considered: (1) B19 virus causes a similar illness, (2) B19 virus infection triggers the onset of an illness caused by another condition, and (3) B19 virus directly causes JRA, adult Still disease, and RA.

In one study involving patients with refractory RA and refractory polyarticular JRA, researchers found that both groups had a significantly higher frequency of IgG B19 virus antibody as determined by enzyme-linked immunosorbent assay (ELISA) than did aged-matched controls.[168] However, when the data in this study were examined, the prevalence of antibody in the control population clearly was less than should be expected. In another study, Kishore and colleagues[133] studied IgM B19 virus antibody by ELISA and found that 28 percent of patients with JRA, 8 percent of controls, and none of the patients with RA had positive values. They interpreted their JRA findings to be triggering either B19 virus infections or perhaps intercurrent infections in patients with established JRA. In a provocative study, Takahashi and coworkers[261] found B19 virus DNA in the synovial tissues of 30 of 39 patients with RA. The data suggested that the virus identified in synovial tissue was active and led to their conclusion that B19 virus is involved in the initiation and perpetuation of RA synovitis. In contrast, Nikkari and associates[193, 195] in Finland performed extensive studies and noted that chronic rheumatoid-like arthropathies triggered by B19 virus occasionally occur. However, their data do not support a general role for B19 virus in the etiology or pathogenesis of RA.

Tyndall and colleagues[268] noted an adult woman with erosive polyarthritis associated with B19 virus infection, and Samii and coworkers[230] reported two adults with bilateral carpal tunnel syndrome associated with B19 virus infection. Berg and associates[22] could find no association with either IgG or IgM antibody to B19 virus and fibromyalgia in a study of 26 adult women and matched controls.

The following other rheumatic and vasculitic syndromes have been noted in association with parvovirus B19 infection: fibromyalgia, systematic lupus erythematosus, Kawasaki disease, leukocytoclastic vasculitis, polyarteritis nodosa, Wegener granulomatosis, chronic fatigue syndrome, systemic sclerosis, giant-cell arteritis, transient anticardiolipin syndrome, hemophagocytic syndrome and Raynaud phenomenon.†

INFECTION IN IMMUNOCOMPROMISED PATIENTS

Some immunodeficient patients suffer chronic B19 virus infections.‡ These patients have persistent anemia caused by continuous lysis of red cell precursors. This problem has been noted most commonly in children with acute lymphocytic leukemia.[42, 65, 140, 146]

Other immune deficiency states include Nezelof syndrome, acute myeloid leukemia, chronic myeloid leukemia, Burkitt lymphoma, lymphoblastic lymphoma, myelodysplastic syndrome, astrocytoma, Wilms tumor, human immunodeficiency virus infection, severe combined immunodeficiency, bone marrow transplantation, other organ transplants, systemic lupus erythematosus, and patients receiving

*See references 28, 82, 103, 107, 109, 118, 125, 152, 163, 180, 183, 262, 266, 270, 283, 295, 299.
†See references 28, 103, 109, 125, 180, 183, 264, 270, 283, 298.
‡See references 45, 83, 99, 109, 124, 125, 133, 168, 171, 193, 196, 214, 250, 254, 261.

*See references 26, 37, 109, 124, 155, 168, 186, 196, 214, 250, 261, 269, 286.
†See references 54, 81, 89, 104, 117, 125, 130, 191, 192, 220, 298.
‡See references 5, 24, 27, 38, 49, 65, 98, 109, 114, 124, 140, 141, 146, 159, 179, 181, 194, 197, 210, 232, 241, 242, 294, 296.

chemotherapy. The immune deficiency in the aforementioned conditions can be a primary event or a secondary event related to treatment.

Patients with chronic anemia have high persistent concentrations of B19 virus in their serum, although the values (10^8 particles per milliliter) are less than those seen in primary infections (10^{10} to 10^{11} particles per milliliter) in healthy individuals and in patients with hemoglobinopathies.

Viremia and anemia may, if untreated, persist for years. Fatigue and pallor are the most common clinical symptoms, and other findings of B19 virus infection, such as exanthem and arthralgia, rarely occur. Because of immunodeficiency, IgM antibody studies generally are not useful in making the diagnosis. Therefore, the diagnosis of persistent B19 virus infection depends on demonstration of specific B19 antigen or DNA in blood.

INTRAUTERINE INFECTION

Although a large epidemiologic study of an outbreak of erythema infectiosum more than 35 years ago failed to reveal evidence of teratogenicity, virologic and serologic studies conducted during the last decade indicate that B19 virus crosses the placenta and causes infection in the fetus.* Infection in pregnancy results in fetal hydrops, fetal death, and miscarriage. To determine the rate and outcome of fetal infection that occurs after infection in pregnant women, a large prospective study was performed in England during a 3½-year period from January 1985 to June 1988,[215] and more recently, from 1992 to 1995, a second study was performed.[167] These two studies included 427 pregnant women with B19 virus infection; 367 infants survived, and 129 of them had follow-up examinations at 7 to 10 years of age.[167] The excess rate of fetal loss occurred only during the first 20 weeks of gestation, and it was 9 percent. Seven cases of fetal hydrops occurred, and three of these fetuses survived; two of the three received intrauterine transfusions. None of the surviving infants in the two studies had abnormalities attributable to B19 virus infection, and no later effects were found at 7 to 10 years of age. Of the infants exposed in utero after 20 weeks' gestation, more than half were infected, but no clinical effects were identified.

In a study in Connecticut related to a large outbreak of erythema infectiosum in which 39 infected pregnant women were monitored, two miscarriages occurred.[223] Fetal loss caused by B19 virus infection was estimated to be 5 percent. In another study in Spain, fetal loss occurred in only 1 of 60 women with B19 virus infection during pregnancy.[95]

Koch and colleagues[138] performed follow-up examinations on 19 infants born to mothers who had serologically confirmed B19 virus infections between the 4th and 38th weeks of gestation. In none of these infants did hydrops develop during pregnancy, and all were normal after birth. One child, whose mother had erythema infectiosum at approximately the 20th week of gestation, had a persistent asymptomatic infection for at least the first 7 months of life. Donders and coworkers[69] noted a child in whom a sonogram demonstrated fetal hydrops at 30 weeks' gestation. Cordocentesis revealed a hemoglobin concentration of 2.4 g/dL. One week later, a hydropic 1550-g infant was delivered by cesarean section. The baby's bone marrow showed an arrest in erythropoiesis, with giant pronormoblasts. The baby received multiple transfusions for the first 4 months of life, and B19 viral DNA was identified in blood at 19 weeks of age. At 2 years of age, this child was found to be clinically, hematologically, and immunologically normal.

In contrast to the case just noted, Brown and associates[34] reported a baby with a similar exposure and delivery history who had persistent anemia and, in spite of therapy, was transfusion-dependent at 4 years of age. In addition, Brown and associates reported two other infants who had received intrauterine transfusions for fetal hydrops and had persistent anemia after birth.

At the present time, a large number of babies who were exposed to B19 virus in utero have been studied, with convincing evidence of specific congenital malformations.[131, 177, 215, 222, 223, 290] However, van Elsacker-Niele and associates[272] noted B19 virus infection in cells other than those of the erythroid series in two aborted fetuses. Ocular malformation was found in one, and evidence of extensive inflammatory reactions in all fetal and placental tissues was noted in both.

Tiesson and colleagues[263] reported an aborted fetus with a bilateral cleft lip, alveolus, and palate; micrognathia; and webbed joints. In another aborted fetus, ocular abnormalities similar to those seen in congenital rubella were noted.[284] In a newborn with anemia, blueberry muffin rash, and hepatomegaly, parvovirus B19 virus gene sequences were found in the liver and placenta.[245]

NEUROLOGIC ILLNESS

Two children with encephalitis in association with erythema infectiosum were noted in the era before discovery of the causative role of B19 virus in erythema infectiosum.[19, 101] In the present era, occasional cases of aseptic meningitis and encephalitis have been reported in association with B19 virus infection in both children and adults.[44, 105, 109, 110, 124, 142, 199, 255, 258] These cases have been documented by the demonstration of specific B19 virus IgM antibody or the presence of B19 viral DNA in cerebrospinal fluid.

Other neuralgic illnesses associated with B19 virus infection include postinfectious neuralgic amyotrophy,[205] Guillain-Barré syndrome,[169] acute bilateral carpal tunnel syndrome,[230] and numbness and tingling of the fingers in seven nurses.[299] Five of these nurses had erythema infectiosum, and in the other two the only manifestation of infection was numbness and tingling. All cases in this study were diagnosed by the demonstration of specific B19 virus IgM antibody during an outbreak of erythema infectiosum in Buffalo, New York, in 1987.

MYOCARDITIS

Myocarditis in association with parvovirus B19 infection has been observed in five children and four adults.[75, 190, 206, 227] Infection of the heart also has been noted in eight fetuses. Enders and associates[75] described two children with life-threatening myocarditis. One of these children died, and the second received a cardiac transplant. The illnesses in both these children occurred in the spring (April), and one had joint pain and urticarial lesions on the flexor surfaces of both arms, erythematous macules on the abdomen and upper part of the chest, and purpuric lesions on the back. Both children had B19 viral DNA identified in the heart and B19-specific IgM antibody.

Nigro and colleagues[190] noted three young children, aged 7, 12, and 18 months, with acute lymphocytic myocarditis

*See references 3–5, 30, 34, 38, 43, 69, 74, 91, 92, 95, 108, 109, 121, 124, 131, 134, 136, 138, 139, 164, 167, 170, 199, 207, 215, 222–224, 229, 248, 263, 271, 272, 289–291, 296, 302.

and parvovirus B19 infection. Two of these children had full cardiac recoveries, but chronic persistent myocarditis developed in the other child.

ACUTE HEPATITIS

Acute hepatitis has been noted as a manifestation of B19 virus infection. Yoto and coworkers[293] described seven children with acute hepatitis in association with B19 virus infection. They carefully studied and ruled out other common causes of acute hepatitis. Sokal and associates[251] reported fulminant hepatitis in four children younger than 5 years of age in association with parvovirus B19 infection. Their patients had a distinct clinical pattern with low serum bilirubin concentrations and rapid recovery of liver function without transplantation.

OTHER ILLNESSES

One adult patient had chronic red cell aplasia for a 10-year period that was treated with regular blood transfusions.[147] After diagnosis of persistent B19 virus infection, the patient was treated with intravenous immunoglobulin (IVIG), which resulted in an apparent cure. A presumably immunologically normal woman had recurrent episodes of paresthesia over the course of a 4-year period in conjunction with persistent B19 virus DNA in her blood.[80] Evidence of persistent infection in immunologically normal patients has been noted in other studies.[127, 182]

Kerr and associates[126] studied 53 patients who had contracted acute B19 virus illnesses. Seven of those studied had B19 virus DNA demonstrated in serum specimens 26 to 65 months after their acute illnesses. All seven were women, and four were asymptomatic. Of the other three, one had chronic hemolytic anemia, one had persistent arthralgia of the knees, and the last had arthralgia and chronic fatigue syndrome. Jacobson and colleagues[120] described an 18-year-old woman with chronic fatigue syndrome and chronic B19 virus infection. Her condition improved after administration of IVIG. Faden and associates[80] described a nurse with recurrent episodes of paresthesia who had B19 virus DNA demonstrated in her sera for almost a 4-year period. This woman also had persistent serum IgM antibody to B19 virus.

Tsuda and coworkers[265] described five young adults with cervical lymphadenopathy associated with B19 virus infection. All had fever, one had arthralgia, and all had leukopenia. Morinet and colleagues[174] described a 27-year-old man with pseudoappendicitis or acute mesenteric lymphadenitis and serologic evidence of B19 virus infection. A 16-month-old boy with peripheral facial palsy, parotitis, and intraparotid lymphadenitis had evidence of parvovirus B19 IgM antibody and IgG antibody seroconversion.[162]

Two adult patients with pneumonia, severe respiratory distress, and parvovirus B19 infection have been described.[175, 282]

Diagnosis

DIFFERENTIAL DIAGNOSIS

Because the exanthem of erythema infectiosum is unique, its diagnosis should be easy. During epidemics, no difficulties should arise, but sporadic cases can be a problem. In the differential diagnosis, rubella and scarlet fever are of most concern. Because rubella virus has been recovered from some patients with illness thought to be erythema infectiosum[19] and because an erythema infectiosum–like illness was observed in volunteers who underwent intranasal administration of a rubella virus strain recovered from a patient with erythema infectiosum–like illness,[231] this diagnostic possibility always should be considered. When the risk of development of congenital rubella is a possibility, rubella-specific diagnostic tests should be performed (see Chapter 177).

Erythema infectiosum can be differentiated from scarlet fever by the usual lack of pharyngitis in the former and a positive culture for *Streptococcus pyogenes* in the latter. Other differential diagnostic considerations are other infectious exanthems (see Chapter 65), collagen vascular diseases, drug reactions, and allergic responses to environmental substances. Although a presumptive diagnosis of erythema infectiosum may be made by exclusion of other etiologic possibilities, a definitive diagnosis can be made only by specific serologic tests or the identification of B19 antigens or DNA in blood or tissue specimens.

Aplastic crisis in a patient with chronic hemolytic anemia can be diagnosed by finding a hemoglobin concentration that is 2 g/dL or more below the steady-state value for that patient, together with a reticulocyte count either less than 0.2 percent of the steady-state value or elevated above the steady-state value (indicative of hyperplasia of erythrocyte precursors in the recovery phase). Although B19 virus infection is the most common cause of aplastic crisis, moderate to severe degrees of hypoplasia may be associated with systemic bacterial infections (e.g., *Salmonella*, pneumococcal) or marrow-suppressive drugs (e.g., chloramphenicol).[166, 239]

SPECIFIC DIAGNOSIS

Several tests have been developed and refined that allow a reliable serologic diagnosis of acute and past B19 virus infection and demonstration of B19 virus in blood and tissues.* IgM and IgG antibody can be detected by enzyme immunoassay, hemadherence, radioimmunoassay, or immunofluorescence; antigen can be detected by DNA hybridization, PCR, or electron microscopy.

In a normal host, acute or recent infection is determined best by demonstration of specific IgM antibody. In immunocompromised patients with suspected acute or chronic infection, the diagnosis is made by detection of antigen in blood. Similarly, detection of antigen also can be performed early in aplastic crisis and to study aborted fetal tissues.

Past infection and immunity to B19 virus are determined by demonstration of specific serum IgG antibody.

Some caution should be observed in accepting the results of IgM serology and antigen detection in unusual clinical circumstances. The sensitivity and specificity of the various serologic tests vary, and additional false-positive and false-negative results can be expected, depending on the skill of workers in individual laboratories.[39, 57] Antigen-detection systems can be contaminated, and such contamination may not be discernible by conventional controls. When the results of tests on specimens from patients with unusual illnesses are positive, repeating the tests in a different laboratory is worthwhile.

Söderlund and associates[249] reported an IgG avidity assay that is highly sensitive and specific for the identification of recent primary infection with parvovirus B19. Persistent

---

*See references 5, 10, 15, 32, 39, 40, 46, 55, 57, 66, 76, 86, 113, 129, 135, 137, 173, 189, 228, 234, 236, 259, 281, 301.

infection may be determined by the presence of IgG antibody to NS1.[276]

Treatment and Prognosis

No specific treatment of B19 virus infection exists. Symptomatic therapy for erythema infectiosum rarely is necessary, especially in children. Starch baths may be helpful in reducing pruritus. Arthralgia or arthritis may be troublesome and may be treated with analgesics.

Patients with aplastic crisis may require transfusion of erythrocytes to raise the peripheral hemoglobin concentration.

The outlook in virtually all cases of erythema infectiosum is excellent. If patients with aplastic crisis receive transfusions with packed erythrocytes when necessary, the prognosis for these patients also is excellent. If B19 virus infection occurs during pregnancy, the pregnancy should be monitored carefully. At delivery, examination of cord blood or blood from the neonate for detection of virus and IgM antibody will reveal whether the virus has crossed the placenta and infected the fetus. When it has occurred, the child should be examined carefully for any defect and monitored for some years to exclude the possibility of development of delayed sequelae.

Some researchers have suggested that pregnant women with symptomatic B19 virus infection be observed for fetal aplastic crisis by monitoring maternal serum for elevated levels of alpha-fetoprotein.[41] If elevated levels are found, serial ultrasonography can be performed to detect hydrops fetalis. Fetal hydrops can be treated with in utero transfusions.[226] However, this approach is considered risky because of the demonstration of extensive infection in aborted fetuses and the potential for congenital malformation.

Therapeutic abortion is not indicated in pregnant women with documented B19 virus infection.

Immunocompromised patients with chronic B19 virus infection can be treated successfully with IVIG preparations,[26, 37, 68, 109, 124, 140, 241] as can other patients without demonstrated immune deficiencies who have chronic infections.[80, 120] Although the amount of specific B19 virus antibody varies among different IVIG products, all contain significant concentrations.[68] No formal treatment studies have been performed, and several different treatment programs have been used. Even though some cures have been achieved with single-dose IVIG therapy, I favor an initial 4-day course with 500 mg/kg/day. After the patient has received treatment, the viremia should cease and clinical improvement should occur. Some immunocompromised patients have required repeated treatment courses.

Prevention

B19 virus is spread by the oral and respiratory routes, and virus shedding during routine infection occurs when patients are not aware of their illness. Because B19 virus infections occur in outbreaks, the virus can be widespread in a community, with many infections going unrecognized.

Patients with erythema infectiosum do not need to be isolated because they have passed their period of infectivity. Although patients with aplastic crisis also usually are past the period of virus shedding, they should be isolated because some will be shedding virus at the time of initial evaluation. All patients with chronic infection should be considered contagious until treated with IVIG and demonstrated to be nonviremic.

Pregnant women are of particular concern during an outbreak.[43, 92] Seropositivity caused by parvovirus infection is approximately 50 percent in women of child-bearing age, so no risk exists in approximately half of those who might become exposed. Determining an IgG antibody titer can allay the fear in those who are antibody-positive. Cartter and associates[43] examined occupational risk factors for B19 virus infection in pregnant women. They found the following rates of infection: school teachers, 16 percent; daycare workers, 9 percent; homemakers, 9 percent; and women working outside the home, 4 percent. In another study, Gillespie and colleagues[92] found the greatest risk for infection in school and daycare personnel. These results suggest that in certain circumstances (in older women and women with past fertility problems), having women in high-risk occupations avoid the workplace during the outbreak period might be reasonable.

Technologic advances have led to the development of recombinant experimental vaccines that show considerable promise for effective prevention.[20, 59] These vaccines could be useful in selected populations, such as patients with hemoglobinopathies and seronegative women of child-bearing age.

REFERENCES

1. Abuhammour, W., Abdel-Haq, N., and Asmar, B.: Picture of the month. Petechial eruption with parvovirus B19 infection. Arch. Pediatr. Adolesc. Med. *153*:87–88, 1999.
2. Adler, S. P., Manganello, A. M. A., Koch, W. C., et al.: Risk of human parvovirus B19 infections among school and hospital employees during endemic periods. J. Infect. Dis. *168*:361–368, 1993.
3. Ager, E. A., Chin, T. D. Y., and Poland, J. D.: Epidemic erythema infectiosum. N. Engl. J. Med. *275*:1326–1331, 1966.
4. Anand, A., Gray, E. S., Brown, T., et al.: Human parvovirus infection in pregnancy and hydrops fetalis. N. Engl. J. Med. *316*:183–186, 1987.
5. Anderson, L. J.: Human parvoviruses. J. Infect. Dis. *161*:603–608, 1990.
6. Anderson, L. J., Tsou, C., Parker, R. A., et al.: Detection of antibodies and antigens of human parvovirus B19 by enzyme-linked immunosorbent assay. J. Clin. Microbiol. *24*:522–526, 1986.
7. Anderson, M. J., and Cohen, B. J.: Human parvovirus B19 infections in United Kingdom 1984–86. Lancet *1*:738–739, 1987.
8. Anderson, M. J., Davis, L. R., Hodgson, J., et al.: Occurrence of infection with a parvovirus-like agent in children with sickle cell anemia during a two-year period. J. Clin. Pathol. *35*:744–749, 1982.
9. Anderson, M. J., Higgins, P. G., Davis, L. R., et al.: Experimental parvovirus infection in man. J. Infect. Dis. *152*:257–265, 1985.
10. Anderson, M. J., Jones, S. E., and Minson, A. C.: Diagnosis of human parvovirus infection by dot-blot hybridization using cloned viral DNA. J. Med. Virol. *15*:163–172, 1985.
11. Anderson, M. J., Kidd, I. M., and Morgan-Capner, P.: Human parvovirus and rubella-like illness. Lancet *2*:663, 1985.
12. Anderson, M. J., Lewis, E., Kidd, I. M., et al.: An outbreak of erythema infectiosum associated with human parvovirus infection. J. Hyg. *93*: 85–93, 1984.
13. Andrewes, C. H., Pereira, H. G., and Wildy, P.: *Parvoviridae*. *In* Andrewes, C. H., Pereira, H. G., and Wildy, D. (eds.): Viruses of Vertebrates. London, Bailliere Tindall, 1978, pp. 255–271.
14. Auriemma, P. R.: Erythema infectiosum: Report on a familial outbreak. Am. J. Public Health *44*:1450–1454, 1954.
15. Azzi, A., Zakrzewska, K., Gentilomi, G., et al.: Detection of B19 parvovirus infections by a dot-blot hybridization assay using a digoxigenin-labelled probe. J. Virol. Methods *27*:125–134, 1990.
16. Bagot, M., and Revuz, J.: Papular-purpuric "gloves and socks" syndrome: Primary infection with parvovirus B19? J. Am. Acad. Dermatol. *25*:341–342, 1991.
17. Balfour, H. H., Jr.: Erythema infectiosum (fifth disease): Clinical review and description of 91 cases seen in an epidemic. Clin. Pediatr. (Phila.) *8*:721–727, 1969.
18. Balfour, H. H., Jr., May, D. B., Rotte, T. C., et al.: A study of erythema infectiosum: Recovery of rubella virus and echovirus-12. Pediatrics *50*:285–290, 1972.
19. Balfour, H. H., Jr., Schiff, G. M., and Bloom, J. E.: Encephalitis associated with erythema infectiosum. J. Pediatr. *77*:133–136, 1970.
20. Bansal, G. P., Hatfield, J. A., Dunn, F. E., et al.: Candidate recombinant vaccine for human B19 parvovirus. J. Infect. Dis. *167*:1034–1044, 1993.
21. Bard, J. W., and Perry, H. O.: Erythema infectiosum. Arch. Dermatol. *93*:49–53, 1966.

22. Berg, A. M., Naides, S. J., and Simms, R. W.: Established fibromyalgia syndrome and parvovirus B19 infection. J. Rheumatol. *20*:1941–1943, 1993.
23. Berns, K. I.: *Parvoviridae* and their replication. *In* Fields, B. N., and Knipe, D. M. (eds.): Virology. 2nd ed., Vol. 2. New York, Raven Press, 1990, pp. 1743–1764.
24. Bertoni, E., Rosati, A., Zanazzi, M., et al.: Unusual incidence of aplastic anemia due to B19 parvovirus infection in renal transplant recipients. Transplant. Proc. *29*:818–819, 1997.
25. Bessis, D., Lamaury, I., Jonquet, O., et al.: Human parvovirus B19 induced papular-purpuric "gloves and socks" syndrome. Eur. J. Dermatol. *4*:133–134, 1994.
26. Bloom, M. E., and Young, N. S.: Parvoviruses. *In* Knipe, D. M., and Howley, P. M. (eds.): Virology. 4th ed., Vol. 2. Philadelphia, Lippincott Williams & Wilkins, 2001, pp. 2361–2379.
27. Borkowski, J., Amrikachi, M., and Hudnall, S. D.: Fulminant parvovirus infection following erythropoietin treatment in a patient with acquired immunodeficiency syndrome. Arch. Pathol. Lab. Med. *124*:441–445, 2000.
28. Boruchoff, S. E., Woda, B. A., Pihan, G. A., et al.: Parvovirus B19–associated hemophagocytic syndrome. Arch. Intern. Med. *150*:897–899, 1990.
29. Boysen, G.: Erythema infectiosum. Acta Paediatr. *31*:211–224, 1944.
30. Brandenburg, H., Los, F. J., and Cohen-Overbeek, T. E.: A case of early intrauterine parvovirus B19 infection. Prenatal Diagn. *16*:75–77, 1996.
31. Brass, C., Elliott, L. M., and Stevens, D. A.: Academy rash: A probable epidemic of erythema infectiosum (fifth disease). J. A. M. A. *248*:568–572, 1982.
32. Brown, C. S., van Bussel, M., Wassenaar, A. L. M., et al.: An immunofluorescence assay for the detection of parvovirus B19 IgG and IgM antibodies based on recombinant viral antigen. J. Virol. Methods *29*:53–62, 1990.
33. Brown, K. E., Anderson, S. M., and Young, N. S.: Erythrocyte P antigen: Cellular receptor for B19 parvovirus. Science *262*:114–117, 1993.
34. Brown, K. E., Green, S. W., de Mayolo, J. A., et al.: Congenital anaemia after transplacental B19 parvovirus infection. Lancet *343*:895–896, 1994.
35. Brown, K. E., Hibbs, J. R., Gallinella, G., et al.: Resistance to parvovirus B19 infection due to lack of virus receptor (erythrocyte P antigen). N. Engl. J. Med. *330*:1192–1196, 1994.
36. Brown, K. E., Mori, J., Cohen, B. J., et al.: In vitro propagation of parvovirus B19 in primary foetal liver culture. J. Gen. Virol. *72*:741–745, 1991.
37. Brown, K. E., Young, N. S., and Liu, J. M.: Molecular, cellular and clinical aspects of parvovirus B19 infection. Crit. Rev. Oncol. Hematol. *16*:1–31, 1994.
38. Brown, T., Anand, A., Ritchie, L. D., et al.: Intrauterine human parvovirus infection and hydrops fetalis. Lancet *2*:1033–1034, 1984.
39. Bruu, A. L., and Nordb, S. A.: Evaluation of five commercial tests for detection of immunoglobulin M antibodies to human parvovirus B19. J. Clin. Microbiol. *33*:1363–1365, 1995.
40. Carrière, C., Boulanger, P., and Delsert, C.: Rapid and sensitive method for the detection of B19 virus DNA using the polymerase chain reaction with nested primers. J. Virol. Methods *44*:221–234, 1993.
41. Carrington, D., Whittle, M. J., Gibson, A. A. M., et al.: Maternal serum alpha fetoprotein: A marker of fetal aplastic crisis during intrauterine human parvovirus infection. Lancet *1*:433–435, 1987.
42. Carstensen, H., Ornvold, K., and Cohen, B. J.: Human parvovirus B19 infection associated with prolonged erythroblastopenia in a leukemic child. Pediatr. Infect. Dis. *8*:56, 1989.
43. Cartter, M. L., Farley, T. A., Rosengren, S., et al.: Occupational risk factors for infection with parvovirus B19 among pregnant women. J. Infect. Dis. *163*:282–285, 1991.
44. Cassinotti, P., Schultze, D., Schlageter, P., et al.: Persistent human parvovirus B19 infection following an acute infection with meningitis in an immunocompetent patient. Eur. J. Clin. Microbiol. Infect. Dis. *12*:701–704, 1993.
45. Cassinotti, P., Siegl, G., Michel, B. A., et al.: Presence and significance of human parvovirus B19 DNA in synovial membranes and bone marrow from patients with arthritis of unknown origin. J. Med. Virol. *56*:199–204, 1998.
46. Cassinotti, P., Weitz, M., and Siegl, G.: Human parvovirus B19 infections: Routine diagnosis by a new nested polymerase chain reaction assay. J. Med. Virol. *40*:228–234, 1993.
47. Caul, E. O., Usher, M. J., and Burton, P. A.: Intrauterine infection with human parvovirus B19: A light and electron microscopy study. J. Med. Virol. *24*:55–66, 1988.
48. Chargin, L., Sobel, N., and Goldstein, H.: Erythema infectiosum: Report of an extensive epidemic. Arch. Dermatol. Syph. *47*:467–477, 1942.
49. Chernak, E., Dubin, G., Henry, D., et al.: Infection due to parvovirus B19 in patients infected with human immunodeficiency virus. Clin. Infect. Dis. *20*:170–173, 1995.
50. Cherry, J. D.: Newer viral exanthems. Adv. Pediatr. *16*:233–286, 1969.
51. Cherry, J. D.: Parvovirus infections in children and adults. Adv. Pediatr. *46*:245–269, 1999.
52. Chorba, T., Coccia, P., Holman, R. C., et al.: The role of parvovirus B19 in aplastic crisis and erythema infectiosum (fifth disease). J. Infect. Dis. *154*:383–393, 1986.
53. Clarke, H. C.: Erythema infectiosum: An epidemic with a probable posterythema phase. Can. Med. Assoc. J. *130*:603–604, 1984.
54. Clewley, J. P.: Biochemical characterization of a human parvovirus. J. Gen. Virol. *65*:241–244, 1984.
55. Clewley, J. P., Cohen, B. J., and Field, A. M.: Detection of parvovirus B19 DNA, antigen, and particles in the human fetus. J. Med. Virol. *23*:367–376, 1987.
56. Coe, H. C., and Kelly, F. L.: Erythema infectiosum. Calif. West. Med. *36*:39–40, 1932.
57. Cohen, B. J., and Bates, C. M.: Evaluation of 4 commercial test kits for parvovirus B19–specific IgM. J. Virol. Methods *55*:11–25, 1995.
58. Cohen, B. J., Mortimer, P. P., and Pereira, M. S.: Diagnostic assays with monoclonal antibodies for the human serum parvovirus-like virus (SPLV). J. Hyg. (Camb.) *91*:113–130, 1983.
59. Collett, M. S., and Young, N. S.: Prospects for a human B19 parvovirus vaccine. Rev. Med. Virol. *4*:91–103, 1994.
60. Condon, F. J.: Erythema infectiosum: Report of an areawide outbreak. Am. J. Public Health *49*:528–535, 1959.
61. Conway, S. P., Cohen, B. J., Field, A. M., et al.: A family outbreak of parvovirus B19 infection with petechial rash in a 7-year-old boy. J. Infect. *15*:110–112, 1987.
62. Cooper, C. L., and Choudhri, S. H.: Photo quiz II. Leukocytoclastic vasculitis secondary to parvovirus B19 infection. Clin. Infect. Dis. *26*:849, 989, 1998.
63. Cossart, Y. E., Field, A. M., Cant, B., et al.: Parvovirus-like particles in human sera. Lancet *1*:72–73, 1975.
64. Cotmore, S., and Tattersall, P.: Characterization and molecular cloning of a human parvovirus genome. Science *226*:1161–1165, 1984.
65. Coulombel, L., Morinet, F., Mielot, F., et al.: Parvovirus infection, leukemia, and immunodeficiency. Lancet *1*:101–102, 1989.
66. Cubel, R. C. N., Oliveira, S. A., Brown, D. W. G., et al.: Diagnosis of parvovirus B19 infection by detection of specific immunoglobulin M antibody in saliva. J. Clin. Microbiol. *34*:205–207, 1996.
67. Deiss, V., Tratschin, J. D., Weitz, M., et al.: Cloning of the human parvovirus B19 genome and structural analysis of its palindromic termini. Virology *175*:247–254, 1990.
68. Dockrell, D. H., Poland, G. A., Jones, M. F., et al.: Variability in parvovirus B19 IgG levels in intravenous immunoglobulin samples. Diagn. Microbiol. Infect. Dis. *26*:133–135, 1996.
69. Donders, G. G. G., Van Lierde, S., Van Elsacker-Niele, A. M. W., et al.: Survival after intrauterine parvovirus B19 infection with persistence in early infancy: A two-year follow-up. Pediatr. Infect. Dis. J. *13*:234–236, 1994.
70. Drago, F., Semino, M., Rampini, P, Rebora, A.: Parvovirus B19 infection associated with acute hepatitis and a purpuric exanthem. Br. J. Dermatol. *141*:160–161, 1999.
71. Duncan, J. R., Capellini, M. D., Anderson, M. J., et al.: Aplastic crisis due to parvovirus infection in pyruvate kinase deficiency. Lancet *2*:14–16, 1983.
72. Dunnet, W. N., Thorm, B. T., and Ayling, R. G.: Food poisoning from oysters. C. D. R. *36*:3, 1984.
73. Edelson, R. N., and Altman, R.: Erythema infectiosum: A statewide outbreak. J. Med. Soc. N. J. *67*:805–809, 1970.
74. Eis-Hubinger, A. M., Dieck, D., Schild, R, et al. Parvovirus B19 infection in pregnancy. Intervirology *47*:178–184, 1998.
75. Enders, G., Dotch, J., Bauer, J, et al.: Life-threatening parvovirus B19–associated myocarditis and cardiac transplantation as possible therapy: Two case reports. Clin. Infect. Dis. *26*:355–358, 1998.
76. Erdman, D. D., Durigon, E. L., and Holloway, B. P.: Detection of human parvovirus B19 DNA PCR products by RNA probe hybridization enzyme immunoassay. J. Clin. Microbiol. *32*:2295–2298, 1994.
77. Erdman, D. D., Durigon, E. L., Wang, Q.-Y., et al.: Genetic diversity of human parvovirus B19: Sequence analysis of the VP1/VP2 gene from multiple isolates. J. Gen. Virol. *77*:2767–2774, 1996.
78. Eriksson, B. M., Stromberg, A., and Kreuger, A.: Human parvovirus B19 infection with severe anemia affecting mother and son. Scand. J. Infect. Dis. *20*:335–337, 1988.
79. Escherich, T.: Discussion. Comptes-rendus du XII Congres International de Medecin. Moscow, S. P. Yakovlev, *3*:133, 1898.
80. Faden, H., Gary, G. W., and Anderson, L. J.: Chronic parvovirus infection in a presumably immunologically healthy woman. Clin. Infect. Dis. *15*:595–597, 1992.
81. Ferri, C., Zakrzewska, K., Longombardo, G., et al. : Parvovirus B19 infection of bone marrow in systemic sclerosis patients. Clin. Exp. Rheumatol. *17*:718–720, 1999.
82. Foreman, N. K., Oakhill, A., and Caul, E. O.: Parvovirus-associated thrombocytopenic purpura. Lancet *2*:1426–1427, 1988.
83. Foto, F., Saag, K. G., Scharosch, L. L., et al.: Parvovirus B19–specific DNA in bone marrow from B19 arthropathy patients: Evidence for B19 virus persistence. J. Infect. Dis. *167*:744–748, 1993.
84. Fox, M. J., and Clark, J. M.: Erythema infectiosum. Am. J. Dis. Child. *73*:453–457, 1947.
85. Franssila, R., Hokynar, K., and Hedman, K.: T helper cell–mediated in vitro responses of recently and remotely infected subjects to a candidate recombinant vaccine for human parvovirus b19. J. Infect. Dis. *183*: 805–809, 2001.

86. Fridell, E., Trojnar, J., and Wahren, B.: A new peptide for human parvovirus B19 antibody detection. Scand. J. Infect. Dis. *21*:597–603, 1989.
87. Fried, R. I.: Erythema infectiosum: Fifth disease, a clinical note. Ohio St. Med. J. *47*:1027–1028, 1951.
88. Fukada, K., Matumoto, K., Takakura, F., et al.: Four putative subtypes of human parvovirus B19 based on amino acid polymorphism in the C-terminal region of non-structural protein. J. Med. Virol. *62*:60–69, 2000.
89. Gabriel, S. E., Espy, M., Erdman, D. D., et al. : The role of parvovirus B19 in the pathogenesis of giant cell arteritis: A preliminary evaluation. Arthritis Rheum. *42*:1255–1258, 1999.
90. García-Tapia, A. M., del Alamo, C. F. G., Girón, J. A., et al.: Spectrum of parvovirus B19 infection: Analysis of an outbreak of 43 cases in Cadiz, Spain. Clin. Infect. Dis. *21*:1424–1430, 1995.
91. Gentilomi, G., Zerbini, M., Gallinella, G., et al. : B19 parvovirus induced fetal hydrops: Rapid and simple diagnosis by detection of B19 antigens in amniotic fluids. Prenat. Diagn. *18*:363–368, 1998.
92. Gillespie, S. M., Cartter, M. L., Asch, S., et al.: Occupational risk of human parvovirus B19 infection for school and day-care personnel during an outbreak of erythema infectiosum. J. A. M. A. *263*:2061–2065, 1990.
93. Goldman, F., Rotbart, H., Gutierrez, K., et al.: Parvovirus-associated aplastic crisis in a patient with red blood cell glucose-6-phosphate dehydrogenase deficiency. Pediatr. Infect. Dis. *9*:593–594, 1990.
94. Gowda, N., Rao, S. P., Cohen, B., et al.: Human parvovirus infection in patients with sickle cell disease with and without hypoplastic crisis. J. Pediatr. *110*:81–84, 1987.
95. Gratacós, E., Torres, P. J., Vidal, J., et al.: The incidence of human parvovirus B19 infection during pregnancy and its impact on perinatal outcome. J. Infect. Dis. *171*:1360–1363, 1995.
96. Greenwald, P., and Bashe, W. J., Jr.: An epidemic of erythema infectiosum. Am. J. Dis. Child. *107*:30–34, 1964.
97. Grimmer, H., and Joseph, A.: An epidemic of infectious erythema in Germany. Arch. Dermatol. *80*:283–285, 1959.
98. Gyllensten, K., Sönnerborg, A., Jorup-Rönström, C. J., et al.: Parvovirus B19 infection in HIV-1 infected patients with anemia. Infection *22*:356–358, 1994.
99. Hajeer, A. H., MacGregor, A. J., Rigby, A. S., et al.: Influence of previous exposure to human parvovirus B19 infection in explaining susceptibility to rheumatoid arthritis: An analysis of disease discordant twin pairs. J. Rheum. Dis. *53*:137–139, 1994.
100. Halasz, C. L. G., Cormier, D., and Den, M.: Petechial glove and sock syndrome caused by parvovirus B19. J. Am. Acad. Dermatol. *27*:835–838, 1992.
101. Hall, C. B., and Horner, F. A.: Encephalopathy with erythema infectiosum. Am. J. Dis. Child. *131*:65–67, 1977.
102. Hammon, W. D., and Enders, J. F.: A virus disease of cats, principally characterized by aleucocytosis, enteric lesions and the presence of intranuclear inclusion bodies. J. Exp. Med. *69*:327–352, 1939.
103. Hanada, T., Koike, K., Takeya, T., et al.: Human parvovirus B19–induced transient pancytopenia in a child with hereditary spherocytosis. Br. J. Haematol. *70*:113–115, 1988.
104. Harel, L., Straussberg, R., Rudich, H., et al.: Raynaud's phenomenon as a manifestation of parvovirus B19 infection: Case reports and review of parvovirus B19 rheumatic and vasculitic syndromes. Clin. Infect. Dis. *30*:500–503, 2000.
105. Haseyama, K., Kudoh, T., Yoto, Y., et al.: Detection of human parvovirus B19 DNA in cerebrospinal fluid. Pediatr. Infect. Dis. J. *16*:324–326, 1997.
106. Hauswirth, W. W.: Autonomous parvovirus DNA structure and replication. *In* Berns, K. I. (ed.): The Parvoviruses. London, Plenum Press, 1983, pp. 129–152.
107. Heegaard, E. D., Hasle, H., Clausen, N., et al.: Parvovirus B19 infection and Diamond-Blackfan anaemia. Acta Paediatr. *85*:299–302, 1996.
108. Heegaard, E. D., Hasle, H., Skibsted, L., et al.: Congenital anemia caused by parvovirus B19 infection. Pediatr. Infect. Dis. J. *19*:1216–1218, 2000.
109. Heegaard, E. D., and Hornsleth, A.: Parvovirus: The expanding spectrum of disease. Acta Paediatr. *84*:109–117, 1995.
110. Heegaard, E. D., Peterslund, N. A., and Hornsleth, A.: Parvovirus B19 infection associated with encephalitis in a patient suffering from malignant lymphoma. Scand. J. Infect. Dis. *27*:631–633, 1995.
111. Hemauer, A., von Poblotzki, A., Gigler, A., et al. : Sequence variability among different parvovirus B19 isolates. J. Gen. Virol. *77*:1781–1785, 1996.
112. Herrick, T. P.: Erythema infectiosum: A clinical report of 74 cases. Am. J. Dis. Child. *31*:486–495, 1926.
113. Hicks, K. E., Beard, S., Cohen, B. J., et al.: A simple and sensitive DNA hybridization assay used for the routine diagnosis of human parvovirus B19 infection. J. Clin. Microbiol. *33*:2473–2475, 1995.
114. Higashida, K., Kobayashi, K., Sugita, K., et al.: Pure red blood cell aplasia during azathioprine therapy associated with parvovirus B19 infection. Pediatr. Infect. Dis. J. *16*:1093–1095, 1997.
115. Higgins, C. S., and Anderson, M. J.: Acute parvovirus infection associated with chronic arthritis. Unpublished data.
116. Hoffman, E.: Erythema infectiosum (groszflecken oder ringelroteln). Dtsch. Med. Wochenschr. *1*:777–779, 1916.
117. Holm, J. M., Hansen, L. K., and Oxhøj, H.: Kawasaki disease associated with parvovirus B19 infection. Eur. J. Pediatr. *154*:633–634, 1995.
118. Inoue, S., Kinra, N. K., Mukkamala, S., et al.: Parvovirus B19 infection: Aplastic crisis, erythema infectiosum and idiopathic thrombocytopenic purpura. Pediatr. Infect. Dis. *10*:251–253, 1991.
119. International Committee on Taxonomy of Viruses: Virus taxonomy update. Arch. Virol. *133*:491–495, 1993.
120. Jacobson, S. K., Daly, J. S., Thorne, G. M., et al.: Chronic parvovirus B19 infection resulting in chronic fatigue syndrome: Case history and review. Clin. Infect. Dis. *24*:1048–1051, 1997.
121. Jensen, I. P., Schou, O., and Vestergaard, B. F.: The 1994 human parvovirus B19 epidemic in Denmark: Diagnostic and epidemiological experience. A. P. M. I. S. *106*:843–848, 1998.
122. Johansen, J. N., Christensen, L. S., Zakrzewska, K., et al.: Typing of European strains of parvovirus B19 by restriction endonuclease analyses and sequencing: Identification of evolutionary lineages and evidence of recombination of markers from different lineages. Virus Res. *53*:215–223, 1998.
123. Kelleher, J. H., Luban, N. L. C., Mortimer, P. P., et al.: The human serum "parvovirus": A specific cause of aplastic crisis in hereditary spherocytosis. J. Pediatr. *102*:720–722, 1983.
124. Kerr, J. R.: Parvovirus B19 infection. Eur. J. Clin. Microbiol. Infect. Dis. *15*:10–29, 1996.
125. Kerr, J. R.: Pathogenesis of human parvovirus B19 in rheumatic disease. Ann. Rheum. Dis. *59*:672–683, 2000.
126. Kerr, J. R., Curran, M. D., Moore, J. E., et al.: Parvovirus B19 infection—persistence and genetic variation. Scand. J. Infect. Dis. *27*: 551–557, 1995.
127. Kerr, J. R., Curran, M. D., Moore, J. E., et al.: Persistent parvovirus B19 infection. Lancet *345*:1118, 1995.
128. Kerr, P. S., and Marsh, E. H.: Outbreak of erythema infectiosum in Elmsford, N.Y. Am. J. Public Health *23*:1271–1274, 1933.
129. Kim, E. C., Durigon, E. L., Erdman, D. D., et al.: Chemiluminescent microwell hybridization assay for direct detection of human parvovirus B19 DNA. J. Virol. Methods *50*:349–354, 1994.
130. Kim Jacobson, S., Daly, J. S., Thorne, G. M., et al.: Chronic parvovirus B19 infection resulting in chronic fatigue syndrome: Case history and review. Clin. Infect. Dis. *24*:1048–1051, 1997.
131. Kinney, J. S., Anderson, L. J., Farrar, J., et al.: Risk of adverse outcomes of pregnancy after human parvovirus B19 infection. J. Infect. Dis. *157*:663–667, 1988.
132. Kiraz, S., Ertenli, I., Benekli, M., et al. : Parvovirus B19 infection in Behçet's disease. Clin. Exp. Rheumatol. *14*:71–73, 1996.
133. Kishore, J., Misra, R., Gupta, D., et al.: Raised IgM antibodies to parvovirus B19 in juvenile rheumatoid arthritis. Indian J. Med. Res. *107*:15–18, 1998.
134. Knott, P. D., Welply, G. A. C., and Anderson, M. J.: Serologically proven intrauterine infection with parvovirus. B. M. J. *289*:1660, 1984.
135. Koch, W. C.: A synthetic parvovirus B19 capsid protein can replace viral antigen in antibody-capture enzyme immunoassays. J. Virol. Methods *55*:67–82, 1995.
136. Koch, W. C., and Adler, S. P.: Human parvovirus B19 infections in women of childbearing age and within families. Pediatr. Infect. Dis. *8*:83–87, 1989.
137. Koch, W. C., and Adler, S. P.: Detection of human parvovirus B19 DNA by using the polymerase chain reaction. J. Clin. Microbiol. *28*:65–69, 1990.
138. Koch, W. C., Adler, S. P., and Harger, J.: Intrauterine parvovirus B19 infection may cause an asymptomatic or recurrent postnatal infection. Pediatr. Infect. Dis. J. *12*:747–750, 1993.
139. Koch, W.C., Harger, J. H., Barnstein, B., et al.: Serologic and virologic evidence for frequent intrauterine transmission of human parvovirus B19 with a primary maternal infection during pregnancy. Pediatr. Infect. Dis. J. *17*:489–494, 1998.
140. Koch, W. C., Massey, G., Russell, C. E., et al.: Manifestations and treatment of human parvovirus B19 infection in immunocompromised patients. J. Pediatr. *116*:355–359, 1990.
141. Koduri, P. R., Kumapley, R., Khokha, N. D., et al.: Red cell aplasia caused by parvovirus B19 in AIDS: Use of i.v. immunoglobulin. Ann. Hematol. *75*:67–68, 1997.
142. Koduri, P. R., and Naides, S. J.: Aseptic meningitis caused by parvovirus B19. Clin. Infect. Dis. *21*:1053, 1995.
143. Komatsuda, A., Ohtani, H., Nimura, T., et al.: Endocapillary proliferative glomerulonephritis in a patient with parvovirus B19 infection. Am. J. Kidney Dis. *36*:851–854, 2000.
144. Koziol, D. E., Kurtzman, G., Ayub, J., et al.: Nosocomial human parvovirus B19 infection: Lack of transmission from a chronically infected patient to hospital staff. Infect. Control Hosp. Epidemiol. *13*:343–348, 1992.
145. Kurtzman, G. J., Cohen, B. J., Field, A. M., et al.: Immune response to B19 parvovirus and an antibody defect in persistent viral infection. J. Clin. Invest. *84*:1114–1123, 1989.
146. Kurtzman, G. J., Cohen, B., Meyers, P., et al.: Persistent B19 parvovirus infection as a cause of severe chronic anaemia in children with acute lymphocytic leukaemia. Lancet *2*:1159–1162, 1988.

147. Kurtzman, G., Frickhofen, N., Kimball, J., et al.: Pure red-cell aplasia of ten years' duration due to persistent parvovirus B19 infection and its cure with immunoglobulin therapy. N. Engl. J. Med. *321*:519–523, 1989.
148. Langnas, A. N., Markin, R. S., Cattral, M. S., et al.: Parvovirus B19 as a possible causative agent of fulminant liver failure and associated aplastic anemia. Hepatology *22*:1661–1665, 1995.
149. Lauer, B. A., MacCormack, J. N., and Wilfert, C.: Erythema infectiosum: An elementary school outbreak. Am. J. Dis. Child. *130*:252–254, 1976.
150. Lawton, A. L., and Smith, R. E.: Erythema infectiosum: A clinical study of an epidemic in Branford, Conn. Arch. Intern. Med. *47*:28–41, 1931.
151. Lefrère, J. J., Couroucé, A. M., Girot, R., et al.: Human parvovirus and thalassaemia. J. Infect. *13*:45–49, 1986.
152. Lefrère, J. J., Couroucé, A. M., and Kaplan, C.: Parvovirus and idiopathic thrombocytopenic purpura. Lancet *1*:279, 1989.
153. Lefrère, J. J., Couroucé, A. M., Muller, J. Y., et al.: Human parvovirus and purpura. Lancet *2*:730, 1985.
154. Lies, W., III, and Morgan, S. K.: Erythema infectiosum (fifth disease): Report of an outbreak. J. Med. Assoc. Ala. *32*:331–332, 1963.
155. Longo, G., Luppi, M., Bertesi, M., et al.: Still's disease, severe thrombocytopenia, and acute hepatitis associated with acute parvovirus B19 infection. Clin. Infect. Dis. *26*:994–995, 1998.
156. Lowenthal, E. A., Wells, A., Emanuel, P. D., et al.: Sickle cell acute chest syndrome associated with parvovirus B19 infection: Case series and review. Am. J. Hematol. *51*:207–213, 1996.
157. Lyon, C. C.: Severe acral pruritus associated with parvovirus B19 infection. Br. J. Dermatol. *139*:153–154, 1998.
158. Macartney, L., McCandlish, I. A. P., Thompson, H., et al.: Canine parvovirus enteritis 2: Pathogenesis. Vet. Rec. *115*:453–460, 1984.
159. Malarme, M., Vandervelde, D., and Brasseur, M.: Parvovirus infection, leukemia and immunodeficiency. Lancet *1*:1457, 1989.
160. Mallouh, A. A., and Qudah, A.: Acute splenic sequestration together with aplastic crisis caused by human parvovirus B19 in patients with sickle cell disease. J. Pediatr. *122*:593–595, 1993.
161. Mallouh, A. A., and Qudah, A.: An epidemic of aplastic crisis caused by human parvovirus B19. Pediatr. Infect. Dis. J. *14*:31–34, 1995.
162. Martinon-Torres, F., Seara, M. J. F., Del Rio Pastoriza, I., et al.: Parvovirus B19 infection complicated by peripheral facial palsy and parotitis with intraparotid lymphadenitis. Pediatr. Infect. Dis. J. *18*:307–308, 1999.
163. McClain, K., Estrov, Z., Chen, H., et al.: Chronic neutropenia of childhood: Frequent association with parvovirus infection and correlations with bone marrow culture studies. Br. J. Haematol. *85*:57–62, 1993.
164. McNamara, P. J., and Ramanan, R.: Survival of a preterm neonate with late onset hydrops fetalis due to parvovirus B19 infection. Acta Paediatr. *87*:1088–1089, 1998.
165. McOmish, F., Yap, P. L., Jordan, A., et al.: Detection of parvovirus B19 in donated blood: A model system for screening by polymerase chain reaction. J. Clin. Microbiol. *321*:323–328, 1993.
166. Megas, H., Papidiki, E., and Constantinides, B.: *Salmonella* septicemia and aplastic crisis in a patient with sickle cell anemia. Acta Paediatr. *50*:517–521, 1961.
167. Miller, E., Fairley, C. K., Cohen, B. J., et al.: Immediate and long term outcome of human parvovirus B19 infection in pregnancy. Br. J. Obstet. Gynaecol. *105*:174–178, 1998.
168. Mimori, A., Misaki, Y., Hachiya, T., et al.: Prevalence of antihuman parvovirus B19 IgG antibodies in patients with refractory rheumatoid arthritis and polyarticular juvenile rheumatoid arthritis. Rheumatol. Int. *14*:87–90, 1994.
169. Minohara, Y., Koitabashi, Y., Kato, T., et al.: A case of Guillain-Barré syndrome associated with human parvovirus B19 infection. J. Infect. *36*:327–328, 1998.
170. Miyagawa, S., Takahashi, Y., Nagai, A., et al.: Angio-oedema in a neonate with IgG antibodies to parvovirus B19 following intrauterine parvovirus B19 infection. Br. J. Dermatol. *143*:428–430, 2000.
171. Moore, T. L., Parvovirus-associated arthritis. Curr. Opin. Rheumatol. *12*:289–294, 2000.
172. Moore, W. F.: Erythema infectiosum: Review, and report of two cases. Hawaii Med. J. *16*:35–36, 1956.
173. Mori, J., Field, A. M., Clewley, J. P., et al.: Dot blot hybridization assay of B19 virus DNA in clinical specimens. J. Clin. Microbiol. *27*:459–464, 1989.
174. Morinet, F., Monsuez, J. J., Roger, P., et al.: Parvovirus B19 associated with pseudoappendicitis. Lancet *2*:1466, 1987.
175. Morris, C. N., and Smilack, J. D.: Parvovirus B19 infection associated with respiratory distress. Clin. Infect. Dis. *27*:900–901, 1998.
176. Mortimer, P. P.: Hypothesis: The aplastic crisis of hereditary spherocytosis is due to a single transmissible agent. J. Clin. Pathol. *36*:445–448, 1983.
177. Mortimer, P. P., Cohen, B. J., Buckley, M. M., et al.: Human parvovirus and the fetus. Lancet *2*:1012, 1985.
178. Mortimer, P. P., Luban, N. L. C., Kelleher, J. F., et al.: Transmission of serum parvovirus like virus by clotting factor concentrates. Lancet *2*:482–484, 1983.
179. Moudgil, A., Shidban, H., Nast, C. C., et al.: Parvovirus B19 infection–related complications in renal transplant recipients: Treatment with intravenous immunoglobulin. Transplantation *64*:1847–1850, 1997.
180. Muir, K., Todd, W. T. A., Watson, W. H., et al.: Viral-associated haemophagocytosis with parvovirus B19–related pancytopenia. Lancet *339*:1139–1140, 1992.
181. Musiani, M., Zerbini, M., Gentilomi, G., et al.: Persistent B19 parvovirus infections in haemophilic HIV-1 infected patients. J. Med. Virol. *46*:103–108, 1995.
182. Musiani, M., Zerbini, M., Gentilomi, G., et al.: Parvovirus B19 clearance from peripheral blood after acute infection. J. Infect. Dis. *172*:1360–1363, 1995.
183. Mustafa, M. M., and McClain, K. L.: Diverse hematologic effects of parvovirus B19 infection. Pediatr. Clin. North Am. *43*:809–821, 1996.
184. Muzyczka, N., and Berns, K. I.: *Parvoviridae:* The viruses and their replication. *In* Knipe, D. M. and Howley, P. M. (eds): Virology. 4th ed., Vol. 2. Philadelphia, Lippincott Williams & Wilkins, 2001, pp. 2327–2359.
185. Naides, S. J.: Erythema infectiosum (fifth disease) occurrence in Iowa. Am. J. Public Health *78*:1230–1231, 1988.
186. Naides, S. J., and Field, E. H.: Transient rheumatoid factor positivity in acute human parvovirus B19 infection. Arch. Intern. Med. *148*:2587–2589, 1988.
187. Naides, S. J., Howard, E. J., Swack, N. S., et al.: Parvovirus B19 infection inhuman immunodeficiency virus type 1–infected persons failing or intolerant to zidovudine therapy. J. Infect. Dis. *168*:101–105, 1993.
188. Naides, S. J., Piette, W., Veach, L. A., et al.: Human parvovirus B19 induced vesiculopustular skin eruption. Am. J. Med. *84*:968–972, 1988.
189. Nascimento, J. P., Hallam, N. F., Mori, J., et al.: Detection of B19 parvovirus in human fetal tissues by in situ hybridisation. J. Med. Virol. *33*:77–82, 1991.
190. Nigro, G., Bastianon, V., Colloridi, V., et al.: Human parvovirus B19 infection in infancy associated with acute and chronic lymphocytic myocarditis and high cytokine levels: Report of 3 cases and review. Clin. Infect. Dis. *31*:65–69, 2000.
191. Nigro, G., Piazze, J., Taliani, G., et al.: Postpartum lupus erythematosus associated with parvovirus B19 infection. J. Rheumatol. *24*:968–970, 1997.
192. Nigro, G., Zerbini, M., Krysztofiak, A., et al.: Active or recent parvovirus B19 infection in children with Kawasaki disease. Lancet *343*:1260–1261, 1994.
193. Nikkari, S., Luukkainen, R., Möttönen, T., et al.: Does parvovirus B19 have a role in rheumatoid arthritis? Ann. Rheum. Dis. *53*:106–111, 1994.
194. Nikkari, S., Mertsola, J., Korvenranta, H., et al.: Wegener's granulomatosis and parvovirus B19 infection. Arthritis Rheum. *37*:1707–1708, 1994.
195. Nikkari, S., Roivainen, A., Hannonen, P., et al.: Persistence of parvovirus B19 in synovial fluid and bone marrow. Ann. Rheum. Dis. *54*:597–600, 1995.
196. Nocton, J. J., Miller, L. C., Tucker, L. B., et al.: Human parvovirus B19–associated arthritis in children. J. Pediatr. *122*:186–190, 1993.
197. Nour, B., Green, M., Michaels, M., et al.: Parvovirus B19 infection in pediatric transplant patients. Transplantation *56*:835–838, 1993.
198. Nunoue, T., Koike, T., Koike, R., et al.: Infection with human parvovirus B19 aplasia of the bone marrow and a rash in hereditary spherocytosis. J. Infect. *14*:67–70, 1987.
199. Okumura, A., and Ichikawa, T.: Aseptic meningitis caused by human parvovirus B19. Arch. Dis. Child. *68*:784–785, 1993.
200. Ongradi, J., Becker, K., Horvath, A., et al.: Simultaneous infection by human herpesvirus 7 and human parvovirus B19 in papular-purpuric gloves-and-socks syndrome. Arch. Dermatol. *136*:672, 2000.
201. Ozawa, K., Kurtzman, G., and Young, N.: Replication of the B19 parvovirus in human bone marrow cell cultures. Science *233*:883–886, 1986.
202. Pattison, J. R.: Parvoviruses: Medical and biological aspects. *In* Fields, B. N., and Knipe, D. M. (eds.): Virology. 2nd ed., Vol. 2. New York, Raven Press, 1990, pp. 1765–1782.
203. Paver, W. K., Caul, E. O., Ashley, C. R., et al.: A small virus in human feces. Lancet *1*:664–665, 1973.
204. Paver, W. K., and Clarke, S. K. R.: Comparison of human fecal and serum parvovirus-like viruses. J. Clin. Microbiol. *4*:67–70, 1976.
205. Pellas, F., Olivares, J. P., Zandotti, C., et al.: Neuralgic amyotrophy after parvovirus B19 infection. Lancet *342*:503–504, 1993.
206. Peschgens, T., Merz, U., Steidel, K., et al.: Parvovirus B19–assoziierte myokarditis bei einem 7-monate-alten kind. Padiatr. Grenzgeb. *32*:527–530, 1994.
207. Petrikovsky, B. M., Baker, D., and Schneider, E.: Fetal hydrops secondary to human parvovirus infection in early pregnancy. Prenat. Diagn. *16*:342–344, 1996.
208. Phillips, I. E.: Erythema infectiosum: Outbreak in Bristol, Tennessee-Virginia area. Arch. Dermatol. Syph. *67*:628–629, 1953.
209. Phillips, I. E.: Erythema infectiosum: Clinical and epidemiological observations. South. Med. J. *47*:253–257, 1954.
210. Pillay, D., Patou, G., Griffiths, P. D., et al.: Secondary parvovirus B19 infection in an immunocompromised child. Pediatr. Infect. Dis. J. *10*:623–624, 1991.

211. Pillay, D., Patou, G., Hurt, S., et al.: Parvovirus B19 outbreak in a children's ward. Lancet *339*:107–109, 1992.
212. Plummer, F. A., Hammond, G. W., Forward, K., et al.: An erythema infectiosum–like illness caused by human parvovirus infection. N. Engl. J. Med. *313*:74–79, 1985.
213. Potter, C. G., Potter, A. C., Hatton, C. S. R., et al.: Variation of erythroid and myeloid precursors in the marrow and peripheral blood of volunteer subjects infected with human parvovirus (B19). J. Clin. Invest. *79*:1486–1492, 1987.
214. Pouchot, J., Ouakil, H., Debin, M. L., et al.: Adult Still's disease associated with acute human parvovirus B19 infection. Lancet *341*:1280–1281, 1993.
215. Public Health Laboratory Service Working Party on Fifth Disease: Prospective study of human parvovirus (B19) infection in pregnancy. B. M. J. *300*:1166–1170, 1990.
216. Rao, K. R. P., Patel, A. R., Anderson, M. J., et al.: Infection with a parvovirus-like virus and aplastic crisis in chronic hemolytic anemia. Ann. Intern. Med. *98*:930–932, 1983.
217. Rao, S. P., Miller, S. T., and Cohen, B. J.: Transient aplastic crisis in patients with sickle cell disease. Am. J. Dis. Child. *146*:1328–1330, 1992.
218. Rector, J. M.: Erythema infectiosum: Clinical observations during an epidemic. J. Pediatr. *15*:540–545, 1939.
219. Reid, D. M., Reid, T. M. S., Brown, T., et al.: Human parvovirus-associated arthritis: A clinical and laboratory description. Lancet *2*:422–425, 1985.
220. Reitblat, T., Drogenikov, T., Sigalov, I., et al.: Transient anticardiolipin antibody syndrome in a patient with parvovirus B19 infection. Am. J. Med. *109*:512–513, 2000.
221. Rivier, G., Gerster, J. C., Terrier, P., et al.: Parvovirus B19–associated monoarthritis in a 5-year-old boy. J. Rheumatol. *22*:766–767, 1995.
222. Rodis, J. F., Hovick, T. J., Jr., Quinn, D. L., et al.: Human parvovirus infection in pregnancy. Obstet. Gynecol. *72*:733–738, 1988.
223. Rodis, J. F., Quinn, D. L., Gary, G. W., Jr., et al.: Management and outcomes of pregnancies complicated by human B19 parvovirus infection: A prospective study. Am. J. Obstet. Gynecol. *163*:1168–1171, 1990.
224. Rogers, B. B., Singer, D. B., Mak, S. K., et al.: Detection of human parvovirus B19 in early spontaneous abortuses using serology, histology, electron microscopy, in situ hybridization, and the polymerase chain reaction. Obstet. Gynecol. *81*:402–408, 1993.
225. Saarinen, U. M., Chorba, T. L., Tattersall, P., et al.: Human parvovirus B19–induced epidemic acute red cell aplasia in patients with hereditary hemolytic anemia. Blood *67*:1411–1417, 1986.
226. Sahakian, V., Weiner, C. P., Naides, S. J., et al.: Intrauterine transfusion treatment of nonimmune hydrops fetalis secondary to human parvovirus B19 infection. Am. J. Obstet. Gynecol. *164*:1090–1091, 1991.
227. Saint-Martin, J., Choulot, J. J., Bonnaud, E., et al.: Myocarditis caused by parvovirus. J. Pediatr. *116*:1007–1008, 1990.
228. Salimans, M. M. M., Holsappel, S., van de Rijke, F. M., et al.: Rapid detection of human parvovirus B19 DNA by dot-hybridization and the polymerase chain reaction. J. Virol. Methods *23*:19–28, 1989.
229. Saller, D. N., Rogers, B. B., and Canick, J. A.: Maternal serum biochemical markers in pregnancies with fetal parvovirus B19 infection. Prenat. Diagn. *13*:467–471, 1993.
230. Samii, K., Cassinotti, P., de Freudenreich, J., et al.: Acute bilateral carpal tunnel syndrome associated with human parvovirus B19 infection. Clin. Infect. Dis. *22*:162–164, 1996.
231. Schiff, G., Linnemann, C., Balfour, H., et al.: Challenge study with rubella virus isolated from a patient with erythema infectiosum. Clin. Res. *19*:675, 1971.
232. Schleuning, M., Jager, G., Holler, E., et al.: Human parvovirus B19–associated disease in bone marrow transplantation. Infection *27*:114–117, 1999.
233. Schwarz, T. F., Bruns, R., Schröder, C., et al.: Human parvovirus B19 infection associated with vascular purpura and vasculitis. Infection *17*:170–171, 1989.
234. Schwarz, T. F., Jäger, G., Holzgreve, W., et al.: Diagnosis of human parvovirus B19 infections by polymerase chain reaction. Scand. J. Infect. Dis. *24*:691–696, 1992.
235. Schwarz, T. F., Nerlich, A., Hottentr{umlaut a}ger, B., et al.: Parvovirus B19 infection of the fetus: Histology and in situ hybridization. Am. J. Clin. Pathol. *96*:121–126, 1991.
236. Schwarz, T. F., Roggendorf, M., and Deinhardt, F.: Human parvovirus B19: ELISA and immunoblot assays. J. Virol. Methods *20*:155–168, 1988.
237. Schwarz, T. F., Wiersbitzky, S., and Pambor, M.: Case report: Detection of parvovirus B19 in a skin biopsy of a patient with erythema infectiosum. J. Med. Virol. *43*:171–174, 1994.
238. Semble, E. L., Agudelo, C. A., and Pegram, P. S.: Human parvovirus B19 arthropathy in two adults after contact with childhood erythema infectiosum. Am. J. Med. *83*:560–562, 1987.
239. Serjeant, G. R., Mason, J., Topley, J. M., et al.: Outbreak of aplastic crisis in sickle cell anemia associated with parvovirus-like agent. Lancet *2*:595–597, 1981.
240. Serjeant, G. R., Serjeant, B. E., Thomas, P. W., et al.: Human parvovirus infection in homozygous sickle cell disease. Lancet *341*:1237–1240, 1993.
241. Seyama, K., Kobayashi, R., Hasle, H., et al.: Parvovirus B19–induced anemia as the presenting manifestation of X- linked hyper-IgM syndrome. J. Infect. Dis. *178*:318–324, 1998.
242. Sharma, V. R., Fleming, D. R., and Slone, S. P.: Pure red cell aplasia due to parvovirus B19 in a patient treated with rituximab. Blood *96*: 1184–1186, 2000.
243. Shaw, H. L. K.: Erythema infectiosum. Am. J. Med. Sci. *129*:16–22, 1905.
244. Shneerson, J. M., Mortimer, P. P., and Vandervelde, E. M.: Febrile illness due to a parvovirus. B. M. J. *2*:1580, 1980.
245. Silver, M. M., Hellmann, J., Zielenska, M., et al.: Anemia, blueberry-muffin rash, and hepatomegaly in a newborn infant. J. Pediatr. *128*:579–586, 1996.
246. Smith, E. H.: An epidemic of erythema infectiosum, "the fifth disease." Arch. Pediatr. *46*:456–458, 1929.
247. Smith, P. T., Landry, M. L., Carey, H., et al.: Papular-purpuric gloves and socks syndrome associated with acute parvovirus B19 infection: Case report and review. Clin. Infect. Dis. *27*:164–168, 1998.
248. Smoleniec, J. S., Pillal, M., Caul, E. O., et al.: Subclinical transplacental parvovirus B19 infection: An increased fetal risk? Lancet *343*:1100–1101, 1994.
249. Söderlund, M., Brown, C. S., Cohen, B. J., et al.: Accurate serodiagnosis of B19 parvovirus infections by measurement of IgG avidity. J. Infect. Dis. *171*:710–713, 1995.
250. Söderlund, M., von Essen, R., Haapasaari, J., et al.: Persistence of parvovirus B19 DNA in synovial membranes of young patients with and without chronic arthropathy. Lancet *349*:1063–1065, 1997.
251. Sokal, E. M., Melchior, M., Cornu, C., et al.: Acute parvovirus B19 infection associated with fulminant hepatitis of favourable prognosis in young children. Lancet *352*:1739–1741, 1998.
252. Srivastava, A., Bruno, E., Briddell, R., et al.: Parvovirus B19–induced perturbation of human megakaryocytopoiesis in vitro. Blood *76*:1997–2004, 1990.
253. Srivastava, A., and Lu, L.: Replication of B19 parvovirus in highly enriched hematopoietic progenitor cells from normal human bone marrow. J. Virol. *62*:3059–3063, 1988.
254. Stahl, H. D., Pfeiffer, R., Von Salis-Soglio, G., et al. : Parovirus B19–associated mono- and oligoarticular arthritis may evolve into a chronic inflammatory arthropathy fulfilling criteria for rheumatoid arthritis or spondylarthropathy. Clin. Rheumatol. *19*:510–511, 2000.
255. Stein, A., Berthet, B., and Raoult, D.: Prolonged fever caused by parvovirus B19–induced meningitis: Case report and review. Clin. Infect. Dis. *29*:446–447, 1999.
256. Stricker, G.: Die neue Kindersenche in der Umgebung von Giessen (erythema infectiosum). Z. Prakt. Aerzte *40*:121, 1899.
257. Summers, J., Jones, S. E., and Anderson, M. J.: Characterization of the agent of erythrocyte aplasia as a human parvovirus. J. Gen. Virol. *64*:2527–2532, 1983.
258. Suzuki, N., Terada, S., and Inoue, M.: Neonatal meningitis with human parvovirus B19 infection. Arch. Dis. Child. *73*:196–197, 1995.
259. Tabrizi, S. N., Chen, S., Borg, A. J., et al.: Use of polymerase chain reaction for detection of human parvovirus B19. J. Infect. Dis. *170*: 1047–1048, 1994.
260. Takahashi, T., Ozawa, K., Takahashi, K., et al.: Susceptibility of human erythropoietic cells to B19 parvovirus in vitro increases with differentiation. Blood *75*:603–610, 1990.
261. Takahashi, Y., Murai, C., Shibata, S., et al.: Human parvovirus B19 as a causative agent for rheumatoid arthritis. Proc. Natl. Acad. Sci. U. S. A. *95*:8227–8232, 1998.
262. Tchernia, G., Morinet, F., Congard, B., et al.: Diamond Blackfan anaemia: Apparent relapse due to B19 parvovirus. Eur. J. Pediatr. *152*:209–210, 1993.
263. Tiessen, R. G., van Elsacker-Niele, A. M. W., Vermeij-Keers, C., et al.: A fetus with a parvovirus B19 infection and congenital anomalies. Prenat. Diagn. *14*:173–176, 1994.
264. Tschamer, A.: Ueber ortliche Rotheln. Jahrb. Kinderheilk. *29*:372–374, 1889.
265. Tsuda, H., Maeda, Y., and Nakagawa, K.: Parvovirus B19–related lymphadenopathy. Br. J. Haematol. *85*:631–632, 1993.
266. Tsuda, H., Maeda, Y., Nakagawa, K., et al. : Parvovirus B19–associated haemophagocytic syndrome with prominent neutrophilia. Br. J. Haematol *86*:413–414, 1994.
267. Turton, J., Appleton, H., and Clewley, J. P.: Similarities in nucleotide sequence between serum and faecal human parvovirus DNA. Epidemiol. Infect. *105*:197–201, 1990.
268. Tyndall, A., Jelk, W., and Hirsch, H. H.: Parvovirus B19 and erosive polyarthritis. Lancet *343*:480–481, 1994.
269. Ueno, Y., Umadome, H., Shimodera, M., et al.: Human parvovirus B19 and arthritis. Lancet. *341*:1280, 1993.
270. Uike, N., Miyamura, T., Obama, K., et al.: Parvovirus B19–associated haemophagocytosis in Evans syndrome: Aplastic crisis accompanied by severe thrombocytopenia. Br. J. Haematol. *84*:530–532, 1993.
271. Valeur-Jensen, A. K., Pedersen, C. B., Westergaard, T., et al.: Risk factors for parvovirus B19 infection in pregnancy. J. A. M. A. *281*:1099–1105, 1999.

272. van Elsacker-Niele, A. M. W., Salimans, M. M. M., Weiland, H. T., et al.: Fetal pathology in human parvovirus B19 infection. Br. J. Obstet. Gynaecol. *96*:768–775, 1989.
273. Veraldi, S., Mancuso, R. Rizzitelli, G., et al.: Henoch-Schönlein syndrome associated with human parvovirus B19 primary infection. Eur. J. Dermatol. *9*:232–233, 1999.
274. Viguier, M., Guillevin, L., and Laroche, L.: Treatment of parvovirus B19–associated polyarteritis nodosa with intravenous immune globulin. N. Engl. J. Med. *344*:1481–1482, 2001.
275. von Poblotzki, A., Gerdes, C., Reischl, U., et al., Lymphoproliferative responses after infection with human parvovirus B19. J. Virol. *70*:7327–7330, 1996.
276. von Poblotzki, A., Hemauer, A., Gigler, A., et al.: Antibodies to the nonstructural protein of parvovirus B19 in persistently infected patients: Implications for pathogenesis. J. Infect. Dis. *172*:1356–1359, 1995.
277. Wadlington, W. B.: Erythema infectiosum: Report of an epidemic. J. Tenn. St. Med. Assoc. *50*:1–5, 1957.
278. Wadlington, W. B.: Erythema infectiosum. J. A. M. A. *192*:58–60, 1965.
279. Wadlington, W. B.: Erythema infectiosum (fifth disease). Am. J. Dis. Child. *110*:443–444, 1965.
280. Wadlington, W. B., and Riley, H. D., Jr.: Arthritis and hemolytic anemia following erythema infectiosum. J. A. M. A. *203*:473–475, 1968.
281. Wang, Q. Y., and Erdman, D. D.: Development and evaluation of capture immunoglobulin G and M hemadherence assays by using human type O erythrocytes and recombinant parvovirus B19 antigen. J. Clin. Microbiol. *33*:2466–2467, 1995.
282. Wardeh, A. and Marik, P.: Acute lung injury due to parvovirus pneumonia. J. Intern. Med. *244*:257–260, 1998.
283. Watanabe, M., Shimamoto, Y., Yamaguchi, M., et al.: Viral-associated haemophagocytosis and elevated serum TNF-alpha with parvovirus-B19–related pancytopenia in patients with hereditary spherocytosis. Clin. Lab. Haematol. *16*:179–182, 1994.
284. Weiland, H. T., Vermey-Keers, C., Salimans, M. M. M., et al.: Parvovirus B19 associated with fetal abnormality. Lancet *1*:682–683, 1987.
285. Werner, G. H., Brachman, P. S., Ketler, A., et al.: A new viral agent associated with erythema infectiosum. Ann. N. Y. Acad. Sci. *67*:338–345, 1956–1957.
286. White, D. G., Woolf, A. D., Mortimer, P. P., et al.: Human parvovirus arthropathy. Lancet *2*:419–421, 1985.
287. Wierenga, K. J., Pattison, J. R., Brink, N., et al.: Glomerulonephritis after human parvovirus infection in homozygous sickle-cell disease. Lancet *346*:475–476, 1995.
288. Wilcox, K. R., and Evans, A. S.: Erythema infectiosum: Report of an outbreak in Marshfield, Wisconsin. Wis. Med. J., March 1958.
289. Willekes, C., Roumen, F. J. M. E., Van Elsacker-Niele, A. M. W., et al.: Human parvovirus B19 infection and unbalanced translocation in a case of hydrops fetalis. Prenat. Diagn. *14*:181–185, 1994.
290. Woernle, C. H., Anderson, L. J., Tattersall, P., et al.: Human parvovirus B19 infection during pregnancy. J. Infect. Dis. *156*:17–20, 1987.
291. Yaegashi, N., Okamura, K., Tsunoda, A., et al.: A study by means of a new assay of the relationship between an outbreak of erythema infectiosum and non-immune hydrops fetalis caused by human parvovirus B19. J. Infect. *31*:195–200, 1995.
292. Yee, T. T., Cohen, B. J., Pasi, K. J., et al.: Transmission of symptomatic parvovirus B19 infection by clotting factor concentrate. Br. J. Haematol. *93*:457–459, 1996.
293. Yoto, Y., Kudoh, T., Haseyama, K., et al.: Human parvovirus B19 infection associated with acute hepatitis. Lancet *347*:868–869, 1996.
294. Yoto, Y., Kudoh, T., Suzuki, N., et al.: Retrospective study on the influence of human parvovirus B19 infection among children with malignant diseases. Acta Haematol. *90*:8–12, 1993.
295. Yoto, Y., Kudoh, T., Suzuki, N., et al.: Thrombocytopenia induced by human parvovirus B19 infections. Eur. J. Haematol. *50*:255–257, 1993.
296. Young, N.: Hematologic and hematopoietic consequences of B19 parvovirus infection. Semin. Hematol. *25*:159–172, 1988.
297. Young, N. S., Mortimer, P. P., Moore, J. G., et al.: Characterization of a virus that causes transient aplastic crisis. J. Clin. Invest. *73*:224–230, 1984.
298. Yufu, Y., Matsumoto, M., Miyamura, T., et al.: Parvovirus B19–associated haemophagocytic syndrome with lymphadenopathy resembling histiocytic necrotizing lymphadenitis (Kikuchi's disease). Br. J. Haematol. *96*:868–871, 1997.
299. Zachoval, R., Kroener, M., Brommer, M., et al.: Numbness and tingling of fingers associated with parvovirus B19 infection. J. Infect. Dis. *161*:354–355, 1990.
300. Zahorsky, J.: An epidemic of erythema infectiosum. Am. J. Dis. Child. *28*:261–262, 1924.
301. Zerbini, M., Gibellini, D., Musiani, M., et al.: Automated detection of digoxigenin-labelled B19 parvovirus amplicons by a capture hybridization assay. J. Virol. Methods *55*:1–9, 1995.
302. Zerbini, M., Musiani, M., Gentilomi, G., et al.: Symptomatic parvovirus B19 infection of one fetus in a twin pregnancy. Clin. Infect. Dis. *17*:262–263, 1993.
303. Zuckerman, S. N.: Erythema infectiosum, with report of an epidemic in San Francisco. Arch. Pediatr. *57*:168–176, 1940.

SUBSECTION **2**

PAPILLOVIRIDAE

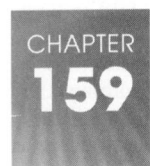

Human Polyomaviruses and Papillomaviruses

JOHN A. VANCHIERE ■ GAIL J. DEMMLER

Until 2000, the polyomaviruses and papillomaviruses made up the virus family *Papovaviridae,* defined as small viruses containing double-stranded DNA that replicate in the nucleus of infected cells and share the ability to cause malignant transformation of a variety of cell types. They are now classified into two distinct families, *Polyomaviridae* and *Papillomaviridae.* Human polyomaviruses are 45 nm in diameter with a genome approximately 5200 base pairs in length; papillomaviruses are somewhat larger, 55 nm in diameter with a genome approximately 8000 base pairs in length. The genomic organization of the polyomaviruses and papillomaviruses differs in that polyomaviruses use both DNA strands to encode proteins whereas papillomaviruses use just one DNA strand. Viruses in both families cause infection in immunocompetent and immunodeficient hosts and also have been associated with malignancies.

Human Polyomaviruses

The human polyomaviruses, JC virus (JCV) and BK virus (BKV), and the simian virus 40 (SV40), which is also able to infect humans, represent a unique group of viruses that generally have been thought to cause disease rarely and only in immunocompromised patients. However, a growing body of evidence supports the idea that these ubiquitous agents may be associated with disease in immunocompetent patients. Polyomaviruses derive their name from "poly," meaning many, and "oma," which refers to their ability to induce tumors. Their colorful history and critical role in the elucidation of fundamental cellular and molecular pathways render them important tools from a research point of view. The recent finding of polyomaviruses associated with several human cancers and renal disease has brought them to the foreground of clinical medicine, but relatively little is known of their potential to cause disease. Our knowledge of the role of polyomaviruses in human disease is growing because of technologic advances in molecular biology, and the next decade will probably establish clinically important associations involving these viruses.

HISTORY

The recognition of progressive multifocal leukoencephalopathy (PML) as a clinical entity in 1958 marks the beginning of our knowledge of the human polyomaviruses.[11] Edward P. Richardson, Jr., a neuropathologist at Massachusetts General Hospital in Boston, and his colleagues described three cases of progressive neurologic disease in patients receiving chemotherapy for leukemia. At autopsy, they found many foci of demyelination, including oligodendrocytes with intranuclear inclusions and astrocytes that were enlarged with bizarre nuclear changes.[11] Richardson subsequently reported a larger series of PML cases and proposed a viral etiology associated with immune suppression.[224] In 1965, papovavirus-like particles were observed by electron microscopy of brain tissue from patients with PML, and in 1971, JCV, the etiologic agent of PML, was isolated from primary human fetal glial cell cultures that had been inoculated with a brain extract from a patient with PML.[196, 310] In the same year, another human polyomavirus, BKV, was cultivated from the urine of a renal transplant patient.[87] Each virus was named with the initials of the patient from whom it was isolated.

SV40, the prototype polyomavirus, was isolated in 1960 by Sweet and Hilleman as a contaminant of secondary rhesus monkey kidney cell cultures that were used to produce early polio vaccines.[274] Additionally, several early adenovirus vaccines and a respiratory syncytial virus vaccine were contaminated with SV40.[140, 171] Interestingly, although rhesus monkey kidney cells showed no cytopathic effect, when supernatants from vaccine cultures were used to inoculate green monkey kidney cells, a pronounced cytopathic effect was observed, thus giving rise to the original name of SV40, vacuolating virus. By that time, millions of doses of both live and killed preparations of polio vaccine containing SV40 had been given to humans in the United States and Europe. Soon after its identification, the demonstration that SV40 induced tumors in neonatal rodents prompted great concern about its potential effects in humans.[91] Serologic studies showed that the formaldehyde-inactivated (Salk or IPV) poliovirus vaccine, but not the live attenuated (Sabin or OPV) poliovirus vaccine, induced high-titer, SV40-specific antibody responses.[89] Although the OPV preparations contained higher titers of infectious SV40 virus, they failed to induce virus-specific antibodies in vaccinees despite prolonged shedding in stool.[167] A 30-year follow-up of infants inadvertently exposed to SV40 between 1955 and 1962 via an OPV preparation showed no excess risk of cancer.[268] Since the 1960s, the mechanism of SV40-induced tumorigenesis has been intensely studied, and as a result of SV40-related research, we have knowledge of many facets of cell and molecular biology, including transcriptional regulation, alternative splicing, eukaryotic DNA replication, tumor suppressor proteins, nuclear localization signals, and viral effects on cell cycle control.[50]

VIROLOGY

Polyomaviruses are classified in the family *Polyomaviridae*. Twelve polyomaviruses are known, each with a limited host range in which one or several closely related species are infected.[250, 139] JCV and BKV infect only humans, and SV40 infects both humans and monkeys. The nucleotide sequence of JCV has 75 percent overall homology with BKV and 69 percent homology with SV40.[304]

The polyomavirus genome can be divided into structural, nonstructural, and regulatory regions. The structural (late) region of the viral genome encodes VP1, VP2, and VP3, the capsid proteins that envelop the viral genome. VP1 is the major capsid protein and accounts for more than 70 percent of the virion mass; it participates in host-cell recognition and stimulation of the host immune response. VP2 and VP3 are smaller, less abundant capsid proteins. The nonstructural (early) region of the polyomavirus genome encodes the large T antigen, the best studied of the polyomavirus proteins; this antigen initiates viral DNA replication, stimulates cellular entry into S phase, and influences cellular and viral transcription. The small t antigen is produced by alternative splicing of the early viral mRNA and promotes G_1 cell cycle progression; it is not required for viral growth in cultured cells. The large T antigen of SV40 is responsible for the transformation of cells in vivo and in vitro, although small t antigen appears to be required under certain growth conditions. Large T antigen is a multifunctional protein that contains binding sites for the cellular pRb and p53 proteins. By binding to pRb, the large T antigen allows E2F-mediated progression of the cell cycle, thus providing the right environment for replication of viral DNA, and through its association with p53, a cellular tumor suppressor protein, the large T antigen blocks p53-induced cellular gene expression, thereby leading to genomic instability and survival of damaged cells.[34] The large T antigens of JCV and BKV, similarly, can interact with a variety of cellular proteins, including the p53 and pRb family proteins.[111] The regulatory region of the polyomavirus genome contains both the origin of replication and the viral promoter. The origin is recognized by the large T antigen, in concert with host-cell factors, including cellular DNA polymerase, and viral DNA replication is initiated. Both early and late viral transcription is mediated by cellular RNA polymerase. T-antigen binding to viral DNA autoregulates the production of early mRNA and, by interaction with cellular factors, stimulates late transcription. Polyomaviruses have either an archetypal (single enhancer) or rearranged (complex) regulatory region that may influence the ability of a particular strain to cause disease by virtue of its effect on replication efficiency.[37, 111]

EPIDEMIOLOGY

Serologic data, screening of environmental samples, and the worldwide distribution of PML cases among immune-suppressed individuals suggest that human polyomaviruses are endemic throughout the world[25, 75, 195] (Fig. 159–1). The prevalence of antibodies against polyomaviruses increases with age, beginning in early childhood. BKV seroconversion

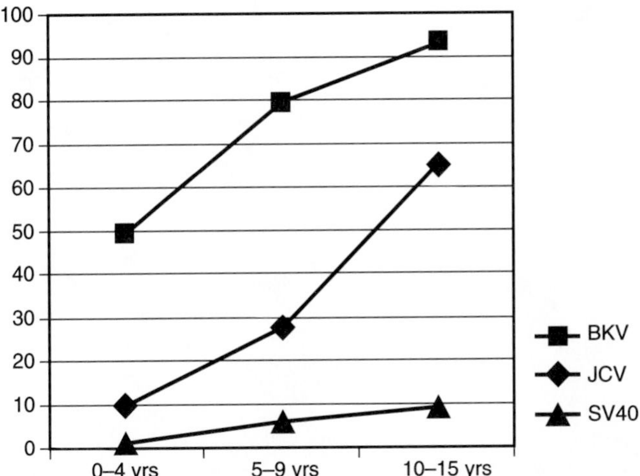

FIGURE 159–1 ■ Seroprevalence estimates for JC virus (◆), BK virus (■), and SV40 (▲) in childhood. (Data from Lednicky, J. A., and Butel, J. S.: Polyomaviruses and human tumors: A brief review of current concepts and interpretations. Front. Biosci. *4*:D153–D164, 1999.)

occurs in 50 percent of children by the time they reach the age of 3 to 4 years, and JCV antibodies are acquired by 50 percent of children by the age of 10 to 14 years.[195, 250] The prevalence of antibodies in humans directed against SV40 has not been studied well; one study observed that the presence of antibody increased with age, with approximately 10 percent of the population being seropositive for SV40 by young adulthood.[36] Population-based seroprevalence data suggest that more than 80 percent of adults have been infected with JCV, BKV, or both viruses.[74, 195, 208, 250] BKV seroconversion has been associated with mild upper respiratory tract illnesses in children, and BKV viruria has been reported in a child with acute tonsillitis.[93, 94, 273]

Humans are the only known reservoir for JCV and BKV, whereas SV40 primarily is a simian virus that has crossed species from monkeys to humans. Polyomaviruses persist in the kidney and, to a lesser degree, in B lymphocytes and oligodendrocytes in both humans (JCV and BKV) and monkeys (SV40).[61, 63, 133, 183] The exact mechanism of transmission of JCV and BKV is not known, but they are suspected of being acquired by the respiratory route, perhaps after being excreted in urine.[111] SV40 was introduced inadvertently into humans as a contaminant of early polio vaccines; however, such direct exposure cannot account for the SV40 seropositivity in children born more recently than 1962, thus suggesting modern human-to-human spread of the virus. In the pediatric population, a recent SV40 seroprevalence survey found nearly 6 percent of hospitalized children with antibodies to SV40.[36] Among kidney transplant patients in the cohort, 40 percent had evidence of SV40 infection, but whether such infection was related to immunosuppressive medications or the underlying kidney disease was not clear.[36]

In immunocompetent individuals, persistence of JCV and BKV in the kidney apparently is asymptomatic, with intermittent shedding of JCV in urine more frequently than BKV.[2, 249] Viral DNA (JCV or BKV) can be found in 30 to 50 percent of kidney samples from immunocompetent adults taken at surgery or autopsy, and JCV or BKV is excreted in the urine of approximately 20 percent of healthy adults.[43, 107, 285] The frequency of polyomavirus excretion in urine varies with age, being more common in older adults.

JCV also is lymphotropic, and the finding of JCV in plasma and peripheral blood mononuclear cells generally correlates with immune status in that it is noted less frequently in immunocompetent patients and increases in frequency in human immunodeficiency virus (HIV)-infected patients with lower CD4 counts.[56, 84, 126] An SV40 seroprevalence study in HIV-infected patients found no difference between patients and age-matched HIV-uninfected controls,[113] thus implying that SV40 infection may not be related to immune status. Several conditions, including pregnancy and systemic lupus erythematosus, are associated with excretion of BKV or JCV in urine.[159, 272, 278, 279] The immunologic and virologic factors regulating initiation and maintenance of persistence are unknown.

CLINICAL MANIFESTATIONS

Central Nervous System Manifestations

PML is a clinical syndrome characterized by progressive neurologic impairment in immunocompromised patients. In PML, the host immune system fails to maintain viral latency; JCV replicates in and lyses oligodendroglia and causes destruction of cerebral white matter in a multifocal or patchy distribution. PML is the sentinel acquired immunodeficiency syndrome (AIDS)–defining illness in approximately 5 percent of adults, and its incidence in HIV-infected adults may be greater than 25 percent.[17] PML occurs less commonly in HIV-infected children than in adults. Other immunosuppressed individuals who are at high risk for PML include patients receiving chemotherapy, solid organ or bone marrow transplant (BMT) recipients, and those with primary T-cell defects.

Clinical manifestations of PML can include behavior changes; blindness, deafness, and other cranial nerve dysfunctions; motor and cognitive deficits; and incoordination as a result of cerebellar involvement.[18] The onset of symptoms usually is insidious, and associated systemic signs such as fever and headache are uncommon. Progression of symptoms occurs over a period of several weeks to months, and the condition is inevitably fatal. The diagnosis of PML is largely clinical and based on the history, physical examination, and characteristic findings on neuroimaging studies. Computed tomography and magnetic resonance imaging of the brain show focal demyelination and white matter edema with relative sparing of the gray matter. The magnetic resonance image of a child with AIDS and PML is shown in Figure 159–2.[173] Cerebrospinal fluid (CSF) analysis usually is normal in patients with PML, probably partly a result of impairment or depletion (or both) of T lymphocytes.[18] BKV also has been associated with neurologic dysfunction in AIDS patients, though much less frequently than has JCV.[31, 289] In addition, BKV encephalitis has been reported in a patient without known immunodeficiency in association with polyomavirus seroconversion.[297]

Renal Manifestations

Polyomaviruria is a common occurrence in immunocompetent adults and may be so in children as well. Hemorrhagic cystitis related to BKV viruria has been reported in several non-immunosuppressed children, but no other nonmalignant diseases have been linked to polyomavirus infection in immunocompetent children.[235] Urinary excretion of BKV occurs in about a third of renal transplant and BMT patients, and BK viremia also may be present.[156] Post-transplant polyomaviruria is due predominantly to reactivation of latent infection and occurs more commonly in patients who receive organs from a seropositive donor. Excretion of BKV usually occurs in the first 2 to 3 months after transplantation. In

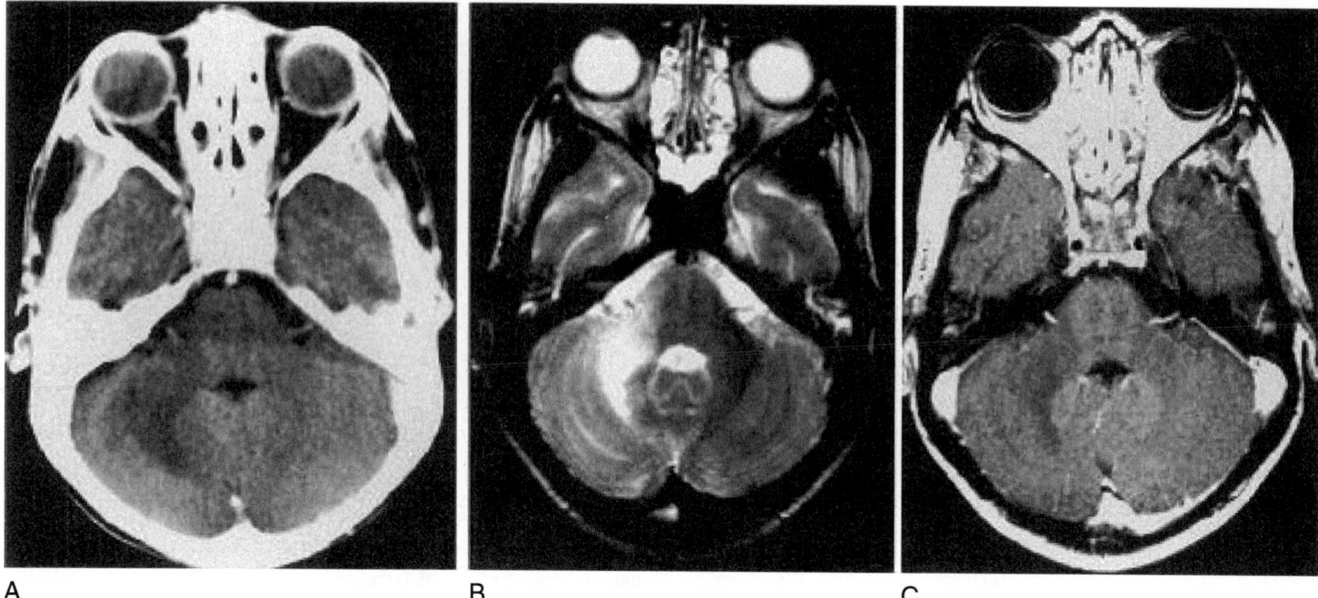

FIGURE 159–2 ■ *A,* Contrast-enhanced brain computed tomogram of a child with progressive multifocal leukoencephalopathy showing low-density, nonenhancing right-sided cerebellar white matter lesion without a mass effect. *B,* On T2-weighted magnetic resonance imaging (MRI), the lesion produces high signal without a mass effect or edema. *C,* The lesion gives low signal on T1-weighted MRI and fails to enhance with intravenous contrast. (From Morriss, M. C., Rutstein, R. M., Rudy, B., et al.: Progressive multifocal leukoencephalopathy in an HIV-infected child. Neuroradiology *39*:142–144, 1997.)

renal transplant recipients, BKV viruria is associated with ureteral ulceration and stenosis, sometimes requiring surgical intervention to prevent or relieve obstructive nephropathy. The prognostic significance of polyomaviruses in renal transplant patients has become a topic of great interest as managing immunosuppression to balance allograft rejection and infectious complications has become more sophisticated. A large serologic study of JCV and BKV infection after renal transplantation found no association with adverse outcomes, and a more recent analysis failed to relate polyomaviruria in kidney transplant recipients with rejection episodes.[4, 210] However, recent case reports linking polyomavirus infection and allograft failure have re-opened the issue.[199, 214] In one case series of biopsy-proven interstitial nephritis in adult renal allograft recipients, 19 of 22 patients had increased serum creatinine at 11.5 ± 13.0 months post-transplant.[214] Allograft biopsy to exclude acute rejection and drug toxicity was performed. Intranuclear viral inclusions and mononuclear inflammatory infiltrates were common histopathologic findings. Antirejection therapy was associated with graft loss in 8 of 12 patients, whereas a reduction in immunosuppression was associated with graft survival and clearance of viruria in 3 of 6 patients. A smaller study in Europe had similar findings.[184] Prospective studies of polyomaviruria and allograft biopsy findings have not been completed in children or adults, and care should be exercised in attributing renal allograft dysfunction to polyomaviruses because both cytomegalovirus (CMV) and adenovirus infections, as well as rejection and drug toxicity, can produce similar findings.

Polyomaviruria, especially that involving BKV, is a common finding in adult BMT recipients; it occurred in over half the patients in several studies and usually appears 2 to 8 weeks after transplantation.[7, 10, 248] The same researchers have linked BKV viruria with hemorrhagic cystitis in BMT recipients.[7, 9, 223] The temporal relationship of BKV infection in comparison to other viral infections after BMT is shown in Figure 159–3.

Interstitial nephritis caused by BKV has been described in children with various immune deficiencies, including hyper-IgM immunodeficiency and AIDS.[53, 227] Renal dysfunction is a common finding in AIDS patients, but its etiology has not been linked to polyomaviruses as it has in monkeys concurrently infected with simian immunodeficiency virus and SV40.[254] Several studies of Balkan endemic nephropathy have associated this enigmatic disease in Eastern Europe with polyomaviruses, but further study is needed to establish

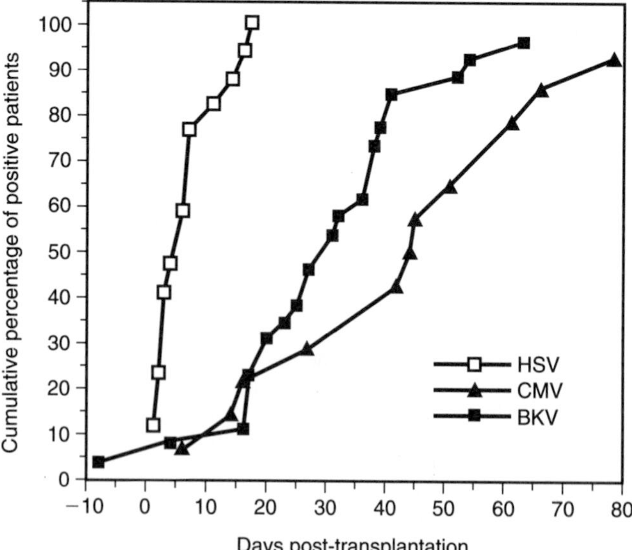

FIGURE 159–3 ■ Cumulative percentages of bone marrow transplant recipients positive for BK virus (■; $n = 26$), herpes simplex virus (□; $n = 22$), and cytomegalovirus (▲; $n = 14$) by the first day of detection. (From Arthur, R. R., Shah, K. V., Charache, P., et al.: BK and JC virus infections in recipients of bone marrow transplants. J. Infect. Dis. *158*:563–569, 1988.)

a causal link.[181, 267] One large pediatric study observed an association between SV40 seropositivity and renal transplantation and detected SV40 sequences in renal biopsy specimens, thus suggesting a possible (but still unproven) role for SV40 in pediatric renal disease.[35, 36]

Other Manifestations

In spite of the contention that polyomaviruses are transmitted primarily in respiratory secretions, little evidence has indicated that such transmission is accompanied by clinical disease of the respiratory tract. Several case reports of BKV-associated pulmonary disease have been published, uniformly in the setting of severe immunosuppression and with poor outcomes.[53, 236, 289] Interstitial pneumonitis in a patient with severe immune compromise should raise the suspicion of the possibility of polyomavirus-associated disease, but other viral pathogens such as CMV and adenovirus should be considered first.

BKV-associated retinal necrosis in an AIDS-infected patient has been described, as have elevated hepatic transaminase levels in association with BKV viruria and detection of BKV in normal liver specimens.[31, 106, 125, 192] The clinical significance of these manifestations is unknown.

Malignancies

The polyomaviruses are named for their ability to induce tumors in laboratory animals. Their association with human tumors was noted first in 1974 when Soriano and colleagues isolated SV40 from a metastatic malignant melanoma in a patient with SV40 neutralizing antibodies.[259] SV40 T antigen and capsid antigen were detected in lung, liver, and muscle metastases of the patient, but not in normal tissue.[259] Since that time, polyomaviruses have been linked to a variety of neoplasms in humans, frequently analogous to the tumor types produced in rodents. SV40 T antigen or DNA has been detected in a significant number of meningiomas, ependymomas, choroid plexus tumors, astrocytomas, pleural mesotheliomas, and osteosarcomas.[8, 115] Several recent studies have reported the presence of SV40 in non-Hodgkin lymphomas.[162, 225, 295] In the case of pleural mesotheliomas, which also have been associated with asbestos exposure, the presence of SV40 has been shown to be a negative prognostic indicator.[211] Perhaps the viral infection is acting as a cofactor, along with the carcinogen asbestos, in leading to an adverse outcome. In one study, JCV DNA was found in 11 of 23 pediatric medulloblastomas, and JCV T antigen was detected by immunohistochemistry in 4 of 16 samples tested.[130] JCV has recently been detected in colorectal cancers and in normal tissue samples from the human gastrointestinal tract.[134, 222] The significance of these findings is unclear at the present time, but of note is that SV40 has been detected in association with human cancers much more frequently than have JCV and BKV. A study of bone marrow aspirates and white blood cells from pediatric patients with leukemia failed to find evidence of polyomaviruses.[257]

LABORATORY DIAGNOSIS

Even though the presumptive diagnosis of polyomavirus infection primarily is a clinical one, some laboratory techniques can be helpful in making the diagnosis in the proper clinical circumstances. Serologic tests and viral culture are of little use clinically because these tests are laborious and rarely available. Polyomaviruses in urine could be considered normal flora, much like CMV detected in urine after infancy. Histologic study of urinary sediment can reveal "decoy cells," or uroepithelial cells with characteristic polyomavirus inclusions, which is presumptive evidence of polyomavirus-associated nephritis in renal transplant patients.[76] Detection of specific polyomavirus DNA from urine samples is of little significance, whereas polymerase chain reaction (PCR) detection from blood samples may correlate with nephritis.[185] Suspicious histologic changes in biopsy material should be confirmed with a polyomavirus-specific test, either PCR or immunohistochemistry, because polyomavirus-associated changes are difficult to distinguish from acute rejection and CMV-associated disease.

Detection of JCV DNA in CSF by PCR is the diagnostic test of choice for suspected PML.[104, 126, 239, 282] In adult patients with AIDS and neurologic symptoms, PCR amplification of JCV DNA from CSF is 99 percent predictive of PML, whereas brain biopsy has a slightly lower sensitivity.[57] On gross examination, tissue typical of PML has been described as "worm-eaten," and microscopic examination reveals multiple foci of demyelination with enlarged oligodendroglia, giant astrocytes, and an intense phagocytic infiltration.[292] Immunohistochemical techniques and other nucleic acid detection methods also can be used to confirm the diagnosis of PML.[120] JC viremia is a general indicator of immune suppression and is a common finding in HIV-infected patients without PML.[126]

TREATMENT AND PREVENTION

At the present time, no specific antiviral agents are available for the treatment of polyomavirus disease or polyomavirus-associated tumors. Gentle reduction of immune suppression is indicated in renal transplant patients with proven, symptomatic polyomavirus disease because such reduction may allow the host immune system to restore viral latency. In HIV-infected patients, initiation of highly active antiretroviral therapy (HAART) can help alleviate the symptoms of PML.[65, 209, 283] Despite administration of HAART, PML still will develop in some HIV-infected patients.[280] This phenomenon may be related to incomplete immune reconstitution, especially in adults. Cidofovir has been used successfully in conjunction with HAART in patients with AIDS and PML, but its benefit above that of HAART and in non-AIDS patients has not been determined.[168, 234] Given the ubiquity and generally benign nature of polyomavirus infections, as well as the paucity of information about the nature of their transmission and clinical significance, specific efforts to prevent polyomavirus transmission are not indicated at this time.

Human Papillomaviruses

The human papillomaviruses (HPVs) are responsible for a variety of benign, yet bothersome cutaneous proliferations, including common skin warts. However, HPVs also have been associated with serious, even life-threatening illnesses, including genitourinary cancer and respiratory papillomatosis. Our current understanding of the complex role that HPVs play in these diverse clinical conditions remains incomplete, and management of these diseases remains an ongoing challenge.

HISTORY

Warts or papillomas have been recognized for centuries to occur at a variety of different body sites, including the skin, genital tract, oral cavity, conjunctiva, and respiratory tract. Their infectious nature has been suspected by clinicians for many decades and has been the product of much folklore. The viral etiology of warts was discovered scientifically, however, in 1907, when human volunteers were inoculated experimentally with a cell-free extract prepared from wart tissue.[47] These early experiments also suggested that warts could be transmitted from person to person. When electron microscopy became available in the 1940s, virus particles were visualized within many of these clinical sites, initially in skin warts and subsequently in genital warts, thereby confirming the viral etiology of these lesions. However, despite the abundance of virus particles seen in some lesions such as skin warts, virologic investigation of the disease processes was hampered by the inability to propagate papillomaviruses in cell culture or laboratory animals. The limited amount of information available from the study of virus particles obtained directly from wart tissue led to speculation, in the 1960s, that HPVs were composed of a single virus type. Scientists further theorized that the specific body site and epithelium involved, rather than the virus type, were responsible for the characteristic morphology and disease process.[229] With the advent of molecular biologic techniques in the 1970s, however, more than 70 different types of HPV were recognized, and researchers quickly recognized that specific clinical diseases were associated with infection with specific HPV types. Most recently, HPV infection of the genital tract has emerged as one of the most prevalent sexually transmitted infections, and the link to some squamous cell carcinomas of the cervix has been strengthened. In addition, at least two mucosal HPV types appear to produce respiratory papillomatosis in pediatric patients. Finally, the role of some cutaneous HPV types in the evolution of squamous cell carcinoma from wart lesions in patients with epidermodysplasia verruciformis (EV) recently has been elucidated. Challenges for the future revolve around developing effective treatment strategies because current measures are palliative, at best, and most lesions recur. New antiviral chemotherapeutic agents are being developed, and immunomodulators such as interferon provide promise for the treatment of serious disease caused by HPVs.

TABLE 159–1 ■ MAJOR HUMAN PAPILLOMAVIRUS GENES

Gene	Protein Products and Function
Early (E) Region	
E1	Viral regulatory protein that initiates viral DNA replication
E2	Viral regulatory protein that controls replication and inhibits or activates early transcription of the viral genome
E3	Unknown
E4	A late viral protein that controls viral maturation; expressed in terminally differentiated keratinocytes
E5	Major transforming protein; causes cellular proliferation
E6	Major transforming oncoprotein; associates with the cellular target, p53, a tumor suppressor protein, and promotes its proteolytic degradation; causes cellular proliferation and perturbation of keratinocyte differentiation
E7	Major transforming protein; associates with the cellular target pRB and inactivates its cell cycle restriction function; causes cellular proliferation and perturbation of keratinocyte differentiation
E8	Unknown; ? regulates viral DNA replication
Late (L) Region	
L1	Major structural viral capsid protein
L2	Minor structural viral capsid protein

VIROLOGY

The family *Papillomaviridae* contains the HPVs, which are small, nonenveloped viruses with a diameter of about 55 nm. They have a capsid composed of 72 capsomers arranged in icosahedral symmetry and a genome composed of double-stranded circular DNA that is approximately 8 kb in length. The complete nucleotide sequence is available for some HPVs, and partial information is available for all HPV types. The genome is divided into three regions—early, late, and regulatory—and many nucleotide sequences are shared between types. The early region is approximately 4.5 kb in length, contains eight open-reading frames (E1 to E8), and encodes genes that produce the proteins required for viral DNA replication and cellular transformation (Table 159–1). The late region is approximately 2.5 kb in length, contains two open-reading frames (L1 and L2), and codes for major and minor capsid structural proteins. The regulatory or long control region is located between the early and late regions. It is approximately 1 kb in length and contains the origin of replication and many control elements for viral transcription and replication.[204] The virus appears to replicate solely in the nucleus of the cell in association with low-molecular-weight histones. Because the HPV genome codes for only 10 proteins, it does not have a viral protease, DNA polymerase, or other enzymes involved in nucleotide metabolism and, therefore, requires many host-cell enzymes and cellular differentiation factors to complete its viral replicative life cycle.

The life cycle of HPVs is integrated intimately with the life cycle and maturation of epithelial cells. Initial virus infection probably occurs in the basal keratinocyte, with early transcription of the viral genome regulated by the E2 protein. Cellular proliferation and perturbation of keratinocyte differentiation then are induced by the E6 and E7 proteins. The cells are stimulated in the S phase of the cell cycle, and host enzymes for DNA synthesis are used by the virus to complete viral DNA replication. After double-stranded DNA is produced, L1 and L2, the major and minor capsid proteins, and E4, a late-associated structural protein whose gene is located in the early region of the genome, are synthesized. During the final stages of cellular keratinocyte differentiation, the final stages of virus production also occur with the assembly of complete viral particles. However, progeny viruses are not released until dead keratinocytes are sloughed from the epithelial surface.

Papillomaviruses display a high degree of species, tissue, and cellular specificity. HPVs appear to infect only humans, and most animal papillomaviruses also do not infect other species. In addition, they primarily infect the surface squamous epithelium of the skin or mucosa, and specific viral types appear to have a preference for either skin or mucosa, as well as for specific body sites. However, some HPV types recently have been detected in transitional and cuboidal epithelium in the anogenital tract. More than 70 types of HPV have been recognized by DNA homology studies, and they fall naturally into two main groups: cutaneous and mucosal (Table 159–2). The cutaneous HPVs contain types from a variety of benign skin warts, as well as more than 15 types recovered from a small group of patients with a rare

TABLE 159–2 ■ HUMAN PAPILLOMAVIRUS TYPES AND ASSOCIATED CLINICAL CONDITIONS

Condition	Usual Location	Morphology	HPV Type
Cutaneous (Skin) Warts			
Common (verruca vulgaris)	Hands, lips, extremities	Multiple, dome shaped	2, 4
Plantar (verruca plantaris)	Bottom of feet	Single, painful	1
Flat (verruca plana)	Arms, face, knees	Multiple	3, 10, 28, 41
Filiform	Face, neck	Multiple, thread-like	2, 4
Mosaic	Feet, hands	Multiple, superficial	7
Butcher's	Hands	Multiple, dome shaped	7
Epidermodysplasia verruciformis	Face, trunk, extremities	Multiple flat warts or reddish-brown plaques	5, 8, 9, 12, 14, 15, 17, 19–25, 36–38, 47, 49
Immunosuppressed patients	Face, trunk, extremities	Dome-shaped or epidermodysplasia verruciformis-like plaques; may be persistent or progressive	1–5, 8, 10, 20, 23, 28, 49
Mucosal (Anogenital) Warts			
Subclinical	Cervix	Asymptomatic	6, 11, 13, 16, 18, 30–35, 39, 40, 42–45, 51–59
Condylomata acuminata	Cervix, vulva, urethra, anus, penis, scrotum	Multiple exophytic, pink, gray	6, 11, 16
Flat condylomata	Cervix	Asymptomatic, flat plaques	6, 11, 16, 18, 31
Giant condylomata acuminata (Buschke-Löwenstein tumors)	Perirectal area	Large, tumor-like	6, 11
Bowenoid papulosis	Penis, vulva, perirectal area	Multiple, large	16
Cervical cancer	Cervix	Asymptomatic; pigmented papillomas; erythematous or white plaques; ulcerations; mass lesion	Strong association: 16, 18, 31, 45 Moderate association: 30, 33, 35, 39, 51, 52, 56, 58, 59, 68 Weak association: 6, 11, 26, 34, 40, 43, 44, 53–55, 57, 62, 66, 74
Vulvar cancer	Vulva	Asymptomatic; pigmented papillomas; erythematous or white plaques; ulcerations; mass lesion	16
Penile cancer	Penis	Painless, ulcerative mass lesion	16
Anal cancer	Perianal area, anal canal	Asymptomatic; pigmented papillomas; erythematous or white plaques; ulcerations; mass lesion	16, 18, 31
Ovarian cancer	Ovaries	Unknown	6?, 16?, 18?
Mucosal (Other) Warts			
Respiratory papillomatosis	Larynx, trachea, bronchi, lungs	Multiple papillomas	6, 11
Nasal and paranasal papillomas	Nose, paranasal sinuses	Single or multiple papillomas	6, 11, 57, 57b
Focal epithelial hyperplasia (Heck disease)	Oral cavity	Discrete, multiple nodules	13, 32
Oral cavity papillomas	Gums, buccal mucosa, soft palate, tonsils	Single or multiple papillomas	6, 11, 16
Conjunctival papillomas	Conjunctivae	Single or multiple papillomas	6, 11, 16
Giant-cell hepatitis	Liver	Unknown	6?

dermatologic disorder—epidermodysplasia verruciformis (EV). The mucosal HPVs occur mainly in the genital tract but also infect and produce disease at other mucosal sites such as the respiratory tract, oral cavity, and conjunctiva. The mucosal HPVs also can be subgrouped into low-, high-, and intermediate- or moderate-risk types, depending on the frequency with which they are found in invasive cancers.[20, 146, 265, 290]

Propagation of HPVs in monolayer cell culture to yield full viral particles has not been possible yet, probably because full epithelial cell differentiation and keratinization of squamous epithelial cells are required for the virus to replicate completely, and such differentiation is not achieved in conventional cell culture. Therefore, other methods have been developed to study the biology of HPVs. For example, research laboratories have propagated a few papillomaviruses successfully by inoculating virion extracts into susceptible tissue and transplanting this tissue into athymic nude mice.[129] Molecular assays of viral transformation with cloned HPV DNA have been used to define the viral genes involved in the induction of cellular proliferation and transformation. Rabbit papillomavirus animal models also have been used to study the function of E5 protein. In addition, the three-dimensional structure of the important viral proteins, such as E2 and potentially E6 and E7, have been determined by x-ray crystallography and multidimensional nuclear magnetic resonance spectroscopy.

Induction of cellular proliferation is the hallmark of infection with the papillomaviruses. Warts, for example, arise when a cell or a small group of cells in the basal cell layer of the epithelium are infected with an HPV type. The viral DNA replicates in an episomal or small circular form and stimulates the cells to proliferate and produce a self-limited tumor, also called a papilloma, or wart. In a wart, all layers of the normal epithelium are present, except with the addition of hyperplasia of the prickle cell layer, a condition called acanthosis. Hyperkeratosis is common in cutaneous warts but usually is absent in mucosal warts. Viral particles are produced in the differentiated, uppermost granular layers of the epithelium, where the viral cytopathic effect (koilocytosis) characteristic of HPVs is displayed. Benign lesions express both early and late genes, but if the lesion progresses to malignancy, expression of the capsid antigens and production of viral particles are inhibited, and only early-region transcripts and proteins are detectable. When invasive cancer occurs, the viral DNA usually is integrated into the cellular genome. Another unique characteristic of the HPVs is the presence of latent or persistent viral genome in apparently normal cells. Such persistence probably accounts for the recurrence of both genital and laryngeal papillomas, even after apparently successful treatment and prolonged disease-free periods.[72, 264]

EPIDEMIOLOGY

The papillomaviruses are widespread in nature, and infection with HPVs occurs in people of all ages from all parts of the world. These viruses infect squamous epithelium at several body sites, and individual HPV types display marked specificity for a particular site. Infection appears to be transmitted through fomites, moisture, and minor skin trauma in the case of cutaneous warts; by sexual intercourse in the case of genital warts and condyloma; and during birth through an infected maternal birth canal in patients with juvenile-onset respiratory papillomatosis. In addition, HPV DNA has been detected in aerosolized smoke and vapor during laser and electrocautery treatment of patients with cutaneous and genital warts and laryngeal papillomatosis, and anecdotal reports of possible transmission from patient to surgeon have appeared.[1, 71, 86, 237, 238] The incubation period for most infections varies from 3 weeks to as long as 8 months, with an average of approximately 3 months. In respiratory papillomatosis, the incubation period may be 5 years or longer and, with cervical cancer, 10 years or longer. Infection with HPVs may be asymptomatic. Some may produce benign, barely noticeable warts; others may produce recurrent or growing lesions that are life-threatening and resistant to treatment; and a few infections may progress to invasive, even fatal cancer. The outcome of an infection with HPV is influenced by several factors, including virus type, location of the lesion, immunologic status of the host, environmental and infectious cofactors, and the nature of the epithelium that has been infected.

Cutaneous warts are rare findings in children younger than 5 years but are relatively common in older children, adolescents, and young adults. In fact, as many as 10 percent of school-age children may have warts at some site on their bodies at any given time, and as many as 50 percent of individuals may have had cutaneous warts at some time during their life. Certain activities, such as the use of public swimming pools and tattooing, or certain occupations, such as butchers, handlers of meat, poultry, and fish, and workers in slaughterhouses, appear to have an increased risk of acquiring cutaneous warts.[58, 118, 144, 231, 281] Most warts regress within 2 years, presumably because the host mounts a cell-mediated immune response. Warts may increase in number and size, however, if the individual is immunocompromised, is pregnant, or has the rare familial disorder EV. The genotypes of HPV recovered from skin warts correlate, though not absolutely, with the morphology and body site of the wart. For example, HPV-1 is associated with deep plantar warts, HPV-2 with common skin warts, HPV-3 and HPV-10 with flat skin warts, and HPV-7 with butcher's warts, whereas a large number of different HPV types can be recovered from patients with EV (see Table 159–2).

Infection of the genital tract with HPVs also appears to occur commonly, but its prevalence varies widely according to the population studied and the criteria used to define infection. For example, an estimated 1 to 2 percent of sexually active individuals have external anogenital warts, or condyloma acuminatum. However, when cytologic methods to detect subclinical disease are used, as many as 10 percent of sexually active women have been shown to have HPV-related disease of the cervix. Even higher prevalence rates have been observed when highly sensitive molecular techniques that detect both asymptomatic infection and disease are used. For instance, one study of young university women found that 46 percent were positive for at least one HPV type when extremely sensitive PCR-based methods were used.[14] Furthermore, studies suggest that as many as 75 percent of women have been infected with HPV at some time during their life.[243, 275] In contrast, older women appear to have a lower prevalence of HPV infection than younger women do, even when sensitive molecular methods are used.[166, 240] Not all genital infections with HPV may be transmitted sexually, however, because HPV DNA also has been detected on medical instruments and on the underwear of patients with genital HPV disease, thus suggesting that genital tract HPVs may be transmitted in certain circumstances by fomites, similar to cutaneous warts.[70, 71]

Most epidemiologic studies suggest that HPV infection of the genital tract is a sexually transmitted disease and that age and the number of lifetime sexual partners both are independent risk factors for infection.[172] Of particular concern is the high and apparently increasing prevalence of cervical HPV infection in adolescents. In fact, recent epidemiologic evidence suggests that infection with HPV is the most common sexually transmitted disease in adolescent women. For example, in one study of more than 600 adolescents who attended three urban clinics in Colorado, 24 percent of the patients had evidence of HPV infection (15% with clinically apparent genital warts, 36% with subclinical HPV infection detected cytologically, and 49% with subclinical infection detected by the presence of HPV DNA in cervical tissue).[114] In another study of sexually active adolescents, an incidence rate of 29 percent was observed during a 13.3-month study period.[228] Whether this high prevalence of HPV infection represents persistent infection with the same HPV genotype or reinfection with a new genotype remains controversial. For example, one study in Panama showed that the proportion of women with HPV infection increased in accordance with the number of consecutive specimens tested (21 to 82% in a cohort of high-risk subjects sampled monthly for at least six visits) and suggested that persistent HPV infection with periodic viral shedding was the most likely explanation.[215] In contrast, other studies have shown that detection of the same HPV DNA genotype on a second examination is unusual and suggested that spontaneous regression or resolution occurred, followed by reinfection with a new type of HPV.[187, 228] The importance of the "male factor" in HPV infection of young women has been shown recently. Young women were more likely to be infected with

HPV if their male sexual partners were older or of black race or Hispanic ethnicity, if they had high numbers of sexual partners, and if they participated in high-risk behavior such as having sex while intoxicated and lack of seat belt use.[33]

Epidemiologic observations show a strong link between HPV infection and cervical cancer because they both have characteristics of a sexually transmitted disease. For instance, the number of lifetime sexual partners is a risk factor for both HPV infection and cervical cancer.[33] Furthermore, cervical carcinoma is more likely to develop in women with a history of genital warts than in women with a negative history, and it is significantly more likely to develop in women married to men in whom cancer of the penis develops.[77, 95] Associations also have been found between specific genotypes of HPV infection and the presence of invasive cervical cancer. HPV types 16, 18, 31, and 45 are associated strongly with cervical cancer; HPV types 33, 35, 39, 51, 52, 56, 58, 59, and 68 have a moderate association with cervical cancer; and HPV types 6, 11, 26, 42, 43, 44, 53, 54, 55, 62, and 66 rarely have been seen in cancerous lesions of the cervix.[251] In addition, cohort studies have shown that the presence of HPV DNA precedes the development of pre-invasive cervical lesions.[217] However, despite strong circumstantial evidence and compelling laboratory documentation of the role that HPV plays in cervical cancer, HPV infection alone appears to be neither sufficient nor necessary for cervical cancer to develop. The disease still may be multifactorial in etiology and involve cofactors such as demography, genetics, socioeconomic status, race and ethnicity, age, nutrition and other dietary factors, pregnancy and parity, hormonal exposure, use of oral contraceptives, smoking, immune status, and the presence of other sexually transmitted infections and diseases.[172, 217, 251, 253]

Like cervical cancer in women, the HPVs are associated with squamous intraepithelial lesions and anal canal tumors in men. More than 80 percent of anal cancer specimens have HPV DNA detected in this tissue.[80] Although anal cancer is rare in men, certain risk factors have been identified, including HIV infection, a homosexual or bisexual lifestyle, and the practice of receptive anal intercourse.[78, 198] More than 90 percent of HIV-positive homosexual men will have anal HPV infection, and as many as 73 percent will have infection with more than one HPV type at a single time.[198] HPV-16 is the most commonly detected HPV type, but almost all types have been identified in this clinical setting.

Another potential consequence of genital infection with HPV is perinatal transmission of the virus from mother to infant. Genital HPVs, including the high-risk genotypes 16 and 18 and the lower-risk genotypes 6 and 11, may be transmitted from mother to infant, presumably by passage through an infected birth canal, although ascending infection and postnatal acquisition also are possibilities.[39, 197] HPV DNA has been detected in buccal and genital cells obtained from infants born to mothers infected with HPV-16 and HPV-18, and pregnant women with a high viral load of HPV DNA in cervical cells are more likely to transmit HPV infection to their newborn infants than are mothers with a low viral load.[121] Furthermore, a recent study has demonstrated that HPV DNA may persist for at least 6 months in perinatally infected infants.[39] In fact, infection of the oral mucosa appears to be a common event in healthy adults and children. DNA from HPV-6 and HPV-16 has been detected by PCR in 17 and 23 percent of oral mucosa samples from adults and in 24 and 19 percent of oral samples from preschool children, respectively.[117] The consequences of infection of the oral mucosa with genital-type and other HPVs range from asymptomatic infection to a variety of oral, respiratory, and ocular lesions. For example, HPV types 6, 11, 16, and 18 have been seen in leukoplakia, lichen planus, oral papillomas, squamous cell carcinoma of the tongue, and verrucous carcinoma of the larynx.[30, 59, 151] Dysplastic and malignant lesions of the ocular conjunctiva and cornea also have been associated with HPV-16.[163] HPV-6 and HPV-11 have been linked to juvenile- and adult-onset laryngeal papillomatosis.[178] Circumstantial evidence implicating perinatal transmission of HPV as a cause of respiratory papillomatosis includes retrospective analyses that have shown an association between juvenile laryngeal papillomatosis and genital warts in the mother at the time of delivery.[16, 51, 213] Juvenile laryngeal papillomatosis also appears to be uncommon in children delivered by cesarean section.[247] It also must be noted, however, that this disease has a bimodal age distribution. Although the peak incidence of the disease occurs between birth and 5 years of age, almost half the patients with HPV-associated laryngeal papillomatosis are seen for the first time in adulthood.[49]

CLINICAL MANIFESTATIONS

Cutaneous Warts

Common cutaneous skin warts, or verrucae, have variable morphology and may appear at any location on the skin.[42, 251] Common skin warts, or verrucae vulgares, usually are well-demarcated, dome-shaped papules with multiple conical projections (papillomatosis) that give the surface of the wart a rough appearance and texture. Common warts generally occur on the hands, especially the dorsum, but they also are seen frequently between the fingers, periungually, and on the palms and soles. They occasionally may be mosaic and spread superficially over the skin, or they may be filiform in morphology and appear as thread-like warts on the face and neck. They most commonly are associated with HPV-2 and HPV-4. Butcher's warts, a form of cutaneous wart seen in meat and poultry handlers who suffer repeated minor trauma to the hands, are associated with HPV-7. Plantar warts, also called verrucae plantares, occur most commonly in adolescents and young adults. They are generally single lesions and have a highly thickened corneal layer, or hyperkeratosis, with areas of punctate bleeding. They also are painful because they typically are found on pressure-bearing points on the plantar surface of the foot or the palms of the hand. They usually are associated with HPV-1. Flat warts, or verrucae planae, in contrast, do not have papillomatosis or hyperkeratosis, and they often are multiple. These warts are more common findings in young children and occur most frequently on the arms, face, and knees. HPV types 3, 10, 28, and 41 have been associated with flat warts.[42, 251] Although the clinical appearance of cutaneous warts almost always is diagnostic, the differential diagnosis includes other viral skin disorders, such as molluscum contagiosum, and other infectious diseases, such as actinomycosis, blastomycosis, sporotrichosis, leishmaniasis, chronic vegetating pyoderma, atypical mycobacterial infection (e.g., swimming pool granuloma), and tuberculosis verrucosa cutis (warty tuberculosis). Giant verrucae or warts also must be differentiated from squamous cell carcinoma.

Epidermodysplasia Verruciformis

EV, a rare skin disorder initially manifested in infancy or early childhood, is characterized by the inability to resolve HPV-induced, cutaneous wart-like lesions.[153] Seen worldwide, this disease is familial, and a history of parental consanguinity is noted in approximately 10 percent of reported cases, thus implying a genetic basis for the disease. Although both autosomal recessive and X-linked recessive forms of inheritance have been observed, the precise genetic defect or mode of inheritance remains elusive.[6, 55, 153, 251] Patients with EV also have both nonspecific and HPV-specific defects in cell-mediated immunity, especially T-cell defects, and some patients will have developmental disabilities.[52, 92, 112, 152, 154, 155] Although the lesions seen with EV are polymorphic, two clinical types of warts are seen primarily in these patients: flat warts and red or reddish-brown macular plaques. Both the flat warts and plaques appear first on the face, trunk, and extremities. They slowly become confluent and then appear to disseminate. Occasionally, the plaques may be achromatic with pigmented borders and resemble pityriasis versicolor.

Malignant transformation develops in 30 to 50 percent of patients with EV and occurs during adulthood, usually decades after the initial manifestation in childhood. Therefore, long-term, careful clinical follow-up of children in whom EV is diagnosed is important. The malignant transformation occurs in multiple foci in the reddish-brown plaque lesions, especially in areas that are exposed frequently to sunlight or other ultraviolet light, such as the forehead. It also is more likely to occur if the patient is infected with the highly oncogenic HPV types 5, 8, or 47. The tumors that result usually are slow growing, yet locally destructive. Histopathologically, they may appear as an in situ or invasive carcinoma.[112] They generally do not metastasize unless exposed to co-carcinogens such as x-irradiation.[194] The skin cancers in EV patients, though a serious and challenging clinical entity, also provide an excellent example and scientific model to study host factors such as genetic defects, the infecting type of HPV, and environmental factors such as ultraviolet light in the genesis of malignant transformation and the development of cancer.[251]

Patients with EV may be infected with multiple types of HPV, including HPV-3 and HPV-10, which are associated with flat warts in healthy individuals.[153, 251] The HPV types most commonly associated with lesions in EV patients, however, are 5, 8, 17, and 20, types not usually seen in the general population. Other HPV types associated with this disorder are 9, 12, 14, 15, 19 to 25, 36 to 38, 47, and 49. The EV-associated HPV types that have a high oncogenic potential are 5, 8, and 47 because they appear in more than 90 percent of skin carcinomas in EV patients, whereas HPV types 14, 20, 21, and 25 appear to have low oncogenic potential because they usually are detected only in benign skin lesions of patients with EV. It is likely that healthy individuals are infected asymptomatically with many of the HPV types seen in the lesions of patients with EV and that an immunologic defect probably allows the HPV infection to produce a chronic disease process. For example, HPV-8 antibodies have been found in healthy individuals, and HPV-5 DNA and HPV-8 DNA have been detected in refractory warts and skin carcinoma in immunocompromised patients such as renal allograft recipients.[97, 148, 205, 263]

The appearance of EV-like skin lesions also may be seen in individuals who are immunocompromised as a result of HIV infection, as well as in transplant recipients, those receiving cancer chemotherapy, and other immunosuppressed patients.* These lesions may appear as brownish plaques, like typical EV lesions, or they may be morphologically similar to flat or common cutaneous warts. Skin warts in immunocompromised patients may be single or multiple, and they may persist or progress. These patients also have a high risk of developing squamous cell carcinoma, and the risk increases with exposure to sunlight or ultraviolet light, as well as with immunosuppression of long duration.[189, 291] A variety of HPV types have been identified in patients who are immunosuppressed. For example, all the main types of HPV (1 to 4, 28) associated with skin warts in the general population have been detected in immunosuppressed patients. In addition, HPV types 5, 8, 10, 20, 23, 28, and 49, which are associated primarily with EV, have been detected, either alone or in combination, in immunosuppressed patients, especially renal transplant recipients.[153]

*See references 19, 32, 67, 212, 232, 233, 256, 261, 284, 291.

Infections of the Male and Female Genital Tract

Genital tract infection with the mucosal HPVs probably is the most prevalent sexually transmitted infection caused by a viral pathogen, and because of its link to cervical, penile, and anal cancer, such infection most likely imposes far greater morbidity on the general population than does cutaneous infection with HPVs. Genital tract infection with HPVs may be latent, active yet asymptomatic, manifested as genital warts or condyloma, or associated with various stages of cervical cytologic and histologic abnormalities, including low- and high-grade squamous intraepithelial lesions, carcinoma in situ, and invasive carcinoma. Pregnancy, immunosuppression, and especially HIV infection have been associated with an increased prevalence of HPV infection and disease in both men and women.[78, 101]

Asymptomatic or subclinical infection occurs in as many as 10 percent of females older than 15 years, and the rates may be as high as 30 percent in some sexually active adolescent populations and over 90 percent in homosexual HIV-positive men. All genital HPVs (types 6, 11, 13, 16, 18, 30 to 35, 39, 40, 42 to 45, and 51 to 59) are involved.[198, 251, 301] The outcome of infection with a genital HPV is variable and includes resolution of the infection and elimination of viral DNA, viral persistence with no cytologic abnormalities, transient cytologic abnormalities that resolve completely in a few months, cytologic abnormalities that persist, and cytologic abnormalities that progress to in situ or invasive cervical cancer. Although the frequencies of these different outcomes of genital HPV infection are not known precisely, complete resolution of the infection appears to be the most frequent occurrence, whereas invasive cancer is the rarest outcome.[109, 176, 303] Whether reinfection with the same strain of HPV can occur is unknown. However, viral persistence appears to be likely in older women and HIV-infected individuals with cancer-related HPVs, especially types 16, 18, and 33.[108, 176, 251, 270] Subclinical HPV infections do not cause symptoms and may be detectable only with sensitive molecular techniques that detect HPV DNA. Subclinical HPV infection also may produce subtle flat lesions that can be detected only by acetic acid treatment followed by colposcopy of the cervix.

The most common clinical manifestation of HPV infection of the genital tract is condyloma acuminatum, or genital warts. These warts usually are caused by infection with HPV-6 and HPV-11 and occasionally HPV-16. They generally are multiple; exophytic; pink, purplish, or gray; and papular or pedunculated lesions composed of short or long fronds of connective tissue covered by acanthotic squamous epithelium. In females, they involve the vaginal introitus, vulva, perineum, cervix, urethra, and anus. The lesions usually are asymptomatic, but they may cause itching, burning, or pain. During pregnancy, genital warts may increase in number and size and regress after delivery. In males, genital warts occur on the penis, scrotum, perineum, and anus. They generally are asymptomatic but may cause itching, burning, and dyspareunia. Adult and adolescent women and men, as well as children, with external anogenital warts also may have HPV infection at internal cervical-vaginal or intra-anal mucosal sites.[99, 110, 123, 124] In addition to typical papillary warts, flat condylomata may occur, especially in the cervix. These flat warts are difficult to visualize with the naked eye, and their detection may be aided by colposcopy. Flat condylomata usually are caused by HPV types 6, 11, 16, 18, and 31 and may progress to low- and high-grade cervical intraepithelial lesions.[251] Infection with HIV increases the risk for development of HPV infection and HPV-associated genital lesions and neoplasms in adult men and women, and, therefore, patients should be examined carefully for these conditions.[48, 198, 270, 293] Whether HIV infection increases the risk for HPV infection or disease in adolescents and children also is a concern but is unclear at this time.[230, 266] In addition, immunosuppression from chemotherapy and transplantation is associated with an increased risk for acquisition of HPV-associated genital infection, disease, and malignant transformation. In a renal transplant recipient, a novel HPV type 74 was discovered recently and subsequently detected in as many as 5 percent of renal transplant recipients.[145] In adolescents, anogenital warts may develop within 1 to 2 months after consensual sexual activity, as well as after sexual assault.[122] Infants and children also may have anogenital warts, which may result from sexual abuse or from perinatal transmission.[54, 99, 100] The risk of development of genital warts in a sexually abused child is not identified clearly; however, approximately half the cases of genital warts in children reported in the literature appear to be related to sexual abuse. In addition, molecular techniques have shown that anogenital warts in children contain HPV DNA from types 6, 11, or 16, the same types responsible for genital warts in adults, whereas HPV DNA from types 1, 2, and 4, which cause common cutaneous warts, has not been found in anogenital warts in children.[54] Anogenital warts in children are more likely to be acquired by sexual abuse than by perinatal transmission if the child is older than 2 years because this period is outside the plausible incubation period of perinatal transmission of HPV. Rapid progression of anogenital warts has been described in children with recent varicella infection. The differential diagnosis of anogenital warts includes other infectious diseases such as condyloma latum associated with secondary syphilis and molluscum contagiosum, as well as noninfectious disorders such as epithelial papillae, enlarged sebaceous glands or sebaceous cysts, seborrheic keratosis, lentigo, pigmented nevi, skin tags, hemorrhoids, Crohn disease, and carcinoma.

Giant condylomata acuminata may occur on the penis, vulva, or perirectal area. These giant tumor-like lesions also are called Buschke-Löwenstein tumors and condylomatous carcinoma and were reported first by Buschke in Germany in 1896. The growth of these lesions is indolent and rarely may cause inguinal lymphadenopathy, fistulous tracts, inflammation, fibrosis, and hemorrhage of the surrounding tissues. Histologically, these lesions are benign and appear similar to typical anogenital warts. However, progression to dysplasia and carcinoma has been documented. Buschke-Löwenstein tumors are associated with HPV-6 and HPV-11, in contrast to invasive genital carcinomas, which most commonly are associated with HPV-16 and HPV-18.[186]

Progression of HPV-induced anogenital condylomatous lesions to dysplasia or invasive carcinoma is well documented but unusual.[132, 217, 298] Most anogenital carcinomas probably arise from infection with high-risk HPV-16 and HPV-18 because more than 70 percent of human cervical cancers contain DNA from HPV-16 or HPV-18.[132, 216] This epidemiologic observation complements in vitro studies that document the transforming properties of these viral types.[251, 300] Other risks and cofactors for development of cervical cancer also have been identified, and it is likely that progression from subclinical infection to carcinoma is multifactorial.[251] Invasive cervical cancer appears to evolve in a progressive cascade of cervical epithelial abnormalities that recently have been reclassified. These abnormalities currently are referred to as low-grade and high-grade squamous intraepithelial lesions. The category low-grade squamous intraepithelial lesion includes subclinical HPV infection, condyloma, and what was known formerly as grade 1 cervical intraepithelial neoplasia, or mild dysplasia. In the high-grade squamous intraepithelial lesion category, most or all of the thickness of the cervical epithelium is replaced by abnormal cells or microinvasive carcinoma. This category includes what previously was referred to as grades 2 and 3 cervical intraepithelial neoplasia, or moderate to severe dysplasia, and carcinoma in situ. If not detected and treated, high-grade squamous intraepithelial lesions may evolve into invasive carcinoma, breach the basement membrane, and metastasize to regional lymph nodes and other parts of the body. The HPV types that have a strong association with invasive cervical cancer are 16, 18, 31, and 45, whereas types 33, 35, 39, 51, 52, 56, 58, 59, and 68 are associated only moderately with cervical cancer. The remaining types (6, 11, 26, 43, 44, 53 to 55, 62, and 66) rarely have been associated with cancer. Cervical cancer usually is asymptomatic and detected by cytologic screening. However, patients with advanced invasive cervical cancer may have abnormal menstrual bleeding or pain. The lesions also may be visible by direct visual inspection and appear as pigmented papillomas, erythematous plaques, or leukoplakic lesions or, if further advanced, as ulcerations or large masses. Squamous carcinoma of the penis is a quite rare occurrence, especially in countries that practice routine newborn circumcision. However, when penile cancer does occur, it usually is manifested as a painless, slowly enlarging ulcerative mass.

Bowenoid papulosis is another manifestation of HPV infection of the anogenital tract (see Fig. 65–20). It typically occurs in adults younger than 40 years and is characterized by multiple, large maculopapular lesions that are erythematous and reddish, purplish, or brownish, with a smooth, velvety surface. These lesions may regress spontaneously or persist. Bowenoid papulosis is associated with HPV-16 and histologically appears to be high-grade squamous intraepithelial lesions or squamous cell carcinoma in situ. Bowen disease, on the other hand, is seen in patients older than 40 years and causes single, reddish, scaling or crusting lesions that histologically also appear to be high-grade squamous intraepithelial lesions.[298]

Traditionally, cervical dysplasia and carcinoma have been considered disorders of middle-aged and older women. However, during the past 10 to 20 years, the prevalence of HPV infection and abnormal cervical cytology in young women and adolescents has increased. For example, recent studies suggest 18 to 53 percent prevalence rates for HPV infection in sexually active adolescents, with high-risk HPV-16 and HPV-18 being the most common types detected.[114] The prevalence of cervical low- and high-grade squamous intraepithelial lesions detected by Papanicolaou smear in adolescents also appears to have increased from 3 percent in the 1970s to 18 percent in the 1990s.[230] These alarming observations should alert physicians who care for adolescents and suggest that an epidemic of cervical cancer may occur in the near future.

Recurrent Respiratory Papillomatosis

Recurrent respiratory papillomatosis (RRP) is a rare, histologically benign, yet paradoxically life-threatening, condition caused by HPV-6 and HPV-11.[81] Worldwide, it probably is the most common tumor of the larynx in children, with an incidence of 0.1 to 2.8 per 100,000 observed.[258, 288] In the United States, the estimated incidence in children is 0.6 per 100,000, with the condition newly diagnosed in an estimated 1500 patients each year.[177, 288] The disease may be seen in both children and adults. Approximately two thirds of cases of RRP are seen in children, and in this population it also may be called juvenile-onset recurrent respiratory papillomatosis (JORRP). Approximately a fourth of the cases in children will be present before they reach 1 year of age, half by 5 years of age, and the remaining by 11 years of age. Adult-onset RRP usually is manifested in patients between 20 and 40 years of age, but occasionally it may be seen in adolescents.[81, 251]

Circumstantial evidence suggests that infants and children with JORRP most likely acquire HPV perinatally during passage through an HPV-infected birth canal. For example, 30 to 60 percent of mothers of children with JORRP have a history of genital warts, as compared with less than 5 percent of mothers of children who do not have JORRP.[201, 213] Furthermore, children with JORRP rarely are born by cesarean section. In fact, significant risk factors for JORRP include vaginal delivery, being firstborn, and maternal age younger than 20 years.[252] HPV-6 and HPV-11, most commonly associated with JORRP, also are responsible for most of the genital warts seen in women.[69, 251] HPV DNA has been detected in the oropharynx of infants born to mothers with genital HPV infection.[251] However, RRP develops in only a small proportion of infants born to mothers with genital warts or subclinical HPV infection. The mode of transmission of HPV-6 and HPV-11 in adult-onset RRP is unknown. The most common initial symptom of RRP and JORRP is hoarseness or a change in voice. Infants and toddlers may have a hoarse cry, stridor, airway obstruction, respiratory distress, or difficulty in phonation. They also may have a croup-like illness. The most common site for RRP and JORRP is the true vocal cord of the larynx. Supraglottic and subglottic extension of the lesions also may occur. In addition, the disease may involve the trachea, bronchi, palate, nasopharynx, paranasal sinuses, and lungs. When the lungs are involved, pulmonary nodules, atelectasis, and secondary bacterial pneumonia may occur (Fig. 159–4). The disease also may produce permanent lung damage with bronchiectasis and cavitations (Fig. 159–5). In approximately 2 to 3 percent of patients, progression to invasive squamous papillomatosis and even malignant transformation to squamous cell carcinoma will occur, with invasion of the soft tissues of the neck, esophagus, and lung parenchyma (Fig. 159–6). The incidence increases to 14 percent in patients who received the radiation therapy that commonly was used until 1970 to treat RRP.[88, 157, 242] Smoking and severe, recurrent disease also appear to increase the risk for development of malignant transformation in adolescents and adults. In addition, sudden and unexpected death may occur from airway obstruction if the lesions obstruct the laryngeal lumen.[260] The clinical course of RRP and JORRP is highly variable and characterized by common and unpredictable remissions and exacerbations, even despite apparently successful removal of the lesions.

Nasal and Paranasal Papillomas

Nasal papillomas or warts are rare tumors that may develop at any age, including childhood, and may occur as solitary lesions or in combination with papillomas elsewhere in the respiratory tract.[29, 221] Histologically, they usually resemble the laryngeal papillomas seen in RRP. They most commonly are caused by HPV-6 and HPV-11, although HPV types 16, 57, and 57b also have been detected in nasal papillomas. Cocaine snorting is one risk factor for the development of nasal papillomas.[245] Papillomas also may involve the paranasal sinuses.[29, 221]

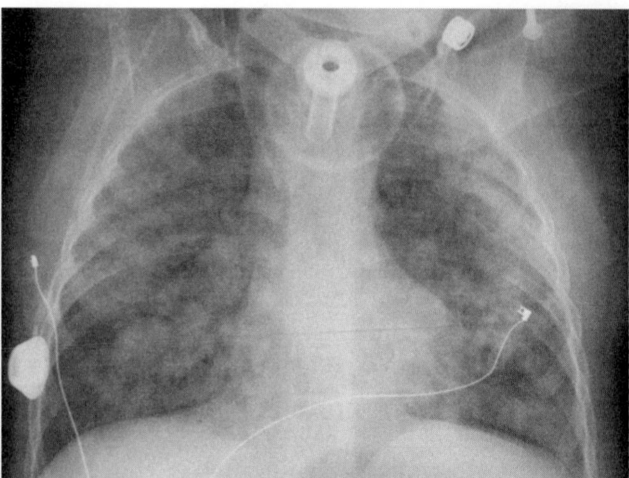

FIGURE 159–4 ■ Chest radiograph of a 6-year-old girl with severe, recurrent, and progressive respiratory papillomatosis since 1 year of age.

Papillomas and Cancers of the Oral Cavity

Papillomas or warts in the oral cavity are heterogeneous etiologically and may be caused by cutaneous HPV types that are associated with warts on the skin, as well as by mucosal HPV types that are associated with genital warts. For example, focal epithelial hyperplasia, also called Heck disease, is a rare, yet well-defined clinical condition of the oral mucosa that is associated with HPV-13 and HPV-32 and infects

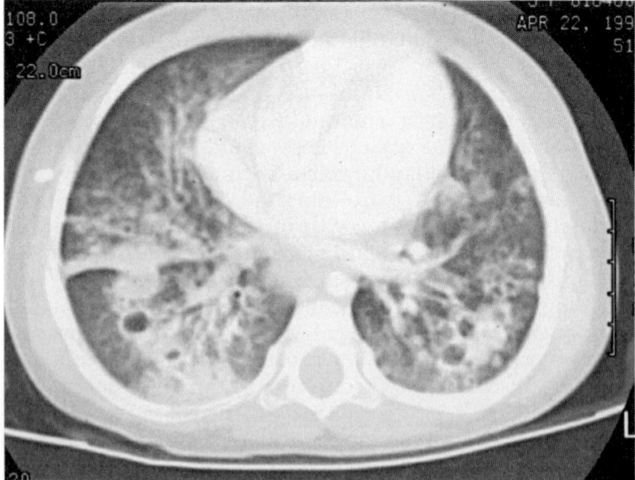

FIGURE 159–5 ■ Chest computed tomograph of a 6-year-old girl with severe, recurrent, and progressive respiratory papillomatosis. The tomograph shows pulmonary nodules, bronchiectasis, and cavitations.

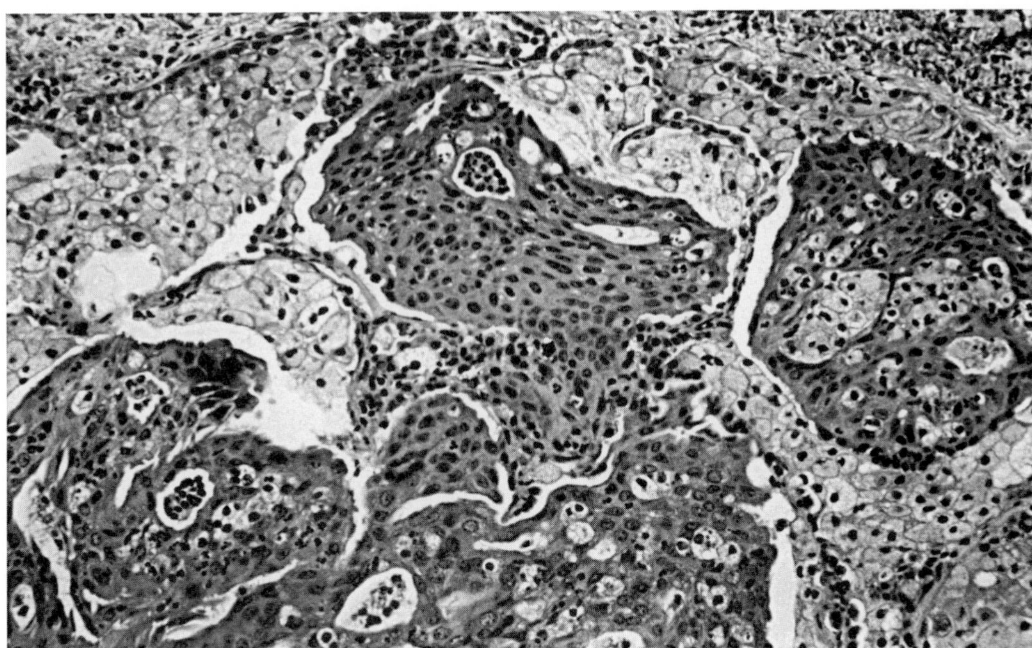

FIGURE 159–6 ■ Lung biopsy tissue (hematoxylin and eosin stain, 50× original magnification, light microscopy) from a 6-year-old girl with severe, progressive, recurrent respiratory papillomatosis. This tissue demonstrates invasive squamous papillomatosis. The squamous cells are growing along preformed pulmonary structures, but no evidence of malignancy is apparent at this time because of the absence of invasion of lung tissue. (Courtesy of Dr. Claire Langston, Department of Pathology, Baylor College of Medicine and Texas Children's Hospital, Houston, Texas.)

only the oral cavity.[251, 276] It occurs worldwide but is most prevalent in Central and South America, Alaska, and Greenland. Focal epithelial hyperplasia may develop in children or adults and often clusters in families or geographic regions.[191] The lesions are discrete, multiple, elevated nodules readily visible on the oral mucosa. They may persist for years or resolve spontaneously. They do not, however, appear to undergo malignant transformation, nor do they appear to metastasize to other parts of the body. Warts caused by HPV-2, the same type associated with verrucae vulgares, or common cutaneous warts of the skin, may occur on the lips and on the mucosa of the oral cavity.[68] Oral papillomas involving the gums, buccal mucosa, soft palate, and tonsils also may be caused by HPV-6, HPV-11, and HPV-16, which primarily are associated with genital warts, or condylomata acuminata.[179, 251] Recently, HPV-16 antibodies were found to be associated with squamous cell carcinoma of the head and neck, and HPV-16 DNA was detected in oropharyngeal and tongue cancers, thus suggesting that HPV may play a role in these cancers.[170]

Conjunctival Papillomas

Conjunctival papillomas occur in all age groups but are exceedingly rare. They may be asymptomatic initially and then cause a constant foreign body sensation or chronic conjunctivitis. When large, they appear as pink mulberry- or cauliflower-like growths that may cause pain or interfere with lid closure. In most children and some adults, they appear to be caused by HPV-6 and HPV-11, which characteristically infect the genital tract and, therefore, may be transmitted during birth, similar to RRP.[135, 164] HPV-16, another HPV that commonly infects the genital tract, also has been associated with conjunctival and lacrimal sac carcinoma in adults.[150, 163]

Gastrointestinal Papillomas and Cancer

Tonsillar and oropharyngeal carcinomas may contain HPV DNA, and patients with head and neck cancers, including cancer of the tongue and oropharynx, may be seropositive for HPV type 16, an oncogenic HPV.[170] Esophageal infection with HPV may be asymptomatic or produce papillomas that cause dysphagia.[12] HPV DNA has been detected in esophageal brush specimens of HIV-infected individuals who did not have proliferative mucosal lesions at the time of endoscopy.[286] In addition, HPVs, along with a variety of cofactors, may be involved in the genesis of esophageal carcinoma.[41] Similarly, HPV DNA has been detected in tissue samples from patients with colon cancer, but with unclear implications regarding their role.[251] The association of HPVs with anal warts, anal squamous intraepithelial lesions, and anal cancer, however, appears to be strong. Infection with HPV types 16, 18, and 31 most commonly occurs, but mere infection with these specific HPV types does not appear to be sufficient for the development of cancer. Similar to cervical cancer, cofactors such as other sexually transmitted diseases, chemical carcinogens (e.g., tobacco), and HIV infection and AIDS also may be involved in the pathogenesis of anal cancer.[81, 131, 186, 198]

Liver Disease

Recent reports also have suggested that HPVs may play a role in liver disease. For example, HPV DNA, especially HPV-6, has been detected by sensitive molecular techniques in the liver of patients with neonatal giant-cell hepatitis, postinfantile giant-cell hepatitis, post–liver transplantation giant-cell hepatitis, and primary hepatocellular carcinoma.[62, 200, 246] However, the pathogenic role of HPV in these diseases, though an intriguing possibility, remains unproven at this time.

Other Cancers

The potential role of HPVs in the pathogenesis of a variety of unusual cancers has been explored by a variety of investigators using different approaches, with conflicting results. Therefore, the role of HPVs in these cancers remains unproven at this time. For example, HPV DNA from types 6, 16, and 18 has been detected in tissue from some but not all patients with ovarian carcinoma.[251, 287] HPVs also have been detected in tissue from patients with cancer of the endometrium, urethra, urinary bladder, and prostate, with unclear pathogenic implications.[251]

LABORATORY DIAGNOSIS

The typical appearance of verrucae vulgares on the skin and condylomata acuminata in the anogenital area in otherwise healthy individuals usually is sufficient to make the clinical diagnosis of these HPV-associated illnesses. However, laboratory confirmation of HPV-associated lesions may be necessary for unusual manifestations in healthy individuals, for immunocompromised patients, and for patients with suspected malignant lesions. Methods commonly and traditionally used in viral diagnosis, such as cell culture, serology, and electron microscopy, have limited clinical utility in detecting HPV infection, whereas a variety of molecular methods, used alone or in combination, have proved quite useful in research and clinical settings. Cytologic and histologic approaches also are helpful in diagnosing HPV-associated cancers.

Electron Microscopy

Virions with typical papillomavirus morphology can be detected in abundance in cutaneous warts but are difficult to detect in tissue from patients with RRP, JORRP, genital warts, or histologically diagnosed cancers.

Cell Culture

None of the papillomaviruses has been propagated in cell culture monolayer. Therefore, the routine viral cultures available in most diagnostic virology laboratories will not detect the presence of HPVs. Research laboratories have shown that HPV-1, when inoculated into skin keratinocytes or respiratory tract–derived epithelial cells, will replicate its DNA transiently in an episomal form over several serial passages. However, viral capsid proteins and intact viral particles are not produced.[46] Other research laboratories have inoculated cervical tissue with extracts of HPV-11 virions obtained from condyloma acuminatum lesions and later transplanted the tissue beneath the renal capsule of athymic nude mice.[129] After several months, viral cytopathic effects have been seen, and viral capsid antigen and complete viral particles were produced. Clearly, these research methods need refinement before routine cultivation of HPVs becomes available to the clinician.

Serology

The inability to cultivate papillomaviruses routinely has hampered significantly the development of serologic tests to detect and study the humoral responses to infection with HPVs. Therefore, routine serologic assays to detect group- and type-specific antibody to HPVs are not available to the clinician. However, research laboratories continue to study the humoral response to HPV by a variety of methods. For example, serologic studies using purified virions of HPV-1 from plantar warts and HPV-11 obtained from mouse xenograft systems have revealed associations between seropositivity and clinical symptoms of infection with these HPV types.[26–29, 45, 128, 206, 262, 294] Other studies of the serologic response to HPV have used recombinant DNA methods to clone and express late-region L1 and L2 proteins with bacterial fusion proteins.[73, 90, 116, 306, 307] Most recently, investigators have used vaccinia virus or baculovirus expression systems to produce virion-like particles composed primarily of viral capsids of HPV types 1, 6, 11, and 16.[38, 96, 136, 180, 226, 271] However, serologic assays that use intact virions or virion-like particles, though technically the most successful to date, apparently still have problems with sensitivity and specificity. Persistent, high-titer humoral responses are not detected in HPV infections, and in contrast to other sexually transmitted viral infections (e.g., herpes simplex virus, HIV, hepatitis B virus infections), seroconversion does not appear to be a clearly defined marker for primary HPV infection. Cross-reactivity between HPV types also appears to occur and limits the specificity of current assays. In addition to efforts to delineate the virus-specific humoral responses to HPV infection and HPV-associated cancers by measuring antibodies to HPV capsid proteins and HPV transforming proteins, studies evaluating serologic markers as predictors of invasive genital tract disease and ultimate survival also are being conducted.[271]

Colposcopy

Colposcopy is an important procedure to perform in women with abnormal Papanicolaou smears or external anogenital warts. It also may be used to diagnose asymptomatic, flat cervical warts in women whose sexual partners have external anogenital warts or to monitor women who are considered to be at high risk for acquisition of genital HPV infection for other reasons. The urethral meatus, penis, scrotum, and anus of males also may be inspected with a colposcope. Gynecologists, urologists, and family practitioners, as well as pediatricians who are specialists in adolescent medicine, usually perform the procedure. Briefly, the cervix and vulva in females or the urethral meatus, penis, scrotum, and anus in males are visualized under magnification with a colposcope to identify lesions, with special attention paid to their topography, the presence of abnormal whitening, and their vascular architecture. The area then is soaked in dilute acetic acid (3 to 5%) and visualized again for the presence of previously undetected lesions that appear as whitened plaques. Whitening after acetic acid application, however, is not specific for HPV infection or disease, and biopsy is required for definitive diagnosis. Colposcopic examination of the cervix not only gives a more accurate assessment of the anatomic extent of suspicious lesions or neoplasia but also allows the colposcopist to direct biopsies of suspicious areas accurately. Tissue biopsy specimens then may be sent for histologic examination and detection of HPV DNA by molecular techniques.

Cytology

Obtaining and staining exfoliated cervical cells via the Papanicolaou method is a routine procedure that detects most HPV infections and has reduced the incidence of invasive squamous cell carcinoma of the cervix dramatically. It should be performed routinely in all sexually active females, including adolescents. Cytologic analysis also has been evaluated as a screening examination of exfoliated urethral cells from males and in the urine of both men and women, but with less success and acceptance than with cervical cell screening.[180] Papanicolaou smear screening, however, is limited by the expertise of the physician who obtains the specimen and the pathologist who performs the cytologic analysis.[175] For example, because most cervical neoplasia arises at the junction of the squamous and columnar epithelium of the cervix (transformation zone), care must be taken to obtain cells from this region. Interobserver variability also exists among pathologists who read Papanicolaou smears. Furthermore, Papanicolaou smears are not as sensitive as colposcopy for detecting cervical cancer, and a negative Papanicolaou smear does not eliminate the diagnosis in women at high risk for cervical cancer. Therefore, women with anogenital warts and those who are immunosuppressed should undergo colposcopic examination to detect subclinical cervical lesions and not just be evaluated with a Papanicolaou smear.

The cytologic abnormality that is specific and characteristic of HPV infection is the presence of koilocytosis (derived from the Greek word *koilos,* which means "hollow" or "cavity") or koilocytotic cells that display fat, swollen, wrinkled, or raisinoid nuclei surrounded by a halo. Other abnormalities, including dyskeratosis, parakeratosis, and hyperkeratosis, may occur but are considered secondary or nonspecific. The prevalence of cytologic abnormalities in women screened by Papanicolaou smears consistently has been estimated at 2 to 3 percent. Most abnormalities, however, resolve spontaneously in 3 to 6 months, but some persist and rarely may progress to cervical squamous cell carcinoma. If the infection progresses to disease, the koilocytosis typically diminishes, and the cells begin to display dysplastic changes and nuclear abnormalities. These abnormalities currently are graded into two categories: (1) low-grade squamous intraepithelial lesions, which include very mild dysplasia and the former grade 1 cervical intraepithelial neoplasia, and (2) high-grade squamous intraepithelial lesions, which include moderate to severe dysplasia and carcinoma in situ and the former grades 2 and 3 cervical intraepithelial neoplasia.[182]

Histology

HPV infection may occur in histologically normal tissue and be detected only by molecular methods that detect viral DNA. Benign and asymptomatic HPV infection also may cause koilocytosis, the typical histologic feature of HPV infection that has specific nuclear and cytoplasmic characteristics. Condyloma acuminatum lesions display not only koilocytosis but also other histopathologic characteristics of active HPV infection, such as hyperkeratosis, parakeratosis, acanthosis, and lengthening of the rete pegs. Atypical features, including mitotic figures above the basal layer, dysplastic cells, and single-cell keratinization, suggest dysplasia such as bowenoid papulosis. Precancerous and cancerous lesions of the cervix and penis also may be graded as low-grade or high-grade squamous intraepithelial lesions and invasive squamous cell carcinoma.

Histologic examination of tissue for the presence of HPV-associated disease may be augmented in certain circumstances by the detection of shared, genus-specific HPV capsid antigens that may be identified by immunohistochemistry with immunoperoxidase-labeled antibodies raised to bovine papillomavirus capsid antigen. This procedure is usually successful in identifying HPV antigens in low-grade squamous intraepithelial lesions but rarely detects antigen in high-grade squamous intraepithelial lesions because of the biology of HPV expression in these cancerous cells. Similarly, it is unusual to detect HPV antigens by this method in cutaneous or anogenital warts or other HPV-associated cancers. In addition, the utility of this method for typing the HPV infection currently is limited because unique, type-specific HPV capsid antigens are available only in research laboratories.[305]

Molecular Methods That Detect Human Papillomavirus DNA

HPV DNA may be detected in tissue by several methods, including dot-blot, slot-blot, Southern blot, and in situ hybridization assays and by amplification procedures such as PCR. HPV DNA has been detected by these methods in the majority of HPV-associated neoplasms, as well as in a significant proportion of asymptomatic individuals, including women with normal Papanicolaou smears. The variability of HPV DNA detection between studies is great and appears to be influenced by the population studied, the frequency and type of sampling, and the sensitivity and specificity of the molecular methods used. Because type-specific antisera are not available for HPVs, the diagnosis of type-specific HPV infection or disease requires molecular DNA methods.

SOUTHERN BLOT HYBRIDIZATION

Southern blot hybridization is considered the reference standard for detection of HPV DNA in clinical samples. In this assay, nucleic acid is extracted from the sample, which is usually fresh tissue or exfoliated cervical cells, and digested or cleaved into smaller fragments by restriction enzymes. These fragments then are separated by gel electrophoresis and transferred onto special filter paper. Hybridization with radiolabeled probes directed against specific HPV DNA sequences then is performed. Advantages of Southern blot hybridization include good sensitivity (approximately 10^5 DNA copies) and specificity and the ability to distinguish HPV types easily. Disadvantages of this method include the need for special equipment and expertise. It also is technically expensive and time-consuming and requires a large sample of tissue that is destroyed during the DNA isolation procedure.

DOT- AND SLOT-BLOT HYBRIDIZATION

Dot- and slot-blot hybridization apply extracted DNA from a sample directly onto a specific area (dot or slot) of filter paper, with the gel electrophoresis and transfer steps of Southern hybridization being bypassed. The filter paper is incubated with a solution containing a complementary probe, followed by stringency washes to remove any unhybridized probe.[14, 305] Detection of successful hybridization is by autoradiography if a ^{32}P-labeled probe is used or by colorimetric reaction if an enzyme-labeled probe is used. Advantages of dot-blot hybridization include commercial availability of some assays, ease of performance, rapid turnaround time, and low cost. Its sensitivity and specificity generally are slightly below those of Southern blot analysis, but the method is sufficiently sensitive to detect HPV DNA in cytologically normal as well as abnormal cervical samples, and its use, in combination with Papanicolaou smear, has been advocated to improve identification of women at high risk for development of cervical cancer.[98, 174] Dot-blot hybridization may be performed on tissue samples or cervical swabs collected in special sample transport medium or buffer, and its utility in screening urine for HPV DNA also has been explored.[180] Moreover, typing of HPV DNA may be performed by dot-blot hybridization methods. For example, one commercial kit, by using a combination of radiolabeled probe mixtures, delineates as many as seven types of HPV by category group: types 6/11, 16/18, and 31/33/35.[98, 174, 296] In addition, probes to detect almost all HPV types have been developed in a variety of research laboratories.

A novel, non-radioactive, chemiluminescent liquid hybridization assay (hybrid capture assay) is commercially available and detects as many as 14 HPV types divided into high-risk (types 16, 18, 31, 33, 35, 45, 51, 52, 56) and low-risk (types 6, 11, 42, 43, 44) groups based on association with cervical cancer.[241] This DNA hybrid capture assay is relatively rapid and simple to perform and is unique because it provides quantitative data that reflect viral concentration.

IN SITU HYBRIDIZATION

In situ tissue hybridization assays are performed directly on fresh or fixed tissue sections or on cytologic specimens and have the unique advantage of allowing the examiner to correlate histopathologic abnormalities with the location of HPV DNA. They may be performed with radioactive or enzyme-labeled probes. The sensitivity of many in situ hybridization assays is less than that of Southern blot assays, especially if enzyme-labeled probes are used.[40, 188, 277, 305] Commercial reagents and kits are available. However, this methodology remains technically challenging.

DNA AMPLIFICATION ASSAYS

DNA amplification systems, primarily PCR based, recently have been applied to detect HPV DNA in clinical samples. Current PCR methodology uses oligonucleotide primers and a thermostable DNA polymerase known as *Taq* polymerase to drive a reaction that allows the exponential production of copies of a target piece of DNA. This target DNA is detected preliminarily by gel electrophoresis and confirmed with a complementary radioactive or enzyme-labeled probe. Numerous strategies have been explored. However, many laboratories now use PCR amplification with degenerate or consensus primers that are capable of recognizing a portion of one of the late genes from a broad spectrum of papillomaviruses. The popular MY09 (primer for the negative strand)/MY11 (primer for the positive strand) primer system amplifies a 450–base pair target region located in the HPV L1 open-reading frame; this site contains both conserved regions common to most or all papillomaviruses and divergent regions that appear to be unique for each HPV DNA type.[158] Amplification and detection by the MY9/MY11 primers in a PCR assay identifies HPV DNA, which can be confirmed by using "generic" HPV probe mixes. Typing of known HPV types then can be performed with type-specific HPV probes that are labeled oligonucleotides composed of sequences complementary to each viral type. Alternatively, restriction fragment length polymorphism or sequence analysis can be performed on the PCR product to identify new HPV types that are unable to be typed with the available type-specific probes.[22, 190, 202, 203]

HPV DNA detection by PCR-based methods can be performed on a variety of specimens, including fresh or fixed tissue, exfoliated urethral and cervical cells, and urine, and the machinery and reagents needed to perform the testing are readily available.[299] However, to perform the tests properly and avoid the pitfalls of false-positive reactions from contamination of specimens, a well-designed laboratory facility and technical personnel who are experienced in PCR-based diagnostics and rigidly adhere to carryover precautions are necessary. In addition, internal reaction controls must be used to evaluate sample processing amplification and control for false-negative reactions caused by inadequate DNA recovery and PCR reaction failures. Variations on the traditional PCR methodology to detect HPV DNA also have been reported. For example, single- and double-tube nested PCR tests, extremely sensitive methods that detect very low copy number levels of DNA, have detected and typed EV-associated HPVs in cutaneous cancers from renal transplant recipients and have been used to study HPVs associated with genital infection and cancer.[21, 308]

Both the major advantage and the major disadvantage of detection of HPV DNA by PCR-based methods is extreme sensitivity, which theoretically is estimated to be 1 DNA copy but practically has been observed to be between 10 and 100 DNA copies. Though useful as a research tool to study the epidemiology of HPV infection, the clinical application of this and other DNA detection methods for HPV infection and disease is evolving. For example, by using traditional methods of Papanicolaou smear screening, colposcopy, and biopsy, the prevalence of cytologic, colposcopic, and histologic abnormalities of the cervix in the general population consistently has been estimated to be between 2 and 3 percent.[305] However, a wide range of prevalence, between 7 and 82 percent for detection of HPV infection by molecular methods, has been reported; the prevalence varies according to the population studied and the methodology used, but PCR-based methods in high-risk groups have the highest prevalence rates.[14, 123, 147, 215, 304, 309] The recognition that HPVs, especially high-risk types 16 and 18, are associated with cervical and other cancers suggests that detection of HPV DNA may be used as an adjunct to cytologic screening by Papanicolaou smear and offers the potential opportunity to identify women with cervical neoplasia who have false-negative Papanicolaou smears. On the other hand, the significance of the presence of HPV DNA, even if it is from a high-risk type, in histologically normal tissue is unclear, and the presence of HPV DNA, no matter what type, in histologically abnormal tissue does not influence management at this time. Further studies are needed to explore and resolve the clinical role of DNA-based diagnostics in the management of HPV infections.

TREATMENT

Most cutaneous and mucosal HPV-associated warts and lesions in healthy individuals will regress spontaneously in 1 to 2 years. Treatment may be desirable if the lesions are large, multiple, or recurrent; if they cause pain or discomfort; or if they are undesirable cosmetically. Treatment is mandatory if the lesions are life-threatening, such as laryngeal papillomas that obstruct the airway, and cervical cancer. A variety of treatment strategies are available, but none produces a universally effective or permanent cure. Rather, current approaches focus on reduction of the clinically apparent lesion, and most require repetitive application. Clinically significant HPV-associated lesions also usually require the additional expertise of a specialist. For example, a dermatologist should be consulted to assist in the management of a patient with severe recalcitrant cutaneous warts, a gynecologist and oncologist for patients with cervical cancer, an ophthalmologist for a patient with conjunctival papillomas, and an otolaryngologist and pulmonologist for children and adults with severe RRP. These specialists are likely to know the currently available treatment regimens most effective for each patient's HPV clinical manifestation. The role of the infectious diseases specialist in the management of HPV-associated disease is evolving and may become more prominent as HPV-specific antiviral chemotherapy becomes available for clinical trial and eventually for routine clinical use in patients. Current standard therapies focus on physical, surgical, or chemical destruction of the clinical manifestation of the HPV infection, such as the wart or papilloma.

Surgical techniques used to treat papillomas include traditional local excision by knife, cryotherapy with liquid nitrogen or dry ice, electrocautery and curettage, and ultrasonication.[13, 23, 24, 119, 160, 255] Newer ablative surgical techniques that use carbon dioxide laser vaporization and flash-lamp pulsed dye laser therapy allow more precise and complete removal of visible papillomas and are becoming widely used to treat genital and laryngeal papillomas.[70, 219, 269] Surgical excision by knife remains the initial mainstay of many HPV diseases, however, because it provides tissue for a histopathologic diagnosis, as well as removal or debulking of large lesions. Ablation by cryotherapy with liquid nitrogen, electrocautery, or laser vaporization may be used to remove small, single, or multiple lesions or be performed in combination with surgery for large or difficult lesions.[169] These surgical therapies also may release viral antigens and produce local and systemic immunologic stimulation that may assist in eradicating the lesions. Disadvantages of these physical methods of wart and papilloma removal include pain, scarring, and disfigurement. These methods also are relatively invasive and impractical for patients with disseminated disease. Furthermore, recurrent treatments usually are necessary. In addition, laser vapors contain HPV DNA and may be a vehicle for spreading the infection in the patient or to the treating physician or surgeon, and, thus, the vapors or smoke plume should be contained.[86] Recurrence of lesions after treatment occurs commonly and most likely is due to the presence of HPV DNA sequences in clinically and histologically normal epithelium adjacent to and beyond the treatment area.[72]

Warts and papillomas also may be disrupted physically and removed by using chemical ablatives applied topically to the lesion. Simple organic acids such as bichloracetic and trichloracetic acid or salicylic acid applied twice daily for several days have shown some success in the localized treatment of skin and genital warts.[82] They are caustic substances that produce a white slough that peels off, and they can be applied weekly until the lesion is destroyed.[82] Antimitotic agents such as the traditional podophyllin or the newer preparation podophyllotoxin can be applied twice daily for several weeks. Antimetabolites such as bleomycin, cantharidin, and 5-fluorouracil also have shown efficacy when administered locally once or twice a week because they inhibit the cellular proliferation induced by HPV infection.[127, 207] These topical chemicals usually are easy to apply to skin and genital warts, but they also may cause local pain, redness, swelling, irritation, blisters, and scarring.[127] Moreover, they are not virus-specific, and recurrences are common. They also are impractical for extensive lesions and may be toxic if used in certain circumstances. For example, they may damage the cornea if used to treat conjunctival papillomas, and they should not be used on pregnant women.[169] The systemically administered antitumor agent methotrexate also has been administered to individual patients with disseminated HPV disease, with variable success.

Immunomodulation is another treatment strategy for HPV-associated disease. A systemic immunologic response probably is responsible for the spontaneous regression frequently observed in cutaneous and mucosal warts. Therefore, stimulation of the immune system with immunomodulators also may produce remission in patients with HPV-associated disease. Interferons have antiviral, antiproliferative, and immunomodulating properties. More than 10 years' clinical research experience has accrued in treating HPV-associated disease with interferon administered topically, intralesionally, or systemically by subcutaneous injection. Both lymphoblastoid (a) and fibroblast (b) interferon have been used with some success to treat patients with genital warts and respiratory papillomatosis topically, locally, and systemically.[66, 79, 83, 218, 244, 251] However, interferon-g has not been shown to be beneficial. Both recombinant and natural-source interferon-a preparations have been demonstrated in placebo-controlled trials to be effective and are approved by the U.S. Food and Drug Administration for the intralesional treatment of genital warts.[66, 79] A 25- to 30-gauge needle is used to inject approximately 0.1 mL (1×10^6 U) at the base of up to five warts at a time for a total dose of 5×10^6 U at each visit. This dose is repeated two to three times weekly for 3 weeks. Maximal effect usually is seen within 4 to 8 weeks. Repeat injections may be given if the warts are persistent or recurrent. Interferon therapy also may be effective if used alone or in combination with laser surgery to treat patients with RRP.[103, 105, 138, 139, 149] Fever, headache, chills, and myalgias frequently occur with local and systemic interferon treatment. Severe and persistent fatigue, nausea, and leukopenia are other fairly common adverse reactions, especially with systemically administered interferon. Systemic natural leukocyte interferon also causes regression of warts and reduction of the virus load in tissues in patients with EV.[5] Cimetidine, an immunomodulator that alters lymphocyte function, has been used in an attempt to treat children with recalcitrant cutaneous warts.[193] Contact and systemic immunotherapy with a variety of agents also has been tried as an alternative treatment of HPV-associated disease, but with variable success.[251]

Retinoids and retinoic acid, which are analogues of vitamin A, can regulate the growth and differentiation of malignant, premalignant, and even normal cells.[220] Clinically, they have a documented effect against squamous cell carcinoma.[142, 143] For these reasons, anecdotal reports and small series of patients have emerged in which retinoic acid was used to treat HPV-associated disease, especially RRP. In these reports, retinoids have been used with varying success, primarily as adjuvant agents with surgical therapy, to treat adult patients with severe, refractory RRP.[3, 15, 64] The combination of interferon and retinoic acid has been shown to be synergistic against breast cancer cells in vitro and potentially may be useful in refractory cases of RRP.[161]

Specific HPV antiviral chemotherapy is a promising direction for the future. The ideal anti-HPV drug would eliminate existing lesions swiftly and safely, eradicate latent HPV DNA to prevent recurrences, and permit the development of natural immunity against future reinfection and disease. Unique aspects of HPV infection and disease, however, make designing specific antiviral therapies a challenge. For example, HPV disease usually is focal, the virus is involved intricately in the cell's life cycle, and HPV has great diversity with more than 70 genotypes. The inability to grow HPVs readily in cell culture also hampers our ability to study the antiviral properties and cellular toxicities of candidate compounds. Molecular assays that isolate individual viral functions, therefore, have been used to evaluate the ability of antiviral compounds to inhibit each individual step in the virus life cycle. Furthermore, animal models for HPV-associated disease are lacking. Despite these challenges, the in vitro antiviral activity and clinical efficacy of a variety of compounds have been studied. For example, ribavirin, a nucleoside analogue with a broad antiviral spectrum, has been used in clinical trials for the treatment of laryngeal papillomatosis.[165] Cidofovir, a newly licensed antiviral compound to treat serious disease caused by CMV, also is being studied in patients with HPV-associated genital papillomas and RRP. In addition, novel strategies such as antisense oligonucleotides and therapeutic DNA vaccines may be investigated in the near future.

PREVENTION

Prevention of HPV infection and disease involves two potential approaches: behavioral strategies and vaccines. Prevention of genital HPV infection includes the use of barrier methods, such as condoms, to reduce transmission between sexual partners. Hospital infection control policies should address the potential transmissibility of HPV from patients to health care workers during laser vaporization and electrocautery therapy. Care should be taken to wear protective mask and eye wear and to use appropriate and well-functioning suction devices during these procedures.

There appears to be substantial medical and industry interest in the development of prophylactic vaccines to prevent HPV infection and therapeutic vaccines to treat HPV-associated disease; however, several challenges for the design of HPV vaccines exist. For example, a successful vaccine probably would need to induce broad-spectrum immunity that covers all HPV types. Studies of the immunogenicity and efficacy of new HPV vaccines should appraise whether natural HPV infection induces strong and lasting systemic or local immunity to reinfection. In addition, few animal models are suitable for HPV vaccine studies and none for cervical cancer, which is the main impetus for vaccine development. Finally, HPV infection and disease are confined primarily to the epithelial surface. Therefore, a successful vaccine probably should be able to induce protective secretory IgA, especially in the genital tract.

Despite these challenges, vaccines suitable for prophylaxis are in the research and developmental stages. Most efforts to produce an HPV vaccine have focused on L1, the major capsid protein and primary constituent of the surface of the mature HPV particle.[85] Large quantities of conformationally correct viral capsid proteins L1 and L2 have been produced as noninfectious, "virus-like" particles in the baculovirus and vaccinia virus expression systems, and some forms have been shown to induce neutralizing antibodies in animal model systems.[44, 102, 141] Most recently, a novel polynucleotide DNA vaccine that contains DNA encoding the major capsid protein L1 has been developed. It also appears to be a promising vaccine that could protect humans against HPV infection and simplify the production of a multivalent vaccine by combining plasmids that encode the capsid proteins of different HPV types.[60] Therapeutic vaccines most likely would need to induce cytotoxic T-cell responses against viral antigens such as the major capsid protein L1 and E6 and E7, the major transforming proteins. These vaccines may be possible in the near future if research and development continue.

REFERENCES

1. Abramson, A. L., DiLorenzo, T. P., and Steinberg, B. M.: Is papillomavirus detectable in the plume of laser-treated laryngeal papilloma? Arch. Otolaryngol. Head Neck Surg. *116*:604–607, 1990.
2. Agostini, H. T., Ryschkewitsch, C. F., and Stoner, G. L.: Genotype profile of human polyomavirus JC excreted in urine of immunocompetent individuals. J. Clin. Microbiol. *34*:159–164, 1996.
3. Alberts, D. S., Coulthard, S. W., and Meyskens, F. L., Jr.: Regression of aggressive laryngeal papillomatosis with 13-cis-retinoic acid (Accutane). J. Biol. Response Mod. *5*:124–128, 1986.
4. Andrews, C. A., Shah, K. V., Daniel, R. W., et al.: A serological investigation of BK virus and JC virus infections in recipients of renal allografts. J. Infect. Dis. *158*:176–181, 1988.
5. Androphy, E. J.: Papillomaviruses and interferon. Ciba Found. Symp. *120*:221–234, 1986.
6. Androphy, E. J., Dvoretzky, I., and Lowy, D. R.: X-linked inheritance of epidermodysplasia verruciformis. Genetic and virologic studies of a kindred. Arch. Dermatol. *121*:864–868, 1985.
7. Apperley, J. F., Rice, S. J., Bishop, J. A., et al.: Late-onset hemorrhagic cystitis associated with urinary excretion of polyomaviruses after bone marrow transplantation. Transplantation *43*:108–112, 1987.
8. Arrington, A. S., and Butel, J. S.: SV40 and human tumors. *In* Khalili, K., and Stoner, G. L. (eds.): The Human Polyomaviruses JC, BK, and SV40: Molecular and Clinical Perspectives. New York, John Wiley & Sons, 2000.
9. Arthur, R. R., Shah, K. V., Baust, S. J., et al.: Association of BK viruria with hemorrhagic cystitis in recipients of bone marrow transplants. N. Engl. J. Med. *315*:230–234, 1986.
10. Arthur, R. R., Shah, K. V., Charache, P., et al.: BK and JC virus infections in recipients of bone marrow transplants. J. Infect. Dis. *158*:563–569, 1988.
11. Astrom, K.-E., Mancall, E. L., and Richardson, E. P., Jr.: Progressive multifocal leukoencephalopathy. Brain *81*:93–111, 1958.
12. Baehr, P., and McDonald, G.: Infections of the esophagus. *In* Surawicz, C., and Owen, R. (eds.): Gastrointestinal and Hepatic Infections. Philadelphia, W. B. Saunders, 1995, pp. 3–33.
13. Bashi, S. A.: Cryotherapy versus podophyllin in the treatment of genital warts. Int. J. Dermatol. *24*:535–536, 1985.
14. Bauer, H. M., Ting, Y., Greer, C. E., et al.: Genital human papillomavirus infection in female university students as determined by a PCR-based method. J. A. M. A. *265*:472–477, 1991.
15. Bell, R., Hong, W. K., Itri, L. M., et al.: The use of cis-retinoic acid in recurrent respiratory papillomatosis of the larynx: A randomized pilot study. Am. J. Otolaryngol. *9*:161-164, 1988.
16. Bennett, R. S., and Powell, K. R.: Human papillomaviruses: Associations between laryngeal papillomas and genital warts. Pediatr. Infect. Dis. J. *6*:229–232, 1987.
17. Berger, J. R., and Levy, R. M.: The neurologic complications of human immunodeficiency virus infection. Med. Clin. North Am. *77*:1–23, 1993.
18. Berger, J. R., Pall, L., Lanska, D., et al.: Progressive multifocal leukoencephalopathy in patients with HIV infection. J. Neurovirol. *4*:59–68, 1998.
19. Berger, T. G., Sawchuk, W. S., Leonardi, C., et al.: Epidermodysplasia verruciformis–associated papillomavirus infection complicating human immunodeficiency virus disease. Br. J. Dermatol. *124*:79–83, 1991.
20. Bergeron, C., Barrasso, R., Beaudenon, S., et al.: Human papillomaviruses associated with cervical intraepithelial neoplasia. Great diversity and distinct distribution in low- and high-grade lesions. Am. J. Surg. Pathol. *16*:641–649, 1992.
21. Berkhout, R. J., Tieben, L. M., Smits, H. L., et al.: Nested PCR approach for detection and typing of epidermodysplasia verruciformis–associated human papillomavirus types in cutaneous cancers from renal transplant recipients. J. Clin. Microbiol. *33*:690–695, 1995.
22. Bernard, H. U., Chan, S. Y., Manos, M. M., et al.: Identification and assessment of known and novel human papillomaviruses by polymerase chain reaction amplification, restriction fragment length polymorphisms, nucleotide sequence, and phylogenetic algorithms. J. Infect. Dis. *170*:1077–1085, 1994.
23. Billingham, R. P., and Lewis, F. G.: Laser versus electrical cautery in the treatment of condylomata acuminata of the anus. Surg. Gynecol. Obstet. *155*:865–867, 1982.
24. Birch, H., and Mankart, H.: Ultrasound for juvenile laryngeal papillomas. Arch. Otolaryngol. *77*:603–608, 1963.
25. Bofill-Mas, S., Pina, S., and Girones, R.: Documenting the epidemiologic patterns of polyomaviruses in human populations by studying their presence in urban sewage. Appl. Environ. Microbiol. *66*:238–245, 2000.
26. Bonnez, W., Da Rin, C., Rose, R. C., et al.: Use of human papillomavirus type 11 virions in an ELISA to detect specific antibodies in humans with condylomata acuminata. J. Gen. Virol. *72*:1343–1347, 1991.
27. Bonnez, W., Da Rin, C., Rose, R. C., et al.: Evolution of the antibody response to human papillomavirus type 11 (HPV-11) in patients with condyloma acuminatum according to treatment response. J. Med. Virol. *39*:340–344, 1993.
28. Bonnez, W., Kashima, H. K., Leventhal, B., et al.: Antibody response to human papillomavirus (HPV) type 11 in children with juvenile-onset recurrent respiratory papillomatosis (RRP). Virology *188*:384–387, 1992.
29. Brandsma, J. L., Abramson, A., and Sciubba, J.: Papillomavirus infections of the nose. *In* Steinberg, B., Brandsma, J. L., and Taichman, L. B. (eds.): Papillomaviruses and Cancer Cells. New York, Cold Spring Harbor Laboratory, 1987, pp. 301–308.
30. Brandsma, J. L., Steinberg, B. M., Abramson, A. L., et al.: Presence of human papillomavirus type 16 related sequences in verrucous carcinoma of the larynx. Cancer Res. *46*:2185–2188, 1986.
31. Bratt, G., Hammarin, A. L., Grandien, M., et al.: BK virus as the cause of meningoencephalitis, retinitis and nephritis in a patient with AIDS. A. I. D. S. *13*:1071–1075, 1999.
32. Bunney, M. H., Barr, B. B., McLaren, K., et al.: Human papillomavirus type 5 and skin cancer in renal allograft recipients. Lancet *2*:151–152, 1987.
33. Burk, R. D., Ho, G. Y., Beardsley, L., et al.: Sexual behavior and partner characteristics are the predominant risk factors for genital human papillomavirus infection in young women. J. Infect. Dis. *174*:679–689, 1996.

34. Butel, J. S.: Viral carcinogenesis: Revelation of molecular mechanisms and etiology of human disease. Carcinogenesis *21*:405–426, 2000.
35. Butel, J. S., Arrington, A. S., Wong, C., et al.: Molecular evidence of simian virus 40 infections in children. J. Infect. Dis. *180*:884–887, 1999.
36. Butel, J. S., Jafar, S., Wong, C., et al.: Evidence of SV40 infections in hospitalized children. Hum. Pathol. *30*:1496–1502, 1999.
37. Butel, J. S., and Lednicky, J. A.: Cell and molecular biology of simian virus 40: Implications for human infections and disease. J. Natl. Cancer Inst. *91*:119–134, 1999.
38. Carter, J. J., Hagensee, M., Taflin, M. C., et al.: HPV-1 capsids expressed in vitro detect human serum antibodies associated with foot warts. Virology *195*:456–462, 1993.
39. Cason, J., Kaye, J. N., Jewers, R. J., et al.: Perinatal infection and persistence of human papillomavirus types 16 and 18 in infants. J. Med. Virol. *47*:209–218, 1995.
40. Caussy, D., Orr, W., Daya, A. D., et al.: Evaluation of methods for detecting human papillomavirus deoxyribonucleotide sequences in clinical specimens. J. Clin. Microbiol. *26*:236–243, 1988.
41. Chang, F., Syrjanen, S., Wang, L., et al.: Infectious agents in the etiology of esophageal cancer. Gastroenterology *103*:1336–1348, 1992.
42. Chen, S. L., Tsao, Y. P., Lee, J. W., et al.: Characterization and analysis of human papillomaviruses of skin warts. Arch. Dermatol. Res. *285*:460–465, 1993.
43. Chesters, P. M., Heritage, J., and McCance, D. J.: Persistence of DNA sequences of BK virus and JC virus in normal human tissues and in diseased tissues. J. Infect. Dis. *147*:676–684, 1983.
44. Christensen, N. D., Hopfl, R., DiAngelo, S. L., et al.: Assembled baculovirus-expressed human papillomavirus type 11 L1 capsid protein virus-like particles are recognized by neutralizing monoclonal antibodies and induce high titres of neutralizing antibodies. J. Gen. Virol. *75*:2271–2276, 1994.
45. Christensen, N. D., Kreider, J. W., Shah, K. V., et al.: Detection of human serum antibodies that neutralize infectious human papillomavirus type 11 virions. J. Gen. Virol. *73*:1261–1267, 1992.
46. Christian, C., Reddel, R., and Gerwin, B.: Infection of cultured human cells of respiratory tract origin with human papillomavirus type 1. *In* Steinberg, B., Brandsma, J. L., and Taichman, L. B. (eds.): Papillomaviruses and Cancer Cells. New York, Cold Spring Harbor Laboratory, 1987, pp. 301–308.
47. Ciuffo, G.: Innesto positivo con filtrato di verruca vulgare. G. Ital. Mal. Venereol. *48*:12–17, 1907.
48. Clark, R. A., Brandon, W., Dumestre, J., et al.: Clinical manifestations of infection with the human immunodeficiency virus in women in Louisiana. Clin. Infect. Dis. *17*:165–172, 1993.
49. Cohen, S. R., Geller, K. A., Seltzer, S., et al.: Papilloma of the larynx and tracheobronchial tree in children. A retrospective study. Ann. Otol. Rhinol. Laryngol. *89*:497–503, 1980.
50. Cole, C. N.: *Polyomavirinae*: The viruses and their replication. *In* Fields, B. N., Knipe, D. M., Howley, P. M., et al.: (eds.): Fields Virology. Philadelphia, Lippincott-Raven, 1996, pp. 1997–2025.
51. Cook, T. A., Brunschwig, J. P., Butel, J. S., et al.: Laryngeal papilloma: Etiologic and therapeutic considerations. Ann. Otol. Rhinol. Laryngol. *82*:649–655, 1973.
52. Cooper, K. D., Androphy, E. J., Lowy, D., et al.: Antigen presentation and T-cell activation in epidermodysplasia verruciformis. J. Invest. Dermatol. *94*:769–776, 1990.
53. Cubukcu-Dimopulo, O., Greco, A., Kumar, A., et al.: BK virus infection in AIDS. Am. J. Surg. Pathol. *24*:145–149, 2000.
54. Davis, A. J., and Emans, S. J.: Human papilloma virus infection in the pediatric and adolescent patient. J. Pediatr. *115*:1–9, 1989.
55. Deau, M. C., Favre, M., and Orth, G.: Genetic heterogeneity among human papillomaviruses (HPV) associated with epidermodysplasia verruciformis: Evidence for multiple allelic forms of HPV5 and HPV8 E6 genes. Virology *184*:492–503, 1991.
56. Degener, A. M., Pietropaolo, V., Di Taranto, C., et al.: Detection of JC and BK viral genome in specimens of HIV-1 infected subjects. New Microbiol. *20*:115–122, 1997.
57. De Luca, A., Cingolani, A., Linzalone, A., et al.: Improved detection of JC virus DNA in cerebrospinal fluid for diagnosis of AIDS-related progressive multifocal leukoencephalopathy. J. Clin. Microbiol. *34*:1343–1346, 1996.
58. De Peuter, M., De Clercq, B., Minette, A., et al.: An epidemiological survey of virus warts of the hands among butchers. Br. J. Dermatol. *96*:427–431, 1977.
59. de Villiers, E. M., Weidauer, H., Otto, H., et al.: Papillomavirus DNA in human tongue carcinomas. Int. J. Cancer *36*:575–578, 1985.
60. Donnelly, J. J., Martinez, D., Jansen, K. U., et al.: Protection against papillomavirus with a polynucleotide vaccine. J. Infect. Dis. *173*:314–320, 1996.
61. Dorries, K., Vogel, E., Gunther, S., et al.: Infection of human polyomaviruses JC and BK in peripheral blood leukocytes from immunocompetent individuals. Virology *198*:59–70, 1994.
62. Drut, R., Gomez, M. A., Drut, R. M., et al.: Human papillomavirus (HPV)-associated neonatal giant cell hepatitis (NGCH). Pediatr. Pathol. Lab. Med. *16*:403–412, 1996.
63. Dubois, V., Dutronc, H., Lafon, M. E., et al.: Latency and reactivation of JC virus in peripheral blood of human immunodeficiency virus type 1–infected patients. J. Clin. Microbiol. *35*:2288–2292, 1997.
64. Eicher, S. A., Taylor-Cooley, L. D., and Donovan, D. T.: Isotretinoin therapy for recurrent respiratory papillomatosis. Arch. Otolaryngol. Head Neck Surg. *120*:405–409, 1994.
65. Elliot, B., Aromin, I., Gold, R., et al.: 2.5 year remission of AIDS-associated progressive multifocal leukoencephalopathy with combined antiretroviral therapy. Lancet *349*:850, 1997.
66. Eron, L. J., Judson, F., Tucker, S., et al.: Interferon therapy for condylomata acuminata. N. Engl. J. Med. *315*:1059–1064, 1986.
67. Euvrard, S., Chardonnet, Y., Pouteil-Noble, C., et al.: Association of skin malignancies with various and multiple carcinogenic and noncarcinogenic human papillomaviruses in renal transplant recipients. Cancer *72*:2198–2206, 1993.
68. Eversole, L. R., Laipis, P. J., and Green, T. L.: Human papillomavirus type 2 DNA in oral and labial verruca vulgaris. J. Cutan. Pathol. *14*:319–325, 1987.
69. Ferenczy, A.: HPV-associated lesions in pregnancy and their clinical implications. Clin. Obstet. Gynecol. *32*:191–199, 1989.
70. Ferenczy, A., Bergeron, C., and Richart, R. M.: Human papillomavirus DNA in fomites on objects used for the management of patients with genital human papillomavirus infections. Obstet. Gynecol. *74*:950–954, 1989.
71. Ferenczy, A., Bergeron, C., and Richart, R. M.: Human papillomavirus DNA in CO_2 laser-generated plume of smoke and its consequences to the surgeon. Obstet. Gynecol. *75*:114–118, 1990.
72. Ferenczy, A., Mitao, M., Nagai, N., et al.: Latent papillomavirus and recurring genital warts. N. Engl. J. Med. *313*:784–788, 1985.
73. Firzlaff, J. M., Kiviat, N. B., Beckmann, A. M., et al.: Detection of human papillomavirus capsid antigens in various squamous epithelial lesions using antibodies directed against the L1 and L2 open reading frames. Virology *164*:467–477, 1988.
74. Flaegstad, T., Ronne, K., Filipe, A. R., et al.: Prevalence of anti BK virus antibody in Portugal and Norway. Scand. J. Infect. Dis. *21*:145–147, 1989.
75. Flaegstad, T., Traavik, T., and Kristiansen, B. E.: Age-dependent prevalence of BK virus IgG and IgM antibodies measured by enzyme-linked immunosorbent assays (ELISA). J. Hyg. (Lond.) *96*:523–528, 1986.
76. Fogazzi, G. B., Cantu, M., and Saglimbeni, L.: 'Decoy cells' in the urine due to polyomavirus BK infection: Easily seen by phase-contrast microscopy. Nephrol. Dial. Transplant. *16*:1496–1498, 2001.
77. Franceschi, S., Doll, R., Gallwey, J., et al.: Genital warts and cervical neoplasia: An epidemiological study. Br. J. Cancer *48*:621–628, 1983.
78. Friedman, H. B., Saah, A. J., Sherman, M. E., et al.: Human papillomavirus, anal squamous intraepithelial lesions, and human immunodeficiency virus in a cohort of gay men. J. Infect. Dis. *178*:45–52, 1998.
79. Friedman-Kien, A. E., Eron, L. J., Conant, M., et al.: Natural interferon alfa for treatment of condylomata acuminata. J. A. M. A. *259*:533–538, 1988.
80. Frisch, M., Glimelius, B., van den Brule, A. J., et al.: Sexually transmitted infection as a cause of anal cancer. N. Engl. J. Med. *337*:1350–1358, 1997.
81. Gabbott, M., Cossart, Y. E., Kan, A., et al.: Human papillomavirus and host variables as predictors of clinical course in patients with juvenile-onset recurrent respiratory papillomatosis. J. Clin. Microbiol. *35*:3098–3103, 1997.
82. Gabriel, G., and Thin, R. N.: Treatment of anogenital warts. Comparison of trichloracetic acid and podophyllin versus podophyllin alone. Br. J. Vener. Dis. *59*:124–126, 1983.
83. Gall, S. A., Hughes, C. E., and Trofatter, K.: Interferon for the therapy of condyloma acuminatum. Am. J. Obstet. Gynecol. *153*:157–163, 1985.
84. Gallia, G. L., Houff, S. A., Major, E. O., et al.: Review: JC virus infection of lymphocytes—revisited. J. Infect. Dis. *176*:1603–1609, 1997.
85. Galloway, D. A.: Human papillomavirus vaccines: A warty problem. Infect. Agents Dis. *3*:187–193, 1994.
86. Garden, J. M., O'Banion, M. K., Shelnitz, L. S., et al.: Papillomavirus in the vapor of carbon dioxide laser–treated verrucae. J. A. M. A. *259*:1199–1202, 1988.
87. Gardner, S. D., Field, A. M., Coleman, D. V., et al.: New human papovavirus (B.K.) isolated from urine after renal transplantation. Lancet *1*:1253–1257, 1971.
88. Gaylis, B., and Hayden, R. E.: Recurrent respiratory papillomatosis: Progression to invasion and malignancy. Am. J. Otolaryngol. *12*:104–112, 1991.
89. Gerber, P.: Patterns of antibodies to SV40 in children following the last booster with inactivated poliomyelitis vaccines. Proc. Soc. Exp. Biol. Med. *125*:1284–1287, 1967.
90. Ghim, S. J., Jenson, A. B., and Schlegel, R.: HPV-1 L1 protein expressed in cos cells displays conformational epitopes found on intact virions. Virology *190*:548–552, 1992.
91. Girardi, A. J., Sweet, B. H., Slotnick, V. B., et al.: Development of tumors in hamsters inoculated in the neonatal period with vacuolating virus, SV40. Proc. Soc. Exp. Biol. Med. *109*:649–660, 1962.
92. Glinski, W., Obalek, S., Jablonska, S., et al.: T cell defect in patients with epidermodysplasia verruciformis due to human papillomavirus type 3 and 5. Dermatologica *162*:141–147, 1981.

93. Goudsmit, J., Baak, M. L., Sleterus, K. W., et al.: Human papovavirus isolated from urine of a child with acute tonsillitis. B. M. J. *283*:1363–1364, 1981.
94. Goudsmit, J., Wertheim-van, D. P., van Strien, A., et al.: The role of BK virus in acute respiratory tract disease and the presence of BKV DNA in tonsils. J. Med. Virol. *10*:91–99, 1982.
95. Graham, S., Priore, R., Graham, M., et al.: Genital cancer in wives of penile cancer patients. Cancer *44*:1870–1874, 1979.
96. Greer, C. E., Wheeler, C. M., Ladner, M. B., et al.: Human papillomavirus (HPV) type distribution and serological response to HPV type 6 virus–like particles in patients with genital warts. J. Clin. Microbiol. *33*:2058–2063, 1995.
97. Gross, G., Ellinger, K., Roussaki, A., et al.: Epidermodysplasia verruciformis in a patient with Hodgkin's disease: Characterization of a new papillomavirus type and interferon treatment. J. Invest. Dermatol. *91*:43–48, 1988.
98. Guerrero, E., Daniel, R. W., Bosch, F. X., et al.: Comparison of ViraPap, Southern hybridization, and polymerase chain reaction methods for human papillomavirus identification in an epidemiological investigation of cervical cancer. J. Clin. Microbiol. *30*:2951–2959, 1992.
99. Gutman, L. T., St. Claire, K. K., Everett, V. D., et al.: Cervical-vaginal and intraanal human papillomavirus infection of young girls with external genital warts. J. Infect. Dis. *170*:339–344, 1994.
100. Gutman, L. T., St. Claire, K., Herman-Giddens, M. E., et al.: Evaluation of sexually abused and nonabused young girls for intravaginal human papillomavirus infection. Am. J. Dis. Child. *146*:694–699, 1992.
101. Hagensee, M. E., Kiviat, N., Critchlow, C. W., et al.: Seroprevalence of human papillomavirus types 6 and 16 capsid antibodies in homosexual men. J. Infect. Dis. *176*:625–631, 1997.
102. Hagensee, M. E., Olson, N. H., Baker, T. S., et al.: Three-dimensional structure of vaccinia virus–produced human papillomavirus type 1 capsids. J. Virol. *68*:4503–4505, 1994.
103. Haglund, S., Lundquist, P. G., Cantell, K., et al.: Interferon therapy in juvenile laryngeal papillomatosis. Arch. Otolaryngol. *107*:327–332, 1981.
104. Hammarin, A. L., Bogdanovic, G., Svedhem, V., et al.: Analysis of PCR as a tool for detection of JC virus DNA in cerebrospinal fluid for diagnosis of progressive multifocal leukoencephalopathy. J. Clin. Microbiol. *34*:2929–2932, 1996.
105. Healy, G. B., Gelber, R. D., Trowbridge, A. L., et al.: Treatment of recurrent respiratory papillomatosis with human leukocyte interferon. Results of a multicenter randomized clinical trial. N. Engl. J. Med. *319*:401–407, 1988.
106. Hedquist, B. G., Bratt, G., Hammarin, A. L., et al.: Identification of BK virus in a patient with acquired immune deficiency syndrome and bilateral atypical retinitis. Ophthalmology *106*:129–132, 1999.
107. Heritage, J., Chesters, P. M., and McCance, D. J.: The persistence of papovavirus BK DNA sequences in normal human renal tissue. J. Med. Virol. *8*:143–150, 1981.
108. Hildesheim, A., Schiffman, M. H., Gravitt, P. E., et al.: Persistence of type-specific human papillomavirus infection among cytologically normal women. J. Infect. Dis. *169*:235–240, 1994.
109. Ho, G. Y., Bierman, R., Beardsley, L., et al.: Natural history of cervicovaginal papillomavirus infection in young women. N. Engl. J. Med. *338*:423–428, 1998.
110. Horn, J. E., McQuillan, G. M., Shah, K. V., et al.: Genital human papillomavirus infections in patients attending an inner-city STD clinic. Sex. Transm. Dis. *18*:183–187, 1991.
111. Imperiale, M. J.: The human polyomaviruses, BKV and JCV: Molecular pathogenesis of acute disease and potential role in cancer. Virology *267*:1–7, 2000.
112. Jablonska, S., Biczysko, W., Jakubowicz, K., et al.: The ultrastructure of transitional states to Bowen's disease and invasive Bowen's carcinoma in epidermodysplasia verruciformis. Dermatologica *140*: 186–194, 1970.
113. Jafar, S., Rodriguez-Barradas, M., Graham, D. Y., et al.: Serological evidence of SV40 infections in HIV-infected and HIV-negative adults. J. Med. Virol. *54*:276–284, 1998.
114. Jamison, J. H., Kaplan, D. W., Hamman, R., et al.: Spectrum of genital human papillomavirus infection in a female adolescent population. Sex. Transm. Dis. *22*:236–243, 1995.
115. Jasani, B., Cristaudo, A., Emri, S. A., et al.: Association of SV40 with human tumors. Semin. Cancer Biol. *11*:49–61, 2001.
116. Jenison, S. A., Yu, X. P., Valentine, J. M., et al.: Human antibodies react with an epitope of the human papillomavirus type 6b L1 open reading frame which is distinct from the type-common epitope. J. Virol. *63*:809–818, 1989.
117. Jenison, S. A., Yu, X. P., Valentine, J. M., et al.: Evidence of prevalent genital-type human papillomavirus infections in adults and children. J. Infect. Dis. *162*:60–69, 1990.
118. Jennings, L. C., Ross, A. D., and Faoagali, J. L.: The prevalence of warts on the hands of workers in a New Zealand slaughterhouse. N. Z. Med. J. *97*:473–476, 1984.
119. Jensen, S. L.: Comparison of podophyllin application with simple surgical excision in clearance and recurrence of perianal condylomata acuminata. Lancet *2*:1146–1148, 1985.
120. Jochum, W., Weber, T., Frye, S., et al.: Detection of JC virus by anti-VP1 immunohistochemistry in brains with progressive multifocal leukoencephalopathy. Acta Neuropathol.(Berl.) *94*:226–231, 1997.
121. Kaye, J. N., Cason, J., Pakarian, F. B., et al.: Viral load as a determinant for transmission of human papillomavirus type 16 from mother to child. J. Med. Virol. *44*:415–421, 1994.
122. Kellogg, N. D., and Parra, J. M.: The progression of human papillomavirus lesions in sexual assault victims. Pediatrics *96*:1163–1165, 1995.
123. Kiviat, N. B., Koutsky, L. A., Paavonen, J. A., et al.: Prevalence of genital papillomavirus infection among women attending a college student health clinic or a sexually transmitted disease clinic. J. Infect. Dis. *159*:293–302, 1989.
124. Kjaer, S. K., Dahl, C., Engholm, G., et al.: Case-control study of risk factors for cervical neoplasia in Denmark. II. Role of sexual activity, reproductive factors, and venereal infections. Cancer Causes Control *3*:339–348, 1992.
125. Knepper, J. E., and diMayorca, G.: Cloning and characterization of BK virus–related DNA sequences from normal and neoplastic human tissues. J. Med. Virol. *21*:289–299, 1987.
126. Koralnik, I. J., Boden, D., Mai, V. X., et al.: JC virus DNA load in patients with and without progressive multifocal leukoencephalopathy. Neurology *52*:253–260, 1999.
127. Krebs, H. B.: Treatment of genital condylomata with topical 5-fluorouracil. Dermatol. Clin. *9*:333–341, 1991.
128. Kreider, J. W., Howett, M. K., Leure-Dupree, A. E., et al.: Laboratory production in vivo of infectious human papillomavirus type 11. J. Virol. *61*:590–593, 1987.
129. Kreider, J. W., Howett, M. K., Lill, N. L., et al.: In vivo transformation of human skin with human papillomavirus type 11 from condylomata acuminata. J. Virol. *55*:369–376, 1986.
130. Krynska, B., Del Valle, L., Croul, S., et al.: Detection of human neurotropic JC virus DNA sequence and expression of the viral oncogenic protein in pediatric medulloblastomas. Proc. Natl. Acad. Sci. U. S. A. *96*:11519–11524, 1999.
131. Kuypers, J., and Kiviat, N.: Anal papillomavirus infections. *In* Surawicz, C., and Owen, R. (eds.): Gastrointestinal and Hepatic Infections. Philadelphia, W. B. Saunders, 1995, pp. 279–285.
132. Labropoulou, V., Diakomanolis, E., Dailianas, S., et al.: Genital papillomavirus in Greek women with high-grade cervical intraepithelial neoplasia and cervical carcinoma. J. Med. Virol. *48*:80–87, 1996.
133. Lafon, M. E., Dutronc, H., Dubois, V., et al.: JC virus remains latent in peripheral blood B lymphocytes but replicates actively in urine from AIDS patients. J. Infect. Dis. *177*:1502–1505, 1998.
134. Laghi, L., Randolph, A. E., Chauhan, D. P., et al.: JC virus DNA is present in the mucosa of the human colon and in colorectal cancers. Proc. Natl. Acad. Sci. U. S. A. *96*:7484–7489, 1999.
135. Lass, J. H., Grove, A. S., Papale, J. J., et al.: Detection of human papillomavirus DNA sequences in conjunctival papilloma. Am. J. Ophthalmol. *96*:670–674, 1983.
136. Le Cann, P., Touze, A., Enogat, N., et al.: Detection of antibodies against human papillomavirus (HPV) type 16 virions by enzyme-linked immunosorbent assay using recombinant HPV 16 L1 capsids produced by recombinant baculovirus. J. Clin. Microbiol. *33*:1380–1382, 1995.
137. Lednicky, J. A., and Butel, J. S.: Polyomaviruses and human tumors: A brief review of current concepts and interpretations. Front. Biosci. *4*:D153–D164, 1999.
138. Leventhal, B. G., Kashima, H. K., Mounts, P., et al.: Long-term response of recurrent respiratory papillomatosis to treatment with lymphoblastoid interferon alfa-N1. Papilloma Study Group. N. Engl. J. Med. *325*:613–617, 1991.
139. Leventhal, B. G., Kashima, H. K., Weck, P. W., et al.: Randomized surgical adjuvant trial of interferon alfa-n1 in recurrent papillomatosis. Arch. Otolaryngol. Head Neck Surg. *114*:1163–1169, 1988.
140. Lewis, A. M. J., Levine, A. S., Crumpacker, C. S., et al.: Studies of nondefective adenovirus 2–simian virus 40 hybrid viruses. V. Isolation of additional hybrids which differ in their simian virus 40–specific biological properties. J. Virol. *11*:655–664, 1973.
141. Lin, Y. L., Borenstein, L. A., Ahmed, R., et al.: Cottontail rabbit papillomavirus L1 protein–based vaccines: Protection is achieved only with a full-length, nondenatured product. J. Virol. *67*:4154–4162, 1993.
142. Lippman, S. M., Kessler, J. F., Al Sarraf, M., et al.: Treatment of advanced squamous cell carcinoma of the head and neck with isotretinoin: A phase II randomized trial. Invest. New Drugs *6*:51–56, 1988.
143. Lippman, S. M., and Meyskens, F. L., Jr.: Treatment of advanced squamous cell carcinoma of the skin with isotretinoin. Ann. Intern. Med *107*:499–502, 1987.
144. Long, G. E., and Rickman, L. S.: Infectious complications of tattoos. Clin. Infect. Dis. *18*:610–619, 1994.
145. Longuet, M., Cassonnet, P., and Orth, G.: A novel genital human papillomavirus (HPV), HPV type 74, found in immunosuppressed patients. J. Clin. Microbiol. *34*:1859–1862, 1996.
146. Lorincz, A. T., Reid, R., Jenson, A. B., et al.: Human papillomavirus infection of the cervix: Relative risk associations of 15 common anogenital types. Obstet. Gynecol. *79*:328–337, 1992.

147. Lorincz, A. T., Schiffman, M. H., Jaffurs, W. J., et al.: Temporal associations of human papillomavirus infection with cervical cytologic abnormalities. Am. J. Obstet. Gynecol. *162*:645–651, 1990.
148. Lutzner, M. A., Orth, G., Dutronquay, V., et al.: Detection of human papillomavirus type 5 DNA in skin cancers of an immunosuppressed renal allograft recipient. Lancet *20*:422–424, 1983.
149. Lyons, G. D., Schlosser, J. V., Lousteau, R., et al.: Laser surgery and immunotherapy in the management of laryngeal papilloma. Laryngoscope *88*:1586–1588, 1978.
150. Madreperla, S. A., Green, W. R., Daniel, R., et al.: Human papillomavirus in primary epithelial tumors of the lacrimal sac. Ophthalmology *100*:569–573, 1993.
151. Maitland, N. J., Cox, M. F., Lynas, C., et al.: Detection of human papillomavirus DNA in biopsies of human oral tissue. Br. J. Cancer *56*:245–250, 1987.
152. Majewski, S., and Jablonska, S.: Epidermodysplasia verruciformis: Immunological and clinical aspects. Curr. Top. Microbiol. Immunol. *186*:157–175, 1994.
153. Majewski, S., and Jablonska, S.: Epidermodysplasia verruciformis as a model of human papillomavirus-induced genetic cancer of the skin. Arch. Dermatol. *131*:1312–1318, 1995.
154. Majewski, S., Malejczyk, J., Jablonska, S., et al.: Natural cell-mediated cytotoxicity against various target cells in patients with epidermodysplasia verruciformis. J. Am. Acad. Dermatol. *22*:423–427, 1990.
155. Majewski, S., Skopinska-Rozewska, E., Jablonska, S., et al.: Partial defects of cell-mediated immunity in patients with epidermodysplasia verruciformis. J. Am. Acad. Dermatol. *15*:966–973, 1986.
156. Major, E. O.: Human polyomaviruses. *In* Knipe, D. M., and Howley, P. (eds.): Fields Virology. Philadelphia, Lippincott-Raven, 2001, pp. 2175–2196.
157. Majoros, M., Parkhill, E., and Devine, K.: Papillomas of the larynx in children: A clinicopathologic study. Am. J. Surg. *108*:470–475, 1964.
158. Manos, M. M., Ting, Y., and Wright, D.: The use of polymerase chain reaction amplification for the detection of genital human papillomaviruses. Cancer Cells *7*:209–214, 1989.
159. Markowitz, R. B., Eaton, B. A., Kubik, M. F., et al.: BK virus and JC virus shed during pregnancy have predominantly archetypal regulatory regions. J. Virol. *65*:4515–4519, 1991.
160. Marres, E. H., Wentges, R. T., and Brinkman, W. F.: Cryosurgical treatment of juvenile laryngeal papillomatosis. Laryngoscope *76*:1979–1982, 1966.
161. Marth, C., Daxenbichler, G., and Dapunt, O.: Synergistic antiproliferative effect of human recombinant interferons and retinoic acid in cultured breast cancer cells. J. Natl. Cancer Inst. *77*:1197–1202, 1986.
162. Martini, F., Dolcetti, R., Gloghini, A., et al.: Simian-virus-40 footprints in human lymphoproliferative disorders of HIV⁻ and HIV⁺ patients. Int. J. Cancer *78*:669–674, 1998.
163. McDonnell, J. M., Mayr, A. J., and Martin, W. J.: DNA of human papillomavirus type 16 in dysplastic and malignant lesions of the conjunctiva and cornea. N. Engl. J. Med. *320*:1442–1446, 1989.
164. McDonnell, P. J., McDonnell, J. M., Kessis, T., et al.: Detection of human papillomavirus type 6/11 DNA in conjunctival papillomas by in situ hybridization with radioactive probes. Hum. Pathol. *18*:1115–1119, 1987.
165. McGlennen, R. C., Adams, G. L., Lewis, C. M., et al.: Pilot trial of ribavirin for the treatment of laryngeal papillomatosis. Head Neck *15*:504–512, 1993.
166. Melkert, P. W., Hopman, E., van den Brule, A. J., et al.: Prevalence of HPV in cytomorphologically normal cervical smears, as determined by the polymerase chain reaction, is age-dependent. Int. J. Cancer *53*:919–923, 1993.
167. Melnick, J. L., and Stinebaugh, S.: Excretion of vacuolating SV-40 virus (papova virus group) after ingestion as a contaminant of oral poliovaccine. Proc. Soc. Exp. Biol. Med. *109*:965–968, 1962.
168. Meylan, P. R. A., Vuadens, P., Maeder, P., et al.: Monitoring the response of AIDS-related progressive multifocal leukoencephalopathy to HAART and cidofovir by PCR for JC virus DNA in the CSF. Eur. Neurol. *41*:172–174, 1999.
169. Miller, D. M., Brodell, R. T., and Levine, M. R.: The conjunctival wart: Report of a case and review of treatment options. Ophthalmic Surg. *25*:545–548, 1994.
170. Mork, J., Lie, A. K., Glattre, E., et al.: Human papillomavirus infection as a risk factor for squamous-cell carcinoma of the head and neck. N. Engl. J. Med. *344*:1125–1131, 2001.
171. Morris, J. A., Johnson, K. M., Aulisio, C. G., et al.: Clinical and Serologic responses in volunteers given vacuolating virus (SV40) by respiratory route. Proc. Soc. Exp. Biol. Med. *108*:56–59, 1961.
172. Morrison, E. A.: Natural history of cervical infection with human papillomaviruses. Clin. Infect. Dis. *18*:172–180, 1994.
173. Morriss, M. C., Rutstein, R. M., Rudy, B., et al.: Progressive multifocal leukoencephalopathy in an HIV-infected child. Neuroradiology *39*:142–144, 1997.
174. Moscicki, A. B., Palefsky, J. M., Gonzales, J., et al.: The association between human papillomavirus deoxyribonucleic acid status and the results of cytologic rescreening tests in young, sexually active women. Am. J. Obstet. Gynecol. *165*:67–71, 1991.
175. Moscicki, A. B., Palefsky, J. M., Gonzales, J., et al.: Colposcopic and histologic findings and human papillomavirus (HPV) DNA test variability in young women positive for HPV DNA. J. Infect. Dis. *166*:951–957, 1992.
176. Moscicki, A. B., Shiboski, S., Broering, J., et al.: The natural history of human papillomavirus infection as measured by repeated DNA testing in adolescent and young women. J. Pediatr. *132*:277–284, 1998.
177. Mounts, P., and Kashima, H.: Association of human papillomavirus subtype and clinical course in respiratory papillomatosis. Laryngoscope *94*:28–33, 1984.
178. Mounts, P., Shah, K. V., and Kashima, H.: Viral etiology of juvenile- and adult-onset squamous papilloma of the larynx. Proc. Natl. Acad. Sci. U. S. A. *79*:5425–5429, 1982.
179. Naghashfar, Z., Sawada, E., Kutcher, M. J., et al.: Identification of genital tract papillomaviruses HPV-6 and HPV-16 in warts of the oral cavity. J. Med. Virol. *17*:313–324, 1985.
180. Nahhas, W. A., Marshall, M. L., Ponziani, J., et al.: Evaluation of urinary cytology of male sexual partners of women with cervical intraepithelial neoplasia and human papilloma virus infection. Gynecol. Oncol. *24*:279–285, 1986.
181. Nastac, E., Stoian, M., Hozoc, M., et al.: Prevalence of hemagglutination-inhibiting antibodies to BK virus in patients with endemic Balkan nephropathy. Virologie *33*:169–170, 1982.
182. National Cancer Institute Workshop: The 1988 Bethesda system for reporting cervical/vaginal cytologic diagnoses. J. A. M. A. *262*:931–940, 1998.
183. Newman, J. S., Baskin, G. B., and Frisque, R. J.: Identification of SV40 in brain, kidney and urine of healthy and SIV-infected rhesus monkeys. J. Neurovirol. *4*:394–406, 1998.
184. Nickeleit, V., Hirsch, H. H., Binet, I. F., et al.: Polyomavirus infection of renal allograft recipients: From latent infection to manifest disease. J. Am. Soc. Nephrol. *10*:1080–1089, 1999.
185. Nickeleit, V., Klimkait, T., Binet, I. F., et al.: Testing for polyomavirus type BK DNA in plasma to identify renal-allograft recipients with viral nephropathy. N. Engl. J. Med. *342*:1309–1315, 2000.
186. Noffsinger, A., Witte, D., and Fenoglio-Preiser, C. M.: The relationship of human papillomaviruses to anorectal neoplasia. Cancer *70*:1276–1287, 1992.
187. Nuovo, G. J., and Pedemonte, B. M.: Human papillomavirus types and recurrent cervical warts. J. A. M. A. *263*:1223–1226, 1990.
188. Nuovo, G. J., and Richart, R. M.: A comparison of slot blot, southern blot, and in situ hybridization analyses for human papillomavirus DNA in genital tract lesions. Obstet. Gynecol. *74*:673–678, 1989.
189. Obalek, S., Favre, M., Szymanczyk, J., et al.: Human papillomavirus (HPV) types specific of epidermodysplasia verruciformis detected in warts induced by HPV3 or HPV3-related types in immunosuppressed patients. J. Invest. Dermatol. *98*:936–941, 1992.
190. Ong, C. K., Bernard, H. U., and Villa, L. L.: Identification of genomic sequences of three novel human papillomavirus sequences in cervical smears of Amazonian Indians. J. Infect. Dis. *170*:1086–1088, 1994.
191. Oraetiruys-Clausen, F.: Rare oral viral disorder (molluscum contagiosum, localized keratoacanthoma, verrucae, condyloma acuminatum, and focal epithelial hyperplasia). Oral Surg. Oral Med. Oral Pathol. *34*:604–618, 1972.
192. O'Reilly, R. J., Lee, F. K., Grossbard, E., et al.: Papovavirus excretion following marrow transplantation: Incidence and association with hepatic dysfunction. Transplant. Proc. *13*:262–266, 1981.
193. Orlow, S. J., and Paller, A.: Cimetidine therapy for multiple viral warts in children. J. Am. Acad. Dermatol. *28*:794–796, 1993.
194. Ostrow, R. S., Bender, M., Niimura, M., et al.: Human papillomavirus DNA in cutaneous primary and metastasized squamous cell carcinomas from patients with epidermodysplasia verruciformis. Proc. Natl. Acad. Sci. U. S. A *79*:1634–1638, 1982.
195. Padgett, B. L., and Walker, D. L.: Prevalence of antibodies in human sera against JC virus, an isolate from a case of progressive multifocal leukoencephalopathy. J. Infect. Dis. *127*:467–470, 1973.
196. Padgett, B. L., Walker, D. L., ZuRhein, G. M., et al.: Cultivation of papova-like virus from human brain with progressive multifocal leucoencephalopathy. Lancet *1*:1257–1260, 1971.
197. Pakarian, F., Kaye, J., Cason, J., et al.: Cancer associated human papillomaviruses: Perinatal transmission and persistence. Br. J. Obstet. Gynaecol. *101*:514–517, 1994.
198. Palefsky, J. M., Holly, E. A., Ralston, M. L., et al.: Prevalence and risk factors for human papillomavirus infection of the anal canal in human immunodeficiency virus (HIV)-positive and HIV-negative homosexual men. J. Infect. Dis. *177*:361–367, 1998.
199. Pappo, O., Demetris, A. J., Raikow, R. B., et al.: Human polyoma virus infection of renal allografts: Histopathologic diagnosis, clinical significance, and literature review. Mod. Pathol. *9*:105–109, 1996.
200. Pappo, O., Yunis, E., Jordan, J. A., et al.: Recurrent and de novo giant cell hepatitis after orthotopic liver transplantation. Am. J. Surg. Pathol. *18*:804–813, 1994.
201. Pastner, B., Baker, D., and Jackman, E.: Human papillomaviruses. *In* Gonik, B. (ed.): Viral Diseases in Pregnancy. New York, Springer-Verlag, 1994, pp. 185–195.

202. Peyton, C. L., Jansen, A. M., Wheeler, C. M., et al.: A novel human papillomavirus sequence from an international cervical cancer study. J. Infect. Dis. *170*:1093–1095, 1994.
203. Peyton, C. L., and Wheeler, C. M.: Identification of five novel human papillomavirus sequences in the New Mexico triethnic population. J. Infect. Dis. *170*:1089–1092, 1994.
204. Pfister, H.: Biology and biochemistry of papillomaviruses. Rev. Physiol. Biochem. Pharmacol. *99*:111–181, 1984.
205. Pfister, H., Iftner, T., and Fuchs, P. G.: Papillomaviruses from epidermodysplasia verruciformis patients and renal allograft recipients. *In* Howley, P. M., and Broker, T. R. (eds.): Papillomaviruses: Molecular and Clinical Aspects. New York, Liss, 1985, pp. 85–100.
206. Pfister, H., and zur Hausen, H.: Seroepidemiological studies of human papilloma virus (HPV-1) infections. Int. J. Cancer *21*:161–165, 1978.
207. Phelps, W. C., and Alexander, K. A.: Antiviral therapy for human papillomaviruses: Rationale and prospects. Ann. Intern. Med. *123*:368–382, 1995.
208. Portolani, M., Marzocchi, A., Barbanti-Brodano, G., et al.: Prevalence in Italy of antibodies to a new human papovavirus (BK virus). J. Med. Microbiol. *7*:543–546, 1974.
209. Power, C., Nath, A., Aoki, F. Y., et al.: Remission of progressive multifocal leukoencephalopathy following splenectomy and antiretroviral therapy in a patient with HIV infection. N. Engl. J. Med. *336*:661–662, 1997.
210. Priftakis, P., Bogdanovic, G., Tyden, G., et al.: Polyomaviruria in renal transplant patients is not correlated to the cold ischemia period or to rejection episodes. J. Clin. Microbiol. *38*:406–407, 2000.
211. Procopio, A., Strizzi, L., Vianale, G., et al.: Simian virus-40 sequences are a negative prognostic cofactor in patients with malignant pleural mesothelioma. Genes Chromosomes Cancer *29*:173–179, 2000.
212. Prose, N. S., Knebel-Doeberitz, C., Miller, S., et al.: Widespread flat warts associated with human papillomavirus type 5: A cutaneous manifestation of human immunodeficiency virus infection. J. Am. Acad. Dermatol. *23*:978–981, 1990.
213. Quick, C. A., Watts, S. L., Krzyzek, R. A., et al.: Relationship between condylomata and laryngeal papillomata. Clinical and molecular virological evidence. Ann. Otol. Rhinol. Laryngol. *89*:467–471, 1980.
214. Randhawa, P. S., Finkelstein, S., Scantlebury, V., et al.: Human polyomavirus-associated interstitial nephritis in the allograft kidney. Transplantation *67*:103–109, 1999.
215. Reeves, W. C., Arosemena, J. R., Garcia, M., et al.: Genital human papillomavirus infection in Panama City prostitutes. J. Infect. Dis. *160*:599–603, 1989.
216. Reeves, W. C., Brinton, L. A., Garcia, M., et al.: Human papillomavirus infection and cervical cancer in Latin America. N. Engl. J. Med. *320*:1437–1441, 1989.
217. Reeves, W. C., Rawls, W. E., and Brinton, L. A.: Epidemiology of genital papillomaviruses and cervical cancer. Rev. Infect. Dis. *11*:426–439, 1989.
218. Reichman, R. C., Oakes, D., Bonnez, W., et al.: Treatment of condyloma acuminatum with three different interferon-alpha preparations administered parenterally: A double-blind, placebo-controlled trial. J. Infect. Dis. *162*:1270–1276, 1990.
219. Reid, R.: Superficial laser vulvectomy. I. The efficacy of extended superficial ablation for refractory and very extensive condylomas. Am. J. Obstet. Gynecol. *151*:1047–1052, 1985.
220. Repucci, A., DiLorenzo, T. P., and Abramson, A.: In vitro modulation of human laryngeal papilloma cell differentiation by retinoic acid. Otolaryngol. Head Neck Surg. *105*:528–532, 1991.
221. Respler, D. S., Jahn, A., Pater, A., et al.: Isolation and characterization of papillomavirus DNA from nasal inverting (schneiderian) papillomas. Ann. Otol. Rhinol. Laryngol. *96*:170–173, 1987.
222. Ricciardiello, L., Laghi, L., Ramamirtham, P., et al.: JC virus DNA sequences are frequently present in the human upper and lower gastrointestinal tract. Gastroenterology *119*:1228–1235, 2000.
223. Rice, S. J., Bishop, J. A., Apperley, J., et al.: BK virus as cause of haemorrhagic cystitis after bone marrow transplantation. Letter. Lancet *2*:844–845, 1985.
224. Richardson, E. P., Jr.: Progressive multifocal leukoencephalopathy. N. Engl. J. Med. *265*:815–823, 1961.
225. Rizzo, P., Carbone, M., Fisher, S. G., et al.: Simian virus 40 is present in most United States human mesotheliomas, but it is rarely present in non-Hodgkin's lymphoma. Chest *116*(Suppl.):470–473, 1999.
226. Rose, R. C., Bonnez, W., Reichman, R. C., et al.: Expression of human papillomavirus type 11 L1 protein in insect cells: In vivo and in vitro assembly of viruslike particles. J. Virol. *67*:1936–1944, 1993.
227. Rosen, S., Harmon, W., Krensky, A. M., et al.: Tubulo-interstitial nephritis associated with polyomavirus (BK type) infection. N. Engl. J. Med. *308*:1192–1196, 1983.
228. Rosenfeld, W. D., Rose, E., Vermund, S. H., et al.: Follow-up evaluation of cervicovaginal human papillomavirus infection in adolescents. J. Pediatr. *121*:307–311, 1992.
229. Rowson, K. E., and Mahy, B. W.: Human papova (wart) virus. Bacteriol. Rev. *31*:110–131, 1967.
230. Roye, C. F.: Abnormal cervical cytology in adolescents: A literature review. J. Adolesc. Health *13*:643–650, 1992.
231. Rudlinger, R., Bunney, M. H., Grob, R., et al.: Warts in fish handlers. Br. J. Dermatol. *120*:375–381, 1989.
232. Rudlinger, R., and Grob, R.: Papillomavirus infection and skin cancer in renal allograft recipients. Lancet *1*:1132–1133, 1989.
233. Rudlinger, R., Smith, I. W., Bunney, M. H., et al.: Human papillomavirus infections in a group of renal transplant recipients. Br. J. Dermatol. *115*:681–692, 1986.
234. Sadler, M., Chinn, R., Healy, J., et al.: New treatments for progressive multifocal leukoencephalopathy in HIV-1–infected patients. A. I. D. S. *12*:533–535, 1998.
235. Saitoh, K., Sugae, N., Koike, N., et al.: Diagnosis of childhood BK virus cystitis by electron microscopy and PCR. J. Clin. Pathol. *46*:773–775, 1993.
236. Sandler, E. S., Aquino, V. M., Goss-Shohet, E., et al.: BK papova virus pneumonia following hematopoietic stem cell transplantation. Bone Marrow Transplant. *20*:163–165, 1997.
237. Sawchuk, W. S., and Felten, R. P.: Infectious potential of aerosolized particles. Arch. Dermatol. *125*:1689–1692, 1989.
238. Sawchuk, W. S., Weber, P. J., Lowy, D. R., et al.: Infectious papillomavirus in the vapor of warts treated with carbon dioxide laser or electrocoagulation: Detection and protection. J. Am. Acad. Dermatol. *21*:41–49, 1989.
239. Schatzl, H. M., Sieger, E., Jager, G., et al.: Detection by PCR of human polyomaviruses BK and JC in immunocompromised individuals and partial sequencing of control regions. J. Med. Virol. *42*:138–145, 1994.
240. Schiffman, M. H.: Recent progress in defining the epidemiology of human papillomavirus infection and cervical neoplasia. J. Natl. Cancer Inst. *84*:394–398, 1992.
241. Schiffman, M. H., Kiviat, N. B., Burk, R. D., et al.: Accuracy and interlaboratory reliability of human papillomavirus DNA testing by hybrid capture. J. Clin. Microbiol. *33*:545–550, 1995.
242. Schnadig, V. J., Clark, W. D., Clegg, T. J., et al.: Invasive papillomatosis and squamous carcinoma complicating juvenile laryngeal papillomatosis. Arch. Otolaryngol. Head Neck Surg. *112*:966–971, 1986.
243. Schneider, A., Kirchhoff, T., Meinhardt, G., et al.: Repeated evaluation of human papillomavirus 16 status in cervical swabs of young women with a history of normal Papanicolaou smears. Obstet. Gynecol. *79*:683–688, 1992.
244. Schonfeld, A., Nitke, S., Schattner, A., et al.: Intramuscular human interferon-beta injections in treatment of condylomata acuminata. Lancet *1*:1038–1042, 1984.
245. Schuster, D. S.: Snorters' warts. Arch. Dermatol. *123*:571–1987.
246. Scinicariello, F., Sato, T., Lee, C. S., et al.: Detection of human papillomavirus in primary hepatocellular carcinoma. Anticancer Res. *12*:763–766, 1992.
247. Shah, K., Kashima, H., Polk, B. F., et al.: Rarity of cesarean delivery in cases of juvenile-onset respiratory papillomatosis. Obstet. Gynecol. *68*:795–799, 1986.
248. Shah, K. V.: Polyomaviruses. *In* Fields, B. N., Knipe, D. M., Howley, P. M., et al.: (eds.): Fields Virology. Philadelphia, Lippincott-Raven, 1996, pp. 2027–2043.
249. Shah, K. V., Daniel, R. W., Strickler, H. D., et al.: Investigation of human urine for genomic sequences of the primate polyomaviruses simian virus 40, BK virus, and JC virus. J. Infect. Dis. *176*:1618–1621, 1997.
250. Shah, K. V., Daniel, R. W., and Warszawski, R. M.: High prevalence of antibodies to BK virus, an SV40-related papovavirus, in residents of Maryland. J. Infect. Dis. *128*:784–787, 1973.
251. Shah, K. V., and Howley, P. M.: Papillomaviruses. *In* Fields, B., Knipe, D., and Howley, P. M. (eds.): Fields Virology. Philadelphia, Lippincott-Raven, 1996, pp. 2077–2109.
252. Shah, K. V., Stern, W. F., Shah, F. K., et al.: Risk factors for juvenile onset recurrent respiratory papillomatosis. Pediatr. Infect. Dis. J. *17*:372–376, 1998.
253. Shen, C. Y., Ho, M. S., Chang, S. F., et al.: High rate of concurrent genital infections with human cytomegalovirus and human papillomaviruses in cervical cancer patients. J. Infect. Dis. *168*:449–452, 1993.
254. Simon, M. A., Ilyinskii, P. O., Baskin, G. B., et al.: Association of simian virus 40 with a central nervous system lesion distinct from progressive multifocal leukoencephalopathy in macaques with AIDS. Am. J. Pathol. *154*:437–446, 1999.
255. Singleton, G. T., and Adkins, W. Y.: Cryosurgical treatment of juvenile laryngeal papillomatosis. An eight year experience. Ann. Otol. Rhinol. Laryngol. *81*:784–790, 1972.
256. Slawsky, L. D., Gilson, R. T., Hockley, A. J., et al.: Epidermodysplasia verruciformis associated with severe immunodeficiency, lymphoma, and disseminated molluscum contagiosum. J. Am. Acad. Dermatol. *27*: 448–450, 1992.
257. Smith, M. A., Strickler, H. D., Granovsky, M., et al.: Investigation of leukemia cells from children with common acute lymphoblastic leukemia for genomic sequences of the primate polyomaviruses JC virus, BK virus, and simian virus 40. Med. Pediatr. Oncol. *33*:441–443, 1999.
258. Solomon, D., Smith, R. R., Kashima, H. K., et al.: Malignant transformation in non-irradiated recurrent respiratory papillomatosis. Laryngoscope *95*:900–904, 1985.

259. Soriano, F., Shelburne, C. E., and Gokcen, M.: Simian virus 40 in a human cancer. Nature *249*:421–424, 1974.
260. Sperry, K.: Lethal asphyxiating juvenile laryngeal papillomatosis. A case report with human papillomavirus in situ hybridization analysis. Am. J. Forensic Med. Pathol. *15*:146–150, 1994.
261. Stark, L. A., Arends, M. J., McLaren, K. M., et al.: Prevalence of human papillomavirus DNA in cutaneous neoplasms from renal allograft recipients supports a possible viral role in tumour promotion. Br. J. Cancer *69*:222–229, 1994.
262. Steele, J. C., and Gallimore, P. H.: Humoral assays of human sera to disrupted and nondisrupted epitopes of human papillomavirus type 1. Virology *174*:388–398, 1990.
263. Steger, G., Olszewsky, M., Stockfleth, E., et al.: Prevalence of antibodies to human papillomavirus type 8 in human sera. J. Virol. *64*:4399–4406, 1990.
264. Steinberg, B. M., Topp, W. C., Schneider, P. S., et al.: Laryngeal papillomavirus infection during clinical remission. N. Engl. J. Med. *308*:1261–1264, 1983.
265. Stellato, G., Nieminen, P., Aho, H., et al.: Human papillomavirus infection of the female genital tract: Correlation of HPV DNA with cytologic, colposcopic, and natural history findings. Eur. J. Gynaecol. Oncol. *13*:262–267, 1992.
266. St Louis, M. E., Icenogle, J. P., Manzila, T., et al.: Genital types of papillomavirus in children of women with HIV-1 infection in Kinshasa, Zaire. Int. J. Cancer *54*:181–184, 1993.
267. Stoian, M., Hozoc, M., Iosipenco, M., et al.: Serum antibodies to papova viruses (BK and SV 40) in subjects from the area with Balkan endemic nephropathy. Virologie *34*:113–117, 1983.
268. Strickler, H. D., Rosenberg, P. S., Devesa, S. S., et al.: Contamination of poliovirus vaccine with SV40 and the incidence of medulloblastoma. Med. Pediatr. Oncol. *32*:77–78, 1999.
269. Strong, M. S., Vaughan, C. W., Cooperband, S. R., et al.: Recurrent respiratory papillomatosis: Management with the CO_2 laser. Ann. Otol. Rhinol. Laryngol. *85*:508–516, 1976.
270. Sun, X. W., Kuhn, L., Ellerbrock, T. V., et al.: Human papillomavirus infection in women infected with the human immunodeficiency virus. N. Engl. J. Med. *337*:1343–1349, 1997.
271. Sun, Y., Eluf-Neto, J., Bosch, F. X., et al.: Human papillomavirus-related serological markers of invasive cervical carcinoma in Brazil. Cancer Epidemiol. Biomarkers Prev. *3*:341–347, 1994.
272. Sundsfjord, A., Osei, A., Rosenqvist, H., et al.: BK and JC viruses in patients with systemic lupus erythematosus: Prevalent and persistent BK viruria, sequence stability of the viral regulatory regions, and nondetectable viremia. J. Infect. Dis. *180*:1–9, 1999.
273. Sundsfjord, A., Spein, A. R., Lucht, E., et al.: Detection of BK virus DNA in nasopharyngeal aspirates from children with respiratory infections but not in saliva from immunodeficient and immunocompetent adult patients. J. Clin. Microbiol. *32*:1390–1394, 1994.
274. Sweet, B. H., and Hilleman, M. R.: The vacuolating virus, S.V.$_{40}$. Proc. Soc. Exp. Biol. Med. *105*:420–427, 1960.
275. Syrjanen, K., Hakama, M., Saarikoski, S., et al.: Prevalence, incidence, and estimated life-time risk of cervical human papillomavirus infections in a nonselected Finnish female population. Sex. Transm. Dis. *17*:15–19, 1990.
276. Syrjanen, S.: Human papillomavirus infections in the oral cavity. *In* Syrjanen, K., Gissmann, L., and Koss, L. (eds.): Papillomaviruses and Human Disease. New York, Springer-Verlag, 1987, pp. 104–137.
277. Syrjanen, S., Partanen, P., Mantyjarvi, R., et al.: Sensitivity of in situ hybridization techniques using biotin- and ^{35}S-labeled human papillomavirus (HPV) DNA probes. J. Virol. Methods *19*:225–238, 1988.
278. Taguchi, F., Hara, K., Kajioka, J., et al.: Isolation of BK virus from a patient with systemic lupus erythematosus (SLE). Microbiol. Immunol. *23*:1131–1132, 1979.
279. Taguchi, F., Hara, K., and Nagaki, D.: BK papovavirus in urine of a patient with systemic lupus erythematosus. Letter. Acta Virol. *22*:513, 1978.
280. Tantisiriwat, W., Tebas, P., Clifford, D. B., et al.: Progressive multifocal leukoencephalopathy in patients with AIDS receiving highly active antiretroviral therapy. Clin. Infect. Dis. *28*:1152–1154, 1998.
281. Taylor, S. W.: A prevalence study of virus warts on the hands in a poultry processing and packing station. J. Soc. Occup. Med. *30*:20–23, 1980.
282. Telenti, A., Aksamit, A. J. J., Proper, J., et al.: Detection of JC virus DNA by polymerase chain reaction in patients with progressive multifocal leukoencephalopathy. J. Infect. Dis. *162*:858–861, 1990.
283. Teofilo, E., Gouveia, J., Brotas, V., et al.: Progressive multifocal leukoencephalopathy regression with highly active antiretroviral therapy. A. I. D. S. *12*:449–1998.
284. Tieben, L. M., Berkhout, R. J., Smits, H. L., et al.: Detection of epidermodysplasia verruciformis–like human papillomavirus types in malignant and premalignant skin lesions of renal transplant recipients. Br. J. Dermatol. *131*:226–230, 1994.
285. Tominaga, T., Yogo, Y., Kitamura, T., et al.: Persistence of archetypal JC virus DNA in normal renal tissue derived from tumor-bearing patients. Virology *186*:736–741, 1992.
286. Trottier, A. M., Coutlee, F., Leduc, R., et al.: Human immunodeficiency virus infection is a major risk factor for detection of human papillomavirus DNA in esophageal brushings. Clin. Infect. Dis. *24*:565–569, 1997.
287. Trottier, A. M., Provencher, D., Mes-Masson, A. M., et al.: Absence of human papillomavirus sequences in ovarian pathologies. J. Clin. Microbiol. *33*:1011–1013, 1995.
288. Ushikai, M., Fujiyoshi, T., Kono, M., et al.: Detection and cloning of human papillomavirus DNA associated with recurrent respiratory papillomatosis in Thailand. Jpn. J. Cancer Res. *85*:699–703, 1994.
289. Vallbracht, A., Lohler, J., Gossmann, J., et al.: Disseminated BK type polyomavirus infection in an AIDS patient associated with central nervous system disease. Am. J. Pathol. *143*:29–39, 1993.
290. van den Brule, A. J., Walboomers, J. M., Du, M. M., et al.: Difference in prevalence of human papillomavirus genotypes in cytomorphologically normal cervical smears is associated with a history of cervical intraepithelial neoplasia. Int. J. Cancer *48*:404–408, 1991.
291. Van der Leest, R. J., Zachow, K. R., Ostrow, R. S., et al.: Human papillomavirus heterogeneity in 36 renal transplant recipients. Arch. Dermatol. *123*:354–357, 1987.
292. Vazeux, R., Cumont, M., Girard, P. M., et al.: Severe encephalitis resulting from coinfections with HIV and JC virus. Neurology *40*:944–948, 1990.
293. Vernon, S. D., Holmes, K. K., and Reeves, W. C.: Human papillomavirus infection and associated disease in persons infected with human immunodeficiency virus. Clin. Infect. Dis. *21*(Suppl. 1):121–124, 1995.
294. Viac, J., Chomel, J. J., Chardonnet, Y., et al.: Incidence of antibodies to human papillomavirus type 1 in patients with cutaneous and mucosal papillomas. J. Med. Virol. *32*:18–21, 1990.
295. Vilchez, R. A., Madden, C. R., Kozinetz, C. A., et al.: Association of simian virus 40 and non-Hodgkin lymphoma. Lancet *359*:817–823, 2002.
296. ViraPap and ViraType HPV DNA typing kit manuals and product information, 1989.
297. Voltz, R., Jager, G., Seelos, K., et al.: BK virus encephalitis in an immunocompetent patient. Arch. Neurol. *53*:101–103, 1997.
298. von Krogh, G.: Clinical relevance and evaluation of genitoanal papilloma virus infection in the male. Semin. Dermatol. *11*:229–240, 1992.
299. Vossler, J. L., Forbes, B. A., and Adelson, M. D.: Evaluation of the polymerase chain reaction for the detection of human papillomavirus from urine. J. Med. Virol. *45*:354–360, 1995.
300. Vousden, K.: Mechanisms of transformation by HPV. *In* Stern, P., and Stanley, M. (eds.): Human Papillomaviruses and Cervical Cancer: Biology and Immunology. Oxford, Oxford University Press, 1994, pp. 92–116.
301. Walboomers, J. M., Husman, A., and van den Brule, A. J.: Detection of genital human papillomavirus infections: Critical review of methods and prevalence studies in relation to cervical cancer. *In* Stern, P., and Stanley, M. (eds.): Human Papillomaviruses and Cervical Cancer: Biology and Immunology. Oxford, Oxford University Press, 1994, pp. 41–71.
302. Walker, D. L., and Frisque, R. J.: The biology and molecular biology of JC virus. *In* Salzman, N. P. (ed.): The Papovaviridae. Vol. 1. The polyomaviruses. New York, Plenum Press, 1986, pp. 327–377.
303. Wallin, K. L., Wiklund, F., Angstrom, T., et al.: Type-specific persistence of human papillomavirus DNA before the development of invasive cervical cancer. N. Engl. J. Med. *341*:1633–1638, 1999.
304. Ward, P., Parry, G. N., Yule, R., et al.: Human papillomavirus subtype 16a. Lancet *2*:170, 1989.
305. Wilbur, D. C., and Stoler, M. H.: Testing for human papillomavirus: Basic pathobiology of infection, methodologies, and implications for clinical use. Yale J. Biol. Med. *64*:113–125, 1991.
306. Yaegashi, N., Jenison, S. A., Batra, M., et al.: Human antibodies recognize multiple distinct type-specific and cross-reactive regions of the minor capsid proteins of human papillomavirus types 6 and 11. J. Virol. *66*:2008–2019, 1992.
307. Yaegashi, N., Jenison, S. A., Valentine, J. M., et al.: Characterization of murine polyclonal antisera and monoclonal antibodies generated against intact and denatured human papillomavirus type 1 virions. J. Virol. *65*:1578–1583, 1991.
308. Ylitalo, N., Bergstrom, T., and Gyllensten, U.: Detection of genital human papillomavirus by single-tube nested PCR and type-specific oligonucleotide hybridization. J. Clin. Microbiol. *33*:1822–1828, 1995.
309. Young, L. S., Bevan, I. S., Johnson, M. A., et al.: The polymerase chain reaction: A new epidemiological tool for investigating cervical human papillomavirus infection. B. M. J. *298*:14–18, 1989.
310. Zu, R. G., and Chou, S.-M.: Particles resembling papova viruses in human cerebral demyelination disease. Science *148*:1477–1479, 1965.

MISCELLANEOUS SLOW VIRUSES AND PRION-RELATED DISEASES

CHAPTER 160 Transmissible Spongiform Encephalopathies (Creutzfeldt-Jakob Disease, Gerstmann-Sträussler-Scheinker Disease, Kuru, Fatal Familial Insomnia, New Variant Creutzfeldt-Jakob Disease)

WILLIAM J. BRITT

The group of diseases classified as transmissible spongiform encephalopathies (TSEs) represents a subset of diseases that have been termed cerebral amyloidoses or cerebral proteopathies.[185, 225] These diseases have in common the deposition of insoluble, proteinaceous aggregates in the central nervous system (CNS), and they are manifested by relentlessly progressive cortical dysfunction (Table 160–1). The protein aggregates characteristic of these diseases are composed of polymeric fibrils of a host-encoded protein deposited in several different regions of the CNS but often present in other organ systems. The symptoms associated with the spongiform encephalopathies are thought to arise from cellular and end-organ dysfunction caused by the abnormal deposition of an insoluble isoform of a normal cellular protein, PrP^c.[28, 66, 185] However, because the physiologic function of this cellular protein remains incompletely defined, at least some of the symptoms associated with these diseases possibly are caused by loss of normal PrP^c function. The TSEs share several clinical features with other types of cerebral amyloidosis, and the insoluble protein aggregates have biophysical properties similar to those of the plaques found in Alzheimer disease. In contrast to these latter diseases, the TSEs can, by definition, be transmitted by parenteral inoculation or by other less efficient routes such as ingestion of the material in contaminated tissue from the nervous system.

TABLE 160–1 ■ NATURALLY OCCURRING TRANSMISSIBLE SPONGIFORM ENCEPHALOPATHIES

Host	Disease
Human	Kuru
	Creutzfeldt-Jakob disease
	Sporadic
	Familial
	Infectious
	Variant Creutzfeldt-Jakob disease
	Gerstmann-Sträussler-Scheinker syndrome
	Fatal familial insomnia
Sheep, goats	Scrapie
Mink	Transmissible mink encephalopathy
Deer, elk	Chronic wasting disease
Cattle	Bovine spongiform encephalopathy
Cats	Feline spongiform encephalopathy

Until late in the 20th century, TSEs were diseases of domestic livestock. Scrapie, a disease of sheep, was described first in the mid-1700s.[31] Farmers had recognized early that the agent responsible for scrapie was communicable and instituted control measures that included isolation and destruction of affected animals and herds.[5] Even though farmers were aware of the communicability of scrapie among herds of sheep, its transmissibility was not demonstrated formally until 1936.[76] Some 10 years later, an outbreak of scrapie developed in a flock of sheep that were inoculated with a vaccine for louping that was ill prepared from the CNS tissue of sheep that had been exposed to scrapie.[31] Together, these reports provided definitive evidence of the transmissible nature of scrapie. The term *slow virus disease* was coined by veterinarians to describe the natural history of a curious group of diseases in domestic animals, such as scrapie, that were characterized by a prolonged incubation period lasting up to years and progressive clinical deterioration that was relentless once symptoms appeared.[206] This term was used to describe this group of diseases until the 1980s, when investigators began to realize that, although the agent responsible for the spongiform changes in scrapie-infected mice was transmissible, it could not be classified as a conventional virus.

A decade earlier, observational and laboratory studies of kuru, a progressive cerebellar ataxia and dementia that occurred predominantly in adolescent and young adults of the Fore tribe in Papua New Guinea, provided an important clue in the search for the etiology of this group of diseases.[2] The natural history of this disease was described initially by Zigas and Gajdusek and was noted to be associated with the ritual cannibalism practiced by this tribe. In 1959, an astute veterinary neuropathologist, William Hadlow, observed a striking similarity in the spongiform changes seen in the brains of patients with kuru and the brains of sheep with scrapie and suggested that these two diseases could be caused by similar mechanisms, possibly a transmissible agent.[105]

With the knowledge that kuru possibly was caused by a transmissible agent, Gajdusek and coworkers eventually demonstrated that the clinical and histopathologic findings of kuru could be transmitted to chimpanzees and other nonhuman primates by inoculation of brain tissue from patients with kuru.[89–91, 186] Interestingly, Gajdusek and coworkers initially thought that the experiment failed because the animals did not become symptomatic until nearly 2 years after inoculation, and later reports from this same laboratory indicated that nearly 20 years elapsed between inoculation and the development of disease in some chimpanzees.[12, 31]

Subsequent studies by other investigators have demonstrated that brain homogenates from patients with Creutzfeldt-Jakob disease (CJD), Gerstmann-Sträussler-Scheinker disease (GSS), fatal familial insomnia (FFI), and, most recently, variant Creutzfeldt-Jakob disease (vCJD) can transmit spongiform changes to nonhuman primates.[20, 97] The discovery by Prusiner and colleagues that the etiologic agent of scrapie was an isoform of a normal host protein, PrP^c (alternatively referred to as the prion protein), that could transmit disease in the absence of nucleic acid initially was met with great skepticism and even today continues to evoke debate.[61, 181]

During the ensuing decades, the hypothesis that a protein could promote the formation of a polymeric fibrillary, insoluble plaque without the requirement of nucleic acid encoding an infectious agent protein has been supported by studies from numerous laboratories. This hypothesis represented a paradigm shift in biology, and Prusiner was awarded a Nobel Prize in 1997 for his groundbreaking studies of prion diseases. Interestingly, approximately 20 years earlier, Gajdusek also was awarded a Nobel Prize for his description of the transmissible nature of kuru and similar diseases of the CNS.

The most recent chapter in the TSE saga has been the appearance of mad cow disease (bovine spongiform encephalopathy [BSE]) in Great Britain in the mid-1980s, and by the late 1990s nearly 200,000 diseased animals had died.[44] Mad cow disease has been discovered in cattle in several European countries and most recently in Japan. Of greatest concern has been its apparent transmission to more than 100 individuals in Great Britain and at least 3 in France.[44] Although cases of BSE have not been reported in the United States, a significant increase in TSE in elk and deer has been reported recently in wild game farms in Colorado, thus raising the possibility that this TSE also could enter domestic cattle in the United States. Because of concern that large numbers of human cases may eventually develop secondary to contamination of food products and pharmaceutical reagents with BSE, substantial interest has developed in the study of TSEs.

Epidemiology

The natural history of TSE is described most frequently in the context of the epidemiology of CJD. Three different modes of disease acquisition have been described: (1) sporadic, (2) inherited mutations in the cellular gene encoding PrP (genetic), and (3) acquisition after exogenous exposure to prion-contaminated material, such as after neurologic procedures (infectious). Little is known about genetic or environmental factors that contribute to the development of sporadic forms of these diseases, although numerous epidemiologic studies have claimed associations ranging from ingestion of mutton to exposure to blood products after surgery.[3, 34, 72, 161] Extensive studies in cases of CJD have revealed numerous genetic mutations in the cellular gene encoding the normal cellular prion protein PrP^c that are associated with the development of disease, and these mutations have been defined as genetic causes of CJD and other TSEs (see the next section).

In addition, genetic polymorphisms in both the cellular gene encoding PrP^c and other host genes could predispose to the development of sporadic cases of CJD, including other reported TSEs. Polymorphisms in methionine at position 129 in the coding sequence of PrP^c is the genetic abnormality most commonly recognized in association with sporadic CJD.[175] Homozygosity for the methionine codon corresponding to amino acid position 129 of PrP^c is seen in approximately 64 to 81 percent of patients with sporadic CJD, yet it is present in only approximately 39 percent of the general population.[1, 235] Interestingly, valine homozygosity at this position has been associated more frequently with the onset of CJD in patients younger than 40 years of age.[1] Furthermore, retrospective analysis of a small number of kuru patients has revealed that all were homozygous for methionine at position 129 and all had more rapidly progressive disease with a shorter incubation period than did other kuru patients from this cohort.[151] The codon at position 129 also appears to modulate the clinical course of inherited TSEs such as FFI, and patients homozygous for methionine at position 129 have been reported to have a more rapid clinical course than that of patients heterozygous at this codon.[168] Polymorphisms in PrP^c, including those that occur at position 129, have not been associated with the development of vCJD after exposure to material that is contaminated by BSE; in fact, all human cases in Great Britain have been homozygous for methionine at position 129.[124]

Sporadic CJD is the most common TSE in humans and accounts for approximately 85 percent of all cases of CJD.[34] It occurs worldwide at a rate of approximately 1 case per 10^6 population.[34] CJD is a disease of late middle age, with a mean age at onset of 55 to 65 years. The range of reported cases of CJD is from 20 to 84 years of age; however, vCJD has been reported in adolescents.[23, 33, 167] Little evidence exists for case-to-case transmission of CJD, with the obvious exception of cases resulting from iatrogenic transmission.[58] Vertical transmission has not been reported in studies of human CJD. Anecdotal reports of CJD developing in the spouses of individuals with CJD have raised the possibility of horizontal transmission.[36] Alternatively, disease in spouses could result from shared environmental exposure. Very recently, sporadic cases of non-CJD TSE previously thought to be caused solely by genetic mutations have been reported, thus extending the spectrum of sporadic TSEs in humans.[152, 162] With the exception of cases that can be linked to an inherited genetic mutation, no epidemics of CJD have been reported, an observation that led British epidemiologists to suspect a link between what initially was thought to be an increased frequency of CJD in young adults and the outbreak of BSE in the British Isles.[5, 11, 74, 100, 222, 232]

Genetic mutations in the cellular prion gene PrP^c can result in a variety of inherited TSEs, and such mutations probably account for the reported outbreaks of TSE in isolated populations. Because of the relatively late onset of disease, even in patients with well-characterized mutations in PrP^c, the possibility that TSEs were inherited diseases of the CNS was not considered until more recent studies of the host-cell origin of prions and the discovery that a cellular gene encoded the pathogenic protein PrP^c. Estimates from various studies suggest that between 5 and 15 percent of cases of CJD may arise from mutations in the cellular PrP^c gene.[34] Genetic linkage studies have demonstrated that TSEs are inherited as an autosomal dominant trait, an observation consistent with several studies in families with FFI and GSS.[18, 120, 164] Defined mutations in the PrP^c gene have been shown to account for the increased rate of TSE in either geographically or ethnically isolated population such as Libyan-born Jews, an ethnic group with an incidence of TSE nearly 40 times greater than that observed in other populations.[5, 89, 99, 121, 132, 165, 208]

A large number of mutations in PrP^c have been described (>20), and they appear to be scattered throughout the gene. Reported mutations include both point mutations in the coding sequence resulting in amino acid substitutions and larger octapeptide insertions.[51, 58, 98, 122, 189, 227] Although specific mutations in PrP^c are by definition not present in cases of sporadic CJD, mutations likely contribute to the development of CJD in these individuals. In most cases, disease secondary to a genetic mutation in PrP^c develops in middle age, which suggests that although these diseases exhibit autosomal dominant inheritance, the genetic background of the host contributes significantly to the various phenotypes observed in patients with TSE.

Although farmers and neuropathologists were well aware that scrapie was transmissible, the possibility that human TSEs also were transmissible was not demonstrated until Gajdusek and coworkers defined the natural history of kuru in the Fore tribe in Papua New Guinea.[2] Kuru was seen most frequently in adolescents and young adults of both sexes, but only in older women. The disease was a common occurrence in this tribe, with an incidence of 1 percent, and was a significant cause of death in this population.[2] Gajdusek performed a detailed observational study of the Fore people, including their ritualistic cannibalism of the dead. This ritual included homogenization of the brain of dead relatives in bamboo cylinders with crude hand tools. The brain reportedly was ingested as well as smeared over the body by relatives and other members of the tribe. During most of their childhood, Fore children remained with their mothers and other women of the village, including the time spent preparing the brains of dead relatives for ritual cannibalism. The agent responsible for kuru was thought to be acquired during this time of exposure, either by ingestion of contaminated brain material or through skin abrasions that were present because of the nearly universal scabies infestation.

Gajdusek and coworkers hypothesized that kuru was caused by an infectious agent and injected homogenates prepared from the brain of a deceased kuru patient into nonhuman primates; after an incubation period of more than 2 years, a disease similar to kuru was observed in the experimental animals.[12] After transmissibility of kuru was demonstrated in experimental animals, several other TSEs were shown to be transmissible to nonhuman primates and other experimental animals.[39, 69, 97, 214, 217] Subsequent studies have demonstrated that kuru can be transmitted to nonhuman primates by the oral ingestion of contaminated tissue.[95] Although the origin of the TSE agent responsible for kuru in the Fore tribe is unknown, the most plausible explanation is that a spontaneous mutation in the cellular PrP^c gene resulted in a case of TSE in the Fore tribe, which then was propagated in this closed population by cannibalism. After ritual cannibalism was stopped, new cases of the disease disappeared, and the last case of kuru in an individual younger than 30 years of age was reported in 1985.[2] Interestingly, one reported case of kuru developed some 40 years after exposure to infectious material, a dramatic illustration of the prolonged incubation period of these diseases.[13]

Before the 1980s, cases of TSE occurring during childhood and adolescence, with the exception of kuru, were either extremely rare or not recognized. In the late 1980s, cases of TSE resembling CJD were reported in young adults who as children had received injections of human growth hormone prepared from cadaveric pituitary glands.[26, 35, 37] The practice of pooling pituitary glands from large numbers of cadavers was thought to have increased the risk of contamination of the preparation with prions from donors with unrecognized CJD. More than 100 cases of TSE occurring after the injection of contaminated growth hormone preparations have been reported.[58] Whether new cases of TSE will develop in adults given cadaveric growth hormone before the mid-1980s is uncertain, but the mean incubation period of 12 years in documented cases has suggested that the occurrence of significant numbers of new cases is unlikely.[41]

Other sources of TSE include dura grafts, corneal transplants, and contaminated stereotactic neurosurgical equipment.[35, 75, 80, 108, 118, 136, 171] An alarming case of TSE occurred in a chimpanzee after the use of a stereotactic electrode that 2 years previously had been used in a procedure involving a patient with CJD. Because this electrode had been decontaminated numerous times with conventional sterilization methods before use in this experimental animal, this case illustrated the potential for iatrogenic transmission of TSE to humans undergoing neurosurgical procedures.[96]

Studies of experimental models of TSEs, primarily scrapie in mice, have shown that the infectious titer of the scrapie agent is amplified in the spleen and regional lymph nodes and enters the CNS by a blood-borne route or by infection of the peripheral nervous system.[135, 137, 139, 149, 158] In addition, recent studies in mice have demonstrated that brain tissue from animals injected with hamster scrapie can harbor the infectious agent for a prolonged period without evidence of disease.[191] Even during a period of inactive persistence and replication, the scrapie prion could be detected, thus suggesting that transmission of prion disease by contaminated blood products or surgical instruments may occur even if screening assays for the detection of TSE are mandated.

To further cloud the issue, other investigators have postulated that less virulent strains of prions can attenuate the virulence of other strains of prions, which then can be transmitted readily during asymptomatic periods.[160] After transmission to a secondary host, the phenotype of the more virulent strain can be expressed. These studies have raised the possibility that TSEs could be acquired by the transfusion of blood and blood products obtained from infected hosts.[150] However, considerable controversy exists regarding the transmissibility of TSE by blood and blood products. Investigators have argued that the risk is exceedingly small based on experimental studies in rodents and epidemiologic studies of patients who routinely receive blood products, such as hemophiliacs.[27, 30, 83, 84, 195, 219, 233] Despite these and experimental data from animal studies, the Food and Drug Administration has recommended a very conservative policy for blood and blood products. In addition to exclusion of donors who have symptoms consistent with TSEs, individuals who have lived or visited Great Britain and other countries with BSE for a cumulative period of 3 months during the interval from 1980 to 1996 should not donate blood (www.redcross.org/services/biomed/blood/learn/eligibl.html).

With the possible exception of kuru, little evidence suggesting that TSEs such as CJD could be acquired by the ingestion of contaminated tissue was available.[34] This claim was challenged in the early 1990s by reports of several young adults with CJD in Great Britain.[74, 232] Analysis of the rates of acquisition of CJD in England revealed that its incidence was approximately 15-fold higher than that of previous years based on surveillance studies from previous decades.[44] In the years preceding the startling increase in the rate of CJD, the cattle industry in Great Britain was in the midst of a rapidly spreading epidemic of BSE, a disease ultimately shown to be a TSE.[111, 230] A similar disease had been noted in domestic cats, as well as in animals housed in zoos and fed British beef and beef by-products.[20, 67] The first case of human disease thought to be associated with BSE was termed vCJD, and it was described approximately 10 years after the first cases of BSE were reported in cows.[232] During the ensuing years, investigators have closed the circle of evidence, and the current consensus is that vCJD represents the transmission of BSE to humans, presumably by the ingestion of contaminated meat or by-products from BSE-infected cattle. These by-products include many common household and medical products, such as gelatin in food products and pharmaceutical capsules, bullion cubes used for food preparation, and a wide variety of beef-containing foodstuff.

Although the origin of BSE is far from settled, most investigators consider that changes in the rendering of beef carcasses for use as a protein supplement in animal feed led to the epidemic. Before the late 1970s, beef carcasses were heated and treated with hydrocarbons such as chloroform to delipidate the homogenate.[28, 79, 216, 230] Omitting the hydrocarbon delipidation step apparently decreased the inactivation of bovine prions, thus allowing the introduction of this agent into the food products of British cattle. The epidemic began slowly in cattle, with the first case verified in 1986; by the mid-1990s, however, more than 3500 new cases of BSE were being reported each year. As a result of the BSE epidemic, 200,000 diseased cattle died and nearly 4.5 million cattle were slaughtered preemptively to curtail the epidemic.[4, 44, 238]

As noted earlier, transmission to humans was suggested first in 1995 after reports of CJD in three young adults, and by 1996, additional cases of CJD in young adults were thought to have been caused by exposure to beef from cows infected with BSE.[65] Of the initial 20 human cases, only 1 individual was older than 40 years, with the mean age of human cases being 28 years.[184, 239] Additional evidence from in vitro studies of the prion thought to be responsible for BSE and vCJD and from animal inoculation studies strongly argued that vCJD represented human infection with the agent responsible for BSE.[47, 70, 115, 148] Because the BSE epidemic was recognized initially in 1985, researchers have argued that the incubation period is approximately 10 years. Based on studies of kuru and experimental animal models of TSE, this estimate is dependent on exposure, genetic susceptibility, and as yet other unrecognized risk factors.[57, 153] For this and other reasons, mathematic projections of the extent of the human epidemic have been based on theoretic estimates of exposure rates, possible dose-dependent incubation periods, and as yet undefined host genes that may alter susceptibility to TSE.

Even though most of these variables cannot be quantified, some investigators have argued that the epidemic of vCJD in humans has peaked and that the 100 or so cases of vCJD that have resulted from contaminated beef will be the extent of human disease associated with BSE.[73, 94] In contrast, other models of the current data suggest that as many as 100,000 people may be affected. Perhaps the most compelling argument against such a large number of human cases has been the slowly evolving epidemic of vCJD in humans, with the number of new cases declining over the last several years, although several investigators have contested this hypothesis.[5, 44, 93, 231]

Pathology and Pathogenesis

Although the histopathologic features of TSEs have been described exhaustively, the pathogenesis of these diseases remains unknown because the nature of the etiologic agent remains controversial. The initial claim that TSE resulted from a transmissible protein was met with great skepticism. Almost all existing experimental studies had been performed with the agent responsible for scrapie in sheep adapted for growth in mice. Years of experimental study indicated that this agent was not a conventional virus. Based on studies involving inactivation of the agent by ultraviolet radiation, researchers argued that the scrapie agent did not contain nucleic acid. The findings from several laboratories indicated that if the scrapie agent contained nucleic acid, its coding sequence was limited sufficiently to preclude it from encoding any replicative functions.[14, 15, 183] In addition, other workers demonstrated that the infectivity of the scrapie agent could be eliminated or significantly reduced by treatment with agents that denatured proteins, such as guanidine hydrochloride, sodium hypochlorite (bleach), and proteases.[181] Thus, the agent was postulated to be an infectious protein.[103, 163, 181]

In a seminal series of experiments, Prusiner and coworkers isolated an infectious fraction from a scrapie-infected hamster brain homogenate and obtained a partial amino acid sequence.[19, 187] This fundamental finding led to identification of the scrapie prion (PrP^c) and eventually the finding that a cellular gene, PrP^c, present on chromosome 20, encoded the transmissible agent responsible for scrapie.[10, 62, 207] The protein product of this gene, PrP^c, is a small membrane-associated glycoprotein that is covalently linked to cellular membranes, including the plasma membrane, by a phosphoinositol linkage.[107, 209–211]

Once the protein encoded by the PrP^c gene had been identified and linked to scrapie and other TSEs, researchers thought that the pathogenesis of these diseases would be elucidated quickly. However, their pathogenesis continues to be uncertain, perhaps because of the inability to assign a function to the normal protein product PrP^c.

A variety of functions have been proposed for the normal nonpathogenic isoform of cellular PrP^c, yet transgenic mice lacking the gene encoding PrP^c have normal life spans and exhibit only minor variation in normal sleep patterns.[50, 71, 188] Most interestingly, these mice are completely resistant to prion disease regardless of the source of exposure, a finding that is consistent with the hypothesis that PrP^c is necessary for the disease process associated with scrapie and other TSEs.[49] Normal cellular PrP^c is a glycoprotein that is secreted and displayed on the cell surface; it can be released by treating cellular membranes with phospholipases.[211] Genetic mutations in the cellular PrP^c gene appear to predispose the protein to assume other topologies, including a transmembrane form.[109, 110] This latter form is postulated to play an important role in the neurodegeneration associated with accumulation of the misfolded forms of PrP^c.[110] The conformation of the normal cellular form of PrP^c is primarily alpha-helical and is susceptible to protease digestion. In contrast to the alpha-helical form of PrP^c, the pathogenic form, PrP^{sc} (scrapie prion protein), exists in an extended beta-sheet and is characteristically insoluble and partially resistant to protease digestion (PrP protease-resistant [PrP^{res}]). The partial resistance of PrP^{res} to proteinase K digestion is a property of PrP^{res} that allows pathogenic prions to be detected in tissue specimens.[200, 203, 220, 221] Conversion of PrP^c to PrP^{res} is a central paradigm of the prion hypothesis and is thought to occur either as a result of a process similar to the nucleation of crystal formation by seeding the normal cellular pool of PrP^c with PrP^{res} or, alternatively, as a result of the template-directed misfolding of a normal cellular protein. Thus, PrP^{res} can be viewed as a transmissible infectious agent that catalyzes conversion of the normal cellular protein to a form associated with cell death in the CNS and, eventually, disease in the host.

The process by which a misfolded host protein leads to loss of normal function and disease in humans has several well-studied precedents in human biology, such as cystic fibrosis.[64, 102, 104, 236] In addition, diseases associated with the accumulation of cellular proteins such as amyloid are well described. In the case of TSEs, the proposed mechanism for the generation of pathogenic prions, as noted earlier, is the conformational change from a predominance of alpha-helical structures to an extended beta-sheet. In vitro cell-free systems and studies from kindred with inherited TSEs such as GSS and FFI have shown that exposure to a misfolded prion protein such as PrP^{res} can result in this conversion.[53, 88, 129, 183, 185, 200, 229] Interestingly, the pathogenic form of the prion, PrP^{res}, is derived from the mutant allele in individuals heterozygous for this allele, a finding consistent with its autosomal dominant mode of inheritance in GSS and FFI.[60]

An estimate of the energetics required for the change in conformation of PrP^c to PrP^{res} has argued that this conversion is unfavorable and that a mutant template or perhaps a chaperone protein (protein X) must be present for this conversion reaction to proceed at a finite rate.[17, 56, 133, 142, 218] However, even in the face of an extremely slow conversion reaction, the change in protein conformation essentially is irreversible and results in an accumulation of the insoluble and protease-resistant PrP^{res} protein. More recent arguments have been put forth that certain conformations of PrP^c favor conversion to the pathogenic forms of PrP^{res}, thus providing additional constraints on the expression of disease that could explain the non-PrP^c genetic contributions to disease susceptibility, as well as providing a final common pathway for genetic and infectious forms of the disease.[109, 110]

Interestingly, several studies have argued that the relative abundance of different protease fragments generated after protease K treatment of PrP^{res} may reflect different distributions of disease in the CNS, thus providing additional diversity in disease phenotype attributed to this single small protein.[166, 176, 177] Once the pathogenic form of the prion (PrP^{res}) begins to accumulate, additional newly synthesized molecules are converted to PrP^{res} and clinical symptoms develop, depending on the site of cell loss in the CNS. Accumulation of the PrP^{res} isoform probably involves a combination of newly synthesized PrP^{res} and decreased clearance of the misfolded aggregate.

Recent studies have suggested that failure to clear the misfolded pathogenic isoform may ultimately be the major pathway leading to the accumulation of PrP^{res} and disease.[199] Finally, one should note that several studies have linked copper binding to the product of PrP^c and oxidation of the prion protein.[130, 193, 204, 237] Alternatively, a copper-containing prion complex localized to the synaptic junction could protect normal synapses from oxidants or perhaps play a direct role in copper metabolism or transport.[24, 130] Loss of normal prion function by misfolding then could lead to neuronal loss. The importance of these newly described characteristics of PrP^c remains undefined at this time.

The challenge of a self-replicating protein to existing paradigms of molecular biology and genetics was noted quickly by biologists and biochemists. Previously, several investigators had demonstrated clearly that distinctive strains of the scrapie agent existed and that these strains induced definable and reproducible disease phenotypes in experimental animals.[16, 22, 45, 46, 135] These well-accepted and reproducible studies strongly argued for the presence of a genetic program in the scrapie agent that most likely was encoded by nucleic acid. More recently, several studies have suggested that the phenotypic behavior of scrapie strains may be dependent entirely on the pathogenic conformation that PrP^c assumes when exposed to pathogenic forms of PrP^{res}, which in turn are dependent themselves on post-translational modifications, thus providing an explanation for the phenotypic behavior of different strains of scrapie.[17, 199, 223]

A second characteristic of the etiologic agents of TSE was a so-called species barrier. This phenotype was noted when scrapie agents from sheep first were adapted to mice and subsequently to other species such as hamsters. As an example, researchers have shown that more than 1000 lethal doses of BSE (as defined in cattle) must be given to a mouse to induce disease.[228] Interestingly, the species barrier not only contributes to the resistance of species to infection with prions derived from other species but also can lengthen the mean incubation period in a population. The species barrier often is invoked to explain the rarity of TSE even in populations repeatedly exposed to TSE from other species, such as humans exposed to scrapie-infected sheep and possibly the relatively low number of human cases of vCJD that develop after exposure to beef contaminated with BSE.[65] Only recently has a coherent explanation for the restriction of transmission of prion disease between species been proposed. This restriction appears to be related to the efficiency with which exogenous prions interact with endogenous host-derived PrP^c to form PrP^{res}.[119, 143, 192]

However, considerable gaps in knowledge of the infectious agent responsible for TSEs still remain and have contributed to the controversy that surrounds the infectious protein hypothesis.[61] Perhaps most confusing has been the observation that protease-resistant prions (PrP^{res}) that appear biochemically identical to pathogenic PrP^{res} derived from infected brain tissue can be produced in cell-free systems in vitro, but to date these preparations cannot transmit disease to uninfected animals unless supplemented with brain tissue derived from diseased animals.[113]

The pathway leading from ingestion of PrP^{res} tissue to deposition in the CNS has been shown to require local replication in lymphoid tissue, which is thought to be followed by blood-borne dissemination to the nervous system.[71, 112, 137, 139] Other studies have demonstrated that expression of PrP^{res} in the peripheral nervous system is sufficient to transmit disease, thus suggesting that direct hematogenous dissemination to the brain is not necessary for transmission of TSE.[190] The high titer of infectious prions found in the liver and the spleen, as well as in lymphoid tissue such as the tonsils and in other lymphoid tissues of the oropharynx and gut, suggests that the titer of the infecting PrP^{res} is amplified in these tissues before spread to the CNS.

Recent studies that have documented the presence of PrP^{res} in the appendix 8 months before the onset of TSE are consistent with this proposed mode of spread to the CNS.[117] B lymphocytes initially were thought to be a likely candidate for the cell type that transmitted PrP^{res} to the CNS; however, recent studies have provided data inconsistent with this mechanism of transmission.[7, 25, 68, 139, 169, 170, 205] Several studies have suggested that follicular dendritic cells in lymphoid tissue probably are sites of prion replication and may direct the prion to the CNS. Other investigators have suggested that as yet unidentified host-cell molecules may provide the necessary interactions with the prion molecule that permit their trafficking with migratory myeloid cells and, ultimately, their entry into the CNS. Candidate molecules included components of the complement system based on the study of PrP^{sc} in transgenic mice lacking specific components of the complement system.[140]

Although inoculation of a susceptible host with prion-contaminated cadaveric growth hormone or the use of contaminated instruments during neurosurgical procedures clearly can transmit CJD, the route of infection leading to vCJD has been assumed to be through the oral ingestion of contaminated beef, based on studies in nonhuman primates.[20] Studies have demonstrated that other TSEs, including kuru, can be transmitted by the oral ingestion of infectious material, but only after the ingestion of large inocula, and extended incubation periods often are required.[95] In studies in mice, researchers have demonstrated that the oral ingestion of 10 g of BSE-infected cow brain can infect and kill most mice.[9] Even though extrapolating from these data to determine a comparable dose required for human infection will be difficult, these findings demonstrate that the BSE agent can be transmitted by oral ingestion.

The pathologic findings of TSE include the hallmark of a triad of histologic findings: (1) neuronal loss, (2) proliferation of reactive astrocytes, and (3) status spongiosis.[13] Status spongiosus is a descriptive term for degeneration of neurons and collapse of the cortical cytoarchitecture leading to vacuolation of the neuropil.[13] Amyloid plaques are observed in some patients.[13, 138, 146] Whether the distribution of spongiform lesions is related to the pathogenesis of these disorders or merely reflects the duration of disease before the onset of clinical symptoms is unknown; however, some TSEs such as FFI exhibit a preponderance of histopathologic changes in specific locations such as the thalamus.[13, 106, 164, 178] Recent descriptions of the neuropathology of vCJD have suggested that distinctive histopathologic changes allow cases of vCJD to be distinguished easily from CJD. Such changes include a distinctive plaque containing a central amyloid core and a fibrillary periphery with extensive spongiform changes in the immediate periphery of the plaque.[87, 124] The surrounding spongiform changes are proximal to the plaque, and the remaining neuropil is relatively intact.[124] These findings are unique to vCJD cases and are not seen in sporadic CJD cases outside Great Britain.[47, 125] Histopathologic lesions also have been described in the cerebral and cerebellar cortices, the basal ganglia, the thalamus, and the brain stem.[124] Involvement of the cerebellum appears to be more common in vCJD than in reported cases of sporadic CJD. Finally, electron-microscopic studies of plaques from vCJD brain tissue have suggested subtle, but recognizable, differences in plaques from patients with vCJD and those with CJD.[87]

Clinical Manifestations

Only the clinical manifestation of sporadic CJD and vCJD are discussed here because the other TSEs such as GSS and FFI are diseases that are unlikely to be encountered in pediatrics (Table 160–2). Interested readers are referred to discussions of these diseases in adults.[32, 85, 92, 98, 154, 157, 164] Clinical signs and symptoms during the early stages of CJD are somewhat subtle, often complex, and include both motor and sensory dysfunction. Abnormalities in gait and vision and complaints of headache, dizziness, and paresthesias are noted often.[27, 155, 156, 199] Psychointellectual dysfunction, including loss of memory, speech abnormalities, anxiety, and depression, also often are initial complaints of patients in the early stages of CJD.[32, 42, 156] Neurologic abnormalities may include corticospinal tract dysfunction manifested as hyperreflexia, spasticity, and extensor plantar reflexes. Visual disturbances include visual field abnormalities and, in some cases, cortical blindness. Seizures are not a frequent clinical symptom of patients with CJD. Other less common findings include evidence of autonomic system dysfunction and, rarely, lower motor neuron disease.[172, 201] Although death secondary to complications associated with the vegetative state usually occurs within 1 year of the onset of symptoms, a small percentage of patients may exhibit a prolonged disease course.[42]

The clinical symptoms of vCJD are distinct from those of sporadic CJD, and because this disease has been reported in an adolescent, these symptoms could be encountered by pediatricians. The age range for reported cases of vCJD is 16 to 48 years, a distribution clearly outside that of sporadic CJD.[59, 232, 239] Symptoms associated with this TSE have included psychiatric and sensory disturbances such as

TABLE 160–2 ■ HUMAN TRANSMISSIBLE ENCEPHALOPATHIES

Disease	Acquisition	Clinical Features
Kuru	Ingestion/percutaneous inoculation with contaminated CNS tissue during ritual cannibalism in Fore tribe in New Guinea. Last case reported in 1985	Bimodal age distribution with disease in adolescents and older adults. Adolescents presented with ataxia and dementia with prominent cerebellar involvement. Rapidly progressive disease
Creutzfeldt-Jakob disease	Sporadic cases account for 85% of reported cases of CJD; approximately 15% are secondary to defined mutation in PrP^c, and an unknown number are secondary to infection. Well-documented cases occur after neurosurgical procedures and injection of cadaveric growth hormone	Classic manifestation of dementia and sensory abnormalities, followed by loss of motor function. Rapid progression of symptoms with death usually occurring <1 yr after onset. Disease of late middle age except in cases acquired after iatrogenic transmission
Variant Creutzfeldt-Jakob disease	Acquired through exposure to beef or beef by-products contaminated with BSE. Route of acquisition unknown but presumed to be oral	Manifestations similar to those for CJD, but disease progresses more slowly, with death occurring >12 mo after symptoms develop. Mean age of cases approximately 28 yr, with documented cases in adolescents
Gerstmann-Stäussler-Scheinker syndrome	Autosomal dominant inheritance with documented point mutations in PrP^c gene	Disease of middle age, with mean age of 45 yr at onset. Motor abnormalities and progressive dementia
Familial fatal insomnia	Autosomal dominant inheritance with point mutations in PrP^c gene. Sporadic cases also reported recently	Disease of middle age. Manifestations include insomnia, dysautonomia, and motor dysfunction

BSE, bovine spongiform encephalopathy; CJD, Creutzfeldt-Jakob disease; CNS, central nervous system.

dysesthesias and paresthesias with electromyographic evidence of denervation. Psychiatric symptoms included anxiety, depression, anorexia, social withdrawal, and other nonspecific complaints. As the disease progresses, more familiar findings of TSE develop and include pyramidal tract dysfunction, rigidity, cerebellar dysfunction, and myoclonus. Visual disturbances also have been described late in the disease. The duration of illness has exceeded 1 year in most patients with vCJD, and illness occurs after development of complications associated with the vegetative state.

Diagnosis

The diagnosis of CJD and vCJD requires a high index of suspicion and, in the case of vCJD, a history compatible with exposure to contaminated beef or beef by-products or possibly a previous neurosurgical procedure. Routine laboratory findings are nonspecific and not helpful. No evidence has been found of systemic or CNS inflammation; thus, routine laboratory analysis of cerebrospinal fluid (CSF) often is nondiagnostic. More recently, assays for specific CSF proteins, such as the 14-3-3 complex first observed on two-dimensional polyacrylamide gels, may provide helpful laboratory evidence of CJD or vCJD.[101, 123, 240–242] Other surrogates for the diagnosis of CJD and vCJD have been proposed, but none has sufficient specificity to provide a definitive diagnosis.[131, 173, 174, 226] Definitive premortem diagnosis requires biopsy tissue, and histopathologic diagnosis can be facilitated by use of PrP^{res}-specific antibodies in both immunocytochemistry and Western blot formats.* Importantly, the use of monoclonal antibodies specific for PrP^{res} has permitted a more thorough understanding of the distribution of prions in CNS and non-CNS tissue in patients with TSEs.[82, 114, 116, 127, 138] More recently, Hill and coworkers have reported that tonsillar biopsy followed by detection of PrP^{res} by both Western blot and immunocytochemistry could be used to diagnose vCJD disease.[114, 116] If confirmed, this approach could eliminate the need of CNS biopsy tissue for the diagnosis of prion disease.

Imaging in patients with suspected prion disease has been extremely helpful in making the diagnosis of these rare diseases. Although computed tomography may reveal a variety of structural abnormalities, none is sufficiently specific to be considered diagnostic. In contrast, several investigators have claimed that increased T2 signals from magnetic resonance imaging (MRI) of the striatum and thalamus are specific for prion diseases, especially vCJD.[8, 86, 203] Other investigators have suggested that abnormal signals originating from the pulvinar in the thalamus are distinctive for vCJD and should be considered diagnostic.[234] Similarly, electroencephalographic (EEG) tracings from patients with CJD and vCJD are characteristic but not diagnostic. The classic findings are synchronous bilateral biphasic or triphasic periodic sharp waves on a background of generalized slowing.[21, 63, 202, 212] The lack of characteristic EEG tracings and MRI findings should cast doubt on the diagnosis of CJD or vCJD, especially several months after the onset of clinical symptoms.

Prevention and Treatment

Because effective treatment of TSEs has not been defined yet, prevention of disease remains the goal of current medical practice. Infection developing after exposure during neurosurgical procedures, including dural grafting and placement of stereotactic electrodes, and infection after exposure to contaminated CNS tissue in the form of growth hormone or gonadotropic hormone preparations and after corneal grafting are well-known, and the modes of transmission of TSEs in most cases are preventable. Transmission by blood and blood products has not been reported, but the American Red Cross has placed restrictions on donors who may have been exposed to agents associated with TSEs. Cases of TSE that develop after exposure to human feces, urine, or mucosal secretions have not been reported, and, therefore, the current universal precautions used in health care settings should suffice to prevent nosocomial transmission during the routine care of patients with a TSE. Inactivation of tissue and fluid suspected of being contaminated with prions is problematic. Early studies indicated that subjecting prion-containing brain tissue to temperatures in excess of 360° C resulted in only approximately a 90 percent reduction in infectivity.[40] In addition, CJD has been transmitted from paraffin-embedded tissue sections.[38] Several different approaches for decontaminating prion-contaminated tissue and instruments have been proposed.[43, 48, 159, 194, 198, 215] Suffice it to say that the concentration of prions in lymphoid and nervous tissue should be emphasized to anyone in contact with patients with TSEs, and material that may be contaminated with prions should be handled in a rigorous manner to ensure safe disposal.

As noted earlier, no known treatment of TSE exists. In vitro models of PrP^c folding have suggested that a variety of agents may limit the production of pathogenic forms of PrP^{res} in neuroblastoma cells in vitro. Such agents include derivatives of Congo red, polyene antibiotics related to amphotericin B, branched polyamines, and phenothiazines.[52, 54, 77, 78, 180, 213] To date, no evidence has shown that any of these proposed therapies would be effective in treating human TSEs. Interestingly, at least two recent reports have suggested that antiprion antibodies may offer a therapeutic approach to TSEs. In these reports, researchers contend that antiprion antibodies directed at cell surface PrP^c prevented infection of susceptible cells and also eliminated infection in a chronically infected cell line.[81, 145, 179] These findings suggest that impaired clearance of misfolded PrP^c contributes to disease in animals infected with PrP^{res} and that passive antibody therapy potentially could cure similar infections in vivo.

*See references 6, 48, 55, 124, 126, 147, 178, 196, 224, 242.

REFERENCES

1. Alperovitch, A., Zerr, I., Pocchiari, M., et al.: Codon 129 prion protein genotype and sporadic Creutzfeldt-Jakob disease. Lancet *353*:1673–1674, 1999.
2. Alpers, M. P.: Epidemiology and clinical aspects of kuru. *In* Prusiner, S. B., and McKinley, M. (eds.): Prions: Novel Infectious Pathogens Causing Scrapie and Creutzfeldt-Jakob Disease. San Diego, CA, 1987.
3. Alter, M., Hoenig, E., and Pratzon, G.: Creutzfeldt-Jakob disease: Possible association with eating brains. N. Engl. J. Med. *296*:820–821, 1977.
4. Anderson, R. M., Donnelly, C. A., Ferguson, N. M., et al.: Transmission dynamics and epidemiology of BSE in British cattle. Nature *382*:779–788, 1996.
5. Andrews, N. J., Farrington, C. P., Cousens, S. N., et al.: Incidence of variant Creutzfeldt-Jakob disease in the UK. Lancet *356*:481–482, 2000.
6. Armstrong, R. A., Cairns, N. J., and Lantos, P. L.: Spatial pattern of prion protein deposits in patients with sporadic Creutzfeldt-Jakob disease. Neuropathology *21*:19–24, 2001.
7. Aucouturier, P., Geissmann, F., Damotte, D., et al.: Infected splenic dendritic cells are sufficient for prion transmission to the CNS in mouse scrapie. J. Clin. Invest. *108*:703–708, 2001.
8. Bahn, M. M., Kido, D. K., Lin, W., and Pearlman, A. L.: Brain magnetic resonance diffusion abnormalities in Creutzfeldt-Jakob disease. Arch. Neurol. *54*:1411–1415, 1997.
9. Barlow, R. M., Middleton, D. J.: Dietary transmission of bovine spongiform encephalopathy to mice. Vet. Rec. *126*:111–112, 1990.

10. Basler, K., Oesch, B., Scott, M., et al.: Scrapie and cellular PrP isoforms are encoded by the same chromosomal gene. Cell *46*:417–428, 1986.
11. Bateman, D., Hilton, D., Love, S., et al.: Sporadic Creutzfeldt-Jakob disease in a 18-year-old in the UK. Lancet *346*:1155–1156, 1995.
12. Beck, E., Daniel, P. M., Alpers, M., et al.: Experimental "kuru" in chimpanzees: A pathological report. Lancet *2*:1056–1059, 1966.
13. Bell, J. E., and Ironside, J. W.: Neuropathology of spongiform encephalopathies in humans. Br. Med. Bull. *49*:738–777, 1993.
14. Bellinger-Kawahara, C., Cleaver, J. E., Diener, T. O., and Prusiner, S. B.: Purified scrapie prions resist inactivation by UV irradiation. J. Virol. *61*:159–166, 1987.
15. Bellinger-Kawahara, C., Diener, T. O., McKinley, M. P., et al.: Purified scrapie prions resist inactivation by procedures that hydrolyze, modify, or shear nucleic acids. Virology *160*:271–274, 1987.
16. Belt, P. B., Muileman, I. H., and Schreuder, B. E.: Identification of five allelic variants of the sheep PrP gene and their association with natural scrapie. J. Gen. Virol. *76*:509–517, 1995.
17. Bessen, R. A., Kocisko, D. A., Raymond, G. J., et al.: Non-genetic propagation of strain-specific properties of scrapie prion protein. Nature *375*:698–700, 1995.
18. Boellaard, J. W., Brown, P., and Tateishi, J.: Gerstmann-Sträussler-Scheinker disease—the dilemma of molecular and clinical correlations. Clin. Neuropathol. *18*:271–85, 1999.
19. Bolton, D. C., McKinley, M. P., and Prusiner, S. B.: Identification of a protein that purifies with the scrapie prion. Science *218*:1309–1311, 1982.
20. Bons, N., Mestre-Frances, N., Belli, P., et al.: Natural and experimental oral infection of nonhuman primates by bovine spongiform encephalopathy agents. Proc. Natl. Acad. Sci. U. S. A. *96*:4046–4051, 1999.
21. Bortone, E., Bettoni, L., Giorgi, C., et al.: Reliability of EEG in the diagnosis of Creutzfeldt-Jakob disease. Electroencephalogr. Clin. Neurophysiol. *90*:323–330, 1994.
22. Bossers, A., Schreuder, B. E., Muileman, I. H., et al.: PrP genotype contributes to determining survival times of sheep with natural scrapie. J. Gen. Virol. *77*:2669–2673, 1996.
23. Britton, T. C., al-Sarraj, S., Shaw, C., et al.: Sporadic Creutzfeldt-Jakob disease in a 16-year-old in the UK. Lancet *346*:1155, 1995.
24. Brown, D. R.: Copper and prion disease. Brain Res. Bull. *55*:165–173, 2001.
25. Brown, K. L., Stewart, K., Ritchie, D., et al.: Follicular dendritic cells in scrapie pathogenesis. Arch. Virol. Suppl. *16*:13–21, 2000.
26. Brown, P.: Human growth hormone therapy and Creutzfeldt-Jakob disease: A drama in three acts. Pediatrics *81*:85–92, 1988.
27. Brown, P.: Can Creutzfeldt-Jakob disease be transmitted by transfusion? Curr. Opin. Hematol. *2*:472–477, 1995.
28. Brown, P.: On the origins of BSE. Lancet *352*:252–253, 1998.
29. Brown, P.: Transmission of spongiform encephalopathy through biological products. Dev. Biol. Stand. *93*:73–78, 1998.
30. Brown, P.: The risk of blood-borne Creutzfeldt-Jakob disease. Dev. Biol. Stand. *102*:53–59, 2000.
31. Brown, P., and Bradley, R.: 1755 and all that: A historical primer of transmissible spongiform encephalopathy. B. M. J. *317*:1688–1692, 1998.
32. Brown, P., Cathala, F., Castaigne, P., and Gajdusek, D. C.: Creutzfeldt-Jakob disease: Clinical analysis of a consecutive series of 230 neuropathologically verified cases. Ann. Neurol. *20*:597–602, 1986.
33. Brown, P., Cathala, F., Labauge, R., et al.: Epidemiologic implications of Creutzfeldt-Jakob disease in a 19 year-old girl. Eur. J. Epidemiol. *1*:42–47, 1985.
34. Brown, P., Cathala, F., Raubertas, R. F., et al.: The epidemiology of Creutzfeldt-Jakob disease: Conclusion of a 15-year investigation in France and review of the world literature. Neurology *37*:895–904, 1987.
35. Brown, P., Cervenakova, L., Goldfarb, L. G., et al.: Iatrogenic Creutzfeldt-Jakob disease: An example of the interplay between ancient genes and modern medicine. Neurology *44*:291–293, 1994.
36. Brown, P., Cervenakova, L., McShane, L., et al.: Creutzfeldt-Jakob disease in a husband and wife. Neurology *50*:684–688, 1998.
37. Brown, P., Gajdusek, D. C., Gibbs, C. J., Jr., and Asher, D. M.: Potential epidemic of Creutzfeldt-Jakob disease from human growth hormone therapy. N. Engl. J. Med. *313*:728–731, 1985.
38. Brown, P., Gibbs, C. J., Jr., Gajdusek, D. C., et al.: Transmission of Creutzfeldt-Jakob disease from formalin-fixed, paraffin-embedded human brain tissue. N. Engl. J. Med. *315*:1614–1615, 1986.
39. Brown, P., Gibbs, C. J., Jr., Rodgers-Johnson, P., et al.: Human spongiform encephalopathy: The National Institutes of Health series of 300 cases of experimentally transmitted disease. Ann. Neurol. *35*:513–529, 1994.
40. Brown, P., Liberski, P. P., Wolff, A., and Gajdusek, D. C.: Resistance of scrapie infectivity to steam autoclaving after formaldehyde fixation and limited survival after ashing at 360 degrees C: Practical and theoretical implications. J. Infect. Dis. *161*:467–472, 1990.
41. Brown, P., Preece, M., Brandel, J. P., et al.: Iatrogenic Creutzfeldt-Jakob disease at the millennium. Neurology *55*:1075–1081, 2000.
42. Brown, P., Rodgers-Johnson, P., and Cathala, F.: Creutzfeldt-Jakob disease of long duration: Clinicopathological characteristics, transmissibility, and differential diagnosis. Ann. Neurol. *16*:295–304, 1984.
43. Brown, P., Rohwer, R. G., Green, E. M., et al.: Effect of chemicals, heat, and histopathologic processing on high-infectivity hamster-adapted scrapie virus. J. Infect. Dis. *145*:683–687, 1982.
44. Brown, P., Will, R. G., Bradley, R., et al.: Bovine spongiform encephalopathy and variant Creutzfeldt-Jakob disease: Background, evolution, and current concerns. Emerg. Infect. Dis. *7*:6–16, 2001.
45. Bruce, M. E., and Dickinson, A. G.: Biological evidence that scrapie agent has an independent genome. J. Gen. Virol. *68*:79–89, 1987.
46. Bruce, M. E., McConnell, I., Fraser, H., and Dickinson, A. G.: The disease characteristics of different strains of scrapie in Sinc congenic mouse lines: Implications for the nature of the agent and host control of pathogenesis. J. Gen. Virol. *72*:595–603, 1991.
47. Bruce, M. E., Will, R. G., Ironside, J. W., et al.: Transmissions to mice indicate that 'new variant' CJD is caused by the BSE agent. Nature *389*:498–501, 1997.
48. Budka, H., Aguzzi, A., Brown, P., et al.: Tissue handling in suspected Creutzfeldt-Jakob disease (CJD) and other human spongiform encephalopathies (prion diseases). Brain Pathol. *5*:319–322, 1995.
49. Bueler, H., Aguzzi, A., Sailer, A., et al.: Mice devoid of PrP are resistant to scrapie. Cell *73*:1339–1347, 1993.
50. Bueler, H., Fischer, M., Lang, Y., et al.: Normal development and behaviour of mice lacking the neuronal cell-surface PrP protein. Nature *356*:577–582, 1992.
51. Carlson, G. A., Hsiao, K., Oesch, B., et al.: Genetics of prion infections. Trends Genet. *7*:61–65, 1991.
52. Caspi, S., Halimi, M., Yanai, A., et al.: The anti-prion activity of Congo red. Putative mechanism. J. Biol. Chem. *273*:3484–3489, 1998.
53. Caughey, B.: Interactions between prion protein isoforms: The kiss of death? Trends Biochem. Sci. *26*:235–242, 2001.
54. Caughey, B., Ernst, D., and Race, R. E.: Congo red inhibition of scrapie agent replication. J. Virol. *67*:6270–6272, 1993.
55. Caughey, B., Horiuchi, M., Demaimay, R., and Raymond, G. J.: Assays of protease-resistant prion protein and its formation. Methods Enzymol. *309*:122–133, 1999.
56. Caughey, B., Kocisko, D. A., Raymond, G. J., and Lansbury, P. T.: Aggregates of scrapie-associated prion protein induce the cell-free conversion of protease-sensitive prion protein to the protease-resistant state. Chem. Biol. *2*:807–817, 1995.
57. Cervenakova, L., Goldfarb, L. G., Garruto, R., et al.: Phenotype-genotype studies in kuru: Implications for new variant Creutzfeldt-Jakob disease. Proc. Natl. Acad. Sci. U. S. A. *95*:13239–13241, 1998.
58. Chapman, J., Brown, P., Rabey, J. M., et al.: Transmission of spongiform encephalopathy from a familial Creutzfeldt-Jakob disease patient of Jewish Libyan origin carrying the PRNP codon 200 mutation. Neurology *42*:1249–1250, 1992.
59. Chazot, G., Broussolle, E., Lapras, C., et al.: New variant of Creutzfeldt-Jakob disease in a 26-year-old French man. Lancet *347*:1181, 1996.
60. Chen, S. G., Parchi, P., Brown, P., et al.: Allelic origin of the abnormal prion protein isoform in familial prion diseases. Nat. Med. *3*:1009–1015, 1997.
61. Chesebro, B.: BSE and prions: Uncertainties about the agent. Science *279*:42–43, 1998.
62. Chesebro, B., Race, R., Wehrly, K., et al.: Identification of scrapie prion protein-specific mRNA in scrapie-infected and uninfected brain. Nature *315*:331–333, 1985.
63. Chiofalo, N., Fuentes, A., and Galvez, S.: Serial EEG findings in 27 cases of Creutzfeldt-Jakob disease. Arch. Neurol. *37*:143–145, 1980.
64. Choo-Kang, L. R., and Zeitlin, P. L.: Type I, II, III, IV, and V cystic fibrosis transmembrane conductance regulator defects and opportunities for therapy. Curr. Opin. Pulm. Med. *6*:521–529, 2000.
65. Collinge, J.: Variant Creutzfeldt-Jakob disease. Lancet *354*:317–323, 1999.
66. Collinge, J.: Prion diseases of humans and animals: Their causes and molecular basis. Annu. Rev. Neurosci. *24*:519–550, 2001.
67. Collinge, J., Beck, J., Campbell, T., et al.: Prion protein gene analysis in new variant cases of Creutzfeldt-Jakob disease. Lancet *348*:56, 1996.
68. Collinge, J., and Hawke, S.: B lymphocytes in prion neuroinvasion: Central or peripheral players? Letter. Nat. Med. *4*:1369–1370, 1998.
69. Collinge, J., Palmer, M. S., Sidle, K. C., et al.: Transmission of fatal familial insomnia to laboratory animals. Lancet *346*:569–570, 1995.
70. Collinge, J., Sidle, K. C., Meads, J., et al.: Molecular analysis of prion strain variation and the aetiology of 'new variant' CJD. Nature *383*:685–690, 1996.
71. Collinge, J., Whittington, M. A., Sidle, K. C., et al.: Prion protein is necessary for normal synaptic function. Nature *370*:295–297, 1994.
72. Collins, S., Law, M. G., Fletcher, A., et al.: Surgical treatment and risk of sporadic Creutzfeldt-Jakob disease: A case-control study. Lancet *353*:693–697, 1999.
73. Cousens, S. N., Vynnycky, E., Zeidler, M., et al.: Predicting the CJD epidemic in humans. Nature *385*:197–198, 1997.
74. Cousens, S. N., Zeidler, M., Esmonde, T. F., et al.: Sporadic Creutzfeldt-Jakob disease in the United Kingdom: Analysis of epidemiological surveillance data for 1970–96. B. M. J. *315*:389–395, 1997.
75. Creutzfeldt-Jakob disease associated with cadaveric dura mater grafts—Japan, January 1979–May 1996. M. M. W. R. Morb. Mortal. Wkly. Rep. *46*:1066–109, 1997.

76. Cuille, J., Chelle, P. L.: Pathologie animale la maladie dile tremblante du mouton est-elle inoculable. C. R. Acad. Sci. *203*:1552–1554, 1936.
77. Demaimay, R., Harper, J., Gordon, H., et al.: Structural aspects of Congo red as an inhibitor of protease-resistant prion protein formation. J. Neurochem. *71*:2534–2541, 1998.
78. Demaimay, R., Race, R., and Chesebro, B.: Effectiveness of polyene antibiotics in treatment of transmissible spongiform encephalopathy in transgenic mice expressing Syrian hamster PrP only in neurons. J. Virol. *73*:3511–3513, 1999.
79. Di Martino, A., Safar, J., Gibbs, C. J.: The consistent use of organic solvents for purification of phospholipids from brain tissue effectively removes scrapie infectivity. Biologicals *22*:221–225, 1994.
80. Duffy, P., Wolf, J., Collins, G., et al.: Possible person-to-person transmission of Creutzfeldt-Jakob disease. Letter. N. Engl. J. Med. *290*:692–693, 1974.
81. Enari, M., Flechsig, E., and Weissmann, C.: Scrapie prion protein accumulation by scrapie-infected neuroblastoma cells abrogated by exposure to a prion protein antibody. Proc. Natl. Acad. Sci. U. S. A. *98*:9295–9299, 2001.
82. Esiri, M. M., Carter, J., and Ironside, J. W.: Prion protein immunoreactivity in brain samples from an unselected autopsy population: Findings in 200 consecutive cases. Neuropathol. Appl. Neurobiol. *26*:273–284, 2000.
83. Evatt, B.: Creutzfeldt-Jakob disease and haemophilia: Assessment of risk. Haemophilia *6*:94–99, 2000.
84. Evatt, B., Austin, H., Barnhart, E., et al.: Surveillance for Creutzfeldt-Jakob disease among persons with hemophilia. Transfusion *38*:817–820, 1998.
85. Farlow, M. R., Yee, R. D., and Dlouhy, S. R.: Gerstmann-Sträussler-Scheinker disease. I. Extending the clinical spectrum. Neurology *39*:1446–1452, 1989.
86. Finkenstaedt, M., Szudra, A., Zerr, I., et al.: MR imaging of Creutzfeldt-Jakob disease. Radiology *199*:793–798, 1996.
87. Fournier, J. G., Kopp, N., Streichenberger, N., et al.: Electron microscopy of brain amyloid plaques from a patient with new variant Creutzfeldt-Jakob disease. Acta Neuropathol. *99*:637–642, 2000.
88. Gabizon, R., Telling, G., Meiner, Z., et al.: Insoluble wild-type and protease-resistant mutant prion protein in brains of patients with inherited prion disease. Nat. Med. *2*:59–64, 1996.
89. Gajdusek, D. C., and Gibbs, C. J., Jr.: Transmission of two subacute spongiform encephalopathies of man (kuru and Creutzfeldt-Jakob disease) to New World monkeys. Nature *230*:588–591, 1971.
90. Gajdusek, D. C., and Gibbs, C. J., Jr.: Transmission of kuru from man to rhesus monkey *(Macaca mulatta)* 8 and one-half years after inoculation. Nature *240*:351, 1972.
91. Gajdusek, D. C., Gibbs, C. J., Jr., and Alpers, M.: Transmission and passage of experimental "kuru" to chimpanzees. Science *155*:212–214, 1967.
92. Gallassi, R., Morreale, A., Montagna, P., et al.: Fatal familial insomnia: Behavioral and cognitive features. Neurology *46*:935–939, 1996.
93. Ghani, A. C., Ferguson, N. M., and Donnelly, C. A.: Predicted vCJD mortality in Great Britain. Nature *406*:583–584, 2000.
94. Ghani, A. C., Ferguson, N. M., Donnelly, C. A., et al.: Epidemiological determinants of the pattern and magnitude of the vCJD epidemic in Great Britain. Proc. R. Soc. Lond. B Biol. Sci. *265*:2443–2452, 1998.
95. Gibbs, C. J., Jr., Amyx, H. L., Bacote, A., et al.: Oral transmission of kuru, Creutzfeldt-Jakob disease, and scrapie to nonhuman primates. J. Infect. Dis. *142*:205–208, 1980.
96. Gibbs, C. J., Asher, D. M., Kobrine, A., et al.: Transmission of Creutzfeldt-Jakob disease to a chimpanzee by electrodes contaminated during neurosurgery. J. Neurol. Neurosurg. Psychiatry *57*:757–758, 1994.
97. Gibbs, C. J., Gajdusek, D. C., Asher, D. M., et al.: Creutzfeldt-Jakob disease (spongiform encephalopathy): Transmission to the chimpanzee. Science *161*:388–389, 1968.
98. Goldfarb, L. G., Brown, P., McCombie, W. R., et al.: Transmissible familial Creutzfeldt-Jakob disease associated with five, seven, and eight extra octapeptide coding repeats in the PRNP gene. Proc. Natl. Acad. Sci. U. S. A. *88*:10926–10930, 1991.
99. Goldfarb, L. G., Korczyn, A. D., Brown, P., et al.: Mutation in codon 200 of scrapie amyloid precursor gene linked to Creutzfeldt-Jakob disease in Sephardic Jews of Libyan and non-Libyan origin. Lancet *336*:637–638, 1990.
100. Gore, S. M.: Commentary: Age related exposure of patients to the agent of BSE should not be downplayed. B. M. J. *315*:395–396, 1997.
101. Green, A. J., Thompson, E. J., Stewart, G. E., et al.: Use of 14-3-3 and other brain-specific proteins in CSF in the diagnosis of variant Creutzfeldt-Jakob disease. J. Neurol. Neurosurg. Psychiatry *70*:744–748, 2001.
102. Gregersen, N., Bross, P., and Jorgensen, M. M.: Defective folding and rapid degradation of mutant proteins is a common disease mechanism in genetic disorders. J. Inherit. Metab. Dis. *23*:441–447, 2000.
103. Griffith, J. S.: Self-replication and scrapie. Nature *215*:1043–1044, 1967.
104. Haardt, M., Benharouga, M., Lechardeur, D., et al.: C-terminal truncations destabilize the cystic fibrosis transmembrane conductance regulator without impairing its biogenesis. A novel class of mutation. J. Biol. Chem. *274*:21873–21877, 1999.
105. Hadlow, W. J.: Scrapie and kuru. Lancet *2*:289, 1959.
106. Hainfellner, J. A., Liberski, P. P., Guiroy, D. C., et al.: Pathology and immunocytochemistry of a kuru brain. Brain Pathol. *7*:547–553, 1997.
107. Hay, B., Barry, R. A., Lieberburg, I., et al.: Biogenesis and transmembrane orientation of the cellular isoform of the scrapie prion protein [published erratum appears in Mol Cell Biol *7*:2035, 1987]. Mol. Cell. Biol. *7*:914–920, 1987.
108. Heckmann, J. G., Lang, C. J., Petruch, F., et al.: Transmission of Creutzfeldt-Jakob disease via a corneal transplant. J. Neurol. Neurosurg. Psychiatry *63*:388–390, 1997.
109. Hegde, R. S., Mastrianni, J. A., Scott, M. R., et al.: A transmembrane form of the prion protein in neurodegenerative disease. Science *279*:827–834, 1998.
110. Hegde, R. S., Tremblay, P., Groth, D., et al. Transmissible and genetic prion diseases share a common pathway of neurodegeneration. Nature *402*:822–826, 1999.
111. Heim, D., and Wilesmith, J. W.: Surveillance of BSE. Arch. Virol. Suppl. *16*:127–133, 2000.
112. Heppner, F. L., Christ, A. D., Klein, M. A., et al.: Transepithelial prion transport by M cells. Nat. Med. *7*:976–977, 2001.
113. Hill, A. F., Antoniou, M., and Collinge, J.: Protease-resistant prion protein produced in vitro lacks detectable infectivity. J. Gen. Virol. *80*:11–14, 1999.
114. Hill, A. F., Butterworth, R. J., Joiner, S., et al.: Investigation of variant Creutzfeldt-Jakob disease and other human prion diseases with tonsil biopsy samples. Lancet *353*:183–189, 1999.
115. Hill, A. F., Desbruslais, M., Joiner, S., et al.: The same prion strain causes vCJD and BSE. Nature *389*:448–450, 526, 1997.
116. Hill, A. F., Zeidler, M., Ironside, J., and Collinge, J.: Diagnosis of new variant Creutzfeldt-Jakob disease by tonsil biopsy. Lancet *349*:99–100, 1997.
117. Hilton, D. A., Fathers, E., Edwards, P., et al.: Prion immunoreactivity in appendix before clinical onset of variant Creutzfeldt-Jakob disease. Lancet *352*:703–704, 1998.
118. Hogan, R. N., Brown, P., Heck, E., and Cavanagh, H. D.: Risk of prion disease transmission from ocular donor tissue transplantation. Cornea *18*:2–11, 1999.
119. Horiuchi, M., Priola, S. A., Chabry, J., and Caughey, B.: Interactions between heterologous forms of prion protein: Binding, inhibition of conversion, and species barriers. Proc. Natl. Acad. Sci. U. S. A. *97*:5836–5841, 2000.
120. Hsiao, K., Dlouhy, S. R., Farlow, M. R., et al.: Mutant prion proteins in Gerstmann-Sträussler-Scheinker disease with neurofibrillary tangles. Nat. Genet. *1*:68–71, 1992.
121. Hsiao, K., Meiner, Z., Kahana, E., et al.: Mutation of the prion protein in Libyan Jews with Creutzfeldt-Jakob disease. N. Engl. J. Med. *324*:1091–1097, 1991.
122. Hsiao, K., and Prusiner, S. B.: Inherited human prion diseases. Neurology *40*:1820–1827, 1990.
123. Hsich, G., Kenney, K., and Gibbs, C. J.: The 14-3-3 brain protein in cerebrospinal fluid as a marker for transmissible spongiform encephalopathies. N. Engl. J. Med. *335*:924–930, 1996.
124. Ironside, J. W.: Pathology of variant Creutzfeldt-Jakob disease. Arch. Virol. Suppl. *16*:143–151, 2000.
125. Ironside, J. W., and Bell, J. E.: Florid plaques and new variant Creutzfeldt-Jakob disease. Lancet *350*:1475, 1997.
126. Ironside, J. W., Hilton, D. A., Ghani, A., et al.: Retrospective study of prion-protein accumulation in tonsil and appendix tissues. Lancet *355*:1693–1694, 2000.
127. Ironside, J. W., Head, M. W., Bell, J. E., et al.: Laboratory diagnosis of variant Creutzfeldt-Jakob disease. Histopathology *37*:1–9, 2000.
128. Ironside, J. W., Sutherland, K., Bell, J. E., et al.: A new variant of Creutzfeldt-Jakob disease: Neuropathological and clinical features. Cold Spring Harb. Symp. Quant. Biol. *61*:523–530, 1996.
129. Jackson, G. S., and Collinge, J.: Prion disease—the propagation of infectious protein topologies. Microbes Infect. *2*:1445–1449, 2000.
130. Jackson, G. S., Murray, I., Hosszu, L. L., et al.: Location and properties of metal-binding sites on the human prion protein. Proc. Natl. Acad. Sci. U. S. A. *98*:8531–8535, 2001.
131. Jimi, T., Wakayama, Y., Shibuya, S., et al.: High levels of nervous system–specific proteins in cerebrospinal fluid in patients with early stage Creutzfeldt-Jakob disease. Clin. Chim. Acta *211*:37–46, 1992.
132. Kahana, E., Alter, M., Braham, J., and Sofer, D.: Creutzfeldt-Jakob disease: Focus among Libyan Jews in Israel. Science *183*:90–91, 1974.
133. Kaneko, K., Zulianello, L., Scott, M., et al.: Evidence for protein X binding to a discontinuous epitope on the cellular prion protein during scrapie prion propagation. Proc. Natl. Acad. Sci. U. S. A. *94*:10069–10074, 1997.
134. Kimberlin, R. H., and Walker, C. A.: Intraperitoneal infection with scrapie is established within minutes of injection and is non-specifically enhanced by a variety of different drugs. Arch. Virol. *112*:103–114, 1990.
135. Kimberlin, R. H., Walker, C. A., and Fraser, H.: The genomic identity of different strains of mouse scrapie is expressed in hamsters and preserved on reisolation in mice. J. Gen. Virol. *70*:2017–2025, 1989.

136. Kimura, K., Nonaka, A., Tashiro, H., et al.: Atypical form of dural graft associated Creutzfeldt-Jakob disease: Report of a postmortem case with review of the literature. J. Neurol. Neurosurg. Psychiatry *70*:696–699, 2001.
137. Kitamoto, T., Muramoto, T., Mohri, S., et al.: Abnormal isoform of prion protein accumulates in follicular dendritic cells in mice with Creutzfeldt-Jakob disease. J. Virol. *65*:6292–6295, 1991.
138. Kitamoto, T., Tateishi, J., Tashima, T., et al.: Amyloid plaques in Creutzfeldt-Jakob disease stain with prion protein antibodies. Ann. Neurol. *20*:204–208, 1986.
139. Klein, M. A., Frigg, R., Flechsig, E., et al.: A crucial role for B cells in neuroinvasive scrapie. Nature *390*:687–690, 1997.
140. Klein, M. A., Kaeser, P. S., Schwarz, P., et al.: Complement facilitates early prion pathogenesis. Nat. Med. *7*:488–492, 2001.
141. Klitzman, R. L., Alpers, M. P., and Gajdusek, C.: The natural incubation period of kuru and the episodes of transmission in three clusters of patients. Neuroepidemiology *3*:3–20, 1984.
142. Kocisko, D. A., Come, J. H., Priola, S. A., et al.: Cell-free formation of protease-resistant prion protein. Nature *370*:471–474, 1994.
143. Kocisko, D. A., Priola, S. A., Raymond, G. J., et al.: Species specificity in the cell-free conversion of prion protein to protease-resistant forms: A model for the scrapie species barrier. Proc. Natl. Acad. Sci. U. S. A. *92*:3923–3927, 1995.
144. Korth, C., May, B. C., Cohen, F. E., and Prusiner, S. B.: Acridine and phenothiazine derivatives as pharmacotherapeutics for prion disease. Proc. Natl. Acad. Sci. U. S. A. *98*:9836–9841, 2001.
145. Korth, C., Streit, P., and Oesch, B.: Monoclonal antibodies specific for the native, disease-associated isoform of the prion protein. Methods Enzymol. *309*:106–122, 1999.
146. Lantos, P. L.: From slow virus to prion: A review of transmissible spongiform encephalopathies. Histopathology *20*:1–11, 1992.
147. Lantos, P. L., McGill, I. S., Janota, I., et al.: Prion protein immunocytochemistry helps to establish the true incidence of prion diseases. Neurosci. Lett. *147*:67–71, 1992.
148. Lasmezas, C. I., Fournier, J. G., Nouvel, V., et al.: Adaptation of the bovine spongiform encephalopathy agent to primates and comparison with Creutzfeldt-Jakob disease: Implications for human health. Proc. Natl. Acad. Sci. U. S. A. *98*:4142–4127, 2001.
149. Lavelle, G. C., Sturman, L., and Hadlow, W. J.: Isolation from mouse spleen of cell populations with high specific infectivity for scrapie virus. Infect. Immun. *5*:319–323, 1972.
150. Lee, D. C., Stenland, C. J., Miller, J. L., et al.: A direct relationship between the partitioning of the pathogenic prion protein and transmissible spongiform encephalopathy infectivity during the purification of plasma proteins. Transfusion *41*:449–455, 2001.
151. Lee, H. S., Brown, P., Cervenakova, L., et al.: Increased susceptibility to Kuru of carriers of the PRNP 129 methionine/methionine genotype. J. Infect. Dis. *183*:192–196, 2001.
152. Liberski, P. P., Barcikowska, M., Cervenakova, L., et al.: A case of sporadic Creutzfeldt-Jakob disease with a Gerstmann-Sträussler-Scheinker phenotype but no alterations in the PRNP gene. Acta Neuropathol. *96*:425–430, 1998.
153. Lloyd, S. E., Onwuazor, O. N., Beck, J. A., et al.: Identification of multiple quantitative trait loci linked to prion disease incubation period in mice. Proc. Natl. Acad. Sci. U. S. A. *98*:6279–6283, 2001.
154. Lugaresi, E., Medori, R., Montagna, P., et al.: Fatal familial insomnia and dysautonomia with selective degeneration of thalamic nuclei. N. Engl. J. Med. *315*:997–1003, 1986.
155. MacKnight, C., and Rockwood, K.: Bovine spongiform encephalopathy and Creutzfeldt-Jakob disease: Implications for physicians. C. M. A. J. *155*:529–536, 1996.
156. Mandell, A. M., Alexander, M. P., and Carpenter, S.: Creutzfeldt-Jakob disease presenting as isolated aphasia. Neurology *39*:55–58, 1989.
157. Manetto, V., Medori, R., Cortelli, P., et al.: Fatal familial insomnia: Clinical and pathologic study of five new cases. Neurology *42*:312–319, 1992.
158. Manuelidis, E. E., Gorgacs, E. J., and Manuelidis, L.: Viremia in experimental Creutzfeldt-Jakob disease. Science *200*:1069–1071, 1978.
159. Manuelidis, L.: Decontamination of Creutzfeldt-Jakob disease and other transmissible agents. J. Neurovirol. *3*:62–65, 1997.
160. Manuelidis, L., and Yun Lu, Z.: Attenuated Creutzfeldt-Jakob disease agents can hide more virulent infections. Neurosci. Lett. *293*:163–166, 2000.
161. Masters, C. L., Harris, J. O., Gajdusek, D. C., et al.: Creutzfeldt-Jakob disease: Patterns of worldwide occurrence and the significance of familial and sporadic clustering. Ann. Neurol. *5*:177–188, 1979.
162. Mastrianni, J. A., Nixon, R., Layzer, R., et al.: Prion protein conformation in a patient with sporadic fatal insomnia. N. Engl. J. Med. *340*:1630–1638, 1999.
163. McKinley, M. P., Bolton, D. C., and Prusiner, S. B.: A protease-resistant protein is a structural component of the scrapie prion. Cell *35*:57–62, 1983.
164. Medori, R., Tritschler, H. J., LeBlanc, A., et al.: Fatal familial insomnia, a prion disease with a mutation at codon 178 of the prion protein gene. N. Engl. J. Med. *326*:444–449, 1992.
165. Meiner, Z., Gabizon, R., and Prusiner, S. B.: Familial Creutzfeldt-Jakob disease. Codon 200 prion disease in Libyan Jews. Medicine (Baltimore) *76*:227–237, 1997.
166. Monari, L., Chen, S. G., Brown, P., et al.: Fatal familial insomnia and familial Creutzfeldt-Jakob disease: Different prion proteins determined by a DNA polymorphism. Proc. Natl. Acad. Sci. U. S. A. *91*:2839–2842, 1994.
167. Monreal, J., Collins, G. H., Masters, C. L., et al.: Creutzfeldt-Jakob disease in an adolescent. J. Neurol. Sci. *52*:341–350, 1981.
168. Montagna, P., Cortelli, P., Avoni, P., et al.: Clinical features of fatal familial insomnia: Phenotypic variability in relation to a polymorphism at codon 129 of the prion protein gene. Brain Pathol. *8*:515–520, 1998.
169. Montrasio, F., Cozzio, A., Flechsig, E., et al.: B lymphocyte–restricted expression of prion protein does not enable prion replication in prion protein knockout mice. Proc. Natl. Acad. Sci. U. S. A. *98*:4034–4037, 2001.
170. Montrasio, F., Frigg, R., Glatzel, M., et al.: Impaired prion replication in spleens of mice lacking functional follicular dendritic cells. Science *288*:1257–1259, 2000.
171. Nakamura, Y., Yanagawa, H., Kitamoto, T., and Sato, T.: Epidemiologic features of 65 Creutzfeldt-Jakob disease patients with a history of cadaveric dura mater transplantation in Japan. Epidemiol. Infect. *125*:201–205, 2000.
172. Nomura, E., Harada, T., Kurokawa, K., et al.: Creutzfeldt-Jakob disease associated with autonomic nervous system dysfunction in the early stage. Intern. Med. *36*:492–496, 1997.
173. Otto, M., Stein, H., Szudra, A., et al.: S-100 protein concentration in the cerebrospinal fluid of patients with Creutzfeldt-Jakob disease. J. Neurol. *244*:566–570, 1997.
174. Otto, M., Wiltfang, J., Schutz, E., et al.: Diagnosis of Creutzfeldt-Jakob disease by measurement of S100 protein in serum: Prospective case-control study. B. M. J. *316*:577–582, 1998.
175. Palmer, M. S., Dryden, A. J., Hughes, J. T., and Collinge, J.: Homozygous prion protein genotype predisposes to sporadic Creutzfeldt-Jakob disease. Nature *352*:340–342, 1991.
176. Parchi, P., Castellani, R., Cortelli, P., et al.: Regional distribution of protease-resistant prion protein in fatal familial insomnia. Ann. Neurol. *38*:21–29, 1995.
177. Parchi, P., Chen, S. G., Brown, P., et al.: Different patterns of truncated prion protein fragments correlate with distinct phenotypes in P102L Gerstmann-Sträussler-Scheinker disease. Proc. Natl. Acad. Sci. U. S. A. *95*:8322–8327, 1998.
178. Parchi, P., Giese, A., Capellari, S., et al.: Classification of sporadic Creutzfeldt-Jakob disease based on molecular and phenotypic analysis of 300 subjects. Ann. Neurol. *46*:224–33, 1999.
179. Peretz, D., Williamson, R. A., Kaneko, K., et al.: Antibodies inhibit prion propagation and clear cell cultures of prion infectivity. Nature *412*:739–743, 2001.
180. Perrier, V., Wallace, A. C., Kaneko, K., et al.: Mimicking dominant negative inhibition of prion replication through structure-based drug design. Proc. Natl. Acad. Sci. U. S. A. *97*:6073–6078, 2000.
181. Prusiner, S. B.: Novel proteinaceous infectious particles cause scrapie. Science *216*:136–144, 1982.
182. Prusiner, S. B.: Molecular biology and genetics of neurodegenerative diseases caused by prions. Adv. Virus Res. *41*:241–280, 1992.
183. Prusiner, S. B.: Molecular biology and pathogenesis of prion diseases. Trends Biochem. Sci. *21*:482–487, 1996.
184. Prusiner, S. B.: Prion diseases and the BSE crisis. Science *278*:245–251, 1997.
185. Prusiner, S. B.: Shattuck lecture—neurodegenerative diseases and prions. N. Engl. J. Med. *344*:1516–1526, 2001.
186. Prusiner, S. B., Gajdusek, C., and Alpers, M. P.: Kuru with incubation periods exceeding two decades. Ann. Neurol. *12*:1–9, 1982.
187. Prusiner, S. B., Groth, D. F., Bolton, D. C., et al.: Purification and structural studies of a major scrapie prion protein. Cell *38*:127–134, 1984.
188. Prusiner, S. B., Groth, D., Serban, A., et al.: Ablation of the prion protein (PrP) gene in mice prevents scrapie and facilitates production of anti-PrP antibodies. Proc. Natl. Acad. Sci. U. S. A. *90*:10608–10612, 1993.
189. Prusiner, S. B., and Scott, M. R.: Genetics of prions. Annu. Rev. Genet. *31*:139–175, 1997.
190. Race, R., Oldstone, M., and Chesebro, B.: Entry versus blockade of brain infection following oral or intraperitoneal scrapie administration: Role of prion protein expression in peripheral nerves and spleen. J. Virol. *74*:828–833, 2000.
191. Race, R., Raines, A., Raymond, G. J., et al.: Long-term subclinical carrier state precedes scrapie replication and adaptation in a resistant species: Analogies to bovine spongiform encephalopathy and variant Creutzfeldt-Jakob disease in humans. J. Virol. *75*:10106–10112, 2001.
192. Raymond, G. J., Hope, J., Kocisko, D. A., et al.: Molecular assessment of the potential transmissibilities of BSE and scrapie to humans. Nature *388*:285–288, 1997.
193. Requena, J. R., Groth, D., Legname, G., et al.: Copper-catalyzed oxidation of the recombinant SHa(29-231) prion protein. Proc. Natl. Acad. Sci. U. S. A. *98*:7170–7175, 2001.

194. Richard, M., Biacabe, A. G., Perret-Liaudet, A., et al.: Protection of personnel and environment against Creutzfeldt-Jakob disease in pathology laboratories. Clin. Exp. Pathol. *47*:192–200, 1999.
195. Ricketts, M. N., Cashman, N. R., Stratton, E. E., and ElSaadany, S.: Is Creutzfeldt-Jakob disease transmitted in blood? Emerg. Infect. Dis. *3*:155–163, 1997.
196. Roberts, G. W., Lofthouse, R., Brown, R., et al.: Prion-protein immunoreactivity in human transmissible dementias. N. Engl. J. Med. *315*:1231–1233, 1986.
197. Roos, R., Gajdusek, D. C., and Gibbs, C. J., Jr.: The clinical characteristics of transmissible Creutzfeldt-Jakob disease. Brain *96*:1–20, 1973.
198. Rutala, W. A., and Weber, D. J.: Creutzfeldt-Jakob disease: Recommendations for disinfection and sterilization. Clin. Infect. Dis. *32*:1348–1356, 2001.
199. Safar, J., Cohen, F. E., and Prusiner, S. B.: Quantitative traits of prion strains are enciphered in the conformation of the prion protein. Arch. Virol. Suppl. *16*:227–235, 2000.
200. Safar, J., Wille, H., Itri, V., et al.: Eight prion strains have PrP(Sc) molecules with different conformations. Nat. Med. *4*:1157–1165, 1998.
201. Salazar, A. M., Masters, C. L., Gajdusek, D. C., et al.: Syndromes of amyotrophic lateral sclerosis and dementia: Relation to transmissible Creutzfeldt-Jakob disease. Ann. Neurol. *14*:17–26, 1983.
202. Schlenska, G. K., and Walter, G. F.: Temporal evolution of electroencephalographic abnormalities in Creutzfeldt-Jakob disease. J. Neurol. *236*:456–460, 1989.
203. Schreuder, B. E., van Keulen, L. J., Vromans, M. E., et al.: Preclinical test for prion diseases. Nature *381*:563, 1996.
204. Shaked, Y., Rosenmann, H., Hijazi, N., et al.: Copper binding to the PrP isoforms: A putative marker of their conformation and function. J. Virol. *75*:7872–7874, 2001.
205. Shlomchik, M. J., Radebold, K., Duclos, N., et al.: Neuroinvasion by a Creutzfeldt-Jakob disease agent in the absence of B cells and follicular dendritic cells. Proc. Natl. Acad. Sci. U. S. A. *98*:9289–9294, 2001.
206. Sigurdsson, B.: Rida, a chronic encephalitis of sheep, with general remarks on infections which develop slowly and some of their special characteristics. Br. Vet. J. *110*:341–354, 1954.
207. Sparkes, R. S., Simon, M., Cohn, V. H., et al.: Assignment of the human and mouse prion protein genes to homologous chromosomes. Proc. Natl. Acad. Sci. U. S. A. *83*:7358–7362, 1986.
208. Spudich, S., Mastrianni, J. A., Wrensch, M., et al.: Complete penetrance of Creutzfeldt-Jakob disease in Libyan Jews carrying the E200K mutation in the prion protein gene. Mol. Med. *1*:607–613, 1995.
209. Stahl, N., Baldwin, M. A., Burlingame, A. L., and Prusiner, S. B.: Identification of glycoinositol phospholipid linked and truncated forms of the scrapie prion protein. Biochemistry *29*:8879–8884, 1990.
210. Stahl, N., Borchelt, D. R., Hsiao, K., and Prusiner, S. B.: Scrapie prion protein contains a phosphatidylinositol glycolipid. Cell *51*:229–240, 1987.
211. Stahl, N., Borchelt, D. R, and Prusiner, S. B.: Differential release of cellular and scrapie prion proteins from cellular membranes by phosphatidylinositol-specific phospholipase C. Biochemistry *29*:5405–5412, 1990.
212. Steinhoff, B. J., Racker, S., Herrendorf, G., et al.: Accuracy and reliability of periodic sharp wave complexes in Creutzfeldt-Jakob disease. Arch. Neurol. *53*:162–166, 1996.
213. Supattapone, S., Wille, H., Uyechi, L., et al.: Branched polyamines cure prion-infected neuroblastoma cells. J. Virol. *75*:3453–3461, 2001.
214. Tateishi, J., Brown, P., Kitamoto, T., et al.: First experimental transmission of fatal familial insomnia. Nature *376*:434–435, 1995.
215. Tateishi, J., Tashima, T., and Kitamoto, T.: Practical methods for chemical inactivation of Creutzfeldt-Jakob disease pathogen. Microbiol. Immunol. *35*:163–166, 1991.
216. Taylor, D. M., Fernie, K., McConnell, I., et al.: Solvent extraction as an adjunct to rendering: The effect on BSE and scrapie agents of hot solvents followed by dry heat and steam. Vet. Rec. *143*:6–9, 1998.
217. Telling, G. C., Scott, M., Hsiao, K. K., et al.: Transmission of Creutzfeldt-Jakob disease from humans to transgenic mice expressing chimeric human-mouse prion protein. Proc. Natl. Acad. Sci. U. S. A. *91*:9936–9940, 1994.
218. Telling, G. C., Scott, M., Mastrianni, J., et al.: Prion propagation in mice expressing human and chimeric PrP transgenes implicates the interaction of cellular PrP with another protein. Cell *83*:79–90, 1995.
219. Turner, M.: The risk of transmission of nvCJD by blood transfusion and the potential benefits of leucodepletion. Transfus. Sci. *19*:331–332, 1998.
220. van Keulen, L. J., Schreuder, B. E., Meloen, R. H., et al.: Immunohistochemical detection and localization of prion protein in brain tissue of sheep with natural scrapie. Vet. Pathol. *32*:299–308, 1995.
221. van Keulen, L. J., Schreuder, B. E., Meloen, R. H., et al.: Immunohistochemical detection of prion protein in lymphoid tissues of sheep with natural scrapie. J. Clin. Microbiol. *34*:1228–1231, 1996.
222. Verity, C. M., Nicoll, A., Will, R. G., et al.: Variant Creutzfeldt-Jakob disease in UK children: A national surveillance study. Lancet *356*:1224–1227, 2000.
223. Wadsworth, J. D., Hill, A. F., Joiner, S., et al.: Strain-specific prion-protein conformation determined by metal ions. Nat. Cell. Biol. *1*:55–59, 1999.
224. Wadsworth, J. D., Joiner, S., Hill, A. F., et al.: Tissue distribution of protease resistant prion protein in variant Creutzfeldt-Jakob disease using a highly sensitive immunoblotting assay. Lancet *358*:171–180, 2001.
225. Walker, L. C., and LeVine, H.: The cerebral proteopathies: Neurodegenerative disorders of protein conformation and assembly. Mol. Neurobiol. *21*:83–95, 2000.
226. Weber, T., Otto, M., Bodemer, M., and Zerr, I.: Diagnosis of Creutzfeldt-Jakob disease and related human spongiform encephalopathies. Biomed. Pharmacol. *51*:381–387, 1997.
227. Weber, T., Tumani, H., Holdorff, B., et al.: Transmission of Creutzfeldt-Jakob disease by handling of dura mater. Lancet *341*:123–124, 1993.
228. Wells, G. A., Hawkins, S. A., Green, R. B., et al.: Preliminary observations on the pathogenesis of experimental bovine spongiform encephalopathy (BSE): An update. Vet. Rec. *142*:103–106, 1998.
229. Westaway, D., Carlson, G. A., and Prusiner, S. B.: On safari with PrP: Prion diseases of animals. Trends Microbiol. *3*:141–147, 1995.
230. Wilesmith, J. W.: Bovine spongiform encephalopathy. Vet. Rec. *122*:614, 1988.
231. Will, R. G., Cousens, S. N., and Farrington, C. P.: Deaths from variant Creutzfeldt-Jakob disease. Lancet *353*:979, 1999.
232. Will, R. G., Ironside, J. W., Zeidler, M., et al.: A new variant of Creutzfeldt-Jakob disease in the UK. Lancet *347*:921–925, 1996.
233. Will, R. G., and Kimberlin, R. H.: Creutzfeldt-Jakob disease and the risk from blood or blood products. Vox Sang. *75*:178–180, 1998.
234. Will, R. G., Zeidler, M., Stewart, G. E., et al.: Diagnosis of new variant Creutzfeldt-Jakob disease. Ann. Neurol. *47*:575–582, 2000.
235. Windl, O., Dempster, M., Estibeiro, J. P., et al.: Genetic basis of Creutzfeldt-Jakob disease in the United Kingdom: A systematic analysis of predisposing mutations and allelic variation in the PRNP gene. Hum. Genet. *98*:259–264, 1996.
236. Wine, J. J.: The genesis of cystic fibrosis lung disease. J. Clin. Invest. *103*:309–312, 1999.
237. Wong, B. S., Chen, S. G., Colucci, M., et al.: Aberrant metal binding by prion protein in human prion disease. J. Neurochem. *78*:1400–1408, 2001.
238. Woolhouse, M. E., and Anderson, R. M.: Understanding the epidemiology of BSE. Trends Microbiol. *5*:421–424, 1997.
239. Zeidler, M., Johnstone, E. C., Bamber, R. W., et al.: New variant Creutzfeldt-Jakob disease: Psychiatric features. Lancet *350*:908–910, 1997.
240. Zerr, I., Bodemer, M., Gefeller, O., et al.: Detection of 14-3-3 protein in the cerebrospinal fluid supports the diagnosis of Creutzfeldt-Jakob disease. Ann. Neurol. *43*:32–40, 1998.
241. Zerr, I., Bodemer, M., Otto, M., et al.: Diagnosis of Creutzfeldt-Jakob disease by two-dimensional gel electrophoresis of cerebrospinal fluid. Lancet *348*:846–849, 1996.
242. Zerr, I., Pocchiari, M., Collins, S., et al.: Analysis of EEG and CSF 14-3-3 proteins as aids to the diagnosis of Creutzfeldt-Jakob disease. Neurology *55*:811–815, 2000.

ADENOVIRIDAE

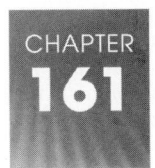

CHAPTER 161 Adenoviruses

JAMES D. CHERRY

Adenoviruses, which are responsible for a varied array of illnesses in children,* are associated most commonly with respiratory illness and gastroenteritis, but cardiac, neurologic, cutaneous, urinary, and lymphatic manifestations also occur frequently. Although many of the clinical manifestations of adenoviral infections are distinctive, the specific viral etiologic agent rarely is recognized by physicians.

Adenoviruses first were noted in explant cultures of human adenoid tissue; this finding, plus the observation of their apparent general affinity for lymphatic tissue, led to their name.[112, 115, 131, 359]

History

The first adenoviral strains were not isolated until 1953, when tissue culture techniques became available, although epidemic disease caused by adenoviruses had been observed throughout the first half of that century. Epidemic keratoconjunctivitis first was noted and reported in Austria by several physicians in 1889.[2, 135, 346, 367, 390] Major outbreaks of epidemic keratoconjunctivitis were reported in Bombay in 1901, in Madras in 1920 and 1928, in Hawaii in 1941, and on the West Coast of the United States in 1942.[177, 191, 192, 234, 448]

Epidemics of illness such as pharyngoconjunctival fever have been observed throughout this century. Béal[16] in 1907 was the first to report the syndrome; in the 1920s, epidemics associated with swimming in public pools and in lakes were noted in Germany and the United States.[12, 317] Initial studies by Rowe and colleagues[359] revealed cytopathic changes in explant tissue cultures of human adenoids that had been removed surgically. Fluid from these cultures caused distinctive cytopathologic changes in other tissue cultures, and antiserum prepared in hyperimmunized rabbits neutralized the effect. In 1954, Hilleman and Werner[189] isolated similar cytopathic agents from the throat washings of military recruits with febrile acute respiratory disease. Shortly thereafter, epidemic keratoconjunctivitis and pharyngoconjunctival fever were seen to be illnesses of adenoviral etiology.[89, 92–94, 213]

Initially, adenoviruses were known by the following names: adenoid degeneration (AD) agent because of its recovery in human adenoid tissue explants[359]; respiratory illness patient number 67 (RI-67) agent, which was recovered from a military recruit with primary atypical pneumonia during an epidemic of acute respiratory disease[188, 189]; adenoidal-pharyngeal-conjunctival (APC) agent[202]; and acute respiratory disease (ARD) agent.[72] In 1956, early investigators in the field selected the term *adenovirus* for the new group of viruses. The name suggested the characteristic involvement of lymphadenoid tissue, as well as the tissue from which the organism was first isolated.[112]

Because of considerable morbidity and major economic considerations relating to adenoviral epidemic respiratory disease in military recruits, the development of vaccines received attention early. Initially, inactivated vaccines were produced, and they achieved some degree of success.[161, 187, 249] Later, live viral preparations grown in diploid human fibroblast tissue culture became available and proved quite successful in control of specific adenoviral infections in the military services.[103, 104, 153, 249, 354, 382, 406–409]

In 1975, enteric adenoviruses (adenovirus types 40 and 41) first were reported.[123, 369, 436] They were demonstrated by electron microscopy and subsequently were shown to be a significant cause of diarrhea in children.[39, 68, 240, 282, 337, 405, 416, 419]

Properties of the Virus

CLASSIFICATION

Adenoviruses that infect humans are placed in the family *Adenoviridae* and the genus *Mastadenovirus*.[120, 195, 275, 371] At present, 49 immunologically distinct adenoviral types have been recovered from humans.* Additional adenoviral types have been isolated from monkeys, cattle, dogs, mice, and chickens.[179, 181–183] Mammalian adenoviruses have a common generic antigen that can be identified by complement fixation and enzyme-linked immunosorbent assay (ELISA).[215, 327, 351, 438] Individual serotypes are identified by neutralization.[167, 168, 232]

Adenoviruses originally were subclassified on the basis of four hemagglutination patterns with rat and rhesus monkey red blood cells.[355] This subclassification is updated in Table 161–1. In 1962, researchers found that adenovirus type 12 could cause tumors in hamsters, and soon thereafter, investigators realized that adenoviruses also could be classified by their oncogenic potential in rodents.[200, 411] Grouping by oncogenic potential was similar, with few exceptions, to grouping by hemagglutination properties: hemagglutination group I organisms had moderate oncogenic potential, group II and group III organisms had low or no potential, and group IV organisms had high oncogenic potential.[145, 196, 207]

*See references 1, 39, 41, 62, 111, 131, 197, 361, 383, 419.

*See references 97, 98, 120, 180–183, 185, 186, 197, 230, 368, 431, 433, 439.

TABLE 161–1 ■ SEPARATION OF HUMAN ADENOVIRUSES INTO SUBGROUPS BY ABILITY TO AGGLUTINATE RHESUS MONKEY AND RAT ERYTHROCYTES

Subgroup	Characteristic	Type
I	Complete agglutination of monkey erythrocytes	3, 7, 11, 14, 16, 21, 34, 35
II	Complete agglutination of rat erythrocytes	8–10, 13, 15, 17, 19, 20, 22–30, 32, 33, 36–39, 42–49
III	Partial agglutination of rat erythrocytes	1, 2, 4–6, 40, 41
IV	No or little agglutination of monkey or rat erythrocytes	12, 18, 31

Data from references 179, 185, 190, 191, 221, 230, 249, 306, 307, 368, 440.

Adenoviruses also have been subclassified (A to F) on the basis of the percentage of guanine plus cytosine in their DNA and other biochemical and biophysical criteria[185, 230, 334, 368, 430–432] (Table 161–2). In general, subgroup A organisms are the same as hemagglutination group IV; subgroup B, the same as hemagglutination group I; subgroups C, E, and F, the same as hemagglutination group III; and subgroup D, the same as hemagglutination group II. Restriction enzyme analysis has resulted in genome typing of specific adenoviral serologic types.[255] In particular, numerous genotypes of adenovirus type 7 have been identified, and the severity of disease may relate to genotype.

PHYSICAL PROPERTIES

Adenoviruses are nonenveloped DNA viruses 65 to 80 nm in diameter.[120, 145, 195, 196, 207, 237, 275] The virion consists of a protein capsid composed of 252 capsomeres and a nucleoprotein core that contains the DNA viral genome and two to four internal proteins.[340] The virion is roughly spherical in the form of an icosahedron; each of the 20 sides is an equilateral triangle, with the vertices of each converging in groups of 5 and resulting in 12 pentagonal vertices.[39, 131, 195] Each vertex capsomere contacts five other capsomeres and is designated a penton. Each penton contains a base plate and a rodlike projection, the fiber. The virion has 240 nonvertex capsomeres that occur in groups of 6 and are known as hexons.[237, 307, 418] Hexons contain the generic complement-fixing antigen.[131] Each capsomere has a diameter of 8 nm and a central hole 2 to 3 nm in diameter.[443] The capsomeres constitute 87 percent of the dry weight of the virion.

The central core of the virion, which accounts for 12 to 14 percent of its dry weight, is composed of linear double-stranded DNA (molecular mass, 23.85×10^6 d for adenovirus type 2) and two to four basic proteins.[136, 196, 443]

Adenoviruses are highly stable in general.[100, 131, 143, 207, 251] They are resistant to lipid solvents and retain activity at pH ranging from 2 to 10.

At 24° C, maximal infectivity is maintained between pH 6 and 9.5. Adenoviruses are stable at room temperature for 2 weeks, at 36° C for 7 days, and for at least 70 days at 4° C. Infectivity is destroyed by heating to 56° C for 30 minutes. Sodium dodecyl sulfate (0.25%) inactivates virus by disruption of the capsid.[237]

TABLE 161–2 ■ GROUPING OF HUMAN ADENOVIRAL SEROTYPES BASED ON BIOCHEMICAL AND BIOPHYSICAL CRITERIA

Subgroup	Adenovirus Type(s)	Location and Manifestations of Infection
A	12, 18, 31	Gastrointestinal; may cause disease in children
B:1	3, 7, 16, 21	Respiratory, eye, and gastrointestinal symptomatic infections
B:2	11, 14, 34, 35	Urinary and respiratory; symptomatic urinary tract infections (particularly in immunosuppressed patients) and symptomatic respiratory infections
C	1, 2, 5, 6	Respiratory and gastrointestinal; symptomatic respiratory infections and hepatitis in immunosuppressed patients
D	8–10, 13, 15, 17, 19, 20, 22–30, 32, 33, 36–39, 42–49	Eye and gastrointestinal; symptomatic eye infections, gastrointestinal infections in HIV-infected patients
E	4	Symptomatic eye and respiratory infections
F	40, 41	Symptomatic gastrointestinal infections

Data from references 185, 196, 230, 249, 334, 368, 404, 431.

ANTIGENIC COMPOSITION

The antigenic determinants of adenoviruses are contained on the protein structural subunits (hexons, pentons, and fibers).[418] The hexon antigen (alpha component) carries the generic antigenic component that is common to all mammalian adenoviruses and is measured by complement fixation or ELISA. Another hexon antigen (epsilon component) reacts with neutralizing antibodies lacking hemagglutination-inhibiting activity. The antigen related to viral fiber also induces type-specific neutralizing antibody for some adenoviral types. Minor antigens are related to the pentons. One of them (the cell-detaching factor) causes rounding and clumping of tissue culture cells.

Gerna and associates,[142] using the immunoperoxidase antibody technique, found that the early antigens of all serotypes belonging to one group (see Table 161–1) react strongly with all type-specific immune sera of the same group.

TISSUE CULTURE GROWTH

Although adenoviruses can be grown in a wide variety of cells of human epithelial origin, primary or diploid cultures of human embryonic kidney are preferable for the recovery of agents from clinical specimens.[251] Continuous cell lines such as HeLa and HEp-2 also are quite sensitive.[176, 207, 360] Adenoviruses will grow in monkey kidney tissue culture, but evolution of the cytopathic effect is considerably slower than that occurring in cells of human origin. In addition, the cytopathic effect is more variable in monkey kidney tissue culture, and many isolates will be missed.

Enteric adenoviruses have been detected in human feces by electron microscopy.* These enteric adenoviruses, identified as types 40 and 41, usually do not grow in standard tissue culture systems. Both viral types will grow in Graham 293 cells (a human embryonic kidney cell line transformed

*See references 39, 82, 97, 215, 229, 345, 350, 416, 431, 438.

by adenovirus type 5); type 40 also will grow in tertiary monkey kidney cells, and some strains of type 41 will grow in HEp-2, Chang conjunctiva cells, and tertiary cynomolgus cells.[400, 433] Grabow and associates[154] noted that the PLC/PRG/5 cell line was 100 times more sensitive to a laboratory strain of adenovirus type 41 and 10 times more sensitive to a laboratory strain of adenovirus type 40 than Graham 293 cells were.

Specimens for viral culture may be obtained from the eye, pharynx, blood, lungs, pleural and pericardial fluids, liver, stool, intestinal epithelium, lymph nodes, cerebrospinal fluid (CSF), brain, urine, and renal tissue. For best isolation rates, clinical specimens should be inoculated in cell culture within 6 hours of collection. Tissue culture tubes are incubated best at 37° C, and rolling offers no advantage over stationary incubation.[251] Although the cytopathic effect has considerable variability, the most consistent finding is marked rounding and clumping of cells, often in grapelike clusters.[340, 343] Cytopathic effect may be noted as early as 1 to 2 days after inoculation, but it may be delayed as long as 4 weeks. Use of the shell viral technique, in which infected cells in a specimen are centrifuged onto HEp-2 tissue culture cells, yields positive cultures in 1 to 2 days.[113] The cytopathic effect characteristically is followed by detachment of the entire cell sheet from the glass of the tissue culture tube within 2 to 4 days.[158, 177, 328, 357, 360]

VIRUS MULTIPLICATION

Initial attachment of adenoviruses to cells is relatively slow, with up to 6 hours required.[90, 144, 207] The fiber protein of the virus mediates attachment to the cellular receptor.[372] An important adenovirus receptor is the coxsackievirus and adenovirus receptor (CAR) protein. It is a high-affinity receptor for all adenoviral subgroups except subgroup B. Penetration into the host cell occurs rapidly, either by phagocytosis or by direct entry through the plasma membrane.[207, 259] The eclipse period with adenoviruses varies from 11 to 21 hours, depending on the serotype.[144, 207] During eclipse, viral DNA uncoating requires approximately 2 hours when determined biochemically.[207] After uncoating, the viral DNA rapidly enters the nucleus of the cell and dissociates from its internal protein.[90, 145, 259] After the eclipse period, viral DNA accumulates, often doubling the content of the infected cell and becoming a part of the typical inclusion bodies of the infected cells.[145]

Characteristic cytopathic changes in tissue culture, as demonstrated by light microscopy of hematoxylin and eosin–stained material or by electron microscopy, appear as early as 8 to 24 hours after infection occurs.[35, 37, 167] Two types of intranuclear alterations may be seen. In the first, early, small, discrete eosinophilic inclusions are observed. They gradually enlarge, become more prominent, and then form a large crystalline central mass surrounded by a clear zone or halo.[35, 151] This type of early cytopathic effect appears to occur in cells that contain only small amounts of infectious virus.[36] The second type of intranuclear alteration, which generally is a later occurrence, consists of large basophilic intranuclear inclusions.[35] Occasionally, giant forms measuring greater than 14 mm across are noted.[35] These mature inclusions may expand the nucleus of the cell greatly so that the cell's DNA content is 10 times higher than that of an uninfected cell. They contain a large amount of viral antigen and infective virus. Cytopathic changes vary considerably with the different adenoviral serotypes.[37, 237]

In general, virus remains within the nucleus of intact, infected cells, with less than 1 percent of the total virus content of a culture being free within the extracellular fluid at any one time.[237]

ANIMAL SUSCEPTIBILITY

Human adenoviruses usually do not produce clinical illness in laboratory animals, although infections with several different serotypes have occurred in selected animals.[207] When adenoviral strains were administered intranasally to young, "pathogen-free," colostrum-deprived pigs or 1-month-old cotton rats, pneumonia developed in the animals, and intranuclear inclusions were observed microscopically in their lungs.[207, 316] An adenovirus type 5 strain was given intravenously to a rabbit, and the virus was recovered from the animal's spleen when removed 2 months later. Many adenoviral strains will propagate in a variety of different animal tissue cultures. In addition, in some cultures, marked cytopathic effects are observed, but little infectious virus is produced.

ADENO-ASSOCIATED VIRUSES

Adeno-associated viruses are a group of small, defective, single-stranded, DNA-containing, virus-like particles that replicate in tissue culture only in the presence of adenoviruses.[30, 90, 131, 207, 228, 383] Four serologic types have been identified; however, only types 2 and 3 have been recovered from humans.[131, 237] These agents have been isolated from throat and anal swab specimens of children from whom adenoviral strains also were isolated.[30] Approximately 30 percent of children have complement-fixing antibody to adeno-associated virus types 2 and 3; most of these children have had evidence of adenoviral infection as well.[31] Neutralizing antibody to adeno-associated virus types 2 and 3 is noted in the sera of 60 to 80 percent of children 8 to 14 years of age.[322] The specific relevance of adeno-associated viruses is unknown.

Epidemiology

GENERAL PREVALENCE

Adenoviral infections account for 2 to 5 percent of all respiratory illnesses.[51, 69, 75, 129, 130, 329] In children, adenoviruses are estimated to be responsible for 2 to 24 percent of respiratory viral illnesses,[41, 51, 55, 57, 194, 257, 267] and they are implicated in 5 to 11 percent of upper respiratory tract infections, 4 to 10 percent of cases of pharyngitis, 3 to 9 percent of cases of croup, 5 to 11 percent of cases of bronchitis, 2 to 10 percent of cases of bronchiolitis, and 4 to 10 percent of cases of pneumonia.[41, 55–57, 132, 293, 324] Enteric adenoviral infections are the cause of 5 to 15 percent of acute diarrheal illnesses in children.[68, 82, 254, 282, 337, 345, 416, 419] Specific categories of illness caused by adenoviruses vary with respect to viral serotype, patient age, socioeconomic status, and environmental conditions.[53, 76, 164, 175, 216, 451] Adenoviruses have a predilection for infants and children younger than 5 years of age who spend portions of their days in closed environments, such as daycare centers, orphanages, and other institutions.[20, 23, 53, 169, 258, 429] Epidemics of disease caused by adenoviral infection have been associated with swimming pools, daycare centers, resident schools, certain industries, hospitals, physicians' offices, and young recruits in early basic military training.* Adenoviruses are recovered commonly from

*See references 64, 86, 213, 214, 236, 252, 269, 315, 325, 335, 349, 380, 414, 453.

children in tropical countries and in situations characterized by crowding, such as lower socioeconomic settings.[53, 57, 70, 216, 451]

AGE INCIDENCE AND PREVALENCE

Although adenoviral infections occur in all age groups, the incidence of infection generally is related inversely to age.[76, 237] More than 90 percent of newborn infants have transplacentally acquired complement-fixing adenoviral serum antibody.[298, 391] Most infants have neutralizing antibody to one or more of the common adenoviral types, which appears to be protective during the first 6 months of life. When adenoviral infection does occur in a neonate, it is often severe and occasionally fatal.[7, 456] By the sixth month of life, only 14 percent of infants have demonstrable adenoviral complement-fixing antibody. By the time children reach 1 year of age, complement-fixing adenoviral antibody is observed in 44 to 50 percent of the sera tested.[202, 301]

The incidence of adenoviral infection peaks in infants and children between 6 months and 5 years of age.[280, 329] By the time that they are 5 years of age, 70 to 80 percent of children have neutralizing antibody to adenovirus types 1 and 2, and 50 percent have antibody to adenovirus type 5.[99, 129, 202, 210, 323, 329, 421]

Adenoviral infections also occur commonly in grade-school and junior-high-school children, but the incidence diminishes in high-school adolescents. Adenoviral infections occur in only 1 to 2 percent of college students, and they are noted infrequently in civilian adults.[114, 116, 117, 157, 393] Approximately 1 percent of adults with respiratory infectious illness will have adenoviral infection; in hospitalized adults, the incidence is approximately 4 percent.[157] The most common adenoviral respiratory infections in children are caused by types 1, 2, 3, and 5.[20, 421, 427, 429] Types 6 and 7 are the next most frequent isolates associated with childhood respiratory infection. Adenovirus types 40 and 41 are the most common causes of diarrhea.[68, 239, 254]

MILITARY RECRUITS

Epidemic adenoviral disease occurs commonly in military recruits, with virtually all illness developing during the first 8 weeks of basic training.[127, 274, 423, 424] The attack rate has varied between 40 and 90 percent.[127, 158, 266, 422] Adenoviruses account for 30 to 70 percent of acute respiratory disease, 67 percent of common cold-like illnesses, 62 to 77 percent of cases of acute febrile pharyngitis and tonsillitis, 67 percent of cases of bronchitis, and 24 percent of cases of pneumonia.[26, 128] Some adenoviral infections are associated with minimal or no symptoms.[128, 158]

GEOGRAPHIC DISTRIBUTION

Adenoviral infections have been noted throughout the world.* Epidemic, endemic, and sporadic infections all occur.

SEASONAL PATTERNS

Sporadic infections with adenoviruses occur throughout the year.[129, 133, 150, 190, 201, 257, 267, 286, 293] Epidemic adenoviral respiratory disease is most common in the winter, spring, and early summer.* Seasonal patterns depend on serotypes, population groups, and exposure. Epidemics of disease in military recruits commonly associated with adenovirus types 4 and 7 occur most frequently in the winter and spring.[32, 127, 128, 187] Pharyngoconjunctival fever epidemics have been noted most commonly in the summer months in school-age children in association with summer camps or swimming pools.[269, 426, 443] No seasonal pattern has been identified for adenoviral gastroenteritis.[82, 229, 350, 416]

HOST AND SOCIAL FACTORS

The overall incidence of adenoviral illnesses is higher in males.[76, 177] In a study involving 3313 adenovirus isolates, the male-female ratio was 1.3:1.[76]

Susceptibility to adenoviral infection apparently does not vary by race. More severe disease has been noted in infants of native and Indian populations in New Zealand and Canada.[19, 152] However, the relationship of these findings to socioeconomic conditions was not identified initially.

The incidence of adenoviral infection is greatest in lower socioeconomic population groups.[216] Spread of infection has been observed in daycare centers, schools, children's homes, hospitals, clinics, physicians' offices, and certain industrial settings.† Acute, overwhelming illness, including bronchiolitis and pneumonia with severe pulmonary residua, has been reported in neonates, small infants, and occasionally, adults.[7, 175, 253] Adenoviral infections are a significant problem in immunocompromised hosts; when they occur, they frequently are severe and occasionally are fatal.‡

SPREAD OF INFECTION

Adenoviruses frequently are isolated from the conjunctiva, throat, and stool. Despite the ease of virus isolation, the effectiveness of spread of infection in the general population varies considerably.[57] Adenovirus types 1, 2, 3, 5, and 7 are effective spreaders; however, they are not as highly contagious as are varicella, measles, and influenza viruses.[56, 57] Close contact appears to be necessary for infection to spread from one person to another.[391] Illness does not spread rapidly in the usual school setting but does spread dramatically in closed environments.[23, 56, 169, 201] Although adenovirus type 4 spreads less effectively in the general population, spread is rapid in nonimmune military recruits who live in close contact with each other.[65] In an outbreak of adenovirus type 7 in a children's home, 84 percent of the residents were shown to be infected.

Transmission of virus occurs by droplets reaching the conjunctiva, nose, or throat or, alternatively, by the fecal-oral route. In volunteer studies, adenoviruses have been shown to spread by small-droplet aerosols and to a lesser degree by large droplets.[9, 77, 78] Adenovirus type 4 has been recovered from room air and cough samples of patients with the virus in their throats.[10]

In epidemics of pharyngoconjunctival fever, the virus appears to spread from contaminated swimming pool water to the eyes of recipients. Epidemics of keratoconjunctivitis have occurred as a result of contact with contaminated ophthalmic instruments and fingers.[14, 92, 188, 213, 214, 223, 236, 286, 385]

*See references 55, 59, 85, 118, 126, 131, 134, 136, 152, 175, 184, 190, 205, 210, 212, 216, 223, 228, 235–237, 241, 244, 286, 287, 321, 373, 376, 386, 390, 391, 395, 401, 414, 420–423, 426, 443, 450, 451.

*See references 32, 38, 131, 169, 193, 210, 241, 321, 339, 421, 424.

†See references 20, 23, 25, 64, 164, 167, 214, 315, 325, 337, 380, 419, 453.

‡See references 50, 52, 84, 91, 124, 159, 260, 278, 311, 384, 456.

In daycare centers, orphanages, and the military, transmission probably occurs most commonly through small-droplet aerosols in crowded quarters.[335] An alternative in children is the fecal-oral route. Enteric adenoviruses have been identified in fecal specimens for approximately 8 days after the onset of gastroenteritis.[229]

Family members may excrete adenoviruses in their feces intermittently for prolonged periods after initial infection.[41, 129] In one study, 20 percent of persons excreted adenoviruses in stool for longer than 3 months. Intrahousehold spread appears to continue as long as susceptible family members are present.[129] Infants born into households in which household members are adenoviral fecal excreters often become infected, presumably through the fecal-oral route. In general, 50 percent of susceptible household members will experience infection, although the rate varies inversely with age and also depends on the serotype of adenovirus. Reinfection with specific adenoviral serotypes occurs, but most are asymptomatic or associated with only minimal illness.

Nosocomial spread of both respiratory and enteric adenoviruses is a common occurrence and has been the cause of fatal illnesses in infants and immunocompromised patients.[3, 101, 122, 238, 380, 456]

Pathogenesis and Pathology

Adenoviral infections usually are acute and self-limited, and, therefore, opportunities to study the pathogenesis and pathologic process have been infrequent. Study of the pathologic mechanisms has been performed in human volunteers, tissue and organ culture systems, and recent murine model systems and by examination of specimens from persons dying of adenoviral disease.

VIRAL INFECTION

In general, the characteristics of adenoviral infection depend on the host and the serotype of the agent.* In most respiratory illnesses, initial viral infection occurs in the respiratory tract and involves the mucous membranes of the nose, oropharynx, and conjunctiva. Adenoviral agents have been isolated from sputum and oral secretions from 2 days before the onset of clinical illness up to 8 days after the onset of symptoms. Deeper respiratory involvement of the trachea, pleurae, and lungs may result from initial small-particle aerosol, from progression of local infection, or perhaps as a result of viremia. Gastrointestinal infection in conjunction with respiratory infection also occurs early and probably is the result of swallowed virus. Stool isolates of respiratory viral types frequently are noted concomitantly with respiratory tract infection. However, in contrast to the upper respiratory infection, the virus may persist for a long time in the lower gastrointestinal tract. Infection with enteric adenoviral types is presumed to involve intestinal epithelial cells. In one fatal infection, adenoviral antigen was demonstrated in jejunal cells.[345, 437]

In experimental studies with aerosolized adenovirus type 4, recovery of virus from throat specimens occurred on day 5 or 6, progressed to a maximal concentration at day 11 or 12, and was seen uncommonly after day 20. Maximal recovery of adenovirus type 4 from anal specimens occurred on day 13 and continued for longer than 3 weeks. Adenovirus types 26 and 27 inoculated into the conjunctiva resulted in short-term isolation of virus from the eyes on days 3 to 7 and, less frequently, from the throat on day 4.[222] Viral isolation from the rectum was a common finding beginning at the end of the first week. Maximal fecal shedding occurred during the second and third weeks.

Adenoviruses may invade the bloodstream early in disease, as evidenced by the occurrence of maculopapular, morbilliform, or petechial exanthems (or any combination of such rashes), as well as by recovery of virus from multiple organs such as the brain, kidney, urinary bladder, lymphoid tissue, and liver and at postmortem examination.* The virus has been cultured from the mononuclear cells of heparinized blood.[6]

PATHOLOGY

Early pathologic changes are observed in the epithelium of the respiratory tract. The severity of adenoviral involvement varies with the different serotypes. In tracheal organ cultures, the growth of adenovirus type 7 was characterized by an initial focal cytopathologic effect at 100 hours that quickly progressed to involve the whole epithelium.[80] Frequently, the cilia of incision-bearing cells were noted to be intact. In contrast to the findings with adenovirus type 7, a type 12 strain resulted in only a mild cytopathologic effect on the organ culture system.[80]

Microscopic examination of autopsy material from patients dying of adenoviral pneumonia revealed a loss of cilia in the tracheal epithelium, proliferation of other respiratory epithelial cells, and the presence of intranuclear inclusions.[18, 25, 45, 58, 134, 441, 444, 446, 457] In severe pneumonia, total destruction with necrotizing bronchitis, bronchiolitis, and pneumonia is observed (Fig. 161–1). Mononuclear cellular infiltration is seen, and hyaline membranes and necrosis are present. Cilia and goblet cells are absent, and muscle fiber bundles and elastic fibers are dispersed. Frequently, epithelial cells have a characteristic appearance with adenoviral infection. These infected cells are enlarged grossly and lose nuclear membranes; the nuclear material has migrated into the cytoplasm.[336] Blood vessels show edema, filament separation of their walls, and occasionally, thrombosis.[457]

On histologic examination, adenoviral inclusions are characterized by small eosinophilic and larger basophilic intranuclear bodies.[18, 134, 298, 387]

Hepatic involvement in adenoviral infection has been reported frequently.[2, 10, 25, 52, 134, 336, 384] In addition to isolation of virus from the liver, focal areas of liver necrosis accompanied by characteristic hepatic intranuclear inclusions have been demonstrated.[2, 52, 456] Electron-microscopic examination has revealed adenoviral particles within the intranuclear inclusions.[2, 25, 336, 441, 456] Hematogenous spread to the central nervous system (CNS) has been observed.[376] Most patients with adenoviral CNS infection have had an associated pneumonia.[81, 376] In CNS disease, the brain is edematous and congested. On microscopic examination, a perivascular accumulation of lymphocytes is noted, along with gigantic nuclear inclusions in the cortical neurons. Viral particles within these nuclear inclusions have been observed by electron microscopy.[67]

In epidemic keratoconjunctivitis caused by adenovirus type 8, the walls of the conjunctival vessels are damaged, and aneurysms are present. The surrounding conjunctival connective tissue is edematous. The virus has been suggested to penetrate the cornea along nerves deep into the

*See references 25, 41, 45, 71, 147–149, 298, 336, 387, 436, 447.

*See references 6, 7, 25, 33, 45, 58, 152, 160, 163, 261, 271.

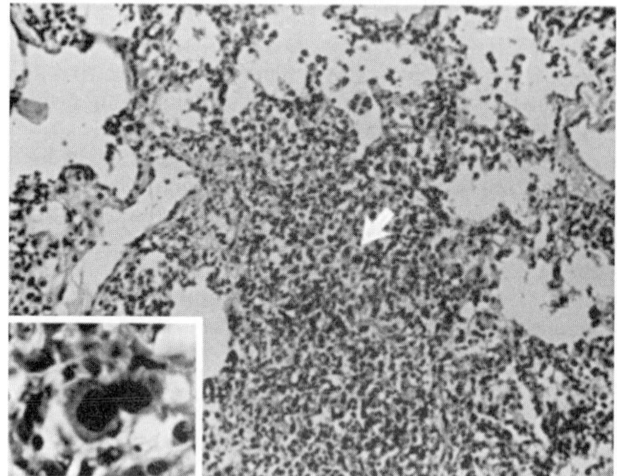

FIGURE 161–1 ■ The lung of a 17-month-old infant with adenoviral pneumonia. The infant died 10 days after the onset of illness, with no other contributing disease. The adenovirus isolated was not typed. A patchy pneumonia is present, and the *arrow* indicates two cells with nuclear inclusions. *Inset,* Two similar cells with typical adenoviral nuclear inclusions at higher magnification (hematoxylin and eosin staining, ×190; inset, ×770). (Courtesy of Dr. David D. Porter, Department of Pathology, David Geffen School of Medicine at UCLA.)

epithelial layers in a manner similar to that occurring in herpes simplex virus infection.[428]

Adenoviral strains have been isolated from and intranuclear inclusions have been demonstrated in renal tubular epithelium, lymph nodes, muscle, and gastrointestinal epithelium.[22, 52, 437, 454–456]

IMMUNOLOGIC EVENTS

The local response in adenoviral infection depends on the site of viral inoculation, the method of transmission, the viral serotype, the concentration of the inoculum, and the antibody status of the host. Three days after infection, when virus can be recovered from the nasopharynx, marked transudation of proteins from serum into the respiratory tract occurs, along with the production of secretory IgA antibody.[273] Approximately 7 days after the onset of illness, serum-neutralizing, hemagglutination-inhibiting, and complement-fixing antibodies appear.[90, 250] At the same time, the nasal secretions contain specific IgA and IgG antibody.[24] In general, neutralizing antibody is the most sensitive indicator of adenoviral infection, hemagglutination-inhibiting antibody is less sensitive, and complement-fixing antibody is the least sensitive.[236, 337] Antibody titers peak in 2 to 3 weeks; complement-fixing antibody declines in 2 to 3 months but may persist for up to a year.[90] Neutralizing antibody persists for a longer period and is measurable in many instances for periods of up to 10 years. Reinfection with the same adenoviral serotype is rare because of type-specific immunity.[21, 358]

Although alterations in leukocytes are not common findings, a decrease in lymphocytes has been observed before or at the onset of clinical illness and an increase in neutrophils early in the disease, followed by a decrease later. Neutropenia may develop in severe disseminated illness and is attributed to a direct toxic effect of virus on leukocytes, marrow reserves, or both.[102] The erythrocyte sedimentation rates of children have been normal or elevated to 55 mm/hr.[390, 391]

Studies by Ginsberg and associates[147–149] in murine adenoviral pneumonia model systems noted that tumor necrosis factor–α, interleukin-1, and interleukin-6 were elaborated during the first 2 to 3 days of infection. However, only tumor necrosis factor–α played an early role in the initial phase of pathogenesis. The second phase of the inflammatory response is caused by the infiltration of cytotoxic T cells.

Mistchenko and colleagues[281] studied cytokines and adenovirus-specific circulating immune complexes in 38 children with adenoviral infections. They placed the patients into three groups based on the severity of their respiratory illnesses: moderate illness, severe illness, and fatal illness. Serum interleukin-1 was not detected in children with moderate illness but was found in 7 of 12 with severe illness and in 13 of the 16 children who died. Tumor necrosis factor–α was frequently present in the sera of fatal cases, it was not present in the sera of moderately ill children, and it was present in the sera of only 2 of 12 patients with severe but nonfatal illness. Interleukin-8 was noted in all sera, but values were highest in children with fatal illness. Serum immune complexes (IgG containing) were found in 7 of the 16 children who died. Finally, patients with increased concentrations of interleukin-6, interleukin-8, and tumor necrosis factor–α were those with hypoperfusion, febrile peaks, seizures, and a manifestation of septic shock. Five of 10 children with severe or fatal illness had serum autoantibodies specific for smooth muscle.

Matsubara and associates[270] noted the participation of peripheral blood $CD8^+$ T cells and $HLA\text{-}DR^+$, $CD8^+$ T cells in children with adenoviral infection. One child with a severe adenoviral type 7 pneumonia had a marked increase in $HLA\text{-}DR^+$ $CD8^+$ T cells, serum levels of interferon-γ, and peripheral blood interferon-γ–producing T cells.

Clinical Manifestations

Adenoviral infections are exceedingly common events, and the spectrum of disease is quite broad (Table 161–3). As noted in Table 161–3, some specific adenoviral diseases exist; however, the overall majority of infections involve a variety of anatomically associated illnesses. In many instances, similar illnesses are caused by other respiratory viruses, and the clinical spectra of the various adenoviral serotypes frequently overlap. Certain specific adenoviral types do have clinical characteristics that facilitate etiologic diagnosis, however.

RESPIRATORY TRACT

Common Cold

Although adenoviruses frequently receive etiologic consideration in colds, they are, in fact, associated only rarely with this illness.[217] One report associated adenovirus with 3 percent of common colds in children,[329] and in another study, 6.4 percent of children with coryza had adenoviral isolates.[111] Respiratory tract infections with adenoviruses usually are associated with fever and, frequently, with some degree of pharyngitis; therefore, when strict clinical criteria are applied, they do not qualify as colds.[201, 393] Occasionally, adenoviruses, particularly types 1, 2, 3, 5, and 7, have been recovered from patients with typical colds.

Nasopharyngitis, Pharyngitis, and Tonsillitis

Adenoviral pharyngitis is an acute illness characterized by fever, sore throat, extensive exudative tonsillitis, and often, cervical adenopathy.[111, 217, 287, 383] In two studies involving

TABLE 161–3 ■ CLINICAL SPECTRUM OF ADENOVIRAL INFECTIONS

System/Organ	Illness Category	Epidemic Occurrence	Frequency	Adenoviral Type(s)
Respiratory	Common cold	No	Rare	1, 2, 3, 5, 7
	Nasopharyngitis, pharyngitis, and tonsillitis	Yes	Common	1,* 2,* 3,* 4, 5,* 7,* 7a, 14, 15, (21/H21+35)†
	Acute respiratory disease	Yes (in military recruits)	Very common	2, 3, 4,* 5, 7,* 8, 11, 14, 21
	Acute laryngotracheitis	No	Occasional	1, 2, 3, 5, 6, 7
	Acute bronchiolitis	No	Occasional	3, 7, 21
	Pneumonia (civilian population)	Yes	Common	1, 2, 3,* 4, 5, 7,* 7a, * 8, 11, 21,* (21/H21 + 35),† 35
	Atypical pneumonia in military recruits	Yes	Common	4,* 7,* 21
	Pertussis-like syndrome	No	Rare	1, 2, 3, 5, 12, 19
	Bronchiolitis obliterans	No	Rare	7i, 21
	Unilateral hyperlucent lung	No	Rare	7, 21
Eye	Acute follicular conjunctivitis	Yes	Common	1, 2, 3, 4, 6, 7, 9, 10, 11, 15, 16, 17, 19, 20, 22, 34, 37
	Pharyngoconjunctival fever	Yes	Common	1, 2,* 3,* 4,* 5, 6, 7,* 7a,* 8, 14,* 37
	Epidemic keratoconjunctivitis	Yes	Occasional	2, 3, 4, 5, 7, 8,* 10, 11, 13, 14, 15, 16, 17, 19, 23, 29, 37
Skin	Morbilliform and rubelliform exanthem	Rare	Occasional	3, 4, 7, 7a
	Roseola-like	No	Occasional	1, 2
	Stevens-Johnson syndrome	No	Rare	7
	Petechial exanthem	No	Rare	7
Genitourinary	Acute hemorrhagic cystitis	No	Rare	7, 11, 21,
	Nephritis	No	Rare	3, 4, 7a
	Orchitis	No	Rare	Unknown
	Oculogenital syndrome	Yes	Rare	19, 37
Gastrointestinal	Gastroenteritis	Yes	Common	1, 2, 3,* 5, 7,* 11, 12, 15, 17, 31,* 32, 33, 40,* 41*
	Mesenteric lymphadenitis	No	Rare	1, 2, 3, 5, 7
	Intussusception	No	Rare	1, 2, 3, 5, 6, 7
	Appendicitis	No	Rare	1, 2, 7
	Hepatitis	No	Rare	1, 2, 3, 5,* 7, (11+35/H11+35)†
Heart	Myocarditis	No	Rare	7, 7a, 21
	Pericarditis	No	Rare	7
Neurologic	Encephalitis and meningitis	No	Rare	1, 2, 3, 5, 6, 7, 11, 12, 32
Joint	Arthritis	No	Rare	7
Auditory	Deafness	No	Rare	3
Endocrine	Thyroiditis	No	Rare	Unknown

*Most common.
†Intermediate strain.

74 children with adenoviral pharyngitis, Ruuskanen and associates[361, 362] described the pharyngeal findings. Most commonly, only mild inflammation and redness were observed. When exudates were present, they found them to be thick and membranous, thin and follicular, or thin and spotty; most typical were follicular and spotty exudates. Associated symptoms include malaise, headache, myalgia, chills, and cough. In infants and preschool children, nasal congestion and discharge are noticeable and abdominal pain is a common complaint.[421] Children with adenoviral acute febrile pharyngitis also frequently have laryngotracheitis, bronchitis, or pneumonia.[451] The usual duration of illness varies from 5 to 7 days, although occasionally, symptoms persist well into the second week.[361]

Acute febrile pharyngitis is the most common adenoviral illness in children and is particularly important as an epidemic illness in closed environments.[23, 383, 391, 450] For example, in an epidemic in a children's home, 63 percent of the residents were infected with adenovirus type 7a.[169] Moffet and colleagues[287] noted that adenoviruses were the etiologic agents most commonly recovered from hospitalized preschool children with febrile exudative pharyngitis; 23 percent of the children studied had adenoviral infections. In a university student health service study, 2.4 percent of illnesses with acute febrile pharyngitis were caused by adenoviruses.[297] Adenoviruses account for 37 to 75 percent of nonstreptococcal pharyngitis in military recruits.

In children, 86 percent of cases of febrile pharyngitis are associated with adenovirus types 1, 2, 3, 5, and 7.[169, 201, 287]

On occasion, adenovirus types 7a, 9, 14, 15, and the intermediate strain 21/H21+35[186, 383, 391] also have been noted in association with pharyngitis. In military recruits, adenovirus types 4 and 7 are the main etiologic agents.

Acute Respiratory Disease

ARD is an epidemic disease that occurs predominantly in military recruit populations. This illness was studied extensively during World War II by the Commission on Acute Respiratory Diseases, and although individual cases were quite undifferentiated, the epidemiologic aspects of the outbreaks clearly indicated a specific etiologic agent.[72, 146, 383, 394, 414, 420] The disease is an acute, febrile respiratory illness of short duration with constitutional and localized respiratory symptoms.[139] After an incubation period of 5 to 7 days, fever (mean temperature, 39.5° C), pharyngitis, laryngitis, tracheitis, and a nonproductive cough develop.[29, 88, 146, 323] The initial dry, hacking cough may progress to paroxysms. Malaise, myalgia, chills, headache, dizziness, rhinitis, conjunctivitis, abdominal pain, and local cervical lymphadenopathy are common complaints.[88] The inflammatory process may spread to the bronchi, the bronchioles, and the parenchyma of the lungs. In epidemics, as many as 67 percent of those affected wheeze and have other evidence of small airway obstruction; pneumonia occurs in 10 to 20 percent.[187, 253, 290] The illness gradually resolves over the course of an 8- to 36-day period.[133] Early in the illness, the total white blood cell count may be slightly elevated, with a small increase in the percentage of polymorphonuclear leukocytes.

In experimental, aerosol-induced ARD, the incubation period ranged between 6 and 13 days.[78] Typical illness included fever to 39°C, rhinitis, prostration, malaise, myalgia, and headache. Pneumonia occurred occasionally. The virus was recovered from throat culture specimens 5 days after inoculation, from the nose at 6 days, and after 9 days in fecal specimens. Serum-neutralizing antibody responses occurred between the third and fourth weeks. All ill volunteers had leukopenia and an elevated erythrocyte sedimentation rate during the illness.

The syndrome occurs most commonly in military recruits early in basic training; illness has been documented in as many as 90 percent of new trainees within the first 8 weeks of arrival at a training site.[187] The usual etiologic agents are adenovirus types 4 and 7. Occasionally, epidemics have been associated with adenovirus types 3, 11, 14, and 21,[131] and sporadic cases have been noted in connection with adenovirus types 2, 5, and 8.[187, 323] The peak seasons of illness are winter and spring.[187]

Because of the magnitude of the problem of ARD in military recruits, live attenuated adenoviral vaccines against type 4 and 7 were developed and used in all branches of the U.S. military beginning in the early 1970s.[15, 156] These vaccines were used successfully until the early 1990s, when production delays occurred; subsequently, in 1995, the vaccine manufacturer stopped production. Since early 1999, no vaccine has been available, and epidemic disease has returned to military training bases. Although illness may occur in civilian adults, it is an uncommon event and not epidemic. In volunteer studies, subjects with serum antibody to a particular adenoviral type are protected against disease with that type of intranasal inoculation.[21, 78]

Epidemic ARD has not been described in children. However, a sporadic comparative illness, usually clinically identified as acute bronchitis, is commonly the result of adenoviral infection.[451] Adenovirus type 7 is the etiologic agent most frequently found in these cases.

Acute Laryngotracheitis

On occasion, adenoviruses have been implicated as a cause of acute laryngotracheitis. In general, croup caused by adenoviruses is not severe and frequently is manifested only as a barking, brassy cough. Laryngotracheitis often is seen in association with febrile pharyngitis, bronchiolitis, and pneumonia.[416] Epidemics have not been observed. Adenovirus types 1, 2, 3, 5, 6, and 7 have been implicated as etiologic agents.

Acute Bronchiolitis

Adenoviruses account for approximately 5 percent of cases of bronchiolitis in infants.[444] The bronchiolitis caused by adenoviral infection is sporadic and usually similar to illness associated with other viral agents. Occasionally, adenoviral bronchiolitis occurring early in infancy has been fatal or has resulted in serious residual lung damage and chronic disease.[435] This severe illness has been associated with serotypes 3, 7, and 21.

Pneumonia

YOUNG CHILDREN. Adenoviruses are common isolates in children with pneumonia. Their overall frequency in the causation of nonbacterial pneumonia in children is less than that of respiratory syncytial virus and parainfluenza virus type 3, but an alarming number of fatal illnesses have been noted. Severe and fatal illnesses in infants and young children have been noted in association with adenovirus types 1, 2, 3, 4, 5, 7, 7a, 7h, 7i, 8, 19, 21, 35, and the intermediate strain 21/H21+35.* The more severe cases of pneumonias have been linked to types 3, 7, and 21.[378, 446] Adenoviral pneumonia has been epidemic and sporadic.[58, 65]

Severe pneumonia occurs most commonly in neonates and young children 3 to 18 months of age.† The onset of illness is acute, with persistent cough and fever (>39° C). On physical examination, moderate to severe dyspnea is apparent, as is the associated tachypnea. Inspiratory and expiratory wheezes and rales are heard on auscultation. Other signs and symptoms include lethargy, diarrhea and vomiting, pharyngitis, and occasionally, conjunctivitis. Extrapulmonary complications that occur commonly are meningitis, encephalitis, seizures, splenomegaly, hepatomegaly and hepatitis, myocarditis, nephritis, bleeding tendency, and exanthems.[25, 45, 58, 74, 244, 376, 378, 387, 390] Chest radiographs reveal diffuse infiltrates, which usually are bilateral and may be bronchial, peribronchial, or interstitial.[18, 244, 442] Hyperinflation and lobar collapse occur frequently.[152] Rarely, pleural effusions or mediastinal lymphadenopathy has been described.[244] In surviving infants, symptoms persist for 2 to 4 weeks, and radiographic changes resolve slowly, frequently being present at the 3-week follow-up examination.[58, 65, 378] Recovery often is gradual, and exacerbations occur commonly.[209, 321]

Serious sequelae often result from adenoviral lower respiratory disease, particularly in association with adenovirus types 3, 7, 7a, and 21.[11, 19, 152, 209, 244, 378] These sequelae include bronchiectasis, bronchiolitis obliterans, and unilateral hyperlucent lung.[11, 19, 244, 264, 284, 332, 378, 444] An estimated 14 to 60 percent of children with documented adenoviral lower respiratory tract disease have some degree of permanent pulmonary sequelae.[152, 244, 377, 378] In a study of 27 children conducted 10 years after they had documented adenoviral type 7 pneumonia, 12 had radiographic evidence of bronchiectasis or residual pulmonary changes; 16 children had abnormal pulmonary function studies.[377]

Maček and associates[263] have suggested that persistent adenoviral infections may be the cause of chronic airway obstructive disease in children. They noted adenoviral antigen in bronchoalveolar lavage specimens from 31 of

*See references 6, 18, 19, 25, 44, 45, 58, 65, 96, 101, 138, 152, 189, 209, 218, 219, 231–233, 241, 246, 261, 271, 284, 285, 295, 310, 321, 332, 333, 347, 376, 378, 387, 390, 446.

†See references 18, 19, 25, 44, 45, 74, 101, 152, 218, 233, 244, 271, 333, 347.

34 patients with chronic disease but in no bronchoalveolar specimens from a control group.

On occasion, severe and fatal adenoviral pneumonia has been related to malnutrition, environmental crowding, or a preceding severe viral disease such as measles.[11, 18, 19, 152, 241, 298, 378]

Severe adenoviral pneumonia associated with adenovirus types 3 and 7 also has been reported occasionally in previously healthy adults.[326, 335, 381] One adult had severe pneumonia caused by adenovirus type 21 that was associated with myalgia, rhabdomyolysis, and myoglobinuria.[447]

ATYPICAL PNEUMONIA IN MILITARY RECRUITS. Approximately 7 to 20 percent of cases of pneumonia in military recruits are associated with adenoviral infection.[47, 128, 141] Primary atypical adenoviral pneumonia commonly occurs in the winter months and generally is caused by adenovirus types 4, 7, and 21.[128] The illness is associated with fever, cough, sore throat, rhinorrhea, and chest pain. Other common symptoms include nausea, vomiting, myalgia, headache, and diarrhea. On physical examination, rales and pharyngitis are noted in almost all cases. Rhinitis and generalized lymphadenopathy are observed in approximately half of those afflicted, and occasionally, conjunctivitis is noted. Chest radiographs reveal a bilaterally mottled appearance, most prominent in the lower lobes; they remain abnormal for 4 to 36 days.[47] Although serum cold agglutinins are observed, titers of 1:32 or higher are noted in only 18 percent of patients.[47, 141]

Fatal pneumonia, absolute leukopenia, and disseminated disease have been reported in four previously healthy military trainees. Adenovirus type 7 was the etiologic agent in three of these cases, and the fourth illness was caused by adenovirus type 4.[106, 253]

PERTUSSIS-LIKE SYNDROME. A pertussis-like illness has been noted in association with several adenoviruses, including types 1, 2, 3, 5, 12, and 19.[71, 73, 169, 300, 313] The illness occurs commonly in infants younger than 36 months. The onset of illness is insidious and initially suggestive of a cold. The cough becomes progressively worse and by 1 to 2 weeks is paroxysmal. Severe recurrent episodes of paroxysms result in the production of mucus, post-tussive fatigue, and vomiting.[73] Approximately 50 percent of children have a typical whoop, and cyanosis occurs with paroxysms. Peripheral leukocytosis with white blood cell counts ranging from 25,000 to 125,000 cells/mm^3 with lymphocytosis and thrombocytosis is the usual finding.[71, 313] The recovery time ranges from 4 to 10 weeks from the onset of illness.[73] Radiologic evidence of bronchiolitis is present in most children; interstitial pneumonia occurs occasionally. In my opinion, most and probably all these pertussis-like illnesses are indeed *Bordetella pertussis* infections in which adenovirus is a co-infecting agent.

BRONCHIOLITIS OBLITERANS. Bronchiolitis obliterans is a chronic bronchiolitis that initially was described in 1901 by Lange.[245] It has been noted to occur after measles, influenza, and pertussis and after the inhalation of toxic substances.[11, 19, 444] Adenovirus types 2, 7, 7i, and 21 have resulted in a bronchiolitis obliterans–type chronic illness.[11, 19, 284, 332, 435, 444] These adenoviruses cause a severe necrotizing bronchiolitis that heals with fibrosis and predominantly obliterates the small airways.19 The onset of disease is characterized by an acute febrile illness, cough, and respiratory distress. Disease may wax and wane for several weeks or months and is associated with recurrent episodes of atelectasis, pneumonia, and wheezing. Although some children recover from these episodes, the remainder have chronic pulmonary disease, including irreversible atelectasis, bronchiectasis, or hyperlucent lung syndrome.[19, 435, 444]

UNILATERAL HYPERLUCENT LUNG. Unilateral hyperlucent lung is a well-defined syndrome characterized by increased translucency of all or part of one lung, along with a reduction in lung size.[83, 264] The unilateral hyperlucency is associated with a decrease in the size and number of pulmonary vessels, as observed on pulmonary angiograms, and an absence of peripheral filling at bronchography.[264] Although the disease may have a number of etiologies, including pneumonia secondary to other viruses, it has been noted to occur after severe necrotizing bronchiolitis and pneumonia caused by adenovirus types 7 and 21.[264, 444]

EYE

Acute Follicular Conjunctivitis

Acute follicular conjunctivitis is the most common and benign of the adenoviral infections of the eye. The infection in this disease is confined to the eye, generally is unilateral, and is manifested by follicular lesions on the conjunctival surface. Symptoms occur after an incubation period of 5 to 7 days and include lacrimation, itching, burning, a foreign body sensation, and conjunctival erythema.[99] Examination shows erythema and lymphoid follicular hyperplasia in the conjunctiva in association with serous drainage and increased lacrimation. Occasionally, adenopathy of the preauricular lymph nodes is seen. Symptoms resolve in 10 days to 3 weeks, with recovery usually complete.[77, 99] Adenovirus types 1, 2, 3, 4, 6, 7, 9, 10, 11, 15, 16, 17, 19, 20, 22, 34, and 37 have been isolated from the eyes of afflicted patients.[34, 74, 99, 366, 371, 415]

Pharyngoconjunctival Fever

Pharyngoconjunctival fever is presented in detail in Chapter 12.

Epidemic Keratoconjunctivitis

Epidemic keratoconjunctivitis is caused most commonly by adenovirus type 8, but it also has resulted from infection with adenovirus types 2, 3, 4, 5, 7, 10, 11, 13, 14, 15, 16, 17, 19, 22, 23, 29, and 37.* Currently, adenovirus type 37 is the virus most commonly recovered from patients with epidemic keratoconjunctivitis in the United States and Europe. The most severe disease is associated with adenovirus types 5, 8, and 19.[87]

The illness occurs most commonly in adults, but a few cases of disease in children have been reported.[170, 286, 401] It has no seasonal pattern. Although transmission of the viral agent from the respiratory tract to the eye occurs in sporadic cases, the usual method of viral spread is by contaminated ophthalmic instruments and eye solutions, hand-to-eye contact by medical personnel and others, swimming pools, or hands or fomites in close contact situations, such as in families and in industry.† The incubation period is typically 5 to 10 days but ranges from as short a period as 2 days to as long as 2 weeks.[89, 236] The initial symptom is generally unilateral, acute, follicular conjunctivitis that suggests a foreign body. Photophobia, lacrimation, discharge, hyperemia, and edema of the conjunctiva are notable. Preauricular adenopathy occurs in as many as 90 percent of patients, and

*See references 14, 34, 49, 78, 87, 89, 92, 94, 95, 118, 164, 166, 170, 213, 214, 223, 224, 227, 286, 288, 303, 305, 366, 385, 389, 402, 450.
†See references 14, 49, 87, 89, 92, 125, 213, 236, 269, 286, 288, 401, 434.

50 percent of those afflicted have pharyngitis and rhinitis. Spread to the other eye may occur in 2 to 7 days. Seven to 10 days after onset of the disease, the conjunctivitis resolves, and painful, superficial, punctate epithelial opacities appear in the center of the cornea. These lesions frequently extend subepithelially and then heal, with subepithelial infiltrates left behind that may persist for months. In severe cases, hazy vision may continue for several years.[14]

An infantile form of epidemic keratoconjunctivitis has been described that usually affects infants younger than 2 years of age. This pseudomembranous or membranous conjunctivitis generally is accompanied by high fever, pharyngitis, otitis media, diarrhea, and vomiting. Preauricular lymphadenopathy typically is absent.[401]

Virus can be recovered from the eye for a usual period of approximately 2 weeks but has been detected for 2 to 3 years in patients with chronic papillary conjunctivitis.[87, 331] In acute illness, conjunctival scrapings obtained during the first 10 days of infection reveal characteristic inclusion bodies when they are Giemsa-stained.[205] Virus-specific fluorescent antibody staining is diagnostic in epidemic keratoconjunctivitis.[370] Preparations of corneal and conjunctival epithelia reveal adenoviral particles when examined with the electron microscope.[94]

SKIN

Adenovirus types 1, 2, 3, 4, 7, and 7a, plus several unknown types, have been noted in connection with exanthematous disease.[61] The cutaneous manifestation most commonly associated with adenoviral infection is an erythematous maculopapular rash that appears while the child is febrile. In many instances, children with this illness have been thought to have either measles or rubella.[241] In most adenoviral infections with exanthems, other clinical findings more characteristic of adenoviruses, such as conjunctivitis, rhinitis, pharyngitis, and lymphadenopathy, also are present. In some instances, the exanthem truly is morbilliform with a characteristic confluence, but Koplik spots do not occur.

A widespread erythematous rash often is present early in the course of severe pneumonia in infants.[152] Chany and colleagues[58] noted a measles-like rash in five patients who died of adenovirus type 7a pneumonia. One report describes a child with an adenovirus type 7 infection and illness suggestive of meningococcemia.[363] This patient had fever, vomiting, diarrhea, and a petechial exanthem.

On several occasions, illness characterized by fever and defervescence and then the appearance of a maculopapular rash suggesting the diagnosis of roseola infantum has been observed.[126, 136, 211, 212, 302] Adenoviral infections also are confused with rubella. However, the respiratory symptoms and the degree of fever associated with adenoviral infection should clarify the diagnosis. With rubella, respiratory complaints and fever are minimal. On occasion, severe disease with Stevens-Johnson syndrome has been noted. Such patients frequently have pneumonia, and the illness is quite similar to that caused by *Mycoplasma pneumoniae*.

Lähdeaho and associates[243] have noted that serum antibodies to the E1b protein–derived peptides of the enteric adenovirus type 40 are associated with dermatitis herpetiformis.

GENITOURINARY TRACT

Acute Hemorrhagic Cystitis

Acute hemorrhagic cystitis is an uncommon manifestation of adenoviral infection and is characterized by a sudden onset of dysuria and frequency, with hematuria developing 12 to 24 hours later.[247, 248, 291, 292, 294, 308] Occasionally, fever, suprapubic pain, and enuresis occur. Antecedent upper respiratory infection is noted in some children. Symptoms persist for a few days to 2 weeks, with the usual duration being approximately 5 days. Acute hemorrhagic cystitis has been reported in both the United States and Japan. It occurs primarily in children, most often boys, and usually is associated with adenovirus type 11. Occasionally, adenovirus types 7 and 21 have been implicated. Adenoviral antigen has been identified by immunofluorescence in exfoliated bladder cells. Although no sequelae have been reported, the long-term prognosis is unknown.[291]

Nephritis

Hematuria occasionally has been reported in infants with severe pneumonia and disseminated adenoviral infection. Red blood cells and, at times, red blood cell casts in the urine also have been noted in some children with upper respiratory illnesses caused by adenoviruses and specifically in patients with pharyngoconjunctival fever associated with adenovirus types 3, 4, and 7a.[383, 388, 421, 426] In one instance, a young boy had a maculopapular and petechial exanthem and thrombocytopenia associated with adenovirus type 7 infection. Hematuria also was noted.

Orchitis

Orchitis developed in one child who had a 5-day history of pain and fever, erythema, and swelling of the right testicle.[299] The testicular involvement resolved in several days, and the illness was associated with a 16-fold rise in adenoviral complement-fixation antibody titer.

Oculogenital Syndrome

In 1977, Laverty and associates[247] reported a woman who in addition to having pharyngoconjunctival fever, had cervicitis and paresthesia of the legs; a type 19 adenovirus was recovered from this woman's cervix. In Perth, Australia, adenovirus type 19 was recovered from the genital tracts of 59 men and women being examined for genital herpes simplex virus infection in a sexually transmitted disease clinic.[205] Several of the patients also had conjunctivitis, and in two, adenovirus type 19 was isolated from conjunctival specimens. Similar oculogenital illnesses have been noted in association with adenoviral types 2, 8, and 37.[54, 366, 397]

Hemolytic-Uremic Syndrome

Two 2-year-old children with hemolytic-uremic syndrome in association with adenoviral infections have been described.[28]

Hemorrhagic Fever with Renal Syndrome

A 22-year-old woman with an adenovirus type 11 infection and hemorrhagic fever with renal syndrome has been reported.[417]

GASTROINTESTINAL TRACT

Gastroenteritis

Infantile diarrhea has been associated with epidemic and sporadic adenoviral diseases such as acute upper respiratory infection, severe pneumonia, and pharyngoconjunctival fever.[126, 244, 383, 392, 437] Outbreaks of diarrhea characterized by acute abdominal pain followed by diarrhea, nausea and vomiting, fever, headache, and pharyngitis have been associated with adenovirus type 3 and 7 infections.[140, 391] Other symptoms occurring in patients with diarrhea include conjunctivitis, rhinitis, pharyngotonsillitis, hepatomegaly, and cervical adenitis.[392] In two patients who had diarrhea and upper respiratory illness in association with adenovirus type 15 infection, viral particles were visualized within the nuclei of mucosal cells at autopsy by electron microscopy.[107]

The widespread use of electron microscopy for the study of rotavirus diarrhea led to the finding of previously unrecognized adenoviruses that were fastidious and could not be grown in routine cell cultures.[123, 369] These adenoviruses, now identified as types 40 and 41, subsequently were shown to be important causes of gastroenteritis in children.* In enteric adenoviral infection, diarrhea is the most prominent symptom.[416] In children with adenovirus type 40 infection, Uhnoo and colleagues[416] found that the mean duration was 8.6 days, whereas in those infected with adenovirus type 41, it was 12.2 days. Most illnesses occur in children younger than 3 years of age: the mean age for adenovirus type 40 diarrhea was 15.2 months, whereas it was 28.3 months in type 41 illnesses. Most patients had mild vomiting that lasted approximately 2 days. When compared with illnesses caused by established respiratory adenoviruses, fever occurred less commonly, was less severe, and had a shorter duration in enteric adenoviral infections. Upper respiratory symptoms and signs, such as pharyngitis, coryza, cough, and otitis media, were observed in 21 percent of children with enteric adenoviral infection. Brandt and colleagues[40] noted that dual infections with respiratory viruses (such as respiratory syncytial virus and enteric adenoviruses) are common occurrences, so caution should be observed in attributing respiratory symptoms to enteric adenoviruses.

Yolken and Franklin[452] found that enteric adenoviruses were an important cause of nosocomial diarrhea in infants who had previously undergone gastrointestinal surgery for necrotizing enterocolitis.

Mesenteric Lymphadenitis

Adenoviral serotypes 1, 2, 3, 5, and 7 have been recovered from lymph nodes and the appendix in cases of mesenteric lymphadenitis.[22, 33, 235] Patients with mesenteric lymphadenitis often have abdominal pain and other symptoms similar to those of acute appendicitis. Pharyngitis is a frequently related finding. Mesenteric adenitis often is associated with concurrent or recent adenoviral illness.[74, 341] Frequently, the peak incidence of mesenteric lymphadenitis occurs when adenoviral illness is common in the community.

Intussusception

The suggestion that adenoviruses could be an etiologic factor in intussusception arose because these agents frequently can be recovered from throat, stool, and mesenteric lymph node specimens obtained from children who undergo surgery for intussusception.† Most children with intussusception were younger than 2 years of age; some had preceding respiratory symptoms.[356, 454] Adenovirus serotypes 1, 2, 3, 5, 6, and 7 have been implicated. Typical adenoviral intranuclear inclusions have been demonstrated in cells in stool, intestinal epithelia (ileum), and the appendix by electron microscopy.[309, 454, 455] Mesenteric lymph nodes often are enlarged at surgery.[455] Antibody titer rises to adenoviruses have been noted in children after undergoing intussusception. Investigators have suggested that bowel wall hypermotility caused by direct viral involvement or by hypertrophy of lymphatic tissue is the lead point for the intussusception.[22, 70, 139, 309, 339, 356, 454, 455]

Appendicitis

Adenoviruses have been associated with both acute and chronic appendicitis.[33] Right iliac fossa abdominal pain in conjunction with sore throat is a common finding. The virus has been isolated from the appendix and mesenteric lymph nodes at surgery. During acute infection, lymphoid follicles of the ileum, appendix, and mesenteric lymph nodes are infected with virus. In chronic infection, adenovirus remains in cells; on microscopic examination, slight inflammation is seen in the appendix.

Hepatitis

Hepatitis in association with adenoviral infection has been reported many times in small infants, in children with overwhelming disseminated disease, and in immunocompromised patients.[2, 10, 25, 45, 52, 232, 456] In one study, 27 of 30 persons thought to have sporadic infectious hepatitis were found to be infected with adenovirus type 5.[171] Adenovirus types 1, 2, and 3 were isolated from the stool specimens of 12 children younger than 3 years in an outbreak of infectious hepatitis on a Native American reservation in Arizona.[172]

In one report, three children with severe, fatal adenovirus type 7 pneumonia had associated findings that simulated Reye syndrome: lethargy, diarrhea, seizures, elevated CSF pressure, myocarditis, hepatitis, and disseminated intravascular coagulation.[242] Edwards and colleagues[110] reported three children with Reye syndrome and adenoviral infection. They suggested that adenoviruses might be an important agent in initiating the syndrome.

HEART

Myocarditis

In children, myocarditis has been noted in association with severe pneumonia and disseminated disease caused by adenovirus types 7, 7a, and 21.[174] Similar cardiac involvement has been seen in military recruits with severe acute respiratory disease.[58, 65, 174, 383]

The use of polymerase chain reaction (PCR) assays has led to recognition of adenovirus as the etiology of many cases of acute myocarditis.[42, 162, 262, 268]

Pericarditis

Pericarditis has been associated with severe adenoviral pneumonia. In a patient with adenovirus type 7 pneumonia, electrocardiographic changes consistent with pericarditis were demonstrated, and the virus was isolated in high titer from pericardial fluid at postmortem examination.[298] Recently, Mistchenko and coworkers[283] reported a 10-month-old boy with fatal pericarditis caused by adenovirus type 7. In serum and pericardial fluid from this child, interleukin-6,

*See references 390, 43, 68, 239, 240, 282, 312, 337, 350, 405, 416, 419.

†See references 22, 27, 70, 139, 199, 309, 335, 356, 454, 455.

tumor necrosis factor–a, and adenovirus-specific immune complexes were identified.

NEUROLOGIC

Although CNS disease in adenoviral infection is an uncommon finding, a variety of clinical manifestations have been observed. Both meningitis and encephalitis have been noted as the major manifestations of adenoviral infection or in association with severe disease at other body sites.[306, 310] Adenovirus types 1, 2, 3, 5, 6, 7, 12, and 32, in isolated instances, have been recovered from both brain and CSF.* In two children with respiratory and CNS symptoms, adenoviruses were recovered from spinal fluid.[119] One child was convalescing from herpes zoster and the other from varicella. Adenovirus type 7 was recovered from tissue cultures of brain from an elderly patient with chronic schizophrenia.[261] In another instance, adenovirus type 32 was recovered from the brain of a man with lymphosarcoma and subacute encephalitis.[67, 353] In an epidemic of adenoviral infection caused by type 7, 25 percent of the hospitalized patients had symptoms referable to the CNS.[376, 378] Many of the patients died; those who survived had little residual effect. Too few cases are reported in the literature to predict the prognosis of CNS disease in children accurately. An adenovirus type 2 was isolated from a muscle biopsy specimen from a patient with inclusion-body myositis.[279]

INFECTION IN IMMUNOCOMPROMISED HOSTS

Adenovirus types 1, 2, 4, 5, 6, 7, 7a, 11, 29, 31, 32, 34, and 35 have been recovered from children and adults who were immunocompromised by immunodeficiency diseases, malignancies, steroid therapy, immunosuppressive therapy, radiation therapy, and transplantation procedures.†

Baldwin and colleagues[13] studied the outcome and clinical course of 105 adenovirus infections in 100 patients after they received bone marrow transplants. The incidence was higher in unrelated donor than in matched sibling donor transplants. Diarrhea and fever were the most common initial findings. Six deaths were attributed to the adenoviral infections; five of the six patients had pneumonia, and four had associated graft-versus-host disease. Three additional patients had severe disease.

In a study involving 532 recipients of hematopoietic stem cell transplants, a 12 percent incidence of adenoviral infection was noted.[198] Forty-one patients had infections classified as "invasive," and mortality was 76 percent in this group. Recipients of allogeneic transplants were more likely to have adenoviral infections than were autologous stem cell recipients.

The most common manifestation of adenoviral infection in pediatric patients with bone marrow transplants at St. Jude Children's Research Hospital was hemorrhagic cystitis, followed by gastroenteritis, pneumonitis, and liver failure.[165]

Shirali and coworkers[374] noted that demonstration of the adenoviral genome in endomyocardial biopsy specimens of heart transplant recipients was a predictor of graft loss in children. Scattered reports have found an association between adenoviral infection and viruria and hemorrhagic cystitis in patients with renal transplants.[121, 245] A fatal case of subacute meningoencephalitis caused by an adenovirus has been described in a bone marrow transplant patient.[91]

In many instances, a fulminant, bacterial, sepsis-like picture with high fever, cough, and lethargy is associated with adenoviral infection in compromised patients.[456] Severe pneumonia often is demonstrated, both clinically and radiologically, and hepatic involvement with disseminated intravascular coagulation also is a frequent occurrence. Fatalities are reported, and recovery often is slow.

OTHER MANIFESTATIONS

Arthritis

Arthritis has been noted in association with adenovirus type 7 infection.[318] The illness was characterized by fever, acute respiratory symptoms, erythematous macular rash, aseptic meningitis, and inflammatory arthritis of both knees.

Thyroiditis

In 1964, Swann[396] reported five patients with acute thyroiditis and thyroid enlargement in whom serologic study revealed greater than fourfold titer rises in adenoviral complement-fixing antibody.

Deafness

Deafness of sudden onset was reported in an adult with a 2-day history of sore throat, low-grade fever, rhinorrhea, and cough. Adenovirus type 3 was isolated from the patient's throat, and a greater than fourfold rise in neutralizing antibody titer to this virus was observed.[208]

CONGENITAL AND NEONATAL INFECTIONS

Neonatal and congenital adenoviral infections reflect disseminated infection with the involvement of multiple organs.[1, 44, 66, 233, 314, 390] Major manifestations include hepatosplenomegaly, progressive pneumonia, hepatitis, and thrombocytopenia. Towbin and colleagues[410] reported intrauterine adenoviral myocarditis manifested as nonimmune hydrops fetalis. Illnesses frequently appear initially as an early-onset sepsis syndrome. An infant has been reported with a congenital pleural effusion from which type 3 adenovirus was recovered.[277]

A recent study by Couroucli and associates[79] has noted an association between adenoviral infection and bronchopulmonary dysplasia (BPD). They found a significant increase in the frequency of adenovirus genome in tracheal aspirates from patients with BPD versus controls.

Diagnosis

DIFFERENTIAL DIAGNOSIS

The differential diagnosis of adenoviral infection must be subcategorized on the basis of the major clinical manifestations. In many instances, because of specific clinical symptoms such as pharyngoconjunctival fever or epidemic keratoconjunctivitis, the adenoviral etiology can be suspected strongly. With other, more general respiratory diseases such as pharyngitis, bronchitis, croup, bronchiolitis, and pneumonia, the adenoviral etiology cannot be established on

*See references 60, 74, 81, 119, 137, 226, 319, 330, 353, 376, 390, 395.

†See references 2, 13, 17, 50, 52, 67, 84, 91, 124, 159, 165, 180, 206, 225, 260, 297, 304, 311, 320, 353, 373–375, 379, 384, 412, 441, 456.

clinical grounds. Fever in adenoviral respiratory infections tends to be higher than that occurring in parainfluenza and respiratory syncytial viral infections but similar to that in influenza A and B viral infections.[342] High and prolonged fever occurs as commonly in adenoviral infections as it does in bacterial respiratory infections.

In pharyngitis, adenoviral infection must be differentiated both from other viral diseases, such as those caused by Epstein-Barr, parainfluenza, and influenza viruses and enteroviruses, and from streptococcal disease. In a young child, follicular pharyngitis is more likely to be caused by adenoviral than by streptococcal infection.

Adenoviral pneumonia in young children frequently is not distinguishable on clinical grounds from that caused by bacteria. In older children and adolescents, in particular, adenoviral pneumonia often can be differentiated from bacterial disease by its bilateral nature. Differentiating adenoviral illness from disease caused by *M. pneumoniae* is more difficult; however, cold agglutinin titers generally are higher and more persistently positive in mycoplasmal disease.

Adenoviral eye disease must be differentiated from that caused by viruses of the herpes group, *Chlamydia* spp., and bacteria, including *Neisseria gonorrhoeae*.

Diarrhea caused by enteric adenoviruses can be differentiated from other viral diarrheas by electron microscopy, by identification with ELISA, and by specific culture of the enteric agents in Graham 293 cell culture. Enteric bacterial and parasitic agents also must be considered in the differential diagnosis.

The high, relatively prolonged fever occurring in association with lymphadenopathy, exanthem, and enanthem noted with adenoviral infection often causes confusion with Kawasaki disease.[63] Because Kawasaki disease must be treated early with intravenous immunoglobulin, adenoviral infections should be considered early and appropriate studies performed.

SPECIFIC DIAGNOSIS

Adenoviral infection can be diagnosed specifically by viral isolation in an appropriate tissue culture system or by a direct antigen-detection assay. Most adenoviral types can be recovered from clinical specimens in primary or diploid cultures of human embryonic kidney.[251] The enteric viral types 40 and 41 can be grown in Graham 293 cells.[400, 433] The rapidity of detection of adenoviruses by culture is enhanced by centrifugation of specimens in shell vials or plastic-welled plates.[108, 113, 265]

Direct identification of adenoviruses in respiratory secretions by radioimmunoassay, immunofluorescence techniques, and ELISA now is performed widely.[46, 265, 276, 344, 361, 362, 364, 403] However, in general, the sensitivity, when compared with that of virus isolation, is relatively low; on the other hand, the specificity is high (>95%). Rapid techniques for the identification of enteric adenoviruses in general have been sensitive and specific.[4, 155, 178, 365, 416, 445] However, in newborns, false-positive results with a latex agglutination test have been reported.[204] Several techniques using DNA probes have been studied for the rapid identification of both respiratory and enteric adenoviral infection.[48, 203, 399] PCR assay also is useful for the rapid detection of adenoviral infection but generally lacks the sensitivity of culture.[5, 109, 173, 206, 289, 320] PCR assay is particularly useful for the identification of adenovirus DNA in formalin-fixed, paraffin-embedded tissues and other biopsy and postmortem specimens.[162, 262, 268, 374, 413]

Acute infection also can be diagnosed serologically by the expression of specific IgM serum antibody.[276] Infection can be confirmed serologically by the demonstration of a rise in antibody titer in two sequential serum samples. Antibody response to the adenovirus group antigen can be detected by complement fixation or ELISA. Type-specific antibodies can be determined by neutralization, ELISA, or hemagglutination inhibition.

Treatment

During the febrile period of illness, adequate hydration should be maintained and excessive activity discouraged. The fever may be controlled with acetaminophen. In children with eye involvement, careful attention should be paid to the possibility of secondary bacterial infection. If local purulence develops, cultures should be taken and topical antimicrobial therapy started. The use of steroid-containing ophthalmic ointments should be avoided.

In a number of instances, immunocompromised patients with disseminated adenoviral infection have been treated with ribavirin administered intravenously, and successful outcomes have been reported.[8, 220, 256, 272, 296, 449] In one instance, a loading dose of 30 mg/kg/day divided into three doses was followed by maintenance therapy with 15 mg/kg/day.[272] Cidofovir was used successfully in treating a 17-year-old boy who had received a stem cell transplant and had severe adenoviral gastroenteritis.[348]

Human fibroblast-derived interferon, applied topically, was used to treat epidemic adenovirus keratoconjunctivitis in a comparative trial.[352] The duration of illness was reduced in the patients treated with interferon, but many of the control patients received dexamethasone. A child with combined immunodeficiency and severe, diffuse adenovirus type 7a pneumonia improved dramatically after receiving a large dose of high-titer adenovirus type 7a immune serum globulin.[84]

Prevention

Serious incapacitating epidemics caused by adenoviruses in military recruits in basic training led to the development of adenoviral vaccines.[7, 249] The initial vaccines were formalin-inactivated preparations of monkey kidney tissue culture–grown virus and were administered parenterally.[6, 161, 187] These vaccines achieved only limited success because of variable degrees of potency in different vaccine lots.[19] An inactivated adenoviral vaccine that contained types 3, 4, and 7 was prepared in monkey tissue culture for trial in children.[425] Three doses of this vaccine resulted in high levels of neutralizing antibody to the three viral types, and this antibody persisted in most infants for at least 1 year. Many of the initial lots of inactivated adenoviral vaccine were found to contain live simian adenoviruses that were capable of producing neoplasms in suckling hamsters. Because of this finding, inactivated vaccine trials were discontinued. Next, a live attenuated adenovirus type 4 vaccine that was cultivated in human diploid tissue culture was developed and administered orally by enteric-coated capsule to volunteers.[161] Asymptomatic gastrointestinal infection occurred, and a good serum-neutralizing antibody response was elicited.[161, 382, 386] Most recipients of live oral vaccine excrete virus in stool for several days to a month after vaccination. With military use of the vaccine, shedding in stool was not associated with transmission of the virus to nonimmune contacts.[290] In other studies of married couples and families with children, virus was transmitted to nonimmune contacts.[290, 386] Transmission usually occurred without illness.[290]

The administration of live, enteric-coated, type 4 and 7 adenovirus vaccine resulted in a significant decrease in the incidence of ARD in military recruits.[105, 153, 398] Unfortunately adenoviral vaccines no longer are available, and the incidence of ARD in military recruits again is a significant problem.[14, 156] Few attempts have been made to protect children with live adenoviral vaccines. In one study, live enteric-coated adenovirus type 4 vaccine was given to children 5 to 11 years of age. Asymptomatic gastrointestinal infection resulted from administration of the vaccine.

Prognosis

The overall prognosis of adenoviral infection generally is excellent. Secondary bacterial complications, if untreated, can result in the prolongation of illness and permanent sequelae in some instances. The prognosis of adenoviral infection in the very young and in immunocompromised patients must be guarded.

REFERENCES

1. Abzug, M. J., and Levin, M. J.: Neonatal adenovirus infection: Four patients and review of the literature. Pediatrics *87*:890–896, 1991.
2. Adler, H.: Keratitis sub-epithelialis. Centralbl. Prakt. Augenheilk. *13*:289–295, 1889.
3. Adrian, T., Wigans, R., and Richter, J.: Gastroenteritis in infants, associated with a genome type of adenovirus 31 and with combined rotavirus and adenovirus 31 infection. Eur. J. Pediatr. *146*:38–40, 1987.
4. Ahluwalia, G. S., Scott-Taylor, T. H., Klisko, B., et al.: Comparison of detection methods for adenovirus from enteric clinical specimens. Diagn. Microbiol. Infect. Dis. *18*:161–166, 1994.
5. Allard, A., Girones, R., Juto, P., et al.: Polymerase chain reaction for detection of adenoviruses in stool samples. J. Clin. Microbiol. *28*:2659–2667, 1990.
6. Andiman, W. A., Jacobson, R. I., and Tucker, G.: Leukocyte-associated viremia with adenovirus type 2 in an infant with lower-respiratory-tract disease. N. Engl. J. Med. *297*:100–101, 1977.
7. Angella, J. J., and Connor, J. D.: Neonatal infection caused by adenovirus type 7. J. Pediatr. *72*:474–478, 1968.
8. Arav-Boger, R., Echavarria, M., Forman, M., et al.: Clearance of adenoviral hepatitis with ribavirin therapy in a pediatric liver transplant recipient. Pediatr. Infect. Dis. *19*:1097–1100, 2000.
9. Artenstein, M. S., Miller, W. S., Lamson, T. H., et al.: Large-volume air sampling for meningococci and adenoviruses. Am. J. Epidemiol. *87*:567–577, 1968.
10. Aterman, K., Embil, J., Easterbrook, K. B., et al.: Liver necrosis, adenovirus type 2 and thymic dysplasia. Virchows Arch. *360*:155–171, 1973.
11. Azizirad, H., Polgar, G., Borns, P. F., et al.: Bronchiolitis obliterans. Clin. Pediatr. (Phila.) *14*:572–584, 1975.
12. Bahn, C. A.: Swimming bath conjunctivitis. New Orleans Med. Surg. J. *79*:586–590, 1927.
13. Baldwin, A., Kingman, H., Darville, M., et al.: Outcome and clinical course of 100 patients with adenovirus infection following bone marrow transplantation. Bone Marrow Transplant. *26*:1333–1338, 2000.
14. Barnard, D. L., Hart, J. C. D., Marmion, V. J., et al.: Outbreak in Bristol of conjunctivitis caused by adenovirus type 8, and its epidemiology and control. B. M. J. *2*:165–169, 1973.
15. Barraza, E. M., Ludwig, S. L., Gaydos, J. C., et al.: Reemergence of adenovirus type 4 acute respiratory disease in military trainees: Report of an outbreak during a lapse in vaccination. J. Infect. Dis. *179*:1531–1533, 1999.
16. Béal, R.: Sur une forme particulaire de conjonctivité aigue avec follicules. Annales D'Oculistique, Jan. 1907, pp. 1–33.
17. Beby-Defaux, A., Maille, L., Chabot, S., et al.: Fatal adenovirus type 7b infection in a child with Smith-Lemli-Opitz syndrome. J. Med. Virol. *65*:66–69, 2001.
18. Becroft, D. M. O.: Histopathology of fatal adenovirus infection of the respiratory tract in young children. J. Clin. Pathol. *20*:561–569, 1967.
19. Becroft, D. M. O.: Bronchiolitis obliterans, bronchiectasis, and other sequelae of adenovirus type 21 infection in young children. J. Clin. Pathol. *24*:72–82, 1971.
20. Bell, J. A., Huebner, R. J., Rosen, L., et al.: Illness and microbial experiences of nursery children at junior village. Am. J. Hyg. *74*:267–292, 1961.
21. Bell, J. A., Ward, T. G., Huebner, R. J., et al.: Studies of adenoviruses (APC) in volunteers. Am. J. Public Health *46*:1130–1146, 1956.
22. Bell, T. M., and Steyn, J. H.: Viruses in lymph nodes of children with mesenteric adenitis and intussusception. B. M. J. *1*:700–702, 1962.
23. Bell, T. M., Turner, G., Macdonald, A., et al.: Type-3 adenovirus infection. Lancet *2*:1327–1329, 1960.
24. Bellanti, J. A., Artenstein, M. S., Brandt, B. L., et al.: Immunoglobulin responses in serum and nasal secretions after natural adenovirus infections. J. Immunol. *103*:891–898, 1969.
25. Benyesh-Melnick, M., and Rosenberg, H. S.: The isolation of adenovirus type 7 from a fatal case of pneumonia and disseminated disease. J. Pediatr. *64*:83–87, 1964.
26. Berge, T. O., England, B., Mauris, C., et al.: Etiology of acute respiratory disease among service personnel at Fort Ord, California. Am. J. Hyg. *62*:283–294, 1955.
27. Bhisitkul, D. M., Todd, K. M., and Listernick, R.: Adenovirus infection and childhood intussusception. Am. J. Dis. Child. *146*:1331–1333, 1992.
28. Blachar, Y., Leibovitz, E., and Levin, S.: The interferon system in two patients with hemolytic uremic syndrome associated with adenovirus infection. Acta Paediatr. *79*:108–109, 1990.
29. Blacklock, J. W. S.: Section of pathology with section of epidemiology and preventive medicine: Discussion on adenovirus infections. Proc. R. Soc. Med. *50*:753–755, 1957.
30. Blacklow, N. R., Hoggan, M. D., Kapikian, A. Z., et al.: Epidemiology of adenovirus-associated virus infection in a nursery population. Am. J. Epidemiol. *88*:368–378, 1968.
31. Blacklow, N. R., Hoggan, M. D., Sereno, M. S., et al.: A seroepidemiologic study of adenovirus-associated virus infection in infants and children. Am. J. Epidemiol. *94*:359–366, 1971.
32. Bloom, H. H., Forsyth, B. R., Johnson, K. M., et al.: Patterns of adenovirus infections in Marine Corps personnel. I. A 42-month survey in recruit and nonrecruit populations. Am. J. Hyg. *80*:328–342, 1964.
33. Bonard, E. C., and Paccaud, M. F.: Abdominal adenovirosis and appendicitis. Helv. Med. Acta *33*:164–171, 1966.
34. Boniuk, M., Phillips, C. A., and Friedman, J. B.: Chronic adenovirus type 2 keratitis in man. N. Engl. J. Med. *273*:924–925, 1965.
35. Boyer, G. S., Denny, F. W., Jr., and Ginsberg, H. S.: Sequential cellular changes produced by types 5 and 7 adenoviruses in HeLa cells and in human amniotic cells: Cytological studies aided by fluorescein-labelled antibody. J. Exp. Med. *110*:827–843, 1959.
36. Boyer, G. S., Denny, F. W., Jr., Miller, I., et al.: Correlation of production of infectious virus with sequential stages of cytologic alteration in HeLa cells infected with adenoviruses types 5 and 7. J. Exp. Med. *112*:865–882, 1960.
37. Boyer, G. S., Leuchtenberger, C., and Ginsberg, H. S.: Cytological and cytochemical studies of HeLa cells infected with adenoviruses. J. Exp. Med. *105*:195–214, 1957.
38. Brandt, C. D., Kim, H. W., Jeffries, B. C., et al.: Infections in 18,000 infants and children in a controlled study of respiratory tract disease. II. Variation in adenovirus infections by year and season. Am. J. Epidemiol. *95*:218–227, 1972.
39. Brandt, C. D., Kim, H. W., Rodriguez, W. J., et al.: Adenoviruses and pediatric gastroenteritis. J. Infect. Dis. *151*:437–443, 1985.
40. Brandt, C. D., Kim, H. W., Rodriguez, W. J., et al.: Simultaneous infections with different enteric and respiratory tract viruses. J. Clin. Microbiol. *23*:177–179, 1986.
41. Brandt, C. D., Kim, H. W., Vargosko, A. J., et al.: Infections in 18,000 infants and children in a controlled study of respiratory tract disease. I. Adenovirus pathogenicity in relation to serologic type and illness syndrome. Am. J. Epidemiol. *90*:484–500, 1969.
42. Briassoulis, G., Papadopoulos, G., Zavras, N., et al.: Cardiac troponin I in fulminant adenovirus myocarditis treated with a 24-hour infusion of high-dose intravenous immunoglobulin. Pediatr. Cardiol. *21*:391–394, 2000.
43. Brown, M.: Laboratory identification of adenoviruses associated with gastroenteritis in Canada from 1983 to 1986. J. Clin. Microbiol. *28*: 1525–1529, 1990.
44. Brown, M., Rossier, E., Carpenter, B., et al.: Fatal adenovirus type 35 infection in newborns. Pediatr. Infect. Dis. J. *10*:955–956, 1991.
45. Brown, R. S., Nogrady, B., Spence, L., et al.: An outbreak of adenovirus type 7 infection in children in Montreal. Can. Med. Assoc. J. *108*:434–439, 1973.
46. Bruckova, M., Grandien, M., Pettersson, C. A., et al.: Use of nasal and pharyngeal swabs for rapid detection of respiratory syncytial virus and adenovirus antigens by enzyme-linked immunosorbent assay. J. Clin. Microbiol. *27*:1867–1869, 1989.
47. Bryant, R. E., and Rhoades, E. R.: Clinical features of adenoviral pneumonia in Air Force recruits. Am. Rev. Respir. Dis. *96*:717–723, 1967.
48. Buitenwerf, J., Louwerens, J. J., and DeJong, J. C.: A simple and rapid method for typing adenoviruses 40 and 41 without cultivation. J. Virol. Methods *10*:39–44, 1985.
49. Burns, R. P., and Potter, M. H.: Epidemic keratoconjunctivitis due to adenovirus type 19. Am. J. Ophthalmol. *81*:27–29, 1976.
50. Cames, B., Rahler, J., Burtomboy, G., et al.: Acute adenovirus hepatitis in liver transplant recipients. J. Pediatr. *120*:33–37, 1992.
51. Carballal, G., Videla, C. M., Alejandra Espinosa, M., et al.: Multicentered study of viral acute lower respiratory infections in children from four cities of Argentina, 1993–1994. J. Med. Virol. *64*:167–174, 2001.

52. Carmichael, G. P., Jr., Zahradnik, J. M., Moyer, G. H., et al.: Adenovirus hepatitis in an immunosuppressed adult patient. Am. J. Clin. Pathol. *71*:352–355, 1979.
53. Cesario, T. C., Kriel, R. L., Caldwell, G. G., et al.: Epidemiologic observations of virus infections in a closed population of young children. Am. J. Epidemiol. *94*:457–466, 1971.
54. Cevenini, R., Donati, M., Landini, M. P., et al.: Adenovirus associated with an oculo-genital infection. Microbiologica *2*:425–427, 1979.
55. Chanock, R. M., Chambon, L., Chang, W., et al.: WHO respiratory disease survey in children: A serological study. Bull. World Health Organ. *37*:363–369, 1967.
56. Chanock, R. M., Mufson, M. A., and Johnson, K. M.: Comparative biology and ecology of human virus and mycoplasma respiratory pathogens. Prog. Med. Virol. *7*:208–252, 1965.
57. Chanock, R. M., and Parrott, R. H.: Acute respiratory disease in infancy and childhood: Present understanding and prospects for prevention. Pediatrics *36*:21–39, 1965.
58. Chany, C., Lepine, P., Lelong, M., et al.: Severe and fatal pneumonia in infants and young children associated with adenovirus infections. Am. J. Hyg. *67*:367–378, 1958.
59. Chapple, P. J.: A survey of antibodies to adenovirus 8 and coxsackievirus A21 in human sera. Bull. World Health Organ. *34*:243–248, 1966.
60. Chatterjee, N. K., Samsonoff, W. A., Balasubramaniam, N., et al.: Isolation and characterization of adenovirus 5 from the brain of an infant with fatal cerebral edema. Clin. Infect. Dis. *31*:830–833, 2000.
61. Cherry, J. D.: Newer viral exanthems. Adv. Pediatr. *16*:233–286, 1969.
62. Cherry, J. D.: Newer respiratory viruses. Their role in respiratory illnesses of children. Adv. Pediatr. *20*:225–290, 1973.
63. Cherry, J. D.: Unpublished observation.
64. Chiba, S., Nakata, S., Nakamura, I., et al.: Outbreak of infantile gastroenteritis due to type 40 adenovirus. Lancet *2*:954–957, 1983.
65. Chin-Hsien, T.: Adenovirus pneumonia epidemic among Peking infants and preschool children in 1958. Chin. Med. J. *80*:331–339, 1960.
66. Chiou, C. C., Soong, W. J., Hwang, B., et al.: Congenital adenoviral infection. Pediatr. Infect. Dis. J. *13*:664–665, 1994.
67. Chou, S. M., Roos, R., Burrell, R., et al.: Subacute focal adenovirus encephalitis. J. Neuropathol. Exp. Neurol. *32*:34–50, 1973.
68. Christensen, M. L.: Human viral gastroenteritis. Clin. Microbiol. Rev. *2*: 51–89, 1989.
69. Claesson, B. A., Trollfors, B., Brolin, I., et al.: Etiology of community-acquired pneumonia in children based on antibody responses to bacterial and viral antigens. Pediatr. Infect. Dis. J. *8*:856–861, 1989.
70. Clarke, E. J., Phillips, I. A., and Alexander, E. R.: Adenovirus infection in intussusception in children in Taiwan. J. A. M. A. *208*:1671–1674, 1969.
71. Collier, A. M., Connor, J. D., and Irving, W. R., Jr.: Generalized type 5 adenovirus infection associated with the pertussis syndrome. J. Pediatr. *69*:1073–1078, 1966.
72. Commission on Acute Respiratory Diseases: Acute respiratory disease among new recruits. Am. J. Public Health *36*:439–450, 1946.
73. Connor, J. D.: Evidence for an etiologic role of adenoviral infection in pertussis syndrome. N. Engl. J. Med. *283*:390–394, 1970.
74. Connor, J. D., Buchta, R. M., DeGenaro, F., Jr., et al.: Potpourri of adenoviral infections. West. J. Med. *120*:55–61, 1974.
75. Cooney, M. K., Hall, C. E., and Fox, J. P.: The Seattle Virus Watch. III. Evaluation of isolation methods and summary of infections detected by virus isolations. Am. J. Epidemiol. *96*:286–305, 1972.
76. Cooper, R. J., Hallett, R., Tullo, A. B., et al.: The epidemiology of adenovirus infections in Greater Manchester, UK 1982–96. Epidemiol. Infect. *125*:333–345, 2000.
77. Couch, R. B., Cate, T. R., Douglas, R. G., Jr., et al.: Effect of route of inoculation on experimental respiratory viral disease in volunteers and evidence for airborne transmission. Bacteriol. Rev. *30*:517–529, 1966.
78. Couch, R. B., Cate, T. R., Fleet, W. F., et al.: Aerosol-induced adenoviral illness resembling the naturally occurring illness in military recruits. Am. Rev. Respir. Dis. *93*:529–535, 1965.
79. Couroucli, X. I., Welty, S. E., Ramsay, P. L., et al.: Detection of microorganisms in the tracheal aspirates of preterm infants by polymerase chain reaction: Association of adenovirus infection with bronchopulmonary dysplasia. Pediatr. Res. *47*:225–232, 2000.
80. Craighead, J. E.: Cytopathology of adenoviruses types 7 and 12 in human respiratory epithelium. Lab. Invest. *22*:553–557, 1970.
81. Crandell, R. A., Dowdle, W. R., Holcomb, T. M., et al.: A fatal illness associated with two viruses: An intermediate adenovirus type (21–26) and influenza A2. J. Pediatr. *72*:467–473, 1968.
82. Cukor, G., and Blacklow, N. R.: Human viral gastroenteritis. Microbiol. Rev. *48*:157–179, 1984.
83. Cumming, G. R., Macpherson, R. I., and Chernick, V.: Unilateral hyperlucent lung syndrome in children. J. Pediatr. *78*:250–260, 1971.
84. Dagan, R., Schwartz, R. H., Insel, R. A., et al.: Severe diffuse adenovirus 7a pneumonia in a child with combined immunodeficiency: Possible therapeutic effect of human immune serum globulin containing specific neutralizing antibody. Pediatr. Infect. Dis. *3*:246–250, 1984.
85. D'Ambrosio, E., Del Grosso, N., Chicca, A., et al.: Neutralizing antibodies against 33 human adenoviruses in normal children in Rome. J. Hyg. (Camb.) *89*:155–161, 1982.
86. D'Angelo, L. J., Hierholzer, J. C., Keenlyside, R. A., et al.: Pharyngoconjunctival fever caused by adenovirus type 4: Report of a swimming pool–related outbreak with recovery of virus from pool water. J. Infect. Dis. *140*:42–47, 1979.
87. Darougar, S., Quinlan, M. P., Gibson, J. A., et al.: Epidemic keratoconjunctivitis and chronic papillary conjunctivitis in London due to adenovirus type 19. Br. J. Ophthalmol. *61*:76–85, 1977.
88. Dascomb, H. E., and Hilleman, M. R.: Clinical and laboratory studies in patients with respiratory disease caused by adenoviruses (RI-APC-ARD agents). Am. J. Med. *21*:161–174, 1956.
89. Davidson, S. I.: Epidemic kerato-conjunctivitis: Report of an outbreak which resulted in ward cross-infection. Br. J. Ophthalmol. *48*:573–580, 1964.
90. Davis, B. D., Dulbecco, R., Eisen, H. N., et al.: Microbiology. Hagerstown, Harper & Row, 1973, pp. 1222–1236.
91. Davis, D., Henslee, P. J., and Markesbery, W. R.: Fatal adenovirus meningoencephalitis in a bone marrow transplant patient. Ann. Neurol. *23*:385–389, 1988.
92. Dawson, C., and Darrell, R.: Infections due to adenovirus type 8 in the United States. I. An outbreak of epidemic keratoconjunctivitis originating in a physician's office. N. Engl. J. Med. *268*:1031–1033, 1963.
93. Dawson, C., Darrell, R., Hanna, L., et al.: Infections due to adenovirus type 8 in the United States. II. Community-wide infection with adenovirus type 8. N. Engl. J. Med. *268*:1034–1037, 1963.
94. Dawson, C. R., Hanna, L., and Togni, B.: Adenovirus type 8 infections in the United States. IV. Observations on the pathogenesis of lesions in severe eye disease. Arch. Ophthalmol. *87*:258–268, 1972.
95. Dawson, C. R., O'Day, D., and Vastine, D.: Adenovirus 19, a cause of epidemic keratoconjunctivitis, not acute hemorrhagic conjunctivitis. N. Engl. J. Med. *293*:45–46, 1975.
96. Day, A. S., McGregor, D. O., Henderson, S. J., et al.: Fatal adenoviral disease in siblings. Pediatr. Infect. Dis. J. *17*:83–85, 1998.
97. de Jong, J. C., Wigand, R., Kidd, A. H., et al.: Candidate adenoviruses 40 and 41: Fastidious adenoviruses from human infant stool. J. Med. Virol. *11*:215–231, 1983.
98. de Jong, J. C., Wigand, R., Wadell, G., et al.: Adenovirus 37: Identification and characterization of a medically important new adenovirus type of subgroup D. J. Med. Virol. *7*:105–118, 1981.
99. Denny, F. W., Jr.: Viruses newly isolated from the upper respiratory tract. Pediatr. Clin. North Am. *7*:295–314, 1960.
100. Denny, F. W., Jr., and Ginsberg, H. S.: Certain biological characteristics of adenovirus types 5, 6, 7, and 14. J. Immunol. *86*:567–574, 1961.
101. deSilva, L. M., Colditz, P., and Wadell, G.: Adenovirus type 7 infections in children in New South Wales, Australia. J. Med. Virol. *29*:28–32, 1989.
102. Douglas, R. G., Jr., Alford, R. H., Cate, T. R., et al.: The leukocyte response during viral respiratory illness in man. Ann. Intern. Med. *64*:521–530, 1966.
103. Dudding, B. A., Bartelloni, P. J., Scott, R. M., et al.: Enteric immunization with live adenovirus type 21 vaccine. Infect. Immun. *5*:295–299, 1972.
104. Dudding, B. A., Top, F. H., Jr., Scott, R. M., et al.: An analysis of hospitalizations for acute respiratory disease in recruits immunized with adenovirus type 4 and type 7 vaccines. Am. J. Epidemiol. *95*: 141–147, 1972.
105. Dudding, B. A., Top, F. H., Jr., Winter, P. E., et al.: Acute respiratory disease in military trainees: The Adenovirus Surveillance Program, 1966–1971. Am. J. Epidemiol. *97*:187–198, 1973.
106. Dudding, B. A., Wagner, S. C., Zeller, J. A., et al.: Fatal pneumonia associated with adenovirus type 7 in three military trainees. N. Engl. J. Med. *286*:1289–1292, 1972.
107. Duncan, I. B. R.: Adenovirus type 15 and human thyroid tissue-culture. Lancet *1*:829–830, 1960.
108. Durepaire, N., Ranger-Rogez, S., and Denis, F.: Evaluation of rapid culture centrifugation method for adenovirus detection in stools. Diagn. Microbiol. Infect. Dis. *24*:25–29, 1996.
109. Echavarria, M. S., Ray, S. C., Ambinder, R., et al.: PCR detection of adenovirus in bone marrow transplant recipient: Hemorrhagic cystitis as a presenting manifestation of disseminated disease. J. Clin. Microbiol. *37*:686–689, 1999.
110. Edwards, K. M., Bennett, S. R., Garner, W. L., et al.: Reye's syndrome associated with adenovirus infections in infants. Am. J. Dis. Child. *139*:343–346, 1985.
111. Edwards, K. M., Thompson, J., Paolini, J., et al.: Adenovirus infections in young children. Pediatrics *76*:420–424, 1985.
112. Enders, J. F., Bell, J. A., Dingle, J. H., et al.: "Adenoviruses": Group name proposed for new respiratory-tract viruses. Science *124*:119–120, 1956.
113. Espy, M. J., Hierholzer, J. C., and Smith, T. F.: The effect of centrifugation on the rapid detection of adenovirus in shell vials. Am. J. Clin. Pathol. *88*:358–360, 1987.
114. Evans, A. S.: Acute respiratory disease in University of Wisconsin students. N. Engl. J. Med. *256*:377–384, 1957.
115. Evans, A. S.: Latent adenovirus infections of the human respiratory tract. Am. J. Hyg. *67*:256–266, 1958.

116. Evans, A. S.: Adenovirus infections in children and young adults: With comments on vaccination. N. Engl. J. Med. *259*:464–468, 1958.
117. Evans, A. S., and Dick, E. C.: Acute pharyngitis and tonsillitis in University of Wisconsin students. J. A. M. A. *190*:699–708, 1964.
118. Farkas, E., Jancso, A., and Radnot, M.: Clinical and virologic studies: On the first widespread outbreak of epidemic keratoconjunctivitis in Hungary. Am. J. Ophthalmol. *60*:78–82, 1965.
119. Faulkner, R., and Van Rooyen, C. E.: Adenoviruses types 3 and 5 isolated from the cerebrospinal fluid of children. Can. Med. Assoc. J. *87*: 1123–1125, 1962.
120. Fenner, F.: Classification and nomenclature of viruses. Intervirology *7*:1–115, 1976.
121. Fiala, M., Payne, J. E., Berne, T. V., et al.: Role of adenovirus type 11 in hemorrhagic cystitis secondary to immunosuppression. J. Urol. *112*:595–597, 1974.
122. Finn, A., Anday, E., and Talbot, G. H.: An epidemic of adenovirus 7a infection in a neonatal nursery: Course, morbidity, and management. Infect. Control Hosp. Epidemiol. *9*:398–404, 1988.
123. Flewett, T. H., Bryden, A. S., Davies, H., et al.: Epidemic viral enteritis in a long-stay children's ward. Lancet *1*:4–5, 1975.
124. Flomenberg, P., Babbitt, J., Drobyski, W. R., et al.: Increasing incidence of adenovirus disease in bone marrow transplant recipients. J. Infect. Dis. *169*:775–781, 1994.
125. Ford, E., Nelson, K. E., and Warren, D.: Epidemiology of epidemic keratoconjunctivitis. Epidemiol. Rev. *9*:244–261, 1987.
126. Forssell, P., Halonen, H., Stenstrom, R., et al.: An adenovirus epidemic due to types 1 and 2. Ann. Pediatr. Fenn. *8*:35–44, 1962.
127. Forsyth, B. R., Bloom, H. H., Johnson, K. M., et al.: Patterns of adenovirus infections in Marine Corps personnel. II. Longitudinal study of successive advanced recruit training companies. Am. J. Hyg. *80*: 343–355, 1964.
128. Forsyth, B. R., Bloom, H. H., Johnson, K. M., et al.: Etiology of primary atypical pneumonia in a military population. J. A. M. A. *191*:92–96, 1965.
129. Fox, J. P., Brandt, C. D., Wassermann, F. E., et al.: The virus watch program: A continuing surveillance of viral infections in metropolitan New York families. VI. Observations of adenovirus infections: Virus excretion patterns, antibody response, efficiency of surveillance, patterns of infection, and relation to illness. Am. J. Epidemiol. *89*:25–50, 1969.
130. Fox, J. P., Hall, C. E., and Cooney, M. K.: The Seattle virus watch. VII. Observations of adenovirus infections. Am. J. Epidemiol. *105*:362–386, 1977.
131. Foy, H. M.: Adenoviruses. *In* Evans, A. S. (ed.): Viral Infections of Humans: Epidemiology and Control. 3rd ed. New York, Plenum, 1989, pp. 77–94.
132. Foy, H. M., Cooney, M. K., Maletzky, A. J., et al.: Incidence and etiology of pneumonia, croup and bronchiolitis in preschool children belonging to a prepaid medical care group over a four-year period. Am. J. Epidemiol. *97*:80–92, 1973.
133. Foy, H. M., Cooney, M. K., McMahan, R., et al.: Viral and mycoplasmal pneumonia in a prepaid medical care group during an eight-year period. Am. J. Epidemiol. *97*:93–102, 1973.
134. Freiman, I., Super, M., Joosting, A. C. C., et al.: An epidemic of adenovirus type 7 bronchopneumonia in Bantu children. Afr. Med. J. *45*: 107–109, 1971.
135. Fuchs, E.: Keratitis punctata superficialis. Wien. Klin. Wochenschr. *2*:837–841, 1889.
136. Fukumi, H., Nishikawa, F., Kokuku, Y., et al.: Isolation of adenovirus from an exanthematous infection resembling roseola infantum. Jpn. J. Med. Sci. Biol. *10*:87–91, 1957.
137. Gabrielson, M. O., Joseph, C., and Hsiung, G. D.: Encephalitis associated with adenovirus type 7 occurring in a family outbreak. J. Pediatr. *68*:142–144, 1966.
138. Garcia, A. G. P., Fonseca, M. E. F., DeBonis, M., et al.: Morphological and virological studies in six autopsies of children with adenovirus pneumonia. Mem. Inst. Oswaldo Cruz *88*:141–147, 1993.
139. Gardner, P. S., Knox, E. G., Court, S. D. M., et al.: Virus infection and intussusception in childhood. B. M. J. *2*:697–700, 1962.
140. Gardner, P. S., McGregor, C. B., and Dick, K.: Association between diarrhoea and adenovirus type 7. B. M. J. *1*:91–93, 1960.
141. George, R. B., Ziskind, M. M., Rasch, J. R., et al.: *Mycoplasma* and adenovirus pneumonias: Comparison with other atypical pneumonias in a military population. Ann. Intern. Med. *65*:931–942, 1966.
142. Gerna, G., Cattaneo, E., Revello, M. G., et al.: Grouping of human adenoviruses by early antigen reactivity. J. Infect. Dis. *145*:678–682, 1982.
143. Ginsberg, H. S.: Characteristics of the new respiratory viruses (adenoviruses). II. Stability to temperature and pH alterations. Proc. Soc. Exp. Biol. Med. *93*:48–52, 1956.
144. Ginsberg, H. S.: Characteristics of the adenoviruses. III. Reproductive cycle of types 1 to 4. J. Exp. Med. *107*:133–152, 1958.
145. Ginsberg, H. S.: Adenoviruses. Am. J. Clin. Pathol. *57*:771–776, 1972.
146. Ginsberg, H. S., Gold, E., Jordan, W. S., Jr., et al.: Relation of the new respiratory agents to acute respiratory diseases. Am. J. Public Health *45*:915–922, 1955.
147. Ginsberg, H. S., Horswood, R. L., Chanock, R. M., et al.: Role of early genes in pathogenesis of adenovirus pneumonia. Proc. Natl. Acad. Sci. U. S. A. *87*:6191–6195, 1990.
148. Ginsberg, H. S., Moldawer, L. L., Sehgal, P. B., et al.: A mouse model for investigating the molecular pathogenesis of adenovirus pneumonia. Proc. Natl. Acad. Sci. U. S. A. *88*:1651–1655, 1991.
149. Ginsberg, H. S., and Prince, G. A.: The molecular basis of adenovirus pathogenesis. Infect. Agents Dis. *3*:1–8, 1994.
150. Glezen, W. P., Loda, F. A., Clyde, W. A., Jr., et al.: Epidemiologic patterns of acute lower respiratory disease of children in a pediatric group practice. J. Pediatr. *78*:397–406, 1971.
151. Godman, G. C., Morgan, C., Brietenfeld, P. M., et al.: A correlative study by electron and light microscopy of the development of type 5 adenovirus. II. Light microscopy. J. Exp. Med. *112*:383–401, 1960.
152. Gold, R., Wilt, J. C., Adhikari, P. K., et al.: Adenoviral pneumonia and its complications in infancy and childhood. J. Can. Assoc. Radiol. *20*:218–224, 1969.
153. Gooch, W. M., and Mogabgab, W. J.: Simultaneous oral administration of live adenovirus 4 and 7 vaccines: Protection and lack of emergency of other types. Arch. Environ. Health *25*:388–394, 1972.
154. Grabow, W. O. K., Puttergill, D. L., and Bosch, A.: Propagation of adenovirus types 40 and 41 in the PLC/PRF/5 primary liver carcinoma cell line. J. Virol. Methods *37*:201–208, 1992.
155. Grandien, M., Pettersson, C. A., Svensson, L., et al.: Latex agglutination test for adenovirus diagnosis in diarrheal disease. J. Med. Virol. *23*:311–316, 1987.
156. Gray, G. C., Goswami, P. R., Malasig, M. D., et al.: Adult adenovirus infections: Loss of orphaned vaccines precipitates military respiratory disease epidemics. Clin. Infect. Dis. *31*:663–670, 2000.
157. Grayston, J. T., Lashof, J. C., Loosli, C. G., et al.: Adenoviruses. III. Their etiological role in acute respiratory diseases in civilian adults. J. Infect. Dis. *103*:93–101, 1958.
158. Grayston, J. T., Woolridge, R. L., Loosli, C. G., et al.: Adenovirus infections in naval recruits. J. Infect. Dis. *104*:61–70, 1957.
159. Green, W. R., Greaves, W. L., Frederick, W. R., et al.: Renal infection due to adenovirus in a patient with human immunodeficiency virus infection. Clin. Infect. Dis. *18*:989–991, 1994.
160. Gresser, I., and Kibrick, S.: Isolation of vaccinia virus and type 1 adenovirus from urine. N. Engl. J. Med. *265*:743–744, 1961.
161. Griffin, J. P., and Greenberg, B. H.: Live and inactivated adenovirus vaccines: Clinical evaluation of efficacy in prevention of acute respiratory disease. Arch. Intern. Med. *125*:981–986, 1970.
162. Griffin, L. D., Kearney, D., Ni, J., et al.: Analysis of formalin-fixed and frozen myocardial autopsy samples for viral genome in childhood myocarditis and dilated cardiomyopathy with endocardial fibroelastosis using polymerase chain reaction (PCR). Cardiovasc. Pathol. *4*:3–11, 1995.
163. Gutekunst, R. R., and Heggie, A. D.: Viremia and viruria in adenovirus infections: Detection in patients with rubella or rubelliform illness. N. Engl. J. Med. *264*:374–378, 1961.
164. Guyer, B., O'Day, D. M., Hierholzer, J. C., et al.: Epidemic keratoconjunctivitis: A community outbreak of mixed adenovirus type 8 and type 19 infection. J. Infect. Dis. *132*:142–150, 1975.
165. Hale, G. A., Heslop, H. E., Krance, R. A., et al.: Adenovirus infection after pediatric bone marrow transplantation. Bone Marrow Transplant. *23*:277–282, 1999.
166. Hara, J., Ishibashi, T., Fujimoto, F., et al.: Adenovirus type 10 keratoconjunctivitis with increased intraocular pressure. Am. J. Ophthalmol. *90*:481–484, 1980.
167. Harford, C. G., Hamlin, A., Parker, E., et al.: Electron microscopy of HeLa cells infected with adenoviruses. J. Exp. Med. *104*:443–453, 1956.
168. Harnett, G. B., and Newnham, W. A.: Isolation of adenovirus type 19 from the male and female genital tracts. Br. J. Vener. Dis. *57*:55–57, 1981.
169. Harris, D. J., Wulff, H., Ray, C. G., et al.: Viruses and disease. III. An outbreak of adenovirus type 7a in a children's home. Am. J. Epidemiol. *93*:399–402, 1971.
170. Harrison, H. R., Howe, P., Minnich, L., et al.: A cluster of adenovirus 19 infections with multiple clinical manifestations. J. Pediatr. *94*:917–919, 1979.
171. Hartwell, W. V., Love, G. J., and Eidenbock, M. P.: Adenovirus in blood clots from cases of infectious hepatitis. Science *152*:1390, 1966.
172. Hatch, M. H., and Siem, R. A.: Viruses isolated from children with infectious hepatitis. Am. J. Epidemiol. *84*:495–509, 1966.
173. Henderson, Y. C., Liu, T. J., and Clayman, G. L.: A simple and sensitive method for detecting adenovirus in serum and urine. J. Virol. Methods *71*:51–56, 1998.
174. Henson, D., and Mufson, M. A.: Myocarditis and pneumonitis with type 21 adenovirus infection: Association with fatal myocarditis and pneumonitis. Am. J. Dis. Child. *121*:334–339, 1971.
175. Herbert, F. A., Wilkinson, D., Burchak, E., et al.: Adenovirus type 3 pneumonia causing lung damage in childhood. Can. Med. Assoc. J. *116*: 274–276, 1977.
176. Herbert, H.: Superficial punctate keratitis associated with an encapsulated bacillus. Ophthalmol. Rev. *20*:339–345, 1901.

177. Herrmann, E. C., Jr.: Experiences in laboratory diagnosis of adenovirus infections in routine medical practice. Mayo Clin. Proc. *43*:635–644, 1968.
178. Herrmann, J. E., Perron-Henry, D. M., and Blacklow, N. R.: Antigen detection with monoclonal antibodies for the diagnosis of adenovirus gastroenteritis. J. Infect. Dis. *155*:1167–1171, 1987.
179. Hierholzer, J. C.: Further subgrouping of the human adenoviruses by differential hemagglutination. J. Infect. Dis. *128*:541–550, 1973.
180. Hierholzer, J. C., Atuk, N. O., and Gwaltney, J. M., Jr.: New human adenovirus isolated from a renal transplant recipient: Description and characterization of candidate adenovirus type 34. J. Clin. Microbiol. *1*:366–376, 1975.
181. Hierholzer, J. C., and Bingham, P. G.: Vero microcultures for adenovirus neutralization tests. J. Clin. Microbiol. *7*:499–506, 1978.
182. Hierholzer, J. C., Gamble, W. C., and Dowdle, W. R.: Reference equine antisera to 33 human adenovirus types: Homologous and heterologous titers. J. Clin. Microbiol. *1*:65–74, 1975.
183. Hierholzer, J. C., Kemp, M. C., Gary, G. W., Jr., et al.: New human adenovirus associated with respiratory illness: Candidate adenovirus type 39. J. Clin. Microbiol. *16*:15–21, 1982.
184. Hierholzer, J. C., Pumarola, A., Rodriguez-Torres, A., et al.: Occurrence of respiratory illness due to an atypical strain of adenovirus type 11 during a large outbreak in Spanish military recruits. Am. J. Epidemiol. *99*:434–442, 1974.
185. Hierholzer, J. C., Stone, Y. O., and Broderson, J. R.: Antigenic relationships among the 47 human adenoviruses determined in reference horse antisera. Arch. Virol. *121*:179–197, 1991.
186. Hierholzer, J. C., Torrence, A. E., and Wright, P. F.: Generalized viral illness caused by an intermediate strain of adenovirus (21/H21+35). J. Infect. Dis. *141*:281–288, 1980.
187. Hilleman, M. R.: Epidemiology of adenovirus respiratory infections in military recruit populations. Ann. N. Y. Acad. Sci. *67*:262–272, 1957.
188. Hilleman, M. R., Tousimis, A. J., and Werner, J. H.: Biophysical characterization of the RI (RI-67) viruses. Proc. Soc. Exp. Biol. Med. *89*: 587–593, 1955.
189. Hilleman, M. R., and Werner, J. H.: Recovery of new agent from patients with acute respiratory illness. Proc. Soc. Exp. Biol. Med. *85*:183–188, 1954.
190. Hillis, W. D., Cooper, M. R., and Bang, F. B.: Adenovirus infections in West Bengal. I. Persistence of viruses in infants and young children. Indian J. Med. Res. *61*:1–9, 1973.
191. Hogan, M. J., and Crawford, J. W.: Epidemic keratoconjunctivitis (superficial punctate keratitis, keratitis subepithelialis, keratitis maculosa, keratitis nummularis): With a review of the literature and a report of 125 cases. Am. J. Ophthalmol. *25*:1059–1078, 1942.
192. Holmes, W. J.: Epidemic infectious conjunctivitis. Hawaii Med. J. *1*:11–12, 1941.
193. Holzel, A., Parker, L., Patterson, W. H., et al.: Virus isolations from throats of children admitted to hospital with respiratory and other diseases: Manchester 1962–1964. B. M. J. *1*:614–619, 1965.
194. Horn, M. E. C., Brain, E., Gregg, I., et al.: Respiratory viral infection in childhood: A survey in general practice, Roehampton 1967–1972. J. Hyg. (Camb.) *74*:157–168, 1975.
195. Horne, R. W., Brenner, S., Waterson, A. P., et al.: The icosahedral form of an adenovirus. J. Mol. Biol. *1*:84–86, 1959.
196. Horwitz, M. S.: *Adenoviridae* and their replication. *In* Fields, B. N., Knipe, D. M., Chanock, R. M., et al.: Virology. 2nd ed. New York, Raven Press, 1990, pp. 1679–1721.
197. Horwitz, M. S.: Adenoviruses. *In* Knipe, D. M., and Howley, P. M. (eds.): Virology. 4th ed. Philadelphia, Lippincott Williams & Wilkins, 2001, pp. 2301–2326.
198. Howard, D. S., Phillips, G. L., II, Reece, D. E., et al.: Adenovirus infections in hematopoietic stem cell transplant recipients. Clin. Infect. Dis. *29*:1494–1501, 1999.
199. Hsu, H. Y., Kao, C. L., Huang, L. M., et al.: Viral etiology of intussusception in Taiwanese childhood. Pediatr. Infect. Dis. J. *17*:893–898, 1998.
200. Huebner, R. J., Casey, M. J., Chanock, R. M., et al.: Tumors induced in hamsters by a strain of adenovirus type 3: Sharing of tumor antigens and neoantigens with those produced by adenovirus type 7 tumors. Proc. Natl. Acad. Sci. U. S. A. *54*:381–388, 1965.
201. Huebner, R. J., Rowe, W. P., and Chanock, R. M.: Newly recognized respiratory tract viruses. Annu. Rev. Microbiol. *12*:49–76, 1958.
202. Huebner, R. J., Rowe, W. P., Ward, T. G., et al.: Adenoidal-pharyngeal-conjunctival agents: A newly recognized group of common viruses of the respiratory system. N. Engl. J. Med. *251*:1077–1086, 1954.
203. Hypia, T.: Detection of adenovirus in nasopharyngeal specimens by radioactive and nonradioactive DNA probes. J. Clin. Microbiol. *21*:730–733, 1985.
204. Ieven, M., Van Reempts, P., Overmeier, B. V., et al.: A pseudoepidemic of adenoviruses in a neonatal care unit. Diagn. Microbiol. Infect. Dis. *18*:157–159, 1994.
205. Imre, G., Korchmaros, I., Geck, P., et al.: Antigenic specificity of inclusion bodies in epidemic keratoconjunctivitis. Ophthalmologica *148*:7–12, 1964.
206. Inderlied, C., and Church, J. A.: Adenovirus viremia in human immunodeficiency virus–infected children. Pediatr. Infect. Dis. J. *16*:413–415, 1997.
207. Jackson, G. G., and Muldoon, R. L.: Viruses causing common respiratory infection in man. IV. Reoviruses and adenoviruses. J. Infect. Dis. *128*: 811–866, 1973.
208. Jaffe, B. F., and Maassab, H. F.: Sudden deafness associated with adenovirus infection. N. Engl. J. Med. *276*:1406–1408, 1967.
209. James, A. G., Lang, W. R., Liang, A. Y., et al.: Adenovirus type 21 bronchopneumonia in infants and young children. J. Pediatr. *95*:530–533, 1979.
210. Jansson, E., and Wager, O.: Adenovirus antibodies in patients with respiratory infection. Ann. Med. Intern. Fenn. *50*:221–227, 1961.
211. Jansson, E., Wager, O., Forssell, P., et al.: An exanthema subitum–like rash in patients with adenovirus infection. Ann. Paediatr. Fenn. *7*:3–11, 1961.
212. Jansson, E., Wager, O., Forssell, P., et al.: Epidemic occurrence of adenovirus type 7 infection in Helsinki. Ann. Paediatr. Fenn. *8*:24–34, 1962.
213. Jawetz, E.: The story of shipyard eye. B. M. J. *1*:873–876, 1959.
214. Jernigan, J. A., Lowry, B. S., Hayden, F. G., et al.: Adenovirus type 8 epidemic keratoconjunctivitis in an eye clinic: Risk factors and control. J. Infect. Dis. *167*:307–313, 1993.
215. Johansson, M. E., Uhnoo, I., Kidd, A. H., et al.: Direct identification of enteric adenovirus, a candidate new serotype, associated with infantile gastroenteritis. J. Clin. Microbiol. *12*:95–100, 1980.
216. Joncas, J., Moisan, A., and Pavilanis, V.: Incidence of adenovirus infection: A family study. Can. Med. Assoc. J. *87*:52–58, 1962.
217. Jordan, W. S., Jr., Badger, G. F., Curtiss, C., et al.: A study of illness in a group of Cleveland families. X. The occurrence of adenovirus infections. Am. J. Hyg. *64*:336–348, 1956.
218. Kajon, A. E., Murtagh, P., Franco, S. G., et al.: A new genome type of adenovirus 3 associated with severe lower acute respiratory infection in children. J. Med. Virol. *30*:73–76, 1990.
219. Kajon, A. E., and Wadell, G.: Molecular epidemiology of adenoviruses associated with acute lower respiratory disease of children in Buenos Aires, Argentina (1984–1988). J. Med. Virol. *36*:292–297, 1992.
220. Kapelushnik, J., Or, R., Delukina, M., et al.: Intravenous ribavirin therapy for adenovirus gastroenteritis after bone marrow transplantation. J. Pediatr. Gastroenterol. Nutr. *21*:110–112, 1995.
221. Kasel, J. A., Banks, P. A., Wigand, R., et al.: An immunologic classification of heterotypic antibody responses to adenoviruses in man. Proc. Soc. Exp. Biol. Med. *119*:1162–1165, 1965.
222. Kasel, J. A., Evans, H. E., Spickard, A., et al.: Conjunctivitis and enteric infection with adenovirus types 26 and 27: Responses to primary, secondary and reciprocal cross-challenges. Am. J. Hyg. *77*:265–282, 1963.
223. Kasova, V., Brackova, M., Kotelensky, F., et al.: Isolation of adenovirus type 29 from an outbreak of epidemic keratoconjunctivitis. Acta Virol. *21*:173, 1977.
224. Keenlyside, R. A., Hierholzer, J. C., and D'Angelo, L. J.: Keratoconjunctivitis associated with adenovirus type 37: An extended outbreak in an ophthalmologist's office. J. Infect. Dis. *147*:191–198, 1983.
225. Keller, E. W., Rubin, R. H., Black, P. H., et al.: Isolation of adenovirus type 34 from a renal transplant recipient with interstitial pneumonia. Transplantation *23*:188–191, 1977.
226. Kelsey, D. S.: Adenovirus meningoencephalitis. Pediatrics *61*:291–293, 1978.
227. Kemp, M. C., Hierholzer, J. C., Cabradilla, C. P., et al.: The changing etiology of epidemic keratoconjunctivitis: Antigenic and restriction enzyme analyses of adenovirus types 19 and 37 isolated over a 10-year period. J. Infect. Dis. *148*:24–33, 1983.
228. Kendall, E. J. C., Cook, G. T., and Stone, D. M.: Acute respiratory infections in children: Isolation of Coxsackie B virus and adenovirus during a survey in a general practice. B. M. J. *2*:1180–1184, 1960.
229. Kidd, A. H., Cosgrove, B. P., Brown, R. A., et al.: Faecal adenoviruses from Glasgow babies: Studies on culture and identity. J. Hyg. (Camb.) *88*:463–474, 1982.
230. Kidd, A. H., Jonsson, M., Garwicz, D., et al.: Rapid subgenus identification of human adenovirus isolates by a general PCR. J. Clin. Microbiol. *34*:622–627, 1996.
231. Kim, K. S.: Fatal pneumonia caused by adenovirus type 35. Am. J. Dis. Child. *135*:473–475, 1981.
232. Kim, Y. J., Schmidt, N. J., and Mirkovic, R. R.: Isolation of an intermediate type of adenovirus from a child with fulminant hepatitis. J. Infect. Dis. *152*:844, 1985.
233. Kinney, J. S., Hierholzer, J. C., and Thibeault, D. W.: Neonatal pulmonary insufficiency caused by adenovirus infection successfully treated with extracorporeal membrane oxygenation. J. Pediatr. *125*:110–112, 1994.
234. Kirkpatrick, H.: An epidemic of macular keratitis. Br. J. Ophthalmol. *4*:16–20, 1920.
235. Kjellen, L., Sterner, G., and Svedmyr, A.: On the occurrence of adenoviruses in Sweden. Acta Paediatr. *46*:164–176, 1957.
236. Kjer, P., and Mordhorst, C. H.: Studies on an epidemic of keratoconjunctivitis caused by adenovirus type 8. II. Clinical and epidemiological aspects. Acta Ophthalmol. *39*:984–992, 1961.

237. Knight, V., and Kasel, J. A.: Adenoviruses. *In* Knight, V. (ed.): Viral and Mycoplasmal Infections of the Respiratory Tract. Philadelphia, Lea & Febiger, 1973, pp. 65–86.
238. Koneru, B., Jaffe, R., Esquivel, C. O., et al.: Adenoviral infections in pediatric liver transplant recipients. J. A. M. A. *258*:489–492, 1987.
239. Kotloff, K. L., Losonsky, G. A., Morris, J. G., Jr., et al.: Enteric adenovirus infection and childhood diarrhea: An epidemiologic study in three clinical settings. Pediatrics *84*:219–225, 1989.
240. Krajden, M., Brown, M., Petrasek, A., et al.: Clinical features of adenovirus enteritis: A review of 127 cases. Pediatr. Infect. Dis. J. *9*:636–641, 1990.
241. Kuei-Fang, J., Ying, T., Yu-Ch'un, L., et al.: The role of adenovirus in the etiology of infantile pneumonia and pneumonia complicating measles. Chin. Med. J. *81*:141–146, 1962.
242. Ladisch, S., Lovejoy, F. H., Hierholzer, J. C., et al.: Extrapulmonary manifestations of adenovirus type 7 pneumonia simulating Reye syndrome and the possible role of an adenovirus toxin. J. Pediatr. *95*:348–355, 1979.
243. Lähdeaho, M. L., Parkkonen, P., Reunala, T., et al.: Antibodies to E1b protein–derived peptides of enteric adenovirus type 40 are associated with celiac disease and dermatitis herpetiformis. Clin. Immunol. Immunopathol. *69*:300–305, 1993.
244. Lang, W. R., Howden, C. W., Laws, J., et al.: Bronchopneumonia with serious sequelae in children with evidence of adenovirus type 21 infection. B. M. J. *1*:73–79, 1969.
245. Lange, W.: Über eine eigentumliche Erkrankung der kleinen Bronchien und Bronchiolen. Dtsch. Arch. Klin. Med. *70*:342, 1901.
246. Larrañaga, C., Kajon, A., Villagra, E., et al.: Adenovirus surveillance on children hospitalized for acute lower respiratory infections in Chile (1988–1996). J. Med. Virol. *60*:342–346, 2000.
247. Laverty, C. R., Russell, P., Black, J., et al.: Adenovirus infection of the cervix. Acta Cytol. *21*:114–117, 1977.
248. Lee, H. J., Pyo, J. W., Choi, E. H., et al.: Isolation of adenovirus type 7 from the urine of children with acute hemorrhagic cystitis. Pediatr. Infect. Dis. J. *15*:633–634, 1996.
249. Lee, S. G., and Hung, P. P.: Vaccines for control of respiratory disease caused by adenoviruses. Rev. Med. Virol. *3*:209–216, 1993.
250. Lehrich, J. R., Kasel, J. A., and Rossen, R. D.: Immunoglobulin classes of neutralizing antibody formed after human inoculation with soluble adenoviral antigens. J. Immunol. *97*:654–662, 1966.
251. Lennette, E. H., and Schmidt, N. J. (eds.): Diagnostic Procedures for Viral and Rickettsial Infections. 4th ed. New York, American Public Health Association, 1969, pp. 205–225.
252. Levandowski, R. A., and Rubenis, M.: Nosocomial conjunctivitis caused by adenovirus type 4. J. Infect. Dis. *143*:28–31, 1981.
253. Levin, S., Dietrich, J., and Guillory, J.: Fatal nonbacterial pneumonia associated with adenovirus type 4: Occurrence in an adult. J. A. M. A. *201*:155–157, 1967.
254. Lew, J. F., Glass, R. I., Petric, M., et al.: Six-year retrospective surveillance of gastroenteritis viruses identified at 10 electron microscopy centers in the United States and Canada. Pediatr. Infect. Dis. J. *9*: 709–714, 1990.
255. Li, Q. G., and Wadell, G.: Analysis of 15 different genome types of adenovirus type 7 isolated on five continents. J. Virol. *60*:331–335, 1986.
256. Liles, W. C., Cushing, H., Holt, S., et al.: Severe adenoviral nephritis following bone marrow transplantation. Bone Marrow Transplant. *12*: 409–412, 1993.
257. Loda, F. A., Clyde, W. A., Jr., Glezen, W. P., et al.: Studies on the role of viruses, bacteria, and *M. pneumoniae* as causes of lower respiratory tract infections in children. J. Pediatr. *72*:161–176, 1968.
258. Loda, F. A., Glezen, W. P., and Clyde, W. A., Jr.: Respiratory disease in group day care. Pediatrics *49*:428–437, 1972.
259. Lonberg-Holm, K., and Philipson, L.: Early events of virus-cell interaction in an adenovirus system. J. Virol. *4*:323–338, 1969.
260. Londergan, T. A., and Walzak, M. P.: Hemorrhagic cystitis due to adenovirus infection following bone marrow transplantation. J. Urol. *151*:1013–1014, 1994.
261. Lord, A., Sutton, R. N. P., and Corsellis, J. A. N.: Recovery of adenovirus type 7 from human brain cell cultures. J. Neurol. Neurosurg. Psychiatry *38*:710–712, 1975.
262. Lozinki, G. N., Davis, G., Kraus, H. F., et al.: Adenovirus myocarditis: Retrospective diagnosis by gene amplification from formalin-fixed paraffin-embedded tissues. Hum. Pathol. *25*:831–834, 1994.
263. Maček, V., Sorli, J., Kopriva, S., et al.: Persistent adenoviral infection and chronic airway obstruction in children. Am. J. Respir. Crit. Care Med. *150*:7–10, 1994.
264. Macpherson, R. I., Cumming, G. R., and Chernick, V.: Unilateral hyperlucent lung: A complication of viral pneumonia. J. Can. Assoc. Radiol. *20*:225–231, 1969.
265. Mahafzah, A. M., and Landry, M. L.: Evaluation of immunofluorescent reagents, centrifugation, and conventional cultures for the diagnosis of adenovirus infection. Diagn. Microbiol. Infect. Dis. *12*:407–411, 1989.
266. Maisel, J. C., Pierce, W. E., Crawford, Y. E., et al.: Virus pneumonia and adenovirus infection: A reappraisal. Am. J. Hyg. *75*:56–68, 1962.
267. Maletzky, A. J., Cooney, M. K., Luce, R., et al.: Epidemiology of viral and mycoplasmal agents associated with childhood lower respiratory illness in a civilian population. J. Pediatr. *78*:407–414, 1971.
268. Martin, A. B., Webber, S., Fricker, F. J., et al.: Acute myocarditis. Rapid diagnosis by PCR in children. Circulation *90*:330–339, 1994.
269. Martone, W. J., Hierholzer, J. C., Keenlyside, R. A., et al.: An outbreak of adenovirus type 3 disease at a private recreation center swimming pool. Am. J. Epidemiol. *111*:229–237, 1980.
270. Matsubara, T., Inoue, T., Tashiro, N., et al.: Activation of peripheral blood $CD8^+$ T cells in adenovirus infection. Pediatr. Infect. Dis. J. *19*: 766–768, 2000.
271. Matsuoka, T., Naito, T., Kubota, Y., et al.: Disseminated adenovirus (type 19) infection in a neonate: Rapid detection of the infection by immunofluorescence. Acta Paediatr. *79*:568–571, 1990.
272. McCarthy, A. J., Bergin, M., DeSilva, L. M., et al.: Intravenous ribavirin therapy for disseminated adenovirus infection. Pediatr. Infect. Dis. J. *14*: 1003–1004, 1995.
273. McCormick, D. P., Wenzel, R. P., Davies, J. A., et al.: Nasal secretion protein responses in patients with wild-type adenovirus disease. Infect. Immun. *6*:282–288, 1972.
274. McNamara, M. J., Pierce, W. E., Crawford, Y. E., et al.: Patterns of adenovirus infection in the respiratory diseases of naval recruits: A longitudinal study of two companies of naval recruits. Am. Rev. Respir. Dis. *86*:485–494, 1962.
275. Melnick, J. L.: Taxonomy of viruses, 1976. Prog. Med. Virol. *22*:211–221, 1976.
276. Meurman, O., Ruuskanen, O., and Sarkkinen, H.: Immunoassay diagnosis of adenovirus infections in children. J. Clin. Microbiol. *18*:1190–1195, 1983.
277. Meyer, K., Girgis, N., and McGravey, V.: Adenovirus associated with congenital pleural effusion. J. Pediatr. *107*:433–435, 1985.
278. Michaels, M. G., Green, M., Wald, E. R., et al.: Adenovirus infection in pediatric liver transplant recipients. J. Infect. Dis. *165*:170–174, 1992.
279. Mikol, J., Felten-Papaiconomou, A., Ferchal, F., et al.: Inclusion-body myositis: Clinicopathological studies and isolation of an adenovirus type 2 from muscle biopsy specimen. Ann. Neurol. *11*:576–581, 1982.
280. Miller, D. G., Gabrielson, M. O., and Horstmann, D. M.: Clinical virology and viral surveillance in a pediatric group practice: The use of double-seeded tissue culture tubes for primary virus isolation. Am. J. Epidemiol. *88*:245–256, 1968.
281. Mistchenko, A. S., Diez, R. A., Mariani, A. L., et al.: Cytokines in adenoviral disease in children: Association of interleukin-6, interleukin-8, and tumor necrosis factor alpha levels with clinical outcome. J. Pediatr. *124*:714–720, 1994.
282. Mistchenko, A. S., Huberman, K. H., Gomez, J. A., et al.: Epidemiology of enteric adenovirus infection in prospectively monitored Argentine families. Epidemiol. Infect. *109*:539–546, 1992.
283. Mistchenko, A. S., Maffey, A. F., Casal, G., et al.: Adenoviral pericarditis: High levels of interleukin-6 in pericardial fluid. Pediatr. Infect. Dis. J. *14*:1007–1009, 1995.
284. Mistchenko, A. S., Robaldo, J. F., Rosman, F. C., et al.: Fatal adenovirus infection with new genome type. J. Med. Virol. *54*:233–236, 1998.
285. Mitchell, L. S., Taylor, B., Reimels, W., et al.: Adenovirus 7a: A community-acquired outbreak in a children's hospital. Pediatr. Infect. Dis. J. *19*:996–1000, 2000.
286. Mitsui, Y., Hanna, L., Hanabusa, J., et al.: Association of adenovirus type 8 with epidemic keratoconjunctivitis. Arch. Ophthalmol. *61*:891–898, 1959.
287. Moffet, H. L., Siegel, A. C., and Doyle, H. K.: Nonstreptococcal pharyngitis. J. Pediatr. *73*:51–60, 1968.
288. Mordhorst, C. H., and Kjer, P.: Studies on an epidemic of keratoconjunctivitis caused by adenovirus type 8. I. Virus isolation in human amniotic cells, and serological observations. Acta Ophthalmol. *39*:974–983, 1961.
289. Morris, D. J., Cooper, R. J., Barr, T., et al.: Polymerase chain reaction for rapid diagnosis of respiratory adenovirus infection. J. Infect. *32*:113–117, 1996.
290. Mueller, R. E., Muldoon, R. L., and Jackson, G. G.: Communicability of enteric live adenovirus type 4 vaccine in families. J. Infect. Dis. *119*:60–66, 1969.
291. Mufson, M. A., and Belshe, R. B.: A review of adenoviruses in the etiology of acute hemorrhagic cystitis. J. Urol. *115*:191–194, 1976.
292. Mufson, M. A., Belshe, R. B., Horrigan, T. J., et al.: Cause of acute hemorrhagic cystitis in children. Am. J. Dis. Child. *126*:605–609, 1973.
293. Mufson, M. A., Krause, H. E., Mocega, H. E., et al.: Viruses, *Mycoplasma pneumoniae* and bacteria associated with lower respiratory tract disease among infants. Am. J. Epidemiol. *91*:192–202, 1970.
294. Mufson, M. A., Zollar, L. M., Mankad, V. N., et al.: Adenovirus infection in acute hemorrhagic cystitis. Am. J. Dis. Child. *121*:281–285, 1971.
295. Munoz, F. M., Piedra, P. A., Demmler, G. L.: Disseminated adenovirus disease in immunocompromised and immunocompetent children. Clin. Infect. Dis. *27*:1194–1200, 1998.
296. Murphy, G. F., Wood, D. P., Jr., McRoberts, J. W., et al: Adenovirus associated haemorrhagic cystitis treated with intravenous ribavirin. J. Urol. *149*:565–566, 1993.

297. Myerowitz, R. L., Stalder, H., Oxman, M. N., et al.: Fatal disseminated adenovirus infection in a renal transplant recipient. Am. J. Med. *59*:591–598, 1975.
298. Nahmias, A. J., Griffith, D., and Snitzer, J.: Fatal pneumonia associated with adenovirus type 7. Am. J. Dis. Child. *114*:36–41, 1967.
299. Naveh, Y., and Friedman, A.: Orchitis associated with adenoviral infection. Am. J. Dis. Child. *129*:257–258, 1975.
300. Nelson, K. E., Gavitt, F., Batt, M. D., et al.: The role of adenoviruses in the pertussis syndrome. J. Pediatr. *86*:335–341, 1975.
301. Nemir, R. L., O'Hare, D., Goldstein, S., et al.: Adenovirus complement-fixing antibody titers from birth through the first year of life: A longitudinal study. Pediatrics *32*:497–500, 1963.
302. Neva, F. A., and Enders, J. F.: Isolation of a cytopathogenic agent from an infant with a disease in certain respects resembling roseola infantum. J. Immunol. *72*:315–321, 1954.
303. Newland, J. C., and Cooney, M. K.: Characteristics of an adenovirus type 19 conjunctivitis isolate and evidence for a subgroup associated with epidemic conjunctivitis. Infect. Immun. *21*:303–309, 1978.
304. Niemann, T. H., Trigg, M. E., Winick, N., et al.: Disseminated adenoviral infection presenting as acute pancreatitis. Hum. Pathol. *24*:1145–1148, 1993.
305. Noda, M., Miyamoto, Y., Ikeda, Y., et al.: Intermediate human adenovirus type 22/H10, 19, 37 as a new etiological agent of conjunctivitis. J. Clin. Microbiol. *29*:1286–1289, 1991.
306. Norrby, E.: Biological significance of structural adenovirus components. Curr. Top. Microbiol. *43*:1–43, 1968.
307. Norrby, E.: The structural and functional diversity of adenovirus capsid components. J. Gen. Virol. *5*:221–236, 1969.
308. Numazaki, Y., Kumasaka, T., Yano, N., et al.: Further study on acute hemorrhagic cystitis due to adenovirus type 11. N. Engl. J. Med. *289*: 344–347, 1973.
309. Numazaki, Y., Yano, N., Ikeda, M., et al.: Adenovirus infection in intussusception of Japanese infants. Jpn. J. Microbiol. *17*:87–89, 1973.
310. Odio, C., McCracken, G. H., Jr., and Nelson, J. D.: Disseminated adenovirus infection: A case report and review of literature. Pediatr. Infect. Dis. *2*:46–48, 1984.
311. Ohori, N. P., Michaels, M. G., Jaffe, R., et al.: Adenovirus pneumonia in lung transplant recipients. Hum. Pathol. *26*:1073–1079, 1995.
312. Oishi, I., Yamazaki, K., Minekawa, Y., et al.: Three-year survey of the epidemiology of rotavirus, enteric adenovirus, and some small spherical viruses including "Osaka-agent" associated with infantile diarrhea. Biken J. *28*:9–19, 1985.
313. Olson, L. C., Miller, G., and Hanshaw, J. B.: Acute infectious lymphocytosis presenting as a pertussis-like illness: Its association with adenovirus type 12. Lancet *1*:200–201, 1964.
314. Osamura, T., Mizuta, R., Yoshioka, H., et al.: Isolation of adenovirus type 11 from the brain of a neonate with pneumonia and encephalitis. Eur. J. Pediatr. *152*:496–499, 1993.
315. Pacini, D. L., Collier, A. M., and Henderson, F. W.: Adenovirus infections and respiratory illnesses in children in group day care. J. Infect. Dis. *156*:920–927, 1987.
316. Pacini, D. L., Dubovi, E. J., and Clyde, W. A., Jr.: A new animal model for human respiratory tract disease due to adenovirus. J. Infect. Dis. *150*:92–97, 1984.
317. Paderstein, R.: Was ist schwimmbad-konjunktivitis? Klin. Monatsbl. Augenheilk. *74*:634–642, 1925.
318. Panush, R. S.: Adenovirus arthritis. Arthritis Rheum. *17*:534–536, 1974.
319. Papapetropoulou, M. and Vantarakis, A. C.: Detection of adenovirus outbreak at a municipal swimming pool by nested PCR amplification. J. Infect. *36*:101–103, 1998.
320. Parizhskaya, M., Walpusk, J., Mazariegos, G., et al.: Enteric adenovirus infection in pediatric small bowel transplant recipients. Pediatr. Dev. Pathol. *4*:122–128, 2001.
321. Parker, W. L., Wilt, J. C., and Stakiw, W.: Adenovirus infections. Can. J. Public Health *52*:246–251, 1961.
322. Parks, W. P., Boucher, D. W., Milnick, J. L., et al.: Seroepidemiological and ecological studies of the adenovirus-associated satellite viruses. Infect. Immun. *2*:716–722, 1970.
323. Parrott, R. H.: Newly isolated viruses in respiratory disease. Pediatrics *20*:1066–1083, 1957.
324. Parrott, R. H.: Viral respiratory tract illnesses in children. Bull. N. Y. Acad. Med. *39*:629–648, 1963.
325. Parrott, R. H., Rowe, W. P., Huebner, R. J., et al.: Outbreak of febrile pharyngitis and conjunctivitis associated with type 3 adenoidal-pharyngeal-conjunctival virus infection. N. Engl. J. Med. *251*: 1087–1090, 1954.
326. Pearson, R. D., Hall, W. J., Menegus, M. A., et al.: Diffuse pneumonitis due to adenovirus type 21 in a civilian. Chest *78*:107–109, 1980.
327. Pereira, H. G.: Typing of adenoidal-pharyngeal-conjunctival (APC) viruses by complement-fixation. J. Pathol. Bacteriol. *72*:105–109, 1956.
328. Pereira, H. G.: A protein factor responsible for the early cytopathic effect of adenoviruses. Microbiology *6*:601–611, 1958.
329. Pereira, M. S.: Adenovirus infections. Postgrad. Med. J. *49*:798–801, 1973.
330. Pereira, M. S., and MacCallum, F. O.: Infection with adenovirus type 12. Lancet *1*:198–199, 1964.
331. Pettit, T. H., and Holland, G. N.: Chronic keratoconjunctivitis associated with ocular adenovirus infection. Am. J. Ophthalmol. *88*:748–751, 1979.
332. Pichler, M. N., Reichenbach, J., Schmidt, H., et al.: Severe adenovirus bronchiolitis in children. Acta Paediatr. *89*:1387–1392, 2000.
333. Piedra, P. A., Kasel, J. A., Norton, H. J., et al.: Description of an adenovirus type 8 outbreak in hospitalized neonates born prematurely. Pediatr. Infect. Dis. J. *11*:460–465, 1992.
334. Pina, M., and Green, M.: Biochemical studies on adenovirus multiplication. IX. Chemical and base composition analysis of 28 human adenoviruses. Proc. Natl. Acad. Sci. U. S. A. *54*:547–551, 1965.
335. Pingleton, S. K., Pingleton, W. W., Hill, R. H., et al.: Type 3 adenoviral pneumonia occurring in a respiratory intensive care unit. Chest *73*:554–555, 1978.
336. Pinkerton, H., and Carroll, S.: Fatal adenovirus pneumonia in infants: Correlation of histologic and electron microscopic observations. Am. J. Pathol. *65*:543–548, 1971.
337. Poerregaard, A., Hjelt, K., Genner, J., et al.: Role of enteric adenoviruses in acute gastroenteritis in children attending day-care centres. Acta Paediatr. *79*:370–371, 1990.
338. Portnoy, B., Salvatore, M. A., Hanes, B., et al.: The sensitivity of the complement fixation test for the detection of adenovirus infections in infants and children with lower respiratory disease. Am. J. Epidemiol. *86*:362–372, 1967.
339. Potter, C. W.: Adenovirus infection as an aetiological factor in intussusception of infants and young children. J. Pathol. Bacteriol. *88*:263–274, 1964.
340. Prage, L., Pettersson, U., and Philipson, L.: Internal basic proteins in adenovirus. Virology *36*:508–511, 1968.
341. Prince, R. L.: Evidence for an aetiological role for adenovirus type 7 in the mesenteric adenitis syndrome. Med. J. Aust. *2*:56–57, 1979.
342. Putto, A., Ruuskanen, O., and Meurman, O.: Fever in respiratory virus infections. Am. J. Dis. Child. *140*:1159–1163, 1986.
343. Rafajko, R. R.: Differences in cytopathic effects of adenovirus in monkey kidney tissue culture. Proc. Soc. Exp. Biol. Med. *119*:975–982, 1965.
344. Ray, C. G., and Minnich, L. L.: Efficiency of immunofluorescence for rapid detection of common respiratory viruses. J. Clin. Microbiol. *25*:355–357, 1987.
345. Retter, M., Middleton, P. J., Tam, J. S., et al.: Enteric adenoviruses: Detection, replication, and significance. J. Clin. Microbiol. *10*:574–578, 1979.
346. Reuss, V. A.: Keratitis maculosa. Wien. Klin. Wochenschr. *2*:665–666, 1889.
347. Reynolds, M. A., Hart, C. A., Sills, J. A., et al.: Two cases of adenovirus type 1 pneumonia: Diagnosis by direct electron microscopy and culture. Pediatr. Infect. Dis. *5*:105–107, 1986.
348. Ribaud, P., Scieux, C., Freymuth, F., et al.: Successful treatment of adenovirus disease with intravenous cidofovir in an unrelated stem-cell transplant recipient. Clin. Infect. Dis. *28*:690–691, 1999.
349. Richmond, S. J., Caul, E. O., Dunn, S. M., et al.: An outbreak of gastroenteritis in young children caused by adenoviruses. Lancet *1*:1178–1180, 1979.
350. Rodriguez, W. J., Kim, H. W., Brandt, C. D., et al.: Fecal adenoviruses from a longitudinal study of families in metropolitan Washington, D.C.: Laboratory, clinical, and epidemiologic observations. J. Pediatr. *107*:514–520, 1985.
351. Roggendorf, M., Wigand, R., Deinhardt, F., et al.: Enzyme-linked immunosorbent assay for acute adenovirus infection. J. Virol. Methods *4*:27–35, 1982.
352. Romano, A., Revel, M., Guarari-Rotman, D., et al.: Use of human fibroblast-derived (beta) interferon in the treatment of epidemic adenovirus keratoconjunctivitis. J. Interferon Res. *1*:95–100, 1980.
353. Roos, R., Chou, S. M., Basnight, M., et al.: Isolation of an adenovirus 32 strain from human brain in a case of subacute encephalitis. Proc. Soc. Exp. Biol. Med. *139*:636–640, 1972.
354. Rose, H. M., Lamson, R. H., and Buescher, E. L.: Adenoviral infection in military recruits: Emergence of type 7 and 21 infections in recruits immunized with type 4 oral vaccine. Arch. Environ. Health *21*:356–361, 1970.
355. Rosen, L.: A hemagglutination-inhibition technique for typing adenoviruses. Am. J. Hyg. *71*:120–128, 1959.
356. Ross, J. G., Potter, C. W., and Zachary, R. B.: Adenovirus infection in association with intussusception in infancy. Lancet *2*:221–223, 1962.
357. Rowe, W. P., Hartley, J. W., Roizman, B., et al.: Characterization of a factor formed in the course of adenovirus infection of tissue cultures causing detachment of cells from glass. J. Exp. Med. *108*:713–729, 1958.
358. Rowe, W. P., and Huebner, R. J.: Present knowledge of the clinical significance of the adenoidal-pharyngeal-conjunctival group of viruses. Am. J. Trop. Med. Hyg. *5*:453–460, 1956.
359. Rowe, W. P., Huebner, R. J., Gilmore, L. K., et al.: Isolation of a cytopathogenic agent from human adenoids undergoing spontaneous degeneration in tissue culture. Proc. Soc. Exp. Biol. Med. *84*:570–573, 1955.
360. Rowe, W. P., Huebner, R. J., Hartley, J. W., et al.: Studies of the adenoidal-pharyngeal-conjunctival (APC) group of viruses. Am. J. Hyg. *61*:197–218, 1955.

361. Ruuskanen, O., Meurman, O., and Sarkkinen, J.: Adenoviral diseases in children: A study of 105 hospital cases. Pediatrics *76*:79–83, 1985.
362. Ruuskanen, O., Sarkkinen, H., Meurman, O., et al.: Rapid diagnosis of adenoviral tonsillitis: A prospective clinical study. J. Pediatr. *104*:725–728, 1984.
363. Sahler, O. J. Z., and Wilfert, C. M.: Fever and petechiae with adenovirus type 7 infection. Pediatrics *53*:233–235, 1974.
364. Salomòn, H. E., Grandien, M., Avila, M. M., et al.: Comparison of three techniques for detection of respiratory viruses in nasopharyngeal aspirates from children with lower acute respiratory infections. J. Med. Virol. *28*:159–162, 1989.
365. Sanekata, T., Taniguchi, K., Demura, M., et al.: Detection of adenovirus type 41 in stool samples by a latex agglutination method. J. Immunol. Methods *127*:235–239, 1990.
366. Schaap, G. J. P., de Jong, J. C., van Bijsterveld, O. P., et al.: A new intermediate adenovirus type causing conjunctivitis. Arch. Ophthalmol. *97*:2336–2338, 1979.
367. Schloesser, C.: Comments on keratitis punctata. Centralbl. Prakt. Augenheilk. *13*:360, 1889.
368. Schnurr, D., and Dondero, M. E.: Two new candidate adenovirus serotypes. Intervirology *36*:79–83, 1993.
369. Schoub, B. D., Koornhof, H. L., Lecatsas, G., et al.: Virus in acute summer gastroenteritis in black infants. Lancet *1*:1093–1094, 1975.
370. Schwartz, H. S., Vastine, D. W., Yamashiroya, H., et al.: Immunofluorescent detection of adenovirus antigen in epidemic keratoconjunctivitis. Invest. Ophthalmol. *15*:199–207, 1976.
371. Severe, J. L., and Traub, R. G.: Conjunctivitis with follicles associated with adenovirus type 22. N. Engl. J. Med. *266*:1375–1376, 1962.
372. Shenk, T. E.: Adenoviruses. *In* Knipe, D. M. and Howley, P. M. (eds.): Virology. 4th ed. Philadelphia, Lippincott Williams & Wilkins, 2001, pp. 2265–2300.
373. Shields, A. F., Hackman, R. C., Fife, K. H., et al.: Adenovirus infections in patients undergoing bone-marrow transplantation. N. Engl. J. Med. *312*:529–533, 1985.
374. Shirali, G. S., Ni, J., Chinnock, R. E., et al.: Association of viral genome with graft loss in children after cardiac transplantation. N. Engl. J. Med. *344*:1498–1503, 2001.
375. Siegal, F. P., Dikman, S. H., Arayata, R. B., et al.: Fatal disseminated adenovirus 11 pneumonia in an agammaglobulinemic patient. Am. J. Med. *71*:1062–1067, 1981.
376. Simila, S., Jouppila, R., Salmi, A., et al.: Encephalomeningitis in children associated with an adenovirus type 7 epidemic. Acta Paediatr. *59*:310–316, 1970.
377. Simila, S., Linna, O., Lanning, P., et al.: Chronic lung damage caused by adenovirus type 7: A ten-year follow-up study. Chest *80*:127–131, 1981.
378. Simila, S., Ylikorkala, O., and Wasz-Hockert, O.: Type 7 adenovirus pneumonia. J. Pediatr. *79*:605–611, 1971.
379. Simsir, A., Greenebaum, E., Nuovo, G., et al.: Late fatal adenovirus pneumonitis in a lung transplant recipient. Transplantation *65*:592–594, 1998.
380. Singh-Naz, N., Brown, M., and Ganeshananthan, M.: Nosocomial adenovirus infection: Molecular epidemiology of an outbreak. Pediatr. Infect. Dis. J. *12*:922–925, 1993.
381. Smith, R. H.: Fatal adenovirus infection with misleading positive serology for infectious mononucleosis. Lancet *1*:299–300, 1979.
382. Smith, T. J., Buescher, E. L., Top, F. H., Jr., et al.: Experimental respiratory infection with type 4 adenovirus vaccine in volunteers: Clinical and immunological responses. J. Infect. Dis. *122*:239–248, 1970.
383. Sohier, R., Chardonnet, Y., and Prunieras, M.: Adenoviruses: Status of current knowledge. Prog. Med. Virol. 7:253–325, 1965.
384. South, M. A., Dolen, J., Beach, D. K., et al.: Fatal adenovirus hepatic necrosis in severe combined immune deficiency. Pediatr. Infect. Dis. *1*:416–419, 1982.
385. Sprague, J. B., Hierholzer, J. C., Currier, R. W., II, et al.: Epidemic keratoconjunctivitis: A severe industrial outbreak due to adenovirus type 8. N. Engl. J. Med. *289*:1341–1346, 1973.
386. Stanley, E. D., and Jackson, G. G.: Spread of enteric live adenovirus type 4 vaccine in married couples. J. Infect. Dis. *119*:51–59, 1969.
387. Steen-Johnsen, J., Orstavik, I., and Attramadal, A.: Severe illnesses due to adenovirus type 7 in children. Acta Paediatr. *58*:157–163, 1969.
388. Steigbigel, R. T., LaScolea, L. J., Jr., and Marx, G.: Renal hematuria associated with adenovirus 7a infection. Am. J. Dis. Child. *132*:208–210, 1978.
389. Stellwag, V. K.: A peculiar form of corneal inflammation. Wien. Klin. Wochenschr. *August*:613–614, 1889.
390. Sterner, G.: Infections with adenovirus type 7 in children and their relationship to acute respiratory disease. Acta Paediatr. *48*:287–298, 1959.
391. Sterner, G.: Adenovirus infection in childhood: An epidemiological and clinical survey among Swedish children. Acta Paediatr. *142*:5–30, 1962.
392. Sterner, G., Gerzen, P., Ohlson, M., et al.: Acute respiratory illness and gastroenteritis in association with adenovirus type 7 infections. Acta Paediatr. *50*:457–468, 1961.
393. Stovin, S.: Sporadic acute respiratory infections in adults with special reference to adenovirus infections. J. Hyg. *56*:404–414, 1958.
394. Stuart-Harris, C. H.: The adenoviruses and respiratory disease in man. Lectures on the Scientific Basis of Medicine *8*:148–164, 1958–1959.
395. Sutton, R. N. P., Pullen, H. J. M., Blackledge, P., et al.: Adenovirus type 7: 1971–74. Lancet *2*:987–991, 1976.
396. Swann, N. H.: Acute thyroiditis: Five cases associated with adenovirus infection. Metabolism *13*:908–910, 1964.
397. Swenson, P. D., Lowens, M. S., Celum, C. L., et al.: Adenovirus types 2, 8 and 37 associated with genital infections in patients attending a sexually transmitted disease clinic. J. Clin. Microbiol. *33*:2728–2731, 1995.
398. Takafuji, E. T., Gaydos, J. C., Allen, R. G., et al.: Simultaneous administration of live, enteric-coated adenovirus types 4, 7, and 21 vaccines: Safety and immunogenicity. J. Infect. Dis. *140*:48–53, 1979.
399. Takiff, H. E., Seidlin, M., Krause, P., et al.: Detection of enteric adenoviruses by dot-blot hybridization using a molecularly cloned viral DNA probe. J. Med. Virol. *16*:107–118, 1985.
400. Takiff, H. E., Straus, S. E., and Garon, C. F.: Propagation and in vitro studies of previously non-cultivable enteral adenoviruses in 293 cells. Lancet *2*:832–834, 1981.
401. Tanaka, C.: Epidemic keratoconjunctivitis in Japan and the Orient. Am. J. Ophthalmol. *43*:46–50, 1957.
402. Tanaka, C.: A study of the relationship between adenovirus and epidemic keratoconjunctivitis. Arch. Ophthalmol. *59*:49–54, 1958.
403. Thiele, G. M., Okano, M., and Purtilo, D. T.: Enzyme-linked immunosorbent assay (ELISA) for detecting antibodies in sera of patients with adenovirus infection. J. Virol. Methods *23*:321–332, 1989.
404. Tiemessen, C. T., and Kidd, A. H.: The subgroup F adenoviruses. J. Gen. Virol. *76*:481–497, 1995.
405. Tiemessen, C. T., Wegerhoff, F. O., Erasmus, M. J., et al.: Infection by enteric adenoviruses, rotaviruses, and other agents in a rural African environment. J. Med. Virol. *28*:176–182, 1989.
406. Top, F. H., Jr.: Control of adenovirus acute respiratory disease in U.S. Army trainees. Yale J. Biol. Med. *48*:185–195, 1975.
407. Top, F. H., Jr., Buescher, E. L., Bancroft, W. H., et al.: Immunization with live types 7 and 4 adenovirus vaccines. II. Antibody response and protective effect against acute respiratory disease due to adenovirus type 7. J. Infect. Dis. *124*:155–160, 1971.
408. Top, F. H., Jr., Dudding, B. A., Russell, P. K., et al.: Control of respiratory disease in recruits with types 4 and 7 adenovirus vaccines. Am. J. Epidemiol. *94*:142–146, 1971.
409. Top, F. H., Jr., Grossman, R. A., Bartelloni, P. J., et al.: Immunization with live types 7 and 4 adenovirus vaccines. I. Safety, infectivity, and potency of adenovirus type 7 vaccine in humans. J. Infect. Dis. *124*:148–154, 1971.
410. Towbin, J. A., Griffin, L. D., Martin, A. B., et al: Intrauterine adenoviral myocarditis presenting as nonimmune hydrops fetalis: Diagnosis by polymerase chain reaction. Pediatr. Infect. Dis. J. *13*:144–150, 1994.
411. Trentin, J. J., Yabe, Y., and Taylor, G.: The quest for human cancer viruses. Science *137*:835–849, 1962.
412. Trifajova, J., Bruckova, M., Ryc, M., et al.: Type 5 adenovirus isolated from urine of patient with Hodgkin's disease. J. Hyg. Epidemiol. Microbiol. Immunol. *25*:321–323, 1981.
413. Turner, P. C., Bailey, A. S., Cooper, R. J., et al.: The polymerase chain reaction for detecting adenovirus DNA in formalin-fixed, paraffin-embedded tissue obtained post mortem. J. Infect. *27*:43–46, 1993.
414. Tyrrell, D. A. J., Balducci, D., and Zaiman, T. E.: Acute infections of the respiratory tract and the adenoviruses. Lancet *2*:1326–1330, 1956.
415. Uchio, E., Matsuura, N., Takeuchi, S., et al.: Acute follicular conjunctivitis caused by adenovirus type 34. Am. J. Ophthalmol. *128*:680–686, 1999.
416. Uhnoo, I., Wadell, G., Svensson, L., et al.: Importance of enteric adenoviruses 40 and 41 in acute gastroenteritis in infants and young children. J. Clin. Microbiol. *20*:365–372, 1984.
417. Usami, T., Mugiya, S., Ushima, T., et al.: Systematic infection resembling hemorrhagic fever with the renal syndrome caused by adenoviral type 11. J. Urol. *157*:617–618, 1997.
418. Valentine, R. C., and Pereira, H. G.: Antigens and structure of the adenovirus. J. Mol. Biol. *13*:13–20, 1965.
419. Van, R., Wun, C. C., O'Ryan, M. L., et al.: Outbreaks of human enteric adenovirus types 40 and 41 in Houston day care centers. J. Pediatr. *120*:516–520, 1992.
420. Van Der Veen, J.: Infections with adenovirus in Europe. Soc. Belge Med. Trop. Ann. *38*:891–904, 1958.
421. Van Der Veen, J.: The role of adenoviruses in respiratory disease. Am. Rev. Respir. Dis. *88*:167–180, 1963.
422. Van Der Veen, J., and Dijkman, J. H.: Association of type 21 adenovirus with acute respiratory illness in military recruits. Am. J. Hyg. *76*:149–159, 1962.
423. Van Der Veen, J., and Kok, G.: Isolation and typing of adenoviruses recovered from military recruits with acute respiratory disease in the Netherlands. Am. J. Hyg. *65*:119–129, 1957.
424. Van Der Veen, J., Oei, K. G., and Arbarbanal, M. F. W.: Patterns of infections with adenovirus types 4, 7, and 21 in military recruits during a 9-year survey. J. Hyg. (Camb.) *67*:255–268, 1969.
425. Van Der Veen, J., Van Zaane, D. J., Sprangers, M. A., et al.: Homotypic and heterotypic antibody response in infants to adenovirus vaccine. Arch. Gesamte. Virusforsch. *21*:320–333, 1967.

426. Van Der Veen, J., and Ven Der Ploeg, G.: An outbreak of pharyngoconjunctival fever caused by types 3 and 4 adenovirus at Waalwijk, The Netherlands. Am. J. Hyg. *68*:95–105, 1958.
427. Vargosko, A. J., Kim, H. W., Parrott, R. H., et al.: Recovery and identification of adenovirus in infections of infants and children. Bacteriol. Rev. *29*:487–495, 1965.
428. Vass, Z.: Histological findings in epidemic keratoconjunctivitis. Acta Ophthalmol. *42*:119–121, 1964.
429. Vihma, L.: Surveillance of acute viral respiratory diseases in children. Acta Paediatr. *192*:27–41, 1969.
430. Wadell, G.: Classification of human adenoviruses by SDS polyacrylamide gel electrophoresis of structural polypeptides. Intervirology *11*:47–57, 1979.
431. Wadell, G.: Molecular epidemiology of human adenoviruses. Curr. Top. Microbiol. Immunol. *110*:191–220, 1984.
432. Wadell, G., Hammarskhold, M. L., Winberg, G., et al.: Genetic variability of adenoviruses. Ann. N. Y. Acad. Sci. *354*:16–42, 1980.
433. Wadell, G., Sundell, G., and de Jong, J. C.: Characterization of candidate adenovirus 37 by SDS–polyacrylamide gel electrophoresis of virion polypeptides and DNA restriction site mapping. J. Med. Virol. *7*: 119–125, 1981.
434. Warren, D., Nelson, K. E., Farrar, J. A., et al.: A large outbreak of epidemic keratoconjunctivitis: Problems in controlling nosocomial spread. J. Infect. Dis. *160*:938–943, 1989.
435. Wenman, W. M., Pagtakhan, R. D., Reed, M. H., et al.: Adenovirus bronchiolitis in Manitoba: Epidemiologic, clinical, and radiologic features. Chest *81*:605–609, 1982.
436. White, G. P. B., and Stancliffe, D.: Viruses and gastroenteritis. Lancet *2*:703, 1975.
437. Whitelaw, A., Davies, H., and Parry, J.: Electron microscopy of fatal adenovirus gastroenteritis. Lancet *1*:361, 1977.
438. Wigand, R., Baumeister, H. G., Maass, G., et al.: Isolation and identification of enteric adenoviruses. J. Med. Virol. *11*:233–240, 1983.
439. Wigand, R., Gelderblom, H., and Wadell, G.: New human adenovirus (candidate adenovirus 36), a novel member of subgroup D. Arch. Virol. *64*:225–233, 1980.
440. Wigand, R., and Keller, D.: Relationship of human adenoviruses 12, 18 and 31 as determined by hemagglutination inhibition. J. Med. Virol. *2*:137–142, 1978.
441. Wigger, H. J., and Blanc, W. A.: Fatal hepatic and bronchial necrosis in adenovirus infection with thymic alymphoplasia. N. Engl. J. Med. *275*:870–874, 1966.
442. Wildin, S. R., Chonmaitree, T., and Swischuk, L. E.: Roentgenographic features of common pediatric viral respiratory tract infections. Am. J. Dis. Child. *142*:43–46, 1988.
443. Wilt, J. C., and Stackiw, W.: Adenovirus infections in Manitoba. Can. Med. Assoc. J. *102*:269–272, 1970.
444. Wohl, M. E. B., and Chernick, V.: Bronchiolitis. Am. Rev. Respir. Dis. *118*:759–781, 1978.
445. Wood, D. J., Bijlsma, K., de Jong, J. C., et al.: Evaluation of a commercial monoclonal antibody–based enzyme immunoassay for detection of adenovirus types 40 and 41 in stool specimens. J. Clin. Microbiol. *27*:1155–1158, 1989.
446. Wright, H. T., Beckwith, J. B., and Gwinn, J. L.: A fatal case of inclusion body pneumonia in an infant infected with adenovirus type 3. J. Pediatr. *64*:528–533, 1964.
447. Wright, J., Couchonnal, G., and Hodges, G. R.: Adenovirus type 21 infection: Occurrence with pneumonia, rhabdomyolysis, and myoglobinuria in an adult. J. A. M. A. *241*:2420–2421, 1979.
448. Wright, R. E.: Superficial punctate keratitis. Br. J. Ophthalmol. *14*:257–291, 1930.
449. Wulffraat, N., Geelan, S., van Dijken, P., et al.: Recovery from adenovirus pneumonia in a severe combined immunodeficiency patient treated with intravenous ribavirin. Transplantation *59*:927, 1995.
450. Yin-Coggrave, M.: Isolation of adenoviruses from cases of epidemic keratoconjunctivitis in Singapore. Am. J. Ophthalmol. *55*:575–583, 1963.
451. Yodfat, Y., and Nishmi, M.: Successive overlapping outbreaks of febrile pharyngitis and pharyngoconjunctival fever, associated with adenovirus types 2 and 7, in a kibbutz. Isr. J. Med. Sci. *10*:1505–1509, 1974.
452. Yolken, R. H., and Franklin, C. C.: Gastrointestinal adenovirus: An important cause of morbidity in patients with necrotizing enterocolitis and gastrointestinal surgery. Pediatr. Infect. Dis. *4*:42–47, 1985.
453. Yolken, R. H., Lawrence, F., Leister, F., et al.: Gastroenteritis associated with enteric type adenovirus in hospitalized infants. J. Pediatr. *101*: 21–26, 1982.
454. Yunis, E. J., Atchison, R. W., Michaels, R. H., et al.: Adenovirus and ileocecal intussusception. Lab. Invest. *33*:347–351, 1975.
455. Yunis, E. J., and Hashida, Y.: Electron microscopic demonstration of adenovirus in appendix vermiformis in a case of ileocecal intussusception. Pediatrics *51*:566–570, 1973.
456. Zahradnik, J. M., Spencer, M. J., and Porter, D. D.: Adenovirus infection in the immunocompromised patient. Am. J. Med. *68*:725–732, 1980.
457. Zinserling, A.: Peculiarities of lesions in viral and mycoplasmal infections of the respiratory tract. Virchows Arch. *356*:259–273, 1972.

SUBSECTION 5

HEPATOVIRIDAE

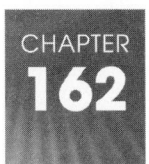

Hepatitis B and D Viruses

ANNEMARIE BRODERICK ■ MAUREEN M. JONAS

HEPATITIS B

Biology of the Hepatitis B Virus

Hepatitis B virus (HBV) is the prototype of a family of DNA viruses called *hepadnaviruses* (hepatotropic DNA viruses). This group consists of enveloped, coated DNA viruses with similar structure and genome organization. All primarily infect the livers of their respective hosts, and all can cause acute and chronic infections. Hepatitis B virus is the most studied member of the family that also includes the woodchuck hepatitis virus (WHV), the ground squirrel hepatitis virus, the duck hepatitis virus (DHV), and hepatitis viruses found in herons, Ross's geese, and arctic squirrels.[145] The WHV and DHV share approximately 70 percent sequence homology with HBV but do not infect humans.[150] The use of these animal models has facilitated the study of hepadnavirus structure and replication, supplementing information obtained from infected humans and cloning studies.

Three types of particles are found in the sera of HBV-infected people by immune electron microscopy after precipitation with antibodies to the viral envelope. All three types share a common surface antigen, hepatitis B surface antigen

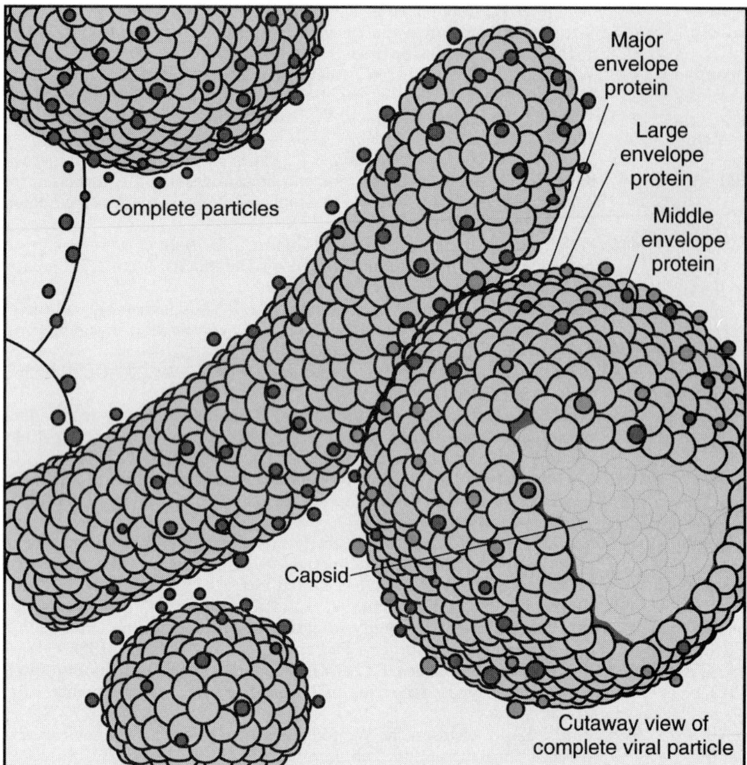

FIGURE 162–1 ■ The three forms of HBV surface antigen: whole virions, rods, and proteins. A cutaway view of the whole virion shows the three envelope proteins: major, middle, and large. (From Mutchnik, M. G.: Acute and chronic hepatitis B. In Feldman, M., and Maddrey, W. C. (eds): The Liver. Philadelphia, Current Medicine, 1996.)

(HBsAg), but only one, the Dane particle, contains viral DNA and therefore is capable of replication. The particles without nucleic acid are of two shapes: a filament, 20 nm in width and ranging from 50 to 1000 nm in length; and a sphere, also of 20 nm diameter. These shapes are illustrated in Figure 162–1. The Dane particle or whole virion is 42 nm in diameter and contains a core, or nucleocapsid, enclosing the DNA. The outer shell is composed of large amounts of hepatitis B surface proteins in a lipoprotein envelope, which is derived from host cells. Inside this shell is found the nucleocapsid, an icosahedral structure composed of 240 core protein subunits with regular penetrating channels (Fig. 162–2). The nucleocapsid proteins are detected serologically as hepatitis B core antigen (HBcAg). This nucleocapsid is 25 to 27 nm in diameter, and within it are contained the viral genome and polymerase. HBV e antigen (HBeAg) is a soluble antigen produced from the same open reading frame as is HBcAg, but, unlike core antigen, e antigen is secreted into serum, where it is thought to have a role in induction of tolerance to HBV. The viral genome is composed of double-stranded circular DNA that can be relaxed or closed depending on the stage in the reproduction cycle.[150] This DNA, which is 3.2 kilobase pairs in size, encodes four overlapping open reading frames (ORFs) that overlap with other regulatory *cis*-acting sequences such as promoters, enhancers, and polyadenylation and genome packaging signals.

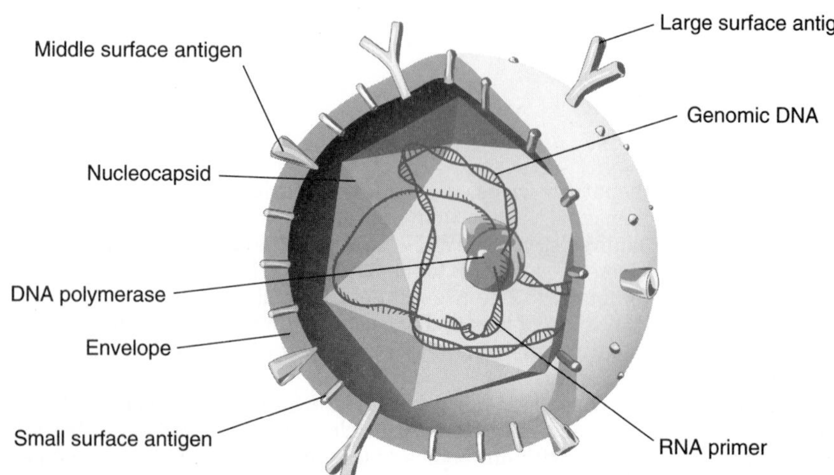

FIGURE 162–2 ■ Schematic diagram of the intact HBV virion. (Courtesy of GlaxoSmithKline, Research Triangle Park, NC.)

The subviral particles (spheres and filaments) are composed of envelope proteins and host-derived lipid components.[145] These particles are abundant in the serum of infected individuals (10^6 to 10^{14} particles per milliliter), and they are highly immunogenic, stimulating the production of neutralizing antibodies. One hypothesis is that they absorb neutralizing antibodies, thus shielding the intact virion from the host immune response. Subviral particles were used to produce the first effective HBV vaccine.[165]

MOLECULAR VIROLOGY

The viral genome, as noted previously, contains four ORFs in its circular DNA. The DNA strands are not completely symmetric; the minus strand is shorter, leading to a region of single-stranded DNA. This gap can be filled by the virus's own polymerase when required. The four genes are *S* for the surface or envelope gene; *P* for the viral polymerase gene; *C* for the core gene, which encodes nucleocapsid protein; and *X* for the X gene. The surface proteins synthesized by HBV are termed the large, middle, and major proteins and are type II transmembrane proteins that can form multimers. Transcription initiated at the *pre-S1*, *pre-S2,* or *S* epitopes leads to formation of these three proteins. Although antibodies to S protein alone will provide protection against HBV infection, epitopes of *pre-S1* also can stimulate neutralizing antibody production.[101] A group of antigens used for subtyping HBV strains in epidemiologic studies is found in association with S proteins. Analysis of subdeterminants of HBsAg has revealed four major serotypes of HBV, *adw*, *adr*, *ayw*, and *ayr,* thus allowing differentiation of HBV infections from different sources. The "a" determinant is found in all isolates. Antibody to hepatitis B surface antigen (anti-HBs) is directed against this determinant and provides protection against all serotypes.

Seven HBV genotypes have been identified by use of polymerase chain reaction (PCR)–restriction fragment length polymorphism analysis of the complete viral genome.[106] They have been designated A through G, and worldwide distribution varies. Type D occurs more commonly in Mediterranean regions, whereas type F occurs more commonly in the Central and Latin Americas.[117] A study of 187 patients with chronic HBV infection revealed the following marked regional variations in genotype: North Europeans, 63 percent A; South Europeans and Middle Easterners, 96 percent D; Africans, 53 percent A, 27 percent D, 20 percent E; East Asians, 14 percent A, 43 percent B, and 43 percent C.[106] HBV genotypes may have important clinical differences, although reports are only anecdotal at present. HBV infection with genotype C was found in Taiwanese adults to be associated with more severe liver disease and hepatocellular carcinoma (HCC) in those older than the age of 50 years, whereas genotype B is associated with HCC in those younger than 50 years of age.[85] An association of genotype with response to interferon-α (IFN-α) treatment also has been suggested.[86] A recent study from Taiwan analyzed the responses of 58 patients with chronic HBV infection genotypes B and C to treatment with IFN-α. The patients with genotype C had higher aminotransferases at baseline. After a 48-week follow-up period, only 15 percent of those with genotype C were HbeAg- and HBV DNA-negative, as compared with 42 percent of those with genotype B.

HBV polymerase consists of two major domains tethered by an intervening spacer region. Elucidating the structure and biochemistry of hepadnavirus polymerases has proved difficult because they require cellular factors, which are lost during extraction from cells, for enzymatic activity.[126] The ORF that encodes the *P* gene overlaps to a large extent with the core protein ORF; indeed, both proteins are translated from the same mRNA.[27]

The core gene encodes the viral capsid proteins that combine to form the core particles. The core proteins combine first into dimers; 120 dimers unite to form a shell 36 nm in diameter.[45] The hepatitis B core antigen appears to be phosphorylated within cells and becomes dephosphorylated upon export.[161] The main role of core proteins is enclosure of viral DNA, but they also play a role in the cytolysis of infected cells when expressed on the cell surface.[103] Mutations in the core gene, the pre-core region, and the promoter for *C* have become clinically important.

Mutations affecting all ORFs of the HBV genome have been described. Most viral genomes carry more than one mutation, and most individuals are infected with more than one variant. Some of the mutations are thought to contribute to viral latency, low-level infection, severity of liver disease, and vaccine escape. The group best studied is the pre-core mutants, which result in lack of HBeAg production, even in the presence of active viral replication, the so-called e-minus HBV infection. In contrast to the situation in patients with wild-type virus, in whom absence of HBeAg usually signifies absent HBV replication and mild liver disease (see later), in e-minus infection, HBV DNA levels are high, antibody to hepatitis B e antigen (anti-HBe) is detected, and liver disease may be severe. Sporadic cases and outbreaks of fulminant HBV infection have been attributed to pre-core mutants. Mutations in the *S* or *pre-S* gene, which encode envelope protein, have been reported in patients infected after vaccination and in individuals who receive monoclonal antibody to HBV after liver transplantation. This variant contains a missense mutation in the *a* determinant of the surface antigen. Subsequently, these mutants were demonstrated in chronic HBV carriers even without these immune pressures. This mutation causes an infection in which HBsAg is undetectable but in which HBeAg and HBV-DNA are found, in contrast to the typical serologic pattern (see later).

The role of X protein is not yet fully understood, but it is required for establishment of infection in vivo although not for transfection of cells in vitro.[18, 36] X protein is involved in transcriptional activation during viral replication[103] and also has been shown to transactivate the promoters of other viruses such as human immunodeficiency virus (HIV) and human T-lymphotropic virus type 1.[139]

VIRAL LIFE CYCLE OVERVIEW

Like retroviruses, hepadnaviruses replicate by means of reverse transcription of an RNA intermediate[163] (i.e., the flow of genetic information is from DNA to RNA to DNA). After binding of the virus to receptors on the cell surface, virion nucleocapsids are delivered to the cytoplasm, where they translocate to the nucleus. There the genomic DNA is converted to the cccDNA form (a nuclear pool of viral covalently closed circular DNA that serves as a template for the reverse transcription). This form of DNA is transcribed by host RNA polymerase II, and the resulting RNAs are translated to originate the *P, C, S/pre-S,* and *X* gene products. These viral pregenomic RNAs then are encapsidated into the cytoplasm with the *P* gene product. DNA synthesis then is initiated, and the RNA template is degraded. After minus-strand synthesis and subsequent plus-strand synthesis are completed, the progeny cores then bud into intracellular membranes and acquire their glycoprotein envelope. The enveloped virions are secreted by vesicular transport.

Nucleocapsids are exported from the hepatocyte cytoplasm toward the cell membrane, where they become invested with surface proteins bound in the membrane bilayer, resulting in budding of mature virions into the bloodstream. Although HBV can infect numerous tissues, including spleen, kidney, peripheral blood mononuclear cells, and pancreas, the virus replicates exclusively in the liver. This is the sole site of replication because the tissue-specific viral promoter and enhancer are in liver cells.

No efficient tissue culture technique supports HBV infection. In the cell culture systems presently available, such as primary duck hepatocytes infected with DHV and immortalized human hepatoma cell lines such as HepG2 and HuH7 and chick LMH, the viral replicative cycle is not cytopathic. The infected hepatocytes are normal morphologically and display growth rates identical to those of uninfected controls.[17, 141]

VIRAL BINDING AND CELL ENTRY

Studies of the early phases of the viral life cycle have been conducted using primarily DHV. The binding reaction has two components: one is of low affinity and is nonsaturable, and the second is of high affinity and saturable.[91] At 37° C, cell entry and viral infection occur. After binding, the virus must fuse with the host cell membrane. This phenomenon appears to occur by a pH-independent mechanism. The binding and entry processes are slow, with maximal infection occurring after 16 hours of cell exposure to the inoculum.[131] The pre-S proteins appear to be involved primarily in the cell fusion interactions.[91] Monoclonal antibodies to these proteins prevent infection of primary duck hepatocytes.[91] The pre-S proteins also appear to determine the narrow spectrum of the viral host determination (i.e., if the virus entry process is bypassed by transfection into heterologous cells, viral replication of heron HBV is able to replicate normally in duck cells, which normally are not susceptible to this virus).

The cellular receptors for the hepadnaviruses are not known. The hepatotropism of HBV infection is presumed to be caused by the presence of a specific receptor, although none has been identified.[150] Many proteins, such as apolipoprotein H[44] and endonexin 2 (a phospholipid-binding protein), bind to the HBV envelope glycoproteins, particularly S protein.[70] Receptors for pre-S proteins still have not been identified, and the biologic significance of these findings is yet to be determined. The mechanisms by which viral DNA is delivered to the nucleus after entry also are unclear.

In the nucleus, viral DNA is transformed to the cccDNA, a process that entails repair of the single-stranded gap, removal of the 5′-terminal structures, and covalent ligation of the strands.[2] Host mechanisms appear to contribute greatly to this process.[94]

VIRAL TRANSCRIPTION

Several viral transcripts have been identified, but their function in the viral life cycle remains uncertain. These transcripts are either genomic or subgenomic and are able to translate specific viral gene products. Genomic RNAs can serve as both templates for viral DNA synthesis and messages for ORF *pre-C, C,* and *P* translation. Subgenomic RNAs function as mRNAs for the translation of the envelope and X proteins. Several viral promoters originate the viral transcripts. They are the genomic RNAs,[72] the L protein mRNA (*pre-S1* promoter),[26] the M and S protein mRNAs (*S* promoter),[26] the X protein mRNA (*X* promoter), and the core (C) or pregenomic RNA. Two genomic regions appear to function as enhancer elements of the viral promoters: enhancer I *(EnI)* and enhancer II *(EnII)*.[36, 37] *EnI* is located between the *S* and *X* coding regions, and it up-regulates all viral promoters.[74] *EnII* has been shown so far to up-regulate the *S* promoter.[111] Deletion of any of the enhancers decreases viral transcription significantly.

GENOMIC REPLICATION

The ORF *P* region of hepadnaviruses encodes for the viral polymerases. Considerable similarities exist between this region and the coding regions for retroviral reverse transcriptases.[171] Changes in ORF *P* inactivate viral DNA synthesis.[13] However, unlike retroviruses, hepadnaviruses do not have integrases; therefore, no homologies exist between ORF *P* and reverse-transcribing regions for integrases (and for proteases as well).[122] The first step in HBV genomic replication is the encapsidation of the genomic RNA template.[164] The pregenomic RNA is encapsidated into the core particle.[55] In order to package this small RNA portion into the capsid, both C protein and *P* gene products are required.[71] Encapsidation of polymerase occurs by binding of the P protein to the RNA that will be packaged.[11] Single-stranded pregenomic RNA is converted to partially duplex virion DNA through reverse transcription. The P protein interacts with the 5′ end of the pregenomic RNA.

Reverse transcription then is initiated by P at the 5′ stem-loop, with minus-strand DNA being extended by three to four nucleotides. P then is attached covalently to the new DNA, and both are transferred to the 3′ copy of the direct repeat 1 (DR1), with the DNA being extended. While the minus strand is being elongated, pregenomic RNA is degraded by the RNaseH of P. P then reaches the 5′ end of the template, where an RNA oligomer is formed. This oligomer translocates and anneals to direct repeat 2 (DR2), where it serves as a primer for plus-strand DNA synthesis. The plus strand is elongated to the 5′ end of the minus-strand DNA template. A second template transfer then occurs, with complementary sequences at the 3′ end of the minus-strand DNA enabling the genome to become circular.[168]

VIRAL ASSEMBLY AND RELEASE

The 20-nm subviral particles are assembled between the endoplasmic reticulum and the Golgi apparatus.[79] These 20-nm particles contain predominantly S proteins, which are synthesized in the endoplasmic reticulum.[68] In addition, these particles may contain M subunits but generally do not have L proteins.[69] The assembly process is encoded totally in the S domain.[102] Assembled particles are transported through the secretory pathway and traverse the Golgi complex.[88, 162] The S protein carries out the entire assembly process without the involvement of other viral proteins.[2] Therefore, subviral particles containing only envelope proteins are released. In vitro studies have shown that overexpression of L proteins gives rise to filamentous viral particles in the endoplasmic reticulum.[39] The overabundance of L, M, and S aggregates apparently is cytopathic to hepatocytes in vitro. Similar cytopathic features have been seen in human infections with HBV, yet the role of envelope protein expression in hepatocyte injury remains to be determined.[2]

The assembly of the Dane particle differs from the assembly of the 20-nm particles in that all three proteins, L, M, and S, are present.[69] Studies of HepG2 cell lines transfected with HBV mutants have shown that no virus budding occurs if the envelope proteins are not present (mutations in *S*) and that for virion formation and release, both L and S proteins are needed.[24] M proteins apparently are not necessary for viral assembly.

VIRAL PERSISTENCE

Nuclear cccDNA appears to be crucial to viral persistence. Hepatocytes that harbor this form of viral genome are the only ones that produce virus.[2] As mentioned earlier, the replicative cycle of HBV is not cytopathic to hepatocytes, and, therefore, infected cells multiply normally. The cytoplasmic mechanism of reverse transcription, which delivers the cccDNA and consequently delivers this product to the nucleus, must therefore be passed on to progeny cells. When HBV DNA is integrated into the cell chromosome, viral DNA may be rearranged, although whether this happens before or after integration is unclear. This rearrangement may lead to disruption of viral genes, especially the core and polymerase genes, whereas the coding regions and promoters for the envelope proteins remain intact.[137]

Immunopathogenesis

Individuals infected with hepatitis B show tremendous variation in clinical and immunologic responses. HBV is not directly cytopathic, and the variability in liver damage is due to host immune responses. Although HBV preferentially infects hepatocytes and replicates therein, it can infect other liver cells, such as cholangiocytes, as well as cells in extrahepatic tissue. Examples include peripheral blood lymphocytes, pancreatic acinar cells, cornea, spleen, thyroid gland, kidney, adrenal gland, and smooth muscle.[116]

Responses to HBV infection and the likelihood of developing chronic infection are dependent on both the person's age at the time of developing infection and immune competence. Ninety percent of infants born to mothers who are HBeAg-positive become chronically infected with HBV, compared with only 5 percent of those infected as adults. The production of antibodies to pre-S and S antigens by B cells, as well as cytotoxic T-lymphocyte (CTL) responses, mediates recovery from acute HBV infection. Individuals who clear HBV have a strong polyclonal human leukocyte antigen (HLA) class I restricted CTL response to multiple epitopes in the HBV envelope, nucleocapsid, and polymerase regions. This CTL response can be reactivated many years after clearance of all detectable evidence of HBV infection.[107]

Infants infected perinatally are at the highest risk for development of chronic HBV infection. During childhood, those infected as neonates characteristically have high circulating levels of HBV DNA but low disease activity, with very low rates of HBeAg seroconversion, either spontaneously or after treatment with IFN.[107] In children in Taiwan with chronic HBV infection, the HBeAg positivity rate decreases spontaneously from 100 percent in infancy to 76 percent at age 10 to 14 years.[31]

Researchers have offered numerous hypotheses as to why this immune tolerance develops in neonates. One theory proposes that transplacental passage of HBeAg induces $CD4^+$ anergy and, therefore, no CTL responses to HbeAg occur. However, HbeAg-specific T-cell proliferation eventually is detected in those who subsequently seroconvert, rendering clonal deletion an unlikely mechanism.[107] Defective interleukin-2 production has been demonstrated in children who have chronic HBV, although whether it is a cause or consequence of chronic infection is not yet clear.[67]

The development of chronic infection is a failure of host immune responses. As the virus replicates within hepatocytes, viral antigens appear on the cell surface. Subsequently, cytotoxic T lymphocytes directed against HBcAg infiltrate the liver and cause hepatocyte necrosis.[50] In addition, HBV interferes with the production of cytokines, especially IFNs, that would otherwise elicit class II major histocompatibility complex (MHC) antigen expression and enhance viral clearance. For reasons not fully understood, both the HBV-specific CTL response and the $CD4^+$ helper T-cell response are weak in chronic HBV infection. However, HBeAg, produced in large amounts in chronic HBV infection, and HBsAg share T-cell epitopes. HBeAg may enter the thymus and induce immune tolerance to both HBsAg and HBeAg by decreasing the production of HBV-specific cytotoxic T lymphocytes. However, these cells can be reactivated in patients who undergo a spontaneous or IFN-induced HBeAg seroconversion.[134]

The distribution of HBcAg within hepatocytes of chronically infected individuals with and without active inflammation is different. In the former, HBcAg is present in a higher concentration in the cytoplasm than in the nucleus, whereas the reverse is true in the latter. The HBcAg in the cytoplasm may act as target for hepatocytolysis.[40] How HBcAg moves from the nucleus and cytoplasm has not been established, although it is regulated by the cell cycle. The localization of HBV DNA within the cell also varies by cell cycle; if the cell is proliferating, likely no HBV DNA will be found in the cytoplasm. The location of HBsAg on the cell surface or within the hepatocyte varies as well. Membrane staining of HBsAg on hepatocytes is a marker of active replication in chronic HBV infection, and concordance with serum HBV DNA levels exists.[40]

Fulminant hepatitis is seen in fewer than 1 percent of infected individuals and has a high mortality rate. It is characterized by a brisk immune response and viral clearance. Those who survive clear HBV and do not have chronic HBV infection. A higher incidence of fulminant hepatitis occurs in those patients infected with HBV mutants that do not produce the HBeAg, suggesting either an increased rate of replication or lack of immune detection of the mutant HBV.[97] HBV mutants arise during reverse transcription of RNA, and three main types of mutations produce HBV mutants that can replicate:

1. Mutations of the *S* gene are found in infants born to HbsAg-positive mothers who develop HBV infection despite HBV vaccination. In 41 such children studied in Singapore, HBV had a single amino acid substitution at position 145 of glycine for arginine of the *a* determinant.[127]
2. Mutations of the core promoter blocks production of HbeAg; thus, these patients could be HbeAg-negative, which usually would imply that HBV no longer is actively replicating, but actually they are HBV DNA-positive, implying ongoing active viral replication.[183]
3. Mutation of the *P* gene can lead to antiviral resistance.

Apart from the *S* gene mutants, the clinical significance of HBV mutants in children has not been studied widely.

Diagnosis

ACUTE INFECTION

The clinical and serologic events that typify acute HBV infection are depicted in Figure 162–3. When signs and

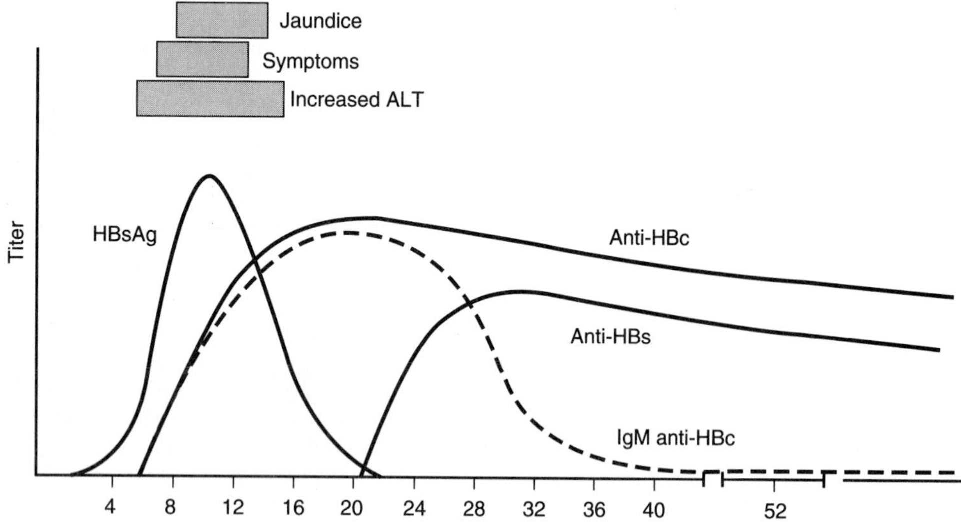

FIGURE 162–3 ■ Clinical and serologic features of acute HBV infection. HBsAg is detectable within 4 weeks and reaches a peak value at 12 weeks. This coincides with the onset of jaundice. HBeAg becomes detectable at the same time. Anti-HBc IgM is detected from 6 to 8 weeks and peaks at 20 weeks. It then declines, but anti-HBc IgG persists. Upon resolution of acute infection, the serum contains anti-HBc, IgG type, and anti-HBs.

symptoms of hepatitis develop, HBsAg is detectable in serum. At about the same time, HBeAg, a marker of active viral replication, also is present. Shortly afterward, antibody to hepatitis B core antigen (anti-HBc) is made; this early antibody is predominantly of the immunoglobulin M (IgM) class. Thus, the diagnosis of acute HBV infection is made by detection of HBsAg and IgM anti-HBc; although HBeAg confirms active replication, its presence need not be sought to confirm the diagnosis. After several weeks, HBeAg levels decline, and anti-HBe develops. Shortly thereafter, HbsAg disappears from serum, and the only serologic marker during this phase may be the IgM anti-HBc. Antibody to the surface antigen, anti-HBs, appears as the level of HBsAg wanes; after approximately 4 months, HBsAg is undetectable and anti-HBs is present, representing resolution of the acute infection. At about the same time, IgM anti-HBc also disappears, and anti-HBc then is predominantly of the IgG class. Therefore, after resolution of acute HBV infection, an individual's serum contains anti-HBc, IgG type, and anti-HBs.

CHRONIC INFECTION

The clinical and serologic features of chronic HBV infection are depicted in Figure 162–4. Chronic HBV infection is defined by persistence of HBsAg for more than 6 months; typically, it persists for many years. In these patients, anti-HBs does not develop, although anti-HBc is present, predominantly of the IgG class. Therefore, the diagnosis of chronic HBV infection entails documentation of presence of HBsAg for at least 6 months or detection of HBsAg and anti-HBc, not IgM. In chronic HBV infection, HBeAg persists for variable periods of time, often many years, indicating ongoing viral replication. In some patients, replication may cease, and viral DNA may become integrated into the hepatocyte genome. Loss of HBeAg and eventual appearance of anti-HBe usually accompany this event. Occasionally, a low level of anti-HBs is found in individuals with chronic HBV infection (HBsAg$^+$); this antibody, present in low titer, is directed at a heterotypic subdeterminant of the surface antigen and

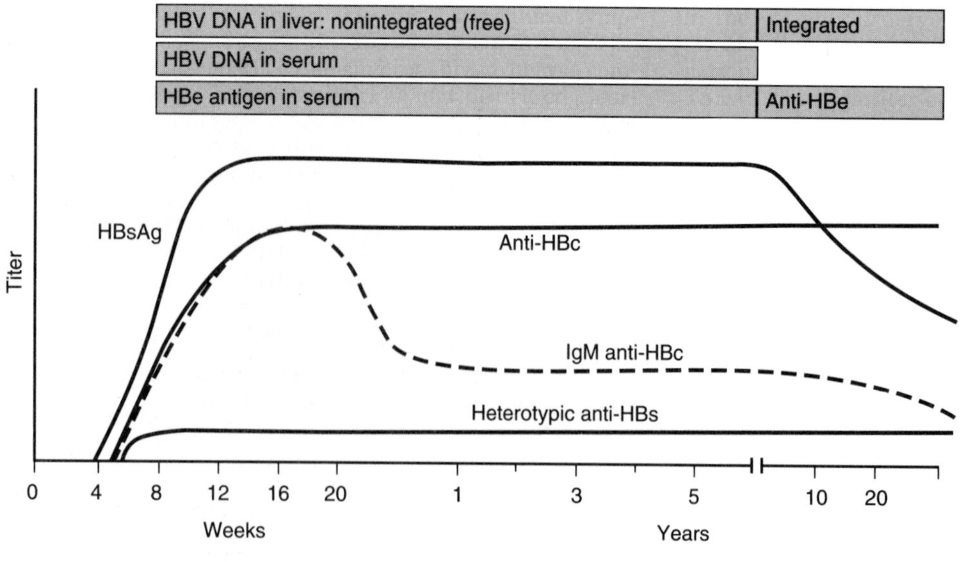

FIGURE 162–4 ■ Clinical and serologic features of chronic HBV infection. HBsAg, HBeAg, and anti-HBc are detectable and may persist for years. HBeAg to antibody seroconversion is associated with disappearance of HBV DNA from serum. The diagnosis of chronic HBV infection is dependent on finding HBsAg for at least 6 months or the combination of HBsAg and anti-HBc of the IgG class.

TABLE 162–1 ■ SEROLOGIC DIAGNOSIS OF HEPATITIS B

	Acute Infection	Chronic Infection	Resolved Infection	Vaccinated
HBsAg	+	+	–	–
Anti-HBc (total)	+	+	+	–
Anti-HBc (IgM)	+	–	–	–
Anti-HBs	–	–	+	+

HBsAg, hepatitis B surface antigen; anti-HBc, antibody to hepatitis B core antigen; anti-HBs, antibody to hepatitis B surface antigen; +, positive; –, negative.

is not protective. A further guide to the serologic diagnosis of acute and chronic HBV infection can be found in Table 162–1.

Replicating HBV virus produces HBV DNA, which may be detected in blood or serum. Quantitative assays of HBV DNA are very useful to follow response to treatment, but the assay used should be consistent because they are not interchangeable. Four major assays based on different molecular biology techniques are available commercially. The liquid hybridization assay (Abbott Laboratories, Abbott Park, IL) can detect as little as 2 picograms of HBV DNA (about 30,000 virion equivalents) per milliliter of serum and involves the denaturation of HBV DNA and the hybridization of radioactive HBV DNA probes. The hybridized samples are eluted and counted by a scintillation counter. The branched-chain DNA (bDNA) assay (Quantiplex, Chiron Diagnostics, Emeryville, CA) also is in common use. The branching refers to the binding of amplifier oligonucleotides, leading to "branched DNA." Two other assays in use are a PCR assay (Amplicor HBV, Roche Diagnostics, Indianapolis, IN) and an RNA-DNA hybrid assay (Abbott Laboratories/ Digene, Abbott Park, IL) that requires only 30 μL of serum.

Histopathologic Features

The purposes of obtaining a liver biopsy in HBV infection are to quantify the severity of changes, to rule out other causes of liver disease, and to allow a comparison of changes after treatment. In typical acute viral hepatitis, obtaining liver biopsy usually is not required or indicated. If performed, the findings are liver cell degeneration and necrosis, with lobular disarray. The acute injury to hepatocytes is manifested as both ballooning and acidophilic degeneration, either of which can resolve or progress to cell death. Inflammatory cell infiltration and liver cell regeneration are also seen.[75]

The histopathologic nomenclature of chronic HBV has changed since the 1990s. The older terms of chronic active, chronic persistent, and chronic lobular hepatitis have been replaced by one term, *chronic hepatitis*. It is characterized by limiting plate piecemeal necrosis, or interface hepatitis, and fibrosis, which may progress to architectural distortion of lobules and eventual cirrhosis.[75] Chronic hepatitis can be caused by viral hepatitis B or C as well as autoimmune, metabolic, and cryptogenic disorders.[82] Chronic HBV is characterized by "ground-glass cells" (Fig. 162–5*A*), hepatocytes containing HBsAg, most easily identified by staining with orcein, Victoria blue, or aldehyde fuschin. However, these cells also are found in other liver diseases, and the pattern of staining is important. In hepatitis B, ground-glass cells are found either singly or in clusters arranged in a haphazard pattern. Ground-glass cells are found in a panacinar pattern in liver of patients receiving phenobarbitone or phenytoin. "Sanded" liver nuclei are caused by accumulation of HBcAg and generally are identified by electron microscopy[82] or immunoperoxidase techniques (see Fig. 162–5*B*).

A histopathologic grading system, the Knodell-Ishak score, is used to allow standardization and meaningful comparisons of histopathologic interpretation in chronic hepatitis. Four histopathologic features—periportal with or without bridging necrosis, intralobular degeneration and focal necrosis, portal inflammation, and fibrosis—each are scored using specific criteria.[92] This system has proved reproducible and now is in common use. It has replaced the older nomenclature.[23] This systematic classification is useful in estimating progression of disease and response to therapy and for comparing outcomes of therapeutic trials.

Epidemiology

HBV infection occurs throughout the world, although marked geographic differences in rates of both acute and chronic infection exist. An estimated 360 million individuals

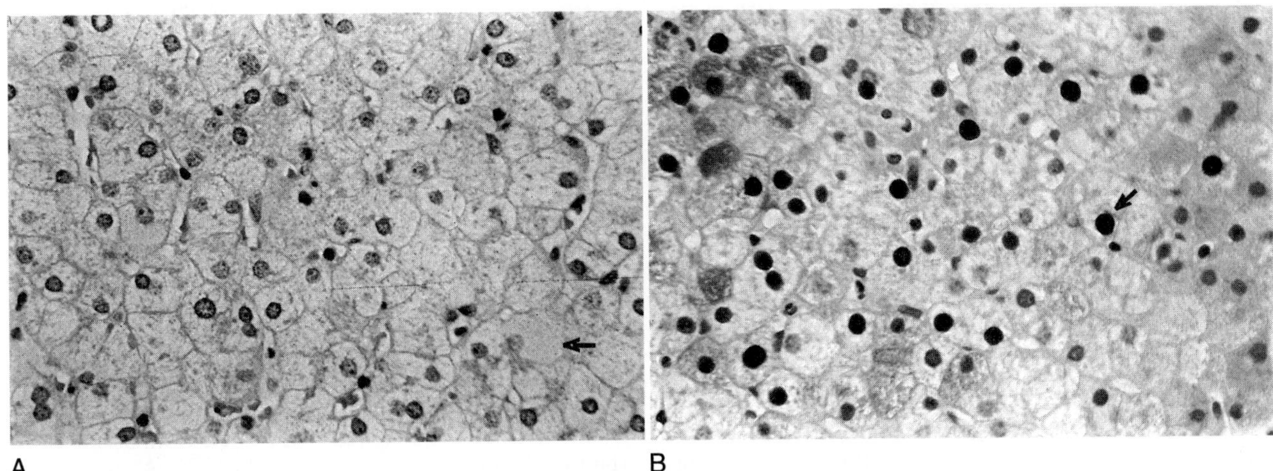

FIGURE 162–5 ■ *A*, Photomicrograph of a liver biopsy speimen from a child with chronic HBV infection. Ground-glass hepatocytes *(arrow)* are demonstrated. (Hematoxylin and eosin stain; original magnification ×20.) *B*, Photomicrograph of the liver of a child with chronic HBV infection. The darkly stained nuclei *(arrow)* contain HBcAg. (Immunoperoxidase stain for HBcAg; original magnification ×20.)

(approximately 5 percent of the world's population) are infected worldwide.[114] Fifty-five to 92 million people are expected to die between 45 and 55 years of age from HBV-related chronic liver disease or primary hepatocellular cancer.[58]

Areas of high, intermediate, and low endemicity, as reflected by the number of carriers, have been identified. Highly endemic areas are those in which more than 8 percent of the population is infected. Examples include Southeast Asia, Africa, Commonwealth of Independent States, and China. More than 70 percent of the world's population lives in these high-endemicity areas. The Middle East, Central and South America, and parts of Eastern Europe are examples of intermediate-endemicity regions, where infection is found in 2 to 7 percent of the population. The United States, Australia, and Western Europe are areas of low endemicity, with chronic infection rates of less than 2 percent of the total population.[174] In areas of low endemicity, acute infections occur more commonly in adults, which, although causing significant morbidity, are less likely to result in chronic carriage than are asymptomatic infections in children.

In the United States, the prevalence of chronic HBV infection (HBsAg positive) among the general population, based on the National Health and Nutrition Examination Surveys (NHANES) III survey, is estimated at 0.42 percent. NHANES III was conducted from 1988 to 1994 and revealed that 5.5 percent of the U.S. population had evidence of either past or chronic infection with HBV.[119] The rates among ethnic groups varied, with non-Hispanic blacks having the highest rates (12.8 percent) compared with non-Hispanic whites (2.8 percent) and Mexican Americans (4.8 percent). The strongest predictors of HBV infection were non-Hispanic black ethnicity, increased number of sexual partners, foreign birth, cocaine use, and having less than a high school education.[119]

HBV may be transmitted vertically, horizontally, parenterally, or sexually. Vertical transmission of HBV occurs in the perinatal setting when an infected mother transmits the infection to her child. Horizontal transmission occurs among children in groups of high endemicity who were not infected at birth. This form of transmission occurs in households of an infected family member, in which other members acquire HBV without sexual or overt contact with contaminated bodily fluid. In adolescents and adults, infection is transmitted by contaminated blood or other bodily fluids through percutaneous or mucous membrane routes. Examples are intravenous drug use; occupational exposure to blood; sexual contact, especially in men who have sex with men; and nosocomial infections from contaminated shared equipment.[114]

In countries where HBV infection is highly endemic, perinatal or vertical transmission is a very common occurrence, whereas in regions of low endemicity, sexual transmission occurs more commonly. If a mother tests positive for both HBeAg and HBsAg, the risk for transmission of HBV to her child is 85 to 90 percent without immunoprophylaxis.[10] The most common risk factors for HBV infection in the United States were examined in the 1992–1993 sentinel counties study.[152] These risk factors were heterosexual exposure to a person with hepatitis or having multiple sexual partners (41 percent), intravenous drug use (15 percent), household contact (4 percent), and employment as a healthcare worker (1 percent).

Within the United States, the number of reported cases of acute hepatitis B decreased more than 50 percent between 1990 and 1998 (21,102 to 10,258 reported cases).[7] However, less than one third of adults have symptoms, implying that the number of people exposed is far greater than the reported cases.[115] Nonetheless, the decrease in the number of acute infections is considered real because during this decade, elimination strategies such as screening of pregnant women, universal immunization of infants, and catch-up immunization of older children and those in high-risk groups were implemented. The experience from Taiwan, the first country to implement mass vaccination against HBV, is even more encouraging. Since 1986, all newborns have been vaccinated against HBV. The program has been extended to other children and adults, leading to a 10-fold decrease in the chronic infection rate.[33] After approximately 10 years, a significant decrease in the incidence of hepatocellular carcinoma in children was reported.[29] Current vaccination recommendations are discussed later in this chapter.

Researchers have estimated that only 45 percent of the expected 20,000 HbsAg-positive women giving birth in the United States between 1993 and 1996 were identified.[156] This low figure may be due to numerous factors; women likely to be infected often do not receive prenatal care, or women may be tested but the information not conveyed to the place of birth or to the pediatrician caring for the child.[10] Attention to this aspect of care is extremely important because the reduction in rate of transmission from mother to child with use of hepatitis B immunoglobulin (HBIG) and hepatitis B vaccine is 90 percent.[84]

HBsAg can be found the breast milk of HBV-infected mothers. However, in studies performed in Taiwan and England, breast feeding by HbsAg-seropositive mothers did not seem to increase significantly the risk for neonatal acquisition of HBV infection.[129] Effective immunoprophylaxis should allow for safe breast feeding in this setting.

Natural History

Adults who have an acute HBV infection and who are immunocompetent have less than a 5 percent risk for development of chronic HBV infection,[80] compared with a greater than 90 percent risk in vertically infected neonates. If an infected person has other medical problems, such as end-stage renal disease requiring hemodialysis, or is co-infected with HIV, the risk for development of chronic HBV infection increases. If chronic HBV infection develops in an adult, the prognosis is dependent on whether active HBV replication and liver histologic changes are present or whether the adult is "immunologically tolerant" of the infection. Approximately 50 percent of adult chronic carriers have evidence of ongoing viral replication, and 15 to 20 percent of these individuals develop cirrhosis within 5 years.[176] However, the remaining adult chronic HBV carriers have normal aminotransferase values and normal or nearly normal liver histology. After 7- to 11-year follow-up of such patients, only 2 percent were found to have histologic progression of liver disease, and 15 percent had become HBsAg-negative.[48] The risk for development of hepatocellular carcinoma is increased in all HBV chronic carriers but especially those with active viral replication.[14]

The natural history of chronic HBV infection in children has been examined in several populations. Most Chinese children, in whom chronic HBV usually is perinatally acquired, remain HBeAg-positive, with very high levels of viral replication, yet only minimal clinical liver disease.[108, 109] In contrast, children in the West with chronic HBV infection frequently clear HBeAg and HBV DNA from serum during the first two decades.[21] Those who lose HBeAg tend to have higher alanine aminotransferase (ALT) levels early in life, indicating more active liver disease. Some of the children become seronegative for HBsAg as well, and reactivation of viral replication is observed only rarely. These differences are ascribed to the older age at acquisition of HBV in the Western children, associated with a more efficient immune response. These observations influence the management and counseling of children with chronic HBV infection as well as the design and interpretation of therapeutic trials.

Extrahepatic manifestations of both acute and chronic HBV infection occur more commonly in adults. As many as 25 percent of adults with acute HBV infection have extrahepatic manifestations such as arthralgias and even serum-like sickness. Vasculitides can develop in both acute and chronic HBV infection, and examples include polyarteritis nodosa, renal disease, and mononeuritis.[118] Occasionally, a chronically infected child presents with extrahepatic disease, such as membranoproliferative glomerulonephritis.[90, 160]

CARCINOGENESIS

HCC is a recognized sequela of chronic infection with HBV; worldwide, most cases of HCC are linked to HBV infection. In Taiwan, the incidence of HCC in chronically infected individuals is 200 to 812 cases per 100,000 person-years, compared to 10 to 30 cases per 100,000 person-years in the general population. With liver cirrhosis secondary to chronic HBV infection, the incidence increases to 1000 to 5000 cases per 100,000 person-years (1 to 5 percent per year).[34] The lifetime risk for development of HCC in a chronic HBsAg carrier is estimated at 40 to 50 percent.[14]

Almost 100 percent of woodchucks chronically infected with WHV develop HCC within 3 years.[95] The detection of integrated HBV sequences in both human HCC and animal models led to numerous hypotheses regarding the mechanisms leading to HCC. Current hypotheses center on the integration of viral DNA into host genome, which may be associated with activation of oncogenes, deactivation of tumor suppressor genes, or other genetic instability. The finding that HCC cells in an individual HBV carrier contain HBV DNA in discrete rather than random sites, indicating clonal expansion of tumor cells, supports this theory. In general terms, the integrated HBV may affect genes locally by replacing or activating genes by insertional mutagenesis, or HBV may affect more distant genes by means of gene products that can be diffused.[132] Integration of HBV occurs at random sites on host hepatocyte chromosomes rather than at one fixed site. HCC tissue can itself contain a variety of chromosomal abnormalities, such as polyploidy, allelic imbalance, and translocations.[128] More than a dozen genes have been implicated in HCC, not only suggesting heterogeneity of genetic etiologic factors but also indicating that an accumulation of genetic mutations is required for HCC to develop.

Although many mutations are found in HCC, they can be clustered into four main pathways. The first is that of tumor suppressor or DNA damage repair genes typified by *p53*. A mutation in *p53* is detected in approximately 30 percent of HCC tumors, although this figure varies in different geographic regions, being more common in China and less so in Europe. The rate of *p53* mutation is increased by exposure to aflatoxin.[128] A second pathway is that of cell cycle control, the *RB1* pathway. An example is the retinoblastoma gene, which is mutated in about 15 percent of HCC tumors.[182] The third pathway involves transforming growth factor-β (TGF-β). One of the receptors for this cytokine, mannose-6-phophate/insulin-like growth factor-2 receptor, is mutated in approximately one third of HCC tumors. This receptor is involved in the activation of TGF-β, which inhibits growth and induces apoptosis in hepatocytes. The final pathway associated with transformation of a normal hepatocyte to a malignant one is the β-catenin and adenomatosis polyposis coli *(APC)* gene system, which is involved in signal transduction. The E-adherin gene, which produces a protein that forms complexes with β-catenin, frequently is mutated in HCC.[154]

Abnormalities in hepatocyte regulatory genes may be activated by the integration of HBV X protein (HBx). HBx can function as a transcription activator, protease inhibitor, and effector of cell signaling pathways. Two other HBV proteins, middle hepatitis B virus surface protein and the large hepatitis B virus protein, share similar properties.[132]

The frequency and significance of integration of viral DNA into the host genome are unresolved issues in childhood HBV infection; some studies have shown early integration, whereas others describe it as a rare event.[12, 30, 65, 149, 177, 180] Although HCC is detected most often after at least 20 years of chronic HBV infection, cases in children as young as 8 months old have been reported.[64, 167, 179] Childhood HCC associated with HBV infection has been described in both Asian[32, 167] and Western[64, 130] populations. Because most cases are reported retrospectively, data regarding incidence are not available. No guidelines have been developed for prospective monitoring of children with chronic HBV infection for development of HCC, although periodic measurement of serum alpha-fetoprotein levels and hepatic ultrasounds are recommended in adults.

The exact mechanism of HCC carcinogenesis caused by chronic HBV infection is not understood fully, and a universal gene or final common pathway has not been identified. The interplay of hepatocyte injury caused by HBV infection, coupled with the need for hepatocyte regeneration to retain organ function, sets the milieu for gene mutations to accumulate and the eventual development of HCC. Prevention of HBV infection and eradication of existing infection remain the most effective measures to prevent HCC.

Hepatitis B in Special Populations

HEPATITIS B AND HUMAN IMMUNODEFICIENCY VIRUS CO-INFECTION

The prevalence and course of HBV in adults who are co-infected with HIV has been examined in numerous studies. Of 181 HIV-infected adults in Greece, 71.8 percent of the men who have sex with men and 91.7 percent of intravenous drug users had evidence of HBV infection.[54] In a study from Australia conducted between 1985 and 1989, men with HIV infection were more likely to have chronic HBV infection than were HIV-negative men.[19] No evidence has been found for direct interaction between HBV and HIV. HIV and HBV co-infected individuals have higher circulating levels of HBV DNA but not worse hepatic necroinflammation.[41] Spontaneous HBeAg–to–anti-HBe seroconversion rarely occurs in this group. Special considerations for treatment and immunization are discussed in the appropriate subsections.

HEPATITIS B IN SOLID ORGAN TRANSPLANT RECIPIENTS

Chronic HBV infection became a relative contraindication to liver transplantation after initial poor results. In the 1970s and 1980s, more than 80 percent of patients became reinfected quickly, and 55 percent died within 60 days of surgery. Patients who had recurrence of HBV infection after liver transplantation developed a characteristic histologic lesion, termed *fibrosing cholestatic hepatitis*, which eventually led to loss of the allograft.[15] The demonstration in the 1990s that HBIG is efficacious in decreasing infection of the allograft has allowed successful transplantation. The use of long-term HBIG decreases the risk for recurrence to 30 percent at 12 months and increases patient survival to greater than 90 percent at 12 months after transplantation.[144] The allograft reinfection rate is even lower if the patient does not have active HBV replication at the time of transplantation. The cost of HBIG is a major factor; each weekly dose costs more than $3000 (U.S.), and duration of therapy appears to be lifelong. The addition of nucleoside analogues to the use of HBIG after transplantation is discussed later, and this strategy may offer savings in both cost and convenience.

HBV infection (acute and chronic) is the sixth most common indication for liver transplantation in the United States,[175] but rarely does a child with HBV need a liver transplant. Of 215 children who underwent transplantation between 1986 and 1992 at a major French center, only 4 had HBV-associated disease.[113]

The role of HBV infection in the course of other solid organ transplants has been examined. In one study, all HBV-infected patients who received heart transplants developed chronic infection. However, HBV-associated liver disease did not appear to progress rapidly.[112] The chronic HBV infection had little effect on 5-year survival after the heart transplantation.[112] In a study from Taiwan, overall patient and allograft survival after kidney transplantation were not affected by HBV infection, despite increased hepatic morbidity.[78] Of the 113 patients who received a kidney transplant between 1986 and 1998, 20 patients were HbsAg positive, and 9 were positive for both HBsAg and HCV antibody. Of the 20 who were infected with HBV alone, 4 developed fulminant hepatic failure and died within 2 years of renal transplantation, 2 developed cirrhosis, and 2 others developed hepatocellular carcinoma.[78] Overall, however, the 5-year survival was not dissimilar in those infected with HBV and those not infected.

Treatment

Treatment for acute hepatitis B is purely supportive, and most patients recover fully. The role of antiviral therapy in fulminant HBV infection has not been studied systematically. Treatment, when indicated, is directed at those with chronic HBV infection. In this setting, the long-term goals of therapy are eradication of HBV and improvement or regression of liver disease. Shorter-term goals for an individual course of treatment include cessation or decrease in viral replication as indicated by loss of HBeAg and loss of HBV DNA from serum, clearance of HBsAg, normalization of liver histopathology, and normalization of aminotransferase values.

To date, no agents fulfill all of these goals effectively in most patients. Children and adults have differences in immune tolerance and rate of progression of liver disease because of differences of age at and mode of infection. Therefore, studies of treatments for chronic HBV in adults cannot be extrapolated directly to children. In addition, the timing and choice of therapeutic agent are crucial because children in different areas of the world may respond differently to therapy at different points in their infections.

A potential candidate for treatment should have serologic evidence of HBV infection for at least 6 months. The serologic criteria include detectable serum HBsAg, HbeAg, or HBV DNA (in case of eAg-negative HBV infection.) A liver biopsy should be obtained before the start of therapy to provide evidence of chronic hepatitis, to stage the disease, and to rule out other processes. In most studies performed before the high prevalence of eAg negative infections, seroconversion from HBeAg to anti-HBe in serum was used as the primary outcome variable for response to therapy. Spontaneous rates of HBeAg clearance in children younger than 3 years are very low (less than 2 percent per year) and increase with age. In children older than 6 years of age, the yearly clearance rates vary from 14.3 to 35.3 percent.[31] Therapeutic trial results must be compared with the "background rate" of spontaneous seroconversion.

Two medications are approved for treatment of chronic HBV in adults, IFN-α and lamivudine. IFN-α first was reported as a successful treatment for chronic HBV in 1976,[66] and recombinant IFN-α-2B was approved by the U.S. Food and Drug Administration in 1992 for adults and in 1998 for children with chronic HBV. Lamivudine initially was used as treatment of HIV infection and was found to have antiviral effect for HBV.

IFNs are a family of cytokines with immunomodulatory, antiproliferative, and direct antiviral actions. The three types of IFN are α, β, and γ. IFN-α has been the primary form used in this setting. It induces the display of HLA class I molecules on hepatocyte membranes, which in turn promotes lysis by $CD8^+$ cytotoxic lymphocytes. At the same time, it directly inhibits viral protein synthesis.[103] IFN-α is available in several forms, including IFN-α-2a, IFN-α-2b, and lymphoblastoid IFN-α. Only IFN-α–2a and -2b have been licensed in the United States for use in children.

Treatment of children in Western countries leads to loss of HBV DNA or HBeAg seroconversion in 20 to 58 percent, as compared with 8 to 17 percent outcome in control children.[173] Success rates are not as high for treatment of children in Asian countries, most of whom were perinatally infected; only 3 to 17 percent cleared HBV DNA or seroconverted HBeAg to anti-Hbe.[100] These differences in treatment responses are thought to be related to age at development of infection. However, in a large multinational, randomized control trial of IFN-α-2b, no differences were found in loss of HBsAg between children born in Asian countries (22%) and those from Europe and North America (26%) if aminotransferase values were elevated.[158] If only children with elevated aminotransferases are selected for treatment with IFN-α, then children younger than 13 years of age with intermediate HBV DNA levels (10 to 200 pg/mL by Abbott radioimmunoassay) are most likely to have a good response, regardless of ethnicity.[158]

Higher doses of IFN-α (10 megaunits/m^2) are not associated with higher clearance rates, although treatment for 6 months seems to improve outcome.[173] In the multinational randomized controlled trial referenced previously, children received 6 megaunits/m^2 of IFN-α-2b three times a week for 6 months. However, the dose of IFN-α-2b had to be reduced because of bone marrow suppression or fever in 23 percent of children. In this study, serum HBeAg and HBV DNA became negative in 26 percent of treated children and 11 percent of controls. In children who responded to therapy, liver histology improved, and serum aminotransferase values normalized.[157] Prednisone priming (i.e., a course of steroids immediately before IFN-α treatment) has been proposed to induce an acute exacerbation of hepatitis B, thereby rendering the patient more susceptible to IFN. However, a dual-center, double-blind randomized trial of lymphoblastoid IFN-α with or without steroid pretreatment showed no improvement in HBeAg-to-HBeAb seroconversion rate over that of IFN-α alone.[63]

Reported studies of IFN-α included children older than 18 months of age, without hepatitis C and HIV co-infections because these may alter treatment algorithms. Children with evidence of active immunologic responses to HBV (i.e., low levels of viral replication [HBV DNA] and high ALT values [greater than twice normal]) are more likely to have a response to therapy with IFN-α.[172] Children who acquired disease by vertical transmission are more likely to have established immune tolerance and may be less likely to respond to treatment. Children with very low HBV DNA levels may be in the process of spontaneous seroconversion; therefore, an expectant policy may be prudent.

Ten percent of treated adults and children lose HbsAg, compared with 1 percent of untreated patients.[96, 158] Long-term (1.1 to 11.5 years) follow-up of adult responders to IFN-α showed a significantly reduced incidence of hepatocellular carcinoma compared with either treated nonresponders or control patients. HCC was detected in 1 of the 67 treated patients and in 4 of the 34 untreated patients.[105] Reports of long-term outcomes in treated children are very few, but in a report from Turkey, none of 23 children with chronic HBV infection and elevated aminotransferases who failed to respond to IFN-α developed cirrhosis or HCC at a mean follow-up of 4.5 years.[93] The role of retreatment of nonresponders has been addressed in a few studies. In a series from Europe, 9 of 27 nonresponder adults retreated with IFN α-2a (9 million units thrice weekly for 6 months) cleared HBV DNA and HbeAg, compared with 3 of 30 control patients.[25] An open-label pilot study of IFN-β in HBV-infected children who did not respond to IFN-α suggested some possible benefit.[140]

Side effects of IFN-α include a transient influenza-like syndrome (fever, myalgia, headache, arthralgia, and anorexia) that occurs in virtually all patients at the start of therapy. Bone marrow suppression, especially neutropenia, is a common side effect, seen in 39 percent of children in one series.[81] Changes in personality, irritability, and temper tantrums are reported more frequently in children than in adults.[81, 158] These problems resolve once treatment is withdrawn. Epistaxis not associated with thrombocytopenia or prolonged prothrombin time, febrile seizures, and marked elevation of aminotransferases have been reported. Quality of life is impaired in children during IFN therapy compared with their pretreatment levels because of medication side effects and fear of injections. However, within 3 months of cessation of treatment, these effects are reversed.[81] Therapy in children seldom is discontinued because of side effects.

Two meta-analyses of treatment of chronic HBV in children with IFN-α have been conducted.[172, 173] Each report concludes that treatment leads to a higher rate of HBeAg to anti-Hbe seroconversion than would occur spontaneously. Randomized control trials may be analyzed for "number to treat" (i.e., the number of children requiring treatment in order to have a therapeutic response in one patient). If only children with ALT values twice normal are considered, 2.5 children need to be treated for one to clear HBV DNA. However if all infected children are treated, then 7.1 children would require therapy to clear HBV DNA from one child.[172] Approximately two thirds of children treated with IFN-α show no sustained response to therapy.

Lamivudine (2′,3′-dideoxycytosine), also known as 3TC, is an oral nucleoside analogue. It is triphosphorylated intracellularly to an active intermediate that is incorporated into the growing DNA chain, thereby terminating the chain and inhibiting viral replication. Preliminary studies of lamivudine in Chinese adults who were chronic HBsAg carriers revealed that 4 weeks of treatment with lamivudine suppressed HBV DNA concentration to less than 90 percent of its pretreatment level. This effect was reversed at the cessation of treatment.[99] Two large, randomized, controlled studies of lamivudine as initial treatment for chronic HBV infection, one from Hong Kong[98] and the other from the United States,[53] showed serologic, biochemical, and histologic evidence of benefit. In the American study, treatment was of 52 weeks' duration, and 32 percent of 61 patients treated lost HbeAg, versus 11 percent of controls. This response was sustained to at least 4 months after the cessation of therapy. Of treated patients, 17 percent lost HBeAg, developed HBe antibodies, and had undetectable levels of HBV DNA, compared with 6 percent of control patients. Prolonging treatment with lamivudine to 18 months increased the loss of HBeAg to 38 percent and seroconversion to 21 percent.[52] However, prolonged treatment increases the risk for emergence of mutation in the HBV polymerase gene at the YMDD locus, as reported in 10 of the 23 patients treated for 18 months. Of these, only 3 had evidence of virologic breakthrough (detectable HBV DNA).[52] This mutation arises because of a methionine-to-valine or a methionine-to-isoleucine switch in the C domain of the HBV polymerase.[170] The long-term significance of YMDD variants of HBV is not clear. However, once lamivudine monotherapy is stopped, wild-type virus reappears.[60] Treatment with lamivudine also improves liver histology and decreases the rate of progression to hepatic fibrosis.[53] Based on the observation that both therapeutic response and development of resistant mutants increase in frequency with treatment time, the optimal duration of lamivudine therapy has not been defined.

Clinical experience with lamivudine for children with HBV infection is limited. A recent dose-ranging study of the pharmacokinetics, safety, and preliminary efficacy was conducted in multiple centers in Europe and Canada. It showed that lamivudine was well tolerated and that a dose of 3 mg/kg once daily in children 2 to 12 years of age and of 100 mg daily in those older than 12 years of age provided levels of exposure and trough concentrations similar to those in adults receiving 100 mg daily. The decrease in HBV DNA at 4 weeks was of a magnitude similar to that seen in adults.[159] Long-term benefits are not known.

Lamivudine has been associated with nausea, vomiting, headaches, abdominal discomfort, diarrhea, and fatigue in adults; these symptoms usually are mild and transient.[43] Symptomatic elevation in serum lipase also has been reported, but this elevation was not noted in the multicenter study of safety and dosing of lamivudine in children. Indeed, no serious side effects were reported in this study.[159] Because lamivudine is excreted by the kidneys, the dose should be reduced in patients with renal failure. Upon cessation of therapy in adults, 25 percent of treated patients had elevations of serum ALT of up to three times baseline, as compared with 8 percent of placebo-treated patients. This "lamivudine withdrawal flare" rarely may progress to jaundice and incipient liver failure, as noted in 2 of 41 patients in a Dutch study.[73] Therefore, monitoring patients closely after a course of lamivudine is important.

Because lamivudine is tolerated so well, many patients, including those with advanced liver disease in whom IFN is contraindicated, can be considered for treatment. Researchers have suggested that the medication should be continued until HBeAg disappears from the serum, anti-HBe appears, or, if neither occurs, HBV DNA becomes persistently undetectable. Transplant recipients may develop fulminant hepatitis with YMDD mutants; therefore, the drug should be used cautiously in this group.[60] Although as an oral medication with a satisfactory safety profile lamivudine is an attractive medication for children, its efficacy in children has not been demonstrated. As in adults, the optimal duration of therapy has not been defined.

Preliminary studies of combination therapy with IFN-α and lamivudine did not show an increase in the rate of

HBeAg-to-HBeAb seroconversion.[121] However, in a larger series of patients, the combination of these agents led to seroconversion rates of 29 percent at week 52 compared with 19 percent in those treated with IFN-α alone and 18 percent with lamivudine monotherapy.[146]

A variety of nucleoside and nucleotide analogues with proven efficacy against HIV, cytomegalovirus, and herpes simplex virus have been shown to have antiviral activity against HBV. One example is famciclovir, the prodrug of penciclovir, a purine nucleoside analogue used for short-term treatment of varicella-zoster virus and herpes simplex virus infections. It has proven efficacy both in vivo and in vitro against HBV. In a 1-year, randomized, placebo-controlled, multicenter study in adults with chronic HBV, it led to a modest suppression of viral replication (9% of treated patients became HBeAg negative versus 3% of controls) and a significant improvement in liver histology scores.[49] Its use for chronic HBV infection in children has not been reported. Other analogues in various stages of testing against chronic HBV infection include lobucavir, adefovir, and emtricitabine.

Immunomodulatory therapies such as pre-S/S peptide vaccination and DNA vaccination have shown benefit in cell lines and animal models but have not been used yet in humans.[38, 138]

Patients with HBV who also are infected with HIV or who are immunosuppressed after organ transplantation respond poorly to IFN therapy because of high levels of viremia and depressed cell-mediated immunity. Therefore, therapeutic interest has focused on alternative agents. Lamivudine has been shown to be well tolerated in those adults with HBV and HIV receiving highly active retroviral therapy, with a reduction in HBV DNA. However, of 18 adults treated for 6 months, only 2 had HBeAg seroconversion.[16]

As stated previously, HBV infection is likely to recur after liver transplantation. The rapid graft loss that results has led to the development of strategies for prevention and the treatment of recurrent HBV infection. Administration of HBIG reduces graft reinfection from 75 to 35 percent after orthotopic liver transplantation. Lamivudine used before and after transplantation also can decrease HBV activity; however, YMDD mutants are likely to appear with prolonged therapy and can lead to hepatitis and liver failure in immunosuppressed patients.[60] This group of HBV-infected patients may benefit from newer combinations of antiviral agents.

In individuals with chronic HBV infection who undergo cytotoxic or immunosuppressive therapy for other conditions, viral replication may be enhanced, leading to an increase in the number of infected hepatocytes. When the cytotoxic therapy or immunosuppression is withdrawn, immune function is restored, and destruction of hepatocytes that can lead to acute hepatitis or even liver failure is rapid. Lamivudine has been used with some success in this group.[178]

The child most likely to be treated successfully with today's agents is one who acquired HBV beyond infancy, has evidence of immune responsiveness to HBV, and has mild to moderate inflammatory changes on liver biopsy. The child ideally has no other medical problems, and child and family can comply with the regimen and monitoring.

Immunoprophylaxis

A comprehensive strategy to prevent HBV infection, both acute hepatitis B and the sequelae of chronic HBV infection, must eliminate transmission that occurs during infancy a nd childhood as well as during adolescence and adulthood. HBV transmission cannot be prevented through vaccinating only the groups at highest risk of developing infection. Routine visits for prenatal and well-child care can be used to target hepatitis B prevention. A comprehensive prevention strategy currently recommended by the Centers for Disease Control and Prevention (CDC) includes (1) prenatal testing of pregnant women for HBsAg to identify newborns who require immunoprophylaxis for the prevention of perinatal infection and to identify household contacts who should be vaccinated, (2) routine vaccination of all newborn infants, (3) catch-up vaccination of older children and adolescents, and (4) vaccination of adults at high risk for development of infection[4] (Table 162–2).

Two types of products are available for prophylaxis against HBV infection. HBIG provides temporary (3 to 6 months) protection by means of passive immunity and is indicated only in certain postexposure settings. Hepatitis B vaccine evokes active immunity against HBV and is recommended for both preexposure and postexposure prophylaxis.

HEPATITIS B IMMUNOGLOBULIN

HBIG is prepared from plasma known to contain a high titer of anti-HBs. The human plasma from which HBIG is prepared is screened for antibodies to HIV, and the process used to prepare HBIG inactivates and eliminates HIV from the final product; no evidence has been found that HIV can be transmitted by HBIG. HBIG is used in the postexposure

TABLE 162–2 ■ RECOMMENDED USE OF HEPATITIS B VACCINES

Age	No. of Doses	Schedule	Dose: Recombivax HB (10 μg/mL)	Dose: Engerix-*B* (20 μg/mL)
Infants of HBsAg-negative mothers	3	0–2, 1–4, and 6–18 mo	5 μg (0.5 mL)	10 μg (0.5 mL)
Infants of HBsAg-positive mothers	3	HBIG and vaccine within 12 hr, then vaccine at 1–2 and 6 mo	5 μg (0.5 mL)	10 μg (0.5 mL)
Children and adolescents aged 1 to 19 yr	3	0, 1–2, and 4–6 mo	5 μg (0.5 mL)	10 μg (0.5 mL)
Adolescents aged 11 to 15 yr	2	0 and 4–6 mo	10 μg (1.0 mL)	NA
Adults aged >20 yr	3	0, 1–2, and 4–6 mo	10 μg (1.0 mL)	20 μg (1.0 mL)
Immunocompromised adults	3	0, 1, and 6 mo	40 μg (1.0 mL)*	NA
	4	0, 1, 2, and 6 mo	NA	40 μg (2.0 mL)

*This is a special formulation of Recombivax HB.
From Vaccine Use. NIH Publication No. 00-425, July 1998.

prophylaxis of newborns of HBV-infected women and for susceptible individuals with sexual, needle-stick, or mucosal exposures. It is administered intramuscularly. The dose for infants with perinatal HBV exposure is 0.5 mL. The dose for adults is 0.06 mL/kg body weight. Efficacy ranges from 70 to 95 percent.[10] HBIG in large doses is used after liver transplantation in HBV-infected patients to prevent infection of the allograft.

HEPATITIS B VACCINE

The two licensed recombinant vaccines are produced by using *Saccharomyces cerevisiae* (common baker's yeast), into which a plasmid containing the gene for HBsAg has been inserted. Purified HBsAg is obtained by lysis of the yeast cells and separation of HBsAg by biochemical and biophysical techniques. Hepatitis B vaccines are packaged to contain 10 to 40 μg of HBsAg protein/mL after adsorption to aluminum hydroxide (0.5 mg/mL). The two vaccines available in the United States are Recombivax HB (Merck and Company, Inc, West Point, PA) and Energix-B (SmithKline Beecham Biologicals, Pittsburgh, PA).

The recommended series of three intramuscular doses of HBV vaccine (see Table 162–2) induces a protective antibody response (anti-HBs) in more than 90 percent of healthy adults and in more than 95 percent of infants, children, and adolescents. HBV vaccine should be administered into the deltoid muscles of adults and children or the anterolateral thigh muscles of neonates and infants; the immunogenicity is substantially lower when injections are administered into the buttocks. When HBV vaccine is administered to infants at the same time as are other vaccines, separate sites in the anterolateral thigh may be used for the multiple injections.

The vaccination schedule used most often for adults and children has been three intramuscular injections, the second and third administered 1 and 6 months, respectively, after the first. Each of the two available vaccines has been evaluated to determine the age-specific dose at which an optimal antibody response is achieved. The recommended doses vary by product and the recipient's age and are outlined in Table 162–2.

Perinatal transmission of HBV can be prevented effectively if the HBsAg-positive mother is identified and if her infant receives appropriate immunoprophylaxis. Administration of HBIG and the first dose of HBV vaccine within 12 hours of birth prevents 90 percent of perinatal infections.[84] Serologic testing of infants who receive immunoprophylaxis to prevent perinatal infection should be performed to identify the 5 percent of infants who become HBV carriers despite these measures. Testing for anti-HBs and HBsAg in children 12 to 15 months of age determines the success of vaccination and, in the case of failure, identifies HBV carriers or infants who may require treatment or revaccination. The following are the current recommendations as to timing of immunizations for infants in the United States[8]:

1. Infants born to HbsAg-negative mothers should receive the first vaccine dose by 2 months of age, the second at least 1 month later, and the third at least 4 months after the first dose and 2 months after the second. The third dose should not be given before the child reaches 6 months of age. Testing for serologic response is not necessary and is not recommended.
2. Infants born to HbsAg-positive mothers should receive 0.5 mL of HBIG and the first dose of HBV vaccine within 12 hours of birth, administered intramuscularly at separate sites. The infant should receive the second dose at 2 months and the third at 6 months of age. Premature infants of HBV-infected women should receive vaccine in the same schedule. Testing for serologic response (HBsAg and anti-HBs) should be done when the child is 12 to 15 months of age.
3. Infants born to mothers whose HBsAg status is unknown should receive the first dose of vaccine within 12 hours of birth. Meanwhile, a maternal blood sample should be sent for HBsAg testing. If positive, HBIG should be given as soon as possible (not later than 1 week of age). The infant then should complete the routine vaccination schedule.
4. In addition, the American Academy of Pediatrics and the Advisory Committee on Immunization Practices (ACIP) guidelines recommend that all nonimmunized children begin HBV vaccination at any visit.
5. For older children and adolescents aged 11 to 15 years, the routine three-dose schedule may be used, but a two-dose schedule of vaccination also has been approved, using the Recombivax HB vaccine. The adult dose (1.0 mL) is administered to the adolescent, and the second dose is given 4 to 6 months later. Short-term (2-year) follow-up in groups immunized by either schedule showed similar rates of anti-HBs decline. Of emphasis is that a lower dose of vaccine is used in the three-dose schedule, and if the original dose is not known, the full three-dose schedule should be used.[6]
6. Immunization also should be offered to high-risk groups until universal childhood immunization has created an immune adult population. Table 162–3 summarizes the groups who should be considered for HBV vaccination.

In a three-dose schedule, increasing the interval between administrations of the first and second doses of hepatitis B vaccine has little effect on immunogenicity or final antibody titer. The third dose confers optimal protection, acting as a booster dose. Longer intervals between the last two doses (4 to 12 months) result in higher final titers of anti-HBs

TABLE 162–3 ■ HIGH-RISK GROUPS TARGETED FOR HEPATITIS B VACCINATION

Group	Special Considerations
Workers with occupational exposure risk	Workplace policies in event of potential exposure should be in place as well.
Hemodialysis patients	Should be immunized early in the disease course to increase the response rate.
Recipients of clotting factor concentrates	Blood donors are screened for hepatitis B virus infection.
Household and sexual contacts	
International travelers	If a stay of longer than 6 months in an endemic area is anticipated *or* for those planning shorter stays but for whom sexual contacts or blood transfusion is possible.
Sexually active men who have sex with men and all sexually active people with multiple partners or unprotected intercourse	Most recent infections in the United States are through sexual transmission.
Injecting drug users and sexual partners	Clean needle programs are adjunct to immunization.
Prison inmates	
Adopted children	All internationally adopted children should be screened for hepatitis B surface antigen. If the child is seropositive, the adoptive family should be immunized.

antibodies. Larger vaccine doses or an increased number of doses is required to induce protective antibody in many hemodialysis patients and other immunocompromised persons (e.g., those who take immunosuppressive drugs or who are infected with HIV). Children with end-stage renal disease respond better than do adults to HBV immunization. Ninety percent of pediatric chronic dialysis patients and 100 percent of children vaccinated before beginning hemodialysis became anti-HBs positive in one study.[59] An immunocompromised person who has previously shown an adequate anti-HBs antibody titer that then falls to less than 10 mIU/mL should receive a booster dose.

Performing postvaccination serologic testing is not necessary after routine vaccination of infants, children, or adolescents. Testing for immunity is advised only for patients whose subsequent clinical management depends on knowledge of their immune status (e.g., infants born to HBsAg-positive mothers, hemodialysis patients and staff, patients with HIV infection). Postvaccination testing also should be considered for those at occupational risk who may have exposures from injuries with sharp instruments because knowledge of their antibody response helps determine appropriate postexposure prophylaxis.

When revaccinated, 15 to 25 percent of people who do not respond to the primary vaccine series produce an adequate antibody response after one additional dose, and 30 to 50 percent do so after three additional doses.[83] Therefore, revaccination should be considered for people who do not respond to the initial series. The duration of vaccine-induced immunity has been evaluated in long-term follow-up studies of both adults and children. A 12-year follow-up of a prospective randomized trial of recombinant yeast vaccine versus plasma-derived vaccine without booster doses in 318 children was performed in Hong Kong. Outcomes measured were anti-HBs titers and protection from HBV infection. At 12 years, anti-HBs was greater than 10 mIU/mL in 80 percent of children who completed a three-dose schedule of either type of vaccine. However, even without a detectable anti-HBs titer, no child became HBsAg positive. The authors concluded that a three-dose schedule produced long-term immunity and that booster doses were not required because of effective anamnestic response.[181]

In general, follow-up studies of children vaccinated at birth to prevent perinatal HBV infection have shown that a continued high level of protection from chronic HBV infections lasts at least 5 years.[153]

VACCINE SIDE EFFECTS AND ADVERSE REACTIONS

Hepatitis B vaccines have been shown to be safe for both adults and children. Pain at the injection site (3–29%) and a temperature greater than 37.7° C (1–6%) have been the side effects most frequently reported, but they were reported no more frequently among vaccinees than among subjects receiving a placebo.[166] Anaphylaxis is the only serious adverse event; this event occurs rarely, at a rate of about 1 per 600,000 vaccine doses.[5]

In the United States, surveillance of adverse reactions has shown a possible association between Guillain-Barré syndrome and receipt of the first dose of plasma-derived hepatitis B vaccine (CDC, unpublished data). Guillain-Barré syndrome was reported at a low rate (0.5 per 100,000 vaccinees), no deaths were reported, and all cases were among adults. However, plasma-derived HBV vaccine no longer is in use. An estimated 2.5 million adults received one or more doses of recombinant hepatitis B vaccine during the period 1986 to 1990. Available data from reporting systems for adverse events do not indicate an association between recombinant vaccine and Guillain-Barré syndrome (CDC, unpublished data).

Reports of multiple sclerosis (MS) developing after vaccination for HBV led to concern that the vaccine might cause MS in previously healthy subjects. This theory was refuted in a nested control study of two large cohorts of nurses in the United States that compared the HBV immunization histories of each of 192 women who developed MS with five healthy controls and one woman with breast cancer. No association was found.[9] In a case crossover study using the European MS database, recent vaccination against HBV, tetanus, or influenza did not appear to increase the short-term risk for relapse in MS.[42]

Vaccines are prepared with thimerosal, sodium ethylmercuric thiosalicylate, to prevent bacterial and fungal contamination. This preservative has aroused great public concern regarding mercury toxicity and the amount of mercury exposure relative to body weight. Infants were considered at greater risk for mercury poisoning from thimerosal-containing vaccines. No adverse outcomes have been associated clearly with thimerosal use, but nonetheless, in 1999, a joint statement was issued by the American Academy of Pediatrics, the American Academy of Family Physicians, the Advisory Committee on Immunization Practices, and the U.S. Public Health Service. These four bodies called for the national goal of removal of thimerosal from vaccines and the performance of studies to establish any relationship between exposure to thimerosal and health effects. HBV vaccination in newborns was suspended temporarily in 1999 until thimerosal-free vaccines became available, unless the mother was infected with HBV. Two thimerosal-free HBV vaccines now are available in the United States for use in infants. Hence, parents can be reassured about the lack of exposure to mercury in HBV vaccines.

A study from Taiwan has demonstrated a reduction in hepatocellular incidence secondary to vaccination use.[28] Universal introduction of hepatitis B vaccination in childhood in Taiwan and other countries will take many years to demonstrate its full efficacy, but benefits will continue for many generations to come.[1]

HBV vaccine in infants and children is very important for the prevention of new infection. However, an important concern is other general aspects of prevention of HBV transmission. The leading cause of HBV transmission in the United States today is engagement in high-risk activities by adolescent and adult populations. Attendance at social programs that address high-risk activities should be encouraged.

RECOMMENDATIONS TO PREVENT HOUSEHOLD TRANSMISSION

When a person is found to have acute or chronic HBV, immunization of household contacts is recommended. Guidance on universal precautions should be provided. Parents of infected children and siblings should learn to treat bodily fluids, especially blood, as potentially infectious. All bloody emissions and blood-soiled items should be handled with gloves, and any blood-stained items should be either cleaned with bleach or disposed of carefully. Both the infected person and others in the house should cover skin abrasions with waterproof bandages. Razors and toothbrushes never should be shared. If needle sharps are in use, they should be secured and disposed of according to local guidelines. Schools, workplaces, and health care providers should practice universal precautions for all individuals regardless of whether HBV status is known.

HEPATITIS D

Hepatitis D virus (HDV) is a subviral particle, unique in the animal world, that requires a helper virus, HBV, to cause infection. As a subviral particle, HDV, which also is known as the delta agent or virus, does not encode its own envelope protein and requires HBV to produce its envelope and to become an infectious virion. HDV first was described in 1977 when a new antigen was described in the hepatocytes of patients infected with HBV. Transmission experiments demonstrated that the antigen was indeed a new virus.[135] Infection with HDV and HBV can be contracted at the same time (co-infection), or HDV infection can be contracted as a new infection in a person previously infected with HBV (superinfection). HDV has three genotypes and geographic variation in both incidence and genotype distribution.[151] Genotype IIb predominates in Okinawa, Japan,[143] whereas genotype I predominates in Europe and the United States.[151] The relationship between HDV genotype and clinical outcome has not been studied except in Rhodes, Greece, where low-sequence diversity in HDV genotype I has been associated with a mild course of disease.[151]

Virology

HDV is a spherical particle with a diameter of 36 nm.[120] When the envelope is degraded, a nucleocapsid containing hepatitis D antigen (HDAg) and the HDV RNA genome is released. The two forms of HDAg are the small s-HDAg, which is 195 amino acids in length and is required for replication, and the larger l-HDAg, which is 214 amino acids long, is required for virion assembly, and inhibits HDV replication.[120] s-HDAg is a nuclear protein that undergoes phosphorylation by protein kinase C, and inhibitors of protein kinase C inhibit HDV replication in cell culture systems.[35] The ratio of the two forms of HDAg found in patients may vary.

The HDV RNA genome is single stranded and circular, with a length of 1679 nucleotides. It is the smallest genome of any animal virus.[169] During viral replication, the genomic RNA serves as a template for complementary RNA, which in turn is a template for more genomic RNA. A host-derived RNA polymerase is required.[169] Each copy of the genome and antigenome contains ribozyme activity that cleaves RNA and is required for HDV replication.[120] Posttranscriptional modification of the RNA leads to the production of the l-HDAg in addition to the s-HDAg already transcribed.[35, 169]

To leave the host cell, HDV RNA and HDAg must be packaged into virions. The l-HDAg undergoes isoprenylation of a cysteine residue near its C terminus to allow virion assembly. Inhibition of this isoprenylation interferes with viral production by preventing interaction with HBsAg.[35] Once this interaction occurs, HBsAg and host cell membrane lipids enclose HVD RNA, l-HDAg, and s-HDAg to form a virion. Noninfectious HDV particles, which contain only l-HDAg and HBsAg, can be found in serum.[120]

Epidemiology

The epidemiology of HDV parallels that of HBV, for obvious reasons. Modes of transmission of HDV also are similar to those for HBV and include direct or indirect parenteral exposure to blood or body fluids and sexual and perinatal transmission. Sexual transmission is less efficient than that of HBV, as evidenced by the relatively low frequency of HDV in homosexual men.[147] Perinatal transmission can occur but seldom does because HBV carrier mothers also infected with HDV usually are anti-HBe positive and thus less infectious. Intrafamilial transmission of HDV has been demonstrated in endemic areas, such as southern Italy, by means of a combined epidemiologic and molecular study, which demonstrated that within family units, the HDV strains were nearly identical.[123]

The geographic differences in HDV endemicity in the world are great, and four levels have been characterized. Highest endemicity (more than 20% of asymptomatic HBV carriers, more than 60% of HBV carriers with chronic liver disease) is seen in the poorest areas in northern South America and Africa as well as in Romania.[30] In these populations, HDV superinfection in HBV carriers is a significant cause of chronic liver disease and has caused outbreaks of fulminant hepatitis. In these areas, HDV infection is seen commonly in both children and adults, and intrahousehold transmission has been implicated. Parts of the Middle East, Africa, some Pacific Islands, and parts of Asia report intermediate HDV endemicity (10–20% of asymptomatic HBV carriers, 30–60% of HBV carriers with chronic liver disease). Infection in these regions occurs predominantly in adults, and outbreaks are uncommon occurrences, but HDV is an important cause of chronic liver disease. Low endemicity (3–9% of asymptomatic HBV carriers, 10–25% of HBV carriers with chronic liver disease) is observed in most developed countries, including the United States, but subpopulations in these countries, such as parenteral drug abusers and prostitutes, have a high infection rate. In areas of low HBV endemicity, transmission of HDV appears to be mainly by the percutaneous route, with higher rates of HDV found in intravenous drug users and hemophiliacs than in other HBV high-risk groups. HDV is considered only a moderately important cause of chronic liver disease in developed countries.[177] Finally, for as yet unexplained reasons, certain subpopulations have a high carriage rate of HBV, but virtually no HDV infection; they include Native Americans, Eskimos, and residents of some Asian countries.

Within the U.S. blood donor population, the prevalence of HDV is low; only 1.4 to 8 percent of donors are infected or have evidence of prior infection.[3] Estimates from the CDC for 1990 indicate that among the about 250,000 yearly cases of acute HBV infection, 7500 simultaneously acquire HDV infection. An estimated 70,000 carriers of HDV are in the United States, where about 1000 deaths per year are caused by chronic HDV and 35 by fulminant HDV. In certain regions, the prevalence of HDV infection appears to be decreasing. In Italy, the prevalence of HDV infection in patients who are HBsAg carriers decreased from 23 percent in 1987 to 14 percent in 1992 and to 8.3 percent in 1997.[61, 142] Corresponding data for the United States are not available.

Immunopathogenesis

Unlike HBV, HDAg is found only in the liver or serum.[62] The mechanism by which HDV infection leads to hepatic injury has not been elucidated. Despite some evidence that HDV can be directly cytopathic, cytopathic viruses seldom result in chronic infections. In addition, some HDV carriers have no evidence of hepatic cell damage. Both cellular and humoral components of the host immune system are involved in the response to HDV, although the relative contribution of each is controversial. Investigations into the humoral response to HDV demonstrated that HDAg contains epitopes or immunogenic domains to which sera from acutely infected humans and woodchucks react. The predominantly recognized epitopes are not exposed on the virion surface; thus, antibodies that recognize these epitopes cannot neutralize virus particles, which may explain why no association exists between the humoral response and clinical outcome.[120] Autoantibodies, especially liver-kidney microsomal type 3 antibodies and anti–basal cell layer antibody, are found occasionally in people with HDV infection. The significance of these antibodies is unclear, but they may play a role in some of the immunopathogenesis of HDV.

Cellular immune responses to HDV also have been demonstrated. $CD4^+$ and $CD8^+$ lymphocytes have been found in liver of patients infected with HDV. These cells may either contribute to hepatitis or aid in control of HDV infection.[120] Studies have shown that patients with HDV superinfection of chronic HBV who had peripheral $CD4^+$ cells that reacted to four epitopes on HDAg were seronegative for HDV IgM, implying inactive disease.[124] Such $CD4^+$ T-cell clones produce IFN-γ and may be directly cytopathic. Individuals without these specific $CD4^+$ cells had active HDV disease.[125] These epitopes are in highly conserved regions of HDV, which is encouraging for the prospect of vaccine development.

An unusual mechanism of HDAg presentation by hepatocytes has been reported. The processing of HDAg peptide appears to occur outside the cell, where the peptide is cleaved into smaller fragments that bind to class II MHC molecules of all three HLA types found on hepatocytes and mononuclear cells. This form of antigen presentation could have many possible effects on T-cell responses: amplification of T-cell response to HDAg, stimulation of cytotoxic T cells to kill uninfected hepatocytes, or exhaustion of T-cell responses to HDAg, allowing infected cells to escape detection.[120]

The relationship of HBV infection status to pathogenesis of HDV also is unclear. In patients with active HBV replication (i.e., HBV DNA and HBeAg seropositive), HDV viremia is high.[136] Conversely, in HBV and HDV carriers without liver disease or with minimal inflammatory hepatic lesions, markers of HBV replication are absent, and HDV viremia is low.[20, 136] In co-infected liver transplant recipients, HDV reinfection can occur without evidence of active HBV replication, but necroinflammatory activity does not develop until HBV infection is reactivated.[47]

Diagnosis

Establishing the diagnosis of either acute or chronic HBV infection is a prerequisite for the diagnosis of HDV infection, which is made by detection of antibody to HDV (anti-HDV). Assays for both IgM and IgG anti-HDV are available. HDV infection may occur at the same time as does HBV infection, a pattern that is termed co-infection. If it occurs and the individual has acute, resolving hepatitis B, the HDV infection also will resolve.[51] In this instance, anti-HDV is found in the IgM form during the acute illness and persists for 2 to 6 weeks. Subsequently, IgG anti-HDV is found in serum, but it also diminishes to undetectable levels when the HBV infection resolves (Fig. 162–6). In HDV superinfection of an individual chronically infected with HBV, both IgM and IgG anti-HDV are detected. Most often, superinfection with HDV leads to chronic HDV infection, diagnosed by persistence of both IgM and IgG anti-HDV (Fig. 162–7). Anti-HDV becomes predominantly IgG after about 6 weeks and persists if infection does not resolve; titers correlate well with ongoing viral replication.

Detection of HDAg and measurement of HDV RNA by the PCR technique are primarily research tools. HDAg is found in serum during the incubation period but decreases after this stage. This test is of limited clinical usefulness because time of testing is key to interpreting the result. HDV RNA detected in serum by PCR assay is both an early marker of acute infection and an indication of viral replication in chronic infection.[76] HDV-RNA also may be detected in liver by in situ reverse transcriptase PCR assay.

Histopathologic features of HDV infection are very similar to those of isolated HBV infection (see earlier). HDAg can be identified in nuclei and, to a lesser extent, in the cytoplasm of infected hepatocytes.

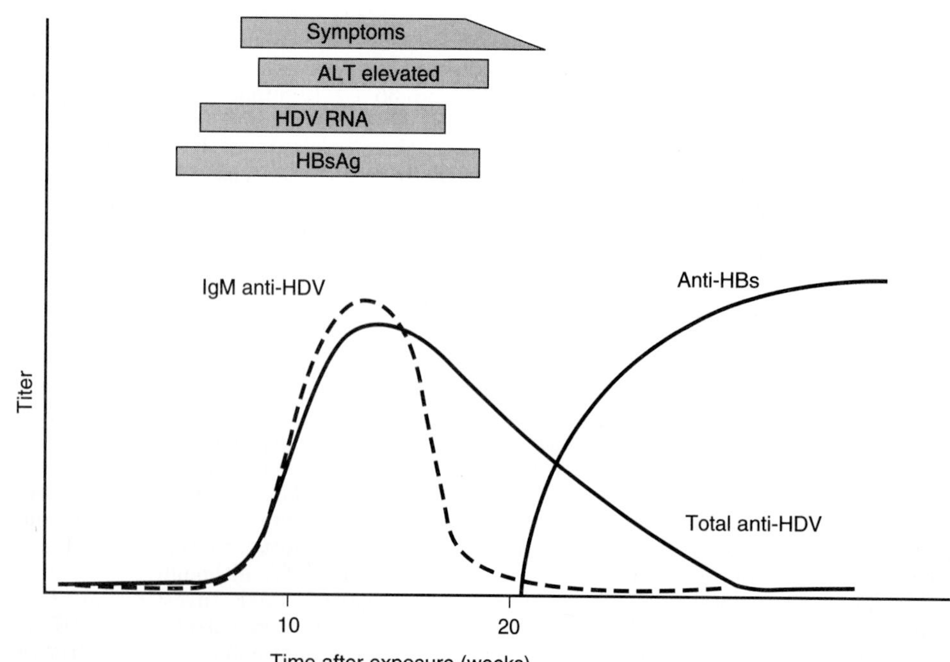

FIGURE 162–6 ■ Serologic events during HBV and HDV co-infection, which resolves. After exposure to both viruses, HBsAg and HDV RNA can be detected shortly before the onset of symptoms. Serum alanine aminotransferase (ALT) is elevated for the duration of detectable serum HDV RNA and HBsAg. Serum IgM anti-HDV rises when symptoms are present and falls as HDV infection resolves and anti-HBs titer becomes elevated. When both infections have resolved, anti-HBs is detectable in serum, but total anti-HDV is very low.

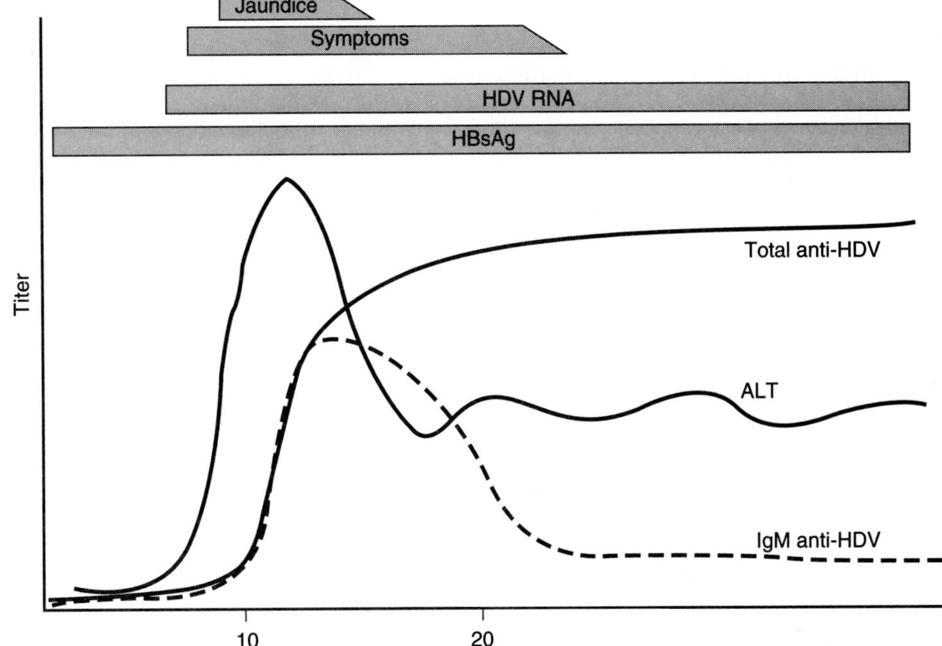

FIGURE 162–7 ■ Serologic events during HBV and HDV superinfection. If an individual already infected with HBV is infected with HDV, there is a marked elevation of alanine aminotransferase (ALT) coincident with onset of symptoms and onset of jaundice. HDV RNA can also be detected at the onset of symptoms. ALT levels fluctuate over the next few months as IgM anti-HDV decreases and total anti-HDV rises. Throughout the course of HDV superinfection, HBsAg remains detectable.

Clinical Features

In areas of high HDV endemicity, HDV co-infections have no major impact on the natural history of acute HBV infection. However, in areas of low endemicity, co-infection may induce severe or even fulminant hepatitis. In general, co-infection with HDV does not have clinical features that distinguish it from HBV infection alone. Symptoms develop 2 months after exposure, are similar to those of acute HBV infection, and usually resolve by 4 months after exposure. However, two peaks in aminotransferases often are noted, a pattern that is unusual in HBV infection alone. The infections resolve together.[51] Co-infection with both viruses does not increase the risk for development of chronic HBV infection.[110]

HDV superinfections in individuals with chronic HBV infection have different manifestations. HDV infection becomes persistent in most individuals (Fig. 162–8), and the predominant clinical pattern of chronic HDV infection varies by geographic location. In the United States and Europe, HDV superinfection leads to chronic liver disease in more than 90 percent of cases, whereas in some Pacific Island and African populations, most individuals with chronic HDV are asymptomatic.[136] When chronic liver disease does occur, the progression to cirrhosis is rapid; in studies in both adults and children, cirrhosis has been noted to occur in as few as 2 to 10 years. The cirrhosis associated with HDV infection has two patterns: in a minority of patients, especially the high-risk drug users, it progresses rapidly to hepatic failure and portal hypertension. In others, more stable cirrhosis occurs, with little inflammatory component, compatible with prolonged survival.[22] In a small minority of those who are superinfected, a self-limited hepatitis develops, and subsequently both HBV and HDV infections are cleared. HDV infection has been demonstrated to lead to

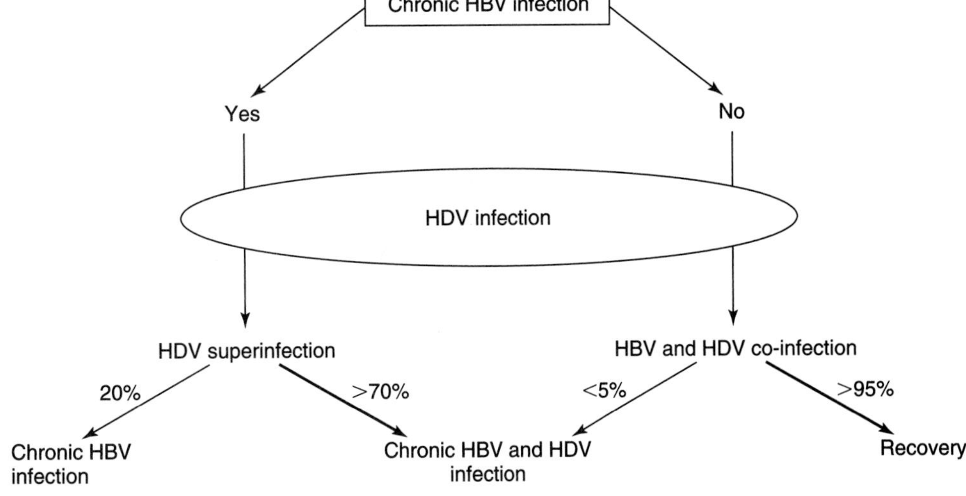

FIGURE 162–8 ■ Outcomes of HBV and HDV superinfection and co-infection. When a person already infected with HBV becomes infected with HDV, there is a greater than 70 percent chance of becoming chronically infected with both HDV and HBV. In contrast, if a person acquires HBV and HDV de novo, there is a less than 5 percent chance of chronic HBV and HDV infection.

HCC at a younger age and a higher rate than does HBV infection alone.[136]

Children with HDV infection follow a course similar to that of adults. In one European series, the subset of children chronically infected with HBV who also had HDV had more advanced liver disease, and the prevalence of HDV infection increased in parallel with the activity of hepatitis. During the study period, disease progressed more rapidly in children infected with both viruses.[56] Testing for HDV infection is recommended in any child with chronic HBV and unusually severe liver disease or an acute exacerbation of stable liver disease.

HDV infection after liver transplantation can appear without apparent HBV reinfection of either the graft or serum. However, use of PCR assay and buoyant density analysis has demonstrated that low levels of HBV infection do in fact occur in patients with recurrent HDV, and this replication of HBV is sufficient to permit replication of HDV. The HDV virion found in such infections shares the characteristics of typical HDV infection.[155]

Treatment

Although several antiviral agents have been studied, the only treatment that has had any beneficial effect in HDV infection is IFN-α. Trials in adults, in both Europe and the United States, have shown that treatment with either 9 million units three times weekly or 5 million units daily of IFN-α results in normalization of serum aminotransferase levels, decrease or disappearance of HDV-RNA from serum, and improvement in hepatic inflammation in about 50 percent of cases.[57] However, most patients relapsed with hepatitis shortly after treatment was discontinued. Response maintained after treatment was noted primarily in individuals who became HbsAg negative. No factors predictive of response have been identified. Prognosis in nonresponders and in those who relapse has been poor. Currently, no recommendations have been established regarding the use of IFN-α for the treatment of chronic HDV infection in children; reported series in total describe only 17 children. Results in seven children from Greece were disappointing. The children were treated with IFN-α, 3 million units/m^2 of body surface area three times a week for 1 year. All remained anti-HDV IgM positive, and 4 of 7 had persistent HDV RNA in serum. A significant reduction in serum aminotransferase values was noted after 1 year of treatment, but no significant improvement occurred in the liver histology.[46] A study of 8 children from Germany also found no effect of IFN-α on replication of HDV. However, serum aminotransferase values improved, and children underwent earlier anti-HBe seroconversion compared with historical controls.[148] In the sole report from the United States, seroconversion of HBeAg to anti-HBe and normalization of aminotransferase levels was reported in one of two HBV and HDV co-infected children treated with IFN.[87]

No cases of successful therapy of HDV in children using nucleoside analogues have been reported, but one case of successful famciclovir treatment in an adult who had developed HDV and HBV infections after liver transplantation has been reported. This patient cleared HDAg and HBV DNA within 18 days of initiation of therapy and at 3 months became HBsAg negative.[89] Lamivudine has been shown to have no effect on either HDV viremia or liver disease activity in chronic HDV infection.[133]

Some children and adults require liver transplantation for management of end-stage HDV-associated liver disease. Patients co-infected with HDV and HBV have lower rates of HBV infection of the allograft than do those in patients with isolated HBV infection. These data were reported in a series of 58 patients with HBV, of whom 25 also had HDV infection and who underwent liver transplantation between 1984 and 1996 in Belgium. Fifty-two patients survived longer than 3 months, and median follow-up was 74 months. HDV infection improved survival at 5 years, 96 ± 4 percent compared with 63 ± 10 percent for those infected with HBV alone.[104] As yet, no explanation has been given for the better outcome of transplantation in individuals who have both HBV and HDV infections. Administration of HBIG is required before and after transplantation, as in those patients with HBV infection alone.

Immunoprophylaxis

Passive or active immunization specifically against HDV infection is not available. HDAg itself is highly immunogenic, but antibodies are not neutralizing. Description of a T-cell response to several HDV epitopes in individuals with less severe disease activity has stimulated speculation about possible vaccine development, but studies are preliminary. A DNA-based HDV vaccine successfully induced cellular responses in an animal model and also was successful when used with a HBV vaccine.[77] At the present time, individuals with chronic HBV infection, who are the same people at risk for acquiring HDV, cannot be protected from HDV except by avoidance of high-risk behaviors and exposures. However, prevention of HBV infection in susceptible individuals will prevent HDV co-infection and will be the most important mechanism for decreasing the prevalence of HDV infection in a population. The current strategy aimed at decreasing susceptibility to HBV infection by universal immunization of newborns and catch-up immunization of older children and adolescents should reduce substantially the risk for subsequent development of HDV infection during young adulthood. In Italy, the decrease in HDV prevalence in those with chronic HBV infection from 23 percent in 1987 to 8.3 percent in 1997 has lead to speculation that chronic HDV may be a "vanishing disease."[61]

REFERENCES

1. Abraham, P., Mistry, F. P., Bapat, M. R., et al.: Evaluation of a new recombinant DNA hepatitis B vaccine (Shanvac-B). Vaccine *17*:1125–1129, 1999.
2. Acs, G., Sells, M. A., Purcell, R. H., et al.: Hepatitis B virus produced by transfected Hep G2 cells causes hepatitis in chimpanzees. Proc. Natl. Acad. Sci. U. S. A. *84*:4641–4644, 1987.
3. Alter, M. J., and Mast, E. E.: The epidemiology of viral hepatitis in the United States. *In* Martin, P., and Friedman, L. (eds.): Gastroenterology Clinics of North America: Viral Hepatitis. Philadelphia, W. B. Saunders, 1994, pp. 437–455.
4. Anonymous: Update: Recommendations to prevent hepatitis B virus transmission—United States. M. M. W. R. Morb. Mortal. Wkly. Rep. *48*:33–4, 1999.
5. Anonymous: Update: Vaccine side effects, adverse reactions, contraindications, and precautions. Recommendations of the Advisory Committee on Immunization Practices (ACIP). M. M. W. R. Morb. Mortal. Wkly. Rep. *45*:1–35., 1996.
6. Anonymous: Alternate two-dose Hepatitis B vaccination schedule for adolescents aged 11–15 years. M. M. W. R. Morb. Mortal. Wkly. Rep. *49*:261, 2000.
7. Anonymous: Summary of notifiable diseases, United States, 1998. M. M. W. R. Morb. Mortal. Wkly. Rer. *47*:2–92, 1999.
8. Anonymous: Recommended childhood immunization schedule—United States, 1998. M. M. W. R. Morb. Mortal. Wkly. Rep. *47*:8–12, 1998.
9. Ascherio, A., Zhang, S. M., Hernan, M. A., et al.: Hepatitis B vaccination and the risk of multiple sclerosis. N. Engl. J. Med. *344*:327–332, 2001.
10. Barr, D., Hershow, R., Furner, S., et al.: Assessing prenatal hepatitis B screening in Illinois with an inexpensive study design adaptable to other jurisdictions. Am. J. Public Health *89*:19–24, 1999.

11. Bartenschlager, R., and Schaller, H.: Hepadnaviral assembly is initiated by polymerase binding to the encapsidation signal in the viral RNA genome. EMBO. J. *11*:3413–3420, 1992.
12. Bartolome, J., Moraleda, G., Ruiz-Moreno, M., et al.: Hepatitis B virus DNA patterns in the liver of children with chronic hepatitis B. J. Med. Virol. *31*:195–199, 1990.
13. Bavand, M., Feitelson, M., and Laub, O.: The hepatitis B virus-associated reverse transcriptase is encoded by the viral pol gene. J. Virol. *63*:1019–1021, 1989.
14. Beasley, R. P.: Hepatitis B virus. The major etiology of hepatocellular carcinoma. Cancer *61*:1942–1956, 1988.
15. Benner, K. G., Lee, R. G., Keeffe, E. B., et al.: Fibrosing cytolytic liver failure secondary to recurrent hepatitis B after liver transplantation. Gastroenterology *103*:1307–1312, 1992.
16. Bernabeu-Wittel, M.: Hepatitis B replication decreases in HIV co-infected patients treated with lamivudine. Abstract. Hepatology *28*:724A, 1998.
17. Bishop, N., Civitico, G., Wang, Y. Y., et al.: Antiviral strategies in chronic hepatitis B virus infection. I. Establishment of an in vitro system using the duck hepatitis B virus model. J. Med. Virol. *31*:82–89, 1990.
18. Blum, H. E., Zhang, Z. S., Galun, E., et al.: Hepatitis B virus X protein is not central to the viral life cycle in vitro. J. Virol. *66*:1223–1227, 1992.
19. Bodsworth, N. J., Cooper, D. A., and Donovan, B.: The influence of human immunodeficiency virus type 1 infection on the development of the hepatitis B virus carrier state. J. Infect. Dis. *163*:1138–1140, 1991.
20. Bonino, F., Brunetto, M. R., and Negro, F.: Factors influencing the natural course of HDV hepatitis. Prog. Clin. Biol. Res. *364*:137–146, 1991.
21. Bortolotti, F., Cadrobbi, P., Crivellaro, C., et al.: Long-term outcome of chronic type B hepatitis in patients who acquire hepatitis B virus infection in childhood. Gastroenterology *99*:805–810, 1990.
22. Bortolotti, F., DiMarco, V., Vajro, P., et al.: Long-term evolution of chronic delta hepatitis in children. J. Pediatr. *122*:736–738, 1993.
23. Brunt, E. M.: Grading and staging the histopathological lesions of chronic hepatitis: The Knodell histology activity index and beyond. Hepatology *31*:241–246, 2000.
24. Bruss, V., and Ganem, D.: The role of envelope proteins in hepatitis B virus assembly. Proc. Natl. Acad. Sci. U. S. A. *88*:1059–1063, 1991.
25. Carreno, V., Marcellin, P., Hadziyannis, S., et al.: Retreatment of chronic hepatitis B e antigen-positive patients with recombinant interferon alfa-2a. The European Concerted Action on Viral Hepatitis (EUROHEP). Hepatology *30*:277–282, 1999.
26. Chang, H. K., and Ting, L. P.: The surface gene promoter of the human hepatitis B virus displays a preference for differentiated hepatocytes. Virology *170*:176–183, 1989.
27. Chang, L. J., Pryciak, P., Ganem, D., and Varmus, H. E.: Biosynthesis of the reverse transcriptase of hepatitis B viruses involves de novo translational initiation not ribosomal frameshifting. Nature *337*:364–368, 1989.
28. Chang, M. H., Chen, C. J., Lai, M. S., et al.: Universal hepatitis B vaccination in Taiwan and the incidence of hepatocellular carcinoma in children. Taiwan Childhood Hepatoma Study Group. N. Engl. J. Med. *336*:1906–1907, 1997.
29. Chang, M. H., Chen, C. J., Lai, M. S., et al.: Universal hepatitis B vaccination in Taiwan and the incidence of hepatocellular carcinoma in children. Taiwan Childhood Hepatoma Study Group. N. Engl. J. Med. *336*:1855–1859, 1997.
30. Chang, M. H., Chen, P. J., Chen, J. Y., et al.: Hepatitis B virus integration in hepatitis B virus-related hepatocellular carcinoma in childhood. Hepatology *13*:316–320, 1991.
31. Chang M-H, Sung J-L, Lee C-Y, et al.: Factors affecting clearance of hepatitis B e antigen in hepatitis B surface antigen carrier children. J. Pediatr. *115*:385–390, 1989.
32. Cheah, P. L., Looi, L. M., Lin, H. P., and Yap, S. F.: Childhood primary hepatocellular carcinoma and hepatitis B virus infection. Cancer *65*:174–176, 1990.
33. Chen, H. L., Chang, M. H., Ni, Y. H., et al.: Seroepidemiology of hepatitis B infection in children: Ten years of mass vaccination in Taiwan. J. A. M. A. *276*:1802–1803, 1996.
34. Chen, P. J., and Chen, D. S.: Hepatitis B virus infection and hepatocellular carcinoma: Molecular genetics and clinical perspectives. Semin. Liver Dis. *19*:253–62, 1999.
35. Chen, P. J., Wu, H. L., Wang, C. J., et al.: Molecular biology of hepatitis D virus: Research and potential for application. J Gastroenterol. Hepatol. *12*:S188–192, 1997.
36. Chen, S. T., La Porte, P., and Yee, J. K.: Mutational analysis of hepatitis B virus enhancer 2. Virology *196*:652–659, 1993.
37. Chen, S. T., Su, H., and Yee, J. K.: Repression of liver-specific hepatitis B virus enhancer 2 activity by adenovirus E1A proteins. J. Virol. *66*:7452–7460, 1992.
38. Cheng, K. C.: Selective synthesis and secretion of particles composed of the hepatitis B virus middle surface protein directed by a recombinant vaccinia virus: Induction of antibodies to pre-S and S epitopes. J. Virol. *61*:1286–1290, 1987.
39. Chisari, F. V., Filippi, P., Buras, J., et al.: Structural and pathological effects of synthesis of hepatitis B virus large envelope polypeptide in transgenic mice. Proc. Natl. Acad. Sci. U. S. A. *84*:6909–6913, 1987.
40. Chu, C. M., and Liaw, Y. F.: Natural history of chronic hepatitis B virus infection: An immunopathological study. J. Gastroenterol. Hepatol. *12*:S218–222, 1997.
41. Colin, J. F., Cazals-Hatem, D., Loriot, M. A., et al.: Influence of human immunodeficiency virus infection on chronic hepatitis B in homosexual men. Hepatology *29*:1306–1310, 1999.
42. Confavreux, C., Suissa, S., Saddier, P., et al.: Vaccinations and the risk of relapse in multiple sclerosis. Vaccines in Multiple Sclerosis Study Group. N. Engl. J. Med. *344*:319–326, 2001.
43. Conjeevaram, H. S.: Therapy for chronic hepatitis B: Nucleoside analogues in adult and pediatric patients. Acta. Gastroenterol. Belg. *61*:224–227, 1998.
44. Control, C. F. D.: Hepatitis B virus: A comprehensive strategy for the eliminating transmission in the United states through universal childhood vaccination. Recommendations of the Immunization Practices Advisory Committee (ACIP). M. M. W. R. Morb. Mortal. Wkly. Rep. *40*:1–25, 1991.
45. Crowther, R. A., Kiselev, N. A., Bottcher, B., et al.: Three-dimensional structure of hepatitis B virus core particles determined by electron cryomicroscopy. Cell *77*:943–950, 1994.
46. Dalekos, G. N., Galanakis, E., Zervou, E., et al.: Interferon-alpha treatment of children with chronic hepatitis D virus infection: The Greek experience. Hepatogastroenterology *47*:1072–1076, 2000.
47. David, E., Rahier, J., Pucci, A., et al.: Recurrence of hepatitis D (delta) in liver transplants: Histopathological aspects. Gastroenterology *104*:1122–1128, 1993.
48. de Franchis, R., Meucci, G., Vecchi, M., et al.: The natural history of asymptomatic hepatitis B surface antigen carriers. Ann. Intern. Med. *118*:191–194, 1993.
49. De Man, R. A., Marcellin, P., Habal, F., et al.: A randomized, placebo-controlled study to evaluate the efficacy of 12-month famciclovir treatment in patients with chronic hepatitis B e antigen-positive hepatitis B. Hepatology *32*:413–417, 2000.
50. Desmet, V. J.: Immunopathology of chronic viral hepatitis. Hepatogastroenterology *38*:14–21, 1991.
51. Di Bisceglie, A. M., and Negro, F.: Diagnosis of hepatitis delta virus infection. Hepatology *10*:1014–1016, 1989.
52. Dienstag, J. L., Schiff, E. R., Mitchell, M., et al.: Extended lamivudine retreatment for chronic hepatitis B: Maintenance of viral suppression after discontinuation of therapy. Hepatology *30*:1082–1087, 1999.
53. Dienstag, J. L., Schiff, E. R., Wright, T. L., et al.: Lamivudine as initial treatment for chronic hepatitis B in the United States. N. Engl. J. Med. *341*:1256–1263, 1999.
54. Dimitrakopoulos, A., Takou, A., Haida, A., et al.: The prevalence of hepatitis B and C in HIV-positive Greek patients: Relationship to survival of deceased AIDS patients. J. Infect. *40*:127–131, 2000.
55. Enders, G. H., Ganem, D., and Varmus, H. E.: 5′-Terminal sequences influence the segregation of ground squirrel hepatitis virus RNAs into polyribosomes and viral core particles. J. Virol. *61*:35–41, 1987.
56. Farci, P., Barbera, C., Navone, C., et al.: Infection with the delta agent in children. Gut *26*:4–7, 1985.
57. Farci, P., Mandas, A., Coiana, A., et al.: Treatment of chronic hepatitis D with interferon alfa-2a. N. Engl. J. Med. *330*:88–94, 1994.
58. Fenner, F.: Candidate viral diseases for elimination or eradication. Bull. W. H. O. *76*:68–70, 1998.
59. Fivush, B. A.: Immunization guidelines for pediatric renal disease. Semin. Nephrol. *18*:256–263, 1998.
60. Fontana, R.: Antivirals in hepatitis B. Clin. Perspect. Gastroenterol. July/August, 207–213, 1999.
61. Gaeta, G., Stroffolini, T., Chiaramonte, M., et al.: Chronic hepatitis D: A vanishing disease? An Italian multicenter study. Hepatology *32*:824–827, 2000.
62. Gerken, G., and Meyer zum Buschenfelde, K. H.: Chronic hepatitis delta virus (HDV) infection. Hepatogastroenterology *38*:29–32, 1991.
63. Giacchino, R., Main, J., Timitilli, A., et al.: Dual-centre, double-blind, randomised trial of lymphoblastoid interferon alpha with or without steroid pretreatment in children with chronic hepatitis B. Liver *15*:143–148, 1995.
64. Giacchino, R., Navone, C., Facco, F., et al.: HBV-DNA-related hepatocellular carcinoma occurring in childhood: Report of three cases. Dig. Dis. Sci. *36*:1143–1146, 1991.
65. Goto, Y., Yoshida, J., Kuzushima, K., et al.: Patterns of hepatitis B virus DNA integration in liver tissue of children with chronic infections. J. Pediatr. Gastroenterol. Nutr. *16*:70–74, 1993.
66. Greenberg, H. B., Pollard, R. B., Lutwick, L. I., et al.: Effect of human leukocyte interferon on hepatitis B virus infection in patients with chronic active hepatitis. N. Engl. J. Med. *295*:517–522, 1976.
67. Guida, S., Fiore, M., Scotese, I., et al.: Defective interleukin-2 production in children with chronic hepatitis B: Role of adherent cells. J. Pediatr. Gastroenterol. Nutr. *24*:312–316, 1997.
68. Gunther, S., Meisel, H., Reip, A., et al.: Frequent and rapid emergence of mutated pre-C sequences in HBV from e-antigen positive carriers who seroconvert to anti-HBe during interferon treatment. Virology *187*:271–279, 1992.

69. Heermann, K. H., Goldmann, U., Schwartz, W., et al.: Large surface proteins of hepatitis B virus containing the pre-s sequence. J. Virol. *52*:396–402, 1984.
70. Hertogs, K., Leenders, W. P., Depla, E., et al.: Endonexin II, present on human liver plasma membranes, is a specific binding protein of small hepatitis B virus (HBV) envelope protein. Virology *197*:549–557, 1993.
71. Hirsch, R. C., Lavine, J. E., Chang, L. J., et al.: Polymerase gene products of hepatitis B viruses are required for genomic RNA packaging as well as for reverse transcription. Nature *344*:552–555, 1990.
72. Honigwachs, J., Faktor, O., Dikstein, R., et al.: Liver-specific expression of hepatitis B virus is determined by the combined action of the core gene promoter and the enhancer. J. Virol. *63*:919–924, 1989.
73. Honkoop, P., de Man, R. A., Niesters, H. G., et al.: Acute exacerbation of chronic hepatitis B virus infection after withdrawal of lamivudine therapy. Hepatology *32*:635–639, 2000.
74. Hu, K. Q., and Siddiqui, A.: Regulation of the hepatitis B virus gene expression by the enhancer element I. Virology *181*:721–726, 1991.
75. Huang, S. N., Tsai, S. L., Liaw, Y. P.: Histopathology and pathobiology of hepatropic virus-induced liver injury. J. Gastroenterol. Hepatol. 1997:S195–S217, 1997.
76. Huang, Y. H., Wu, J. C., Sheng, W. Y., et al.: Diagnostic value of anti-hepatitis D virus (HDV) antibodies revisited: A study of total and IgM anti-HDV compared with detection of HDV-RNA by polymerase chain reaction. J. Gastroenterol. Hepatol. *13*:57–61, 1998.
77. Huang, Y. H., Wu, J. C., Tao, M. H., et al.: DNA-based immunization produces Th1 immune responses to hepatitis delta virus in a mouse model. Hepatology *32*:104–110, 2000.
78. Huo, T. I., Yang, W. C., Wu, J. C., et al.: Impact of hepatitis B and C virus infection on the outcome of kidney transplantation in Chinese patients. Chung Hua I Hsueh Tsa Chih (Taipei) *63*:93–100, 2000.
79. Huovila, A. P., Eder, A. M., and Fuller, S. D.: Hepatitis B surface antigen assembles in a post-ER, pre-Golgi compartment. J. Cell Biol. *118*:1305–1320, 1992.
80. Hyams, K. C.: Risks of chronicity following acute hepatitis B virus infection. Clin. Infect. Dis. *20*:992, 1995.
81. Iorio, R., Pensati, P., Botta, S., et al.: Side effects of alpha-interferon therapy and impact on health-related quality of life in children with chronic viral hepatitis. Pediatr. Infect. Dis. J. *16*:984–90, 1997.
82. Ishak, K.: Chronic hepatitis: Morphology and nomenclature. Mod. Pathol. *7*:690–713, 1994.
83. Jilg, W., Schmidt, M., and Deinhardt, F.: Immune response to hepatitis B revaccination. J. Med. Virol. *24*:377–384, 1988.
84. Jonas, M. M., Reddy, R. K., DeMedina, M., and Schiff, E. R.: Hepatitis B infection in a large municipal obstetrical population: Characterization and prevention of perinatal transmission. Am. J. Gastroenterol. *85*:277–280, 1990.
85. Kao, J. H., Chen, P. J., Lai, M. Y., and Chen, D. S.: Hepatitis B genotypes correlate with clinical outcomes in patients with chronic hepatitis B. Gastroenterology *118*:554–559, 2000.
86. Kao, J. H., Wu, N. H., Chen, P. J., et al.: Hepatitis B genotypes and the response to interferon therapy. J. Hepatol. *33*:998–1002, 2000.
87. Kay, M. H., Wyllie, R., Deimler, C., et al.: Alpha interferon therapy in children with chronic active hepatitis B and delta virus infection. J. Pediatr. *123*:1001–1004, 1993.
88. Kelly, R. B.: Pathways of protein secretion in eukaryotes. Science *230*:25–32, 1985.
89. Klein, M., Geoghegan, J., Schmidt, K., et al.: Conversion of recurrent delta-positive hepatitis B infection to seronegativity with famciclovir after liver transplantation. Transplantation *64*:162–163, 1997.
90. Kleinknecht, C., Levy, M., Peix, A., et al.: Membranous glomerulonephritis and hepatitis B surgace antigen in children. J. Pediatr. *95*:946–952, 1979.
91. Klingmuller, U., and Schaller, H.: Hepadnavirus infection requires interaction between the viral pre-S domain and a specific hepatocellular receptor. J. Virol. *67*:7414–7422, 1993.
92. Knodell, R. G., Ishak, K. G., Black, W. C., et al: Formulation and application of a numerical scoring system for assessing histological activity in asymptomatic chronic active hepatitis. Hepatology *1*:431–435, 1981.
93. Kocak, N. G. F., Slatik, I. N., Ozen, H., and Yuce, A.: Long term prognosis of interferon nonresponder children with hepatitis B. Am. J. Gastroenterol. *95*:1841, 2000.
94. Kock, J., and Schlicht, H. J.: Analysis of the earliest steps of hepadnavirus replication: Genome repair after infectious entry into hepatocytes does not depend on viral polymerase activity. J. Virol. *67*:4867–4874, 1993.
95. Korba, B. E., Wells, F. V., Baldwin, B., et al.: Hepatocellular carcinoma in woodchuck hepatitis virus-infected woodchucks: Presence of viral DNA in tumor tissue from chronic carriers and animals serologically recovered from acute infections. Hepatology *9*:461–470, 1989.
96. Korenman, J., Baker, B., Waggoner, J., et al.: Long-term remission of chronic hepatitis B after alpha-interferon therapy. Ann. Intern. Med. *114*:629–634, 1991.
97. Kosake, Y., Takase, K., Kojima, M., et al.: Fulminant hepatitis B: Induction by the hepatitis B virus mutants defective in the precore region and incapable of encoding e antigen. Gastroenterology *100*:1087–1094, 1991.
98. Lai, C.-L., Chien R-N., Leung, N. W. Y., et al.: A one-year trial of lamivudine for chronic hepatitis B. N. Engl. J. Med. *339*:61–68, 1998.
99. Lai, C.-L., Ching, C-K., Tung, A. K. M., et al.: Lamivudine is effective in suppressing hepatitis B virus DNA in Chinese hepatitis B surface antigen carriers: A placebo-controlled trial. Hepatology *25*:241–244, 1997.
100. Lai, C. L., Lok, A. S., Lin, H. J., et al.: Placebo-controlled trial of recombinant alpha2-interferon in Chinese HBsAg-carrier children. Lancet *2*:877–880, 1987.
101. Lambert, V., Fernholz, D., Sprengel, R., et al.: Virus-neutralizing monoclonal antibody to a conserved epitope on the duck hepatitis B virus pre-S protein. J. Virol. *64*:1290–1297, 1990.
102. Laub, O., Rall, L. B., Truett, M., et al.: Synthesis of hepatitis B surface antigen in mammalian cells: Expression of the entire gene and the coding region. J. Virol. *48*:271–280, 1983.
103. Lee, W. M.: Hepatitis B virus infection. N. Engl. J. Med. *337*:1733–1745, 1997.
104. Lerut, J. P., Donataccio, M., Ciccarelli, O., et al.: Liver transplantation and HBsAg-positive postnecrotic cirrhosis: Adequate immunoprophylaxis and delta virus co-infection as the significant determinants of long-term prognosis. J. Hepatol. *30*:706–714, 1999.
105. Lin, S. M., Sheen, I. S., Chien, R. N., et al.: Long-term beneficial effect of interferon therapy in patients with chronic hepatitis B virus infection. Hepatology *29*:971–975, 1999.
106. Lindh, M., Andersson, A. S., and Gusdal, A.: Genotypes, nt 1858 variants, and geographic origin of hepatitis B virus: Large-scale analysis using a new genotyping method. J. Infect. Dis. *175*:1285–1293, 1997.
107. Lok, A. S.: Hepatitis B infection: Pathogenesis and management. J. Hepatol. *32*:89–97, 2000.
108. Lok, A. S. F., and Lai, C. L.: A longitudinal follow-up of asymptomatic hepatitis B surface antigen-positive Chinese children. Hepatology *8*:1130–1133, 1988.
109. Lok, A. S. F., Lai, C. L., Su, P. C., et al.: Treatment of chronic hepatitis B with interferon: Experience in Asian patients. Semin. Liver Dis. *9*:249–253, 1989.
110. London, W., and Evan, A.: The epidemiology of hepatitis viruses B, C and D. Clin. Lab. Med. *16*:251–271, 1996.
111. Lopez-Cabrera, M., Letovsky, J., Hu, K. Q., and Siddiqui, A.: Transcriptional factor C/EBP binds to and transactivates the enhancer element II of the hepatitis B virus. Virology *183*:825–829, 1991.
112. Lunel, F., Cadranel, J. F., Rosenheim, M., et al.: Hepatitis virus infections in heart transplant recipients: Epidemiology, natural history, characteristics, and impact on survival. Gastroenterology *119*:1064–1074, 2000.
113. Lykavieris, P., Fabre, M., Yvart, J., and Alvarez, F.: HBV infection in pediatric liver transplantation. J. Pediatr. Gastroenterol. Nutr. *16*:321–327, 1993.
114. Maddrey, W. C.: Hepatitis B: An important public health issue. J. Med. Virol. *61*:362–366, 2000.
115. Margolis, H. S.: Hepatitis B virus infection. Bull. W. H. O. *76*:152–153, 1998.
116. Mason, A., Wick, M., White, H., and Perrillo, R.: Hepatitis B virus replication in diverse cell types during chronic hepatitis B virus infection. Hepatology *18*:781–789, 1993.
117. Mbayed, V., Lopez, J. L., Telenta, P. F. S., et al.: Distribution of hepatitis B genotypes in two different pediatric populations from Argentina. J. Clin. Microbiol. *36*:3362–3365, 1998.
118. McMahon, B. J., Heyward, W. L., Templin, D. W., et al.: Hepatitis B-associated polyarteritis nodosa in Alaskan Eskimos: Clinical and epidemiologic features and long-term follow-up. Hepatology *9*:97–101, 1989.
119. McQuillan, G. M., Coleman, P. J., Kruszon-Moran, D., et al.: Prevalence of hepatitis B virus infection in the United States: The National Health and Nutrition Examination Surveys, 1976 through 1994. Am. J. Public Health *89*:14–18, 1999.
120. Modahl, L. E., and Lai, M. M.: Hepatitis delta virus: The molecular basis of laboratory diagnosis. Crit. Rev. Clin. Lab. Sci. *37*:45–92, 2000.
121. Mutimer, D., Naoumov, N., Honkoop, P., et al.: Combination alpha-interferon and lamivudine therapy for alpha-interferon-resistant chronic hepatitis B infection: Results of a pilot study. J. Hepatol. *28*:923–929, 1998.
122. Nassal, M., Galle, P. R., and Schaller, H.: Proteaselike sequence in hepatitis B virus core antigen is not required for e antigen generation and may not be part of an aspartic acid-type protease. J. Virol. *63*:2598–2604, 1989.
123. Niro, G. A., Casey, J. L., Gravinese, E., et al.: Intrafamilial transmission of hepatitis delta virus: Molecular evidence. J. Hepatol. *30*:564–569, 1999.
124. Niro, G. A., Smedile, A., Andriulli, A., et al.: The predominance of hepatitis delta virus genotype I among chronically infected Italian patients. Hepatology *25*:728–734, 1997.
125. Nisini, R. P. M., Accapezzato, D., Bonino, F., et al.: Human CD4$^+$ T-cell response to hepatitis delta virus: Identification of multiple epitpopes and characterization of T-helper cytokine profiles. J. Virol. *71*:2241–2251, 1997.
126. Oberhaus, S. M., and Newbold, J. E.: Detection of DNA polymerase activities associated with purified duck hepatitis B virus core particles by using an activity gel assay. J. Virol. *67*:6558–6566, 1993.

127. Oon, C-J., Zhao, Y., Goh, K-T., et al.: Molecular epidemiology of hepatitis B virus variants in Singapore. Vaccine *13*:699–702, 1995.
128. Ozturk, M.: Genetic aspects of hepatocellular carcinogenesis. Semin. Liver Dis. *19*:235–242, 1999.
129. Pickering, L.: 2000 Red Book: Report of the Committee of Infectious Disease. 25th ed. Elk Grove Village, IL, American Academy of Pediatrics, 2000, pp. 98–101.
130. Pontisso, P., Basso, G., Perilongo, G., et al.: Does hepatitis B virus play a role in primary liver cancer in children of Western countries? Cancer Detect. Prevent. *15*:363–368, 1991.
131. Pugh, J. C., and Summers, J. W.: Infection and uptake of duck hepatitis B virus by duck hepatocytes maintained in the presence of dimethyl sulfoxide. Virology *172*:564–572, 1989.
132. Rabe, C., and Caselmann, W. H.: Interaction of hepatitis B virus with cellular processes in liver carcinogenesis. Crit. Rev. Clin. Lab. Sci. *37*:407–429, 2000.
133. Rayes, N., Seehofer, D., Hopf, U., et al.: Comparison of famciclovir and lamivudine in the long-term treatment of hepatitis B infection after liver transplantation. Transplantation *71*:96–101, 2001.
134. Rehermann, B., Lau, D., Hoofnagle, J. H., and Chisari, F. V.: Cytotoxic T lymphocyte responsiveness after resolution of chronic hepatitis B virus infection. J. Clin. Invest. *97*:1655–1665, 1996.
135. Rizzetto, M.: The delta agent. Hepatology *3*:729–737, 1983.
136. Rizzetto, M.: Hepatitis delta virus disease: An overview. Prog. Clin. Biol. Res. *382*:425–430, 1993.
137. Rogler, C. E., and Summers, J.: Novel forms of woodchuck hepatitis virus DNA isolated from chronically infected woodchuck liver nuclei. J. Virol. *44*:852–863, 1982.
138. Rollier, C., Charollois, C., Jamard, C., et al.: Early life humoral response of ducks to DNA immunization against hepadnavirus large envelope protein. Vaccine *18*:3091–3096, 2000.
139. Rossner, M. T.: Review: Hepatitis B virus X-gene product: A promiscuous transcriptional activator. J. Med. Virol. *36*:101–117, 1992.
140. Ruíz-Moreno, M., Fernández, P., Leal, A., et al.: Pilot interferon-β trial in children with chronic hepatitis B who had previously not responded to interferon-alfa therapy. Pediatrics *99*:222–225, 1997.
141. Rumin, S., Gripon, P., Le Seyec, J., et al.: Long-term productive episomal hepatitis B virus replication in primary cultures. J. Viral Hepat. *3*:227–238, 1996.
142. Sagnelli, E., Stroffolini, T., Ascione, A., et al.: Decrease in HDV endemicity in Italy. J. Hepatol. *26*:20–24, 1997.
143. Sakugawa, H., Nakasone, H., Nakayoshi, T., et al.: Hepatitis delta virus genotype IIb predominates in an endemic area, Okinawa, Japan. J. Med. Virol. *58*:366–372, 1999.
144. Samuel, D., Muller, R., Alexander, G., et al.: Liver transplantation in European patients with the hepatitis B surface antigen. N. Engl. J. Med. *329*:1842–1847, 1993.
145. Scaglioni, P. P., Melegari, M., and Wands, J. R.: Recent advances in the molecular biology of hepatitis B virus. Baillieres Clin. Gastroenterol. *10*:207–225, 1996.
146. Schalm, S. W., Heathcote, J., Cianciara, J., et al.: Lamivudine and alpha interferon combination treatment of patients with chronic hepatitis B infection: A randomised trial. Gut *46*:562–568, 2000.
147. Scharsschmidt, B., Hed, M., and Hollander, H.: Hepatitis B in patients with HIV infection: Relationship to AIDS and patient survival. Ann. Intern. Med. *117*:837, 1992.
148. Schneider, A., Habermehl, P., Gerner, P., et al.: Alpha-interferon treatment in HBeAg positive children with chronic hepatitis B and associated hepatitis D. Klin. Padiatr. *210*:363–365, 1998.
149. Scotto, J., Hadchouel, M., Hery, C., et al.: Hepatitis B virus DNA in children's liver diseases: Detection by blot hybridisation in liver and serum. Gut *24*:618–624, 1983.
150. Seeger, C., and Mason, W. S.: Hepatitis B virus biology. Microbiol. Mol. Biol. Rev. *64*:51–68, 2000.
151. Shakil, A. O., Hadziyannis, S., Hoofnagle, J. H., et al.: Geographic distribution and genetic variability of hepatitis delta virus genotype I. Virology *234*:160–167, 1997.
152. Shapiro, C. N.: Epidemiology of hepatitis B. Pediatr. Infect. Dis. J. *12*:433–437, 1993.
153. Shih, H. H., Chang, M. H., Hsu, H. Y., et al.: Long term immune response of universal hepatitis B vaccination in infancy: A community-based study in Taiwan. Pediatr. Infect. Dis. J. *18*:427–432, 1999.
154. Slagle, B. L., Zhou, Y. Z., Birchmeier, W., and Scorsone, K. A.: Deletion of the E-cadherin gene in hepatitis B virus-positive Chinese hepatocellular carcinomas. Hepatology *18*:757–762, 1993.
155. Smedile, A., Casey, J. L., Cote, P. J., et al.: Hepatitis D viremia following orthotopic liver transplantation involves a typical HDV virion with a hepatitis B surface antigen envelope. Hepatology *27*:1723–1729, 1998.
156. Smith, N., Yusuf, H., and Averhoff, F.: Surveillance and prevention of hepatitis B virus transmission. Am. J. Public Health *89*:11–13, 1999.
157. Sokal, E. M.: Viral hepatitis throughout infancy to adulthood. Acta Gastroenterol. Belg. *61*:170–174, 1998.
158. Sokal, E. M., Conjeevaram, H. S., Roberts, E. A., et al.: Interferon alfa therapy for chronic hepatitis B in children: A multinational randomized controlled trial. Gastroenterology *114*:988–995, 1998.
159. Sokal, E. M., Roberts, E. A., Mieli-Vergani, G., et al.: A dose ranging study of the pharmacokinetics, safety, and preliminary efficacy of lamivudine in children and adolescents with chronic hepatitis B. Antimicrob. Agents Chemother. *44*:590–597, 2000.
160. Southwest Pediatric Nephrology Study Group: Hepatitis B surface antigenemia in North American children with membranous glomerulonephropathy. J. Pediatr. *106*:571–578, 1985.
161. Standring, D. N., Ou, J. H., Masiarz, F. R., and Rutter, W. J.: A signal peptide encoded within the precore region of hepatitis B virus directs the secretion of a heterogeneous population of e antigens in *Xenopus* oocytes. Proc. Natl. Acad. Sci. U. S. A. *85*:8405–8409, 1988.
162. Stibbe, W., and Gerlich, W. H.: Structural relationships between minor and major proteins of hepatitis B surface antigen. J. Virol. *46*:626–628, 1983.
163. Summers, J., and Mason, W. S.: Replication of the genome of a hepatitis B-like virus by reverse transcription of an RNA intermediate. Cell *29*:403–415, 1982.
164. Summers, J., O'Connell, A., and Millman, I.: Genome of hepatitis B virus: Restriction enzyme cleavage and structure of DNA extracted from Dane particles. Proc. Natl. Acad. Sci. U. S. A. *72*:4597–4601, 1975.
165. Szmuness, W., Stevens, C. E., Harley, E. J., et al.: Hepatitis B vaccine: Demonstration of efficacy in a controlled clinical trial in a high-risk population in the United States. N. Engl. J. Med. *303*:833–841, 1980.
166. Szmuness, W., Stevens, C. E., Harley, E. J., et al.: Hepatitis B vaccine: Demonstration of efficacy in a controlled clinical trial in a high-risk population in the United States. N. Engl. J. Med. *303*:833–841, 1980.
167. Tanaka, T., Miyamoto, H., Hino, O., et al.: Primary hepatocellular carcinoma with hepatitis B virus-DNA-integration in a 4-year-old boy. Hum. Pathol. *17*:202, 1986.
168. Tavis, J. E., Perri, S., and Ganem, D.: Hepadnavirus reverse transcription initiates within the stem-loop of the RNA packaging signal and employs a novel strand transfer. J. Virol. *68*:3536–3543, 1994.
169. Taylor, J. M.: Replication of human hepatitis delta virus: Influence of studies on subviral plant pathogens. Adv. Virus Res. *54*:45–60, 1999.
170. Tipples, G. A., Ma, M. M., Fischer, K. P., et al.: Mutation in HBV RNA-dependent DNA polymerase confers resistance to lamivudine *in vivo*. Hepatology *24*:714–717, 1996.
171. Toh, H., Hayashida, H., and Miyasa, T.: Sequence homology between retrovirla reverse transcriptase and putatuve polymerase of hepatitis B virus and cauliflower mosaic virus. Nature *305*:827–829, 1983.
172. Torre, D., and Tambini, R.: Interferon-alpha therapy for chronic hepatitis B in children: a meta-analysis. Clin. Infect. Dis. *23*:131–137, 1996.
173. Vajro, P., Tedesco, M., Fontanella, A., et al.: Prolonged and high dose recombinant interferon alpha-2b alone or after prednisone priming accelerates termination of active viral replication in children with chronic hepatitis B infection. Pediatr. Infect. Dis. J. *15*:223–231, 1996.
174. Van Damme, P., and Vellinga, A.: Epidemiology of hepatitis B and C in Europe. Acta Gastroenterol. Belg. *61*:175–182, 1998.
175. Vierling, J. M., and Brownstein, A. P.: Hepatitis B: An appropriate indication for liver transplantation. Hepatitis B Liver Transplant Symposium, American Liver Foundation, Tucson, AZ 1998.
176. Weissberg, J. I., Andres, L. L., Smith, C. I., et al.: Survival in chronic hepatitis B: An analysis of 379 patients. Ann. Intern. Med. *101*:613–616, 1984.
177. Wirth, S., Keller, K-M., Schaefer, E., and Zabel, B.: Hepatitis B virus DNA in liver tissue of chronic HBsAg carriers in childhood and its relationship to other viral markers. J. Pediatr. Gastroenterol. Nutr. *14*:431–435, 1992.
178. Wong, J. B.: Interferon treatment for chronic hepatitis B or C infection: Costs and effectiveness. Acta Gastroenterol. Belg. *61*:238–242, 1998.
179. Wu, T. C., Tong, M. J., Hwang, B., et al.: Primary hepatocellular carcinoma and hepatitis B infection during childhood. Hepatology *7*:46–48, 1987.
180. Yaginuma, K., Kobayashi, H., Kobayashi, M., et al.: Multiple integration site of hepatitis B virus DNA in hepatocellular carcinoma and chronic active hepatitis tissues from children. J. Virol. *61*:1808–1813, 1987.
181. Yuen, M. F., Lim, W. L., Cheng, C. C., et al.: Twelve-year follow-up of a prospective randomized trial of hepatitis B recombinant DNA yeast vaccine versus plasma-derived vaccine without booster doses in children. Hepatology *29*:924–927, 1999.
182. Zhang, X., Xu, H. J., Murakami, Y., et al.: Deletions of chromosome 13q, mutations in retinoblastoma 1, and retinoblastoma protein state in human hepatocellular carcinoma. Cancer Res. *54*:4177–4182, 1994.
183. Zuckerman, A. J., and Zuckerman, J. N.: Molecular epidemiology of hepatitis B virus mutants. J. Med. Virol. *58*:193–195, 1999.

HERPESVIRIDAE

CHAPTER 163 Herpes Simplex Viruses 1 and 2

ANN M. ARVIN

The family of eight human herpesviruses includes herpes simplex virus (HSV) types 1 and 2; cytomegalovirus (CMV); Epstein-Barr virus; varicella-zoster virus (VZV); and human herpesviruses 6, 7, and 8. This chapter deals with infections caused by HSV-1 and HSV-2 acquired after the neonatal period.

Herpes derives from the word meaning "to creep" in Greek. Initially, this term referred to cutaneous, spreading lesions in general and included the classic description of fever blisters recorded by Hippocrates and Herodotus. In the 1700s, Astrus described genital herpes lesions, and by the 1800s, the term *herpes* usually was restricted to poxvirus and herpesvirus lesions. Cultivation of HSV on rabbit cornea by Gruter (1912) differentiated HSV from VZV. Subsequent work differentiated the antigenic, biologic, and epidemiologic characteristics of HSV-1 and HSV-2.[289]

HSV-1 is the prototype of the alpha-herpesvirus subfamily, which includes HSV-2 and VZV.[206, 289] These viruses share the characteristic of neurotropism and establish latency in sensory ganglia; persistence is associated with periodic reactivation and reappearance of infectious virus at mucocutaneous sites. Understanding HSV-1 and HSV-2 infections requires knowing that most infected individuals do not have any clinical manifestations, either at the time of initial acquisition or during episodes of reactivation. The next step is to recognize that when HSV-1 or HSV-2 causes disease, as opposed to HSV infection, the illness may range from minor, such as "fever blisters," to life-threatening, as exemplified by HSV encephalitis. As with all herpesviruses, the immune status of the host is an important determinant of disease severity, as is whether infection is primary or recurrent. Proper management of HSV-1 and HSV-2 infection depends on clinical recognition of the common and atypical syndromes caused by these viruses and knowledge of the laboratory methods that are useful for proving the diagnosis. Attention to the clinical and laboratory diagnosis of HSV infection is important because oral antiviral treatment is safe and often benefits healthy children and early antiviral therapy reduces the risk of severe or fatal infections developing in immunocompromised patients. When misused, some therapies, such as corticosteroids for ocular HSV infection, may worsen the outcome. HSV-1 infections in children of all ages and HSV-2 infections in adolescents are among the most common treatable viral illnesses encountered in pediatric practice.

The Viruses

HSV-1 and HSV-2 virions consist of an icosahedral protein capsid enclosing a core of double-stranded DNA, surrounded by a protein tegument, and enclosed in a lipid-containing envelope.[206] The HSV genome codes for more than 100 proteins. The genomic DNA of HSV-1 and HSV-2 has substantial sequence homology (approximately 50%), but the viruses also have unique sequences that encode variant proteins, and they differ biologically in their patterns of replication in vitro and in vivo. Tegument proteins are located between the capsid and the viral envelope. The phospholipid-rich viral envelope is acquired when the virion buds through regions of the nuclear membrane that have been modified by the insertion of viral proteins. The envelope has glycoproteins that are important targets of the humoral and cellular immune responses (gB, gC, gD, and gG). The glycoproteins gE and gI function as immunoglobulin Fc receptors, and gC is a complement receptor. Most glycoproteins are found in both HSV-1 and HSV-2 and exhibit a high degree of amino acid similarity. The glycoprotein G of HSV-2 is larger than its HSV-1 homologue and has unique sites that are recognized by virus-specific host responses. Whereas both forms of HSV can infect either oral or genital sites, HSV-1 usually is a cause of infections of oral mucocutaneous sites (above the waist), and most genital mucocutaneous infections (below the waist) are caused by HSV-2.[76, 289] HSV-1 also is more likely to recur at oral sites and HSV-2 reactivates in the genital area, even in persons who were infected initially at both oral and genital sites with HSV-1 or HSV-2.[148]

HSV attaches to and penetrates cells via glycoproteins D and B by using specific cell surface receptors called herpesvirus entry molecules, and entry is facilitated by interactions with heparin sulfate proteoglycans. After the virion enters the cell, an orderly expression of immediate early or alpha genes occurs that triggers viral gene transcription and inhibits host cell function, early or beta viral genes that encode regulatory proteins and DNA replication enzymes, and, finally, late or gamma genes that encode structural proteins. Replication of viral DNA and accumulation of structural proteins allow virion capsid assembly in the cell nucleus and envelopment by modified cellular membranes that are incorporated into the virion envelope when viruses egress. Infectious virions are released from the infected cell or can spread to adjacent cells via membrane fusion. Human HSV replicates in tissue culture cells derived from many mammalian species, as well as in embryonated hens' eggs and various laboratory animals, including rodents, rabbits, and primates. Lack of restriction of the host range in infectivity distinguishes HSV-1 and HSV-2 from the other human herpesviruses. HSV-1 and HSV-2 infections progress rapidly in cell culture and cause relatively characteristic focal cytopathologic effects; confirmation that these effects are caused by HSV can be accomplished by staining the infected cells with specific antisera or monoclonal antibodies that differentiate HSV-1 from HSV-2 and from other viral pathogens.

HSV isolates can be analyzed further by using the technique of DNA endonuclease restriction analysis, in which viral DNA is recovered from infected cells, digested enzymatically, and analyzed in gels to determine the pattern of DNA fragments resulting from enzymatic digestion. Epidemiologically unrelated HSV isolates can be differentiated by using multiple restriction enzymes to digest viral DNA, which reveals a unique "viral fingerprint," or by genomic sequencing. These methods are useful for molecular epidemiologic studies to confirm the relatedness of viruses recovered from different sites or at different times in the same individual or to document transmission to another individual, such as mother to infant or infant to infant in nurseries; this technique has shown that apparent "outbreaks" of encephalitis were instead random, unrelated case clusters.[42, 110, 160]

Like other herpesviruses, HSV-1 and HSV-2 have gene products that facilitate the avoidance of immune surveillance during primary infection, latency, and reactivation. These mechanisms include elaboration of virally encoded IgG Fc receptors and complement receptors that bind host immune components; down-regulation of major histocompatibility complex (MHC) class I antigen, which prevents CD8+ T-cell recognition of infected cells; interference with up-regulation of MHC class II molecules by interferon-γ, which inhibits CD4+ T-cell–mediated adaptive immune responses; and inhibition of the lytic activity of natural killer cells.

Transmission

Infectious HSV-1 and HSV-2 virions are released into the oral or genital secretions of infected but asymptomatic persons who are experiencing primary or recurrent infection. This phenomenon is referred to as viral shedding or excretion and results in periodic opportunities for the virus to be transferred to susceptible contacts. Though not widely understood, most HSV-1 and HSV-2 transmission is caused by these silent infections, which are common, and transmission occurs with equivalent frequency regardless of whether the individual who is shedding the virus has ever had symptoms of oral or genital herpes.

Although HSV-1 and HSV-2 are highly infectious after inoculation of mucocutaneous sites, they are not transmitted casually from person to person. The enveloped virions are relatively unstable outside mammalian cells, and close interpersonal contact usually is required for transfer of infectious virus particles. In most circumstances, transmission requires direct apposition of infected with uninfected mucous membranes or skin during intimate contact such as kissing or sexual contact. Outbreaks associated with gingivostomatitis have occurred at daycare centers.[144, 231] If the uninfected, exposed skin or mucous membranes are damaged, the risk of transmission appears to be enhanced. Although skin is less susceptible to direct inoculation than the mucous membranes are, transmission via skin inoculation may be increased by local trauma. For example, affected areas are more susceptible in burn patients[88] and infants with diaper rash, and children with eczema are at risk for contracting serious disseminated HSV infections (Kaposi varicelliform eruption).[287] HSV-1 transfer that occurs between wrestlers (herpes gladiatorum)[236] and between rugby players (herpes rugbeiorum or "scrum-pox")[239, 290] probably occurs after the abrasion of saliva-contaminated skin. One outbreak at a wrestling camp involved 60 of 175 participants.[29, 113] Health care workers may acquire HSV infections of the paronychial region (herpetic whitlow), presumably from direct contact of ungloved hands with oropharyngeal secretions.[97, 208] Medical personnel may transfer HSV to their patients and be responsible for subsequent outbreaks of gingivostomatitis. Children may acquire HSV whitlow in the course of primary HSV-1 gingivostomatitis through nail biting or thumb sucking. When herpetic whitlow develops in persons who are not health care workers, HSV-2 is the most common cause and often is associated with primary genital HSV infection.[99] The usual route of transmission to newborns is by exposure during passage through an HSV-infected birth canal. Genital and anal HSV infections are transmitted through direct contact with infected genitalia or from oral-genital or oral-anal contact.

Newly acquired HSV-1 and HSV-2 infections are associated with shedding of very high titers of infectious virus, whether symptomatic or not. In addition, active recurrent HSV-1 or HSV-2 lesions contain substantial titers of virus, which may increase the likelihood of transmission during close contact with a susceptible individual. The incidence of transmission is 5 to 15 percent per year in individuals who are HSV-1– and HSV-2–seronegative or HSV-1–seropositive but HSV-2–seronegative and whose sexual partners have recurrent genital herpes.[168, 169] In additional couple studies, transmission occurred in 10 percent of partners, with higher transmission from men (17%) than from women (4%). In women lacking antibodies to HSV-1 and HSV-2, transmission was 32 percent; if they had antibodies to type 1, it was 9 percent.[169] Studies of long-term patients by HSV-2–specific serology show that many individuals remain uninfected despite long-term contact with a person who has HSV-2 infection.[144] The extent to which HSV-1 immunity protects against HSV-2 infection is not clear, but the evidence is that symptoms of new HSV-2 infection may be prevented if the exposed individual has HSV-1 immunity, whereas subclinical infection often is not blocked.[36, 42] Information about whether HSV-1 or HSV-2 acquired earlier interferes with the acquisition of infection by unrelated HSV-1 or HSV-2 strains is limited, but a few individuals with multiple sexual partners have been found to shed HSV-2 viruses that are genetically distinct. HSV has been isolated from the hands of patients with oral lesions and has been shown to persist for several hours on inanimate objects or in distilled water. Nonetheless, inanimate sources are not implicated as important reservoirs of HSV persistence and spread.[183, 273] HSV transmission from transplanted organs[77] and inseminated donor sperm has been reported.[173]

When HSV-1 and HSV-2 shedding has been evaluated prospectively in seropositive individuals with or without a history of symptoms, the usual frequency of detection of virus in oral or genital secretions is approximately 1 to 2 percent.[9, 283, 289] Rates of asymptomatic shedding may be higher after recent reactivation in individuals with symptomatic recurrences. In patients with known genital herpes, silent excretion has been documented as often as 10 percent of the time when they appear to be lesion-free. Twelve percent of women with primary HSV-1 genital infection and 18 percent with primary genital HSV-2 infection subsequently shed virus asymptomatically, especially in the first 3 months after resolution of the primary infection.[135] Two percent of women attending a sexually transmitted disease clinic shed HSV-2 asymptomatically.[143] In partner studies, 70 percent of HSV-2 transmissions were associated with sexual contact during periods of asymptomatic viral shedding.[169] Investigation of HSV-1 transmission is less extensive, but the high prevalence of asymptomatic HSV-1 infection in the population and its acquisition in early childhood suggests a similar pattern of spread by exposure to virus present in oral secretions from asymptomatic individuals.

Epidemiology

Understanding HSV epidemiology requires distinguishing between the prevalence of infection, which is high, and the frequency of HSV-related disease, which is low. HSV-1 and HSV-2 are only infectious for the human host under usual, natural circumstances. Molecular genetic analysis indicates that the HSV genome has evolved in parallel with the evolution of *Homo sapiens* from primate ancestors. These viruses maintain their persistence in the human population through their capacity to persist and reactivate in the individual host. The prevalence of HSV-1 and HSV-2 is a consequence of efficient transmission to susceptible close contacts and the continuous presence of a large pool of infected persons in the population. Because HSV-1 and HSV-2 are not cleared after primary infection but instead establish latency and reactivate frequently in an infected host, opportunities for viral spread to new susceptible persons are extremely common. HSV-1 and HSV-2 infections are ubiquitous and global in their distribution. Seroepidemiologic studies have shown that HSV infections are found in all human populations, even in the most remote and isolated communities. HSV-1 and HSV-2 have no seasonal pattern because the mechanism of transmission is by intimate contact, which occurs year-round. Individuals who have been infected with HSV-1 or HSV-2 remain a reservoir for infectious virus throughout their lifetime and, as intermittent shedders, are a source of virus for spread to susceptible contacts. Most transmission is from asymptomatic infection, and most acquisition is asymptomatic. For example, the rate of subclinical shedding of HSV-2 in individuals with no reported history of genital herpes was similar to that in subjects with such a history (3.0% versus 2.7%).[282] Shedding of HSV-1 in oral secretions is equally prevalent.

When symptoms of a new HSV-1 infection do occur, the source of the infection rarely is identified because the susceptible individual usually has many infected contacts. Furthermore, the first symptomatic episodes of HSV-1 or HSV-2 often represent reactivations of earlier infections.

The average age at acquisition and the prevalence of HSV-1 and HSV-2 infections are influenced by the virus type. Although neonatal HSV infections are acquired from maternal genital infection and most often are caused by HSV-2, HSV-1 acquisition predominates in childhood. Depending on social and economic factors, 40 to 60 percent of young children are seropositive by 5 years of age, with somewhat higher rates of acquisition in lower socioeconomic groups. Earlier acquisition of HSV-1 may be influenced particularly by whether the mother, or other major caregivers, has HSV-1 infection. Attendance in child care centers, which bring children together in close contact, may increase the likelihood of HSV-1 acquisition at an earlier age.[146, 231] Acquisition of HSV-1 continues with age at an average rate of 1 to 2 percent per year throughout the childhood and adult years; by later ages, 70 to 90 percent of individuals have been infected by HSV-1.[244] Seroepidemiologic studies of higher socioeconomic groups have reported HSV-1 infection in 30 to 46 percent of university students.[96] Because transmission of HSV-2 is associated with sexual activity, the prevalence of HSV-2 begins to increase with adolescence. Now that serologic methods can be used to differentiate HSV-1 and HSV-2 infection, the seroprevalence of HSV-2 in adults has been shown to range from 20 to 80 percent. The comprehensive National Health and Nutritional Examination Survey (NHANES) investigation of HSV-2 epidemiology in the United States documented a 30 percent increase in prevalence from the 1970s to the 1990s, which has resulted in HSV-2 infection in about 20 percent of adults.[87, 95] An increasing frequency of HSV-2 infection was observed in all ages above 12 years, including teenagers of all ethnicities, and its prevalence rose fivefold in white teenagers. High HSV-2 infection rates are documented in higher as well as lower socioeconomic groups.[36, 143, 144, 262] Rates are consistently higher in women than in men, regardless of other variables, and in individuals with more sexual partners.

Changes in the epidemiology of symptomatic HSV-2 infection have been suggested by rising numbers of medical visits for genital herpes. Approximately 300,000 new cases occur each year in the United States. The extent to which the increase in symptomatic cases of HSV-2 infection reflects a true increase in the prevalence of HSV-2 or a higher likelihood that HSV-2 infection will result in symptoms is not certain; for example, a decrease in the number of young adults with HSV-1 infection acquired in childhood could be associated with loss of cross-reactive HSV immunity and an increased risk for development of symptomatic genital herpes. A higher risk of contracting genital HSV infection is associated with lower socioeconomic status, early age at first intercourse, increased numbers of sexual partners, female sex, previous marriage, urban living, black race, and a history of other sexually transmitted diseases.[87, 126]

Symptomatic disease occurs in a minority of individuals with newly acquired infection, with an estimated incidence of 10 to 20 percent or less. However, silent infections can give rise to symptoms that appear months or years later as a result of viral reactivation. The epidemiology of HSV-1 or HSV-2 reactivation as a cause of symptomatic illness depends on the prevalence of these infections in the population as a whole, but it also is influenced by host factors that perturb the balance between the virus and the infected individual. For example, HSV-related symptoms may be triggered by exposure to sunlight (ultraviolet), febrile illnesses, immunosuppression from illness or necessary therapies, and other variables. These variables are cofactors that affect the frequency of HSV-related disease within the infected cohort but not the epidemiologic pattern of infection.

Pathogenesis and Pathology

HSV-1 and HSV-2 exhibit particular tropism for cells of ectodermal origin, including skin and neuronal cells. Initial viral replication is thought to occur at the portal of entry, usually in mucous membranes or skin.[289] In symptomatic cases, the incubation period for primary infection appears to vary from 2 to 20 days. In contrast to varicella, HSV viremia is difficult to detect in a normal host, although it may be found in some immunocompromised patients.[108, 252] If mucocutaneous lesions are induced during primary or recurrent infection, the pathologic cell changes caused by HSV-1 or HSV-2 replication include cytoplasmic enlargement and nuclear alterations; in addition, the cell fusion may lead to the formation of multinucleate giant cells. The nuclei of infected cells often have eosinophilic intranuclear inclusions and marginated nuclear chromatin. As the cells manifest injury, a local inflammatory response ensues, intercellular edema develops, and vesicles form in the affected area. The vesicles become visible as they enlarge and usually are surrounded by an erythematous margin. At later stages, the vesicles become pustular and then dry and crust. HSV lesions typically are superficial and do not scar. Vesicles that form on mucous membranes are transient, with rapid sloughing of the superficial layer, and they usually are seen first as shallow ulcers.

HSV-1 and HSV-2 have a characteristic ability to establish latency in neurons of the sensory ganglia by mechanisms that as yet are unidentified. The viruses persist in this latent state for various intervals; reactivation induces viral replication with the production of infectious virus at mucosal or other sites. Evidence related to a possible neural site for latent HSV was presented nearly 80 years ago when Cushing reported the appearance of herpetic vesicles in the trigeminal distribution after rhizotomy of the trigeminal nerve and destruction of the sensory ganglion.[189, 289] Persons who have recurrent HSV infections frequently describe tingling sensations, itching, and burning at the site of recurrence beginning several hours before the appearance of clusters of vesicles. Persons who have recurrent genital herpes may experience severe shooting pain in their legs and even urinary retention before and in connection with recurrent genital herpes infections. Occasionally, recurrent HSV skin eruptions may occur in a zosteriform pattern and in a distribution reflecting the sensory innervation of a particular dermatome.

Replication at the portal of entry appears to result in infection of sensory nerve endings, followed by transport of the virus to the dorsal root ganglia along neuronal axons. Latency is established regardless of whether the primary infection is symptomatic, and it appears to be an invariable consequence of HSV infection with either virus type.[22, 204, 206] HSV-1 and HSV-2 persist in neuronal cells of the sensory ganglia, with substantial numbers of these cells harboring latent virus, as demonstrated by the detection of latency-associated transcripts. The latency-associated transcripts overlap the viral genes *ICPO* and *ICP34.5* in an antisense direction.[63, 206, 233, 253] The role of these transcripts in the establishment or maintenance of latency remains to be clarified. The presence of latency-associated transcripts appears to be necessary for efficient reactivation of viral production in vivo.[191] Viral particles are not produced in latently infected cells. HSV-1 persists most predominantly in the cranial nerve ganglia, whereas HSV-2 latency occurs in the lumbosacral ganglia. Cocultivation techniques have been used to recover HSV from the dorsal root ganglia innervating the areas of skin in which persons have experienced recurrent herpes lesions. HSV-1 has been found in trigeminal ganglia, and HSV-2 has been recovered from sacral ganglia.[24] Once latency is established in the sensory ganglia, antiviral drugs cannot eradicate the latent virus from infected neurons. Because the latent virus does not multiply, it is not susceptible to drugs that affect viral DNA synthesis, such as acyclovir. When reactivation is triggered, HSV-1 or HSV-2 is transported back down axons to mucocutaneous sites, where they replicate and infectious virus is released into secretions.[22, 63, 204, 206] Individuals with symptomatic recurrent HSV infections almost always have HSV lesions in the identical or a directly adjacent site. Reactivation is not prevented by adaptive immunity, although whether symptoms occur may be influenced by the host response.

The stimulus for reactivation of latent virus may be provided by iatrogenic or naturally occurring episodes of immunosuppression and by endocrine (such as menstruation) or exogenous factors (such as trauma, sun, acupuncture, emotional stress). Ultraviolet irradiation of persons who have a history of recurrent oral herpes reliably induces recurrence either quickly (within 48 hours) or 2 to 7 days later.[245] Skin subject to recurrent HSV infection has been transplanted elsewhere on the body and exchanged with skin taken from the site of graft placement and previously not involved in HSV infections. Subsequent recurrence of HSV infection was found to be localized to the original site, not to the original skin. These studies and others strongly suggest that latent virus does not reside in skin cells.

Primary HSV infection elicits humoral and cellular immunity, which can be detected shortly after the appearance of lesions in individuals in whom symptoms develop. Based on animal models and some human studies, the initial host response is mediated by innate, nonspecific mechanisms, followed by the acquisition of virus-specific adaptive immunity.[209] The nonspecific response consists of mobilization of polymorphonuclear leukocytes and monocytes to the site of infection, release of interferon-α and other cytokines, and activation of macrophages and natural killer cells. The innate response is followed by the production of antiviral antibodies that mediate virus neutralization, complement fixation, and cellular or complement cytotoxicity. Induction of specific cellular immunity is detected by measuring T-cell recognition of HSV proteins in proliferation and cytotoxicity assays, interleukin-2 and interferon-γ production, and a positive delayed hypersensitivity skin test reaction. Failure of virus-specific cell-mediated immunity to develop, as may occur in newborns and children with genetic immunodeficiencies, immunocompromised children, and other high-risk populations, can be associated with life-threatening dissemination of HSV-1 or HSV-2. If HSV disseminates, these viruses can infect and destroy cells in many organs (e.g., the lungs, liver, adrenals, and brain), with catastrophic effects.

Symptomatic HSV-1 and HSV-2 recurrences are less severe than are primary lesions in immunologically intact persons. In persons previously infected with one type of virus (e.g., HSV-1), new infections with the second type (e.g., HSV-2) more often are silent or the symptoms are less severe than in a host who has never been infected with either virus. When re-infection with unrelated strains has been identified, symptoms also have been mild and, without molecular analysis of viral DNA, would be attributed to reactivation of endogenous virus.[45] The immune response to symptomatic reactivation is not associated with a significant increase in the production of antibody, although fourfold rises and re-emergence of IgA and IgM antiviral antibody may occur. Natural killer cell activity and cytokine production increase, and relative defects in these and HSV-specific T-cell responses may predispose to frequent or severe symptomatic recurrences, but definitive associations have not been established. Patients who have diseases or are being treated with agents that reduce cell-mediated immunity, such as those undergoing antitumor chemotherapy or individuals with acquired immunodeficiency syndrome (AIDS), often have frequent HSV recurrences that are longer in duration and more severe, but dissemination rarely occurs. Nonetheless, no evidence suggests a specific immunodeficiency in otherwise healthy persons who have symptomatic HSV recurrences.

Viral encephalitis is the most severe consequence of HSV infection in an otherwise healthy host. HSV-1 is the pathogen in almost all these cases, and the pathologic mechanism is thought to be ascending infection along neuronal pathways from the cranial nerve ganglia to the brain.[67] Encephalitis may accompany or develop after primary HSV infection, but it also occurs as a consequence of reactivation of latent virus. When the virus reaches brain parenchymal cells, it replicates efficiently and induces widespread hemorrhagic necrosis and vascular compromise. HSV encephalitis has been associated with an acute-phase elevation in β_2-microglobulin, neopterin, interleukin-6, and interferon-γ in cerebrospinal fluid (CSF).[17, 18] During convalescence, increased levels of soluble CD8, β_2-microglobulin, neopterin, and specific anti-HSV IgG have been detected. How these markers relate to disease pathogenesis is not established yet.

Clinical Manifestations

Most HSV-1 and HSV-2 infections do not cause symptoms, but when infection is symptomatic, the clinical manifestations usually are self-limited and not severe. If symptoms occur, the disease associated with primary infection tends to be much more extensive than are the minor, localized lesions at mucocutaneous junctions caused by viral reactivation. Nonetheless, prospective studies document that new HSV infections can be as mild as symptomatic recurrences, and, as a result, definitive differentiation of primary from recurrent infection is not possible with clinical criteria.

GINGIVOSTOMATITIS

Gingivostomatitis is the most common form of HSV-induced primary illness in children. A history of such symptoms has been reported in as little as 1 percent to as many as 31 percent of seropositive children, the higher percentage being from a study involving the Navajo Indians. It usually is seen in young children between 10 months and 3 years of age. In those younger than 10 months, residual maternal antibody probably modifies or prevents the appearance of recognizable symptoms in association with primary HSV-1 infection. Although acute gingivostomatitis caused by HSV is a relatively infrequent occurrence, it is sufficiently common that most pediatricians become familiar with the condition and learn to distinguish this infection from herpangina.[187, 289]

The illness begins with irritability and fever. Despite these systemic symptoms, HSV is not cultured from the blood during this period.[108] The infant usually refuses to eat and may refuse fluids. Thereafter, vesicular lesions appear around and on the lips, along the gingiva, on the anterior of the tongue, and on the anterior (hard) portion of the palate (Figs. 163–1 and 163–2). The vesicles break down rapidly, and when seen, lesions usually appear as 1- to 3-mm shallow gray ulcers on an erythematous base. The gums are erythematous, mildly swollen, and ulcerated. They may appear friable and frequently bleed on contact. The child experiences extreme discomfort, cannot or will not eat, and if fluids are refused as well, may require hospitalization to ensure adequate hydration. The risk of dehydration is compounded by the fever that usually accompanies this syndrome. Vesicles often extend around the lips and chin or down the neck in an immunologically intact child. The child often has a foul smell to the breath (fetor oris). The lesions bleed easily and may become covered with a black crust. The cervical and submental nodes are usually swollen and tender. The clinical signs continue to evolve for 4 to 5 days, and the process of resolution requires at least an additional week. In an analysis of the natural history of HSV gingivostomatitis in 36 children, oral lesions persisted for an average of 12 days, most children had extraoral lesions, fever lasted for 2 to 6 days, and difficulty taking liquids was noted for 4 to 10 days. The duration of viral shedding was 7 days (range, 2 to 12 days).[4] Herpetic epiglottitis[35] and acute otitis media[51] are unusual complications.

HSV gingivostomatitis is differentiated from herpangina, a manifestation of enteroviral infection, by the predominance of ulcers in the anterior and posterior portions of the oropharynx; herpangina usually causes posterior pharyngeal ulcers. In addition, unlike HSV infection, herpangina often has a more acute onset, a shorter duration, and seasonal occurrence.[187] Whereas enterovirus-associated hand, foot, and mouth disease can be manifested as oral ulcers and a vesicular eruption on the distal portions of extremities, the bilateral distribution should differentiate it from HSV gingivostomatitis and concurrent HSV autoinoculation to a digit. Severe Stevens-Johnson syndrome (erythema multiforme) may mimic HSV infection, but the generalized macular rash accompanied by "bull's-eye" lesions is characteristic of erythema multiforme. Rarely, recurrent HSV infection can be associated with erythema multiforme, as discussed later. Impetigo may be confused with the lesions of HSV infection, and misdiagnosis is re-enforced because *Staphylococcus aureus* colonization of skin may be identified in bacterial cultures and be considered causative.

Parents and caregivers are familiar with "cold sores" or "fever blisters" but may not know that these lesions are caused by HSV. Because HSV infection may be thought of as a sexually transmitted disease, the physician is advised

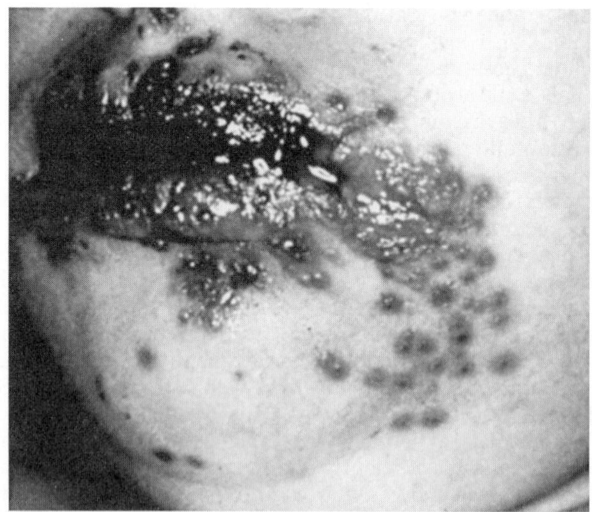

FIGURE 163–1 ■ Primary HSV gingivostomatitis in a normal toddler: ulcerative-vesicular stage. (Courtesy of Dr. Theodore Rosen, Department of Dermatology, Baylor College of Medicine, Houston.)

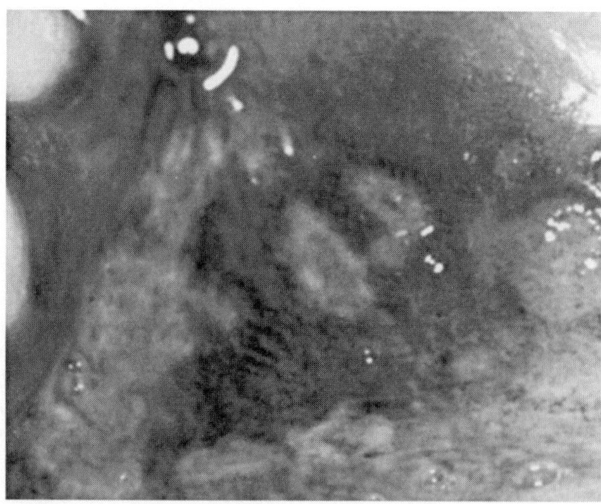

FIGURE 163–2 ■ Primary HSV gingivostomatitis in a 6-year-old demonstrating involvement of the oral mucosa with ulcers.

to anticipate confusion and anxiety when making the diagnosis of HSV oral infection and to address these concerns by explaining the normal mode of acquisition of oral HSV infection in young children.

In adolescents, primary HSV-1 infection initially may be seen as a posterior, occasionally exudative pharyngitis.[167] The characteristic findings are shallow tonsillar ulcers with a gray exudate. In this setting, HSV infection must be differentiated from streptococcal and Epstein-Barr virus infection and rarely from diphtheria, acute human immunodeficiency virus (HIV) infection, and tularemia-induced pharyngitis. In one study of college students of a higher socioeconomic level, HSV was the most common etiologic agent of acute pharyngitis (24%).[98] A more recent study of 613 college students with upper respiratory complaints documented an incidence of 5.7 percent with positive HSV cultures. Twelve of the 35 students with positive cultures had vesicular lesions on the lips, throat, or gums, and 29 of the 35 had a primary diagnosis of pharyngitis that was indistinguishable from other causes of pharyngitis.[169] In some cases, acute pharyngitis is caused by HSV-2; the symptoms and clinical course appear to be similar, and viral cultures are required to identify the type of infecting virus. This information may be useful prognostically inasmuch as recurrent HSV-2 infection at oral sites is an extremely rare occurrence, although these individuals may have recurrent genital infections.

VULVOVAGINITIS

Primary herpetic vulvovaginitis occurs rarely in infants and children. HSV-1 may cause this clinical syndrome, perhaps if inadvertently introduced when the genital area is touched by a caregiver with HSV on the hands. Progression of the infection may be limited to a few lesions, or it may resemble symptomatic primary genital herpes caused by HSV-2. Obtaining cultures to identify the type of infecting virus is important because HSV-1 infection is not expected to recur and HSV-2 infection may reflect sexual abuse of the child. As is true of other potentially sexually transmitted diseases, genital HSV infection in young children warrants a careful and sensitive appraisal of the circumstances that may have led to the infection. Also useful is knowing that some children infected with HSV-2 in the newborn period have had genital lesions later in childhood.

Pediatricians are likely to encounter genital herpes in their adolescent patients. Reports about the incidence of genital herpes in which data are given for subgroups of children and adolescents are limited, but a rate of 3 per 100,000 in the 10- to 14-year-old age group and 76 per 100,000 in the 15- to 19-year-old age group was reported in a Minnesota study of a predominantly white, middle-class population of northern European ethnicity.[52] The NHANES report described the prevalence in 12- to 19-year-old subjects as 5.6 percent.[87] In one study of 379 adolescents aged 14 to 19 years who were treated at a sexually transmitted disease or urban community clinic, 12 percent had HSV-2 antibodies and only 22 percent of these patients had a history of genital herpes. HSV-2 seropositivity correlated with African-American race or female gender but with not condom use, the number of sexual partners in the previous 2 months, or a previous history of a sexually transmitted disease, thus indicating that prevalence was related to demographic rather than behavioral variables.[260]

In contrast to earlier concepts, prospective studies have documented that many infections are subclinical and that new genital HSV-2 infections have a wide range of manifestations.[153] Variation is common with respect to the extent and severity of lesions; whether the lesions are bilateral or localized; the presence or absence of systemic symptoms such as malaise, myalgia, headache, and fever; dysuria; and regional lymphadenopathy. Symptoms can be mild enough to suggest recurrent infection or may be those of severe, "classic" primary genital herpes. In such cases in adults, local genital symptoms include severe pain (in 95% of men and 99% of women), itching, dysuria (44% of men and 83% of women), vaginal or urethral discharge, and tender inguinal adenopathy (80%). The lesions begin as vesicles or pustules and progress to wet ulcers and then to healing ulcers with or without crusts (Figs. 163–3 to 163–5). Crusting usually occurs only on squamous epithelium. Lesions tend to last for 2 to 3 weeks before complete healing (mean, 19 days). They

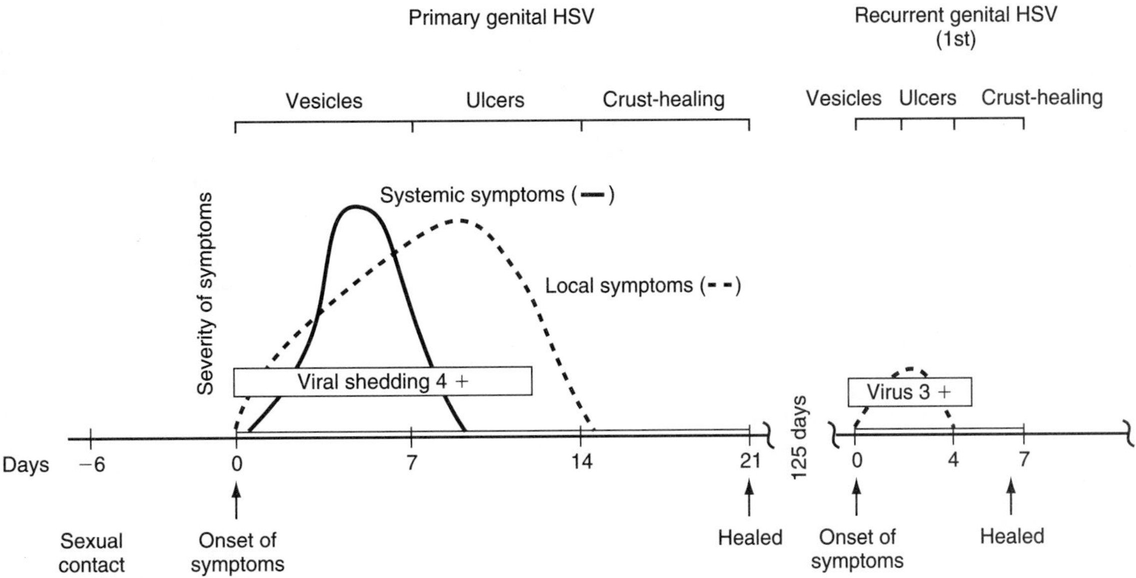

FIGURE 163–3 ■ Graphic representation of the course of primary and recurrent HSV genital infection. The days illustrated are for average cases.

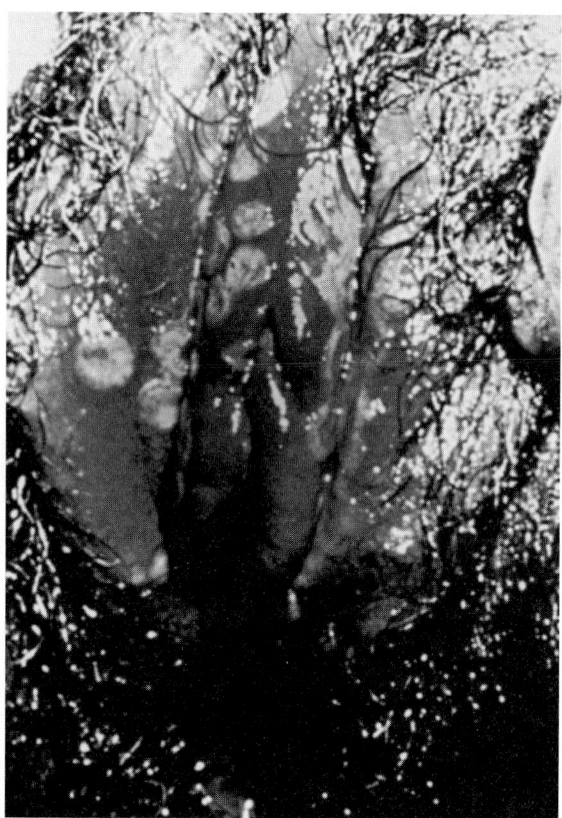

FIGURE 163–4 ■ Primary genital herpes in a female. (Courtesy of Dr. Theodore Rosen, Department of Dermatology, Baylor College of Medicine, Houston.)

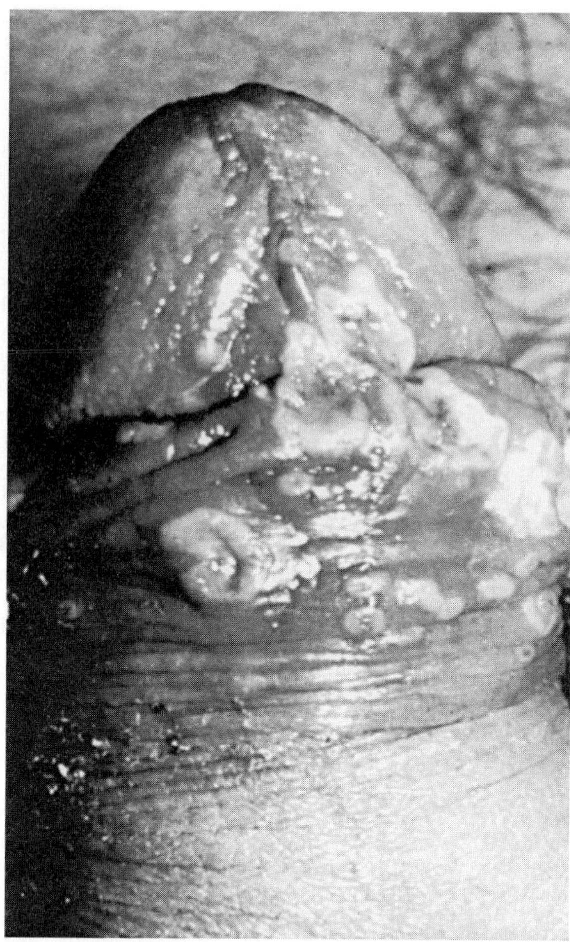

FIGURE 163–5 ■ Primary genital HSV infection in a male. (Courtesy of Dr. Theodore Rosen, Department of Dermatology, Baylor College of Medicine, Houston.)

may spread in a wavelike fashion from the initial site to the thighs, buttocks, and urethra. Virus shedding generally persists for 1 to 2 weeks or longer. Some primary infections are associated with atypical lesions (e.g., fissures, furuncles, excoriations), and extragenital lesions, typically on the buttocks, may be observed.[30, 143]

When evaluating potential primary genital herpes in a sexually active adolescent, the history may reveal recent contact with a partner who has known recurrent genital herpes. When exposure can be documented, the incubation period is estimated to be 2 to 14 days. However, most of these episodes will not be associated with a known exposure. In addition, recognizing that as many as two thirds of first reported episodes of symptomatic genital herpes actually are caused by reactivation is important. In these cases, the exposure may have occurred months or years before the signs of HSV-2 infection appear. In some adult series, 50 to 60 percent of persons without a history of HSV infection can identify symptoms consistent with previous infection after careful instruction about the typical signs, but many have not had any previous episodes.[151] HSV-1 accounts for 5 to 25 percent of primary genital HSV infections in the United States, whereas as many as 50 percent of cases diagnosed in other geographic areas, such as England and Japan, are caused by HSV-1. Indications are that HSV-1 is becoming a more common primary genital isolate in the United States. Patients who have primary HSV-1 genital infections may have lesions elsewhere (25%), typically on the hands and face.[30]

Primary genital HSV-2 infections may be associated with viral meningitis. This complication is manifested as fever, stiff neck, headache, and photophobia with a CSF lymphocytic cellular response and usually a normal glucose level.[115, 268] HSV-2 can be isolated from CSF in the early phase of the illness. HSV-2–associated meningitis differs from HSV-1 encephalitis in that it is almost always mild, self-limited, and not associated with neurologic residua.

Other complications of primary HSV genital infection include sacral autonomic nervous dysfunction, which is manifested as poor rectal sphincter tone, constipation, sacral anesthesia, urinary retention, or impotence; extragenital lesions, which occur more commonly in women and occur on the buttocks, groin, thighs, or less commonly, the fingers or conjunctiva, usually in the second week of disease; secondary yeast infections in women; and pharyngitis, which usually is associated with fever, malaise, myalgia, headache, tender anterior cervical adenopathy, and a mildly erythematous to diffusely ulcerative or exudative posterior pharyngitis. Most of these patients have throat cultures positive for HSV. HSV has been associated uncommonly with acute salpingitis[157] and inguinal lymphadenitis.[265] Of critical importance has been the association of previous HSV infection with an increased incidence of HIV infection, perhaps because the genital ulcers of HSV facilitate HIV transmission.[251]

Transmission to the newborn is a complication of primary or recurrent genital herpes in women of child-bearing age. This complication is discussed in Chapter 73.

Genital herpes creates significant psychologic difficulties for many patients. Whereas many people cope well with the illness and the likelihood of recurrent disease, a syndrome of profound depression, poor self-esteem, complete abstention from sexual activities, and general withdrawal develops in some. This reaction, or "leper syndrome," must be anticipated and discussed in a sensitive and caring manner. Information about the high prevalence of these infections in the population may be helpful, with emphasis on the fact that most infected people do not realize that they are infected and shed the virus intermittently, just like those who have had symptoms. Self-help groups of persons who have genital herpes exist in many parts of the United States and can be contacted through the American Social Health Association, Herpes Resource Center, P.O. Box 13827, Research Triangle Park, NC, 27709, and the American Herpes Foundation.

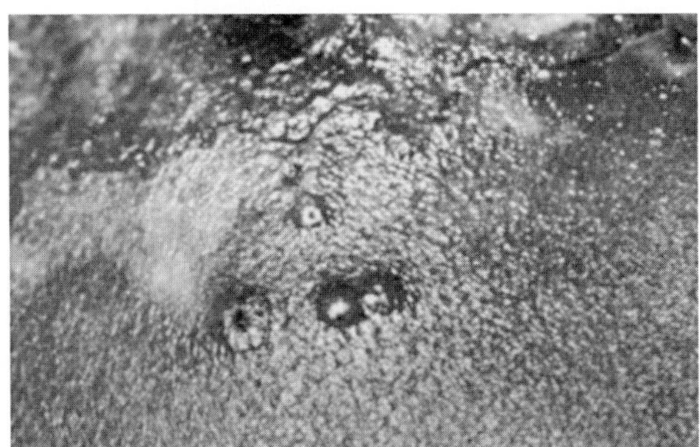

FIGURE 163–7 ■ Secondary HSV infection at a burn site in a 2-year-old. Note the vesicles at the border of the burn.

OTHER PRIMARY SKIN INFECTIONS

Mucocutaneous junction areas are common sites of HSV infection, and damaged skin often provides a portal of entry for HSV. Vesicular lesions spread throughout the affected skin, usually crusting and resolving in about 1 week. The illness accompanying eczema herpeticum can be severe (Fig. 163–6) and even fatal, although in most cases it resolves without specific therapy and leaves no sequelae. Similar widespread herpetic lesions may occur in skin altered by thermal or chemical burns. In this situation, a secondary fever may occur, usually 1 to several weeks after the initial insult. Careful inspection of the burn site or adjacent normal tissue may reveal vesicles (Fig. 163–7) or nonspecific ulcerative lesions. Without therapy, several of these patients have died of disseminated HSV infection.[88] A similar syndrome occurs rarely in children after simple skin abrasions (Fig. 163–8). Herpetic recurrences may follow in these cases, but recurrences are localized to the area of skin that was affected initially. HSV infection can be severe as a secondary infection at the site of common diaper rash.[124]

Herpetic whitlow is a painful, erythematous, swollen lesion that occurs on the terminal phalanx, sometimes associated with a damaged cuticle.[27, 97, 208] The fingers (69%) and thumb (21%) are involved most frequently.[97] Less commonly, the palm may be the site of inoculation and major involvement.[225] The digit is swollen, and the painful white swelling appears to be filled with pus but, when opened for drainage, is found to contain little fluid and no purulent material. The white appearance is caused by the presence of necrotic epithelial cells. Occasionally, the whitlow, which may persist for 7 to 10 days, initially is accompanied by a few vesicles that may give a clue to the etiologic agent of the primary infection. Less commonly, the whitlow is associated with fever, lymphadenopathy, and lymphangitis.[221]

Whitlow is seen in four typical situations. Most commonly, infants with primary herpetic gingivostomatitis autoinoculate their fingers (Fig. 163–9). At times, whitlow is

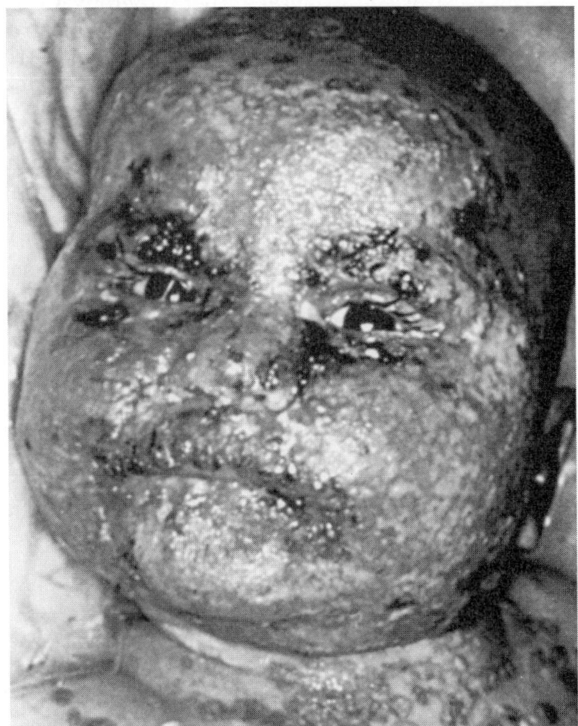

FIGURE 163–6 ■ Extensive HSV infection in an infant with atopic eczema (Kaposi varicelliform eruption). (Courtesy of Dr. Theodore Rosen, Department of Dermatology, Baylor College of Medicine, Houston.)

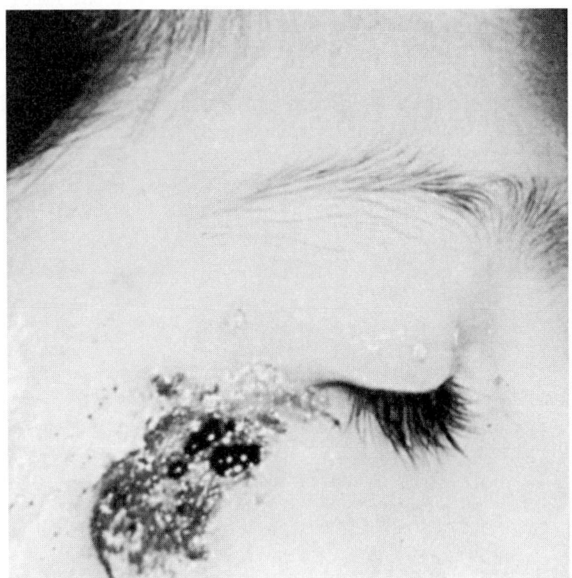

FIGURE 163–8 ■ Facial HSV infection in a young girl after a mild abrasion. (Courtesy of Dr. Johnie Frazier, Department of Pediatrics, University of Texas Medical School, Houston.)

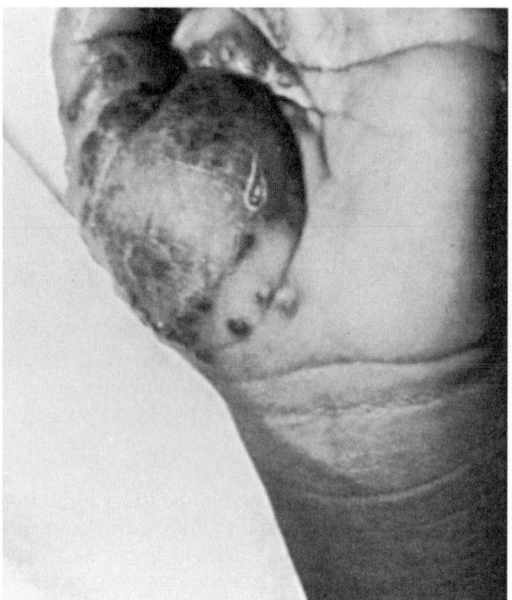

FIGURE 163–9 ■ Extensive herpetic whitlow in a toddler with oral HSV infection.

encountered in infants without obvious oral disease, and sometimes it may be caused by adults kissing their children's fingers. In these settings, the viral isolate almost always is HSV-1.[27, 97] In sexually active patients, the whitlow more commonly is a manifestation of concurrent genital disease, which should be sought by appropriate history and physical examination.[99] These infections are caused most frequently by HSV-2. In the fourth setting, persons such as dentists, respiratory therapists, nurses, and pediatricians who examine oral cavities or handle secretion-contaminated material without wearing gloves are at risk for acquiring herpetic whitlow[84] (Fig. 163–10). In addition, the same poor medical practice facilitates transfer of HSV to other patients, especially in intensive care settings.[2]

Herpetic whitlow often is confused with a bacterial felon or paronychia, and such confusion may lead to the incorrect intervention of incision and drainage. This procedure is not indicated and is not beneficial for the management of herpetic whitlow, which should be treated with oral acyclovir. Needle aspiration and culture provide the diagnosis of whitlow, and initiation of antiviral therapy can be based on the clinical signs.

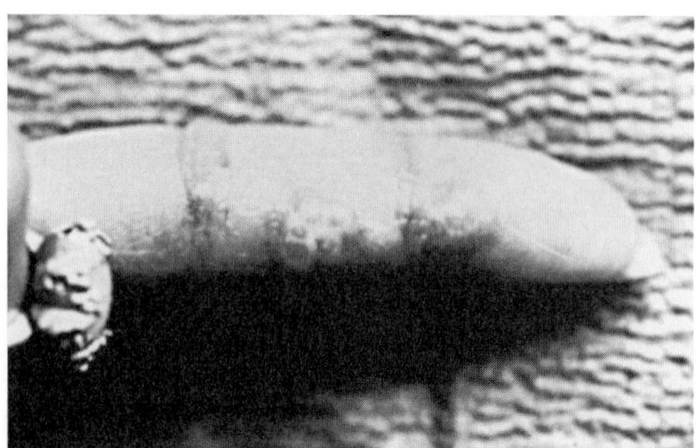

FIGURE 163–10 ■ Recurrent herpetic whitlow in a pediatrician.

In several sports, cutaneous (especially facial) HSV infection is a hazard, particularly in sports with close physical contact such as wrestling (herpes gladiatorum) and rugby (scrum-pox, derived from the line-up of rugby players, the "scrum" or "scrummage").[29, 113, 236, 239, 290] Often, the initial lesions are diagnosed as impetigo, unless HSV is considered. HSV infection develops in approximately 3 percent of wrestlers in high school, typically on the head and neck but also on the extremities and trunk and in the eyes.[113]

INFECTION OF THE EYE

Primary infection of the eye by HSV may be manifested as blepharitis or follicular conjunctivitis. The symptoms often are accompanied by pre-auricular lymphadenopathy, corneal injection, watering, discharge, itching, lid swelling, and in a third of cases, malaise and fever. If restricted to the conjunctivae, the infection (which can be accompanied by vesicular herpetic lesions elsewhere on the face or in the nose or mouth) usually resolves without sequelae or specific features. Herpetic infection of the eye may, however, progress to involve the cornea, with far more serious potential consequences. For this reason, an ophthalmologic consultant always should examine and evaluate these cases.

Corneal involvement by HSV may be manifested initially by minute vesicles at the corneal margin. Progression of the corneal infection (best seen with the use of topical fluorescein dye) is marked by the appearance of branching lesions (a dendritic pattern) or the less diagnostic irregular (ameboid or geographic) ulcer.[28, 64] The child complains of severe photophobia accompanied in some cases by blurred vision, chemosis, and lacrimation. Primary eye infection may include stromal involvement, uveitis, and rarely retinitis.[188] Retinitis is manifested as multiple whitish-yellow, punctate retinal lesions. Spontaneous healing, which generally requires 2 to 3 weeks, can be speeded by topical antiviral therapy. Corticosteroids are contraindicated. The risk of visual impairment caused by direct viral damage, immunopathologic reactions, or both is enhanced greatly with recurrences. With each bout of infection, the corneal ulcers become more extensive and can result in scarring and impairment of sight. Herpetic infection of the eye recurs in approximately 32 percent of patients who have primary symptomatic infection and is more common in younger patients.[298] Recurrences may be manifested as blepharitis, follicular conjunctivitis with or without lid lesions, or ulcers and keratitis, which more often are accompanied by ulcerations deeper into the corneal stroma (diskiform or necrotizing keratitis) with resultant extensive scarring, irregular astigmatism, and even corneal perforation.[298] Children who have dendritic ulcers have a better prognosis for good vision than do those with geographic or diskiform keratitis.[28] Rarely, in normal and immunocompromised patients (especially those with AIDS), HSV eye infection may result in acute retinal necrosis,[90] and very infrequently, an oculoglandular syndrome of conjunctivitis and adenopathy may be caused by HSV infection.[47]

INFECTIONS OF THE CENTRAL NERVOUS SYSTEM

HSV is the most common identifiable cause of serious or life-threatening sporadic encephalitis. It accounts for 2 to 5 percent of all cases of encephalitis in the United States and for as many as 20 percent of all cases with an etiologic diagnosis (60–70% of cases of encephalitis have no established cause).[199] With the advent of immunization for measles, mumps, rubella, and varicella, the relative incidence of HSV in cases of encephalitis has increased, although absolute numbers remain stable in children.[140, 177, 199] The case-fatality rate associated with untreated HSV encephalitis is approximately 70 percent,[295] and survivors generally have severe and permanent neurologic disability. Both HSV-1 and HSV-2 have been implicated in the etiology of central nervous system (CNS) infection by HSV, but typical HSV encephalitis is caused by HSV-1.[62, 224, 289] Spread of HSV-1 to the CNS seems to proceed via either neurogenic pathways or hematogenous dissemination or perhaps through the cribriform plate from infected nasopharyngeal mucosa during primary infection. Recurrent infection probably results from spread via sensory neurons. HSV-2 meningitis is not associated with brain parenchymal infection; whether the infection is a consequence of hematogenous delivery or spread along neuronal pathways is not known.

Although HSV encephalitis may involve virtually any area of the brain, this infection has a striking tendency to involve the orbital region of the frontal lobes and, with particular frequency, portions of the temporal lobes. Johnson and Mims have suggested that the predilection of HSV to involve regions of the brain governing olfaction suggests that a pathogenetic pathway proceeds from the nasal-respiratory mucosa via the olfactory bulbs and along the subsequent tracts into the brain.[127] Other researchers have suggested that reactivated virus travels from the trigeminal ganglia via the fifth nerve fibers to the meninges of the anterior and middle fossae.[68] More recent studies in children involving diagnosis by polymerase chain reaction (PCR) assay and magnetic resonance imaging (MRI) have defined cases with more diffuse cerebral involvement.[226, 289]

HSV encephalitis must be differentiated from HSV meningitis, which usually is caused by HSV-2 and is a complication of primary genital infection. In HSV meningitis, symptoms and signs of meningitis, including headache, photophobia, and stiff neck, appear before or shortly after genital lesions are noted. The signs are similar to those of other acute viral meningitides such as enteroviral meningitis. This syndrome may occur in children as well as adults.[73] HSV-2 meningitis may develop less commonly in the absence of genital lesions[228] or rarely in neonates.[227] Seizures and focal CNS findings usually are absent. Examination of CSF reveals lymphocytosis (with 300 to 2600 white blood cells) and may demonstrate low glucose levels. In cases of HSV meningitis, in contrast to HSV encephalitis, the virus can be cultured from the CSF,[11, 62, 115] and HSV PCR assay also may be diagnostic.[228] Recovery was usually complete without specific therapy, but with the availability of effective antiviral agents, HSV meningitis should be treated with acyclovir. HSV meningitis may reappear with genital recurrences. Studies using PCR DNA detection analysis have shown that HSV is the major agent responsible for benign recurrent lymphocytic meningitis, also known as Mollaret meningitis.[266] These adult patients had three to nine attacks of recurrent lymphocytic meningitis with 48 to 1600 cells per liter, normal glucose, and protein concentrations of 41 to 240 mg/dL in CSF. PCR analysis detected HSV-2 and, less commonly, HSV-1. Acute viral meningitis caused by reactivation of HSV-1 also has been described in a pre-adolescent child.[58]

HSV encephalitis is a highly lethal disease caused by HSV-1 in 93 to 96 percent of cases.[20, 178, 289, 292, 296] It may be a result of primary (30%) or recurrent (70%) infection.[178, 289] Although no specific data exist, researchers have suggested that HSV encephalitis is more likely to be associated with primary infection in younger persons because new infections occur more commonly in this age group. One report suggests that primary infection is more likely to be associated with fatal encephalitis. Of 113 cases of biopsy-documented HSV encephalitis, 31 percent occurred in patients younger than 20 years, and 6 to 10 percent of patients were between 6 months and 10 years of age.[241, 242] Unlike most other common forms of viral meningoencephalitis such as enterovirus or arbovirus infection, HSV encephalitis is not seasonal. It is an acute illness characterized by fever, malaise, irritability, and nonspecific symptoms lasting 1 to 7 days, with progression to the signs and symptoms of CNS involvement in 3 to 7 days and, finally, to coma and death (Table 163–1). A biphasic illness consisting of initial improvement followed by worsening may occur. The signs of HSV encephalitis resemble those of other viral encephalitides, with initial fever and altered behavior.[112] Meningeal signs are uncommon. No correlation exists between isolation of HSV from sites extrinsic to the CNS (such as the oropharynx or genital tract) and the diagnosis of HSV encephalitis.[178, 290] Thus, the presence of oral or genital lesions is of no help in the diagnosis or exclusion of HSV encephalitis. Nonetheless, if a patient has HSV encephalitis, identical viruses have been isolated from the brain and oral secretions.[293]

The CSF generally reveals pleocytosis with as many as 2000 white blood cells/mm^3 but usually (80% of the time) more than 50/mm^3. In 90 percent of cases, more than 60 percent of the cells are lymphocytes. Early in infection, neutrophils may predominate. In 75 to 85 percent of cases, red blood cells, reflecting the hemorrhagic necrosis, are seen in the CSF. Between 5 and 25 percent of patients have hypoglycorrhachia, and 80 to 88 percent have elevated protein levels in the CSF (median, 80 mg/dL), which rise to striking levels as the disease progresses. Two to 3 percent of patients with early HSV encephalitis have normal CSF.[141, 178] Repeat analysis of the CSF usually reveals abnormalities consistent with encephalitis. HSV almost never is cultured from lumbar spinal fluid and has been grown rarely from ventricular fluid.[89] Thus, whereas CSF examination is helpful, it is not at all diagnostic of HSV encephalitis. When the CSF of patients with HSV encephalitis is compared with that of patients undergoing biopsy for suspected HSV, but with another resultant diagnosis, no differentiating characteristics of the CSF are found that could allow one to predict HSV infection accurately. HSV DNA can be detected in the CSF of patients who have HSV encephalitis by the use of PCR assay.[6, 19, 70, 149, 210, 270]

Neurodiagnostic tests have been of limited assistance. Probably one of the most useful is the electroencephalogram

TABLE 163–1 ■ HISTORICAL AND CLINICAL FINDINGS IN HSV ENCEPHALITIS

Historical Finding	Initial Clinical Finding (%)
Alteration of consciousness	97
Fever	81
Headache	67
Persistent seizures	71
Personality change	46
Vomiting	33
Hemiparesis	24
Memory loss	92
Personality changes	85
Dysphasia	76
Autonomic dysfunction	60
Ataxia	40
Seizures	38
Focal	28
Generalized	10
Cranial nerve defects	32
Visual field loss	14
Papilledema	14

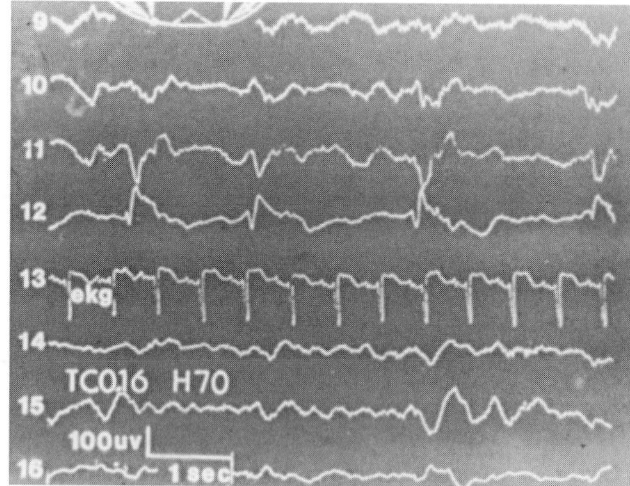

FIGURE 163–11 ■ Electroencephalogram in a 9-month-old with HSV encephalitis. Note the paroxysmal discharges, in lead 12 especially.

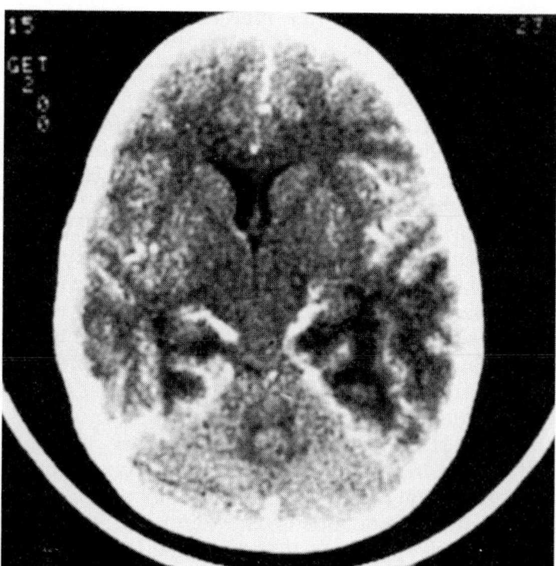

FIGURE 163–12 ■ Computed tomographic scan 1 week after the onset of HSV encephalitis in a 6-year-old. Note the bilateral temporal low-density areas with dye enhancement and the greater mass effect on the patient's left side than on the right side.

(EEG)[40] (Fig. 163–11). A "typical" pattern of unilateral or bilateral (poor prognosis) periodic focal spikes against a background of slow (flattened) activity (paroxysmal lateral epileptiform discharges [PLEDs]) has been associated with HSV encephalitis. These findings are suggestive but not pathognomonic. Other findings include large-amplitude, irregular, slow activity; sharp waves; and variable spikes. In 80 to 90 percent of patients, the EEG is not only abnormal but also localizing. In many cases in the pediatric and adult age groups, the EEG may be one of the earliest localizing laboratory tests.[71, 103, 139] Less commonly, the results of a radionuclide or computed tomography (CT) scan are abnormal and localizing (50–60% of cases).[130, 158] CT results may be characteristic late in illness and consist of low-density, contrast-enhanced lesions in the temporal area, mass effect, edema, and hemorrhage (Fig. 163–12); early in the illness, when diagnosis is critical, CT results more often are unremarkable.[103, 139, 175] Indeed, abnormal CT results are a poor prognostic factor.[175] Reports suggest that MRI findings may be abnormal at initial evaluation for HSV encephalitis because of its high sensitivity to changes in brain water content[233] (Fig. 163–13). MRI is more sensitive than is CT for detection of HSV encephalitis.[69] Findings include hyperintensity of the temporal areas on T2-weighted images with gadolinium enhancement.

Focal abnormalities in HSV encephalitis are significantly more likely to be observed on EEG, CT, MRI, or radionuclide brain scan than are those in other illnesses confused with it. All these findings are biased by the current concept of HSV encephalitis as a focal encephalitis, with very few biopsy data

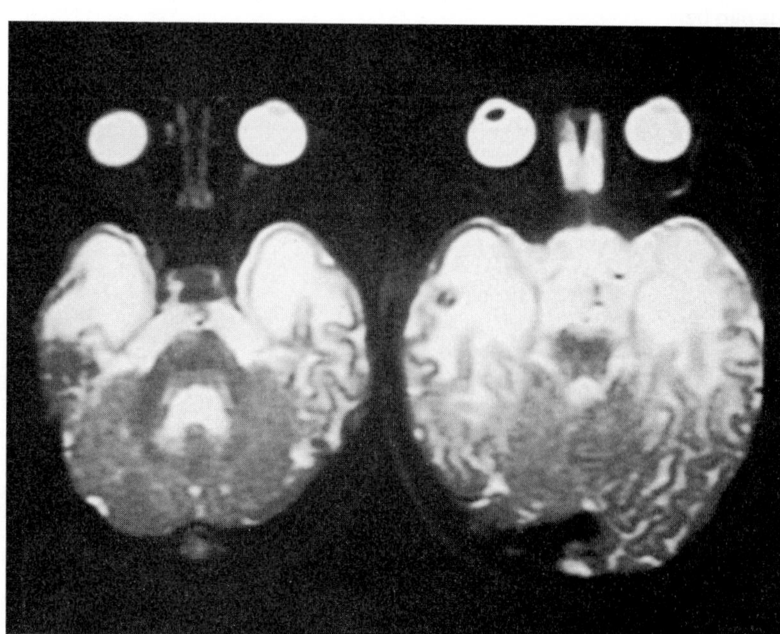

FIGURE 163–13 ■ Magnetic resonance image in a patient with HSV encephalitis. Note the increased signal intensity bilaterally in the temporal lobes. (From Kohl, S.: Herpes simplex virus encephalitis in children. Pediatr. Clin. North Am. *35*:465–483, 1988.)

available on the etiology of nonfocal encephalitis. Whether a significant number of cases of HSV encephalitis are milder and nonfocal is unknown because few of them ever come to brain biopsy or even careful retrospective serologic diagnosis. Studies using MRI and PCR technology have identified cases with multifocal brain involvement[226] or mild clinical courses.[70]

Clinical and laboratory evaluation of patients with suspected HSV encephalitis is valuable only for increasing the index of suspicion, not for confirming the diagnosis of HSV encephalitis. In one series of 24 children with HSV encephalitis diagnosed by PCR assay and compared with 38 children in whom HSV encephalitis was excluded by PCR assay, no significant differences were found in clinical manifestations at onset or in CSF cell counts, protein, or glucose.[122] However, more children with HSV encephalitis had localizing findings detected by CT (75% versus 31%), whereas 36 percent of those without encephalitis had EEG abnormalities as opposed to no EEG abnormalities detected in those with HSV encephalitis. The differential diagnosis of this condition is relatively large, with many treatable conditions (Table 163–2). Especially in the pediatric age range, the ability to discriminate HSV encephalitis from other etiologic agents mimicking it is poor (50% in the national collaborative series in 71 patients younger than 20 years and 42% in a smaller series of 12 patients younger than 12 years).[139] Confirmation of the specific diagnosis of HSV encephalitis remains essential, both to provide optimal aggressive therapy for that condition and, of equal importance, to achieve a diagnosis for the 50 to 60 percent of patients without HSV infection, roughly 16 percent of whom would benefit from other specific therapies.[71, 139, 175, 292] In most cases, the diagnosis can be established by PCR analysis of CSF.[6, 19, 105, 149, 210, 226, 228, 275] Large studies show PCR analysis to be 98 percent sensitive and 94 percent specific when compared with brain biopsy.[149] Some of the 6 percent "false-positive" results probably were due to poor handling of the biopsy tissue for culture. PCR analysis may yield positive results by 1 day after the onset of symptoms.[105] However, a negative PCR result at the onset of symptoms does not exclude the diagnosis. PCR primers must be chosen to detect HSV-2, as well as HSV-1, because 4 to 6 percent of HSV encephalitis cases may be caused by HSV-2.[20]

TABLE 163–2 ■ DIFFERENTIAL DIAGNOSIS OF HSV ENCEPHALITIS

Infections	Noninfectious Disorders
Fungal	Tumor
Especially *Cryptococcus*	Vascular disease
Bacterial	Arteriovenous malformations
Abscess, cerebritis	Toxins
Listeria monocytogenes meningitis	Alcoholic encephalopathy
	Leukemia
Lyme disease	Cerebral infarction
Subdural, epidural empyema	Andrenal leukodystrophy
Tuberculosis	
Bacterial endocarditis	
Meningococcal meningitis	
Protozoal	
Toxoplasmosis	
Amebic	
Rickettsial	
Viral	
Mumps virus	
Coxsackievirus, echovirus	
Arbovirus (especially St. Louis, California, and eastern and western equine encephalitis)	
Postinfluenzal encephalitis	
Reye syndrome	
Lymphocytic choriomeningitis virus	
Rabies virus	
Epstein-Barr virus	
Human herpesvirus 6	
Rubella virus	
Cytomegalovirus	
Adenovirus	
Tick-borne encephalitis virus	
Powassan virus	
Subacute sclerosing encephalitis (measles virus)	
Progressive multifocal leuko-encephalopathy	

If PCR results are negative in a patient who has symptoms and signs of HSV encephalitis, brain biopsy may be contemplated. The risk associated with brain biopsy is low. In the national collaborative study of 432 biopsies, 6 complications occurred (hemorrhage in 3 patients and poorly controlled brain edema in 3, for a 1.4% complication rate).[292] Roughly 2 to 3 percent of brain biopsies yielded false-negative results, usually because of biopsy of the wrong site.[292] Decision analysis suggests that obtaining a biopsy is especially critical in a patient with low CSF glucose levels.[223]

Although it is a research tool at present, quantitative PCR analysis may have value as a prognostic tool and as a method of assessing the response to antiviral therapy in patients with HSV encephalitis.[74] In 16 patients, those with high copy numbers of HSV DNA in CSF tended to have abnormal CT scans, be older, and have more severe sequelae. HSV DNA levels were found to decrease during acyclovir therapy in seven patients; the exception was a patient whose copy numbers increased and who subsequently had a fatal infection.

A less acute form of HSV encephalitis in immunocompromised patients has been reported. Also less commonly, HSV has been implicated in brain stem encephalitis.[81] Relapse occurs in approximately 5 percent of treated patients.[139] Choreoathetosis may be an initial sign of relapse.[283] Reports of a post-herpetic encephalomyelitis caused by a probable autoimmune or demyelinating etiologic factor are being seen increasingly frequently[1, 136]; moreover, virus-positive recurrence of HSV encephalitis has been described months after patients have undergone apparently successful therapy.[72] These consequences can be differentiated and documented only by PCR analysis or, if necessary, brain biopsy and appropriate tissue histologic examination and culture.

INFECTION OF THE GASTROINTESTINAL TRACT IN NORMAL HOSTS

Whereas infection of visceral organs is well recognized in immunocompromised hosts, case reports of such infection in apparently healthy persons are less common. Nonetheless, HSV esophagitis has been described in these patients, including several children who were 11 months to 17 years of age.[12, 25, 92, 174, 186] HSV-1 is the usual pathogen, and the syndrome is associated with primary infection.[92] The initial symptoms include fever, severe odynophagia, retrosternal and subxiphoid pain, and an inability to eat. Skin lesions generally are absent. Esophagoscopy reveals ulcerations and fibrinous and, at times, hemorrhagic exudate. Distal involvement may be more extensive than the proximal esophageal findings suggest. Double-contrast esophagography may be diagnostic, although endoscopy and biopsy usually are necessary for making a definitive diagnosis.[94] Symptoms generally remit in 5 to 7 days after nonspecific therapy such as antacids, H_2-blockers, and hydration.[12, 174, 205]

HSV infection can be manifested as an anorectal infection in males who have sex with males.[101, 196] This syndrome occasionally affects women practicing passive anal intercourse. In most series of HSV proctitis, the younger persons are adolescent males involved in passive anal intercourse. Initial symptoms include severe anorectal pain, discharge, tenesmus, hematochezia, and, in particular, fever, difficulty urinating, sacral paresthesias, constipation, and (in 50–70% of patients) ulcers or vesicles in the perianal or distal rectal area.[101] The duration of symptoms is 2 to 3 weeks. Primary HSV infection accounts for proctitis in this group in 25 to 30 percent of cases. Syphilis and infection with *Giardia lamblia, Entamoeba histolytica, Campylobacter fetus, Shigella*, other enteric bacteria, and *Neisseria gonorrhoeae* also must be considered in the differential diagnosis of this entity. Appropriate cultures and histologic analysis are crucial for establishing a specific diagnosis.

HSV is a rare cause of hepatitis in an immunocompetent host, but it has been reported in children.[23] In a review of the literature describing 35 patients who had HSV-associated hepatitis, only 14 percent had no underlying condition. The remainder had various immunocompromising conditions such as transplantation, steroid administration, pregnancy, burns, primary immunodeficiency, or cancer. These patients tended to have fulminant hepatic necrosis, extremely elevated serum transaminase levels, disseminated intravascular coagulation, and a mortality rate of 86 percent.[49] In a prospective study of healthy young adults who had genital herpes (primary or recurrent), 14 percent had mild elevations in liver enzyme tests.

RECURRENT INFECTIONS

HSV-1 and HSV-2 have the characteristic capacity of herpesviruses to establish latency and undergo episodes of reactivation despite the presence of an apparently adequate immune response. Persistence is facilitated because latent infection of neurons occurs in an immunologically "privileged" site. Reactivation of HSV infection with viral shedding usually causes no lesions. HSV can be recovered from the pharynx and genital sites of asymptomatic persons. It has been found in the tears of persons with a history of recurrent ophthalmic disease, even in the absence of eye lesions or symptoms. All HSV-2–seropositive women from whom vaginal secretion samples were obtained for more than 100 days had documented asymptomatic viral shedding, and shedding occurred on 1 percent of the days on which cultures were obtained.[282]

Patterns of HSV reactivation include asymptomatic reactivation after silent primary infection, asymptomatic reactivation after symptomatic primary infection, and symptomatic recurrence after either silent or symptomatic primary infection. The risk of having symptomatic recurrences may be higher in individuals who have symptomatic primary infections. When reactivation causes disease, the clinical manifestations of recurrent HSV infection depend on the area involved. Most HSV recurrences are milder than the primary illness, although patients may have symptomatic recurrences without having had clinically apparent primary disease. Recurrent infection in a normal host also may be more severe than the primary infection. This pattern is particularly evident in HSV infection of the eye, in which recurrent illness is associated with deep stromal damage and scarring.[193] This enhanced severity may be related to a greater extent to a more exuberant immune response than to viral damage. HSV encephalitis, which may be a manifestation of viral reactivation, certainly is devastating.[178, 289]

The most common manifestation of recurrent HSV infection is herpes labialis ("cold sores," "fever blisters"). Recurrences were observed in 25 to 50 percent of persons who had symptomatic primary HSV-1 oral infection, but in only 24 percent of those who had primary HSV-2 oral infection.[148] The mean rate of recurrence after symptomatic primary HSV-1 infection in adults is approximately 0.1 per month. These recurrences often are associated with a variety of febrile illnesses, local trauma, sun, or menstruation.[21, 246, 248] Whether acquisition of HSV-1 in childhood is less likely to be associated with recurrent herpes labialis is not known.

Most persons with herpes labialis experience a prodrome (pain, burning, tingling, or itching) at the site that lasts a few hours to several days. Subsequently, an orderly progression ensues from papules (lasting 12 to 36 hours) to vesicles (usually gone by 48 hours) and finally to ulcers and crusting (lasting 2 to 4 days) (Fig. 163–14). The typical lesion is 35 to 80 mm in size. Most outbreaks are healed by 5 to 10 days (mean, 200 hours). Most pain occurs during the vesicular stage. Virus is isolated readily from vesicles (80–90% of the time) and less commonly from ulcers and crusts (34% of the time). Maximal virus titers (10^7 to 10^8) in lesions are detected in the first day or two, and virus generally is not isolated after 120 hours.[21, 248] Virus also may be detected in the saliva and on the hands of persons with herpes labialis.[273]

Recurrences tend to affect the same location or closely related areas. In general, they occur on the lips, mucocutaneous junction, or other parts of the face. Recurrent lesions found inside the mouths of normal hosts rarely are caused by HSV and more likely are aphthous lesions. When HSV recurrences are within the mouth, they tend to be on tissue adjacent to bone, such as the gums or palate, and not on the

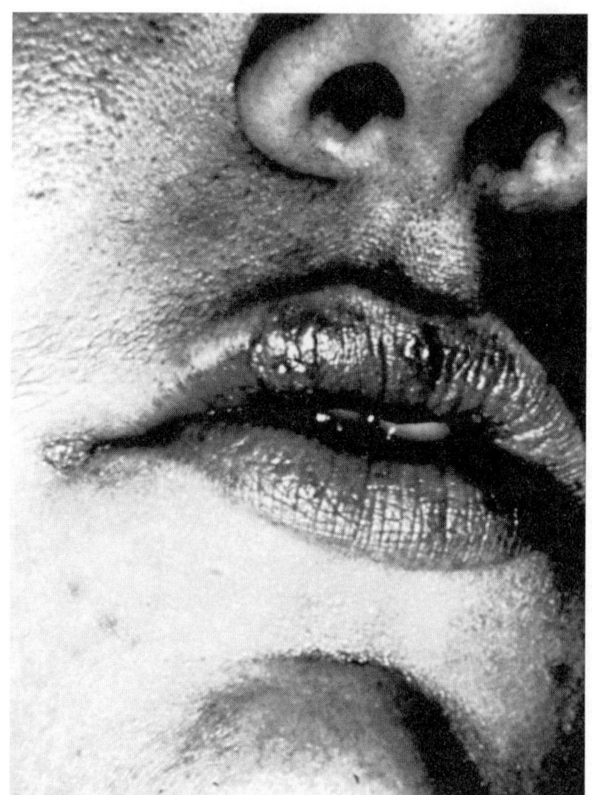

FIGURE 163–14 ■ Recurrent herpes labialis (cold sore) in an adolescent.

lips or buccal mucosa.[245] A differential diagnosis of the condition also includes pemphigus, lichen planus, ulcers caused by cyclic neutropenia, and ulcers associated with celiac disease, ulcerative colitis, Crohn disease, pernicious anemia, and Behçet syndrome.

Recurrent genital herpes is the second most common manifestation of HSV. Studies have elucidated several factors that increase the risk of having recurrent genital disease after symptomatic primary genital infection. Recurrence rates are much higher after primary HSV-2 (90%) than after having primary HSV-1 (25–55%) infection.[148, 200] The mean rate of recurrence is 0.02 to 0.1 per month after primary genital HSV-1 and 0.3 per month after primary HSV-2 genital infection.[148, 200] Recurrences are more common in men than in women and after a recurrent lesion than after a first attack.[200]

Only 5 to 12 percent of persons who have recurrent genital herpes have constitutional symptoms. Local symptoms include pain (average, 4 to 6 days), itching, dysuria (10–30%), adenopathy (20–30%), lesions (average, 50 to 60 mm) lasting 4 to 5 days until crusting, and healing by 9 to 11 days (range, 4 to 29 days) (see Fig. 163–3). Symptoms in females tend to be more severe than those in males. Virus is shed for an average of 3 to 4 days (but in some cases as long as 20 days). Virus generally is shed with titers of 10^2 to 10^4 per lesion. In dry areas, vesicles are seen, but in wet areas, the vesicles rapidly break down into ulcers. Symptoms generally are milder and of shorter duration than those in primary genital disease.[41] New crops of lesions commonly occur during the course of recurrence. The severity of recurrence is quite variable; in some cases, several discrete recurrences blend into a single, prolonged recurrence, and, in rare cases, patients have almost continuous recurrences.[106] In one study of patients who were HSV-2–seropositive with no history of genital herpes, 62 percent had recognized herpetic lesions at later evaluation.[282] Recurrences in the previously asymptomatic group were shorter (3 versus 5 days) and less frequent (3.0 per year versus 8.2 per year) when the pattern of recurrence in this cohort was compared with that of subjects with a known history of genital herpes.

With the advent of endonuclease restriction analysis, researchers have clear evidence that, whereas most recurrences represent endogenous reactivation of the same latent virus, re-infection with a new homologous virus (i.e., HSV-2 and new HSV-2) as well as heterologous virus (i.e., HSV-2 and then HSV-1 or vice versa) is possible.[45] How common this occurrence is remains to be ascertained and must depend to some degree on the sexual activity and number of partners of the persons studied.[230]

Other cutaneous recurrences may develop at each anatomic site of primary infection. HSV infection may recur on the face or trunk in a typical dermatome distribution, such as that associated with VZV. Indeed, frequent repeated attacks of zosteriform-like lesions on any part of the body in a normal host suggest HSV and not VZV infection.

ERYTHEMA MULTIFORME

Erythema multiforme is thought to be an immune-mediated, "allergic" response to recurrent HSV infection.[86, 119, 172, 185, 286] It has been associated with the presence of human leukocyte DQw3 antigen.[129] In several series, approximately 15 to nearly 100 percent of patients who have erythema multiforme, especially those who have recurrent erythema multiforme, gave a history of recurrent HSV infection before the skin eruption, which may be macular or urticarial.[119] In one series, 5 of 80 patients who had recurrent oral HSV infection experienced a rash (presumably erythema multiforme) 8 to 14 days after the onset of a cold sore.[248] Studies in adults and children have documented HSV antigen-antibody immune complexes and HSV DNA (detected by PCR analysis and in situ hybridization) in the skin of patients who had erythema multiforme after having HSV infection.[37, 38, 185] In a series of 20 children who had erythema multiforme (10 who had antecedent herpes), 16 were documented to have HSV DNA at the site of the rash.[286] The skin manifestations may last 14 to 21 days, and therapy generally is directed toward the allergic and not the viral component of the illness. Suppression of HSV recurrences prevents the associated episodes of erythema multiforme. Indeed, suppressive treatment of erythema multiforme with acyclovir, even in the absence of recurrent HSV infection, completely suppresses clinical manifestations.[232, 264] In one series, the syndrome developed in 12 children at a mean age of 8 years within 4 days after the appearance of herpes labialis lesions, and symptoms lasted for an average of 10 days; nine children had recurrent erythema multiforme, with an average of 2.6 episodes per year.[286] Detection of HSV by PCR assay of skin biopsy tissue was described in all cases. None of three children given acyclovir suppressive therapy had recurrences during treatment for at least 6 months, but erythema multiforme with recurrent HSV developed in one child when use of the drug was discontinued, thus supporting a causative role for HSV in the syndrome.

HSV INFECTION IN IMMUNOCOMPROMISED HOSTS

As the practice of pediatrics continues to include more patients with severe acquired immunodeficiency states brought about by increasingly intensive therapy for malignancies, expanding application of bone marrow and organ transplantation, and HIV infection, the prevalence of severe HSV infection in immunocompromised hosts is increasing. Table 163–3 lists conditions associated with unusually severe HSV infections. HSV infection in the neonatal period is discussed in Chapter 73. Aside from the several cases of HSV encephalitis in patients with agammaglobulinemia (who also had concomitant infections with enterovirus),[161] common links in these varied groups are either skin abnormalities (eczema, burns) or immunologic defects, primarily in the cell-mediated components of the immune system.[33, 88, 114, 192, 254, 267] The critical defects have not been defined and may involve one or a combination of inadequate functions (e.g., of $CD4^+$ T cells, $CD8^+$ T cells, natural killer cells, macrophage antigen processing, or other factors).

The incidence of severe HSV infection in children with diseases that predispose them to these complications (see Table 163–3) is defined poorly but, in limited series, was similar to that seen in adults.[91, 289] Most infections are caused by reactivation, as would be expected given the relative frequency of primary and recurrent infections. In series of pediatric or adult patients who have received renal, bone marrow, or cardiac transplants, 70 to 90 percent of seropositive persons excrete HSV, usually from the oropharynx and generally at the time of peak immunosuppression (in the first month after transplantation).[179] Of 68 children who underwent renal transplantation, a herpesvirus was isolated in 43 percent, with 28 percent of the isolates being HSV.[269] HSV in cardiac transplant cases causes symptomatic illness in 45 to 85 percent of seropositive patients, depending on the intensity of immunosuppression. HSV was the virus most commonly isolated in children who underwent bone marrow transplantation (23%).[284] HSV has been suggested to be one of the etiologic agents of interstitial pneumonitis that develops

TABLE 163–3 ■ CONDITIONS CONTRIBUTING TO UNUSUALLY SEVERE HSV INFECTIONS

Newborn period
Malnutrition
Malignancy
Immunosuppressive therapy
Antineoplastic
Transplantation
Corticosteroids or adrenocorticotropic hormone
Primary immunodeficiency
Agammaglobulinemia
Wiskott-Aldrich syndrome
Ataxia-telangiectasia
Severe combined immunodeficiency syndrome
Nucleoside phosphorylase deficiency
Thymoma and hypogammaglobulinemia
Common variable agammaglobulinemia
Chronic mucocutaneous candidiasis
Natural killer cell defect
Acquired immunodeficiency syndrome
Pregnancy
Burns
Trauma
Skin abnormalities
Atopic eczema
Bullous impetigo
Burns
Darier disease
Ichthyosiform erythroderma
Pemphigus
Viral infection
Measles
Pertussis
Tuberculosis
Severe bacterial infection
Haemophilus meningitis
Sarcoidosis

after bone marrow transplantation.[182, 198] In children with leukemia, HSV infection occurs more commonly in those with myelocytic leukemia than in those with lymphocytic leukemia, and the risk of developing infection increases with neutropenia and chemotherapy. HSV infection was the most common serious viral infection in children with leukemia. Whereas most infections occurred during periods of remission, on a per-day basis, the risk of developing infection was seven times higher during induction.[299] Of 24 patients who died of infection during remission in the St. Jude's series, 2 (8%) had HSV (1 with disseminated disease, 1 with encephalitis). In Africa, patients suffering from underlying malnutrition and concomitant measles infection may contract fatal disseminated HSV infection; such events rarely occur in industrialized nations.[26, 132, 267]

Chronic mucocutaneous ulcers (persisting for more than 1 month), bronchitis, pneumonitis, and esophagitis caused by HSV are conditions that have been used to categorize the severity of HIV infection.[203] Chronic HSV mucocutaneous disease or widespread organ involvement was the AIDS-defining condition in 7 of 789 (0.9%) HIV-infected children.[272] In series of children with AIDS, 5 to 29 percent experienced HSV opportunistic infection.[91] Chronic ulcerative HSV lesions often develop in children with HIV infection, although first episodes did not result in disseminated infection.[220] Notably, many of these children also had perianal ulcers from which HSV-1 was isolated. In HIV-infected patients, illnesses caused by HSV usually involved chronic mucocutaneous ulcers or extension to the lungs, bronchi, or esophagus. Dissemination is a rare occurrence.[13] Multiple recurrences of infection are common as the immunodeficiency worsens. In patients with AIDS, HSV rarely causes a typical[109, 277] or more indolent[7] encephalitis. HSV usually does not result in mortality in HIV-infected patients, but it causes significant morbidity.[134] HSV genital ulcer disease increases the risk of acquisition of HIV.[118]

Several major syndromes are attributable to HSV in immunocompromised patients, with some overlap and occasionally progression from one to the other. The first and most common manifestation is a local, chronic, often extensive cutaneous or mucocutaneous infection. The second form is infection involving a single organ (e.g., esophagitis or pneumonitis). The most serious illness is characterized by more widespread dissemination involving distant areas of skin or visceral organs (e.g., the lungs, liver, adrenals) and the CNS. Although data are limited, disseminated disease probably most often represents primary infection except in the most severely immunocompromised patients. More localized syndromes may be a manifestation of either primary infection or recurrent illness.

The typical localized HSV infection begins in the mouth or about the lips, often appearing innocuously as an ordinary herpes labialis recurrence. Over the course of several days, the papules and vesicles progress to bullae, often with hemorrhagic fluid. The bullae or vesicles evolve into huge, chronic, bloody, coalescing, ulcerated, oozing lesions eroding into the subcutaneous tissue and occasionally destroying underlying structures. The tissue is malodorous, and the lesions are painful (Fig. 163–15). The lip and palate are the sites most commonly affected. Oral lesions account for approximately 60 percent of HSV infections in children undergoing transplantation.[269] A similar syndrome, usually caused by HSV-2 infection, may be seen in the perianal or vaginal area and is one of the characteristic syndromes that occur in males who have sex with males who are infected with AIDS (Fig. 163–16). Untreated, the lesions may lead to death because of local destruction and hemorrhage, or they may regress as the immune status of the host improves or as antiviral chemotherapy is administered. A syndrome of herpetic geometric glossitis has been reported in HIV-infected patients.[104] Affected patients have a tender tongue accompanied by dorsal longitudinal crossed and branching fissures.

Extensive HSV skin infections may occur in patients with burns, eczema, pemphigus, or abrasions, often with

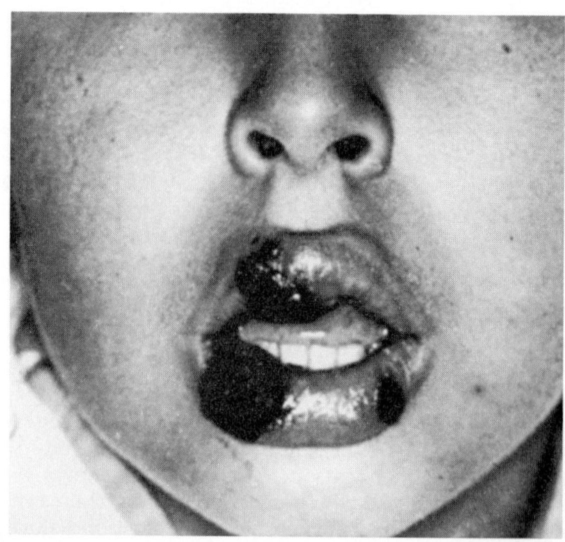

FIGURE 163–15 ■ Chronic, hemorrhagic HSV infection in a girl with leukemia and a bone marrow transplant.

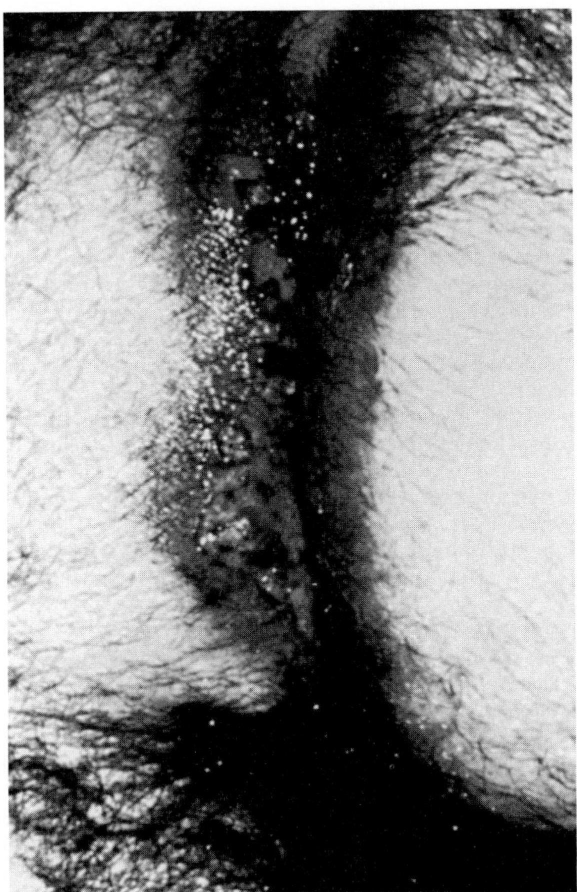

FIGURE 163–16 ■ HSV proctitis and rectal infection in a male homosexual with AIDS. (Courtesy of Dr. Victor Fainstein, Department of Internal Medicine, M. D. Anderson Cancer Center, Houston.)

conversion of second-degree tissue damage to third-degree damage (see Figs. 163–6 and 163–7). Of 179 children with eczema, herpes skin infections developed in 10, 7 of whom required hospitalization.[66] Though rare, local infection may progress to dissemination in some cases, possibly as a result of the more severe immunodeficiency occurring with several of these conditions. The widespread necrotizing lesions are known commonly as Kaposi varicelliform eruption or eczema herpeticum (see Fig. 163–6). The predisposition to severe HSV-1 infection in children with atopic eczema appears to be due to the cutaneous abnormalities because these children have T-cell responses to HSV, as well as high HSV IgG antibody titers.[102]

These lesions must be differentiated from bacterial infections caused by gram-positive or gram-negative organisms, chronic fungal infections (as seen with *Mucor* or *Blastomyces*), other viral infections (vaccinia, varicella), mycobacterial infection, and various noninfectious lesions such as pyoderma gangrenosum, chemotherapy-induced ulcers, or Sweet syndrome. HSV is the agent associated most commonly with oral lesions in immunocompromised patients.[91]

HSV esophagitis rarely has been reported in normal children,[25] but it is a relatively common finding in immunocompromised patients. Pathologic studies have suggested that approximately 25 percent of cases of autopsy-proven esophagitis (1–6% of all autopsies) are secondary to HSV infection (14 of 55 cases).[181] Underlying conditions included burns, aplastic anemia, malignancies, transplantation, a variety of other serious medical problems, and postoperative trauma induced by nasogastric tubes.[46, 164, 181] Twenty to 50 percent of these patients have HSV involvement elsewhere (the lungs, trachea, and less commonly, the skin). The esophagitis may be asymptomatic or associated with dysphagia, odynophagia, epigastric discomfort, and retrosternal pain. Characteristic findings in the esophagus are ulcers with raised granular margins. The ulcers often are covered with fibrinous exudate and, in advanced cases, are confluent, with progression to complete mucosal loss in large segments of the esophagus. Typically, visceral herpes infection is not suspected before death, but uncommonly, involvement of adjacent gastric tissue can be documented. Diagnostic evaluation should include a barium swallow, which may demonstrate edema, nodules, and ulceration of the esophagus; however, barium studies cannot differentiate HSV from other etiologic agents of esophagitis. Esophagoscopy accompanied by biopsy and viral culture is diagnostic and helps exclude other common causes of this syndrome, including *Candida,* CMV, and possibly other fungi and bacteria or chemotherapy-induced changes.[46, 181]

HSV pneumonia is an unusual condition, but lung involvement has been described in immunocompromised hosts. This diagnosis rarely is made ante mortem, and it occurs almost exclusively in immunocompromised patients. In one series of 1000 consecutive autopsies,[180] HSV pneumonia was identified in 10 cases. HSV pulmonary infection occurred in 3 percent of children after renal transplantation.[269] In most adult cases, the process is a result of endogenous viral mucocutaneous reactivation and involvement of lung tissue by contiguous spread, which causes focal pneumonia (60% of the time), or involvement by hematogenous spread from an oral or genital site, which results in diffuse pneumonitis.[198] Although the largest series was composed primarily of adult patients, three of the patients were 7 years of age or younger (with Down syndrome and congestive heart failure, rhabdomyosarcoma, and pneumococcal pneumonia and a seizure disorder).[120] Patients had cough, dyspnea, fever, and hypoxia, and 50 percent had rales. Most had other concomitant pulmonary infections with bacteria, *Candida, Aspergillus,* and CMV. HSV pneumonia cannot be diagnosed by the association of upper airway cultures and radiographic abnormalities. It must rest on an aggressive approach using culture and histopathologic examination of involved lung tissue obtained by either biopsy or bronchoscopy.[242]

HSV meningoencephalitis is not a common occurrence in immunocompromised patients. It may occur as a component of widely disseminated disease, or it may be a localized condition. Several cases have been reported in patients who had agammaglobulinemia in association with concomitant enteroviral infection of the brain.[161] The meningoencephalitis may be fulminant, such as occurs in a normal host.[161] An interesting case that followed an atypical subacute course accompanied by bilateral brain involvement has been reported in an anergic patient who had Hodgkin disease. Although HSV does not appear to have a predilection for CNS infection in immunocompromised hosts, patients with AIDS are an exception and may have ascending myelitis, acute transverse myelitis, and encephalitis.[91, 94, 109, 277]

Hepatitis caused by HSV has been reported most commonly after solid organ or bone marrow transplantation[125, 134, 135, 145] and during pregnancy.[133] Signs include fever, abdominal pain, and elevated liver enzyme levels. Hepatitis usually occurs during the first 3 weeks after transplantation, unless prophylactic acyclovir is given. Mortality is very high (67–100%). In at least one case, orthotopic liver transplantation resulted in survival.[237]

The most severe form of HSV in an immunocompromised host is widely disseminated disease that can involve the liver, adrenals, lungs, spleen, kidney, and often the brain. In a large series from South Africa and Kenya,[26, 132, 267] measles and severe malnutrition were frequent cofactors (83%) in children 2 to 25 months of age who had widely disseminated HSV infection. These illnesses represented fatal primary infections. Similar syndromes have been described; they and other underlying conditions are listed in Table 163–3. Dissemination has been reported coincident with pertussis, *Haemophilus influenzae* meningitis,[123] and other bacterial infections.[26] Disseminated HSV infection occurred in 10 percent and 25 percent of children who had HSV infection and who underwent bone marrow and renal transplantation, respectively.[178, 284]

The clinical manifestation of disseminated HSV usually is one of initial fever and skin or mucocutaneous involvement in 80 percent of cases, but instead of healing as expected, the infection disseminates. The cutaneous dissemination may involve a widespread vesicular eruption that looks much like varicella, or it may involve more local, large hemorrhagic vesicles and bullae. Involvement of the major target organs, as noted previously, gives rise to syndromes of hepatitis, pneumonia, shock, bleeding, disseminated intravascular coagulopathy, seizures, coma, renal failure, hypothermia, and death in days to weeks. Laboratory examination may reveal leukopenia, thrombocytopenia, elevated liver function test values, hyponatremia, azotemia, pneumonitis, hypoglycemia, CSF pleocytosis, abnormal EEG results, and electrocardiographic abnormalities. Death occurs commonly in this syndrome (90%), even after the institution of antiviral chemotherapy. Because the liver often is involved and biopsy may be precluded by the tenuous condition of the patient, HSV infection should be considered in all high-risk groups (see Table 163–3) with fulminant hepatitis.

Neonatal herpes simplex virus infection is discussed in Chapter 73.

Diagnosis

Clinical findings may suggest a probable diagnosis of HSV infection, but obtaining a definitive laboratory diagnosis is necessary or useful in many circumstances.[10] Accurate laboratory diagnosis requires attention to obtaining the correct specimens necessary for identifying the etiology of the clinical syndrome. Appropriate interpretation of the laboratory results is the second critical factor. Evaluation of mucocutaneous lesions in high-risk patients guides the use of antiviral therapy if the lesion is herpetic. However, because HSV often is shed in immunosuppressed and otherwise healthy individuals, finding HSV in oropharyngeal secretions does not mean that the clinical condition is caused by HSV. In general, the virus must be isolated from the relevant tissue for confirmation of the diagnosis. The test selected also is important (e.g., HSV is rarely found in spinal fluid cultures of patients with HSV encephalitis), and detection of viral DNA by PCR assay or, if necessary, brain biopsy is required to prove the diagnosis and to exclude other treatable etiologies. Laboratory diagnosis also is valuable when HSV infections are not life-threatening. For example, proving that a genital lesion is caused by HSV-1 or HSV-2 facilitates making decisions about antiviral therapy and allows initiating appropriate counseling about the risk of recurrences and measures that may reduce HSV transmission to contacts.

VIRAL CULTURE

The gold standard of HSV diagnosis remains recovery of infectious virus in tissue culture. HSV grows rapidly (mean, 2 to 3 days; high-titer samples, 12 to 24 hours; low-titer samples, 5 to 7 days) and produces a typical cytopathic effect (Fig. 163–17). Human diploid cells (WI-38 or human embryonic lung cells) and primate cells (Vero) are used by most diagnostic laboratories. A tentative diagnosis can be made in 95 percent of cases by the cell types infected and the typical cytopathogenic effect. High-titer specimens of VZV or CMV occasionally cause confusion. Sensitivity can be improved by centrifugation of specimens directly onto cell monolayers; a more rapid result can be obtained by using shell vial cultures combined with antigen-detection methods.[83, 121, 271]

Definitive identification of the infecting virus is accomplished by using HSV-1– and HSV-2–specific antisera or monoclonal antibodies or by endonuclease restriction patterns. HSV-1 and HSV-2 also have biologic differences (replication in chicken embryo cells, effects on baby mice, allantoic membrane pock morphology, and sensitivity to various chemicals). Cocultivation of ganglia tissue along with permissive cells remains the standard technique for detecting latent virus, but this technique has little application in clinical medicine.[22, 24]

DIRECT DETECTION OF HSV-INFECTED CELLS

Direct detection methods allow making a diagnosis of HSV infection rapidly when mucocutaneous lesions are present or when tissue sections from infected organs are examined.[10, 65, 176, 229] Direct immunofluorescence or immunoperoxidase staining of cells taken from mucocutaneous lesions is the procedure used most commonly. Specimens are obtained by exposing the base of the lesion, scraping to remove cells, and transferring the cells to a glass slide. The use of fluorescein-conjugated monoclonal antibodies to HSV to stain lesion scrapings yields sensitivities, when compared with viral culture isolation, in the range of 78 to 88 percent with few

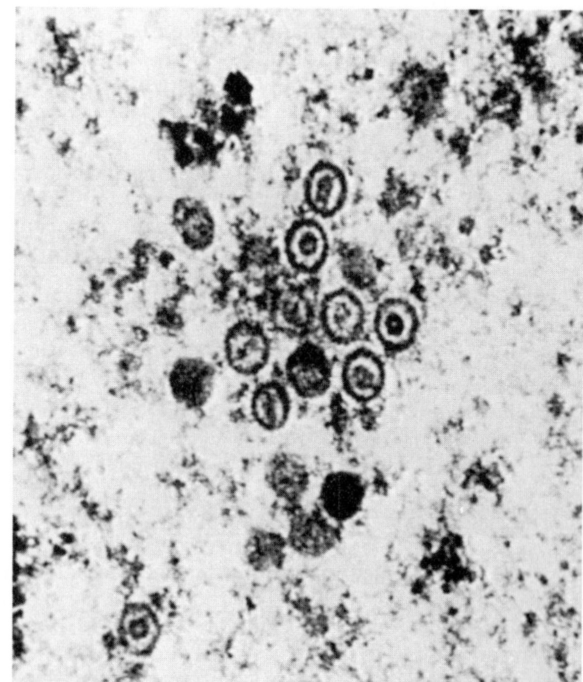

FIGURE 163–17 ■ Electron-microscopic demonstration of HSV particles in a brain biopsy specimen from a 9-month-old with HSV encephalitis.

false-positive reactions.[184] Nonetheless, a sample for viral culture should be obtained when the lesion scraping is performed so that the direct detection result can be confirmed. Direct detection methods should not be used to test secretion specimens for asymptomatic shedding, cells from the CSF of patients with suspected encephalitis, or cells from oropharyngeal or tracheal aspirate or bronchoalveolar lavage samples. HSV antigens can be detected directly in clinical specimens by enzyme-linked immunosorbent assays (ELISAs), immunoperoxidase assays, hemagglutination assays, or avidin-biotin enzyme conjugate assays.[5, 39, 57, 184, 229] Sensitivities range from 70 to 95 percent with specificities of 65 to 95 percent when compared with viral culture. None of these methods is reliable for detecting asymptomatic HSV shedding.[276] Except for sporadic reports, antigen-detection tests for HSV in CSF have been unsuccessful and should not be used.[137]

Nonspecific methods such as Papanicolaou (Pap) staining or the Tzanck test have been used in the past to suggest possible HSV infection. Even though these methods may show cytologic changes in specimens obtained from suspected HSV lesions, the diagnosis of HSV should not rely on these methods in current practice because rapid, specific methods are available. Although cytologic examination of HSV lesions reveals typical giant cells and, less commonly, Cowdry type A intranuclear inclusions, these changes also are seen with CMV and VZV. Some series report finding cytologic changes in 80 percent of culture-positive specimens if the examiner is experienced, but other series find such changes in only 40 percent. A negative Tzanck or Pap smear does exclude the diagnosis of HSV infection in critical situations such as infections in newborns, patients with encephalitis, or immunosuppressed patients. Electron microscopy of vesicular fluid or tissue preparations may reveal the characteristic virus of the herpes family (Fig. 163–18). However, the microscopist cannot differentiate HSV from other herpesviruses, and this diagnostic approach rarely is available as a rapid method. Because selection of antiviral drugs for herpesviruses requires specific identification of the infecting virus (e.g., HSV must be differentiated from CMV in the brain, lungs, or liver because therapy differs), nonspecific methods have limited clinical value.

POLYMERASE CHAIN REACTION ASSAYS

PCR assays involve repeated amplification of targeted regions of HSV DNA by the design of primers that will anneal to denatured DNA and produce millions of copies of the DNA sequence.[19, 50, 210] The sensitivity of PCR methods can permit the detection of fewer than 10 copies of the viral genome in a sample. PCR has been applied successfully to the diagnosis of HSV infection.[6, 19, 117, 165, 210, 218] However, the extreme sensitivity of PCR renders it prone to false-positive results in the event of poor technique or specimen contamination. In clinical laboratories that have proper experience with PCR and when appropriate controls are used in the assay, PCR assay is the method of choice for detection of low copy numbers of HSV DNA and for detection of HSV DNA in CSF for the diagnosis of HSV encephalitis.[19, 210, 270] Sequential testing by PCR assay has rendered the use of brain biopsy unnecessary in most situations.[149] PCR also has been used to demonstrate prolonged presence of HSV DNA in genital lesions.[56] The sensitivity of the PCR method appears to be adequate for detecting asymptomatic shedding of HSV, although a positive PCR result does not indicate necessarily the presence of infectious virus.[55, 111] A negative PCR result does not exclude the diagnosis of HSV because specimens obtained early in the clinical course of some infections may be negative and clinical specimens often contain inhibitors of PCR.[48, 111, 202] HSV PCR has potential value for testing the CSF of patients with suspected herpes encephalitis.[105, 131, 195, 210, 228, 241] HSV DNA was detected by PCR in the CSF of 53 (98%) of 54 patients with biopsy-proven herpes simplex encephalitis and was detected in all 18 CSF specimens obtained before brain biopsy from patients with proven herpes encephalitis.[149] However, clinicians must recognize that PCR may be negative early in the course of HSV encephalitis. HSV PCR also has utility when the clinical diagnosis is difficult to make, as illustrated by the detection of HSV in vitreous fluid and in unusual mucocutaneous lesions in patients with AIDS.[59, 154] Primers for both HSV-1 and HSV-2 can be included in the PCR reaction to allow simultaneous detection and typing of the infecting virus.[270]

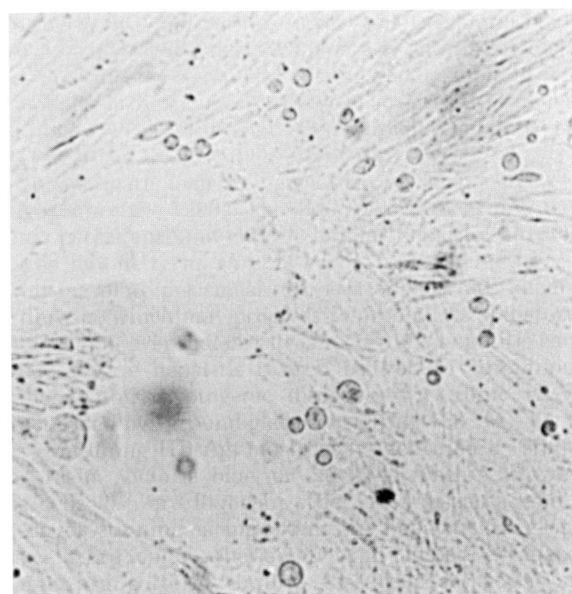

FIGURE 163–18 ■ Culture of HSV on human fibroblasts demonstrating disruption of the cell monolayer and rounding and enlargement of cells to show the cytopathogenic effect.

DNA hybridization with radiolabeled or biotinylated probes also can be used to detect directly HSV in pathologic specimens.[79, 86, 93] This technique may detect virus or incomplete viral DNA or RNA in latency or in sites with low levels of productive infection.

SEROLOGIC DIAGNOSIS

In contrast to methods that detect the virus (viral culture) or viral DNA (PCR assay) or proteins (direct antigen detection), serologic methods have limited value for the clinical diagnosis of HSV infection. With standard methods, demonstration of the presence of IgG antibodies to HSV in serum means that the individual has acquired HSV-1 or HSV-2, or both, at some time in the recent (2 to 4 weeks) or distant (many years) past. Because these viruses cause persistent infection, the presence of HSV antibodies signifies only that the individual has latent HSV-1 or HSV-2 (or both) in sensory ganglia and that the virus can be expected to reactivate and be shed in secretions intermittently. Many serologic methods can be used to assess HSV IgG immune status to document whether an individual is infected with HSV, and most are sensitive. HSV serologic testing generally is performed by using commercial ELISA or latex agglutination procedures.[93] However, practitioners must understand that the extensive cross-reactivity between HSV-1 and HSV-2 antibodies renders differentiating past HSV-1 from past HSV-2 infection impossible with any of these methods.[14, 15, 93, 262] Serologic reports that list HSV-1 and HSV-2 antibody titers separately are misleading, but they often are provided without the necessary explanation about the lack of sensitivity for identifying the patient's infection status.

Recently, some laboratories have begun to use validated serologic methods that circumvent the problem of cross-reactivity between HSV-1 and HSV-2 antibodies. These specialized serologic methods can be used to show whether the individual has infection with HSV-1, HSV-2, or both, but not when the infection was acquired. If paired sera are available, showing seroconversion to HSV-2 even when the patient has HSV-1 infection may be possible.[14, 36, 80, 126, 143] These methods use Western blot (immunoblot) analysis to demonstrate reactivity with type-specific viral proteins. For example, the fact that the gG of HSV-1 differs significantly from the HSV-2 homologue permits detection of type-specific IgG and IgM antibodies.[14, 116, 262] When one of these methods was evaluated in patients with HSV-2 infection proved by viral culture and Western blot analysis, its sensitivity for detection of HSV-2 antibody was 96 percent and its specificity was 98 percent.[16] Although these HSV type-specific serologic tests have become available through commercial diagnostic laboratories, practitioners must confirm that the laboratory is using such a method and not the "standard" ELISA or other tests that are commonly—and misleadingly—reported as though HSV-1 and HSV-2 antibodies have been identified accurately.

If the patient is seronegative at the onset of symptoms or at the initial evaluation, primary HSV infection can be documented by using any of the standard ELISA methods to show seroconversion with paired sera.[138] However, again, the serotype of HSV responsible for the seroconversion cannot be determined with most commercial serologic tests. Serologic tests also are not useful for evaluating possible recurrent HSV because recurrences often are not accompanied by a significant rise in antibody titer. Determining HSV IgG antibody titers in paired sera is not helpful because titers may vary more than fourfold in the absence of viral reactivation. Testing for IgM antibodies does not improve the serologic diagnosis; HSV IgM assays cannot be used to distinguish primary from recurrent infection because reactivation also can induce the production of IgM antibody. In addition, HSV IgM antibody assays are difficult to standardize, and false-positive results occur commonly, even when effort is made to fractionate serum IgG and IgM before testing.

Local production of HSV IgG in CSF samples can be used to document HSV encephalitis in some patients, but a 2- to 4-week interval is required to demonstrate this change,[178] and it cannot be used to guide antiviral therapy.[19, 137, 242, 275] Testing CSF for HSV IgM antibodies has no demonstrated diagnostic value.

GENETIC ANALYSIS FOR MOLECULAR EPIDEMIOLOGY

HSV DNA from epidemiologically unrelated isolates has a specific cleavage pattern, or "fingerprint," when digested by endonuclease restriction enzymes and subjected to electrophoresis in a gel[44] (Fig. 163–19). These methods can be used to type the virus and demonstrate relatedness or differences among isolates obtained from different sites in the same person during one illness or from the same site over

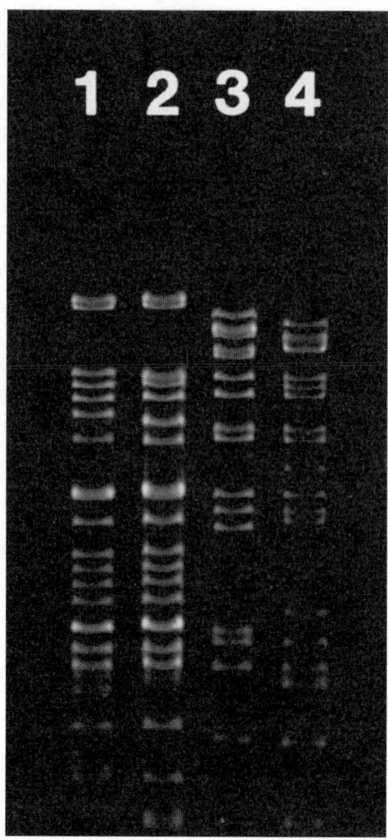

FIGURE 163–19 ■ Electrophoretic separation of the DNA fragments of four HSV isolates by size, produced by restriction endonuclease enzyme digestion using the BamHI enzyme. Lanes 1 and 2 are two different HSV-2 clinical isolates, whereas lanes 3 and 4 are two different HSV-1 clinical isolates. The origin of the gel is at the top. (Courtesy of Dr. Saul Kit, Division of Biochemical Virology, Baylor College of Medicine, Houston.)

time for the purpose of evaluating apparent "outbreaks" or nosocomial transmission.[44, 45, 110, 160, 293] This method has improved the understanding of HSV-1 and HSV-2 epidemiology, investigation of the possibility of exogenous re-infection versus recurrence, and the possibility that individuals may harbor more than one latent virus "strain." To be sure of identity, several restriction enzymes must be used to test each isolate. Thus, this method is valuable for epidemiologic purposes, but it is time consuming and requires special expertise beyond that of most viral diagnostic laboratories.

DRUG SUSCEPTIBILITY TESTING

Although not in general use, antiviral drug susceptibility testing of HSV isolates is becoming available in many centers. With the availability of specific antiviral therapy and evolving mechanisms of viral drug resistance, the clinician must rely increasingly on sensitivity tests that resemble the in vitro minimal inhibitory concentration tests used for bacteria. Evolving clinical data are providing meaningful values for "sensitive and resistant" virus, although the specific numbers vary by assay. In general, a median infectious dose (ID_{50}) of more than 3 μg/mL for acyclovir and more than 100 μg/mL for foscarnet denotes a resistant isolate.[54, 216] Rapid screening tests that take 3 to 4 days to perform are being developed.[215] In addition, detection of HSV enzyme characteristics, such as thymidine kinase–negative

HSV isolates, which are therefore resistant to acyclovir, can be useful. In an immunocompromised patient, in particular, failure to respond to antiviral therapy should alert the clinician to the need for viral susceptibility testing.

Prognosis, Complications, and Sequelae

Most HSV infections occurring beyond the fetal and neonatal periods cause minor morbidity but very rarely are life-threatening. The introduction of antiviral drugs that inhibit HSV replication has changed the management and outcome of these infections during the past 20 years. Even before these drugs were available, eczema herpeticum resolved without sequelae in most cases. Despite antiviral therapy, HSV encephalitis can be fatal or be associated with serious consequences ranging from moderate to extensive and permanent neurologic disability. The case-fatality rate for untreated encephalitis may be as high as 75 percent,[295] and progressive neurologic damage may occur.[72, 107, 137] In a series of PCR-diagnosed cases, a Glasgow Coma Scale score higher than 11 was associated with a poor outcome, and the youngest cohort, those younger than 3 years, had higher morbidity and mortality rates.[122] Genital herpes causes significant physical and psychologic morbidity. In immunocompromised patients, disseminated HSV infection can result in fatal or serious illness. Although early studies suggested that cervical cancer was triggered by HSV, better methods have excluded HSV as a cause of malignant transformation. HSV is one of the most common infectious causes of blindness in the developed countries.

Treatment

HSV-1 and HSV-2 infections are treated with acyclovir or related drugs. Acyclovir is a nucleoside analogue that is a competitive inhibitor of HSV DNA polymerase, and it terminates DNA chain elongation. Acyclovir is an inactive agent; inhibition of viral DNA synthesis by blocking viral DNA polymerase and DNA chain elongation requires phosphorylation of acyclovir. HSV-1 and HSV-2 viral thymidine kinases are much more active than mammalian cell kinases are, and acyclovir becomes a specific antiviral agent in the presence of viral thymidine kinase.

Because the oral bioavailability of acyclovir is only approximately 20 percent, efficacy with oral administration requires high and frequent dosing. Concentrations of acyclovir achieved in CSF are approximately 50 percent of plasma levels. Acyclovir is excreted by glomerular filtration, so doses must be reduced for patients with impaired renal function. Acyclovir has been an exceptionally safe drug in clinical practice, but adverse reactions, including rash, nausea, vomiting, diarrhea, abdominal pain, and headache, can occur. Neurotoxicity may occur with an overdose, usually when the dose is not adjusted for poor renal clearance. Acyclovir also can cause acute renal insufficiency by precipitation in the renal tubules in dehydrated patients with high plasma concentrations or by rapid infusion of the drug. Valacyclovir, the L-valine ester of acyclovir, is converted to acyclovir[274] and has much higher bioavailability after oral administration, with plasma concentrations similar to those obtained after intravenous administration of acyclovir. Famciclovir is an oral prodrug of penciclovir[195]; it also is well absorbed orally and is metabolized to the active form on absorption. The major advantage of these agents is that less frequent dosing is required than with acyclovir. HSV-1 and HSV-2 seldom are resistant to acyclovir or the related drugs, but resistance can occur in immunocompromised patients who receive prolonged antiviral therapy. However these doses have not been tested in children. HSV isolates resistant to acyclovir usually have mutations in viral thymidine kinase. Foscarnet or, in some cases, cidofovir is an alternative for treatment of acyclovir-resistant HSV.[34]

ORAL HSV INFECTION

Although the published experience is limited, the use of oral acyclovir for children with gingivostomatitis is appropriate and can be expected to modify the duration of symptoms if it is initiated early in the clinical course. Several small placebo-controlled trials of primary herpes gingivostomatitis in young children have been described.[7, 78] In one study, the pain and hypersalivation resolved more quickly in acyclovir-treated patients.[78] In a larger study, symptoms resolved more rapidly with a 10-day course of oral acyclovir (600 mg/m^2 four times a day); differences were observed in drooling (4 versus 8 days with placebo), gum swelling (5 versus 7 days), speed of intraoral lesion healing (6 versus 8 days), appearance of new lesions (57% versus 94%), and viral shedding in saliva (4 versus 10 days). Therapy had no effect on the subsequent development of cold sores.[3] A comparison of oral acyclovir suspension, 15 mg/kg five times a day for 7 days, or placebo, started within 72 hours, documented that drug recipients had a shorter duration of oral lesions (median of 4 versus 10 days [difference, 6 days; 95% confidence interval, 4.0 to 8.0]) and earlier resolution of other symptoms, including fever (1 versus 3 days [2 days, 0.8 to 3.2]), extraoral lesions (0 versus 5.5 days [5.5 days, 1.3 to 4.7]), difficulty eating (4 versus 7 days [3 days, 1.31 to 4.69]), and difficulty drinking (3 versus 6 days [3 days, 1.1 to 4.9]).[3] Treatment also decreased the period of viral shedding (1 versus 5 days [4 days, confidence interval, 2.9 to 5.1]). Symptomatic therapy includes antipyretics and oral hydration. The use of oral anesthetics is not recommended and has resulted in self-injury as a result of children's chewing on anesthetized oral mucosa or lips.

Although the duration of symptoms is shorter with recurrences, children with frequent or severe recurrences may benefit from treatment with oral acyclovir given as soon as new lesions appear. Topical acyclovir has been licensed for the treatment of recurrent oral herpes labialis based on experience in adults. However, its benefits on clinical symptoms are minimal. If treatment is indicated, oral acyclovir is the best option. Several studies have produced conflicting results regarding the use of topical acyclovir for the treatment of oral herpes recurrences. Topical acyclovir can decrease the duration of HSV shedding from 2 to 3 days with placebo treatment to 1 to 2 days,[249] and the effect on symptoms is either none[290] or subtle (1 less day with vesicles and a 2- to 3-day acceleration of healing). Although no controlled studies have been conducted, acyclovir therapy should be used for the treatment of rare cases of HSV esophagitis in normal hosts.[92]

HSV KERATITIS

Children with HSV keratitis should be referred for immediate evaluation by an ophthalmologist who is familiar with this illness and its progressive, sight-threatening forms and with optimal antiviral therapy. The use of cycloplegic and anti-inflammatory agents, which may be necessary, requires specialized experience. Five topical preparations have been shown to have a beneficial effect on HSV keratitis and probably other superficial ocular HSV infections such as conjunctivitis and blepharitis.[159] These preparations include idoxuridine (Stoxil), vidarabine (Vira-A), trifluridine (Viroptic), acyclovir, and interferon. Orally administered acyclovir also has been used to treat dendritic keratitis, with effects that were similar to those achieved with topical acyclovir in the treatment of dendritic corneal ulceration. Several series suggest that oral acyclovir is therapeutic in patients who have stromal keratitis or keratouveitis.[155, 234, 273] When given in conjunction with topical antiviral therapy, the response to oral acyclovir was good even in those who had failed topical therapy.[235] Oral therapy also is useful for prophylaxis against viral reactivation in those who require corticosteroids for the treatment of stromal keratitis.

HSV ENCEPHALITIS

Intravenous acyclovir (10 mg/kg per dose three times a day for 14 to 21 days) is the drug of choice for HSV encephalitis beyond the neonatal period. Two well-controlled clinical studies in Sweden and the United States that compared vidarabine with acyclovir (30 mg/kg/day in three divided doses for 10 to 12 days) provided evidence that acyclovir is significantly more effective than is vidarabine in treating HSV encephalitis.[242, 290] In the Swedish study, the early mortality rate was 19 percent in the acyclovir-treated group and 50 percent in the vidarabine-treated group.[242] The National Institutes of Health collaborative study[290] generated similar data. As was observed in the earlier vidarabine studies,[295] younger age and less severe neurologic signs at initiation of therapy markedly influence the outcome of HSV encephalitis treated with acyclovir. Lethargic patients have a 15 percent mortality rate, whereas comatose patients have a 40 percent mortality rate. The use of long-term therapy remains controversial.[107, 137, 289]

In addition to antiviral therapy, intensive care is required for optimizing the outcome of these patients. Fluid management for the prevention of overhydration is critical. Often, direct measurement of intracranial pressure is necessary for effective monitoring of increased pressure and treatment with diuretic agents. The use of steroids is common but remains controversial and unstudied; viral replication does not appear to be more extensive as a consequence of steroid therapy. Anticonvulsant therapy for management of the often severe and prolonged seizures, as well as ventilatory support, is usually necessary at some time during the illness.

GENITAL HSV INFECTION

Oral acyclovir is the drug of choice for HSV genital infection. Although topical acyclovir was the first antiviral therapy used to treat genital herpes, it has been replaced by the oral agent. Some benefit was observed with the topical drug, but it is difficult to use, and its effectiveness is limited when compared with oral acyclovir; treatment decreased the mean duration of viral shedding (4.1 versus 7.0 days with placebo) and time to crusting of lesions (7.1 versus 10.5 days).[61] In the treatment of recurrent genital disease, topical acyclovir generally tended to have a minor effect on the duration of viral shedding (from 1 to 2 days in treated patients compared with 2 to 3 days in placebo recipients), with little or no effect on symptoms.[163, 201] These results were not improved markedly with immediate use of topical ointment. Early studies in which intravenous acyclovir was given to patients with primary genital HSV infection also were performed.[60, 171] When used in a placebo-controlled, double-blind study at a dose of 5 mg/kg every 8 hours for 5 days, acyclovir decreased the duration of viral shedding (2 versus 8 to 13 days in placebo-treated patients), shortened local and systemic symptoms by 2 to 5 days, and decreased the time to healing by 7 to 12 days. Complications such as extragenital lesions or urinary retention were reduced significantly.[59, 197]

Oral acyclovir has therapeutic effects on both primary and recurrent HSV infection in adults and should be given to adolescents with these infections. The major effect of intravenous acyclovir therapy on the first episode of genital HSV infection is seen in those who have true primary disease, as opposed to those who have HSV-1 immunity and are experiencing new HSV-2 infection.[190] The intravenous route of administration has been replaced by oral therapy with acyclovir and related agents. In either case, optimal benefit requires early intervention. In a double-blind, placebo-controlled study of patients who had primary genital infection, acyclovir in a dose of 200 mg five times per day for 5 to 10 days significantly reduced viral shedding (1 to 6 days versus 13 to 15 days with placebo), lesion formation after 48 hours (0–4% versus 43–44%), the duration of lesions (10 to 12 versus 16 to 21 days), and the duration and severity of symptoms.[43] In similar studies of adult patients who had recurrent genital HSV infection, acyclovir (200 mg five times per day for 5 days) decreased the duration of virus shedding (1 to 2 versus 2 to 4 days), time to healing (5 to 6 versus 6 to 7 days), and development of new lesions (2–10% versus 19–25%), especially when administered early in the recurrence.

In these short-term studies in which patients were cautioned regarding hydration, no significant side effects were observed. Furthermore, no cytogenetic effects were noted.[53] Studies of virus from either placebo or acyclovir recipients showed that 4 to 15 percent of viruses isolated after therapy were more resistant to acyclovir, regardless of therapy.[54] Neither oral nor intravenous acyclovir reduces the rate of recurrence when used to treat either primary or recurrent genital infection. Oral acyclovir is the drug of choice for patients who have primary genital HSV infection, HSV proctitis,[207] and frequent recurrent disease. Intravenous acyclovir should be reserved for patients who have severe local or systemic symptoms or complications such as urinary retention or aseptic meningitis syndrome.[190]

In adults, valacyclovir administered two times a day was as efficacious as acyclovir administered five times a day in the treatment of recurrent genital herpes. Similarly, famciclovir administered two times a day was found to be efficacious in the treatment of genital HSV infection, but it has not been compared with standard acyclovir or valacyclovir treatment.[170, 211, 212, 256]

Symptomatic therapy for HSV lesions should be directed toward reduction of local discomfort, promotion of healing, and prevention of autoinoculation and superinfection. Nonspecific creams and ointments probably delay healing and increase the risk of occurrence of maceration and infection. Keeping lesions clean and dry probably is the most important local measure. Urinating sometimes is painful and can be made less so by urinating into a bathtub or sitz bath. Some experts advise Burow solution sitz baths or short compress treatments. Prolonged soaking delays healing.

MUCOCUTANEOUS HSV INFECTION IN IMMUNOCOMPROMISED HOSTS

Acyclovir and related drugs given orally or intravenously are the agents of choice for serious mucocutaneous HSV-1 or HSV-2 infection in high-risk hosts. Early initiation of treatment provides the best outcome. Given the limited oral bioavailability of acyclovir, higher plasma concentrations can be achieved with valacyclovir or famciclovir, but clinical experience with these drugs is limited in children. If the infection is considered potentially life-threatening, intravenous acyclovir is the treatment of choice. Therapeutic responses to HSV infection in immunocompromised hosts have been difficult to study because of the variable nature of the disease. The experience with vidarabine demonstrated the benefits of antiviral therapy initially. In a randomized, controlled, crossover study of mucocutaneous HSV infection, vidarabine (10 mg/kg/day intravenously in a 12-hour infusion) was shown to decrease pain and induce defervescence in patients older than 40 years. In none of the 85 patients in this study did visceral dissemination of HSV develop. However, these observations are of historical interest now because the drug is not available and has been replaced by acyclovir. Acyclovir ointment appears to have some minor effects on pain, viral shedding, and time to complete healing of lesions in immunocompromised persons with mild, non–life-threatening mucocutaneous HSV infection,[294] but oral acyclovir is more effective for mild illness.

Patients who have more severe illness should be cared for in a hospital setting with the intravenous preparation. Intravenous acyclovir has been analyzed extensively in immunocompromised patients who have mucocutaneous HSV infection.[91, 289] When used early, acyclovir arrests the progression of infection. In several double-blind, placebo-controlled studies, acyclovir has been shown to be highly effective. It decreased the time to cessation of new lesions (1 versus 3 days with placebo), time to lesion crusting (3 to 7 versus 9 to 14 days), time to lesion healing (12 to 14 versus 18 to 28 days), cessation of pain (4 to 10 versus 7 to 16 days), and termination of viral shedding (3 versus 14 to 17 days).[280] Acyclovir administered intravenously is the most effective agent and the drug of choice for treating HSV in an immunocompromised host. The dosage is 250 mg/m^2 or 5 mg/kg every 8 hours infused over a 1-hour period. In patients with severe disease, the dose may be doubled. The major toxic effect has been renal, with a reversible obstructive nephropathy and transient rises in serum creatinine levels (5–10% of patients). Adequate hydration usually prevents this problem. Dosage guidelines have been established in patients who have impaired renal function (Table 163–4). One to 5 percent of patients may experience nausea and vomiting. Less commonly (1%), reversible neurologic symptoms (lethargy, agitation, tremor, disorientation, coma, transient hemiparesthesia) and laboratory abnormalities (abnormal EEG, increased CSF myelin basic protein) have developed in bone marrow transplant patients. These patients usually had received interferon and CNS chemoprophylaxis for leukemia.[279] Other less serious problems include phlebitis (14%) and hives (5%).

Several studies have focused on the use of oral acyclovir in this patient population.[258] The 50 percent virus-inhibiting concentration (IC_{50}) of acyclovir generally is 0.1 to 0.5 μg/mL for HSV-1 and 0.5 to 2 μg/mL for HSV-2. Many studies use molar concentrations; in the case of acyclovir, the dose in micromoles divided by 4 equals the dose in micrograms per milliliter. Whereas peak serum levels with intravenous acyclovir vary from 8 to 15 μg/mL, the levels achieved with oral therapy are considerably lower (1 to 2 μg/mL). In preliminary studies of relatively small populations of immunocompromised adults, oral acyclovir at doses of 200 mg five times per day effectively promoted the healing of lesions and inhibited viral shedding.[258] Pediatric studies have used oral doses of 600 mg/m^2 given four times per day.[261] The relative efficacies of oral and intravenous acyclovir have not been compared in this setting. The choice of route of administration requires clinical judgment about the degree of immunosuppression, assessment for evidence of dissemination, and frequent re-evaluation if oral drug is given.

TABLE 163–4 ■ GUIDELINES FOR USE OF ACYCLOVIR IN PATIENTS WITH RENAL IMPAIRMENT*

Creatinine Clearance (mL/min/1.7 m^2)	Dose (mg/kg)	Dosing Interval (hr)
50	5	8
25–50	5	12
10–25	5	24
0–10	2.5	24

*A dose (5 mg/kg) should be administered after each dialysis session in patients undergong hemodialysis.

To date, all studies of acyclovir in immunosuppressed patients have documented the propensity of recurrent lesions to reappear when therapy is withdrawn. Whether acyclovir reduces the humoral and cellular immune responses to HSV is not certain[278]; more likely, these patients remain subject to HSV recurrences because adaptive immunity is reconstituted as a consequence of the underlying disease.

Neonatal herpes simplex infection is discussed in Chapter 73.

ACYCLOVIR-RESISTANT HSV INFECTION

After more than a decade of use, acyclovir remains an effective antiviral compound. In immunocompetent hosts, acyclovir resistance has been a rare problem, even with prolonged courses of suppressive therapy. Mutant, thymidine kinase–negative virus strains have been recovered in 3 to 10 percent of patients treated with acyclovir, but acyclovir-resistant virus also can be recovered in placebo-treated patients, thus indicating that subpopulations of HSV are present in the lesions.[54] Thymidine kinase–negative HSV recurrences in immunocompromised patients have been documented well, with demonstration of the ability of these viruses to establish latency and recur. These viral mutants are less virulent in animal models, and patients who were culture-positive for such mutants often have thymidine kinase–positive HSV isolates recovered from lesions during their next recurrence.[240]

Acyclovir-resistant virus occasionally has been shed by immunocompetent patients before, during, or after receiving therapy, yet it usually has not been associated with treatment failure.[142, 156, 259] In pretreatment patients, 3.6 percent of isolates (31 of 870) were resistant to acyclovir (not inhibited by 3 μg/mL).[56] A similar percentage (3.1%) of resistant isolates was recovered from 663 immunocompetent patients after acyclovir therapy.[54] An immunocompetent patient was reported who had an acyclovir-resistant virus containing an altered thymidine kinase that caused multiple recurrences of genital herpes unresponsive to acyclovir therapy.[140] To date, these occurrences are rare in the immunocompetent patient population.

Drug resistance occasionally is a problem in the acyclovir-treated immunocompromised population. Many cases of acyclovir-resistant virus causing local invasive disease and, less commonly, dissemination and even acyclovir-unresponsive meningoencephalitis have been reported.[91, 94, 162, 214] Recurrences with acyclovir-resistant HSV-1 may be encountered, as described in a child with Wiskott-Aldrich syndrome.[219] Of the three mechanisms of altered sensitivity of HSV to acyclovir (absent thymidine kinase [TK–], altered thymidine kinase [TK^A], and altered viral DNA polymerase), the TK$^-$ type is encountered in the vast majority of cases.[54, 91, 94] These viruses cannot phosphorylate acyclovir and convert it to the active triphosphate. Among marrow transplant recipients receiving multiple courses of acyclovir, acyclovir-resistant virus was recovered from 2 percent of patients during initial therapy and from 9 percent after treatment for a second recurrence. In a tertiary care center, acyclovir resistant, clinically significant virus was recovered from 5 percent of immunocompromised patients (usually after receiving acyclovir) but from no immunocompetent hosts.[82] Illness caused by acyclovir-resistant viruses was more severe in pediatric patients and occurred more commonly in very immunocompromised patients such as those with AIDS or those who had undergone bone marrow transplantation.[82] Among bone marrow transplant receipients and AIDS patients who were tested after receiving acyclovir therapy, 18 percent (105 of 582) had isolates that were acyclovir-resistant.[54] In vitro viral susceptibility of HSV has been highly associated with clinical response to acyclovir in HIV-infected patients.[216]

In addition, acyclovir-resistant isolates are resistant to ganciclovir, which also requires phosphorylation. Foscarnet (40 mg/kg every 8 hours) has been used and was associated with an excellent clinical response and cessation of viral shedding.[258] The most common side effects of foscarnet are nephrotoxicity (azotemia), alterations in serum calcium and phosphorus, and neutropenia, observed in 10 to 25 percent of patients.[128, 214] In an immunocompromised patient who has HSV infection unresponsive to acyclovir, foscarnet therapy is indicated. Viral susceptibility testing may aid in clinical management.[217]

More recently, in patients receiving chronic or multiple courses of foscarnet, foscarnet-resistant HSV isolates (IC_{50} >100 μg/mL) have been recovered from lesions failing to respond to foscarnet.[216, 217] Of note, these lesions often responded to acyclovir, alone or in combination with foscarnet.[217] Perhaps the mutation in DNA polymerase responsible for foscarnet resistance was in an area not related to acyclovir activity. Other experimental strategies used to treat acyclovir-resistant viruses have included high-dose, continuous-infusion acyclovir (1.5 to 2.0 mg/kg/hr) or the use of intravenous cidofovir.[150, 243] In the case of acyclovir- and foscarnet-resistant viruses, topical 3-hydroxy-2-phosphonomethoxypropyl cytosine (HPMPC or eidofovir) or a combination of topical trifluorothymidine and interferon-α[32, 213, 219] has been used successfully in patients who have chronic mucocutaneous lesions.

Prevention

INFECTION CONTROL

Because HSV infection is ubiquitous in the human population and intermittent asymptomatic shedding is extremely common, preventing transmission of HSV is difficult. HSV is sensitive to heat and lipid solvents, so the use of antiseptics, soap and hot water, or chlorine decreases the risk of transfer of virus in settings such as the home, spas, pools, wrestling meets, and hospitals. In addition, appropriate use of gloves by all health care personnel in contact with potentially infected body secretions or rashes should decrease the acquisition and nosocomial spread of HSV. These recommendations are all part of universal body substance precaution policies. Condoms may diminish the passage of infectious HSV. The use of cesarean section for preventing neonatal HSV is discussed in Chapter 73.

Health care providers should wear gloves and wash carefully before and after contact with respiratory or genital tract secretions. Parents and caretakers of infants with eczema or severe diaper rash should be especially careful to avoid making direct or indirect contact of this altered skin with an active HSV lesion. Burn patients should be protected against exposure to or direct contact with personnel or visitors who have active HSV lesions. Immunosuppressed patients with evidence of HSV infection usually are experiencing reactivation of latent virus. Primary HSV infections in immunosuppressed persons, as in neonates, may be especially severe, and protecting these susceptible patients against exposure to HSV lesions is important. Wrestlers and rugby players who have exposed skin lesions caused by HSV should be excluded from competition.

IMMUNOPROPHYLAXIS

The development of vaccines is a long-term objective, with significant potential to ameliorate the disease burden associated with HSV-1 and HSV-2.[8] However, attempts to create effective HSV vaccines have met with limited success to date.[168] In one early report, a vaccine containing the recombinant glycoprotein D of HSV-2 (gD_2) was used in patients who had established recurrent genital HSV infections, and vaccine recipients had a third fewer genital herpes recurrences than those experienced by placebo recipients during the study year.[255] However, experience with the use of recombinant vaccines to prevent primary HSV infection has yielded mixed results. Recombinant HSV-2 gD_2 and gB_2 have been demonstrated to induce high humoral and cell-mediated immune responses in seronegative and seropositive recipients.[152] Some vaccines may protect some women who have no HSV immunity at baseline.[31] Although animal data suggest successful immunomodulation with various agents such as bacille Calmette-Guérin, interleukin-2, or immune serum, these strategies have not been effective in humans. Agents such as bacille Calmette-Guérin, smallpox vaccine, lysine, and many other compounds have been shown to be ineffective and at times dangerous. No adequate controlled trials of high-dose intravenous immune globulin as an intervention to suppress frequently recurring genital herpes have been reported, and this method is not likely to be effective because these patients have high titers of HSV-specific antibodies.[166]

CHEMOPROPHYLAXIS

Intramuscular human interferon-α administered before and after surgery on the trigeminal nerve root significantly decreased the incidence of HSV shedding and clinical reactivation.[189] In similar studies, interferon had no significant effect on HSV shedding or reactivation in renal transplant patients.[50] Intravenous acyclovir has been shown to prevent the reactivation of HSV almost completely in immunosuppressed patients receiving a bone marrow transplant or antileukemic chemotherapy. Therapy usually is begun at the onset of immunosuppression and continued for 1½ to 3 months. HSV is reactivated in 50 to 70 percent of these adult patients. Oral acyclovir administered chronically also markedly suppressed recurrence in immunodeficient patients.[222, 263] In children undergoing bone marrow transplantation, acyclovir in dosages of 500 mg/m^2/day in three divided doses for 3 weeks, then 250 mg/m^2/day for 3 months orally, suppressed HSV infection. The use of prophylactic acyclovir is indicated in HSV-seropositive, immunosuppressed pediatric patients.

Oral acyclovir (200 mg two to five times per day) administered chronically can nearly completely prevent the reactivation of genital HSV in patients with frequent recurrences. Recurrences decreased by 50 to 70 percent, and the time to recurrence changed from 14 to 25 days in patients receiving placebo and from 100 to 125 days in those receiving acyclovir.[75, 259] Breakthrough recurrences tended to be mild and to have less viral shedding and rarely were caused by acyclovir-resistant virus. When acyclovir was discontinued (after 12 to 15 weeks of administration), HSV recurrences reverted to the pretreatment frequency. Higher doses of acyclovir suppressed recurrences in patients experiencing a "breakthrough" with more conventional doses. In patients receiving therapy for 5 years, the number of recurrences declined from the first year (1.7) to the fifth year (0.8).[100] Twenty to 25 percent of patients are recurrence-free for 4 to 5 years.[100] After prophylactic therapy ended, suppressive therapy no longer was warranted in some patients because of longer periods between recurrences.[85, 256] Patients who had resistant virus had re-isolation of acyclovir-sensitive virus. Thus, acyclovir suppressed recurrences without eliminating latent virus. A study has reported that acyclovir does not seem to change the rate of asymptomatic viral shedding.[257] A more recent study has demonstrated that acyclovir (400 mg twice a day) resulted in a 95 percent reduction in subclinical viral shedding when compared with placebo in women with genital herpes.[281] Side effects of chronic acyclovir therapy are limited to an increase in mean corpuscular erythrocyte volume and hemoglobin concentration without anemia or megaloblastic changes and to asthenia and mild gastrointestinal upset.[259] Valacyclovir and famciclovir can be used to effectively suppress frequently recurring genital herpes, although these drugs are more expensive for this indication than is acyclovir.[170] Oral herpetic recurrences were prevented in skiers given a brief course of acyclovir during their ski trip.[247]

Experience with acyclovir prophylaxis for HSV reactivation in children is limited. Prophylactic oral acyclovir (30 to 60 mg/kg/day in three to five doses for 1 week) has been shown to decrease seroconversion effectively and to eradicate symptomatic cases of HSV gingivostomatitis in a nursery setting in which outbreaks of HSV primary infection were occurring.[147, 194] Suppression has been effective in infants with frequent recurrences of HSV-2 after neonatal HSV-2 infection and has been safe. To date, up to 10 years of suppressive therapy in adults has not resulted in serious side effects[85, 100, 256] or an increase in the problem of drug-resistant HSV in a healthy host.

Acknowledgment

The author thanks Steve Kohl for the opportunity to base this chapter on his comprehensive discussion of HSV infections from the previous edition.

REFERENCES

1. Abramson, J. S., Roach, E. S., and Levy, H. B.: Postinfectious encephalopathy after treatment of herpes simplex encephalitis with acyclovir. Pediatr. Infect. Dis. *3*:146–147, 1984.
2. Adams, G., Stover, B. H., Keenlyside, R. A., et al.: Nosocomial herpetic infections in a pediatric intensive care unit. Am. J. Epidemiol. *113*:126–132, 1981.
3. Amir, J., Harel, L., Smetana, Z., and Varsano, I.: Treatment of herpes simplex gingivostomatitis with acyclovir in children: A randomised double blind placebo controlled study. B. M. J. *314*:1800–1803, 1997.
4. Amir, J., Harel, L., Smetana, Z., and Varsano, I.: The natural history of primary herpes simplex type 1 gingivostomatitis in children. Pediatr. Dermatol. *16*:259–263, 1999.
5. Amir, J. R., Straussberg, L., Harel, L., et al.: Evaluation of a rapid enzyme immunoassay for the detection of herpes simplex virus antigen in children with herpetic gingivostomatitis. Pediatr. Infect. Dis. J. *15*:627–629, 1996.
6. Ando, Y., Kimura, H., Miwata, H., et al.: Quantitative analysis of herpes simplex virus DNA in cerebrospinal fluid of children with herpes simplex encephalitis. J. Med. Virol. *41*:170–173, 1993.
7. Aoki, F. Y., Law, B. J., Hammond, G. W., et al.: Acyclovir suspension for treatment of acute herpes simplex virus gingivostomatitis in children: A placebo-controlled, double-blind trial. Abstract. Presented at the 33rd Interscience Conference on Antimicrobial Agents and Chemotherapy, New Orleans, LA, 1993, p. 399.
8. Arvin, A. M.: Genital herpesvirus infections: Rationale for a vaccine strategy. *In* Hitchcok, P. J., MacKay, H. T., Wasserheit, J. N., and Binder, R. (eds.): Sexually Transmitted Diseases and Adverse Outcomes of Pregnancy. Washington, DC, American Society for Microbiology, 1999, pp. 259–267.
9. Arvin, A. M., Hensleigh, P. A., Au, D. S., et al.: Failure of antepartum maternal cultures to predict the infant's risk of exposure to herpes simplex virus at delivery. N. Engl. J. Med. *315*:796–800, 1986.
10. Arvin, A. M., and Prober, C. G.: Herpes simplex virus type 2, a persistent problem. N. Engl. J. Med. *337*:1158–1159, 1997.
11. Arvin, A. M., and Prober, C. G.: Herpes simplex viruses. *In* Murphy, P. (ed.): Manual of Clinical Microbiology. 7th ed. Washington, DC, American Society for Microbiology, 1998, pp. 878–887.
12. Ashenburg, C., Rothstein, F. C., and Dahms, B. B.: Herpes esophagitis in the immunocompetent child. J. Pediatr. *108*:584–587, 1986.
13. Ashkenazi, S., and Kohl, S.: Nervous system abnormalities in pediatric HIV infection and AIDS. Semin. Pediatr. Infect. Dis. *1*:94–106, 1990.
14. Ashley, R., Cent, A., Maggs, V., et al.: Inability of enzyme immunoassays to discriminate between infections with herpes simplex virus types 1 and 2. Ann. Intern. Med. *115*:520–526, 1991.
15. Ashley, R. L., Eagleton, M., Pfeiffer, N.: Ability of a rapid serology test to detect seroconversion to herpes simplex virus type 2 glycoprotein g soon after infection. J. Clin. Microbiol. *37*:1632–1633, 1999.
16. Ashley, R. L., Wald, A., and Eagleton, M.: Premarket evaluation of the POCkit HSV-2 type-specific serologic test in culture-documented cases of genital herpes simplex virus type 2. Sex. Transm. Dis. *27*:266–269, 2000.
17. Aurelius, E., Andersson, B., Forsgren, M., et al.: Cytokines and other markers of intrathecal immune response in patients with herpes simplex encephalitis. J. Infect. Dis. *170*:678–680, 1994.
18. Aurelius, E., Fosgren, M., Skoldenberg, B., et al.: Persistent intrathecal immune activation in patients with herpes simplex encephalitis. J. Infect. Dis. *168*:1248–1252, 1993.
19. Aurelius, E., Johansson, B., Skoldenberg, B., et al.: Rapid diagnosis of herpes simplex encephalitis by nested polymerase chain reaction assay of cerebrospinal fluid. Lancet *337*:189–192, 1991.
20. Aurelius, E., Johansson, B., Skoldenberg, B., et al.: Encephalitis in immunocompetent patients due to herpes simplex virus type 1 or 2 as determined by type-specific polymerase chain reaction and antibody assays of cerebrospinal fluid. J. Med. Virol. *39*:179–186, 1993.
21. Bader, C., Crumpacker, C. S., Schnipper, L. E., et al.: The natural history of recurrent facial-oral infection with herpes simplex virus. J. Infect. Dis. *138*:897–905, 1978.
22. Baringer, J. R.: Recovery of herpes simplex virus from human trigeminal ganglions. N. Engl. J. Med. *291*:828, 1974.
23. Barton, L. L., Weaver-Woodard, S., Gutierrez, J. A., and Lee, D. M.: Herpes simplex virus hepatitis in a child: Case report and review. Pediatr. Infect. Dis. J. *18*:1026–1028, 1999.
24. Bastian, F. O., Rabson, A. S., Yee, C. L., et al.: Herpes-virus hominis: Isolation from human trigeminal ganglion. Science *178*:306–307, 1972.
25. Bastian, J. F., and Kaufman, I. A.: Herpes simplex esophagitis in a healthy 10-year-old boy. J. Pediatr. *100*:426–427, 1982.
26. Becker, W. B., Kipps, A., and McKenzie, D.: Disseminated herpes simplex virus infection: Its pathogenesis based on virological and pathological studies in 33 cases. Am. J. Dis. Child. *115*:1–8, 1968.
27. Behr, J. T., Daluga, D. J., Light, T. R., et al.: Herpetic infections in the fingers of infants. Report of five cases. J. Bone Joint Surg. Am. *69*:137–139, 1987.
28. Beigi, B., Algawi, K., Foley-Nolan, A., et al.: Herpes simplex keratitis in children. Br. J. Ophthalmol. *78*:458–460, 1994.
29. Belongia, E. A., Goodman, J. L., Holland, E. J., et al.: An outbreak of herpes gladiatorum at a high-school wrestling camp. N. Engl. J. Med. *325*:906–910, 1991.
30. Benedetti, J. K., Zeh, J., Selke, S., et al.: Frequency and reactivation of nongenital lesions among patients with genital herpes simplex virus. Am. J. Med. *98*:237–242, 1995.
31. Bernstein, D. L., and Stanberry, L. R.: Herpes simplex virus vaccines. Vaccine *17*:1681–1689, 1999.
32. Birch, C. J., Tyssen, D. P., Tachedjian, G., et al.: Clinical effects and in vitro studies of trifluorothymidine combined with interferon-α for treatment of drug-resistant and sensitive herpes simplex virus infections. J. Infect. Dis. *166*:108–112, 1992.
33. Biron, C. A., Byron, K. S., and Sullivan, J. L.: Severe herpes virus infections in an adolescent without natural killer cells. N. Engl. J. Med. *320*:1731–1735, 1989.
34. Blot, N., Schneider, P., Young, P., et al.: Treatment of an acyclovir and foscarnet-resistant herpes simplex virus infection with cidofovir in a child after an unrelated bone marrow transplant. Bone Marrow Transplant. *26*:903–905, 2000.
35. Bogger-Goren, S.: Acute epiglottitis caused by herpes simplex virus. Pediatr. Infect. Dis. J. *6*:1133–1134, 1987.

36. Breinig, M. K., Kingsley, L. A., Armstrong, J. A., et al.: Epidemiology of genital herpes in Pittsburgh: Serologic, sexual and racial correlates of apparent and inapparent herpes simplex infections. J. Infect. Dis. *162*:299–305, 1990.
37. Brice, S. L., Krzemien, D., Weston, W. L., et al.: Detection of herpes simplex virus DNA in cutaneous lesions of erythema multiforme. J. Invest. Dermatol. *93*:183–187, 1989.
38. Brice, S. L., Stockert, S. S., Jester, J. D., et al.: Herpes simplex virus–associated erythema multiforme in children. Abstract. Clin. Res. *38*:182, 1990.
39. Brinker, J. P., and Herrmann, J. E.: Comparison of three monoclonal antibody–based enzyme immunoassays for detection of herpes simplex virus in clinical specimens. Eur. J. Clin. Microbiol. Infect. Dis. *14*:314–317, 1995.
40. Brodtkorb, E., Lindqvist, M., Johnson, M., et al.: Diagnosis of herpes simplex encephalitis: A comparison between electroencephalography and computed tomography findings. Acta Neurol. Scand. *66*:462–471, 1982.
41. Brown, Z. A., Benedetti, J. D., and Watts, D. H.: A comparison between detailed and simple histories in the diagnosis of genital herpes complicating pregnancy. Am. J. Obstet. Gynecol. *172*:1299–1303, 1995.
42. Bryson, Y., Dillon, M., Bernstein, D. I., et al.: Risks of acquisition of genital herpes simplex virus type 2 in sex partners of persons with genital herpes: A prospective couple study. J. Infect. Dis. *167*:942–946, 1993.
43. Bryson, Y. J., Dillon, M., Lovett, M., et al.: Treatment of first episodes of genital herpes simplex virus infection with oral acyclovir. A randomized double-blind controlled trial in normal subjects. N. Engl. J. Med. *308*: 916–921, 1983.
44. Buchman, T. G., Roizman, B., Adams, G., et al.: Restriction endonuclease fingerprinting of herpes simplex virus DNA: A novel epidemiological tool applied to a nosocomial outbreak. J. Infect. Dis. *138*:488–498, 1978.
45. Buchman, T. G., Roizman, B., and Nahmias, A. J.: Demonstration of exogenous genital reinfection with herpes simplex virus type 2 by restriction endonuclease fingerprinting of viral DNA. J. Infect. Dis. *140*:295–304, 1979.
46. Buss, D. H., and Scharyj, M.: Herpesvirus infection of the esophagus and other visceral organs in adults: Incidence and clinical significance. Am. J. Med. *66*:457–462, 1979.
47. Caputo, G. M., and Byck, H.: Concomitant oculoglandular and ulceroglandular fever due to herpes simplex type 1. Am. J. Med. *93*:577–580, 1992.
48. Cassinotti, P., Mietz, H., and Siegl, G.: Suitability and clinical application of a multiplex nested PCR assay for the diagnosis of herpes simplex virus infections. J. Med. Virol. *50*:75–81, 1996.
49. Chase, R. A., Pottage, J. C., Jr., Haber, M. H., et al.: Herpes simplex viral hepatitis in adults: Two case reports and review of the literature. Rev. Infect. Dis. *9*:329–333, 1987.
50. Cheeseman, S. H., Rubin, R. H., Stewart, J. A., et al.: Controlled clinical trial of prophylactic human-leukocyte interferon in renal transplantation. Effect on cytomegalovirus and herpes simplex virus infections. N. Engl. J. Med. *300*:1345–1349, 1979.
51. Chonmaitree, T., Owen, M., Patel, J., et al.: Presence of cytomegalovirus and herpes simplex virus in middle ear fluids from children with acute otitis media. Clin. Infect. Dis. *15*:650–653, 1992.
52. Chuang, T.-Y., Su, W. P. D., Perry, H. O., et al.: Incidence and trend of herpes progenitalis. A 15-year population study. Mayo Clin. Proc. *58*:436–441, 1983.
53. Clive, D., Corey, L., Reichman, R. C., et al.: A double-blind, placebo-controlled cytogenetic study of oral acyclovir in patients with recurrent genital herpes. J. Infect. Dis. *164*:753–757, 1991.
54. Collins, P., and Ellis, M. N.: Sensitivity monitoring of clinical isolates of herpes simplex virus to acyclovir. J. Med. Virol. *1*(Suppl.):58–66, 1993.
55. Cone, R. W., Hobson, A. C., Brown, Z., et al.: Frequent detection of genital herpes simplex virus DNA by polymerase chain reaction among pregnant women. J. A. M. A. *272*:792–796, 1994.
56. Cone, R. W., Hobson, A. C., Palmer, J., et al.: Extended duration of herpes simplex virus DNA in genital lesions detected by the polymerase chain reaction. J. Infect. Dis. *164*:757–760, 1991.
57. Cone, R. W., Swenson, P. D., Hobson, A. C., et al: Herpes simplex virus detection from genital lesions: A comparative study using antigen detection (HerpChek) and culture. J. Clin. Microbiol. *31*:1774–1776, 1993.
58. Conway, J. H., Weinberg, K. A., Ashley, R. L., et al.: Viral meningitis in a preadolescent child caused by reactivation of latent herpes simplex (type 1). Pediatr. Infect. Dis. J. *16*:627–629, 1997.
59. Cunningham, E. T., Jr., Short, G. A., Irvine, A. R., et al.: Acquired immunodeficiency syndrome–associated herpes simplex virus retinitis. Clinical description and use of a polymerase chain reaction–based assay as a diagnostic tool. Arch. Ophthalmol. *114*:834–840, 1996.
60. Corey, L., Fife, K. H., Benedetti, J. K., et al.: Intravenous acyclovir for the treatment of primary genital herpes. Ann. Intern. Med. *98*:914–921, 1983.
61. Corey, L., Nahmias, A. J., and Guinan, M. E.: A trial of topical acyclovir in genital herpes simplex virus infection. N. Engl. J. Med. *306*:1313–1319, 1982.
62. Craig, C., and Nahmias, A. J.: Different patterns of neurologic involvement with herpes simplex virus types 1 and 2: Isolation of herpes simplex virus type 2 from the buffy coat of two adults with meningitis. J. Infect. Dis. *127*:365–372, 1973.
63. Croen, K. D., Ostrove, S. M., Dragovic, L., et al.: Characterization of herpes simplex virus type 2 latency-associated transcription in human sacral ganglia and in cell culture. J. Infect. Dis. *163*:23–28, 1991.
64. Darougar, S., Wishart, M. S., and Viswalingam, N. D.: Epidemiological and clinical features of primary herpes simplex virus ocular infection. Br. J. Ophthalmol. *69*:2–6, 1985.
65. Dascal, A., Chan-Thim, J., Morahan, M., et al.: Diagnosis of herpes simplex virus infection in a clinical setting by a direct enzyme immunoassay kit. J. Clin. Microbiol. *27*:700–704, 1989.
66. David, T. J., and Langson, M.: Herpes simplex infection in atopic eczema. Arch. Dis. Child. *60*:338–343, 1985.
67. Davis, L. E., and Johnson, R. T.: An explanation for the localization of herpes simplex encephalitis? Ann. Neurol. *5*:2–5, 1979.
68. Davis, L. E., and McLaren, L. C.: Relapsing herpes simplex encephalitis following antiviral therapy? Ann. Neurol. *13*:192–195, 1983.
69. Demaeral, P. H., Wilms, G., Robberecht, W., et al.: MRI of herpes simplex encephalitis. Neuroradiology *34*:490–493, 1992.
70. DeVincenzo, J. P., and Thorne, G.: Mild herpes simplex encephalitis diagnosed by polymerase chain reaction: A case report and review. Pediatr. Infect. Dis. J. *13*:662–664, 1994.
71. DiSclafani, A., Kohl, S., and Ostrow, P. T.: The importance of brain biopsy in suspected herpes simplex encephalitis. Surg. Neurol. *17*:101–106, 1982.
72. Dix, R. D., Baringer, J. R., Panitch, H. S., et al.: Recurrent herpes simplex encephalitis: Recovery of virus after Ara-A treatment. Ann. Neurol. *13*:196–200, 1983.
73. Do, A. N., Green, P. A., and Demmler, G. J.: Herpes simplex type 2 meningitis and associated genital lesions in a three-year-old child. Pediatr. Infect. Dis. J. *13*:1014–1016, 1994.
74. Domingues, R. B., Lakeman, F. D., Mayo, M. S., and Whitley, R. J.: Application of competitive PCR to cerebrospinal fluid samples from patients with herpes simplex encephalitis. J. Clin. Microbiol. *36*:2229–2234, 1998.
75. Douglas, J. M., Critchlow, C., and Benedetti, J.: A double-blind study of oral acyclovir for suppression of recurrences of genital herpes simplex virus infection. N. Engl. J. Med. *310*:1551–1556, 1984.
76. Dowdle, W. R., Nahmias, A. J., Harwell, R. W., et al.: Association of antigenic type of herpesvirus hominis with site of viral recovery. J. Immunol. *99*:774–780, 1967.
77. Drummer, J. S., Armstrong, J., Somers, J., et al.: Transmission of infection with herpes simplex virus by renal transplantation. J. Infect. Dis. *155*:202–206, 1987.
78. Ducoulombier, H., Cousin, J., Dewilde, A., et al.: A controlled clinical trial versus placebo of acyclovir in the treatment of herpetic gingivostomatitis in children [in French]. Ann. Pediatr. (Paris) *35*:212–216, 1988.
79. Eglin, R. P., Lehner, T., and Subak-Sharpe, J. H.: Detection of RNA complementary to herpes-simplex virus in mononuclear cells from patients with Behçet's syndrome and recurrent oral ulcers. Lancet *2*:1356–1361, 1982.
80. Eis-Hübinger, A. M., Däumer, M., Matz, B., and Schneweis, K. E.: Evaluation of three glycoprotein G2–based enzyme immunoassays for detection of antibodies to herpes simplex virus type 2 in human sera. J. Clin. Microbiol. *37*:1242–1246, 1999.
81. Ellison, P. H., and Hanson, P. A.: Herpes simplex: A possible cause of brain stem encephalitis. Pediatrics *59*:240–243, 1977.
82. Englund, J. A., Zimmerman, M. E., Swierhosz, E. M., et al.: Herpes simplex virus resistant to acyclovir: A study in a tertiary care center. Ann. Intern. Med. *112*:416–422, 1990.
83. Espy, M., and Smith, T. F.: Detection of herpes simplex virus in conventional tube cell cultures and in shell vials with a DNA probe kit and monoclonal antibodies. J. Clin. Microbiol. *26*:22–24, 1988.
84. Fedler, H. M., and Long, S. S.: Herpetic whitlow. Epidemiology, clinical characteristics, diagnosis and treatment. Am. J. Dis. Child. *137*:861–863, 1983.
85. Fife, K. H., Crumpacker, C. S., and Mertz, G. J.: Recurrence and resistance patterns of herpes simplex virus following cessation of greater than or equal to 6 years of chronic suppression with acyclovir. J. Infect. Dis. *169*:1338–1341, 1994.
86. Fiumara, N. J., and Solomon, J.: Recurrent herpes simplex virus infections and erythema multiforme: A report of three patients. Sex. Transm. Dis. *10*:144–147, 1983.
87. Fleming, D. T., McQuillan, G. M., Johnson, R. E., et al.: Herpes simplex virus type 2 in the United States, 1976 to 1994. N. Engl. J. Med. *337*:1105–1111, 1997.
88. Foley, F. D., Greenwald, K. A., Nash, G., et al.: Herpesvirus infection in burned patients. N. Engl. J. Med. *282*:652–656, 1970.
89. Frank, A. L., and Tucker, G.: Isolation of herpes simplex type 1 from ventricular fluid of an infant with encephalitis. J. Pediatr. *92*:601–602, 1978.
90. Freeman, W. R., Thomas, E. L., Rao, N. A., et al.: Demonstration of herpes group virus in acute retinal necrosis syndrome. Am. J. Ophthalmol. *102*:701–709, 1986.
91. Frenck, R. W., and Kohl, S.: Herpes simplex virus in the immunocompromised child. *In* Patrick, C. C. (ed.): Infections in Immunocompromised Infants and Children. New York, Churchill Livingstone, 1992, pp. 603–624.

92. Galbraith, J. C. T., and Shafran, S.: Herpes simplex esophagitis in the immunocompetent patient: Report of four cases and review. Clin. Infect. Dis. *14*:894–901, 1992.
93. Garland, S. M., Lee, T. N., Ashley, R. L., et al.: Automated microneutralization: Method and comparison with Western blot for type-specific detection of herpes simplex antibodies in two pregnant populations. J. Virol. Methods *55*:285–294, 1995.
94. Gateley, A., Gander, R. M., Johnson, P. C., et al.: Herpes simplex virus type 2 meningoencephalitis resistant to acyclovir in a patient with AIDS. J. Infect. Dis. *116*:711–720, 1990.
95. Genital herpes infections, United States, 1966–1984. M. M. W. R. Morb. Mortal. Wkly. Rep. *35*:402–404, 1986.
96. Gibson, J. J., Hornung, C. A., Alexander, G. R., et al.: A cross-sectional study of herpes simplex virus types 1 and 2 in college students: Occurrence and determinants of infection. J. Infect. Dis. *162*:306–312, 1990.
97. Gill, M. J., Arlette, J., and Buchan, K.: Herpes simplex virus infection of the hand. A profile of 79 cases. Am. J. Med. *84*:89–93, 1988.
98. Glezen, W. P., Fernald, G. W., and Lohr, J. A.: Acute respiratory disease of university students with special reference to the etiologic role of herpesvirus hominis. Am. J. Epidemiol. *101*:111–121, 1975.
99. Glogau, R., Hanna, L., and Jawetz, E.: Herpetic whitlow as part of genital virus infection. J. Infect. Dis. *136*:689–692, 1977.
100. Goldberg, L. H., Kaufman, R., Kurtz, T. O., et al.: Long-term suppression of recurrent genital herpes with acyclovir: A 5-year benchmark. Arch. Dermatol. *129*:582–587, 1993.
101. Goodell, S. E., Quinn, T. C., Mkrtichian, E., et al.: Herpes simplex virus proctitis in homosexual men: Clinical, sigmoidoscopic, and histopathological features. N. Engl. J. Med. *308*:868–871, 1983.
102. Goodyear, H. M., McLeish, P., Randall, S., et al.: Immunological studies of herpes simplex virus infection in children with atopic eczema. Br. J. Dermatol. *134*:85–93, 1996.
103. Greenberg, S. B., Taber, L., Septimus, E., et al.: Computerized tomography in brain-biopsy-proven herpes simplex encephalitis: Early normal results. Arch. Neurol. *38*:58–59, 1981.
104. Grossman, M. E., Stevens, A. W., and Cohen, P. R.: Brief report: Herpetic geometric glossitis. N. Engl. J. Med. *329*:1859–1860, 1993.
105. Guffond, T., Dewilde, A., Lobert, P. E., et al.: Significance and clinical relevance of the detection of herpes simplex virus DNA by polymerase chain reaction in cerebrospinal fluid from patients with presumed encephalitis. Clin. Infect. Dis. *18*:744–749, 1994.
106. Guinan, M. E., MacCalman, J., Kern, E. R., et al.: The course of untreated recurrent genital herpes simplex infection in 27 women. N. Engl. J. Med. *304*:759–763, 1983.
107. Gutman, L. T., Wilfert, C. M., and Eppes, S.: Herpes simplex virus infection in children: Analysis of cerebrospinal fluid and progressive neurodevelopmental deterioration. J. Infect. Dis. *154*:415–421, 1986.
108. Halperin, S. A., Shehab, Z., Thacker, D., et al.: Absence of viremia in primary herpetic gingivostomatitis. Pediatr. Infect. Dis. *2*:452–453, 1983.
109. Hamilton, R. L., Achim, C., Grafe, M. R., et al.: Herpes simplex virus brainstem encephalitis in an AIDS patient. Clin. Neuropathol. *14*:45–50, 1995.
110. Hammer, S. M., Buchman, T. G., D'Angelo, L. J., et al.: Temporal cluster of herpes simplex encephalitis: Investigation by restriction endonuclease cleavage of viral DNA. J. Infect. Dis. *141*:436–440, 1980.
111. Hardy, D. A., Arvin, A. M., Yasukawa, L. L., et al.: The successful identification of asymptomatic genital herpes simplex infection at delivery using the polymerase chain reaction. J. Infect. Dis. *162*:1031–l035, 1990.
112. Hargrave, D. R., and Webb, D. W.: Movement disorders in association with herpes simplex virus encephalitis in children: A review. Dev. Med. Child Neurol. *40*:640–642, 1998.
113. Herpes gladiatorum at a high school wrestling camp—Minnesota. M. M. W. R. Morb. Mortal. Wkly. Rep. *39*:69–71, 1990.
114. Herrod, H. G.: Chronic mucocutaneous candidiasis in childhood and complications of non-*Candida* infection: A report of the pediatric immunodeficiency study group. J. Pediatr. *116*:377–382, 1990.
115. Hevron, J. E.: Herpes simplex virus type 2 meningitis. Obstet. Gynecol. *49*:622–624, 1977.
116. Ho, D. W., Field, P. R., Irving, W. L., et al.: Detection of immunoglobulin M antibodies to glycoprotein G-2 by Western blot (immunoblot) for diagnosis of initial herpes simplex virus type 2 genital infections. J. Clin. Microbiol. *31*:3157–3164, 1993.
117. Hobson, A., Wald, A., Wright, N., and Corey, L.: Evaluation of a quantitative competitive PCR assay for measuring herpes simplex virus DNA content in genital tract secretions. J. Clin. Microbiol. *35*:548–552, 1997.
118. Hook, E. W. I., Cannon, R. O., Nahmras, A. J., et al.: Herpes simplex virus infection as a risk factor for human immunodeficiency virus infection in heterosexuals. J. Infect. Dis. *165*:251–255, 1992.
119. Huff, J. C., and Weston, W. L.: Recurrent erythema multiforme. Medicine (Baltimore) *68*:133–140, 1989.
120. Hull, H. F., Blumhagen, J. D., Benjamin, D., et al.: Herpes simplex viral pneumonitis in childhood. J. Pediatr. *104*:211–215, 1984.
121. Hursh, D. A., Wendt, S. F., Lee, C. F., et al.: Detection of herpes simplex virus by using A549 cells in centrifugation culture with a rapid membrane enzyme immunoassay. J. Clin. Microbiol. *27*:1695–1696, 1989.
122. Ito, Y., Ando, Y., Kimura, H., et al.: Polymerase chain reaction–proved herpes simplex encephalitis in children. Pediatr. Infect. Dis. J. *17*:29–32, 1998.
123. Jaworski, M. A., Moffatt, M. E. K., and Ahronheim, G. A.: Disseminated herpes simplex associated with *H. influenzae* infection in a previously healthy child. J. Pediatr. *96*:426–429, 1980.
124. Jenson, H. B., and Shapiro, E. D.: Primary herpes simplex virus infection of a diaper rash. Pediatr. Infect. Dis. J. *6*:1136–1138, 1987.
125. Johnson, J. R., Egaas, S., Gleaves, C. A., et al.: Hepatitis due to herpes simplex virus in marrow-transplant recipients. Clin. Infect. Dis. *14*:38–45, 1992.
126. Johnson, R. E., Nahmias, A. J., Magder, L. S., et al.: A seroepidemiologic survey of the prevalence of herpes simplex virus type 2 infection in the United States. N. Engl. J. Med. *321*:7–12, 1989.
127. Johnson, R. T., and Mims, C. A.: Pathogenesis of viral infections of the nervous system. N. Engl. J. Med. *278*:23–30, 1968.
128. Jones, T. J., and Paul, R.: Disseminated acyclovir-resistant herpes simplex virus type 2 treated successfully with foscarnet. J. Infect. Dis. *171*:508–509, 1995.
129. Kampgen, E., Bung, G., and Wank, R.: Association of herpes simplex virus–induced erythema multiforme with the human leukocyte antigen DQw3. Arch. Dermatol. *124*:1372–1375, 1988.
130. Kao, C. H., Wang, S. J., Mak, S. C., et al.: Viral encephalitis in children: Detection with technetium-99mm HMPAO brain single-photon emission CT and its value in prediction of outcome. Am. J. Neuroradiol. *15*:1369–1373, 1994.
131. Kimberlin, D. W., Lakeman, F. D., Arvin, A. M., et al.: Application of the polymerase chain reaction to the diagnosis and management of neonatal herpes simplex virus disease. National Institute of Allergy and Infectious Diseases Collaborative Antiviral Study Group. J. Infect. Dis. *174*:1162–1167, 1996.
132. Kipps, A., Becker, W., Wainwright, J., et al.: Fatal disseminated primary herpes virus infection in children: Epidemiology based on 93 non-neonatal cases. S. Afr. Med. J. *41*:647–651, 1967.
133. Klein, N. A., Mabie, W. C., Shaver, D. C., et al.: Herpes simplex virus hepatitis in pregnancy: Two patients successfully treated with acyclovir. Gastroenterology *100*:239–244, 1991.
134. Kline, M. W., Bohannon, B., Kozinetz, C. A., et al.: Characteristics of human immunodeficiency virus–associated mortality in pediatric patients with vertically transmitted infection. Pediatr. Infect. Dis. J. *11*:676–677, 1992.
135. Koelle, D. M., Benedetti, J., Langenberg, A., et al.: Asymptomatic reactivation of herpes simplex virus in women after the first episode of genital herpes. Ann. Intern. Med. *116*:433–437, 1992.
136. Koenig, H., Rabinowitz, S. G., Day, E., et al.: Postinfectious encephalomyelitis after successful treatment of herpes simplex encephalitis with adenine arabinoside: Ultrastructural observations. N. Engl. J. Med. *300*:1089–1093, 1979.
137. Kohl, S.: Herpes simplex virus encephalitis in children. Pediatr. Clin. North Am. *35*:465–483, 1988.
138. Kohl, S., Adam, E., Matson, D. O., et al.: Kinetics of human antibody responses to primary genital herpes simplex virus infection. Intervirology *18*:164–168, 1982.
139. Kohl, S., and James, A. R.: Herpes simplex virus encephalitis during childhood: The importance of brain biopsy diagnosis. J. Pediatr. *107*:212–215, 1985.
140. Koskiniemi, M., and Vaheri, A.: Effect of measles, mumps, rubella vaccination on patterns of encephalitis in children. Lancet *1*:31–34, 1989.
141. Koskiniemi, M., Vaheri, A., and Taskinen, E.: Cerebrospinal fluid alterations in herpes simplex virus encephalitis. Rev. Infect. Dis. *6*:608–619, 1984.
142. Kost, R. G., Hill, E. L., Tigges, M., et al.: Brief report: Recurrent acyclovir-resistant genital herpes in an immunocompetent patient. N. Engl. J. Med. *329*:1777–1782, 1993.
143. Koutsky, L. A., Stevens, C. E., Holmes, K. K., et al.: Underdiagnosis of genital herpes by current clinical and viral-isolation procedures. N. Engl. J. Med. *326*:1533–1539, 1992.
144. Kulhanjian, J. A., Soroush, V., Au, D. S., et al.: Identification of women at unsuspected risk of contracting primary herpes simplex virus type 2 infections during pregnancy. N. Engl. J Med. *326*:916–20, 1992.
145. Kusne, S., Schwartz, M., Breinig, M. K., et al.: Herpes simplex virus hepatitis after solid organ transplantation in adults. J. Infect. Dis. *163*:1001–1007, 1991.
146. Kuzushima, K., Kimura, H., Kino, Y., et al.: Clinical manifestations of primary herpes simplex virus type 1 infection in a closed community. Pediatrics *87*:152–158, 1991.
147. Kuzushima, K., Kudo, T., Kimura, H., et al.: Prophylactic oral acyclovir in outbreaks of primary herpes simplex virus type 1 infection in a closed community. Pediatrics *89*:379–383, 1992.
148. Lafferty, W. E., Coombs, R. W., Benedetti, J., et al.: Recurrences after oral and genital herpes simplex infection: Influence of site of infection and viral type. N. Engl. J. Med. *316*:1444–1449, 1987.
149. Lakeman, F. D., and Whitley, R. J.: Diagnosis of herpes simplex encephalitis: Application of polymerase chain reaction to cerebrospinal

fluid from brain-biopsied patients and correlation with disease. J. Infect. Dis. *171*:857–863, 1995.
150. Lalezari, J. P., Drew, H. L., Glutzer, E., et al.: Treatment with intravenous (S)-1-[3-hydroxy-2-(phosphonylmethoxy)propyl]cytosine of acyclovir-resistant mucocutaneous infection with herpes simplex virus in a patient with AIDS. J. Infect. Dis. *170*:570–572, 1994.
151. Langenberg, A., Benedetti, J., Jenkins, J., et al.: Development of clinically recognizable genital lesions among women previously identified as having "asymptomatic" herpes simplex virus type 2 infection. Ann. Intern. Med. *110*:882–887, 1989.
152. Langenberg, A. G., Burke, R. L., Adair, S. F., et al.: A recombinant glycoprotein vaccine for herpes simplex type 2: Safety and efficacy. Ann. Intern. Med. *122*:889–898, 1995.
153. Langenberg, A. G., Corey, L., Ashley, R. L., et al.: A prospective study of new infections with herpes simplex virus type 1 and type 2. N. Engl. J. Med. *341*:1432–1438, 1999.
154. Langtry, J. A., Ostlere, L. S., Hawkins, D. A., and Staughton, R. C.: The difficulty in diagnosis of cutaneous herpes simplex virus infection in patients with AIDS. Clin. Exp. Dermatol. *19*:224–226, 1994.
155. Lee, S. Y., and Pavan-Langston, D.: Role of acyclovir in the treatment of herpes simplex virus keratitis. Int. Ophthalmol. Clin. *34*:9–18, 1994.
156. Lehrman, S. N., Douglas, J. M., Corey, L., et al.: Recurrent genital herpes and suppressive oral acyclovir therapy: Relation between clinical outcome and in vitro drug sensitivity. Ann. Intern. Med. *104*:786–790, 1986.
157. Lehtinen, M., Runtala, I., Teisala, K., et al.: Detection of herpes simplex virus in women with acute pelvic inflammatory disease. J. Infect. Dis. *152*:78–82, 1985.
158. Leonard, J. R., Moran, C. J., Cross, D. T., 3rd, et al.: MR imaging of herpes simplex type 1 encephalitis in infants and young children: A separate pattern of findings. A. J. R. Am. J. Roentgenol. *174*:1651–1655, 2000.
159. Liesegang, T. J.: Classification of herpes simplex virus keratitis and anterior uveitis. Cornea *18*:127–143, 1999.
160. Linnemann, C. C., Buchman, T. G., Light, I. J., et al.: Transmission of herpes simplex virus type 1 in a nursery for the newborn: Identification of viral isolates by DNA "fingerprinting." Lancet *1*:964–966, 1978.
161. Linnemann, C. C., May, D. B., Schubert, W. K., et al.: Fatal viral encephalitis in children with X-linked hypogammaglobulinemia. Am. J. Dis. Child. *126*:100–103, 1973.
162. Ljungman, P., Ellis, M. N., Hackman, R. C., et al.: Acyclovir-resistant herpes simplex virus causing pneumonia after marrow transplantation. J. Infect. Dis. *162*:244–248, 1990.
163. Luby, J. P., Gnann, J. W., Alexander, W. J., et al.: A collaborative study of patient-initiated treatment of recurrent genital herpes with topical acyclovir or placebo. J. Infect. Dis. *150*:1–6, 1984.
164. Lumbreras, C., Fernandez, I., Velosa, J., et al.: Infectious complications following pancreatic transplantation: Incidence, microbiological and clinical characteristics, and outcome. Clin. Infect. Dis. *20*:514–520, 1995.
165. Martin A. B., Webber, S., Fricker, F. J., et al.: Acute myocarditis: Rapid diagnosis by PCR in children. Circulation *90*:330–339, 1994.
166. Masci, S., DeSimone, C., Famularo, G., et al.: Intravenous immunoglobulins suppress the recurrences of genital herpes simplex virus: A clinical and immunological study. Immunopharmacol. Immunotoxicol. *17*:33–47, 1995.
167. McMillan, J. A., Weiner, L. B., Higgins, A. M., et al.: Pharyngitis associated with herpes simplex virus in college students. Pediatr. Infect. Dis. J. *12*:280–284, 1993.
168. Mertz, G. J., Ashley, R., Burke, R. L., et al.: Double-blind, placebo-controlled trial of a herpes simplex virus type 2 glycoprotein vaccine in persons at high risk for genital herpes infection. J. Infect. Dis. *116*:653–660, 1990.
169. Mertz, G. J., Benedetti, J., Ashley, R., et al.: Risk factors for the sexual transmission of genital herpes. Ann. Intern. Med. *116*:197–202, 1992.
170. Mertz, G. J., Loveless, M. O., Krauss, S. J., et al.: Famciclovir for suppression of recurrent genital herpes. Abstract. Presented at the 34th Interscience Conference on Antimicrobial Agents and Chemotherapy, Orlando, FL, 1994, p. 11.
171. Mindel, A., Adler, M. W., Sutherland, S., et al.: Intravenous acyclovir treatment for primary genital herpes. Lancet *1*:697–700, 1982.
172. Molin, L.: Oral acyclovir prevents herpes simplex virus–associated erythema multiforme. Br. J. Dermatol. *116*:109–111, 1987.
173. Moore, D. E., Ashley, R. L., Zarutskie, P. W., et al.: Transmission of genital herpes by donor insemination. J. A. M. A. *261*:3441–3443, 1989.
174. Moore, D. J., Davidson, G. P., and Binns, G. F.: Herpes simplex oesophagitis in young children. Med. J. Aust. *144*:716–717, 1986.
175. Morawetz, R. B., Whitley, R. J., and Murphy, D. M.: Experience with brain biopsy for suspected herpes encephalitis: A review of forty consecutive cases. Neurosurgery *12*:654–657, 1983.
176. Moseley, R. D., Corey, L., Benjamin, D., et al.: Comparison of viral isolation, direct immunofluorescence, and indirect immunoperoxidase techniques for detection of genital herpes simplex virus infection. J. Clin. Microbiol. *13*:913–918, 1981.
177. Nahmias, A. J., and Whitley, R. J.: Herpes simplex virus encephalitis in pediatrics. Pediatr. Rev. *2*:259–266, 1981.
178. Nahmias, A. J., Whitley, R. J., Visintine, A. N., et al.: Herpes simplex virus encephalitis: Laboratory evaluations and their diagnostic significance. J. Infect. Dis. *145*:829–836, 1982.
179. Naraqi, S., Jackson, G. G., Jonasson, O., et al.: Prospective study of prevalence, incidence, and source of herpesvirus infections in patients with renal allografts. J. Infect. Dis. *136*:531–540, 1977.
180. Nash, G.: Necrotizing tracheobronchitis and bronchopneumonia consistent with herpetic infection. Hum. Pathol. *3*:283–291, 1972.
181. Nash, G., and Ross, J. S.: Herpetic esophagitis, a common cause of esophageal ulceration. Hum. Pathol. *5*:339–345, 1974.
182. Neiman, P. E., Reeves, W., Ray, G., et al.: A prospective analysis of interstitial pneumonia and opportunistic viral infection among recipients of allogeneic bone marrow grafts. J. Infect. Dis. *136*:754–767, 1977.
183. Nerurkar, L. S., West, F., May, M., et al.: Survival of herpes simplex virus in water specimens collected from hot tubs in spa facilities and on plastic surfaces. J. A. M. A. *250*:3081–3083, 1983.
184. Ogburn, J. R., Hoffpauir, J. T., Cole, E., et al.:. Evaluation of new transport medium for detection of herpes simplex virus by culture and direct enzyme-linked immunosorbent assay. J. Clin. Microbiol. *32*:3082–3084, 1994.
185. Orton, P. W., Huff, J. C., Tonnesen, M. G., et al.: Detection of a herpes simplex viral antigen in skin lesions of erythema multiforme. Ann. Intern. Med. *101*:48–50, 1984.
186. Owensby, L. C., and Stammer, J. L.: Esophagitis associated with herpes simplex infection in an immunocompetent host. Gastroenterology *74*:1305–1306, 1978.
187. Parrott, R. H., Wolf, S. I., Nudelman, J., et al.: Clinical and laboratory differentiation between herpangina and infectious (herpetic) gingivostomatitis. Pediatrics *14*:122–129, 1954.
188. Pavan-Langston, D., and Brockhurst, R. J.: Herpes simplex panuveitis: A clinical report. Arch. Ophthalmol. *81*:783–787, 1969.
189. Pazin, G. J., Armstrong, J. A., Lam, M. T., et al.: Prevention of reactivated herpes simplex infection by human leukocyte interferon after operation on the trigeminal root. N. Engl. J. Med. *301*:225–230, 1979.
190. Peacock, J. E., Kaplowitz, L. G., Sparling, P. F., et al.: Intravenous acyclovir therapy of first episodes of genital herpes: A multicenter double-blind, placebo controlled trial. Am. J. Med. *85*:301–306, 1988.
191. Perng, G. C., Dunkel, E. C., Geary, P. A., et al.: The latency-associated gene of herpes simplex virus type 1 (HSV-1) is required for efficient in vivo spontaneous reactivation of HSV-1 from latency. J. Virol. *68*:8045–8055, 1994.
192. Pien, F. D., Smith, T. F., Anderson, C. F., et al.: Herpesviruses in renal transplant patients. Transplantation *16*:489–495, 1973.
193. Poirier, R. H.: Herpetic ocular infections of childhood. Arch. Ophthalmol. *98*:704–706, 1980.
194. Prober, C. G., and Enzmann D. R.: Early diagnosis and management of herpes simplex encephalitis. Pediatr. Infect. Dis. J. *15*:387–388, 1996.
195. Puchhammer-Stoeckl, E., Heinz, F. X., Kundi, M, et al.:. Evaluation of the polymerase chain reaction for diagnosis of herpes simplex virus encephalitis. J. Clin. Microbiol. *31*:146–148, 1993.
196. Quinn, T. C., Corey, L., Chaffee, R. G., et al.: The etiology of anorectal infections in homosexual men. Am. J. Med. *71*:395–406, 1981.
197. Quinnan, G. V., Masur, H., Rook, A. H., et al.: Herpes virus infections in the acquired immune deficiency syndrome. J. A. M. A. *252*:72–77, 1984.
198. Ramsey, P. G., Fife, K. H., Hackman, R. C., et al.: Herpes simplex virus pneumonia: Clinical, virologic, and pathologic features in 20 patients. Ann. Intern. Med. *97*:813–820, 1982.
199. Rantala, H., and Uhari, M.: Occurrence of childhood encephalitis: A population based study. Pediatr. Infect. Dis. J. *8*:426–430, 1989.
200. Reeves, W. C., Corey, L., Adams, H. G., et al.: Risk of recurrence after first episodes of genital herpes: Relation to HSV type antibody response. N. Engl. J. Med. *305*:315–319, 1981.
201. Reichman, R. C., Badger, G. J., Guinan, M. E., et al.: Topically administered acyclovir in the treatment of recurrent herpes simplex genitalis: A controlled trial. J. Infect. Dis. *147*:336–340, 1983.
202. Revello, M. G. F., Baldanti, A., Sarasini, D., et al.: Quantitation of herpes simplex virus DNA in cerebrospinal fluid of patients with herpes simplex encephalitis by the polymerase chain reaction. Clin. Diagn. Virol. *7*:183–191, 1997.
203. 1994 Revised classification system for human immunodeficiency virus infection in children less than 13 years of age. M. M. W. R. Morb. Mortal. Wkly. Rep. *43*:1–10, 1994.
204. Rock, D. L., and Fraser, N. W.: Detection of HSV-1 genome in central nervous system of latently infected mice. Nature *302*:523, 1983.
205. Rogers, M. F., Thomas P. A., Starcher, E. T., et al.: Acquired immunodeficiency syndrome in children: Report of the Centers for Disease Control national surveillance, 1982 to 1985. Pediatrics *79*:1008–1014, 1987.
206. Roizman, B.: Herpes simplex viruses and their replication. *In* Knipe, D., and Howley, P. (eds.): Fields Virology. Philadelphia, Lippincott-Raven, 1995, pp. 2231–2296.
207. Rompalo, A. M., Mertz, G. J., and Davis, L. G.: Oral acyclovir for treatment of first episode herpes simplex virus proctitis. J. A. M. A. *19*:2879–2881, 1988.

208. Rosato, F. E., Rosato, E. F., and Plotkin, S. A.: Herpetic paronychia: An occupational hazard of medical personnel. N. Engl. J. Med. *283*:804–805, 1970.
209. Rouse, B. T., and Lopez, C. (eds.): Immunobiology of Herpes Simplex Infection. Boca Raton, FL, C.R.C. Press, 1984.
210. Rowley, A. H., Whitley, R. J., Lakeman, F. O., et al.: Rapid detection of herpes-simplex virus DNA in cerebrospinal fluid of patients with herpes simplex encephalitis. Lancet *335*:440–441, 1990.
211. Sacks, S. L., Aoki, F. Y., Diaz-Mitoma, F., et al.: Patient-initiated treatment of recurrent genital herpes with oral famciclovir: A Canadian multicenter, placebo-controlled, dose-ranging study. Abstract. Presented at the 34th Interscience Conference on Antimicrobial Agents and Chemotherapy, Orlando, FL, 1994, p. 11.
212. Sacks, S. L., Aoki, F. Y., Diaz-Mitoma, F., et al.: Patient-initiated, twice-daily oral famciclovir for early recurrent genital herpes: A randomized, double-blind multicenter trial. Canadian Famciclovir Study Group. J. A. M. A. *276*:44–49, 1996.
213. Sacks, S. L., Shafran, S. D., Diaz-Mitoma, F., et al.: A multicenter phase I/II dose escalation study of single-dose cidofovir gel for treatment of recurrent genital herpes. Antimicrob. Agents Chemother. *42*:2996–2999, 1998.
214. Safrin, S., Crumpaker, C., Chatis, P., et al.: A controlled trial comparing foscarnet with vidarabine for acyclovir-resistant, mucocutaneous herpes simplex in the acquired immunodeficiency syndrome. N. Engl. J. Med. *325*:551–555, 1991.
215. Safrin, S., Elbeik, T., and Mills, J.: A rapid screen test for in vitro susceptibility of clinical herpes simplex virus isolates. J. Infect. Dis. *169*:879–882, 1994.
216. Safrin, S., Elbeik, T., Phan, L., et al.: Correlation between response to acyclovir and foscarnet therapy and in vitro susceptibility results from isolates of herpes simplex virus from human immunodeficiency virus–infected patients. Antimicrob. Agents Chemother. *38*:1246–1250, 1994.
217. Safrin, S., Kemmerly, S., Plotkin, B., et al.: Foscarnet-resistant herpes simplex virus in patients with AIDS. J. Infect. Dis. *169*:193–196, 1994.
218. Safrin, S., Shaw, H., Bolan, G., et al.: Comparison of virus culture and the polymerase chain reaction for diagnosis of mucocutaneous herpes simplex virus infection. Sex. Transm. Dis. *24*:176–80, 1997.
219. Saijo, M., Suzutani, T., Murono, K., et al.: Recurrent aciclovir-resistant herpes simplex in a child with Wiskott-Aldrich syndrome. Br. J. Dermatol. *139*:311–314, 1998.
220. Salvini, F., Carminati, G., Pinzani, R., et al.: Chronic ulcerative herpes simplex virus infection in HIV-infected children. A. I. D. S. Patient Care S. T. D. S. *11*:421–428, 1997.
221. Sands, M., and Brown, R.: Herpes simplex lymphangitis: Two cases and a review of the literature. Arch. Intern. Med. *148*:2066–2067, 1988.
222. Saral, R., Ambinder, R. F., Burns, W. H., et al.: Acyclovir prophylaxis against herpes simplex virus infection in patients with leukemia: A randomized, double-blind, placebo-controlled study. Ann. Intern. Med. *99*:773–776, 1983.
223. Sawyer, J., Ellner, J., and Ransohoff, D. F.: To biopsy or not to biopsy in suspected herpes simplex encephalitis: A quantitative analysis. Med. Decis. Making *8*:95–101, 1988.
224. Schauseil-Zipf, U., Harden, A., Hoare, R. D., et al.: Early diagnosis of herpes simplex encephalitis in childhood: Clinical, neurophysiological and neuroradiological studies. Eur. J. Pediatr. *138*:154–161, 1982.
225. Schleiss, M. R., and Fong, W.: Primary palmar herpes simplex virus 1 infection in a ten-year-old girl. Pediatr. Infect. Dis. J. *11*:338–339, 1992.
226. Schlesinger, Y., Buller, R. S., Brunstrom, J. E., et al.: Expanded spectrum of herpes simplex encephalitis in childhood. J. Pediatr. *126*:234–241, 1995.
227. Schlesinger, Y., and Storch, G. A.: Herpes simplex meningitis in infancy. Pediatr. Infect. Dis. J. *13*:141–144, 1994.
228. Schlesinger, Y., Tebas, P., Gaudreault-Keener, M., et al.: Herpes simplex virus type 2 meningitis in the absence of genital lesions: Improved recognition with use of the polymerase chain reaction. Clin. Infect. Dis. *20*:842–848, 1995.
229. Schmidt, N. J., Dennis, J., Devlin, V., et al.: Comparison of direct immunofluorescence and direct immunoperoxidase procedures for detection of herpes simplex virus antigen in lesion specimens. J. Clin. Microbiol. *18*:445–448, 1983.
230. Schmidt, O. W., Fife, K. H., and Corey, L.: Reinfection is an uncommon occurrence in patients with symptomatic recurrent genital herpes. J. Infect. Dis. *149*:645–646, 1984.
231. Schmitt, D. L., Johnson, D. W., and Henderson, F. W.: Herpes simplex type 1 infections in group day care. Pediatr. Infect. Dis. J. *10*:729–734, 1991.
232. Schofield, J. K., Tatnall, F. M., and Leigh, I. M.: Recurrent erythema multiforme: Clinical features and treatment in a large series of patients. Br. J. Dermatol. *128*:542–545, 1993.
233. Schroth, G., Gawehn, J., Thron, A., et al.: Early diagnosis of herpes simplex encephalitis by MRI. Neurology *37*:179–183, 1987.
234. Schwab, I. R.: Oral acyclovir in the management of herpes simplex ocular infection. Ophthalmology *95*:423–430, 1988.
235. Schwartz, G. S., and Holland, E. J.: Oral acyclovir for the management of herpes simplex virus keratitis in children. Ophthalmology *107*:278–282, 2000.
236. Selling, B., and Kibrick, S.: An outbreak of herpes simplex among wrestlers (herpes gladiatorum). N. Engl. J. Med. *270*:979–982, 1964.
237. Shanley, C. J., Braun, D. K., Brown, K., et al.: Fulminant hepatic failure secondary to herpes simplex virus hepatitis: Successful outcome after orthotopic liver transplantation. Transplantation *59*:145–149, 1995.
238. Shepp, D. H., Dandiker, P. S., and Meyers, J. D.: Treatment of varicella-zoster virus infection in severely immunocompromised patients: A randomized comparison of acyclovir and vidarabine. N. Engl. J. Med. *314*:208–212, 1986.
239. Shute, P., Jeffries, D. J., and Maddocks, A. C.: Scrumpox caused by herpes simplex virus. B. M. J. *2*:1629, 1979.
240. Sibrack, C. D., Gutman, L. T., Wilfert, C. M., et al.: Pathogenicity of acyclovir-resistant herpes simplex virus type 1 from an immunodeficient child. J. Infect. Dis. *146*:673–682, 1982.
241. Skoldenberg, B.: Herpes simplex encephalitis. Scand. J. Infect. Dis. Suppl. *100*:8–13, 1996.
242. Skoldenberg, B., Alestig, K., Burman, L., et al.: Acyclovir versus vidarabine in herpes encephalitis: Randomized, multicentre study in consecutive Swedish patients. Lancet *2*:707–711, 1984.
243. Snoeck, R., Andrei, G., Gerard, M., et al.: Successful treatment of progressive mucocutaneous infection due to acyclovir- and foscarnet-resistant herpes simplex virus with (S)-1-(3-hydroxy-2-phosphonylmethyloxypropyl) cytosine (HPMPC). Clin. Infect. Dis. *18*:570–578, 1994.
244. Spicher, V. M., Bouvier, P., Schlegel-Haueter, S. E., et al.: Epidemiology of herpes simplex virus in children by detection of specific antibodies in saliva. Pediatr. Infect. Dis. J. *20*:265–272, 2001.
245. Spruance, S. L.: Pathogenesis of herpes simplex labialis: Excretion of virus in the oral cavity. J. Clin. Microbiol. *19*:675–679, 1984.
246. Spruance, S. L., Freeman, D. J., and Stewart, J. C. B.: The natural history of ultraviolet radiation–induced herpes simplex labialis and response to therapy with peroral and topical formulations of acyclovir. J. Infect. Dis. *163*:728–734, 1991.
247. Spruance, S. L., Hamill, M. L., Hoge, W. S., et al.: Acyclovir prevents reactivation of herpes simplex labialis in skiers. J. A. M. A. *260*:1597–1599, 1988.
248. Spruance, S. L., Overall, J. C., Kern, E. R., et al.: The natural history of recurrent herpes simplex labialis: Implication for antiviral therapy. N. Engl. J. Med. *297*:69–75, 1977.
249. Spruance, S. L., Schnipper, L. E., Overall, J. C., Jr., et al.: Treatment of herpes simplex labialis with topical acyclovir in polyethylene glycol. J. Infect. Dis. *146*:85–90, 1982.
250. Spruance, S. L., Stewart, J. C. B., Rowe, N. H., et al.: Treatment of recurrent herpes simplex labialis with oral acyclovir. J. Infect. Dis. *161*:185–190, 1990.
251. Stamm, W. E., Handsfield, H. H., Rompalo, A. M., et al.: The association between genital ulcer disease and acquisition of HIV infection in homosexual men. J. A. M. A. *260*:1429–1433, 1988.
252. Stanberry, L. R., Floyd-Reising, S. A., Connelly, B. L., et al.: Herpes simplex viremia: Report of eight pediatric cases and review of the literature. Clin. Infect. Dis. *18*:401–407, 1994.
253. Stevens, J. G., and Cook, M. L.: Latent herpes simplex virus in spinal ganglia of mice. Science *173*:843, 1971.
254. St. Geme, J. W., Prince, J. T., Burke, B. A., et al.: Impaired cellular resistance to herpes-simplex virus in Wiskott-Aldrich syndrome. N. Engl. J. Med. *273*:229–234, 1965.
255. Straus, S. E., Corey, L., Burke, R. L., et al.: Placebo-controlled trial of vaccination with recombinant glycoprotein D of herpes simplex virus type 2 for immunotherapy of genital herpes. Lancet *343*:1460–1463, 1994.
256. Straus, S. E., Croen, K. D., Sawyer, M. H., et al.: Acyclovir suppression of frequently recurring genital herpes: Efficacy and diminished need during successive years of treatment. J. A. M. A. *260*:2227–2230, 1988.
257. Straus, S. E., Seidlin, M., Takiff, H. E., et al.: Effect of oral acyclovir treatment on symptomatic and asymptomatic virus shedding in recurrent genital herpes. Sex. Transm. Dis. *16*:107–113, 1989.
258. Straus, S. E., Smith, H. A., Brickman, C., et al.: Acyclovir for chronic mucocutaneous herpes simplex virus infection in immunosuppressed patients. Ann. Intern. Med. *96*:270–277, 1982.
259. Straus, S. E., Takiff, H. E., Seidlin, M., et al.: Suppression of frequently recurring genital herpes: A placebo-controlled double-blind trial of oral acyclovir. N. Engl. J. Med. *310*:1545–1550, 1984.
260. Sucato, G., Celum, C., Dithmer, D., et al.: Demographic rather than behavioral risk factors predict herpes simplex virus type 2 infection in sexually active adolescents. Pediatr. Infect. Dis. J. *20*:422–426, 2001.
261. Sullender, W. M., Arvin, A. M., Diaz, P. S., et al.: Pharmacokinetics of acyclovir suspension in infants and children. Antimicrob. Agents Chemother. *31*:1722–1726, 1987.
262. Sullender, W. M., Yasukawa, L. L., Schwartz, M., et al.: Type specific antibodies to herpes simplex virus type 2 (HSV-2) glycoprotein G in pregnant women, infants exposed to maternal HSV 2 infections at delivery, and infants with neonatal herpes. J. Infect. Dis. *157*:164–171, 1988.

263. Tang, I. Y. S., Maddax, M. S., Veremis, S. A., et al.: Low-dose oral acyclovir for prevention of herpes simplex virus infection during OKT3 therapy. Transplant. Proc. *21*:1758–1760, 1989.
264. Tatnall, F. M., Schofield, J. K., and Leigh I. M.: A double-blind, placebo-controlled trial of continuous acyclovir therapy in recurrent erythema multiforme. Br. J. Dermatol. *132*:267–270, 1995.
265. Taxy, J. B., Tillaw, I., and Goldman, P. M.: Herpes simplex lymphadenitis. Arch. Pathol. Lab. Med. *109*:1043–1044, 1985.
266. Tedder, D. G., Ashley, R., Tyler, K. L., et al.: Herpes simplex virus infection as a cause of benign recurrent lymphocytic meningitis. Ann. Intern. Med. *121*:334–338, 1994.
267. Templeton, A. C.: Generalized herpes simplex in malnourished children. J. Clin. Pathol. *23*:24–30, 1970.
268. Terni, M., Caccialanza, P., Cassai, E., et al.: Aseptic meningitis in association with herpes progenitalis. N. Engl. J. Med. *285*:503–505, 1971.
269. Trachtman, H., Weiss, R. A., Spigland, I., et al.: Clinical manifestations of herpesvirus infections in pediatric renal transplant recipients. Pediatr. Infect. Dis. J. *4*:480–486, 1985.
270. Troendle-Atkins, J., Demmler, G. J., and Buffone, G. J.: Rapid diagnosis of herpes simplex virus encephalitis by using the polymerase chain reaction. J. Pediatr. *123*:376–380, 1993.
271. Tse, P., Aarnaes, S. L., de la Meza, L. M., and Peterson, E. M.: Detection of herpes simplex virus by 8 h in shell vial cultures with primary rabbit kidney cells. J. Clin. Microbiol. *27*:199–200, 1989.
272. Turner, B. J., Denison, M., Eppes, S. C., et al.: Survival experience of 789 children with the acquired immunodeficiency syndrome. Pediatr. Infect. Dis. J. *12*:310–320, 1993.
273. Turner, R., Shehab, Z., Osborne, K., et al.: Shedding and survival of herpes simplex virus from "fever blisters." Pediatrics *70*:547–549, 1982.
274. Tyring, S. K., Douglas, J. M., Jr., Corey, L., et al.: A randomized, placebo-controlled comparison of oral valacyclovir and acyclovir in immunocompetent patients with recurrent genital herpes infections. The Valaciclovir International Study Group. Arch. Dermatol. *134*:185–191, 1998.
275. Uren, E. C., Johnson, P. D., Montanaro, J., et al.: Herpes simplex virus encephalitis in pediatrics: Diagnosis by detecting antibodies and DNA in cerebrospinal fluid. Pediatr. Infect. Dis. J. *12*:1001–1006, 1993.
276. Verano, L., and Michalski, F. J.: Comparison of a direct antigen enzyme immunoassay, Herpchek, with cell culture for detection of herpes simplex virus from clinical specimens. J. Clin. Microbiol. *33*:1378–1379, 1995.
277. Vital, C., Monlun, E., Vital, A., et al.: Concurrent herpes simplex virus type 1 necrotizing encephalitis, cytomegalovirus ventriculoencephalitis and cerebral lymphoma in an AIDS patient. Acta Neuropathol. *89*:105–108, 1995.
278. Wade, J. C., Day, L. M., Crowley, J. J., et al.: Recurrent infection with herpes simplex virus after marrow transplantation: Role of the specific immune response and acyclovir treatment. J. Infect. Dis. *149*:750–756, 1984.
279. Wade, J. C., and Meyers, J. D.: Neurologic symptoms associated with parenteral acyclovir treatment after marrow transplantation. Ann. Intern. Med. *98*:921–925, 1983.
280. Wade, J. C., Newton, B., McLaren, C., et al.: Intravenous acyclovir to treat mucocutaneous herpes simplex virus infection after marrow transplantation: A double-blind trial. Ann. Intern. Med. *96*:265–269, 1982.
281. Wald, A., Zeh, J., Barnum, G., et al.: Suppression of subclinical shedding of herpes simplex virus type 2 with acyclovir. Ann. Intern. Med. *124*:8–15, 1996.
282. Wald, A., Zeh, J., Selke, S., et al.:. Reactivation of genital herpes simplex virus type 2 infection in asymptomatic seropositive persons. N. Engl. J. Med. *342*:844–850, 2000.
283. Wang, H. S., Kuo, M. F., Huang, S. C., et al.: Choreoathetosis as an initial sign of relapsing of herpes simplex encephalitis. Pediatr. Neurol. *11*:341–345, 1994.
284. Wasserman, R., August, C. S., and Plotkin, S. A.: Viral infections in pediatric bone marrow transplant patients. Pediatr. Infect. Dis. J. *7*:109–115, 1988.
285. Waugh, M. A.: Anorectal herpesvirus hominis infection in men. J. Am. Vener. Dis. Assoc. *3*:68–70, 1976.
286. Weston, W. L., Brice, S. L., Jester, J. D., et al.: Herpes simplex virus in childhood erythema multiforme. Pediatrics *89*:32–34, 1992.
287. Wheeler, C. E., Jr., and Abele, D. C.: Eczema herpeticum, primary and recurrent. Arch. Dermatol. *93*:162–173, 1966.
288. White, W. B., and Grant-Kels, J. M.: Transmission of herpes simplex virus type 1 infection in rugby players. J. A. M. A. *252*:533–535, 1984.
289. Whitley. R. J.: Herpes simplex viruses. *In* Roizman, B., Knipe, D., and Howley, P. (eds.): Fields Virology. Philadelphia, Lippincott-Raven, 1995, p. 2296.
290. Whitley, R. J., Alford, C. A., Hirsch, M. S., et al.: Vidarabine versus acyclovir therapy in herpes simplex encephalitis. N. Engl. J. Med. *314*:144–149, 1986.
291. Whitley, R. J., and Arvin, A. M.: Herpes simplex virus infection. *In* Remington, J., and Klein, J. (eds.): Infectious Diseases of the Fetus and Newborn. 4th ed. Philadelphia, W. B. Saunders, 1995, pp. 354–372.
292. Whitley, R. J., Cobbs, C. G., Alford, C. A., Jr., et al.: Diseases that mimic herpes simplex encephalitis: Diagnosis, presentation, and outcome. J. A. M. A. *262*:234–239, 1989.
293. Whitley, R. J., Lakeman, A. D., Nahmias, A., et al.: DNA restriction-enzyme analysis of herpes simplex virus isolates obtained from patients with encephalitis. N. Engl. J. Med. *307*:1060–1062, 1982.
294. Whitley, R. J., Levin, M., Marton, N., et al.: Infections caused by herpes simplex virus in the immunocompromised host: Natural history and topical acyclovir therapy. J. Infect. Dis. *150*:323–329, 1984.
295. Whitley, R. J., Soong, S. J., Dolin, R., et al.: Adenine arabinoside therapy of biopsy-proved herpes simplex encephalitis. N. Engl. J. Med. *297*:289–294, 1977.
296. Whitley, R. J., Soong, S. J., Linneman, C., Jr., et al.: Herpes simplex encephalitis: Clinical assessment. J. A. M. A. *247*:317–320, 1982.
297. Wilhelmus, K. R., Beck, R. W., Moke, P. S., et al.: Acyclovir for the prevention of recurrent herpes simplex virus eye disease. The Herpetic Eye Disease Study Group. N. Engl. J. Med. *339*:300–306, 1998.
298. Wishart, M. S., Darougar, S., and Viswalingam, N. D.: Recurrent herpes simplex virus ocular infection: Epidemiological and clinical features. Br. J. Ophthalmol. *71*:669–672, 1987.
299. Wood, D. J., and Corbitt, G.: Viral infections in childhood leukemia. J. Infect. Dis. *152*:266–273, 1985.
300. Yamamoto, L. Y., Tedder, D. G., Ashley, R., et al.: Herpes simplex virus type 1 DNA in cerebrospinal fluid of a patient with Mollaret's meningitis. N. Engl. J. Med. *325*:1082–1085, 1991.

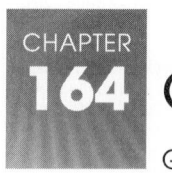

CHAPTER 164 Cytomegalovirus

GAIL J. DEMMLER

Cytomegalovirus (CMV) is a ubiquitous agent that commonly infects persons of all ages from all parts of the world and from all socioeconomic and cultural backgrounds. Although most CMV infections are asymptomatic, certain patient groups are at risk for acquiring serious, even life-threatening illness. Discerning which role CMV is playing in a particular patient requires a thorough understanding of the epidemiology, virology, and pathophysiology of the virus and can be difficult, even for the most experienced clinicians.

History

The recorded history of CMV probably began in 1881, when Ribbert described and then in 1904 reported "protozoan-like cells" in the organs of an infant who died of presumed congenital syphilis.[221] In 1921, Goodpasture and Talbot[112] hypothesized that these swollen cells, or "cytomegalia," were host cells that had been injured by a virus. During the first half of the 20th century, CMV was recognizable only by the pathologic changes that it produced in infected cells, and because these cells frequently were seen in the salivary glands of animals and humans, CMV originally was called the salivary gland virus.

In 1956, human CMV first was isolated in tissue culture by three independent investigators, Rowe, Smith, and Weller.[227, 242, 283] Because several human and animal viruses subsequently were found to replicate in salivary glands, the descriptive name *cytomegalovirus* was proposed by Weller in 1960. The ability to cultivate CMV in tissue culture led to the development of serologic techniques, which in the 1960s and 1970s resulted in many important clinical and epidemiologic observations. For example, CMV was found to commonly infect people of all ages throughout the world. By 1962, CMV was established as a significant pathogen of the fetus and newborn that was capable of producing a spectrum of clinical manifestations and neurologic sequelae.[282] In 1966, Kaariainen and colleagues[143] presented evidence supporting CMV as a cause of post-transfusion mononucleosis syndrome.

The molecular biology of the virus was explored during the 1970s and 1980s and continues to be studied by many investigators. In addition, during the 1970s and 1980s, CMV emerged as a major cause of morbidity and mortality in immunosuppressed patients, especially those who underwent organ or marrow transplantation or who had acquired immunodeficiency syndrome (AIDS). In 1976, the first clinical trial of the live attenuated CMV vaccine Towne 125 was reported; since then, more than 500 renal allograft recipients, as well as healthy young men and women, have received the vaccine under investigational protocols.[98, 201] In addition, research on a subunit vaccine based on glycoproteins of the virus began in the 1980s, and in the 1990s, recombinant vaccines were developed and tested in human volunteers. CMV infection has become a treatable disease, with two specific antiviral agents, ganciclovir (licensed in 1989) and foscarnet (licensed in 1991), now available to clinicians to treat seriously ill patients.

Virology

CMV is a member of the *Herpesviridae* family of DNA viruses. This family contains many important human pathogens and is subdivided into three subfamilies: (1) *Alphaherpesvirinae,* fast-growing, cytolytic viruses that are latent in neurons and include herpes simplex virus (HSV) types 1 and 2 and varicella-zoster virus (VZV); (2) *Betaherpesvirinae,* slow-growing, cytomegalic viruses that contain the CMVs; and (3) *Gammaherpesvirinae,* herpesviruses that preferentially grow in lymphocytes and sometimes transform them into malignant states. This subfamily includes Epstein-Barr virus and, tentatively, the newly recognized human herpesviruses 6, 7, and 8.

CMV is the largest member of *Herpesviridae.* The genome is double-stranded DNA 240 kb in size (150×10^6 d; guanine + cytosine [G+C] content, 58 percent), and it has a unique long sequence and a unique short sequence, both of which are bounded by repetitive sequences that are inverted relative to each other. The genome, therefore, can assume four isomeric forms. The viral particle has a 110-nm icosahedral capsid composed of 162 capsomeres. The entire virion is enclosed by a lipid envelope, which yields a final diameter of approximately 200 nm.[258]

Replication of CMV is slow when compared with that of HSV. Whereas it takes herpes simplex only 4 to 8 hours to produce infectious progeny virus, CMV requires at least 24 hours. The CMV genome is transcribed slowly in a regulated sequence; on the basis of the appearance of different classes of CMV-specific proteins, the replicative cycle can be divided into three periods: immediate-early, early, and late. The immediate-early period is defined as the first 4 hours after infection. During this period, specific segments of the DNA genome undergo restricted transcription, and certain regulatory proteins are produced that allow the virus to take control of host-cell macromolecular synthesis. The early period of replication begins after the immediate-early phase and persists for almost 20 hours. This period is characterized by replication of viral DNA, synthesis of infected cell proteins, and production of progeny virus. The late period usually is considered to occur 24 hours after infection. During this period, the structural components of the virus are produced, and infectious virus is released from the cell. Monoclonal antibodies against the various immediate-early, early, and late proteins produced by CMV have been used as rapid viral diagnostic tools.

CMV has no distinct serotypes. However, strain relatedness or differences can be determined by molecular analysis of viral DNA. Restriction enzyme analysis of DNA extracted from CMV isolates that are linked epidemiologically (for example, serial isolates from the same person, mother-infant pairs, or family members experiencing temporally related CMV infections) shows identical or similar DNA fragment–mapping patterns. This technique or modifications of this technique have been applied to the epidemiology of CMV in a variety of patients, such as transplant recipients, congenitally infected infants, and patients whose CMV was transmitted from person to person in hospitals, daycare centers, and residences. More recent studies have used polymerase chain reaction (PCR) methodology to determine whether CMV genotypes exist by showing differences in the *a* sequence, major immediate-early (MIE), glycoprotein B (gB or UL55), and the UL144 regions of the viral genome.[21] Four gB genotypes have been characterized recently, and studies suggest that adverse outcomes after CMV infection may be linked to infection with a specific gB genotype. Infection with the CMV gB3 genotype appears to be associated more commonly with fatal infections in bone marrow transplant recipients, and CMV gB2 and gB4 genotypes appear to be more often fatal in patients with AIDS.[103, 211] At this time, all known gB genotypes appear to cause congenital CMV infection, but no relationship between gB genotypes and congenital CMV infection and disease or sequelae has been found.[21]

Epidemiology

Seroepidemiologic studies have shown that infection with CMV occurs commonly and usually is inapparent.[300] The incidence of CMV infection does not appear to be seasonal. However, the prevalence of CMV IgG antibody is influenced by many factors, including the age, geographic location, cultural and socioeconomic status, and child-rearing practices of the group. For example, in developed countries such as the United Kingdom and the United States, the prevalence of CMV antibody is 40 to 60 percent in adult populations of middle-upper socioeconomic status and more than 80 percent in lower socioeconomic status groups.[118, 254, 299] In contrast, in developing countries, 80 percent of children acquire CMV by the time that they reach 3 years of age, and almost all persons have been infected by adulthood.[11, 14, 278] Studies on the age-related prevalence of infection with CMV in the United States suggest three periods of increased acquisition: early childhood, adolescence, and the child-bearing years.[11, 284, 298]

INFANTS AND CHILDREN

Approximately 1 percent of all newborns are born congenitally infected with CMV; ranges of 0.2 to 2.5 percent are reported.[228] Maternal CMV infection that is either primary or recurrent during pregnancy can result in an infant who is infected congenitally with CMV. However, the rate of intrauterine infection with recurrent infection in the mother is less than 1 percent, whereas transmission to the fetus occurs in 40 to 50 percent of mothers who are infected primarily with CMV during pregnancy.[254] Although most newborns congenitally infected with CMV are asymptomatic, symptoms and sequelae are much more likely to occur in infants congenitally infected as a result of the mother's primary infection during pregnancy than in infants congenitally infected from a recurrent maternal infection.

CMV also can be transmitted perinatally from a mother to her infant. The virus can be shed in the mother's cervicovaginal secretions, urine, saliva, and breast milk. The most common and most efficient routes of perinatal transmission are ingestion or aspiration of cervicovaginal secretions at the time of delivery or ingestion of breast milk after delivery. CMV-seropositive mothers frequently shed CMV in their breast milk, and as many as 53 percent of children who are breast-fed with milk that contains infectious virus can become infected with CMV.[85] These infections usually are benign in normal-term infants but may be extremely serious in preterm, very low-birth-weight neonates.[169, 276] In addition, as many as 57 percent of babies whose mothers shed CMV at or around the time of delivery become infected with CMV.[220]

Children not congenitally or perinatally infected with CMV may be infected during the toddler or preschool years. The acquisition of CMV by children between 1 and 3 years of age is influenced by home exposure to the virus, by the socioeconomic status of the family, and by group daycare exposure. Weller and Hanshaw[282] suggested that the child-rearing practices in Sweden, where group daycare was common practice, accounted for the relatively high prevalence of CMV infection in Swedish children when compared with children in the United States and Great Britain, where daycare centers were not common at that time.

Pass and colleagues[191] first reported the prevalence of CMV in daycare centers in the United States in 1982.[191] They found that 51 percent of children who attended a daycare center in Alabama excreted CMV in their saliva or urine. In this study, the prevalence of CMV excretion varied with age; 83 percent of children 13 to 24 months of age shed virus as opposed to only 9 percent of children younger than 1 year. Pass and colleagues concluded that the high prevalence of CMV infection probably was due to horizontal spread between the children in daycare. Subsequent studies have confirmed a high prevalence of CMV excretion in children in daycare centers across the United States. Overall prevalence rates of 22 to 57 percent have been observed, with the highest prevalence of active CMV infection (29–78%) found in children 1 to 3 years of age.[1, 140, 179, 191, 193, 194] Children who attend daycare centers also shed high titers of virus (up to 10^5 median tissue culture infective dose per milliliter), with a mean duration of viral shedding of 13 months in urine and 7 months in saliva.[179] This prolonged, generally asymptomatic shedding of large quantities of virus, coupled with mobility and the less than hygienic daily habits notorious in toddler-aged children, no doubt facilitates the transmission of CMV in daycare centers.

Several studies support the idea that the high prevalence of CMV infection in young children who attend daycare centers is due to horizontal transmission; these studies used molecular fingerprinting techniques to show that infected children in contact with each other shed strains of CMV with similar or identical restriction enzyme banding patterns and that predominant strains of CMV appeared to circulate over a given period in a given daycare center.[1, 2, 134] Reinfection with a genetically different strain of CMV also has been observed and may be important in child-to-child transmission of CMV in the daycare center environment.[5] The importance of horizontal spread of CMV has been shown in special care centers for mentally retarded children as well.[238] CMV also has been isolated from plastic toys and from the hands of daycare center workers.[90, 134, 191]

Current epidemiologic evidence suggests that CMV-infected children may transmit the virus to the daycare center workers who care for them.[2, 4] In addition, children who attend daycare centers may transmit CMV to their CMV-seronegative parents. In one study of parents of children who attended one of three daycare centers in Alabama, 14 of 67 parents (21%) whose children attended daycare seroconverted, as compared with none of 31 parents whose children were cared for at home.[195] Excretion of CMV by the child clearly was a key risk factor for parental seroconversion because none of the seroconversions occurred in parents whose children attended the daycare center but did not shed CMV. Moreover, this study revealed a strong trend toward a greater risk of acquiring CMV infection (seroconversion rate, 45%) in the parents of children 18 months or younger. Additional evidence implicating young children who attend daycare centers as a source of CMV infection for their parents was provided by a study in Virginia daycare centers, in which the parents of children in daycare shed CMV strains identical to the strains shed by their children.[3] Furthermore, CMV strains from daycare settings, when transmitted from toddlers to their pregnant mothers, may be the source of congenital infection.[180]

Whereas early childhood the most is probably rapid period of acquisition of CMV, annual seroconversion rates of only 3 to 6.2 percent have been observed in older children 3 to 10 years of age in the United States, thus reflecting an age-related plateau in the acquisition of CMV. One identified risk factor for the acquisition of CMV infection in a school-age child has been recent or active CMV infection in a family member.[298]

ADOLESCENTS

In support of these early findings, a seroepidemiologic study of CMV infection in sexually active adolescent females found a strong association between indicators of sexual activity and serologic evidence of CMV infection and concluded that sexual activity was an important risk factor for the acquisition of CMV infection in adolescent girls.[49, 245] Early cross-sectional epidemiologic studies of CMV implied a gradual increase in CMV antibody prevalence during the teenage years, and this period of rapid acquisition was attributed to the intimate physical contact that is so common during the teenage years.[11, 226] However, these studies were conducted primarily in lower socioeconomic groups. In a seroepidemiologic study of several groups in Houston on the acquisition of CMV infection in late childhood and adolescence, the prevalence of antibody increased with age in subjects of nonwhite races, as it did according to previous studies, but the prevalence of antibody in subjects of white race did not increase with age.[284]

Vertical transmission of CMV acquired during the teenage years may result in congenital infection with CMV in infants born to teenage mothers. In 1984, Kumar and colleagues[154] studied primary CMV infection in more than 3000 pregnant adolescents in Ohio. They found that 57 percent were CMV-seropositive, that 1 percent of susceptible pregnant adolescents acquired CMV, and that if primary CMV infection occurred during pregnancy, the risk of intrauterine transmission was 50 percent. Information provided by the National Registry for CMV Disease and the National Center for Health Statistics suggests that adolescents who are pregnant actually may be at higher risk than are older mothers for giving birth to an infant with congenital CMV disease because 34 percent of mothers who give birth to a baby with congenital CMV disease are younger than 20 years; however, this age group represents only 16 percent of the mothers giving birth in the United States.[68, 135]

INTRAFAMILIAL TRANSMISSION

CMV also can be transmitted within the family setting. Evidence for intrafamilial transmission of CMV has been provided in the form of case reports, seroepidemiologic studies, and accounts in which molecular analysis of CMV strains was used to trace the transmission of CMV in family members or extended family members with temporally related CMV infections. In most studies, the index case was a child; when a CMV-infected child entered a household, attack rates were 47 to 53 percent.[264, 295]

Three patterns of intrafamilial transmission have been observed: transmission between siblings, transmission between parents, and transmission between children and parents. Additional support for the intrafamilial transmission of CMV has been provided by published studies in which molecular analysis was performed on CMV isolates from family members or extended family members who experienced temporally related CMV infections. In each of these studies, restriction enzyme analysis of viral DNA from CMV isolates in family members showed that the strain of CMV was the same within each family.[83, 196, 252] New molecular techniques based on PCR amplification of a hypervariable region of the CMV genome also have corroborated the observation that genetically similar strains of CMV can be transmitted between family members over the course of time.[246]

SEXUAL TRANSMISSION

CMV also appears to be transmitted by heterosexual and homosexual contact. The evidence to support sexual transmission is anecdotal, virologic, serologic, and molecular and, when taken together, suggests that sexual transmission of CMV is important in certain groups. However, because the virus is shed in saliva, cervicovaginal secretions, and semen, which form of intimate contact results in transmission between sex partners is unclear.[71, 158, 220]

Several observations support the idea that CMV can be transmitted sexually. For example, CMV antibody prevalence increases with age, CMV antibody is more prevalent in sexually active women than in celibate women, CMV antibody is associated with indices of sexual activity such as recent infection with *Chlamydia trachomatis* or *Neisseria gonorrhoeae,* and a strikingly high annual incidence (37%) of primary CMV infection has been observed in young women with a recent first sexual experience.[50, 60, 67, 141, 245, 289] In addition, in a longitudinal study of the site-specific shedding of CMV in human immunodeficiency virus (HIV)-seropositive homosexual and bisexual men, CMV was cultured from semen more frequently than from other body sites or fluids.[223] Moreover, molecular analysis of viral DNA has shown strains of CMV isolated from sex partners to be identical in most cases analyzed.[71, 124]

Infection of the genital tract can recur by reactivation of an endogenous strain or by reinfection with an exogenous or different strain of CMV.[245] The consequences of such reinfections are unknown but may have important implications, especially if a CMV vaccine is used to control congenital CMV disease in the future.

NOSOCOMIAL TRANSMISSION

CMV can be transmitted in the hospital setting by transfusion of blood products, by bone marrow and organ transplantation, and, rarely, by person-to-person transmission. Despite numerous studies that have used serologic, virologic, and molecular epidemiologic techniques, transmission of CMV from a CMV-infected patient to a health care worker has not been documented.[6, 17, 22, 33, 73, 84, 132] Therefore, even though health care workers are exposed to CMV-infected patients, their risk of acquiring CMV appears to be no greater than that of the general population. In addition, unlike homes and daycare centers, hospitals routinely perform rigorous infection control procedures, including universal precautions, which probably accounts for the relatively low risk of acquiring CMV, as well as other infections, in the hospital setting. However, infant-to-infant transmission has been shown to occur, albeit infrequently, in crowded hospital units with a high prevalence of CMV excretion in patients.[73, 248] CMV also can survive on plastic surfaces and has been cultured from inanimate objects in contact with CMV-infected patients in the hospital setting.[73, 208]

Blood products are a well-established source of CMV infection, and donor-to-recipient transmission of CMV has been documented by restriction enzyme analysis of viral DNA.[267] Post-transfusion CMV mononucleosis can be seen in adults who receive large volumes of fresh whole blood.[143] In addition, 15 to 17 percent of CMV-seronegative neonates who receive blood products from CMV-seropositive donors acquire CMV.[296] Post-transfusion CMV infection in newborns, especially premature infants, can cause a syndrome of shock, lymphocytosis, and pneumonitis; CMV infection also appears to hasten the progression to bronchopulmonary dysplasia in these patients.[232, 296]

CMV apparently is transmitted in the residual leukocytes found in whole blood, packed red blood cells, and platelet fractions, as well as by pure leukocyte transfusions. The risk of post-transfusion CMV infection developing is approximately 3 percent per unit transfused, and the risk of symptomatic infection is much higher in CMV-seronegative recipients than in CMV-seropositive recipients.

IMMUNOSUPPRESSED PATIENTS

Primary and reactivation infections, as well as reinfection with CMV, occur commonly in organ and marrow transplant recipients. Active infection with CMV occurs in almost all organ and marrow transplant recipients and usually is manifested clinically and virologically 30 to 90 days after transplantation. Rarely, CMV retinitis can occur years after transplantation and generally is associated with chronic CMV viremia.[96] CMV can be transmitted to the recipient by the transplanted organ, by transfused blood products, and, theoretically, also by intimate contact with persons actively infected with CMV.

Infections with CMV are primary when they occur in CMV-seronegative recipients who receive transplants or blood products from CMV-seropositive donors. Recipients who are CMV-seropositive pretransplant can experience reactivation of their own endogenous strain of CMV. In addition, CMV-seropositive transplant recipients may be superinfected by strains of CMV present in the donor organ.[53] In fact, in one study of renal transplant recipients in the United Kingdom, proven superinfection with the donor's strain of CMV was more common than proven reactivation of the recipient's strain of virus.[121] Although reactivation, reinfection, and primary CMV infection all can produce symptoms in immunosuppressed transplant recipients, primary CMV infections are much more likely to be severe and even fatal.[206]

The type of transplant also appears to influence the type of CMV disease expressed. For example, the most severe and lethal form of CMV interstitial pneumonitis is seen in bone marrow transplant recipients, especially those experiencing a graft-versus-host reaction. CMV pneumonia also is a common occurrence after heart, lung, or renal transplantation, and severe CMV hepatitis is a special problem after liver transplantation.

The iatrogenic immunosuppression essential for graft maintenance probably is responsible for the common occurrence of reactivation infection after transplantation, as well as the increased incidence of severe and symptomatic infection seen after primary CMV infection in transplant recipients. Cytotoxic drugs such as cyclophosphamide and azathioprine, in addition to corticosteroids, have been associated with reactivation of latent CMV infection, and the addition of antilymphocyte globulin to an immunosuppressive regimen can increase the morbidity of CMV infections.[197] The use of cyclosporine as the primary immunosuppressive agent, even in conjunction with corticosteroids, does not appear to reduce the risk of acquiring CMV infection when compared with a regimen of azathioprine and corticosteroids; however, it may decrease the incidence of severe, symptomatic CMV disease in some transplant recipients.[82] The use of OKT3 to treat rejection in certain transplant patients increases the risk for dissemination in those with primary CMV infection.[240]

The frequency and morbidity of CMV infection in patients with malignancies are not as high as in patients who have undergone marrow and organ transplantation; however, the use of chemotherapy, especially for leukemias, is associated with significant CMV disease, particularly pneumonitis and persistent fever with viral dissemination. CMV-seropositive patients receiving immunosuppressive therapy for connective tissue disease also can have significant reactivation infection with CMV.[78]

The progressive and profound immunosuppression in adults and children with AIDS also is associated with CMV infection and disease. Although the source of CMV infection in adults with AIDS most likely is heterosexual or homosexual contact, sources of CMV infection in young children with AIDS have not been determined. One can hypothesize, however, that many of these infections are acquired from the mother, either congenitally or perinatally. Infants infected perinatally with HIV who also acquire CMV congenitally appear to be at significant risk for rapid progression of disease in the first 18 months of life, as well as for debilitating neurologic disease.[79, 153, 235] Patients with AIDS also may be infected with multiple strains of CMV.[81, 249]

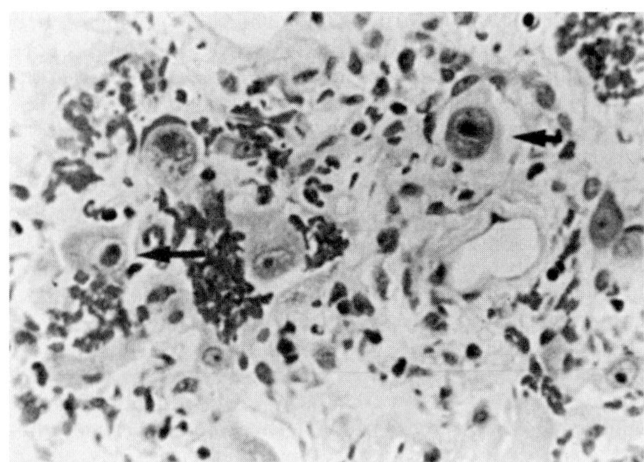

FIGURE 164–1 ■ Typical cytomegalic inclusion cells seen in lung tissue obtained by open lung biopsy from a bone marrow transplant recipient with fatal cytomegalovirus pneumonitis (×640). (Courtesy of Dr. Milton J. Finegold, Department of Pathology, Texas Children's Hospital, Houston.)

Pathology, Pathogenesis, and Immunity

CMV infection causes characteristic type A Cowdry intranuclear inclusions and massive enlargement of the affected cells (Fig. 164–1). It is this property of "cytomegaly" from which CMV acquired its name. The cytomegalic cells (25 to 40 μm in diameter) are two to four times larger than normal cells, and the nucleus usually is more than 10 μm in diameter. The intranuclear inclusion also is large (up to 10 μm in diameter) and is surrounded by an intranuclear halo and then the nuclear membrane, which gives a characteristic "owl's eye" appearance. Basophilic, granular, intracytoplasmic inclusions (2 to 4 μm in diameter) also may be present in cells that have intranuclear inclusions. These large cells represent productive virus infection, and both the nuclear and cytoplasmic inclusions contain viral nucleocapsids and express virus-specific antigens.[129] These cytomegalic cells frequently are associated with epithelial cells, and their presence generally indicates a productive and symptomatic infection with CMV. Cells also may be infected latently with CMV. These cells may express virus-specific antigen and contain viral nucleic acid without producing typical cytomegaly or a cytopathic effect. The significance of these cells must be considered carefully within the clinical context of the patient.

With severe, disseminated CMV disease, involvement can be seen in virtually all organ systems. The salivary glands are infected commonly in both symptomatic and asymptomatic infections, and the ductal epithelium usually is the site of pathologic involvement. The kidneys also are infected commonly in both symptomatic and asymptomatic CMV infection. In the kidneys, cytomegalic cells are most pronounced in the proximal tubules and interstitial cellular infiltrates, and even immune complex deposits can be seen in the glomeruli.

CMV infection often causes prolonged viruria, but it rarely results in significant renal dysfunction. In the lungs, cytomegalic cells are seen in alveolar and bronchial epithelium and are associated with mononuclear cell inflammation. Pulmonary alveolar macrophages also may express viral antigen and contain CMV DNA. The brain parenchyma can be involved, and a variety of pathologic processes can be observed and include sensorineural hearing loss. Other organs that can be infected or diseased with CMV include the liver, pancreas, adrenals, eyes, lymph nodes, heart, skin, bone, male and female genital tracts, esophagus, stomach, intestine, and placenta.

Infections with CMV can be latent and nonproductive, productive yet asymptomatic, or productive and symptomatic. Therefore, determining whether a patient is "sick with CMV" or "sick from CMV" sometimes is difficult. Viral strain differences have not been shown to date to influence pathogenicity. However, immune responses, including maturity of the immune response, appear to be a major factor in virulence of the infection because CMV disease occurs more frequently in fetuses, premature neonates, transplant recipients, and patients with AIDS than in older healthy infants, children, and adults with acquired CMV infection.

The cell-mediated immune response, both specific and nonspecific, is thought to be important in host defense against CMV. The nonspecific immune mechanisms of natural killer cells and interferon production occur soon after the development of CMV infection, when early antigens are being produced and before infectious virus is released from the cell. The generation of cytotoxic T cells against CMV early antigens probably is the most important specific host immune response to CMV, and patients who are defective in this T-cell response are at high risk for acquiring serious CMV disease.[119]

Clinical and laboratory evidence also supports the concept of CMV as an immunosuppressive agent. The proliferative response of T cells to stimulation with mitogens and CMV antigen is suppressed in patients with CMV mononucleosis, and immunosuppressed patients with active CMV disease commonly have other opportunistic infections.[222] In addition, CMV pneumonitis in bone marrow transplant recipients has been hypothesized to result from host cell–mediated events produced in response to chronic viral replication.[301] Homology between certain CMV proteins and class I and II major histocompatibility complex products has been observed. This "molecular mimicry" implies that the severe tissue destruction seen in CMV pneumonitis may be partly an autoimmune phenomenon in these patients.

Humoral immunity, on the other hand, does not appear to be a key factor in the host's defense against CMV infection. For example, the fetus can be infected via intrauterine transmission as a result of reactivation of CMV infection in a woman who is CMV seropositive before pregnancy, and infants commonly are infected perinatally from infected cervicovaginal secretions or breast milk in the presence of passive maternal antibody.[254] In addition, CMV-seropositive transplant recipients can be reinfected with a new strain of CMV from the donor organ, and viruria and viremia occur in transplant recipients despite high titers of neutralizing antibody against the specific strain of CMV.[53, 54] The presence of CMV antibody, therefore, should be considered a marker of previous or current infection with the virus rather than a measure of immunity per se.

Although humoral immunity does not appear to prevent infection with CMV, it does appear to lessen the severity of symptoms associated with the infection. Infants congenitally infected with CMV as a result of reactivation infection in their mother almost always are asymptomatic, whereas perinatally infected infants rarely have significant symptoms. Primary infections in transplant recipients are more likely to be symptomatic than is reinfection or reactivation. One hypothesis regarding how CMV eludes host humoral defenses is that the virus binds to the host protein β_2-microglobulin and masks the antigenic determinants that are important for neutralization by antibody.[172]

Clinical Manifestations

CONGENITAL INFECTIONS

Annually, 30,000 to 40,000 babies are born with congenital CMV infection. Of these babies, as many as 10 percent have severe, classic "cytomegalic inclusion disease" characterized by intrauterine growth retardation, jaundice, hepatosplenomegaly, thrombocytopenia with petechiae and purpura, pneumonia, and severe central nervous system (CNS) damage with microcephaly, intracerebral calcifications, chorioretinitis, and sensorineural hearing loss (see Fig. 65–21). Another 5 percent have atypical involvement such as ventriculomegaly, periventricular leukomalacia, periventricular cystic malformations with or without calcifications, strabismus, optic atrophy, long bone osteitis characterized by fine vertical metaphyseal striations, isolated and transient thrombocytopenia and petechiae, cutaneous vasculitis, hemolytic anemia, ascites, and chronic hepatitis.[58] As many as 90 percent of these infants who are symptomatic at birth later have neurologic sequelae or progressive deafness. However, the range of severity of these sequelae appears to be broad, and severity may be predicted by head circumference and computed tomographic findings at birth.[31, 186]

The differential diagnosis of symptomatic congenital CMV disease includes congenital toxoplasmosis, congenital HSV infection, congenital syphilis, congenital rubella syndrome, congenital infection with lymphocytic choriomeningitis virus, and congenital HIV infection. In addition, noninfectious causes, such as genetic disorders, metabolic disease, and maternal exposure to drugs and toxins, should be considered.

Most infants who are infected congenitally with CMV are asymptomatic at birth. However, 10 to 17 percent of these infants later may have unilateral or bilateral deafness or differences in higher-level auditory function.[61, 254, 288] Progressive or late-onset hearing loss also may occur in these infants, thus rendering it likely that universal newborn hearing screening programs will miss rather than detect many of these children.[100] Small retinal lesions may occur as well.[58] Earlier studies suggested that developmental problems may occur in asymptomatically infected children, but more recent studies suggest that cognitive outcome appears to be normal when compared with uninfected children.[146]

Very low-birth-weight infants who are infected congenitally with CMV may experience pulmonary and systemic deterioration temporally associated with steroid therapy.[270]

PERINATAL INFECTIONS

Perinatally acquired infections in healthy infants usually are manifested when the child is between 4 and 16 weeks of age, but most such infections are asymptomatic. However, as many as one third of infants exposed to CMV perinatally may have signs and symptoms of disease associated with CMV infection, most often self-limited lymphadenopathy, hepatosplenomegaly, hepatitis, or pneumonitis.[156] Perinatally acquired infection with CMV also can cause a viral, sepsis-like syndrome or severe, protracted pneumonitis that has been associated with the development of bronchopulmonary dysplasia in premature infants.[169, 232] These infections, however, do not appear to cause neurodevelopmental sequelae or deafness.[157] The differential diagnosis includes other perinatally acquired infections such as *Chlamydia* pneumonitis, hepatitis B virus infection, and infection with HIV, as well as postnatally acquired infections with enteroviruses, adenovirus, and a variety of bacterial pathogens.

MONONUCLEOSIS SYNDROME

CMV-induced mononucleosis occurs as a primary infection in both immunocompetent and immunosuppressed persons and, occasionally, as a reactivation infection in immunosuppressed patients. It can result from person-to-person transmission of the virus, as well as from transmission by blood products or by organ or marrow transplantation. Though originally described in adults and most often occurring in patients between 20 and 40 years of age, it also can be seen in adolescents, children, and even infants.[167, 190] Typical CMV-induced mononucleosis is characterized by fever and strikingly severe malaise of approximately 1 to 4 weeks' duration, peripheral lymphocytosis with atypical lymphocytes, and mildly elevated liver enzymes. In some patients, headache, myalgias, and abdominal pain with diarrhea are prominent symptoms. In premature infants with transfusion-acquired CMV mononucleosis, shock, hepatosplenomegaly, pneumonitis, thrombocytopenia, and renal failure are prominent manifestations.[296] In contrast to Epstein-Barr virus–induced mononucleosis, CMV-induced mononucleosis rarely causes pharyngitis, tonsillitis, or significant splenomegaly, and it does not result in production of heterophile antibodies.[59, 133] However, like Epstein-Barr virus–induced mononucleosis, it can be associated with a morbilliform rash after ampicillin administration, an elevated erythrocyte sedimentation rate, polyclonal hypergammaglobulinemia, and the production of other antibodies such as rheumatoid factor, cold agglutinins, and antinuclear antibodies. Complications rarely occur but include interstitial pneumonitis, myocarditis, pericarditis, hemolytic anemia, thrombocytopenia with or without petechiae or purpura, hemophagocytic syndrome, arthralgias and arthritis, maculopapular rashes, adrenal insufficiency, splenic infarction, ulcerative colitis and proctitis, Guillain-Barré syndrome, and meningoencephalitis.[48, 59, 64, 95, 133, 151, 152, 162] Severe, icteric hepatitis, as well as granulomatous hepatitis, also can occur, but hepatic necrosis and liver failure caused by CMV have not been documented convincingly in normal hosts.[29, 59, 133, 152, 218]

The differential diagnosis of CMV-induced mononucleosis includes mononucleosis induced by other viruses such as Epstein-Barr virus, hepatitis A or B virus, and HIV. In addition, acquired toxoplasmosis can produce a mononucleosis syndrome in healthy persons.

INTERSTITIAL PNEUMONITIS

CMV is a major cause of interstitial pneumonia in both adults and children who are immunosuppressed because of congenital immunodeficiency, AIDS, organ or marrow transplantation, or malignancy. In recipients of bone marrow transplants, CMV accounts for 17 to 70 percent of cases of interstitial pneumonitis in adult patients but only 10 percent of cases in patients younger than 21 years.[281] Pneumonia also can occur in apparently immunocompetent young infants with perinatally acquired CMV infection and in healthy adults with CMV-induced mononucleosis.[148, 156, 253, 285] Whereas the pneumonia in immunocompetent hosts almost always is benign and self-limited, CMV pneumonia in immunosuppressed patients is a serious, often fatal illness, especially in bone marrow transplant recipients, who have a mortality rate of up to 90 percent. It also can be particularly troublesome after pediatric heart and lung transplantation.[185] CMV pneumonitis usually occurs 1 to 3 months after transplantation and begins with symptoms of fever and a dry, nonproductive cough. It then can progress over the course of 1 to 2 weeks to dyspnea, retractions, wheezing, and hypoxia, which require ventilatory support. It may occur as the only disease manifestation or be part of a disseminated CMV infection. The radiographic appearance of CMV pneumonia usually is diffuse, interstitial infiltrates, but peribronchial infiltrates with hyperinflation and nodular

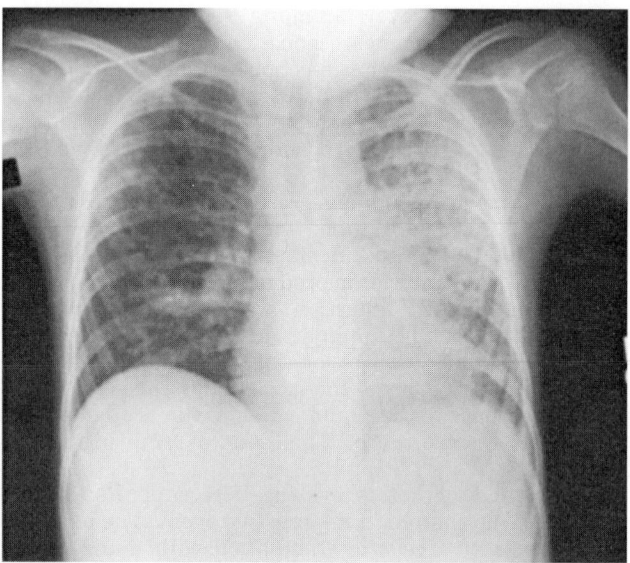

FIGURE 164–2 ■ Chest radiograph of a bone marrow transplant recipient with rapidly fatal cytomegalovirus pneumonitis. An open lung biopsy specimen showed numerous cytomegalic inclusion cells, exhibited cytomegalovirus early antigens by immunoperoxidase staining, and grew cytomegalovirus after inoculation into tissue culture.

pulmonary infiltrates also have been described[148, 265] (Fig. 164–2). Co-infection with other pathogens, especially gram-negative enteric bacteria and fungal pathogens in transplant recipients and *Pneumocystis carinii* in patients with AIDS, can occur.[277]

Congenitally infected infants also may be born with CMV pneumonitis, which often is severe enough to require ventilatory support and usually is part of a multisystem CMV disease process. Very low-birth-weight infants who are infected congenitally with CMV may experience CMV pneumonitis in temporal association with steroid therapy.[270]

The differential diagnosis of CMV pneumonitis in immunocompromised patients, including neonates, is extensive and includes infection with other viruses, such as HSV, VZV, measles virus, respiratory syncytial virus, influenza A and B viruses, parainfluenza viruses, and adenoviruses; bacterial pneumonia caused by a variety of gram-positive and gram-negative organisms; infection with protozoa, such as *P. carinii* and *Toxoplasma gondii; Chlamydia* and *Mycoplasma*; and fungal pneumonia, caused especially by *Candida* and *Aspergillus*. Noninfectious causes of pneumonitis, such as pulmonary hemorrhage, aspiration pneumonia, rejection, and pulmonary damage from chemotherapeutic agents, also should be considered.

RETINITIS AND OTHER EYE ABNORMALITIES

Chorioretinitis, as well as optic atrophy, cortical blindness, and strabismus, occurs in 17 to 41 percent of newborns with symptomatic congenital CMV infection and rarely in children born with asymptomatic congenital CMV infection.[30, 58, 228] Although most retinal lesions in congenitally infected infants appear to be inactive at birth, some observations suggest that progression of preexisting lesions and late-onset new lesions resulting in vision loss may occur rarely in both symptomatic and asymptomatic congenitally infected infants.[30] Retinitis does not seem to be a prominent part of perinatally acquired infection.[157] CMV retinitis once was a rare manifestation of CMV disease in solid organ transplant recipients undergoing chronic immunosuppression for more than a year and in patients receiving chemotherapy for malignancy.[96] In the 1980s, CMV retinitis emerged as a common manifestation of CMV disease in patients with severe immunosuppression, especially bone marrow transplant recipients and patients with AIDS. It probably is a result of hematogenous spread of the virus to the retina, with continued local viral replication. Despite the common occurrence of CMV retinitis in adults with AIDS, however, it rarely has been reported in children with AIDS.[163]

CMV produces characteristic white, perivascular infiltrates and hemorrhage, with a necrotic, rapidly progressive retinitis. It descriptively has been called cottage cheese retinitis and ketchup or brushfire retinitis.[28] Early, peripheral retinitis can be asymptomatic, or the complaints may be minimal and nonspecific; it is especially difficult to ascertain in infants and young children. It does not cause eye pain, photophobia, or conjunctivitis. Once the retinitis has progressed, it can cause blurred vision, decreased visual acuity, visual field defects, and blindness. Young children and infants who have suffered visual loss as a result of CMV retinitis may exhibit strabismus or failure to fix and follow objects within their visual field. CMV retinitis also can progress rapidly to total blindness if the macula is involved. Immunosuppressed children with CMV disease should receive regular expert ophthalmologic examinations to monitor for the development of sight-threatening retinitis. Early diagnosis may allow prompt institution of antiviral therapy, which may be sight saving.[163]

The funduscopic appearance of CMV retinitis usually is characteristic. However, in patients in whom the appearance of the retina is not typical or in whom the retinitis has progressed despite specific antiviral treatment, other causes of retinal lesions that should be considered include cotton-wool spots associated with hypertension, diabetes, connective tissue disease, anemia and leukemia, ocular toxoplasmosis, and candidal infection of the retina, as well as syphilis, HSV infection, lymphocytic choriomeningitis virus infection, and VZV infection. Detection of the virus by culture or its DNA by a PCR-based method in vitreous fluid may help in the diagnosis of difficult or atypical patients.[93]

Although chorioretinitis is the most common ocular manifestation of CMV disease, CMV also has been associated with other unusual eye abnormalities. In congenitally infected infants, microphthalmos, anophthalmia, optic nerve hypoplasia and coloboma, optic nerve atrophy, Peter anomaly, and irregular retinal pigment have been observed.[104] CMV also has been isolated from tears and has been associated with conjunctivitis in patients with CMV mononucleosis and AIDS, as well as with corneal epithelial keratitis and disk neovascularization.[160]

HEPATITIS

CMV hepatitis in bone marrow, heart, and lung transplant recipients, in patients with cancer or AIDS, and even in healthy persons experiencing a primary CMV infection usually is manifested as mild hepatomegaly and mildly elevated serum hepatic enzyme levels. It commonly occurs in conjunction with fever, thrombocytopenia, and lymphopenia or lymphocytosis. Jaundice and hyperbilirubinemia usually do not occur, severe hepatitis or cirrhosis is exceedingly rare, and hepatic necrosis and liver failure caused by CMV hepatitis have not been documented convincingly in these patients. CMV infection also has been associated with granulomatous hepatitis.[29, 2187] In addition, CMV hepatitis is a unique and prominent problem in children who have undergone liver transplantation.[35] Most CMV hepatitis occurs 1 to 2 months after transplantation, but it may be noted as early as 2 weeks or as long as 4 months after transplantation.[37] It is more common and more severe after a primary CMV infection and is associated with liver transplantation using a CMV-seropositive donor and the use of OKT3 antibodies for severe rejection.[240] CMV hepatitis in liver transplant recipients is characterized by prolonged fever, leukopenia, thrombocytopenia, elevated liver enzymes, hyperbilirubinemia, and liver failure. Distinguishing between CMV hepatitis and acute rejection often is difficult, even with a liver biopsy, and the two commonly coexist. CMV infection also has been associated with ascending cholangitis, chronic rejection, and the vanishing bile duct syndrome in liver transplant recipients.[37, 187]

Infants with congenital CMV disease also may have hepatitis. The liver usually is smooth and nontender and commonly extends 3 to 5 cm below the right costal margin. Ascites may be present prenatally and may persist postnatally for 1 to 2 weeks. The hepatomegaly usually resolves by the time that the infant is 3 months of age, and persistence beyond 1 year is highly unusual. Mild hepatitis generally is present, and transaminase levels in neonatal hepatitis caused by CMV rarely exceed 300 IU. Hyperbilirubinemia is present at birth in approximately a third of newborns with congenital CMV and may be striking, with conjugated (direct) bilirubin levels up to 30 mg/dL.[135] The abnormal results of liver function tests gradually resolve over the course of the first few weeks of life, and chronic hepatitis as a result of congenital infection with CMV is an unusual occurrence.

The differential diagnosis of CMV hepatitis includes other causes of viral hepatitis, including hepatitis A, B, and C, Epstein-Barr virus, HSV, enterovirus, and adenovirus, as well as toxoplasmosis, other infections such as bacterial ascending cholangitis, and noninfectious causes such as ischemic injury, vascular thrombosis, hemolysis, rejection, and hepatitis induced by drugs or toxins. In newborns with a significant and persistent direct hyperbilirubinemia, the diagnosis of biliary atresia should be considered as well.

GASTROINTESTINAL DISEASE

Serious gastrointestinal disease causing esophagitis, gastritis, gastroenteritis, pyloric and small bowel obstruction, duodenitis, colitis, proctitis, pancreatitis, hemorrhage, and acalculous cholecystitis has been associated with CMV infection in immunocompromised persons, especially patients with AIDS and those who have undergone bone marrow, kidney, intestinal, or liver transplantation.[10, 74–76, 165, 188, 199, 208, 216, 272] Rarely, self-limited CMV gastroenteritis, colitis, and proctitis have been associated with CMV mononucleosis syndrome in apparently normal individuals.[59, 133, 209] Characteristic signs and symptoms in infants and children include nausea, vomiting, dysphagia, epigastric pain and tenderness, delayed gastric emptying, watery guaiac-positive stools or gastrointestinal hemorrhage, and disaccharide and monosaccharide intolerance. Severe disease may cause dehydration and failure to thrive. Endoscopy with biopsy is required for definitive diagnosis and usually shows linear, localized, or punctate ulcers. Hemorrhagic lesions or diffuse erosion can occur in severe disease. Characteristic cytomegalic inclusion cells can be seen in the gastrointestinal endothelium, epithelium, and glandular tissue; CMV may be cultured from stool or biopsy specimens; or CMV DNA may be detected by PCR-based methods.[111] In addition, these patients often are viremic and occasionally have evidence of disseminated CMV infection with involvement of the lungs and retina.

The differential diagnosis of CMV colitis includes infection with other viruses, especially HSV and adenovirus, and infection with bacteria, particularly *Salmonella, Shigella, Campylobacter,* and *Yersinia,* as well as *Clostridium difficile* and *Mycobacterium avium–intracellulare*. Parasitic infection with *Cryptosporidium, Giardia,* and amebae also should be excluded. The differential diagnosis of CMV esophagitis and gastritis includes HSV infection, *Candida* esophagitis, reflux esophagitis, and peptic ulcer disease.

MENINGOENCEPHALITIS AND OTHER NEUROLOGIC DISORDERS

CNS involvement is well described and occurs relatively commonly in infants with symptomatic congenital CMV infection. Although the severity of damage to the CNS during congenital infection varies greatly, postmortem examination of severely affected infants has demonstrated necrotizing encephalitis, especially in the deep periventricular structures, and scattered areas of necrosis and inclusion-bearing cells. Although direct viral infection of neural structures probably plays a major role in CNS disease in congenital CMV infection, infectious vasculitis also may occur. In addition, because congenital CMV disease can be associated with marked thrombocytopenia, intracranial hemorrhage can contribute to CMV-related CNS injury.[20, 43, 125, 275] Clinical manifestations of this disease process include microcephaly, cerebral palsy, intracerebral calcifications, seizures, hemiparesis, developmental delay, ventriculomegaly, paraventricular cysts, intraventricular strands, periventricular leukomalacia, lissencephaly-pachygyria, porencephaly, meningoencephalitis, and sensorineural deafness (Fig. 164–3). Remarkably, despite the well-documented neuropathology in congenital disease, isolation of CMV from the cerebrospinal fluid (CSF) of a congenitally infected child is an extremely unusual finding.[139] CMV DNA has been detected in the CSF of congenitally infected infants, and its presence at birth appeared to identify infants at risk for a poor neurodevelopmental outcome.[15]

The differential diagnosis of symptomatic congenital CMV infection with neurologic disease includes congenital toxoplasmosis, congenital HSV infection, congenital rubella syndrome, congenital infection with lymphocytic choriomeningitis virus, brain tumors such as craniopharyngioma, and calcified hematoma. In addition, congenital CMV disease involving the CNS also may be mimicked by genetic disorders such as tuberous sclerosis, Sturge-Weber syndrome, and Aicardi syndrome; metabolic conditions such as hyperthyroidism; α_1-antitrypsin deficiency; galactosemia; peroxisome disorders such as Zellweger syndrome, neonatal adrenoleukodystrophy, and infantile Refsum disease; urea cycle deficiencies; organic acidemias; and liposomal storage disorders.[19] Maternal exposure to drugs and toxins, especially isotretinoin, cocaine, and alcohol, also are included in the differential diagnosis. The presence or absence of intracerebral calcification, as well as the pattern of calcifications when present, may be helpful in distinguishing among these disorders. Additionally, the appropriate microbiologic studies, chromosome analysis, metabolic studies, and drug screens should be performed.

In postnatal life, CMV meningoencephalitis appears to be rare yet well documented.[18] It may occur as a complication of CMV mononucleosis, as an isolated manifestation of primary CMV infection in a normal host, or as a primary or recurrent infection in an immunocompromised patient. Symptoms include headache, photophobia, nuchal rigidity, memory deficits, and inability to concentrate. CSF findings include mild mononuclear pleocytosis and slightly elevated protein. Although the virus is isolated from the CSF and brain parenchyma exceedingly rarely, neuropathologic findings of intranuclear inclusions and microglial nodules are characteristic.

CMV encephalitis may complicate adult immunocompromised transplant recipients, and recognition of CMV encephalitis in patients with AIDS is growing.[24] As many as 50 percent of patients with AIDS may have evidence of CMV infection of the CNS at postmortem examination.[182] CMV has been reported to cause a subacute, occasionally progressive, encephalitis in patients with AIDS and has been implicated as a cofactor in the pathogenesis of the AIDS dementia complex seen in both adults and children.[63, 128, 178, 243, 287] In this disease, CMV may be isolated from CSF, or CMV DNA may be detected in the fluid or brain by PCR-based methods.[114] In children, this syndrome is characterized by weakness, confusion, and loss of developmental milestones.

The differential diagnosis of CMV encephalitis and meningoencephalitis in a normal host includes primarily other neurotropic viruses such as HSV, Epstein-Barr virus, VZV, enterovirus, and arboviruses. Neurosyphilis and tuberculous meningitis also should be considered. In immunocompromised patients, especially those with AIDS, the following should be added to the differential diagnosis of CNS infection: progressive multifocal leukoencephalopathy

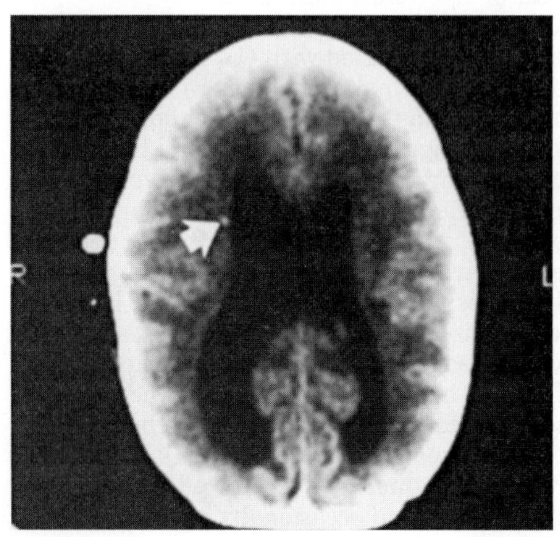

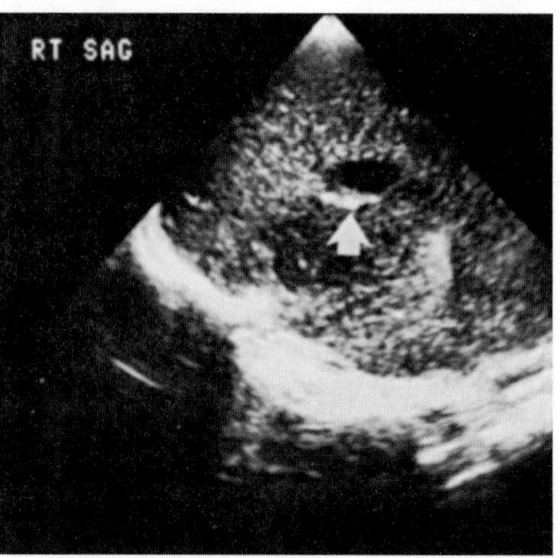

FIGURE 164–3 ■ Computed tomographic scan *(left)* and ultrasound examination *(right)* of the head of an infant with congenital cytomegalovirus disease. Both tests showed moderate asymmetric enlargement of the lateral ventricles with punctate periventricular calcifications.

caused by papovavirus; HIV encephalitis; fungal CNS infection caused by *Cryptococcus neoformans*, *Candida* spp., *Aspergillus*, or *Histoplasma*; protozoal infections with *T. gondii* and, rarely, *P. carinii* and *Strongyloides stercoralis*; bacterial infections with *M. avium–intracellulare* and *Nocardia asteroides*; noninfectious diseases such as primary cerebral lymphoma and lymphomatoid granulomatosis; and vascular complications such as hemorrhage and infarction.[12] Of importance is to remember that in immunosuppressed patients, more than one of these conditions can coexist in the CNS.

CMV also can invade the peripheral nervous system and cause a painful peripheral neuropathy in patients with AIDS.[105, 225, 274] Ascending paralysis caused by myelitis, with or without vasculitis or necrosis, also can occur and may appear similar to Guillain-Barré syndrome.[274] In addition, CMV polyradiculopathy has been described in adult patients with AIDS and may occur in older children. This disease usually begins with leg pain and sacral paresthesias and may progress to weakness and flaccid paralysis. The CSF characteristically has a polymorphonuclear pleocytosis and moderately elevated protein.[149] The association of CMV infection with infantile spasms, Guillain-Barré syndrome, Charcot-Marie-Tooth disease, Huntington disease, Alzheimer disease, myasthenia gravis, and neuropsychiatric diseases (e.g., schizophrenia) has been reported, but a definite causal relationship between CMV and these diseases remains to be proved.[18]

DEAFNESS AND OTHER EAR DISORDERS

Hearing loss is present at birth in approximately 25 to 50 percent of infants with symptomatic congenital CMV infection and in about 15 percent of infants with asymptomatic congenital CMV infection.[135] Given that congenital CMV infection affects 30,000 to 40,000 infants annually in the United States, this congenital infection probably is the most common cause of nonhereditary sensorineural deafness. Progression or fluctuation of the hearing loss occurs in at least two thirds of these children through the preschool years, and continued progression may occur through the school age and adolescent years.[101, 288] Although CMV has been detected in the endolabyrinth of infants who died of congenital CMV disease, whether this progressive deafness is caused by continued viral replication in the inner ear, reinfection with a new strain of virus, or a complex cascade of immunopathologic events still is unclear.[66] Mondini dysplasia of the temporal bones has been seen in infants with congenital CMV infection, but the importance of this observation relative to the pathogenesis of the progressive hearing loss commonly seen in congenitally infected infants is unknown at this time.[25]

CMV has been isolated from the middle ear effusions of healthy and immunocompromised children with otitis media.[52, 87] In addition, CMV infection, defined serologically, has been associated with sudden-onset deafness, acute labyrinthitis, and Meniere syndrome.[260, 290] Older children who were born with asymptomatic congenital CMV infection also may exhibit differences in higher auditory function, even though they do not have sensorineural or conductive hearing loss.[61]

MYOCARDITIS AND OTHER CARDIOVASCULAR DISORDERS

Myocarditis has been described as a rare complication of severe congenital CMV disease and CMV mononucleosis in presumably healthy adults and children.[266, 279, 291] CMV myocarditis also has been seen in renal and heart transplant recipients, usually as part of a disseminated CMV infection and associated with graft rejection treated with high-dose immunosuppressive therapy.[110, 207, 236] Patients can have heart failure, cardiomegaly, electrocardiographic abnormalities, and poor left ventricular function on echocardiography; cytomegalic inclusion cells and the presence of CMV DNA can be documented by myocardial biopsy.

The association of CMV infection with other cardiac disorders such as congenital heart block, structural cardiac anomalies, and pericarditis is anecdotal, and a cause-and-effect relationship is not well documented.[145] CMV coronary endotheliitis with superimposed thrombosis and myocardial infarction has been described in adult heart transplant recipients and was reported in an infant who died of disseminated CMV disease with an apical ventricular aneurysm.[177, 230] CMV infection also has been postulated to play a role in the pathogenesis of atherosclerosis and coronary artery disease in both normal persons and heart transplant recipients.[116, 171, 173]

ENDOCRINE SYSTEM

Histopathologic evidence of involvement of the organs of the endocrine system is described well in both congenital and postnatally acquired disseminated CMV infections.[129] Endocrine disorders such as Graves disease and diabetes insipidus have been associated with congenital CMV infection, but these reports may represent coincidental findings.[174, 229] Longitudinal studies are required to determine whether the autoimmune endocrinopathies in children with congenital rubella parallel the findings in children with congenital CMV infection. CMV infection also has been associated with autoimmune type 1 diabetes, although a specific cause-and-effect relationship has not been established.[189] In addition, immunosuppressed patients, especially persons with AIDS, may manifest clinical endocrinopathies caused by CMV infection, such as adrenal insufficiency and adrenal necrosis.[117] CMV inclusions also have been found in the pituitary gland of patients with AIDS, all of whom showed evidence of CMV encephalitis or disseminated infection elsewhere in the body.[94] Moreover, involvement of the thyroid and parathyroid glands with CMV has been reported in adults with AIDS.[102]

GENITOURINARY SYSTEM

Disease of the male and female genitourinary system as a result of CMV has been reported, and adult patients with AIDS may have symptomatic epididymitis and cystitis caused by CMV.[27, 210, 262] CMV also commonly yet asymptomatically infects the cervicovaginal secretions and semen of both healthy and immunosuppressed adults.[141, 158]

SKIN

Cutaneous manifestations of CMV infection are well described and can occur with both congenital and acquired CMV infection.[162] Infants with symptomatic congenital infection may have nonpalpable petechiae, purpura, or bruises, usually as a result of thrombocytopenia. Violaceous or dark, magenta-colored infiltrative papules or nodules, called "blueberry muffin" lesions, also may occur, but these lesions are more characteristic of congenital rubella syndrome. The skin lesions associated with acquired CMV infection are usually localized cutaneous ulcers or a widespread, exanthematous, maculopapular eruption, although vesiculobullous lesions also have been described.[198] CMV mononucleosis syndrome in adults and children may be accompanied by a maculopapular, rubelliform rash that may be pruritic. In addition, ampicillin-associated rashes may occur with CMV mononucleosis. CMV also may cause a cutaneous, leukoblastic vasculitis.[231] Well-demarcated, ulcerated lesions that show histopathologic evidence of CMV infection may be seen in immunocompromised patients after transplantation or in those who suffer from AIDS. Finally, CMV may play a role in the neoplastic process in Kaposi sarcoma, but definitive proof of a causal relationship remains to be shown.

UNUSUAL ASSOCIATIONS

CMV infection, either congenital or acquired, has been detected in association with a wide variety of conditions, including defects in tooth structure and the formation of enamel, portal vein thrombosis associated with protein S and protein C deficiency, unexplained fevers in burn patients, bacterial sepsis in burn patients, congenital eventration of the diaphragm, inguinal hernia, and fatal *Staphylococcus epidermidis* infection in very low-birth-weight infants.[13, 26, 144, 155, 166, 255] However, given the common occurrence of CMV infection, these associations may be coincidental rather than part of a cause-and-effect relationship.

Laboratory Diagnosis

DETECTION OF THE INFECTIOUS AGENT

CMV can be isolated in tissue culture with fibroblast cell lines such as human foreskin fibroblasts and human embryonic lung fibroblasts.[234] Specimens that contain a high titer of virus, such as those from congenitally infected infants, may show growth in 24 hours. Some specimens, such as those from persons with acquired asymptomatic infection, may require as long as 6 weeks for detectable growth, but most cultures grow in 1 to 2 weeks. CMV has been isolated from a variety of specimens, including urine, saliva, nasopharyngeal and sinus washings, conjunctiva, tears, middle ear fluid, breast milk, semen, cervicovaginal secretions, stool, CSF, white blood cells, amniotic fluid, bronchial lavage samples, and biopsy or autopsy specimens. All samples for virus isolation (except blood, which should be at room temperature) should be held at 4° C (on wet ice or in a refrigerator) until processed in the virology laboratory. Specimens for isolation of virus should be inoculated within hours of collection for an optimal isolation rate. Although isolation of CMV proves that a productive infection is present, it does not confirm an etiologic relationship with the disease process and requires careful interpretation within the patient's clinical context.

An adaptation of tissue culture that now is popular in viral diagnostic laboratories is a low-speed centrifugation enhancement, monoclonal antibody culture technique, also called shell vial assay. In this test, inoculated tissue culture cells in small vials are stained with a fluorescein-conjugated monoclonal antibody to either an early or a late CMV antigen (or both). Cells infected with CMV exhibit nuclear and membrane fluorescence 18 to 72 hours after inoculation. This rapid viral diagnostic technique is especially reliable with urine and bronchoalveolar lavage specimens and has been applied with variable results to blood and tissue specimens.[109] However, maximal sensitivity and specificity are obtained when shell vials are used as an adjunct to and not in place of routine tissue culture. CMV-infected cells also can be detected by direct immunofluorescence on exfoliated cells in bronchoalveolar lavage specimens or in frozen tissue specimens.[123] This procedure, however, requires a laboratory experienced in direct immunofluorescence technique.

Detection of CMV DNA by traditional DNA-DNA hybridization methods and, more recently, by PCR-based methods now is available in many laboratories. These very sensitive tests may be used to detect and quantify CMV DNA in a variety of samples and are useful for diagnosing or predicting CMV disease.[40, 47, 65, 70, 108, 243, 245, 251]

The clinical utility of PCR-based diagnostic tests is evolving, but they do appear to have value in the diagnosis of CMV disease. For example, detection of CMV DNA in the CSF of patients with AIDS seems to be a reliable diagnostic method for detection of CMV infection of the CNS, and detection of CMV DNA in the CSF of newborns with congenital CMV disease correlates with poor neurodevelopmental outcome.[15, 57, 114, 293] Similarly, detection of CMV DNA by PCR in vitreous fluid provides persuasive evidence that a patient's retinitis is CMV related.[82] CMV DNA also may be detected in the white blood cells of patients with CMV infection, and detection of CMV DNA in the plasma or serum of selected groups of patients, such as newborns and immunocompromised patients, appears to correlate with disease severity and viral dissemination.[181, 239, 250, 251]

Another use for PCR-based diagnosis of CMV infection is the very early diagnosis of CMV infection in high-risk patients such as transplant recipients before the development of potentially fatal CMV disease such as pneumonitis. This approach may allow preemptive antiviral therapy to be initiated at a time when CMV infection appears active but before overt disease is detected.[39, 294] The role of CMV DNA detection by PCR assay in monitoring a patient's response to antiviral therapy, however, appears to be limited because CMV DNA persists for long periods after the resolution of CMV-related clinical symptoms in many patients.[106]

CMV antigen also may be detected in the white blood cells of patients with CMV infection and disease, and this CMV antigenemia test is used by some clinical laboratories as a rapid screen for CMV viremia. It is relatively easy to perform, and the degree of antigenemia may be quantitated to monitor response to antiviral therapy.[106]

Exfoliated cells in urine or bronchoalveolar lavage specimens or cells in tissue obtained by biopsy can be examined for histologic evidence of CMV infection. Cells that are infected productively with CMV are enlarged, have type A Cowdry intranuclear inclusions, and occasionally have perinuclear inclusions. The appearance of these cells is characteristic and has been likened to owl's eyes. Immunohistochemical staining can be used to augment the detection of these typical cells. The presence of these cells correlates with the presence of active CMV disease and may be useful clinically.

SEROLOGY

Standard serologic techniques also can be applied to the diagnosis of CMV infections. CMV IgG antibody can be determined in serum by several different methods, including complement fixation, hemagglutination inhibition, indirect fluorescent antibody assay, anticomplement immunofluorescence assay, enzyme-linked immunosorbent assay (ELISA), and latex agglutination and neutralization tests. ELISA and the indirect fluorescent antibody assay are used most commonly in clinical virology laboratories. The presence of CMV IgG antibody in a single serum specimen implies that the patient at some time has been infected with CMV. On the other hand, a negative IgG antibody determination is good evidence against current or past CMV infection because CMV antibody usually is present at the time of infection and persists for life. Severely immunocompromised patients, especially bone marrow transplant recipients, however, can lose their ability to make IgG antibody and become CMV seronegative, even though they are infected actively with CMV. This occurrence has a poor prognosis and usually is a terminal event. Primary infection with CMV is documented best by clear seroconversion from negative to positive CMV IgG antibody. A fourfold rise in CMV IgG antibody titer is not diagnostic of a primary infection because reactivation infection also can cause titers to fluctuate. In addition, the height of the titer or ELISA index in a single serum specimen is not diagnostic.

CMV IgM antibody can be determined in serum by radioimmunoassay, indirect fluorescent antibody assay, or ELISA. Both the indirect fluorescent antibody assay and ELISA are used commonly in clinical laboratories, although some indirect fluorescent antibody assays have a considerable false-positive rate. Accurate interpretation of CMV IgM antibody results requires knowledge of the methods used and careful consideration of the clinical context to exclude diseases that produce cross-reacting antibody or polyclonal responses. Test methods also should remove rheumatoid factor from the test serum, a common cause of false-positive IgM reactions. If the test is performed properly, the presence of CMV IgM antibody implies a current or recent primary CMV infection. In healthy adults, CMV IgM antibody usually persists for 6 weeks and may be present for as long as 3 to 6 months after the primary infection.[72] Western blot assays using viral structural proteins separated from purified viral particles or from recombinant viral proteins appear to be sensitive and specific for detection of CMV IgM. Currently, these tests are available only in research or reference laboratories.[159] A recently developed test called the CMV IgG avidity index also may be used to time a suspected primary infection with CMV. A low avidity index (30%) suggests a recent primary infection, usually within 3 months, whereas a high avidity index (>60%) suggests a past or recurrent CMV infection.[115] In immunocompromised adults experiencing clinically significant reactivation infection with CMV, CMV IgM antibody may be detected for prolonged periods.[183] The sensitivity and specificity of CMV IgM antibody determination in diagnosing acquired, primary CMV infection or clinically significant reactivation infection in infants and children have not been studied systematically, although clinicians frequently use this test for this purpose.

LABORATORY DIAGNOSIS OF SPECIFIC CLINICAL SYNDROMES

Congenital Infection

Viral culture is the diagnostic test of choice when considering congenital infection with CMV.[68] The diagnosis is established by isolation of the virus from urine or saliva in the first 1 to 2 weeks of life. Urine cultures obtained after 3 weeks of life must be interpreted cautiously because perinatally acquired and transfusion-acquired infections with CMV may be manifested as early as 3 weeks of age.[232] Detection of nuclear inclusion–bearing renal epithelial cells in urinary sediment collected in the first 2 weeks of life also implies the presence of congenital infection. This technique is insensitive, however, when compared with tissue culture and is important only historically. Detection of CMV DNA in the urine, serum, or CSF of newborns by DNA hybridization or DNA amplification techniques also correlates with congenital infection and disease but may be less sensitive than is viral isolation.[15, 38, 70, 181]

The diagnosis of fetal intrauterine CMV disease also may be established by isolation of the virus from amniotic fluid or detection of CMV DNA by PCR amplification in amniotic fluid obtained at least 2 weeks after the suspected time of maternal primary infection. Fetal condition also can be determined by serial fetal ultrasound examinations.[77, 131, 219] Fetal blood samples that show the presence of CMV IgM antibody, thrombocytopenia, or leukopenia or elevated liver function test results also provide supportive evidence of CMV-associated fetal disease. Prenatal screening of pregnant women and prenatal diagnosis of congenital CMV infection should be accompanied by prenatal counseling by personnel knowledgeable about all the possible outcomes that can occur and all the options that are available to the parents and physician.[88]

Standard serologic tests also can be applied to diagnose congenital infection with CMV, but this approach is cumbersome and retrospective. The absence of CMV IgG antibody in cord blood rules out congenital infection, whereas its presence may imply passive transfer from the mother or indicate a congenital infection. Serial serologic specimens also can be obtained when the infant is 1, 3, and 6 months of age. If CMV IgG antibody levels disappear during the infant's first months of life, congenital infection is ruled out. However, if CMV IgG antibody persists, the infant either was infected congenitally or acquired CMV infection perinatally or postnatally. The presence of CMV IgM antibody in cord or infant blood collected in the first 3 weeks of life suggests the diagnosis of congenital CMV infection.[120, 256] However, CMV IgM antibody may be insensitive (22%) when compared with urine CMV culture for the diagnosis of congenital infection, according to one study.[181]

Perinatal and Postnatal Infection

The diagnosis of perinatal infection with CMV is difficult to make but is documented best by a negative CMV viral culture and CMV IgM antibody level at birth, a positive viral culture and CMV IgM antibody at 8 to 16 weeks of age, and persistence of CMV IgG antibody. Postnatal primary CMV infection is diagnosed by CMV IgG seroconversion, the presence of CMV IgM antibody, and viral shedding in saliva, urine, and other body fluids.

Cytomegalovirus Syndromes in Immunocompromised Hosts

In immunocompromised patients, determining whether serologic or virologic evidence of active CMV infection correlates with disease is difficult because CMV commonly is shed from saliva, urine, and respiratory tract secretions in these patients without clear evidence of a disease process. Therefore, detection of a productive virus infection in the organ system suspected to be involved usually is necessary to establish the diagnosis of CMV disease in an immunocompromised patient. For example, interstitial pneumonitis caused by CMV is documented best by an open lung biopsy specimen that shows characteristic CMV histopathology and positive viral culture. Detection of CMV in bronchoalveolar

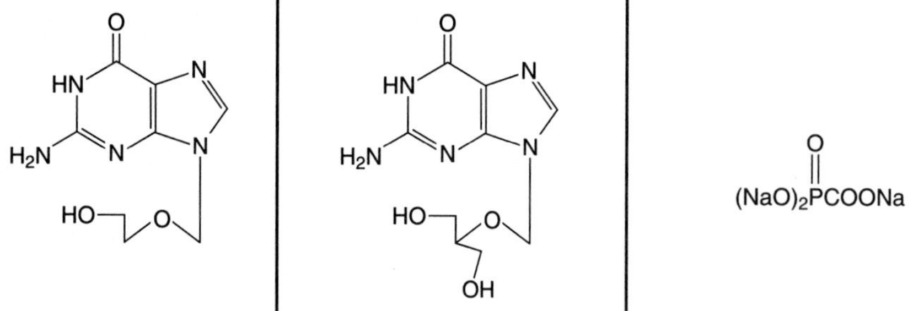

O
HN N
H_2N N N
HO O

9-[(2-Hydroxyethoxy) methyl]guanine
Acyclovir

O
HN N
H_2N N N
HO O
OH

9-[(1,3-Dihydroxy-2-propoxy)methyl]guanine
Ganciclovir

O
‖
$(NaO)_2PCOONa$

Trisodium phosphonoformate
Foscarnet

FIGURE 164–4 ■ Structures of acyclovir, ganciclovir, and foscarnet.

lavage specimens also correlates with lung biopsy results.[108] Similarly, the diagnosis of CMV hepatitis or colitis is documented best by the presence of cytomegalic inclusion cells, isolation of CMV, or detection of CMV DNA from biopsy specimens. In addition, viremia often precedes or accompanies serious disease, such as CMV pneumonitis in bone marrow transplant recipients or CMV retinitis or colitis in patients with AIDS.[251, 273]

Prospective monitoring of high-risk adult patients by serial CMV cultures of urine, blood, or bronchial lavage samples, serial blood samples to test for evidence of CMV antigenemia or DNAemia, and collection of serum to detect seroconversion by serologic testing usually are indicated because they may allow early administration of preemptive therapy with a specific antiviral agent, such as ganciclovir, at a time when CMV infection is active but before overt disease develops.[233, 271]

Treatment

Antiviral agents with activity against CMV include ganciclovir, valganciclovir, cidofovir, and foscarnet[9, 42, 44, 161, 224, 261] (Fig. 164–4). Acyclovir and valacyclovir also may have limited activity against CMV under certain conditions. In addition, biologicals such as immunoglobulin and CMV hyperimmune globulin may benefit selected patients, and novel approaches such as adoptive immunotherapy also are being investigated. Treatment is beneficial for immunocompromised hosts, controversial for newborns with serious CMV disease, and currently usually not indicated for normal hosts with asymptomatic or mildly symptomatic CMV infection.

Treatment of CMV-associated disease, such as retinitis, pneumonitis, hepatitis, colitis, esophagitis, or encephalitis, in immunocompromised hosts usually involves a 2- to 3-week period of induction therapy with an intravenous antiviral medication, usually ganciclovir.* In special circumstances, such as suspected drug resistance, foscarnet or cidofovir may be indicated.[89, 263] The induction period should be accompanied by clinical improvement and a virologic response. If the host is expected to remain severely immunocompromised after receiving successful induction therapy, maintenance therapy at a reduced dosage schedule, three to five times a week administered intravenously or orally, is indicated through the expected period of immune suppression. In patients with AIDS, oral or intravenous maintenance therapy usually is continued indefinitely.[80] In adult patients with AIDS who have refractory CMV retinitis, treatment with a ganciclovir implant may augment systemic therapy, but published experience evaluating this approach in children is not available.[45, 269] Recently, one study showed that valganciclovir, the new orally bioavailable prodrug of ganciclovir, appears to be as effective as is intravenous ganciclovir for induction therapy for CMV retinitis.[168] If despite administration of antiviral therapy CMV disease persists or progresses or if a virologic response does not occur, drug resistance should be considered. Resistance to ganciclovir has been documented most commonly in patients with AIDS, but it also can occur in patients with malignancies and in transplant recipients.[55, 136] Most ganciclovir-resistant CMV strains have a mutation in the UL97 phosphotransferase gene, but specific mutations in the UL54 DNA polymerase gene also may occur alone or in combination with UL97 mutations. Most ganciclovir-resistant CMV strains exhibit cross-resistance to cidofovir, and strains simultaneously resistant to ganciclovir, cidofovir, and foscarnet also rarely may occur.[56, 263]

The administration of ganciclovir along with intravenous immunoglobulin or CMV hyperimmune globulin to bone marrow transplant recipients with CMV pneumonitis has been shown to increase survival over that of historical controls who were treated with a variety of other antiviral regimens, including ganciclovir alone, immunoglobulin alone, acyclovir, vidarabine, and interferon. However, differences in the method of diagnosis of CMV pneumonitis, the duration of illness, and treatment regimens between study subjects and historical controls obscure interpretation of these studies.[86, 213] Nonetheless, CMV-associated interstitial pneumonitis in bone marrow transplant recipients may be an immunopathologic process, and combination therapy may prevent active virus replication (ganciclovir) while blunting the immune response to viral antigens already expressed on CMV-infected cells (immunoglobulin).[237] In contrast, a small pilot study showed that the addition of CMV hyperimmune globulin did not appear to enhance the efficacy of ganciclovir treatment in patients with AIDS-associated CMV retinitis.[138]

Standard immunoglobulin or CMV hyperimmune globulin should not be used alone for the treatment of established

*See references 41, 62, 74, 92, 99, 122, 137, 147, 164, 165, 170, 247, 280.

CMV infections in immunocompromised patients.[212] The combination of high-dose corticosteroids with ganciclovir does not appear to improve survival in bone marrow transplant recipients with biopsy-proven CMV pneumonitis.[214] On the other hand, a regimen combining ganciclovir with hematopoietic growth factor may decrease marrow toxicity.

Treatment of infants with symptomatic congenital CMV infection remains controversial at this time. Anecdotal reports have shown clinical and virologic improvement in congenitally infected newborns treated with ganciclovir.[130, 184, 217, 270] A multicenter phase I/II study of the pharmacokinetics, antiviral effects, and safety of intravenous ganciclovir was conducted in 47 newborns with symptomatic congenital CMV disease and neurologic involvement.[268, 286, 302] In this study, a 6-mg/kg dose of ganciclovir administered by a 1-hour infusion every 12 hours for a period of 6 weeks produced a significant reduction in the quantity of urinary virus excretion; however, viral shedding recurred when ganciclovir treatment was discontinued. Neutropenia, thrombocytopenia, and elevated liver enzymes also were observed. Limited clinical follow-up in 30 of the original 47 infants showed hearing loss improved or stabilized in 16 percent of the treated infants. Subsequently, a phase III, multicenter, randomized clinical trial enrolled 100 infants and was completed in 1999.[150] In this study, ganciclovir treatment in the newborn period appeared to have an impact on hearing loss by slightly improving hearing, maintaining normal hearing, or preventing hearing deterioration, as measured when the infants reached 6 and 12 months of age. Because only 44 percent of the enrolled infants were assessed in follow-up, a long-term follow-up study of these infants is ongoing to determine whether the beneficial effect lasts through childhood and adolescence. In addition to an effect on hearing loss, treatment provided more rapid resolution of hepatitis, when present, and improved short-term growth in weight and head circumference. Not known from this study is whether treatment influences the vision, cognitive outcome, or development of motor disabilities in these children. Currently, the difficult decision to administer antiviral therapy to a newborn with congenital CMV disease remains at the discretion of the clinician. Short-term antiviral therapy is likely to benefit infants who have multisystem disease with viremia, pneumonia, or active sight-threatening retinitis. In these clinical circumstances, a reduction in viral load should improve the infant's clinical condition and resolve end-organ disease. However, the sustained effect of short-term treatment on long-term sequelae, such as hearing loss and neurodevelopmental disabilities, is not clear at this time. A longer duration of therapy, perhaps with an oral antiviral agent such as valganciclovir, possibly will improve or prevent the development of long-term sequelae in these infants. In addition to specific antiviral therapy, management of congenitally infected infants includes supportive care and seizure control. If thrombocytopenia is severe and persistent, platelet transfusions and immunoglobulin also may be of benefit. Long-term management includes serial hearing tests to detect progressive or late-onset hearing loss, developmental assessments to evaluate for cognitive and motor disabilities, and ophthalmologic follow-up if abnormalities were present in the newborn period.[288]

Prevention

Prevention of CMV disease is important because it causes significant morbidity and mortality in a variety of patients. In immunocompromised hosts, it also is associated with the development of other complications, such as opportunistic co-infections and graft rejection in transplant recipients, and it increases resource utilization in transplant programs. In premature newborns, potentially fatal viral sepsis syndromes can occur. Furthermore, congenital infection is a leading cause of deafness and developmental disabilities in children. Approaches to the prevention of CMV disease include the use of CMV-seronegative blood products, selection of CMV-seronegative donors for transplant recipients, passive immunoprophylaxis with immunoglobulin, prophylactic or preemptive use of antiviral agents, active immunization with a CMV vaccine, and behavioral strategies.

BLOOD PRODUCT, HUMAN MILK, AND TRANSPLANT DONOR SELECTION

Transplant recipients who are CMV seronegative and receive solid organ or bone marrow transplants from CMV-seropositive donors are at significant risk for acquiring symptomatic primary CMV infection. Therefore, whenever possible, CMV-seronegative recipients should receive transplants from CMV-seronegative donors, and all blood product transfusions should be from CMV-seronegative donors.

Infection with CMV in seriously ill CMV-seronegative neonates can be prevented by using blood products from CMV-seronegative donors or by using frozen deglycerolized red blood cells.[34, 296] Saline-washed red blood cells, however, do not appear to prevent the acquisition of CMV infection in neonates, even though as many as 90 percent of the leukocytes can be removed by this method.[69] An alternative method of preparing leukocyte-depleted blood, filtration through a cotton-wool filter, appears to prevent post-transfusion acquisition of CMV infection in neonates.[107] Many institutions now provide CMV-seronegative or leukocyte-depleted blood products routinely to all neonates or to all low-birth-weight neonates, regardless of the CMV serostatus of the mother. Because ingestion of CMV-positive breast milk by premature infants has been associated with illness, donor selection or pretreatment of human milk administered to extremely premature infants may reduce the risk of acquisition of CMV-associated disease in these infants, although clinical trials to prove this hypothesis have not been published yet.[169, 276]

PASSIVE IMMUNOPROPHYLAXIS

Although immunoglobulin or CMV hyperimmune globulin should not be used alone for the treatment of established CMV disease in immunocompromised patients, these preparations may be used to prevent the acquisition of serious CMV disease in selected immunocompromised patients. Passive immunization remains controversial, however, partly because studies have used different dosages (100 to 200 mg/kg) administered at varying intervals (1 week before transplantation and every 1 to 3 weeks after transplantation) for varying lengths of time (60 to 120 days). CMV immunoglobulin has been shown to decrease the incidence of symptomatic CMV disease from 60 to 21 percent in CMV-seronegative renal transplant recipients who received a kidney from a CMV-seropositive donor.[244] CMV immunoprophylaxis also has decreased the incidence of CMV pneumonitis in CMV-seronegative bone marrow transplant recipients who did not receive granulocyte transfusions.[32, 175, 292] The use of immunoglobulin in pregnant women to prevent or ameliorate CMV infection in the fetus has not been studied, and its use cannot be recommended at this time.

PROPHYLAXIS AND EARLY PREEMPTIVE THERAPY WITH ANTIVIRAL AGENTS

The prophylactic use of antiviral agents in transplant recipients has been evaluated and in some studies appears to reduce the incidence of serious CMV disease. However, this approach remains controversial because no regimen has been shown to completely prevent the acquisition of CMV infection or disease.[199] For example, acyclovir is used by some clinicians as prophylaxis for CMV disease in organ transplant recipients, despite evidence that acyclovir is inactive against most strains of CMV and CMV disease occurs despite such prophylaxis.[241] In one study, intravenous administration of acyclovir, 500 mg/m^2 of body surface area per dose every 8 hours for 5 days before and 30 days after transplantation, to CMV-seropositive bone marrow transplant recipients appeared to reduce the incidence of CMV disease.[176] High-dose oral acyclovir administered 1 day before and for 12 weeks after transplantation also has been shown to reduce the incidence of CMV disease and infection in renal transplant recipients.[23]

The prophylactic administration of human leukocyte interferon-α has been shown to reduce the incidence of severe CMV disease in renal transplant recipients, but it has no apparent benefit in bone marrow transplant recipients, and it is not used routinely in any patient population.[51, 127, 215] Many clinicians currently favor the prophylactic use of ganciclovir in transplant recipients at high risk for acquiring serious CMV disease. Prophylaxis treatment regimens vary, however, and it is difficult to make recommendations about which regimen, if any, is best. Most solid organ transplant recipients appear to benefit from intravenous ganciclovir, 5 to 10 mg/kg/day administered once or twice daily for 2 to 6 weeks post-transplantation, usually followed by continuing antiviral prophylaxis with acyclovir or a reduced dose of ganciclovir. Prophylactic ganciclovir does not appear, however, to benefit adult lung transplant patients in most published studies. Similarly, administering a short 2-week course of ganciclovir near the time of transplantation, without continuing antiviral prophylaxis, does not appear to reduce significantly the incidence of CMV disease in most solid organ transplant recipients studied.[16] The impact of intravenous immunoglobulin or CMV hyperimmune globulin, when given with a prophylactic antiviral agent, on the incidence of CMV disease in solid organ recipients is unclear. However, many clinicians administer it concomitantly with an antiviral agent when attempting to prevent CMV disease in certain high-risk transplant recipients. In bone marrow transplant recipients, the administration of ganciclovir prophylaxis after marrow engraftment reduced CMV disease but did not seem to reduce overall mortality significantly. In addition, ganciclovir-treated bone marrow transplant recipients experienced prolonged neutropenia.[113]

The strategy of preemptive antiviral therapy has certain advantages over strategies that either treat only patients with overt clinical disease or administer prophylactic antiviral agents to many patients at risk, only a few of whom appear to benefit. In addition, preemptive or very early antiviral treatment strategies include viral surveillance of blood, urine, and respiratory samples. Viral surveillance of these samples can be by standard viral culture, viral antigen detection, viral nucleic acid detection by PCR assay, or a combination of these tests. Detection of CMV viremia and culture-positive bronchoalveolar lavage samples have correlated with the development of serious CMV disease in transplant recipients.[39] At least two studies of bone marrow transplant recipients now have documented the efficacy of early intervention with intravenous ganciclovir therapy at the time that positive CMV surveillance cultures were obtained but before clinical disease developed.[113, 233] This strategy also appears efficacious in solid organ transplant recipients.[241] Another approach to preemptive therapy that does not entail viral surveillance techniques is to administer an antiviral agent, such as ganciclovir, during times of rejection, when CMV reactivation is likely to occur. This approach has been modestly successful in high-risk renal transplant recipients.[126]

ACTIVE IMMUNIZATION

Prevention of acquisition of CMV disease through active immunization should be a priority for the 21st century.[259] Pregnant women and their fetuses, as well as transplant recipients, would benefit greatly if a safe, effective CMV vaccine became widely available. The ideal CMV vaccine should be safe, effective, immunogenic, and cost-effective. It should prevent the development of primary CMV infection without causing chronic persistent infection. The vaccine also should not be capable of infecting the fetus, and it should not be oncogenic.

In 1975, Plotkin and associates[203] characterized and reported a candidate CMV vaccine strain, Towne 125, that was isolated originally from the urine of a congenitally infected infant named Towne. Since then, more than 500 subjects, including renal transplant recipients and healthy adult male and female volunteers, have received the investigational Towne 125 vaccine.[46, 98, 142, 201–203, 205, 257] Studies of these subjects showed that Towne 125 is attenuated and relatively safe and that it induces humoral and cellular immunity in both healthy and immunosuppressed subjects.

The vaccine also appeared to be protective in a randomized, placebo-controlled study of 91 immunosuppressed renal transplant recipients.[202] In this study, 30 CMV-seronegative vaccine recipients received a kidney from a CMV-seropositive donor, and the incidence of severe CMV disease was significantly lower in the vaccine group than in the placebo group. However, the CMV infection rate did not differ significantly among the groups, and members of both groups experienced mild to moderate CMV disease. Subsequent studies have confirmed that CMV-seronegative renal transplant recipients who receive a live attenuated CMV vaccine are more resistant to serious CMV disease.[204] Whether a CMV vaccine given to CMV-seronegative women of child-bearing age before pregnancy will protect the fetus from intrauterine infection or disease is not known, but studies that may answer this question are in progress.

Another novel vaccine strategy being investigated is the development of mutant hybrid strains of CMV that combine the safety of the Towne strain with another CMV strain to produce enhanced immunogenicity and possibly, however, also enhanced virulence.[8, 200] Other investigators have evaluated subunit vaccines for CMV that contain purified glycoprotein B (gB) complexed with a powerful adjuvant.[36, 91, 192] Most recently, the cellular immune system has been targeted by "DNA vaccines" that encode gB and appear to induce protective cellular immunity against CMV. Finally, adoptive immunotherapy using sensitized T cells may be available soon in clinical trials.

BEHAVIORAL STRATEGIES TO PREVENT PRIMARY CYTOMEGALOVIRUS INFECTION

When faced with the current complexities associated with the development of a CMV vaccine and the challenges of administering effective antiviral therapy, some investigators suggest that an alternative practical option for prevention of

CMV infection during pregnancy is education of young women of child-bearing age.[297] Reliable, relatively inexpensive serologic evaluation is available, so all women contemplating pregnancy should know their CMV serologic status. In addition, because epidemiologic studies have shown a major source of CMV infection to be close contact with young children, women who are CMV seronegative should be aware that a high percentage of young children are infected actively with CMV and that while pregnant, they should exercise good hygienic practices when in close contact with young children, especially those who attend daycare centers or are known to have an active CMV infection. In fact, some studies have shown that the incidence of child-to-parent transmission of CMV may be reduced by interventions that identify susceptible pregnant women and educate them about increasing protective behavior such as handwashing and decreasing risky behavior for acquiring CMV such as kissing on the mouth and sharing eating utensils.[7, 97] In addition, CMV can be transmitted from husband to wife, and if the spouse experiences a CMV mononucleosis syndrome, a CMV-seronegative woman may wish to consider avoiding pregnancy for an individualized period.[71]

REFERENCES

1. Adler, S. P.: The molecular epidemiology of cytomegalovirus transmission among children attending a daycare center. J. Infect. Dis. *152*:760–767, 1985.
2. Adler, S. P.: Cytomegalovirus transmission among children in daycare, their mothers and caretakers. Pediatr. Infect. Dis. *7*:279–285, 1988.
3. Adler, S. P.: Molecular epidemiology of cytomegalovirus: Viral transmission among children attending a daycare center, their parents, and caretakers. J. Pediatr. *116*:366–372, 1988.
4. Adler, S. P.: Cytomegalovirus and child daycare: Evidence for an increased infection rate among day-care workers. N. Engl. J. Med. *321*:1290–1296, 1989.
5. Adler, S. P.: Molecular epidemiology of cytomegalovirus: A study of factors affecting transmission among children at three day-care centers. Pediatr. Infect. Dis. J. *10*:584–590, 1991.
6. Adler, S. P., Baggett, J., Wilson, M., et al.: Molecular epidemiology of cytomegalovirus in a nursery: Lack of evidence for nosocomial transmission. J. Pediatr. *108*:117–123, 1986.
7. Adler, S. P., Finney, J. W., Manganello, A. M., et al.: Prevention of child-to-mother transmission of cytomegalovirus by changing behaviors: A randomized controlled trial. Pediatr. Infect. Dis. J. *15*:240–246, 1996.
8. Adler, S. P., Hempfling, S. H., Starr, S. E., et al.: Safety and immunogenicity of the Towne strain cytomegalovirus vaccine. Pediatr. Infect. Dis. J. *17*:200–207, 1998.
9. Akeeson-Johansson, A., Lernestedt, J. O., Rigden, O., et al.: Sensitivity of cytomegalovirus to intravenous foscarnet treatment. Bone Marrow Transplant. *1*:215–220, 1986.
10. Alexander, J. A., Cuellar, R. E., Fadden, R. J., et al.: Cytomegalovirus infection of the upper gastrointestinal tract before and after liver transplantation. Transplantation *46*:378–382, 1988.
11. Alford, C. A., Stagno, S., Pass, R. F., et al.: Epidemiology of cytomegalovirus infections. *In* Nahmias, A. J., Dowdle, W. R., and Schinazi, R. F. (eds.): The Human Herpesviruses: An Interdisciplinary Perspective. New York, Elsevier North Holland, 1987, pp. 159–171.
12. Anders, K., Steinsapir, K. D., Iverson, D. J., et al.: Neuropathologic findings in the acquired immunodeficiency syndrome (AIDS). Clin. Neuropathol. *5*:1–20, 1986.
13. Arav-Boger, R., Reif, S., and Bujanover, Y.: Portal vein thrombosis caused by protein C and protein S deficiency associated with cytomegalovirus infection. J. Pediatr. *126*:586–588, 1995.
14. Ashraf, S. J., Parande, C. M., and Arya, S. C.: Cytomegalovirus antibodies of patients in the Gizen area of Saudi Arabia. J. Infect. Dis. *152*:1351, 1985.
15. Atkins, J. T., Demmler, G. J., Williamson, W. D., et al.: Polymerase chain reaction to detect cytomegalovirus DNA in the cerebrospinal fluid of neonates with congenital infection. J. Infect. Dis. *169*:1334–1337, 1994.
16. Bailey, T. C., Trulock, E. P., Ettinger, N. A., et al.: Failure of prophylactic ganciclovir to prevent cytomegalovirus disease in recipients of lung transplants. J. Infect. Dis. *165*:548–552, 1992.
17. Balcarek, K. B., Bagley, R., Cloud, G. A., et al.: Cytomegalovirus infection among employees in a children's hospital: No evidence for increased risk associated with patient care. J. A. M. A. *263*:840–844, 1990.
18. Bale, J. F.: Human cytomegalovirus infection and disorders of the nervous system. Arch. Neurol. *41*:310–320, 1984.
19. Bale, J.: Conditions mimicking congenital infections. Semin. Pediatr. Neurol. *1*:63–67, 1994.
20. Bale, J. F., Bray, P. F., and Bell, W. E.: Neuroradiographic abnormalities in congenital cytomegalovirus infection. Pediatr. Neurol. *1*:42–47, 1985.
21. Bale, J. F., Murph, J. R., Demmler, G. J., et al.: Intrauterine cytomegalovirus infection and glycoprotein B genotypes. J. Infect. Dis. *182*:933–936, 2000.
22. Balfour, C. L., and Balfour, H. H.: Cytomegalovirus is not an occupational risk for nurses in renal transplant and neonatal units: Results of a prospective surveillance study. J. A. M. A. *256*:1909–1914, 1986.
23. Balfour, H. H., Chace, B. A., Stapleton, J. T., et al.: A randomized, placebo-controlled trial of oral acyclovir for the prevention of cytomegalovirus disease in recipients of renal allografts. N. Engl. J. Med. *320*:1381–1387, 1989.
24. Bamborschke, S., Wullen, T., Huber, M., et al.: Early diagnosis and successful treatment of acute cytomegalovirus encephalitis in a renal transplant recipient. J. Neurol. *239*:205–208, 1992.
25. Bauman, N. M., Kirby-Keyser, L. J., Dolan, K. D., et al.: Mondini dysplasia and congenital cytomegalovirus infection. J. Pediatr. *124*:71–78, 1994.
26. Becraft, D.: Prenatal cytomegalovirus infection and muscular deficiency (eventration) of the diaphragm. J. Pediatr. *94*:74–75, 1979.
27. Benson, M. C., Kaplan, M. S., O'Toole, K., et al.: A report of cytomegalovirus cystitis and a review of other genitourinary manifestations of the acquired immune deficiency syndrome. J. Urol. *140*:153–154, 1988.
28. Bloom, J. N., and Palestine, A. G.: The diagnosis of cytomegalovirus retinitis. Ann. Intern. Med. *109*:963–969, 1988.
29. Bonkowsky, H. L., Lee, R. V., and Klatskin, G.: Acute granulomatous hepatitis: Occurrence in cytomegalovirus mononucleosis. J. A. M. A. *233*:1284–1288, 1975.
30. Boppana, S., Amos, C., Britt, W., et al.: Late onset and reactivation of chorioretinitis in children with congenital cytomegalovirus infection. Pediatr. Infect. Dis. J. *13*:1139–1142, 1994.
31. Boppana, S. B., Fowler, K. B., Vaid, Y., et al.: Neuroradiographic findings in the newborn period and long-term outcome in children with symptomatic congenital cytomegalovirus infection. Pediatrics *99*: 409–414, 1997.
32. Bowden, R. A., Sayers, S., Flournoy, N., et al.: Cytomegalovirus immune globulin and seronegative blood products to prevent primary cytomegalovirus infection after marrow transplantation. N. Engl. J. Med. *16*:1006–1010, 1986.
33. Brady, M. T.: Cytomegalovirus infections: Occupational risk for health professionals. Am. J. Infect. Control *14*:197–203, 1986.
34. Brady, M. T., Milam, J. D., Anderson, D. C., et al.: Use of deglycerolized red blood cells to prevent post transfusion infection with cytomegalovirus in neonates. J. Infect. Dis. *150*:334–339, 1984.
35. Breinig, M. K., Zitelli, B., Starzl, T. E., et al.: Epstein-Barr virus, cytomegalovirus, and other viral infections in children after liver transplantation. J. Infect. Dis. *156*:273–279, 1987.
36. Britt, W. J., Vugler, L., Butfiloski, E. J., et al.: Cell surface expression of human cytomegalovirus (HCMV) gp 55–116(gB): Use of HCMV-recombinant vaccinia virus–infected cells in analysis of the human neutralizing antibody response. J. Virol. *64*:1079–1085, 1990.
37. Bronsther, O., Makowka, L., Jaffe, R., et al.: Occurrence of cytomegalovirus hepatitis in liver transplant patients. J. Med. Virol. *24*:423–434, 1988.
38. Buffone, G. J., Demmler, G. J., Schimbor, C. M., et al.: DNA hybridization assay for congenital cytomegalovirus infection. J. Clin. Microbiol. *26*:2184–2186, 1988.
39. Buffone, G. J., Frost, A., Samo, T., et al.: The diagnosis of CMV pneumonitis in lung and heart/lung transplant patients by PCR compared with traditional laboratory criteria. Transplantation *56*:342–347, 1993.
40. Buffone, G. J., Schimbor, C. M., Demmler, G. J., et al.: Detection of cytomegalovirus in urine by nonisotopic DNA hybridization. J. Infect. Dis. *154*:163–166, 1986.
41. Buhles, W. C., Mastre, J. B., Tinker, A. J., et al.: Ganciclovir treatment of life- or sight-threatening cytomegalovirus infection: Experience in 314 immunocompromised patients. Rev. Infect. Dis. *10*(Suppl.):495–506, 1988.
42. Butler, K., DeSmet, M., Husson, R. N., et al.: Treatment of aggressive cytomegalovirus retinitis with ganciclovir in combination with foscarnet in a child infected with human immunodeficiency virus. J. Pediatr. *120*:483–486, 1992.
43. Butt, W., Mackey, R. J., deCrespigny, L. C., et al.: Intracranial lesions of congenital cytomegalovirus infection detected by ultrasound scanning. Pediatrics *73*:611–614, 1984.
44. Cacoub, P., Deray, G., Baumelou, A., et al.: Acute renal failure induced by foscarnet: 4 cases. Clin. Nephrol. *29*:315–318, 1988.
45. Cantrill, H. L., Henry, K., Melroe, N. H., et al.: Treatment of cytomegalovirus retinitis with intravitreal ganciclovir. Ophthalmology *96*:367–374, 1989.
46. Carney, W. P., Hirsch, M. S., Iacoviello, V. R., et al.: T-lymphocyte subsets and proliferative responses following immunization with cytomegalovirus vaccine. J. Infect. Dis. *147*:958–960, 1983.

47. Cassol, S. A., Poon, M. C., Pal, R., et al.: Primer-mediated enzymatic amplification of cytomegalovirus (CMV) DNA: Application to the early diagnosis of CMV infection in marrow transplant recipients. J. Clin. Invest. *83*:1109–1115, 1989.
48. Chanarin, I., and Walford, D. M.: Thrombocytopenic purpura in cytomegalovirus mononucleosis. Lancet *2*:238–239, 1973.
49. Chandler, S. H., Handsfield, H. H., and McDougall, J. K.: Isolation of multiple strains of cytomegalovirus from women attending a clinic for sexually transmitted diseases. J. Infect. Dis. *155*:655–660, 1987.
50. Chandler, S. H., Holmes, K. K., Wentworth, B. B., et al.: The epidemiology of cytomegaloviral infection in women attending a sexually transmitted disease clinic. J. Infect. Dis. *152*:597–605, 1985.
51. Cheeseman, S. H., Rubin, R. H., Stewart, J. A., et al.: Controlled clinical trial of prophylactic human leukocyte interferon in renal transplantation. N. Engl. J. Med. *300*:1345–1349, 1979.
52. Chonmaitree, T., Owen, M. J., Pater, J., et al.: Presence of cytomegalovirus and herpes simplex virus in middle ear fluids from children with acute otitis media. Clin. Infect. Dis. *15*:650–653, 1992.
53. Chou, S.: Acquisition of donor strains of cytomegalovirus by renal transplant recipients. N. Engl. J. Med. *314*:1418–1423, 1986.
54. Chou, S.: Neutralizing antibody responses to reinfecting strains of cytomegalovirus in transplant recipients. J. Infect. Dis. *160*:16–21, 1989.
55. Chou, S., Guentzel, S., Michels, K. R., et al.: Frequency of UL97 phosphotransferase mutations related to ganciclovir resistance in clinical cytomegalovirus isolates. J. Infect Dis. *172*:238–242, 1995.
56. Chou, S., Marousek, G., Guentzel, S., et al.: Evolution of mutations conferring multidrug resistance during prophylaxis and therapy for cytomegalovirus disease. J. Infect. Dis. *176*:786–789, 1997.
57. Cinque, P., Vago, L., and Brytling, M.: Cytomegalovirus infection of the central nervous system in patients with AIDS: Diagnosis by DNA amplification from cerebrospinal fluid. J. Infect. Dis. *166*:1408–1411, 1992.
58. Coats, D. K., Demmler, G. J., Paysse, E. A., et al.: Ophthalmologic findings in children with congenital cytomegalovirus infection. J. A. A. P. O. S. *4*:110–116, 2000.
59. Cohen, J. I., and Corey, G. R.: Cytomegalovirus infection in the normal host. Medicine (Baltimore) *64*:100–114, 1985.
60. Collier, A. C., Handsfield, H. H., Roberts, P. L., et al.: Cytomegalovirus infection in women attending a sexually transmitted disease clinic. J. Infect. Dis. *162*:46–51, 1990.
61. Connolly, P. K., Jerger, S., Williamson, W. D., et al.: Evaluation of higher-level auditory function in children with asymptomatic congenital cytomegalovirus infection. Am. J. Otol. *13*:185–193, 1992.
62. Crumpacker, C., Marlowe, S., Zhang, J. L., et al.: Treatment of cytomegalovirus pneumonia. Rev. Infect. Dis. *10*(Suppl.):538–546, 1988.
63. Curless, R. G., Scott, G. B., Post, M. J., et al.: Progressive cytomegalovirus encephalopathy following congenital infection in an infant with acquired immunodeficiency syndrome. Childs Nerv. Syst. *3*:255–257, 1987.
64. Danish, E. H., Dahms, B. B., and Kumar, M. L.: Cytomegalovirus-associated hemophagocytic syndrome. Pediatrics *75*:280–283, 1985.
65. Dankner, W. M., McCutchan, J. A., Richman, D. D., et al.: Localization of human cytomegalovirus in peripheral blood leukocytes by in situ hybridization. J. Infect. Dis. *161*:31–36, 1990.
66. Davis, G. L., Spector, G. J., Strauss, M., et al.: Cytomegalovirus endolabyrinthitis. Arch. Pathol. Lab. Med. *101*:118–121, 1977.
67. Davis, L. E., Stewart, J. A., and Garvin, S.: Cytomegalovirus infection: A seroepidemiologic comparison of nuns and women from a venereal disease clinic. Am. J. Epidemiol. *102*:327–330, 1975.
68. Demmler, G. J.: Summary of a workshop on surveillance for congenital CMV disease. Rev. Infect. Dis *13*:315–329, 1991.
69. Demmler, G. J., Brady, M. T., Bijou, H., et al.: Post-transfusion cytomegalovirus infection in neonates: Role of saline-washed red blood cells. J. Pediatr. *108*:762–765, 1986.
70. Demmler, G. J., Buffone, G. J., Schimbor, C. M., et al.: Detection of cytomegalovirus in urine from newborns by using polymerase chain reaction DNA amplification. J. Infect. Dis. *158*:1177–1184, 1988.
71. Demmler, G. J., O'Neil, G. W., O'Neil, J. H., et al.: Transmission of cytomegalovirus from husband to wife. J. Infect. Dis. *154*:545–546, 1986.
72. Demmler, G. J., Six, H. R., Hurst, S. M., et al.: Enzyme-linked immunosorbent assay for the detection of IgM-class antibodies to cytomegalovirus. J. Infect. Dis. *153*:1152–1154, 1986.
73. Demmler, G. J., Yow, M. D., Spector, S. A., et al.: Nosocomial cytomegalovirus infections in two hospitals caring for infants and children. J. Infect. Dis. *156*:9–16, 1987.
74. Dietrich, D. T., Chachoua, A., Francois, L., et al.: Ganciclovir treatment of gastrointestinal infections caused by cytomegalovirus in patients with AIDS. Rev. Infect. Dis. *10*(Suppl.):532–537, 1988.
75. Dimmick, J. E., and Bove K. E.: Cytomegalovirus infection of the bowel in infancy: Pathogenetic and diagnostic significance. Pediatr. Pathol. *2*:95–102, 1984.
76. Dolgin, S. E., Larsen, J. G., Shah, K. D., et al.: CMV enteritis causing hemorrhage and obstruction in an infant with AIDS. J. Pediatr. Surg. *25*:696–698, 1990.
77. Donner, C., Liesnard, C., Congent, J., et al.: Prenatal diagnosis of 52 pregnancies at risk for congenital cytomegalovirus infection. Obstet. Gynecol. *82*:481–486, 1993.
78. Dowling, J. N., Saslow, A. R., Armstrong, J. A., et al.: Cytomegalovirus infection in patients receiving immunosuppressive therapy for rheumatologic disorders. J. Infect. Dis. *133*:399–408, 1976.
79. Doyle, M., Atkins, J.-T., and Rivera-Matos, I. R.: Congenital cytomegalovirus infection in infants infected with human immunodeficiency virus type 1. Pediatr. Infect. Dis. J. *15*:1102–1106, 1996.
80. Drew, W. L., Ives, D., Lalezari, J. P., et al.: Oral ganciclovir as maintenance treatment for cytomegalovirus retinitis in patients with AIDS. N. Engl. J. Med. *333*:615–620, 1995.
81. Drew, W. L., Sweet, E. S., Miner, R. C., et al.: Multiple infections by cytomegalovirus in patients with acquired immunodeficiency syndrome: Documentation by Southern blot hybridization. J. Infect. Dis. *150*:952–953, 1984.
82. Dummer, J. S., White, L. T., Ho, M., et al.: Morbidity of cytomegalovirus infection in recipients of heart-lung transplants who received cyclosporine. J. Infect. Dis. *152*:1182–1191, 1985.
83. Dworsky, M., Lakeman, A., and Stagno, S.: Cytomegalovirus transmission within a family. Pediatr. Infect. Dis. *3*:236–238, 1984.
84. Dworsky, M. E., Weoch, K., Cassady, G., et al.: Occupational risk for primary cytomegalovirus infection among pediatric health-care workers. N. Engl. J. Med. *309*:950–953, 1983.
85. Dworsky, M., Yow, M., Stagno, S., et al.: Cytomegalovirus infection of breast milk and transmission in infancy. Pediatrics *72*:295–300, 1983.
86. Emanuel, D., Cunningham, I., Jules-Elysee, K., et al.: Cytomegalovirus pneumonia after bone marrow transplantation successfully treated with the combination of ganciclovir and high-dose intravenous immune globulin. Ann. Intern. Med. *109*:777–782, 1988.
87. Embil, J. A., Goldbloom, A. L., and McFarlane, E. S.: Isolation of cytomegalovirus from middle ear effusion. J. Pediatr. *107*:435–436, 1985.
88. Enders, G., Bader, V., Lindemann, L., et al.: Prenatal diagnosis of congenital cytomegalovirus infection in 189 pregnancies with known outcome. Prenat. Diagn. *21*:326–377, 2001.
89. Erice, A., Chou, S., Biron, K. K., et al.: Progressive disease due to ganciclovir-resistant cytomegalovirus in immunocompromised patients. N. Engl. J. Med. *320*:289–293, 1989.
90. Faix, R. G.: Survival of cytomegalovirus on environmental surfaces. J. Pediatr. *106*:649–652, 1985.
91. Farrar, G. H., Bull, J. R., and Greenaway, P. J.: Prospects for the clinical management of human cytomegalovirus infections. Vaccine *4*:217–224, 1986.
92. Felsenstein, E., D'Amico, D. J., Hirsch, M. S., et al.: Treatment of cytomegalovirus retinitis with 9-[2-hydroxy-1-(hydroxymethyl)ethoxymethyl]guanine. Ann. Intern. Med. *103*:377–380, 1985.
93. Fenner, T. E., Garweg, J., Hufert, F. T., et al.: Diagnoses of human cytomegalovirus-induced retinitis in human immunodeficiency virus type-1–infected subjects by using the polymerase chain reaction. J. Clin. Microbiol. *29*:2621–2622, 1991.
94. Ferreiro, J., and Vinters, H. V.: Pathology of the pituitary gland in patients with the acquired immune deficiency syndrome (AIDS). Pathology *20*:211–215, 1988.
95. Fiala, M., and Kattlove, H.: Cytomegalovirus mononucleosis with severe thrombocytopenia. Ann. Intern. Med. *79*:450–451, 1973.
96. Fiala, M., Payne, J. E., Berne, T. V., et al.: Epidemiology of cytomegalovirus infection after transplantation and immunosuppression. J. Infect. Dis. *132*:421–433, 1975.
97. Finney, J. W., Miller, K. M., and Adler, S. P.: Changing protective and risky behaviors to prevent child-to-parent transmission of cytomegalovirus. J. Appl. Behav. Anal. *26*:471–472, 1993.
98. Fleisher, G. R., Starr, S. E., Friedman, H. M., et al.: Vaccination of pediatric nurses with live attenuated cytomegalovirus. Am. J. Dis. Child. *136*:294–296, 1982.
99. Flores-Aguilar, J., Huang, J. S., Wiley, C. A., et al.: Long-acting therapy of viral retinitis with (S)-1-(3-hydroxy-2-phosphorylmethoxypropyl) cytosine. J. Infect. Dis. *169*:642–647, 1994.
100. Fowler, K. B., Dahle, A. J., Boppana, S. B., et al.: Newborn hearing screening: Will children with hearing loss caused by congenital cytomegalovirus infection be missed? J. Pediatr. *135*:60–64, 1999.
101. Fowler, K. B., McCollister, F. P., Dahle, A. J., et al.: Progressive of fluctuating sensorineural hearing loss in children with asymptomatic congenital cytomegalovirus infection. J. Pediatr. *130*:626–630, 1997.
102. Frank, T. S., LiVolsi, V. A., and Connor, A. M.: Cytomegalovirus infection of the thyroid in immunocompromised adults. Yale J. Biol. Med. *60*:1–8, 1987.
103. Fries, B. C., Chou, S., Boeckh, M., et al.: Frequency distribution of cytomegalovirus envelope glycoprotein genotypes in bone marrow transplant recipients. J. Infect. Dis. *169*:769–774, 1994.
104. Frenkel, L. D., Keys, M. P., Hefferen, S. J., et al.: Unusual eye abnormalities associated with congenital cytomegalovirus infection. Pediatrics *5*:763–766, 1980.
105. Fuller, G. N., Jacobs, J. M., and Guiloff, R. J.: Association of painful peripheral neuropathy in AIDS with cytomegalovirus infection. Lancet *2*:937–940, 1989.
106. Gerna, G., Zipeto, D., Parea, M., et al.: Monitoring of human cytomegalovirus infections and ganciclovir treatment in heart transplant

recipients by determination of viremia, antigenemia and DNAemia. J. Infect. Dis. *164*:488–498, 1991.
107. Gilbert, G. L., Hudson, I. L., Hayes, K., et al.: Prevention of transfusion-acquired cytomegalovirus infection in infants by blood filtration to remove leukocytes. Lancet *1*:1228–1231, 1989.
108. Gleaves, C. A., Myerson, D., Bowden, R. A., et al.: Direct detection of cytomegalovirus from bronchoalveolar lavage samples by using a rapid in situ DNA hybridization assay. J. Clin. Microbiol. *27*:2429–2432, 1989.
109. Gleaves, C. A., Smith, T. F., Shuster, E. A., et al.: Comparison of standard tube and shell vial cell culture techniques for the detection of cytomegalovirus in clinical specimens. J. Clin. Microbiol. *21*:217–221, 1985.
110. Gonwa, T. A., Capehart, J. E., Pilcher, J. W., et al.: Cytomegalovirus myocarditis as a cause of cardiac dysfunction in a heart transplant. Transplantation *47*:197–199, 1989.
111. Goodgame, R. W., Genta, R. M., Estrada, R., et al.: Frequency of positive tests for cytomegalovirus in AIDS patients: Endoscopic lesions compared with normal mucosa. Am. J. Gastroenterol. *88*:338–343, 1993.
112. Goodpasture, E. Q., and Talbot, F. B.: Concerning the nature of "protozoan-like" cells in certain lesions of infancy. Am. J. Dis. Child. *21*:415–425, 1921.
113. Goodrich, J. M., Mori, M., Gleaves, C., et al.: Early treatment with ganciclovir to prevent cytomegalovirus disease after allogeneic bone marrow transplantation. N. Engl. J. Med. *325*:1601–1607, 1991.
114. Gozlan, J., Salord, J. M., Roullet, E., et al.: Rapid detection of cytomegalovirus DNA in cerebrospinal fluid of AIDS patients with neurologic disorders. J. Infect. Dis. *166*:1416–1421, 1992.
115. Grangeot-Keros, L., Mayaux, M. J., Lebon, P., et al.: Value of cytomegalovirus (CMV) IgG avidity index for the diagnosis of primary CMV infection in pregnant women. J. Infect. Dis. *175*:944–950, 1997.
116. Grattan, M. T., Moreno-Cabral, C. E., Starnes, V. A., et al.: Cytomegalovirus infection is associated with cardiac allograft rejection and atherosclerosis. J. A. M. A. *261*:3561–3566, 1989.
117. Greene, L. W., Cole, W., Greene, J. B., et al.: Adrenal insufficiency as a complication of the acquired immunodeficiency syndrome. Ann. Intern. Med. *101*:497–498, 1984.
118. Griffiths, P. D., and Baboonian, C.: A prospective study of primary cytomegalovirus infection during pregnancy: Final report. Br. J. Obstet. Gynaecol. *92*:307–315, 1984.
119. Griffiths, P. D., and Grundy, J. E.: Molecular biology and immunology of cytomegalovirus. Biochem. J. *241*:313–324, 1987.
120. Griffiths, P. D., Stagno, S., Pass, R. F., et al.: Congenital cytomegalovirus infection: Diagnostic and prognostic significance of the detection of specific immunoglobulin M antibodies in cord serum. Pediatrics *69*:544–549, 1982.
121. Grundy, J. E., Super, M., Sweny, P., et al.: Symptomatic cytomegalovirus infection in seropositive kidney recipients: Reinfection with donor virus rather than reactivation of recipient virus. Lancet *1*:132–135, 1988.
122. Gudnason, T., Belani, K. K., and Balfour, H. H.: Ganciclovir treatment of cytomegalovirus disease in immunocompromised children. Pediatr. Infect. Dis. *8*:436–440, 1989.
123. Hackman, R. C., Myerson, D., Meyers, J. D., et al.: Rapid diagnosis of cytomegalovirus pneumonia by tissue immunofluorescence with a murine monoclonal antibody. J. Infect. Dis. *151*:325–329, 1985.
124. Handsfield, H. H., Chandler, S. H., Caine, V. A., et al.: Cytomegalovirus infection in sex partners: Evidence for sexual transmission. J. Infect. Dis. *151*:344–348, 1985.
125. Hayward, J. C., Titelbaum, D. S., Clancy, R. R., et al.: Lissencephaly-pachygyria associated with congenital cytomegalovirus infection. J. Child. Neurol. *6*:109–114, 1991.
126. Hibberd, P. L., Tokoff-Rubin, N. E., Conti, D., et al.: Preemptive ganciclovir therapy to prevent cytomegalovirus disease in cytomegalovirus antibody–positive renal transplant recipients. Ann. Intern. Med. *123*:18–26, 1995.
127. Hirsch, M. S., Schooley, R. T., Cosimi, A. B., et al.: Effects of interferon-alpha on cytomegalovirus reactive syndromes in renal transplant recipients. N. Engl. J. Med. *308*:1489–1493, 1983.
128. Ho, D. D., Bredesen, D. E., Vinters, H. V., et al.: The acquired immunodeficiency sydrome (AIDS) dementia complex. Ann. Intern. Med. *111*:400–410, 1989.
129. Ho, M.: Characteristics of cytomegalovirus. *In* Greenough, W. B., and Merigan, T. C. (eds.): Cytomegalovirus Biology and Infection: Current Topics in Infectious Disease. New York, Plenum, 1982, pp. 9–32.
130. Hocker, J. R., Cook, L. N., Addams, G., et al.: Ganciclovir therapy of congenital cytomegalovirus pneumonia. Pediatr. Infect. Dis. J. *9*: 743–744, 1990.
131. Hohlfeld, P., Vial, Y., Maillard-Grignon, C., et al.: Cytomegalovirus fetal infections. Obstet. Gynecol. *78*:615–618, 1991.
132. Hokeberg, I., Olding-Stenkvist, E., Grillner, L., et al.: No evidence of hospital-acquired cytomegalovirus infection in a pregnant pediatric nurse using restriction endonuclease analysis. Pediatr. Infect. Dis. J. 7:812–814, 1988.
133. Horwitz, C. A., Henle, W., Henle, G., et al.: Clinical and laboratory evaluation of cytomegalovirus-induced mononucleosis in previously healthy individuals. Medicine (Baltimore) *65*:124–134, 1986.
134. Hutto, C., Little, E. A., Ricks, R., et al.: Isolation of cytomegalovirus from toys and hands in a daycare center. J. Infect. Dis. *154*:527–530, 1986.
135. Istas, A. S., Demmler, G. J., Dobbins, J. G., et al.: Surveillance for congenital cytomegalovirus disease: A report from the National Congenital Cytomegalovirus Disease Registry. Clin. Infect. Dis. *20*:665–670, 1995.
136. Jacobs, D. A., Enger, C., Dunn, J. P., et al.: Cytomegalovirus retinitis and viral resistance: Ganciclovir resistance. J. Infect. Dis. *177*:770–773, 1998.
137. Jacobson, M. A., and Mills, J.: Serious cytomegalovirus disease in the acquired immunodeficiency syndrome (AIDS). Ann. Intern. Med. *108*:585–594, 1988.
138. Jacobson, M. A., O'Donnel, J. J., Rousell, R., et al.: Failure of adjunctive cytomegalovirus immune globulin to improve efficacy of ganciclovir in patients with acquired immunodeficiency syndrome and cytomegalovirus retinitis: A phase 1 study. Antimicrob. Agents Chemother. *34*:176–178, 1990.
139. Jamison, R. M., and Hathorn, A. W.: Isolation of cytomegalovirus from cerebrospinal fluid of a congenitally infected infant. Am. J. Dis. Child. *132*:63–64, 1978.
140. Jones, L. A., Duke-Duncan, P. M., and Yeager, A. S.: Cytomegaloviral infections in infant-toddler centers: Centers for the developmentally delayed versus regular daycare. J. Infect. Dis. *151*:953–955, 1985.
141. Jordan, M. C., Rousseau, W. E., Noble, G. R., et al.: Association of cervical cytomegalovirus with venereal disease. N. Engl. J. Med. *288*:932–934, 1973.
142. Just, M., Buergin-Wolff, A., Emoedi, G., et al.: Immunization trials with live attenuated cytomegalovirus Towne 125. Infection *3*:111–114, 1975.
143. Kaariainen, L., Klemola, E., and Paloheimo, J.: Rise of cytomegalovirus antibodies in an infectious-mononucleosis–like syndrome after transfusion. B. M. J. *1*:1270–1272, 1966.
144. Kagan, R. J., Naragi, S., Matsuda, T., et al.: Herpes simplex virus and cytomegalovirus infections in burned patients. J. Trauma *25*:40–45, 1985.
145. Karn, K., Julian, T. M., and Ogburn, P. L.: Fetal heart block associated with congenital cytomegalovirus infection: A case report. J. Reprod. Med. *29*:278–280, 1984.
146. Kashden, J., Frison, S., Fowler, K. B., et al.: Intellectual assessment of children with asymptomatic congenital cytomegalovirus infection. J. Dev. Behav. Pediatr. *19*:254–259, 1998.
147. Keay, S., Petersen, E., Icenogle, T., et al.: Ganciclovir treatment of serious cytomegalovirus infection in heart and heart-lung transplant recipients. Rev. Infect. Dis. *10*(Suppl.):563–572, 1988.
148. Kim, Y. J., Gururaj, V. J., and Mirkovic, R. R.: Concomitant diffuse nodular pulmonary infiltration in an infant with cytomegalovirus infection. Pediatr. Infect. Dis. *1*:173–176, 1982.
149. Kim, Y. S., and Hollander, H.: Polyradiculopathy due to cytomegalovirus: Report of two cases in which improvement occurred after prolonged therapy and review of the literature. Clin. Infect. Dis. *17*:32–37, 1993.
150. Kimberlin, D. W., Lin, C.-Y., Sanchez, P., et al.: Effect of ganciclovir therapy on hearing in symptomatic congenital cytomegalovirus disease involving the central nervous system: A randomized, controlled trial. J. Pediatr. *143*:17–26, 2003.
151. Klemola, E., Stenstrom, R., and von Essen, R.: Pneumonia as a clinical manifestation of cytomegalovirus infection in previously healthy adults. Scand. J. Infect. Dis. *4*:7–10, 1972.
152. Klemola, E., von Essen, R., Henle, G., et al.: Infectious mononucleosis–like disease with negative heterophil agglutination test: Clinical features in relations to Epstein-Barr virus and cytomegalovirus and antibodies. J. Infect. Dis. *121*:608–614, 1970.
153. Kovacs, A., Schluchter, M., Easley, K., et al.: Cytomegalovirus infection and HIV-1 disease progression in infants born to HIV-1 infected mothers. N. Engl. J. Med. *341*:77–84, 1999.
154. Kumar, M. L., Gold, E., Jacobs, I. B., et al.: Primary cytomegalovirus infection in adolescent pregnancy. Pediatrics *74*:493–500, 1984.
155. Kumar, M. L., Jenson, H. B., Dahms, B. B.: Fatal *Staphylococcal epidermidis* infections in very low-birth-weight infants with cytomegalovirus infection. Pediatrics *76*:110–114, 1985.
156. Kumar, M. L., Nankervis, G. A., Cooper, A. R., et al.: Postnatally acquired cytomegalovirus infections in infants of CMV-excreting mothers. J. Pediatr. *104*:669–673, 1984.
157. Kumar, M. L., Nankervis, G. A., Jacobs, I. B., et al.: Congenital and postnatally acquired cytomegalovirus infections: Long-term follow-up. J. Pediatr. *104*:674–679, 1984.
158. Lang, D. J., and Kummer, J. F.: Cytomegalovirus in semen: Observations in selected populations. J. Infect. Dis. *132*:472–473, 1975.
159. Lazarotto, T., Maine, G. T., Dalmonte, P., et al.: A novel Western blot test containing both viral and recombinant proteins for anti-cytomegalovirus immunoglobulin MN detection. J. Clin. Microbiol. *35*:393–397, 1997.
160. Lee, R. W., and Ai, E.: Disc neovascularization in patients with AIDS and cytomegalovirus retinitis. Retina *11*:305–308, 1991.
161. Lehoang, P., Giarard, B., Robinet, M., et al.: Foscarnet in the treatment of cytomegalovirus retinitis in acquired immunodeficiency syndrome. Ophthalmology *96*:865–874, 1989.

162. Lesher, J. L.: Cytomegalovirus infections and the skin. J. Am. Acad. Dermatol. *18*:1333–1338, 1988.
163. Levin, A. V., Zeichner, S., Duker, J. S., et al.: Cytomegalovirus retinitis in an infant with acquired immunodeficiency syndrome. Pediatrics *84*:683–687, 1989.
164. Levin, M.: Current approaches to the prevention and treatment of cytomegalovirus disease after bone marrow transplantation: An overview. Semin. Hematol. *27*:1–4, 1990.
165. Lim, W., Kahn, E., Gupta, A., et al.: Treatment of cytomegalovirus enterocolitis with ganciclovir in an infant with acquired immunodeficiency syndrome. Pediatr. Infect. Dis. *7*:354–357, 1988.
166. Linneman, C. C., and MacMillan, B. G.: Viral infections in pediatric burn patients. Am. J. Dis. Child. *135*:750–753, 1981.
167. Lui, W. Y., and Chang, W. K.: Cytomegalovirus mononucleosis in Chinese infants. Arch. Dis. Child. *47*:643, 1972.
168. Martin, D. F., Sierra-Madero, J., Walmsley, S., et al.: A controlled trial of valganciclovir as induction therapy for cytomegalovirus retinitis. N. Engl. J. Med. *346*:1119–1126, 2002.
169. Maschmann, J., Hamprecht, K., Dietz, K., et al.: Cytomegalovirus infection of extremely low-birth weight infants via breast milk. Clin. Infect. Dis. *33*:1998–2002, 2000.
170. Matthews, T., and Boehme, R.: Antiviral activity and mechanism of action of ganciclovir. Rev. Infect. Dis. *10*(Suppl.):490–494, 1988.
171. McDonald, K., Rector, T. S., Braunlin, E. A., et al.: Association of coronary artery disease in cardiac transplant recipients with cytomegalovirus infection. Am. J. Cardiol. *64*:359–362, 1989.
172. McKeating, J. A., Griffiths, P. D., and Grundy, J. E.: Cytomegalovirus in urine specimens has host beta 2 microglobulin bound to the viral envelope: A mechanism of evading the host immune response. J. Gen. Virol. *68*:785–792, 1987.
173. Melnick, J. L., Adam, E., and DeBakey, M. E.: Possible role of cytomegalovirus in atherogenesis. J. A. M. A. *263*:2204–2207, 1990.
174. Mena, W., Royal, S., Pass, R. F., et al.: Diabetes insipidus associated with symptomatic congenital cytomegalovirus infection. J. Pediatr. *122*: 911–913, 1993.
175. Meyers, J. D., Leszcynski, J., Zaia, J., et al.: Prevention of cytomegalovirus infection by cytomegalovirus immune globulin after marrow transplantation. Ann. Intern. Med. *98*:442–446, 1983.
176. Meyers, J. D., Reed, E. C., Shepp, D. H., et al.: Acyclovir for prevention of cytomegalovirus infection and disease after allogeneic marrow transplantation. N. Engl. J. Med. *318*:70–75, 1988.
177. Millett, R., Tomita, T., Marshall, H. E., et al.: Cytomegalovirus endomyocarditis in a transplanted heart. Arch. Pathol. Lab. Med. *115*:511–515, 1991.
178. Morgello, S., Cho, E. S., Nielsen, S., et al.: Cytomegalovirus encephalitis in patients with acquired immunodeficiency syndrome: An autopsy study of 30 cases and a review of the literature. Hum. Pathol. *18*:289–297, 1987.
179. Murph, J. R., and Bale, J. F.: The natural history of acquired cytomegalovirus infection among children in group daycare. Am. J. Dis. Child. *142*:843–846, 1988.
180. Murph, J. R., Souze, I. E., Dawson, J. D., et al.: Epidemiology of congenital cytomegalovirus infection: maternal risk factors and molecular analysis of cytomegalovirus strains. Am. J. Epidemiol. *47*:940–947, 1998.
181. Nelson, C. T., Istas, A. S., Wilkerson, M. K., et al.: Polymerase chain reaction detection of cytomegalovirus DNA in serum as a diagnostic test for congenital cytomegalovirus infection. J. Clin. Microbiol. *33*: 3317–3318, 1995.
182. Nielsen, S. L., Petito, C. K., Urmacher, C. D., et al.: Subacute encephalitis in acquired immune deficiency syndrome: A postmortem study. Am. J. Clin. Pathol. *82*:678–682, 1984.
183. Nielsen, S. L., Sorensen, I., and Anderson, H. K.: Kinetics of specific immunoglobulins M, E, A and G in congenital, primary and secondary cytomegalovirus infection studied by antibody-capture enzyme-linked immunosorbent assay. J. Clin. Microbiol. *26*:654–661, 1988.
184. Nigro, G., Scholz, H., and Bartman, U.: Ganciclovir therapy for symptomatic congenital cytomegalovirus infection in infants: A two-regimen experience. J. Pediatr. *124*:318–322, 1994.
185. Noyes, B. E., Kurland, G., Orenstein, D. M., et al.: Experience with pediatric lung transplantation. J. Pediatr. *124*:261–268, 1994.
186. Noyola, D. F., Demmler, G. J., Nelson, C. T., et al.: Early predictors of neurodevelopmental outcome in symptomatic congenital cytomegalovirus infection. J. Pediatr. *138*:325–331, 2001.
187. O'Grady, J. G., Sutherland, S., Harvey, R. Y., et al.: Cytomegalovirus infection and donor/recipient HLA antigens: Interdependent co-factors in pathogenesis of vanishing bile duct syndrome after liver transplantation. Lancet *2*:302–305, 1988.
188. Ong, E. L., Ellis, M. E., Tweele, D., et al.: *Cytomegalovirus cholecystitis* and colitis associated with the acquired immunodeficiency syndrome. J. Infect. Dis. *18*:73–75, 1989.
189. Pak, C. Y., McArthur, R., Eun, H. M., et al.: Association of cytomegalovirus infection with autoimmune type 1 diabetes. Lancet *2*:1–4, 1988.
190. Pannuti, C. S., Vilasboas, L. S., Angelo, M., et al.: Cytomegalovirus mononucleosis in children and adults: Differences in clinical presentation. Scand. J. Infect. Dis. *17*:153–156, 1985.
191. Pass, R. F., August, A. M., Dworsky, M., et al.: Cytomegalovirus infection in a day-care center. N. Engl. J. Med. *307*:477–479, 1982.
192. Pass, R. F., Duliege, A.-M., Boppana, S., et al.: A subunit cytomgalovirus vaccine based on recombinant envelope glycoprotein B and a new adjuvant. J. Infect. Dis. *180*:990–995, 1999.
193. Pass, R. F., and Hutto, S. C.: Group daycare and cytomegaloviral infections of mothers and children. Rev. Infect. Dis. *8*:599–605, 1986.
194. Pass, R. F., Hutto, S. C., Reynolds, D. W., et al.: Increased frequency of cytomegalovirus infection in children in group daycare. Pediatrics *74*:121–126, 1984.
195. Pass, R. F., Hutto, S. C., Ricks, R., et al.: Increased rate of cytomegalovirus infection among parents of children attending day-care centers. N. Engl. J. Med. *314*:1414–1418, 1986.
196. Pass, R. F., Little, E. A., Stagno, S., et al.: Young children as a probable source of maternal congenital cytomegalovirus infection. N. Engl. J. Med. *316*:1366–1370, 1987.
197. Pass, R. F., Whitley, R. J., Diethelm, A. G., et al.: Cytomegalovirus infection in patients with renal transplants: Potentiation by antithymocyte globulin and an incompatible graft. J. Infect. Dis. *142*:9–17, 1980.
198. Patterson, J. W., Broecker, A. H., Kornstein, M. J., et al.: Cutaneous cytomegalovirus infection in a liver transplant patient: Diagnosis by in situ DNA hybridization. Am. J. Dermatopathol. *10*:524–530, 1988.
199. Paya, C.: Prevention of cytomegalovirus disease in recipients of solid organ transplants. Clin. Infect. Dis. *32*:596–603, 2001.
200. Plotkin, S. A.: Vaccination against cytomegalovirus, the challenging demon. Pediatr. Infect. Dis. J. *18*:313–326, 1999.
201. Plotkin, S. A., Farquhar, J., and Hornberger, E.: Clinical trials of immunization with the Towne 125 strain of human cytomegalovirus. J. Infect. Dis. *134*:470–475, 1976.
202. Plotkin, S. A., Friedman, H. M., Fleisher, G. R., et al.: Towne-vaccine–induced prevention of cytomegalovirus disease after renal transplants. Lancet *1*:528–530, 1984.
203. Plotkin, S. A., Furukawa, T., Zygraich, N., et al.: Candidate cytomegalovirus strain for human vaccination. Infect. Immun. *12*:521–527, 1975.
204. Plotkin, S. A., Higgins, R., Kurtz, J. B., et al.: Multicenter trial of Towne strain attenuated virus vaccine in seronegative renal transplant recipients. Transplantation *58*:1176–1178, 1994.
205. Plotkin, S. A., Smiley, M. L., Friedman, H. M., et al.: Prevention of cytomegalovirus disease by Towne strain live attenuated vaccine. Birth Defects *20*:271–287, 1984.
206. Pollard, R. B.: Cytomegalovirus infections in renal, heart, heart-lung and liver transplantation. Pediatr. Infect. Dis. *7*(Suppl.):97–102, 1988.
207. Powell, K. F., Bellamy, A. R., Catton, M. G., et al.: Cytomegalovirus myocarditis in a heart transplant recipient: Sensitive monitoring of viral DNA by the polymerase chain reaction. J. Heart Transplant. *8*:465–470, 1989.
208. Proujansky, R., Orenstein, S. R., Kocoshis, S. A., et al.: Cytomegalovirus gastroenteritis after liver transplantation. J. Pediatr. *113*:700–703, 1988.
209. Rabinowitz, M., Bassan, I., and Robinson, M. J.: Sexually transmitted cytomegalovirus proctitis in a woman. Am. J. Gastroenterol. *83*:885–887, 1988.
210. Randazzo, R. F., Hulette, C. M., Gottlieb, M. S., et al.: Cytomegaloviral epididymitis in a patient with the acquired immune deficiency syndrome. J. Urol. *136*:1095–1097, 1986.
211. Rasmussen, L., Hong, C., Zipeto, D., et al.: Cytomegalovirus gB genotype distribution differs in human immunodeficiency virus–infected patients and immunocompromised allograft recipients. J. Infect. Dis. *175*:179–184, 1997.
212. Reed, E. C., Bowden, R. A., Dandliker, P. S., et al.: Efficacy of cytomegalovirus immunoglobulin in marrow transplant recipients with cytomegalovirus pneumonia. J. Infect. Dis. *156*:641–644, 1987.
213. Reed, E. C., Bowden, R. A., Dandliker, P. S., et al.: Treatment of cytomegalovirus pneumonia with ganciclovir and intravenous cytomegalovirus immune globulin in patients with bone marrow transplants. Ann. Intern. Med. *109*:783–788, 1988.
214. Reed, E. C., Dandliker, P. S., Meyers, J. D., et al.: Treatment of cytomegalovirus pneumonia with 9-[2-hydroxy-1-(hydroxymethyl)-ethoxymethyl]guanine and high dose corticosteroids. Ann. Intern. Med. *105*:214–215, 1986.
215. Reed, E. C., and Meyers, J. D.: Treatment of cytomegalovirus infection: Diagnosis and treatment of viral infections. Clin. Lab. Med. *7*:831–852, 1987.
216. Reed, E. C., Wolford, J. L., Kopecky, K. J., et al.: Ganciclovir for the treatment of cytomegalovirus gastroenteritis in bone marrow transplant patients. Ann. Intern. Med. *112*:505–510, 1990.
217. Reigstad, H., Bjerknes, R., Markestad, T., et al.: Ganciclovir therapy of congenital cytomegalovirus disease. Acta Paediatr. *81*:707–708, 1992.
218. Reller, L. B.: Granulomatous hepatitis associated with acute cytomegalovirus infection. Lancet *1*:20–22, 1973.
219. Revello, M. G., Baldanti, F., Furione, M., et al.: Polymerase chain reaction for prenatal diagnosis of congenital human cytomegalovirus infection. J. Med. Virol. *47*:462–466, 1995.
220. Reynolds, D. W., Stagno, S., Hosty, T. S., et al.: Maternal CMV excretion and perinatal infection. N. Engl. J. Med. *289*:4–7, 1973.

221. Ribbert, H.: Ueber protozoanartige Zellen in der neire eines syphilitischen Neugeborenen und in der Parotis von Kindern. Zentralbl. Allg. Pathol. *15*:945–948, 1904.
222. Rinaldo, C. R., Carney, W. P., Richter, B. S., et al.: Mechanisms of immunosuppression of cytomegalovirus mononucleosis. J. Infect. Dis. *141*:488–495, 1980.
223. Rinaldo, C. R., Kingsley, L. A., Ho, M., et al.: Enhanced shedding of cytomegalovirus in semen of human immunodeficiency virus–seropositive homosexual men. J. Clin. Microbiol. *30*:1148–1155, 1992.
224. Ringden, O., Lonnqvist, B., Paulin, T., et al.: Pharmacokinetics, safety and preliminary clinical experiences using foscarnet in the treatment of cytomegalovirus infections in bone marrow and renal transplant recipients. J. Antimicrob. Chemother. *17*:378–387, 1986.
225. Robert, M. E., Geraghty, J. J., Miles, S. A., et al.: Severe neuropathy in a patient with acquired immune deficiency syndrome (AIDS): Evidence for widespread cytomegalovirus infection of peripheral nerve and human immunodeficiency virus–like immunoreactivity of anterior horn cells. Acta Neuropathol. *79*:255–261, 1989.
226. Rosenthal, S. L., Stanberry, L. R., Biro, F. M., et al.: Seroprevalence of herpes simplex virus types 1 and 2 and cytomegalovirus in adolescents. Clin. Infect. Dis. *24*:135–139, 1997.
227. Rowe, W. P., Hartley, J. W., Waterman, S., et al.: Cytopathogenic agent resembling human salivary gland virus recovered from tissue cultures of human adenoids. Proc. Soc. Exp. Biol. Med. *92*:418–424, 1956.
228. Saigal, S., Luny, K. O., Larke, R., et al.: The outcome in children with congenital cytomegalovirus infection. Am. J. Dis. Child. *136*:896–901, 1982.
229. Salisbury, S., and Embil, J. A.: Graves disease following congenital cytomegalovirus infection. J. Pediatr. *92*:954–955, 1978.
230. Sanchez, G. R., Neches, W. H., and Jaffe, R.: Myocardial aneurysm in association with disseminated cytomegalovirus infection. Pediatr. Cardiol. *2*:63–65, 1982.
231. Sandler, A., and Snedeker, J. D.: Cytomegalovirus infection in an infant presenting with cutaneous vasculitis. Pediatr. Infect. Dis. *6*:422–423, 1987.
232. Sawyer, M. H., Edwards, D. K., and Spector, S. A.: Cytomegalovirus infection and bronchopulmonary dysplasia in premature infants. Am. J. Dis. Child. *141*:303–305, 1987.
233. Schmidt, G. M., Horak, D. A., and Niland, J. C.: A randomized, controlled trial of prophylactic ganciclovir for cytomegalovirus pulmonary infection in recipients of allogeneic bone marrow transplants. N. Engl. J. Med. *324*:1005–1011, 1991.
234. Schmidt, N. J., and Emmons, R. W.: Diagnostic Procedures for Viral, Rickettsial and Chlamydial Infections. 6th ed. Washington, D.C., American Public Health Association, 1989, pp. 321–378.
235. Scott, G. B., Buck, B. E., Letterman, J. G., et al.: Acquired immunodeficiency syndrome in infants. N. Engl. J. Med. *310*:76–81, 1984.
236. Shabtai, M., Luft, B., Waltzer, W. C., et al.: Massive cytomegalovirus pneumonia and myocarditis in a renal transplant recipient: Successful treatment with DHPG. Transplant. Proc. *20*:562–563, 1988.
237. Shanley, J. D., Via, C. S., Sharrow, S. O., et al.: Interstitial pneumonitis during murine cytomegalovirus infection and graft-versus-host reaction. Transplantation *44*:658–662, 1987.
238. Shen, C., Chang, W., Chang, S., et al.: Cytomegalovirus transmission in special-care centers for mentally retarded children. Pediatrics *91*:79–82, 1993.
239. Shibata, D., Martin, W. J., Appleman, M. D., et al.: Detection of cytomegalovirus DNA in peripheral blood of patients infected with human immunodeficiency virus. J. Infect. Dis. *158*:1185–1192, 1988.
240. Singh, N., Dummer, J. S., Kusne, S., et al.: Infections with cytomegalovirus and other herpesviruses in 121 liver transplant recipients: Transmission by donated organ and the effect of OKT3 antibodies. J. Infect. Dis. *158*:124–131, 1988.
241. Singh, N., Yu, V., Mieles, L., et al.: High-dose acyclovir compared with short-course preemptive ganciclovir therapy to prevent cytomegalovirus disease in liver transplant recipients. Ann. Intern. Med. *120*:375–381, 1994.
242. Smith, M. G.: Propagation in tissue cultures of a cytopathogenic virus from human salivary gland virus (SGV) disease. Proc. Soc. Exp. Biol. Med. *92*:424–430, 1956.
243. Snider, W. D., Simpson, D. M., Nielsen, S., et al.: Neurological complications of acquired immune deficiency syndrome: Analysis of 50 patients. Ann. Neurol. *14*:403–418, 1984.
244. Snydman, D. R., Werner, B. G., Heinze-Lacey, B., et al.: Use of cytomegalovirus immune globulin to prevent cytomegalovirus disease in renal transplant recipients. N. Engl. J. Med. *317*:1049–1054, 1987.
245. Sohn, Y. M., Oh, M. K., Balcarek, K. B., et al.: Cytomegalovirus infection in sexually active adolescents. J. Infect. Dis. *163*:460–463, 1991.
246. Sokol, D. M., Demmler, G. J., and Buffone, G. J.: Rapid epidemiologic analysis of cytomegalovirus by using polymerase chain reaction amplification of the L-S junction region. J. Clin. Microbiol. *30*:839–844, 1992.
247. Sommadossi, J. P., Bevan, R., Ling, T., et al.: Clinical pharmacokinetics of ganciclovir in patients with normal and impaired renal function. Rev. Infect. Dis. *10*(Suppl.):507–514, 1988.
248. Spector, S. A.: Transmission of cytomegalovirus among infants in hospital documented by restriction-endonuclease-digestion analyses. Lancet *1*:378–381, 1983.
249. Spector, S. A., Hirata, K. K., and Neuman, T. R.: Identification of multiple cytomegalovirus strains in homosexual men with acquired immunodeficiency syndrome. J. Infect. Dis. *150*:953–956, 1984.
250. Spector, S. A., Merrill, R., Wolf, D., et al.: Detection of human cytomegalovirus in plasma of AIDS patients during acute visceral disease by DNA amplification. J. Clin. Microbiol. *30*:2359–2365, 1992.
251. Spector, S. A., Rua, J. A., Spector, D. H., et al.: Detection of human cytomegalovirus in clinical specimens by DNA-DNA hybridization. J. Infect. Dis. *150*:121–126, 1984.
252. Spector, S. A., and Spector, D. H.: Molecular epidemiology of cytomegalovirus infections in premature twin infants and their mother. Pediatr. Infect. Dis. *1*:405–409, 1982.
253. Stagno, S., Brasfield, D. M., Brown, M. B., et al.: Infant pneumonitis associated with cytomegalovirus, *Chlamydia, Pneumocystis,* and *Ureaplasma:* A prospective study. Pediatrics *68*:322–329, 1981.
254. Stagno, S., Pass, R. F., Dworsky, M. E., et al.: Congenital cytomegalovirus infection: The relative importance of primary and recurrent maternal infection. N. Engl. J. Med. *306*:945–949, 1982.
255. Stagno, S., Pass, R. F., Thomas, J. P., et al.: Defects of tooth structure in congenital cytomegalovirus infection. Pediatrics *69*:646–648, 1982.
256. Stagno, S., Tinker, M. K., Elrod, C., et al.: Immunoglobulin M antibodies detected by enzyme-linked immunosorbent assay and radioimmunoassay in the diagnosis of cytomegalovirus infections in pregnant women and newborn infants. J. Clin. Microbiol. *21*:930–935, 1985.
257. Starr, S. E., Glazer, J. P., Friedman, H. M., et al.: Specific cellular and humoral immunity after immunization with live Towne strain cytomegalovirus vaccine. J. Infect. Dis. *143*:585–589, 1981.
258. Stinski, M. F.: Cytomegalovirus and its replication. *In* Fields, B. N. (ed.): Virology. 2nd ed. New York, Raven Press, 1990, pp. 1959–1980.
259. Stratton, K. R., Durch, J. S., and Lawrence, R. S.: Vaccines for the 21st Century: A Tool for Decision Making. Report of the Committee to Study Priorities for Vaccine Development; Division of Health Promotion and Disease Prevention. Washington, D. C., Institute of Medicine, National Academy of Sciences, National Academy Press, 1999.
260. Strauss, M.: Human cytomegalovirus labyrinthitis. Am. J. Otolaryngol. *11*:292–298, 1990.
261. Studies of Ocular Complications of AIDS Research Group, in collaboration with the AIDS Clinical Trials Group: Mortality in patients with the acquired immunodeficiency syndrome treated with either foscarnet or ganciclovir for cytomegalovirus retinitis. N. Engl. J. Med. *326*:213–220, 1992.
262. Subietas, A., Deppisch, L. M., and Astarloa, J.: Cytomegalovirus oophoritis: Ovarian cortical necrosis. Hum. Pathol. *8*:285–292, 1977.
263. Sullivan, V., Coen, D. M.: Isolation of foscarnet-resistant human cytomegalovirus patterns of resistance and sensitivity to other antiviral drugs. J. Infect. Dis. *164*:781–784, 1991.
264. Taber, L. H., Frank, A. L., Yow, M. D., et al.: Acquisition of cytomegaloviral infections in families with young children: A serologic study. J. Infect. Dis. *151*:948–952, 1985.
265. Tanner, D. D., Buckley, P. J., Hong, R., et al.: Fatal cytomegalovirus bronchiolitis in a patient with Nezelof's syndrome. Pediatrics *65*:98–102, 1980.
266. Tiula, E., and Leinikki, P.: Fatal cytomegalovirus infection in a previously healthy boy with myocarditis and consumption coagulopathy as presenting signs. Scand. J. Infect. Dis. *4*:57–60, 1972.
267. Tolpin, M. D., Stewart, J. A., Warren, D., et al.: Transfusion transmission confirmed by restriction endonuclease analysis. J. Pediatr. *107*:953–956, 1985.
268. Trang, J. M., Kidd, L., Gruber, W., et al.: Linear single-dose pharmacokinetics of ganciclovir in newborns with congenital cytomegalovirus infections. Clin. Pharmacol. Ther. *53*:15–21, 1993.
269. Ussery, F. M., Gibson, S. R., Conklin, R. H., et al.: Intravitreal ganciclovir in the treatment of AIDS-associated cytomegalovirus retinitis. Ophthalmology *95*:640–648, 1988.
270. Vallejo, J. G., Englund, J. A., Garcia-Prats, J. A., et al.: Ganciclovir treatment of steroid-associated cytomegalovirus disease in a congenitally infected neonate. Pediatr. Infect. Dis. J. *13*:239–240, 1994.
271. Van der Bij, W., and Speich, R.: Management of cytomegalovirus infection and disease after solid organ transplantation. Clin. Infect. Dis. *33*(Suppl. 1):533–537, 2001.
272. Victoria, M. S., Nangia, B. S., and Jindrak, K.: Cytomegalovirus pyloric obstruction in a child with acquired immunodeficiency syndrome. Pediatr. Infect. Dis. *4*:550–552, 1985.
273. Vilmer, E., Mazeron, M. C., Rabian, C., et al.: Clinical significance of cytomegalovirus viremia in bone marrow transplantation. Transplantation *40*:30–35, 1985.
274. Vinters, H. V., Kwok, M. K., Ho, H. W., et al.: Cytomegalovirus in the nervous system of patients with the acquired immune deficiency syndrome. Brain *112*:245–268, 1989.
275. Virnig, N. L., and Balfour, H. H.: Hemiatrophy and hemiparesis in a patient with congenital cytomegalovirus infection. Am. J. Dis. Child. *129*:1359–1360, 1975.
276. Vochem, M., Hamprecht, K., Jahn, G., et al.: Transmission of cytomegalovirus to preterm infants through breast milk. Pediatr. Infect. Dis. J. *17*:53–57, 1998.

277. Wang, N. S., Huang, S. N., and Thurkbeck, W. M.: Combined *Pneumocystis carinii* and cytomegalovirus infection. Arch. Pathol. *90*:529–594, 1970.
278. Wang, P. S., and Evans, A. S.: Prevalence of antibodies to Epstein-Barr virus and cytomegalovirus in sera from a group of children in the People's Republic of China. J. Infect. Dis. *153*:150–152, 1986.
279. Waris, E., Rasanen, P., Kreus, K. E., et al.: Fatal cytomegalovirus disease in a previously healthy adult. Scand. J. Infect. Dis. *4*:61–67, 1972.
280. Watson, F. S., O'Connell, J. B., Amber, I. J., et al.: Treatment of cytomegalovirus pneumonia in heart transplant recipients with 9(1,3-dihydroxy-2-propoxymethyl)-guanine (DHPG). J. Heart Transplant. *7*:102–105, 1988.
281. Weiner, R. S., Bortin, M. M., Gale, R. P., et al.: Interstitial pneumonitis after bone marrow transplantation. Ann. Intern. Med. *104*:168–175, 1986.
282. Weller, T. H., and Hanshaw, J. B.: Virological and clinical observation of cytomegalic inclusion disease. N. Engl. J. Med. *266*:1233–1344, 1962.
283. Weller, T. H., Macauley, J. C., Craig, J. M., et al.: Isolation of intranuclear inclusion–producing agents from infants with illnesses resembling cytomegalic inclusion disease. Proc. Soc. Exp. Biol. Med. *94*:4–12, 1957.
284. White, N. H., Yow, M. D., Demmler, G. J., et al.: Prevalence of cytomegalovirus antibody in subjects between the ages of 6 and 22 years. J. Infect. Dis. *159*:1013–1017, 1989.
285. Whitley, R. J., Brasfield, D., Reynolds, D. W., et al.: Protracted pneumonitis in young infants associated with perinatally acquired cytomegaloviral infection. J. Pediatr. *89*:16–22, 1976.
286. Whitley, R. J., Cloud, G., Gruber, W., et al.: Ganciclovir treatment of symptomatic congenital cytomegalovirus infection: Results of a phase II study. J. Infect. Dis. *175*:1080–1086, 1997.
287. Wiley, C. A., Schrier, R. D., Denaro, F. J., et al.: Localization of cytomegalovirus proteins and genome during fulminant central nervous system infection in an AIDS patient. J. Neuropathol. Exp. Neurol. *45*:127–139, 1986.
288. Williamson, W. D., Demmler, G. J., Percy, A. K., et al.: Progressive hearing loss in infants with asymptomatic congenital cytomegalovirus infection. Pediatrics *90*:862–866, 1992.
289. Wilmott, F. E.: Cytomegalovirus in female patients attending a VD clinic. Br. J. Vener. Dis. *51*:278–280, 1975.
290. Wilson, W. R.: The relationship of the herpesvirus family to sudden hearing loss: A prospective clinical study and literature review. Laryngoscope *96*:870–877, 1986.
291. Wink, K., and Schmitz, H.: Cytomegalovirus myocarditis. Am. Heart J. *100*:667–677, 1980.
292. Winston, D. J., Pollard, R. B., Ho, W. G., et al.: Cytomegalovirus immune plasma in bone marrow transplant recipients. Ann. Intern. Med. *97*:11–18, 1982.
293. Wolf, D. G., and Spector, S. A.: Diagnosis of human cytomegalovirus central nervous system disease in AIDS patients by DNA amplification from cerebrospinal fluid. J. Infect. Dis. *166*:1412–1415, 1992.
294. Wolf, D. G., and Spector, S. A.: Early diagnosis of human cytomegalovirus disease in transplant recipients by DNA amplification in plasma. Transplantation *56*:330–334, 1993.
295. Yeager, A.: Transmission of cytomegalovirus to mothers by infected infants: Another reason to prevent transfusion-acquired infections. Pediatr. Infect. Dis. *2*:295–297, 1983.
296. Yeager, A. S., Grumet, F. C., Hafleigh, E. B., et al.: Prevention of transfusion-acquired cytomegalovirus infections in newborn infants. J. Pediatr. *98*:281–287, 1981.
297. Yow, M. D.: Congenital cytomegalovirus disease: A NOW problem. J. Infect. Dis. *159*:163–167, 1989.
298. Yow, M. D., White, N. H., Taber, L. H., et al.: Acquisition of cytomegalovirus infection from birth to 10 years: A longitudinal serologic study. J. Pediatr. *110*:37–42, 1987.
299. Yow, M. D., Williamson, D. W., Leeds, L. J., et al.: Epidemiologic characteristics of cytomegalovirus infection in mothers and their infants. Am. J. Obstet. Gynecol. *158*:1189–1195, 1988.
300. Zaia, J. A.: Epidemiology and pathogenesis of cytomegalovirus disease. Semin. Hematol. *27*:1–4, 1990.
301. Zaloga, G. P., Chernow, B., and Eil, C.: Hypercalcemia and disseminated cytomegalovirus infection in the acquired immunodeficiency syndrome. Ann. Intern. Med. *102*:331–332, 1985.
302. Zhou, X.-S., Gruber, W., Demmler, G., et al.: Population pharmacokinetics of ganciclovir in newborns with congenital cytomegalovirus infections. Antimicrob. Agents Chemother. *40*:2202–2205, 1996.

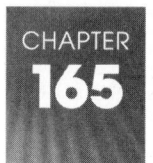

CHAPTER 165 Epstein-Barr Virus

CHARLES T. LEACH ■ CIRO V. SUMAYA

Epstein-Barr virus (EBV) is an extremely common herpesvirus that is the etiologic agent of classic infectious mononucleosis (IM). Evidence that the virus also plays a principal role in the development of certain lymphoproliferative diseases and epithelial malignancies is increasing. Its ability to remain in a dormant (latent) state after infection allows reactivation and recurrence of disease, especially under immunosuppressive conditions. Unfortunately, antiviral agents have little effect on EBV-associated diseases. Eventually, vaccination may provide protection for persons at highest risk for development of severe disease manifestations.

This chapter reviews progress in understanding the immunobiology of EBV and its disease associations. Enhanced understanding of EBV is leading to newer diagnostic methods and improved management of EBV-associated diseases.

History

One can identify four distinct periods of history related to IM and its etiologic agent EBV[116, 400]: (1) early descriptions of IM, (2) identification of the heterophile antibody test associated with IM, (3) discovery of EBV in Burkitt lymphoma (BL) cells, and (4) the association of acute EBV infection with heterophile-positive IM.

Credit for the original description of a disease consistent with what now is called *infectious mononucleosis* commonly is given to a German physician named Pfeiffer, who in 1889 described relatively mild illness characterized by fever and lymphadenopathy[349]; later, his report was translated into English.[293] The illness came to be known as "Drüsenfieber," or glandular fever. Although some cases of glandular fever were typical of what now is recognized as IM, certain characteristics of this illness, including its predominance in children and familial clustering, did not fit. In England, glandular fever and IM have become synonymous, yet many experts consider glandular fever to be a different illness.

In the early 1900s, numerous case descriptions of illnesses epidemiologically and clinically compatible with IM appeared.[58, 173, 220] However, because the illness now recognized as IM had not yet been described and these illnesses were suggestive of leukemia, most of them were reported erroneously as acute leukemia with spontaneous cure. Although the term *infectious mononucleosis* first was used in one of these case reports,[220] the illness was not distinguished from leukemia until Sprunt and Evans published their landmark paper in 1920.[420] These authors described a series of patients with clinical syndromes consistent with typical IM, including classic hematologic findings. A subsequent report by Downey and McKinlay provided a more detailed description of the hematologic manifestations.[103]

Although most cases of IM could be identified by hematologic and clinical findings, not until a specific serologic test was identified, in 1932, could classic IM be better defined. In the course of investigating heterophile antibodies in serum from patients with rheumatic fever and other diseases, Paul and Bunnell[343] noted very high titers of heterophile antibodies in serum from a control patient. Further investigation revealed that the control patient was a medical student with IM. Evaluation of sera from three other patients confirmed the presence of high titers of heterophile antibodies during acute IM.

In 1958, Dennis Burkitt, an English surgeon, described 38 cases of "round-cell sarcoma" developing in children and adolescents living in one region of Uganda, Africa.[56] Eventually, the tumors were determined to represent lymphomas, not sarcomas. Although a new mosquito-borne infectious disease was suspected as the culprit initially, Epstein and colleagues[110] eventually were able to cultivate and evaluate tumor cells by electron microscopy; they noted particles with ultrastructural characteristics similar to those of herpes simplex virus (HSV), which had been described a few years earlier. Further work established this virus as the fourth human herpesvirus (after herpes simplex 1, herpes simplex 2, and cytomegalovirus [CMV]). Although its taxonomic name is *human herpesvirus type 4,*[313] most scientists and physicians continue to use its historic name.

The association between this new herpesvirus and IM was noted serendipitously in 1968 when an IM-like illness developed in a technician working in the laboratory of the Henles.[187] Stored, pre-illness serum from this technician contained neither heterophile nor EBV antibodies, but both heterophile and EBV antibodies appeared 6 days after the onset of symptoms. In addition, virus was cultivated from the technician's peripheral blood cells. Subsequent testing of serial specimens from other patients with IM also demonstrated seroconversion to EBV in all cases. This work, as well as studies from Yale University,[117, 327] among others, firmly established EBV as the cause of IM. Investigators subsequently showed that EBV has the capacity to transform ("immortalize") human B lymphocytes in vitro, which allowed the derivation of EBV-transformed B-lymphoblastoid cell lines capable of being propagated indefinitely in tissue culture.[188, 352]

Virology: Structure and Genome

The structure of EBV is typical for a member of the herpesvirus family: it displays an inner core of DNA surrounded by a nucleocapsid, tegument, and an envelope.[108] Within the inner core, which measures approximately 45 nm, exist 170,000 to 175,000 base pairs of double-stranded DNA coding for nearly 100 viral proteins. The surrounding nucleocapsid displays icosahedral symmetry (162 capsomeres) and measures approximately 100 to 110 nm in diameter. Outside the capsid lies the tegument, which consists of amorphous proteinaceous material, and it in turn is surrounded by the viral envelope. The complete virion measures approximately 150 to 220 nm.

The entire EBV genome has been sequenced.[31] The structure of EBV is characteristic of all the herpesviruses, with short and long sections of "unique" sequences (U_s and U_L, respectively) separated by a major internal repeat region (IR_1) generally consisting of 6 to 12 direct repeats of a 3-kb sequence. The virus also has numerous other regions of repeated nucleotide sequences, including direct repeat of a 0.5-kb sequence at its termini.

Molecular Biology

Much of the early information regarding the molecular biology of EBV comes from laboratory strains derived from BL tumor cell lines (e.g., HR-1[197]) and marmoset lymphoid cell lines transformed by viral strains infecting human beings (e.g., B95-8[312]).

REPLICATION

To infect cells, EBV uses a cell surface receptor (CR2, CD21) found primarily on B lymphocytes and nasopharyngeal epithelial cells[411, 478] and less commonly on other cells.[235, 303, 476] This receptor is the same as the surface moiety functioning as the receptor for the third component of serum complement (the C3d receptor).[127] The major histocompatibility complex (MHC) class II protein functions as a cofactor for this virus-receptor interaction.[276] The initial and predominantly replicative (lytic) EBV infection probably occurs in epithelial cells of the oropharynx and adjacent structures,[413, 469] with virus then transmitted to circulating B cells passing through these lymphoepithelial tissues. After entering the B lymphocyte, the virus is transported through the cytoplasm and is stripped of its envelope in endocytic vesicles.[324] Subsequently, the viral genome circularizes and is maintained in the cell nucleus as a multicopy plasmid.[282] Spontaneous replication occurs in only a small proportion of latently infected B cells. In contrast, after infection of epithelial cells, active replication occurs and leads to lysis and death of the cell. Proteins synthesized during viral replication are important for viral gene regulation, replication of the genome, production of mature particles, and modulation of the immune system.

The EBV antigens responsible for the antibody responses used for diagnostic purposes have been mapped to various portions of the genome. Viral capsid antigens (VCAs) are the primary structural proteins in viral capsids and are found in replicating cells.[107, 185] EBV early antigens (EAs) consist of more than 15 proteins coded by genes distributed throughout the genome.[227] The EBV nuclear antigen (EBNA), traditionally defined by anticomplement immunofluorescence,[365] corresponds to six virally encoded proteins found in the nucleus of an EBV-infected cell.[227] The major EBNA protein is encoded by the *Bam*HI "K" restriction fragment of the B95-8 strain of EBV.[438] This EBNA-1 (or K-EBNA) encodes a DNA-binding protein that attaches to a specific portion of the EBV genome (*ori*-P) responsible for the replication of EBV episomal DNA within mammalian cells.[474, 475] By tethering EBV plasmids to cellular chromosomes, the EBNA-1 protein appears to play a key role in effecting faithful replication of the genome.[239] Coding sequences for the lytic origins of replication (*ori*Lyt) occur twice in the EBV genome.

LATENCY

Latently infected B cells are the primary reservoir of EBV in the body. In a typical healthy EBV-seropositive adult, between 1 and 50 B cells per million are infected with EBV, and this condition remains relatively constant over many years.[27] Although as many as 100 gene products may be expressed during active viral replication, only 11 are expressed during viral latency. In this way, the virus limits cytotoxic T-cell recognition of EBV-infected cells. The EBV gene products expressed during latency include three membrane proteins (latent membrane proteins [LMPs] 1, 2A, and 2B), six nuclear proteins (EBV nuclear antigens [EBNAs] 1, 2, 3A, 3B, 3C, and a leader protein [EBNA-LP]), and two small nontranslated RNA molecules (EBV-encoded RNA [EBER] 1 and 2).[480]

Based on in vitro genetic and somatic cell hybrid experiments, three different patterns of latent gene expression occur in EBV-infected cells from patients with lymphoproliferative diseases.[83, 480] Type I latency, typically observed in cells derived from BL and gastric carcinoma, exhibits the most limited repertoire: only EBNA-1 and the EBERs are expressed.[156, 386] Type II latency is found in non–B-cell tumors such as nasopharyngeal carcinoma (NPC), Hodgkin disease (HD), and certain T-cell lymphomas.[118, 309, 338, 479] Besides expression of EBNA-1 and EBERs, these cells also express three latent membrane proteins (LMP-1, LMP-2A, LMP-2B). Patients with IM, post-transplant lymphoproliferative disease (PTLD), and X-linked lymphoproliferative disease (XLPD) have a broad pattern of latent gene expression (type III) wherein all 11 known genes associated with latency are expressed.[446, 477] Some studies have indicated that B cells latently infected in EBV-seropositive healthy persons display a fourth pattern characterized by the expression of LMP-2, EBERs, and, usually, EBNA-1 genes.[83, 360, 448] Although these expression pattern categories may be useful for histopathologic characterization, an important note is that significant heterogeneity can occur in histopathologically similar tumors.

TRANSFORMATION

In vitro, resting human B cells infected with EBV develop into lymphoblastoid cell lines. These cells are described as immortalized or transformed because instead of following one of two normal pathways (differentiation or apoptosis [programmed cell death]), they proliferate continuously. Current evidence suggests that EBV proteins coded by six latency-associated genes are essential for this cell transformation process: EBNA-1, EBNA-2, EBNA-3A, EBNA-3C, EBNA-LP, and LMP-1.[122] The remaining latency-associated viral gene products, although not essential for transformation, are involved in the initiation and maintenance of cell transformation.

EBV generally transforms relatively mature B lymphocytes secreting a complete immunoglobulin product (heavy chain plus light chain).[53, 332] EBV also is capable of infecting and transforming B cells in earlier stages of development (e.g., pre-B cells [producing only mu chains] and lymphoid precursors lacking immunoglobulin gene rearrangement).[139, 140, 241] Tumor cells and cell lines from BLs are B cells that generally express small amounts of immunoglobulin, which may be detected as surface immunoglobulin molecules, cytoplasmic/secreted molecules, or both. The major heavy-chain isotype expressed by Burkitt tumors appears to be mu chain (IgM), although other isotypes can be observed.[332] Similarly, the EBV-infected cells observed in the blood of persons with mononucleosis and the tumor cells found in immunodeficient hosts with EBV-associated lymphoproliferative diseases and lymphoma are B lymphocytes; these EBV-infected cell populations may include cells producing any of the major classes of human immunoglobulin (IgG, IgA, or IgM).[53, 332, 376, 377] EBV-related malignant lymphoproliferations in immunosuppressed patients may be polyclonal, oligoclonal, or monoclonal; the lymphoproliferations probably are polyclonal at first but eventually progress to monoclonality.[94] BLs, on the other hand, always appear to be monoclonal at initial evaluation.[39, 332]

EBV SUBTYPES

The two subtypes of EBV (EBV-1 and EBV-2) described are based on genomic differences in several latent genes.[387, 396] Seroepidemiologic and virologic studies have suggested geographic differences in the prevalence of these two subtypes, with both types found widely in central Africa and elsewhere, but type 1 predominating in Western countries. In vitro, type 2 viruses appear less vigorous in their ability to transform lymphoblastoid cell lines.[371] Most EBV-infected persons harbor one subtype, but immunocompromised persons may be co-infected with both type 1 and type 2 strains. No substantial evidence supports the view that any one subtype is responsible for specific lymphoproliferative diseases; instead, the viruses identified in EBV-associated malignancies generally appear to reflect the recognized geographic differences.

Immunopathogenesis

INFECTIOUS MONONUCLEOSIS

EBV elicits a wide range of immunologic responses in humans, partly because of its propensity to infect B lymphocytes. In a normal host, the immunologic effects probably are responsible for most EBV-associated disease manifestations. Both cellular and humoral immunity develops in response to EBV infection. Detection of humoral antibodies directed against viral capsid and nuclear proteins is important for the diagnosis of acute infection. However, the responsibility for effective control of EBV infection lies primarily with the cellular immune elements.

Two to 7 weeks after exposure, up to 20 percent of circulating B lymphocytes become infected during primary EBV infection, although 1 percent is typical.[375] A brisk cellular immune response ensues. In the acute stage, proliferating EBV-infected B cells are controlled principally by natural killer T cells, helper ($CD4^+$) T cells, and cytotoxic-suppressor ($CD8^+$) T cells.[370] In adults, the proliferation of $CD8^+$ T cells causes a temporary inversion of the normal $CD4^+/CD8^+$ T-cell ratio; however, $CD8^+$ T-lymphocyte expansion is less marked in children.[460] After this T-cell response, the number of EBV-infected B cells falls dramatically during the next 4 to 6 weeks to concentrations of approximately 1 per million circulating B cells.[378] During convalescence, HLA-restricted cytotoxic T lymphocytes keep EBV in check, primarily by targeting the latently expressed EBNA-3 protein.[442]

During the acute stages of IM, despite a brisk immune system response to EBV, widespread and extensive impairment in general cell-mediated and humoral immunity also is present. For example, low or absent delayed-type hypersensitivity reactions develop in response to tuberculin and other antigens.[170, 296] In addition, T cells from patients with IM display unusually weak proliferative responses when exposed to recall antigens (e.g., *Candida albicans*, tetanus toxoid).[315, 445] Although EBV-specific cytotoxic and suppressor T cells appear during acute infection, the T-cell response primarily is nonspecific and HLA unrestricted.[247, 248, 340, 366] Furthermore, a polyclonal humoral response occurs during acute EBV infection.[384] Each B cell committed to one isotype continues to produce that isotype after EBV transformation, thereby leading to secretion of all classes of immunoglobulins, though primarily IgM.[439, 470]

Once primary infection occurs, EBV, like other herpesviruses, is able to persist in a latent state in a human host throughout that person's lifetime. This ability indicates that EBV exerts some influence on the immune response to prevent its complete eradication. Indeed, several mechanisms for eluding the immune system have been observed. For example, the EBNA-1 protein contains a spacer region consisting of multiple Gly-Ala repeats that inhibit protein processing and MHC class I recognition of cells expressing EBNA-1.[273] In addition, one viral protein (BARF1) serves as a soluble receptor for colony-stimulating factor type 1 (CSF-1). CSF-1 normally stimulates the production of interferon-α (IFN-α) by monocytes, but the presence of BARF1 soaks up CSF-1 and prevents CSF-1–triggered production of IFN-α. EBV also encodes a viral cytokine (BCRF1) with 70 percent similarity to a human cytokine (interleukin-10 [IL-10]) that is important in the immune response.[316] In vitro studies have revealed that BCRF1 mimics IL-10 by inhibiting the secretion of IFN-γ from peripheral blood mononuclear cells.[210] IFN-γ plays an important role in stimulating protective responses to viruses.

EBV-ASSOCIATED TUMORS

In normal hosts, cellular immune responses are adequate for control and sequestration of EBV-infected cells. However, cellular immune deficiency may allow uncontrolled proliferation of EBV-infected B cells during primary or reactivated EBV infection. Such an excessive EBV-associated B-cell production may be histologically pleomorphic (such as B-cell lymphoproliferative diseases) or relatively uniform (monomorphic, such as B-cell lymphomas). In organ transplant recipients, no consistent chromosomal translocations are associated with the lymphomas. Many of these lesions regress once immunosuppressive therapy after transplantation is withdrawn.[477] In rare, severe cases, B cells harboring EBV DNA and expressing EBNA may become disseminated throughout the body as plasmacytoid cells visible on peripheral blood smears and as B-lymphoid cells potentially invading all organs of the body. Life-threatening EBV infections also may be correlated with an overly strong virus-induced T-cell proliferation that might cause autoaggressive activity producing hypogammaglobulinemia or other major organ dysfunctions.[38]

The pathogenesis of EBV-associated malignant disorders in some settings may be multifactorial and involve a mixture of virologic, genetic, and environmental factors. NPC, which predominantly occurs in a specific geographic locale, has been linked serologically with EBV.[189, 199] The identification of epithelial cells as potential targets for EBV infection, thereby allowing a lytic (productive) infection, has strengthened this relationship.[413] Further studies have revealed that NPC is a monoclonal proliferation that develops subsequent to EBV infection, with EBV gene products required for tumor growth.[341] However, NPC also clearly has a genetic association inasmuch as strong linkage to a specific HLA type exists.[277] Furthermore, early EBV gene expression can affect profoundly the growth of infected cells, with full malignant potential reached when mutations occur on chromosomes 3 or 9 (presumably affecting tumor suppressor genes).[211, 212] These mutations possibly result from adverse environmental conditions (e.g., exposure to chemical carcinogens such as the volatile nitrosamines in salted fish[484]).

The EBV genome and expression of EBNA-1 are present in virtually all BL cells derived from African patients with BL (endemic BL), with the genome existing as circular episomes. In contrast, less than 30 percent of cases of "sporadic" BL (occurring in Europe and the United States) contain EBV DNA.[215, 485] BL cells, but not the lymphoid cells found in IM, exhibit characteristic chromosomal alterations thought to be associated with enhanced malignant potential. Approximately 90 percent of BL tumors exhibit a reciprocal translocation involving the long arms of chromosomes 8 and 14, t(8;14); most of the remainder have t(8;2) and t(8;22).[250, 388] These translocations place the c-*myc* oncogene under the control of an immunoglobulin promoter,[90, 444] which results in transcriptional deregulation and overexpression of the c-*myc* oncogene.[88, 265] Therefore, the evolution of endemic BL appears to be a multistep process involving malaria-induced B-cell proliferation, EBV infection, c-*myc* gene rearrangement and activation, and probably other elements.[96, 97, 249, 331, 409]

Lymphoproliferative disease (PTLD) may develop in organ and bone marrow transplant recipients during the intense immunosuppression after graft placement. PTLDs span a spectrum of lymphoproliferation from polyclonal disease to monoclonal, monomorphic disease that often is difficult to distinguish from the typical malignant lymphomas developing in patients with intact immune systems. No proof exists that an orderly progression leading to malignant lymphoma occurs; however, one model for the pathogenesis of PTLD proposes that defective immune surveillance after transplantation allows polyclonal proliferation of EBV-infected cells displaying a type III latency pattern (similar to that observed in IM).[83] Subsequently, genetic mutations at various loci (e.g., c-*myc*, p53) may allow progression to full malignant lymphoma.[95]

Histopathology[89, 153, 449]

INFECTIOUS MONONUCLEOSIS

Because IM typically is benign and the diagnosis is based primarily on clinical and serologic findings, histopathologic examination of tissues seldom is required. However, histopathologic information is available on some tissues (e.g., lymph nodes, tonsils, spleen) from unusual cases and from patients requiring surgery. For patients in whom lymphoproliferative disease and other serious manifestations of EBV infection develop, a larger amount of information is available from a broader range of tissues.

Lymph nodes are enlarged diffusely during acute IM. Histologically, active lymphoid follicles are noted, with lymphoid proliferation extending to the sinuses, blood vessels, trabecula, and capsule. The capsule remains intact despite substantial hyperplasia. The lymphoid response consists primarily of T and B immunoblasts, typically with a pleomorphic pattern and frequent mitoses indicative of rapid cell turnover. Other cells identifiable in lymph node tissues include a substantial number of small lymphocytes, large atypical lymphocytes, plasma cells, histiocytes, and eosinophils. Micronecrosis may be present, although it is less extensive than that observed with herpes lymphadenitis. Tonsillar tissue also contains an active lymphoproliferative response, but with more prominent follicles and extensive necrosis.

The spleen is enlarged two to three times its normal weight during acute IM, primarily as a result of hyperplasia of the red pulp. Like lymph nodes, the cellularity principally is from immunoblasts with substantial pleomorphism. Hemorrhage, primarily subcapsular in location, is identified commonly. The liver typically shows minimal disease, with infiltration by lymphocytes and monocytes occurring principally in the portal areas and possibly minor degenerative changes taking place in hepatocytes. Bone marrow may appear relatively normal during IM, but some series have reported hypercellularity and small granulomata. From the relatively few cases of central nervous system (CNS) disease associated with EBV infection, histopathology reveals lymphocytic infiltration of the meninges.[10] Less common findings include demyelination, degeneration, focal hemorrhage, congestion, and edema.

EBV-ASSOCIATED LYMPHOPROLIFERATIVE DISEASES

The most common form of non-Hodgkin lymphoma (NHL) is BL, which consists of sheets of small noncleaved cells that are histologically uniform. Most arise from a single infected cell (monoclonality). The majority of CNS NHL tumors display large-cell morphology, with virtually all containing monoclonal EBV DNA. In PTLD, a wide range of histologic findings may be noted. At one extreme, one finds a more pleomorphic response arising from numerous infected cells (polyclonality). At the other end is observed frank malignant lymphoma.[87]

HD tissues are characterized by the presence of Reed-Sternberg cells admixed with lymphocytes and other reactive cells. Reed-Sternberg cells are large (15 to 45 μm), multinucleated cells probably derived from B or T cells. These cells exhibit strongly stained nucleoli surrounded by a characteristic clear area resembling a halo. A classification system with four distinctive histologic categories based on the predominant cell type and characteristics of the background cellularity has been devised for HD.[179] These four types are (1) lymphocyte predominant, (2) nodular sclerosing, (3) mixed (most strongly associated with EBV), and (4) lymphocyte depleted. The nodular sclerosing variety is the form most commonly observed in children.

OTHER EBV-ASSOCIATED DISEASES

The tissues involved in hemophagocytic lymphohistiocytosis (HLH) typically include the bone marrow, spleen, liver, and lymph nodes, but the skin or brain may be affected as well.[128] In the bone marrow, hypocellularity often is noted. Activated macrophages (or "histiocytes") appearing "stuffed" are observed engulfing all bone marrow cellular elements or their precursors or fragments, including erythrocytes, leukocytes, and platelets.[128, 374, 467]

Of the three histopathologic categories of epithelial tumors in the nasopharynx, the most common form is the undifferentiated variety, which is associated most strongly with EBV. Examination of these tumors reveals undifferentiated squamous cells with substantial infiltration by lymphocytes. Malignant cells consistently contain multiple copies of monoclonal EBV DNA within episomes, and several EBV proteins are expressed.

Tissues affected by oral hairy leukoplakia (predominantly in patients with acquired immunodeficiency syndrome [AIDS]) reveal keratin or parakeratin projections, mild hyperparakeratosis and acanthosis, ballooning and hyperplasia of the prickle-cell layer, and only a sparse inflammatory cell infiltrate in the subepithelial connective tissue.[154]

The principal histologic findings in pulmonary tissue from children infected with human immunodeficiency virus (HIV) and lymphocytic interstitial pneumonitis are lymphoid nodules and diffuse infiltration of the alveolar septa and peribronchiolar regions by lymphocytic cells, including lymphocytes, plasma cells, plasmacytoid lymphocytes, and immunoblasts.[19] Some lymphoid nodules may be observed as well. The infiltrating lymphocytes consist of B cells and T cells.[238] Necrosis is not observed, and blood vessels are not affected.

Epidemiology

SEROPREVALENCE

Epidemiologic studies of EBV were stimulated by the development of reagents for the detection of specific anti-EBV antibodies in serum in the mid-1960s.[185] Specifically, tests detecting antibodies to VCA (long lasting, early in infection) and EA (short duration, early in infection) were used. Henle and Henle, using an immunofluorescence method, first noted a high prevalence of EBV VCA antibodies (100%) in patients with BL, but they also discovered a relatively high prevalence (85%) in normal adults.[185] Subsequent studies in American[146, 186, 354, 429] and British[348] populations have now established that 80 to 95 percent of adults have serologic evidence of past EBV infection, with most infections occurring during infancy and childhood.

The age at initial (primary) infection varies markedly in different cultural and socioeconomic settings, a fact that has great pertinence to manifestations of disease associated with primary infection. In developing countries, EBV infection generally occurs at an early age, with 80 to 100 percent of children becoming infected by 3 to 6 years of age. In these settings, most children with primary EBV infection have clinically silent or mild disease.[44, 132, 430] In privileged communities and in industrialized countries, primary infection with EBV occurs later in life. In these settings and for reasons that are unclear, primary infection in older age groups, for example, individuals between 10 and 30 years of age, is more likely to induce clinical symptoms, most often a mononucleosis syndrome. An IM case rate of 50 to 75 percent associated with primary EBV infection was documented in U. S. college students.[326] An unexpectedly high rate of IM also has been noted along with eventual primary EBV infection in siblings of a pediatric case of IM.[434]

INCIDENCE

The incidence of IM from population-based studies ranges between 50 and 100 cases per 100,000 population.[117, 182, 184] These studies indicate that the highest incidence rates for IM occur in the age group 15 to 19 years. Although one report described a modest seasonal change for IM,[182] most studies have indicated no seasonal predilection.[184, 399] IM consistently has developed at a higher rate in persons of white race than in other ethnic groups.[182] In one study, IM developed in males at a rate slightly higher than in females.[184]

VIRAL SHEDDING

The initial indication that EBV was shed in oropharyngeal secretions came from Chang and Golden in 1971 when they identified a "leukocyte-transforming agent" in throat washings from four of eight adults with IM.[70] Although EBV was suspected, specific laboratory tests could not confirm it. Other investigators using more specific identification methods clearly established EBV as the leukocyte-transforming agent.[147, 283, 311] Subsequent studies in healthy populations have indicated the following*: (1) most children and adults with acute IM shed EBV in their oropharynx, (2) between 6 and 20 percent of the general population shed EBV in the oropharynx, (3) oropharyngeal shedding may be intermittent or continuous, and (4) high concentrations of EBV in oropharyngeal secretions are associated with high concentrations of EBV in B lymphocytes in the peripheral blood but not with concentrations of EBV-specific serum antibodies.

In addition to the oropharynx, EBV DNA (detected by polymerase chain reaction [PCR]) may be found in the urine of persons during and for several months after an episode of IM.[259] A second site of EBV shedding, the uterine cervix, has been described by Sixbey and associates.[412]

TRANSMISSION

COMMON MODES OF TRANSMISSION. Reports in the first half of the 20th century, before widespread acceptance and use of the heterophile antibody test, suggested the occurrence of epidemics of IM.[172, 333, 447] However, researchers generally thought that the criteria used in most of these reports for the diagnosis of IM were inadequate to convince one that the outbreaks were indeed associated with EBV.[202] Attempts to experimentally infect humans with EBV collected from the oropharyngeal secretions, blood, urine, and feces of patients with IM generally failed.[113, 114, 329, 417] These experiments, conducted before the development of specific EBV antibody tests, presumably were unsuccessful because most experimental subjects were immune as a result of previous EBV infection.

Intimate sharing of oral secretions is thought to play a major role in the transmission of EBV.[115, 202] The fact that EBV infection is extremely common worldwide, especially in underdeveloped regions, suggests that the virus is spread relatively efficiently in the general population. Surprisingly, outbreaks of EBV infection are uncommon events. However, transmission of EBV, even among close contacts of a person with acute EBV infection, may occur slowly. Studies of families of index cases of IM have indicated that EBV is not transmitted efficiently.[67, 133, 184] Furthermore, Chang reported a lack of EBV transmission from a man with IM to his EBV-seronegative wife, even after 16 months of follow-up.[66] In addition, data from a family study indicated that after the index IM episode, EBV antibodies developed (seroconversion) in only 35 percent of the nonimmune sibling contacts after an average observation period of 5.6 contact months.[434] Nonetheless, this same study also noted that the eventual seroconversion event in siblings was more likely to be associated with an IM episode than would be expected in the general population.[434]

Evidence has shown that EBV replicates in oropharyngeal epithelial cells,[413] with subsequent infection of B cells possibly occurring as a result of contact with these cells.[5] More recent studies indicate that latent and productive EBV infection occurs in lymphoid cells on the surface of the tonsillar epithelium and within the crypt, but not in epithelial cells.[12] Thus, transmission of EBV from person to person may be due to transfer of virus from persistently infected EBV lymphoid cells; EBV-infected epithelial cells may not be required for this phenomenon.[330] The incubation period for typical EBV-associated IM is imprecise but is estimated at 30 to 50 days.[133, 202]

*See references 69, 71, 100, 124, 152, 311, 328, 431, 433, 434, 436, 473.

TRANSMISSION VIA BLOOD PRODUCTS, TRANSPLANTED ORGANS. Transmission of EBV via blood transfusion has been reported,[3, 133, 148, 194, 202, 307, 452] but it occurs much less commonly than transmission of CMV. High levels of immunity, transfer of neutralizing antibodies during transfusion, and limited survival of B cells may account for the rarity of this occurrence.[193] In transplant patients, the donor organ may rarely transmit EBV to the recipient.[50, 63, 405]

INTRAUTERINE AND PERINATAL TRANSMISSION. Because most females reaching child-bearing age already have been infected with EBV, primary infections during pregnancy occur infrequently.[131, 216, 263] Therefore, the risk of fetal transmission is difficult to study. One prospective study of primary infections occurring during pregnancy (silent or symptomatic) indicated no adverse fetal outcomes and, when studied, no viral transmission to the fetus.[130] Moreover, Chang and colleagues[69, 73] could find only one EBV-infected specimen among 2696 samples of cord blood lymphocytes. On the other hand, case reports suggest that rare instances of intrauterine transmission may occur.[54, 151, 233] Higher EBV exposure has been reported in infants residing in nurseries.[72] Moreover, detection of EBV in the uterine cervix[412] raises the possibility of venereal or perinatal transmission, but this theory is yet undocumented.

Clinical Syndromes Associated with EBV Infection

SILENT, NONSPECIFIC INFECTIONS

Similar to other lymphotropic human herpesviruses, primary EBV infection in children typically is silent but may result in mild clinical symptoms. Nonspecific clinical symptoms may include prolonged low-grade fever with or without lymphadenopathy, cough, rhinorrhea, and pharyngitis.

INFECTIOUS MONONUCLEOSIS[68, 104, 126, 203, 432]

The signs and symptoms of classic IM develop in most adolescents and adults, as well as some young children, when they experience a primary (initial) EBV infection.

PRODROME. In most persons with IM, a prodrome develops during the end of the incubation period. This prodrome lasts 2 to 5 days and is followed immediately by the full-blown manifestations of IM. Prodromal symptoms typically are mild and may consist of malaise, fatigue, and possibly fever. At this stage, differentiation from other viral infections is difficult.

ACUTE PHASE. The classic clinical features of IM are fever, sore throat, malaise, and fatigue, and physical examination reveals lymphadenopathy and tonsillopharyngitis (Table 165–1). The fever usually begins rather abruptly, ranges from 38° C to 40.5° C (usually <39° C), is more prominent in the afternoon and evening, and persists for 1 to 2 weeks. Occasionally, the fever may last 4 to 5 weeks. Lymphadenopathy occurs in more than 90 percent of children and adults and typically involves the anterior and posterior cervical lymph nodes (Fig. 165–1). Affected nodes are moderately enlarged in a symmetric manner. However, generalized lymphadenopathy is also characteristic and involves the occipital, supraclavicular, axillary, epitrochlear, and inguinal chains. Like other causes of viral lymphadenitis, the lymph nodes in patients with IM may be slightly tender, but they generally are nontender, nonerythematous, and

TABLE 165–1 ■ CLINICAL MANIFESTATIONS OF INFECTIOUS MONONUCLEOSIS IN CHILDREN AND ADULTS

	Frequency (%)		
Sign or Symptom	**Age <4 yr***	**Age 4–16 yr***	**Adults (Range)†**
Lymphadenopathy	94	95	93–100
Fever	92	100	63–100
Sore throat or tonsillopharyngitis	67	75	70–91
Exudative tonsillopharyngitis	45	59	40–74
Splenomegaly	82	53	32–51
Hepatomegaly	63	30	6–24
Cough or rhinitis	51	15	5–31
Rash	34	17	0–15
Abdominal pain or discomfort	17	0	2–14
Eyelid edema	14	14	5–34

*From reference 435.
†From references 104, 115, 205, 299.

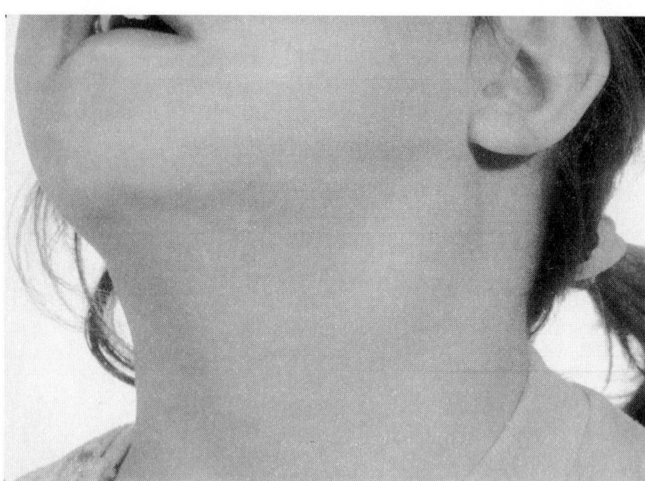

FIGURE 165–1 ■ Anterior cervical lymphadenopathy in an 8 year-old child with infectious mononucleosis. (Courtesy of Dr. James Brien, Scott and White Hospital, Temple, TX.)

discrete. Lymphadenopathy is most prominent during weeks 2 to 4 of the illness. Tonsillopharyngitis develops during the first week of illness and usually resolves rather abruptly the next week. Although mild symptoms occur in some patients, most have substantial symptomatology. Exudative pharyngitis, similar to that found with *Streptococcus pyogenes* pharyngitis, occurs in approximately half of patients (Fig. 165–2). *S. pyogenes* is present in the posterior pharyngeal region of 5 percent of patients with IM and probably represents carriage rather than simultaneous bacterial tonsillopharyngitis.

Splenomegaly occurs in approximately 50 percent of patients with IM, but more frequently in younger children. Usually only the tip of the spleen is palpable, with maximal size developing by the end of the second week of illness. The splenomegaly typically resolves by the third or fourth week. Hepatomegaly occurs in approximately 60 percent of young children with IM and less commonly in older age groups. However, silent inflammation of the liver is a common finding. Cough and rhinitis are noted frequently in young children with IM, perhaps as a result of other concurrent viral infections. Rash (unassociated with antibiotic administration) develops in less than 15 percent of adults with IM but occurs more commonly in children and adolescents (18–34%).[432] The strong correlation in young adults between the administration of ampicillin and the subsequent development of a rash is not observed in children with IM, possibly because of the overall increased incidence of cutaneous manifestations in children with IM. Children are more likely than are adults to have abdominal pain, failure to thrive, otitis media, and recurrent tonsillopharyngitis preceding or following IM.[432] A palatal enanthem is present in approximately one third of adults, but it is a nonspecific finding. Eyelid edema also is described in as many as one third of adults but occurs less commonly (15%) in children.[432]

RESOLUTION PHASE. The acute phase of IM lasts several days to 3 to 4 weeks, with gradual and uneventful resolution. Occasionally, biphasic illness is observed, with recrudescence of acute symptoms after significant improvement. Organomegaly may persist for 1 to 3 months. The

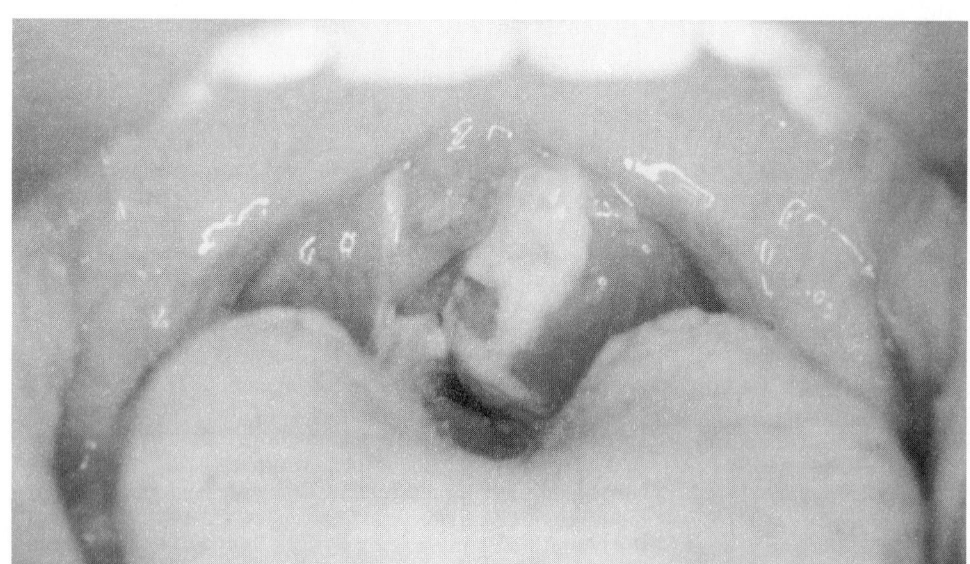

FIGURE 165–2 ■ Exudative pharyngitis in an 8-year-old child with infectious mononucleosis. (Courtesy of Dr. James Brien, Scott and White Hospital, Temple, TX.)

severe fatigue usually resolves within 3 to 4 weeks, but several months may be required for persons with IM to fully resume their pre-illness activity levels.

CHRONIC ACTIVE DISEASE

Chronic active EBV infections are somewhat controversial and not well characterized, but most authorities do recognize their existence in rare patients. After having an IM-like illness, these patients do not recover fully and have continuous or intermittent signs and symptoms persisting for a year or more. These chronic manifestations typically include fever, hepatosplenomegaly, headaches, malaise, and fatigue. In more severe cases, which can be fatal, neurologic disease (e.g., encephalitis), hematologic disease (e.g., hemophagocytosis), and disease localized to other organs (e.g., myocarditis, pneumonitis) can develop.[2] One distinctive characteristic of these patients is the extremely high antibody titers against EBV replicative antigens, including VCA and EA, and low or absent responses to EBNA. Predominantly lytic EBV strains with impaired immortalization capacity are thought to play a role in the pathogenesis of this disorder.[402] Chronic active EBV infection should not be confused with chronic fatigue disorder, which has no clear association with EBV.

HEMOPHAGOCYTIC LYMPHOHISTIOCYTOSIS

Hemophagocytosis, first described in 1939, is a pathologic condition consisting of engulfment of bone marrow cellular elements (erythrocytes, leukocytes, platelets, and their precursors) by activated macrophages (Fig. 165–3). HLH (also called hemophagocytosis syndrome) is characterized primarily by fever, pancytopenia, splenomegaly, and hemophagocytosis in lymphoreticular tissue (bone marrow, spleen, and lymph nodes). Since the initial description of its association with viral infections in 1979,[374] numerous viral infections, including EBV, have been linked with HLH.[367, 428] Hereditary forms of HLH exist, most prominently those occurring in children with XLPD.[319] A disseminated form of EBV infection with features of HLH may develop in these patients. Most other cases are sporadic. Current evidence indicates that cytokines play a central role in the development of this syndrome.[128] Monocytes in HLH are activated by high levels of cytokines elaborated by helper T cells. These activating cytokines include tumor necrosis factor–α, IFN-γ, and other cytokines. Untreated EBV-associated HLH carries a high mortality rate. Recent small series indicate improved survival after chemotherapy or bone marrow transplantation (see "Treatment").[33, 218]

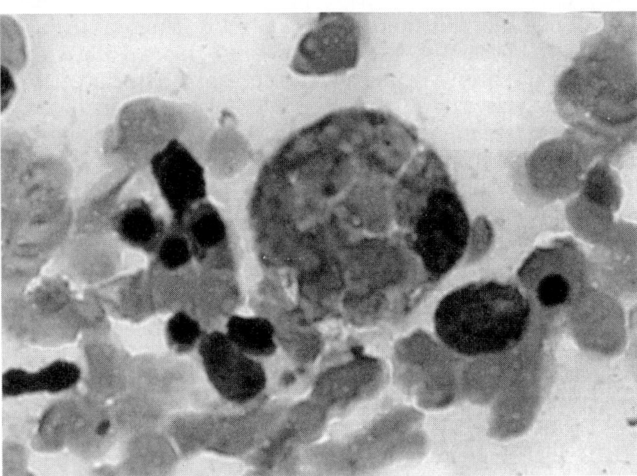

FIGURE 165–3 ■ Bone marrow from an 18-year-old woman with Epstein-Barr virus–associated hemophagocytic lymphohistiocytosis revealing a macrophage *(center)* filled with phagocytosed red blood cells. (From Blood 93:1991, 1999. Photo courtesy of Lindsey Baden, M.D., and Frank Evangelista, M.D., Beth Israel Deaconess Medical Center, Departments of Medicine and Pathology, 330 Brookline Ave., SL-435, Boston.)

MALIGNANCIES ASSOCIATED WITH EBV

NASOPHARYNGEAL CARCINOMA. NPC occurs primarily in adults in southern China, but it may be seen in Greenland, Alaska, and the Mediterranean regions as well; the tumor is extremely rare in Western countries.[119] In endemic regions, children younger than 16 years account for only 1 to 2 percent of all cases of NPC, whereas in the United States, the rate is higher (10%).[219] Common symptoms of children with NPC include cervical lymphadenopathy (usually bilateral), nasal congestion, epistaxis, and recurrent otitis media.[26, 99, 219] At initial evaluation, children with NPC are more likely than are adults to have locoregional disease.[26, 219]

BURKITT LYMPHOMA. Endemic BL is a rapidly progressive and fatal tumor that predominantly affects young children in central Africa and Papua New Guinea[56] (Fig. 165–4). Approximately 60 percent of African patients with BL have jaw masses, with abdominal masses being second most common.[482] Less common sites include the CNS and the eye. Non-African patients with BL are most likely to have abdominal masses initially. In some patients with BL and some with congenital or acquired immunodeficiencies (including AIDS), CNS involvement is present or eventually develops and is characterized by intracranial mass lesions of lymphomatous cells or a cerebrospinal fluid (CSF) pleocytosis consisting of malignant cells, or both.[16, 482, 483]

HODGKIN DISEASE. The association of EBV with HD is based primarily on serologic studies[272, 320] and identification of EBV DNA in Reed-Sternberg cells (the malignant cells characteristic of HD).[22, 461] The differential incidence distribution of HD in children throughout the world agrees with the age at first EBV infection: it increases in adolescence in developed countries and increases in early childhood in developing countries.[167, 230] Virtually all cases of HD in developing countries are associated with the presence of EBV, whereas the virus is present in less than 50 percent of patients with HD in developed countries.[8, 195, 357] However, in developed countries, EBV is strongly associated with HD in children younger than 10 years and in tumors displaying the mixed-cellularity variant.[23, 195, 338] HD rarely occurs in children

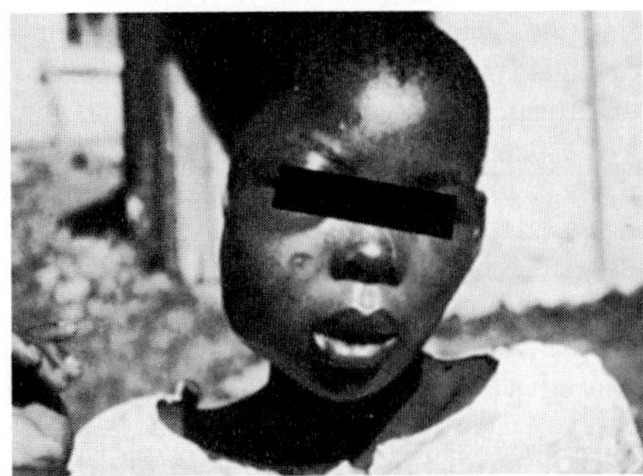

FIGURE 165–4 ■ African boy with Burkitt lymphoma involving the jaw. (Courtesy of Dr. George Miller, Yale University.)

younger than 5 years in Western countries, but it is seen more commonly at younger ages in developing countries. The precise pathogenetic mechanisms for EBV-associated HD are unknown, but evidence indicates that LMP-1 and LMP-2 proteins may play a role.[129] Patients typically have cervical or supraclavicular lymphadenopathy, as well as mediastinal adenopathy (occasionally with obstructive symptoms).[213] Constitutional symptoms such as fever, nightsweats, and weight loss develop in approximately one fourth of patients with HD, and these symptoms worsen the prognosis.

LYMPHOPROLIFERATIVE DISEASE IN IMMUNODEFICIENT PATIENTS. Persons with various types of immunodeficiency are at increased risk for the development of potentially fatal EBV-related PTLDs, B lymphomas, and severe atypical EBV infections. One should keep in mind, however, that IM and other forms of EBV infections in immunocompromised children and adults usually run a course similar to that in immunocompetent persons; actually, even in immunosuppressed (and post-transplantation) subjects, more EBV infections are clinically silent.[192, 200]

TRANSPLANTATION. Children immunosuppressed for organ transplantation (with steroids, azathioprine, anti–T-cell antibodies, mycophenolate, cyclosporine, tacrolimus, or combinations thereof) have an increased risk of developing EBV-related lymphoproliferative syndromes and B lymphomas.[200, 253, 418] Ho and colleagues reported a greater frequency of lymphoproliferative lesions in pediatric transplant recipients (4%) than in adult transplant recipients (0.8%).[200] Pediatric organ transplant recipients are thought to have an increased risk for development of EBV-related disorders because when compared with adult transplant recipients, they are more likely to be seronegative for EBV at transplantation and primary infection is more likely to progress to lymphoproliferative and other severe EBV-associated disorders in these patients.[200, 201] In addition, EBV-associated lymphoproliferative disorders may develop in children with immunodeficiency disease who have received cultured thymus[48] or bone marrow transplantation.[405]

As has been documented recently in young patients with AIDS, subsequent EBV-associated smooth muscle tumors (e.g., leiomyosarcomas) have been found to develop in some patients undergoing organ transplantation.[266, 379]

OTHER MALIGNANCIES. Fatal T-cell lymphomas with evidence of EBV-driven oncogenesis now have been described in several patients.[237, 426] Increasing data also indicate that gastric carcinomas, particularly of the undifferentiated type and in the Japanese, are linked to EBV.[408] Furthermore, EBV has been implicated in the genesis of carcinomas of the thymus,[275] salivary gland,[362] parotid gland,[393] and larynx.[51]

PRIMARY IMMUNODEFICIENCY. Overwhelming primary EBV infection, seen rarely in immunocompetent patients, occurs more commonly in children with certain primary immunodeficiency disorders, most notably, boys with XLPD.[359, 427] These patients typically have features consistent with IM, but fulminant disease leading to death subsequently develops. Widespread uncontrolled lymphoproliferation is found at autopsy, and causes of death include acute hemorrhage, meningoencephalitis, secondary bacterial infection, and liver failure.[319] Survivors usually have hypogammaglobulinemia, and B-cell lymphomas may develop later.

Patients with a wide variety of other congenital immunodeficiencies, including severe combined immunodeficiency syndrome, Wiskott-Aldrich syndrome, ataxia-telangiectasia, Chédiak-Higashi syndrome, common variable immunodeficiency, and other congenital immunodeficiencies, also are at risk for EBV-associated lymphoproliferative disease.

EBV AND HUMAN IMMUNODEFICIENCY VIRUS

Several studies have indicated that underlying HIV infection is responsible for abnormal responses to EBV infections. These findings probably are attributable to the relative ineffectiveness of T cells from AIDS patients in controlling EBV-infected lymphocytes.[45] In HIV-infected adults, these unusual reactions include exaggerated antibody responses to certain EBV antigens, including VCA and EA,[363] and enhanced oropharyngeal shedding of EBV.[7] In one recent study in children, little difference was found in anti-VCA IgG titers, although slightly higher anti–EA-D titers were noted in HIV-infected patients than in healthy controls.[229] Oropharyngeal shedding of EBV occurred more commonly in younger HIV-infected children, and children whose HIV disease progressed more rapidly had a substantially higher rate of excretion.[229] In another study, EBV infection developed in HIV-infected children at an earlier age and was more likely to involve hepatosplenomegaly.[345] Whether EBV directly contributes to the progression of immune deficiency in these patients is a matter of conjecture, although in vitro studies do indicate that some EBV proteins (e.g., LMP, BZLF1) are able to transactivate HIV-1.[176, 295]

Studies have shown clearly that certain lymphoproliferative and other diseases develop in HIV-infected patients at rates higher than those in healthy persons. These diseases include NHL, body cavity lymphoma, HD, smooth muscle tumors, lymphocytic interstitial pneumonitis, and oral hairy leukoplakia.

NHL is the most common malignancy occurring in children with AIDS.[301] In a recent study, approximately one third of these tumors contained EBV DNA.[304] EBV is associated most strongly with primary CNS lymphomas in AIDS patients,[289] although this tumor accounts for less than 10 percent of NHL cases in children.[304] NHL invariably occurs in patients with AIDS who have profound immune suppression (e.g., CD4+ concentration <50 cells/µL). Pediatric AIDS patients with NHL typically have systemic symptoms of fever and weight loss. Signs of extranodal disease include hepatosplenomegaly, abdominal distention, jaundice, and bone marrow involvement, and, rarely, CNS symptoms.[302]

Body cavity lymphoma is a rare malignancy that occurs almost exclusively in adult patients with AIDS, but also in some children.[264] Patients typically have immunoblastic lymphomatous effusions without solid tumors in body cavities such as the peritoneum and pleura. More than 85 percent of these nonsolid tumors are associated with human herpesvirus 8; however, EBV also is identified frequently in tumor cells from these patients and may be clonal. The precise role that EBV plays in the pathogenesis of these unusual tumors is unknown.

Leiomyosarcoma is a malignant tumor of smooth muscle tissue that is an extremely rare finding in healthy patients, but it is the second most common malignancy in children with AIDS.[301] EBV may be responsible for this unusually high incidence of smooth muscle tumors found in children with AIDS.[228, 303] Leiomyosarcoma tissue from patients with AIDS has high concentrations of EBV (CD21) receptors.[228, 303] Moreover, all pediatric AIDS cases wirh leiomyosarcoma contain clonal EBV DNA and express EBERs and EBNA-1.[228, 303] Leiomyosarcoma may develop in any smooth muscle tissue in AIDS patients, but more typically it is noted first in the gastrointestinal tract and lungs.

Lymphocytic interstitial pneumonitis is a PTLD that occurs primarily in children with AIDS.[17] In 1997, it accounted for 17 percent of AIDS-defining illnesses in children.[198] Although serologic and virologic evidence points to an association with EBV,[17, 242, 390] the exact role that EBV plays in this lymphoid proliferation is unclear at present. Radiographically, diffuse interstitial infiltrates are noted. The course of disease is variable, with some children remaining stable for long periods and others exhibiting a slow, but relentless progression to chronic lung disease typified by tachypnea, cough, wheezing, and hypoxemia. Advanced disease is characterized by clubbing, wasting, cor pulmonale, and bronchiectasis.

Oral hairy leukoplakia is a nonmalignant squamous cell proliferation that develops in the oropharynx of patients with AIDS. Though common in adults with AIDS, it occurs in less than 5 percent of HIV-infected children.[292] EBV DNA and virus replication can be detected within epithelial cells,[155, 415] with defective variants possible.[143] Oral hairy leukoplakia lesions are manifested as nonremovable gray or white plaques on the lateral surface of the tongue; they often have vertical corrugations and a shaggy or "hairy" appearance when dry.[403]

Complications

Acute EBV infection in a healthy child or adolescent, regardless of whether it is associated with typical IM, rarely is complicated by serious illness. The most frequent complications, exanthems and mild hepatitis, more appropriately are considered part of the normal disease spectrum. More serious complications involving major organs have been reported regularly since the first description of IM as a distinct clinical entity, but they remain rare (for review, see elsewhere[6, 226, 347, 432]). Most complications, including the more severe ones, are transient.

In one prospective study,[432] significant complications involving mainly the pulmonary, neurologic, and hematologic systems were noted in approximately 20 percent of children with IM. Thrombocytopenia with hemorrhagic manifestations, severe airway obstruction, and neurologic complications developed in children with IM more frequently than in adults; jaundice occurred less frequently.

EXANTHEMS

AMPICILLIN RASH. Historically, patients with IM were treated frequently with antibiotics, primarily for suspected streptococcal pharyngitis or bacterial lymphadenitis. Soon after the release of ampicillin, reports linked the antibiotic with the occurrence of exanthems in patients with IM. Two large case series have indicated that administration of ampicillin (or amoxicillin) precipitates an exanthem in most (95% to 100%) adolescents and adults with EBV-associated IM[339, 358]; it is less common in children with IM.[432] This phenomenon has become known as the "ampicillin rash" associated with IM. The rash usually develops 5 to 10 days after treatment is initiated and resolves within a few days of discontinuation. Characteristically, the cutaneous lesions are maculopapular and pruritic and involve the trunk, face, and extremities[339] (Fig. 165–5). A rash also may develop in patients with IM treated with other β-lactam antibiotics, but such rashes do not represent hypersensitivity reactions.

OTHER EXANTHEMS. An exanthem will develop in approximately 3 to 15 percent of persons with IM not treated with β-lactam antibiotics.[30, 203, 232, 299, 364, 432] These rashes are maculopapular but can be urticarial, scarlatiniform, or erythema multiforme–like. Though most commonly associated with hepatitis B, some cases of Gianotti-Crosti syndrome (papular acrodermatitis of childhood) also have been related to primary EBV infection.[207]

CARDIAC

Mild electrocardiographic abnormalities (mostly nonspecific ST and T wave changes) have been observed in 6 to 16 percent of adults with IM.[104, 204] Abnormalities usually are noted during the second or third week of illness and disappear by the fourth week, but they may persist longer. Serious cardiac complications occur extremely rarely; fatal myocarditis has been well documented in one adolescent in association with IM.[138]

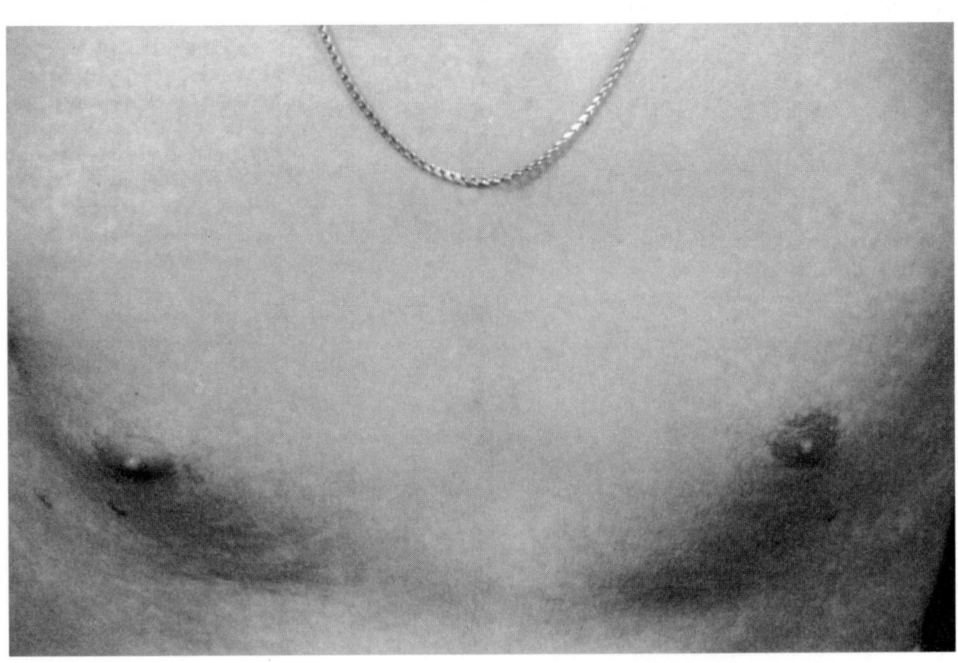

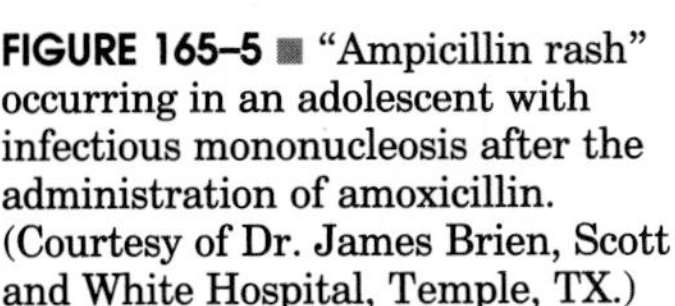

FIGURE 165–5 ■ "Ampicillin rash" occurring in an adolescent with infectious mononucleosis after the administration of amoxicillin. (Courtesy of Dr. James Brien, Scott and White Hospital, Temple, TX.)

HEMATOLOGIC

HEMOLYTIC ANEMIA. Hemolytic anemia occurs in 1 to 3 percent of patients with IM,[205, 432] and many cases have been reported in children with previously unrecognized hemoglobinopathies. The anemia typically develops during the second or third week of illness and resolves in 1 to 2 weeks. Corticosteroid therapy may hasten resolution.[145]

APLASTIC ANEMIA. This anemia is a rare complication of IM, with only scattered case reports in the literature.[158, 262, 456] Steroids have been beneficial,[158] but bone marrow transplantation has been necessary in some cases.[274] Fatalities have been recorded, usually in association with pancytopenia.[1, 456]

THROMBOCYTOPENIA. Thrombocytopenia occurs in 25 to 50 percent of patients with IM[60, 61] and probably is immune mediated. Platelet counts usually return to normal levels 4 to 6 weeks after the onset of illness. Severe thrombocytopenia (platelet counts $<20 \times 10^3/mm^3$) occurs rarely, with fewer than 40 cases identified in a recent review.[351] These authors noted a complication rate of 27 percent and a mortality rate of 5 percent associated with severe thrombocytopenia.

NEUTROPENIA. Mild to moderate neutropenia occurs frequently during IM.[59, 62] Neutrophil counts typically reach their lowest values during the third and fourth weeks of illness but may persist for another month or more. Although severe neutropenia (absolute neutrophil count <200) and agranulocytosis are rare events, with patients recovering uneventfully, death from overwhelming bacterial infection has been reported.[323] Antineutrophil antibodies elicited during EBV-induced polyclonal antibody stimulation are probably the source.[401]

PANCYTOPENIA. Pancytopenia has been reported to develop in a small number of children and adults with IM.[262] Fatalities attributable to overwhelming bacterial infection have occurred.[224, 456]

GASTROINTESTINAL TRACT

SPLEEN. Detectable splenomegaly develops in as many as 50 percent of patients with IM, with one study demonstrating splenic enlargement by ultrasound in 100 percent of patients hospitalized with IM.[102] Patients with a palpable spleen are at risk for spontaneous rupture. In the United States, spontaneous rupture of the spleen occurs in an estimated 1 in every 1000 adults with IM[121, 294]; the rate of splenic rupture in children is unknown but probably is lower. Rupture typically occurs during the first to third week of illness and is heralded by abdominal pain. Signs of hypovolemia occur frequently and include orthostasis, tachycardia, and syncope. Pain in the left shoulder (Kehr sign)[287] caused by diaphragmatic irritation from blood is observed in approximately 50 percent of patients with splenic rupture; right shoulder and subscapular pain may develop as well.[397] Splenic abscess has been described in a child with IM.[78]

To reduce the risk of splenic rupture, physicians customarily caution patients against engaging in strenuous physical activity and contact sports during recovery from the acute illness and for the period of significant organomegaly. Recommendations for reduced activity vary between 3 weeks and 6 months. Rutkow[391] has recommended that nonathletes wait 2 to 3 months and athletes wait 6 months before resuming regular activity. Most cases of splenic rupture require emergency splenectomy.[121] In an effort to maintain hematologic and immunologic competence, selected patients with splenic rupture who meet certain requirements, including hemodynamic stability with low transfusion requirements and a normal level of consciousness, may be managed with medical therapy.[25]

LIVER. Mild, subclinical inflammation of the liver is not an unusual event during IM, as mentioned previously. Rarely, more serious cases of hepatic disease have been described, including two children with fulminant hepatic failure.[98, 141, 252, 285, 291, 297] Chronic hepatitis also has been reported.[443]

OTHER. Other gastrointestinal diseases associated with IM include pancreatitis and cholecystitis.[183, 252, 279]

NEUROLOGIC

Acute neurologic disorders develop in 1 to 5 percent of persons with IM.[42, 203, 410] Neurologic complications usually occur at the height of the typical manifestations of IM, but they also may develop during the resolution phase. In addition, some reports document neurologic disease as a heralding event, before the development of typical IM, or even as the sole manifestation of EBV infection, especially in children.[47, 101, 111, 318] The most common neurologic complications include those occurring in the CNS, such as aseptic meningitis, meningoencephalitis, encephalitis, and Guillain-Barré syndrome; however, other central and peripheral neurologic complications have been described. The pathophysiology of CNS manifestations is not well established. Possible mechanisms include direct viral invasion, immunologic mechanisms, and inflammation.

ENCEPHALITIS AND ASEPTIC MENINGITIS. EBV frequently affects the CNS, yet most patients exhibit no symptoms. CSF pleocytosis occurs in approximately one fourth of patients with typical IM, and electroencephalographic abnormalities are noted in a third.[346] In two large series of patients with encephalitis, EBV was responsible for 2 to 5 percent of cases,[244, 251] and EBV caused 8 percent of cases of focal encephalitis.[465] Clinical findings in EBV encephalitis include fever, headache, vomiting, seizures, alteration in mental status, irritability, disorientation, lethargy, and, occasionally, a comatose state. Symptoms suggestive of schizophrenia, such as delusions, hallucinations, and extreme agitation, are seen occasionally. Patients with aseptic meningitis typically complain of a stiff neck, headache, fever, and vomiting. CSF findings in these patients include lymphocytic pleocytosis (usually <200 cells/μL, with atypical lymphocytes occasionally observed), mildly elevated protein levels, and normal glucose. EBV antibodies, EBV DNA, and even EBV itself have been identified in the CSF or brain tissue of persons with EBV-associated neurologic complications.[175, 217, 234, 344] Some reports suggest that the immune dysregulation caused by primary EBV infection may act as a triggering mechanism for the development of measles-associated subacute sclerosing meningoencephalitis.[123, 206]

OTHER CNS MANIFESTATIONS. EBV-associated cerebellitis is a rare occurrence that primarily develops in children and young adults.[81, 85, 111, 150] Full recovery occurs within weeks to months. Cranial nerve palsies, singly or in combination, also occur rarely; the facial nerve is involved most commonly.[290, 310] Other manifestations of cranial nerve involvement include optic neuritis,[136] deafness,[111, 466] and ophthalmoplegia.[395] Some cases of brain stem encephalitis have been reported.[334, 406]

NON-CNS NEUROLOGIC COMPLICATIONS. Outside the CNS, Guillain-Barré syndrome (ascending polyradiculoneuritis) is the most common complication of EBV infection.[159, 160, 369] Other non-CNS neurologic complications of IM include peripheral neuropathy,[105] autonomic dysfunction,[472] hemiplegia,[32] and transverse myelitis.[451]

RENAL

Silent abnormalities of the urine sediment, including proteinuria and microscopic hematuria, occur commonly in patients with IM.[203, 267] However, clinically significant renal disease is an extremely rare event. Tubulointerstitial disease and nephrotic syndrome have been observed most commonly.[46, 149] Acute renal failure with and without rhabdomyolysis has been reported.[137, 269]

RESPIRATORY TRACT

AIRWAY OBSTRUCTION. Severe airway obstruction occurs in 1 to 5 percent of children and adults with IM. Alpert and Fleisher[6] observed severe airway obstruction in one fourth of children admitted for complications of IM. Patients typically have severe tonsillopharyngitis with progressive symptoms of airway obstruction, usually in association with dysphagia and odynophagia. The intense inflammation and hypertrophy of lymphoid tissue in the Waldeyer ring and surrounding areas probably are responsible for the airway obstruction.[168] Management of airway obstruction has included systemic corticosteroids, tonsillectomy, tracheostomy, and nasopharyngeal airway placement, as well as general supportive measures such as humidification and elevation of the head of the bed.[416, 468] Nonsurgical management, including the administration of systemic steroids, is usually beneficial, although tonsillectomy may be necessary in refractory cases.[416, 424, 468] With the widespread availability of intensive care and mechanical ventilation, mortality from this complication is much lower than previously observed.

NECK ABSCESSES. Cervical and peritonsillar abscesses have been described in association with IM.[57, 177, 231, 463] This uncommon complication occurs after severe tonsillopharyngitis in patients with IM and typically is caused by bacteria found in the oral cavity, including alpha-hemolytic streptococci and anaerobes. Appropriate management includes administration of antibiotics and surgical drainage. Some concern exists that corticosteroid treatment of incipient airway obstruction may predispose to the development of an abscess.[57, 177] On the other hand, abscesses may develop in the absence of previous corticosteroid therapy.[144, 355]

PULMONARY DISEASE. Radiographic evidence of pulmonary infiltrates occurs in 0 to 5 percent of patients with IM,[104, 260] yet significant symptomatology rarely is present.[104, 203, 260] Some cases of IM with pulmonary disease may represent co-infection with other etiologic agents.[18, 125] However, several immunocompetent adults (but few children) with acute EBV infection have been reported to have pulmonary disease seemingly unrelated to other organisms.[82, 174, 335] Typically, unilateral or bilateral interstitial infiltrates are observed, and pleural effusions may be present.[106, 454] In some cases, EBV has been detected in lung tissue.[421, 457] Recovery is the rule, although mechanical ventilation may be necessary.

PSYCHIATRIC

CHRONIC FATIGUE. In the early 1980s, a chronic debilitating disorder (now designated chronic fatigue syndrome) began receiving increased publicity and purportedly was linked etiologically to EBV.[236, 425] The syndrome occurs more commonly in middle-aged women and is characterized primarily by chronic debilitating fatigue, as well as low-grade fever, mild lymphadenopathy, pharyngitis, neuropsychologic problems, and other symptoms. The association with EBV was drawn mainly from epidemiologic features and some abnormal EBV-specific immune responses. Variable general immunologic abnormalities have been described in some cases. However, no consistency exists in these findings, and a plausible pathogenetic association has not been demonstrated. Most experts today do not regard EBV as a major etiologic agent in the development of this syndrome, although it may play a contributory role along with other viruses (e.g., human herpesvirus 6, CMV). More information on this topic is found in Chapter 83.

"ALICE-IN-WONDERLAND" SYNDROME. This unusual syndrome, technically termed "metamorphopsia," is a visual illusion manifested as a distortion in size, form, movement, or color, and it is associated most commonly with migraine headaches, epilepsy, and hallucinogenic drugs. Copperman first described its association with IM in 1977,[86] and other similar cases also have been described.[79, 112, 257, 258] Onset may occur during or soon after resolution of the clinical IM symptoms, and it may resolve within 4 to 6 weeks. Visual-evoked potentials suggest diminished cerebral perfusion in affected cases.[257]

MISCELLANEOUS COMPLICATIONS

Other complications purportedly associated with IM or primary EBV infection include recurrent tonsillitis,[458] sinusitis,[437] periorbital cellulitis,[437] and ocular disease.[300]

Diagnosis

GENERAL LABORATORY FINDINGS

Patients with IM typically have an absolute lymphocytosis (>50% lymphocytes, with total leukocytes >5000/μL), prominent atypical lymphocytes (usually >10% of total leukocytes), and a positive test result for Paul-Bunnell heterophile antibodies (positive "differential heterophile"). The atypical lymphocytes observed in the blood of mononucleosis patients (Fig. 165–6) predominantly consist of activated T lymphocytes responding to the B-cell infection.[342] Although often considered a hallmark of IM, atypical lymphocytes also may be observed in association with CMV infection, toxoplasmosis, measles, mumps, roseola, rubella, drug reactions, and other conditions.[76, 471]

For a typical uncomplicated case of IM, a specific diagnosis of EBV infection is unnecessary, with a complete blood count and differential and a heterophile antibody test being sufficient for diagnostic testing. These tests are uncommonly normal early in the disease course and thus may need to be repeated during the first 3 to 4 weeks before diagnostic results are achieved. The clinician should be aware that very young (<4 years) patients with primary EBV infection frequently have a negative heterophile test.[433]

Heterophile antibodies classically were measured as sheep erythrocyte agglutinins.[343] Beef, ox, and horse red blood cells

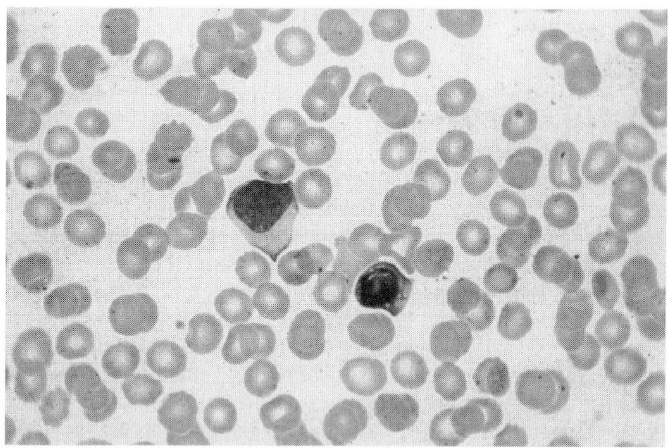

FIGURE 165–6 ■ Atypical lymphocytes in the peripheral blood of a patient with infectious mononucleosis. (Courtesy of Dr. Margaret Gulley, University of North Carolina, Chapel Hill, NC.)

also are agglutinated by the heterophile antibodies found in the serum of IM patients, but these heterophile antibodies do not bind to guinea pig kidney antigen extracts. These properties of mononucleosis heterophile antibodies distinguish them from the naturally occurring Forssman heterophile antibodies and from the heterophile antibodies found in serum sickness and other conditions. Thus, traditional tests for Paul-Bunnell heterophile antibodies involve absorption of the test serum with beef or ox red blood cells (which remove Paul-Bunnell heterophile antibodies) and guinea pig extract (which does not remove them). Tests in current use (e.g., Mono-Test, Mono-Diff, Mono-Spot) typically use horse red blood cells, which provide a more sensitive assay than do sheep erythrocytes. However, when horse erythrocyte agglutination tests are performed, the specificity of a positive results always should be confirmed by absorption of the serum with at least guinea pig kidney extract or, preferably, both guinea pig kidney extract and beef (or ox) red blood cells. Materials for the absorption steps are included in many, but not all, of the kits available commercially. Another heterophile antibody test, the beef (or ox) erythrocyte hemolysin assay, does not require absorption of the test sera but is somewhat less sensitive than is horse erythrocyte agglutination testing. Other tests[134, 171, 270, 381] using purified forms of heterophile antigen do not seem to offer any significant advantage over the rapid slide test with horse erythrocyte agglutination.

Other laboratory tests in patients with severe mononucleosis syndromes or in those with atypical clinical manifestations may indicate involvement of major organs, but such involvement rarely is associated with severe complications (see the previous section "Complications"). These laboratory abnormalities include elevated transaminase levels, mild hemolytic anemia, and neutropenia.

EBV ANTIBODIES

The diagnosis of EBV infection by specific laboratory testing should be reserved for patients with (1) atypical manifestations, (2) lymphoproliferative diseases, (3) severe illness, (4) negative heterophile tests, and (5) prolonged or serious illness. In most cases, serologic testing is the preferred mode of obtaining a specific viral diagnosis. Isolation of virus (see "Virus Isolation," later) is labor intensive and not widely available. Furthermore, after having acute EBV infection, individuals not uncommonly shed virus in the pharynx throughout their lifetimes, so identification of virus does not indicate acute infection necessarily. Other laboratory methods demonstrating high concentrations of actively replicating virus (such as antigen testing or quantitative PCR) may be more useful in associating EBV infection with disease (Table 165–2).

Evolution of the serologic response to EBV antigens after an acute EBV infection is depicted in Figure 165–7. By the time of clinical evaluation for IM and probably other forms of primary EBV infection, an appreciable antibody response to EBV VCA has developed in most persons.[189, 433] In the case of primary infections (e.g., IM), the initial serum sample often contains both IgG and IgM antibodies to VCA. Most children also have (or they will shortly develop) antibodies to the EA complex; these antibodies sometimes are measured separately as antibodies to the restricted (R) or diffuse (D) components.[132, 433] Antibodies to the EA-R component are limited to the cytoplasm of the cell line used for testing, whereas antibodies to the EA-D component are displayed in both the nucleus and cytoplasm. The EA-D pattern is

TABLE 165–2 ■ SUMMARY OF LABORATORY TESTS FOR EBV-ASSOCIATED DISEASES

Detection of	Test	Purpose
Antibodies	Heterophile antibody	Detect heterophile antibodies indicating infectious mononucleosis (more reliable in patients >4 yr old)
	EBV antibodies	Measure antibody response to viral proteins in serum samples; distinguish acute from remote infection
EBV DNA and RNA	Southern blot	Assess clonality of lesions with respect to EBV DNA structure; distinguish latent from replicative infection
	In situ hybridization	
	RNA (EBERs)	Identify EBER transcripts in specific cell types within histologic lesions
	DNA	Identify EBV DNA in specific cell types within histologic lesions
	PCR	Detect and quantitate EBV DNA in blood or CSF to diagnose and monitor disease
EBV proteins	Immunohistochemistry	Identify EBV protein expression in specific cell types within histologic lesions; distinguish latent from replicative infection based on expression profiles
EB virus	Virus culture	Detect infectious virions or latently infected B cells; impractical for routine clinical use
	Electron microscopy	Identify whole virions representing replicative infection; impractical for routine clinical use

CSF, cerebrospinal fluid; EBER, EBV-encoded RNA.
Adapted from Gulley, M.L.: Molecular diagnosis of Epstein-Barr virus-related diseases. J. Mol. Diagn. *3*:1-10, 2001.

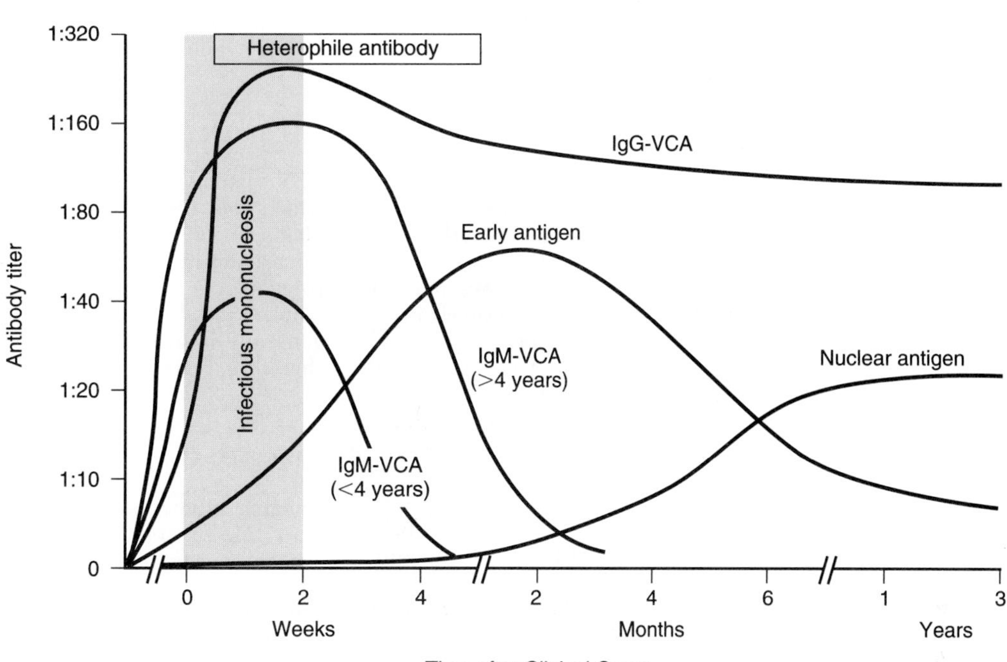

FIGURE 165–7 ■ Schematic representation of the evolution of antibodies to various Epstein-Barr virus antigens in patients with infectious mononucleosis. The titers are geometric mean values expressed as reciprocals of the serum dilution. The minimal titer tested for viral capsid antigen (VCA) and early antigen (EA) antibodies was 1:10, and for Epstein-Barr nuclear antigen (EBNA) it was 1:2.5. The IgM response to capsid antigen was divided because of the significant differences noted according to age. (From Jenson, H. B., Ench, Y., and Sumaya, C. V.: Epstein-Barr virus. *In* Rose, N. R., de Macario, E. C., Folds, J. D., et al. [eds.]: Manual of Clinical Laboratory Immunology. 5th ed. Washington, D.C., American Society for Microbiology, 1997, pp. 634–643.)

observed most commonly in adults and children with IM and NPC, whereas EA-R may be seen in children and adults with asymptomatic EBV infection or BL, certain immunodeficient subjects, and occasionally very young children with IM.[227] During the early phase of primary infection, most persons do not have detectable antibodies to EBNA; a few have marginally detectable anti-EBNA titers. Thus, the serologic diagnosis of recent or current primary EBV infection typically consists of a positive IgG and IgM anti-VCA response and negative anti-EBNA, with positive results in the anti-EA assay.

When a disease is not a consequence of primary infection but may be related to persistent or reactivated EBV infection (e.g., BL, NPC, some lymphomas of immunocompromised hosts, some chronic or atypical illnesses), the following serologic profile may be observed: positive IgG anti-VCA, often in high titer; usually negative IgM anti-VCA; often elevated anti-EA titer; and a positive anti-EBNA assay (though sometimes at low titer and occasionally undetectable).[178, 190, 191, 227, 359, 427]

IgM antibodies to VCA typically disappear within 2 to 3 months, and IgG antibodies to EA usually disappear within 6 to 12 months after infection[433] (see Fig. 165–2). IgG anti-VCA and anti-EBNA antibodies persist for life and are indicative of a chronic virus-carrying state.[433] Some studies also have shown the persistence of anti-EA antibodies for several years after an acute EBV infection and the occasional appearance of anti-EA antibodies in healthy seropositive persons; however, the clinical or virologic importance of this finding is not clear. Of note is that males with XLPD frequently have no or low levels of EBV antibodies in response to EBV infection.[394] Heterophile antibodies may persist for months and sometimes for a year or more in persons who have recovered from IM; they remain detectable longer (usually more than a year) when the more sensitive horse erythrocyte agglutination and a quantitative method for determining the antibody response are used.

Some studies[298, 372, 382] suggest that monitoring for decreases in anti-EBNA antibodies, in addition to such increased immunologic mediators as IL-4 and soluble CD23 and increased circulating EBV (see later, "EBV Antigens"), may be useful in providing early serologic signs of EBV-associated tumor development in organ and bone marrow transplant recipients.

Molecular cloning of subregions of the EBV genome into high-expression plasmid vectors presently is being used to generate large amounts of pure proteins containing EBV-encoded polypeptide sequences for use in immunoblot and enzyme-linked immunosorbent assay–based tests.[55, 65, 120, 196, 298, 372, 382] These methods are beginning to yield potentially better methods for EBV serodiagnosis. Although some tests approved by the Food and Drug Administration are available commercially, they have not been tested widely on children's sera. Because of this observation and some published data[271] suggesting problems in interpretation, the results of these test kits in this age group should be viewed with caution.

Reliable performance and interpretation of the traditional immunofluorescence assays used in EBV serology require specialized training and the use of appropriate standards and controls in the clinical laboratory. New developments in serologic testing should expand the understanding and definition of interactions between EBV and humans in various states of health and disease. Nonetheless, establishing a correlation between results obtained with the new tests and those obtained by traditional methods will be important.

EBV NUCLEIC ACID (DNA OR RNA)

In immunocompromised patients, the serologic response to EBV antigens may be incomplete, lacking, or otherwise not helpful. In such situations, demonstrating EBV nucleic acid in tissue sections or in blood may be necessary for diagnostic purposes.[9] Methods include Southern blotting, in situ hybridization, and detection of EBV DNA by PCR.[165] Besides their utility as diagnostic aids, these tests also are useful for epidemiologic and pathogenetic purposes relevant to EBV infection.

Southern blot hybridization has been very helpful in demonstrating the association of EBV with disease.[16, 462] Although it is not as sensitive as PCR, Southern blotting has the advantage of providing additional information regarding the monoclonality of EBV-associated lesions, detection of lytic EBV processes, and recognition of viral integration into the genome.[154, 166, 169, 361]

Because of their ubiquity in EBV-infected cells (as many as 10^6 copies per cell), detection of EBERs in tissues by in situ RNA hybridization is becoming a standard method for detecting and localizing latent EBV in tissues.[37, 165, 289] Probes for detection of EBERs ("riboprobes") are labeled conveniently by immunoperoxidase methods. Detection of EBV DNA by in situ hybridization also can be performed,[52] although DNA detection is less sensitive because of the lower copy numbers per cell in comparison to EBERs.

Amplification of EBV DNA by PCR has emerged as an important test for the diagnosis and treatment of several EBV-associated diseases. In adult patients with AIDS and primary CNS lymphomas, detection of EBV DNA in CSF has high sensitivity and specificity in most studies.[20, 37, 80, 91, 165, 289] PCR for EBV in CSF, possibly in combination with certain imaging studies,[20] may be sufficient for the diagnosis of CNS lymphoma and could preclude performing brain biopsy, which can be associated with complications. On the other hand, lumbar puncture in patients with cerebral lesions also must be considered carefully because of the risk for cerebral herniation.

In organ transplant recipients, quantitative PCR for EBV DNA in peripheral blood serves as a useful tool for the diagnosis of PTLD and as a marker during follow-up.[34, 209, 372, 380, 385, 398] In these studies, levels of EBV DNA in blood typically are low in healthy control subjects, high in those with PTLD or other EBV-associated diseases, and intermediate in asymptomatic organ transplant patients. With successful management, EBV DNA concentrations typically diminish to baseline levels.[209, 380] Although negative predictive values for these tests are higher than 90 percent, positive predictive values are substantially lower. Further studies are needed to establish quantitative laboratory standards for diagnosing and monitoring EBV-associated PTLD.

Quantitative PCR also may be useful for diagnosing and monitoring other EBV-associated malignancies, including NPC,[286] HD,[268] and NHL.[423] Larger studies are necessary to better define the role of EBV viral load testing in these diseases.

EBV PROTEINS

Immunofluorescent techniques may be used to detect the presence of cells carrying EBV proteins in touch imprints of biopsy material or in frozen sections of cryopreserved tissue.[154, 289, 353, 477] Most commonly, tissues are examined for VCA, EBNA-1, and LMP-1 proteins with the use of mouse monoclonal antibodies.

VIRUS ISOLATION

EBV from blood or oropharyngeal specimens (rarely, other specimens) can be isolated in tissue culture with a transformation assay.[227] For oropharyngeal specimens, the test requires incubation with fresh cord blood mononuclear cells for as long as 6 weeks. Transforming virus can be identified in peripheral blood by incubating mononuclear cells in the presence of cyclosporine (for inhibition of cytotoxic T cells, which can suppress the growth of EBV-positive B cells). An end-point dilution assay may be used to quantitate the amount of EBV within blood specimens.[378] Virus isolation tests are used primarily for research purposes and are not widely available.

ELECTRON MICROSCOPY

EBV virions also may be detected by electron microscopy, which has been used in patients with oral hairy leukoplakia,[222] NPC,[24] and other EBV-associated lesions. The ultrastructural features of EBV virions, however, are indistinguishable from those of other herpesviruses, and confirmatory tests usually are necessary. Electron microscopy generally is available only at larger research centers and, therefore, is impractical for routine diagnostic testing.

IMAGING STUDIES

Imaging studies are seldom necessary in typical patients with IM. In one study of patients hospitalized with IM, the most common findings on chest radiography were splenomegaly (47%), hilar adenopathy (13%), and interstitial infiltrates (5%).[260] Imaging studies are used more commonly for evaluation of EBV-associated neurologic disease, especially in immunocompromised patients. Patients with EBV-associated encephalitis usually have normal neuroimaging results.[101] However, some patients may display diffuse swelling or patchy low-density lesions by computed tomography (CT), and magnetic resonance imaging (MRI) may reveal increased signal on T2-weighted images, as well as atrophy.[101, 407] Contrast CT scans of primary cerebral lymphoma in patients with AIDS typically reveal large (2 to 6 mm) lesions occurring anywhere in the cerebrum with diffuse and homogeneous enhancement[441]; however, some overlap exists with findings observed in other diseases such as cerebral toxoplasmosis. Thallium 201 single-photon emission CT (SPECT), in conjunction with MRI and PCR testing of CSF for EBV DNA, may be useful in distinguishing CNS lymphomas from toxoplasmosis in AIDS patients.[20]

DIFFERENTIAL DIAGNOSIS

INFECTIOUS MONONUCLEOSIS. EBV causes an estimated 80 to 95 percent of IM syndromes.[435] Numerous agents have been associated with heterophile-negative IM. CMV is responsible for most cases of heterophile-negative IM with typical clinical and hematologic findings.[208] Certain features of CMV mononucleosis may help distinguish it from EBV (e.g., less common sore throat and lymphadenopathy, less intense atypical lymphocytosis, and prominent splenomegaly), but these characteristics have considerable overlap with EBV-associated IM. Serologic testing consistent with acute CMV infection in the absence of characteristic EBV serologic findings confirms the diagnosis. The remainder of cases may be attributable to infection with *Toxoplasma gondii*, adenoviruses, rubella virus, and hepatitis A virus. Acute HIV syndrome also may mimic IM. However, in children with non-EBV IM, the etiology frequently remains elusive. In heterophile-negative children with mononucleosis and both the clinical and hematologic characteristics of the syndrome, the most likely known agents are EBV and CMV.

OTHER EBV-ASSOCIATED DISORDERS. EBV-associated HLH may be confused with IM, systemic connective tissue disorders, septicemia, and certain hematologic malignancies.[218] CNS lymphomas in patients with AIDS are difficult to distinguish from cerebral toxoplasmosis based on clinical findings and imaging studies. Historically, a negative *T. gondii* serum antibody test eliminates toxoplasmosis, whereas a positive test may necessitate a trial of antitoxoplasmic therapy. Response within a week suggests toxoplasmosis, but a nonresponse indicates the need for stereotactic brain biopsy to establish a diagnosis. Identification of EBV DNA in CSF by PCR may help confirm the diagnosis of lymphoma.

Treatment

INFECTIOUS MONONUCLEOSIS

SUPPORTIVE CARE. Support, including rest, fluids, and antipyretics, is all that is required for uncomplicated IM. Although studies dating back to the 1950s have demonstrated a beneficial effect of corticosteroids in reducing the symptoms associated with IM (e.g., fever, pharyngitis, lymphadenitis), most physicians use corticosteroids cautiously, if at all.[305] This decision is based on the unknown long-term consequences of such therapy, including a potential deleterious effect on the immune system. Nonetheless, small series and anecdotal reports suggest that some severely symptomatic patients (e.g., high fever, severe pharyngitis) may benefit from short-term courses of corticosteroids.[14, 40, 49] In practice, corticosteroids are used most commonly for patients with complicated illnesses (e.g., with stridor from massively enlarged tonsils or paratracheal adenopathy, or for those with hematologic or neurologic complications) (see "Complications").

ANTIVIRAL TREATMENT. Numerous antiviral agents inhibit EBV replication in vitro. Such agents include acyclovir, penciclovir, ganciclovir, and other nucleoside analogues.[29, 84, 92, 281] None of these agents is capable of eliminating latent EBV present as episomes in infected cells. Five randomized, placebo-controlled trials of acyclovir (with or without corticosteroids) in adolescents and adults with IM demonstrated no beneficial effect in resolving the clinical signs and symptoms associated with illness, as well as no reduced rate of complications.[13, 15, 337, 453, 455] Recently, a meta-analysis substantiated these findings.[450] Acyclovir did reduce the rate of EBV shedding in the oropharynx significantly, albeit temporarily.[450]

OTHER EBV-ASSOCIATED DISEASES

Providing details regarding the treatment of EBV-associated lymphoproliferative diseases, including lymphomas, is beyond the scope of this chapter. However, a brief overview of treatment of the principal diseases is provided.

X-LINKED LYMPHOPROLIFERATIVE DISEASE. Limited success has been achieved with allogeneic hematopoietic stem cell transplantation in males with XLPD, in whom fulminant primary EBV infection may develop.[161, 459] Now that the gene defect in XLPD has been identified, consideration may be given to a gene therapeutic approach. Further studies of the function of the *SH2D1A* gene, as well as the consequences of its dysregulation, are necessary before this approach can be safely evaluated.[392] No therapeutic measure has been successful once disseminated EBV develops in these patients.

HEMOPHAGOCYTIC LYMPHOHISTIOCYTOSIS. Early studies using non–etoposide-containing regimens were largely unsuccessful in significantly reducing the high mortality associated with HLH.[21] Recently, chemotherapeutic regimens that include etoposide (toxic to macrophages) have reduced the mortality rate significantly. More recently, corticosteroids have been added to etoposide regimens, with enhanced remission rates.[74, 218] For refractory cases, bone marrow transplantation has been successful.[33, 180, 218]

POST-TRANSPLANT LYMPHOPROLIFERATIVE DISEASE. The most effective therapy for PTLD in transplant recipients is reduction of immunosuppression to allow more effective control of EBV infection by the cell-mediated immune system. Hayashi and colleagues noted a 58 percent response rate to curtailment of immunosuppression in a group of pediatric transplant recipients.[181] However, decisions concerning immunosuppression reduction must be weighed against the risk of graft rejection and must be performed carefully. If such measures cannot be performed or are unsuccessful, other therapies may be considered. IFN-α has induced complete remissions in some studies,[93, 278] but relapses and graft rejection have occurred. The use of anti–B-cell monoclonal antibodies (anti-CD20, anti-CD21, and anti-CD23) is an attractive form of treatment and has been used in several series with good success.[41, 314] For example, Milpied and associates[314] noted a response rate of 65 percent in a group of 32 solid organ transplant recipients with PTLD who were treated with anti-CD20 antibody (rituximab). Most patients tolerate treatment well, although tumor lysis syndrome may occur during treatment of bulky disease and hypogammaglobulinemia may persist for several months. Conventional NHL chemotherapy has been successful in one series of patients with PTLD[181]; in contrast, two other reports describe increased toxicity and mortality associated with infection when standard doses are used.[322, 440] A low-dose chemotherapy regimen consisting of cyclophosphamide and prednisone is being evaluated.[35, 162] A new experimental therapy using EBV-specific cytotoxic T lymphocytes also is being investigated in allogeneic bone marrow transplant recipients.[383]

B-CELL LYMPHOMA. Endemic (African) BLs, which are highly associated with EBV,[255] are treated primarily with cyclophosphamide-based chemotherapy.[256, 481] Favorable responses were observed recently by Labrecque and coworkers in patients with tumors expressing lytic genes.[256] Treatment of sporadic BL also is based primarily on multiagent chemotherapy that includes cyclophosphamide.[280]

B-cell lymphomas in patients with AIDS are extremely difficult to treat, primarily because of the underlying extreme host immune deficiency. Early regimens using standard chemotherapeutic regimens were largely failures, with survival rates lower than those of untreated patients; most patients died of opportunistic infections, drug toxicity, and resistant tumors. Alternative therapeutic strategies have improved outcomes for this malignancy, yet mortality remains substantial.[284] These strategies have included lower doses of standard drugs,[240] continuous infusion of chemotherapy,[419] hematopoietic growth factors,[261] novel immunotherapies (e.g., IL-2),[43] and adoptive immunotherapy,[464] as well as improved management of opportunistic infections and HIV.

Virtually all AIDS-related primary CNS lymphomas are associated with EBV infection. Historically, radiation therapy in conjunction with corticosteroids was used for treatment, but with disappointing survival rates. More recently, combined-modality treatment with radiation and chemotherapy has been investigated but with poor outcomes.[135] A minority of healthier patients with AIDS may respond better to combined-modality regimens.[64] Improved immunologic function as a result of highly active antiretroviral therapy also shows some promise for improving outcome.[306] Moreover, Slobod and colleagues[414] recently reported successful treatment with hydroxyurea, a ribonucleotide reductase inhibitor capable of purging EBV episomes from cells in vitro, in two AIDS patients with primary CNS lymphoma.[77] Larger clinical trials of hydroxyurea for CNS lymphomas and possibly other EBV-associated malignancies are anticipated.

HODGKIN DISEASE. Historically, children with HD were treated with high-dose radiation. However, high rates of skeletal growth inhibition and secondary malignancies were noted in survivors, so new trials using lower involved-field radiation in conjunction with multiagent chemotherapy were conducted. These trials form the basis for combination treatment regimens used currently in growing children.[214, 356] Although the presence or absence of EBV in tumor (more likely in mixed-cellularity types) currently plays no role in pretherapy staging, some recent studies suggest improved outcomes for patients with EBV-positive tumors.[317, 321]

NASOPHARYNGEAL CARCINOMA. NPCs are sensitive to radiotherapy as well as chemotherapy. Surgery is not usually an option because of the location of the primary tumor, although it is needed for persistent or recurrent lymph node disease. For early localized disease, radiotherapy generally is indicated, whereas combined-modality treatment (radiation and chemotherapy) may be considered for more advanced disease.[4] Children failing treatment have a high rate of distant metastases, principally to bone.[26, 219]

CHRONIC ACTIVE DISEASE. Treatment modalities for chronic active EBV infection have varied widely because the rarity of this disease precludes performing proper clinical trials. Resolution of symptoms has been reported in case reports involving antiviral drugs (e.g., acyclovir, ganciclovir),[221] immunomodulatory agents (e.g., corticosteroids, intravenous immune globulin, cytokines),[142, 243] adoptive transfer of cytotoxic T cells,[254] etoposide,[336] or combinations thereof.

HIV-ASSOCIATED DISEASES (See Chapter 193). Oral hairy leukoplakia generally does not require therapy because patients typically are asymptomatic and the lesions have no malignant potential. Some lesions have responded to antiretroviral[350] and antiherpesviral agents,[325, 368] although recurrences are common. Treatment strategies for lymphocytic interstitial pneumonitis are not well defined. Supportive care, including supplemental oxygen, may be necessary. Suppression of HIV with effective antiretroviral agents also is logical to improve immune function and minimize the potential direct effect of HIV. Although no controlled studies have documented the value of antiretrovirals, benefit is suggested by the declining prevalence of lymphocytic interstitial pneumonitis in children with AIDS since antiretrovirals were introduced (prevalence of 28% in 1988 and 10% in 1996).[198] Uncontrolled studies also suggest a beneficial effect from corticosteroids,[28, 389] and this therapy is now generally recommended.[19, 308] No controlled studies have evaluated antiherpesviral drugs (e.g., acyclovir) for lymphocytic interstitial pneumonitis.

Prognosis

The prognosis for healthy persons with IM is extremely good, with mortality considered a rare occurrence. In a series of 30 fatal cases of IM, Lukes and Cox found splenic rupture, Guillain-Barré syndrome, hemorrhage, and secondary infection to be the most common causes of death.[288] In Penman's study of 20 documented deaths,[347] predominantly of young adults, the causes of death (in order of frequency) were neurologic complications, splenic rupture, secondary infection, hepatic failure, and myocarditis. EBV-induced aplastic anemia, a rare but dreaded hematologic complication, now is thought to have a better prognosis for eventual recovery if the patient can be supported successfully through the acute stages.[36, 262]

The prognosis for patients with EBV-associated lymphoproliferative diseases is variable and depends on the immunologic status of the patient and the type of lymphoproliferation. A registry of 161 males with XLPD indicated a mortality rate of 70 percent by the age of 10 years and 100 percent by the age of 40.[157] HLH has a greater than 90 percent fatality rate without treatment; most deaths are caused by hemorrhage, overwhelming infection, disseminated intravascular coagulation, or multiorgan failure.[75, 225] Even with reduced immunosuppression, PTLD occurring after solid organ transplantation carries a mortality rate of 40 to 60 percent,[200, 422] with higher mortality rates (>85%) in bone marrow transplant recipients.[404] The prognosis for healthy children with NHL generally is good, with 5-year relative survival rates of 80 percent.[373] However, the prognosis for AIDS patients with NHL is poor. In adults with AIDS, median survival is 1 to 8 months for CNS lymphomas[246] (virtually all of which are EBV associated) and 7 months for non-CNS lymphomas. Childhood HD generally has a very good prognosis, with 5-year survival rates greater than 90 percent.[373]

In most studies, children with NPC have long-term survival rates similar to those of adults (approximately 50%); whether adjuvant chemotherapy improves the long-term outcome is not clear.[26, 219]

Prevention

EBV is shed regularly in saliva, and, therefore, infection control policies are difficult to develop. In addition, mechanisms for EBV transmission are not well understood, and EBV outbreaks occur rarely, if at all. For these reasons, no more than standard infection control precautions are recommended for patients hospitalized with EBV infections, including IM.[11] Although transfusion-associated EBV infection occurs rarely, persons with recent EBV infection or mononucleosis-like illnesses are urged to refrain from donating blood.[11]

Efforts continue in the development of an EBV vaccine. Because of concern over the administration of a vaccine with unknown long-term consequences, including malignancy, most efforts have focused on the development of subunit EBV vaccines. A subunit vaccine containing the EBV gp350/220 protein has proved effective in preventing EBV infection in an experimental animal model.[109] More recently, a gp350 vaccine evaluated in Chinese patients elicited good antibody responses and provided some protection from EBV infection.[163] A similar vaccine has been developed in the United States,[223] with phase I clinical trials under way. Another vaccine containing EBV latent antigens also is being investigated.[245] An effective vaccine could be considered for persons at high risk for developing EBV-associated lymphoproliferative disease and cancer, such as patients with AIDS, those with XLPD, and organ transplant recipients.

REFERENCES

1. Ahronheim, G. A., Auger, F., Joncas, J. H., et al.: Primary infection by Epstein-Barr virus presenting as aplastic anemia. N. Engl. J. Med. *309*:313–314, 1983.
2. Alfieri, C., and Tanner, J.: Chronic-active Epstein-Barr virus infections. Herpes *5*:12–14, 1998.
3. Alfieri, C., Tanner, J., Carpentier, L., et al.: Epstein-Barr virus transmission from a blood donor to an organ transplant recipient with recovery of the same virus strain from the recipient's blood and oropharynx. Blood *87*:812–817, 1996.

4. Ali, H., and al-Sarraf, M.: Nasopharyngeal cancer. Hematol. Oncol. Clin. North Am. *13*:837–847, 1999.
5. Allday, M. J., and Crawford, D. H.: Role of epithelium in EBV persistence and pathogenesis of B-cell tumours. Lancet *1*:855–857, 1988.
6. Alpert, G., and Fleisher, G. R.: Complications of infection with Epstein-Barr virus during childhood: A study of children admitted to the hospital. Pediatr. Infect. Dis. *3*:304–307, 1984.
7. Alsip, G. R., Ench, Y., Sumaya, C. V., et al.: Increased Epstein-Barr virus DNA in oropharyngeal secretions from patients with AIDS, AIDS-related complex, or asymptomatic human immunodeficiency virus infections. J. Infect. Dis. *157*:1072–1076, 1988.
8. Ambinder, R. F., Browning, P. J., Lorenzana, I., et al.: Epstein-Barr virus and childhood Hodgkin's disease in Honduras and the United States. Blood *81*:462–467, 1993.
9. Ambinder, R. F., and Mann, R. B.: Detection and characterization of Epstein-Barr virus in clinical specimens. Am. J. Pathol. *145*:239–252, 1994.
10. Ambler, M., Stoll, J., Tzamaloukas, A., et al.: Focal encephalomyelitis in infectious mononucleosis. A report with pathological description. Ann. Intern. Med. *75*:579–583, 1971.
11. American Academy of Pediatrics: Epstein-Barr virus infections (infectious mononucleosis). *In* Pickering, L. K. (ed.): Red Book 2000: Report of the Committee on Infectious Diseases. 25th ed. Elk Grove Village, IL, American Academy of Pediatrics, 2000, pp. 238–240.
12. Anagnostopoulos, I., Hummel, M., Kreschel, C., et al.: Morphology, immunophenotype, and distribution of latently and/or productively Epstein-Barr virus–infected cells in acute infectious mononucleosis: Implications for the interindividual infection route of Epstein-Barr virus. Blood *85*:744–750, 1995.
13. Andersson, J., Britton, S., Ernberg, I., et al.: Effect of acyclovir on infectious mononucleosis: A double-blind, placebo-controlled study. J. Infect. Dis. *153*:283–290, 1986.
14. Andersson, J., and Ernberg, I.: Management of Epstein-Barr virus infections. Am. J. Med. *85*:107–115, 1988.
15. Andersson, J., Skoldenberg, B., Henle, W., et al.: Acyclovir treatment in infectious mononucleosis: A clinical and virological study. Infection *15*(Suppl.):14–20, 1987.
16. Andiman, W., Gradoville, L., Heston, L., et al.: Use of cloned probes to detect Epstein-Barr viral DNA in tissues of patients with neoplastic and lymphoproliferative diseases. J. Infect. Dis. *148*:967–977, 1983.
17. Andiman, W. A., Eastman, R., Martin, K., et al.: Opportunistic lymphoproliferations associated with Epstein-Barr viral DNA in infants and children with AIDS. Lancet *2*:1390–1393, 1985.
18. Andiman, W. A., McCarthy, P., Markowitz, R. I., et al.: Clinical, virologic, and serologic evidence of Epstein-Barr virus infection in association with childhood pneumonia. J. Pediatr. *99*:880–886, 1981.
19. Andiman, W. A., and Shearer, W. T.: Lymphoid interstitial pneumonitis. *In* Pizzo, P. A., and Wilfert, C. M. (eds.): Pediatric AIDS: The Challenge of HIV Infection in Infants, Children, and Adolescents. 3rd ed. Baltimore, Williams & Wilkins, 1998, pp. 323–334.
20. Antinori, A., De Rossi, G., Ammassari, A., et al.: Value of combined approach with thallium-201 single-photon emission computed tomography and Epstein-Barr virus DNA polymerase chain reaction in CSF for the diagnosis of AIDS-related primary CNS lymphoma. J. Clin. Oncol. *17*:554–560, 1999.
21. Arico, M., Janka, G., Fischer, A., et al.: Hemophagocytic lymphohistiocytosis. Report of 122 children from the International Registry. FHL Study Group of the Histiocyte Society. Leukemia *10*:197–203, 1996.
22. Armstrong, A. A., Alexander, F. E., Cartwright, R., et al.: Epstein-Barr virus and Hodgkin's disease: Further evidence for the three disease hypothesis. Leukemia *12*:1272–1276, 1998.
23. Armstrong, A. A., Alexander, F. E., Paes, R. P., et al.: Association of Epstein-Barr virus with pediatric Hodgkin's disease. Am. J. Pathol. *142*:1683–1688, 1993.
24. Arnold, W., and Huth, F.: Light and electron microscopic investigations of nasopharyngeal carcinomas with regard to the viral etiology of these tumors. J. Cancer Res. Clin. Oncol. *94*:87–109, 1979.
25. Asgari, M. M., and Begos, D. G.: Spontaneous splenic rupture in infectious mononucleosis: A review. Yale J. Biol. Med. *70*:175–182, 1997.
26. Ayan, I., and Altun, M.: Nasopharyngeal carcinoma in children: Retrospective review of 50 patients. Int. J. Radiat. Oncol. Biol. Phys. *35*:485–492, 1996.
27. Babcock, G. J., Decker, L. L., Volk, M., et al.: EBV persistence in memory B cells in vivo. Immunity *9*:395–404, 1998.
28. Bach, M. C.: Zidovudine for lymphocytic interstitial pneumonia associated with AIDS. Lancet *2*:796, 1987.
29. Bacon, T. H., and Boyd, M. R.: Activity of penciclovir against Epstein-Barr virus. Antimicrob. Agents Chemother. *39*:1599–1602, 1995.
30. Baehner, R. L., and Shuler, S. E.: Infectious mononucleosis in childhood: Clinical expressions, serologic findings, complications, prognosis. Clin. Pediatr. (Phila.) *6*:393–399, 1967.
31. Baer, R., Bankier, A. T., Biggin, M. D., et al.: DNA sequence and expression of the B95-8 Epstein-Barr virus genome. Nature *310*:207–211, 1984.
32. Baker, F. J., Kotchmar, G. S., Jr., Foshee, W. S., et al.: Acute hemiplegia of childhood associated with Epstein-Barr virus infection. Pediatr. Infect. Dis. *2*:136–138, 1983.
33. Baker, K. S., DeLaat, C. A., Steinbuch, M., et al.: Successful correction of hemophagocytic lymphohistiocytosis with related or unrelated bone marrow transplantation. Blood *89*:3857–3863, 1997.
34. Baldanti, F., Grossi, P., Furione, M., et al.: High levels of Epstein-Barr virus DNA in blood of solid-organ transplant recipients and their value in predicting posttransplant lymphoproliferative disorders. J. Clin. Microbiol. *38*:613–619, 2000.
35. Balfour, I. C., Wall, D., Luisiri, A., et al.: Cyclophosphamide/prednisone for combination immunosuppression and therapy of lymphoproliferative disease. J. Heart Lung Transplant. *18*:492–495, 1999.
36. Baranski, B., Armstrong, G., Truman, J. T., et al.: Epstein-Barr virus in the bone marrow of patients with aplastic anemia. Ann. Intern. Med. *109*:695–704, 1988.
37. Barletta, J. M., Kingma, D. W., Ling, Y., et al.: Rapid in situ hybridization for the diagnosis of latent Epstein-Barr virus infection. Mol. Cell. Probes *7*:105–109, 1993.
38. Baumgarten, E., Herbst, H., Schmitt, M., et al.: Life-threatening infectious mononucleosis: Is it correlated with virus-induced T cell proliferation? Clin. Infect. Dis. *19*:152–156, 1994.
39. Bechet, J. M., Fialkow, P. J., Nilsson, K., et al.: Immunoglobulin synthesis and glucose-6-phosphate dehydrogenase as cell markers in human lymphoblastoid cell lines. Exp. Cell Res. *89*:275–282, 1974.
40. Bender, C. E.: The value of corticosteroids in the treatment of infectious mononucleosis. J. A. M. A. *199*:529–531, 1967.
41. Benkerrou, M., Jais, J. P., Leblond, V., et al.: Anti–B-cell monoclonal antibody treatment of severe posttransplant B-lymphoproliferative disorder: Prognostic factors and long-term outcome. Blood *92*:3137–3147, 1998.
42. Bernstein, T. C., and Wolff, H. G.: Involvement of the nervous system in infectious mononucleosis. Ann. Intern. Med. *33*:1120–1138, 1950.
43. Bernstein, Z. P., Porter, M. M., Gould, M., et al.: Prolonged administration of low-dose interleukin-2 in human immunodeficiency virus–associated malignancy results in selective expansion of innate immune effectors without significant clinical toxicity. Blood *86*:3287–3294, 1995.
44. Biggar, R. J., Henle, W., Fleisher, G., et al.: Primary Epstein-Barr virus infections in African infants. I. Decline of maternal antibodies and time of infection. Int. J. Cancer *22*:239–243, 1978.
45. Birx, D. L., Redfield, R. R., and Tosato, G.: Defective regulation of Epstein-Barr virus infection in patients with acquired immunodeficiency syndrome (AIDS) or AIDS-related disorders. N. Engl. J. Med. *314*:874–879, 1986.
46. Blowey, D. L.: Nephrotic syndrome associated with an Epstein-Barr virus infection. Pediatr. Nephrol. *10*:507–508, 1996.
47. Bonforte, R. J.: Convulsion as a presenting sign of infectious mononucleosis. Am. J. Dis. Child. *114*:429–432, 1967.
48. Borzy, M. S., Hong, R., Horowitz, S. D., et al.: Fatal lymphoma after transplantation of cultured thymus in children with combined immunodeficiency disease. N. Engl. J. Med. *301*:565–568, 1979.
49. Brandfonbrener, A., Epstein, A., Wu, S., et al.: Corticosteroid therapy in Epstein-Barr virus infection. Effect on lymphocyte class, subset, and response to early antigen. Arch. Intern. Med. *146*:337–339, 1986.
50. Breinig, M. K., Zitelli, B., Starzl, T. E., et al.: Epstein-Barr virus, cytomegalovirus, and other viral infections in children after liver transplantation. J. Infect. Dis. *156*:273–279, 1987.
51. Brichacek, B., Hirsch, I., Sibl, O., et al.: Association of some supraglottic laryngeal carcinomas with EB virus. Int. J. Cancer *32*:193–197, 1983.
52. Brousset, P., Butet, V., Chittal, S., et al.: Comparison of in situ hybridization using different nonisotopic probes for detection of Epstein-Barr virus in nasopharyngeal carcinoma and immunohistochemical correlation with anti–latent membrane protein antibody. Lab. Invest. *67*:457–464, 1992.
53. Brown, N. A., and Miller, G.: Immunoglobulin expression by human B lymphocytes clonally transformed by Epstein Barr virus. J. Immunol. *128*:24–29, 1982.
54. Brown, Z. A., Stenchever, M. A.: Infectious mononucleosis and congenital anomalies. Am. J. Obstet. Gynecol. *131*:108–109, 1978.
55. Buisson, M., Fleurent, B., Mak, M., et al.: Novel immunoblot assay using four recombinant antigens for diagnosis of Epstein-Barr virus primary infection and reactivation. J. Clin. Microbiol. *37*:2709–2714, 1999.
56. Burkitt, D. P.: A sarcoma involving the jaws in African children. Br. J. Surg. *46*:218–223, 1958.
57. Burstin, P. P., and Marshall, C. L.: Infectious mononucleosis and bilateral peritonsillar abscesses resulting in airway obstruction. J. Laryngol. Otol. *112*:1186–1188, 1998.
58. Cabot, R. C.: The lymphocytosis of infection. Am. J. Med. Sci. *145*:335–339, 1913.
59. Cantow, E. F., and Kostinas, J. E.: Studies on infectious mononucleosis. IV. Changes in the granulocytic series. Am. J. Clin. Pathol. *46*:43–47, 1966.
60. Cantow, E. F., and Kostinas, J. E.: Studies on infectious mononucleosis. III. Platelets. Am. J. Med. Sci. *251*:664–667, 1966.
61. Carter, R. L.: Platelet levels in infectious mononucleosis. Blood *25*:817–821, 1965.
62. Carter, R. L.: Granulocyte changes in infectious mononucleosis. J. Clin. Pathol. *19*:279–283, 1966.
63. Cen, H., Breinig, M. C., Atchison, R. W., et al.: Epstein-Barr virus transmission via the donor organs in solid organ transplantation: Polymerase chain reaction and restriction fragment length polymorphism analysis of IR2, IR3, and IR4. J. Virol. *65*:976–980, 1991.

64. Chamberlain, M. C.: Long survival in patients with acquired immune deficiency syndrome–related primary central nervous system lymphoma. Cancer *73*:1728–1730, 1994.
65. Chan, K. H., Luo, R. X., Chen, H. L., et al.: Development and evaluation of an Epstein-Barr virus (EBV) immunoglobulin M enzyme-linked immunosorbent assay based on the 18-kilodalton matrix protein for diagnosis of primary EBV infection. J. Clin. Microbiol. *36*:3359–3361, 1998.
66. Chang, R. S.: What is the determinant for susceptibility to infectious mononucleosis? N. Engl. J. Med. *292*:1298, 1975.
67. Chang, R. S.: Interpersonal transmission of EB-virus infection. N. Engl. J. Med. *293*:454–455, 1975.
68. Chang, R. S.: Infectious Mononucleosis. Boston, G. K. Hall, 1980.
69. Chang, R. S., and Blankenship, W.: Spontaneous in vitro transformation of leukocytes from a neonate. Proc. Soc. Exp. Biol. Med. *144*:337–339, 1973.
70. Chang, R. S., and Golden, H. D.: Transformation of human leucocytes by throat washing from infectious mononucleosis patients. Nature *234*:359–360, 1971.
71. Chang, R. S., Lewis, J. P., Reynolds, R. D., et al.: Oropharyngeal excretion of Epstein-Barr virus by patients with lymphoproliferative disorders and by recipients of renal homografts. Ann. Intern. Med. *88*:34–40, 1978.
72. Chang, R. S., Rosen, L., and Kapikian, A. Z.: Epstein-Barr virus infections in a nursery. Am. J. Epidemiol. *113*:22–29, 1981.
73. Chang, R. S., and Seto, D. S.: Perinatal infection by Epstein-Barr virus. Lancet *2*:201, 1979.
74. Chen, J. S., Lin, K. H., Lin, D. T., et al.: Longitudinal observation and outcome of nonfamilial childhood haemophagocytic syndrome receiving etoposide-containing regimens. Br. J. Haematol. *103*:756–762, 1998.
75. Chen, R. L., Lin, K. H., Lin, D. T., et al.: Immunomodulation treatment for childhood virus-associated haemophagocytic lymphohistiocytosis. Br. J. Haematol. *89*:282–290, 1995.
76. Chin, T. D.: Diagnosis of infectious mononucleosis. South. Med. J. *69*:654–658, 1976.
77. Chodosh, J., Holder, V. P., Gan, Y. J., et al.: Eradication of latent Epstein-Barr virus by hydroxyurea alters the growth-transformed cell phenotype. J. Infect. Dis. *177*:1194–1201, 1998.
78. Chulay, J. D., and Lankerani, M. R.: Splenic abscess. Report of 10 cases and review of the literature. Am. J. Med. *61*:513–522, 1976.
79. Cinbis, M., and Aysun, S.: Alice in Wonderland syndrome as an initial manifestation of Epstein-Barr virus infection. Br. J. Ophthalmol. *76*:316, 1992.
80. Cinque, P., Brytting, M., Vago, L., et al.: Epstein-Barr virus DNA in cerebrospinal fluid from patients with AIDS-related primary lymphoma of the central nervous system. Lancet *342*:398–401, 1993.
81. Cleary, T. G., Henle, W., and Pickering, L. K.: Acute cerebellar ataxia associated with Epstein-Barr virus infection. J. A. M. A. *243*:148–149, 1980.
82. Cloney, D. L., Kugler, J. A., Donowitz, L. G., et al.: Infectious mononucleosis with pleural effusion. South. Med. J. *81*:1441–1442, 1988.
83. Cohen, J. I.: Epstein-Barr virus infection. N. Engl. J. Med. *343*:481–492, 2000.
84. Colby, B. M., Shaw, J. E., Elion, G. B., et al.: Effect of acyclovir [9-(2-hydroxyethoxymethyl)guanine] on Epstein-Barr virus DNA replication. J. Virol. *34*:560–568, 1980.
85. Connelly, K. P., and DeWitt, L. D.: Neurologic complications of infectious mononucleosis. Pediatr. Neurol. *10*:181–184, 1994.
86. Copperman, S. M.: "Alice in Wonderland" syndrome as a presenting symptom of infectious mononucleosis in children: A description of three affected young people. Clin. Pediatr. (Phila.) *16*:143–146, 1977.
87. Craig, F. E., Gulley, M. L., and Banks, P. M.: Posttransplantation lymphoproliferative disorders. Am. J. Clin. Pathol. *99*:265–276, 1993.
88. Croce, C. M., Tsujimoto, Y., Erikson, J., et al.: Chromosome translocations and B cell neoplasia. Lab. Invest. *51*:258–267, 1984.
89. Custer, R. P., and Smith, E. B.: The pathology of infectious mononucleosis. Blood *3*:830–857, 1948.
90. Dalla-Favera, R., Bregni, M., Erikson, J., et al.: Human c-myc onc gene is located on the region of chromosome 8 that is translocated in Burkitt lymphoma cells. Proc. Natl. Acad. Sci. U. S. A. *79*:7824–7827, 1982.
91. d'Arminio Monforte, A., Cinque, P., Vago, L., et al.: A comparison of brain biopsy and CSF-PCR in the diagnosis of CNS lesions in AIDS patients. J. Neurol. *244*:35–39, 1997.
92. Datta, A. K., Hood, R. E.: Mechanism of inhibition of Epstein-Barr virus replication by phosphonoformic acid. Virology *114*:52–59, 1981.
93. Davis, C. L., Wood, B. L., Sabath, D. E., et al.: Interferon-alpha treatment of posttransplant lymphoproliferative disorder in recipients of solid organ transplants. Transplantation *66*:1770–1779, 1998.
94. Delecluse, H. J., and Hammerschmidt, W.: The genetic approach to the Epstein-Barr virus: From basic virology to gene therapy. Mol. Pathol. *53*:270–279, 2000.
95. Delecluse, H. J., Kremmer, E., Rouault, J. P., et al.: The expression of Epstein-Barr virus latent proteins is related to the pathological features of post-transplant lymphoproliferative disorders. Am. J. Pathol. *146*:1113–1120, 1995.
96. de-The, G.: Is Burkitt's lymphoma related to perinatal infection by Epstein-Barr virus? Lancet *1*:335–338, 1977.
97. de-The, G., Geser, A., Day, N. E., et al.: Epidemiological evidence for causal relationship between Epstein-Barr virus and Burkitt's lymphoma from Ugandan prospective study. Nature *274*:756–761, 1978.
98. Deutsch, J., Wolf, H., Becker, H., et al.: Demonstration of Epstein-Barr virus DNA in a previously healthy boy with fulminant hepatic failure. Eur. J. Pediatr. *145*:94–98, 1986.
99. Deutsch, M., Mercado, R., Jr., and Parsons, J. A.: Cancer of the nasopharynx in children. Cancer *41*:1128–1133, 1978.
100. Diaz-Mitoma, F., Preiksaitis, J. K., Leung, W. C., et al.: DNA-DNA dot hybridization to detect Epstein-Barr virus in throat washings. J. Infect. Dis. *155*:297–303, 1987.
101. Domachowske, J. B., Cunningham, C. K., Cummings, D. L., et al.: Acute manifestations and neurologic sequelae of Epstein-Barr virus encephalitis in children. Pediatr. Infect. Dis. J. *15*:871–875, 1996.
102. Dommerby, H., Stangerup, S. E., Stangerup, M., et al.: Hepatosplenomegaly in infectious mononucleosis, assessed by ultrasonic scanning. J. Laryngol. Otol. *100*:573–579, 1986.
103. Downey, H., and McKinlay, C. A.: Acute lymphadenosis compared with acute lymphatic leukemia. Arch. Intern. Med. *32*:82–112, 1923.
104. Dunnet, W. N.: Infectious mononucleosis. B. M. J. *1*:1187–1191, 1963.
105. Dussaix, E., Le Touze, P., and Tardieu, M.: Neuropathy of the brachial plexus complicating infectious mononucleosis in an 18-month-old child. Arch. Fr. Pediatr. *43*:129–130, 1986.
106. Eaton, O. M., Little, P. F., and Silver, H. M.: Infectious mononucleosis with pleural effusion: Review of the literature. Arch. Intern. Med. *115*:87–89, 1965.
107. Epstein, M. A., and Achong, B. G.: Specific immunofluorescence test for the herpes-type EB virus of Burkitt lymphoblasts, authenticated by electron microscopy. J. Natl. Cancer. Inst. *40*:593–607, 1968.
108. Epstein, M. A., and Achong, B. G.: Morphology of the virus and of virus-induced cytopathologic changes. *In* Epstein, M. A., and Achong, B. G. (eds.): The Epstein-Barr Virus. New York, Springer-Verlag, 1979, pp. 23–37.
109. Epstein, M. A., Morgan, A. J., Finerty, S., et al.: Protection of cottontop tamarins against Epstein-Barr virus–induced malignant lymphoma by a prototype subunit vaccine. Nature *318*:287–289, 1985.
110. Epstein, M. S., Achong, B. G., and Barr, Y. M.: Virus particles in cultured lymphoblasts from Burkitt's lymphoma. Lancet *1*:702–703, 1964.
111. Erzurum, S., Kalavsky, S. M., and Watanakunakorn, C.: Acute cerebellar ataxia and hearing loss as initial symptoms of infectious mononucleosis. Arch. Neurol. *40*:760–762, 1983.
112. Eshel, G. M., Evov, A., Lahat, E., et al.: Alice in Wonderland syndrome, a manifestation of acute Epstein-Barr virus infection. Pediatr. Infect. Dis. J. *6*:68, 1987.
113. Evans, A. S.: Experimental attempts to transmit infectious mononucleosis to man. Yale J. Biol. Med. *20*:19–26, 1947.
114. Evans, A. S.: Further experimental attempts to transmit infectious mononucleosis to man. J. Clin. Invest. *29*:508–512, 1950.
115. Evans, A. S.: Infectious mononucleosis in University of Wisconsin students: Report of a five-year investigation. Am. J. Hyg. *71*:342–362, 1960.
116. Evans, A. S.: The history of infectious mononucleosis. Am. J. Med. Sci. *267*:189–195, 1974.
117. Evans, A. S., Niederman, J. C., and McCollum, R. W.: Seroepidemiologic studies of infectious mononucleosis with EB virus. N. Engl. J. Med. *279*:1121–1127, 1968.
118. Fahraeus, R., Fu, H. L., Ernberg, I., et al.: Expression of Epstein-Barr virus–encoded proteins in nasopharyngeal carcinoma. Int. J. Cancer *42*:329–338, 1988.
119. Fandi, A., Altun, M., Azli, N., et al.: Nasopharyngeal cancer: Epidemiology, staging, and treatment. Semin. Oncol. *21*:382–397, 1994.
120. Farber, I., Hinderer, W., Rothe, M., et al.: Serological diagnosis of Epstein-Barr virus infection by novel ELISAs based on recombinant capsid antigens p23 and p18. J. Med. Virol. *63*:271–276, 2001.
121. Farley, D. R., Zietlow, S. P., Bannon, M. P., et al.: Spontaneous rupture of the spleen due to infectious mononucleosis. Mayo Clin. Proc. *67*:846–853, 1992.
122. Farrell, P. J.: Epstein-Barr virus immortalizing genes. Trends Microbiol. *3*:105–109, 1995.
123. Feorino, P. M., Humphrey, D., Hochberg, F., et al.: Mononucleosis-associated subacute sclerosing panencephalitis. Lancet *2*:530–532, 1975.
124. Ferbas, J., Rahman, M. A., Kingsley, L. A., et al.: Frequent oropharyngeal shedding of Epstein-Barr virus in homosexual men during early HIV infection. A. I. D. S. *6*:1273–1278, 1992.
125. Fermaglich, D. R.: Pulmonary involvement in infectious mononucleosis. J. Pediatr. *86*:93–95, 1975.
126. Finch, S. C.: Clinical symptoms and signs of infectious mononucleosis. *In* Carter, R. L., and Penman, H. G. (eds.): Infectious Mononucleosis. Oxford, Blackwell, 1969, pp. 19–46.
127. Fingeroth, J. D., Weis, J. J., Tedder, T. F., et al.: Epstein-Barr virus receptor of human B lymphocytes is the C3d receptor CR2. Proc. Natl. Acad. Sci. U. S. A. *81*:4510–4514, 1984.
128. Fisman, D. N.: Hemophagocytic syndromes and infection. Emerg. Infect. Dis. *6*:601–608, 2000.
129. Flavell, K. J., and Murray, P. G.: Hodgkin's disease and the Epstein-Barr virus. Mol. Pathol. *53*:262–269, 2000.
130. Fleisher, G., and Bologonese, R.: Infectious mononucleosis during gestation: Report of three women and their infants studied prospectively. Pediatr. Infect. Dis. *3*:308–311, 1984.

131. Fleisher, G., and Bologonese, R.: Epstein-Barr virus infections in pregnancy: A prospective study. J. Pediatr. *104*:374–379, 1984.
132. Fleisher, G., Henle, W., Henle, G., et al.: Primary infection with Epstein-Barr virus in infants in the United States: Clinical and serologic observations. J. Infect. Dis. *139*:553–558, 1979.
133. Fleisher, G. R., Pasquariello, P. S., Warren, W. S., et al.: Intrafamilial transmission of Epstein-Barr virus infections. J. Pediatr. *98*:16–19, 1981.
134. Fletcher, M. A., Lo, T. M., Levey, B. A., et al.: Immunochemical studies of infectious mononucleosis. VI. A radioimmunoassay for the detection of infectious mononucleosis heterophile antibody and antigen. J. Immunol. Methods *14*:51–58, 1977.
135. Forsyth, P. A., Yahalom, J., and DeAngelis, L. M.: Combined-modality therapy in the treatment of primary central nervous system lymphoma in AIDS. Neurology *44*:1473–1479, 1994.
136. Frey, T.: Optic neuritis in children: Infectious mononucleosis as an etiology. Doc. Ophthalmol. *34*:183–188, 1973.
137. Friedman, B. I., and Libby, R.: Epstein-Barr virus infection associated with rhabdomyolysis and acute renal failure. Clin. Pediatr. (Phila.) *25*:228–229, 1986.
138. Frishman, W., Kraus, M. E., Zabkar, J., et al.: Infectious mononucleosis and fatal myocarditis. Chest *72*:535–538, 1977.
139. Fu, S. M., and Hurley, J. N.: Human cell lines containing Epstein-Barr virus but distinct from the common B cell lymphoblastoid lines. Proc. Natl. Acad. Sci. U. S. A. *76*:6637–6640, 1979.
140. Fu, S. M., Hurley, J. N., McCune, J. M., et al.: Pre-B cells and other possible precursor lymphoid cell lines derived from patients with X-linked agammaglobulinemia. J. Exp. Med. *152*:1519–1526, 1980.
141. Fuhrman, S. A., Gill, R., Horwitz, C. A., et al.: Marked hyperbilirubinemia in infectious mononucleosis. Analysis of laboratory data in seven patients. Arch. Intern. Med. *147*:850–853, 1987.
142. Fujisaki, T., Nagafuchi, S., and Okamura, T.: Gamma-interferon for severe chronic active Epstein-Barr virus. Ann. Intern. Med. *118*:474–475, 1993.
143. Gan, Y. J., Shirley, P., Zeng, Y., et al.: Human oropharyngeal lesions with a defective Epstein-Barr virus that disrupts viral latency. J. Infect. Dis. *168*:1349–1355, 1993.
144. Ganzel, T. M., Goldman, J. L., and Padhya, T. A.: Otolaryngologic clinical patterns in pediatric infectious mononucleosis. Am. J. Otolaryngol. *17*:397–400, 1996.
145. Gelati, G., Verucchi, G., Chiodo, F., et al.: Hemolytic anemia as a complication of Epstein-Barr virus infection: A report of two cases. J. Exp. Pathol. *3*:485–489, 1987.
146. Gerber, P., and Birch, S. M.: Complement-fixing antibodies in sera of human and nonhuman primates to viral antigens derived from Burkitt's lymphoma cells. Proc. Natl. Acad. Sci. U. S. A. *58*:478–484, 1967.
147. Gerber, P., Lucas, S., Nonoyama, M., et al.: Oral excretion of Epstein-Barr virus by healthy subjects and patients with infectious mononucleosis. Lancet *2*:988–989, 1972.
148. Gerber, P., Walsh, J. H., Rosenblum, E. N., et al.: Association of EB-virus infection with the post-perfusion syndrome. Lancet *1*:593–595, 1969.
149. Gilboa, N., Wong, W., Largent, J. A., et al.: Association of infectious mononucleosis with nephrotic syndrome. Arch. Pathol. Lab. Med. *105*:259–262, 1981.
150. Gohlich-Ratmann, G., Wallot, M., Baethmann, M., et al.: Acute cerebellitis with near-fatal cerebellar swelling and benign outcome under conservative treatment with high dose steroids. Eur. J. Paediatr. Neurol. *2*:157–162, 1998.
151. Goldberg, G. N., Fulginiti, V. A., Ray, C. G., et al.: In utero Epstein-Barr virus (infectious mononucleosis) infection. J. A. M. A. *246*:1579–1581, 1981.
152. Golden, H. D., Chang, R. S., Prescott, W., et al.: Leukocyte-transforming agent: Prolonged excretion by patients with mononucleosis and excretion by normal individuals. J. Infect. Dis. *127*:471–473, 1973.
153. Gowing, N. F.: Infectious mononucleosis: Histopathologic aspects. Pathol. Annu. *10*:1–20, 1975.
154. Greenspan, D., Greenspan, J. S., Conant, M., et al.: Oral "hairy" leucoplakia in male homosexuals: Evidence of association with both papillomavirus and a herpes-group virus. Lancet *2*:831–834, 1984.
155. Greenspan, J. S., Greenspan, D., Lennette, E. T., et al.: Replication of Epstein-Barr virus within the epithelial cells of oral "hairy" leukoplakia, an AIDS-associated lesion. N. Engl. J. Med. *313*:1564–1571, 1985.
156. Gregory, C. D., Rowe, M., and Rickinson, A. B.: Different Epstein-Barr virus–B cell interactions in phenotypically distinct clones of a Burkitt's lymphoma cell line. J. Gen. Virol. *71*:1481–1495, 1990.
157. Grierson, H., and Purtilo, D. T.: Epstein-Barr virus infections in males with the X-linked lymphoproliferative syndrome. Ann. Intern. Med. *106*:538–545, 1987.
158. Grishaber, J. E., McClain, K. L., Mahoney, D. H., Jr., et al.: Successful outcome of severe aplastic anemia following Epstein-Barr virus infection. Am. J. Hematol. *28*:273–275, 1988.
159. Grose, C., and Feorino, P. M.: Epstein-Barr virus and Guillain-Barré syndrome. Lancet *2*:1285–1287, 1972.
160. Grose, C., Henle, W., Henle, G., et al.: Primary Epstein-Barr-virus infections in acute neurologic diseases. N. Engl. J. Med. *292*:392–395, 1975.
161. Gross, T. G., Filipovich, A. H., Conley, M. E., et al.: Cure of X-linked lymphoproliferative disease (XLP) with allogeneic hematopoietic stem cell transplantation (HSCT): Report from the XLP registry. Bone Marrow Transplant. *17*:741–744, 1996.
162. Gross, T. G., Hinrichs, S. H., Winner, J., et al.: Treatment of post-transplant lymphoproliferative disease (PTLD) following solid organ transplantation with low-dose chemotherapy. Ann. Oncol. *9*:339–340, 1998.
163. Gu, S. Y., Huang, T. M., Ruan, L., et al.: First EBV vaccine trial in humans using recombinant vaccinia virus expressing the major membrane antigen. Dev. Biol. Stand. *84*:171–177, 1995.
164. Gulley, M. L.: Molecular diagnosis of Epstein-Barr virus–related diseases. J. Mol. Diagn. *3*:1–10, 2001.
165. Gulley, M. L., Eagan, P. A., Quintanilla-Martinez, L., et al.: Epstein-Barr virus DNA is abundant and monoclonal in the Reed-Sternberg cells of Hodgkin's disease: Association with mixed cellularity subtype and Hispanic American ethnicity. Blood *83*:1595–1602, 1994.
166. Gulley, M. L., Raphael, M., Lutz, C. T., et al.: Epstein-Barr virus integration in human lymphomas and lymphoid cell lines. Cancer *70*:185–191, 1992.
167. Gutensohn, N., and Cole, P.: Epidemiology of Hodgkin's disease in the young. Int. J. Cancer *19*:595–604, 1977.
168. Gutgesell, H. P.: Acute airway obstruction in infectious mononucleosis. Pediatrics *47*:141–143, 1971.
169. Gutierrez, M. I., Bhatia, K., and Magrath, I.: Replicative viral DNA in Epstein-Barr virus associated Burkitt's lymphoma biopsies. Leuk. Res. *17*:285–289, 1993.
170. Haider, S., Coutinho, M., Emond, R. T., et al.: Tuberculin anergy and infectious mononucleosis. Lancet *2*:74, 1973.
171. Halbert, S. P., Anken, M., Henle, W., et al.: Detection of infectious mononucleosis heterophil antibody by a rapid, standardized enzyme-linked immunosorbent assay procedure. J. Clin. Microbiol. *15*:610–616, 1982.
172. Halcrow, J. P., Owen, L. M., and Rodger, N. O.: Infectious mononucleosis, with an account of an epidemic in an E.M.S. hospital. B. M. J. *2*:443–447, 1943.
173. Hall, A. J.: A case resembling acute lymphocytic leukemia ending in complete recovery. Proc. R. Soc. Med. *8*:15–19, 1915.
174. Haller, A., von Segesser, L., Baumann, P. C., et al.: Severe respiratory insufficiency complicating Epstein-Barr virus infection: Case report and review. Clin. Infect. Dis. *21*:206–209, 1995.
175. Halsted, C. C., and Chang, R. S.: Infectious mononucleosis and encephalitis: Recovery of EB virus from spinal fluid. Pediatrics *64*:257–258, 1979.
176. Hammarskjold, M. L., and Simurda, M. C.: Epstein-Barr virus latent membrane protein transactivates the human immunodeficiency virus type 1 long terminal repeat through induction of NF-kappa B activity. J. Virol. *66*:6496–6501, 1992.
177. Handler, S. D., and Warren, W. S.: Peritonsillar abscess: A complication of corticosteroid treatment in infectious mononucleosis. Int. J. Pediatr. Otorhinolaryngol. *1*:265–268, 1979.
178. Hanto, D. W., Gajl-Peczalska, K. J., Frizzera, G., et al.: Epstein-Barr virus (EBV) induced polyclonal and monoclonal B-cell lymphoproliferative diseases occurring after renal transplantation. Clinical, pathologic, and virologic findings and implications for therapy. Ann. Surg. *198*:356–369, 1983.
179. Harris, N. L., Jaffe, E. S., Stein, H., et al.: A revised European-American classification of lymphoid neoplasms: A proposal from the International Lymphoma Study Group. Blood *84*:1361–1392, 1994.
180. Hasegawa, D., Sano, K., Kosaka, Y., et al.: A case of hemophagocytic lymphohistiocytosis with prolonged remission after syngeneic bone marrow transplantation. Bone Marrow Transplant. *24*:425–427, 1999.
181. Hayashi, R. J., Kraus, M. D., Patel, A. L., et al.: Posttransplant lymphoproliferative disease in children: Correlation of histology to clinical behavior. J. Pediatr. Hematol. Oncol. *23*:14–18, 2001.
182. Heath, C. W., Jr., Brodsky, A. L., and Potolsky, A. I.: Infectious mononucleosis in a general population. Am. J. Epidemiol. *95*:46–52, 1972.
183. Hedstrom, S. A., and Belfrage, I.: Acute pancreatitis in two cases of infectious mononucleosis. Scand. J. Infect. Dis. *8*:124–126, 1976.
184. Henke, C. E., Kurland, L. T., and Elveback, L. R.: Infectious mononucleosis in Rochester, Minnesota, 1950 through 1969. Am. J. Epidemiol. *98*:483–490, 1973.
185. Henle, G., and Henle, W.: Immunofluorescence in cells derived from Burkitt's lymphoma. J. Bacteriol. *91*:1248–1256, 1966.
186. Henle, G., Henle, W., Clifford, P., et al.: Antibodies to Epstein-Barr virus in Burkitt's lymphoma and control groups. J. Natl. Cancer Inst. *43*:1147–1157, 1969.
187. Henle, G., Henle, W., and Diehl, V.: Relation of Burkitt's tumor–associated herpes-type virus to infectious mononucleosis. Proc. Natl. Acad. Sci. U. S. A. *59*:94–101, 1968.
188. Henle, W., Diehl, V., Kohn, G., et al.: Herpes-type virus and chromosome marker in normal leukocytes after growth with irradiated Burkitt cells. Science *157*:1064–1065, 1967.
189. Henle, W., and Henle, G.: Evidence for an oncogenic potential of the Epstein-Barr virus. Cancer Res. *33*:1419–1423, 1973.

190. Henle, W., and Henle, G.: Epidemiologic aspects of Epstein-Barr virus (EBV)-associated diseases. Ann. N. Y. Acad. Sci. *354*:326–331, 1980.
191. Henle, W., and Henle, G.: Epstein-Barr virus–specific serology in immunologically compromised individuals. Cancer Res. *41*:4222–4225, 1981.
192. Henle, W., and Henle, G.: Immunology of Epstein-Barr virus. *In* Roizman, B. (ed.): The Herpesviruses. New York, Plenum, 1982, pp. 209–252.
193. Henle, W., and Henle, G.: Epstein-Barr virus and blood transfusions. Prog. Clin. Biol. Res. *182*:201–209, 1985.
194. Henle, W., Henle, G., Scriba, M., et al.: Antibody responses to the Epstein-Barr virus and cytomegaloviruses after open-heart and other surgery. N. Engl. J. Med. *282*:1068–1074, 1970.
195. Herbst, H., Stein, H., and Niedobitek, G.: Epstein-Barr virus and CD30[+] malignant lymphomas. Crit. Rev. Oncog. *4*:191–239, 1993.
196. Hinderer, W., Lang, D., Rothe, M., et al.: Serodiagnosis of Epstein-Barr virus infection by using recombinant viral capsid antigen fragments and autologous gene fusion. J. Clin. Microbiol. *37*:3239–3244, 1999.
197. Hinuma, Y., and Grace, J. T.: Cloning of immunoglobulin-producing human leukemic and lymphoma cells in long-term cultures. Exp. Biol. Med. *124*:107–111, 1967.
198. HIV/AIDS surveillance report. *9*:1–44, 1997.
199. Ho, H. C., Ng, M. H., Kwan, H. C., et al.: Epstein-Barr-virus–specific IgA and IgG serum antibodies in nasopharyngeal carcinoma. Br. J. Cancer *34*:655–660, 1976.
200. Ho, M., Jaffe, R., Miller, G., et al.: The frequency of Epstein-Barr virus infection and associated lymphoproliferative syndrome after transplantation and its manifestations in children. Transplantation *45*:719–727, 1988.
201. Ho, M., Miller, G., Atchison, R. W., et al.: Epstein-Barr virus infections and DNA hybridization studies in posttransplantation lymphoma and lymphoproliferative lesions: The role of primary infection. J. Infect. Dis. *152*:876–886, 1985.
202. Hoagland, R. J.: The transmission of infectious mononucleosis. Am. J. Med. Sci. *229*:262–272, 1955.
203. Hoagland, R. J.: The clinical manifestations of infectious mononucleosis: A report of two hundred cases. Am. J. Med. Sci. *240*:21–29, 1960.
204. Hoagland, R. J.: Mononucleosis and heart disease. Am. J. Med. Sci. *248*:1–6, 1964.
205. Hoagland, R. J.: Infectious Mononucleosis. New York, Grune & Stratton, 1967.
206. Hochberg, F. H., Lehrich, J. R., Richardson, E. P., Jr., et al.: Mononucleosis-associated subacute sclerosing panencephalitis. Acta Neuropathol. *34*:33–40, 1976.
207. Hofmann, B., Schuppe, H. C., Adams, O., et al.: Gianotti-Crosti syndrome associated with Epstein-Barr virus infection. Pediatr. Dermatol. *14*:273–277, 1997.
208. Horwitz, C. A., Henle, W., Henle, G., et al.: Heterophil-negative infectious mononucleosis and mononucleosis-like illnesses. Laboratory confirmation of 43 cases. Am. J. Med. *63*:947–957, 1977.
209. Hoshino, Y., Kimura, H., Kuzushima, K., et al.: Early intervention in post-transplant lymphoproliferative disorders based on Epstein-Barr viral load. Bone Marrow Transplant. *26*:199–201, 2000.
210. Hsu, D. H., de Waal Malefyt, R., Fiorentino, D. F., et al.: Expression of interleukin-10 activity by Epstein-Barr virus protein BCRF1. Science *250*:830–832, 1990.
211. Huang, D. P., Lo, K. W., Choi, P. H., et al.: Loss of heterozygosity on the short arm of chromosome 3 in nasopharyngeal carcinoma. Cancer Genet. Cytogenet. *54*:91–99, 1991.
212. Huang, D. P., Lo, K. W., van Hasselt, C. A., et al.: A region of homozygous deletion on chromosome 9p21–22 in primary nasopharyngeal carcinoma. Cancer Res. *54*:4003–4006, 1994.
213. Hudson, M. M., and Donaldson, S. S.: Hodgkin's disease. Pediatr. Clin. North Am. *44*:891–906, 1997.
214. Hudson, M. M., and Donaldson, S. S.: Treatment of pediatric Hodgkin's lymphoma. Semin. Hematol. *36*:313–323, 1999.
215. Hummel, M., Anagnostopoulos, I., Korbjuhn, P., et al.: Epstein-Barr virus in B-cell non-Hodgkin's lymphomas: Unexpected infection patterns and different infection incidence in low- and high-grade types. J. Pathol. *175*:263–271, 1995.
216. Icart, J., Didier, J., Dalens, M., et al.: Prospective study of Epstein Barr virus (EBV) infection during pregnancy. Biomedicine *34*:160–163, 1981.
217. Imai, S., Usui, N., Sugiura, M., et al.: Epstein-Barr virus genomic sequences and specific antibodies in cerebrospinal fluid in children with neurologic complications of acute and reactivated EBV infections. J. Med. Virol. *40*:278–284, 1993.
218. Imashuku, S., Hibi, S., Ohara, T., et al.: Effective control of Epstein-Barr virus–related hemophagocytic lymphohistiocytosis with immunochemotherapy. Blood *93*:1869–1874, 1999.
219. Ingersoll, L., Woo, S. Y., Donaldson, S., et al.: Nasopharyngeal carcinoma in the young: A combined M.D. Anderson and Stanford experience. Int. J. Radiat. Oncol. Biol. Phys. *19*:881–887, 1990.
220. Ireland, R. A., Baetjer, W. A., Ruhrah, J.: A case of lymphatic leukemia with apparent cure. J. A. M. A. *65*:948–949, 1915.
221. Ishida, Y., Yokota, Y., Tauchi, H., et al.: Ganciclovir for chronic active Epstein-Barr virus infection. Lancet *341*:560–561, 1993.
222. Itin, P. H., Bircher, A. J., Litzisdorf, Y., et al.: Oral hairy leukoplakia in a child: Confirmation of the clinical diagnosis by ultrastructural examination of exfoliative cytologic specimens. Dermatology *189*:167–169, 1994.
223. Jackman, W. T., Mann, K. A., Hoffmann, H. J., et al.: Expression of Epstein-Barr virus gp350 as a single chain glycoprotein for an EBV subunit vaccine. Vaccine *17*:660–668, 1999.
224. Jain, S., and Sherlock, S.: Infectious mononucleosis with jaundice, anaemia, and encephalopathy. B. M. J. *3*:138–139, 1975.
225. Janka, G., Imashuku, S., Elinder, G., et al.: Infection- and malignancy-associated hemophagocytic syndromes. Secondary hemophagocytic lymphohistiocytosis. Hematol. Oncol. Clin. North Am. *12*:435–444, 1998.
226. Jenson, H. B.: Acute complications of Epstein-Barr virus infectious mononucleosis. Curr. Opin. Pediatr. *12*:263–268, 2000.
227. Jenson, H. B., Ench, Y., and Sumaya, C. V.: Epstein-Barr virus. *In* Rose, N. R., de Macario, E. C., Folds, J. D., et al. (eds.): Manual of Clinical Laboratory Immunology. 5th ed. Washington, D.C., American Society for Microbiology, 1997, pp. 634–643.
228. Jenson, H. B., Leach, C. T., McClain, K. L., et al.: Benign and malignant smooth muscle tumors containing Epstein-Barr virus in children with AIDS. Leuk. Lymphoma *27*:303–314, 1997.
229. Jenson, H. B., McIntosh, K., Pitt, J., et al.: Natural history of primary Epstein-Barr virus infection in children of mothers infected with human immunodeficiency virus type 1. J. Infect. Dis. *179*:1395–1404, 1999.
230. Johansson, B., Klein, G., Henle, W., et al.: Epstein-Barr virus (EBV)-associated antibody patterns in malignant lymphoma and leukemia. I. Hodgkin's disease. Int. J. Cancer *6*:450–462, 1970.
231. Johnsen, T., Katholm, M., and Stangerup, S. E.: Otolaryngological complications in infectious mononucleosis. J. Laryngol. Otol. *98*:999–1001, 1984.
232. Joncas, J., Chiasson, J. P., Turcotte, J., et al.: Studies on infectious mononucleosis. III. Clinical data, serologic and epidemiologic findings. C. M. A. J. *98*:848–854, 1968.
233. Joncas, J. H., Alfieri, C., Leyritz-Wills, M., et al.: Simultaneous congenital infection with Epstein-Barr virus and cytomegalovirus. N. Engl. J. Med. *304*:1399–1403, 1981.
234. Joncas, J. H., Chicoine, L., Thivierge, F., et al.: Epstein-Barr virus antibodies in the cerebrospinal fluid. A case of infectious mononucleosis with encephalitis. Am. J. Dis. Child. *127*:282–285, 1974.
235. Jondal, M., and Klein, G.: Surface markers on human B and T lymphocytes. II. Presence of Epstein-Barr virus receptors on B lymphocytes. J. Exp. Med. *138*:1365–1378, 1973.
236. Jones, J. F., Ray, C. G., Minnich, L. L., et al.: Evidence for active Epstein-Barr virus infection in patients with persistent, unexplained illnesses: Elevated anti–early antigen antibodies. Ann. Intern. Med. *102*:1–7, 1985.
237. Jones, J. F., Shurin, S., Abramowsky, C., et al.: T-cell lymphomas containing Epstein-Barr viral DNA in patients with chronic Epstein-Barr virus infections. N. Engl. J. Med. *318*:733–741, 1988.
238. Joshi, V. V., Oleske, J. M., Minnefor, A. B., et al.: Pathologic pulmonary findings in children with the acquired immunodeficiency syndrome: A study of ten cases. Hum. Pathol. *16*:241–246, 1985.
239. Kanda, T., Otter, M., and Wahl, G. M.: Coupling of mitotic chromosome tethering and replication competence in Epstein-Barr virus–based plasmids. Mol. Cell. Biol. *21*:3576–3588, 2001.
240. Kaplan, L. D., Straus, D. J., Testa, M. A., et al.: Low-dose compared with standard-dose m-BACOD chemotherapy for non-Hodgkin's lymphoma associated with human immunodeficiency virus infection. N. Engl. J. Med. *336*:1641–1648, 1997.
241. Katamine, S., Otsu, M., Tada, K., et al.: Epstein-Barr virus transforms precursor B cells even before immunoglobulin gene rearrangements. Nature *309*:369–372, 1984.
242. Katz, B. Z., Berkman, A. B., and Shapiro, E. D.: Serologic evidence of active Epstein-Barr virus infection in Epstein-Barr virus–associated lymphoproliferative disorders of children with acquired immunodeficiency syndrome. J. Pediatr. *120*:228–232, 1992.
243. Kawa-Ha, K., Franco, E., Doi, S., et al.: Successful treatment of chronic active Epstein-Barr virus infection with recombinant interleukin-2. Lancet *1*:154, 1987.
244. Kennard, C., and Swash, M.: Acute viral encephalitis: Its diagnosis and outcome. Brain *104*:129–148, 1981.
245. Khanna, R., Moss, D. J., and Burrows, S. R.: Vaccine strategies against Epstein-Barr virus–associated diseases: Lessons from studies on cytotoxic T-cell–mediated immune regulation. Immunol. Rev. *170*:49–64, 1999.
246. Khoo, V. S., and Liew, K. H.: Acquired immunodeficiency syndrome–related primary cerebral lymphoma. Clin. Oncol. (R. Coll. Radiol.) *11*:6–14, 1999.
247. Klein, E., Ernberg, I., Masucci, M. G., et al.: T-cell response to B-cells and Epstein-Barr virus antigens in infectious mononucleosis. Cancer Res. *41*:4210–4215, 1981.
248. Klein, E., Masucci, M. G., Berthold, W., et al.: Lymphocyte-mediated cytotoxicity toward virus-induced tumor cells; natural and activated killer lymphocytes in man. *In* Essex, M., Todaro, G., and zur Hausen, H. (eds.): Viruses in Naturally Occurring Cancers. Cold Spring Harbor Conferences on Cell Proliferation. Cold Spring Harbor, NY, Cold Spring Harbor Laboratory, 1980, pp. 1187–1197.

249. Klein, G.: Lymphoma development in mice and humans: Diversity of initiation is followed by convergent cytogenetic evolution. Proc. Natl. Acad. Sci. U. S. A. *76*:2442–2446, 1979.
250. Klein, G.: The role of gene dosage and genetic transpositions in carcinogenesis. Nature *294*:313–318, 1981.
251. Kolski, H., Ford-Jones, E. L., Richardson, S., et al.: Etiology of acute childhood encephalitis at The Hospital for Sick Children, Toronto, 1994–1995. Clin. Infect. Dis. *26*:398–409, 1998.
252. Koutras, A.: Epstein-Barr virus infection with pancreatitis, hepatitis and proctitis. Pediatr. Infect. Dis. *2*:312–313, 1983.
253. Kurland, G., and Orenstein, D. M.: Complications of pediatric lung and heart-lung transplantation. Curr. Opin. Pediatr. *6*:262–271, 1994.
254. Kuzushima, K., Yamamoto, M., Kimura, H., et al.: Establishment of anti–Epstein-Barr virus (EBV) cellular immunity by adoptive transfer of virus-specific cytotoxic T lymphocytes from an HLA-matched sibling to a patient with severe chronic active EBV infection. Clin. Exp. Immunol. *103*:192–198, 1996.
255. Labrecque, L. G., Lampert, I., Kazembe, P., et al.: Correlation between cytopathological results and in situ hybridisation on needle aspiration biopsies of suspected African Burkitt's lymphomas. Int. J. Cancer *59*:591–596, 1994.
256. Labrecque, L. G., Xue, S. A., Kazembe, P., et al.: Expression of Epstein-Barr virus lytically related genes in African Burkitt's lymphoma: Correlation with patient response to therapy. Int. J. Cancer *81*:6–11, 1999.
257. Lahat, E., Berkovitch, M., Barr, J., et al.: Abnormal visual evoked potentials in children with "Alice in Wonderland" syndrome due to infectious mononucleosis. J. Child Neurol. *14*:732–735, 1999.
258. Lahat, E., Eshel, G., and Arlazoroff, A.: "Alice in Wonderland" syndrome and infectious mononucleosis in children. J. Neurol. Neurosurg. Psychiatry *53*:1104, 1990.
259. Landau, Z., Gross, R., Sanilevich, A., et al.: Presence of infective Epstein-Barr virus in the urine of patients with infectious mononucleosis. J. Med. Virol. *44*:229–233, 1994.
260. Lander, P., and Palayew, M. J.: Infectious mononucleosis—a review of chest roentgenographic manifestations. J. Can. Assoc. Radiol. *25*:303–306, 1974.
261. Laporte, J. P., Lesage, S., Woler, M., et al.: Administration of three cytokines instead of bone marrow transplantation in an HIV+ patient with high-grade lymphoma. Eur. J. Haematol. *53*:123–125, 1994.
262. Lazarus, K. H., Baehner, R. L.: Aplastic anemia complicating infectious mononucleosis: A case report and review of the literature. Pediatrics *67*:907–910, 1981.
263. Le, C. T., Chang, R. S., and Lipson, M. H.: Epstein-Barr virus infections during pregnancy. A prospective study and review of the literature. Am. J. Dis. Child. *137*:466–468, 1983.
264. Leach, C. T., Frantz, C., Head, D. R., et al.: Human herpesvirus-8 (HHV-8) associated with small non-cleaved cell lymphoma in a child with AIDS. Am. J. Hematol. *60*:215–221, 1999.
265. Leder, P., Battey, J., Lenoir, G., et al.: Translocations among antibody genes in human cancer. Science *222*:765–771, 1983.
266. Lee, E. S., Locker, J., Nalesnik, M., et al.: The association of Epstein-Barr virus with smooth-muscle tumors occurring after organ transplantation. N. Engl. J. Med. *332*:19–25, 1995.
267. Lee, S., and Kjellstrand, C. M.: Renal disease in infectious mononucleosis. Clin. Nephrol. *9*:236–240, 1978.
268. Lei, K. I., Chan, L. Y., Chan, W. Y., et al.: Quantitative analysis of circulating cell-free Epstein-Barr virus (EBV) DNA levels in patients with EBV-associated lymphoid malignancies. Br. J. Haematol. *111*:239–246, 2000.
269. Lei, P. S., Lowichik, A., Allen, W., et al.: Acute renal failure: Unusual complication of Epstein-Barr virus–induced infectious mononucleosis. Clin. Infect. Dis. *31*:1519–1524, 2000.
270. Levey, B. A., Lo, T. M., Caldwell, K. E., et al.: Latex test for serodiagnosis of infectious mononucleosis. J. Clin. Microbiol. *11*:256–262, 1980.
271. Levine, D., Tilton, R. C., Parry, M. F., et al.: False positive EBNA IgM and IgG antibody tests for infectious mononucleosis in children. Pediatrics *94*:892–894, 1994.
272. Levine, P. H., Ablashi, D. V., Berard, C. W., et al.: Elevated antibody titers to Epstein-Barr virus in Hodgkin's disease. Cancer *27*:416–421, 1971.
273. Levitskaya, J., Sharipo, A., Leonchiks, A., et al.: Inhibition of ubiquitin/proteasome-dependent protein degradation by the Gly-Ala repeat domain of the Epstein-Barr virus nuclear antigen 1. Proc. Natl. Acad. Sci. U. S. A. *94*:12616–12621, 1997.
274. Levy, M., Kelly, J. P., Kaufman, D. W., et al.: Risk of agranulocytosis and aplastic anemia in relation to history of infectious mononucleosis: A report from the International Agranulocytosis and Aplastic Anemia Study. Ann. Hematol. *67*:187–190, 1993.
275. Leyvraz, S., Henle, W., Chahinian, A. P., et al.: Association of Epstein-Barr virus with thymic carcinoma. N. Engl. J. Med. *312*:1296–1299, 1985.
276. Li, Q., Spriggs, M. K., Kovats, S., et al.: Epstein-Barr virus uses HLA class II as a cofactor for infection of B lymphocytes. J. Virol. *71*:4657–4662, 1997.
277. Liebowitz, D.: Nasopharyngeal carcinoma: The Epstein-Barr virus association. Semin. Oncol. *21*:376–381, 1994.
278. Liebowitz, D., Anastasi, J., Hagos, F., et al.: Post-transplant lymphoproliferative disorders (PTLD): Clinicopathologic characterizations and response to immunomodulatory therapy with interferon-alpha. Ann. Oncol. 7(Suppl. 3):28, 1996.
279. Lifschitz, C., and LaSala, S.: Pancreatitis, cholecystitis, and choledocholithiasis associated with infectious mononucleosis. Clin. Pediatr. (Phila.) *20*:131, 1981.
280. Lilleyman, J. S., and Pinkerton, C. R.: Lymphoblastic leukaemia and non-Hodgkin's lymphoma. Br. Med. Bull. *52*:742–763, 1996.
281. Lin, J. C., Smith, M. C., and Pagano, J. S.: Comparative efficacy and selectivity of some nucleoside analogs against Epstein-Barr virus. Antimicrob. Agents Chemother. *27*:971–973, 1985.
282. Lindahl, T., Adams, A., Bjursell, G., et al.: Covalently closed circular duplex DNA of Epstein-Barr virus in a human lymphoid cell line. J. Mol. Biol. *102*:511–530, 1976.
283. Lipman, M., Andrews, L., Niederman, J., et al.: Direct visualization of enveloped Epstein-Barr herpesvirus in throat washing with leukocyte-transforming activity. J. Infect. Dis. *132*:520–523, 1975.
284. Little, R. F., Yarchoan, R., and Wilson, W. H.: Systemic chemotherapy for HIV-associated lymphoma in the era of highly active antiretroviral therapy. Curr. Opin. Oncol. *12*:438–444, 2000.
285. Lloyd-Still, J. D., Scott, J. P., and Crussi, F.: The spectrum of Epstein-Barr virus hepatitis in children. Pediatr. Pathol. *5*:337–351, 1986.
286. Lo, Y. M., Chan, L. Y., Chan, A. T., et al.: Quantitative and temporal correlation between circulating cell-free Epstein-Barr virus DNA and tumor recurrence in nasopharyngeal carcinoma. Cancer Res. *59*:5452–5455, 1999.
287. Lowenfels, A. B.: Kehr's sign—a neglected aid in rupture of the spleen. N. Engl. J. Med. *274*:1019, 1966.
288. Lukes, R. J., and Cox, F. H.: Clinical and morphologic findings in 30 fatal cases of infectious mononucleosis. Am. J. Pathol. *34*:586, 1958.
289. MacMahon, E. M., Glass, J. D., Hayward, S. D., et al.: Epstein-Barr virus in AIDS-related primary central nervous system lymphoma. Lancet *338*:969–973, 1991.
290. Maddern, B. R., Werkhaven, J., Wessel, H. B., et al.: Infectious mononucleosis with airway obstruction and multiple cranial nerve paresis. Otolaryngol. Head Neck Surg. *104*:529–532, 1991.
291. Madigan, N. P., Newcomer, A. D., Campbell, D. C., et al.: Intense jaundice in infectious mononucleosis. Mayo Clin. Proc. *48*:857–862, 1973.
292. Magalhaes, M. G., Bueno, D. F., Serra, E., et al.: Oral manifestations of HIV positive children. J. Clin. Pediatr. Dent. *25*:103–106, 2001.
293. Major, R H.: Classic Descriptions of Disease, with Biographical Sketches of the Authors. Springfield, IL, Charles C Thomas, 1945.
294. Maki, D. G., and Reich, R. M.: Infectious mononucleosis in the athlete. Diagnosis, complications, and management. Am. J. Sports Med. *10*:162–173, 1982.
295. Mallon, R., Borkowski, J., Albin, R., et al.: The Epstein-Barr virus BZLF1 gene product activates the human immunodeficiency virus type 1 5′ long terminal repeat. J. Virol. *64*:6282–6285, 1990.
296. Mangi, R. J., Niederman, J. C., Kelleher, J. E., et al.: Depression of cell-mediated immunity during acute infectious mononucleosis. N. Engl. J. Med. *291*:1149–1153, 1974.
297. Markin, R. S., Linder, J., Zuerlein, K., et al.: Hepatitis in fatal infectious mononucleosis. Gastroenterology *93*:1210–1217, 1987.
298. Martinez, O. M., Villanueva, J. C., Lawrence-Miyasaki, L., et al.: Viral and immunologic aspects of Epstein-Barr virus infection in pediatric liver transplant recipients. Transplantation *59*:519–524, 1995.
299. Mason, W. R., and Adams, E. K.: Infectious mononucleosis: An analysis of 100 cases with particular attention to diagnosis, liver function tests and treatment of selected cases with prednisone. Am. J. Med. Sci. *236*:447–459, 1958.
300. Matoba, A. Y.: Ocular disease associated with Epstein-Barr virus infection. Surv. Ophthalmol. *35*:145–150, 1990.
301. McClain, K. L.: Epstein-Barr virus lymphoproliferative diseases. Semin. Pediatr. Infect. Dis. 7:1–8, 1996.
302. McClain, K. L., Joshi, V. V., and Murphy, S. B.: Cancers in children with HIV infection. Hematol. Oncol. Clin. North Am. *10*:1189–1201, 1996.
303. McClain, K. L., Leach, C. T., Jenson, H. B., et al.: Association of Epstein-Barr virus with leiomyosarcomas in young people with AIDS. N. Engl. J. Med. *332*:12–18, 1995.
304. McClain, K. L., Leach, C. T., Jenson, H. B., et al.: Molecular and virologic characteristics of lymphoid malignancies in children with AIDS. J. Acquir. Immune Defic. Syndr. *23*:152–159, 2000.
305. McGowan, J. E., Chesney, P. J., Crossley, K. B., et al.: Guidelines for the use of systemic glucocorticosteroids in the management of selected infections. Working Group on Steroid Use, Antimicrobial Agents Committee, Infectious Diseases Society of America. J. Infect. Dis. *165*:1–13, 1992.
306. McGowan, J. P., and Shah, S.: Long-term remission of AIDS-related primary central nervous system lymphoma associated with highly active antiretroviral therapy. A. I. D. S. *12*:952–954, 1998.
307. McMonigal, K., Horwitz, C. A., Henle, W., et al.: Post-perfusion syndrome due to Epstein-Barr virus: Report of two cases and review of the literature. Transfusion *23*:331–335, 1983.
308. McSherry, G. D.: Human immunodeficiency-virus–related pulmonary infections in children. Semin. Respir. Infect. *11*:173–183, 1996.

309. Meijer, C. J., Jiwa, N. M., Dukers, D. F., et al.: Epstein-Barr virus and human T-cell lymphomas. Semin. Cancer Biol. *7*:191–196, 1996.
310. Mendonca, D.: A case of infectious mononucleosis presenting with a bilateral facial palsy. J. Laryngol. Otol. *85*:981–982, 1971.
311. Miller, G., Niederman, J. C., and Andrews, L. L.: Prolonged oropharyngeal excretion of Epstein-Barr virus after infectious mononucleosis. N. Engl. J. Med. *288*:229–232, 1973.
312. Miller, G., Shope, T., Lisco, H., et al.: Epstein-Barr virus: Transformation, cytopathic changes, and viral antigens in squirrel monkey and marmoset leukocytes. Proc. Natl. Acad. Sci. U. S. A. *69*:383–387, 1972.
313. Miller, M. J.: Viral taxonomy. Clin. Infect. Dis. *29*:731–733, 1999.
314. Milpied, N., Vasseur, B., Parquet, N., et al.: Humanized anti-CD20 monoclonal antibody (rituximab) in post transplant B-lymphoproliferative disorder: A retrospective analysis on 32 patients. Ann. Oncol. *11*(Suppl. 1):113–116, 2000.
315. Moody, C. E., Casazza, B. A., Christenson, W. N., et al.: Lymphocyte transformation induced by autologous cells. VIII. Impaired autologous mixed lymphocyte reactivity in patients with acute infectious mononucleosis. J. Exp. Med. *150*:1448–1455, 1979.
316. Moore, K. W., Vieira, P., Fiorentino, D. F., et al.: Homology of cytokine synthesis inhibitory factor (IL-10) to the Epstein-Barr virus gene BCRFI. Science *248*:1230–1234, 1990.
317. Morente, M. M., Piris, M. A., Abraira, V., et al.: Adverse clinical outcome in Hodgkin's disease is associated with loss of retinoblastoma protein expression, high Ki67 proliferation index, and absence of Epstein-Barr virus-latent membrane protein 1 expression. Blood *90*:2429–2436, 1997.
318. Mozes, B., Pines, A., Werner, D., et al.: Grand-mal as the major presenting symptom of infectious mononucleosis. J. Neurol. Neurosurg. Psychiatry *47*:569–570, 1984.
319. Mroczek, E. C., Weisenburger, D. D., Grierson, H. L., et al.: Fatal infectious mononucleosis and virus-associated hemophagocytic syndrome. Arch. Pathol. Lab. Med. *111*:530–535, 1987.
320. Mueller, N., Evans, A., Harris, N. L., et al.: Hodgkin's disease and Epstein-Barr virus. Altered antibody pattern before diagnosis. N. Engl. J. Med. *320*:689–695, 1989.
321. Murray, P. G., Billingham, L. J., Hassan, H. T., et al.: Effect of Epstein-Barr virus infection on response to chemotherapy and survival in Hodgkin's disease. Blood *94*:442–447, 1999.
322. Nalesnik, M. A., Makowka, L., and Starzl, T. E.: The diagnosis and treatment of posttransplant lymphoproliferative disorders. Curr. Probl. Surg. *25*:365–472, 1988.
323. Neel, E. U.: Infectious mononucleosis. Death due to agranulocytosis and pneumonia. J. A. M. A. *236*:1493–1494, 1976.
324. Nemerow, G. R., and Cooper, N. R.: Early events in the infection of human B lymphocytes by Epstein-Barr virus: The internalization process. Virology *132*:186–198, 1984.
325. Newman, C., and Polk, B. F.: Resolution of oral hairy leukoplakia during therapy with 9-(1,3-dihydroxy-2-propoxymethyl)guanine (DHPG). Ann. Intern. Med. *107*:348–350, 1987.
326. Niederman, J. C., Evans, A. S., Subrahmanyan, L., et al.: Prevalence, incidence and persistence of EB virus antibody in young adults. N. Engl. J. Med. *282*:361–365, 1970.
327. Niederman, J. C., McCollum, R. W., Henle, G., et al.: Infectious mononucleosis. Clinical manifestations in relation to EB virus antibodies. J. A. M. A. *203*:205–209, 1968.
328. Niederman, J. C., Miller, G., Pearson, H. A., et al.: Infectious mononucleosis. Epstein-Barr-virus shedding in saliva and the oropharynx. N. Engl. J. Med. *294*:1355–1359, 1976.
329. Niederman, J. C., and Scott, R. B.: Studies on infectious mononucleosis: Attempts to transmit the disease to human volunteers. Yale J. Biol. Med. *38*:1–10, 1965.
330. Niedobitek, G., Agathanggelou, A., Herbst, H., et al.: Epstein-Barr virus (EBV) infection in infectious mononucleosis: Virus latency, replication and phenotype of EBV-infected cells. J. Pathol. *182*:151–159, 1997.
331. Niedobitek, G., Meru, N., and Delecluse, H. J.: Epstein-Barr virus infection and human malignancies. Int. J. Exp. Pathol. *82*:149–170, 2001.
332. Nilsson, K.: The nature of lymphoid cell lines and their relationship to the virus. *In* Epstein, M. A., and Achong, B. G. (eds.): The Epstein-Barr Virus. New York, Springer-Verlag, 1979, pp. 225–295.
333. Nolan, R. A.: Report of so-called epidemic of glandular fever (infectious mononucleosis). U. S. Navy Med. Bull. *33*:479–483, 1935.
334. North, K., de Silva, L., and Procopis, P.: Brain-stem encephalitis caused by Epstein-Barr virus. J. Child Neurol. *8*:40–42, 1993.
335. Offit, P. A., Fleisher, G. R., Koven, N. L., et al.: Severe Epstein-Barr virus pulmonary involvement. J. Adolesc. Health Care *2*:121–125, 1981.
336. Okano, M.: Therapeutic approaches for severe Epstein-Barr virus infection. Pediatr. Hematol. Oncol. *14*:109–119, 1997.
337. Pagano, J. S., Sixbey, J. W., and Lin, J. C.: Acyclovir and Epstein-Barr virus infection. J. Antimicrob. Chemother. *12*:113–121, 1983.
338. Pallesen, G., Hamilton-Dutoit, S. J., Rowe, M., et al.: Expression of Epstein-Barr virus latent gene products in tumour cells of Hodgkin's disease. Lancet *337*:320–322, 1991.
339. Patel, B. M.: Skin rash with infectious mononucleosis and ampicillin. Pediatrics *40*:910–911, 1967.
340. Patel, P. C., and Menezes, J.: Epstein-Barr virus (EBV)–lymphoid cell interactions. II. The influence of the EBV replication cycle on natural killing and antibody-dependent cellular cytotoxicity against EBV-infected cells. Clin. Exp. Immunol. *48*:589–601, 1982.
341. Pathmanathan, R., Prasad, U., Sadler, R., et al.: Clonal proliferations of cells infected with Epstein-Barr virus in preinvasive lesions related to nasopharyngeal carcinoma. N. Engl. J. Med. *333*:693–698, 1995.
342. Pattengale, P. K., Smith, R. W., and Perlin, E.: Atypical lymphocytes in acute infectious mononucleosis. Identification by multiple T and B lymphocyte markers. N. Engl. J. Med. *291*:1145–1148, 1974.
343. Paul, J. R., and Bunnell, W. W.: The presence of heterophile antibodies in infectious mononucleosis. Am. J. Med. Sci. *183*:90–104, 1932.
344. Pedneault, L., Katz, B. Z., and Miller, G.: Detection of Epstein-Barr virus in the brain by the polymerase chain reaction. Ann. Neurol. *32*:184–192, 1992.
345. Pedneault, L., Lapointe, N., Alfieri, C., et al.: Natural history of Epstein-Barr virus infection in a prospective pediatric cohort born to human immunodeficiency virus–infected mothers. J. Infect. Dis. *177*:1087–1090, 1998.
346. Pejme, J.: Infectious mononucleosis: A clinical and haemotological study of patients and contacts, and a comparison with healthy subjects. Acta Med. Scand. Suppl. *413*:1–83, 1964.
347. Penman, H. G.: Fatal infectious mononucleosis: A critical review. J. Clin. Pathol. *23*:765–771, 1970.
348. Pereira, M. S., Blake, J. M., and Macrae, A. D.: EB virus antibody at different ages. B. M. J. *4*:526–527, 1969.
349. Pfeiffer, E.: Drusenfieber. Jahrb. Kinderheilkd. *29*:257–264, 1889.
350. Phelan, J. A., and Klein, R. S.: Resolution of oral hairy leukoplakia during treatment with azidothymidine. Oral Surg. Oral Med. Oral Pathol. *65*:717–720, 1988.
351. Pipp, M. L., Means, N. D., Sixbey, J. W., et al.: Acute Epstein-Barr virus infection complicated by severe thrombocytopenia. Clin. Infect. Dis. *25*:1237–1239, 1997.
352. Pope, J. H., Horne, M. K., and Scott, W.: Transformation of foetal human leukocytes in vitro by filtrates of a human leukaemic cell line containing herpes-like virus. Int. J. Cancer *3*:857–866, 1968.
353. Poppema, S., van Imhoff, G., Torensma, R., et al.: Lymphadenopathy morphologically consistent with Hodgkin's disease associated with Epstein-Barr virus infection. Am. J. Clin. Pathol. *84*:385–390, 1985.
354. Porter, D. D., Wimberly, I., and Benyesh-Melnick, M.: Prevalence of antibodies to EB virus and other herpesviruses. J. A. M. A. *208*:1675–1679, 1969.
355. Portman, M., Ingall, D., Westenfelder, G., et al.: Peritonsillar abscess complicating infectious mononucleosis. J. Pediatr. *104*:742–744, 1984.
356. Potter, R.: Paediatric Hodgkin's disease. Eur. J. Cancer *35*:1466–1474, 1999.
357. Preciado, M. V., De Matteo, E., Diez, B., et al.: Epstein-Barr virus (EBV) latent membrane protein (LMP) in tumor cells of Hodgkin's disease in pediatric patients. Med. Pediatr. Oncol. *24*:1–5, 1995.
358. Pullen, H., Wright, N., and Murdoch, J. M.: Hypersensitivity reactions to antibacterial drugs in infectious mononucleosis. Lancet *2*:1176–1178, 1967.
359. Purtilo, D. T., Tatsumi, E., Manolov, G., et al.: Epstein-Barr virus as an etiological agent in the pathogenesis of lymphoproliferative and aproliferative diseases in immune deficient patients. Int. Rev. Exp. Pathol. *27*:113–183, 1985.
360. Qu, L., and Rowe, D. T.: Epstein-Barr virus latent gene expression in uncultured peripheral blood lymphocytes. J. Virol. *66*:3715–3724, 1992.
361. Raab-Traub, N., and Flynn, K.: The structure of the termini of the Epstein-Barr virus as a marker of clonal cellular proliferation. Cell *47*:883–889, 1986.
362. Raab-Traub, N., Rajadurai, P., Flynn, K., et al.: Epstein-Barr virus infection in carcinoma of the salivary gland. J. Virol. *65*:7032–7036, 1991.
363. Rahman, M. A., Kingsley, L. A., Breinig, M. K., et al.: Enhanced antibody responses to Epstein-Barr virus in HIV- infected homosexual men. J. Infect. Dis. *159*:472–479, 1989.
364. Rea, T. D., Russo, J. E., Katon, W., et al.: Prospective study of the natural history of infectious mononucleosis caused by Epstein-Barr virus. J. Am. Board Fam. Pract. *14*:234–242, 2001.
365. Reedman, B. M., and Klein, G.: Cellular localization of an Epstein-Barr virus (EBV)-associated complement-fixing antigen in producer and non-producer lymphoblastoid cell lines. Int. J. Cancer *11*:499–520, 1973.
366. Reinherz, E. L., O'Brien, C., Rosenthal, P., et al.: The cellular basis for viral-induced immunodeficiency: Analysis by monoclonal antibodies. J. Immunol. *125*:1269–1274, 1980.
367. Reisman, R. P., and Greco, M. A.: Virus-associated hemophagocytic syndrome due to Epstein-Barr virus. Hum. Pathol. *15*:290–293, 1984.
368. Resnick, L., Herbst, J. S., Ablashi, D. V., et al.: Regression of oral hairy leukoplakia after orally administered acyclovir therapy. J. A. M. A. *259*:384–388, 1988.
369. Ricker, W., Blumberg, A., Peters, C. H., et al.: The association of the Guillain-Barré syndrome with infectious mononucleosis with a report of two fatal cases. Blood *2*:217–226, 1947.
370. Rickinson, A. B., and Moss, D. J.: Human cytotoxic T lymphocyte responses to Epstein-Barr virus infection. Annu. Rev. Immunol. *15*:405–431, 1997.

371. Rickinson, A. B., Young, L. S., and Rowe, M.: Influence of the Epstein-Barr virus nuclear antigen EBNA 2 on the growth phenotype of virus-transformed B cells. J. Virol. *61*:1310–1317, 1987.
372. Riddler, S. A., Breinig, M. C., and McKnight, J. L.: Increased levels of circulating Epstein-Barr virus (EBV)-infected lymphocytes and decreased EBV nuclear antigen antibody responses are associated with the development of posttransplant lymphoproliferative disease in solid-organ transplant recipients. Blood *84*:972–984, 1994.
373. Ries, L. A. G., Eisner, M. P., Kosary, C. L., et al.: SEER Cancer Statistics Review, 1973–1998 [cited 30 November 2001]. Available from URL: http://seer.cancer.gov/Publications/CSR1973_1998/ 2001.
374. Risdall, R. J., McKenna, R. W., Nesbit, M. E., et al.: Virus-associated hemophagocytic syndrome: A benign histiocytic proliferation distinct from malignant histiocytosis. Cancer *44*:993–1002, 1979.
375. Robinson, J., Smith, D., and Niederman, J.: Mitotic EBNA-positive lymphocytes in peripheral blood during infectious mononucleosis. Nature *287*:334–335, 1980.
376. Robinson, J. E., Brown, N., Andiman, W., et al.: Diffuse polyclonal B-cell lymphoma during primary infection with Epstein-Barr virus. N. Engl. J. Med. *302*:1293–1297, 1980.
377. Robinson, J. E., Smith, D., and Niederman, J.: Plasmacytic differentiation of circulating Epstein-Barr virus–infected B lymphocytes during acute infectious mononucleosis. J. Exp. Med. *153*:235–244, 1981.
378. Rocchi, G., de Felici, A., Ragona, G., et al.: Quantitative evaluation of Epstein-Barr-virus–infected mononuclear peripheral blood leukocytes in infectious mononucleosis. N. Engl. J. Med. *296*:132–134, 1977.
379. Rogatsch, H., Bonatti, H., Menet, A., et al.: Epstein-Barr virus–associated multicentric leiomyosarcoma in an adult patient after heart transplantation: Case report and review of the literature. Am. J. Surg. Pathol. *24*:614–621, 2000.
380. Rogers, B. B., Sommerauer, J., Quan, A., et al.: Epstein-Barr virus polymerase chain reaction and serology in pediatric post-transplant lymphoproliferative disorder: Three-year experience. Pediatr. Dev. Pathol. *1*:480–486, 1998.
381. Rogers, R., Windust, A., and Gregory, J.: Evaluation of a novel dry latex preparation for demonstration of infectious mononucleosis heterophile antibody in comparison with three established tests. J. Clin. Microbiol. *37*:95–98, 1999.
382. Rooney, C. M., Loftin, S. K., Holladay, M. S., et al.: Early identification of Epstein-Barr virus–associated post-transplantation lymphoproliferative disease. Br. J. Haematol. *89*:98–103, 1995.
383. Rooney, C. M., Smith, C. A., Ng, C. Y., et al.: Infusion of cytotoxic T cells for the prevention and treatment of Epstein-Barr virus–induced lymphoma in allogeneic transplant recipients. Blood *92*:1549–1555, 1998.
384. Rosen, A., Gergely, P., Jondal, M., et al.: Polyclonal Ig production after Epstein-Barr virus infection of human lymphocytes in vitro. Nature *267*:52–54, 1977.
385. Rowe, D. T., Qu, L., Reyes, J., et al.: Use of quantitative competitive PCR to measure Epstein-Barr virus genome load in the peripheral blood of pediatric transplant patients with lymphoproliferative disorders. J. Clin. Microbiol. *35*:1612–1615, 1997.
386. Rowe, M., Rowe, D. T., Gregory, C. D., et al.: Differences in B cell growth phenotype reflect novel patterns of Epstein-Barr virus latent gene expression in Burkitt's lymphoma cells. EMBO J. *6*:2743–2751, 1987.
387. Rowe, M., Young, L. S., Cadwallader, K., et al.: Distinction between Epstein-Barr virus type A (EBNA 2A) and type B (EBNA 2B) isolates extends to the EBNA 3 family of nuclear proteins. J. Virol. *63*:1031–1039, 1989.
388. Rowley, J. D.: Identification of the constant chromosome regions involved in human hematologic malignant disease. Science *216*:749–751, 1982.
389. Rubinstein, A., Bernstein, L. J., Charytan, M., et al.: Corticosteroid treatment for pulmonary lymphoid hyperplasia in children with the acquired immune deficiency syndrome. Pediatr. Pulmonol. *4*:13–17, 1988.
390. Rubinstein, A., Morecki, R., Silverman, B., et al.: Pulmonary disease in children with acquired immune deficiency syndrome and AIDS-related complex. J. Pediatr. *108*:498–503, 1986.
391. Rutkow, I. M.: Rupture of the spleen in infectious mononucleosis: A critical review. Arch. Surg. *113*:718–720, 1978.
392. Sadelain, M., and Kieff, E.: Why commonplace encounters turn to fatal attraction. Nat. Genet. *20*:103–104, 1998.
393. Saemundsen, A. K., Albeck, H., Hansen, J. P., et al.: Epstein-Barr virus in nasopharyngeal and salivary gland carcinomas of Greenland Eskimoes. Br. J. Cancer *46*:721–728, 1982.
394. Sakamoto, K., Freed, H. J., and Purtilo, D. T.: Antibody responses to Epstein-Barr virus in families with the X-linked lymphoproliferative syndrome. J. Immunol. *125*:921–925, 1980.
395. Salazar, A., Martinez, H., and Sotelo, J.: Ophthalmoplegic polyneuropathy associated with infectious mononucleosis. Ann. Neurol. *13*:219–220, 1983.
396. Sample, J., Young, L., Martin, B., et al.: Epstein-Barr virus types 1 and 2 differ in their EBNA-3A, EBNA-3B, and EBNA-3C genes. J. Virol. *64*:4084–4092, 1990.
397. Sargison, K. D., Cole, T. P., and Kyle, J.: Traumatic rupture of the spleen. Br. J. Surg. *55*:506–508, 1968.
398. Savoie, A., Perpete, C., Carpentier, L., et al.: Direct correlation between the load of Epstein-Barr virus–infected lymphocytes in the peripheral blood of pediatric transplant patients and risk of lymphoproliferative disease. Blood *83*:2715–2722, 1994.
399. Sawyer, R. N., Evans, A. S., Niederman, J. C., et al.: Prospective studies of a group of Yale University freshmen. I. Occurrence of infectious mononucleosis. J. Infect. Dis. *123*:263–270, 1971.
400. Schooley, R. T.: Etiology. *In* Schlossberg, D. (ed.): Infectious Mononucleosis. Clinical Topics in Infectious Disease, 2nd ed. New York, Springer-Verlag, 1989, pp. 1–7.
401. Schooley, R. T., Densen, P., Harmon, D., et al.: Antineutrophil antibodies in infectious mononucleosis. Am. J. Med. *76*:85–90, 1984.
402. Schwarzmann, F., von Baehr, R., Jager, M., et al.: A case of severe chronic active infection with Epstein-Barr virus: Immunologic deficiencies associated with a lytic virus strain. Clin. Infect. Dis. *29*:626–631, 1999.
403. Scully, C., Laskaris, G., Pindborg, J., et al.: Oral manifestations of HIV infection and their management. I. More common lesions. Oral Surg. Oral Med. Oral Pathol. *71*:158–166, 1991.
404. Shapiro, R. S., McClain, K., Frizzera, G., et al.: Epstein-Barr virus associated B cell lymphoproliferative disorders following bone marrow transplantation. Blood *71*:1234–1243, 1988.
405. Shearer, W. T., Ritz, J., Finegold, M. J., et al.: Epstein-Barr virus–associated B-cell proliferations of diverse clonal origins after bone marrow transplantation in a 12-year-old patient with severe combined immunodeficiency. N. Engl. J. Med. *312*:1151–1159, 1985.
406. Shian, W. J., and Chi, C. S.: Fatal brainstem encephalitis caused by Epstein-Barr virus. Pediatr. Radiol. *24*:596–597, 1994.
407. Shian, W. J., and Chi, C. S.: Epstein-Barr virus encephalitis and encephalomyelitis: MR findings. Pediatr. Radiol. *26*:690–693, 1996.
408. Shibata, D., Tokunaga, M., Uemura, Y., et al.: Association of Epstein-Barr virus with undifferentiated gastric carcinomas with intense lymphoid infiltration. Lymphoepithelioma-like carcinoma. Am. J. Pathol. *139*:469–474, 1991.
409. Shiramizu, B., Barriga, F., Neequaye, J., et al.: Patterns of chromosomal breakpoint locations in Burkitt's lymphoma: Relevance to geography and Epstein-Barr virus association. Blood *77*:1516–1526, 1991.
410. Silverstein, A., Steinberg, G., and Nathanson, M.: Nervous system involvement in infectious mononucleosis. The heralding and-or major manifestation. Arch. Neurol. *26*:353–358, 1972.
411. Sixbey, J. W., Davis, D. S., Young, L. S., et al.: Human epithelial cell expression of an Epstein-Barr virus receptor. J. Gen. Virol. *68*:805–811, 1987.
412. Sixbey, J. W., Lemon, S. M., and Pagano, J. S.: A second site for Epstein-Barr virus shedding: The uterine cervix. Lancet *2*:1122–1124, 1986.
413. Sixbey, J. W., Nedrud, J. G., Raab-Traub, N., et al.: Epstein-Barr virus replication in oropharyngeal epithelial cells. N. Engl. J. Med. *310*:1225–1230, 1984.
414. Slobod, K. S., Taylor, G. H., Sandlund, J. T., et al.: Epstein-Barr virus–targeted therapy for AIDS-related primary lymphoma of the central nervous system. Lancet *356*:1493–1494, 2000.
415. Snijders, P. J., Schulten, E. A., Mullink, H., et al.: Detection of human papillomavirus and Epstein-Barr virus DNA sequences in oral mucosa of HIV-infected patients by the polymerase chain reaction. Am. J. Pathol. *137*:659–666, 1990.
416. Snyderman, N. L., and Stool, S. E.: Management of airway obstruction in children with infectious mononucleosis. Otolaryngol. Head Neck Surg. *90*:168–170, 1982.
417. Sohier, R., Lepine, P., and Sautter, V.: Recherches sur de la transmission experimentale de la mononucleose infectieuse au singe et a l'homme. Ann. Inst. Pasteur (Paris) *65*:50–62, 1940.
418. Sokal, E. M., Caragiozoglou, T., Lamy, M., et al.: Epstein-Barr virus serology and Epstein-Barr virus–associated lymphoproliferative disorders in pediatric liver transplant recipients. Transplantation *56*:1394–1398, 1993.
419. Sparano, J. A., Wiernik, P. H., Leaf, A., et al.: Infusional cyclophosphamide, doxorubicin, and etoposide in relapsed and resistant non-Hodgkin's lymphoma: Evidence for a schedule-dependent effect favoring infusional administration of chemotherapy. J. Clin. Oncol. *11*:1071–1079, 1993.
420. Sprunt, T. P., and Evans, F. A.: Mononuclear leukocytosis in reaction to acute infections (infectious mononucleosis). Bull Johns Hopkins Hosp. *31*:410–417, 1920.
421. Sriskandan, S., Labrecque, L. G., and Schofield, J.: Diffuse pneumonia associated with infectious mononucleosis: Detection of Epstein-Barr virus in lung tissue by in situ hybridization. Clin. Infect. Dis. *22*:578–579, 1996.
422. Starzl, T. E., Nalesnik, M. A., Porter, K. A., et al.: Reversibility of lymphomas and lymphoproliferative lesions developing under cyclosporin-steroid therapy. Lancet *1*:583–587, 1984.
423. Stevens, S. J., Pronk, I., and Middeldorp, J. M.: Toward standardization of Epstein-Barr virus DNA load monitoring: Unfractionated whole blood as preferred clinical specimen. J. Clin. Microbiol. *39*:1211–1216, 2001.
424. Stevenson, D. S., Webster, G., and Stewart, I. A.: Acute tonsillectomy in the management of infectious mononucleosis. J. Laryngol. Otol. *106*:989–991, 1992.
425. Straus, S. E., Tosato, G., Armstrong, G., et al.: Persisting illness and fatigue in adults with evidence of Epstein-Barr virus infection. Ann. Intern. Med. *102*:7–16, 1985.

426. Su, I. J., Hsieh, H. C., Lin, K. H., et al.: Aggressive peripheral T-cell lymphomas containing Epstein-Barr viral DNA: A clinicopathologic and molecular analysis. Blood *77*:799–808, 1991.
427. Sullivan, J. L.: Epstein-Barr virus and the X-linked lymphoproliferative syndrome. Adv. Pediatr. *30*:365–399, 1983.
428. Sullivan, J. L., Woda, B. A., Herrod, H. G., et al.: Epstein-Barr virus–associated hemophagocytic syndrome: Virological and immunopathological studies. Blood *65*:1097–1104, 1985.
429. Sumaya, C. V.: Epidemiologic study of a leukocyte-transforming agent in a general population. J. Clin. Microbiol. *2*:520–523, 1975.
430. Sumaya, C. V.: Primary Epstein-Barr virus infections in children. Pediatrics *59*:16–21, 1977.
431. Sumaya, C. V.: Epstein-Barr virus serologic testing: Diagnostic indications and interpretations. Pediatr. Infect. Dis. *5*:337–342, 1986.
432. Sumaya, C. V., and Ench, Y.: Epstein-Barr virus infectious mononucleosis in children. I. Clinical and general laboratory findings. Pediatrics *75*:1003–1010, 1985.
433. Sumaya, C. V., and Ench, Y.: Epstein-Barr virus infectious mononucleosis in children. II. Heterophil antibody and viral-specific responses. Pediatrics *75*:1011–1019, 1985.
434. Sumaya, C. V., and Ench, Y.: Epstein-Barr virus infections in families: The role of children with infectious mononucleosis. J. Infect. Dis. *154*:842–850, 1986.
435. Sumaya, C. V., and Ench, Y.: Childhood infectious mononucleosis not associated with Epstein-Barr virus. Abstract. Pediatr. Res. *21*:336A, 1987.
436. Sumaya, C. V., Henle, W., Henle, G., et al.: Seroepidemiologic study of Epstein-Barr virus infections in a rural community. J. Infect. Dis. *131*:403–408, 1975.
437. Sumaya, C. V., and Neerhout, R. C.: Sinusitis and periorbital infections complicating infectious mononucleosis. Am. J. Dis. Child. *130*:777, 1976.
438. Summers, W. P., Grogan, E. A., Shedd, D., et al.: Stable expression in mouse cells of nuclear neoantigen after transfer of a 3.4-megadalton cloned fragment of Epstein-Barr virus DNA. Proc. Natl. Acad. Sci. U. S. A. *79*:5688–5692, 1982.
439. Sutton, R. N., Reynolds, K., Almond, J. P., et al.: Immunoglobulins and EB virus antibodies in infectious mononucleosis. Clin. Exp. Immunol. *13*:359–366, 1973.
440. Swinnen, L. J., Mullen, G. M., Carr, T. J., et al.: Aggressive treatment for postcardiac transplant lymphoproliferation. Blood *86*:3333–3340, 1995.
441. Taiwo, B. O.: AIDS-related primary CNS lymphoma: A brief review. A. I. D. S. Read. *10*:486–491, 2000.
442. Tan, L. C., Gudgeon, N., Annels, N. E., et al.: A re-evaluation of the frequency of $CD8^+$ T cells specific for EBV in healthy virus carriers. J. Immunol. *162*:1827–1835, 1999.
443. Tanaka, K., Shimada, M., Sasahara, A., et al.: Chronic hepatitis associated with Epstein-Barr virus infection in an infant. J. Pediatr. Gastroenterol. Nutr. *5*:467–471, 1986.
444. Taub, R., Kirsch, I., Morton, C., et al.: Translocation of the c-myc gene into the immunoglobulin heavy chain locus in human Burkitt lymphoma and murine plasmacytoma cells. Proc. Natl. Acad. Sci. U. S. A. *79*:7837–7841, 1982.
445. ten Napel, C. H., and The, T. H.: Lymphocyte reactivity in infectious mononucleosis. J. Infect. Dis. *141*:716–723, 1980.
446. Thomas, J. A., Hotchin, N. A., Allday, M. J., et al.: Immunohistology of Epstein-Barr virus–associated antigens in B cell disorders from immunocompromised individuals. Transplantation *49*:944–953, 1990.
447. Tidy, H. L., and Daniel, E. C.: Glandular fever and infective mononucleosis, with an account of an epidemic. Lancet *2*:9–13, 1923.
448. Tierney, R. J., Steven, N., Young, L. S., et al.: Epstein-Barr virus latency in blood mononuclear cells: Analysis of viral gene transcription during primary infection and in the carrier state. J. Virol. *68*:7374–7385, 1994.
449. Tindle, B. H.: Pathology of infectious mononucleosis. *In* Schlossberg, D. (ed.): Infectious Mononucleosis. New York, Springer-Verlag, 1989, pp. 126–141.
450. Torre, D., and Tambini, R.: Acyclovir for treatment of infectious mononucleosis: A meta-analysis. Scand. J. Infect. Dis. *31*:543–547, 1999.
451. Tsutsumi, H., Kamazaki, H., Nakata, S., et al.: Sequential development of acute meningoencephalitis and transverse myelitis caused by Epstein-Barr virus during infectious mononucleosis. Pediatr. Infect. Dis. J. *13*:665–667, 1994.
452. Turner, A. R., MacDonald, R. N., and Cooper, B. A.: Transmission of infectious mononucleosis by transfusion of pre-illness plasma. Ann. Intern. Med. *77*:751–753, 1972.
453. Tynell, E., Aurelius, E., Brandell, A., et al.: Acyclovir and prednisolone treatment of acute infectious mononucleosis: A multicenter, double-blind, placebo-controlled study. J. Infect. Dis. *174*:324–331, 1996.
454. Vander, J. B.: Pleural effusion in infectious mononucleosis. Ann. Intern. Med. *41*:146–151, 1954.
455. van der Horst, C., Joncas, J., Ahronheim, G., et al.: Lack of effect of peroral acyclovir for the treatment of acute infectious mononucleosis. J. Infect. Dis. *164*:788–792, 1991.
456. van Doornik, M. C., van 'T Veer-Korthof, E. T., and Wierenga, H.: Fatal aplastic anaemia complicating infectious mononucleosis. Scand. J. Haematol. *20*:52–56, 1978.
457. Veal, C. F., Carr, M. B., and Briggs, D. D.: Diffuse pneumonia and acute respiratory failure due to infectious mononucleosis in a middle-aged adult. Am. Rev. Respir. Dis. *141*:502–504, 1990.
458. Veltri, R. W., Sprinkle, P. M., and McClung, J. E.: Epstein-Barr virus associated with episodes of recurrent tonsillitis. Arch. Otolaryngol. *101*:552–556, 1975.
459. Vowels, M. R., Tang, R. L., Berdoukas, V., et al.: Brief report: Correction of X-linked lymphoproliferative disease by transplantation of cord-blood stem cells. N. Engl. J. Med. *329*:1623–1625, 1993.
460. Weigle, K. A., Sumaya, C. V., and Montiel, M. M.: Changes in T-lymphocyte subsets during childhood Epstein-Barr virus infectious mononucleosis. J. Clin. Immunol. *3*:151–155, 1983.
461. Weiss, L. M., Movahed, L. A., Warnke, R. A., et al.: Detection of Epstein-Barr viral genomes in Reed-Sternberg cells of Hodgkin's disease. N. Engl. J. Med. *320*:502–506, 1989.
462. Weiss, L. M., Strickler, J. G., Warnke, R. A., et al.: Epstein-Barr viral DNA in tissues of Hodgkin's disease. Am. J. Pathol. *129*:86–91, 1987.
463. Westmore, G. A.: Cervical abscess: A life-threatening complication of infectious mononucleosis. J. Laryngol. Otol. *104*:358–359, 1990.
464. Wheatley, G. H., 3rd, McKinnon, K. P., Iacobucci, M., et al.: Dendritic cells improve the generation of Epstein-Barr virus–specific cytotoxic T lymphocytes for the treatment of posttransplantation lymphoma. Surgery *124*:171–176, 1998.
465. Whitley, R. J., Cobbs, C. G., Alford, C. A., Jr., et al.: Diseases that mimic herpes simplex encephalitis. Diagnosis, presentation, and outcome. NIAD Collaborative Antiviral Study Group. J. A. M. A. *262*:234–239, 1989.
466. Williams, L. L., Lowery, H. W., and Glaser, R.: Sudden hearing loss following infectious mononucleosis: Possible effect of altered immunoregulation. Pediatrics *75*:1020–1027, 1985.
467. Woda, B. A., and Sullivan, J. L.: Reactive histiocytic disorders. Am. J. Clin. Pathol. *99*:459–463, 1993.
468. Wohl, D. L., and Isaacson, J. E.: Airway obstruction in children with infectious mononucleosis. Ear Nose Throat J. *74*:630–638, 1995.
469. Wolf, H., Haus, M., and Wilmes, E.: Persistence of Epstein-Barr virus in the parotid gland. J. Virol. *51*:795–798, 1984.
470. Wollheim, F. A., and Williams, R. C., Jr.: Studies on the macroglobulins of human serum. I. Polyclonal immunoglobulin class M (IgM) increase in infectious mononucleosis. N. Engl. J. Med. *274*:61–67, 1966.
471. Wood, T. A., and Frenkel, E. P.: The atypical lymphocyte. Am. J. Med. *42*:923–936, 1967.
472. Yahr, M. D., and Frontera, A. T.: Acute autonomic neuropathy: Its occurrence in infectious mononucleosis. Arch. Neurol. *32*:132–133, 1975.
473. Yao, Q. Y., Rickinson, A. B., and Epstein, M. A.: A re-examination of the Epstein-Barr virus carrier state in healthy seropositive individuals. Int. J. Cancer *35*:35–42, 1985.
474. Yates, J., Warren, N., Reisman, D., et al.: A cis-acting element from the Epstein-Barr viral genome that permits stable replication of recombinant plasmids in latently infected cells. Proc. Natl. Acad. Sci. U. S. A. *81*:3806–3810, 1984.
475. Yates, J. L., Warren, N., and Sugden, B.: Stable replication of plasmids derived from Epstein-Barr virus in various mammalian cells. Nature *313*:812–815, 1985.
476. Yefenof, E., Bakacs, T., Einhorn, L., et al.: Epstein-Barr virus (EBV) receptors, complement receptors, and EBV infectibility of different lymphocyte fractions of human peripheral blood. I. Complement receptor distribution and complement binding by separated lymphocyte subpopulations. Cell. Immunol. *35*:34–42, 1978.
477. Young, L., Alfieri, C., Hennessy, K., et al.: Expression of Epstein-Barr virus transformation–associated genes in tissues of patients with EBV lymphoproliferative disease. N. Engl. J. Med. *321*:1080–1085, 1989.
478. Young, L. S., Clark, D., Sixbey, J. W., et al.: Epstein-Barr virus receptors on human pharyngeal epithelia. Lancet *1*:240–242, 1986.
479. Young, L. S., Dawson, C. W., Clark, D., et al.: Epstein-Barr virus gene expression in nasopharyngeal carcinoma. J. Gen. Virol. *69*:1051–1065, 1988.
480. Young, L. S., Dawson, C. W., and Eliopoulos, A. G.: The expression and function of Epstein-Barr virus encoded latent genes. Mol. Pathol. *53*:238–247, 2000.
481. Ziegler, J. L.: Chemotherapy of Burkitt's lymphoma. Cancer *30*:1534–1540, 1972.
482. Ziegler, J. L.: Burkitt's lymphoma. N. Engl. J. Med. *305*:735–745, 1981.
483. Ziegler, J. L., Beckstead, J. A., Volberding, P. A., et al.: Non-Hodgkin's lymphoma in 90 homosexual men. Relation to generalized lymphadenopathy and the acquired immunodeficiency syndrome. N. Engl. J. Med. *311*:565–570, 1984.
484. Zou, X. N., Lu, S. H., and Liu, B.: Volatile *N*-nitrosamines and their precursors in Chinese salted fish—a possible etological factor for NPC in china. Int. J. Cancer *59*:155–158, 1994.
485. zur Hausen, H., Schulte-Holthausen, H., Klein, G., et al.: EBV DNA in biopsies of Burkitt tumours and anaplastic carcinomas of the nasopharynx. Nature *228*:1056–1058, 1970.

CHAPTER

166 Human Herpesviruses 6, 7, and 8

CHARLES GROSE

Before 1986, five human herpesviruses (HHVs) were known. They included herpes simplex virus (HSV) types 1 (oral) and 2 (genital), cytomegalovirus (CMV), varicella-zoster virus (VZV), and Epstein-Barr virus (EBV). The herpesviruses are important pathogens causing a variety of childhood diseases that are described in other chapters of this textbook. An inherent characteristic of herpesviruses is their ability to form a latent infection, in which the viral genome continues to reside within the host. When the virus reactivates, it often causes further symptoms and signs. Thus, herpesviruses cause a spectrum of illnesses during the lifetime of the infected human host. During the last decades of the 20th century, three novel herpesviruses were discovered. Two of them have been designated HHV-6 and HHV-7, whereas the newest member of the family tentatively has been called either Kaposi sarcoma–associated herpesvirus (KSHV) or HHV-8. The viruses and the diseases they cause are described in this chapter.

Human Herpesviruses 6 and 7

One unexpected consequence of the epidemic of acquired immunodeficiency syndrome (AIDS) was the discovery of a new human DNA virus. The virus was first isolated from the white blood cells of six patients with lymphoproliferative disorders, two of whom had AIDS.[27] The virus was propagated by subsequent infection of phytohemagglutinin-stimulated human leukocytes. Further electron-microscopic characterization of the cultured virus demonstrated similarities to a herpesvirus, including (1) an icosahedral capsid composed of 162 capsomers covered by a lipid membrane and (2) an enveloped particle with a diameter of 200 nm (Fig. 166–1). Because the virus was isolated originally from B lymphocytes, the agent was designated human B-lymphotropic virus (HBLV). However, this apparent tropism for B lymphocytes was not confirmed by other investigators, who found that the virus preferentially infected T lymphocytes and not B lymphocytes.[17] When they analyzed the virally infected cells with monoclonal antibodies, they discovered that most of the cells exhibited the T-cell–associated CD4 molecule. Thus, the initial designation of HBLV was changed to HHV-6.

The DNA sequence and the deduced amino acid sequence of a major portion of the HHV-6 genome have been published.[7] Calculation of the percentage of amino acid identity shared by HHV-6 proteins with those in other herpesviruses revealed that HHV-6 proteins most closely resembled those of human CMV. The strains of HHV-6 have been divided into group A and group B. The HHV-6 isolates related to prototype strain U1102 have been called group A, whereas those related to strain Z29 have been designated group B. In 1990, while searching for additional strains of HHV-6, Frenkel and coworkers[13] isolated a new T-lymphotropic herpesvirus that was designated HHV-7. HHV-7 is related closely at a genetic level to HHV-6 and to a lesser degree to CMV.[7] All three of these agents are subclassified as beta-herpesviruses.

Most persons contract their primary HHV-6 infection before reaching the age of 5 years; adult populations from the United States, Sweden, and Japan have a seroprevalence rate above 80 percent.[3] In infants and young children, group B strains of HHV-6 appear to be a major cause of the disease roseola (exanthem subitum). Roseola is discussed at greater length in Chapter 66. Children also may contract a primary HHV-6 infection without manifesting a rash. After acute infection, HHV-6 forms a latent infection, probably in T lymphocytes. Endogenous virus reactivates in adults with immunosuppressive disorders, such as AIDS, although reactivation has not been associated with a specific disease entity. Seronegative recipients of organ transplants may acquire a primary HHV-6 infection from latent virus in the donor organ. In a small number of infants, acute HHV-7 infection appears to cause a roseola illness much like that of acute HHV-6 infection.

DISEASES CAUSED BY HHV-6 AND HHV-7

Soon after the HHV-6 agent was discovered, virologists investigated the seroprevalence of this infection among the U.S. population. Several hundred sera collected before blood donation by healthy adults from Minneapolis and Kansas City were screened for antibodies to HHV-6; 81 to 88 percent of the samples had detectable levels of antiviral reactivity. These results clearly showed that most adults in the

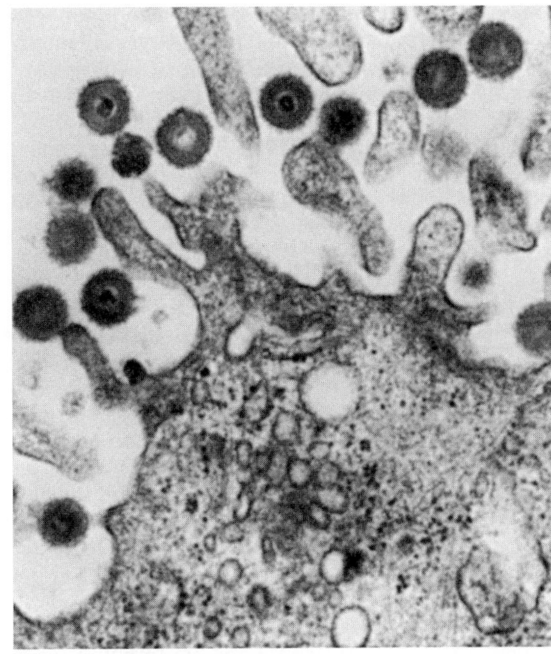

FIGURE 166–1 ■ Electron micrograph of cultured mononuclear cells infected with HHV-6. Several enveloped viral particles are visible in the extracellular area. (Courtesy of Dr. Y. Asano.)

United States had prior exposure to HHV-6 infection.[25] In a similar serologic survey in Sweden, 97 percent of adults had detectable HHV-6 antibody.[16] Further studies in a pediatric population in the state of North Carolina demonstrated that most newborn infants had maternally derived anti–HHV-6 antibody, which disappeared by 3 months of age.[25] Thereafter, many young children quickly acquired de novo antibody produced in response to exposure to the infectious agent.[25] The rate of seropositivity reached 100 percent in some studies in young American children,[3] and in Sweden the percentage was approximately 60 percent at 1 year of age and 85 percent at 5 years of age.[16]

A Japanese study further delineated the nature of the illness associated with acute HHV-6 infection in young children.[36] HHV-6 was cultured from the peripheral blood leukocytes of four infants with presumed roseola (exanthem subitum); each subject was 6 months of age and had an acute febrile illness followed by a concurrent fall in temperature and the onset of a rash. The blood samples were collected during the febrile stage of the disease. In a subsequent paper by the same group, two infants (6 and 7 months of age) were described who developed HHV-6 infection *without* a rash.[29] Both infants had been seen by physicians because of a 2- to 3-day history of high fever (38.5° C to 39.5° C). The only abnormal clinical finding was congestion of the throat. In both cases, the temperature rapidly returned to normal around day 3 of illness, but no rash was ever observed. Cultures of peripheral blood cells from both infants were positive for HHV-6.[29] Further seroprevalence studies performed in Japan showed that most Japanese (86%) contracted HHV-6 infection by the age of 24 months.[37] Thereafter, the increase in seropositivity among the childhood populations was small. The earlier statistics suggest that HHV-6 infection goes unrecognized in most children.

Primary HHV-6 infection has been implicated in a few cases of severe hepatitis. The first case was that of a 21-year-old patient with cystic fibrosis who received a liver transplant.[35] The recipient lacked antibodies to HHV-6, and the organ donor was seropositive. Two weeks after transplantation, the recipient developed fever and grand mal seizures; her hepatic function deteriorated. HHV-6 was cultured from her peripheral blood cells, and herpesviral particles were seen by electron-microscopic examination of a liver biopsy specimen. The patient also developed antibodies to HHV-6 by day 16 after transplantation. The apparent source of infection was the donor liver, from which HHV-6 presumably was reactivated after transplantation. She gradually recovered her hepatic function over the course of several weeks.

A fatal case of fulminant HHV-6 hepatitis has been reported in a 3-month-old boy.[5] The infant was admitted to a hospital because of fever, jaundice, convulsions, and loss of consciousness. His serum bilirubin concentration, liver transaminases, and blood ammonia level were elevated markedly. Within 7 days, he became comatose and died. As part of the diagnostic evaluation, HHV-6 was cultured from his mononuclear cells. Furthermore, HHV-6 DNA was detected in biopsy samples of liver and brain, which were obtained immediately after death. A serum sample drawn before death showed reactivity to HHV-6. On the other hand, the child had no serologic evidence of acute infection with hepatitis A, B, or C or with any other HHV.

Thus, these two case reports suggest that HHV-6 can cause severe hepatitis in infants and nonimmune recipients of an organ from an HHV-6–seropositive donor. The virus also may have been the etiologic agent of encephalitis in these two patients.

In one retrospective review of roseola in association with acute HHV-6 infection, the signs and symptoms were tabulated.[3] The study population included 94 boys and 82 girls, who ranged in age from 3 weeks to 18 months (Table 166–1). As would be predicted, the two most common clinical findings were fever and rash. The temperature often rose to 39° C, and fever persisted for 2 to 4 days. The rash usually appeared when the fever lessened; the rash was papular in 54 percent, macular in 40 percent, and maculopapular in the remainder of the children. The exanthem typically persisted for 3 to 4 days and was not followed by desquamation. Diarrhea was a surprisingly frequent occurrence, but it was not severe. An enanthem called Nagayama spots in Japan consisted of papules on the mucosa of the soft palate and uvula. Of the total study group, 8 percent developed febrile seizures. More severe central nervous system (CNS) complications have been documented in children not enrolled in this study. Four children have been diagnosed with HHV-6 encephalitis, all with abnormal electroencephalograms. One of the four children died, and the other three had permanent neurologic sequelae. In the United States in particular, acute HHV-6 infection also appears to be associated with concurrent acute otitis media.[25]

Reactivation of previous HHV-6 infection has been demonstrated in some healthy children and adults who contracted a second herpes-type infection, such as primary EBV infection (infectious mononucleosis) or primary CMV infection.[16] A similar serologic survey was performed in 10 renal transplant recipients who initially were HHV-6 seropositive.[20] After transplantation, all 10 showed greater than fourfold rises in antibody to HHV-6. Only 2 of the 10 developed a febrile illness, and both of them also had primary CMV infection. More recent evidence suggests that HHV-6 infection in combination with CMV infection may worsen post-transplantation pneumonitis previously thought to be associated solely with CMV infection. HHV-6 does not appear to be related causally to Kawasaki disease.[21]

Whether HHV-7 causes a distinct illness has been the subject of many medical investigations since 1990. In general, HHV-7 antibody is acquired by mid-childhood, but there appears to be no corresponding sentinel illness. However, in two infants with roseola, both isolation of HHV-7 and seroconversion to HHV-7 were documented; in addition, another five children with roseola were found to have undergone seroconversion to HHV-7.[33] HHV-7 also has been isolated from one infant with an acute febrile illness.[24] Therefore, in a small number of young children, acute HHV-7 infection may be associated with fever and sometimes a roseola rash.

TABLE 166–1 ■ SELECTED FEATURES IN ROSEOLA ASSOCIATED WITH INFECTION IN CHILDREN

Clinical Findings	%
Prodromal symptoms	14
Fever above 37.5° C	98
Rash	98
Diarrhea	68
Nagayama spots	65
Cough	50
Cervical adenopathy	31
Edematous eyelids	30
Bulging fontanelle	26
Convulsions	8

Data modified from Asano Y., and Grose, C.: Human herpesvirus type 6 infections. *In* Glaser, R., and Jones, J. (eds.): Herpesvirus Infections. New York, Marcel Dekker, 1994, pp. 227–244.

NEUROLOGIC COMPLICATIONS

In the preceding paragraphs, CNS symptoms were mentioned briefly. In a large series of clinical studies performed in Japan, seizures were a common feature of acute HHV-6 infection.[30, 39] In one series of 105 young children with acute febrile convulsions, 21 had evidence of primary HHV-6 infection, as assayed by either isolation of virus from blood or seroconversion of HHV-6 antibodies. When the age of the patient was assessed, HHV-6 infection was found in 13 of 23 seizure patients younger than 1 year of age; thus, the seizure group with HHV-6 infection was significantly younger than the seizure group without HHV-6 infection. In addition, the frequency of clustering seizures, long-lasting seizures, partial seizures, and postictal paralysis in children having their first febrile convulsion episode was significantly higher in those with primary HHV-6 infection than in those without HHV-6 infection.

In studies from Japan, assays for HHV-6 and HHV-7 DNA were performed on cerebrospinal fluid samples from 43 children with CNS symptoms.[38] All children had symptoms compatible with aseptic meningitis. HHV-6 DNA was detected in the peripheral blood cells of 15 and in the cerebrospinal fluid of 7; all were HHV-6 variant B. HHV-7 DNA was detected in the peripheral blood cells of 28 and in the cerebrospinal fluid of 6 patients. Thus, the clinical study demonstrated that both HHV-6 and HHV-7 can invade the CNS or, alternatively, frequently reactivate within the CNS during childhood neurologic disease. Yet, further longitudinal studies are required to determine to what extent HHV-6 or HHV-7 infection is the etiologic agent of a particular neurologic disease.

PATHOGENESIS OF HHV-6 AND HHV-7 INFECTION

The pathogenesis of HHV-6 infection certainly includes a viremia while the child is asymptomatic; the total duration of the incubation period is not well defined but may be approximately 10 days. The prodrome, which signals the end of the incubation period, includes 2 to 4 days of fever, which precedes the onset of the rash.[4] During this period, virtually 100 percent of peripheral blood cell cultures are positive for HHV-6. By day 3 or 4, when the rash first appears, the viremia is abating. Between 5 and 7 days after the onset of the fever (or 2 to 4 days after appearance of exanthem), viremia persists in less than 20 percent of the children. Viremia is absent later in convalescence. The serologic response to virus infection is undetectable before the onset of rash but first appears coincidentally with the exanthem.

The mothers of infants with HHV-6 infection have been studied to determine whether they are the source of the infectious agent.[40] Because most mothers are seropositive, the possibility exists that HHV-6 infection could reactivate in the mother, who would then transmit the infection to her child, possibly through exchange of saliva. Cultures of peripheral blood mononuclear cells and saliva specimens of 14 mothers of infected infants failed to yield conclusive results. However, in another study, HHV-6 DNA was detected in the vaginal secretions of young adult women, so perinatal HHV-6 transmission remains a possibility.[15]

In contrast with HHV-6, HHV-7 seropositivity occurs in childhood but after the first 2 years of life. HHV-7 transmission has been investigated in large multigenerational Japanese families living in the same household.[32] The results indicated that HHV-7 is transmitted gradually from older generation to younger generation (Fig. 166–2). Transmission often occurs in childhood before the child enters a traditional primary school at age 6 years. Either parent can transmit the virus. A reasonable explanation for this pattern of transmission is exchange of infectious saliva among family members living in the same household during many years.

RELATIONSHIP OF HHV-6 INFECTION TO ACQUIRED IMMUNODEFICIENCY SYNDROME

HHV-6 was first isolated from patients with immunosuppressive disorders, including infection with human immunodeficiency virus (HIV) type 1. An immediate question, therefore, was the relationship of HHV-6 infection to AIDS. In spite of extensive searches conducted since 1986, no specific syndrome related to HHV-6 infection in patients with AIDS has been identified. In HIV-negative homosexual men, no difference in HHV-6 antibody status was noted.[12, 28] Because we now know that most persons first contract roseola as young children, expression of HHV-6 in adults with AIDS probably represents a reactivation of a latent HHV-6 infection. Similar reactivations have been documented with the other herpesviruses (HSV-1, HSV-2, CMV, EBV, and VZV) in the same population of severely immunosuppressed patients.

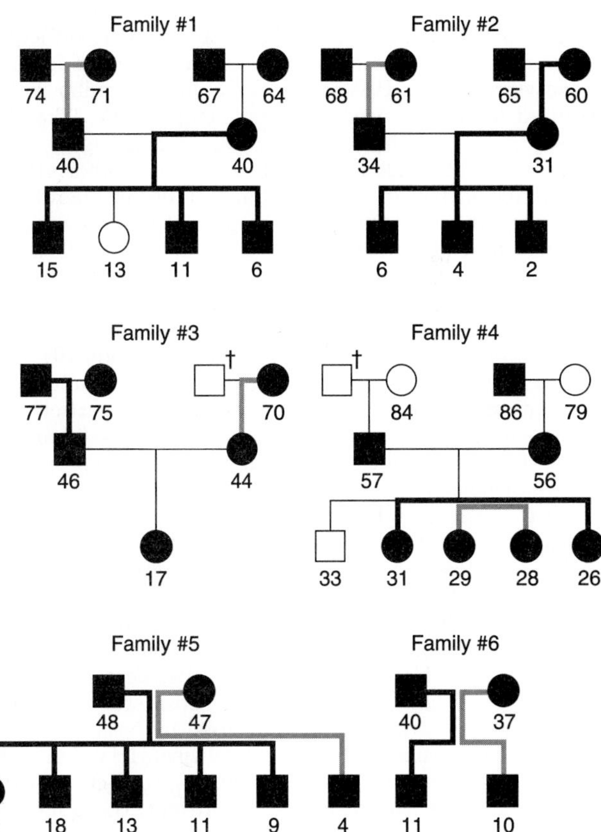

FIGURE 166–2 ■ Pedigrees of six families with HHV-7 infection. All families resided in Okayama, Japan. Males and females are indicated as boxes and circles, respectively. Persons from whom HHV-7 was isolated are shaded. A person who was already deceased is marked †. Members who have similar HHV-7 DNA restriction patterns are connected with bold lines. Numbers under the boxes and circles indicate ages. (From Takahashi, Y., Yamada, M., Nakamura, J., et al.: Transmission of human herpesvirus 7 through multigenerational families in the same household. Pediatr. Infect. Dis. J. *16*:975–978, 1997.)

HHV-6 may play a more subtle role in the pathogenesis of HIV-1 infection than first was imagined. The two viruses appear to infect a similar or overlapping subset of lymphocytes. The phenotypes of the T cells infected by HHV-6 have been determined to be both $CD4^{+}CD8^{+}$ and $CD4^{+}CD8^{-}$.[31] Both HIV-1 and HHV-6 productively can infect the same $CD4^{+}$ T lymphocyte under experimental conditions in the laboratory.[18, 19] HHV-6 could be a cofactor in the pathogenesis of AIDS.[14]

DIAGNOSIS

Infection with HHV-6 can be diagnosed by several means, including (1) measurement of antibody, (2) isolation of virus, (3) detection of viral antigen, and (4) detection of viral DNA. The first method (i.e., the traditional approach for diagnosis of virus infection) usually requires acute and convalescent serum samples for determination of a fourfold or greater rise in titer of virus-specific IgG antibody. Finding IgM specific for HHV-6 in a single serum sample also would indicate an acute infection in a young child. The titer of IgG antibody rises during reactivation of the virus in adults, but whether IgM antibody to HHV-6 appears regularly at the same time is not known. HHV-6 antibodies usually have been measured by an indirect immunofluorescence method, although neutralization tests also have been performed.[3, 4, 12, 16, 25, 29, 35]

Isolation of HHV-6 was the original technique for identification of this herpesvirus.[27] The method is more difficult to perform than are those methods commonly used for most herpesviruses (e.g., HSV, CMV, VZV) but is similar to that required for isolation of the lymphotropic EBV. The virus usually is isolated in a cell substrate consisting of mononuclear cells obtained from cord blood of a newborn infant. The source of virus in the patient also is the peripheral blood mononuclear cell population. The patient's blood sample is obtained in a heparinized tube, and the mononuclear cells are separated in a density gradient (e.g., Ficoll-Hypaque medium). Cells from the patient are cocultured with cord blood cells in enriched medium supplemented with human interleukin-2.[29] The cultures are observed periodically under light microscopy. If the balloon-like cells are examined by electron microscopy, numerous herpesviral particles are seen, as illustrated in Figure 166–1. Thus, HHV-6 harbored in a patient's mononuclear cells can infect and be propagated in cord blood cells.

Viral genome can be detected in infected tissues by DNA hybridization techniques.[35] Viral DNA also can be detected in tissue samples by polymerase chain reaction. In one fatal case of HHV-6 infection,[5] DNA was extracted from postmortem liver and brain samples and amplified by polymerase chain reaction with an HHV-6 primer. On direct gel electrophoresis, HHV-6–specific DNA was detected in both the liver and the brain specimens. These studies indicate that HHV-6 infection can be diagnosed by both traditional and newer molecular techniques. Likewise, HHV-7 infection usually is diagnosed by isolation of virus or detection of viral DNA in samples from patients. At present, these methods are available mainly in research laboratories.

TREATMENT OF HHV-6 INFECTION

In most instances of HHV-6 infection in healthy children, treatment with antiviral medication is not indicated. Recovery is complete within a few days after onset of the rash, and sequelae rarely occur. However, HHV-6 disease in immunocompromised persons may be more persistent or severe. Many immunocompromised persons also are receiving antiviral medication for other herpesvirus infections and, therefore, may have suppressed HHV-6 infection unbeknownst to physician or patient. Several groups have analyzed the in vitro sensitivity of HHV-6 to four antiviral drugs: acyclovir, ganciclovir, phosphonoformic acid, and zidovudine.[1, 26] The first three compounds have been used in treatment of other herpesvirus infections, and the fourth is a therapy for HIV infection. Multiplication of HHV-6 in cell culture is inhibited readily by ganciclovir at a concentration of 2 to 10 µmol/L, easily achievable levels in humans. This effect is of interest because ganciclovir inhibits human CMV to a similar degree; as mentioned earlier, CMV and HHV-6 are related closely at a genomic level. Phosphonoformic acid (foscarnet) at a concentration of 66 µmol/L also is effective against HHV-6 infection. On the other hand, HHV-6 is affected by acyclovir only at concentrations of 50 to 100 µmol/L, considerably higher levels than those required for treatment of HSV-1, HSV-2, and VZV infections and possibly toxic in humans. Likewise, zidovudine has no effect on this herpesvirus. At present, none of these antiviral drugs has been approved specifically for treatment of HHV-6 infections.

Kaposi Sarcoma Herpesvirus (Human Herpesvirus 8)

Yet another consequence of the HIV epidemic in the 1980s was the appearance of Kaposi sarcoma in many people with AIDS. The increase in Kaposi sarcoma was especially puzzling because the tumor occurred more frequently in people who acquired HIV by sexual transmission rather than by infusion of infected blood products, such as factor VIII in hemophiliac patients. The question often arose whether a second infectious agent was involved in the etiology of Kaposi sarcoma. The answer to that question was provided by a report published in late 1994. The authors announced the identification of novel herpesvirus-like DNA sequences collected from patients with AIDS in New York.[9] The viral DNA was called Kaposi sarcoma–associated herpesvirus (KSHV). Others have suggested that the agent be called human herpesvirus 8 (HHV-8).

The authors of the original KSHV report discovered the herpesvirus-like DNA sequences by using a combination of genetic techniques, including amplification of DNA by polymerase chain reaction and subsequent representational difference analysis.[9] Thereby, they were able to identify and characterize unique DNA sequences in Kaposi sarcoma that were absent from nonmalignant tissue from the same patient. One such sequence was called KS330*Bam,* and this 330–base pair piece of DNA showed close homology to regions of the genome of herpesvirus saimiri, a simian herpesvirus, and to a lesser degree to EBV, the agent that causes infectious mononucleosis. A second DNA fragment called KS631*Bam* was homologous to another region in the herpesvirus saimiri genome. In their study, the authors located one or both of these herpesvirus-like DNA sequences in 20 of 27 different samples of Kaposi sarcoma tissue. The investigators oncluded that they had discovered DNA of a previously unknown herpesvirus within Kaposi sarcoma tissues.

Their results were confirmed quickly by other groups. In one study from California, investigators detected the KS330*Bam* DNA sequence in 13 of 13 biopsy specimens of Kaposi sarcoma from patients with AIDS.[2] This study also found the same sequence in the peripheral blood cells collected from 10 of the 13 patients but not in the blood samples of 20 patients with no history of Kaposi sarcoma. A third study from France found the herpesvirus-like DNA in biopsy specimens from five patients with Mediterranean-type Kaposi sarcoma; all five patients were HIV seronegative.[11] In subsequent studies, HHV-8 DNA has been detected in most Kaposi sarcomas in HIV-seropositive individuals as well as in most Kaposi sarcomas (classical) in HIV-seronegative individuals, often residing in the Mediterranean area.

The authors of the original KSHV report subsequently found the herpesvirus-like DNA sequences in body cavity–based lymphomas from patients with AIDS.[8] HHV-8 DNA also has been found in the B-cell lymphoproliferative disorder known as multicentric Castleman disease.[6] Of equal importance, the unusual herpesvirus-like sequences were not found in several other lymphomas or leukemias (e.g., small-lymphocyte lymphoma, monocytoid B-cell lymphoma, follicular lymphoma, diffuse large-cell lymphoma, Burkitt lymphoma, lymphoblastic lymphoma, anaplastic large-cell lymphoma, multiple myeloma, hairy-cell leukemia, acute lymphoblastic leukemia, cutaneous T-cell lymphoma, or post-transplantation lymphoproliferative disorder).

TRANSMISSION OF HHV-8 INFECTION

One of the most perplexing aspects of HHV-8 epidemiology is the mode of transmission. That the seroprevalence is high among a population of adult men who have sex with men is well known.[22] Yet, the question remains whether larger segments of the population are infected on a worldwide basis, and, in particular, whether children are infected. To answer this question, several HHV-8 seroepidemiology studies were surveyed. Two studies provide partial answers to the question of childhood infection.

The first study was performed in a village in French Guiana, South America, among 1337 individuals of African origin.[23] They ranged in age from 2 to 91 years. The serologic data indicated that HHV-8 seropositivity was strongly age dependent. Among 14 children aged 2 to 14 years, 3 of 146 were positive; aged 5 to 9 years, 14 of 278 were positive; aged 10 to 14 years, 31 of 232 were positive; aged 15 to 19 years, 24 of 149 were positive; aged 20 to 29 years, 38 of 236 were positive; aged 30 to 39 years, 16 of 120 were positive; aged 40 to 49 years, 19 of 70 were positive; and older than 50 years, 32 of 106 were positive. These seroprevalence data clearly show a gradual acquisition of infection during early childhood, with a stepwise increment from approximately 5 to 12 percent at age 10 years.

HIV infection did not play a role in likelihood of transmission because HIV infection is not common in this village. Instead, extensive analyses of intrafamilial relationships demonstrated a highly significant familial correlation in HHV-8 seropositivity between mother and child (especially when children were younger than 10 years) and between siblings. The correlation was highest when the siblings had an age difference less than 5 years. By contrast, no evidence of dependence between spouses or between father and child was found.

The low HHV-8 seroprevalence in children younger than 5 years has been seen in other smaller studies in developing countries and strongly suggests that intrauterine transmission is a rare event. Similarly, breast-feeding is an unlikely mode of spread. The most likely mechanism is exchange of saliva between mother and child, for example, by premastication of food. Similarly, young siblings closely matched in age may eat from the same container and thereby exchange saliva with food. Of interest, a similarity in transmission appears to exist between HHV-8 and HHV-7, when HHV-7 was studied in multigenerational Japanese households (see Fig. 166–2).

A second large HHV-8 seroepidemiology analysis was performed in Israel.[10] The incidence of classic Kaposi sarcoma in Israel is among the highest in the developed world. Because of this statistic, the investigators undertook a study to ascertain the HHV-8 seroprevalence in Israel and also to investigate HHV-8 intrafamilial transmission. The study population included 1648 healthy blood donors determined to be positive for hepatitis B antigen and 2403 family members.

The seroprevalence data showed that 9 percent of children aged 2 to 14 years and 9 percent of adolescents and young adults aged 15 to 24 years were HHV-8 seropositive. Seroprevalence in older adults ranged from 12 to 18 percent. HHV-8 positivity was more likely to occur in children when at least one of the parents was positive compared with children with neither parent positive. The most important predictor of a child's HHV-8 seropositivity status was maternal seropositivity. Further, a child's likelihood of having HHV-8 seropositivity was heightened when the mother's anti–HHV-8 titer was especially elevated.

Unlike the study in French Guiana, the study in Israel determined that HHV-8 was transmitted between spouses. The Israeli investigators speculated that factors associated with hepatitis B infection may favor HHV-8 transmission. Further, they also found that carriers of hepatitis B infection were more likely to have higher anti–HHV-8 titers. In the Israeli population, no association was found with prior surgery, blood transfusion, intravenous drug abuse, or HIV status.

These two large seroepidemiological studies demonstrate that HHV-8 is spread by nonsexual means in children in many countries around the world. In these same countries, HHV-8 seropositivity commonly occurs in adult populations, regardless of their HIV status.[34] The most reasonable hypothesis is that the virus is contained within saliva. In the United States and the United Kingdom, however, HHV-8 seroprevalence is considered to be extremely low in young children. Only in the HIV-seropositive adult population is HHV-8 coinfection commonplace. Extensive studies have been performed in the United States among men who have sex with men and who were HHV-8 seropositive.[22] HHV-8 DNA was detected in 60 percent of mucosal samples collected from 50 men, whereas only 1 percent of anal or genital samples were positive in the same test. The investigators concluded that oral exposure to saliva containing HHV-8 is a potential risk factor for acquisition of HHV-8 infection among men who have sex with men. Obviously, this study does not address the issue of the very low HHV-8 seroprevalence in children in the United States and the United Kingdom, but the study does emphasize that infectious saliva is a likely mode of transmission. In the United States, among adult nonimmigrant heterosexual populations, only a small percentage are HHV-8 seropositive; no common source of infection is apparent within this group.

REFERENCES

1. Agut, H., Collandre, H., Aubin, J. T., et al.: In vitro sensitivity of human herpesvirus-6 to antiviral drugs. Res. Virol. *140*:219–228, 1989.
2. Ambroziak, J. A., Blackbourn, D. J., Herndier, B. G., et al.: Herpes-like sequences in HIV-infected and uninfected Kaposi's sarcoma patients. Science *268*:582–583, 1995.
3. Asano, Y., and Grose, C.: Human herpesvirus type 6 infections. *In* Glaser, R., and Jones, J. (eds.): Herpesvirus Infections. New York, Marcel Dekker, 1994, pp. 227–244.
4. Asano, Y., Yoshikawa, T., Suga, S., et al.: Viremia and neutralizing antibody response in infants with exanthem subitum. J. Pediatr. *114*:535–539, 1989.
5. Asano, Y., Yoshikawa, T., Suga, S., et al.: Fatal fulminant hepatitis in an infant with herpesvirus-6 infection Lancet *1*:862–863, 1990.
6. Ascoli, V., Signoretti, S., Onetti-Muda, A., et al.: Primary effusion lymphoma in HIV-infected patients with multicentric Castleman's disease. J. Pathol. *193*:200–209, 2001.
7. Berneman, Z. N., Dharam, V. A., Ge, L., et al.: Human herpesvirus 7 is a T-lymphotropic virus and is related to, but significantly different from,

human herpesvirus 6 and human cytomegalovirus. Proc. Natl. Acad. Sci. U. S. A. *89*:10552–10556, 1992.
8. Cesarman, E., Chang, Y., Moore, P. S., et al.: Kaposi's sarcoma–associated herpesvirus-like DNA sequences in AIDS-related body-cavity-based lymphomas. N. Engl. J. Med. *332*:1186–1191, 1995.
9. Chang, Y., Cesarman, E., Pessin, M. S., et al.: Identification of herpesvirus-like DNA sequences in AIDS-associated Kaposi's sarcoma. Science *266*:1865–1869, 1994.
10. Davidovici, B., Karakis, I., Bourboulia, D., et al.: Seroepidemiology and molecular epidemiology of Kaposi's sarcoma–associated herpesvirus among Jewish population groups in Israel. J. Natl. Cancer Inst. *93*:194–202, 2001.
11. Dupin, N., Grandadam, M., Calvez, V., et al.: Herpesvirus-like DNA sequences in patients with Mediterranean Kaposi's sarcoma. Lancet *345*:761–762, 1995.
12. Fox, J., Briggs, M., and Tedder, R. S.: Antibody to human herpesvirus 6 in HIV-1 positive and negative homosexual men. Lancet *2*:396–397, 1988.
13. Frenkel, N., Schirmer, E. C., Wyatt, L. S., et al.: Isolation of a new herpesvirus from CD4+ T cells. Proc. Natl. Acad. Sci. U. S. A. *87*:748–752, 1990.
14. Horvat, R. T., Wood, C., and Balachandran, N.: Transactivation of human immunodeficiency virus promoter by human herpesvirus 6. J. Virol. *63*:970–973, 1989.
15. Leach, C. T., Newton, E. R., McParlin, S., et al.: Human herpesvirus 6 infection of the female genital tract. J. Infect. Dis. *169*:1281–1283, 1994.
16. Linde, A., Dahl, H., Wahren, B., et al.: IgG antibodies to human herpesvirus-6 in children and adults both in primary Epstein-Barr virus and cytomegalovirus infections. J. Virol. Methods *21*:117–123, 1988.
17. Lopez, C., Pellett, P., Stewart, J., et al.: Characteristics of human herpesvirus-6. J. Infect. Dis. *157*:1271–1273, 1988.
18. Lusso, P., Markham, P. D., Tschachler, E., et al.: In vitro cellular tropism of human B-lymphotropic virus (human herpesvirus-6). J. Exp. Med. *167*:1659–1670, 1988.
19. Lusso, P., Ensoli, B., Markham, P. D., et al.: Productive dual infection of human CD4+ T lymphocytes by HIV-1 and HHV-6. Nature *337*:370–373, 1989.
20. Morris, D. J., Littler, E., Arrand, J. R., et al.: Human herpesvirus 6 infection in renal transplant recipients. N. Engl. J. Med. *320*:1560–1561, 1989.
21. Okano, M., Luka, J., Thiele, G. M., et al.: Human herpesvirus 6 infection and Kawasaki disease. J. Clin. Microbiol. *27*:2379–2380, 1989.
22. Pauk, J., Huang, M. L., Brodie, S. J., et al.: Mucosal shedding of human herpesvirus 8 in men. N. Engl. J. Med. *343*:1369–1377, 2000.
23. Plancoulaine, S., Abel, L., van Beveren, M., et al.: Human herpesvirus 8 transmission from mother to child between siblings in an endemic population. Lancet *356*:1062–1065, 2000.
24. Portolani, M., Cermelli, C., Mirandola, P., et al.: Isolation of human herpesvirus 7 from an infant with febrile syndrome. J. Med. Virol. *45*:282–283, 1995.
25. Pruksananonda, P., Hall, C. B., Insel, R. A., et al.: Primary human herpesvirus 6 infection in young children. N. Engl. J. Med. *326*: 1445–1450, 1992.
26. Russler, S. K., Tapper, M. A., and Carrigan, D. R.: Susceptibility of human herpesvirus 6 to acyclovir and ganciclovir. Lancet *2*:382, 1989.
27. Salahuddin, S. Z., Ablashi, D. V., Markham, P. D., et al.: Isolation of a new virus, HBLV, in patients with lymphoproliferative disorders. Science *234*:596–601, 1986.
28. Spira, T. J., Bozemann, L. H., Sanderlin, K. C., et al.: Lack of correlation between human herpesvirus-6 infection and the course of human immunodeficiency virus infection. J. Infect. Dis. *161*:567–570, 1990.
29. Suga, S., Yoshikawa, T., Asano, Y., et al.: Human herpesvirus-6 infection (exanthem subitum) without rash. Pediatrics *83*:1003–1006, 1989.
30. Suga, S., Suzuki, K., Ihira, M., et al.: Clinical characteristics of febrile convulsions during primary HHV-6 infection. Arch. Dis. Child. *82*:62–66, 2000.
31. Takahashi, K., Sonoda, S., Higashi, K., et al.: Predominant CD4 T-lymphocyte tropism of human herpesvirus 6–related virus. J. Virol. *63*:3161–3163, 1989.
32. Takahashi, Y., Yamada, M., Nakamura, J., et al.: Transmission of human herpesvirus 7 through multigenerational families in the same household. Pediatr. Infect. Dis. J. *16*:975–978, 1997.
33. Tanaka, K., Kondo, T., Torigoe, S., et al.: Human herpesvirus 7: Another causal agent for roseola (exanthem subitum). J. Pediatr. *125*:1–5, 1994.
34. Vitale, F., Viviano, E., Perna, A. M., et al.: Serological and virological evidence of non-sexual transmission of human herpesvirus type 8 (HHV8). Epidemiol. Infect. *125*:671–675, 2000.
35. Ward, K. N., Gray, J. J., and Efstathious, S.: Brief report: Primary human herpesvirus 6 infection in a patient following liver transplantation from a seropositive donor. J. Med. Virol. *28*:69–72, 1989.
36. Yamanishi, K., Okuno, T., Shiraki, K., et al.: Identification of human herpesvirus-6 as a causal agent for exanthem subitum. Lancet *1*:1065–1067, 1988.
37. Yoshikawa, T., Suga, S., Asano, Y., et al.: Distribution of antibodies to a causative agent of exanthem subitum (human herpesvirus-6) in healthy individuals. Pediatrics *84*:675–677, 1989.
38. Yoshikawa, T., Ihira, M., Suzuki, K., et al.: Invasion by human herpesvirus 6 and human herpesvirus 7 of the central nervous system in patients with neurological signs and symptoms. Arch. Dis. Child. *83*:170–171, 2000.
39. Yoshikawa, T., and Asano, Y.: Central nervous system complications in human herpesvirus-6 infection. Brain Dev. *22*:307–314, 2000.
40. Yoshiyama, H., Suzuki, E., Yoshida, T., et al.: Role of human herpesvirus 6 infection in infants with exanthem subitum. Pediatr. Infect. Dis. J. *9*:71–74, 1990.

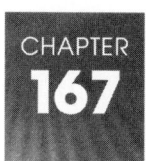

Varicella-Zoster Virus

ANNE A. GERSHON

Varicella-zoster virus (VZV) causes two diseases, varicella (chickenpox) and zoster (shingles). Varicella, the primary infection, usually occurs in childhood and is manifested as a pruritic rash accompanied by fever and other systemic signs and symptoms that often are of a mild to moderate nature. Zoster is primarily a disease of adults, although it can occur in children. It develops in a setting of low cell-mediated immunity (CMI) to VZV, such as occurs with normal aging or after disease or the use of various therapies such as steroids, cancer chemotherapy, organ transplantation, and irradiation. During varicella, VZV establishes a latent infection in sensory nerve ganglia; zoster results when latent VZV reactivates and returns from the ganglion to infect the skin and produce a unilateral dermatomal eruption.

The origin of the nomenclature "chickenpox" is uncertain, but it may have come from the French *pois chiche* (chick pea) or from the farmyard fowl (in Old English, *cicen*, and in Middle High German, *kuchen*).[25] *Herpes* is the Greek word meaning "to creep," and *zoster* comes from the Greek and Latin word meaning "girdle" or "belt."

The Organism

VZV is an alpha-herpesvirus. It has a DNA core surrounded by a nucleocapsid composed of 162 hexagonal capsomeres that form an icosahedron with a diameter of approximately 100 nm.[29] A tegument surrounds this structure, which in turn is surrounded by a lipid-containing envelope. Enveloped virions have a diameter of approximately 200 nm.

The genome of VZV has been sequenced; it contains 68 open-reading frames (ORFs).[30] The linear, double-stranded DNA consists of a long unique segment, U_L, and a short unique sequence, U_S, flanked by internal and terminal repeats.[32, 35, 132] The genome of the Oka vaccine strain also has been sequenced, and the molecular basis for attenuation of the strain is being investigated.[2, 62, 98]

Five ORFs (genes 4, 21, 29, 62, and 63) have been detected in human sensory ganglia during latent VZV infection.[30, 75] VZV is synthesized by an orderly cascade of gene expression consisting of immediate early (IE), early, and, finally, late lytic structural genes. The genes detectable during latent infection are IE and early genes for the most part; one postulation is that cellular immunity to VZV normally can control early replication of the virus so that productive or lytic infection does not occur.[75]

During productive infection, VZV synthesizes more than 30 polypeptides; the function of most of these polypeptides remains unknown, but some are structural and others are nonstructural and presumably have regulatory action. VZV synthesizes at least seven glycoproteins (g) termed gB, gC, gE, gH, gI, gK, and gL.[28, 65, 90] These glycoproteins correspond to those of herpes simplex virus (HSV), but unlike HSV, VZV has no equivalent of gD, which is the major glycoprotein of HSV. The major glycoprotein of VZV is gE. The VZV glycoproteins not only provide structure for the virion but also play roles in infectivity such as mediating adhesion and promoting entry into uninfected cells of the host. The glycoproteins also are antigenic, as is the tegument, and immune responses are directed toward these structures.

Just one antigenic type of VZV has been identified, and only minor differences in DNA exist among the various VZV isolates.[106] Wild-type VZV DNA can be distinguished from that of vaccine-type virus by restriction enzyme analysis of DNA from cultured virus or by polymerase chain reaction (PCR).[2, 62, 95]

VZV replicates in the nuclei of infected cells, where the DNA core and capsid are synthesized. The capsid is enveloped by a complex process, after which it traverses the cell in cytoplasmic vesicles.[59] In vitro, VZV grows rather slowly and is highly cell associated; its synthetic pathway entraps it in endosomic vesicles, where it is inactivated before it can be released. In vivo, however, infectious VZV is released from cells and is highly contagious; VZV avoids the endosomal route in vivo and exits from cells by the secretory pathway.

VZV has an extremely limited host range and infects mostly primates. Hairless guinea pigs may be infected with VZV; the illness produced is extremely mild, and latent infection occurs only infrequently, but specific immune responses can be demonstrated.[109] A rat model of latent VZV infection has been described.[31]

Transmission

VZV is spread by the airborne route[97] and requires direct contact with an infected individual for transmission. In varicella, VZV is transmitted from the skin and the respiratory tract. VZV is isolated readily from skin lesions, but isolating the virus from the respiratory tract is extremely difficult.[111, 135] Spread of VZV from varicella patients before the onset of rash in closed communities has been reported, however, thus implicating respiratory spread.[63] VZV DNA has been detected by PCR in the nasopharynx of children during the pre-eruptive and early stages of varicella.[89, 123] Investigations of leukemic recipients of live attenuated varicella vaccine have implicated spread of VZV from skin. No transmission to siblings from vaccinees who had no rash was found, but a 14 percent transmission rate occurred when siblings were exposed to a child who had a vaccine-associated skin rash.[136] Taken together, these observations suggest that VZV can spread from skin lesions as well as from the respiratory tract. Epidemiologic studies suggest that transmission is most likely to take place in the early stages of varicella.[108]

Zoster is not transmissible per se, but the vesicular lesions of zoster contain infectious VZV and can transmit varicella to other individuals.[22, 92] Zoster is thought to be less contagious than is varicella, and whether VZV is spread from the respiratory tract of patients with zoster is unknown.

Epidemiology

VZV infections occur worldwide, and both sexes are affected equally. The virus spreads less efficiently in countries with tropical climates than in those with temperate climates,[91] thereby resulting in a high rate of susceptibility in adults reared in tropical countries. In the prevaccine era, approximately 3.8 million cases of chickenpox, an entire birth cohort, occurred annually in the United States. In the United States in the prevaccine era, 8 to 9 percent of children between the ages of 1 and 9 years contracted the illness annually.[116] These data were collected before the time that many children began to attend daycare facilities; exposure to VZV in the daycare setting may lead to earlier acquisition of disease. The impact of daycare, however, may never be fully known in the United States because live attenuated varicella was licensed for general use in 1995 and already is making an impact on the epidemiology of chickenpox.[124]

The link between varicella and zoster was recognized first almost 100 years ago when von Bokay appreciated that cases of varicella often occurred after exposure to a patient with zoster.[140] Early in the 20th century, medical investigators inoculated vesicular fluid from zoster patients into varicella-susceptible children, who then contracted chickenpox.[22, 92] Weller first successfully isolated VZV in vitro, gave the virus its name, and demonstrated that the viruses isolated from patients with varicella and zoster are identical.[145] Garland proposed that zoster is the result of reactivation of latent VZV.[41] Hope-Simpson presciently recognized the importance of the immune system in preventing reactivation of VZV; he postulated that zoster results when immunity to VZV wanes with age.[78] The importance of declining CMI to VZV has been identified in the pathogenesis of zoster.[7, 73] With the use of molecular techniques for DNA analysis, researchers have established that the DNA of the viruses causing varicella and zoster is the same, and autopsies have revealed that latent VZV is detectable in nuclei of the neurons and satellite cells of the sensory ganglia of individuals with a past history of varicella.[27, 103–105] Researchers also have shown that zoster is not acquired by contact with patients who have zoster or chickenpox.[47] Zoster develops in approximately 15 percent of the varicella-immune population during their lifetime.[78]

Varicella is highly contagious; clinical infection will develop in 80 to 90 percent of susceptible individuals exposed in a household.[119] Secondary varicella cases in a family usually are more severe than are the primary cases.[119] Approximately 75 percent of adults with no past history of varicella have detectable antibodies to VZV,[96] thus indicating that subclinical varicella can occur. One epidemiologic study suggests that its incidence is approximately 5 percent.[119]

Subclinical zoster also may occur, and zoster with dermatomal pain and no rash has been described. Increases in VZV immune responses and episodes of viremia shown by PCR in asymptomatic individuals suggest silent reactivation.[52, 66, 152] Asymptomatic shedding of VZV is not known to occur.

Second attacks of varicella are uncommon occurrences but may occur more frequently in the immunocompromised than in immunologically normal individuals.[54, 86] Immunologic boosting to VZV occurs commonly on re-exposure to the virus.[5, 54] Whether boosting is necessary for long-term maintenance of immunity to VZV is not known.

Adults and children older than 2 years of age with zoster usually have a history of a previous attack of varicella.[78] Zoster is a rare occurrence in childhood, but the incidence is increased in young children who had varicella either in utero or before reaching their second birthday.[34] Chickenpox in the first year of life increases the risk of developing childhood zoster by a relative factor between roughly 3 and 21,[68] possibly because of immaturity of the immune response to VZV in young infants. According to published reports,[43] infants with congenital varicella syndrome are at greatly increased risk, as high as 18 percent in the first few years of life, for the development of zoster at an early age.

The incidence of zoster in a population begins to increase sharply at approximately 50 years of age.[78] This increased incidence of zoster with advancing age is associated with and presumably caused by the relative loss of CMI to VZV that occurs naturally with aging.[14, 23]

Zoster develops with increased frequency in patients with neoplasms and after organ transplantation[100]; in severely immunocompromised patients with zoster, disseminated infection with viremia also may occur.[37] Spinal trauma, irradiation, and corticosteroid therapy may be additional precipitating factors. Children who are infected with human immunodeficiency virus (HIV) and have CD4 levels less than 15 percent when varicella develops are at great risk for the development of zoster; in one published series, the incidence was 70 percent.[48]

On occasion, however, zoster may develop in healthy young adults who are not immunocompromised, presumably from a transient fall in CMI to VZV caused by a stimulus such as another viral infection or stress. Because zoster does not develop in all immunocompromised persons, deficiency of CMI to VZV is a necessary, but not sufficient, requirement for this illness. The distribution of lesions in chickenpox, which primarily involves the trunk and head, is reflected in a proportionately greater representation of these regions in the dermatomal lesions of zoster.[130] Zoster may recur, either in the same dermatome or in a different dermatome; the chance of recurrent zoster developing is similar to the chance of having a first attack for a particular age group.[78]

Varicella occurs most commonly in the winter and early spring. In contrast, zoster occurs equally during all seasons of the year.

Pathogenesis

The incubation period of varicella ranges from 10 to 23 days (average of 14 days).[63] During the incubation period, VZV is thought to spread to regional lymph nodes, undergo multiplication, and cause a primary low-grade viremic phase after approximately 5 days that spreads the virus to the viscera, where further multiplication of VZV occurs. This process results in the second and greater viremic phase, which delivers the virus to the skin, where it causes the characteristic skin rash.[67] VZV can be isolated from blood cultures either a few days before the onset of rash or within 1 to 2 days after onset in immunocompetent children.[8]

The skin lesions of VZV infection begin as macules and progress rapidly to papules, vesicles, pustules, and scabs. Histologic changes in the skin lesions are similar for chickenpox and zoster. The hallmarks of each disease are multinucleated giant cells and intranuclear inclusions. In varicella, they are localized primarily in the dermis and epidermis, where ballooning degeneration of cells in the deeper layers is accompanied by intercellular edema. As the edema progresses, the cornified layers and basal layers separate to form a thin-roofed vesicle. An exudate of mononuclear cells is seen in the dermis.[1, 145] In zoster, in addition to skin lesions that resemble those of varicella, a mononuclear inflammatory infiltrate is present in the dorsal root ganglion of the affected dermatome. Hemorrhagic necrosis of ganglion cells and demyelination of the corresponding axon also may be present.[36, 76, 103]

Both humoral and CMI responses to VZV develop within a few days after the onset of varicella. Peak antibody levels are attained 4 to 8 weeks after onset, remain high for approximately 6 months, and then decline. Positive IgG VZV antibody titers are detectable in healthy adults for decades after their case of varicella.[51, 129, 151] After active immunization against varicella, antibody titers are lower than after natural infection but persist for as long as 20 years in healthy vaccinees immunized as children.[9, 146] Serum IgG, IgA, and IgM develop after occurrences of both varicella and zoster. Zoster occurs despite high levels of specific antibodies, but significantly higher titers develop during convalescence and are indicative of an anamnestic response to VZV in this secondary infection.[20, 138]

CMI responses are thought to play the major role in host defense against the virus. CMI to VZV can be demonstrated in vitro by stimulation of lymphocytes with VZV antigens,[72, 155] by an intradermal skin test,[96] and by specific lysis of histocompatible target cells by cytotoxic T cells.[6] Natural killer cell and antibody-dependent cellular toxicity to VZV also have been described.[81] The CMI responses of normal subjects with remote clinical evidence of varicella are characterized by occasional high activity in the absence of symptoms, thus suggesting either exposure to VZV with boosting of the immune response or subclinical reactivation of the virus. CMI reactions remain positive for years after a case of varicella, although this response may wane in many individuals older than 50 years of age.[14, 23] The predominant cell in vesicular lesions is the polymorphonuclear leukocyte (PMN). PMNs may play a role in generating interferon in vesicular lesions, which may be a factor in recovery.[131]

Exactly how immunity to varicella and zoster is mediated is unclear. Because patients with isolated agammaglobulinemia do not experience either severe or recurrent varicella, researchers long presumed that CMI is more important in host defense than is humoral immunity. We now recognize that T-cell cytotoxicity is crucial in recovery from VZV infection.[4, 6] The response or responses that prevent clinical illness after reinfection with VZV are presumed to be those of cytotoxic T lymphocytes, but antibodies also may play a role. Specific antibodies must have some importance because varicella-zoster immune globulin (VZIG) can be used to prevent or modify varicella in exposed susceptible persons. However, the issues are not straightforward. Varicella may develop in young infants after exposure despite detectable transplacental antibody titers,[11] and modified cases of breakthrough varicella have developed in vaccinated leukemic children despite the presence of humoral and CMI responses as determined by lymphocyte stimulation on exposure to VZV.[50, 55] Still, clinical illness is far less likely to develop in individuals with detectable antibody titers or positive CMI responses (or both) at exposure to VZV than in those without antibodies. Some forms of CMI and antibodies both probably play roles in host defense against VZV.

Nosocomial Varicella

Nosocomial varicella may be a serious and expensive problem in hospitals, where both patients and employees may be susceptible to chickenpox.[64, 71, 143] Because varicella-susceptible hospital employees may serve as vectors for the spread of VZV to susceptible patients, serologic testing of employees for immunity to chickenpox if they have no past history of clinical varicella and offering vaccine to those who are susceptible are appropriate measures.

The risk of horizontal transmission occurring in maternity wards or the newborn nursery after hospital exposure to an adult or child is surprisingly low.[43] A few episodes of nursery transmission of varicella have been reported,[40, 49, 70] but the low incidence of such transmission may be a result of the fact that many infants are in isolettes. Furthermore, most hospital employees and most mothers and their newborn infants have antibodies to VZV and are at low risk for the development of clinical illness. Even in low-birth-weight infants, antibodies to VZV usually are detectable.[107, 118]

Clinical Manifestations: Varicella

Varicella is a highly contagious, usually self-limited systemic infection characterized by fever and a generalized pruritic rash lasting approximately 5 days. A prodromal phase in children is unusual, but malaise and fever for 1 to 2 days before the onset of rash is a common manifestation in adults.[25] The rash is more intense on the trunk and head than on the extremities, and it typically evolves as a series of "crops" over the course of 1 to 2 days in normal hosts. Most children with varicella have 250 to 500 superficial skin lesions, many of which are vesicular[119] (Fig. 167–1). Not uncommonly, a few lesions may develop in the mouth, conjunctiva, or other mucosal sites. Residual scarring is exceptional but can occur, and depigmented areas of skin may occur in dark-skinned patients. A self-limited increase in hepatic transaminase levels without jaundice is not an uncommon occurrence during varicella.[113] Rarely, thrombocytopenia and neutropenia may transiently occur transiently with varicella. More severe infections are more likely to develop in adults than in children, presumably because of lower CMI responses to VZV in adults than children.[42, 110] Newborn infants who acquire varicella from their mothers in the few days before delivery also are at risk for acquisition of severe varicella because of immaturity of the CMI response.[43]

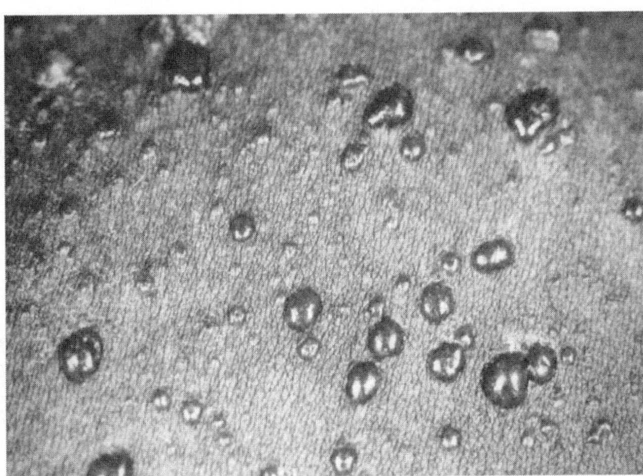

FIGURE 167–1 ■ Typical skin lesions of varicella.

COMPLICATIONS OF VARICELLA

The most frequent complication of varicella in normal hosts is bacterial superinfection of the skin, lungs, or bones, most often by *Staphylococcus aureus* or group A beta-hemolytic streptococci.[19, 153] Central nervous system complications, which may precede or follow varicella, include transient cerebellar ataxia, severe cerebral encephalitis, aseptic meningitis, and transverse myelitis.[83, 85] Encephalopathy as a sequela of Reye syndrome has become a rare complication because aspirin no longer is recommended for children with varicella. Other complications of chickenpox encountered less commonly include arthritis, glomerulonephritis, myocarditis, and purpura fulminans.[145]

Varicella may be severe and even fatal in immunocompromised patients, including those with an underlying malignancy or congenital or acquired deficits in CMI, such as patients who have undergone organ transplantation or have underlying HIV infection, and in children receiving high doses of corticosteroids for any reason[39] (Fig. 167–2). These patients may be susceptible to progressive varicella, with continuing fever and the development of new vesicular lesions for 2 weeks or longer. Their skin lesions characteristically are large, umbilicated, and hemorrhagic, and primary varicella pneumonia is a frequent complication. Alternatively, in some immunocompromised patients, an acute form of varicella with disseminated intravascular coagulation develops and is rapidly fatal, at times before antiviral therapy can be instituted. A 30 percent rate of dissemination with a 7 percent fatality rate was reported in leukemic children in whom chickenpox developed in the pre-antiviral drug era.[38] Severe varicella has been observed in children with underlying HIV infection, especially those classified as having acquired immunodeficiency syndrome (AIDS).[87] In most HIV-infected children, however, mild to moderate forms of varicella develop, although the illness generally is more severe than that in otherwise healthy children.[48] Varicella does not seem to be a cofactor for clinical progression of HIV infection to AIDS, but in approximately 5 percent of these

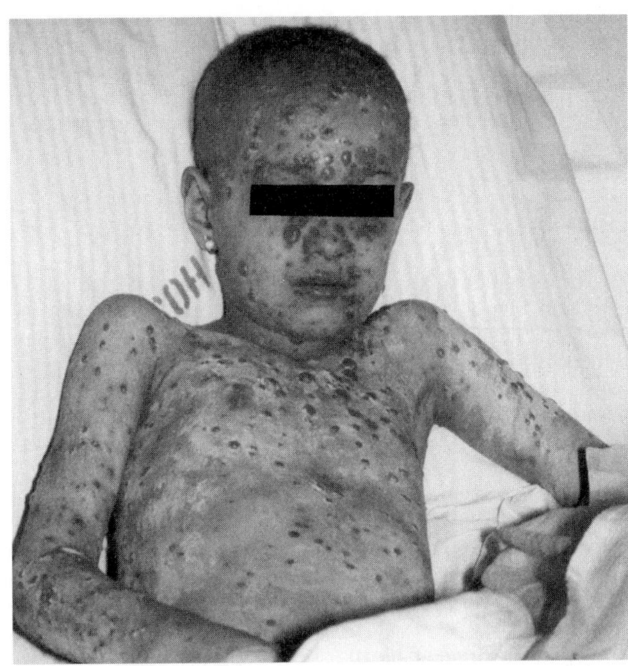

FIGURE 167–2 ■ Progressive varicella in a 9-year-old child with underlying leukemia.

children, chronic wart-like hyperkeratotic VZV lesions may develop, presumably a chronic form of zoster.[3]

Primary varicella pneumonia accounts for many of the fatalities ascribed to varicella, particularly in immunocompromised patients, adults, and neonates.[112] In male military recruits with varicella, radiographic evidence of pneumonia was found in 16 percent.[144] Symptoms include fever, cough, and dyspnea. Other common symptoms and signs are cyanosis, rales, hemoptysis, and chest pain. The chest radiograph typically reveals a diffuse nodular or miliary pattern, most pronounced in the perihilar region.[134] Blood gas analyses and pulmonary function tests indicate a diffusion defect that may persist in some cases for months after recovery.[18] The availability of antiviral chemotherapy has improved greatly the outcome of this complication.

CONGENITAL VARICELLA SYNDROME

LaForet and Lynch in 1947 were the first to describe an infant with multiple congenital anomalies after maternal chickenpox.[94] The infant had hypoplasia of the right lower extremity, clubfoot, absent deep tendon reflexes on the right, cerebral cortical atrophy, cerebellar aplasia, chorioretinitis, torticollis, insufficiency of the anal and vesical sphincters, and cicatricial cutaneous lesions on the left lower extremity, which are now recognized to be typical. In 1974, Srabstein and colleagues rediscovered this syndrome. Their report of another case and review of the literature concluded that, although the virus could not be isolated from affected infants, the congenital syndrome consisted of a typical constellation of birth defects as originally described by LaForet and Lynch.[128] This syndrome occurs after maternal VZV infection in the first or second trimester of pregnancy; approximately 2 percent of the offspring of pregnancies complicated by varicella are affected. Approximately 75 affected infants have been described in the literature; 95 percent occurred after maternal varicella and 5 percent after maternal zoster. In the prevaccine era, approximately 40 affected infants were thought to be born yearly in the United States.[43]

Cicatricial scars of the skin, the most prominent stigmata, are reported in more than 60 percent of cases.[43] Other frequent abnormalities include chorioretinitis, microphthalmos, Horner syndrome, cataract, nystagmus, hypoplastic limbs, cortical atrophy or mental retardation (or both), and early death.

Clinical Manifestations: Zoster

Zoster usually begins as a localized unilateral vesicular skin eruption involving one to three dermatomal segments (Fig. 167–3). The skin lesions resemble those of varicella but tend more toward confluence and are likely to be painful, especially in adults. Zoster generally is a milder disease in children than in adults.

COMPLICATIONS OF ZOSTER

Between 25 and 50 percent of persons older than 50 years of age in whom zoster develops may experience protracted pain, or post-herpetic neuralgia (PHN), after healing of the rash. Pain may persist for months to years and is described as aching, jabbing, or boring. The cause of PHN is unknown. Children rarely experience PHN; both the incidence and duration of PHN are related directly to increasing age.[60, 61]

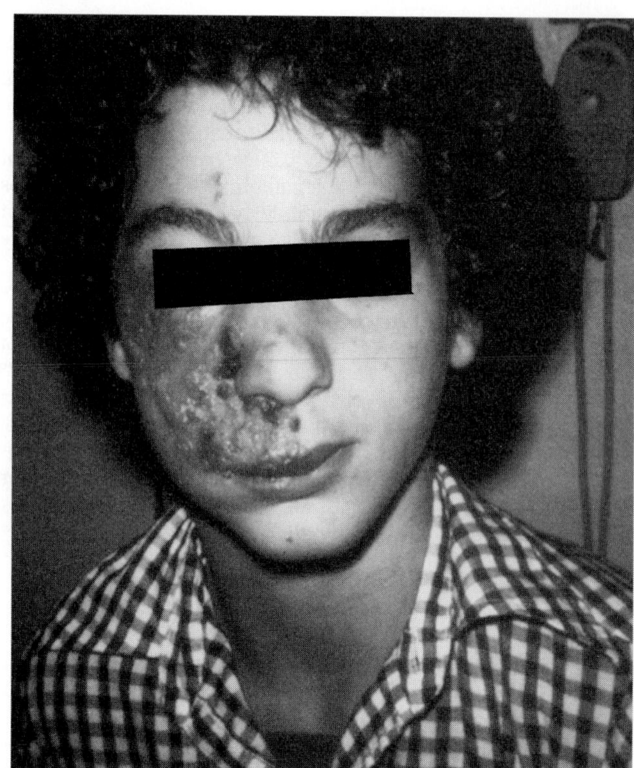

FIGURE 167–3 ■ Zoster in an otherwise healthy 10-year-old boy.

Zoster may be particularly severe and common after bone marrow transplantation; in the first year after undergoing transplantation, 20 to 70 percent of patients develop zoster.[44]

Diagnosis

CLINICAL DIAGNOSIS OF VARICELLA AND ZOSTER

Making a clinical diagnosis of VZV infection usually is not difficult because the vesicular rash is so characteristic. In questionable cases of varicella, epidemiologic information, such as a history of recent exposure to varicella or zoster and subsequent transmission of varicella to another person, may be useful. The differential diagnosis of varicella includes generalized HSV infection, rickettsial pox, impetigo, allergic reactions including Stevens-Johnson syndrome and poison ivy, and insect bites.

In one study of zoster, 13 percent of clinically diagnosed cases were proved by culture to be caused by HSV infection.[88] The unilateral rash of zoster most frequently appears on the trunk or face. The trigeminal nerve, most commonly the ophthalmic branch, is an especially significant site because the eye may be involved.

LABORATORY DIAGNOSIS

Laboratory diagnosis of VZV infection is facilitated by the presence of VZV in superficial skin lesions, where it is easily accessible for testing. The diagnosis is made best by the demonstration of specific viral antigens in skin scrapings or isolation of VZV from skin vesicles by immunofluorescence with a commercial monoclonal antibody to VZV that is conjugated to fluorescein.[56] This diagnostic method is highly sensitive and rapid and can be completed within approximately an hour.

The diagnosis also may be made by culture of virus from skin lesions. Vesicular fluid for culture should be obtained as early in the course of illness as possible for successful virus isolation. Within several days after the onset of varicella, vesicular fluid no longer is likely to be infectious, although viable VZV may be present in zoster lesions for a longer period, especially in immunocompromised patients. VZV cannot be isolated from skin lesions that have become pustular or dry. Isolation of VZV is a slow method because approximately 48 hours is required before the first signs of a viral cytopathic effect are seen. Virus isolation is less sensitive than immunofluorescence staining because infectious virus persists for a shorter time in vesicles and is more labile than are viral antigens. VZV rarely is isolated from cerebrospinal fluid (CSF) and respiratory secretions. Isolation of VZV or demonstration of viral antigen in material obtained from skin or other lesions or autopsy tissue is diagnostic of a current infection with VZV because, unlike other herpesviruses, no known carrier state or shedding of VZV by asymptomatic individuals exists. For the diagnosis of VZV infection, PCR testing of skin scrapings, vesicular fluid, respiratory secretions, and CSF has been used successfully.[16, 95, 101, 102]

Numerous serologic tests, including the fluorescent antibody to membrane antigen (FAMA) method,[151, 154] latex agglutination,[57, 129] and enzyme-linked immunosorbent assay (ELISA), are useful for measuring antibodies to VZV.[95, 122] Antibody to VZV develops within a few days after the onset of varicella, persists for many years, and is present before the onset of zoster. VZV infections may be documented by a fourfold or greater rise in VZV antibody titer in acute and convalescent serum specimens. Specific IgM in one serum specimen suggests recent VZV infection.[20] Persistence of VZV antibody beyond 8 months of age is highly suggestive of intrauterine varicella.[49] Immunity to varicella is very likely if a positive antibody titer to VZV is demonstrated on a single serum sample. However, serologic methods, particularly commercial ELISA assays, may fail to identify individuals who have been immunized.[129]

The value of serologic procedures for the diagnosis of zoster is limited. Heterologous increases in antibody titer against VZV in patients with HSV infection who previously had varicella may occur and has been ascribed to antigens common to the two viruses.[46]

Treatment

Traditionally, nonspecific measures, such as frequent bathing to discourage bacterial skin infection, antihistamines given orally, calamine lotion applied locally, oatmeal baths to decrease itching, and cutting fingernails short to discourage scratching have been used to treat varicella. Fever is controlled best with acetaminophen rather than aspirin, which may predispose to Reye syndrome.[74]

Useful specific antiviral therapy for VZV became available in the mid-1980s with the introduction of acyclovir, an inhibitor of DNA polymerase and a DNA chain terminator. The antiviral effect of acyclovir depends on its being phosphorylated in the body by virus-induced thymidine kinases, which accounts for its relative lack of toxicity.[149]

Patients with severe or potentially severe VZV infections should be treated with intravenous acyclovir (30 mg/kg/day for adults and adolescents and 1500 mg/m^2/day for children, both given in three divided doses). Orally administered acyclovir is less reliable for immunocompromised patients because only approximately 20 percent of this formulation is absorbed from the gastrointestinal tract and no data on its efficacy in high-risk patients have been published. Because acyclovir is excreted by the kidneys, patients with a creatinine clearance less than 50 mL/min/1.73 m^2 should receive one half to one third of this dosage. Intravenous acyclovir is infused for at least 1 hour, with maintenance fluids given both before and during the infusion. Providing adequate hydration is important to prevent renal damage from precipitation of the drug in the renal tubules. Other adverse effects of acyclovir include phlebitis, rash, nausea, and neurologic manifestations such as headache and tremor. In general, however, acyclovir is extremely well tolerated.

Early intravenous therapy should be instituted for patients at high risk for development of severe VZV infection, such as leukemic children and those who have undergone organ or bone marrow transplantation, to prevent the dissemination of VZV.[126, 148] Not only may this therapy be potentially lifesaving in immunocompromised patients, but it also prevents considerable morbidity from VZV infection. Children thought to be somewhat less immunocompromised, such as those with HIV infection but without AIDS, may be given a treatment trial with oral acyclovir under close medical supervision. For such patients not doing well, intravenous therapy should be started promptly. In zoster patients, the use of intravenous acyclovir is associated with more rapid healing of skin lesions and resolution of acute pain than if no specific treatment is given.[150]

Considerable controversy has ensued about the role of orally administered acyclovir for the treatment of varicella and zoster in otherwise healthy children because most of these infections are self-limited. Customarily, however, adults, who are at greater risk for development of severe infection, are treated. Oral dosages used are 80 mg/kg/day (in four divided doses) for children and 4 g/day (in five divided doses) for adults. Double-blind, placebo-controlled studies in healthy children given oral acyclovir at 80 mg/kg/day for 5 days or placebo beginning within 24 hours of the onset of varicella rash have revealed that the number of chickenpox skin lesions is reduced significantly by acyclovir. A modest benefit was derived from acyclovir; children who received it had fever for approximately 1 day less, but they did not return to school any more rapidly, nor did they have fewer complications of chickenpox.[13, 33]

Some evidence indicates that early administration of oral acyclovir may decrease the acute pain associated with zoster.[80] However, the need to administer specific therapy for zoster in otherwise healthy children for whom pain is not a particular problem rarely occurs.

A newer drug, penciclovir, has an action similar to that of acyclovir.[77] It is administered as famciclovir, a prodrug that when given orally is converted rapidly to penciclovir in the body. A major advantage of famciclovir is that it is administered only three times a day (1500 mg/day for an adult) whereas acyclovir is given four to five times daily. Penciclovir has an antiviral action similar to that of acyclovir. One study suggests that famciclovir given to elderly patients with zoster early in the course of infection decreases the duration of PHN, though not its incidence.[137] No data regarding whether varicella may be treated successfully with famciclovir exist, nor have any data on the use of famciclovir in immunocompromised patients or in children been published.

The prodrug of acyclovir, valacyclovir, also is given orally, reaches blood levels that are approximately three to four times higher than those of acyclovir, and has been shown in one study to be superior to acyclovir for treating zoster.[15] Neither valacyclovir nor famciclovir is licensed in the United States for use in children.

Of concern about the potential widespread use of acyclovir is that drug resistance may develop. At present, resistance is less a problem with VZV than with HSV, but VZV resistant to acyclovir has been reported in a few patients with underlying AIDS.[82] Foscarnet was licensed by the Food and Drug Administration for the treatment of VZV infections that are resistant to acyclovir and famciclovir. Foscarnet inhibits the synthesis of VZV DNA polymerase.[120, 121, 127] Intravenous foscarnet is given at a dosage of 180 mg/kg/day in two divided doses, adjusted according to renal function. The main toxicity of foscarnet is renal damage and electrolyte imbalance.[44]

Prognosis

The prognosis of varicella and zoster is excellent in children without underlying health problems. The outlook for immunocompromised patients receiving antiviral chemotherapy also is good, especially if treatment is begun at an early stage of the illness. In general, zoster carries a better prognosis than varicella does, possibly because it is a secondary infection. If the disease is diagnosed promptly, complications such as bacterial superinfections usually can be treated successfully with antimicrobials. In the prevaccine era, despite the availability of antiviral therapy and passive immunization, the Centers for Disease Control and Prevention (CDC) estimated that approximately 100 deaths from varicella occurred annually in the United States, mostly in children with no previous health problems. An epidemiologic study of more than 250,000 health maintenance organization records indicated that the rates of varicella in adolescents and young adults and the complication and hospitalization rates had increased in recent years by a factor of approximately 5.[24] The widespread use of varicella vaccine in the United States is expected to decrease sharply the morbidity and mortality rates from this illness.

Prevention

VZV is such an infectious agent that general measures are not useful for prevention of varicella in susceptible individuals. Some protection, however, can be acchieved by isolation of hospitalized patients, particularly in rooms with negative-pressure ventilation. Hospitalized patients with active VZV infection should be admitted to a private room, and hospital personnel and visitors should wash their hands before and after entering the room and wear masks, gowns, and gloves while in it. The CDC now recommends postexposure vaccination for healthy varicella-susceptible exposed individuals.[117]

PASSIVE IMMUNIZATION AGAINST VARICELLA WITH VZIG

Varicella-susceptible children at high risk for development of severe chickenpox should be passively immunized if they are closely exposed to someone with VZV infection. Administration of VZIG may be a lifesaving measure for a high-risk susceptible child; it may modify varicella or prevent it.

VZIG is a licensed product that is distributed in Massachusetts by the Massachusetts Public Health Biological Laboratory and elsewhere by the American Red Cross. Although VZIG has been shown to be effective when given within 3 days and perhaps as long as 5 days, it should be administered as soon as possible.[53] The dose is 1.25 mL (1 vial or 125 U) for every 10 kg of body weight, with a maximal dosage of 6 mL (5 vials or 625 U) intramuscularly. The cost of a vial is approximately $75. VZIG should be re-administered to high-risk susceptible individuals who are closely re-exposed 3 weeks after a first exposure.

VZIG is used for the prevention of severe varicella in varicella-susceptible children who have been closely exposed to varicella or zoster and are at high risk for development of severe or fatal chickenpox. This population includes immunocompromised children with cancer, newborn infants whose mothers have active varicella at the time of delivery, and hospitalized premature infants. Children at high risk should be considered to be susceptible to varicella if they have no history of having had chickenpox. False-positive antibody tests may occur in immunocompromised children, and, therefore, susceptible children may be identified serologically as immune; hence, a history of illness is a preferred indication of these patients' immune status. VZIG should be administered to VZV-exposed adults only if they have been proved serologically to be susceptible to chickenpox because most adults with a negative history of varicella actually are immune.

Patients with HIV infection, especially those with AIDS, have some increased risk for development of severe varicella, and their management should be similar to that of immunocompromised children with regard to VZIG. Even children who are receiving intravenous globulin for treatment of HIV infection should receive VZIG if they have no past history of varicella and close exposure has occurred.

Infants whose mothers have an onset of chickenpox 5 days or less before delivery or within 48 hours after delivery should be given 1 vial of VZIG as soon as possible after birth.[43] The transplacental route of infection and the immaturity of the immune system probably account for the severity of varicella in these infants.[43] Attack rates for varicella as high as 50 percent in infants exposed to mothers who have varicella have been reported despite the administration of VZIG.[43, 115] Passively immunized infants should be observed closely, but usually they can be managed as outpatients. Intravenous acyclovir should be reserved for the rare, passively immunized infant with varicella in whom an extensive skin rash (more than 200 vesicles) or possible pneumonia develops.[12]

Administration of VZIG to full-term infants who are exposed to VZV after they are 48 hours old is not necessary. VZIG is optional for newborn infants (under 1 week old) if their siblings at home have active varicella. Infants exposed to VZV after birth almost always have mild varicella. Although the reported mortality rate from varicella in children younger than 1 year of age is four times that in older children, both rates are exceedingly low, 8 per 100,000 cases and 2 per 100,000 cases, respectively.[114] The mortality rate for adults and for leukemic children receiving chemotherapy, in contrast, is 20 and 1000 times higher, respectively.[116]

VZIG is not useful to treat or prevent zoster, and whether giving VZIG to pregnant varicella-susceptible women who have been exposed to VZV will protect their fetus from congenital varicella syndrome is not known.

ACTIVE IMMUNIZATION AGAINST VARICELLA

Live attenuated varicella vaccine was developed in Japan almost 30 years ago. It was licensed in the United States in 1995 for healthy children and adults who are susceptible to varicella and has proved to be an extremely safe and well-tolerated vaccine.[17, 125] The most frequent adverse reaction is a mild rash that develops several weeks after vaccination in 5 percent of healthy children.[51, 58, 125, 146] These rashes usually are not serious, even in immunocompromised children, although the potential for transmission of the vaccine virus exists.[21, 136] The risk of transmission is present while the vaccinee has a rash, and it was found to be at least four times less than the chance of transmission of the wild-type virus from vaccinated children with underlying leukemia.[136] In healthy vaccinees, however, transmission of vaccine virus to others has proved to be an exceedingly rare occurrence, with only three documented instances after the distribution of as many as 20 million doses of vaccine in the United States.[125] Again, transmission occurred only when the vaccinee had a rash.

The risk from wild-type VZV is greater than the risk from vaccine-type VZV. After weighing the potential risks and benefits, immunization is recommended for hospital workers and persons whose varicella-susceptible family members are immunocompromised or pregnant.[117] Varicella is given generally to only healthy persons. Conceivably, immunocompromised individuals inadvertently exposed to a vaccinee with rash could be given VZIG. Individuals in whom an extensive VZV rash develops within 2 to 3 weeks after immunization are likely to have wild-type infection.[125] In such situations, PCR and restriction fragment length polymorphism (RFLP) analysis can be used to differentiate between wild-type and vaccine-type VZV.[95]

Live attenuated varicella vaccine is highly protective in healthy and immunocompromised children and in healthy adults, but not all vaccinees are protected completely. Approximately 10 to 20 percent may have a modified breakthrough illness after intimate exposure. Varicella vaccine has been virtually 100 percent effective in preventing severe varicella.[50, 125] The vaccine is highly effective in adults; after two doses, more than 75 percent of adults are completely protected from varicella.[45, 58, 122] In contrast, approximately 85 percent of healthy children are protected after only one dose of vaccine.[26, 84, 93, 139, 146, 147] Breakthrough varicella, however, almost always is a modified illness with fewer than 50 skin lesions and minimal systemic signs in children as well as adults. In one study, children with breakthrough varicella missed on average only 2 days of school.[142]

Loss of VZV antibodies occurs rarely in healthy vaccinated children, small numbers of whom have been monitored for as long as 20 years after immunization.[9, 84, 146] Booster doses of vaccine may be given safely to persons who have lost detectable antibodies, but whether boosters provide additional protective immunity is unknown.[51, 58, 141] Vaccinated leukemic children have a lower risk for acquisition of zoster than do their counterparts who have had natural infection, possibly because they have fewer opportunities for the development of latent infection.[72]

Many states now require varicella vaccination for children to attend daycare or school. In geographic areas where vaccine use in children younger than 3 years of age is 70 percent or more, the incidence of varicella has decreased sharply, not only in the vaccinated but in all age groups, a process indicative of herd immunity.[124] Postexposure prophylaxis with vaccine now is recommended by the CDC.

DRUG PROPHYLAXIS

Prophylaxis of varicella in exposed persons may be achieved by the administration of acyclovir.[10, 79, 99, 133] This approach is not recommended often, however, because the optimal dosage and timing of administration have not been studied in large groups of children, nor is it known whether long-term maintenance of immunity exists in all children. In the United States, prevention of varicella by vaccination is a preferable approach. Long-term acyclovir therapy may be used to prevent the development of zoster in patients who have undergone bone marrow transplantation; however, its value is questionable because zoster commonly develops after administration of acyclovir is stopped.[69]

REFERENCES

1. Annunziato, P., Lungu, O., Panagiotidis, C., et al.: Varicella-zoster virus proteins in skin lesions: Implications for a novel role of ORF29p in chickenpox. J. Virol. *74*:2005, 2000.
2. Argaw, T., Cohen, J., Klutch, M., et al.: Nucleotide sequences that distinguish Oka vaccine from parental Oka and other varicella-zoster virus isolates. J. Infect. Dis. *181*:1153, 2000.
3. Aronson, J., McSherry, G., Hoyt, L., et al.: Varicella in children with HIV infection. Pediatr. Infect. Dis. J. *11*:1004, 1992.
4. Arvin, A., Koropchak, C., Sharp, M., et al.: The T-lymphocyte response to varicella-zoster viral proteins. Adv. Exp. Med. Biol. *278*:71, 1990.
5. Arvin, A., Koropchak, C. M., and Wittek, A. E.: Immunologic evidence of reinfection with varicella-zoster virus. J. Infect. Dis. *148*:200, 1983.
6. Arvin, A. M.: Cell-mediated immunity to varicella-zoster virus. J. Infect. Dis. *166*(Suppl.):35, 1992.
7. Arvin, A. M., Pollard, R. B., Rasmussen, L., et al.: Selective impairment in lymphocyte reactivity to varicella-zoster antigen among untreated lymphoma patients. J. Infect. Dis. *137*:531, 1978.
8. Asano, Y., Itakura, N., Hiroishi, Y., et al.: Viremia is present in incubation period in nonimmunocompromised children with varicella. J. Pediatr. *106*:69, 1985.
9. Asano, Y., Suga, S., Yoshikawa, T., et al.: Experience and reason: Twenty year follow up of protective immunity of the Oka live varicella vaccine. Pediatrics *94*:524, 1994.
10. Asano, Y., Yoshikawa, T., Suga, S., et al.: Postexposure prophylaxis of varicella in family contact by oral acyclovir. Pediatrics *92*:219, 1993.
11. Baba, K., Yabuuchi, H., Takahashi, M., et al.: Immunologic and epidemiologic aspects of varicella infection acquired during infancy and early childhood. J. Pediatr. *100*:881, 1982.
12. Bakshi, S., Miller, T. C., Kaplan, M., et al.: Failure of VZIG in modification of severe congenital varicella. Pediatr. Infect. Dis. *5*:699, 1986.
13. Balfour, H. H., Kelly, J. M., Suarez, C. S., et al.: Acyclovir treatment of varicella in otherwise healthy children. J. Pediatr. *116*:633, 1990.
14. Berger, R., Florent, G., and Just, M.: Decrease of the lympho-proliferative response to varicella-zoster virus antigen in the aged. Infect. Immun. *32*:24, 1981.
15. Beutner, K. R., Friedman, D. J., Forszpaniak, C., et al.: Valaciclovir compared with acyclovir for improved therapy for herpes zoster in immunocompetent adults. Antimicrob. Agents Chemother. *39*:1546, 1995.
16. Bezold, G., Volkenandt, M., Gottlober, P., et al.: Detection of HSV and VZV in clinical swabs: Frequent inhibition of PCR as determined by internal controls. Mol. Diagn. *5*:279, 2001.
17. Black, S., Shinefield, H., Ray, P., et al.: Post marketing evaluation of the safety and effectiveness of varicella vaccine. Pediatr. Infect. Dis. *18*:1041, 1999.
18. Bocles, J. S., Ehrenkranz, N. J., and Marks, A.: Abnormalities of respiratory function in varicella pneumonia. Ann. Intern. Med. *60*:183, 1964.
19. Bradley, J. S., Schlievert, P. M., and Sample, T. G.: Streptococcal toxic shock–like syndrome as a complication of varicella. Pediatr. Infect. Dis. J. *10*:77, 1991.
20. Brunell, P., Gershon, A. A., Uduman, S. A., et al.: Varicella-zoster immunoglobulins during varicella, latency, and zoster. J. Infect. Dis. *132*:49, 1975.
21. Brunell, P. A., Shehab, Z., Geiser, C., et al.: Administration of live varicella vaccine to children with leukemia. Lancet *2*:1069, 1982.
22. Bruusgaard, E.: The mutual relation between zoster and varicella. Br. J. Dermatol. Syph. *44*:1, 1932.
23. Burke, B. L., Steele, R. W., Beard, O. W., et al.: Immune responses to varicella-zoster in the aged. Arch. Intern. Med. *142*:291, 1982.
24. Choo, P. W., Donahue, J. G., Manson, J. E., et al.: The epidemiology of varicella and its complications. J. Infect. Dis. *172*:706, 1995.
25. Christie, A. B.: Chickenpox. *In* Infectious Diseases: Epidemiology and Clinical Practice, Edinburgh, E. & S. Livingstone, 1969.
26. Clements, D., Moreira, S. P., Coplan, P., et al.: Postlicensure study of varicella vaccine effectiveness in a day-care setting. Pediatr. Infect. Dis. J. *18*:1047, 1999.
27. Croen, K. D., Ostrove, J. M., Dragovic, L. Y., et al.: Patterns of gene expression and sites of latency in human ganglia are different for varicella-zoster and herpes simplex viruses. Proc. Natl. Acad. Sci. U. S. A. *85*:9773, 1988.
28. Davison, A., Edson, C., Ellis, R., et al.: New common nomenclature for glycoprotein genes of varicella-zoster virus and their products. J. Virol. *57*:1195, 1986.
29. Davison, A. J.: Varicella-zoster virus. The Fourteenth Fleming Lecture. J. Gen. Virol. *72*:475, 1991.

30. Davison, A. J., and Scott, J. E.: The complete DNA sequence of varicella-zoster virus. J. Gen. Virol. *67*:1759, 1986.
31. Debrus, S., Sadzot-Delvaux, C., Nikkels, A. F., et al.: Varicella-zoster virus gene 63 encodes an immediate-early protein that is abundantly expressed during latency. J. Virol. *69*:3240, 1995.
32. Dumas, A. H., Geelen, J. L. M. C., Weststrate, M. W., et al.: XbaI, PstI, and BglII restriction enzyme maps of the two orientations of the varicella-zoster virus genome. J. Virol. *39*:390, 1981.
33. Dunkel, L., Arvin, A., Whitley, R., et al.: A controlled trial of oral acyclovir for chickenpox in normal children. N. Engl. J. Med. *325*:1539, 1991.
34. Dworsky, M., Whitely, R., and Alford, C.: Herpes zoster in early infancy. Am. J. Dis. Child. *134*:618, 1980.
35. Ecker, J. R., and Hyman, R. W.: Varicella zoster virus DNA exists as two isomers. Proc. Natl. Acad. Sci. U. S. A. *79*:156, 1982.
36. Esiri, M., and Tomlinson, A.: Herpes zoster: Demonstration of virus in trigeminal nerve and ganglion by immunofluorescence and electron microscopy. J. Neurol. Sci. *15*:35, 1972.
37. Feldman, S., Chaudhary, S., Ossi, M., et al.: A viremic phase for herpes zoster in children with cancer. J. Pediatr. *91*:597, 1977.
38. Feldman, S., Hughes, W., and Daniel, C.: Varicella in children with cancer: 77 cases. Pediatrics *80*:388, 1975.
39. Feldman, S., and Lott, L.: Varicella in children with cancer: Impact of antiviral therapy and prophylaxis. Pediatrics *80*:465, 1987.
40. Friedman, C. A., Temple, D. M., Robbins, K. K., et al.: Outbreak and control of varicella in a neonatal intensive care unit. Pediatr. Infect. Dis. J. *13*:152, 1994.
41. Garland, J.: Varicella following exposure to herpes zoster. N. Engl. J. Med. *228*:336, 1943.
42. Gershon, A.: Varicella-zoster virus: Prospects for control. Adv. Pediatr. Infect. Dis. *10*:93, 1995.
43. Gershon, A.: Chickenpox, measles, and mumps. *In* Remington, J., and Klein, J. (eds.): Infections of the Fetus and Newborn Infant. 5th ed. Philadelphia, W. B. Saunders, 2001.
44. Gershon, A.: Zoster in immunosuppressed patients. *In* Watson, C. P. N., and Gershon, A. (eds.): Herpes Zoster and Postherpetic Neuralgia. Amsterdam, Elsevier, 2001, p. 107.
45. Gershon, A. A., LaRussa, P., and Steinberg, S.: Live attenuated varicella vaccine: Current status and future uses. Semin. Pediatr. Infect. Dis. *2*:171, 1991.
46. Gershon, A., LaRussa, P., and Steinberg, S.: Varicella-zoster virus. *In* Murray, P. R. (ed.): Manual of Clinical Microbiology. Washington, DC, American Society for Microbiology, 1995, p. 895.
47. Gershon, A., LaRussa, P., Steinberg, S., et al.: The protective effect of immunologic boosting against zoster: An analysis in leukemic children who were vaccinated against chickenpox. J. Infect. Dis. *173*:450, 1996.
48. Gershon, A., Mervish, N., LaRussa, P., et al.: Varicella-zoster virus infection in children with underlying HIV infection. J. Infect. Dis. *176*:1496, 1997.
49. Gershon, A., Raker, R., Steinberg, S., et al.: Antibody to varicella-zoster virus in parturient women and their offspring during the first year of life. Pediatrics *58*:692, 1976.
50. Gershon, A. A., and Steinberg, S.: Persistence of immunity to varicella in children with leukemia immunized with live attenuated varicella vaccine. N. Engl. J. Med. *320*:892, 1989.
51. Gershon, A. A., and Steinberg, S.: Live attenuated varicella vaccine: Protection in healthy adults in comparison to leukemic children. National Institute of Allergy and Infectious Diseases. J. Infect. Dis. *161*:661, 1990.
52. Gershon, A., Steinberg, S., Borkowsky, W., et al.: IgM to varicella-zoster virus: Demonstration in patients with and without clinical zoster. Pediatr. Infect. Dis. *1*:164, 1982.
53. Gershon, A., Steinberg, S., and Brunell, P.: Zoster immune globulin: A further assessment. N. Engl. J. Med. *290*:243, 1974.
54. Gershon, A. A., Steinberg, S., Gelb, L., et al.: Clinical reinfection with varicella-zoster virus. J. Infect. Dis. *149*:137, 1984.
55. Gershon, A. A., Steinberg, S., Gelb, L., et al.: Live attenuated varicella vaccine: Efficacy for children with leukemia in remission. J. A. M. A. *252*:355, 1984.
56. Gershon, A., Steinberg, S., and LaRussa, P.: Varicella-zoster virus. *In* Lennette, E. H. (ed.): Laboratory Diagnosis of Viral Infections. 2nd ed. New York, Marcel Dekker, 1992, p. 749.
57. Gershon, A., Steinberg, S., and LaRussa, P.: Detection of antibodies to varicella-zoster virus by latex agglutination. Clin. Diag. Virol. *2*:271, 1994.
58. Gershon, A. A., Steinberg, S., LaRussa, P., et al.: Immunization of healthy adults with live attenuated varicella vaccine. J. Infect. Dis. *158*:132, 1988.
59. Gershon, A., Zhu, Z., Sherman, D. L., et al.: Intracellular transport of newly synthesized varicella-zoster virus: Final envelopment in the trans-Golgi network. J. Virol. *68*:6372, 1994.
60. Gilden, D. H., Dueland, A. N., Cohrs, R., et al.: Postherpetic neuralgia. Neurology *41*:1215, 1991.
61. Gilden, D. H., Kleinschmidt-DeMasters, B. K., LaGuardia, J. J., et al.: Neurologic complications of the reactivation of varicella-zoster virus. N. Engl. J. Med. *342*:635, 2000.
62. Gomi, Y., Imagawa, T., Takahashi, M., et al.: Oka varicella vaccine is distinguishable from its parental virus in DNA sequence of open reading frame 62 and its transactivation activity. J. Med. Virol. *61*:497, 2000.
63. Gordon, J. E.: Chickenpox: An epidemiologic review. Am. J. Med. Sci. *244*:362, 1962.
64. Gray, G. C., Palinkas, L. A., and Kelley, P. W.: Increasing incidence of varicella hospitalizations in United States Army and Navy personnel: Are today's teenagers more susceptible? Should recruits be vaccinated? Pediatrics *86*:867, 1990.
65. Grose, C.: Glycoproteins encoded by varicella-zoster virus: Biosynthesis, phosphorylation, and intracellular trafficking. Annu. Rev. Microbiol. *44*:59, 1990.
66. Grose, C., and Litwin, V.: Immunology of the varicella-zoster glycoproteins. J. Infect. Dis. *157*:877, 1988.
67. Grose, C. H.: Variation on a theme by Fenner. Pediatrics *68*:735, 1981.
68. Guess, H., Broughton, D. D., Melton, L. J., et al.: Epidemiology of herpes zoster in children and adolescents: A population-based study. Pediatrics *76*:512, 1985.
69. Guidelines for preventing opportunistic infections among hematopoietic stem cell transplant recipients. M. M. W. R. Recommen. Rep. *49*(RR-10):1–125, 2000.
70. Gustafson, T. L., Shehab, Z., and Brunell, P.: Outbreak of varicella in a newborn intensive care nursery. Am. J. Dis. Child. *138*:548, 1984.
71. Haiduven-Griffeths, D., and Fecko, H.: Varicella in hospital personnel: A challenge for the infection control practitioner. Am. J. Infect. Control *15*:207, 1987.
72. Hardy, I. B., Gershon, A., Steinberg, S., et al.: Incidence of zoster after live attenuated varicella vaccine. Paper presented at the International Conference on Antimicrobial Agents and Chemotherapy, 1991, Chicago.
73. Hardy, I. B., Gershon, A., Steinberg, S., et al.: The incidence of zoster after immunization with live attenuated varicella vaccine. A study in children with leukemia. N. Engl. J. Med. *325*:1545, 1991.
74. Haverkos, H. W., Amsel, Z., and Drotman, D. P.: Adverse virus-drug interactions. Rev. Infect. Dis. *13*:697, 1991.
75. Hay, J., and Ruyechan, W. T.: Varicella-zoster virus: A different kind of herpesvirus latency? Semin. Virol. *5*:241, 1994.
76. Head, H., Campbell, A. W.: The pathology of herpes zoster and its bearing on sensory localization. Brain *23*:353, 1900.
77. Hodge, R. A. V.: Review: Antiviral portrait series, Number 3. Famciclovir and penciclovir. The mode of action of famciclovir including its conversion to penciclovir. Antiviral Chem. Chemother. *4*:67, 1993.
78. Hope-Simpson, R. E.: The nature of herpes zoster: A long term study and a new hypothesis. Proc. R. Soc. Med. *58*:9, 1965.
79. Huang, Y.-C., Lin, T.-Y., and Chiu, C.-H.: Acyclovir prophylaxis of varicella after household exposure. Pediatr. Infect. Dis. J. *14*:152, 1995.
80. Huff, J. C., Bean, B., Balfour, H. H., et al.: Therapy of herpes zoster with oral acyclovir. Am. J. Med. *85*(2A):84, 1988.
81. Ihara, T., Starr, S., Ito, M., et al.: Human polymorphonuclear leukocyte–mediated cytotoxicity against varicella-zoster virus–infected fibroblasts. J. Virol. *51*:110, 1984.
82. Jacobson, M. A., Berger, T. G., and Fikrig, S.: Acyclovir-resistant varicella-zoster virus infection after chronic oral acyclovir therapy in patients with the acquired immunodeficiency syndrome. Ann. Intern. Med. *112*:187, 1990.
83. Jenkins, R. B.: Severe chickenpox encephalopathy. Am. J. Dis. Child. *110*:137, 1965.
84. Johnson, C., Stancin, T., Fattlar, D., et al.: A long-term prospective study of varicella vaccine in healthy children. Pediatrics *100*:761, 1997.
85. Johnson, R., and Milbourn, P. E.: Central nervous system manifestations of chickenpox. Can. Med. Assoc. J. *102*:831, 1970.
86. Junker, A. K., Angus, E., and Thomas, E.: Recurrent varicella-zoster virus infections in apparently immunocompetent children. Pediatr. Infect. Dis. J. *10*:569, 1991.
87. Jura, E., Chadwick, E., Josephs, S. H., et al.: Varicella-zoster virus infections in children infected with human immunodeficiency virus. Pediatr. Infect. Dis. J. *8*:586, 1989.
88. Kalman, C. M., and Laskin, O. L.: Herpes zoster and zosteriform herpes simplex virus infections in immunocompetent adults. Am. J. Med. *81*:775, 1986.
89. Kido, S., Ozaki, T., Asada, H., et al.: Detection of varicella-zoster virus (VZV) DNA in clinical samples from patients with VZV by the polymerase chain reaction. J. Clin. Microbiol. *29*:76, 1991.
90. Kinchington, P. R., and Cohen, J. I.: Viral proteins. *In* Arvin, A. M., and Gershon, A. A. (eds.): Varicella-Zoster Virus: Virology and Clinical Management. Cambridge, Cambridge University Press, 2000, p. 74.
91. Kjersem, H., and Jepsen, S.: Varicella among immigrants from the tropics, a health problem. Scand. J. Soc. Med. *18*:171, 1990.
92. Kundratitz, K.: Experimentelle Ubertragung von Herpes Zoster auf den Mensschen und die Beziehungen von Herpes Zoster zu Varicellen. Monatss. Kinder. *29*:516, 1925.
93. Kuter, B. J., Weibel, R. E., Guess, H. A., et al.: Oka/Merck varicella vaccine in healthy children: Final report of a 2-year efficacy study and 7-year follow-up studies. Vaccine *9*:643, 1991.
94. LaForet, E. G., and Lynch, L. L.: Multiple congenital defects following maternal varicella. N. Engl. J. Med. *236*:534, 1947.
95. LaRussa, P., Lungu, O., Hardy, I., et al.: Restriction fragment length polymorphism of polymerase chain reaction products from vaccine and wild-type varicella-zoster virus isolates. J. Virol. *66*:1016, 1992.

96. LaRussa, P., Steinberg, S., Seeman, M. D., et al.: Determination of immunity to varicella by means of an intradermal skin test. J. Infect. Dis. *152*:869, 1985.
97. Leclair, J. M., Zaia, J., Levin, M. J., et al.: Airborne transmission of chickenpox in a hospital. N. Engl. J. Med. *302*:450, 1980.
98. Lim, S. M., Song, S. W., Kim, S. L., et al.: Comparison between of the attenuated BR-Oka and the wild type strain of varicella zoster virus (VZV) on the DNA level. Arch. Pharm. Res. *23*:418, 2000.
99. Lin, T. Y., Huang, Y. C., Ning, H. C., et al.: Oral acyclovir prophylaxis of varicella after intimate contact. Pediatr. Infect. Dis. J. *16*:1162, 1997.
100. Locksley, R. M., Flournoy, N., Sullivan, K. M., et al.: Infection with varicella-zoster virus after marrow transplantation. J. Infect. Dis. *152*:1172, 1985.
101. Loparev, V. N., Argaw, T., Krause, P., et al.: Improved identification and differentiation of varicella-zoster virus (VZV) wild type strains and an attenuated varicella vaccine strain using a VZV open reading frame 62–based PCR. J. Clin. Microbiol. *38*:3156, 2000.
102. Loparev, V. N., McCaustland, K., Holloway, B. P., et al.: Rapid genotyping of varicella-zoster virus vaccine and wild type strains with fluorophore-labeled hybridization probes. J. Clin. Microbiol. *38*:4315, 2000.
103. Lungu, O., Annunziato, P., Gershon, A., et al.: Reactivated and latent varicella-zoster virus in human dorsal root ganglia. Proc. Natl. Acad. Sci. U. S. A. *92*:10980–10984, 1995.
104. Lungu, O., Panagiotidis, C., Annunziato, P., et al.: Aberrant intracellular localization of varicella-zoster virus regulatory proteins during latency. Proc. Natl. Acad. Sci. U. S. A. *95*:7080–7085, 1998.
105. Mahalingham, R., Wellish, M., Dueland, A. N., et al.: Localization of herpes simplex virus and varicella zoster virus DNA in human ganglia. Ann. Neurol. *31*:444, 1992.
106. Martin, J. H., Dohner, D., Wellinghoff, W. J., et al.: Restriction endonuclease analysis of varicella-zoster vaccine virus and wild type DNAs. J. Med. Virol. *9*:69, 1982.
107. Mendez, D., Sinclair, M. B., Garcia, S., et al.: Transplacental immunity to varicella-zoster virus in extremely low birthweight infants. Am. J. Perinatol. *9*:236, 1992.
108. Moore, D. A., and Hopkins, R. S.: Assessment of a school exclusion policy during a chickenpox outbreak. Am. J. Epidemiol. *133*:1161, 1991.
109. Myers, M., and Connelly, B. L.: Animal models of varicella. J. Infect. Dis. *166*(Suppl.):48, 1992.
110. Nader, S., Bergen, R., Sharp, M., et al. Comparison of cell-mediated immunity (CMI) to varicella-zoster virus (VZV) in children and adults immunized with live attenuated varicella vaccine. J. Infect. Dis. *171*:13, 1995.
111. Ozaki, T., Matsui, Y., Asano, Y., et al.: Study of virus isolation from pharyngeal swabs in children with varicella. Am. J. Dis. Child. *143*:1448, 1989.
112. Pearson, H. E.: Parturition varicella-zoster. Obstet. Gynecol. *23*:21, 1964.
113. Pitel, P. A., McCormick, K. L., Fitzgerald, E., et al:. Subclinical hepatic changes in varicella infection. Pediatrics *65*:631, 1980.
114. Preblud, S., Bregman, D. J., and Vernon, L. L.: Deaths from varicella in infants. Pediatr. Infect. Dis. *4*:503, 1985.
115. Preblud, S., Nelson, W. L., Levin, M., et al.: Modification of congenital varicella infection with VZIG. Paper presented at the Interscience Conference on Antimicrobial Agents and Chemotherapy, 1986, New Orleans, LA.
116. Preblud, S. R.: Varicella: Complications and costs. Pediatrics *76*(Suppl.):728, 1986.
117. Prevention of varicella. Update recommendations of the Advisory Committee on Immunization Practices (ACIP). M. M. W. R. Recomm. Rep. *48*(RR-6):1, 1999.
118. Raker, R., Steinberg, S., Drusin, L., et al.:. Antibody to varicella-zoster virus in low birth weight infants. J. Pediatr. *93*:505, 1978.
119. Ross, A. H., Lencher, E., and Reitman, G.: Modification of chickenpox in family contacts by administration of gamma globulin. N. Engl. J. Med. *267*:369, 1962.
120. Safrin, S., Berger, T., Gilson, I., et al.: Foscarnet therapy in five patients with AIDS and acyclovir-resistant varicella-zoster infection. Ann. Intern. Med. *115*:19, 1991.
121. Safrin, S., Crumpacker, C., Chatis, P., et al.: A controlled trial comparing foscarnet with vidarabine for acyclovir-resistant mucocutaneous herpes simplex in the acquired immunodeficiency syndrome. N. Engl. J. Med. *325*:551, 1991.
122. Saiman, L., LaRussa, P., Steinberg, S., et al.: Persistence of immunity to varicella-zoster virus vaccination among health care workers. Infect. Control Hosp. Epidemiol. *22*:279, 2001.
123. Sawyer, M. H., Wu, Y. N., Chamberlin, C. J., et al.: Detection of varicella-zoster virus DNA in the oropharynx and blood of patients with varicella. J. Infect. Dis. *166*:885, 1992.
124. Seward, J. F., Watson, B. M., Peterson, C. L., et al.: Varicella disease after introduction of varicella vaccine in the United States, 1995–2000. J. A. M. A. *287*:606, 2002.
125. Sharrar, R. G., LaRussa, P., Galea, S., et al.: The postmarketing safety profile of varicella vaccine. Vaccine *19*:916, 2000.
126. Shepp, D. H., Dandliker, P. S., and Meyers, J. D.: Treatment of varicella-zoster virus infection in severely immunocompromised patients: A randomized comparison of acyclovir and vidarabine. N. Engl. J. Med. *314*:208, 1986.
127. Smith, K., Kahlter, D. C., Davis, C., et al.: Acyclovir-resistant varicella zoster responsive to foscarnet. Arch. Dermatol. *127*:1069, 1991.
128. Srabstein, J. C., Morris, N., Larke, B., et al.: Is there a congenital varicella syndrome? J. Pediatr. *84*:239, 1974.
129. Steinberg, S., and Gershon, A.: Measurement of antibodies to varicella-zoster virus by using a latex agglutination test. J. Clin. Microbiol. *29*:1527, 1991.
130. Stern, E. S.: The mechanism of herpes zoster and its relation to chickenpox. Br. J. Dermatol. Syph. *49*:264, 1937.
131. Stevens, D., Ferrington, R., Jordan, G., et al.: Cellular events in zoster vesicles: Relation to clinical course and immune parameters. J. Infect. Dis. *131*:509, 1975.
132. Straus, S. E., Aulakh, H. S., Ruyechan, W. T., et al.: Structure of varicella-zoster virus DNA. J. Virol. *40*:516, 1981.
133. Suga, S., Yoshikawa, T., Ozaki, T., et al.: Effect of oral acyclovir against primary and secondary viraemia in incubation period of varicella. Arch. Dis. Child. *69*:639, 1993.
134. Triebwasser, J. H., Harris, R. E., Bryant, R. E., et al.: Varicella pneumonia in adults. Report of seven cases and a review of the literature. Medicine (Baltimore) *46*:409, 1967.
135. Trlifajova, J., Bryndova, D., and Ryc, M.: Isolation of varicella-zoster virus from pharyngeal and nasal swabs in varicella patients. J. Hyg. Epidemiol. Microbiol. Immunol. *28*:201, 1984.
136. Tsolia, M., Gershon, A., Steinberg, S., et al.: Live attenuated varicella vaccine: Evidence that the virus is attenuated and the importance of skin lesions in transmission of varicella-zoster virus. J. Pediatr. *116*:184, 1990.
137. Tyring, S., Barbarash, R. A., Nahlik, J. E., et al.: Famciclovir for the treatment of acute herpes zoster: Effects on acute disease and post herpetic neuralgia. Ann. Intern. Med. *123*:89, 1995.
138. Uduman, S. A., Gershon, A. A., and Brunell, P. A.: Should patients with zoster receive zoster immune globulin. J. A. M. A. *234*:1049, 1975.
139. Vazquez, M., LaRussa, P., Gershon, A., et al.: The effectiveness of the varicella vaccine in clinical practice. N. Engl. J. Med. *344*:955, 2001.
140. von Bokay, J.: Über den aetiologischen Zusammenhang der Varizellen mit gewissen Fallen von Herpes Zoster. Wien Klin. Wochenschr. *22*:1323, 1909.
141. Watson, B., Boardman, C., Laufer, D., et al.: Humoral and cell-mediated immune responses in healthy children after one or two doses of varicella vaccine. Clin. Infect. Dis. *20*:316, 1995.
142. Watson, B. M., Piercy, S. A., Plotkin, S. A., et al.: Modified chickenpox in children immunized with the Oka/Merck varicella vaccine. Pediatrics *91*:17, 1993.
143. Weber, D. J., Rutala, W. A., and Hamilton, H.: Prevention and control of varicella-zoster infections in healthcare facilities. Infect. Control Hosp. Epidemiol. *17*:694, 1996.
144. Weber, D. M., and Pellecchia, J. A.: Varicella pneumonia: Study of prevalence in adult men. J. A. M. A. *192*:572, 1965.
145. Weller, T. H.: Varicella and herpes zoster: Changing concepts of the natural history, control, and importance of a not-so-benign virus. N. Engl. J. Med. *309*:1362, 1983.
146. White, C. J., Kuter, B. J., Hildebrand, C. S., et al.: Varicella vaccine (VARIVAX) in healthy children and adolescents: Results from clinical trials, 1987 to 1989. Pediatrics *87*:604, 1991.
147. White, C. J., Kuter, B. J., Ngai, A., et al.: Modified cases of chickenpox after varicella vaccination: Correlation of protection with antibody response. Pediatr. Infect. Dis. J. *11*:19, 1992.
148. Whitley, R.: Therapeutic approaches to varicella-zoster virus infections. J. Infect. Dis. *166*(Suppl.):51, 1992.
149. Whitley, R. J., Middlebrooks, M., and Gnann, J. W.: Acyclovir: The past ten years. Adv. Exp. Med. Biol. *278*:243, 1990.
150. Whitley, R. J., and Straus, S.: Therapy for varicella-zoster virus infections: Where do we stand. Infect. Dis. Clin. Pract. *2*:100, 1993.
151. Williams, V., Gershon, A., and Brunell, P.: Serologic response to varicella-zoster membrane antigens measured by indirect immunofluorescence. J. Infect. Dis. *130*:669, 1974.
152. Wilson, A., Sharp, M., Koropchak, C., et al.: Subclinical varicella-zoster virus viremia, herpes zoster, and T lymphocyte immunity to varicella-zoster viral antigens after bone marrow transplantation. J. Infect. Dis. *165*:119, 1992.
153. Wilson, G., Talkington, D., Gruber, W., et al.: Group A streptococcal necrotizing fasciitis following varicella in children: Case reports and review. Clin. Infect. Dis. *20*:1333, 1995.
154. Zaia, J., and Oxman, M.: Antibody to varicella-zoster virus–induced membrane antigen: Immunofluorescence assay using monodisperse glutaraldehyde-fixed target cells. J. Infect. Dis. *136*:519, 1977.
155. Zaia, J. A., Leary, P. L., and Levin, M. J.: Specificity of the blastogenic response of human mononuclear cells to herpes antigens. Infect. Immun. *20*:646, 1978.

POXVIRIDAE

CHAPTER 168 Smallpox (Variola Virus)

JAMES D. CHERRY

Smallpox was a dreaded febrile exanthematous disease caused by the orthopoxvirus variola virus.[3–8, 14] After an extensive decade-long World Health Organization (WHO) program to eradicate smallpox, the world was certified free of smallpox in 1979.[46] This chapter reviews the history and clinical manifestations of smallpox. Virology and smallpox vaccination are presented in Chapter 169.

History[8, 11, 12, 14, 15, 24, 25, 45]

Evidence suggests that endemic smallpox was occurring before 1500 BC. Three mummies dating from the 18th to the 20th dynasties in Egypt had pustular lesions all over their bodies.[14] Reliable written accounts of smallpox first appeared during the fourth century. Smallpox was differentiated from measles in 340 AD by Ko Hung in China. At that time in China, smallpox was an established endemic disease that had come from the west 300 years earlier. During the period from 340 to 1000 AD, the disease was described in Egypt, India, Korea, Japan, southern Europe, and North Africa. A major contribution to the spread of smallpox was the great Islamic expansion across North Africa and into Spain in the seventh and eighth centuries.

By the year 1000, smallpox probably was endemic in populated areas of Europe, Asia, and the African Mediterranean countries. Smallpox was established further in northern Europe by the population movements related to the Crusades. By the 16th century, smallpox was a serious disease in Europe, as indicated by death statistics in Geneva, London, and Sweden. In London during the 17th century, approximately 10 percent of the yearly deaths were attributed to smallpox.

The disease was introduced into the American colonies in 1507 and into Mexico soon thereafter. Epidemics of smallpox posed serious problems for the colonists, as well as for the Native Americans. These epidemics also may have been important in certain stages of the American Revolution.[5, 16] Smallpox persisted in the United States and Mexico until the 1940s and 1950s, respectively, despite concerted efforts to eliminate the problem.

Soon after recognition of this disease, the Chinese are reported to have made efforts to prevent it. The technique used presumably was variolation, the intentional intranasal or intracutaneous inoculation of susceptible persons with vesicular fluid or crusts from smallpox patients. This technique apparently originated in China and subsequently was used in many countries, including the United States. As recently as 1968 and 1969, isolated instances of variolation were noted in remote areas of Africa and Asia.[16, 25]

After making his observations in 1796 on the immunity against smallpox that was conferred by inoculation with material obtained from cowpox lesions, Jenner extended his research to include intentional and deliberate exposure of some of those immunized with cowpox. This strategy provided convincing evidence of solid protection against smallpox.[28] Encouraged by the results, he predicted in 1801 the ultimate eradication of smallpox, a remarkable prediction indeed.[16, 19]

The Intensified Smallpox Eradication Program of the WHO, established in 1967, initiated remarkable progress toward total global eradication of this disease.[24] Several factors responsible for this rapid progress included emphasis on surveillance of disease, with containment rather than routine vaccination; improved vaccines and vaccination technology; and sound administrative and fiscal support.[16, 17, 22, 24, 32] Of the more than 30 countries in 1967 in which smallpox was endemic, the disease persisted in only 5 in 1975 and in 2 in 1977. The world's last case of endemic smallpox occurred on October 31, 1977, in Merca, Somalia.[10] A year later, in 1978, a photographer working at the University of Birmingham in England was infected with a laboratory strain of smallpox virus and died.[43]

After the world eradication of smallpox, the World Health Assembly in 1980 recommended that all countries cease vaccination.[46] Subsequently, a WHO expert committee recommended that all laboratories throughout the world destroy their stocks of variola virus or transfer them into either of two WHO reference laboratories.[23] The laboratories were the Russian State Research Center on Virology and Biotechnology, Koltsovo, Novosibirsk Region, and the Centers for Disease Control and Prevention (CDC) in Atlanta, Georgia.[4] Reportedly, all countries complied with this recommendation.

The WHO committee at a later date recommended that all variola virus stocks be destroyed by 1999, and the World Health Assembly concurred with this recommendation.[6] In 1998, a committee of the Institute of Medicine reviewed the possible importance of retaining variola virus for research purposes.[27] In May 1999, the World Health Assembly agreed to postpone the destruction of all variola stocks until 2002.[18]

In the early 1990s, evidence revealed that during the previous 10 years the Soviet government apparently had developed a successful program to produce variola virus for use as a biologic weapon.[23, 41] In the late 1990s, concern increased with regard to bioterrorism and, in particular, with the possibility that Russian expertise and equipment might have fallen into non-Russian hands because financial support for laboratories and workers had declined.

Smallpox has the dubious distinction of being used as a biologic weapon almost 250 years ago.[11] In the French and Indian Wars (1754 to 1767), British forces sent smallpox-contaminated blankets and handkerchiefs to the Indians surrounding Fort Pitt in the summer of 1763.

Etiology

Smallpox is caused by variola virus, an orthopoxvirus.[15, 24, 35] The virus particles are brick shaped and measure 250 to 300 × 200 to 250 × 100 nm; the size and shape are similar for all orthopoxviruses. The distinctive appearance is helpful in rapidly identifying members of this virus group by electron microscopy of vesicular fluid or crusts. The virus is stable when dried and may remain viable for long periods in dried crusts and indefinitely under freeze-drying techniques in the laboratory. It is propagated readily on the chorioallantoic membrane of embryonated eggs and in a variety of mammalian cell cultures.

Epidemiology

In infected patients, variola virus was found in respiratory secretions and in vesicular fluid from skin lesions. Transmission most often took place after close personal contact, but airborne spread also could occur.[24, 23, 44] Patients with smallpox were most infectious from the onset through the first 7 to 10 days of rash.

All persons were susceptible to smallpox unless they previously had been infected with variola virus itself or with cowpox or vaccinia virus. Thus, the occurrence of smallpox depended entirely on the presence of a source of infection and effective exposure of susceptible persons. The age distribution of cases varied in individual countries, largely depending on vaccination practices. Preschool children often were not vaccinated and thus had the greatest prevalence of disease.

The seasonal influence was substantial and perhaps is shown best by the spread of disease after the winter and spring introduction of smallpox into Europe; spread of infection was more than 30 times as great after the introduction of infection into European nations between December and May, in contrast to substantially less frequent spread after introduction between June and November.[26]

Substantial contrast in case-fatality rates was recognized in different geographic areas; these differences did not seem to depend on the supportive care available and did not appear to be related to ethnic or specific resistance factors. The only logical explanation for these different rates was substantial differences in the virulence of the virus prevalent in the regions. The mildest form of smallpox, described as variola minor, or alastrim, was prevalent in Brazil, Ethiopia, and adjacent countries. Case-fatality rates of 1 percent or less were customary, and permanent residual scarring and blindness were most unusual occurrences. In other areas of Africa and Indonesia, the disease appeared to be of intermediate severity, whereas on the Indian subcontinent, case-fatality rates were as high as 30 percent, with residual permanent scarring, blindness, and other sequelae occurring frequently in those who survived the acute illness.[16]

Pathology

The characteristic pathologic lesions affected the skin and mucous membranes. They involved the deeper layers of the skin and progressed through macular, papular, vesicular, and pustular stages, with the subsequent formation of crusts. Lesions similar to those on the skin also were found in the lower respiratory and gastrointestinal tracts.

Secondary bacterial infection occurred frequently and often affected the skin and lungs. Hemorrhagic complications (hemorrhagic smallpox) were not uncommon events.

Clinical Manifestations[12, 24, 31]

After an incubation period of between 7 and 17 days, the disease began abruptly with fever (temperatures between 38.9° C and 40.5° C [102° F and 105° F]), headache, and marked malaise.[6a] Backache and muscle pain were prominent symptoms. Nausea, vomiting, and abdominal pain also were present.

After these prodromal signs and symptoms were present for 2 to 4 days, the fever usually decreased, and the characteristic cutaneous eruption appeared. The rash was most extensive on the face and extremities, and the individual lesions passed through the stages of macules and papules; by the third or fourth day, they clearly were vesicular. Lesions in a single area of the body were characteristically at the same stage of development.

By the sixth day, the vesicular fluid usually was cloudy and the individual pustules frequently were umbilicated. Pustules often converged and become confluent. By the 10th day, the individual lesions began to dry and formed characteristic crusts that remained intact for several days before they were shed. The patient's temperature customarily fell during the early appearance of the rash, although the fever usually returned. Significant fever after the 10th or 12th day of disease suggested the presence of bacterial superinfection.

Although most cases were similar to this description, which was characteristic of the ordinary type of smallpox, other clinical variations were described. The hemorrhagic type was the most severe form, with a case-fatality rate that approached 100 percent. In this form, hemorrhagic manifestations appeared during the prodromal stage, with extensive cutaneous extravasation of blood and bleeding from the various body orifices. Death usually occurred within the first week of illness, and frequently, few typical diagnostic lesions appeared on the skin surfaces before death. Fortunately, this form of disease occurred in only 2 or 3 percent of the total cases of variola major in Asia, and it rarely was seen elsewhere.

A flat variety had been reported in approximately 6 percent of cases observed in India. In this variety, the cutaneous lesions remained flat and soft to touch, in contrast to the ordinary variety; these lesions characteristically resolved without pustulation. This form was associated with case-fatality rates of 75 to 96 percent.[16]

A modified form of disease occurred almost exclusively in previously vaccinated persons. Although the prodromal illness often was severe, skin lesions were few, evolved rapidly, and were more superficial; the prognosis was excellent.

The mildest form of the disease, alastrim or variola minor, was caused by a specific variola virus with less pathogenicity in humans. Serious forms of the illness, as with variola major, were unusual. The skin lesions tended to be superficial, and the clinical course resembled that of varicella, with the exception of the distribution of cutaneous lesions. They involved the face and extremities, in contrast to the characteristic central body distribution of varicella. Residual scarring, if it occurred at all, usually reflected secondary bacterial infection of individual lesions.

In recently vaccinated persons, asymptomatic infection with variola virus after exposure had been demonstrated by increases in antibody titer against the virus when acute and convalescent sera were tested. This event was uncommon and of neither clinical nor epidemiologic significance.

Complications included hemorrhagic events and various secondary bacterial infections, including impetigo, pneumonia, empyema, and otitis media. Nephritis and arthritis with permanent joint changes were described.

Differential Diagnosis

The typical course, the characteristic cutaneous lesions, and the presence of other cases after contact 7 to 17 days earlier left little doubt of the etiologic agent. Varicella presented the greatest problem in differential diagnosis, particularly from the variola minor or alastrim form of the disease, but the distribution of cutaneous lesions for each was characteristic. Generalized vaccinia or eczema vaccinatum was distinguished by a history of exposure to vaccinia virus, previous skin lesions, and the distribution of the rash. Impetigo (especially the bullous variety caused by staphylococcal infection), scabies, secondary syphilis, and yaws were other considerations. Usually, little difficulty was encountered clinically in distinguishing among these infections.

Monkeypox resembled smallpox clinically, but it occurred only in central and western Africa, primarily in the Democratic Republic of Congo. Specific laboratory procedures were required for diagnosis.[26]

Other conditions that were included in the differential diagnosis included erythema multiforme, pityriasis rosea, measles, rickettsialpox, disseminated herpes simplex infection, syphilis, enteroviral exanthems, and bacterial, viral, and rickettsial petechial and purpuric rashes.

Specific Diagnosis

Several laboratory procedures are available to provide specific and accurate diagnosis.

Vesicular fluid, crusts, or scrapings from skin lesions reveal the characteristic brick-shaped viral particles of the variola-vaccinia virus group when examined by electron microscopy. These orthopoxviruses differ in appearance from the herpesviruses, which in the past were the agents most frequently confused with smallpox. Electron microscopy is precise and rapid and is preferred when facilities for this examination are available.[9] Smallpox virus DNA also can be identified rapidly by polymerase chain reaction (PCR).[12, 13, 30, 39] PCR has an advantage over electron microscopy in that it can specifically distinguish smallpox virus from the orthopoxviruses.

Orthopoxviruses may be recovered and propagated on the chorioallantoic membrane of embryonated eggs or in tissue culture.[12] Recovery of the virus requires more time (3 to 7 days) than the direct antigen-detection tests do, but it provides the specific active virus required for differentiation among the various orthopoxvirus types.[36, 38]

Infection also can be determined serologically by using acute-phase and convalescent-phase sera in enzyme-linked immunosorbent assays, Western blotting, or virus neutralization assays.[12]

Treatment

Therapy primarily was supportive and symptomatic. The skin was kept clean, the bed linen was changed at regular intervals, and local or systemic therapy was provided for treatment of the frequent bacterial complications. Attention given to appropriate fluid and nutritional support was required.

Methisazone, convalescent smallpox serum, and vaccinia immune globulin (VIG) were effective in preventing the disease after exposure, but no evidence showed that these agents altered the course of the disease once symptoms occurred.[29] Idoxuridine was used for corneal lesions.[5]

At the present time, methisazone is not available, and the supply of VIG is very limited. Recent studies with the antiviral cidofovir indicate that this agent may be useful for the treatment of smallpox.[7]

Prevention

ACTIVE IMMUNIZATION

Many strains of vaccinia virus were used in the effective prophylaxis of smallpox. In 1967, at least 15 strains were in use in various countries.[1] In the late 1960s and 1970s, most vaccinations were performed with the New York City Board of Health strain or the Lister (Elstree) strain, which were similar. They were prepared by the freeze-drying process, and inoculation was performed best with use of a bifurcated needle, with 5 (for primary immunization) to 15 (for revaccination) punctures within a small (5 mm in diameter) area of the skin of the upper left deltoid region. The vaccination site was not to be covered tightly, although a loose, dry dressing was applied during the height of the reaction for decreasing the possibility of transferring the vaccinia virus by fingers to the eye or to skin lesions, such as insect bites or impetigo lesions, and so on. A small, but definite risk of complications, both local and neurologic, was associated with vaccination.[33, 37] Other aspects of immunization in the present era are presented in Chapter 169.

The Advisory Committee on Immunization Practices (ACIP) in June of 2001 made recommendations for the use of smallpox vaccine to protect persons who may need to work with orthopoxviruses and to prepare for a possible bioterrorism attack. Before the terrorist attacks in the Fall of 2001, the Department of Health and Human Services undertook a program to increase public health preparedness by attempting to expand the existing stockpiles of smallpox vaccine through the purchase of vaccine produced in cell culture. The additional purchase of vaccine was initiated to address the perceived vulnerability to future terrorist attacks, including those that may involve biologic agents. This additional vaccine, when added to the capability of diluting the smallpox vaccine stored at the CDC, along with vaccine discovered in the inventory of a pharmaceutical manufacturer is sufficient to immunize the entire population of the United States. Recent studies have shown that the current supply of vaccine is viable and in good titer. However, attempts to dilute the vaccine to titers less than 10^7 pfu/mL may reduce the rate of successful vaccination.[18a, 18b]

The primary strategy used to control an outbreak of smallpox and interdict the transmission of virus has been known as a surveillance and containment (ring vaccination) strategy. This strategy identifies infected persons through intensive surveillance and subsequently both isolates the individuals with the disease and vaccinates household and close contacts of the infected patient. Vaccination also would be recommended under this scenario for contacts of the primary contact with the patient (so-called secondary contacts). This strategy was instrumental in the eradication of smallpox as a naturally occurring disease. Depending upon the size of any smallpox outbreak and the availability of resources for rapid and thorough contact tracing, ring vaccination was supplemented previously in areas with identified smallpox cases to include voluntary vaccination of all those individuals without vaccine contraindications. This strategy was pursued to expand the ring of immune individuals within an outbreak area and reduce further the chance of any secondary transmission of smallpox to patients occurring before they could be identified and isolated.

Most recently, the ACIP reconsidered its recommendations for the use of smallpox vaccine. In so doing, they considered the following factors: the level of disease risk or threat, the expected severe adverse reactions to vaccination, the supply of vaccinia immune globulin that might be available, vaccine supply, vaccine deployment, and vaccination capacity at the state and local levels. In addition to these factors, the following additional assumptions were made: (1) vaccine currently is available only under an investigational new drug protocol and requires appropriate informed consent, patient follow-up, and oversight administratively by federal, state, and local public health officials; (2) based on the information available at the time of their meeting, the risk for smallpox occurring as a result of a deliberate release by terrorists was considered to be low although not zero; (3) the epidemiology of person-to-person transmission after a bioterrorism release of smallpox would be consistent with prior experience; (4) vaccinia vaccine and vaccine immune globulin would be available for use in sufficient supply and handled and administered appropriately; and (5) appropriate screening for contraindications to vaccination would be implemented and would include both vaccinated persons and their contacts, and recommended precautions would be taken to minimize the risks of adverse events occurring among vaccinees as well as among their close contacts; (6) health care workers and others would be afforded protection from infection through appropriate infection control measures, including use of appropriate personal protective equipment; and (7) surveillance and containment was considered the strategy for control and containment of smallpox and, furthermore, state and local health departments were presumed to have the capacity to vaccinate their entire population of their areas within a period of several weeks if so indicated.

The CDC has developed protocols to permit rapid, simultaneous delivery of smallpox vaccine to every state in United States territory within 12 to 24 hours. Smallpox response planning at the federal level now has been conveyed to state and local health departments in order to address the rapid distribution of the vaccine if vaccination programs are suggested.

The CDC currently recommends that cases of febrile rash illnesses for which smallpox is considered in the differential diagnosis should be reported immediately to local or state health departments, or both. After evaluation is performed by local or state health departments, if smallpox laboratory diagnostics are considered necessary, the CDC Rash Illness Evaluation Team should be consulted at 770-488-7100 or 404-639-2888. At this time, laboratory confirmation for smallpox is available routinely only at the CDC. Both a clinical consultation and a preliminary laboratory diagnosis can be completed within a period of 8 to 24 hours.

To assist the public health and other medical personnel in evaluating the possibility of smallpox in patients who present with febrile rash illnesses, the CDC has developed a rash illness assessment algorithm. Copies of this algorithm are available from state health departments and may be viewed on the CDC web site at *http://www.cdc.gov/nip/small pox/poster-protocol.pdf*. Orders for copies of this poster can be made over the internet at *https://www2.cdc.gov/nchstp_od/PIWeb/niporderform.asp*. Updated additional information can be found on the CDC interim smallpox response plan and guidelines at the following website: *http://www.bt.cdc.gov/DocumentsApp/Smallpox/RPG/index.asp*.

Medical evaluation of the current risks of smallpox compared to the potential risks of vaccine complications was such that the ACIP concluded that under current conditions and in the absence of a case of smallpox or a confirmed smallpox bioterrorism threat, vaccination of the general population was not recommended because they considered the potential benefits of vaccination did not outweigh the risks of vaccine complications. It is possible, however, that a decision to immunize the population of the United States may be made based on other than solely medical facts to include the threat of economic disruption should a case of smallpox be reported in the United States.

Smallpox vaccination was recommended for persons predesignated by the appropriate bioterrorism and public health authorities to be responsible for direct patient contact and investigation of the initial cases of smallpox. They further recommended that to enhance public health preparedness in response for smallpox control, specific teams of the federal, state, and local levels should be established to investigate and facilitate the diagnostic work-up of the initial suspect case of smallpox and to initiate control measures. Designated smallpox response teams might include persons designated as medical team leader, public health advisor, medical epidemiologists, disease investigators, diagnostic laboratory scientists, nurse vaccinators, and other security personnel. Such teams also may include medical personnel who would assist in the evaluation of suspected smallpox cases.

The ACIP recommended that each state and territorial plan include no less than one smallpox response team. Considerations for additional teams should take into account population and geographic considerations and should be developed in accordance with federal, state and local bioterrorism plans. Moreover, smallpox vaccination was recommended for selected persons predesignated by the appropriate bioterrorism and public health authorities who would provide care for smallpox cases in health care facilities to which such cases would be referred.

The risk of adverse events occurring with vaccinia (smallpox) vaccine is presumed potentially to be at least as severe and frequent as those that occurred during the era when universal vaccinia vaccination was performed (Figs. 168–1 through 168–5; see Color Plates I and II). One might suspect that the number of adverse reactions may be increased in frequency in the current era compared to the 1960s and 1970s because a larger proportion of the population of the United States and the world may have an inherited or acquired form of immunodeficiency or may be receiving a variety of agents that suppress the immune system. Acquired immunodeficiency disease (AIDS) is a new disease that has appeared since the discontinuation of use of smallpox vaccine. Individuals with AIDS might be unusually susceptible to adverse reactions from smallpox vaccine. Moreover, survivors of many forms of cancer, through the use of immunosuppressive agents and radiations, are much more prevalent today than in the era when universal vaccination was carried out.

The number of adverse events per million doses of primary smallpox vaccination and revaccination is reported in Table 168–1. The rates described are based on surveys of vaccination complications that occurred in the late 1960s in the United States. Whether the growth of vaccine in tissue culture rather than on calf skin will change the neurotropism of vaccinia virus is not known. The high prevalence of

TABLE 168–1 ■ RATES OF REPORTED COMPLICATIONS ASSOCIATED WITH VACCINIA VACCINATION (CASES/MILLION VACCINATIONS)

Age (yr) and Status Total*	Inadvertent Inoculation	Generalized Vaccinia	Eczema Vaccinatum	Progressive Vaccinia	Postvaccinial Encephalitis	Total
			Primary			
<1	507.0	394.4	14.1	—†	42.3	1549.3
1–4	577.3	233.4	44.2	3.2	9.5	1261.8
5–19	371.2	139.7	34.9	—	8.7	855.9
>/20	606.1	212.1	30.3	—	—	1515.2
Overall Rates	529.2	241.5	38.5	1.5	12.3	1253.8
			Revaccination			
<1	—	—	—	—	—	—
1–4	109.1	—	—	—	—	200.0
5–19	47.7	9.9	2.0	—	—	85.5
>/20	25.0	9.1	4.5	6.8	4.5	113.6
Overall Rates	42.1	9.0	3.0	3.0	2.0	108.2

*Rates of overall complications by age group include complications not provided in this table, including severe local reactions, bacterial superinfection of the vaccination site, and erythema multiforme.

†No instances of this complication were identified during the 1968 10-state survey.

From Lane, J. M., Ruben, F. L., Neff, J. M., and Millar, J. D.: Complications of smallpox vaccination, 1968: Results of 10 statewide surveys. J. Infect. Dis. *122*: 303–309, 1970.

immunosuppression in the United States today as compared to the late 1960s might render the rates of vaccinia necrosum higher than those which occurred in 1968. The rate of postvaccinial encephalitis in adults was difficult to document in the 1960s because very few adults were primary vaccinees. Studies performed in Europe showed higher rates of postvaccinial encephalitis in adults than in young children.

Inadvertent inoculation at sites other than those at which the vaccine was administered was the most frequent complication and accounted for nearly one half of all complications of primary vaccination or revaccination (see Fig. 168–2). Most of these lesions healed without therapy. Vaccinia immune globulin was useful for cases of ocular implantation.

Progressive vaccinia, a potentially fatal complication of vaccination, occurred almost exclusively in immunocompromised individuals (see Fig. 168–5).

Approximately 15 to 25 percent of vaccinees who developed postvaccinial encephalitis died, and an additional 25 percent had permanent neurologic sequelae. Most of the deaths caused by vaccination were the results of postvaccinial encephalitis or progressive vaccinia.

The CDC also has prepared estimates derived from vaccinia immune globulin distribution data from the 1960s of the population at risk and estimates of the proportion of at-risk vaccinees and contacts who would develop severe adverse reactions. Using two different methods for calculation, vaccinia immune globulin needs were estimated to be approximately 80/1,000,000 persons in a postevent vaccination scenario. If vaccination were provided pre-event, the risk of adverse events might be lower because vaccination could be deferred for patients with a contraindication to such immunization. Individuals who are immunocompromised because of cancer or the therapy of this disorder, who are known to have infection with the human immunodeficiency virus, or who may be receiving immunosuppressive therapy for any other reason could be identified readily and vaccination deferred in these cases.

PASSIVE IMMUNIZATION AND ANTIVIRAL PROTECTION

Transient protection after exposure was provided by VIG when available.[29] Because this material was often in short supply, the use of methisazone was considered, although this drug was not licensed and was available only on special request. When used prophylactically, methisazone provided some measure of protection. Vomiting was a frequent side effect, and dosing presented problems in some persons.

CONTROL OF SOURCES OF INFECTION

All known contacts of cases needed to be vaccinated or revaccinated promptly and kept under surveillance until at least 17 days transpired after the last contact with a known case. When fever developed in such persons, prompt isolation was required until the nature of the illness was determined. All personnel in contact with an index case or involved in the surveillance of contacts needed to be vaccinated or revaccinated.

Environmental isolation and disinfection precautions also were required because the virus persisted in crusts for many months. Proper double wrapping and disinfection of all articles leaving the patient's room were necessary. Precautions also were required to prevent transfer of crusts by the shoes or clothing of personnel to areas outside the isolation unit. Isolation precautions for the patient were necessary until all crusts had been shed. After recovery or death of the patient, terminal disinfection of the room was required.

CONCERN REGARDING SMALLPOX IN THE 21ST CENTURY

Increased concern relating to biologic terrorism occurred during the last decade, and the events of September 11, 2001, and immediately thereafter brought home the potential reality of this threat for the present and future.[2, 7, 20, 21, 23, 34, 42] As of 2002, only approximately 20 percent of the U.S. population has any immunity to smallpox.[20] The only antiviral available, which is unproven but may be effective, is cidofovir.[7, 23] New tissue culture–derived vaccines are being developed.[7, 40]

REFERENCES

1. Arita, I.: The control of vaccine quality in the smallpox eradication programme: International Symposium on Smallpox Vaccine, Bilthoven. Symp. Series Immunobiol. Standards *19*:79–87, 1972.

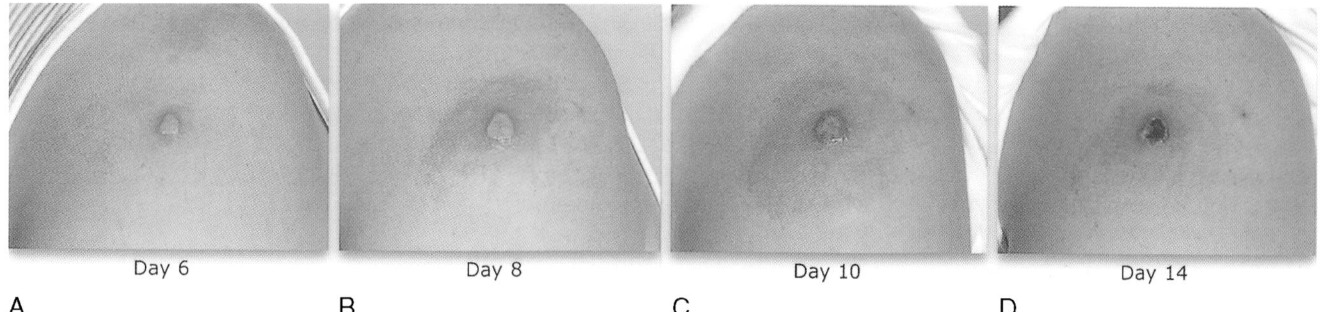

FIGURE 168–1 ■ *A–D,* Typical sequential appearance of the response ("take") following primary smallpox vaccination in a child.

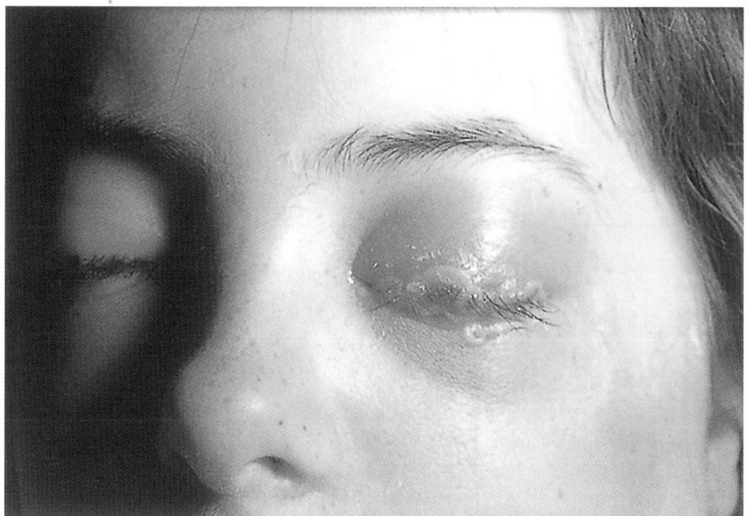
FIGURE 168–2 ■ Accidental implantation of vaccinia virus, after primary vaccination, by autoinoculation or contact transfer.

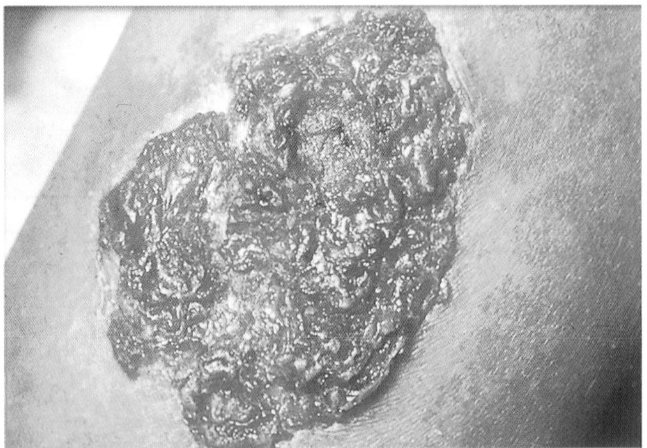

FIGURE 168–3 ■ Secondary bacterial infection at the site of primary vaccination.

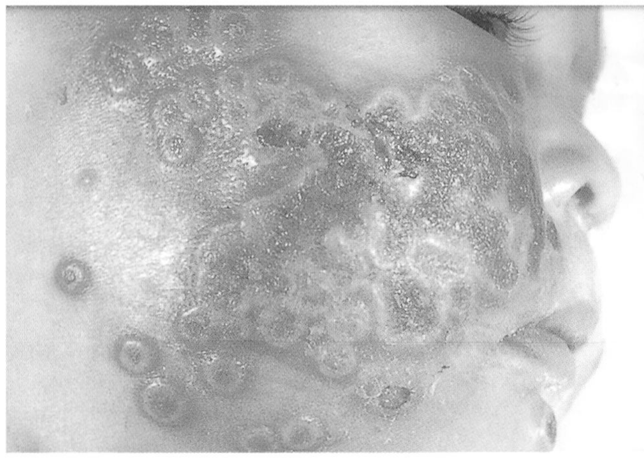

FIGURE 168–4 ■ Eczema vaccinatum. Accidental implantation of vaccinia virus in a child with eczema.

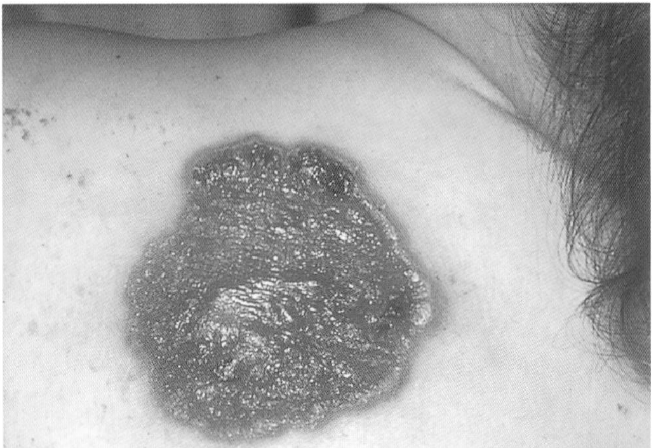

FIGURE 168–5 ■ Progressive vaccinia in an immunocompromised person who was inadvertently vaccinated.

2. Barbera, J., Macintyre, A., Gostin, L., et al.: Large-scale quarantine following biological terrorism in the United States. J. A. M. A. *286*:2711–2717, 2001.
3. Behbehani, A. M.: The smallpox story: Historical perspective. Globally eradicated today, smallpox once killed scores of people over thousands of years. A. S. M. News *57*:571–576, 1991.
4. Beman, J. G., and Arita, I.: The confirmation and maintenance of smallpox eradication. N. Engl. J. Med. *303*:1263–1273, 1980.
5. Benenson, A. S.: Smallpox. *In* Wehrle, P. F., and Top, F. H. (eds.): Communicable and Infectious Diseases. 9th ed. St. Louis, C. V. Mosby, 1982, pp. 577–588.
6. Breman, J. G., and Henderson, D. A.: Poxvirus dilemmas: Monkeypox, smallpox and biological terrorism. N. Engl. J. Med. *339*:556–559, 1998.
6a. Breman, J. G., and Henderson, D. A.: Diagnosis and management of smallpox. N. Engl. J. Med. *346*:1300–1308, 2002.
7. Cohen, J., and Marshall, E.: Vaccines for biodefense: A system in distress. Science *294*:498–501, 2001.
8. Crosby, A. W.: Smallpox. *In* Kiple, K. F. (ed.): The Cambridge World History of Human Diseases. New York, Cambridge University Press, 1993, pp. 1008–1013.
9. Cruickshank, J. G., Bedson, H. S., and Watson, D. H.: Electron microscopy in the rapid diagnosis of smallpox. Lancet *2*:527, 1966.
10. Deria, A., Jezek, Z., Markvart, K., et al.: The worlds last endemic case of smallpox: Surveillance and containment measures. Bull. World Health Organ. *58*:279–283, 1980.
11. d'Errico, P.: Jeffrey Amherst and smallpox blankets. Lord Jeffrey Amherst's letters discussing germ warfare against American Indians. http://www.nativeweb.org/pages/legal/amherst/lord_jeff.html 11/6/01.
12. Esposito, J. J., and Fenner, F.: Poxviruses. *In* Knipe, D. M., and Howley, P. M. (eds.): Fields Virology, 4th ed. Philadelphia, Lippincott Williams & Wilkins, 2001, pp. 2885–2920.
13. Esposito, J. J., and Massung, R. F.: Poxvirus infections in humans. *In* Murray, P. R., Tenover, F., Baron, E. J. (eds.): Clinical Microbiology. Washington, DC, American Society of Microbiology, 1995, pp. 1131–1138.
14. Fenner, F.: Smallpox, "the most dreadful scourge of the human species." Its global spread and recent eradication (2). Med. J. Aust. 141:728–735, 1984.
15. Fenner, F.: Poxviruses. *In* Fields, B. N., Knipe, D. M., Howley, P. M., et al. (eds.): Fields Virology. 3rd ed. Philadelphia, Lippincott-Raven, 1996, pp. 2673–2702.
16. Fenner, F., Henderson, D. A., Arita, I., et al.: Smallpox and Its Eradication. Geneva, World Health Organization, 1988.
17. Foege, W. H., Millar, J. D., and Lane, J. M.: Selective epidemiologic control in smallpox eradication. Am. J. Epidemiol. *94*:311–315, 1971.
18. Fox, J. L.: Current topics: World Health Assembly delaying smallpox destruction. A. S. M. News. *65*:464–465, 1999.
18a. Frey, S. E., Couch, R. B., Tacket, C. O., et al.: Clinical responses to undiluted and diluted smallpox vaccine. N. Engl. J. Med. *346*:1265–1274, 2002.
18b. Frey, S. E., Newman, F. K., Cruz, J., et al.: Dose-related effects of smallpox vaccine. N. Engl. J. Med. *346*:1275–1280, 2002.
19. Henderson, D. A.: Eradication of smallpox: The critical year ahead. Proc. R. Soc. Med. *66*:493–500, 1973.
20. Henderson, D. A.: The looming threat of bioterrorism. Science *283*:1279–1282, 1996.
21. Henderson, D. A.: Countering the posteradication threat of smallpox and polio. Clin. Infect. Dis. *34*:79–83, 2002.
22. Henderson, D. A., Arita, I., and Shafa, E.: Studies of the bifurcated needle and recommendations for its use. Document SE/72.5. Geneva, Smallpox Eradication Unit of WHO, 1972.
23. Henderson, D. A., Inglesby, T. V., Bartlett, J. G., et al.: Smallpox as a biological weapon: Medical and public health management. J. A. M. A. *281*:2127–2137, 1999.
24. Henderson, D. A., and Moss, B.: Smallpox and vaccinia. *In* Plotkin, S. A., and Orenstein, W. A. (eds.): Vaccines. 3rd ed. Philadelphia, W. B. Saunders, 1999, pp. 74–97.
25. Hopkins, D. R.: Princes and Peasants: Smallpox in History. Chicago, University of Chicago Press, 1983.
26. Human monkeypox: The past five years. W. H. O. Chron. *38*:227–29, 1984.
27. Institute of Medicine: Assessment of future scientific need for live variola virus. Washington, DC, National Academy Press, 1999.
28. Jenner, E.: The origin of the vaccine inoculation. London, D. N. Shury, 1801. Cited in Crookshank, E. M.: History and Pathology of Vaccination. Vol. II. 1889, p. 276.
29. Kempe, C. H., Berge, T. O., and England, B.: Hyperimmune gamma globulin, source, evaluation, and use of prophylaxis and therapy. Pediatrics *18*:177, 1956.
30. Knight, J. C., Massung, R. F., and Esposito, J. J.: Polymerase chain reaction identification of smallpox virus. *In* Becker, Y., and Darai, G. (eds.): PCR: Protocols for Diagnosis of Human and Animal Viral Disease. Heidelberg, Germany, Springer-Verlag, 1995, pp. 297–302.
31. Krugman, S., and Ward, R.: Smallpox and vaccinia. *In* Krugman, S., and Ward, R. (eds.): Infectious Disease of Children. 4th ed. St. Louis, C. V. Mosby, 1968, pp. 314–334.
32. Ladnyi, I. D., Ziegler, P., and Kima, F.: A human infection caused by monkeypox virus in Basankusu Territory, Democratic Republic of the Congo. Bull. World Health Organ. *46*:593–597, 1972.
33. Lane, J. M., and Millar, J. D.: Risks of smallpox vaccination complications in the United States. Am. J. Epidemiol. *93*:238, 1971.
34. Meltzer, M. I., Damon, I., LeDuc, J. W., et al.: Modeling potential responses to smallpox as a bioterrorist weapon. Emerg. Infect. Dis. *7*:595–969, 2001.
35. Moss, B.: Poxviridae: The viruses and their replication. *In* Knipe, D. M., and Howley, P. M. (eds.): Fields Virology. 4th ed., Vol. 2. Philadelphia, Lippincott Williams & Wilkins, 2001, pp. 2849–2883.
36. Nakano, J. H., and Bingham, P. G.: Smallpox, vaccinia, and human infections with monkeypox virus. *In* Lennette, E. H., Spaulding, E. H., and Truant, J. P. (eds.): Manual of Clinical Microbiology. 2nd ed. Washington, DC, American Society for Microbiology, 1974, pp. 782–794.
37. Neff, J., Millar, J. D., Roberto, R. R., et al.: Smallpox vaccination by intradermal jet injection. III. Evaluation in a well vaccinated population. Bull. World Health Organ. *41*:771–778, 1969.
38. Nizamuddin, M., and Dumbell, K. R.: A simple laboratory test to distinguish the virus of smallpox from that of alastrim. Lancet *1*:68, 1961.
39. Ropp, S. L., Knight, J. C., Massung, R. F., et al.: PCR strategy for identification and differentiation of smallpox and other orthopoxviruses. J. Clin. Microbiol. *33*:2069–2076, 1995.
40. Rosenthal, S. R., Merchlinsky, M., Kleppinger, C., et al.: Developing new smallpox vaccines. Emerg. Infect. Dis. *7*:920–926, 2001.
41. Stone, R.: Down to the wire on bioweapons talks. Science *293*:414–416, 2001.
42. Tucker, J. B.: Historical trends related to bioterrorism: An empirical analysis. Emerg. Infect. Dis. *5*:498–504, 1999.
43. Wehrle, P. F.: Smallpox eradication: A global appraisal. J. A. M. A. *240*:1977–1979, 1978.
44. Wehrle, P. F., Posch, J., Richter, K. H., et al.: Airborne smallpox in a German hospital. Bull. World Health Organ. *43*:669–679, 1970.
45. White, P. J., and Shackelford, P. G.: Edward Jenner, MD, and the scourge that was. Am. J. Dis. Child. *137*:864–869, 1983.
46. World Health Organization: The Global Eradication of Smallpox. Final Report of the Global Commission for the Certification of Smallpox Eradication. History of International Public Health No. 4. Geneva, World Health Organization, 1980.

CHAPTER 169

Other Poxviruses

JAMES D. CHERRY

Smallpox, which is caused by variola virus (see Chapter 168), was the most important human poxvirus disease, but this disease has been eradicated from the world. Today, only one human poxvirus, molluscum contagiosum virus, causes specific human illness. In addition, nine other poxviruses can cause human infections. Eight of these viruses are acquired zoonotically, and the other, vaccinia, is a laboratory virus that is acquired iatrogenically.

Properties of the Viruses

CLASSIFICATION

The family *Poxviridae* has two subfamilies: *Chordopoxvirinae* (vertebrate poxviruses) and *Entomopoxvirinae* (insect poxviruses).[25, 55] Eight genera are included in the *Chordopoxvirinae* subfamily, and four of these genera contain species that infect humans (Table 169–1).

TABLE 169–1 ■ POXVIRUSES THAT CAN CAUSE HUMAN ILLNESS

Genus	Species
Orthopoxvirus	Variola virus
	Monkeypox virus
	Vaccinia virus
	Cowpox virus
Parapoxvirus	Orf virus
	Bovine papular stomatitis virus
	Pseudocowpox virus
Yatapoxvirus	Tanapoxvirus
	Yabapoxvirus
Molluscipoxvirus	Molluscum contagiosum virus

STRUCTURE[4, 55]

Poxviruses are the largest animal viruses and are discernible by light microscopy. In general, by electron microscopy, orthopoxviruses appear brick shaped, with a length of 350 nm and a width of 270 nm. They contain double-stranded DNA genomes that vary from 130 to 300 kbp, depending on the particular species. A 30-nm lipoprotein bilayer (envelope) surrounds the virus core. The envelope contains seven or more distinct glycoproteins. Parapoxvirus organisms have a different structure than do *Orthopoxvirus, Yatapoxvirus,* and *Molluscipoxvirus* organisms. They are ovoid and vary from 260 × 160 nm for orf virus to 300 × 190 nm for pseudocowpox virus.

Specific Viruses and Their Illnesses

MONKEYPOX VIRUS[3, 34, 38–40, 44, 56]

Monkeypox virus was isolated first from sick laboratory primates in Copenhagen in 1958.[67] It was found to be the cause of a smallpox-like illness in humans in western and central Africa in 1970. Human disease occurs in a large geographic area from Sierra Leone in the west to the Democratic Republic of Congo (formerly Zaire) in the east.[38] Illness is usually sporadic, with animals as the source in 72 percent of cases and human-to-human transmission in the remaining 28 percent. Numerous different monkeys and other primates, as well as rodents, are thought to be the source of human cases.

Jezek and associates[40] studied 282 patients in the Democratic Republic of Congo and found that 50 percent were 4 years of age or younger and 93 percent were 14 years or younger. The clinical features of human monkeypox virus infection are similar to those of smallpox, but the overall illness tends to be less severe. Smallpox vaccination markedly lessens the severity of the illness. Illness usually starts with fever for 1 to 3 days before the onset of rash. The fever is accompanied by severe headache, backache, general malaise, and prostration.

The rash usually appears first on the face. Similar to smallpox lesions, the lesions develop and progress together in the same body region through the stages of macules, papules, vesicles, and pustules. Most patients have discrete lesions; 23 percent have semiconfluent, and 7 percent have confluent lesions. Most patients have mucous membrane involvement, and conjunctivitis occurs commonly. Lymphadenopathy, particularly of the submaxillary and cervical lymph nodes, is significant but not a usual finding in smallpox.

The overall duration of illness is 2 to 4 weeks. Complications include secondary bacterial infection of the skin; pneumonia; vomiting, diarrhea, and dehydration; keratitis and corneal ulceration; septicemia; and encephalitis. The death rate in nonvaccinated patients was 11 percent in the study reported by Jezek and associates,[40] and all deaths occurred in children 8 years of age or younger. One case of congenital monkeypox infection has been reported.[38] This child's mother had typical illness on August 12, 1983, and the child was born prematurely on September 23, 1983. At birth, the child had generalized skin lesions; the child died 6 weeks later of malnutrition.

In May 2003, cases of monkeypox in humans were noted for the first time in the Western Hemisphere. As of June 11, 2003, 50 cases had been noted in four states (New Jersey, Indiana, Wisconsin, and Illinois). The sources of these human infections were ill pet prairie dogs (CDC unpublished data).

COWPOX VIRUS

In Europe, a disease with ulcers on the teats of cows (cowpox disease) has been recognized for hundreds of years.[25] Milkers who milked cows that were infected often got similar ulcers on their hands, and milkmaids who had contracted cowpox were known to be immune to smallpox. This observation led Edward Jenner in May 1796 to inoculate James Phipps, an 8-year-old boy, with cowpox material obtained from a lesion on a local dairy maid.[2, 35, 36, 38] After experimental challenge with material from a smallpox lesion, smallpox did not develop in Phipps.

Studies during the last 30 years indicate that bovine cowpox is not a common illness and cows are not the natural reservoir of the virus in nature.[1, 2, 4] The virus is distributed geographically throughout western Europe, and the reservoir hosts are wild rodents.

Baxby[1] reported 12 human illnesses caused by cowpox virus. Five of the patients were exposed to infected cows, and the other seven had no direct contact with cattle. All the patients, however, lived in or had visited a rural area before the onset of illness. Of 10 patients in whom lesions were described, 6 had lesions on the hand only, 3 had lesions on the chin or face only, and 1 had involvement of both the face and hand. Most patients had local edema, lymphadenitis, and fever. The lesions were confused with anthrax in two instances.

An 18-year-old man who was immunocompromised suffered a fatal infection with a cowpox-like virus that was acquired from a cat with a skin lesion on an anterior paw.[20]

VACCINIA VIRUS

Vaccinia virus is the live immunizing antigen successfully used in the global program to eradicate smallpox. This orthopoxvirus is different from cowpox virus, the agent that Jenner and others used for vaccination in the early 19th century. Vaccinia virus has been used for vaccination for more than 100 years. Restriction endonuclease studies indicate that strains of vaccinia virus from different parts of the world are similar to each other and distinctly different from cowpox virus.[25] The origin of vaccinia virus is unknown.[4] Four hypotheses regarding its origin are that (1) it evolved from variola virus through continual passage in the skin of cows or humans, (2) it evolved from cowpox virus through continual passage in the skin of animals, (3) it is a hybrid between cowpox virus and variola virus, and (4) it is a virus from an animal (the natural host) that is now extinct.

Vaccinia virus causes outbreaks of disease in buffaloes in India.[4, 25] However, the animal infection is thought to have resulted originally from contact of buffaloes with vaccinated humans during smallpox eradication programs rather than from the virus being a primary buffalo pathogen. More recently, in Brazil, skin lesions on dairy cows and their milkers that resemble cowpox have been found to be caused by a single strain of vaccinia virus.[21] This virus, designated Cantagalo virus (CTGV), is similar to a smallpox vaccine strain used in the region 20 years ago. Researchers have suggested that the original vaccinia virus persisted in an indigenous animal, accumulated polymorphisms, and recently emerged in cattle and milkers as CTGV.

Because of the original success of the smallpox eradication program, routine vaccinia vaccination in the United States was discontinued in 1971.[6, 15] In 1976, the recommendation for routine vaccination of health care workers also was discontinued.[14] In 1982, the only active licensed producer of vaccinia vaccine in the United States discontinued production for general use, and in 1983, distribution to civilian populations was discontinued.[9]

For several years, all military personnel continued to be vaccinated routinely. Although more recently only selected groups of military personnel were vaccinated against smallpox, with the initiation of action in Iraq and the concurrent threat of biological warfare, all troops designated for military action in that area were given smallpox vaccinations.

Since January 1982, smallpox vaccination has not been required for international travelers, and International Certificates of Vaccination no longer include smallpox vaccination.[71]

In 1980, the Advisory Committee on Immunization Practices (ACIP) recommended the use of vaccinia vaccine to protect laboratory workers from possible infection while working with nonvariola orthopoxviruses (e.g., vaccinia, monkeypox).[13] In 1984, these recommendations were included in guidelines for biosafety in microbiologic and biomedical laboratories.[64] These guidelines expanded the recommendation to include persons working in animal care areas where studies with orthopoxviruses were being conducted and recommended that these workers have documented evidence of satisfactory smallpox vaccination within the preceding 3 years. The Centers for Disease Control and Prevention (CDC) has provided vaccinia vaccine for these laboratory workers since 1983.[10]

Because studies of recombinant vaccinia virus vaccines have advanced to the stage of clinical trials, health care workers (e.g., physicians, nurses) and veterinarians now may be exposed to vaccinia and recombinant vaccinia viruses and should be considered for vaccinia vaccination.[28, 33]

Vaccinia Vaccine

The vaccinia vaccine currently licensed in the United States is a lyophilized preparation of infectious vaccinia virus (official name, smallpox vaccine, dried; produced in the 1970s as Dryvax by Wyeth Laboratories and available only from the CDC). The vaccine was prepared from calf lymph with a seed virus derived from the New York City Board of Health (NYCBOH) strain of vaccinia; it has a concentration of 10^8 pock-forming units per milliliter. Vaccine is administered by using the multiple-puncture technique with a bifurcated needle.

After percutaneous administration of a standard dose of vaccinia vaccine, neutralizing or hemagglutination-inhibition antibody develops in more than 95 percent of primary vaccinees (i.e., persons receiving their first dose of vaccine) at a titer of 1:10 or higher.[16] Neutralizing antibody titers of 1:10 or higher are found in 75 percent of persons for 10 years after receiving second doses and up to 30 years after receiving three doses of vaccine.[24, 52] The level of antibody required for protection against vaccinia infection is not known. However, when the response to revaccination is used as an indication of immunity, less than 10 percent of persons with neutralizing titers of 1:10 or higher exhibit a primary-type response at revaccination as compared with more than 30 percent of persons with titers of less than 1:10.[54] Recent studies have shown that the current supply of vaccine is viable and in good titer. However, attempts to dilute the vaccine to titers less than 10^7 pfu/mL, in order to extend the current supply, may reduce the rate of successful vaccination.[28a, 28b]

In the present era with concerns relating to smallpox as a bioterrorism agent, more precise knowledge about the duration of immunity in previously vaccinated persons is critical.[17] In this regard, a study performed in Liverpool, England, in 1902 to 1903 is of interest. In this study, researchers found that the smallpox case-fatality rate in adults older than 50 years who had been vaccinated in infancy was 5.5 percent, whereas it was 50 percent in similar aged adults who had not been vaccinated. Similar, but better, protection was noted in younger adults, and in general, adults who had been vaccinated as infants had less severe disease than did those who had not been vaccinated.

Recombinant Vaccinia Virus

Vaccinia virus is the prototype of the genus *Orthopoxvirus*. It is a double-stranded DNA virus that has a broad host range under experimental conditions and rarely is isolated from animals outside the laboratory.[4, 21, 25, 27] Many strains of vaccinia virus exist and have different levels of virulence for humans and animals. For example, the Temple of Heaven and Copenhagen vaccinia strains are highly pathogenic in animals, whereas the NYCBOH strain, from which the Wyeth vaccine was derived, has relatively low pathogenicity.[26]

Vaccinia virus can be engineered genetically to contain and express foreign DNA without impairing the ability of the virus to replicate. Such foreign DNA can encode protein antigens that induce protection against one or more infectious agents. Recombinant vaccinia viruses have been engineered to express the immunizing antigens of many viruses, bacteria, parasites, and tumors of veterinary and medical importance.[18, 28, 33, 34, 45, 62, 63, 72]

Recombinant vaccinia viruses have been created from several strains of vaccinia virus. In the United States, most recombinants have been made from either the NYCBOH strain or a mouse neuroadapted derivative, the WR strain. Some recombinants have been made from the Copenhagen and Lister vaccinia strains, which are more pathogenic in animals than the NYCBOH strain is. Animal studies generally suggest that recombinants may be no more pathogenic than is the parent strain of vaccinia virus. However, no consistently reliable laboratory marker or animal test predicts the attenuation of vaccinia virus or a particular recombinant for humans.[59] Laboratory-acquired infections with vaccinia or recombinant viruses have been reported.[41, 58, 61] However, because no surveillance system has been established to monitor laboratory workers, the risk of acquiring infection in persons who handle virus cultures or materials contaminated with these viruses is not known.

With the initiation of human and veterinary trials of recombinant vaccines, physicians, nurses, veterinarians, and other personnel who are exposed to recipients of these vaccines could be exposed to both vaccinia and recombinant agents. This exposure could occur from contact with dressings contaminated with the virus or through exposure to the vaccine. The risk of transmission of recombinant viruses to exposed health care workers is unknown. To date, no reports of transmission to health care personnel from vaccine recipients have been published. If appropriate infection control precautions are observed, health care workers probably are at less risk of acquiring infection than laboratory workers are because of the smaller volume and lower titer of virus in clinical specimens than in laboratory material.[30, 70] However, because of the potential for transmission of vaccinia or recombinant vaccinia viruses to such persons, the ACIP suggests that health care personnel who have direct contact with contaminated dressings or other infectious material from volunteers in clinical studies be considered for vaccination.

Laboratory and other health care personnel who work with viral cultures or other infective material always should observe appropriate biosafety guidelines and adhere to published infection control procedures.[30, 65, 70]

Vaccine Use

Vaccinia vaccine is recommended for laboratory workers who directly handle (1) cultures or (2) animals contaminated or infected with vaccinia, recombinant vaccinia viruses, or other orthopoxviruses that infect humans (e.g., monkeypox, cowpox). Other health care workers (e.g., physicians, nurses) whose contact with these viruses is limited to contaminated material (e.g., dressings) but who adhere to appropriate infection control measures are at lower risk of inadvertently acquiring infection than are laboratory workers. However, because a theoretic risk of infection does exist, vaccination may be considered for this group. Because of the low risk of infection, vaccination is not recommended for persons who do not handle virus cultures or materials directly or who do not work with animals contaminated or infected with these viruses.

According to available data on the persistence of neutralizing antibody after vaccination, persons working with vaccinia, recombinant vaccinia viruses, or other nonvariola orthopoxviruses should be revaccinated every 10 years.

Since September 11, 2001, and the emergence of major concerns relating to smallpox as a bioterrorism agent, new tissue culture–grown smallpox vaccines are being developed and tested. Plans are to stockpile sufficient vaccine to protect the entire population. New strategies for vaccine use are being planned. At present, increasing the use of vaccines in the military and in other public servants is advisable (see Chapter 168). However, unless smallpox again becomes a national or international problem, routine use of vaccine is not indicated.[2a, 25a]

Side Effects and Adverse Reactions

A papule develops at the site of vaccination 2 to 5 days after percutaneous administration of vaccinia vaccine to a nonimmune person (i.e., primary vaccination). The papule becomes vesicular and then pustular and reaches its maximal size in 8 to 10 days. The pustule dries and forms a scab, which separates within 14 to 21 days after vaccination and leaves a typical scar. Primary vaccination can produce swelling and tenderness of regional lymph nodes beginning 3 to 10 days after vaccination and persisting for 2 to 4 weeks after the skin lesion has healed. Maximal viral shedding occurs 4 to 14 days after vaccination, but vaccinia can be recovered from the site of vaccination until the scab separates from the skin.[32, 46]

Fever occurs commonly after vaccinia vaccination. As many as 70 percent of children have 1 or more days with a temperature of 37.8° C (100° F) or higher 4 to 14 days after receiving primary vaccination,[16, 54] and 15 to 20 percent have temperatures of 38.9° C (102° F) or higher. After revaccination, 35 percent of children have temperatures of 37.8° C (100° F) or higher and 5 percent have temperatures of 38.9° C (102° F) or higher.[32] Fever occurs less commonly in adults than in children after vaccination or revaccination.[32]

An erythematous or urticarial rash may occur approximately 10 days after receipt of primary vaccination. The vaccinee usually is afebrile, and the rash resolves spontaneously within 2 to 4 days. Rarely, bullous erythema multiforme (Stevens-Johnson syndrome) occurs.[31]

Inadvertent inoculation at other sites, the most frequent complication of vaccinia vaccination, accounts for approximately one half of all complications of primary vaccination and revaccination. Inadvertent inoculation usually results from autoinoculation of vaccine virus transferred from the site of vaccination. The most common sites involved are the face, eyelid, nose, mouth, genitalia, and rectum. Most lesions heal without specific therapy, but vaccinia immune globulin (VIG) may be useful for cases of ocular implantation (see "Treatment of Complications of Vaccinia Vaccine").

Generalized vaccinia in persons without any underlying illness is characterized by a vesicular rash of varying extent. The rash generally is self-limited and requires little or no therapy, except in patients whose conditions appear to be toxic or in those who have a serious underlying illness.

More severe complications of vaccinia vaccination include eczema vaccinatum, progressive vaccinia, and postvaccinial encephalitis. These complications occur at least 10 times more often in primary vaccinees than in revaccinees and more frequently in infants than in older children and adults.[48–50]

Eczema vaccinatum is a localized or systemic dissemination of vaccinia virus in persons who have eczema or a history of eczema and other chronic or exfoliative skin conditions (e.g., atopic dermatitis). The illness often is mild and self-limited but may be severe and occasionally fatal. The most serious cases in vaccine recipients occur in primary vaccinees and appear to be independent of the activity of the underlying eczema.[68] Severe cases also have been observed after contact infection.

Progressive vaccinia (vaccinia necrosum) is a severe, potentially fatal illness characterized by progressive necrosis in the area of vaccination, often with metastatic lesions. It occurs almost exclusively in persons with cellular immunodeficiency.

The most serious complication is postvaccinial encephalitis. Most frequently, it affects primary vaccinees younger than 1 year of age. Fifteen to 25 percent of affected vaccinees with this complication die, and 25 percent have permanent neurologic sequelae.[31, 49, 50]

Death after vaccinia vaccination rarely occurs, with approximately 1 to 2 deaths per million primary vaccinations and 0.1 death per million revaccinations. Death most often is the result of postvaccinial encephalitis or progressive vaccinia.

Vaccinia may be transmitted when a recently vaccinated person has contact with a susceptible person. In the CDC's 10-state survey of complications of smallpox vaccination, the risk of transmission to contacts was 27 infections per million total vaccinations; 44 percent of these contact cases occurred in children 5 years of age or younger.[50] Since 1980, several cases of contact transmission of vaccinia from vaccinated military recruits have been reported and include six cases transmitted by a single vaccine recipient.[7, 8, 12]

More than 60 percent of cases of contact transmission result in uncomplicated inadvertent inoculation. Approximately 30 percent result in eczema vaccinatum, which may be fatal.[50] Eczema vaccinatum may be more severe in contacts than in vaccinated persons, possibly because of simultaneous multiple inoculation at several sites.[19, 49] Contact transmission rarely results in postvaccinial encephalitis or vaccinia necrosum.

Precautions and Contraindications

Before administering vaccinia vaccine, the physician should obtain a careful history to document the absence of contraindications to vaccination in both vaccinees and household contacts of vaccinees. Special effort should be made to identify vaccinees and household contacts who have eczema, a history of eczema, or immunodeficiencies. Vaccinia vaccine should not be administered if these conditions are present in a possible recipient or in most instances if they are present in household contacts.

Specific precautions and contraindications include a history or the presence of eczema, pregnancy, altered immunocompetence, infection with human immunodeficiency virus, and allergies to vaccine components. The reader is referred to the CDC for more complete information on contraindications.[6]

Prevention of Contact Transmission of Vaccinia

Vaccinia virus may be cultured from the site of primary vaccination beginning at the time that a papule develops (2 to 5 days after vaccination) until the scab separates from the skin lesion (14 to 21 days after vaccination). During this time, care must be taken to prevent spread of the virus to another area of the body or to another person. Present recommendations state that the vaccination site should be covered at all times with a porous bandage until the scab has separated and the underlying skin has healed.[6] An occlusive bandage should not be used. The vaccination site should be kept dry. When the vaccinee bathes, the site should be covered with an impermeable bandage.

Vaccinated health care workers may continue to have contact with patients, including those with immunodeficiencies, as long as the vaccination site is covered and good handwashing technique is maintained.

Semipermeable polyurethane dressings (e.g., Op-Site) are effective barriers to vaccinia and recombinant vaccinia viruses.[18] However, exudate may accumulate beneath the dressing, so care must be taken to prevent viral contamination when the dressing is removed. In addition, accumulation of fluid beneath the dressing may increase maceration of the vaccination site. Accumulation of exudate may be decreased by first covering the vaccination with dry gauze and then applying the dressing over the gauze. To date, experience with this type of containment dressing has been limited to research protocols, and further investigation is needed.

Of interest is that the aforementioned recommendations differ considerably from recommendations made before the discontinuation of routine smallpox vaccination.[47] Specifically, dressings were not recommended for the reason that secondary infections were more likely to occur when dressings were used because the vaccine was not sterile. My opinion is that the present dressing recommendations prolong the duration of the vaccination lesion and, therefore, prolong the period of contagion. At present, care should be taken to not dress vaccination sites excessively, and sites should be examined daily for signs of maceration and possible secondary bacterial infection.

The most important measure to prevent inadvertent implantation and contact transmission from vaccinia vaccination is thorough handwashing after changing the bandage or after any other contact with the vaccination site.

Treatment of Complications of Vaccinia Vaccine

The only product currently available for the treatment of complications of vaccinia vaccination is VIG. VIG is an isotonic sterile solution of the immunoglobulin fraction of plasma from persons vaccinated with vaccinia vaccine. It is effective for the treatment of eczema vaccinatum and some cases of progressive vaccinia and may be useful in the treatment of ocular vaccinia resulting from inadvertent implantation. VIG also is recommended for severe generalized vaccinia if the patient has a toxic condition or a serious underlying disease. VIG is of no benefit in the treatment of postvaccinial encephalitis.

The recommended dose for the treatment of complications is 0.6 mL/kg of body weight. VIG must be administered intramuscularly and should be administered as early as possible after the onset of symptoms. Because therapeutic doses of VIG may be large (e.g., 42 mL for a person weighing 70 kg), the product should be given in divided doses over a 24- to 36-hour period. Doses may be repeated, usually at intervals of 2 to 3 days, until recovery begins (e.g., no new lesions appear).

The CDC is the only source of VIG for civilians.

An adult patient with progressive vaccinia is reported to have benefited with the administration of ribavirin and VIG.[36, 43] Cidofovir also may prove useful for the treatment of vaccinia complications.

Misuse of Vaccinia Vaccine

Vaccinia vaccine never should be used therapeutically for any reason. No evidence exists that it has any value in the treatment or prevention of recurrent herpes simplex virus infection, warts, or any disease other than that caused by human orthopoxviruses.[42] Misuse of vaccinia vaccine to treat herpesvirus infections has been associated with severe complications.[11, 66]

Vaccinia Vaccine Availability

The CDC is the only source of vaccinia vaccine and VIG for civilians. The CDC provides vaccinia vaccine to protect laboratory and other health care personnel whose occupations place them at risk of exposure to vaccinia and other closely related orthopoxviruses, including vaccinia recombinants.

ORF VIRUS

Orf virus is a member of the genus *Parapoxvirus* (see Table 65–1). Infection with orf virus causes the disease by the same name (orf), which also is called ecthyma contagiosum.[25] The reservoir host of orf virus is sheep, and the virus enjoys worldwide distribution. Orf is an occupationally acquired disease, and most cases occur in adults.[29, 51] Human disease is characterized by single or multiple lesions that most often are located on the hands. The lesions last approximately 35 to 40 days and progress through six stages[51]: maculopapular, 1 to 7 days; target, 7 to 14 days; acute, 14 to 21 days; regenerative, 21 to 28 days; papillomatous, 28 to 35 days; and regressive, 35 to 40 or more days. Patients may have low-grade fever and regional lymphadenitis. Two patients with a widespread papulovesicular eruption, fever, malaise, and lymphadenopathy have been described.[69] A giant orf granuloma developed at the site of a rope burn in a 12-year-old boy who lived on a farm.[57]

OTHER PARAPOXVIRUSES

Human infections with pseudocowpox virus and bovine papular stomatitis virus are, like orf, occupational diseases. Pseudocowpox infections occur on the hands of milkers, and infections with bovine papular stomatitis virus occur on the hands of veterinarians and others with close contact.[5, 25, 53] The lesions of milker's nodule are relatively painless, but they may be pruritic; they are red initially and then become purple. They are firm, do not ulcerate, and last 4 to 6 weeks. The lesions from bovine papular stomatitis virus are wart-like and last 3 to 4 weeks.

Humans also have been infected with the parapoxviruses of camels and seals.[60]

YATAPOXVIRUSES

Tanapox virus and Yabapoxvirus are two monkey viruses that cause human infection[22, 23, 25, 37] (see Table 65–1). Tanapox in humans first was observed along the Tana River in Kenya in 1957, and outbreaks also were studied in the Democratic Republic of Congo.[25] Yabapoxvirus was isolated first from tumors in monkeys in Nigeria. This virus has caused illness in animal handlers in primate centers in the United States, but human infections have not been identified in the field in Africa.

Outbreaks of tanapox in Africa have involved both children and adults.[37] The illness starts with fever, headache, backache, and mild prostration. Skin lesions occur 2 to 4 days after the onset of illness. Individual lesions start with itching followed by the development of a pock-like lesion. At 7 days, the lesion is approximately 10 mm in diameter with surrounding erythema. Local lymphadenitis and regional lymphadenitis occur.

The lesions ulcerate during the second week of illness and last approximately 6 weeks. Most patients have a single lesion, but some have 2 to 10. The prognosis usually is good, but secondary bacterial infection can occur.

MOLLUSCUM CONTAGIOSUM VIRUS

In contrast to the other poxviruses discussed in this chapter, which are zoonotic agents, molluscum contagiosum virus is a human virus that is a common cause of human skin lesions[25] (see Chapter 67 and Table 65–1). The virus has not been grown in cell culture as yet, and it does not cause infection in experimental animals.

Although the virus has not been cultivated in the laboratory, large amounts of virus can be extracted from human lesions. Analysis of viral DNA from lesions in patients from different parts of the world indicates that two major subtypes and a third, rare subtype exist.

The clinical aspects of molluscum contagiosum virus infection are presented in Chapter 67.

Diagnosis and Differential Diagnosis

Because all but two viruses presented in this chapter are zoonotic agents, careful attention must be given to geographic location and animal exposure. All these diseases are characterized by local lesions, so virus is readily available for direct identification and culture. All poxviruses can be identified by examination of material from lesions by electron microscopy. All viruses except molluscum contagiosum virus grow in one or more tissue culture systems, the chorioallantoic membrane of embryonated eggs, or both. Unusual agents should be referred to specific reference laboratories for species identification.

REFERENCES

1. Baxby, D.: Is cowpox misnamed? A review of 10 human cases. B. M. J. *1*:1379–1381, 1977.
2. Bennett, M., and Baxby, D.: Cowpox. J. Med. Microbiol. *45*:157–158, 1996.
2a. Bicknall, W. J.: The case for voluntary smallpox vaccination (editorial). N. Engl. J. Med. *346*:1323–1324, 2002.
3. Breman, J. G., Ruti, K., Steniowski, M. V., et al.: Human monkeypox, 1970–79. Bull. World Health Organ. *58*:165–182, 1980.
4. Buller, R. M. L., and Palumbo, G. J.: Poxvirus pathogenesis. Microbiol. Rev. *55*:80–122, 1991.
5. Carson, C. A., and Kerr, K. M.: Bovine papular stomatitis with apparent transmission to man. J. Am. Vet. Med. Assoc. *151*:183–187, 1987.
6. Centers for Disease Control: Vaccinia (smallpox) vaccine: Recommendations of the Immunization Practices Advisory Committee (ACIP). M. M. W. R. Recomm. Rep. *40*(RR-14):1–10, 1991.
7. Centers for Disease Control: Contact spread of vaccinia from a National Guard vaccinee—Wisconsin. M. M. W. R. Morb. Mortal. Wkly. Rep. *34*:182–183, 1985.
8. Centers for Disease Control: Contact spread of vaccinia from a recently vaccinated Marine—Louisiana. M. M. W. R. Morb. Mortal. Wkly. Rep. *33*:37–38, 1984.
9. Centers for Disease Control: Smallpox vaccine no longer available for civilians—United States. M. M. W. R. Morb. Mortal. Wkly. Rep. *32*(29):387, 1983.
10. Centers for Disease Control: Smallpox vaccine available for protection of at-risk laboratory workers. M. M. W. R. Morb. Mortal. Wkly. Rep. *32*:543, 1983.
11. Centers for Disease Control: Vaccinia necrosum after smallpox vaccination—Michigan. M. M. W. R. Morb. Mortal. Wkly. Rep. *31*(36):501–502, 1982.
12. Centers for Disease Control: Vaccinia outbreak—Newfoundland. M. M. W. R. Morb. Mortal. Wkly. Rep. *30*(36):453–455, 1981.
13. Centers for Disease Control: Smallpox vaccine: Recommendation of the Immunization Practices Advisory Committee. M. M. W. R. Morb. Mortal. Wkly. Rep. *29*:417–420, 1980.

14. Centers for Disease Control: Recommendation of the Immunization Practices Advisory Committee (ACIP): Smallpox vaccination of hospital and health personnel. M. M. W. R. Morb. Mortal. Wkly. Rep. *25*:9, 1976.
15. Centers for Disease Control: Public Health Service recommendations on smallpox vaccination. M. M. W. R. Morb. Mortal. Wkly. Rep. *20*:339, 1971.
16. Cherry, J. D., McIntosh, K., Connor, J. D., et al.: Primary percutaneous (smallpox) vaccination. J. Infect. Dis. *135*:145–154, 1977.
17. Cohen, J.: Smallpox vaccinations: How much protection remains? Science *294*:985, 2001.
18. Cooney, E. L., Collier, A. C., Greenberg, P. D., et al.: Safety of and immunological response to a recombinant vaccinia virus vaccine expressing HIV envelope glycoprotein. Lancet *337*:567–572, 1991.
19. Coperman, P. W. M., and Wallace, H. J.: Eczema vaccinatum. B. M. J. *2*:906, 1964.
20. Czerny, C. P., Zeller-Lue, C., Eis-Hübinger, A. M., et al.: Characterization of a cowpox-like orthopox virus which had caused a lethal infection in man. Arch. Virol. *13*:13–24, 1997.
21. Damaso, C. R. A., Esposito, J. J., Condit, R. C., et al.: An emergent poxvirus from humans and cattle in Rio de Janeiro State: Cantagalo virus may derive from Brazilian smallpox vaccine. Virology *277*:439–449, 2000.
22. Downie, A. W., and Espaa, C.: A comparative study of tanapox and yaba viruses. J. Gen. Virol. *19*:37–49, 1973.
23. Downie, A. W., Taylor-Robinson, C. H., Caunt, A. E., et al.: Tanapox: A new disease caused by a pox virus. B. M. J. *1*:363–368, 1971.
24. El-Ad, B., Roth, Y., Winder, A., et al.: The persistence of neutralizing antibodies after revaccination against smallpox. J. Infect. Dis. *161*:446–448, 1990.
25. Esposito, J. J., and Fenner, F.: Poxviruses. *In* Knipe, D. M., and Howley, P. M. (eds.): Fields Virology, 4th ed. Philadelphia, Lippincott Williams & Wilkins, 2001, pp. 2885–2920.
25a. Fauci, A. S.: Smallpox vaccination policy—the need for dialogue (editorial). N. Engl. J. Med. *346*:1319–1320, 2002.
26. Fenner, F., Henderson, D. A., Arita, I., et al.: Smallpox and Its Eradication. Geneva, World Health Organization, 1988, pp. 581–583.
27. Fenner, F., Wittek, R., and Dumbell, K. R.: The Orthopoxviruses. San Diego, Academic, 1989, pp. 10–13.
28. Flexner, C., and Moss, B.: Vaccinia virus as a live vector for expression of immunogens. *In* Levine, M. M., Woodrow, G. C., Kaper, J. B., et al. (eds.): New Generation Vaccines. 2nd ed. New York, Marcel Dekker, 1997, pp. 297–314.
28a. Frey, S. E., Couch, R. B., Tacket, C. O., et al.: Clinical responses to undiluted and diluted smallpox vaccine. N. Engl. J. Med. *346*:1265–1274, 2002.
28b. Frey, S. E., Newman, F. K., Cruz, B. S., et al.: Dose-related effects of smallpox vaccine. N. Engl. J. Med. *346*:1275–1280, 2002.
29. Ganske, J. G., Miller, S. H., and Demuth, R. J.: Ecthyma contagiosum (orf). Plast. Reconstr. Surg. *68*:779–780, 1981.
30. Garner, J. S., and Simmons, B. P.: Guideline for isolation precautions in hospitals. Infect. Control *4*(Suppl.):245–325, 1983.
31. Goldstein, J. A., Neff, J. M., Lane, J. M., et al.: Smallpox vaccination reactions, prophylaxis and therapy of complications. Pediatrics *55*:342–347, 1975.
32. Graham, B. S., Belshe, R., Clements, M. L., et al.: HIV–GP-160 recombinant vaccinia vaccination of vaccinia-naive adults followed by RGP160 booster. Abstract. Paper presented at the Sixth International Conference on AIDS, June 1991, Florence, Italy.
33. Henderson, D. A., and Moss, B.: Smallpox and vaccinia. *In* Plotkin, S. A., and Orenstein, W. A. (eds.): Vaccines. 3rd ed. Philadelphia, W. B. Saunders, 1999, pp. 74–97.
34. Hutin, Y. J. F., Williams, R. J., Malfait, P., et al.: Outbreak of human monkeypox, Democratic Republic of Congo, 1996–1997. Emerg. Infect. Dis. *7*:434–438, 2001.
35. Jenner, E.: An Inquiry into the Causes and Effects of the Variolae Vaccinae, a Disease Discovered in Some of the Western Counties of England, Particularly Gloucestershire, and Known by the Name of the Cowpox. London, Sampson Low, 1798.
36. Jenner, E.: Further Observations on the Variolae Vacciniae or Cowpox. London, Sampson Low, 1799.
37. Jezek, Z., Arita, I., Szczeniowski, M., et al.: Human tanapox in Zaire: Clinical and epidemiological observations on cases confirmed by laboratory studies. Bull. World Health Organ. *63*:1027–1035, 1985.
38. Jezek, Z., and Fenner, F.: Human monkeypox. *In* Melnick, J. L. (ed.): Monographs in Virology. Vol. 17. Basel, Karger, 1988, pp. 1–140.
39. Jezek, Z., Marennikova, S. S., Mutumbo, M., et al.: Human monkeypox: A study of 2,510 contacts of 214 patients. J. Infect. Dis. *154*:551–555, 1986.
40. Jezek, Z., Szczeniowski, M., Paluku, K. M., et al.: Human monkeypox: Clinical features of 282 patients. J. Infect. Dis. *156*:293–298, 1987.
41. Jones, L., Ristow, S., Yima, T., et al.: Accidental human vaccination with vaccinia virus expressing nucleoprotein gene. Nature *319*:543, 1986.
42. Kern, A. B., and Schiff, B. L.: Smallpox vaccination in the management of recurrent herpes simplex: A controlled evaluation. J. Invest. Dermatol. *33*:99–102, 1959.
43. Kesson, A. M., Ferguson, J. K., Rawlinson, W. D., et al.: Progressive vaccinia treated with ribavirin and vaccinia immune globulin. Clin. Infect. Dis. *25*:911–914, 1997.
44. Khodakevich, L., Jezek, Z., and Messinger, D.: Monkeypox virus: Ecology and public health significance. Bull. World Health Organ. *66*:747–752, 1988.
45. Kieny, M. P., Lathe, R., Drillien, R., et al.: Expression of rabies virus glycoprotein from a recombinant vaccinia virus. Nature *312*:163–166, 1984.
46. Koplan, J. P., and Marton, K. I.: Smallpox vaccination revisited: Some observations on the biology of vaccinia. Am. J. Trop. Med. Hyg. *24*:656–663, 1975.
47. Krugman, S., and Ward, R.: Smallpox and vaccinia. *In* Infectious Disease of Children. 4th ed. St. Louis, C. V. Mosby, 1968, pp. 314–334.
48. Lane, J. M., Miller, J. D., and Neff, J. M.: Smallpox and smallpox vaccination policy. Annu. Rev. Med. *22*:251–272, 1971.
49. Lane, J. M., Ruben, F. L., Neff, J. M., et al.: Complications of smallpox vaccination, 1968: National surveillance in the United States. N. Engl. J. Med. *281*:1201–1207, 1969.
50. Lane, J. M., Ruben, F. L., Neff, J. M., et al.: Complications of smallpox vaccination, 1968: Results of ten statewide surveys. J. Infect. Dis. *122*:303–309, 1970.
51. Leavell, U. W., Jr., McNamara, M. J., Muelling, R., et al.: Orf: Report of 19 human cases with clinical and pathological observations. J. A. M. A. *204*:657–664, 1968.
52. Lublin-Tennenbaum, T., Katzenelson, T., El-Ad, E., et al.: Correlation between cutaneous reaction in vaccinees immunized against smallpox and antibody titer determined by plaque neutralization test and ELISA. Viral Immunol. *3*:19–25, 1990.
53. McEvoy, J. D. S., and Allan, B. C.: Isolation of bovine papular stomatitis virus from humans. Med. J. Aust. *1*:1254–1256, 1972.
54. McIntosh, K., Cherry, J. D., Benenson, A. S., et al.: Standard percutaneous (smallpox) revaccination of children who received primary percutaneous vaccination. J. Infect. Dis. *135*:155–166, 1977.
55. Moss, B.: *Poxviridae:* The viruses and their replication. *In* Fields, B. N., Knipe, D. M., Howley, P. M., et al. (eds.): Fields Virology. 4th ed. Philadelphia, Lippincott-Raven, 1996, pp. 2637–2671.
56. Mutombo, M. W., Arita, I., and Jezek, Z.: Human monkeypox transmitted by a chimpanzee in a tropical rain-forest area of Zaire. Lancet *1*:735–737, 1983.
57. Pether, J. V. S., Guerrier, C. J. W., Jones, S. M., et al.: Giant orf in a normal individual. Br. J. Dermatol. *115*:497–499, 1986.
58. Pike, R. M.: Laboratory-associated infections: Summary and analysis of 3,921 cases. Health Lab. Sci. *102*:105–114, 1976.
59. Recombinant vaccinia viruses as live virus vectors for vaccine antigens: Memorandum from a W. H. O./USPHS/NIBSC meeting. Bull. World Health Organ. *63*:471–477, 1985.
60. Robinson, A. J., and Lyttle, D. J.: Parapoxviruses: Their biology and potential as recombinant vaccines. *In* Binns, M. M., and Smith, G. L. (eds.): Recombinant Poxviruses. Boca Raton, FL, C. R. C. Press, 1992, pp. 285–327.
61. Shimojo, J.: Virus infections in laboratories in Japan. Bibl. Haematol. *40*:771–773, 1975.
62. Smith, G. L., Mackett, M., and Moss, B.: Infectious vaccinia virus recombinants that express hepatitis B virus surface antigen. Nature *302*:490–495, 1983.
63. Smith, G. L., Murphy, B. R., and Moss, B.: Construction and characterization of an infectious vaccinia virus that expresses the influenza hemagglutinin gene and induces resistance to influenza virus infection in hamsters. Proc. Natl. Acad. Sci. U. S. A. *80*:7155–7159, 1983.
64. U.S. Department of Health and Human Services: Biosafety in Microbiological and Biomedical Laboratories. 1st ed. Washington, D.C., U. S. Govt. Printing Office, HHS Publication No. (NIH) 88–8395, 1984, p. 66.
65. U.S. Department of Health and Human Services: Biosafety in Microbiological and Biomedical Laboratories. 2nd ed. Washington, D.C., U. S. Govt. Printing Office, HHS Publication No. (NIH) 88–8396, 1984, pp. 78–79.
66. U.S. Food and Drug Administration: Inappropriate use of smallpox vaccine. F. D. A. Drug Bull. *12*(2):12, 1982.
67. von Magnus, P., Andersen, E. K., Petersen, K. B., et al.: A pox-like disease in cynomolgus monkeys. Acta Pathol. Microbiol. Scand. *46*:156–176, 1959.
68. Waddington, E., Bray, P. T., Evans, A. D., et al.: Cutaneous complications of mass vaccination in South Wales 1962. Trans. St. Johns Hosp. Dermatol. Soc. *50*:22–42, 1964.
69. Wilkinson, J. D.: Orf: A family with unusual complications. Br. J. Dermatol. *97*:447–450, 1977.
70. Williams, W. W.: Guideline for infection control in hospital personnel. Infect. Control *4*(Suppl.):326–349, 1983.
71. World Health Organization: Smallpox vaccination certificates. Wkly. Epidemiol. Rec. *39*:305, 1981.
72. Zagury, D., Leonard, R., Fouchard, M., et al.: Immunization against AIDS in humans. Nature *326*:249–250, 1987.

RNA VIRUSES

SUBSECTION **1**

PICORNAVIRIDAE

CHAPTER

170 Enteroviruses and Parechoviruses

JAMES D. CHERRY

Enteroviruses—coxsackieviruses, echoviruses, polioviruses, and newer enteroviruses—and parechoviruses are responsible for significant and frequent human illnesses with protean clinical manifestations.* Enteroviruses and parechoviruses are two genera of the family *Picornaviridae.* Coxsackieviruses, echoviruses, and polioviruses first were categorized together and named in 1957 by a committee sponsored by the National Foundation for Infantile Paralysis[579]; the human alimentary tract was thought to be the natural habitat of these agents. They are grouped together because of similarities in physical, biochemical, and molecular properties, as well as shared features in their epidemiology and pathogenesis and the many disease syndromes that they cause.

History

Poliomyelitis, the first enteroviral disease to be recognized and the most important one, has a long history.[661] The earliest record is an Egyptian stele of the 18th dynasty (1580 to 1350 BC), which shows a young priest with a withered, shortened leg, the characteristic deformity of paralytic poliomyelitis.[377, 573] Michael Underwood,[830] a London pediatrician, published the first medical description in 1789 in *A Treatise on Diseases of Children.* During the 19th century, many reports appeared in Europe and the United States describing small clusters of cases of "infantile paralysis." The authors were puzzled about the nature of the affliction; not until the 1860s and 1870s was the spinal cord firmly established as the seat of the pathologic process. The contagious nature of poliomyelitis was not appreciated until the latter part of the 19th century. Medin, a Swedish pediatrician, was the first to describe the epidemic nature of poliomyelitis (1890), and his pupil Wickman worked out the basic principles of the epidemiology.[866]

The virus first was isolated in monkeys by Landsteiner and Popper in 1908.[498] The availability of a laboratory animal assay system opened up many avenues of research that in the ensuing 40 years led to the demonstration that an unrecognized intestinal infection was the usual one and the paralytic disease a relatively uncommon event.

Coxsackieviruses and echoviruses have had a shorter history. Epidemic pleurodynia was described clinically in 1735 by Hannaeus more than 200 years before the coxsackieviral etiology of this disease was discovered.[339] In 1948, Dalldorf and Sickles[198] first reported the isolation of a coxsackievirus after inoculation of suckling mice.

In 1949, Enders and associates[233] described the growth of poliovirus 2 in tissue culture, and their techniques paved the way for recovery of a large number of other cytopathic viruses. Most of these "new" viruses failed to produce illness in laboratory animals. Because the relationships of many of these newly recovered agents to human disease were unknown, they were called orphan viruses.[572] Later, several agents were grouped together and called *e*nteric *c*ytopathogenic *h*uman *o*rphan viruses, or echoviruses.

Live attenuated poliovirus vaccines became available 40 years ago, and the most notable advance during the last 15 years has been a dramatic reduction in worldwide poliomyelitis as a result of the global immunization initiative.[174, 392, 809] The last case of confirmed paralytic polio in the Western Hemisphere caused by a wild-type virus strain occurred in 1991.[708]

The Viruses

MORPHOLOGY AND CLASSIFICATION[247, 576–578, 580, 687, 727]

The enteroviruses are single-stranded RNA viruses belonging to the family *Picornaviridae* (pico = small). They are grouped together because they share certain physical, biochemical, and molecular properties. On electron micrographs, the viruses are seen as 30-nm particles that consist of naked protein capsids constituting approximately 70 to 75 percent of the particles and dense central cores (nucleoid) of RNA. Enterovirus capsids are composed of four structural proteins: VP1, VP2, VP3, and VP4. The capsid shell has icosahedral symmetry with 20 triangular faces and 12 vertices. The shell is formed by VP1, VP2, and VP3; VP4 lies on its inner surface.

The three surface proteins (VP1, VP2, VP3) have no sequence homology, but they have the same topology.[687] Specifically, they form an eight-stranded antiparallel β-barrel that is wedge shaped and composed of two antiparallel β-sheets. The amino acid sequences in the loops that connect the β-strands and the N- and C-terminal sequences that extend from the β-barrel domain of VP1, VP2, and VP3 give each enterovirus its distinct antigenicity.

The coat proteins protect the RNA genome from nucleases and are important determinants of host range and tropism. They determine antigenicity, and they deliver the RNA genome into the cytoplasm of new host cells.

*See references 137, 139, 140, 197, 326, 463, 527, 572, 576, 758, 859–862, 864.

TABLE 170–1 ■ ORIGINAL CLASSIFICATION OF HUMAN ENTEROVIRUSES: ANIMAL AND TISSUE CULTURE SPECTRUM*

		Cytopathic Effect		Illness and Pathology	
Virus	**Antigenic Types**†	Monkey Kidney Tissue Culture	Human Tissue Culture	Suckling Mouse	Monkey
Polioviruses	1–3	+	+	–	+
Coxsackieviruses A	1–24‡	–	–	+	–
Coxsackieviruses B	1–6	+	+	+	–
Echoviruses	1–34§	+	±	–	–

*Many enteroviral strains have been isolated that do not conform to these categories.
†New types, beginning with type 68, were assigned enterovirus type numbers instead of coxsackievirus or echovirus numbers. Types 68 through 71 were identified.
‡Type 23 was found to be the same as echovirus 9.
§Echovirus 10 was reclassified as a reovirus; echovirus 28 was reclassified as a rhinovirus.
Modified from Cherry, J. D.: Enteroviruses. *In* Remington, J. S., and Klein, J. O. (eds.): Infectious Diseases of the Fetus and Newborn Infant. 3rd ed. Philadelphia, W. B. Saunders, 1990, pp. 325–366.

The genome of enteroviruses is a single-stranded, positive-sense RNA molecule.[679] It contains a 5′ noncoding region that is followed by a single long open-reading frame, a short 3′ noncoding region, and a poly(a) tail. The four capsid proteins (VP1 to VP4) and seven nonstructural proteins (2A, 2B, 2C, 3A, 3B, 3C, 3D) result from a cleaved, long polyprotein that was translated from genomic RNA.

Viral components and complete virions are formed in the cytoplasm of infected cells. If the rate of virus assembly is rapid and many particles are formed in one area, crystallization may occur.

The original classification of human enteroviruses is shown in Table 170–1. The enteroviral subgroups were differentiated from each other by their different effects in tissue culture and animals. Although these differentiating factors are still useful, many strains now have been isolated that do not conform to such rigid specificities. For example, several coxsackievirus A strains grow and have a cytopathic effect in monkey kidney tissue cultures, and some echovirus strains cause paralysis in mice. The enteroviruses characterized more recently were assigned enterovirus-type numbers instead of coxsackievirus or echovirus numbers. The prototype enteroviral strains Fermon, Toluca-1, J670/71, and BrCr were assigned enteroviral numbers 68 through 71, respectively. Enteroviral types are identified definitively by neutralization with type-specific antisera.

Studies of the viral genome of echoviruses 22 and 23 found that they were distinctly different from other enteroviruses, and hence, they have been placed in the new genus *Parechovirus;* they are parechoviruses types 1 and 2.[687, 782, 783] Parechoviruses contain only three capsid polypeptides: VP1, VP2, and VP0, which is the uncleared precursor to VP2 plus VP4.

Complete or partial genetic sequence data are available for all enteroviruses.[209, 460, 653, 677, 679, 683, 687] In general, sequence comparisons partially support the classic subgrouping of enteroviruses as noted in Table 170–1. However, in many instances, genetic relationships do not correlate with the original subdivisions.[405, 653, 679] All prototype human enterovirus strains fall into one of five genomically identified clusters.[399, 405, 653, 679] Presented in Table 170–2 is the species designation by genetic analysis for the original enteroviral types.

The cellular receptors and co-receptors for attachment of selected enteroviruses and parechoviruses in the replication cycle are presented in Table 170–3. After attachment, the replication cycle takes 5 to 10 hours and occurs in the cytoplasm.

CHARACTERISTICS AND HOST SYSTEMS[576, 580, 653]

Enteroviruses are relatively stable viruses in that they retain activity for several days at room temperature and can be stored indefinitely at ordinary freezer temperatures (–20° C). They are inactivated quickly by heat (>56° C), formaldehyde, chlorination, and ultraviolet light.

Enteroviral strains grow rapidly when adapted to susceptible host systems and cause cytopathology in 2 to 7 days. The typical tissue culture cytopathic effect is shown in Figure 170–1; characteristic pathologic findings in mice are shown in Figures 170–2 and 170–3. Final titers of virus recovered in the laboratory vary markedly among different viral strains and the host system used; typically, concentrations of 10^3 to 10^7 infectious doses per 0.1 mL of tissue culture fluid or tissue homogenate are obtained. Unadapted viral strains frequently require long periods of incubation. In both tissue culture and suckling mice, evidence of growth usually is visible. Blind passage occasionally is necessary for the cytopathology to become apparent.

Although many different primary and secondary tissue culture systems support the growth of various enteroviruses, primary rhesus monkey kidney cultures generally are accepted to have the most inclusive spectrum.[94] Other simian kidney tissue cultures, however, also have the same broad spectrum. Tissue cultures of human origin have a

TABLE 170–2 ■ GENOMIC CLASSIFICATION OF ENTEROVIRUSES*

Species Designation	Original Enteroviral Type
Poliovirus (PV)	Poliovirus types 1, 2, 3
Human enterovirus A (HEV-A)	Coxsackievirus A types 2–8, 10, 12, 14, 16 Enterovirus type 71
Human enterovirus B (HEV-B)	Coxsackievirus type A9 Coxsackievirus types B1–B6 Echovirus types 1–9, 11–21, 24–27, 29–33 Enterovirus type 69
Human enterovirus C (HEV-C)	Coxsackievirus A types 1, 11, 13, 15, 17–22, 24
Human enterovirus D (HEV-D)	Enterovirus types 68, 70

*Data from Ishiko, H., Shimada, Y., Yonaha, M., et al.: Molecular diagnosis of human enteroviruses by phylogeny-based classification by use of the VP4 sequence. J. Infect. Dis. *185:*744–754, 2002; and Pallansch, M. A., and Roos, R. P., Enteroviruses: Polioviruses, coxsackieviruses, and newer enteroviruses. *In* Knipe, D. M., and Howley, P. M. (eds.): Fields Virology. Vol. 1. Philadelphia, Lippincott Williams & Wilkins, 2001, pp. 723–775.

TABLE 170–3 ■ CELL RECEPTORS AND CO-RECEPTORS FOR SELECTED ENTEROVIRUSES AND PARECHOVIRUSES

Virus Type	Receptor	Co-receptor
Polioviruses 1–3	Pvr	
Coxsackievirus A13, A18	Icam-1	
Coxsackievirus A21	Decay-accelerating factor (CDSS)	Icam-1
Coxsackievirus A9	$\alpha_v\beta_3$ (vitronectin receptor)	
Coxsackievirus B1–B6	CAR (coxsackievirus-adenovirus receptor) or decay-accelerating factor (CDSS)	$\alpha_v\beta_6$-Integrin
Echoviruses 1, 8	$\alpha_2\beta_1$-Integrin (V1a-2)	β_2-Microglobulin
Echoviruses 3, 6, 7, 11–13, 20, 21, 29, 33	Decay-accelerating factor (CDSS)	β_2-Microglobulin
Enteroviruses 70	Decay-accelerating factor (CDSS)	
Parechovirus 1	$\alpha_v\beta_1$, $\alpha_v\beta_3$ (vitronectin receptor)	

From Racaniello, V. R.: *Picornaviridae*: The viruses and their replication. *In* Knipe, D. M., and Howley, P. M. (eds.): Fields Virology. Vol. 1. Philadelphia, Lippincott Williams & Wilkins, 2001, pp. 685–722.

more limited spectrum, but several echovirus types have shown more consistent primary isolation in human than in monkey kidney culture. A satisfactory system for the primary recovery of enteroviruses from clinical specimens would include primary rhesus, cynomolgus, or African green monkey kidney; a diploid, human embryonic lung fibroblast cell strain; rhabdomyosarcoma cell line tissue cultures; and intraperitoneal and intracerebral inoculation of suckling mice younger than 24 hours.[57, 346, 359, 576, 580]

ANTIGENIC CHARACTERISTICS[573, 575, 576, 580, 653]

Although some minor cross-reactions exist between several coxsackievirus and echovirus types, common group antigens of diagnostic importance have not been defined well. Heat treatment of virions and the use of synthetic peptides have produced antigens with broad enteroviral reactivity.[810, 811] These antigens have been used in enzyme-linked immunosorbent assay (ELISA) and complement-fixation (CF) tests to determine IgG and IgM enteroviral antibodies and for antigen detection. In one study, Terletskaia-Ladwig and colleagues[811] reported the identification of patients infected with enteroviruses by the use of an IgM enzyme immunoassay (EIA). This test used heat-treated coxsackievirus B5 and echovirus 9 as antigens, and it identified patients infected with echoviruses 4, 11, and 30. The sensitivity of the test was 35 percent. In another study involving heat-treated virus or synthetic peptides, the respective sensitivities were 67 and 62 percent.[810] However, both tests lacked

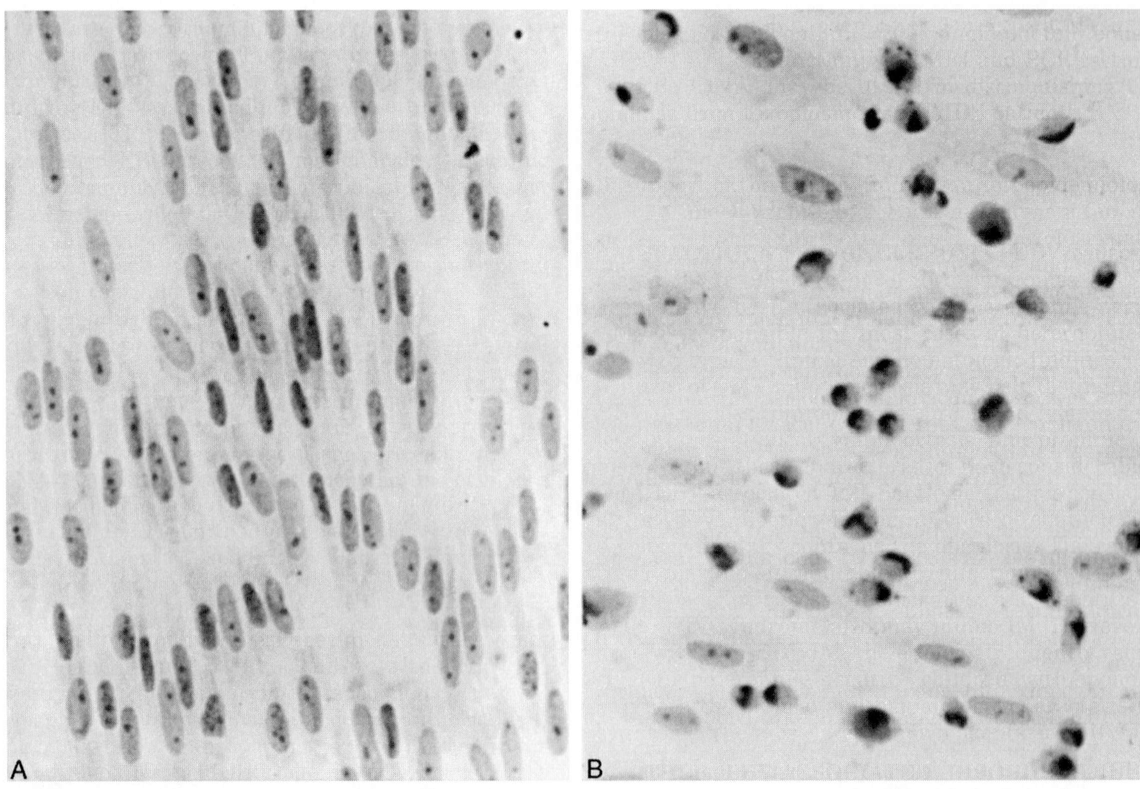

FIGURE 170–1 ■ Fetal rhesus monkey kidney tissue culture (HL-8). *A,* Uninoculated tissue culture. *B,* Echovirus 11 cytopathic effect. (From Cherry, J. D.: Enteroviruses. *In* Remington, J. S., and Klein, J. O. [eds.]: Infectious Diseases of the Fetus and Newborn Infant. Philadelphia, W. B. Saunders, 1976.)

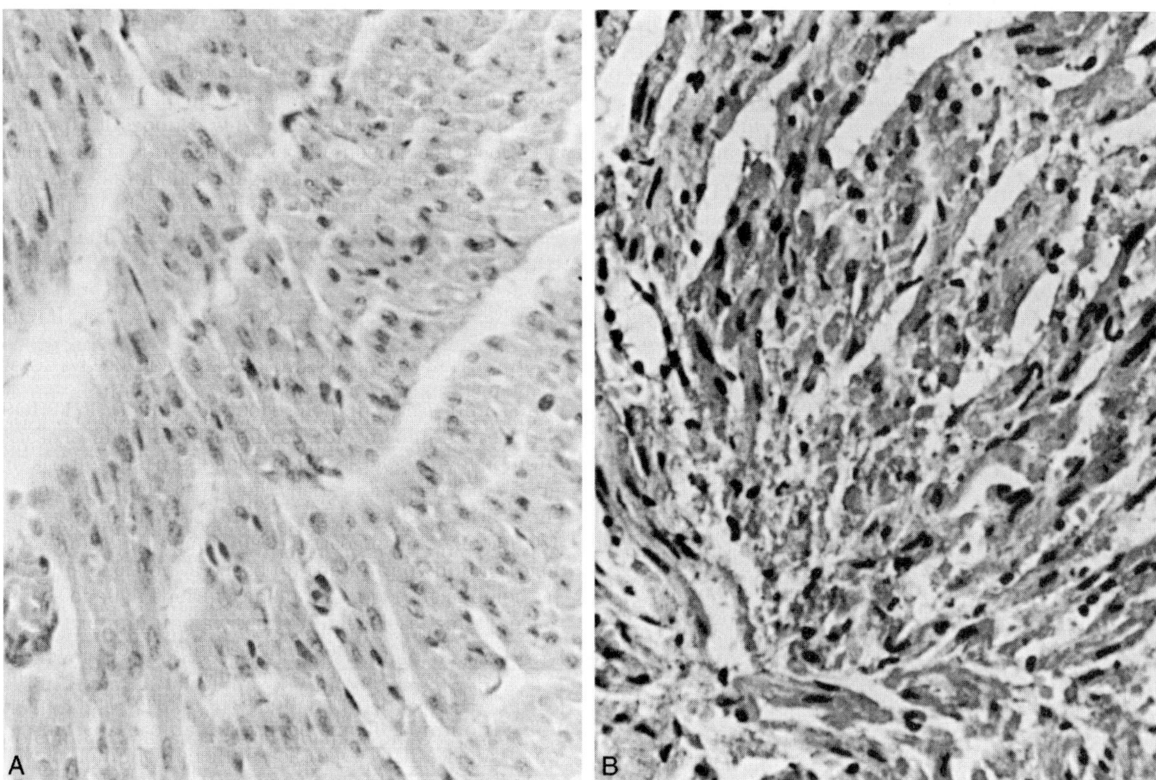

FIGURE 170–2 ■ Suckling mouse myocardium. *A,* Normal suckling mouse myocardium. *B,* Myocardium of a suckling mouse infected with coxsackievirus B1. (From Cherry, J. D.: Enteroviruses. *In* Remington, J. S., and Klein, J. O. [eds.]: Infectious Diseases of the Fetus and Newborn Infant. Philadelphia, W. B. Saunders, 1976.)

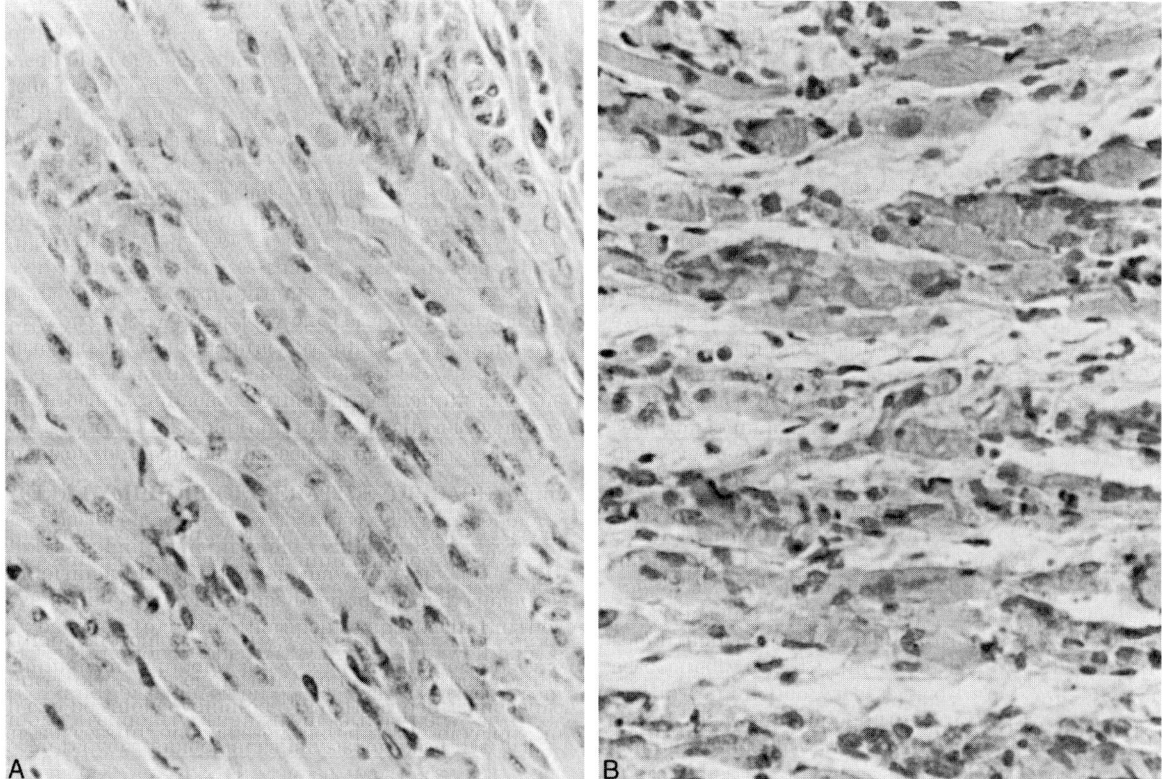

FIGURE 170–3 ■ Suckling mouse skeletal muscle. *A,* Normal suckling mouse skeletal muscle. *B,* Skeletal muscle of a mouse infected with coxsackievirus A16. (From Cherry, J. D.: Enteroviruses. *In* Remington, J. S., and Klein, J. O. [eds.]: Infectious Diseases of the Fetus and Newborn Infant. Philadelphia, W. B. Saunders, 1976.)

specificity. Intratypic strain differences are common findings, and some strains (prime strains) are neutralized poorly by antisera to prototype viruses. In animals, these prime strains induce antibodies that neutralize the specific prototype viruses, however.

The identification of polioviral, coxsackieviral, and echoviral types by neutralization in suckling mice or tissue culture with antiserum pools is relatively well defined. Neutralization is induced by the epitopes on structural proteins VP1, VP2, and VP3; in particular, several epitopes are clustered on VP1. Prime strains do cause diagnostic difficulty because frequently they are not neutralized by the reference antisera, which is a particular problem with echoviruses 4, 9, and 11 and enterovirus 71. If these types or other possible prime strains are suspected, in some instances this problem can be overcome by using antisera in less diluted concentrations or antisera prepared against several different strains of problem viruses. Recently, Kubo and associates[488] have been able to type enteroviral isolates not identified through neutralization by nucleotide sequence analysis of the VP4 gene. They specifically identified prime strains of echovirus 18 and enterovirus 71. Sequence analysis of the VP1 gene also is useful for typing enteroviral prime strains not identified by neutralization.[641]

HOST RANGE

Humans are the only natural hosts of polioviruses, coxsackieviruses, and echoviruses.[289] However, enteroviruses have been recovered in nature from sewage, flies, swine, dogs, a calf, a budgerigar, a fox, mussels, and oysters.[139] In addition, serologic evidence of infection with enteroviruses similar to human strains has been noted in chimpanzees, cattle, rabbits, a fox, a chipmunk, and a marmot.[139] Infection of these animals probably results from direct contact with an infected human or human excreta. Eighteen genetically distinct enteroviruses have been isolated from nonhuman primates.[678] Of 10 of these strains, 7 were related closely genetically to human enteroviruses, whereas the other 3 were related only distantly. Contamination of shellfish also is interesting because in addition to their possible role in human infection, they offer a source of enteroviral storage during cold-weather periods.[139] Contaminated food is another possible source of human infection.[139]

Epidemiology

TRANSMISSION

Humans are the only natural hosts of human polioviruses, coxsackieviruses, and echoviruses.[197, 289, 463, 572, 631, 758, 860, 862] Spread is from person to person by the fecal-oral and possibly the oral-oral (respiratory spread) route. Swimming and wading pools may serve as a means of spread of enteroviruses during the summertime.[458] Oral-oral transmission by way of the contaminated hands of health care personnel and transmission by fomites have been documented in a chronic care pediatric ward.[424] Enteroviruses have been recovered from trapped flies, and such carriage probably contributes to the spread of human infection, particularly in lower socioeconomic populations that have poor sanitary facilities.[139]

Children are the main susceptible cohort; they are immunologically susceptible, and their unhygienic habits facilitate spread. Spread is from child to child (via feces to skin to mouth) and then within family groups. Recovery of enteroviruses is related inversely to age, but the prevalence of specific antibodies is related directly to age. The incidence of infection and the prevalence of antibodies do not differ between boys and girls.

GEOGRAPHIC DISTRIBUTION AND SEASON

Enteroviruses have a worldwide distribution.[139, 258, 289] Neutralizing antibodies for specific viral types have been noted in serologic surveys throughout the world, and most strains have been recovered in worldwide isolation studies. In any given area, frequent fluctuations occur in predominant types. Epidemics probably depend on newly susceptible individuals in the population rather than reinfection; they may be localized and sporadic and may vary in etiology from place to place in the same year. Pandemic waves of infection also occur.

In temperate climates, enteroviral infections occur primarily in the summer and fall, but in the tropics, they are prevalent all year.[139, 289, 575] A basic concept in understanding their epidemiology concerns the far greater frequency of unrecognized infection than clinical disease, as illustrated by poliomyelitis, which remained an epidemiologic mystery until researchers appreciated that unrecognized infections were the main source of contagion. Serologic surveys were instrumental in elucidating the problem: in populations living in conditions of poor sanitation and hygiene, epidemics did not occur, but wide dissemination of polioviruses was confirmed by demonstrating the presence of specific antibodies to all three types in almost 100 percent of children by the time that they reached 5 years of age.

Epidemics of poliomyelitis first began to appear in Europe and the United States during the latter part of the 19th century; they continued with increasing frequency in the economically advanced countries until the introduction of effective vaccines in the 1950s and 1960s.[81, 165, 377, 661] The evolution from endemic to epidemic follows a characteristic pattern beginning with collections of a few cases, then endemic rates that are higher than usual, followed by severe epidemics with high attack rates. The age group attacked in endemic areas and in early epidemics is the youngest, with more than 90 percent of paralytic cases beginning in children younger than 5 years of age. Once this pattern of epidemicity begins, it is irreversible unless preventive vaccination is performed.

As epidemics recur over a period of years, a shift in age incidence occurs whereby relatively fewer cases are in the youngest children; the peak often occurs in the 5- to 14-year-old group, and an increasing proportion of cases develop in young adults. These changes are correlated with socioeconomic factors and improved standards of hygiene: when children are protected from immunizing infections in the first few years of life, the pool of susceptible persons builds up, and introduction of a virulent strain often is followed by an epidemic.[377] The extensive use of vaccines in the past 40 years has resulted in the elimination of paralytic poliomyelitis from large geographic areas, but the disease remains endemic in various parts of the world. Although seasonal periodicity is distinct in temperate climates, some viral activity does take place during the winter months.[139] Infection and the acquisition of postinfection immunity occur with greater intensity and at earlier ages in crowded, economically deprived populations with less efficient sanitation.

Molecular techniques have allowed study of the genotypes of specific viral types in populations over the course of time.[213, 406, 525, 611] For example, Mulders and colleagues[611] studied the molecular epidemiology of wild poliovirus 1 in

Europe, the Middle East, and the Indian subcontinent. They found that four major genotypes were circulating. Two genotypes were found predominantly in eastern Europe, a third genotype was circulating mainly in Egypt, and the fourth genotype was dispersed widely. All four genotypes were found in Pakistan.

PREVALENCE OF DIFFERENT TYPES

The epidemiologic behavior of coxsackieviruses and echoviruses parallels that of polioviruses, in which unrecognized infections far outnumber those with distinctive symptoms. The agents are disseminated widely throughout the world, and outbreaks caused by one or another type occur regularly. They tend to be localized, with different agents being prevalent in different years. In the late 1950s, however, echovirus 9 had a far wider circulation; it swept through a large part of the world and infected not only children but also young adults. This behavior has been repeated occasionally with other enteroviruses: after a long absence, a particular agent returns and circulates among the susceptible persons of different ages who have been born since the last epidemic. Other agents remain endemic in a given area and surface as sporadic cases and occasionally in small outbreaks. Multiple types requently are factive at the same time, although one agent commonly is predominant in a given locality.

Listed in Table 170–4 are the five most prevalent nonpolio enterovirus isolations per year in the United States from 1961 through 1999.[11, 116, 120, 121, 139, 792] Most patients from whom viruses were isolated had neurologic illnesses. Other enteroviruses also possibly were prevalent but did not cause clinical disease severe enough to induce physicians to submit

TABLE 170–4 ■ PREDOMINANT TYPES OF NONPOLIO ENTEROVIRAL ISOLATIONS IN THE UNITED STATES: 1961 TO 1999*

	Five Most Common Viral Types Per Year				
	First	Second	Third	Fourth	Fifth
1961	Coxsackievirus B5	Coxsackievirus B2	Coxsackievirus B4	Echovirus 11	Echovirus 9
1962	Coxsackievirus B3	Echovirus 9	Coxsackievirus B2	Echovirus 4	Coxsackievirus B5
1963	Coxsackievirus B1	Coxsackievirus A9	Echovirus 9	Echovirus 4	Coxsackievirus B4
1964	Coxsackievirus B4	Coxsackievirus B2	Coxsackievirus A9	Echovirus 4	Echovirus 6, coxsackievirus B1
1965	Echovirus 9	Echovirus 6	Coxsackievirus B2	Coxsackievirus B5	Coxsackievirus B4
1966	Echovirus 9	Coxsackievirus B2	Echovirus 6	Coxsackievirus B5	Coxsackievirus A9, A16
1967	Coxsackievirus B5	Echovirus 9	Coxsackievirus A9	Echovirus 6	Coxsackievirus B2
1968	Echovirus 9	Echovirus 30	Coxsackievirus A16	Coxsackievirus B3	Coxsackievirus B4
1969	Echovirus 30	Echovirus 9	Echovirus 18	Echovirus 6	Coxsackievirus B4
1970	Echovirus 3	Echovirus 9	Echovirus 6	Echovirus 4	Coxsackievirus B4
1971	Echovirus 4	Echovirus 9	Echovirus 6	Coxsackievirus B4	Coxsackievirus B2
1972	Coxsackievirus B5	Echovirus 4	Echovirus 6	Echovirus 9	Coxsackievirus B3
1973	Coxsackievirus A9	Echovirus 9	Echovirus 6	Coxsackievirus B2	Coxsackievirus B5, echovirus 5
1974	Echovirus 11	Echovirus 4	Echovirus 6	Echovirus 9	Echovirus 18
1975	Echovirus 9	Echovirus 4	Echovirus 6	Coxsackievirus A9	Coxsackievirus B4
1976	Coxsackievirus B2	Echovirus 4	Coxsackievirus B4	Coxsackievirus A9	Coxsackievirus B3, echovirus 6
1977	Echovirus 6	Coxsackievirus B1	Coxsackievirus B3	Echovirus 9	Coxsackievirus A9
1978	Echovirus 9	Echovirus 4	Coxsackievirus A9	Echovirus 30	Coxsackievirus B4
1979	Echovirus 11	Echovirus 7	Echovirus 30	Coxsackievirus B2	Coxsackievirus B4
1980	Echovirus 11	Coxsackievirus B3	Echovirus 30	Coxsackievirus B2	Coxsackievirus A9
1981	Echovirus 30	Echovirus 9	Echovirus 11	Echovirus 3	Coxsackievirus A9, echovirus 5
1982	Echovirus 11	Echovirus 30	Echovirus 5	Echovirus 9	Coxsackievirus B5
1983	Coxsackievirus B5	Echovirus 30	Echovirus 20	Echovirus 11	Echovirus 24
1984	Echovirus 9	Echovirus 11	Coxsackievirus B5	Echovirus 30	Coxsackievirus B2, A9
1985	Echovirus 11	Echovirus 21	Echovirus 6, 7†		Coxsackievirus B2
1986	Echovirus 11	Echovirus 4	Echovirus 7	Echovirus 18	Coxsackievirus B5
1987	Echovirus 6	Echovirus 18	Echovirus 11	Coxsackievirus A9	Coxsackievirus B2
1988	Echovirus 11	Echovirus 9	Coxsackievirus B4	Coxsackievirus B2	Echovirus 6
1989	Coxsackievirus B5	Echovirus 9	Echovirus 11	Coxsackievirus B2	Echovirus 6
1990	Echovirus 30	Echovirus 6	Coxsackievirus B2	Coxsackievirus A9	Echovirus 11
1991	Echovirus 30	Echovirus 11	Coxsackievirus B1	Coxsackievirus B2	Echovirus 7
1992	Echovirus 11	Echovirus 30	Echovirus 9	Coxsackievirus B1	Coxsackievirus A9
1993	Echovirus 30	Coxsackievirus B5	Coxsackievirus A9	Echovirus 7	Coxsackievirus B3
1994	Coxsackievirus B2	Coxsackievirus B3	Echovirus 6	Echovirus 30	Enterovirus 71
1995	Echovirus 9	Echovirus 11	Coxsackievirus A9	Coxsackievirus B2	Echovirus 30, coxsackievirus B5
1996	Coxsackievirus B5	Echovirus 17	Echovirus 6	Coxsackievirus A9	Coxsackievirus B4
1997	Echovirus 30	Echovirus 6	Echovirus 7	Echovirus 11	Echovirus 18
1998	Echovirus 30	Echovirus 9	Echovirus 11	Coxsackievirus B3	Echovirus 6
1999	Echovirus 11	Echovirus 16	Echovirus 9	Echovirus 14	Echovirus 25

*The majority of patients from whom viruses were isolated had neurologic illnesses.[11, 116, 120, 121, 139, 279, 792]
†Third and fourth place tie.

specimens for study. In addition, probably many coxsackievirus A infections, even in epidemic situations, went undiagnosed because suckling mouse inoculation was not performed. Although 62 nonpolio enteroviral types and 2 parechovirus types have been identified, of interest is that in the 39 years covered in Table 170–4, only 24 different virus types are noted. In the earlier years, echovirus 9 was most common, with echoviruses 6 and 11 and coxsackieviruses B2 and B4 being the next most common. Since 1990, echoviruses 30 and 11 have been the most frequent circulating viral types. Interestingly, in 1999, three of the five most common viral types (echoviruses 14, 16, and 25) were new to the list.

Similar data for the most common enteroviral isolates in Spain from 1988 to 1997 and in Belgium from 1980 to 1994 are available.[216, 824] The enterovirus isolated most frequently in both countries was echovirus 30. In 1997 and 1998, major epidemic disease caused by enterovirus 71 occurred in Taiwan, Malaysia, Australia, and Japan.[91, 127, 369, 481, 565]

Even though the use of live polioviral vaccine has eliminated epidemic poliomyelitis in the United States, determining the effect that polio vaccine viruses has had on enteroviral ecology has been difficult. In 1970, polioviruses accounted for only 6 percent of the total number of enteroviral isolations from patients with neurologic illnesses.[139] Although the figures are not directly comparable, more than one third of the enteroviral isolations in 1962 from similar patients were polioviruses.[139] However, Horstmann and colleagues[378] studied specimens from sewage and asymptomatic children during the vaccine era and noted that the number of yearly polioviral isolations (presumably vaccine strains) was greater than the number of nonpolioviral enteroviruses. The prevalence of vaccine viruses apparently did not affect the seasonal epidemiology of other enteroviruses.

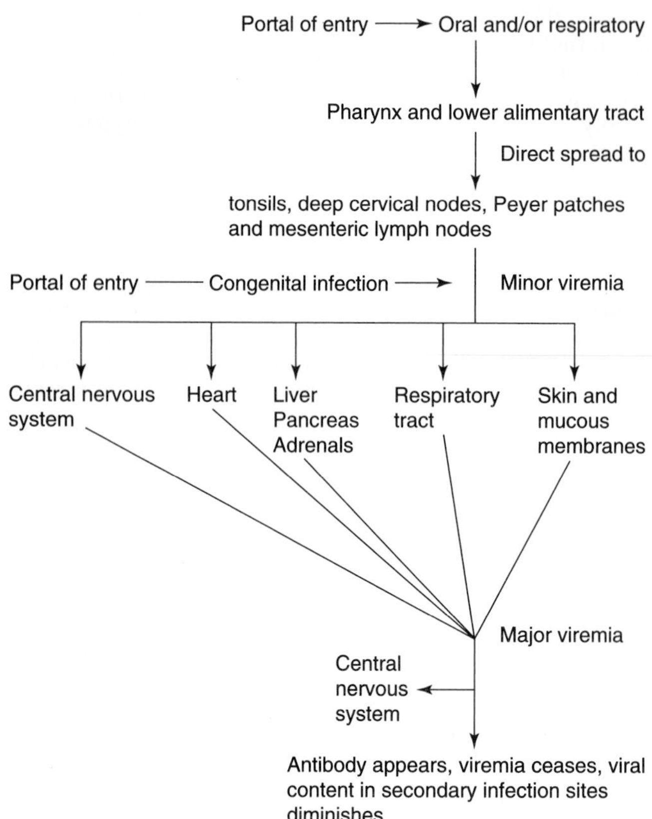

FIGURE 170–4 ■ Pathogenesis of enteroviral infections. (Modified from Cherry, J. D.: Enteroviruses. *In* Remington, J. S., and Klein, J. O. [eds.]: Infectious Diseases of the Fetus and Newborn Infant. Philadelphia, W. B. Saunders, 1976.)

Pathogenesis and Pathology

EVENTS DURING PATHOGENESIS[81, 139, 140, 576, 653, 731]

Figure 170–4 diagrams the events of pathogenesis. After initial acquisition of virus by the oral or respiratory route, implantation occurs in the pharynx and the lower alimentary tract. Within 1 day, the infection extends to the regional lymph nodes. On approximately the third day, minor viremia occurs and results in the involvement of many secondary infection sites. In congenital infections, infection is initiated during the minor viremia phase. Multiplication of virus in secondary infection sites coincides with the onset of clinical symptoms. Illness can vary from minor infections to fatal ones. Major viremia occurs during the period of multiplication of virus in secondary infection sites; this period usually lasts from the third to the seventh day of infection. In many echovirus and coxsackievirus infections, central nervous system (CNS) involvement apparently occurs at the same time as other secondary organ involvement. Occasionally, the CNS symptoms of enteroviral infections are delayed, thus suggesting that seeding occurred later in association with the major viremic phase.

Cessation of viremia correlates with the appearance of serum antibody. The viral concentration in secondary infection sites begins to diminish on approximately the seventh day. However, infection continues in the lower intestinal tract for prolonged periods.

In Figure 170–5, clinical and subclinical events in polioviral infections are presented. By 3 to 5 days after exposure, virus can be recovered from blood, the throat, and feces. This finding may be accompanied by symptoms of the "minor illness," or the infection may be unrecognized clinically. The end of the period of viremia coincides with the appearance of antibodies and the onset of clinical signs of CNS involvement. The available evidence favors blood as the main pathway of CNS invasion in natural disease, but experimental infections in monkeys indicate that the virus can travel along the axons of peripheral nerves. Possibly, when tonsillectomy is performed on a child with inapparent poliovirus infection, the virus enters the nerve fibers exposed during surgery and spreads to the cranial nerve nuclei in the brain, thereby resulting in bulbar paralysis.

FACTORS THAT AFFECT PATHOGENESIS

The pathogenesis and pathology of enteroviral infections depend on the virulence, tropism, and inoculum concentration of virus, as well as on many specific host factors. Enteroviruses obviously have marked differences in both tropism and virulence. Although some generalizations can be made with regard to tropism, marked differences occur even among strains of specific viral types. Differences in the virulence of specific enteroviral types may be the result of recombination among enteroviruses or point mutations.[693, 707, 743]

Van Eden and associates[836] studied 17 families during an outbreak of poliomyelitis caused by type 1 virus in the Netherlands, and their findings suggested that HLA-related genetic factors were important in the occurrence of paralytic disease.

Enterovirus infections in the fetus and neonate generally are thought to be more severe than are similar infections in

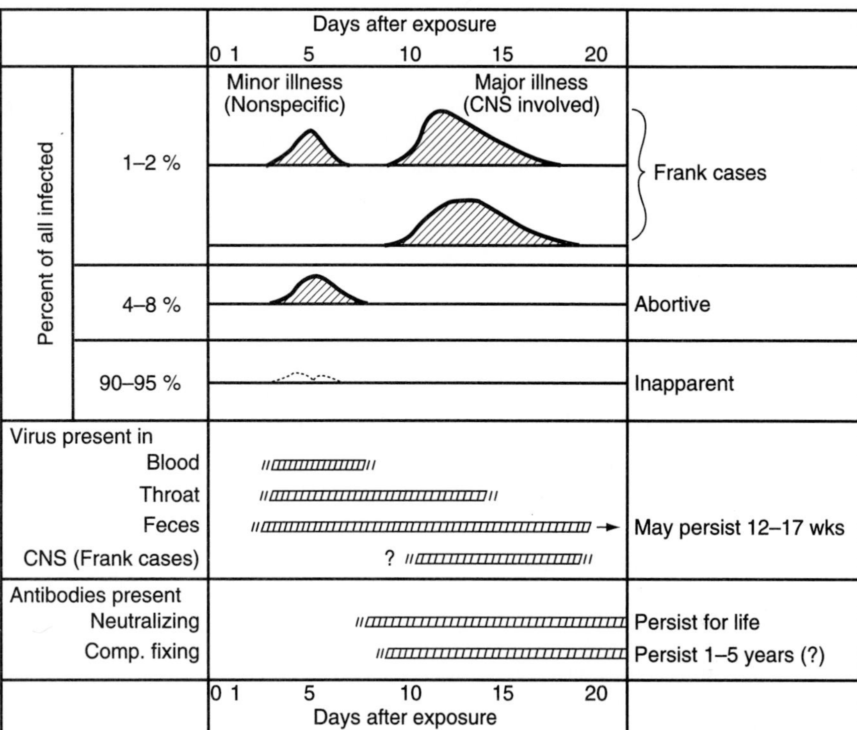

FIGURE 170–5 ■ The course of clinical and subclinical forms of poliovirus infection in relation to the presence of virus and the development of antibodies. (From Bodian, D., and Horstmann, D. M.: Poliomyelitis. *In* Horsfall, F. L., and Tamm, I. [eds.]: Viral and Rickettsial Infections of Man. 4th ed. Philadelphia, J. B. Lippincott, 1965, pp. 430–473.)

older persons, which undoubtedly is the case with coxsackievirus B infection and probably also with coxsackievirus A and echovirus infections. Although the reasons for this increased severity are unknown, several aspects of neonatal immune mechanisms have been suggested. In addition, the similarity of coxsackievirus B infections in suckling mice to those in human neonates has provided a useful animal model system. Heinberg and associates[353] compared coxsackievirus B1 infections in 24-hour-old suckling mice with similar infection in older mice. They noted that adult mice produced interferon in all infected tissues, whereas suckling mice produced only small amounts of interferon in the liver. They thought that the difference in outcome of coxsackievirus B1 infection in suckling and older mice could be explained by the inability of cells of the immature animals to elaborate interferon.

Other researchers suggest that the increased susceptibility of suckling mice to severe coxsackievirus infections is related to the transplacentally acquired, increased concentrations of adrenocortical hormones.[55, 82] Kunin[491] has suggested that the difference in age-specific susceptibility might be explained at the cellular level. He has shown that a variety of tissues of newborn mice bind coxsackievirus B3 whereas tissues of adult mice are virtually inactive in this regard.[490, 491] The progressive loss of receptor-containing cells with increasing age may be the mechanism that accounts for less severe infections in older animals.

In the past, researchers assumed that specific pathology in various organs and tissues in enteroviral infections was caused by the direct cytopathic effect and tropism of a particular virus. In more recent years, however, a large number of studies using murine model systems have suggested that host immune responses contribute to the pathology.* These studies suggest that T-cell–mediated processes and virus-induced autoimmunity cause both acute and chronic tissue damage. In contrast, other studies suggest that the primary viral cytopathic effect is responsible for the tissue damage and that the various T-cell responses are a reaction to the damage and not the cause of the damage.[564]

During the last 40 years, the clinical manifestations caused by several enteroviral serotypes have changed. For example, echovirus 11 infection initially was noted in association with exanthem and aseptic meningitis in children. More recently, it has been found to be the cause of severe sepsis-like illness in neonates. These phenotypic changes in disease expression may be the result of recombination among enteroviruses.[459, 743]

PATHOLOGY

The clinical signs of enteroviral infection vary widely, so wide variations in pathology also exist. Because pathologic material generally is available only from patients with fatal illness, this section discusses only the more severe manifestations. Worth emphasizing, however, is that these fatal infections account for just a small portion of all enteroviral infections. The pathologic findings in children with milder infections, such as nonspecific febrile illness, have not been described.

Coxsackieviruses A

Records of severe illness associated with coxsackieviruses A are rare. Gold and colleagues,[306] in a study of sudden unexpected death in infants, recovered coxsackievirus A4 from the brains of three children. In none of these patients were histologic abnormalities noted in the brain or spinal cord. An adult with a fatal coxsackievirus A7 infection had diffuse pancarditis and organized pneumonitis.[41]

*See references 27, 135, 281, 284, 357, 360, 371, 436, 499, 653, 655, 685, 694, 713, 762, 877.

Coxsackieviruses B

Of the nonpolio enteroviruses, coxsackieviruses B have been associated most frequently with severe and catastrophic disease. The most common findings in these cases have been myocarditis, meningoencephalitis, or both. Involvement of the adrenals, pancreas, liver, and lungs also has been noted.

HEART.[139, 242, 287, 878] Grossly, the heart usually is enlarged, with dilatation of the chambers and flabby musculature. Microscopically, the pericardium frequently contains some inflammatory cells along with thickening and edema, and the endocardium may have focal infiltrations of inflammatory cells. The myocardium (Fig. 170–6) is congested and contains infiltrations of inflammatory cells (lymphocytes, mononuclear cells, reticulum cells, histiocytes, plasma cells, and polymorphonuclear and eosinophil leukocytes). Involvement of the myocardium often is patchy and focal but occasionally diffuse. The muscle shows loss of striation as well as edema and eosinophilic degeneration. Muscle necrosis without extensive cellular infiltration is a common finding.

BRAIN AND SPINAL CORD.[139, 242, 597, 878] The meninges are congested, edematous, and occasionally mildly infiltrated with inflammatory cells. Lesions in the brain and spinal cord are focal rather than diffuse but frequently involve many different areas. The lesions consist of areas of eosinophilic degeneration of cortical cells, clusters of mononuclear and glial cells (Fig. 170–7), and perivascular cuffing. Two children with fatal coxsackieviral B infection (types 2 and 4) had, in addition to typical inflammatory encephalitic lesions, widespread multifocal areas of liquefaction necrosis without inflammation.[235]

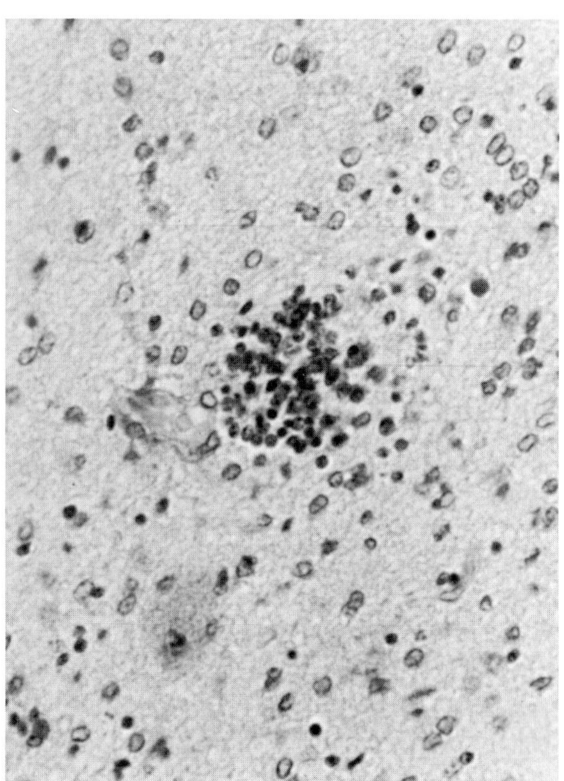

FIGURE 170–7 ■ Coxsackievirus B4 encephalitis in a 9-day-old infant with focal infiltration of mononuclear and glial cells. (From Cherry, J. D.: Enteroviruses. *In* Remington, J. S., and Klein, J. O. [eds.]: Infectious Diseases of the Fetus and Newborn Infant. Philadelphia, W. B. Saunders, 1976.)

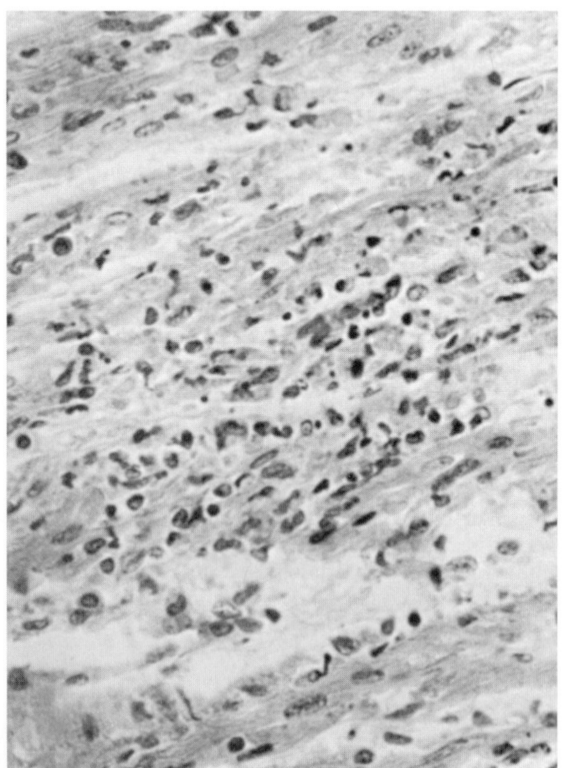

FIGURE 170–6 ■ Coxsackievirus B4 myocarditis in a 9-day-old infant. Note the myocardial necrosis and mononuclear cellular infiltration. (From Cherry, J. D.: Enteroviruses. *In* Remington, J. S., and Klein, J. O. [eds.]: Infectious Diseases of the Fetus and Newborn Infant. Philadelphia, W. B. Saunders, 1976.)

OTHER ORGANS.[10, 139, 288, 597, 878] The lungs frequently have areas of mild focal pneumonitis with peribronchiolar mononuclear cellular infiltration. The liver often is engorged and occasionally contains isolated foci of liver cell necrosis and mononuclear infiltration. In the pancreas, occasional focal degeneration of islet cells occurs. Congestion has been observed in the adrenal glands, along with mild to severe cortical necrosis; inflammatory cells are present.

Echoviruses

Though frequently responsible for illness, until relatively recently echoviruses rarely were associated with fatal infection. Interestingly, in several different reports with eight different echovirus types, hepatic necrosis was a major pathologic finding.[76, 139, 291, 334, 588, 606, 884] Massive hepatic necrosis has been seen with echoviruses 3, 6, 7, 9, 11, 14, 19, and 21. At autopsy, one infant with echovirus 6 infection had cloudy and thickened leptomeninges, liver necrosis, adrenal and renal hemorrhage, and mild interstitial pneumonitis.[139] One infant with echovirus 9 infection had an enlarged and congested liver with marked central necrosis,[139] and another with this virus had interstitial pneumonitis without liver involvement.[139] Three infants with echovirus 11 infection had renal and adrenal hemorrhage and small vessel thrombi in the renal medulla and in both the medulla and inner cortex of the adrenals.[615] These patients' livers were normal. Two infants, one with echovirus 6 and the other with echovirus 31 infection, had only extensive pneumonia.[88, 139]

Enteroviruses

The brain of a child who died of acute encephalitis caused by enterovirus 71 infection has been examined.[889] Grossly, the brain appeared normal, but microscopically, it revealed typical features of acute encephalitis consisting of perivascular cuffing with mixed inflammatory cells, neuronophagia, and inflammatory nodules.

Polioviruses[81, 165]

The neuropathy of poliomyelitis usually is pathognomonic; only certain cells and areas of the neuraxis are susceptible to the virus. Neuronal damage is caused directly by virus multiplication, but not all affected neurons are killed. The injury may be reversible, and function may be restored within 3 to 4 weeks after onset. Little histologic evidence of meningeal reaction exists. Perivascular cuffing and some interstitial glial infiltration are present. Histologic sections generally reveal more widespread lesions than would be estimated from the clinical findings. Scattered neurons may undergo considerable destruction without clinical disability.

Regions in which neuronal lesions occur are (1) the spinal cord (anterior horn cells chiefly and to a lesser degree the intermediate and dorsal horn and dorsal root ganglia), (2) the medulla (vestibular nuclei, cranial nerve nuclei, and the reticular formation that contains the vital centers), (3) the cerebellum (nuclei in the roof and vermis only), (4) the midbrain (chiefly the gray matter but also the substantia nigra and occasionally the red nucleus), (5) the thalamus and hypothalamus, (6) the pallidum, and (7) the cerebral cortex (motor cortex). The viruses spare the following areas: (1) the entire cerebral cortex except the motor area, (2) the cerebellum except the vermis and deep midline nuclei, and (3) the white matter of the spinal cord. This distribution of lesions permits a histologic diagnosis of poliomyelitis.

Extraneural pathology usually is a secondary phenomenon. Bronchopulmonary changes such as aspiration pneumonia, atelectasis, and purulent bronchitis may occur because of impaired coughing and decreased thoracic movement. Cardiovascular changes may result in hypertension, cardiac failure, and pulmonary edema. Prolonged immobilization leads to negative nitrogen and calcium balance, along with urinary lithiasis, renal failure, hypertension with encephalopathy, and convulsions. Treatment itself may cause untoward complications, such as urinary tract infection (after catheterization), decubitus ulcers, and psychotic disturbances. Ulcerations in the alimentary tract may result in serious bleeding and occasional perforation. Respiratory failure culminates in respiratory acidosis and anoxic changes.

Clinical Manifestations—Nonpolio Enteroviruses and Parechoviruses

Nonpolio enteroviral and parechoviral infections are exceedingly common occurrences, and the spectrum of disease is protean (Tables 170–5 through 170–18). Many of the clinical-virologic associations listed in Tables 170–5 through 170–18 are based on a limited number of cases. Because coxsackieviruses and echoviruses frequently are carried asymptomatically in the gastrointestinal tract for relatively long periods, some of the observed illnesses and the viruses concomitantly recovered may not have a cause-and-effect relationship. However, repeated observations since the 1960s have supported many virus-illness associations, even though their occurrence has been sporadic.

Few specific enterovirus or parechovirus diseases exist, but, rather, a variety of interrelated syndromes and anatomically associated illnesses. Many illnesses and syndromes can be caused by different viral types, and most types are capable of inducing a variety of clinical syndromes. On the other hand, certain specific coxsackieviral and echoviral types have clinical characteristics that facilitate an etiologic diagnosis.

During the last 2 decades, few careful studies have been conducted in which specific clinical findings have been correlated with individual enteroviral types. This paucity has been fostered by the expense of serotyping and the lack of use of suckling mice inoculation for virus isolation. The increased use of polymerase chain reaction (PCR) during the last decade also has contributed to the lack of identification of disease manifestations by specific viral type, which is unfortunate because the clinical manifestations caused by specific viral types are not constant and disease severity varies by specific enteroviral type.

ASYMPTOMATIC INFECTION

Because researchers have known that 90 to 95 percent of poliovirus infections are not recognized clinically, they have assumed that most infections with enteroviruses and parechoviruses are asymptomatic. This opinion also is strengthened by the fact that these viruses can be recovered frequently from the stools of normal children. However, relatively few data are available on the rate of asymptomatic infection with nonpolio enteroviruses and parechoviruses. All too frequently, isolation of enteroviruses and parechoviruses from stool is equated with asymptomatic infection, which is an error because illness, if it takes place, occurs shortly after the acquisition of virus and is short lived; a particular infection may have been associated with a nonspecific illness 2 or 3 months before collection of a stool specimen obtained in a surveillance program. Unfortunately, in several studies involving controlled population groups in which accurate clinical expression rates could have been determined, clinical observations apparently were of secondary importance to the investigators.[139, 289, 290, 292, 480] The data available suggest differences in clinical expression among coxsackieviral and echoviral types.

Table 170–5 lists the approximate frequency of asymptomatic infections with selected coxsackieviruses and echoviruses. As can be seen, the rates vary among the group as a whole and even within specific types. Overall, approximately half and perhaps more of all nonpolio enteroviral infections appear to be associated with clinical manifestations. In general, the more carefully clinical symptoms are examined, the smaller the percentage of truly asymptomatic infections. Clinical expression also is related inversely to age. With coxsackievirus A16, asymptomatic infection occurs in only approximately 10 percent of children younger than 5 years, whereas rates are higher in older children and adults.[8, 139] Sabin[730] reported no asymptomatic infections in infants with echovirus 18, and Nishmi and Yodfat[639] noted less than 20 percent of infections without illness in children younger than 8 years during an echovirus 4 epidemic. At the other extreme, Clemmer and associates[173] reported that 96 percent of infections with coxsackievirus B3 were asymptomatic. In other studies, the illness rate of coxsackievirus B3 has been 60 to 75 percent.

NONSPECIFIC FEBRILE ILLNESS (Table 170–6)

Nonspecific febrile illness is the most common manifestation of coxsackieviral and echoviral infection. All viral types

TABLE 170–5 ■ APPROXIMATE FREQUENCIES OF ASYMPTOMATIC INFECTION WITH SELECTED COXSACKIEVIRUSES AND ECHOVIRUSES

	Asymptomatic Infection Frequency (%)
Coxsackieviruses	
A	50
A16	50
B	20
B2	11-50
B3	25-96
B4	30-70
B5	5-40
Echoviruses	50
4	Uncommon—60
6	Rare
9	15-60
18	Rare-20
20	33
25	30
30	50

From Cherry, J. D.: Enteroviruses: Polioviruses (poliomyelitis), coxsackieviruses, echoviruses, and enteroviruses. *In* Feigin, R. D., and Cherry, J. D. (eds.): Textbook of Pediatric Infectious Diseases. 2nd ed. Philadelphia, W. B. Saunders, 1987, pp. 1729–1790.

cause this clinical finding, but its frequency varies considerably among the individual viruses.

The onset of illness usually is abrupt, without a prodrome. In young children, the initial finding is fever and associated malaise. In older children, headache generally is noted. The temperature ranges between 38.3° and 40° C (101° and 104° F) and has a mean duration of 3 days. In some instances, the fever is biphasic: it occurs for 1 day, is absent for 2 to 3 days, and then recurs for an additional 2 to 4 days. In many young children, the only manifestation of illness is fever, and its presence is discovered by chance by a parent.

Malaise and anorexia often are related to the degree of temperature elevation, as is headache in older patients. Sore throat is a common complaint, but an inflamed pharynx is not seen on examination. Nausea and vomiting occasionally occur at the onset of illness, as does mild abdominal discomfort. One or two loose stools may be noted. Generalized myalgia also is observed, and children complain of a scratchy feeling in the throat.

Physical examination usually yields benign findings. Minimal conjunctivitis, injection of the pharynx, and cervical lymphadenitis may be present. The duration of illness varies from 24 hours to approximately 6 days, with an average of 3 to 4 days. The white blood cell count is normal.

Enteroviruses, particularly coxsackieviruses A, are significant causes of febrile convulsions in young children.[381]

RESPIRATORY MANIFESTATIONS (see Table 170–6)

Common Cold

Although numerous coxsackieviruses and echoviruses have been recovered from children with mild upper respiratory infections, only rarely do the illnesses qualify as common colds. (The common cold is an acute illness with nasal stuffiness, rhinitis, no objective evidence of pharyngitis, and no or minimal fever.) In most instances, significant fever (temperature >38.3° C [>101° F]) is associated with enteroviral infections and usually some degree of pharyngitis.

Coxsackievirus A21 is the only enterovirus that clearly qualifies as a common cold virus.[139, 426] This agent has produced epidemics of mild respiratory illness in military populations. In adult volunteers, instillation of this virus in the nose has resulted in the common cold syndrome. Epidemic disease has not been observed in children. Other viruses that have been associated with the common cold syndrome include echoviruses 2 and 20 and coxsackieviruses B1, B2, B3, B4, B5, and A24.[139]

Pharyngitis (Pharyngitis, Tonsillitis, Tonsillopharyngitis, and Nasopharyngitis)

Pharyngitis is a common clinical manifestation of coxsackieviral and echoviral infection. Probably all enteroviruses on

TABLE 170–6 ■ ENTEROVIRUSES AND PARECHOVIRUSES NOTED IN ASSOCIATION WITH NONSPECIFIC FEBRILE ILLNESS AND RESPIRATORY DISEASE

	Virus Types		
Clinical Categories	Coxsackieviruses A	Coxsackieviruses B	Enteroviruses and Parechoviruses (PE)
Nonspecific febrile illness	All types	All types	All types
Common cold	Mainly 21, 24; rarely other types	Mainly 1–5; rarely 6	Mainly 2, 20; rarely other types
Pharyngitis (pharyngitis, tonsillitis, tonsillopharyngitis, and nasopharyngitis)	Probably all types; mainly 9	Probably all types; mainly 1-5	Probably all types; mainly 2, 4, 6, 9, 11, 16, 19, 25, 30, 71
Herpangina	1-10, 16, 22	1-5	6, 9, 11, 16, 17, 25, PE 1
Lymphonodular pharyngitis	10		
Stomatitis and other lesions in the anterior of the mouth	5, 9, 10, 16	2, 5	9, 11, 20, 71
Parotitis	Coxsackievirus A not typed	3, 4	70
Croup	9	4, 5	4, 11, 21
Bronchitis		1,4	8, 12–14
Bronchiolitis and infectious asthma	Many types	Many types	Many types
Pneumonia	9, 16	1–6	6, 7, 9, 11, 12, 19, 20, 30, PE 1
Pleurodynia	1, 2, 4, 6, 9, 16	1–6	1–3, 6–9, 11, 12, 14, 16–19, 24, 25, 30 PE 2

occasion cause mild pharyngitis. The most common coxsackieviruses and echoviruses associated with pharyngitis are coxsackieviruses A9, B1, B2, B3, B4, and B5; echoviruses 2, 4, 6, 9, 11, 16, 19, 25, and 30; and enterovirus 71.* Pharyngitis in coxsackievirus and echovirus infections frequently is associated with other clinical findings such as meningitis, pleurodynia, and exanthem. These other manifestations become more important than pharyngitis in individual cases in the minds of parents as well as clinicians.

Pharyngitis caused by coxsackieviruses and echoviruses usually is abrupt in onset without a prodrome. Although pharyngeal involvement is present at the onset of disease, the initial complaint is most often fever. The temperature usually ranges between 38.3° and 40° C (101° and 104° F), but higher temperatures are not unusual. In general, fever tends to be more pronounced in younger patients. Young children have malaise and anorexia. School-age children complain of headache and myalgia. Sore throat, coryza and vomiting, diarrhea, or a combination thereof also may be noted.

Examination of the tonsils and pharynx shows varying degrees of erythema. In some cases, only injection is noted, whereas in others, severe pharyngitis with patches of exudate is seen. The usual duration of uncomplicated coxsackieviral or echoviral pharyngitis is 3 to 6 days. Routine laboratory study is of minimal value in enteroviral pharyngitis; the total white blood cell count may be normal or slightly elevated with a normal differential determination. Throat culture rules out disease caused by group A streptococci.

Other Intraoral Manifestations

HERPANGINA. See Chapter 11.

ACUTE LYMPHONODULAR PHARYNGITIS. In 1962, Steigman and colleagues[786] reported a unique enanthem associated with coxsackievirus A10 infection. The lesions had the typical distribution of herpangina; they were papular, discrete, 3 mm in diameter, and surrounded by a zone of erythema. The lesions were white to yellow and persisted for 6 to 10 days. This entity has not been reported again, although coxsackievirus A10 has been noted in association with hand, foot, and mouth syndrome.[139, 759]

STOMATITIS AND OTHER LESIONS IN THE ANTERIOR OF THE MOUTH. The main enteroviral cause of stomatitis and ulcerative lesions in the anterior of the mouth is coxsackievirus A16, and the clinical entity is the hand, foot, and mouth syndrome. This condition is presented in detail later in this chapter. Worth mentioning here, however, is that occasionally, enanthem occurs without the exanthem and that this enanthem also has been associated with other coxsackieviruses (A5, A9, A10, B2, B5), echovirus 33, and enterovirus 71.[139, 203, 217, 252, 526, 759]

In echovirus 9 infection, Tyrrell and colleagues[829] reported six children with a unique enanthem: painless whitish dots, ulcers, or vesicles were noted on the buccal surfaces near the Stensen duct. They also noted the occasional occurrence of similar lesions under the tongue.

Deseda-Tous and colleagues[208] reported an adolescent with hemorrhagic vesicular lesions on the pharynx, mucosal surfaces, and tongue in association with an echovirus 11 infection. Clarke and Stott[168] observed reddish macules on the buccal mucosa of a patient with echovirus 20 infection, and Cherry and Jahn[144] noted one child with hand, foot, and mouth syndrome in whom the buccal lesions suggested Koplik spots, although the lesions were larger and more yellow in this patient.

Parotitis

Parotitis in association with herpangina and coxsackievirus A infection was reported in 1957 by Howlett and associates.[384] In 1960, Kraus[486] described two additional cases, and Bertaggia and associates[77] and Winsser and Altieri[876] noted parotitis in association with coxsackieviruses B3 and B4, respectively. Three patients with acute hemorrhagic conjunctivitis and parotitis caused by enterovirus 70 also have been reported.[748]

Croup

In large studies of respiratory illness in young children, croup is associated sporadically with coxsackieviral and echoviral infection.[131, 139, 262, 297, 863] In general, these illnesses are mild when compared with croup caused by parainfluenza and influenza viruses.

An outbreak of croup associated with echovirus 11 in a day nursery has been reported.[667] In this instance, 17 of 53 ill children were found to be infected with the U strain of echovirus 11. A subsequent study noted the same virus in four children with croup.[668] Croup also is reported in outbreaks of coxsackievirus B5 infection.[39, 183] Other specific agents associated with croup include coxsackieviruses A9 and B4 and echoviruses 4 and 21.[139]

Bronchitis

An acute febrile illness with cough, rhonchi, and referred breath sounds occasionally is a sporadic manifestation of enteroviral infection. A specific association of coxsackieviruses B1 and B4, echoviruses 8, 12, 13, and 14, and parechovirus 1 has been found.[131, 139, 183, 224, 226]

Bronchiolitis and Infectious Asthma

Coxsackieviruses and echoviruses have been associated sporadically with bronchiolitis, infectious asthma, and the precipitation of asthmatic attacks in atopic children.[131, 139, 224, 262, 297, 318, 373, 863] Epidemic disease has not been observed, and the illnesses usually have been mild.

Pneumonia

In general studies of respiratory infections in children, sporadic coxsackieviruses and echoviruses have been noted in 1 to 7 percent of patients with pneumonia and positive viral cultures.[131, 139, 262, 297] Specific virus types include coxsackieviruses A9, A16, B1, B2, B3, B4, B5, and B6; echoviruses 6, 7, 9, 11, 12, 19, 20, and 30; and enterovirus 71.*

In only three instances can an outbreak of pneumonia caused by specific viruses be suggested to have occurred. During the summer of 1959, Lerner and colleagues[516] noted that 3 of 15 children infected with coxsackievirus A9 had pneumonia. An interesting note is that the three patients with pneumonia had a vesicular rash. The illness in one child was fatal.

*See references 139, 146–148, 185, 237, 335, 349, 446, 447, 455, 463, 513, 515, 604, 729, 733, 773.

*See references 139, 185, 224, 251, 293, 413, 446, 516, 596, 749, 773, 861.

Eckert and associates[224] observed six children with coxsackievirus B1 infection and pneumonia during the summer of 1963. These illnesses were not described further, although the mean white blood cell count in 12 children who had lower respiratory infections with coxsackieviruses B was reported as 11,383 with a normal differential. All children were hospitalized.

Goldwater[307] reported a coxsackievirus B6 outbreak in south Australia during the summer of 1992 to 1993. Twenty-seven patients had pneumonia associated with high fever and severe cough that lasted several weeks.

In addition to the fatal case of coxsackievirus A9 infection described by Lerner and colleagues,[516] deaths occurred with coxsackieviruses B1, B5, and A16.[251, 413, 885]

Pleurodynia (Bornholm Disease)[40, 139, 197, 312, 326, 463, 595, 800, 850]

Epidemic pleurodynia is an illness that first was noted over 250 years ago by Hannaeus, a Danish physician.[339] Not until the late 19th century, however, did the illness receive further attention in the medical literature. At this time, several epidemics in Scandinavian countries were described.[139, 192, 250] Although Finsen referred to the disease as pleurodynia, others who designated outbreaks used eographic names, such as Skien disease, Bamle disease, Drangedral disease, and Bornholm disease, or descriptive names such as epidemic myalgia, devil's grippe, epidemic diaphragmatic spasm, or epidemic benign pleurisy.[312] In 1933, Sylvest[800] published the classic monograph on the subject, and from this paper the name Bornholm disease (from Bornholm Island, a Danish island in the Baltic Sea) came to be associated with the illness. The enteroviral etiology of epidemic pleurodynia was established in 1949.[191, 857]

Historically, pleurodynia is an epidemic disease, but sporadic cases do occur. A characteristic incubation period of approximately 4 days is followed by a sudden onset of fever and pain. The pain typically is located in the chest or upper part of the abdomen and is muscular in origin and of variable intensity. Occasionally, the pain occurs in other areas of the body. Frequently, the pain is excruciatingly severe and sudden and is associated with profuse sweating, so the patient may appear pale and as though in shock. The pain is spasmodic, with durations varying from a few minutes to several hours. Most commonly, the spasmodic periods last approximately 15 to 30 minutes. During spasms, respirations usually are rapid, shallow, and grunting, suggestive of pneumonia or pleural inflammation. Coughing, sneezing, or deep breathing makes the pain worse. Older children and adults describe the pain as stabbing or knifelike. An older person often fears that a heart attack is occurring.

When pain localizes in the abdomen, it frequently is crampy and suggests colic in a younger child. The child may double over and refuse to walk or move. Occasionally, the abdominal pain in association with a pale, sweaty, shock-like appearance suggests acute intestinal obstruction. Splinting and guarding of the abdomen also lead to a consideration of appendicitis and peritonitis.

The fever and pain usually last 1 to 2 days. Frequently, however, the illness is biphasic; after the initial febrile period, the patient is asymptomatic for several days, and then the pain and fever recur. Rarely, patients have several recurrent episodes over the course of several weeks. In these patients, fever is less prominent.

Some degree of tenderness is present in the areas of pain, but frank myositis with muscle swelling is not observed. Pleural friction rubs may be noted on auscultation, and they may appear and disappear with the coming and going of pain episodes.

In epidemics, both children and adults are afflicted, but most cases occur in persons younger than 30 years. Most children have other symptoms of enteroviral infection, such as anorexia, nausea, vomiting, headache, and sore throat. Routine laboratory study is not very helpful. The white blood cell count varies considerably, but an increased percentage of polymorphonuclear neutrophils and band forms is a frequent finding. The erythrocyte sedimentation rate also is inconsistent; normal to extremely high values may be observed. The chest radiograph most often is normal.

Complications in pleurodynia are uncommon. Aseptic meningitis has been noted in some patients, and adult men have experienced orchitis. Cardiac involvement—myocarditis and pericarditis—also may complicate pleurodynia.

The major etiologic agents in epidemic pleurodynia are coxsackieviruses B3 and B5.[40, 139, 389, 729, 755, 773] Other viruses associated with epidemic disease include coxsackieviruses B1 and B2 and echoviruses 1 and 6.[30, 139, 219] Agents associated with sporadic occurrences of pleurodynia include coxsackieviruses A1, A2, A4, A6, A9, A16, B1, B2, B3, B4, B5, and B6; echoviruses 1, 2, 3, 6, 7, 8, 9, 11, 12, 14, 16, 17, 18, 19, 24, 25, and 30; and parechovirus 2.*

In recent years, pleurodynia rarely has been reported. Because the enteroviruses that cause pleurodynia still circulate, cases probably are overlooked or misdiagnosed. An outbreak caused by coxsackievirus B1 in football players at a public high school was reported.[400] Unfortunately, no clinical data were presented.

Gastrointestinal Manifestations

Gastrointestinal manifestations occur commonly in coxsackieviral and echoviral infections.† Clinical manifestations in addition to vomiting and diarrhea are varied; an outline is given in Table 170–7.

Early studies paid particular attention to diarrheal disease in children. However, when specific studies of infantile diarrhea were undertaken, the enteroviral association was far from clear.[56, 139, 311, 657, 780, 896] The correlation of infection and disease in these studies was compromised by the fact that the main source of culture in study patients and controls was from stool; persistent infection in the bowel rendered separation of controls and ill patients impossible.

At present, all coxsackieviruses and echoviruses frequently have one or more gastrointestinal symptoms as part of their general illness. The intensity and spectrum do vary among the specific agents, however, and also among strains of particular viral types. In a review of World Health Organization (WHO) virus reports covering a 4-year period, Assaad and Cockburn[33] found that the main clinical sign or symptom was gastrointestinal in 12 percent of coxsackieviral and 6.8 percent of echoviral infections. In another analysis, Assaad and Borecka[32] noted 16 deaths during the period 1967 to 1975 in those with coxsackievirus and echovirus infections in which the principal clinical association was gastrointestinal.

In a 20-year survey in Wisconsin, Nelson and colleagues[625] noted that gastrointestinal symptoms occurred in approximately a third of all patients from whom they recovered nonpolio enteroviruses. Morens and colleagues[599]

*See references 58, 139, 183, 219, 336, 441, 468, 562, 595, 798.

†See references 32, 33, 139, 159, 197, 326, 373, 463, 500, 552, 555, 560, 562, 572, 595, 598, 599, 631, 690, 758, 780, 859, 860, 862.

TABLE 170–7 ■ ENTEROVIRUSES AND PARECHOVIRUSES NOTED IN ASSOCIATION WITH GASTROINTESTINAL COMPLAINTS

	Virus Types		
Clinical Categories	Coxsackieviruses A	Coxsackieviruses B	Enteroviruses and Parechoviruses (PE)
Gastrointestinal, not specified	2, 4, 5, 6, 7, 9, 10, 14, 16	1–5	1–9, 11, 12, 14, 16–21, 24, 25, 30, 71, PE 1, 2
Nausea and vomiting	9, 16	2–5	2, 4, 6, 9, 11, 16, 18–20, 30, PE 1
Diarrhea	1, 9, 16	2–5	3, 4, 6, 7, 9, 11–14, 16–21, 25, 30, PE 1
Constipation	9	3–5	4, 6, 9, 11
Abdominal pain	9, 16	2–5	4, 6, 9, 11, 18, 19, 30
Pseudoappendicitis			1, 8, 14
Peritonitis		1	
Mesenteric adenitis		5	7, 9, 11
Appendicitis		2, 5	
Intussusception		3	7, 9
Hepatitis	4, 9, 10, 20, 24	1–5	1, 3, 4, 6, 7, 9, 11, 14, 20, 21, 30
Reye syndrome	2	4	14, PE 1
Pancreatitis	9	3–5	
Diabetes mellitus		1–5	

reported that in 4 percent of patients from whom nonpolio enteroviruses were recovered during the 1971 to 1975 period, gastrointestinal disease was the major diagnosis. Horn and coworkers,[373] studying respiratory viral infections, noted that 21.2 percent of subjects from whom enteroviruses were recovered had gastrointestinal complaints.

Vomiting

Vomiting is a common manifestation of infection with many coxsackieviral and echoviral types, but it rarely is the major complaint of the patient or the parent.* The frequency of vomiting during outbreaks of illness caused by coxsackieviruses and echoviruses depends on the specific types of virus and the major manifestation during a particular outbreak. Table 170–8 presents the frequency of vomiting by viral type. In 14 different enteroviral types, vomiting has been noted as a significant aspect of the illness during disease outbreaks. Except for coxsackievirus A16 infections—hand, foot, and mouth syndrome—in which it was an uncommon complaint, vomiting occurs in approximately 50 percent of all cases in epidemic enteroviral disease. Vomiting is noted most commonly in meningitis and least commonly in pleurodynia and uncomplicated exanthematous disease.

Diarrhea

Diarrhea occurs commonly in coxsackieviral and echoviral infections, but it usually is just one of many manifestations of the systemic illness.† Specific studies of diarrheal disease in infants and children have had varied results; some studies indicate an enteroviral etiology, whereas others reveal that coxsackieviruses and echoviruses have been recovered from well children at the same prevalence.

*See references 8, 31, 139, 146, 148, 154, 185, 186, 206, 245, 246, 312, 329, 335, 336, 341, 443, 446, 447, 455, 466, 474, 513, 544, 546, 639, 671, 676, 697, 709, 726, 730, 733, 742, 773, 819, 850, 854, 865, 872, 873.

†See references 8, 30, 31, 71, 93, 95, 139, 144, 183–186, 206, 245, 246, 308, 311, 326, 335, 336, 341, 446, 447, 455, 463, 474, 495, 506, 513, 544, 552, 555, 560, 617, 658, 662, 671, 674, 680, 690–692, 709, 729, 730, 758, 780, 781, 808, 819, 860, 862, 873, 896, 897.

Ramos-Alvarez and Olarte[691] carried out an extensive study of diarrheal disease in Mexico City and noted that echoviruses were recovered eight times more frequently from children with diarrhea than from control, nondiarrheal children. They found that echoviruses 6 and 19 predominated, but types 3, 7, 9, 12, 14, 18, and 21 also were recovered. Pelon and colleagues[662] noted an association between coxsackieviruses B4 and B5 and acute diarrhea; they observed a 42 percent coxsackievirus B isolation rate in children with acute diarrhea and a corresponding rate of only 12 percent in those without diarrhea. Goodwin and associates[311] noted echoviruses in the stools of children with diarrhea at twice the rate observed in normal children. In a study by Yow and colleagues,[896, 897] no association was found between enteroviruses and infantile diarrhea. Echoviruses were recovered twice as frequently from children ill with diarrhea as from children without gastrointestinal illness.[897] In Canada, McLean and colleagues[560] could find no association between enteroviral infection and gastroenteritis. In a large study of diarrhea in India, coxsackieviruses A9, B3, and B6 and echoviruses 12 and 21 were recovered more commonly from ill patients than from children without diarrhea.[617]

In several studies of specific diarrhea outbreaks, the afflicted persons have been noted to be actively infected with a particular virus type. Goldwater and Laws[308] observed three children younger than 6 months who were infected with echovirus 19 and had gastroenteritis without other signs or symptoms. Klein and colleagues[474] recovered echovirus 11 from the blood of two laboratory workers with acute gastroenteritis. Diarrhea occurred in three of nine volunteers given echovirus 11.[95] Eichenwald and associates[227] and Cramblett and colleagues[183] reported epidemic diarrhea caused by echovirus 18 in neonates. An outbreak of diarrhea associated with coxsackievirus A1 was noted in 7 of 14 bone marrow transplant recipients during a 3-week period.[821]

Table 170–9 presents the frequency of diarrhea in outbreaks of specific coxsackieviral and echoviral illnesses. Diarrhea varied with regard to the viruses represented and in different studies with the same agents. Diarrhea in enteroviral disease rarely is severe. In most instances, loose stools occur for a 2- to 4-day period. The stools rarely are watery, never are bloody, and at most number 6 to 8 per day.

TABLE 170–8 ■ FREQUENCY OF VOMITING IN OUTBREAKS OF ILLNESS CAUSED BY COXSACKIEVIRUSES AND ECHOVIRUSES

Virus Type	Age Group (yr)	Vomiting (%)	Main Characteristics of Outbreak	References
Coxsackievirus A9	Mainly children	60–73	Meningitis	139
	Children	14–20	Rash	139, 516
Coxsackievirus A16	Children and adults	3–15	Hand, foot, and mouth syndrome	8, 709
Coxsackievirus B2	Mainly children	50	Meningitis	139
	Mainly children	18–66	Febrile, respiratory	139
Coxsackievirus B3	Adults and children	33	Pleurodynia	139
	Children	9	Febrile, respiratory	139
	Mainly children	25	Fever, diarrhea	244
Coxsackievirus B4	Mainly children	27	Nonspecific febrile	245
Coxsackievirus B5	Adults and children	31–37	Pleurodynia	312, 773
	Adults and children	50–95	Meningitis	139, 154, 329, 726
	Mainly children	25–33	Nonspecific febrile	154, 726, 873
	Children	45	Febrile, respiratory	742
	Mainly children	100	Hepatosplenic syndrome	773
	Children	40	Rash	146
Echovirus 2	Children	12	Respiratory, rash	139
Echovirus 4	Mainly children	70–90	Meningitis	447, 697
	Mainly children	9–50	Epidemic disease including meningitis, minor illness	139, 639
Echovirus 6	Mainly children	55–98	Meningitis	341, 446, 466, 494, 854
	Mainly children	50–75	Epidemic disease including meningitis	139, 873
Echovirus 9	0–4	64–71	Rash, meningitis	139, 733
	5–9	81–83		
	10–19	61–92		
	>20	20–38		
	Mainly children	39–95	Rash, meningitis	139, 676, 854, 865
	Mainly children	26	Pharyngitis	139
	Mainly children	71	Epidemic disease including meningitis	139
Echovirus 11	Not specified	100	Febrile, respiratory	139
Echovirus 16	Children	30	Rash	335
Echovirus 19	<0.5	25	Meningitis, upper respiratory, nonspecific febrile	139
	0.5–2	31		
	3–5	37		
	6–12	68		
	13–18	61		
	19–25	53		
	26+	43		
Echovirus 20	Children	67	Febrile, respiratory	185
Echovirus 30	Mainly children	15–91	Meningitis	316, 443, 671, 819
	<5	50	Febrile, respiratory	139
	>5	70		

Constipation

Some degree of constipation is a rather frequent occurrence in many acute infectious illnesses, but its evaluation is rendered difficult by the subjective nature of the complaint. In coxsackievirus and echovirus diseases, a short period of constipation may be associated with fever, vomiting, and anorexia early in the course of the illness. This period frequently is followed by mild diarrhea.[95] As noted in Table 170–7, constipation has been reported specifically as a symptom with four coxsackieviral and four echoviral types. Constipation is a particularly common event in children with enteroviral meningitis; it occurs in 10 to 40 percent of cases.[139, 245, 246, 446, 447, 493]

Abdominal Pain

Abdominal pain is a common complaint in many coxsackieviral and echoviral infections. Table 170–10 lists the frequency of occurrence of abdominal pain and the main characteristic of the illness by virus type. Approximately 10 percent of patients with coxsackievirus A16 hand, foot, and mouth syndrome complain of abdominal pain. In about a quarter of patients, many coxsackieviruses and echoviruses associated with meningitis cause abdominal pain.

The magnitude of abdominal pain as a clinical complaint in coxsackieviral and echoviral infections varies considerably. For example, in aseptic meningitis, headache and other neurologic complaints overshadow the abdominal symptoms. In other situations, fever and abdominal pain are diagnostically troublesome because of the possibility of a surgical abdomen (discussed further in the next paragraph). The pain most frequently is periumbilical; it may be either constant or colicky. The fever is most often higher than 38.3° C (101° F).

Peritonitis, Pseudoperitonitis, Appendicitis, Pseudo-obstruction, Mesenteric Adenitis, and Intussusception

Occasionally, coxsackieviruses and echoviruses are associated with illnesses that suggest severe abdominal involvement. Liebman and St. Geme[522] described two children with abdominal findings suggestive of acute appendicitis (semirigid, tender abdomen, rebound tenderness, rectal tenderness) who had associated infections with echoviruses 1 and 14. McLean[559] described a surgical abdomen in one child with coxsackievirus B1 infection. In this case, virus was recovered from the peritoneal exudate; at surgery, this boy

TABLE 170–9 ■ FREQUENCY OF DIARRHEA IN OUTBREAKS OF ILLNESS CAUSED BY COXSACKIEVIRUSES AND ECHOVIRUSES

Virus Type	Age Group (yr)	Diarrhea (%)	Main Characteristics of Outbreak	References
Coxsackievirus A9	Adults and children	7–100	Fever, rash	139, 515
Coxsackievirus A16	Mainly children	4–33	Hand, foot, and mouth syndrome	8, 144, 513, 712
Coxsackievirus B2	Mainly children	9–56	Febrile, respiratory	139
	Mainly children	12	Meningitis	544
Coxsackievirus B3	Mainly children	2–5	Pleurodynia	139
	Children	11	Meningitis	183
	Mainly children	54	Nonspecific febrile	244
Coxsackievirus B4	Children	9	Meningitis	184
	Mainly children	8	Febrile, respiratory	246
Coxsackievirus B5	<1	21	Meningitis and febrile, respiratory	674
	1–9	15		
	10–29	3		
	Mainly children	5–9	Meningitis	139, 183, 873
Echovirus 4	Mainly children	5–75	Meningitis	447, 506, 730
	Mainly children	65	Nonspecific febrile	506
Echovirus 6	Mainly children	6–12	Meningitis	
Echovirus 9	0–4	14	Meningitis, rash	139, 341, 446, 730
	5–9	10		
	10–19	8		
	<20	0		
	Mainly children	3–40	Meningitis	139, 186, 730
	Children	15	Rash, fever	215
	Mainly children	5–15	Respiratory	139
Echovirus 11	Adults	33–100	Gastrointestinal	95, 474
	Mainly infants	40	Nonspecific febrile	71
Echovirus 13	Children	11	Respiratory	139
Echovirus 16	Children	20	Rash	335
Echovirus 17	<1–4	100	Fever, diarrhea	139
Echovirus 18	Infants	100	Diarrhea	228
Echovirus 19	<2	30	Meningitis	139
	2–4	7		
	5–11	7		
	12–17	0		
	>18	9		
	Mainly children	3	Meningitis	308
	Mainly children	10	Respiratory	184, 308
	Mainly children	9	Diarrhea	318
Echovirus 20	Children	100	Respiratory, enteric	185
Echovirus 30	<5	12	Meningitis	139
	>5	5		
	Adults and children	7–10	Meningitis	336, 671, 819

was found to have peritonitis, but his appendix was normal. Thomas[812] reported a 5-year-old boy with coxsackievirus B5 infection who at surgery was found to have excessive clear peritoneal fluid and markedly enlarged mesenteric lymph nodes. A pregnant woman with acute abdominal pain and rebound tenderness associated with echovirus 8 infection has been described.[660]

Tobe[817] has shown in immunofluorescence studies the presence of coxsackievirus B2 and B5 antigens in the mucous membranes and mesenteric lymph nodes of patients with appendicitis more often than in similar studies in control subjects. He has suggested that the viral infection acts as a trigger for the appendicitis. Bell and Steyn[63] recovered echoviruses 7 and 9 from the mesenteric lymph nodes of children with intussusception.

Hepatitis*

Marked liver involvement is not a rare finding in disseminated coxsackieviral and echoviral infections in neonates.[140] The association of hepatitis and enteroviral infection in older children is defined less clearly but probably occurs more commonly than generally realized based on the number of individual cases reported. Caution must be exercised in accepting enteroviruses as the exclusive etiologic agent of hepatitis, however, because hepatitis A virus infection has been ruled out in only a few of the available studies.

Morris and associates[604] described an illness suggestive of a coxsackieviral or echoviral infection in an 18-month-old child who had hyperbilirubinemia and abnormal liver function test results. From this child, coxsackievirus A4 was recovered from blood during the acute illness, and a rise in neutralizing antibody titer to the isolated virus was demonstrated. Chang and Weinstein[130] reported a 3-year-old boy with pharyngitis, urinary abnormalities, and neurologic symptoms who had elevated liver enzyme values (aspartate transaminase of 1600 and alanine transaminase of 1180). Coxsackievirus A9 was recovered from this child's cerebrospinal fluid (CSF), and the child's antibody response to this agent was significant. Coxsackievirus A20 has been associated with clinical hepatitis, and simultaneous infections with coxsackievirus A24 and hepatitis A virus have been demonstrated.[756]

*See references 9, 124, 130, 197, 380, 463, 500, 505, 546, 598, 599, 604, 651, 749, 756, 758, 773, 796, 839, 847.

TABLE 170–10 ■ FREQUENCY OF ABDOMINAL PAIN IN OUTBREAKS OF ILLNESS CAUSED BY COXSACKIEVIRUSES AND ECHOVIRUSES

Virus Type	Age Group (yr)	Abdominal Pain (%)	Main Characteristics of Outbreak	References
Coxsackievirus A9	Mainly children	7	Meningitis	139
	Children	20	Rash	148
Coxsackievirus A16	Mainly children	12	Hand, foot, and mouth syndrome	516, 709
Coxsackievirus B2	Mainly children	22	Meningitis	544
Coxsackievirus B3	Children and adults	25–90	Pleurodynia	139
Coxsackievirus B4	Children and adults	10	Meningitis	139
	Mainly children	36	Febrile, respiratory	246
Coxsackievirus B5	Mainly children	10	Meningitis	139
	Children	13	Febrile, respiratory	742
	Children and adults	23–67	Pleurodynia	312, 729, 773
Echovirus 4	Mainly children	28–50	Meningitis	139, 447
	Mainly children	13	Febrile, respiratory	639
Echovirus 6	Mainly children	17–43	Meningitis	139, 341, 446, 466
Echovirus 9	0–4	28	Meningitis, rash	139, 154, 513, 733
	5–9	30		
	10–19	25		
	≥20	0		
Echovirus 11	Adults	38	Gastrointestinal	95
Echovirus 16	Children	20	Rash	335
Echovirus 19	<0.5	3	Meningitis	139
	0.5–2	3		
	3–5	27		
	6–12	38		
	13–18	13		
	19–25	9		
	26+	3		
Echovirus 30	Mainly children	17	Meningitis	443, 819

An adult with a coxsackievirus B1 infection had both myocarditis and liver involvement.[9] A similar illness caused by coxsackievirus B3 in a 19-year-old woman has been described.[796] An 11-month-old boy had a Reye-like syndrome in conjunction with coxsackievirus B2 infection.[449] Reye syndrome has been associated with echovirus 3 infection.[347] Siegel and colleagues[773] described a hepatosplenic syndrome in which 15 patients had hepatomegaly and coxsackievirus B5 infection. These patients, most of whom were children, had otherwise typical enteroviral illnesses. Liver function studies were performed in only three instances, and their results were normal.

Echoviruses 1, 3, 4, 6, 7, 9, 11, 14, 20, 21, and 30 have been associated with hepatitis.[139, 390, 463, 542, 595, 749] Hepatomegaly occurs commonly in enteroviral infections.[139, 144, 244, 495, 516] During the period 1971 through 1975, more than 7000 cases of nonpolio enterovirus infection were reported to the Viral Diseases Division at the Centers for Disease Control and Prevention (CDC).[599] In this group were 13 cases of hepatitis and 6 of Reye syndrome; coxsackieviruses A2 and B4 and echoviruses 14 and 22 were associated with the latter illness.

Pancreatitis

One of the effects of coxsackievirus B in suckling mice is extensive infection in the pancreas. As with other similarities of infection between suckling mice and human neonates, generalized coxsackievirus B infection in neonates also is accompanied frequently by extensive pancreatic damage. In contrast, pancreatic involvement in older children and adults is not a common occurrence.[105, 613, 618, 832] Coxsackieviruses B3, B4, B5, and A9 have been noted.

Diabetes Mellitus

A possible relationship between juvenile diabetes mellitus and the seasonal occurrence of coxsackievirus B4 was suggested in 1969 by Gamble and Taylor.[277] In a second study, Gamble and associates[276] noted higher titers of coxsackievirus B4 antibodies in insulin-dependent diabetic patients within 3 months of the onset of disease than in normal subjects or long-term diabetics.

Since the 1960s, many studies in animal models and children have looked at the relationship between juvenile-onset, type 1 insulin-dependent diabetes mellitus (IDDM) and coxsackieviruses B.* Between 1973 and 1984, 10 case-control studies examined the prevalence of antibody to various coxsackieviruses B in patients with IDDM and controls. In eight of these studies, the prevalence was greater in the patients with IDDM. In three of these studies, IgM antibody to the coxsackieviruses B was examined, and in each the prevalence was greater in the patients with IDDM than in controls. A Finnish study noted that patients with IDDM were more likely to have IgA antibodies to coxsackievirus B4 than were controls.[396]

Helfand and associates[354] performed a well-done case-control study of IDDM. They found that new-onset cases in patients 13 to 18 years of age were more likely than controls to be IgM antibody–positive for 9 of 14 enterovirus serotypes. The serotypes were coxsackieviruses B2, B3, B4, B5, and B6; coxsackievirus A9; and echoviruses 9, 30, and 34.

Cudworth and colleagues[189] noted a correlation between HLA type BW15 and coxsackieviruses B1, B2, B3, and B4 antibodies in IDDM patients.

In 1979, Yoon and colleagues[894] reported the recovery of coxsackievirus B4 from the pancreas of a previously healthy 10-year-old boy who died after being in a diabetic coma.

Clements and coworkers[171] noted that 9 of 14 serum samples from children with new-onset diabetes were positive for enterovirus RNA by PCR. In contrast, only 4 percent of

*See references 21, 34, 43, 44, 125, 171, 189, 210, 266, 344, 354, 362, 367, 437, 440, 470, 530–532, 585, 652, 754, 760, 815, 834, 871.

serum samples from control children had evidence of enterovirus RNA.

In the murine model, See and Tilles[760] found that a diabetogenic strain of coxsackievirus B4 infection resulted in persistent detection of viral RNA in the pancreases of most infected mice. This persistence of antigen was associated with chronic islet cell inflammation and elevated islet cell antibody levels. Stimulated peritoneal macrophages caused lysis of islet cells either directly or by an antibody-dependent mechanism. A study in prediabetic children found that the presence of enterovirus RNA in serum was a risk factor for beta-cell autoimmunity and type 1 diabetes.[532] Glutamic acid decarboxylase (GAD_{65}) is one of the major beta-cell target antigens in the autoimmune beta-cell damaging process that leads to the development of IDDM.[530] Antibody and cellular immunity cross-reactivity exists between GAD_{65} and the 2C protein of coxsackievirus B4.[34, 530] The results of several studies suggest that enteroviral infections are associated with the development of beta-cell autoimmunity and the eventual destruction of islet cells.[367, 531] Time periods from enteroviral infection to the development of beta-cell autoimmunity and the eventual development of IDDM from beta-cell destruction have a great range that perhaps explains the lack of a more specific seasonally related onset of IDDM. A case of neonatal type 1 diabetes associated with a maternal echovirus 6 infection has been reported.[652]

EYE FINDINGS

Acute Hemorrhagic Conjunctivitis*

Although conjunctivitis has been a frequent finding in nonpolio enteroviral illnesses for 50 years, its occurrence as a dominant complaint has been observed only during the last 35 years. In June 1969, Chatterjee and associates[132] noted an epidemic of acute hemorrhagic conjunctivitis in Accra, Ghana. This disease was nicknamed Apollo 11 disease because it coincided with the time of the Apollo 11 moon landing. Since 1969, many epidemics of acute hemorrhagic conjunctivitis have been described. In most epidemics, enterovirus 70 has been the etiologic agent, but similar epidemics have been caused by a variant of coxsackievirus A24.[166] In recent years, this virus has been the cause of more epidemics than enterovirus 70 has.[117, 303, 697] Most epidemics have occurred in tropical and semitropical countries; however, outbreaks have been observed in Minnesota, Moscow, London, and other European cities.[492, 892] In the continental United States, epidemic disease has occurred in Florida and North Carolina.[115] During epidemics, all age groups are affected, but the highest attack rate is in school-age children.[851]

Acute hemorrhagic conjunctivitis has a sudden onset with severe eye pain and associated photophobia, blurred vision, lacrimation, erythema, and congestion of the eye, as well as edema and chemosis of the lids.[363] Subconjunctival hemorrhages of varying size and frequently a transient punctate epithelial keratitis, conjunctival follicles, and preauricular lymphadenopathy are present. The eye discharge initially is serous but becomes mucopurulent with secondary bacterial infection. Systemic symptoms, including fever, are rare. Within 2 to 3 days after the onset of illness, patients note some improvement, and recovery is usually complete in 7 to 12 days. In a study in American Samoa, researchers found that illness caused by coxsackievirus A24 was somewhat different from that caused by enterovirus 70.[746] In cases caused by coxsackievirus A24, conjunctival hemorrhage was less severe and upper respiratory and systemic symptoms were more common. In a study in American Samoa of disease caused by enterovirus 70, researchers found that children 2 to 10 years of age had the highest attack rate and that antibody from previous infection gave only partial protection against symptomatic reinfection.[75]

Occasionally, findings suggestive of pharyngoconjunctival fever have been noted. A small percentage of patients have had a poliomyelitis-like illness or polyradiculomyeloneuropathy after having enterovirus 70 acute hemorrhagic conjunctivitis.[317, 844]

Epidemics are explosive, with spread mainly by the eye-hand-fomite-eye route.

*See references 75, 117, 139, 303, 317, 326, 363, 482, 746.

Conjunctivitis Associated with Other Enteroviral Illness

Conjunctivitis is a common minor manifestation of enteroviral illness with several specific agents. Table 170–11 presents the frequency of occurrence of conjunctivitis in selected outbreaks of disease caused by coxsackieviruses and echoviruses. Conjunctivitis was most prevalent in coxsackievirus B3 and B5 and echovirus 9 and 30 infections. In addition to the outbreaks reported in Table 170–11, conjunctivitis has been noted in isolated illnesses associated with echoviruses 1, 6, and 20.[463]

Photophobia

As might be expected, photophobia occurs commonly in aseptic meningitis caused by coxsackieviruses and echoviruses. During epidemic meningitis, researchers have noted it with the following viruses: coxsackievirus A9 and echoviruses 3, 4, 6, 7, 9, 19, and 30.* It is most common with echovirus 9 and 30 infections, but the incidence of this complaint varies greatly in different reports. In one echovirus 30 outbreak, 80 percent of the patients studied had photophobia.[819] On average, 20 percent of patients with meningitis have remarkable photophobia. Photophobia also is associated with pleurodynia caused by coxsackievirus B infections.[729, 850]

Other Eye Findings

Nodular lesions on the palpebral conjunctiva were observed in some patients with coxsackievirus A10 infection and lymphonodular pharyngitis.[786] A corneal ulcer occurred in one patient with hand, foot, and mouth syndrome,[537] and optic neuritis has been described in a boy with pleurodynia; in this latter case, the enteroviral etiology was not confirmed in the laboratory.[827] Periorbital edema was observed in one patient with echovirus 9 meningitis. An adult woman with panuveitis associated with coxsackievirus B3 infection has been described.[257] Monofocal outer retinitis in a 36-year-old man with hand, foot, and mouth syndrome has been described.[330] Sore eyes and other unspecified eye complaints also have been noted frequently with coxsackieviral and echoviral infections.[139, 240, 255, 329, 506, 536, 627, 744, 750]

CARDIOVASCULAR MANIFESTATIONS

Pericarditis and Myocarditis

Pericarditis, myocarditis, or both have been noted in association with 27 different nonpolio enteroviruses. The relative

*See references 62, 139, 312, 318, 442, 443, 446, 447, 466, 513, 542, 671, 819.

TABLE 170–11 ■ FREQUENCY OF CONJUNCTIVITIS IN OUTBREAKS OF ILLNESS CAUSED BY COXSACKIEVIRUSES AND ECHOVIRUSES

Virus Type	Age Group	Conjunctivitis (%)	Main Characteristics of Illness	References
Coxsackievirus A9	Children	20	Pharyngitis, rash	516
Coxsackievirus A16	Mainly children	0–18	Hand, foot, and mouth syndrome	132, 537, 709
Coxsackievirus B2	Mainly children	2	Nonspecific febrile, respiratory	139
Coxsackievirus B3	Children	2–42	Upper respiratory	139
Coxsackievirus B4	Children	25	Upper respiratory	139
Coxsackievirus B5	Mainly children	7–50	Rash, meningitis, hepatosplenic, respiratory, pleurodynia	147, 183, 729, 742
Echovirus 2	Children	25	Rhinorrhea	139
Echovirus 4	Children	Rare	Meningitis	542
Echovirus 9	Mainly children	13–30	Rash, meningitis	114, 139, 733
Echovirus 11	Children	15	Rash	147
Echovirus 16	Children	6–10	Rash	335, 629
Echovirus 30	Mainly children	10–60	Meninigitis, nonspecific fever	139, 336, 819

importance of the different serotypes is presented in Table 170–12. The coxsackieviruses B have been implicated most frequently in heart disease. Coxsackievirus B5 has been the most common causative agent, but types 2, 3, and 4 also have been implicated frequently. Of the echoviruses, type 6 has been associated most often with cardiac involvement, but the clinical findings with this agent have been described in only a few cases.

With coxsackievirus B cardiac disease, hepatitis, pneumonia, nephritis, meningitis, and orchitis have been occasional associated findings. Occasionally, arrhythmias are the only clinical manifestations of myocarditis.[145, 826] Constrictive pericarditis occurs occasionally.[553] The mortality rate of acute coxsackieviral and echoviral heart disease is unknown, but it is significant. Unfortunately, in the present era, proper virologic study rarely is performed in nonfatal disease.

In the only published follow-up study, researchers found that patients who survived acute coxsackievirus myocarditis usually recovered completely without any residual disability.[794]

The early descriptions of coxsackievirus B infection with myocarditis in the 1950s and early 1960s indicated acute, usually fulminant illnesses in which a coxsackievirus B serotype could be recovered from multiple sites such as the throat, stool, and CSF, as well as from the heart and other organs at autopsy.[287, 462, 464, 835] Coxsackieviruses B originally were isolated from suckling mice, and the infection in these mice caused acute, overwhelming fatal infections involving multiple organs, including the heart.[197, 430] Coxsackievirus B infections in mice were studied in mouse model systems in the 1950s and 1960s, and researchers found that infections in older mice were affected markedly by the virus strain, mouse genetics, and drugs.[82, 383, 469] During the last 3 decades, studies in mouse model systems have become more sophisticated but still depend on specific coxsackievirus B strains and specific mouse strains.*

More recent studies in mouse model systems have noted the progression of acute coxsackievirus B infection to chronic infection and cardiomyopathy.[19, 370, 439, 551, 685, 700] During the last 2 decades, acute, subacute, and chronic cardiomyopathy in patients has been studied by antigen-detection techniques and newer serologic methods.* Bowles and colleagues[87] found coxsackievirus B nucleic acid sequences in myocardial biopsy samples from several patients with cardiomyopathy. Muir and colleagues[610] detected enterovirus-specific IgM antibodies in the sera of nine patients with chronic relapsing pericarditis. Fujioka and coworkers[269] reported positive enteroviral PCR results from endomyocardial biopsy specimens in 6 of 31 patients (19%) with dilated cardiomyopathy. Andréoletti and collaborators[22] noted enterovirus RNA in 18 of 25 samples from the heart tissue of patients with dilated cardiomyopathy or ischemic cardiomyopathy. However, in two other well-controlled studies, enteroviral RNA could not be identified in endomyocardial biopsy samples or in heart tissue from patients undergoing heart transplantation.[175, 523] In 1994, Muir and Archard[607] and Melchers and associates[571] reviewed the evidence for persistent enteroviral infection in chronic medical conditions, including idiopathic dilated cardiomyopathy. Muir and Archard concluded that persistent enterovirus infection is associated causally with chronic medical conditions, whereas Melchers and colleagues found no clear evidence for enteroviral persistence and the subsequent development of chronic medical conditions.

During the last 7 years, additional studies in humans have been performed, and they again have had mixed results with regard to the role of coxsackievirus B in the etiology of chronic cardiomyopathy. The general theme in most contemporary mouse model studies is that damage to the myocardium is not caused by the direct cytopathic effect of the virus but is caused by the cellular immune response of the host. Unfortunately, the mouse model data and the less than definitive data from human studies have led cardiologists and others to think that the model systems are representative of human disease.[243, 528] In spite of publications that suggest otherwise, my opinion is that no convincing evidence has shown that persistent enteroviral cardiac infections occur in persons with normal immune systems. Also questionable is whether primary enteroviral cardiac infections play a significant role in the later development of dilated cardiomyopathy. No adequate follow-up studies of survivors of acute enteroviral myocarditis or pericarditis have been conducted. Levi and colleagues[517] compared follow-up cardiac data on 10 adults who had acute myocarditis associated with coxsackieviral infections 42 to 68 months previously with similar cardiac data from normal age- and

*See references 19, 101, 104, 162, 281, 282, 284, 285, 287, 300, 357, 360, 370, 387, 388, 439, 461, 467, 473, 499, 535, 551, 564, 626, 645, 655, 685, 700, 703, 704, 710, 761, 762, 823, 825, 877.

*See references 18, 20, 22, 28, 175, 204, 269, 352, 521, 523, 571, 607, 608, 610.

TABLE 170–12 ■ NONPOLIO ENTEROVIRUSES AND PARECHOVIRUSES ASSOCIATED WITH PERICARDITIS AND MYOCARDITIS

Virus Type	Age Group or Age of Individual Patients	Etiologic Importance*	Heart Involvement: Pericarditis	Heart Involvement: Myocarditis	Heart Involvement: Unspecified	Other Aspects of Illness	References
Coxsackievirus A1	Infants and adults	±	+	+			139, 321
A2	Adults	±			+		33, 139
A4	Mainly children	+	+	+		Sudden infant death	33, 306, 322, 852
A5	—	±	+				837
A7	Adults	±	+	+		Hand, foot, and mouth syndrome	41
A8	—	±			+		321
A9	Mainly infants	+		+		High fatality rate	322
A10	—	±			+		33
A16	Infants	±		+		High fatality rate	139, 885
Coxsackievirus B1	Infants, children, and adults	++	+	+		Rare hepatitis	9, 30, 33, 98, 139, 206, 321, 463, 562, 625, 712, 753, 860
B2	Infants, children, and adults	+++	+	+		Occasional pneumonia	30, 33, 97, 98, 139, 206, 248, 326, 380, 463, 483, 562, 625, 712, 753, 758, 852, 860
B3	Infants, children,and adults	+++	+	+		Rare hepatitis	33, 38, 61, 97, 98, 139, 206, 326, 380, 463, 483, 519, 625, 712, 758, 796, 849, 852, 860
B4	Infants, children, and adults	+++	+	+		Occasional pneumonia; myocardial calcifications; rare hepatitis, orchitis, nephritis, hemolytic uremic syndrome	30, 33, 38, 48, 90, 96–98, 139, 206, 248, 326, 380, 463, 483, 625, 698, 712, 798, 826, 829, 852
B5	Infants, children, and adults	++++	+	+		Occasional pneumonia, pleurodynia, and meningitis; rare orchitis	30, 32, 40, 84, 98, 139, 294, 312, 351, 356, 483, 529, 562, 602, 625, 644, 670, 674, 681, 753, 758, 852, 856, 860, 873
Echovirus 1	Adolescents	±	+	+			33, 750, 860
4	—	±			+		33, 570
6	Children and adults	++	+				33, 58, 139, 860
7	Children and adults	±			+		33, 139, 595
8	Adolescents	±	+				139, 428, 441
9	Children and adults	+	+	+			33, 139, 145, 519, 570, 593, 852
11	Children and adults	+			+		33, 58, 139, 712
14	—	±			+		595, 837
17	—	±			+		33
19	Children and adults	±	+	+			58, 139
25	Children	±		+			58, 59
30	—	±			+		33, 519
Enterovirus 71		±		+		Encephalitis	369
Parechovirus 1	Children	±		+			543, 728

*++++ = most common; ± = rare.

sex-matched subjects. No statistically significant differences in the two groups were found in the seven tests evaluated. Orinius[650] performed cardiac examinations on 53 adults who had coxsackievirus B infections 2 to 11 years previously. The initial diagnoses in these 53 patients were meningitis in 33 cases, encephalitis in 3 cases, pleurodynia in 6 cases, pericarditis in 2 cases, and nonspecific complaints in 9 cases. Of this group, the "possibility of cardiomyopathy was established" in two (4%) cases. Interestingly, the two patients who had had pericarditis were normal at follow-up.

Sainani and associates[734] performed follow-up studies on 20 adults and 2 teenagers who had coxsackievirus B myocarditis or pericarditis and found that 5 (23%) patients had chronic heart failure. Unfortunately, the duration of time since the primary illness of the patients is not presented. Bergström and colleagues[70] performed follow-up examinations on five patients (two teenagers and three adults) who had had enteroviral myopericarditis and found that none had significant complaints or physical signs. No follow-up data are available for neonates, infants, and children who have had enteroviral myocarditis.

In 1954, Stürup[794] reported a follow-up study of patients admitted to the hospital in 1930 to 1932 with pleurodynia. Of nine patients evaluated, including four who had had acute pericarditis, none had constructive pericarditis.

Other Cardiac Manifestations

Several investigators have studied the possible association of coxsackievirus B infection and myocardial infarction.* In many instances, patients with infarction have been demonstrated to have concomitant coxsackievirus B infection.† In controlled studies, the results have varied. Nikoskelainen and associates[637] noted that 9 of 59 patients with acute myocardial infarction had coxsackievirus B infection, whereas in the control group of 38 patients without infarction, only 1 patient had evidence of infection. Similarly, Nicholls and Thomas[632] found that 26 percent of patients had infections, but no infections were found in the control subjects. In contrast, five other studies failed to show an increased rate of infection in patients with myocardial infarction when compared with controls.[319, 324, 647, 673, 880] However, two of these studies were performed during a nonenteroviral season,[673, 880] and in a third study, little coxsackievirus B activity occurred in the community during the study period.[319] In analyzing the available studies, coxsackievirus B infection would appear to have a role in myocardial infarction. In one coxsackievirus B5 infection, inferolateral wall myocardial necrosis occurred, but coronary arteriography did not demonstrate obstruction.[207]

Chandy and associates[128] presented data in which antibody to group B coxsackieviruses was related to rheumatic-like valvular heart disease, and Burch and associates[98] demonstrated coxsackievirus B antigens in rheumatic lesions of the heart. Limson and colleagues[524] could find no association between group B coxsackieviruses and rheumatic fever. Soboleva and associates[778] noted an association between coxsackievirus A13 and rheumatic fever; they reported seven children with concomitant streptococcal and coxsackievirus A13 infection. Children with fulminant enterovirus 71 infection have been noted to have acute left ventricular dysfunction.[127, 129, 385]

*See references 319, 324, 502–504, 592, 632, 637, 673, 880, 882.
†See references 319, 324, 502, 503, 592, 632, 637, 647, 880, 882.

GENITOURINARY MANIFESTATIONS

Orchitis and Epididymitis

Group B coxsackieviruses are second only to mumps as causative agents of orchitis.* Coxsackievirus B5 is the virus associated most commonly with this disease, although coxsackieviruses B2 and B4 also have been implicated on many occasions. In almost all instances, the orchitis is a secondary event in enteroviral infections. The most common association is with pleurodynia. The illness frequently is biphasic: fever and pleurodynia initially and then apparent recovery followed by orchitis approximately 2 weeks after onset. Many patients also have epididymitis. In epidemics of disease caused by group B coxsackieviruses, the occurrence of testicular involvement varies considerably. Generally, orchitis occurs infrequently, but in one coxsackievirus B2 outbreak, 17 percent of postpubertal males had orchitis, and 7 percent also had epididymitis.[139] Orchitis also is associated frequently with pericarditis and myocarditis. In one instance, coxsackievirus B5 was recovered from a testicular biopsy specimen.[181]

In virtually all instances, testicular involvement has occurred in postpubertal patients, with most cases appearing in young adults. In addition to coxsackieviruses B2, B4, and B5, other enteroviruses have been implicated: coxsackieviruses B1 and B3[139, 463] and echoviruses 6, 9, and 11.[463, 858] Meningitis and exanthem have been associated with orchitis.

Nephritis

Scattered cases of nephritis associated with nonpolio enteroviral infections have been reported. Bayatpour and colleagues[53] noted acute glomerulonephritis in a 9-year-old boy with an extensive coxsackievirus B4 infection. This child had a concomitant rise in anti-streptolysin O titer. Yuceoglu and associates[898] reported twins with echovirus 9 infection and acute glomerulonephritis; Burch and Colcolough[96] observed a patient with progressive fatal pancarditis and nephritis in whom coxsackievirus B4 antigen was found in the kidneys. Mesangiolytic glomerulonephritis associated with an echovirus 6 infection has been described in an infant with immune deficiency.[386]

Other Genitourinary Findings

Hemolytic-uremic syndrome has been associated with virologic or serologic evidence of infection with coxsackieviruses A4, A9, B2, B3, B4, and B5 and echovirus 22.[35, 296, 648, 698, 699] Other abnormal renal or urinary findings in nonpolio enteroviral infections include acute oliguric renal failure with coxsackievirus B5[29]; pyuria, hematuria, or proteinuria with echoviruses 1, 6, and 9 and coxsackievirus B5[139, 446, 513, 733, 750]; and hemorrhagic cystitis.[599]

A 7-year-old girl with coxsackievirus A10 infection had vaginal ulcerative lesions,[586] and Wassermann test results have been falsely positive with echovirus 9 and coxsackievirus B5 infections.[684]

HEMATOLOGIC FINDINGS

Acute Infectious Lymphocytosis[327, 379]

In 1968, Horwitz and Moore[379] described an outbreak of infectious lymphocytosis during which 27 mentally retarded children were studied. The mean white blood cell count of the study group patients was 57,200; lymphocytes accounted

*See references 30, 139, 181, 264, 326, 463, 599, 758, 798, 860.

for at least 50 percent of the total in all cases. Approximately half the patients had low-grade fever, and 15 of 27 had moderate diarrhea. A nontypeable enterovirus suggestive of coxsackievirus group A was recovered from the ill patients, and neutralizing antibody to a strain (EVU-16) of the isolated virus developed in 31 percent of the patients in whom serologic studies were performed.

MUSCLE AND JOINT MANIFESTATIONS

Arthritis

During the period 1971 to 1975, during which enteroviruses were recovered from 7075 persons in the United States, nine instances of rheumatic disease were reported[599]; though not clearly specified, 3 patients apparently had arthritis. Blotzer and Myers[79] noted an adult with echovirus 9 infection and the concomitant onset of arthritis that persisted for 3 months. Echovirus 9 has been recovered from the synovial fluid of a man with acute monocytic arthritis,[489] and one adult and one adolescent had serologic evidence of coxsackievirus B4 infection in association with the onset of rheumatoid arthritis–like illness.[395]

Myositis

Because group A coxsackieviruses routinely cause myositis in suckling mice, a reasonable approach is to suspect a similar clinical manifestation in people. Myalgia is a common complaint as well in illnesses caused by many coxsackieviruses and echoviruses.[30, 139, 264, 336, 494, 562] However, at present, almost no direct evidence (demonstration of virus in muscle) or indirect evidence (elevations in muscle enzymes) of muscle involvement in routine enteroviral illnesses exists. Of the nine patients with rheumatic disease noted by Morens and colleagues,[599] six apparently had myositis; in one instance, coxsackievirus A2 was implicated, and in another patient with polymyositis, coxsackievirus A9 was the related agent. Three patients with echovirus 18 infection and polymyositis have been reported.[457] Acute rhabdomyolysis in one adult and myositis, myoglobinemia, and myoglobinuria in another adult have been associated with echovirus 9 infection.[419, 434] Christensen and associates[164] noted that children with dermatomyositis were more likely to have serum antibody to one or more coxsackieviruses B than were control children. Chou and Gutmann[160] noted enterovirus-like particles in the muscles of two patients with fatal dermatomyositis; Tang and colleagues[806] demonstrated coxsackievirus A9 in the muscles of an 11-year-old girl with chronic myopathy. Using both PCR and dot-blot hybridization assays, Fox and colleagues[261] could not find evidence of persistent enteroviral infection in 32 adults with inflammatory muscle disease (1 patient with dermatomyositis and 31 patients with polymyositis).

SKIN MANIFESTATIONS

Nonpolio enteroviruses as a group are a common cause of a variety of skin manifestations.[137, 861, 864] In the summer and fall, they are the leading cause of exanthems. Variation in the clinical expression rate of exanthem and in the age of the host is marked among the various viral types. In general, dermatologic expression is related inversely to the age of the infected patient. The frequency of exanthem and common associated illnesses by viral type are presented in Table 170–13.

Coxsackievirus A2

Rash associated with coxsackievirus A2 has occurred rarely. Febrile illness with exanthem in conjunction with coxsackievirus A2 infection was observed in Cincinnati in 1957; no details of this outbreak have been presented.[730] Assaad and Cockburn[33] reviewed approximately 15,000 enteroviral illnesses for the period 1967 to 1970 that were reported to the WHO and noted that in 45 instances, skin or mucous membrane lesions associated with coxsackievirus A2 infection were the main clinical manifestations.

Coxsackievirus A3

One case has been reported, but no details are available.[595]

Coxsackievirus A4 (see Fig. 65–15)

Exanthem has been noted infrequently with coxsackievirus A4 infection.[33, 143, 256, 604, 900] However, many cases may be missed because this virus grows poorly in tissue culture and suckling mouse inoculation rarely is used in present-day diagnostic laboratories. Six children were observed in one outbreak.[256] All patients initially had herpangina, and then the exanthem appeared concurrently with or after defervescence. It initially was erythematous, maculopapular, and discrete. In some children, the rash resolved within 4 days, but in others it progressed and became vesicular. The vesicular lesions occurred in crops, spread to the extremities but not the palms and soles, and were yellowish, opaque, and 5 to 10 mm in size. They persisted for 1 to 2 weeks and regressed with a brownish discoloration. The lesions easily were confused with resolving bug bites.

Other manifestations of coxsackievirus A4 infection include an exanthem suggesting combined scarlet fever and rubella,[286] a maculopapular rash that cleared with desquamation,[604] and an anaphylactoid, purpura-like rash (see Fig. 65–15).[143]

Coxsackievirus A5

During the 4-year period studied by Assaad and Cockburn,[33] coxsackievirus A5 was second only to coxsackievirus A16 in the number of instances in which exanthem or mucous membrane involvement was the main clinical manifestation. Even with this apparent frequency, most instances of exanthem have been sporadic rather than part of an outbreak of exanthematous disease. The most common finding is the hand, foot, and mouth syndrome, which is not clinically discernible from that caused by coxsackievirus A16.[188, 252, 256] In one patient, the virus was recovered from vesicular fluid.[252]

Coxsackievirus A7

Coxsackievirus A7 was recovered from one child with a morbilliform rash and aseptic meningitis.[320] An adult with a fatal coxsackievirus 7 infection had pancarditis, pneumonia, and hand, foot, and mouth syndrome.[41]

Coxsackievirus A9 (see Figs. 65–12 and 65–14)

Coxsackievirus A9 is a common cause of exanthem.* In contrast to coxsackievirus A16 and echovirus 9, in which rates of clinical exanthem expression are high, the rate of skin

*See references 33, 139, 143, 148, 375, 391, 429, 432, 468, 516, 599, 643, 870.

TABLE 170–13 ■ FREQUENCY OF EXANTHEM IN OUTBREAKS OF ILLNESS CAUSED BY ENTEROVIRUSES AND PARECHOVIRUSES

Virus Type	Age Group	Occurrence of Rash	Characteristics of Rash	Associated Manifestations	References
Coxsackievirus A2	Children	Rare	Maculopapular	Fever	33, 730
A4	Children	Rare	Maculopapular, vesicular	Fever, herpangina, hepatitis	33, 143, 256, 604, 900
A5	Mainly children	Occasional	Hand, foot, and mouth syndrome	Fever	33, 188, 252, 256
A7	Children and adults	Rare	Morbilliform; hand, foot, and mouth syndrome	Meningitis, pneumonia, pancarditis	41, 320
A9	Mainly children	4%	Maculopapular, vesicular, urticarial, petechial; hand, foot, and mouth syndrome	Fever, meningitis, pneumonia	33, 139, 143, 148, 375, 391, 429, 432, 468, 516, 599, 643, 869
A10	Mainly children	Occasional	Hand, foot, and mouth syndrome	Fever	33, 99, 139, 170, 217, 518
A16	Children and adults	88%, <5 yr 38%, 5–12 yr 11%, adults	Hand, foot, and mouth syndrome	Fever	8, 14, 25, 30, 33, 93, 139, 143, 144, 236, 256, 267, 286, 304, 305, 364–366, 518, 537, 538, 567, 600, 616, 706, 709, 816
B1	Children	Occasional	Maculopapular, vesicular	Fever, meningitis	33, 139, 142, 143, 203, 533
B2	Children	Rare	Maculopapular, vesicular, petechial	Fever, herpangina, meningitis	30, 33, 256
B3	Mainly children	Occasional	Maculopapular, vesicular, petechial	Fever, hepatosplenomegaly	30, 33, 103, 139, 179, 244, 342, 389, 515
B4	Mainly children	Occasional	Maculopapular, vesicular, urticarial	Fever, respiratory	139, 246, 447, 465
B5	Mainly children	10%	Maculopapular, petechial, urticarial	Fever, meningitis	33, 84, 139, 146, 179, 206, 329, 350, 625, 640, 670, 674, 742, 773, 789, 793, 799, 873, 887
B6	Children and adults	20%	Morbilliform	Pneumonia	307
Echovirus 1	Children	Rare	Maculopapular	Conjunctivitis	554
2	Children	Rare	Macular, maculopapular	Fever, pharyngitis	139, 733, 784
3	Children	Rare	Petechial	Fever, meningitis	33, 347, 376
4	Mainly children	10–20%	Macular, maculopapular, petechial	Fever, meningitis	139, 142, 225, 274, 447, 506, 542, 639, 697, 781
5	Infants and adults	Occasional	Macular	Fever	292, 764
6	Mainly children	Rare	Maculopapular, macular, papulopustular, vesicular	Fever, meningitis	33, 446, 549, 561, 566, 840, 842, 873
7	Children	Occasional	Maculopapular	Fever, meningitis	33, 417, 554
9	Children and adults	57%, <5 yr 41%, 5–9 yr 6%, >10 yr	Maculopapular, petechial, vesicular	Fever, meningitis	33, 68, 139, 169, 177, 186, 201, 240, 253, 275, 278, 348, 375, 415, 429, 438, 463, 465, 476, 493, 510, 536, 563, 599, 625, 636, 676, 682, 695, 725, 733, 779, 790, 803, 865
11	Mainly children	Occasional	Maculopapular,vesicular, urticarial	Fever, meningitis	33, 95, 139, 147, 208, 758
13	Children	Rare	Maculopapular		372
14	Mainly children	Rare	Maculopapular, scarlatiniform	Fever, meningitis	33, 733
16	Children	Occasional	Roseola-like	Fever, herpangina	137, 180, 335, 627–630
17	Children	Occasional	Macular, maculopapular, papulovesicular	Fever, diarrhea, herpangina, meningitis	33, 93, 142, 149
18	Children and adults	Occasional, 1epidemic	Rubelliform	Fever, meningitis	457, 569, 599, 625
19	Children and adults	Occasional	Maculopapular	Fever, meningitis, upper respiratory	176, 184, 308
25	Children	Occasional	Maculopapular, hemangioma-like	Fever, pharyngitis	59, 603, 622
30	Children and adults	Occasional	Macular, maculopapular	Fever, meningitis	33, 139, 443, 819, 888
32	Children	Rare	Hemangioma-like	Fever	141
33	—	Rare	—	Meningitis	445, 454
Enterovirus 71	Children	Occasional	Macular, maculopapular, vesicular; hand, foot, and mouth syndrome	Fever, meningitis, encephalitis, paralytic disease	12, 293, 407, 456, 574, 587
Parechovirus 1	Infants	Rare	Morbilliform	Respiratory	72

manifestations in coxsackievirus A9 infection is low. A review of 259 coxsackievirus A9 infections in 1970 revealed an exanthem rate of 4 percent.[139] Most cases of coxsackievirus A9 exanthem occur sporadically, although a few outbreaks have been described.[148, 515, 643]

Skin manifestations in coxsackievirus A9 infection have been interesting and varied. The most common rash illness is characterized by fever and an erythematous, maculopapular rash that starts on the face and neck and spreads to the trunk and extremities. Aseptic meningitis is a common associated finding.

In 1960, Lerner and colleagues[516] reported on 11 children with exanthem associated with coxsackievirus A9 infection. Six had vesicular lesions, and two patients had associated viral pneumonia. Since 1960, vesicular exanthem has been noted on several occasions.[139, 148, 391] Most commonly, illnesses have been described as hand, foot, and mouth syndrome, but when the reports were analyzed, the rashes were vesicular but not always in a peripheral pattern.

Papular urticaria and large urticarial lesions have been an occasional manifestation of coxsackievirus A9 infection[143, 148] (see Fig. 65–12). Other manifestations include Stevens-Johnson syndrome and a severe illness simulating meningococcemia[143, 599] (see Fig. 65–14).

Coxsackievirus A10

The most common exanthematous illness associated with coxsackievirus A10 infection is the hand, foot, and mouth syndrome.[99, 139, 170, 217, 408, 518] Stevens-Johnson syndrome has been associated with coxsackievirus A10 infection in one instance,[139] and a child with ulcerative genital lesions also has been reported.[586]

Coxsackievirus A16 (see Figs. 65–9, 65–10, 65–11, and 65–16)

In the WHO review of enteroviral infections for the 4-year period 1967 through 1970, coxsackievirus A16 was associated with almost half of all skin or mucous membrane diseases. Coxsackievirus A16 is the major cause of hand, foot, and mouth syndrome (see Figs. 65–9, 65–10, and 65–11). Of historical interest is that hand, foot, and mouth syndrome apparently was a new clinical entity in 1956.[642] It was noted in sporadic outbreaks until approximately 1963, and since that time it has been a regularly recurring disease throughout the world.* Serologic data suggest that coxsackievirus A16 was not in wide circulation until about 1963.[144]

The symptoms and signs of coxsackievirus A16 hand, foot, and mouth syndrome are recorded in Table 170–14. All illnesses have a typically enteroviral pattern with a short incubation period (4 to 6 days) and a summer and fall seasonal pattern. The clinical expression rate of the enanthem-exanthem complex is high: close to 100 percent in young children, 38 percent in schoolchildren, and 11 percent in adults.[600] Exanthem occurs more commonly in children, but in adults, the rash occurs more frequently with coxsackievirus A16 than with any of the other enteroviral agents.

Illness is ushered in with a mild prodromal fever, anorexia, malaise, and frequently a sore mouth. Enanthem occurs 1 to 2 days after the onset of fever, and the exanthem appears shortly thereafter. Of the cutaneous lesions, oral lesions are present more consistently than lesions of the skin. Because of this prevalence, illness, particularly in adults, is identified mistakenly as aphthous stomatitis (canker sores) or herpes simplex virus (HSV) infection. The intraoral lesions are ulcerative and average approximately 4 to 8 mm in size. The tongue and buccal mucosa are involved most frequently.

As noted in Table 170–14, the hands are involved more commonly than are the feet. Buttock lesions also occur frequently, but they usually do not progress to vesiculation. The lesions on the hands and feet generally are vesicular and vary in size from 3 to 7 mm; they typically occur more commonly on the dorsal surfaces but frequently on the palms and soles as well. The vesicles contain virus, but cytologic examination usually does not reveal diagnostic findings. They clear by absorption of the fluid in approximately 1 week.

Of considerable interest is the frequent association of coxsackievirus A16 with subacute, chronic, and recurring skin lesions.[236, 623] Evans and Waddington[236] described an 84-year-old woman with chronic recurring skin lesions of more than 2 years' duration. Nankervis and associates[623] noted both subacute and recurring lesions in children. Higgins and Crow[364] reported a 31-year-old woman with Darier disease who had a Kaposi varicelliform eruption caused by coxsackievirus A16, and a similar illness was noted in a 1-year-old boy with eczema.[616]

One child with a Gianotti-Crosti–like eruption (papular acrodermatitis of childhood) associated with coxsackievirus A16 infection has been described.[414]

TABLE 170–14 ■ SYMPTOMS AND SIGNS OF COXSACKIEVIRUS A16 ILLNESS (HAND, FOOT, AND MOUTH SYNDROME)*

Symptoms and Signs	Percentage of Cases	
Enanthem		90
Buccal	61	
Tongue	44	
Palate, uvula, anterior pillars	36	
Gums	15	
Exanthem		64
Hands	52	
Feet	31	
Buttocks	31	
Legs	13	
Arms	10	
Face	5	
Sore mouth or throat		67
Malaise		61
Anorexia		52
Fever		42
Submandibular and/or cervical adenitis		22
Coryza		11
Cough		11
Diarrhea		10
Nausea and vomiting		3

*Data from references 14, 144, 256, 267, 537, 567, 706, 709.
From Cherry, J. D.: Newer viral exanthems. Adv. Pediatr. *16*:233–286, 1969.

Coxsackievirus B1

Exanthem occasionally occurs in coxsackievirus B1 infections.[33, 139, 142, 143, 203, 533] The most common cutaneous finding is an erythematous maculopapular eruption that is discrete. Two children with illnesses suggestive of hand, foot, and mouth syndrome have been observed.[143]

*See references 8, 14, 25, 30, 93, 139, 144, 163, 236, 256, 267, 286, 302, 304, 305, 364–366, 518, 537, 538, 567, 600, 623, 706, 709, 816.

Coxsackievirus B2

Coxsackievirus B2–associated exanthem is rare. Maculopapular, vesicular, and petechial lesions have been noted.[30, 33, 256]

Coxsackievirus B3

Exanthem occasionally is reported as a sporadic event in coxsackievirus B3 infections, and in one instance, a small outbreak occurred.[30, 33, 103, 179, 245, 342, 389, 515, 899] Erythematous maculopapular eruptions occur most commonly, but petechial rash illnesses suggestive of meningococcemia also have been observed. Hand, foot, and mouth syndrome has been observed in one child,[515] and another had a more generalized vesicular eruption. An adult with recurrent hand, foot, and mouth syndrome had a rise in neutralizing antibody titer to coxsackievirus B3.[179]

Coxsackievirus B4

Although cutaneous manifestations with coxsackievirus B4 were noted as frequently as were those associated with coxsackieviruses B1, B2, and B3,[33, 139] few clinical descriptions exist.[447, 465] Morbilliform, petechial, and urticarial rashes have been described.

Coxsackievirus B5

Of the group B coxsackieviruses, type B5 is noted most frequently to have skin manifestations.* The rash usually is maculopapular; petechial lesions are observed occasionally, and one child with urticaria has been reported.[146] Several children studied by Cherry and colleagues[146] had a roseola-like illness pattern. During outbreaks of coxsackievirus B5 illness, approximately 10 percent of young children have an exanthem. Many patients have concomitant aseptic meningitis. One adult patient with recurrent hand, foot, and mouth syndrome had serologic evidence of coxsackievirus B5 infection.

Coxsackievirus B6

Goldwater[307] identified 97 children and adults with coxsackievirus B6 infection. The most prominent finding in these cases was cough and pneumonia. Twenty patients had exanthems; the rash was morbilliform and associated with high fever and cough.

Echovirus 1

Exanthem and conjunctivitis have been associated with echovirus 1 infection in several children.[554]

Echovirus 2

Exanthem occasionally occurs with echovirus 2 infection.[139, 733, 784] The rash has been erythematous macular in some instances but usually is maculopapular and discrete. Most children have had associated fever and pharyngitis.

Echovirus 3

Exanthem was noted in 2 of 29 children with echovirus 3 infection.[347] In both instances, the rashes were petechial; most patients in this outbreak had aseptic meningitis. Details of other echovirus 3 infections and exanthems are lacking.[33, 376]

Echovirus 4

Echovirus 4 is a common cause of epidemic aseptic meningitis, and exanthem is an associated finding in 10 to 20 percent of pediatric cases.[143, 254, 274, 447, 506, 542, 639, 697, 781] The rash is usually macular or maculopapular, has its onset 1 to 3 days after the initial fever, and lasts 1 to 2 days. A child with a petechial rash has been noted.[447]

Echovirus 5

One major outbreak of echovirus 5 infection with exanthem has been described.[292] This outbreak, which involved a maternity unit, resulted in a macular rash in 36 percent of the infants and 14 percent of the mothers. The rash was most prominent on the limbs and buttocks, appeared 24 to 36 hours after the onset of fever, and lasted 2 days. Selwyn and Howitt[764] reported a child who had a macular rash with a zoster distribution. A neonate with sepsis-like illness and exanthem has been described.[332]

Echovirus 6

Although echovirus 6 has been one of the more prevalent enteroviruses during the last 30 years, it has been associated only sporadically with exanthematous disease. The following manifestations have been observed: morbilliform,[840] maculopapular,[561, 873] macular,[549] and papulopustular exanthems[446]; Stevens-Johnson syndrome[842]; and pityriasis rosea in an adult and a child.[446] Meade and Chang[566] reported an interesting zoster-like eruption in a 7-year-old boy in whom echovirus 6 was recovered from several bullae.

Echovirus 7

Echovirus 7 has been associated occasionally with exanthem.[33, 417, 595] In one outbreak of aseptic meningitis, 5 of 13 patients had erythematous maculopapular rashes that occurred during fever.[417] One child with a discrete maculopapular rash and thrombocytopenia has been described.[554] A 37-year-old woman with echovirus 7 infection, leukocytoclastic vasculitis, and palpable purpura has been reported.[153]

Echovirus 9 (see Fig. 65–13)

For more than 40 years, echovirus 9 has been the most prevalent nonpolio enterovirus, and exanthem is a common clinical manifestation (Table 170–15).* Nonspecific febrile illness and aseptic meningitis are the usual major manifestations of echovirus 9 infection. Exanthem occurs in approximately a third of cases. The prevalence of exanthem is related inversely to age; 57 percent of children younger than 5 years have a rash, whereas only 6 percent of those older than 10 years have similar cutaneous findings.[513] The rash usually is rubelliform, but in addition or as the sole manifestation, petechiae are common findings. Rash and fever generally appear at approximately the same time, and frequently the illness closely mimics meningococcemia. The rash usually lasts approximately 3 to 5 days. In one instance, the rash progressed to a vesicular stage.[510]

---

*See references 33, 84, 139, 146, 179, 206, 329, 350, 640, 670, 674, 742, 773, 789, 793, 799, 873.

*See references 33, 68, 139, 169, 177, 186, 201, 240, 253, 268, 275, 278, 309, 348, 375, 415, 429, 438, 463, 465, 476, 493, 510, 536, 563, 599, 636, 676, 682, 695, 725, 733, 779, 790, 803, 865.

TABLE 170–15 ■ SIGNS AND SYMPTOMS IN ECHOVIRUS 9 DISEASE*

Sign or Symptom	Percentage of Cases
Fever	92
Headache	85
Nuchal rigidity	83
Nausea and vomiting	71
Pain (neck, back, trunk)	44
Exanthem	35
Nonexudative pharyngitis	28
Cough	24
Sore throat	20
Cervical lymphadenopathy	18
Coryza	18
Abdominal pain	17
Photophobia	16

*Modified from references 68, 201, 240, 253, 275, 415, 493, 510, 725, 779, 865.
From Cherry, J. D.: Newer viral exanthems. Adv. Pediatr. *16*:233–286, 1969.

Echovirus 11

Exanthem occasionally occurs with echovirus 11 infection, and it varies considerably in appearance.[33, 95, 139, 147, 208, 758] The most notable lesions have been bug bite–like vesicles and urticaria.[147] A child with subacute recurrent vesicular lesions[147] and an adult woman with a disseminated vesicular eruption have been reported.[208]

Echovirus 13

One child with a maculopapular eruption has been described.[372]

Echovirus 14

Echovirus 14 is a rare cause of exanthem, and few details are available.[33, 733] One child with a scarlatiniform eruption and aseptic meningitis has been reported.[733]

Echovirus 16

The first of the enteroviral exanthematous diseases to be described was that caused by echovirus 16. It initially was studied by Neva and colleagues,[628, 629] and the illness was called Boston exanthem. Two outbreaks of echovirus 16 infection with exanthem were documented by Neva and colleagues in 1951 and 1954[627, 630] and another in Paris in 1960.[180] Since then, Boston exanthem has been reported only once. Seven cases were observed in 1974.[335]

The exanthem associated with echovirus 16 infection is erythematous, maculopapular, and discrete and similar to that of other enteroviral infections. What has been unique with echovirus 16 infection is the relationship of rash to fever. Frequently, the illness is roseola-like in that the rash occurs at the time of or after defervescence.[137, 335] Ulcerative lesions on the soft palate and tonsillar pillars (herpangina) sometimes have been observed.

Echovirus 17

Rash is an occasional occurrence in echovirus 17 infection.[33, 93, 143, 149] In one outbreak, transient erythematous rashes were noted.[93] In cases that I have studied, papular, maculopapular, and papulovesicular lesions were noted; two patients had herpangitic enanthems, and one had aseptic meningitis.[143, 149]

Echovirus 18

Kennett and associates[457] described an extensive epidemic of echovirus 18 infection in which aseptic meningitis with or without exanthem was the major finding. In 15 patients, exanthem was the chief complaint. The rash was described as rubelliform. Most patients were children, but adults also had exanthem.

Echovirus 19

In one extensive epidemic of echovirus 19 infection, exanthem was a common occurrence.[176] Fifty percent of children younger than 6 months had exanthem, and many of these infants presented a picture of septicemia with peripheral circulatory failure. Rash occurred in adults and older children, but the percentage decreased with age. The rash usually was erythematous, maculopapular, and discrete. It started on the face and upper part of the trunk and spread to the extremities. Fever occurred in all cases, and meningitis and signs of upper respiratory tract involvement were noted commonly.

In another outbreak of echovirus 19 infection, 33 percent of those infected had exanthem,[308] whereas in an outbreak studied by Cramblett and colleagues,[184] exanthem was a rare finding.

Echovirus 21

A 19-day-old infant with aseptic meningitis and rash has been reported.[158]

Echovirus 24

A 4-month-old infant had rash and aseptic meningitis as a result of echovirus 24 infection.[158]

Echovirus 25

Echovirus 25 has been associated with an array of different skin manifestations.[59, 141, 328, 603, 622] In one epidemic of febrile pharyngitis, approximately a third of the patients had exanthem.[603] The rash most often was maculopapular and discrete, but occasionally it displayed a morbilliform confluence. The rash most frequently occurred during the period of defervescence.

Of considerable interest are two children with acute hemangioma-like lesions.[141] The lesions were erythematous and papular and surrounded by a 1- to 4-mm-wide halo of blanched-appearing skin. The center of each lesion had a bright red dot that suggested a dilated capillary or terminal arteriole. The whole lesion would blanch with pinpoint pressure in its middle.

Echovirus 30

Echovirus 30 is a common cause of epidemic aseptic meningitis, and exanthem occasionally is noted concomitantly. The rash is macular or maculopapular.[33, 139, 402, 443, 508, 819, 888]

Echovirus 32

Two children with echovirus 32 infection and hemangioma-like lesions were described by Cherry and colleagues.[141]

Some lesions seemed to be composed of many dilated capillaries; they easily blanched with pressure.

Echovirus 33

Four patients with aseptic meningitis and echovirus 33 infection also have had exanthem.[445, 454] Two adults have had vesicular lesions that suggested HSV infection.[203]

Enterovirus 71

Kennett and associates[456] studied 49 patients with enterovirus 71 infection and noted exanthem in 11. Six patients had aseptic meningitis, and in five, rash was the predominant complaint. The exanthems varied: some were erythematous maculopapular, some vesicular, and some a combination of lesions. Two children had hand, foot, and mouth syndrome, and one child had a florid, diffuse erythematous rash. Outbreaks of hand, foot, and mouth syndrome caused by enterovirus 71 have been observed in Japan, Sweden, Australia, the United States, Taiwan, and Malaysia.* In many cases, varied neurologic manifestations also occurred.

Parechovirus 1

A morbilliform rash was noted in three infants with respiratory disease and parechovirus 1 infection.[72]

Clinical Exanthematous Manifestations and Syndromes

The major clinical exanthematous manifestations and syndromes of coxsackieviruses and echoviruses are presented in Table 170–16. Unusual findings include hemangioma-like lesions with echoviruses 25 and 32, anaphylactoid purpura with coxsackievirus A4 and echoviruses 9 and 18, zoster-like rash with echoviruses 5 and 6, pityriasis-like rash with echovirus 6, and chronic or recurrent rash with coxsackievirus A16 and echovirus 11.

NEUROLOGIC MANIFESTATIONS

Neurologic illness is a frequent manifestation of infection with most enteroviruses and parechoviruses. The most common illness is aseptic meningitis, but encephalitis and other manifestations also occur. The prevalence of nonpolio enteroviruses and parechoviruses in the various clinical syndromes is presented in Table 170–17.

Aseptic Meningitis

Aseptic meningitis caused by enteroviruses occurs both in epidemics and as isolated cases. The etiologic agents most often associated with epidemic disease are presented in Table 170–18. Epidemic disease has occurred most commonly with coxsackievirus B5 and echoviruses 4, 6, 9, and 30. In general, illness occurs more frequently in children, but if a specific outbreak is large, adults also are involved. Virtually all patients have fever and pharyngitis; other respiratory manifestations occur commonly. Rash is a frequent occurrence but varies with the specific viral agents. Between a third and a half of all patients with echovirus 9 meningitis have exanthem. Abdominal pain is a common complaint in patients with epidemic enteroviral aseptic meningitis.

*See references 127, 129, 293, 369, 385, 407, 481, 565, 574, 651, 889.

Except for rash, herpangina, pleurodynia, or myocarditis, little else occurs clinically to help identify the etiology in a sporadic case of aseptic meningitis. Initial symptoms include fever, headache, malaise, nausea, and vomiting. The headache usually is frontal or generalized; adolescents and adults frequently note retrobulbar pain. Pain in the neck, back, and legs occurs commonly. Abdominal pain is noted in approximately a fifth of patients, but this symptom varies with the specific etiologic viral type. Photophobia is a common occurrence.

Physical examination reveals a temperature in the range of 38° to 40° C (100.4° to 104° F). Skin rash occurs often and most commonly is erythematous, maculopapular, and discrete. Frequently, particularly with echovirus 9 infection, the rash is petechial and suggests meningococcemia. Hand, foot, and mouth syndrome is a common event in cases of aseptic meningitis caused by enterovirus 71 infection.[127, 129, 369, 481, 565] Pharyngitis occurs frequently. Generalized muscle stiffness or spasm usually is observed, although the degree varies considerably; the Kernig and Brudzinski signs are positive in less than half the cases. Deep tendon reflexes usually are normal. In one study, 9 percent of children with enteroviral meningitis had the syndrome of inappropriate secretion of antidiuretic hormone.[136] The onset of this syndrome was noted 36 hours after admission to the hospital, and it usually lasted less than 2 days.

Examination of CSF reveals considerable variation among patients and in the same patient on repeated examination. CSF leukocyte counts vary from a few cells to a few thousand per cubic millimeter; the median is in the range of 100 to 500 cells/mm^3. The percentage of neutrophils also varies greatly. Initial examinations frequently reveal a predominance of neutrophils, but rarely more than 90 percent, as seen in bacterial disease. Usually, between 30 and 60 percent neutrophils is found on initial examination. Repeated examinations of CSF demonstrate an increasing percentage of mononuclear cells. Dagan and colleagues[193] observed that the rate of isolation of virus from the CSF in enteroviral meningitis was directly proportional to the number of leukocytes in the fluid.

CSF protein levels usually are elevated mildly, and glucose concentrations usually are normal; hypoglycorrhachia rarely occurs.[36, 151, 229, 495, 545, 765, 774, 776, 795] Occasionally, the CSF findings suggest tuberculosis meningitis with mononuclear pleocytosis, hypoglycorrhachia, and elevated protein levels.[541] A child with coxsackievirus B4 meningitis had eosinophils in the CSF.[150] The results of other routine laboratory studies such as the white blood cell count occasionally are abnormal but not helpful diagnostically.

The duration of illness varies significantly. In most patients, the temperature returns to normal within 4 to 6 days, and disability as a result of neurologic involvement lasts 1 to 2 weeks. Occasionally, the pattern of illness is biphasic: an initial period with fever, headache, nausea, vomiting, and muscle aches and pains of a few days' duration followed by general recovery and then return to the same symptoms plus more pronounced neurologic involvement.

Wilfert and associates[868] performed a longitudinal assessment of children who had enteroviral meningitis early in life and found that receptive language functioning was significantly worse than that of children in a control group without meningitis. In another study, Sells and colleagues[763] examined the long-term effects of CNS enteroviral infection in 19 children. Of this group, 11 were free of detectable abnormalities, 5 had possible defects, and 3 had definite neurologic sequelae. In more recent studies, patients who have

TABLE 170–16 ■ CLINICAL EXANTHEMATOUS MANIFESTATIONS OF ENTEROVIRUSES

	Associated Viral Agents and Prevalence of Manifestations			
Clinical Manifestations	**Virus Subgroup**	**Common**	**Occasional**	**Rare**
Macular rash	Coxsackievirus A			
	B		1, 2, 5	
	Echovirus and enterovirus		2, 4, 5, 13, 14, 17, 19, 30	18, 71
Maculopapular rash	Coxsackievirus A	9	2, 4, 5, 10, 16	6, 7
	B		1–5	
	Echovirus and enterovirus	4, 9	2, 5–7, 11, 16–19, 25, 30, 71	1, 3, 13, 14, 27, 33
Vesicular rash	Coxsackievirus A	5, 16	8–10	4, 7
	B			1–3, 5
	Echovirus and enterovirus		11	6, 9, 17, 71
Petechial or purpuric rash	Coxsackievirus A	9	4	
	B		2–5	
	Echovirus	9	4, 7	3
Urticarial rash	Coxsackievirus A	9	16	
	B		4, 5	
	Echovirus		11	
Erythema multiforme or Stevens-Johnson syndrome	Coxsackievirus A		9	10, 16
	B			4, 5
	Echovirus			6, 11
Exanthem and meningitis	Coxsackievirus A		2, 9	7
	B		1, 2, 4, 5	
	Echovirus and enterovirus	4, 9	6, 11, 17, 18, 25, 30	3, 14, 33, 71
Exanthem and pneumonia	Coxsackievirus A		9	7
	B		6	1
	Echovirus			9, 11
Hand, foot, and mouth syndrome	Coxsackievirus A	16	5, 10	7, 9
	B			1, 3, 5
	Echovirus and enterovirus	71		
Hemangioma-like lesions	Coxsackievirus A			
	B			
	Echovirus			25, 32
Herpangina and exanthem	Coxsackievirus A		4	9
	B			2
	Echovirus		16, 17	
Roseola-like illness	Coxsackievirus A			6, 9
	B		5	1, 2, 4
	Echovirus		16, 25	9, 11, 27, 30
Anaphylactoid purpura	Coxsackievirus A			4
	B			
	Echovirus			9, 18
Zoster-like rash	Coxsackievirus A			
	B			
	Echovirus			5, 6
Pityriasis-like rash	Coxsackievirus A			
	B			6
	Echovirus			
Chronic or recurrent rash	Coxsackievirus A	16		
	B			
	Echovirus			11

had meningitis have performed as well as controls in follow-up developmental evaluations.[69, 714, 719]

Encephalitis

In the United States, an average of approximately 2500 cases of encephalitis per year are reported to the CDC.[114] Of this group, only approximately 2 percent demonstrate an enteroviral etiology. However, the seasonal pattern of disease and the absence of arboviral activity in many geographic locations suggest that 500 to 1000 cases of enteroviral encephalitis actually occur each year in the United States. The prevalence of coxsackieviruses and echoviruses as etiologic agents in encephalitis is presented in Table 170–17. Echovirus 9 is the most frequent cause of enteroviral encephalitis. Other enteroviral types commonly associated are echoviruses 4, 6, 11, and 30 and coxsackievirus B5. Echoviruses 4, 6, and 11 have been noted most frequently over a long period.

In general, the prognosis in encephalitis caused by enteroviral infection is good, but fatalities do occur. The viral types that have been isolated from the brain or CSF in fatal cases are coxsackieviruses B3 and B6; echoviruses 2, 9, 17, and 25; and enterovirus 71.[326, 463]

Paralysis

Paralysis caused by anterior horn cell disease occasionally results from infection with nonpolio enteroviruses. In contrast to the prevalence of poliovirus, which in the prevaccine era resulted in epidemic paralytic disease, paralysis caused by nonpolio enteroviruses usually is a sporadic event.

TABLE 170–17 ■ NEUROLOGIC MANIFESTATIONS OF NONPOLIO ENTEROVIRUSES AND PARECHOVIRUSES*

	Associated Viral Agents and Prevalence of Manifestations				
Clinical Manifestations	Virus Subgroup	Common	Occasional	Rare	References
Aseptic meningitis	Coxsackievirus A	9	7	1–6, 8, 10, 11–14, 16–18, 21, 22, 24	12, 13, 68, 74. 112, 122, 127, 129, 139, 201, 223, 232, 240, 253, 274, 275, 309, 326, 331, 338, 355, 369, 415, 417, 421, 429, 452, 453, 463, 481, 493, 507, 508, 513, 557, 561, 565, 574, 575, 595, 601, 705, 714, 719, 725, 730, 758, 765, 768, 779, 833, 841, 865, 869, 888
	B	2, 4, 5	1, 3	6	
	Echovirus	4, 6, 9, 30, 33, 71	3, 11, 12, 14, 16, 18, 19, 25, 31	1, 2, 5, 7, 8, 15, 17, 20–24, 26, 27, 29, 32	
Encephalitis	Coxsackievirus A		9	2, 4–7, 10, 16	127, 129, 139, 326, 350, 369, 407, 463, 481, 485, 496, 565, 590, 595, 752
	B	5	1, 2, 4	3	
	Echovirus	4, 6, 9, 11, 30, 71	3, 25	1, 2, 5, 7, 8, 12, 13, 14, 15, 17–24, 27, 31, 33, 71	12, 719
Paralysis (lower motor neuron involvement)	Coxsackievirus A		4, 7, 9	2, 5, 6, 10, 11, 14, 21, 24	2, 4, 6, 10, 12, 14, 20, 33, 127, 129, 133, 139, 159, 199, 220, 249, 254, 293, 301, 323, 325, 326, 349, 369, 407, 463, 481, 484, 537–539, 565, 574, 672, 696, 739, 758, 785, 843, 844, 892, 899
	B		2, 3	1, 4–6	
	Echovirus	70, 71	9, 11, 30	1–4, 6–8, 12, 14, 16–19, 22, 25, 27, 31, 70, 71	
Guillain-Barré syndrome and transverse myelitis	Coxsackievirus A		9	2, 4, 5, 6, 19	12, 45, 60, 62, 78, 206, 249, 286, 314, 317, 411, 423, 462, 463, 511, 565, 739, 802, 831
	B			1, 4	
	Echovirus		6, 70	5, 7, 19, 22	
Cerebellar ataxia	Coxsackievirus A		9	4, 7	
	B			3, 4	66, 244, 326, 335, 407, 463, 549, 556, 619, 900
	Echovirus		6, 9, 71	16	
Peripheral neuritis	Coxsackievirus A				
	B				758
	Echovirus		9		
Neurologic sequelae and other neurologic illness	Coxsackievirus A		3	9	
	B		3	2, 4	123, 127, 129, 369, 463, 481, 565, 663, 711, 758, 763, 845, 846, 883
	Echovirus	71	9	19, 25, 30, 33	

*Parechoviruses 1 and 2 are listed as echoviruses 22 and 23, respectively.
Enteroviruses 70 and 71 are listed under echovirus.

TABLE 170–18 ■ COXSACKIEVIRUSES AND ECHOVIRUSES ASSOCIATED WITH EPIDEMIC ASEPTIC MENINGITIS

Virus Type	Age Group	Common Nonneurologic Findings	References
Coxsackievirus A7	Children and adults	Fever	320
A9	Mainly children	Fever, rash, pharyngitis	139, 516
B1	Mainly children	Fever, pharyngitis	139
B2	Children and adults	Fever, pharyngitis, rhinitis, abdominal pain, diarrhea	139, 544
B3	Children and adults	Fever, pharyngitis, conjunctivitis	139
B4	Children and adults	Fever, pharyngitis, rash, conjunctivitis	139, 246
B5	Mainly children	Fever, pharyngitis, rash, pleurodynia, abdominal pain, diarrhea, rhinitis, myocarditis	40, 139, 146, 154, 329, 559, 674, 726, 793, 799, 801
Echovirus 3	Children	Fever, rash	347
4	Mainly children	Fever, pharyngitis, abdominal pain, rash, conjunctivitis	139, 255, 274, 442, 447
6	Children and adults	Fever, pharyngitis, abdominal pain, pleurodynia, cardiac involvement	139, 341, 446, 466, 494
	Children	Fever, rash	417
9	Mainly children	Fever, rash, abdominal pain, pharyngitis	139, 201, 253, 268, 309, 348, 415, 438, 493, 536, 638, 682, 725, 733, 779, 790, 820, 854, 862
11	Mainly children	Fever, upper respiratory, pneumonia	572
13	Mainly children	Fever	122
16	Children	Fever, rash	335
18	Children and adults	Fever, rash	457
19	Mainly children	Fever, upper respiratory, rash	176, 308
25	Children and adults	Fever, rash	59
30	Children and adults	Fever, pharyngitis, rhinitis, conjunctivitis, rash, abdominal pain	139, 316, 336, 443, 671, 888
31	Children and adults	Fever	507
33	Children and adults	Fever, rash	445, 454
Enterovirus 71	Mainly children	Fever, rash	127, 129, 369, 456, 481, 565

Coxsackievirus A7 has been associated with outbreaks of paralytic disease on three occasions.[323, 325, 843] Many cases of illness similar to poliomyelitis have occurred during outbreaks and epidemics of illness caused by enterovirus 71.[12, 199, 293, 349, 407, 574, 739] Paralytic disease also has been noted during epidemics of acute hemorrhagic conjunctivitis caused by enterovirus 70.[844, 892]

Guillain-Barré Syndrome and Transverse Myelitis

As Table 170–17 shows, many coxsackieviruses and echoviruses apparently have been associated with Guillain-Barré syndrome. In general, no specific viral types appear to cause the disease. Rather, the disease occurs sporadically in association with the prevalent enteroviral types.

Other Neurologic Illnesses (see Table 170–17)

Cerebellar ataxia has been associated with coxsackieviruses A4, A7, A9, B3, and B4 and echoviruses 6, 9, and 16. Scott[758] specifically comments on peripheral neuritis with echovirus 9 infection. Coxsackievirus A9 has been associated with focal encephalitis and acute hemiplegia on two occasions,[123, 139] and echovirus 25 infection was noted in a 5-year-old boy with focal encephalitis and subacute hemichorea.[663] Coxsackievirus B4 was isolated from the spinal fluid of a 22-year-old woman with intracranial hypertension,[883] and postencephalitis Parkinson syndrome occurring after coxsackievirus B2 meningoencephalitis has been described.[845] Two children with coxsackievirus B3 infections have had a syndrome of opsoclonus-myoclonus.[487] A 4-year-old boy with “Alice in Wonderland” syndrome (complex symptoms of perceptual distortion) associated with coxsackievirus B1 infection has been described.[846]

Phillips and colleagues[669] and Barrett and associates[47] noted the simultaneous occurrence of enteroviral and St. Louis encephalitis viral infection in the same community. In six instances, dual infections occurred, and the afflicted children tended to have more serious illnesses.

Multiple attacks of enteroviral aseptic meningitis in the same individuals have been noted occasionally.[477, 620]

From molecular techniques and antibody prevalence data, chronic enteroviral infections have been suggested to play a role in the chronic fatigue and postviral fatigue syndromes.[24, 102, 172, 607, 895] However, these findings have not been confirmed by other investigators.[571, 584, 797] Woodall and associates[881] found conserved enteroviral sequences in spinal cords from subjects with sporadic motor neuron disease and from one patient with possible familial motor neuron disease. Berger and associates[67] noted enterovirus RNA sequences in spinal cord specimens from 13 of 17 patients with amyotrophic lateral sclerosis, but Portlance Walker and colleagues[675] could not duplicate these findings in a study of 20 spinal cord specimens from similar patients. Behan and associates[54] looked for picornavirus RNA in biopsy specimens from 41 patients with inflammatory myopathy, but all results were negative.[54]

Simonsen and coworkers[775] noted an outbreak of vertigo in Wyoming in August 1992 in which IgM antibody studies suggested an enteroviral etiology.

SUDDEN INFANT DEATH

Balduzzi and Greendyke[42] recovered coxsackievirus A5 from the stool of a 1-month-old child who experienced sudden infant death. In a similar investigation of sudden infant death, Gold and associates[306] recovered coxsackievirus A4 from the brains of three babies. Coxsackievirus A8 also was recovered from the stool of a child in whom anorexia was noted on the day before death. Coxsackievirus B3 was recovered at the autopsy of an infant who died suddenly on the eighth day of life.[42] Morens and colleagues[599] noted sudden infant death eight times in association with enteroviral infection; parechovirus was found on two occasions. In a subgroup of infants with sudden unexplained death in whom the "clinical, biologic, and histologic" findings suggested viral infection, evidence of enterovirus infection was found more commonly than in infants without findings of viral infection.[315] Specifically, enteroviral RNA was detected in the respiratory tract in 54 percent of the viral infection group and in none of the group without findings suggestive of viral infection. These results were supported by IgM antibodies to coxsackieviruses B in 56 percent of the first group and in none of the second group.

In five instances of cot death in one study, echovirus 11 was isolated from the lungs in two cases, from the myocardium in one case, and from the nose or feces in the other two cases.[76]

CHRONIC ENTEROVIRAL INFECTIONS IN IMMUNOCOMPROMISED PATIENTS

Patients with cell-mediated and combined immunodeficiencies are susceptible to chronic and often fatal infections with many viruses.[271] Patients with agammaglobulinemia and normal cell-mediated function generally survive infections with these same viruses. Enteroviruses are the exception, however, in that chronic, unusual infections with a variety of enteroviruses have been reported.* The most common illness is meningoencephalitis, but arthritis and polymyositis are other frequent findings. Echovirus 11 has been the most common cause of chronic infection, but the following other enteroviruses also have been causative: echoviruses 2, 3, 5, 7, 9, 15, 17, 18, 19, 24, 25, 29, 30, and 33; coxsackieviruses A11, A15, B2, and B3; and parechovirus 1.[558] Enteroviruses have been recovered from many other body sites, such as the liver, heart, lung, pancreas, lymph nodes, bone marrow, muscle, throat, and stool, in addition to the CSF.

Several patients with X-linked agammaglobulinemia have had polymyositis- or dermatomyositis-like syndromes caused by echovirus infections; the following echoviruses have been implicated: types 2, 3, 5, 9, 11, 17, 19, 24, 25, 30, and 33.[46, 187, 568]

A 15-year-old boy with X-linked agammaglobulinemia and chronic arthritis caused by echovirus 11 has been reported.[7] Three children with X-linked hyper-IgM syndrome and persistent enteroviral meningoencephalitis have been described.[190] Persistent enteroviral infections of the CNS have been reported in pediatric and adult patients infected with human immunodeficiency virus.[222, 654] Enteroviral infections have caused deaths in bone marrow transplant recipients.[23, 272]

CONGENITAL INFECTIONS

Abortion

Landsman and associates[497] studied 2631 pregnancies during an echovirus 9 epidemic and could find no difference in antibody to echovirus 9 in women who aborted and in those who delivered term infants. A similar study in Finland revealed no increase in the abortion rate in women infected in early pregnancy with echovirus 9.[695] Although coxsackieviral infections occur commonly, epidemics with specific viral types involving large populations have not been studied.

Two women with coxsackievirus A16 hand, foot, and mouth syndrome had spontaneous abortions.[646] In one instance, coxsackievirus A16 was recovered from the products of conception. Frisk and Diderholm[265] found that 33 percent of women with abortions had IgM antibody to coxsackieviruses B whereas only 8 percent of controls had similar antibody. In a second, larger study, the same research group confirmed their original findings.[37]

Congenital Malformations

In a large prospective study, Brown and Karunas[92] made a serologic search for selected maternal enteroviral infections in association with congenital malformations. Sera from 630 mothers of infants with anomalies and from 1164 mothers of children without defects were studied carefully. Specifically, serologic evidence of infection with coxsackieviruses B1, B2, B3, B4, B5, and A9 and with echoviruses 6 and 9 was sought during the first trimester and during the last 6 months of pregnancy. In this study, infants were examined for 113 specific abnormalities; these anomalies were grouped into 12 categories for analysis. The investigators demonstrated a positive correlation between maternal infection and infant anomaly with coxsackieviruses B2, B3, B4, and A9. The overall anomaly rate associated with first-trimester infection with coxsackievirus B4 was significantly higher than that in controls. Maternal coxsackievirus B2 infection throughout pregnancy, coxsackievirus B4 infection during the first trimester of pregnancy, and infection with at least one of the five group B coxsackieviruses during pregnancy all were associated with urogenital anomalies when compared with controls. Coxsackievirus A9 infection was associated with digestive anomalies and coxsackieviruses B3 and B4 with cardiovascular defects. When coxsackieviruses B were analyzed as a group (B1 to B5), an overall association with congenital heart disease was found; the likelihood of having cardiovascular anomalies was increased when maternal infection with two or more coxsackieviruses B occurred.

Gauntt and colleagues[283] found that ventricular fluid from 4 of 28 babies with severe anatomic defects contained neutralizing antibody to one or more coxsackievirus B types. In one case, specific IgM antibody to coxsackievirus B6 was demonstrated.

In a serologic study in Scotland, Ross and colleagues[715] found no association between maternal coxsackievirus B infection and fetal developmental anomalies. Elizan and associates[230] were unable to find any relationship between maternal infection with coxsackieviruses B and congenital CNS malformations. In three studies, no association between maternal echovirus 9 infection and congenital malformation was noted.[476, 497, 695]

Prematurity and Stillbirth

Bates[51] reported an 8-month-old stillborn fetus with calcific pancarditis and hydrops fetalis at autopsy. Fluorescent antibody study revealed coxsackievirus B3 antigen in the myocardium. Burch and colleagues[97] noted three stillborn infants who had fluorescent antibody evidence of coxsackievirus B myocarditis, one each with coxsackieviruses B2, B3, and B4. They also noted a premature boy who had histologic and immunofluorescent evidence of cardiac infection with coxsackieviruses B2, B3, and B4; he lived only 24 hours.

Freedman[263] reported the occurrence of a full-term stillbirth in a woman infected with echovirus 11. Because the baby had no pathologic or virologic evidence of infection,

*See references 7, 46, 80, 178, 187, 190, 218, 221, 234, 333, 361, 558, 721, 838, 853, 855.

Freedman attributed the event to a secondary consequence of maternal infection caused by fever and dehydration rather than primary transplacental infection. In another stillbirth in which echovirus 11 was recovered from amniotic fluid, the fetus was found to have evidence of focal encephalitis, massive adrenal hemorrhage, and diffuse subarachnoid hemorrhage.[777] Echovirus 27 was recovered from amniotic fluid in an intrauterine fetal death at 28 weeks' gestation.[632] A 26-week, 1300-g stillborn fetus with hydrocephalitis, fibrotic peritonitis, and hepatosplenomegaly was noted by PCR and immunohistochemical study to have an enterovirus 71 infection.[161]

NEONATAL INFECTIONS

Epidemiology and Pathogenesis

Neonatal infection with coxsackieviruses and echoviruses can result from transplacental viral transmission, contact infection during birth, and human-to-human contact after birth. Transplacental passage of coxsackieviruses and echoviruses at term has been noted on many occasions. Benirschke[64] studied the placentas in three cases of congenital coxsackievirus B disease and could find no histologic evidence of infection. In 1956, Kibrick and Benirschke[464] reported the first case of intrauterine infection with coxsackievirus B3. In this instance, the infant was delivered by cesarean section and became symptomatic several hours after birth. Brightman and associates[89] recovered coxsackievirus B5 from the placenta and rectum of a premature infant. No histologic abnormalities of the placenta were noted.

Berkovich and Smithwick[73] noted an asymptomatic neonate who had specific IgM parechovirus 1 antibody in cord blood, thus suggesting intrauterine infection with this virus. Hughes and colleagues[390] reported a newborn infant with echovirus 14 infection who had markedly elevated IgM (190 mg/dL) on the sixth day of life. This child probably also was infected in utero. In addition, echovirus 19 has been noted in a transplacentally acquired infection.[666] Other evidence of intrauterine infection has been presented for coxsackieviruses A4, B1, B2, B3, B4, and B5 and echoviruses 9, 11, and 19.*

There is little definitive evidence for either ascending infection or contact infection during birth with coxsackieviruses or echoviruses. However, transmission of infection during the birth process seems probable.[149, 444] The fecal carriage rate of enteroviruses in asymptomatic adult patients varies between 0 and 6 percent or higher in different population groups.[139] Cherry and colleagues[149] noted that in 2 of 55 mothers (4%), enteroviruses were present in feces shortly after delivery. Coxsackievirus B5 was recovered from the cervices of four women with febrile illnesses during the third trimester of pregnancy.[702] Echovirus 11 was isolated from the cervix of a mother whose baby became ill on the third day of life with a fatal echovirus 11 necrotizing hepatitis.[701]

Several epidemics with coxsackieviruses and echoviruses in newborn nurseries have been studied.[89, 106, 581, 615] Brightman and associates[89] observed an epidemic of coxsackievirus B5 in a premature nursery. Their data suggested that the virus was introduced into this nursery by an asymptomatic infant who had been infected in utero. Secondary infections occurred in 12 babies and 2 nurses. The timing of the secondary cases suggested that three generations had occurred and that the nurses had been infected during the second generation. The investigators suggested that the infection had spread from infant to infant and from infant to nurse.

Javett and associates[418] reported an acute epidemic of myocarditis associated with coxsackievirus B3 infection in a Johannesburg maternity home. Unfortunately, no epidemiologic investigation or search for asymptomatic infected infants was performed. However, in analyzing the dates of onset of the illnesses, single infections apparently occurred for five generations and then five children became ill within a 3-day period.

Kipps and colleagues[472] carried out epidemiologic investigations in two coxsackievirus B3 nursery epidemics. In the first epidemic, the initial infection probably was transmitted from a mother to her baby; this baby then was the source of five secondary cases in newborn infants and one illness in a nurse. Four of the five secondary cases were located on one side of the nursery, but only one cot was close to that of the index baby, and this cot did not adjoin the cots of the three other contact cases. In the second outbreak, a baby who also was infected by his mother probably introduced the virus into the nursery. The three secondary cases were geographically far removed from the primary case.

Cramblett and colleagues[182] reported an outbreak of echovirus 11 disease in four infants in an intensive care nursery. All infants were in enclosed incubators, and three patients became ill within 24 hours; the fourth child became ill 4 days later. Echovirus 11 was recovered from two members of the nursery staff. These data suggest that transmission from personnel to infants occurred because of inadequate washing of hands.

In another outbreak in an intensive care unit, the initial patient was transferred to the nursery because of severe echovirus 11 disease.[615] After transfer, the senior house officer and a psychologist in the unit were infected. The investigators inferred that these infected personnel spread the disease by respiratory droplet to nine other babies. In another echovirus 11 nursery outbreak, Mertens and colleagues[581] found that the infection spread through close contact between infected newborns and the nurses in the unit. Spread of infection was interrupted with the installation of vigorous hygienic and isolation measures. In an echovirus 11 outbreak in an intermediate care unit, Kinney and colleagues[471] found that gavage feeding, mouth care, and being a twin were risk factors for acquiring illness.

Many other instances of isolated nursery infections and small outbreaks with coxsackieviruses and echoviruses have been reported. The most consistent source of original nursery infection seems to be transmission from a mother to her baby,* but virus can be introduced into the nursery by personnel.[403, 501, 799]

In a longitudinal study of neonatal enteroviral infections carried out during the summer and fall of 1981, Jenista and associates[420] found that the nonpolio enterovirus infection rate was 12.8 percent. Lower socioeconomic status and lack of breast-feeding were found to be risk factors for acquiring infection. Nonpolio enteroviral infections were determined to be a significant cause for re-admission of the cohort neonates to the hospital. During a community outbreak of echovirus 11 disease, Modlin and colleagues[591] found that passive transplacental passage of antibody to neonates prevented the development of severe disease but not mucosal infection.

*See references 51, 65, 83, 139, 149, 342, 433, 444, 540, 666.

*See references 25, 49, 134, 139, 140, 151, 176, 200, 229, 238, 335, 404, 495, 527, 545, 589, 615, 686, 799.

Clinical Manifestations

Coxsackieviral and echoviral infections in neonates result in a wide variety of clinical manifestations ranging from asymptomatic infection to fatal encephalitis and myocarditis.[140] Unfortunately, in more recent years, enteroviral illnesses have not been examined by specific viral type but in a more generic fashion.[4, 5, 751] An overview by illness category and prevalence is presented in Table 170–19.

INAPPARENT INFECTION. Although inapparent infection probably occurs occasionally with many different enteroviruses, little documentation of this assumption exists. Cherry and colleagues[149] studied 590 normal neonates during a 6-month period and noted only one asymptomatic infection. This child was infected in utero or immediately thereafter with coxsackievirus B2. The mother had an upper respiratory illness 10 days before delivery.

During a survey of perinatal viral infections, 44 babies were found to be infected with parechovirus 1 in the study period May to December 1966.[409] The prevalence of virus and the incidence of new infections during this period were fairly uniform. No illness was attributed to parechovirus 1 infection, and the virus disappeared from the nursery in mid-December. Asymptomatic infections with parechovirus 1 have been noted on two other occasions.[72, 621] Infections without evidence of illness also have been noted with coxsackieviruses A9, B1, B4, and B5 and echoviruses 3, 5, 9, 11, 13, 14, 20, 30, and 31.[139, 140, 228, 239, 292, 410, 420, 605]

MILD, NONSPECIFIC FEBRILE ILLNESS. In a review of 338 enteroviral infections in early infancy, 9 percent were classified as nonspecific febrile illnesses.[598] Illness may be sporadic or part of an outbreak with a specific viral type. In the latter case the clinical manifestations vary, depending on the viral type: some infants have aseptic meningitis and other signs and symptoms, whereas others simply have nonspecific fever. Specific viruses related to nonspecific fever are listed in Table 170–19. Although by definition illness in this category is mild, being aware that viral infection may be extensive is important. When sought, virus may be isolated from the blood, urine, and spinal fluid of infants with mild illnesses.[49, 412]

SEPSIS-LIKE ILLNESS. The main diagnostic problem in neonatal enteroviral infections is differentiation of bacterial from viral disease. Even in an infant with mild nonspecific fever, bacterial disease must be considered strongly. The sepsis-like illness described here always is alarming. Illness is characterized by fever, poor feeding, abdominal distention, irritability, rash, lethargy, and hypotonia.[335, 495] Other findings include diarrhea, vomiting, seizures, and apnea. In severe, frequently fatal illnesses, most often caused by echovirus 11 infection, jaundice, hepatitis, disseminated intravascular coagulation, thrombocytopenia, and hypotension occur.[433, 588, 606, 701]

Sepsis-like illness is a common occurrence. Morens[598] noted its presence in one fifth of 338 enteroviral infections in infants. In an attempt to differentiate bacterial from viral disease, Lake and associates[495] studied 27 infants with enteroviral infection. White blood cell counts were not helpful because the total count, the number of neutrophils, and the number of band form neutrophils were elevated in most cases. Of most importance were historical data. Most mothers had suffered a recent, febrile, viral-like illness. In addition, other factors often associated with bacterial sepsis, such as prolonged rupture of membranes, prematurity, and low Apgar scores, were unusual findings in the enteroviral infection group. Bone marrow failure developed in a newborn baby boy with a sepsis-like illness caused by echovirus 11 infection.[807] The neutropenia resolved spontaneously, and the thrombocytopenia normalized after treatment with intravenous immunoglobulin (IVIG).

Abzug reviewed the prognosis in 16 neonates who had a sepsis-like illness with hepatitis and coagulopathy.[3] The case-fatality rate was 31 percent. In addition to having hepatitis and coagulopathy, the five fatal cases had myocarditis and three had encephalitis. The follow-up of six survivors noted normalization of liver function and platelet counts and the absence of subsequent significant medical problems.

RESPIRATORY ILLNESS. Respiratory complaints generally are overshadowed by other manifestations of neonatal enteroviral disease. Only 7 percent of 338 enteroviral infections in early infancy were classified as respiratory illness in one study.[598] Herpangina has been observed and photographed only once; Chawareewong and associates[134] noted several infants with herpangina and coxsackievirus A5 infection.

Hercík and colleagues[358] reported an epidemic of respiratory illness in 22 neonates associated with echovirus 11 infection. All these infants had rhinitis and pharyngitis, 50 percent had laryngitis, and 32 percent had interstitial pneumonitis. Berkovich and Pangan[72] studied respiratory illnesses in premature infants and reported 64 babies with illness, 18 of whom had virologic or serologic evidence of parechovirus 1 infection. In addition, many had high but constant levels of serum antibody to parechovirus 1. Some of these latter infants probably also were infected with parechovirus 1. The children with proven parechovirus 1 infection could not be differentiated clinically from those without evidence of such infection. Ninety percent of the infants had coryza, and 39 percent had radiographic evidence of pneumonia.

Except for echoviruses 11 and parechovirus 1, respiratory illness associated with enteroviruses has occurred sporadically. The following other viruses have been noted: coxsackieviruses A5, A9, B1, B4, and B5 and echoviruses 9, 17, 18, 19, 20, 22, and 31. In the review by Morens,[598] only 7 of 338 enteroviral infections of infancy were classified as pneumonia.

Eichenwald and Kostevalov[228] recovered echovirus 20 from four full-term infants younger than 8 days. Although these infants were asymptomatic, they were found to be colonized extensively with staphylococci, and they disseminated these organisms into the air around them. Because of this ability to disseminate staphylococci, they were called *cloud babies*. The investigators thought that these cloud babies contributed to the epidemic spread of staphylococci in the nursery. Because active staphylococcal dissemination occurred only when echovirus 20 could be recovered from the nasopharynx, viral-bacterial synergistic activity was thought to be present.

GASTROINTESTINAL MANIFESTATIONS. Significant gastrointestinal illness occurs in approximately 7 percent of enteroviral infections of infancy.[598] Vomiting and diarrhea occur commonly but usually are only part of the overall illness complex and not the major manifestations. In 1958, Eichenwald and associates[227] described epidemic diarrhea associated with echovirus 18 infection. In a nursery unit of premature infants, 12 of 21 babies were mildly ill. Neither temperature elevation nor hypothermia occurred. Six infants were lethargic and listless, and moderate abdominal distention developed in two. The diarrhea lasted from 1 to 5 days; they had five or six watery, greenish stools per day, occasionally expelled explosively. In two infants, a small amount of blood, but no mucus or pus cells, was noted in their stools. Five other babies in another nursery also had

TABLE 170–19 ■ MAJOR MANIFESTATIONS OF NEONATAL NONPOLIO ENTEROVIRAL AND PARECHOVIRAL* INFECTIONS

Specific Involvement	Common	Rare	References
Inapparent Infection	Echo 22	Cox A9, B1, B2, B4, B5 Echo 3, 5, 9, 11, 14, 20, 30, 31	73, 139, 149, 228, 239, 292, 410, 605, 621
Mild, nonspecific, febrile illness	Cox B5 Echo 5, 11, 33	Cox B1–B4, A9, A16 Echo 4, 7, 9, 17	25, 49, 71, 85, 139, 149, 200, 229, 292, 345, 412, 445, 527, 594, 615 771, 828
Sepsis-like illness	Cox B2–B5 Echo 5, 11, 16	Cox B1, A9 Echo 2–4, 6, 9, 14,19, 21, 22, 23	5, 26, 76, 83, 139, 140, 155, 176, 182, 200, 241, 306, 334, 433, 444, 495, 527, 545, 581, 588, 606, 615, 666, 701, 741, 745, 788, 799, 885
Respiratory illness (general)	Echo 11, 22	Cox B1, B4, B5, A9 Echo 9, 17	149, 358, 390, 410
Herpangina		Cox A5	134
Coryza		Cox A9 Echo 11, 17, 19, 22	73, 184, 358, 621, 752
Pharyngitis		Cox B4 Echo 11, 17, 18	71, 358, 569, 741, 771
Laryngotracheitis or bronchitis		Cox B1, B4 Echo 11	224, 358, 597
Pneumonia		Cox B4, A9 Echo 9, 11, 17, 22, 31	73, 139, 155, 200, 241, 358, 410, 582, 818, 876
Cloud baby		Echo 20	228
Gastrointestinal			
Vomiting or diarrhea	Echo 5, 17, 18	Cox B1, B2, B5 Echo 4, 6, 8, 9, 11, 16, 19, 21, 22	71, 139, 176, 227, 228, 241, 292, 343, 358, 410, 527, 582, 690, 741, 799
Hepatitis	Echo 11, 19	Cox A9, B1, B4 Echo 6, 9, 14, 21	139, 140, 380, 433, 463, 588, 606, 885
Pancreatitis		Cox B3, B4, B5	479, 876
Necrotizing enterocolitis		Cox B2, B3	495
Cardiovascular			
Myocarditis and pericarditis	Cox B1–B4	Cox B5, A9 Echo 11, 19	48, 97, 139, 227, 240, 286, 334, 380, 394, 404, 410, 418, 444, 462, 464, 465, 472, 594, 597, 804, 828, 885
Skin	Cox B5 Echo 5, 17, 22	Cox B1 Echo 4, 9, 11, 16, 18	73, 85, 139, 143, 146, 182, 292, 335, 444, 527, 569, 582, 640, 741
Neurologic			
Aseptic meningitis	Cox B2–B5 Echo 3, 9, 11, 17	Cox A9, A14, B1 Echo 1, 14, 21, 30 Entero 71	73, 85, 139, 140, 146, 182, 212, 228, 241, 334, 342, 347, 348, 429, 444, 545, 581, 582, 640, 751, 752, 757, 788, 799
Encephalitis	Cox B1–B4	Cox B5 Echo 9, 23	151, 238, 239, 348, 745, 757, 885
Paralysis		Cox B2	429
Sudden infant death		Cox B3, A4, A5, A8 Echo 22	42, 306, 599

*Parechoviruses 1 and 2 are listed in this table as echoviruses 22 and 23, respectively.

similar diarrheal illness. Echovirus 18 was recovered from all ill infants.

In 22 infants with epidemic respiratory disease caused by echovirus 11, all had vomiting as a manifestation of the illness.[358] Linnemann and colleagues[527] noted vomiting in 36 percent and diarrhea in 7 percent of neonates with echoviral infection. In another study, Lake and associates[495] found diarrhea in 81 percent and vomiting in 33 percent of neonates with nonpolio enteroviral infections.

Hepatitis is an important neonatal nonpolio enteroviral illness. Morens[598] noted that 2 percent of neonates with clinically severe enteroviral disease had hepatitis. Lake and colleagues[495] observed that hepatomegaly was present in 37 percent of neonates with enteroviral infection, and hepatosplenomegaly was observed by Hercík and associates[358] in 12 of 22 newborns with echovirus 11 respiratory illness.

Severe hepatitis, frequently with hepatic necrosis, has been noted with echoviruses 6, 9, 11, 14, 19, and 21.* Echovirus 11 most often has been associated with severe and usually fatal hepatitis; findings include disseminated intravascular coagulation and thrombocytopenia, as well as apnea, lethargy, poor feeding, and jaundice.

Philip and Larson[666] reported three catastrophic neonatal echovirus 19 infections that resulted in hepatic necrosis and massive terminal hemorrhage. One infant, infected in utero, was symptomatic at birth. The Apgar score was 3, and multiple petechiae were observed. Generalized ecchymoses and apneic episodes occurred, and the infant died at 3.5 hours of age. Thrombocytopenia was noted, and echovirus 19 was isolated from the brain, liver, spleen, and lymph nodes. The other two infants who died of echovirus 19 infection were twins. They were normal during the first 3 days of life but then became mildly cyanotic and lethargic. Shortly thereafter, apneic episodes occurred, and jaundice and petechiae developed. Both twins became oliguric, and they died on the eighth and ninth days of life with severe, terminal gastrointestinal bleeding. Both twins were thrombocytopenic, and virus was recovered from systemic sites in both.

Pancreatitis was noted in three of four newborns with coxsackievirus B5 meningitis[479] and in a coxsackievirus B4 infection at autopsy.[876] In other fatal coxsackievirus B infections, pancreatic involvement has been detected, but clinical manifestations rarely have been observed.

Lake and associates[495] reported three infants with necrotizing enterocolitis. Coxsackievirus B3 was recovered from two of these infants and coxsackievirus B2 from the third.

CARDIOVASCULAR MANIFESTATIONS. In contrast to enteroviral cardiac disease in children and adults, in which pericarditis is a common finding, neonatal disease usually always involves the heart muscle. Most cases of neonatal myocarditis are caused by coxsackievirus B infection, and nursery outbreaks have occurred on several occasions. In 1961, Kibrick[462] reviewed the clinical findings in 45 cases of neonatal myocarditis; his findings are summarized in Table 170–20. Of interest is that many of the early experiences, particularly in South Africa, involved catastrophic nursery epidemics. Since the observation in 1972 of five newborns with echovirus 11 infection and myocarditis, no other nursery epidemics have been reported.[214]

The illness caused by coxsackieviruses B most commonly was abrupt in onset, with symptoms of listlessness, anorexia, and fever. A biphasic pattern was noted in approximately a third of the patients. Progression was rapid, and signs of circulatory failure appeared in a 2-day period.

*See references 71, 83, 139, 140, 334, 390, 433, 588, 606, 666.

TABLE 170–20 ■ SIGNS AND SYMPTOMS IN NEONATAL COXSACKIEVIRUS B MYOCARDITIS

Category	Frequency (%)
Feeding difficulty	84
Listlessness	81
Cardiac signs	81
Respiratory distress	75
Cyanosis	72
Fever	70
Pharyngitis	64
Hepatosplenomegaly	53
Biphasic course	35
Central nervous system signs	27
Hemorrhage	13
Jaundice	13
Diarrhea	8

Modified from Kibrick, S.: Viral infections of the fetus and newborn. Perspect. Virol. *2*:140–159, 1961.

If death did not occur, recovery occasionally was rapid but usually took place gradually over an extended period. Most patients had cardiac findings such as tachycardia, cardiomegaly, electrocardiographic changes, and transitory systolic murmurs. Many patients showed signs of respiratory distress and cyanosis. Approximately a third of the infants had signs suggesting neurologic involvement. Of the 45 cases analyzed by Kibrick,[462] only 12 survived.

In an echovirus 11 nursery outbreak reported by Drew,[214] 5 of 10 babies had tachycardia out of proportion to their fever. Three of these babies had electrocardiograms; supraventricular tachycardia was noted in all, and ST-segment depression was observed in two of the records. Supraventricular tachycardia also has occurred with coxsackievirus B infection.[410] Echovirus 19 has been associated with myocarditis, and coxsackievirus A9 was noted in a child with pericarditis.[184, 804]

In recent years, neonatal myocarditis caused by enteroviruses has been seen less commonly than it was in the 1950s and early 1960s. In his review, Morens[598] noted only 2 instances among 248 severe neonatal enteroviral illnesses.

EXANTHEM. Exanthem as a manifestation of neonatal enteroviral infection has been reported with coxsackieviruses B1 and B5 and echoviruses 4, 5, 9, 11, 16, 17, and 18 and parechovirus 1. In most instances, rash is just a minor manifestation of severe neonatal disease. In 27 infants studied by Lake and colleagues,[495] 41 percent had exanthem. Cutaneous manifestations generally commence between the third and fifth days of illness. The rash usually is macular or maculopapular. Petechial lesions are noted occasionally. Surprisingly, vesicular lesions have not been described, nor has any rash illness in neonates been associated with coxsackievirus A16. Hall and associates[335] reported two neonates with echovirus 16 infections in which the illnesses were roseola-like. The patients had fever for 2 and 3 days, defervescence, and then the appearance of a maculopapular rash.

NEUROLOGIC MANIFESTATIONS. As noted in Table 170–19, neurologic illness has been associated with coxsackieviruses B1, B2, B3, B4, and B5 and many echoviruses as well. In neonates, differentiation of meningitis from meningoencephalitis is usually difficult. Meningoencephalitis occurs commonly in infants with sepsis-like illness, and postmortem studies reveal many infants with disseminated viral disease (heart, liver, adrenal glands) in addition to CNS involvement. In Moren's review,[598] 50 percent of the enteroviral infection patients analyzed had encephalitis or meningitis.

The initial clinical findings in neonatal meningitis or meningoencephalitis are similar to those in nonspecific febrile illness or sepsis-like illness. Most often, the child is normal and then becomes febrile, anorectic, and lethargic. Jaundice frequently is noted in newborns, and vomiting occurs in neonates of all ages. Less common findings include apnea, tremulousness, and general increased tonicity. Seizures occur occasionally.

Examination of CSF reveals considerable variation in protein, glucose, and cellular values. In seven newborns with meningitis caused by coxsackievirus B5 studied by Swender and colleagues,[799] the mean CSF protein value was 244 mg/dL and the highest value was 480 mg/dL. The mean CSF glucose value was 57 mg/dL, and one of the seven infants had pronounced hypoglycorrhachia (a value of 12 mg/dL). The mean CSF leukocyte count in the seven babies was 1069 cells/mm,^{3} with 67 percent polymorphonuclear cells. The highest cell count was 4526 cells/mm^3 with 85 percent polymorphonuclear cells. In another study involving 28 children younger than 2 months in which coxsackievirus B5 was the implicated pathogen, 36 percent of the infants had CSF leukocyte counts of 500 cells/mm^3 or greater.[545] In this same study, only 13 percent of the infants had CSF protein values of 120 mg/dL or greater; 12 percent of the infants had glucose values less than 40 mg/dL.

In summary, one must stress that the CSF findings in neonatal nonpolio enteroviral infections frequently are similar to those in bacterial disease. In particular, the most consistent finding in bacterial disease, hypoglycorrhachia, is noted in approximately 10 percent of newborns with enteroviral meningitis.[151, 229, 495, 545, 799]

Johnson and associates[429] reported a 1-month-old boy with right-sided facial paralysis and loss of abdominal reflexes. The facial paralysis persisted through convalescence; the reflexes returned to normal within 2 weeks. The boy was infected with coxsackievirus B2.

Clinical Manifestations—Polioviruses[15, 81, 138, 140, 165, 382]

When a susceptible person has had effective contact with a poliovirus, one of several responses may occur in the following order of frequency: (1) inapparent infection, (2) minor illness (abortive poliomyelitis), (3) nonparalytic poliomyelitis (aseptic meningitis), and (4) paralytic poliomyelitis.

Paralytic poliomyelitis is the most dramatic expression of the infection and the only one clinically recognizable as caused by a poliovirus; it accounts for not more than 1 to 2 percent of infections during epidemics and considerably less under endemic conditions (see Fig. 170–5). The aseptic meningitis syndrome is similarly infrequent; nonspecific "minor illness" is estimated to occur in 4 to 8 percent, and 90 to 95 percent of those infected have inapparent infections. Factors that determine the type of clinical response are poorly understood, but the degree of virulence of the virus and certain host characteristics are important.

Age has a significant effect on patterns of infection; older patients are more likely to have severe paralytic disease and a higher mortality rate. Pregnancy increases the risk, probably primarily because of hormonal factors but also because of the fact that pregnant women may be exposed more to young children, who are the main sources of contagion. Tonsillectomy in the presence of inapparent infection can precipitate bulbar poliomyelitis; evidence also suggests that tonsillectomy at any time in the past results in enhanced susceptibility to the bulbar form of the disease. Recent diphtheria-tetanus-pertussis vaccination increases the likelihood of development of paralysis; the site of injection and the site of paralysis appear to be correlated. Physical exertion and trauma around the time of onset also increase the risk for severe paralysis, especially in adults.

MINOR ILLNESS (ABORTIVE POLIOMYELITIS)

The minor illness is mild and nonspecific, with low-grade fever, malaise, anorexia, and sore throat. Physical examination reveals no significant abnormalities, CSF is normal, and recovery occurs within 24 to 72 hours. The illness often is so mild that it goes unrecognized, and patients rarely are seen by a physician.

NONPARALYTIC POLIOMYELITIS (ASEPTIC MENINGITIS)

The onset of nonparalytic poliomyelitis is associated with vague malaise followed by fever, headache, aching of the muscles, and sometimes hyperesthesia and paresthesia. Anorexia, nausea, vomiting, constipation, or diarrhea also may be present. The temperature rises to 37.8° to 39.5° C (101° to 103° F); stiffness of the neck, back, and hamstrings soon appears.

Approximately two thirds of affected children have a short symptom-free interlude between the first phase (minor illness) and the second phase (CNS or major illness). This two-phase course occurs less commonly in adults, in whom the evolution of symptoms is more insidious. Nuchal and spinal rigidity is necessary for the diagnosis of nonparalytic poliomyelitis during the second phase.

Physical examination reveals nuchal-spinal signs and changes in superficial and deep reflexes. With cooperative patients, the nuchal-spinal signs are sought first by active tests. The child is asked to sit up unassisted. If doing so causes undue effort, if the knees flex upward, and if the patient writhes a bit from side to side while sitting up and uses the hands on the bed for the tripod supporting position, unmistakable spinal rigidity is present. Still sitting, the patient is asked to flex chin to chest and is observed for nuchal rigidity. Alternatively, from the supine position with the knees held down gently, the patient is asked to sit up and kiss the knees. If the knees draw up sharply or if the maneuver cannot be completed adequately, the patient has stiffness of the spine caused by muscle spasm. If the diagnosis still is uncertain, attempts should be made to elicit the Kernig and Brudzinski signs. Gentle forward flexion of the occiput and neck elicits nuchal rigidity, which may precede spinal rigidity. Head drop may be demonstrated by placing the hands under the patient's shoulders and raising the trunk. Normally, the head follows the plane of the trunk, but in poliomyelitis, it often falls backward limply. The frequency of the head-drop sign, even in nonparalytic poliomyelitis, with no subsequent residuals indicates that it is not caused by true paresis of the neck flexors. In struggling infants, distinguishing voluntary resistance from clinically important involuntary nuchal rigidity may be difficult. One may place the infant's shoulders flush with the edge of the table, support the weight of the occiput in the hand, and then flex the head anteriorly. Nuchal rigidity that persists during this maneuver may be interpreted as involuntary. When not closed, the anterior fontanel also may be tense or bulging.

In the early stages, the reflexes are normally active and remain so unless paralysis supervenes. Changes in reflexes, either increased or depressed, may precede weakness by

12 to 24 hours; hence, detecting such changes is important, especially in nonparalytic patients managed at home. The superficial reflexes (i.e., cremasteric and abdominal and the reflexes of the spinal and gluteal muscles) are usually the first to be diminished. The spinal and gluteal reflexes are elicited by tapping segmentally downward on each side of the spine and buttocks. These reflexes may disappear before the abdominal and cremasteric ones do. Changes in the deep tendon reflexes, whether exaggerated or depressed, generally occur 8 to 24 hours after depression of the superficial reflexes and indicate impending paresis of the extremities.

Laboratory findings consist of a normal or slightly elevated white blood cell count and the characteristic CSF changes of aseptic meningitis: approximately 20 to 300 cells, predominantly lymphocytes, a normal glucose level, and normal or slightly elevated protein. If a spinal tap is performed in the first few hours after onset, a predominance of polymorphonuclear leukocytes may be seen, but it shifts in 6 to 12 hours to more than 90 percent lymphocytes. If no further progression of clinical signs occurs, the disease remains nonparalytic, the temperature falls to normal, and signs of meningeal irritation gradually disappear. Recovery ensues in 3 to 10 days, depending on the severity of the illness.

PARALYTIC POLIOMYELITIS

The manifestations of paralytic poliomyelitis are those enumerated earlier for nonparalytic poliomyelitis plus weakness in one or more muscle groups, either skeletal or cranial. Patients in whom paralysis is destined to develop often wear an anxious expression; they are extremely alert, restless, and flushed and appear acutely ill. The fever is higher than that in abortive disease, and the patient may have intense muscle pain. Shortly before actual muscle weakness is detected, the superficial and deep reflexes often diminish or disappear on the affected side. Frequently, a symptom-free interlude of several days occurs between the initial illness phase and the recurrence of symptoms that culminate in paralysis.

The onset of paralysis may be extraordinarily sudden and progress in a few hours to complete loss of motion in one or more extremities. Asymmetric involvement is typical in milder cases. More gradual spread of weakness also occurs and may continue over a period of 3 to 5 days. Bladder paralysis of 1 to 3 days' duration develops in approximately 20 percent of patients, and bowel atony is noted commonly, occasionally to the point of paralytic ileus. In general, when the fever subsides, no further paralysis is likely to occur. The lower limbs are affected more commonly than are the upper, but in severe cases, quadriplegia and loss of function of the intercostal, abdominal, and trunk muscles with resultant respiratory difficulty may ensue. The superficial and deep reflexes in the affected limbs are lost; twitching of the muscles and diffuse fasciculations may be seen transiently. Sensory abnormalities are rare occurrences.

Flaccid paralysis is the most obvious clinical expression of the neuronal changes. The ensuing muscular atrophy is caused by denervation plus the atrophy of disuse. The pain, spasticity, nuchal and spinal rigidity, and hypertonia early in the illness probably are caused by lesions in the brain stem, spinal ganglia, and posterior columns. Respiratory and cardiac arrhythmias, blood pressure and vasomotor changes, and the like reflect damage to vital centers in the medulla.

On physical examination, the distribution of paralysis characteristically is spotty. To detect mild muscular weakness, one often must apply gentle resistance in opposition to the muscle group being tested. The spinal form has weakness of some of the muscles of the neck, abdomen, trunk, diaphragm, thorax, or extremities. The bulbar form is characterized by weakness in the motor distribution of one or more cranial nerves, with or without dysfunction of the vital centers of respiration and circulation. Patients with bulbar disease often are extremely agitated, even delirious, or they may become stuporous. The 10th cranial nerve nuclei are involved most commonly and result in paralysis of the pharynx, soft palate, and vocal cords. Facial paralysis occurs less commonly; it usually is asymmetric and involves only selected muscle groups. Ocular palsies are unusual findings.

Components of both the bulbar and spinal forms occur together in bulbospinal poliomyelitis. In the encephalitic form of the disease, irritability, disorientation, drowsiness, and coarse tremors not explained by inadequate ventilation are noted. Even during poliomyelitis epidemics, this form can be recognized only if some peripheral or cranial nerve paralysis coexists or ensues. Hypoxia and hypercapnia caused by inadequate ventilation from respiratory insufficiency may produce disorientation without true encephalitis.

Numerous components acting together may result in insufficiency in ventilation (Table 170–21). The most serious consequences are hypoxia and hypercapnia, which may produce profound effects on many other systems. Respiratory insufficiency should be detected early to diminish its widespread effects, and because the situation may shift rapidly, continued clinical evaluation is essential. Despite weakness of the respiratory muscles, the patient may respond with so much respiratory effort that normal alveolar ventilation is maintained. In fact, the increased effort (associated with anxiety and fear) actually may produce overventilation at the outset and result in respiratory alkalosis. Such effort is fatiguing and soon leads to respiratory failure.

For clarity, certain terms characterizing patterns of disease need definition: (1) *Pure spinal poliomyelitis with respiratory insufficiency* refers to tightness, weakness, or paralysis of the respiratory muscles (chiefly the diaphragm and intercostals) without discernible clinical involvement of the cranial nerves or vital centers. The cervical and thoracic spinal cord segments chiefly are involved. (2) *Pure bulbar poliomyelitis* refers to paralysis of the motor cranial nerve

TABLE 170–21 ■ COMMON SOURCES OF HYPOXIA AND HYPERCAPNIA IN POLIOMYELITIS

1. Cranial nerves IX to XII involved with
   a. Pharyngeal paralysis and pooling of secretions
   b. Laryngeal involvement—either spasm of laryngeal muscles of paralysis of vocal cords
   c. Lingual paralysis
   d. Tracheal accumulation of secretions from inability to cough
   e. Aspiration of vomitus
2. Vital center involvement with
   a. Inefficient, irregular respiration
   b. Cardiovascular disturbance
   c. Hyperpyrexia causing increased oxygen consumption
3. Cervical and spinal cord involvement causing paresis of the primary and accessory muscles of respiration
4. Pulmonary complications, viz., pneumonia, atelectasis, and edema
5. Contributory factors
   a. Panic
   b. Gastric dilatation
   c. Sedation
   d. Inadequate equipment, viz., small-bore tracheostomy tubes, unsuitable respirator settings, and the like

From Cherry, J. D.: Enteroviruses. *In* Behrmon, R. E., and Vaughan, V. C. (eds.): Nelson Textbook of Pediatrics. 12th ed. Philadelphia, W. B. Saunders, 1983, pp. 791–804.

nuclei with or without involvement of the vital centers that control respiration, circulation, and body temperature. Involvement of the 9th, 10th, and 12th cranial nerves is most important because it results in paralysis of the pharynx, tongue, and larynx with consequent airway obstruction. (3) *Bulbospinal poliomyelitis with respiratory insufficiency* refers to involvement of the respiratory muscles with coexisting bulbar paralysis.

The clinical findings resulting from involvement of the respiratory muscles are (1) an anxious expression; (2) inability to speak without frequent pauses, which results in short, jerky, "breathless" sentences and can be demonstrated by asking the child to count numbers serially; (3) increased respiratory rate; (4) movement of the alae nasi and the accessory muscles of respiration; (5) inability to cough or sniff with full depth; (6) paradoxical abdominal movements caused by diaphragmatic immobility from spasm or weakness of one or both leaves; and (7) relative immobility of the intercostal spaces, which may be segmental, unilateral, or bilateral. When the arms are weak and especially when deltoid paralysis occurs, one should beware of impending respiratory paralysis because the phrenic nerve nuclei are in adjacent areas of the spinal cord. Observing the patient's capacity for thoracic breathing while the abdominal muscles are splinted manually can be performed to assess minor degrees of paresis. Light manual splinting of the thoracic cage helps in evaluating the effectiveness of diaphragmatic movement.

The clinical findings of bulbar poliomyelitis with respiratory difficulty (other than paralysis of the extraocular, facial, and masticatory muscles) include (1) a nasal twang to the voice or cry as a result of palatal and pharyngeal weakness (hard consonant words such as "cookie" or "candy" bring out this condition best); (2) an inability to swallow smoothly, which results in an accumulation of saliva in the pharynx and indicates partial immobility (holding the larynx lightly and asking the patient to swallow confirms the immobility); (3) accumulated pharyngeal secretions, which may cause irregular respiration because each inspiration must be "planned" and cannot be "subconscious" in view of the risk of aspirating; the respirations thus may appear interrupted and abnormal even to the point of falsely simulating intercostal or diaphragmatic weakness; (4) the impossibility of effective coughing, with resultant constant fatiguing efforts to clear the throat; (5) nasal regurgitation of saliva and fluids caused by palatal paralysis, with an inability to separate the oropharynx from the nasopharynx during swallowing; (6) deviation of the palate, uvula, or tongue; (7) involvement of vital centers, as manifested by an irregularity in the rate, depth, and rhythm of respiration; by cardiovascular alterations that include changes in blood pressure (especially increased), alternate flushing and mottling of the skin, and cardiac arrhythmias; and by rapid changes in body temperature; (8) paralysis of one or both vocal cords, which causes hoarseness, aphonia, and ultimately asphyxia unless recognized by laryngoscopy and managed by immediate tracheostomy; and (9) the "rope sign," an acute angulation between the chin and larynx caused by weakness of the hyoid muscles (the hyoid bone is pulled posteriorly, which narrows the hypopharyngeal inlet).

Myocardial failure sometimes develops secondary to pulmonary complications or as a result of acute myocarditis.

The initial manifestation of poliovirus infection on occasion can resemble that of Guillain-Barré syndrome.[893]

Congenital Infections

ABORTION. Poliomyelitis is associated with an increased incidence of abortion. Horn[374] noted 43 abortions in 325 pregnancies complicated by maternal poliomyelitis. Abortion was related directly to the severity of the maternal illness, including the degree of fever during the acute phase of illness. However, abortion also has occurred in association with mild nonparalytic poliomyelitis. Siegel and Greenberg[772] noted that fetal death occurred in 14 of 30 instances (46.7%) of maternal poliomyelitis during the first trimester. Kaye and associates[450] reviewed the literature in 1953 and recorded 19 abortions in 101 cases of poliomyelitis in pregnancy. In a small study in Evanston Hospital, the abortion rate in maternal poliomyelitis was little different from the expected rate.[86]

CONGENITAL MALFORMATIONS. Although isolated instances of congenital malformation and maternal poliomyelitis have been noted, little statistical evidence supports the suggestion that polioviruses are teratogens. In their review of the literature, Kaye and colleagues[450] noted 6 anomalies in 101 infants born to mothers with poliomyelitis during pregnancy. In the reviews of Horn,[374] Bates,[52] and Siegel and Greenberg,[772] no evidence of maternal polioviral infection–induced anomalies was found. Similarly, no evidence suggests that infection with poliovirus vaccine during pregnancy causes congenital malformations.[343]

PREMATURITY AND STILLBIRTH. In Horn's study[374] of 325 pregnancies, 9 infants died in utero. In each instance, the mother was critically ill with poliomyelitis. Horn[374] also noted that 45 infants weighed less than 6 lb, and 17 of them had a birth weight less than 5 lb. These low-birth-weight infants were born predominantly to mothers who had poliomyelitis early in pregnancy. In New York City, Siegel and Greenberg[772] also noted an increase in prematurity after maternal poliomyelitis infection. It was related specifically to maternal paralytic poliomyelitis.

Neonatal Infections

GENERAL. In the excellent review by Bates[52] in 1955, 58 cases of poliomyelitis in infants younger than 1 month were described. Although complete data were not available on many of the cases, 51 had paralysis, died of their disease, or both. Of the total number of infants on whom they had clinical data, only one had nonparalytic disease. More than half the cases were secondary to maternal disease. Because others have noted congenital infection without symptomatic maternal infection, infection in the mother probably was the source for an even greater percentage of the neonatal illnesses. The incubation period of neonatal poliomyelitis has not been established, and, therefore, determining how many of the babies were infected in utero is difficult. Probably, most illnesses that occurred within the first 5 days of life were congenital.

Most of the neonates had symptoms of fever, anorexia or dysphagia, and listlessness. Almost half the infants noted in this review died, and of those surviving, 48 percent had residual paralysis.

INFECTION ACQUIRED IN UTERO. Elliott and associates[231] described an infant girl in whom "complete flaccidity" was noted at birth. This child's mother had had mild paralytic poliomyelitis, with the onset of minor illness occurring 19 days before the infant's birth. Fetal movements had ceased 6 days before delivery, thus suggesting that paralysis had occurred at this time. On examination, the baby was severely atonic; when supported under the back, she was passively opisthotonic. Respiratory efforts were abortive and confined to the accessory muscles; laryngoscopy revealed complete flaccidity in the larynx.

Johnson and Stimson[425] reported a case in which the mother's probable abortive infection occurred 6 weeks before the birth of the baby. The baby initially was thought to be normal but apparently underwent no medical examination until the fourth day of life. At this time, the physician noted right hemiplegia. On the following day, a more complete examination revealed lateral bulging of the right side of the abdomen accompanied by crying and maintenance of the lower extremities in a frog leg position. Adduction and flexion at the hips were weak, and the knee and ankle jerks were absent. Laboratory studies were unremarkable except for examination of CSF. It revealed 20 lymphocytes and a protein level of 169 mg/dL. During a 6-month period, this child's paralysis gradually improved and resulted in only residual weakness of the left lower extremity.

Paresis of the left arm was noted shortly after birth in another child with apparent transplacentally acquired poliomyelitis.[534] At 2 days of age, the baby was quadriplegic, but patellar reflexes were present and the child had no respiratory or swallowing difficulties. This child had pneumonia at 3 weeks of age, but otherwise, general neurologic improvement occurred. Examination at 8 weeks of age revealed bilateral atrophy of the shoulder girdle muscles. The CSF in this case had 63 leukocytes/mm^3, 29 percent of them polymorphonuclear cells, and a protein concentration of 128 mg/dL.

All three of the infants just discussed apparently were infected in utero several days before birth. Their symptoms were exclusively neurologic; fever, irritability, and vomiting did not occur.

POSTNATALLY ACQUIRED INFECTION. In contrast to infections acquired in utero, those acquired postnatally are more typical of classic poliomyelitis. Shelokov and Weinstein[769] described a child who was asymptomatic at birth. The onset of minor symptoms in the mother occurred 3 weeks before and the onset of major symptoms occurred 1 day before delivery. On the sixth day of life, the infant suddenly became ill with watery diarrhea. He looked grayish and pale. On the following day, he was irritable, lethargic, and limp and had a temperature of 38° C. Mild opisthotonos and weakness of both lower extremities developed. He was responsive to sound, light, and touch. The CSF had an elevated protein level and an increased number of leukocytes. His condition worsened during a total period of 3 days, and then gradual improvement began. At 1 year of age, he had severe residual paralysis of the right leg and moderate weakness in the left leg.

Baskin and associates[50] described two infants with neonatal poliomyelitis. The first child, whose mother had severe poliomyelitis at the time of delivery, was well for 3 days and then had a temperature of 38.3° C. On the fifth day of life, the boy became listless and cyanotic. Examination of CSF revealed a protein level of 300 mg/dL and 108 leukocytes/mm^3. His condition worsened, and extreme flaccidity, irregular respiration, and progressive cyanosis developed; he died on the seventh day of life. The second infant was a boy who was well until he was 8 days old but then became listless with a temperature of 38.3° C. During the next 5 days, flaccid quadriplegia developed, as did irregular, rapid, and shallow respirations and an inability to swallow. The child died on the 14th day of life. Acute poliomyelitis had developed in his mother 6 days before the onset of his symptoms.

Abramson and colleagues[2] reported four children with neonatal poliomyelitis, two of whom died. In three of the children, the illnesses were typical of acute poliomyelitis in older children. The other child died at 13 days of age with generalized paralysis. The onset of his illness was difficult to define, and he was never febrile.

Bates[52] described infants with acute poliomyelitis and clinical illnesses similar to those that occur in older persons.

Diagnosis and Differential Diagnosis

CLINICAL DIAGNOSIS

Clinical differentiation of enteroviral disease frequently is thought to be impossible. Although treatable bacterial illnesses always should be considered and treated first, also true is that when all the circumstances of a particular illness are considered, enteroviral diseases can be suspected on clinical grounds. The most important factors in clinical diagnosis are the season of the year, geographic location, exposure, incubation period, and clinical symptoms.

In temperate climates, enteroviral prevalence is distinctly seasonal, so disease usually is seen in the summer and fall. Enteroviral disease is less likely to occur in the winter. In the tropics, enteroviruses are prevalent throughout the year, and the season, therefore, is not diagnostically helpful.

As with all infectious illnesses, knowledge of exposure and incubation time is important. A careful history of maternal illness is critical in neonatal disease. For example, nonspecific, mild febrile illness in a mother that occurs in the summer and fall should warn of the possibility of severe neonatal illness. Specific findings (i.e., aseptic meningitis, pleurodynia, herpangina, pericarditis, myocarditis) should alert the clinician to enteroviral illnesses. The short incubation period of enteroviral infections should be considered.

LABORATORY DIAGNOSIS

Virus Isolation and Detection Techniques

Most viral diagnostic laboratories have facilities for the recovery of most enteroviruses that cause illness. A three-tissue culture system that includes primary monkey kidney, a diploid, human embryonic lung fibroblast cell strain, and the RD cell line allow the isolation of virtually all coxsackieviruses B and echoviruses and some coxsackieviruses A (e.g., coxsackieviruses A9 and A16). In a study in which Buffalo green monkey kidney cells and subpassage of primary human embryonic kidney cells were used in addition to primary monkey kidney and human diploid fibroblast (MRC-5) cells, the enterovirus recovery rate was increased 11 percent.[157] For a complete diagnostic isolation spectrum, suckling mouse inoculation also should be performed.

Proper selection and handling of specimens are most important in the isolation of viruses. Enteroviral infections tend to be generalized, so collection of material from multiple sites is important; specimens should be collected from any or all of the following: nasopharynx, throat, stool, blood, urine, CSF, and any other body fluids that are available. Swabs from the nose, throat, and rectum should be placed in a carrying medium containing a small amount of protein. Hanks balanced salt solution with 2 percent agamma calf serum and antibiotics is satisfactory. Fluid specimens should be collected in sterile vials; specimens of postmortem material are collected best in vials that contain carrying medium. In general, specimens should be refrigerated immediately after collection and during transportation to the laboratory. Of importance is that the specimens not be exposed to sunlight during transportation. If an extended period will elapse before a specimen is processed in the laboratory, shipping and storing it frozen are advisable.

Contrary to popular belief, tissue culture evidence of enteroviral growth takes only a few days in many cases and less than a week in most.[316] The use of spin amplification, the shell vial technique, and monoclonal antibodies has been shown to reduce the time of detection in enteroviral cultures significantly.[478, 822] After isolation of an enterovirus, type identification is performed conventionally by neutralization, and this process, unfortunately, frequently takes a long time.

Nucleic acid techniques with cDNA and RNA probes have been shown to be useful for direct identification of enteroviruses.[107, 202, 397, 664, 717, 718, 720] Of most importance today, however, has been the development of numerous PCR techniques. Since 1990, innumerable reports have described enteroviral PCR methods and their use in identifying enterovirus RNA in clinical specimens.* PCR has proved most useful for the direct identification of enteroviruses in the CSF of patients with meningitis.[723, 747, 805, 813, 891] When compared with culture of CSF specimens, PCR is more rapid and sensitive, and the specificity is equal.

PCR also has proved useful in the identification of enteroviruses in blood, urine, and throat specimens.[6, 17, 100, 633, 767] Particularly impressive are the findings of Byington and associates.[100] Using PCR on specimens of blood and CSF, they found that more than 25 percent of infants admitted to the hospital for suspected sepsis in 1997 had nonpolio enterovirus infections. Based on this study and the work of Adréoletti and coworkers,[17] I believe that the general workup for febrile children hospitalized for possible sepsis should include PCR for enteroviruses in both blood and CSF, if available. A shortcoming of PCR is that enterovirus RNA is identified but a specific enteroviral type is not. Because of this shortcoming, I recommend that conventional culture be performed in addition to PCR.

Enteroviral RNA also has been identified in numerous tissue specimens from patients with chronic medical conditions such as idiopathic dilated cardiomyopathy. However, as discussed earlier ("Cardiovascular Manifestations"), the possibility of a lack of specificity (false-positive results) is a concern. Polioviruses can be separated from other enteroviruses, and poliovirus vaccine strains can be identified rapidly by PCR.[1, 152, 225, 890]

Serology

Except in special circumstances, the use of serologic techniques for the primary diagnosis of suspected enteroviral infection is impractical. Standard serologic study depends on the demonstration of a rise in antibody titer to a specific virus as an indication of infection with that agent. Although ELISA, hemagglutination inhibition, and CF take only a short time to perform, these tests can be carried out only after the collection of a second, convalescent-phase blood specimen. These tests also are impractical in searching for the cause of a specific illness in a child because of the existence of so many antigenically different enteroviruses. As noted previously ("Antigenic Characteristics"), group antigens can be produced that allow serologic diagnosis by IgM EIA and CF, but these tests lack specificity.[740, 810, 811]

In the evaluation of a patient with a suspected enteroviral infection, serum should be collected as soon as possible after the onset of illness and then again 2 to 4 weeks later. This serum should be stored frozen. In most clinical situations, performing serologic tests on the collected serum is not necessary because demonstration of a rise in antibody titer in the serum of an infant from whom a specific virus has been isolated from a body fluid obviously is superfluous. However, collected serum can be useful diagnostically if the prevalence of specific enteroviruses in a community is known. In this situation, looking for antibody titer changes to a selected number of viral types is relatively easy. More rapid diagnosis can be made with a single serum sample if a search for specific IgM enteroviral antibody is made.[126, 156, 280, 298, 299, 310, 771, 901]

Unfortunately, no enterovirus IgM antibody tests are commercially available. Commercial laboratories do offer enteroviral CF antibody panels. However, these tests are expensive, and their results in the clinical setting almost always are meaningless unless acute- and convalescent-phase sera are analyzed.

Histology

Enteroviral infections have no specific histologic findings such as those seen in cytomegalovirus or HSV infection. However, tissues can be examined for specific enteroviral antigens by immunofluorescence and for RNA by PCR.[97, 124, 547]

DIFFERENTIAL DIAGNOSIS

The differential diagnosis of enteroviral infection depends on the clinical manifestations. In general, the most important considerations relate to bacterial diseases such as those commonly associated with pharyngitis, pneumonia, pericarditis, meningitis, and septicemia. Other viruses must be considered with upper respiratory illnesses, gastrointestinal infections, rashes, encephalitis, and neonatal illness.

Paralytic poliomyelitis usually presents no diagnostic problem in the presence of an outbreak, but sporadic cases are another matter, especially in countries such as the United States, where the disease (except for the vaccine-associated form) has disappeared and many pediatricians have never seen a case. Rarely, other enteroviruses have been shown to cause paralytic syndromes that are indistinguishable from poliomyelitis.

Several other diseases must be considered in the differential diagnosis of sporadic cases of paralytic illness. Guillain-Barré syndrome is the most common and difficult differential problem. Fever, headache, and meningeal signs usually occur less commonly in Guillain-Barré syndrome; the paralysis characteristically is symmetric, and sensory changes are common findings. Also in Guillain-Barré syndrome, the CSF contains few cells but a significant elevation in protein concentration. Other illnesses confused with paralytic poliomyelitis include peripheral neuritis (postinjection, toxic, herpes zoster), arboviral infection, rabies, tetanus, botulism, and tick paralysis.

Treatment

SPECIFIC THERAPY

No specific therapy for any enteroviral infection presently is approved for use in the United States. In severe, catastrophic, and generalized neonatal infection, in all probability the baby received no specific antibody for the particular virus from the mother. In this situation, administering immunoglobulin to the infant probably is advisable because high titers of neutralizing antibody to many enteroviruses frequently are present in immunoglobulin.[161, 194] Little

*See references 1, 6, 17, 22, 100, 152, 171, 172, 175, 225, 261, 269, 313, 337, 398, 523, 548, 571, 607, 633, 688, 716, 719, 723, 744, 751, 766, 767, 770, 797, 805, 813, 879, 890, 891.

evidence supports the claim that this therapy is beneficial; however, it can be expected to stop further organ seeding secondary to continued viremia. Intravenous or intraventricular injection of immunoglobulin with IVIG and administration of hyperimmune plasma have been useful on some occasions and not others in the treatment of enteroviral infection in patients with agammaglobulinemia.*

Abzug and associates[4] performed a small but controlled study in which nine enterovirus-infected neonates received IVIG and seven similarly infected infants received supportive care. In this study, no significant difference was found in clinical scores, antibody values, or the magnitude of viremia and viruria in those treated versus control infants. However, five infants received IVIG with a high neutralizing antibody titer (>1:800) to their individual viral isolates, and they experienced more rapid cessation of viremia and viruria. A neonate with disseminated echovirus 11 infection and hepatitis, pneumonitis, meningitis, disseminated intravascular coagulation, decreased renal function, and anemia who survived after receiving a large dose of IVIG and supportive care has been described.[431] Administering IVIG to older children with life-threatening enteroviral infection also seems reasonable. A specific recommended dosage is unknown, but 400 mg/kg/day for 4 days or 2 g/kg in one dose has been used.

Jantausch and associates[416] reported an infant with a disseminated echovirus 11 infection who survived after receiving maternal plasma transfusions. A neonate with fulminant echovirus 11 infection survived after undergoing orthotopic liver transplantation.[167]

The antiviral drug pleconaril offers promise for the treatment of enteroviral infections.[451, 665, 722, 724] This drug is a novel compound that integrates into the capsid of enteroviruses. It prevents the virus from attachment to cellular receptors and the uncoating and subsequent release of viral RNA into the host cell. In a double-blinded, placebo-controlled study of 39 patients with enteroviral meningitis, a statistically significant shortening of disease duration was noted: from 9.5 days in controls to 4.0 days in drug recipients.[722] Pleconaril also has been used on a compassionate-release basis for the treatment of patients with life-threatening infection.[724] The following categories of enteroviral illness have been treated: chronic meningoencephalitis in patients with agammaglobulinemia or hypogammaglobulinemia, neonatal sepsis, myocarditis, poliomyelitis (wild type or vaccine associated), encephalitis, and bone marrow transplant patients. Although these treatments have not had control arms, favorable clinical responses have been observed in 22 of 36 treated patients, including 12 of 18 patients with chronic meningoencephalitis.

In severe illnesses such as neonatal myocarditis or encephalitis, one frequently is tempted to administer corticosteroids. Although some workers have thought that this therapy has been beneficial in treating coxsackieviral myocarditis, I believe that corticosteroids should not be given during acute enteroviral infection. The deleterious effects of these agents in coxsackieviral infection of mice are particularly persuasive factors in this opinion.[82, 469] Immunosuppressive therapy for myocarditis of unknown etiology with prednisone and cyclosporine or azathioprine was evaluated in a controlled trial of 111 adults, but no beneficial effect was observed.[550]

Because the possibility of bacterial sepsis cannot be ruled out in many instances of enteroviral infection, antibiotics frequently should be administered for the most likely potential pathogens. Care in the selection and administration of antibiotics is urged so that drug toxicity is not added to the problems of the patient.

*See references 7, 80, 187, 221, 234, 333, 361, 558, 568, 838, 855.

NONSPECIFIC THERAPY

Mild, Nonspecific Febrile Illness

In patients in whom fever is the only symptom, careful observation is important. Many patients who eventually become severely ill initially have 2 to 3 days of fever without other localized findings. Care should be taken to administer adequate fluids to febrile infants, and excessive elevation of temperature should be prevented if possible.

Myocarditis

Myocarditis has no specific therapy. However, congestive heart failure and arrhythmias occur, and they should be treated by the usual methods. In administering digitalis to patients with enteroviral myocarditis, paying careful attention to the initial dosage is most important because the heart often is extremely sensitive; frequently, only small amounts of digoxin are necessary.

Meningoencephalitis

In patients with meningoencephalitis, convulsions, cerebral edema, and disturbances in fluid and electrolyte balance all occur frequently and respond to treatment. Seizures are treated best with phenobarbital, phenytoin, or lorazepam. Cerebral edema can be treated with urea, mannitol, or large doses of corticosteroids. As noted, the use of corticosteroids in patients with active enteroviral infection seems unwise because the local benefit might be outweighed by the overall deleterious effects. Fluids should be monitored closely, and serum electrolyte levels should be determined frequently because inappropriate antidiuretic hormone secretion is a common occurrence.

Poliomyelitis

The broad principles of management are to allay fear, minimize the ensuing skeletal deformities, anticipate and meet complications in addition to the neuromusculoskeletal ones, and prepare the child and family for the prolonged treatment that may be required and for permanent disability when it seems likely. Patients with the nonparalytic and mildly paralytic forms may be treated at home.

Most patients with paralytic poliomyelitis require hospitalization. A calm atmosphere is desired. Suitable body alignment is necessary to avoid excessive skeletal deformity. A neutral position with the feet at a right angle, knees slightly flexed, and hips and spine straight is achieved by the use of boards, sandbags, and occasionally, light splint shells. Active and passive motion is indicated as soon as the pain has disappeared. The orthopedist and physiatrist should see these patients as early in the illness as possible and assume responsibility before fixed deformities develop.

Management of pure bulbar poliomyelitis consists essentially of maintaining the airway and avoiding all risks of inhalation of saliva, food, or vomitus. Gravity drainage of accumulated secretions is favored by the head-low (foot of the bed elevated 20 to 25 degrees) prone position with the face to one side. Aspirators with rigid or semirigid tips are preferred for direct oral and pharyngeal use, and soft flexible catheters may be used for nasopharyngeal aspiration. Fluid and electrolyte balance is maintained best by intravenous infusion because tube or oral feeding in the first few days may incite vomiting. After the initial few days, sips of sterile water may be given from a spoon, with increments as indicated by the ability to swallow. In addition to close observation for respiratory insufficiency, blood pressure should be recorded at least twice daily. Hypertension is not an uncommon occurrence and occasionally leads to hypertensive encephalopathy. Patients with pure bulbar poliomyelitis may require tracheostomy because of vocal cord paralysis or constriction of the hypopharynx. Most patients with pure bulbar poliomyelitis who recover have little residual impairment; some patients exhibit mild dysphagia and occasional vocal fatigue with slurring of speech.

Impaired ventilation must be recognized early; mounting anxiety, restlessness, and fatigue are early indications for prompt intervention. Tracheostomy is indicated for some patients with pure bulbar poliomyelitis, spinal respiratory muscle paralysis, and bulbospinal paralysis. Unlike other patients on whom tracheostomy is performed, these patients generally are unable to cough, sometimes for many months. Frequent and swift endotracheal aspiration under aseptic conditions is necessary. Mechanical ventilation often is needed. Patients are fully conscious and aware; terrifying procedures are performed best with an outward atmosphere of calm. Explaining the procedure and having the parents on hand may be helpful. A reduction in thoracic compliance occurs early, and higher than expected pressure gradients may be required to achieve adequate ventilation. Weaning a patient from dependency on respiratory assistance is a torturous process, as is total musculoskeletal rehabilitation. Motivation of the patient and the team of personnel is paramount.

Prognosis

The prognosis for nonpolio enteroviral infections is excellent in the great majority of instances. Virtually all morbidity and mortality are related to cardiac and neurologic disease in older children and to these diseases plus general disseminated infection with hepatitis in neonates.

The prognosis for poliomyelitis varies with the degree of muscle involvement. In patients with mild muscle weakness, complete recovery is the rule. If paralysis is present, recovery of muscle function continues for a period of approximately 18 months to 2 years. By 3 months, about 60 percent of the ultimate improvement has been achieved, and by 6 months, 80 percent. The final result depends on the extent and localization of nerve cell damage.

Respiratory failure is responsible for most of the deaths in paralytic poliomyelitis. With the many recent improvements in techniques for handling this complication, the overall mortality rate has been reduced to approximately 4 percent; with the bulbar form and in adults, it still may be as high as 10 percent.

Occasionally, new neuromuscular symptoms develop later in life in patients who have had paralytic poliomyelitis.[108, 195, 196, 427, 689, 814, 874, 875] Although the cause of this late-onset weakness and muscle atrophy (postpolio syndrome) is not understood completely, it is most likely the result of routine attrition of anterior horn cells associated with aging rather than persistent neural infection with polioviruses. However, specific immunopathologic mechanisms possibly play a role in some instances.[295]

Leparc-Goffart and associates[509] presented data suggesting the presence of poliovirus-specific genomic sequences in the CSF of patients with postpolio syndrome. However, Muir and colleagues,[609] who performed similar studies, found no association of chronic neurologic disease with the presence of enteroviral RNA in CSF.

Prevention

NONPOLIO ENTEROVIRAL INFECTIONS

Attenuated and inactivated viral vaccines for enteroviruses other than polioviruses are not available. However, if a virulent enteroviral type were to emerge, a specific vaccine for active immunization probably could be developed.

Passive protection with IVIG may be useful in preventing disease. In practice, however, it would seem worthwhile only for sudden and virulent nursery outbreaks. For example, if several cases of myocarditis occurred in a nursery, administering IVIG to all babies in the nursery would seem reasonable. Pooled human immunoglobulin in most instances can be expected to contain antibodies against coxsackieviruses B1, B2, B3, B4, and B5, as well as several coxsackieviruses A and echoviruses.[194] Therefore, this procedure would offer protection to infants without transplacentally acquired specific antibody who had not become infected yet. Immune serum has been useful in the management of three nursery enteroviral outbreaks.[106, 614, 659]

POLIOVIRAL INFECTIONS

In the United States, the total annual number of paralytic cases fell from an average of 16,000 in the 5 years before the introduction of vaccine to approximately 10 cases per year between 1980 and 1984. The experience in 1979, however, when 26 paralytic cases were reported, served as a reminder that virulent polioviruses still could surface in susceptible persons.[111, 113] Most of the 1979 cases occurred in Pennsylvania and several other states in Amish population groups who had not been immunized. A similar epidemic in Connecticut in 1972 involved a pocket of unimmunized students in a Christian Science school.[109] These outbreaks reflected the fact that poliomyelitis was still occurring in many parts of the world. The possibility of the introduction of virulent strains was ever present, and only through continued and extensive immunization programs could the disease be prevented from reappearing in epidemic form.[377]

The remarkable overall record of the decline in paralytic poliomyelitis in the United States was a result of the development and use of two effective vaccines.[377] Inactivated poliovirus vaccine, the first to be licensed, was used extensively beginning in 1955 and considerably reduced the incidence of the disease, although epidemics continued to occur. Live attenuated oral poliovirus vaccine, licensed in 1961 and 1962, subsequently was recommended as the method of choice in the United States based on its superiority in terms of immunogenic capacity, ability to induce local IgA antibody in the oropharynx and intestinal tract and thus provide greater resistance to reinfection, and ease of administration. Oral poliovirus vaccine gradually supplanted inactivated poliovirus vaccine, and between 1973 and 1978, it was the only vaccine available. Its extraordinary effectiveness at that time, despite reaching only 65 percent of children younger than 5 years with the recommended three doses, suggested that the capacity of the attenuated strains to spread contributes to a much higher immunization rate than was indicated by vaccination statistics. The potential impact of such spread on the immunity of the population was illustrated by the observations of Fox and Hall,[260] who conducted long-term virologic surveillance of middle-income families in Seattle. Polioviruses (vaccine strains) accounted for 50 percent of the 2937 viral isolates from healthy children, their parents, and others in the community. In an analysis of 611 of the poliovirus isolates, researchers found that 75.6 percent were from vaccinees, 10.5 percent were from vaccinee contacts, and 14 percent were from persons without recent known contact with vaccine or a vaccinee. These findings provided a vivid picture of the pervasiveness of the attenuated strains and their continuous circulation in the population. This feature also was supported by the almost invariable recovery of polioviruses from weekly samples of sewage that were collected throughout the year in urban communities.[378]

Despite its striking success, the oral vaccine had some problems. One was greatly reduced seroconversion rates when the vaccine was given to children living in the tropics: as few as 50 percent had satisfactory responses, in contrast to the more than 95 percent response rate in the United States and similar countries.[211, 575] Viral interference from other enteroviruses played some role, and the presence of an inhibitory substance in the oropharynx that prevented significant multiplication of the vaccine strains also has been involved. The seroconversion problem was lessened by using pulse immunization programs.[422, 732] For example, the strategy of national annual vaccination days twice a year, 2 months apart, was successful in developing countries.

Another problem with oral poliovirus vaccine—and the major problem in the United States—was the occurrence of a small number of vaccine-associated cases of poliomyelitis.[377, 575] The immunogenic effectiveness of the vaccine depends on multiplication of the attenuated strains in the intestinal tract. Because no poliovirus strain is completely stable, the progeny of vaccine strains undergo a certain degree of mutation, which rarely resulted in increased virulence and vaccine-associated cases in recipients and their contacts, most often their parents.

Since 1980, no indigenous cases of wild poliovirus disease have occurred in the United States.[119, 791] From 1980 to 1989, 80 cases of vaccine-associated paralytic poliomyelitis and 5 cases of imported disease were reported. The overall rate of vaccine-associated paralytic poliomyelitis was 1 case per 2.5 million doses of distributed vaccine; the risk for recipients was 1 case per 6.8 million doses, and for household contacts it was 1 case per 6.4 million doses. Of the 80 cases, 30 occurred in vaccinees, 32 occurred in household contacts, 4 were community acquired, and 14 occurred in immunologically abnormal persons.

Further analysis revealed that the risk associated with the first dose of vaccine was 1 case per 700,000 doses, but it was only 1 case per 6.9 million for subsequent doses; for vaccine recipients, the calculated risks were 1 case per 1.4 million initial doses and 1 case per 41.5 million subsequent doses. The calculated risks for contact cases were 1 case per 1.9 million initial doses of vaccine and 1 case per 13.8 million subsequent doses.

Immunodeficient children are at particular risk of acquiring vaccine-associated paralytic poliomyelitis.[110, 791] From 1969 through 1976, 11 percent of vaccine-associated cases occurred in immunodeficient patients; 10 of 11 of these patients were children and younger than 1 year. From 1980 to 1989, 18 percent of vaccine-associated paralytic poliomyelitis cases occurred in immunodeficient patients.[791]

Although the risks mentioned earlier were considered acceptable in view of the benefits provided, the question raised repeatedly since the 1970s was whether the United States should return to the use of inactivated poliovirus vaccine, which does not carry a risk of acquiring paralytic disease and has been highly successful in several small European countries in which more than 95 percent of the population had been immunized.[259, 270, 368, 435, 448, 612, 656, 735–738, 791]

The problem was reviewed in detail by a committee of the Institute of Medicine (IOM) of the National Academy of Sciences, which reported its recommendations in April 1977.[635] The conclusion was that given the situation in the United States, in which not more than 65 percent of susceptible children were vaccinated at that time, oral poliovirus vaccine should continue to be the principal vaccine for routine immunization. Inactivated poliovirus vaccine, on the other hand, should be provided for two groups: immunodeficient persons, because of their greatly enhanced risk of acquiring vaccine-associated disease after receiving the oral vaccine, and adults receiving primary immunization, because of their greater susceptibility to paralytic disease. Also suggested was that the inactivated vaccine be available as an alternative for those who prefer it. In addition, a single dose of trivalent oral poliovirus vaccine was suggested for all entrants into the seventh grade of school as a means of added protection for later years when they became parents.

In January 1988, a panel appointed by the IOM again reviewed policy options for vaccination against poliomyelitis in the United States.[401] The IOM panel concluded that no change in policy should be recommended at that time. However, they did recommend that a new enhanced inactivated poliovirus vaccine replace the old vaccine when inactivated vaccine was indicated. They also suggested that when a new enhanced diphtheria-tetanus-pertussis inactivated poliovirus vaccine became available, a regimen of two or more doses of it followed by the oral vaccine be considered.

In 1996, the U.S. polio vaccine immunization program was evaluated extensively by both the Advisory Committee on Immunization Practices (ACIP) and the Committee on Infectious Diseases of the American Academy of Pediatrics (AAP). The ACIP recommended that sequential administration of inactivated poliovirus vaccine followed by oral poliovirus vaccine be the schedule of choice in the United States.[649] The schedule consisted of two doses of the inactivated vaccine at 2 and 4 months of age and two doses of the oral vaccine at 12 to 18 months and 4 to 6 years of age. Both committees indicated that schedules that include all the doses of each vaccine also were acceptable.[340, 649] At the present time, an all-inactivated polio vaccination schedule is recommended in the United States.[16] It is a four-dose schedule with doses at 2 and 4 months, 6 to 18 months, and 4 to 6 years. The reader is advised to consult the recommendations of the ACIP and the AAP, as well as the manufacturers' literature, for full consideration of the contraindications and indications for polio vaccines.

Routine primary poliovirus vaccination of adults older than 18 years is not conducted in the United States. However, adults at risk of exposure to wild polioviruses (laboratory workers, international travelers, health care workers) should be immunized. For the vaccination of adults, inactivated poliovirus vaccine is recommended.

Patients with immunodeficiency diseases should not be given oral poliovirus vaccine; live virus also should not be used in households in which an immunodeficient person resides.

GLOBAL ERADICATION OF POLIOMYELITIS

The WHO established the Expanded Program on Immunization (EPI) in 1974.[393, 849, 886] Afterward, the use of oral poliovirus vaccine in developing countries vastly increased. In 1980 in Brazil, researchers demonstrated that mass administration of the oral vaccine on National Immunization Days (NIDs) led to a dramatic reduction in poliomyelitis.[205] This demonstration led in 1985 to the targeted eradication of polio from the Western Hemisphere by 1990. This campaign was successful in that the last confirmed case of paralytic polio caused by wild poliovirus occurred in 1991 in Peru.[113] In September 1994, an international commission convened by the Pan American Health Organization certified that indigenous transmission of wild poliovirus had been interrupted in the Americas.[118]

In 1988, the World Health Assembly established the objective of global polio eradication by 2000.[393] This program was based on four strategies recommended by the WHO: (1) maintenance of high vaccination coverage levels among children with at least three doses of oral poliovirus vaccine; (2) development of sensitive systems of epidemiologic and laboratory surveillance, including use of the standard WHO case definition (a confirmed case of polio is defined as acute flaccid paralysis and at least one of the following: laboratory-confirmed wild poliovirus infection, residual paralysis of 60 days, death, or no follow-up investigation at 60 days); (3) administration of supplementary doses of oral poliovirus vaccine to all young children (usually those younger than 5 years) during NIDs to rapidly interrupt poliovirus transmission; and (4) "mopping up" vaccination campaigns—localized campaigns targeted at high-risk areas where wild poliovirus transmission is most likely to persist at low levels. NIDs are mass campaigns over the course of a short period (days to weeks) during which two doses of oral poliovirus vaccine are administered to all children in the target age group regardless of previous vaccination history, with an interval of 4 to 6 weeks between doses.

From 1985 through 1990, worldwide routine vaccination coverage levels increased from 47 to 85 percent and stabilized at 80 to 81 percent from 1991 to 1994.[119] From 1985 through 1994, the number of cases reported annually decreased 84 percent, from 39,361 to 6241. The number of countries reporting polio cases decreased steadily from 1985 (99 of 196 [51%]) to 1988 (88 of 196 [45%]) and 1994 (51 of 214 [24%]). In addition, the number of countries reporting zero polio cases increased from 1985 (84 [43%]) to 1988 (104 [53%]) and 1994 (145 [68%]). The number of countries with endemic polio that conducted NIDs each year increased from 15 in 1988 to 37 as of April 14, 1995; 24 additional countries scheduled their first NIDs for later in 1995.

At the beginning of the 21st century, NIDs had been conducted in every country in the world with endemic polio. In 1999, 7141 cases of poliomyelitis were reported worldwide. These cases occurred in 30 countries, mainly in south Asia and central Africa. By the end of 2000, fewer than 3500 cases occurred in endemic areas throughout the world, and wild type 2 poliovirus has not been detected since October 1999.[809] At the close of 2001, the area of endemic poliomyelitis had been reduced to 10 countries, with fewer than 1000 cases reported.[624]

Despite substantial progress toward global eradication of polio, several challenges remain, including (1) increasing vaccination levels in unvaccinated subpopulations; (2) preventing the reintroduction of wild poliovirus into polio-free areas by eliminating reservoirs in polio-endemic countries (particularly in the Indian subcontinent); (3) increasing the awareness of donor agencies and governments in industrialized countries of the substantial financial and humanitarian benefits of global eradication of polio, thus engendering support from unaffected countries beyond that already provided by organizations such as Rotary International; (4) encouraging all countries that remain polio-endemic to make polio eradication a high priority, including the implementation of NIDs and the initiation of acute flaccid paralysis surveillance; and (5) providing support to vaccination program managers for training to develop managerial skills for implementing and maintaining effective vaccination and surveillance programs in all countries.[119] The success of the polio eradication initiative will depend on finding solutions to these financial, managerial, political, and technical challenges.

The present goal for global eradication of poliomyelitis is the year 2005. Recent world events and new knowledge relating to reversion of polio vaccine strains and recombination of polio vaccine strains with nonpolio enteroviruses has led to the realization that decisions related to discontinuation of immunization after world eradication are exceedingly complex.[459, 624, 809, 879]

REFERENCES

1. Abraham, R., Chonmaitree, T., McCombs, J., et al.: Rapid detection of poliovirus by reverse transcription and polymerase chain amplification: Application for differentiation between poliovirus and nonpoliovirus enteroviruses. J. Clin. Microbiol. *31*:395–399, 1993.
2. Abramson, H., Greenberg, M., and Magee, M. C.: Poliomyelitis in the newborn infant. J. Pediatr. *43*:167–173, 1953.
3. Abzug, M. J.: Prognosis for neonates with enterovirus hepatitis and coagulopathy. Pediatr. Infect. Dis. J. *20*:758–763, 2001.
4. Abzug, M. J., Keyserling, H. L., Lee, M. L., et al.: Neonatal enterovirus infection: Virology, serology and effects of intravenous immune globulin. Clin. Infect. Dis. *20*:1201–1206, 1995.
5. Abzug, M. J., Levin, M. J., and Rotbart, H. A.: Profile of enterovirus disease in the first two weeks of life. Pediatr. Infect. Dis. J. *12*:820–824, 1993.
6. Abzug, M. J., Loeffelholz, M., and Rotbart, H. A.: Diagnosis of neonatal enterovirus infection by polymerase chain reaction. J. Pediatr. *126*:447–450, 1995.
7. Ackerson, B. R., Raghunathan, R., Keller, M. A., et al.: Echovirus 11 arthritis in a patient with X-linked agammaglobulinemia. Pediatr. Infect. Dis. J. *6*:485–488, 1987.
8. Adler, J. L., Mostow, S. R., Mellin, H., et al.: Epidemiologic investigation of hand, foot, and mouth disease. Infection caused by coxsackievirus A16 in Baltimore, June through September 1968. Am. J. Dis. Child. *120*:309–313, 1970.
9. Agranat, A. L.: A near-fatal case of Coxsackie B myocarditis (with pericarditis) in an adult. S. Afr. Med. J. *35*:831–832, 1961.
10. Ahmad, N., and Abraham, A. A.: Pancreatic isleitis with Coxsackie virus B5 infection. Hum. Pathol. *13*:661–662, 1982.
11. Alexander, J. P., and Anderson, L. J. (Respiratory and Enterovirus Branch, Centers for Disease Control): Personal communication, 1990.
12. Alexander, J. P., Jr., Baden, L., Pallansch, M. A., et al.: Enterovirus 71 infections and neurologic disease: United States, 1977–1991. J. Infect. Dis. *169*:905–908, 1994.
13. Alexander, J. P., Jr., Chapman, L. E., Pallansch, M. A., et al.: Coxsackievirus B2 infection and aseptic meningitis: A focal outbreak among members of a high school football team. J. Infect. Dis. *167*:1201–1205, 1993.
14. Alsop, J., Flewett, T. H., and Foster, J. R.: "Hand-foot-and-mouth disease" in Birmingham in 1959. B. M. J. *2*:1708–1711, 1960.
15. American Academy of Pediatrics: Poliovirus infections. *In* Peter, G. (ed.): 1994 Red Book: Report of the Committee on Infectious Diseases. 23rd ed. Elk Grove Village, IL, American Academy of Pediatrics, 1994, pp. 379–386.
16. American Academy of Pediatrics: Poliovirus infections. *In* Pickering, L. K. (ed.): 2000 Red Book: Report of the Committee on Infectious Diseases. 25th ed. Elk Grove Village, IL, American Academy of Pediatrics, 2000, pp. 465–470.
17. Andréoletti, L., Blassel-Damman, N., Dewilde, A., et al.: Comparison of use of cerebrospinal fluid, serum, and throat swab specimens in diagnosis of enteroviral acute neurological infection by a rapid RNA detection PCR assay. J. Clin. Microbiol. *36*:589–591, 1998.
18. Andréoletti, L., Bourlet, T., Moukassa, D., et al.: Enteroviruses can persist with or without active viral replication in cardiac tissue of patients with end-stage ischemic or dilated cardiomyopathy. J. Infect. Dis. *182*:1222–1227, 2000.
19. Andréoletti, L., Hober, D., Becquart, P., et al.: Experimental CVB3-induced chronic myocarditis in two murine strains: Evidence of interrelationships between virus replication and myocardial damage in persistent cardiac infection. J. Med. Virol. *52*:206–214, 1997.
20. Andréoletti, L., Hober, D., Decoene, C., et al.: Detection of enteroviral RNA by polymerase chain reaction in endomyocardial tissue of patients with chronic cardiac diseases. J. Med. Virol. *48*:53–59, 1996.

21. Andréoletti, L., Hober, D., Hober-Vandenberghe, C., et al.: Detection of Coxsackie B virus RNA sequences in whole blood samples from adult patients at the onset of type I diabetes mellitus. J. Med. Virol. *52*:121–127, 1997.
22. Andréoletti, L., Wattre, P., Decoene, C., et al.: Detection of enterovirus-specific RNA sequences in explanted myocardium biopsy specimens from patients with dilated or ischemic cardiomyopathy. Clin. Infect. Dis. *21*:1315–1317, 1995.
23. Aquino, V. M., Farah, R. A., Lee, M. C., et al.: Disseminated Coxsackie A9 infection complicating bone marrow transplantation. Pediatr. Infect. Dis. J. *15*:1053–1054, 1996.
24. Archard, L. C., Bowles, N. E., Behan, P. O., et al.: Postviral fatigue syndrome: Persistence of enterovirus RNA in muscle and elevated creatinine kinase. J. R. Soc. Med. *81*:326–329, 1988.
25. Archibald, E., and Purdham, D. R.: Coxsackievirus type: A16 infection in a neonate. Arch. Dis. Child. *54*:649, 1979.
26. Arnon, R., Naor, N., Davidson, S., et al.: Fatal outcome of neonatal echovirus 19 infection. Pediatr. Infect. Dis. J. *10*:788–789, 1991.
27. Arola, A., Kalimo, H., Ruuskanen, O., et al.: Experimental myocarditis induced by two different coxsackievirus B3 variants: Aspects of pathogenesis and comparison of diagnostic methods. J. Med. Virol. *47*:251–259, 1995.
28. Arola, A., Kallajoki, M., Ruuskanen, O., et al.: Detection of enteroviral RNA in end-stage dilated cardiomyopathy in children and adolescents. J. Med. Virol. *56*:364–371, 1998.
29. Aronson, M. D., and Phillips, C. A.: Coxsackievirus B5 infections in acute oliguric renal failure. J. Infect. Dis. *132*:302–306, 1975.
30. Artenstein, M. S., Cadigan, F. C., Jr., and Buescher, E. L.: Clinical and epidemiological features of Coxsackie group B virus infections. Ann. Intern. Med. *63*:597–603, 1965.
31. Ash, I.: Large epidemic outbreak of vomiting associated with meningism and exanthem. B. M. J. *1*:316–318, 1958.
32. Assaad, F., and Borecka, I.: Nine-year study of WHO virus reports on fatal viral infections. Bull. World Health Organ. *55*:445–453, 1977.
33. Assaad, F., and Cockburn, W. C.: Four-year study of WHO virus reports on enteroviruses other than poliovirus. Bull. World Health Organ. *46*:329–336, 1972.
34. Atkinson, M. A., Bowman, M. A., Campbell, L., et al.: Cellular immunity to a determinant common to glutamate decarboxylase and Coxsackie virus in insulin-dependent diabetes. J. Clin. Invest. *94*:2125–2129, 1994.
35. Austin, T. W., and Ray, C. G.: Coxsackie virus group B infections and the hemolytic-uremic syndrome. J. Infect. Dis. *127*:698–701, 1973.
36. Avner, E. D., Satz, J., and Plotkin, S. A.: Hypoglycorrhachia in young infants with viral meningitis. J. Pediatr. *87*:833–834, 1975.
37. Axelson, C., Bondestam, K., Frisk, G., et al.: Coxsackie B virus infection in women with miscarriage. J. Med. Virol. *39*:282–285, 1993.
38. Ayuthya, P. S. N., Jayavasu, J., and Pongpanich, B.: Coxsackie group B virus and primary myocardial disease in infants and children. Am. Heart J. *88*:311–314, 1974.
39. Babb, J. M., Stoneman, M. E. R., and Stern, H.: Myocarditis and croup caused by Coxsackie virus type B5. Arch. Dis. Child. *36*:551–556, 1961.
40. Bain, H. W., McLean, D. M., and Walker, S. J.: Epidemic pleurodynia (Bornholm disease) due to Coxsackie B-5 virus: The interrelationship of pleurodynia, benign pericarditis and aseptic meningitis. Pediatrics *27*:889–903, 1961.
41. Baker, D. A., and Phillips, C. A.: Fatal hand-foot-and-mouth disease in an adult caused by coxsackievirus A7. J. A. M. A. *242*:1065, 1979.
42. Balduzzi, P. C., and Greendyke, R. M.: Sudden unexpected death in infancy and viral infection. Pediatrics *38*:201–206, 1966.
43. Banatvala, J. E.: Insulin-dependent (juvenile onset, type 1) diabetes mellitus: Coxsackie B viruses revisited. Prog. Med. Virol. *34*:33–54, 1987.
44. Banatvala, J. E., Bryant, J., Schernthaner, G., et al.: Coxsackie B, mumps, rubella, and cytomegalovirus specific IgM responses in patients with juvenile-onset insulin-dependent diabetes mellitus in Britain, Austria, and Australia. Lancet *1*:1409–1412, 1985.
45. Barak, Y., and Schwartz, J. F.: Acute transverse myelitis associated with ECHO type 5 infection. Am. J. Dis. Child. *142*:128, 1988.
46. Bardelas, J. A., Winkelstein, J. A., Tsai, S. T., et al.: Fatal ECHO 24 infection in a patient with hypogammaglobulinemia: Relationship to dermatomyositis-like syndrome. J. Pediatr. *90*:396–399, 1977.
47. Barrett, F. F., Yow, M. D., and Phillips, C. A.: St. Louis encephalitis in children during the 1964 Houston epidemic. J. A. M. A. *193*:381–385, 1965.
48. Barson, W. J., Craenen, J., Hosier, D. M., et al.: Survival following myocarditis and myocardial calcification associated with infection by Coxsackie virus B4. Pediatrics *68*:79–81, 1981.
49. Barton, L. L.: Febrile neonatal illness associated with echo virus type 5 in the cerebrospinal fluid. Clin. Pediatr. (Phila.) *16*:383–385, 1977.
50. Baskin, J. L., Soule, E. H., and Mills, S. D.: Poliomyelitis of the newborn: Pathologic changes in two cases. Am. J. Dis. Child. *80*:10–21, 1950.
51. Bates, H. R.: Coxsackie virus B3 calcific pancarditis and hydrops fetalis. Am. J. Obstet. Gynecol. *106*:629–630, 1970.
52. Bates, T.: Poliomyelitis in pregnancy, fetus, and newborn. Am. J. Dis. Child. *90*:189–195, 1955.
53. Bayatpour, M., Zbitnew, A., Dempster, G., et al.: Role of coxsackievirus B4 in the pathogenesis of acute glomerulonephritis. Can. Med. Assoc. J. *109*:873–875, 1973.
54. Behan, W. M. H., Gow, J. W., Simpson, K., et al.: Search for picornaviruses at onset of inflammatory myopathy. J. Clin. Pathol. *49*:592–594, 1996.
55. Behbehani, A. A., Sulkin, S. E., and Wallis, C.: Factors influencing susceptibility of mice to Coxsackie virus infection. J. Infect. Dis. *110*:147–154, 1962.
56. Behbehani, A. M., and Wenner, H. A.: Infantile diarrhea: A study of the etiologic role of viruses. Am. J. Dis. Child. *111*:623–629, 1966.
57. Bell, E. J., and Cosgrove, B. P.: Routine enterovirus diagnosis in a human rhabdomyosarcoma cell line. Bull. World Health Organ. *58*:423–428, 1980.
58. Bell, E. J., and Grist, N. R.: Echoviruses, carditis and acute pleurodynia. Lancet *1*:326–328, 1970.
59. Bell, E. J., Grist, N. R., and Russell, S. J. M.: Echovirus 25 infections in Scotland, 1961–64. Lancet *2*:464–466, 1965.
60. Bell, E. J., and Russell, S. J. M.: Acute transverse myelopathy and ECHO-2 virus infection. Lancet *2*:1226–1227, 1963.
61. Bell, J. F., and Meis, A.: Pericarditis in infection due to Coxsackie virus group B, type 3. N. Engl. J. Med. *261*:126–128, 1959.
62. Bell, T. M., Clark, N. S., and Chambers, W.: Outbreak of illness associated with E.C.H.O. type 7 virus. B. M. J. *2*:292–294, 1963.
63. Bell, T. M., and Steyn, J. H.: Viruses in lymph nodes of children with mesenteric adenitis and intussusception. B. M. J. *2*:700–702, 1962.
64. Benirschke, K.: Viral infection of the placenta. *In* Viral Etiology of Congenital Malformations, May 19–20, 1967. Washington, D.C., U.S. Government Printing Office, 1968.
65. Benirschke, K., and Pendleton, M. E.: Coxsackie virus infection: An important complication of pregnancy. Obstet. Gynecol. *12*:305–309, 1958.
66. Berg, R., and Jelke, H.: Acute cerebellar ataxia in children associated with Coxsackie viruses group B. Acta Paediatr. Scand. *54*:497–502, 1965.
67. Berger, M. M., Kopp N., Vital, C., et al.: Detection and cellular localization of enterovirus RNA sequences in spinal cord of patients with ALS. Neurology *54*:20–25, 2000.
68. Berglund, A., Böttiger, M., Johnson, T., et al.: Outbreak of aseptic meningitis with rubella-like rash probably caused by ECHO virus type 9. Arch. Ges. Virusforsch. *8*:294–305, 1958.
69. Bergman, I., Painter, M. J., and Wald, E. R.: Outcome in children with enteroviral meningitis during the first year of life. J. Pediatr. *110*:705–709, 1987.
70. Bergström, K., Erikson, U., Nordbring, F., et al.: Acute non-rheumatic myopericarditis: A follow-up study. Scand. J. Infect. Dis. *2*:7–16, 1970.
71. Berkovich, S., and Kibrick, S.: ECHO 11 outbreak in newborn infants and mothers. Pediatrics *33*:534–540, 1964.
72. Berkovich, S., and Pangan, J.: Recoveries of virus from premature infants during outbreaks of respiratory disease: The relation of ECHO virus type 22 to disease of the upper and lower respiratory tract in the premature infant. Bull. N. Y. Acad. Med. *44*:377–387, 1968.
73. Berkovich, S., and Smithwick, E. M.: Transplacental infection due to ECHO virus type 22. J. Pediatr. *72*:94–96, 1968.
74. Berlin, L. E., Rorabaugh, M. L., Heldrich, F., et al.: Aseptic meningitis in infants less than 2 years of age: Diagnosis and etiology. J. Infect. Dis. *168*:888–892, 1993.
75. Bern, C., Pallansch, M. A., Gary, H. E., Jr., et al.: Acute hemorrhagic conjunctivitis due to enterovirus 70 in American Samoa: Serum-neutralizing antibodies and sex-specific protection. Am. J. Epidemiol. *136*:1502–1506, 1992.
76. Berry, P. J., and Nagington, J.: Fatal infection with echovirus 11. Arch. Dis. Child. *57*:22–29, 1982.
77. Bertaggia, A., Meneghetti, F., and Carretta, M.: Observations on a case of parotitis due to Coxsackie virus B3. G. Mal. Infekt. *28*:188–189, 1976.
78. Biren, V. P., and Meitens, C.: Nachweis einer coxsackie B2-infektion bei polyradikulitis (Guillain-Barré syndrom) Ann. Paediatr. *204*:312–322, 1965.
79. Blotzer, J. W., and Myers, A. R.: Echovirus-associated polyarthritis: Report of a case with synovial fluid and synovial histologic characterization. Arthritis Rheum. *21*:978–981, 1978.
80. Bodensteiner, J. B., Morris, H. H., Howell, J. T., et al.: Chronic ECHO type 5 virus meningoencephalitis in X-linked hypogammaglobulinemia: Treatment with immune plasma. Neurology *29*:815–819, 1979.
81. Bodian, D., and Horstmann, D. M.: Poliomyelitis. *In* Horsfall, F. L., and Tamm, I. (eds.): Viral and Rickettsial Infections of Man. 4th ed. Philadelphia, J. B. Lippincott, 1965, pp. 430–473.
82. Boring, W. D., Angevine, D. M., and Walker, D. L.: Factors influencing host-virus interactions. I. A comparison of viral multiplication and histopathology in infant, adult, and cortisone-treated adult mice infected with the Conn-5 strain of Coxsackie virus. J. Exp. Med. *102*:753–766, 1955.
83. Bose, C. L., Gooch, W. M., Sanders, G. O., et al.: Dissimilar manifestations of intrauterine infection with Echovirus II in premature twins. Arch. Pathol. Lab. Med. *107*:361–363, 1983.
84. Bottiger, M., Johnsson, T., and von Zeipel, G.: Family infections with acute pericarditis and myocarditis by Coxsackie virus B5. Arch. Ges. Virusforsch. *13*:153–155, 1963.

85. Bowen, G. S., Fisher, M. C., Deforest, A., et al.: Epidemic of meningitis and febrile illness in neonates caused by ECHO type II virus in Philadelphia. Pediatr. Infect. Dis. *2*:359–363, 1983.
86. Bowers, V. M., Jr., and Danforth, D. N.: The significance of poliomyelitis during pregnancy: An analysis of the literature and presentation of 24 new cases. Am. J. Obstet. Gynecol. *65*:34–39, 1953.
87. Bowles, N. E., Richardson, P. J., Olsen, E. G. J., et al.: Detection of Coxsackie B virus–specific RNA sequences in myocardial biopsy samples from patients with myocarditis and dilated cardiomyopathy. Lancet *1*:1120–1122, 1986.
88. Boyd, M. T., Jordan, S. W., and Davis, L. E.: Fatal pneumonitis from congenital echovirus type 6 infection. Pediatr. Infect. Dis. *6*:1138–1139, 1987.
89. Brightman, V. J., Scott, T. F. M., Westphal, M., et al.: An outbreak of Coxsackie B-5 virus infection in a newborn nursery. J. Pediatr. *69*:179–192, 1966.
90. Brodie, H. R., and Marchessault, V.: Acute benign pericarditis caused by Coxsackie virus group B. N. Engl. J. Med. *262*:1278–1280, 1960.
91. Brown, B. A., Oberste, M. S., Alexander, Jr. J. P., et al.: Molecular epidemiology and evolution of enterovirus 71 strains isolated from 1970 to 1998. J. Virol. *73*:9969–9975, 1999.
92. Brown, G. C., and Karunas, R. S.: Relationship of congenital anomalies and maternal infection with selected enteroviruses. Am. J. Epidemiol. *95*:207–217, 1972.
93. Brown, J. M., Wright, J. A., and Ogden, W. S.: Hand, foot, and mouth disease. B. M. J. *1*:58, 1964.
94. Bryden, A. S.: Isolation of enteroviruses and adenoviruses in continuous simian cell lines. Med. Lab. Sci. *49*:60–65, 1992.
95. Buckland, F. E., Bynoe, M. L., Philipson, L., et al.: Experimental infection of human volunteers with the U-virus, A strain of ECHO virus type 11. J. Hyg. *57*:274–284, 1959.
96. Burch, G. E., and Colcolough, H. L.: Progressive Coxsackie viral pancarditis and nephritis. Ann. Intern. Med. *71*:963–970, 1969.
97. Burch, G. E., Sun, S. C., Chu, K. C., et al.: Interstitial and coxsackievirus B myocarditis in infants and children. J. A. M. A. *203*:1–8, 1968.
98. Burch, G. E., Sun, S. C., Colcolough, H. L., et al.: Coxsackie B viral myocarditis and valvulitis identified in routine autopsy specimens by immunofluorescent techniques. Am. Heart J. *74*:13–23, 1967.
99. Burry, J. N., Moore, B., and Mattner, C.: Hand, foot and mouth disease in South Australia. Med. J. Aust. *2*:587–589, 1968.
100. Byington, C. L., Taggart, W., Carroll, K. C., et al.: A polymerase chain reaction–based epidemiologic investigation of the incidence of nonpolio enteroviral infections in febrile and afebrile infants 90 days and younger. Pediatrics *103*:E27, 1999.
101. Cabinian, A. E., Kiel, R. J., Smith, S., et al.: Modification of exercise-aggravated coxsackievirus B3 murine myocarditis by T lymphocyte suppression in an inbred model. J. Lab. Clin. Med. *115*:454–462, 1990.
102. Calder, B. D., Warnock, P. J., McCartney, R. A., et al.: Coxsackie B viruses and the post-viral syndrome: A prospective study in general practice. J. R. Coll. Gen. Pract. *37*:11–14, 1987.
103. Canby, J. P.: Petechiae and fever: Infection with Coxsackie virus group B, type 3—Case report. Clin. Pediatr. (Phila.) *2*:187–188, 1963.
104. Cao, Y., Schnurr, D. P., and Schmidt, N. J.: Differing cardiotropic and myocarditic properties of group B type 4 coxsackievirus strains. Arch. Virol. *80*:119–130, 1984.
105. Capner, P., Lendrum, R., Jeffries, D. J., et al.: Viral antibody studies in pancreatic disease. Gut *16*:866–870, 1975.
106. Carolane, D. J., Long, A. M., McKeever, P. A., et al.: Prevention of spread of echovirus 6 in a special care baby unit. Arch. Dis. Child. *60*:674–676, 1985.
107. Carstens, J. M., Tracy, S., Chapman, N. M., et al.: Detection of enteroviruses in cell cultures by using in situ transcription. J. Clin. Microbiol. *30*:25–35, 1992.
108. Cashman, N. R., Maselli, R., and Wollmann, R. L.: Late denervation in patients with antecedent paralytic poliomyelitis. N. Engl. J. Med. *317*:7–12, 1987.
109. Centers for Disease Control and Prevention: Follow-up on poliomyelitis, Connecticut, New York, Massachusetts, New Hampshire. M. M. W. R. Morb. Mortal. Wkly. Rep. *21*:365–366, 1972.
110. Centers for Disease Control and Prevention: Poliomyelitis surveillance summary 1974–1976. Issued October 1977.
111. Centers for Disease Control and Prevention: Follow-up on poliomyelitis—United States, Canada, Netherlands. M. M. W. R. Morb. Mortal. Wkly. Rep. *28*:345–346, 1979.
112. Centers for Disease Control and Prevention: Aseptic meningitis surveillance: Annual summary 1976. Atlanta, U. S. Department of Health, Education and Welfare. Issued January 1979.
113. Centers for Disease Control and Prevention: Annual summary 1979: Reported morbidity and mortality in the United States. M. M. W. R. Morb. Mortal. Wkly. Rep. *28*:1–119, 1980.
114. Centers for Disease Control and Prevention: Encephalitis surveillance, annual summary 1978. Issued May 1981.
115. Centers for Disease Control and Prevention: Acute hemorrhagic conjunctivitis—Florida, North Carolina. M. M. W. R. Morb. Mortal. Wkly. Rep. *30*(40):501–502, 1982.
116. Centers for Disease Control and Prevention: Enterovirus surveillance—United States, 1985. M. M. W. R. Morb. Mortal. Wkly. Rep. *34*(32): 494–495, 1985.
117. Centers for Disease Control and Prevention: Acute hemorrhagic conjunctivitis—Mexico. M. M. W. R. Morb. Mortal. Wkly. Rep. *38*(18): 327–329, 1989.
118. Centers for Disease Control and Prevention: Certification of poliomyelitis eradication—The Americas, 1994. M. M. W. R. Morb. Mortal. Wkly. Rep. *43*(39):720–722, 1994.
119. Centers for Disease Control and Prevention: Progress toward global poliomyelitis eradication, 1985–1994. M. M. W. R. Morb. Mortal. Wkly. Rep. *44*(14):273–275, 281, 1995.
120. Centers for Disease Control and Prevention: Nonpolio enterovirus surveillance—United States, 1993–1996. M. M. W. R. Morb. Mortal. Wkly. Rep. *46*:748–750, 1997.
121. Centers for Disease Control and Prevention: Enterovirus surveillance—United States, 1997–1999. M. M. W. R. Morb. Mortal. Wkly. Rep. *49*(40):913–916, 2000.
122. Centers for Disease Control and Prevention: Echovirus type 13—United States, 2001. M. M. W. R. Morb. Mortal. Wkly. Rep. *50*(36):777–780, 2001.
123. Chalhub, E. G., Devivo, D. C., Seigel, B. A., et al.: Coxsackie A9 focal encephalitis associated with acute infantile hemiplegia and porencephaly. Neurology *27*:574–579, 1977.
124. Chambon, M., Delage, C., Bailly, J. L., et al.: Fatal hepatic necrosis in a neonate with echovirus 20 infection: Use of the polymerase chain reaction to detect enterovirus in liver tissue. Clin. Infect. Dis. *24*:523–524, 1997.
125. Champsaur, H. F., Bottazzo, G. F., Bertrams, J., et al.: Virologic, immunologic, and genetic factors in insulin-dependent diabetes mellitus. J. Pediatr. *100*:15–20, 1982.
126. Chan, D., and Hammond, G. W.: Comparison of serodiagnosis of group B coxsackievirus infections by an immunoglobulin M capture enzyme immunoassay versus microneutralization. J. Clin. Microbiol. *21*:830–834, 1985.
127. Chan, L. G., Parashar, U. D., Lye, M. S., et al.: Deaths of children during an outbreak of hand, foot, and mouth disease in Sarawak, Malaysia: Clinical and pathological characteristics of the disease. For the Outbreak Study Group. Clin. Infect. Dis. *31*:678–683, 2000.
128. Chandy, K. G., John, T. J., Mukundan, P., et al.: Coxsackie B antibodies in "rheumatic" valvular heart disease. Lancet *1*:381, 1979.
129. Chang, L. Y., Lin, T. Y., Hsu, K. H., et al.: Clinical features and risk factors of pulmonary oedema after enterovirus-71–related hand, foot, and mouth disease. Lancet *354*:1682–1686, 1999.
130. Chang, T. W., and Weinstein, L.: Infection of the nervous system by Coxsackie A9 virus. Bull. Tufts N. E. Med. Ctr. *6*:181–193, 1960.
131. Chanock, R. M., and Parrott, R. H.: Acute respiratory disease in infancy and childhood: Present understanding and prospects for prevention. Pediatrics *36*:21–39, 1965.
132. Chatterjee, S., Quarcoopome, C. O., and Apenteng, A.: Unusual type of epidemic conjunctivitis in Ghana. Br. J. Ophthalmol. *54*:628, 1970.
133. Chaves, S. S., Lobo, S., Kennett, M., et al.: Coxsackie virus A24 infection presenting as acute flaccid paralysis. Lancet *357*:605, 2001.
134. Chawareewong, S., Kiangsiri, S., Lokaphadhana, K., et al.: Neonatal herpangina caused by Coxsackie A-5 virus. J. Pediatr. *93*:492–494, 1978.
135. Chehadeh, W., Weill, J., Vantyghem, M. C., et al.: Increased level of interferon-alpha in blood of patients with insulin-dependent diabetes mellitus: Relationship with coxsackievirus B infection. J. Infect. Dis. *181*:1929–1939, 2000.
136. Chemtob, S., Reece, E. R., and Mills, E. L.: Syndrome of inappropriate secretion of antidiuretic hormone in enteroviral meningitis. Am. J. Dis. Child. *139*:292–294, 1985.
137. Cherry, J. D.: Newer viral exanthems. Adv. Pediatr. *116*:233–286, 1969.
138. Cherry, J. D.: Enteroviruses. *In* Behrman, R. E., and Vaughan, V. C. (eds.): Nelson Textbook of Pediatrics. 12th ed. Philadelphia, W. B. Saunders, 1983, pp. 791–804.
139. Cherry, J. D.: Enteroviruses: Polioviruses (poliomyelitis), coxsackieviruses, echoviruses, and enteroviruses. *In* Feigin, R. D., and Cherry, J. D. (eds.): Textbook of Pediatric Infectious Diseases. 2nd ed. Philadelphia, W. B. Saunders, 1987, pp. 1729–1790.
140. Cherry, J. D.: Enteroviruses. *In* Remington, J. S., and Klein, J. O. (eds.): Infectious Diseases of the Fetus and Newborn Infant. 3rd ed. Philadelphia, W. B. Saunders, 1990, pp. 325–366.
141. Cherry, J. D., Bobinski, J. E., Horvath, F. L., et al.: Acute hemangioma-like lesions associated with ECHO viral infections. Pediatrics *44*: 498–502, 1969.
142. Cherry, J. D., and Jahn, C. L.: Concomitant enterovirus infection, smallpox vaccination, and exanthem. J. Pediatr. *67*:679–681, 1965.
143. Cherry, J. D., and Jahn, C. L.: Virologic studies of exanthems. J. Pediatr. *68*:204–214, 1966.
144. Cherry, J. D., and Jahn, C. L.: Hand, foot, and mouth syndrome: Report of six cases due to Coxsackie virus, group A, type 16. Pediatrics *37*:637–643, 1966.
145. Cherry, J. D., Jahn, C. L., and Meyer, T. C.: Paroxysmal atrial tachycardia associated with ECHO 9 virus infection. Am. Heart J. *73*:681–686, 1967.

146. Cherry, J. D., Lerner, A. M., Klein, J. O., et al.: Coxsackie B5 infections with exanthems. Pediatrics *31*:455–462, 1963.
147. Cherry, J. D., Lerner, A. M., Klein, J. O., et al.: Echo 11 virus infections associated with exanthems. Pediatrics *32*:509–516, 1963.
148. Cherry, J. D., Lerner, A. M., Klein, J. O., et al.: Coxsackie A9 infections with exanthems: With particular reference to urticaria. Pediatrics *31*:819–823, 1963.
149. Cherry, J. D., Soriano, F., and Jahn, C. L.: Search for perinatal viral infection: A prospective, clinical, virologic, and serologic study. Am. J. Dis. Child. *116*:245–250, 1968.
150. Chesney, J. C., Hoganson, G. E., and Wilson, M. H.: CSF eosinophilia during an acute Coxsackie B4 viral meningitis. Am. J. Dis. Child. *134*:703, 1980.
151. Chesney, P. J., Quennec, P., and Clark, C.: Hypoglycorrhachia and Coxsackie B3 meningoencephalitis. Am. J. Clin. Pathol. *70*:947–948, 1978.
152. Chezzi, C.: Rapid diagnosis of poliovirus infection by PCR amplification. J. Clin. Microbiol. *34*:1722–1725, 1996.
153. Chia, J. K., and Bold, E. J.: Life-threatening leukocytoclastic vasculitis with pulmonary involvement due to echovirus 7. Clin. Infect. Dis. *27*:1326–1327, 1998.
154. Chin, T. D. Y., Lehan, P. H., Rubin, H., et al.: Epidemiological studies of aseptic meningitis caused by Coxsackie virus B5. Am. J. Public Health *48*:1193–1200, 1958.
155. Cho, C. T., Janelle, J. G., and Behbehani, A.: Severe neonatal illness associated with Echo 9 virus infection. Clin. Pediatr. (Phila.) *12*:304–305, 1973.
156. Chomel, J. J., Thouvenot, D., Fayol, V., et al.: Rapid diagnosis of echovirus type 33 meningitis by specific IgM detection using an enzyme linked immunosorbent assay (ELISA). J. Virol. Methods *10*:11–19, 1985.
157. Chonmaitree, T., Ford, C., Sanders, C., et al.: Comparison of cell cultures for rapid isolation of enteroviruses. J. Clin. Microbiol. *26*:2576–2580, 1988.
158. Chonmaitree, T., Menegus, M. A., and Powell, K. R.: The clinical relevance of "CSF viral culture": A two-year experience with aseptic meningitis in Rochester, N.Y. J. A. M. A. *247*:1843–1847, 1982.
159. Chonmaitree, T., Menegus, M. A., Schervish-Swierkosz, E. M., et al.: Enterovirus 71 infection: Report of an outbreak with two cases of paralysis and a review of the literature. Pediatrics *67*:489–493, 1981.
160. Chou, S. M., and Gutmann, L.: Picornavirus-like crystals in subacute polymyositis. Neurology *20*:205–213, 1970.
161. Chow, K. C., Lee, C. C., Lin, T. Y., et al.: Congenital enterovirus 71 infection: A case study with virology and immunohistochemistry. Clin. Infect. Dis. *31*:509–512, 2000.
162. Chow, L. H., Gauntt, C. J., and McManus, B. M.: Differential effects of myocarditic variants of coxsackievirus B3 in inbred mice. A pathologic characterization of heart tissue damage. Lab. Invest. *64*:55–64, 1991.
163. Christen, A. G., Crandell, R. A., and Kerstein, M. H.: Hand-foot-and-mouth disease in a father and son. Oral Surg. Oral Med. Oral Pathol. *24*:427–432, 1967.
164. Christensen, M. L., Pachman, L. M., Schneiderman, R., et al.: Prevalence of Coxsackie B virus antibodies in patients with juvenile dermatomyositis. Arthritis Rheum. *29*:1365–1370, 1986.
165. Christie, A. B.: Acute poliomyelitis. *In* Christie, A. B. (ed.): Infectious Diseases: Epidemiology and Clinical Practice. 2nd ed. Edinburgh, Churchill Livingstone, 1974, pp. 567–614.
166. Christopher, S., Theogaraj, S., Godbole, S., et al.: An epidemic of acute hemorrhagic conjunctivitis due to coxsackievirus A24. J. Infect. Dis. *146*:16–19, 1982.
167. Chuang, E., Maller, E. S., Hoffman, M. A., et al.: Successful treatment of fulminant echovirus 11 infection in a neonate by orthotopic liver transplantation. J. Pediatr. Gastroenterol. Nutr. *17*:211–214, 1993.
168. Clarke, A., and Stott, J.: E.C.H.O. type 20. B. M. J. *1*:900–901, 1961.
169. Clarke, M., Hunter, M., McNaughton, G. A., et al.: Seasonal aseptic meningitis caused by Coxsackie and Echo viruses: Toronto, 1957. Can. Med. Assoc. J. *81*:5–8, 1959.
170. Clarke, S. K. R., Morley, T., and Warin, R. P.: Hand, foot, and mouth disease. B. M. J. *1*:58, 1964.
171. Clements, G. B., Galbraith, D. N., and Taylor, K. W.: Coxsackie B virus infection and onset of childhood diabetes. Lancet *346*:221–223, 1995.
172. Clements, G. B., McGarry, F., Nairn, C., et al.: Detection of enterovirus-specific RNA in serum: The relationship to chronic fatigue. J. Med. Virol. *45*:156–161, 1995.
173. Clemer, D. I., Li, F., LeBlanc, D. R., et al.: An outbreak of subclinical infection with coxsackievirus B3 in southern Louisiana. Am. J. Epidemiol. *83*:123–129, 1966.
174. Cochi, S. L., Hull, H. F., Sutter, R. W., et al.: Commentary: The unfolding story of global poliomyelitis eradication. J. Infect. Dis. *175*(Suppl. 1):1–3, 1997.
175. Cochrane, H. R., May, F. E. B., Ashcroft, T., et al.: Enteroviruses and idiopathic dilated cardiomyopathy. J. Pathol. *163*:129–131, 1991.
176. Codd, A. A., Hale, J. H., Bell, T. M., et al.: Epidemic of echovirus 19 in the north-east of England. J. Hyg. (Camb.) *76*:307–317, 1976.
177. Constable, F. L., and Howitt, L. F.: Outbreak of E.C.H.O. type 9 infection in a children's home. B. M. J. *1*:1483–1486, 1961.
178. Cooper, J. B., Pratt, W. R., English, B. K., et al.: Coxsackievirus B3 producing fatal meningoencephalitis in a patient with X-linked agammaglobulinemia. Am. J. Dis. Child. *137*:82–83, 1983.
179. Coucke, C., Kint, A., and Gabriel, P.: Hand, foot and mouth disease in the adult subject. Dermatologica *153*:272–276, 1976.
180. Couvreur, J., Cook, C. M., Chany, C., et al.: Une épidémie d'exanthème B virus ECHO de type 16 en milieu hospitalier avec bilan d'une enqu{circumflex e}te longitudinale. Arch. Ges. Virusforsch. *13*:215–232, 1963.
181. Craighead, J. E., Mahoney, E. M., Carver, D. H., et al.: Orchitis due to Coxsackie virus group B, type 5: Report of a case with isolation of virus from the testis. N. Engl. J. Med. *267*:498–500, 1962.
182. Cramblett, H. G., Haynes, R. E., Azimi, P. H., et al.: Nosocomial infection with echovirus type 11 in handicapped and premature infants. Pediatrics *51*:603–607, 1973.
183. Cramblett, H. G., Moffet, H. L., Black, J. P., et al.: Coxsackie virus infections: Clinical and laboratory studies. J. Pediatr. *64*:406–414, 1964.
184. Cramblett, H. G., Moffet, H. L., Middleton, G. K., Jr., et al.: Echo 19 virus infections: Clinical and laboratory studies. Arch. Intern. Med. *110*:574–579, 1962.
185. Cramblett, H. G., Rosen, L., Parrott, R. H., et al.: Respiratory illness in six infants infected with a newly recognized echo virus. Pediatrics *21*:168–176, 1958.
186. Crawford, M., Macrae, A. D., and O'Reilly, J. N.: An unusual illness in young children associated with an enteric virus. Arch. Dis. Child. *31*:182–188, 1956.
187. Crennan, J. M., Van Scoy, R. E., McKenna, C. H., et al.: Echovirus poliomyelitis in patients with hypogammaglobulinemia. Am. J. Med. *81*:35–42, 1986.
188. Crow, K. D., Warin, R., and Wilkinson, D. S.: Hand, foot, and mouth disease. B. M. J. *2*:1267–1268, 1963.
189. Cudworth, A. G., White, G. B. B., Woodrow, J. C., et al.: Etiology of juvenile-onset diabetes: A prospective study. Lancet *1*:385–388, 1977.
190. Cunningham, C. K., Bonville, C. A., Ochs, H. D., et al.: Enteroviral meningoencephalitis as a complication of X-linked hyper IgM syndrome. J. Pediatr. *134*:584–588, 1999.
191. Curnen, E. C., Shaw, E. W., and Melnick, J. L.: Disease resembling non-paralytic poliomyelitis associated with a virus pathogenic for infant mice. J. A. M. A. *141*:894–901, 1949.
192. Daae, A.: Epidemi i drangedal af akut muskelrheumatisme udbredt ved smitte. Norsk Mag. F. Laegevidensk. *2 n. s.*:409–413, 529–542, 1872.
193. Dagan, R., Jenista, J. A., and Menegus, M. A.: Association of clinical presentation, laboratory findings, and virus serotypes with the presence of meningitis in hospitalized infants with enterovirus infection. J. Pediatr. *113*:975–978, 1988.
194. Dagan, R., Prather, S. L., Powell, K. R., et al.: Neutralizing antibodies to non-polio enteroviruses in human immune serum globulin. Pediatr. Infect. Dis. *2*:454–456, 1983.
195. Dalakas, M. C., Elder, G., Hallett, M., et al.: A long-term follow-up study of patients with post-poliomyelitis neuromuscular symptoms. N. Engl. J. Med. *314*:959–963, 1986.
196. Dalakas, M. C., Sever, J. L., Madden, D. L., et al.: Late postpoliomyelitis muscular atrophy: Clinical, virologic, and immunologic studies. Rev. Infect. Dis. *6*(Suppl.):562–567, 1984.
197. Dalldorf, F., and Melnick, J. L.: Coxsackie viruses. *In* Horsfall, F. L., and Tamm, I. (eds.): Viral and Rickettsial Infections of Man. Philadelphia, J. B. Lippincott, 1965, pp. 474–512.
198. Dalldorf, G., and Sickles, G. M.: An unidentified, filtrable agent isolated from the feces of children with paralysis. Science *108*:61–62, 1948.
199. DaSilva, E. E., Winkler, M. T., and Pallansch, M. A.: Role of enterovirus 71 in acute flaccid paralysis after the eradication of poliovirus in Brazil. Emerg. Infect. Dis. *2*:231–233, 1996.
200. Davies, D. P., Hughes, C. A., MacVicar, J., et al.: Echovirus-11 infection in a special-care baby unit. Lancet *1*:96–97, 1979.
201. Davies, J. W., McDermott, A., and Severs, D.: Epidemic virus meningitis due to echo 9 virus in Newfoundland. Can. Med. Assoc. J. *79*:162–167, 1958.
202. De, L., Nottay, B., Yang, C. F., et al.: Identification of vaccine-related polioviruses by hybridization with specific RNA probes. J. Clin. Microbiol. *33*:562–571, 1995.
203. Dechamps, C., Peigue-Lafeuille, H. H., Laveran, H., et al.: Four cases of vesicular lesions in adults caused by enterovirus infections. J. Clin. Microbiol. *26*:2182–2183, 1988.
204. de Leeuw, N., Melchers, W. J. G., Balk, A. H. M. M., et al.: No evidence for persistent enterovirus infection in patients with end-stage idiopathic dilated cardiomyopathy. J. Infect. Dis. *178*:256–259, 1998.
205. DeQuadros, C. A., Andrus, J. K., Olive, J. M., et al.: Eradication of poliomyelitis: Progress in the Americas. Pediatr. Infect. Dis. J. *10*:222–229, 1991.
206. Dery, P., Marks, M. I., and Shapera, R.: Clinical manifestations of coxsackievirus infections in children. Am. J. Dis. Child. *128*:464–468, 1974.
207. Desa'neto, A., Bullington, J. D., Bullington, R. H., et al.: Coxsackie B5 heart disease: Demonstration of inferolateral wall myocardial necrosis. Am. J. Med. *68*:295–298, 1980.

208. Deseda-Tous, J., Bryatt, P. H., and Cherry, J. D.: Vesicular lesions in adults due to echovirus 11 infections. Arch. Dermatol. *113*:1705–1706, 1977.
209. Diedrich, S., Driesel, G., and Schreier, E.: Sequence comparison of echovirus type 30 isolates to other enteroviruses in the 5′ noncoding region. J. Med. Virol. *46*:148–152, 1995.
210. Dippe, S. E., Bennett, P. H., Miller, M., et al.: Lack of causal association between Coxsackie B4 virus infection and diabetes. Lancet *1*:1314–1318, 1975.
211. Domok, I., Balayan, M. S., Fayinka, O. A., et al.: Factors affecting the efficacy of live poliovirus vaccine in warm climates. Bull. World Health Organ. *51*:333–347, 1974.
212. Dömök, I., and Molnar, E.: An outbreak of meningoencephalomyocarditis among newborn infants during the epidemic of Bornholm disease in 1958 in Hungary. II. Aetiological findings. Ann. Pediatr. *194*:102–114, 1960.
213. Drebot, M. A., Nguan, C. Y., Campbell, J. J., et al.: Molecular epidemiology of enterovirus outbreaks in Canada during 1991–1992: Identification of echovirus 30 and coxsackievirus B1 strains by amplicon sequencing. J. Med. Virol. *44*:340–347, 1994.
214. Drew, J. H.: ECHO 11 virus outbreak in a nursery associated with myocarditis. Aust. Paediatr. J. *9*:90–95, 1973.
215. Drouhet, V.: Enterovirus infection and associated clinical symptoms in children. Ann. Inst. Pasteur *98*:562–568, 1960.
216. Druyts-Voets, E.: Epidemiological features of entero non-poliovirus isolations in Belgium 1980–94. Epidemiol. Infect. *119*:71–77, 1997.
217. Duff, M. F.: Hand-foot-and-mouth syndrome in humans: Coxsackie A10 infections in New Zealand. B. M. J. *2*:661–664, 1968.
218. Dunn, J. J., Romero, J. R., Wasserman, R., et al.: Stable enterovirus 5′ nontranslated region over a 7-year period in a patient with agammaglobulinemia and chronic infection. J. Infect. Dis. *182*:298–301, 2000.
219. Duxbury, A. E., and Warner, P.: Epidemiological and laboratory investigations on Bornholm disease in Adelaide, 1957. Med. J. Aust. *1*:518–523, 1958.
220. Duxbury, A. E., White, J., Lipscomb, B. M., et al.: Illness simulating paralytic poliomyelitis associated with Coxsackie group A type 4 virus infection. Med. J. Aust. *2*:709–711, 1961.
221. Dwyer, J. M., and Erlendsson, K.: Intraventricular gamma-globulin for the management of enterovirus encephalitis. Pediatr. Infect. Dis. J. *7*:S30–S33, 1988.
222. Dyer, J. R., Edis, R. H., and French, M. A.: Enterovirus associated neurological disease in an HIV-1 infected man. J. Neurovirol. *4*:569–571, 1998.
223. Eckert, G. L., Barron, A. L., and Karzon, D. T.: Aseptic meningitis due to ECHO virus type 18. Am. J. Dis. Child. *99*:1–3, 1960.
224. Eckert, H. L., Portnoy, B., Salvatore, M. A., et al.: Group B, Coxsackie virus infection in infants with acute lower respiratory disease. Pediatrics *39*:526–531, 1967.
225. Egger, D., Pasamontes, L., Ostermayer, M., et al.: Reverse transcription multiplex PCR for differentiation between polio- and enteroviruses from clinical and environmental samples. J. Clin. Microbiol. *33*:1442–1447, 1995.
226. Ehrnst, A., and Eriksson, M.: Epidemiological features of type 22 echovirus infection. Scand. J. Infect. Dis. *25*:275–281, 1993.
227. Eichenwald, H. F., Ababio, A., Arky, A. M., et al.: Epidemic diarrhea in premature and older infants caused by Echo virus type 18. J. A. M. A. *166*:1563–1566, 1958.
228. Eichenwald, H. F., and Kostevalov, O.: Immunologic responses of premature and full-term infants to infection with certain viruses. Pediatrics *25*:829–839, 1960.
229. Eilard, T., Kyllerman, M., Wennerblom, I., et al.: An outbreak of Coxsackie virus type B2 among neonates in an obstetrical ward. Acta Paediatr. Scand. *63*:103–107, 1974.
230. Elizan, T. S., Ajero-Froechlich, L., Fabiyi, A., et al.: Viral infection in pregnancy and congenital CNS malformations in man. Arch. Neurol. *20*:115–119, 1969.
231. Elliott, G. B., McAllister, J. E., and Alberta, C.: Fetal poliomyelitis. Am. J. Obstet. Gynecol. *72*:896–902, 1956.
232. Elvin-Lewis, M., and Melnick, J. L.: ECHO 11 viruses associated with aseptic meningitis. Proc. Soc. Exp. Biol. Med. *102*:647–649, 1959.
233. Enders, J. R., Weller, T. H., and Robbins, F. C.: Cultivation of the Lansing strain of poliomyelitis virus in cultures of various human embryonic tissues. Science *109*:85–87, 1949.
234. Erlendsson, K., Swartz, T., and Dwyer, J. M.: Successful reversal of echovirus encephalitis in X-linked hypogammaglobulinemia by intraventricular administration of immunoglobulin. N. Engl. J. Med. *312*:351–353, 1985.
235. Estes, M. L., and Rorke, L. B.: Liquefactive necrosis in Coxsackie B encephalitis. Arch. Pathol. Lab. Med. *110*:1090–1092, 1986.
236. Evans, A. D., and Waddington, E.: Hand, foot and mouth disease in South Wales, 1964. Br. J. Dermatol. *79*:309–317, 1967.
237. Evans, A. S., and Dick, E. C.: Acute pharyngitis and tonsillitis in University of Wisconsin students. J. A. M. A. *190*:699–708, 1964.
238. Farmer, K., MacArthur, B. A., and Clay, M. M.: A follow-up study of 15 cases of neonatal meningoencephalitis due to Coxsackie virus B5. J. Pediatr. *87*:568–571, 1975.
239. Farmer, K., and Patten, P. T.: An outbreak of Coxsackie B5 infection in a special care unit for newborn infants. N. Z. Med. J. *68*:86–89, 1968.
240. Faulkner, R. S., MacLeod, A. J., and Van Rooyen, C. E.: Virus meningitis: Seven cases in one family. Can. Med. Assoc. J. *77*:439–444, 1957.
241. Faulkner, R. S., and Van Rooyen, C. E.: Echovirus type 17 in the neonate. Can. Med. Assoc. J. *108*:878–882, 1973.
242. Fechner, R. E., Smith, M. G., and Middelkamp, J. N.: Coxsackie B virus infection of the newborn. Am. J. Pathol. *42*:493–505, 1963.
243. Feldman, A. M., and McNamara, D.: Myocarditis. N. Engl. J. Med. *343*:1388–1398, 2000.
244. Feldman, W., and Larke, R. P. B.: Acute cerebellar ataxia associated with the isolation of coxsackievirus type A9. Can. Med. Assoc. J. *106*:1104–1105, 1972.
245. Felici, A., Archetti, I., Russi, F., et al.: Contribution to the study of diseases caused by the Coxsackie B group of viruses in Italy. III. Arch. Ges. Virusforsch. *11*:592–598, 1961.
246. Felici, A., and Gregorig, B.: Contribution to the study of diseases in Italy caused by the Coxsackie B group of viruses. II. Epidemiological, clinical and virological data obtained in the course of a summer outbreak caused by Coxsackie B4 virus. Arch. Ges. Virusforsch. *9*:317–328, 1959.
247. Fenner, F.: Classification and nomenclature of viruses: Second report of the International Committee on Taxonomy of Viruses. Intervirology *7*:1–115, 1976.
248. Ferreira, A. G., Jr., Ferriera, S. M. A. G., Gomes, M. L. C., Linhares, A. C.: Enteroviruses as a possible cause of myocarditis, pericarditis, and dilated cardiomyopathy in Belem, Brazil. Braz. J. Med. Biol. Res. *28*:869–874, 1995.
249. Figueroa, J. P., Ashley, D., King, D., et al.: An outbreak of acute flaccid paralysis in Jamaica associated with echovirus type 22. J. Med. Virol. *29*:315–319, 1989.
250. Finsen, J.: Iagttagelser sygdomsforholdeme i Island (Afhandling for den medicinske doktorgrad ved Kobenhavns Universitet). Copenhagen, C. A. Reitzels, 1874, pp. 145–151.
251. Flewett, T. H.: Histological study of two cases of Coxsackie B virus pneumonia in children. J. Clin. Pathol. *18*:743–746, 1965.
252. Flewett, T. H., Warin, R. P., and Clarke, S. K. R.: Hand, foot, and mouth disease associated with Coxsackie A5 virus. J. Clin. Pathol. *16*:53–55, 1963.
253. Flugsrud, L., Abrahamsen, A. M., and Lahelle, O.: An outbreak of aseptic meningitis associated with a virus related to ECHO type 9. Acta Med. Scand. *112*:129–135, 1958.
254. Foley, J. F., Chin, T. D. Y., and Gravelle, C. R.: Paralytic disease due to infection with echo virus type 9. N. Engl. J. Med. *260*:924–926, 1959.
255. Forbes, J. A.: Meningitis in Melbourne due to E.C.H.O. virus. Part I. Clinical aspects. Med. J. Aust. *1*:246–248, 1958.
256. Forman, M. L., and Cherry, J. D.: Enanthems associated with uncommon viral syndromes. Pediatrics *41*:873–882, 1968.
257. Förster, W., Bialasiewicz, A. A., and Busse, H.: Coxsackievirus B3-associated panuveitis. Br. J. Ophthalmol. *77*:182–183, 1993.
258. Fox, J. P.: Epidemiological aspects of Coxsackie and ECHO virus infections in tropical areas. Am. J. Public Health *54*:1134–1142, 1964.
259. Fox, J. P.: Eradication of poliomyelitis in the United States: A commentary on the Salk reviews. Rev. Infect. Dis. *2*:277–281, 1980.
260. Fox, J. P., and Hall, C. E.: Viruses in families. Littleton, PSG Publishing, 1980, pp. 190–195.
261. Fox, S. A., Finklestone, E., Robbins, P. D., et al.: Search for persistent enterovirus infection of muscle in inflammatory myopathies. J. Neurol. Sci. *125*:70–76, 1994.
262. Foy, H. M., Cooney, M. K., Maletzky, A. J., et al.: Incidence and etiology of pneumonia, croup and bronchiolitis in preschool children belonging to a prepaid medical care group over a four-year period. Am. J. Epidemiol. *97*:80–92, 1973.
263. Freedman, P. S.: Echovirus 11 infection and intrauterine death. Lancet *1*:96–97, 1979.
264. Freij, L., Norrby, R., and Olsson, B.: A small outbreak of Coxsackie B5 infection with two cases of cardiac involvement and orchitis followed by testicular atrophy. Acta Med. Scand. *187*:177–181, 1970.
265. Frisk, G., and Diderholm, H.: Increased frequency of Coxsackie B virus IgM in women with spontaneous abortion. J. Infect. *24*:141–145, 1992.
266. Frisk, G., and Diderholm, H.: Antibody responses to different strains of Coxsackie B4 virus in patients with newly diagnosed type I diabetes mellitus or aseptic meningitis. J. Infect. *34*:205–210, 1997.
267. Froeschle, J. E., Nahmias, A. J., Feorino, P. M., et al.: Hand, foot, and mouth disease (Coxsackie A16) in Atlanta. Am. J. Dis. Child. *114*:278–283, 1967.
268. Frothingham, T. E.: Echo virus type 9 associated with three cases simulating meningococcemia. N. Engl. J. Med. *259*:484–485, 1958.
269. Fujioka, S., Koide, H., Kitaura, Y., et al.: Molecular detection and differentiation of enteroviruses in endomyocardial biopsies and pericardial effusions from dilated cardiomyopathy and myocarditis. Am. Heart J. *131*:760–765, 1996.
270. Fulginiti, V. A.: The problems of poliovirus immunization. Hosp. Pract. *15*:61–67, 1980.
271. Galama, J. M. D.: Enteroviral infections in the immunocompromised host. Rev. Med. Microbiol. *8*:33–40, 1997.

272. Galama, J. M. D., DeLeeuw, N., Wittebol, S., et al.: Prolonged enteroviral infection in a patient who developed pericarditis and heart failure after bone marrow transplantation. Clin. Infect. Dis. *22*:1004–1008, 1996.
273. Galama, J. M. D., Vogels, M. T. E., Jansen, G. H., et al.: Antibodies against enteroviruses in intravenous Ig preparations: Great variation in titres and poor correlation with the incidence of circulating serotypes. J. Med. Virol. *53*:273–276, 1997.
274. Gallacher, K., Ghosh, K., Patel, A., et al.: An outbreak of echovirus type 4 infections and its implications for diagnosis and management in general practice. J. Infect. *26*:321–324, 1993.
275. Galpine, J. F., Clayton, T. M., Ardley, J., et al.: Outbreak of aseptic meningitis with exanthem. B. M. J. *1*:319–321, 1958.
276. Gamble, D. R., Kinsley, M. L., FitzGerald, M. G., et al.: Viral antibodies in diabetes mellitus. B. M. J. *3*:627–630, 1969.
277. Gamble, D. R., and Taylor, K. W.: Seasonal incidence of diabetes mellitus. B. M. J. *3*:631–633, 1969.
278. Garnett, D. G., Burlingham, A., and Van Zwanenberg, D.: Outbreak of aseptic meningitis of virus origin in East Suffolk. Lancet *1*:500–502, 1957.
279. Gary, H. (Respiratory and Enteric Viruses Branch, Centers for Disease Control and Prevention): Personal communication. 1996.
280. Gaudin, O.-G., Pozzetto, B., Aouni, M., et al.: Detection of neutralizing IgM antibodies in the diagnosis of enterovirus infections. J. Med. Virol. *28*:200–205, 1989.
281. Gauntt, C. J., Arizpe, H. M., Higdon, A. L., et al.: Molecular mimicry, anti–coxsackievirus B3 neutralizing monoclonal antibodies, and myocarditis. J. Immunol. *154*:2983–2995, 1995.
282. Gauntt, C. J., Gomez, P. T., Grant, J. A., et al.: Characterization and myocarditic capabilities of coxsackievirus B3 variants in selected mouse strains. J. Virol. *52*:598–605, 1984.
283. Gauntt, C. J., Gudvangen, R. J., Brans, Y. W., et al.: Coxsackievirus group B antibodies in the ventricular fluid of infants with severe anatomic defects in the central nervous system. Pediatrics *76*:64–68, 1985.
284. Gauntt, C. J., Higdon, A. L., Arizpe, H. M., et al.: Epitopes shared between coxsackievirus B3 (CVB3) and normal heart tissue contribute to CVB3-induced murine myocarditis. Clin. Immunol. Immunopathol. *68*:129–134, 1993.
285. Gauntt, C. J., Higdon, A., Bowers, D., et al.: What lessons can be learned from animal model studies in viral heart disease? Scand. J. Infect. Dis. *88*(Suppl.):49–65, 1993.
286. Gear, J.: Coxsackie virus infections in southern Africa. Yale J. Biol. Med. *34*:289–303, 1961/1962.
287. Gebhard, J. R., Perry, C. M., Harkins, S., et al.: Coxsackievirus B3–induced myocarditis: Perforin exacerbates disease, but plays no detectable role in virus clearance. Am. J. Pathol. *153*:417–428, 1998.
288. Gear, J. H. S.: Coxsackie virus infections of the newborn. Prog. Med. Virol. *1*:106–121, 1958.
289. Gelfand, H. M.: The occurrence in nature of the Coxsackie and ECHO viruses. Progr. Med. Virol. *3*:193–244, 1961.
290. Gelfand, H. M., Holguin, A. H., Marchetti, G. E., et al.: A continuing surveillance of enterovirus infections in healthy children in six United States cities. I. Viruses isolated during 1960 and 1961. Am. J. Hyg. *78*:358–375, 1963.
291. Georgieff, M. K., Johnson, D. E., Thompson, T. R., et al.: Fulminant hepatic necrosis in an infant with perinatally acquired echovirus 21 infection. Pediatr. Infect. Dis. J. *6*:71–73, 1987.
292. German, L. J., McCracken, A. W., and Wilkie, K. M.: Outbreak of febrile illness associated with E. C. H. O. virus type 5 in a maternity unit in Singapore. B. M. J. *1*:742–744, 1968.
293. Gilbert, G. L., Dickson, K. E., Waters, M. J., et al.: Outbreak of enterovirus 71 infection in Victoria, Australia, with a high incidence of neurologic involvement. Pediatr. Infect. Dis. J. *7*:484–488, 1988.
294. Gillett, R. L.: Acute benign pericarditis and the Coxsackie viruses. N. Engl. J. Med. *261*:838–845, 1959.
295. Ginsberg, A. H., Gale, M. J., Jr., Rose, L. M., et al.: T-cell alterations in late postpoliomyelitis. Arch. Neurol. *46*:497–501, 1989.
296. Glasgow, L. A., and Balduzzi, P.: Isolation of Coxsackie virus group A, type 4, from a patient with hemolytic-uremic syndrome. N. Engl. J. Med. *273*:754–756, 1965.
297. Glezen, W. P., Loda, F. A., Clyde, W. A., Jr., et al.: Epidemiologic patterns of acute lower respiratory disease of children in a pediatric group practice. J. Pediatr. *78*:397–406, 1971.
298. Glimaker, M., Samuelson, A., Magnius, L., et al.: Early diagnosis of enteroviral meningitis by detection of specific IgM antibodies with a solid-phase reverse immunosorbent test (SPRIST) and μ-capture EIA. J. Med. Virol. *36*:193–201, 1992.
299. Glimaker, M., Ehrnst, A., Magnius, L., et al.: Early diagnosis of enteroviral meningitis by a solid-phase reverse immunosorbent test and virus isolation. Scand. J. Infect. Dis. *22*:519–526, 1990.
300. Godeny, E. K., and Gauntt, C. J.: Involvement of natural killer cells in coxsackievirus B3–induced murine myocarditis. J. Immunol. *137*: 1695–1702, 1986.
301. Godtfredsen, A., and Hansen, B.: A case of mild paralytic disease due to Echo virus type 11. Acta Pathol. Microbiol. Scand. *53*:111–116, 1961.
302. Goh, K. T., Doraisingham, S., Tan, J. L., et al.: An outbreak of hand, foot, and mouth disease in Singapore. Bull. World Health Organ. *60*:965–969, 1982.
303. Goh, K. T., Ooi, P. L., Miyamura, K., et al.: Acute haemorrhagic conjunctivitis: Seroepidemiology of coxsackievirus A24 variant and enterovirus 70 in Singapore. J. Med. Virol. *31*:245–247, 1990.
304. Gohd, R. S., and Faigel, H. C.: Hand-foot-and-mouth disease resembling measles: A life-threatening disease: Case report. Pediatrics *37*:644–648, 1966.
305. Gohd, R. S., and Gordon, W.: Endemic nature of coxsackievirus A-16. Bacteriol. Proc. *108*:152, 1967.
306. Gold, E., Carver, D. H., Heinberg, H., et al.: Viral infection: A possible cause of sudden, unexpected death in infants. N. Engl. J. Med. *264*:53–60, 1961.
307. Goldwater, P. N.: Immunoglobulin M capture immunoassay in investigation of coxsackievirus B5 and B6 outbreaks in South Australia. J. Clin. Microbiol. *33*:1628–1631, 1995.
308. Goldwater, P. N., and Laws, J.: Echovirus 19 outbreak in Auckland, 1975–76. N. Z. Med. J. *597*:319–322, 1977.
309. Gondo, K., Kusuhara, K., Take, H., et al.: Echovirus type 9 epidemic in Kagoshima, southern Japan: Seroepidemiology and clinical observation of aseptic meningitis. Pediatr. Infect. Dis. J. *14*:787–791, 1995.
310. Gong, C. M., Ho, D. W. T., Field, P. R., et al.: Immunoglobulin responses to echovirus type 11 by enzyme linked immunosorbent assay: Single-serum diagnosis of acute infection by specific IgM antibody. J. Virol. Methods *9*:209–221, 1984.
311. Goodwin, M. H., Jr., Love, G. J., Mackel, D. C., et al.: Observations on the association of enteric viruses and bacteria with diarrhea. Am. J. Trop. Med. Hyg. *16*:178–185, 1967.
312. Gordon, R. B., Lennette, E. H., and Sandrock, R. S.: The varied clinical manifestations of Coxsackie virus infections: Observations and comments on an outbreak in California. Arch. Intern. Med. *103*:63–75, 1959.
313. Gorgievski-Hrisoho, M., Schumacher, J. D., Vilimomovic, N., et al.: Detection by PCR of enteroviruses in cerebrospinal fluid during a summer outbreak of aseptic meningitis in Switzerland. J. Clin. Microbiol. *36*:2408–2412, 1998.
314. Graber, D., Fossoud, C., Grouteau, E., et al.: Acute transverse myelitis and Coxsackie A9 virus infection. Pediatr. Infect. Dis. J. *13*:77, 1994.
315. Grangeot-Keros, L., Broyer, M., Briand, E., et al.: Enterovirus in sudden unexpected deaths in infants. Pediatr. Infect. Dis. J. *15*:123–128, 1996.
316. Gravelle, C. R., Noble, G. R., Feltz, E. T., et al.: An epidemic of echovirus type 30 meningitis in an Arctic community. Am. J. Epidemiol. *99*:368–374, 1974.
317. Green, I. J., Hung, T. P., and Sung, S. M.: Neurologic complications with elevated antibody titer after acute hemorrhagic conjunctivitis. Am. J. Ophthalmol. *80*:832–834, 1975.
318. Gregg, I.: The role of viral infection in asthma and bronchitis. *In* Proudfoot, A. T. (ed.): Symposium on Viral Diseases. Edinburgh, Royal College of Physicians, 1975, pp. 82–98.
319. Griffiths, P. D., Hannington, G., and Booth, J. C.: Coxsackie B virus infections and myocardial infarction. Lancet *1*:1387–1389, 1980.
320. Grist, N. R.: Further studies of Coxsackie A7 virus infection in the west of Scotland. Lancet *2*:261–263, 1965.
321. Grist, N. R., and Bell, E. J.: Coxsackie virus heart disease. B. M. J. *3*:556, 1968.
322. Grist, N. R., and Bell, E. J.: Coxsackie viruses and the heart. Am. Heart J. *77*:295–300, 1969.
323. Grist, N. R., and Bell, E. J.: Enteroviral etiology of the paralytic poliomyelitis syndrome: Studies before and after vaccination. Arch. Environ. Health *21*:382–387, 1970.
324. Grist, N. R., and Bell, E. J.: A six-year study of Coxsackie virus B infections in heart disease. J. Hyg. *73*:165–172, 1974.
325. Grist, N. R., and Bell, E. J.: Paralytic poliomyelitis and nonpolio enteroviruses: Studies in Scotland. Rev. Infect. Dis. *6*(Suppl.):385–386, 1984.
326. Grist, N. R., Bell, E. J., and Assaad, F.: Enteroviruses in human disease. Prog. Med. Virol. *24*:114–157, 1978.
327. Grose, C., and Horwitz, M. S.: Characterization of an enterovirus associated with acute infectious lymphocytosis. J. Gen. Virol. *30*:347–355, 1976.
328. Guidotti, M. B.: An outbreak of skin rash by echovirus 25 in an infant home. J. Infect. *6*:67–70, 1983.
329. Guthrie, N.: Coxsackie B5 meningitis: Report of an outbreak in a high school football squad. J. Tenn. State Med. Assoc. *55*:355–356, 1962.
330. Haamann, P., Kessel, L., and Larsen, M.: Monofocal outer retinitis associated with hand, foot, and mouth disease caused by coxsackievirus. Am. J. Ophthalmol. *129*:552–553, 2000.
331. Habel, K., Silverberg, R. J., and Shelokov, A.: Isolation of enteric viruses from cases of aseptic meningitis. Ann. N. Y. Acad. Sci. *67*:223–229, 1957.
332. Haddad, J., Gut, J. P., Wendling, M. J., et al.: Enterovirus infections in neonates: A retrospective study of 21 cases. Eur. J. Med. *2*:209–214, 1993.
333. Hadfield, M. G., Seidlin, M., Houff, S. A., et al.: Echovirus meningomyeloencephalitis with administration of intraventricular immunoglobulin. J. Neuropathol. Exp. Neurol. *44*:520–529, 1985.

334. Halfon, N., and Spector, S. A.: Fatal echovirus type 11 infections. Am. J. Dis. Child. *135*:1017–1020, 1981.
335. Hall, C. B., Cherry, J. D., Hatch, M. H., et al.: The return of Boston exanthem. Am. J. Dis. Child. *131*:323–326, 1977.
336. Hall, C. E., Cooney, M. K., and Fox, J. P.: The Seattle virus watch program. I. Infection and illness experience of virus watch families during a communitywide epidemic of echovirus type 30 aseptic meningitis. Am. J. Public Health *60*:1456–1465, 1970.
337. Halonen, P., Rocha, E., Hierholzer, J., et al.: Detection of enteroviruses and rhinoviruses in clinical specimens by PCR and liquid-phase hybridization. J. Clin. Microbiol. *33*:648–653, 1995.
338. Hammon, W. M., Yohn, D. S., Ludwig, E. H., et al.: A study of certain nonpoliomyelitis and poliomyelitis enterovirus infections: Clinical and serologic associations. J. A. M. A. *167*:727–734, 1958.
339. Hannaeus, G.: Dissertation. Copenhagen, 1735.
340. Hanneman, R. E.: Personal communication, 1996.
341. Hanninen, P., and Pohjonen, R.: Echovirus type 6 meningitis: Clinical and virological observations during an epidemic in Turku in 1968. Scand. J. Infect. Dis. *3*:121–125, 1971.
342. Hanson, L. A., Lundgren, S., Lycke, E., et al.: Clinical and serological observations in cases of Coxsackie B3 infections in early infancy. Acta Paediatr. Scand. *55*:577–583, 1966.
343. Harjulehto, T., Aro, T., Hovi, T., et al.: Congenital malformations and oral poliovirus vaccination during pregnancy. Lancet *1*:771–772, 1989.
344. Härkönen, T., Puolakkainen, M., Sarvas, M., et al.: Picornavirus proteins share antigenic determinants with heat shock proteins 60/65. J. Med. Virol. *62*:383–391, 2000.
345. Hart, E. W., Brunton, G. B., Taylor, C. E. D., et al.: Infection of newborn babies with ECHO virus type 5. Lancet *2*:402, 1962.
346. Hatch, M. H., and Marchetti, G. E.: Isolation of echoviruses with human embryonic lung fibroblast cells. Appl. Microbiol. *22*:736–737, 1971.
347. Haynes, R. E., Cramblett, H. G., Hilty, M. D., et al.: Echo virus type 3 infections in children: Clinical and laboratory studies. J. Pediatr. *80*:589–595, 1972.
348. Haynes, R. E., Cramblett, H. G., and Kronfol, H. J.: Echovirus 9 meningoencephalitis in infants and children. J. A. M. A. *208*:1657–1660, 1969.
349. Hayward, J. C., Gillespie, S. M., Kaplan, K. M., et al.: Outbreak of poliomyelitis-like paralysis associated with enterovirus 71. Pediatr. Infect. Dis. J. *8*:611–616, 1989.
350. Heathfield, K. W. G., Pilsworth, R., Wall, B. J., et al.: Coxsackie B5 infections in Essex, 1965, with particular reference to the nervous system. Q. J. Med. *144*:579–595, 1967.
351. Hedlung, P., Lycke, E., and Tibblin, G.: The association of acute benign pericarditis in adults with Coxsackie B5 virus infection. Arch. Ges. Virusforsch. *13*:156–159, 1963.
352. Heim, A., Grumbach, I., Hake, S., et al.: Enterovirus heart disease of adults: A persistent, limited organ infection in the presence of neutralizing antibodies. J. Med. Virol. *53*:196–204, 1997.
353. Heinberg, H., Gold, E., and Robbins, F. C.: Differences in interferon content in tissues of mice of various ages infected with Coxsackie B1 virus. Proc. Soc. Exp. Biol. Med. *115*:947–953, 1964.
354. Helfand, R. F., Gary, H. E., Jr., Freeman, C. V., et al.: Serologic evidence of an association between enteroviruses and the onset of type 1 diabetes mellitus. J. Infect. Dis. *172*:1206–1211, 1995.
355. Helfand, R. F., Khan, A. S., Pallansch, M. A., et al.: Echovirus 30 infection and aseptic meningitis in parents of children attending a child care center. J. Infect. Dis. *169*:1133–1137, 1994.
356. Helin, M., Savola, J., and Lapinleimu, K.: Cardiac manifestations during a Coxsackie B5 epidemic. B. M. J. *3*:97–99, 1968.
357. Henke, A., Huber, S., Stelzner, A., et al.: The role of CD8+ T lymphocytes in coxsackievirus B3–induced myocarditis. J. Virol. *69*:6720–6728, 1995.
358. Hercík, L., Huml, M., Mimra, J., et al.: Epidemien der respirationstrakterkrankungen bei neugeborenen durch ECHO 11-virus. Zentralbl. Bakteriol. *213*:18–27, 1970.
359. Herrmann, E. C., Jr.: Experience in providing a viral diagnostic laboratory compatible with medical practice. Mayo Clin. Proc. *42*:112–123, 1967.
360. Herskowitz, A., Beisel, K. W., Wolfgram, L. J., et al.: Coxsackievirus B3 murine myocarditis: Wide pathologic spectrum in genetically defined inbred strains. Hum. Pathol. *16*:671–673, 1985.
361. Hertel, N. T., Pedersen, F. K., and Heilmann, C.: Coxsackie B3 virus encephalitis in a patient with agammaglobulinemia. Eur. J. Pediatr. *148*:642–643, 1989.
362. Hierholzer, J. C., and Farris, W. A.: Follow-up of children infected in a coxsackievirus B-3 and B-4 outbreak: No evidence of diabetes mellitus. J. Infect. Dis. *129*:741–746, 1974.
363. Hierholzer, J. C., Killiard, K. A., and Esposito, J. J.: Serosurvey for "acute hemorrhagic conjunctivitis" virus (enterovirus 70) antibodies in the southeastern United States, with review of the literature and some epidemiologic implications. Am. J. Epidemiol. *102*:533–544, 1975.
364. Higgins, P. G., and Crow, K. D.: Recurrent Kaposi's varicelliform eruption in Darier's disease. Br. J. Dermatol. *88*:391–394, 1973.
365. Higgins, P. G., Ellis, E. M., Boston, D. G., et al.: Hand, foot and mouth disease, 1963–64: A study of cases and family contacts. Mo. Bull. Ministry Health (London) *24*:38–45, 1965.
366. Higgins, P. G., and Warin, R. P.: Hand, foot, and mouth disease: A clinically recognizable virus infection seen mainly in children. Clin. Pediatr. (Phila.) *6*:373–376, 1967.
367. Hiltunen, M., Hyöty, H., Knip, M., et al.: Islet cell antibody seroconversion in children is temporally associated with enterovirus infections. Childhood Diabetes in Finland (DiMe) Study Group. J. Infect. Dis. *175*:554–560, 1997.
368. Hinman, A. R., Koplan, J. P., Orenstein, W. A., et al.: Live or inactivated poliomyelitis vaccine: An analysis of benefits and risks. Am. J. Public Health *78*:291–295, 1988.
369. Ho, M., Chen, E. R., Hsu, K. H., et al.: An epidemic of enterovirus 71 infection in Taiwan. Taiwan Enterovirus Epidemic Working Group. N. Engl. J. Med. *341*:929–935, 1999.
370. Hober, D., Andreoletti, L., Shen, L., et al.: Coxsackievirus B3–induced chronic myocarditis in mouse: Use of whole blood culture to study the activation of TNF alpha–producing cells. Microbiol. Immunol. *40*:837–845, 1996.
371. Hober, D., Chehadeh, W., Bouzidi, A., et al.: Antibody-dependent enhancement of coxsackievirus B4 infectivity of human peripheral blood mononuclear cells results in increased interferon-alpha synthesis. J. Infect. Dis. *184*:1098–1108, 2001.
372. Hooft, C., Nihoul, E., Lambert, Y., et al.: Clinical findings during an Echo virus type 13 endemic infection. Helv. Paediatr. Acta *18*:230–239, 1963.
373. Horn, M. E. C., Brain, E., Gregg, I., et al.: Respiratory viral infection in childhood: A survey in general practice, Roehampton 1967–1972. J. Hyg. (Camb.) *74*:157–168, 1975.
374. Horn, P.: Poliomyelitis in pregnancy: A 20-year report from Los Angeles County, California. Obstet. Gynecol. *6*:121–137, 1955.
375. Horstmann, D. M.: The new ECHO viruses and their role in human disease. Arch. Intern. Med. *102*:155–162, 1958.
376. Horstmann, D. M.: Viral exanthems and enanthems. Pediatrics *41*:867–870, 1968.
377. Horstmann, D. M.: The poliomyelitis story: A scientific hegira. Yale J. Biol. Med. *58*:79–90, 1985.
378. Horstmann, D. M., Emmons, J., Gimpel, L., et al.: Enterovirus surveillance following a community-wide oral poliovirus vaccination program: A seven-year study. Am. J. Epidemiol. *97*:173–186, 1973.
379. Horwitz, M. S., and Moore, G. T.: Acute infectious lymphocytosis: An etiologic and epidemiologic study of an outbreak. N. Engl. J. Med. *279*:399–404, 1968.
380. Hosier, D. M., and Newton, W. A., Jr.: Serious Coxsackie infection in infants and children: Myocarditis, meningoencephalitis and hepatitis. Am. J. Dis. Child. *96*:251–267, 1958.
381. Hosoya, M., Sato, M., Honzumi, K., et al.: Association of nonpolio enteroviral infection in the central nervous system of children with febrile seizures. Pediatrics *107*:E12, 2001.
382. Howe, H. A., and Wilson, J. L.: Poliomyelitis. *In* Rivers, T. M., and Horsfall, F. L., Jr. (eds.): Viral and Rickettsial Infections of Man. Philadelphia, J. B. Lippincott, 1959, pp. 432–518.
383. Howes, D. W.: Studies of coxsackieviruses: Comparison of age-susceptibility relationships in mice. Aust. J. Exp. Biol. *32*:253–264, 1954.
384. Howlett, J. G., Somlo, F., and Kalz, F.: A new syndrome of parotitis with herpangina caused by the Coxsackie virus. Can. Med. Assoc. *77*:5–7, 1957.
385. Huang, F. L., Jan, S. L., Chen, P. Y., et al.: Left ventricular dysfunction in children with fulminant enterovirus 71 infection: An evaluation of the clinical course. Clin. Infect. Dis. *34*:1020–1024, 2002.
386. Huang, T. W., and Wiegenstein, L. M.: Mesangiolytic glomerulonephritis in an infant with immune deficiency and echovirus infection. Arch. Pathol. Lab. Med. *101*:125–128, 1977.
387. Huber, S. A., and Lodge, P. A.: Coxsackievirus B-3 myocarditis in BALB/c mice. Evidence for autoimmunity to myocyte antigens. Am. J. Pathol. *116*:21–29, 1984.
388. Huber, S. A., Mortensen, A., and Moulton, G.: Modulation of cytokine expression by CD4+ T cells during coxsackievirus B3 infections of BALB/c mice initiated by cells expressing the gamma delta + T-cell receptor. J. Virol. *70*:3039–3044, 1996.
389. Huebner, R. J., Risser, J. A., Bell, J. A., et al.: Epidemic pleurodynia in Texas: A study of 22 cases. N. Engl. J. Med. *248*:267–274, 1953.
390. Hughes, J. R., Wilfert, C. M., Moore, M., et al.: Echovirus 14 infection associated with fatal neonatal hepatic necrosis. Am. J. Dis. Child. *123*:61–67, 1972.
391. Hughes, R. O., and Roberts, C.: Hand, foot, and mouth disease associated with Coxsackie A9 virus. Lancet *2*:751–752, 1972.
392. Hull, H. F.: Progress towards global polio eradication. Dev. Biol. *105*:3–7, 2001.
393. Hull, H. F., Ward, N. A., Hull, B. P., et al.: Paralytic poliomyelitis: Seasoned strategies, disappearing disease. Lancet *343*:1331–1337, 1994.
394. Hurley, R., Norman, A. P., and Pryse-Davies, J.: Massive pulmonary hemorrhage in the newborn associated with Coxsackie B virus infection. B. M. J. *3*:636–637, 1969.
395. Hurst, N. P., Martynoga, A. G., Nuki, G., et al.: Coxsackie B infection and arthritis. B. M. J. *286*:605–607, 1983.
396. Hyöty, H., Huupponen, T., Kotola, L., et al.: Humoral immunity against viral antigens in type 1 diabetes: Altered IgA-class immune response

against Coxsackie B4 virus. Acta Pathol. Microbiol. Immunol. Scand. *94*:83–88, 1986.
397. Hyypiä, T.: Identification of human picornaviruses by nucleic acid probes. Mol. Cell. Probes *3*:329–343, 1989.
398. Hyypiä, T., Auvinen, P., and Maaronen, M.: Polymerase chain reaction for human picornaviruses. J. Gen. Virol. *70*:3261–3268, 1989.
399. Hyypiä, T., Hovi, T., Knowles, N. J., et al.: Classification of enteroviruses based on molecular and biological properties. J. Gen. Virol. *78*:1–11, 1997.
400. Ikeda, R. M., Kondrack, S. F., Drabkin, P. D., et al.: Pleurodynia among football players at a high school: An outbreak associated with coxsackievirus B1. J. A. M. A. *270*:2205–2206, 1993.
401. Institute of Medicine: An Evaluation of Poliomyelitis Vaccine Policy Options. IOM Publication 88–04. Washington, D.C., National Academy of Sciences, 1988.
402. Irvine, D. H., Irvine, A. B. H., and Gardner, P. S.: Outbreak of E. C. H. O. virus type 30 in a general practice. B. M. J. *4*:774–776, 1967.
403. Isaacs, D., Dobson, S. R. M., Wilkinson, A. R., et al.: Conservative management of an echovirus 11 outbreak in a neonatal unit. Lancet *1*:543–545, 1989.
404. Isacsohn, M., Eidelman, A. I., Kaplan, M., et al.: Neonatal coxsackievirus group B infections: Experience of a single department of neonatology. Isr. J. Med. Sci. *30*:371–374, 1994.
405. Ishiko, H., Shimada, Y., Yonaha, M., et al.: Molecular diagnosis of human enteroviruses by phylogeny-based classification by use of the VP4 sequence. J. Infect. Dis. *185*:744–754, 2002.
406. Ishiko, H., Takeda, N., Miyamura, K., et al.: Phylogenetic analysis of a coxsackievirus A24 variant: The most recent worldwide pandemic was caused by progenies of a virus prevalent around 1981. Virology *187*:748–759, 1992.
407. Ishimaru, Y., Nakano, S., Yamaoka, K., et al.: Outbreaks of hand, foot, and mouth disease by enterovirus 71: High incidence of complication disorders of central nervous system. Arch. Dis. Child. *55*:583–588, 1980.
408. Itagaki, A., Ishihara, J., Mochida, K., et al.: A clustering outbreak of hand, foot, and mouth disease caused by Coxsackie virus A10. Microbiol. Immunol. *27*:929–935, 1983.
409. Jack, I., Grutzner, J., Gray, N., et al.: A survey of prenatal virus disease in Melbourne, July 21, 1967. Personal communication.
410. Jack, I., and Townley, R. R. W.: Acute aseptic myocarditis of newborn infants, due to Coxsackie viruses. Med. J. Aust. *2*:265–268, 1961.
411. Jackson, A. L.: A clinical study of the Landry-Guillain-Barré syndrome with reference to aetiology, including the role of Coxsackie virus infections. S. Afr. J. Lab. Clin. Med. *7*:121–137, 1961.
412. Jahn, C. L., and Cherry, J. D.: Mild neonatal illness associated with heavy enterovirus infection. N. Engl. J. Med. *274*:394–395, 1966.
413. Jahn, C. L., Felton, O. L., and Cherry, J. D.: Coxsackie B1 pneumonia in an adult. J. A. M. A. *189*:236–237, 1964.
414. James, W. D., Odom, R. B., and Hatch, M. H.: Gianotti-Crosti–like eruption associated with coxsackievirus A16 infection. J. Am. Acad. Dermatol. *6*:862–866, 1982.
415. Jamieson, W. M., Kerr, M., and Sommerville, R. G.: Echo type-9 meningitis in east Scotland. Lancet *1*:581–583, 1958.
416. Jantausch, B. A., Luban, N. L. C., Duffy, L., et al.: Maternal plasma transfusion in the treatment of disseminated neonatal echovirus 11 infection. Pediatr. Infect. Dis. J. *14*:154–155, 1995.
417. Jarvis, W. R., and Tucker, G.: Echovirus type 7 meningitis in young children. Am. J. Dis. Child. *135*:1009–1012, 1981.
418. Javett, S. N., Heymann, S., Mundel, B., et al.: Myocarditis in the newborn infant. J. Pediatr. *48*:1–22, 1956.
419. Jehn, U. W., and Fink, M. K.: Myositis, myoglobinemia, and myoglobinuria associated with enterovirus Echo 9 infection. Arch. Neurol. *37*:457–458, 1980.
420. Jenista, J. A., Powell, K. R., and Menegus, M. A.: Epidemiology of neonatal enterovirus infection. J. Pediatr. *104*:685–690, 1984.
421. Jhala, C. I., Draper, J., and Walcher, D. N.: Aseptic meningitis syndrome due to virus Echo type 23. Am. J. Dis. Child. *102*:868–870, 1961.
422. John, T. J., Pandian, R., Gadomski, A., et al.: Control of poliomyelitis by pulse immunisation in Vellore, India. B. M. J. *286*:31–32, 1983.
423. Johnson, D. A., and Eger, A. W.: Myelitis associated with an echovirus. J. A. M. A. *201*:637–638, 1967.
424. Johnson, I., Hammond, G. W., and Verma, M. R.: Nosocomial Coxsackie B4 virus infections in two chronic-care pediatric neurological wards. J. Infect. Dis. *151*:1153–1156, 1985.
425. Johnson, J. F., and Stimson, P. M.: Clinical poliomyelitis in the early neonatal period. J. Pediatr. *40*:733–737, 1956.
426. Johnson, K. M., Bloom, H. H., Forsyth, B., et al.: Relative role of identifiable agents in respiratory disease. II. The role of enteroviruses in respiratory disease. Am. Rev. Respir. Dis. *88*:240–245, 1962.
427. Johnson, R. T.: Late progression of poliomyelitis paralysis: Discussion of pathogenesis. Rev. Infect. Dis. *6*(Suppl.):568–570, 1984.
428. Johnson, R. T., Portnoy, B., Rogers, N. G., et al.: Acute benign pericarditis: Virologic study of 34 patients. Arch. Intern. Med. *108*:823–832, 1961.
429. Johnson, R. T., Shuey, H. E., and Buescher, E. L.: Epidemic central nervous system disease of mixed enterovirus etiology. I/II. Clinical and epidemiologic description. Am. J. Hyg. *71*:321–330, 331–341, 1960.
430. Johnsson, T., and Lundmark, C.: A hispathological study of Coxsackie virus infections in mice. Arch. Ges. Virusforsch. *6*:262–281, 1955.
431. Johnston, J. M., and Overall, J. C., Jr.: Intravenous immunoglobulin in disseminated neonatal echovirus 11 infection. Pediatr. Infect. Dis. J. *8*:254–256, 1989.
432. Joncas, J. H., Podoski, M. O., and Pavilanis, V.: Rash associated with Coxsackie A9 infection. Can. Med. Assoc. J. *95*:372–373, 1966.
433. Jones, M. J., Kolb, M., Votava, H. J., et al.: Intrauterine echovirus type 11 infection. Mayo Clin. Proc. *55*:509–512, 1980.
434. Josselson, J., Pula, T., and Sadler, J. H.: Acute rhabdomyolysis associated with an echovirus 9 infection. Arch. Intern. Med. *140*:1671–1672, 1980.
435. Judelsohn, R.: Changing the US polio immunization schedule would be bad public health policy. Pediatrics *98*:115–116, 1996.
436. Juhela, S., Hyöty, H., Hinkkanen, A., et al.: T cell responses to enterovirus antigens and to beta-cell autoantigens in unaffected children positive for IDDM-associated autoantibodies. J. Autoimmun. *12*:269–278, 1999.
437. Juhela, S., Hyöty, H., Roivainen, M., et al.: T-cell responses to enterovirus antigens in children with type 1 diabetes. Diabetes *49*:1308–1313, 2000.
438. Kahlmeter, O.: Clinical aspects of Echo viruses. Ciba Found. Symp. *7*:24–36, 1959.
439. Kandolf, R., Klingel, K., Zell, R., et al.: Molecular mechanisms in the pathogenesis of enteroviral heart disease: Acute and persistent infections. Clin. Immunol. Immunopathol. *68*:153–158, 1993.
440. Kang, Y., Chatterjee, N. K., Nodwell, M. J., et al.: Complete nucleotide sequence of a strain of Coxsackie B4 virus of human origin that induces diabetes in mice and its comparison with nondiabetogenic Coxsackie B4 JBV strain. J. Med. Virol. *44*:353–361, 1994.
441. Kantor, F. S., and Hsiung, G. D.: Pleurodynia associated with Echo virus type 8. N. Engl. J. Med. *266*:661–663, 1962.
442. Kaplan, G. J., Bender, T. R., Clark, P. S., et al.: Echovirus type 4 meningitis and related febrile illness: Epidemiologic study of an outbreak in two Eskimo communities in 1970. Am. J. Epidemiol. *96*:74–85, 1972.
443. Kaplan, G. J., Clark, P. S., Bender, T. R., et al.: Echovirus type 30 meningitis and related febrile illness: Epidemiologic study of an outbreak in an Eskimo community. Am. J. Epidemiol. *92*:257–265, 1970.
444. Kaplan, M. H., Klein, S. W., McPhee, J., et al.: Group B coxsackievirus infections in infants younger than three months of age: A serious childhood illness. Rev. Infect. Dis. *5*:1019–1032, 1983.
445. Kapsenberg, J. G.: ECHO virus type 33 as a cause of meningitis. Arch. Ges. Virusforsch. *23*:144–147, 1968.
446. Karzon, D. T., and Barron, A. L.: An epidemic of aseptic meningitis syndrome due to Echo virus type 6. I. Correlation of enterovirus isolation with illness. II. Clinical study. III. Sequelae. Pediatrics *29*:409–417, 418–431, 432–437, 1962.
447. Karzon, D. T., Eckert, G. L., Barron, A. L., et al.: Aseptic meningitis epidemic due to Echo 4 virus. Am. J. Dis. Child. *101*:610–622, 1961.
448. Katz, S. L.: Poliovaccine policy: Time for a change. Pediatrics *98*:116–117, 1996.
449. Kaul, A., Cohen, M. E., Broffman, G., et al.: Reye-like syndrome associated with Coxsackie B2 virus infection. J. Pediatr. *94*:67–69, 1979.
450. Kaye, B. M., Rosner, D. C., and Stein, I., Sr.: Viral diseases in pregnancy and their effect upon the embryo and fetus. Am. J. Obstet. Gynecol. *65*:109–118, 1953.
451. Kearns, G. L., Bradley, J. S., Jacobs, R. F., et al.: Single dose pharmacokinetics of pleconaril in neonates. Pediatric Pharmacology Research Unit Network. Pediatr. Infect. Dis. J. *19*:833–839, 2000.
452. Kelen, A. E., Lesiak, J. M., and Labzoffsky, N. A.: Sporadic occurrence of Echo virus types 27 and 31 associated with aseptic meningitis in Ontario. Can. Med. Assoc. J. *91*:1266–1268, 1964.
453. Kelen, A. E., Lesiak, J. M., and Labzoffsky, N. A.: An outbreak of aseptic meningitis due to Echo 25 virus. Can. Med. Assoc. J. *90*:1349–1351, 1964.
454. Kelen, A. E., Lesiak, J. M., and Labzoffsky, N. A.: Occurrence of echovirus 33 infections in Ontario. Can. Med. Assoc. J. *98*:985–987, 1968.
455. Kendall, E. J. C., Cook, G. T., and Stone, D. M.: Acute respiratory infections in children: Isolation of Coxsackie B virus and adenovirus during a survey in a general practice. B. M. J. *2*:1180–1184, 1960.
456. Kennett, M. L., Birch, C. J., Lewis, F. A., et al.: Enterovirus type 71 infection in Melbourne. Bull. World Health Organ. *51*:609–615, 1974.
457. Kennett, M. L., Ellis, A. W., Lewis, F. A., et al.: An epidemic associated with echovirus type 18. J. Hyg. (Camb.) *70*:325–334, 1972.
458. Keswick, B. H., Gerba, C. P., and Goyal, S. M.: Occurrence of enteroviruses in community swimming pools. Am. J. Public Health *71*:1026–1030, 1981.
459. Kew, O., Morris-Glasgow, V., Landaverde, M., et al.: Outbreak of poliomyelitis in Hispaniola associated with circulating type 1 vaccine-derived poliovirus. Science *296*:356–359, 2002.
460. Kew, O. M., Mulders, M. N., Lipskaya, G. Y., et al.: Molecular epidemiology of polioviruses. Virology *6*:401–414, 1995.
461. Khatib, R., Chason, J. L., Silberberg, B. K., et al.: Age-dependent pathogenicity of group B coxsackieviruses in Swiss-Webster mice: Infectivity for myocardium and pancreas. J. Infect. Dis. *141*:394–403, 1980.

462. Kibrick, S.: Viral infections of the fetus and newborn. Perspect. Virol. *2*:140–159, 1961.
463. Kibrick, S.: Current status of Coxsackie and ECHO viruses in human disease. Prog. Med. Virol. *6*:27–70, 1964.
464. Kibrick, S., and Benirschke, K.: Acute aseptic myocarditis and meningoencephalitis in the newborn child infected with Coxsackie virus group B, type 3. N. Engl. J. Med. *255*:883–889, 1956.
465. Kibrick, S., and Enders, J. F.: Disease due to Echo virus type 9 in Massachusetts. N. Engl. J. Med. *259*:482–484, 1958.
466. Kibrick, S., Melendex, L., and Enders, J. F.: Clinical associations of enteric viruses with particular reference to agents exhibiting properties of the Echo group. Ann. N. Y. Acad. Sci. *67*:311–325, 1957.
467. Kiel, R. J., Smith, F. E., Chason, J., et al.: Coxsackievirus B3 myocarditis in C3H/HeJ mice: Description of an inbred model and the effect of exercise on virulence. Eur. J. Epidemiol. *5*:348–350, 1989.
468. Kilbourne, E. D., and Goldfield, M.: Coxsackie viruses and "virus-like" diseases of the adult: A three-year study in a contagious disease hospital. Am. J. Med. *21*:175–183, 1956.
469. Kilborne, E. D., Wilson, C. B., and Perrier, D.: The induction of gross myocardial lesions by a Coxsackie (pleurodynia) virus and cortisone. J. Clin. Invest. *35*:362–370, 1956.
470. King, M. L., Shaikh, A., Bidwell, D., et al.: Coxsackie B virus specific IgM responses in children with insulin-dependent (juvenile-onset; type 1) diabetes mellitus. Lancet *1*:1397–1399, 1983.
471. Kinney, J. S., McCray, E., Kaplan, J. E., et al.: Risk factors associated with echovirus 11′ infection in a hospital nursery. Pediatr. Infect. Dis. J. *5*:192–197, 1986.
472. Kipps, A., Naude, W. duT., Don, P., et al.: Coxsackie virus myocarditis of the newborn: Epidemiological features. Med. Proc. *4*:401–406, 1958.
473. Kishimoto, C., Kitazawa, M., Hiraoka, Y., et al.: Extracellular matrix remodeling in coxsackievirus B3 myocarditis. Clin. Immunol. Immunopathol. *85*:47–55, 1997.
474. Klein, J. O., Lerner, A. M., and Finland, M.: Acute gastroenteritis associated with Echo virus, type 11. Am. J. Med. Sci. *240*:749–753, 1960.
475. Kleinman, H., Ramras, D. G., Cooney, M. K., et al.: Aseptic meningitis due to Echo virus type 7. N. Engl. J. Med. *267*:1116–1121, 1962.
476. Kleinman, H., Rogers, D., Ellwood, P. M., Jr., et al.: Epidemic of ECHO 9 aseptic meningitis in Minnesota, 1957. Univ. Minn. Med. Bull. *29*:306, 1958.
477. Klemola, E., and Lapinleimu, K.: Multiple attacks of aseptic meningitis in the same individual. B. M. J. *1*:1087–1090, 1964.
478. Klespies, S. L., Cebula, D. E., Kelley, C. L., et al.: Detection of enteroviruses from clinical specimens by spin amplification shell vial culture and monoclonal antibody assay. J. Clin. Microbiol. *34*:1465–1467, 1996.
479. Koch, V. F., Enders-Ruckle, G., and Wokittel, E.: Coxsackie B-5 infektionen mit signifikanter antikorperentwicklung bei neugeborenen. Arch. Kinderheilk. *165*:245–258, 1962.
480. Kogon, A., Spigland, I., Frothingham, T. E., et al.: The virus watch program: A continuing surveillance of viral infections in metropolitan New York families. VII. Observations on viral excretion, seroimmunity, intrafamilial spread and illness association in Coxsackie and Echovirus infections. Am. J. Epidemiol. *89*:51–61, 1969.
481. Komatsu, H., Shimizu, Y., Takeuchi, Y., et al.: Outbreak of severe neurologic involvement associated with enterovirus 71 infection. Pediatr. Neurol. *20*:17–23, 1999.
482. Kono, R.: Apollo 11 diseases or acute hemorrhagic conjunctivitis: A pandemic of a new enterovirus infection of the eyes. Am. J. Epidemiol. *101*:383–390, 1975.
483. Koontz, C. H., and Ray, C. G.: The role of Coxsackie group B virus infections in sporadic myopericarditis. Am. Heart J. *82*:750–758, 1971.
484. Kopel, F. B., Shore, B., and Hodes, H. L.: Nonfatal bulbospinal paralysis due to ECHO 4 virus. J. Pediatr. *67*:588–594, 1965.
485. Koskiniemi, M., Paetau, R., and Linnavuori, K.: Severe encephalitis associated with disseminated echovirus 22 infection. Scand. J. Infect. Dis. *21*:463–466, 1989.
486. Kraus, N. S.: La parotite da virus Coxsackie. Estratto Minerva Med. *51*:1379–1381, 1960.
487. Kuban, K. C., Ephros, M. A., Freeman, R. L., et al.: Syndrome of opsoclonus-myoclonus caused by Coxsackie B3 infection. Ann. Neurol. *13*:69–71, 1983.
488. Kubo, H., Iritani, N., and Seto, Y.: Molecular classification of enteroviruses not identified by neutralization tests. Emerg. Infect. Dis. *8*:298–304, 2002.
489. Kujala, G., and Newman, J. H.: Isolation of echovirus type 11 from synovial fluid in acute monocytic arthritis. Arthritis Rheum. *28*:98–99, 1985.
490. Kunin, C. M.: Virus-tissue union and the pathogenesis of enterovirus infections. J. Immunol. *88*:556–569, 1962.
491. Kunin, C. M.: Cellular susceptibility to enteroviruses. Bacteriol. Rev. *28*:382–390, 1964.
492. Kuritsky, J. N., Weaver, J. H., Bernard, K. W., et al.: An outbreak of acute hemorrhagic conjunctivitis in central Minnesota. Am. J. Ophthalmol. *96*:449–452, 1983.
493. LaForest, R. A., McNaughton, G. A., Beale, A. J., et al.: Outbreak of aseptic meningitis (meningoencephalitis) with rubelliform rash: Toronto, 1956. Can. Med. Assoc. J. *77*:1–4, 1957.
494. Lahelle, O.: Aseptic meningitis caused by Echo virus. J. Hyg. *55*:475–484, 1957.
495. Lake, A. M., Lauer, B. A., Clark, J. C., et al.: Enterovirus infections in neonates. J. Pediatr. *89*:787–791, 1976.
496. Landry, M. L., Ponseca, S. N. S., Cohen, S., et al.: Fatal enterovirus type 71 infection: Rapid detection and diagnostic pitfalls. Pediatr. Infect. Dis. J. *14*:1095–1100, 1995.
497. Landsman, J. B., Grist, N. R., and Ross, C. A. C.: Echo 9 virus infection and congenital malformations. Br. J. Prev. Soc. Med. *18*:152–156, 1964.
498. Landsteiner, K., and Popper, E.: Übertragung der poliomyelitis acuta auf affen. Z. Immun. Forsch. *2*:377–390, 1909.
499. Lane, J. R., Neumann, D. A., Lafond-Walker, A., et al.: Role of IL-1 and tumor necrosis factor in Coxsackie virus–induced autoimmune myocarditis. J. Immunol. *151*:1682–1690, 1993.
500. Lansky, L. L., Krugman, S., and Hug, G.: Anicteric Coxsackie B hepatitis. J. Pediatr. *94*:64–65, 1979.
501. Lapinleimu, K., and Kaski, U.: An outbreak caused by coxsackievirus B5 among newborn infants. Scand. J. Infect. Dis. *4*:27–30, 1972.
502. Lau, R. C. H.: Coxsackie B virus infection in acute myocardial infarction and adult heart disease. Med. J. Aust. *2*:520–522, 1982.
503. Lau, R. C. H.: Coxsackie B virus infections in New Zealand patients with cardiac and noncardiac diseases. J. Med. Virol. *11*:131–137, 1983.
504. Lau, R. C. H.: Coxsackie B virus–specific IgM responses in coronary care unit patients. J. Med. Virol. *18*:193–198, 1986.
505. Leggiadro, R. J., Chwatsky, D. N., and Zucker, S. W.: Echovirus 3 infection associated with anicteric hepatitis. Am. J. Dis. Child. *136*:843, 1982.
506. Lehan, P. H., Chick, E. W., Doto, I. L., et al.: An epidemic illness associated with a recently recognized enteric virus (Echo virus type 4). I. Epidemiologic and clinical features. Am. J. Hyg. *66*:63–75, 1957.
507. Lennette, E. H., Magoffin, R. L., and Knouf, E. G.: Viral central nervous system disease: An etiologic study conducted at the Los Angeles County General Hospital. J. A. M. A. *179*:687–695, 1962.
508. Leonardi, G. P., Greenberg, A. J., Costello, P., et al.: Echovirus type 30 infection associated with aseptic meningitis in Nassau County, New York, USA. Intervirology *36*:53–56, 1993.
509. Leparc-Goffart, I., Julien, J., Fuchs, F., et al.: Evidence of presence of poliovirus genomic sequences in cerebrospinal fluid from patients with postpolio syndrome. J. Clin. Microbiol. *34*:2023–2026, 1996.
510. Lepow, M. L., Carver, D. H., and Robbins, F. C.: Clinical and epidemiologic observations on enterovirus infection in a circumscribed community during an epidemic of Echo 9 infection. Pediatrics *26*:12–26, 1960.
511. Lepow, M. L., Carver, D. H., Wright, H. T., Jr., et al.: A clinical, epidemiologic and laboratory investigation of aseptic meningitis during the four-year period 1955–1958. I. Observations concerning etiology and epidemiology. N. Engl. J. Med. *266*:1181–1187, 1962.
512. Lepow, M. L., Coyne, N., Thompson, L. B., et al.: A clinical, epidemiologic and laboratory investigation of aseptic meningitis during the four-year period 1955–1958: II. The clinical disease and its sequelae. N. Engl. J. Med. *266*:1188–1193, 1962.
513. Lerner, A. M., Klein, J. O., Cherry, J. D., et al.: New viral exanthems. N. Engl. J. Med. *269*:678–686, 736–740, 1963.
514. Lerner, A. M., Klein, J. O., and Finland, M.: A laboratory outbreak of infections with Coxsackie virus group A, type 9. N. Engl. J. Med. *263*:1302–1304, 1960.
515. Lerner, A. M., Klein, J. O., and Finland, M.: Infection with Coxsackie virus group B, type 3, with vesicular eruption: Report of two cases. N. Engl. J. Med. *263*:1305, 1960.
516. Lerner, A. M., Klein, J. O., Levin, H. S., et al.: Infections due to Coxsackie virus group A, type 9, in Boston, 1959, with special reference to exanthems and pneumonia. N. Engl. J. Med. *263*:1265–1272, 1960.
517. Levi, G. F., Proto, C., Quadri, A., et al.: Coxsackie virus heart disease and cardiomyopathy. Am. Heart J. *93*:419–421, 1977.
518. Levin, S., Measroch, V., Pech, W., et al.: Hand-foot-and-mouth disease. S. Afr. Med. J. *55*:502–504, 1962.
519. Lewes, D., Rainford, D. J., and Lane, W. F.: Symptomless myocarditis and myalgia in viral and *Mycoplasma pneumoniae* infections. Br. Heart J. *36*:924–932, 1974.
520. Lewis, H. M., Parry, J. V., Parry, R. P., et al.: Role of viruses in febrile convulsions. Arch. Dis. Child. *54*:869–876, 1979.
521. Li, Y., Bourlet, T., Andreoletti, L., et al.: Enteroviral capsid protein VP1 is present in myocardial tissues from some patients with myocarditis or dilated cardiomyopathy. Circulation *101*:231–234, 2000.
522. Liebman, W. M., and St. Geme, J. W., Jr.: Enteroviral pseudoappendicitis. Am. J. Dis. Child. *120*:77–78, 1970.
523. Liljeqvist, J. A., Bergstrom, T., Holmstrom, S., et al.: Failure to demonstrate enterovirus aetiology in Swedish patients with dilated cardiomyopathy. J. Med. Virol. *39*:6–10, 1993.
524. Limson, B. M., Chan, V. F., Guzman, S. V., et al.: Occurrence of infection with group B coxsackievirus in rheumatic and nonrheumatic Filipino children. J. Infect. Dis. *140*:415–418, 1979.
525. Lin, K.-H., Wang, H.-L., Sheu, M.-M., et al.: Molecular epidemiology of a variant of coxsackievirus A24 in Taiwan: Two epidemics caused by

phylogenetically distinct viruses from 1985 to 1989. J. Clin. Microbiol. *31*:1160–1166, 1993.

526. Lindenbaum, J. E., Van Dyck, P. C., and Allen, R. G.: Hand, foot and mouth disease associated with coxsackievirus group B. Scand. J. Infect. Dis. *7*:161–163, 1975.
527. Linnemann, C. C., Jr., Steichen, J., Sherman, W. G., et al.: Febrile illness in early infancy associated with ECHO virus infection. J. Pediatr. *84*:49–54, 1974.
528. Liu, P., Wang, E. E. L., and Sole, M.: Viral, myocarditis: Changing concepts in pathogenesis and implications in diagnosis and treatment. Cardiovasc. Pathol. *22*:47–257, 1993.
529. Longson, M., Cole, F. M., and Davies, D.: Isolation of a Coxsackie virus group B, type 5, from the heart of a fatal case of myocarditis in an adult. J. Clin. Pathol. *22*:654–658, 1969.
530. Lönnrot, M., Hyöty, H., Knip, M., et al.: Antibody cross-reactivity induced by the homologous regions in glutamic acid decarboxylase (GAD65) and 2C protein of coxsackievirus B4. Childhood Diabetes in Finland Study Group. Clin. Exp. Immunol. *104*:398–405, 1996.
531. Lönnrot, M., Korpela, K., Knip, M., et al.: Enterovirus infection as a risk factor for beta-cell autoimmunity in a prospectively observed birth cohort: The Finnish Diabetes Prediction and Prevention Study. Diabetes *49*:1314–1318, 2000.
532. Lönnrot, M., Salminen, K., Knip, M., et al.: Enterovirus RNA in serum is a risk factor for beta-cell autoimmunity and clinical type 1 diabetes: A prospective study. Childhood Diabetes in Finland (DiMe) Study Group. J. Med. Virol. *61*:214–220, 2000.
533. Lycke, E., Hiltigardh, A., and Redin, B.: Coxsackie B1 virus and febrile illness with rash. Lancet *1*:1097, 1959.
534. Lycke, E., and Nilsson, L. R.: Poliomyelitis in a newborn due to intrauterine infection. Acta Paediatr. *51*:661–664, 1962.
535. Lyden, D. C., and Huber, S. A.: Aggravation of coxsackievirus, group B, type 3–induced myocarditis and increase in cellular immunity to myocyte antigens in pregnant BALB/c mice and animals treated with progesterone. Cell. Immunol. *187*:462–472, 1984.
536. MacLeod, A. J., Faulkner, R. S., and Van Rooyen, C. E.: Echo-9 virus infections in eastern Canada: Clinical and laboratory studies. Can. Med. Assoc. J. *78*:661–665, 1958.
537. Magoffin, R. L., Jackson, E. W., and Lennette, E. H.: Vesicular stomatitis and exanthem: A syndrome associated with Coxsackie virus, type A16. J. A. M. A. *175*:441–445, 1961.
538. Magoffin, R. L., and Lennette, E. H.: Nonpolioviruses and paralytic disease. Calif. Med. *97*:1–7, 1962.
539. Magoffin, R. L., Lennette, E. H., and Schmidt, N. J.: Association of Coxsackie viruses with illnesses resembling mild paralytic poliomyelitis. Pediatrics *28*:602–613, 1961.
540. Makower, H., Skurska, Z., and Halazinska, L.: On transplacental infection with Coxsackie virus. Texas Rep. Biol. Med. *16*:346–353, 1958.
541. Malcolm, B. S., Eiden, J. J., and Hendley, J. O.: ECHO virus type 9 meningitis simulating tuberculous meningitis. Pediatrics *65*:725–726, 1980.
542. Malherbe, H., Harwin, R., and Smith, A. H.: An outbreak of aseptic meningitis associated with Echo virus type 4. S. Afr. Med. J. *31*:1261–1264, 1957.
543. Maller, H. M., Powars, D. F., Horowitz, R. E., et al.: Fatal myocarditis associated with Echo virus, type 22, infection in a child with apparent immunological deficiency. J. Pediatr. *71*:204–210, 1967.
544. Marchessault, V., Pavilanis, V., Podoski, M. O., et al.: An epidemic of aseptic meningitis caused by Coxsackie B type 2 virus. Can. Med. Assoc. J. *85*:123–126, 1961.
545. Marier, R., Rodriguez, W., Chloupek, R. J., et al.: Coxsackievirus B5 infection and aseptic meningitis in neonates and children. Am. J. Dis. Child. *129*:321–325, 1975.
546. Marks, M. I., Joncas, J. H., and Mauer, S. M.: Fatal hepatitis in siblings: Isolation of coxsackievirus B5 and herpes simplex virus. Can. Med. Assoc. J. *102*:1391–1401, 1970.
547. Martin, A. B., Webber, S., Fricker, F. J., et al.: Acute myocarditis. Rapid diagnosis by PCR in children. Circulation *90*:330–339, 1994.
548. Martino, T. A., Sole, M. J., Penn, L. Z., et al.: Quantitation of enteroviral RNA by competitive polymerase chain reaction. J. Clin. Microbiol. *31*:2634–2640, 1993.
549. Marzetti, G., and Midulla, M.: Acute cerebellar ataxia associated with Echo type 6 infection in two children. Acta Paediatr. Scand. *56*:547–551, 1967.
550. Mason, J. W., O'Connell, J. B., Herskowitz, A., et al.: A clinical trial of immunosuppressive therapy for myocarditis. The Myocarditis Treatment Trial Investigators. N. Engl. J. Med. *333*:269–275, 1995.
551. Matsumori, A., and Kawai, C.: Coxsackie virus B3 perimyocarditis in BALB/c mice: Experimental model of chronic perimyocarditis in the right ventricle. J. Pathol. *131*:97–106, 1980.
552. Matsuura, K., Hasegawa, S., Nakayama, T., et al.: Epidemiological studies on echovirus type 18 infection in Toyama Prefecture. Microbiol. Immunol. *27*:359–368, 1983.
553. Matthews, J. D., Cameron, S. J., and George, M.: Constrictive pericarditis following Coxsackie virus infection. Thorax *25*:624–626, 1970.
554. Matumoto, M.: Newer respiratory disease viruses in Japan and some Far Eastern countries. Am. Rev. Respir. Dis. *88*:46–55, 1963.
555. McAllister, R. M.: Echo virus infections. Pediatr. Clin. North Am. *7*:927–945, 1960.
556. McAllister, R. M., Hummeler, K., and Coriell, L. L.: Report of a case with isolation of type 9 ECHO virus from the cerebrospinal fluid. N. Engl. J. Med. *261*:1159–1162, 1959.
557. McIntyre, J. P., and Keen, G. A.: Laboratory surveillance of viral meningitis by examination of cerebrospinal fluid in Cape Town, 1981–9. Epidemiol. Infect. *111*:357–371, 1993.
558. McKinney, R. E., Jr., Katz, S. L., and Wilfert, C. M.: Chronic enteroviral meningoencephalitis in agammaglobulinemic patients. Rev. Infect. Dis. *9*:334–356, 1987.
559. McLean, D. M.: Patterns of infection with enteroviruses. J. Pediatr. *54*:823–828, 1959.
560. McLean, D. M., Catiyanonda, K., Ladyman, S. R., et al.: Gastroenteritis of infants in two Canadian communities. Can. Med. Assoc. J. *102*:1247–1251, 1970.
561. McLean, D. M., Larke, R. P. B., Cobb, C., et al.: Mumps and enteroviral meningitis in Toronto, 1966. Can. Med. Assoc. J. *96*:1355–1361, 1967.
562. McLean, D. M., Larke, R. P. B., McNaughton, G. A., et al.: Enteroviral syndromes in Toronto, 1964. Can. Med. Assoc. J. *92*:658–661, 1965.
563. McLean, D. M., and Melnick, J. L.: Association of mouse pathogenic strain of Echo virus type 9 with aseptic meningitis. Proc. Soc. Exp. Biol. Med. *94*:656–660, 1957.
564. McManus, B. M., Chow, L. H., Wilson, J. E., et al.: Direct myocardial injury by enterovirus: A central role in the evolution of murine myocarditis. Clin. Immunol. Immunopathol. *68*:159–169, 1993.
565. McMinn, P., Stratov, I., Nagarajan, L., et al.: Neurological manifestations of enterovirus 71 infection in children during an outbreak of hand, foot, and mouth disease in Western Australia. Clin. Infect. Dis. *32*:236–242, 2001.
566. Meade, R. H., and Chang, T. W.: Zoster-like eruption due to echovirus 6. Am. J. Dis. Child. *133*:283–284, 1979.
567. Meadow, S. R.: Hand, foot, and mouth diseases. Arch. Dis. Child. *40*:560–564, 1965.
568. Mease, P. J., Ochs, H. D., and Wedgwood, R. J.: Successful treatment of echovirus meningoencephalitis and myositis-fasciitis with intravenous immune globulin therapy in a patient with X-linked agammaglobulinemia. N. Engl. J. Med. *304*:1278–1281, 1981.
569. Medearis, D. N., Jr., and Kramer, R. A.: Exanthem associated with Echo virus type 18 viremia. J. Pediatr. *55*:367–373, 1959.
570. Meehan, W. F., and Bertrand, C. A.: Ventricular tachycardia associated with echovirus infection. J. A. M. A. *212*:1701–1703, 1970.
571. Melchers, W., Zoll, J., van Kuppeveld, F., et al.: There is no evidence for persistent enterovirus infections in chronic medical conditions in humans. Rev. Med. Virol. *4*:235–243, 1994.
572. Melnick, J. L.: Echoviruses. *In* Horsfall, J. R., and Tamm, I. (eds.): Viral and Rickettsial Infections of Man. Philadelphia, J. B. Lippincott, 1965, pp. 513–545.
573. Melnick, J. L.: Portraits of viruses: The picornaviruses. Intervirology *20*:61–100, 1983.
574. Melnick, J. L.: Enterovirus type 71 infections: A varied clinical pattern sometimes mimicking paralytic poliomyelitis. Rev. Infect. Dis. *6*(Suppl.):387–390, 1984.
575. Melnick, J. L.: Enteroviruses. *In* Evans, A. S. (ed.): Viral Infections on Humans: Epidemiology and Control. 3rd ed. New York, Plenum Medical, 1989, pp. 191–263.
576. Melnick, J. L.: Enteroviruses: Polioviruses, coxsackieviruses, echoviruses and newer enteroviruses. *In* Fields, B. N., and Knipe, D. M. (eds.): Virology. 2nd ed. New York, Raven Press, 1990, pp. 549–605.
577. Melnick, J. L.: My role in the discovery and classification of the enteroviruses. Annu. Rev. Microbiol. *50*:1–24, 1996.
578. Melnick, J. L., Cockburn, W. C., Dalldorf, G., et al.: Picornavirus group. Virology *19*:114–116, 1963.
579. Melnick, J. L., Dalldorf, G., Enders, J. F., et al.: The enteroviruses. Am. J. Public Health *47*:1556–1566, 1957.
580. Melnick, J. L., and Wenner, H. A.: Enteroviruses. *In* Lennette, E. H., and Schmidt, N. J. (eds.): Diagnostic Procedures for Viral and Rickettsial Infections. 4th ed. New York, American Public Health Association, 1969.
581. Mertens, T., Hager, H., and Eggers, H. J.: Epidemiology of an outbreak in a maternity unit of infections with an antigenic variant of echovirus 11. J. Med. Virol. *9*:81–91, 1982.
582. Miller, D. G., Gabrielson, M. O., Bart, K. J., et al.: An epidemic of aseptic meningitis, primarily among infants, caused by echovirus 11-prime. Pediatrics *41*:77–90, 1978.
583. Miller, M. A., Sutter, R. W., Strebel, P. M., et al.: Cost-effectiveness of incorporating inactivated poliovirus vaccine into the routine childhood immunization schedule. J. A. M. A. *276*:967–971, 1996.
584. Miller, N. A., Carmichael, H. A., Calder, B. D., et al.: Antibody to Coxsackie B virus in diagnosing postviral fatigue syndrome. B. M. J. *302*:140–141, 1991.
585. Mirkovic, R. R., Varma, S. K., and Yoon, J. W.: Incidence of coxsackievirus B type 4 (CB4) infections concomitant with onset of insulin-dependent diabetes mellitus. J. Med. Virol. *14*:9–16, 1984.

586. Mitchell, S. C., and Dempster, G.: The finding of genital lesions in a case of Coxsackie virus infection. Can. Med. Assoc. J. *72*:117–119, 1955.
587. Miwa, C., Ohtani, M., Watanabe, H., et al.: Epidemic of hand, foot, and mouth disease in Gifu Prefecture in 1978. Jpn. J. Med. Sci. Biol. *33*:167–180, 1980.
588. Modlin, J. F.: Fatal echovirus 11 disease in premature neonates. Pediatrics *66*:775–780, 1980.
589. Modlin, J. F.: Perinatal echovirus infection: Insights from a literature review of 61 cases of serious infection and 16 outbreaks in nurseries. Rev. Infect. Dis. *8*:918–926, 1986.
590. Modlin, J. F., Dagan, R., Berlin, L. E., et al.: Focal encephalitis with enterovirus infections. Pediatrics *88*:841–845, 1991.
591. Modlin, J. F., Polk, B. F., Horton, P., et al.: Perinatal echovirus infection: Risk of transmission during a community outbreak. N. Engl. J. Med. *305*:368–371, 1981.
592. Mokhtar, M. O. E.-H., Banatvala, J. E., and Coltart, D. J.: Coxsackie-B-virus–specific IgM responses in patients with cardiac and other diseases. Lancet *2*:1160–1162, 1980.
593. Monif, G. R. G., Lee, C. W., and Hsiung, G. D.: Isolated myocarditis with recovery of Echo type 9 virus from the myocardium. N. Engl. J. Med. *277*:1353–1355, 1967.
594. Montgomery, J., Gear, J., Prinsloo, F. R., et al.: Myocarditis of the newborn: An outbreak in a maternity home in southern Rhodesia associated with Coxsackie group-B virus infection. S. Afr. Med. J. *29*:608–612, 1955.
595. Moore, M.: Enteroviral disease in the United States, 1970–1979. J. Infect. Dis. *146*:103–108, 1982.
596. Moore, M. L., Hooser, L. E., Davis, E. V., et al.: Sudden unexpected death in infancy: Isolations of ECHO type 7 virus. Proc. Soc. Exp. Biol. Med. *116*:231–234, 1964.
597. Moossy, J., and Geer, J. C.: Encephalomyelitis, myocarditis and adrenal cortical necrosis in Coxsackie B3 virus infection: Distribution of the central nervous system lesions. Arch. Pathol. *70*:614–622, 1960.
598. Morens, D. M.: Enteroviral disease in early infancy. J. Pediatr. *92*:374–377, 1978.
599. Morens, D. M., Zweighaft, R. M., and Bryan, J. M.: Nonpolio enterovirus disease in the United States, 1971–1975. Int. J. Epidemiol. *8*:49–54, 1979.
600. Morgante, O., Wilkinson, D., Burchak, E. C., et al.: Outbreak of hand-foot-and-mouth disease among Indian and Eskimo children in a hospital. J. Infect. Dis. *125*:587–597, 1972.
601. Mori, I., Matsumoto, K., Hatano, M., et al.: An unseasonable winter outbreak of echovirus type 30 meningitis. J. Infect. *31*:219–223, 1995.
602. Morita, H., Kitaura, Y., Deguchi, H., et al.: Coxsackie B5 myopericarditis in a young adult: Clinical course and endomyocardial biopsy findings. Jpn. Circ. J. *47*:1077–1083, 1983.
603. Moritsugu, Y., Sawada, K., Hinohara, M., et al.: An outbreak of type 25 echovirus infection with exanthem in an infant home near Tokyo. Am. J. Epidemiol. *87*:599–608, 1968.
604. Morris, J. A., Elisberg, B. L., Pond, W. L., et al.: Hepatitis associated with Coxsackie virus group A, type 4. N. Engl. J. Med. *267*:1230–1233, 1962.
605. Moscovici, C., and Maisel, J.: Intestinal viruses of newborn and older prematures. Am. J. Dis. Child. *101*:771–777, 1961.
606. Mostoufizadeh, M., Lack, E. E., Gang, D. L., et al.: Postmortem manifestations of echovirus 11 sepsis in five newborn infants. Hum. Pathol. *14*:818–823, 1983.
607. Muir, P., and Archard, L. C.: There is evidence for persistent enterovirus infections in chronic medical conditions in humans. Rev. Med. Virol. *4*:245–250, 1994.
608. Muir, P., Nicholson, F., Illavia, S. J., et al.: Serological and molecular evidence of enterovirus infection in patients with end-stage dilated cardiomyopathy. Heart *76*:243–249, 1996.
609. Muir, P., Nicholson, F., Spencer, G. T., et al.: Enterovirus infection of the central nervous system of humans: Lack of association with chronic neurological disease. J. Gen. Virol. *77*:1469–1476, 1996.
610. Muir, P., Nicholson, F., Tilzey, A. J., et al.: Chronic relapsing pericarditis and dilated cardiomyopathy: Serological evidence of persistent enterovirus infection. Lancet *1*:804–806, 1989.
611. Mulders, M. N., Lipskaya, G. Y., van der Avoort, H. G. A. M., et al.: Molecular epidemiology of wild poliovirus type 1 in Europe, the Middle East, and the Indian subcontinent. J. Infect. Dis. *171*:1399–1405, 1995.
612. Murdin, A. D., Barreto, L., and Plotkin, S.: Inactivated poliovirus vaccine: Past and present experience. Vaccine *14*:735–746, 1996.
613. Murphy, A. M., and Simmul, R.: Coxsackie B4 virus infections in New South Wales during 1962. Med. J. Aust. *2*:443–445, 1964.
614. Nagington, J., Gandy, G., Walker, J., et al.: Use of normal immunoglobulin in an echovirus 11 outbreak in a special-care baby unit. Lancet *2*:443–446, 1983.
615. Nagington, J., Wreghitt, T. G., Gandy, G., et al.: Fatal echovirus 11 infections in outbreak in special-care baby unit. Lancet *2*:725–728, 1978.
616. Nahmias, A. J., Froeschle, J. E., Feorino, P. M., et al.: Generalized eruption in a child with eczema due to coxsackievirus A16. Arch. Dermatol. *97*:147–148, 1968.
617. Nair, E., and Kalra, S. L.: Cytopathic enteroviruses in Delhi area. I. From cases of diarrhoea and healthy controls. Indian J. Med. Res. *57*:141–148, 1968.
618. Nakao, T.: Coxsackie viruses and diabetes. Lancet *2*:1423, 1971.
619. Nakao, T., and Horino, K.: Clinical and virological studies of acute cerebellar ataxia in childhood. Tohoku J. Exp. Med. *101*:47–53, 1970.
620. Nakao, T., and Miura, R.: Recurrent virus meningitis. Pediatrics *47*:773–776, 1971.
621. Nakao, T., Miura, R., and Sato, M.: ECHO virus type 22 infection in a premature infant. Tohoku J. Exp. Med. *102*:61–68, 1970.
622. Nakao, T., and Morita, M.: Exanthem associated with ECHO 25 virus. Jika Rinsho *18*:772–773, 1965.
623. Nankervis, G., Starr, J., and Gold, E.: Hand, foot and mouth syndrome in a group of families. Program for the Society for Pediatric Research, May 3–4, 1968, p. 152.
624. Nathanson, N., and Fine, P.: Virology. Poliomyelitis eradication—a dangerous endgame. Science *296*:269–270, 2002.
625. Nelson, D., Hiemstra, H., Minor, T., et al.: Non-polio enterovirus activity in Wisconsin based on a 20-year experience in a diagnostic virology laboratory. Am. J. Epidemiol. *109*:352–361, 1979.
626. Neu, N., Beisel, K. W., Traystman, M. D., et al.: Autoantibodies specific for the cardiac myosin isoform are found in mice susceptible to coxsackievirus B3–induced myocarditis. J. Immunol. *138*:2488–2492, 1987.
627. Neva, F. A.: A second outbreak of Boston exanthem disease in Pittsburgh during 1954. N. Engl. J. Med. *254*:838–843, 1956.
628. Neva, F. A., and Enders, J. F.: Cytopathogenic agents isolated from patients during an unusual epidemic exanthem. J. Immunol. *72*:307–314, 1954.
629. Neva, F. A., Feemster, R. F., and Gorbach, I. J.: Clinical and epidemiological features of an unusual epidemic exanthem. J. A. M. A. *155*:544–548, 1954.
630. Neva, F. A., and Zuffante, S. M.: Agents isolated from patients with Boston exanthem disease during 1954 in Pittsburgh. J. Lab. Clin. Med. *50*:712–779, 1957.
631. News and Notes: Epidemiology: Echovirus infections. B. M. J. *3*:594, 1970.
632. Nicholls, A. C., and Thomas, M.: Coxsackie virus infection in acute myocardial infarction. Lancet *1*:883–884, 1977.
633. Nielsen, J. L., Berryman, G. K., and Hankins, G. D. V.: Intrauterine fetal death and the isolation of echovirus 27 from amniotic fluid. J. Infect. Dis. *158*:501–502, 1988.
634. Nielsen, L. P., Modlin, J. F., and Rotbart, H. A.: Detection of enteroviruses by polymerase chain reaction in urine samples of patients with aseptic meningitis. Pediatr. Infect. Dis. J. *15*:625–627, 1996.
635. Nightingale, E. O.: Recommendations for a national policy on poliomyelitis vaccination. N. Engl. J. Med. *297*:249–253, 1977.
636. Nihoul, E., Quersin-Thiry, L., and Weynants, A.: ECHO virus type 9 as the agent responsible for an important outbreak of aseptic meningitis in Belgium. Am. J. Hyg. *66*:102–118, 1957.
637. Nikoskelainen, J., Kalliomaki, J. L., Lapinleimu, K., et al.: Coxsackie B virus antibodies in myocardial infarction. Acta Med. Scand. *214*:29–32, 1983.
638. Nishmi, M., Morr, J., Abrahamov, A., et al.: A winter outbreak of Echo virus type 9 meningitis in Jerusalem, with cases of a simultaneous mixed pneumococcal-viral infection. Israel J. Med. Sci. *7*:1240–1247, 1971.
639. Nishmi, M., and Yodfat, Y.: An outbreak among kibbutz children of a febrile illness associated with Echo virus type 4. Isr. J. Med. Sci. *6*:535–539, 1970.
640. Nogen, A. G., and Lepow, M. L.: Enteroviral meningitis in very young infants. Pediatrics *40*:617–626, 1967.
641. Norder, H., Bjerregaard, L., and Magnius, L. O.: Homotypic echoviruses share aminoterminal VP1 sequence homology applicable for typing. J. Med. Virol. *63*:35–44, 2001.
642. Norton, H.: Report of an outbreak of "hand-foot-and-mouth disease" in Sydney. Med. J. Aust. *2*:570, 1961.
643. Novack, A., Feldman, H. A., Wang, S. S., et al.: A community-wide coxsackievirus A9 outbreak. J. A. M. A. *202*:862–866, 1967.
644. Null, F. C., Jr., and Castle, C. H.: Adult pericarditis and myocarditis due to Coxsackie virus group B, type 5. N. Engl. J. Med. *261*:937–942, 1959.
645. O'Connell, J. B., Reap, E. A., and Robinson, J. A.: The effects of cyclosporine on acute murine Coxsackie B3 myocarditis. Circulation *73*:353–359, 1986.
646. Ogilvie, M. M., and Tearne, C. F.: Spontaneous abortion after hand-foot-and-mouth disease caused by Coxsackie virus A16. B. M. J. *281*:1527–1528, 1980.
647. O'Neill, D., McArthur, J. D., Kennedy, J. A., et al.: Coxsackie B virus infection in coronary care unit patients. J. Clin. Pathol. *36*:658–661, 1983.
648. O'Regan, S., Robitaille, P., Mongeau, J. G., et al.: The hemolytic uremic syndrome associated with echo 22 infection. Clin. Pediatr. (Phila.) *19*:125–127, 1980.
649. Orenstein, W. A.: Personal communication, 1996.
650. Orinius, E.: The late cardiac prognosis after Coxsackie-B infection. Acta. Med. Scand. *183*:235–237, 1968.

651. O'Shaughnessey, W. J., and Buechner, H. A.: Hepatitis associated with a Coxsackie B5 virus infection during late pregnancy. J. A. M. A. *179*:71–72, 1962.
652. Otonkoski, T., Roivainen, M., Vaarala, O., et al.: Neonatal type I diabetes associated with maternal echovirus 6 infection: A case report. Diabetologia *43*:1235–1238, 2000.
653. Pallansch, M. A., and Roos, R. P.: Enteroviruses: Polioviruses, coxsackieviruses, echoviruses, and newer enteroviruses. *In* Knipe, D. M., Howley, P. M. (eds.): Fields Virology. Vol. 1. Philadelphia, Lippincott Williams & Wilkins, 2001, pp. 723–775.
654. Palomba, E., and Tovo, P. A.: Persistent fever as the only manifestation of chronic coxsackievirus B4 infection in the brain of a human immunodeficiency virus type 1–infected child. Clin. Infect. Dis. *28*:912–913, 1999.
655. Paque, R. E.: Role of anti-idiotypic antibodies in induction, regulation, and expression of coxsackievirus-induced myocarditis. Prog. Med. Virol. *39*:204–227, 1992.
656. Paradiso, P. R.: The future of polio immunization in the United States: Are we ready for change? Pediatr. Infect. Dis. J. *15*:645–649, 1996.
657. Parks, W. P., Queiroga, L. T., and Melnick, J. L.: Studies on infantile diarrhea in Karachi, Pakistan. II. Multiple virus isolations from rectal swabs. Am. J. Epidemiol. *85*:469–478, 1967.
658. Parrott, R. H.: The clinical importance of group A Coxsackie viruses. Ann. N. Y. Acad. Sci. *67*:230–241, 1957.
659. Pasic, S., Jankovic, B., Abinun, M., et al.: Intravenous immunoglobulin prophylaxis in an echovirus 6 and echovirus 4 nursery outbreak. Pediatr. Infect. Dis. J. *16*:718–720, 1997.
660. Paterson, W. G., and Smith, I. W.: An unusual acute abdomen in pregnancy: An Echo 8 virus infection. Practitioner *203*:337–339, 1969.
661. Paul, J. R.: A History of Poliomyelitis. New Haven, Yale University Press, 1971.
662. Pelon, W., Villarejos, V. M., Rhim, J. S., et al.: Coxsackie group B virus infection and acute diarrhoea occurring among children in Costa Rica. Arch. Dis. Child. *4*:636–641, 1966.
663. Peters, A. C. B., Vielvoye, G. J., Versteeg, J., et al.: Echo 25 focal encephalitis and subacute hemichorea. Neurology *29*:676–681, 1979.
664. Petitjean, J., Freymuth, F., Kopecka, H., et al.: Detection of enteroviruses in cerebrospinal fluids: Enzymatic amplification and hybridization with a biotinylated riboprobe. Mol. Cell. Probes *8*:15–22, 1994.
665. Pevear, D. C., Tull, T. M., Seipel, M. E., et al.: Activity of pleconaril against enteroviruses. Antimicrob. Agents. Chemother. *43*:2109–2115, 1999.
666. Philip, A. G. S., and Larson, E. J.: Overwhelming neonatal infection with ECHO 19 virus. J. Pediatr. *82*:391–397, 1973.
667. Philipson, L.: Association between a recently isolated virus and an epidemic of upper respiratory disease in a day nursery. Arch. Ges. Virusforsch. *8*:204–215, 1958.
668. Philipson, L., and Wesslen, T.: Recovery of a cytopathogenic agent from patients with non-diphtheritic croup and from day-nursery children. Arch. Ges. Virusforsch. *8*:77–94, 1958.
669. Phillips, C. A., Melnick, J. L., Barrett, F. F., et al.: Dual virus infections. Simultaneous enteroviral disease and St. Louis encephalitis. J. A. M. A. *197*:169–172, 1966.
670. Plager, H., Beebe, R., and Miller, J. K.: Coxsackie B-5 pericarditis in pregnancy. Arch. Intern. Med. *110*:735–738, 1962.
671. Plager, H., and Deibel, R.: Echo 30 virus infections: Outbreak in New York State. N. Y. State J. Med. *70*:391–393, 1970.
672. Plager, H., and Harrison, F. F.: Paralysis associated with ECHO virus type 9. N. Y. State J. Med. *61*:798–800, 1961.
673. Ponka, A., Jalanki, H., Ponka, T., et al.: Viral and mycoplasmal antibodies in patients with myocardial infarction. Ann. Clin. Res. *13*:429–432, 1981.
674. Pope, J. G., and Pollock, T. M.: Coxsackie B5 virus infections during 1965: A report to the Director of the Public Health Laboratory Service from various laboratories in the United Kingdom. B. M. J. *4*:575–577, 1967.
675. Portlance Walker, M., Schlaberg, R., Hays, A. P.: Absence of echovirus sequence in brain and spinal cord in amyotropic lateral sclerosis patients. Ann. Neurol. *49*:249–253, 2001.
676. Portnoy, B., Leedom, J. M., Hanes, B., et al.: Aseptic meningitis associated with ECHO virus type 9 infection: With special reference to variability by sex and incidence of paralytic sequelae. Calif. Med. *102*:261–267, 1965.
677. Pöyry, T., Hyypiä, T., Horsnell, C., et al.: Molecular analysis of coxsackievirus A16 reveals a new genetic group of enteroviruses. Virology *202*:962–967, 1994.
678. Pöyry, T., Kinnunen, L., Hovi, T., et al.: Relationships between simian and human enteroviruses. J. Gen. Virol. *80*:635–638, 1999.
679. Pöyry, T., Kinnunen, L., Hyypiä, T., et al.: Genetic and phylogenetic clustering of enteroviruses. J. Gen. Virol. *77*:1699–1717, 1996.
680. Prakash, C. V.: Entero-viruses in infantile diarrhoea in India. I. Investigations carried out in Bombay. Indian J. Med. Res. *250*:343–347, 1962.
681. Price, R. A., Garcia, J. H., and Rightsel, W. A.: Choriomeningitis and myocarditis in an adolescent with isolation of Coxsackie B-5 virus. Am. J. Clin. Pathol. *53*:825–883, 1970.
682. Prince, J. T., St. Geme, J. W., Jr., and Scherer, W. F.: ECHO-9 virus exanthema. J. A. M. A. *167*:691–696, 1958.
683. Pulli, T., Koskimies, P., and Hyypiä, T.: Molecular comparison of coxsackie A virus serotypes. Virology *212*:30–38, 1995.
684. Quaife, R. A., and Gostling, J. V. T.: False positive Wassermann reaction associated with evidence of enterovirus infection. J. Clin. Pathol. *24*:120–121, 197.
685. Rabausch-Starz, I., Schwaiger, A., Grünewald, K., et al.: Persistence of virus and viral genome in myocardium after coxsackievirus B3–induced murine myocarditis. Clin. Exp. Immunol. *96*:69–74, 1994.
686. Rabkin, C. S., Telzak, E. E., Ho, M. S., et al.: Outbreak of echovirus 11 infection in hospitalized neonates. Pediatr. Infect. Dis. J. *7*:186–190, 1988.
687. Racaniello, V. R.: *Picornaviridae*: The viruses and their replication. *In* Knipe, D. M., and Howley, P. M. (eds.): Fields Virology. Vol. 1, Philadelphia, Lippincott Williams & Wilkins, 2001, pp. 685–722.
688. Ramers, C., Billman, G., Hartin, M., et al.: Impact of a diagnostic cerebrospinal fluid enterovirus polymerase chain reaction test on patient management. J. A. M. A. *283*:2680–2685, 2000.
689. Ramlow, J., Alexander, M., LaPorte, R., et al.: Epidemiology of the post-polio syndrome. Am. J. Epidemiol. *136*:769–786, 1992.
690. Ramos-Alvarez, M.: Cytopathogenic enteric viruses associated with undifferentiated diarrheal syndromes in early childhood. Ann. N. Y. Acad. Sci. *67*:326, 1957.
691. Ramos-Alvarez, M., and Olarte, J.: Diarrheal diseases of children: The occurrence of enteropathogenic viruses and bacteria. Am. J. Dis. Child. *107*:218–231, 1964.
692. Ramos-Alvarez, M., and Sabin, A. B.: Enteropathogenic viruses and bacteria: Role in summer diarrheal diseases of infancy and early childhood. J. A. M. A. *167*:147–156, 1958.
693. Ramsingh, A. I., and Collins, D. N.: A point mutation in the VP4 coding sequence of coxsackievirus B4 influences virulence. J. Virol. *69*:7278–7281, 1995.
694. Ramsingh, A. I., Lee, W. T., Collins, D. N., et al.: T cells contribute to disease severity during coxsackievirus B4 infection. J. Virol. *73*:3080–3086, 1999.
695. Rantasalo, I., Pentitinen, K., Saxen, L., et al.: Echo 9 virus antibody status after an epidemic period and the possible teratogenic effect of the infection. Ann. Paediatr. Fenn. *6*:175–184, 1960.
696. Ranzenhofer, E. R., Dizon, F. C., Lipton, M. M., et al.: Clinical paralytic poliomyelitis due to Coxsackie virus group A, type 7. N. Engl. J. Med. *259*:182, 1958.
697. Ray, C. G., McCollough, R. H., Doto, I. L., et al.: Echo 4 illness: Epidemiological, clinical and laboratory studies of an outbreak in a rural community. Am. J. Epidemiol. *84*:253–267, 1966.
698. Ray, C. G., Portman, J. N., Stamm, S. J., et al.: Hemolytic-uremic syndrome and myocarditis: Association with coxsackievirus B infection. Am. J. Dis. Child. *122*:418–420, 1971.
699. Ray, C. G., Tucker, V. L., Harris, D. J., et al.: Enteroviruses associated with the hemolytic-uremic syndrome. Pediatrics *46*:378–388, 1970.
700. Reyes, M. P., Ho, K. L., Smith, F., et al.: A mouse model of dilated-type cardiomyopathy due to coxsackievirus B3. J. Infect. Dis. *144*:232–236, 1981.
701. Reyes, M. P., Ostrea, E. M., Jr., Roskamp, J., et al.: Disseminated neonatal echovirus 11 disease following antenatal maternal infection with a virus-positive cervix and virus-negative gastrointestinal tract. J. Med. Virol. *12*:155–159, 1983.
702. Reyes, M. P., Zalenski, D., Smith, F., et al.: Coxsackievirus-positive cervices in women with febrile illnesses during the third trimester of pregnancy. Am. J. Obstet. Gynecol. *155*:159–161, 1986.
703. Rezkalla, S., Khatib, G., and Khatib, R.: Coxsackievirus B3 murine myocarditis: Deleterious effects of nonsteroidal anti-inflammatory agents. J. Lab. Clin. Med. *107*:393–395, 1986.
704. Rezkalla, S. H., Raikar, S., and Kloner, R. A.: Treatment of viral myocarditis with focus on captopril. Am. J. Cardiol. *77*:634–637, 1996.
705. Rice, S. K., Heinl, R. E., Thornton, L. L., et al.: Clinical characteristics, management strategies, and cost implications of a statewide outbreak of enterovirus meningitis. Clin. Infect. Dis. *20*:931–937, 1995.
706. Richardson, H. B., Jr., and Leibovitz, A.: Hand, foot, and mouth disease in children. J. Pediatr. *67*:6–12, 1965.
707. Rinehart, J. E., Gomez, R. M., and Roos, R. P.: Molecular determinants for virulence in coxsackievirus B1 infection. J. Virol. *71*:3986–3991, 1997.
708. Robbins, F. C., and de Quadros, C. A.: Certification of the eradication of indigenous transmission of wild poliovirus in the Americas. J. Infect. Dis. *175*(Suppl):281–285, 1997.
709. Robinson, C. R., Doane, F. W., and Rhodes, A. J.: Report of an outbreak of febrile illness with pharyngeal lesions and exanthem, Toronto, summer 1957: Isolation of group A Coxsackie virus. Can. Med. Assoc. J. *79*:615–621, 1958.
710. Robinson, J. A., O'Connell, J. B., Roeges, L. M., et al.: Coxsackie B3 myocarditis in athymic mice. Proc. Soc. Exp. Biol. Med. *166*:80–91, 1981.
711. Roden, V. J., Cantor, H. E., O'Connor, D. M., et al.: Acute hemiplegia of childhood associated with Coxsackie A9 viral infection. J. Pediatr. *86*:56–58, 1975.

712. Rodriguez-Torres, R., Lin, J. S., and Berkovich, S.: A sensitive electrocardiographic sign in myocarditis associated with viral infection. Pediatrics *43*:846–851, 1969.
713. Roivainen, M., Knip, M., Hyöty, H., et al.: Several different enterovirus serotypes can be associated with prediabetic autoimmune episodes and onset of overt IDDM. Childhood Diabetes in Finland (DiMe) Study Group. J. Med. Virol. *56*:74–78, 1998.
714. Rorabaugh, M. L., Berlin, L. E., Heldrich, F., et al.: Aseptic meningitis in infants younger than 2 years of age: Acute illness and neurologic complications. Pediatrics *92*:206–211, 1993.
715. Ross, C. A. C., Bell, E. J., Kerr, M. M., et al.: Infective agents and embryopathy in the west of Scotland 1966–70. Scot. Med. J. *17*:252–258, 1972.
716. Rotbart, H. A.: Diagnosis of enteroviral meningitis with the polymerase chain reaction. J. Pediatr. *117*:85–89, 1990.
717. Rotbart, H. A.: Enzymatic RNA amplification of the enteroviruses. J. Clin. Microbiol. *28*:438–442, 1990.
718. Rotbart, H. A.: Nucleic acid detection systems for enteroviruses. Clin. Microbiol. Rev. *4*:156–168, 1991.
719. Rotbart, H. A.: Enteroviral infections of the central nervous system. Clin. Infect. Dis. *20*:971–981, 1995.
720. Rotbart, H. A., Abzug, M. J., and Levin, M. J.: Development and application of RNA probes for the study of picornaviruses. Mol. Cell. Probes *2*:65–73, 1988.
721. Rotbart, H. A., Kinsella, J. P., and Wasserman, R. L.: Persistent enterovirus infection in culture-negative meningoencephalitis: Demonstration by enzymatic RNA amplification. J. Infect. Dis. *161*:787–791, 1990.
722. Rotbart, H. A., O'Connell, J. F., and McKinlay, M. A.: Treatment of human enterovirus infections. Antiviral. Res. *38*:1–14, 1998.
723. Rotbart, H. A., Sawyer, M. H., Fast, S., et al.: Diagnosis of enteroviral meningitis by using PCR with a colorimetric microwell detection assay. J. Clin. Microbiol. *32*:2590–2592, 1994.
724. Rotbart, H. A., and Webster, A. D.: Treatment of potentially life-threatening enterovirus infections with pleconaril. Clin. Infect. Dis. *32*:228–235, 2001.
725. Rotem, C. E.: Meningitis of virus origin. Lancet *1*:502–504, 1957.
726. Rubin, H., Lehan, P. H., Doto, I. L., et al.: Epidemic infection with Coxsackie virus group B, type 5. I. Clinical and epidemiologic aspects. N. Engl. J. Med. *258*:255–263, 1958.
727. Rueckert, R. R.: *Picornaviridae* and their replication. *In* Fields, B. N., and Knipe, D. M. (eds.): Virology. 2nd ed. New York, Raven Press, 1990, pp. 507–548.
728. Russell, S. J. M., and Bell, E. J.: Echoviruses and carditis. Lancet *1*:784–785, 1970.
729. Ryder, D. E., Doane, F. W., Zbitnew, A., et al.: Report of an outbreak of Bornholm disease, with isolation of Coxsackie B5 virus: Toronto, 1958. Can. J. Public Health *50*:265–269, 1959.
730. Sabin, A. B.: Role of ECHO viruses in human disease. *In* Rose, H. M. (ed.): Viral Infections of Infancy and Childhood. New York, Hoeber-Harper, 1960, pp. 78–100.
731. Sabin, A. B.: Poliomyelitis. *In* Braude A. I. (ed.): Medical Microbiology and Infectious Diseases. Philadelphia, W. B. Saunders, 1981, pp. 1348–1365.
732. Sabin, A. B.: Oral poliovirus vaccine: History of its development and use and current challenge to eliminate poliomyelitis from the world. J. Infect. Dis. *151*:420–436, 1985.
733. Sabin, A. B., Krumbiegel, E. R., and Wigand, R.: ECHO type 9 virus disease: Virologically controlled clinical and epidemiologic observations during a 1957 epidemic in Milwaukee with notes on concurrent similar diseases associated with Coxsackie and other ECHO viruses. Prog. Pediatr. *96*:197–219, 1958.
734. Sainani, G. S., Krompotic, E., and Slodki, S. J.: Adult heart disease due to the Coxsackie virus B infection. Medicine (Baltimore) *47*:133–147, 1968.
735. Salk, D.: Polio immunization policy in the United States: A new challenge for a new generation. Am. J. Public Health *78*:296–300, 1988.
736. Salk, D.: Eradication of poliomyelitis in the United States. I. Live virus vaccine-associated and wild poliovirus disease. Rev. Infect. Dis. *2*:228–242, 1980.
737. Salk, D.: Eradication of poliomyelitis in the United States. II. Experience with killed poliovirus vaccine. Rev. Infect. Dis. *2*:243–257, 1980.
738. Salk, D.: Eradication of poliomyelitis in the United States. III. Poliovaccines. Practical considerations. Rev. Infect. Dis. *2*:258–273, 1980.
739. Samuda, G. M., Chang, W. K., Yeung, C. Y., et al.: Monoplegia caused by enterovirus 71: An outbreak in Hong Kong. Pediatr. Infect. Dis. J. *6*:206–208, 1987.
740. Samuelson, A., Glimåker, M., Skoog, E., et al.: Diagnosis of enteroviral meningitis with IgG-EIA using heat-treated virions and synthetic peptides as antigens. J. Med. Virol. *40*:271–277, 1993.
741. Sanders, D. Y., and Cramblett, H. G.: Viral infections in hospitalized neonates. Am. J. Dis. Child. *116*:251–256, 1968.
742. Sanders, D. Y., Powell, R. V., and Smith, A.: Outbreak of Coxsackie B5 virus in a children's home. South. Med. J. *62*:474–476, 1969.
743. Santti, J., Hyypiä, T., Kinnunen, L., et al.: Evidence of recombination among enteroviruses. J. Virol. *73*:8741–8749, 1999.
744. Saslaw, S., Wooley, C. F., and Anderson, G. R.: Aseptic meningitis syndrome: Report of eleven cases with cerebrospinal fluid isolation of enteroviruses. Arch. Intern. Med. *105*:69–75, 1960.
745. Sato, K., Yamashita, T., Sakae, K., et al.: A new-born baby outbreak of echovirus type 33 infection. J. Infect. *37*:123–126, 1998.
746. Sawyer, L. A., Hershow, R. C., Pallansch, M. A., et al.: An epidemic of acute hemorrhagic conjunctivitis in American Samoa caused by coxsackievirus A24 variant. Am. J. Epidemiol. *130*:1187–1198, 1989.
747. Sawyer, M. H., Holland, D., Aintablian, N., et al.: Diagnosis of enteroviral central nervous system infection by polymerase chain reaction during a large community outbreak. Pediatr. Infect. Dis. J. *13*:177–182, 1994.
748. Saxena, R. C., Bhatia, M., and Chaturvedi, U. C.: Recent epidemic conjunctivitis in Lucknow: A clinical study. Orient. Arch. Ophthalmol. *10*:253–257, 1982.
749. Schleissner, L. A., and Portnoy, B.: Hepatitis and pneumonia associated with ECHO virus, type 9, infection in two adult siblings. Ann. Intern. Med. *68*:1315–1319, 1968.
750. Schleissner, L. A., and Portnoy, B.: Spectrum of ECHO virus 1 disease in a young diabetic. Chest *63*:457–459, 1973.
751. Schlesinger, Y., Sawyer, M. H., and Storch, G. A.: Enteroviral meningitis in infancy: Potential role for polymerase chain reaction in patient management. Pediatrics *94*:157–162, 1994.
752. Schmidt, N. J., Lennette, E. H., and Ho, H. H.: An apparently new enterovirus isolated from patients with disease of the central nervous system. J. Infect. Dis. *129*:304–309, 1974.
753. Schmidt, N. J., Magoffin, R. L., and Lennette, E. H.: Association of group B coxsackieviruses with cases of pericarditis, myocarditis, or pleurodynia by demonstration of immunoglobulin M antibody. Infect. Immun. *8*:341–348, 1973.
754. Schmidt, W. A. K., Brade, L., Muntefering, H., et al.: Course of Coxsackie B antibodies during juvenile diabetes. Med. Microbiol. Immunol. *164*:291–298, 1978.
755. Schoub, B. D., Johnson, S., McAnerney, J. M., et al.: Epidemic coxsackie B virus infection in Johannesburg, South Africa. J. Hyg. (Camb.) *95*:447–455, 1985.
756. Schultz, W. W., and Weiss, E.: Demonstration of specific antibodies to a Coxsackie-like virus in patients of a hepatitis outbreak. Am. J. Epidemiol. *110*:124–131, 1979.
757. Schürmann, W., Statz, A., Mertens, T., et al.: Two cases of coxsackie B2 infection in neonates: Clinical, virological, and epidemiological aspects. Eur. J. Pediatr. *140*:59–63, 1983.
758. Scott, T. F. M.: Clinical syndromes associated with entero virus and reo virus infections. Adv. Virus Res. *8*:165–197, 1962.
759. Seddon, J. H., and Duff, M. F.: Hand-foot-and-mouth disease: Coxsackie virus types A5, A10 and A16 infections. N. Z. Med. J. *74*:368–373, 1971.
760. See, D. M., and Tilles, J. G.: Pathogenesis of virus-induced diabetes in mice. J. Infect. Dis. *171*:1131–1138, 1995.
761. Seko, Y., Matsuda, H., Kato, K., et al.: Expression of intercellular adhesion molecule-1 in murine hearts with acute myocarditis caused by coxsackievirus B3. J. Clin. Invest. *91*:1327–1336, 1993.
762. Seko, Y., Yoshifumi, E., Yagita, H., et al.: Restricted usage of T-cell receptor Va genes in infiltrating cells in murine hearts with acute myocarditis caused by Coxsackie virus B3. J. Pathol. *178*:330–334, 1996.
763. Sells, C. J., Carpenter, R. L., and Ray, C. G.: Sequelae of central nervous system enterovirus infections. N. Engl. J. Med. *293*:1–4, 1975.
764. Selwyn, S., and Howitt, L. F.: A mosaic of enteroviruses: Poliovirus, Coxsackie, and Echo infections in a group of families. Lancet *2*:548–551, 1962.
765. Severien, C., Jacobs, K. H., and Schoenemann, W.: Marked pleocytosis and hypoglycorrhachia in Coxsackie meningitis. Pediatr. Infect. Dis. J. *13*:322–323, 1994.
766. Severini, G. M., Mestroni, L., Falaschi, A., et al.: Nested polymerase chain reaction for high-sensitivity detection of enteroviral RNA in biological samples. J. Clin. Microbiol. *31*:1345–1349, 1993.
767. Sharland, M., Hodgson, J., Davies, E. G., et al.: Enteroviral pharyngitis diagnosed by reverse transcriptase–polymerase chain reaction. Arch. Dis. Child. *74*:462–463, 1996.
768. Shelokov, A., and Habel, K.: Viremia in Coxsackie B meningitis. Proc. Soc. Exp. Biol. Med. *94*:782–784, 1957.
769. Shelokov, A., and Weinstein, L.: Poliomyelitis in the early neonatal period: Report of a case of possible intrauterine infection. J. Pediatr. *38*:80–84, 1951.
770. Shimizu, H., Schnurr, D. P., and Burns, J. C.: Comparison of methods to detect enteroviral genome in frozen and fixed myocardium by polymerase chain reaction. Lab. Invest. *71*:612–616, 1994.
771. Sieber, O. F., Jr., Kilgus, A. H., Fulginiti, V. A., et al.: Immunological response of the newborn infant to Coxsackie B-4 infection. Pediatrics *40*:444–446, 1967.
772. Siegel, M., and Greenberg, M.: Poliomyelitis in pregnancy: Effect on fetus and newborn infant. J. Pediatr. *49*:280–288, 1956.
773. Siegel, W., Spencer, F. J., Smith, D. J., et al.: Two new variants of infection with Coxsackie virus group B, type 5, in young children: A syndrome of lymphadenopathy, pharyngitis and hepatomegaly or splenomegaly, or both, and one of pneumonia. N. Engl. J. Med. *268*:1210–1216, 1963.
774. Silver, T. S., and Todd, J. K.: Hypoglycorrhachia in pediatric patients. Pediatrics *58*:67–71, 1976.
775. Simonsen, L., Khan, A. S., Gary, H. E., Jr., et al.: Outbreak of vertigo in Wyoming: Possible role of an enterovirus infection. Epidemiol. Infect. *117*:149–157, 1996.

776. Singer, J. I., Maur, P. R., Riley, J. P., et al.: Management of central nervous system infections during an epidemic of enteroviral aseptic meningitis. J. Pediatr. *96*:559–563, 1980.
777. Skeels, M. R., Williams, J. J., and Ricker, F. M.: Perinatal echovirus infection. N. Engl. J. Med. *305*:1529–1530, 1981.
778. Soboleva, V. D., Lozovskaya, L. S., Alekseyeva, V. B., et al.: Coxsackie A13 virus in the foci of rheumatism. J. Hyg. Epidemiol. Microbiol. Immunol. (Praha) *22*:195–202, 1978.
779. Solomon, P., Weinstein, L., Chang, T. W., et al.: Epidemiologic, clinical, and laboratory features of an epidemic of type 9 Echo virus meningitis. J. Pediatr. *55*:609–619, 1959.
780. Sommerville, R. G.: Enteroviruses and diarrhea in young persons. Lancet *2*:1347–1349, 1958.
781. Spudis, E. V., and Cramblett, H. G.: ECHO 4 meningoencephalitis. Arch. Neurol. *12*:404–409, 1965.
782. Stanway, G., and Hyypia, T.: Parechoviruses. J. Virol. *73*:5249–5254, 1999.
783. Stanway, G., Joki-Korpela, P., and Hyypia, T.: Human parechoviruses—biology and clinical significance. Rev. Med. Virol. *10*:57–69, 2000.
784. Steigman, A. J.: Poliomyelitis properties of certain non-polio viruses: Enteroviruses and Heine-Medin disease. J. Mt. Sinai Hosp. *25*:391–404, 1958.
785. Steigman, A. J., and Lipton, M. M.: Fatal bulbospinal paralytic poliomyelitis due to ECHO 11 virus. J. A. M. A. *174*:178–179, 1960.
786. Steigman, A. J., Lipton, M. M., and Braspennickx, H.: Acute lymphonodular pharyngitis: A newly described condition due to Coxsackie A virus. J. Pediatr. *61*:331–336, 1962.
787. Steinhoff, M. C.: Viruses and diarrhea: A review. Am. J. Dis. Child. *132*:302–307, 1978.
788. Steinmann, J., and Albrecht, K.: Echovirus 11-epidemie bei fruhgeborenen auf einer neonatal-intensive-station. Zentrabl. Baktiol. *259*: 284–293, 1985.
789. Stern, H.: Aetiology of central nervous system infections during prevalence of poliovirus and Coxsackie virus: Some clinical manifestations of Coxsackie virus infections. B. M. J. *1*:1061–1066, 1961.
790. Stones, P. B.: Isolation of ECHO virus type 9 during an outbreak of meningo-encephalitis. B. M. J. *2*:1514, 1958.
791. Strebel, P. M., Sutter, R. W., Cochi, S. L., et al.: Epidemiology of poliomyelitis in the United States one decade after the last reported case of indigenous wild virus–associated disease. Clin. Infect. Dis. *14*:568–579, 1992.
792. Strikas, R. A., Anderson, L. J., and Parker, R. A.: Temporal and geographic patterns of isolates of nonpolio enterovirus in the United States, 1970–1983. J. Infect. Dis. *153*:346–351, 1986.
793. Ström, J.: Coxsackie B5 infection causing serous meningitis with exanthema and benign pericarditis with myocarditis in two siblings. Acta Paediatr. Suppl. *135*:197–202, 1962.
794. Stürup, H.: The long-term prognosis of acute non-specific pericarditis: A follow-up examination including cases of dry pleurisy from an epidemic of Bornholm disease (myalgia epidemica) in 1930–32. Dan. Med. Bull. *1*:89–91, 1954.
795. Sumaya, C. V., and Corman, L. I.: Enteroviral meningitis in early infancy: Significance in community outbreaks. Pediatr. Infect. Dis. *1*:151–154, 1982.
796. Sun, N. C., and Smith, V. M.: Hepatitis associated with myocarditis: Unusual manifestation of infection with Coxsackie virus group B, type 3. N. Engl. J. Med. *274*:190–193, 1966.
797. Swanink, C. M. A., Melchers, W. J. G., van der Meer, J. W. M., et al.: Enteroviruses and the chronic fatigue syndrome. Clin. Infect. Dis. *19*:860–864, 1994.
798. Swann, N. H.: Epidemic pleurodynia, orchitis, and myocarditis in an adult due to Coxsackie virus, group B, type 4. Ann. Intern. Med. *54*:1008–1013, 1961.
799. Swender, P. T., Shott, R. J., and Williams, M. L.: A community and intensive care nursery outbreak of coxsackievirus B5 meningitis. Am. J. Dis. Child. *127*:42–45, 1974.
800. Sylvest, E.: Epidemic Myalgia: Bornholm Disease. Translated by H. Andersen. London, Oxford University Press, 1934.
801. Syverton, J. T., McLean, D. M., da Silva, M. M., et al.: Outbreak of aseptic meningitis caused by Coxsackie B5 virus: Laboratory, clinical, and epidemiologic study. J. A. M. A. *164*:2015–2019, 1957.
802. Takahashi, S., Miyamoto, A., Oki, J., et al.: Acute transverse myelitis caused by ECHO virus type 18 infection. Eur. J. Pathol. *154*:378–380, 1995.
803. Takos, M. J., Weil, M., and Sigel, M. M.: Outbreak of ECHO 9 exanthema traced to a children's party. Am. J. Dis. Child. *100*:360–364, 1960.
804. Talsma, M., Vegting, M., and Hess, J.: Generalised coxsackie A9 infection in a neonate presenting with pericarditis. Br. Heart. J. *52*:683–685, 1984.
805. Tanel, R. E., Kao, S.-Y., Niemiec, T. M., et al.: Prospective comparison of culture vs genome detection for diagnosis of enteroviral meningitis in childhood. Arch. Pediatr. Adolesc. Med. *150*:919–924, 1996.
806. Tang, T. T., Sedmak, G. V., Siegesmund, K. A., et al.: Chronic myopathy associated with coxsackievirus type A9: A combined electron microscopical and viral isolation study. N. Engl. J. Med. *292*:608–611, 1975.
807. Tarcan, A., Özbek, N., and Gürakan, B.: Bone marrow failure with concurrent enteroviral infection in a newborn. Pediatr. Infect. Dis. J. *20*:719–721, 2001.
808. Tateno, I., Suzuki, S., Kagawa, S., et al.: On an Echo-like agent constantly recoverable from volunteers given Niigata strain of acute epidemic gastroenteritis. Jpn. J. Exp. Med. *26*:125–128, 1956.
809. Technical Consultative Group to the World Health Organization on the Global Eradication of Poliomyelitis: "Endgame" issues for the global polio eradication initiative. Clin. Infect. Dis. *34*:72–77, 2002.
810. Terletskaia-Ladwig, E., Metzger, C., Schalasta, G., Enders, G.: A new enzyme immunoassay for the detection of enteroviruses in faecal specimens. J. Med. Virol. *60*:439–445, 2000.
811. Terletskaia-Ladwig, E., Metzger, C., Schalasta, G., Enders, G.: Evaluation of enterovirus serological tests IgM-EIA and complement fixation in patients with meningitis, confirmed by detection of enteroviral RNA by RT-PCR in cerebrospinal fluid. J. Med. Virol. *61*:221–227, 2000.
812. Thomas, H. M., Jr.: Acute viral peritonitis due to group B Coxsackie viruses. Md. State Med. J. *11*:282–285, 1962.
813. Thoren, A., and Widell, A.: PCR for the diagnosis of enteroviral meningitis. Scand. J. Infect. Dis. *26*:249–254, 1994.
814. Thorsteinsson, G.: Management of postpolio syndrome. Mayo Clin. Proc. *72*:627–638, 1997.
815. Tian, J., Lehmann, P. V., and Kaufman, D. L.: T cell cross-reactivity between coxsackievirus and glutamate decarboxylase is associated with a murine diabetes susceptibility allele. J. Exp. Med. *180*:1979–1984, 1994.
816. Tindall, J. P., and Callaway, J. L.: Hand-foot-and-mouth disease: It's more common than you think. Am. J. Dis. Child. *124*:372–375, 1972.
817. Tobe, T.: Inapparent virus infection as a trigger of appendicitis. Lancet *1*:1343–1346, 1965.
818. Toce, S. S., and Keenan, W. K.: Congenital echovirus 11 pneumonia in association with pulmonary hypertension. Pediatr. Infect. Dis. J. *7*:360–361, 1988.
819. Torphy, D. E., Ray, C. G., Thompson, R. S., et al.: An epidemic of aseptic meningitis due to Echo-virus type 30: Epidemiologic features and clinical and laboratory findings. Am. J. Public Health *60*:1447–1455, 1970.
820. Toth, M., Osvoth, P., Galambos, M., et al.: Kindergarten outbreak of an exanthematous disease caused by echo-virus type 9. Acta Paediatr. Hung. *5*:235–239, 1964.
821. Townsend, T. R., Bolyard, E. A., Yolken, R. H., et al.: Outbreak of coxsackie A1 gastroenteritis: A complication of bone-marrow transplantation. Lancet *1*:820–823, 1982.
822. Trabelsi, A., Grattard, F., Nejmeddine, M., et al.: Evaluation of an enterovirus group-specific anti-VP1 monoclonal antibody, 5-D8/1, in comparison with neutralization and PCR for rapid identification of enteroviruses in cell culture. J. Clin. Microbiol. *33*:2454–2457, 1995.
823. Tracy, S., Höfling, K., Pirruccello, S., et al.: Group B coxsackievirus myocarditis and pancreatitis: Connection between viral virulence phenotypes in mice. J. Med. Virol. *62*:70–81, 2000.
824. Trallero, G., Casas, I., Tenorio, A., et al.: Enteroviruses in Spain: Virological and epidemiological studies over 10 years (1988–97). Epidemiol. Infect. *124*:497–506, 2000.
825. Traystman, M. D., Chow, L. H., McManus, B. M., et al.: Susceptibility to Coxsackievirus B3–induced chronic myocarditis maps near the murine Tcr alpha and Myhc alpha loci on chromosome 14. Am. J. Pathol. *138*:721–726, 1991.
826. Tubman, T. R. J., Craig, B., and Mulholland, H. C.: Ventricular tachycardia associated with coxsackie B4 virus infection. Acta Paediatr. Scand. *79*:572–575, 1990.
827. Turnbull, D. C.: Optic neuritis: Associated with Bornholm disease. Am. J. Ophthalmol. *46*:81–83, 1958.
828. Tuuteri, L., Lapinleimu, K., and Meurman, L.: Fatal myocarditis associated with Coxsackie B3 infection in the newborn. Ann. Paediatr. Fenn. *9*:56–64, 1963.
829. Tyrrell, D. A. J., Lane, R. R., Snell, B., et al.: Clinical and laboratory studies of a syndrome characterized by meningitis and an exanthem, caused by a virus related to ECHO 9. *In* Rose, H. M. (ed.): Viral Infections of Infancy and Childhood. New York, Hoeber-Harper, 1960, pp. 101–118.
830. Underwood, M.: A Treatise on the Diseases of Children. 2nd ed. London, J. Mathews, 1789.
831. Urano, T., Kawase, T., Kodaira, K., et al.: Gullain-Barré syndrome associated with Echo virus type 7 infections. Pediatrics *45*:294–295, 1970.
832. Ursing, B.: Acute pancreatitis in Coxsackie B infection. B. M. J. *3*:524–525, 1973.
833. Utz, J. P., and Shelokov, A. I.: Coxsackie B virus infection: Presence of virus in blood, urine and cerebrospinal fluid. J. A. M. A. *168*:264–267, 1958.
834. Vague, P., Vialettes, B., Prince, M. A., et al.: Coxsackie B viruses and autoimmune diabetes. N. Engl. J. Med. *305*:1157–1158, 1981.
835. Van Creveld, S.: Virus myocarditis in infancy—acute phase and possible late sequels. *In* Rose, H. M. (ed.): Viral Infections of Infancy and Childhood: A Symposium of the Section on Microbiology. The New York Academy of Medicine. New York, Paul B. Hoeber, 1960, pp. 33–54.
836. Van Eden, W., Persijn, G. G., Bikkerk, H., et al.: Differential resistance to paralytic poliomyelitis controlled by histocompatibility leukocyte antigens. J. Infect. Dis. *147*:422–426, 1983.

837. Van Loon, G. R., and Masson, A. M.: Viral pericarditis: A report of five cases. Can. Med. Assoc. J. *99*:163–168, 1968.
838. Van Maldergem, L., Mascart, F., Ureel, D., et al.: Echovirus meningoencephalitis in X-linked hypogammaglobulinemia. Acta Paediatr. Scand. *78*:325–326, 1989.
839. Verboon-Maciolek, M. A., Swanink, C. M. A., Krediet, T. G., et al.: Severe neonatal echovirus 20 infection characterized by hepatic failure. Pediatr. Infect. Dis. J. *16*:524–527, 1997.
840. Verlinde, J. D., Van Tongeren, H. A. E., Wilterdink, J. B., et al.: "Biak fever": An epidemic illness associated with Echo 6 virus. Trop. Geogr. Med. *11*:276–280, 1959.
841. Vieth, U. C., Kunzelmann, M., Diedrich, S., et al.: An echovirus 30 outbreak with a high meningitis attack rate among children and household members at four day-care centers. Eur. J. Epidemiol. *25*:655–658, 1999.
842. Von Zeipel, G., and Svedmyr, A.: A study of the association of Echo viruses to aseptic meningitis. Arch. Ges. Virusforsch. *7*:355–368, 1957.
843. Voroshilova, M. K., and Chumakov, M. P.: Poliomyelitis-like properties of AB-IV Coxsackie A7 group of viruses. Prog. Med. Virol. *2*:106–170, 1959.
844. Wadia, N. H., Katrak, S. M., Misra, V. P., et al.: Polio-like motor paralysis associated with acute hemorrhagic conjunctivitis in an outbreak in 1981 in Bombay, India: Clinical and serologic studies. J. Infect. Dis. *147*:660–668, 1983.
845. Walters, J. H.: Postencephalitic Parkinson syndrome after meningoencephalitis due to Coxsackie virus group B, type 2. N. Engl. J. Med. *263*:744–747, 1960.
846. Wang, S.-M., Liu, C.-C., Chen, Y.-J., et al.: Alice in Wonderland syndrome caused by coxsackievirus B1. Pediatr. Infect. Dis. J. *15*:470–471, 1996.
847. Wang, S.-M., Liu, C.-C., Yang, Y.-J., et al.: Fatal coxsackievirus B infection in early infancy characterized by fulminant hepatitis. J. Infect. *37*:270–273, 1998.
848. Ward, C.: Severe arrhythmias in coxsackievirus B3 myopericarditis. Arch. Dis. Child. *53*:174–176, 1978.
849. Ward, N. A., Milstien, J. B., Hull, H. F., et al.: The WHO-EPI initiative for the global eradication of poliomyelitis. Biologicals *21*:327–333, 1993.
850. Warin, J. F., Davies, J. B. M., Sanders, F. K., et al.: Oxford epidemic of Bornholm disease, 1951. B. M. J. *1*:1345–1351, 1953.
851. Waterman, S. H., Casas-Benabe, R., Hatch, M. H., et al.: Acute hemorrhagic conjunctivitis in Puerto Rico, 1981–1982. Am. J. Epidemiol. *120*:395–403, 1984.
852. Waterson, A. P.: Virological investigations in congestive cardiomyopathy. Postgrad. Med. J. *54*:505–507, 1978.
853. Webster, A. D. B., Rotbart, H. A., Warner, T., et al.: Diagnosis of enterovirus brain disease in hypogammaglobulinemic patients by polymerase chain reaction. Clin. Infect. Dis. *17*:657–661, 1993.
854. Wehrle, P. F., Judge, M. E., Parizeau, M. C., et al.: Disability associated with ECHO virus infections. N. Y. State J. Med. *59*:3941–3945, 1959.
855. Weiner, L. S., Howell, J. T., Langford, M. P., et al.: Effect of specific antibodies on chronic echovirus type 5 encephalitis in a patient with hypogammaglobulinemia. J. Infect. Dis. *140*:858–863, 1979.
856. Weinstein, S. B.: Acute benign pericarditis associated with Coxsackie virus group B, type 5. N. Engl. J. Med. *257*:265–267, 1957.
857. Weller, T. H., Enders, J. F., Buckingham, M., et al.: The etiology of epidemic pleurodynia: A study of two viruses isolated from a tropical outbreak. J. Immunol. *65*:337–346, 1950.
858. Welliver, R. C., and Cherry, J. D.: Aseptic meningitis and orchitis associated with echovirus 6 infection. J. Pediatr. *92*:239–240, 1978.
859. Wenner, H. A.: The Echo viruses. Ann. N. Y. Acad. Sci. *10*:398–412, 1962.
860. Wenner, H. A.: The enteroviruses. Am. J. Clin. Pathol. *57*:751–761, 1972.
861. Wenner, H. A.: Virus diseases associated with cutaneous eruptions. Prog. Med. Virol. *16*:269–336, 1973.
862. Wenner, H. A., and Behbehani, A. M.: ECHO viruses. Monogr. Virol. *1*:1–72, 1968.
863. Wenner, H. A., Christodoulopoulou, G., Weston, J., et al.: The etiology of respiratory illnesses occurring in infancy and childhood. Pediatrics *31*:4–17, 1963.
864. Wenner, H. A., and Lou, T. Y.: Virus diseases associated with cutaneous eruptions. Prog. Med. Virol. *5*:219–294, 1963.
865. Wesslén, T., Eriksson, S., Ehinger, A., et al.: Epidemic of aseptic meningitis associated with Echo virus type 9. Arch. Ges. Virusforsch. *8*:183–191, 1958.
866. Wickman, I.: On the epidemiology of Heine-Medin's disease. Rev. Infect. Dis. *2*:319–327, 1980.
867. Wilfert, C. M., Buckley, R. H., Mohanakumar, T., et al.: Persistent and fatal central nervous system echovirus infections in patients with agammaglobulinemia. N. Engl. J. Med. *296*:1485–1489, 1977.
868. Wilfert, C. M., Thompson, R. J., Jr., Sunder, T. R., et al.: Longitudinal assessment of children with enteroviral meningitis during the first three months of life. Pediatrics *67*:811–815, 1981.
869. Wilkins, A. J. W., Kotze, D. M., Melvin, J., et al.: Meningo-encephalitis due to Coxsackie B virus in Southern Rhodesia. S. Afr. Med. J. *29*:25–28, 1955.
870. Willems, W. R., Hornig, C., Bauer, H., et al.: A case of Coxsackie A9 virus infection with orchitis. J. Med. Virol. *3*:137–140, 1978.
871. Wilson, C., Connolly, J. H., and Thomson, D.: Coxsackie B2 virus infection and acute-onset diabetes in a child. B. M. J. *1*:1008–1009, 1977.
872. Wilt, J. C., Medovy, H., Besant, D., et al.: Aseptic meningitis in Manitoba, 1957. Can. Med. Assoc. J. *78*:839–842, 1958.
873. Wilt, J. C., Parker, W. L., Owens, A. L., et al.: Enterovirus infections in Manitoba. 1959. Can. Med. Assoc. J. *83*:839–843, 1960.
874. Windebank, A. J., Litchy, W. J., Daube, J. R., et al.: Late effects of paralytic poliomyelitis in Olmsted County, Minnesota. Neurology *41*:501–507, 1991.
875. Windebank, A. J., Litchy, W. J., Daube, J. R., et al.: Lack of progression of neurologic deficit in survivors of paralytic polio: A 5-year prospective population-based study. Neurology *46*:80–84, 1996.
876. Winsser, J., and Altieri, R. H.: A three-year study of Coxsackie virus, group B infection in Nassau County. Am. J. Med. Sci. *247*:269–273, 1964.
877. Wolfgram, L. J., and Rose, N. R.: Coxsackievirus infection as a trigger of cardiac autoimmunity. Immunol. Res. *8*:61–80, 1989.
878. Wong, S. N., Tam, A. Y. S., Ng, T. H., et al.: Fatal coxsackie B1 virus infection in neonates. Pediatr. Infect. Dis. J. *8*:638–641, 1989.
879. Wood, D. J., Sutter, R. W., and Dowdle, W. R.: Stopping poliovirus vaccination after eradication: issues and challenges. Bull. World Health Organ. *78*:347–357, 2000.
880. Wood, S. F., Rogen, A. S., Bell, E. J., et al.: Role of coxsackie B viruses in myocardial infarction. Br. Heart J. *40*:523–525, 1978.
881. Woodall, C. J., Riding, M. H., Graham, D. J., et al.: Sequences specific for enterovirus detected in spinal cord from patients with motor neurone disease. B. M. J. *308*:1541–1543, 1994.
882. Woods, J. D., Nimmo, M. J., and Mackay-Scollay, E. M.: Acute transmural myocardial infarction associated with active Coxsackie virus B infection. Am. Heart J. *89*:283–287, 1975.
883. Wooley, C. F.: Intracranial hypertension associated with recovery of a Coxsackie virus from the cerebrospinal fluid. Neurology *110*:572–574, 1960.
884. Wreghitt, T. G., Sutehall, G. M., King, A., et al.: Fatal echovirus 7 infection during an outbreak in a special care baby unit. J. Infect. *19*:229–236, 1989.
885. Wright, H. T., Jr., Landing, B. H., Lennette, E. H., et al.: Fatal infection in an infant associated with Coxsackie virus group A, type 16. N. Engl. J. Med. *268*:1041–1044, 1963.
886. Wright, P. F., Kim-Farley, R. J., de Quadros, C. A., et al.: Strategies for the global eradication of poliomyelitis by the year 2000. N. Engl. J. Med. *325*:1773–1779, 1991.
887. Yaffee, H. S.: Erythema multiforme caused by Coxsackie B5: A possible association with epidemic pustular stomatitis of children. Arch. Dermatol. *82*:737–739, 1960.
888. Yamashita, K., Miyamura, K., Yamadera, S., et al.: Epidemics of aseptic meningitis due to echovirus 30 in Japan. Jpn. J. Med. Sci. Biol. *47*:221–239, 1994.
889. Yan, J.-J., Wang, J.-R., Liu, C.-C., et al.: An outbreak of enterovirus 71 infection in Taiwan 1998: A comprehensive pathological, virological, and molecular study on a case of fulminant encephalitis. J. Clin. Virol. *17*:13–22, 2000.
890. Yang, C.-F., De, L., Holloway, B. P., et al.: Detection and identification of vaccine-related polioviruses by the polymerase chain reaction. Viral Res. *20*:159–179, 1991.
891. Yerly, S., Guervaix, A., Simonet, V., et al.: Rapid and sensitive detection of enteroviruses in specimens from patients with aseptic meningitis. J. Clin. Microbiol. *34*:199–201, 1996.
892. Yin-Murphy, M.: Acute hemorrhagic conjunctivitis. Prog. Med. Virol. *29*:23–44, 1984.
893. Yohannan, M. D., Ramia, S., and Al Frayh, A. R. S.: Acute paralytic poliomyelitis presenting as Guillain-Barré syndrome. J. Infect. *22*:129–133, 1991.
894. Yoon, J.-W., Austin, M., Onodera, T., et al.: Virus-induced diabetes mellitus: Isolation of a virus from the pancreas of a child with diabetic ketoacidosis. N. Engl. J. Med. *300*:1173–1179, 1979.
895. Yousef, G. E., Bell, E. J., Mann, G. F., et al.: Chronic enterovirus infection in patients with postviral fatigue syndrome. Lancet *1*:146–150, 1988.
896. Yow, M. D., Melnick, J. L., Blattner, R. J., et al.: Enteroviruses in infantile diarrhea. Am. J. Hyg. *77*:283–292, 1963.
897. Yow, M. D., Melnick, J. L., Phillips, C. A., et al.: An etiologic investigation of infantile diarrhea in Houston during 1962 and 1963. Am. J. Epidemiol. *83*:255–261, 1966.
898. Yuceoglu, A. M., Berkovich, S., and Minkowitz, S.: Acute glomerulonephritis associated with ECHO virus type 9 infection. J. Pediatr. *69*:603–609, 1966.
899. Yui, L. A., and Gledhill, R. F.: Limb paralysis as a manifestation of coxsackie B virus infection. Dev. Med. Child Neurol. *33*:427–438, 1991.
900. Zanetti, A. R.: Enterovirus associated sporadic cases and epidemics. Annali Sclavo *19*:187–192, 1977.
901. Zuniga, M. D. R., Reichardt, J., Braun, W., et al.: Detection of IgM antibodies against Coxsackie B viruses by a western blot technique. Acta Virol. *37*:1–10, 1993.

CHAPTER 171

Rhinoviruses

ROBERT L. ATMAR

In 1954, the first recognized rhinovirus (RV) (type 1A) was isolated in monkey kidney cell culture by Mogabgab and associates[214, 231] from a recruit at Great Lakes Naval Training Center (Chicago) during an outbreak of afebrile common colds in his training company. Independently, Price and colleagues[239] reported the isolation of an antigenically identical virus from nurses and children with colds. In 1963, the RVs were so named because of their association with illnesses of the nasal passages.[287]

Before these actual virus isolations, evidence suggested that viruses cause the common cold. Despite indications that some cold-like illnesses could be complicated by bacterial infections,[25, 73, 80, 296] bacteria-free nasal filtrates from persons with apparent symptomatic respiratory infections clearly were able to initiate these illnesses. Kruse,[184] in 1914, first demonstrated transmission with apparently sterile filtrates, and in the late 1920s, his results were confirmed in a series of experiments in humans and chimpanzees by Dochez and associates.[80] In the 1930s, workers from this latter laboratory reported growth of the agent in tissue culture and embryonated eggs, but their results were not confirmed.[9] In the 1940s and 1950s, Andrewes and colleagues[8] at the Common Cold Unit in Salisbury, England, and Dingle and the members of the U.S. Armed Forces Commission on Acute Respiratory Diseases were able to transmit colds from person to person with apparently sterile filtrates.[58] Jackson and colleagues[163] performed similar experiments in Chicago and also demonstrated immunity. In 1953, the Salisbury researchers reported isolation of an agent, DC, in serially passaged filtrates of tubed tissue cultures of human embryonic lungs, the virus being detected by its ability to produce colds in humans.[7] (Although these results could not be substantiated at the time, a virus *was* present; in 1968, the DC filtrates were found to contain RV-9.[60])

The next major advance in growing common cold viruses took place in the late 1950s in Salisbury. Tyrrell and Parsons[288] inoculated human embryonic kidney cells with nasal filtrates and incubated the cultures under conditions simulating those of the nasal passages (e.g., 33° C, neutral pH, and in a roller drum for aeration). Six distinct types of RVs (types 1B to 6)[65] were isolated by observing cytopathic effects.[275] Shortly thereafter, Hamparian and coworkers[65, 133, 178] isolated 18 RVs (types 7 to 12 and 18 to 29) by using a semicontinuous diploid cell strain obtained by Hayflick and Moorhead[139] from human fetal lung cultures. The use of Hayflick's cell lines greatly accelerated the isolation and characterization of "new" RVs, and now, 100 serotypes (or 101 if RV-1A and RV-1B are counted as two serologic entities) officially have been identified.[132] More remain untyped, but the number of additional serotypes seems limited.[132, 175, 216]

Although the RVs are associated primarily with mild upper respiratory tract disease, they also may be involved in bronchitis, sinusitis, and, on occasion, pneumonia in all age groups. They seem to be precipitants of "infectious asthma" attacks. RVs cause approximately 30 to 50 percent of all acute respiratory illness.[65, 98]

The Organism

GENERAL DESCRIPTION

Rhinovirus is one of four genera of human pathogens in the family *Picornaviridae.*[292] *Enterovirus* includes polioviruses, coxsackieviruses, and echoviruses; *Parechovirus* includes two serotypes formerly identified as echovirus types 22 and 23; and hepatitis A virus is the single member of *Hepatovirus.*[292] Like the other picornaviruses, the RVs are small (30 nm), nonenveloped (therefore, resistant to lipid solvents such as ether and chloroform), and icosahedral (20-sided, hexagonal in cross section), with a genome consisting of single-stranded RNA (molecular weight, 2.5×10^6) 7210 nucleotides long.[292] A picornavirus can be thought of as an RNA genome surrounded by a 20-sided protein coat (the capsid) (Fig. 171–1). The RNA alone is infectious and can serve as a messenger.

RVs differ from enteroviruses in being rendered noninfectious at an acidity below pH 5 and by their higher buoyant density in cesium chloride.

The genomes of RVs demonstrate much cross-homology.[89] Several RVs, including RV-1B, RV-2, RV-14, RV-16, and RV-89, have been sequenced completely.[89, 156, 187, 262, 267] RV-1B and RV-2 are minor receptor group RVs, and their protein homologies are close: 74 to 94 percent. On the other hand, RV-14 proteins are related nearly as closely to those in the poliovirus and enterovirus groups as to those in the RVs.[157, 166, 267] Researchers have shown in nucleic acid hybridization experiments that cDNA to a segment near the

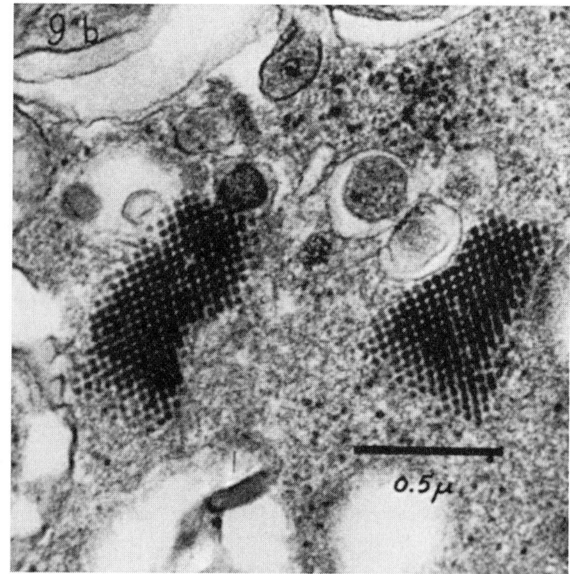

FIGURE 171–1 ■ Rhinovirus type 2 in human fetal lung cells. Note the hexagonal virus crystals closely packed in a rectangular lattice (×40,000). (From Kawana, R., and Matsumoto, I.: Electron microscopic study of rhinovirus replication in human fetal lung cells. Jpn. J. Microbiol. *15*:207–217, 1971.)

5′ end of the RV genome reacts with the genomes of many different picornaviruses (rhinoviruses and enteroviruses).[3, 24] The interrelationships of viruses in these two genera will become clearer as more sequence data are obtained.

STRUCTURE OF THE VIRION

Knowledge of the structure of the RVs and some of the other picornaviruses is increasing with determination of the capsid structures in atomic detail for five serotypes, RV-1A, RV-2, RV-3, RV-14, and RV-16.[12, 24, 149, 180, 251, 252, 293, 306] The thin (5 nm) protein capsid has an undulating exterior marked by 12 vertices (the icosahedral fivefold axis) equally spaced over the surface. Surrounding these vertices is a steep (2.5 nm deep), narrow canyon. For the known 101 RV serotypes, only three different receptor binding sites exist: 90 serotypes bind to intracellular adhesion molecule-1 (ICAM-1, the major receptor group), 10 other serotypes bind to members of the low-density lipoprotein receptor family (LDL-R, the minor receptor group), and 1 serotype (type 87) binds to an as yet unidentified receptor.[1, 114, 289]

ICAM-1 binds to the base of the canyon of RVs in the major receptor group.[251, 253, 289] Virus-neutralizing antibody prevents virus attachment to cells by adhering to serospecific sites and blocking the cell receptor from access to its binding site at the canyon base. These antibody sites may directly overlap ICAM-1 binding sites, or they may be separate from the ICAM-1 binding sites but at a point sufficiently close to allow the binding site to be blocked by steric hindrance.[46, 264] Binding of the major receptor group RVs to ICAM-1 leads to destabilization of the virus capsid and uncoating of the viral RNA.[115]

The LDL-R family binds to a different site for the minor receptor group of RVs than that recognized by ICAM-1. The binding site for these RVs is the small star-shaped dome above the canyon on the icosahedral fivefold axis. Attachment of minor receptor group viruses to LDL-R does not lead to virus uncoating, in contrast to what is seen with binding of major receptor group RVs to ICAM-1. Instead, internalization into acidic endosomal compartments is required for uncoating of minor receptor group RVs.[147]

A pocket of unknown function whose walls are lined by 17 amino acids that vary with each RV type has been found at the base of the canyon.[10] A variety of organic molecules have been determined to bind in this pocket; when these molecules are bound, either the virus is prevented from uncoating (necessary to release viral RNA for its translation to viral protein) or the cell receptor is prevented from docking in the canyon.[99, 235] Numerous drugs made by several different drug companies in the United States, Europe, and Japan have been developed to exploit the antipicornavirus potentialities of this pocket, and the sensitivity of the RVs to these drugs has been used as an additional means of classifying the RVs (into inhibitor groups A and B).[10, 11] One group of these drugs, the WIN compounds synthesized by Sterling-Winthrop, has had wide scientific exposure[203]; however, clinical trials have been discouraging.[279, 285] One disadvantage of these compounds is that the various RV serotypes vary widely in sensitivity to these organic molecules.[10] Another problem has been failure to attain effective concentrations of drug at the site of infection.

VIRUS REPLICATION

Replication of the RVs is similar to that of the enteroviruses.[244] After attachment to the cellular receptor, the virus undergoes endocytosis and RNA is released. Genomic viral RNA functions as messenger RNA and attaches to ribosomes, which stimulates its translation by host enzymes into a single long polyprotein. This polyprotein is cleaved by viral proteases to yield viral RNA polymerase, capsid proteins, proteases, and proteins to halt the synthesis of host proteins and other products. Under laboratory conditions, infectious virus first is formed after approximately 2 hours and reaches a maximum of approximately 1000 infectious particles per cell at approximately 7 hours. Infectious virus is, however, a minority of the virus-like particles formed; only approximately 1 in 200 are complete viruses capable of replicating in cell culture. All viral replication occurs in the cytoplasm, and viruses are released by cell lysis.[244]

HOST RANGE

Animals

RVs have been isolated from natural infections in only cattle, chimpanzees, and humans.[195, 292] Just two bovine RV serotypes have been reported, and they may cause infections ranging from subclinical to overt respiratory disease in epizootics; no evidence of human infection has been reported.[249] Chimpanzees and humans both are infected with human RVs; however, chimpanzee infections are subclinical.[75, 260] A natural, subclinical outbreak of RV-31 in chimpanzees has been reported in a primate center.[74, 75]

Many attempts have been made to infect a wide variety of animals with human RVs, but other than the chimpanzee, only the gibbon has been susceptible, and it is not reliably so.[75] A type 2 RV was adapted to grow in a mouse cell line (L cells), and the adapted virus was shown to grow in a mouse model.[304] Equine “RVs” have been described, but these viruses belong to different picornavirus genera.[223, 292]

Cell and Tissue Cultures

The spectrum of tissue culture cells infected by human RVs also is narrow.[62, 185] For initial isolation, human embryonic diploid cells generally are used (Fig. 171–2), although for some RV types, an especially sensitive strain[59] of a continuous cell line, HeLa, serves as well or better.[62, 185] Some RVs grow only in human organ cultures and, perhaps, some only in living human beings.[185]

The first RV (RV-1A) was propagated in primary cell culture from primate kidneys (rhesus monkey cell cultures are used most commonly); surprisingly, chimpanzee kidney cell cultures do not propagate RVs.[71] However, most RVs propagate on original isolation only in cells of human origin, and they are called H strains; others also can be isolated in monkey kidney cell cultures and are called M strains. After laboratory propagation, all RVs seem adaptable to the RV-sensitive HeLa cell strain.[59] HeLa-grown RVs attain much higher titers than those in the primary human diploid cells used for initial isolation.

ANTIGENIC PROPERTIES

An outstanding characteristic of RV is its great antigenic diversity; at least 101 serotypes exist.[132] Evidence has shown, however, that the number of additional serotypes may be limited.[98, 132, 175, 216] Certain serotypes cross-react, but little evidence indicates that this cross-reaction could be exploited in vaccination.[61, 96, 213]

RVs often are poor antigens. Significant (fourfold or greater) increases in serum antibody may not develop in as many as 50 percent of patients from whom RVs are isolated, and the levels attained are often low.[96–98]

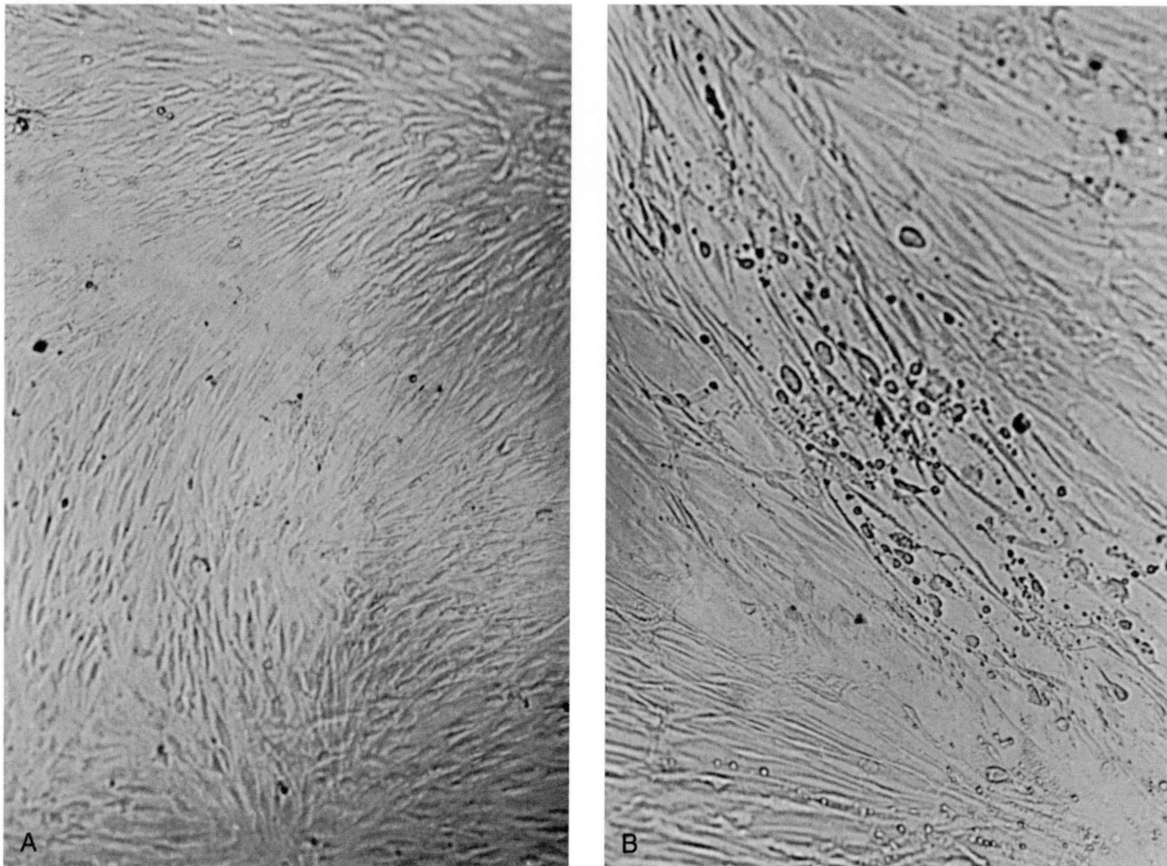

FIGURE 171–2 ■ *A,* Normal human diploid (fetal tonsil) cell sheet. *B,* Cell sheet infected for 2 days with rhinovirus type 16. The rounded and misshapen cells are characteristic. (Courtesy of Dr. David M. Warshauer, University of Wisconsin, Madison.)

RVs may be undergoing continuous antigenic change.[213] Sufficiently marked antigenic variation has been found for RV-22 and RV-51 to interfere with their typing; however, this drift does not seem to predict a continuing proliferation of RV types.[98, 216, 258, 270]

Epidemiology and Transmission

SEASONAL DISTRIBUTION

During the usual September through May "cold season," RV infections often are predominant at both ends, early fall and mid to late spring (Figs. 171–3 and 171–4). They are also important causes of summer colds. This seasonal pattern seems general because similar findings have been reported from families in Charlottesville, Virginia; Seattle, Washington; and elsewhere.[21, 97, 98, 119, 145, 197] In the Southern Hemisphere, a similar seasonal pattern occurs, but during opposing months.[169] The general spring-summer-fall seasonal predominance of the RVs does not mean that RVs are absent during the remainder of the year; they are found in varying degrees year-round.[65, 97, 98, 121, 197, 216, 217, 247]

CYCLING AND CIRCULATION OF INDIVIDUAL RHINOVIRUS TYPES

Unlike most respiratory viruses (e.g., parainfluenza types 1 and 3 and respiratory syncytial virus [RSV]), individual RV types seldom repeat within a population from year to year. Several serotypes usually circulate simultaneously,[134] frequently coincident with other respiratory viruses.[72, 151, 217] The various respiratory viruses circulate simultaneously within the neighborhood, as well as within the larger community. In 24 neighboring families in Madison, Wisconsin (Eagle Heights) (see Fig. 171–4), 14 different RV types plus several nontypable RVs were found during the 2 academic years 1963 to 1965. Only one type (RV-15) was found both years. The other common respiratory viruses also were present.

Several respiratory viruses may circulate concurrently among close neighbors or even within a family. As an example, from March to May 1963, RV-43 and RV-55, one nontypable RV, parainfluenza types 1 and 3, chickenpox, and poliomyelitis types 2 and 3 (from a community vaccination program) circulated through 10 Eagle Heights families studied in a 12-unit apartment building (Fig. 171–5). In two families, RV-43 and RV-55 were present simultaneously.

The combination of many RV types and nearly annual recycling of other respiratory agents can produce a veritable welter of different viral infections in individual families (Fig. 171–6).

CIRCULATION WITHIN SCHOOLROOMS

The mechanism of respiratory virus dissemination throughout the community may be the schoolroom or similar environments. In a Chicago nursery population, Beem[28]

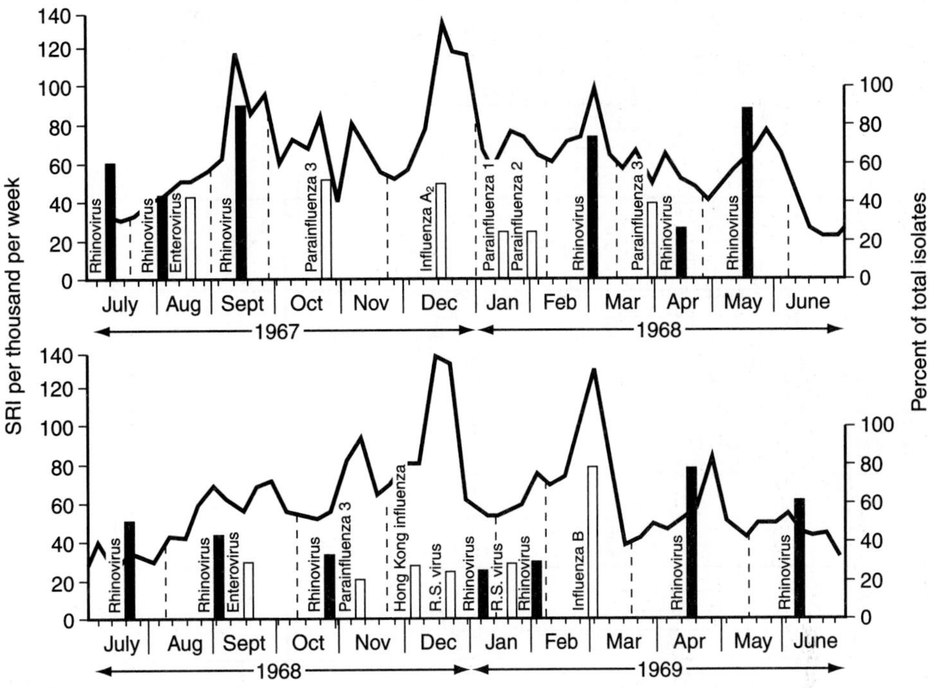

FIGURE 171–3 ■ Incidence of total symptomatic respiratory infection and predominant isolates in metropolitan Tecumseh, Michigan (population 10,000), 1967 to 1969. RS, respiratory syncytial. (Adapted from Monto, A. S., and Cavallaro, J. J.: The Tecumseh study of respiratory illness. II. Patterns of occurrence of infection with respiratory pathogens, 1965–1969. Am. J. Epidemiol. *94*:280–289, 1971.)

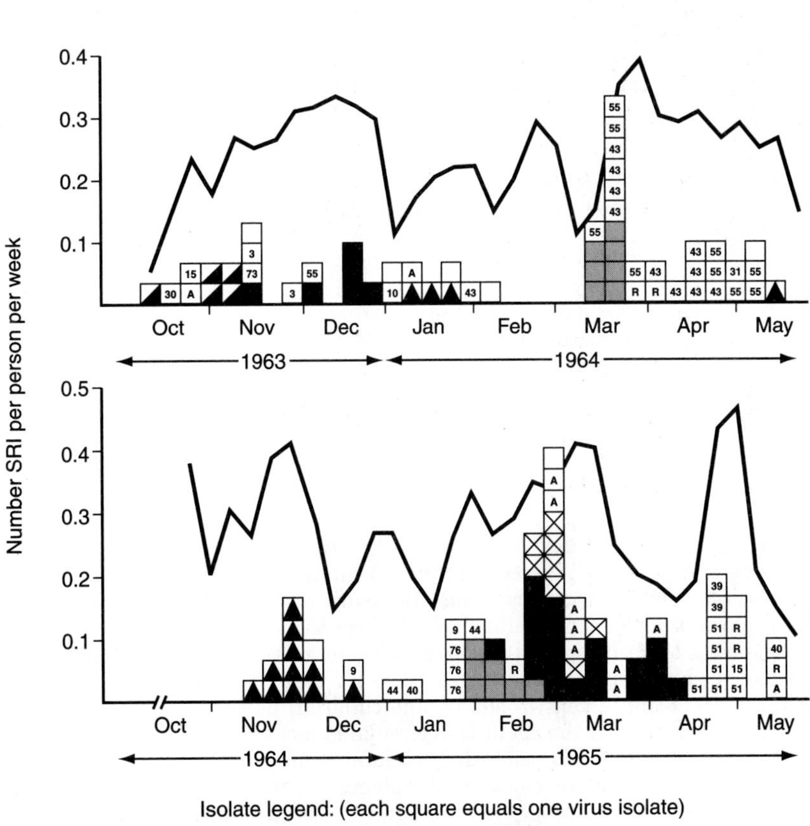

FIGURE 171–4 ■ Rhinoviruses and other respiratory viruses associated with symptomatic respiratory infection in three neighboring apartment buildings in Eagle Heights, a University of Wisconsin housing village in Madison, Wisconsin (24 to 26 families, about 100 persons), 1963 to 1965.

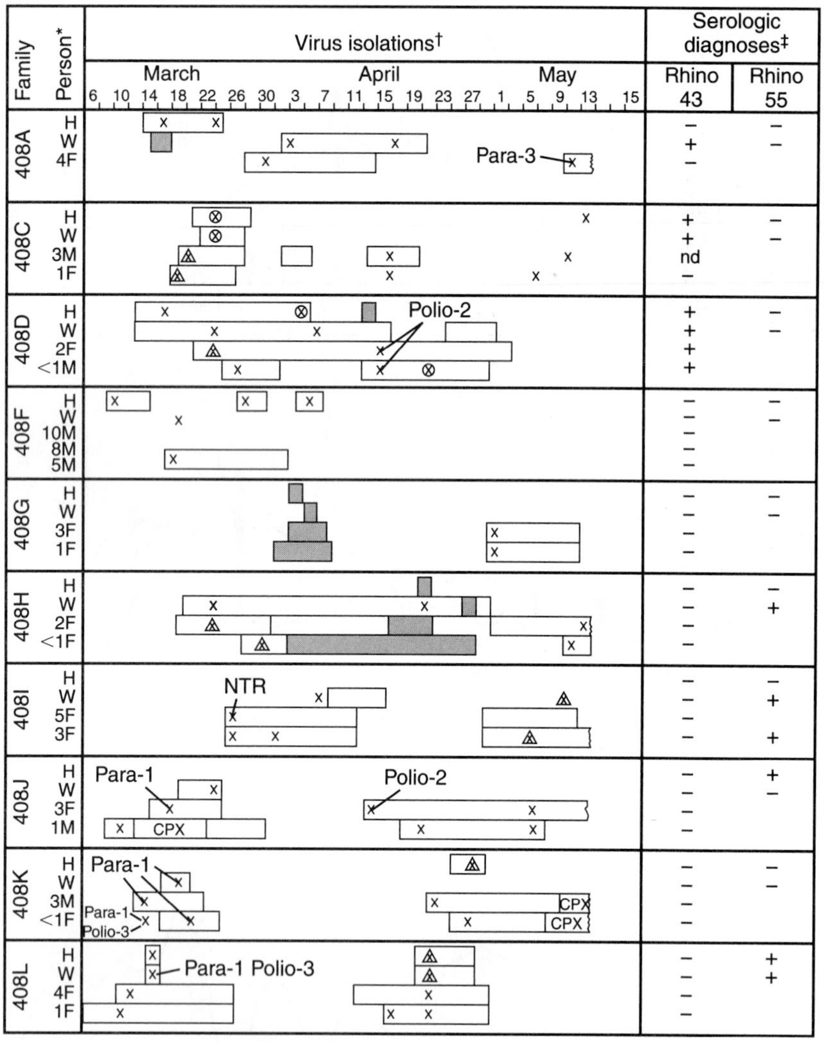

*H = Husband; W = Wife; 6M = 6-year-old male; 4F = 4-year-old female; etc.

†Legend:

- □ Respiratory illness
- ■ Gastroenteritis
- x Throat specimen taken
- ⊗ Rhinovirus 43 isolate
- ⚠ Rhinovirus 55 isolate

Para = Parainfluenza
Polio = Poliomyelitis
NTR = Non-typable rhinovirus
CPX = Chickenpox (clin. diag.)

‡A fourfold or greater rise in neutralization titer between the pre- and post-epidemic sera; nd = Not done

FIGURE 171–5 ■ Distribution of respiratory viruses in one Eagle Heights apartment building, Madison, Wisconsin, March 6 to May 15, 1964. (Adapted from Dick, E. C., Blumer, C. R., and Evans, A. S.: Epidemiology of infections with rhinovirus types 43 and 55 in a group of University of Wisconsin student families. Am. J. Epidemiol. *86*:386–400, 1967.)

observed that some RV types spread extensively and involved as many as 77 percent of the 22 children studied. He observed similar widespread infection with RSV but not with parainfluenza and influenza viruses. In an upper middle-class Madison second-grade schoolroom, results were similar but not identical (Fig. 171–7). The RV types studied infected 18 to 55 percent of susceptible children; however, influenza B virus was the agent that circulated most widely.

Although several RV types usually circulate concurrently, all types present are not equal in prevalence. In the aforementioned Chicago nursery school study,[28] 14 different serotypes were isolated during the academic year 1962 to 1963, but 10 of the serotypes did not spread at all. Only three types disseminated widely, and they infected more than 40 percent of the children. Likewise, in the 1963 to 1965 Madison Eagle Heights Village study (see Fig. 171–4), 14 RV types were isolated, but only 3 types (RV-43, RV-51, and RV-55) were "spreaders." Similar patterns of serologic prevalence have been reported from laboratories in Tecumseh, Michigan,[217] New York City, Seattle,[97, 98] and Charlottesville.[145]

PREDOMINATING RHINOVIRUS TYPES

Although the pattern of predominating RV types within a circumscribed population and a defined time frame seem to be well-established, a predominance of serotypes over large geographic areas or over many years does not seem to occur. This phenomenon has been studied exhaustively in widely separated locations and over many years: the Gulf South from 1962 to 1970, Tecumseh from 1966 to 1971 and from

Apartment	63–64	64–65
APT C; 2,1 Child	E11, R43, R55, Vla	INF A_2, P–1, R44
APT D; 2 Child	RS, R43, R55, R–NT	INF A_2, RS, R15
APT G; 2,3 Child	E11, RS	P–1, P–3, RS, R51
APT H; 2 Child	RS, R55	Ad2, P–3, R40, R44, R51
APT K; 2 Child	P–1, R55	NOT DONE
APT L; 2,4 Child	P–1, RS, R55	INF A_2, P–1, RS, R44
APT A; 1 Child	E11, P–3, R43, R55	NOT DONE
APT B	NOT	DONE
APT E; 3 Child	NOT DONE	P–3
APT F; 4,2 Child	E11, R15	INF A_2, P–3, RS, R9, R44, R51
APT I; 2 Child	E11, R55	INF A_2, Ad8, R40, R44, R–NT
APT J; 2 Child	Ad2, P–1, R55, Vla	R51

FIGURE 171–6 ■ Viral infections in a single Eagle Heights apartment building, Madison, Wisconsin, 1963 to 1965. Ad, adenovirus; E, echovirus; INF A_2, influenza A (H2N2); NT, nontypable; P, parainfluenza; R, rhinoviruses; RS, respiratory syncytial; Vla, unidentified virus-like agent. Numbers after letters refer to type (e.g., RV55, rhinovirus type 55). See Figure 171–9 for apartment arrangement.

1976 to 1981, and Seattle from 1965 to 1969 and from 1975 to 1979.[97, 98, 212, 213, 216, 218] Although "common types" (usually the isolation of at least five to eight strains of a serotype during the period studied) occurred during each period and at each place, different types were "common" findings in different places and times. For example, at Tecumseh, Monto and colleagues,[216, 218] during two 6-year study periods, obtained 475 RV isolates covering 70 serotypes (out of a possible 89 at that time[173]), but only RV-1B, RV-10, RV-28, and RV-58 were isolated in both periods. However, they were not particularly common because only 16, 22, 15, and 18 isolates, respectively, of these four types were found during the 12 years. As shown in Figures 171–4 and 171–8, in the neighboring state of Wisconsin from 1963 to 1965, the common types were RV-43, RV-51, and RV-55, completely different from those in Michigan. Finally, the late John Fox sifted data from family populations surveyed by him and others in New York City, Seattle, and Tecumseh.[97, 98] He found only four common serotypes (RV-1B, RV-12, RV-15, and RV-38) from among 802 isolates. Dominant RV serotypes often appear to occur locally over relatively short periods but do not extend for decades or over the nation, at least in the United States.

	Viral agent	Number of susceptible students*	Number infected (%)
1968	Non-typeable 'M' Rhinovirus	19	7 (37%)
	Rhinovirus 19	17	3 (18%)
	Rhinovirus 36	11	6 (55%)
	Parainfluenza 3	2	2 (100%)
	Respiratory syncytial	N.D.	5
1968–69	Rhinovirus 6	24	9 (37%)
	Influenza B	0	13
	Respiratory syncytial	3	8

*Number with neutralizing antibody titers ≤1:8 at the onset of study

FIGURE 171–7 ■ Attack rates of several respiratory viruses within a Madison, Wisconsin, second-grade classroom of 26 students, three semesters, 1968 to 1969.

Person-to-Person Transmission

EPIDEMIOLOGIC OBSERVATIONS

Individual RV serotypes often disseminate with surprising difficulty, as has been noted previously in Eagle Heights Village (see Figs. 171–4 and 171–8), a Madison elementary school (see Fig. 171–7), and a Chicago nursery school.[28] At least within family populations, the most common finding is that a specific RV serotype does not spread from the index case. Hendley and associates,[145] in a study of 19 families in Charlottesville, found that RVs from 10 of 22 index cases did not spread at all and that in only seven families did dissemination to at least one other person take place. In only 4 of the 19 families did further sequential spread occur. Fox and associates,[97, 98] in a surveillance of more than 200 Seattle families, found intrafamily secondary attack rates in susceptible individuals (no homotypic antibody) to be 44 percent from 1965 to 1969 and 28 percent from 1975 to 1979. In both periods, children younger than 5 years had the highest secondary attack rate, 60 percent and 30 percent, respectively. Monto and Johnson[215, 219] reported similar findings in 48 Panamanian families: with five RV isolates used as antigens, the secondary attack rate varied from 10.5 to 56 percent.

In Madison, Wisconsin, interfamily and intrafamily dissemination of the three "spreading" RV types, RV-43, RV-51, and RV-55, was examined in the 24 to 26 neighboring families in Eagle Heights Village (see Figs. 171–4, 171–5, 171–8,

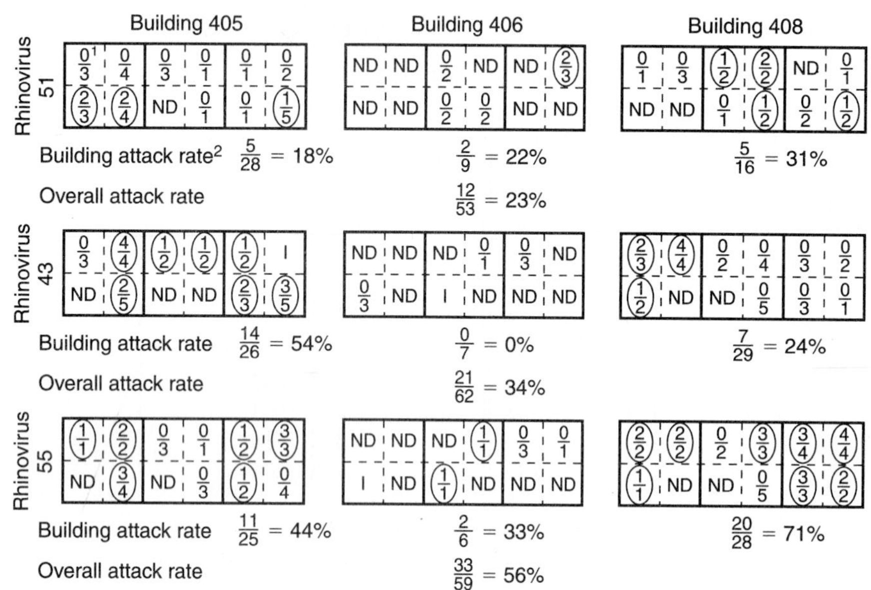

[1]No. diagnosed cases/no. susceptibles (no detectable antibody)

[2]As diagnosed by either virus isolation and/or a fourfold or greater serologic response

FIGURE 171–8 ■ Attack rates of three "spreading" rhinoviruses in three neighboring Eagle Heights apartment buildings, Madison, Wisconsin. I, all members immune; ND, not done; O, family with one or more infected members.

and 171–9). These 3 serotypes were the only ones of 14 to spread beyond the index family. RV-51 attacked 23 percent of susceptible individuals, and many family members and close neighbors remained uninfected. RV-43 infected 34 percent of susceptible individuals; in one building (408), only the families in a single-end fourplex became infected. On the other hand, RV-55 caused a miniepidemic in buildings 405 and 408, with a 71 percent attack rate attained in the latter; several families had all members infected. RV dissemination seemed to focus on the fourplex, probably because in the winter months the children played in the hallways and stairs connecting the fourplex apartments (see Fig. 171–9). Nevertheless, even the spreading RVs left many susceptible individuals untouched among next-door fourplex neighbors and within many families.

As part of the same study, surveillance was performed for Asian influenza (influenza A [H2N2]), which attacked the population during the winter of 1964 to 1965 (see Fig. 171–4), and for parainfluenza type 1. Although intrafamily attack rates of Asian influenza often were 100 percent, many persons and families remained uninfected by this usually epidemic virus (Fig. 171–10). The occupants of building 408 had an attack rate of 74 percent, nearly identical to that associated with RV-55 the previous year. The spread of parainfluenza type 1 was much like that of RV-51 (see Figs. 171–8 and 171–10).

The erratic spreading patterns of these five viruses in Eagle Heights Village were perplexing. Although certainly these agents were capable of 100 percent infection of family members and, occasionally, of near neighbors, a most provocative fact was that they—even Asian influenza virus—so often were not transmitted at all.

Determination of the reason for such erratic spreading patterns can be sought in well-controlled chain-of-infection experiments with human volunteers. Performing such experiments with a virulent influenza virus would not be ethical; however, RVs are one of the few viruses with which healthy, adult humans can be infected safely. RV transmission experiments from several laboratories are described next.

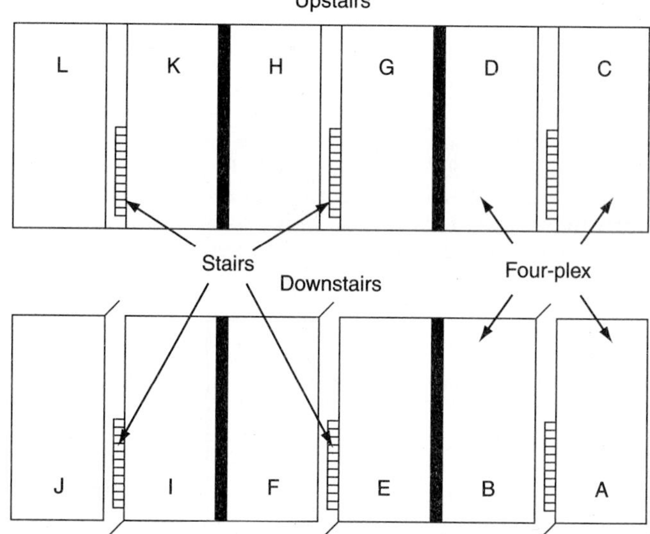

FIGURE 171–9 ■ Apartment arrangement in an Eagle Heights Village apartment building, Madison, Wisconsin. Each 12-unit building is divided into three fourplexes: two apartments upstairs and two apartments downstairs, accessible inside the unit by stairs. Access to the other fourplexes is only through doors to the outside.

PERSON-TO-PERSON TRANSMISSION TO HUMAN VOLUNTEERS

Experiments with Nasal Secretions from Persons with Colds of Unknown Etiology

Experimentation with common colds in human volunteers began at England's Common Cold Unit in Salisbury shortly after World War II.[283, 284] However, most of the transmission trials at this unit were performed with nasal secretions before discovery of most of the respiratory viruses, and the results

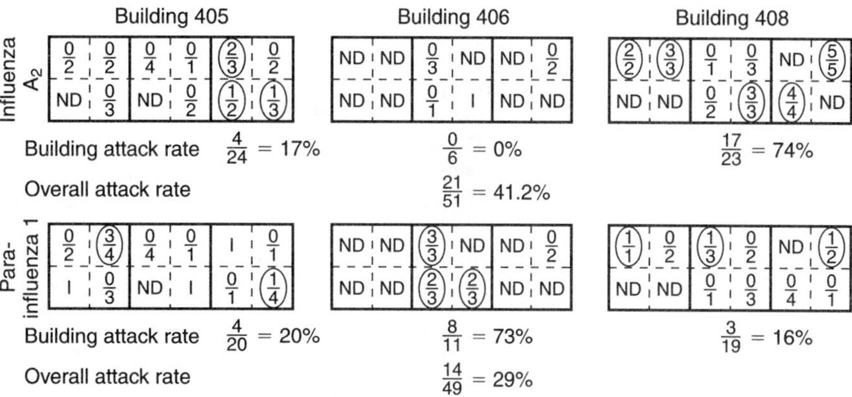

FIGURE 171–10 ■ Attack rates of two myxoviruses in three neighboring Eagle Heights apartment buildings, Madison, Wisconsin. I, all members immune; ND, not done; O, family with one or more infected members.

are difficult to interpret. (Adenoviruses were cultivated first about 1953, followed by parainfluenza viruses, RSVs, RVs [1956], and coronaviruses [1965].) Nonetheless, the general findings of these early experiments were correct; the usual common cold often is surprisingly difficult to transmit.[283]

Early Experiments with Rhinovirus Colds

Even in pure culture, the RVs retained their uncertainty of transmission. Couch and colleagues,[63, 66] trying to repeat a successful coxsackievirus A21 aerosol transmission experiment with RV-15, attained no transmission after housing 15 donors (persons infected intranasally with laboratory-grown virus) with 12 recipients (persons without antibody to the donor's virus) for 26 days. At approximately the same time, the Madison laboratory performed transmission trials with RV-55 and RV-16 in a series of experiments ranging in duration from a 1- to 1.5-minute kiss to a 3-day weekend in a dormitory room. In 26 donors and 33 recipients, only two transmissions occurred, one from a 1.5-minute kiss and the other from a weekend in a dormitory.[67] Only when young married student couples were used was a substantial rate attained; among 24 couples, 9 donor spouses infected their mates, for a transmission rate of 38 percent.[68]

Median Human Infectious Dose for Rhinovirus

Judging from RV challenge experiments with laboratory-grown virus administered by nosedrops or aerosol, less than one median tissue culture infective dose ($TCID_{50}$) can initiate infection.[67, 81] Much more (2000 times) is required when placed on the tongue or dried just outside the anterior nares (10,000 times).[67] How accurately these conditions approach the natural state is not known.[143]

Characteristics of a "Good" Rhinovirus Transmitter

In the experiments with married couples, "successful" donors shed enough virus to contaminate their environment, exhibited signs and symptoms of a moderate to severe cold, and spent many hours at home with their spouses.[68] As an example of the effect of high virus shedding, intracouple transmission rates were 71 percent for donors with nasopharyngeal RV titers of 5000 to more than 80,000 $TCID_{50}$, 33 percent for those with 1000 to 5000 $TCID_{50}$, and only 18 percent for those with less (p = .025). Illustrative of both shedding and production of sufficient nasal secretions was contamination of the hands with RV: donors whose hands were assayed for virus and who transmitted infections to their spouses all had RV on their hands, whereas none of the nontransmitters did (p = .03). The amount of time spent together seemed important in transmission (p = .025) (Table 171–1). Nonetheless, many infected spouses who spent hours of direct contact with their partners did not transmit the infection.

Some Early Conclusions

The preceding findings both in epidemiologic studies and in human volunteers suggest that in general, attending a concert or a motion picture with those who have even obvious signs of colds is unlikely to result in infection. (On the other hand, students who spend day after day in classrooms may have a higher chance of acquiring infection [see Fig. 171–7].) In addition, a relatively short stay (a few hours) among friends or relatives with RV-caused colds is not likely to cause

TABLE 171–1 ■ RELATIONSHIP OF THE CAPACITY OF ARTIFICIALLY INFECTED DONORS TO TRANSMIT RHINOVIRUS TYPE 16 TO THEIR SPOUSES TO THE NUMBER OF HOURS SPENT TOGETHER AND TO THE NUMBER OF HOURS OF DIRECT CONTACT

		Number of Hours†	
Donor*	**Transmission**	**In the Same Air Space‡**	**In Direct Contact§**
A	+	149	10
B	–	142	13
C	+	138	20
D	+	127	39
E	+	122	5
F	–	112	21
G	–	112	12
H	–	105	19
I	–	103	26
J	–	86	6
K	–	63	12

*Listed in order of the number of hours in the same air space, greatest to least. The larger the number of hours spent together, the greater the likelihood of transmission (two-sample Wilcoxon rank test, p =.025).
†During the 7-day period after artificial infection. The total possible number of hours is 168.
‡When the couples were home together.
§Embracing, kissing, and so forth.
Adapted from D'Alessio, D.J., Peterson, J.A., Dick, C.R., et al.: Transmission of experimental rhinovirus colds in volunteer married couples. J. Infect. Dis. *133*:28–36, 1976.

infection, even with brief embracing. Moreover, evidence from a group practice in Massachusetts shows that pediatricians' waiting rooms may *not* be places where respiratory viruses commonly are transferred.[192] These conclusions come with a caveat, however, in that direct experience is with only RVs. Respiratory illnesses in which cough is a large component, such as influenza and measles, can result in substantial dissemination, even in a pediatric clinic.[30, 47, 113]

Route-of-Transmission Experiments

Because RVs and perhaps other respiratory viruses often seem to spread with relative difficulty under many normal circumstances, the route of transmission becomes important because controlling the transmission of respiratory viruses in various habitats such as schoolrooms and families may be feasible by blocking transmission routes.

Since the early 1970s, much human volunteer experimentation on RV transmission routes has been conducted, chiefly at the University of Virginia, England's Common Cold Unit, and the laboratory at the University of Wisconsin. Gwaltney and Hendley[122] at Charlottesville focused on the possibility that RV colds were disseminated via direct or indirect hand contact. Interest in this approach had been provoked by their inadvertently passing RVs from infected to noninfected persons through the vehicle of an ethanol-sterilized nasal speculum. Subsequently, they observed a lot of nose picking and eye rubbing among Department of Medicine Grand Rounds participants and Sunday school attendees[146] (infection through conjunctival swabs had been reported previously[37]). They then showed that RV-39 retained infectivity for several hours on various surfaces and could be found on the hands of RV-39–infected persons. They concluded that RV transmission might occur via self-inoculation by environmentally contaminated hands and demonstrated, in human volunteers, RV-39 self-inoculation from an environmental source.[146]

The Charlottesville team subsequently conducted a series of three experiments that, when combined with their previous "self-inoculation" results, greatly influenced the medical community.[41, 64, 124, 146, 167] In two of the experiments, groups of recipients were exposed to RV-infected donors (the RV used was an untypable strain, HH) in circumstances wherein they were exposed naturally in separate closed rooms to large-particle (12 recipients) or small-particle (10 recipients) aerosols produced by donors during periods of 45 minutes (large particles) or 3 days (small particles). One of the large-particle aerosol recipients was infected, whereas no one exposed to small-particle aerosols was. (These essentially negative transmission rates by aerosol exposure were not surprising[122] because as noted previously, Couch[64] had been unsuccessful doing so via the airborne route over a period of 26 days and the Madison laboratory attained only one RV transmission among 11 recipients after 3 days' exposure in a dormitory.[67]) The third group of Charlottesville recipients was exposed to RV by inoculating themselves with the donor's nasal mucus. The donors blew their noses into their hands. The recipients then stroked the donors' contaminated hands for 10 seconds and then inoculated themselves by deliberately placing their fingers, two or three times, on their nasal and conjunctival mucosa. This inoculation procedure was repeated on 3 successive days. Eleven of the 15 hand contact recipients (73%) were infected with the donors' RV. The authors concluded that transmission by the hand contact/self-inoculation route was much more efficient than the aerosol route was and "may be an important natural route of RV transmission."[124] One deficiency of this experiment was that donors and recipients shared the same air space over a measured—often brief—period during which fresh nasal mucus was transferred from the donor to the recipient. Nonetheless, Gwaltney did achieve a high rate of RV transmission with nasal secretions, something that had not been accomplished readily in more "natural" experiments.[63, 67] Also in support of hand transmission was the observation in the aforementioned married couple experiments that the ability to transmit was correlated significantly with the presence of RV on the donors' hands.[68] As a result of these various pieces of evidence and lack of compelling evidence to the contrary, hand-to-hand or fomite transmission became the accepted route for RV contagion.[41, 64, 87, 276] However, the evidence for hand transmission either was deduced or was contrived (i.e., indirect nose-to-nose mucus transfer); no actual natural transmission of RV by hand contact had been demonstrated.[79, 266]

In later experiments, the Charlottesville group demonstrated approximately 50 percent transmission via fomites by using the same hand contact/self-inoculation method described earlier, except that either a coffee cup handle or a plastic tile was interposed between donors' and recipients' hands.[123]

At England's Common Cold Unit, Reed[245] investigated the likelihood of natural hand-contact transmission among residents (roommates) of several housing units, 38 of whom had been infected with RV-2. Reed[245] found that 16 of the donors had RV on their fingers, but that none was transmitted to the fingers of their 18 roommates, even though virus could be recovered from some (6 of 40) objects recently handled by RV-2–infected donors. Reed also found that none of 29 virus transfers from virus dried on the fingers could pass through a fomite to a recipient; the conclusion was that "spread of colds is unlikely to occur via objects contaminated by the hands of the virus shedder. . . ."

The laboratory at Wisconsin continued its attempts to devise a natural transmission model to examine routes of transmission and, potentially, methods for interruption of transmission. Although the results of the transmission experiment with married couples were illuminating, the system itself had one great deficiency as an experimental model: the participants could not be observed during their interaction periods.[68] A model was needed in which donors and recipients could be monitored at all times. Ultimately, the scheme for such a system was suggested by two virologic-epidemiologic events in Antarctica, one from a few summer seasons (1975 to 1980) in which Dick and associates studied respiratory virus dissemination in an isolated Antarctic population and the other from a human volunteer experiment conducted in an Antarctic field party from England's Common Cold Unit.[150, 261, 295] Both experiences suggested that high natural transmission rates after just a few days of exposure could be achieved only in an environment with a high donor-to-recipient ratio and in a population density such as might be found in the classrooms and dormitories of a boarding school. Accordingly, a model was devised whereby donors (with the qualities of a "good" transmitter as described earlier) and recipients interacted during waking hours by playing cards and board and video games and engaging in communal studying.[68] During the night, donors and recipients bunked together in the same or an adjoining room. With such an arrangement, graduate student monitors recorded activities and all clinical signs 24 hours a day. These artifices were successful; with 8 donors and 12 to 16 recipients, a 50 percent recipient attack rate usually was attained over a 12-hour period and a 100 percent rate over the course of a week.[167, 207] Informally, this model, a fully observed monotypic RV miniepidemic, was named "Antarctic Hut," from its origins.[144]

Route-of-Transmission "Blocking" Experiments

Using the Antarctic Hut model, a series of four RV-16 route-of-transmission blocking experiments were conducted to determine whether the virus was spread by hand contact, aerosol, or both.[79, 167] The first three experiments lasted 12 hours, with 8 donors and 12 recipients; the donor-recipient interaction was through playing variants of stud and draw poker (Fig. 171–11). This interaction mode facilitated both aerosol and fomite–hand contact transmission. Half the recipients were blocked completely from any hand contact/self-inoculation by wearing arm restraints (see Fig. 171–11). Evidently, little transmission was due to hand or fomite contact because the RV-16 infection rate in the restrained recipients was only slightly lower than in the unrestrained recipients, 56 versus 67 percent, an insignificant reduction (p = .494). The fourth experiment, involving aerosol blocking, commenced immediately after the third. The poker game continued in the original room with eight donors alone, and all the equipment from the third experiment, including the cards (which literally were gummy from the previous 12-hour game), poker chips, pencils, and so forth, was moved to an identical room across the hall. The continuing eight-donor poker game in the room used for the third experiment was refurnished with poker implements. Subsequently, 12 new recipients entered the second room, began playing poker with the now heavily used cards and other paraphernalia, and made exaggerated hand-to-nose self-inoculation movements. Aerosol transmission was blocked effectively by the two brick walls between the rooms. Once each hour, the cards, poker chips, and other portables were exchanged between the donor and recipient rooms to maintain a freshly contaminated supply of fomites in the recipient room. The result was extremely surprising; not 1 of the 12 "fomite recipients" caught RV-16. Judging from the results of these four Antarctic Hut experiments in which fomite–hand contact and aerosol transmission were blocked alternately, aerosol transmission clearly seemed the predominant route, at least for RV-16 among student poker players at the University of Wisconsin. A few months after the 1987 publication of these results, an editorial appeared in *The Lancet* titled "Splints Don't Stop Colds—Surprising!"[79, 266] It concluded that " . . it looks as though coughs and sneezes *do* spread these diseases more than sticky fingers."

Subsequently, a set of experiments was conducted to determine how RV-16 had disappeared along the five-step fomite transmission chain from nose to hand to fomite to hand to nose.[168] The experiments were a more elaborate version of Reed's previous studies,[245] and the same results were noted. The virus seemed to disappear precipitously at each step in the chain; 10^6 $TCID_{50}$ of RV-16 in the donor's nose was reduced to 0 to 64 $TCID_{50}$ on the card-playing implements, and then the virus nearly disappeared on reaching the recipients' hands.

Putting the results of these various experiments together, natural transmission of RVs via the hand contact/self-inoculation route seems unlikely *unless* the virus actually is suspended in fresh mucus, in which case little virus is lost in transit.[168, 245] However, judging from the foregoing experiments, wet mucus seems to be passed infrequently from one adult to another, as was predicted by Reed.[245]

What is clear is that rhinovirus illnesses may be transmitted by both the hand contact and aerosol routes. Certainly, the evidence presented in favor of the aerosol route as predominant should *not* discourage anyone from careful handwashing, especially around small children, in whom transmission by virus in wet mucus indeed could occur.

Interruption of Transmission

The Virginia team[119, 144] performed a blocking experiment in the field in which mothers of families attempted to prevent hand contact/self-inoculation by dipping their fingers in iodine. The results of this 1979 to 1982 study were reported twice as segments of two general reviews on RV transmission, and the results differed somewhat in the two publications. In the first presentation, the mothers with iodinated fingers had a lower illness rate than the did placebo mothers

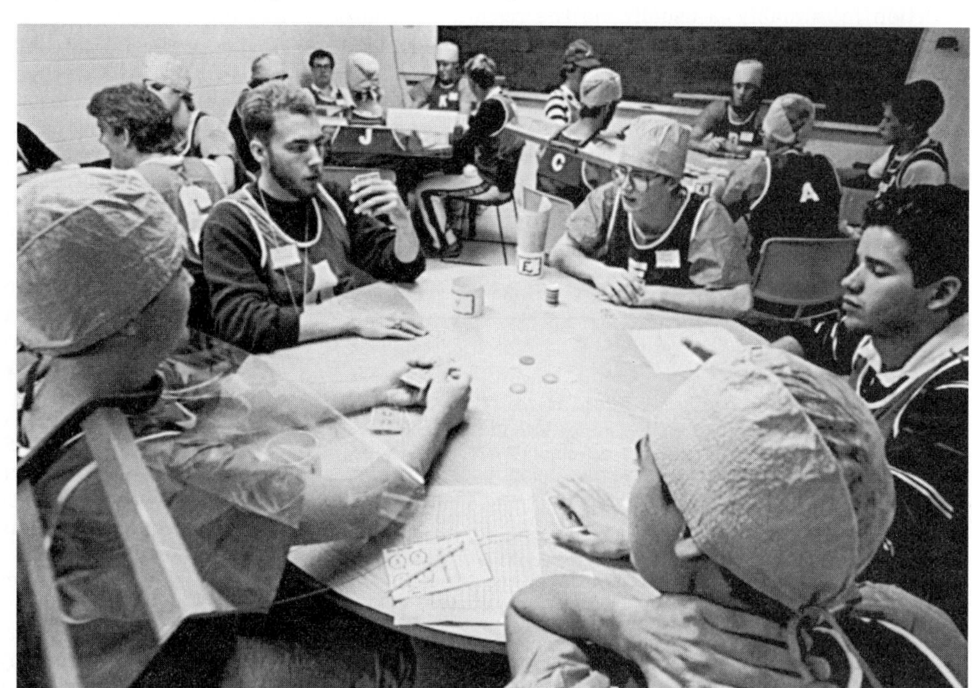

FIGURE 171–11 ■ A typical "Antarctic Hut" transmission experiment in progress using stud and draw poker as the interaction promoter. At each of four tables are two "donors" (infected with rhinovirus type 16) and three "recipients" (no antibody to rhinovirus type 16) (wearing surgical scrub suits). This particular experiment is one in which hand contact/self-inoculation transmission is blocked in 6 of the 12 recipients by wearing Thatcher collars. The collars block hand contact transmission by preventing touching of the face by the hands; therefore, virus can pass from donors to recipients only by aerosol.

from 1979 to 1981, but not in 1982.[119] In the second review, the illness rate during the 4 years was reported as being 40 percent lower in the mothers with iodinated fingers than in the placebo mothers, and the difference was significant ($p = .047$).[144] Commendably, the authors speak directly to the difficulty of conducting and interpreting such investigations.[144]

The Madison group also examined transmission interruption methods to prevent spread from person to person. As part of a general investigation of the epidemiology of respiratory viruses in an isolated (ca. 200 persons) Antarctic population at McMurdo Station in 1979, use of an iodinated facial tissue developed by the S. C. Johnson Company (Johnson's Wax) of Racine, Wisconsin, was successful in interrupting transmission.[76, 261, 295] Three days after all personnel began copious use of these tissues, the incidence of respiratory illness dropped rapidly and significantly ($p < .01$); in fact, respiratory illness nearly disappeared from the base.[78] Although this effect was striking, the trial could be controlled only historically. However, the apparent success was sufficient to interest the Kimberly-Clark Corporation, makers of Kleenex tissues, in applying virucidal facial tissue technology to interrupt RV-16 transmission in the Antarctic Hut model. Kimberly-Clark soon made available a nontoxic, highly virucidal facial tissue. The tissues completely stopped transmission of RV-16, in comparison to transmission rates of 42 and 75 percent in control recipients using ordinary cotton handkerchiefs ($p < .001$) (Table 171–2).[77] Kimberly-Clark test-marketed these tissues under the brand name "Avert," but their sales were below expectations. Subsequently, two field trials of Avert in families were conducted in Charlottesville and Tecumseh, with reductions in transmission of 5 to 39 percent.[93, 193] These results were disappointing but not unexpected. Changing established habits of personal nasal sanitation was not easy in the highly supervised, well-motivated adults in Antarctica; it may be impossible in unsupervised children.

Pathogenesis and Host Factors

GENERAL COURSE OF INFECTION

Infection presumably is usually via the respiratory route, although infection by the conjunctival route has been demonstrated.[37, 146] To infect via the respiratory tract, a mucus blanket approximately 200 times the width of the RV and propelled forward by continuously beating cilia must be penetrated by as yet unknown means.[143] (Possibly, it is a formidable barrier and may account for the difficulty of RV transmission.) Nonetheless, when given intranasally by pipette, only 1 $TCID_{50}$ is needed to initiate infection.[67, 81] The incubation period for a cold normally is 2 to 3 days, but up to 7 days has been reported.[83, 145] Ciliary dysfunction can predispose to respiratory infection.[32, 39] RVs replicate well in the upper respiratory tract (see later), and substantial evidence indicates that they replicate in the lower respiratory tract as well.[108, 130, 229, 230]

TABLE 171–2 ■ APPARENT COMPLETE INTERRUPTION BY VIRUCIDAL TISSUES OF RHINOVIRUS TYPE 16 (RV-16) TRANSMISSION*

	Cotton Hand'cfs.	Virucidal Tissues		Cotton Hand'cfs.
	Exp. A	Exp. B	Exp. C	Exp. D
Recipients who "caught" RV-16 colds/total (%)†	5/12 (42)	0/12	0/12	9/12 (75)

*In each of four experiments, eight volunteers with RV-16 colds played poker for 12 hours with 12 other volunteers (without RV-16 antibody) and for nasal sanitation used either ordinary cotton handkerchiefs (Hand'cfs) (experiments A and D) or virucidal tissues (B and C). Three-ply Kleenex tissues were treated, per 100 g, with 9.1 g of citric acid, 4.5 g of malic acid, and 1.8 g of sodium lauryl sulfate. Cotton or paper handkerchiefs were used to clear nasal passages, smother coughs and sneezes, and wipe surfaces. Virucidal tissues were used carefully and copiously.

†Diagnosed by at least one isolation of RV-16 or a fourfold rise in antibody to RV-16 in the convalescent serum sample or both.

Adapted from Dick, E.C., Hossain, S.U., Mink, K.A., et al.: Interruption of transmission of rhinovirus colds among human volunteers using virucidal handkerchiefs. J. Infect. Dis. *153*:352–356, 1986.

RVs may be shed in large amounts (1000 to 1,000,000 infectious particles per milliliter of nasal washing) during the first 2 to 3 days of a cold and may be produced for 2 to 3 weeks thereafter.[79, 81, 83, 207] However, the effect on cells of the nasopharyngeal cavity seems benign despite much local reaction to the virus, which results in the usual signs and symptoms of a cold. Systematic studies of RV-inoculated human volunteers at the University of Virginia demonstrated that damage to the respiratory epithelium was slight, although a few sloughed ciliated epithelial cells did contain RV antigen.[280, 299] RV was recovered only at focal sites in the nose and nasopharynx at the time of maximal symptoms, and in situ hybridization studies demonstrated evidence of RV infection in only a minority of epithelial cells.[18, 27, 301] Furthermore, using primary monolayer cultures of ciliated and nonciliated epithelial cells, Winther and associates[300] demonstrated that RV, coronavirus, influenza A virus, and adenovirus all grow well in these cell cultures; however, RV and coronavirus produced no discernible cytopathic effect, whereas influenza virus and adenovirus nearly destroyed the cell sheet by 96 hours.

Because the RVs seem to cause only mild pathologic changes in cells of the respiratory tract, attention has turned to various immunologic or inflammatory substances as possible causes of symptomatic illness.[277] Researchers have known for some years that peripheral blood neutrophils increase in the first 2 to 3 days of illness in RV-infected volunteers.[42, 277] Phagocytes (neutrophils and monocytes) also have been demonstrated in large numbers in the nasal secretions of RV-infected symptomatic human volunteers.[190] Although the microbe-killing ability of phagocytes is well known, these cells in themselves also could cause cold symptoms through the release of various toxic products, such as superoxide and hydrogen peroxide, during the respiratory burst.[35, 273] In fact, increasing numbers of leukocytes in the peripheral blood correlate with increased symptoms, and in infected non-ill human volunteers, the white blood cell count does not increase.[277] More recently, an association has been noted between the nasal levels of two proinflammatory mediators involved in granulocyte regulation, granulocyte colony-stimulating factor (G-CSF) and interleukin-8 (IL-8), and blood and nasal neutrophilia have been identified.[109, 226] Nasal IL-8 levels also correlate with the severity of clinical symptoms.[116, 282]

Increased nasal levels of other inflammatory mediators (e.g., IL-1β, IL-6, RANTES [regulated on activation, normal T cell expressed and secreted], kinins) have been associated with more severe clinical symptoms.[222, 226, 240, 241, 308] Furthermore, topical nasal administration of IL-6 or bradykinin leads to development of some of the symptoms of the common cold.[104, 242] At least some of these inflammatory responses appear to be dependent on an activation pathway regulated by nuclear factor kB (NF-kB).[307, 308] Resolution of clinical symptoms may be caused by the elaboration of inhibitors of inflammation, such as IL-1 receptor antagonist.[305] These inflammatory mediators may serve as a target for the development of drugs to relieve the symptoms of RV infection, although the use of a specific kinin inhibitor did not lead to clinical improvement.[120, 148]

IMMUNITY CAUSED BY SERUM ANTIBODY

Serum antibody to the various RV types develops with age (presumably from repeated infections), and by adulthood, antibody may be detected against approximately 50 percent of RV types tested.[121] The presence of serum antibody correlates positively with immunity, and resistance to infection and the degree of disease expression are related to the amount of antibody present.[4, 5, 36] As examples, in the Eagle Heights families, 21 of 75 persons (28%) without antibody were infected with either RV-43 or RV-55, whereas only 5 of 35 (14%) with homologous antibody to either of these agents were infected.[72] No one was infected who had homologous serum antibody levels above 1:16. Similar results were observed in the Charlottesville and Seattle families.[97, 98, 145] However, large doses can overwhelm antibody. At the clinical center of the National Institute of Allergy and Infectious Diseases, where human volunteers were used, 1000 $TCID_{50}$ was found to infect persons with serum antibody titers up to 1:256.[43] Judging from the paucity of reports of natural infections in persons with serum antibody titers greater than 1:16, virus inocula in naturally contracted cases must be low.

IMMUNITY CAUSED BY ANTIBODY IN NASAL SECRETIONS

At the National Institutes of Health, researchers found that intranasal administration of RV vaccine produced both serum and nasal antibody, whereas two intramuscular injections of this vaccine produced little, if any, nasal antibody.[44] When the volunteers given the vaccine intranasally were challenged with approximately 100 $TCID_{50}$ of homologous RV, they were protected significantly against both clinical illness and infection, whereas those administered the same vaccine intramuscularly remained susceptible.[233]

On the other hand, other investigators who used the same vaccine preparation but gave it subcutaneously in three injections found nasal antibody responses in 21 of 46 (45%) volunteers.[84] They discovered that when compared with unimmunized, antibody-free controls, challenge of these volunteers with 3 $TCID_{50}$ of virus produced significantly less virus shedding and reduced the duration and severity of illness. Possibly, this lower infectious dose more closely approximates a natural situation. This study also showed that protection against infection with the low virus challenge correlated with the magnitude of serum antibody and not with the presence of secretory antibody. The relative roles of serum and secretory antibody in RV infections are still unsettled.

ANTIBODY APPEARANCE OVER THE COURSE OF INFECTION

A general pattern of the development of humoral (secretory and serum) antibody has emerged from several studies.[36, 86, 250] Approximately 24 hours after infection, a sharp increase in nasal IgA secretion occurs. When symptoms begin approximately 48 hours after infection, rhinorrhea commences, and the transudate is composed of significant amounts of IgG. After approximately 1 week and after the actual episode of illness, virus-specific antibody, predominantly IgA, appears in the nasal passages, tears, and the parotid saliva. Serum antibody (usually IgG but occasionally IgM) also begins to be formed at 1 week and rises to peak levels at 1 month. Both serum and secretory antibody appears sooner and rises more rapidly in persons with detectable neutralizing antibody in their pre-infection serum specimens. Antibody has been detected in nasal secretions and serum approximately 1 year after infection and, judging from the high proportion of the adult population with antibody to many RV serotypes, probably lasts much longer.[34, 121]

CELL-MEDIATED IMMUNITY

As noted previously, evidence that neutrophils increase both in the peripheral blood and in the nasopharynx during the first few days of an RV cold is substantial.[42, 298] Evidence that peripheral blood lymphocytes actually decrease in the first 2 to 3 days of an RV cold and that migration of lymphocytes into the nasal secretions increases at this time also exists.[42, 190] As noted earlier, specific humoral antibody usually is not present in the serum or nasopharynx this early in the illness, which suggests that these in situ nasopharyngeal lymphocytes, through cell-mediated immunity, play an important role in controlling RV proliferation. Hsia and colleagues[155] examined the ability of peripheral blood lymphocytes to liberate various cytokines (IL-2 and interferon-γ) and participate in other cellular immune processes (cytotoxicity and antigen-stimulated blastogenesis) during the early days of RV colds in experimentally infected human volunteers. They found that during infection, all these cell-mediated immunity activities were increased significantly when compared with pre-infection levels. Of special interest was their observation that the cellular ability to liberate higher levels of IL-2 correlated inversely and significantly ($p < .02$) with virus shedding and nasal mucus production. Cross-reactive T-cell epitopes are shared by RVs, and T cells isolated from peripheral blood and from tonsillar tissue proliferate and secrete a variety of cytokines (interferon-γ, IL-2, IL-4, IL-5) after exposure to RV antigens.[107, 136, 297] Thus, activation of T cells may contribute not only to virus clearance but also to airway inflammation.[107]

INTERFERENCE AMONG RHINOVIRUSES

Interference in infection with heterotypic RV serotypes, which lasts between 5 and 16 weeks, has been reported in human volunteers.[94] Complete resistance to infection has been observed after inoculation with as much as 2000 $TCID_{50}$ of RV-16 (administered by nasopharyngeal spray) in a subject with an unsuspected "wild" RV (not typed) infection present at the time of inoculation.[189] However, epidemiologic studies in a nursery school population,[28] a military population,[248] and a family population[211] showed sequential heterotypic RV infections occurring frequently, sometimes at intervals as short as 2 days. In the family population, one subject was infected by three different RVs within a 30-day period. The factor or factors responsible for the interference observed in the experimental human infection model have not been identified.

Simultaneous infection with an RV and other respiratory viruses, including influenza A and B viruses, coronaviruses, parainfluenza type 1, RSV, adenoviruses, various enteroviruses, or other RV serotypes, also has been reported.[88, 98, 188]

INFLUENCE OF A COLD ENVIRONMENT ON THE COURSE OF INFECTION

Exposure to cold temperatures is thought to either initiate or exacerbate respiratory infections. In fact, chilling animals has been shown to increase the severity and frequency of viral infection.[294] However, investigation of the effects of chilling on humans infected with "common cold viruses" and with RV-15 has not demonstrated significant effects.[85] In the RV-15 experiments, the conditions were realistic. The subjects (men) were cooled sufficiently in air to cause shivering for approximately an hour or were immersed in water long enough to cause a decline in rectal temperature.

EFFECT OF AGE AND SEX

A much higher prevalence of RV infection is found in infants and young children than in older persons. In Seattle,[97] the RV infection rate in children 0 to 5 years of age was nearly twice that of older children and adults (0.77 versus 0.41 infections per person per year, respectively); in Tecumseh,[218] the isolation rate in the 1- to 4-year-old group was far higher than that in any other age bracket. The high attack rates in these young children were not unexpected because less than 10 percent of them had antibody to any of the 56 RV types[121] and children ordinarily are subjected continuously to the family-like environment so conducive to transmission of RVs. In especially crowded populations, attack rates may be high. In an Alaskan Eskimo village, 70 percent of 395 children were infected during a spring outbreak of RV-16 infection.[303]

The frequency of infection with RV generally declines throughout life. Beginning at the age of school attendance, the number of RV infections declines gradually from 1 to 2 per year to 0.25 per year in the age group older than 60 years.[121, 220] Results from most laboratories have found that persons 20 to 30 years of age account for an exception to the general decline in incidence with age[97, 145, 217, 220]; RV infections as well as infections with other respiratory pathogens increase during this period of life. Because the increase is especially marked in mothers,[97, 145] it probably is due to respiratory illness in small children being transferred to parents.

In Tecumseh, the number of respiratory illnesses per year was consistently higher for females than for males (3 to >60 years of age).[220] If one assumes that RVs account for a similar proportion of disease in each gender, this finding would indicate that females generally have more RV infections. As noted earlier, women with young children clearly seem to have more RV infections than do others in their age group. In Seattle,[97] mothers had 1.5 times more RV infections than fathers did, and in Charlottesville, females of child-bearing age had approximately 1.2 times more RV illness than males did.[121]

EFFECT OF PSYCHOSOCIAL FACTORS

Numerous psychosocial factors have been shown to influence susceptibility to RV infection, primarily in the experimental human infection model. Increased psychologic stress, as measured by numerous stress indices, was associated with an increased susceptibility to infection and an increased likelihood of developing illness.[56, 57] In contrast, having a more diverse societal network (increased number of social ties) was associated with resistance to infection and illness.[55] Antibody-negative (serum antibody levels <1:2) subjects were equally susceptible to infection regardless of the degree of stress or number of social ties, although these factors did influence the likelihood of clinical illness developing.[55, 56] Increased stress in working adults also was associated with an increased risk of having a natural common cold.[272]

Clinical Manifestations

Consonant with their benign cytopathology in the respiratory tract, RV infections in any age group usually cause only mild upper respiratory tract illness—that is, common colds.[64] Investigators estimate that RVs cause 30 to 50 percent of common colds, at least in adults.[194] In healthy adults, RV infections usually are so innocuous that human volunteers can be infected safely with these agents to study their epidemiology, pathogenesis, and control with experimental drugs.[64, 144, 167, 207, 284] However, even in adults, development of serious illness is possible: RV-associated, radiograph-positive, atypical pneumonia has been described in military trainees[105] and in adults with underlying illnesses, especially immunocompromised adults and those with diseases of the respiratory tract.*

Nonetheless, children, particularly the very young, are the ones most likely to be subject to serious, sometimes fatal RV-caused illness. As an example of a fatal outcome, a report from Los Angeles described an 11-month-old infant with mild asthma who died, totally unexpectedly during sleep, of apparent acute asthma and interstitial pneumonitis caused by RV-47 (isolated from lung and blood specimens).[186] The authors wrote a special plea to other physicians to be alert for similar exigencies in their own patients. In this respect, two deaths of infants from possible rhinoviremia, one of which occurred during a cold, and six "cot" deaths, diagnosed as bronchiolitis/pneumonia and from which RVs were isolated, may suggest that RV involvement in fatal illnesses in infants is more common than realized.[247, 290]

At least in theory, generalized illness with viremia seems possible with RV infections; the RVs are a division of the larger picornavirus group, which contains many viruses capable of generalized and fatal infection and whose genomes have considerable homology with the RVs (see "Structure of the Virion").[228]

SPECTRUM OF RESPIRATORY DISEASE

Early Studies: Severe Disease in Young Children

Investigators have known since discovery of the first RV serotypes that these viruses cause considerably more severe illness in children than in adults. In 1959 and 1960, Hamparian, Hilleman, and their associates[134, 246] conducted a clinical and virologic investigation of 15 children (younger than 8 years) and 20 adults from the Philadelphia area who had acute respiratory disease and from whom RVs (then called coryzaviruses) had been isolated (Table 171–3). The 20 adults all had typical upper respiratory illness, some with low-grade fever (peak of 37.3° C [99.2° F]). In contrast, 60 percent of the children had temperatures higher than 37.7° C (100° F), 20 percent had otitis, and 53 percent (eight children) exhibited one or more signs of lower respiratory tract involvement. One had laryngotracheitis (croup); one, bronchitis; two, asthmatic bronchitis; and one, bronchopneumonia. The last infant was 2 months old, and crepitant rales were heard over the right side of the chest anteriorly and posteriorly; the chest cleared in 2 days.

*See references 23, 91, 102, 105, 110, 129, 198, 224, 268, 269.

TABLE 171–3 ■ SIGNS AND SYMPTOMS OF RESPIRATORY ILLNESS IN 20 ADULTS AND 15 CHILDREN (2 MONTHS TO 8 YEARS OF AGE) WITH RHINOVIRUS INFECTIONS, 1959–1960, PHILADELPHIA*

Sign or Symptom	Adults	Children
Fever†	4 (20%)	9 (60%)
Eye, ear, nose, and throat		
Rhinorrhea	18 (90%)	10 (67%)
Purulent nasal discharge	4 (20%)	1 (7%)
Pharyngitis	10 (50%)	5 (33%)
Conjunctival infection	2 (10%)	1 (7%)
Anterior cervical lymphadenopathy	1 (5%)	8 (53%)
Hoarseness	4 (20%)	0
Croup	0	1 (7%)
Infection of the tympanic membrane	0	3 (20%)
Chest		
Cough	8 (40%)	15 (100%)
Dyspnea	0	4 (27%)
Refractions	0	3 (20%)
Rhonchi	0	7 (47%)
Rales	0	2 (13%)
Wheezing	0	4 (27%)

*The children were from the outpatient clinics and wards of the Children's Hospital of Philadelphia, and the adults were employees of Merck and Company, Inc., Rahway, N.J.

†In adults, 37.2° C (99° F) or above by mouth: The peak was 37.3° C (99.2° F). In children, 37.7° C (100° F) or above by rectum; range, 37° C (98.6° F) to 39.1° C (102.4° F); mean 37.9° C (100.4° F).

Adapted from Reilly, C.M., Hoch, S.M., Stokes, J., Jr., et al.: Clinical and laboratory findings in cases of respiratory illness caused by coryzaviruses. Ann. Intern. Med. *57*:515–525, 1962.

Shortly thereafter, in 1963, the Eagle Heights Village study of young student families began.[72] The epidemiologic aspects of this investigation have been described previously (see "Epidemiology and Transmission"). Daily home clinical surveillance was performed, and although the illnesses generally were so mild that the participants did not see a physician, the same differential severity between adults and children was noted (Table 171–4). With all viruses, including RVs, children were much more likely to be febrile and their symptoms were much more likely to last longer. Overall, however, RV-caused illnesses were milder than those caused by other viruses.

A thorough investigation of infants and young children hospitalized with lower respiratory disease at Madison General Hospital was conducted at the same time[49] (Table 171–5). A virus was cultured from 38 percent of these patients, and RVs predominated (11 of 27 isolates). These children (average age, <1 year) with RV infections were seriously ill: the mean temperature was 39.4° C (103° F), and eight had bronchopneumonia. Six of the virus-infected children yielded a bacterial pathogen in predominance in throat cultures. Five of them, beta-hemolytic *Streptococcus* in one, *Streptococcus pneumoniae* in two, and *Haemophilus influenzae* in two, were present coincidentally with the RV isolates. All the RV-associated cases had antecedent milder respiratory symptoms, especially coryza.

Rhinovirus Preeminence in the Respiratory Disease of Larger Populations

Two large populations, one a general medical practice in Roehampton, near London, England,[151] and the other a group of families in Tecumseh, a small town in the United States near Detroit,[217] were assayed for the various respiratory viruses in illnesses of differing severity. Each had a pediatric population base of 900 or more. RVs easily were the most common cause of respiratory illness in either population (Table 171–6): 26.3 percent of isolates in England and 38.1 percent in Michigan.

In both populations, RVs frequently were associated with lower respiratory tract illness (Table 171–7); the proportion was much higher in the Roehampton clinic. The major RV diagnosis in lower respiratory tract[151] disease was wheezy bronchitis: 42 percent of all RV isolates in Roehampton and 15 percent in Tecumseh.[216] Otherwise, the severity of disease associated with RV infection often was milder; in Roehampton, none of the RV isolates were from children with bronchiolitis or pneumonia, whereas 8.4 percent of the RSV isolates were associated with one of these diagnoses. In Tecumseh, restriction of activity was an important differential marker for etiology in that only 24.3 percent of those with RV illness curtailed their normal activities whereas the percentages often were double that for the other respiratory

TABLE 171–4 ■ COMPARISON OF THE CLINICAL ILLNESS ATTRIBUTABLE TO RHINOVIRUSES WITH THAT ATTRIBUTABLE TO OTHER RESPIRATORY VIRUSES OBTAINED FROM 24 FAMILIES (89 PERSONS) IN THE UNIVERSITY OF WISCONSIN'S EAGLE HEIGHTS VILLAGE, 1963–1965*

				Percentage with				
				Fever (°C)†				
Virus	Age Group	Number of Patients	Average Duration of Illness (Days)	37.7–38.3	<38.3	*Cough*	*Nasal Discharge*	*Sore Throat*
Rhinovirus	Children	26	11	15	4	73	92	15
	Adults	25	9	8	4	68	96	56
Respiratory syncytial	Children	21	10	37	20	90	95	9
	Adults	1	8	0	0	100	100	0
Parainfluenza 1	Children	7	9	0	27	57	100	29
	Adults	6	8	17	0	33	83	67
Parainfluenza 3	Children	10	6	30	60	70	90	40
	Adults	1	6	0	0	0	100	100
Influenza	Children	2	10	100	100	100	100	50
	Adults	3	8	33	66	100	67	67

*The 42 children surveyed varied evenly in age from younger than 1 to 7 years; only 3 were older than 7.

†The temperature range 37.7° C to 38.3° C is 100° F to 101° F; less than 38.3° C is less than 101° F.

Adapted from Dick, E.C., Blumer, C.R., and Evans, A.S.: Epidemiology of infections with rhinovirus types 43 and 55 in a group of University of Wisconsin student families. Am J. Epidemiol. *86*:386–400, 1967.

TABLE 171–5 ■ CLINICAL FINDINGS IN 11 CHILDREN HOSPITALIZED WITH SEVERE PULMONARY DISEASE IN MADISON, WISCONSIN, FROM WHOM RHINOVIRUSES WERE ISOLATED, JANUARY THROUGH MAY 15, 1964

	Patients										
	A	*B*	*C*	*D*	*E*	*F*	*G*	*H*	*I*	*J**	*K*
Clinical Findings											
Age (yr)	6/12	6/12	7	4-6/12	1	5	8/12	5/12	5/12	2/12	2
Sex	M	M	M	M	F	F	M	M	F	M	F
History											
Cough	+	+	+				+		+		+
Coryza	+				+	+	+	+	+	+	+
Respiratory distress	+	+		+			+	+		+	
Antibiotics before study	+					+	+	+		+	
Physical Findings											
Highest											
Temp (°C)	39.7	40	38.2	39.4	40.5	38.7	40.1	39.3	40.2	38.1	38.3
Temp (°F)	103.6	104	100.8	103	105	101.8	104.2	102.8	104.4	100.6	101
Tonsillitis or pharyngitis				+		+					
Hoarseness or croup											+
Tachypnea	+	+	+					+		+	+
Chest refractions	+							+		+	
Rhonchi							+	+		+	+
Rales			+				+				
Wheezing	+	+	+					+			
Laboratory Studies											
Initial leukocyte count (1000 × mm^3)	10	15.5	8.7	11.4	19.8	10	10.7	7.3	30.5	13	11.2
Neutrophils (%)	42	55	93	77	74	79	49	69	72	73	75
Pneumonitis on chest radiographs	+	+		+		+	+	+	+	+	
Throat culture†	Pn	NF	HI	St	NF	NF	HI	NF	NF	Pn	NF
Diagnosis	BP Br	BP Br	Bron	BP Tons	URI UTI	BP Tons OM	BP	BP	BP	BP Atel	Cr

*Hospitalized since birth with choanal atresia. Right upper lobe pneumonia and atelectasis were present for 1 month before study.
†Only the predominant organism is recorded. Pn indicates *Streptococcus pneumoniae*: NP, normal flora: HI, *Haemophilus influenzae*; St, beta-hemolytic *Streptococcus*; Br, bronchiolitis; BP, bronchopneumonia; Bron, bronchitis; Tons, tonsillitis; URI, upper respiratory infection; UTI, urinary tract infection; OM, otitis media; Atel, atelectasis; CR, croup.
Adopted from Cherry, J.D., Diddams, J.A., and Dick, E.C.: Rhinovirus infections in hospitalised children. Arch. Environ. Health *14*:390–396, 1967.

viruses, varying from 42 percent for RSV to 63 percent for influenza B virus.

Rhinovirus Infections in Hospitalized Children

In Bristol, England, in 1971, 377 infants hospitalized for respiratory disease yielded 199 (53%) viral diagnoses.[165] RSV was predominant and accounted for 79 percent of the diagnoses, but RVs were second at 12 percent (23 patients). Half of the RV diagnoses were in infants with bronchiolitis or pneumonia. RV illnesses were comparable in severity to those caused by RSV. One 4-month-old with RV-associated bronchopneumonia died. Except for the absence of deaths, similar results were found in 102 hospitalized children in Colorado, where the etiologic diagnosis rate was 85 percent.[227]

Serious RV infections in young children have been reported from several locations, and some of these outbreaks have allowed direct comparisons between RV and RSV infection. In the intensive care nursery of Strong Memorial Hospital in Rochester, New York, eight infants 2 weeks to 6 months of age became nosocomially infected, four with RV and four with RSV, in early February 1980.[291] One of the RV isolates was from an asymptomatic baby. All seven symptomatic babies had a dramatic and sudden onset of respiratory illness that included cyanosis, apnea, labored respirations, increased nasal or tracheal secretions, tachypnea, and lethargy. Wheezing, tachycardia, irritability, and cardiac arrest each occurred in a single infant. None of the signs and symptoms differentiated RV and RSV illnesses.

At St. Anna Children's Hospital in Vienna, Austria, from 1984 to 1986, Kellner and colleagues[177] compared the clinical features of RV and RSV infection in 519 children 10 days to 3 years of age (median age, 6.6 months). Viral pathogens were detected in 227 (44%) of the children, and of these, 119 (23%) were RSV and 60 (12%) were RV. The physical findings (Table 171–8) and the clinical diagnosis (Table 171–9) of the children with RV or RSV infection were alike, except that RV infections were more likely than were RSV infections to be associated with upper respiratory tract infection.

Several retrospective reviews of clinical and laboratory records also have implicated RVs as probable causes of lower respiratory illness in infants. In 1982 and 1983, Krilov and associates[183] found 32 RV-infected children who had significant signs of pulmonary disease in Boston hospitals, half with radiologic evidence of new focal infiltrates. From 1984 to 1988, Abzug and associates[2] examined all virus-positive cultures from pneumonias in neonates younger than 30 days in Denver hospitals. The definition of pneumonia was strict and included new infiltrates on chest radiographs plus

TABLE 171–6 ■ RHINOVIRUSES AND OTHER RESPIRATORY VIRUSES ISOLATED FROM SOME ENGLISH AND AMERICAN CHILDREN YOUNGER THAN 15 YEARS WITH SYMPTOMATIC RESPIRATORY INFECTIONS

Agent	Roehampton England*†	Tecumseh, Michigan U.S.A.‡§
Rhinoviruses	162 (26.3)‖	82 (38.1)
Parainfluenza	111 (18.0)	56 (26.0)
Influenza A and B	89 (14.5)	34 (15.8)
Respiratory syncytial virus	56 (9.1)	19 (8.8)
Adenoviruses	45 (7.3)	9 (4.1)
Enteroviruses	66 (10.7)	15 (6.9)
Other agents	58‡¶ (9.4)	—
Double isolates	27** (4.4)	—
Total isolates	614	215

*Results from a general practice clinic (919 children) during 1968 to 1972 Roehampton is a London residential suburb.
†Adapted from Horn, M.E.C., Brain, E., Gregg, I., et al.: Respiratory viral infection in childhood: A survery in general practice, Roehampton 1967–1972. J. Hyg. (Camb.) *74*:157–168, 1975.
‡Results from surveillance (472 children) during 1966 to 1969. Tecumseh is a city of about 10,000, located approximately 50 miles southwest of Detroit.
§Adapted from Monto, A.S., and Cavalloro, J.J.: The Tecumseh study of respiratory illness. II. Patterns of occurrence of infection with respiratory pathogens, 1965–1969. Am. J. Epidemiol. *94*:280–289, 1971.
‖Percentage of total isolates.
¶Mumps 3; herpes simplex, 17: *Mycoplasma pneumoniae*, 37: psittacosis (serologic diagnosis), 1.
**Includes nine rhinoviruses.

TABLE 171–7 ■ ASSOCIATION OF RHINOVIRUSES WITH UPPER AND LOWER RESPIRATORY INFECTION IN SOME ENGLISH CHILDREN (ROEHAMPTON[128]) AND AMERICAN FAMILIES (TECUMSEH[184])*

	Percentage of Rhinovirus Isolates	
	Roehampton	*Tecumseh*†
Upper respiratory infection	47	71
Lower respiratory infection	53	21

*See Table 171–6 for virus isolation data and population description.
†Includes rhinovirus isolates from both children and adults (82 isolates from children and 58 isolates from adults).

several typical physical signs. Forty patients were found; RSV was isolated from slightly more than half the cases, and RVs and enteroviruses, at six isolates each, were the second most frequent. McMillan and colleagues[204] identified 48 pediatric patients who had RV infections and were admitted (n =40) or treated in the emergency center (n =8) at their institution in Syracuse, New York, between 1985 and 1989. Most of them (n = 41) were younger than 1 year, and almost half (n = 20) had a clinical picture of bronchiolitis. Suspected sepsis (n = 9) was the next most common diagnosis. Kim and Hodinka[179] identified 93 pediatric patients with RV infection who were evaluated in the emergency center (n = 5) or admitted (n = 88) to their hospital in Philadelphia between 1990 and 1996. Most of them (n = 67) were younger than 1 year. An acute respiratory illness was the most common clinical finding (n = 78, 84%), with fever and suspected sepsis being the next most common (n = 13, 14%). A second viral or bacterial pathogen was identified in eight (9%) of the subjects. Many of the subjects (n = 62, 67%) had an underlying condition such as prematurity or reactive airway disease. The authors concluded that RV infection was associated with severe lower respiratory illness and the need for hospitalization and could be a complicating factor in patients with underlying conditions.[179] Chidekel and colleagues[50] examined 40 patients with bronchopulmonary dysplasia and noted 8 episodes of worsening lung disease in 6 infants associated with RV infection. The findings and clinical course of these infants were similar to those noted in other infants infected with RSV, although the need for mechanical ventilation was greater in association with RSV infection.

Glezen and colleagues[111] performed a prospective study to evaluate the occurrence of respiratory virus infection in subjects with respiratory or cardiac disorders admitted to three hospitals in Houston, Texas, between 1991 and 1995. RV infections were identified in 51 subjects from a total of 1198 evaluated illnesses; 6 of them were associated with a second respiratory virus infection.[92] In children younger than 5 years, asthma exacerbation, bronchiolitis, and suspected sepsis were the most common clinical findings, whereas in older children and young adults, almost all subjects had an exacerbation of asthma. In older adults, a complication of an underlying disease (asthma, chronic obstructive lung disease, congestive heart failure) or pneumonia was diagnosed. In this prospective study, RV infections were an important cause of lower respiratory tract illness in all age groups.[92]

Two infants hospitalized at the Children's National Medical Center in Washington, D.C., a 1-month-old girl with bacteriologically negative pertussis syndrome and a 6-month-old boy with a prolonged and life-threatening asthma attack, yielded RVs from the lower respiratory tract by bronchoalveolar lavage.[259] No other pathogens were recovered. An infant with underlying cardiovascular abnormalities and transfusion-associated graft-versus-host disease was found to have pneumonia at autopsy. RV was isolated from the lung, and immunohistochemistry showed RV antigen in alveolar cells in the lung.[160]

Despite the foregoing evidence that RVs can be an important cause of severe lower respiratory tract disease, large studies in Chapel Hill, North Carolina,[70] Huntington, West Virginia,[29] and Tucson, Arizona,[302] by experienced investigators yielded the usual respiratory viruses in appropriate numbers, but only 1 to 3 percent were RVs. These studies may represent the importance of RV-caused disease in these populations fairly, but negative cultures do not necessarily mean the absence of RVs. These viruses are difficult to grow, even in supposedly sensitive cell cultures, and often only a few organisms are present in the specimen (Table 171–10).

In summary, evidence is accumulating that RVs can cause serious lower respiratory illness, especially in young children. In some populations, they may be second to RSV in importance and cause comparably severe signs and symptoms.

Asthma

A specific lower respiratory illness in which the RVs clearly appear important, perhaps most important, is "wheezy bronchitis" or "infectious asthma." (No clinical term that describes the illnesses in which infection and wheezing are present is accepted widely.[142] In this chapter, these two foregoing terms and others always are used in an attempt to reflect the individual investigator's meaning and preference.) The association between RVs and these illnesses first was noted by Horn, Gregg, and their associates[151–153] as part of their previously described 1967 to 1972 Roehampton study of ill children (see Table 171–6). Forty-two percent of the 162 RV isolates at Roehampton were from children with attacks of wheezy bronchitis, approximately

TABLE 171–8 ■ PHYSICAL FINDINGS IN YOUNG CHILDREN* WITH RESPIRATORY ILLNESS AT THE TIME OF THEIR ADMISSION TO ST. ANNA CHILDREN'S HOSPITAL, VIENNA, AUSTRIA, 1984-1986—COMPARISON BETWEEN RHINOVIRUS (RV) AND RESPIRATORY SYNCYTIAL VIRUS (RSV) INFECTIONS

Physical Findings	All Patients† (*n* = 519)	RSV (*n* = 119)	RV (*n* = 60)
Stridor during expiration	67 (13%)	15 (13%)	10 (16%)
Cyanosis	18 (3%)	4 (3%)	2 (3%)
Swollen cervical glands	87 (17%)	17 (14%)	9 (15%)
Red throat	344 (66%)	75 (63%)	41 (68%)
Nasal flaring	75 (14%)	29 (16%)	11 (18%)
Crepitations	20 (4%)	7 (6%)	2 (3%)
Chest radiograph (positive)	260 (50%)	79 (66%)	35 (58%)
Wheezing	113 (22%)	30 (25%)	13 (22%)
Moist rales	174 (34%)	43 (36%)	22 (36%)
Dry rales	49 (9%)	13 (11%)	5 (8%)
Respiratory rate/min			
Median (range)	43 (10-96)	40 (10-84)	36 (10-64)
Body temperature			
Median (range)	38.4° C (36.4° C-41.8° C)	39.9° C (36.8° C-41.0° C)	38.5° C (36.9° C-41.0° C)
Duration of illness			
Median (range)	11.6 days (2-45)	10.5 days (4-12)	12.8 days (3-31)

*Ten days to 3 years of age (median age, 6.6 months).
†One hundred twelve (21%) children had upper respiratory tract, and 342 (66%) had lower respiratory tract illnesses: 471 (91%) were inpatients, and 48 (9%) were outpatients.
Adapted from Kellner, G., Popow-Kraupp, T., Kundi, M., et al.: Clinicial manifestations of respiratory tract infections due to respiratory syncytial virus and rhinoviruses in hospitalized children. Acta Paediatr. Scand. *78*:390–394, 1989.

TABLE 171–9 ■ CLINICAL DIAGNOSIS OF RESPIRATORY ILLNESSES OF YOUNG CHILDREN* AT ST. ANNA CHILDREN'S HOSPITAL, VIENNA, AUSTRIA, 1984-1986—COMPARISON BETWEEN RHINOVIRUS (RV) AND RESPIRATORY SYNCYTIAL VIRUS (RSV) INFECTIONS

Clinical Diagnosis	All Patients (n = 519)	RSV (n = 119)	RV (n = 60)
Upper respiratory tract infection			
Rhinitis	65 (12%)	4 (3%)	5 (9%)
Otitis media	10 (2%)	0	2 (3%)
Epiglottitis	6 (1%)	1 (1%)	2 (3%)
Pharyngitis	23 (4%)	3 (2%)	4 (6%)
Laryngitis	8 (2%)	1 (1%)	2 (3%)
Other diseases	25 (5%)	0	1(2%)
Total	137 (26%)	9 (7%)	16 (26%)†
Lower respiratory tract infection			
Croup	14 (3%)	4 (3%)	4 (6%)
Tracheobronchitis	100 (19%)	46 (39%)	16 (27%)
Bronchitis	24 (5%)	3 (2%)	0
Obstructive bronchitis‡	78 (15%)	28 (24%)	8 (14%)
Pneumonia	126 (24%)	29 (25%)	15 (25%)
Other diseases	40 (8%)	0	1 (2%)
Total	382 (74%)	110 (93%)	44 (74%)

*See footnotes to Table 171–8.
†RVs were more likely to cause upper respiratory tract infection ($p < .01$).
‡This diagnosis included children with expiratory wheeze and evidence of air trapping. In a later paper, this same definition was used for wheezy bronchitis.[145]
Adapted from Kellner, G., Popow-Kraupp, T., Kundi, M., et. al.: Clinical manifestations of respiratory tract infections due to respiratory syncytial virus and rhinoviruses in hospitalized children. Acta Paediatr. Scand. *78*:390–394, 1989.

twice the percentage of other viruses causing this syndrome. Many of these children were known to be subject to recurrent episodes.

During the later years (1971 to 1972) of this period, the Madison laboratory performed a longitudinal clinical and microbial study (children were sampled at least twice weekly for viral and once monthly for bacterial culture) of 16 nonatopic children with "infectious asthma" and 15 of their normal siblings. A clear temporal relationship was found between (1) the onset of symptomatic respiratory infection, (2) an asthmatic episode, and (3) the presence of viruses, predominantly RVs, in the pharynx[209, 210] (Fig. 171–12). Precipitation of an asthmatic episode occurred much more frequently during severe symptomatic respiratory infections than during mild ones. RVs caused an asthma attack in 14 of 15 severe symptomatic respiratory infections but in only 1 of 6 mild ones. Subclinical infections never precipitated an attack. Except for one instance in which *H. influenzae* may have caused asthma, bacterial infections were not associated with asthma attacks, even when they were accompanied by severe symptomatic respiratory infection. (Note that the severe group A streptococcal infections in subjects CC and P did not precipitate asthma, whereas severe RV-49 infections in these two children caused more than three asthma attacks that were sufficiently incapacitating for the child to stay home from school.[210]) The asthmatic siblings seemed especially susceptible to symptomatic infection; total infections of probable viral etiology ($p <.02$), known viral infections ($p <.01$), and RV-caused symptomatic respiratory infections ($p <.01$) all were significantly greater in the asthmatic than in the nonasthmatic siblings.[208]

A somewhat similar year-long prospective investigation was conducted in England[162] in 30 preschool children with histories of recurrent respiratory infection often accompanied by wheezing, as well as in their unaffected siblings. The children with recurring infections had approximately twice

TABLE 171–10 ■ QUANTITY OF VIRUS FOUND IN 87 THROAT SWAB SQUEEZINGS FROM CHILDREN 3 TO 11 YEARS OF AGE, MADISON, WISCONSIN, 1971–1972*

	Per 0.1 mL
1 $TCID_{50}$ or less†	22
>1 to ≤50 $TCID_{50}$	46
≥50 to <50 $TCID_{50}$	14
>50 to <500 $TCID_{50}$	5

*Fourteen rhinovirus types are represented.
†Median tissue culture infective doses.

the number of illnesses and viruses isolated than the controls did. Their illnesses also were much more severe, and they often involved the lower respiratory tract. RVs were heavily preponderant, at 57 percent of the isolates, and were associated with wheezy bronchitis four times more often than RSVs were. Atopic children, as measured by positive skin testing and raised serum IgE levels, did not seem especially subject to development of recurrent infection.

At the University of Colorado, McIntosh and associates[201, 202] demonstrated in 1973 the importance of other respiratory viruses in asthma; later, they suggested that RSV is the major agent associated with asthma in children younger than 4 years and that RVs are preeminent in older children and adults.[201, 202] Subsequent reports have demonstrated the importance of RVs in older children, as well as in many younger children. As examples of RVs in younger children, in recurrent asthmatic patients seen at the pediatric allergy unit in Oslo, Norway, from 1981 to 1983, most of the acute bronchial asthma cases were RV associated (45%), with RSV being second (19%).[38] Twenty-nine percent of those in the virus-infected group were between 2 and 3 years of age, with the incidence gradually decreasing to 1 percent in adolescents 15 years of age. Also illustrative of RV in the very young is the prospective study of the 30 English preschool children with recurrent wheezing infections described earlier, in which RVs were most important in children whose mean age was 2.2 years.[162] Mertsola and colleagues[206] in Turku, Finland, examined children with wheezy bronchitis (mean age, 3.2 years) and found RVs and coronaviruses to be most important. The comparative importance of RSV and RV in asthma in infants (median age, 6.6 months) with probable wheezy bronchitis (see "Obstructive bronchitis" in Table 171–9) was examined from 1984 to 1986 by Viennese investigators; 28 isolates yielded RSV, and only 8 yielded RV.[176] In a later paper from this group covering 1986 to 1990, 179 RSV isolates and 49 RVs were recovered from these hospitalized infants; most of the RVs were recovered from infants with some wheezing.[175] Only three had pneumonia without wheezing.

A cohort of 9- to 11-year-old children with asthma was evaluated from April 1989 to May 1990.[170, 172] Nucleic acid

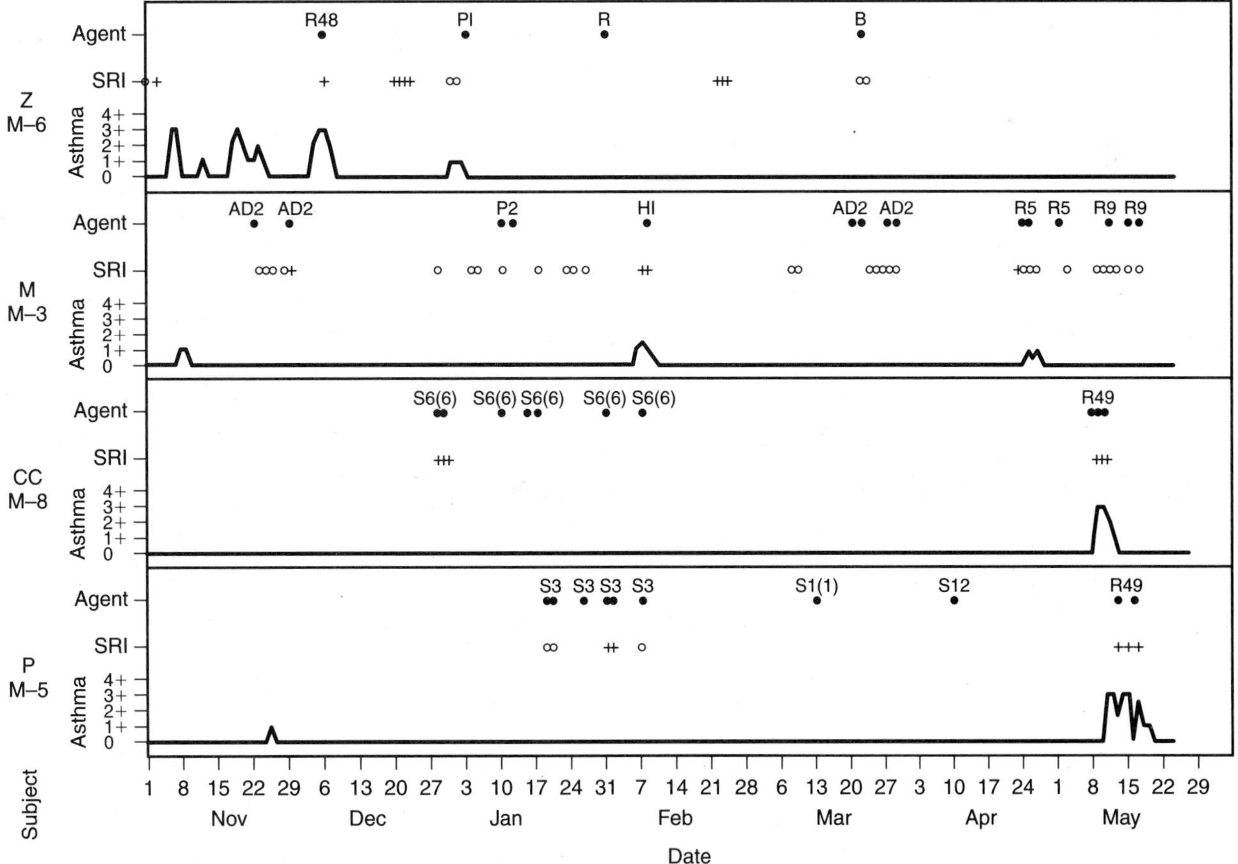

FIGURE 171–12 ■ Temporal relationship among asthma, symptomatic respiratory infection (SRI), and infectious agent in four children with "infectious" asthma. AD, adenovirus; B, influenza B; HI, *Haemophilus influenzae*; P, parainfluenza; R, rhinovirus; S, group A *Streptococcus*; open circle, mild; +, severe (fever or more than one sign or symptom). Numbers after R and P indicate type; numbers after S indicate T type (M type, if typable, is in parentheses). (Adapted from Minor, T. D., Dick, E. C., DeMeo, A. N., et al.: Viruses as precipitants of asthmatic attacks in children. J. A. M. A. *227*:292–298, 1974.)

detection methods (reverse transcriptase–polymerase chain reaction [RT-PCR]) were used in addition to traditional culture methods to identify RV infections. Respiratory viruses were detected in 80 to 85 percent of illness episodes (the rate depended on the definition of illness), and RVs were present in approximately half the illnesses. The occurrence of respiratory viral infections in this cohort correlated strongly with hospital admissions for both children and adults in the same geographic area.[171] RVs also have been associated with exacerbations of asthma in adults, though at a somewhat lower frequency (as many as 33% of episodes).[23, 224]

Viral infection is an important risk factor for wheezing in children of all ages who are receiving emergency care.[90] RSV infection and passive tobacco smoke exposure were associated most frequently with wheezing illness in young children (<2 years). Thirty-one percent of children older than 2 years had an accompanying viral infection, usually an RV infection, and were more likely to have IgE antibody to inhalant allergens than were the younger children. This study illustrates the dichotomy of etiologies for wheezing illness in the pediatric age group: RSV infection is the predominant cause in infants, and atopy combined with viral infection, usually RV infection, is the main cause in older children.

Two groups serotyped the RVs isolated from children with wheezy bronchitis and found no types to be particularly "asthmagenic"; the Viennese group identified 12 serotypes, and the Madison group reported 21.[175, 208–210] Only three serotypes overlapped: RV-1B, RV-20, and RV-32. Therefore, a total of 30 different RV serotypes precipitated asthmatic attacks.

The mechanism of bronchospasm in virus-infected patients with wheezy bronchitis has generated much speculation and research. Especially provocative is RV-caused wheezing because RVs were thought to be unable to replicate well at the temperature of the lower respiratory tract.[135, 283, 288] More recent data have shown that RVs can replicate at the higher temperatures of the lower respiratory tract and that they can be found in the lower airways.[108, 130, 160, 229, 230] Whether the virus-associated bronchospasm is caused by local viral growth or by replication in the upper respiratory tract has not been resolved, although the former seems to be more likely.[106] RV infection clearly induces the production of numerous proinflammatory cytokines, and an increased number of inflammatory cells has been demonstrated in the lower respiratory tract in association with RV infection.[101, 106] The presence of activated cytotoxic T cells in the lower airways has been suggested to be a contributory factor leading to asthma-associated mortality.[225] Animal models also suggest the possibility that reflex neurogenic pathways might be activated in association with respiratory viral infection and lead to bronchoconstriction. The pathogenesis of respiratory virus–induced bronchospasm is an area of active research, with the hope that preventive or therapeutic intervention strategies can be developed.

Otitis Media

Although acute otitis media is chiefly a bacterial disease, with approximately two thirds of middle ear fluid specimens yielding *S. pneumoniae, H. influenzae,* or both and *Moraxella catarrhalis* and other bacteria playing lesser roles, otitic involvement often is preceded or accompanied by a putative viral upper respiratory tract illness.[14, 16, 119, 181, 255] Most bacterial pathogens found in middle ear fluid are colonizers of the nasopharynx, and bacterial infection of the middle ear is considered to be a direct extension from that area.[181, 191] Clear and comprehensive evidence for viral extension from the nasopharynx to the middle ear has been established. Sarkkinen and coworkers,[257] using antigen-detection techniques on middle ear fluid and nasopharyngeal secretions, found RSV, adenovirus, and parainfluenza viruses in either the middle ear fluid or the nasopharyngeal secretions of 58 of 131 children (44%) with acute otitis media. Twenty-four of these children had viruses in middle ear fluid, and only 1 of the 24 did not have the same viral antigen in both the middle ear fluid and nasopharyngeal secretions. Most of the sampling was conducted during a local epidemic of RSV infection, and the curve of RSV detection in the middle ear fluid and nasopharyngeal secretions followed the pattern of the RSV epidemic curve. Other investigators have found similar relationships between the viruses in middle ear fluid and nasopharyngeal secretions.[51, 182]

Gwaltney[118] isolated one RV from culture of 16 middle ear fluid specimens in 1971. In 1986, Chonmaitree and colleagues[51] reported three RV isolates in 84 middle ear fluid specimens; then Arola,[13] as part of his 1990 M.D. thesis, performed a thorough investigation of the role of RVs in this illness.[14–17, 255] In 1987 to 1988, nasopharyngeal secretions were taken from 363 patients (mean age, 2.5 years) with acute otitis media, and viruses were detected in 154 (42%); surprisingly, RV predominated over RSV, 24 versus 13 percent.[14] RVs were isolated all through the year, but the usual fall and spring peaks were observed. Patients with RSV infection generally were sicker, with higher fever ($p < .05$) and more severe cough ($p < .01$), but the appearance of the tympanic membrane was similar in both patients with RV and those with RSV. The usual bacterial pathogens were cultured from 82 percent of the nasopharyngeal secretions, and after 2 days of antimicrobial treatment, fever and earache were reduced sharply in nearly all patients; however, in those with concomitant viral infections, respiratory symptoms remained a week or more with declining intensity. In comparison with RV, cough was particularly long lasting in patients with RSV.

Arola and collaborators[16] attempted to detect virus in both the nasopharyngeal secretions (116 cases) and middle ear fluid (143 cases) of patients with acute otitis media (mean age, 1.5 years) and were successful in 33 (28%) and 16 (11%), respectively. RVs were the predominant isolate, with 21 (18%) in nasopharyngeal secretions and 11 (8%) in middle ear fluid. Fifty-three percent of the patients harbored a bacterial pathogen in middle ear fluid. In the RV-positive group in whom both viral and bacterial cultures were performed, six of nine middle ear fluid specimens yielded no bacterial pathogens; that is, RV was the only pathogen found. Unfortunately, they were not able to serotype the RVs to determine whether the same serotype was present in both the nasopharyngeal secretions and middle ear fluid.

More recent studies have found evidence of RVs in middle ear effusion with RT-PCR methods. Pitkaranta and colleagues[237] isolated respiratory viruses from the middle ear effusions of 30 percent of 100 children who had otitis media with effusion. RVs constituted approximately two thirds of the respiratory viruses identified. Bacterial pathogens were identified in 35 percent of the samples, and both bacteria and viruses were found in 11 percent. A criterion for selection was the absence of an upper respiratory tract illness within the preceding week, so whether the presence of RV RNA represented evidence of ongoing or past infection is unclear. Blomqvist and colleagues[31] found RV RNA in middle ear effusions from 41 percent of children with otitis media in the first 2 years of life.

Although in general, the presence of both bacterial and viral pathogens in middle ear fluid does not interfere with the effectiveness of antibacterial therapy, in those specific patients whose acute otitis media is refractory to treatment, it may.[17] When measured against a comparison group of 66 "normal" acute otitis media cases (controls), 22 refractory cases harbored significantly ($p < .05$) more (68% versus 41%) viral pathogens than the controls did. In addition, when only the middle ear fluid of these groups was examined for the presence of viruses, refractory cases had virus in 32 percent of samples versus 15 percent in controls. RVs were the dominant virus in both groups. Bacterial pathogens were grown from the middle ear fluid of 4 of the 22 in the poor-responder group, and all harbored concomitant respiratory viruses, 2 of them RVs; only 1 of the 4 bacteria was resistant to the antibacterial agent used in therapy. These investigators also examined patients in the 66-patient control group who were refractory to treatment and found significantly more ($p < .05$) viruses in the middle ear fluid of this group than in those with a good response to therapy. The authors concluded that the presence of viruses in the middle ear fluid of children with acute otitis media can delay response to antibacterial therapy.

Chonmaitree and associates[52] in Galveston, Texas, also investigated the role of viruses in middle ear fluid as agents that may interfere with antibacterial therapy. In their initial report, viruses were cultured from the middle ear fluid of 11 of 58 children (19%); RSV and RV were the most frequent viruses isolated at 3 each. Of the patients in whom therapy failed, significantly more ($p < .05$) harbored viruses as well, and of those whose bacteria were susceptible to the treatment antibiotic, significantly more were combined viral-bacterial infections. In two subsequent reports, the highest rate of poor bacteriologic outcome occurred when RV was isolated from middle ear fluid; seven of nine instances of RV infection resulted in bacteriologic treatment failure.[271]

These studies from Finland and Texas suggest that viruses, including RVs, may play a role in acute otitis media, especially in prolonging the response to antimicrobial treatment. Perhaps pertinently, McBride and associates[200] at the Universities of Pittsburgh and Virginia used RV-infected human volunteers and found that the eustachian tube became occluded in 50 percent of the volunteers and that abnormal middle ear pressure was present for as long as 10 days. These studies were extended by Buchman and colleagues,[33] who inoculated 60 volunteers with RV-39. Middle ear pressures of less than −100 mm H_2O were noted in 22 subjects (37%). In two of the three who had pressures less than −100 mm H_2O, upper respiratory illness with middle ear effusion developed. In this study, the otologic manifestations of experimental RV infection were extended to include otitis media.

Arola and colleagues[15] examined the role of viruses in 61 children (mean age, 3.2 years) with subacute or chronic asymptomatic otitis media with effusion. Five RVs and one adenovirus were found in the middle ear fluid. In addition, bacterial pathogens were isolated from the patient with adenovirus infection and from two of the RV patients. None of these patients with otitis media and effusion were ill with an upper respiratory tract infection at the time that the specimen was obtained, and the effusion had endured 30 to 60 days before myringotomy was performed.

Sinusitis

RVs can cause a clinical syndrome of rhinosinusitis that appears similar to that caused by bacterial infection. Gwaltney and colleagues[125] performed computed tomography of the sinuses on adults with acute common colds (<4 days' duration). RV infection was documented by culture in 27 percent. Radiographic abnormalities included mucosal thickening and air-fluid levels. The signs and symptoms resolved without antibiotic therapy, thus suggesting that the radiographic signs were caused by an acute viral infection. Few attempts have been made to recover viruses directly from the sinuses. In two reports from Virginia, 140 aspirates obtained by direct puncture of the maxillary sinuses yielded 86 positive specimens, only 12 of which contained viruses. Seven of them were RVs, and the remainder were influenza A or parainfluenza viruses.[126, 131] Five of the viruses were isolated in conjunction with bacterial pathogens. In a more recent study, Pitkaranta and associates[236] used RT-PCR to identify RVs in 50 percent of adults with acute community-acquired sinusitis. Because the signs and symptoms of viral rhinosinusitis and bacterial sinusitis can be difficult to distinguish, the American Academy of Pediatrics has developed clinical practice guidelines for the diagnosis and treatment of bacterial sinusitis.[54]

Rhinovirus Infections in Nonindustrialized Populations

Not many RV surveillance studies have been conducted in nonindustrialized populations, but those that have reveal some unique findings. In the spring of 1967, Wulff and associates[303] observed an outbreak of RV-16 and RV-29 infection in a 93-family (429 children) Eskimo population in Bethel, Alaska. The RV-16 outbreak, the larger of the two, was analyzed thoroughly. The investigators found 37 RV-16 isolates, but only 19 of them were from ill children; therefore, nearly half, 18 children, had subclinical infections. The ill children often were only mildly so; 12 had common colds, and only 1 had bronchitis and 1 had pneumonia. RV-16 spread widely in the population under study, with 70 percent of antibody-free children demonstrating a fourfold or greater serologic response. Eighty-five of the 93 families were infected with RV-16, and the 8 families that escaped infection had only 1 to 3 children each. The amount of RV dissemination was not especially surprising because it was not much higher than that of RV-55 in Eagle Heights Village (see Fig. 171–8), but surprisingly half the RV infections were subclinical.

Much subclinical RV infection also was reported in a surveillance of 136 preschool children in two small villages (combined population of 1750 in 1982) on an island in the Melanesian nation of Vanuatu, a group of 80 islands located in the South Pacific approximately midway between Australia and Fiji.[274] RVs by far were the predominant viruses (21 isolates), and all were type 16 and all caused subclinical infection. In addition, pneumococci often were found in conjunction with these symptomless RV-16 cases and rarely otherwise.

These two examples of a high rate of subclinical RV infection are unusual judging by experience in more industrialized societies. Surveillance of a year-long (1971 to 1972), twice-weekly sampling of 32 children 3 to 11 years of age in Madison produced much different results.[208, 210] As depicted in Figure 171–12 and Table 171–11, only 11 (0.8%) cases of asymptomatic shedding occurred all year. On the other hand, all of these children were members of at least middle-class families, and some continental U.S. populations may be analogous to those in underdeveloped nations. Gwaltney[121] notes that the rate of overall inapparent RV infection in the continental United States may approach 25 percent.

However, as emphatically described in reviews by Chretien and associates[53] and by Graham,[112] asymptomatic infection with respiratory viruses is not the major problem of families in communities and nations struggling to raise their children in healthy environments. Graham[112] has estimated that worldwide, 98 to 99 percent of deaths from acute respiratory disease occur in the developing nations. A study of children 5 years or younger was conducted in such a nation,

TABLE 171–11 ■ RHINOVIRUSES AND OTHER VIRAL AND BACTERIAL PATHOGENS ISOLATED DURING PERIODS OF RESPIRATORY ILLNESS AND WHEN ILLNESS-FREE FROM 33 MIDDLE-CLASS CHILDREN 3 TO 11 YEARS OF AGE (AVERAGE AGE, 6 YEARS)—MADISON, WISCONSIN, 1971-1972*

	1971–1972 (Nov–Feb)	1972 (Mar–May)	Total
Illness-Free	753	566	1319
Agents Isolated			
Rhinoviruses	4 (0.5)†	7 (1.2)	11 (0.8)
Other viruses‡	10 (1.3)	6 (1.1)	16 (1.2)
Bacterial pathogens§	14 (1.9)	4 (0.7)	18 (1.4)
Total	28 (3.7)	17 (3.0)	45 (3.4)
Respiratory Illness	305	195	500
Agents Isolated			
Rhinoviruses	13 (4.3)	57 (29.2)	70 (14)
Other viruses	44 (14.4)	14 (7.2)	58 (11.6)
Bacterial pathogens	35 (11.5)	10 (5.1)	45 (9.0)
Total	92 (30.2)	81 (41.5)	173 (34.6)

*Throat swabs were taken twice weekly and inoculated into three cell lines and a sheep blood agar plate.[175,177]

†Percent isolation rate (i.e., 4/753, 0.5%).

‡Adenoviruses, influenza viruses A and B, parainfluenza virus, herpes simplex virus, and enteroviruses. Coronaviruses would not have been isolated; the fact that they often are midwinter viruses may account for the relatively low isolation rate for 1971-1972.

§Chiefly group A streptococci in more than 100 colonies per pour plate.

Kenya.[140] Eight hundred twenty-two children with severe acute respiratory disease were examined etiologically by modern cell culture techniques. Fifty-four percent of the children yielded viruses (444 isolates), with enterovirus by far being the most common (162 isolates), followed by RSV (98 isolates) and the RVs (54 isolates). Half the RV isolates were also culture-positive for possible bacterial pathogens, and 11 RV isolates were from infants younger than 3 months. The authors conclude that RVs may be significant respiratory pathogens in Kenya.

RVs were found to be prevalent in a 29-month household-based study in an impoverished urban population in Fortaleza, Brazil; 175 children younger than 5 weeks in 63 families were surveyed for clinical illness and respiratory viruses.[69] The study yielded two major findings: (1) the burden of respiratory illness in these children was so continuous that assigning beginning and ending dates was impossible, and (2) RVs, by far the most common virus isolated, accounted for 46 percent of all viruses obtained. RV was dominant in all age groups, but overwhelmingly so in children 0 to 6 months of age. In this age group, only RV and parainfluenza virus were isolated, in a ratio of approximately seven RVs to one parainfluenza virus. The role of RVs in nonindustrialized nations must be assessed carefully; for example, what proportion of RVs in this study in Brazil were just "innocent bystanders," as found in the subclinical infections in Bethel and Vanuatu (see previous discussion)?

Diagnosis of Infection

RV infections cannot be diagnosed solely on the basis of clinical grounds because they cause such a wide spectrum of respiratory illness, particularly in infants and children. However, because of the characteristic spring-summer-fall seasonal pattern of the RVs, tentatively assigning an RV etiology in cases of mild to moderate respiratory illness during these months is not unreasonable.

Obtaining a culture of the etiologic agent and interpreting the meaning of a positive specimen can be difficult with the RVs. These viruses often propagate unpredictably, even in relatively sensitive diploid cell cultures such as WI-38 and FT cells or in Ohio strain HeLa cells,[19, 59, 62, 65, 121, 295] and often these cells are highly variable in their susceptibility.[121] Isolation of RV from children is hampered by the common practice of relying on a throat swab. Inocula from many throat swabs contain one tissue culture infectious virus particle or less and seldom contain infectious particles by the hundreds (see Table 171–10). Hendley and colleagues[145] found nasal specimens to be superior for RV studies, and diagnostic rhinovirologists from many nations successfully use nasal aspirates.[127, 154, 175, 176, 206] Specimens should be placed in cell culture as soon as possible and without previous freezing and thawing (however, refrigeration [4° C] overnight results in little loss). If freezing is necessary and dry ice is used, great care must be taken to avoid contamination of the specimen with sublimed carbon dioxide because the resultant carbonic acid rapidly kills the virus. Cell cultures should be incubated at 33°C and slowly rolled. Evidence of virus growth usually is seen between 2 days and 2 weeks. Once a cytopathic effect is evident, standard techniques for identification are used.[72, 121, 154, 177, 210, 216] Because of the technical difficulties in isolating RVs, before initiating etiologic studies of viral respiratory illness, specimen collection and culture procedures should be developed carefully in collaboration with an experienced respiratory virologist.

RVs are known to be found in the absence of symptoms, but infrequently, at least in industrialized nations. Cherry[48] compiled shedding data from well children who were part of nine independent studies (1798 specimens) and found the total subclinical shedding rate to be 3 percent. RV shedding from well children was 5 percent or less in eight of these studies but was 11 percent in the remaining survey of a Chicago nursery school population.[28] Only 11 (0.8%) of 1319 specimens from healthy Madison children 3 to 11 years of age yielded an RV by culture (see Table 171–11). However, the rate of subclinical RV shedding is known to be high, up to 50 percent, in some Third World populations, so healthy control specimens should be obtained when possible to measure background RV carriage rates.[274, 303]

RVs can be isolated year-round, but the highest RV incidence usually is during the spring-fall-summer months in both hemispheres.*

As described early in this chapter, RVs have many base sequences in common among the RNA genomes of the various serotypes, especially in the noncoding region at the 5′ end. Several laboratories have taken advantage of this observation by designing RT-PCR assays for the detection of RVs. Some assays do not distinguish RVs from enteroviruses, whereas others are RV-specific.[103, 128, 158, 161] In a clinical study of children with acute respiratory illnesses, Johnston and colleagues[172] detected RV by PCR in 146 of 292 samples (50%) that yielded RV in only 47 (16%) by standard culture. PCR was thus three times more sensitive than was culture for detecting RV infection. Additional studies have confirmed the superiority of RT-PCR assays over culture methods for the detection of RVs.[6, 23, 159] RT-PCR assays also can be used to classify picornavirus isolates as enteroviruses or RVs; Atmar and Georghiou[22] found 100 percent concordance between PCR results and acid lability testing.

*See references 21, 98, 121, 145, 167, 183, 197, 216, 234, 247.

Prevention and Treatment

Prevention and treatment are addressed thoroughly in Chapter 8 and elsewhere, and only measures peculiar to the RVs are added here.[40, 194] Although some protection after the use of inactivated vaccines has been demonstrated,[84, 232] the existence of at least 101 serotypes limits the prospect of a vaccine being developed. However, based on the observation that cross-reacting antigenic groupings exist among the RVs, developing a vaccine that targets these epitopes may be possible.[61]

The most effective RV cold preventive described to date that has been demonstrated to be effective for natural RV colds in Australia and the United States is interferon-α, a protein produced as part of the host's natural antiviral defense and now produced for experimentation by genetic recombinant methods.[87, 137] It was administered by nasal spray to other members of the family after symptoms appeared in the index case; 80 percent of the secondary RV colds were prevented. However, interferon given in this fashion does not seem to be effective against other respiratory viruses; for example, in a follow-up study in Seattle, interferon-α did not reduce the incidence of colds when administered in a protocol identical to that used in the previous family studies, chiefly because RV infections were in the minority.[82, 87, 100, 137] RVs often have a decided seasonality, so rapid diagnosis of the index case by PCR would be helpful to determine when interferon-α could be used effectively to stop intrafamily spread. A combination of rapid diagnosis and family prophylaxis with interferon-α could be most helpful in families such as those with asthmatic children, in whom RV infection may be serious (see "Clinical Manifestations"). The disadvantage of interferon prophylaxis is that prolonged intranasal administration (>7 days) or repeated treatment produces an inflammatory response consisting of nasal stuffiness, ulceration, and blood-tinged discharge.[256]

Numerous antiviral agents that have in vitro activity against RVs have been developed. The section in this chapter on structure of the virion describes the development of some of these agents, which was made possible by taking advantage of current detailed knowledge of RV structure and specific cell receptors. Several of these preparations, including capsid binding agents, soluble receptor (soluble ICAM-1), and antibody to the receptor (ICAM-1), have been tested in clinical trials, but development of most of these agents has not been pursued for a variety of reasons[26, 281] (reviewed by Arruda and Hayden[20]). More recently, another capsid binding agent, pleconaril, has been found to have in vitro antiviral activity against many enteroviruses and RVs, and phase III clinical trials on naturally acquired colds have demonstrated some reduction in the severity and duration of several respiratory symptoms.[138] Another anti-RV drug, AG7088, which is a potent, irreversible inhibitor of viral 3C protease, also is being developed and has reached clinical trial.[199, 278] Further studies of both these agents, especially in children, will be needed to determine their potential benefits.

Colds usually are treated symptomatically with mild nonsteroidal anti-inflammatory drugs, sympathomimetics (e.g., phenylpropanolamine), and antihistamines; they are discussed in Chapter 8.[265] Anticholinergic agents (e.g., topical ipratropium bromide) and first-generation antihistamines reduce rhinorrhea, whereas second-generation ("nonsedating") antihistamines have no effect. The efficacy of the first-generation antihistamines may result from their ability to block muscarinic as well as histaminic receptors and to cross the blood-brain barrier.[221] Sympathomimetics decrease nasal obstruction, although topical administration may lead to rebound nasal obstruction. Nonsteroidal anti-inflammatory agents decrease the severity of some of the systemic symptoms associated with colds (e.g., malaise, headache).[278] A combination of antiviral and antimediator preparations may provide effective therapy.[120] A variety of other treatments, including vitamin C, *Echinacea,* intranasal humidified air, and zinc lozenges, have been reported to have some clinical benefit, although for many of these agents the data are conflicting.[45, 95, 141, 164, 196, 205, 238, 278, 286] Almost all clinical evaluations of symptomatic and alternative therapies have been performed in adults; very few data exist on the utility of such therapy in children.[196, 263]

The use of oral or inhaled corticosteroids appears to enhance the shedding of viable virus.[117, 243] One potential consequence of their use, seen in a study of pediatric patients with a common cold syndrome, is a significant increase in the risk for acute otitis media in RV-infected subjects.[254] Thus, steroids do not have a role in the treatment of RV infections. Similarly, no role exists for the use of antibiotic therapy in uncomplicated RV infection.

Acknowledgment

The author would like to acknowledge the contributions of Elliot C. Dick, Stanley L. Inhorn, and W. Paul Glezen, who contributed to this chapter in previous editions of the text.

REFERENCES

1. Abraham, G., and Colonno, R. J.: Many rhinovirus serotypes share the same cellular receptor. J. Virol. *51*:340–345, 1984.
2. Abzug, M. J., Beam, A. C., Gyorkos, E. A., et al.: Viral pneumonia in the first month of life. Pediatr. Infect. Dis. J. *9*:881–885, 1990.
3. Al-Nakib, W., Stanway, G., Forsyth, M., et al.: Detection of human rhinoviruses and their molecular relationship using cDNA probes. J. Med. Virol. *20*:289–296, 1986.
4. Alper, C. M., Doyle, W. J., Skoner, D. P., et al.: Pre-challenge antibodies moderate infection rate, and signs and symptoms in adults experimentally challenged with rhinovirus type 39. Laryngoscope *106*:1298–1305, 1996.
5. Alper, C. M., Doyle, W. J., Skoner, D. P., et al.: Pre-challenge antibodies moderate disease expression in adults experimentally exposed to rhinovirus strain Hanks. Clin. Infect. Dis. *27*:119–128, 1998.
6. Andreweg, A. C., Bestebroer, T. M., Huybreghs, M., et al.: Improved detection of rhinoviruses in clinical samples by using a newly developed nested reverse transcription-PCR assay. J. Clin. Microbiol. *37*:524–530, 1999.
7. Andrewes, C. H., Chaproniere, D. M., Gompels, A. E. H., et al.: Propagation of common-cold virus in tissue cultures. Lancet *2*:546–547, 1953.
8. Andrewes, C. H., Lovelock, J. E., and Sommerville, T.: An experiment on the transmission of colds. Lancet *1*:25–27, 1951.
9. Andrewes, C. H., and Oakley, W. G.: The common cold wins the first round. St. Bartholomew's Hosp. J. *40*:74–75, 1933.
10. Andries, K., Dewindt, B., Snoeks, J., et al.: Two groups of rhinoviruses revealed by a panel of antiviral compounds present sequence divergence and differential pathogenicity. J. Virol. *64*:1117–1123, 1990.
11. Andries, K., Dewindt, B., Snoeks, J., et al.: A comparative test of fifteen compounds against all known human rhinovirus serotypes as a basis for a more rational screening program. Antiviral Res. *16*:213–225, 1991.
12. Arnold, E., and Rossmann, M. G.: Analysis of the structure of a common cold virus, human rhinovirus 14, refined at a resolution of 3.0 Å. J. Mol. Biol. *211*:763–801, 1990.
13. Arola, M.: Respiratory Viruses in Otitis Media. M.D. Thesis. Turku, Finland, Departments of Pediatrics and Virology, University of Turku, 1990.
14. Arola, M., Ruuskanen, O., Ziegler, T., et al.: Clinical role of respiratory virus infection in acute otitis media. Pediatrics *86*:848–855, 1990.
15. Arola, M., Ziegler, T., Puhakka, H., et al.: Rhinovirus in otitis media with effusion. Ann. Otol. Rhinol. Laryngol. *99*:451–453, 1990.
16. Arola, M., Ziegler, T., Ruuskanen, O., et al.: Rhinovirus in acute otitis media. J. Pediatr. *113*:693–695, 1988.
17. Arola, M., Ziegler, T., and Ruuskanen, O.: Respiratory virus infection as a cause of prolonged symptoms in acute otitis media. J. Pediatr. *116*:697–701, 1990.
18. Arruda, E., Boyle, T. R., Winther, B., et al.: Localization of rhinovirus replication in the upper respiratory tract by in situ hybridization. J. Infect. Dis. *171*:1329–1333, 1995.
19. Arruda, E., Crump, C. E., Rollins, B. E., et al.: Comparative susceptibilities of human embryonic fibroblasts and HeLa cells for isolation of human rhinoviruses. J. Clin. Microbiol. *34*:1277–1279, 1996.

20. Arruda, E., and Hayden, F. G.: Clinical studies of antiviral agents for picornaviral infections. *In* Jeffries, D. J., and de Clerq, E. (eds.): Antiviral Chemotherapy. New York, John Wiley & Sons, 1995, pp. 321–355.
21. Arruda, E., Pitakaranta, A., Witek, T. J., Jr., et al.: Frequency and natural history of rhinovirus infections in adults during autumn. J. Clin. Microbiol. *35*:2864–2868, 1997.
22. Atmar, R. L., and Georghiou, P. R.: Classification of respiratory tract picornavirus isolates as enteroviruses or rhinoviruses by using reverse transcription–polymerase chain reaction. J. Clin. Microbiol. *31*:2544–2546, 1993.
23. Atmar, R. L., Guy, E., Guntupalli, K. K., et al.: Respiratory tract viral infections in inner-city asthmatic adults. Arch. Intern. Med. *158*:2453–2459, 1998.
24. Auvinen, P.: Common and specific sequences in picornaviruses. Mol. Cell. Probes *4*:273–284, 1990.
25. Baker, J. W., Hong, R., Dick, E. C., et al.: Asthma, IgA deficiency, and respiratory infections. J. Allergy Clin. Immunol. *58*:713–721, 1976.
26. Bangham, C. R. M., and McMichael, A. J.: Nosing ahead in the cold war. Nature *344*:16, 1990.
27. Bardin, P. G., Johnston, S. L., Sanderson, G., et al.: Detection of rhinovirus infection of the nasal mucosa by oligonucleotide in situ hybridization. Am. J. Respir. Cell Mol. Biol. *10*:207–213, 1994.
28. Beem, M. O.: Acute respiratory illness in nursery school children: A longitudinal study of the occurrence of illness and respiratory viruses. Am. J. Epidemiol. *90*:30–44, 1969.
29. Belshe, R. B., Van Voris, L. P., and Mufson, M. A.: Impact of viral respiratory diseases on infants and young children in a rural and urban area of southern West Virginia. Am. J. Epidemiol. *117*:467–474, 1983.
30. Bloch, A. B., Orenstein, W. A., Ewing, W. M., et al.: Measles outbreak in a pediatric practice: Airborne transmission in an office setting. Pediatrics *75*:676–683, 1985.
31. Blomqvist, S., Roivainen, M., Puhakka, T., et al.: Virological and serological analysis of rhinovirus infections during the first two years of life in a cohort of children. J. Med. Virol. *66*:263–268, 2002.
32. Boat, T. F., and Carson, J. L.: Ciliary dysmorphology and dysfunction: Primary or acquired? N. Engl. J. Med. *323*:1700–1702, 1990.
33. Buchman, C. A., Doyle, W. J., Skoner, D., et al.: Otologic manifestations of experimental rhinovirus infection. Laryngoscope *104*:1295–1299, 1994.
34. Buscho, R. F., Perkins, J. C., Knopf, H. L. S., et al.: Further characterization of the local respiratory tract antibody response induced by intranasal instillation of inactivated rhinovirus 13 vaccine. J. Immunol. *108*:169–177, 1972.
35. Busse, W. W., Vrtis, R. F., and Dick, E. C.: The role of viral infections in intrinsic asthma: Activation of neutrophil inflammation. Agents Actions Suppl. *28*:41–56, 1989.
36. Butler, W. T., Waldmann, T. A., Rossen, R. D., et al.: Changes in IgA and IgG concentrations in nasal secretions prior to the appearance of antibody during viral respiratory infection in man. J. Immunol. *105*:584–591, 1970.
37. Bynoe, M. L., Hobson, D., Horner, J., et al.: Inoculation of human volunteers with a strain of virus isolated from a common cold. Lancet *1*:1194–1196, 1961.
38. Carlsen, K. H., Orstavik, I., Leegaard, J., et al.: Respiratory virus infections and aeroallergens in acute bronchial asthma. Arch. Dis. Child. *59*:310–315, 1984.
39. Carson, J. L., Collier, A. M., and Hu, S. S.: Acquired ciliary defects in nasal epithelium of children with acute viral upper respiratory infections. N. Engl. J. Med. *312*:463–468, 1985.
40. Casey, M. J., and Dick, E. C.: Acute respiratory infections. *In* Casey, M. J., Foster, C., and Hixson, E. G. (eds.): Winter Sports Medicine. Philadelphia, F. A. Davis, 1990, pp. 112–128.
41. Cate, T. R.: Self-control of the common cold? Ann. Intern. Med. *88*:569–570, 1978.
42. Cate, T. R., Couch, R. B., Fleet, W. F., et al.: Production of tracheobronchitis in volunteers with rhinovirus in a small-particle aerosol. Am. J. Epidemiol. *81*:95–105, 1965.
43. Cate, T. R., Couch, R. B., and Johnson, K. M.: Studies with rhinoviruses in volunteers: Production of illness, effect of naturally acquired antibody, and demonstration of a protective effect not associated with serum antibody. J. Clin. Invest. *43*:56–67, 1964.
44. Cate, T. R., Rossen, R. D., Douglas, R. G., Jr., et al.: The role of nasal secretion and serum antibody in the rhinovirus common cold. Am. J. Epidemiol. *84*:352–363, 1966.
45. Chalmers, T. C.: Effects of ascorbic acid on the common cold. Am. J. Med. *58*:532–536, 1975.
46. Che, Z., Olson, N. H., Leippe, D., et al.: Antibody-mediated neutralization of human rhinovirus 14 explored by means of cryoelectron microscopy and x-ray crystallography of virus-Fab complexes. J. Virol. *72*:4610–4622, 1998.
47. Chen, R. T., Goldbaum, G. M., Wassilak, S. G. F., et al.: An explosive point-source measles outbreak in a highly vaccinated population: Modes of transmission and risk factors for disease. Am. J. Epidemiol. *129*:173–182, 1989.
48. Cherry, J. D.: Newer respiratory viruses: Their role in respiratory illnesses of children. Adv. Pediatr. *20*:225–290, 1973.
49. Cherry, J. D., Diddams, J. A., and Dick, E. C.: Rhinovirus infections in hospitalized children. Arch. Environ. Health *14*:390–396, 1967.
50. Chidekel, A. S., Rosen, C. L., and Bazzy, A. R.: Rhinovirus infection associated with serious lower respiratory illness in patients with bronchopulmonary dysplasia. Pediatr. Infect. Dis. J. *16*:43–47, 1997.
51. Chonmaitree, T., Howie, V. M., and Truant, A. L.: Presence of respiratory viruses in middle ear fluids and nasal wash specimens from children with acute otitis media. Pediatrics *77*:698–702, 1986.
52. Chonmaitree, T., Owen, M. J., and Howie, V. M.: Respiratory viruses interfere with bacteriologic response to antibiotic in children with acute otitis media. J. Infect. Dis. *162*:546–549, 1990.
53. Chretien, J., Holland, W., Macklem, P., et al.: Acute respiratory infections in children: A global public-health problem. N. Engl. J. Med. *310*:982–984, 1984.
54. Clinical practice guideline: Management of sinusitis. Pediatrics *108*:798–808, 2001.
55. Cohen, S., Doyle, W. J., Skoner, D. P., et al.: Social ties and susceptibility to the common cold. J. A. M. A. *277*:1940–1944, 1997.
56. Cohen, S., Frank, E., Doyle, W. J., et al.: Types of stressors that increase susceptibility to the common cold in healthy adults. Health Psychol. *17*:214–223, 1998.
57. Cohen, S., Tyrrell, D. A. J., and Smith, A. P.: Psychological stress and susceptibility to the common cold. N. Engl. J. Med. *325*:606–612, 1991.
58. Commission on Acute Respiratory Diseases: Experimental transmission of minor respiratory illness to human volunteers by filter-passing agents. I. Demonstration of two types of illness characterized by long and short incubation periods and different clinical features. J. Clin. Invest. *26*: 957–973, 1947.
59. Conant, R. M., and Hamparian, V. V.: Rhinoviruses: Basis for a numbering system. I. HeLa cells for propagation and serologic procedures. J. Immunol. *100*:107–113, 1968.
60. Conant, R. M., Hamparian, V. V., Stott, E. J., et al.: Identification of rhinovirus strain D. C. Nature *217*:1264, 1968.
61. Cooney, M. K., Fox, J. P., and Kenny, G. E.: Antigenic groupings of 90 rhinovirus serotypes. Infect. Immun. *37*:642–647, 1982.
62. Cooney, M. K., and Kenny, G. E.: Demonstration of dual rhinovirus infection in humans by isolation of different serotypes in human heteroploid (HeLa) and human diploid fibroblast cell cultures. J. Clin. Microbiol. *5*:202–207, 1977.
63. Couch, R. B.: Personal communication, 1978.
64. Couch, R. B.: The common cold: Control? J. Infect. Dis. *150*:167–173, 1984.
65. Couch, R. B.: Rhinoviruses. *In* Knipe, D. M., Howley, P. M., Griffin, D. E., et al. (eds.): Fields Virology. 4th ed., Vol. 1. Philadelphia, Lippincott Williams & Wilkins, 2001, pp. 777–797.
66. Couch, R. B., Douglas, R. G., Jr., Lindgren, K. M., et al.: Airborne transmission of respiratory infection with coxsackievirus A type 21. Am. J. Epidemiol. *91*:78–86, 1970.
67. D'Alessio, D. J., Meschievitz, C. K., Peterson, J. A., et al.: Short-duration exposure and the transmission of rhinoviral colds. J. Infect. Dis. *150*:189–194, 1984.
68. D'Alessio, D. J., Peterson, J. A., Dick, C. R., et al.: Transmission of experimental rhinovirus colds in volunteer married couples. J. Infect. Dis. *133*:28–36, 1976.
69. de Arruda N. E., Hayden, F. G., McAuliffe, J. F., et al.: Acute respiratory viral infections in ambulatory children of urban northeast Brazil. J. Infect. Dis. *164*:252–258, 1991.
70. Denny, F. W., and Clyde, W. A., Jr.: Acute lower respiratory tract infections in nonhospitalized children. J. Pediatr. *108*:635–646, 1986.
71. Dick, E. C.: Chimpanzee kidney tissue cultures for growth and isolation of viruses. J. Bacteriol. *86*:573–576, 1963.
72. Dick, E. C., Blumer, C. R., and Evans, A. S.: Epidemiology of infections with rhinovirus types 43 and 55 in a group of University of Wisconsin student families. Am. J. Epidemiol. *86*:386–400, 1967.
73. Dick, E. C., and Carr, D. L.: *Haemophilus influenzae*. Arch. Environ. Health *13*:450–453, 1966.
74. Dick, E. C., and Dick, C. R.: A subclinical outbreak of human rhinovirus 31 infection in chimpanzees. Am. J. Epidemiol. *88*:267–272, 1968.
75. Dick, E. C., and Dick, C. R.: Natural and experimental infections of nonhuman primates with respiratory viruses. Lab. Anim. Sci. *24*:177–181, 1974.
76. Dick, E. C., Gavinski, S. S., Mahl, M. C., et al.: A virucidal handkerchief for helping prevent transmission of respiratory infection at McMurdo Station and Scott Base during the winter fly-in period. Antarctic J. U. S. *14*:189–190, 1979.
77. Dick, E. C., Hossain, S. U., Mink, K. A., et al.: Interruption of transmission of rhinovirus colds among human volunteers using virucidal paper handkerchiefs. J. Infect. Dis. *153*:352–356, 1986.
78. Dick, E. C., Jennings, L. C., Meschievitz, C. K., et al.: Possible modification of the normal winter fly-in respiratory disease outbreak at McMurdo Station. Antarctic J. U. S. *15*:173–174, 1980.
79. Dick, E. C., Jennings, L. C., Mink, K. A., et al.: Aerosol transmission of rhinovirus colds. J. Infect. Dis. *156*:442–448, 1987.
80. Dochez, A. R., Shibley, G. S., and Mills, K. C.: Studies in the common cold. IV. Experimental transmission of the common cold to anthropoid apes and human beings by means of a filtrable agent. J. Exp. Med. *52*:701–716, 1930.

81. Douglas, R. G., Jr.: Pathogenesis of rhinovirus common colds in human volunteers. Ann. Otol. Rhinol. Laryngol. *79*:563–571, 1970.
82. Douglas, R. G., Jr.: The common cold: Relief at last? N. Engl. J. Med. *314*:114–115, 1986.
83. Douglas, R. G., Jr., Cate, T. R., Gerone, P. J., et al.: Quantitative rhinovirus shedding patterns in volunteers. Am. Rev. Respir. Dis. *94*:159–167, 1966.
84. Douglas, R. G., Jr., and Couch, R. B.: Parenteral inactivated rhinovirus vaccine: Minimal protective effect. Proc. Soc. Exp. Biol. Med. *139*:899–902, 1972.
85. Douglas, R. G., Jr., Lindgren, K. M., and Couch, R. B.: Exposure to cold environment and rhinovirus common cold: Failure to demonstrate effect. N. Engl. J. Med. *279*:742–747, 1968.
86. Douglas, R. G., Jr., Rossen, R. D., Butler, W. T., et al.: Rhinovirus neutralizing antibody in tears, parotid saliva, nasal secretions and serum. J. Immunol. *99*:297–303, 1967.
87. Douglas, R. M., Moore, B. W., Milles, H. B., et al.: Prophylactic efficacy of intranasal alpha-2 interferon against rhinovirus infections in the family setting. N. Engl. J. Med. *314*:65–70, 1986.
88. Drews, A. L., Atmar, R. L., Glezen, W. P., et al.: Dual respiratory virus infections. Clin. Infect. Dis. *25*:1421–1429, 1997.
89. Duechler, M., Skern, T., Sommergruber, W., et al.: Evolutionary relationships within the human rhinovirus genus: Comparison of serotypes 89, 2, and 14. Proc. Natl. Acad. Sci. U. S. A. *84*:2605–2609, 1987.
90. Duff, A. L., Pomeranz, E. S., Gelber, L. E., et al.: Risk factors for acute wheezing in infants and children: Viruses, passive smoke, and IgE antibodies to inhalant allergens. Pediatrics *92*:535–540, 1993.
91. Eadie, M. B., Stott, E. J., and Grist, N. R.: Virological studies in chronic bronchitis. B. M. J. *2*:671–673, 1966.
92. El-Sahly, H. M., Atmar, R. L., Glezen, W. P., et al.: Spectrum of clinical illness in hospitalized patients with "common cold" virus infections. Clin. Infect. Dis. *31*:96–100, 2000.
93. Farr, B. M., Hendley, J. O., Kaiser, D. L., et al.: Two randomized controlled trials of virucidal nasal tissues in the prevention of natural upper respiratory infections. Am. J. Epidemiol. *128*:1162–1172, 1988.
94. Fleet, W. F., Couch, R. B., Cate, T. R., et al.: Homologous and heterologous resistance to rhinovirus common cold. Am. J. Epidemiol. *82*:185–196, 1965.
95. Forstall, G. J., Macknin, M. L., Yen-Lieberman, B. R., et al.: Effect of inhaling heated vapor on symptoms of the common cold. J. A. M. A. *271*:1109–1111, 1994.
96. Fox, J. P.: Is a rhinovirus vaccine possible? Am. J. Epidemiol. *103*:345–354, 1976.
97. Fox, J. P., Cooney, M. K., and Hall, C. E.: The Seattle virus watch. V. Epidemiologic observations of rhinovirus infections, 1965–1969, in families with young children. Am. J. Epidemiol. *101*:122–143, 1975.
98. Fox, J. P., Cooney, M. K., Hall, C. E., et al.: Rhinoviruses in Seattle families, 1975–1979. Am. J. Epidemiol. *122*:830–846, 1985.
99. Fox, M. P., Otto, M. J., and McKinlay, M. A.: Prevention of rhinovirus and poliovirus uncoating by WIN 51711, a new antiviral drug. Antimicrob. Agents Chemother. *30*:110–116, 1986.
100. Foy, H. M., Fox, J. P., and Cooney, M. K.: Efficacy of alpha$_2$-interferon against the common cold. N. Engl. J. Med. *315*:513–514, 1986.
101. Fraenkel, D., Bardin, P., Sanderson, G., et al.: Lower airway inflammation during rhinovirus colds in normal and asthmatic subjects. Am. J. Respir. Crit Care Med. *151*:879–886, 1995.
102. Frick, W. E., and Busse, W. W.: Respiratory infections: Their role in airway responsiveness and pathogenesis of asthma. Clin. Chest Med. *9*:539–549, 1988.
103. Gama, R. E., Horsnell, P. R., Hughes, P. J., et al.: Amplification of rhinovirus specific nucleic acids from clinical samples using the polymerase chain reaction. J. Med. Virol. *28*:73–77, 1989.
104. Gentile, D. A, Yokitis, J., Angelini, B. L., et al.: Effect of intranasal challenge with interleukin-6 on upper airway symptomatology and physiology in allergic and nonallergic patients. Ann. Allergy Asthma Immunol. *86*:531–536, 2001.
105. George, R. B., and Mogabgab, W. J.: Atypical pneumonia in young men with rhinovirus infections. Ann. Intern. Med. *71*:1073–1078, 1969.
106. Gern, J. E., and Busse, W. W.: Association of rhinovirus infections with asthma. Clin. Microbiol. Rev. *12*:9–18, 1999.
107. Gern, J. E., Dick, E. C., Kelly, E. A. B., et al.: Rhinovirus-specific T cells recognize both shared and serotype-restricted viral epitopes. J. Infect. Dis. *175*:1108–1114, 1997.
108. Gern, J. E., Galagan, D. M., Jarjour, N. N., et al.: Detection of rhinovirus RNA in lower airway cells during experimentally induced infection. Am. J. Respir. Crit. Care Med. *155*:1159–1161, 1997.
109. Gern, J. E., Vrtis, R., Grindle, K. A., et al. Relationship of upper and lower airway cytokines to outcome of experimental rhinovirus infection. Am. J. Respir. Crit. Care Med. *162*:2226–2231, 2000.
110. Ghosh, S., Champlin, R., Couch, R., et al.: Rhinovirus infections in myelosuppressed adult blood and marrow transplant recipients. Clin. Infect. Dis. *29*:528–532, 1999.
111. Glezen, W. P., Greenberg, S. B., Atmar, R. L., et al.: Impact of respiratory virus infections on persons with chronic underlying conditions. J. A. M. A. *283*:499–505, 2000.
112. Graham, N. M. H.: The epidemiology of acute respiratory infections in children and adults: A global perspective. Epidemiol. Rev. *12*:149–178, 1990.
113. Gregg, M. B.: The epidemiology of influenza in humans. Ann. N. Y. Acad. Sci. *353*:45–53, 1980.
114. Greve, J. M., Davis, G., Meyer, A. M., et al.: The major human rhinovirus receptor is ICAM-1. Cell *56*:839–847, 1989.
115. Greve, J. M., Forte, C. P., Marlor, C. W., et al.: Mechanisms of receptor-mediated rhinovirus neutralization defined by two soluble forms of ICAM-1. J. Virol. *65*:6015–6023, 1991.
116. Grunberg, K., Timmers, M. C., Smits, H. H., et al.: Effect of experimental rhinovirus colds on airway hyperresponsiveness to histamine and interleukin-8 in nasal lavage in asthmatic subjects in vivo. Clin. Exp. Allergy *27*:36–45, 1997.
117. Gustafson, L. M., Proud, D., Hendley, J. O., et al.: Oral prednisone therapy in experimental rhinovirus infections. J. Allergy Clin. Immunol. *97*:1009–1114, 1996.
118. Gwaltney, J. M., Jr.: Virology of middle ear. Ann. Otol. *80*:365–370, 1971.
119. Gwaltney, J. M., Jr.: Understanding and controlling rhinovirus colds. *In* de la Maza, L. M., and Peterson, E. M. (eds.): Medical Virology. Vol. 4. Hillsdale, NJ, Lawrence Erlbaum, 1985, pp. 233–251.
120. Gwaltney, J. M., Jr.: Combined antiviral and antimediator treatment of rhinovirus colds. J. Infect. Dis. *166*:776–782, 1992.
121. Gwaltney, J. M., Jr.: Rhinoviruses. *In* Evans, A. S., and Kaslow, R. A. (eds.): Viral Infections of Humans: Epidemiology and Control. 4th ed. New York, Plenum, 1997, pp. 815–838.
122. Gwaltney, J. M., Jr., and Hendley, J. O.: Rhinovirus transmission: One if by air, two if by hand. Am. J. Epidemiol. *107*:357–361, 1978.
123. Gwaltney, J. M., Jr., and Hendley, J. O.: Transmission of experimental rhinovirus infection by contaminated surfaces. Am. J. Epidemiol. *116*:828–833, 1982.
124. Gwaltney, J. M., Jr., Moskalski, P. B., and Hendley, J. O.: Hand-to-hand transmission of rhinovirus colds. Ann. Intern. Med. *88*:463–467, 1978.
125. Gwaltney, J. M., Jr., Phillips, C. G., Miller, R. D., et al.: Computed tomographic study of the common cold. N. Engl. J. Med. *330*:25–30, 1994.
126. Gwaltney, J. M., Jr., Sydnor, A., Jr., and Sande, M. A.: Etiology and antimicrobial treatment of acute sinusitis. Ann. Otol. Rhinol. Laryngol. *90*(Suppl. 84):68–71, 1981.
127. Hall, C. B., and Douglas, R. G., Jr.: Clinically useful method for the isolation of respiratory syncytial virus. J. Infect. Dis. *131*:1–5, 1975.
128. Halonen, P., Rocha, E., Hierholzer, J., et al.: Detection of enteroviruses and rhinoviruses in clinical specimens by PCR and liquid-phase hybridization. J. Clin. Microbiol. *33*:648–653, 1995.
129. Halperin, S. A., Eggleston, P. A., Beasley, P., et al.: Exacerbations of asthma in adults during experimental rhinovirus infection. Am. Rev. Respir. Dis. *132*:976–980, 1985.
130. Halperin, S. A., Eggleston, P. A., Hendley, J. O., et al.: Pathogenesis of lower respiratory tract symptoms in experimental rhinovirus infection. Am. Rev. Respir. Dis. *128*:806–810, 1983.
131. Hamory, B. H., Sande, M. A., Sydnor, A., Jr., et al.: Etiology and antimicrobial therapy of acute maxillary sinusitis. J. Infect. Dis. *139*:197–202, 1979.
132. Hamparian, V. V., Colonno, R. J., Cooney, M. K., et al.: A collaborative report: Rhinoviruses—extension of the numbering system from 89 to 100. Virology *159*:191–192, 1987.
133. Hamparian, V. V., Ketler, A., and Hilleman, M. R.: Recovery of new viruses (coryzaviruses) from cases of common cold in human adults. Proc. Soc. Exp. Biol. Med. *108*:444–453, 1961.
134. Hamparian, V. V., Leagus, M. B., Hilleman, M. R., et al.: Epidemiologic investigations of rhinovirus infections. Proc. Soc. Exp. Biol. Med. *117*: 469–476, 1964.
135. Hamre, D.: Rhinoviruses. *In* Melnick, J. L. (ed.): Monographs in Virology. Vol. 1. Basel, Karger, 1968.
136. Hastings, G. Z., Rowlands, D. J., and Francis, M. J.: Proliferative responses of T cells primed against human rhinovirus to other rhinovirus serotypes. J. Gen. Virol. *72*:2947–2952, 1991.
137. Hayden, F. G., Albrecht, J. K., Kaiser, D. L., et al.: Prevention of natural colds by contact prophylaxis with intranasal alpha 2-interferon. N. Engl. J. Med. *314*:71–75, 1986.
138. Hayden, F. G., Kim, K., Hudson, S., et al.: Pleconaril treatment provides early reduction of symptom severity in viral respiratory infection (VRI) due to picornaviruses. Abstract 414. Clin. Infect. Dis. *33*:1159, 2001.
139. Hayflick, L., and Moorhead, P. S.: The serial cultivation of human diploid cell strains. Exp. Cell Res. *25*:585–621, 1961.
140. Hazlett, D. T. G., Bell, T. M., Tukei, P. M., et al.: Viral etiology and epidemiology of acute respiratory infections in children in Nairobi, Kenya. Am. J. Trop. Med. Hyg. *39*:632–640, 1988.
141. Hemila, H., and Herman, Z. S.: Vitamin C and the common cold: A retrospective analysis of Chalmers' review. J. Am. Coll. Nutr. *14*: 116–123, 1995.
142. Henderson, F. W., Clyde, W. A., Jr., Collier, A. M., et al.: The etiologic and epidemiologic spectrum of bronchiolitis in pediatric practice. J. Pediatr. *95*:183–190, 1979.
143. Hendley, J. O.: Rhinovirus colds: Immunology and pathogenesis. Eur. J. Respir. Dis. *64*(Suppl. 128):340–343, 1983.

144. Hendley, J. O., and Gwaltney, J. M., Jr.: Mechanisms of transmission of rhinovirus infections. Epidemiol. Rev. *10*:242–258, 1988.
145. Hendley, J. O., Gwaltney, J. M., Jr., and Jordan, W. S., Jr.: Rhinovirus infections in an industrial population. IV. Infections within families of employees during two fall peaks of respiratory illness. Am. J. Epidemiol. *89*:184–196, 1969.
146. Hendley, J. O., Wenzel, R. P., and Gwaltney, J. M., Jr.: Transmission of rhinovirus colds by self-inoculation. N. Engl. J. Med. *288*:1361–1364, 1973.
147. Hewat, E. A., Neumann, E., Conway, J. F., et al.: The cellular receptor to human rhinovirus 2 binds around the 5-fold axis and not in the canyon: A structural view. EMBO J. *19*:6317–6325, 2000.
148. Higgins, P. G., Barrow, G. I., and Tyrrell, D. A. J.: A study of the efficacy of the bradykinin antagonist, NPC 567, in rhinovirus infections in human volunteers. Antiviral Res. *14*:339–344, 1990.
149. Hogle, J. M., Chow, M., and Filman, D. J.: Three-dimensional structure of poliovirus at 2.9 Å resolution. Science *229*:1358–1365, 1985.
150. Holmes, M. J., Reed, S. E., Stott, R. J., et al.: Studies of experimental rhinovirus type 2 infections in polar isolation and in England. J. Hyg. (Camb.) *76*:379–393, 1976.
151. Horn, M. E. C., Brain, E., Gregg, I., et al.: Respiratory viral infection in childhood: A survey in general practice, Roehampton 1967–1972. J. Hyg. (Camb.) *74*:157–168, 1975.
152. Horn, M. E., Brain, E. A., Gregg, I., et al.: Respiratory viral infection and wheezy bronchitis in childhood. Thorax *34*:23–28, 1979.
153. Horn, M. E. C., and Gregg, I.: Role of viral infection and host factors in acute episodes of asthma and chronic bronchitis. Chest *63*(Suppl.): 44–48, 1973.
154. Horn, M. E., Reed, S. E., and Taylor, P.: Role of viruses and bacteria in acute wheezy bronchitis in childhood: A study of sputum. Arch. Dis. Child. *54*:587–592, 1979.
155. Hsia, J., Goldstein, A. L., Simon, G. L., et al.: Peripheral blood mononuclear cell interleukin-2 and interferon-γ production, cytotoxicity, and antigen-stimulated blastogenesis during experimental rhinovirus infection. J. Infect. Dis. *162*:591–597, 1990.
156. Hughes, P. J., North, C., Jellis, C. H., et al.: The nucleotide sequence of human rhinovirus 1B: Molecular relationships within the Rhinovirus genus. J. Gen. Virol. *69*:49–58, 1988.
157. Hughes, P. J., North, C., Minor, P. D., et al.: The complete nucleotide sequence of coxsackievirus A21. J. Gen. Virol. *70*:2943–2952, 1989.
158. Hyypia, T., Auvinen, P., and Maaronen, M.: Polymerase chain reaction for human picornaviruses. J. Gen. Virol. *70*:3261–3268, 1989.
159. Hyppia, T., Puhakka, T., Ruuskanen, O., et al.: Molecular diagnosis of human rhinovirus infections: Comparison with virus isolation. J. Clin. Microbiol. *36*:2081–2083, 1998.
160. Imakita, M., Shiraki, K., Yutani, C., et al.: Pneumonia caused by rhinovirus. Clin. Infect. Dis. *20*:611–612, 2000.
161. Ireland, D. C., Kent, J., and Nicholson, K. G.: Improved detection of rhinoviruses in nasal and throat swabs by seminested RT-PCR. J. Med. Virol. *40*:96–101, 1993.
162. Isaacs, D., Clarke, J. R., Tyrrell, D. A. J., et al.: Selective infection of lower respiratory tract by respiratory viruses in children with recurrent respiratory tract infections. B. M. J. *284*:1746–1748, 1982.
163. Jackson, G. G., Dowling, H. F., and Anderson, T. O.: Neutralization of common cold agents in volunteers by pooled human globulin. Science *128*:27–28, 1958.
164. Jackson, J. L., Peterson, C., and Lesho, E.: A meta-analysis of zinc salts lozenges and the common cold. Arch. Intern. Med. *157*:2373–2376, 1997.
165. Jacobs, J. W., Peacock, D. B., Corner, B. D., et al.: Respiratory syncytial and other viruses associated with respiratory disease in infants. Lancet *1*:871–876, 1971.
166. Jenkins, O., Booth, J. D., Minor, P. D., et al.: The complete nucleotide sequence of coxsackievirus B4 and its comparison to other members of the Picornaviridae. J. Gen. Virol. *68*:1835–1848, 1987.
167. Jennings, L. C., and Dick, E. C.: Transmission and control of rhinovirus colds. Eur. J. Epidemiol. *3*:327–335, 1987.
168. Jennings, L. C., Dick, E. C., Mink, K. A., et al.: Near disappearance of rhinovirus along a fomite transmission chain. J. Infect. Dis. *158*:888–892, 1988.
169. Jennings, L. C., MacDiarmid, R. D., and Miles, J. A. R.: A study of acute respiratory disease in the community of Port Chalmers I. Illnesses within a group of selected families and the relative incidence of respiratory pathogens in the whole community. J. Hyg. (Camb.) *81*:49–66, 1978.
170. Johnston, S. L., Pattemore, P. K., Sanderson, G., et al.: Community study of role of viral infections in exacerbations of asthma in 9–11 year old children. B. M. J. *310*:1225–1228, 1995.
171. Johnston, S. L., Pattemore, P. K., Sanderson, G., et al.: The relationship between upper respiratory infections and hospital admission for asthma: A time-trend analysis. Am. J. Respir. Crit. Care Med. *154*:654–660, 1996.
172. Johnston, S. L., Sanderson, G., Pattemore, P. K., et al.: Use of polymerase chain reaction for diagnosis of picornavirus infection in subjects with and without respiratory symptoms. J. Clin. Microbiol. *31*:111–117, 1993.
173. Kapikian, A. Z., Conant, R. M., Hamparian, V. V., et al.: Rhinoviruses: Extension of the numbering system. Virology *43*:524–526, 1971.
174. Kawana, R., and Matsumoto, I.: Electron microscopic study of rhinovirus replication in human fetal lung cells. Jpn. J. Microbiol. *15*: 207–217, 1971.
175. Kellner, G., Popow-Kraupp, T., Binder, C., et al.: Respiratory tract infections due to different rhinovirus serotypes and the influence of maternal antibodies on the clinical expression of the disease in infants. J. Med. Virol. *35*:267–272, 1991.
176. Kellner, G., Popow-Kraupp, T., Kundi, M., et al.: Contribution of rhinoviruses to respiratory viral infections in childhood: A prospective study in a mainly hospitalized infant population. J. Med. Virol. *25*: 455–469, 1988.
177. Kellner, G., Popow-Kraupp, T., Kundi, M., et al.: Clinical manifestations of respiratory tract infections due to respiratory syncytial virus and rhinoviruses in hospitalized children. Acta Paediatr. Scand. *78*:390–394, 1989.
178. Ketler, A., Hamparian, V. V., and Hilleman, M. R.: Characterization and classification of ECHO 28-rhinovirus-coryzavirus agents. Proc. Soc. Exp. Biol. Med. *110*:821–831, 1962.
179. Kim, J. O., and Hodinka, R. L.: Serious respiratory illness associated with rhinovirus infection in a pediatric population. Clin. Diagn. Virol. *10*:57–65, 1998.
180. Kim, S., Smith, T. J., Chapman, M. S., et al.: Crystal structure of human rhinovirus serotype 1A (HRV1A). J. Mol. Biol. *210*:91–111, 1989.
181. Klein, B. S., Dollette, F. R., and Yolken, R. H.: The role of respiratory syncytial virus and other viral pathogens in acute otitis media. J. Pediatr. *101*:16–20, 1982.
182. Klein, J. O.: Microbiology of otitis media. Ann. Otol. Rhinol. Laryngol. *89*(Suppl. 68):98–101, 1980.
183. Krilov, L., Pierik, L., Keller, E., et al.: Association of rhinoviruses with lower respiratory tract disease in hospitalized patients. J. Med. Virol. *19*:345–352, 1986.
184. Kruse, V. W.: The causative agent of coughs and colds: From the Hygienic Institute of the University of Leipzig. Muenchner Med. Wochenschr. *61*:1547, 1914.
185. Larson, H. E., Reed, S. E., and Tyrrell, D. A. J.: Isolation of rhinoviruses and coronaviruses from 38 colds in adults. J. Med. Virol. *5*:221–229, 1980.
186. Las Heras, J., and Swanson, V. L.: Sudden death of an infant with rhinovirus infection complicating bronchial asthma: Case report. Pediatr. Pathol. *1*:319–323, 1983.
187. Lee, W. M., Wang, W., and Rueckert, R. R.: Complete sequence of the RNA genome of human rhinovirus 16, a clinically useful common cold virus belonging to the ICAM-1 receptor group. Virus Genes *9*:177–181, 1995.
188. Lefkowitz, L. B., Jr., and Jackson, G. G.: Dual respiratory infection with parainfluenza and rhinovirus: The pathogenesis of transmitted infection in volunteers. Am. Rev. Respir. Dis. *93*:519–528, 1966.
189. Lemanske, R. F., Jr., Dick, E. C., Swenson, C. A., et al.: Rhinovirus upper respiratory infection increases airway hyperreactivity and late asthmatic reactions. J. Clin. Invest. *83*:1–10, 1989.
190. Levandowski, R. A., Weaver, C. W., and Jackson, G. G.: Nasal-secretion leukocyte populations determined by flow cytometry during acute rhinovirus infection. J. Med. Virol. *25*:423–432, 1988.
191. Li, F., Browning, G. F., Studdert, M. J., et al.: Equine rhinovirus 1 is more closely related to foot-and-mouth disease virus than to other picornaviruses. Proc. Natl. Acad. Sci. U. S. A. *93*:990–995, 1996.
192. Lobovits, A. M., Freeman, J., Goldmann, D. A., et al.: Risk of illness after exposure to a pediatric office. N. Engl. J. Med. *313*:425–428, 1985.
193. Longini, I. M., Jr., and Monto, A. S.: Efficacy of virucidal nasal tissues in interrupting familial transmission of respiratory agents: A field trial in Tecumseh, Michigan. Am. J. Epidemiol. *128*:639–644, 1988.
194. Lowenstein, S. R., and Parrino, T. A.: Management of the common cold. Adv. Intern. Med. *32*:207–234, 1987.
195. Lupton, H. W., Smith, M. H., and Frey, M. L.: Identification and characterization of a bovine rhinovirus isolated from Iowa cattle with acute respiratory tract disease. Am. J. Vet. Res. *41*:1029–1034, 1980.
196. Macknin, M. L., Piedmonte, M., Calendine, C., et al.: Zinc gluconate lozenges for treating the common cold in children. A randomized controlled trial. J. A. M. A. *279*:1962–1967, 1998.
197. Makela, M. J., Puhakka, T., Ruuskanen, O., et al.: Viruses and bacteria in the etiology of the common cold. J. Clin. Microbiol. *36*:539–542, 1998.
198. Malcolm, E., Arruda, E., Hayden, F. G., et al.: Clinical features of patients with acute respiratory illness and rhinovirus in their bronchoalveolar lavages. J. Clin. Virol. *21*:9–16, 2001.
199. Matthews, D. A., Dragovich, P. S., Webber, S. E., et al.: Structure-assisted design of mechanism-based irreversible inhibitors of human rhinovirus 3C protease with potent antiviral activity against multiple rhinovirus serotypes. Proc. Natl. Acad. Sci. U. S. A. *96*:11000–11007, 1999.
200. McBride, T. P., Doyle, W. J., Hayden, F. G., et al.: Alterations of the eustachian tube, middle ear, and nose in rhinovirus infection. Arch. Otolaryngol. Head Neck Surg. *115*:1054–1059, 1989.

201. McIntosh, K.: Bronchiolitis and asthma: Possible common pathogenetic pathways. J. Allergy Clin. Immunol. *57*:595–604, 1976.
202. McIntosh, K., Ellis, E. F., Hoffman, L. S., et al.: The association of viral and bacterial respiratory infections with exacerbations of wheezing in young asthmatic children. J. Pediatr. *82*:578, 1973.
203. McKinlay, M. A., Frank, J. A., Jr., Benziger, D. P., et al.: Use of WIN 51711 to prevent echovirus type 9–induced paralysis in suckling mice. J. Infect. Dis. *154*:676–681, 1986.
204. McMillan, J. A., Weiner, L. B., Higgins, A. M., et al.: Rhinovirus infection associated with serious illness among pediatric patients. Pediatr. Infect. Dis. J. *12*:321–325, 1993.
205. Melchart, D., Walther, E., Linde, K., et al.: Echinacea root extracts for the prevention of upper respiratory tract infections. A double-blind, placebo-controlled randomized trial. Arch. Fam. Med. *7*:541–545, 1998.
206. Mertsola, J., Ziegler, T., Ruuskanen, O., et al.: Recurrent wheezy bronchitis and viral respiratory infections. Arch. Dis. Child. *66*:124–129, 1991.
207. Meschievitz, C. K., Schultz, S. B., and Dick, E. C.: A model for obtaining predictable natural transmission of rhinoviruses in human volunteers. J. Infect. Dis. *150*:195–201, 1984.
208. Minor, T. E., Baker, J. W., Dick, E. C., et al.: Greater frequency of viral respiratory infections in asthmatic children as compared with their nonasthmatic siblings. J. Pediatr. *85*:472–477, 1974.
209. Minor, T. E., Dick, E. C., Baker, J. W., et al.: Rhinovirus and influenza type A infections as precipitants of asthma. Am. Rev. Respir. Dis. *113*:149–153, 1976.
210. Minor, T. E., Dick, E. C., DeMeo, A. N., et al.: Viruses as precipitants of asthmatic attacks in children. J. A. M. A. *227*:292–298, 1974.
211. Minor, T. E., Dick, E. C., Peterson, J. A., et al.: Failure of naturally acquired rhinovirus infections to produce temporal immunity to heterologous serotypes. Infect. Immun. *10*:1192–1193, 1974.
212. Mogabgab, W. J.: Prospects for the control of pneumonias. Infect. Dis. Rev. *4*:41–71, 1976.
213. Mogabgab, W. J., Holmes, B. J., and Pollock, B.: Antigenic relationships of common rhinovirus types from disabling upper respiratory illnesses: International Symposium on Immunity to Infections of the Respiratory System in Man and Animals, London, 1974. Dev. Biol. Stand. *28*:400–411, 1975.
214. Mogabgab, W. J., and Pelon, W.: Problems in characterizing and identifying an apparently new virus found in association with mild respiratory disease in recruits. Ann. N. Y. Acad. Sci. *67*:403–412, 1957.
215. Monto, A. S.: A community study of respiratory infections in the tropics. III. Introduction and transmission of infections within families. Am. J. Epidemiol. *88*:69–79, 1968.
216. Monto, A. S., Bryan, E. R., and Ohmit, S.: Rhinovirus infections in Tecumseh, Michigan: Frequency of illness and number of serotypes. J. Infect. Dis. *156*:43–49, 1987.
217. Monto, A. S., and Cavallaro, J. J.: The Tecumseh study of respiratory illness. II. Patterns of occurrence of infection with respiratory pathogens, 1965–1969. Am. J. Epidemiol. *94*:280–289, 1971.
218. Monto, A. S., and Cavallaro, J. J.: The Tecumseh study of respiratory illness. IV. Prevalence of rhinovirus serotypes, 1966–1969. Am. J. Epidemiol. *96*:352–360, 1972.
219. Monto, A. S., and Johnson, K. M.: A community study of respiratory infections in the tropics. II. The spread of six rhinovirus isolates within the community. Am. J. Epidemiol. *88*:55–68, 1968.
220. Monto, A. S., and Ullman, B. M.: Acute respiratory illness in an American community. J. A. M. A. *227*:164–169, 1974.
221. Muether, P. S., and Gwaltney, J. M., Jr.: Variant effect of first- and second-generation antihistamines as clues to their mechanism of action on the sneeze reflex in the common cold. Clin. Infect. Dis. *33*:1483–1488, 2001.
222. Naclerio, R. M., Proud, D., Lichtenstein, L. M., et al.: Kinins are generated during experimental rhinovirus colds. J. Infect. Dis. *157*:133–142, 1988.
223. Newman, J. F. E., Rowlands, D. J., Brown, F., et al.: Physico-chemical characterization of two serologically unrelated equine rhinoviruses. Intervirology *8*:145–154, 1977.
224. Nicholson, K. G., Kent, J., and Ireland, D. C.: Respiratory viruses and exacerbations of asthma in adults. B. M. J. *307*:982–986, 1993.
225. O'Sullivan, S., Cormican, L., Faul, J. L., et al.: Activated, cytotoxic CD8+ T lymphocytes contribute to the pathology of asthma death. Am. J. Respir. Crit. Care Med. *164*:560–564, 2001.
226. Pacifico, L., Iacobini, M., Viola, F., et al.: Chemokine concentrations in nasal washings of infants with rhinovirus illnesses. Clin. Infect. Dis. *31*:834–838, 2000.
227. Paisley, J. W., Lauer, B. A., McIntosh, K., et al.: Pathogens associated with acute lower respiratory tract infection in young children. Pediatr. Infect. Dis. *3*:14–19, 1984.
228. Pallansch, M. A., and Roos, R. P.: Enteroviruses: polioviruses, coxsackieviruses, echoviruses, and newer enteroviruses. *In* Knipe, D. M., Howley, P. M., Griffin, D. E., et al. (eds.): Fields Virology. 4th ed., Vol. 1. Philadelphia, Lippincott Williams & Wilkins, 2001, pp. 723–776.
229. Papadopoulos, N. G., Bates, P. J., Bardin, P. G., et al: Rhinoviruses infect the lower airways. J. Infect. Dis. *181*:1780–1784, 2000.
230. Papadopoulos, N. G., Sanderson, G., Hunter, J., et al.: Rhinoviruses replicate effectively at lower airway temperatures. J. Med. Virol. *58*: 100–104, 1999.
231. Pelon, W., Mogabgab, W. J., Phillips, I. A., et al.: Cytopathic agents isolated from recruits with mild respiratory illnesses. Abstract. Bacteriol. Proc. 1956, p. 67.
232. Perkins, J. C., Tucker, D. N., Knopf, H. L. S., et al.: Evidence for protective effect of an inactivated rhinovirus vaccine administered by the nasal route. Am. J. Epidemiol. *90*:319–326, 1969.
233. Perkins, J. C., Tucker, D. N., Knopf, H. L. S., et al.: Comparison of protective effect of neutralizing antibody in serum and nasal secretions in experimental rhinovirus type 13 illness. Am. J. Epidemiol. *90*:519–526, 1969.
234. Person, D. A., and Herrmann, E. C., Jr.: Experiences in laboratory diagnosis of rhinovirus infections in routine medical practice. Mayo Clin. Proc. *45*:517–526, 1970.
235. Pevear, D. C., Fancher, M. J., Felock, P. J., et al.: Conformational change in the floor of the human rhinovirus canyon blocks absorption to HeLa cell receptors. J. Virol. *63*:2002–2007, 1989.
236. Pitkaranta, A., Arruda, E., Malmberg, H., et al.: Detection of rhinovirus in sinus brushings of patients with acute community-acquired sinusitis by reverse transcription-PCR. J. Clin. Microbiol. *35*:1791–1793, 1997.
237. Pitkaranta, A., Jero, J., Arruda, E., et al.: Polymerase chain reaction–based detection of rhinovirus, respiratory syncytial virus, and coronavirus in otitis media with effusion. J. Pediatr. *133*:390–394, 1998.
238. Prasad, A. S., Fitzgerald, J. T., Bao, B., et al.: Duration of symptoms and plasma cytokine levels in patients with the common cold treated with zinc acetate. A randomized, double-blind, placebo-controlled trial. Ann. Intern. Med. *133*:245–252, 2000.
239. Price, W. H., Emerson, H., Ibler, I., et al.: Studies of the JH and 2060 viruses and their relationship to mild upper respiratory disease in humans. Am. J. Hyg. *69*:224–249, 1959.
240. Proud, D., Gwaltney, J. M., Jr., Hendley, J. O., et al.: Increased levels of interleukin-1 are detected in nasal secretions of volunteers during experimental rhinovirus colds. J. Infect. Dis. *169*:1007–1013, 1994.
241. Proud, D., Naclerio, R. M., Gwaltney, J. M., et al.: Kinins are generated in nasal secretions during natural rhinovirus colds. J. Infect. Dis. *161*:120–123, 1990.
242. Proud, D., Reynolds, C. J., Lacapra, S., et al.: Nasal provocation with bradykinin induces symptoms of rhinitis and a sore throat. Am. Rev. Respir. Dis. *137*:613–616, 1988.
243. Puhakka, T., Makela, M. J., Malmstrom, K., et al.: The common cold effects of intranasal fluticasone propionate treatment. J. Allergy Clin. Immunol. *101*:726–731, 1998.
244. Racaniello, V. R.: Picornaviridae: The viruses and their replication. *In* Knipe, D. M., Howley, P. M., Griffin, D. E., et al. (eds.): Fields Virology. 4th ed., Vol. 1. Philadelphia, Lippincott Williams & Wilkins, 2001, pp. 685–722.
245. Reed, S. E.: An investigation of the possible transmission of rhinovirus colds through indirect contact. J. Hyg. (Camb.) *75*:249–258, 1975.
246. Reilly, C. M., Hoch, S. M., Stokes, J., Jr., et al.: Clinical and laboratory findings in cases of respiratory illness caused by coryzaviruses. Ann. Intern. Med. *57*:515–525, 1962.
247. Roebuck, M. O.: Rhinoviruses in Britain 1963–1973. J. Hyg. (Camb.) *76*:137–146, 1976.
248. Rosenbaum, M. J., De Berry, P., Sullivan, E. J., et al.: Epidemiology of the common cold in military recruits with emphasis on infections by rhinovirus types 1A, 2, and two unclassified rhinoviruses. Am. J. Epidemiol. *93*:183–193, 1971.
249. Rosenquist, B. D., and Allen, G. K.: Effect of bovine fibroblast interferon on rhinovirus infection in calves. Am. J. Vet. Res. *51*:870–873, 1990.
250. Rossen, R. D., Kasel, J. A., and Couch, R. B.: The secretory immune system: Its relation to respiratory viral infection. Prog. Med. Virol. *13*:194–238, 1971.
251. Rossmann, M. G.: The canyon hypothesis: Hiding the host cell receptor attachment site on a viral surface from immune surveillance. J. Biol. Chem. *264*:14587–14590, 1989.
252. Rossmann, M. G., Arnold, E., Erickson, J. W., et al.: Structure of a human common cold virus and functional relationship to other picornaviruses. Nature *317*:145–153, 1985.
253. Rossmann, M. G., and Palmenberg, A. C.: Conservation of the putative receptor attachment site in picornaviruses. Virology *164*:373–382, 1988.
254. Ruohola, A., Heikkinen, T., Waris, M., et al.: Intranasal fluticasone propionate does not prevent acute otitis media during viral upper respiratory infection in children. J. Allergy Clin. Immunol. *106*:467–471, 2000.
255. Ruuskanen, O., Arola, M., Putto-Laurila, A., et al.: Acute otitis media and respiratory virus infections. Pediatr. Infect. Dis. J. *8*:94–99, 1989.
256. Samo, T. C., Greenberg, S. B., Couch, R. B., et al.: Efficacy and tolerance of intranasally applied recombinant leukocyte A interferon in normal volunteers. J. Infect. Dis. *148*:535–542, 1983.
257. Sarkkinen, H., Ruuskanen, O., Meurman, O., et al.: Identification of respiratory virus antigens in middle ear fluids of children with acute otitis media. J. Infect. Dis. *151*:444–448, 1985.
258. Schieble, J. H., Lennette, E. H., and Fox, V. L.: Antigenic variation of rhinovirus type 22. Proc. Soc. Exp. Biol. Med. *133*:329–333, 1970.

259. Schmidt, H. J., and Fink, R. J.: Rhinovirus as a lower respiratory tract pathogen in infants. Pediatr. Infect. Dis. J. *10*:700–702, 1991.
260. Shipkowitz, N. L., Bower, R. R., Schleicher, J. B., et al.: Antiviral activity of a bis-benzimidazole against experimental rhinovirus infections in chimpanzees. Appl. Microbiol. *23*:117–122, 1972.
261. Shult, P. A., Polyak, F., Dick, E. C., et al.: Adenovirus 21 infection in an isolated Antarctic station: Transmission of the virus and susceptibility of the population. Am. J. Epidemiol. *133*:599–607, 1991.
262. Skern, T., Sommergruber, W., Blaas, D., et al.: Human rhinovirus 2: Complete nucleotide sequence and proteolytic processing signals in the capsid protein region. Nucleic Acids Res. *13*:2111–2126, 1985.
263. Smith, M. B. H., and Feldman, W.: Over-the-counter cold medications: A critical review of clinical trials between 1950 and 1991. J. A. M. A. *269*:2258–2263, 1993.
264. Smith, T. J., Chase, E. S., Schmidt, T. J., et al.: Neutralizing antibody to human rhinovirus 14 penetrates the receptor-binding canyon. Nature *383*:350–354, 1996.
265. Sperber, S. J., and Hayden, F. G.: Chemotherapy of rhinovirus colds. Antimicrob. Agents Chemother. *32*:409–419, 1988.
266. Splints don't stop colds—surprising! Lancet *1*:277–278, 1988.
267. Stanway, G., Hughes, P. J., Mountford, R. C., et al.: The complete nucleotide sequence of a common cold virus: Human rhinovirus 14. Nucleic Acids Res. *12*:7859–7875, 1984.
268. Stenhouse, A. C.: Rhinovirus infection in acute exacerbations of chronic bronchitis: A controlled prospective study. B. M. J. *3*:461–463, 1967.
269. Stott, E. J., Grist, N. R., and Eadie, M. B.: Rhinovirus infections in chronic bronchitis: Isolation of eight possibly new rhinovirus serotypes. J. Med. Microbiol. *1*:109–117, 1968.
270. Stott, E. J., and Walker, M.: Antigenic variation among strains of rhinovirus type 51. Nature *224*:1311–1312, 1969.
271. Sung, B. S., Chonmaitree, T., Broemeling, L. D., et al.: Association of rhinovirus infection with poor bacteriologic outcome of bacterial-viral otitis media. Clin. Infect. Dis. *17*:38–42, 1993.
272. Takkouche, B., Regueira, C., and Gestal-Otero, J. J.: A cohort study of stress and the common cold. Epidemiology *12*:345–349, 2001.
273. Taussig, L. M., Busse, W. W., Lemen, R. J., et al.: Models of infectious airway injury in children. Am. Rev. Respir. Dis. *137*:979–984, 1988.
274. Taylor, R., Fauran, C., Berry, P., et al.: The prevalence of viruses and bacteria in the respiratory tract of pre-school children from a Vanuatu village community and the relationship with certain environmental variables. Papua New Guinea Med. J. *31*:19–27, 1988.
275. Taylor-Robinson, D., and Tyrrell, D. A. J.: Serotypes of viruses (rhinoviruses) isolated from common colds. Lancet *1*:452–454, 1962.
276. Thomas, P.: The common cold. Med. World News *32*:24–30, 1991.
277. Turner, R. B.: The role of neutrophils in the pathogenesis of rhinovirus infections. Pediatr. Infect. Dis. J. *9*:832–835, 1990.
278. Turner, R. B.: The treatment of rhinovirus infections: Progress and potential. Antiviral Res. *49*:1–14, 2001.
279. Turner, R. B., Dutkow, F. J., Goldstein, N. J., et al.: Efficacy of oral WIN 54954 for prophylaxis of experimental rhinovirus infection. Antimicrob. Agents Chemother. *37*:297–300, 1993.
280. Turner, R. B., Hendley, J. O., and Gwaltney, J. M., Jr.: Shedding of infected ciliated epithelial cells in rhinovirus colds. J. Infect. Dis. *145*:849–853, 1982.
281. Turner, R. B., Wecker, M. T., Pohl, G., et al.: Efficacy of tremacamra, a soluble intercellular adhesion molecule 1, for experimental rhinovirus infection. A randomized clinical trial. J. A. M. A. *281*:1797–1804, 1999.
282. Turner, R. B., Weingand, K. W., Yeh, C.-Y., et al.: Association between interleukin-8 concentration in nasal secretions and severity of symptoms of experimental rhinovirus colds. Clin. Infect. Dis. *26*:840–846, 1998.
283. Tyrrell, D. A. J.: Common Colds and Related Diseases. Baltimore, Williams & Wilkins, 1965.
284. Tyrrell, D.: The origins of the Common Cold Unit. J. R. Coll. Physicians Lond. *24*:137–140, 1990.
285. Tyrrell, D. A. J., and Al-Nakib, W.: Prophylaxis and treatment of rhinovirus infections. *In* DeClercq, E. (ed.): Clinical Use of Antiviral Drugs. Boston, Martinus Nijhoff, 1988, pp. 241–276.
286. Tyrrell, D., Barrow, I., and Arthur, J.: Local hyperthermia benefits natural and experimental common colds. B. M. J. *298*:1280–1283, 1989.
287. Tyrrell, D. A. J., and Chanock, R. M.: Rhinoviruses: A description. Science *141*:152–153, 1963.
288. Tyrrell, D. A. J., and Parsons, R.: Some virus isolations from common colds: Cytopathic effects in tissue cultures. Lancet *1*:239, 1960.
289. Uncapher, C. R., DeWitt, C. M., and Colonno, R. J.: The major and minor group receptor families contain all but one human rhinovirus serotype. Virology *180*:814–817, 1991.
290. Urquhart, G. E. D., and Stott, E. J.: Rhinoviraemia. B. M. J. *4*:28–30, 1970.
291. Valenti, W. M., Clarke, T. A., Hall, C. B., et al.: Concurrent outbreaks of rhinovirus and respiratory syncytial virus in an intensive care nursery: Epidemiology and associated risk factors. J. Pediatr. *100*:722–726, 1982.
292. Van Regenmortel, M. H. V., Fauquet, C. M., Bishop, D. H. L., et al.: Virus Taxonomy. Seventh Report of the International Committee on Taxonomy of Viruses. New York, Academic, 2000, pp. 657–678.
293. Verdaguer, N., Blaas, D., and Fita I.: Structure of human rhinovirus serotype 2 (HRV2). J. Mol. Biol. *300*:1179–1194, 2000.
294. Walker, D. L., and Boring, W. D.: Factors influencing host-virus interactions. III. Further studies on alteration of coxsackie virus infection in adult mice by environmental temperature. J. Immunol. *80*:39–44, 1958.
295. Warshauer, D. M., Dick, E. C., Mandel, A. D., et al.: Rhinovirus infections in an isolated Antarctic station: Transmission of the viruses and susceptibility of the population. Am. J. Epidemiol. *129*:319–340, 1989.
296. Webster, L. T., and Clow, A. D.: The association of pneumococci, *H. influenzae* and *Streptococcus hemolyticus* with coryza, pharyngitis, and sinusitis in man. J. Exp. Med. *55*:445–453, 1932.
297. Wimalasundera, S. S., Katz, D. R., and Chain, B. M.: Characterization of the T cell response to human rhinovirus in children: implications for understanding the immunopathology of the common cold. J. Infect. Dis. *176*:755–759, 1997.
298. Winther, B., Brofeldt, S., Christensen, B., et al.: Light and scanning electron microscopy of nasal biopsy material from patients with naturally acquired common colds. Acta Otolaryngol. (Stockh.) *97*:309–318, 1984.
299. Winther, B., Farr, B., Turner, R. B., et al.: Histopathologic examination and enumeration of polymorphonuclear leukocytes in the nasal mucosa during experimental rhinovirus colds. Acta Otolaryngol. Suppl. (Stockh.) *413*:19–24, 1984.
300. Winther, B., Gwaltney, M. J., Jr., and Hendley, J. O.: Respiratory virus infection of monolayer cultures of human nasal epithelial cells. Am. Rev. Respir. Dis. *141*:839–845, 1990.
301. Winther, B., Gwaltney, M. J., Jr., Mygind, N., et al.: Sites of rhinovirus recovery after point inoculation of the upper airway. J. A. M. A. *256*:1763–1767, 1986.
302. Wright, A. L., Taussig, L. M., Ray, C. G., et al.: The Tucson children's respiratory study. II. Lower respiratory tract illness in the first year of life. Am. J. Epidemiol. *129*:1232–1246, 1989.
303. Wulff, H., Noble, G. R., Maynard, J. E., et al.: An outbreak of respiratory infection in children associated with rhinovirus types 16 and 29. Am. J. Epidemiol. *90*:304–311, 1969.
304. Yin, F. H., and Lomax, N. B.: Establishment of a mouse model for human rhinovirus infection. J. Gen. Virol. *67*:2335–2340, 1986.
305. Yoon, H. J., Zhu, Z., Gwaltney, J. M., Jr., et al.: Rhinovirus regulation of IL-1 receptor antagonist in vivo and in vitro: A potential mechanism of symptom resolution. J. Immunol. *162*:7461–7469, 1999.
306. Zhao, R., Pevear, D. C., Kremer, M. J., et al.: Human rhinovirus 3 at 3.0 A resolution. Structure *4*:1205–1220, 1996.
307. Zhu, Z., Tang, W., Gwaltney, J. M., Jr., et al.: Rhinovirus stimulation of interleukin-8 in vivo and in vitro: Role of NF-kB. Am. J. Physiol. *273*:L814–L824, 1997.
308. Zhu, Z., Tang, W., Ray, A., et al.: Rhinovirus stimulation of interleukin-6 in vivo and in vitro: Evidence for nuclear factor kB–dependent transcriptional activation. J. Clin. Invest. *97*:421–430, 1996.

CHAPTER

172 Hepatitis A Virus

BETH P. BELL ■ CRAIG N. SHAPIRO ■ HAROLD S. MARGOLIS

History

Hepatitis A has been recognized as a clinical entity for centuries, and large epidemics of jaundice occurred during military campaigns in ancient and modern times. During the past several decades, epidemiologic and clinical studies defined the infectious nature of the disease, which led to the differentiation of "infectious hepatitis," now designated hepatitis A.[113, 136] Before 1970, attempts to isolate a virus associated with hepatitis A were uniformly unsuccessful, and information concerning the clinical course of infection, the fecal-oral route of transmission, and the efficacy of immunoglobulin in preventing disease was obtained from studies conducted in humans.[136, 138, 295] In 1973, hepatitis A virus (HAV) was identified by immune electron microscopy in stool samples of patients with hepatitis A.[80] This discovery led to the development of serologic tests that differentiate acute and resolved infections, characterization of the virus, definition of pathogenetic events during infection, and further definition of the epidemiology of HAV infection. In contrast to the other hepatitis viruses, HAV has been propagated in cell culture,[52, 209, 284] which has led to the development and licensure of vaccines shown to be highly efficacious in preventing infection and disease in immunized individuals.[120, 206, 283]

Properties

CLASSIFICATION

HAV is a 27-nm, nonenveloped, positive-sense RNA virus belonging to the family *Picornaviridae.* Although HAV initially was classified in the genus *Enterovirus,* nucleotide analysis indicates that HAV is distinct from all other picornaviruses.[155, 291] When compared with other enteroviruses, HAV has essentially no nucleotide or amino acid homology, does not have an intestinal replication phase, replicates slowly in cell culture and rarely produces a cytopathic effect, and is relatively resistant to inactivation by heating.[49] For these reasons, HAV has been reclassified in a separate genus designated *Hepatovirus.*[177, 291]

GENOMIC ORGANIZATION AND GENETIC VARIATION

The HAV genome is composed of single-stranded, positive-sense RNA containing approximately 7500 nucleotides. HAV genomic organization and replication are similar to those of polio and other picornaviruses: (1) the 5′ end is not translated, appears to contain an internal ribosomal entry site, and has a covalently linked protein (VPg); (2) sequences for structural proteins are located toward the 5′ end, followed by sequences encoding nonstructural proteins, including proteases and RNA polymerases; and (3) the viral RNA encodes a single polyprotein from which functional structural and nonstructural proteins are cleaved proteolytically.[155, 285, 291] Each capsid structural motif is composed of three major polypeptides (VP1, VP2, and VP3) of 22,000 to 33,000 d that form an outer shell with icosahedral symmetry. Based on nucleotide sequence, a fourth polypeptide, VP4 (2500 d), should be encoded but has not been identified in mature virions.[291]

HAV exists as a single serotype. The neutralization site appears to be conformational and derived from epitopes located on VP1 and VP3 as identified by neutralizing monoclonal antibodies.[183, 201] A high degree of nucleotide conservation exists among geographically diverse human HAV isolates. However, nucleotide variation in VP1 and VP3 has been used to define four human HAV genotypes, and this genetic variation has proved useful in identifying clusters and linking apparently sporadic cases.[60, 115, 215] In addition, HAVs that appear to be restricted in their primary replication to Old World monkeys have been isolated.[184, 267] These viruses represent at least three genotypes not identified in humans.[215]

HAV replicates more slowly in cell culture than do other picornaviruses, with wild-type virus requiring many weeks of adaptation before infectious foci or HAV antigen is detected.[21, 153, 237] HAV produces a high ratio of defective to complete (infectious) virus both in cell culture and during infection.[29, 291] Cell culture adaptation is associated with mutations in nonstructural proteins and the 5′-nontranslated region.[72, 73] Cell culture–adapted HAV rarely produces a cytopathic effect, although cytopathic strains have been isolated and serve as a useful model for laboratory studies.[50, 186] Adaptation also results in loss of virulence (attenuation) when evaluated in the chimpanzee model of infectivity.[125]

The HAV virion appears to be extremely stable, although the molecular determinants of this characteristic are not known. HAV is stable in the environment, with only a 100-fold decline in infectivity when stored for longer than 4 weeks at room temperature.[49, 170, 171, 199] The virus retains infectivity when treated with nonionic detergents, organic solvents, and low pH at 38° C for 90 minutes.[49] HAV is more resistant than is poliovirus to heat in that it is inactivated only partially at 60° C for 1 hour[49]; temperatures of 85 to 95° C for 1 minute are required for complete inactivation of HAV in foods such as shellfish.[49, 176] HAV is inactivated completely by formalin (0.02% at 37° C for 72 hours) but appears to be relatively resistant to free chlorine, especially when the virus is associated with organic matter.[162, 235] For general-purpose disinfection, a 1:1 dilution of 6 percent sodium hypochlorite (the household bleach available in the United States is 5% sodium hypochlorite) or 500 μg/mL free chlorine with 1-minute contact time should inactivate HAV in most situations.[170]

Epidemiology

ROUTES OF TRANSMISSION

Routes of HAV transmission are determined by the timing and location of virus replication, circulation, and excretion during infection. HAV replicates in the liver, is excreted in bile, and is found in highest concentration in stool (up to

10^8 infectious particles per milliliter).[259] The highest concentration in stool occurs during the 2-week period before jaundice develops or liver enzymes become elevated, followed by a rapid decline after jaundice appears[80, 242, 259] (Fig. 172–1). Children and infants may shed HAV for longer periods than adults do. Through the use of polymerase chain reaction (PCR) to amplify viral nucleic acid, HAV RNA has been detected in the stool of infected neonates for as long as 6 months after infection, and some studies have shown excretion in older children and adults 1 to 3 months after the onset of clinical illness.[120, 217, 293] Chronic shedding of HAV does not occur; however, virus may be present in stool during relapsing illness (see the section on relapsing hepatitis A).[241] Viremia occurs during the prodromal stage of infection and extends through the period of liver enzyme elevation (see Fig. 172–1), with virus concentrations several orders of magnitude less than those in stool.[28, 43, 137, 151] In experimentally infected animals, HAV can be detected in saliva during periods of peak excretion in stool,[43] but transmission by saliva has not been demonstrated.

Detection of HAV antigen in stool by enzyme immunoassay (EIA) or detection of HAV RNA in serum or stool by PCR cannot delineate whether an infected person is infectious because these assays may detect defective as well as infectious viral particles. Nucleic acid amplification by immunocapture PCR requires the presence of intact virus,[30, 124] and HAV RNA may be detected in stool for months with immunocapture PCR. However, the period of infectivity appears to be shorter than the period when HAV RNA can be detected in stool. Data from epidemiologic studies suggest that peak infectivity occurs during the 2 weeks before the onset of symptoms. For practical purposes, both children and adults with hepatitis A can be assumed to be noninfectious 1 week after jaundice appears.

Because of the high concentration of virus in the stool of infected persons, HAV transmission occurs primarily by the fecal-oral route, usually by person-to-person transmission in households and extended-family settings and between sexual contacts.[246] Person-to-person transmission results in high rates of infection in young children in developing countries and is the predominant mode of transmission in the United States, particularly during community-wide outbreaks, as well as in outbreaks in childcare centers.[15] HAV can remain infectious in the environment,[171] and fecal contamination of food or water can result in common-source outbreaks. HAV has been transmitted by transfusion, but such transmission occurs rarely because the blood donation must occur during the early prodromal stage of the disease or from an asymptomatic person who is viremic.[151] Nucleic acid amplification tests such as PCR assay now are applied to screening of blood and source plasma. These assays are sufficiently sensitive to remove most units that have HAV. Transmission has not been associated with saliva.

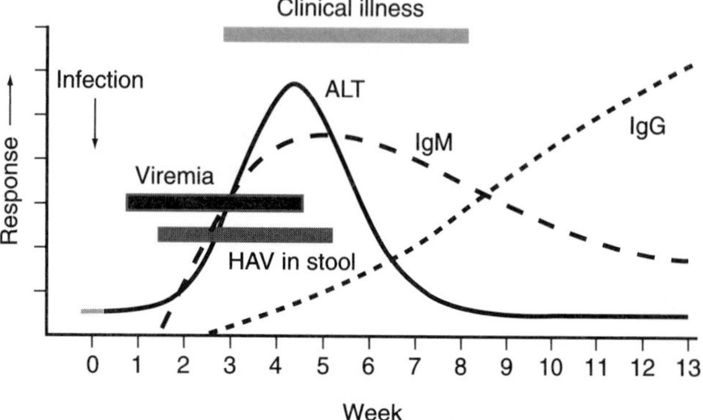

FIGURE 172–1 ■ Immunologic, virologic, and biochemical events during the course of a typical hepatitis A virus (HAV) infection. ALT, alanine aminotransferase.

Two published case reports have described intrauterine transmission of HAV during the first trimester that resulted in fetal meconium peritonitis.[148, 172] After delivery, both infants were found to have a perforated ileum. The risk of transmission to newborns by pregnant women in whom hepatitis A develops in the third trimester of pregnancy appears to be low.[264] However, newborns who acquire HAV infection in this manner or from a transfusion usually are asymptomatic, and the infection is detected by the development of hepatitis A in hospital staff or other persons having contact with the infant.[217, 280]

PATTERNS OF DISEASE WORLDWIDE

Worldwide, the endemicity of HAV infection differs markedly among and within countries (Fig. 172–2). Patterns of HAV infection can be differentiated, each being characterized by distinct age-specific profiles of prevalence of antibody to HAV (anti-HAV), incidence of hepatitis A, and prevailing environmental (hygienic and sanitary) and socioeconomic conditions[15, 102] (Fig. 172–3).

In areas with a high endemic pattern of infection, represented by the least developed countries (i.e., parts of Africa, Asia, and Central and South America), poor socioeconomic conditions allow HAV to spread readily (see Fig. 172–2). Most persons are infected as young children, and essentially the entire population is infected before reaching adolescence, as demonstrated by the age-specific prevalence of anti-HAV[12, 51, 268] (see Fig. 172–3). Because virtually all HAV infections occur in age groups in which asymptomatic infection predominates, reported disease rates may be low and outbreaks rare.

In areas of intermediate endemicity, HAV is not transmitted as readily because of better sanitary and living conditions, and the predominant age of infection is older than that in high-endemic areas[39] (see Figs. 172–2 and 172–3). Paradoxically, the overall incidence and average age of reported cases often increase because high levels of virus circulate in a population that includes many susceptible older children, adolescents, and young adults, in whom symptoms are likely to develop with HAV infection.[99] Large common-source outbreaks also can occur because of the relatively high rate of virus transmission and the large number of susceptible persons, especially among those of higher socioeconomic levels. Such an outbreak occurred in Shanghai in 1988, with more than 300,000 cases associated with the consumption of contaminated clams.[105] Nonetheless, person-to-person transmission in community-wide epidemics continues to account for much of the disease in these countries.

Shifts in age-specific prevalence patterns indicating a transition from high to intermediate endemicity are occurring in many parts of the world (see Fig. 172–3). As this transition occurs, marked variations in hepatitis A epidemiology are seen among countries and within countries and cities, with some areas displaying a pattern typical of high endemicity and others of intermediate endemicity (see Fig. 172–2).* Considerable hepatitis A–related morbidity and associated costs can occur, even in developing countries. Hepatitis A is reported to account for 50 to 60 percent of all

*See references 13, 15, 56, 89, 99, 119, 140, 141, 202, 203, 258, 269, 279.

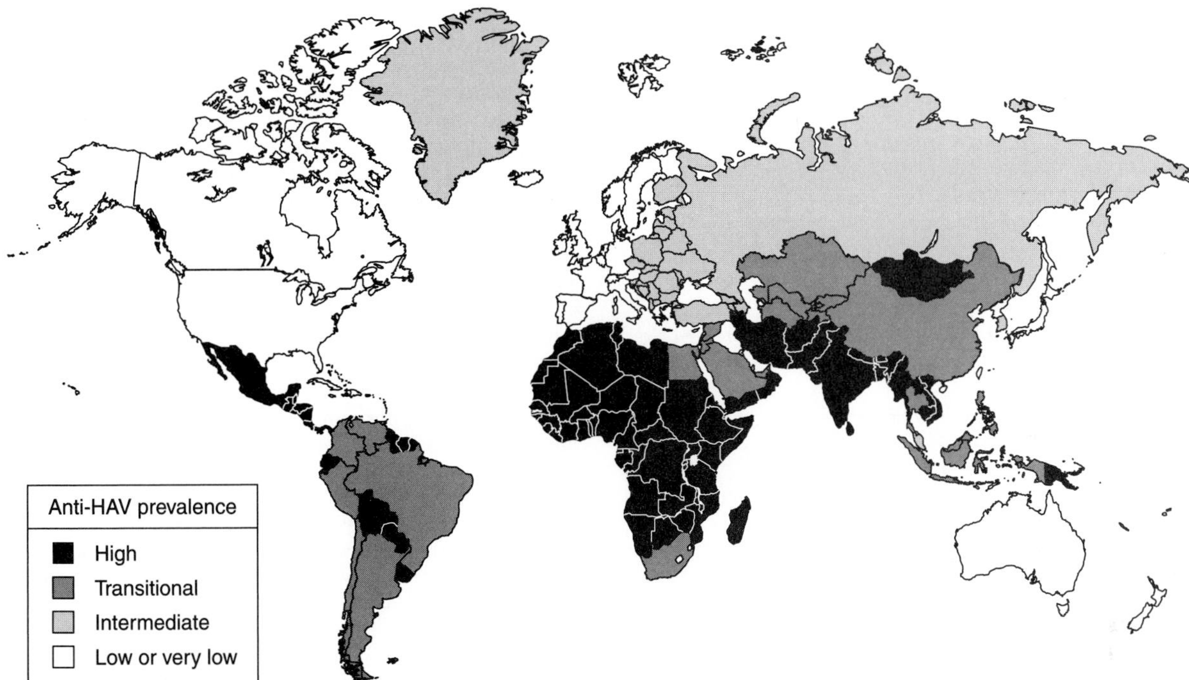

FIGURE 172–2 ■ Geographic distribution of patterns of endemicity of hepatitis A virus (HAV) infection. The distribution was generalized from the best available data.

acute viral hepatitis cases among children in Pakistan, and 232 children with fulminant hepatic failure secondary to hepatitis A were admitted to one tertiary care referral hospital in Karachi during a 9-year period.[226] Hepatitis A was the etiology of the fulminant hepatitis of two thirds of the children treated at two hospitals in Argentina during a 15-year period, and in one of these hospitals performing liver transplantation, a third of the liver transplantations in children were required because of fulminant hepatitis A.[40]

In most areas of North America and western Europe, sanitary and hygienic conditions are such that the endemicity of HAV infection is low (see Figs. 172–2 and 172–3). Relatively fewer children are infected, and disease often occurs in the context of community-wide and childcare center outbreaks and occasionally as common-source outbreaks.[17, 93, 207, 227, 261] In some regions (e.g., Scandinavia), the endemicity of HAV infection is very low and disease occurs almost exclusively in defined risk groups, such as travelers returning from areas where HAV infection is endemic or injecting drug users.[26]

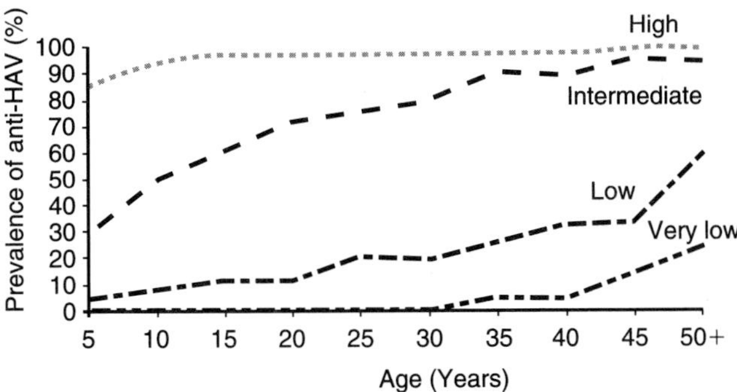

FIGURE 172–3 ■ Patterns of hepatitis A virus (HAV) infection worldwide.

PATTERNS OF DISEASE IN THE UNITED STATES

During the past several decades, the incidence of hepatitis A has displayed a cyclic pattern, with large nationwide epidemics occurring approximately every 10 to 15 years; the last peak occurred in 1995 (Fig. 172–4). However, even between these epidemics, disease rates are relatively high. In 1997, 30,021 cases were reported to the Centers for Disease Control and Prevention (CDC).[253] Furthermore, incidence models indicate that most infections are not detected. One such analysis estimated an average of 271,000 infections per year during 1980 to 1999, 10.4 times the reported number of cases.[6]

The incidence of hepatitis A has varied by age, race/ethnicity, and geographic region. Historically, the highest rates were reported in children 5 to 14 years of age, with approximately a third of cases occurring in children younger than 15 years.[35, 36] Because many children have unrecognized asymptomatic infection, they probably represent a major reservoir for HAV transmission. Incidence models indicate that more than half of HAV infections occur in children younger than 10 years, most of whom are 0 to 4 years old.[6] Among racial and ethnic groups, before the use of hepatitis A vaccine, rates in American Indians and Alaska Natives were more than 10 times the rate in other racial and ethnic groups, and rates in Hispanics were approximately three times higher than in non-Hispanics.[205]

Analysis of national surveillance data over time indicates that the incidence of hepatitis A has displayed striking regional variation, with the highest rates and the majority of cases consistently occurring in a limited number of states and counties concentrated in the western and southwestern United States (Fig. 172–5). Although rates in these areas fluctuated from year to year, they consistently remained above the national average. Cases in residents of the 11 states—representing 22 percent of the U.S. population—in which the average annual incidence of hepatitis A was

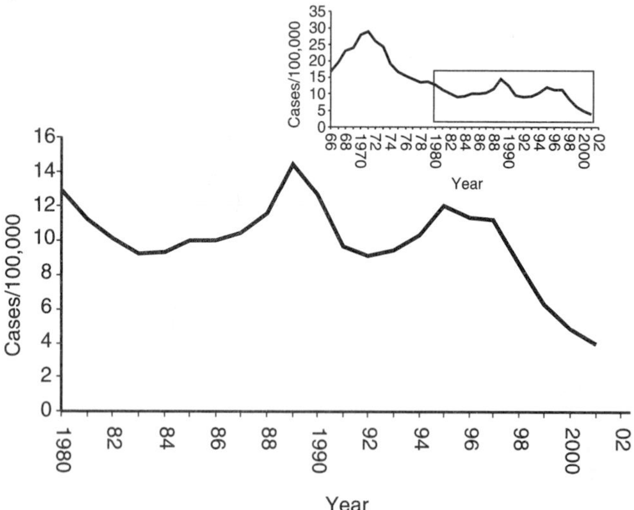

FIGURE 172–4 ■ Hepatitis A incidence rates (per 100,000 population) based on cases reported to the Centers for Disease Control and Prevention (1966–2001).

20 cases or more per 100,000 during 1987 to 1997 (twice the national average of about 10 per 100,000) accounted for an average of 50 percent of the reported cases (Table 172–1). An additional 18 percent of cases occurred in residents of states with average annual rates above the national average but less than twice the national average during this time (see Table 172–1).

Data from disease surveillance systems indicate that the source of infection most commonly reported is household or sexual contact with a person who has hepatitis A (15–25% of reported cases).[17, 36] Approximately 10 to 15 percent of reported cases occur in employees and children who attend childcare centers and members of their households, but these cases are attributed to contact within the childcare center without requiring a known contact with hepatitis A or even identifying a case of hepatitis A in the center.[17, 36] International travel (5–7%) and suspected food- or waterborne outbreaks (2–5%) each account for a small proportion of cases.[36, 227] One third of cases among returning international travelers are in children, and Mexico is the most common (>80%) destination (CDC, unpublished data). Cyclic outbreaks occur in men who have sex with men and users of injecting and noninjecting drugs.[17, 45, 88, 106, 114, 222] During outbreak years, this exposure can account for as many as 10 percent of nationally reported cases (CDC, unpublished data). Nearly 50 percent of patients with hepatitis A do not have a recognized source of infection[36] but may be contacts of persons, especially children, with asymptomatic infection.

Most cases of hepatitis A in the United States occur in the context of community-wide epidemics, during which infection is transmitted from person to person in households and extended family settings.[17] Once initiated, these epidemics often persist for several years and have proved difficult to control,[197, 233] even when attempts are made to rapidly vaccinate some portion of the population.[8, 47] Children play an important role in HAV transmission. In communities with historically the highest hepatitis A rates, as exemplified by American Indian and Alaska Native communities, the pattern of transmission was similar to that found in countries with an intermediate endemicity of HAV infection (see the section on patterns of disease worldwide).[33, 59, 145, 232, 289] Asymptomatic transmission occurred in susceptible young children at low levels during interepidemic periods until a cohort of susceptible children became large enough to sustain a

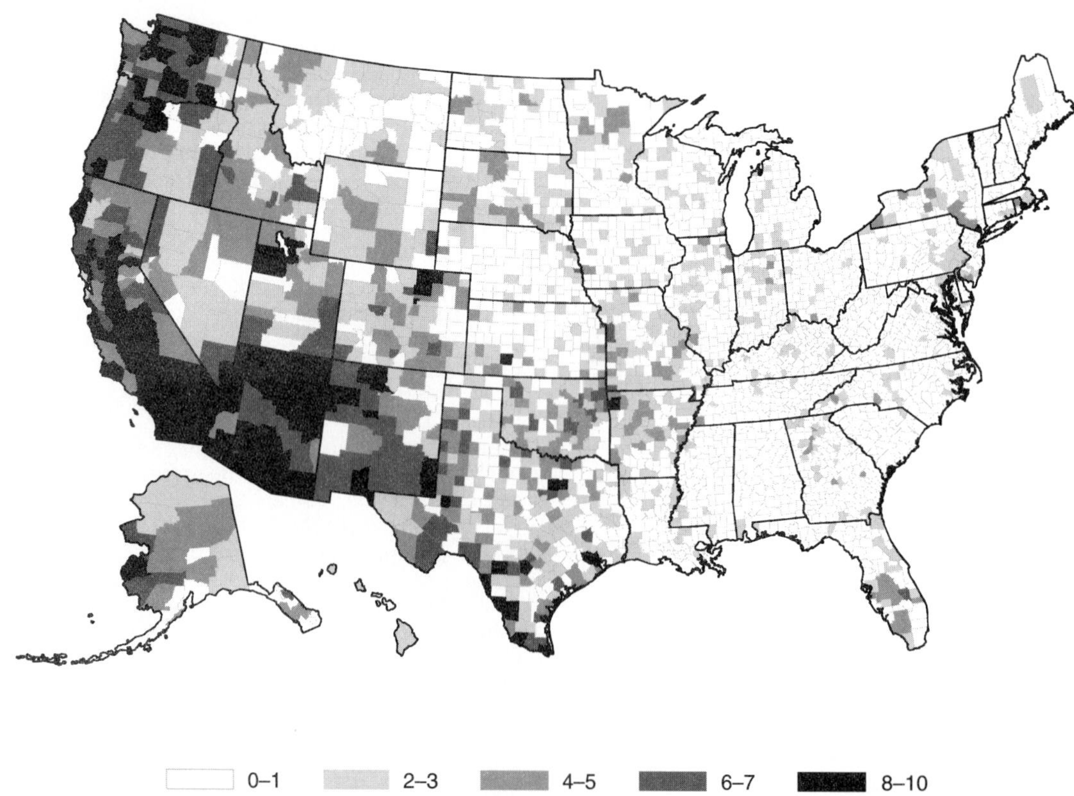

FIGURE 172–5 ■ Number of years that the reported incidence of hepatitis A exceeded 10 cases per 100,000 population (approximately the U.S. average), by county (1987–1997).

TABLE 172–1 ■ OCCURRENCE OF HEPATITIS A IN STATES WITH AVERAGE REPORTED INCIDENCE OF ≥10 CASES PER 100,000 POPULATION—1987-1997*

State	Rate (per 100,000)†	Cumulative Average No. of Cases/Year‡	Cumulative % Cases	Cumulative % Population§
Arizona	48	1,852	7	2
Alaska	45	2,137	8	2
Oregon	40	3,297	12	3
New Mexico	40	3,916	14	4
Utah	33	4,519	16	5
Washington	30	6,007	21	7
Oklahoma	24	6,786	24	8
South Dakota	24	6,953	25	8
Idaho	21	7,172	26	9
Nevada	21	7,449	27	10
California	20	13,706	50	22
Missouri	19	14,706	54	24
Texas	16	17,587	64	31
Colorado	16	18,138	56	33
Arkansas	14	18,483	67	34
Montana	11	18,576	68	34
Wyoming	11	18,627	68	34

*The overall U.S. rate during 1987 to 1997 was 10.8/100,000 population.
†Children living in areas (states, counties, communities) where the rate was 20 or more cases per 100,000 population should be vaccinated routinely. Children living in areas where the rate was 10 or more cases per 100,000 population but no fewer than 20 cases per 100,000 population should be considered for routine vaccination.
‡Approximately 37% of cases were among persons < aged 20 years.
§Estimate for 1997, U.S. Census.

community-wide outbreak.[232, 243] Asymptomatic transmission among children also is important in sustaining outbreaks in areas with consistently elevated rates (see Table 172–1). During community-wide outbreaks, serologic studies of members of households with an adult case and no identified source have found that 25 to 40 percent of contacts younger than 6 years had serologic evidence of having had recent HAV infection (CDC, unpublished data).[246] In one of these studies, 52 percent of households of adults without an identified source of infection included a child younger than 6 years, and the presence of a young child was associated with household transmission of HAV.[246] In this study, transmission chains were identified as involving as many as six generations and more than 20 cases.

As determined by the Third National Health and Nutrition Examination Survey conducted during 1988 to 1994, approximately one third of the U.S. population has serologic evidence of previous HAV infection.[206] Anti-HAV prevalence is related directly to age—it ranges from 9 percent in children 6 to 11 years of age to 75 percent in persons older than 70 years—and it is related inversely to income. The prevalence of anti-HAV is higher in Mexican Americans (70%) than in non-Hispanic blacks (39%) and whites (23%).

EPIDEMIOLOGY OF HEPATITIS A IN SPECIFIC SETTINGS

Childcare Centers

The role of children with asymptomatic infection has been recognized in outbreaks in childcare centers since the 1970s.[228] Because infection in children is usually mild or asymptomatic, these outbreaks often are not recognized until adult contacts (usually parents) become ill.[104] Outbreaks rarely occur in centers that do not have children in diapers, and they are more common in larger centers.[104] Both poor hygiene in these children and the need for staff to handle and change diapers contribute to spread. Despite the occurrence of outbreaks when HAV is introduced into a childcare center, studies of childcare center employees do not show a significantly increased prevalence of HAV infection in comparison to control populations.[85, 122] Occasionally, outbreaks in childcare centers can be the source of more extensive transmission within a community.[52, 103, 274] However, it is likely that most disease within childcare centers reflects transmission from the community.

Other Groups and Settings

Hepatitis A cases in schoolchildren usually reflect disease that has been acquired in the community. However, multiple cases among children within a school may indicate a common-source outbreak.[115] Historically, HAV infection was endemic in institutions for the developmentally disabled, but with smaller facilities and improved conditions, the incidence and prevalence of infection have decreased, and outbreaks rarely are reported in the United States.[254]

During the past 2 decades, outbreaks have been reported with increasing frequency in illicit drug users in North America, Australia, and Europe.[106, 109, 114, 116, 190, 222, 231] In the United States, these outbreaks often have occurred in the context of a large community-wide outbreak, and in the past decade, they frequently have involved users of injected and noninjected methamphetamine, who may account for as many as 30 percent of reported cases in these communities during outbreaks.[17, 114, 116] Cross-sectional serologic surveys have demonstrated that injecting drug users have a higher prevalence of anti-HAV than the general U.S. population does.[121, 278] Transmission among injecting drug users probably occurs through both percutaneous and fecal-oral routes.[116]

Hepatitis A outbreaks in men who have sex with men have been reported frequently, most recently in urban areas in the United States, Canada, England, and Australia.[45, 88, 110, 252] These outbreaks may occur in the context of an outbreak in the larger community.[17] Some studies conducted during outbreaks and seroprevalence surveys among men who have sex with men have identified specific sex practices associated with illness, whereas others have not demonstrated such associations.[45, 46, 108, 126, 278]

Transfusion-related hepatitis A rarely occurs because HAV does not result in chronic infection and blood donors are screened for elevated aminotransferase levels. Currently, nucleic acid amplification tests also are used to screen blood and source plasma and are sufficiently sensitive to remove most units that contain HAV. However, outbreaks have been reported in Europe and the United States in patients who received factor VIII and factor IX concentrates prepared by solvent-detergent treatment to inactivate lipid-containing viruses.[164, 245] HAV is resistant to solvent-detergent treatment, and contamination presumably occurred from plasma donors with hepatitis A who donated during the incubation period. The risk of acquiring infection in patients with hemophilia is not known, although data from one serologic survey of hemophiliac patients suggest that they may be at increased risk for acquisition of HAV infection.[161] Transmission related to blood transfusions also has resulted in nosocomial outbreaks in neonatal intensive care units.[129, 189, 217] Hepatitis A has been reported in adult cancer patients treated with lymphocytes incubated in serum from a donor with HAV infection.[281]

Nosocomial transmission from adult patients to health care workers usually has been associated with fecal incontinence of the patient.[97, 195] Such transmission is a rare event, however, because most patients with hepatitis A are hospitalized after the onset of jaundice, when infectivity is low.[242] Health care workers have not been found to have an increased prevalence of anti-HAV in comparison to control populations in serologic surveys conducted in the United States.[92]

Persons from developed countries who travel to developing countries with a high, transitional, or intermediate endemicity of HAV infection are at substantial risk of acquiring hepatitis A[249] (see Fig. 172–2). In prospective studies, the risk of HAV infection occurring in travelers who do not receive immunoglobulin was found to be 3 to 5 per 1000 per month of stay,[250] on the same order of magnitude as that for malaria and higher than that for cholera or typhoid. The risk may be higher among travelers staying in areas with poor hygienic conditions,[142] it varies according to the region and the length of stay, and it appears to be increased even among travelers who reported staying in urban areas or luxury hotels.[249] In some European countries, returning international travelers with hepatitis A account for a substantial proportion of reported cases (16 to 40%).[38, 286] In the United States, approximately 5 percent of reported cases occur in persons with a history of recent international travel; children account for approximately a third of these cases (CDC, unpublished data).[36]

Food-borne hepatitis A outbreaks are recognized relatively infrequently in the United States and are associated most commonly with contamination of food during preparation by a food handler with HAV infection. Implicated foods include those not cooked after handling, such as sandwiches and salads, glazed pastries, ice, and cold drinks, as well as partially cooked foods.* Control of these outbreaks usually requires intensive public health effort.[54] However, persons who work as food handlers are not at increased risk for acquiring hepatitis A because of their occupation. Food contaminated before retail distribution, such as shellfish harvested from polluted water and lettuce or fruits contaminated at the growing or processing stage, has been recognized increasingly as the source of hepatitis A outbreaks.[60, 61, 66, 115, 187, 193, 204, 213, 216] Water-borne hepatitis A outbreaks are extremely rare events and are related to sewage contamination or inadequate treatment of water.[19, 23, 27, 31, 63, 87]

*See references 34, 54, 84, 101, 143, 160, 168, 179, 182, 196, 244, 282.

Pathogenesis and Pathology

PATHOLOGY

The light microscopic findings in acute hepatitis A, which include inflammatory cell infiltration, hepatocellular necrosis, and liver cell regeneration, are common to all forms of acute viral hepatitis. These histologic findings vary with the stage and severity of hepatitis. Early biopsy specimens generally show portal infiltration by lymphocytes, plasma cells, and periodic acid–Schiff positive macrophages.[67, 260] Spotty or focal necrosis is seen commonly, as evidenced by balloon degeneration, shrinkage, and fragmentation of hepatocytes.[67] HAV antigen is found primarily in the cytoplasm of hepatocytes, but it also can be found in liver macrophages. However, because HAV infection is self-limited and does not result in chronic liver disease, liver biopsy rarely is indicated (see the section on treatment).

Differences have been noted in the light microscopic findings of hepatitis A and other forms of viral hepatitis, particularly hepatitis B. In addition to degeneration of hepatocytes in the perivenular area, periportal inflammation and destruction of hepatocytes adjacent to the portal area may be more pronounced than in hepatitis B.[1, 194, 260] Findings in some patients, including extension of the inflammatory infiltration from the periportal area into the hepatic parenchyma and disruption of the limiting plate, may be difficult to distinguish from chronic hepatitis.[1, 67] Cholestasis may be more prominent than in hepatitis B.[223]

The histologic findings in fulminant hepatitis A are indistinguishable from those in other forms of fulminant viral hepatitis. Examination of pathologic specimens shows massive hepatic necrosis, abnormal architecture of surviving hepatocytes, and a diffuse inflammatory response.[132] Viral antigen can be found in pathologic specimens.

CELLULAR IMMUNE RESPONSE

Unlike that of other picornaviruses, infection of cultured cells with wild-type HAV has no cytopathic effect. The general assumption is that HAV infection is also noncytopathic in vivo and, therefore, the cytopathic changes in the liver associated with hepatitis A are immune mediated. This assumption is supported by the finding that symptoms and biochemical evidence of liver injury do not occur at the time of maximal virus replication and fecal shedding (during the late incubation period). Rather, liver injury is associated closely with viral clearance. $CD8^+$, class 1–dependent, cytotoxic, and virus-specific T cells that are capable of producing interferon-γ are present in the circulation and the liver.[83, 270, 271] Additional inflammatory cells, recruited to the site of infection by interferon-γ and other cytokines secreted by $CD8^+$ cells, may be responsible for much of the liver injury. Complement has been shown to bind to HAV capsid proteins, and serum complement levels drop during infection, but whether complement-mediated cellular injury occurs is unclear.[167] The mechanism by which infection is resolved remains uncertain.

HUMORAL IMMUNE RESPONSE

Antibodies directed against conformational epitopes displayed on intact virions as well as empty viral capsids are produced during the later stages of infection (see the section on genomic organization and genetic variation). Virus-specific IgM and IgG and IgA antibodies are present in serum; IgM anti-HAV generally can be detected at the onset of symptoms (see the section on serologic events in acute HAV infection).

Clinical Manifestations

Similar to other forms of viral hepatitis, the clinical manifestations of HAV infection are variable and range from asymptomatic anicteric infection to symptoms of acute hepatitis, including fever, malaise, anorexia, nausea, vomiting, and right upper quadrant pain. The likelihood of having symptomatic HAV infection and the severity of the illness are related to the age of the patient. In early childhood, infection usually is asymptomatic, whereas infection in adulthood generally is accompanied by symptoms. The diagnosis of hepatitis A is a serologic diagnosis because no constellation of symptoms is pathognomonic of the disease.

INCUBATION PERIOD

The average incubation period is 28 to 30 days but can range from 15 to 50 days.[135] The average incubation period has been reported to be shorter in patients who acquired HAV infection by parenteral transmission from contaminated blood products and in chimpanzees infected parenterally than in those infected orogastrically.[167, 234]

SPECTRUM OF ILLNESS

HAV infection, confirmed by the detection of IgM anti-HAV in serum, can be inapparent (asymptomatic, with no elevation in serum aminotransferase levels), subclinical (asymptomatic, with elevation of serum aminotransferase levels), or clinically evident (with symptoms). Specific symptoms of liver dysfunction include jaundice and dark urine caused by hyperbilirubinemia. However, symptomatic hepatitis A without jaundice (anicteric) does occur. Nonspecific symptoms of acute hepatitis A can include fever, myalgia, anorexia, nausea, right upper quadrant pain or discomfort, diarrhea, and pruritus.

Many acute HAV infections, particularly inapparent and subclinical infection and anicteric hepatitis A, are not recognized as cases of viral hepatitis.[246, 292] The frequency of symptoms with acute infection is influenced strongly by age. Children are less likely to have symptomatic infection than adults are, and jaundice rarely occurs in children younger than 6 years.[95] In one report describing outbreaks in several daycare centers, the proportion of infected children without symptoms was 84 percent in children younger than 3 years, 50 percent in children 3 to 4 years of age, and 20 percent in children 5 years or older.[104] Symptoms develop in most adults with acute infection. In a study of two outbreaks among young adult U.S. military personnel, symptoms developed in 76 to 97 percent of infected persons, and approximately 55 percent were icteric.[146]

CLINICAL SIGNS AND SYMPTOMS

In an individual patient, the clinical symptoms of acute hepatitis A are indistinguishable from those caused by other forms of viral hepatitis. Particularly in older children and adults, the onset of illness often is quite abrupt and may consist of fever, myalgia, anorexia, malaise, nausea, intermittent dull abdominal pain, and vomiting. Fever, rarely higher than 102°F, and headache occur more frequently than in other forms of acute viral hepatitis.[255] Many pediatric patients may have diarrhea or, less commonly, upper respiratory symptoms such as cough, sore throat, and runny nose, and the diagnosis of hepatitis A might not be considered in children with predominantly respiratory or gastrointestinal symptoms and transient fever without the typical malaise, fatigue, and anorexia.[82, 149] Dark urine followed by jaundice and light-colored stool, if present, will appear within a few days to a week after onset of the prodromal symptoms.[18, 100, 146, 149] When this icteric phase begins, symptoms often resolve and appetite returns in young children, but older children and adult patients may experience a transient worsening in the prodromal symptoms of anorexia, malaise, and weakness.[132, 181]

In addition to jaundice and scleral icterus, physical findings may include mild hepatomegaly and tenderness, but severe tenderness suggests other diagnoses. The spleen may be palpable in 10 to 20 percent of patients, and posterior cervical adenopathy may be present.[42, 146, 265] Pleural effusions have been reported to occur, do not appear to be associated with more severe disease, and resolve spontaneously.[3] Ascites, peripheral edema, and findings indicative of hepatic encephalopathy suggest the presence of a more severe form of hepatitis (see the section on atypical clinical manifestations and complications of hepatitis A). Ultrasonographic findings in children with uncomplicated hepatitis A have included edema or thickening of the gallbladder wall, abdominal lymphadenopathy, and less commonly, transient ascites and pancreatic abnormalities.[42, 128]

The symptoms of hepatitis A last for several weeks on average and usually not longer than 2 months.[133] Prolonged or relapsing hepatitis A can occur (see the section on relapsing hepatitis A) and, in the case of prolonged hepatitis A, may be associated with genetic markers for autoimmune hepatitis.[77]

LABORATORY ABNORMALITIES

As in other forms of viral hepatitis, during HAV infection, inflammation of the liver is accompanied by abnormalities in serum hepatic enzymes, with increases in serum alanine aminotransferase (ALT), aspartate aminotransferase (AST), alkaline phosphatase, and gamma-glutamyltranspeptidase (GGTP) levels. Elevations of serum ALT and AST occur most consistently and may precede the appearance of symptoms by a week or more (see Fig. 172–1). Peak levels generally occur 3 to 10 days after the onset of symptoms and are between 200 and 5000 IU but can reach as high as 20,000 IU. The level of ALT usually is higher than that of AST because the inflammatory response is destructive, particularly to the plasma membrane, in acute viral hepatitis. ALT is found in the cytosol of the plasma membrane, whereas AST is located mainly in cell mitochondria.[100]

Serum bilirubin levels, though frequently elevated, usually remain below 10 mg/dL and peak 1 to 2 weeks after illness begins. Higher levels can be seen in some patients, especially when HAV infection is complicated by cholestasis (see the section on cholestatic hepatitis A) or hemolysis secondary to an underlying glucose-6-phosphate dehydrogenase (G6PD) deficiency state.[37] In patients with G6PD deficiency, indirect bilirubin may account for more than 50 percent of the total bilirubin. Alkaline phosphatase and 5′-nucleotidase activity usually are elevated only mildly, rarely reaching more than 2 or 3 times the normal level. GGTP levels generally are 3 to 10 times the upper limit of normal.

Serum immunoglobulin levels often are elevated, and IgM levels are frequently higher than those in acute hepatitis B and non-A, non-B hepatitis.[294] In patients without underlying liver disease, the prothrombin time is usually normal. A prolonged prothrombin time, generally associated with severe liver damage, is a prognostic indicator for the development of fulminant hepatitis.[290]

Patients with acute HAV infection usually have a mild lymphocytosis with occasional atypical mononuclear cells.[181] Except for patients who have hemolysis associated with G6PD deficiency, the hematocrit is generally normal.[37, 181]

Apart from patients who have relapsing or cholestatic hepatitis A (see the section on atypical clinical manifestations and complications of hepatitis A), serum bilirubin and aminotransferase levels usually return to normal by 2 to 3 months after the onset of illness in most patients.[133]

SEROLOGIC EVENTS IN ACUTE HEPATITIS A VIRUS INFECTION

Because the pattern and magnitude of symptoms and the hepatic enzyme abnormalities of hepatitis A are not distinctive of hepatitis A, the diagnosis requires serologic detection of specific antibody responses to HAV. Sensitive and specific radioimmunoassays (RIAs) or EIAs show that virtually all patients have detectable IgM anti-HAV during the acute or early convalescent phase of HAV infection[157] (see Fig. 172–1). A small proportion (3%) of patients tested within 3 days of the onset of symptoms may be IgM anti-HAV–negative but become IgM anti-HAV–positive within the initial 2 weeks of illness.[157] During the first 4 to 8 weeks after the onset of symptoms, the titer of IgM anti-HAV in serum is high.[107] Antibody generally disappears within 6 months, although rarely it can be detected for 2 years or longer.[69, 107, 131, 157] IgM anti-HAV may be detectable for a longer period in patients with symptomatic illness than in those with asymptomatic infection.[107, 244]

IgG anti-HAV is present in low titer at or shortly after the onset of acute HAV infection, and the titer rises over the course of several weeks as the IgM anti-HAV titer falls (see Fig. 172–1). IgG anti-HAV remains detectable in serum for the lifetime of the individual and confers lasting protection against disease. Secretory IgA antibodies are detected in a minority of humans or primates with acute HAV infection but are unlikely to provide any significant protection against HAV infection.[247] IgG anti-HAV is transferred passively across the placenta and declines to undetectable levels in most infants by the time they reach 12 to 15 months of age.[80, 159]

Commercially available immunoassays (RIAs or EIAs) either detect total (IgG and IgM) antibody against HAV capsid proteins by using a competitive inhibition (blocking) format or detect IgM antibody to capsid proteins by using an IgM capture format.[150] These assays do not measure the neutralizing antibodies responsible for biologic activity against HAV, but detection of total anti-HAV by conventional assays is correlated with the appearance of neutralizing antibodies.[134, 150] Neutralizing antibodies elicited against one strain of HAV have been shown to have biologic activity against other HAV strains.[152]

When tested in parallel with a World Health Organization anti-HAV reference reagent, the lower limit of detection of commercially available assays is approximately 100 mIU/mL of anti-HAV.[91, 150] Administration of small amounts of immune globulin provides a high level of protection against hepatitis A, although the antibody concentrations achieved by passive immunization with immune globulin or active immunization with vaccine are 10- to 100-fold lower than those produced after natural infection.[150] Antibody concentrations achieved by passive immunization and occasionally by active immunization and known to provide protection against HAV infection both in vivo and in vitro may be below the level of detection of the commercial immunoassays. However, the neutralizing antibody that provides protection in these situations can be detected by assays that measure inhibition of HAV in cell culture (i.e., radioimmunofocus inhibition test or plaque assay).[5, 50, 150, 152] In addition, immunoassays that are more sensitive than the commercially available assays have been developed but generally are available only in research laboratories.

The lower limit of antibody necessary to provide protection against HAV infection is unknown. In vitro studies with cell culture–derived virus suggest that low levels of antibody (e.g., <20 mIU/mL) are neutralizing.[152] Clinical trials that evaluated vaccine efficacy have not provided an estimate of the minimal protective antibody level because vaccine-induced levels of antibody have been very high and few infections have occurred in vaccinees. Experimental studies in chimpanzees indicate that very low levels of passively transferred antibody (<10 mIU/mL) obtained from immunized individuals do not protect against infection but prevent clinical hepatitis and shedding of virus.[210]

Atypical Clinical Manifestations and Complications of Hepatitis A (Table 172–2)

RELAPSING HEPATITIS A

Relapsing hepatitis is a relatively common manifestation of hepatitis A that occurs in approximately 10 percent of patients.[224] One to 4 months after having the initial episode of acute hepatitis, these patients have a second episode; more than one relapse rarely occurs.[96, 224, 263] Patients with relapsing hepatitis A have no distinctive clinical features of their first disease episode. After the first episode, most patients experience a significant improvement in symptoms and biochemical abnormalities. However, the frequency with which serum aminotransferase levels completely normalize during this period has been variable; in one report, normalization occurred in only one of seven patients with relapsing hepatitis A.[263] The relapse episode of hepatitis rarely is more severe than is the initial episode and is accompanied by

TABLE 172–2 ■ ATYPICAL CLINICAL MANIFESTATIONS AND COMPLICATIONS OF HEPATITIS A VIRUS INFECTION

Relapsing hepatitis A[96, 224, 263]
Fulminant hepatitis A[169, 191, 212, 262]
Extrahepatic manifestations
Transient rash or arthralgias[94, 263]
Papular acrodermatitis of childhood[219]
Cutaneous vasculitis[55, 117, 118]
Cryoglobulinemia[117, 118, 224]
Guillain-Barré acute syndrome[255]
Other neurologic syndromes (e.g., myeloradiculopathy, mononeuritis, vertigo, meningoencephalitis)[10, 25, 198, 256]
Renal syndromes (acute renal failure, nephritic syndrome, acute glomerulonephritis)[9, 58, 123]
Pancreatitis[178]
Aplastic anemia and thrombocytopenia[74, 163]
Cholestatic hepatitis A[98, 263]
Hepatitis A triggering autoimmune hepatitis[263, 275]

elevated serum aminotransferase levels (typically to >1000 mIU/mL) and persistence of IgM anti-HAV. Molecular studies have demonstrated the presence of HAV in stool and HAV RNA in serum during relapse, but whether patients are infectious is unknown.[96] The illness usually lasts a total of 16 to 40 weeks and results in full recovery.[96, 224] Although the pathogenesis of relapsing hepatitis is unknown, it most probably is immunologically mediated.[224] Persistent HAV infection with a relapsing clinical course has been reported in patients after they have undergone liver transplantation for fulminant hepatitis A; HAV-specific genomic sequences have been identified in the grafts of these patients.[76, 290]

FULMINANT HEPATITIS A

In the United States, a relatively small proportion of all fulminant hepatitis is caused by hepatitis A.[169, 212, 225, 262] Among patients hospitalized with hepatitis A, the case-fatality rate has been estimated to be 0.14 percent.[100] However, based on all cases of hepatitis A reported in the United States, the case-fatality rate from fulminant hepatitis A is approximately 0.4 percent.[206] Host factors reported to be associated with an increased risk for development of fulminant hepatitis include older age[100, 139] and underlying chronic liver disease.[2, 14, 57, 127, 154, 276] In molecular studies that have examined capsid sequences, fulminant hepatitis A was not associated with viral variants.

Fulminant hepatitis A has no distinctive clinical features that distinguish it from fulminant hepatic failure of other causes. Within approximately 8 weeks of the onset of illness, symptoms of hepatic encephalopathy and marked prolongation of the prothrombin time are noted in patients with no history of previous liver disease.[191] Complications can include cerebral edema, sepsis, gastrointestinal bleeding, and hypoglycemia. The prognosis of fulminant hepatitis A without transplantation is better than that of fulminant disease related to other viral etiologies, and 40 to 70 percent of patients can be expected to recover.[94, 192, 225, 262]

EXTRAHEPATIC MANIFESTATIONS

During acute hepatitis A, transient rash and arthralgias occur in as many as 14 and 19 percent of patients, respectively, particularly during the prodromal period.[94, 263] Urticaria has been reported but occurs less frequently than in acute hepatitis B.[68] Papular acrodermatitis of childhood, the Gianotti-Crosti syndrome, rarely occurs in the United States but has been reported elsewhere in association with HAV infection.[219] The cutaneous lesions, which consist of nonpruritic, symmetric flat papules on the face, extremities, and buttocks, may persist for several weeks before spontaneously resolving.[70]

Other extrahepatic manifestations that occur chiefly in association with cholestatic or relapsing hepatitis A include cutaneous vasculitis and cryoglobulinemia.[55, 117, 118] The vasculitis, manifested as erythematous maculopapular lesions often affecting the lower extremities and buttocks and typically associated with purpura, appears as leukocytoclastic vasculitis and granular deposits of IgM anti-HAV and complement in blood vessel walls in skin biopsy specimens. Cryoglobulinemia includes cryoglobulins composed of IgG and IgM and IgM anti-HAV antibodies.[55, 117, 118, 224] These manifestations resolve spontaneously with resolution of the hepatitis.

In the absence of fulminant disease, neurologic syndromes have been observed only rarely in association with hepatitis A. Guillain-Barré syndrome has been reported to occur 3 days to 2 weeks after the onset of hepatitis A, as have myeloradiculopathy, vertigo, mononeuritis (cranial or peripheral nerve), meningoencephalitis, and exacerbation of multiple sclerosis.[10, 25, 198, 256] Renal complications, including acute renal failure, nephrotic syndrome, and acute glomerulonephritis, also rarely have been reported in children who did not have fulminant disease.[9, 58, 123] Self-limited, mild pancreatitis likewise appears to occur.[178] Reported hematologic complications include aplastic anemia and severe thrombocytopenia.[74, 163]

CHOLESTATIC HEPATITIS A

Cholestatic hepatitis occurs in a small percentage of patients with hepatitis A. These patients are deeply icteric and may have pruritus, fatigue, fever, loose stools, anorexia, dark urine, and weight loss. In two reports of 10 patients with cholestatic hepatitis A, peak serum bilirubin levels generally were higher than 10 mg/dL, with some as high as 38 mg/dL, and remained elevated for 12 to 16 weeks.[98, 263] Serum aminotransferase levels declined but remained elevated during the period of cholestasis. In one of these reports, five patients had prolonged prothrombin times that normalized with the administration of vitamin K.[98]

Cholestatic hepatitis A can be distinguished from obstructive jaundice by normal abdominal ultrasound findings. Conducting further invasive diagnostic procedures such as liver biopsy or direct forms of cholangiography is not necessary in most cases.[224] Although patients will recover completely without therapy, a course of corticosteroids with a gradual taper over a span of at least 4 weeks has been reported to hasten relief of symptoms and resolution of cholestasis.[224]

HEPATITIS A TRIGGERING AUTOIMMUNE HEPATITIS

Several reports have described patients in whom hepatitis A is followed by type 1 autoimmune chronic hepatitis.[211, 263, 275] Laboratory studies demonstrated a T-cell defect in these patients, thus suggesting a genetic predisposition to the development of autoimmune hepatitis that is "triggered" by HAV infection. These patients have required corticosteroid therapy, sometimes for long periods.

Treatment

Hepatitis A has no specific therapy, and because HAV infection is self-limited and does not result in chronic infection or chronic liver disease, treatment generally is supportive. Hospitalization may be necessary for patients who are dehydrated from nausea and vomiting or who have fulminant hepatic failure. Because no conclusive data indicate that bed rest or inactivity influences the course of illness, no restriction of activity is necessary. Similarly, no specific diet is indicated, although many patients may have an intolerance to fatty foods during their illness. Medications, particularly those that have the potential to cause hepatic damage and those that are metabolized by the liver, should be used with caution. The half-life of these latter medications may be prolonged.

For fulminant hepatic failure caused by hepatitis A, small uncontrolled trials conducted among adults suggest that some patients have benefited from prostaglandin E and interferon, and amantadine and ribavirin have shown activity in vitro against HAV.[48, 156, 238] No evidence exists that exchange transfusions, plasmapheresis, or corticosteroids are effective.[75, 100] Liver transplantation is successful in some patients.[248, 262, 290] Persistent HAV infection has been demonstrated in some transplant recipients, but whether it affects survival is unknown.[76] Because survival rates of adult and pediatric patients are relatively high without transplantation and no single factor is predictive of a poor outcome, establishing criteria for choosing candidates for transplantation has been difficult.[94, 192, 262, 273] Reported survival rates after transplantation in patients with fulminant hepatitis from all viral causes range from 40 to 89 percent, depending on the severity of liver failure and other factors.[147, 262, 290]

Prevention

In addition to general measures of good personal hygiene, particularly handwashing, provision of safe drinking water, and proper disposal of sanitary waste, pre-exposure or postexposure immunization with immune globulin and pre-exposure immunization with hepatitis A vaccine can prevent the acquisition of hepatitis A.

IMMUNE GLOBULIN

Immune globulin is a sterile solution of antibodies prepared by a serial cold ethanol precipitation procedure from pooled human plasma that has tested negative for hepatitis B surface antigen, antibody to human immunodeficiency virus (HIV), and antibody to hepatitis C virus.[44] This precipitation procedure has been shown to inactivate hepatitis B virus and HIV.[218] Since 1995, immune globulin prepared in the United States has been required to be negative for hepatitis C virus RNA by PCR amplification or to be produced by a method that ensures additional virus inactivation. When administered before exposure or within 2 weeks after exposure, immune globulin is more than 85 percent effective in preventing hepatitis A by passive transfer of anti-HAV.[130, 180, 251] Whether immune globulin completely prevents infection or leads to asymptomatic infection and the development of persistent anti-HAV (passive-active immunity) probably is related to the amount of time that has elapsed between exposure and administration of immune globulin.[149, 251] Although in recent years immune globulin lots have had slightly lower titers of anti-HAV, probably because of a decreasing prevalence of previous HAV infection in plasma donors, no clinical or epidemiologic evidence of decreased efficacy has been reported.[257]

Household and sexual contacts of patients with hepatitis A should receive immune globulin as soon as possible but no later than 2 weeks after exposure.[206] Aggressive use of immune globulin is indicated to control hepatitis A outbreaks in childcare centers in which hepatitis A is diagnosed in a child or employee[206, 229] (Table 172–3) and in other settings (e.g., hospitals, facilities for developmentally disabled persons) when outbreaks occur.[206] When a food handler is identified with hepatitis A, immune globulin should be administered to other food handlers at the establishment and under limited circumstances to patrons.[34, 206] Once cases are identified that are associated with a food service establishment, it generally is too late to administer immune globulin to patrons because the 2-week postexposure period during which is globulin is effective will have passed.

Immune globulin also may be given to persons who are traveling to countries with high, transitional, or intermediate endemicity of HAV infection (see Fig. 172–2) instead of or in addition to hepatitis A vaccine.[206] Immune globulin should be given to children younger than 2 years who are traveling to such countries because hepatitis A vaccine is not licensed in the United States for children in this age group (see the section on vaccines).[206] Although hepatitis A often is asymptomatic in infants and young children, pre-exposure prophylaxis is indicated to prevent the rare severe cases and transmission to others after returning from abroad.

TABLE 172–3 ■ CONTROL OF HEPATITIS A IN CHILDCARE CENTERS

If hepatitis A is diagnosed in a child or employee at a childcare center or hepatitis A cases are identified within a 6-week period in two or more families using the same center, center attendees and employees should receive immune globulin.
If diapered children are at the childcare center, immune globulin should be given to all children and employees at the center. Immunoglobulin also should be given to newly enrolled children and new employees during the 6 weeks after the last center-associated case is identified.
If no diapered children are at the childcare center, immune globulin should be administered only to classroom contacts (children and staff) of the infected child.
If the child with hepatitis A is an older child with no link to a diapered child, immune globulin for classroom contact only can be considered.
Immune globulin administration to household contacts of diapered children in the childcare center should be considered if three or more family members are affected or if the outbreak is recognized more than 3 weeks after the first child becomes ill.
In areas where routine hepatitis A vaccination of children is recommended, previously unvaccinated children can be vaccinated when they receive postexposure prophylaxis with immune globulin.
Parents should be notified not to transfer their children to another center.
Health care providers should report cases of hepatitis A to local public health authorities and consult with local public health authorities regarding preventive measures.

Adapted from Shapiro, C. N., and Hadler, S.C.: Hepatitis A and hepatitis B virus infections in day care centers. Pediatr. Ann. *20*:435–441, 1991.

For postexposure prophylaxis, 0.02 mL/kg body weight of immune globulin should be administered intramuscularly. For infants and young children, the injection can be administered in the anterolateral aspect of the thigh or the deltoid muscles; for older children and adolescents, the injection should be administered in the deltoid or gluteus, muscles into which a large volume of immune globulin can be injected.[90] If the immune globulin is administered in the gluteus, the injection should be given in the superior-lateral aspect to avoid injuring the sciatic nerve.[90]

For pre-exposure prophylaxis of travelers, the dose of immune globulin is 0.02 mL/kg body weight if travel will be for less than 3 months. Because of the decay of passive immunity over the course of time, a dose of 0.06 mL/kg is necessary for persons who will be abroad for 3 to 5 months, and re-administration every 5 months is necessary for extended trips. Hepatitis A vaccine, if not contraindicated, is probably a better choice for such persons.

Serious adverse events from immune globulin are rare. Because anaphylaxis has been reported after repeated administration to persons with IgA deficiency, these persons should not receive immune globulin.[71] Pregnancy or lactation is not a contraindication to the administration of immune globulin. For infants and pregnant women, a preparation that does not include thimerosal is preferable.

Immune globulin does not interfere with the immune response to oral poliovirus or yellow fever vaccine or, in general, to inactivated vaccines. However, immune globulin can interfere with the immune response to some live attenuated vaccines (e.g., measles-mumps-rubella vaccine [MMR], varicella vaccine). Administration of MMR and varicella vaccines should be delayed for at least 3 months and at least 5 months, respectively, after the administration of immune globulin. Immune globulin should not be given within 2 weeks after the administration of MMR or within 3 weeks of the administration of varicella vaccine, unless the benefits of immune globulin administration are greater than the benefits of vaccination.[90] For travelers younger than 2 years in whom the use of immune globulin may interfere with the administration of other needed vaccines (e.g., MMR, varicella), the use of inactivated hepatitis A vaccine could be considered (see the section on inactivated vaccines).

HEPATITIS A VACCINE

The ability to propagate HAV in cell culture allowed for the development of hepatitis A vaccines. Both inactivated and live attenuated hepatitis A vaccines have been developed by using defined isolates from infected cell lines.[64, 165, 166, 175, 240] However, only inactivated vaccines have been evaluated for efficacy in controlled clinical trials and licensed in the United States, and the live attenuated vaccines evaluated to date do not appear to offer any distinct advantage over inactivated vaccines.[120, 283]

Vaccine Preparation and Performance

Inactivated hepatitis A vaccines are prepared by a method similar to that used to prepare inactivated polio vaccine, by propagation of cell culture–adapted virus in human fibroblasts, purification by ultrafiltration or other methods, formalin inactivation, and adsorption to an aluminum hydroxide adjuvant.[7, 41] Inactivated vaccines using the HM175 strain and the CR326F′ strain have been licensed in pediatric and adult formulations for intramuscular administration and are available in the United States for persons 2 years and older (Table 172–4). One of these vaccines (HM175 strain) is formulated with 2-phenoxyethanol as a preservative, whereas the other is formulated without a preservative (see Table 172–4). The antigen content of one vaccine (CR326F′ strain) is expressed as units of HAV antigen as defined by a standard; the antigen content of the other vaccine (HM175 strain) is determined by reactivity in a quantitative immunoassay for HAV antigen and is expressed as enzyme-linked immunosorbent assay (ELISA) units (ELU) (see Table 172–4).

Two other inactivated hepatitis A vaccines are manufactured and available in parts of Europe.[144, 277] In addition, a combination inactivated hepatitis A and recombinant hepatitis B vaccine is available in the United States for persons 18 years and older; a pediatric formulation is available in Europe, Canada, and other parts of the world.[65, 79]

In extensive studies in children and adults, the inactivated hepatitis A vaccines available in the United States have been found to be highly immunogenic. In general, after one dose of vaccine, 95 to 100 percent of children 2 years or older and adults respond with concentrations of antibody considered to be protective; a second dose given 6 to 18 months later results in a boost in antibody concentration and likely is important for long-term protection.[11, 41, 112, 174, 185] IgM anti-HAV occasionally can be detected by standard assays, primarily if measured soon (i.e., 2 to 3 weeks) after vaccination (CDC, unpublished data).[236, 239]

Studies in children younger than 2 years are limited but suggest that the vaccine is safe and immunogenic for those who do not have passively transferred antibody from previous maternal HAV infection.[200, 230, 266] In studies of infants who received hepatitis A vaccine according to several different schedules, those with passively transferred maternal antibody at the time of vaccination responded, but final antibody concentrations were approximately one third to one tenth those of infants who did not have passively transferred antibody and were vaccinated according to the same schedule.[53, 158, 200, 230, 266] The clinical significance, if any, of these lower antibody concentrations is unknown. One study found that all infants vaccinated in the presence of passively transferred maternal antibody responded to a booster dose given 6 months later with an anamnestic response, thus suggesting that they had been primed by the primary series.[53] However, in another small study, two of six children who had lost detectable antibody did not have an anamnestic response to a booster dose administered approximately 6 years after receiving the primary vaccine series in infancy in the presence of passively transferred antibody.[81] Most infants born to anti-HAV–positive mothers have lost detectable antibody by the time they reach 12 to 15 months of age, and studies are under way to determine a dosage and schedule of hepatitis A vaccine for use in the first 2 years of life.[86, 159]

Inactivated hepatitis A vaccine has been shown to be highly efficacious in preventing clinically apparent disease. In a study of approximately 40,000 Thai children 1 to 16 years of age, the efficacy of inactivated vaccine (HM175 strain) was 94 percent (95% confidence interval, 79 to 99%) after two doses (360 ELU per dose) administered 1 month apart.[120] In a study of another inactivated vaccine (CR326F′ strain) involving approximately 1000 children 2 to 16 years of age in a New York community with high hepatitis A rates, efficacy was 100 percent (lower bound of the 95% confidence interval, 87%) starting 17 days after the administration of one dose (25 U).[283]

Since hepatitis A vaccines became available in the United States in 1995, studies and demonstration projects have evaluated their effectiveness in controlling and preventing the development of hepatitis A in communities. In areas with the highest hepatitis A rates (see Table 172–1), such as

TABLE 172–4 ■ RECOMMENDED DOSES AND SCHEDULES OF HEPATITIS A VACCINES*

Age (yr)	Vaccine	Dose	Volume (mL)	No. Doses	Schedule (mo)†
2–18	HAVRIX	720 ELU	0.5	2	0, 6–12
	VAQTA	25 U	0.5	2	0, 6–18
≥19	HAVRIX	1440 ELU	1.0	2	0, 6–12
	VAQTA	50 U	1.0	2	0, 6–12

ELU, enzyme-linked immunosorbent assay units.
*HAVRIX is manufactured from hepatitis A virus (HAV) strain HM175 by Glaxo SmithKline; VAQTA is manufactured from HAV strain CR326F′ by Merck & Co, Inc.
†Zero months represents timing of the initial dose; subsequent numbers represent months after the initial dose.

American Indian and Alaska Native communities, vaccination of the majority of children—and in some cases adolescents and young adults—resulted in a rapid decline in the incidence of disease, and with ongoing routine vaccination of children, the reduction in incidence of disease has been sustained.[111, 173, 283] In larger, more heterogeneous communities with lower, but consistently elevated hepatitis A rates, interrupting ongoing community-wide epidemics by vaccinating children has proved difficult.[8, 47] First-dose coverage generally has been low (20–45%), and the impact of vaccination often has been limited to vaccinated age groups, which may not represent most cases. In contrast, the results of a demonstration project of ongoing, routine vaccination of children conducted from 1995 to 2000 in a county in California suggest that this strategy can reduce the incidence of hepatitis A markedly over the course of time.[8] During the 6-year-long project, the number of reported cases declined by 94 percent. The four cases reported in 2000 represented the lowest number ever reported in the county since surveillance began in 1966, and the county's 2000 incidence rate was the lowest of any county in California.

Several lines of evidence suggest that hepatitis A vaccine may have some efficacy when administered after exposure to HAV, but definitive studies have not been conducted. Hepatitis A vaccine administered soon after exposure prevented infection in a chimpanzee model.[214] However, only one small randomized trial in humans has been completed, and hepatitis A vaccine was found to be 79 percent efficacious in preventing infection when compared with no treatment.[220] However, the confidence interval was wide (7–95%), and the study did not include a comparison group that received passive postexposure prophylaxis with immune globulin.[16] Because of the demonstrated high efficacy of immune globulin when administered after exposure to HAV, it continues to be recommended by most U.S. advisory groups for postexposure prophylaxis.[4, 206]

Experience to date indicates that the incidence of adverse events after vaccination is comparable to that after the administration of other widely used vaccines. In prelicensure clinical studies in children, the side effects reported most frequently included soreness, tenderness, warmth, or induration at the injection site (4–19%); feeding problems (8%); and headache (4%). Through 1998, more than 6.5 million doses, including more than 2.3 million pediatric doses, were administered to the U.S. civilian population, and more than 65 million doses had been administered worldwide.[206] No serious adverse events in children or adults have been identified that could be definitively ascribed to hepatitis A vaccine.[22, 188] For events for which incidence rates are available, such as Guillain-Barré syndrome, reported rates were not higher than reported background rates.[206]

Antibody has been shown to persist at high levels in vaccinated adults and children for at least 5 to 8 years after vaccination.[78, 272, 288] In one follow-up study, two thirds of infants who did not have passively transferred maternal antibody at the time of vaccination had detectable anti-HAV 6 years later, and all who had lost antibody had an anamnestic response to a booster dose.[81] Estimates based on kinetic models of decline in antibody suggest that the duration of protection could be 20 years or longer.[272, 287, 288]

In some settings, performing prevaccination serologic testing may be considered in an attempt to reduce cost by not vaccinating persons with previous immunity.[32] Testing of children is not indicated because of their expected low prevalence of infection and the lower cost of vaccine for this age group. Testing may be considered for older adolescents in certain population groups with a high prevalence of infection (e.g., American Indians, Alaska Natives), but the cost of testing, vaccine cost, and the likelihood that the person will return for vaccination should take into account. Postvaccination testing is not indicated because of the high rate of response to the vaccine. Furthermore, testing methods that can detect the low anti-HAV concentrations generated by immunization are not licensed for use in the United States.

Vaccine Recommendations and Use

Recommendations for the use of hepatitis A vaccine were issued first by the Advisory Committee on Immunization Practices of the U.S. Public Health Service (Table 172–5),

TABLE 172–5 ■ RECOMMENDATIONS FOR ROUTINE PRE-EXPOSURE USE OF HEPATITIS A VACCINE*

Group	Comments
Children living in communities with consistently high rates of hepatitis A	Includes Alaska, Arizona, California, Idaho, Nevada, New Mexico, Oklahoma, Oregon, South Dakota, Utah, Washington, and selected areas in other states.†‡
International travelers§	Immune globulin may be given in addition to or instead of vaccine; children <2 yr old should receive immune globulin
Men who have sex with men	Includes adolescents
Illicit drug users	Includes adolescents
Persons with chronic liver disease	Increased risk of fulminant hepatitis A with HAV infection
Persons receiving clotting factor concentrates	
Persons who work with HAV in research laboratory settings	

*Hepatitis A vaccine is not licensed for children younger than 2 years.

†Where the average reported hepatitis A incidence from 1987 to 1997 was 20/100,000 population or greater (approximately twice the national average).

‡Routine vaccination also can be considered for children living in Arkansas, Colorado, Missouri, Montana, Texas, Wyoming, and selected areas in other states where the average reported incidence from 1987 to 1997 was 10/100,000 population or higher.

§Persons traveling to Canada, Western Europe, Japan, Australia, or New Zealand are at no greater risk than in the United States.

From Prevention of hepatitis A through active or passive immunization. Recommendation of the Advisory Committee on Immunization Practices (ACIP). M. M. W. R. Recomm. Rep. *48*(RR-12):1–37, 1999.

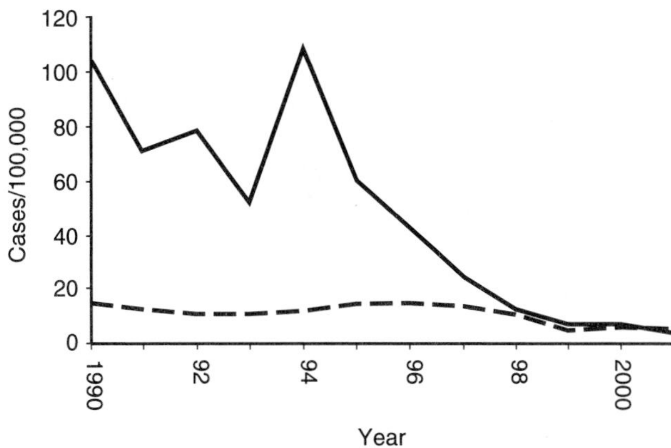

FIGURE 172–6 ■ Hepatitis A incidence rates (per 100,000 populations) among American Indians and Alaska Natives and all other racial/ethnic groups based on cases reported to the Centers for Disease Control and Prevention (1990–2001). The *solid line* represents American Indians and Alaska Natives, and the *dashed line* represents all other groups. Routine hepatitis A vaccination of American Indian and Alaska Native children was recommended by the Advisory Committee on Immunization Practices in 1996.

the American Academy of Pediatrics, and other groups in 1996; they were updated in 1999.[4, 205, 206] To achieve a sustained reduction in the overall incidence of hepatitis A, widespread routine vaccination is needed. Therefore, these recommendations call for routine vaccination of children living in areas where rates of hepatitis A consistently have been elevated, beginning when the children are 2 years or older (see Tables 172–1 and 172–5). Various vaccination strategies that are being used include vaccinating one or more single-age cohorts of children or adolescents, vaccinating children in selected settings (e.g., daycare), and vaccinating children and adolescents over a wide range of ages in a variety of settings, such as when they seek health care for other purposes.

The impact of routine vaccination of children can been seen in areas that historically have had the highest hepatitis A rates (e.g., American Indian communities), where this strategy has been recommended since 1996 (Fig. 172–6). Surveys conducted in 1999 to 2000 indicated vaccination coverage of 50 to 80 percent of preschool- and school-age American Indian and Alaska Native children, thus suggesting that the recommendation for routine vaccination was being implemented.[20] By 2000, the incidence of hepatitis A in American Indians and Alaska Natives had declined by 97 percent when compared with the beginning of the preceding decade and was the same as the overall U.S. rate[20] (see Fig. 172–6).

National surveillance data suggest that routine vaccination of children living in areas with consistently elevated rates, which has been recommended since 1999, has had an impact on the overall incidence of hepatitis A in the United States. The 2001 rate of 3.8 per 100,000 population is a historic low (see Fig. 172–4). Rates declined most dramatically in parts of the country in which routine vaccination of children is recommended (see Table 172–5). When compared with the average rates from 1987 to 1997, the provisional 2001 rate in these states declined by approximately 80 percent versus a 39 percent decrease elsewhere.[221] However, because the incidence of hepatitis A is cyclic, ongoing monitoring of incidence rates will be needed to determine the overall impact of the current strategy.

Vaccination of persons at increased risk of acquiring hepatitis A, including travelers to countries where hepatitis A is endemic, adolescent and adult men who have sex with men, persons who use illegal drugs, those who work with HAV in research settings, and persons who have clotting factor disorders, also is recommended.[206] Vaccination likewise is recommended for persons with chronic liver disease because of the high case-fatality rate among these persons if they acquire hepatitis A.[14]

Considerable interest has been generated in the use of hepatitis A vaccine to control ongoing community-wide epidemics. Implementation of routine vaccination of children, which is recommended for most of the communities that experience these outbreaks, will prevent them in the future. Because of logistic difficulties, accelerated vaccination as an additional measure to control outbreaks should be undertaken with caution (see the section on vaccine preparation and performance). Effort probably is better directed toward sustained routine vaccination of children to maintain high levels of immunity and prevent future epidemics.

Although outbreaks of hepatitis A occur in childcare centers, their frequency is not sufficiently high to warrant routine vaccination of attendees or staff to prevent such outbreaks (see the section on the epidemiology of hepatitis A in specific settings), and little experience has been gained in using vaccine to control outbreaks when they occur.[24] When outbreaks are recognized, aggressive use of immune globulin is effective in limiting transmission (see Table 172–3). In areas where routine vaccination of children is recommended, previously unvaccinated children can be vaccinated when they receive postexposure prophylaxis with immune globulin.[206] In addition, childcare center attendees can be a readily accessible target population for ongoing routine vaccination programs.

Vaccination of successive cohorts of children eventually should result in a sustained reduction in the incidence of disease nationwide and thus provide the opportunity to eliminate HAV transmission. To achieve this goal, vaccination of young children nationwide will be needed. Advances in hepatitis A vaccine development, such as the availability of a vaccine that can be used in the first 2 years of life and combination vaccines that include hepatitis A vaccine, would facilitate this effort.

REFERENCES

1. Abe, H., Beninger, P. R., Ikejiri, N., et al.: Light microscopic findings of liver biopsy specimens from patients with hepatitis type A and comparison with type B. Gastroenterology *82*:938–947, 1982.
2. Akriviadis, E. A., and Redeker, A. G.: Fulminant hepatitis A in intravenous drug users with chronic liver disease. Ann. Intern. Med. *110*:838–839, 1989.
3. Alhan, E., Yildizdas, D., Yapicioglu, H., and Necmi, A.: Pleural effusion associated with acute hepatitis A infection. Letter. Pediatr. Infect. Dis. J. *18*:1111–1112, 1999.
4. American Academy of Pediatrics: Hepatitis A. *In* Pickering, L. K. (ed.): 2000 Red Book: Report of the Committee on Infectious Diseases. 25th ed. Elk Grove Village, IL, American Academy of Pediatrics, 2000, pp. 280–289.
5. Anderson, D. A.: Cytopathology, plaque assay, and heat inactivation of hepatitis A strain HM-175. J. Med. Virol. *22*:35–44, 1987.
6. Armstrong, G. L., and Bell, B. P.: Hepatitis A virus infections in the United States: Model-based estimates and implications for childhood immunization. Pediatrics *109*:839–845, 2002.
7. Armstrong, M. E., Giesa, P. A., Davide, J. P., et al.: Development of the formalin-inactivated hepatitis A vaccine VAQTA from the live attenuated virus strain CR326F. J. Hepatol. *18*(Suppl. 2):20–26, 1993.
8. Averhoff, F., Shapiro, C. N., Bell, B. P., et al.: The effectiveness of routine childhood hepatitis A immunization in the prevention of hepatitis A. J. A. M. A. *286*:2968–2973, 2001.
9. Aydin, A., Mikla, S., Ficicioglu, C., et al.: Nephrotic syndrome associated with hepatitis A virus infection. Letter. Pediatr. Infect. Dis. J. *18*:391, 1999.

10. Azuri, J., Lerman-Sagie, T., Mizrahi, A., and Bujanover, Y.: Guillain-Barré syndrome following serological evidence of hepatitis A in a child. Eur. J. Pediatr. *158*:341–342, 1999.
11. Balcarek, K. B., Bagley, M. R., Pass, R. F., et al.: Safety and immunogenicity of an inactivated hepatitis A vaccine in preschool children. J. Infect. Dis. *171*(Suppl. 1):70–72, 1995.
12. Bartoloni, A., Aquilini, D., Roselli, M., et al.: Prevalence of antibody to hepatitis A virus in the Santa Cruz region of Bolivia. J. Trop. Med. Hyg. *92*:279–281, 1989.
13. Barzaga, N. G.: Hepatitis A shifting epidemiology in South-East Asia and China. Vaccine *18*(Suppl.):61–64, 2000.
14. Bell, B. P.: Hepatitis A and hepatitis B vaccination of patients with chronic liver disease. Acta Gastroenterol. Belg. *63*:359–365, 2000.
15. Bell, B. P.: Global epidemiology of hepatitis A: Implications for control strategies. *In* Margolis, H. S., Alter, M. J., Liang, T. J., and Dienstag, J. L. (eds.): Viral Hepatitis and Liver Disease. London, International Medical Press, 2002, pp. 9–14.
16. Bell, B. P., and Margolis, H. S.: Efficacy of hepatitis A vaccine in prevention of secondary hepatitis A infection. Letter. Lancet *354*:341, 1999.
17. Bell, B. P., Shapiro, C. N., Alter, M. J., et al.: The diverse patterns of hepatitis A epidemiology in the United States. Implications for vaccination strategies. J. Infect. Dis. *178*:1579–1584, 1998.
18. Benenson, M. W., Takafuji, E. T., Bancroft, W. H., et al.: A military community outbreak of hepatitis type A related to transmission in a child care facility. Am. J. Epidemiol. *112*:471–481, 1980.
19. Bergeisen, G. H., Hinds, M. W., and Skaggs, J. W.: A waterborne outbreak of hepatitis A in Meade County, Kentucky. Am. J. Public Health *75*:161–164, 1985.
20. Bialek, S., Thoroughman, D., and Bell, B. P.: Trends in hepatitis A incidence among American Indians, 1990–1999. Antiviral Ther. *5*(Suppl. 1):11, 2000.
21. Binn, L. N., Lemon, S. M., Marchwicki, R. H., et al.: Primary isolation and serial passage of hepatitis A virus strains in primate cell cultures. J. Clin. Microbiol. *20*:28–33, 1984.
22. Black, S., Shinefield, H., Su, L., et al.: Post-marketing safety evaluation of inactivated hepatitis A vaccine (VAQTA, Merck) in 9740 children and adults. Abstract. *In* Program and Abstracts: 38th Interscience Conference on Antimicrobial Agents and Chemotherapy (ICAAC). Washington, DC, American Society for Microbiology, 1998.
23. Bloch, A. B., Stramer, S. L., Smith, D., et al.: Recovery of hepatitis A virus from a water supply responsible for a common source outbreak of hepatitis A. Am. J. Public Health *80*:428–430, 1990.
24. Bonnani, P., Colombai, R., Franchi, G., et al.: Experience of hepatitis A vaccination during an outbreak in a nursery school of Tuscany, Italy. Epidemiol. Infect. *121*:377–380, 1998.
25. Bosch, V. V., Dowling, P. C., and Cook, S. D.: Hepatitis A virus immunoglobulin M antibody in acute neurological disease. Ann. Neurol. *14*:685–687, 1983.
26. Böttiger, M., Christenson, B., and Grillner, L.: Hepatitis A immunity in the Swedish population. A study of prevalence markers in the Swedish population. Scand. J. Infect. Dis. *29*:99–102, 1997.
27. Bowen, G. S., and McCarthy, M.: Hepatitis A associated with a hardware store water fountain and a contaminated well in Lancaster County, Pennsylvania, 1980. Am. J. Epidemiol. *117*:695–705, 1983.
28. Bower, W. A., Nainan, O. V., Han, X., and Margolis, H. S.: Duration of viremia in hepatitis A virus infection. J. Infect. Dis. *182*:12–17, 2000.
29. Bradley, D. W., Fields, H. A., McCaustland, K. A., et al.: Biochemical and biophysical characterization of light and heavy density hepatitis A virus particles: Evidence HAV is an RNA virus. J. Med. Virol. *2*:175–187, 1978.
30. Brown, V. K., and Robertson, B. H.: Immunoselection of clinical specimens containing virus followed by polymerase chain reaction amplification and rapid direct sequencing. Biotechniques *8*:10–12, 1990.
31. Bryan, J. A., Lehmann, J. D., Setiady, I. F., et al.: An outbreak of hepatitis A associated with recreational lake water. Am. J. Epidemiol. *99*:145–154, 1974.
32. Bryan, J. P., and Nelson, M.: Testing for antibody to hepatitis A to decrease the cost of hepatitis A prophylaxis with immune globulin or hepatitis A vaccines. Arch. Intern. Med. *154*:663–668, 1994.
33. Bulkow, L. R., Wainwright, R. B., McMahon, B. J., et al.: Secular trends in hepatitis A virus infection among Alaska Natives. J. Infect. Dis. *168*:1017–1020, 1993.
34. Carl, M., Francis, D. P., and Maynard, J. P.: Food-borne hepatitis A: Recommendation for control. J. Infect. Dis. *148*:1133–1135, 1983.
35. Centers for Disease Control and Prevention: Hepatitis Surveillance Report No. 54. Atlanta, CDC, 1992.
36. Centers for Disease Control and Prevention: Hepatitis Surveillance Report No. 57. Atlanta, CDC, 2000.
37. Chan, T. K., and Todd, D.: Hemolysis complicating viral hepatitis in patients with glucose-6-phosphate dehydrogenase deficiency. B. M. J. *1*:131–133, 1975.
38. Christenson, B.: Epidemiological aspects of acute viral hepatitis A in Swedish travelers to endemic areas. Scand. J. Infect. Dis. *17*:5–10, 1985.
39. Cianciara, J.: Hepatitis A shifting epidemiology in Poland and Eastern Europe. Vaccine *18*(Suppl.):68–70, 2000.
40. Ciocca, M.: Clinical course and consequences of hepatitis A virus infection. Vaccine *18*(Suppl.):71–74, 2000.
41. Clemens, R., Safary, A., Hepburn, A., et al.: Clinical experience with an inactivated hepatitis A vaccine. J. Infect. Dis. *17*(Suppl. 1):44–49, 1995.
42. Cohen, H. A., Amir, J., Frydman, M., et al.: Infection with the hepatitis A virus associated with ascites in children. Am. J. Dis. Child. *146*:1014–1016, 1992.
43. Cohen, J. I., Feinstone, S., and Purcell, R. H.: Hepatitis A virus infection in a chimpanzee: Duration of viremia and detection of virus in saliva and throat swabs. J. Infect. Dis. *160*:887–890, 1989.
44. Cohn, E. J., Oncley, J. L., Strong, L. E., et al.: Chemical, clinical, and immunological studies on the products of human plasma fractionation. I. The characterization of the protein fractions of human plasma. J. Clin. Invest. *23*:417–432, 1944.
45. Cotter, S., Sansom, S., Long, T., et al.: Outbreak of hepatitis A among men who have sex with men: Implications for hepatitis A vaccination strategies. J. Infect. Dis. In press.
46. Coutinho, R. A., Albrecht-Van Lent, P., Lelie, N., et al.: Prevalence and incidence of hepatitis A among male homosexuals. B. M. J. *287*:1743–1745, 1983.
47. Craig, A. S., Sockwell, D. C., Schaffner, W., et al.: Use of hepatitis A vaccine in a communitywide outbreak of hepatitis A. Clin. Infect. Dis. *27*:531–535, 1998.
48. Crance, J. M., Biziagos, E., Passagot, J., et al.: Inhibition of hepatitis A virus replication in vitro by antiviral compounds. J. Med. Virol. *31*:155–160, 1990.
49. Cromeans, T., Nainan, O. V., Fields, H. A. et al.: Hepatitis A and E viruses. *In* Hui, Y. H., Gorham, J. R., Murrell, K. D., et al. (eds.): Foodborne Disease Handbook. New York, Marcel Dekker, 1994, pp. 1–56.
50. Cromeans, T., Sobsey, M. D., and Fields, H. A.: Development of a plaque assay for a cytopathic, rapidly replicating isolate of hepatitis A virus. J. Med. Virol. *22*:45–56, 1987.
51. Coursaget, P., Leboulleux, D., Gharbi, Y., et al.: Etiology of acute sporadic hepatitis in adults in Senegal and Tunisia. Scand. J. Infect. Dis. *27*:9–11, 1995.
52. Daemer, R. J., Feinstone, S. M., Gust, I. D., et al.: Propagation of human hepatitis A virus in African green monkey kidney cell culture: Primary isolation and serial passage. Infect. Immun. *32*:388–393, 1981.
53. Dagan, R., Amir, J., Mijalovsky, A., et al.: Immunization against hepatitis A in the first year of life: Priming despite the presence of maternal antibody. Pediatr. Infect. Dis. J. *19*:1045–1052, 2000.
54. Dalton, C. B., Haddix, A., Hoffman, R. E., and Mast, E. E.: The cost of a food-borne outbreak of hepatitis A in Denver, Colo. Arch. Intern. Med. *156*:1013–1016, 1996.
55. Dan, M., and Yaniv, R.: Cholestatic hepatitis, cutaneous vasculitis and vascular deposits of immunoglobulin M and complement associated with hepatitis A virus infection. Am. J. Med. *89*:103–104, 1990.
56. Das, K., Jain, A., Gupta, S., et al.: The changing epidemiological pattern of hepatitis A in an urban population of India: Emergence of a trend similar to the European countries. Eur. J. Epidemiol. *16*:507–510, 2000.
57. Datta, D., Williams, I., Culver, D., et al.: Association between deaths due to hepatitis A and chronic liver disease, United States, 1981–1997. Antiviral Ther. *5*(Suppl. 1):79, 2000.
58. Demiricin, G., Öner, A., Tinaztepe, K., et al.: Acute glomerulonephritis in hepatitis A virus infection. J. Pediatr. Gastroenterol. Nutr. *27*:86–89, 1998.
59. Dentinger, C., Heinrich, N. L., Bell, B. P., et al.: A prevalence study of hepatitis A virus infection in a migrant community: Is hepatitis A vaccine indicated? J. Pediatr. *138*:705–709, 2001.
60. Dentinger, C. M., Bower, W. A., Nainan, O. V., et al.: An outbreak of hepatitis A associated with green onions. J. Infect. Dis. *183*:1273–1276, 2001.
61. Desenclos, J. A., Klontz, K. C., Wilder, M. H., et al.: A multistate outbreak of hepatitis A caused by the consumption of raw oysters. Am. J. Public Health *81*:1268–1272, 1991.
62. Desenclos, J. A., and MacLafferty, L.: Communitywide outbreak of hepatitis A linked to children in day care centers and with increased transmission in young adult men in Florida, 1988–9. J. Epidemiol. Community Health *47*:269–273, 1993.
63. De Serres, G., Cromeans, T. L., Levesque, B., et al.: Molecular confirmation of hepatitis A virus from well water: Epidemiology and public health implications. J. Infect. Dis. *179*:37–43, 1999.
64. D'Hondt, E.: Possible approaches to develop vaccines against hepatitis A. Vaccine *10*(Suppl. 1):48–52, 1992.
65. Diaz-Mitoma, F., Law, B., and Parsons, J.: A combined vaccine against hepatitis A and B in children and adolescents. Pediatr. Infect. Dis. J. *18*:108–114, 1999.
66. Dienstag, J. L., Lucas, C. R., Gust, I. D., et al.: Mussel-associated viral hepatitis, type A: Serological confirmation. Lancet *1*:561–564, 1976.
67. Dmochowski, L.: Viral type A and type B hepatitis: Morphology, biology, immunology and epidemiology—A review. Am. J. Clin. Pathol. *65*:741–786, 1976.
68. Dollberg, S., Berkun, Y., and Gross-Kisselstein E.: Urticaria in patients with hepatitis A infection. Pediatr. Infect. Dis. J. *10*:702–703, 1991.
69. Dollberg, S., Kerem, E., Klar, A., et al.: Disappearance of IgM antibodies to hepatitis A virus after acute infection in children and adolescents. J. Pediatr. Gastroenterol. Nutr. *10*:307–309, 1990.

70. Draelos, Z. K., Hansen, R. C., and James, W. D.: Gianotti-Crosti syndrome associated with infections other than hepatitis B. J. A. M. A. *256*:2386–2388, 1986.
71. Ellis, E. F., and Henney, C. S.: Adverse reactions following administration of human gamma globulin. J Allergy Clin Immunol *43*:45–54, 1969.
72. Emerson, S. U., Huang, Y. K., McRill, C., et al.: Mutations in both the 2B and 2C genes of hepatitis A virus are involved in adaptation to growth in cell culture. J. Virol. *66*:650–654, 1992.
73. Emerson, S. U., McRill, C., Rosenblum, B., et al.: Mutations responsible for adaptation of hepatitis A virus to efficient growth in cell culture. J. Virol. *65*:4882–4886, 1991.
74. Ertem, D., Acar, Y., Arat, C., and Pehlivanoglu, E.: Thrombotic and thrombocytopenic complications secondary to hepatitis A infection in children. Letter. Am. J. Gastroenterol. *94*:3653–3655, 1999.
75. European Association for the Study of the Liver (EASL): Randomised trial of steroid therapy for acute liver failure. Gut *20*:620–623, 1979.
76. Fagan, E., Yousef, G., Brahm, J., et al.: Persistence of hepatitis A virus in fulminant hepatitis and after liver transplantation. J. Med. Virol. *30*:131–136, 1990.
77. Fainboim, L., Velasco, M. C. C., Marcos, C. Y., et al.: Protracted, but not acute, hepatitis A virus infection is strongly associated with HLA-DRB1*1301, a marker for pediatric autoimmune hepatitis. Hepatology *33*:1512–1517, 2001.
78. Fan, P. C., Chang, M. H., Lee, P. I., et al.: Follow up immunogenicity of an inactivated hepatitis A virus vaccine in healthy children: Results after 5 years. Vaccine *16*:232–235, 1998.
79. FDA approval for a combined hepatitis A and B vaccine. M. M. W. R. Morb. Mortal. Wkly. Rep. *50*(37):806–807, 2001.
80. Feinstone, S. M., Kapikian, A. Z., and Purcell, R. H.: Hepatitis A: Detection by immune electron microscopy of a virus-like antigen association with acute illness. Science *182*:1026–1028, 1973.
81. Fiore, A. E., Shapiro, C. N., Sabin, K. M., et al.: Hepatitis A vaccination of infants: Effect of maternal antibody status on antibody persistence and response to a booster dose. Pediatr. Infect. Dis. J. In press.
82. Fishman, L. N., Jonas, M. M., and Lavine, J. E.: Update on viral hepatitis in children. Pediatr. Clin. North Am. *43*:57–74, 1996.
83. Fleischer, B., Fleischer, S., Maier, K., et al.: Clonal analysis of infiltrating T lymphocytes in liver tissue in viral hepatitis A. Immunology *69*:14–19, 1990.
84. Foodborne hepatitis A: Alaska, Florida, North Carolina, Washington. M. M. W. R. Morb. Mortal. Wkly. Rep. *39*(14):228–232, 1990.
85. Fornasini, M. A., Morrow, A. L., and Pickering, L. K.: Illness and health-related benefits among child daycare providers. Abstract 835. Paper presented at a meeting of the American Pediatric Society and Society for Pediatric Research, Seattle, 1994.
86. Franzen, C., and Frosner, G.: Placental transfer of hepatitis A antibody. N. Engl. J. Med. *304*:427, 1981.
87. Friedman, L. S., O'Brien, T. F., Morse, L. J., et al.: Revisiting the Holy Cross football team hepatitis outbreak (1969) by serological analysis. J. A. M. A. *254*:774–777, 1985.
88. Friedman, M. S., Blake, P. A., Koehler, J. E., et al.: Factors influencing a communitywide campaign to administer hepatitis A vaccine to men who have sex with men. Am. J. Public Health *90*:1942–1946, 2000.
89. Gdalevich, M., Grotto, I., Mandel, Y., et al.: Hepatitis A antibody prevalence among young adults in Israel—the decline continues. Epidemiol. Infect. *121*:477–479, 1998.
90. General recommendations on immunization: Recommendations of the Advisory Committee on Immunization Practices (ACIP). M. M. W. R. Recomm. Rep. *43*(RR-1):1–38, 1994.
91. Gerety, R. J., Smallwood, L. A., Finlayson, J. S., Tabor, E.: Standardization of the antibody to hepatitis A virus (anti-HAV) content of immunoglobulin. Dev. Biol. Stand. *54*:411–416, 1983.
92. Gibas, A., Biewett, D. R., Schoenfeld, D. A., et al.: Prevalence and incidence of viral hepatitis in health workers in the prehepatitis B vaccination era. Am. J. Epidemiol. *136*:603–610, 1992.
93. Gil, A., Gonzalez, A., Dal-Ré, R., et al.: Prevalence of antibodies against varicella zoster, herpes simplex (types 1 and 2), hepatitis B, and hepatitis A viruses among Spanish adolescents. J. Infect. *36*:53–56, 1998.
94. Gimson, A. E. S., White, Y. S., Eddleston, A. L. W. F., et al.: Clinical and prognostic differences in fulminant hepatitis type A, B and non-A, non-B. Gut *24*:1194–1198, 1983.
95. Gingrich, G. A., Hadler, S. C., Elder, H. A., et al.: Serologic investigation of an outbreak of hepatitis A in a rural day-care center. Am. J. Public Health *73*:1190–1193, 1983.
96. Glikson, M., Galun, E., Oren, R., et al.: Relapsing hepatitis A: Review of 14 cases and literature survey. Medicine (Baltimore) *71*:14–23, 1992.
97. Goodman, R. A.: Nosocomial hepatitis A. Ann. Intern. Med. *103*:452–454, 1985.
98. Gordon, S. C., Reddy, K. R., Schiff, L., et al.: Prolonged intrahepatic cholestasis secondary to acute hepatitis A. Ann. Intern. Med. *101*:635–637, 1984.
99. Green, M. S., Colin, B., and Slater, P. E.: Rise in the incidence of viral hepatitis in Israel despite improved socioeconomic conditions. Rev. Infect. Dis. *2*:464–469, 1989.
100. Gust, I. D., and Feinstone, S. M.: History. *In* Gust, I. D., and Feinstone, S. M. (eds.): Hepatitis. Boca Raton, FL, CRC Press, 1988, pp. 1–19.
101. Gustafson, T. L., Hutcheson, R. H., Fricker, R. S., et al.: An outbreak of foodborne hepatitis A: The value of serologic testing and matched case-control analysis. Am. J. Public Health *73*:1191–1201, 1983.
102. Hadler, S. C.: Global impact of hepatitis A virus infection: Changing patterns. *In* Hollinger, F. B., Lemon, S. M., and Margolis, H. S. (eds.): Viral Hepatitis and Liver Disease. Baltimore, Williams & Wilkins, 1991, pp. 14–20.
103. Hadler, S. C., Erben, J. J., Matthews, D., et al.: Effect of immunoglobulin on hepatitis A in day-care centers. J. A. M. A. *249*:48–53, 1983.
104. Hadler, S. C., Webster, H., Erben, J. J., et al.: Hepatitis A in day-care centers: A community-wide assessment. N. Engl. J. Med. *302*: 1222–1227, 1980.
105. Halliday, M. L., Kang, L.-Y., Zhou, T., et al.: An epidemic of hepatitis A attributable to the ingestion of raw clams in Shanghai, China. J. Infect. Dis. *164*:852–859, 1991.
106. Harkness, J., Gildon, B., and Istre, G. R.: Outbreaks of hepatitis A among illicit drug users, Oklahoma, 1984–87. Am. J. Public Health *79*:463–466, 1989.
107. Hatzakis, A., and Hadziyannis, S.: Sex-related differences in immunoglobulin M and total antibody response to hepatitis A observed in two epidemics of hepatitis A. Am. J. Epidemiol. *120*:936–942, 1984.
108. Henning, K. J., Bell, E., Braun, J., and Barker, N.: A community-wide outbreak of hepatitis A: Risk factors for infection among homosexual and bisexual men. Am. J. Med. *99*:132–136, 1995.
109. Hepatitis A among drug abusers. M. M. W. R. Morb. Mortal. Wkly. Rep. *37*(19):297–300, 305, 1988.
110. Hepatitis A among homosexual men: United States, Canada, and Australia. M. M. W. R. Morb. Mortal. Wkly. Rep. *41*(9):155, 161–164, 1992.
111. Hepatitis A vaccination programs in communities with high rates of hepatitis A. M. M. W. R. Morb. Mortal. Wkly. Rep. *46*(26):600–603, 1997.
112. Horng, Y. C., Chang, M. H., Lee, C. Y., et al.: Safety and immunogenicity of hepatitis A vaccine in healthy children. Pediatr. Infect. Dis. J. *12*:359–362, 1993.
113. Huang, S.-N., Lorenz, D., and Gerety, R. J.: Electron and immunoelectron microscopic study on liver tissues of marmosets infected with hepatitis A virus. Lab. Invest. *41*:63–71, 1979.
114. Hutin, Y. J. F., Bell, B. P., Marshall, K. L. E., et al.: Identifying target groups for a potential vaccination program during a hepatitis A communitywide outbreak. Am. J. Public Health *89*:918–921, 1999.
115. Hutin, Y. J. F., Pool, V., Cramer, E. H., et al.: A multistate foodborne outbreak of hepatitis A. N. Engl. J. Med. *340*:595–602, 1999.
116. Hutin, Y. J. F., Sabin, K. M., Hutwagner, L. C., et al.: Multiple modes of hepatitis A virus transmission among methamphetamine users. Am. J. Epidemiol. *152*:186–192, 2000.
117. Ilan, Y., Hillman, M., Oren, R., et al.: Vasculitis and cryoglobulinemia associated with persisting cholestatic hepatitis A virus infection. Am. J. Gastroenterol. *85*:586–587, 1990.
118. Inman, R. D., Hodge, M., Johnston, M. E. A., et al.: Arthritis, vasculitis and cryoglobulinemia associated with relapsing hepatitis A virus infection. Ann. Intern. Med. *105*:700–703, 1986.
119. Innis, B. L., Snitbhan, R., Hoke, C. H., et al.: The declining transmission of hepatitis A in Thailand. J. Infect. Dis. *163*:989–995, 1991.
120. Innis, B. L., Snitbhan, R., Kunasol, P., et al.: Protection against hepatitis A by an inactivated vaccine. J. A. M. A. *271*:1328–1334, 1994.
121. Ivie, K., Spruill, C., and Bell, B. P.: Prevalence of hepatitis A virus infection among illicit drug users, 1993–1994. Antiviral Ther. *5*(Suppl. 1):A.7, 2000.
122. Jackson, L. A., Stewart, L. K., Solomon, S. L., et al.: Risk of infection with hepatitis A, B or C, cytomegalovirus, varicella, or measles among child care providers. Pediatr. Infect. Dis. J. *15*:584–589, 1996.
123. Jamil, S. M., and Massry, S. G.: Acute anuric renal failure in nonfulminant hepatitis A infection. Am. J. Nephrol. *18*:329–332, 1998.
124. Jansen, R. W., Newbold, J. E., and Lemon, S. M.: Combined immunoaffinity cDNA-RNA hybridization assay for detection of hepatitis A virus in clinical specimens. J. Clin. Microbiol. *22*:984–989, 1985.
125. Karron, R. A., Daemer, R., Ticehurst, J., et al.: Studies of prototype live hepatitis A virus vaccines in primate models. J. Infect. Dis. *157*:338–345, 1988.
126. Katz, M. H., Hsu, L., Wong, E., et al.: Seroprevalence of and risk factors for hepatitis A infection among young homosexual and bisexual men. J. Infect. Dis. *175*:1225–1229, 1997.
127. Keefe, E. B.: Is hepatitis A more severe in patients with chronic hepatitis B and other chronic liver diseases? Am. J. Gastroenterol. *90*:201–205, 1995.
128. Klar, A., Branski, D., Nadjari, M., et al.: Gallbladder and pancreatic involvement in hepatitis A. J. Clin. Gastroenterol. *27*:143–145, 1998.
129. Klein, B. S., Michaels, J. A., Ryter, M. W., et al.: Nosocomial hepatitis A: A multi-nursery outbreak in Wisconsin. J. A. M. A. *252*:2716–2721, 1984.

130. Kluge, I.: Gamma-globulin in the prevention of viral hepatitis: A study of the effect of medium-size doses. Acta Med. Scand. *174*:469–477, 1963.
131. Koa, H. W., Ashcavai, M., and Redeker, A. G.: Persistence of hepatitis IgM antibody after acute clinical hepatitis A. Hepatology *4*:933–936, 1984.
132. Koff, R. S.: Viral hepatitis. *In* Walker, W. A., Durie, P. R., Hamilton, J. R., et al. (eds.): Pediatric Gastrointestinal Disease: Pathophysiology, Diagnosis, Management. Philadelphia, B. C. Decker, 1991, pp. 857–874.
133. Koff, R. S.: Clinical manifestations and diagnosis of hepatitis A virus infection. Vaccine *10*:(Suppl. 1):15–17, 1992.
134. Krah, D.: A simplified multiwell plate assay for the measurement of hepatitis A virus infectivity. Biologicals *19*:223–227, 1991.
135. Krugman, S., and Giles, J. P.: Viral hepatitis: New light on an old disease. J. A. M. A. *212*:1019–1029, 1970.
136. Krugman, S., Giles, J. P., and Hammond, J.: Infectious hepatitis: Evidence for two distinctive clinical, epidemiological and immunological types of infection. J. A. M. A. *200*:365–373, 1967.
137. Krugman, S., Ward, R., and Giles, W. P.: The natural history of infectious hepatitis. Am. J. Med. *32*:717–728, 1962.
138. Krugman, S., Ward, R., Giles, J. P., et al.: Infectious hepatitis, study on effect of gamma globulin and on the incidence of apparent infection. J. A. M. A. *174*:823–830, 1960.
139. Kumashiro, R., Sata, M., Suzuki, H., et al.: Clinical study of acute hepatitis type A in patients older than 50 years. Acta Hepatol. Jpn. *29*:457–462, 1988.
140. Kunasol, P., Cooksley, G., Chan, V. F., et al.: Hepatitis A virus: Declining seroprevalence in children and adolescents in Southeast Asia. Southeast Asian J. Trop. Med. Public Health *29*:255–262, 1998.
141. Lagos, R., Potin, M., Muñoz, A., et al.: Anticuerpos séricos contra el virus hepatitis A en sujetos de nivel socioeconómico medio y bajo, en comunas urbanas de Santiago. Rev. Med. Chile *127*:429–436, 1999.
142. Lange, W. R., and Frame, J. D.: High incidence of viral hepatitis among American missionaries in Africa. Am. J. Trop. Med. Hyg. *43*:527–533, 1990.
143. Latham, R. H., and Schable, C. A.: Foodborne hepatitis A at a family reunion. Am. J. Epidemiol. *115*:640–645, 1982.
144. Lea, A. P., and Balfour, L. A.: Virosomal hepatitis A vaccine (strain RG-SB). Biodrugs *7*:232–248, 1997.
145. Leach, C. T., Koo, F. C., Hilsenbeck, S. G., and Jenson, H. B.: The epidemiology of viral hepatitis in children in south Texas: Increased prevalence of hepatitis A along the Texas-Mexico border. J. Infect. Dis. *180*:509–513, 1999.
146. Lednar, W. M., Lemon, S. M., Kirkpatrick, J. W., et al.: Frequency of illness associated with epidemic hepatitis A virus infection in adults. Am. J. Epidemiol. *122*:226–233, 1985.
147. Lee, H., and Vacanti, J. P.: Liver transplantation and its long-term management in children. Pediatr. Clin. North Am. *43*:99–124, 1996.
148. Leikin, E., Lysidiewicz, A., Garry, D., and Tejani, N.: Intrauterine transmission of hepatitis A virus. Obstet. Gynecol. *88*:690–691, 1996.
149. Lemon, S. M.: Type A viral hepatitis: New developments in an old disease. N. Engl. J. Med. *313*:1059–1067, 1985.
150. Lemon, S. M.: Immunologic approaches to assessing the response to inactivated hepatitis A vaccine. J. Hepatol. *18*(Suppl. 2):15–19, 1993.
151. Lemon, S. M.: The natural history of hepatitis A: The potential for transmission by transfusion of blood or blood products. Vox Sang. *67*(Suppl. 4):19–23, 1994.
152. Lemon, S. M., and Binn, L. N.: Serum neutralizing antibody response to hepatitis A virus. J. Infect. Dis. *148*:1033–1039, 1983.
153. Lemon, S. M., Binn, L. N., and Marchwicki, R. H.: Radioimmunofocus assay for quantitation of hepatitis A virus in cell culture. J. Clin. Microbiol. *17*:834–839, 1983.
154. Lemon, S. M., and Shapiro, C. N.: The value of immunization against hepatitis A. Infect. Agents Dis. *1*:38–49, 1994.
155. Lemon, S. M., Whetter, L. E., Chang, K. H., et al.: Recent advances in understanding the molecular virology of hepatoviruses: Contrasts and comparisons with hepatitis C virus. *In* Nishioka, K., Suzuki, H., Mishiro, S., et al. (eds.): Viral Hepatitis and Liver Disease. Tokyo, Springer-Verlag, 1994, pp. 22–27.
156. Levin, S., Leibowitz, E., Torten, J., et al.: Interferon treatment in acute progressive and fulminant hepatitis. Isr. J. Med. Sci. *25*:364–372, 1989.
157. Liaw, Y. F., Yang, C. Y., Chu, C. M., et al.: Appearance and persistence of hepatitis A IgM antibody in acute clinical hepatitis A observed in an outbreak. Infection *14*:156–158, 1986.
158. Lieberman, J. M., Marcy, M., Partridge, S., et al.: Evaluation of hepatitis A vaccine in infants: Effect of maternal antibodies on the antibody response. Abstract 76. *In* Abstracts of the 36th Annual Meeting of the Infectious Diseases Society of America, Denver. Alexandria, VA, Infectious Diseases Society of America, 1998, p. 38.
159. Linder, N., Karetnyi, Y., Gidony, Y., et al.: Decline of hepatitis A antibodies during the first 7 months of life in full-term and preterm infants. Infection *27*:128–131, 1999.
160. Lowry, P. W., Levine, R., Stroup, D. F., et al.: Hepatitis A outbreak on a floating restaurant in Florida, 1986. Am. J. Epidemiol. *129*:155–164, 1989.
161. Mah, M. W., Royce, R. A., Rathouz, P. J., et al.: Prevalence of hepatitis A antibodies in hemophiliacs: Preliminary results from the Southeastern Delta Hepatitis Study. Vox Sang. *67*(Suppl. 1):21–22, 1994.
162. Mahoney, F. J., Farley, T. A., Kelso, K. Y., et al.: An outbreak of hepatitis A associated with swimming in a public pool. J. Infect. Dis. *165*:613–618, 1992.
163. Maiga, M. Y., Oberti, F., Rifflet, H., et al.: Manifestations hématologiques liées au virus de l'hépatite A. Gastroenterol. Clin. Biol. *21*:327–330, 1997.
164. Mannucci, P. M., Gdovin, S., Gringeri, A., et al.: Transmission of hepatitis A to patients with hemophilia by factor VIII concentrates treated with organic solvent and detergent to inactivate viruses. Ann. Intern. Med. *120*:1–7, 1994.
165. Mao, J. S., Dong, D. X., Zhang, H. Y., et al.: Primary study of attenuated live hepatitis A vaccine (H2 strain) in humans. J. Infect. Dis. *159*:621–624, 1989.
166. Mao, J. S., Dong, D. X., Zhang, S. Y., et al.: Further studies of attenuated live hepatitis A vaccine (strain H2) in humans. *In* Hollinger, F. B., Lemon, S. M., and Margolis, H. S. (eds.): Viral Hepatitis and Liver Disease. Baltimore, Williams & Wilkins, 1991, pp. 110–111.
167. Margolis, H. S., Nainan, O. V., Krawczynski, K., et al.: Appearance of immune complexes during experimental hepatitis A infection in chimpanzees. J. Med. Virol. *26*:315–326, 1988.
168. Massoudi, M., Bell, B. P., Paredes, V., et al.: Multiple outbreaks of hepatitis A associated with an infected foodhandler. Public Health Rep. *114*:157–164, 1999.
169. Mathiesen, L. R., Skinoj, P., Nielsen, J. O., et al.: Hepatitis type A, B, and non-A non-B in fulminant hepatitis. Gut *21*:72–77, 1980.
170. Mbithi, J. N., Springthorpe, S., Boulet, J. R., et al.: Survival of hepatitis A virus on human hands and its transfer on contact with animate and inanimate surfaces. J. Clin. Microbiol. *30*:757–763, 1992.
171. McCaustland, K. A., Bond, W. W., Bradley, D. W., et al.: Survival of hepatitis A virus in feces after drying and storage for 1 month. J. Clin. Microbiol. *16*:957–958, 1982.
172. McDuffie, R. S., and Bader, T.: Fetal meconium peritonitis after maternal hepatitis A. Am. J. Obstet. Gynecol. *180*:1031–1032, 1999.
173. McMahon, B. J., Beller, M., Williams, J., et al.: A program to control an outbreak of hepatitis A in Alaska by using an inactivated hepatitis A vaccine. Arch. Pediatr. Adolesc. Med. *150*:733–739, 1996.
174. McMahon, B. J., Williams, J., Bulkow, L., et al.: Immunogenicity of an inactivated hepatitis A vaccine in Alaska Native children and Native and non-Native adults. J. Infect. Dis. *171*:676–679, 1995.
175. Midthun, K., Ellerbeck, E., Gershman, K., et al.: Safety and immunogenicity of a live attenuated hepatitis A virus vaccine in seronegative volunteers. J. Infect. Dis. *163*:735–739, 1991.
176. Millard, J., Appleton, H., and Parry, J. V.: Studies on heat inactivation of hepatitis A virus with special reference to shellfish. Part 1. Procedures for infection and recovery of virus from laboratory-maintained cockles. Epidemiol. Infect. *98*:397–414, 1987.
177. Minor, P. D.: *Picornaviridae*. *In* Franki, R. I. B., Fauquet, C. M., Knudson, D. L., et al.: (eds.): Classification and Nomenclature of Viruses: The Fifth Report of the International Committee on Taxonomy of Viruses. Vienna, Springer-Verlag, 1991, pp. 320–326.
178. Mishra, A., Saigal, S., Gupta, R., et al.: Acute pancreatitis associated with viral hepatitis: A report of six cases with review of the literature. Am. J. Gastroenterol. *94*:2292–2295, 1999.
179. Mishu, B., Hadler, S., Boza, V. A., et al.: Foodborne hepatitis A: Evidence that microwaving reduces risk? J. Infect. Dis. *162*:655–658, 1990.
180. Mosley, J. W., Reisler, D. M., Brachott, D., et al.: Comparison of two lots of immune serum globulin for prophylaxis of infectious hepatitis. Am. J. Epidemiol. *87*:539–550, 1968.
181. Mowat, A. P.: Liver Disorders in Childhood. 3rd ed. Oxford, Butterworth, 1994.
182. Myers, J. D., Romm, F. J., Tihen, W. S., et al.: Foodborne hepatitis A in a general hospital: Epidemiologic study of an outbreak attributed to sandwiches. J. A. M. A. *231*:1049–1053, 1975.
183. Nainan, O. V., Brinton, M. A., and Margolis, H. S.: Identification of amino acids located in the antibody binding sites of human hepatitis A virus. Virology *191*:984–987, 1992.
184. Nainan, O. V., Margolis, H. S., Robertson, B. H., et al.: Sequence analysis of a new hepatitis A virus naturally infecting cynomolgus macaques *(Macaca fascicularis)*. J. Gen. Virol. *72*:1685–1689, 1991.
185. Nalin, D. R.: VAQTA, hepatitis A vaccine, purified, inactivated. Drugs Future *20*:24–29, 1995.
186. Nasser, A. M., and Metcalf, T. G.: Production of cytopathology in FRhK-4 cells by BS-C-1–passaged hepatitis A virus. Appl. Environ. Microbiol. *53*:2967–2971, 1987.
187. Niu, M. T., Polish, L. B., Robertson, B. H., et al.: A multistate outbreak of hepatitis A associated with frozen strawberries. J. Infect. Dis. *166*:518–524, 1992.
188. Niu, M. T., Salive, M., Drueger, C., et al.: Two-year review of hepatitis A vaccine safety: Data from the Vaccine Adverse Event Reporting System (VAERS). Clin. Infect. Dis. *26*:1475–1476, 1998.
189. Noble, R. C., Kane, M. A., Reeves, S. A., et al.: Posttransfusion hepatitis A in a neonatal intensive care unit. J. A. M. A. *252*:2711–2715, 1984.
190. O'Donovan, D., Cooke, R. P. D., Joce, R., et al.: An outbreak of hepatitis A amongst injecting drug users. Epidemiol. Infect. *127*: 469–473, 2001.

191. O'Grady, J. G.: Management of acute and fulminant hepatitis A. Vaccine *10*(Suppl. 1):21–23, 1992.
192. O'Grady, J. G., Alexander, G. J., Hayllar, K. M., et al.: Early indicators of the prognosis in fulminant hepatic failure. Gastroenterology *97*:439–445, 1989.
193. Ohara, H., Naruto, H., Watanabe, W., et al.: An outbreak of hepatitis A caused by consumption of raw oysters. J. Hyg. (Camb.) *91*:163–165, 1983.
194. Okuno, T., Sano, A., Deguchi, T., et al.: Pathology of acute hepatitis A in humans. Comparison with acute hepatitis B. Am. J. Clin. Pathol. *81*:162–169, 1984.
195. Papaevangelou, G. J., Roumeliotou-Karayannis, A. J., and Contoyannis, P. C.: The risk of hepatitis A and B virus infections from patients under care without isolation precautions. J. Med. Virol. 7:143–148, 1981.
196. Parkin, W. E., Marzinsky, P., and Griffin, M. R.: Foodborne hepatitis A associated with cheeseburgers. J. Med. Soc. N. J. *80*:612–615, 1983.
197. Pavia, A. T., Nielson, L., Armington, L., et al.: A communitywide outbreak of hepatitis A in a religious community: Impact of mass administration of immune globulin. Am. J. Epidemiol. *131*:1085–1093, 1990.
198. Pelletier, G., Elghozi, D., Trepo, C., et al.: Mononeuritis in acute viral hepatitis. Digestion *32*:5306, 1985.
199. Peterson, D. A., Wolfe, L. G., Larkin, E. P., et al.: Thermal treatment and infectivity of hepatitis A virus in human feces. J. Med. Virol. *2*:201–206, 1978.
200. Piazza, M., Safary, A., Vegnente, A., et al.: Safety and immunogenicity of hepatitis A vaccine in infants: A candidate for inclusion in the childhood vaccination programme. Vaccine *17*:585–588, 1999.
201. Ping, L.-H., Jansen, R. W., Stapleton, J. T., et al.: Identification of an immunodominant antigenic site involving the capsid protein VP3 of hepatitis A virus. Proc. Natl. Acad. Sci. U. S. A. *85*:8281–8285, 1988.
202. Pinho, J. R. R., Sumita, L. M., Moreira, R. C., et al.: Duality of patterns in hepatitis A epidemiology: A study involving two socioeconomically distinct populations in Campinas, São Paulo State, Brazil. Rev. Inst. Med. Trop. Sao Paulo *40*:105–106, 1998.
203. Poovorawan, Y., Vimolkej, T., Chongsrisawat, V., et al.: The declining pattern of seroepidemiology of hepatitis A virus infection among adolescents in Bangkok, Thailand. Southeast Asian J. Trop. Med. Public Health *28*:154–157, 1997.
204. Portnoy, B. L., Mackowiak, P. A., Caraway, C. T., et al.: Oyster-associated hepatitis failure of shellfish certification programs to prevent outbreaks. J. A. M. A. *233*:1065–1068, 1975.
205. Prevention of hepatitis A through active or passive immunization: Recommendations of the Advisory Committee on Immunization Practices (ACIP). M. M. W. R. Recomm. Rep. *45*(RR-15):1–30, 1996.
206. Prevention of hepatitis A through active or passive immunization: Recommendations of the Advisory Committee on Immunization Practices (ACIP). M. M. W. R. Recomm. Rep. *48*(RR-12):1–37, 1999.
207. Prodinger, W. M., Larcher, C., Sölder, B. M., et al.: Hepatitis A in western Austria—the epidemiological situation before the introduction of active immunization. Infection *22*:53–55, 1994.
208. Provost, P. J., Bishop, R. P., Gerety, R. J., et al.: New findings in live, attenuated hepatitis A vaccine development. J. Med. Virol. *20*:165–175, 1986.
209. Provost, P. J., and Hilleman, M. R.: Propagation of human hepatitis A virus in cell culture in vitro. Proc. Soc. Exp. Biol. Med. *160*:213–221, 1979.
210. Purcell, R. H., D'Hondt, E., Bradbury, R., et al.: Inactivated hepatitis A vaccine: Active and passive prophylaxis in chimpanzees. Vaccine *10*(Suppl.):148–156, 1992.
211. Rahaman, S. M., Chira, P., and Koff, R. S.: Idiopathic autoimmune chronic hepatitis triggered by hepatitis A. Am. J. Gastroenterol. *89*:106–108, 1994.
212. Rakela, J., Redeker, A. G., Edwards, V. M., et al.: Hepatitis A virus infection in fulminant hepatitis and chronic active hepatitis. Gastroenterology *74*:879–882, 1978.
213. Reid, T. M. S., and Robinson, H. G.: Frozen raspberries and hepatitis A. Epidemiol. Infect. *98*:109–112, 1987.
214. Robertson, B. H., D'Hondt, E. H., Spelbring, J., et al.: Effect of postexposure vaccination in a chimpanzee model of hepatitis A virus infection. J. Med. Virol. *43*:249–251, 1994.
215. Robertson, B. H., Jansen, R. W., Khanna, B., et al.: Genetic relatedness of hepatitis A virus strains recovered from different geographical regions. J. Gen. Virol. *73*:1365–1377, 1992.
216. Rosenblum, L. S., Mirkin, I. R., Allen, D. T., et al.: A multifocal outbreak of hepatitis A traced to commercially distributed lettuce. Am. J. Public Health *80*:1075, 1990.
217. Rosenblum, L. S., Villarino, M. E., Nainan, O. V., et al.: Hepatitis A outbreak in a neonatal intensive care unit: Risk factors for transmission and evidence of prolonged viral excretion among preterm infants. J. Infect. Dis. *164*:476–482, 1991.
218. Safety of therapeutic immune globulin preparations with respect to transmission of human T-lymphotropic virus type III/lymphadenopathy-associated virus infection. M. M. W. R. Morb. Mortal. Wkly. Rep. *35*(14):231–233, 1986.
219. Sagi, E. F., Linder, N., and Shouval, D.: Papular acrodermatitis of childhood associated with hepatitis A virus infection. Pediatr. Dermatol. *3*:31–33, 1985.
220. Sagliocca, L., Amoroso, P., Stroffolini, T., et al.: Efficacy of hepatitis A vaccine in prevention of secondary hepatitis A infection: A randomized trial. Lancet *353*:1136–1139, 1999.
221. Samandari, T., Wasley, A., and Bell, B. P.: Evaluating the impact of hepatitis A vaccination in the United States, 1990–2001. Abstract. *In* Proceedings of the 51st Annual Epidemic Intelligence Service (EIS) Conference. Atlanta, Centers for Disease Control and Prevention, 2002.
222. Schade, C. P., and Komorwska, D.: Continuing outbreak of hepatitis A linked with intravenous drug abuse in Multnomah County. Public Health Rep. *103*:452–459, 1988.
223. Scheuer, P. J.: Liver Biopsy Interpretation. 4th ed. London, Bailliere Tindall, 1988.
224. Schiff, E. R.: Atypical clinical manifestations of hepatitis A. Vaccine *10*(Suppl. 1):18–20, 1992.
225. Schiodt, F. V., Atillasoy, E., Shakil, A. O., et al.: Etiology and outcome for 295 patients with acute liver failure in the United States. Liver Transpl. Surg. *5*:29–34, 1999.
226. Shah, U., Habib, Z., and Kleinman, R. E.: Liver failure attributable to hepatitis A virus infection in a developing country. Pediatrics *105*:436–438, 2000.
227. Shapiro, C. N., Coleman, P. J., McQuillan, G. M., et al.: Epidemiology of hepatitis A: Seroepidemiology and risk groups in the USA. Vaccine *10*(Suppl.):59–62, 1992.
228. Shapiro, C., and Hadler, S.: Significance of hepatitis in children in day care. Semin. Pediatr. Infect. Dis. *1*:270–279, 1990.
229. Shapiro, C. N., and Hadler, S. C.: Hepatitis A and hepatitis B virus infections in day care centers. Pediatr. Ann. *20*:435–441, 1991.
230. Shapiro, C. N., Letson, G. W., Kuehn, D., et al.: Effect of maternal antibody on immunogenicity of hepatitis A vaccine in infants. Abstract H61. Paper presented at the Interscience Conference on Antimicrobial Agents and Chemotherapy, Washington, D.C., 1995.
231. Shaw, D. D., Whiteman, D. C., Merritt, A. D., et al.: Hepatitis A outbreaks among illicit drug users and their contacts in Queensland, 1997. Med. J. Aust. *170*:584–587, 1999.
232. Shaw, F. E. J., Shapiro, C. N., Welty, T. K., et al.: Hepatitis transmission among the Sioux Indians of South Dakota. Am. J. Public Health *80*:1091–1094, 1990.
233. Shaw, F. E., Jr., Sudman, J. H., Smith, S. M., et al.: A community-wide epidemic of hepatitis A in Ohio. Am. J. Epidemiol. *123*:1057–1065, 1986.
234. Sherertz, R. J., Russell, B. A., and Reuman, P. D.: Transmission of hepatitis A by transfusion of blood products. Arch. Intern. Med. *144*:1579–1580, 1984.
235. Shi, G. R., Li, S. Q., and Qian, L.: The epidemiological study on a foodborne outbreak of non-A, non-B hepatitis. J. Chin. Med. Univ. *16*:150, 1987.
236. Shouval, D., Ashur, Y., Adler, R., et al.: Single and booster dose responses to an inactivated hepatitis A virus vaccine: Comparison with immune serum globulin prophylaxis. Vaccine *11*:9–14, 1993.
237. Simmonds, R. S., Szucs, G., Metcalf, T. G., et al.: Persistently infected cultures as a source of hepatitis A virus. Appl. Environ. Microbiol. *49*:749–755, 1985.
238. Sinclair, S. B., and Levy, G. A.: Treatment of fulminant viral hepatic failure with prostaglandin E: A preliminary report. Dig. Dis. Sci. *36*:791–800, 1991.
239. Sjogren, M. H., Hoke, C. H., Binn, L. N., et al.: Immunogenicity of an inactivated hepatitis A vaccine. Ann. Intern. Med. *114*:470–471, 1991.
240. Sjogren, M. H., Purcell, R. H., McKee, K., et al.: Clinical and laboratory observations following oral or intramuscular administration of a live attenuated hepatitis A vaccine candidate. Vaccine *10*(Suppl. 1):135–137, 1992.
241. Sjogren, M. H., Tanno, H., Fay, O., et al.: Hepatitis A virus in stool during clinical relapse. Ann. Intern. Med. *106*:221–226, 1987.
242. Skinhoj, P., Mathiesen, L. R., Kryger, P., et al.: Faecal excretion of hepatitis A virus in patients with symptomatic hepatitis A infection. Scand. J. Gastroenterol. *16*:1057–1059, 1981.
243. Smith, P. F., Grabau, J. C., Werzberger, A., et al.: The role of young children in a community-wide outbreak of hepatitis A. Epidemiol. Infect. *118*:243–252, 1997.
244. Snydman, D. R., Dienstag, J. L., Stedt, B., et al.: Use of IgM–hepatitis A antibody testing: Investigating a common source foodborne outbreak. J. A. M. A. *245*:827–830, 1981.
245. Soucie, J. M., Robertson, B. H., Bell, B. P., et al.: Hepatitis A virus infections associated with clotting factor concentrate in the United States. Transfusion *38*:573–579, 1998.
246. Staes, C. J., Schlenker, T. L., Risk, I., et al.: Sources of infection among persons with acute hepatitis A and no identified risk factors during a sustained communitywide outbreak. Pediatrics *106*:e54, 2000.
247. Stapleton, J. T., Lange, D. K., LeDuc, J. W., et al.: The role of secretory immunity in hepatitis A virus infection. J. Infect. Dis. *163*:7–11, 1991.
248. Starzl, T. E., Demetris, A. J., and Van Thiel, D.: Liver transplantation. N. Engl. J. Med. *321*:1014–1022, 1989.
249. Steffen, R., Kane, M. A., Shapiro, C. N., et al.: Epidemiology and prevention of hepatitis A in travelers. J. A. M. A. *272*:885–889, 1994.
250. Steffen, R., Rickenbach, M., Wilhelm, U., et al.: Health problems after travel to developing countries. J. Infect. Dis. *156*:84, 1987.

251. Stokes, J., and Neefe, J. R.: The prevention and attenuation of infectious hepatitis by gamma globulin. J. A. M. A. *127*:144–145, 1945.
252. Stokes, M., Ferson, M. J., and Young, L. C.: Outbreak of hepatitis A among homosexual men in Sydney. Am. J. Public Health *87*:2039–2041, 1997.
253. Summary of notifiable diseases, United States, 1997. M. M. W. R. Morb. Mortal. Wkly. Rep. *46*(54):ii–vii, 3–87, 1998.
254. Szmuness, W., Purcell, R. H., Dienstag, J. L., et al.: Antibody to hepatitis A antigen in institutionalized mentally retarded patients. J. A. M. A. *237*:1702–1705, 1977.
255. Tabor, E.: Clinical presentation of hepatitis A. *In* Gerety, R. J. (ed.): Hepatitis A. New York, Academic Press, 1984, pp. 47–53.
256. Tabor, E.: Guillain-Barré syndrome and other neurologic syndromes in hepatitis A, B, and non-A, non-B. J. Med. Virol. *21*:207–216, 1987.
257. Tankersley, D. L., and Preston, M. S.: Quality control of immune globulins. *In* Krijnen, H. W., Strengers, P. F. W., and VanAken, X. (eds.): Immunoglobulins: Proceedings of an International Symposium. Amsterdam, Central Laboratory of Netherlands Red Cross Transfusion Service, 1988, pp. 381–399.
258. Tapia-Conyer, R., Santos, J. I., Cavalcanti, A. M., et al.: Hepatitis A in Latin America: A changing epidemiological pattern. Am. J. Trop. Med. Hyg. *61*:825–829, 1999.
259. Tassopoulos, N. C., Papaevangelou, G. J., Ticehurst, J. R., et al.: Fecal excretion of Greek strains of hepatitis A virus in patients with hepatitis A and in experimentally infected chimpanzees. J. Infect. Dis. *154*:231–237, 1986.
260. Teixera, M. R., Jr., Weller, I. V. D., Murray, A., et al.: The pathology of hepatitis A in man. Liver *2*:53–60, 1982.
261. Termorshuizen, F., Dorigo-Zetsma, J. W., deMelker, H. E., et al.: The prevalence of antibodies to hepatitis A virus and its determinants in the Netherlands: A population-based survey. Epidemiol. Infect. *124*:459–466, 2000.
262. Tibbs, C. J., and Williams, R.: Liver transplantation for acute and chronic hepatitis. J. Viral Hepatol. *2*:65–72, 1995.
263. Tong, M. J., El-Farra, N. S., and Grew, M. I.: Clinical manifestations of hepatitis A: Recent experience in a community teaching hospital. J. Infect. Dis. *151*(Suppl. 1):15–18, 1995.
264. Tong, M. J., Thursby, M., Rakela, J., et al.: Studies on the maternal-infant transmission of the viruses which cause acute hepatitis. Gastroenterology *80*:999–1004, 1981.
265. Toppet, V., Souayah, H., Delplace, O., et al.: Lymph node enlargement as a sign of acute hepatitis A in children. Pediatr. Radiol. *20*:249–252, 1990.
266. Troisi, C. L., Hollinger, F. B., Krause, D. S., and Pickering, L. K.: Immunization of seronegative infants with hepatitis A vaccine (HAVRIX; SKB): A comparative study of two dosing schedules. Vaccine *15*:1613–1617, 1997.
267. Tsarev, S. A., Emerson, S. U., Balayan, M. S., et al.: Simian hepatitis A virus (HAV) strain AGM-27: Comparison of genome structure and growth in cell culture with other HAV strains. J. Gen. Virol. *72*:1677–1683, 1991.
268. Tsega, E., Mengesha, B., Hansson, B. G., et al.: Hepatitis A, B and delta infection in Ethiopia: A serologic survey with demographic data. Am. J. Epidemiol. *123*:344–351, 1986.
269. Tufenkeji, H.: Hepatitis A shifting epidemiology in the Middle East and Africa. Vaccine *18*(Suppl.):65–67, 2000.
270. Vallbracht, A., Fleischer, S., Maier, K., et al.: Clonal analysis of infiltrating T-lymphocytes in liver tissue in viral hepatitis A. Immunology *69*:14–19, 1990.
271. Vallbracht, A., Maier, K., Stierhof, Y. D., et al.: Liver-derived cytotoxic T cells in hepatitis A virus infection. J. Infect. Dis. *160*:209–217, 1989.
272. Van Herck, K., and van Damme, P.: Inactivated hepatitis A vaccine–induced antibodies: Follow-up and estimates of long-term persistence. J. Med. Virol. *63*:1–7, 2001.
273. Van Thiel, D.: When should the decision to proceed with transplantation actually be made in cases of subfulminant liver failure: At admission to hospital or when a donor organ is made available? J. Hepatol. *17*:1–2, 1993.
274. Venczel, L. V., Desai, M. M., Vertz, P. D., et al.: The role of child care in a community-wide outbreak of hepatitis A. Pediatrics *108*:e78, 2001.
275. Vento, S., Garofano, T., DiPerri, G., et al.: Identification of hepatitis A virus as a trigger for autoimmune chronic hepatitis type I in susceptible individuals. Lancet *337*:1183–1187, 1991.
276. Vento, S., Garofano, T., Renzini, C., et al.: Fulminant hepatitis associated with hepatitis A virus superinfection in patients with chronic hepatitis C. N. Engl. J. Med. *338*:286–290, 1998.
277. Vidor, E., Fritzell, B., and Plotkin, S.: Clinical development of a new inactivated hepatitis A vaccine. Infection *24*:447–458, 1996.
278. Villano, S. A., Nelson, K. E., Vlahov, D., et al.: Hepatitis A among homosexual men and injection drug users: More evidence for vaccination. Clin. Infect. Dis. *25*:726–728, 1997.
279. Wang, L. Y., Cheng, Y. W., Chou, S. J., et al.: Secular trend and geographical variation in hepatitis A infection and hepatitis B carrier rate among adolescents in Taiwan: An island-wide survey. J. Med. Virol. *39*:1–5, 1993.
280. Watson, J. C., Fleming, D. W., Boretta, A. J., et al.: Vertical transmission of hepatitis A resulting in an outbreak in a neonatal intensive care unit. J. Infect. Dis. *167*:567–571, 1993.
281. Weisfuse, I. B., Graham, D. J., Will, M., et al.: An outbreak of hepatitis A among cancer patients treated with interleukin-2 and lymphokine-activated killer cells. J. Infect. Dis. *161*:647–652, 1990.
282. Weltman, A. C., Bennett, N. M., Ackman, D. A., et al.: An outbreak of hepatitis A associated with a bakery, New York, 1994: The 1968 "West Branch, Michigan" outbreak repeated. Epidemiol. Infect. *117*:333–341, 1996.
283. Werzberger, A., Mensch, B., Kuter, B., et al.: A controlled trial of formalin-inactivated hepatitis A vaccine in healthy children. N. Engl. J. Med. *327*:453–457, 1992.
284. Wheeler, C. M., Fields, H. A., Schable, C. A., et al.: Adsorption, purification, and growth characteristics of hepatitis A virus strain HAS-15 propagated in fetal Rhesus monkey kidney cells. J. Clin. Microbiol. *23*:434–440, 1986.
285. Wheeler, C. M., Robertson, B. H., Van Nest, G., et al.: Structure of hepatitis A virion: Peptide mapping of the capsid region. J. Virol. *58*:307–313, 1986.
286. Widell, A., Hansson, B. G., Moestrup, T., et al.: Acute hepatitis A, B and non-A, non-B in a Swedish community studied over a ten-year period. Scand. J. Infect. Dis. *14*:253–259, 1982.
287. Wiedermann, G., Kindi, M., and Ambrosch, F.: Estimated persistence of anti-HAV antibodies after single dose and booster hepatitis A vaccination (0–6 schedule). Acta Trop. *69*:121–125, 1998.
288. Wiens, B. L., Bohidar, N. R., Pigeon, J. G., et al.: Duration of protection from clinical hepatitis A disease after vaccination with VAQTA. J. Med. Virol. *49*:235–241, 1996.
289. Williams, R.: Prevalence of hepatitis A virus antibody among Navajo school children. Am. J. Public Health *76*:282–283, 1986.
290. Williams, R., and Wendon, J.: Indications for orthotopic liver transplantation in fulminant liver failure. Hepatology *20*(Suppl.):5–10, 1994.
291. Wimmer, E., and Murdin, A. D.: Hepatitis A virus and the molecular biology of picornaviruses: A case for a new genus of the family *Picornaviridae*. *In* Hollinger, F. B., Lemon, S. M., and Margolis, H. (eds.): Viral Hepatitis and Liver Disease. Baltimore, Williams & Wilkins, 1991, pp. 31–41.
292. Yang, N. Y., Yu, P. H., Mao, Z. Y., et al.: Inapparent infection of hepatitis A virus. Am. J. Epidemiol. *127*:599–604, 1988.
293. Yotsuyanagi, H., Koike, K., Yasuda, K., et al.: Prolonged fecal excretion of hepatitis A virus in adult patients with hepatitis A as determined by polymerase chain reaction. Hepatology *24*:10–13, 1996.
294. Zhuang, H., Kaldor, J., Locarnini, S. A., et al.: Serum immunoglobulin levels in acute A, B, and non-A, non-B hepatitis. Gastroenterology *82*:549–553, 1982.
295. Zuckerman, A. J.: The history of viral hepatitis from antiquity to the present. *In* Deinhardt, F., and Dienhardt, J. (eds.): Viral Hepatitis: Laboratory and Clinical Science. Vol. 3. New York, Marcel Dekker, 1983, pp. 3–32.

CALICIVIRIDAE

CHAPTER 173 Caliciviruses and Hepatitis E Virus

DAVID O. MATSON

CALICIVIRUSES

Caliciviruses currently include four genera that differ in genomic organization and phylogenetic comparisons of genomic sequence identity. Recent epidemiologic studies have blurred distinctions in the host of origin and ecologic relationships. Taxonomic decisions have resulted in separation of hepatitis E virus (HEV) from the family *Caliciviridae* into an uncertain taxonomic status.[13, 64, 66] Because of its historical relationship to caliciviruses, HEV is treated briefly at the end of this chapter.

Caliciviruses first were recognized to be distinct pathogens in 1932, when outbreaks of a vesicular exanthem restricted to domestic pigs occurred in California (vesicular exanthem of swine virus [VESV] infection, prototype of the *Vesivirus* genus of *Caliciviridae*).[10] The illness initially was thought to be foot and mouth disease (FMD) of cattle, and the potential for confusion between FMD and VESV in an era when rapid diagnostic assays were unavailable led to the designation of VESV as a foreign animal disease and to extensive programs to eradicate the agent. These programs continued for decades and had a major impact on the agricultural industry of the West Coast of the United States. VESV strains, when later visualized by electron microscopy, had distinctive and unique features that led to the name calicivirus (from "chalice," for the virion's surface cups). A program of sterilization of feed and restriction of feed types finally stopped the outbreaks in the 1950s. In the 1970s, the source of the outbreaks was suggested to be marine animals fed to pigs, especially fish meal.[195] The close relationship hypothesized for caliciviruses isolated from marine mammals and VESVs was proved by genome sequencing, which established the hypothesis made in the early 1970s that caliciviruses move between marine and terrestrial reservoirs.[160]

The first recognition of caliciviruses in humans was in 1972, when viral particles were linked to an outbreak of gastroenteritis in schoolchildren, teachers, and their household contacts in Norwalk, Ohio.[1, 105] The Norwalk agent (prototype of the *Norovirus* genus) was round and had a rough particle surface when visualized by electron microscopy, but these features did not permit any definitive classification. Many similar small, round-structured viruses (SRSVs) were described subsequently from outbreaks of gastroenteritis around the world. A few experiments with these outbreak agents suggested that at least some of them had physical properties like those of the known animal caliciviruses.[103]

In the 1970s, investigators using electron microscopy to survey diarrheal stool specimens from children visualized particles whose appearance was similar to the animal caliciviruses previously identified.[5, 126, 142] These "typical" caliciviruses occurred in a small percentage of sporadic diarrhea stool specimens and in a few outbreaks of gastroenteritis, including an outbreak in an orphanage in Sapporo, Japan (prototype of the *Sapovirus* genus).[28] Genomic sequencing has confirmed that the SRSVs and human viruses with typical calicivirus morphology are caliciviruses.[98, 123, 139]

In 1984, a highly fatal, highly contagious hepatitis was observed in European rabbits bred in China.[225] This syndrome spread some 7000 miles across Asia into Europe and reached Spain within 4 years, a dispersal rate of approximately 5 miles per day in a sedentary host. European rabbit populations experienced mortality rates exceeding 90 percent within 3 days of exposure. Typical calicivirus particles were visualized in infected rabbit livers, and this calicivirus, the rabbit hemorrhagic disease virus (RHDV; prototype of the *Lagovirus* genus), eventually was linked to the syndrome.[164, 172]

These summaries illustrate the diversity of the ecologic relationships of the caliciviruses, highlight the broad spectrum of illness (from mild gastroenteritis to fatal hepatitis) associated with members of the family, and indicate how recently many of these widespread caliciviruses have been discovered.

Properties of Caliciviruses

Evidence of human infection has been detected for each of the four calicivirus genera. Each genus is discussed, with special emphasis on human infection.

STRUCTURAL FEATURES OF THE VIRION

The *Caliciviridae* is a family of nonenveloped RNA viruses classified until 1978 within the *Picornaviridae*.[33] The caliciviral genome is a positive-sense, single-stranded RNA molecule of approximately 8000 nucleotides. Caliciviruses have a single structural polypeptide with a molecular weight of approximately 60,000 d.[98] Typical calicivirus virion particles are 40.5 nm in diameter and have an icosahedral symmetry with 32 cup-shaped surface depressions[177] (Fig. 173–1). Distinguishing the identifying features of a calicivirus in a clinical specimen is not always easy (see Fig. 173–1*B*). Staining of particles, particle integrity, and component debris vary among clinical samples. In one orientation, the surface cups combine to generate a Star of David image under the electron microscope (see Fig. 173–1*C*). In another orientation, the depressions are responsible for spike-like projections from the surface (see Fig. 173–1*D*).

Cryoelectron microscopy and x-ray crystallography have resolved the three-dimensional structure of typical and

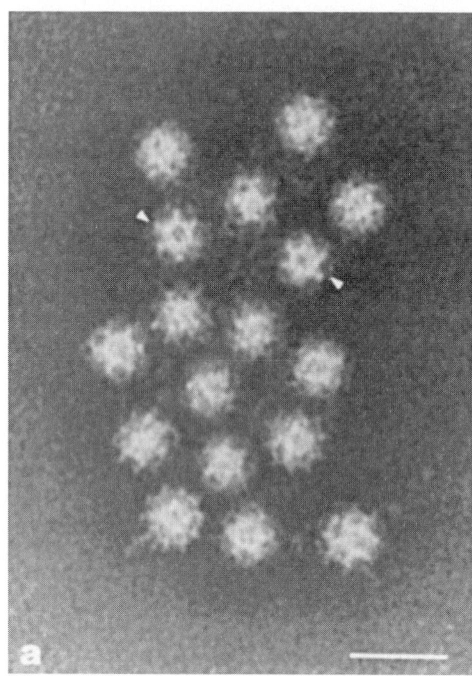

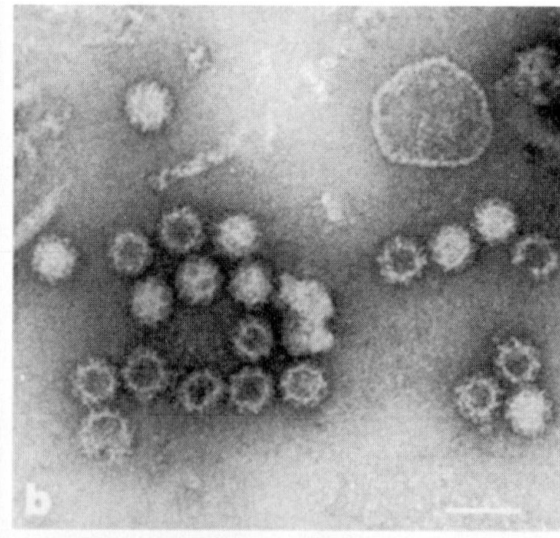

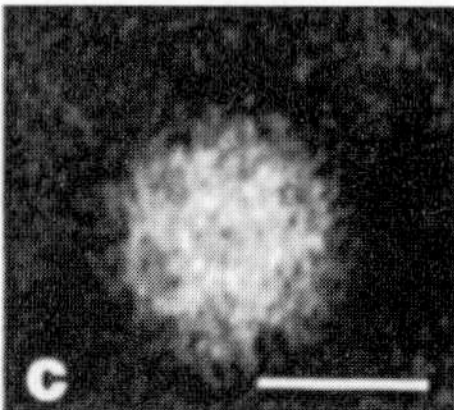

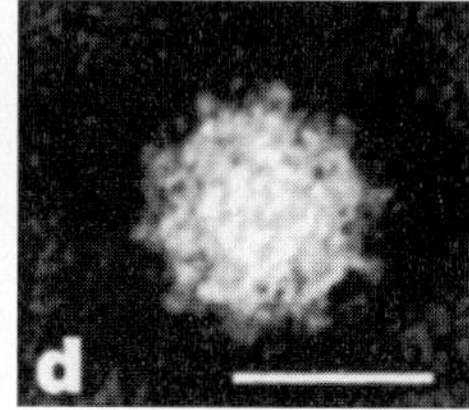

FIGURE 173–1 ■ Human calicivirus particles visualized by electron microscopy. Particles in a preparation of a purified Sapporo/1982/Japan prototype strain show distinct surface cups, and the Star of David pattern is visible on some particles (a, *arrowheads).* Particle staining, particle type, and debris in clinical specimens are variable, which frustrates the recognition of distinct structural features (b, specimen from a child from Houston, Texas, infected with an antigenically distinct *Sapovirus).* Two particles at high magnification show the Star of David pattern (c) and the 10 surface projections (d) characteristic of calicivirus (specimen from a symptomatic child attending a daycare center in Phoenix, Arizona). Bar in *A* and *B* = 50 nm; bar in *C* and *D* = 25 nm.

SRSV morphologic types.[176–178] Typical virion particles have 90 true arches protruding from the surface of a shell that has a diameter of 27 nm. When such particles are visualized by negative-stain electron microscopy, as in a clinical laboratory, the particles are smaller (30 to 35 nm), presumably from desiccation. The arches form surface spikes in some particle orientations, and when the particles are rotated, the compressed two-dimensional image of the three-dimensional particle transforms the walls of the cup-shaped depressions into the distinctive Star of David appearance. SRSVs differ from typical caliciviruses in that they have shorter arches; otherwise, the structures of the two forms are similar.

TAXONOMIC RELATIONSHIPS AMONG THE CALICIVIRUSES

Recent decisions made by the International Committee on Taxonomy of Viruses include the separation of caliciviruses from picornaviruses in 1978,[33] inclusion of HEV in the family in 1995,[34] recognition and naming of distinct calicivirus genera, separation of HEV from the family in 1999,[13, 64, 66] and renaming of the Norwalk-like virus (now *Norovirus)* and Sapporo-like virus (now *Sapovirus)* genera in 2002.[140]

Phylogenetic evaluation of sequence identity among calicivirus strains sorts them according to the same four groups as sorting by genomic organization does (see later).[13] The most informative genomic region for classification of a strain within the family and within a genus is the capsid region, whereas the RNA polymerase gene is conserved sufficiently among the genera to blur distinctions. The strains fall into four genera; each genus also includes multiple clades of uncertain biologic significance (Fig. 173–2).

PROTOTYPE STRAINS AND HOSTS OF ORIGIN

The four calicivirus genera differ in genomic organization and degree of shared sequence identity[13] (Table 173–1). Strains commonly recovered from natural human infections fall into two genera: *Norovirus,* a virtual synonym for SRSVs, which include the Norwalk virus and Snow Mountain virus prototypes, and *Sapovirus,* a virtual synonym for “typical” human caliciviruses. The genera of common animal caliciviruses include *Lagovirus* and *Vesivirus. Lagovirus* prototypes include RHDV and European brown hare syndrome virus. *Vesivirus* prototypes include VESV; feline calicivirus, a cause of hemorrhagic pneumonia in cats; and other strains of marine and terrestrial animal origin. Additional genera may exist because many clinical specimens contain virus particles with structural features of caliciviruses that have been resistant to genomic characterization.

The restriction of *Norovirus* and *Sapovirus* infections to humans has been broken by the finding of Newbury agent and Jena virus, noroviruses of cows, and porcine enteric calicivirus, a *Sapovirus* of pigs.[43, 56, 70, 124, 216] In addition, evidence ranging from conclusive to suggestive supports *Vesivirus* and *Lagovirus* infection in humans. San Miguel sea lion virus serotype 5 (SMSV-5), a *Vesivirus,* produced blisters on the extremities of a laboratory worker, an illness similar to that observed in the original sea lion host.[194] Similar, less conclusive cases of *Vesivirus* illness also have occurred in field biologists working with marine mammals, and anti-*Vesivirus* antibody has been detected in association with non-A-G hepatitis in humans.[203] Other *Vesivirus* strains have caused illness in several primate species.[202] Antibody developed in one person exposed to the *Lagovirus* RHDV in a Mexican outbreak.[68] A case-control study of exposure and prevalence of antibody to RHDV in Australia after continent-wide escape of the virus from Australian Animal Health Laboratory facilities suggested that subclinical human infection was a common occurrence in persons with certain rabbit exposure,[133] although this conclusion is controversial.[22, 23, 143, 196]

GENOMIC ORGANIZATION

The genomic organization among calicivirus genera differs in the number and size of open reading frames (ORFs), the

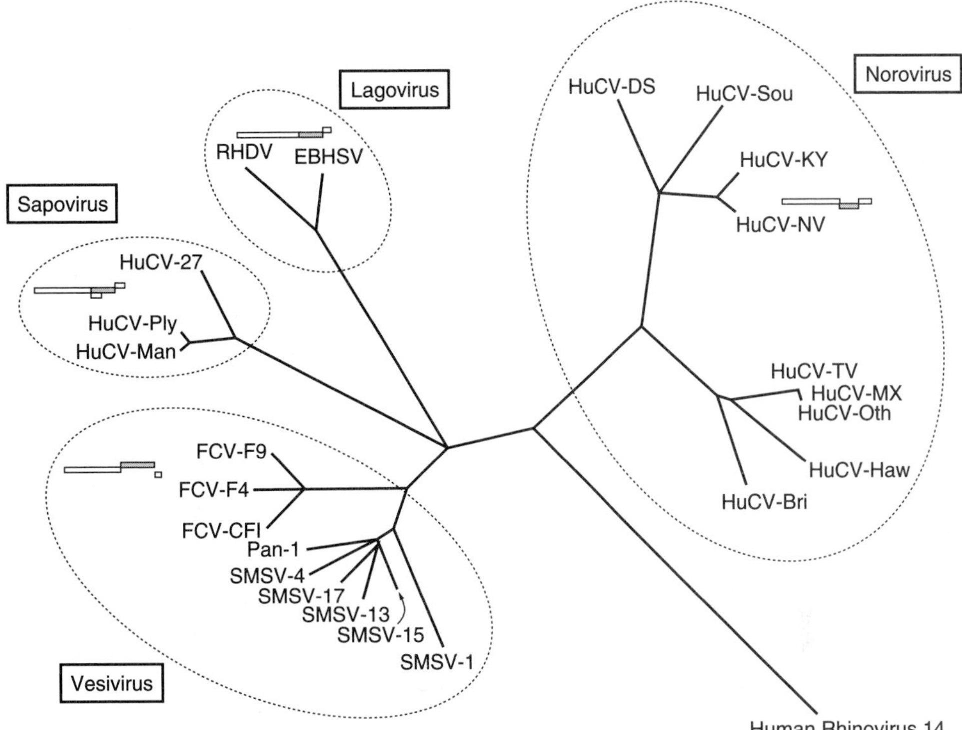

FIGURE 173–2 ■ Distance tree (Fitch-Margoliash method) constructed from the capsid-region nucleic acid sequences of selected caliciviruses by using 1000 bootstrapped dataset replications and the computer program FITCH of PHYLIP 3.5c. The branch points indicated are those appearing in more than 95 percent of the bootstrapped trees. *Ovals* indicate strains with a common genomic organization. Rhinovirus 14 is included as an outgroup. (From Berke, T., Golding, B., Jiang, X., et al.: A phylogenetic analysis of the caliciviruses. J. Med. Virol. *52*:419–424, 1997.)

presence of certain genes, and the need for post-translational cleavage for gene product function[24, 46, 47, 81, 123] (Fig. 173–3). The genome of noroviruses has three ORFs. ORF1 encodes a polyprotein cleaved during replication into a set of nonstructural proteins, ORF2 encodes the capsid protein, and ORF3 encodes a protein that appears to be a minor structural protein.[204] Vesiviruses differ from noroviruses in that a longer genome is present in some vesiviruses (e.g., Pan-1)[181] but not in others (e.g., feline calicivirus)[24] and a longer ORF1 with an additional predicted protein is found at the N terminus. The ORF2 of vesiviruses is longer than that of noroviruses, with the extra nucleotides at the 5′ end of ORF2.[47, 158] This extra sequence encodes a protein fragment that must be post-translationally cleaved to agree with experimental data of *Vesivirus* virion structure.[177] The ORF3 of vesiviruses (≈120 amino acids) is approximately half the size of that of noroviruses (250 to 275 amino acids). In lagoviruses and sapoviruses, the genes found in the ORF1 and ORF2 of noroviruses and vesiviruses are fused into one longer ORF1. A gene comparable to that of ORF3 of noroviruses also is present. An ORF in another frame at the 5′ end of the capsid gene occurs in sapoviruses but not in all *Sapovirus* strains.[91, 123] Consensus amino acid motifs encoded within the proteins are markers for enzymatic and structural functions (2C, 3C, 3D, and PPG) shared with picornaviruses and other viruses with a single-stranded RNA genome.

Caliciviruses synthesize a subgenomic RNA molecule during replication.[146, 159] This subgenomic molecule is plus-sense, begins just before the capsid gene, and extends to the poly-A tail, including ORF3. Each completely sequenced calicivirus genome exhibits conservation of the 5′ end nucleotide sequence of the genome and the 5′ end of the capsid gene. This sequence conservation is high within the same strain

TABLE 173–1 ■ GENERA OF HUMAN AND ANIMAL CALICIVIRUSES

Genus	Known Hosts	Examples
*Norovirus**	Human, cow, pig	Norwalk and Snow Mountain viruses; Jena virus (bovine)
*Sapovirus**	Human, pig	Sapporo caliciviruses 82/Japan, 86/Houston, 90/Houston; Manchester and Plymouth viruses; porcine enteric calicivirus
Lagovirus	Rabbit, hare? pig? dog? human? fox? mouse? bird?	Rabbit hemorrhagic disease virus of Europe, Asia, Australia, New Zealand; European brown hare syndrome virus
Vesivirus	Pig, cat, chimpanzee, sea lion, dolphin, mussel, sea otter, raccoon, Aruba Island rattlesnake	A48; feline caliciviruses F4,CFI, F65, F9; Pan-1, Tur-1; San Miguel sea lion virus types 1 to 17

*Previous names of these genera were Norwalk-like and Sapporo-like viruses; synonyms for *Norovirus* and *Sapovirus* were small, round-structured viruses and typical caliciviruses, respectively.
Data from references 13, 64, 193.

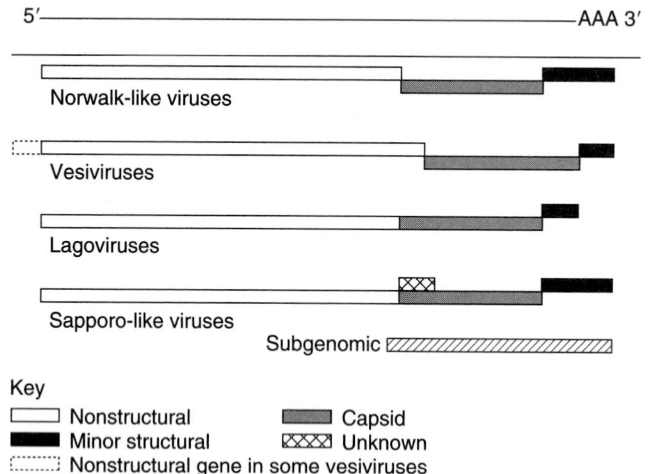

FIGURE 173–3 ■ Genomic organization of calicivirus genera. The genome of *Norovirus* has three open-reading frames (ORFs) that in the 5′ to 3′ direction include a nonstructural polypeptide, the virion capsid gene, and a minor structural protein. The genomes of the other three genera differ from that of noroviruses in the length of the ORFs, including a unique gene at the 5′ end of ORF1 in some vesiviruses and a post-translationally cleaved N terminus of the capsid protein in vesiviruses and sapoviruses. A subgenomic RNA beginning just 5′ of ORF2 and continuing to the poly-A tail is synthesized during replication. Some sequence comparisons suggest that the longer ORF3 of *Norovirus* (and the comparable gene of *Sapovirus)* arose by intragenic recombination.

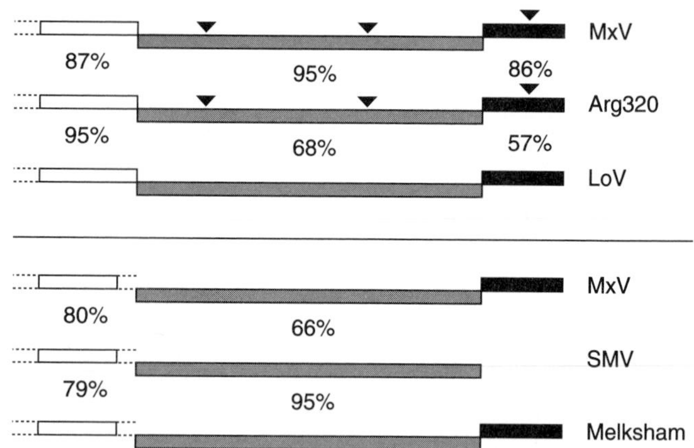

FIGURE 173–4 ■ Sequence comparisons of Argentine calicivirus strain 320 (Arg320; *top)* and Snow Mountain virus (SMV; *bottom),* each with two other noroviruses. Arg320 is significantly closer to Lordsdale virus (LoV) than Mexico virus (M × V) in the RNA polymerase genome region and significantly closer to M × V than LoV in the capsid and ORF3 genes. Deletions/insertions in the capsid and ORF3 genes of Arg320 are shared with M × V, but not LoV. SMSV is equally close to M × V and Melksham virus in the known polymerase region, but much closer to Melksham than M × V in the capsid region. The ORF3 sequence is not available for SMV. *Box shadings* are as in Figure 173–3. (Data from references 79, 93, 132.)

and among strains in the same genus.[115, 132] This terminal and internal conserved sequence probably is a target for binding of the calicivirus RNA polymerase enzyme to initiate the synthesis of full-length genomic and subgenomic RNA, respectively. The conserved sequence also probably favors recombination of RNA among calicivirus strains (see later).

RECOMBINANTS

EVIDENCE FOR RECOMBINATION WITHIN CALICIVIRUSES. With the description of statistically significant phylogenetic clades within calicivirus genera, data were available to recognize strains that might be natural recombinants within caliciviruses. Two examples are the well-characterized Argentine strain 320 (Arg320) and the prototype Snow Mountain virus, recognized to be recombinants when the RNA polymerase and capsid regions of these strains were characterized[79, 93] (Fig. 173–4). In both strains, the change in relative sequence identity took place at the ORF1/ORF2 junction, where sequence conservation at the 5′ end of the genome also occurs (see earlier), thus indicating that the recombination site occurred there. This site also was suggested (see later) to be the break-and-rejoin site for recombination between caliciviruses and picornaviruses. For Arg320, the ORF1 sequence was closest to Lordsdale virus, among the sequenced noroviruses, and the capsid and ORF3 sequences were closest to Mexico virus. A similar change in relative sequence identity also occurred with Snow Mountain virus, as detected when partial polymerase and capsid sequences were compared with reference Mexico and Melksham viruses.

Except for the recombinant genomic structure, the recombinants otherwise are unremarkable, and the strains were recognized only because they initially were characterized in two genomic regions. Recombination may be a mechanism by which caliciviruses quickly escape host immunity, analogous to antigenic shifts in influenza viruses but by a different molecular mechanism. The two potential parental strains of each recombinant are within the range of genetic diversity of strains currently co-circulating. Therefore, the recombination event could have occurred recently but not necessarily during infection of the persons from whom the recombinants were recovered. On the other hand, one would not have difficulty imagining that many calicivirus strains currently in circulation could have derived from recombination events remotely in the past.

POTENTIAL ORIGINS OF RECOMBINANTS WITHIN CALICIVIRUSES. Generation of recombinants within caliciviruses requires certain biologic and molecular attributes. Outbreaks caused by multiple *Norovirus* strains and co-infection with different *Norovirus* strains do occur.[61, 138, 180, 208] Infection of single cells simultaneously by two caliciviruses implies an absence of immune or molecular interference. Calicivirus RNA also must have attributes that permit or favor recombination, such as a site where errors in procession of RNA polymerase can occur. The subgenomic RNA described earlier is the molecule most likely to participate in recombination. The highly conserved 5′ end sequence of the genome and the 5′ end of the capsid gene in noroviruses is an obvious common target for calicivirus RNA polymerase to switch from one RNA molecule to another.

EVIDENCE FOR RECOMBINATION OF CALICIVIRUSES WITH OTHER VIRUS FAMILIES. After sequencing a portion of feline calicivirus strain F9, Neill[157] observed that ORF1 contained significant sequence identity with picornaviruses. This significant identity was concentrated around certain amino acid motifs within ORF1 that are homologous to those within the nonstructural region of picornaviruses and encode, in order, the 2C, 3C, and 3D genes. The order of these motifs and the approximate number of nucleotides between them were the same in both virus families (Fig. 173–5). The capsid gene of caliciviruses also is homologous

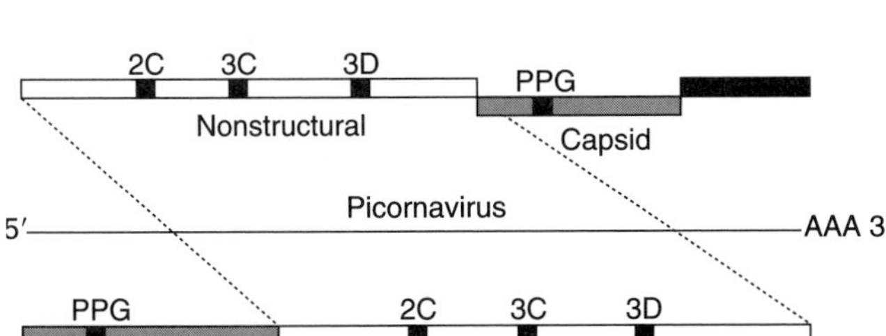

FIGURE 173–5 ■ Genomic organization of caliciviruses and picornaviruses showing the switch in order of nonstructural and structural genes. In caliciviruses, the nonstructural genes are encoded in ORF1; several of the genes were recognized because of the presence of significant sequence identity and consensus motifs like those known for picornaviruses (2C, 3C, and 3D). The capsid gene of caliciviruses is encoded in ORF2 (noroviruses and vesiviruses; see Fig. 173–3), which lies 3′ to the nonstructural genes, and is marked by a "PPG" motif that signals a relatively conserved region between the families. In picornaviruses, this order of nonstructural-structural "gene cassettes" is reversed, with the order and approximate distance of motifs within the nonstructural peptide the same. *Box shadings* are as in Figure 173–3.

to the VP1 to VP4 capsid proteins of picornaviruses to the extent of a shared PPG amino acid motif in a relatively conserved 5′ portion of the capsid gene or genes, formation of capsomeres having polypeptide β-pleated sheets as a core structural element, and formation of a spherical virion capsid by the protein or proteins.[176] These findings led to the hypothesis that at some point in time, the caliciviruses and picornaviruses were/are "recombination partners."[47]

ANTIGENIC PROPERTIES OF THE VIRION

The presence of a single calicivirus capsid protein ought to limit the antigenic complexity of the virion. Despite this limitation, circulating caliciviruses are highly diverse (e.g., see Hohdatsu and colleagues[81]). Assays to detect viral antigen and antiviral antibody have been developed for prototype strains of the genera and for distinct genetic clades within them.[72, 92, 94, 99, 152] Within the limits of testing, analysis of convalescent and hyperimmune antisera does not detect strains across generic boundaries, thus suggesting that different genetic groups represent distinct antigenic groups. Furthermore, epitopes not shared across phylogenetic clades within a genus have been identified.[75,96,226]

Most vesiviruses can be cultivated readily in cell culture, whereas cultivation of viruses in the other genera has been successful for only one animal strain.[56, 195, 198] The vesiviruses include a large number (>40) of serotypes (neutralization types).[195] Similarly, characterization of lagoviruses suggests the existence of serotypes.[162, 222] Determining whether the other genera have similar diversity has not been possible because of the lack of ability to test strains for their neutralization characteristics. Antigenic characterization of caliciviruses is at a primitive level of development.

Norovirus and *Sapovirus* Human Caliciviruses

Noroviruses and sapoviruses share a number of properties. To avoid repetition, I will discuss features common to the genera under each of the following headings and then those distinct to each genus.

EPIDEMIOLOGY

General Prevalence

Serologic studies indicate that *Norovirus* and *Sapovirus* infections occur commonly, with virtually all individuals having antibody by the second decade of life wherever studied. Noroviruses and sapoviruses have been found everywhere that they have been sought and probably have a worldwide distribution. Strains from multiple genetic clades and antigenically distinct strains within each genus co-circulate wherever it has been studied.[91, 138] In the same way, regional differences exist in the prevalence of antibody to specific types.[62, 83, 163, 167, 212]

Noroviruses are known best for causing outbreaks of gastroenteritis in adults, commonly associated with contaminated water and food, particularly shellfish. Noroviruses account for approximately 60 percent of such outbreaks in North America and Europe for which no bacterial or parasitic cause can be found.[53, 67, 80, 88, 112, 114, 148] Studies suggest that large changes in the relative prevalence of *Norovirus* clades have occurred during the past 30 years. For example, prototype Norwalk virus and closely related strains appear to have been the predominant noroviruses in the 1970s in several regions studied.[67] Thereafter, Snow Mountain virus and related strains (in a separate genetic clade within *Norovirus)* have been predominant, and strains within the clade that contains the prototype Norwalk virus are found infrequently (<5%).[63, 95, 96, 131, 212, 219] In addition, some *Norovirus* strains appear to prevail within a community for as short a time as 1 year.[89, 127] The causes of such temporal variation are uncertain, but they at least are related to widespread distribution of contaminated foodstuffs or water (or both) in a pattern like that observed for *Salmonella*.[77] This epidemiologic pattern also suggests the existence of type-common neutralizing epitopes, for individual antigenic types each cause only a small percentage of illness episodes in a region at any time. Contamination events, in which a single type is delivered across a large geographic region in a short period of time with an inoculum large enough to overcome (mild) host resistance, would thus be needed for any one antigenic type to be predominant. Such predominance would be of short duration.

Recombinant norovirus Arg320 and Snow Mountain virus first were recovered from persons with gastroenteritis in Argentina and the United States, respectively.[93, 103] Arg320 also was recovered from outbreaks of gastroenteritis in the United States[99] and the Netherlands.[111] Snow Mountain–like strains occur worldwide. The widespread occurrence of these recombinants in symptomatic persons suggests their ready infectivity, easy transmissibility, sustained virulence after multiple passage in humans, and genetic and ecologic stability.

Unlike the noroviruses, sapoviruses are known primarily from sporadic cases of diarrhea in children, although outbreaks in closed populations do occur.[28, 29, 37, 91, 99, 155] The proportion of outbreaks traced to sapoviruses probably will increase as improved methods for detection of them are applied. Typical caliciviruses visualized in stool specimens by electron microscopy but not yet further characterized probably fall into this genus.[35–37, 41, 142, 165]

Morbidity and Mortality

Cross-sectional surveys of diarrheal stool specimens from children or adults yield *Norovirus* in 0.5 to 16 percent of samples, with the higher values reported by recent studies and achieved by applying more sensitive detection methods.[44, 45, 58, 110, 128, 166, 169–171, 179] Attack rates in outbreaks frequently are high: 20 to 90 percent. These observed attack rates for outbreaks are similar to those from volunteer studies involving a single (low) inoculum of the Norwalk virus prototype, in which 82 percent of volunteers were infected and 56 percent were ill.[60] Secondary attack rates in common-source outbreaks range from 5 to 30 percent.[59] A general tendency is that noroviruses are detected more frequently in cross-sectional studies of subclinical or moderately severe illness than in episodes resulting in hospitalization; this trend is the reverse of that observed for rotaviruses, which are detected more frequently in more severe illness.[169, 171] Death from *Norovirus* illness rarely occurs. Cross-sectional studies in adults are conspicuously absent.[151] In adults, the severity of *Norovirus* infections is greater, and this trend is in part a consequence of an unusual pattern of protective immunity observed for these strains (see later).

Like noroviruses, sapoviruses are identified more frequently in less severe gastroenteritis episodes than in cases resulting in hospitalization. Cross-sectional surveys of gastroenteritis in nonhospitalized children have found sapoviruses in as many as 20 percent of cases.[58, 131, 156, 166, 182, 218] Similar studies of hospitalized children have found sapoviruses in as many as 5 percent of acute gastroenteritis episodes.[171] Death from *Sapovirus* infection is rare but does occur.[55, 135]

Age Incidence and Prevalence

Norovirus infections in developed countries generally have been thought to occur in individuals 4 years or older. This conclusion was derived from comparative serologic studies that revealed large differences in patterns of acquisition of age-specific antibody between developing and developed countries. For example, in Bangladesh, the prevalence of antibody in 4-year-old children was 100 percent, as opposed to a prevalence of 19 percent in children of the same age in the United States.[15, 104] In addition, studies of outbreaks suggested that young children in developed countries were spared.

More recent studies using more sensitive assays have changed these conclusions. For example, among 154 infants 23 months old who participated in a vaccine trial in Finland from 1987 to 1989, 73 percent had anti–Norwalk virus antibody.[122] In England, the prevalence of antibody to Norwalk virus in 1991 and 1992 was 48 percent in 1-year-old toddlers overall, with the prevalence in that age group ranging from 12 to 60 percent in different regions.[62] In South Africa, antibody prevalence in 1992 was 57 percent in 1-year-old children.[212] These results contrast with those from Hokkaido, Japan, where the prevalence of antibody to Norwalk virus in children 1 to 3 years of age was approximately 6 percent.[163] In England and Japan, but not in South Africa, a significant increase in the prevalence of antibody to Norwalk virus was noted in school-age children, in whom it reached 80 percent in England and 70 percent in Japan by the third decade of life.

Children are likely to be infected with multiple *Norovirus* types.[38, 138] Testing of a large population-based collection of sera from two cities in Chile for antibody to prototype Norwalk virus and Mexico virus (a Snow Mountain–like *Norovirus)* suggested that these two viruses had different modes of transmission and that exposure to the two types differed in that population.[167] For example, the overall prevalence of antibody to Norwalk virus was 83 percent and that to Mexico virus was 91 percent in this age-stratified sample of persons living in Santiago, whereas it was 67 percent and 90 percent, respectively, in Punta Arenas $p < .001$ for antibody to Norwalk virus). Consumption of uncooked vegetables was an independent risk factor for the acquisition of antibody to both viruses in Santiago, but only for Mexico virus in Punta Arenas. Consumption of seafood and attendance at childcare centers were independent risk factors for the acquisition of antibody to both viruses in Punta Arenas but not in Santiago. Results of this kind, to which attributes of the person providing serum, other than just age and location, are matched to the results of antibody testing, are needed for a more complete understanding of the modes of transmission and ecologic differences among calicivirus genera. The large differences in the prevalence of age-specific antibody among and within countries suggest that "herd immunity" to neutralizing epitopes specific to such clades can develop in populations. Such differences also suggest that the acquisition of antibody is the result of selected, variable, and cumulative exposure, such as from multistate and multicontinent movement of strains in contaminated food.[3, 100, 121, 184]

Serologic studies confirm that children acquire *Sapovirus* infection soon after birth and that virtually all are infected by the time they reach 4 years of age.[39, 154, 186] Children are infected with multiple *Sapovirus* types during this period.[39, 136, 137] Outbreaks have been described in infants, young children, and adults.[80] The prevalence of antibody to sapoviruses exceeds 70 percent in adults studied in Asia, Australia, Africa, Europe, and North America.[39, 154, 170]

Norovirus and *Sapovirus* outbreaks tend to be recognized in closed populations where common exposure occurs, such as nurseries, childcare centers, schools, hospitals, camps, hotels, and ships.* Outbreaks in young adults in military camps and on deployment, especially navy ships, are a special example because of the increased severity of *Norovirus* illness in young adults.[8, 31, 87, 128, 141, 168, 192] Vehicles of infection in outbreaks include water from regulated and unregulated delivery systems and foods commonly washed, such as salad and fruit.[4, 36] Shellfish are a frequent source of infection. Person-to-person spread also occurs. New infections can occur over the course of several weeks, with the longest outbreak lasting 3 months. Such prolonged or repeated outbreaks have been associated with persistent asymptomatic excretion in food handlers, continual surface contamination at the site, and re-exposure to the same strain from contaminated foods.[27, 28, 37, 40, 155]

Seasonal Patterns

Both sporadic and outbreak-associated *Norovirus* infections have a winter seasonality[58, 65, 150, 171] (Fig. 173–6). This trend has exceptions, however. Infections related to certain foodstuffs will occur when such foodstuffs are harvested and eaten fresh (fruit, salads, shellfish) or processed, shipped, and consumed later (frozen fruits, ice). Infection from exposure related to certain types of recreation, such as swimming, should have a seasonal predominance. In addition, contamination of water supplies should occur more frequently when flooding results in mixing of water and sewage and when shellfish are harvested.[74]

A distinct seasonal prevalence of *Sapovirus*-associated illness is not as apparent, but a winter predominance is suggested from several studies.[136, 170, 171]

PATHOGENESIS AND PATHOLOGY

Viral Infection

The incubation period after exposure to *Norovirus* ranges from 10 to 51 hours, with a mean of 24 hours.[16, 29, 48, 49, 60, 137, 187, 224]

*See references 27, 28, 65, 130, 137, 138, 153, 180, 191, 217.

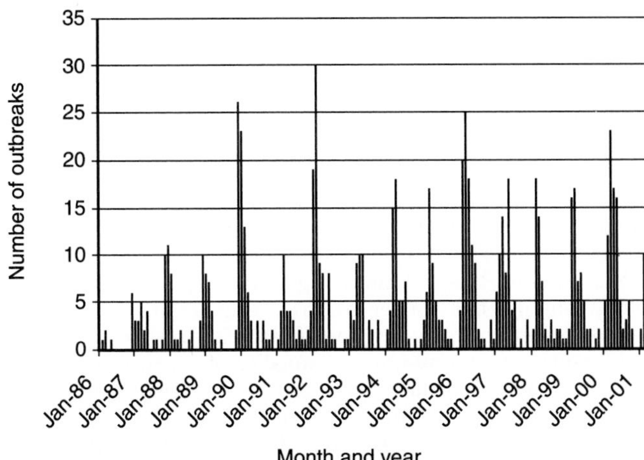

FIGURE 173–6 ■ Seasonality of 840 presumed viral outbreaks in nursing homes for the elderly in Maryland, 1986 to 2000. Detailed analyses of 20 outbreaks found noroviruses in 18. (Data extracted from Fig. 1 in Green, K. Y., Belliot, G., Taylor, J. L., et al.: A predominant role for Norwalk-like viruses as agents of epidemic gastroenteritis in Maryland nursing homes for the elderly. J. Infect. Dis. *185*:133–146, 2002.)

Illness usually lasts 2 to 3 days.[60] Excretion begins as early as 15 hours after the development of infection, peaks at 25 to 72 hours after infection, and persists at least 7 days.[60] Transmission of infection occurs by fecal-oral spread. Noroviruses also have been detected in vomitus, thus suggesting the possibility of spread by aerosol or dispersion of vomitus particles.[25, 109, 187]

Some volunteers administered Norwalk virus prototype had no response, neither illness nor evidence of infection, to the inoculum. These nonresponders have B blood type.[86] Results from binding assays support the role of complex sugar structures that determine blood type specificity in *Norovirus* virion attachment.[129] The absence of these cell surface structures prevents illness because the cell is not infected. These findings complement those suggesting that certain ethnic groups are inherently resistant to infection.[52] Similar information about sapoviruses is lacking.

Pathology

The pathogenic features of *Norovirus* infection have not been determined. The following information is based on studies of porcine and calf enteric caliciviruses.[57, 71, 76] Enteric animal caliciviruses cause lesions in the proximal portion of the small bowel. The first day after inoculation, enterocytes swell along the sides of the microvilli at the base. Damaged enterocytes subsequently slough, with stunted villi left behind. The adjacent villi fuse, which helps maintain the integrity of the intestinal mucosa. Neutrophils and mononuclear cells infiltrate the epithelium. The peak of pathologic abnormalities is 3 to 7 days after inoculation, at which time gradual healing begins to occur, with restoration of normal villus architecture about 10 days after inoculation. Mucosal injury is accompanied by deficiencies of β-galactosidase activity and D-xylose absorption. The capacity for D-xylose absorption recovers by the time that the normal histologic appearance of the villi is restored, but the β-galactosidase deficiency is delayed for an unknown period thereafter. Individual responses to inoculation vary in both the distribution and severity of lesions.

Prototype Norwalk virus causes similar histologic abnormalities, also located in the proximal part of the small bowel.[189] However, the abrupt onset of illness in adults and the consistent finding that individuals with antibody are more likely to be ill than are individuals lacking antibody suggest that an immune mechanism plays a role in illness.

The pathogenic features of *Sapovirus* calicivirus infection in humans have not been determined and are presumed to be the same as those for *Norovirus* caliciviruses.

Immunologic Events

The humoral immune responses to *Norovirus* and *Sapovirus* infection are like those for infection with other virus. Individuals lacking antibodies show a rapid rise in the titer of serum and fecal antibody that persists for months, and individuals with high serum antibody levels are unlikely to mount an antibody response when re-exposed to the virus. Children with anti-*Norovirus* or anti-*Sapovirus* antibody appear to be protected against subsequent infection, at least in the short term.[40, 122, 155] A striking and consistent observation is that adult volunteers inoculated with noroviruses who have higher levels of preexisting serum or fecal antibody are more likely to excrete virus or be ill than are individuals who have low or no preexisting antibody.[60] The mechanism is unknown for this apparent conflict with the usual observation that serum or fecal antibody is a marker for protection against infection.

When the symptom profile of 50 Norwalk virus volunteers was assessed, the increased risk of being symptomatic with higher preexisting antibody titers was statistically significant for ill subjects who had vomiting as the predominant clinical feature.[60] Because vomiting in the gastroenteritis syndrome may result from a process different from that causing diarrhea, this observation suggests an alternative pathogenic mechanism peculiar to the noroviruses. The existence of such an alternative pathogenic mechanism would explain the unusual observation that age-specific morbidity tends to be greatest in adults. One issue unresolved from these studies is whether the antibody assays used in these volunteer studies measured neutralizing or non-neutralizing anti–Norwalk virus antibody. Moreover, asymptomatic infection apparently can occur independent of the absence of attachment structures related to blood type.[60, 86]

CLINICAL MANIFESTATIONS

The clinical manifestations of *Norovirus* and *Sapovirus* are those of acute gastroenteritis.[60, 103, 185] In 50 adult volunteers inoculated with Norwalk virus, diarrhea was noted in 59 percent, nausea in 66 percent, cramps in 66 percent, headache or body ache in 66 percent, vomiting in 39 percent, chills in 24 percent, and fever in 22 percent.[60] This constellation of common symptoms is indistinguishable from those associated with other gastroenteritis pathogens. As is the case for most other viral pathogens, the majority of *Norovirus* and *Sapovirus* infections are likely to be asymptomatic. Extraintestinal infection caused by noroviruses and sapoviruses is unknown.

In 154 hospitalized children with calicivirus infection, vomiting was present in 120 (78%) patients, diarrhea in 102 (66%), and fever in 82 (53%).[171] The prevalence of these symptoms was similar in *Norovirus*- and *Sapovirus*-associated illness. Fever was noted more commonly (76%) in patients younger than 3 months than in older children (45%, $p < .001$). Similarly, vomiting occurred more commonly (86%) in older patients than in patients younger than 3 months (56%, $p < .001$). The median duration of symptoms was 1 day for vomiting (median number of episodes, 6 per day; range, 1 to 35 per day), 2 days for diarrhea (median of 6 stools per day; range, 1 to 50), and 1 day for fever. Conditions associated with hospitalization in these 154 children included dehydration (n = 42, 27%), respiratory symptoms (n = 15, 10%), and seizures (n = 6, 4%). Metabolic acidosis (n = 2), hypoglycemia (n = 1), and hypocalcemia (n = 1) were rare findings. The median cost for an episode of calicivirus-associated illness in these children was $3574 (1999 dollars), more than 90 percent of which was for the cost of hospitalization. These 154 hospitalized children had 191 visits to a physician's office and 45 visits to an emergency room, in addition to the hospital stay.

In direct comparison to rotavirus infection, *Norovirus*- and *Sapovirus*-associated illness was a mean of 2 points, of a 20-point score, less severe than rotavirus-associated illness was.[170, 171] Younger children (<3 months) had less severe illness than older children did (p = .006). The combination of vomiting, diarrhea, and fever occurred more frequently (58% of cases) in rotavirus-associated illness than in calicivirus-associated illness (23%, p < .001). Co-infections with rotavirus increased the severity of calicivirus-associated illness. Children hospitalized for rotavirus illness were older (median age, 408 days) than those hospitalized for calicivirus illness (median age, 257 days; p < .001).

Sapovirus illnesses also usually are indistinguishable from those caused by other gastroenteritis pathogens. A few children who were studied intensively after they were hospitalized for *Sapovirus* illness had prolonged malabsorption, frank rectal bleeding, severe dehydration and acidosis, and transient leukopenia. Three children with combined immunodeficiency and *Sapovirus* infection early in life that resulted in chronic diarrhea and death have been reported.[17, 35] Sapoviruses have been the only identified pathogen in the stool specimens of a few children who died of gastroenteritis, but little information describing the illness or the pathologic findings in these children has been reported.[35, 55]

DIAGNOSIS

Differential Diagnosis

Recognized outbreaks of calicivirus infection have tended to be associated with a rapid onset of symptoms and a broad age range of affected persons, especially if associated with common exposure to water or food. The pattern of symptoms is a fairly good marker for calicivirus-associated outbreaks: a brief duration of illness, 2 to 3 days; vomiting as a prominent symptom in more than 50 percent of the outbreak cases; an incubation period of 24 to 48 hours; a high (30%, usually >50%) secondary attack rate; and cultures of freshly processed stool specimens negative for bacterial, parasitic, or fungal pathogens.[106] When outbreaks have such characteristics, noroviruses will be detected in approximately 80 percent of them. Sapoviruses have been detected with current diagnostic techniques in about 3 to 5 percent of such outbreaks. Stool samples should be submitted to a facility skilled in using individual assays for these pathogens. Caliciviruses are destroyed by repeated freezing and thawing.[37, 85] Therefore, bulk stool samples stored at 4° C and not frozen should be collected early after the development of infection and referred promptly. Consultation with the reference laboratory should precede sample referral.[119]

Specific Diagnosis

Detection methods relying on target nucleic acid amplification are needed for noroviruses and sapoviruses because virus is excreted in stool in low concentration, rarely exceeding 10^6 particles per gram of stool. In addition, assays for antigen detection are highly specific; they apparently do not detect group-specific epitopes on the viruses and probably underestimate the prevalence of noroviruses in a survey.[55] Only a few laboratories routinely perform calicivirus detection assays, and some strains are not detected by the best designed consensus primer oligonucleotides because of genomic sequence diversity among strains.[82, 92, 96, 97, 227] Reverse transcriptase–polymerase chain reaction amplicons from the viral RNA polymerase genomic region are produced most reliably, but conservation among strains within and between genera in this region is sufficiently strong to warrant caution when assigning causality of an outbreak of illness to a particular strain based on the sequence of the (frequently small) amplicons from this region.[11, 13] Paired serum samples may be required to detect and confirm the presence of an etiologic agent.

Vesivirus Caliciviruses

EPIDEMIOLOGY

General Prevalence

Vesiviruses include a large number of animal caliciviruses isolated from many different hosts, including pigs, cows, cats, dogs, sea lions, sea otters, walruses, whales, several snakes, pygmy chimpanzees, and gorillas. These viruses probably have a worldwide distribution in terrestrial and marine environments, although studies of San Miguel calicivirus-like strains are lacking outside North America.[195] Vesiviruses include at least 40 neutralization types (serotypes). The prevalence of these serotypes in different regions has had little study.

Morbidity and Mortality

Vesiviruses cause a variety of severe illnesses in animals. The morbidity and mortality rates of individual strains differ from species to species in experimental infections. One laboratory worker was infected with SMSV-5 and experienced a flulike illness, followed during the next several days by viremia and vesicular exanthem similar to that observed in the original pinniped host.[194] SMSV-5 was visualized in vesicular fluid by electron microscopy and was cultured from the lesions; the genome was amplified and sequenced. The worker also mounted a greater than fourfold serum neutralizing antibody response to SMSV-5. Biologists working with marine mammals had similar illnesses but were studied less intensively than the laboratory worker was.[10, 194, 199]

Host and Social Factors

Although vesiviruses cause a variety of diseases, only a few cause gastroenteritis, a feature common to *Norovirus* and *Sapovirus* caliciviruses.[51] Among the vesiviruses are a number that exhibit a broad range of hosts. For example, SMSV-5 has been found to infect sea lions, seals, opaleye fish, pigs, cattle, and laboratory workers.[193, 201]

PATHOGENESIS AND PATHOLOGY

Viral Infection

Vesiviruses cause infection on mucosal surfaces (pneumonia, aphthous ulcers) and disease after viremia (generalized vesicular eruption, encephalitis, hepatitis, spontaneous abortion). The incubation period after exposure is short: 1 to 4 days.[207] Excretion is variable among species. For three cultivatable vesiviruses, asymptomatic and persistent virus excretion was detected for months after primary infection.[101, 198, 202]

Pathology

The pathogenic features of *Vesivirus* infection are variable and depend on the syndrome of the affected host.

CLINICAL MANIFESTATIONS

The proven clinical manifestations of *Vesivirus* calicivirus infection in humans are limited to a few cases. Because vesiviruses cause a variety of illnesses in animals and these viruses occur naturally in primates, the potential spectrum of illness in humans is broad. Groups at greatest risk of acquiring infection probably would be zoo workers, indigenous populations handling marine mammals, veterinarians, and laboratory workers, but studies of these groups have been limited.[199, 200] Evaluation of donors of blood for transfusion and patients with non-A-G hepatitis has revealed a pattern of increasing prevalence of anti-*Vesivirus* antibody as the certainty of hepatitis in the group increased, as follows: in normal blood donors, anti-*Vesivirus* antibody prevalence was 5 percent; in blood donors whose donation was rejected solely because of elevated liver transaminases, 8 percent; and in patients with non-A-G hepatitis, 19 percent ($p < .001$).[203] Asymptomatic viremia with a San Miguel marine calicivirus type has been detected in one blood donor with anti-*Vesivirus* antibody.[203]

DIAGNOSIS

Many vesiviruses can be cultivated in cell culture, and many are found in sufficiently high concentration in clinical samples to permit the use of electron microscopy and classic virologic methods for detection of infecting viruses. Other strains have resisted cultivation, and molecular techniques have been developed for them.[134, 161, 190] Vesiviruses are heat-labile, and clinical samples should be submitted promptly and unfrozen.

Lagovirus Caliciviruses

EPIDEMIOLOGY

General Prevalence

The prototype *Lagovirus* is RHDV. Lagoviruses include the genetically distinct European brown hare syndrome virus and multiple genetically distinct strains recovered from asymptomatic rabbits.[21, 22, 116, 118, 120, 222] Antigenic diversity occurs in this genus, but the number of serotypes in the genus is unknown, for like noroviruses and sapoviruses, lagoviruses cannot be cultivated in the laboratory.[222] RHDV has been epidemic in Asia and Europe since its first recognition in China in 1984. Rabbits in more than 40 countries have been affected. Disease spreads rapidly and appears to "leap" large distances in a short period. The ability of the virus to spread rapidly across large bodies of water (e.g., the English Channel) suggests that arthropods or other flying vectors have a role in transmission.[26] One outbreak in Mexico was traced to a shipment of rabbit meat from Asia; extensive slaughter of rabbits in Mexico was required to eradicate the agent.[68] Three outbreaks have occurred in North America and Cuba.[84] The source of these outbreaks is unknown.

RHDV was released in 1995 in controlled field studies off the coast of mainland Australia but escaped from the study site the same year and spread on that continent.[90] Subsequently, the virus was introduced illegally into the South Island of New Zealand. Clandestine, deliberate spread in both countries to control exotic European rabbits led to wide dispersal of the agent. These releases occurred despite conflicting evidence of RHDV infection in experimental animals and, subsequently, in humans.[23, 133]

Morbidity and Mortality

RHDV infections are highly fatal (>80%) in wild and domesticated European rabbits. Subclinical infections occur in young rabbits, and immunity from early infection appears to attenuate later exposure. In the food-associated outbreak in Mexico, antibody developed in one human. Zoo workers, rabbit breeders, and foresters would have the largest occupational risk of RHDV exposure. The human infection in the Mexican outbreak apparently was subclinical.[68] Ostensibly subclinical infection also occurred in some persons exposed to rabbits in Australia after escape of the virus there.[133]

Host and Social Factors

The range of hosts of lagoviruses and the host of RHDV before its recognition in rabbits in China are unknown. In Australian studies, numerous Australian animal species challenged with a subimmunogenic dose of RHDV had no antibody response. On the other hand, antibodies did develop in kiwis, mice, dogs, and foxes; in the case of foxes, the serum antibody response was attributable to oral feeding.[32] Natural spread in rabbits is enhanced by their colony breeding behavior.

CLINICAL MANIFESTATIONS AND PATHOGENESIS

The incubation period after exposure is 1 to 3 days.[214] Lagoviruses cause a fatal hepatitis in rabbits and hares that results in disseminated intravascular coagulation and diffuse hemorrhage. Death is rapid: 6 to 12 hours after the onset of illness. RHDV and European brown hare syndrome virus appear to be sufficiently distinct to preclude cross-protection.

DIAGNOSIS

Because the infections in the Mexican worker exposed during the RHDV outbreak and in the workers in Australia who tested antibody-positive apparently were subclinical, the spectrum of potential infection in humans is unknown. Samples from persons with suspected infection should be submitted to reference laboratories after consultation. Diagnosis is possible through immunologic and molecular techniques.

Treatment and Prevention

SPECIFIC MEASURES

No specific treatment of calicivirus infection has been reported. The existence of at least partially effective vaccines for feline calicivirus and RHDV indicates that this prevention method would work for other caliciviruses. A norovirus vaccine incorporating an immunogen-expressed capsid protein that self-assembles into virion-like particles is being developed.[9, 209] Feline interferon and ribavirin inhibit the replication of feline calicivirus (a *Vesivirus)* in feline cell lines.[147, 175] Morpholino antisense oligomers blocked virion production by three *Vesivirus* strains in three cell lines.[205, 206] These antisense compounds have potential for prophylaxis and treatment of illness.[197]

NONSPECIFIC MEASURES

Children with diarrhea are more likely than are children without diarrhea to be excreting enteric viruses, which reflects an association between the incidence of diarrhea and the cleanliness of the environment. This principle is likely to hold for caliciviruses as well. For children in care settings with other children, a few infection control measures are likely to reduce the spread of infection. Such measures include trained personnel, cleanliness of surfaces and food preparation, exclusion of ill or carrier care providers, adequate handwashing, and exclusion or cohorting of ill children.[42, 69] Laboratory workers exposed to caliciviruses should be aware of the risk of acquiring infection.

Prognosis

Understanding of the features of calicivirus infection has increased rapidly since 1990, when molecular tools for studying the viruses became available. The availability of refined diagnostic reagents will permit an accurate assessment of the extent and variety of calicivirus-associated illness. Specific preventive measures are under development, but their potential is clouded by uncertainty about the antigenic and genetic diversity of strains and the strength of cross-protection induced by exposure to one or more strains.

HEPATITIS E VIRUS

Genomic Organization

The genomic organization of HEV is similar to that of sapoviruses; however, in HEV, the spacing of consensus motifs in ORF1, including absence of the 3C motif, differs from that found in the four calicivirus genera. Phylogenetic analysis of the relatively conserved nonstructural genes in ORF1 among the virus families has indicated that HEV is closer to *Togaviridae,* which includes rubella and Sindbis viruses, than to *Caliciviridae* or *Picornaviridae*[13, 64] (Fig. 173–7). Based on these analyses, HEV is conclusively distinct from the four calicivirus genera.[66]

Epidemiology

GENERAL PREVALENCE

Beginning in the 1950s, particularly large outbreaks of hepatitis were reported from southern Asia.[73, 108, 149, 211, 220] Because the outbreaks appeared to result from fecal-oral contamination, they initially were attributed to hepatitis A virus. However, the outbreaks were frequently very large and affected thousands of individuals, had a high mortality rate in pregnant women, and did not show a pattern of person-to-person transmission. In 1987, epidemiologic and laboratory investigation finally succeeded in identifying the cause of these outbreaks to be a new virus, HEV, which was transiently classified in the *Caliciviridae.*[19, 113, 210]

Hepatitis E is known from outbreak and sporadic cases of hepatitis in Asia, Africa, Australia, and Latin America. Known transmission occurs via contaminated drinking water, but the intermittent nature of the outbreaks suggests that additional factors, such as an animal reservoir, may be important. A porcine HEV has been described; it is widespread and closely related to the HEV of humans.[144, 188, 215]

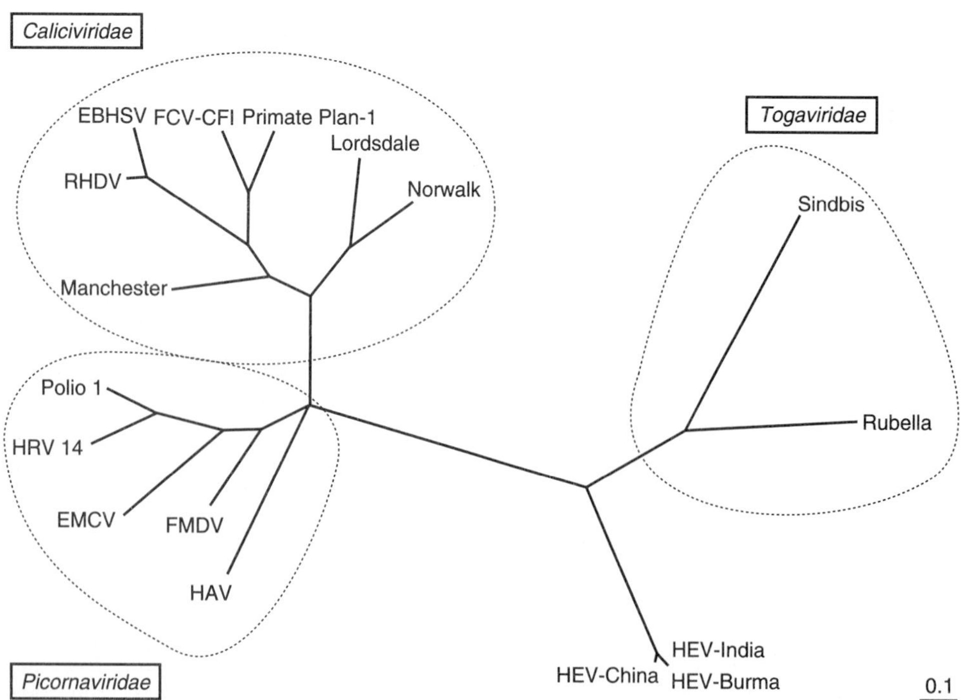

FIGURE 173–7 ■ Phylogenetic relationships of hepatitis E virus with the *Picornaviridae, Caliciviridae,* and *Togaviridae* in the helicase ("2C") region of the genome. Partial gene sequences (200 amino acids) were used for the phylogenetic analysis. The tree was constructed from the nucleic acid alignment by using the maximal likelihood algorithm. (Tree courtesy of T. Berke.)

A distinct HEV also occurs in chickens.[78] Cases have been imported to Europe and North America; based on serosurveys (see later), hepatitis E appears to be endemic in many regions not previously thought to host the agent.

MORBIDITY AND MORTALITY

Hepatitis E causes acute hepatitis, like hepatitis A, with a mortality rate of 0.5 to 3.0 percent in the general population.[221] Mortality is particularly high in pregnant women, with rates approaching 20 to 25 percent. Hepatitis E is the principal cause of enterically transmitted acute hepatitis in some cross-sectional surveys and was shown to occur 10 to 20 times more frequently than does hepatitis A.[30] Whether this trend is general or reflects the waxing and waning occurrence of hepatitis A and E from year to year in some regions will need to be determined from longitudinal studies.

Hepatitis E outbreaks can be intense. During one epidemic period in Kapur, India, 111 hepatitis cases occurred in 2018 members of 343 families, for a hepatitis attack rate of 5.5 percent in the individuals and 24 percent in the households.[2] The pattern of secondary cases suggested that person-to-person spread did not occur. During an epidemic period of 20 months' duration in Somalia, 11,413 cases and 346 deaths occurred among 245,312 persons in 142 villages, for an attack rate of 4.6 percent and a case-fatality rate of 3 percent.[14]

AGE INCIDENCE AND PREVALENCE

Seroepidemiologic studies in endemic regions suggest that HEV infection occurs primarily after the first decade of life.[7, 173, 213] In Pune, India, antibody prevalence was less than 5 percent in individuals in the first decade of life and reached a peak prevalence of 30 to 40 percent in those in the third and fourth decades of life.[7] This rate contrasted with seroprevalence rates for hepatitis A, with which virtually all children were infected by the second decade of life. These patterns were the same in 1982 and 1992, which indicates that no significant changes occurred in virus circulation that might be expected from the acquisition of herd immunity or other factors. In the study from Somalia cited earlier, the infection rate was 5 percent in children 1 to 4 years of age, 13 percent in children 5 to 15 years of age, and 20 percent in older individuals. The female-to-male ratio in cases was 1.5:1.[14]

SEASONAL PATTERNS

A distinct seasonal prevalence of HEV infection is not apparent. Cases are more likely to occur in seasons when flooding results in contamination of drinking water supplies by sewage disposal systems.

HOST AND SOCIAL FACTORS

Risk factors for sporadic cases of hepatitis E have not been described. Person-to-person spread is not a common mode of transmission. Nosocomial transmission has occurred.[183] The incidence of disease is greatest in regions with the poorest water treatment procedures, and the virus has been detected in treated water and sewage.[102] Pigs and rodents probably are enzootic hosts.[6, 107] Molecular and serologic evidence suggests that HEV is epizootic in humans as a result of pig exposure.[50, 145, 174, 188, 215, 223]

Pathogenesis and Pathology

VIRAL INFECTION

The incubation period after exposure is 15 to 60 days, with an average of 40 days.[108, 149] Excretion lasts as long as 14 days at levels detectable by enzyme immunoassay but probably is longer at lower infectious levels because viral antigen persists in the liver for approximately 6 weeks after infection and virus is excreted in bile.[18]

PATHOLOGY

The pathogenic features of HEV infection are those of an acute viral hepatitis and include focal hepatocellular necrosis, cholestatic inflammation, and acidophilic hepatocellular degeneration.[73, 108, 125, 149]

IMMUNOLOGIC EVENTS

Humoral immune responses to HEV infection follow patterns common to many viral illnesses.[18] Individuals lacking antibodies are at increased risk for the development of illness and show a rapid rise in serum antibody titer that persists for months. Individuals with high serum antibody levels are unlikely to mount an antibody response or become ill when re-exposed to the virus. Asymptomatic and subclinical infection is a common occurrence. Cellular immune responses have not been studied.

Immunoglobulin prepared from donors living in endemic regions may protect naive patients from infection, but such preparations have not been standardized for this purpose.[20]

Clinical Manifestations

HEV probably causes a mild gastroenteritis, but the symptoms of that infection would occur weeks before jaundice develops. Longitudinal studies to determine the features of primary infection have not been conducted. HEV-infected patients with hepatitis frequently have malaise (95–100%), anorexia (66–100%), abdominal pain (37–82%), hepatomegaly (10–85%), nausea and vomiting (29–100%), fever (23–97%), and pruritus (14–47%).[108, 149] Resolution of illness occurs 1 to 6 weeks after onset. Chronic disease has not been observed.

Diagnosis

DIFFERENTIAL DIAGNOSIS

Hepatitis E is indistinguishable clinically from hepatitis caused by other viruses and a variety of noninfectious causes. Clinicians should obtain serial blood samples for serologic assays and submit fresh, unfrozen sequential stool specimens to a reference laboratory skilled in the detection of HEV.

SPECIFIC DIAGNOSIS

The pattern of onset of illness, epidemiologic features such as a recent travel history or other exposure, and the presence of serologic markers will help determine that HEV is the cause of an acute hepatitis. Virus is excreted at low levels, and electron microscopy is a poor technique for detection of HEV. Enzyme-linked immunosorbent assays and molecular techniques have been developed for detection of viral antigen and antiviral antibody, as well as for detection of viral nucleic acid in clinical specimens. Specimens for such testing should be submitted to a reference laboratory after consultation.[18, 54]

REFERENCES

1. Adler, J. L., and Zickl, R.: Winter vomiting disease. J. Infect. Dis. *119*:668–673, 1969.
2. Aggarwal, R., and Naik, S. R.: Hepatitis E: Intrafamilial transmission versus waterborne spread. J. Hepatol. *21*:718–723, 1994.
3. Anderson, A. D., Garrett, V. D., Sobel, J., et al.: Multistate outbreak of Norwalk-like virus gastroenteritis associated with a common carrier. Am. J. Epidemiol. *154*:1013–1019, 2001.
4. Appleton, H.: Small round viruses: Classification and role in food-borne infections. *In* Bock, G., and Whelan, J. (eds.): Novel Diarrhoea Viruses. Chichester, England, Wiley, 1987, pp. 238–249.
5. Appleton, H., and Higgins, P. G.: Viruses and gastroenteritis in infants. Lancet *1*:1297, 1975.
6. Arankalle, V. A., Joshi, M. V., Kulkarni, A. M., et al.: Prevalence of anti–hepatitis E virus antibodies in different Indian animal species. J. Viral Hepat. *8*:223–227, 2001.
7. Arankalle, V. A., Tsarev, S. A., Chadha, M. S., et al.: Age-specific prevalence of antibodies to hepatitis A and E viruses in Pune, India, 1982 and 1992. J. Infect. Dis. *171*:447–450, 1995.
8. Arness, M. K., Feighner, B. H., Canham, M. L., et al.: Norwalk-like viral gastroenteritis outbreak in U.S. Army trainees. Emerg. Infect. Dis. *6*:204–207, 2000.
9. Ball, J. M., Hardy, M. E., Atmar, R. L., et al.: Oral immunization with recombinant Norwalk virus–like particles induces a systemic and mucosal immune response in mice. J. Virol. *72*:1345–1353, 1998.
10. Barlough, J. E., Berry, E. S., Skilling, D. E., et al.: The marine calicivirus story. Compendium on Continuing Education for the Practicing Veterinarian *8*:F5–F14, F75–F82, 1986.
11. Berke, T., Golding, B., Jiang, X., et al.: A phylogenetic analysis of the caliciviruses. J. Med. Virol. *52*:419–424, 1997.
12. Berke, T., and Matson, D. O.: Unpublished data.
13. Berke, T., and Matson, D. O.. Reclassification of the Caliciviridae into distinct genera and exclusion of hepatitis E virus from the family on the basis of comparative phylogenetic analysis. Arch. Virol. *145*:1421–1436, 2000.
14. Bile, K., Isse, A., Mohamud, O., et al.: Contrasting roles of rivers and wells as sources of drinking water on attack and fatality rates in a hepatitis E epidemic in Somalia. Am. J. Trop. Med. Hyg. *51*:466–474, 1994.
15. Black, R. E., Greenberg, H. B., Kapikian, A. Z., et al.: Acquisition of serum antibody to Norwalk virus and rotavirus and relation to diarrhea in a longitudinal study of young children in rural Bangladesh. J. Infect. Dis. *145*:483–489, 1982.
16. Blacklow, N. R., Dolin, R., Fedson, D. S., et al.: Acute infectious nonbacterial gastroenteritis: Etiology and pathogenesis. A combined clinical staff conference at the Clinical Center of the National Institutes of Health. Ann. Intern. Med. *76*:993–1008, 1972.
17. Booth, I. W., Chrystie, I. L., Levinsky, R. J., et al.: Protracted diarrhoea, immunodeficiency and viruses. Eur. J. Pediatr. *138*:271–272, 1982.
18. Bradley, D. W.: Hepatitis E virus: A brief review of the biology, molecular virology, and immunology of a novel virus. J. Hepatol. *22*:140–145, 1995.
19. Bradley, D. W., Krawczynski, K., Cook, E. H., et al.: Enterically transmitted non-A, non-B hepatitis: Serial passage of disease in cynomolgus macaques and tamarins and recovery of disease-associated virus-like particles. Proc. Natl. Acad. Sci. U. S. A. *84*:6277–6281, 1987.
20. Bryan, J. P., Tsarev, S. A., Iqbal, M., et al.: Epidemic hepatitis E in Pakistan: Patterns of serologic response and evidence that antibody to hepatitis E virus protects against disease. J. Infect. Dis. *170*:517–521, 1994.
21. Capucci, L., Fusi, P., Lavazza, A., et al.: Detection and preliminary characterization of a new rabbit calicivirus related to rabbit hemorrhagic disease virus but nonpathogenic. J. Virol. *70*:8614–8623, 1996.
22. Capucci, L., and Lavazza, A.: A brief update on rabbit hemorrhagic disease virus. Emerg. Infect. Dis. *4*:343–344, 1998.
23. Carman, J. A., Garner, M. G., Catton, M. G., et al.: Viral haemorrhagic disease of rabbits and human health. Epidemiol. Infect. *121*:409–418, 1998.
24. Carter, M. J., Milton, I. D., Meanger, J., et al.: The complete nucleotide sequence of a feline calicivirus. Virology *190*:443–448, 1992.
25. Chadwick, P. R., Walker, M., and Rees, A. E.: Airborne transmission of a small round structured virus. Lancet *343*:171, 1994.
26. Chasey, D.: Possible origin of rabbit haemorrhagic disease in the United Kingdom. Vet. Rec. *135*:496–499, 1994.
27. Cheesbrough, J. S., Green, J., Gallimore, C. I., et al.: Widespread environmental contamination with Norwalk-like viruses (NLV) detected in a prolonged hotel outbreak of gastroenteritis. Epidemiol. Infect. *125*:93–98, 2000.
28. Chiba, S., Sakuma, Y., Kogasaka, R., et al.: An outbreak of gastroenteritis associated with calicivirus in an infant home. J. Med. Virol. *4*:249–254, 1979.
29. Chiba, S., Sakuma, Y., Kogasaka, R., et al.: Fecal shedding of virus in relation to the days of illness in infantile gastroenteritis due to calicivirus. J. Infect. Dis. *142*:247–249, 1980.
30. Clayson, E. T., Innis, B. L., Myint, K. S., et al.: Short report: Relative risk of hepatitis A and E among foreigners in Nepal. Am. J. Trop. Med. Hyg. *52*:506–507, 1995.
31. Cohen, D., Block, C. S., Ambar, R., et al.: Pilot study of an extended range of potential etiologic agents of diarrhea in the Israel Defense Forces. Isr. J. Med. Sci. *28*::49–51, 1992.
32. Coman, B. J.: Environmental impact associated with the proposed use of rabbit calicivirus disease for integrated rabbit control in Australia. Australia and New Zealand Rabbit Calicivirus Program, Sydney, February 1996.
33. Cooper, P. D., Agol, V. I., Bachrach, H. L., et al.: Picornaviridae: Second report. Intervirology *10*:165, 1978.
34. Cubitt, W. D., Bradley, D., Carter, M., et al.: Caliciviridae. *In* Murphy, F. A., Fauquet, C. M., Bishop, D. H. L., et al. (eds.): The Sixth Report of the International Committee for Taxonomy of Viruses. Vienna, Springer-Verlag, 1995, pp. 359–363.
35. Cubitt, W. D.: Human caliciviruses: Characterization and epidemiology. Dissertation, Middlesex Hospital Medical School, London, 1985.
36. Cubitt, W. D.: The candidate caliciviruses. *In* Bock, G., and Whelan, J. (eds.): Novel Diarrhoea Viruses. Chichester, England, Wiley, 1987, pp. 126–143.
37. Cubitt, W. D., Blacklow, N. R., Herrmann, J. E., et al.: Antigenic relationships between human caliciviruses and Norwalk virus. J. Infect. Dis. *156*:806–814, 1987.
38. Cubitt, W. D., and McSwiggan, D. A.: Calicivirus gastroenteritis in northwest London. Lancet *2*:975–977, 1981.
39. Cubitt, W. D., McSwiggan, D. A.: Seroepidemiological survey of the prevalence of antibodies to a strain of human calicivirus. J. Med. Virol. *21*:361–368, 1987.
40. Cubitt, W. D., McSwiggan, D. A., and Arstall, S.: An outbreak of calicivirus infection in a mother and baby unit. J. Clin. Pathol. *33*:1095–1098, 1980.
41. Cubitt, W. D., Pead, P. J., and Saeed, A. A.: A new serotype of calicivirus associated with an outbreak of gastroenteritis in a residential home for the elderly. J. Clin. Pathol. *34*:924–926, 1981.
42. Cummings, G. D.: Epidemic diarrhea of the newborn from the point of view of the epidemiologist and bacteriologist. J. Pediatr. *30*:706–710, 1947.
43. Dastjerdi, A. M., Green, J., Gallimore, C. I., et al.: The bovine Newbury agent-2 is genetically more closely related to human SRSVs than to animal caliciviruses. Virology *254*:1–5, 1999.
44. De Wit, M. A. S., Koopmans, M. P. G., Kortbeek, L. M., et al.: Gastroenteritis in sentinel general practices, the Netherlands. Emerg. Infect. Dis. *7*:82–91, 2001.
45. De Wit, M. A. S., Koopmans, M. P. G., Kortbeek, L. M., et al.: Etiology of gastroenteritis in sentinel general practices in the Netherlands. Clin. Infect. Dis. *33*:280–288, 2001.
46. Dingle, K. E., Lambden, P. R., Caul, E. O., et al.: Human enteric Caliciviridae: The complete genome sequence and expression of virus-like particles from a genetic group II small round structured virus. J. Gen. Virol. *76*:2349–2355, 1995.
47. Dinulos, M. B., and Matson, D. O.: Recent developments with human caliciviruses. Pediatr. Infect. Dis. J. *13*:998–1003, 1994.
48. Dolin, R., Blacklow, N. R., Dupont, H., et al.: Transmission of acute infectious nonbacterial gastroenteritis to volunteers by oral administration of stool filtrates. J. Infect. Dis. *123*:307–312, 1971.
49. Dolin, R., Blacklow, N. R., Dupont, H., et al.: Biological properties of Norwalk agent of acute infectious nonbacterial gastroenteritis. Proc. Soc. Exp. Biol. Med. *140*:578–583, 1972.
50. Drobeniuc, J., Favorov, M. O., Shapiro, C. N., et al.: Hepatitis E virus antibody prevalence among persons who work with swine. J. Infect. Dis. *184*:1594–1597, 2001.
51. Evermann, J. F., McKeirnan, A. J., Smith, A. W., et al.: Isolation and identification of caliciviruses from dogs with enteric infections. Am. J. Vet. Res. *46*:218–220, 1985.
52. Ewald, D., Franks, C., Thompson, S., et al.: Possible community immunity to small round structured virus gastroenteritis in a rural aboriginal community. Commun. Dis. Intell. *24*:48–50, 2000.
53. Fankhauser, R. L., Noel, J. S., Monroe, S. S., et al.: Molecular epidemiology of "Norwalk-like viruses" in outbreaks of gastroenteritis in the United States. J. Infect. Dis. *178*:1571–1578, 1998.
54. Favorov, M. O., Fields, H. A., Purdy, M. A., et al.: Serologic identification of hepatitis E virus infections in epidemic and endemic settings. J. Med. Virol. *36*:246–250, 1992.
55. Flewett, T. H., and Davies, H.: Caliciviruses in man. Lancet *1*:311, 1976.
56. Flynn, W. T., and Saif, L. J.: Serial propagation of porcine enteric calicivirus-like virus in primary porcine kidney cell cultures. J. Clin. Microbiol. *26*:206–212, 1988.
57. Flynn, W. T., Saif, L. J., and Moorhead, P. D.: Pathogenesis of porcine enteric calicivirus-like virus in four-day-old gnotobiotic piglets. Am. J. Vet. Res. *49*:819–825, 1988.

58. Glass, R. I., Noel, J., Ando, T., et al.: The epidemiology of enteric caliciviruses from humans: A reassessment using new diagnostics. J. Infect. Dis. *181*(Suppl.):254–261, 2000.
59. Goetz, H., Ekdahl, K., Lindbaeck, J., et al.: Clinical spectrum and transmission characteristics of infection with Norwalk-like virus: Findings from a large community outbreak in Sweden. Clin. Infect. Dis. *33*:622–628, 2001.
60. Graham, D. Y., Jiang, X., Tanaka, T., et al.: Norwalk virus infection of volunteers: New insights based on improved assays. J. Infect. Dis. *170*:34–43, 1994.
61. Gray, J. J., Green, J., Cunliffe, C., et al.: Mixed genogroup SRSV infection among a party of canoeists exposed to contaminated recreational water. J. Med. Virol. *52*:425–429, 1997.
62. Gray, J. J., Jiang, X., Morgan-Capner, P., et al.: Prevalence of antibodies to Norwalk virus in England: Detection by enzyme-linked immunosorbent assay using baculovirus-expressed Norwalk virus capsid antigen. J. Clin. Microbiol. *31*:1022–1025, 1993.
63. Green, J., Vinje, J., Gallimore, C. I., et al.: Capsid protein diversity among Norwalk-like viruses. Virus Genes *20*:227–236, 2000.
64. Green, K. Y., Ando, T., Balayan, M. S., et al.: Caliciviridae. *In* van Regenmortel, M. H. V., Fauquet, C. M., Bishop, D. H. L., et al. (eds.): Virus Taxonomy: Classification and Nomenclature of Viruses. Seventh Report of the International Committee on Taxonomy of Viruses. San Diego, Academic Press, 2000, pp. 725–735.
65. Green, K. Y., Belliot, G., Taylor, J. L., et al.: A predominant role for Norwalk-like viruses as agents of epidemic gastroenteritis in Maryland nursing homes for the elderly. J. Infect. Dis. *185*:133–146, 2002.
66. Green, K. Y., Berke, T., and Matson, D. O.: Hepatis E–like viruses. *In* van Regenmortel, M. H. V., Fauquet, C. M., Bishop, D. H. L., et al. (eds.): Virus Taxonomy: Classification and Nomenclature of Viruses. Seventh Report of the International Committee on Taxonomy of Viruses. San Diego, Academic Press, 2000, pp. 735–739.
67. Greenberg, H. B., Valdesuso, J., Yolken, R. H., et al.: Role of Norwalk virus in outbreaks of nonbacterial gastroenteritis. J. Infect. Dis. *139*:564–568, 1979.
68. Gregg, D. A., House, C., Meyer, R., et al.: Viral haemorrhagic disease of rabbits in Mexico: Epidemiology and viral characterization. Rev. Sci. Tech. *10*:435–451, 1991.
69. Gulati, B. R., Allwood, P. B., Hedberg, C. W., et al.: Efficacy of commonly used disinfectants for the inactivation of calicivirus on strawberry, lettuce, and a food-contact surface. J. Food Prot. *64*:1430–1434, 2001.
70. Guo, M., Chang, K. O., Hardy, M. E., et al.: Molecular characterization of a porcine enteric calicivirus genetically related to Sapporo-like human caliciviruses. J. Virol. *73*:9625–9631, 1999.
71. Guo, M., Hayes, J., Cho, K. O., et al.: Comparative pathogenesis of tissue culture–adapted and wild-type Cowden porcine enteric calicivirus (PEC) in gnotobiotic pigs and induction of diarrhea by intravenous inoculation of wild-type PEC. J. Virol. *75*:9239–9251, 2001.
72. Guo, M., Qian, Y., Chang, K. O., et al.: Expression and self-assembly in baculovirus of porcine enteric calicivirus capsids into virus-like particles and their use in an enzyme-linked immunosorbent assay for antibody detection in swine. J. Clin. Microbiol. *39*:1487–1493, 2001.
73. Gupta, D. N., and Smetana, H. F.: The histopathology of viral hepatitis as seen in the Delhi epidemics (1955–56). Indian J. Med. Res. *45*:101–113, 1957.
74. Hafliger, D., Hubner, P., and Luthy, J.: Outbreak of viral gastroenteritis due to sewage-contaminated drinking water. Int. J. Food Microbiol. *54*:123–126, 2000.
75. Hale, A. D., Tanaka, T. N., Kitamoto, N., et al.: Identification of an epitope common to genogroup I "Norwalk-like viruses." J. Clin. Microbiol. *38*:1656–1660, 2000.
76. Hall, G. A., Bridger, J. C., Brooker, B. E., et al.: Lesions of gnotobiotic calves experimentally infected with a calicivirus-like (Newbury) agent. Vet. Pathol. *21*:208–215, 1984.
77. Hall, J. A., Goulding, J. S., Bean, N. H., et al.: Epidemiologic profiling: Evaluating foodborne outbreaks for which no pathogen was isolated by routine laboratory testing: United States, 1982–9. Epidemiol. Infect. *127*:381–387, 2001.
78. Haqshenas, G., Shivaprasad, H. L., Woolcock, P. R., et al.: Genetic identification and characterization of a novel virus related to human hepatitis E virus from chickens with hepatitis-splenomegaly syndrome in the United States. J. Gen. Virol. *82*:2449–2462, 2001.
79. Hardy, M. E., Kramer, S. F., Treanor, J. J., et al.: Human calicivirus genogroup II capsid sequence diversity revealed by analyses of the prototype Snow Mountain agent. Arch. Virol. *142*:1469–1479, 1997.
80. Hedlund, K. O., Rubilar-Abreu, E., and Svensson, L.: Epidemiology of calicivirus infections in Sweden, 1994–1998. J. Infect. Dis. *181*(Suppl.): 275–280, 2000.
81. Hohdatsu, T., Sato, K., Tajima, T., et al.: Neutralizing features of commercially available feline calicivirus (FCV) vaccine immune sera against FCV field isolates. J. Vet. Med. Sci. *61*:299–301, 1999.
82. Honma, S., Nakata, S., Kinoshita-Numata, K., et al.: Evaluation of nine sets of PCR primers in the RNA dependent RNA polymerase region for detection and differentiation of members of the family Caliciviridae, Norwalk virus and Sapporo virus. Microbiol. Immunol. *44*:411–419, 2000.
83. Honma, S., Nakata, S., Numata, K., et al.: Epidemiological study of prevalence of genogroup II human calicivirus (Mexico virus) infections in Japan and Southeast Asia as determined by enzyme-linked immunosorbent assays. J. Clin. Microbiol. *36*:2481–2484, 1998.
84. *http://www.promedmail.org*. Notices of outbreaks in the United States and Cuba on ProMed, 2000–2002.
85. Humphrey, T. J., Cruickshank, J. G., and Cubitt, W. D.: An outbreak of calicivirus associated gastroenteritis in an elderly persons' home: A possible zoonosis? J. Hyg. Camb. *92*:293–299, 1984.
86. Hutson, A. M., Atmar, R. L., Graham, D. Y., et al.: Norwalk virus infection and disease is associated with ABO histo-blood group type. J. Infect. Dis. *185*:1335–1337, 2002.
87. Hyams, K. C., Bourgeois, A. L., Merrell, B. R., et al.: Diarrheal disease during Operation Desert Shield. N. Engl. J. Med. *325*:1423–1428, 1991.
88. Inouye, S., Yamashita, K., Yamadera, S., et al.: Surveillance of viral gastroenteritis in Japan: Pediatric cases and outbreak incidents. J. Infect. Dis. *181*(Suppl.):270–274, 2000.
89. Iritani, N., Set, Y., Haruki, K., et al.: Major change in the predominant type of "Norwalk-like viruses" in outbreaks of acute nonbacterial gastroenteritis in Osaka City, Japan, between April 1996 and March 1999. J. Clin. Microbiol. *38*:2649–2654, 2000.
90. Jarvis, B. D. W.: Rabbit Control and RCD: Dilemmas and Implications. Miscellaneous Series 55. Wellington, Royal Society of New Zealand, 1999.
91. Jiang, X., Berke, T., Zhong, W., et al.: Sapporo-like human caliciviruses are genetically and antigenically diverse. Arch. Virol. *142*:1813–1827, 1997.
92. Jiang, X., Cubitt, D., Hu, J., et al.: Development of a type-specific EIA for detection of Snow Mountain agent–like human caliciviruses in stool specimens. J. Gen. Virol. *76*:2739–2747, 1995.
93. Jiang, X., Espul, C., Zhong, W. M., et al.: Characterization of a novel human calicivirus that may be a naturally occurring recombinant. Arch. Virol. *144*:2377–2387, 1999.
94. Jiang, X., Matson, D. O., Ruiz-Palacios, G. M., et al.: Expression, self-assembly, and antigenicity of a Snow Mountain–like calicivirus capsid protein. J. Clin. Microbiol. *33*:1452–1455, 1995.
95. Jiang, X., Matson, D. O., Velazquez, F. R., et al.: Study of Norwalk-related viruses in Mexican children J. Med. Virol. *47*:309–316, 1995.
96. Jiang, X., Turf, E., Hu, J., et al.: Outbreaks of gastroenteritis in elderly nursing homes and retirement facilities associated with human caliciviruses. J. Med. Virol. *50*:335–341, 1996.
97. Jiang, X., Wang, J., Graham, D. Y., et al.: Detection of Norwalk virus in stool by polymerase chain reaction. J. Clin. Microbiol. *30*:2529–2534, 1992.
98. Jiang, X., Wang, M., Wang, K., et al.: Sequence and genomic organization of Norwalk virus. Virology *195*:51–61, 1993.
99. Jiang, X., Wilton, N., Zhong, W. M., et al.: Diagnosis of human caliciviruses by use of enzyme immunoassays. J. Infect. Dis. *181*(Suppl.):349–359, 2000.
100. Johansson, P. J. H., Torven, M., Hammarlund, A.-C., et al.: Food-borne outbreak of gastroenteritis associated with genogroup I calicivirus. J. Clin. Microbiol. *40*:794–798, 2002.
101. Johnson, R. P., and Povey, R. C.: Feline calicivirus infection in kittens borne by cats persistently infected with the virus. Res. Vet. Sci. *37*:114–119, 1984.
102. Jothikumar, N., Aparna, K., Kamatchiammal, S., et al.: Detection of hepatitis E virus in raw and treated wastewater with the polymerase chain reaction. Appl. Environ. Microbiol. *59*:2558–2562, 1993.
103. Kapikian, A. Z., and Chanock, R. M.: Norwalk group of viruses. *In* Fields, B. N., and Knipe, D. M. (eds.): Virology. New York, Raven Press, 1990, pp. 671–693.
104. Kapikian, A. Z., Greenberg, H. B., Cline, W. L., et al.: Prevalence of antibody to the Norwalk agent by a newly developed immune adherence assay. J. Med. Virol. *2*:281–294, 1978.
105. Kapikian, A. Z., Wyatt, R. G., Dolin, R., et al.: Visualization by immune electron microscopy of a 27-nm particle associated with acute infectious non-bacterial gastroenteritis. J. Virol. *10*:1075–1081, 1972.
106. Kaplan, J. E., Feldman, R., Cambell, D. S., et al.: The frequency of a Norwalk-like pattern of illness in outbreaks of acute gastroenteritis. Am. J. Public Health *72*:1329–1332, 1982.
107. Karetnyi, I. V., Dzhumalieva, D. I., Usmanov, R. K., et al.: The possible involvement of rodents in the spread of viral hepatitis E. Zh. Mikrobiol. Epidemiol. Immunobiol. *4*:52–56, 1993.
108. Khuroo, M. S.: Study of an epidemic of non-A, non-B hepatitis: Possibility of another human hepatitis virus distinct from post-transfusion non-A, non-B type. Am. J. Med. *68*:818–824, 1980.
109. Kilgore, P. E., Belay, E. D., Hamlin, D. M., et al.: A university outbreak of gastroenteritis due to a small round-structured virus: Application of molecular diagnostics to identify the etiologic agent and patterns of transmission. J. Infect. Dis. *173*:787–793, 1996.
110. Kirkwood, C. D., and Bishop, R. F.: Molecular detection of human calicivirus in young children hospitalized with acute gastroenteritis in Melbourne, Australia, during 1999. J. Clin. Microbiol. *39*:2722–2724, 2001.
111. Koopmans, M. D.: Personal communication.
112. Koopmans, M. D., Vinje, J., de Wit, M., et al.: Molecular epidemiology of human enteric caliciviruses in The Netherlands. J. Infect. Dis. *181*(Suppl.):262–269, 2000.

113. Krawcrynski, K., and Bradley, D. W.: Enterically transmitted non-A, non-B hepatitis: Identification of virus-associated antigen in experimentally infected cynomolgus macaques. J. Infect. Dis. *159*:1042–1049, 1989.
114. Kukkula, M., Maunula, L., Silvennoinen, E., et al.: Outbreak of viral gastroentertitis due to drinking water contaminated by Norwalk-like viruses. J. Infect. Dis. *180*:1771–1776, 1999.
115. Lambden, P. R., Liu, B., and Clarke, I. N.: A conserved sequence motif at the 5′ terminus of the Southampton virus genome is characteristic of the Caliciviridae. Virus Genes *10*:149–152, 1995.
116. Laurent, S., Vautherot, J. F., Le Gall, G., et al.: Structural, antigenic and immunogenic relationships between European brown hare syndrome virus and rabbit haemorrhagic disease virus. J. Gen. Virol. *78*:2803–2811, 1997.
117. Lauritzen, A., Jarrett, O., and Sabara, M.: Serological analysis of feline calicivirus isolates from the United States and United Kingdom. Vet. Microbiol. *56*:55–63, 1997.
118. Lavazza, A., Scicluna, M. T., and Capucci, L.: Susceptibility of hares and rabbits to the European brown hare syndrome virus (EBHSV) and rabbit haemorrhagic disease virus (RHDV) under experimental conditions. Zentralbl. Veterinarmed. [B] *43*:401–410, 1996.
119. LeBaron, C. W., Furutan, N. P., Lew, J. F., et al.: Viral agents of gastroenteritis: Public health importance and outbreak management. M. M. W. R. Recomm. Rep. *39*(RR-5):1–24, 1990.
120. Le Gall, G., Huguet, S., Vende, P., et al.: European brown hare syndrome virus: Molecular cloning and sequencing of the genome. J. Gen. Virol. *77*:1693–1697, 1996.
121. Le Guyader, F., Neill, F. H., Estes, M. K., et al.: Detection and analysis of a small round-structured virus strain in oysters implicated in an outbreak of acute gastroenteritis. Appl. Environ. Microbiol. *62*:4268–4272, 1996.
122. Lew, J. F., Valdesuso, J., Vesikari, T., et al.: Detection of Norwalk virus or Norwalk-like virus infections in Finnish infants and young children. J. Infect. Dis. *169*:1364–1367, 1994.
123. Liu, B. L., Clarke, I. N., Caul, E. O., et al.: Human enteric caliciviruses have a unique genome structure and are distinct from the Norwalk-like viruses. Arch. Virol. *140*:1345–1356, 1995.
124. Liu, B. L., Lambden, P. R., Gunther, H., et al.: Molecular characterization of a bovine enteric calicivirus: Relationship to the Norwalk-like viruses. J. Virol. *73*:819–825, 1999.
125. Longer, C. F., Denny, S. L., Caudill, J. D., et al.: Experimental hepatitis E: Pathogenesis in cynomolgus macaques *(Macaca fascicularis)*. J. Infect. Dis. *168*:602–609, 1993.
126. Madeley, C. R., Cosgrove, B. P.: Caliciviruses in man. Lancet *2*:199, 1976.
127. Maguire, A. J., Greeen, J., Brown, D. W. G., et al.: Molecular epidemiology of outbreaks of gastroenteritis associated with small round-structured viruses in East Anglia, United Kingdom, during the 1996–1997 season. J. Clin. Microbiol. *37*:81–89, 1999.
128. Marie-Cardine, A., Gourlain, K., Mouterde, O., et al.: Epidemiology of acute viral gastroenteritis in children hospitalized in Rouen, France. Clin. Infect. Dis. *34*:1170–1178, 2002.
129. Marionneau, S., Ruvoen, N., Le Moullac-Vaidye, B., et al.: Norwalk virus binds to histo-blood group antigens present on gastroduodenal epithelial cells of secretor individuals. J. Gastroenterol. *122*:1967–1977, 2002.
130. Marshall, J. A., Yuen, L. K., Catton, M. G., et al.: Multiple outbreaks of Norwalk-like virus gastroenteritis associated with a Mediterranean-style restaurant. J. Med. Microbiol. *50*:143–151, 2001.
131. Martinez, N., Espul, C., Cuello, H., et al.: Sequence diversity of human caliciviruses recovered from children with diarrhea in Mendoza, Argentina, 1995 to 1998. J. Med. Virol. *67*:289–298, 2002.
132. Matson, D. O.: Unpublished data.
133. Matson, D. O.: Re-analysis of serologic data from the Australian study of human health risks of infection by rabbit hemorrhagic disease virus. *In* Jarvis, B. D. W. (ed.): Rabbit Control and RCD: Dilemmas and Implications. Miscellaneous Series 55. Wellington, Royal Society of New Zealand, 1999, pp. 62–66.
134. Matson, D. O., Berke, T., Dinulos, M. B., et al.: Partial characterization of the genome of nine animal caliciviruses. Arch. Virol. *141*:2443–2456, 1996.
135. Matson, D. O., Estes, M. K.: Unpublished data.
136. Matson, D. O., Estes, M. K., Glass, R. I., et al.: Human calicivirus-associated diarrhea in children attending day care centers. J. Infect. Dis. *159*:71–78, 1989.
137. Matson, D. O., Estes, M. K., Tanaka, T., et al.: Asymptomatic human calicivirus infection in a day care center. Pediatr. Infect. Dis. J. *9*:190–196, 1990.
138. Matson, D. O., Mitchell, D. K., Van, R., et al.: Enteric viral pathogens as causes of outbreaks of diarrhea among children attending day care centers during one year of observation. Pediatr. Res. *37*:826, 1995.
139. Matson, D. O., Zhong, W. M., Nakata, S., et al.: Molecular characterization of a human calicivirus with sequence relationships closer to animal caliciviruses than other known human caliciviruses. J. Med. Virol. *45*:215–222, 1995.
140. Mayo, M. A.: Virus taxonomy—Houston. Arch. Virol. *147*:1071–1076, 2002.
141. McCarthy, M., Estes, M. K., Hyams, K. C.: Norwalk-like virus infection in military forces: Epidemic potential, sporadic disease, and the future direction of prevention and control efforts. J. Infect. Dis. *181*(Suppl.):387–391, 2000.
142. McSwiggan, D. A., Cubitt, W. D., and Moore, W.: Calicivirus associated with winter vomiting disease. Lancet *1*:1215, 1978.
143. Mead, C.: Rabbit hemorrhagic disease. Emerg. Infect. Dis. *4*:344–345, 1998.
144. Meng, X. J., Purcell, R. H., Halbur, P. G., et al.: A novel virus in swine is closely related to the human hepatitis E virus. Proc. Natl. Acad. Sci. U. S. A. *94*:9860–9865, 1997.
145. Meng, X. J., Wiseman, B., Elvinger, F., et al.: Prevalence of antibodies to hepatitis E virus in veterinarians working with swine and in normal blood donors in the United States and other countries. J. Clin. Microbiol. *40*:117–122, 2002.
146. Meyers, G., Wirblich, C., and Thiel, H. J.: Genomic and subgenomic RNAs of rabbit hemorrhagic disease virus are both protein-linked and packaged into particles. Virology *184*:677–686, 1991.
147. Mochizuki, M., Nakatani, H., and Yoshida, M.: Inhibitory effects of recombinant feline interferon on the replication of feline enteropathogenic viruses in vitro. Vet. Microbiol. *39*:145–152, 1994.
148. Morens, D. M., Zweighaft, R. M., Vernon, T. M., et al.: A waterborne outbreak of gastroenteritis with secondary person-to-person spread. Association with a viral agent. Lancet *1*:964–966, 1979.
149. Morrow, R. H., Smetana, H. F., Sai, F. T., et al.: Unusual features of viral hepatitis in Accra, Ghana. Ann. Intern. Med. *68*:250–264, 1968.
150. Mounts, A. W., Ando, T., Koopmans, M., et al.: Cold weather seasonality of gastroenteritis associated with Norwalk-like viruses. J. Infect. Dis. *181*(Suppl.):284–287, 2000.
151. Mounts, A. W., Holman, R. C., Clarke, M. J., et al.: Trends in hospitalizations associated with gastroenteritis among adults in the United States, 1979–1995. Epidemiol. Infect. *123*:1–8, 1999.
152. Nagesha, H. S., Wang, L. F., Hyatt, A. D., et al.: Self-assembly, antigenicity, and immunogenicity of the rabbit haemorrhagic disease virus (Czechoslovakian strain V-351) capsid protein expressed in baculovirus. Arch. Virol. *140*:1095–1108, 1995.
153. Nakata, S., Chiba, S., Terashima, H., et al.: Humoral immunity in infants with gastroenteritis caused by human calicivirus. J. Infect. Dis. *152*:274–279, 1985.
154. Nakata, S., Chiba, S., Terashima, H., et al.: Prevalence of antibody to human calicivirus in Japan and Southeast Asia determined by radioimmunoassay. J. Clin. Microbiol. *22*:519–521, 1985.
155. Nakata, S., Estes, M. K., and Chiba, S.: Detection of human calicivirus antigen and antibody by enzyme-linked immunosorbent assays. J. Clin. Microbiol. *26*:2001–2005, 1988.
156. Nakata, S., Honma, S., Numata, K.-K., et al.: Members of the family Caliciviridae (Norwalk virus and Sapporo virus) are the most prevalent cause of gastroenteritis outbreaks among infants in Japan. J. Infect. Dis. *181*:2029–2032, 2000.
157. Neill, J. D.: Nucleotide sequence of a region of the feline calicivirus genome which encodes picornavirus-like RNA-dependent RNA polymerase, cysteine protease and 2C polypeptides. Virus Res. *17*:145–160, 1990.
158. Neill, J. D.: Nucleotide sequence of the capsid protein gene of two serotypes of San Miguel sea lion virus: Identification of conserved and non-conserved amino acid sequences among calicivirus capsid proteins. Virus Res. *24*:211–222, 1992.
159. Neill, J. D., and Mengeling, W. L.: Further characterization of the virus-specific RNAs in feline calicivirus infected cells. Virus Res. *11*:59–72, 1988.
160. Neill, J. D., Meyer, R. F., and Seal, B. S.: Genetic relatedness of the caliciviruses: San Miguel sea lion and vesicular exanthema of swine viruses constitute a single genotype within the Caliciviridae. J. Virol. *69*:4484–4488, 1995.
161. Neill, J. D., and Seal, B. S.: Development of PCR primers for specific amplification of two distinct regions of the genomes of San Miguel sea-lion and vesicular exanthema of swine viruses. Mol. Cell. Probes *9*:33–37, 1995.
162. Nowotny, N., Bascunana, C. R., Ballagi-Pordany, A., et al.: Phylogenetic analysis of rabbit haemorrhagic disease and European brown hare syndrome viruses by comparison of sequences from the capsid protein gene. Arch. Virol. *142*:657–673, 1997.
163. Numata, K., Nakata, S., Jiang, X., et al.: Epidemiological study of Norwalk virus infections in Japan and Southeast Asia by enzyme-linked immunosorbent assays with Norwalk virus capsid protein produced by the baculovirus expression system. J. Clin. Microbiol. *32*:121–126, 1994.
164. Ohlinger, V. F., and Thiel, H. J.: Identification of the viral haemorrhagic disease virus of rabbits as a calicivirus. Rev. Sci. Tech. *10*:311–323, 1991.
165. Oishi, I., Maeda, A., Yamazaki, K., et al.: Calicivirus detected in outbreaks of acute gastroenteritis in school children. Biken J. *23*:163–168, 1980.
166. O'Ryan, M. L., Mamani, N., Gaggero, A., et al.: Human caliciviruses are a significant pathogen of acute sporadic diarrhea in children of Santiago, Chile. J. Infect. Dis. *182*:1519–1522, 2000.
167. O'Ryan, M. L., Vial, P., Mamani, N., et al.: Assessment of independent risk factors for antibody acquisition to Norwalk and MX caliciviruses in Chilean individuals. Clin. Infect. Dis. *27*:789–795, 1998.

168. Oyofo, B. A., Soderquist, R., Lesmana, M., et al.: Norwalk-like virus and bacterial pathogens associated with cases of gastroenteritis onboard a US Navy ship. Am. J. Trop. Med. Hyg. *61*:904–908, 1999.
169. Pang, X. L., Joensuu, J., and Vesikari, T.: Human calicivirus-associated sporadic gastroenteritis in Finnish children less than two years of age followed prospectively during a rotavirus vaccine trial. Pediatr. Infect. Dis. J. *18*:420–426, 1999.
170. Pang, X. L., Zeng, S. Q., Honma, S., et al.: Effect of rotavirus vaccine on Sapporo virus gastroenteritis in Finnish infants. Pediatr. Infect. Dis. J. *20*:295–300, 2001.
171. Parada, E., Berke, T., Jiang, X., et al.: Clinical characteristics and burden of calicivirus infection among hospitalized children. Submitted for publication.
172. Parra, F., and Prieto, M.: Purification and characterization of a calicivirus as the causative agent of a lethal hemorrhagic disease in rabbits. J. Virol. *64*:4013–4015, 1990.
173. Paul, D. A., Knigge, M. F., Ritter, A., et al.: Determination of hepatitis E virus seroprevalence by using recombinant fusion proteins and synthetic peptides. J. Infect. Dis. *169*:801–806, 1994.
174. Pina, S., Buti, M., Cotrina, M., et al.: HEV identified in serum from humans with acute hepatitis and in sewage of animal origin in Spain. J. Hepatol. *33*:826–833, 2000.
175. Povey, R. C.: In vitro antiviral efficacy of ribavirin against feline calicivirus, feline viral rhinotracheitis virus, and canine parainfluenza virus. Am. J. Vet. Res. *39*:175–178, 1978.
176. Prasad, B. V., Hardy, M. E., Dokland, T., et al.: X-ray crystallographic structure of the Norwalk virus capsid. Science *286*:287–290, 1999.
177. Prasad, B. V. V., Matson, D. O., and Smith, A. W.: Three-dimensional structure of the primate calicivirus. J. Mol. Biol. *240*:256–264, 1994.
178. Prasad, B. V. V., Rothnagel, R., Jiang, X., et al.: Three-dimensional structure of baculovirus-expressed Norwalk virus capsids. J. Virol. *68*:5117–5125, 1994.
179. Reuter, G., Farkas, T., Berke, T., et al.: Genetic diversity of sporadic and outbreak strains of human caliciviruses in Hungary, 1997 to 2000. Orv. Hetil. *143*:351–354, 2002.
180. Reuter, G., Farkas, T., Berke, T., et al.: Molecular epidemiology of human calicivirus gastroenteritis outbreaks in Hungary, 1998 to 2000. J. Med. Virol. *68*:390–398, 2002.
181. Rinehart-Kim, J., Zhong, W.-M., Jiang, X., et al.: Complete nucleotide sequence and genomic organization of a primate calicivirus, Pan-1. Arch. Virol. *144*:199–208, 1999.
182. Robinson, S., Clarke, I. N., Vipond, I. B., et al.: Epidemiology of human Sapporo-like caliciviruses in the South West of England: Molecular characterisation of a genetically distinct isolate. J. Med. Virol. *67*:282–288, 2002.
183. Robson, S. C., Adams, S., Brink, N., et al.: Hospital outbreak of hepatitis E. Lancet *339*:1424–1425, 1992.
184. Sair, A. I., d'Souza, D. H., Moe, C. L., et al.: Improved detection of human enteric viruses in foods by RT-PCR. J. Virol. Methods *100*:57–69, 2002.
185. Sakai, Y., Nakata, S., Honma, S., et al.: Clinical severity of Norwalk virus and Sapporo virus gastroenteritis in children in Hokkaido, Japan. Pediatr. Infect. Dis. J. *20*:849–853, 2001.
186. Sakuma, Y., Chiba, S., Kogasaka, R., et al.: Prevalence of antibody to human calicivirus in general population of northern Japan. J. Med. Virol. 7:221–225, 1981.
187. Sawyer, L. A., Murphy, J. J., Kaplan, J. E., et al.: 25-30-nm virus particle associated with a hospital outbreak of acute gastroenteritis with evidence for airborne transmission. Am. J. Epidemiol. *127*:1261–1271, 1988.
188. Schlauder, G. G., Dawson, G. J., Erker, J. C., et al.: The sequence and phylogenetic analysis of a novel hepatitis E virus isolated from a patient with acute hepatitis reported in the United States. J. Gen. Virol. *79*:447–456, 1998.
189. Schreiber, D. S., Blacklow, N. R., and Trier, J. S.: The mucosal lesion of the proximal small intestine in acute infectious nonbacterial gastroenteritis. N. Engl. J. Med. *288*:1318–1323, 1973.
190. Seal, B. S., Lutze-Wallace, C., Kreutz, L. C., et al.: Isolation of caliciviruses from skunks that are antigenically and genotypically related to San Miguel sea lion virus. Virus Res. *37*:1–12, 1995.
191. Sharp, T. W., Hyams, K. C., Watts, D., et al.: Epidemiology of Norwalk virus during an outbreak of acute gastroenteritis aboard a US aircraft carrier. J. Med. Virol. *45*:61–67, 1995.
192. Sharp, T. W., Thornton, S. A., Wallace, M. R., et al.: Diarrheal disease among military personnel during Operation Restore Hope, Somalia, 1992–1993. Am. J. Trop. Med. Hyg. *52*:188–193, 1995.
193. Smith, A. W.: Virus cycles in aquatic mammals, poikilotherms, and invertebrates. *In* Hurst, C. J. (ed.): Viral Ecology. San Diego, CA, Academic Press, 2000, pp. 447–491.
194. Smith, A. W., Berry, E. S., Skilling, D. E., et al.: In vitro isolation and characterization of a calicivirus causing a vesicular disease of the hands and feet. Clin. Infect. Dis. *26*:434–439, 1998.
195. Smith, A. W., and Boyt, P. M.: Caliciviruses of ocean origin: A review. J. Zoo Wildl. Med. *21*:3–23, 1990.
196. Smith, A. W., Cherry, N. J., and Matson, D. O.: Letter to the editors. A brief update on rabbit hemorrhagic disease virus. Emerg. Infect. Dis. *4*:345–346, 1998.
197. Smith, A. W., Matson, D. O., Stein, D. A., et al.: Antisense treatment of Caliciviridae: An emerging disease agent of animals and humans. Curr. Opin. Mol. Ther. *4*:177–184, 2002.
198. Smith, A. W., Mattson, D. E., Skilling, D. E., et al.: Isolation and partial characterization of a calicivirus from calves. Am. J. Vet. Res. *44*:851–855, 1983.
199. Smith, A. W., Prato, C., and Skilling, D. E.: Caliciviruses infecting monkeys and possibly man. Am. J. Vet. Res. *39*:287–289, 1978.
200. Smith, A. W., Skilling, D. E., Cherry, N., et al.: Calicivirus emergence from ocean reservoirs: Zoonotic and interspecies movements. Emerg. Infect. Dis. *4*:13–20, 1998.
201. Smith, A. W., Skilling, D. E., Dardiri, A. H., et al.: Calicivirus pathogenic for swine: A new serotype isolated from opaleye *Girella nigricans,* an ocean fish. Science *209*:940–941, 1980.
202. Smith, A. W., Skilling, D. E., Ensley, P. K., et al.: Calicivirus isolation and persistence in a pygmy chimpanzee *(Pan paniscus).* Science *221*:79–81, 1983.
203. Smith, A. W., Skilling, D. E., Houghton, M., et al.: Evidence for *Vesivirus* calicivirus infection in association with human hepatitis. Submitted for publication.
204. Sosnovtsev, S. V., and Green, K. Y.: Identification and genomic mapping of the ORF3 and VPg proteins in feline calicivirus virions. Virology *277*:193–203, 2000.
205. Stein, D. A., Skilling, D. E., Berke, T., et al.: Isolation and partial characterization of a calicivirus from a cat with hepatitis and hemorrhagic enteritis. Submitted for publication.
206. Stein, D. A., Skilling, D. E., Iversen, P. L., et al.: Inhibition of *Vesivirus* infections in mammalian cell culture with antisense morpholino oligomers. Antisense Nucleic Acid Drug Dev. *11*:317–325, 2001.
207. Studdert, M. J.: Caliciviruses. Arch. Virol. *58*:157–191, 1978.
208. Sugieda, M., Nakajima, K., and Nakajima, S.: Outbreaks of Norwalk-like virus–associated gastroenteritis traced to shellfish: Coexistence of two genotypes in one specimen. Epidemiol. Infect. *116*:339–346, 1996.
209. Tacket, C. O., Mason, H. S., Losonsky, G., et al.: Human immune responses to a novel Norwalk virus vaccine delivered in transgenic potatoes. J. Infect. Dis. *182*:302–305, 2000.
210. Tam, A. W., Smith, M. W., Guerra, M. E., et al.: Hepatitis E virus (HEV): Molecular cloning and sequencing of the full-length viral genome. Virology *185*:120–131, 1991.
211. Tandon, B. N., Joshi, Y. K., Jain, S. K., et al.: An epidemic of non-A, non-B hepatitis in north India. Indian J. Med. Res. *75*:739–744, 1982.
212. Taylor, M. B., Parker, S., Grabow, W. O. K., et al.: An epidemiological investigation of Norwalk virus infection in South Africa. Epidemiol. Infect. *116*:203–206, 1996.
213. Tsarev, S. A., Tsareva, T. S., Emerson, S. U., et al.: ELISA for antibody to hepatitis E virus (HEV) based on complete open-reading frame-2 protein expressed in insect cells: Identification of HEV in primates. J. Infect. Dis. *168*:369–378, 1993.
214. Ueda, K., Park, J. H., Ochiai, K., et al.: Disseminated intravascular coagulation (DIC) in rabbit haemorrhagic disease. Jpn. J. Vet. Res. *40*:133–141, 1992.
215. van der Poel, W. H., Verschoor, F., van der Heide, R., et al.: Hepatitis E virus sequences in swine related to sequences in humans, The Netherlands. Emerg. Infect. Dis. *7*:970–976, 2001.
216. van der Poel, W. H., Vinje, J., van der Heide, R., et al.: Norwalk-like calicivirus genes in farm animals. Emerg. Infect. Dis. *6*:36–41, 2000.
217. Vinje, J., Altena, S. A., and Koopmans, M. P. G.: The incidence and genetic variability of small round-structured viruses in outbreaks of gastroenteritis in The Netherlands. J. Infect. Dis. *176*:1374–1378, 1997.
218. Vinje, J., Deijl, H., van der Heide, R., et al.: Molecular detection and epidemiology of Sapporo-like viruses. J. Clin. Microbiol. *38*:530–536, 2000.
219. Vinje, J., and Koopmans, M. P.: Molecular detection and epidemiology of small round-structured viruses in outbreaks of gastroenteritis in the Netherlands. J. Infect. Dis. *174*:610–615, 1996.
220. Viswanathan, R.: Infectious hepatitis in Delhi (1955–56): Epidemiology. Indian J. Med. Res. *45*:71–76, 1957.
221. Wattre, P.: Hepatitis E virus. Ann. Biol. Clin. *52*:507–513, 1994.
222. Wirblich, C., Meyers, G., Ohlinger, V. F., et al.: European brown hare syndrome virus: Relationship to rabbit hemorrhagic disease virus and other caliciviruses. J. Virol. *68*:5164–5173, 1994.
223. Wu, J. C., Chen, C. M., Chiang, T. Y., et al.: Clinical and epidemiological implications of swine hepatitis E virus infection. J. Med. Virol. *60*:166–171, 2000.
224. Wyatt, R. G., Dolin, R., Blacklow, N. R., et al.: Comparison of three agents of acute infectious nonbacterial gastroenteritis by cross-challenge in volunteers. J. Infect. Dis. *129*:709–714, 1974.
225. Xu, Z. J., and Chen, W. X.: Viral hemorrhagic disease in rabbits: A review. Vet. Res. Commun. *13*:205–212, 1989.
226. Yoda, T., Terano, Y., Suzuki, Y., et al.: Characterization of monoclonal antibodies generated against Norwalk virus GII capsid protein expressed in *Escherichia coli*. Microbiol. Immunol. *44*:905–914, 2000.
227. Yuen, L. K. W., Catton, M. G., Cox, B. J., et al.: Heminested multiplex reverse transcription–PCR for detection and differentiation of Norwalk-like virus genogroups 1 and 2 in fecal samples. J. Clin. Microbiol. *39*:2690–2694, 2001.

REOVIRIDAE

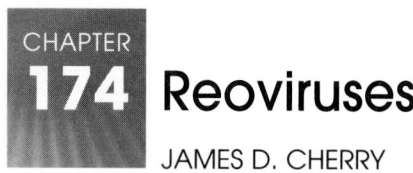

CHAPTER 174 Reoviruses

JAMES D. CHERRY

Reoviruses are ubiquitous in nature, but their role in human disease is vague. After their classification in 1959, numerous reports noted their association with human disease.[58, 70] Since that time, these viruses have been evaluated extensively in laboratory animal studies, but few cases of human disease have been reported during the last 3 decades.

History

On the basis of its cytopathic effect in monkey kidney tissue culture and its recovery from stool specimens at a time of enterovirus surveillance, the first recovered reovirus was designated ECHO virus type 10.[9, 10] This virus and four similar strains were recovered in 1954 from the stools of healthy children in Cincinnati and Mexico.[54, 55] By 1959, researchers were aware that ECHO 10 viral strains appeared to have many characteristics that were different from those of enteroviruses, such as large size and unique cytopathic effect, and they were withdrawn from this grouping. The term *reovirus* was chosen to stress the association of these agents with both the respiratory *(r)* and enteric *(e)* tracts. The *o* for orphan was retained in the designation. In the early 1960s, reoviral infections were noted in association with human illness.[15, 27, 34, 62, 63, 76, 87]

Properties[8, 47, 57, 58, 68, 82–84]

Reoviruses are members of the family *Reoviridae*.[17] This family has numerous double-stranded RNA viruses, including the nonfusogenic mammalian orthoreoviruses commonly referred to as reoviruses that are presented in this chapter.[47, 84] All mammalian reoviruses are related by a common, group-specific, complement-fixing antigen.[66, 83] Three distinct human serotypes can be identified by neutralization or hemagglutination inhibition.[64]

Reovirus particles are composed of an inner protein shell (core) with a diameter of 60 nm that is surrounded by an outer protein shell (outer capsid) measuring 81 nm in diameter.[68] The outer capsid has icosahedral symmetry and is composed of between 92 and 180 hexagonal and pentagonal subunits (capsomers). The genome of orthoreoviruses has a total size of approximately 23,500 base pairs with 10 gene segments: three large (L1, L2, L3), three medium (M1, M2, M3), and four small (S1, S2, S3, S4). These genes encode 12 proteins. The outer capsid is composed of four proteins: sigma-1, sigma-3, lambda-2, and mu-1. Sigma-1 is the reovirus cell-attachment protein against which serotype-specific neutralizing antibodies are developed. This protein also is the hemagglutinin. Sigma-3 protein binds double-stranded RNA and is sensitive to protease degradation. It is a zinc metalloprotein that has effects on translation. Lambda-2 protein is important in particle assembly and mu-1 in cell penetration.

The inner capsid is composed of four proteins: lambda-3, lambda-1, mu-2, and sigma-2. Lambda-3 is an RNA-dependent RNA polymerase. Lambda-1 is a zinc metalloprotein that binds RNA. Mu-2 binds RNA, and sigma-2 binds double-stranded RNA.

The four nonstructural proteins are mu-NS, mu-NSC, sigma-1s, and sigma-NS. Mu-NS is a core-binding protein, and sigma-NS binds single-stranded RNA. The roles of mu-NSC and sigma-1s are unknown.

Reoviruses are moderately heat stable. The half-life at 56° C of a type 3 strain is 1.6 minutes; at 37° C, it is approximately 2.5 hours. Reoviruses are inactivated by visible light in the presence of heterocyclic dyes. They are inactivated by ultraviolet light but are more resistant to this treatment than are RNA viruses with single-stranded nucleic acid. Reoviruses are stable through a wide pH range and also are stable as aerosols, particularly when the relative humidity is high. They are relatively resistant to 3 percent formaldehyde solution, 1 percent hydrogen peroxide, and 1 percent phenol but are inactivated completely by 70 percent ethyl alcohol at room temperature for 1 hour. Brief exposure to 70 percent ethanol is ineffective in disinfecting reoviruses, but brief exposure to 95 percent ethanol or sodium hypochlorite is effective.

Reoviruses replicate with a cytopathic effect in a large number of tissue culture systems of both primate and other animal origins. For recovery from clinical material, monkey kidney tissue culture is satisfactory. Cytopathic effect is enhanced in rolled compared with stationary cultures.[34] Infected cells develop characteristic cytoplasmic inclusions that contain double-stranded RNA, virus-specific proteins, and complete and incomplete viral particles. All three serotypes agglutinate human erythrocytes, and this virus-cell interaction is stable in a wide temperature and pH range.

Of all viruses that naturally infect humans, reoviruses have the broadest host range. They have been recovered from natural infections in cattle, chimpanzees, monkeys, mice, dogs, turkeys, sheep, pigs, chickens, and cats.[11, 20, 22, 39–42, 59, 67, 85, 86] In addition, hemagglutination-inhibiting and neutralizing antibodies to one or more of the three reoviral serotypes have been found in the serum of rabbits, horses, trout, guinea pigs, antelopes, zebras, warthogs, bats, wallabies, quokkas, kangaroos, and several genera of New World monkeys.[46, 61, 64, 66, 74, 75]

Because of their widespread prevalence in nature and the ease of causing infection in laboratory animals, reoviruses have been used widely in pathogenicity studies. The following unique illnesses have been observed: diabetes mellitus in mice; hydrocephalus in hamsters, ferrets, rats, and mice; encephalitis in mice; chronic infection with runting in mice; myocarditis in mice; chronic obstructive jaundice associated with choledochal obliteration in mice; and lymphomas in mice with chronic infection.*

Epidemiology

The serologic data presented in the preceding section of this chapter demonstrate that reoviruses are prevalent infectious agents in the animal world. Similarly, surveys of sera collected from humans indicate worldwide human infection.† The occurrence in nature of identical viruses in many different animals and humans leads to consideration of possible transmission from species to species. At present, this transmission has not been demonstrated.

Reoviruses are recovered frequently from sewage.[16, 26, 30, 36, 40, 48] In San Diego, reoviruses have been recovered more consistently than has any other virus throughout the year from sewage.[16] This finding suggests that reoviral infection is endemic in humans in the San Diego area.

The type 2 hemagglutination-inhibiting antibody prevalence pattern by age in sera collected in Boston from 1959 to 1962 is presented in Table 174–1. Antibody is transmitted transplacentally to the newborn. During the first year of life, this acquired antibody wanes, after which antibody prevalence increases with increasing age. Approximately 50 percent of school-age children have hemagglutination-inhibiting antibody titers to type 2 reovirus greater than or equal to 1:20; approximately 80 percent of adults have similar titers.

The method of transmission of reoviruses is unknown. However, because they are recovered most frequently from the feces, the primary spread probably is by the fecal-oral route, similar to that of enteroviruses. Because the reoviruses are stable in aerosols and because respiratory illness has been associated with reovirus infections, the respiratory route is an additional possibility.

TABLE 174–1 ■ HEMAGGLUTINATION-INHIBITING (H1) ANTIBODIES TO REOVIRUS TYPE 2 IN 253 SERUM SPECIMENS COLLECTED IN BOSTON FROM 1959 TO 1962

Age Group	Percentage with H1 Titer ≥1:20
Premature newborn	68
0–6 months	25
7–12 months	9
13–24 months	27
2–5 years	37
6–10 years	52
11–20 years	54
21–40 years	34
41–60 years	83
>60 years	73

From Lerner, A.M., Cherry, J. D., Klein, J. O., et al.: Infections with reoviruses. N. Engl. J. Med. *267*:947–952, 1962. Reprinted, with permission from The New England Journal of Medicine.

Clinical Manifestations

The role of reoviral infections in human disease is far from clear. In most instances, virologic or serologic evidence of reoviral infection has been a sporadic finding in human illness, so that cause and effect are impossible to establish; one possibility is that the observed illness is caused by an unrecognized infectious agent and the reoviral infection is concomitant but not pathogenic.

The prevalence of antibody to all three reoviral types in humans and the frequency of reovirus isolation from human sewage indicate that human infection is a common occurrence, but the relative paucity of virus recovery during studies of community disease suggests that most infections are inapparent or associated with trivial illness.

UPPER RESPIRATORY ILLNESS

In the winter of 1957, Rosen and colleagues[62] noted an outbreak of infection with reovirus type 1 in nursery children in a welfare institution. Illness was noted in 16 of 22 infected children and was characterized by low-grade fever (rectal temperatures from 38.1° C to 38.6° C [100.6° F to 101.5° F]), rhinorrhea, and pharyngitis. The average duration of fever was 2.2 days; in nine children, the duration was only 1 day. Three children had diarrhea, and three had mild otitis media. In another study conducted at the same institution during the winter of 1955 to 1956, four children with reovirus type 3 infection and illness were noted.[63] One child had a temperature of 38.9° C (102° F), coryza, and tonsillitis; another child had fever (temperature of 38.2° C [100.8° F]), cough, and diarrhea; and two children had only coryza. During another reovirus type 3 outbreak in the fall of 1957, all six infected infants had symptoms. Five children had mild fever, five had coryza, and four had diarrhea. Pharyngitis was not observed in any of the infected children.

Other sporadic instances of similar mild upper respiratory illnesses have been described.[12, 21, 23, 72, 76] In volunteer trials in young adults, reovirus type 1 infection was associated with malaise, rhinorrhea, cough, sneezing, pharyngitis, and headache in some subjects in one study,[60] and cold-like illness was observed in 37 percent of subjects in another trial.[23] In both volunteer studies and natural infection, mild diarrhea occurred with the upper respiratory illness.

PNEUMONIA

Tillotson and Lerner[80] described a 5-year-old girl who had extensive pneumonia and died after 15 days of illness. This child initially had fever, cough, rhinorrhea, and a generalized maculopapular rash. When admitted to the hospital on the tenth day of illness, the child was cyanotic and in marked respiratory distress; rash was present no longer, but mild pharyngitis and conjunctivitis were. A chest radiograph revealed a diffuse confluent pneumonia, and reovirus type 3 was recovered from the lungs, adrenals, liver, spleen, kidney, a lymph node, heart, brain, and blood.

Joske and associates[27] described a 10-month-old girl who died after a respiratory illness of 4 days' duration. A reovirus type 1 was recovered from the stool and brain of this child, and postmortem study revealed interstitial pneumonia, myocarditis, hepatitis, and encephalitis. El-Rai and Evans[15] reported the case of an 18-year-old boy who had fever (temperature of 39.4° C [103° F]), nausea, vomiting, cough, and patchy pneumonia. He had serologic evidence of infection with reovirus type 1. Pneumonia has been noted in another child with reovirus type 3 infection.[76]

*See references 24, 29, 37, 38, 49, 50, 52, 71, 73, 77.

†See references 4–6, 18, 28, 32, 33, 35, 51, 65, 69, 79, 81.

GASTROINTESTINAL MANIFESTATIONS

Mild diarrhea has been noted both in association with upper respiratory illness and as an isolated event.[53, 60, 62, 63, 67] Because reovirus type 3 consistently produces steatorrhea in mice, this clinical manifestation has been sought in illnesses of children and noted in six.[66, 76] Three patients with hepatitis and encephalitis have been described.[27] Zalan and associates[87] have noted two patients in whom abdominal pain and cramps were prominent.

In 1980, Bangaru and associates[1] reported the similarity of induced hepatobiliary injury caused by reovirus type 3 infection in mice and biliary atresia in human infants. Subsequent to this observation, Morecki and colleagues[19, 44, 45] looked for an association between reovirus type 3 infection and biliary atresia in humans. In their first report, they found that 17 of 25 patients (68%) with biliary atresia had antibodies (indirect immunofluorescent antibody technique) to reovirus type 3, whereas similar antibodies were recovered in only 3 of 37 control sera.[44] In a second study, they found that 62 percent of babies with extrahepatic biliary atresia and 52 percent of infants with idiopathic neonatal hepatitis had antibodies to reovirus type 3; only 12 percent of control children had similar antibodies.[19] In an ultrastructural and immunocytochemical study, they found evidence of reovirus type 3 in the porta hepatis of an infant with extrahepatic biliary atresia.[45]

Using similar serologic techniques, Dussaix and associates[13] were unable to find any relationship between reovirus type 3 antibody and either biliary atresia or neonatal hepatitis. They found reovirus type 3 antibody in sera from 45 percent of infants with biliary atresia, 50 percent of infants with neonatal hepatitis, and 50 percent of control infants. Minuk and colleagues[43] found no association between reovirus type 3 infection and idiopathic cholestatic liver disease in adults. Brown and colleagues[7] reported a relatively large study of reovirus type 3 infection and extrahepatic biliary atresia and neonatal hepatitis. They interpreted their data as demonstrating no correlation between the virus and the illnesses studied. However, the geometric mean antibody value in the combined biliary atresia and neonatal hepatitis groups was significantly higher than that of the control group. Richardson and associates[56] reported a study in which they examined the percentage of IgG, IgA, and IgM serum antibodies to reovirus type 3 in 40 infants with extrahepatic biliary atresia, 59 infants with neonatal hepatitis, 61 infants with cholestatic liver disease with causes other than extrahepatic biliary atresia or neonatal hepatitis, and 138 control infants with no liver disease. They found no difference in the prevalence of IgG and IgA antibodies between the groups with liver disease and the control subjects. They did, however, note a greater prevalence of IgM antibody in each of the groups with liver disease compared with the rate in the control group. However, the virus probably could not play a role in such a wide variety of illnesses. Most likely, by some unknown mechanism related to liver disease, the increased prevalence is due to false-positive findings. Steele and associates,[78] using a reverse transcriptase–mediated polymerase chain reaction, found no evidence of reovirus type 3 in preserved tissues from infants with cholestatic liver disease.

EXANTHEM

Exanthem has been a common manifestation of clinically apparent reoviral infections.[15, 27, 33, 80] Lerner and associates[32] noted exanthem in six of seven children infected with reovirus type 2. Predominant symptoms in these patients included fever, malaise, anorexia, and pharyngitis. Two children had adenopathy, and one child had diarrhea. The rash was maculopapular in five patients and vesicular in one child. One child had a measles-like illness with photophobia, conjunctivitis, cervical lymphadenopathy, and a confluent maculopapular rash that lasted approximately 1 week.

Exanthem has been noted in a 5-year-old girl with pneumonia and type 3 reovirus infection, a 28-month-old girl with encephalitis and type 2 infection, and an 18-year-old boy with pharyngitis and cervical and posterior occipital lymph node enlargement and type 2 infection.[15, 27, 80]

NEUROMUSCULAR DISEASE

Joske and colleagues[27] described three cases of hepatitis-encephalitis syndrome with reoviral infections. All these cases had abnormal liver function test results and clinical and laboratory evidence of meningeal and cerebral involvement. One child died, one had mild neurologic residua at the 6-week follow-up, and one recovered without difficulty. Two patients were infected with reovirus type 2 and one with reovirus type 3.

El-Rai and Evans[15] found serologic evidence of reovirus type 2 infection in two children with aseptic meningitis, and Zalan and colleagues[87] described two children with reovirus type 2 infections associated with leg weakness and pain. Johansson and colleagues[25] described a 3-month-old girl with meningitis, diarrhea, vomiting, and fever. Reovirus type 1 was isolated from this child's cerebrospinal fluid, and the child had a fourfold rise in neutralizing antibody to the isolated virus. Krainer and Aronson[31] described a 29-year-old woman who died of disseminated demyelinating encephalomyelitis in which a reovirus was recovered from the cerebrospinal fluid and brain.

OTHER MANIFESTATIONS

A 25-year-old man with Hodgkin disease had persistent reovirus type 1 viruria for a 5-week period, but no associated clinical illness was demonstrated.[13] Reoviruses have been recovered from biopsy material from patients with Burkitt lymphoma.[2, 3] One child with hemorrhagic bullous myringitis was infected with reovirus type 2.[87]

Diagnosis

Because no specific clinical features suggest reoviral infection, virologic and serologic studies are necessary for diagnosis. Reoviruses can be recovered from clinical material in primary monkey kidney tissue culture.[57] Care must be taken in interpreting results, however, because reoviruses can be contaminants of monkey tissue cultures. Cytopathic effect in tissue culture is enhanced by rolling during incubation.[34] Identification of virus is made by neutralization; the distinctive cytopathic effect should be helpful in selecting strains for study with reovirus antisera. Paired serum specimens can be examined for antibody titer rise to reoviruses by neutralization, indirect immunofluorescent antibody technique, enzyme-linked immunosorbent assay, or hemagglutination inhibition.

REFERENCES

1. Bangaru, B., Morecki, R., Glaser, J. H., et al.: Comparative studies of biliary atresia in the human newborn and reovirus-induced cholangitis in weaning mice. Lab. Invest. *43*:456–462, 1980.

2. Bell, T. M., Massie, A., Ross, M. G. R., et al.: Further isolations of reovirus type 3 from cases of Burkitt's lymphoma. B. M. J. *1*:1514–1517, 1966.
3. Bell, T. M., Massie, A., Ross, M. G. R., et al.: Isolation of a reovirus from a case of Burkitt's lymphoma. B. M. J. *1*:1212–1213, 1964.
4. Berger, R. H., and Brody, J. A.: Reovirus antibody patterns in Alaska. Am. J. Epidemiol. *86*:724–735, 1967.
5. Bricout, F. J. R., and Duval, J.: Pouvoir pathogéne et diffusion des reovirus. Ann. Pediatr. *41*:43–48, 1965.
6. Brown, P. K., and Taylor-Robinson, D.: Respiratory virus antibodies in sera of persons living in isolated communities. Bull. World Health Organ. *34*:895–900, 1966.
7. Brown, W. R., Sokol, R. J., Levin, M. J., et al.: Lack of correlation between infection with reovirus 3 and extrahepatic biliary atresia or neonatal hepatitis. J. Pediatr. *113*:670–676, 1988.
8. Cohen, J. A., Williams, W. V., Weiner, D. B., et al.: Reoviruses. *In* von Regenmortel, M. H. V., and Neurath, A. R. (eds.): Immunochemistry of Viruses, II: The Basis for Serodiagnosis and Vaccines. New York, Elsevier Science, 1990, pp. 381–401.
9. Committee on the ECHO Viruses. Science *122*:1187, 1955.
10. Committee on the Enteroviruses. Am. J. Public Health *47*:1556, 1957.
11. Csiza, C. K.: Characterization and serotyping of three feline reovirus isolates. Infect. Immun. *9*:159–166, 1974.
12. deLavergne, E., Olive, D., and LeMoyne, M. T.: Les reovirus: Les difficultés de la mise en évidence de leur pouvoir pathogéne chez l'homme. Presse Med. *73*:951–956, 1965.
13. Dussaix, E., Hadchouel, M., Tardieu, M., et al.: Biliary atresia and reovirus type 3 infection. N. Engl. J. Med. *310*:658, 1984.
14. Edmonson, J. H., Millian, S. J., Goodenow, M., et al.: Persistent viruria due to reovirus in a patient treated for Hodgkin's disease in a protected environment. J. Infect. Dis. *121*:438–441, 1970.
15. El-Rai, F. M., and Evans, A. S.: Reovirus infections in children and young adults. Arch. Environ. Health *7*:700–704, 1963.
16. England, B.: Concentration of reovirus and adenovirus from sewage and effluents by protamine sulfate (Salmine) treatment. Appl. Microbiol. *24*:510–512, 1972.
17. Fenner, F.: Classification and nomenclature of viruses: Second report of the International Committee on Taxonomy of Viruses. Intervirology *7*:34, 1976.
18. George, S., and John, T. J.: Reovirus antibodies in human sera in South India. Indian J. Med. Res. *58*:1680–1685, 1970.
19. Glaser, J. H., Balistreri, W. F., and Morecki, R.: Role of reovirus type 2 in persistent infantile cholestasis. J. Pediatr. *105*:912–915, 1984.
20. Hartley, J. W., Rowe, W. P., and Huebner, R. J.: Recovery of reoviruses from wild and laboratory mice. Proc. Soc. Exp. Biol. Med. *108*:390–395, 1961.
21. Hilleman, M. R., Hamparian, V. V., Ketler, A., et al.: Acute respiratory illnesses among children and adults. J. A. M. A. *180*:445–453, 1962.
22. Hull, R. N., Minner, J. R., and Smith, J. W.: New viral agents recovered from tissue cultures of monkey kidney cells. I. Origin and properties of cytopathogenic agents S.V.1, S.V.2, S.V.4, S.V.5, S.V.6, S.V.11, S.V.12, and S.V.15. Am. J. Hyg. *63*:204–215, 1956.
23. Jackson, G. G., Muldoon, R. L., and Cooper, G. S.: Reovirus type 1 as an etiologic agent of the common cold. J. Clin. Invest. *40*:1051, 1961.
24. Jenson, A. B., Rabin, E. R., Phillips, C. A., et al.: Reovirus encephalitis in newborn mice: An electron microscopic and virus assay study. Am. J. Pathol. *47*:223–239, 1965.
25. Johansson, P. J., Sveger, T., Ahlfors, K., et al.: Reovirus associated with meningitis. Scand. J. Infect. Dis. *28*:117–120, 1996.
26. Jopkiewics, T. K., Krzeminska, K., and Stachowska, Z.: Virologic survey of sewage in the city of Bydgoszcz [English summary]. Przegl. Epidemiol. *22*:521–527, 1968.
27. Joske, R. A., Keall, D. D., Leak, P. J., et al.: Hepatitis-encephalitis in humans with reovirus infection. Arch. Intern. Med. *113*:811–816, 1964.
28. Kalra, S. L., Nair, E., and Nair, C. M. G.: Reovirus antibodies in Delhi. Indian J. Med. Res. *57*:1–4, 1969.
29. Kilham, L., and Margolis, G.: Hydrocephalus in hamsters, ferrets, rats, and mice following inoculations with reovirus type 1. I. Virologic studies. Lab. Invest. *21*:183–188, 1969.
30. Knocke, K. W., Pittler, H., and Hoepken, W.: Nachweis von Reovirus in Abwassern [English summary]. Zentralbl. Bakteriol. Parasitol. Infektionskr. Hyg. *203*:417–421, 1967.
31. Krainer, L., and Aronson, B. E.: Disseminated encephalomyelitis in humans with recovery of hepato-encephalitis virus (HEV). J. Neuropathol. Exp. Neurol. *18*:339–342, 1969.
32. Leers, W. D., and Rozee, K. R.: A survey of reovirus antibodies in sera of urban children. Can. Med. Assoc. J. *94*:1040–1042, 1966.
33. Lerner, A. M., Cherry, J. D., Klein, J. O., et al.: Infections with reoviruses. N. Engl. J. Med. *267*:947–952, 1962.
34. Lerner, A. M., Cherry, J. D., and Finland, M.: Enhancement of cytopathic effects of reoviruses in rolled cultures of rhesus kidney. Proc. Soc. Exp. Biol. Med. *110*:727–729, 1962.
35. Levy, J. A., Tanabe, E., and Curnen, E. C.: Occurrence of reovirus antibodies in healthy African children and in children with Burkitt's lymphoma. Cancer *21*:53–57, 1968.
36. Malherbe, H. H., and Strickland-Cholmley, M.: Quantitative studies on viral survival in sewage purification processes. *In* Berg, G. (ed.): Transmission of Viruses by the Water Route. New York, John Wiley & Sons, 1967, pp. 379–387.
37. Maratos-Flier, E.: Reovirus and endocrine cells. Curr. Top. Microbiol. Immunol. *233*:85–89, 1998.
38. Margolis, G., and Kilham, L.: Hydrocephalus in hamsters, ferrets, rats, and mice following inoculations with reovirus type I. II. Pathologic studies. Lab. Invest. *21*:189–192, 1969.
39. Massie, E. L., and Shaw, E. D.: Reovirus type 1 in laboratory dogs. Am. J. Vet. Res. *27*:783–787, 1966.
40. Matsuura, K., Ishikura, M., Nakayama, T., et al.: Ecological studies on reovirus pollution of rivers in Toyama Prefecture. II. Molecular epidemiological study of reoviruses isolated from river water. Microbiol. Immunol. *37*:305–310, 1993.
41. McFerran, J. B., Nelson, R., and Clarke, J. K.: Isolation and characterization of reoviruses isolated from sheep. Arch. Ges. Virusforsch. *40*:72–81, 1973.
42. McFerran, J. B., and Connor, T.: A reovirus isolated from a pig. Res. Vet. Sci. *11*:388–390, 1970.
43. Minuk, G. Y., Paul, R. W., and Lee, P. W. K.: The prevalence of antibodies to reovirus type 3 in adults with idiopathic cholestatic liver disease. J. Med. Virol. *16*:55–60, 1985.
44. Morecki, R., Glaser, J. H., Cho, S., et al.: Biliary atresia and reovirus type 3 infection. N. Engl. J. Med. *307*:481–484, 1982.
45. Morecki, R., Glaser, J. H., Johnson, A. B., et al.: Detection of reovirus type 3 in the porta hepatis of an infant with extrahepatic biliary atresia: Ultrastructural and immunocytochemical study. Hepatology *4*:1137–1142, 1984.
46. Munz, E., Reimann, M., and Ackerman, E.: Serologische Untersuchungen zur Epidemiologie von Reovirus-Infektionen bei Menschen, Nutz- und Wildtieren in Tanzania. Acta Trop. *36*:277–288, 1979.
47. Nibert, M. L., and Schiff, L. A.: Reoviruses and their replication. Virology *2*:1679–1728, 2001.
48. Nupen, E. M.: Virus studies on the Windhoek waste-water reclamation plant (southwest Africa). Water Res. *4*:661–672, 1970.
49. Onodera, T., Jenson, A. B., Yoon, J. W., et al.: Virus-induced diabetes mellitus: Reovirus infection of pancreatic B cells in mice. Science *201*:529–530, 1978.
50. Organ, E. L., and Rubin, D. H.: Pathogenesis of reovirus gastrointestinal and hepatobiliary disease. Curr. Top. Microbiol. Immunol. *233*:67–83, 1998.
51. Pal, S. R., and Agarwal, S. C.: Sero-epidemiological study of reovirus infection amongst the normal population of the Chandigarh area: Northern India. J. Hyg. (Camb.) *66*:519–529, 1968.
52. Phillips, P. A., Keast, D., Walters, M. N.-I., et al.: Murine lymphoma induced by reovirus 3. Pathology *3*:133–138, 1971.
53. Ramos-Alvarez, M., and Sabin, A. B.: Enteropathogenic viruses and bacteria: Role in summer diarrheal diseases of infancy and early childhood. J. A. M. A. *167*:147–156, 1958.
54. Ramos-Alvarez, M., and Sabin, A. B.: Intestinal viral flora of healthy children demonstrable by monkey kidney tissue culture. Am. J. Public Health *46*:295–299, 1956.
55. Ramos-Alvarez, M., and Sabin, A. B.: Characteristics of poliomyelitis and other enteric viruses recovered in tissue culture from healthy American children. Proc. Soc. Exp. Biol. Med. *87*:655–661, 1954.
56. Richardson, S. C., Bishop, R. F., and Smith, A. L.: Reovirus serotype 3 infection in infants with extrahepatic biliary atresia or neonatal hepatitis. J. Gastroenterol. Hepatol. *9*:264–268, 1994.
57. Rosen, L.: Reoviruses. *In* Lennette, E. H., and Schmidt, N. J. (eds.): Diagnostic Procedures for Viral and Rickettsial Infections. 4th ed. New York, American Public Health Association, 1969, pp. 354–363.
58. Rosen, L.: Reoviruses. *In* Wenner, H. A., Behbehani, A. M., and Rosen, L. (eds.): Virology Monographs. New York, Springer-Verlag, 1968, pp. 74–107.
59. Rosen, L., Abinati, F. R., and Hovis, J. F.: Further observations on the natural infection of cattle with reoviruses. Am. J. Hyg. *77*:38–48, 1963.
60. Rosen, L., Evans, H. E., and Spickard, A.: Reovirus infections in human volunteers. Am. J. Hyg. *77*:29–37, 1963.
61. Rosen, L.: Reoviruses in animals other than man. Ann. N. Y. Acad. Sci. *101*:461–465, 1962.
62. Rosen, L., Hovis, J. F., Mastrota, F. M., et al.: An outbreak of infection with a type 1 reovirus among children in an institution. Am. J. Hyg. *71*:266–274, 1960.
63. Rosen, L., Hovis, J. F., Mastrota, F. M., et al.: Observations on a newly recognized virus (Abney) of the reovirus family. Am. J. Hyg. *71*:258–265, 1960.
64. Rosen, L.: Serologic grouping of reoviruses by hemagglutination inhibition. Am. J. Hyg. *71*:242–249, 1960.
65. Ruiz-Gomez, J., Faingezicht-Gutman, I., and Sosa-Martinez, J.: Virus reo: Investigación de anticuerpos en individuos de diferentes edades. Bol. Med. Hosp. Infant (Mex.) *22*:359–363, 1965.
66. Sabin, A. B.: Reoviruses: A new group of respiratory and enteric viruses formerly classified as ECHO type 10 is described. Science *130*:1387–1389, 1959.
67. Sabin, A. B.: The significance of viruses recovered from the intestinal tracts of healthy infants and children. Ann. N. Y. Acad. Sci. *66*:226–230, 1956.

68. Schiff, L. A., and Fields, B. N.: Reoviruses and their replication. *In* Fields, B. N., Knipe, D. M., Chanock, R. M., et al. (eds.): Fields' Virology. 2nd ed. New York, Raven Press, 1990, pp. 1275–1306.
69. Schmidt, J., Tauchnitz, C., and Kühn, O.: Untersuchungen über das Vorkommen hämagglutinationschemmender Antikörper gegen die Reovirustypen 1 und 2 in der Bevölkerung. Z. Hyg. Infektionskr. *150*:269–279, 1965.
70. Scott, T. F. M.: Clinical syndromes associated with entero virus and reo virus infections. Adv. Virus Res. *8*:165–197, 1962.
71. Sherry, B., and Blum, M. A.: Multiple viral core proteins are determinants of reovirus-induced acute myocarditis. J. Virol. *68*:8461–8465, 1994.
72. Stanley, N. F.: Reoviruses. Br. Med. Bull. *23*:150–155, 1967.
73. Stanley, N. F., Leak, P. J., Walter, M. N. I., et al.: Murine infection with reovirus. II. The chronic disease following reovirus type 3 infection. Br. J. Exp. Pathol. *95*:142–149, 1964.
74. Stanley, N. F., Leak, P. J., Grieve, G. M., et al.: The ecology and epidemiology of reovirus. Aust. J. Exp. Biol. Med. Sci. *42*:373–384, 1964.
75. Stanley, N. F., and Leak, P. J.: The serologic epidemiology of reovirus infection with special reference to the Rottnest Island quokka *(Setonix brachyurus)*. Am. J. Hyg. *78*:82–88, 1963.
76. Stanley, N. F.: Reovirus: A ubiquitous orphan. Med. J. Aust. *2*:815–818, 1961.
77. Stanley, N. F., Dorman, D. C., and Ponsford, J.: Studies on the pathogenesis of a hitherto undescribed virus (hepato-encephalomyelitis) producing unusual symptoms in suckling mice. Aust. J. Exp. Biol. Med. Sci. *31*:147–160, 1953.
78. Steele, M. I., Marshall, C. M., Lloyd, R. E., et al.: Reovirus 3 not detected by reverse transcriptase mediated polymerase chain reaction analysis of preserved tissue from infants with cholestatic liver disease. Hepatology *21*:697–702, 1995.
79. Taylor-Robinson, D.: Respiratory virus antibodies in human sera from different regions of the world. Bull. World Health Organ. *32*:833–847, 1965.
80. Tillotson, J. R., and Lerner, A. M.: Reovirus type 3 associated with fatal pneumonia. N. Engl. J. Med. *276*:1060–1063, 1967.
81. Toth, M., and Honty, A.: Age-incidence of haemagglutination-inhibiting antibodies to reovirus types 1, 2 and 3. Acta Microbiol. Acad. Sci. Hung. *13*:119–126, 1966.
82. Tyler, K. L., and Fields, B. N.: Reoviruses. *In* Fields, B. N., Knipe, D. M., Chanock, R. M., et al. (eds.): Fields' Virology. 2nd ed. New York, Raven Press, 1990, pp. 1307–1328.
83. Tyler, K. L., and Fields, B. N.: *Reoviridae:* A brief introduction. *In* Fields, B. N., Knipe, D. M., Chanock, R. M., et al. (eds.): Virology. 2nd ed. New York, Raven Press, 1990, pp. 1271–1273.
84. Tyler, K. L.: Mammalian reoviruses. Virology. *2*:1729–1745, 2001.
85. Walker, E. R., Friedman, M. H., and Olson, N. O.: Electron microscopic study of an avian reovirus that causes arthritis. J. Ultrastruct. Res. *41*:67–79, 1972.
86. Wooley, R. E., Dees, T. A., Cromack, A. S., et al.: Infectious enteritis of turkeys: Characterization of two reoviruses isolated by sucrose density gradient centrifugation from turkeys with infectious enteritis. Am. J. Vet. Res. *33*:157–164, 1972.
87. Zalan, E., Leers, W. D., and Labzoffsky, N. A.: Occurrence of reovirus infection in Ontario. Can. Med. Assoc. J. *87*:714–715, 1962.

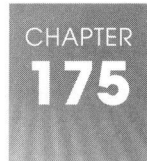

CHAPTER 175 Orbiviruses and Coltiviruses

THEODORE F. TSAI

Viruses in the genera Orbivirus and Coltivirus differ from others in the family *Reoviridae* structurally, in physicochemical properties, and by their arthropod mode of transmission.[2, 4, 43] More than 100 orbiviruses are classified into 14 serogroups defined by relationships in complement fixation, agar gel precipitation, and immunofluorescent assays. Additional serocomplex relationships are recognized, whereas individual viruses are differentiated by neutralization tests. Orbiviruses are principally animal pathogens (e.g., the bluetongue viruses); only viruses in the Kemerovo, Orungo, Lebombo, and Changuinola serogroups have been shown to cause human illness. Three coltiviruses are recognized to be human pathogens: Colorado tick fever (CTF) virus, Salmon River virus, and WX-3 virus (provisional). Banna virus recently has been reclassified as a Seadornavirus.[2]

The orbiviruses are spherical nonenveloped viruses with two protein shells: an outer shell (capsid) approximately 86 nm in diameter and an inner shell (core) 69 nm in diameter. The inner core VP7 protein, arranged in trimers, contains group-reactive antigens, and the outer capsid VP2 or VP5 proteins bear serotype-specific antigens. The viruses are acid-labile, and some exhibit sensitivity to lipid solvents. The double-stranded RNA viral genome is composed of 10 segments associated with viral structural and nonstructural proteins. Their complete nucleotide sequences and coding assignments have been determined for a bluetongue virus, and partial information is available for others. In general, reassortments of genomic segments among viruses within serogroups are viable, but not between groups, thus validating the broad serogroup classification. The genetic relationships (e.g., RNA hybridization) among viruses within serogroups diverge from the antigenic relationships in some instances, which provides an additional basis for taxonomic classification.

The coltiviruses resemble the orbiviruses in size and in having two capsids. Virions have a smoother surface morphology, and the genome is organized into 12 RNA segments.[43] The taxon was established from the genus Orbivirus in 1991.

Colorado Tick Fever Virus

CTF is an acute tick-borne febrile illness caused by the eponymous coltivirus.[5, 12, 17, 18]

Eyach virus, isolated from *Ixodes* ticks in France and Germany; S6-1403, isolated in California from a gray squirrel; and mosquito strains from Indonesia are related to, but distinct from, CTF virus and have not been associated with human disease.[4, 27] The closely related Salmon River virus was isolated from a viremic person with a CTF-like illness who most likely acquired her infection while camping on the middle fork of Idaho's Salmon River. Most CTF-like illnesses in Idaho and Montana are likely to be infections with Salmon River virus (unpublished observations, T. F. Tsai). RNA hybridization studies of CTF viral strains from a 33-year interval found minor heterogeneity, thus suggesting that a single gene pool has been maintained by mixing of viral strains and by constraints on viral replication within tick vectors and vertebrate hosts. A wide variety of small and large mammals are infected naturally with the virus, but clinical illness develops only in humans. Experimental infection of rhesus monkeys, hamsters, and mice produces hematologic changes similar to those occurring in human infections.[20]

EPIDEMIOLOGY

Cases occur principally in association with the habitats and activity patterns of the wood tick *Dermacentor andersoni*. Most cases occur in May and June, when adult ticks are most active, but infections from March to November have been reported. Infections are acquired principally in the western part of the United States and Canada in the known geographic distribution of the vector[7, 10–12] (Fig. 175–1). CTF viral antibodies have been found in serosurveys in South Korea, but no viral isolates have been recovered (unpublished observations, C. H. Calisher).

In rare cases, CTF has occurred in persons who had not traveled to areas of known risk, such as those exposed to ticks brought home on the clothing of family members and, in one case, by transfusion.[33, 37, 41, 42]

CTF virus is maintained in a 2- to 3-year cycle among small mammals, principally rodents, and *D. andersoni* ticks[5, 12, 18] (Fig. 175–2). Once infected in the larval stage, ticks remain infected through the nymphal and adult stages (trans-stadial transmission). Larvae are infected by viremic rodents. After molting, they carry the virus through the winter, and as nymphs, they infect other rodents and renew the cycle of transmission the following spring. Humans become infected incidentally by the bite of infected adult ticks.

The least chipmunk *(Eutamias minimus)*, the golden-mantled ground squirrel *(Spermophilus lateralis)*, and the porcupine *(Erethizon dorsatum)* appear to be the primary hosts for larval, nymphal, and adult *D. andersoni*; secondary hosts include rock mice *(Peromyscus maniculatus)*, meadow voles *(Microtus pennsylvanicus)*, and pine squirrels *(Tamiasciurus hudsonicus)*.[6]

D. andersoni is found exclusively in the high plains and in mountainous terrain between 4000 and 10,000 ft in altitude in the geographic distribution previously mentioned. The specific microhabitats where infected ticks are most prevalent are south-facing slopes with open stands of ponderosa pine, moderate shrubs, and rocky surfaces that provide favorable habitats for the intermediate rodent hosts.[6, 32] Both male and female adult ticks can transmit infection to humans, and the period of attachment required for transmission of the virus may be very brief.

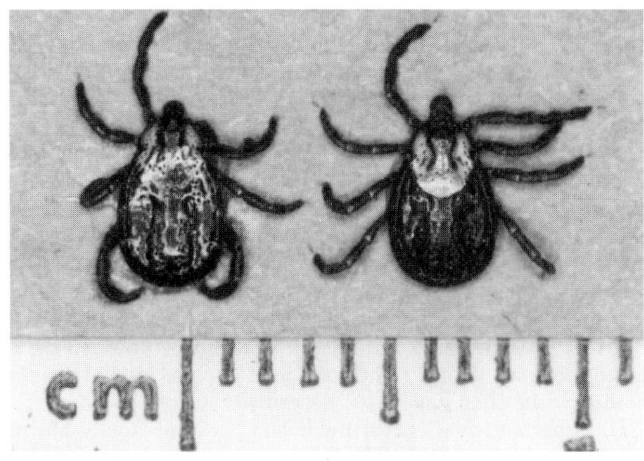

FIGURE 175–2 ■ Adult male *(left)* and female *(right)* *Dermacentor andersoni* ticks. Both can transmit Colorado tick fever virus.

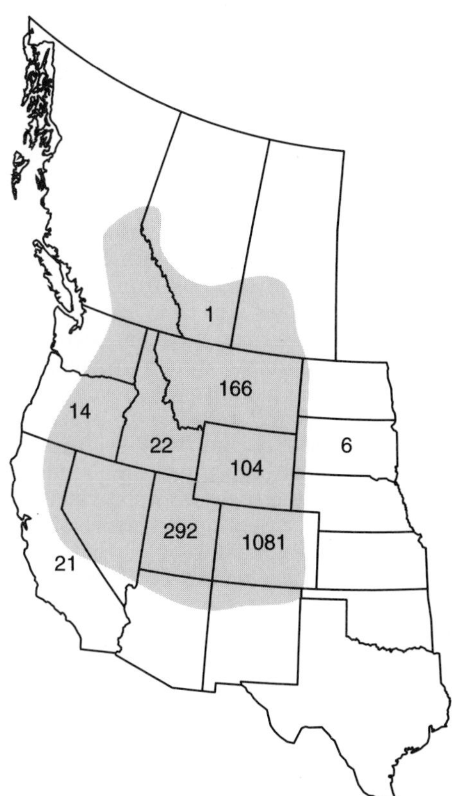

FIGURE 175–1 ■ Geographic distribution of *Dermacentor andersoni* ticks and reported cases of Colorado tick fever, 1980 to 1991.

CLINICAL MANIFESTATIONS

A history of a tick bite or tick exposure is given by more than 90 percent of patients.[21] The incubation period usually is 3 to 4 days, with a range of 0 to 14 days after known exposure to a tick.[21] The onset typically is abrupt, with fever, chills, malaise, headache, retro-orbital pain, myalgia, lumbar pain, and hyperesthesia. Nausea, vomiting, and abdominal pain occur less frequently. Upper respiratory symptoms usually are absent, although conjunctival injection may develop. Lymphadenopathy and hepatosplenomegaly are found in some patients. Maculopapular and petechial eruptions have been observed in 5 to 12 percent of cases.[40]

The disease classically is diphasic with an initial attack lasting 2 to 3 days followed by an equal interval of defervescence and a second and rarely a third recurrence. However, this saddleback pattern is absent in more than 50 percent of cases. Symptoms resolve several days after the second bout of fever, but prolonged asthenia lasting for several weeks is a typical finding, especially in adults.[21]

Leukopenia is a hallmark of the illness. The mean initial leukocyte count is $3900/mm^3$, which diminishes to a nadir 5 to 6 days after the onset of illness, often during the period of remission. A left shift with an absolute neutropenia and relative lymphocytosis is a usual finding. Examination of bone marrow aspirates shows maturational arrest in the granulocytic series, with absent mature forms and numerous metamyelocytes and myelocytes. Megakaryocytes are depleted, and a reduced peripheral platelet count ($<150{,}000/mm^3$) is found in most patients; however, thrombocytopenia rarely reaches a level of clinical significance.[25, 31]

Uncomplicated recovery is the rule. Epididymo-orchitis, pneumonitis, hepatitis, and pericarditis have been reported as complications, but the most serious complications are encephalitis and hemorrhage,[15, 19, 21, 23, 30] which have been reported nearly exclusively in children younger than 10 years.[10, 21, 38, 40] Three deaths have been reported, all in children who exhibited signs of generalized bleeding accompanied by a reduced platelet count.[9, 21] Examination of the bone marrow in one child disclosed a generalized depression of myeloid and erythroid elements and a marked reduction in megakaryocytes. Central nervous system signs consistent with meningitis and encephalitis have been reported in both children and adults. Examination of cerebrospinal fluid disclosed elevated protein and mononuclear cell pleocytosis in the few cases that have been described.

D. andersoni is a vector for both CTF and Rocky Mountain spotted fever (RMSF).[4] Although dual isolation of CTF virus and *Rickettsia rickettsii* from the same tick has not been reported, a concurrent rickettsial infection could not be discounted in all of the previously mentioned fatal cases attributed to CTF. Furthermore, a dual infection could develop in an individual exposed to more than one tick.

CTF virus is teratogenic in experimentally infected mice, but few clinical data are available on the teratogenic potential of the virus in humans.[22] One pregnant woman aborted 2 weeks after having an illness, and in an infant delivered 6 days after the onset of CTF in the mother, a febrile illness with leukopenia developed at 3 days of age, thus indicating a possible vertically acquired infection. In a single reported instance, a second attack of CTF has been documented, which indicates that immunity may not be permanent.[21]

The combined historical elements of tick exposure and outdoor activity in an enzootic area should suggest the diagnosis in patients with a spring-summer grippe-like illness. In a controlled study, abdominal pain, pharyngitis, and rash were less common symptoms in patients with CTF than in patients with other acute illnesses in the same season. Although RMSF occurs rarely in the states in which CTF is prevalent, the possibility of this potentially fatal disease should be considered in the differential diagnosis. Helpful differentiating features include the rarity of a petechial rash in CTF and its biphasic course. Tick-borne relapsing fever also follows a remitting course, but it has a more acute and toxic onset; splenomegaly occurs commonly, and remission is by crisis. The geographic distribution of the diseases overlaps; however, human encounters with the argasid (soft) tick vectors of relapsing fever (*Ornithodoros* ticks) are likely to occur in cabins and other protected areas.

PATHOPHYSIOLOGY

Experimental infection of rhesus monkeys, rodents, and human marrow cells in vitro has shown that CTF virus infects the erythropoietic elements (erythroblasts to reticulocytes) at an early stage of infection.[13, 14, 20, 26, 35, 37] After the infected cells mature and are released into the peripheral circulation, the virus persists intracellularly, where it has been identified by electron microsoopy.[14, 35] CTF virus has been cultured from circulating erythrocytes for up to 120 days after the onset of illness.[24] Red cell survival evidently is not shortened, and infected cells circulate in the presence of neutralizing antibody. Prolonged viremia has not been associated with either a protracted or a more severe course of illness. Infected CD34$^+$ progenitor cells and impaired mononuclear cell production of colony-stimulating factors may contribute to the acute aregenerative cytopenia.[36] High levels of serum interferon-γ correlate with fever during the acute phase of illness.[1]

LABORATORY DIAGNOSIS

Direct immunofluorescent examination of blood smears for intraerythrocytic viral antigen is an accessible and rapid approach to laboratory diagnosis.[13] However, polymerase chain reaction analysis and viral culture of blood samples are more sensitive.[3, 25] Ninety-six percent of all cases diagnosed by seroconversion are identified by isolation of virus from acute or convalescent blood samples in baby mice or Vero or BHK cells.[8, 13] Freezing and thawing the clot should be avoided. Virus has been isolated from a blood clot that had been refrigerated for 14 months. Serologic diagnosis by demonstration of fourfold rises in neutralizing, complement-fixation, immunofluorescent, or enzyme-linked immunosorbent assay antibody is confirmatory.[3] Neutralizing antibody rises slowly; only a third of patients had detectable neutralizing antibody 10 days after onset, but fourfold rises appeared within 30 days of onset in 92 percent.

TREATMENT

No specific therapy is available. Because thrombocytopenia may occur and hemorrhage is a reported complication in children, antipyretics that interfere with coagulation should not be used.

PREVENTION

Repellents containing permethrin should be sprayed on clothing, and repellents containing diethyltoluamide (DEET) should be applied to exposed skin (Table 175–1). Long pants should be tucked into socks, and shirts should be worn tucked into slacks. Clothing, gear, and skin should be inspected frequently for attached ticks. Light-colored clothing facilitates such inspections. One case of human-to-human transmission by transfusion of infected blood has been reported.[41] Persons with documented CTF should be prohibited from donating blood until the often prolonged viremia has cleared.[37]

Banna and WX-3 Viruses

Banna and WX-3 viruses have been associated with febrile illness and encephalitis in China. Both have 12 RNA segments and are antigenically distinct from the CTF, S6-1403, and Eyach viruses (coltiviruses from the Rocky Mountain region, California, and Germany). Banna virus was isolated from encephalitis patients in Yunnan province in southern China and later from 98 patients with fever, headache, and arthralgias from Xinjiang province in western China.[28] WX-3 and nine related strains that segregate into four distinct RNA electropherotypes were isolated from *Culex tritaeniorhychnus* mosquitoes in Gansu province and the suburbs of Beijing in 1991.[39] Serologic evidence of recent infection with the strains was found in 50 percent of encephalitis patients in Henan province and in 17 percent of patients in Jiangsu province, suggesting that these coltiviruses may be a leading cause of summer viral encephalitis after Japanese encephalitis. Details of the clinical illness and epidemiology of infection have not been reported.

Kemerovo and Related Viruses

The Kemerovo serogroup contains more than 50 chiefly tick-borne viruses divided into four serocomplexes. Only

TABLE 175–1 ■ PRECAUTIONS TO MINIMIZE POTENTIAL ADVERSE REACTIONS FROM REPELLENTS

Repellents should be applied only to exposed skin and/or clothing (as directed on the product label). Do not use under clothing.
Never use repellents over cuts, wounds, or irritated skin.
Avoid mucosal contact—don't apply to eyes and mouth, and apply sparingly around ears. When using sprays, do not spray directly onto face; spray on hands first and then apply to face.
Do not allow children to handle this product, and do not apply to children's hands. When using on children, apply to your own hands and then put it on the child.
Do not spray in enclosed areas. Avoid breathing a repellent spray. Avoid ingestion, and do not use it near food.
Use just enough repellent to cover exposed skin and/or clothing. Heavy application and saturation are unnecessary for effectiveness; if biting insects do not respond to a thin film of repellent, apply a bit more.
After returning indoors, wash treated skin with soap and water or bathe. This is particularly important when repellents are used repeatedly in a day or on consecutive days. Also, wash treated clothing before wearing it again.
Pregnant and nursing women should minimize the use of repellents.
If you suspect that you or your child is reacting to an insect repellent, discontinue use, wash the treated skin, and then call your local poison control center. If/when you go to a doctor, take the repellent with you.
Specific medical information about the active ingredients in repellents and other pesticides is available at the National Pesticide Telecommunications Network (NPTN) at 1-800-858-7378. NPTN operates from 6:30 AM to 4:30 PM (Pacific Time) 9:30 AM to 7:30 PM (Eastern Time) 7 days a week.

Adapted from U.S. Environmental Protection Agency recommendations available at http://www.epa.gov/pesticides/factsheets/chemicals/deet/htm.

Kemerovo, Tribec, and Lipovnik viruses have been associated with human illness. Kemerovo virus was isolated from the cerebrospinal fluid of two encephalitis patients and from ticks in the Kemerovo region of Russia; seroconversion was demonstrated in 10 other meningoencephalitis patients with tick bites and in whom Russian spring-summer encephalitis was excluded.[7, 29] The virus is transmitted in an *Ixodes persulcatus*–rodent cycle. Lipovnik virus has been reported in neurologic infections in the former Czechoslovakia, where flaviviral tick-borne encephalitis (TBE) is endemic; one study showed seroconversion to Lipovnik virus in half the patients with encephalitis who were studied, including some with suspected dual infection with TBE virus.[29] This finding seems plausible because both viruses are transmitted by *Ixodes ricinus* ticks, and multiple exposure to singly infected ticks or infection with a dually infected tick may be possible. In addition, serologic evidence of Lipovnik or Tribec infection was reported in patients with chronic polyradiculoneuritis; however, spirochetal infection was not ruled out in these cases.

On the basis of serologic rises in patients with acute febrile illness diagnosed clinically as RMSF, a Kemerovo-related virus is suspected to occur in the southwestern region of the United States. Patients with a history of a tick bite or tick exposure, whose sera were negative for *R. rickettsii,* demonstrated fourfold or greater changes in immunofluorescent titers to Lipovnik and Six Gun City viruses (Kemerovo group). Rises in immunofluorescent antibody titers to 128 to 512 suggested recent infection with a Kemerovo-related virus, possibly a novel agent or related to rabbit syncytium virus, which is enzootic in the United States. The patients had acute febrile illnesses with myalgia, vomiting, and severe abdominal pain, along with leukopenia, thrombocytopenia, and anemia, similar to RMSF. No agent has been isolated, but neither was the possibility of *Ehrlichia* infection excluded. Serologic evidence of infection was found in a cotton rat in the vicinity of one case. The syndrome tentatively is called Oklahoma tick fever.

Orungo Virus

Orungo virus is unrelated antigenically to the other orbiviruses. Infection is prevalent in western, central, and eastern Africa and apparently is transmitted in a sylvatic monkey–*Aedes* mosquito cycle similar to that of yellow fever. Human-to-human transmission by *Anopheles* mosquitoes is speculated to occur. The virus has been isolated from patients with fever and headache, and serologic evidence of infection has been reported in outbreaks of illness characterized by fever, headache, myalgia, nausea, and vomiting. Seroconversion has been observed in patients studied during yellow fever outbreaks, presumably because of concurrent transmission of the viruses. The virus also was isolated from the blood of a child with convulsions and flaccid paralysis.[16, 34]

Lebombo Virus

Lebombo virus is not grouped antigenically. The virus first was isolated from *Aedes circumluteolus* mosquitoes in South Africa. Subsequently, the virus was recovered from a Nigerian child with nonspecific febrile illness; the virus also was isolated from rodents and mosquitoes in Nigeria.[34]

Changuinola Virus

Changuinola virus belongs to an antigenic complex of 12 principally phlebotomine-borne orbiviruses. The virus is transmitted in Panama among forest mammals and *Phlebotomus* flies. Only one human case has been reported—a nonspecific febrile illness in a mosquito catcher.

REFERENCES

1. Ater, J. L., Overall, J. C., Yeh, T. J., et al.: Circulating interferon and clinical symptoms in Colorado tick fever. J. Infect. Dis. *151*:966, 1985.
2. Attoui, H., Billoir, F., Biagini, P., et al.: Complete sequence determination and genetic analysis of Banna virus and Kadipiro virus: Proposal for assignment to a new genus (Seadornavirus) within the family *Reoviridae.* J. Gen. Virol. *81*:1507–1515, 2000.
3. Attoui, H., Billoir, F., Bruey, J. M., et al.: Serologic and molecular diagnosis of Colorado tick fever viral infections. Am. J. Trop. Med. Hyg. *59*:763–768, 1998.
4. Attoui, H., Charrel, R. N., Billoir, F., et al.: Comparative sequence analysis of American, European and Asian isolates of viruses in the genus Coltivirus. J. Gen. Virol. *79*:2481–2489, 1998.
5. Burgdorfer, W.: Tick-borne diseases in the United States: Rocky Mountain spotted fever and Colorado tick fever: A review. Acta Trop. *34*:103, 1977.
6. Carey, A. B., McLean, R. B., and Maupin, G. O.: The structure of a Colorado tick fever ecosystem. Ecol. Monogr. *50*:131–151, 1980.
7. Chumakov, M. P., Karpovich, L. G., Sarmanova, E. S., et al.: Report on the isolation from *Ixodes persulcatus* ticks and from patients in western Siberia of a virus differing from the agent of tick-borne encephalitis. Arch. Virol. 7:82–83, 1993.
8. Earnest, M. P., Breckinridge, J. C., Barr, R. J., et al.: Colorado tick fever: Clinical and epidemiologic features and evaluation of diagnostic methods. Rocky Mtn. Med. J. *68*:60–62, 1971.
9. Eklund, C. M., and Kennedy, R. C.: Preliminary studies of pathogenesis of Colorado tick fever virus infection in mice. *In* Libikova, H. (ed.): Biology of Viruses of the Tick-Borne Encephalitis Complex. London, Academic, 1962, pp. 286–293.
10. Eklund, C. M., Kennedy, R. C., and Casey, M.: Colorado tick fever. Rocky Mtn. Med. J. *58*:21–25, 1961.

11. Eklund, C. M., Kohls, G. M., and Brennan, J. M.: Distribution of Colorado tick fever and virus-carrying ticks. J. A. M. A. *157*:335–337, 1955.
12. Emmons, R. W.: Ecology of Colorado tick fever. Annu. Rev. Microbiol. *42*:49, 1988.
13. Emmons, R. W., and Lennette, E. H.: Immunofluorescent staining in the laboratory diagnosis of Colorado tick fever. J. Lab. Clin. Med. *68*:923–929, 1966.
14. Emmons, R. W., Oshiro, L. S., Johnson, H. N., et al.: Intra-erythrocytic location of Colorado tick fever virus. J. Gen. Virol. *17*:185–195, 1972.
15. Emmons, R. W., and Schade, H. I.: Colorado tick fever simulating acute myocardial infarction. J. A. M. A. *222*:87–88, 1972.
16. Familusi, J. B., Moore, D. L., Fomufod, A. K., et al.: Virus isolates from children with febrile convulsions in Nigeria: A correlation study of clinical and laboratory observations. Clin. Pediatr. (Phila.) *11*:272–276, 1972.
17. Florio, L., Mugrage, E. R., and Stewart, M. O.: Colorado tick fever. Ann. Intern. Med. *25*:466–471, 1946.
18. Florio, L., Stewart, M. O., and Mugrage, E. R.: The etiology of Colorado tick fever. J. Exp. Med. *83*:1–10, 1946.
19. Fraser, C. H., and Schiff, D. W.: Colorado tick fever encephalitis. Pediatrics *29*:187–190, 1962.
20. Gerloff, R. K., and Larson, C. L.: Experimental infection of rhesus monkeys with Colorado tick fever virus. Am. J. Pathol. *35*:1043–1054, 1959.
21. Goodpasture, H. C., Poland, J. D., Francy, D. B., et al.: Colorado tick fever: Clinical, epidemiologic and laboratory aspects of 228 cases in Colorado in 1973–1974. Ann. Intern. Med. *88*:303–310, 1978.
22. Harris R. E., Morahan, P., and Coleman, P.: Teratogenic effects of Colorado tick fever virus in mice. J. Infect. Dis. *131*:397–402, 1975.
23. Hierholzer, W. J., Jr., and Barry, D. W.: Colorado tick fever pericarditis. J. A. M. A. *217*:825, 1971.
24. Hughes, L. E., Casper, E. A., and Clifford, C. M.: Persistence of Colorado tick fever virus in red blood cells. Am. J. Trop. Med. Hyg. *23*:530–532, 1974.
25. Johnson, A. J., Karabatsos, N., and Lanciotti, R. S.: Detection of Colorado tick fever virus by using reverse transcriptase PCR and application of the technique in laboratory diagnosis. J. Clin. Microbiol. *35*:1203–1208, 1997.
26. Johnson, E. S., Napoli, V. M., and White, W. C.: Colorado tick fever as a hematologic problem. Am. J. Clin. Pathol. *34*:118–124, 1960.
27. Karabatos, N., Poland, J. D., Emmons, R. W., et al.: Antigenic variants of Colorado tick fever virus. J. Virol. *68*:1463, 1987.
28. Li, Q. P., Shei, S. T., Hua, C., et al.: First isolation of 8 strains of new orbivirus (Banna) from patients with innominate fever in Xinjiang. Endemic Dis. Bull. *7*:77–82, 1993.
29. Libikova, H., Heinz, F., Ujhazyova, D., et al.: Orbiviruses of the Kemerovo complex and neurological diseases. Med. Microbiol. Immunol. *116*:255–263, 1978.
30. Loge, R. V.: Acute hepatitis associated with Colorado tick fever. West. J. Med. *142*:91, 1985.
31. Markovitz, A.: Thrombocytopenia in Colorado tick fever. Arch. Intern. Med. *111*:307–308, 1963.
32. McLean, R. G., Shriner, R. B., Pokorny, K. S., et al.: The ecology of Colorado tick fever in Rocky Mountain National Park in 1974. III. Habitats supporting the virus. Am. J. Trop. Med. Hyg. *40*:86, 1989.
33. Midoneck, S. R., Richard, J., and Murray, H. W.: Colorado tick fever in a resident of New York City. Arch. Fam. Med. *3*:731–732, 1994.
34. Moore, D. E., Causey, O. R., and Carey, D. E.: Arthropod-borne viral infections of man in Nigeria, 1964–1970. Ann. Trop. Med. Parasitol. *69*:49–64, 1975.
35. Oshiro, L. S., Dondero, D. V., Emmons, R. W., et al.: The development of Colorado tick fever virus within cells of the haemopoietic system. J. Gen. Virol. *39*:73–79, 1978.
36. Philip, C. S., Callaway, C., Chu, M. C., et al.: Replication of Colorado tick fever virus within human hematopoietic progenitor cells. J. Virol. *67*:2389–2395, 1993.
37. Philip, R. N., Casper, E. A., Cory, J., et al.: The potential for transmission of arboviruses by blood transfusion with particular references to Colorado tick fever. *In* Greenwalt, T. J., and Jamieson, G. A. (eds.): Transmissible Disease and Blood Transfusion. New York, Grune & Stratton, 1975, pp. 175–195.
38. Silver, H. K., Meiklejohn, G., and Kempe, C. H.: Colorado tick fever. Am. J. Dis. Child. *101*:30–36, 1961.
39. Song, L. T., Chen, B. Q., and Zhao, Z. J.: Isolation and identification of new members of Coltivirus from mosquitoes collected in China. J. Clin. Exp. Virol. China *9*:7–10, 1995.
40. Spruance, S. L., and Bailey, A.: Colorado tick fever. Arch. Intern. Med. *131*:288–293, 1973.
41. Transmission of Colorado tick fever virus by blood transfusion—Montana. M. M. W. R. Morb. Mortal. Wkly. Rep. *24*:422–427, 1975.
42. Tsai, T. F.: Arboviral infections in the United States. Infect. Dis. Clin. North Am. *5*:73–102, 1991.
43. Van Rejenmortel, M. H., Fauguet, C. M., Bishop, D. H. L., et al. (Eds.): Virus Taxonomy. Classification and Nomenclature of Viruses. Seventh Report of the International Committee on Taxonomy of Viruses. San Diego, Academic, 2000.

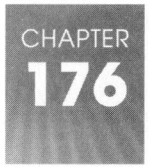

CHAPTER 176 Rotaviruses

DAVID I. BERNSTEIN ■ RICHARD L. WARD

Rotaviruses are recognized as the single most important cause of severe infantile gastroenteritis worldwide.[108, 179, 220] In the United States alone, these viruses are estimated to cause between 24,000 and 110,000 hospitalizations in young children annually[152, 191, 192, 275, 390] and between 20 and 40 deaths.[152, 191, 192] Direct medical costs associated with rotavirus disease in the United States have been estimated to be between $100 and $400 million annually,[9, 275] with an additional $1 billion in nonmedical expenses.[452] On a world scale, rotaviruses are estimated to be responsible for nearly 1 million deaths each year.[206, 220] For these reasons, rotaviruses have received a high priority as a target for vaccine development.[206, 378]

Transmissions of rotaviruses occur by the fecal-oral route, providing a highly efficient mechanism for universal exposure that has circumvented differences in regional and national cultural practices and public health standards. The symptoms associated with rotavirus disease typically are diarrhea and vomiting accompanied by fever, nausea, anorexia, cramping, and malaise that can be mild and of short duration or produce severe dehydration.[219, 224, 240, 361, 388, 395, 425, 455] Severe disease occurs primarily in young children, most commonly between 6 and 24 months of age. Approximately 90 percent of children in both developed and developing countries experience a rotavirus infection by the time they reach 3 years of age.[219, 220] Rotavirus infection normally provides short-term protection and immunity against subsequent severe illnesses but does not provide lifelong immunity; furthermore, numerous cases of sequential illnesses have been reported.* Neonates also can experience rotavirus infections, and they occur endemically in some settings but are typically asymptomatic.[26, 28, 170, 178, 303, 355] These neonatal infections have been reported to reduce the morbidity associated with a subsequent rotavirus infection.[26, 28]

*See references 28, 31, 63, 79, 104, 139, 254, 274, 336, 379, 505.

Rotavirus illnesses also occur in adults[114, 135, 200, 232, 389, 497] and the elderly,[93, 271, 424] but as with other sequential rotavirus infections, the symptoms usually are mild.

Because of the frequent occurrence of rotavirus infections and the reduced severity of illness typically associated with sequential infections, a realistic goal for a rotavirus vaccine may be to protect against severe disease. Several vaccine candidates have been developed and evaluated in infants, with promising results.* Incorporation of an effective rotavirus vaccine into the infant immunization schedule in developed countries could reduce hospitalizations due to dehydrating diarrhea in young children by 40 to 60 percent.[378] More important, worldwide use of such a vaccine could decrease by approximately 10 to 20 percent the total number of deaths caused by diarrhea.[108, 206, 378] Until an effective vaccine is available, control of rotavirus disease is limited to nonspecific methods, particularly rehydration therapy for replacement of body fluids and electrolytes.

History

Viruses with morphologic features later associated with rotaviruses were observed first by electron microscopy in 1963 in intestinal tissues and rectal swab specimens from mice and monkeys.[2, 269] These agents, called epizootic diarrhea of infant mice virus and simian agent 11, respectively, were described as 70-nm particles that had a wheel-like appearance. Hence, they were later designated "rota" viruses from the Latin word for wheel.[126, 504] In 1969, Mebus and colleagues[289] demonstrated the presence of these particles in stools of calves with diarrhea, thus associating these viruses with a diarrheal disease in cattle. The correlation between these viruses and human diarrheal disease was reported first in 1973 by Bishop and colleagues.[29] They used electron microscopy to examine biopsy specimens of duodenal mucosa from children with acute gastroenteritis. Within a short time, these and other investigators confirmed the association between the presence of rotavirus in feces and acute gastroenteritis.[30, 51, 100, 125, 223] In addition to their distinctive morphologic features, these human viruses along with their animal rotavirus counterparts later were shown to share a group antigen[221, 500] and have been classified as members of the *Rotavirus* genus within the *Reoviridae* family.[280] In 1980, particles that were indistinguishable morphologically from established rotavirus strains but lacked the common group antigen were discovered in pigs.[35, 399] This finding subsequently led to the identification of rotaviruses belonging to six additional groups (B to G) based on a common group antigen, with the original rotavirus strains classified as group A.[400] Only groups A to C have been associated with human diseases, and most known cases of rotavirus gastroenteritis have been caused by group A strains. However, nongroup A rotaviruses have been associated with large outbreaks in China[204] and Japan,[243, 278] which suggests that they could become major pathogens in the future. This suggestion is supported by seroepidemiology data showing high prevalence of group C rotavirus antibody in different countries.[208, 315, 385, 451]

Properties

Visualization of the rotavirus particle by conventional electron microscopy revealed a double-shelled structure with icosahedral symmetry.[117, 193, 272] The outer shell is composed of two structural proteins, VP4 and VP7, which form capsomers that radiate from the inner capsid composed of the major structural protein VP6.[119, 220] This inner shell surrounds a core containing the viral genome and three additional structural proteins, VP1, VP2, and VP3.

Much greater structural definition was obtained by cryo-electron microscopy (Fig. 176–1). This technique showed that the rotavirus core is surrounded by a third protein shell composed of VP2,[366, 417] which can self-assemble into corelike particles when it is expressed in insect cells by a baculovirus recombinant.[91, 516] Thus, the mature rotavirus particle contains three protein shells with radii of 21 to 26.5 nm (inner shell), 26.5 to 35 nm (intermediate shell), and 35 to 38 nm (outer shell). Detailed analysis of the outer shell suggests that it is composed primarily of the VP7 glycoprotein (780 molecules/virus), which contains 132 aqueous channels that are positioned over 132 channels within the perforated VP6 intermediate shell, also composed of 780 molecules/virus.[368, 507] Sixty dimers of the VP4 protein, 20 nm in length, are anchored to the VP6 shell and form spikelike projections as they extend through and 11 to 12 nm beyond the VP7 shell.[365, 366, 417, 506] Thus, the full diameter of the mature rotavirus particle, including the VP4 spikes, is approximately 100 nm.

Further examination of the rotavirus structure by cryo-electron microscopy has indicated that the inner shell composed of VP2 molecules not only encloses the viral genome but interacts with it as well.[367] This interaction has been found to cause significant conformational changes in the VP2 structure. Furthermore, VP1 and VP3 have been proposed to form a complex below the VP2 layer that interacts with ordered portions of the genome.[367] This interaction appears to be a prerequisite for transcription and capping of new mRNAs by VP1 and VP3, respectively, on initiation of

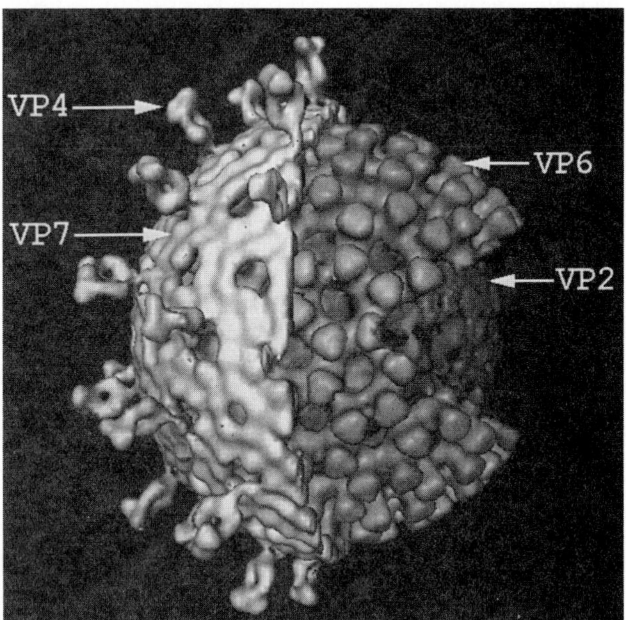

FIGURE 176–1 ■ Computer-generated image of the triple-shelled rotavirus particle obtained by cryoelectron microscopy. The cut-away diagram shows the outer capsid composed of VP4 spikes and VP7 shell, intermediate VP6 shell, and inner VP2 shell surrounding the core containing the 11 double-stranded RNA segments and VP1 and VP3 proteins. (Courtesy of Dr. B. V. V. Prasad, Baylor College of Medicine, Houston, TX.)

*See references 19, 22, 25, 70, 74, 133, 244, 295, 470, 473.

TABLE 176–1 ■ SIZES OF ROTAVIRUS GENE SEGMENTS AND PROPERTIES OF ENCODED PROTEINS

RNA Segment	No. of Base Pairs	Encoded Protein	Molecular Weight of Protein ($\times 10^{-4}$)	Properties of Protein
1	3300	VP1	12.5	Inner core protein RNA binding RNA transcriptase
2	2700	VP2	10.2	Inner capsid protein RNA binding
3	2600	VP3	9.8	Inner core protein Guanylyltransferase
4	2360	VP4	8.7	Outer capsid protein Hemagglutinin Neutralization protein Receptor binding Fusogenic protein
5	1600	NSP1	5.9	Nonstructural protein RNA binding Contains zinc fingers
6	1360	VP6	4.5	Intermediate capsid protein Group and subgroup antigen
7	1100	NSP3	3.5	Nonstructural protein RNA binding Translational control (?)
8	1060	NSP2	3.7	Nonstructural protein RNA binding
9	1060	VP7	3.7	Outer capsid glycoprotein Neutralization protein
10	750	NSP4	2.0	Nonstructural glycoprotein Transmembrane protein Enterotoxin
11	660	NSP5	2.2	Nonstructural protein Phosphorylated

the rotavirus replication cycle in an infected cell.[247] Finally, the amino terminus of VP2 has been reported to be necessary for the encapsidation of VP1 and VP3.[248, 515]

The genome of rotavirus is composed of 11 segments of double-stranded RNA that encode the six structural proteins—VP1 to 4, VP6, and VP7—and five nonstructural proteins designated NSP1 to NSP5.[119] Each segment encodes one known rotavirus protein, the functions of which have been investigated but, in some cases, remain poorly defined.* The genome segments range in size from approximately 660 to 3300 base pairs, and their encoded proteins, whose known functions are briefly described in Table 176–1, have molecular weights of approximately 22,000 to 125,000.

The RNA genome segments of rotavirus can be extracted from viral particles and separated by polyacrylamide gel electrophoresis into 11 distinct bands visualized by ethidium bromide or silver staining (Fig. 176–2). Each rotavirus strain has a characteristic RNA profile or electropherotype, a property that has been used extensively in epidemiologic studies of these viruses.† The characteristic RNA electrophoretic pattern of group A rotaviruses consists of four size classes containing segments 1 to 4, 5 and 6, 7 to 9, and 10 and 11. RNA segments of strains belonging to less well characterized rotavirus groups (i.e., groups B to G) also can be separated into four size classes, but the distribution of segments within these classes differs from group to group.[36, 350, 398, 400]

*See references 33, 119, 202, 226, 257, 270, 343, 362, 463, 466, 469.
†See references 214, 310, 333, 360, 386, 387, 411, 435, 458, 484.

Replication

Rotaviruses are activated by cleavage of the outer capsid VP4 protein by trypsin-like proteases into proteins VP5* and VP8*, which remain virus associated.[8, 76, 118, 120, 258] After attachment to receptors on the cytoplasmic membrane* through association with protein VP8*,[106, 263, 264, 291, 393, 514] the activated virion either passes directly through this membrane or is taken within a vesicle into the cytoplasm.[141, 217, 255, 432, 433] Either during membrane penetration[92, 433] or soon thereafter, the outer capsid proteins are removed, thus stimulating the RNA-dependent RNA polymerase (i.e., the VP1 transcriptase) associated with the inner shell to synthesize the 11 viral mRNAs that are capped by VP3 and subsequently translated into viral proteins.[116, 131, 186, 246, 273, 343, 346, 362, 469] Once viral proteins accumulate within the cytoplasm, large inclusions or viroplasms are formed in which the assembly of virion precursors is initiated.[4, 7] The earliest particles detected contain the complete complement of single-stranded plus-sense RNAs (i.e., one molecule of each mRNA) together with VP1, VP3, NSP1, NSP2, NSP3, and NSP5.[142, 343] This initial replication intermediate then loses its NSP1 proteins and becomes a core replication intermediate with the addition of VP2. Still later, core replication intermediates become double-shelled particles with the addition of VP6 and loss of most of the remaining nonstructural proteins. During these assembly steps, an RNA polymerase (replicase) associated with the replication intermediates

*See references 14, 68, 140, 175, 176, 187, 212, 259, 290, 292, 431, 513.

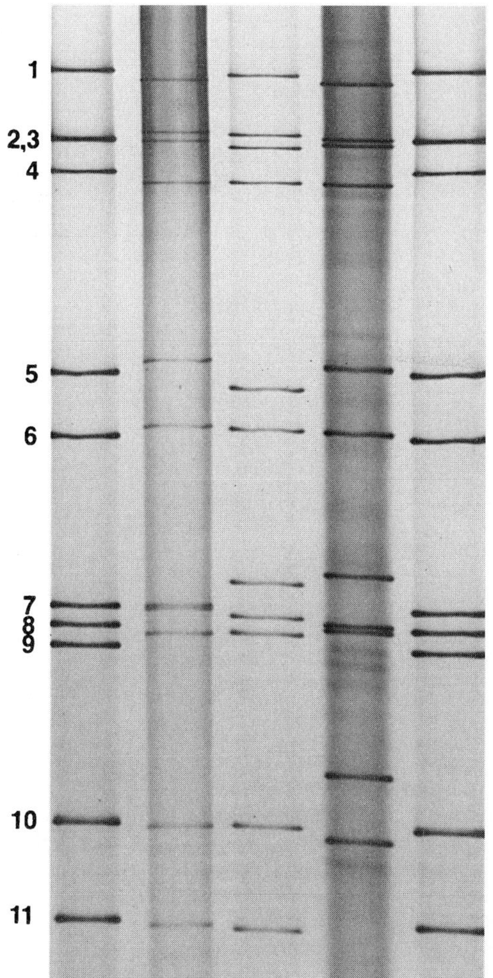

FIGURE 176–2 ■ Polyacrylamide gel electrophoretic patterns of genomic RNAs obtained from group A human rotaviruses and visualized by silver staining. The patterns demonstrate the characteristic four size classes of RNA separated into groups of four, two, three, and two segments each. Human rotavirus strains included (from left to right) lane 1, Wa; lane 2, 248 strain; lane 3, 456 strain; lane 4, DS-1; lane 5, Wa.

uses the single-stranded mRNAs within the particles as a template for minus-strand synthesis and formation of the double-stranded RNA genome segments.[62, 270, 344, 345, 347, 498] The double-shelled particles then associate with VP4 and bud into the rough endoplasmic reticulum after their transient association with the NSP4 transmembrane glycoprotein.[60, 265, 293, 318, 363, 439] The other rotavirus glycoprotein VP7, which becomes sequestered within the rough endoplasmic reticulum, then is added to complete the formation of mature viral particles.[78, 265, 266, 364, 430] These mature viruses accumulate within the lumen of the rough endoplasmic reticulum until cell lysis occurs. In cell culture, maximum production of infectious rotaviruses is found at approximately 12 hours after infection is initiated.[75]

Classification of Rotavirus

ELECTROPHEROTYPES AND GENOGROUPS

A variety of classification schemes have been used to characterize rotaviruses for epidemiologic purposes. Each scheme, however, is intertwined with a unique property of viruses with segmented genomes, that is, the ability to form reassortants. During the rotavirus replication cycle, newly formed plus-sense viral mRNAs are free within the viroplasm before incorporation into replication intermediates in the first stages of virion assembly.[370] From these genomic precursors, the appropriate number and combination of segments are selected for assembly of progeny virions. Co-infection of cells with more than one virion permits reassortment of the mRNAs from both parents. If co-infection is with different strains of virus, reassortment of mRNAs results in progeny that are genetic mosaics of the co-infecting strains (Fig. 176–3). These new strains, or reassortants, are identified by their specific array of genome segments, usually through their electrophoretic mobilities during polyacrylamide gel electrophoresis (i.e., electropherotypes). The properties of the new virus strains depend on which segments are inherited from which parent and the functional behavior of each particular combination of segments and their protein products.

Rotavirus reassortants form readily in cell culture[143, 161, 370, 460, 485, 486, 488] and in co-infected experimental animals,[45, 154] which is responsible, at least partially, for the variety of rotavirus strains found in nature.[158, 252, 448, 496, 512] Reassortant formation between rotavirus strains is not a universal phenomenon, however. For example, no evidence that reassortants form between strains belonging to different rotavirus groups has been found.[508] Even within group A rotaviruses, severe limitations exist within strain combinations that are capable of forming stable reassortants, limitations that appear to be related directly to the degree of genetic variation between strains.[370, 485]

One outcome of restricted reassortant formation between rotavirus strains is the concept of genetic families[134] or genogroups.[309] A genogroup is composed of rotavirus strains with gene segments that form interstrain RNA-RNA hybrids of sufficient stability to migrate as defined bands during polyacrylamide gel electrophoresis.[309] Thus, members of a genogroup share a high degree of genetic relatedness and have significantly less genetic homology with members of other genogroups. Because rotavirus genogroups appear to be species specific,[128, 308, 309] interspecies transmission of rotaviruses should be detectable readily by genogroup analyses. Almost all human rotaviruses belong to the Wa or DS-1 genogroup,[134, 307, 496] a designation developed from these prototype strains. The concept of genogroup has been used extensively to determine the origin of rotaviruses causing human infections and disease, particularly to detect viruses or reassortants with gene segments of animal origin.[47, 95, 97, 99, 112, 300, 305, 306, 459]

SEROTYPES

Both outer capsid proteins of rotavirus, VP4 and VP7, contain neutralization epitopes, and thereby both are involved in determination of serotype.[166, 168, 198, 216, 320] Serotyping was based originally solely on differences in the VP7 protein because animals hyperimmunized with rotaviruses develop most neutralizing antibody to this protein. Cross-neutralization studies conducted with these hyperimmune sera readily separated the strains into VP7 serotypes.[199, 502] When researchers later found that VP4 could, in some cases, be the dominant neutralization protein,[71, 354, 490, 493] a dual serotyping scheme was required. Although VP7 serotypes could be determined readily by cross-neutralization studies, determination was more difficult to make for VP4.[156, 267, 339, 419, 436] Therefore, two numeric systems were devised to classify the

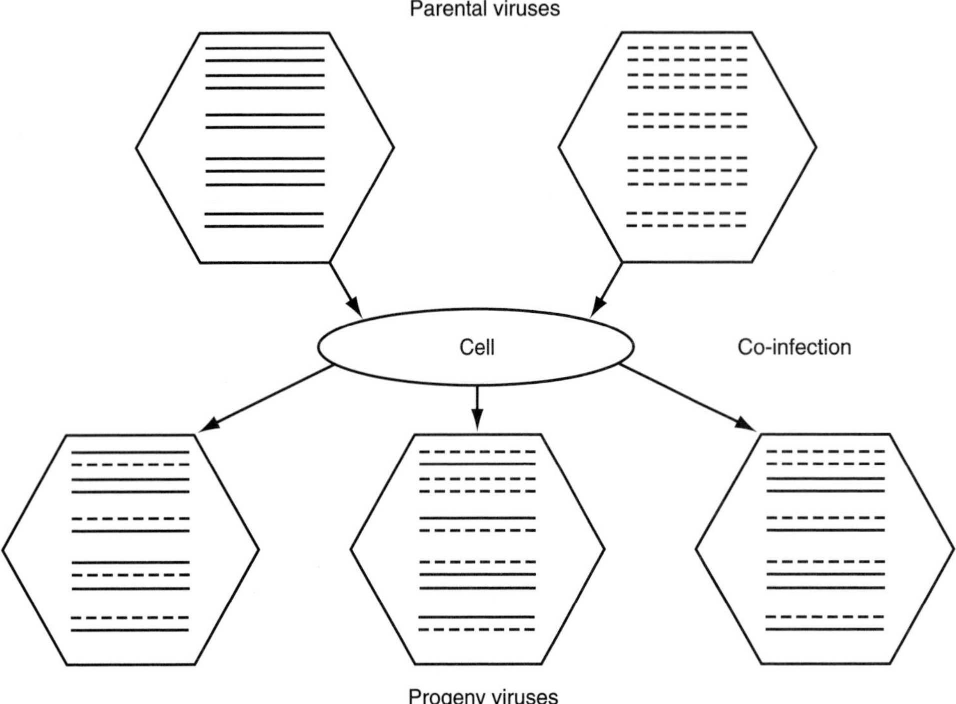

FIGURE 176–3 ■ Diagram of the formation of reassortant progeny rotaviruses after co-infection of a cell with two different (parental) strains of rotavirus.

VP4 protein in rotavirus strains. One is based on comparative nucleic hybridization and sequence analyses (genotypes),[119, 144, 160] and the second is based on neutralization (serotypes) with use of antisera against baculovirus-expressed VP4 proteins[156] or reassortants with specific VP4 genes.[419]

Rotavirus classification based on VP4 and VP7 designates P type and G type to describe the protease sensitivity and glycosylated structure of these two proteins, respectively.[119] Until very recently, 14 G types[119] and 20 P types[145] had been identified. However, Rao and colleagues[371] have isolated new bovine strains in India that appear to represent both a new G type and P type on the basis of sequence analyses. Human rotaviruses belonging to 11 G serotypes have been isolated,[148] but most have been identified as G1, G2, G3, or G4, and strains belonging to these G types commonly have been designated serotype 1, 2, 3, or 4, respectively.[220] The severity of illness caused by viruses belonging to these four serotypes has varied little if at all.[13, 17, 373] Likewise, 7 P genotypes have been found in humans, but almost all illnesses have been associated with P genotypes 4 and 8.[220] However, other G and P types have been the types most frequently isolated in some settings; particularly G serotype 9 strains have been found worldwide, sometimes representing a large fraction of the isolates.[94, 96, 145, 301, 369, 404, 428, 445]

GENETIC LINKAGE

If the G and P types of rotaviruses found in humans could associate freely because of reassortant formation, investigators anticipated that the combinations of types for these proteins would be generated randomly, which, however, clearly is not the case. For example, G1[P8] and G2[P4] rotaviruses similar to the prototype Wa and DS-1 strains, respectively, frequently are isolated but belong to two distinct genogroups of human rotaviruses.[309] Therefore, they rarely should form reassortants, an assumption that has been substantiated through analyses of numerous rotavirus strains.

Other associations between gene segments also have been found. The VP6 protein or group antigen can be divided into two subgroups (I and II) on the basis of antigenic differences within this protein.[167, 437] Almost all G2 and G8 human rotaviruses belong to subgroup I, whereas G1, G3, G4, and G9 human rotaviruses belong almost solely to subgroup II.[72, 146, 199, 386, 435] G3 also is a common serotype in animal strains, but in contrast to results found with G3 human strains, almost all G3 animal rotaviruses belong to subgroup I. In addition, subgroup I human, but not animal, strains have been found to have a characteristic "short" electropherotype associated with an inversion in the migration order of segments 10 and 11.[215, 242] Thus, distinct genetic linkages have been found by serotype, genotype, subtype, and electropherotype analysis as well as by genogroup determination.

Cross-Species Rotavirus Infections

Rotaviruses have an extremely wide host range, but natural cross-species infections, particularly those between animals and humans, may be rare occurrences. However, numerous human isolates appear to be animal strains or animal-human rotavirus reassortants, as determined by genogroup and sequence analyses.[47, 95, 97, 99, 112, 300, 305, 306, 459] The importance of these strains in human disease may be limited. Researchers have suggested, however, that once adapted to replication in humans, such strains may become important human pathogens.[309]

The property of host restriction has been used extensively to develop rotavirus vaccines for humans from naturally attenuated bovine and simian rotaviruses. Oral immunization of infants with these experimental live virus vaccines has resulted in low levels of intestinal replication and partial protection against human rotavirus illnesses.[19, 70, 74, 133, 244, 295, 470, 473] Thus, the barrier of host restriction can be bypassed sufficiently under these controlled conditions to permit the development of protective immune responses in a heterologous host. Experimental studies in animals have shown that intestinal replication of rotaviruses in heterologous species generally is limited, and if shedding of progeny viruses is detectable, it often occurs only when animals are inoculated with very high doses of the heterologous viruses.[45, 53, 84, 123, 283, 325, 494, 495]

The basis for host-range restriction is unknown and probably involves the collective properties of at least several genes. When reassortants between a murine and a simian rotavirus were used in a mouse model, however, a significant linkage to host-range restriction was associated with gene 5 encoding NSP1.[45] Other studies also report nonrandom selection of gene 5 in progeny after co-infection of cells in culture[161] and in mice,[154] suggesting a possible growth advantage associated with this gene. This gene also shows a high amount of sequence divergence among rotaviruses of different species,[119] which supports its possible role in host restriction. Of note, however, is that in a study in which the NSP1 gene from a bovine rotavirus that produces an abortive infection in pigs was substituted in a porcine rotavirus that replicates productively in pigs, the new reassortant still demonstrated productive replication in piglets.[40] Thus, NSP1 is not the only determinant of host range.

Epidemiology of Rotavirus

AGE-DEPENDENT SUSCEPTIBILITY TO ROTAVIRUS DISEASE

In addition to restrictions in interspecies transmission of rotaviruses, age restrictions are associated with rotavirus disease. In animals, rotavirus illness appears to be limited to the first days or weeks of life. Mice are susceptible to rotavirus disease only for their first 15 days of life but can experience a rotavirus infection for their entire lifetime.[286] Similarly, piglets and calves are most susceptible to rotavirus diarrhea during their first days of life.[37, 233] In contrast, severe human rotavirus disease occurs most commonly in patients between 6 and 24 months of age (Fig. 176–4),[220, 391, 484] but milder rotavirus illnesses occur throughout our lifetimes.

Causes for the reduced severity of rotavirus disease before 6 months and after the first years of life are subjects of intense investigation. Possibly, nonimmunologic, age-dependent changes that occur within the intestine, including an observed decrease in virus-specific receptors on enterocytes between suckling and adult mice, could account for this reduced severity.[384] A similar suggestion has been made for calves.[465] This suggestion also may explain why human infants are more susceptible to rotavirus illnesses than are older children or adults. Decreased concentrations of proteases needed to cleave the VP4 protein in intestinal secretions of newborns relative to older infants also could help explain the resistance of neonates to rotavirus disease.[250]

Neonatal rotavirus infections are common occurrences and appear to be endemic in some newborn nurseries.[28, 355, 386] On the basis of sequence analyses, researchers proposed that neonatal strains possess unique VP4 genes, which have been classified as genotype [P6].[119, 130, 155] Because neonatal rotavirus infections also typically are asymptomatic, rotaviruses containing [P6] VP4 genes were designated neonatal or asymptomatic strains. Further epidemiologic studies have shown that these descriptions are not totally accurate, however; asymptomatic neonatal infections sometimes are caused by non-[P6] strains,[97, 98] and many symptomatic infections of older infants in some settings are caused by [P6] strains.[94–96, 145, 301, 369, 428, 445] Therefore, why most neonatal rotavirus infections are caused by [P6] strains and whether the [P6] genotype is in any way responsible for the asymptomatic phenotype of these infections remain unclear.

The onset of rotavirus disease in infants has been reported to coincide with the decline of maternal antibody

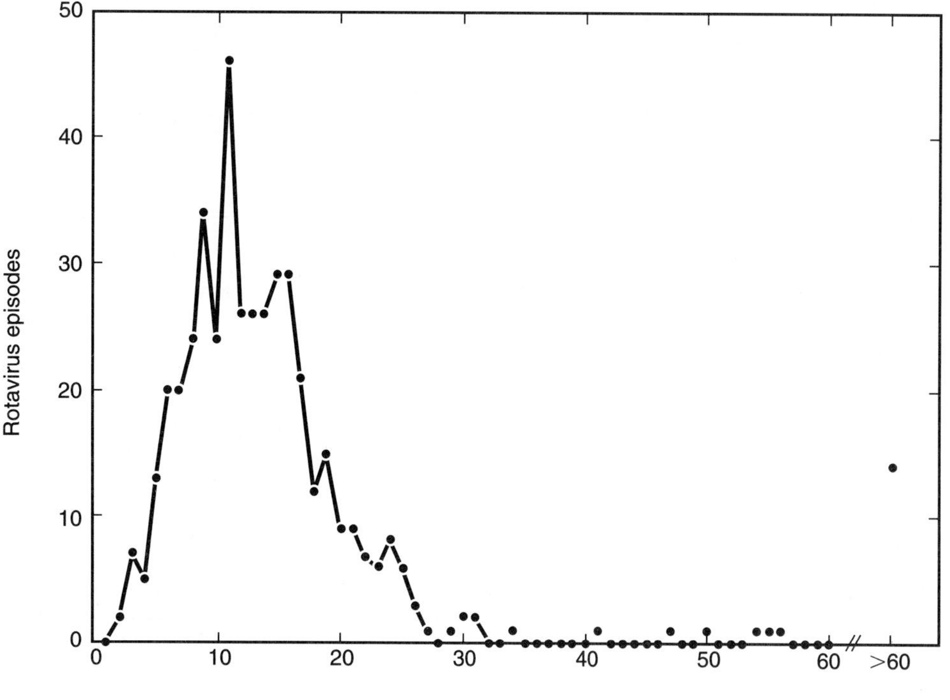

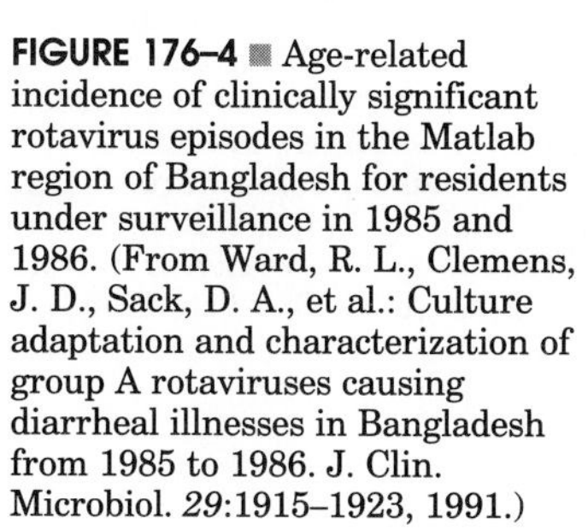
FIGURE 176–4 ■ Age-related incidence of clinically significant rotavirus episodes in the Matlab region of Bangladesh for residents under surveillance in 1985 and 1986. (From Ward, R. L., Clemens, J. D., Sack, D. A., et al.: Culture adaptation and characterization of group A rotaviruses causing diarrheal illnesses in Bangladesh from 1985 to 1986. J. Clin. Microbiol. *29*:1915–1923, 1991.)

titers to low concentrations.[519] Therefore, the commonly asymptomatic nature of neonatal rotavirus infections may be due, at least partially, to protection from transplacental antibody that may persist for the first months of life.[24] Mechanisms by which transplacental maternal antibody might protect against intestinal infection are unclear. Passive transfer of neutralizing antibody to the intestine of both humans and animals is associated with protection,[38, 103, 113, 189, 401, 410, 418, 420] but circulating antirotavirus IgG appears to confer little if any protection in animals.[323, 420, 421] Possibly, maternal IgG in humans is taken into the intestine where it neutralizes rotaviruses before infection. Regardless of why rotavirus infection of neonates typically is asymptomatic, these infections have been found to reduce the severity of rotavirus illnesses in older infants.[26, 28] For these reasons, two rotavirus strains obtained from neonates have been developed as vaccine candidates,[12, 295] and two others obtained more recently from India[97, 99] have been evaluated in phase I safety studies (unpublished results).

The reduced severity of rotavirus disease in older children and adults is probably due primarily to immune responses stimulated by previous rotavirus infections. In developed as well as in developing countries, almost all humans experience at least one rotavirus infection by the time they reach 3 years of age, and circulating rotavirus antibody remains detectable indefinitely.[219, 220] Protection against rotavirus infection and disease in adults has been correlated with titers of both circulating and intestinal rotavirus antibody.[163, 225, 481, 482] Although these antibodies have not been established as the effectors of protection, their presence indicates a natural infection that has elicited a protective immune response.

ROTAVIRUS SEASONALITY AND SOURCES OF EPIDEMIC STRAINS

As with other respiratory and enteric viruses, distinct seasonality is associated with rotavirus disease.[88, 179, 223, 238] It is particularly evident in temperate climates, where rotaviruses probably are responsible for the large increase in diarrheal deaths found during the winter season.[152, 191, 192, 249] The seasonality of rotavirus disease is less apparent in tropical climates but is still more prevalent in the drier, cooler months.[179] The cause for the seasonality of rotavirus disease is a topic of considerable interest but remains unknown.

The transmission of rotavirus infections is thought to be fecal-oral, with little evidence of airborne transmission. Yet a unique pattern of rotavirus infections that follows the general direction of the prevailing winds is observed annually in North America.[249] These infections begin in Mexico and the southwestern United States in mid to late fall and travel systematically across the continent, ending in the northeastern United States and Maritime Provinces of Canada in the spring (Fig. 176–5). Until recently, it was the only description of a repetitive geographic sequence for the seasonal epidemic activity of a viral agent. However, a similar pattern of rotavirus spread was reported for western Europe, where the seasonal peak started in Spain in January and ended in the more northern countries in March.[238] These annual events, including wind movements, have no satisfactory explanations. The phenomenon appears to be independent of latitude, which argues against temperature-dependent associations and humidity. Furthermore, the electropherotypes and serotypes of isolates found in different geographic locations can vary,[480] a counterindication for

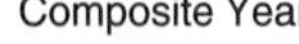

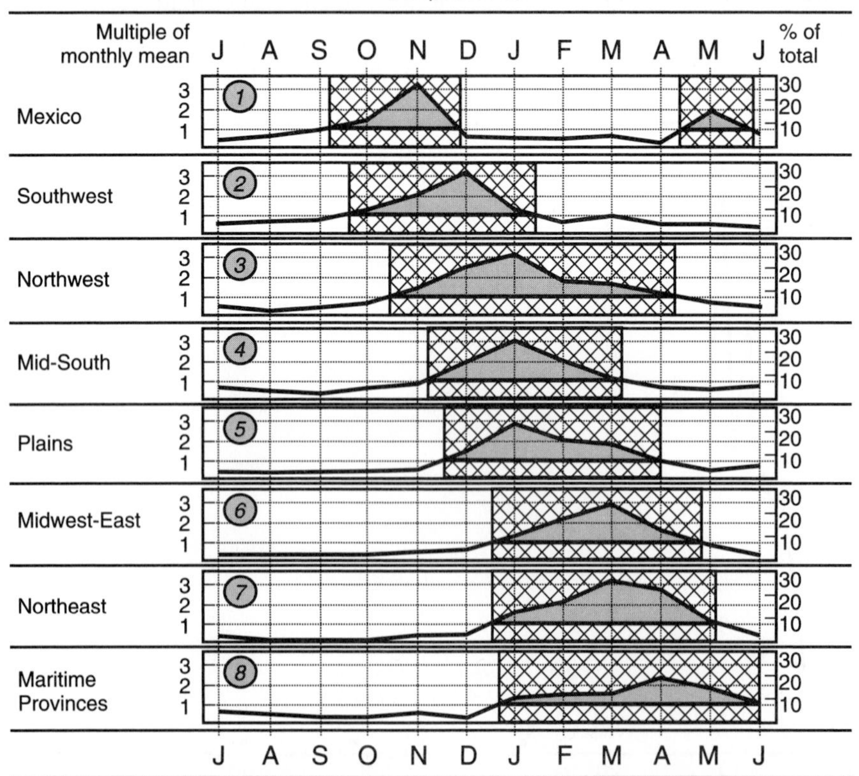

FIGURE 176–5 ■ West-to-east movement of annual rotavirus epidemics in North America based on a monthly average of rotavirus illnesses between 1984 and 1988. Results are from 88 centers in Canada, Mexico, and the United States. (From LeBaron, C. W., Lew, J., Glass, R. I., et al.: Annual rotavirus epidemic patterns in North America. J. A. M. A. *264*:983–988, 1990.)

a gradual, physical transmission of rotavirus infections as a wave to the north and east.

Because rotavirus illnesses occur with seasonal regularity and decrease to almost undetectable levels during the off-season, the virus must be retained in a less active state during most of each year. Retention of human rotavirus in animal reservoirs between seasons is unlikely because of the low interspecies transmissibility associated with this virus, as already discussed. Therefore, the virus may continue to replicate at low levels in humans until conditions are favorable for the annual epidemic. The occasional rotavirus illnesses that occur in the off-season support the suggestion that humans are a reservoir. Also possible is that the virus survives in the environment that provides continuous exposure throughout the year but results in sustained rotavirus illnesses only during seasonal epidemics. Rotaviruses are shed in extremely high concentrations (i.e., approximately 10^{11} particles/g of human feces),[489] retain their infectivities for many months at ambient temperatures,[121, 229, 297] and are detectable readily on environmental surfaces.[55] Therefore, the environment could be a reservoir for human rotavirus and a possible source for the initiation of seasonal epidemics.

To provide clues about the origin of rotavirus strains responsible for epidemics, many extensive studies have been performed to characterize the circulating viruses, primarily using electropherotypes and serotypes. From these studies, investigators have determined that rotavirus strains in a specific locale can vary little over sequential seasons or change dramatically, even within a single season.[360, 386, 411, 435, 484] Furthermore, multiple strains often are present within a region at any period during an epidemic. Because gene reassortment can be extensive after co-infection with rotavirus,[96, 158, 252, 345, 370] identifying the source of new strains within a defined geographic area is difficult. They could be derived from outside sources, they could be obtained from local reservoirs, or they could arise by gene reassortment of circulating strains. Clearly, if the source of virus responsible for initiating annual rotavirus epidemics could be identified, much would be learned about the epidemiology of rotavirus.

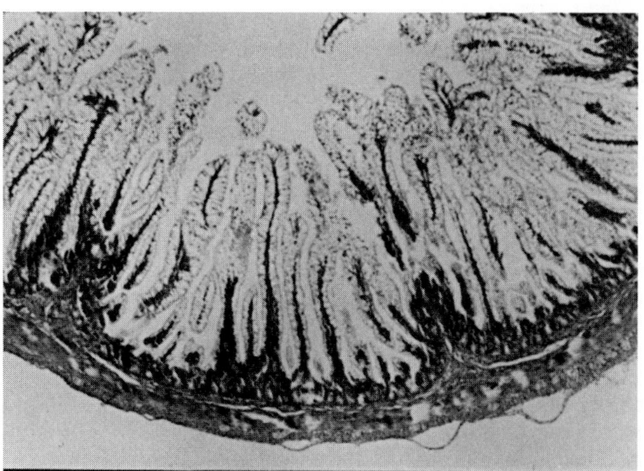

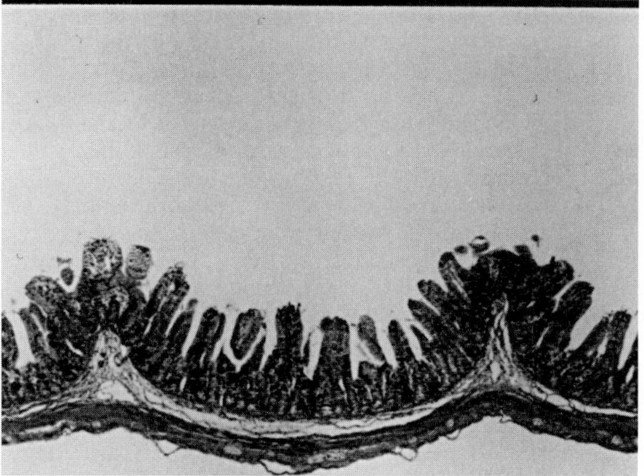

FIGURE 176–6 ■ *Top*, Normal histologic appearance of ileum from an 8-day-old gnotobiotic pig (hematoxylin and eosin stain). Normal mature vacuolate absorptive cells cover the villi. *Bottom*, Ileum from an 8-day-old gnotobiotic pig after oral inoculation with virulent human rotavirus (Wa strain). Severe villous atrophy and early crypt hyperplasia are evident (hematoxylin and eosin stain). (Courtesy of Dr. L. A. Ward, Ohio Agricultural Research and Development Center, The Ohio State University, Wooster, OH.)

Pathology and Pathogenesis

HISTOLOGIC AND STRUCTURAL CHANGES IN INTESTINAL VILLI

After fecal-oral transmission of rotavirus, infection is initiated in the upper intestine and typically leads to a series of histologic and physiologic changes. These changes have been examined extensively, particularly through experimental infections of animals (Fig. 176–6). Studies in calves revealed that rotavirus infection caused the villus epithelium to change from columnar to cuboidal, which resulted in shortening and stunting of the villi.[287, 288, 349] The cells at the villus tips became denuded, while in the underlying lamina propria, the numbers of reticulum-like cells increased and mononuclear cell infiltration was observed. The infection started at the proximal end of the small intestine and advanced distally. The most pronounced changes usually, but not always,[446] were associated with the proximal small intestine. When bovine rotaviruses of different virulence were compared, a low-virulence strain infected the proximal small intestine poorly but infected more villus enterocytes in the mid and distal intestine than did the high-virulence strain.[41, 181] Although the low-virulence strain replicated in these cells and caused cytopathic effects, it did not damage intestinal structure or affect function. Similar observations were made after piglets were infected with rotavirus.[81, 165, 348, 440]

The pathology of murine rotavirus infection also has been examined in several studies, and the results are similar to those found in larger animals.[3, 11, 16, 80, 241, 256, 338, 423] Many of these studies have been conducted with heterologous rotavirus strains that require infection with many times more virus because of the restricted replication of these viruses in mice.[16, 45, 123, 169, 325, 495] The histologic changes induced by these heterologous strains are similar to those found after murine rotavirus infection, even though viral replication is limited after oral inoculation with these viruses. Studies with the mouse model also have revealed a potential hazard associated with the possible use of heterologous viruses as vaccine candidates. Although replication of the homologous strains appeared to be restricted to the intestine, oral inoculation of either mice with severe combined immune deficiency (SCID) or normal mice with a simian rotavirus resulted in its spread to the liver and induction of hepatitis.[456, 457] Because of evidence for abnormal liver function during natural rotavirus infection in humans,[171, 173, 239] this observation has caused concern about the use of animal strains as vaccine candidates. However, no significant alteration of liver function has been associated with any rotavirus vaccine candidate after extensive investigations, even though most candidates have been derived from animal rotavirus strains. As discussed in detail in a later section, however, use of the same simian rotavirus strain in combination with three monoreassortants of this virus as a vaccine in infants was found to increase the incidence of intussusception in the week after administration of the first dose of vaccine.[335] This occurrence necessitated the removal of the vaccine from the market.

A few studies have examined the pathologic changes in the intestines of humans, but the results appeared to be similar to those found in animals.[193, 434] Tissue tropism for rotavirus infection in humans also appeared to be restricted normally to villi of the small intestine. Sporadic instances of nongastrointestinal rotavirus-associated disease, including the association with abnormal liver function mentioned before, as well as respiratory and nervous system involvement have been reported.* However, because no consistent evidence of extraintestinal replication of rotavirus has been forthcoming, the general assumption is that rotavirus pathology is strictly intestinal.

As with host-range restriction, the molecular basis for pathogenicity has not been established. Offit and coworkers[321] reported that the virulence of reassortants generated between heterologous rotaviruses and tested in a mouse model correlated with the presence of the VP4 protein from the more virulent virus. Neither rotavirus strain used in this study (a simian and a bovine strain) replicated efficiently in mice, however, which suggested that the observation may have limited applicability. A later study with murine-simian rotavirus reassortants revealed no association between the VP4 protein and virulence.[45] In that study, the strongest association between virulence and a gene product was with NSP1, a nonstructural protein.

Associations between virulence and specific gene segments also were examined in piglets. Virulence variants that appeared to differ only in their VP4 genes were isolated from the feces of an infected pig.[39, 52] To eliminate the possibility that virulence was determined by other gene products, the VP4 gene of the virulent strain was transferred into the avirulent strain by reassortment.[438] This transfer caused the avirulent strain to become virulent.[43] In another study with reassortants between a virulent porcine virus and a human strain attenuated for piglets, investigators found that the porcine rotavirus genes encoding VP3, VP4, VP7, and NSP4 were required for virulence in piglets.[196] Whether either of these observations has general applicability or pertains only to a limited combination of rotavirus strains because of specific interactions between their proteins remains to be determined. Passage of a porcine rotavirus in piglets was reported to increase its virulence dramatically,[39] whereas passage of a virulent porcine rotavirus in cell culture attenuated this virus.[454] Thus, the associations between specific rotavirus genes and virulence can be altered readily by natural selection through mutation.

MECHANISMS OF DIARRHEA

Although rotaviruses cause severe diarrhea in numerous species, including humans, the mechanisms responsible have not been determined and may be due to multiple factors. An early study in piglets indicated that net sodium and calcium fluxes were not different between control and infected animals, but glucose-mediated sodium absorption was diminished by rotavirus infection.[101] On the basis of this and other physiologic changes, the authors concluded that retarded differentiation of uninfected enterocytes that migrated at an accelerated rate from the crypts after the virus had invaded villus cells was responsible for absorptive abnormalities. Another study with piglets led to the conclusion that destruction of the villus tip cells causes carbohydrate malabsorption and osmotic diarrhea.[162] In mice, researchers reported that carbohydrate malabsorption did not occur as in piglets, and, therefore, crypt cell secretions may be the cause of fluid loss.[82] Additional studies in animals and humans concerning changes in the absorption of macromolecules across the intestinal surface after rotavirus infection have revealed no general pattern.[165, 188, 205, 317] Uptake of some molecules, such as horseradish peroxidase and 2-rhamnose, is increased; uptake of other molecules, such as lactulose and D-xylose, is decreased. Therefore, the relationship between the absorptive properties of intestinal mucosa induced by rotavirus infection and development of diarrhea remains unclear.

The importance of virus replication for induction of rotavirus diarrhea also has been challenged. Inoculation of mice with heterologous rotaviruses had been observed to produce diarrhea only when mice were inoculated with large quantities of these viruses, and in these cases, diarrhea occurred despite a lack of efficient viral replication.[45, 325, 495] Subsequently, inoculation with a large number of inactivated particles from a heterologous rotavirus was reported also to result in diarrhea.[415] The authors suggested that rotavirus attachment or entry into cells was sufficient to induce diarrhea in this model and that the mechanism of rotavirus-induced diarrhea was consistent with a viral toxin–like effect exerted during virus-cell contact.

Diarrhea also has been induced in infant mice and rats by intraperitoneal inoculation with the rotavirus NSP4 protein as well as with a 22–amino acid peptide derived from this protein.[10, 299] Investigators observed that this protein and its peptide caused an increase in calcium concentration in insect cells when added exogenously.[443] In subsequent experiments, NSP4 and its peptide were found to increase the levels of intracellular calcium[444] by activating a calcium-dependent signal transduction pathway that mobilizes transport of this ion from the endoplasmic reticulum.[111, 443] Further reports suggest that NSP4 possesses membrane destabilization activity[46, 442] that may result from increased intracellular calcium concentrations, resulting in cytoskeleton disorganization and cell death.[48, 49, 352, 353] Thus, binding NSP4 to intestinal epithelium after its release from infected cells may contribute to altered ion transport and diarrhea. Whether it is a major mechanism of diarrhea occurring after rotavirus infection remains to be determined. Some additional studies in mice support a role for NSP4 as a cause of diarrhea,[195, 517] whereas others indicate that mutations in NSP4 are not responsible for attenuation of rotavirus in either mice or humans,[6, 251, 492] thus questioning its importance as a cause of diarrhea in nature.

Immunity

Much has been learned about the immune response to rotavirus, but the key question of what provides protection from infection or disease remains unanswered. Rotavirus infections clearly induce a humoral immune response beginning with production of IgM antibodies and later including IgA and IgG antibody.[102, 172, 281, 381] Infection also induces local, intestinal antibodies that are predominantly IgA but also include IgG and IgM initially.[21, 90, 102, 172, 276, 281, 381] After infection in mice, as many as 50 percent of all IgA cells in the

*See references 185, 194, 213, 227, 236, 253, 279, 302, 313, 403, 456, 457, 462, 499, 510, 518.

lamina propria of the intestine can be rotavirus specific.[416] Cell-mediated immunity, including lymphoproliferative responses, also is detected easily after infection in animals and humans,[329, 330, 447] and a brisk cytolytic T-cell response ($CD8^+$) has been found in the intestine and spleen of infected mice.[326, 327]

The most immunogenic protein appears to be VP6. Thus, antibodies measured by enzyme-linked immunosorbent assay (ELISA) are directed mainly at this protein and may not be neutralizing.[414] Some evidence suggests, however, that IgA antibodies directed at VP6 can be protective by as yet incompletely understood mechanisms.[54] Antibodies directed at either the VP4 or the VP7 proteins can neutralize virus and provide protection when they are given passively to animals.[277, 331] Although numerous problems are associated with measuring the VP4- and VP7-specific responses in humans,[319] the preponderance of information suggests that after infection, the predominant response appears to be to the VP4 protein,[50, 490, 493] whereas VP7 antibodies were noted more commonly after vaccination with a poorly replicating vaccine, WC3.[20, 487] Both VP4 and VP7 proteins can induce both type-specific and cross-reactive serotype responses, although most of the VP7 responses are type-specific, whereas those directed at VP4, especially the VP5* region, are more likely to be cross-reactive.[156, 164, 267, 298, 436] These findings have important implications for vaccine development, as will be discussed.

Rotavirus-specific cytotoxic T lymphocytes recognize VP7 better than VP4 and are not serotype specific.[322, 326] Adoptive transfer of splenic lymphocytes from mice infected with homologous or heterologous rotavirus strains can protect suckling mice.[328] Protection is major histocompatibility complex restricted and appears to depend on the presence of $CD8^+$ lymphocytes. Similarly, $CD8^+$ splenic or intraepithelial lymphocytes obtained from the intestine of rotavirus-infected mice can eliminate the chronic rotavirus shedding seen in SCID mice.[110] Adoptive transfer of $CD8^+$ cells from mice immunized with baculovirus recombinants expressing VP1, VP4, VP6, or VP7 also can terminate the chronic shedding in SCID mice.[109] Studies revealed that adoptive transfer of splenic $CD4^+$ cells from either naive or rotavirus-immunized mice resolved shedding in chronically infected, immunodeficient Rag-2 mice (unpublished results). Therefore, either $CD8^+$ or $CD4^+$ T cells are capable of resolving rotavirus infections. Possible roles of these cells in resolution or prevention of human rotavirus infections remain to be determined.

An obvious place to begin to understand rotavirus immunity is to determine the effectiveness of previous rotavirus infections in prevention of subsequent infections and disease. The important questions relate not only to the degree of protection but also to whether protection is serotype specific. As discussed earlier in this chapter, multiple serotypes of human rotavirus are based on neutralization epitopes on the VP4 (P serotypes) and VP7 (G serotypes) outer capsid proteins. Thus, protection may be limited to those strains that share neutralization epitopes, or it may be associated with the development of other B- or T-cell immune responses to shared epitopes.

Many investigators have reported that natural rotavirus infections produce incomplete protection, but little doubt exists that previous infections protect against severe reinfections.* In a large study, protection from both rotavirus reinfection and rotavirus diarrhea increased with each new infection.[467] Sequential infections even with the same serotype have been reported, however. In the initial study reporting rotavirus disease with reinfection by the same serotype, the investigators noted that protection of young children in a Japanese orphanage lasted 6 months then declined after 1 year.[63] This study noted a close correlation between titers of serotype-specific antibody and protection. Animal studies also support a role for serotype-specific infection. Thus, in a study with piglets, immunization with reassortant viruses containing either the VP4 or the VP7 protein of the same serotype was protective, whereas immunization with reassortants containing heterotypic genes for these proteins was not protective.[197] In other studies using mice, this association was not as clear,[495] and protection was better correlated to serum and intestinal levels of IgA.[123, 283, 286]

Although, as discussed earlier, reinfections with rotavirus appear to be common occurrences, other studies have shown protection that lasts at least 1 year.[23, 28, 480] Neonates infected within the first 2 weeks of life were protected against severe disease but not against reinfection in one study.[28] In another, infants who developed a symptomatic or an asymptomatic rotavirus infection during the first year of study were protected against contracting a subsequent rotavirus illness or even an asymptomatic reinfection during the following year.[23] Similarly, when the placebo recipients of a large vaccine trial were observed, a natural rotavirus infection in the first year was found to be 93 percent protective against a symptomatic reinfection in the second year.[480] This protection occurred even though the G1 strains that circulated during the first year were responsible for only 66 percent of rotavirus disease in the second year. Other studies conducted in less developed countries and in daycare centers have not shown the same degree of protection.[31, 79, 274, 379, 467] Differences in these studies may be due to the variation in circulating strains, the dose of exposure, or the duration of protection.

Protection has been correlated to both serum and stool antibody titers produced after natural rotavirus infection.[31, 63, 79, 89, 276, 337, 467, 468, 481] In one study, serum antibody levels, especially IgA, were found to be a marker for protection.[468] Reports of a correlation with serotype-specific neutralizing antibody and protection[63, 337] have not been supported in other larger studies.[190, 483, 519] In the largest study, which was conducted in Bangladesh during a 2-year period when four major G serotypes circulated, the titers of both homologous and heterologous neutralizing antibody were significantly lower in patients with acute rotavirus disease than in matched control subjects.[483] However, further analysis could not find a correlation with serotype-specific neutralizing antibody. Thus, protection seemed to be correlated better with the magnitude of the response rather than with specific neutralizing responses. Similarly, animal studies in both calves and mice have shown that protection can occur in the absence of virus-specific neutralizing antibodies in the serum, feces, or intestinal washes.[42, 283, 285, 495, 501]

Some results from rotavirus vaccine trials also fail to support a role for serum neutralizing antibody and protection. Thus, immunization with heterologous animal rotavirus vaccines has provided protection in some studies without inducing serum neutralizing antibody to human serotypes.[69, 471] In other studies that failed to demonstrate overall efficacy, protection was seen in those who developed the highest antibody titers to the heterologous vaccine,[24, 491] again implicating the magnitude of the response rather than specific neutralizing antibody titers. These measures of serum antibody possibly are a marker for the true protective responses in the intestine.

*See references 23, 28, 31, 63, 79, 104, 139, 274, 336, 379, 394, 467, 468, 480, 505.

Studies evaluating the protective role of previous infections and the mechanism of protection have used adults in challenge studies. Although essentially all adults have been infected previously with rotavirus, they are susceptible to reinfection and mild disease on natural exposure.[200, 497] Initial challenge studies revealed an association between the preinoculation titer of serotype-specific neutralizing serum antibody and protection.[225] These studies later were extended to show a correlation between VP7 antibody and protection but failed to establish a relationship between intestinal antibodies and protection.[163] When similar studies were conducted with a larger group of adults, the correlation between both serum and intestinal antibody became clearer.[481, 482] The most significant correlations were found to be between serum rotavirus IgG and shedding and between intestinal neutralizing antibody and illness. However, some subjects with high titers of antibody became infected and ill, whereas some subjects with low titers appeared to be protected.

Animal models also have proved useful for examining protective immune responses. Initially, large animals, such as piglets and calves, were used, whereas mouse models were limited to the study of passive protection because mice are susceptible to rotavirus diarrhea only for the first 15 days of life. These studies have been extended to the study of protection from infection with adult mice, which allows evaluation of both passive and active immunization.[494]

Initial studies of passive immunization, including cross-fostering studies in mice, found that gastrointestinal but not circulating antibodies were protective and that secretory IgA was more effective than was IgG at providing protection.[38, 262, 323, 401, 410, 418] Animals can be protected with antibodies directed at either VP4 or VP7.[324, 331] Similarly, active immunization against both homotypic and heterotypic challenge has been demonstrated in mice, calves, pigs, and rabbits.[42, 83, 85, 197, 285, 495, 501] Protection has been seen after both oral and parenteral immunization, although what provides protection is not clear. In studies of mice, although no correlation could be found between protection and either serum or intestinal neutralizing antibody, levels of serum or fecal rotavirus IgA did correlate with protection.[123, 283] The use of these models has been extended to gene knockout mice to distinguish the role of $CD8^+$ cells and antibody in protection. These studies have particular relevance to vaccines. These studies indicated that $CD8^+$ cytolytic cells are important for resolution of an infection, but only antibody could provide protection from a subsequent challenge.[136–138, 282] Reports have indicated that antibody may be important for complete resolution of a rotavirus infection as well as for protection against subsequent infection.[284, 464] The levels, location, and targets of this protective antibody, as well as the proteins against which it is directed, are of immediate importance, provided the results found in mice are relevant to larger animals and humans.

Information on protective immune responses continues to become available and should prove useful in the development of rotavirus vaccines. The absence, to date, of a reliable immunologic marker of protection continues to render vaccine trials more difficult, however.

Vaccines

The development of rotavirus vaccines is a high priority for public health institutions.[206, 378] Cost-effectiveness analyses have shown that a rotavirus immunization program would be cost-effective from the perspective of society and the health care system.[452] On the basis of the contention that protection from rotavirus is achieved best by inducing local intestinal immune responses, vaccine efforts have been directed mostly at the development of live attenuated rotavirus vaccines.[86, 129, 151] Most of these efforts have concentrated on the use of animal rotavirus strains, labeled the jennerian approach[222, 337] because it relies on the natural attenuation of animal viruses in humans for safety and largely heterotypic immune responses for protection. Human rotavirus genes have been introduced into these animal strains by creating reassortant viruses as described earlier to increase the relatedness of the vaccine to human rotaviruses. This approach has been labeled the modified jennerian approach.[129] Table 176–2 lists some of the major efficacy trials conducted to date.

Just 10 years after the identification of rotavirus as an agent of severe diarrhea, the first vaccine trials were performed.[471] The initial study used RIT 4237, a bovine rotavirus. Since then, other vaccine candidates, including a rhesus monkey rotavirus (RRV or MMU 18006), another bovine rotavirus (WC3), and animal-human reassortants using RRV and WC3 have been evaluated. Less extensive studies also have been performed with use of neonatal human viruses M37 and RV3[12, 132, 477] that are thought to be naturally attenuated. Results of safety and efficacy trials of a human rotavirus strain 89–12, attenuated by multiple passages in tissue culture, also have been reported.[22, 25] Serial passage also was used to attenuate two strains from India that are natural reassortants,[18] and cold adaptation also has been used to attenuate human strains.[73]

The initial studies of RIT vaccine produced variable results. The vaccine was safe and effective in Finland, providing a protective efficacy of approximately 50 percent against all disease and a greater than 80 percent protection against severe disease.[470, 472, 473] However, later studies in developing countries were disappointing,[105, 183, 244] showing little or no efficacy. Similarly, the vaccines failed to provide protection in a study performed on the Navajo reservation in Arizona.[407]

The WC3 rotavirus vaccine similarly is of bovine origin and also appears to be free of side effects. It replicates poorly in humans, but infants develop a neutralizing antibody response to WC3 and both rotavirus IgA and IgG antibody.[24] The initial studies conducted in Philadelphia appeared promising,[69] but later trials in Cincinnati[24] and in less developed countries[147] did not show significant protection. This vaccine virus was used then to make reassortants containing rotavirus genes encoding the VP7 and VP4 proteins of human serotypes discussed later.[73]

RRV has undergone more trials than any of the other vaccine candidates. RRV replicates better in humans than the bovine vaccine strains do, perhaps because it is a G3 serotype, but it also produces mild side effects, including low-grade fever and mild diarrhea, especially when it is given to older children who have lost maternal antibodies.[261, 357, 474] RRV induces serum rotavirus IgG and IgA, intestinal rotavirus IgA, and RRV neutralizing antibody but not G1-specific neutralizing antibody.[66, 262, 357] Protection with this vaccine has been inconsistent, ranging from greater than 50 percent, even in developing countries,[127, 268, 356, 375] to moderate (20–50%),[376, 475] to nonexistent.[66, 407] Some evidence suggests that protection is better against G3 than G1 outbreaks,[86, 129] but the evidence is not conclusive.

Because of the belief that homotypic immunity might increase the protection seen with rotavirus vaccines and because of a lack of consistent protection with the animal strains, most recent efforts have been directed toward creating reassortant vaccines that contain the VP7 or the VP7 and VP4 encoding genes of human rotavirus strains, with the remainder of the genes from an animal strain.

TABLE 176–2 ■ SELECTED VACCINE STUDIES

Vaccine	Country	No. of Subjects	No. of Doses	Protection* (Overall/ Severe Disease)	Reference
RTT 4237	Finland	178	1	50/88	473
	Finland	328	2	58/82	472
	Rwanda	245	3	0/0	105
	Gambia	185	3	0/37	183
	Peru	391	3	40/75	244
WC3	USA (Philadelphia, PA)	104	1	43/89	69
	USA (Cincinnati, OH)	206	1	17/41	24
	Central African Republic	472	2	0/36	147
RRV	USA (Rochester, NY)	176	1	0/0	66
	Venezuela	247	1	68/100	127
	Finland	200	1	38/67	475
	Venezuela	320	1	64/90	356
	USA (Rochester, NY)	223	1	66/N.D.	268
	USA (Indian Reservation)	321	1	0/N.D.	407
RRV/Human Reassortants					
RRV G1	Finland	359	1	67/N.D.	476
RRV G2	Finland			66/N.D.	
RRV G1	USA (Rochester, NY)	223	1	77/N.D.	268
RRV G1	USA	898	3	69/73	19
RRV TV				64/82	
RRV G1	USA	1187	3	54/69	374
RRV TV				49/80	
RRV TV	Finland	2273	3	66/91	211
RRV TV	Venezuela	2207	3	48/88	358
WC3 Reassortants					
WC3 G1	USA (Rochester, NY)	325	3	64/87	449
WC3 TV	USA	417	3	73/73	74
89–12					
89–12	USA	215	2	89/100	22

*Measured in the first year after vaccination.
N. D., not done.

As discussed earlier, these proteins were chosen because they induce neutralizing antibody. The segmented genome of rotavirus renders production of these reassortant rotaviruses that contain mostly gene segments from the attenuated animal strain with one or two segments originating from human strains relatively easy. One goal of this strategy is to create a multivalent vaccine containing viruses with human rotavirus genes representing the main human serotypes.

Reassortant vaccines have been developed with both RRV[294, 296] and WC3[22, 70, 449] as the animal strain. The RRV/human VP7 rotavirus reassortants contain 10 genes from RRV and a single human rotavirus gene that specifies the neutralization protein VP7 (Fig. 176–7). A monovalent RRV vaccine containing the G1 VP7 reassortant and a bivalent preparation containing the G1 and G2 reassortants initially were evaluated.[268, 476] The tetravalent preparation was the one licensed in 1998, however. This vaccine contains RRV and reassortants with the VP7 genes of G1, G2, or G4 serotypes. The G3 serotype virus of this vaccine is RRV. Vaccination produces a rotavirus IgG and IgA serum antibody response, but neutralizing antibodies are produced predominantly to RRV rather than to the human serotypes.[19, 354, 374] This finding appears to be consistent with the experiments showing that VP4 rather than VP7 is more immunogenic after natural infection.[490, 493]

Extensive evaluations of the tetravalent RRV reassortant were completed before licensure.[19, 211, 358, 374] In two large trials conducted at centers across the United States,[19, 374] the tetravalent vaccine was found to be safe, with the subjects having a slight increase in temperature after the first dose. The efficacy of the vaccine against rotavirus disease for the first year was 49 to 64 percent, whereas during a 2-year follow-up, it was 57 percent. Protection increased with severity scores to a level of about 80 percent for severe disease. Vaccination also significantly decreased the number of medical office visits for rotavirus gastroenteritis or dehydration. Vaccination appeared to provide protection against both G1 and G3 serotypes. Similar results were reported from Finnish studies except that fever occurred somewhat more commonly and efficacy was somewhat enhanced.[211] Protection similar to that seen in the U.S. studies also was provided by the vaccine when it was used in a less developed country, Venezuela.[358]

For these reasons, the vaccine was licensed in the United States in 1998 and recommended for general use in all infants.[5] However, less than 1 year after licensing, 15 cases of intussusception that occurred shortly after vaccination were reported to the Vaccine Adverse Events Reporting System (VAERS).[57] Thirteen of these cases occurred after the patient received the first dose of vaccine, and 12 occurred within 1 week of vaccination. After this report, approximately 100 cases of intussusception after receipt of rotavirus vaccine were reported to VAERS. Further review of this and other data led the American Academy of Pediatrics Advisory Committee on Immunization Practices

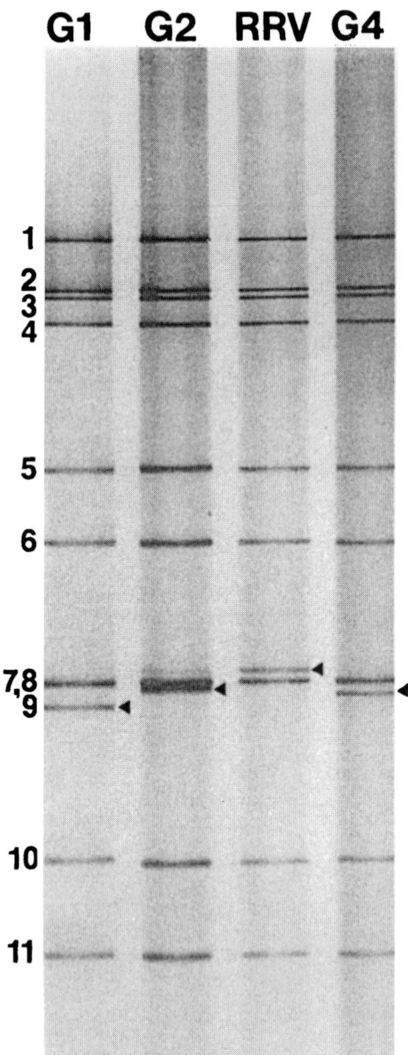

FIGURE 176–7 ■ Polyacrylamide gel electrophoretic patterns of the genome segments from RRV and the G1, G2, and G4 reassortant strains that compose the tetravalent RRV-based vaccine. The strains all contain 10 RRV genes and differ only in the gene segment encoding the VP7 pattern, which migrates in the seventh (RRV) or ninth (reassortants) position, as designated by arrowheads.

to conclude that an association exists between receipt of the vaccine and development of intussusception and to withdraw the recommendation for use.[1, 58] The vaccine has therefore beenwithdrawn by the manufacturer pending further review.

In one report, investigators assessed the association between RRV-TV and intussusception among infants between 1 and 12 months of age.[304] A case-controlled analysis of data from 19 states revealed an increased risk of development of intussusception from 3 to 14 days after receipt of the first dose of vaccine (adjusted odds ratio 21.7). A smaller risk also existed after receipt of the second dose of vaccine. Researchers estimated that one case of intussusception attributable to vaccination with RRV would occur for every 4670 to 9474 infants vaccinated. The exact excess burden of intussusception during the life of the child has yet to be defined, however, and the risk may be lower than the original estimates, approaching 1 per 10,000 to 12,000.[235a, 240a, 358a, 417a] The relationship, if any, between wild-type rotavirus infection and intussusception is discussed in the clinical section.

WC3-based reassortants also have been evaluated. A monovalent vaccine containing the VP7 protein of a human G1 rotavirus provided 64 percent efficacy against all symptomatic rotavirus disease and 87 percent efficacy against more severe disease during a predominantly serotype G1 outbreak in Rochester.[468] The WC3-based reassortant quadrivalent vaccine includes both VP7 and VP4 human rotavirus gene substitutions[74] with G1, G2, G3, or P[8] substitutions and most other segments from WC3. In studies conducted at multiple centers in the United States, it was shown to be safe, with only a slight increase in diarrhea after receipt of the first dose.[74] The vaccine was 73 percent effective against all cases of rotavirus gastroenteritis and 73 percent effective against more severe cases.[74] Several other multicenter trials have been conducted with a multivalent WC3 reassortant vaccine, but results are not available. Large safety trials are under way with a WC3-based vaccine as well.

Evaluations of an attenuated human strain, 89–12, also have been published.[22, 25] Strain 89–12 is a G1P[8] strain initially obtained from an infant with rotavirus gastroenteritis in Cincinnati, Ohio. The isolate was attenuated by multiple passages in tissue culture and shown to be safe.[25] Results of a multicenter efficacy trial showed that two doses of this vaccine provided 89 percent protection against any rotavirus disease, and protection from more serious diseases was 100 percent. Further trials of this vaccine are under way.

Other approaches to rotavirus vaccines, including the use of attenuated human viruses, also are being evaluated. The initial evaluation of M37, a strain isolated from an asymptomatic newborn, showed reduced immunogenicity and a lack of efficacy.[132, 477] Similarly, evaluations of another neonatal strain (RV3) showed the vaccine virus replicated poorly and induced an immune response in only a minority of recipients.[12] The use of cold-adapted vaccines also has undergone limited clinical evaluation.[73, 129] Preclinical studies have included the use of virus-like particles[87, 334] that appeared to be protective in mice but not in pigs.[511] DNA vaccines[61, 65] and subunit vaccines, including VP7, VP4, and VP6,[64, 479] also have shown some promise.

Clinical Manifestations

Rotavirus is the most common cause of dehydrating diarrhea in children in the United States and worldwide and infects nearly every child in the first few years of life.[108, 179, 219, 220] Approximately 20 percent of summer diarrhea is associated with rotavirus infection, compared with approximately 70 to 80 percent of winter cases.[429] At the peak of rotavirus infection in Cincinnati, approximately 90 percent of admissions for gastroenteritis are secondary to rotavirus infection (unreported observation). In a surveillance study of diarrhea across the United States, the percentage of specimens positive for rotavirus increased from 6 percent in October to 36 percent in February.[56] In the United States, more than 1 million cases of severe diarrhea are caused annually by rotavirus, resulting in 20 to 40 deaths.[152, 153, 191, 192, 231] In one study,[275] researchers estimated that 8.5 per 1000 children per year are hospitalized in the United States for rotavirus illness in the first 2 years of life. More recently, estimates are that between 1 in 25 and 1 in 57 children younger than 5 years are hospitalized, and 1 in 21 required an emergency department visit because of diarrhea.[340, 341] On the basis of a conservative estimate by the Centers for Disease Control and Prevention of 55,000 hospitalizations for rotavirus diarrhea in the United States, 1 in 73 children would be hospitalized.[153] A worldwide estimated 870,000 deaths are associated with rotavirus infection.[108, 206, 220] The incidence of rotavirus infections is highest in children between 6 and 24 months of age,[391] but the age may be lower in less developed countries.[180, 373] Adults, including elderly patients, also are susceptible to reinfection, which can cause mild disease.[93, 114, 200, 232, 271, 389, 497]

After an incubation period of approximately 2 to 4 days, an abrupt onset of vomiting and diarrhea occurs. Vomiting may precede the diarrhea in approximately half the cases.[177] The disease usually is self-limited, lasting 4 to 8 days, although the duration of symptoms ranged between 2 and 22 days in a Guatemalan study.[505] When hospitalization is required, the stay usually is brief, with an average of 4 days and a range of 2 to 14 days.[388] Recovery generally is complete, but persistent diarrhea associated with lactose intolerance has been described.[15, 230]

In general, rotavirus infections are more severe than are those caused by other viral gastrointestinal agents.[32, 388] In developing countries, 20 to 40 percent of hospitalizations for diarrhea are due to rotavirus infections,[108] whereas in the United States, rotavirus is estimated to account for between one third and two thirds of admissions for diarrhea in children.[34, 390] Vomiting, dehydration, and hospitalization occur significantly more often in patients infected with rotavirus than in those with other causes of diarrhea.[388, 455] In one study,[388] vomiting and diarrhea also lasted longer in patients infected with rotavirus (2.6 versus 0.9 days and 5.0 versus 2.6 days, respectively). In another study, the severity score for rotavirus diarrhea was almost twice that of disease having other causes.[394] However, rotavirus infections also frequently can be asymptomatic,[373, 519] and a carrier state has been defined.[59] Reports of neonatal infections that are asymptomatic in selected settings also are common.[26, 28, 170, 178, 303, 355]

Other clinical findings associated with rotavirus infections include fever, abdominal distress, and mild dehydration. Fever occurs commonly during rotavirus illness, with estimates of between 45 and 84 percent of patients.[240, 388, 429, 455] Dehydration caused by rotavirus reportedly was more likely to be isotonic than was dehydration caused by other agents,[388] although one fourth of the patients infected with rotavirus presented with hypernatremic dehydration in another study.[240] Other findings include irritability and pharyngeal or tympanic membrane erythema. Numerous reports associate respiratory symptoms, such as cough, pharyngitis, otitis media, and pneumonia, with rotavirus infections, but the relationship of these symptoms to rotavirus is unclear, and the ability to isolate rotavirus from respiratory secretions has varied among studies.[177, 253, 388, 408, 518] Laboratory findings are related mostly to the extent of dehydration and can include elevated blood urea nitrogen and evidence of mild metabolic acidosis.

The diarrheal stools usually are loose and watery, with as many as 10 stools per day. Mucus is found in approximately 20 percent of stools, but blood and fecal leukocytes seldom are found.[203, 359] The peak viral shedding in stools occurs on about day 3 of illness.[100, 478] When evaluated by polymerase chain reaction (PCR), the duration of rotavirus shedding ranged from 4 to 57 days in hospitalized patients.[380] Approximately half of the children shed for fewer than 10 days and 70 percent for fewer than 20 days. In Guatemala, prolonged viral shedding also has been reported for as long as 5 weeks and is associated with immunodeficiency.[274, 409]

Other clinical manifestations associated either etiologically or incidentally with rotavirus infection include encephalitis and meningitis[213, 227, 403, 462, 499]; various upper and lower respiratory infections, including otitis media, laryngitis, pharyngitis, and pneumonia[253, 314, 388, 408, 518]; Kawasaki syndrome[279]; sudden infant death syndrome[510]; hepatic abscess[173]; and pancreatitis.[313] Elevated liver function test results also have been reported during rotavirus infection.[171, 173, 239] Perhaps the strongest link is to neonatal necrotizing enterocolitis.[228, 392] However, the difficulty of false-positive reactions obtained with some ELISA tests in neonates must be considered.[67, 372, 450] Rotavirus infections can be more severe in immunosuppressed persons, including bone marrow transplant recipients, patients infected with human immunodeficiency virus, and those who are malnourished,[115, 150, 209, 218, 509] and they may spread to the liver and kidney.[150]

The relationship between intussusception and natural rotavirus infection is of great interest because of the reported link between the tetravalent RRV vaccine and intussusception (discussed in the section on vaccines). Several studies have investigated the possible infectious etiology of intussusception.[27, 77, 201, 237, 302, 312] These studies are small and mostly uncontrolled and have yielded conflicting results regarding rotavirus, although most investigators conclude that rotavirus infections are not a major cause of intussusception. In contrast, adenoviruses have been recovered consistently.[27, 77, 201, 312] The best argument against a major role for rotavirus as a cause of intussusception is a lack of seasonal variation for intussusception as opposed to the clear peak for rotavirus infection in winter and fall, as described in this chapter.[60a, 60b, 342, 377]

Laboratory Diagnosis

Rotavirus infection cannot be diagnosed on the basis of clinical presentation, even in combination with stool examination and nonspecific laboratory tests. Therefore, specific tests have been developed. Findings suggestive of rotavirus infection include a mildly febrile illness with vomiting and watery diarrhea that is occurring in the winter months in temperate climates, especially in patients 6 to 24 months of age. The presence of more severe dehydration also is suggestive. In the initial epidemiologic studies, electron microscopy was used for identification because of the large number of particles present in stools ($>10^{10}$) and the characteristic appearance of rotavirus. This technique largely has been replaced by enzyme immunoassay–based and latex agglutination tests, for which kits are available commercially. Both tests have good sensitivity compared with electron microscopy.[107, 115, 149, 235, 441] One problem noted in the past was false-positive results in neonatal stools with certain ELISA kits.[67, 372, 450] Inclusion of a rotavirus-negative capture antibody as a control in these kits should eliminate these false-positive reactions.

Rotavirus also can be grown in tissue culture,[184, 489, 503] although the methods used for routine viral cultures do not detect rotavirus. The serotype (G type) of cultured strains, and sometimes virus in stools, can be identified by use of monoclonal antibodies.[224] DNA probes[245, 426] and reverse transcription–PCR can be used to identify genotypes as a surrogate for serotypes.[144, 159] Electrophoresis of extracted RNA also can identify rotavirus by its characteristic 11 segments and is used to define electropherotypes.[214, 387, 411] All these methods have proved useful as epidemiologic tools and in vaccine studies. Identification of electropherotypes is especially useful for epidemiologic studies because it allows identification of specific strains.

Rotavirus infection, both symptomatic and asymptomatic, also can be identified by changes in rotavirus antibody. ELISA assays are used most commonly to measure serum IgM, IgA, and IgG levels as well as stool and intestinal antibodies. Specific neutralizing titers also can be measured for each serotype of rotavirus by plaque reduction[199, 502] or focus reduction assays.[20, 44] One ELISA-based antigen reduction neutralization assay has been found to be better suited for the analyses of large numbers of specimens.[234] Serologic detection of infection is more difficult in the first months of life because of the presence of maternal antibodies. Detection of rotavirus IgA, which does not cross the placenta, has been used as a marker for previous infection in the first months of life.

Treatment

Treatment of rotavirus gastroenteritis is aimed largely at restoring the proper fluid balance in dehydrated patients. Emphasis has shifted from intravenous rehydration to oral rehydration with glucose-electrolyte solutions. The glucose in the solution enhances sodium and, therefore, water absorption in the intestine.[311] Several studies have shown the utility of this approach for treatment of rotavirus gastroenteritis.[397, 405, 406] The solution accepted by the World Health Organization contains 30 mEq/L of sodium, 30 mEq/L of potassium, and 30 mEq/L of bicarbonate, which is similar to other oral rehydrating solutions available commercially. Should oral rehydration efforts fail, or in cases of severe dehydration and shock, fluid should be administered intravenously.

Other experimental approaches to treatment are based on the success of passive oral therapy in animals. Chronic rotavirus shedding has been treated successfully with human milk that contained rotavirus antibody.[409] Treatment and prophylaxis of normal children with immune colostrum, immunoglobulin, or milk from rotavirus-immunized cows also have been evaluated with some success.[103, 189, 260, 453] The treatment of normal children with one dose of human serum immunoglobulin given orally was reported to be effective in reducing the mean duration of diarrhea, viral excretion, and hospital stay,[174] and prophylaxis with bovine antibody–supplemented formula decreased the number of days with rotavirus diarrhea.[453] Trials of bismuth subsalicylate also have been conducted with some reported success,[124, 422] as have trials with probiotics.[396]

Racecadotril (acetorphan), an enkephalinase inhibitor with antisecretory and antidiarrheal properties that decreases intestinal hypersecretion but not motility by preventing the breakdown of endogenous enkephalinase in the gastrointestinal tract, has been shown to be effective in the treatment of diarrhea in adults and children.[182, 402] In one study, oral treatment with racecadotril decreased stool output by 46 percent in boys 3 to 35 months of age with watery diarrhea. A similar decrease was seen in boys with rotavirus infection.[402]

Nongroup A Rotaviruses

As described earlier, rotaviruses can be classified into seven groups (A to G). All seven groups are associated with diarrhea in animals, although only groups A, B, and C have been associated with disease in humans.[400] Of these, group A causes most illness. However, major epidemics of group B rotavirus have been reported in China.[122, 204] Seroprevalence studies have identified group B rotavirus infections in Hong Kong, Myanmar, Thailand, Australia, Canada, England, Sweden, Africa, and the United States, although the prevalence is lower than that in the epidemic regions of China.[400] Group C infections have been reported largely from Japan,[278, 243, 332, 461] but they also have been detected in the United States.[210] Unlike group A rotavirus, group C rotavirus appears to cause disease predominantly in children older than 3 years and in adults.[122, 243, 278, 316, 332] Group C rotavirus infections may be distributed widely, although the exact extent of infection has been limited by the poor assays that were available. The development of ELISA[207, 451] and PCR[157, 316] assays should improve diagnosis, however. Evidence of infection has been reported in Asia, Australia, Europe, Central and South America,[351, 400, 451] and the United States.[210, 315, 427] Recent serologic evidence has shown infection rates of 30 to 43 percent in England and the United States.[208, 385]

Outbreaks caused by water-borne or food-borne spread of group B rotavirus in China[204] and group C rotavirus in Japan have been reported, although person-to-person spread also has been implicated.[122] As discussed before, outbreaks usually involve older children and adults,[122, 243, 316, 332] but infants apparently can be infected.[210] Group C rotaviruses have been associated with extrahepatic biliary atresia.[382, 412] Most recently, group C rotavirus RNA was detected in liver specimens from 10 of 20 patients with biliary atresia, but no controls.[383] If infection is suspected, the diagnosis is suggested by electron-microscopic detection of the typical rotavirus particles with a negative test result for rotavirus by the routine assays that detect only group A rotaviruses. The detection of typical RNA migration patterns by polyacrylamide gel electrophoresis of RNA also is suggestive. PCR and ELISA assays have been reported.[157, 207, 316, 413, 451]

REFERENCES

1. Abramson, J. S., Baker, C. J., Fisher, M. C., et al.: Possible association of intussusception with rotavirus vaccination. American Academy of Pediatrics. Committee on Infectious Diseases. Pediatrics *104*:575, 1999.
2. Adams, W. R., and Kraft, L. M.: Epizootic diarrhea of infant mice: Identification of the etiologic agent. Science *141*:359–360, 1963.
3. Adams, W. R., and Kraft, L. M.: Electron microscopic study of the intestinal epithelium of mice infected with the agent of epizootic diarrhea of infant mice (EDIM virus). Am. J. Pathol. *51*:39–60, 1967.
4. Altenburg, B. C., Graham, D. Y., and Estes, M. K.: Ultrastructural study of rotavirus replication in cultured cells. J. Gen. Virol. *46*:75–85, 1980.
5. American Academy of Pediatrics, Committee on Infectious Diseases: Prevention of rotavirus disease: Guidelines for use of rotavirus vaccine. Pediatrics *102*:1483–1491, 1998.
6. Angel, J., Tang, B., Feng, N., et al.: Studies of the role for NSP4 in the pathogenesis of homologous murine rotavirus diarrhea. J. Infect. Dis. *177*:455–458, 1998.
7. Aponte, C., Poncet, D., and Cohen, J.: Recovery and characterization of a replicase complex in rotavirus-infected cells by using a monoclonal antibody against NSP2. J. Virol. *70*:985–991, 1996.
8. Arias, C. F., Romero, P., Alvarez, V., and Lopez, S.: Trypsin activation pathway of rotavirus infectivity. J. Virol. *70*:5832–5839, 1996.
9. Avendano, P., Matson, D. O., Long, J., et al.: Costs associated with office visits for diarrhea in infants and toddlers. Pediatr. Infect. Dis. J. *12*:897–902, 1993.
10. Ball, J. M., Peng, T., and Estes, M. K.: Rotavirus nonstructural protein, NSP4, induces diarrhea. Abstract. American Society for Virology, Austin, TX, July 8–12, 1995, p. 146.
11. Banfield, W. G., Kasnic, G., and Blackwell, J. H.: Further observations on the virus of epizootic diarrhea of infant mice: An electron microscopic study. Virology *36*:411–417, 1968.
12. Barnes, G. L., Lund, J. S., Adams, L., et al.: Phase I trial of a candidate rotavirus vaccine (RV3) derived from a human neonate. J. Paediatr. Child. Health *33*:300–304, 1997.
13. Barnes, G. L., Unicomb, L., and Bishop, R. F.: Severity of rotavirus infection in relation to serotype, monotype and electropherotype. J. Paediatr. Child. Health *28*:54–57, 1992.
14. Bass, D. M., and Greenberg, H. B.: Strategies for the identification of icosahedral virus receptors. J. Clin. Invest. *89*:3–9, 1992.
15. Beattie, R. M., Vieira, M. C., Phillips, A. D., et al.: Carbohydrate intolerance after rotavirus gastroenteritis: A rare problem in the 1990s. Arch. Dis. Child. *72*:446, 1995.
16. Bell, L. M., Clark, H. F., O'Brien, E. A., et al.: Gastroenteritis caused by human rotaviruses (serotype three) in a suckling mouse model. Proc. Soc. Exp. Biol. Med. *184*:127–132, 1987.

17. Bern, C., Unicomb, L., Gentsch, J. R., et al.: Rotavirus diarrhea in Bangladeshi children: Correlation of disease severity with serotypes. J. Clin. Microbiol. *30*:3234–3238, 1992.
18. Bernstein, D. I.: Rotavirus vaccine, current status and future prospects. BioDrugs *14*:275–344, 2000.
19. Bernstein, D. I., Glass R., Rodgers, G., et al.: Evaluation of rhesus rotavirus monovalent and tetravalent reassortant vaccines in U.S. children. J. A. M. A. *273*:1191–1196, 1995.
20. Bernstein, D. I., Kacica, M. A., McNeal, M. M., et al.: Local and systemic antibody response to rotavirus WC3 vaccine in adult volunteers. Antiviral Res. *12*:293–300, 1989.
21. Bernstein, D. I., McNeal, M. M., Schiff, G. M., et al.: Induction and persistence of local anti-rotavirus antibody in relation to serum antibodies. J. Med. Virol. *28*:90–95, 1989.
22. Bernstein, D. I, Sack, D. A., Rothstein, E., et al.: Efficacy of live, attenuated, human rotavirus vaccine 89–12 in infants: A randomised placebo-controlled trial. Lancet *354*:287–290, 1999.
23. Bernstein, D. I., Sander, D. S., Smith, V., et al.: Protection from rotavirus reinfection: Two-year prospective study. J. Infect. Dis. *164*:277–283, 1991.
24. Bernstein, D. I., Smith, V., Sander, D., et al.: Evaluation of WC3 rotavirus vaccine and correlates of protection in healthy infants. J. Infect. Dis. *162*:1055–1062, 1990.
25. Bernstein, D. I., Smith, V. E., Sherwood, J. R., et al.: Safety and immunogenicity of live, attenuated human rotavirus vaccine 89–12. Vaccine *16*:381–387, 1998.
26. Bhan, M. K., Lew, J. F., Sazawal, S., et al.: Protection conferred by neonatal rotavirus infection against subsequent rotavirus diarrhea. J. Infect. Dis. *168*:282–287, 1993.
27. Bhisitkul, D. M., Todd, K. M., and Listernick, R.: Adenovirus infection and childhood intussusception. Am. J. Dis. Child. *146*:1331–1333, 1992.
28. Bishop, R., Barnes, G., Cipriani, E., et al.: Clinical immunity after neonatal rotavirus infection: A prospective longitudinal study in young children. N. Engl. J. Med. *309*:72–76, 1983.
29. Bishop, R. F., Davidson, G. P., Holmes, I. H., et al.: Virus particles in epithelial cells of duodenal mucosa from children with acute gastroenteritis. Lancet *2*:1281–1283, 1973.
30. Bishop, R. F., Davidson, G. P., Holmes, I. H., et al.: Detection of a new virus by electron microsocpy of faecal extracts from children with acute gastroenteritis. Lancet *1*:149–151, 1974.
31. Black, R., Greenberg, H., Kapikian, A., et al.: Acquisition of serum antibody to Norwalk virus and rotavirus in relation to diarrhea in a longitudinal study of young children in rural Bangladesh. J. Infect. Dis. *145*:483–489, 1982.
32. Black, R. E., Merson, M. H., Huq, I., et al.: Incidence and severity of rotavirus and *Escherichia coli* diarrhoea in rural Bangladesh: Implications for vaccine development. Lancet *1*:141–143, 1981.
33. Both, G. W., Bellamy, A. R., and Mitchell, D. B.: Rotavirus protein structure and function. Curr. Top. Microbiol. Immunol. *185*:67–105, 1994.
34. Brandt, C. D., Kim, H. W., Rodriguez, W. J., et al.: Gastroenteritis—a human reovirus-like agent infection during the 1975–76 outbreak: An electron microscopic study. Clin. Proc. Child. Hosp. *33*:21–26, 1977.
35. Bridger, J. C.: Detection by electron microscopy of caliciviruses, astroviruses and rotavirus-like particles in the faeces of piglets with diarrhoea. Vet. Rec. *107*:532, 1980.
36. Bridger, J. C.: Novel rotaviruses in animals and man. Ciba Found. Symp. *128*:5–23, 1987.
37. Bridger, J. C.: A definition of bovine rotavirus virulence. J. Gen. Virol. *75*:2807–2812, 1994.
38. Bridger, J. C., and Brown, J. F.: Development of immunity to porcine rotavirus in piglets protected from disease by bovine colostrum. Infect. Immun. *31*:906–910, 1981.
39. Bridger, J. C., Burke, B., Beards, G. M., et al.: The pathogenicity of two porcine rotaviruses differing in their in vitro growth characteristics and gene 4. J. Gen. Virol. *73*:3011–3015, 1992.
40. Bridger, J. C., Dhaliwal, W., Adamson, M. J. V., and Howard, C. R.: Determinants of rotavirus host range restriction—a heterologous bovine NSP1 gene does not affect replication kinetics in the pig. Virology *245*:47–52, 1998.
41. Bridger, J. C., Hall, G. A., and Parsons, K. R.: A study of the basis of virulence variation of bovine rotaviruses. Vet. Microbiol. *33*:169–174, 1992.
42. Bridger, J., Oldham, G., Howard, C., et al.: In vivo depletion of CD8$^+$ but not CD4$^+$ or BOWC1$^+$ lymphocytes increases primary rotavirus excretion in calves. Abstract. Fourth International Symposium of Double-Stranded RNA Viruses, Scottsdale, AZ, 1987, pp. S6–S7.
43. Bridger, J. C., Tauscher, G. I., and Desselberger, U.: Viral determinants of rotavirus pathogenicity in pigs: Evidence that the fourth gene of a porcine rotavirus confers diarrhea in the homologous host. J. Virol. *72*:6929–6931, 1998.
44. Bridger, J. C., and Woode, G. N.: Neonatal calf diarrhoea: Identification of a reovirus-like (rotavirus) agent in faeces by immunofluorescence and immune electron microscopy. Br. Vet. J. *131*:528–535, 1975.
45. Broome, R. L., Vo, P. T., Ward, R. L., et al.: Murine rotavirus genes encoding outer capsid proteins VP4 and VP7 are not major determinants of host range restriction and virulence. J. Virol. *67*:2448–2455, 1993.
46. Browne, E. P., Bellamy, A. R., and Taylor, J. A.: Membrane-destabilizing activity of rotavirus NSP4 is mediated by a membrane-proximal amphipathic domain. J. Gen. Virol. *81*:1955–1959, 2000.
47. Browning, G. F., Snodgrass, D. R., Nakagomi, O., et al.: Human and bovine serotype G8 rotaviruses may be derived by reassortment. Arch. Virol. *125*:121–128, 1992.
48. Brunet, J.-P., Cotte-Laffitte, J., Linxe, C., et al.: Rotavirus infection induces an increase in intracellular calcium concentration in human intestinal epithelial cells: Role in microvillar actin alteration. J. Virol. *74*:2323–2332, 2000.
49. Brunet, J.-P, Jourdan, N., Cotte-Lafitte, J., et al.: Rotavirus infection induces cytoskeleton disorganization in human intestinal epithelial cells: Implication of an increase in intracellular calcium concentration. J. Virol. *74*:10801–10806, 2000.
50. Brussow, H., Offit, P., Gerna, G., et al.: Polypeptide specificity of antiviral serum antibodies in children naturally infected with human rotavirus. J. Virol. *64*:4130–4136, 1990.
51. Bryden, A. S., Davies, H. A., Hadley, R. E., et al.: Rotavirus enteritis in the West Midlands during 1974. Lancet *2*:241–243, 1975.
52. Burke, B., McCrae, M. A., and Desselberger, U.: Sequence analysis of two porcine rotaviruses differing in growth in vitro and in pathogenicity: Distinct VP4 sequences and conservation of NS53, VP6 and VP7 genes. J. Gen. Virol. *75*:2205–2212, 1994.
53. Burns, J. W., Krishnaney, A. A., Vo, P. T., et al.: Analyses of homologous rotavirus infection in the mouse model. Virology *207*:143–153, 1995.
54. Burns, J. W., Sindat-Pajouh, M., Krishnaney, A. A., and Greenberg, H. B.: Protective effect of rotavirus VP6-specific IgA monoclonal antibodies that lack neutralizing activity. Science *272*:104–107, 1996.
55. Butz, A. M., Fosarelli, P., Dick, J., et al.: Prevalence of rotavirus on high-risk fomites in daycare facilities. Pediatrics *92*:202–205, 1993.
56. Centers for Disease Control: Rotavirus surveillance: United States, 1989–1990. M. M. W. R. *40*:80–87, 1991.
57. Centers for Disease Control: Intussusception among recipients of rotavirus vaccine—United States, 1998–1999. M. M. W. R. Morb. Mortal. Wkly. Rep. *48*:577–581, 1999.
58. Centers for Disease Control: Withdrawal of rotavirus vaccine recommendation. M. M. W. R. Morb. Mortal. Wkly. Rep. *48*:1007, 1999.
59. Champosaur, H., Questiaux, E., Prevot, J., et al.: Rotavirus carriage asymptomatic infection and disease in the first two years of life. I. Virus shedding. J. Infect. Dis. *149*:667–674 1984.
60. Chan, W.-K., Au, K.-S., and Estes, M. K.: Topography of the simian rotavirus nonstructural glycoprotein (NS28) in the endoplasmic reticulum membrane. Virology *164*:435–442, 1988.
60a. Chang, E. J., Zangwill, K. M., Lee, H., et al.: Lack of association between rotavirus infection and intussusception: Implications for use of attenuated rotavirus vaccines. Pediatr. Infect. Dis. J. *21*:97–102, 2002.
60b. Chang, H. G., Smith, P. F., Ackelsberg, J., et al.: Intussusception, rotavirus diarrhea, and rotavirus vaccine use among children in New York state. Pediatrics *108*:54–60, 2001.
61. Chen, S. C., Fynan, E. F., Robinson, H. L., et al.: Protective immunity induced by rotavirus DNA vaccines. Vaccine *15*:899–902, 1997.
62. Chen, D., and Patton, J.T.: Rotavirus RNA replication requires a single-stranded 3′ end for efficient minus-strand synthesis. J. Virol. *72*: 7387–7396, 1998.
63. Chiba, S., Nakata, S., Urasawa, T., et al.: Protective effect of naturally acquired homotypic and heterotypic rotavirus antibodies. Lancet *1*:417–421, 1986.
64. Choi, A. H., Basu, M., McNeal, M. M., et al.: Antibody-independent protection against rotavirus infection of mice stimulated by intranasal immunization with chimeric VP4 or VP6 protein. J. Virol. *73*:7574–7581, 1999.
65. Choi, A. H., Basu, M., Rae, M. N., et al.: Particle-bombardment-mediated DNA vaccination with rotavirus VP4 or VP7 induces high levels of serum rotavirus IgG but fails to protect mice against challenge. Virology *250*:230–240, 1998.
66. Christy, C., Madore, P., Pichichero, M., et al.: Field trials of rhesus rotavirus vaccine in infants. Pediatr. Infect. Dis. J. *7*:645–650, 1988.
67. Chrystie, I. L., Totterdell, B. M., and Banatvala, J. E.: False positive rotazyme tests on faecal samples from babies. Lancet *2*:1028, 1983.
68. Ciarlet, M., and Estes, M.K.: Human and most animal rotavirus strains do not require the presence of sialic acid on the cell surface for efficient infectivity. J. Gen. Virol. *80*:943–948, 1999.
69. Clark, H., Borian, F., Bell, L., et al.: Protective effect of WC3 vaccine against rotavirus diarrhea in infants during a predominantly serotype 1 rotavirus season. J. Infect. Dis. *158*:570–587, 1988.
70. Clark, H. F., Borian, F. E., Modesto, K., et al.: Serotype 1 reassortant of bovine rotavirus WC3 strain, strain W179–9, induces a polytypic antibody response in infants. Vaccine *8*:327–332, 1990.
71. Clark, H. F., Borian, F. E., and Plotkin, S. A.: Immune protection of infants against rotavirus gastroenteritis by a serotype 1 reassortant of bovine rotavirus WC3. J. Infect. Dis. *161*:1099–1104, 1990.
72. Clark, H. F., Hoshino, Y., Bell, L. M., et al.: Rotavirus isolate WI61 representing a presumptive new human serotype. J. Clin. Microbiol. *25*:1757–1762, 1987.

73. Clark, H. F., Offit, P. A., Ellis, R. W., et al.: The development of multivalent bovine rotavirus (strain WC3) reassortant vaccine for infants. J. Infect. Dis. *174*(Suppl.):S73–S80, 1996.
74. Clark, H., White, C. J., Offit, P. A., et al.: Preliminary evaluation of safety and efficacy of quadrivalent human-bovine reassortant rotavirus vaccine (QHBRV). Pediatr. Res. *37*:172A, 1995.
75. Clark, S. M., Barnett, B. B., and Spendlove, R. S.: Production of high-titer bovine rotavirus with trypsin. J. Clin. Microbiol. *9*:413–417, 1979.
76. Clark, S. M., Roth, J. R., Clark, M. L., et al.: Trypsin enhancement of rotavirus infectivity: Mechanism of enhancement. J. Virol. *39*:816–822, 1981.
77. Clarke, E. J., Jr., Phillips, I. A., and Alexander, E. R.: Adenovirus infection in intussusception in children in Taiwan. J. A .M. A. *208*:1671–1674, 1969.
78. Clarke, M. L., Lockett, L. J., and Both, G. W.: Membrane binding and endoplasmic reticulum retention sequences of rotavirus VP7 are distinct: Role of carboxy-terminal and other residues in membrane binding. J. Virol. *69*:6473–6478, 1995.
79. Clemens, J. D., Ward, R. L., Rao, M. R., et al.: Seroepidemiologic evaluation of antibodies to rotavirus as correlates of the risk of clinically significant rotavirus diarrhea in rural Bangladesh. J. Infect. Dis. *165*:161–165, 1992.
80. Coelho, K. I. R., Bryden, A. S., Hall, C., et al.: Pathology of rotavirus infection in suckling mice: A study by conventional histology, immunofluorescence, ultrathin sections, and scanning electron microscopy. Ultrastruct. Pathol. *2*:59–69, 1981.
81. Collins, J. E., Benfield, D. A., and Duimstra, J. R.: Comparative virulence of two porcine group-A rotavirus isolates in gnotobiotic pigs. Am. J. Vet. Res. *50*:827–835, 1989.
82. Collins, J., Starkey, W. G., Wallis, T. S., et al.: Intestinal enzyme profiles in normal and rotavirus-infected mice. J. Pediatr. Gastroenterol. Nutr. *7*:264–272, 1988.
83. Conner, M. E., Crawford, S. E., Barone, C., et al.: Rotavirus vaccine administered parenterally induces protective immunity. J. Virol. *67*:6633–6641, 1993.
84. Conner, M. E., Estes, M. K., and Graham, D. Y.: Rabbit model of rotavirus infection. J. Virol. *62*:1625–1633, 1988.
85. Conner, M., Gilger, M., Estes, M., et al.: Serologic and mucosal immune response to rotavirus infection in the rabbit model. J. Virol. *65*:2562–2571, 1991.
86. Conner, M. E., Matson, D. O., and Estes, M. K.: Rotavirus vaccines and vaccination potential. *In* Ramig, R. F. (ed.): Rotaviruses. Berlin, Springer-Verlag, 1994, pp. 285–337.
87. Conner, M. E., Zarley, C. D., Hu, B., et al.: Virus-like particles as a rotavirus subunit vaccine. J. Infect. Dis. *174*(Suppl.):S88–S92, 1996.
88. Cook, S. M., Glass, R. I., LeBaron, C. W., et al.: Global seasonality of rotavirus infections. Bull. World Health Organ. *68*:171–177, 1990.
89. Coulson, B. S., Grimwood, K., Hudson, I. L., et al.: Role of coproantibody in clinical protection of children during reinfection with rotavirus. J. Clin. Microbiol. *30*:1678–1684, 1992.
90. Coulson, B. S., Grimwood, K., Masendycz, P. J., et al.: Comparison of rotavirus immunoglobulin A coproconversion with other indices of rotavirus infection in a longitudinal study in childhood. J. Clin. Microbiol. *28*:1367–1374, 1990.
91. Crawford, S. E., Labbé, M., Cohen, J., et al.: Characterization of virus-like particles produced by the expression of rotavirus capsid proteins in insect cells. J. Virol. *68*:5945–5952, 1994.
92. Cuadras, M. A., Arias, C. F., and Lopez, S.: Rotaviruses induce an early membrane permeabilization of MA104 cells and do not require a low intracellular Ca^{2+} concentration to initiate their replication cycle. J. Virol. *71*:9065–9074, 1997.
93. Cubitt, W. D., and Holzel, H.: An outbreak of rotavirus infection in a long-stay ward of a geriatric hospital. J. Clin. Pathol. *33*:306–308, 1980.
94. Cubitt, W. D., Steele, A. D., and Iturriza, M.: Characterisation of rotaviruses from children treated at a London hospital during 1996: Emergence of strains G9P2A[6] and G3P2A[6]. J. Med. Virol. *61*:150–154, 2000.
95. Cunliffe, N. A., Gentsch, J. R., Kirkwood, C. D., et al.: Molecular and serologic characterization of novel serotype G8 human rotavirus strains detected in Blantyre, Malawi. Virology *274*:309–320, 2000.
96. Cunliffe, N. A., Gondwe, J. S., Broadhead, R. L., et al.: Rotavirus G and P types in children with acute diarrhea in Blantyre, Malawi, from 1997 to 1998: Predominance of novel P[6]G8 strains. J. Med. Virol. *57*:308–312, 1999.
97. Das, M., Dunn, S. J., Woode, G. N., et al.: Both surface proteins (VP4 and VP7) of an asymptomatic neonatal rotavirus strain (I321) have high levels of sequence identity with the homologous proteins of a serotype 10 bovine rotavirus. Virology *194*:374–379, 1993.
98. Das, B. K., Gentsch, J. R., Cicirello, H. G., et al.: Characterization of rotavirus strains from newborns in New Delhi, India. J. Clin. Microbiol. *32*:1820–1822, 1994.
99. Das, B. K., Gentsch, J. R., Hoshino, Y., et al.: Characterization of the G serotype and genogroup of New Delhi newborn rotavirus strain 116E. Virology *197*:99–107, 1993.
100. Davidson, G. P., Bishop, R. F., Townley, R. R. W., et al.: Importance of a new virus in acute sporadic enteritis in children. Lancet *1*:242–245, 1975.
101. Davidson, G. P., Gall, D. G., Petric, M., et al.: Human rotavirus enteritis induced in conventional piglets: Intestinal structure and transport. J. Clin. Invest. *60*:1402–1409, 1977.
102. Davidson, G. P., Hogg, R., and Kirabakaran, C: Serum and intestinal immune response to rotavirus enteritis in children. Infect. Immun. *40*:447–452, 1983.
103. Davidson, G. P., Whyte, P. B. D., Daniels, E., et al.: Passive immunization of children with bovine colostrum containing antibodies to human rotavirus. Lancet *2*:709–712, 1989.
104. DeChamps, C., Laveran, H., Peigue-Lafeville, H., et al.: Sequential rotavirus infections: Characterization of serotypes and electropherotypes. Res. Virol. *142*:39–45, 1991.
105. DeMol, P., Zissis, G., Tubzler, J. P., et al.: Failure of live attenuated oral rotavirus vaccine. Lancet *2*:108, 1986.
106. Denisova, E., Dowling, W., LaMonica, R., et al.: Rotavirus capsid protein VP5 permeabilizes membranes. J. Virol. *73*:3147–3153, 1999.
107. Dennehy, P. H., Schutzbank, T. E., and Thorne, G. M.: Evaluation of an automated immunodiagnostic assay, VIDAS Rotavirus, for detection of rotavirus in fecal specimens. J. Clin. Microbiol. *32*:825–827, 1994.
108. De Zoysa, I., and Feachem, R. G.: Interventions for the control of diarrhoeal diseases among young children: Rotavirus and cholera immunization. Bull. World Health Organ. *63*:569–583, 1985.
109. Dharakul, T., Labbé, M., Cohen, J., et al.: Immunization with baculovirus-expressed recombinant rotavirus proteins VP1, VP4, VP6 and VP7 induces $CD8^+$ T lymphocytes that mediate clearance of chronic rotavirus infection in SCID mice. J. Virol. *65*:5928–5932, 1991.
110. Dharakul, T., Rott, L., and Greenberg, H.: Recovery from chronic rotavirus infection in mice with severe combined immunodeficiency: Virus clearance mediated by adoptive transfer of immune $CD8^+$ T lymphocytes. J. Virol. *64*:4375–4382, 1990.
111. Dong, Y., Zeng, C. Q. Y., Ball, J. M., et al.: The rotavirus enterotoxin NSP4 mobilizes intracellular calcium in human intestinal cells by stimulating phospholipase C–mediated inositol 1,4,5-trisphosphate production. Proc. Natl. Acad. Sci. U. S. A. *94*:3960–3965, 1997.
112. Dunn, S. J., Greenberg, H. B., Ward, R. L., et al.: Serotypic and genotypic characterization of human serotype 10 rotaviruses from asymptomatic neonates. J. Clin. Microbiol. *31*:165–169, 1993.
113. Ebina, T., Ohta, M., Kanamaru, Y., et al.: Passive immunizations of suckling mice and infants with bovine colostrum containing antibodies to human rotavirus. J. Med. Virol *38*:117–123, 1992.
114. Echeverria, P., Blacklow, N. R., Cukor, G. G., et al.: Rotavirus as a cause of severe gastroenteritis in adults. J. Clin. Microbiol. *18*:663–667, 1983.
115. Eiden, J., Losonsky, G. A., Johnson, J., et al.: Rotavirus RNA variation during chronic infection of immunocompromised children. Pediatr. Infect. Dis. *4*:632–637, 1985.
116. Ericson, B. L., Graham, D. Y., Mason, B. B., et al.: Identification, synthesis and modifications of simian rotavirus SA11 polypeptides in infected cells. J. Virol. *42*:825–839, 1982.
117. Esparza, J., and Gil, F.: A study on the ultrastructure of human rotavirus. Virology *91*:141–150, 1978.
118. Espejo, R. T., Lopez, S., and Arias, C. F.: Structural polypeptides of simian rotavirus SA11 and the effect of trypsin. J. Virol. *37*:156–160, 1981.
119. Estes, M. K., and Cohen, J.: Rotavirus gene structure and function. Microbiol. Rev. *53*:410–449, 1989.
120. Estes, M. K., Graham, D. Y., and Mason, B. B.: Proteolytic enhancement of rotavirus infectivity: Molecular mechanisms. J. Virol. *39*:879–888, 1981.
121. Estes, M. K., Graham, D. Y., Smith, E. M., et al.: Rotavirus stability and inactivation. J. Gen. Virol. *43*:403–409, 1979.
122. Fang Z.-Y., Ye, Q., Ho, M.-S., et al.: Investigation of an outbreak of adult diarrhea rotavirus in China. J. Infect. Dis. *160*:948–953, 1989.
123. Feng, N., Burns, J. W., Bracy, L., et al.: Comparison of mucosal and systemic humoral immune responses and subsequent protection in mice orally inoculated with a homologous or a heterologous rotavirus. J. Virol. *68*:7766–7773, 1994.
124. Figueroa-Qunitanilla, D., Salazar-Lindo, E., Sack, R. B., et al.: A controlled trial of bismuth subsalicylate in infants with acute watery diarrheal disease. N. Engl. J. Med. *328*:1653–1658, 1993.
125. Flewett, T. H., Bryden, A. S., and Davies, H.: Virus particles in gastroenteritis. Lancet *2*:1497, 1973.
126. Flewett, T. H., Bryden, A. S., Davies, H., et al.: Relation between viruses from acute gastroenteritis of children and newborn calves. Lancet *2*:61–63, 1974.
127. Flores, J., Gonzalez, M., Perez, M., et al.: Protection against severe rotavirus diarrhoea by rhesus rotavirus vaccine in Venezuelan infants. Lancet *1*:882–884, 1987.
128. Flores, J., Hoshino, Y., Boeggeman, E., et al.: Genetic relatedness among animal rotaviruses. Arch. Virol. *87*:273–285, 1986.
129. Flores, J., and Kapikian, A. Z.: Vaccines against rotavirus. *In* Woodrow, G. C., and Levine M. M. (eds.): New Generation Vaccines. New York, Marcel Dekker, 1990, pp. 765–788.
130. Flores, J., Midthun, K., Hoshino, Y., et al.: Conservation of the fourth gene among rotaviruses recovered from asymptomatic newborn infants and its possible role in attenuation. J. Virol. *60*:972–979, 1986.

131. Flores, J., Myslinski, J., Kalica, A. R., et al.: In vitro transcription of two human rotaviruses. J. Virol. *43*:1032–1037, 1982.
132. Flores, J., Perez-Schael, I., Blanco, M., et al.: Comparison of reactogenicity and antigenicity of M37 rotavirus vaccine and rhesus-rotavirus-based quadrivalent vaccine. Lancet *2*:330–334, 1990.
133. Flores, J., Perez-Schael, I., Gonzalez, M., et al.: Protection against severe rotavirus diarrhoea by rhesus rotavirus vaccine in Venezuelan infants. Lancet *1*:882–884, 1987.
134. Flores, J., Perez, I., White, L., et al.: Genetic relatedness among human rotaviruses as determined by RNA hybridization. Infect. Immun. *37*:648–655, 1982.
135. Ford-Jones, E. L., Wang, E., Petric, M., et al.: Hospitalization for community-acquired, rotavirus-associated diarrhea. Arch. Pediatr. Adolesc. Med. *154*:578–587, 2000.
136. Franco, M. A., and Greenberg, H. B.: Immunity to rotavirus infection in mice. J. Infect. Dis. *179*:S466–S469, 1999.
137. Franco, M. A., and Greenberg, H. B.: Role of B cells and cytotoxic T lymphocytes in clearance of and immunity to rotavirus infection in mice. J. Virol. *69*:7800–7806, 1995.
138. Franco, M. A., Tin, C., and Greenberg, H. B.: $CD8^+$ T cells can mediate almost complete short-term and partial long-term immunity to rotavirus in mice. J. Virol. *71*:4165–4170, 1997.
139. Friedman, M., Gaul, A., Sarov, B., et al.: Two sequential outbreaks of rotavirus gastroenteritis: Evidence of symptomatic and asymptomatic reinfection. J. Infect. Dis. *158*:814–822, 1988.
140. Fukudome, K., Yoshie, O., and Konno, T.: Comparison of human, simian, and bovine rotaviruses for requirement of sialic acid in hemagglutination and cell adsorption. Virology *172*:196–205, 1989.
141. Fukuhara, N., Yoshie, O., Kitaoka, S., et al.: Role of VP3 in human rotavirus internalization after target cell attachment via VP7. Virology *62*:2209–2218, 1988.
142. Gallegos, C. O., and Patton, J. T.: Characterization of rotavirus replication intermediates: A model for the assembly of single-shelled particles. Virology *172*:616–627, 1989.
143. Garbarg-Chenon, A., Bricout, F., and Nicolas, J. C.: Study of genetic reassortments between two human rotaviruses. Virology *139*:358–365, 1984.
144. Gentsch, J. R., Glass, R. I., Woods, P., et al.: Identification of group A rotavirus gene 4 types by polymerase chain reaction. J. Clin. Microbiol. *30*:1365–1373, 1992.
145. Gentsch, J. R., Woods, P.A., Ramachandran, M., et al.: Review of G and P typing results from a global collection of rotavirus strains: Implications for vaccine development. J. Infect. Dis. *174*:S30–S36, 1996.
146. Georges-Courbot, M. C., Beraud, A. M., Beards, G. M., et al.: Subgroups, serotypes, and electropherotypes of rotavirus isolated from children in Bangui, Central African Republic. J. Clin. Microbiol. *26*:668–671, 1988.
147. Georges-Courbot, M., Monges, J., Siopathis, M., et al.: Evaluation of the efficacy of a low-passage bovine rotavirus (strain WC3) vaccine in children in Central Africa. Res. Virol. *142*:405–411, 1991.
148. Gerna, G., Steele, A. D., Hoshino, Y., et al.: A comparison of the VP7 gene sequences of human and bovine rotaviruses. J. Gen. Virol. *75*:1781–1784, 1994.
149. Gilchrist, M. J. R., Bretl, T. S., Moultney, et al.: Comparison of seven kits for detection of rotavirus in fecal specimens with a sensitive, specific enzyme immunoassay. Diagn. Microbiol. Infect. Dis. *8*:221–228, 1987.
150. Gilger, M. A., Matson, D. O., Conner, M. E., et al.: Extraintestinal rotavirus infections in children with immunodeficiency. J. Pediatr. *120*:912–917, 1992.
151. Glass, R. I., Gentsch, J. R., and Smith, J. C.: Rotavirus vaccines: Success by reassortment? Science *265*:1389–1391, 1994.
152. Glass, R. I., Lew, J. F., Gangarosa, R. E., et al.: Estimates of morbidity and mortality rates for diarrheal diseases in American children. J. Pediatr. *118*:S27–S33, 1991.
153. Glass, R. I., Kilgore, P. E., Holman, R. C., et al.: The epidemiology of rotavirus diarrhea in the United States: Surveillance and estimates of disease burden. J. Infect. Dis. *174*:S5–S11, 1996.
154. Gombold, J. L., and Ramig, R. F.: Analysis of reassortment of genome segments in mice mixedly infected with rotaviruses SA11 and RRV. J. Virol. *57*:110–116, 1986.
155. Gorziglia, M., Hoshino, Y., Buckler-White, A., et al.: Conservation of amino acid sequence of VP8 and cleavage region of 84-kDa outer capsid protein among rotaviruses recovered from asymptomatic neonatal infection. Proc. Natl. Acad. Sci. U. S. A. *83*:7039–7043, 1986.
156. Gorziglia, M., Larralde, G., Kapikian, A. Z., et al.: Antigenic relationships among human rotaviruses as determined by outer capsid protein VP4. Proc. Natl. Acad. Sci. U. S. A. *87*:7155–7159, 1990.
157. Gouvea, V., Allen, J. R., Glass, R. I., et al.: Detection of group B and C rotaviruses by polymerase chain reaction. J. Clin. Microbiol. *29*:519–523, 1991.
158. Gouvea, V., and Brantley, M.: Is rotavirus a population of reassortants? Trends Microbiol. *3*:159–162, 1995.
159. Gouvea, V., Ramirez, C., Li, B., et al.: Restriction endonuclease analysis of the VP7 genes of human and animal rotaviruses. J. Clin. Microbiol. *31*:917–923, 1993.
160. Gouvea, V., Santos, N., and Timenetsky, M. C.: VP4 typing of bovine and porcine group A rotaviruses by PCR. J. Clin. Microbiol. *32*:1333–1337, 1994.
161. Graham, A., Kudesia, G., Allen, A. M., et al.: Reassortment of human rotavirus possessing genome rearrangements with bovine rotavirus: Evidence of host cell selection. J. Gen. Virol. *68*:115–122, 1987.
162. Graham, D. Y., Sackman, J. W., and Estes, M. K.: Pathogenesis of rotavirus-induced diarrhea: Preliminary studies in miniature swine piglet. Dig. Dis. Sci. *29*:1028–1035, 1984.
163. Green, K. Y., and Kapikian, A. Z.: Identification of VP7 epitopes associated with protection against human rotavirus illness or shedding in volunteers. J. Virol. *66*:548–553, 1992.
164. Green, K. Y., Sarasini, A., Qian, Y., et al.: Genetic variation in rotavirus serotype 4 subtypes. Virology *188*:362–368, 1992.
165. Greenberg, H. B., Clark, H. F., and Offit, P. A.: Rotavirus pathology and pathophysiology. Curr. Top. Microbiol. Immunol. *185*:255–283, 1994.
166. Greenberg, H. B., Flores, J., Kalica, A. R., et al.: Gene coding assignments for growth restriction, neutralization and subgroup specificities of the W and DS-1 strains of human rotavirus. J. Gen. Virol. *64*:313–320, 1983.
167. Greenberg, H. B., McAuliffe, V., Valdesuso, J., et al.: Serological analysis of the subgroup protein of rotaviruses, using monoclonal antibodies. Infect. Immun. *39*:91–99, 1983.
168. Greenberg, H. B., Valdesuso, J., Van Wyke, K., et al.: Production and preliminary characterization of monoclonal antibodies directed at two surface proteins of rhesus rotavirus. J. Virol. *47*:267–275, 1983.
169. Greenberg, H. B., Vo, P. T., and Jones, R.: Cultivation and characterization of three strains of murine rotavirus. J. Virol. *57*:585–590, 1986.
170. Grillner, L., Broberger, U., Chrystie, I., et al.: Rotavirus infections in newborns: An epidemiological and clinical study. Scand. J. Infect. Dis. *17*:349–355, 1985.
171. Grimwood, K., Coakley, J. C., Hudson, I. L., et al.: Serum aspartate amino-transferase levels after rotavirus gastroenteritis. J. Pediatr. *112*:597–600, 1988.
172. Grimwood, K., Lund, J., Coulson, B., et al.: Comparison of serum and mucosal antibody responses following severe acute rotavirus gastroenteritis in young children. J. Clin. Microbiol. *26*:732–738, 1988.
173. Grunow, J. E., Dunton, S. F., and Wanter, J. L.: Human rotavirus–like particle in a hepatic abscess. J. Pediatr. *106*:73–76, 1985.
174. Guarino, A., Canani, R. B., Russo, S., et al.: Oral immunoglobulins for treatment of acute rotaviral gastroenteritis. Pediatrics *93*:12–61, 1994.
175. Guerrero, C. A., Zarate, S., Corkidi, G., et al.: Biochemical characterization of rotavirus receptors in MA104 cells. J. Virol. *74*:9362–9371, 2000.
176. Guo, C.-T., Nakagomi, O., Mochizuki, M., et al.: Ganglioside GM_{1a} on the cell surface is involved in the infection by human rotavirus KUN and MO strains. J. Biochem. *126*:683–688, 1999.
177. Haffejee, I. E.: The pathophysiology, clinical features and management of rotavirus diarrhoea. Q. J. Med. *288*:289–299, 1991.
178. Haffejee, I. E.: Neonatal rotavirus infections. Rev. Infect. Dis. *13*:957–962, 1991.
179. Haffejee, I. E.: The epidemiology of rotavirus infections: A global perspective. J. Pediatr. Gastroenterol. Nutr. *20*:275–286, 1995.
180. Haffejee, I. E., and Moosa, A.: Rotavirus studies in Indian (Asian) South African infants with acute gastroenteritis. I. Microbiological and epidemiological aspects. Ann. Trop. Paediatr. *10*:165–172, 1990.
181. Hall, G. A., Bridger, J. C., Parsons, K. R., et al.: Variation in rotavirus virulence: A comparison of pathogenesis in calves between two rotaviruses of different virulence. Vet. Pathol. *30*:223–233, 1993.
182. Hamza, H., Ben Khalifa, H., Baumer, P., et al.: Racecadotril versus placebo in the treatment of acute diarrhoea in adults. Aliment. Pharmacol. Ther. *13*:15–19, 1999.
183. Hanlon, P., Marsh, V., Shenton, F., et al.: Trial of an attenuated bovine rotavirus vaccine (RIT 4237) in Gambian infants. Lancet *1*:1342–1345, 1987.
184. Hasegawa, A., Matsuno, S., Inouye, S., et al.: Isolation of human rotaviruses in primary cultures of monkey kidney cells. J. Clin. Microbiol. *16*:387–390, 1982.
185. Hattori, H., Torii, S., Nagafuji, H., et al.: Benign acute myositis associated with rotavirus gastroenteritis. J. Pediatr. *121*:748–749, 1992.
186. Helmberger-Jones, M., and Patton, J. T.: Characterization of subviral particles in cells infected with simian rotavirus SA11. Virology *155*:655–665, 1986.
187. Hewish, M. J., Takada, Y., and Coulson, B. S.: Integrins $\alpha_2\beta_1$ and $\alpha_4\beta_1$ can mediate SA11 rotavirus attachment and entry into cells. J. Virol. *74*:228–236, 2000.
188. Heyman, M., Corthier, G., Petit, A., et al.: Intestinal absorption of macromolecules during viral enteritis: An experimental study on rotavirus-infected conventional and germ-free mice. Pediatr. Res. *22*:72–78, 1987.
189. Hilpert, H., Brussow, H., Mietens, C., et al.: Use of bovine milk concentrate containing antibody to rotavirus to treat rotavirus gastroenteritis in infants. J. Infect. Dis. *156*:158–166, 1987.
190. Hjelt, K., Graubelle, P. C., Paerregaard, A., et al.: Protective effect of preexisting rotavirus-specific immunoglobulin against naturally acquired rotavirus infection in children. J. Med. Virol. *21*:39–47, 1987.
191. Ho, M.-S., Glass, R. I., Pinsky, P. F., et al.: Rotavirus as a cause of diarrheal morbidity and mortality in the United States. J. Infect. Dis. *158*:1112–1116, 1988.

192. Ho, M.-S., Glass, R. I., Pinsky, P. F., et al.: Diarrheal deaths in American children. Are they preventable? J. A. M. A. *260*:3281–3285, 1988.
193. Holmes, I. H., Ruck, B. J., Bishop, R. F., et al.: Infantile enteritis viruses: Morphogenesis and morphology. J. Virol. *16*:937–943, 1975.
194. Honeyman, M. C., Coulson, B. S., Stone, N. L., et al.: Association between rotavirus infection and pancreatic islet autoimmunity in children at risk of developing type 1 diabetes. Diabetes *49*:1319–1324, 2000.
195. Horie, Y., Nakagomi, O., Koshimura, Y., et al.: Diarrhea induction by rotavirus NSP4 in the homologous mouse model system. Virology *262*:398–407, 1999.
196. Hoshino, Y., Saif, L. J., Kang, S.-Y., et al.: Identification of group A rotavirus genes associated with virulence of a porcine rotavirus and host range restriction of a human rotavirus in the gnotobiotic piglet model. Virology *209*:274–280, 1995.
197. Hoshino, Y., Saif, L., Sereno, M., et al.: Infection immunity of piglets to either VP3 or VP7 outer capsid protein confers resistance to challenge with a virulent rotavirus bearing the corresponding antigen. J. Virol. *62*:744–748, 1988.
198. Hoshino, Y., Sereno, M. M., Midthun, K., et al.: Independent segregation of two antigenic specificities (VP3 and VP7) involved in neutralization of rotavirus infectivity. Proc. Natl. Acad. Sci. U. S. A. *82*:8701–8704, 1985.
199. Hoshino, Y., Wyatt, R. G., Greenberg, H. B., et al.: Serotypic similarity and diversity of rotaviruses of mammalian and avian origin as studied by plaque-reduction neutralization. J. Infect. Dis. *149*:694–702, 1984.
200. Hrdy, D. B.: Epidemiology of rotaviral infection in adults. Rev. Infect. Dis. *9*:461–469, 1987.
201. Hsu, H. Y., Kao, C. L., Huang, L. M., et al.: Viral etiology of intussusception in Taiwanese childhood. Pediatr. Infect. Dis. *17*:893–898, 1998.
202. Hua, J., Chen, X., and Patton, J. T.: Deletion mapping of the rotavirus metalloprotein NS53 (NSP1): The conserved cysteine-rich region is essential for virus-specific RNA binding. J. Virol. *68*:3990–4000, 1994.
203. Huicho, L., Sanchez, D., Contreras, M., et al.: Occult blood and fecal leukocytes as screening tests in childhood infectious diarrhea: An old problem revisited. Pediatr. Infect. Dis. J. *12*:474–477, 1993.
204. Hung, T.: Rotavirus and adult diarrhea. Adv. Virus Res. *35*:193–218, 1988.
205. Ijaz, M. K., Sabara, M. I., Frenchick, P. J., et al.: Assessment of intestinal damage in rotavirus infected neonatal mice by a D-xylose absorption test. J. Virol. Methods *18*:153–157, 1987.
206. Institute of Medicine: Prospects for immunizing against rotavirus. *In* New Vaccine Development: Establishing Priorities: Diseases of Importance in Developing Countries. Vol. 2. Washington, D.C., National Academy Press, 1986, pp. 308–318.
207. James, V. L., Lambden, P. R., Caul, E. O., and Clarke, I. N.: Enzyme-linked immunosorbent assay based on recombinant human group C rotavirus inner capsid protein (VP6) to detect human group C rotaviruses in fecal samples. J. Clin. Microbiol. *36*:3178–3181, 1998.
208. James, V. L., Lambden, P. R., Caul, E. O., et al.: Seroepidemiology of human group C rotavirus in the U.K. J. Med. Virol. *52*:86–91, 1997.
209. Jarvis, W. R., Middleton, P. J., and Gelfand, E. W.: Significance of viral infections in severe combined immunodeficiency disease. Pediatr. Infect. Dis. *2*:187–192, 1983.
210. Jiang, B., Dennehy, P. H., Spangenberger, S., et al.: First detection of group C rotavirus in fecal specimens of children with diarrhea in the United States. J. Infect. Dis. *172*:45–50, 1995.
211. Joensuu, J., Koskenniemi, E., Pang, X. L., and Vesikari, T.: Randomised placebo-controlled trial of rhesus-human reassortant rotavirus vaccine for prevention of severe rotavirus gastroenteritis. Lancet *350*:1205–1209, 1997.
212. Jolly, C. L., Beisner, B. M., and Holmes, I. H.: Rotavirus infection of MA104 cells is inhibited by *Ricinus* lectin and separately expressed single binding domains. Virology *275*:89–97, 2000.
213. Jones, P. D., Roddick, L. G., and Wilkinson, I. A.: Rotavirus and seizures. Med. J. Aust. *162*:223, 1995.
214. Kalica, A. R., Garon, C. F., Wyatt, R. G., et al.: Differentiation of human and calf reovirus-like agents associated with diarrhea using polyacrylamide gel electrophoresis of RNA. Virology *74*:86–92, 1976.
215. Kalica, A. R., Greenberg, H. B., Espejo, R. T., et al.: Distinctive ribonucleic acid patterns of human rotavirus subgroups 1 and 2. Infect. Immun. *33*:958–961, 1981.
216. Kalica, A. R., Greenberg, H. B., Wyatt, R. G., et al.: Genes of human (strain Wa) and bovine (strain UK) rotavirus that code for neutralization and subgroup antigens. Virology *112*:385–390, 1981.
217. Kaljot, T. K., Shaw, R. D., Rubin, D. H., et al.: Infectious rotavirus enters cells by direct cell membrane penetration, not by endocytosis. J. Virol. *62*:1136–1144, 1988.
218. Kanfer, E. J., Abrahamson, G., Taylor, J., et al.: Severe rotavirus-associated diarrhoea following bone marrow transplantation: Treatment with oral immunoglobulin. Bone Marrow Transplant. *14*:651–652, 1994.
219. Kapikian, A. Z.: Viral gastroenteritis. J. A. M. A. *269*:627–630, 1993.
220. Kapikian, A. Z., and Chanock, R. M.: Rotaviruses. *In* Fields, B. N., Knipe, D. M., Chanock, R. M., et al. (eds.): Virology. 2nd ed., Vol. 2. New York, Raven Press, 1990, pp. 1353–1404.
221. Kapikian, A. Z., Cline, W. L., Kim, H. W., et al.: Antigenic relationships among five reovirus-like (RVL) agents by complement fixation (CF) and development of new substitute CF antigens for the human RVL agent of infantile gastroenteritis. Proc. Soc. Exp. Biol. Med. *152*:535–539, 1976.
222. Kapikian, A. Z., Flores, J., Hoshino, Y., et al.: Rotavirus: The major etiologic agent of severe infantile diarrhea may be controllable by a "Jennerian" approach to vaccination. J. Infect. Dis. *153*:815–822, 1986.
223. Kapikian, A. Z., Kim, H. W., Wyatt, R. G., et al.: Reovirus-like agent in stools: Association with infantile diarrhea and development of serologic tests. Science *185*:1049–1053, 1974.
224. Kapikian, A. Z., Kim, H. W., Wyatt, R. G., et al.: Human reovirus-like agent as the major pathogen associated with "winter" gastroenteritis in hospitalized infants and young children. N. Engl. J. Med. *294*:965–972, 1976.
225. Kapikian, A. Z., Wyatt, R. G., Levine, M. M., et al.: Oral administration of human rotavirus to volunteers: Induction of illness and correlates of resistance. J. Infect. Dis. *147*:95–106, 1983.
226. Kattoura, M. D., Chen, Z., and Patton, J. T.: The rotavirus RNA-binding protein NS35 (NSP2) forms 10S multimers and interacts with the viral RNA polymerase. Virology *202*:803–813, 1994.
227. Keidan, I., Shif, I., Keren, G., et al.: Rotavirus encephalopathy: Evidence of central nervous system involvement during rotavirus infection. Pediatr. Infect. Dis. J. *11*:773–775, 1992.
228. Keller, K. M., Schmidt, H., Wirth, S., et al.: Differences in the clinical and radiologic patterns of rotavirus and non-rotavirus necrotizing enterocolitis. Pediatr. Infect. Dis. J. *10*:734–738, 1991.
229. Keswick, B. H., Pickering, L. K., Dupont, H. L., et al.: Survival and detection of rotaviruses on environmental surfaces in day care centers. Appl. Environ. Microbiol. *46*:813–816, 1983.
230. Khoshoo, V., Bhan, M. K., Jayashree, S., et al.: Rotavirus infection and persistent diarrhea in young children. Lancet *2*:1314–1315, 1990.
231. Kilgore, P. E., Holman, R. C., Clarke, M. J., and Glass, R. I.: Trends of diarrheal disease-associated mortality in U.S. children, 1968 through 1991. J. A. M. A. *274*:1143–1148, 1995.
232. Kim, H. W., Brandt, C. D., Kapikian, A. Z., et al.: Human reovirus-like agent infection: Occurrence in adult contacts of pediatric patients with gastroenteritis. J. A. M. A. *238*:404–407, 1977.
233. Kirstein, C. G., Clare, D. A., and Lecce, J. G.: Development of resistance of enterocytes to rotavirus in neonatal agammaglobulinemic piglets. J. Virol. *55*:567–573, 1985.
234. Knowlton, D. R., Spector, D. M., and Ward, R. L.: Development of an improved method for measuring neutralizing antibody to rotavirus. J. Virol. Methods *33*:127–134, 1991.
235. Kohli, E., Pothier, P., Denis, F., et al.: Multicentre evaluation of a new commercial latex agglutination test using a monoclonal antibody for rotavirus detection. Eur. J. Clin. Microbiol. Infect. Dis. *8*:251–253, 1989.
235a. Kombo, L. A., Gerber, M. A., Pickering, L. K., et al.: Intussusception, infection, and immunization: Summary of a workshop on rotavirus. Pediatrics *108*:E37, 2001.
236. Konno, T., Suzuki, H., Kutsuzawa, T., et al.: Human rotavirus and intussusception. N. Engl. J. Med. *297*:945, 1977.
237. Konno, T., Suzuki, H., Kutsuzawa, T., et al.: Human rotavirus infection in infants and young children with intussusception. J. Med. Virol. *2*:265–269, 1978.
238. Koopmans, M., and Brown, D.: Seasonality and diversity of group A rotaviruses in Europe. Acta Paediatr. Suppl. *426*:14–19, 1999.
239. Kovacs, A., Chan, L., Hotrakitya, C., et al.: Serum transaminase elevations in infants with rotavirus gastroenteritis. J. Pediatr. Gastroenterol. Nutr. *5*:873–877, 1986.
240. Kovacs, A., Chan, L., Hotrakitya, C., et al.: Rotavirus gastroenteritis. Am. J. Dis. Child. *141*:161–166, 1987.
240a. Kramarz, P., Franee, F. K., Destefano, F., et al.: Population-based study of rotavirus vaccination and intussusception. Pediatr. Infect. Dis. J. *20*:410–416, 2001.
241. Kubelka, C. F., Marchevsky, R. S., Stephens, P. R. S., et al.: Murine experimental infection with rotavirus SA-11: Clinical and immunohistological characteristics. Exp. Toxicol. Pathol. *45*:433–438, 1993.
242. Kutsuzawa, T., Konno, T., Suzuki, H., et al.: Two distinct electrophoretic migration patterns of RNA segments of human rotaviruses prevalent in Japan in relation to their serotypes. Microbiol. Immunol. *26*:271–273, 1982.
243. Kuzuya, M., Fujii, R., Hamano, M., et al.: Survey of human group C rotaviruses in Japan during the winter of 1992 to 1993. J. Clin. Microbiol. *36*:6–10, 1998.
244. Lanata, C., Black, R., Del Aguila, R., et al.: Protection of Peruvian children against rotavirus diarrhea of specific serotypes by one, two or three doses of the RIT 4237 attenuated bovine rotavirus vaccine. J. Infect. Dis. *159*:452–459, 1989.
245. Larralde, G., and Flores, J.: Identification of gene alleles among human rotaviruses by polymerase chain reaction derived probes. Virology *179*:469–473, 1990.
246. Lawton, J. A., Estes, M. K., and Prasad, B. V. V.: Three-dimensional visualization of mRNA release from actively transcribing rotavirus particles. Nat. Struct. Biol. *4*:118–121, 1997.
247. Lawton, J. A., Estes, M. A., and Prasad, B. V. V.: Identification and characterization of a transcription pause site in rotavirus. J. Virol. *75*:1632–1642, 2001.

248. Lawton, J. A., Zeng, C. Q. Y., Mukherjee, S. K., et al.: Three-dimensional structural analysis of recombinant rotavirus-like particles with intact and amino-terminal-deleted VP2: Implications for the architecture of the VP2 capsid layer. J. Virol. *71*:7353–7360, 1997.
249. LeBaron, C. W., Lew, J., Glass, R. I., et al.: Annual rotavirus epidemic patterns in North America. J. A. M. A. *264*:983–988, 1990.
250. Lebenthal, E., and Lee, P. C.: Development of functional response in human exocrine pancreas. Pediatrics *66*:556–560, 1980.
251. Lee, C.-N., Wang, Y.-L., Kao, C.-L., et al.: NSP4 gene analysis of rotaviruses recovered from infected children with and without diarrhea. J. Clin. Microbiol. *38*:4471–4477, 2000.
252. Leite, J. P. G., Alfieri, A. A., Woods, P. A., et al.: Rotavirus G and P types circulating in Brazil: Characterization by RT-PCR, probe hybridization, and sequence analysis. Arch. Virol. *141*:2365–2374, 1996.
253. Lewis, H. M., Parry, J. V., Davies, H. A., et al.: A year's experience of the rotavirus syndrome and its association with respiratory illness. Arch. Dis. Child. *54*:339–346, 1979.
254. Linares, A., Gabbay, Y., Mascarenhas, J., et al.: Epidemiology of rotavirus subgroups and serotypes in Belem, Brazil: A three-year study. Ann. Inst. Pasteur/Virol. *139*:89–99, 1988.
255. Liprandi, F., Moros, Z., Gerder, M., et al.: Productive penetration of rotavirus in cultured cells induces coentry of the translation inhibitor α-sarcin. Virology *237*:430–438, 1997.
256. Little, L. M., and Shadduck, J. A.: Pathogenesis of rotavirus infection in mice. Infect. Immun. *38*:755–763, 1982.
257. Liu, M., Mattion, N. M., and Estes, M. K.: Rotavirus VP3 expressed in insect cells possesses guanylyltransferase activity. Virology *188*:77–84, 1992.
258. Lopez, S., Arias, C. F., Bell, J. R., et al.: Primary structure of the cleavage site associated with trypsin enhancement of rotavirus SA11 infectivity. Virology *144*:11–19, 1985.
259. Lopez, S., Espinosa, R., Isa, P., et al.: Characterization of a monoclonal antibody directed to the surface of MA104 cells that blocks the infectivity of rotaviruses. Virology *273*:160–168, 2000.
260. Losonsky, G. A., Johnson, G. P., Winkelstein, J. A., et al.: The oral administration of human serum immunoglobulin in immunodeficiency patients with viral gastroenteritis: A pharmacokinetic and functional analysis. J. Clin. Invest. *76*:2362–2367, 1985.
261. Losonsky, G. A., Rennels, M. B., Kapikian, A. Z., et al.: Safety, infectivity, transmissibility, and immunogenicity of rhesus rotavirus vaccine (MMU 18006) in infants. Pediatr. Infect. Dis. *5*:25, 1986.
262. Losonsky, G., Vonderfecht, S., Eiden, J., et al.: Homotypic and heterotypic antibodies for prevention of experimental rotavirus gastroenteritis. J. Clin. Microbiol. *24*:1041–1044, 1986.
263. Ludert, J. E., Feng, N., Yu, J. H., et al.: Genetic mapping indicates that VP4 is the rotavirus cell attachment protein in vitro and in vivo. J. Virol. *70*:487–493, 1996.
264. Ludert, J. E., Mason, B. B., Angel, J., et al.: Identification of mutations in the rotavirus protein VP4 that alter sialic-acid-dependent infection. J. Gen. Virol. *79*:725–729, 1998.
265. Maass, D. R., and Atkinson, P. H.: Rotavirus proteins VP7, NS28, and VP4 form oligomeric structures. J. Virol. *64*:2632–2641, 1990.
266. Maass, D. R., and Atkinson, P. H.: Retention by the endoplasmic reticulum of rotavirus VP7 is controlled by three adjacent amino-terminal residues. J. Virol. *68*:366–378, 1994.
267. Mackow, E. R., Shaw, R. D, Matsui, S. M., et al.: The rhesus rotavirus gene encoding VP3: Location of amino acids involved in homologous and heterologous rotavirus neutralization and identification of a putative fusion region. Proc. Natl. Acad. Sci. U. S. A. *85*:645–649, 1988.
268. Madore, H., Christy, C., Pichichero, M., et al.: Field trial of rhesus rotavirus or human-rhesus rotavirus reassortant vaccine of VP7 serotype 3 or 1 specificity in infants. J. Infect. Dis. *166*:235–243, 1992.
269. Malherbe, H. H., Harwin, R., and Ulrich, M.: The cytopathic effect of vervet monkey viruses. S. Afr. Med. J. *37*:407–411, 1963.
270. Mansell, E. A., and Patton, J. T.: Rotavirus RNA replication: VP2, but not VP6, is necessary for viral replicase activity. J. Virol. *64*:4988–4996, 1990.
271. Marrie, T. J., Lee, S. H. S., Faulkner, R. S., et al.: Rotavirus infection in a geriatric population. Arch. Intern. Med. *142*:313–316, 1982.
272. Martin, M. L., Palmer, E. L., and Middleton, P. J.: Ultrastructure of infantile gastroenteritis virus. Virology *68*:146–153, 1975.
273. Mason, B. B., Graham, D. Y., and Estes, M. K.: In vitro transcription and translation of simian rotavirus SA11 gene products. J. Virol. *33*:1111–1121, 1980.
274. Mata, L., Simhon, A., Urrutia, J. J., et al.: Epidemiology of rotavirus in a cohort of 45 Guatemalan Mayan Indian children observed from birth to the age of three years. J. Infect. Dis. *148*:452–461, 1980.
275. Matson, D. O., and Estes, M. K.: Impact of rotavirus infection at a large pediatric hospital. J. Infect. Dis. *162*:598–604, 1990.
276. Matson, D. O., O'Ryan, M. L., Herrera, I., et al.: Fecal antibody responses to symptomatic and asymptomatic rotavirus infections. J. Infect. Dis. *167*:577–583, 1993.
277. Matsui, S., Offit, P., Vo, P., et al.: Passive protection against rotavirus-induced diarrhea by monoclonal antibodies to the heterotypic neutralization domain of VP7 and the VP8 fragment of VP4. J. Clin. Microbiol. *27*:780–782, 1989.
278. Matsumoto, K., Hatano, M., Kobayashi, K., et al.: An outbreak of gastroenteritis associated with acute rotaviral infection in school children. J. Infect. Dis. *160*:611–615, 1989.
279. Matsuno, S., Utagawa, E., and Sugiura, A.: Association of rotavirus infection with Kawasaki syndrome. J. Infect. Dis. *148*:177, 1983.
280. Matthews, R. E. F.: The classification and nomenclature of viruses: Summary of results of meetings of The International Committee on Taxonomy of Viruses in The Hague, September, 1978. Intervirology *11*:133–135, 1979.
281. McLean, B., Sonza, S., and Holmes, I. H.: Measurement of immunoglobulin A, G and M class rotavirus antibodies in serum and mucosal secretions. J. Clin. Microbiol. *12*:314–319, 1980.
282. McNeal, M. M., Barone, K. S., Rae, M. N., et al.: Effector functions of antibody and $CD8^+$ cells in resolution of rotavirus infection and protection against reinfection in mice. Virology *214*:387–397, 1995.
283. McNeal, M. M., Broome, R. L., and Ward, R. L.: Active immunity against rotavirus infection in mice is correlated with viral replication and titers of serum rotavirus IgA following vaccination. Virology *204*:642–650, 1994.
284. McNeal, M. M., Rae, M. N., and Ward, R. L.: Evidence that resolution of rotavirus infection in mice is due to both CD4 and CD8 cell-dependent activities. J. Virol. *71*:8735–8742, 1997.
285. McNeal, M. M., Sheridan, J., and Ward, R.: Active protection against rotavirus infection of mice following intraperitoneal immunization. Virology *191*:150–157, 1992.
286. McNeal, M. M., and Ward, R. L.: Long-term production of rotavirus antibody and protection against reinfection following a single infection of neonatal mice with murine rotavirus. Virology *211*:474–480, 1995.
287. Mebus, C. A.: Reovirus-like calf enteritis. Dig. Dis. *21*:592–598, 1976.
288. Mebus, C. A., Stair, E. L., Underdahl, N. R., et al.: Pathology of neonatal calf diarrhea induced by a reo-like virus. Vet. Pathol. *8*:490–505, 1974.
289. Mebus, C. A., Underdahl, N. R., Rhodes, M. B., et al.: Calf diarrhea (scours): Reproduced with a virus from a field outbreak. Univ. Nebraska Res. Bull. *233*:1–16, 1969.
290. Mendez, E., Arias, C. F., and Lopez, S.: Binding to sialic acids is not an essential step for the entry of animal rotaviruses to epithelial cells in culture. J. Virol. *67*:5253–5259, 1993.
291. Mendez, E., Arias, C. F., and Lopez, S.: Interactions between the two surface proteins of rotavirus may alter the receptor-binding specificity of the virus. J. Virol. *70*:1218–1222, 1996.
292. Mendez, E., Lopez, S., Cuadras, M. A., et al.: Entry of rotaviruses is a multistep process. Virology *263*:450–459, 1999.
293. Meyer, J. C., Bergmann, C. C., and Bellamy, A. R.: Interaction of rotavirus cores with the nonstructural glycoprotein NS28. Virology *171*:98–107, 1989.
294. Midthun, K., Greenberg, H., Hoshino, Y., et al.: Reassortant rotaviruses as potential live rotavirus vaccine candidates. J. Virol. *53*:949–954, 1985.
295. Midthun, K., Halsey, N. A., Jett-Goheen, M., et al.: Safety and immunogenicity of human rotavirus vaccine strain M37 in adults, children, and infants. J. Infect. Dis. *164*:792–796, 1991.
296. Midthun, K., Hoshino, Y., Kapikian, A., et al.: Single gene substitution rotavirus reassortants containing the major neutralization protein (VP7) of human rotavirus serotype 4. J. Clin. Microbiol. *24*:822–826, 1986.
297. Moe, K., and Shirley, J. A.: The effect of relative humidity and temperature on the survival of human rotavirus in faeces. Arch. Virol. *72*:179–186, 1982.
298. Morita, Y., Taniguchi, K., Urasawa, T., et al.: Analysis of serotype-specific neutralization epitopes on VP7 of human rotavirus by the use of neutralizing monoclonal antibodies and antigenic variants. J. Gen. Virol. *69*:451–458, 1988.
299. Morris, A. P., Scott, J. K., Ball, J. M., et al.: NSP4 elicits age-dependent diarrhea and Ca^{2+}-mediated I^- influx into intestinal crypts of CF mice. Am. J. Physiol. *277*:G431–G444, 1999.
300. Mphahlele, M. J., Peenze, I., and Steele, A. D.: Rotavirus strains bearing the VP4 P[14] genotype recovered from South African children with diarrhoea. Arch. Virol. *144*:1027–1034, 1999.
301. Mphahlele, M. J., and Steele, A. D.: Relative frequency of human rotavirus VP4 (P) genotypes recovered over a ten-year period from South African children with diarrhea. J. Med. Virol. *47*:1–5, 1995.
302. Mulcahy, D. L., Kamath, K. R., de Silva, L. M., et al.: A two-part study of the aetiological role of rotavirus in intussusception. J. Med. Virol. *9*:51–55, 1982.
303. Murphy, A. M., Albrey, M. B., and Hay, P. J.: Rotavirus infections in neonates. Lancet *2*:452–453, 1975.
304. Murphy, T. V., Gargiullo, P. M., Massoudi, M. S., et al.: Intussusception among infants given an oral rotavirus vaccine. N. Engl. J. Med. *344*:564–572, 2001.
305. Nakagomi, O., Isegawa, Y., Ward, R. L., et al.: Naturally occurring dual infection with human and bovine rotaviruses as suggested by the recovery of G1P8 and G1P5 rotaviruses from a single patient. Arch. Virol. *137*:381–388, 1994.
306. Nakagomi, O., Mochizuki, M., Aboudy, Y., et al.: Hemagglutination by a human rotavirus isolate as evidence for transmission of animal rotaviruses to humans. J. Clin. Microbiol. *30*:1011–1013, 1992.

307. Nakagomi, O., and Nakagomi, T.: Molecular evidence for naturally occurring single VP7 gene substitution reassortant between human rotaviruses belonging to two different genogroups. Arch. Virol. *119*:67–81, 1991.
308. Nakagomi, O., and Nakagomi, T.: Genetic diversity and similarity among mammalian rotaviruses in relation to interspecies transmission of rotavirus. Arch. Virol. *120*:43–55, 1991.
309. Nakagomi, O., and Nakagomi, T.: Interspecies transmission of rotaviruses studied from the perspective of genogroup. Microbiol. Immunol. *37*:337–348, 1993.
310. Nakata, S., Gatheru, Z., Ukae, S., et al.: Epidemiological study of the G serotype distribution of Group A rotaviruses in Kenya from 1991 to 1994. J. Med. Virol. *58*:296–303, 1999.
311. Nalin, D. R., Levine, M. M., Mata, L., et al.: Comparison of sucrose with glucose in oral therapy of infant diarrhea. Lancet *2*:277–279, 1978.
312. Nicolas, J. C., Ingrand, D., Fortier, B., and Bricout, F.: A one-year virological survey of acute intussusception in childhood. J. Med. Virol. *9*:267–271, 1982.
313. Nigro, G.: Pancreatitis with hypoglycemia-associated convulsions following rotavirus gastroenteritis. J. Pediatr. Gastroenterol. Nutr. *12*:280–282, 1991.
314. Nigro, G., and Midulla, M.: Acute laryngitis associated with rotavirus gastroenteritis. J. Infect. Dis. *7*:81–82, 1983.
315. Nilsson, M., Sigstam, G., and Svensson, L.: Antibody prevalence and specificity to group C rotavirus in Swedish sera. J. Med. Virol. *60*:210–215, 2000.
316. Nilsson, M., Svenungsson, B., Hedlund, K. O., et al.: Incidence and genetic diversity of group C rotavirus among adults. J. Infect. Dis. *182*:678–684, 2000.
317. Noone, C., Menzies, I. S., Banatvala, J. E., et al.: Intestinal permeability and lactose hydrolysis in human rotaviral gastroenteritis assessed simultaneously by noninvasive differential sugar permeation. Eur. J. Clin. Invest. *16*:217–225, 1986.
318. O'Brien, J. A., Taylor, J. A., and Bellamy, A. R.: Probing the structure of rotavirus NSP4: A short sequence at the extreme C terminus mediates binding to the inner capsid particle. J. Virol. *74*:5388–5394, 2000.
319. Offit, P. A.: Rotaviruses: Immunological determinants of protection against infection and disease. Adv. Virus Res. *44*:161–202, 1994.
320. Offit, P. A., and Blavat, G.: Identification of the two rotavirus genes determining neutralization specificities. J. Virol. *57*:376–378, 1986.
321. Offit, P. A., Blavat, G., Greenberg, H. B., et al.: Molecular basis of rotavirus virulence: Role of gene segment 4. J. Virol. *57*:46–49, 1986.
322. Offit, P., Boyle, D., Both, G., et al.: Outer capsid glycoprotein VP7 is recognized by cross-reactive rotavirus-specific cytotoxic T lymphocytes. Virology *184*:563–568, 1991.
323. Offit, P., and Clark, H.: Protection against rotavirus-induced gastroenteritis in a murine model by passively acquired gastrointestinal but not circulating antibodies. J. Virol. *54*:58–64, 1985.
324. Offit, P., Clark, H., Blavat, G., et al.: Reassortant rotaviruses containing structural proteins VP3 and VP7 from different parents induce antibodies protective against each parental serotype. J. Virol. *60*:491–496, 1986.
325. Offit, P., Clark, H., Kornstein, M., et al.: A murine model for oral infection with a primate rotavirus (simian SA11). J. Virol. *51*:233–236, 1984.
326. Offit, P. A., and Dudzik, K.: Rotavirus-specific cytotoxic T lymphocytes cross-react with target cells infected with different rotavirus serotypes. J. Virol. *62*:127–131, 1988.
327. Offit, P. A., and Dudzik, K.: Rotavirus-specific cytotoxic T lymphocytes appear at the intestinal mucosal surface after rotavirus infection. J. Virol. *63*:3507–3512, 1989.
328. Offit, P., and Dudzik, K.: Rotavirus-specific cytotoxic T lymphocytes passively protect against gastroenteritis in suckling mice. J. Virol. *64*:6325–6328, 1990.
329. Offit, P. A., Hoffenberg, E. J., Pia, E. S., et al.: Rotavirus-specific helper T cell responses in newborns, infants, children and adults. J. Infect. Dis. *165*:1107–1111, 1992.
330. Offit, P. A., Hoffenberg, E. J., Santos, N., et al.: Rotavirus-specific humoral and cellular immune response after primary symptomatic infection. J. Infect. Dis. *167*:1436–1440, 1993.
331. Offit, P., Shaw, R., and Greenberg, H.: Passive protection against rotavirus-induced diarrhea by monoclonal antibodies to surface proteins VP3 and VP7. J. Virol. *58*:700–703, 1986.
332. Oishi, I., Yamazaki, K., and Minekawa, Y.: An occurrence of diarrheal cases associated with group C rotavirus in adults. Microbiol. Immunol. *37*:505–509, 1993.
333. O'Mahony, J., Foley, B., Morgan, S., et al.: VP4 and VP7 genotyping of rotavirus samples recovered from infected children in Ireland over a 3-year period. J. Clin. Microbiol. *37*:1699–1703, 1999.
334. O'Neal, C. M., Crawford, S. E., Estes, M. K., et al.: Rotavirus virus-like particles administered mucosally induce protective immunity. J. Virol. *71*:8707–8717, 1997.
335. Orenstein, J.: Update on intussusception. Contemp. Pediatr. *17*:180–191, 2000.
336. O'Ryan, M., Matson, D., Estes, M., et al.: Molecular epidemiology of rotavirus in young children attending day care centers in Houston. J. Infect. Dis. *162*:810–816, 1990.
337. O'Ryan, M. L., Matson, D. O., Estes, M. K., et al.: Anti-rotavirus G type–specific and isotype-specific antibodies in children with natural rotavirus infections. J. Infect. Dis. *169*:504–511, 1994.
338. Osborne, M. P., Haddon, S. J., Spencer, A. J., et al.: An electron microscopic investigation of time-related changes in the intestine of neonatal mice infected with murine rotavirus. J. Pediatr. Gastroenterol. Nutr. *7*:236–248, 1988.
339. Padilla-Noriega, L., Fiore, L., Rennels, M. B., et al.: Humoral immune responses to VP4 and its cleavage products VP5* and VP8* in infants vaccinated with rhesus rotavirus. J. Clin. Microbiol. *30*:1392–1397, 1992.
340. Parashar, U. D., Chung, M. A., Holman, R. C., et al.: Use of state hospital discharge data to assess the morbidity from rotavirus diarrhea and to monitor the impact of a rotavirus immunization program: A pilot study in Connecticut. Pediatrics *104*:489–494, 1999.
341. Parashar, U. D., Holman, R. C., Bresee, J. S., et al.: Epidemiology of diarrheal disease among children enrolled in four West Coast health maintenance organizations. Pediatr. Infect. Dis. J. *17*:605–611, 1998.
342. Parashar, U. D., Holman, R. C., Cummings, K. C., et al.: Trends in intussusception-associated hospitalizations and deaths among U.S. infants. Pediatrics *106*:1413–1421, 2000.
343. Patton, J. T.: Rotavirus replication. Curr. Top. Microbiol. Immunol. *185*:107–127, 1994.
344. Patton, J. T., Chnaiderman, J., and Spencer, E.: Open reading frame in rotavirus mRNA specifically promotes synthesis of double-stranded RNA: Template size also affects replication efficiency. Virology *264*:167–180, 1999.
345. Patton, J. T., Jones, M. T., Kalbach, A. N., et al.: Rotavirus RNA polymerase requires the core shell protein to synthesize the double stranded RNA genome. J. Virol. *71*:9618–9626, 1997.
346. Patton, J. T., and Spencer, E.: Genomic replication and packaging of segmented double-stranded RNA viruses. Virology *277*:217–225, 2000.
347. Patton, J. T., Wentz, M., Xiaobo, J., and Ramig, R. F.: *cis*-Acting signals that promote genome replication in rotavirus mRNA. J. Virol. *70*:3961–3971, 1996.
348. Pearson, G. R., and McNulty, M. S.: Ultrastructural changes in small intestinal epithelium of neonatal pigs infected with pig rotavirus. Arch. Virol. *59*:127–136, 1979.
349. Pearson, G. R., McNulty, M. S., and Logan, E. F.: Pathological changes in the small intestine of neonatal calves naturally infected with reo-like virus (rotavirus). Vet. Rec. *102*:454–458, 1978.
350. Pedley, S., Bridger, J. C., Chasey, D., et al.: Definition of two new groups of atypical rotaviruses. J. Gen. Virol. *67*:131–137, 1986.
351. Penaranda, M. E., Cubitt, W. D., Sinarachatanant, P., et al.: Group C rotavirus infections in patients with diarrhea in Thailand, Nepal, and England. J. Infect. Dis. *160*:392–397, 1989.
352. Perez, J. F., Chemello, M. E., Liprandi, F., et al.: Oncosis in MA104 cells is induced by rotavirus infection through an increase in intracellular Ca^{2+} concentration. Virology *252*:17–27, 1998.
353. Perez, J. F., Ruiz, M.-.C., Chemello, M. E., and Michelangeli, F.: Characterization of a membrane calcium pathway induced by rotavirus infection in cultured cells. J. Virol. *73*:2481–2490, 1999.
354. Perez-Schael, I., Blanco, M., Vilar, M., et al.: Clinical studies of a quadrivalent rotavirus vaccine in Venezuelan infants. J. Clin. Microbiol. *28*:553–558, 1990.
355. Perez-Schael, I., Daoud, G., White, L., et al.: Rotavirus shedding by newborn children. J. Med. Virol. *14*:127–136, 1984.
356. Perez-Schael, I., Garcia, D., Gonzalez, M., et al.: Prospective study of diarrheal diseases in Venezuelan children to evaluate the efficacy of rhesus rotavirus vaccine. J. Med. Virol. *30*:219–229, 1990.
357. Perez-Schael, I., Gonzalez, M., Daoud, N., et al.: Reactogenicity and antigenicity of the rhesus rotavirus vaccine MMU 18006 in Venezuelan children. J. Infect. Dis. *155*:34, 1987.
358. Perez-Schael, I., Guntinas, M. J., Perez, M., et al.: Efficacy of the rhesus rotavirus–based quadrivalent vaccine in infants and young children in Venezuela. N. Engl. J. Med. *337*:1181–1187, 1997.
358a. Peter, G., Myers, M. G.: National Vaccine Advisory Committee: National Vaccine Program Office. Intussusception, rotavirus, and oral vaccines: Summary of a workshop. Pediatrics *110*:E67, 2002.
359. Pickering, L. K., DuPont, H. L., Olarte, J., et al.: Fecal leukocytes in enteric infections. Am. J. Clin. Pathol. *68*:562–565, 1977.
360. Pipittajan, P., Kasempimolporn, S., Ikegami, N., et al.: Molecular epidemiology of rotaviruses associated with pediatric diarrhea in Bangkok, Thailand. J. Clin. Microbiol. *29*:617–624, 1991.
361. Pitson, G. A., Grimwood, K., Coulson, B. S., et al.: Comparison between children treated at home and those requiring hospital admission for rotavirus and other enteric pathogens associated with acute diarrhea in Melbourne, Australia. J. Clin. Microbiol. *24*:395–399, 1986.
362. Pizarro, J. L., Sandino, A. M., Pizarro, J. M., et al.: Characterization of rotavirus guanylyltransferase activity associated with polypeptide VP3. J. Gen. Virol. *72*:325–332, 1991.
363. Poruchynsky, M. A., and Atkinson, P. H.: Rotavirus protein rearrangements in purified membrane-enveloped intermediate particles. J. Virol. *65*:4720–4727, 1991.

364. Poruchynsky, M. A., Tyndall, C., Both, G. W., et al.: Deletions into an NH_2-terminal hydrophobic domain result in secretion of rotavirus VP7, a resident endoplasmic reticulum membrane glycoprotein. J. Cell Biol. *101*:2199–2209, 1985.
365. Prasad, B. V. V., Burns, J. W., Marietta, E., et al.: Localization of VP4 neutralization sites in rotavirus by three-dimensional cryo-electron microscopy. Nature *343*:476–479, 1990.
366. Prasad, B. V. V., and Chiu, W.: Structure of rotavirus. Curr. Top. Microbiol. Immunol. *185*:9–29, 1994.
367. Prasad, B. V. V., Rothnagel, R., Zeng, C. Q.-Y., et al.: Visualization of ordered genomic RNA and localization of transcriptional complexes in rotavirus. Nature *382*:471–473, 1996.
368. Prasad, B. V. V., Wang, G. J., Clerx, J. P. M., et al.: Three-dimensional structure of rotavirus. J. Mol. Biol. *199*:269–275, 1988.
369. Ramachandran, M., Gentsch, J. R., Parashar, U. D., et al.: Detection and characterization of novel rotavirus strains in the United States. J. Clin. Microbiol. *36*:3223–3229, 1998.
370. Ramig, R. F., and Ward, R. L.: Genomic segment reassortment in rotaviruses and other Reoviridae. Adv. Virus Res. *39*:163–207, 1991.
371. Rao, C. D., Gowda, K., and Reddy, B. S. Y.: Sequence analysis of VP4 and VP7 genes of nontypeable strains identifies a new pair of outer capsid proteins representing novel P and G genotypes in bovine rotaviruses. Virology *276*:104–113, 2000.
372. Ratnam, S., Tobin, A. M., Flemming, J. B., et al.: False positive rotazyme results. Lancet *1*:345–346, 1984.
373. Raul-Velazquez, F., Calva, J. J., Lourdes-Guerrero, M., et al.: Cohort study of rotavirus serotype patterns in symptomatic and asymptomatic infections in Mexican children. Pediatr. Infect. Dis. J. *12*:54–61, 1993.
374. Rennels, M. B., Glass, R. I., Dennehy, P. H., et al.: Safety and efficacy of high-dose rhesus-human reassortant rotavirus vaccines—report of the National Multicenter Trial. Pediatrics *97*:7–13, 1996.
375. Rennels, M., Losonsky, G., Levine, M., et al.: Preliminary evaluation of the efficacy of rhesus rotavirus vaccine strain MMU 18006 in young children. Pediatr. Infect. Dis. J. *5*:587–588, 1986.
376. Rennels, M., Losonsky, G., Young, A., et al.: An efficacy trial of the rhesus rotavirus vaccine in Maryland. Am. J. Dis. Child. *144*:601–604, 1990.
377. Rennels, M. B., Parashar, U. D., Holman, R. C., et al.: Lack of an apparent association between intussusception and wild or vaccine rotavirus infection. Pediatr. Infect. Dis. J. *17*:924–925, 1998.
378. Research priorities for diarrhoeal diseases vaccines: Memorandum from a WHO meeting. Bull. World Health Organ. *69*:667–676, 1991.
379. Reves, R., Hossain, M., Midthun, K., et al.: An observational study of naturally acquired immunity to rotavirus diarrhea in a cohort of 363 Egyptian children. Am. J. Epidemiol. *130*:981–988, 1989.
380. Richardson, S., Grimwood, K., Gorrell, R., et al.: Extended excretion of rotavirus after severe diarrhoea in young children. Lancet *351*:1844–1848, 1998.
381. Riepenhoff-Talty, M., Bogger-Goren, S., Li, P., et al.: Development of serum and intestinal antibody response to rotavirus after naturally acquired rotavirus infection in man. J. Med. Virol. *8*:215–222, 1981.
382. Riepenhoff-Talty, M., Gouvea, V., Evans, M. J., et al.: Group C rotavirus (ROTA C) detected by liquid hybridization on PCR products of liver samples from four infants with extrahepatic biliary atresia (EHBA). *In* Program and Abstracts of the IXth International Congress of Virology, Glasgow, 1993.
383. Riepenhoff-Talty, M., Gouvea, V., Evans, M. J., et al.: Detection of group C rotavirus in infants with extrahepatic biliary atresia. J. Infect. Dis. *174*:8–15, 1996.
384. Riepenhoff-Talty, M., Lee, P. C., Carmody, P. J., et al.: Age-dependent rotavirus-enterocyte interactions. Proc. Soc. Exp. Biol. Med. *170*:146–154, 1982.
385. Riepenhoff-Talty, M., Morse, K., Wang, C. H., et al.: Epidemiology of group C rotavirus infection in Western New York women of childbearing age. J. Clin. Microbiol. *35*:486–488, 1997.
386. Rodger, S. M., Bishop, R. F., Birch, C., et al.: Molecular epidemiology of human rotaviruses in Melbourne, Australia, from 1973 to 1979, as determined by electrophoresis of genome ribonucleic acid. J. Clin. Microbiol. *13*:272–278, 1981.
387. Rodger, S. M., and Holmes, I. H.: Comparison of the genomes of simian, bovine, and human rotaviruses by gel electrophoresis and detection of genomic variation among bovine isolates. J. Virol. *30*:839–846, 1979.
388. Rodriguez, W. J., Kim, H. W., Arrobio, J. O., et al.: Clinical features of acute gastroenteritis associated with human reovirus–like agent in infants and young children. J. Pediatr. *91*:188–193, 1977.
389. Rodriguez, W. J., Kim, H. W., Brandt, C. D., et al.: Common exposure outbreak of gastroenteritis due to type 2 rotavirus with high secondary attack rate within families. J. Infect. Dis. *140*:353–357, 1979.
390. Rodriquez, W. J., Kim, H. W., Brandt, C., et al.: Rotavirus gastroenteritis in the Washington, D.C., area. Am. J. Dis. Child. *134*:777–779, 1980.
391. Rodriguez, W. J., Kim, H. W., Brandt, C. D., et al.: Longitudinal study of rotavirus infection and gastroenteritis in families served by a pediatric medical practice: Clinical and epidemiologic observations. Pediatr. Infect. Dis. J. *6*:170–176, 1987.
392. Rotbart, H. A., Nelson, W. L., Glode, M. P., et al.: Neonatal rotavirus associated necrotizing enterocolitis: Case control study and prospective surveillance during an outbreak. J. Pediatr. *112*:87–93, 1988.
393. Ruggeri, F. M., and Greenberg, H. B.: Antibodies to the trypsin cleavage peptide VP8 neutralize rotavirus by inhibiting binding of virions to target cells in culture. J. Virol. *65*:2211–2219, 1991.
394. Ruuska, T., and Vesikari, T.: A prospective study of acute diarrhoea in Finnish children from birth to $2^1/_2$ years of age. Acta Paediatr. Scand. *80*:500–507, 1991.
395. Ryder, R. W., Sack, D. A., Kapikian, A. Z., et al.: Enterotoxigenic *Escherichia coli* and reovirus-like agent in rural Bangladesh. Lancet *1*:659–662, 1976.
396. Saavedra, J.: Probiotics and infectious diarrhea. Am. J. Gastroenterol. *95*:S16–S18, 2000.
397. Sack, D. A., Chowdhury, A. M. A. K., Eusof, A., et al.: Oral hydration in rotavirus diarrhoea: A double blind comparison of sucrose with glucose electrolyte solution. Lancet *2*:280–283, 1978.
398. Saif, L. J.: Nongroup A rotaviruses. *In* Saif, L. J., and Theil, K. W. (eds.): Viral Diarrheas of Man and Animals. Boca Raton, CRC Press, 1990, pp. 73–95.
399. Saif, L. J., Bohl, E. H., Theil, K. W., et al.: Rotavirus-like, calicivirus-like, and 23-nm virus-like particles associated with diarrhea in young pigs. J. Clin. Microbiol. *12*:105–111, 1980.
400. Saif, L. J., and Jiang, B.: Nongroup A rotaviruses of humans and animals. Curr. Top. Microbiol. Immunol. *185*:339–371, 1994.
401. Saif, L. J., Redman, D. R., Smith, K. L., et al.: Passive immunity to bovine rotavirus in newborn calves fed colostrum supplements from immunized or non-immunized cows. Infect. Immun. *41*:1118–1131, 1983.
402. Salazar-Lindo, E., Santisteban-Ponce, J., Chea-Woo, E., and Gutierrez, M.: Racecadotril in the treatment of acute watery diarrhea in children. N. Engl. J. Med. *343*: 463–467, 2000.
403. Salmi, T. T., Arstila, P., and Koivkko, A.: Central nervous system involvement in patients with rotavirus gastroenteritis. Scand. J. Infect. Dis. *10*:29–31, 1978.
404. Santos, N., Lima, R. C. C., Pereira, C. F. A., and Gouvea, V.: Detection of rotavirus types G8 and G10 among Brazilian children with diarrhea. J. Clin. Microbiol. *36*:2727–2729, 1998.
405. Santosham, M., Burns, B., Nadkarni, V., et al.: Oral rehydration therapy for acute diarrhea in ambulatory children in the United States: A double-blind comparison of four different solutions. Pediatrics *76*:159–166, 1985.
406. Santosham, M., Daum, R. S., Dillman, L., et al: Oral rehydration therapy of infantile diarrhea: A controlled study of well-nourished children hospitalized in the United States and Panama. N. Engl. J. Med. *306*:1070–1076, 1982.
407. Santosham, M., Letson, G. W., Wolff, M., et al.: A field study of the safety and efficacy of two candidate vaccines in a Native American population. J. Infect. Dis. *163*:483–487, 1991.
408. Santosham, M., Yolken R. H., Quiroz, E., et al.: Detection of rotavirus in respiratory secretions of children with pneumonia. J. Pediatr. *103*:58, 1983.
409. Saulsbury, F. T., Winkelstein, J. A., and Yolken, R. H.: Chronic rotavirus infection in immunodeficiency. J. Pediatr. *97*:661–665, 1980.
410. Schaller, J. P., Saif, L. J., Cordle, C. T., et al.: Prevention of human rotavirus–induced diarrhea in gnotobiotic piglets using bovine antibody. J. Infect. Dis. *165*:623–630, 1992.
411. Schnagl, R. D., Rodger, S. M., and Holmes, I. H.: Variation in human rotavirus electropherotypes occurring between rotavirus gastroenteritis epidemics in central Australia. Infect. Immun. *33*:17–21, 1981.
412. Schreiber, R. A., and Kleinman, R. E.: Genetics, immunology, and biliary atresia: An opening or a division? J. Pediatr. Gastroenterol. Nutr. *16*:111–113, 1993.
413. Sen, A., Kobayashi, N., Das, S., et al.: Amplification of various genes of human group B rotavirus from stool specimens by RT-PCR. J. Clin. Virol. *17*:177–181, 2000.
414. Shaw, R., Groene, W., Mackow, E., et al.: VP4-specific intestinal antibody response to rotavirus in a murine model of heterotypic protection. J. Virol. *65*:3052–3059, 1991.
415. Shaw, R. D., Hempson, S. J., and Mackow, E. R.: Rotavirus diarrhea is caused by nonreplicating viral particles. J. Virol. *69*:5946–5950, 1995.
416. Shaw, R., Merchant, A., Groene, W., et al.: Persistence of intestinal antibody response to heterologous rotavirus infection in a murine model beyond 1 year. J. Clin. Microbiol. *31*:188–191, 1993.
417. Shaw, A. L., Rothnagel, R., Chen, D., et al.: Three-dimensional visualization of the rotavirus hemagglutinin structure. Cell *74*:693–701, 1993.
417a. Simonsen, L., Morens, D., Elixhauser, A., et al.: Effect of rotavirus vaccination programme on trends in admission of infants to hospital for intussusception. Lancet *358*:224–229, 2001.
418. Snodgrass, D., Fahey, K., Wells, P., et al.: Passive immunity in calf rotavirus infections: Maternal vaccination increases and prolongs immunoglobulin G1 antibody secretion in milk. Infect. Immun. *28*:344–349, 1980.
419. Snodgrass, D. R., Hoshino, Y., Fitzgerald, T. A., et al.: Identification of four VP4 serological types (P serotypes) of bovine rotavirus using viral reassortants. J. Gen. Virol. *73*:2319–2325, 1992.

420. Snodgrass, D. R., and Wells, P. W.: Rotavirus infection in lambs: Studies on passive protection. Arch. Virol. *52*:201–205, 1976.
421. Snodgrass, D., and Wells, P.: Passive immmunity in rotaviral infections. J. Am. Vet. Med. Assoc. *173*:565–568, 1978.
422. Soriano-Brucher, H. E., Avendano, P., O'Ryan, M., et al.: Use of bismuth subsalicylate in acute diarrhea in children. Rev. Infect. Dis. *12*:S51–S56, 1990.
423. Starkey, W. G., Collins, J., Wallis, T. S., et al.: Kinetics, tissue specificity and pathological changes in murine rotavirus infection of mice. J. Gen. Virol. *67*:2625–2634, 1986.
424. Steel, H. M., Garnham, S., Beards, G. M., et al.: Investigation of an outbreak of rotavirus infection in geriatric patients by serotyping and polyacrylamide gel electrophoresis (PAGE). J. Med. Virol. *37*:132–136, 1992.
425. Steele, A. D., Bos, P., and Alexander, J. J.: Clinical features of acute infantile gastroenteritis associated with human rotavirus subgroups I and II. J. Clin. Microbiol. *26*:2647–2649, 1988.
426. Steele, A. D., Garcia D., Sears J., et al.: Distribution of VP4 gene alleles in human rotaviruses by using probes to the hyperdivergent region of the VP4 gene. J. Clin. Microbiol. *31*:1735–1740, 1993.
427. Steele, A. D., James, V. L.: Seroepidemiology of human group C rotavirus in South Africa. J. Clin. Microbiol. *37*:4142–4144, 1999.
428. Steele, A. D., van Niekerk, M. C., and Mphahlele, M. J.: Geographic distribution of human rotavirus VP4 genotypes and VP7 serotypes in five South African regions. J. Clin. Microbiol. *33*:1516–1519, 1995.
429. Steinhoff, M. C.: Rotavirus: The first five years. J. Pediatr. *96*:611–622, 1980.
430. Stirazaker, S. C., and Both, G. W.: The signal peptide of the rotavirus glycoprotein VP7 is essential for its retention in the ER as an integral membrane protein. Cell *56*:741–747, 1989.
431. Superti, F., and Donelli, G.: Gangliosides as binding sites in SA-11 rotavirus infection of LLC-MK2 cells. J. Gen. Virol. *72*:2467–2474, 1991.
432. Suzuki, H., Kitaoka, S., Konno, T., et al.: Two modes of human rotavirus entry into MA104 cells. Arch. Virol. *85*:25–34, 1985.
433. Suzuki, H., Kitaoka, S., Sato, T., et al.: Further investigation on the mode of entry of human rotavirus into cells. Arch. Virol. *91*:135–144, 1986.
434. Suzuki, H., and Konno, T.: Reovirus-like particles in jejunal mucosa of a Japanese infant with acute infectious non-bacterial gastroenteritis. Tohoku J. Exp. Med. *115*:199–221, 1975.
435. Svensson, L., Uhnoo, I., Grandien, M., et al.: Molecular epidemiology of rotavirus infections in Uppsala, Sweden, 1981: Disappearance of a predominant electropherotype. J. Med. Virol. *18*:101–111, 1986.
436. Taniguchi, K., Maloy, W., Nishikawa, K., et al.: Identification of cross-reactive and serotype 2–specific neutralization epitopes on VP3 of human rotavirus. J. Virol. *62*:2421–2426, 1988.
437. Taniguchi, K., Urasawa, T., Urasawa, S., et al.: Production of subgroup-specific monoclonal antibodies to an enzyme-linked immunosorbent assay for subgroup determination. J. Med. Virol. *14*:115–125, 1984.
438. Tauscher, G. I., and Desselberger, U.: Viral determinants of rotavirus pathogenicity in pigs: Production of reassortants by asynchronous co-infection. J. Virol. *71*:853–857, 1997.
439. Taylor, J. A., O'Brien, J. A., and Yeager, M.: The cytoplasmic tail of NSP4, the endoplasmic reticulum–localized non-structural glycoprotein of rotavirus, contains distinct virus binding and coiled coil domains. EMBO J. *15*:4469–4476, 1996.
440. Theil, K. W., Bohl, E. H., Cross, R. F., et al.: Pathogenesis of porcine rotaviral infection in experimentally inoculated gnotobiotic pigs. Am. J. Vet. Res. *39*:213–220, 1978.
441. Thomas, E. E., Puterman, M. L., Kawano, E., et al.: Evaluation of seven immunoassays for detection of rotavirus in pediatric stool samples. J. Clin. Microbiol. *26*:1189–1193, 1988.
442. Tian, P., Ball, J. M., Zeng, C. Q. Y., and Estes, M. K.: The rotavirus non-structural glycoprotein NSP4 possesses membrane destabilization activity. J. Virol. *70*:6973–6981, 1996.
443. Tian, P., Estes, M. K., Hu, Y., et al.: The rotavirus nonstructural glycoprotein NSP4 mobilizes Ca^{2+} from the endoplasmic reticulum. J. Virol. *69*:5763–5772, 1995.
444. Tian, P., Hu, Y., Schilling, W. P., et al.: The nonstructural glycoprotein of rotavirus affects intracellular calcium levels. J. Virol. *68*:251–257, 1994.
445. Timenetsky, M. C. S. T., Santos, N., and Gouvea, V.: Survey of rotavirus G and P types associated with human gastroenteritis in São Paulo, Brazil, from 1986 to 1992. J. Clin. Microbiol. *32*:2622–2624, 1994.
446. Torres-Medina, A.: Effect of combined rotavirus and *Escherichia coli* in neonatal gnotobiotic calves. Am. J. Vet. Res. *45*:643–651, 1984.
447. Totterdell, B. M., Banatvala, J. E., Chrystie, I. L., et al.: Systemic lymphoproliferative responses to rotavirus. J. Med. Virol. *25*:37–44, 1988.
448. Trabelsi, A., Peenze, I., Pager, C., et al.: Distribution of rotavirus VP7 serotypes and VP4 genotypes circulating in Sousse, Tunisia, from 1995 to 1999: Emergence of natural human reassortants. J. Clin. Microbiol. *38*:3415–3419, 2000.
449. Treanor, J. J., Clark, H. F., Pichichero, M., et al.: Evaluation of the protective efficacy of a serotype 1 bovine-human rotavirus reassortant vaccine in infants. Pediatr. Infect. Dis. J. *14*:301–307, 1995.
450. Troonen, H.: False positive rotazyme results. Lancet *1*:345, 1984.
451. Tsunemitsu, H., Jiang, B., and Saif, L. J.: Detection of group C rotavirus antigens and antibodies in animals and humans by ELISA. J. Clin. Microbiol. *30*:2129–2134, 1992.
452. Tucker, A. W., Haddix, A. C., Bresee, J. S., et al.: Cost-effectiveness analysis of a rotavirus immunization program for the United States. J. A. M. A. *279*:1371–1376, 1998.
453. Turner, R. B., and Kelsey, D. K.: Passive immunization for prevention of rotavirus illness in healthy infants. Pediatr. Infect. Dis. J. *12*:718–722, 1993.
454. Tzipori, S., Unicomb, L., Bishop, R., et al.: Studies on attenuation of rotavirus: A comparison in piglets between virulent virus and its attenuated derivative. Arch. Virol. *109*:197–205, 1989.
455. Uhnoo, I., Olding-Stenkvist, E., and Kreuger, A.: Clinical features of acute gastroenteritis associated with rotavirus, enteric adenoviruses, and bacteria. Arch. Dis. Child. *61*:732–738, 1986.
456. Uhnoo, I., Riepenhoff-Talty, M., Chegas, P., et al.: Effect of malnutrition on extraintestinal spread of rotavirus and development of hepatitis in mice. Nutr. Res. *10*:1419–1429, 1990.
457. Uhnoo, I., Riepenhoff-Talty, M., Dharakul, T., et al.: Extramucosal spread and development of hepatitis with rhesus rotavirus in immunodeficient and normal mice. J. Virol. *64*:361–368, 1990.
458. Unicomb, L. E., Podder, G., Gentsch, J. R., et al.: Evidence of high-frequency genomic reassortment of Group A rotavirus strains in Bangladesh: Emergence of Type G9 in 1995. J. Clin. Microbiol. *37*:1885–1891, 1999.
459. Urasawa, S., Hasegawa, A., Urasawa, T., et al.: Antigenic and genetic analyses of human rotaviruses in Chiang Mai, Thailand: Evidence for a close relationship between human and animal rotaviruses. J. Infect. Dis. *166*:227–234, 1992.
460. Urasawa, S., Urasawa, T., and Taniguchi, K.: Genetic reassortment between two human rotaviruses having different serotype and subgroup specificities. J. Gen. Virol. *67*:1551–1559, 1986.
461. Ushijima, H., Honma, H., Mukoyama, A., et al.: Detection of group C rotaviruses in Tokyo. J. Med. Virol. *27*:299–303, 1989.
462. Ushiyima, H., Tajima, T., Tagaya, M., et al.: Rotavirus and central nervous system. Brain.Dev. *6*:215, 1984.
463. Valenzuela, S., Pizarro, J., Sandino, A. M., et al.: Photoaffinity labeling of rotavirus VP1 with 8-azido-ATP: Identification of the viral RNA polymerase. J. Virol. *65*:3964–3967, 1991.
464. VanCott, J. L., McNeal, M. M., Flint, J., et al.: Role for T cell–independent B cell activity in the resolution of primary rotavirus infection in mice. Eur. J. Immunol. *31*:3380-3387, 2001.
465. Varshney, K. C., Bridger, J. C., Parsons, K. R., et al.: The lesions of rotavirus infection in 1- and 10-day-old gnotobiotic calves. Vet. Pathol. *32*:619–627, 1995.
466. Vasquez, M., Sandino, A. M., Pizarro, J. M., et al.: Function of rotavirus VP3 polypeptide in viral morphogenesis. J. Gen. Virol. *74*:937–941, 1993.
467. Velazquez, F. R., Matson, D. O., Calva, J. J., et al.: Rotavirus infection in infants as protection against subsequent infections. N. Engl. J. Med. *335*:1022–1028, 1996.
468. Velazquez, F. R., Matson, D. O., Guerrero, M. L., et al.: Serum antibody as a marker of protection against natural rotavirus infection and disease. J. Infect. Dis. *182*:1602–1609, 2000.
469. Vende, P., Piron, M., Castagne, N., and Poncet, D.: Efficient translation of rotavirus mRNA requires simultaneous interaction of NSP3 with the eukaryotic translation initiation factor eIF4G and the mRNA 3′ end. J. Virol. *74*:7064–7071, 2000.
470. Vesikari, T.: Clinical trials of live oral rotavirus vaccines: The Finnish experience. Vaccine *11*:255–261, 1993.
471. Vesikari, T., Isolauri, E., Delem, A., et al.: Immunogenicity and safety of live oral attenuated bovine rotavirus vaccine strain RIT 4237 in adults and young children. Lancet *2*:807–811, 1983.
472. Vesikari, T., Isolauri, E., Delem, A., et al.: Clinical efficacy of the RIT 4237 live attenuated bovine rotavirus vaccine in infants vaccinated before a rotavirus epidemic. J. Pediatr. *107*:189–194, 1985.
473. Vesikari, T., Isolauri, E., D'Hondt, E., et al.: Protection of infants against rotavirus diarrhoea by RIT 4237 attenuated bovine rotavirus strain vaccine. Lancet *1*:977–981, 1984.
474. Vesikari, T., Kapikian, A. Z., Delem, A., et al.: A comparative trial of rhesus monkey (RRV-1) and bovine (RIT 4237) oral rotavirus vaccines in young children. J. Infect. Dis. *153*:832, 1986.
475. Vesikari, T., Rautanen, T., Varis, T., et al.: Rhesus rotavirus candidate vaccine: Clinical trial in children vaccinated between 2 and 5 months of age. Am. J. Dis. Child. *144*:285–289, 1990.
476. Vesikari, T., Ruuska, T., Green, K., et al.: Protective efficacy against serotype 1 rotavirus diarrhea by live oral rhesus-human reassortant rotavirus vaccines with human rotavirus VP7 serotype 1 or 2 specificity. Pediatr. Infect. Dis. J. *11*:535–542, 1992.
477. Vesikari, T., Ruuska, T., Koivu, H., et al.: Evaluation of the M37 human rotavirus vaccine in 2- to 6-month-old infants. Pediatr. Infect. Dis. J. *10*:912–917, 1991.
478. Vesikari, T., Sarkkinen, H. K., and Maki, M.: Quantitative aspects of rotavirus excretion in childhood. Acta Pediatr. Scand. *70*:717–721, 1981.

479. Wang, L., Huang, J. A., Nagesha, H. S., et al.: Bacterial expression of the major antigenic regions of porcine rotavirus VP7 induces a neutralizing immune response in mice. Vaccine *17*:2636–2645, 1999.
480. Ward, R. L., Bernstein, D. I., and U.S. Rotavirus Vaccine Efficacy Group: Protection against rotavirus disease following natural rotavirus infection. J. Infect. Dis. *169*:900–904, 1994.
481. Ward, R. L., Bernstein, D. I., Shukla, R., et al.: Effects of antibody to rotavirus on protection of adults challenged with a human rotavirus. J. Infect. Dis. *159*:79–88, 1989.
482. Ward, R. L., Bernstein, D. I., Shukla, R., et al.: Protection of adults rechallenged with a human rotavirus. J. Infect. Dis. *161*:440–445, 1990.
483. Ward, R. L., Clemens, J. D., Knowlton, D. R., et al.: Evidence that protection against rotavirus diarrhea after natural infection is not dependent on serotype-specific neutralizing antibody. J. Infect. Dis. *166*:1251–1257, 1992.
484. Ward, R. L., Clemens, J. D., Sack, D. A., et al.: Culture adaptation and characterization of group A rotaviruses causing diarrheal illnesses in Bangladesh from 1985 to 1986. J. Clin. Microbiol. *29*:1915–1923, 1991.
485. Ward, R. L., and Knowlton, D. R.: Genotypic selection following co-infection of cultured cells with subgroup 1 and subgroup 2 human rotaviruses. J. Gen. Virol. *70*:1691–1699, 1989.
486. Ward, R. L., Knowlton, D. R., and Greenberg, H. B.: Phenotypic mixing during coinfection of cells with two strains of human rotavirus. J. Virol. *62*:4358–4361, 1988.
487. Ward, R. L., Knowlton, D. R., Greenberg, H. B., et al.: Serum neutralizing antibody to VP4 and VP7 proteins in infants following vaccination with WC3 bovine rotavirus. J. Virol. *64*:2687–2691, 1990.
488. Ward, R. L., Knowlton, D. R., and Hurst, P.-F. L.: Reassortant formation and selection following coinfection of cultured cells with subgroup 2 human rotaviruses. J. Gen. Virol. *69*:149–162, 1988.
489. Ward, R. L., Knowlton, D. R., and Pierce, M. J.: Efficiency of human rotavirus propagation in cell culture. J. Clin. Microbiol. *19*:748–753, 1984.
490. Ward, R., Knowlton, D., Schiff, G., et al.: Relative concentrations of serum neutralizing antibody to VP3 and VP7 proteins in adults infected with a human rotavirus. J. Virol. *62*:1543–1549, 1988.
491. Ward, R. L., Knowlton, D. R., Zito, E. T., et al.: Serologic correlates of immunity in a tetravalent reassortant rotavirus vaccine trial. J. Infect. Dis. *176*:570–577, 1997.
492. Ward, R. L., Mason, B. B., Bernstein, D. I., et al.: Attenuation of a human rotavirus vaccine candidate did not correlate with mutations in the NSP4 protein gene. J. Virol. *71*:6267–6270, 1997.
493. Ward, R. L., McNeal, M. M., Sander, D. S., et al.: Immunodominance of the VP4 neutralization protein of rotavirus in protective natural infections of young children. J. Virol. *67*:464–468, 1993.
494. Ward, R. L., McNeal, M. M., and Sheridan, J. F.: Development of an adult mouse model for studies on protection against rotavirus. J. Virol. *64*:5070–5075, 1990.
495. Ward, R. L., McNeal, M. M., and Sheridan, J.: Evidence that active protection following oral immunization of mice with live rotavirus is not dependent on neutralizing antibody. Virology *188*:57–66, 1992.
496. Ward, R. L., Nakagomi, O., Knowlton, D. R., et al.: Evidence for natural reassortants of human rotaviruses belonging to different genogroups. J. Virol. *64*:3219–3225, 1990.
497. Wenman, W. M., Hinde, D., Feltham, S., et al.: Rotavirus infection in adults. N. Engl. J. Med. *301*:303–306, 1979.
498. Wentz, M. J., Patton, J. T., and Ramig, R. F.: The 3′-terminal consensus sequence of rotavirus mRNA is the minimal promoter of negative-strand RNA synthesis. J. Virol. *70*:7833–7841, 1996.
499. Wong, C. J., Price, Z., and Bruckner, D. A.: Aseptic meningitis in an infant with rotavirus gastroenteritis. Pediatr. Infect. Dis. *3*:244–246, 1984.
500. Woode, G. N., Bridger, J. C., Jones, J. M., et al.: Morphological and antigenic relationships between viruses (rotaviruses) from acute gastroenteritis of children, calves, piglets, mice, and foals. Infect. Immun. *14*:804–810, 1976.
501. Woode, G., Zheng, S., Rosen, B., et al.: Protection between different serotypes of bovine rotavirus in gnotobiotic calves: Specificity of serum antibody and coproantibody responses. J. Clin. Microbiol. *25*:1052–1058, 1987.
502. Wyatt, R. G., Greenberg, H. B., James, W. D., et al.: Definition of human rotavirus serotypes by plaque reduction assay. Infect. Immun. *37*:110–115, 1982.
503. Wyatt, R. G., James, H. D., Jr., Pittman, A. L., et al.: Direct isolation in cell culture of human rotaviruses and their characterization into four serotypes. J. Clin. Microbiol. *18*:310–317, 1983.
504. Wyatt, R. G., Kalica, A. R., Mebus, C. A., et al.: Reovirus-like agents (rotaviruses) associated with diarrheal illness in animals and man. *In* Pollard, M. (ed.): Perspectives in Virology. New York, Raven Press, 1978, pp. 121–145.
505. Wyatt, R. G., Yolken, R. H., Urrutia, J. J., et al.: Diarrhea associated with rotavirus in rural Guatemala: A longitudinal study of 24 infants and young children. Am. J. Trop. Med. Hyg. *28*:325–328, 1979.
506. Yeager, M., Berriman, J. A., Baker, T. S., et al.: Three-dimensional structure of the rotavirus haemagglutinin VP4 by cryo-electron microscopy and difference map analysis. EMBO J. *13*:1011–1018, 1994.
507. Yeager, M., Dryden, K. A., Olson, N. H., et al.: Three-dimensional structure of rhesus rotavirus by cryo-electron microscopy and image reconstruction. J. Cell Biol. *110*:2133–2144, 1990.
508. Yolken, R., Arango-Jaramillo, S., Eiden, J., et al.: Lack of genomic reassortment following infection of infant rats with group A and group B rotaviruses. J. Infect. Dis. *158*:1120–1123, 1988.
509. Yolken, R. H., Bishop, C. A., Townsend, T. R., et al.: Infectious gastroenteritis in bone-marrow transplant recipients. N. Engl. J. Med. *306*:1009–1012, 1982.
510. Yolken, R. H., and Murphy, M.: Sudden infant death syndrome associated with rotavirus infection. J. Med. Virol. *10*:291–296, 1982.
511. Yuan, L., Geyer, A., Hodgins, D. C., et al.: Intranasal administration of 2/6-rotavirus-like particles with mutant *Escherichia coli* heat-labile toxin (LT-R192G) induces antibody-secreting cell responses but not protective immunity in gnotobiotic pigs. J. Virol. *74*:8843–8853, 2000.
512. Zao, C.-L., Yu, W.-N., Kao, C.-L., et al.: Sequence analysis of VP1 and VP7 genes suggests occurrence of a reassortant of G2 rotavirus responsible for an epidemic of gastroenteritis. J. Gen. Virol. *80*:1407–1415, 1999.
513. Zarate, S., Espinosa, R., Romero, P., et al.: Integrin $\alpha_2\beta_1$ mediates the cell attachment at the rotavirus neuraminidase resistant variant nar3. Virology *278*:50–54, 2000.
514. Zarate, S., Espinosa, R., Romero, P., et al.: The VP5 domain of VP4 can mediate attachment of rotaviruses to cells. J. Virol. *74*:593–599, 2000.
515. Zeng, C. Q. Y., Estes, M. K., Charpilienne, A., and Cohen, J.: The N terminus of rotavirus VP2 is necessary for encapsidation of VP1 and VP3. J. Virol. *72*:201–208, 1998.
516. Zeng, C. Q. Y., Labbé, M., Cohen, J., et al.: Characterization of rotavirus VP2 particles. Virology *201*:55–65, 1994.
517. Zhang, M., Zeng, C. Q. Y., Dong, Y., et al.: Mutations in rotavirus nonstructural glycoprotein NSP4 are associated with altered virus virulence. J. Virol. *72*:3666–3672, 1998.
518. Zheng, B. J., Chang, R. X., Ma, G. Z., et al.: Rotavirus infection of the oropharynx and respiratory tract in young children. J. Med. Virol. *34*:29–37, 1991.
519. Zheng, B. J., Lo, S. K. F., Tam, J. S. L., et al.: Prospective study of community-acquired rotavirus infection. J. Clin. Microbiol. *27*:2083–2090, 1989.

TOGAVIRIDAE

CHAPTER 177 Rubella Virus

JAMES D. CHERRY

Rubella (German measles) is a generally mild, exanthematous, infectious illness in which morbidity and mortality in children usually are minimal. However, infection in pregnancy may result in fetal infection as well, and this usually is associated with considerable adversity for the developing infant. The rubella virus has only one known type.

History

In ancient history, rubella as a disease is lost among the other prominent exanthematous diseases (i.e., scarlet fever, measles, and smallpox). In an extensive review, Griffith[190] suggested that rubella was known to the early Arabian physicians under the name *al-hamikah;* they considered rubella a form of measles, however. Two German physicians, de Bergen in 1752 and Orlow in 1758, usually are credited with providing the first clinical descriptions of rubella as a specific entity.[190, 525] In early writings, rubella generally was called *Rötheln.*[149, 525] However, because of the great interest of German physicians in the disease during the period from the mid-18th to the mid-19th centuries, the name *German measles* frequently was used in other countries.

In 1866, a Scottish physician named Veale described 30 cases of German measles. In his paper, he gave the illness its present name, rubella. His opinion was that the German name Rötheln was too harsh and foreign and that other possible names—rubeola notha and rosalia idiopathica—were too long for general use and could be confused with measles.[149, 501] Other historical synonyms of rubella include rubeola, rubeola sine catarrho, rubeola epidemica, rubeola morbillosa, rubeola scarlatinosa, rosania, roseola, roseola epidemica, rosalia, scarlatina morbillosa, scarlatina hybrida, morbilli scarlatinosi, feuer masern, roséole, roséole idiopathique, rubéole, rougéole fausse, French measles, false measles, bastard measles, hybrid measles, and bastard scarlatina.[190]

In 1881 at the International Congress of Medicine in London, a consensus was reached that rubella was a distinct disease. Rubella was thought to be similar in some respects but not identical to measles or scarlatina. By the beginning of the 20th century, the clinical description of rubella was complete, except that joint manifestations had received curiously little notation.[14, 106, 149, 190, 311, 409, 486]

Rubella gained its present-day importance in 1941 when Gregg,[189] an Australian ophthalmologist, reported congenital defects in babies of mothers who had rubella during early pregnancy. In spite of considerable skepticism, Gregg's observations were confirmed quickly by Swan and colleagues[469, 470] in Australia and other investigators in the United States and the United Kingdom.[135, 386, 392, 525] By 1947, 28 communications describing 500 children with severe congenital defects associated with maternal rubella had appeared in the literature.[525]

In 1938, Hiro and Tasaka[225] demonstrated that rubella was a disease of viral etiology by transmission of disease to humans via the subcutaneous injection of filtered nasal washings. In 1942, Habel[197] was able to infect monkeys with nasal washings and blood from human cases. In 1962, rubella virus first was propagated in the laboratory; two investigative teams, Weller and Neva[524] and Parkman and colleagues,[353] using different techniques, reported the growth of rubella virus in tissue culture.

The isolation of rubella virus in 1962 paved the way for definitive study of the 1964 rubella pandemic. The results of extensive virologic, serologic, and epidemiologic investigation were presented at a Rubella Symposium in May 1965.[259] After the isolation of rubella virus in tissue culture, an intensive worldwide effort to develop vaccines was mounted. The accumulation of these experiences resulted in an extensive body of knowledge related to rubella and rubella immunization that was presented at the International Conference on Rubella Immunization in February 1969.[260] Live attenuated rubella virus vaccines were licensed for use in mid-1969 in the United States.[261, 310] In the 33-year period since vaccine licensure and its universal use in the United States, the yearly occurrence of rubella has fallen from 40,000 cases to fewer than 300.[63, 66, 67, 69, 70, 375, 385, 531]

Properties

CLASSIFICATION

Rubella virus is placed in the *Rubivirus* genus of the family *Togaviridae.*[143, 418, 535] At present, it is the only species in this genus. The virus is similar physiochemically to the other member of its family (alphavirus) but is unrelated serologically. Rubella virus has no invertebrate host (a characteristic of all alphaviruses), and humans are the only known vertebrate host.

PHYSICAL PROPERTIES

The rubella virion is spherical with a diameter of 60 to 70 nm, and it consists of a capsid protein (C) and two glycoproteins (E1 and E2).[77, 276, 293, 362, 418, 535] E1 (relative molecular weight, 58,000) and E2 (relative molecular weight, 42,000 to 47,000) are glycosylated and are located on the viral surface membrane. E1 is the viral hemagglutinin that is found on 5- to 6-nm surface projections.[227, 362] The nucleocapsid has a diameter of 30 to 40 nm and is composed of polypeptide (C protein) and the genomic RNA. The nucleic acid of rubella virus is single-stranded RNA with a molecular weight of 3.2 to 3.8 × 10^6.[427] The outer coat of the virus (envelope) is lipoprotein in nature with host-cell lipid and virus-specified polypeptides.

Rubella virus is relatively sensitive to heat; it generally has been found to lose infectivity within 30 minutes at 56° C.[141, 354, 367] However, Kistler and Sapatino[253] observed that some infectivity persists even after heating for 60 minutes at 70° C. At 37° C in the presence of 2 percent serum, 90 percent is inactivated in 3 hours.[354] At 4° C, with protein stabilization, viral titers are maintained for 7 or more days. The virus is stable indefinitely at −60° C and below but labile at normal (−10° to −20° C) refrigeration temperatures. When stabilized with protein, the virus can survive several rapid freeze-thaw cycles without significant loss of titer.[412]

Rubella virus is sensitive to ultraviolet light. In 1 hour, a high-titer cell-free virus suspension was inactivated by an intensity of 1350 μW/cm^2; on the other hand, a tissue culture suspension of virus was not inactivated completely when it was exposed to a similar intensity of radiation.[253] Rubella virus is sensitive to visible light, and this photosensitivity can be potentiated by the basic dye proflavine.[43]

The virus also is sensitive to pH extremes of less than 6.8 and greater than 8.1.[74] The following chemicals rapidly inactivate rubella virus: ether, acetone, chloroform, deoxycholate, formalin, β-propiolactone, ethylene oxide, free chlorine, and 70 percent alcohol.[367] It is resistant to thimerosal.

ANTIGENIC COMPOSITION

Rubella virus infection of tissue culture cells results in the production of infectious virus that can be neutralized by specific antiserum. Specific viral antibodies can be identified by hemagglutination inhibition (HI), complement fixation (CF), precipitation in gel, platelet aggregation, passive hemagglutination (PH), single radial hemolysis, latex agglutination (LA), enzyme-linked immunosorbent assay (ELISA), and immunofluorescence.* Neutralization and HI identify antibodies that inhibit specific biologic functions of the virus, whereas the other assays identify only the formation of antigen-antibody complexes. The E1 glycoprotein is the predominant erythrocyte-binding and neutralization site of the virus.[488, 518] Weak neuraminidase activity also has been associated with purified rubella virus.[22]

In 1967, Stewart and associates[461] reported that tissue culture–grown rubella virus produced hemagglutination of erythrocytes from chickens that were younger than 1 day and from one goose and one lamb, but no hemagglutination was observed with adult chicken, guinea pig, and other red cell preparations commonly used. Subsequently, techniques involving careful control of test system diluents have revealed that red cells from many different animals are agglutinated by rubella virus.[281, 420] Viral hemagglutinin is stable at −20° C for months and at 4° C for several weeks but is destroyed rapidly by heat.[166, 199]

Sever and colleagues[435] first demonstrated that supernatant fluid from primary African green monkey kidney (AGMK) and RK-13 rabbit kidney tissue cultures contained useful complement-fixing antigens. Two distinct rubella complement-fixing antigens exist.[422] One of the antigens is similar in size and weight to both the hemagglutinin and infectious virus; the other "soluble" antigen is smaller, with a buoyant density of 1.08 g/mL. The soluble antigen is noninfectious and does not contain nucleic acid.[367] Rubella complement-fixing antigens retain their antigenicity after ether treatment.

Two major small-particle antigens have been identified in the medium of tissue culture–infected cells by immunodiffusion.[273, 274, 423] These two soluble antigens are structural components of the virion, and natural infection with rubella virus results in the formation of serum precipitating antibodies. These antigens have been designated theta and iota. Their importance lies in the fact that antibody to the iota antigen rarely is noted in the serum of recipients of some rubella vaccines; therefore, they may be of value in studying vaccine-induced immunity.[59, 275]

The E1 glycoprotein is the dominant surface molecule of rubella virus.[78] It is the main target of the humoral antibody response for both detection and elimination of the virus. HI and neutralization sites have been localized to a small segment of the E1 glycoprotein ($E1_{245}$ to $E1_{285}$).

Seventeen T-cell epitopes have been identified with the lymphoproliferation assay.[78, 322] They involve the capsid protein and E1 and E2 glycoproteins.

Molecular analysis of rubella virus epidemiology from 1961 to 1997 in North America, Europe, and Asia found no major antigenic variation.[159]

TISSUE CULTURE GROWTH

Rubella virus grows in many different tissue cultures, including cell strains, cell lines, and primary cells.[113, 296, 297, 354, 367, 534, 535] Cell sources include mature and embryonic tissue from humans and other primates, rabbits, swine, dogs, birds, hamsters, and cattle. In tissue culture, rubella virus growth can be identified by either cytopathic effect or the ability to produce interference of the growth of another tissue culture–susceptible virus.

The method used most commonly for primary isolation of rubella virus from clinical material is the interference technique with primary AGMK cells.[353] In this system, nonadapted rubella virus grows readily but does not produce a cytopathic effect. Infection is demonstrated in AGMK tissue culture by the failure of a typical enterovirus cytopathic effect to occur after challenge of the culture with echovirus 11 or another suitable enterovirus. A common alternative to the AGMK–echovirus 11 interference system for primary isolation of rubella virus is use of the RK-13 rabbit kidney cell line, in which infection can be identified by cytopathic effect. For laboratory study and determination of neutralizing antibody, many different cell lines (such as RK-13, BHK-21, and LLC-MK2) can be used. The highest titers of rubella virus are produced in the BHK-21 and Vero cell lines.

Kinetic studies in tissue culture indicate that virus adsorption is complete within 90 minutes and the eclipse period lasts approximately 12 hours. The first new virus noted is cell associated, and it is followed in 2 to 4 hours by extracellular virus. In primary cell culture, titers of both cell-associated and free virus reach 10^3 $TCID_{50}$/mL by the fourth day; are not attained until approximately the 17th day. In all cell systems, chronic infection occurs but is limited in some cultures by the cytopathic effect. Rubella virus induces the formation of plaques in several cell lines.

*See references 30, 36, 76, 79, 80, 133, 134, 145, 156, 221, 274, 275, 294, 358, 367, 405, 406, 498, 535, 544.

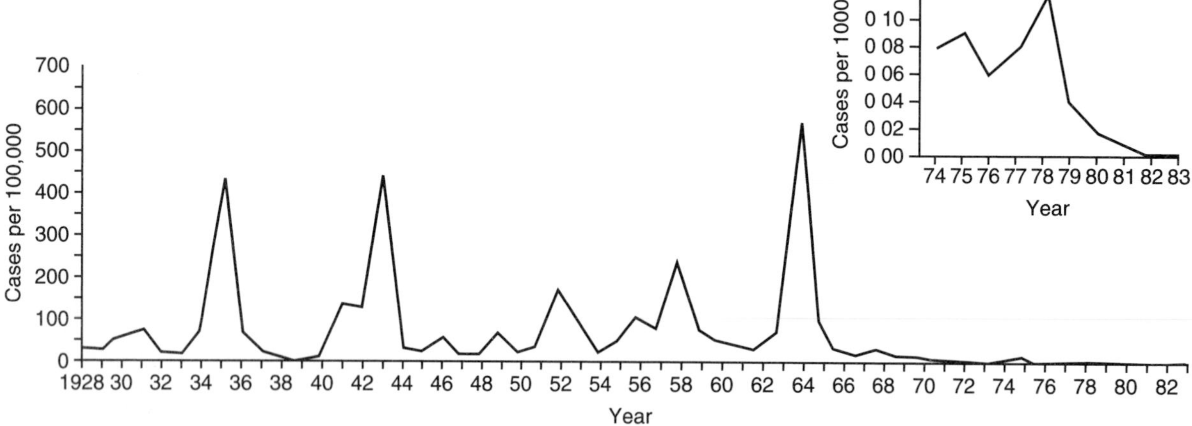

FIGURE 177–1 ■ Rubella incidence in 10 selected areas (Maine, Rhode Island, Connecticut, New York City, Ohio, Illinois, Wisconsin, Maryland, Washington, and Massachusetts) of the United States, 1928 to 1983. (From Rubella and congenital rubella surveillance, 1983. M. M. W. R. CDC Surveill. Summ. *33*[4]:1SS–10SS, 1984.)

ANIMAL SUSCEPTIBILITY

Although natural infection is known to occur only in humans, several other primates have been infected experimentally.[296, 354, 367] In addition to primates, rabbits, hamsters, ferrets, guinea pigs, and suckling mice all have been infected with rubella virus.

Epidemiology

In contrast to measles and other diseases with clearly apparent dramatic cycles, knowledge of rubella epidemiology has been acquired primarily during the last 70 years. Major events during this period that stimulated epidemiologic interest were the observation of teratogenicity in 1941,[189] isolation of the virus in the early 1960s,[353, 524] and the pandemic of 1964. Unfortunately, rubella was not a reportable disease in the United States until 1966, so considerable gaps exist in the available information. At present, we are in a new epidemiologic era because of the widespread use of rubella vaccine. Predicting the incidence of rubella today must take into account the extent and method of vaccine use in the population under surveillance.

INCIDENCE AND PREVALENCE

Epidemic Behavior

The epidemic pattern of rubella in selected areas of the United States in the prevaccine and early vaccine eras is presented in Figure 177–1. The number of reported cases of rubella and congenital rubella syndrome by year in the vaccine era are presented in Figure 177–2. It generally is stated that the rubella epidemic cycle is one of 6- to 9-year intervals, with each cycle consisting of a build-up and fall in incidence over a 3- to 4-year period.[233, 234] However, a close look at Figure 177–1 suggests that the basic pattern in the prevaccine era was a 3.6-year cycle. Of the 11 peaks from 1928 to 1968, all but 2 occurred in a 2- to 4-year span, with a median of 3 years. Over and above the 3-year cycle is the better known 6- to 9-year cycle of major disease. Pandemics occurred in the periods 1941 to 1944 and 1963 to 1965.

Since the introduction and widespread use of rubella vaccine in the United States, epidemic rubella has occurred only once on a national scale[63, 65, 385] (see Fig. 177–2). In 1991, 1401 and 47 cases of rubella and congenital rubella syndrome, respectively, were reported. However, in countries in which universal childhood immunization had not been carriedout, periodic epidemics continued to occur. Epidemic rubella was documented in the former Czechoslovakia in 1972; in Australia in 1969 to 1970 and 1975 to 1976; in Israel in 1972, 1979, and 1983; in Japan in 1975 to 1977; in Brazil in 1981; and in the United Kingdom in 1971 to 1973, 1978, and 1983.*

The incidence of rubella varies with the epidemic cycle, the number of susceptible people within a population group, and the intrapersonal contact within the group. In closed populations such as military training centers and institutions for the mentally handicapped, the attack rate after the introduction of disease approaches 100 percent in susceptible individuals.[236, 237, 277] Introduction of disease in the family also affects virtually all susceptible persons.[167, 168] In community epidemics, attack rates in susceptible people are estimated to range from 50 to 90 percent.

Age Groups

The age distribution of reported rubella cases and estimated incidence rates in Illinois, Massachusetts, and New York City for 1966 through 1968 and the entire United States for 1985 through 1987[69] are presented in Table 177–1. In the period immediately before the introduction of vaccine (1966 to 1968), the attack rate was highest in the 5- to 9-year-old age group, and the incidence was high in preschool-age children. The overall reduction in the rate of rubella from the prevaccine era to 1987 was 99.2 percent. However, 50.2 percent of the cases reported in the period 1985 through 1988 were in persons older than 19 years; in the prevaccine period (1966 through 1968), the percentage in this age group was 10.2. In 1999, 75 percent of the reported cases occurred in persons older than 19 years.[385] During the last 21 years, outbreaks of rubella have occurred in prisons,[72] in colleges and universities,[71] in hospitals,[73, 374, 463] at worksites,[70, 181, 385] in communities with high foreign-born populations,[385] and among the Amish in six areas of the United States.[67]

Because rubella was not a reportable disease in the United States until 1966, few age-specific incidence or

*See references 148, 180, 206, 232, 305, 410, 450, 471, 472.

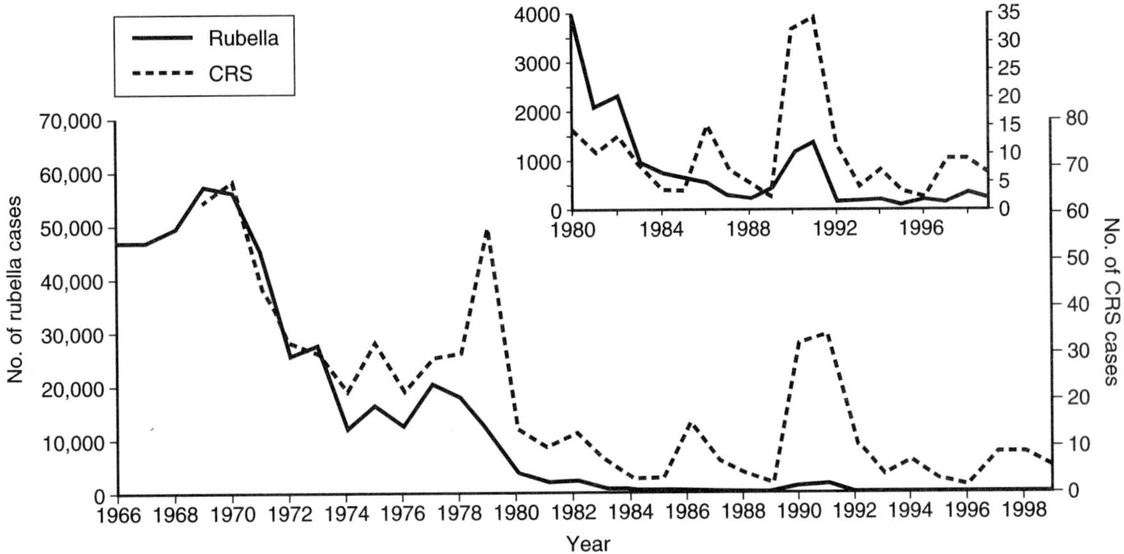

FIGURE 177–2 ■ Number of reported cases of rubella and congenital rubella syndrome (CRS) in the United States from 1966 to 1998. (From Reef, S. E., Frey, T. K., Theal, K., et al.: The changing epidemiology of rubella in the 1990s on the verge of elimination and new challenges for control and prevention. J. A. M. A. *287*:464–472, 2002. Copyright 2002, American Medical Association.)

prevalence data relating to epidemic disease are available. In Table 177–2, age-specific attack rates are presented for two communities during epidemic rubella in 1964.[96] The attack rate curves during epidemic rubella in 1964 are similar to the curve for the prevaccine nonepidemic period from 1966 to 1968 seen in Table 177–1. The overall attack rate during the 1964 epidemic in the two communities was 23 percent. Eighty-six percent of the cases occurred in children younger than 15 years. In 1999, 272 cases of rubella were reported in the United States, and of the 269 with known ages, only 14 percent occurred in children younger than 15 years.[385]

TABLE 177–1 ■ AGE DISTRIBUTION OF REPORTED RUBELLA CASES AND ESTIMATED INCIDENCE RATES*—ILLINOIS, MASSACHUSETTS, AND NEW YORK CITY, 1966–1968,† AND TOTAL UNITED STATES, 1985–1987†

	1966–1968 Average‡		1985–1987 Average§		
Age Group (yr)	**%**	**Rate**	**%**	**Rate**	**Rate change‖ (%) 1966–1987**
<5	21.6	63.3	24.8	0.6	-99.1
5–9	38.5	101.3	11.8	0.3	-99.7
10–14	17.0	44.0	5.2	0.1	-99.7
15–19	12.7	35.7	8.0	0.2	-99.5
≥20	10.2	3.7	50.2	0.1	-96.5
Total	100.0	24.3	100.0	0.2	-99.2

*Reported cases per 100,000 population. Patients with unknown age are excluded.
†Average annual figures over a 3-year period.
‡Represents prevaccine years. National age data were not available before 1975 and were not reported consistently (i.e., >75% of cases) until 1980.
§Total United States data (1986 population projections) are used for 1985–1987; because the overall number of reported rubella cases currently is small, fluctuations (such as the epidemic in New York City in 1985) in only these three reporting areas skewed the data for this period.
‖Based on actual rates.
From Centers for Disease Control: Rubella and congenital rubella syndrome—United States 1985–1988. M. M. W. R. Morb. Mortal. Wkly. Rep. *38*: 173–178, 1989.

Antibody prevalence by age group in the prevaccine era in the St. Louis area is presented in Figure 177–3.[84] As can be seen, rubella HI antibody prevalence went from less than 10 percent in children younger than 3 years to almost 80 percent in pre-adolescents. Surveys of adolescents and young women of child-bearing age conducted before 1969 generally have indicated an immunity rate (HI antibody titer ≥1:8) of approximately 75 to 85 percent.[97]

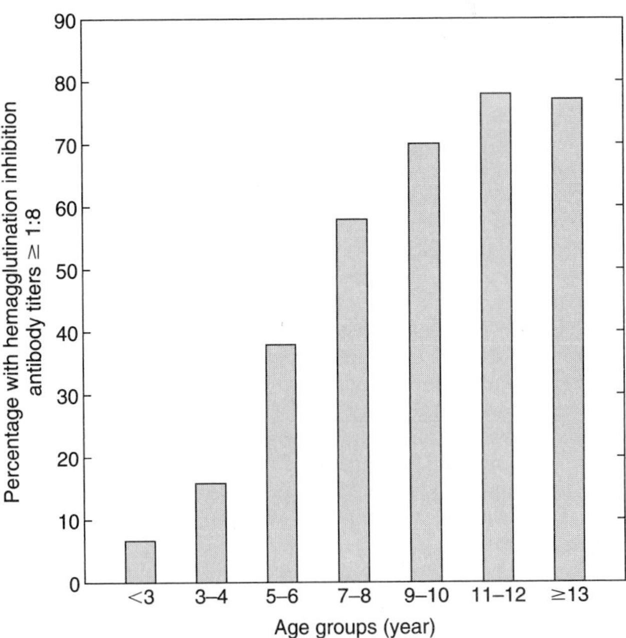

FIGURE 177–3 ■ Percentage of children with rubella hemagglutination-inhibition antibody titers of 1:8 or greater in a St. Louis study in 1969. (From Cherry, J. D.: Rubella: Past, present and future. Volta Rev. *76*:461–465, 1974. Reprinted with permission from The Volta Review. Copyright 1974 by the Alexander Graham Bell Association for the Deaf, 3417 Volta Place, NW, Washington, DC 20007.)

TABLE 177–2 ■ AGE-SPECIFIC ATTACK RATES IN TWO COMMUNITIES DURING EPIDEMIC RUBELLA IN 1964

	Doraville, Georgia			Kingston, Tennessee		
Age Group (yr)	**Total Population**	**Cases**	**Attack Rate (%)**	**Total Population**	**Cases**	**Attack Rate (%)**
0–4	87	32	36.8	69	30	43.5
5–9	206	104	50.5	127	90	70.9
10–14	208	59	28.4	127	68	53.5
15–19	78	9	11.5	90	25	27.8
20+	427	11	2.6	487	19	3.9
Unknown	8	—	—			
Total	1014	215	21.2	900	232	25.8

From Communicable Disease Center: Morbidity and Mortality Weekly Report *13*:349–360, 1964.

Immunity to rubella as indicated by the curve in Figure 177–3 obviously is affected by epidemic periods. With epidemic disease, the curve itself most probably maintains the same slope, but it moves to the left; antibody prevalence in each age group of children increases significantly (perhaps 10 to 30%). However, studies in the prevaccine era on sera from young adults indicate that the percentage of susceptible persons in this age group is affected only slightly by epidemic disease.[97, 148, 432, 438, 534] In a survey of sera from 600 pregnant women in 1962, Sever and associates[438] noted that 17.5 percent had no detectable antibody. In a similar study in 1966 in which the mean age was slightly less (23.6 versus 25.6 years), the percentage without detectable antibody was 7.8. Other surveys of rubella antibody in the sera of young adults acquired after the 1964 pandemic indicate a susceptibility rate in the 15 to 20 percent range, similar to pre-1964 data.[97, 430, 438]

Effect of Vaccination

Rubella vaccine was licensed for use in the United States and many other countries in 1969, and it has been used extensively for more than 30 years.[68, 375, 385, 517] The immunization effort in the United States initially focused on children.[97, 260, 261] A secondary goal was to immunize seronegative postpubertal girls and women of child-bearing age, but little effort was extended in this area until 1978. The overall effect of the immunization effort in the United States on the young adult population is difficult to interpret. As noted in Table 177–1 and subsequent data, the reported number of cases and the incidence of rubella decreased significantly from the prevaccine period until the present.[63, 385, 517] A marked reduction in the number of reported cases of congenital rubella also has occurred since 1969 (see Fig. 177–2). However, the actual number of cases and the incidence of rubella in adolescents and young adults did not decrease until 1981, and 58.2 percent of all patients in the period 1985 through 1987 were 15 years of age (see Table 177–1). Also alarming was the marked upswing in the number of congenital rubella cases in 1990 and 1991.[66, 385] Antibody survey data reported between 1981 and 1993 indicate that 5 to 25 percent of the adolescent and young adult population in the United States was susceptible to rubella.* In four studies in which rubella antibody prevalence was analyzed by the vaccination status of the participants, differences were significant.[269, 316, 347, 391] Between 87 and 96 percent of vaccinated persons had rubella antibody, whereas only 70 to 80 percent of nonvaccinated persons had antibody.

The most recent U.S. serosurvey data found the following seropositive rates by age group: 6 to 11 years, 91.8 percent; 12 to 19 years, 82.6 percent; 20 to 29 years, 84.6 percent; 30 to 39 years, 88.7 percent; 40 to 49 years, 92.5 percent; 50 to 59 years, 93.7 percent; and 60 years and older, 95.7 percent.[131] In this survey, persons born from 1970 to 1974 were found to have the lowest rate of seropositivity (78%).

In contrast to the immunization program in the United States, which focused on children and elimination of epidemic rubella, immunization efforts in the United Kingdom and many other countries were aimed at girls 11 to 14 years of age and selective immunization of women of child-bearing age. This approach would not be expected to disrupt the epidemic pattern of rubella but only decrease disease in young adult women. Serologic surveys in the United Kingdom indicate a significant reduction in the number of seronegative persons in the target population.[92, 200, 316–318, 396, 483] In one study in which 10,000 serum samples were analyzed, 93 to 96 percent of females born after 1956 (who would have been offered rubella vaccine in school) were found to have antibody, whereas only 80 to 89 percent of those born before 1954 were found to have antibody.[92] In spite of the high level of antibody prevalence in women of child-bearing age, rubella infection in pregnancy and congenital rubella continued to be a major problem in the United Kingdom.[318, 483] From 1971 to 1982, 625 cases of congenital rubella were reported, and from 1974 to 1981, 3273 women had their pregnancies terminated because of rubella infection or contact with a person with rubella in England and Wales.[483]

In Finland, where initial immunization in 1975 involved 11- to 13-year-old girls, and since 1982, when a two-dose program involving all children was started, the susceptibility rate in 1992 for 16- to 19-year-old females was 3 to 5 percent, whereas for males it was 30 percent.[495]

In Sweden, the initial immunization program, which began in 1973, targeted school girls, susceptible women after pregnancy, and women at special risk; their second program, which began in 1982, was a universal two-dose schedule at 18 months and 12 years.[46] The rate of susceptibility in pregnant women in Sweden decreased from 12 percent in 1975 to below 2 percent in 1994.

Congenital Rubella

Congenital rubella was not a reportable disease in the United States until 1966, so good data on incidence and prevalence during epidemics of rubella are not available.

*See references 114, 126, 156, 249, 269, 347, 348, 391, 425, 459, 464, 509.

In the 1964 to 1965 rubella epidemic in the United States, 20,000 cases of congenital rubella occurred, 5000 therapeutic abortions were performed, excess fetal wastage of 6250 was reported, and an excess of 2100 neonatal deaths occurred.[97]

Estimates of the risk of acquiring congenital rubella after maternal infection vary considerably in different studies. In general, studies performed before 1964, which included nonepidemic periods, tended to underestimate the risk, whereas early retrospective studies after epidemics resulted in high incidence values.[149] Clearly, however, the individual risk of acquiring congenital rubella depends on the month of pregnancy in which maternal infection occurs. Sallomi[404] analyzed eight published studies that met his rigid criteria and noted the following rates of anomalies by gestational age when maternal infection occurred: weeks 1 to 4, 61 percent; weeks 5 to 8, 26 percent; and weeks 9 to 12, 8 percent. In pregnancies complicated by rubella in weeks 1 to 8, only 36 percent ended in normal live births, 39 percent ended in abortion or stillbirth, and 25 percent produced gross fetal anomalies. Peckham[357] noted that 85 percent of infants born to mothers infected during the first 8 weeks of pregnancy had detectable defects during the first 4 years of life. Infection at other times during pregnancy revealed the following rates of detectable defects: 9 to 12 weeks, 52 percent; 13 to 20 weeks, 16 percent; and after 20 weeks, no defect. Other studies indicate a risk of malformation of 3 percent and a risk of abortion and stillbirth of 4 percent when conception-rubella intervals are greater than 12 weeks.[94]

Infection with rubella virus confers lifelong immunity against clinical illness, but asymptomatic reinfection does occur. Asymptomatic reinfection is noted commonly in pregnant women, but it generally has not been considered a risk to the fetus. However, in rare instances, reinfection has resulted in severely damaged babies.[1, 24, 56, 115, 390, 520]

TRANSMISSION

Rubella infection generally is assumed to be spread by the respiratory route. Although definitive evidence supporting this assumption is not available, data from volunteer projects and study of natural disease strongly support this view.[187, 219, 416] Infected persons regularly shed large concentrations of virus in the nose and throat, and droplets of secretions are released into the environment, which allows respiratory-to-respiratory transmission. Also possible is that the initial hosts may contaminate their own hands and then transmit the infectious agent to environmental surfaces or directly to contacts. In this circumstance, new hosts can acquire infection via the fomite-hand-respiratory or hand-hand-respiratory route.

In experimental transmission studies, Green and colleagues[187] noted that efficient transmission of infection to susceptible persons required prolonged, repeated contact; after a brief, single contact, only 1 in 5 children acquired disease, whereas of 17 subjects with prolonged, repeated contact, all but 1 were infected. Although the period of communicability has never been determined accurately, almost 100 years ago the period of infectivity was noted to precede the eruptive phase of illness.[190] Volunteer studies indicate that virus is present in nasopharyngeal secretions from 7 days before to 14 days after the onset of rash.[187, 219] Maximal shedding and presumably maximal transmissibility occur for an 11-day period of 5 days before to 6 days after the appearance of rash. Infants with congenital rubella shed virus from the nose and throat for many months and have been responsible for the spread of virus to susceptible contacts.[235, 414]

SEASONAL PATTERNS

Rubella is a winter and spring disease, with the largest number of cases occurring in March, April, and May in the United States.[96, 97] This seasonal pattern occurs in years with both a high and a low incidence of rubella. Presumably, some transmission and sporadic illness occur throughout the year in large urban areas.

GEOGRAPHIC DISTRIBUTION

Although clinical rubella has gone unrecognized in many countries in Africa, Asia, and South and Central America, serologic surveillance indicates its presence throughout the world.[94] In remote islands, rubella may not be endemic, so large segments of the population may be susceptible.[49, 223] In these locales, the introduction of rubella results in epidemic infection that involves approximately 90 percent of the susceptible population. In populated areas of the world, rubella is both endemic and epidemic, and between 80 and 90 percent of the adult population has serum rubella antibody.[94] An interesting note is that in several well-populated large islands (Jamaica, Taiwan, Barbados, Trinidad, Hawaii, and Japan) that are not remote, a smaller percentage of the total population has antibody, and rubella is not endemic.[94, 140, 168, 185]

OTHER FACTORS

Sex

The incidence of clinical rubella is similar in boys and girls.[96, 97] In adults, more cases of rubella are reported in women.[97] This finding possibly is the result of interest and concern related to congenital rubella rather than a true difference on the basis of sex. Of interest is that in rubella vaccine trials, girls have been noted to have higher geometric mean convalescent-phase antibody titers than boys do.[314, 451]

Mitchell and associates[324] studied the IgG, IgM, and IgA antibody responses in men and women to rubella virus structural proteins (E1, E2, and C). IgA E2 antibodies did not develop in men, but they did in women. Men had lower IgG antibody to E2, an earlier onset of E1-specific IgG and IgM antibodies, and a greater proportion of total antibody against E1 than women did. In a more recent study, Mitchell[321] reported that men had a more rapid cell-mediated immune response to whole inactivated rubella virus and a panel of rubella virus peptides after reimmunization than women did.

Genetics

Hattis and associates[215] showed that individuals differ in their ability to transmit rubella. During a rubella epidemic, they noted a small number of persons who had high potential for transmitting virus to susceptible persons ("spreaders"). Most persons demonstrated only minimal virus transmission ("nonspreaders"). Honeyman and colleagues[228, 230] suggested that the ability to spread rubella virus is favored by the cell surface antigen HL-A1 or the combination HL-A1 and HL-A8. In a rubella vaccine trial, Spencer and associates[451] noted that 44 percent of persons with high rubella HI antibody titer (≥1:512) responses had HL-A28. In this study, a high convalescent-phase geometric mean antibody titer also was noted to occur in subjects with the AB blood type.

Pathology and Pathogenesis

VIRAL INFECTION

The sequence of events in uncomplicated, postnatally acquired rubella is presented in Table 177–3. Although much is known about rubella infection in humans, considerable gaps regarding specific events exist.[187, 217–219, 416] Estimates for the timing of events in rubella infection (see Table 177–3) have come from volunteer inoculation studies. In many instances, artificial inoculation has resulted in a reduction in the length of the incubation period of clinical disease. This finding suggests that the size of inoculum is important in the initial generation of human infection. It also helps explain the rather wide boundaries of the incubation period noted in many clinical studies.[190, 311, 409]

The primary site of infection is the respiratory epithelium of the nasopharynx. Initial infection of the respiratory epithelium apparently is minor; a more important event is early spread of virus to the regional lymphatics. In volunteers given 100 $TCID_{50}$ of rubella virus intranasally, viral multiplication at the respiratory site was noted on the third day.[416] After viremia, extensive nasopharyngeal infection occurs. In persons who have received either attenuated or unattenuated virus via the subcutaneous route, nasopharyngeal shedding in varying concentration always occurs.[85, 86, 187, 416] Concentrations of virus generally are greater in specimens collected from the nose than from the throat.

Viremia peaks just before the onset of exanthem and disappears shortly thereafter. In contrast, virus continues to be present consistently in the nasopharynx for a 6-day period after the onset of rash and occasionally for an additional week thereafter.[187] In addition to the blood and nasopharynx, other sites from which rubella virus has been recovered are the lymph nodes,[165] urine,[416] cerebrospinal fluid,[455] conjunctival sac,[218] breast milk,[53] synovial fluid,[222] and lungs.[440] Rubella virus was recovered from the skin of rubella patients at sites with rash and without rash.[217, 218]

TABLE 177–3 ■ THE SEQUENCE OF RUBELLA VIRAL INFECTION IN UNCOMPLICATED PRIMARY DISEASE

Day	Event
0	Rubella virus from the respiratory secretions of an infected person comes in contact with the epithelial surface of the nasopharynx of a susceptible person. Localized infection in the respiratory epithelium is established, and virus spreads via lymphatics and possibly by transient viremia to regional lymph nodes
1–22	Viral replication in localized areas of the nasopharynx and regional lymph nodes
3–8	First evidence of nasopharyngeal viral shedding
6–20	Viremia (virus free in serum and associated with leukocytes)
8–14	Establishment of infection in the skin and other viremic sites, including generalized nasopharyngeal involvement
10–17	Maximal viremia and viruria
10–24	Maximal nasopharyngeal viral shedding
17–19	Viremia decreases and then ceases. Viral content at viremic sites rapidly diminishes

From references 187, 217–219, 416.

IMMUNOLOGIC EVENTS

Antibody

After having natural or vaccine rubella viral infection, patients regularly have an antibody response. Serum antibodies to different rubella viral antigens can be measured by HI, CF, neutralization, immunofluorescence, precipitation, radioimmunoassay, ELISA, single radial hemolysis, PH, LA, and platelet aggregation.* In natural postnatal rubella infection, HI and neutralizing antibodies appear 14 to 18 days after exposure, at the time of the rash. HI antibody titers usually peak approximately 2 weeks after the onset of clinical illness, stay at a high level for several weeks, decrease about fourfold over a year's time, and then generally persist for life. Immunofluorescence, ELISA, radioimmunoassay, and LA reveal antibody patterns similar to those determined by HI.[221] Antibody detected by PH does not appear until 3 to 4 weeks after the onset of illness, and that detected by single radial hemolysis is delayed until 1 to 2 weeks after onset. In an Amazon Indian tribe, the geometric mean rubella HI antibody titer 12 years after infection, with no intercurrent rubella exposure, was 1:33.[37] The pattern of the neutralizing antibody response is similar to the HI antibody response, except that the peak is delayed slightly. Brody and colleagues[49] noted that all but 10 percent of an island population had rubella neutralizing antibody 22 years after the time of epidemic illness.

CF antibody first appears approximately a week after HI and neutralizing antibody, peaks approximately 1 month after illness, and in general does not persist as long as does either HI or neutralizing antibody. Occasionally, the CF antibody response is delayed and appears 1 month after the exanthem, with peak titers 2 to 5 months later. Sever and colleagues[436] noted CF antibodies in only 44 percent of persons with neutralizing antibody who were studied 10 to 20 years after illness. The use of an antigen prepared by alkaline extraction has increased the sensitivity of CF, but low levels of antibody still are best identified by HI or neutralization.[367, 421]

After natural infection, precipitating antibodies develop to both theta and iota antigen.[274] Antibody to theta antigen appears early, parallels HI antibody, and is persistent. In contrast, the response to iota antigen is delayed, with a slow rise in concentration during a 2- to 3-month period. Five years after infection, anti-iota antibody cannot be detected.

After immunization, the antibody response pattern varies according to the type of vaccine used.[38, 275, 344, 369, 370, 415, 512] With RA 27/3 vaccine, the serum antibody response is similar to that after natural disease, except that the peak HI and neutralizing antibody titers attained usually are lower. Serum antibody responses noted after HPV-77 and Cendehill vaccine viral infection are different from those found after natural infection in that CF and anti-iota antibodies are noted only irregularly and then in minimal concentration.

Primary rubella virus infection, either naturally acquired or vaccine induced, is characterized by the initial appearance of antibody in the IgM and IgG serum components.[27, 35, 108, 122, 196, 355, 356, 456] In general, the IgM-specific response is short-lived and not detectable more than 8 weeks after the onset of infection. Occasionally, it has been detected in the serum for extended periods.

IgA nasal HI and neutralizing antibodies also occur regularly after natural viral infection. After immunization, the nasal antibody response varies with the type of vaccine and

*See references 13, 36, 79, 144, 183, 221, 275, 279, 294, 308, 309, 320, 336, 358, 367, 433, 435, 502, 506, 544.

the route of administration.[8, 107, 110, 344, 367] After subcutaneous immunization with HPV-77 vaccine, rubella-specific nasal IgA antibody is a rare finding; it occurs in most subjects who receive RA 27/3 vaccine administered intranasally and in approximately half of those given this vaccine by the subcutaneous route.

Specific Cell-Mediated Responses

Rubella-specific, cell-mediated lymphocyte responses regularly occur after infection with rubella virus.* Steele and associates,[458] using an in vitro lymphocyte-mediated cytotoxicity assay, first noted that lymphocytes from persons who previously had rubella caused cell destruction in a tissue culture chronically infected with rubella virus. Rubella antigen–specific, cell-mediated immunity also has been demonstrated in lymphocyte cultures by blast transformation, production of migration-inhibition factor, and production of interferon.[55, 229, 332, 449, 478, 504, 505] With vaccination, rubella-specific, cell-mediated immunity first was noted to occur 7 days after immunization, with peak responses at 3 weeks.[504, 505] Honeyman and associates[220] noted that the rubella antigen–specific, cell-mediated response commenced 1 week before the humoral immune response in both natural and vaccine-induced rubella viral infection. They also noted that the cell-mediated response was of greater magnitude and duration after natural disease than after immunization. Rossier and associates[398] studied cloistered nuns and noted that specific cell-mediated immunity to rubella virus persisted until 79 years of age in the probable absence of reinfection.

Morag and colleagues[332] demonstrated the specific appearance of cell-mediated immunity in tonsillar lymphoid tissue after natural infection or intranasal immunization with rubella vaccine. This responsiveness was conspicuously low after vaccination by the subcutaneous route. In most instances, the presence of cell-mediated responsiveness correlates with the presence of antibody; specific rubella lymphocyte transformation has been noted in the absence of antibody, however.[449] The magnitude of the rubella-specific, cell-mediated response is suppressed during pregnancy.[478]

McCarthy and colleagues[298] identified potential determinants of human cellular immunity to rubella virus by using synthetic peptides representing well-defined sequences of rubella virus structural proteins. They used the following peptide subsequences: two capsid domains (C_1 to C_{29} and C_{64} to C_{97}), a glycoprotein E1 domain ($E1_{202}$ to $E1_{283}$), and a glycoprotein E2 domain ($E2_{31}$ to $E2_{105}$). All but the C_{64} to C_{97} subsequences stimulated specific lymphoproliferative responses in peripheral blood mononuclear cells in 25 to 50 percent of immune subjects. The immunodominant T-proliferative epitope (C_{14} to C_{29}) was recognized by only 50 percent of the peripheral blood mononuclear cells of the study population. Relatively immunodominant T-cell epitopes vary among different persons.

Using a lymphocyte proliferation assay, Mitchell and associates[323] reported positive cell-mediated immune responses to 16 peptides, including 6 that contained antibody neutralization domains after revaccination.

Nonspecific Responses

A large number of nonspecific, immunologically related responses can be demonstrated during rubella virus infections. Niwa and Kanoh[339] performed a comprehensive study of these responses in 85 children and adults during a rubella epidemic. They noted a decreased number of total leukocytes, neutrophils, and T cells initially, which returned to normal values within 1 week. Some patients had slightly elevated levels of serum IgM, and total hemolytic complement was elevated in 12 of 30 patients. Marked increases in C4 and C9 also were present. In addition, they noted a marked insensitivity to dinitrochlorobenzene and purified protein derivatives in many patients. Atypical lymphocytes, autoantibodies, and reduced blastogenesis as measured by phytohemagglutinin stimulation were noted in some patients. Other studies consistently have demonstrated a reduction in the lymphocyte response to PHA.[52, 58, 169, 241, 266, 289, 300] In general, this reduction lasts less than 1 month, and infections with attenuated strains of rubella vaccine virus are less immunosuppressive than are infections with unattenuated rubella virus.

Hyypiä and colleagues[241] noted that during rubella virus infection, the proportion of suppressor-cytotoxic T cells was increased and the proportion of helper-inducer T cells was decreased. Polyclonal activation of B cells was associated with these findings.[242]

Zaknun and coworkers[541] noted a marked increase in urine neopterin levels in two children with acute rubella. Their levels increased dramatically 4 days before the onset of exanthem.

FETAL EVENTS

Viral Infection

A considerable amount of information about fetal infection became available from extensive studies during the 1964 rubella epidemic,* and further information has been obtained more recently from both natural and vaccine viral infections.[40, 123, 132, 268, 364, 429, 499, 539] In spite of the number and extent of investigations performed to date, we know little about virus transmission to the fetus in maternal infections in the latter half of pregnancy.

With maternal infection during the first trimester, placental infection regularly occurs and often persists throughout the remainder of the pregnancy. In the therapeutic abortion studies of Alford and associates,[7] fetal infection occurred in approximately 50 percent of placental infections. However, other studies have revealed almost identical isolation rates from both placental and fetal tissue.[383, 477] Persistent infection is the usual outcome of first-trimester fetal infection. This fetal infection usually involves multiple organs, and virus can be isolated at birth regularly from the throat, rectum, and urine.[235, 365]

Little is known about events in second- and third-trimester maternal rubella infection. Most probably, placental infection is a regular occurrence, and transmission of virus to the infant in utero also may occur regularly. Because few infants have defects when born after maternal rubella infection in the second and third trimesters, a careful search for rubella infection in these infants by virologic or serologic methods rarely has been conducted. Random studies seem to indicate that rubella virus often infects the fetus after the first trimester, and occasionally the infection becomes persistent.[109, 123, 208, 235, 328, 507, 528] Other studies have failed to show virologic or serologic evidence of infection in

*See references 78, 220, 229, 247, 286, 289, 298, 321–323, 324, 332, 350, 397, 398, 449, 458, 504, 505.

*See references 7, 61, 87, 102, 103, 128, 205, 208–211, 235, 326–330, 365, 383, 414, 417, 462, 529.

infants in whom maternal rubella occurred in the second and third trimesters.[87, 329, 462]

With maternal rubella infection, the cervix also is involved, so fetal infection could occur by the ascending route as well as by primary placental infection.[429, 499] In addition, fetal infection has resulted from maternal disease that occurred before conception.[147, 529, 539]

Rubella virus can be recovered regularly after birth from infants with congenital rubella. The percentage of infants with persistent infection decreases over the first year of life; by the first birthday, between 10 and 20 percent of children still shed virus in nasopharyngeal secretions.[102, 383] Rawls and colleagues[383] were unable to isolate virus from the throats of 15 congenitally infected infants after they reached 18 months of age, and Sever and Monif[437] and Cooper and Krugman[102] were unable to demonstrate persistence of nasopharyngeal virus in older children. A 4.5-year-old boy with congenital rubella was found on one occasion to be shedding rubella virus in the throat.[441]

Immunologic Findings

SPECIFIC ANTIBODY. Humoral antibody in a congenitally infected fetus is acquired transplacentally from the mother and is produced actively by the fetus. In a normal maternal-fetal relationship, transport of antibody to the fetus is minimal until the midpoint of the second trimester (16 to 20 weeks).[6, 7] With first-trimester maternal infection (transplacentally acquired), rubella antibody titers in serum amount to only approximately 5 percent of maternal values. The fetal immune system becomes functional during the second trimester,[270] and small amounts of specific rubella fetal IgM antibody can be detected. From the midpoint of pregnancy, antibody levels in the developing fetus rise so that at birth, the maternal and infant values are similar. Although the values of total antibody are similar, the composition is different. Maternal antibody at the time of delivery usually is composed entirely of IgG. In contrast, the infant titer consists of fetal IgM, presumably fetal IgG, and occasionally fetal IgA and transplacentally derived maternal IgG.

Long-term rubella antibody patterns in congenitally infected infants after birth are different from those of their mothers or from those of a group of children with acquired disease.[100, 207, 251, 490] Cooper and colleagues[100] monitored a group of 223 mothers of children with congenital rubella and noted that at the end of 5 years, all still had detectable HI antibody and the geometric mean titer for the group had undergone a fourfold reduction. In contrast, 5-year follow-up of the congenitally infected infants revealed a 16-fold decline in geometric mean titer; 8 of 29 infants had serum HI antibody titers less than 1:8 when examined at 5 years of age. Other investigators have observed similar declines in rubella antibody titers of congenitally infected infants.[207, 251, 490]

Another unique aspect of rubella antibody in congenitally infected infants is the persistence of specific IgM. Cradock-Watson and colleagues[111] studied 40 infants with congenital rubella and noted that IgM antibody persisted for approximately 6 months in most cases and for up to 2 years in a few children. de Mazancourt and colleagues[118] studied the antibody response to rubella virus structural proteins in infants with congenital rubella syndrome and found that the immunoprecipitation patterns were different from those in sera from postnatally infected adults. The sera from congenitally infected infants had little or no C-specific antibody, occasionally only antibody to E1 was precipitated, E1 protein was precipitated in relative excess of E2 protein, and the relative amount of E2 antibody was greater than antibody to E1.

SPECIFIC CELL-MEDIATED IMMUNITY. Rubella-specific, cell-mediated immune responses have been studied in children with congenital rubella by the following assays: lymphocyte-mediated cytotoxicity, lymphocyte transformation, lymphocyte interferon production, and leukocyte migration-inhibition factor production.[54, 164] By all methods of study, infants with congenital rubella have decreased rubella-specific, cell-mediated responses when compared with persons who previously had acquired rubella postnatally. Buimovici-Klein and associates[54] noted that the degree of suppression correlated with the time of in utero infection: the earlier in pregnancy the maternal infection, the greater the depression of specific cell-mediated responses. In the study of an infant with late-onset congenital rubella syndrome, Verder and associates[503] noted decreased activity of killer and natural killer cells and alloreactive direct cytotoxic cells. Their data indicated that defective cytotoxic effector cell function was the primary cause for failure to eliminate virus in the illness.

NONSPECIFIC RESPONSES. Desmyter and colleagues[121] noted that infants with congenital rubella produced normal amounts of interferon after receiving measles immunization. They also found that the clinical response and antibody development in these measles-vaccinated children were similar to those in normal children. Lebon and associates[271] noted that sera collected from rubella-infected fetuses and infants with congenital rubella contain an acid-labile interferon. Michaels[312] observed that infants with congenital rubella who still were shedding virus in their throat or urine had depressed antibody responses to diphtheria and tetanus toxoids. White and colleagues[527] reported decreased in vitro lymphocyte blast transformation responses to vaccinia and diphtheria toxoid antigens in children with congenital rubella in comparison to normal children. They also noted depressed skin reactivity to intradermal *Candida* antigen in the congenital rubella group. Buimovici-Klein and associates[54] observed a marked reduction in lymphocyte transformation after PHA stimulation in their congenital rubella group. The most marked defect was seen in children in whom maternal rubella occurred during the first 8 weeks of pregnancy.

PATHOLOGY

Postnatally Acquired Disease

Almost no data on the histologic findings in uncomplicated rubella are available, but, occasionally, postmortem tissue has been studied from patients with encephalitis. Giuliani and associates[178] studied lymph nodes from rubella patients and noted edema, reticulum cell hyperplasia, and loss of the usual follicular morphologic features. Sherman and associates[440] reported six cases of rubella encephalitis and noted the autopsy findings in three cases. They specifically searched all organs for inclusion bodies, syncytial giant cells, focal cellular necrosis, and unusual proliferative changes, but none were found. Only mild, nonspecific, follicular hyperplasia in the spleen and lymph nodes was seen. Histologic examination of the brain of a 7-year-old girl who died of encephalitis revealed diffuse swelling, nonspecific degeneration, and a sparse, mononuclear perivascular and meningeal exudate.

A synovial biopsy specimen in a woman with rubella arthritis revealed scattered areas of fibrinopurulent exudate and synovial cell hyperplasia; inflammatory cell infiltration composed mainly of lymphocytic cells was present, and vascularity was increased.[540]

TABLE 177–4 ■ PATHOLOGIC FINDINGS IN CONGENITAL RUBELLA

Anatomic Location or System	Gross and Microscopic Findings	References
Placenta	Perivascular mononuclear cellular infiltration in the decidua Edema, fibrosis, and necrosis of villi; cytoplasmic inclusion bodies noted in swollen Hofbauer cells in villous stroma Perivasculitis, endovasculitis, and perivascular fibrosis also noted	349
Generalized growth retardation	Subnormal number of cells in many organs	337
Nervous system	Chronic meningitis with infiltrates of large mononuclear cells, lymphocytes, and plasma cells in the leptomeninges Vascular degeneration, ischemic lesions, and retardation of myelinization throughout brain	393, 394, 445, 479
Eye	Lens: cataract, cortical liquefaction, and spherophakia Iris and ciliary body: necrosis of ciliary body, iridocyclitis, iris atrophy, and pigmentation defects Retina: posterior pigmentary disturbances Cornea: usually normal; occasional endothelial degeneration Optic nerve: posterior bowing	42
Ear	Hemorrhage in fetal cochlea resulting in epithelial necrosis Inflammatory cells in stria vascularis Adhesions between Reissner membrane and tectorial membrane Sacculocochlear degeneration of Scheibe (strial atrophy, collapse of Reissner membrane, atrophy of organ of Corti, rolled-up tectorial membranes, and collapse and degeneration of sacculus) noted after birth	160, 161, 515
Cardiovascular	Common heart defects in order of frequency: patent ductus arteriosus, pulmonary artery stenosis, ventricular septal defect, and atrial septal defect (These rubella-induced lesions do not differ from similar non-rubella-induced lesions.) Myocarditis with swelling of muscle fibers and loss of striations; necrosis Intimal proliferation of major arteries	4, 136, 154, 255, 256, 519
Pulmonary	Chronic interstitial pneumonia with large mononuclear cells, lymphocytes, and plasma cells within interstitial spaces and alveoli	255, 363, 445
Liver	Hyalinization and swelling of hepatocytes, hematopoiesis, and multinucleated giant cells Bile stasis	138, 139, 460, 465
Skin	Purpuric lesion: focal areas of erythropoiesis in dermis and upper subcutaneous adipose tissue Chronic reticulated rash: acute and chronic inflammatory cells and histiocytes in dermis Edema in dermal papillae	60, 254
Bone	Thinning of metaphyseal trabeculae and decrease in number of osteoblasts and osteoclasts Many plasma cells in metaphyses and cartilaginous epiphyses and around vessels Occasional giant cells with cytoplasmic inclusions Thinning of cartilage	384, 400, 428, 526
Muscle	Focal abnormalities: very small fibers with darkly staining nuclei and muscle bundles containing empty connective tissue tubes	452
Teeth	Necrosis of enamel-forming epithelial cells	193, 485
Hematologic	Transient thrombocytopenia with decreased megakaryocytes in bone marrow; increased platelet adhesiveness and platelet agglutinins Lymph node consistent with histiocytosis; unorganized cell mass made up of mononuclear cells with dense round nuclei and irregularly shaped cytoplasm	28, 91, 372, 381
Immunologic	Spleen: fibrosis Loss of normal architecture and absence of germinal centers in spleen and lymph nodes; dysgammaglobulinemia usually with decreased IgG and IgA and elevated IgM	91, 202, 371, 388

Congenital Infection

In contrast to postnatal rubella, the pathologic process of congenital infection has been studied extensively.* Table 177–4 summarizes the main pathologic findings by anatomic location or system in congenital rubella. As noted, defects in congenital rubella result from both specific cell damage and cellular deficiency. Although specific cellular necrosis is important in certain early lesions such as in the inner ear, of greater overall importance are the secondary effects of generalized vascular damage. Also of presumed major importance is the noncytolytic cellular infection characteristic of rubella virus. It results in mitotic arrest and a reduction in total cells in many organs.

*See references 4, 5, 28, 42, 50, 60, 91, 103, 127, 136–139, 154, 160, 161, 193, 203–205, 248, 254–256, 283, 327, 330, 337, 349, 363, 371, 372, 381, 384, 388, 393, 394, 400, 428, 445, 446, 452, 460, 465, 479, 485, 515, 519, 526, 538.

Clinical Manifestations

POSTNATAL ILLNESS*

Although clinical rubella is a distinctive exanthematous disease, its features are not as clearly discernible as are those of measles or chickenpox. The exanthematous illnesses caused by enteroviruses, adenoviruses, and other common respiratory viruses often are clinically similar or identical to those of rubella (see Chapter 65). Because of these other viral illnesses that simulate rubella, descriptions of clinical rubella made before the availability of modern virologic diagnostic techniques are not always accurate, particularly when rubella in infants and young children is described because exanthems caused by other viruses occur most commonly in these age groups. Unfortunately, in spite of the availability of a vast amount of clinical material during the rubella epidemic of 1964, most clinical knowledge relating to postnatally acquired rubella was formulated before the present virologic era.

Incubation Period

Although prodromal complaints and lymphadenopathy frequently precede the exanthem in rubella, the incubation period in most studies has been calculated as being from the time of exposure to the onset of rash. Almost a century ago, Michael[311] reviewed the incubation periods in 59 different reports and noted a variation of 5 days to 4 weeks. However, in most reports, the minimal incubation time was 14 days or more and the maximum was 17 to 21 days. The mean incubation period from modern reviews is considered to be 18 ± 3 days.

In carefully controlled studies, Green and colleagues[187] noted an incubation time of 13 to 15 days to the onset of rash after the intramuscular inoculation of serum from rubella-infected patients and a longer incubation time (16 to 21 days) in cases acquired by contact with ill patients. In similar volunteer studies in young adults, Schiff and colleagues[416] noted that the onset of rash occurred 11 to 12 days after the administration of 100 $TCID_{50}$ of tissue culture–grown rubella virus. The investigators attributed this shorter incubation period to a larger inoculum than that occurring in natural transmission.

Prodromal Period

Complaints before the onset of rash in rubella vary with age. In young children, the first evidence of disease usually is the appearance of rash. Occasionally, mild coryza and diarrhea precede the exanthem in younger patients. In contrast to the lack of prodrome in children, adolescents and adults usually have symptoms before the onset of rash.[81, 146, 192] In one study, 94 percent of college students with rubella had prodromal complaints. In decreasing order of frequency, the reported symptoms were eye pain, sore throat, headache, swollen glands, fever, aches, chills, anorexia, and nausea.[146] Gross and associates[192] reported prodromal upper respiratory complaints, including malaise, cough, sore throat, red eyes, and runny nose, in 65 percent of an infected adolescent study group.

Prodromal symptoms usually precede the onset of rash by 1 to 5 days. In the studies of Green and associates involving volunteers,[187] the onset of lymphadenopathy commonly was noted 5 to 7 days before the onset of rash. In contrast, Schiff and colleagues[416] observed the appearance of lymphadenopathy only 1 day before the appearance of rash; fever was noted 1 to 4 days before the onset of rash, and most of the volunteers also had malaise and sore throat. Pain on lateral and upward eye movement occurs commonly and occasionally is distressing.[81, 146]

Exanthem Period

The rubella exanthem appears first on the face. Spread of the rash is centrifugal from the head toward the hands and feet. The progression, extent, and duration of the exanthem vary considerably. In a typical case, the rash involves the entire body during the first 24 hours, begins to fade on the face during the second day, and has disappeared from the body by the end of the third day. The characteristic rash is erythematous, maculopapular, and discrete (see Fig. 65–3). Its appearance on an adolescent's face occasionally is confused initially with an exacerbation of acne. Frequently, the rash is only macular with a scarlatiniform appearance. In some patients, the rash is present for less than a day, although sometimes it persists for 5 days or more. Particularly in adults, the exanthem frequently is pruritic. This complaint is troublesome because it often leads the patient as well as the physician to attribute the rash to an allergic cause rather than rubella virus infection.

Occasionally, the exanthem progresses to confluence with a morbilliform appearance. In these cases, the rash usually is less coppery and pinker than that in measles and heals without desquamation or brownish discoloration. The typical picture of erythema infectiosum (slapped-cheek appearance and reticular rash) has been observed in rubella-infected patients. Balfour and associates[20] reported eight children with erythema infectiosum from whom rubella virus was recovered concurrently and two additional children with serologic evidence of rubella infection. The preliminary results of volunteer studies with a virus recovered from one of the patients in this study produced a slapped-cheek appearance but a nonreticulated rash in four of five men. One 3-year-old child from whom the author recovered rubella virus had typical erythema infectiosum.[81] A 14-month-old girl had a roseola-like illness and arthritis.[222]

In the volunteer studies of Schiff and associates,[416] the rash was noted to be pink-red and maculopapular. It appeared initially on the face, chest, upper part of the arms, and shoulders and then spread rapidly over the abdomen, back, and thighs. It developed into an erythematous blush on the face and abdomen. The median duration was 3 days, with extremes of 2 and 5 days. No pruritus was noted.

Rubella infection without rash is a rather common occurrence. In some patients, the infection is without symptoms; in other persons, careful questioning reveals prodromal symptoms, and lymphadenopathy is found on examination. Green and associates[187] noted that about 25 percent of exposed children who became infected had subclinical infection. In an intensive study of 46 susceptible children and adults, all but 1 subject had clinical symptoms with infection[431]; 60 percent of the group had both rash and characteristic posterior auricular or suboccipital lymphadenopathy, and 40 percent had lymphadenopathy without rash. In another study of rubella in an institution for retarded children, Horstmann and associates[237] noted that only approximately half the children who became infected had a rash. Of nine children without rash, significant posterior auricular lymph node enlargement developed in five. Buescher[51] reported a subclinical-to-clinical infection ratio in a military recruit population of 6.5:1.

*See references 81, 82, 146, 149, 187, 190, 263, 267, 311, 409, 416, 489, 525.

Lymphadenopathy is a major clinical manifestation of rubella. The most characteristic enlargement occurs in the suboccipital and posterior auricular nodes, but generalized involvement occurs as well. In the volunteer studies of Schiff and colleagues,[416] the lymph node enlargement usually lasted between 5 and 8 days. In two outbreak studies involving adolescents and young adults, posterior auricular and suboccipital lymphadenopathy was noted in all patients with rash.[146, 192] In contrast to these findings, Landrigan and associates[267] noted that only 47 percent of children and 58 percent of adolescents had similar lymph node enlargement during epidemic rubella illness. Although a frequent suggestion is that the finding of exanthem and suboccipital lymphadenopathy is pathognomonic for rubella, this suggestion is incorrect. In young children, similar involvement is common with enteroviral and adenoviral infections. In adolescents and young adults, the association more strongly indicates rubella, but infectious mononucleosis, *Mycoplasma pneumoniae* infection, acquired toxoplasmosis, and other possibilities also must be considered.

The occurrence of fever in rubella varies; when it does develop, the temperature usually is elevated only minimally. In children with experimentally induced rubella, Krugman and Ward[262] noted that 5 of 13 had temperatures of 38° C (100.4° F) or higher. Two children had maximal temperatures of 38.5° C (101.6° F). Schiff and colleagues[416] noted that all nine infected volunteers had fever with a median duration of 5 days. Landrigan and associates[267] found fever in 74 percent of children and only 47 percent of adolescents; Gross and coworkers[192] observed fever in only 6 of 17 adolescents. Occasionally, children with apparent rubella have been noted to have markedly elevated temperatures. Few such cases have undergone virologic study, so some doubt must be raised whether the illnesses were induced by rubella virus or were caused by other viral agents more commonly associated with marked febrile responses, such as enteroviruses and adenoviruses. I have seen an 8-year-old boy with virologically and serologically confirmed rubella with a temperature of 40° C (104° F) on the day before the appearance of his rash. The 14-month-old girl with arthritis described by Hildebrandt and Maassab[222] had a temperature as high as 40.5° C (105° F).

In 1898, Forchheimer[150] described what he thought was the enanthem of German measles. He described pinhead-sized macular lesions with a rose-red color on the soft palate and uvula that appeared at approximately the time of the exanthem and lasted less than 24 hours. This exanthem has not been identified in children examined by me; however, petechial lesions on the soft palate and uvula have been seen occasionally. Mild pharyngitis is not an uncommon occurrence. Other symptoms and signs in rubella include mild conjunctivitis, sore throat, coryza, cough, and headache.

The duration of illness in uncomplicated rubella varies considerably. Most patients would continue normal activity if the rash were not present. In general, full return to normal activity occurs within 3 days. A small number of adults are bothered by persistent headache, eye pain, and pruritus for 7 to 10 days.

The white blood cell (WBC) count in rubella tends to be low. Schiff and colleagues[416] found leukopenia in all nine volunteers. In these subjects, leukopenia paralleled the fever pattern, with onset 24 hours before the rash manifested and persistence for 4 to 5 days. Before rubella could be confirmed by both specific serologic and virologic methods, many experts thought that rubella could be confirmed accurately by characteristics of the WBC count.[224, 240] Leukopenia was found at the onset of disease; the total count rose to a high-normal value during a 10-day period. Relative neutropenia was noted by Hynes[240] in many patients; one patient had a neutrophil count of 868 cells/mm^3 on the first day of illness. Plasma cells, Türk cells, or both were noted in acute rubella in all cases studied by Hynes[240] and Hillenbrand.[224] A Türk cell is a developing plasma cell that is 25 to 40 µm in diameter and contains a 15- to 30-µm nucleus. The nucleus has two to five prominent nucleoli and a well-defined, light reticulum. The cytoplasm often is vacuolated. Twenty-five percent of the patients studied by Hynes[240] had elevated erythrocyte sedimentation rates during the first week of illness.

Complications

JOINT INVOLVEMENT. The incidences of reported arthritis and arthralgia vary considerably in different studies.[32, 75, 170, 192, 246, 267, 444, 494, 525] In general, both arthralgia and arthritis occur more commonly in adults than in prepubertal children. Women are afflicted more often than are men. In a large outbreak in Bermuda in 1971, 42 percent of 125 patients studied complained of joint pain or discomfort.[246] Three patients had swelling of the joints. The prevalence of joint symptoms increased from 18 percent in the 0- to 9-year-old age group by approximately 20 percent increments per decade; 73 percent of those older than 30 years had symptoms. Joint complaints generally were more common in females than in males older than 10 years. This difference was most marked in the 10- to 20-year-old age group. Landrigan and associates[267] studied the location of joint symptoms in adolescents and found that the fingers were involved most often; the knees and wrists also were implicated commonly.

Yanez and associates[540] studied 11 patients with rubella arthritis. In all instances, multiple joints were involved. The onset of arthritis occurred 1 to 6 days after the beginning of the exanthem and lasted 3 to 28 days (mean, 9 days). The erythrocyte sedimentation rate was elevated in three of seven cases, and one patient had markedly positive latex test results. The WBC count was below 5000 cells/mm^3 in five of seven patients. One woman had bilateral carpal tunnel syndrome. Four children with transient carpal tunnel syndrome accompanying rubella virus infection have been reported.[39] Panush[352] noted serum hypocomplementemia with rubella arthritis in a 25-year-old woman.

The possibility that rubella viral infection is related to rheumatoid arthritis has been studied on several occasions.[45, 117, 292, 345, 543] Martenis and colleagues[292] reported a 21-year-old woman in whom rheumatoid arthritis developed after typical rubella with arthritis. Deinard and associates[117] found that all serum specimens from 80 patients with rheumatoid arthritis contained rubella HI antibody. In contrast, only 86 percent of an equal number of nonarthritic controls and a group of persons with other forms of arthritis had measurable rubella antibody titers. Ogra and associates[345] noted that patients with juvenile rheumatoid arthritis had IgM and IgG serum rubella antibody levels that were four to six times higher than those observed in controls during rubella infection. They also noted specific staining for rubella virus antigen in the synovial fluid of 33 percent of these patients with juvenile rheumatoid arthritis. Grahame and associates[182] repeatedly recovered rubella virus from the synovial fluid of six patients with inflammatory oligoarthritis or polyarthritis over a 2-year period.

NEUROLOGIC MANIFESTATIONS. Encephalitis is a rare complication of rubella.* Sherman and colleagues[440] noted

*See references 3, 26, 47, 90, 98, 116, 130, 291, 307, 338, 395, 440, 455, 511, 532.

6 cases of encephalitis in an epidemic during the spring of 1964 that involved approximately 30,000 children. This rate of encephalitis (1 per 5000 cases) is similar to the rate of 1 per 6000 noted in Detroit in 1942.[291] Rubella encephalitis is clinically similar to encephalitis from measles virus infection but is thought to be less severe. Mortality and morbidity rates have varied considerably. Sherman and colleagues[440] noted that three of six children studied in Pittsburgh died of this complication during the spring of 1964, whereas in Atlanta during the same epidemic period, six patients recovered uneventfully.

The onset of encephalitis most often occurs 2 to 4 days after the appearance of rash, but occasionally, rash and neurologic symptoms occur at the same time; in other instances, the appearance of encephalitis is delayed as much as 1 week after the onset of illness. Examination of cerebrospinal fluid usually reveals mild pleocytosis (20 to 100 cells/mm^3), with most cells being lymphocytes. The protein content is normal or slightly elevated, and the sugar concentration is normal.

Kenny and associates[250] studied seven survivors of rubella encephalitis 1 year after illness and could find no significant loss of intellectual function. Five of the seven had abnormalities on electroencephalography, and two patients had minor neurologic abnormalities. Gibbs and colleagues[174] found abnormal electroencephalographic tracings in 6 of 45 children with uncomplicated rubella.

Other neurologic complications associated with rubella include progressive panencephalitis, carotid artery thrombosis, myelitis, optic neuritis, Guillain-Barré syndrome, and peripheral neuritis.*

Of particular interest is the common occurrence of numbness, tingling, and other symptoms consistent with neuritis during rubella infection. Cuetter and John[112] studied 20 patients with complaints of neuritis accompanying rubella and could find no objective sensory deficits or nerve conduction abnormalities.

Wolinsky and colleagues[536] and Lebon and Lyon[272] described a slowly progressive and fatal nervous system disorder with rubella that was similar to subacute sclerosing panencephalitis.

THROMBOCYTOPENIA. Thrombocytopenic purpura occurs in rubella at an incidence of 1 per 3000 cases.[28] Children are afflicted more frequently than are adults, and girls are affected more often than are boys.[20, 195, 243, 285, 333, 351, 457, 516] The median interval between the onset of exanthem and the occurrence of purpura is approximately 4 days. Occasionally, rash and purpura develop simultaneously; often, however, the hemorrhagic manifestations do not become apparent until 2 weeks after the exanthem. The illness usually is self-limited, but its duration varies from a few days to several months; although deaths caused by hemorrhagic complications have occurred, recovery is the general rule.

OTHER COMPLICATIONS. Myocarditis and pericarditis are rare complications of rubella.[165] A 30-year-old woman was noted to have erythema multiforme exudativum and arthritis with apparent clinical rubella.[162] In an outbreak that involved 46 military recruits, testicular pain was a complaint in 25 percent.[419]

During a rubella epidemic in Japan in 1976 in which 79 patients were studied, 71 percent were noted to have mild catarrhal or follicular conjunctivitis.[206] Six patients had epithelial keratitis that persisted for 2 to 7 days. Seventeen patients had preauricular lymph node swelling in association with their eye findings. During the same epidemic, 13 cases of hemolytic anemia (including 2 cases of hemolytic-uremic syndrome) were noted after rubella virus infection.[493] During a rubella epidemic in Japan, Sugaya and colleagues[467] found that 7.5 percent of 241 patients had liver involvement.

*See references 3, 18, 75, 98, 163, 212, 216, 226, 403, 484, 533, 536, 537.

CONGENITAL RUBELLA

From Gregg's original observation in 1941 of congenital defects in babies born to mothers who had rubella during early pregnancy until the pandemic of 1964, congenital rubella syndrome was considered to include only some combination of abnormalities involving the eyes, ears, brain, and heart. However, observations in 1964, supported by new virologic and serologic techniques, revealed a far more complex congenital rubella syndrome picture: rubella syndrome was expanded to include many new anatomic findings and to acknowledge the reality of chronic persistent infection.

Congenital rubella is the result of in utero fetal infection, which usually occurs during the first 12 weeks of pregnancy. The fetal infection generally is subacute or chronic and may result in abortion; stillbirth; congenital malformations; active processes at birth such as thrombocytopenia, encephalitis, or hepatitis; and, rarely, infected infants without defects. Table 177–5 summarizes the clinical findings in congenital rubella, an estimation of their frequency, and their main characteristics.

General: Infant Death and Growth Retardation*

The most common manifestation of congenital rubella, readily apparent at birth, is generalized growth retardation. Between 50 and 85 percent of all babies weigh less than 2500 g, although gestational age is normal. Virtually all babies with intrauterine growth retardation have one or more other stigmata of congenital rubella. After birth, babies with intrauterine growth retardation often demonstrate continued growth retardation. In some instances, the failure to thrive is severe. Others show a normal growth pattern, but the child is proportionally small. The mortality rate of children with congenital rubella is high during the first year of life, with death specifically related to congenital pneumonia, heart defects and myocarditis, hepatitis, thrombocytopenia, encephalitis, immune deficiency, and failure to thrive.

Eye Findings†

Approximately one third of all babies with congenital rubella have cataracts. Cataracts may be bilateral or unilateral and are either central in location with a surrounding clear zone or diffuse. In most instances, cataracts are present at birth, but occasionally they are not observed until later in infancy. Retinopathy consisting of pigmentary defects occurs commonly in congenital rubella and is useful diagnostically, but it rarely adversely affects visual acuity. Microphthalmos occurs relatively commonly and usually is unilateral. Cataracts frequently are associated with microphthalmos.

Congenital glaucoma occurs in approximately 5 percent of congenitally infected infants. This defect usually is present at birth, but often it is overlooked. Early diagnosis is important if sight is to be preserved.

*See references 17, 104, 155, 186, 207, 235, 256, 278, 287, 303, 313, 355, 366, 401, 402, 404, 417, 434, 446, 479.

†See references 17, 29, 42, 95, 99, 104, 137, 155, 172, 179, 186, 207–209, 235, 255–258, 303, 335, 346, 399–401, 411, 417, 426, 434, 446, 479, 485, 489, 491.

TABLE 177–5 ■ FREQUENCY AND MAIN CHARACTERISTICS OF CLINICAL FINDINGS IN CONGENITAL RUBELLA VIRUS INFECTION

Clinical Findings	Frequency (%)	Main Characteristics	Selected References
General			
In utero death	10–30	Spontaneous abortion; stillbirth	186, 207, 404
Intrauterine growth retardation	50–85	Generalized effect	89, 154, 155, 207, 209, 235, 256, 278, 287, 303, 366, 400, 401, 417, 446, 479
Extrauterine growth retardation	10	Failure to thrive	209, 278, 303, 313, 355, 479
Neonatal and infant deaths	10	Due to pneumonia, heart disease, hepatitis, thrombocytopenia, failure to thrive, immune deficiency, encephalitis	104, 186, 207, 256, 401, 417, 479
Eye			
Cataracts	35	Present at birth	17, 29, 42, 104, 155, 172, 186, 207, 209, 235, 255, 256, 303, 335, 401, 411, 417, 445, 479, 489, 491
Retinopathy	35	Present at birth; usually does not cause problems with vision	42, 95, 103, 172, 186, 207, 235, 257, 258, 303, 489, 491
Microphthalmos	5	Usually associated with cataract	42, 137, 172, 235, 256, 401, 426, 479
Glaucoma	5	Usually present at birth	42, 103, 207, 209, 235, 256, 401, 426, 434
Cloudy cornea	Rare	Usually present at birth; resolves spontaneously	42, 209
Severe myopia	Rare	Usually present at birth; defect may progress	99
Hypoplasia of the iris	Rare	Present at birth	42, 399
Strabismus	5	Associated with other eye defects	208, 303, 346
Iridocyclitis	Rare	Transient; associated with other eye defects	445
Auditory			
Nerve deafness	80–90	May be bilateral or unilateral; moderate or severe; often not recognized early	17, 44, 119, 137, 155, 186, 194, 207, 209, 265, 303, 319, 361, 366, 417, 434, 489, 491, 496
Central deafness	5	Often associated with other central nervous system defects	205
Middle ear damage	5	Usually associated with nerve deafness	389
Intraoral, Nasal, and Facial			
Cleft palate or lip	Rare		137, 186, 417
Dental abnormalities	Rare		60, 193, 303
Micrognathia	Rare		233, 417
Chronic rhinitis	Rare	Transitory finding	366
High-arched palate	Rare		207
Neurologic			
Motor defects	10	Associated with mental and other neurologic defects	303, 434, 542
Hyperirritability (tremors)	Rare	Transitory finding	394
Microcephaly	Rare		17, 209, 235, 303, 434, 479, 514, 530
Mental retardation	10–20	Associated with other stigmata	99, 186, 205, 207, 301, 434, 466
Full anterior fontanelle	10	Transitory finding related to meningoencephalitis	101, 401
Meningoencephalitis	10–20	Transitory finding but may last for 1 yr	120, 209, 255, 256, 366, 401, 445, 479
Spastic diplegia and quadriparesis	Rare	Associated with other stigmata	101, 120
Seizures	Rare	Frequently transitory and related to meningoencephalitis	120, 210, 303, 366
Hypotonia	Rare	Transitory defect	119, 120
Brain calcification	Rare		361, 363, 445, 479
Cerebral arterial stenosis	Rare		205
Anencephaly	Rare		417
Encephalocele	Rare		417
Meningomyelocele	Rare		466
Behavior disorders	10–20	Frequently related to deafness	99, 119
Central language disorders	5		142, 186, 523
Autism	5		99, 142, 205
Aqueductal occlusion and/or hydrocephalus	Rare		186, 407
Poor balance	Rare		119, 542
Progressive panencephalitis	Very rare	Has onset during adolescence	487, 522
Cardiovascular			
Patent ductus arteriosus	30	Frequently associated with other defects	17, 29, 137, 155, 207, 209, 214, 244, 255, 328, 434, 445, 479, 491, 519
Pulmonary arterial hypoplasia, supravalvular stenosis, valvular stenosis, and peripheral branch stenosis	25	Frequently associated with other defects	155, 207, 209, 214, 244, 434, 443, 491, 519

(Continued)

TABLE 177–5 ■ FREQUENCY AND MAIN CHARACTERISTICS OF CLINICAL FINDINGS IN CONGENITAL RUBELLA VIRUS INFECTION—cont'd

Clinical Findings	Frequency (%)	Main Characteristics	Selected References
Aortic stenosis	2–5		154, 214, 442, 508, 519
Ventricular and atrial septal defects	2–5		29, 137, 434, 491, 519
Tetralogy of Fallot	2–5		137, 209
Myocarditis and myocardial necrosis	10		4, 137, 255, 256, 328, 479, 519
Intimal fibromuscular proliferation of many arteries	5		136
Ventricular aneurysm	Rare		500
Pulmonary			
Interstitial pneumonitis	5–10	May be acute, subacute, or chronic	41, 137, 209, 255, 256, 328, 361, 363, 366, 417, 445, 479, 530
Tracheoesophageal fistula	Rare		417
Respiratory distress	Rare	Secondary to acute pneumonia	303
Gastrointestinal			
Esophageal atresia	Rare		235
Hepatitis	5–10	Associated with other evidence of disseminated disease	17, 137, 139, 209, 326, 327, 460, 479
Obstructive jaundice	5		255, 256, 328, 394, 445
Chronic diarrhea	Rare	Related to failure to thrive and immune deficiency	366, 479
Pancreatitis	Rare	May lead to diabetes in later life	57, 125
Jejunal or rectal atresia	Rare		137
Genitourinary			
Undescended testicle	Rare	Cause-and-effect relationship with rubella infection in doubt	303, 445
Polycystic kidney, ectopic kidney, renal agenesis, or bilobed kidney	Rare	Cause-and-effect relationship with rubella infection in doubt	136, 137, 306
Hypospadias	Rare	Cause-and-effect relationship with rubella infection in doubt	42, 155, 445
Duplication of ureter	Rare	Cause-and-effect relationship with rubella infection in doubt	29
Renal artery stenosis	Rare		302
Hydroureter and hydronephrosis	Rare	Cause-and-effect relationship with rubella in doubt	394
Inguinal hernia	Rare	Cause-and-effect relationship with rubella in doubt	210, 361, 434, 445
Nephritis and nephrocalcinosis	Rare		445, 479
Testicular agenesis	Rare	Cause-and-effect relationship with rubella in doubt	137
Orthopedic			
Bone radiolucencies	10–20	Radiolucencies in metaphyses of long bones	209, 303, 361, 372, 380, 384, 400, 401, 428, 514, 526, 530
Pathologic fractures	Rare		400
Bone deformities	Rare		81, 186, 284
Clubfoot	Rare		417
Myositis	Rare	Transitory defect	452
Skin			
Dermal erythropoiesis (blueberry muffin syndrome)	5	Transitory defect; usually associated with severe disease	254
Chronic rash	Rare		60, 203
Dermatoglyphic abnormalities	5		2, 9, 377
Dimples	Rare		201
Endocrine			
Diabetes mellitus	Rare		153, 245, 304
Thyroid disorder	Rare		99
Precocious puberty	Rare		99
Growth hormone deficiency	Rare		376
Hematologic			
Thrombocytopenic purpura	5–10	Usually associated with severe disease with high death rate; transitory	17, 28, 29, 33, 103, 155, 209, 235, 256, 264, 303, 361, 366, 372, 380, 381, 400, 401, 417, 434, 510
Hemolytic anemia	Rare	Transitory	325, 361, 381
Hypoplastic anemia	Rare	Transitory	101, 264
Extramedullary hematopoiesis	5–10	Usually associated with severe disease	479
Immunologic			
Thymic hypoplasia	Rare		205
Dysgammaglobulinemia	Rare		94, 202, 371, 388, 446
Asplenia	Rare		234

TABLE 177–5 ■ FREQUENCY AND MAIN CHARACTERISTICS OF CLINICAL FINDINGS IN CONGENITAL RUBELLA VIRUS INFECTION—cont'd

Clinical Findings	Frequency (%)	Main Characteristics	Selected References
Reticuloendothelial			
Generalized lymphadenopathy	10		101, 155, 203, 479
Hepatosplenomegaly	10–20	Usually associated with severe disease; transitory	29, 256, 372, 401, 417, 434
Genetic			
Chromosomal abnormalities	Rare	Cause-and-effect relationship with rubella not established	12, 342

Auditory Defects*

Sensorineural deafness is the most common manifestation of congenital rubella; almost all patients have some degree of hearing impairment. The hearing loss usually is bilateral but may be unilateral. Frequently, the only manifestation of congenital infection is deafness. An important note is that deafness is overlooked frequently in infancy, and children incorrectly are considered to be mentally retarded. All children born to mothers who had rubella during the first half of pregnancy should undergo hearing evaluation several times during the first 5 years of life, regardless of whether they have other manifestations of congenital infection.

Neurologic Findings†

Between 10 and 20 percent of all infants with congenital rubella have active meningoencephalitis at birth. Manifestations of this infection include one or more of the following: a full anterior fontanelle, irritability, hypotonia, seizures, lethargy, and head retraction and arching of the back. Cerebrospinal fluid examination reveals elevated protein and mild pleocytosis. Later neurologic disease, such as mental and motor retardation, can be related to the severity and persistence of the initial meningoencephalitis. Active central nervous system infection has been demonstrated for a year or more.

Behavior disorders occur commonly in children with deafness and often cannot be associated with apparent meningoencephalitis. Congenital rubella children with generalized growth retardation and a proportionally small head size often have normal intelligence. In contrast, the prognosis for mental development in a child with true microcephaly is poor.

Chronic progressive panencephalitis has developed in a small number of adolescents with congenital rubella, similar to measles-related subacute sclerosing panencephalitis.

Cardiovascular Findings‡

In severe congenital rubella with multisystem involvement, myocarditis occurs and often is a cause of death. Of the structural defects of the heart, patent ductus arteriosus is the most common. It may be the only lesion noted, but two thirds of patients have other lesions as well. Pulmonary artery stenosis is the next most common defect. It may involve the main pulmonary artery or its branches. Pulmonary valvular stenosis is the third most frequent defect. Pulmonic valvular or arterial stenosis and patent ductus arteriosus commonly occur together.

Other Manifestations*

The other manifestations of congenital rubella can be separated into three categories: manifestations related to active persistent infection, structural defects, and delayed manifestations of congenital rubella.

MANIFESTATIONS RELATED TO PERSISTENT INFECTION. This category encompasses a broad constellation of clinical events that largely were unknown before the pandemic of 1964. Collectively, they frequently are called the expanded congenital rubella syndrome and include interstitial pneumonitis, hepatitis, nephritis, bone radiolucencies, myositis, dermal erythropoiesis, chronic rash, thrombocytopenic purpura, hemolytic and hypoplastic anemia, immunologic deficiency, generalized lymphadenopathy, hepatosplenomegaly, meningoencephalitis, and myocarditis. Most infants with the expanded rubella syndrome clinically have low birth weight; exanthem caused by thrombocytopenia, dermal erythropoiesis, or both; hepatosplenomegaly; and jaundice. Radiographs usually reveal long-bone radiolucencies. Respiratory distress caused by both diffuse pulmonary disease and myocarditis occurs commonly, and meningoencephalitis usually is evident. The duration of chronic infection in these babies varies. Approximately 20 percent of survivors still are shedding virus at 1 year of age. Between 10 and 20 percent of babies with hepatosplenomegaly and thrombocytopenia die during the first year of life.

CONGENITAL ANOMALIES. Other than deafness, eye defects, and cardiac anomalies, which have been discussed previously, the association of other malformations with congenital rubella infection is less well established. Malformations such as tracheoesophageal fistula, jejunal atresia, inguinal hernia, and others recorded in Table 177–5 occur frequently without evidence of in utero infection. Because they are noted only sporadically in babies born after maternal rubella, they possibly are chance associations rather than cause-and-effect relationships.

DELAYED MANIFESTATIONS. The following delayed manifestations of congenital rubella that were not present in

*See references 17, 44, 119, 137, 155, 186, 194, 205, 207, 209, 265, 303, 319, 361, 366, 389, 417, 434, 489, 491, 496.

†See references 17, 18, 99, 101, 119, 120, 142, 186, 205, 207, 209, 235, 255, 256, 303, 361, 363, 365, 394, 395, 399, 401, 404, 407, 417, 434, 445, 466, 479, 487, 514, 522, 523, 530, 532.

‡See references 4, 17, 136, 137, 154, 155, 207, 209, 214, 236, 244, 255, 256, 328, 434, 442, 443, 445, 479, 491, 508, 519.

*See references 2, 9, 12, 17, 28, 29, 33, 41, 42, 57, 60, 81, 93, 94, 99, 101, 104, 125, 136, 137, 139, 153, 155, 176, 186, 201–203, 205, 209, 210, 235, 245, 254–256, 264, 284, 304, 325–328, 342, 361, 363, 366, 371, 372, 376, 381, 384, 388, 394, 400–402, 417, 428, 434, 439, 445, 446, 452, 460, 465, 479, 510, 514, 526, 530.

early life have been noted: endocrinopathies, deafness, ocular damage, vascular effects, and progressive rubella panencephalitis.[439] Of particular importance is the association between endocrine abnormalities and autoimmunity.[93] In one study of 201 deaf adolescents with congenital rubella, 23.3 percent had positive thyroid microsomal or thyroglobulin antibodies, and of these patients, 19.6 percent had thyroid gland dysfunction. Patients with congenital rubella have an increased incidence of insulin-dependent diabetes mellitus.[176]

Diagnosis

DIFFERENTIAL DIAGNOSIS

Postnatally Acquired Disease (see also Chapter 65)

Because no pathognomonic finding in rubella exists, the clinical diagnosis in an individual case often is difficult to make. However, as with other exanthematous diseases, the key to diagnosis is careful elicitation of historical data. Rubella is an epidemic disease with a high clinical rate of expression of exanthem. Therefore, it is unusual, when proper investigation is carried out, not to find the contact case or other cases in the community. Season also is an important consideration. Rubella generally occurs in the winter and spring, whereas enteroviral exanthems, which are the greatest masqueraders in young children, occur mainly in the summer and fall.

The incubation period also is important in separating German measles from exanthems caused by common enteroviruses or respiratory viruses. In rubella, the incubation period is long (18 ± 3 days), whereas in the other illnesses, the period usually is short (from 3 to 7 days). Age is important. Today, rubella mainly is an illness of adolescents and young adults, and enteroviral exanthems are uncommon occurrences at these ages.

The nature of fever is useful in making the diagnosis of rubella. Fever greater than 38.5° C (101.5° F) is unusual in rubella but common with enteroviral exanthems, measles, and *M. pneumoniae* infection. Generally, a past history of rubella infection is not particularly reliable. However, if a past illness can be documented by year, season, and symptoms, accurate information may be obtained. Useful characteristics of the rubella exanthem are its mild, erythematous, maculopapular, and discrete nature; marked pruritus in adolescents and adults; and an acneiform appearance on the face in adolescents.

Although suboccipital and posterior auricular lymphadenopathy often is thought by some investigators to be pathognomonic, its presence in nonrubella exanthems often leads to undue concern. In general, in a young child, suboccipital and posterior auricular lymphadenopathy occurs as commonly with enteroviral illnesses as with rubella. In young adults, however, this lymphadenopathy is much more useful because the enteroviral differential consideration is less of a problem. Similar lymphadenopathy does occur with acquired toxoplasmosis, infectious mononucleosis, and *M. pneumoniae* infection. A major problem in the differential diagnosis in adults is allergy. However, fever (even low grade), lymphadenopathy, headache, and eye pain, which are common events in rubella, should occur rarely in contact or other simple allergies.

Congenital Rubella

Making the diagnosis of congenital rubella in known maternal exposure generally is not difficult. However, examining an apparently normal child at periodic intervals during the first few years of life is important so that deafness and subtle neurologic defects are not missed. The diagnosis of congenital rubella after an uneventful pregnancy is more difficult to make. All babies with evidence of intrauterine growth retardation or stigmata suggestive of congenital infection should undergo virologic and serologic study for rubella, as well as for other infectious agents. Determination of the amount of serum IgM also can be useful in the study of babies with intrauterine growth retardation or babies born to mothers in whom rubella or other infection was suspected to have occurred during pregnancy.[462] Values greater than 21 mg/dL during the first week of life strongly indicate congenital infection; normal values do not rule out congenital infection, however.

SPECIFIC DIAGNOSIS

Postnatally Acquired Disease

Rubella viral infection can be diagnosed specifically by isolation of virus from nasal or throat specimens in AGMK or other sensitive tissue culture systems; by the observation of a significant change in value of HI, ELISA, immunofluorescence, CF, or neutralizing antibody in two sequential serum samples; or by the demonstration of specific rubella IgM antibody in a single serum sample. Most often today, the diagnosis of rubella is attempted by the use of a single serum test for identifying rubella IgM antibody.* Determination of rubella-specific IgM antibody in saliva 7 to 42 days after the onset of illness also has been shown to be both sensitive and specific.[379] Although practical, one should realize that the specificity and sensitivity of all routinely used tests are not 100 percent. False-positive results occur all too frequently and commonly lead to unnecessary interventions. When the diagnosis is critical, such as with suspected rubella in pregnancy, a wise approach is to study IgG antibody in paired sera collected 1 to 2 weeks apart in addition to determining IgM antibody.

HI has been the standard serologic diagnostic test, and demonstration of a fourfold or greater titer rise is reliable evidence of rubella infection. Today, however, HI rarely is available to the clinician. The usual test available is ELISA, and in most commercial laboratories the ability to determine a significant change in value from the acute phase to the convalescent phase should be questioned.

Congenital Rubella

The best method for definitive diagnosis of congenital rubella is viral isolation. Specimens for viral culture should be obtained from the nose, throat, urine, buffy coat of blood, and cerebrospinal fluid. Because of transplacental passage of maternal IgG, establishment of the diagnosis of congenital rubella in the neonatal period by serologic methods is fraught with difficulty. Usually, specific rubella IgM antibody can be demonstrated with presently available techniques. In questionable cases, follow-up studies comparing infant and maternal antibody values often establish the diagnosis. If the infant's value is the result solely of transplacentally acquired antibody, it should drop fourfold to eightfold by 3 months of age and continue to fall to nondetectable values by 6 to 8 months of age. However, the antibody value in some congenital infections also may fall, so

*See references 11, 21, 30, 31, 62, 76, 80, 107, 134, 145, 152, 173, 177, 231, 290, 309, 334, 356, 424, 447, 502.

disappearance of antibody in serum does not rule out in utero infection completely.

The retrospective diagnosis of congenital rubella in late infancy and the second year of life has been difficult to make. However, researchers have shown that affected children have low avidity of specific IgG antibody and, therefore, a retrospective diagnosis of congenital rubella can be made by specific avidity assays.[220] Also useful for the serologic diagnosis of congenital rubella during the prenatal and newborn periods are rubella-IgG-peptide–enzyme immunoassay and rubella-immunoblot.[301] Newborns who were infected during the first 12 weeks of gestation have reduced levels of antibodies directed at both the linear E1 epitope (SP15) and the topographic E2 epitope.

Fetal rubella can be diagnosed in amniotic fluid samples by reverse transcription–polymerase chain reaction.[387, 474]

Qualitative Demonstration of Rubella Antibody

The original screening method for rubella antibody was HI. Today, HI has been replaced by more rapid and easier tests involving enzyme immunoassay, erythrocyte agglutination, and LA. In general, all are both highly sensitive and specific.[79, 144]

Treatment

POSTNATALLY ACQUIRED DISEASE

Uncomplicated Rubella

No specific therapy is necessary or indicated for uncomplicated rubella. Starch baths may be useful in adults with troublesome pruritus. Of importance is that affected patients understand that they are contagious and that transmission of infection to a pregnant woman could have serious consequences.

Complications of Rubella

Occasionally, arthritis can be severe in adults. When weight-bearing joints are affected, rest is encouraged. Symptoms readily respond to aspirin therapy; corticosteroids are not indicated. In rubella encephalitis, care is supportive, with adequate maintenance of fluids and electrolytes.

Thrombocytopenia usually is self-limited; however, severe bleeding has occurred on occasion. Splenectomy is not indicated. Corticosteroid therapy often is used, but with little evidence of specific benefit in rubella-infected patients. In patients who do not recover rapidly and in those with severe bleeding, treatment with intravenous immunoglobulin should be considered.

MANAGEMENT OF EXPOSED PREGNANT WOMEN

Ideally, all pregnant women should have received rubella vaccine previously or been shown to have rubella antibody by an appropriate serologic test. If a pregnant woman is exposed to a person with rubella and the history of previous immunization or antibody presence is unknown, an immediate blood specimen should be obtained and a rubella antibody test performed. If antibody to rubella is demonstrated, no action is necessary. Susceptible rubella-exposed women should undergo careful clinical observation for fever, lymphadenopathy, or exanthem for a 4-week period. If illness occurs, a nasal specimen should be cultured for rubella virus and serum should be examined for rubella IgM antibody. A second serum specimen should be submitted for rubella antibody examination. If illness occurs, a specimen should be collected 1 to 2 weeks later; if the woman has no illness, the second serum should be collected 6 to 8 weeks after the exposure. If rubella antibody seroconversion is noted or specific IgM antibody is demonstrated, the risk of fetal infection and malformation is considerable. Because false-positive rubella IgM antibody test results are not rare occurrences, all tests that yield positive results should be repeated for confirmation (by another assay and in another laboratory if possible). The patient should be so advised and therapeutic abortion contemplated.

In situations of known exposure of a susceptible pregnant woman in which therapeutic abortion is not possible and exposure can be documented to have taken place within 72 hours, my opinion is that 20 mL of immunoglobulin should be administered immediately. The use of immunoglobulin is controversial, but in certain controlled situations, it has been effective in preventing disease.[49, 315, 413, 497]

MANAGEMENT OF PREGNANT WOMEN WITH AN EXANTHEM THOUGHT TO BE RUBELLA

In this circumstance, if previous rubella serologic study results are available, they are extremely useful. If previous serum antibody has been noted, the mother should be reassured that the present illness is not likely to be rubella. However, because false-positive rubella screening results do occur, a wise approach is to carry out rubella serologic study and, when possible, also viral culture. An acute-phase serum should be examined for rubella-specific IgM antibody. A second serum specimen should be collected 1 to 2 weeks after disappearance of the rash. If rubella antibody rose significantly or IgM antibody was demonstrated, it is highly likely that congenital infection has occurred and that anomalies may result. Again, a wise approach is to confirm IgM-positive test results. In this circumstance, the woman should be counseled regarding therapeutic abortion.

If a previous serum rubella antibody value is not available, a serum sample should be collected immediately and another 2 to 3 weeks later. These sera should be examined as paired specimens for rubella antibody and analyzed for specific rubella IgM antibody. If a rubella antibody rise is demonstrated or the presence of rubella IgM is noted, one must assume that an acute rubella viral infection has occurred, and the patient should be advised about the risk of congenital infection and the possibility of therapeutic abortion.

MANAGEMENT OF CHILDREN WITH CONGENITAL RUBELLA

Isolation Procedures

Most babies with congenital rubella still are infected actively at the time of birth, are contagious, and, therefore, should be placed in isolation. Room isolation and urine precautions are the major necessities. The isolated baby should be cared for only by persons known to be seropositive for rubella. Because rubella viral shedding has been known to occur for a year or more in some babies, isolation of infants with congenital rubella should be continued for this duration unless repeated viral cultures have proved negative.

After discharge from the hospital, no special precautions are necessary in the household setting. However, the parents should be advised of the potential risk to pregnant visitors.

Neonatal Period

As noted, the clinical manifestations of congenital rubella are varied, and in many infants, no symptoms are manifested during the first few months of life. In these apparently asymptomatic infants, no particular management problems are encountered. In other neonates, symptoms of continued viral infection are readily apparent and frequently are severe. In these infants, the following findings are important: pneumonia, thrombocytopenia, eye findings, heart defects, hyperbilirubinemia, and hepatosplenomegaly.

Although purpura and petechiae secondary to thrombocytopenia may be impressively severe in these infants, true hemorrhagic difficulties have not been a major problem. Corticosteroid therapy does not seem to be indicated, but considering treatment with intravenous immunoglobulin might be worthwhile. Careful evaluation of the eyes is important. Of immediate concern is the search for corneal clouding because its presence probably indicates infantile glaucoma. Cataracts and retinopathy also should be sought carefully. Infants with glaucoma should be referred immediately for ophthalmologic evaluation and therapy. Children with cataracts or retinopathy also should be referred, but therapy for cataracts is best delayed until a later age.

Respiratory distress secondary to extensive viral involvement should be managed similar to other neonatal respiratory disease: assisted ventilation and careful attention to arterial blood gas values and pH. Although jaundice secondary to congenital rubella infection rarely is severe, standard criteria for the treatment of hyperbilirubinemia should be followed. Hepatosplenomegaly may be marked in some instances but is of no therapeutic concern.

Cardiac evaluation should be the same as in affected infants without rubella. Specifically, congestive cardiac failure should be treated vigorously; in malignant conditions (patent ductus arteriosus, coarctation of the aorta), lifesaving surgery should be contemplated.

Long-Term Problems

DEAFNESS. Hearing disability is the most frequent abnormality after infection with congenital rubella; more than 80 percent of infected infants have some degree of hearing disability. In many instances, deafness is the only clinical manifestation of congenital rubella, and, because of the difficulty in making this diagnosis in early infancy, the diagnosis frequently is delayed. However, early diagnosis of deafness and institution of proper educational programs are the most productive measures in the long-term management of children with congenital rubella. All too frequently, poor medical advice has been responsible for the delay in making an appropriate diagnosis and providing therapy. Any time that a mother suspects that her child is deaf, specific audiometric testing should be performed. Many general practitioners, pediatricians, and even otolaryngologists think that hearing cannot be tested in infants. This concept must be discouraged vigorously; at proper centers, a severely deaf child can be recognized in virtually all instances.

If deafness is diagnosed, the child should be referred immediately to a training program. Information about training programs can be obtained from the Alexander Graham Bell Association for the Deaf, Inc., 3417 Volta Place, N.W., Washington, DC 20007, *http://www.agbell.org;* and The John Tracy Clinic, Inc., 806 West Adams Boulevard, Los Angeles, CA 90007, *http://www.johntracyclinic.org*. In virtually all instances, severely deaf children should be enrolled in an education program before or during the second year of life, and the child should be fitted with a proper auditory amplification device. Although deafness in congenital rubella is sensorineural, a surprising finding is that conduction defects also are noted in many older children. For these children, other aspects of otolaryngologic care may be indicated.

EYE PROBLEMS. All children with eye problems (cloudy cornea, glaucoma, cataracts, retinitis, strabismus) should be referred at an early age for ophthalmologic evaluation. Glaucoma needs immediate attention. Decisions about cataract surgery should be left to the discretion of the ophthalmologist but, in general, are well deferred until after the end of the first year. Retinopathy, though frequently impressive on ophthalmoscopic examination, rarely causes much visual defect. Strabismus is managed as it is in children without rubella. Advice on eye problems in congenital rubella can be obtained from the American Foundation for the Blind, Inc., 11 Penn Plaza, Suite 300, New York, NY 10001, *http://www.afb.org*.

HEART PROBLEMS. Congenital heart disease secondary to in utero rubella infection should be managed as heart disease is in children without rubella. Of importance is that the children be referred to cardiac centers where sophisticated diagnostic techniques and cardiac surgery facilities are available for correctable lesions.

MUSCULOSKELETAL PROBLEMS. Isolated musculoskeletal defects are relatively uncommon findings in congenital rubella. However, when the symptoms indicate, referral to a cerebral palsy clinic is useful, both for specific therapeutic modalities and for the camaraderie of group therapy for the children as well as the parents.

CENTRAL NERVOUS SYSTEM PROBLEMS. Careful analysis of the data available suggests that many infants who have been labeled retarded actually are children with auditory or visual defects who have not had proper diagnosis and training for their handicaps. No child with congenital rubella should be labeled mentally subnormal until extensive audiologic and ophthalmologic investigations and perhaps specific therapy have been performed. Probably only approximately 10 percent of all congenitally infected rubella children have a central nervous system defect that precludes normal development.

IMMUNOLOGIC DEFECTS. A small number of children with congenital rubella have been noted to have specifically low levels of serum IgG. These infants have systemic continued viral infection and in general do poorly. Although outcome studies are not available, administering immune serum globulin (intramuscular or intravenous immunoglobulin) to these infants periodically seems prudent.

MULTIPLE HANDICAPS. All too frequently, children infected in utero with rubella virus suffer from one or more of the handicaps mentioned. Care of these infants and children requires many different resources and modalities of therapy. Frequently, the physician is the one who is called on to coordinate both the diagnostic and the long-term educational efforts that are necessary for optimal progress of an affected child. In addition to the Alexander Graham Bell Association for the Deaf, The John Tracy Clinic, and the American Foundation for the Blind, already mentioned, the following agencies may be helpful to physicians or the parents of congenital rubella children: United Cerebral Palsy Research and Educational Foundation, Inc., 1600 L Street N.W., Suite 700, Washington, D.C. 20036-5602, *http://www.ucpa.org;* Easter Seal Research Foundation, 230 West Monroe Street, Suite 1800, Chicago, IL 60606, *http://www.easter-seals.org;* The Arc of the U.S., 1010 Wayne Avenue, Suite 650, Silver Spring, MD

20910, *http://www.thearc.org;* and Maternal and Child Health Division, Department of Health and Human Services, Parklawn Building, 5600 Fishers Lane, Rockville, MD 20852, *http://www.hrsa.gov.*

Prevention

ACTIVE IMMUNIZATION: LIVE ATTENUATED RUBELLA VIRUS VACCINE

At present, the one-attenuated rubella virus vaccine is available for use in the United States (RA 27/3 strain grown in WI38 human embryonic lung tissue culture). Vaccination can be expected to produce antibodies in more than 95 percent of those immunized.[15, 19, 282, 368, 415, 451, 512, 517, 521] Antibody titers after RA 27/3 vaccination are slightly lower than those after natural infection, but they have been demonstrated to persist for an 11- to 15-year period with a pattern similar to that occurring after natural infection, even in the absence of re-exposure to rubella virus.[38, 238, 368]

Because of universal immunization, rubella in the United States is currently at an all-time low, but indigenous cases still occur.[64, 66, 385] Finland's vigorous two-dose immunization program has resulted in the elimination of indigenous rubella.[359, 360]

Recommendations for Use

For complete information regarding rubella immunization, the reader is referred to the most recent recommendations of the Immunization Practices Advisory Committee of the U.S. Public Health Service,[15, 63, 68, 517] the recommendations of the Committee on Infectious Diseases of the American Academy of Pediatrics,[10] and the vaccine manufacturer's product information.

Rubella vaccine is recommended for all children 12 months of age or older, adolescents, and adults, particularly women, unless otherwise contraindicated. Vaccination of children protects them from rubella and thus prevents them from subsequently spreading it. Vaccinating susceptible postpubertal women confers individual protection from rubella-induced fetal injury. Vaccinating adolescents or adults in population groups such as those in colleges, places of employment, or military bases protects them from rubella and reduces the chance of epidemics occurring in partially immune groups.

Rubella vaccine should not be administered to infants younger than 1 year because persisting maternal antibodies may interfere with seroconversion. When rubella vaccine is part of a combination vaccine that includes measles antigen, it should be administered to children approximately 12 to 15 months of age. A second dose of measles-mumps-rubella vaccine is recommended at school entry. Children who have not received rubella vaccine at the optimal age should be vaccinated promptly. Because a history of rubella is not a reliable indicator of immunity, all children for whom vaccine is not contraindicated should be vaccinated.

Vaccinating all unimmunized prepubertal children and adolescents, as well as adult women in the child-bearing age group, must be emphasized. Because of the theoretic risk to the fetus, females of child-bearing age should receive vaccine only if they are not pregnant and understand that they should not become pregnant for 3 months after vaccination.

Educational and training institutions such as colleges, universities, and military bases should seek proof of rubella immunity (a positive serologic test or documentation of previous rubella vaccination) from all students and employees in the child-bearing age. Nonpregnant women who lack proof of immunity should be vaccinated unless contraindications exist.

For the protection of susceptible female patients and female employees, persons working in hospitals and clinics who might contract rubella from infected patients or who, if infected, might transmit rubella to pregnant patients either should have serologically demonstrated immunity to rubella or should receive the vaccine.

Routine premarital serologic testing for rubella immunity would enhance efforts to identify susceptible women before pregnancy. Prenatal or antepartum screening for rubella susceptibility should be undertaken and vaccine administered in the immediate postpartum period—before hospital discharge. Previous administration of anti-Rho(D) immunoglobulin (human) or blood products is not a contraindication to vaccination; however, 6- to 8-week postvaccination serologic testing should be performed for confirmation of seroconversion in those few who have received the globulin or blood products. Obtaining laboratory evidence of seroconversion in other vaccinees is not necessary.

No evidence has shown that live rubella virus vaccine given after exposure prevents illness or that vaccinating a person incubating rubella is harmful. However, because a single exposure may not result in infection and postexposure vaccination would protect a person in the event of future exposure, vaccination is recommended unless otherwise contraindicated.

Adverse Reactions

Vaccination in young children rarely is associated with any symptoms. Occasionally, rash, lymphadenopathy, mild fever, and upper respiratory symptoms have been observed.

More severe reactions have been noted rarely in children but have been an occasional problem in adults. Most of these complications were reported in association with the previously available vaccines, but complications with the RA 27/3 vaccine also have been noted.[19, 129] Particularly troublesome are arthralgia and arthritis.* These complaints occur most commonly in adults. Arthralgia develops in approximately 25 percent of susceptible postpubertal females after RA 27/3 vaccination, and approximately 10 percent have been reported to have arthritis-like signs and symptoms.[34, 191, 373] Infrequently, chronic or recurrent arthralgia, sometimes with arthritis or neurologic symptoms, including paresthesias, carpal tunnel syndrome, and blurred vision, reportedly have developed in susceptible vaccinees, primarily adult women.[68, 239] One group of investigators has reported the frequency of chronic joint symptoms and signs in adult women to be as high as 5 to 11 percent[480–482]; however, other data from the United States and other countries suggest that such complications caused by RA 27/3 vaccine are rare or perhaps nonexistent.[105, 151, 158, 213, 341, 448, 453]

Other complications, mainly with vaccines other than RA 27/3, include polyneuropathies (catcher's crouch, carpal tunnel syndrome, neuritis, and myeloradiculoneuritis),[83, 88, 175, 198, 252, 340, 408] marked lymphadenopathy,[81] and vasculitis and myositis.[204]

Geiger and associates[171] noted a persistent rubella virus infection in a 16-year-old boy with acute lymphoblastic leukemia in remission who was vaccinated. The virus was

*See references 16, 25, 88, 105, 184, 280, 331, 343, 373, 454, 473, 475, 476, 480–482, 513.

identified in the patient's peripheral blood mononuclear cells 8 months after immunization. In contrast, persistent infection could not be demonstrated in 10 children with symptomatic human immunodeficiency virus type 1 infection.[157]

Contraindications

Live rubella virus vaccine is contraindicated in pregnancy; in individuals with altered immune states such as immunodeficiency, leukemia, lymphoma, and generalized malignancy; or in patients treated with steroids, alkylating drugs, antimetabolites, and radiation. In addition, rubella vaccination should not be performed during febrile illnesses or when viral interference from another agent might preclude a "take" from the rubella immunization. Rubella immunization also, in most instances, should be deferred for 3 months after the administration of blood products, including immune serum globulin.

Inadvertent Rubella Immunization in Pregnancy

From January 1971 to April 1989, the Centers for Disease Control and Prevention followed to term 321 known rubella-susceptible pregnant women who had been vaccinated with rubella vaccine within 3 months before or 3 months after conception.[68] Ninety-four women received HPV-77 or Cendehill vaccine, 1 received a vaccine of unknown strain, and 226 received RA 27/3 vaccine. None of the 324 infants born to these women had malformations compatible with congenital rubella, but 5 of the infants had serologic evidence of subclinical infection.

PASSIVE IMMUNIZATION

The use of immunoglobulin for the prevention of rubella has been controversial for many years.* However, my opinion is that its use is indicated in certain circumstances. The specific indication for immune serum globulin is for the prevention of rubella in a woman thought to be susceptible to rubella who is in the first 20 weeks of pregnancy. If the exposure can be documented clearly as one to a specific, single person with rubella and immunoglobulin is given within 72 hours of that exposure, prevention of both maternal disease and congenital infection is likely. On the other hand, if the exposure were more general in nature (e.g., a schoolteacher exposed to a child or children in the school setting), the woman probably was exposed for a considerable time before realization of that exposure. Therefore, administration of immunoglobulin probably will be too late (well into the incubation period of her disease and after viremia), so congenital infection is unlikely to be prevented. The dose of immunoglobulin for the prevention of rubella during pregnancy is 20 mL intramuscularly.

QUARANTINE AND DISEASE CONTAINMENT

Patients with rubella should not have contact with susceptible persons until the rash has disappeared. Rubella containment is a vital part of the prevention policy in the United States today. Rubella is a reportable disease, and compliance is the obligation of all physicians and other health care professionals. Rubella reporting enables public health workers to organize vaccination programs so that small outbreaks of disease can be prevented from developing into major epidemics.

*See references 23, 48, 124, 188, 288, 295, 299, 315, 413, 497.

REFERENCES

1. Aboudy, Y., Fogel, A., Barnea, B., et al.: Subclinical reinfection during pregnancy followed by transmission of virus to the fetus. J. Infect. *34*:273–276, 1997.
2. Achs, R., Harper, R. T., and Siegel, M.: Unusual dermatoglyphic findings associated with rubella embryopathy. N. Engl. J. Med. *274*:148–150, 1966.
3. Aguado, J. M., Posada, I., Gonzalez, M., et al.: Meningoencephalitis and polyradiculoneuritis in adults: Don't forget rubella. Clin. Infect. Dis. *17*:785–786, 1993.
4. Ainger, L. E., Lawyer, N. G., and Fitch, C. W.: Neonatal rubella myocarditis. Br. Heart J. *28*:691–697, 1966.
5. Alford, B. R.: Rubella: La bête noire de la médecine. Laryngoscope *78*:1623–1659, 1968.
6. Alford, C. A., Jr.: Studies on antibody in congenital rubella infections. I. Physicochemical and immunologic investigations of rubella-neutralizing antibody. Am. J. Dis. Child. *110*:455–463, 1964.
7. Alford, C. A., Jr., Neva, F. A., and Weller, T. H.: Virologic and serologic studies on human products of conception after maternal rubella. N. Engl. J. Med. *271*:1275–1281, 1964.
8. Al-Nakib, W., Best, J. M., and Banatvala, J. E.: Rubella-specific serum and nasopharyngeal immunoglobulin responses following naturally acquired and vaccine-induced infection: Prolonged persistence of virus-specific IgM. Lancet *1*:182–185, 1975.
9. Alter, M., and Schulenberg, R.: Dermatoglyphics in the rubella syndrome. J. A. M. A. *197*:685–688, 1966.
10. American Academy of Pediatrics: Rubella. *In* Pickering L. K. (ed.): 2000 Red Book: Report of the Committee on Infectious Diseases. 25th ed. Elk Grove Village, IL, American Academy of Pediatrics, 2000, pp. 495–500.
11. Ankerst, J., Christensen, P., Kjellen, L., et al.: A routine diagnostic test for IgA and IgM antibodies to rubella virus: Absorption of IgG with *Staphylococcus aureus*. J. Infect. Dis. *130*:268–273, 1974.
12. Ansari, B. M., and Mason, M. K.: Chromosomal abnormality in congenital rubella. Pediatrics *59*:13–15, 1977.
13. Appleton, P. N., and Macrae, A. D.: Comparison of radial haemolysis with haemagglutination inhibition in estimating rubella antibody. J. Clin. Pathol. *31*:479–482, 1978.
14. Atkinson, I. E.: Rubella (Rotheln). Am. J. Med. Sci. *93*:17–34, 1887.
15. Atkinson, W. L., Pickering, L. K., Schwartz, B., et al.: General recommendations on immunization: recommendations of the Advisory Committee on Immunization Practices (ACIP) and the American Academy of Family Physicians (AAFP). M. M. W. R. Recomm. Rep. *51*(RR-2):1–359, 2002.
16. Austin, S. M., Altman, R., Barnes, E. K., et al.: Joint reactions in children vaccinated against rubella. Study I: Comparison of two vaccines. Am. J. Epidemiol. *95*:53–66, 1972.
17. Avery, G. B., Monif, G. G. R., Sever, J. L., et al.: Rubella syndrome after inapparent maternal illness. Am. J. Dis. Child. *110*:444–446, 1965.
18. Bailey, G.: Carpal-tunnel syndrome. B. M. J. *1*:1207, 1962.
19. Balfour, H. H., Jr., Balfour, C. L., Edelman, C. K., et al.: Evaluation of Wistar RA27/3 rubella virus vaccine in children. Am. J. Dis. Child. *130*:1089–1091, 1976.
20. Balfour, H. H., Jr., May, D. B., Rotte, T. C., et al.: A study of erythema infectiosum: Recovery of rubella virus and echovirus-12. Pediatrics *50*:285–290, 1972.
21. Banatvala, J. E., Best, J. M., Bertrand, J., et al.: Serological assessment of rubella during pregnancy. B. M. J. *3*:247–250, 1970.
22. Bardeletti, G., Kessler, N., and Aymard-Henry, M.: Morphology, biochemical analysis and neuraminidase activity of rubella virus. Arch. Virol. *49*:175–186, 1975.
23. Barenberg, L. H., Levy, W., Greenstein, N. M., et al.: Prophylactic use of human serum against contagion in a pediatric ward: Further observations, with special reference to measles and rubella. Am. J. Dis. Child. *63*:1101–1109, 1942.
24. Barfield, W., Gardner, R., Lett, S., et al.: Congenital rubella reinfection in a mother with anti-cardiolipin and anti-platelet antibodies. Pediatr. Infect. Dis. J. *16*:249–250, 1997.
25. Barnes, E. K., Altman, R., Austin, S. M., et al.: Joint reactions in children vaccinated against rubella. Study II: Comparison of three vaccines. Am. J. Epidemiol. *95*:59–66, 1972.
26. Barraclough, W. W.: German measles encephalomyelitis. Can. Med. Assoc. J. *36*:511–513, 1937.
27. Baublis, J. V., and Brown, G. C.: Specific response of the immunoglobulins to rubella infection. Proc. Soc. Exp. Biol. Med. *128*:206–210, 1968.
28. Bayer, W. L., Sherman, F. E., Michaels, R. H., et al.: Purpura in congenital and acquired rubella. N. Engl. J. Med. *273*:1362–1366, 1390–1391, 1965.

29. Bellanti, J. A., Artenstein, M. S., Olson, L. C., et al.: Congenital rubella: Clinicopathologic, virologic, and immunologic studies. Am. J. Dis. Child. *110*:464–471, 1965.
30. Bellany, K., Rousseau, S. A., and Gardner, P. S.: The development of an M antibody capture ELISA for rubella IgM. J. Virol. Methods *14*:243–251, 1986.
31. Bellin, E., Safyer, S., and Braslow, C.: False-positive IgM-rubella enzyme linked immunoassay in three first trimester pregnant patients. Pediatr. Infect. Dis. J. *9*:671–672, 1990.
32. Bennett, R. A., and Copeman, W. S. C.: Notes on rubella: With special reference to certain rheumatic sequelae. B. M. J. *1*:924–926, 1940.
33. Berge, T., Brunnhage, F., and Nilsson, L. R.: Congenital hypoplastic thrombocytopenia in rubella embryopathy. Acta Paediatr. (Stockh.) *52*:349–352, 1963.
34. Best, J. M., Banatvala, J. E., and Bowen, J. M.: New Japanese rubella vaccine: Comparative trials. B. M. J. *3*:221–224, 1974.
35. Best, J. M., Banatvala, J. E., and Watson, D.: Serum IgM and IgG response in postnatally acquired rubella. Lancet *2*:65–68, 1969.
36. Birch, C. J., Glaun, B. P., Hunt, V., et al.: Comparison of passive haemagglutination and haemagglutination-inhibition techniques for detection of antibodies to rubella virus. J. Clin. Pathol. *32*:128–131, 1979.
37. Black, F. L., Lamm, S. H., Emmons, J. E., et al.: Reactions to rubella vaccine and persistence of antibody in virgin-soil populations after vaccination and wild virus–induced immunization. J. Infect. Dis. *133*:393–398, 1976.
38. Black, F. L., Lamm, S. H., Emmons, J. E., et al.: Durability of antibody titers induced by RA27/3 rubella virus vaccine. J. Infect. Dis. *137*:322–323, 1978.
39. Blennow, G., Bekassy, A. N., Eriksson, M., et al.: Transient carpal tunnel syndrome accompanying rubella infection. Acta Paediatr. Scand. *71*:1025–1028, 1982.
40. Bolognese, R. J., Corson, S. L., Fuccillo, D. A., et al.: Evaluation of possible transplacental infection with rubella vaccination during pregnancy. Am. J. Obstet. Gynecol. *117*:939–941, 1973.
41. Boner, A., Wilmott, R. W., Dinwiddie, R., et al.: Desquamative interstitial pneumonia and antigen-antibody complexes in two infants with congenital rubella. Pediatrics *72*:835–839, 1983.
42. Boniuk, M., and Zimmerman, L. E.: Ocular pathology in the rubella syndrome. Arch. Ophthalmol. *77*:455–473, 1967.
43. Booth, J. C., and Stern, H.: Photodynamic inactivation of rubella virus. J. Med. Microbiol. *5*:515–528, 1972.
44. Borton, T. E., and Stark, E. W.: Audiological findings in hearing loss secondary to maternal rubella. Pediatrics *45*:225–229, 1970.
45. Bosma, T. J., Etherington, J., O'Shea, S., et al.: Rubella virus and chronic joint disease: Is there an association? J. Clin. Microbiol. *36*:3524–3526, 1998.
46. Böttiger, M., and Forsgren, M.: Twenty years' experience of rubella vaccination in Sweden: 10 years of selective vaccination (of 12-year-old girls and of women postpartum) and 13 years of a general two-dose vaccination. Vaccine *15*:1538–1544, 1997.
47. Bradford, R. I. C.: Two cases of rubella meningoencephalitis. B. M. J. *1*:312–313, 1943.
48. Brody, J. A., Sever, J. L., McAllister, R., et al.: Rubella epidemic on St. Paul Island in the Pribilofs, 1963. J. A. M. A. *191*:619–623, 1965.
49. Brody, J. A., Sever, J. L., and Schiff, G. M.: Prevention of rubella by gamma globulin during an epidemic in Barrow, Alaska in 1964. N. Engl. J. Med. *272*:127–129, 1965.
50. Brookhouser, P. E., and Bordley, J. E.: Congenital rubella deafness: Pathology and pathogenesis. Arch. Otolaryngol. *98*:252–257, 1973.
51. Buescher, E. L.: Behavior of rubella virus in adult populations. Arch. Ges. Virusforsch. *16*:470–476, 1965.
52. Buimovici-Klein, E., and Cooper, L. Z.: Immunosuppression and isolation of rubella virus from human lymphocytes after vaccination with two rubella vaccines. Infect. Immun. *25*:352–356, 1979.
53. Buimovici-Klein, E., Hite, R. L., Byrne, T., et al.: Isolation of rubella virus in milk after postpartum immunization. J. Pediatr. *91*:939–941, 1977.
54. Buimovici-Klein, E., Lang, P. B., Ziring, P. R., et al.: Impaired cell-mediated immune response in patients with congenital rubella: Correlation with gestational age at time of infection. Pediatrics *64*:620–626, 1979.
55. Buimovici-Klein, E., Weiss, K. E., and Cooper, L. Z.: Interferon production in lymphocyte cultures after rubella infection in humans. J. Infect. Dis. *135*:380–385, 1977.
56. Bullens, D., Smets, K., Vanhaesebrouck, P.: Congenital rubella syndrome after maternal reinfection. Cin. Pediatr. (Phila.) *39*:113–116, 2000.
57. Bunnell, C. E., and Monif, G. R. G.: Interstitial pancreatitis in the congenital rubella syndrome. J. Pediatr. *80*:465–466, 1972.
58. Cappel, R.: Cell-mediated immunity in experimental rubella infections. Arch. Virol. *47*:375–379, 1975.
59. Cappel, R., Schluederberg, A., and Horstmann, D. M.: Large-scale production of rubella precipitinogens and their use in the diagnostic laboratory. J. Clin. Microbiol. *1*:201–205, 1975.
60. Castrow, F. F., II, and Beukelaer, M. D.: Congenital rubella syndrome: Unusual cutaneous manifestations. Arch. Dermatol. *98*:260–262, 1968.
61. Catalano, L. W., Jr., Fuccillo, D. A., Traub, R. E., et al.: Isolation of rubella virus from placentas and throat cultures of infants: A prospective study after the 1964–65 epidemic. Obstet. Gynecol. *38*:6–14, 1971.
62. Caul, E. O., Smyth, G. W., and Clarke, S. K. R.: A simplified method for the detection of rubella-specific IgM employing sucrose density fractionation and 2-mercaptoethanol. J. Hyg. (Camb.) *73*:329–340, 1974.
63. Centers for Disease Control and Prevention: Control and prevention of rubella: Evaluation and management of suspected outbreaks, rubella in pregnant women, and surveillance for congenital rubella syndrome. M. M. W. R. Recomm. Rep. *50*(RR-12):1–23, 2001.
64. Centers for Disease Control and Prevention: Summary of notifiable diseases, United States, 1998. M. M. W. R. Morb. Mortal. Wkly. Rep. *47*(53):ii–92, 1999.
65. Centers for Disease Control and Prevention: Rubella and congenital rubella syndrome—United States, 1994–1997. M. M. W. R. Morb. Mortal. Wkly. Rep. *46*(16):350–354, 1997.
66. Centers for Disease Control: Increase in rubella and congenital rubella syndrome—United States, 1988–1990. M. M. W. R. Morb. Mortal. Wkly. *40*(6):93–99, 1991.
67. Centers for Disease Control: Outbreaks of rubella among the Amish—United States, 1991. M. M. W. R. Morb. Mortal. Wkly. Rep. *40*(16):264–265, 1991.
68. Centers for Disease Control: Rubella prevention. Recommendations of the Immunization Practices Advisory Committee (ACIP). M. M. W. R. Recomm. Rep. *39*(RR-15):1–18, 1990.
69. Centers for Disease Control: Rubella and congenital rubella syndrome—United States, 1985–1988. M. M. W. R. Morb. Mortal. Wkly. Rep. *38*(11):173–178, 1989.
70. Centers for Disease Control: Rubella outbreak among office workers—New York City. M. M. W. R. Morb. Mortal. Wkly. Rep. *34*(29):455–459, 1985.
71. Centers for Disease Control: Rubella in colleges—United States, 1983–1984. M. M. W. R. Morb. Mortal. Wkly. Rep. *34*(16):228–231, 1985.
72. Centers for Disease Control: Rubella outbreaks in prisons—New York City, West Virginia, California. M. M. W. R. Morb. Mortal. Wkly. Rep. *34*(40):615–618, 1985.
73. Centers for Disease Control: Rubella in hospitals—California. M. M. W. R. Morb. Mortal. Wkly. Rep. *32*(3):37–39, 1983.
74. Chagnon, A., and Laflamme, P.: Effect of acidity on rubella virus. Can. J. Microbiol. *10*:501–503, 1964.
75. Chambers, R. J., and Bywaters, E. G.: Rubella synovitis. Ann. Rheum. Dis. *22*:263–268, 1963.
76. Champsaur, H., Fattal-German, M., and Arranhado, R.: Sensitivity and specificity of viral immunoglobulin M determination by indirect enzyme-linked immunosorbent assay. J. Clin. Microbiol. *26*:328–331, 1988.
77. Chantler, J., Wolinsky, J. S., Tingle, A.: Rubella virus. *In* Knipe, D. M., and Howley, P. M. (eds.): Fields Virology. 4th ed., Vol. 1, Philadelphia, Lippincott Williams & Wilkins, 2001, pp. 963–990.
78. Chaye, H., Ou, D., Chong, P., et al.: Human T- and B-cell epitopes of E1 glycoprotein of rubella virus. J. Clin. Immunol. *13*:93–100, 1993.
79. Chernesky, M. A., DeLong, D. J., Mahony, J. B., et al.: Differences in antibody responses with rapid agglutination tests for the detection of rubella antibodies. J. Clin. Microbiol. *23*:772–776, 1986.
80. Chernesky, M. A., Wyman, L., Mahony, J. B., et al.: Clinical evaluation of the sensitivity and specificity of a commercially available enzyme immunoassay for detection of rubella virus–specific immunoglobulin M. J. Clin. Microbiol. *20*:400–404, 1984.
81. Cherry, J. D.: Unpublished data.
82. Cherry, J. D.: Newer viral exanthems. Adv. Pediatr. *16*:233–286, 1969.
83. Cherry, J. D.: Peripheral pain syndromes following rubella immunization. J. Pediatr. *80*:541–542, 1972.
84. Cherry, J. D.: Rubella: Past, present, and future. Volta Rev. *76*:461–465, 1974.
85. Cherry, J. D., Bobinski, J. E., and Comerci, G. D.: A clinical trial with live attenuated rubella virus vaccine (Cendehill 51 strain). J. Pediatr. *75*:79–86, 1969.
86. Cherry, J. D., Horvath, F. L., Comerci, G. D., et al.: Clinical trials with Cendehill strain attenuated rubella virus vaccine. Antimicrob. Agents Chemother. *9*:357–363, 1970.
87. Cherry, J. D., Soriano, F., and Jahn, C. L.: Search for perinatal viral infection: A prospective, clinical, virologic and serologic study. Am. J. Dis. Child. *116*:245–250, 1968.
88. Chin, J., and Werner, S. B.: Neuritis and arthritis following rubella immunization. J. A. M. A. *215*:485–486, 1971.
89. Chiriboga-Klein, S., Oberfield, S. E., Casullo, A. M., et al.: Growth in congenital rubella syndrome and correlation with clinical manifestations. J. Pediatr. *115*:251–255, 1989.
90. Cifarelli, P. S., and Freireich, A. W.: Rubella encephalitis. N. Y. State J. Med. *66*:1117–1122, 1966.
91. Claman, H. N., Suvatte, V., Githens, J. H., et al.: Histiocytic reaction in dysgammaglobulinemia and congenital rubella. Pediatrics *46*:89–96, 1970.
92. Clarke, M., Boustred, J., Schild, G. C., et al.: Effect of rubella vaccination programme on serological status of young adults in United Kingdom. Lancet *1*:1224–1226, 1979.
93. Clarke, W. L., Shaver, K. A., Bright, G. M., et al.: Autoimmunity in congenital rubella syndrome. J. Pediatr. *104*:370–373, 1984.

94. Cockburn, W. C.: World aspects of the epidemiology of rubella. Am. J. Dis. Child. *118*:112–122, 1969.
95. Collis, W. J., and Cohen, D. N.: Rubella retinopathy: A progressive disorder. Arch. Ophthalmol. *84*:33–35, 1970.
96. Communicable Disease Center: Rubella surveillance summary. M. M. W. R. Morb. Mortal. Wkly. Rep. *13*:351–354, 1964.
97. Communicable Disease Center: Rubella surveillance. June, 1969.
98. Connolly, J. H., Hitchinson, W. M., Allen, I. V., et al.: Carotid artery thrombosis, encephalitis, myelitis and optic neuritis associated with rubella virus infections. Brain *98*:583–594, 1975.
99. Cooper, L. Z.: Congenital rubella in the U.S. Prog. Clin. Biol. Res. *3*:1–22, 1975.
100. Cooper, L. Z., Florman, A. L., Ziring, P. R., et al.: Loss of rubella hemagglutination inhibition antibody in congenital rubella: Failure of seronegative children with congenital rubella to respond to HPV-77 rubella vaccine. Am. J. Dis. Child. *122*:397–403, 1971.
101. Cooper, L. Z., and Krugman, S.: Diagnosis and management: Congenital rubella. Pediatrics *37*:335–338, 1966.
102. Cooper, L. Z., and Krugman, S.: Clinical manifestations of postnatal and congenital rubella. Arch. Ophthalmol. *77*:434–439, 1967.
103. Cooper, L. Z., Preblud, S. R., and Alford, C. A., Jr.: Rubella. *In* Remington, J. S., and Klein, J. O. (eds.): Infectious Diseases of the Fetus and Newborn Infants. Philadelphia, W. B. Saunders, 1995, pp. 268–311.
104. Cooper, L. Z., Ziring, P. R., Ockerse, A. B., et al.: Rubella: Clinical manifestations and management. Am. J. Dis. Child. *118*:18–29, 1969.
105. Cooper, L. Z., Ziring, P. R., Weiss, H. J., et al.: Transient arthritis after rubella vaccination. Am. J. Dis. Child. *118*:218–225, 1969.
106. Corlett, W. T.: A Treatise on the Acute Infectious Exanthemata, Including Rubeola, Rubella, Scarlatina, Varicella and Vaccinia, with Especial Reference to Diagnosis and Treatment. Philadelphia, F. A. Davis, 1902, pp. 348–371.
107. Cradock-Watson, J. E., Bourne, N. S., and Vandervelde, E. M.: IgG, IgA and IgM responses in acute rubella determined by the immunofluorescent technique. J. Hyg. (Camb.) *70*:473–485, 1972.
108. Cradock-Watson, J. E., Macdonald, H., Ridehalgh, M. K. S., et al.: Specific immunoglobulin response in serum and nasal secretions after the administration of attenuated rubella vaccine. J. Hyg. (Camb.) *73*:127–141, 1974.
109. Cradock-Watson, J. E., Ridehalgh, M. K. S., Anderson, M. J., et al.: Fetal infection resulting from maternal rubella after the first trimester of pregnancy. J. Hyg. (Camb.) *85*:381–391, 1980.
110. Cradock-Watson, J. E., Ridehalgh, M. K. S., Bourne, M. S., et al.: Nasal immunoglobulin responses in acute rubella determined by the immunofluorescent technique. J. Hyg. (Camb.) *71*:603–617, 1973.
111. Cradock-Watson, J. E., Ridehalgh, M. K. S., and Chantler, S.: Specific immunoglobulins in infants with the congenital rubella syndrome. J. Hyg. (Camb.) *76*:109–123, 1976.
112. Cuetter, A. C., and John, J. F.: Nerve conduction studies in natural rubella. Ann. Neurol. *1*:199–200, 1977.
113. Cunningham, A. L., and Fraser, J. R. E.: Persistent rubella virus infection of human synovial cells cultured in vitro. J. Infect. Dis. *151*:638–645, 1985.
114. Dales, L. G., and Chin, J.: Public health implications of rubella antibody levels in California. Am. J. Public Health *72*:167–172, 1982.
115. Das, B. D., Lakhani, P., Kurtz, J. B., et al.: Congenital rubella after previous maternal immunity. Arch. Dis. Child. *65*:545–546, 1990.
116. Davison, C., and Friedfeld, L.: Acute encephalomyelitis following German measles. Am. J. Dis. Child. *55*:496–510, 1938.
117. Deinard, A. S., Bilka, P. J., Venters, H. D., et al.: Rubella-antibody titres in rheumatoid arthritis. Lancet *1*:526–528, 1974.
118. de Mazancourt, A., Waxham, M. N., Nicolas, J. C., et al.: Antibody response to the rubella virus structural proteins in infants with the congenital rubella syndrome. J. Med. Virol. *19*:111–122, 1986.
119. Desmond, M. M., Fisher, E. S., Vorderman, A. L., et al.: The longitudinal course of congenital rubella encephalitis in nonretarded children. J. Pediatr. *93*:584–591, 1978.
120. Desmond, M. M., Wilson, G. S., Melnick, J. L., et al.: Congenital rubella encephalitis. J. Pediatr. *71*:311–331, 1967.
121. Desmyter, J., Rawls, W. E., Melnick, J. L., et al.: Interferon in congenital rubella: Response to live attenuated measles vaccine. J. Immunol. *99*:771–777, 1967.
122. Dibbert, H.-J.: Diagnosis of rubella by demonstrating rubella-specific 19 S and 7 S antibodies. Zentralbl. Bakteriol. Hyg. *A234*:145–158, 1976.
123. Division of Maternal and Perinatal Studies, Department of Health, Sydney: Report on pregnancy complicated by wild rubella—Spring, 1971. Med. J. Aust. *2*:545–547, 1973.
124. Doege, T. C., and Kim, K. S. W.: Studies of rubella and its prevention with immune globulin. J. A. M. A. *200*:584–590, 1967.
125. Donowitz, M., and Gryboski, J. D.: Pancreatic insufficiency and the congenital rubella syndrome. J. Pediatr. *87*:241–243, 1975.
126. Dorfman, S. F., and Bowers, C. H., Jr.: Rubella susceptibility among prenatal and family planning clinic populations. Mt. Sinai J. Med. *52*:248–252, 1985.
127. Driscoll, S. G.: Histopathology of gestational rubella. Am. J. Dis. Child. *118*:49–53, 1969.
128. Dudgeon, J. A.: Congenital rubella: Pathogenesis and immunology. Am. J. Dis. Child. *118*:35–44, 1969.
129. Dudgeon, J. A., Marshall, W. C., and Peckham, C. S.: Rubella vaccine trials in adults and children: Comparison of three attenuated vaccines. Am. J. Dis. Child. *118*:237–246, 1969.
130. Dwyer, D. E., Hueston, L., Field, P. R., et al.: Acute encephalitis complicating rubella virus infection. Pediatr. Infect. Dis. J. *11*:238–239, 1992.
131. Dykewicz, C. A., Kruszon-Moran, D., McQuillan, G. M., et al.: Rubella seropositivity in the U.S., 1988–1994. Clin. Infect. Dis. *33*:1279–1286, 2001.
132. Ebbin, A. J., Wilson, M. G., Chandor, S. B., et al.: Inadvertent rubella immunization in pregnancy. Am. J. Obstet. Gynecol. *117*:505–512, 1973.
133. Enders, G., and Knotek, F.: Detection of IgM antibodies against rubella virus: Comparison of two indirect ELISAs and an anti-IgM capture immunoassay. J. Med. Virol. *19*:377–386, 1986.
134. Enders, G., Knotek, F., and Pacher, U.: Comparison of various serological methods and diagnostic kits for the detection of acute, recent, and previous rubella infection, vaccination, and congenital infections. J. Med. Virol. *16*:219–232, 1985.
135. Erickson, C. A.: Rubella early in pregnancy causing congenital malformations of eyes and heart. J. Pediatr. *25*:281–283, 1944.
136. Esterly, J. R., and Oppenheimer, E. H.: Vascular lesions in infants with congenital rubella. Circulation *36*:544–554, 1967.
137. Esterly, J. R., and Oppenheimer, E. H.: Pathological lesions due to congenital rubella. Arch. Pathol. *87*:380–388, 1969.
138. Esterly, J. R., and Oppenheimer, E. H.: The pathologic manifestations of intrauterine rubella infection. Arch. Otolaryngol. *98*:246–248, 1973.
139. Esterly, J. R., Slusser, R. J., Slusser, R. J., et al.: Hepatic lesions in the congenital rubella syndrome. J. Pediatr. *71*:676–685, 1967.
140. Evans, A. S., Cox, F., Nankervis, G., et al.: A health and seroepidemiological survey of a community in Barbados. Int. J. Epidemiol. *3*:167–175, 1974.
141. Fabiyi, A., Sever, J. L., Ratner, N., et al.: Rubella virus: Growth characteristics and stability of infectious virus and complement-fixing antigen. Proc. Soc. Exp. Biol. Med. *122*:392–396, 1966.
142. Feldman, R. B., Pinsky, L., Mendelson, J., et al.: Can language disorder not due to peripheral deafness be an isolated expression of prenatal rubella? Pediatrics *52*:296–299, 1973.
143. Fenner, F.: Classification and nomenclature of viruses: Second report of the International Committee on Taxonomy of Viruses. Intervirology *7*:1–115, 1976.
144. Ferraro, M. J., Kallas, W. M., Welch, K. P., et al.: Comparison of a new, rapid enzyme immunoassay with a latex agglutination test for qualitative detection of rubella antibodies. J. Clin. Microbiol. *25*:1722–1724, 1987.
145. Field, P. R., and Gong, C. M.: Diagnosis of postnatally acquired rubella by use of three enzyme-linked immunosorbent assays for specific immunoglobulins G and M and single radial hemolysis for specific immunoglobulin G. J. Clin. Microbiol. *20*:951–958, 1984.
146. Finklea, J. F., Sandifer, S. H., and Moore, G. T., Jr.: Epidemic rubella at the Citadel. Am. J. Epidemiol. *87*:367–372, 1968.
147. Fleet, W. F., Jr., Benz, E. W., Jr., Karzon, D. T., et al.: Fetal consequences of maternal rubella immunization. J. A. M. A. *227*:621–627, 1974.
148. Fogel, A., Gerichter, C. B., Rannon, L., et al.: Serologic studies in 11,460 pregnant women during the 1972 rubella epidemic in Israel. Am. J. Epidemiol. *103*:51–59, 1976.
149. Forbes, J. A.: Rubella: Historical aspects. Am. J. Dis. Child. *118*:5–11, 1969.
150. Forchheimer, F.: The enanthem of German measles. Trans. Am. Pediatr. Soc. *10*:118–128, 1898.
151. Ford, D. K., Reid, G. D., Tingle, A. J., et al.: Sequential follow up observations of a patient with rubella associated persistent arthritis. Ann. Rheum. Dis. *51*:407–410, 1992.
152. Forghani, B., Schmidt, N. J., and Lennette, E. H.: Demonstration of rubella IgM antibody by indirect fluorescent antibody staining, sucrose density gradient centrifugation and mercaptoethanol reduction. Intervirology *1*:48–59, 1973.
153. Forrest, J. M., Menser, M. A., and Harley, J. D.: Diabetes mellitus and congenital rubella. Pediatrics *44*:445–447, 1969.
154. Fortuin, N. J., Morrow, A. G., and Roberts, W. C.: Late vascular manifestations of the rubella syndrome. Am. J. Med. *51*:134–140, 1971.
155. Franco, S. A., Riley, H. D., Jr., and Chitwood, L. A.: The congenital rubella syndrome. South. Med. J. *63*:825–830, 1970.
156. Fraser, V., Spitznagel, E., Medoff, G., et al.: Results of a rubella screening program for hospital employees: A five-year review (1986–1990). Am. J. Epidemiol. *138*:756–764, 1993.
157. Frenkel, L. M., Nielsen, K., Garakian, A., et al.: A search for persistent measles, mumps, and rubella vaccine virus in children with human immunodeficiency virus type 1 infection. Arch. Pediatr. Adolesc. Med. *148*:57–60, 1994.
158. Frenkel, L. M., Nielsen, K., Garakian, A., et al.: A search for persistent rubella virus infection in persons with chronic symptoms after rubella and rubella immunization and in patients with juvenile rheumatoid arthritis. Clin. Infect. Dis. *22*:287–294, 1996.

159. Frey, T. K., Abernathy, E. S., Bosma, T. J., et al.: Molecular analysis of rubella virus epidemiology across three continents, North America, Europe, and Asia, 1961–1997. J. Infect. Dis. *178*:642–650, 1998.
160. Friedmann, I.: Cochlear pathology in viral disease. Adv. Otorhinolaryngol. *20*:155–177, 1973.
161. Friedmann, I., and Wright, M. I.: Histopathological changes in the foetal and infantile inner ear caused by maternal rubella. B. M. J. *2*:20–23, 1966.
162. Fruehan, A. E.: Erythema multiforme exudativum and arthritis following infection with rubella. N. Y. State J. Med. *63*:859–863, 1963.
163. Fry, J., Dillane, J. B., and Fry, L.: Rubella, 1962. B. M. J. *2*:833–834, 1962.
164. Fucillo, D. A., Steele, R. W., Hensen, S. A., et al.: Impaired cellular immunity to rubella virus in congenital rubella. Infect. Immun. *9*:81–84, 1974.
165. Fujimoto, T., Katoh, C., Hayakawa, H., et al.: Two cases of rubella infection with cardiac involvement. Jpn. Heart J. *20*:227–235, 1979.
166. Furukawa, T., Plotkin, S. A., Sedwick, W. D., et al.: Studies on hemagglutination by rubella virus. Proc. Soc. Exp. Biol. Med. *126*:745–750, 1967.
167. Gale, J. L., Detels, R., Kim, K. S. W., et al.: The epidemiology of rubella on Taiwan. III. Family studies in cities of high and low attack rates. Int. J. Epidemiol. *1*:261–265, 1973.
168. Gale, J. L., Grayston, J. T., Beasley, R. P., et al.: The epidemiology of rubella on Taiwan. II. 1968–1969 epidemic. Int. J. Epidemiol. *1*:253–260, 1973.
169. Ganguly, R., Cusumano, C. L., and Waldman, R. H.: Suppression of cell-mediated immunity after infection with attenuated rubella virus. Infect. Immun. *13*:464–469, 1976.
170. Geiger, J. C.: Epidemic of German measles in a city adjacent to an army cantonment, and its probable relation thereto. J. A. M. A. *70*:1818–1820, 1918.
171. Geiger, R., Fink, F. M., Sölder, B., et al.: Persistent rubella infection after erroneous vaccination in an immunocompromised patient with acute lymphoblastic leukemia in remission. J. Med. Virol. *47*:442–444, 1995.
172. Geltzer, A. I., Guber, D., and Sears, M. L.: Ocular manifestations of the 1964–65 rubella epidemic. Am. J. Ophthalmol. *63*:221–229, 1967.
173. Gerna, G., Zannino, M., Revello, M. G., et al.: Development and evaluation of a capture enzyme-linked immunosorbent assay for determination of rubella immunoglobulin M using monoclonal antibodies. J. Clin. Microbiol. *25*:1033–1038, 1987.
174. Gibbs, F. A., Gibbs, E. L., Carpenter, P. R., et al.: Electroencephalographic abnormality in "uncomplicated" childhood diseases. J. A. M. A. *171*:1050–1055, 1959.
175. Gilmartin, R. C., Jr., Jabbour, J. T., and Duenas, D. A.: Rubella vaccine myeloradiculoneuritis. J. Pediatr. *80*:406–412, 1972.
176. Ginsberg-Fellner, F., Witt, M. E., Fedun, B., et al.: Diabetes mellitus and autoimmunity in patients with the congenital rubella syndrome. Rev. Infect. Dis. 7(Suppl.):170–176, 1985.
177. Gispen, R., Nagel, J., Brand-Saathof, B., et al.: Immunofluorescence test for IgM rubella antibodies in whole serum after absorption with anti-γFc. Clin. Exp. Immunol. *22*:431–437, 1975.
178. Giuliani, G., Angela, G. C., Baglione, L., et al.: German measles: Acute benign viral lymphoreticulosis. The haemato-humoral and histological aspects of rubella. Panminerva Med. *2*:585–602, 1960.
179. Givens, K. T., Lee, D. A., Jones, T., et al.: Congenital rubella syndrome: Ophthalmic manifestations and associated systemic disorders. Br. J. Ophthalmol. *77*:358–363, 1993.
180. Goldwater, P. N., Quiney, J. R., and Banatvala, J. E.: Maternal rubella at St. Thomas' hospital: Is there a need to change British vaccination policy? Lancet *2*:1298–1330, 1978.
181. Goodman, A. K., Friedman, S. M., Beatrice, S. T., et al.: Rubella in the workplace: The need for employee immunization. Am. J. Public Health *77*:725–726, 1987.
182. Grahame, R., Armstrong, R., Simmons, N., et al.: Chronic arthritis associated with the presence of intrasynovial rubella virus. Ann. Rheum. Dis. *42*:2–13, 1983.
183. Granberg, C., and Meurman, O.: Performance of two new enzyme immunoassays for the detection of IgM and IgG antibodies to rubella. Eur. J. Clin. Microbiol. Infect. Dis. *13*:512–516, 1994.
184. Grand, M. G., Wyll, S. A., Gehlbach, S. H., et al.: Clinical reactions following rubella vaccination: A prospective analysis of joint, muscular and neuritis symptoms. J. A. M. A. *220*:1569–1572, 1972.
185. Grayston, J. T., Gale, J. L., and Watten, R. H.: The epidemiology of rubella on Taiwan. I. Introduction and description of the 1957–1958 epidemic. Int. J. Epidemiol. *1*:245–252, 1972.
186. Grayston, J. T., Peng, J. Y., and Lee, G. C. Y.: Congenital abnormalities following gestational rubella in Chinese: Report of a prospective study including five-year follow-up examinations after the 1957–1958 rubella epidemic on Taiwan (Formosa). J. A. M. A. *202*:1–6, 1967.
187. Green, R. H., Balsamo, M. R., Giles, J. P., et al.: Studies of the natural history and prevention of rubella. Am. J. Dis. Child. *110*:348–365, 1965.
188. Green, R. H., Balsamo, M. R., Giles, J. P., et al.: Experimental studies with rubella: Evaluation of gamma globulin for prophylaxis. Arch. Ges. Virusforsch. *16*:513–516, 1965.
189. Gregg, N. M.: Congenital cataract following German measles in the mother. Trans. Ophthalmol. Soc. Aust. *3*:35–46, 1941.
190. Griffith, J. P. C.: Rubella (Rotheln: German measles): With a report of one hundred and fifty cases. Med. Rec. *32*:11–41, 1887.
191. Grillner, L., Hedstrom, E.-E., Bergstrom, H., et al.: Vaccination against rubella of newly delivered women. Scand. J. Infect. Dis. *5*:237–241, 1973.
192. Gross, P. A., Portnoy, B., Mathies, A. W., Jr., et al.: A rubella outbreak among adolescent boys. Am. J. Dis. Child. *119*:326–331, 1970.
193. Guggenheimer, J., Nowak, A. J., and Michaels, R. H.: Dental manifestations of the rubella syndrome. Oral Surg. Oral Med. Oral Pathol. *32*:30–37, 1971.
194. Gumpel, S. M., Hayes, K., and Dudgeon, J. A.: Congenital perceptive deafness: Role of intrauterine rubella. B. M. J. *2*:300–304, 1971.
195. Gunn, W.: A case of rubella complicated by purpura haemorrhagica. Br. J. Child. Dis. *30*:111–117, 1933.
196. Gupta, J. D., Peterson, V. J., and Murphy, A. M.: Differential immune response to attenuated rubella virus vaccine. Infect. Immun. *5*:151–154, 1972.
197. Habel, K.: Transmission of rubella to *Macaca mulatta* monkeys. Public Health Rep. *57*:1126–1139, 1942.
198. Hale, M. S., and Ruderman, J. E.: Carpal tunnel syndrome associated with rubella immunization. Am. J. Phys. Med. *52*:189–193, 1973.
199. Halonen, P. E., Ryan, J. M., and Stewart, J. A.: Rubella hemagglutinin prepared with alkaline extraction of virus grown in suspension culture of BHK-21 cells. Proc. Soc. Exp. Biol. Med. *125*:162–167, 1967.
200. Hambling, M. H.: Effect of a vaccination programme on the distribution of rubella antibodies in women of childbearing age. Lancet *1*:1130–1138, 1975.
201. Hammond, K.: Skin dimples and rubella. Pediatrics *39*:291–292, 1967.
202. Hancock, M. P., Huntley, C. C., and Sever, J. L.: Congenital rubella syndrome with immunoglobulin disorder. J. Pediatr. *72*:636–645, 1968.
203. Hannissian, A. S., and Hashimoto, K.: Paramyxovirus-like inclusions in rubella syndrome. J. Pediatr. *81*:231–237, 1972.
204. Hannissian, A. S., Martinez, A. J., Jabbour, J. T., et al.: Vasculitis and myositis secondary to rubella vaccination. Arch. Neurol. *28*:202–204, 1973.
205. Hanshaw, J. B., and Dudgeon, J. A.: Rubella. *In* Viral Diseases of the Fetus and Newborn. Philadelphia, W. B. Saunders, 1978, pp. 17–96.
206. Hara, J., Fujimoto, F., Ishibashi, T., et al.: Ocular manifestations of the 1976 rubella epidemic in Japan. Am. J. Ophthalmol. *87*:642–645, 1979.
207. Hardy, J. B.: Clinical and developmental aspects of congenital rubella. Arch. Otolaryngol. *98*:230–236, 1973.
208. Hardy, J. B., McCracken, G. H., Jr., Gilkeson, M. R., et al.: Adverse fetal outcome following maternal rubella after the first trimester of pregnancy. J. A. M. A. *207*:2414–2420, 1969.
209. Hardy, J. B., Monif, G. R. G., and Sever, J. L.: Studies in congenital rubella, Baltimore, 1964–65. Bull. Johns Hopkins Hosp. *118*:97–108, 1966.
210. Hardy, J. B., and Sever, J. L.: Indirect inguinal hernia in congenital rubella. J. Pediatr. *73*:416–418, 1968.
211. Hardy, J. B., Sever, J. L., and Gilkeson, M. R.: Declining antibody titers in children with congenital rubella. J. Pediatr. *75*:213–220, 1969.
212. Harrison, B. L.: Neuritis following rubella. B. M. J. *1*:637, 1940.
213. Hart, H., and Marmion, B. P.: Rubella virus and rheumatoid arthritis. Ann. Rheum. Dis. *36*:3–12, 1977.
214. Hastreiter, A. R., Joorabchi, B., Pujatti, G., et al.: Cardiovascular lesions associated with congenital rubella. J. Pediatr. *71*:59–65, 1967.
215. Hattis, R. P., Halstead, S. B., Hermann, K. L., et al.: Rubella in an immunized island population. J. A. M. A. *223*:1019–1021, 1973.
216. Heathfield, K. W. G.: Carpal-tunnel syndrome. B. M. J. *2*:58, 1962.
217. Heggie, A. D.: Pathogenesis of the rubella exanthem: Isolation of rubella virus from the skin. N. Engl. J. Med. *285*:664–666, 1971.
218. Heggie, A. D.: Pathogenesis of the rubella exanthem: Distribution of rubella virus in the skin during rubella with and without rash. J. Infect. Dis. *137*:74–77, 1978.
219. Heggie, A. D., and Robbins, F. C.: Natural rubella acquired after birth: Clinical features and complications. Am. J. Dis. Child. *118*:12–17, 1969.
220. Herne, V., Hedman, K., and Reedik, P.: Immunoglobulin G avidity in serodiagnosis of congenital rubella syndrome. Eur. J. Clin. Microbiol. Infect. Dis. *16*:763–766, 1997.
221. Herrmann, K. L.: Available rubella serologic tests. Rev. Infect. Dis. 7(Suppl.):108–112, 1985.
222. Hildebrandt, H. M., and Maassab, H. F.: Rubella synovitis in a one-year-old patient. N. Engl. J. Med. *274*:1428–1430, 1966.
223. Hillenbrand, F. K. M.: Rubella in a remote community. Lancet *2*:64–66, 1956.
224. Hillenbrand, F. K. M.: The blood picture in rubella: Its place in diagnosis. Lancet *2*:66–68, 1956.
225. Hiro, V. Y., and Tasaka, S.: Die Rotheln sind eine Viruskrankheit. Monatsschr. Kinderheilk. *76*:328–332, 1938.
226. Hodges, G. M.: Neuritis following rubella. B. M. J. *1*:830–831, 1940.
227. Holmes, I. H., Wark, M. C., and Warburton, M. F.: Is rubella an arbovirus? II. Ultrastructural morphology and development. Virology *37*:15–25, 1969.

228. Honeyman, M. C., Dorman, D. C., Menser, M. A., et al.: HL-A antigens in congenital rubella and the role of antigens 1 and 8 in the epidemiology of natural rubella. Tissue Antigens *5*:12–18, 1975.
229. Honeyman, M. C., Forrest, J. M., and Dorman, D. C.: Cell-mediated immune response following natural rubella and rubella vaccination. Clin. Exp. Immunol. *17*:665–671, 1974.
230. Honeyman, M. C., and Menser, M. A.: Ethnicity is a significant factor in the epidemiology of rubella and Hodgkin's disease. Nature *251*:441–442, 1974.
231. Hornsleth, A., Leerhoy, J., Grauballe, P., et al.: Rubella-virus–specific IgM- and IgA-antibodies: The indirect immunofluorescence (IF) technique applied to sera with reduced IgG concentration. Acta Pathol. Microbiol. Scand. [B] *82*:742–744, 1974.
232. Hornstein, L., and Ben-Porath, E.: Rubella antibodies in women of childbearing age during an epidemic and the two years thereafter. Isr. J. Med. Sci. *12*:1189–1193, 1976.
233. Horstmann, D. M.: Problems in measles and rubella. Dis. Mon. *24*:3–52, 1978.
234. Horstmann, D. M.: Rubella. *In* Evans, A. S. (ed.): Viral Infections of Humans: Epidemiology and Control. 3rd ed. New York, Plenum Medical, 1990, pp. 617–631.
235. Horstmann, D. M., Banatvala, J. E., Riordan, J. T., et al.: Maternal rubella and the rubella syndrome in infants: Epidemiologic, clinical, and virologic observations. Am. J. Dis. Child. *110*:408–415, 1965.
236. Horstmann, D. M., Liebhaber, H., LeBouvier, G. L., et al.: Rubella: Reinfection of vaccinated and naturally immune persons exposed in an epidemic. N. Engl. J. Med. *283*:771–778, 1970.
237. Horstmann, D. M., Riordan, J. T., Ohtawara, M., et al.: A natural epidemic of rubella in a closed population: Virological and epidemiological observations. Arch. Ges. Virusforsch. *16*:483–487, 1965.
238. Horstmann, D. M., Schluederberg, A., Emmons, J. E., et al.: Persistence of vaccine-induced immune responses to rubella: Comparison with natural infection. Rev. Infect. Dis. *7*(Suppl.):80–85, 1985.
239. Howson, C. P., Katz, M., Johnston, R. B., Jr., et al.: Chronic arthritis after rubella vaccination. Clin. Infect. Dis. *15*:307–312, 1992.
240. Hynes, M.: Leucocyte count in rubella. Lancet *2*:679–680, 1940.
241. Hyypiä, T., Eskola, J., Laine, M., et al.: B-cell function in vitro during rubella infection. Infect. Immun. *43*:589–592, 1984.
242. Hyypiä, T., Eskola, J., Laine, M., et al.: Polyclonal activation of B cells during rubella infection. Scand. J. Immunol. *21*:615–617, 1985.
243. Jeffries, D. J., Johnson, A. H., and Mowbray, J. F.: Abnormal responses to rubella infection. J. Clin. Pathol. *29*:1003–1006, 1976.
244. Jeresaty, R. M., and Russell, W.: Hepatosplenomegaly and heart disease in the congenital rubella syndrome: Report of eight cases. Pediatrics *39*:36–42, 1967.
245. Johnson, G. M., and Tudor, R. B.: Diabetes mellitus and congenital rubella infection. Am. J. Dis. Child. *120*:453–455, 1970.
246. Judelsohn, R. G., and Wyll, S. A.: Rubella in Bermuda: Termination of an epidemic by mass vaccination. J. A. M. A. *223*:401–406, 1973.
247. Kanra, G. Y., and Vesikari, T.: Cytotoxic activity against rubella-infected cells in the supernatants of human lymphocyte cultures stimulated by rubella virus. Clin. Exp. Immunol. *19*:17–32, 1975.
248. Kelemen, G.: Rubella and deafness. Arch. Otolaryngol. *83*:520–532, 1966.
249. Kelley, P. W., Petrucelli, B. P., Stehr-Green, P., et al.: The susceptibility of young adult Americans to vaccine-preventable infections: A national serosurvey of US army recruits. J. A. M. A. *266*:2724–2729, 1991.
250. Kenny, F. M., Michaels, R. H., and Davis, K. S.: Rubella encephalopathy: Later psychometric, neurologic, and encephalographic evaluation of seven survivors. Am. J. Dis. Child. *110*:374–380, 1965.
251. Kenrick, K. G., Slinn, R. F., Dorman, D. C., et al.: Immunoglobulins and rubella-virus antibodies in adults with congenital rubella. Lancet *1*:548–551, 1968.
252. Kilroy, A. W., Schaffner, W., Fleet, W. F., Jr., et al.: Two syndromes following rubella immunization: Clinical observations and epidemiological studies. J. A. M. A. *214*:2287–2292, 1970.
253. Kistler, G. S., and Sapatino, V.: Temperature- and UV-light resistance of rubella virus infectivity. Arch. Ges. Virusforsch. *38*:11–16, 1972.
254. Klein, H. Z., and Markarian, M.: Dermal erythropoiesis in congenital rubella: Description of an infected newborn who had purpura associated with marked extramedullary erythropoiesis in the skin and elsewhere. Clin. Pediatr. (Phila.) *8*:604–607, 1969.
255. Korones, S. B., Ainger, L. E., Monif, G. R. G., et al.: Congenital rubella syndrome: New clinical aspects with recovery of virus from affected infants. J. Pediatr. *67*:166–181, 1965.
256. Korones, S. B., Ainger, L. E., Monif, G. R. G., et al.: Congenital rubella syndrome: Study of 22 infants. Am. J. Dis. Child. *110*:434–440, 1965.
257. Kresky, B., and Nauheim, J. S.: Rubella retinitis. Am. J. Dis. Child. *114*:305–310, 1967.
258. Krill, A. E.: The retinal disease of rubella. Arch. Ophthalmol. *77*:445–449, 1967.
259. Krugman, S. (ed.): Rubella Symposium. Am. J. Dis. Child. *110*:345–476, 1965.
260. Krugman, S. (ed.): International Conference on Rubella Immunization. Am. J. Dis. Child. *118*:2–410, 1969.
261. Krugman, S.: Present status of measles and rubella immunization in the U.S.: A medical progress report. J. Pediatr. *90*:1–12, 1977.
262. Krugman, S., and Ward, R.: The rubella problem: Clinical aspects, risk of fetal abnormality and methods of prevention. J. Pediatr. *44*:489–498, 1954.
263. Krugman, S., Ward, R., and Katz, S. L.: Rubella (German measles). *In* Infectious Diseases of Children. 6th ed. St. Louis, C. V. Mosby, 1977, pp. 274–292.
264. Lafer, C. Z., and Morrison, A. N.: Thrombocytopenic purpura progressing to transient hypoplastic anemia in a newborn with rubella syndrome. Pediatrics *38*:499–501, 1966.
265. Laguaite, J. K., and Joseph, M.: A study of children with communication problems associated with maternal rubella. South. Med. J. *58*:231–235, 1965.
266. Lalla, M., Vesikari, T., and Virolainen, M.: Lymphoblast proliferation and humoral antibody response after rubella vaccination. Clin. Exp. Immunol. *15*:193–202, 1973.
267. Landrigan, P. J., Stoffels, M. A., Anderson, E., et al.: Epidemic rubella in adolescent boys: Clinical features and results of vaccination. J. A. M. A. *227*:1283–1287, 1974.
268. Larson, H. E., Parkman, P. D., Davis, W. J., et al.: Inadvertent rubella virus vaccination during pregnancy. N. Engl. J. Med. *284*:870–873, 1971.
269. Lawless, M. R., Abramson, J. S., Harlan, J. E., et al.: Rubella susceptibility in sixth graders: Effectiveness of current immunization practice. Pediatrics *65*:1086–1089, 1980.
270. Lawton, A. R., Self, K. S., Royal, S. A., et al.: Ontogeny of B-lymphocytes in the human fetus. Clin. Immunol. Immunopathol. *1*:84–93, 1972.
271. Lebon, P., Daffos, F., Checoury, A., et al.: Presence of an acid-labile alpha-interferon in sera from fetuses and children with congenital rubella. J. Clin. Microbiol. *21*:775–778, 1985.
272. Lebon, P., and Lyon, G.: Non-congenital rubella encephalitis. Lancet *2*:468, 1974.
273. LeBouvier, G. L.: Precipitinogens of rubella virus–infected cells. Proc. Soc. Exp. Biol. Med. *130*:51–54, 1969.
274. LeBouvier, G. L.: Rubella precipitins. *In* International Symposium on Rubella Vaccines, London, 1968. Symposium Series in Immunobiological Standardization. Vol. 11. New York, Karger, 1969, pp. 113–138.
275. LeBouvier, G. L., and Plotkin, S. A.: Precipitin responses to rubella vaccine RA 27/3. J. Infect. Dis. *123*:220–223, 1971.
276. Lee, J. Y., and Bowden, S.: Rubella virus replication and links to teratogenicity. Clin. Microbiol. Rev. *13*:571–587, 2000.
277. Lehane, D. E., Newberg, N. R., and Beam, W. E., Jr.: Evaluation of rubella herd immunity during epidemic. J. A. M. A. *213*:2236–2239, 1970.
278. Lejarraga, H., and Peckham, C. S.: Birthweight and subsequent growth of children exposed to rubella infection in utero. Arch. Dis. Child. *49*:50–54, 1974.
279. Lennette, E. H., Schmidt, N. J., and Magoffin, R. L.: The hemagglutination inhibition test for rubella: A comparison of its sensitivity to that of neutralization, complement-fixation and fluorescent antibody tests for diagnosis of infection and determination of immunity status. J. Immunol. *99*:785–793, 1967.
280. Lerman, S. J., Nankervis, G. A., Heggie, A. D., et al.: Immunologic response, virus excretion, and joint reactions with rubella vaccine: A study of adolescent girls and young women given live attenuated virus vaccine (HPV-77:DE-5). Ann. Intern. Med. *74*:67–73, 1971.
281. Liebhaber, H.: Measurement of rubella antibody by hemagglutination inhibition. I. Variables affecting rubella hemagglutination. J. Immunol. *104*:818–825, 1970.
282. Liebhaber, H., Ingalls, T. H., LeBouvier, G. L., et al.: Vaccination with RA 27/3 rubella vaccine: Persistence of immunity and resistance to challenge after two years. Am. J. Dis. Child. *123*:133–136, 1972.
283. Lindquist, J. M., Plotkin, S. A., Shaw, L., et al.: Congenital rubella syndrome as a systemic infection: Studies of affected infants born in Philadelphia, U. S. A. Med. J. *2*:1401–1406, 1965.
284. Lock, F. R., Gatling, H. B., and Wells, H. B.: Difficulties in the diagnosis of congenital abnormalities: Experience in a study of the effect of rubella on pregnancy. J. A. M. A. *178*:711–714, 1961.
285. Lokietz, H., and Reynolds, F. A.: Postrubella thrombocytopenic purpura: Report of nine new cases and review of published cases. Lancet *85*:226–230, 1965.
286. Lovett, A. E., Hahn, C. S., Rice, C. M., et al.: Rubella virus–specific cytotoxic T-lymphocyte responses: Identification of the capsid as a target of major histocompatibility complex class I–restricted lysis and definition of two epitopes. J. Virol. *67*:5849–5858, 1993.
287. Macfarlane, D. W., Boyd, R. D., Dodrill, C. B., et al.: Intrauterine rubella, head size, and intellect. Pediatrics *55*:797–801, 1975.
288. Macrae, A. D., Mogford, H., Reid, D., et al.: Studies of the effect of immunoglobulin on rubella in pregnancy: Report of the Public Health Laboratory Service Working Party on Rubella. B. M. J. *2*:497–500, 1970.
289. Maller, R., Fryden, A., and Soren, L.: Mitogen stimulation and distribution of T- and B-lymphocytes during natural rubella infection. Acta Pathol. Microbiol. Scand. [C] *86*:93–98, 1978.
290. Mallinson, H., Roberts, C., and White, G. B. B.: Staphylococcal protein A: Its preparation and an application to rubella serology. J. Clin. Pathol. *29*:99–102, 1976.

291. Margolis, F. J., Wilson, J. L., and Top, F. H.: Postrubella encephalomyelitis: Report of cases in Detroit and review of literature. J. Pediatr. *23*:158–165, 1943.
292. Martenis, T. W., Bland, J. H., and Phillips, C. A.: Rheumatoid arthritis after rubella. Arthritis Rheum. *11*:683–687, 1968.
293. Matsumoto, A., and Higashi, N.: Electron microscopic studies on the morphology and the morphogenesis of togaviruses. Ann. Rep. Inst. Virus Res. Kyoto Univ. *17*:11–22, 1974.
294. Matter, L., Gorgievski-Hrisoho, M., and Germann, D.: Comparison of four enzyme immunoassays for detection of immunoglobulin M antibodies against rubella virus. J. Clin. Microbiol. *32*:2134–2139, 1994.
295. McCallin, P. F., Fuccillo, D. A., Ley, A. C., et al.: Gammaglobulin as prophylaxis against rubella-induced congenital anomalies. Obstet. Gynecol. *39*:185–189, 1972.
296. McCarthy, K., and Taylor-Robinson, C. H.: Rubella. Br. Med. Bull. *23*:185–191, 1967.
297. McCarthy, K., Taylor-Robinson, C. H., and Pillinger, S. E.: Isolation of rubella virus from cases in Britain. Lancet *2*:593–598, 1963.
298. McCarthy, M., Lovett, A., Kerman, R. H., et al.: Immunodominant T-cell epitopes of rubella virus structural proteins defined by synthetic peptides. J. Virol. *67*:673–681, 1993.
299. McDonald, J. C., and Peckham, C. S.: Gammaglobulin in prevention of rubella and congenital defect: A study of 30,000 pregnancies. B. M. J. *3*:633–637, 1967.
300. McMorrow, L. E., Vesikari, T., Wolman, S. R., et al.: Suppression of the response of lymphocytes to phytohemagglutinin in rubella. J. Infect. Dis. *130*:464–469, 1974.
301. Meitsch, K., Enders, G., Wolinski, J. S., et al.: The role of rubella-immunoblot and rubella-peptide-EIA for the diagnosis of the congenital rubella syndrome during the prenatal and newborn periods. J. Med. Virol. *51*:280–283, 1997.
302. Menser, M. A., Dorman, D. C., Reye, R. D. K., et al.: Renal-artery stenosis in the rubella syndrome. Lancet *1*:790–792, 1966.
303. Menser, M. A., and Forrest, J. M.: Rubella: High incidence of defects in children considered normal at birth. Med. J. Aust. *1*:123–126, 1974.
304. Menser, M. A., Forrest, J. M., and Bransby, R. D.: Rubella infection and diabetes mellitus. Lancet *1*:57–60, 1978.
305. Menser, M. A., Hudson, J. R., Murphy, A. M., et al.: Epidemiology of congenital rubella and results of rubella vaccination in Australia. Rev. Infect. Dis. 7(Suppl.):37–41, 1985.
306. Menser, M. A., Robertson, S. E. J., Dorman, D. C., et al.: Renal lesions in congenital rubella. Pediatrics *40*:901–904, 1967.
307. Merritt, H. H., and Koskoff, Y. D.: Encephalomyelitis following German measles. Am. J. Med. Sci. *191*:690–696, 1936.
308. Meurman, O. H.: Antibody responses in patients with rubella infection determined by passive hemagglutination, hemagglutination inhibition, complement fixation, and solid-phase radioimmunoassay tests. Infect. Immun. *19*:369–372, 1978.
309. Meurman, O. H., Viljanen, M. K., and Granfors, K.: Solid-phase radioimmunoassay of rubella virus immunoglobulin M antibodies: Comparison with sucrose density gradient centrifugation test. J. Clin. Microbiol. *5*:257–262, 1977.
310. Meyer, H. M., Hopps, H. E., Parkman, P. D., et al.: Control of measles and rubella through use of attenuated vaccines. Am. J. Clin. Pathol. *70*:128–135, 1978.
311. Michael, M.: Rubella: A report of an epidemic of eighty cases. Arch. Pediatr. *25*:598–606, 1908.
312. Michaels, R. H.: Suppression of antibody response in congenital rubella. J. Pediatr. *80*:583–588, 1972.
313. Michaels, R. H., and Kenny, R. M.: Postnatal growth retardation in congenital rubella. Pediatrics *43*:251–259, 1969.
314. Michaels, R. H., and Rogers, K. D.: A sex difference in immunologic responsiveness. Pediatrics *47*:120–123, 1971.
315. Miller, C. H., Dowd, J. M., Rytel, M. W., et al.: Prevention of rubella with γ-globulin. J. A. M. A. *201*:560–561, 1967.
316. Miller, C. L., Miller, E., Sequeira, P. J. L., et al.: Effect of selective vaccination on rubella susceptibility and infection in pregnancy. B. M. J. *291*:1398–1401, 1985.
317. Miller, C. L., Miller, E., and Waight, P. A.: Rubella susceptibility and the continuing risk of infection in pregnancy. B. M. J. *294*:1277–1278, 1987.
318. Miller, K. A., and Zager, T. D.: Rubella susceptibility in an adolescent female population. Mayo Clin. Proc. *59*:31–34, 1984.
319. Miller, M. H., Rabinowitz, M., and Cohen, M.: Pure-tone audiometry in prenatal rubella. Arch. Otolaryngol. *94*:25–29, 1971.
320. Millian, S. J., and Wegman, D.: Rubella serology: Applications, limitations and interpretations. Am. J. Public Health *62*:171–176, 1972.
321. Mitchell, L. A.: Sex differences in antibody- and cell-mediated immune response to rubella re-immunization. J. Med. Microbiol. *48*:1075–1080, 1999.
322. Mitchell, L. A., Décarie, D., Tingle, A. J., et al.: Use of synthetic peptides to map regions of rubella virus capsid protein recognized by human T lymphocytes. Vaccine *12*:639–646, 1994.
323. Mitchell, L. A., Tingle, A. J., Décarie, D., et al.: Identification of rubella virus T-cell epitopes recognized in anamnestic response to RA27/3 vaccine: Associations with boost in neutralizing antibody titer. Vaccine *17*:2356–2365, 1999.
324. Mitchell, L. A., Zhang, T., and Tingle, A. J.: Differential antibody responses to rubella virus infection in males and females. J. Infect. Dis. *166*:1258–1265, 1992.
325. Miyazaki, S., Ohtsuka, M., Ueda, K., et al.: Coombs-positive hemolytic anemia in congenital rubella. J. Pediatr. *94*:759–760, 1979.
326. Monif, G. R. G.: Congenital rubella. *In* Monif, G. R. G. (ed.): Viral Infections of the Human Fetus. London, Macmillan, 1969, pp. 104–132.
327. Monif, G. R. G., Asofsky, R., and Sever, J. L.: Hepatic dysfunction in the congenital rubella syndrome. B. M. J. *1*:1086–1088, 1966.
328. Monif, G. R. G., Avery, G. B., Korones, S. B., et al.: Postmortem isolation of rubella virus from three children with rubella-syndrome defects. Lancet *1*:723–724, 1965.
329. Monif, G. R. G., Hardy, J. B., and Sever, J. L.: Studies in congenital rubella, Baltimore 1964–65. I. Epidemiologic and virologic. Bull. Johns Hopkins Hosp. *118*:85–96, 1966.
330. Monif, G. R. G., Sever, J. L., Schiff, G. M., et al.: Isolation of rubella virus from products of conception. Am. J. Obstet. Gynecol. *91*:1143–1146, 1965.
331. Monto, A. S., Cavallaro, J. J., and Whale, E. H.: Frequency of arthralgia in women receiving one of three rubella vaccines. Arch. Intern. Med. *126*:635–639, 1970.
332. Morag, A., Morag, B., Bernstein, J. M., et al.: In vitro correlates of cell-mediated immunity in human tonsils after natural or induced rubella virus infection. J. Infect. Dis. *131*:409–416, 1975.
333. Morse, E. E., Zinkham, W. H., and Jackson, D. P.: Thrombocytopenic purpura following rubella infection in children and adults. Arch. Intern. Med. *117*:573–579, 1966.
334. Murphy, A. M., Field, P. R., and Collins, E.: The value of specific IgM tests in the early diagnosis of congenital rubella. Med. J. Aust. *2*:290–293, 1978.
335. Murphy, A. M., Reid, R. R., Pollard, I., et al.: Rubella cataracts: Further clinical and virologic observations. Am. J. Ophthalmol. *64*:1109–1119, 1967.
336. Myllyla, G., Vaheri, A., Vesikari, T., et al.: Interaction between human blood platelets, viruses and antibodies. IV. Post-rubella thrombocytopenic purpura and platelet aggregation by rubella antigen-antibody interaction. Clin. Exp. Immunol. *4*:323–332, 1969.
337. Naeye, R. L., and Blanc, W.: Pathogenesis of congenital rubella. J. A. M. A. *194*:1277–1283, 1965.
338. Naveh, Y., and Friedman, A.: Rubella encephalitis successfully treated with corticosteroids. Clin. Pediatr. (Phila.) *14*:286–287, 1975.
339. Niwa, Y., and Kanoh, T.: Immunological behaviour following rubella infection. Clin. Exp. Immunol. *37*:470–476, 1979.
340. Noble, J. S., and Wand, M.: Catcher's crouch and rubella immunization. J. A. M. A. *217*:212, 1971.
341. Norval, M., and Smith, C.: Search for viral nucleic sequences in rheumatoid cells. Ann. Rheum. Dis. *38*:456–462, 1979.
342. Nusbacher, J., Hirschhorn, K., and Cooper, L. Z.: Chromosomal abnormalities in congenital rubella. N. Engl. J. Med. *276*:1409–1413, 1967.
343. Ogra, P. L., and Herd, J. K.: Arthritis associated with induced rubella infection. J. Immunol. *107*:810–813, 1971.
344. Ogra, P. L., Kerr-Grant, D., Umana, G., et al.: Antibody response in serum and nasopharynx after naturally acquired and vaccine-induced infection with rubella virus. N. Engl. J. Med. *285*:1333–1339, 1971.
345. Ogra, P. L., Ogra, S. S., Chiba, Y., et al.: Rubella-virus infection in juvenile rheumatoid arthritis. Lancet *1*:1157–1168, 1975.
346. O'Neill, J. F.: Strabismus in congenital rubella: Management in the presence of brain damage. Arch. Ophthalmol. *77*:450–454, 1967.
347. Orenstein, W. A., Herrmann, K. L., Holmgreen, P., et al.: Prevalence of rubella antibodies in Massachusetts school children. Am. J. Epidemiol. *124*:290–298, 1986.
348. Orenstein, W. A., Heseltine, P. N. R., LeGagnoux, S. J., et al.: Rubella vaccine and susceptible hospital employees: Poor physician participation. J. A. M. A. *245*:711–713, 1981.
349. Ornoy, A., Segal, S., Nishmi, M., et al.: Fetal and placental pathology in gestational rubella. Am. J. Obstet. Gynecol. *116*:949–956, 1973.
350. Ou, D., Chong, P., Tripet, B., et al.: Analysis of T- and B-cell epitopes of capsid protein of rubella virus by using synthetic peptides. J. Virol. *66*:1674–1681, 1992.
351. Ozsoylu, S., Kanra, G., and Savas, G.: Thrombocytopenic purpura related to rubella infection. Pediatrics *62*:567–569, 1978.
352. Panush, R. S.: Serum hypocomplementemia with rubella arthritis: Case report. Mil. Med. *140*:117–118, 1975.
353. Parkman, P. D., Buescher, E. L., and Artenstein, M. S.: Recovery of rubella virus from Army recruits. Proc. Soc. Exp. Biol. Med. *111*:225–230, 1962.
354. Parkman, P. D., Buescher, E. L., Artenstein, M. S., et al.: Studies of rubella. I. Properties of the virus. J. Immunol. *93*:595–617, 1964.
355. Pattison, J. R., Dane, D. S., and Mace, J. E.: Persistence of specific IgM after natural infection with rubella virus. Lancet *1*:185–190, 1975.
356. Pattison, J. R., and Mace, J. E.: The detection of specific IgM antibodies following infection with rubella virus. J. Clin. Pathol. *28*:377–382, 1975.

357. Peckham, C. S.: Clinical and laboratory study of children exposed in utero to maternal rubella. Arch. Dis. Child. *47*:571–577, 1972.
358. Pedneault, L., Zrein, M., Robillard, L., et al.: Comparison of novel synthetic peptide-based DETECT-RUBELLA enzyme immunoassays with enzygnost and IMx for detection of rubella-specific immunoglobulin G. J. Clin. Microbiol. *32*:1085–1087, 1994.
359. Peltola, H., Davidkin, I., Paunio, M., et al.: Mumps and rubella eliminated from Finland. J. A. M. A. *284*:2643–2647, 2000.
360. Peltola, H., Heinonen, O. P., Valle, M., et al.: The elimination of indigenous measles, mumps, and rubella from Finland by a 12-year, two-dose vaccination program. N. Engl. J. Med. *331*:1397–1402, 1994.
361. Peters, E. R., and Davis, R. L.: Congenital rubella syndrome: Cerebral mineralizations and subperiosteal new bone formation as expressions of this disorder. Clin. Pediatr. (Phila.) *5*:743–746, 1966.
362. Pettersson, R. F., Oker-Blom, C., Kalkkinen, N., et al.: Molecular and antigenic characteristics and synthesis of rubella virus structural proteins. Rev. Infect. Dis. *7*(Suppl.):140–149, 1985.
363. Phelan, P., and Campbell, P.: Pulmonary complications of rubella embryopathy. J. Pediatr. *75*:202–212, 1969.
364. Phillips, C. A., Maeck, J. V. S., Rogers, W. A., et al.: Intrauterine rubella infection following immunization with rubella vaccine. J. A. M. A. *213*:624–625, 1970.
365. Phillips, C. A., Melnick, J. L., Yow, M. D., et al.: Persistence of virus in infants with congenital rubella and in normal infants with a history of maternal rubella. J. A. M. A. *193*:1027–1029, 1965.
366. Pineda, R. G., Desmond, M. M., Rudolph, A. J., et al.: Impact of the 1964 rubella epidemic on a clinic population. Am. J. Obstet. Gynecol. *100*:1139–1146, 1968.
367. Plotkin, S. A.: Rubella virus. *In* Lennette, E. H., and Schmidt, N. J. (eds.): Diagnostic Procedures for Viral and Rickettsial Infections. New York, American Public Health Association, 1969, pp. 364–413.
368. Plotkin, S. A., and Buser, F.: History of RA27/3 rubella vaccine. Rev. Infect. Dis. *7*(Suppl.):77–78, 1985.
369. Plotkin, S. A., and Farquhar, J. D.: Immunity to rubella: Comparison between naturally and artificially induced resistance. Postgrad. Med. J. *48*(Suppl. 3):47–59, 1972.
370. Plotkin, S. A., Farquhar, J. D., and Ogra, P. L.: Immunologic properties of RA 27/3 rubella virus vaccine: A comparison with strains presently licensed in the U.S. J. A. M. A. *225*:585–590, 1973.
371. Plotkin, S. A., Klaus, R. M., and Whitley, J. P.: Hypogammaglobulinemia in an infant with congenital rubella syndrome: Failure of 1-adamantanamine to stop virus excretion. J. Pediatr. *69*:1085–1091, 1966.
372. Plotkin, S. A., Oski, F. A., Hartnett, E. M., et al.: Some recently recognized manifestations of the rubella syndrome. J. Pediatr. *67*:182–191, 1965.
373. Polk, B. F., Modlin, J. F., White, J. A., et al.: A controlled comparison of joint reactions among women receiving one of two rubella vaccines. Am. J. Epidemiol. *115*:19–25, 1982.
374. Polk, B. F., White, J. A., DeGirolami, P. C., et al.: An outbreak of rubella among hospital personnel. N. Engl. J. Med. *303*:541–545, 1980.
375. Preblud, S. R., and Alford, C. A., Jr.: Rubella. *In* Remington, J. S., and Klein, J. O. (eds.): Infectious Diseases of the Fetus and Newborn Infant. 3rd ed. Philadelphia, W. B. Saunders, 1990, pp. 196–240.
376. Preece, M. A., Kearney, P. J., and Marshall, W. C.: Growth-hormone deficiency in congenital rubella. Lancet *2*:842–844, 1977.
377. Purvis-Smith, S. G., Howard, P. R., and Menser, M. A.: Dermatoglyphic defects and rubella teratogenesis. J. A. M. A. *209*:1865–1868, 1969.
378. Pustowoit, B., and Liebert, U. G.: Predictive value of serological tests in rubella virus infection during pregnancy. Intervirology *41*:170–177, 1998.
379. Ramsay, M. E., Brugha, R., Brown, D. W. G., et al.: Salivary diagnosis of rubella: A study of notified cases in the United Kingdom, 1991–4. Epidemiol. Infect. *120*:315–319, 1998.
380. Rausen, A. R., London, R. D., Mizrahi, A., et al.: Generalized bone changes and thrombocytopenic purpura in association with intrauterine rubella. Pediatrics *36*:264–267, 1965.
381. Rausen, A. R., Richter, P., Tallal, L., et al.: Hematologic effects of intrauterine rubella. J. A. M. A. *199*:75–78, 1967.
382. Rawls, W. E., Desmyter, J., and Melnick, J. L.: Serological diagnosis and fetal involvement in maternal rubella. J. A. M. A. *203*:627–631, 1968.
383. Rawls, W. E., Phillips, C. A., Melnick, J. L., et al.: Persistent virus infection in congenital rubella. Arch. Ophthalmol. 77:430–433, 1967.
384. Reed, G. B., Jr.: Rubella bone lesions. J. Pediatr. *74*:208–213, 1969.
385. Reef, S. E., Frey, T. K., Theall, K., et al.: The changing epidemiology of rubella in the 1990s. J. A. M. A. *287*:464–472, 2002.
386. Reese, A. B.: Congenital cataract and other anomalies following German measles in the mother. Am. J. Ophthalmol. *27*:483–487, 1944.
387. Revello, M. G., Baldanti, F., Sarasini, A., et al.: Prenatal diagnosis of rubella virus infection by direct detection and semiquantitation of viral RNA in clinical samples by reverse transcription–PCR. J. Clin. Microbiol. *35*:708–713, 1997.
388. Ribon, A., and Wasserman, E.: Immunodeficiency with congenital rubella. Ann. Allergy *32*:35–40, 1974.
389. Richards, C. S.: Middle ear changes in rubella deafness. Arch. Otolaryngol. *80*:48–59, 1964.
390. Robinson, J., Lemay, M., and Vaudry, W. L.: Congenital rubella after anticipated maternal immunity: Two cases and a review of the literature. Pediatr. Infect. Dis. J. *13*:812–815, 1994.
391. Robinson, R. G., Dudenhoeffer, F. E., Holroyd, H. J., et al.: Rubella immunity in older children, teenagers, and young adults: A comparison of immunity in those previously immunized with those unimmunized. J. Pediatr. *101*:188–191, 1982.
392. Rones, B.: The relationship of German measles during pregnancy to congenital ocular defects. Med. Ann. D. C. *13*:285–287, 1944.
393. Rorke, L. B.: Nervous system lesions in the congenital rubella syndrome. Arch. Otolaryngol. *98*:249–252, 1973.
394. Rorke, L. B., and Spiro, A. J.: Cerebral lesions in congenital rubella syndrome. J. Pediatr. *70*:243–255, 1967.
395. Rose, H. D.: Fatal rubella encephalitis. Am. J. Med. Sci. *268*:287–290, 1974.
396. Ross, A. C., and McCartney, A.: Progress of rubella immunity in pregnant women. B. M. J. *1*:1636, 1979.
397. Rossier, E., Phipps, P. H., Polley, J. R., et al.: Absence of cell-mediated immunity to rubella virus 5 years after rubella vaccination. Can. Med. Assoc. J. *116*:481–484, 1977.
398. Rossier, E., Phipps, P. H., Weber, J. M., et al.: Persistence of humoral and cell-mediated immunity to rubella virus in cloistered nuns and in schoolteachers. J. Infect. Dis. *144*:137–141, 1981.
399. Roy, F. H., Hiatt, R. L., Korones, S. B., et al.: Ocular manifestations of congenital rubella syndrome: Recovery of virus from affected infants. Arch. Ophthalmol. *75*:601–607, 1966.
400. Rudolph, A. J., Singleton, E. B., Rosenberg, H. S., et al.: Osseous manifestations of the congenital rubella syndrome. Am. J. Dis. Child. *110*:428–433, 1965.
401. Rudolph, A. J., Yow, M. D., Phillips, C. A., et al.: Transplacental rubella infection in newly born infants. J. A. M. A. *191*:843–845, 1965.
402. Sacks, R., and Habermann, E. T.: Pathological fracture in congenital rubella: A case report. J. Bone Joint Surg. Am. *59*:557–559, 1977.
403. Saeed, A. A., and Lange, L. S.: Guillain-Barré syndrome after rubella. Postgrad. Med. J. *54*:333–334, 1978.
404. Sallomi, S. J.: Rubella in pregnancy: A review of prospective studies from the literature. Obstet. Gynecol. *27*:252–256, 1966.
405. Salmi, A. A.: Gel precipitation reactions between alkaline-extracted rubella antigens and human sera. Acta Pathol. Microbiol. Scand. *76*:271–278, 1969.
406. Salmi, A. A.: Characterization of a structural antigen of rubella virus reacting by gel precipitation. Acta Pathol. Microbiol. Scand. *80*:534–544, 1972.
407. Sarwar, M., Azar-Kia, B., Schechter, M. M., et al.: Aqueductal occlusion in the congenital rubella syndrome. Neurology *24*:198–201, 1974.
408. Schaffner, W., Fleet, W. F., Kilroy, A. W., et al.: Poly-neuropathy following rubella immunization: A follow-up study and review of the problem. Am. J. Dis. Child. *127*:684–687, 1974.
409. Schamberg, J. F., and Kolmer, J. A.: The treatment of measles. *In* Acute Infectious Diseases. 2nd ed. Philadelphia, Lea & Febiger, 1928, pp. 545–573.
410. Schatzmayr, H. G.: Aspects of rubella infection in Brazil. Rev. Infect. Dis. 7(Suppl.):53–55, 1985.
411. Scheie, H. G., Schaffer, D. B., Plotkin, S. A., et al.: Congenital rubella cataracts: Surgical results and virus recovery from intraocular tissue. Arch. Ophthalmol. *77*:440–444, 1967.
412. Schell, K., and Wong, K. T.: Stability and storage of rubella complement-fixing antigen. Nature *212*:621–622, 1966.
413. Schiff, G. M.: Titered lots of immune globulin (Ig): Efficacy in the prevention of rubella. Am. J. Dis. Child. *118*:322–327, 1969.
414. Schiff, G. M., and Dine, M. S.: Transmission of rubella from newborns: A controlled study among young adult women and report of an unusual case. Am. J. Dis. Child. *110*:447–451, 1965.
415. Schiff, G. M., Linnemann, C. C., Shea, L., et al.: Evaluation of RA 27/3 rubella vaccine. J. Pediatr. *85*:379–381, 1974.
416. Schiff, G. M., Sever, J. L., and Huebner, R. J.: Experimental rubella: Clinical and laboratory findings. Arch. Intern. Med. *116*:537–543, 1965.
417. Schiff, G. M., Sutherland, J. M., Light, I. J., et al.: Studies on congenital rubella: Preliminary results on the frequency and significance of presence of rubella virus in the newborn and the effect of γ-globulin in preventing congenital rubella. Am. J. Dis. Child. *110*:441–443, 1965.
418. Schlesinger, S., and Schlesinger, M. J.: *Togaviridae*: The viruses and their replication. *In* Knipe, D. M., and Howley, P. M. (eds.): Fields Virology. 4th ed., Vol. 1. Philadelphia, Lippincott Williams & Wilkins, 2001, pp. 909–911.
419. Schlossberg, D., and Topolosky, M. K.: Military rubella. J. A. M. A. *238*:1273–1274, 1977.
420. Schmidt, N. J., Dennis, J., and Lennette, E. H.: Rubella virus hemagglutination with a wide variety of erythrocyte species. Appl. Microbiol. *22*:469–470, 1971.
421. Schmidt, N. J., and Lennette, E. H.: Complement-fixing and fluorescent antibody responses to an attenuated rubella virus vaccine. Am. J. Epidemiol. *91*:351–354, 1970.

422. Schmidt, N. J., Lennette, E. H., and Gee, P. S.: Demonstration of rubella complement-fixing antigens of two distinct particle sizes by gel filtration of Sephadex G-200. Proc. Soc. Exp. Biol. Med. *123*:758–762, 1966.
423. Schmidt, N. J., and Styk, B.: Immunodiffusion reactions with rubella antigens. J. Immunol. *101*:210–216, 1968.
424. Schmitz, H., Shinizu, H., Kampa, D., et al.: Rapid method to detect rubella immunoglobulin M and immunoglobulin A antibodies. J. Clin. Microbiol. *1*:132–135, 1975.
425. Schum, T. R., Nelson, D. B., Duma, M. A., et al.: Increasing rubella seronegativity despite a compulsory school law. Am. J. Public Health *80*:66–69, 1990.
426. Sears, M. L.: Congenital glaucoma in neonatal rubella. J. Ophthalmol. *51*:744–748, 1967.
427. Sedwick, W. D., and Sokol, F.: Nucleic acid of rubella virus and its replication in hamster kidney cells. J. Virol. *5*:478–481, 1970.
428. Sekeles, E., and Ornoy, A.: Osseous manifestations of gestational rubella in young human fetuses. Am. J. Obstet. Gynecol. *122*:307–312, 1975.
429. Seppala, M., and Vaheri, A.: Natural rubella infection of the female genital tract. Lancet *1*:46–47, 1974.
430. Sever, J. L.: The epidemiology of rubella. Arch. Ophthalmol. *77*:427–429, 1967.
431. Sever, J. L., Brody, J. A., Schiff, G. M., et al.: Rubella epidemic on St. Paul Island in the Pribilofs, 1963. J. A. M. A. *191*:624–626, 1965.
432. Sever, J. L., Fuccillo, D. A., Gilkeson, M. R., et al.: Changing susceptibility to rubella. Obstet. Gynecol. *32*:365–369, 1968.
433. Sever, J. L., Fuccillo, D. A., Gitnick, G. L., et al.: Rubella antibody determinations. Pediatrics *40*:789–797, 1967.
434. Sever, J. L., Hardy, J. B., Nelson, K. B., et al.: Rubella in the collaborative perinatal research study. II. Clinical and laboratory findings in children through 3 years of age. Am. J. Dis. Child. *118*:123–132, 1969.
435. Sever, J. L., Huebner, R. J., Castellano, G. A., et al.: Rubella complement fixation test. Science *148*:385–387, 1965.
436. Sever, J. L., Huebner, R. J., Fabiyi, A., et al.: Antibody responses in acute and chronic rubella. Proc. Soc. Exp. Biol. Med. *122*:513–516, 1966.
437. Sever, J. L., and Monif, G.: Limited persistence of virus in congenital rubella. Am. J. Dis. Child. *110*:452–454, 1965.
438. Sever, J. L., Schiff, G. M., and Huebner, R. J.: Frequency of rubella antibody among pregnant women and other human and animal populations. Obstet. Gynecol. *23*:153–159, 1964.
439. Sever, J. L., South, M. A., and Shaver, K. A.: Delayed manifestations of congenital rubella. Rev. Infect. Dis. 7(Suppl.):164–169, 1985.
440. Sherman, F. E., Michaels, R. H., and Kenny, F. M.: Acute encephalopathy (encephalitis) complicating rubella. J. A. M. A. *192*:675–681, 1965.
441. Shewmon, D. A., Cherry, J. D., and Kirby, S. E.: Shedding of rubella virus in a 4½-year-old boy with congenital rubella. Pediatr. Infect. Dis. *1*:342–343, 1982.
442. Siassi, B., Klyman, G., and Emmanouilides, G. C.: Hypoplasia of the abdominal aorta associated with the rubella syndrome. Am. J. Dis. Child. *120*:476–479, 1970.
443. Simpson, J. W., Nora, J. J., Singer, D. B., et al.: Multiple valvular sclerosis in Turner phenotypes and rubella syndrome. Am. J. Cardiol. *23*:94–97, 1969.
444. Simpson, R. E. H.: Rubella and polyarthritis. B. M. J. *1*:830–831, 1940.
445. Singer, D. B., Rudolph, A. J., Rosenberg, H. S., et al.: Pathology of the congenital rubella syndrome. J. Pediatr. *71*:665–675, 1967.
446. Singer, D. B., South, M. A., Montgomery, J. R., et al.: Congenital rubella syndrome: Lymphoid tissue and immunologic status. Am. J. Dis. Child. *118*:54–61, 1969.
447. Skaug, K., and Gaarer, P. I.: An indirect immunofluorescent antibody test for determination of rubella virus–specific IgM antibodies. Acta Pathol. Microbiol. Scand. [C] *86*:33–35, 1978.
448. Slater, P. E., Ben-Zvi, T., Fogel, A., et al.: Absence of an association between rubella vaccination and arthritis in underimmune postpartum women. Vaccine *13*:1529–1532, 1995.
449. Smith, K. A., Chess, L., and Mardiney, M. R., Jr.: The relationship between rubella hemagglutination inhibition antibody (HIA) and rubella-induced in vitro lymphocyte tritiated thymidine incorporation. Cell. Immunol. *8*:321–327, 1973.
450. Smithells, R. W., Sheppard, S., Holzel, H., et al.: National congenital rubella surveillance programme, 1 July 1971–30 June 1984. B. M. J. *291*:40–41, 1985.
451. Spencer, M. J., Cherry, J. D., Powell, K. R., et al.: Antibody responses following rubella immunization analyzed by HLA and ABO types. Immunogenetics *4*:365–372, 1977.
452. Spiro, A. J., and Rorke, L. B.: Skeletal muscle lesions in congenital rubella syndrome. Am. J. Dis. Child. *112*:427–428, 1966.
453. Spruance, S. L., Metcalf, R., Smith, C. B., et al.: Chronic arthropathy associated with rubella vaccination. Arthritis Rheum. *20*:741–747, 1977.
454. Spruance, S. L., and Smith, C. B.: Joint complications associated with derivatives of HPV-77 rubella virus vaccine. Am. J. Dis. Child. *122*:105–112, 1971.
455. Squadrini, F., Taparelli, F., DeRienzo, B., et al.: Rubella virus isolation from cerebrospinal fluid in postnatal rubella encephalitis. B. M. J. *2*:1329–1330, 1977.
456. Stallman, N. D., Allan, B. C., and Sutherland, C. J.: Prolonged rubella IgM antibody response. Med. J. Aust. *2*:629–631, 1974.
457. Staub, H. P.: Postrubella thrombocytopenic purpura: A report of eight cases with discussion of hemorrhagic manifestations of rubella. Clin. Pediatr. (Phila.) *7*:350–356, 1968.
458. Steele, R. W., Hensen, S. A., Vincent, M. M., et al.: A ^{51}Cr microassay technique for cell-mediated immunity to viruses. J. Immunol. *110*:1502–1510, 1973.
459. Stehr-Green, P. A., Cochi, S. L., Preblud, S. R., et al.: Evidence against increasing rubella seronegativity among adolescent girls. Am. J. Public Health *80*:88, 1990.
460. Stern, H., and Williams, B. M.: Isolation of rubella virus in a case of neonatal giant-cell hepatitis. Lancet *1*:293–295, 1966.
461. Stewart, G. L., Parkman, P. D., Hopps, H. E., et al.: Rubella-virus hemagglutination-inhibition test. N. Engl. J. Med. *276*:554–557, 1967.
462. Stiehm, E. R., Ammann, A. J., and Cherry, J. D.: Elevated cord macroglobulins in the diagnosis of intrauterine infections. N. Engl. J. Med. *275*:971–977, 1966.
463. Storch, G. A., Gruber, C., Benz, B., et al.: A rubella outbreak among dental students: Description of the outbreak and analysis of control measures. Infect. Control *6*:150–156, 1985.
464. Strassburg, M. A., Imagawa, D. T., Fannin, S. L., et al.: A rubella outbreak among hospital employees with exposure to women in early pregnancy. Obstet. Gynecol. *57*:283–288, 1981.
465. Strauss, L., and Bernstein, J.: Neonatal hepatitis in congenital rubella. Arch. Pathol. *86*:317–327, 1968.
466. Streissguth, A. P., Vanderveer, B. B., and Shepard, T. H.: Mental development of children with congenital rubella syndrome. Am. J. Obstet. Gynecol. *108*:391–399, 1970.
467. Sugaya, N., Nirasawa, M., Mitamura, K., et al.: Hepatitis in acquired rubella infection in children. Am. J. Dis. Child. *142*:817–818, 1988.
468. Svenningsen, N. W.: Thrombocytopenia after rubella (report of two cases). Acta Paediatr. Scand. *54*:97–100, 1965.
469. Swan, C., Tostevin, A. L., Mayo, H., et al.: Further observations on congenital defects in infants following infectious diseases during pregnancy, with special reference to rubella. Med. J. Aust. *1*:409–413, 1944.
470. Swan, C., Tostevin, A. L., Moore, B., et al.: Congenital defects in infants following infectious diseases during pregnancy: With special reference to the relationship between German measles and cataract, deaf-mutism, heart disease and microcephaly, and to the period of pregnancy in which the occurrence of rubella is followed by congenital abnormalities. Med. J. Aust. *11*:201–210, 1943.
471. Swartz, T. A.: An extensive rubella epidemic in Israel, 1972: Selected epidemiologic characteristics. Am. J. Epidemiol. *103*:60–66, 1976.
472. Swartz, T. A., Hornstein, L., and Epstein, I.: Epidemiology of rubella and congenital rubella infection in Israel, a country with a selective immunization program. Rev. Infect. Dis. 7(Suppl.):42–46, 1985.
473. Swartz, T. A., Klingberg, W., Goldwasser, R. A., et al.: Clinical manifestations according to age, among females given HPV-77 duck rubella vaccine. Am. J. Epidemiol. *94*:246–251, 1971.
474. Tanemura, M., Suzumori, K., Yagami, Y., et al.: Diagnosis of fetal rubella infection with reverse transcription and nested polymerase chain reaction: A study of 34 cases diagnosed in fetuses. Am. J. Obstet. Gynecol. *174*:578–582, 1996.
475. Thompson, G. R., Ferreyra, A., Brackett, R. G.: Acute arthritis complicating rubella vaccination: Arthritis Rheum. *14*:19–26, 1971.
476. Thompson, G. R., Weiss, J. J., Shillis, J. L., et al.: Intermittent arthritis following rubella vaccination: A three-year follow-up. Am. J. Dis. Child. *125*:526–530, 1973.
477. Thompson, K. M., and Tobin, J. O.: Isolation of rubella virus from abortion material. B. M. J. *1*:264–266, 1970.
478. Thong, Y. H., Steele, R. W., Vincent, M. M., et al.: Impaired in vitro cell-mediated immunity to rubella virus during pregnancy. N. Engl. J. Med. *289*:604–606, 1973.
479. Thorburn, M. J., and Miller, C. G.: Pathology of congenital rubella in Jamaica. Arch. Dis. Child. *42*:389–396, 1967.
480. Tingle, A. J., Allen, M., Petty, R. E., et al.: Rubella associated arthritis. I. Comparative study of joint manifestations associated with natural rubella infection and RA 27/3 rubella immunization. Ann. Rheum. Dis. *45*:110–114, 1986.
481. Tingle, A. J., Chantler, J. K., Pot, K. H., et al.: Postpartum rubella immunization: Association with development of prolonged arthritis, neurological sequelae, and chronic rubella viremia. J. Infect. Dis. *152*:606–612, 1985.
482. Tingle, A. J., Yang, T., Allen, M., et al.: Prospective immunological assessment of arthritis induced by rubella vaccine. Infect. Immun. *40*:22–28, 1983.
483. Tobin, J. O., Sheppard, S., Smithells, R. W., et al.: Rubella in the United Kingdom, 1970–1983. Rev. Infect. Dis. 7(Suppl.):47–52, 1985.
484. Tomlinson, I. W.: Rubella polyneuropathy. Postgrad. Med. J. *51*:30–32, 1975.
485. Tondury, G., and Smith, D.: Fetal rubella pathology. J. Pediatr. *68*:867–879, 1966.
486. Townsend, C. W.: Concerning German measles. Boston Med. Surg. J. *150*:403–404, 1904.

487. Townsend, J. J., Baringer, J. R., Wolinsky, J. S., et al.: Progressive rubella panencephalitis: Late onset after congenital rubella. N. Engl. J. Med. *292*:990–993, 1975.
488. Trudel, M., Nadon, F., Sequin, C., et al.: E1 glycoprotein of rubella virus carries an epitope that binds a neutralizing antibody. J. Virol. Methods *12*:243–250, 1985.
489. Ueda, K., Nishida, Y., Kano, M., et al.: Clinical studies of patients with rubella syndrome occurring in a high incidence in the Ryukyu Islands in 1965: On the diagnostic significance of clinical manifestations. Acta Paediatr. Jpn. *14*:9–16, 1972.
490. Ueda, K., Nishida, Y., Oshima, K., et al.: Seven-year follow-up study of rubella syndrome in Ryukyu with special reference to persistence of rubella hemagglutination inhibition antibodies. Jpn. J. Microbiol. *19*:181–185, 1975.
491. Ueda, K., Nishida, Y., Oshima, K., et al.: Congenital rubella syndrome: Correlation of gestational age at time of maternal rubella with type of defect. J. Pediatr. *94*:763–765, 1979.
492. Ueda, K., Sasaki, F., Tokugawa, K., et al.: The 1976–1977 rubella epidemic in Fukuoka City in Southern Japan: Epidemiology and incidences of complications among 80,000 persons who were school children at 28 primary schools and their family members. Biken J. *27*:161–168, 1984.
493. Ueda, K., Shingaki, Y., Sato, T., et al.: Hemolytic anemia following postnatally acquired rubella during the 1975–1977 rubella epidemic in Japan. Clin. Pediatr. (Phila.) *24*:155–157, 1985.
494. Ueno, Y.: Rubella arthritis: An outbreak in Tokyo. J. Rheumatol. *21*:874–876, 1994.
495. Ukkonen, P.: Rubella immunity and morbidity: Impact of different vaccination programs in Finland 1979–1992. Scand. J. Infect. Dis. *28*:31–35, 1996.
496. Upfold, L. J.: Deafness following rubella in pregnancy. Med. J. Aust. *1*:420–424, 1970.
497. Urquhart, G. E. D., Crawford, R. J., and Wallace, J.: Trial of high-titre human rubella immunoglobulin. B. M. J. *2*:1331–1332, 1978.
498. Vaheri, A., and Vesikari, T.: Small size rubella virus antigens and soluble immune complexes: Analysis by the platelet aggregation technique. Arch. Ges. Virusforsch. *35*:10–24, 1971.
499. Vaheri, A., Vesikari, T., Oker-Blom, N., et al.: Isolation of attenuated rubella-vaccine virus from human products of conception and uterine cervix. N. Engl. J. Med. *286*:1071–1074, 1972.
500. Van der Horst, R. L., and Gotsman, M. S.: Left ventricular aneurysm in rubella heart disease. Am. J. Dis. Child. *120*:248–251, 1970.
501. Veale, H.: History of an epidemic of Rotheln, with observations on its pathology. Edinburgh Med. J. *12*:404–414, 1866.
502. Vejtorp, M., Fanoe, E., and Leerhoy, J.: Diagnosis of postnatal rubella by the enzyme-linked immunosorbent assay for rubella IgM and IgG antibodies. Acta Pathol. Microbiol. Scand. [B] *87*:155–160, 1979.
503. Verder, H., Dickmeiss, E., Haahr, S., et al.: Late-onset rubella syndrome: Coexistence of immune complex disease and defective cytotoxic effector cell function. Clin. Exp. Immunol. *63*:367–375, 1986.
504. Vesikari, T., and Buimovici-Klein, E.: Lymphocyte responses to rubella antigen and phytohemagglutinin after administration of the RA 27/3 strain of live attenuated rubella vaccine. Infect. Immun. *11*:748–753, 1975.
505. Vesikari, T., Kanra, G. Y., Buimovici-Klein, E., et al.: Cell-mediated immunity in rubella assayed by cytotoxicity of supernatants from rubella virus–stimulated human lymphocyte cultures. Clin. Exp. Immunol. *19*:33–43, 1975.
506. Vesikari, T., Vaheri, A., and Leinikki, P.: Antibody response to rubella virion (V) and soluble (S) antigens in rubella infection and following vaccination with live attenuated rubella virus. Arch. Ges. Virusforsch. *35*:25–37, 1971.
507. Vesikari, T., Vaheri, A., Pettay, O., et al.: Congenital rubella: Immune response of the neonate and diagnosis by demonstration of specific IgM antibodies. J. Pediatr. *75*:658–664, 1969.
508. Vince, D. J.: The role of rubella in the etiology of supravalvular aortic stenosis. Can. Med. Assoc. J. *103*:1157–1160, 1970.
509. Vogt, R. L., and Clark, S. W.: Premarital rubella vaccination program. Am. J. Public Health *75*:1088–1089, 1985.
510. Vossaugh, P., Leikin, S., Avery, G., et al.: Neonatal thrombocytopenia in association with rubella. Acta Haematol. *35*:158–162, 1966.
511. Walker, J. M., and Nahmias, A. J.: Neurologic sequelae of rubella infection. Clin. Pediatr. (Phila.) *5*:699–702, 1966.
512. Wallace, R. B., and Isacson, P.: Comparative trial of HPV-77, DE-5 and RA 27/3 live-attenuated rubella vaccines. Am. J. Dis. Child. *124*:536–538, 1972.
513. Wallace, R. B., Libert, P., Ibrahim, M., et al.: Joint symptoms following an area-wide rubella immunization campaign: Report of a survey. Am. J. Public Health *62*:658–661, 1972.
514. Walls, W. L., Altman, D. H., Gair, D. R., et al.: Roentgenological findings in congenital rubella. Clin. Pediatr. (Phila.) *4*:704–708, 1965.
515. Ward, P. H., Honrubia, V., and Moore, B. S.: Inner ear pathology in deafness due to maternal rubella. Arch. Otolaryngol. *87*:40–46, 1968.
516. Warren, H. D., Rogliand, F. T., and Potsubay, S. F.: Thrombocytopenic purpura following rubella. Med. Clin. North Am. *30*:401–404, 1946.
517. Watson, J. C., Hadler, S. C., Dykewicz, C. A., et al.: Measles, mumps, and rubella—vaccine use and strategies for elimination of measles, rubella, and congenital rubella syndrome and control of mumps: Recommendations of the Advisory committee on Immunization Practices. M. M. W. R. Recomm. Rep. *47*(RR-8):1–57, 1998.
518. Waxham, M. N., and Wolinsky, J. S.: Immunochemical identification of rubella virus hemagglutinin. Virology *126*:194–203, 1983.
519. Way, R. C.: Cardiovascular defects and the rubella syndrome. Can. Med. Assoc. J. *97*:1329–1334, 1967.
520. Weber, B., Enders, G., Schlößer, R., et al.: Congenital rubella syndrome after maternal reinfection. Infection *21*:118–121, 1993.
521. Weibel, R. E., Stokes, J., Jr., Buynak, E. B., et al.: Live rubella vaccines in adults and children: HPV-77 and Merck-Benoit strains. Am. J. Dis. Child. *118*:226–229, 1969.
522. Weil, M. L., Itabashi, H. H., Cremer, N. E., et al.: Chronic progressive panencephalitis due to rubella virus simulating subacute sclerosing panencephalitis. N. Engl. J. Med. *292*:994–998, 1975.
523. Weinberger, M. M., Masland, M. W., Asbed, R. A., et al.: Congenital rubella presenting as retarded language development. Am. J. Dis. Child. *120*:125–128, 1970.
524. Weller, T. H., and Neva, F. A.: Propagation in tissue culture of cytopathic agents from patients with rubella-like illness. Proc. Soc. Exp. Biol. Med. *111*:215–225, 1962.
525. Wesselhoeft, C.: Rubella (German measles). N. Engl. J. Med. *236*:943–950, 978–988, 1947.
526. Whalen, J. P., Winchester, P., Krook, L., et al.: Neonatal transplacental rubella syndrome: Its effect on normal maturation of the diaphysis. Am. J. Roentgenol. Rad. Ther. Nucl. Med. *121*:166–172, 1974.
527. White, L. R., Leikin, S., Villavicencio, O., et al.: Immune competence in congenital rubella: Lymphocyte transformation, delayed hypersensitivity, and response to vaccination. J. Pediatr. *73*:229–234, 1968.
528. White, L. R., Sever, J. L., and Alepa, F. P.: Maternal and congenital rubella before 1964: Frequency, clinical features, and search for isoimmune phenomena. J. Pediatr. *74*:198–207, 1969.
529. Whitehouse, W. L.: Rubella before conception as a cause of foetal abnormality. Lancet *1*:139, 1963.
530. Williams, H. J., and Carey, L. S.: Rubella embryopathy: Roentgenologic features. Am. J. Roentgenol. Rad. Ther. Nucl. Med. *97*:92–99, 1966.
531. Williams, N. M., and Preblud, S. R.: Rubella and congenital rubella surveillance, 1983. M. M. W. R. CDC Surveill. Summ. *33*(4):1SS–10SS, 1984.
532. Wingo, S. M.: Encephalomyelitis complicating rubella: Report of a case. U. S. Naval Med. Bull. *45*:546–547, 1945.
533. Witney, E. W.: Neuritis following rubella. B. M. J. *1*:831, 1940.
534. Witte, J. J., Karchmer, A. W., Case, G., et al.: Epidemiology of rubella. Am. J. Dis. Child. *118*:107–111, 1969.
535. Wolinsky, J. S.: Rubella. *In* Fields, B. N., Knipe, D. M., Howley, P. M., et al. (eds.): Fields Virology. 2nd ed. New York, Raven Press, 1990, pp. 815–838.
536. Wolinsky, J. S., Berg, B. O., and Maitland, C. J.: Progressive rubella panencephalitis. Arch. Neurol. *33*:722–723, 1976.
537. Wolinsky, J. S., Dau, P. C., Buimovici-Klein, E., et al.: Progressive rubella panencephalitis: Immunovirological studies and results of isoprinosine therapy. Clin. Exp. Immunol. *35*:397–404, 1979.
538. Wolman, S. R., McMorrow, L. E., Ziring, P. R., et al.: Lack of chromosomal breakage in congenital rubella. Pediatrics *52*:213–220, 1973.
539. Wyll, S. A., and Herrmann, K. L.: Inadvertent rubella vaccination of pregnant women: Fetal risk in 215 cases. J. A. M. A. *225*:1472–1476, 1973.
540. Yanez, J. E., Thompson, G. R., Mikkelsen, W. M., et al.: Rubella arthritis. Ann. Intern. Med. *64*:772–777, 1966.
541. Zaknun, D., Weiss, G., Glatzl, J., et al.: Neopterin levels during acute rubella in children. Clin. Infect. Dis. *17*:521–522, 1993.
542. Zausmer, E.: Congenital rubella: Pathogenesis of motor deficits. Pediatrics *47*:16–26, 1971.
543. Zhang, D., Nikkari, S., Vainionpää, R., et al.: Detection of rubella, mumps, and measles virus genomic RNA in cells from synovial fluid and peripheral blood in early rheumatoid arthritis. J. Rheumatol. *24*:1260–1265, 1997.
544. Zrein, M., Joncas, J. H., Pedneault, L., et al.: Comparison of a whole-virus enzyme immunoassay (EIA) with a peptide-based EIA for detecting rubella virus immunoglobulin G antibodies following rubella vaccination. J. Clin. Microbiol. *31*:1521–1524, 1993.

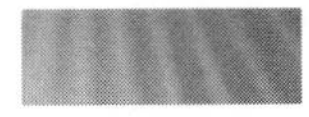

178 Alphaviruses

CHAPTER 178A

Eastern Equine Encephalitis

THEODORE F. TSAI

Eastern equine encephalitis (EEE) is an arthropod-borne viral infection of humans, horses, and other vertebrates that occurs in North and South America. In North America, infections recur in highly focal, primarily coastal locations in association with the habitat of *Culiseta melanura,* the enzootic vector. Birds are the amplifying hosts, and humans and horses are infected incidentally.

Etiologic Agent

EEE virus is an antigenically distinct member of the Alphavirus genus in the *Togaviridae* family. On the basis of nucleotide differences, EEE and Venezuelan equine encephalitis may have diverged 1000 to 2000 years ago, with a subsequent division of EEE virus into North and South American varieties.[7, 42, 44] South American strains can be differentiated by monoclonal antibodies and by short-incubation hemagglutination-inhibition (HI) tests.

North American strains collected over a broad geographic and temporal span demonstrate remarkable genetic stability in one or two major lineages, with minor local divergences occurring within isolated geographic loci. South American strains are genetically heterogeneous. They have been isolated in northward-migrating birds captured in the United States, but they have never been shown to become established.

Ecology

Equine cases have been reported as far north as Quebec, Ontario, and Alberta provinces; in South America, EEE viral activity has been reported from the Caribbean, Mexico, Guatemala, Honduras, Panama, Colombia, Venezuela, Peru, Guyana, and Brazil and as far south as Argentina.[4, 8, 23, 48] The viral transmission cycles in the Caribbean and South America are not well characterized but apparently involve small mammals, birds, and *Culex (Melanoconion)* mosquitoes.[23]

In North America, the distribution of virus activity closely follows the distribution of fresh-water swamps on the Eastern Seaboard, Gulf Coast, and other inland areas and corresponds to the distribution of the principal enzootic vector *C. melanura.*[10, 19, 23] *C. melanura* feeds nearly exclusively on birds, so various epizootic (bridging) vectors are responsible for infecting humans and horses.[20, 27, 30, 32, 46] Numerous species may be involved, including *Coquillettidia perturbans, Aedes sollicitans, Aedes vexans,* and *Aedes canadensis.*

Infection and viremia are subclinical in most native birds, whereas whooping cranes and exotic birds such as emus, house sparrows, ring-necked pheasants, Pekin ducks, and chukar partridges may become ill and die of infection.[3, 12, 13, 47, 51] Outbreaks resulting in thousands of deaths have occurred in commercial pheasant flocks, in some instances perpetuated by cannibalistic pecking or preening of persistently infected quills.[3] Illness and deaths in pigs, goats, calves, rodents, and other mammals also have been reported.[24, 38]

C. melanura is found in and near fresh-water swamps, where larval stages breed in acidic waters associated with mucky peat soils. These foci (from north to south) are found in upland red maple, coastal white cedar, and southern loblolly bay biotypes.[10, 23]

The viral overwintering mechanism has not been elucidated, but the remarkable permanence of endemic foci is a strong argument for overwintering in local reservoirs.[10, 29, 30, 32, 38]

Epidemiology

EEE is a rare sporadic infection, with a median of three cases occurring annually in the United States[34] (Fig. 178–1). The states with the highest rates of infection show an average annual incidence of less than 1 per 10 million (Fig. 178–2). However, these estimates obscure the remarkably consistent and focal distribution of cases on the Atlantic and Gulf Coasts, from Ontario to Texas, and in isolated pockets of activity inland.[4, 8] For example, until 1995, all human cases in Massachusetts had occurred east of Highway 495 in Essex, Norfolk, Plymouth, Bristol, and Middlesex counties; the six southernmost counties account for most of the epizootic activity in New Jersey; and foci of EEE viral activity recur in upstate New York counties near Syracuse, southwestern Michigan, northeastern Indiana, and northeastern Florida.[11, 30] Outbreaks of human cases caused by North American viral strains have been reported from Jamaica, Trinidad, and the Dominican Republic.[5, 16] Isolated epizootics with sporadic human cases have occurred in South America.[48]

Viral transmission, reflected in equine cases, occurs all year in Florida, although the peak incidence is from May to September.[6] Human cases have appeared as early as February and as late as December in Florida, with a peak occurring from June to August. In the Northeast, cases usually appear in late summer, from August to September, and as late as the third week in October.[34]

Cases occur chiefly at the extremes of age. However, serologic studies performed during the New Jersey outbreak disclosed that infection occurs with equal frequency in all age groups, thus indicating that biologic responses to infection rather than factors associated with exposure were responsible for the lower attack rates in young and middle-aged

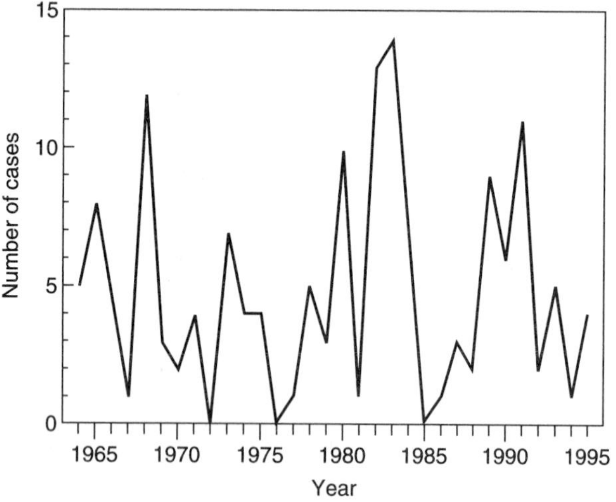

FIGURE 178–1 ■ Reported cases of eastern equine encephalitis by year, 1964 to 1995.

adults.[25] The ratio of inapparent infections to cases was highest in the middle years of life (29:1) and lowest in children younger than 4 years (8:1) and adults older than 55 (16:1).[25]

Family clusters were observed in this epidemic and in the 1947 Louisiana outbreak.[28] In the New Jersey study, family members of cases had twice the rate of inapparent infections as the general population did, and in the southern Louisiana outbreak, two fatal cases and two seropositive members were observed in the same family.[25, 28] Clusters of equine cases on a single premise are reported frequently.

Asymptomatic infections are uncommon occurrences, and long-term residence in an enzootic area leads to only a slight increase in population immunity. For example, even in an unusually active focus in southern New Jersey, only 7 percent of persons who had resided there 45 years or more had neutralizing antibody.[25] In serosurveys of endemic foci in Massachusetts, evidence of past infections was found in 0.5 to 0.7 percent of residents,[43] and a post-epizootic serosurvey of at-risk Connecticut pheasant farmers showed no evidence of infection.[36]

Specific behavioral risk factors have not been described; however, residence or outdoor activity near swampy habitats has been reported anecdotally as a possible contributing factor.

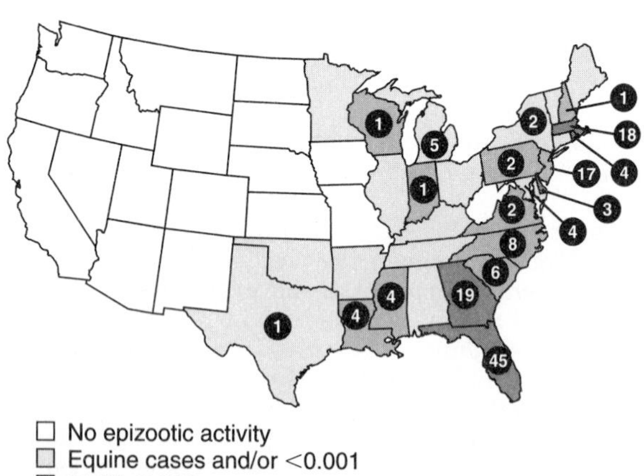

FIGURE 178–2 ■ Reported cases and average annual incidence (per 100,000) of eastern equine encephalitis by State, 1964 to 1995.

Clinical Manifestations

EEE is a fulminant encephalitis with rapid progression to coma and death in one third of patients.* In infants and children, an abrupt onset of fever, irritability, and headache is followed closely by lethargy, confusion, seizures, and coma. The often desperately ill infants may have a bulging fontanelle, meningismus, high temperature, and generalized flaccid or spastic paralysis.[1, 17, 22, 50, 52] Some patients are initially evaluated for status epilepticus. The prodrome in adults and older children usually is brief, with nonspecific symptoms of fever, headache, and dizziness followed by clouding of the sensorium and rapid deterioration to coma. Remarkably, some patients have a prolonged prodrome lasting longer than a week with a waxing and waning course of nonspecific symptoms, which may be associated with a better prognosis.[41, 43, 50] Various neurologic deficits have been described; in some cases, unilateral seizures, hemiparesis, hemiplegia, and aphasia have indicated focal areas of involvement.[15, 39, 41]

The peripheral leukocyte count usually is elevated with a shift to the left. White blood cell counts of 20,000/mm^3 are typical, ranging as high as 60,000 with 55 to 89 percent neutrophils.[43] Cerebrospinal fluid (CSF) usually shows a polymorphonuclear pleocytosis with a total leukocyte count ranging from 500 to 2000/mm^3. The initial neutrophilic pleocytosis of 60 to 100 percent may persist into the second week before shifting to a predominance of mononuclear cells.[44] CSF protein is elevated and glucose is reduced in most cases. Erythrocyte counts higher than 500/mm^3 are found in some cases.

Imaging studies disclose only cerebral edema in three quarters of patients. However, focal rim-enhancing lesions and areas of low alteration with mass effect have been observed on computed tomographic scans in the frontal cortex, thalami, midbrain, and lentiform nuclei.[15, 39, 41] Isointense diffusion-weighted images and hyperintensity on apparent diffusion coefficient images early in illness in one case suggested vasogenic edema in the T2-weighted hyperintense areas.[26] Electroencephalographic tracings with focal or background slowing have been associated with a favorable outcome, whereas disorganized background activity, a burst-suppression pattern, or high-voltage delta slowing have been associated with a poor prognosis.[43]

Mild nonencephalitic illnesses usually are not diagnosed. However, in the 1959 outbreak in New Jersey, fever, headache, nausea, vomiting, and sore throat were common symptoms in 19 patients who had serologic evidence of infection. One third of the patients had illnesses sufficiently severe to motivate them to consult their physicians.[25] Other patients with bladder dysfunction, dysesthesias, weakness, and signs of myelitis have been described.[9, 33] One case of infection during pregnancy has been reported. The third-trimester infection was severe, but the woman recovered from encephalitis and coma and delivered an apparently normal baby. Serologic studies of the neonate's blood were not performed.

Pathology

Pathologic changes in the brain are characterized by lesions in the cortical and deep gray matter, with varying degrees of neuronal loss from mild to extensive focal necrosis.[14, 40] Viral antigen is found predominantly in neurons and only occasionally in astrocytes.[21] Rare viral particles have been identified by electron microscopy in principally extracellular locations.[2, 31] Neutrophils predominate in cellular infiltrates

*See references 1, 2, 11, 15, 17, 18, 21, 26, 35, 39, 41, 43, 50, 52.

in the meninges, vascular cuffs, and foci of tissue damage in the cortex and brain nuclei of patients dying acutely; at later stages, neutrophilic infiltrates are replaced by mononuclear cells.[2, 14, 21, 40] Immunohistochemical examination of one patient disclosed a predominance of helper T cells in perivascular infiltrates, with some B lymphocytes. The most intense inflammatory reaction occurred in areas where antigen-positive neurons were absent, presumably where cell lysis already had occurred. Perivascular macrophages contained cleared viral antigen, but antigen could not be demonstrated in vascular endothelial cells.[21]

Pathogenesis

After peripheral inoculation of experimental animals, local viral replication occurs at a low level or may be undetectable. Viremia develops after this eclipse period, with disseminated infection of the spleen, liver, and kidneys noted in monkeys and guinea pigs and infection of the spleen, heart, and lungs observed in mice. Infectivity can be demonstrated in the brain only after viremia and infection in the viscera are established, thus suggesting that invasion of the central nervous system occurs by hematogenous spread.[40] Neurologic injury is associated with vasogenic edema in the earliest stages and subsequently with viral-induced cytolysis and host inflammatory responses.[26]

The immune response in humans is presumably similar to that observed in experimental alphavirus infections in mice, in which host resistance depends on rapid elaboration of a humoral immune response.

Prognosis and Sequelae

The case-fatality ratio is 33 percent among reported cases and is highest in the elderly; outcome is best in young adults 20 to 59 years of age, in whom the case-fatality rate is 24 percent.[34] Patients with a long prodromal illness (>4 days) have a better prognosis, which is consistent with the protective effect of a peripheral antibody response in the pre-neuroinvasive phase.[43]

Residual neurologic damage is observed more often in young children. In a Florida series, serious sequelae were seen in 4 of 7 survivors younger than 5 years and in 1 of 10 survivors in other age groups.[6] Similar findings were reported in a follow-up of epidemic cases in Massachusetts: seven of eight survivors younger than 3 years had neurologic sequelae, and only one of four surviving adults had residua.[1, 19] Neurologic impairment ranged from mild unilateral spasticity to profound mental retardation, seizure disorders, and quadriplegia.

Diagnosis

A specific laboratory diagnosis usually is made from serologic studies. Isolation of virus from CSF is unusual. The virus should be sought from brain biopsy tissue or autopsy material. EEE virus grows rapidly in a variety of cell lines, including Vero A549 and MRC-5 cells, and causes widespread cytopathic effect in several days.[45] Specific identification of viral isolates can be accomplished rapidly by immunofluorescent or immunoperoxidase techniques. EEE virus has been identified by immunofluorescence and by electron microscopy in brain tissue.[2, 21, 31] Viral antigen in viremic bird blood, infected mosquito pools, and infected equine brains can be detected directly by antigen capture enzyme-linked immunosorbent assay. Polymerase chain reaction analysis of CSF has been reported but has not been evaluated extensively.[44]

Serologic testing is available in many state laboratories. Virus-specific IgM usually can be detected in acute serum and CSF samples.[37] Indirect immunofluorescence, neutralization, and HI are also sensitive procedures. Antibodies are often present in the first week of illness. Neutralizing antibody appears 3 to 4 days after the onset of illness, and HI antibody appears with almost equal rapidity.[25] Both HI and neutralizing antibodies appear to be long lived.[25] Complement-fixing (CF) antibody is slower to rise and can be noted 11 days after onset, with diagnostic fourfold rises often appearing only in the third week after onset.[25] The peaks of both HI and CF titers are observed 3 to 4 weeks after onset.[26] CF antibody declines more rapidly. Measurable CF antibodies were found in approximately 50 percent of persons infected 8 years earlier in one study, although the effects of re-exposure could not be ruled out in this endemic area.[25]

The low prevalence of EEE antibody in the general population suggests that detection of EEE viral antibody in the acute serum of a patient with encephalitis indicates a high probability of that diagnosis. According to the Bayes theorem, if the "rate" of EEE is 1 in every 2000 cases of encephalitis, if HI antibody to EEE is present in 100 percent of cases in the first week of illness, and if the prevalence of HI antibody in the general population is 0.05 percent, the presence of EEE in an encephalitis patient who has demonstrable EEE antibody in a single serum specimen is a certainty. Thus, the probability of the diagnosis is high when specific antibody is found in any (i.e., acute) serum specimen.

Differential Diagnosis

The fulminant clinical course of EEE and the laboratory findings of neutrophilic leukocytosis and polymorphonuclear pleocytosis in the CSF may suggest bacterial cerebritis or meningitis. Because no specific therapy is available, EEE should be a diagnosis of exclusion after effort has been made to diagnose and to treat empirically against bacterial and herpes viral infections.

Treatment

Specific treatment is unavailable. Therapy aimed at supporting cardiorespiratory function, homeostasis of fluid, electrolyte balance, and control of cerebral edema and convulsions may be lifesaving. In a single case, intravenous immunoglobulin and glucocorticoids, given for their potential immunomodulatory effects, were associated with survival in an elderly patient.[26]

Prevention

An effective killed vaccine is licensed for horses, but no human vaccine is licensed. An investigational killed vaccine, available under investigatory permit, is used to protect laboratory personnel. Vaccination of the general public is not feasible as a public health measure because of the low incidence of disease.

Climatologic studies have shown a correlation between outbreaks and heavy rainfall in the summer of an epidemic year and in the preceding fall.[29, 32, 34] Although such predictors would have considerable utility in guiding control measures, outbreaks of EEE have been too few for their validity to be tested. Isolation of Highlands J virus, which shares a common enzootic cycle with EEE virus, often peaks 2 to 3 weeks before the appearance of EEE virus in *C. melanura.*

Surveillance and public health interventions to prevent EEE have been shown to be economic when balanced against the direct and indirect costs of even one human case.[49] Larviciding swampland to control *C. melanura* is difficult because of the large areas involved, the potential toxic effects in fish and other wildlife, and the relative inaccessibility of the larvae. Emergency application of adulticides to control epizootic vectors is indicated when viral, mosquito, and animal surveillance suggests a risk for epizootic transmission. Public health advisories to avoid outdoor activity near enzootic foci and closure of campgrounds and parks in these locations may be necessary when viral transmission indices suggest a high level of risk. The use of repellents and avoidance of outdoor activity 1 to 2 hours after sunset, when many mosquitoes are most active, may reduce the risk of exposure; however, some vector *Aedes* spp. are daytime biters.

REFERENCES

1. Ayres, J. C., and Feemster, R. F.: The sequelae of eastern equine encephalomyelitis. N. Engl. J. Med. *240*:960–962, 1949.
2. Bastian, F. O., Wende, R. D., Singer, D. B., et al.: Eastern equine encephalomyelitis: Histopathologic and ultrastructural changes with isolation of the virus in a human case. Am. J. Clin. Pathol. *64*:10–13, 1975.
3. Beaudette, F. R., Black, J. J., Hudson, C. B., et al.: Equine encephalomyelitis in pheasants from 1947 to 1951. J. Am. Vet. Med. Assoc. *121*:478–483, 1952.
4. Bellavance, R., Rossier, E., and Le Maitre, M. P.: Eastern equine encephalitis in eastern Canada: 1972. Can. J. Public Health *64*:189–190, 1973.
5. Belle, E. A., Grant, L. S., and Thorburn, M. J.: An outbreak of eastern equine encephalomyelitis in Jamaica. II. Laboratory diagnosis and pathology of eastern equine encephalomyelitis in Jamaica. Am. J. Trop. Med. Hyg. *13*:335–341, 1964.
6. Bigler, W. J., Lassing, E. B., Buff, E. E., et al.: Endemic eastern equine encephalomyelitis in Florida: A twenty-year analysis, 1955–1974. Am. J. Trop. Med. Hyg. *25*:884–890, 1976.
7. Brault, A. C., Powers, A. M., Chavez, C. L., et al.: Genetic and antigenic diversity among eastern equine encephalitis viruses from North, Central, and South America. Am. J. Trop. Med. Hyg. *6*:579–586, 1999.
8. Carman, P. S., Artsob, H., Emery S., et al.: Eastern equine encephalitis in a horse from southwestern Ontario. Can. Vet. J. *36*:170–172, 1995.
9. Clarke, D. H.: Two nonfatal human infections with the virus of eastern encephalitis. Am. J. Trop. Med. Hyg. *10*:67–70, 1961.
10. Crans, W. J., Caccamise, D. F., and McNelly, J. R.: Eastern equine encephalomyelitis virus in relation to the avian community of a coastal cedar swamp. J. Med. Entomol. *31*:711–728, 1994.
11. Davenport, D. S., Batts, D. H., and Carter, J. W.: Eastern equine encephalitis in Michigan. Arch. Neurol. *39*:322–323, 1982.
12. Day, J. F., and Stark, L. M.: Eastern equine encephalitis transmission to emus (Dromaius novaehollandiae) in Volusia County, Florida: 1992 through 1994. J. Am. Mosq. Control Assoc. *12*:429–436, 1996.
13. Dein, F. J., Carpenter, J. W., Clark, G. G., et al.: Mortality of captive whooping cranes caused by eastern equine encephalitis virus. J. Am. Vet. Med. Assoc. *9*:1006–1010, 1986.
14. de la Monte, S. M.: Selective vulnerability of particular central nervous system regions to eastern equine encephalitis virus in humans. J. Neuropathol. Exp. Neurol. *44*:358, 1985.
15. Deresiewicz, R. L., Thaler, S. J., Hsu, L., and Zamani, A. A.: Clinical and neuroradiographic manifestations of eastern equine encephalitis. N. Engl. J. Med. *336*:1867–1874, 1997.
16. Eklund, C. M., Bell, J. F., and Brennan, J. M.: Antibody survey following an outbreak of human and equine disease in the Dominican Republic, caused by the eastern strain of equine encephalomyelitis virus. Am. J. Trop. Med. Hyg. *31*:312–328, 1951.
17. Farber, S., Hill, A., Connerly, M. L., et al.: Encephalitis in infants and children. J. A. M. A. *114*:1725–1731, 1940.
18. Feemster, R. F.: Equine encephalitis in Massachusetts. N. Engl. J. Med. *257*:701–704, 1957.
19. Feemster, R. F., and Getting, V. A.: Distribution of the vectors of equine encephalomyelitis in Massachusetts. Am. J. Public Health *31*:791–802, 1941.
20. Feemster, R. F., Wheeler, R. E., Daniels, J. B., et al.: Field and laboratory studies on equine encephalitis. N. Engl. J. Med. *259*:107–113, 1958.
21. Garen, P. D., Tsai, T. F., and Powers, J. M.: Human eastern equine encephalitis: Immunohistochemistry and ultrastructure. Mod. Pathol. *12*:646–652, 1999.
22. Getting, V. A.: Equine encephalomyelitis in Massachusetts. N. Engl. J. Med. *24*:999–1006, 1941.
23. Gibbs, P. J., and Tsai, T.: Eastern encephalitis. *In* Beran, G. (ed.): Handbook of Zoonoses: Section B, Viral. Boca Raton, FL, CRC Press, 1994.
24. Goldfield, M., Sussman, O., Black, H. C., et al.: Arbovirus infection of animals in New Jersey. J. Am. Vet. Med. Assoc. *153*:1780–1787, 1968.
25. Goldfield, M., Taylor, B. F., and Welsh, J. N.: The 1959 outbreak of eastern encephalitis in New Jersey. Am. J. Epidemiol. *87*:18–57, 1968.
26. Golomb, M. R., Durand, M. L., Schaefer, P. W., et al.: A case of immunotherapy-responsive eastern equine encephalitis with diffusion-weighted imaging. Neurology *56*:420–421, 2001.
27. Grady, G. F., Maxfield, H. K., Hildreth, S. W., et al.: Eastern equine encephalitis in Massachusetts, 1957–1976: A prospective study centered upon analyses of mosquitoes. Am. J. Epidemiol. *107*:170–178, 1978.
28. Hauser, G. H.: Human equine encephalomyelitis, eastern type, in Louisiana. New Orleans Med. Surg. J. *100*:551–558, 1948.
29. Hayes, R. O., and Hess, A. D.: Climatological conditions associated with outbreaks of eastern encephalitis. Am. J. Trop. Med. Hyg. *13*:851–858, 1964.
30. Howard, J. J., Grayson, M. A., White, D. J., and Oliver, J.: Evidence for multiple foci of eastern equine encephalitis virus (Togaviridae: Alphavirus) in central New York State. J. Med. Entomol. *33*:421–432, 1996.
31. Kim, J. H., Booss, J., Manvelidis, E. E., et al.: Human eastern equine encephalitis: Electron microscopic study of a brain biopsy. Am. J. Clin. Pathol. *84*:223–227, 1985.
32. Komar, N., and Spielman, A.: Emergence of eastern encephalitis in Massachusetts. Ann. N. Y. Acad. Sci. *740*:157–168, 1995.
33. Lavoie, S. R., Markowitz, S. and Kapadia, S. J.: Eastern equine encephalomyelitis with hematuria and bladder dysfunction. South. Med. J. *86*:812–814, 1993.
34. Letson, G. W., Bailey, R. E., and Pearson, J., et al.: Eastern equine encephalitis (EEE): A description of the 1989 outbreak, recent epidemiologic trends, and the association of rainfall with EEE occurrence. Am. J. Trop. Med. Hyg. *49*:677–685, 1993.
35. Levitt, L. P., Lovejoy, F. H., and Daniels, J. B.: Eastern equine encephalitis in Massachusetts: First human case in 14 years. N. Engl. J. Med. *284*:540, 1971.
36. Liao, S. J.: Eastern equine encephalitis in Connecticut: A serological survey of pheasant farmers. Yale J. Biol. Med. *27*:287–296, 1955.
37. Martin, D. A., Muth, D. A., Brown, T., et al.: Standardization of immunoglobulin M capture enzyme-linked immunosorbent assays for routine diagnosis of arboviral infections. J. Clin. Microbiol. *38*:1823–1826, 2000.
38. McLean, R. G., Frier, G., Parham, G. L., et al.: Investigations of the vertebrate hosts of eastern equine encephalitis during an epizootic in Michigan. Am. J. Trop. Med. Hyg. *34*:1190–1202, 1985.
39. Morse, R. P., Bennish, M. L., and Darras, B. T.: Eastern equine encephalitis presenting with a focal brain lesion. Pediatr. Neurol. *8*:473–475, 1992.
40. Nathanson, N., Stolley, P. D., and Boolukos, P. J.: Eastern equine encephalitis: Distribution of central nervous system lesions in man and rhesus monkeys. J. Comp. Pathol. *79*:109–115, 1969.
41. Piliero, P. J., Brody, J., Zamani, A., et al.: Eastern equine encephalitis presenting as focal neuroradiographic abnormalities: Case report and review. Clin. Infect. Dis. *18*:985–988, 1994.
42. Powers, A. M., Brault, A. C., Shirako, Y., et al.: Evolutionary relationships and systematics of the alphaviruses. J. Virol. *75*:10118–10131, 2001.
43. Przelomski, M. M., O'Rourke, E., Grady, G. F., et al.: Eastern equine encephalitis in Massachusetts: A report of 16 cases 1970–1984. Neurology *38*:736–739, 1988.
44. Sanchez-Seco, M. P., Rosario, D., Quiroz, E., et al.: A generic nested-RT-PCR followed by sequencing for detection and identification of members of the alphavirus genus. J. Virol. Methods *95*:153–161, 2001.
45. Sotomayor, E. A., Josephson, S. L.: Isolation of eastern equine encephalitis virus in A549 and MRC-5 cell cultures. Clin. Infect. Dis. *29*:193–195, 1999.
46. Sudia, W. D., Stamm, D. D., Chamberlain, R. W., et al.: Transmission of eastern equine encephalitis to horses by *Aedes sollicitans* mosquitoes. Am. J. Trop. Med. Hyg. *5*:802–808, 1956.
47. Tengelsen, L. A., Bowen, R. A., Royals, M. A., et al.: Response to and efficacy of vaccination against eastern equine encephalomyelitis virus in emus. J. Am. Vet. Med. Assoc. *218*:1469–1473, 2001.
48. Tikasingh, E. S., Ardoin, P., Everard, C. O. R., et al.: Eastern equine encephalitis in Trinidad, epidemiological investigations following two human cases of South American strain in Santa Cruz. Trop. Geogr. Med. *25*:355–361, 1973.
49. Villari, P., Spielman, A., Komar, N., et al.: The economic burden imposed by a residual case of eastern encephalitis. Am. J. Trop. Med. Hyg. *52*:8–13, 1995.
50. Wesselhoeff, C., Smith, E. C., and Branch, C. F.: Human encephalitis: Eight fatal cases with four due to virus of equine encephalomyelitis. J. A. M. A. *111*:1735–1741, 1938.
51. Williams, S. M., Fulton, R. M., Patterson, J. S., and Reed, W. M.: Diagnosis of eastern equine encephalitis by immunohistochemistry in two flocks of Michigan ring-neck pheasants. Avian Dis. *44*:1012–1016, 2000.
52. Winter, W. D., Jr.: Eastern equine encephalomyelitis in Massachusetts in 1955. N. Engl. J. Med. *255*:262–270, 1956.

CHAPTER **178B**

Western Equine Encephalitis

THEODORE F. TSAI

Western equine encephalitis (WEE) is an endemic and enzootic acute central nervous system (CNS) infection of humans and horses in the western part of the United States, Canada, Mexico, and parts of South America. In North America, *Culex tarsalis,* the principal mosquito vector, also maintains the virus in an avian enzootic cycle.

Etiologic Agent

WEE and other alphaviruses (group A arboviruses) form a genus of principally mosquito-borne viruses in the family *Togaviridae.*[43, 61] Three of the eight viruses constituting the WEE antigenic complex are found in North America: Highlands J, Fort Morgan, and WEE viruses; among them, only WEE virus is a human pathogen. Much of what is known about the molecular biology of alphaviruses has been inferred from studies of the Sindbis (the type species and a member of the WEE complex) and Semliki Forest viruses.

Alphaviruses are small, enveloped, positive-stranded RNA viruses. Virions are spherical and 69 nm in diameter (including the length of their glycoprotein spikes), with a lipid bilayer enveloping a nucleocapsid core containing the 11.7-kb RNA viral genome. Glycoprotein spikes embedded in the viral envelope bind to cell membrane receptors and initiate infection by endocytotic fusion. The viral and lysosomal membranes fuse in a pH-dependent step, and the viral nucleocapsid is released into the cell cytoplasm, where RNA and protein synthesis occurs. The 5′ terminal two thirds of the RNA genome encodes four nonstructural proteins, and the 3′ terminal one third of the RNA genome encodes the three structural proteins. The 30-kd nucleocapsid and two 50-kd glycoproteins—E1 and E2—are translated as a polyprotein from subgenomic 26S RNA. The envelope proteins—E1 and E2—are assembled in trimers of a single E2 protein and an E1 dimer. Eighty such trimer spikes are arranged in an icosahedral lattice on the virion surface.[9] Capsid proteins assemble with the viral genome in the cytoplasm and then bud through the virally modified cell membrane and acquire an envelope.

The E1 glycoprotein possesses a group-reactive hemagglutinin and group-reactive epitopes linked to cross-protection and cell-mediated cytotoxic effects. E1 also mediates viral cellular membrane fusion. Epitopes on E2 are linked to cell receptor recognition, viral neutralization and clearance, and neurovirulence and cellular apoptosis.[18, 65]

Molecular genetic studies indicate that WEE virus arose more than 1000 years ago as a recombinant of eastern equine virus and an ancestral, now extinct, Sindbis-like virus, with the recombinant having acquired the neurotropic potential of eastern equine virus while retaining the antigenic characteristics of the non-neurotropic Sindbis virus.[19, 43, 55, 62, 63] Alphaviruses are thought to have originated in the New World with separate introductions, presumably by birds, to the Old World, resulting in establishment of the present-day Sindbis-like viruses and Semliki Forest–related viruses. Oligonucleotide fingerprints of individual WEE strains generally are similar, and the lineages of other alphaviruses show remarkable stability. A slow rate of evolution, circa 10^{-4} nucleotide changes per year (versus 10^{-2}/yr for other RNA viruses), probably reflects the natural pressure on viruses constrained to replicate in both insect and vertebrate cells.[63]

Ecology

WEE virus is transmitted in an enzootic cycle to mosquitoes, birds, and other vertebrate hosts.[46, 47, 51] Horses and humans are dead-end hosts, but severe CNS infection may develop. Although WEE is a public health and veterinary problem primarily in the western United States and Canada, the geographic range of the virus includes Mexico, Guyana, Brazil, Uruguay, and Argentina. Epizootics in horses, accompanied by small numbers of human cases, were reported in 1972 and 1983 in Argentina, where the virus apparently is transmitted by *Aedes albifasciatus* to introduced European hares and possibly birds. In addition, a distinct sylvatic subtype of WEE virus is transmitted in the subtropical Chaco province.[3, 6]

In the United States, the geographic distribution of the virus and *C. tarsalis,* its principal vector, includes the western and central United States, southern Canada, and Mexico. A related virus—Highlands J virus, isolated from *Culiseta melanura* in the eastern United States—overlaps in its range in the east central part of the United States. Highlands J virus causes encephalitis in horses and possibly in humans.[35]

In the western region of the United States, *C. tarsalis* breeds in ground pools found on pasture lands; in irrigation wastewater; and at the margins of lakes, ponds, marshes, and flooded riversides. Some of these aquatic habitats are shared by birds that participate in the amplification of virus in nature.[46, 47, 51]

The female mosquito becomes infected after feeding on a viremic bird (or mammal). After an extrinsic incubation period of 7 to 9 days, when the virus propagates in the mosquito and the salivary glands become infected, the mosquito can transmit virus to other birds or mammals (amplifying hosts) or to humans and horses (dead-end hosts).

Passerine (perching) birds, especially sparrows and finches, have proved to be particularly important in amplification of the virus. In midsummer, the mosquito shifts its host-seeking activity to mammals. The shift may be influenced by an increase in the defensive behavior of nestling birds, which are its preferred host. The shift corresponds temporally to the appearance of cases in horses and people and appears to be a critical element enabling *C. tarsalis* to function as both an enzootic and an epizootic vector. In California, an auxiliary *Aedes melanimon*–jackrabbit (Lepus californicus) cycle has been demonstrated.

The overwintering mechanism for WEE virus has not been elucidated. However, virus has been recovered from adult *Aedes dorsalis* mosquitoes collected as larvae from a coastal area of California, thus indicating a possible role for vertical transmission of the virus in mosquitoes in some locations. Arguments also have been advanced for viral overwintering in adult mosquitoes and in persistently infected mammals, birds, and poikilotherms (snakes, frogs, and turtles). In Canada, *Aedes* spp. and *Culiseta inorata,* which emerge in the spring before *C. tarsalis* does, have been proposed as early amplifying vectors.[34]

Numerous climatologic and biologic indices with various degrees of predictive value have been shown to correlate with the occurrence of WEE outbreaks; these indices include vector population size, mosquito infection rates, and virus transmission rates to sentinel chickens or wild-caught sparrows. Such transmission indices are monitored in surveillance activities by public health agencies; however, their sensitivity, specificity, and predictive value for forecasting epidemics have been difficult to evaluate because of the sporadic nature of outbreaks.[64] A retrospective analysis of a 21-year experience in California showed correlation between average daily numbers of *C. tarsalis* females and the occurrence of human encephalitis.[41] In a Texas study, house sparrow infection and antibody rates were the best predictors of human disease, and *C. tarsalis* light trap indices were of borderline significance.[25]

Physical measures associated with the incidence of disease in humans or transmission of virus to sentinel species include the ambient air temperature, the snow pack in mountains providing runoff water, the river flow rate, the soil temperature inversion date (the date that the surface soil temperature exceeds the subsurface soil temperature), and the date when 50 or more days of 70° F (21° C) temperature have accumulated. The snow pack and river flow rate are associated with an abundance of irrigation water and flooding, which in turn are associated with the availability of breeding habitats and mosquito population size.[7, 24, 46, 47]

Longitudinal and intraseasonal observations show that high temperatures are associated with a reduced risk of human disease. High ambient air temperature (>89.6° F [32° C]) decreases mosquito survival, adversely affects the competence of *C. tarsalis* to become infected with and transmit WEE virus, and limits host-seeking activity.[50] In a model of global warming, higher temperatures are predicted to move the range of WEE viral transmission northward.[47]

Epidemiology

WEE occurs sporadically and in epidemic form, principally in Canadian provinces and states west of the Mississippi River (Figs. 178–3 and 178–4). Infections occur mainly in rural areas, where water impoundments, irrigated farmland, and naturally flooded sites provide breeding habitats for *C. tarsalis;* however, the increasingly rare interface between vector mosquitoes and humans has resulted in a point seroprevalence of 1 to 2 percent even in locations where the virus is transmitted in an enzootic cycle.[49] The annual median number of cases between 1964 and 1995 was only four, and only four cases were reported between 1988 and 1997, a lower incidence than that for eastern equine encephalitis; however, periodic outbreaks have led to scores or hundreds of cases (see Fig. 178–4).

Recurrent endemic and epidemic transmission was recorded in the Yakima Valley, Washington (1939 to 1942); California's Central Valley (1939 to 1952); the north central states and Canadian provinces, including Minnesota, North and South Dakota, Alberta, Manitoba, and Saskatchewan (1941 and 1975); and the high plains panhandle of Texas (1963 to 1966).[13, 20, 26, 45] The largest outbreak on record, in 1941, resulted in more than 3400 human cases in Minnesota, North and South Dakota, Nebraska, Montana, Alberta, Manitoba, and Saskatchewan; equine cases were estimated to number in the hundreds of thousands. The outbreak centered in North Dakota, where the attack rate for the state was 167 cases per 100,000.[13, 29] In 1952, an

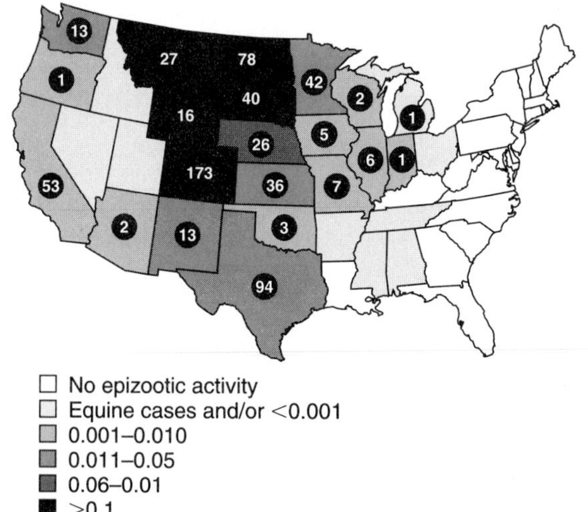

FIGURE 178–3 ■ Reported cases and average annual incidence (per 100,000) of western equine encephalitis by state, 1964 to 1995.

outbreak in California's Central Valley led to 348 reported cases, an incidence of 36 cases per 100,000 residents.[26] More recent outbreaks resulted in 277 cases in the central United States and Manitoba in 1975 and 40 cases in the central and mountain states in 1987.[11, 30, 34]

Most cases occur between June and September (Fig. 178–5), often preceded by cases occurring in horses several weeks earlier. Surveillance of equine cases is a widely used approach to assess the risk for epidemic transmission. However, the low frequency of laboratory-confirmed diagnoses, vaccination, and underreporting limit the precision of equine surveillance as a predictive marker.[42]

Several risk factors for acquiring WEE have been identified:

1. Attack rates usually are highest at the extremes of age[2] (Fig. 178–6). The experience from the 1952 California outbreak showed that one third of cases occurred in infants younger than 1 year.[26, 47] Other reports confirm the bimodal pattern of an elevated risk in infants, a declining risk in children and young adults, and a gradual increase in risk in the elderly.
2. Attack rates in males are twofold higher than those in females in every age group[2] (see Fig. 178–5). Biologic differences in susceptibility to infection may account for the observed disparity in infancy, and greater occupational and recreational exposure outdoors might be responsible for the differences in adults. In the 1981 outbreak in Manitoba, 21 of 25 cases were in males; the 4 affected women were widows who maintained their premises alone.[11]
3. Rural residence is associated with attack rates 1.5 to 5 times higher than those for urban residence (Table 178–1). Counties lying in major river drainage areas and with more irrigated acreage have had the highest incidence of equine and human disease[2] (Fig. 178–7).
4. Agricultural occupation has been suggested as a risk factor in several studies.
5. Length of residence in areas where WEE is endemic is associated inversely with a risk of illness. Acquired immunity, through asymptomatic or mild infection, accumulates with length of residence; in endemic areas, the point prevalence of specific antibody previously approached 20 percent by adulthood.[46, 47]

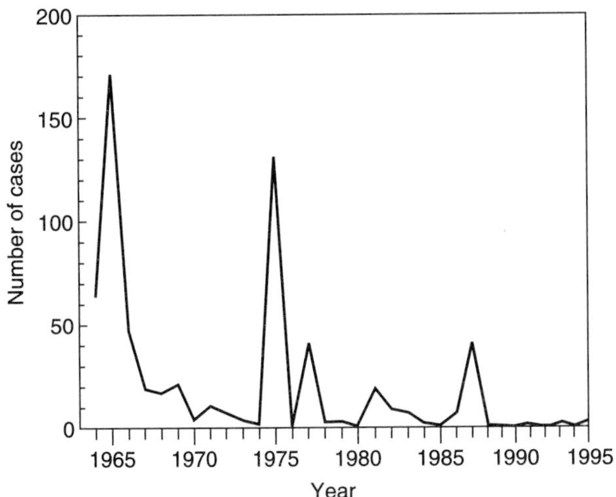

FIGURE 178–4 ■ Reported cases of western equine encephalitis by year, 1964 to 1995.

Clinical Manifestations

The clinical illness ranges from a nonspecific syndrome of headache and fever to aseptic meningitis, meningoencephalitis, and frank encephalitis. The estimated case-infection ratio is 1:58 in children 1 to 4 years of age, but it declines to 1:1150 in adults.[16, 47, 51]

The onset of illness typically is abrupt, with sudden fever, headache, malaise, chills, and nausea and vomiting,[4, 13, 23, 45] occasionally preceded by signs of an upper respiratory infection. Signs of CNS infection gradually become evident as dizziness, drowsiness, increasing headache, stiff neck, and disorientation develop over the course of hours or days. Infants typically have a sudden cessation in feeding, fussiness, fever, and protracted vomiting. The prodromal interval is abbreviated, and convulsions and a lethargic unresponsive state develop rapidly.

On examination, patients appear somnolent and may have signs of meningeal irritation. The sensorium is depressed, and patients may alternate between agitation

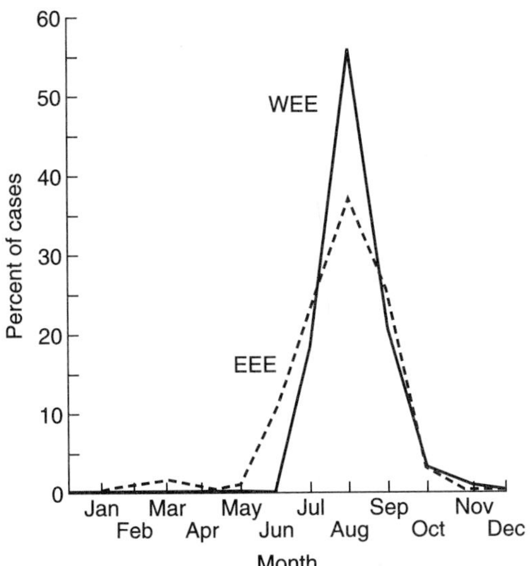

FIGURE 178–5 ■ Reported cases of western and eastern equine encephalitis by month, 1972 to 1989.

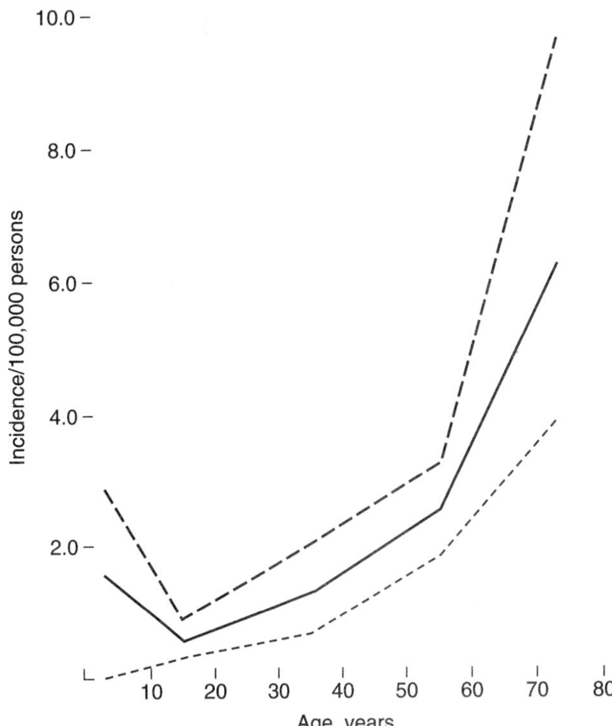

FIGURE 178–6 ■ Age- and sex-specific incidence of western equine encephalitis, Colorado, 1987. ---, male; —, total; ----, female.

and somnolence. Generalized muscular weakness is present, and deep tendon reflexes are diminished. Focal neurologic signs suggesting herpes encephalitis have been reported in anecdotal cases[1, 5]; however, in the 1941 Minnesota outbreak, only 3 of 226 cases reported had unilateral weakness.[13]

In infants, the fontanelle may be tense or bulging, often accompanied by spastic paresis and generalized convulsions. The frequency of seizures is related inversely to age; they occur with greatest frequency in infants younger than 3 months (75 to 80% of cases). In 2- to 4-year-old children, seizures have been reported in 15 percent of cases.[33]

The peripheral leukocyte count is unremarkable. Cerebrospinal fluid (CSF) obtained at an early stage in the illness generally exhibits normal glucose, elevated protein, and a leukocyte count between 10 and 300/mm^3.[30] Mononuclear cells usually predominate.

Five instances of late third-trimester infection in pregnant women have been reported to result in perinatal illness or encephalitis.[10, 33] The women's illnesses had an onset 0 to 10 days before delivery, and the infants became ill on the fifth and sixth postpartum days. Teratogenic effects of infection occurring earlier in gestation have not been reported for WEE virus but are suspected for other group A arboviruses.[36]

Pathology

Specific pathologic changes are confined to the CNS.[4, 30, 39] Grossly, the brain appears normal or may be congested and swollen, with minimal changes observed in the meninges. Microscopic lesions affecting gray and white matter appear throughout the brain but predominate in the basal ganglia. Disseminated small focal abscesses infiltrated with neutrophils are a distinctive feature. The vessels

TABLE 178–1 ■ WESTERN EQUINE ENCEPHALITIS EPIDEMIC ATTACK RATES BY POPULATION DENSITY*

	Minnesota, 1941	Kern County, CA, 1952	Hale County, TX, 1963–1966	Manitoba, 1975
Rural	15.8–22.0	149.2	2.62	10.8
Small town	2.3–5.6			2.4
Urban		28.5	1.0	0.9

*Per 100,000.

appear congested, and small focal hemorrhages or diffuse extravasations of erythrocytes are present along with neutrophilic infiltration of the vascular wall and endarteritis. Vascular lumina may be occluded by endothelial proliferation and swelling.

Extensive patchy areas of demyelination are found throughout the brain. Older lesions appear as sharply circumscribed, punched-out plaques. Secondary microglial reaction in demyelinated areas is minimal.

The spinal cord is affected in the same fashion, with focal, perivascular, and diffuse lesions attracting both polymorphonuclear and mononuclear cells. Lesions predominate in the central gray matter.

Pathogenesis

Peripheral inoculation of experimental animals with WEE virus is followed by viral replication in various extraneural sites before invasion of the CNS (including the peripheral site of inoculation, viscera, muscle, and perhaps vascular endothelial cells).[27, 31, 40, 67]

Host resistance and recovery from infection depend chiefly on an effective antibody response. Antibody contributes to recovery by a variety of means, including viral neutralization and antibody-mediated restriction of viral gene expression.[18, 65] Interferon may contribute to containment of local viral spread in the CNS. Antibodies are

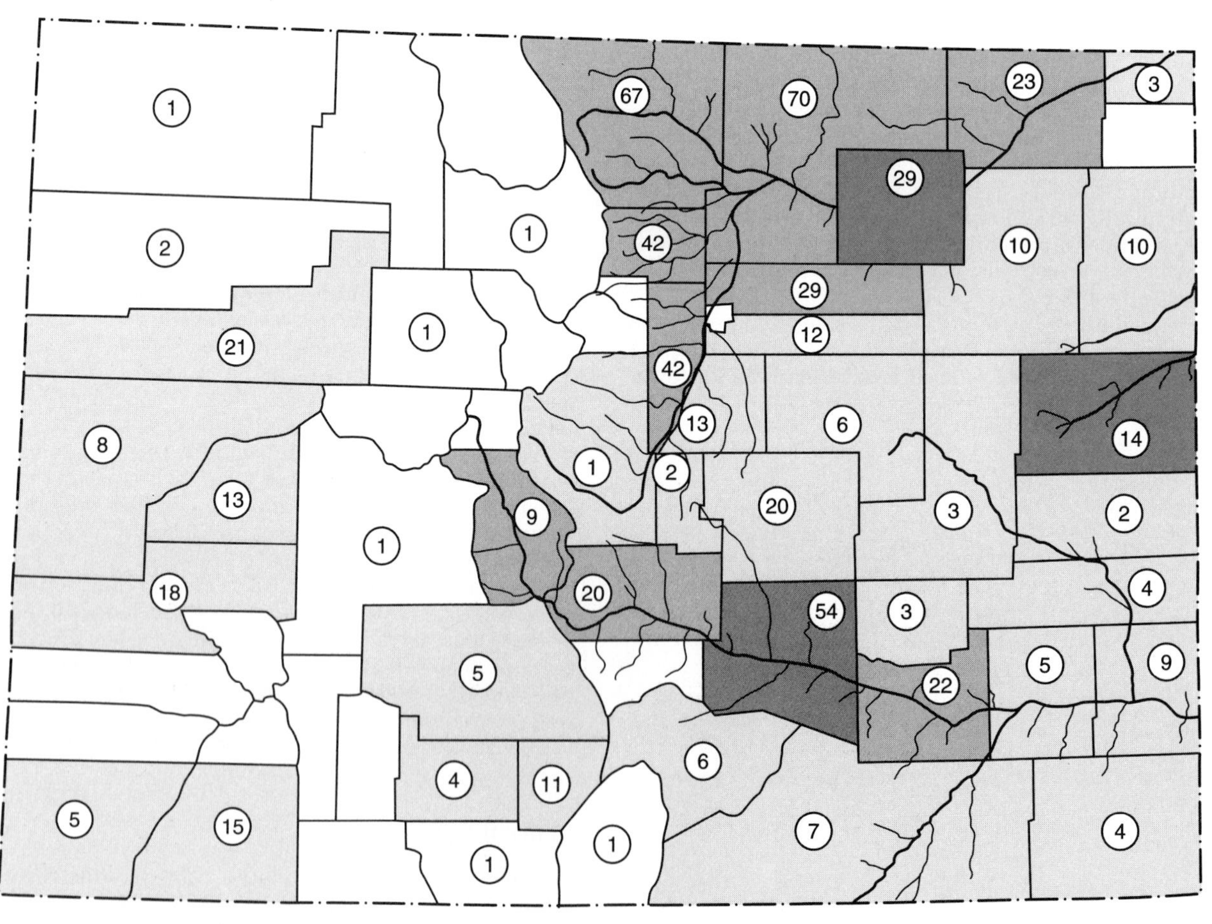

FIGURE 178–7 ■ Reported equine cases and incidence of western equine encephalitis by county, Colorado, 1975 to 1988.

protective and may be cross-protective to other alphaviruses. Antibodies to the E2 glycoprotein typically are virus-specific and associated with neutralization and protection. Antibodies to E1 exhibit greater cross-reactivity with other alphaviruses.[61] Immune serum given to monkeys prophylactically protects them from challenge with WEE virus, and passive protection has been demonstrated in monkeys inoculated with WEE virus and treated with immune serum within 24 hours.[67] However, immunotherapy in monkeys is uniformly unsuccessful in preventing death once signs of CNS infection have appeared. In guinea pigs peripherally inoculated with WEE virus, immunotherapy given within 24 to 48 hours of inoculation leads to survival of some animals and delayed death in others.[40] In one human case, passive immunization led to a delayed antibody response and was followed by the development of parkinsonism.[17]

The age-dependent virulence of specific Sindbis virus strains has been linked to the immaturity of the suckling mouse T- and B-cell repertoire. Fibroblasts from newborn but not weanling mice are susceptible to Sindbis virus infection, and viral infection of immature mouse neurons leads to apoptotic cell death. Mature neurons are protected against apoptosis by induction of the *bcl-2* oncogene, whose products convert the infection to a persistent nonlytic infection. Viral persistence in the brain of recovered mice is modulated by antibody.[18]

Prognosis

Major neurologic sequelae of WEE, including quadriplegia, hemiplegia, spasticity, intracerebral calcifications, developmental delay in children, and epilepsy, have been reported in approximately 13 percent of cases.[12, 14, 23, 68] The risk of serious neurologic sequelae developing in infants is triple that of other age groups, and 30 percent of recovered infants younger than 1 year remain seriously impaired.[14, 16, 60] In infants younger than 1 year, convulsions during the acute phase of illness were associated with a greater risk of poor long-term outcome, including continued seizures. Multiple intracranial calcifications were observed in one recovered infant with persistent seizures.[59] Minor psychiatric or neurologic deficits remained in approximately one fourth of children and adults monitored for 18 months after infection.[14] Central apnea has been reported as a complication of encephalitis in two adult cases.[66]

Parkinson syndrome has been a residual effect in at least 15 cases of adults surviving WEE.[17, 38, 57, 58] Its onset may be immediate or delayed for several years after recovery from the illness. Two retrospective investigations of patients with idiopathic Parkinson disease found no difference between cases and controls in seroprevalence to several arboviruses, including WEE virus.

The case-fatality rate in reported cases in the United States from 1955 to 1978 was 3 to 4 percent. In outbreaks in the central portion of the United States and Canada in 1941, 1975, and 1981, approximately 7 to 9 percent of patients died, with higher fatality rates in the elderly.

Diagnosis

Virus rarely can be recovered from blood or CSF, but it can be isolated readily from the brain of fatal cases. In a few attempts, WEE virus has been isolated from brain biopsy material; in principle, rapid diagnosis can be made by immunofluorescent identification of WEE viral antigen in brain biopsy tissue. The virus can be isolated readily in Vero cell culture or in suckling mice.[58] Polymerase chain reaction analysis of CSF has not been evaluated extensively.

IgM capture enzyme-linked immunosorbent assay (ELISA) is the preferred serologic procedure.[32] IgM antibody usually is present in acute serum within a week after the onset of illness, and its presence is presumptive evidence of recent infection. IgM often can be detected in CSF before it can be identified in serum, and its presence, which indicates intrathecal production of antibody, confirms a recent CNS infection.[32] Identification of virus-specific IgM in serum and CSF by immunofluorescence also is possible; however, this approach is somewhat less sensitive than IgM capture ELISA and may be confounded by the effects of rheumatoid factor.

Hemagglutination-inhibition (HI) and neutralizing antibodies are elevated in the first week of illness in most cases, and a diagnostic fourfold rise in titer usually is observed in the second week. Complement-fixing (CF) antibody is slower to rise, with fourfold changes delayed until the third to fifth week after onset. The CF response may be blunted in older patients.[60]

Neutralizing and HI antibody titers have considerable longevity, with minimal decay noted 30 months after onset. In contrast, CF antibody is relatively short lived, and its presence is a useful indicator of recent infection, particularly in endemic areas where long-term residents may have neutralizing and HI antibody from previous exposure. Only two thirds of patients are estimated to show CF antibody 2 years after onset, and less than 15 percent have residual CF antibody after 5 years.[60]

Differential Diagnosis

The clinical findings in patients with encephalitis seldom are sufficiently characteristic that a specific diagnosis can be made on clinical grounds alone. Fever, vomiting, signs of meningeal irritation, and confusion are nonspecific features of encephalitis and cerebral edema. Early symptoms in infants, such as fever, lethargy, and vomiting, may be even less specific.[28]

Furthermore, the peak occurrence of arboviral infection in midsummer to late summer temporally overlaps the seasonal occurrence of other CNS infections by enteroviruses (e.g., echovirus 13, which recently has become epidemic in the United States), leptospires, and free-living amebae. CNS signs may be prominent in other summertime diseases such as Rocky Mountain spotted fever, heat stroke, shigellosis, and lead encephalopathy. High priority should be given to establishing a specific diagnosis of treatable conditions such as herpes and enteroviral infection while bearing in mind that dual arboviral and enteroviral infection has been reported.[5]

Other causes of CNS infection without an established summertime seasonality that also should be considered in the differential diagnosis include fungal, mycobacterial, and partially treated bacterial meningitis; brain abscess and infected subdural collections; bacterial endocarditis; toxoplasmosis; cat-scratch disease; and infections with rabies, mumps, herpes simplex, Epstein-Barr, human herpesvirus 6, adenovirus, lymphocytic choriomeningitis, and human immunodeficiency virus. Parainfectious disorders such as postinfectious viral encephalitis, acute cerebellar ataxia of childhood, mycoplasmal infection, neuroblastoma with opsoclonus, and Reye syndrome also may enter into the differential diagnosis. Vascular disorders formed the largest single group of disorders mimicking herpes encephalitis in several studies. Drugs such as trimethoprim-sulfamethoxazole, penicillin, isoniazid, phenazopyridine, ibuprofen, tolmetin, sulindac, carbamazepine, high doses of bismuth, OKT3 antibody, and vidarabine also may cause aseptic meningitis or encephalopathy.

Because of the potential for their overlapping circumstances of exposure, diethyltoluamide (DEET) encephalopathy should be excluded. DEET-containing insect repellents have been implicated as a cause of seizures and encephalopathy after brief cutaneous exposure (see later).

Valuable clues to the diagnosis of an arbovirus infection are gleaned from a history of travel, residence, or occupational and recreational activities within the appropriate incubation period. Suspected cases should be reported to public health officials.

Treatment

Specific antiviral therapy is not available. Supportive treatment of acutely ill patients includes monitoring of cardiorespiratory function, fluid and electrolyte balance, and intracranial pressure. A case of laboratory infection treated with immune equine serum resulted in recovery; however, acute Parkinson syndrome developed in this patient and coincided temporally with serum sickness resulting from immunotherapy.[17]

Prevention

Killed vaccine prepared in chick embryo fibroblast culture is available in the United States under an investigatory permit for laboratory and field personnel who are at risk for occupational exposure. Effective killed vaccines are available for horses and usually are administered in bivalent or multivalent formulations (with eastern equine encephalitis, Venezuelan equine encephalitis, and influenza viruses). Vaccination of the general public, even in endemic areas, is not a practical consideration because of the low risk of disease. Personal protective measures include avoiding outdoor activity during the hours of peak mosquito activity at dusk and using repellents.

The most effective repellents contain DEET as the active ingredient, but they should be used with caution, especially in children.[7, 8, 15, 21, 44] DEET is absorbed readily through the skin, and encephalopathy was reported in seven children after cutaneous exposure.[7, 53, 54] Three cases were fatal. In one recovered child, encephalopathy and seizures developed after only two applications. In an additional child, seizures and encephalopathy occurred after cutaneous and respiratory exposure to DEET in an automobile with closed windows. Additional cases of seizures in patients who used small quantities of DEET have been reported, but whether these events were coincidental in populations in which the prevalence of DEET use is high is unclear.[8] DEET may have an effect on ammonia metabolism; in one case, encephalopathy occurred in a patient with partial ornithine carbamoyltransferase deficiency.[22] DEET is a proven neurotoxin when ingested; however, the incidence of neurologic side effects after cutaneous exposure is unknown. Nevertheless, avoiding formulations containing DEET in high concentration is prudent; when applied simultaneously with sunscreen, DEET repellency is unhampered but ultraviolet protection may be reduced. The precautions listed in Table 178–2 should be followed to minimize exposure.

Permethrin, a synthetic pyrethroid available as a 0.5 percent aerosol (Permanone), is both insecticidal and a repellent.[8, 15, 56] Permethrin is extremely effective in reducing bites of mosquitoes and ticks when sprayed on clothing and shoes, and it also can be applied to tents, mosquito nets, and other gear.[15, 55] Its use on the skin is not approved, except as treatment of scabies and head lice.

TABLE 178–2 ■ PRECAUTIONS TO MINIMIZE POTENTIAL ADVERSE REACTIONS FROM REPELLENTS

Repellents should be applied only to exposed skin and/or clothing (as directed on the product label). Do not use under clothing.
Never use repellents over cuts, wounds, or irritated skin.
Avoid mucosal contact—don't apply to the eyes and mouth, and apply sparingly around the ears. When using sprays, do not spray directly onto the face; spray on the hands first and then apply to the face.
Do not allow children to handle this product, and do not apply to children's hands. When using on children, apply to your own hands and then put it on the child.
Do not spray in enclosed areas. Avoid breathing a repellent spray.
Avoid ingestion, and do not use it near food.
Use just enough repellent to cover exposed skin and/or clothing. Heavy application and saturation are unnecessary for effectiveness; if biting insects do not respond to a thin film of repellent, apply a bit more.
After returning indoors, wash treated skin with soap and water or bathe. This precaution is particularly important when repellents are used repeatedly in a day or on consecutive days. Also, wash treated clothing before wearing it again.
Pregnant and nursing women should minimize the use of repellents.
If you suspect that you or your child is reacting to an insect repellent, discontinue use, wash treated skin, and then call your local poison control center. If/when you go to a doctor, take the repellent with you.
Specific medical information about the active ingredients in repellents and other pesticides is available at the National Pesticide Telecommunications Network (NPTN) at 1-800-858-7378. The NPTN operates from 6:30 AM to 4:30 PM (Pacific time); 9:30 AM to 7:30 PM (Eastern Time) 7 days a week.

Adapted from U.S. Environmental Protection Agency recommendations available at http://www.epa.gov/pesticides/factsheets/chemicals/deet/htm.

Prevention is focused primarily on interrupting the transmission of virus from mosquitoes to humans. In many localities where WEE is endemic, mosquito abatement districts monitor mosquito populations, virus infection rates in the vector population, or evidence of transmission of virus to wild or sentinel birds and chickens to provide a basis for predicting epidemic transmission and for emergency mosquito control.[37, 52]

As a general rule, *C. tarsalis* densities exceeding 10 to 15 females per trap night and mosquito infection rates greater than 5 to 10 per 1000 signal a risk for epizootic transmission. Evidence of seroconversion in sentinel chickens and observations of equine cases are further indications that human cases may occur.

REFERENCES

1. Anderson, B. A.: Focal neurologic signs in western equine encephalitis. Can. Med. Assoc. J. *130*:1019–1021, 1984.
2. Arboviral infections of the central nervous system: United States, 1987. M. M. W. R. Morb. Mortal. Wkly. Rep. *37*(33):506–508, 513–515, 1988.
3. Aviles, G., Sabattini, M. S., and Mitchell, C. J.: Transmission of western equine encephalomyelitis virus by Argentine *Aedes albifasciatus*. J. Med. Entomol. *29*:850–853, 1992.
4. Baker, A. B., and Noran, H. H.: Western variety of equine encephalitis in man: A clinicopathologic study. Arch. Neurol. Psychiatr. *47*:565–587, 1942.
5. Bia, F. J., Thornton, G. F., Main, A. J., et al.: Western equine encephalitis mimicking herpes simplex encephalitis. J. A. M. A. *244*:367–369, 1980.

6. Bianchi, T. I., Aviles, G., Monath, T. P., et al.: Western equine encephalomyelitis: Virulence markers and their epidemiologic significance. Am. J. Trop. Med. Hyg. *49*:322–328, 1993.
7. Briassoulis, G., Narlioglov, M., Hatzis, T.: Toxic encephalopathy associated with use of DEET insect repellents: A case analysis of its toxicity in children. Hum. Exp. Toxicol. *20*:8–14, 2001.
8. Brown, M., and Herbert, A. M.: Insect repellents: An overview. J. Am. Acad. Dermatol. *35*:243–249, 1997.
9. Cheng, R. H., Kuhn, R. J., Olson, N. H., et al.: Nucleocapsid and glycoprotein organization in an enveloped virus. Cell *80*:621–630, 1995.
10. Copps, S. C., and Giddings, L. E.: Transplacental transmission of western equine encephalitis. Pediatrics *24*:31–33, 1959.
11. Eadie, J. A., and Friesen, B.: Epidemiological study of western equine encephalitis. *In* Sekla, L. (ed.): Western Equine Encephalitis in Manitoba. Winnipeg, Manitoba, 1982, pp. 142–155.
12. Earnest, M. P., Goolishian, H. A., Calverley, J. R., et al.: Neurologic, intellectual, and psychologic sequelae following western encephalitis: A follow-up study of 35 cases. Neurology *21*:969–974, 1971.
13. Eklund, C. M.: Human encephalitis of the western equine type in Minnesota in 1941: Clinical and epidemiological study of serologically positive cases. Am. J. Hyg. *43*:171–193, 1946.
14. Finley, K. H., Longshore, W. A., Jr., Palmer, R. J., et al.: Western equine and St. Louis encephalitis: Preliminary report of a clinical follow-up study in California. Neurology *5*:223–235, 1955.
15. Fradin, M. S.: Mosquitoes and mosquito repellents: A clinician's guide. Ann. Intern. Med. *128*:931–940, 1998.
16. Froeschle, J. E., and Reeves, W. C.: Serologic epidemiology of western equine and St. Louis encephalitis virus infection in California. II. Analysis of inapparent infections in residents of an endemic area. Am. J. Epidemiol. *81*:44–51, 1965.
17. Gold, H., and Hampil, B.: Equine encephalomyelitis in a laboratory technician with recovery. Ann. Intern. Med. *16*:556–569, 1942.
18. Griffin, D. E., and Hardwick, J. M.: Regulators of apoptosis on the road to persistent alphavirus infection. Annu. Rev. Microbiol. *51*:585–592, 1997.
19. Hahn, C. S., Lustig, S., Strauss, E. G., et al.: Western equine encephalitis virus is a recombinant virus. Proc. Natl. Acad. Sci. U. S. A. *85*:5997–6001, 1988.
20. Hammon, W., M., Reeves, W. C., Benner, S. R., et al.: Human encephalitis in the Yakima Valley, Washington, 1942. J. A. M. A. *128*:1133–1139, 1945.
21. Hampers, L. C., Oker, E., Leikin, J. B.: Topical use of DEET insect repellent as a cause of severe encephalopathy in a healthy adult male. Acad. Emerg. Med. *6*:1295–1297, 1999.
22. Heick, H. M. C., Peterson, R. G., Dalpe-Scott, M., et al.: Insect repellent, N,N-diethyl-m-toluamide, effect on ammonia metabolism. Pediatrics *82*:373–376, 1988.
23. Herzon, H., Shelton, J. T., and Bruyn, H. B.: Sequelae of western equine and other arthropod-borne encephalitides. Neurology *7*:535–548, 1957.
24. Hess, A. D., Cherubin, C. E., and LaMotte, L. C.: Relation of temperature to activity of western and St. Louis encephalitis viruses. Am. J. Trop. Med. Hyg. *12*:657–667, 1963.
25. Holden, P., Hayes, R. O., Mitchell, C. J., et al.: House sparrows, *Passer domesticus* (L.), as hosts of arboviruses in Hale County, Texas. I. Field studies, 1965–1969. Am. J. Trop. Med. Hyg. *22*:244–253, 1973.
26. Hollister, A. C., Longshore, W. A., Jr., Dean, B. H., et al.: The 1952 outbreak of encephalitis in California. Epidemiologic aspects. Calif. Med. *79*:84–90, 1953.
27. Hurst, W.: Infection of the Rhesus monkey *(Macaca mulatta)* and the guinea pig with the virus of equine encephalomyelitis. J. Pathol. Bacteriol. *42*:271–302, 1936.
28. Kokernot, R. H., Shinefield, H. R., and Longshore, W. A.: The 1952 outbreak of encephalitis in California: Differential diagnosis. Calif. Med. *79*:73, 1953.
29. Leake, J. P.: Epidemic of infectious encephalitis. Public Health Rep. *56*:1902–1905, 1941.
30. Leech, R. W., Harris, J. C., and Johnson, R. M.: 1975 Encephalitis epidemic in North Dakota and western Minnesota: An epidemiologic, clinical, and neuropathologic study. Minn. Med. *64*:545–548, 1981.
31. Liu, C., Voth, D. W., Rodina, P., et al.: A comparative study of the pathogenesis of western equine encephalitis and eastern equine encephalomyelitis viral infections in mice by intracerebral and subcutaneous inoculations. J. Infect. Dis. *122*:53–63, 1970.
32. Martin, D. A., Muth, D. A., Brown, T., et al.: Standardization of immunoglobulin M capture enzyme-linked immunosorbent assays for routine diagnosis of arboviral infections. J. Clin. Microbiol. *38*:1823–1826, 2000.
33. Medovy, H.: Western equine encephalomyelitis in infants. J. Pediatr. *22*:308, 1943.
34. Medovy, H.: II. The history of western encephalomyelitis in Manitoba. Can. J. Public Health *67*(Suppl. 1):13–14, 1976.
35. Meehan, P. J., Wells, D. L., Paul, W., et al.: Epidemiological features of and public health response to a St. Louis encephalitis epidemic in Florida, 1990–1991. Epidemiol. Infect. *125*:181–188, 2000.
36. Milner, A. R., and Marshall, I. D.: Pathogenesis of in utero infections with abortogenic and nonabortogenic alphaviruses in mice. J. Virol. *50*:66–72, 1984.
37. Mitchell, C. J., Hayes, R. O., Holden, P., et al.: Effects of ultra-low volume applications of malathion in Hale County, Texas. I. Western encephalitis virus activity in treated and untreated towns. J. Med. Entomol. *6*:155–162, 1969.
38. Mulder, D. W., Parrott, M., and Thaler, M.: Sequelae of western equine encephalitis. Neurology *1*:318–327, 1951.
39. Noran, H. H., and Baker, A. B.: Sequels of equine encephalomyelitis. Arch. Neurol. Psychiatr. *49*:398–413, 1943.
40. Olitsky, P. K., Schlesinger, R. W., and Morgan, I. M.: Induced resistance of the central nervous system to experimental infection with equine encephalomyelitis virus. J. Exp. Med. *77*:359–375, 1943.
41. Olson, J. G., Reeves, W. C., Emmons, R. W., et al.: Correlation of *Culex tarsalis* population indices with the incidence of St. Louis encephalitis and western equine encephalomyelitis in California. Am. J. Trop. Med. Hyg. *28*:335–343, 1979.
42. Potter, M. E., Currier, R. W., II, Pearson, J. E., et al.: Western equine encephalomyelitis in horses in the northern Red River Valley, 1975. J. Am. Vet. Med. Assoc. *170*:1396–1399, 1977.
43. Powers, A. M., Brault, A. C., Shirako, Y., et al.: Evolutionary relationships and systematics of the alphaviruses. J. Virol. *75*:10118–10131, 2001.
44. Qiu, H., Jun, H. W., and McCall, J. W.: Pharmacokinetics, formulations and safety of insect repellent N,N-diethyl-3-methylbenzamide (DEET): A review. J. Am. Mosq. Control Assoc. *14*:12–27, 1998.
45. Ray, C. G., Sciple, G. W., Holden, P., et al.: Acute, febrile CNS illnesses in an endemic area of Texas: Epidemiologic and serologic findings, 1965. Public Health Rep. *82*:785–793, 1967.
46. Reeves, W. C.: Epidemiology and Control of Mosquito Borne Arboviruses in California, 1943–1987. Sacramento, California Mosquito Vector Control Association, 1990.
47. Reeves, W. C., and Hammon, W. M.: Epidemiology of the Arthropod-Borne Viral Encephalitides in Kern County, California, 1943–1952. Berkeley, University of California Press, 1962, pp. 1-257.
48. Reeves, W. C., Hardy, J. L., Reisen, W. K., et al.: Potential effect of global warming on mosquito-borne arboviruses. J. Med. Entomol. *31*:323–332, 1994.
49. Reisen, W. K., and Chiles, R. E.: Prevalence of antibodies to western equine encephalomyelitis and St. Louis encephalitis viruses in residents of California exposed to sporadic and consistent enzootic transmission. Am. J. Trop. Med. Hyg. *57*:526–529, 1997.
50. Reisen, W. K., Meyer, R. P., Presser, S. B., et al.: Effect of temperature on the transmission of western equine encephalomyelitis and St. Louis encephalitis viruses by *C. tarsalis*. J. Med. Entomol. *30*:151–160, 1993.
51. Reisen, W. K., and Monath, T. P.: Western equine encephalitis. *In* Monath, T. P. (ed.): The Arboviruses: Epidemiology and Ecology. Vol. 5. Boca Raton, FL, CRC Press, 1990, pp. 89–137.
52. Reisen, W. K., Yoshimura, G., Reeves, W. C., et al.: The impact of aerial applications of ultra-low volume adulticides on *Culex tarsalis* populations (Diptera: Culicidae) in Kern County, California, USA, 1982. J. Med. Entomol. *21*:573–585, 1984.
53. Robbins, P. J., and Cherniack, M. G.: Review of the biodistribution and toxicity of the insect repellent N,N-diethyl-m-toluamide (DEET). J. Toxicol. Environ. Health *18*:503–525, 1986.
54. Roland, E. H., Jan, J. E., and Rigg, J. M.: Toxic encephalopathy in a child after brief exposure to insect repellents. Can. Med. Assoc. J. *132*:155–156, 1985.
55. Rumenapf, T., Strauss, E. G., and Strauss, J. H.: Aura virus is a new world representative of Sindbis-like viruses. Virology *208*:621, 1995.
56. Schreck, C. E., and Kline, D. L.: Personal protection afforded by controlled-release topical repellents and permethrin-treated clothing against natural populations of *Aedes taeniorhynchus*. J. Am. Mosq. Control Assoc. *5*:77–80, 1989.
57. Schultz, D. R., Barthal, J. S., and Garrett, C.: Western equine encephalitis with rapid onset of parkinsonism. Neurology *27*:1095–1096, 1977.
58. Sciple, G. W., Ray, G., LaMotte, L. C., et al.: Western encephalitis with recovery of virus from cerebrospinal fluid. Neurology *17*:169–171, 1967.
59. Somekh, E., Glode, M. P., Reilly, T. T., et al.: Multiple intracranial calcifications after western equine encephalitis. Pediatr. Infect. Dis. *10*:408, 1991.
60. Stallones, R. A., Reeves, W. C., and Lennette, E. H.: Serologic epidemiology of western equine and St. Louis encephalitis virus infection in California. I. Persistence of complement-fixing antibody following clinical illness. Am. J. Hyg. *79*:16–28, 1964.
61. Strauss, J. H., and Strauss, E. G.: The alphaviruses: Gene expression, replication and evolution. Microbiol. Rev. *58*:491, 1994.
62. Weaver, S. C., Hagenbaugh, A., Bellow, L. A., et al.: A comparison of the nucleotide sequences of eastern and western equine encephalomyelitis viruses with those of other alphaviruses and related RNA viruses. Virology *197*:375–390, 1993.
63. Weaver, S. C., Kang, W., Shirako, Y., et al.: Recombinational history and molecular evolution of western equine encephalitis complex alphaviruses. J. Virol. *71*:613–623.

64. Wegbreit, J., and Reisen, W. K.: Relationships among weather, mosquito abundance, and encephalitis virus activity in California: Kern County 1990–98. J. Am. Mosq. Control Assoc. *16*:22–27, 2000.
65. Wesseling, S. L., and Griffin, D. E.: Local cytokine responses during acute and chronic viral infections to the central nervous system. Semin. Virol. *5*:457, 1994.
66. White, D. P., Miller, F., and Erickson, R. W.: Sleep apnea and nocturnal hypoventilation after western equine encephalitis. Am. Rev. Respir. Dis. *127*:132–133, 1983.
67. Wyckoff, R. W. G., and Tesar, W. C.: Equine encephalomyelitis in monkeys. J. Immunol. *37*:329–343, 1939.
68. Zeifert, M., Pennell, W. H., Finley, K. H., et al.: The electroencephalogram following western and St. Louis encephalitis. Neurology *12*:311–319, 1962.

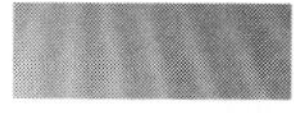

CHAPTER **178C**

Venezuelan Equine Encephalitis

THEODORE F. TSAI

Mosquito-borne Venezuelan equine encephalitis (VEE) arguably is the most important viral zoonosis in Latin America. The disease, known locally as "peste loca," has occurred in combined epizootics and epidemics at regular intervals since the 1920s, sometimes leading to hundreds of thousands of human and equine cases. Between 1935 and 1961, 11 outbreaks were reported, and from 1962 to 1973, epizootics recurred in every year except 1965.[14] The virus was isolated from horse brain in 1938 during an outbreak in Venezuela. Although outbreaks have arisen principally in northern South America, especially from Colombia and Venezuela, in a remarkable period between 1969 and 1971, epizootics and epidemics were reported from Colombia, Venezuela, Ecuador, Peru, all the countries of Central America (except Panama), Mexico, and the state of Texas.[11, 21, 35] Subsequently, no major epizootics/epidemics were recognized until a large outbreak emerged in Venezuela and Colombia in 1995.[24, 31, 32, 38] Molecular phylogenetic analyses performed in the wake of that outbreak suggested that epizootic strains arise spontaneously from sylvatic viral strains circulating silently in nature.[19, 36, 38, 40]

Etiologic Agent

VEE virus is antigenically distinct from other alphaviruses but is itself a complex of antigenically and ecologically distinct viral subtypes[23, 28, 40] (Table 178–3). Epizootic subtypes IAB and IC are so named because they have been associated with major outbreaks in horses. Sylvatic viral subtypes circulate in silent cycles of rodent/bird-mosquito transmission and in general do not cause encephalitis in equines. Both epizootic and sylvatic viral strains cause human illness.

VEE virus is thought to have evolved approximately 1400 years ago from a now extinct ancestral alphavirus in one of two extant lineages of New World alphaviruses represented by eastern equine encephalomyelitis and VEE viruses.[23] Because epizootic VEE viral strains had never been isolated from nature except during epizootics, their reservoirs and the mechanisms by which they emerge to cause outbreaks had remained a puzzle. However, recent molecular phylogenetic analyses have found a close genetic relationship between the epizootic IC and the sylvatic ID strains, thus suggesting that these epizootic strains might arise spontaneously by mutation from naturally circulating ID virus. Other outbreaks have had an iatrogenic source from improperly inactivated equine vaccine.[15, 16, 23, 25, 36, 37, 38]

Comparisons of the attenuated TC-83 vaccine strain of VEE virus and the epizootic IAB parent virus and mutations of virulent infectious clones have shown that changes associated with attenuation occur principally in genes encoding the E2 and E1 glycoproteins, but also in the 5′ nontranslated region.[15, 28] Attenuation is associated with reduced

TABLE 178–3 ■ VIRUSES IN THE VENEZUELAN EQUINE ENCEPHALOMYELITIS COMPLEX

Subtype	Variety	Pattern of Transmission	Location	Transmission Cycle
I	AB	Epizootic	South, Central, and North America	Various mosquitoes and biting insects/equines
	C	Epizootic	Northern South America	Various mosquitoes and biting insects/equines
	D	Enzootic	Ecuador, Panama, Colombia, and Venezuela	*Culex* (*Melanoconion*) *ocossa* and *panocossal* rodents, aquatic birds
	E	Enzootic	Central America	*Culex* (*Melanoconion*) *taeniopus*/ rodents
	F	Enzootic	Brazil	Unknown
II (Everglades)		Enzootic	Southern Florida	*Culex* (*Melanoconion*) *cedeceil*/rodents
III	A			
	Mucambo	Enzootic	South America	*Culex* (*Melanoconion*) portesi/rodents
	B			
	Tonate	Enzootic	South America	Unknown
	Bijou Bridge	Unknown	Western North America	*Oeciacus vicarius*/birds
	C	Enzootic	Peru	Unknown
IV (Pixuna)		Enzootic	Brazil	Unknown
V (Cabassou)		Enzootic	French Guiana	Unknown
VI		Enzootic	Argentina	Unknown

neuroinvasiveness (faster clearance from blood and lower viremia levels), as well as reduced neurovirulence (minimal histopathologic changes after intracerebral inoculation of horses).

VEE virus rapidly produces cytopathic effects in a variety of cell cultures, including Vero, LLC-MK2, and BHK-21, and in primary chicken and duck embryo cells. Epizootic strains cause lethal infections in horses, donkeys, mules, rabbits, and dogs. In certain guinea pig strains, pathogenicity is correlated with equine virulence.

Epidemiology and Ecology

Epizootics and concurrent epidemics of VEE caused by the IAB and IC strains typically have led to thousands and, on at least one occasion, hundreds of thousands of cases in humans and equines. Most such outbreaks have occurred in Venezuela and Colombia and have been caused by IC viruses (see earlier) (Fig. 178–8).[24, 27, 36, 38] The circumstances leading to the emergence of outbreaks are poorly understood, but outbreaks often have occurred in arid areas during years of heavy rainfall and flooding, especially during the dry season.[35] The importance of a nonimmune horse population to amplify the virus has been underscored in the most recent outbreak in 1995, which occurred in areas of Colombia and Venezuela where equine immunizations had lapsed.[24, 31, 32, 38] Equines are the most important vertebrate amplifying host because high levels of viremia develop and are sustained in equines and they provide a large surface area for biting mosquitoes. Numerous species of mosquitoes and other blood-feeding insects, among them *Aedes taeniorhynchus*, a salt marsh mosquito, and *Psorophora confinnis,* found in ground pools, can transmit the virus from horse to horse and from horse to human.[30]

Infections are transmitted rapidly among animals and to people such that outbreaks can disseminate at rates of several miles per day. The epidemic curve of human cases usually follows the equine epizootic by several weeks, and epidemic transmission ceases when the number of susceptible horses has been exhausted by immunization or natural infection.[12, 35]

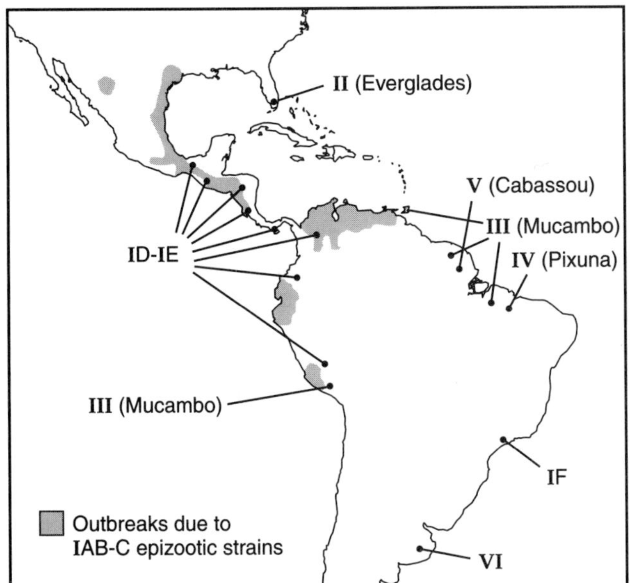

FIGURE 178–8 ■ Locations of Venezuelan equine encephalitis (VEE) outbreaks caused by type IAB-IC epizootic strains and locations where VEE sylvatic subtypes have been recognized.

The role of other animals, including humans, in sustaining epidemic viral transmission has been investigated in urban outbreaks, during which household clustering of cases has been observed, and in recent outbreaks, during which few horses were kept in the community. VEE virus levels in human blood are sufficiently high to infect mosquitoes, and virus also has been isolated from the pharynx of ill persons, indicating the possibility of person-to-person transmission by mosquitoes such as *Aedes aegypti* or by direct close contact.[2, 29] Although such transmission mechanisms may account for some cases, a recent household survey found that rates of apparent secondary transmission were no higher than the underlying community attack rate.[24, 31] Community attack rates of 20 to 50 percent have been recorded, and completion of the course of epidemics in intervals as short as 1 month underscores the considerable force of epidemic transmission.

The series of epizootics beginning in Guatemala in 1969 and reaching Texas in 1971 was caused by an IAB virus that is almost genetically identical to the 1943 Trinidad donkey (epizootic IAB) virus used in inactivated vaccines, thus leading to the conclusion that these outbreaks were iatrogenic and caused by the use of inadequately inactivated equine vaccine.[16, 37] Another outbreak in Argentina was traced to a similar etiology.

In contrast to the epizootic strains, sylvatic VEE viruses are avirulent in horses and cause a low level of viremia after infection, subclinical or mild illness, and minimal inflammatory change after direct intracerebral inoculation.[34] However, outbreaks of enzootic IE-like viruses rarely have caused outbreaks and deaths in horses (e.g., in Chiapas, Mexico, in 1993). The viruses are maintained in mosquitoes, principally *Culex (Melanoconion) taeniopus* in marshy coastal lowlands, in rodents, and in aquatic birds. In coastal lagoons in Panama, ibises (*Endocinus albus*) and spoon-billed ducks (*Cochlearius cochlearius*) appear to serve as intermediate hosts.[1] VEE subtype II virus, the Everglades virus, is enzootic among cotton rats and other small mammals on hammocks in the Everglades swamp and rarely has caused human illness in Florida.[9] The other VEE virus found in the United States, Bijou Bridge virus, is a nonpathogenic virus thought to have evolved from South American subtype III virus transferred as recently as 40 years ago, probably by a migrating bird.

VEE infections caused by sylvatic strains can be considered "diseases of place" that occur sporadically in persons who enter sylvatic habitats where the viruses are maintained.[8] Sporadic cases and rare outbreaks among soldiers in field bivouacs have been reported.[13, 26] Many infections are undoubtedly undiagnosed. Bridge vectors, mosquitoes that feed on mammals in the enzootic transmission cycle and subsequently on humans, usually are responsible for these infections.

Numerous cases and outbreaks of VEE have occurred in laboratories when infective aerosols were generated in laboratory procedures.[17] Laboratory manipulations should be undertaken only in BL-3 laboratories and by immunized personnel.

Clinical Manifestations

The incubation period is brief—2 to 5 days—and in many accounts, the onset of illness was so sudden that it was timed to an exact hour.[17] Fever, chills, headache, myalgia, and malaise are the earliest symptoms, and illness quickly leads to prostration. Photophobia, neck stiffness, backache, conjunctivitis, and sore throat are also common symptoms that occur in approximately one quarter or more of cases. Gastrointestinal complaints, especially nausea and vomiting, and, to a lesser degree, loose stools or diarrhea are reported frequently.[3]

Physical examination discloses severe prostration and few specific findings. The face may appear hyperemic, inflammation of the pharynx is common, and occasionally, tonsillitis, palatal ulcers, or petechiae are observed. The cervical lymph nodes may be enlarged and tender. Conjunctivitis and conjunctival suffusion are noted frequently. Nuchal rigidity can be elicited in 10 percent of cases, more often in children. Despite the disease's name, confusion, agitation, and mild disturbances in consciousness suggesting encephalitis are present in only 5 to 10 percent of cases, and patients with significant neurologic findings, such as cranial nerve palsy, motor weakness and paralysis, seizures, and coma, usually account for less than 5 percent of all cases.[3, 24, 25] In epidemics, neurologic findings and encephalitis occurred more commonly in children; however, sporadic cases, including encephalitis caused by VEE subtype II (Everglades) and III (Tonate) viruses, have occurred in middle-aged or elderly adults.[9, 13] The fatality rate among patients with encephalitis is 10 to 25 percent, or about 0.5 percent of all cases.[24, 25]

In many patients, the illness has an apparently biphasic course, with seizures, projectile vomiting, and ataxia occurring several days after the onset of fever and complete and rapid resolution occurring thereafter. Sequelae such as nervousness, forgetfulness, recurrent headache, and easy fatigability are common and may persist for months or even up to 1 year. Motor abnormalities usually resolve without residual deficit; however, rarely, sensory and motor abnormalities may persist. Long-term effects on psychometric examination have been reported.[18]

Experimental observations in animals suggest that congenital infection may lead to central nervous system anomalies such as porencephaly, micrencephaly, and hydrocephalus.[19] A similar pattern of structural brain abnormalities has been observed in virus culture–positive fetuses aborted during outbreaks.[38, 39] Pancreatic beta-cell infection occurs in experimentally infected animals and has led to speculation that VEE may be followed by diabetes, but epidemiologic studies have failed to find an association.[4, 18]

The principal clinical laboratory finding is leukopenia ($<4500/mm^3$), the nadir of which occurs on the fourth day of illness.[3, 8] After the onset of illness, the absolute neutrophil count declines from normal values to 500 to 2000; total lymphocytes are depressed at the onset of illness and gradually recover after 1 week. The platelet count may be diminished below 100,000 mm^3, and lactate dehydrogenase and hepatic transaminases may be elevated moderately. Cerebrospinal fluid (CSF) shows a lymphocytic pleocytosis of up to several hundred cells, moderately elevated protein, and normal or slightly depressed glucose.

Pathology and Pathogenesis

VEE virus is both lymphotropic and neurotropic.[7, 33] Pathologic changes are observed consistently in the lymph nodes, spleen, lungs, liver, gastrointestinal lymphoid tissue, and brain, with inflammatory infiltrates of mononuclear and polymorphonuclear cells. The lymph nodes and spleen show pronounced lymphoid depletion and necrosis of the germinal centers, along with neutrophilic infiltration and lymphophagocytosis. The selective depletion of lymphoid follicles, with sparing of the paracortical areas and the thymus, suggests that VEE virus principally destroys B cells. These histopathologic changes are reflected in the early lymphopenia seen in the peripheral blood. The liver shows patchy hepatocellular degeneration typical of viral hepatitis. A diffuse interstitial pneumonia with a mixed intraseptal inflammatory cell infiltrate is a consistent finding, and some cases also exhibit intra-alveolar hemorrhage, secondary bronchopneumonia, or both. The brain shows only congestion and edema in most cases. Mild, often focal meningitis and changes associated with encephalitis, perivascular inflammatory infiltrates, and neuronal degeneration are found in a large number of cases.[6, 7] The consistent presence of congestion and edema in various organs and the necrotizing vasculitis seen in some cases suggest that vascular endothelial cells may be a target of infection. This speculation is supported by the observation of VEE viral antigen in the vascular endothelial cells of experimentally infected animals. Secondary immune-mediated destruction of infected vascular endothelia and lymphoid cells may account for delayed clinical manifestations.

Laboratory Diagnosis

VEE virus can be recovered from blood during the first 3 days of illness in at least 75 percent of cases, although isolates have been made after 6 days.[2] Virus also has been recovered from throat swabs in approximately 25 percent of cases.[21] Specimens should be inoculated onto Vero or other susceptible cell cultures, but only in a laboratory with BL-3 level containment because of the risk of laboratory aerosol-associated infection. As an alternative to viral isolation, genomic sequences in acute viremic blood can be detected rapidly and with high sensitivity by polymerase chain reaction. Establishing the subtype of VEE viral isolates is vital because subtypes IAB and IC have a potential for epidemic spread. Isolates can be identified rapidly with subtype-specific monoclonal antibodies.

IgM capture enzyme-linked immunosorbent assay (ELISA) is the recommended serologic procedure. Both serum and CSF specimens can be tested by this means. Elevated viral-specific IgM in a single serum or CSF specimen is diagnostic and often obviates the need for a second paired serum. Alternative available serologic procedures in increasing order of specificity include IgG ELISA, hemagglutination inhibition, complement fixation, and neutralization.

Differential Diagnosis

The self-limited acute febrile illness that characterizes most VEE cases resembles infection caused by dengue, Oropouche, Mayaro, group C bunyaviruses, and various other arboviruses. The epidemic occurrence of cases may suggest dengue or Oropouche fever; however, the absence of rash and hemorrhagic manifestations and an association with equine deaths strongly indicate VEE until disproved. Eastern and western equine encephalitis overlap with VEE in some areas of Latin America, but only sporadic human cases have been recognized. Clinical recognition of sporadic VEE caused by sylvatic viruses is difficult; the diagnosis should be entertained in patients with central nervous system infection and an appropriate exposure history.

Treatment and Prevention

No specific treatment is available. Symptomatic treatment with antipyretics and fluids alone is sufficient in most cases.

In patients with encephalitis, anticonvulsants may be needed, and intensive supportive care, especially early recognition and treatment of secondary pneumonia, may improve the outcome.

Immunization with experimental live attenuated TC-83 vaccine is indicated for laboratory and field personnel with a high risk of exposure to VEE virus.[5, 22] However, the vaccine is immunogenic in only 85 percent of vaccinees, and significant side effects consisting of fever, stiff neck, malaise, and myalgia develop in approximately 20 percent of vaccinees.[10] Previous vaccination with alphaviral vaccines may interfere with response to TC-83, but after immunization with experimental inactivated TC-84 vaccine, antibody will develop in approximately 75 percent of persons who had failed to respond to TC-83.[3, 10, 20] Safer candidate vaccines that may provide better protection against respiratory infection are being investigated.

Immunizing equines with TC-83 vaccine is the best approach to preventing the emergence of outbreaks. Inadequately inactivated vaccine prepared from epizootic IAB strains poses a danger of producing iatrogenic outbreaks and should be used only if appropriate safety and quality assurance standards of vaccine production have been met. Because the live vaccine provides rapid immunity after a single dose, it is the most effective approach in combatting outbreaks. Attenuated vaccine is available commercially in certain Latin American countries, but in the United States, only inactivated vaccine formulated with western and eastern equine encephalitis and equine influenza and tetanus antigens is licensed.

Mosquito control with a combination of larvicides and adulticides may be indicated to mitigate large outbreaks. Taking precautions against mosquito bites, such as using repellents, staying in well-screened or air-conditioned areas when possible, and wearing long-sleeved shirts and long pants, is advised for persons who cannot avoid traveling to areas experiencing epidemics.

REFERENCES

1. Adames, A. J., Dutary, B., Tejera, H., et al.: Relacion entre mosquitos vectores y aves acuaticas en la transmision potencial de dos arbovirus. Rev. Med. Panama *18*:106–119, 1993.
2. Bowen, G. S., and Calisher, C. H.: Virological and serological studies in Venezuelan equine encephalomyelitis in humans. J. Clin. Microbiol. *4*:22–27, 1976.
3. Bowen, G. S., Fashinell, T. R., Dean, P. B., et al.: Clinical aspects of human Venezuelan equine encephalitis in Texas. Bull. Pan. Am. Health Org. *10*:46–57, 1976.
4. Bowen, G. S., Rayfield, E. J., Monath, T. P., et al.: Studies of glucose metabolism in Rhesus monkeys after Venezuelan equine encephalitis virus infection. J. Med. Virol. *6*:227–234, 1980.
5. Burke, D. S., Ramsburg, H. H., and Edelman, R.: Persistence in humans of antibody to subtypes of Venezuelan equine encephalomyelitis (VEE) virus after immunization with attenuated (TC-83) VEE virus vaccine. J. Infect. Dis. *136*:354–359, 1977.
6. Charles, P. C., Walters, E., Margolis, F., et al.: Mechanism of neuroinvasion of Venezuelan equine encephalitis virus in the mouse. Virology *208*:662–671, 1995.
7. de la Monte, S. M., Castro, F., Bonilla, N. J., et al.: The systemic pathology of Venezuelan equine encephalitis virus infection in humans. Am. J. Trop. Med. Hyg. *34*:194–202, 1985.
8. Dietz, W. H., Peralta, P. H., and Johnson, K. M.: Ten clinical cases of human infection with Venezuelan equine encephalomyelitis virus, subtype I-D. Am. J. Trop. Med. Hyg. *28*:329–334, 1979.
9. Ehrenkranz, N. J., and Ventura, A. K.: Venezuelan equine encephalitis virus infection in man. Annu. Rev. Med. *25*:9–14, 1974.
10. Engler, R. J. M., Mangiafico, J. A., Jahrling, P., et al.: Venezuelan equine encephalitis–specific immunoglobulin responses: Live attenuated TC-83 versus inactivated C-84 vaccine. J. Med. Virol. *38*:305–310, 1992.
11. Franck, P. T., and Johnson, K. M.: An outbreak of Venezuelan equine encephalomyelitis in Central America. Am. J. Epidemiol. *94*:487–495, 1971.
12. Gutierrez, V. E., Monath, T. P., Alava, A. A., et al.: Epidemiologic investigations of the 1969 epidemic of Venezuelan encephalitis in Ecuador. Am. J. Epidemiol. *102*:400–413, 1975.
13. Hommell, D., Heraud, J. M., Hulin, A., and Talarmin, A.: Association of Tonate virus (subtype IIIB of the Venezuelan equine encephalitis complex) with encephalitis in a human. Clin. Infect. Dis. *30*:188–190, 2000.
14. Johnson, K. M., and Martin, D. H.: Venezuelan equine encephalitis. Adv. Vet. Sci. Comp. Med. *18*:79–116, 1974.
15. Kinney, R. M., Chang, G.-J., Tsuchiya, K. R., et al.: Attenuation of Venezuelan equine encephalitis virus strain TC-83 is encoded by the 5′-noncoding region and the E2 envelope glycoprotein. J. Virol. *67*:1269–1277, 1993.
16. Kinney, R. M., Tsuchiya, K. R., Sneider, J. M., et al.: Molecular evidence for the origin of the widespread Venezuelan equine encephalitis epizootic of 1969 to 1972. J. Gen. Virol. *73*:3301–3305, 1992.
17. Koprowski, H., and Cox, H. R.: Human laboratory infection with Venezuelan equine encephalomyelitis virus. N. Engl. J. Med. *236*:647–654, 1947.
18. Leon, C. A., Jaramillo, R., Martinez, A., et al.: Sequelae of Venezuelan equine encephalitis in humans: A four-year follow-up. Int. J. Epidemiol. *4*:131–140, 1975.
19. London, W. T., Levitt, N. H., Kent, S. G., et al.: Congenital cerebral and ocular malformations induced in Rhesus monkeys by Venezuelan equine encephalitis virus. Teratology *16*:285–296, 1977.
20. McClain, D. J., Pittman, P. R., Ramsburg, H. H., et al.: Immunologic interference from sequential administration of live attenuated alphavirus vaccines. J. Infect. Dis. *177*:634–641, 1998.
21. Pan American Health Organization: Venezuelan encephalitis. Scientific Publication 243. Proceedings of the Workshop Symposium on Venezuelan Encephalitis Virus, Washington, D.C., 1972, pp. 1–416.
22. Pittman, P. R., Makuch, R. S., Mangiafico, J. A., et al.: Long-term duration of detectable neutralizing antibodies after administration of live-attenuated VEE vaccine and following booster vaccination with inactivated VEE vaccine. Vaccine *14*:337–343, 1996.
23. Powers, A. M., Brault, A. C., Shirako, Y., et al.: Evolutionary relationships and systematics of the alphaviruses. J. Virol. *75*:10118–10131, 2001.
24. Rivas, F., Diaz, L. A., Cardenas, V. M., et al.: Epidemic Venezuelan equine encephalitis in La Guajira, Colombia, 1995. J. Infect. Dis. *175*:828–832, 1997.
25. Rossi, A. L. B.: Rural epidemic encephalitis in Venezuela caused by a group A arbovirus (VEE). Prog. Med. Virol. *9*:176–203, 1967.
26. Sanchez, J. L., Lednar, W. M., Macasaet, F. F., et al.: Venezuelan equine encephalomyelitis: Report of an outbreak associated with jungle exposure. Mil. Med. *149*:618–621, 1984.
27. Sanmartin-Barberi, C., Groot, H., and Osorno-Mesa, E.: Human epidemic in Colombia caused by the Venezuelan equine encephalomyelitis virus. Am. J. Trop. Med. Hyg. *3*:283–293, 1954.
28. Strauss, J. H., and Strauss, E. G.: The alphaviruses: Gene expression, replication and evolution. Microbiol. Rev. *58*:491–562, 1994.
29. Suarez, O. M., and Bergold, G. H.: Investigations of an outbreak of Venezuelan equine encephalitis in towns of eastern Venezuela. Am. J. Trop. Med. Hyg. *17*:875–880, 1968.
30. Sudia, W. D., and Newhouse, V. F.: Epidemic Venezuelan equine encephalitis in North America: A summary of virus-vector-host relationships. Am. J. Epidemiol. *101*:1–58, 1975.
31. Update: Venezuelan equine encephalitis—Colombia, 1995. M. M. W. R. Morb. Mortal. Wkly. Rep. *44*(41):775–777, 1995.
32. Venezuelan equine encephalitis—Colombia, 1995. M. M .W. R. Morb. Mortal. Wkly. Rep. *44*(39):721–724, 1995.
33. Walker, D. H., Harrison, A., Murphy, K., et al.: Lymphoreticular and myeloid pathogenesis of Venezuelan equine encephalitis in hamsters. Am. J. Pathol. *84*:351–370, 1976.
34. Walton, T. E., Alvarez, O., Buckwalter, R. M., et al.: Experimental infection of horses with enzootic and epizootic strains of Venezuelan equine encephalomyelitis virus. J. Infect. Dis. *128*:271–282, 1973.
35. Walton, T. E., and Grayson, M. A.: Venezuelan equine encephalitis. *In* Monath, T. P. (ed.): The Arboviruses: Epidemiology and Ecology. Vol. 4. Boca Raton, FL, CRC Press, 1989, pp. 203–231.
36. Wang, E., Bowen, R. A., Medina, G., et al.: Virulence and viremia characteristics of 1992 epizootic subtype IC Venezuelan equine encephalitis viruses and closely related enzootic subtype ID strains. Am. J. Trop. Med. Hyg. *65*:64–69, 2001.
37. Weaver, S. C., Pfeffer, M., Marriott, K., et al.: Genetic evidence for the origins of Venezuelan equine encephalitis virus subtype IAB outbreaks. Am. J. Trop. Med Hyg. *60*:441–448, 1999.
38. Weaver, S. C., Salas, R., Rico-Hesse, R., et al.: Re-emergence of epidemic Venezuelan equine encephalomyelitis in South America. VEE Study Group. Lancet *348*:436–440, 1999.
39. Wenger, F.: Venezuelan equine encephalitis. Teratology *16*:359–362, 1977.
40. Young, N. A., and Johnson, K. M.: Antigenic variants of Venezuelan equine encephalitis virus: Their geographic distribution and epidemiologic significance. Am. J. Epidemiol. *89*:286–307, 1969.

CHAPTER **178D**

Chikungunya

SCOTT B. HALSTEAD

Chikungunya is a benign, dengue-like syndrome characterized by the abrupt onset of fever, arthralgia, maculopapular rash, and leukopenia. The term in Swahili means "that which bends up" and refers to the characteristic symptom of arthralgia.[47] In historical times, the terms knokkel koorts, abu rokab, mal de genoux, dengue, dyenga, and 3-day fever have been given to epidemics probably caused by chikungunya virus.[9]

The classic account, widely cited as being the initial description of epidemic dengue fever, is that of David Bylon, who was "staads chirurgyn" to the City of Batavia (Jakarta) in the year 1779.[6] Dr. Bylon, who himself contracted the illness, wrote the following:

> It was last May 25, in the afternoon at 5:00 when I noted while talking with two good friends of mine, a growing pain in my right hand, and the joints of the lower arm, which step by step proceeded upward to the shoulder and then continued onto all my limbs; so much so that at 9:00 that same evening I was already in my bed with a high fever. . . .
>
> It's now been three weeks since I . . . was stricken by the illness, and because of that had to stay home for 5 days; but even until today I have continuously pain and stiffness in the joints of both feet, with swelling of both ankles; so much so, that when I get up in the morning, or have sat up for a while and start to move again, I can not do so very well and going up and down stairs is very painful.

This account of a febrile illness of acute onset with involvement of the joints clearly suggests that the disease was chikungunya (see the section on clinical manifestations).

In the same year in Cairo and Alexandria, Egypt, another outbreak of disease occurred that bears a close resemblance to chikungunya.[9, 52]

An important pandemic of "dengue" occurred in the years 1870 to 1873; it appeared first on the East African coast and then on the Arabian coast and in Port Said, Egypt. From there, it was carried to Bombay and Calcutta, India, and Java. The 1870 outbreak led to the discovery that the Swahili word for this disease was *ki-dinga pepo*.[15] The term *denga* or *dyenga* had been used to designate the disease in Africa in an earlier outbreak in 1823. In this pandemic, dengue had spread with the slave trade to the Caribbean, where in 1827 and 1828 an extensive outbreak occurred in the West Indies. In Cuba, the Spanish homonym dengue was used first. Written or serologic evidence exists of chikungunya pandemics in India in 1824 and 1825, 1871 and 1872, 1923, and 1964 and 1965.[9]

Chikungunya virus was isolated first by inoculation of suckling mice from an explosive dengue-like epidemic in Tanganyika in 1952.[48]

Etiologic Agent

CLASSIFICATION

According to epidemiologic criteria, chikungunya virus is arthropod-borne because it is transmitted by several species of mosquito. With the use of antigenic relationships demonstrated by hemagglutination inhibition and complement fixation, chikungunya is placed in the *Alphavirus* genus of the family *Togaviridae*.[30] Antisera prepared to chikungunya virus show strong cross-reactions with o'nyong nyong by complement fixation and virus-dilution neutralization. Mayaro and Semliki Forest viruses, however, demonstrate only weak cross-reactions by hemagglutination inhibition and no reactions by complement fixation with chikungunya antigen. Cross-comparisons by plaque-reduction neutralization tests have shown little relatedness among alphaviruses.[53] Similar results have been obtained by fluorescent antibody technique.

Phylogenetic analysis of the E1 envelope glycoprotein from 18 strains divides chikungunya virus into three distinct genotypes corresponding to their geographic origin.[45] One chikungunya clade consists of viruses from Senegal and Nigeria and represents the West Africa genotype. These viruses had only 78 to 85 percent nucleotide sequence identity to viruses of the Central/East Africa genotype and the closely related Asian genotype. The phyletic grouping is consistent with the introduction of East African strains into Asia within a period 50 to 310 years ago.[45] The African and Asian strains of chikungunya virus are not antigenically separable with the use of mouse immune sera.[41] Although differences in plaque size and heat stability have been described between these strains, these differences might be due to the high number of mouse passages by the prototype African strain. Wild-type strains from all genotypes share the property of autointerference and production of hemorrhagic enteritis (Halstead, S. B., unpublished data, 1965).[20]

MORPHOLOGY

Chikungunya virions are spherical particles approximately 42 nm in diameter.[26] They possess a lipid-containing envelope with fine projections. The central core, approximately 25 to 30 nm in diameter, is roughly hexagonal in cross-section and contains a nucleocapsid of uncertain symmetry. Together with other alphaviruses, the genome is a positive-sense, single-stranded RNA of 12 kb that is messenger active and specifies the viral structural and nonstructural protein, including the polymerase. After an initial round of RNA replication, a subgenomic RNA of approximately 4 kb (26S RNA) is produced. This RNA encodes the viral structural proteins, which include two envelope and capsid proteins.[27] The gene is translated from the 5′ end, where genes for nonstructural proteins are located. Assembly of virus particles at the cell surface occurs by a budding process involving incorporation of the "core" virus precursor into virus particles.[26] Host-cell membranes are modified during infection and contain viral antigen when incorporated into viral envelopes. The protein hemagglutinin spikes are mounted on a phospholipid envelope.

GROWTH

Chikungunya virus produces death in infant mice, rats, and hamsters after intracerebral inoculation. Serial passage of the virus in mice has resulted in selection of a strain with a short incubation period that is lethal to weanling mice.[48] Virus grows to titers of 10^8 to 10^9 infectious doses per milliliter. Low-passage material is highly infectious for humans during routine laboratory handling, and, therefore, appropriate precautions should be taken by laboratory workers.

If a mouse brain seed suspension of low-passage virus is prepared and inoculated into other mice at a 1:5 or 1:10 final concentration, death may be delayed significantly, may be sporadic, or may not occur at all. This difference is due to autointerference.[20] Low-passage strains recovered in suckling mice characteristically demonstrate autointerference when inoculated at dilutions below 1:100.

Chikungunya virus produces a cytopathic effect in primary hamster kidney cells and in BHK-21, BSC-1, Vero, FL, HeLa, and rhesus kidney cells.[30] Virus multiplies in *Aedes aegypti, Aedes vittatus, Aedes albopictus, Anopheles stephensi,* and *Culex fatigans* continuous cell lines and in a cell line derived from *Drosophila.* Plaque assays have been described in LLC-MK2, Vero, and BHK-21 cell and in duck and chick embryos.[30]

Transmission

Chikungunya virus has been recovered from wild *A. aegypti* in Tanzania, Nigeria, India, and Thailand; from *Aedes africanus* in Uganda and Bangui; from *Aedes furcifer-taylori* in South Africa and Senegal; and from *Aedes luteocephalus and Aedes dalzieli* in Senegal.[2, 16, 18, 29, 37, 39] Occasional isolates have been recovered from *Mansonia fuscopennata* in Uganda and from *C. fatigans* in Thailand and Tanzania.

Transmission to humans has been demonstrated with the *A. furcifer-taylori* group; transmission to monkeys or mice has been demonstrated with *A. aegypti, A. albopictus, Aedes calceatus, Aedes triseriatus, Aedes togoi, Aedes pseudoscutellaris, Aedes polynesiensis, Anopheles albinanus, Mansonia africana, Erethmapodites chrysogaster,* and *Aedes apicoargenteus.*[30, 34, 44, 51]

Tesh and colleagues[54] examined *A. albopictus* strains from 13 geographic locations from Hawaii to Africa and found considerable variation in susceptibility to infection by oral feeding. The 50 percent oral infective dose (ID_{50}) of a Hawaiian *A. albopictus* strain for a wild-type virus from India was $10^{5.4}$ plaque-forming units per milliliter. The amount of virus replicated by different mosquito strains varied between $10^{4.6}$ and $10^{7.4}$ plaque-forming units per mosquito. These observations, plus a mathematic model of chikungunya virus transmission developed by deMoor and Steffens,[17] suggest that major factors in determining the endemicity of chikungunya may be arthropod related. Tesh and associates[54] suggested that susceptibility to oral infection and the amount of virus replicated may be under genetic control, whereas deMoor and Steffens[17] found mosquito longevity to be the most important determinant in epidemic transmission of chikungunya.

Serologic studies have demonstrated repeatedly the presence of antibodies in humans throughout the moist forests and semi-arid savannas of East and West Africa.[1, 18, 39, 49] Most recorded chikungunya infections in people occur in areas infested with *A. aegypti.* The epidemiology in these areas is similar to that of other *A. aegypti*–borne diseases and parallels the distribution of the vector. When *A. aegypti* mosquitoes are abundant in occupied dwellings, infection rates can be expected to be highest in women and children who are at home during daylight hours. When *A. aegypti* is found in public buildings, schools, and hospitals, outbreaks may involve persons in occupational patterns. Characteristically, chikungunya pandemics are explosive. Studying *A. aegypti* in laboratory mice, Rao and colleagues[46] documented mechanical transmission. Viremia in humans may be as high as 10^8 infectious doses per milliliter.[46] Because the extrinsic incubation period in *A. aegypti* is relatively long, the explosive nature of chikungunya outbreaks is explained best by mechanical transmission.

Epidemiology

HOST RANGE

Chikungunya virus has the ability to replicate in a broad spectrum of vertebrate species. Newborn mice, hamsters, rats, rabbits, guinea pigs, and kittens all can be infected by subcutaneous inoculation of field strains of chikungunya virus,[11] which produces viremia, sickness, and in most instances, death. Adult rabbits, mice, rats, and chickens inoculated peripherally have an asymptomatic viremia followed by an antibody response. Neutralizing or hemagglutination-inhibition antibodies to chikungunya have been recovered occasionally from sera obtained from ungulates. Attempts to infect cattle, goats, sheep, or horses experimentally failed to produce either viremia or an antibody response.[36] Vervet monkeys and baboons are infected readily. Rhesus monkeys were infected by intravenous and intramuscular inoculation and had viremia titers in excess of 10^7 mouse LD_{50}. *A. aegypti* transmitted virus to rhesus monkeys and could be infected by biting viremic animals.

Chikungunya antibodies have been found in vervet monkeys, baboons, chimpanzees, and red-tailed monkeys in Zimbabwe, South Africa, and Uganda.[33] The zoonotic status of chikungunya virus in Asia has not been studied carefully.

In Africa, zoonotic transmission to subhuman primates is surmised to take place in a wide variety of habitats, with transmission occurring in the forest canopy, at ground level, or both.[35] Chikungunya appears to be enzootic throughout much of eastern, central, southern, and western Africa.[30] Subhuman primate populations are affected in epizootics, which involve critical numbers of the susceptible population, followed by disappearance of the virus. Thus, chikungunya may maintain itself in wildlife populations by constantly moving epizootic activity, in much the same fashion as respiratory and enteric virus infections are maintained in humans. To expect that intercurrent and epidemic human infections in Africa are related to epizootic activity seems reasonable. Many putative or identified chikungunya vectors feed on people as well as subhuman primates.

GEOGRAPHIC DISTRIBUTION

When susceptible human and *A. aegypti* populations are above the threshold level required for transmission, a person-mosquito-person cycle is established. This cycle probably is responsible for most of the large urban outbreaks of chikungunya studied during the past 40 years. In Africa, chikungunya outbreaks have been reported from Uganda, Tanzania, Zimbabwe, South Africa, Angola, Zaire, Nigeria, and Senegal.[30] This distribution best fits the present location of virus research laboratories. A reasonable assumption is that chikungunya is endemic throughout sub-Saharan Africa.

According to historical evidence, chikungunya has spread from the African enzootic focus and caused large pandemics throughout both the Asian and American tropics.[9, 15, 52] Pandemics have swept India in 1824, 1871, 1902, 1923, and 1963 and 1964, with Sri Lanka (formerly Ceylon) involved in 1965.[9] In the 19th century, chikungunya epidemics were reported in the Indonesian archipelago. An extensive serologic survey using the plaque-reduction neutralization test has suggested chikungunya activity possibly during World War II in Kalimantan and Sulawesi, Indonesia. During the late 1950s and early 1960s, chikungunya appears to have established itself endemically in Southeast Asia and was transmitted continuously in urban populations in Thailand, Cambodia, and South Vietnam, possibly into the 1970s.[12, 22, 58] Involvement of urban populations in Burma appears to have been intermittent, with outbreaks recorded in 1963 and from 1970 to 1973.[38] A large chikungunya epidemic affected much of Indonesia in 1983 and 1984 (Slemons, R. D., personal communication) and Burma in 1984 and 1985.[56] Chikungunya virus was isolated in Australia in 1989.[23] Serologic evidence of chikungunya virus infection has been found throughout the Philippines, possibly during World War II; since then, localized outbreaks have occurred in Manila, Philippines, in 1967 and Negros, Philippines, in 1968[3, 8, 32] and as recently as 1986.[14] From 1990 to 1995, chikungunya remained endemic at low levels in Thailand, Myanmar (formerly Burma), and Indonesia.[55] Little or no chikungunya virus infection has been reported in the 20th century in Papua New Guinea, the Solomon Islands, Vanuatu (formerly New Hebrides), the Caroline Islands, the Pacific Islands, or any of the American tropics.[53]

A pertinent question to ask is why is it that chikungunya and dengue viruses, both transmitted by *A. aegypti*, do not have an identical geographic distribution? The question may be answered partially by differences in the transmission of chikungunya and dengue. The threshold for infection of chikungunya virus in *A. aegypti* is relatively high: approximately $10^{5.6}$ mouse infectious doses are required to infect 50 percent of adult females.[54] The infection threshold of female *A. aegypti* for dengue virus is rather similar. However, *A. aegypti* mosquitoes infected with chikungunya virus transmit virus to vertebrates poorly, whereas dengue-infected mosquitoes transmit with great regularity.[19] Thus, transmission of chikungunya virus would be expected to occur only in areas with high human susceptibility rates and consistently high densities of *A. aegypti* and possibly by mechanical transmission.

Clinical Manifestations

The incubation period of chikungunya fever is usually 2 to 4 days. In infants, the disease typically begins with the abrupt onset of fever, followed by flushing of the skin. Febrile convulsions may occur in as many as one third of patients. After 3 to 5 days of fever, a generalized maculopapular rash and lymphadenopathy are noted. Conjunctival injection, swelling of the eyelids, pharyngitis, and symptoms and signs of upper respiratory tract disease are common. No enanthem occurs. Some infants have a biphasic fever curve, and arthralgia may be quite severe, although it is not seen frequently.[4, 10, 21, 28, 43]

In older children, fever develops acutely and is accompanied by headache, myalgia, and arthralgia involving various joints. Residual arthralgia is uncommon. An early macular blush and a maculopapular rash accompany or immediately precede defervescence. At the same time, marked lymphadenopathy occurs. Febrile convulsions are observed commonly. Hemorrhagic findings, including a positive tourniquet test, are rare.[4, 10, 21, 28, 43]

Arthralgia or arthritis is the most conspicuous feature of chikungunya in adults. Usually, patients can identify the precise time and the joint first affected in a chikungunya illness. Swelling and redness of joints and even the pinnae of the ear may occur.[10]

Although dengue and chikungunya illnesses are similar, important distinguishing features are summarized in Tables 178–4 through 178–8 from clinical data obtained from children in Thailand.[21, 43]

Table 178–4 shows the abrupt onset and early severity of chikungunya versus dengue illnesses, many of which came to medical attention only several days after the onset of fever.

Chikungunya virus infections are shorter in duration than dengue virus infections (Table 178–5). Almost half of children with chikungunya had a fever that ended within 72 hours after onset, whereas the median duration of dengue fever was 2 days longer.

Many constitutional signs and symptoms occur with similar frequency in chikungunya and dengue viral infections and cannot be used to differentiate the illnesses clinically (Table 178–6). However, a terminal maculopapular rash, arthralgia or arthritis, and conjunctival injection were more

TABLE 178–4 ■ CHIKUNGUNYA AND DENGUE IN CHILDREN*: COMPARISON OF ONSET OF ILLNESS

	Hospitalized				Outpatient			
	Chikungunya (32 Cases)		*Dengue (523 Cases)*†		*Chikungunya (17 Cases)*		*Primary Dengue (29 Cases)*	
Day of Illness	**Number**	**Percent**	**Number**	**Percent**	**Number**	**Percent**	**Number**	**Percent**
0	8	25	2	0.4	0	0	0	0
1	15	47	44	8	11	65	8	27
2	5	16	67	13	1	6	5	17
3	2	6	145	28	2	12	3	10
4	1	3	148	28	0	0	7	24
5			84	16	3	17	4	14
6			20	4			2	
7	1	3	11	2			7	
8 or more			3	0.6				

*Patients with simultaneous dengue and chikungunya are excluded from analysis.
†Includes primary and secondary infections.
Data from Nimmannitya, S., Halstead, S. B., Cohen, S. N., *et al.*: Dengue and chikungunya virus infection in man in Thailand, 1962-1964. I. Observations on hospitalized patients with hemorrhagic fever. Am. J. Trop. Med. Hyg. *18*:954–971, 1969; and Halstead, S. B., Nimmannitya, S., and Margiotta, M.R.: Dengue and chikungunya virus infection in man in Thailand, 1962–1964. II. Observations on disease in outpatients. Am. J. Trop. Med. Hyg. *18*:972–983, 1969.

TABLE 178–5 ■ CHIKUNGUNYA AND DENGUE IN CHILDREN: COMPARISON OF DURATION OF ILLNESS

Duration of Fever (Days)	Chikungunya (32 Cases)		Dengue (241 Cases)*	
	Number	*Percent*	*Number*	*Percent*
2	11	34.4	8	3.3
3	4	12.5	16	6.6
4	5	15.6	33	13.7
5	5	15.6	52	21.6
6	2	6.3	52	21.6
7	3	9.4	38	15.8
8 or more	2	6.3	42	17.4
	Mean, 4 days		Mean, 5.85 days	

*Includes primary and secondary dengue infections.
After Nimmannitya, S., Halstead, S. B., Cohen, S. N., et al.: Dengue and chikungunya virus infection in man in Thailand, 1962–1964. I. Observations on hospitalized patients with hemorrhagic fever. Am. J. Trop. Med. Hyg. *18*:954–971, 1969.

common symptoms in chikungunya than in dengue (Table 178–7). Shock has been reported infrequently in chikungunya.[10, 50, 57] It was not observed in Thai cases.[43] Changes in taste perception, post-illness bradycardia, and post-illness depression or asthenia are found rarely in chikungunya; these manifestations are distinctive findings in patients with dengue.

Hemorrhagic phenomena rarely occur with chikungunya virus infection. The frequency of hemorrhagic findings in chikungunya and primary and secondary dengue viral infections in Thai children is compared in Table 178–8. The frequency of minor hemorrhagic manifestations in outpatient and inpatient dengue did not differ significantly from that in chikungunya cases. However, petechial rash and spontaneous hematemesis or melena developed in only hospitalized dengue cases.

Pathogenesis and Pathology

The pathologic process of fatal human chikungunya illness has not been studied extensively.[57] Wild-type chikungunya strains produce a hemorrhagic enteritis in mice and hamsters.[20]

Diagnosis

The differential diagnosis includes the viral causes of dengue fever syndrome. In Australia and the western Pacific area, Ross River fever is a frequent cause of epidemic, arthropod-borne, viral arthralgia.

With the use of classic test methods, the diagnosis depends on demonstrating a significant increase in antibody after an illness. Ordinarily, a serum sample collected within 5 days of the onset of fever will not contain hemagglutination-inhibition, complement-fixation, or neutralizing antibodies.[10, 21] Neutralizing and hemagglutination-inhibition antibodies generally are present in samples collected 2 weeks or more after the onset of fever. From a single serum sample collected 7 or more days after onset, detection of antibodies of the IgM class is possible with an IgM capture enzyme-linked immunosorbent assay.[7, 56] Neutralizing antibody can be measured by the virus-dilution method in suckling mice (or weanling mice with use of the Ross high–mouse passage strain) or by the serum-dilution method in any of a variety of tissue cultures or plaque assay techniques.

Virus may be isolated by inoculating acute-phase serum or other suspect materials intracerebrally in 1- to 2-day-old mice or in tissue cultures. On initial passage, death may occur within 2 to 5 days after inoculation. An autointerference phenomenon is noted if low-dilution passages of infected mouse brain are performed. Passage at a 10^{-3} dilution or higher avoids this effect.

Vero cells and suckling mice are equally effective for primary isolation.

TABLE 178–6 ■ CHIKUNGUNYA AND DENGUE IN CHILDREN: COMPARISON OF FREQUENCY OF CLINICAL FINDINGS

	Hospitalized Cases				Outpatient Cases			
	Chikungunya *(32 Cases)*		Dengue* *(142 Cases)*		Chikungunya *(17 Cases)*		Primary Dengue* *(27 Cases)*	
Findings	**Number†**	**Percent**	**Number†**	**Percent**	**Number**	**Percent**	**Number**	**Percent**
Headache	13/19	68	37/83	45	2	12	4	15
Injected pharynx	28/31	90	121/125	97	12	71	27	100
Enanthem	3/27	11	7/84	8	0		0	
Rhinitis	3/31	6	6/47	13	4	24	6	22
Cough	7/30	22	17/79	22	1	6	11	41
Vomiting	19/32	59	73/126	58	6	35	15	56
Constipation	12/30	40	16/30	53	0		4	15
Diarrhea	5/32	16	5/78	6	1	6	1	4
Abdominal pain	6/19	32	38/76	50	3	18	2	7
Lymphadenopathy	8/26	31	32/79	41				
Restlessness	10/30	33	17/79	22				

*Includes primary and secondary dengue infections.
†Number with finding/number with observations recorded.
Adapted from Nimmannitya, S., Halstead, S. B., Cohen, S. N., et al.: Dengue and chikungunya virus infection in man in Thailand, 1962–1964. I. Observations on hospitalized patients with hemorrhagic fever. Am. J. Trop. Med. Hyg. *18*:954–971, 1969; and Halstead, S. B., Nimmannitya, S., and Margiotta, M. R.: Dengue and chikungunya virus infection in man in Thailand, 1962–1964. II. Observations on disease in outpatients. Am. J. Trop. Med. Hyg. *18*:972–983, 1969.

TABLE 178–7 ■ CHIKUNGUNYA AND DENGUE IN CHILDREN: CLINICAL FINDINGS OCCURRING WITH DIFFERENT FREQUENCY

	Chikungunya (32 Cases)		Dengue* (32 Cases)		
Manifestation	*Number*†	*Percent*	*Number*†	*Percent*	**Significance**
Maculopapular rash	19/32	59.4	16/132	12.1	$p < 0.001$
Conjunctival injection	15/27	55.6	20/61	32.8	$0.05 > p < 0.01$
Myalgia/ arthralgia	8/20	40.0	9/75	12.0	$0.05 > p < 0.01$

*Includes primary and secondary dengue infections.
†Number positive/number of observations.
From Nimmannitya, S., Halstead, S. B., Cohen, S. N., et al.: Dengue and chikungunya virus infection in man in Thailand, 1962–1964. I. Observations on hospitalized patients with hemorrhagic fever. Am. J. Trop. Med. Hyg. *18*:954–971, 1969.

Treatment

1. Treatment is supportive.
2. Bed rest is advised during the febrile period. Antipyretics or cold sponging should be used to keep the body temperature below 40° C (104° F).
3. Analgesics or mild sedation may be required to control pain. Post-illness arthritis may require continued treatment with anti-inflammatory agents and graduated physiotherapy.
4. Salicylates, because of their hemorrhagic potential, are contraindicated.
5. Febrile convulsions are treated with phenobarbital given intravenously or orally and continued until the temperature is normal. Severe or intractable convulsions may respond to intravenous diazepam.
6. Children who have lost excessive fluid because of vomiting, fasting, or thirsting and who cannot take oral fluids may require intravenous rehydration. Individuals with severe hemorrhagic phenomena should be studied for underlying hemostatic disorders.

Prognosis

In a few instances, isolation or serologic evidence of recent infection has been obtained in persons with severe hemorrhagic findings or in individuals dying during an acute febrile illness.[10, 28, 40, 50, 57] In addition to hemorrhage, neurologic and myocardial involvement has been reported during chikungunya infection in adults.[10, 13] In adults, arthralgia may persist for weeks, and exercise may prolong this symptom. Typically, pain shifts from joint to joint and is worse in the morning and on first use of the joint. Swelling of ankles, wrists, and fingers occurs frequently. In older patients, the sequelae may resemble rheumatoid arthritis. A post-illness destructive arthropathy has been reported.[5] Chikungunya virus infection might coincide with other pathologic processes and result in death of the individual.[40] Carefully studied, virologically documented cases have shown neither thrombocytopenia nor severe neutropenia.[28] Until more is known of the pathogenesis of chikungunya virus infection, estimating the frequency with which death can be attributed directly to chikungunya fever will be difficult.

Infants with chikungunya may experience residual neurologic deficits after febrile convulsions.

Prevention

Formalin-treated chikungunya virus (Ross strain) grown in African green monkey kidney cells produces a satisfactory immune response and resistance to challenge when administered in three divided doses in monkeys.[24] A vaccine prepared under similar conditions produced hemagglutination-inhibition, complement-fixation, and neutralizing antibody responses in susceptible human volunteers.[25] A comparative study from the same laboratory was made of formalin-inactivated chikungunya vaccines prepared from the virus propagated in African green monkey kidney monolayers and

TABLE 178–8 ■ CHIKUNGUNYA AND DENGUE IN CHILDREN: COMPARISON OF HEMORRHAGIC MANIFESTATIONS

	Chikungunya				Primary Dengue		Secondary Dengue	
	Outpatients (17 Cases)		*Inpatients (32 Cases)*		*Outpatients (27 Cases)*		*Inpatients (135 Cases)*	
Findings	**Number***	**Percent**	**Number***	**Percent**	**Number***	**Percent**	**Number***	**Percent**
Positive tourniquet test	3/17	18.0	24/31	77.4	4/27	14.8	94/112	83.9
Petechiae, scattered	0/17	0	10/32	31.2	4/27	7.4	60/129	46.5
Petechial rash			0/32	0			13/129	10.1
Maculopapular rash	0/17	0	19/32	59.4	2/27	7.4	16/132	12.1
Epistaxis	0/17	0	4/32	12.5	1/27	3.7	20/106	18.9
Gum bleeding			0/32	0			2/135	1.5
Melena/hematemesis	0/17	0	0/32	0	0/27	0	14/119	11.8

*Number positive/number of observations.
After Nimmannitya, S., Halstead, S. B., Cohen, S. N., et al.: Dengue and chikungunya virus infection in man in Thailand, 1962–1964. I. Observations on hospitalized patients with hemorrhagic fever. Am. J. Trop. Med. Hyg. 18:954–971, 1969; and Halstead, S. B., Nimmannitya, S., and Margiotta, M. R.: Dengue and chikungunya virus infection in man in Thailand, 1962–1964. II. Observations on disease in outpatients. Am. J. Trop. Med. Hyg. *18*:972–983, 1969.

concentrated chick embryo suspension cultures.[59] The latter vaccine was significantly more protective to mice against live homologous virus challenge and stimulated the production of four to five times more circulating antibodies than did the vaccine prepared with virus grown in African green monkey kidney cultures. Nakao and Hotta,[42] studying chikungunya grown in BHK-21 cells, found that ultraviolet-inactivated preparations were significantly more immunogenic than were formalin-treated virus. Tween-ether–extracted virus preparations also have been found to be immunogenic. A live attenuated chikungunya vaccine has been developed.[31] In view of the low mortality associated with chikungunya virus infection, commercial production of a chikungunya vaccine is likely to have a low priority.

At present, prevention consists of avoiding mosquito bites. For urban outbreaks in most of the Asian and African tropics, the regimen for individual protection and for chronic and emergency control is the same as has been described for dengue. When other vectors are involved, measures designed to combat *A. aegypti* may fail. In such outbreaks, expert entomologic advice will be needed to design appropriate preventive measures.

For control of mosquitoes, epidemic measures, and health education, see Chapter 179.

REFERENCES

1. Adesina, O. A., and Odelola, H. A.: Ecological distribution of chikungunya haemagglutination-inhibition antibodies in human and domestic animals in Nigeria. Trop. Geogr. Med. *43*:271–275, 1991.
2. Anderson, C. R., Singh, K. R. P., and Sarkar, J. K.: Isolation of chikungunya virus from *Aedes aegypti* fed on naturally infected humans in Calcutta. Curr. Sci. *34*:579–580, 1965.
3. Basaca-Sevilla, V., and Halstead, S. B.: Recent virological studies of haemorrhagic fever and other arthropod-borne virus infections in the Philippines. J. Trop. Med. Hyg. *69*:203–208, 1966.
4. Brighton, S. W., Prozesky, O. W., and de la Harpe, A. L.: Chikungunya virus infection. A retrospective study of 107 cases. S. Afr. Med. J. *63*:313–315, 1983.
5. Brighton, S. W., and Simson, I. W.: A destructive arthropathy following chikungunya virus arthritis—a possible association. Clin. Rheumatol. *3*:253–258, 1984.
6. Bylon, D.: Korte aatekening, wegens eene algemeene ziekte, doorgans genaamd de knokkel-koorts. Verhandelungen van het Bataviaasch Genootschop der Konsten in Wetenschappen. *2*:17–30, 1780.
7. Calisher, C. H., el-Kafrawi, A. O., Al-Deen Mahmud, M. I., et al.: Complex-specific immunoglobulin M antibody patterns in humans infected with alphaviruses. J. Clin. Microbiol. *23*:155–159, 1986.
8. Campos, L. E., San Juan, A., Cenabre, L. C., et al.: Isolation of chikungunya virus in the Philippines. Acta Med. Philippina *5*:152–155, 1969.
9. Carey, D. E.: Chikungunya and dengue: A case of mistaken identity? J. Hist. Med. Allied Sci. *26*:243–262, 1971.
10. Carey, D. E., Myers, R. M., Deranitz, C. M., et al.: The 1964 chikungunya epidemic at Vellore, South India, including observations on concurrent dengue. Trans. R. Soc. Trop. Med. Hyg. *63*:434–445, 1969.
11. Chakravarty, S. K., and Sarkar, J. K.: Susceptibility of newborn and adult laboratory animals to chikungunya virus. Indian J. Med. Res. *57*:1157–1164, 1969.
12. Chastel, C.: Human infections in Cambodia with chikungunya or a closely allied virus. III. Epidemiology. Bull. Soc. Pathol. Exot. *57*:65–82, 1964.
13. Chatterjee, S. N., Chakravarti, S. K., Mitra, A. C., et al.: Virological investigation of cases with neurological complications during the outbreak of haemorrhagic fever in Calcutta. J. Indian Med. Assoc. *45*:314–316, 1965.
14. Chikungunya fever among U.S. Peace Corps volunteers—Republic of the Philippines. M. M. W. R. Morb. Mortal. Wkly. Rep. *35*(36):573–574, 1986.
15. Christie, J.: Remarks on "kidinga Pepo": A peculiar form of exanthematous disease. B. M. J. *1*:577–579, 1872.
16. Cornet, M., and Chateau, R.: Quelques données biologiques sur *Aedes* (Stegomyia) *luteocephalus* (Newstead) en zone de savane soudanienne dans l'ouest du Senegal. Cah. Off. Recherche Sci. Tech. Outre-Mer. Entomol. Méd. Parasitol. *12*:97–109, 1974.
17. deMoor, P. P., and Steffens, F. E.: A computer-simulated model of an arthropod-borne virus transmission cycle, with special reference to chikungunya virus. Trans. R. Soc. Trop. Med. Hyg. *64*:927–934, 1970.
18. Diallo, M., Thonnon, J., Traore-Laminzana, M., et al.: Vectors of chikungunya virus in Senegal: Current data and transmission cycles. Am. J. Trop. Med. Hyg. *60*:281–286, 1999.
19. Gubler, D. J., Nalim, S., Tan, R., et al.: Variation in susceptibility to oral infection with dengue viruses among geographic strains of *Aedes aegypti*. Am. J. Trop. Med. Hyg. *28*:1045–1052, 1979.
20. Halstead, S. B., and Buescher, E. L.: Hemorrhagic disease in rodents infected with virus associated with Thai hemorrhagic fever. Science *134*:475–476, 1961.
21. Halstead, S. B., Nimmannitya, S., and Margiotta, M. R.: Dengue and chikungunya virus infection in man in Thailand, 1962–1964. II. Observations on disease in outpatients. Am. J. Trop. Med. Hyg. *18*:972–983, 1969.
22. Halstead, S. B., Scanlon, J. E., Umpaivit, P., et al.: Dengue and chikungunya virus infection in man in Thailand, 1962–1964. IV. Epidemiologic studies in the Bangkok metropolitan area. Am. J. Trop. Med. Hyg. *18*:987–1021, 1969.
23. Harnett, G. B., and Bucens, M. R.: Isolation of chikungunya virus in Australia. Med. J. Aust. *152*:328–329, 1990.
24. Harrison, V. R., Binn, L. N., and Randall, R.: Comparative immunogenicities of chikungunya vaccines prepared in avian and mammalian tissues. Am. J. Trop. Med. Hyg. *16*:786–791, 1967.
25. Harrison, V. R., Eckels, K. H., Bartelloni, P. J., et al.: Production and evaluation of a formalin-killed chikungunya vaccine. J. Immunol. *107*:643–647, 1971.
26. Higashi, N., Matsumoto, A., Tabata, K., et al.: Electron microscope study of development of chikungunya virus in green monkey kidney stable (VERO) cells. Virology *35*:55–59, 1967.
27. Igarashi, A., Fukuoka, T., Nithiuthai, P., et al.: Structural components of chikungunya virus. Biken J. *13*:93–110, 1970.
28. Jadhav, M., Namboodripad, M., Carman, R. H., et al.: Chikungunya disease in infants and children in Vellore: A report on clinical and haematological features of virologically proved cases. Indian Med. Res. *53*:764–776, 1965.
29. Jupp, P. G., and McIntosh, B. M.: *Aedes furcifer* and other mosquitoes as vectors of chikungunya virus at Mica, northeastern Transvaal, South Africa. J. Am. Mosq. Control Assoc. *6*:415–420, 1990.
30. Karabatsos, N. (ed.): International Catalog of Arbovirus 1985. Ft. Collins, CO, American Society of Tropical Medicine and Hygiene, 1985.
31. Levitt, N. H., Ramsburg, H. H., Hasty, S. E., et al.: Development of an attenuated strain of chikungunya virus for use in vaccine production. Vaccine *4*:157–162, 1986.
32. Macasaet, F. F., Villamil, P. T., Wexler, S., et al.: Epidemiology of arbovirus infections in Negros Oriental. II. Serologic findings of the epidemic in Amlan. J. Philippine Med. Assoc. *45*:311–317, 1969.
33. McIntosh, B. M.: Antibody against chikungunya virus in wild primates in southern Africa. S. Afr. J. Med. Sci. *35*:65–74, 1970.
34. McIntosh, B. M., and Jupp, P. G.: Attempts to transmit chikungunya virus with six species of mosquito. J. Med. Entomol. *7*:615–618, 1970.
35. McIntosh, B. M., Jupp, P. G., and DeSouza, J.: Mosquitoes feeding at two horizontal levels in gallery forest in Natal, South Africa, with reference to possible vectors of chikungunya virus. J. Entomol. Soc. S. Afr. *35*:81–90, 1972.
36. McIntosh, B. M., Paterson, H. E., Donaldson, J. M., et al.: Chikungunya virus: Viral susceptibility and transmission studies with some vertebrates and mosquitoes. S. Afr. J. Med. Sci. *28*:45–52, 1963.
37. McIntosh, B. M., Paterson, H. E., McGillivray, G., et al.: Further studies on the chikungunya outbreak in Southern Rhodesia in 1962. I. Mosquitoes, wild primates and birds in relation to the epidemic. Ann. Trop. Med. Parasitol. *58*:45–51, 1964.
38. Ming, C. K., Thein, S., Thaung, U. T., et al.: Clinical laboratory studies on haemorrhagic fever in Burma, 1970–1972. Bull. World Health Organ. *51*:227–236, 1974.
39. Moore, D. L., Causey, O. R., Reddy, S., et al.: Arthropod-borne viral infections of many in Nigeria, 1964–1970. Ann. Trop. Med. Parasitol. *69*: 49–64, 1975.
40. Munasinghe, D. R., and Rajasuriya, K.: Haemorrhage in Christmas disease following dengue-like fever. Ceylon Med. J. *11*:39–40, 1966.
41. Nakao, E.: Biological and immunological studies on chikungunya virus: A comparative observation of two strains of African and Asian origins. Kobe J. Med. Sci. *18*:133–141, 1972.
42. Nakao, E., and Hotta, S.: Immunogenicity of purified, inactivated chikungunya virus in monkeys. Bull. World Health Organ. *48*:559–562, 1973.
43. Nimmannitya, S., Halstead, S. B., Cohen, S. N., et al.: Dengue and chikungunya virus infection in man in Thailand, 1962–1964. I. Observations on hospitalized patients with hemorrhagic fever. Am. J. Trop. Med. Hyg. *18*:954–971, 1969.
44. Paterson, H. E., and McIntosh, B. M.: Further studies on the chikungunya outbreak in southern Rhodesia in 1962. II. Transmission experiments with the *Aedes furcifertaylori* group of mosquitoes and with a member of the *Anopheles gambiae* complex. Ann. Trop. Med. Parasitol. *58*:52–55, 1964.
45. Powers, A. M., Brault, A. C., Tesh, R. B., et al.: Re-emergence of chikungunya and o'nyong-nyong viruses: Evidence for distinct geographical lineages and distant evolutionary relationships. J. Gen. Virol. *81*:471–479, 2000.
46. Rao, T. R., Devi, P. S., and Singh, K. R. P.: Experimental studies on the mechanical transmission of chikungunya virus by *Aedes aegypti*. Mosq. News *28*:406–408, 1968.

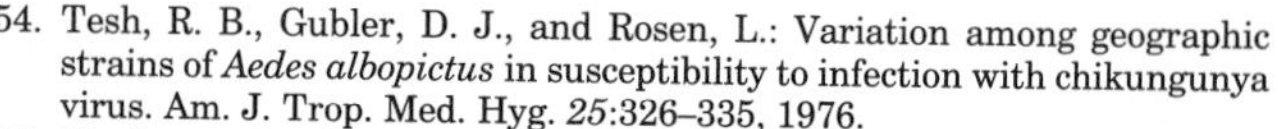

47. Robinson, M. C.: An epidemic of virus disease in Southern Province, Tanganyika Territory, in 1952–1953. I. Clinical features. Trans. R. Soc. Trop. Med. Hyg. *49*:28–32, 1955.
48. Ross, R. W.: The Newala epidemic. III. The virus: Isolation, pathogenic properties and relationship to the epidemic. J. Hyg. *54*:177–191, 1956.
49. Salim, A. R., and Porterfield, J. S.: A serological survey on arbovirus antibodies in the Sudan. Trans. R. Soc. Trop. Med. Hyg. *76*:206–210.
50. Sarkar, J. K., Chatterjee, S. N., Chakrevarti, S. K., et al.: Chikungunya virus infection with haemorrhagic manifestations. Indian J. Med. Res. *53*:921–925, 1965.
51. Shah, K. V., Gilotra, S. K., Gibbs, C. J., Jr., et al.: Laboratory studies of transmission of chikungunya virus by mosquitoes. Indian J. Med. Res. *52*:703–709, 1964.
52. Siler, J. F., Hall, M. W., and Hitchens, A. P.: Dengue: Its history, epidemiology, mechanisms of transmission, etiology, clinical manifestations, immunity and prevention. Philippine J. Sci. *29*:1–305, 1926.
53. Tesh, R. B., Gadjusek, D. C., Garruto, R. M., et al.: The distribution and prevalence of group A arbovirus neutralizing antibodies among human populations in Southeast Asia and the Pacific Islands. Am. J. Trop. Med. Hyg. *24*:664–675, 1975.
54. Tesh, R. B., Gubler, D. J., and Rosen, L.: Variation among geographic strains of *Aedes albopictus* in susceptibility to infection with chikungunya virus. Am. J. Trop. Med. Hyg. *25*:326–335, 1976.
55. Thaikruea, L., Charearnsook, O., Reanphumkarnkit, S., et al.: Chikungunya in Tailand: A re-emerging disease? Southeast Asian J. Trop. Med. Public Health *28*:359–364, 1997.
56. Thein S., La Linn, M., Aaskov, J., et al.: Development of a simple indirect enzyme-linked immunosorbent assay for the detection of immunoglobulin M antibody in serum from patients following an outbreak of chikungunya virus infection in Yangon, Myanmar. Trans. R. Soc. Trop. Med. Hyg. *86*:438–442, 1992.
57. Thiruvengadam, K. V., Kalyanasundaram, V., and Rajgopal, J.: Clinical and pathological studies on chikungunya fever in Madras City. Indian J. Med. Res. *53*:720–728, 1965.
58. Vu-Qui, D., Nguyen-Thi, K. T., and Ly, Q. B.: Antibodies to chikungunya virus in Vietnamese children in Saigon. Bull. Soc. Pathol. Exot. *60*:353–359, 1967.
59. White, A., Berman, S., and Lowenthal, J. P.: Comparative immunogenicities of chikungunya vaccines propagated in monkey kidney monolayers and chick embryo suspension cultures. Appl. Microbiol. *23*:951–952, 1972.

CHAPTER **178E**

Ross River Virus Arthritis

JOHN G. AASKOV

"Epidemics" of a benign disease causing polyarthralgia and rash were first described in Australia in 1927.[51] With the advent of serologic tests able to diagnose Ross River virus infection, epidemic polyarthritis has been recognized as endemic in Australia and some surrounding countries and rarely occurs as epidemics. Approximately 5000 cases of epidemic polyarthritis are reported in Australia each year, with a peak of 7800 cases in 1996.

Some confusion has been generated recently by use of the term *Ross River fever* to describe clinical Ross River virus infections (fever does not develop in more than half of those with clinical disease).[49] Additional confusion has been generated by efforts to call any polyarthritis caused by Australian arboviruses epidemic polyarthritis. Use of the term *epidemic polyarthritis* to describe clinical disease caused by Ross River virus and only Ross River virus has been proposed.

Etiologic Agent

Investigations of an epidemic of polyarthritis in southern Australia in 1956[10, 57] suggested that an alphavirus was the causative agent. This suggestion was confirmed when Ross River virus was isolated from *Aedes vigilax* mosquitoes collected beside Ross River, near Townsville in northern Australia, and shown, on serologic grounds, to be the causative agent of epidemic polyarthritis.[21, 24] Although the first isolation of virus from a human was from a febrile child without arthritis,[20] subsequent use of mosquito cell lines enabled numerous isolations of Ross River virus from epidemic polyarthritis patients in Australia and the Pacific Islands.[8, 54, 59]

Ross River virus is related serologically to Getah and Bebaru viruses in the Semliki Forest virus subgroup.[18] Nucleotide sequencing has confirmed this close relationship among Ross River, Getah, and Semliki Forest viruses.[25] Cryoelectron microscopic studies[14] suggest that the nucleocapsid is approximately 400 Å in diameter and has a T=4 quaternary structure. It is surrounded by a membrane bilayer that is penetrated by 80 spikes, also arranged in a T=4 lattice. Each spike is a trimer of heterodimers of the envelope glycoproteins E1 and E2.

Oligonucleotide mapping and limited nucleotide sequencing suggest that four topotypes of Ross River virus may exist.[46] This finding mirrors the extensive biologic variation (e.g., plaque size, mouse neurovirulence) observed with different isolates.[8, 26, 36] However, how much of this diversity has been generated by passage of virus in the laboratory before study is not clear, and no association has been made between topotype and disease in humans. The virus can be adapted to grow to high titer in the muscle and brain of day-old mice, in which case it causes paralysis and death,[48, 50] and it also grows to high titer in vertebrate and mosquito cell lines.[8]

Transmission and Epidemiology

Ross River virus is endemic in all mainland states of Australia and in Papua New Guinea and possibly in New Caledonia. No disease has been reported from the Pacific island states involved in the 1979–1980 epidemic (Fiji, Samoa, Tonga, Cook Islands)[5, 44, 54, 59] since that time. Sporadic cases, without local virus transmission, have occurred in Europe and the United States in tourists and service personnel returning from Australia.

Isolation of Ross River virus from mosquitoes, especially *A. vigilax*[24, 36] and *Culex annulirostris*,[23, 36] and the widespread occurrence of antibody to the virus in mammals[21, 22] suggested a mammal-mosquito cycle with humans as an incidental host.

However, improved laboratory diagnostic services have shown that clinical infection in humans apparently occurs year-round, although most cases are seen in the late summer and in autumn, and that the majority of patients are city dwellers.[7, 49] Taken together with the explosive spread of disease during the 1979 to 1980 epidemic of Ross River virus infection in the Pacific,[5, 54, 59] this virus appears to be maintained in either of two cycles, mammal-mosquito-mammal or human-mosquito-human, with occasional movement of virus between the two.

Evidence also has been presented of transovarial transmission of Ross River virus in *Aedes* mosquitoes.[43, 45]

Patients may be viremic for up to 7 days after the onset of symptoms,[8, 54] and the incubation time from infection to the onset of symptoms may vary from 1 to 27 days, 7 to 9 days being the usual interval in endemic areas.[29]

In endemic areas, the ratio of subclinical to clinical infection may be as high as 50:1,[7] but during outbreaks, the ratio can be reduced to 4:1 or less.[5, 38] The subclinical infection rate for most of northern Australia is approximately 1.5 percent per annum,[7] but in some areas the rates are much higher.[16, 17]

Infection rates are the same in both sexes, and early reports that clinical disease was more common in females than males[19, 49] are not supported by Australian national data for the last decade. An association between HLA-DR7 and clinical disease also has been observed.[35]

Ross River virus has been shown to cross the placenta in mice[3] and humans.[6] In mice, such crossing may result in extensive postpartum mortality,[3] but in humans, no evidence exists of morbidity or mortality in children infected in utero.

Clinical Manifestations[10, 19, 21, 37, 49]

Epidemic polyarthritis occurs as a mild to severe illness characterized by joint pain, particularly in the knees and the small joints of the hands and feet. Frequently, the joint pain is accompanied by a maculopapular or vesicular rash on the trunk and limbs and sometimes by fever or chills, or both. Sore throat, lymphadenopathy, paresthesia and tenderness of the palms and soles, exanthems, and more rarely, petechiae have been observed. Most patients experience several weeks of painful arthritis, followed by a slow decrease in the severity of symptoms during the 30 to 40 weeks required by most for recovery.[2] Infrequently, symptoms may persist for a year or more,[27] and some patients may experience episodes of severe arthritis during convalescence. In a small proportion of patients (<0.1%), clinical disease may develop without arthritis.[20] Rare cases of glomerulonephritis,[32] hematuria,[11] and central nervous system symptoms[1, 53] accompanying Ross River virus infection in humans also have been reported.

The severity and duration of symptoms are age related, with adults having the most severe and prolonged symptoms. Teenagers may be incapacitated for only a few days and asymptomatic after 1 to 2 weeks.

Pathology

The pathogenesis of epidemic polyarthritis is not understood.

Synovial tissue from patients with epidemic polyarthritis may show a marked mononuclear leukocyte infiltrate with small amounts of fibrin deposition and synovial-cell hyperplasia.[38, 58] No virus or viral antigen has been detected in synovial tissue from patients with epidemic polyarthritis, but a 250-nucleotide fragment of the viral genome was detected by reverse transcription–polymerase chain reaction (RT-PCR) in synovium from 2 of 12 patients 5 weeks after the onset of symptoms.[58] Ross river virus has been shown to replicate for a similar period in human synovial cells maintained at 35°C in vitro.[41] Sindbis virus, which also may cause symptoms similar to those of epidemic polyarthritis, has been found to replicate in the periosteum, tendons, and endosteum within the epiphyses of the long bones of mice adjacent to articular joints.[40] Recovery of virus has not been attempted from these sites in patients with epidemic polyarthritis.

Fluid from affected joints consists almost entirely of mononuclear leukocytes at all stages of disease.[15, 28, 30] Human synovial fibroblasts infected with Ross River virus in vitro demonstrate increased production of mRNA coding for monocyte chemoattractant protein-1 (MCP-1), which recruits and activates monocytes and macrophages.[47]

No evidence of immune complexes or complement activation in arthritic joints has been found, and viral antigen can be detected (in macrophages) for only 5 to 7 days after the onset of symptoms despite the persistence of arthritis for 30 to 40 weeks.[31] No significant levels of anticollagen antibodies could be detected in serum from epidemic polyarthritis patients.[34] Neither anti–Ross River virus antibody levels nor a primary, virus-specific, cell-mediated immune response to Ross River virus infection correlated with the presence or absence of arthritis in human infections.[4] In patients with epidemic polyarthritis, a nonspecific immunologic response (natural killer cells) correlated well with the presence or absence of arthritic symptoms.[2, 4] Functional natural killer cells have been recovered from the knee of a patient with epidemic polyarthritis,[39] and natural killer cells have been found to kill autologous synovial tissue in vitro.[2]

A rash develops in approximately 30 percent of patients with epidemic polyarthritis.[49] The dermis underlying these lesions contains a perivascular infiltrate of $CD8^+$ T cells and some monocytes and macrophages.[33] No immunoglobulin or complement deposition has been observed in these lesions, although Ross River virus antigen was detected in basal epidermal and eccrine duct epithelial cells.[33]

Diagnosis

Most clinical diagnoses of epidemic polyarthritis are confirmed by using an indirect enzyme-linked immunosorbent assay (ELISA)[52] to detect Ross River virus–specific IgM antibodies in serum collected 7 to 10 days after the onset of symptoms. IgM can be detected for approximately 3 months after the onset of disease.[7]

In rare cases (perhaps less than 1 in 5000), anti–Ross River virus IgM antibody production may persist for years. Assays for serum anti–Ross River virus IgA might be an alternative to IgM assays because the duration of IgA production is shorter than for IgM.[13] However, such IgA assays have not been adopted by routine diagnostic laboratories. More recently, indirect ELISA assays that measure the avidity of anti–Ross River virus antibody have been shown to be able to discriminate between recent and old infections with this virus.[42]

Although virus sometimes can be isolated from seronegative, acute-phase sera,[5, 8, 54, 59] this procedure is not performed in most routine diagnostic laboratories. A number of mostly unpublished RT-PCR protocols[56] have been developed for the detection of Ross River virus RNA, but they all are less sensitive than virus isolation for the detection of virus and are not used routinely for the diagnosis of human disease.

Because epidemic polyarthritis is an arthritic disease, care must be taken to avoid false-positive results caused by the presence of rheumatoid factor when using indirect ELISA to detect anti–Ross River virus IgM antibodies. Such precautions include absorbing out IgG or rheumatoid factor before testing sera or performing tests for rheumatoid factor in parallel with ELISA.

Another source of false-positive diagnoses is the production of anti–Ross River virus IgM antibody caused by polyclonal B-cell activation after infection of a host with Epstein-Barr virus, cytomegalovirus, or *Coxiella burnetii.*

Other viral infections to be considered when a patient is suspected of having epidemic polyarthritis include infections with Barmah Forest, Sindbis, Kunjin, or rubella viruses.

Treatment and Prognosis

No specific antiviral therapy is available, although experimental evidence suggests that interferon-γ may ameliorate acute disease.[55] Patients with more severe or more prolonged symptoms have been given either nonsteroidal anti-inflammatory medication or steroids,[12] but the value of such treatment is not clear. Rest, while maintaining mobility and muscle tone, appears to provide significant relief.

Epidemic polyarthritis has not been shown to progress to chronic joint disease.

Prevention

A killed virus vaccine is under development.[9] In urban areas, public health mosquito control programs reduce mosquito numbers, but eliminating mosquito exposure in those with outdoor occupations and pastimes is impossible. Personal protection (insect screening of houses, wearing protective clothing, and applying insect repellents) is the only reliable way to avoid infection.

REFERENCES

1. Aaskov, J. G.: Ross River virus disease. *In* St. George, T. D., and French, E. L. (eds.): Arbovirus Research in Australia. Paper presented at the Second Symposium of the Commonwealth Scientific and Industrial Organisation and Queensland Institute of Medical Research, July 17–19, 1979, p. 166.
2. Aaskov, J. G., Dalglish, D. A., Harper, J. J., et al.: Natural killer (NK) cells in viral arthritis. Clin. Exp. Immunol. *68*:23–32, 1987.
3. Aaskov, J. G., Davies, C. E. A., Tucker, M., et al.: Effect on mice of infection during pregnancy with three Australian arboviruses. Am. J. Trop. Med. Hyg. *30*:198–203, 1981.
4. Aaskov, J. G., Fraser, J. R. E., and Dalglish, D. A.: Specific and nonspecific immunological changes in epidemic polyarthritis in patients. Aust. J. Exp. Biol. Med. Sci. *55*:599–608, 1981.
5. Aaskov, J. G., Mataika, J. U., Lawrence, G. W., et al.: An epidemic of Ross River virus infection in Fiji, 1979. Am. J. Trop. Med. Hyg. *30*:1053–1059, 1981.
6. Aaskov, J. G., Nair, K., Lawrence, G. W., et al.: Evidence for transplacental transmission of Ross River virus in humans. Med. J. Aust. *2*:20–21, 1981.
7. Aaskov, J. G., Ross, P., Davies, C. E. A., et al.: Epidemic polyarthritis in northeastern Australia, 1978–1979. Med. J. Aust. *2*:17–19, 1981.
8. Aaskov, J. G., Ross, P. V., Harper, J. J., et al.: Isolation of Ross River virus from epidemic polyarthritis patients in Australia. Aust. J. Exp. Biol. Med. Sci. *63*:587–597, 1985.
9. Aaskov, J. G., Williams, L., and Yu, S.: A candidate Ross River virus vaccine: Pre-clinical evaluation. Vaccine *15*:1396–1404, 1997.
10. Anderson, S. G., and French, E. L.: An epidemic exanthem associated with polyarthritis in the Murray Valley, 1956. Med. J. Aust. *2*:113–117, 1957.
11. Anstey, N., Currie, B., and Tai, K. S.: Ross River virus disease presenting with hematuria. Southeast Asian J. Trop. Med. Public Health *22*:281–283, 1991.
12. Ashley, D., Watson, R., and Ross, S. A.: Corticosteroids for the complications of Ross River virus infection. Med. J. Aust. *168*:92, 1998.
13. Carter, I. W. J., Fraser, J. R. E., and Cloonan, M. J.: Specific IgA antibody response in Ross River virus infection. Immunol. Cell. Biol. *65*:511–513, 1987.
14. Cheng, R. H., Kuhn, R. J., Olson, N. H., et al.: Nucleocapsid and glycoprotein organisation in an enveloped virus. Cell *80*:621–630, 1995.
15. Clarris, B. J., Doherty, R. L., Fraser, J. R. E., et al.: Epidemic polyarthritis: A cytological, virological and immunochemical study. Aust. N. Z. J. Med. *5*:450–457, 1975.
16. Doherty, R. L.: Arboviruses of Australia. Aust. Vet. J. *48*:172–180, 1972.
17. Doherty, R. L.: Surveys of haemagglutination-inhibiting antibody to arboviruses in Aborigines and other population groups in northern Australia. Trans. R. Soc. Trop. Med. Hyg. *67*:197–205, 1973.
18. Doherty, R. L.: Ross River virus. *In* Karabatsos, N. (ed.): International Catalogue of Arboviruses Including Certain Other Viruses of Vertebrates. 3rd ed. San Antonio, TX, American Society for Tropical Medicine and Hygiene, 1985.
19. Doherty, R. L., Barrett, E. J., Gorman, B. M., et al.: Epidemic polyarthritis in eastern Australia 1959–1970. Med. J. Aust. *1*:5–8, 1971.
20. Doherty, R. L., Carley, J. G., and Best, J. C.: Isolation of Ross River virus from man. Med. J. Aust. *1*:1083–1084, 1972.
21. Doherty, R. L., Gorman, B. M., Whitehead, R. H., et al.: Studies of epidemic polyarthritis: The significance of three group A arboviruses isolated from mosquitoes in Queensland. Australas. Ann. Med. *13*: 22–327, 1964.
22. Doherty, R. L., Gorman, B. M., Whitehead, R. H., et al.: Studies of arthropod-borne virus infections in Queensland. V. Survey of the antibodies to group A arboviruses in man and animals. Aust. J. Exp. Biol. Med. Sci. *44*:365–377, 1966.
23. Doherty, R. L., Standfast, H. A., Domrow, R., et al.: Studies of the epidemiology of arthropod-borne virus infections at Mitchell River Mission, Cape York Peninsula, north Queensland. IV. Arbovirus infections of mosquitoes and mammals, 1967–1969. Trans. R. Soc. Trop. Med. Hyg. *65*:504–513, 1971.
24. Doherty, R. L., Whitehead, R. H., Gorman, B. M., et al.: The isolation of a third group A arbovirus in Australia, with preliminary observations on its relationship to epidemic polyarthritis. Aust. J. Sci. *26*:183–184, 1963.
25. Farragher, S. G., Meek, A. D. J., Rice, C. M., et al.: Genome sequence of a mouse avirulent and a mouse virulent strain of Ross River virus. Virology *163*:509–526, 1988.
26. Fauran, P., Donaldson, M., Harper, J., et al.: Characterisation of Ross River viruses isolated from patients with polyarthritis in New Caledonia and Wallis and Futuna islands. Am. J. Trop. Med. Hyg. *33*:1228–1231, 1984.
27. Fraser, J. R. E.: Epidemic polyarthritis and Ross River virus disease. Clin. Rheum. Dis. *12*:369–388, 1986.
28. Fraser, J. R. E., and Becker, G. J.: Mononuclear cell types in chronic synovial effusions of Ross River virus disease. Aust. N. Z. J. Med. *14*:505, 1984.
29. Fraser, J. R. E., and Cunningham, A. L.: Incubation time of epidemic polyarthritis. Med. J. Aust. *1*:550–551, 1980.
30. Fraser, J. R. E., Cunningham, A. L., Clarris, B. J., et al.: Cytology of synovial effusions in epidemic polyarthritis. Aust. N. Z. J. Med. *11*:168–173, 1981.
31. Fraser, J. R. E., Cunningham, A. L., Mathews, J. D., et al.: Immune complexes and Ross River virus disease (epidemic polyarthritis). Rheumatol. Int. *8*:113–117, 1988.
32. Fraser, J. R. E., Cunningham, A. L., Muller, H. K., et al.: Glomerulonephritis in the acute phase of Ross River virus disease (epidemic polyarthritis). Clin. Nephrol. *29*:149–152, 1988.
33. Fraser, J. R. E., Ratnamohan, A. M., Dowling, J. P. G., et al.: The exanthem of Ross River virus infection: Histology, location of virus antigen and the nature of inflammatory infiltrate. J. Clin. Pathol. *36*:1256–1263, 1983.
34. Fraser, J. R. E., Rowley, M. J., and Tait, B.: Collagen antibodies in Ross River virus disease (epidemic polyarthritis). Rheumatol. Int. *7*:267–269, 1987.
35. Fraser, J. R. E., Tait, T., Aaskov, J. G., et al.: Possible genetic determinants in epidemic polyarthritis caused by Ross River virus infection. Aust. N. Z. J. Med. *10*:597–603, 1980.
36. Gard, G., Marshall, I. D., and Woodroofe, G. M.: Annually recurrent epidemic polyarthritis and Ross River virus activity in a coastal area of New South Wales. II. Mosquitoes, viruses and wildlife. Am. J. Trop. Med. Hyg. *22*:551–560, 1973.
37. Halliday, J. H., and Horan, J. P.: An epidemic of polyarthritis in the Northern Territory. Med. J. Aust. *2*:293–295, 1943.
38. Hawkes, R. A., Boughton, C. R., Naim, H. M., et al.: A major outbreak of epidemic polyarthritis in New South Wales during the summer of 1983–1984. Med. J. Aust. *143*:330–333, 1985.
39. Hazelton, R. A., Hughes, C., and Aaskov, J. G: The inflammatory response in the synovium of a patient with Ross River arbovirus infection. Aust. N. Z. J. Med. *15*:336–339, 1985.
40. Heise, M. T., Simpson, D. A., and Johnston, R. E.: Sindbis-group alphavirus replication in periosteum and endosteum of long bones in adult mice. J. Virol. *74*:9294–9299, 2000.
41. Journeaux, S. F., Brown, W. B., and Aaskov, J. G.: Prolonged infection of human synovial cells with Ross River virus. J. Gen. Virol. *68*:3165–3169, 1987.
42. Kapeleris, J., Lowe, P., Phillips, D., et al.: IgG avidity in the diagnosis of acute Ross River virus infection. Dis. Markers *12*:279–282, 1996.
43. Kay, B. H.: Three modes of transmission of Ross River virus by *Aedes vigilax* (Skuse). Aust. J. Exp. Biol. Med. Sci. *60*:339–344, 1982.
44. Kay, B. H.: Assignment report, WHO Regional Office for the South Pacific, 1983.
45. Lindsay, M. D. A., Broom, A. K., Wright, A. E., et al.: Ross River virus isolations from mosquitoes in arid regions of Western Australia: Implication of vertical transmission as a means of persistence of the virus. Am. J. Trop. Med. Hyg. *49*:686–696, 1993.

46. Lindsay, M. D., Coelen, R. J., and Mackenzie, J. S.: Genetic heterogeneity among isolates of Ross River virus from different geographical regions. J. Virol. *67*:3576–3585, 1995.
47. Mateo, L., Linn, M. L., McColl, S. R., et al.: An arthrogenic alphavirus induces monocyte chemoattractant protein-1 and interleukin-8. Intervirology *43*:55–60, 2000.
48. Mims, C. A., Murphy, F. A., Taylor, W. P., et al.: Pathogenesis of Ross River virus infection in mice. I. Ependymal infection, cortical thinning, and hydrocephalus. J. Infect. Dis. *127*:121–128, 1973.
49. Mudge, P. R., and Aaskov, J. G.: Epidemic polyarthritis in Australia, 1980–1981. Med. J. Aust. *2*:269–273, 1983.
50. Murphy, F. A., Taylor, W. P., Mims, C. A., et al.: Pathogenesis of Ross River virus infection in mice. II. Muscle, heart and brown fat lesions. J. Infect. Dis. *127*:129–138, 1973.
51. Nimmo, J. R.: An unusual epidemic. Med. J. Aust. *1*:549–550, 1928.
52. Oseni, R. A., Donaldson, M. D., Dalglish, D. A., et al.: Detection by ELISA of IgM antibodies to Ross River virus in serum from patients with suspected epidemic polyarthritis. Bull. World Health Organ. *61*:703–708, 1983.
53. Penna, J. E., and Irving, L. G.: Evidence for meningitis in Ross River virus infection. Med. J. Aust. *159*:492–493, 1993.
54. Rosen, L., Gubler, D. J., and Bennett, P. H.: Epidemic polyarthritis (Ross River) virus infection in the Cook Islands. Am. J. Trop. Med. Hyg. *30*:1294–1302, 1981.
55. Seay, A. R., Kern, E. R., and Murray, R. S.: Interferon treatment of experimental Ross River virus polymyositis. Neurology *37*:1189–1193, 1987.
56. Sellner, L. N., Coelen, R. J., and Mackenzie, J. S.: Detection of Ross River virus in clinical samples using a nested reverse transcriptase polymerase chain reaction. Clin. Diagn. Virol. *49*:257–267, 1995.
57. Shope, R. E., and Anderson, S. G.: The virus aetiology of epidemic exanthem and polyarthritis. Med. J. Aust. *1*:156–158, 1960.
58. Soden, M., Vasudevan, H., Roberts, B., et al.: Detection of viral ribonucleic acid and histologic analysis of inflamed synovium in Ross River virus infection. Arthritis Rheum. *43*:365–369, 2000.
59. Tesh, R. B., McLean, R. G., Shrover, D. A., et al.: Ross River virus (Togaviridae: *Alphavirus*) infection (epidemic polyarthritis) in American Samoa. Trans. R. Soc. Trop. Med. Hyg. *75*:426–431, 1981.

CHAPTER **178F**

Other Alphaviral Infections

THEODORE F. TSAI

O'nyong Nyong

The virus name is derived from the Acholi term meaning "very painful and weak," which describes the acute constitutional symptoms and polyarthritis associated with the disease of the same name.[17] The virus is related closely to chikungunya virus, but unlike most arboviruses, it is transmitted by anopheline mosquitoes in an interhuman cycle analogous to that of malaria in rural Africa. Apart from the human-to-human epidemic cycle, the natural transmission cycle and involvement of other vertebrate hosts are largely unknown. The disease first came to attention in, arguably, the largest arboviral epidemic ever recorded. After emerging in Uganda in 1959, the epidemic spread to South and West Africa and produced an estimated 2 million cases before the outbreak died out spontaneously 3 years later. The disease apparently had disappeared from East Africa, although the virus was isolated sporadically from mosquitoes until 1996, when only the second outbreak appeared, in Uganda.[13] In retrospect, the virus had been circulating at low levels in the area several years before this epidemic occurred. Factors underlying emergence of the virus, its natural reservoir, and the reasons for its disappearance only can be surmised, but exhaustion of susceptible human hosts is a likely explanation for the cessation of epidemic transmission. Clinically, the disease is similar to chikungunya, although lymphadenopathy is more pronounced and mimics, in some cases, the enlarged cervical lymph nodes of sleeping sickness.[2] Virus can be isolated from acute-phase blood samples, or the diagnosis can be confirmed serologically by detecting specific IgM. Personal protective measures against malaria (e.g., using bed nets) should be effective against acquiring infection.

Igbo-Ora Fever

Igbo-Ora virus has been determined genetically to be a subtype of o'nyong nyong virus and, like the latter, is transmitted by anopheline mosquitoes and (without adaptation) is nonpathogenic in suckling mice.[21] The viral transmission cycle has not been defined. Sporadic cases and small outbreaks have been reported from Igbo-Ora and Ibadan, Nigeria, the Ivory Coast, and the Central African Republic. Based on a single-case description, the illness consists of fever, polyarthritis, and pharyngitis.

Barmah Forest Fever

Barmah Forest fever occurs only in Australia, where it has been a sporadic and occasionally hyperendemic infection leading to a polyarthropathy indistinguishable from that of Ross River fever.[6, 14, 16] The viral transmission cycle seems to share features with that of Ross River virus; however, independent outbreaks have occurred in locations where both viruses are enzootic, thus indicating differences in their transmission cycles or human susceptibility. Seroprevalence to Barmah Forest virus is generally lower. Anecdotal cases complicated by central nervous system signs and glomerulonephritis have been reported.[12, 16] Serologic diagnosis is straightforward in most cases, with little cross-reaction between the viruses.

Sindbis Fever

Sindbis virus was named after a district north of Cairo, Egypt, where it first was isolated. It is the prototype of an antigenic complex that also includes western equine encephalitis virus and several Sindbis viral subtypes, including Ockelbo and related strains isolated from Scandinavia and the Babanki strain from West Africa. Two genotypes consisting of the South African/Scandinavian strains and the Australian/Asian strains have been defined. The close genetic relationship of the South African and Scandinavian strains indicates a recent introduction to Europe, possibly by a migrating bird.

The virus is distributed widely over four continents, although only sporadic cases have been reported from Asia and Australia. Transmission is endemic and occasionally hyperendemic in Africa and Scandinavia. The virus is transmitted to birds by various species of *Culex* mosquitoes, and humans are infected when virus transmission "spills out" of the enzootic cycle via the intervention of bridging vectors that feed on viremic birds and later on humans.

Endemic infections occur with varying intensity in areas of Africa.[10, 19] Seroprevalence rates range from a few percent to 20 percent in some areas. Outbreaks producing hundreds to thousands of cases have been described. Concurrent transmission with West Nile virus, transmitted in the same avian cycle, is common. In South Africa, transmission occurs during the austral summer from December to April. Infections rarely may be acquired during travel.[4]

An endemic focus in Scandinavia (between 60 and 63 degrees latitude in Sweden) was recognized after a series of outbreaks in 1981 led to several hundred cases in Sweden, Norway, Finland, and adjacent areas of western Russia.[5, 15, 20] Seroprevalence is low, circa 5 percent. By estimating from seroprevalence rates, 600 to 1200 clinical cases may occur annually in Sweden alone. Most cases occur from July to September in middle-aged adults exposed to forested areas while picking berries or mushrooms or during other recreational activities.

Acute arthralgia and rash are the principal features of the illness. They may be preceded by mild fever, headache, and myalgia, but patients may have arthralgia alone. The joints, especially the ankles, wrists, knees, fingers, and toes and less often the hips, shoulders, elbows, neck, and back, are involved symmetrically. The joints appear swollen, and movement is limited. The Achilles and wrist tendons may be inflamed as well, sometimes causing nerve entrapment and paresthesias. Some patients are confined to bed and unable to walk, but typically, the joint pain and stiffness lead to a lesser degree of discomfort and compromised function. A fine papular rash appears on the trunk and extremities (including the palms and soles) but usually spares the face and head, and after a few days the rash has a stained appearance and disappears. Lesions on the hands and feet may vesiculate. Joint symptoms resolve within 3 to 4 months in approximately 60 percent of cases; however, in the remainder, symptoms may persist for 3 to 4 years.[11] Serologic evidence of infection in patients with central nervous system signs has been reported from China.[7]

The illness is not differentiated easily from West Nile fever, which is transmitted under similar epidemiologic circumstances. The diagnosis is confirmed serologically by detecting specific IgM in acute-phase serum samples. IgM is detectable for months in some patients. The virus can be isolated, but not reliably, from acute-phase capillary blood and from skin lesions. Viral genomic products can be detected in skin biopsy samples.[9]

Treatment is symptomatic. Persons who choose to enter sylvatic transmission foci in the summer should apply mosquito repellents and dress appropriately.

Mayaro Fever

Infections are highly prevalent in the forested areas of South and Central America, where Mayaro virus is transmitted among *Haemagogus* mosquitoes, marsupials, and small mammals, somewhat analogous to the jungle cycle of yellow fever. Seroprevalence rates increase with age to higher than 50 percent in native populations in some locations. The virus was isolated first from sporadic fever cases on Trinidad and named after the island's Mayaro district.[1] Outbreaks have occurred in Bolivia, Pará (a state in Brazil), and Surinam, principally in men occupationally exposed to forested sites and in residents of adjoining villages, as well as travelers returning from Central America.[3, 22, 23] The virus is placed in the Semliki Forest antigenic complex; its Una subtype causes arthritis in horses.

The illness consists of acute polyarthritis and rash. Joint swelling, pain, and stiffness principally involve the hands, wrists, ankles, toes, elbows, and knees. The hands may be so swollen that they cannot be closed, and joints of the lower extremities may be so painful that patients limp or are unable to walk. Milder cases may occur, however. The morbilliform rash is difficult to distinguish from rubella, with individual or coalescent papular lesions occurring on the trunk and extremities and usually sparing the face. Rash occurs more often in children than adults. Mild fever, pharyngitis, conjunctivitis, headache, and lymphadenitis occur in some patients. The constitutional symptoms resolve rapidly, but the joint symptoms may wax and wane for several weeks or months. Pneumonitis and renal dysfunction that have been described in some cases may have been caused by concurrent infections. Transient leukopenia usually develops; some patients have had mild elevations in liver enzymes and bilirubin. A fatal case of yellow fever was reported in a patient recovering from Mayaro fever.

The illness is differentiated from other tropical febrile illnesses with rash and musculoskeletal pain by the specific involvement of the joints and the sylvatic setting of exposure. Some patients have features closely resembling rubella. Virus can be isolated from acute-phase blood specimens, but laboratory confirmation by IgM serology is sensitive, specific, and more practical. Symptoms are treated with nonsteroidal anti-inflammatory drugs and rest. Repellents should be used when sylvatic-enzootic foci cannot be avoided.

Semliki Forest Viral Infection

Febrile illnesses with severe persistent headache have been reported from Central and West Africa, where Semliki Forest virus is transmitted principally by forest *Aedes* mosquitoes.[18] The virus appears to be a common cause of infection in horses as well. The MeTri subtype has been implicated serologically in encephalitis cases in Vietnam; its transmission cycle has not been described. A fatal case of encephalitis in a laboratory worker has been reported.[8]

REFERENCES

1. Anderson, C. R., Downs, W. G., Wattley, G. H., et al.: Mayaro virus: A new human disease agent. II. Isolation from blood of patients in Trinidad, B. W. I. Am. J. Trop. Med. Hyg. *6*:1012, 1957.
2. Brighton, S. W., Prozesky, O. W., de la Harpe, A. L.: Chikungunya virus infections: A retrospective study of 107 cases. S. Afr. Med. J. *63*:313–315, 1983.
3. Causey, O. R., and Maroja, O. M.: Mayaro virus: A new human disease agent. III. Investigation of an epidemic of acute febrile illness on the River Guama in Para, Brazil, and isolation of Mayaro virus as causative agent. Am. J. Trop. Med. Hyg. *6*:1017, 1957.
4. Eisenhut, M., Schwarz, T. F., Hegenscheid, B.: Seroprevalence of dengue, chikungunya and Sindbis virus in German aid workers. Infection *27*:82–85, 1999.
5. Espmark, A., and Niklasson, B.: Ockelbo disease in Sweden: Epidemiological, clinical and virological data from the 1982 outbreak. Am. J. Trop. Med. Hyg. *33*:1203, 1984.
6. Flexman, J. P., Smith, D. W., Mackenzie, J. S., et al.: A comparison of the diseases caused by Ross River virus and Barmah Forest virus. Med. J. Aust. *169*:159–163, 1998.
7. Gu, H. X., Artsob, H., Lin, Y. Z., et al.: Arboviruses as aetiological agents of encephalitis in the People's Republic of China. Trans. R. Soc. Trop. Med. Hyg. *86*:198, 1992.
8. Ha, D. Q., Calisher, C. H., Tien, P. H., et al.: Isolation of a newly recognized alphavirus from mosquitoes in Vietnam and evidence for human infection and disease. Am. J. Trop. Med. Hyg. *53*:100, 1995.
9. Horling, J., Vene, S., Franzen, C., et al.: Detection of Ockelbo virus RNA in skin biopsies by polymerase chain reaction. J. Clin. Microbiol. *31*:2004, 1993.
10. Jupp, P. G., Blackburn, N. K., Thompson, D. L., et al.: Sindbis and West Nile virus infection in the Witwatersrand-Pretoria region. S. Afr. Med. J. *70*:218, 1986.

11. Laine, M., Luukkainen, R., Jalava, J., et al.: Prolonged arthritis associated with Sindbis-related (Pogosta) virus infection. Rheumatology (Oxford) *39*:1272–1274, 2000.
12. Katz, I. A., Hale, G. E., Hudson, B. J., et al.: Glomerulonephritis secondary to Barmah Forest virus infection. Med. J. Aust. *167*:21–23, 1997.
13. Kiwanuka, N., Sanders, E. J., Rwaguma, E. B., et al.: O'nyong-nyong fever in south-central Uganda, 1996–1997: Clinical features and validation of a clinical case definition for surveillance purposes. Clin. Infect. Dis. *29*:1243–1250, 1999.
14. Lindsay, M. D. A., Johansen, C. A., Smith, D. W., et al.: An outbreak of Barmah Forest virus disease in the south-west of Western Australia. Med. J. Aust. *162*:291, 1995.
15. Lundstrom, J. O., Vene, S., Espmark, A., et al.: Geographical and temporal distribution of Ockelbo disease in Sweden. Epidemiol. Infect. *106*:567, 1991.
16. Mackenzie, J. B., Chua, K. B., and Daniels, P. W.: Emerging viral diseases of Southeast Asia and the Western Pacific. Emerg. Infect. Dis. *7*:497–504, 2001.
17. Mangi, R. J.: Viral arthritis: The great masquerader. Bull. Rheum. Dis. *43*:5, 1994.
18. Mathiot, C. C., Grimaud, G., Bouquety, G. P., et al.: An outbreak of human Semliki Forest virus infections in Central African Republic. Am. J. Trop. Med. Hyg. *42*:386, 1990.
19. McIntosh, B. M., McGuilivray, G. M., and Dickinson, D. B.: Illness caused by Sindbis and West Nile viruses in South Africa. S. Afr. Med. J. *38*:219, 1964.
20. Niklasson, B., Espmark, A., and Lundstrom, J.: Occurrence of arthralgia and specific IgM antibodies three to four years after Ockelbo disease. J. Infect. Dis. *157*:832, 1988.
21. Olaleye, O. D., Omilabu, S. A., and Fagbami, A. H.: Igbo-Ora virus (an alphavirus isolated in Nigeria): A serological survey for haemagglutination inhibiting antibody in humans and domestic animals. Trans. R. Soc. Trop. Med. Hyg. *82*:905, 1988.
22. Pinheiro, F. P., Freitas, R. B., Travassos da Rosa, J. F. S., et al.: An outbreak of Mayaro virus disease in Belterra, Brazil. I. Clinical and virological findings. Am. J. Trop. Med. Hyg. *30*:674, 1981.
23. Schaeffer, M., Gajdusek, D. C., Lema, A. B., et al.: Epidemic jungle fevers among Okinawan colonists in Bolivian rain forest. I. Epidemiology. Am. J. Trop. Med. Hyg. *8*:372, 1959.

SUBSECTION **5**

FLAVIVIRIDAE

CHAPTER 179 Flaviviruses

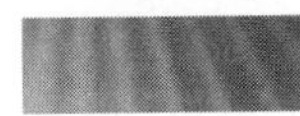

CHAPTER **179A**

St. Louis Encephalitis

THEODORE F. TSAI

St. Louis encephalitis (SLE) has been the most important arboviral infection in the United States because of its potential to occur in massive epidemics. Encephalitis is the principal clinical manifestation, although milder central nervous system (CNS) syndromes do occur, especially in children. The virus is transmitted between birds and *Culex* mosquitoes; humans are incidental hosts.

Etiologic Agent

The SLE virus is a member of the family *Flaviviridae* (group B arboviruses). Characteristics of the virus and its replicative strategy are described in the subchapter Yellow Fever. SLE virus is placed in an antigenic complex with Japanese encephalitis, Murray Valley encephalitis, and West Nile (WN) viruses.

Analysis of the E glycoprotein sequences of strains from the United States and Central and South America has identified three genotypes corresponding to origins in the eastern and western United States and South America. Strains from a more than a 60-year interval diverge by less than 10 percent in the total E gene nucleotide sequence, thus indicating a highly constrained viral adaptation to vector and vertebrate hosts. Strains from the three principal genotypes differ in biologic characteristics, such as the capacity to produce significant viremia in sparrows and virulence in 3-week-old mice.[38] Epidemic-associated strains from the Ohio and Mississippi river basins and Florida are more virulent in mice and produce higher viremia in sparrows, a principal amplifying host, than do strains from the western United States associated with an endemic pattern of transmission. Multiple viral genotypes with distinct biologic characteristics may be transmitted in relatively delimited areas within a region as small as a county in some years and more widely in others.[13, 26]

Ecology

SLE virus is transmitted in an enzootic cycle among birds and *Culex* mosquitoes in three distinct cycles associated with its four principal vector species: *Culex tarsalis* in the western and central United States, *Culex pipiens* and *Culex quinquefasciatus* in the east-central and Atlantic states, and *Culex nigripalpus* in Florida. *Culex salinarius* and *Culex restuans* may have accessory roles in viral amplification and transmission[29, 32, 37, 59] (Fig. 179–1).

In the western United States, *C. tarsalis,* which also is the vector of western equine encephalitis (WEE), serves as both an enzootic and epizootic vector. This species feeds chiefly on birds early in the summer and switches to mammalian hosts,

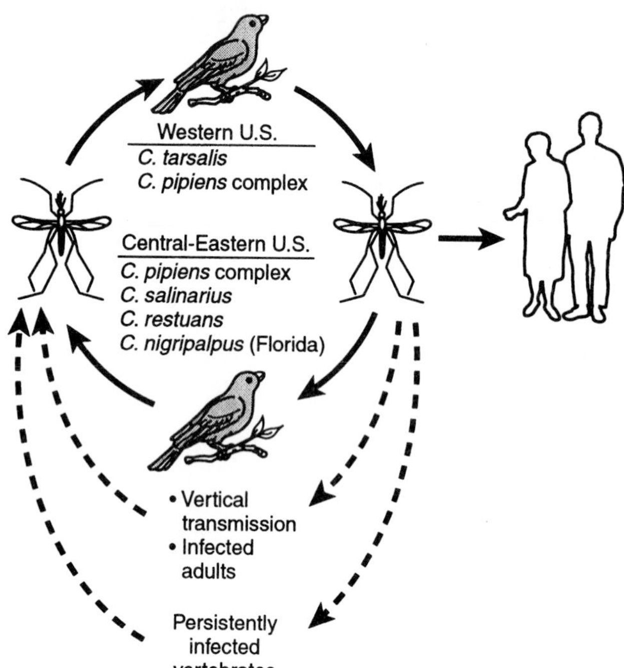

FIGURE 179–1 ■ Transmission cycles of St. Louis encephalitis virus in North America. *Culex* mosquito vectors differ geographically: *C. tarsalis* in the west, *C. pipiens* and *C. quinquefasciatus* in the Ohio and Mississippi valleys, and *C. nigripalpus* in Florida. Epidemics occur when intense viral transmission in the enzootic cycle "spills over" and results in human infections. The viral overwintering mechanism, possibly in mosquitoes or persistently infected vertebrates, has not been proved *(broken lines).*

including humans, in midsummer. Although SLE and WEE viruses coexist in endemic areas of the West, the peak of SLE virus activity appears approximately 2 months later, the relative delay reflecting the higher temperatures required for extrinsic incubation of the virus in vector mosquitoes. Sparrows, finches, and other small birds, and especially their nestlings, are the principal amplifying hosts.[35] Human infections result from encounters with the vector near collections of water along natural and artificial waterways, irrigated farmland, and other breeding sites found chiefly in rural agricultural areas.

In the Ohio and Mississippi valleys and on the Gulf Coast, *C. pipiens* and *C. quinquefasciatus* are, respectively, the enzootic vectors in northern and southern states, with overlapping around the latitude of Memphis. *C. pipiens* does not bite humans readily, and other species, such as *C. restuans* and *C. salinarius,* may be important bridging vectors that infect humans after biting viremic birds.[29, 37, 40] *C. pipiens* complex mosquitoes breed preferentially in polluted water rich in organic material, commonly found in sewage ditches and peridomestic collections of water. Viral amplification occurs in passerine (perching) or columbiforme (pigeon-like) birds (e.g., sparrows, blue jays, doves, other species prolific in residential areas), so both vectors and amplifying hosts are found in close proximity to human dwellings and other sites of human activity.[35] *C. restuans,* which is most active in cool weather, plays a role in viral amplification in early spring and after cool spells in the summer. The mechanism by which the virus overwinters is not known; however, several observations suggest that the virus could persist locally in a resident vertebrate host (e.g., birds, bats), with resumption of viremia contributing to the reinitiation of local transmission in the spring.[2, 52] Other data suggest that the virus could overwinter by transovarial (vertical) transmission in *C. pipiens* complex mosquitoes or in overwintering adult mosquitoes.[5, 40]

C. nigripalpus is both an enzootic and an epizootic vector in Florida.[17, 18, 36] It breeds in a variety of water sources, including ditches, grassy swales, and other temporary collections of water from April to December. In the summer, adult mosquitoes rest during the day in humid vegetated locations and, after sunset, feed actively on birds, thereby amplifying the virus, and also on humans, dogs, cattle, and other mammals, which are dead-end hosts. SLE virus also has been isolated from *C. nigripalpus* in the Caribbean and South America, but transmission cycles in Central and South America are poorly understood.[57] In some areas, the virus is transmitted in a sylvan cycle involving aquatic birds.[1, 57]

The intermittent occurrence of urban SLE outbreaks has been associated with climatic factors, such as an antecedent mild winter, wet spring, and dry hot summer; however, the predictive value of this combination of conditions in foretelling outbreaks has not been evaluated.[37] Snowpack and the resultant availability of irrigation water and an area supportive of mosquito breeding appear to be highly predictive of viral transmission in southern California.[64] In a model of global warming, SLE transmission is predicted to move to northern latitudes and, in existing endemic areas, become seasonal in the spring and fall.[50]

Epidemiology

The epidemiologic patterns of SLE virus transmission reflect human interactions with the virus' reservoirs and its principal mosquito vectors.[28, 29, 37, 59] In western states (Fig. 179–2), perennial transmission of WEE and SLE virus leads to an endemic pattern of transmission, but epidemics are limited by a high level of immunity in the population.[51] Infections occur chiefly in rural areas in association with the habitat of the vector. Combined WEE-SLE outbreaks have taken place typically in rural agricultural areas and their small towns. Recurrent large outbreaks were reported from the Yakima Valley from 1939 to 1942, the Central Valley of California from 1950 to 1959, and the Red River Valley in 1941 and 1975.[27, 37] In 1984, the first urban SLE outbreak in

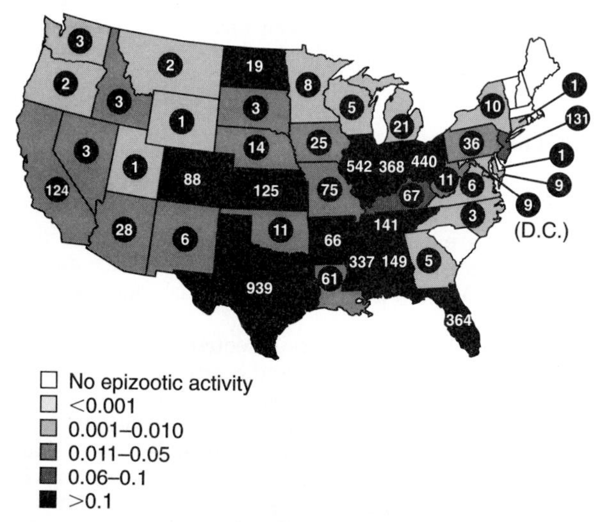

FIGURE 179–2 ■ Reported cases and crude incidence of St. Louis encephalitis per 10,000 by state, 1964 to 1994.

the West led to 27 cases in the urban and suburban areas of Los Angeles and Orange counties; subsequently, surveillance has documented the continued occurrence of sporadic human cases and viral transmission in birds and mosquitoes. A similar outbreak may have occurred a decade earlier in the city of Hermosillo in northern Mexico.[15] Studies in Texas indicated an overlap of urban and rural cycles when an urban outbreak in Dallas followed introduction of the virus to the urban *C. quinquefasciatus* cycle from rural *C. tarsalis*.[24, 28, 29]

In the east-central region of the United States, discrete and occasionally widespread outbreaks occur intermittently, followed by variable, often lengthy periods with no evidence of viral transmission (Fig. 179–3). In some instances, a small premonitory outbreak has been followed by a larger outbreak the next year in the same location, presumably as a result of viral amplification beginning at a higher level in the second of the 2 years. Because virus activity occurs intermittently, the human population is immunologically susceptible, and when the virus is introduced, outbreaks have the potential to become widespread.

Epidemics frequently have occurred in urban locations or their peripheries. In 1975, a nationwide epidemic led to outbreaks in Houston, Chicago, Memphis, and Detroit, as well as smaller outbreaks in rural towns throughout the South and Midwest. Outbreaks in large urban centers generally have been associated with attack rates of less than 40 cases per 100,000 residents.[24, 30, 33, 37, 61, 66]

Epidemic cases often have clustered in more delimited areas where environmental factors are associated with increased mosquito breeding or exposure to mosquitoes. Frequently, these areas are of low socioeconomic status, with dwellings built on open foundations or open sewage ditches being present.[28, 37, 48, 59] In recent urban outbreaks, homelessness and infection with human immunodeficiency virus (HIV) have been the principal risk factors for acquiring SLE.[45, 63] However, in the St. Louis outbreak in 1933, the highest attack rates were in wealthy areas of low housing density, where open sewers, streams, ponds, and weeds were prevalent. In other outbreaks, lush vegetation around houses, which provides shelter for *C. nigripalpus*, and closed sewer systems clogged with grass clippings were factors associated with high attack rates in upper socioeconomic areas.[17, 18, 36]

C. pipiens and *C. quinquefasciatus* are highly domesticated species that bite inside and around houses, and it has followed that an increased risk of infection has been associated with the absence or disrepair of screens and the lack of air conditioning. Epidemic attack rates are 1.2 to 3 times higher in females than males, possibly reflecting increased exposure of females to the peridomestic vector.[33, 37, 61]

In western, *C. tarsalis*–borne outbreaks, in which rural outdoor exposure is a risk factor, attack rates are usually higher in males.[27, 51] A similar observation has been made in Florida, where SLE attack rates are highest in working-age males.[18, 36, 43] *C. quinquefasciatus, C. nigripalpus,* and *C. tarsalis* all are most active in twilight hours, and outdoor activity during these periods is associated with a greater risk of exposure.

Most cases occur in late summer or early fall (Fig. 179–4). However, in Florida, epidemics have continued through mid-December.[18, 36] In the 1975 nationwide epidemic, outbreaks appeared first in the southeastern states in June, followed by an appearance in northern foci later in the summer and fall.[37]

The most important risk factor for acquiring neuroinvasive SLE is advanced age.[30, 37] Age-specific attack rates are lowest in children and rise steadily in adulthood, with attack rates 5 to 40 times higher in persons older than 60 years than in those younger than 10 years. During outbreaks, infections occur uniformly in all age groups, with as many as 300 asymptomatic infections for each clinically apparent case. Therefore, the higher clinical attack rates in the elderly are a function of susceptibility and not exposure.[30, 37] The clinical expression of illness is more severe and the case-fatality rate is also highest in the elderly. The biologic basis for this age-related risk may be immune senescence; however, hypertension and factors associated with cerebrovascular integrity also may be important.[11] Additionally, a secondary peak of increased risk is seen in infants.[61]

In the West, where SLE infections are endemic, an increasing level of immunity associated with length of residence leads to an adult population with lower susceptibility (11% in a recent serosurvey[51]). Consequently, cases often are seen in children and young adults. In a Florida outbreak, immunity to other flaviviruses (mainly from previous

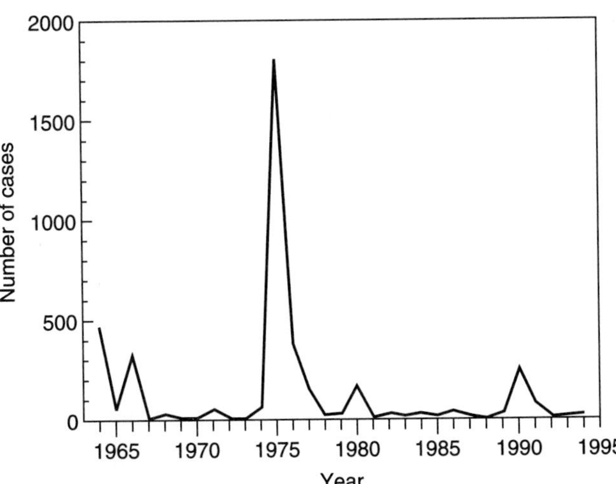

FIGURE 179–3 ■ Reported St. Louis encephalitis cases by year, United States, 1964 to 1994. A nationwide epidemic in 1975 produced more than 2000 cases.

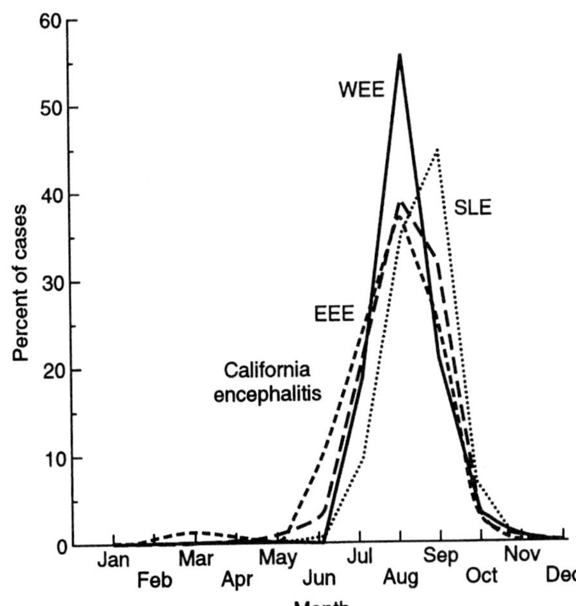

FIGURE 179–4 ■ Reported arboviral encephalitis by etiology and month of onset, United States, 1972 to 1989.

dengue infection) also was shown to protect against the acquisition of SLE.[8]

Sporadic SLE cases acquired in tropical America (Jamaica, Surinam, French Guiana, and northern Argentina) principally have resulted in mild febrile illnesses.[15, 57]

Clinical Manifestations

Clinical manifestations range from a mild "flulike" illness to fatal encephalitis.[9, 49, 54, 66] A case definition that stratifies cases into clinical syndromes of encephalitis, aseptic meningitis, and febrile headache[9] (Table 179–1) has proved useful in surveillance (Fig. 179–5). Although children as a group exhibit milder symptoms, encephalitis develops in more than half of confirmed and presumptive pediatric cases, and 95 percent have objective clinical signs of CNS infection.[6, 7, 66]

SLE cannot be differentiated easily from other viral CNS infections on the basis of clinical features. Photophobia, headache, fever, nausea and vomiting, malaise, and neck stiffness are typical early symptoms. In approximately half of reported cases, an abrupt onset of weakness, incoordination, disturbed sensorium, or other neurologic signs may occur, but equally often, patients have nonspecific symptoms with subtle changes in coordination or mentation during a prodromal phase lasting several days to more than a week. Convulsions have been reported in a third of adult cases.[63]

In addition to fever and signs of meningeal irritation, patients nearly uniformly exhibit alterations in state of consciousness, such as restlessness, confusion, lethargy, delirium, or coma. Neurologic examination usually reveals general weakness, hyperreflexia, and tremulousness, but focal weakness and other deficits are unusual findings. Cranial nerve palsies, especially involving nerves VII, IX, and X, occur in 10 to 25 percent of cases.[9] Clinical signs of increased intracranial pressure have been reported in a few patients. Unusual localizing neurologic signs have been described in patients with involvement of the midbrain, thalamus, or brain stem. In a 4-year-old girl, paralysis of upward gaze was associated with a brain stem infection.[25] Ataxia has been observed in a fourth of the cases in children, and opsoclonus has been reported in several cases in young adults.[20, 21, 63] Convulsions occur in approximately a third of cases.[63] In a series of 26 children with SLE, convulsions were observed in 8, 6 of whom had focal seizures; however, enteroviruses were isolated concurrently in 5 of the 8 patients.[6, 47] In most cases, the fever abates 4 to 7 days after onset, and clinical improvement is evident early in the second week of illness. Polyradiculopathy and transverse myelitis have been reported.[9, 55]

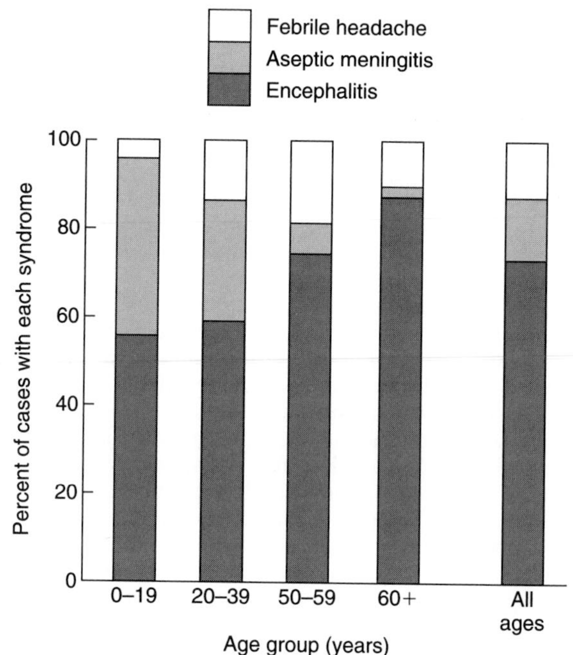

FIGURE 179–5 ■ Distribution of St. Louis encephalitis cases by clinical syndrome and age. Although mortality rates and disease severity increase with age, most cases in children are clinical encephalitis. (Data from Zweighaft, R. M., Rasmussen, C., Brolnitsky, O., et al.: St. Louis encephalitis: The Chicago experience. Am. J. Trop. Med. Hyg. *28*:114–118, 1979.)

TABLE 179–1 ■ DEFINITIONS OF CLINICAL SYNDROMES CAUSED BY ST. LOUIS ENCEPHALITIS

I. Encephalitis* (including meningoencephalitis and encephalomyelitis)
   A. Acute febrile illness (oral temperature ≥37.8° C (≥100° F)
   B. One or more signs in either of the following categories:
      1. Altered level of consciousness (confusion, disorientation, delirium, lethargy, stupor, coma)
      2. Objective signs of neurologic dysfunction (convulsion, cranial nerve palsy, dysarthria, rigidity, paresis, paralysis, abnormal reflexes, tremor)

II. Aseptic meningitis*
   A. Acute febrile Illness
   B. Sign(s) of meningeal irritation (stiff neck with or without positive Kernig or Brudzinski sign)
   C. No objective signs of neurologic dysfunction

III. Febrile headache*
   A. Acute febrile illness
   B. Headache (also may have other systemic symptoms such as nausea or vomiting)
   C. No signs of meningeal irritation or neurologic dysfunction

*Cerebrospinal fluid pleocytosis is present in patients with encephalitis and aseptic meningitis; it also may be found in patients with the syndrome of febrile headache.

From Brinker, K. R., and Monath, T. P.: The acute disease. *In* Monath, T. P. (ed.): St. Louis Encephalitis. Washington, D. C., American Public Health Association, 1980, pp. 503–534.

The peripheral leukocyte count is elevated modestly, with a shift to the left in most patients. Cerebrospinal fluid (CSF) usually contains fewer than 100 leukocytes/mm^3, with a median value between 100 and 200. However, in some cases, fewer than 10 cells and occasionally no cells are discovered in the CSF. An increasing ratio of mononuclear to polymorphonuclear cells is observed on successive examinations. CSF protein rarely exceeds 200 mg/dL, and hypoglycorrhachia is unusual.[9]

In one series, elevated serum aldolase levels suggested a myopathic process, and muscle biopsy and electromyography disclosed lower motor neuron dysfunction, possibly from spinal root involvement. Moderate transaminase elevations have been reported in 19 to 48 percent of adult patients. Decreased serum osmolality attributed to inappropriate secretion of antidiuretic hormone was observed in a fourth to a third of cases in two series.[9, 10]

Urinary incontinence, frequency, or retention and pyuria or proteinuria have been reported in adult patients, and viral antigen was detected on cells in the urinary sediment by immunofluorescence in one report.[31] Lower motor neuron lesions may have been the mechanism for bladder symptoms in some patients.

Electroencephalographic tracings were abnormal in five of six children studied in the 1964 Houston outbreak. One patient had a focal abnormality in the temporal lobe. Five exhibited diffuse changes, two with associated focal discharges and one with a spike abnormality.[6] Electroencephalograms in most adult patients show diffuse generalized slowing, but periodic lateralized epileptiform discharges may be seen; nonconvulsive status epilepticus was reported in one case.[10, 63] Computed tomographic scans may be normal, but magnetic resonance images have disclosed T2-weighted hyperintense abnormalities in the substantia nigra, consistent with edema.[12, 61]

Pathology

Pathologic changes are found predominantly in the midbrain, thalamus, and brain stem, but also in the cerebral cortex and cerebellum. Lesions are observed in the spinal cord in some cases.[53, 56, 58, 65] The leptomeninges are affected to a variable degree with edema, small hemorrhages, and round-cell infiltration.

Perivascular and parenchymal inflammation is prevalent in the brain nuclei and scattered in the white matter of the brain stem and spinal cord and subcortical and deep cerebral areas. Nodular collections of inflammatory cells composed of lymphocytes, microglial cells, and monocytes are found in proximity to or surrounding degenerating neurons characterized by eccentric nuclear displacement, nuclear pyknosis, and cellular contraction. Vascular infiltrations and thrombosis have not been described, as they have in WEE and eastern equine encephalomyelitis. Focal demyelination, which is observed in WEE, has not been characteristic of SLE.

Immunofluorescent examination of frozen sections of brain obtained at autopsy has disclosed widely scattered infected cells in a few samples.[53] Antigen-positive sections corresponded to histopathologically involved areas from which virus was isolated successfully. Transmission electron microscopy has been reported as a novel approach to pathologic diagnosis on tiny tissue fragments.[16]

Pathogenesis

After infection, viral replication occurs locally and in regional lymph nodes. After this eclipse phase, blood-borne (viremic) dissemination ensues, with secondary sites of replication occurring in muscle, endocrine, lymphoreticular, and other tissues and, in less than 1 percent of infections, in the CNS. Vascular endothelial cells may have a role in actively transporting virus from the capillary lumen to the brain and in supporting secondary viral replication.[19] Conditions that compromise cerebrovascular integrity and disrupt the blood-brain barrier may predispose to neuroinvasion; for example, concurrent CNS cysticercosis may be a risk factor for Japanese encephalitis, a related flaviviral infection. Although some experimental studies suggest that CNS invasion occurs through the olfactory epithelium, pathologic studies of Japanese encephalitis cases indicate widespread involvement of the brain stem, deep nuclei, and cortex, most consistent with hematogenous infection.

Recovery from flaviviral encephalitis depends on early intrathecal synthesis of antibodies and viral clearance by macrophages. The inflammatory response in related CNS infections consists of helper-inducer T cells and, to a lesser degree, B lymphocytes infiltrating the perivascular space and parenchyma from the blood. Macrophages and activated microglial cells in the perivascular space and parenchyma, respectively, are responsible for viral clearance. Outcome is determined by the comparative rates of viral spread and neuronal infection, migration of inflammatory cells into the CNS, and the rapidity of the antibody response. Production of interferon is elicited in the brain of human SLE patients, but its role in limiting the spread of virus in the CNS is unclear.[32] The clinical course of SLE in HIV-infected persons has not been significantly different from that of other cases; however, few patients have been studied.

Resistance and susceptibility to some flaviviral infections in mice have been linked to autosomal dominant genes associated with permissiveness to infection and the immune response. Environmental factors that influence susceptibility to flaviviral infection in experimental models include stress from cold or isolation, reticuloendothelial cell blockade, and heavy metal intoxication.

Diagnosis

A laboratory diagnosis of SLE usually is made serologically, although virus has been recovered in the acute phase of illness from blood in six reported instances.[28] Virus should be sought from brain and other organs obtained by biopsy or at autopsy by inoculating Vero cell cultures and suckling mice intracerebrally.[14] Viral antigen has been demonstrated in brain sections examined at autopsy by immunofluorescence and, in one report, in urinary cell sediment.[31, 52] Viral antigen can be detected directly by capture enzyme immunoassay in infected mosquitoes, but the technique has not been evaluated in clinical specimens.[60]

IgM capture enzyme-linked immunosorbent assay (ELISA) is the preferred serologic screening procedure.[39] Intrathecal production of virus-specific IgM reflects recent infection because virus-specific IgM can be detected in serum or CSF in 75 percent or more of specimens obtained within 4 days of onset. In most patients, IgM levels decline in the convalescent sample and disappear approximately 4 months after onset, although IgM persisted at high titer in a few patients for 6 months.[62] In areas where SLE is endemic, virus-specific IgM carried over from the previous transmission season potentially could lead to an erroneous diagnosis. The indirect immunofluorescent antibody procedure offers a similar capacity for rapid diagnosis; however, it is less sensitive than ELISA, and IgM rheumatoid factor can lead to a false-positive result. Positive samples must be tested against both WN and SLE viruses to ascertain the assay's specificity.

Hemagglutination inhibition (HI) and neutralizing antibodies rise rapidly after infection (often within 2 to 5 days after onset), reach a peak in the second week, and persist for years after recovery. An elevated titer (≥80) is presumptive evidence of recent infection. Complement-fixation (CF) antibody may not appear until the second week after onset and rises more slowly and to lower levels. CF antibody declines more rapidly (only half the patients tested 3 years after infection have measurable CF antibody) and is useful as a measure of recent infection. However, its sensitivity was reduced considerably[10] in 20 percent of confirmed cases, specifically in the elderly. HI and CF reactions may reflect cross-reactive WN antibodies and should be confirmed in neutralization tests.

The serologic response in a primary flavivirus infection is usually type-specific, but repeated infections lead to broad heterologous responses that are often difficult to interpret. Human infections with indigenous flaviviruses (e.g., Rio Bravo, Powassan) other than SLE are rare; however, in patients with antecedent yellow fever immunization or infection with dengue virus acquired in areas of the

United States where dengue was previously endemic (e.g., Texas, Florida) or acquired during travel or residence abroad, a broadly reactive flavivirus antibody response may obfuscate the diagnosis. Recent immigrants with preexisting dengue antibodies are the most common source of flaviviral antibodies in most areas of the United States. Incremental increases in specificity are associated with HI, CF, and neutralization assays, but frequently it may not be possible to make a specific diagnosis, even after the completion of cross-neutralization tests.

Differential Diagnosis

In an endemic setting, clinicians should consider SLE principally in the differential diagnosis of patients with aseptic meningitis or acute encephalitis. However, in the context of an outbreak, the diagnostic threshold should be lowered to include patients with less specific findings, especially acute febrile illnesses with headache, and patients who exhibit confusion or are encephalopathic without fever. Increased suspicion of SLE in mildly ill patients should be directed particularly at children and young adults, in whom the infection often is manifested without meningoencephalitis.

The clinical findings of SLE cannot be distinguished easily from those of other CNS infections. However, focal neurologic deficits are less characteristic of SLE and should suggest other diagnoses. The combination of global confusion and tremulousness in SLE may suggest a metabolic encephalopathy, and in elderly patients, the initial manifestations of SLE can overlap the signs and symptoms of a cerebrovascular accident.

WN encephalitis and SLE are virtually identical in their clinical findings, their predilection for the elderly, and other epidemiologic features, including late summer seasonality, urban locus of epidemic transmission, and similar *Culex*-bird transmission cycles, such that individual cases cannot be differentiated except by specific laboratory testing.[34] Although concurrent transmission of the two viruses has not been reported yet in the eastern United States, the geographic overlap of the virus' ranges, especially in Florida, holds this possibility, much as WN and SLE viruses cocirculate in southwest Asia.

The progression of symptoms and localizing signs associated with herpes encephalitis contrasts sharply with the clinical findings in SLE, in which localizing signs are less usual. Enteroviral infections have an overlapping summer seasonality but often are associated with clustering of illnesses in families and other epidemiologic clues of person-to-person spread. Skin eruptions, respiratory symptoms, pericarditis, myocarditis, and conjunctivitis are helpful distinguishing characteristics. Concurrent enterovirus infection and SLE may be associated with an increased risk of convulsions during the acute phase of illness.[6, 47] Enteroviral infections can be confirmed by detecting viral genomic sequences in CSF by polymerase chain reaction, by IgM capture ELISA, or by recovery of virus from stool or CSF. Primary HIV, human herpesvirus–6, and mumps virus infections are other common infections that should be entertained in the differential diagnosis. A third of patients with mumps encephalitis do not have associated parotid gland swelling.

Adenoviral encephalitis is a rare infection in children, more severe than SLE, and sometimes associated with hepatic and other extraneural sites of infection. The presence of lymphoreticular involvement and typical hematologic features should suggest the clinical diagnosis of Epstein-Barr virus infection.

Partially treated bacterial meningitis and parameningeal pyogenic infections are the principal bacterial causes to exclude. Cat-scratch fever can be manifested as fever and encephalopathy mimicking arboviral encephalitis.[44] Convulsions associated with *Shigella* enteritis and ataxia associated with typhoid fever potentially could be interpreted as a primary CNS infection. Tuberculous meningitis is typically a subacute illness; evidence of active extraneural sites of infection should be sought. A low CSF glucose level is a clue to the diagnosis.

In urban areas or where parental occupational exposure may occur, lead intoxication remains an important potential cause of encephalopathy in summer. Hyperthermia associated with sustained exposure to elevated environmental temperature likewise may lead to encephalopathy with convulsions, signs of raised intracranial pressure, and evidence of hepatic dysfunction. This constellation of symptoms also may suggest Reye syndrome. However, Reye syndrome typically occurs in the winter and spring after a respiratory viral infection and is characterized by hypoglycemia and elevated blood ammonia. Patients with salicylism exhibit similar clinical findings, but a history of salicylate ingestion, an elevated anion gap early in the course of illness, and an elevated blood salicylate level should suggest that diagnosis.

Treatment

Supportive therapy, as outlined in the earlier sections, should be aimed at maintaining cardiorespiratory function and fluid and electrolyte balance, controlling convulsions, and monitoring and maintaining normal intracranial pressure.[34] No specific antiviral therapy is available.

Prognosis

The principal risk factor for a fatal outcome is advanced age[9, 28, 30, 37, 61, 62] (see Fig. 179–5). Among all cases reported to the Centers for Disease Control and Prevention from 1955 to 1971, 8 percent died, but the age-specific mortality rate in persons 60 years or older was 19.5 percent. Fatality rates as high as 38 to 80 percent were recorded in the 1933 St. Louis outbreak in patients who were 60 to 89 years of age. Mortality in children has ranged from 2 to 5 percent, with the highest risk in children younger than 5 years. The overall case-fatality rate in an outbreak in Hermosillo, Sonora (involving principally children), was 20 percent.[15] The high fatality rate in this instance is anomalous because fatality rates are usually lower in *C. tarsalis*–borne SLE outbreaks in the West. The role of neurocysticercosis as a risk factor for acquiring SLE should be examined in view of its potential involvement as a risk factor for Japanese encephalitis (see the subchapter Japanese Encephalitis).

In adults, coma, a low CSF leukocyte count (<100 cells/mm^3), and underlying hypertensive vascular disease have been factors associated with a fatal outcome.[11] Risk factors for mortality in children have not been described.

Recovery from SLE is usually complete or associated with soft sequelae such as emotional disturbances, dizziness, headache, memory impairment, and tremor.[4, 22, 42] In one study of 193 cases, 25 percent of children who were 1 to 4 years of age at the time of infection had serious neurologic sequelae, the highest rate of any age group.[46] The incidence of sequelae was 10 percent in children 5 to 9 years of age. Children who were younger than 1 year at the time of infection appeared to be spared any serious sequelae. Deficits in motor and intellectual function were reported in some cases.

TABLE 179–2 ■ PRECAUTIONS TO MINIMIZE POTENTIAL ADVERSE REACTIONS FROM REPELLENTS

Repellents should be applied only to exposed skin and/or clothing (as directed on the product label). Do not use on underclothing.
Never use repellents over cuts, wounds, or irritated skin.
Avoid mucosal contact—do not apply to eyes and mouth and apply sparingly around ears. When using sprays, do not spray directly onto face; spray on hands first and then apply to face.
Do not allow children to handle these products, and do not apply to children's hands. When using on children, apply to your own hands and then put it on the child.
Do not spray in enclosed areas. Avoid breathing a repellent spray.
Avoid ingestion, and do not use it near food.
Use just enough repellent to cover exposed skin and/or clothing. Heavy application and saturation are unnecessary for effectiveness; if biting insects do not respond to a thin film of repellent, apply a bit more.
After returning indoors, wash treated skin with soap and water or bathe, particularly when repellents are used repeatedly in a day or on consecutive days. Also, wash treated clothing before wearing it again.
Pregnant and nursing women should minimize the use of repellents.
If you suspect that you or your child is reacting to an insect repellent, discontinue use, wash the treated skin, and then call your local poison control center. If/when you go to a doctor, take the repellent with you.
Specific medical information about the active ingredients in repellents and other pesticides is available at the National Pesticide Telecommunications Network (NPTN) at 1-800-858-7378. The NPTN operates from 6:30 AM to 4:30 PM Pacific time, 9:30 AM to 7:30 PM Eastern time, 7 days a week.

Adapted from U.S. Environmental Protection Agency recommendations available at http://www.epa.gov/pesticides/factsheets/chemicals/deet/htm.

Convulsions were not a significant residual abnormality. The same cohort monitored at intervals of 6 months to 14 years had no perceptible residual differences in intelligence quotient when compared with the normal population. In a case report, persistent ataxia of the extremities and trunk and dysarthria were reported as residual findings in a 4-year-old patient.[25]

No deleterious effects of SLE on the outcome of pregnancy have been reported. However, infection with Japanese encephalitis virus in the second trimester resulted in transplacental viral transmission and abortion, whereas infection in the third trimester was not associated with fetal damage. In experimentally infected mice, vertical transmission led to learning deficits in congenitally infected pups.[3]

Prevention

Preventive public health efforts have focused on surveillance of viral activity in the enzootic cycle to predict epidemic activity. In many east-central states, weekly serologic surveys of captured wild birds and sentinel chickens are conducted to detect rising seroprevalence rates that reflect viral amplification[40] and an increased risk for human infection. The abundance of female vector mosquitoes and increased viral infection rates in vectors also have been correlated with a risk of epidemic transmission.[64]

When viral activity is elevated, ground and aerial application of insecticides is aimed at reducing the infected adult vector population. If insecticides are applied early enough, viral amplification potentially can be attenuated and epidemic transmission aborted.

Avoiding outdoor activity during the twilight and evening hours, using repellents appropriately (Table 179–2), and repairing screens or installing air conditioners in residences are simple but effective measures that reduce exposure to adult mosquitoes. Improving drainage and removing containers that could serve as mosquito breeding sites are important steps in preventing the disease.

A vaccine is not available. Vaccination of the general public is not a realistic preventive measure because of low attack rates and the intermittent and focal nature of outbreaks. However, if a vaccine or chemoprophylactic were available, selective administration to a targeted population, particularly the elderly, might be appropriate in an outbreak. A WN virus vaccine under development potentially could provide cross-protection against SLE.

REFERENCES

1. Adames, A. J., Dutary, B., Tejera, H., et al.: Relocion entre mosquitos vectores y aves acuaticas en la transmission potencial de dos arbovirus. Rev. Med. Panama *18*:106–119, 1993.
2. Allen, R., Taylor, S. K., and Sulkin, S. E.: Studies of arthropod-borne virus infections in Chiroptera. VIII. Evidence of natural St. Louis encephalitis virus infection in bats. Am. J. Trop. Med. Hyg. *19*:851–859, 1970.
3. Andersen, A. A., and Hanson, R. P.: Intrauterine infection of mice with St. Louis encephalitis virus: Immunological, physiological, neurological, and behavioral effects on progeny. Infect. Immun. *12*:1173–1183, 1975.
4. Azar, G. J., Bond, J. O., Chappell, G. L., et al.: Follow up studies of St. Louis encephalitis in Florida: Sensorimotor findings. Am. J. Public Health *56*:1074–1081, 1966.
5. Bailey, C. L., Eldridge, B. F., Hayes, D. E., et al.: Isolation of St. Louis encephalitis virus from overwintering *Culex pipiens* mosquitoes. Science *199*:1346–1349, 1978.
6. Barrett, F. F., Yow, M. D., and Phillips, C. A.: St. Louis encephalitis in children during the 1964 epidemic. J. A. M. A. *193*:381–385, 1965.
7. Blattner, R. J., and Heys, F. M.: St. Louis encephalitis: Occurrence in children in the St. Louis area during nonepidemic years 1939–1944. J. A. M. A. *129*:854–857, 1945.
8. Bond, J. O., and Hammon, W. M.: Epidemiologic studies of possible cross protection between dengue and St. Louis encephalitis arboviruses in Florida. Am. J. Epidemiol. *92*:321–329, 1970.
9. Brinker, K. R., and Monath, T. P.: The acute disease. *In* Monath, T. P. (ed.): St. Louis Encephalitis. Washington, D.C., American Public Health Association, 1980, pp. 503–534.
10. Brinker, K. R., Paulson, G., Monath, T. P., et al.: St. Louis encephalitis in Ohio, September 1975: Clinical and EEG studies in 16 cases. Arch. Intern. Med. *139*:561–566, 1979.
11. Broun, G. O.: Relationship of hypertensive vascular disease to mortality in cases of St. Louis encephalitis. Med. Bull. St. Louis Univ. *4*:32–37, 1952.
12. Cerna, F., Mehrad, B., Luby, J. P., et al: St. Louis encephalitis and the substantia nigra: MR imaging evaluation. A. J. N. R. Am. J. Neuroradiol. *20*:1281–1283, 1999.
13. Chandler, L. J., Parsons, R., and Randle, Y.: Multiple genotypes of St. Louis encephalitis virus (Flaviviridae: Flavivirus) circulate in Harris County, Texas. Am. J. Trop. Med. Hyg. *64*:12–19, 2001.
14. Coleman, P. H., Lewis, A. L., Schneider, N. J., et al.: Isolations of St. Louis encephalitis virus from postmortem tissues of human cases in the 1962 Florida epidemic. Am. J. Epidemiol. *87*:530–538, 1968.
15. Cortes, A. G., Aquino, M. L. Z., Bahena, J. G., et al.: St. Louis encephalomyelitis in Hermosillo, Sonora, Mexico. Pan Am. Health Organ. Bull. *9*:306–316, 1975.
16. Chu, C. T., Howell, D. N., Morgenlander, J. C., et al.: Electron microscopic diagnosis of human flavivirus encephalitis: Use of confocal microscopy as an aid. Am. J. Surg. Pathol. *23*:1217–1226, 1999.
17. Day, J. F.: Predicting St. Louis encephalitis: Lessons from recent, and not so recent, outbreaks. Annu. Rev. Entomol. *46*:111–138, 2001.
18. Day, J. F., and Stark, L. M.: Frequency of Saint Louis encephalitis virus in humans from Florida, USA: 1990–1999. J. Med. Entomol. *37*:626–633, 2000.
19. Dropulic, B., and Masters, C. L.: Entry of neurotropic arboviruses into the central nervous system: An in vitro study using mouse brain endothelium. J. Infect. Dis. *161*:685–691, 1990.
20. Estrin, W. J.: The serological diagnosis of St. Louis encephalitis in a patient with the syndrome of opsoclonia, body tremulousness, and benign encephalitis. Ann. Neurol. *1*:596–598, 1977.
21. Evans, R. W., and Welch, K.: Opsoclonus in a confirmed case of St. Louis encephalitis. J. Neurol. Neurosurg. Psychiatry *45*:660–661, 1982.
22. Finley, K. H., and Riggs, N.: Convalescence and sequelae. *In* Monath, T. P. (ed.): St. Louis Encephalitis. Washington, D.C., American Public Health Association, 1980, pp. 535–550.

23. Huang, C., Chatterjee, N. K., and Grady, L. J.: Diagnosis of viral infections of the central nervous system. N. Engl. J. Med. *340*:483–484, 1999.
24. Hopkins, C. C., Hollinger, F. B., Johnson, R. F., et al.: The epidemiology of St. Louis encephalitis in Dallas, Texas, 1966. Am. J. Epidemiol. *102*:1–15, 1975.
25. Kaplan, A. M., and Koveleski, J. T.: St. Louis encephalitis with particular involvement of the brain stem. Arch. Neurol. *35*:45–46, 1978.
26. Kramer, L. D., Presser, S. B., Hardy, J. L., and Jackson, A. O.: Genotypic and phenotypic variation of selected Saint Louis encephalitis viral strains isolated in California. Am. J. Trop. Med. Hyg. *57*:222–229, 1997.
27. Longshore, W. A., Stevens, I. M., Hollister, A. C., et al.: Epidemiologic observations on acute infectious encephalitis in California, with special reference to the 1952 outbreak. Am. J. Hyg. *63*:69–86, 1956.
28. Luby, J. P.: St. Louis encephalitis. Epidemiol. Rev. *1*:55–73, 1979.
29. Luby, J. P.: St. Louis encephalitis. *In* Beran, G. W. (ed.): Handbook of Zoonoses. Section B: Viral. 2nd ed. Boca Raton, FL, CRC Press, 1994, p. 47.
30. Luby, J. P., Miller, G., Gardner, P., et al.: The epidemiology of St. Louis encephalitis in Houston, Texas, 1964. Am. J. Epidemiol. *86*:584–597, 1967.
31. Luby, J. P., Murphy, F. K., Gilliam, J. N., et al.: Antigenuria in St. Louis encephalitis. Am. J. Trop. Med. Hyg. *29*:265–268, 1980.
32. Luby, J. P., Stewart, W. E., Sulkin, S. E., et al.: Interferon in human infections with St. Louis encephalitis virus. Ann. Intern. Med. *71*:703–709, 1969.
33. Marfin, A. A., Bleed, D. M., Lofgren, J. P., et al.: Epidemiological aspects of a St. Louis encephalitis epidemic in Jefferson County, Arkansas. Am. J. Trop. Med. Hyg. *49*:30–37, 1993.
34. McCarthy, M.: St. Louis encephalitis and West Nile virus encephalitis. Curr. Treat. Options Neurol. *3*:433–438, 2001.
35. McLean, R. G.: Arboviruses of wild birds and mammals. Bull. Soc. Vector Ecol. *16*:3–16, 1991.
36. Meehan, P. J., Wells, D. L., Paul, W., et al.: Epidemiological features of and public health response to a St. Louis encephalitis epidemic in Florida, 1990–1991. Epidemiol. Infect. *125*:181–188, 2000.
37. Monath, T. P.: Epidemiology. *In* Monath, T. P. (ed.): St. Louis Encephalitis. Washington, D.C., American Public Health Association, 1980, pp. 239–312.
38. Monath, T. P., Cropp, C. B., Bowen, G. S., et al.: Variation in virulence for mice and rhesus monkeys among St. Louis encephalitis virus strains of different origin. Am. J. Trop. Med. Hyg. *29*:948–962, 1980.
39. Monath, T. P., Nystrom, R. R., Bailey, R. E., et al.: Immunoglobulin M antibody capture enzyme-linked immunosorbent assay for diagnosis of St. Louis encephalitis. J. Clin. Microbiol. *20*:784–790, 1984.
40. Monath, T. P., and Tsai, T. F.: St. Louis encephalitis: Lessons from the last decade. Am. J. Trop. Med. Hyg. *37*(Suppl.):40–59, 1987.
41. Naidech, A., and Elliott, D.: St. Louis encephalitis with focal neurological signs. Clin. Infect. Dis. *29*:1334–1335, 1999.
42. Neel, J. L.: Neuropsychiatric sequelae in a case of St. Louis encephalitis. Gen. Hosp. Psychiatry *22*:126–128, 2000.
43. Nelson, D. B., Kappus, K. D., Janowski, J. T., et al.: St. Louis encephalitis, Florida 1977: Patterns of a widespread outbreak. Am. J. Trop. Med. Hyg. *32*:412–418, 1983.
44. Noah, D. L., Bresee, J. S., Gorensek, M. J., et al.: Cluster of five children with acute encephalopathy associated with cat-scratch disease in South Florida. Pediatr. Infect. Dis. J. *14*:866–869, 1995.
45. Okhuysen, P. C., Crane, J. K., and Pappas, J.: St. Louis encephalitis in patients with human immunodeficiency virus infection. Clin. Infect. Dis. *17*:140–141, 1993.
46. Palmer, R. J., and Finley, K. H.: Sequelae of encephalitis: Report of a study after the California epidemic. Calif. Med. *84*:98–100, 1956.
47. Phillips, C. A., Melnick, J. L., Barrett, F. F., et al.: Dual virus infections: Simultaneous enteroviral disease and St. Louis encephalitis. J. A. M. A. *197*:169–172, 1966.
48. Powell, K. E., and Blakey, D. L.: St. Louis encephalitis: The 1975 epidemic in Mississippi. J. A. M. A. *237*:2294–2298, 1977.
49. Quick, D. T., Thompson, J. M., Bond, J. O., et al.: The 1962 epidemic of St. Louis encephalitis in Florida. II. Clinical features of cases in the Tampa Bay area. Am. J. Epidemiol. *81*:415–424, 1965.
50. Reeves, W. C., Hardy, J. L., Reisin, W. K., et al.: Potential effect of global warming on mosquito-borne arboviruses. J. Med. Entomol. *31*:323–332, 1994.
51. Reisen, W. K., and Chiles, R. E.: Prevalence of antibodies to western equine encephalomyelitis and St. Louis encephalitis viruses in residents of California exposed to sporadic and consistent enzootic transmission. Am. J. Trop. Med. Hyg. *57*:526–529, 1997.
52. Reisen, W. K., Kramer, L. D., Chiles, R. E., et al.: Encephalitis virus persistence in California birds: Preliminary studies with house finches. J. Med. Entomol. *38*:393–399, 2001.
53. Reyes, M. G., Gardner, J. J., Poland, J. D., et al.: St. Louis encephalitis: Quantitative histologic and immunofluorescent studies. Arch. Neurol. *38*:329–334, 1981.
54. Riggs, S., Smith, D. L., and Phillips, C. A.: St. Louis encephalitis in adults during the 1964 Houston epidemic. J. A. M. A. *193*:284, 1965.
55. Sanders, M., Blumberg, A., and Haymaker, W.: Polyradiculopathy in man produced by St. Louis encephalitis (SLE). South. Med. J. *69*:1121–1125, 1976.
56. Shinner, J. J.: St. Louis virus encephalomyelitis. Arch. Pathol. *75*:311–322, 1963.
57. Spence, L. P.: St. Louis encephalitis in tropical America. *In* Monath, T. P. (ed.): St. Louis Encephalitis. Washington, D.C., American Public Health Association, 1980, pp. 451–471.
58. Suzuki, M., and Phillips, C. A.: St. Louis encephalitis: A histopathologic study of the fatal cases from the Houston epidemic in 1964. Arch. Pathol. *81*:47–54, 1966.
59. Tsai, T. F.: Arboviral infections in the United States. Infect. Dis. Clin. North Am. *5*:73–102, 1991.
60. Tsai, T. F., Bolin, R. A., Montoya, M., et al.: Detection of St. Louis encephalitis virus antigen in mosquitoes by capture enzyme immunoassay. J. Clin. Microbiol. *25*:370–376, 1987.
61. Tsai, T. F., Canfield, M. A., Reed, C. M., et al.: Epidemiologic aspects of a St. Louis encephalitis outbreak in Harris County, Texas, 1986. J. Infect. Dis. *157*:351–356, 1988.
62. Tsai, T. F., Cobb, W. B., Bolin, R. A., et al.: Epidemiologic aspects of a St. Louis encephalitis outbreak in Mesa County. Am. J. Epidemiol. *126*:460–473, 1987.
63. Wasay, M., Diaz-Arrastia, R., Suss, R. A., et al.: St. Louis encephalitis: A review of 11 cases in a 1995 Dallas, Texas, epidemic. Arch. Neurol. *57*:114–118, 2000.
64. Wegbreit, J., and Reisen, W. K.: Relationships among weather, mosquito abundance, and encephalitis virus activity in California: Kern County 1990–1998. J. Am. Mosq. Control. Assoc. *16*:22–27, 2000.
65. Weil, A.: Histopathology of the central nervous system in epidemic encephalitis (St. Louis epidemic). Arch. Neurol. Psychiatry *31*:1139–1152, 1934.
66. Zweighaft, R. M., Rasmussen, C., Brolnitsky, O., et al.: St. Louis encephalitis: The Chicago experience. Am. J. Trop. Med. Hyg. *28*:114–118, 1979.

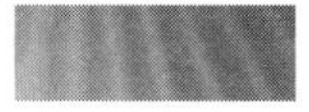

CHAPTER **179B**

Yellow Fever

DUANE J. GUBLER

Yellow fever is a mosquito-borne viral disease of humans and lower primates that occurs naturally in tropical Africa and the Americas (Fig. 179–6). Epidemics, which can occur in both urban and rural areas, often are associated with severe hemorrhagic disease and high fatality rates.

History

Yellow fever first was described as a disease entity in 1648 in the Yucatan, Mexico. It apparently was part of a larger regional epidemic that affected the Caribbean Islands and Central America from Barbados to Mexico from 1647 to 1649.[8] Though first described in the Americas, yellow fever virus, along with its principal urban epidemic mosquito vector *Aedes aegypti,* most likely originated in Africa and was introduced to the New World via the slave trade. During the 17th, 18th, 19th, and early 20th centuries, epidemic yellow fever was a major public health problem. Large epidemics occurred in tropical America, as well as in the United States (as far north as Boston) and Europe (as far north as England).[12] Epidemics occurred primarily in port cities as a result of the primary mode of spread: sailing vessels and commerce.

After transmission by mosquitoes was documented by Reed and the Yellow Fever Commission in Cuba,[11] major

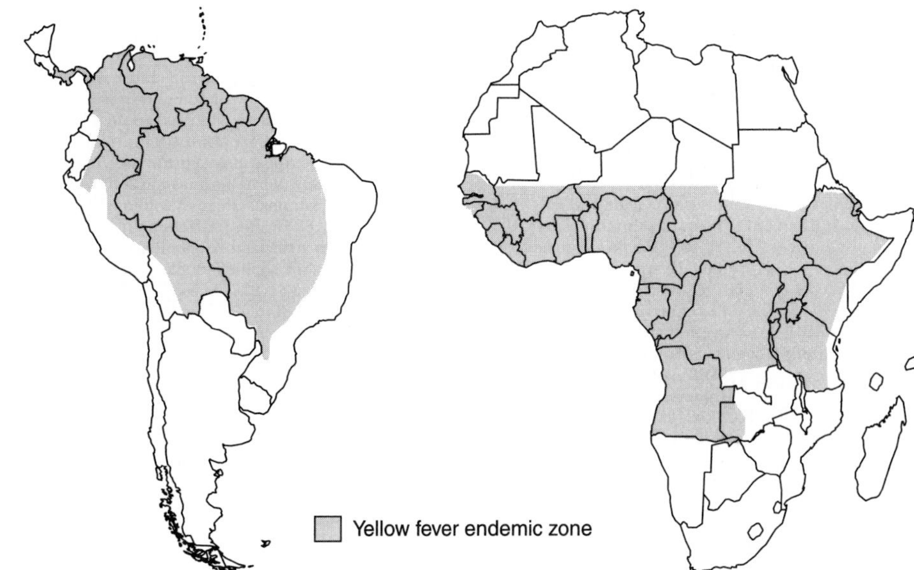

FIGURE 179–6 ■ Geographic distribution of yellow fever in Africa and the Americas.

efforts were undertaken to keep the disease in check by mosquito control. The first yellow fever virus was isolated in 1927. By 1938, an effective live attenuated virus vaccine had been developed. Yellow fever was controlled in the Americas by eradication of the mosquito vector of urban disease, *A. aegypti*, from most Central and South American countries. In West Africa, yellow fever was controlled by mass vaccination programs. The result was the disappearance of major urban epidemics of yellow fever in both Africa and the Americas during the 1950s, 1960s, and 1970s. In the mid-1980s, however, the urban form of disease re-emerged in West Africa, with major epidemics in Nigeria and increased transmission in other countries.[6] Kenya experienced its first epidemic in history in 1993. In the Americas, *A. aegypti* has reinfested most Central and South American countries from which it had been eradicated, and urban centers of the American tropics are at their highest risk for epidemic urban yellow fever in more than 50 years.[1] Thus, the disease continues to be an important public health problem in both Africa and the Americas. Yellow fever has never been recognized in Asia or the Pacific.

Etiologic Agent

Yellow fever is caused by yellow fever virus, the prototype of the genus *Flavivirus,* family *Flaviviridae.* The genus *Flavivirus* contains 68 viruses, which are small (40 to 50 nm in diameter), spherical, and enveloped, with single-stranded RNA about 11 kb in length.[3] Many of the flaviviruses are very closely related antigenically, which has resulted in extensive cross-reactivity in most serologic tests, so a laboratory diagnosis is difficult to make.

Epidemiology

Yellow fever viruses are maintained in natural zoonotic cycles involving lower primates and canopy-dwelling mosquitoes that breed in tree holes in the rain forests of both Africa and the Americas.[6, 8, 12] It is called the jungle or sylvatic cycle of yellow fever. Humans become involved accidentally only when they encroach on this cycle in the forest. Humans thus infected may transport the virus back to a village or city during incubation. If infected persons are fed on by urban *A. aegypti,* the virus then can be transmitted from human to human. Major urban epidemics are transmitted by this highly domesticated mosquito, which lives in close association with humans in most tropical cities of the world.[1]

Yellow fever occurs throughout much of sub-Saharan Africa and tropical America in the sylvatic cycle (see Fig. 179–6). In Africa, cercopithecoid and celobid monkeys are the main vertebrate hosts; infection rarely causes illness and death in these species. Year-round enzootic transmission by *Aedes africanus* occurs in the rain forests. In wet savannah areas bordering the rain forests of western and central Africa, transmission increases during the rainy season and decreases during the dry season. *Aedes furcifer, A. africanus,* and *Aedes leuteocephalus* are the main mosquito vectors in this "zone of emergence," and the virus is transmitted from monkey to monkey, monkey to human, and human to human. In the dry savannah zones, yellow fever activity is intermittent and takes place mainly during the rainy season, but it also occurs in major epidemics in urban areas, where stored water provides the ideal larval habitat for *A. aegypti*. In East Africa, *Aedes simpsoni (Aedes bromeliae)* provides the link between the *A. africanus* sylvatic cycle and humans in areas bordering gallery forests.

In tropical America, howler, spider, squirrel, owl, capuchin, and wooly monkeys all act as vertebrate hosts for yellow fever virus. Mosquitoes of the genus *Haemagogus* are the principal vectors in tropical American rain forests, where they feed in the canopy as well as at ground level. Other mosquito species, such as *Sabethes chloropterus*, *Aedes leucocelaenus*, and *Aedes fulvus,* may play secondary roles. Although most cases have been reported from Bolivia, Brazil, and Peru in recent years, the enzootic zone probably includes the rain forests of at least 10 countries (Colombia, Ecuador, Peru, Bolivia, Brazil, Venezuela, Guyana, Suriname, French Guiana, and Trinidad[14]) and involves "wandering" enzootic transmission among the monkey populations. The humans involved are mainly adult males who work in the forest.

Vertical transmission of yellow fever virus from an infected female mosquito through the eggs to her offspring plays an important role in survival and maintenance of yellow fever virus in enzootic cycles and has been demonstrated in nature in West Africa by isolation of the virus from male *A. furcifer* mosquitoes. Experimentally, *Haemagogus* and *A. aegypti* mosquitoes have been shown to be capable of vertical transmission. This mechanism is thought to be of major importance in survival of the virus during prolonged dry periods in both enzootic regions.

Urban epidemics of yellow fever have reappeared in West Africa in the past 17 years.[10] Unfortunately, surveillance is very poor, and the actual number of cases reported is thought to be grossly underestimated. For example, in Nigeria in 1986 and 1987, the number of reported cases and deaths during epidemics was 2612 and 973, respectively. Seroepidemiologic studies, however, estimated that the actual number of cases and deaths was 130,000 and 29,000, respectively.[10]

In the Americas, the last urban yellow fever epidemic occurred in 1942. Reinvasion of American tropical urban centers by *A. aegypti,* however, has placed more than 300 million susceptible individuals at risk. As might be expected, urban transmission has been reported recently. In 1998, urban transmission of yellow fever was documented in Santa Cruz, Bolivia.[13] Though not comprising a large number of cases, this outbreak underscores the high risk that many tropical urban centers have at the beginning of the 21st century. In addition, six fatal cases of yellow fever in travelers who have visited South America (four cases) or Africa (two cases) in the past 6 years have been confirmed. Three of these cases were U.S. citizens, and three were European. Urban yellow fever epidemics are expected to occur in the Americas in the near future unless vaccination or effective mosquito control programs are implemented.

Yellow fever has never been reported in Asia or the Pacific. The reason is not known, but both variation in mosquito vector competence and partial protection by heterotypic flavivirus antibody have been suggested as reasons why this virus has never become established in that part of the world. If urban epidemics do occur in the American tropics, the virus is expected to move very quickly to this and other permissive areas where urban mosquito vectors are found and cause a major international public health emergency.

Clinical Manifestations

Infection with yellow fever virus causes a spectrum of illness ranging from inapparent infection to severe yellow fever with the classic triad of jaundice, hemorrhage, and albuminuria, which is associated with a high case-fatality rate. Most yellow fever infections are manifested clinically as a mild to severe viral syndrome without symptoms of intoxication; 10 to 20 percent of infections may result in classic yellow fever.[5, 8, 9]

The incubation period may be as long as 13 days but is generally 3 to 6 days.[8] The onset of illness is abrupt, with fever, headache, backache, myalgia, nausea, and other nonspecific signs and symptoms. In mild cases, the illness will last for several days, after which recovery is uneventful and complete. In severe cases, prostration is common, and examination reveals congestion of the skin, conjunctivae, and mucous membranes. The pulse rate usually increases early in the illness, and blood pressure is normal. Leukopenia is a frequent finding, and mild albuminuria may be noted. The temperature is generally between 38.5° and 40° C. Nausea and vomiting are common findings. Minor hemorrhagic manifestations such as epistaxis and bleeding gums may be observed. This period of infection may last for approximately 3 days, at which time the congestion declines and a relative bradycardia may occur despite the elevated temperature (Faget sign). The temperature falls to or below normal, and the patient feels better.

In most patients, this period of remission signals the beginning of convalescence, but in severe cases, it may last only a few hours, at which point the patient enters a period of intoxication characterized by venous congestion and extreme bradycardia despite a secondary rise in temperature. Nausea and vomiting are severe and associated with epigastric pain. Prostration, jaundice, marked albuminuria, and anuria are present. Hemorrhagic manifestations include hematemesis and melena.

The jaundice in some patients is not striking; it is difficult to detect in early disease and often is not detected until after death. The severity of hemorrhagic manifestations also varies greatly, but some hemorrhage can be found in most cases. As indicated earlier, minor hemorrhagic manifestations may be observed in the early stage of illness; severe hemorrhage usually develops late in the illness, although in fulminant cases it may occur as early as the second or third day. Hemorrhage may be so severe that it causes shock and death from blood loss. Albuminuria is one of the most common findings in yellow fever, and it occurs in all but very mild cases. It is present early in the illness and may increase rapidly. The albuminuria probably is related to renal involvement during the period of infection. Anuria, on the other hand, appears to be related to hepatic involvement and never is seen in the absence of other signs of liver infection.

Death may ensue as early as 2 to 4 days after onset but usually occurs after 7 to 10 days of illness in 20 to 50 percent of severe cases. In patients in whom death occurs later, autopsy generally reveals a cause other than yellow fever. Patients with severe infection often have lowered resistance to secondary infection, which may develop at the time of convalescence. Other complications include kidney abscess, pneumonia, subgenerative parotitis, and skin infection. Convalescence usually is rapid and complete except for a general weakness that may last for several weeks. Permanent damage to the liver or kidneys is not apparent.

Pathology

The gross pathology in fatal cases of yellow fever is not striking.[9] The skin, sclerae, serosa, some internal organs, and subcutaneous fat usually have moderate icterus. Serous effusions, edema, and hemorrhages, including petechiae and purpuric lesions on the skin, conjunctivae, mucous membranes, stomach, duodenum, and bladder, are often present. Gastrointestinal hemorrhage may be prominent.

The most characteristic lesions caused by yellow fever virus are seen in the liver, although liver failure is not generally the cause of death. The liver may have a yellowish color and be enlarged and fatty in consistency. In typical cases, marked necrosis of the midzone of the lobule is present. The necrosis extends both centrally and peripherally and on average involves 80 percent of the lobule in fatal cases.[5, 9] The cells bordering the central vein and portal areas usually are spared. Councilman and Torres bodies can be observed in hepatocytes. Little or no inflammatory response occurs, and the reticulin framework is preserved.

The kidneys generally are tense and swollen. Glomerular changes are minor, but acute tubular necrosis and fatty metamorphosis may be significant. Cloudy swelling, degeneration, and fatty infiltration may occur in the myocardial fibers. The spleen and lymph nodes are depleted of lymphocytes, and mononucleocytes or histiocytes accumulate in the follicles of the spleen. Edema and petechiae may be observed in the brain.

Laboratory Findings

Leukopenia and albuminuria are common findings in early disease. In severe cases, prolonged prothrombin and partial thromboplastin times, thrombocytopenia, fibrin split products, and elevated liver enzymes are observed. Total and conjugated serum bilirubin levels are elevated. Albumin levels in urine usually are less than 5 g/L, but in rare cases they may reach 40 g/L. The urine contains bile. Cerebrospinal fluid usually is normal but may be under increased pressure.

Differential Diagnosis

Clinically, yellow fever is difficult to differentiate from many other viral, bacterial, and parasitic infections, including other viral hemorrhagic fevers such as Lassa, Ebola, Marburg, and Rift Valley in Africa; the arenaviruses in the Americas; and dengue hemorrhagic fever in both continents. Other diseases that cause fever and jaundice, such as viral hepatitis, leptospirosis, falciparum malaria, tick-borne relapsing fever, typhus, typhoid, and Q fever, also should be considered in the differential diagnosis. A definitive diagnosis of yellow fever can be made only by using the appropriate laboratory test.

Laboratory Diagnosis

Specific laboratory diagnosis requires isolation of the virus, serologic tests, nucleic acid amplification, or immunohistochemical tests. Virus can be isolated most easily from acute-phase serum taken during the first 4 days of illness, but it has been isolated as long as 14 days after the onset of illness, as well as from the liver after death.[9] The most sensitive method of virus isolation is inoculation of mosquitoes followed by the use of AP-61 cell culture from *Aedes pseudoscutellaris* mosquitoes. Vero cells and inoculation of suckling mice also can be used but are less sensitive. Polymerase chain reaction primer sets can be used to amplify yellow fever–specific nucleic acid sequences from these same tissues with a sensitivity comparable to that of virus isolation. Viral antigen can be demonstrated in the liver by immunohistochemical methods.[2] Either fresh or formalin-fixed tissue can be used with these techniques, which may be performed to establish a virologic diagnosis after virus has been cleared from the blood.

Serologic diagnosis depends on the collection of properly timed acute- and convalescent-phase serum samples to demonstrate a rise in specific antibody. Serologic tests commonly used to diagnose yellow fever include hemagglutination inhibition (HI), complement fixation (CF), and the plaque reduction neutralization test (PRNT), as well as newer tests such as enzyme-linked immunosorbent assay (ELISA) for both IgG and IgM antibodies. The immunofluorescent assay (IFA) is used in some laboratories.

Antibodies detected by HI, PRNT, IFA, and IgM capture ELISA appear within 5 to 7 days after the onset of illness, whereas CF antibodies appear later, usually after 10 to 14 days. HI and PRNT antibodies persist at detectable levels for many years (>50) in most patients, whereas the duration of CF and IgM antibodies is uncertain, but they probably wane to undetectable levels after 12 to 18 months.

PRNT is the most sensitive and specific of the serologic tests. In patients who have had no previous flavivirus infection, this test can be used to make a specific diagnosis of yellow fever, as can IgM capture ELISA. Cross-reaction between yellow fever antigen and antibodies to other related flaviviruses complicates the serodiagnosis of this and other flavivirus diseases. HI, IFA, and IgG ELISA all are nonspecific tests in which considerable cross-reactivity with heterologous flavivirus antibodies occurs.

The use of yellow fever 17D vaccine in disease-endemic areas also may complicate serologic diagnosis. Vaccination induces low-titer (1:10 to 1:40) HI and neutralizing antibodies but no detectable immunofluorescent or CF antibodies. Vaccination also induces IgM antibody, which may remain at detectable levels for as long as 18 months. Vaccination of individuals who have had a previous flavivirus infection induces an anamnestic response of heterotypic flavivirus antibodies at high titer (≥1:1280).

Treatment

Treatment of yellow fever is supportive because no specific therapy exists.[5, 7] Antiviral drugs are not effective. Patients with severe disease requiring hospitalization should have complete bed rest with good nursing care and close monitoring of vital organ functions. Salicylates should be avoided, but mild sedatives may be helpful. Maintaining fluid and electrolyte balance is critical. Guidelines for intensive care of severe yellow fever cases have not been established. Secondary bacterial infections may occur and should be treated with appropriate antibiotics.

Prognosis

Mortality in all yellow fever infections is low (<5%), but in severe cases requiring hospitalization, it may be 20 to 50 percent.[5, 9] The prognosis is poor for patients who enter a period of intoxication with rapidly increasing albuminuria, jaundice, fever, and severe hemorrhage. Patients in the terminal stage of illness usually are somnolent, have below-normal temperatures, and may have intractable hiccups.

Prevention and Control

The most practical and cost-effective method of prevention of yellow fever is vaccination. A single dose of 17D vaccine provides effective, long-term (10 years) protection and should be used in the World Health Organization Expanded Program of Immunization in enzootic countries of Africa and the Americas.

The live, attenuated 17D vaccine is prepared from infected chicken embryos and produces effective immunity in more than 95 percent of recipients.[9] Adverse reactions are rare, but in recent years, such events in elderly persons have been reported increasingly.[4] Infants younger than 4 months have a high risk of encephalitis and should not be vaccinated with the live, attenuated 17D vaccine until they are 9 months of age. Pregnant women also should avoid being vaccinated because vaccine virus may infect the developing fetus, although the risk of adverse events associated with congenital infection is unknown. Finally, the live attenuated 17D vaccine should not be given to persons who are allergic to eggs or to those who are immunodeficient or receiving immunosuppressive drugs.

The other method of preventing yellow fever is mosquito control, especially during epidemic activity. The principal mosquito vector of urban yellow fever, *A. aegypti,* is a highly domesticated species that lives in and around the houses of humans.[1] It breeds primarily in artificial containers that collect rain water or in domestic water storage containers. The most sustainable and effective prevention, therefore, is to control, discard, or chemically treat larval habitats in the domestic environment.[1] This process is labor-intensive but can be done with the help of the citizens in the community.

Some authorities recommend adult mosquito control with insecticide space sprays, primarily ultra-low-volume sprays. Recent field trials, however, have shown this approach to be ineffective unless portable sprayers are used to treat the inside of each dwelling. Because of the excessive cost and lack of efficacy of ultra-low-volume application of insecticides, this method is not recommended.

Patients suspected of having yellow fever should be protected from mosquitoes. The most effective protection is to use a mosquito net on the bed during the acute febrile period of illness. Alternatively, patients can be kept in screened rooms.

REFERENCES

1. Gubler, D. J.: *Aedes aegypti* and *Aedes aegypti*–borne disease control in the 1990's: Top down or bottom up. Am. J. Trop. Med. Hyg. *40*:571–578, 1989.
2. Hall, W. C., Crowell, T. P., Watts, D. M., et al.: Demonstration of yellow fever and dengue antigens in formalin-fixed paraffin-embedded human liver by immunohistochemical analysis. Am. J. Trop. Med. Hyg. *145*:408–417, 1991.
3. Karabatos, N.: International Catalogue of Arboviruses, Including Certain Other Viruses of Vertebrates. San Antonio, TX, American Society of Tropical Medicine and Hygiene, 1985, updated in 2001.
4. Martin, M., Weld, L., Tsai, T., et al.: Advanced age as a risk factor for adverse events temporally associated with yellow fever vaccination. Emerg. Infect. Dis. 7:945–951, 2001.
5. McKee, K. T., and Monath, T. P.: Arboviruses of Africa. *In* Feigin, R. D., and Cherry, J. D. (eds.): Textbook of Pediatric Infectious Diseases. 3rd ed., Vol. 2. Philadelphia, W. B. Saunders, 1990, pp. 1435–1456.
6. Meegan, J. M.: Yellow fever. *In* Beran, G. W., and Steele, J. H. (eds.): Handbook of Zoonoses. 2nd ed. Boca Raton, FL, CRC Press, 1994, pp. 111–124.
7. Monath, T. P.: Yellow fever: A medically neglected disease. Report on a seminar. Rev. Infect. Dis. *9*:165–175, 1987.
8. Monath, T. P.: Yellow fever. *In* Monath, T. P. (ed.): The Arboviruses: Epidemiology and Ecology. Vol. 5. Boca Raton, FL, CRC Press, 1988, pp. 139–231.
9. Monath, T. P.: Yellow fever. *In* Strickland, G. T. (ed.): Hunter's Tropical Medicine. Philadelphia, W. B. Saunders, 1991, pp. 233–238.
10. Nasidi, A., Monath, T. P., DeCock, K., et al.: Urban yellow fever epidemic in western Nigeria, 1987. Trans. R. Soc. Trop. Med. Hyg. *83*:401, 1989.
11. Reed, W.: Recent researches concerning etiology, propagation and prevention of yellow fever, by the United States Army Commission. J. Hyg. *2*:101–119, 1902.
12. Strode, G. K.: Yellow Fever. New York, McGraw Hill, 1951.
13. Van der Stuyft, P. Gianella, A., Pirard, M., et al.: Urbanization of yellow fever in Santa Cruz, Bolivia. Lancet *353*:1558–1562, 1999.
14. [Yellow Fever, 1998–1999.] Wkly. Epidemiol. Rec. *75*(40):322–328, 2000.

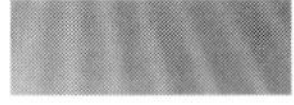

CHAPTER 179C

Dengue and Dengue Hemorrhagic Fever

SCOTT B. HALSTEAD

Dengue fever is an acute febrile illness syndrome caused by several arthropod-borne viruses and characterized by biphasic fever, myalgia or arthralgia, rash, leukopenia, and lymphadenopathy. Synonyms are dengue and breakbone fever. Dengue hemorrhagic fever (DHF), a febrile disease caused by dengue viruses, is characterized by abnormalities in hemostasis and by leakage of fluid and protein from capillaries, which in severe cases results in shock (dengue shock syndrome [DSS]). It is thought to have an immunopathologic basis. Synonyms are hemorrhagic dengue; acute infectious thrombocytopenic purpura; and Philippine, Thai, and Singapore hemorrhagic fever.

The dengue subgroup is composed of four antigenically distinct members.[21, 48, 56, 96] From 1956, according to reports received by the World Health Organization (WHO), dengue viruses were thought to be responsible for more than 5,000,000 hospital admissions and 72,000 deaths in Southeast Asia, southern China, India, Sri Lanka, Pakistan, Cuba, Venezuela, Colombia, Guyana, Brazil, Puerto Rico, and Central America, mostly in vital, healthy children. In Southeast Asian countries, dengue is among the 10 leading causes of death in children 1 to 14 years of age.

The first outbreak that resembled a disease now recognized as dengue fever was described by Benjamin Rush in Philadelphia, Pennsylvania, in 1780.[11, 103] Epidemics probably caused by dengue were common from the 18th to the 20th centuries in inhabitants of the Atlantic coastal areas of the United States and South America, the Caribbean Islands, and the Mississippi basin.[103] Dengue viruses almost certainly were the cause of the 5- and 7-day fevers that occurred in European colonists in tropical Asia.[11] Similar epidemics occurred commonly in settlers in tropical Australia, where in 1905, *Aedes aegypti* was identified as a dengue vector by Bancroft.[72] Ashburn and Craig[103] found the etiologic agent in human blood and showed that it could pass through a diatomaceous earth filter. An intrinsic incubation period of 3 to 8 days in humans, an extrinsic incubation period of 8 to 11 days in mosquitoes, immunity in people and monkeys, and the nonsusceptibility of most domestic animals were demonstrated in the classic studies of Siler and Simmons and their coworkers[103, 104] between 1924 and 1930. When dengue viruses were isolated in laboratory mice in 1943 and 1944, the modern era of dengue research began.[57, 98] Two strains from Hawaii and Papua New Guinea failed to cross-protect humans. From this experiment, researchers recognized the existence of at least two different dengue viruses; they were named dengue virus type 1 and type 2.[97, 98]

During most of the pre-virologic era, dengue viruses were thought to be the cause of a generally benign, self-limited febrile exanthem. However, death, shock, and severe hemorrhagic manifestations accompanied the classic dengue fever outbreaks in Australia in 1897 and for 15 years thereafter. Similar phenomena were recorded in Greece in 1928 and in Formosa in 1931.[35] This "new" syndrome was recognized again in Manila in 1954. It was called Philippine hemorrhagic fever because of a resemblance to the epidemic hemorrhagic fever then occurring in United Nations troops in the Korean Peninsula.[48] In 1956, Philippine hemorrhagic fever was associated with dengue when types 3 and 4 were recovered.[48] It now has become endemic throughout tropical Asia.[35, 43] Since 1967, the terms *dengue hemorrhagic fever* and *dengue shock syndrome* have come into general use.[18]

In 1981, Cuba reported a severe outbreak involving more than 116,000 patients hospitalized within 3 months, 10,000 of whom had DHF/DSS.[63] In 1986, an epidemic of DHF/DSS occurred on Hainan Island, China[80]; in 1988, the Maldive Islands, Sri Lanka, and India were involved.[105, 114] From about 1987, DHF/DSS outbreaks have occurred in Guyana, Venezuela, Brazil, Colombia, Central America, and on a lesser scale, Puerto Rico.[83]

By epidemiologic criteria, dengue viruses are arthropod-borne (arboviruses) because they are transmitted biologically by various members of the genus *Stegomyia*.[72, 75, 103, 104] Gene structure, replicative strategy, and antigenic relatedness place the dengue viruses in the family *Flaviviridae*.[56, 115] At present, 68 members of the flavivirus family have been identified; 29 of them are established as human pathogens.[56] Cross-comparisons by plaque reduction neutralization tests have shown dengue viruses to be an antigenic subgroup with little relationship to other flaviviruses.[21] In addition to their antigenic relatedness and their ability to be transmitted by *Stegomyia,* each type of dengue virus produces a closely similar clinical syndrome in susceptible human beings.[36, 97, 103, 104]

Dengue virions are spherical particles approximately 50 nm in diameter. The central core, approximately 25 nm in diameter, has icosahedral symmetry and contains a single plus strand of RNA. Dengue RNA consists of approximately 11,000 nucleotides coding from the 5′ end for core, premembrane, envelope, and five nonstructural proteins.[34] The envelope, which is studded with poorly resolved projections, is composed of many replicates of the envelope protein (54 kd) embedded in a lipid bilayer. When assembled on the virion, the envelope protein bears epitopes unique to serotypes. Antibodies to these epitopes neutralize by hindering viral entry into cells. Other epitopes are shared between dengue viruses (dengue subgroup antigens) and other flaviviruses (group antigens).

Four clearly defined types exist, as determined by plaque reduction neutralization tests using antibodies raised by infection of monkeys or fluorescent antibody tests using monoclonal antibodies raised in mice.[94] Presumably, the cell attachment receptor differs for each dengue serotype and is blocked by neutralizing antibody.[49] The four types have distinctive genetic structures.[9, 68, 69, 86, 87, 115, 118] Phylogenetic studies suggest that human dengue viruses diverged from four zoonotic dengue types relatively recently, whereas the four zoonotic types evolved from a common ancestor in the more remote past.[115] Different dengue strains cluster in groups that differ genetically (genotypes).[15, 16, 68, 69, 86, 110] Genotypes consist of viruses of similar genetic structure that usually circulate within one geographic area.[16, 69, 110] Genotyping can be used to trace the movement of dengue viruses between the continents. Of particular interest, a strain of dengue type 2 isolated in Jamaica in 1981 and the dengue 2 viruses recovered from 1981 Cuban DHF patients belong to the Southeast Asian genotype.[86, 100] The most sharply divergent genetic differences are among human viruses and strains from Asian and African zoonotic cycles.[86, 115]

Dengue virus can be grown in 1- to 2-day-old mice or hamsters by intracerebral inoculation or in various mosquitoes by oral or parenteral inoculation. High mouse-passaged virus grows and produces deaths in weanling mice. Various tissue cultures of vertebrate and invertebrate origin support dengue virus growth in vitro, as reviewed in the following section.

Transmission

A. aegypti, a daytime-biting mosquito, is the principal vector. All four virus types have been recovered from naturally infected *A. aegypti*.[35, 42] In most tropical areas, *A. aegypti* is highly domesticated and breeds in water stored for drinking, washing, or bathing or in any container collecting fresh water. Dengue viruses also have been recovered from naturally infected *Aedes albopictus,* which breeds outdoors in vegetation.[29, 35, 43, 75] Outbreaks in the Pacific area have been attributed to *Aedes scutellaris* and *Aedes polynesiensis*.

In urban areas, transmission of dengue may be explosive and involve as much as 70 to 80 percent of the population.[103] Because *A. aegypti* has a limited flight range, spread of virus is mainly via mobile viremic human beings.

Dengue viruses replicate in the gut, brain, and salivary glands of infected mosquitoes without apparent harm to adult mosquitoes.[59] Mosquitoes are infectious for a lifetime and as long as 70 days in experimental circumstances.[104] Because female mosquitoes take repeated blood meals, long-lived female mosquitoes have great potency as vectors. Several species of *Stegomyia* and *Toxorhynchites* are infected readily by intrathoracic inoculation, although the threshold of infection by oral feeding is higher.[89, 90] *A. aegypti* and *Culex quinquefasciatus* can transmit dengue mechanically by interrupted feeding.[106] The contribution of mechanical feeding to the spread of dengue virus during epidemics has never been measured, but because of the "skittishness" of *A. aegypti* and its habit of feeding during the day when its intended victim is awake and often moving, interrupted feeding with simultaneous transmission to multiple hosts must occur commonly.

A. aegypti preferentially feeds on people and, hence, is most abundant in and around human habitations. The mosquito preferentially breeds in clean water. Biting activity is reduced at temperatures below a wet bulb temperature of 14° C.[23] Transmission of dengue in temperate countries is interrupted during winter weather, and dengue has not established itself endemically at latitudes above 25 degrees north or south. Breeding sites may be provided by humans through living habits, as in Thailand, where water is stored in and around homes in large earthenware jars.[35, 42] In contrast, *A. aegypti* is not abundant in some parts of India because only small amounts of water are brought to homes from village wells for immediate use. Water in flower vases, household offerings, ant traps, coconut husks, tin cans, and rubber tires may supply breeding sites for *A. aegypti*.[29, 42]

In the tropics, outbreaks of dengue generally coincide with the monsoon season. Eggs, which resist desiccation, are deposited inside water containers above the water line.[42] With the beginning of monsoon rains, a large number of eggs laid outdoors are hatched. Indoor populations do not show seasonal change. Evidence indicates that biting rates increase with increased temperature and relative humidity.[102]

In sylvan settings, dengue virus has been isolated from three subgenera of *Aedes,* namely, *Stegomyia, Diceromyia,* and *Finlaya,* some in circumstances suggesting the occurrence of transovarial transmission. This phenomenon has been demonstrated experimentally, but its contribution to maintenance of virus in a habitat is unknown.[91]

Epidemiology

HOST RANGE

Inoculation of strains of dengue with known human pathogenicity does not produce demonstrable infection in adult chickens, lizards, guinea pigs, rabbits, hamsters, or cotton rats.[101, 103]

Subhuman primates are generally susceptible to infection by dengue viruses. Numerous species belonging to *Macaca, Cercopithecus, Cercocebus, Papio, Hylobates,* and *Pan* can be infected by the bite of virus-infected mosquitoes or by injection of infectious virus preparations.[101, 104] Infection is essentially asymptomatic. Viremia occurs at levels sufficient to infect mosquitoes. Simmons and colleagues[104] were the first to note that wild-caught *Macaca philippinensis* resisted dengue infection whereas *Macaca fuscatus* (Japanese macaque) was susceptible. Work by Rudnick[93] in Malaysia has revealed a jungle cycle of dengue transmission involving canopy-feeding monkeys and *Aedes niveus,* a species that feeds on both monkeys and humans. Although the existence of a jungle dengue cycle in the Malaysian rain forest has been documented, the full geographic range of the subhuman primate zoonotic reservoir is not known. In the early 1980s, an extensive epizootic of dengue virus type 2 apparently occurred and involved subhuman primates over wide areas of West Africa.[88] Genetic and epidemiologic studies have shown that urban human dengue and jungle monkey dengue are relatively compartmentalized.[86, 115] Urban dengue is vectored by anthropophilic mosquitoes, and the virus travels along routes of transportation. *A. aegypti* and susceptible humans are so abundant and so widespread that should dengue viruses be exchanged between humans and monkeys, detection would be extremely difficult. Should urban dengue be eliminated, the reintroduction of virus from jungle cycles could become important.

GEOGRAPHIC DISTRIBUTION

Outbreaks of dengue fever have been documented on every continent except Antarctica.[35] Evidence suggests that human dengue may have originated from enzootic or endemic foci in tropical Asia.[37, 75] The probable spread of *A. aegypti* during historical times from Africa throughout the world provided an ecologic niche quickly occupied by several human viral pathogens: yellow fever, chikungunya, and the dengue viruses. During the 18th and 19th centuries, epidemics occurred in newly settled lands, largely because of the necessity for storage of domestic water in frontier areas. Isolated shipboard or garrison outbreaks often confined to nonindigenous settlers or visitors were reported in Africa, the Indian subcontinent, and Southeast Asia.[11, 72, 103] During World War II, dengue virus infections occurred commonly in combatants of the Pacific War and spread to staging areas not normally infected: Japan, Hawaii, and Polynesia.[38, 97] After its introduction into the Western Hemisphere in 1977,[22] a Southeast Asian genotype, dengue virus type 1, appears to have remained in the region.[86] Dengue is endemic on the larger Caribbean islands and in coastal Central America and the tropical areas of Guyana, Venezuela, Colombia, Ecuador, Peru, and Brazil.[37, 42, 116] A sharp dengue virus type 2 epidemic in Cuba in 1981 led to island-wide *A. aegypti* control and apparent eradication of the virus.[82] In 1986 and 1987, dengue virus type 1 spread through most of coastal Brazil and from there to Paraguay and to Peru and Ecuador.[22, 29, 83] In 1990, more than 9000 dengue cases were reported from Venezuela; 2600 of them were classified as DHF, and 74 deaths were associated with the epidemic.[83] Dengue virus types 1, 2, and 4 were isolated.[83] Shortly thereafter, DHF/DSS caused by dengue type 2 was reported from Brazil and French Guiana.[79, 84] In 1995, dengue virus type 3 was introduced into the region.[53] In 1997, dengue virus type 2 with a Southeast Asian genotype was introduced into Santiago de Cuba and caused a sharp DHF/DSS outbreak observed only in individuals 20 years and older.[33] During the past 20 years, major epidemics of all four dengue serotypes have occurred on several Pacific islands.[29, 37, 38, 42]

Dengue virus types 1 and 2 have been recovered from humans with mild clinical illness in Nigeria in the absence of epidemic disease.[37] In 1983, dengue virus type 3 was isolated in Mozambique.[43] DHF/DSS has not been reported, and even dengue fever outbreaks are rare. In this respect, Africa resembles the situation in Haiti, where multiple dengue serotypes are transmitted at high rates among a predominantly black population, but severe disease is not recognized.[47]

DHF-like disease was described clinically in Thailand beginning in 1950 and in the Philippines from 1953. Cases were confirmed etiologically as dengue in 1958 and 1956, respectively.[48] DHF first was described in Singapore and Malaysia in 1962, Vietnam in 1963, India in 1963, Ceylon (Sri Lanka) in 1965, Indonesia in 1969, Burma (Myanmar), in 1970, China in 1985, and Kampuchea and Laos from about 1985, and major outbreaks have occurred in Sri Lanka and India since 1988, in French Polynesia since 1990, in Pakistan since 1998, and in Bangladesh since 1999.[1, 2, 26, 37, 38, 80, 105, 114, 119] DHF has occurred at consistently high endemicity in Thailand, Burma, and Vietnam and at a lower level in Indonesia.[43] In Thailand, it is the third ranking cause of hospitalization and death in children. Intermittent epidemics have involved Malaysia and the Philippines. The largest epidemic in history occurred in Southeast Asia in 1998, when more than 490,000 hospitalizations and 4000 deaths were reported to the WHO. The sharpest single outbreak involved 116,000 hospitalizations in a 3-month period in Cuba in 1981.[63]

Clinical Manifestations

DENGUE FEVER

Primary infections with dengue virus types 2 and 4 are thought to be largely inapparent, regardless of age.[33, 55, 112, 113] Primary infections with dengue virus types 1 and 3 in adults produce biphasic fever and rash as the most characteristic features of the dengue fever syndrome.[10, 20, 36, 72, 97, 104] Manifestations vary with age and among patients. In infants and young children, the disease may be undifferentiated or characterized by a 1- to 5-day fever, pharyngeal inflammation, rhinitis, and mild cough. A distinctive mean incubation period, duration of illness, or spectrum of clinical findings could characterize disease with different dengue types, although these factors have not been studied carefully. Differences in mild dengue syndromes, hospitalized dengue cases (predominantly during secondary dengue virus infections), and chikungunya illnesses are illustrated in the section on chikungunya (see Tables 179–4 through 179–8).

Chikungunya virus infections produce a dengue fever syndrome. Chikungunya illnesses begin more abruptly than dengue and are of shorter duration. Maculopapular rash, conjunctival injection, and myalgia or arthralgia occur more frequently in chikungunya than in dengue illnesses, but other features associated with both viruses are remarkably similar.[11, 77] DHF syndrome is differentiated from dengue fever by its association with thrombocytopenia and capillary leakage.[120]

In classic dengue fever, after an incubation period of 2 to 7 days, patients experience a sudden onset of fever, which rapidly rises to 39.5° to 41.4° C (103° to 106° F) and is usually accompanied by frontal or retro-orbital headache. Occasionally, back pain precedes the fever. A transient, macular, generalized rash that blanches under pressure may be seen during the first 24 to 48 hours of fever. The pulse rate may be slow in proportion to the degree of fever. Myalgia or bone pain occurs soon after onset and increases in severity. During the second to sixth day of fever, nausea and vomiting are apt to occur, and generalized lymphadenopathy, cutaneous hyperesthesia or hyperalgesia, aberrations in taste, and pronounced anorexia may develop.

One or 2 days after defervescence, a generalized, morbilliform, maculopapular rash appears, with sparing of the palms and soles. It disappears in 1 to 5 days. In some cases, edema of the palms and soles may be noted, and desquamation may occur. About the time of appearance of this second rash, the body temperature, which has fallen to normal, may become elevated slightly and establish the biphasic temperature curve.

Epistaxis, petechiae, and purpuric lesions, though uncommon, may occur at any stage of the disease. Swallowed blood from epistaxis may be passed per rectum or be vomited and could be interpreted as bleeding of gastrointestinal origin. Gastrointestinal bleeding, menorrhagia, and bleeding from other organs have been observed in some dengue fever outbreaks.[85, 111, 117] Very clear evidence argues that peptic ulcer predisposes to gastrointestinal hemorrhage; in some cases, patients may exsanguinate during an otherwise normal dengue fever.[111] This syndrome is confused with DSS and contributes to a misunderstanding of the pathogenesis of DHF/DSS. The mechanism of the hemorrhagic diathesis that commonly occurs with dengue virus infection is not known, but speculation centers on platelet abnormalities.

After the febrile stage, prolonged asthenia, mental depression, bradycardia, and ventricular extrasystoles are noted commonly in adults.[73]

DENGUE HEMORRHAGIC FEVER/DENGUE SHOCK SYNDROME

DHF/DSS is an acute vascular permeability syndrome accompanied by abnormal hemostasis. The incubation period of DHF/DSS is unknown, but presumed to be the same as that of dengue fever. In children, progression of the illness is characteristic.[18, 76, 77, 120] A relatively mild first phase with an abrupt onset of fever, malaise, vomiting, headache, anorexia, and cough may be followed after 2 to 5 days by rapid deterioration and physical collapse. In Thailand, the median day of admission to the hospital after the onset of fever is day 4. In this second phase, the patient usually has cold, clammy extremities, a warm trunk, a flushed face, and diaphoresis. Patients are restless and irritable and complain of midepigastric pain. Frequently, scattered petechiae appear on the forehead and extremities, spontaneous ecchymoses may develop, and easy bruisability and bleeding at sites of venipuncture are common findings. Circumoral and peripheral cyanosis may occur. Respirations are rapid and often labored. The pulse is weak, rapid, and thready, and the heart sounds are faint. The pulse pressure is frequently narrow (≤20 mm Hg); systolic and diastolic pressure may be low or unobtainable. The liver may become palpable two or three fingerbreadths below the costal margin and is usually firm and nontender. Chest radiographs show unilateral (right) or bilateral pleural effusions. Approximately 10 percent of patients have gross ecchymosis or gastrointestinal bleeding. After a 24- or 36-hour period of crisis, convalescence is fairly rapid in children who recover. The temperature may return to normal before or during the stage of shock.

Pathogenesis and Pathology

In rhesus monkeys experimentally infected with dengue virus by subcutaneous inoculation, virus replicates in the skin. Virus disseminated rapidly to regional lymph nodes and then to lymphatic tissue throughout the body.[73] Early in the viremic period, virus could be recovered only from the skin inoculation site and lymph nodes, whereas 2 to 3 days later, evidence of general dissemination to skin and other tissues was found. Virus was recovered from the skin, lymph nodes, and several leukocyte-rich tissues for up to 3 days after termination of viremia. Virus could be recovered from circulating leukocytes and from the skin only at the end of the viremic period. The number of sites from which virus can be recovered increases as the infection progresses. Intracellular infection is terminated abruptly 2 to 3 days after viremia ceases.

In humans, dengue viruses infect and replicate efficiently in intracutaneous Langerhans cells in vitro and in tissue explants.[121] Virus ultimately targets liver parenchymal cells, where infection produces apoptosis, but such cells may not serve as replicative hosts.[51] Late in infection, virus is found associated with circulating B lymphocytes.[58] Fluorescent antibody, virus isolation, and electron-microscopic studies suggest mononuclear phagocytes as major infection hosts.[5, 37–41, 43, 78]

Animals infected initially with dengue virus type 1, 3, or 4 and then with dengue type 2 virus had higher viremia than when the same strain was inoculated into susceptible animals.[39, 41, 43] This phenomenon, in vivo antibody enhancement of dengue virus infection, provides an explanatory hypothesis of the immunopathogenesis of dengue in humans. Epidemiologic, clinical, and virologic studies of DHF/DSS in humans have shown a significant association between severe illness and infection in the presence of circulating dengue antibody, whether passively acquired from the mother or actively acquired from previous infection.[9, 31, 32, 44, 59, 60, 95, 99] This circulating antibody has two biologic activities: neutralization of virus and enhancement of infection.[36, 44] In Thailand, DHF/DSS developed in infants during dengue virus type 2 infection only when maternal neutralizing antibody had catabolized to low titer and infection-enhancing antibodies were left in circulation.[59] Similarly, in a prospective study of dengue virus infection in Thai children, DHF/DSS occurred in children who had circulating enhancing antibodies from a previous single dengue virus infection, but it did not occur in children whose first infection left them with low levels of cross-reactive dengue virus type 2 neutralizing antibody at the time of the second dengue virus infection.[60] A similar mechanism explains the failure of secondary infections to produce DHF/DSS with the American genotype dengue type 2.[116] American genotype dengue 2 viruses are significantly neutralized by human anti–dengue 1, whereas Southeast Asian dengue 2 viruses are not.[62] The full-length sequences of the American and Southeast Asian dengue 2 genomes reveal limited amino acid differences.[68]

In vitro studies of dengue virus type 2 demonstrated enhanced growth in cultures of human mononuclear phagocytes that were supplemented with very small quantities of dengue antibodies.[45] Investigators have proposed that the number of infected mononuclear phagocytes in individuals with naturally or passively acquired antibody may exceed that in nonimmune individuals.[38, 39] In serial blood samples early in the illness in children experiencing secondary dengue infections, enhanced viremia levels predicted severe disease.[113] Vascular permeability is thought to result when infected cells are attacked by activated T lymphocytes, with the subsequent release of vasoactive cytokines.[3, 27, 28, 38, 39, 41, 64, 74, 92] Cytokine production should be quantitatively related to the number of infected target cells. The reduced risk for DHF/DSS in protein-calorie malnourished children[109] and the increased risk for DHF/DSS in girls versus boys are consistent with the hypothesis that a competent immune elimination system must be available to generate the cytokines that produce DHF/DSS.[39–41]

Evidence indicates the existence of a human dengue resistance gene. Epidemiologic studies of the 1981 Cuban outbreak demonstrated a higher risk for DHF/DSS in whites than blacks.[31, 62] A search for DHF/DSS in black children in Haiti revealed no cases despite high dengue type 1, 2, and 4 infection rates and circulation of the Southeast Asian genotype dengue 2 viruses.[47] Several HLA antigens have shown differing frequencies in DHF/DSS cases and controls.[13] Early in the acute stage of secondary dengue virus infection, rapid activation of the complement system occurs.[8, 81] During shock, blood levels of C1q, C3, C4, C5, C6, C7, C8, and C3 proactivator are depressed and C3 catabolic rates are elevated. The blood clotting and fibrinolytic systems are activated. As yet, neither the mediator of vascular permeability nor the complete mechanism of bleeding has been unequivocally identified. The kinin system apparently is not involved. Recent studies suggest a role for tumor necrosis factor, interleukin-2, and interferon-γ.[64, 92] Capillary damage allows fluid, electrolytes, protein, and in some instances, red blood cells to leak into intravascular spaces. This internal redistribution of fluid, together with deficits caused by fasting, thirsting, and vomiting, results in hemoconcentration, hypovolemia, increased cardiac work, tissue hypoxia, metabolic acidosis, and hyponatremia. A mild degree of disseminated intravascular coagulation, plus liver damage and thrombocytopenia, could contribute additively to produce hemorrhage.

If tissue cultures or suckling mice are used for virus recovery, dengue virus is usually absent in tissues at the time of death.[78] If patients experienced a second dengue infection, their tissue suspensions contain large quantities of dengue-neutralizing antibodies. The use of mosquito inoculation techniques improves viral isolation rates.[89, 90, 107] Genetic probes increase viral detection sensitivity still further.[51]

On pathologic examination, usually no gross or microscopic lesions are found that might account for death.[5] In rare instances, death may be caused by gastrointestinal or intracranial hemorrhage. Minimal to moderate hemorrhage is seen in the upper gastrointestinal tract, and petechial hemorrhage occurs frequently in the intraventricular septum of the heart, on the pericardium, and on the subserosal surfaces of major viscera. Focal hemorrhaging is seen occasionally in the lungs, liver, adrenals, and subarachnoid space. The liver usually is enlarged, often with fatty changes. Yellow, watery, at times blood-tinged effusions are present in serous cavities in approximately three fourths of patients. Retroperitoneal tissues are markedly edematous.

On microscopic examination, perivascular edema in soft tissues and widespread diapedesis of red blood cells can be seen. Maturational arrest of megakaryocytes may be noted in the bone marrow,[66] and increased numbers of such megakaryocytes are seen in the capillaries of the lungs, in the renal glomeruli, and in the sinusoids of the liver and spleen. Proliferation of lymphocytoid and plasmacytoid cells, lymphocytolysis, and lymphophagocytosis occur in the spleen and lymph nodes. In the spleen, malpighian corpuscle germinal centers are necrotic. Depletion of lymphocytes occurs in the thymus. In the liver, varying degrees of fatty metamorphosis, focal midzonal necrosis, and hyperplasia of Kupffer cells are present. Non-nucleated cells with vacuolated acidophilic cytoplasm resembling Councilman bodies (apoptotic hepatocytes[51]) are seen in the sinusoids. A mild, proliferative glomerulonephritis is present. Biopsy specimens of the skin rash reveal swelling and minimal necrosis of endothelial cells, subcutaneous deposits of fibrinogen, and in a few cases, dengue antigen in extravascular mononuclear cells and on blood vessel walls.[40, 43]

Diagnosis

DENGUE FEVER

A clinical diagnosis can be made by having a high index of suspicion and knowledge of the geographic distribution and ecology of dengue viruses. Activities of the patient during the period preceding the onset of illness may give important clues to the possibility of infection.

The differential diagnosis includes many viral, respiratory, and influenza-like diseases and the early stages of malaria, typhoid fever, scrub typhus, hepatitis, and leptospirosis. Abortive forms of these latter diseases may never evolve beyond a dengue-like stage. Four arbovirus diseases are dengue-like: chikungunya and o'nyong-nyong fever (togaviruses), West Nile fever (flavivirus), and Oropouche (bunyavirus). Four others are dengue-like but without rash: Colorado tick fever, sandfly fever, Ross River fever, and the mild form of Rift Valley fever. Because of the variation in clinical findings and the multiplicity of possible causative agents, the descriptive term dengue-like disease should be used until a specific etiologic diagnosis is provided by the laboratory.

DENGUE HEMORRHAGIC FEVER/DENGUE SHOCK SYNDROME

According to WHO criteria, DHF is a dengue illness accompanied by thrombocytopenia (<100,000/mm^3) and hemoconcentration (hematocrit >20% of the recovery value). Early detection of vascular permeability remains a diagnostic problem; however, the use of strain-gauge plethysmography documents up to 50 percent higher microvascular permeability in DHF/DSS patients than controls.[4] Pleural or peritoneal effusions are virtually pathognomonic. DSS is diagnosed when these manifestations are accompanied by hypotension or narrow pulse pressure (≤20 mm Hg). In areas endemic for dengue, hemorrhagic fever should be suspected in children with a febrile illness who exhibit shock and hemoconcentration with thrombocytopenia. Hypoproteinemia, hemorrhagic manifestations, and hepatic enlargement are frequent accompanying findings. Because many rickettsial diseases, meningococcemia, and other severe illnesses caused by a variety of agents may produce a similar clinical picture, the diagnosis should be made only when epidemiologic or serologic evidence suggests the possibility of dengue. Hemorrhagic manifestations have been described in other diseases of viral origin, including the arenavirus hemorrhagic fevers of Argentina, Bolivia, and West Africa (Lassa fever); the tick-borne hemorrhagic fevers of India and the former Soviet Union; hemorrhagic fever with renal syndrome, which occurs across northern Eurasia, specifically, from Scandinavia to Korea; and Marburg and Ebola virus infections in central Africa.[54]

Laboratory Studies

An etiologic diagnosis can be made by serologic study of a properly collected serum sample or by isolation of the virus.[52, 120]

Blood should be obtained during or after the febrile period but before 1 month elapses after the onset of illness. The acute-phase serum or plasma collected for virus isolation should be stored optimally at −65° C or colder. Serologic diagnosis depends on a fourfold or greater increase in antibody titer by hemagglutination inhibition, complement fixation, radioimmunoassay, enzyme-linked immunosorbent assay (ELISA), or neutralization. IgM capture ELISA has revolutionized dengue serology, and commercial kits are available.[19] Primary and sequential (secondary) dengue virus infections result in the production of dengue-reactive IgM antibodies, which appear during the acute phase and disappear within 60 days of infection.[52] Secondary or primary dengue virus infections can be confirmed in a single serum specimen by quantitating IgM-IgG antibody ratios. IgG antibody concentrations are abundant in secondary but minimal in primary dengue virus infection. Sequential infection with dengue virus followed by Japanese encephalitis virus, or vice versa, produces relatively specific IgM antibodies to the recent infecting virus.[52]

Numerous techniques are available for the recovery and identification of dengue viruses.[101, 120] Recommendations for general use have been made by a WHO expert committee.[120] Acute-phase serum, mosquito suspensions, or other materials thought to contain dengue virus may be inoculated into suckling mice, which may be examined for sickness or subtle neurologic signs or challenged at 14 days with a neurovirulent dengue virus. Repeated subpassage markedly increases the neurovirulence of dengue virus. Alternatively, materials may be inoculated into any of several tissue cultures of mammalian or mosquito origin and examined for plaques under agar or methylcellulose overlay, for cytopathic effect or resistance to a challenge cytopathic virus by use of a fluid overlay, or for fluorescence or other markers with the use of an appropriate detection system. Intrathoracic inoculation of *A. albopictus, A. aegypti,* or *Toxorhynchites* spp. is a highly sensitive dengue virus recovery system.[89, 90] The presence of virus in mosquitoes may be detected by a fluorescent antibody test, complement fixation, or inoculation of mosquito suspension in tissue culture.

Treatment

DENGUE FEVER

Treatment is supportive. Bed rest is advised during the febrile period. Antipyretics or cold sponging should be used to keep the body temperature below 40° C (104° F). Paracetamol (10–15 mg/kg every 4–6 hours) is the preferred antipyretic agent. Analgesics or mild sedation may be required to control pain. Fluid and electrolyte replacement therapy is required when deficits caused by sweating, fasting, thirsting, vomiting, or diarrhea are present. Because of the risk of Reye syndrome and the dengue hemorrhagic diathesis, aspirin should not be given to reduce fever or control pain.

DENGUE HEMORRHAGIC FEVER/DENGUE SHOCK SYNDROME

Explicit recommendations for management of DSS have been made by a WHO expert committee.[120] These, plus earlier recommendations by Cohen and Halstead[18] and recent studies by Dung and colleagues,[25] are the basis of this section.

No specific antiviral treatment exists, but in DHF/DSS, symptomatic and supportive measures are effective.

The major pathophysiologic abnormality seen in DHF/DSS is an acute increase in vascular permeability that leads to leakage of plasma. Plasma volume studies revealed a reduction of more than 20 percent in severe cases. Supporting evidence of plasma leakage (and consequent hypovolemia) includes a rapid, weak pulse; diaphoresis; cool, pale skin of the extremities; decreased urine output; and direct measurement by strain-gauge plethysmography,[4] pleural effusion on chest radiography, hemoconcentration, and hypoproteinemia. Pleural effusion may not be evident until after fluid resuscitation is started.

In the absence of increased vascular permeability, clinically significant hemoconcentration may result from thirst, dehydration, fever, anorexia, and vomiting. Fluid intake by mouth should be as ample as tolerated. Electrolyte and dextrose solution (as used in diarrheal disease), fruit juice, or both are preferable to plain water. With high fever, a risk of convulsions exists, so antipyretic drugs may be indicated. Salicylates should be avoided because they are known to cause bleeding and acidosis. Acetaminophen is preferable at the following doses: younger than 1 year, 60 mg per dose; 1 to 3 years of age, 60 to 120 mg per dose; 3 to 6 years of age, 120 mg per dose; and 6 to 12 years of age, 240 mg per dose.

Children should be observed closely for early signs of shock. The critical period is the transition from the febrile to the afebrile phase. Frequent hematocrit determinations are essential because they reflect the degree of plasma leakage and the need for administration of intravenous fluid. Hemoconcentration usually precedes changes in blood pressure and pulse. The hematocrit should be determined daily from the third day until the temperature becomes normal for 1 or 2 days.

Oral or parenteral fluid therapy can be administered in an outpatient rehydration unit for correction of dehydration or acidosis or when signs of hemoconcentration are present. The volume of fluid and its composition are similar to the fluids used for the treatment of diarrhea with moderate dehydration. The schedule in Table 179–3 is recommended as a guideline. The fluids should consist of the following:

- One third to half the total fluid as physiologic saline solution.
- Half to two thirds of the remainder as 5 percent glucose in water.
- For acidosis: one fourth of the total fluids should be one-sixth molar sodium bicarbonate.
- Solution for fluid therapy in DHF: lactated Ringer solution, 5 percent glucose in one-half normal physiologic saline solution, 5 percent glucose in one-half lactated Ringer solution, 5 percent glucose in one-third physiologic saline solution.
- Fluids as listed are calculated to be given over a 24-hour period. If the child seems severely dehydrated, half the calculated fluid is given in the first 8 hours and the second half in the next 16 hours. During rapid administration of fluids, watching for signs of cardiac failure is especially important.

TABLE 179–3 ■ FLUID THERAPY*

	mL/kg Body Weight/24 hr		
Weight on Admission	First Day	Second Day	Third Day
<7 kg	220	165	132
7–11 kg	165	132	88
12–18 kg	132	88	88
>18 kg	88	88	88

*See text for composition of fluids.

Written orders should be explicit about the type of solution and the rate of administration. A rough estimate of flow may be derived from the formula

$$\text{mL/hr} = \text{Drops/min} \times 3$$

SHOCK

Patients should be hospitalized and immediately treated when they have any of the following signs and symptoms of shock: restlessness/lethargy, cold extremities and circumoral cyanosis, rapid and feeble pulses, narrowing of pulse pressure (≤20 mm Hg) or hypotension, and a sudden rise in hematocrit or a continuously elevated hematocrit despite the administration of intravenous fluid.

Shock is a medical emergency. Immediate administration of intravenous fluid to expand plasma volume is essential. In children, shock may develop or subside over a 48-hour period, so close observation 24 hours a day is imperative. Patients with similar degrees of severity should be grouped together. Those with shock require intensive 24-hour care by nurses and physicians. Paramedical workers or parents can assist in oral fluid therapy or in surveillance of the rate of intravenous fluid administration and general status of the patient.

Initial fluid therapy with lactated Ringer or isotonic saline solution (20 mL/kg intravenously) infused as rapidly as possible may be required. Positive pressure may be necessary. In continued or profound shock, plasma expanders (6% dextran 70 or 6% hydroxyethylstarch [MW 200,000]) may be given to replace the initial fluid and administered at a rate of 10 to 15 mL/kg/hr or more until improvement in vital signs is apparent. In most cases, not more than 20 to 30 mL/kg of plasma is needed.

Intravenous fluids (5% dextrose, half-normal lactated Ringer or half-normal saline solution) are continued, even after improvement in vital signs and a declining hematocrit. The rate of fluid replacement should be adjusted as judged by the rate of plasma loss. Plasma loss may continue for 24 to 48 hours. Microhematocrit determination is a simple and reliable index for estimating plasma leakage. Monitoring of central venous pressure may be necessary in the management of severe cases of shock that are not easily reversible.

Administration of intravenous fluids should be discontinued when the hematocrit drops to approximately 40 percent and the patient's appetite improves. Good urine flow indicates sufficient circulating volume. In general, fluid therapy is not needed beyond 48 hours after termination of the shock. Extravasated plasma is reabsorbed and causes a further drop in hematocrit after the administration of intravenous fluid is stopped; if more fluid is given, hypervolemia, pulmonary edema, or heart failure may result. Of importance is that a drop in hematocrit at this stage not be viewed as a sign of internal hemorrhage. A strong pulse and blood pressure along with a wide pulse pressure and diuresis are good vital signs at this resorption phase. They rule out the likelihood of the presence of gastrointestinal hemorrhage, which occurs most frequently during the shock stage.

Hyponatremia and, commonly, metabolic acidosis occur. Electrolyte and blood gas determinations should be performed periodically in severely ill patients, as well as in those who do not seem to respond as promptly as expected. These determinations will provide an estimate of the sodium deficit and help determine the presence and degree of acidosis. Acidosis, in particular, may lead to disseminated intravascular coagulation if uncorrected. The use of heparin may be indicated in some of these patients, but extreme caution should be exercised in its use. In general, early volume replacement and early correction of acidosis with sodium bicarbonate result in a favorable outcome, and heparin is not required. Heparin should be reserved for patients with laboratory evidence of consumptive coagulopathy (disseminated intravascular coagulation) or intractable bleeding.

Sedatives are needed in some cases because of marked agitation. Hepatotoxic drugs should be avoided. Chloral hydrate orally or rectally is recommended in a dose of 30 to 50 mg/kg as a single hypnotic dose (maximal dose, 1 g). In patients without pulmonary complications, paraldehyde, 0.1 mL/kg intramuscularly (maximal dose, 10 mL), also may be used.

Oxygen therapy should be given to all patients in shock, but an oxygen mask or tent may increase apprehension.

Blood transfusion is indicated only in patients with severe bleeding (e.g., gastrointestinal bleeding, hematemesis, melena). Fresh whole blood is preferable. Blood grouping and matching for prompt treatment should be carried out as a routine precaution for every patient in shock.

Generally, steroids do not shorten the duration of disease or improve the prognosis in children receiving careful supportive therapy.[108]

Frequent recording of vital signs and determination of hematocrit are important in evaluating the results of treatment. If patients show any signs of shock, vigorous antishock therapy should be instituted promptly. Patients should be monitored constantly until it is reasonably certain that the danger has passed. In practice, the following should be carried out:

1. Pulse, blood pressure, respiratory rate, and temperature should be taken every 15 to 30 minutes or more often, until the shock resolves.
2. Hematocrit or hemoglobin studies should be performed every 2 hours for the first 6 hours and then every 4 hours thereafter until the patient is stable.
3. An accurate record of intake and output, including the type of fluid given, should be made. The frequency and volume of urine output should be recorded.

A pro forma sheet for recording symptoms, signs, and treatment of DHF and DSS cases is useful.

A blinded comparison of four intravenous fluids by Dung and associates[25] provided evidence that the relatively more expensive lactated Ringer solution provides no greater benefit than 0.9 percent saline does. Dextran could contribute to altered hemostasis.[46] Patients with DHF/DSS are resuscitated as though they have diarrhea. A more apt therapeutic analogy may be burn injury or hypovolemia from "third-space" loss in surgery. Of interest would be a trial of small-volume hypertonic saline with or without colloid.[46] The widespread and unstudied use of blood products to treat hemorrhage or simple thrombocytopenia[14] suggests a need for many more careful studies of DHF/DSS resuscitation.[46] In this regard, placebo-controlled or blinded studies are the ideal.[25, 108]

EPIDEMIC DENGUE HEMORRHAGIC FEVER

During epidemics, outpatient and inpatient facilities may be overwhelmed. Under these conditions, only children requiring hospital care should be admitted. A recently elevated body temperature and positive tourniquet test are sufficient to suggest DHF; when possible, a microhematocrit and platelet count should be performed in the outpatient department. Patients with thrombocytopenia and an elevated hematocrit should be sent to a rehydration ward or, if the hematocrit does not fall or rises in the face of fluid therapy, admitted to a hospital. If a patient lives a long distance from the hospital and nearby accommodations are not available, admission for observation may be necessary.

Triage can be performed by properly instructed paramedical workers. Competent laboratory assistance is an essential factor.

Cool extremities, skin congestion, circumoral cyanosis, and a rapid pulse are signs that suggest the need for hospitalization. Patients should be hospitalized until 2 days after the fever terminates.

REGULATORY MEASURES

Dengue diseases are not subject to international quarantine or surveillance regulations. An intensive and effective voluntary reporting system has been devised by the regional offices of the WHO.

Prognosis

All patients suspected of having DHF need not be hospitalized because circulatory failure and shock may develop in only approximately a third of patients. Mild and moderate cases may be treated on an outpatient basis. For the purpose of early recognition of shock, parents should be advised to bring the patient back if evidence of clinical deterioration is noted or such warning signs as restlessness with or without lethargy, severe abdominal pain, cold extremities, and skin congestion occur on or after the third day following the onset of fever.

In most cases, early and effective replacement of lost plasma with plasma, plasma expanders, or fluid and electrolyte solutions (or any combination of these products) results in a favorable outcome. The acute onset of shock and the rapid, often dramatic clinical recovery, together with the fact that no destructive or inflammatory vascular lesions are observed, suggest that the disease is produced by transient functional vascular changes caused by short-acting pharmacologic mediators.

Sequelae in dengue or in DHF have not been studied systematically. Common sequelae of mild and uncomplicated dengue virus infection include bradycardia and ventricular extrasystoles during the convalescent stage, often persisting for several weeks. Profound asthenia with or without mental depression has been described. In DHF/DSS, great care must be taken to reduce invasive procedures for managing shock. Nosocomial infections such as gram-negative sepsis can masquerade as DHF/DSS. Overhydration during the shock resuscitation phase may lead to heart failure and a complicated, stormy post-shock stage. Infrequently, residual brain damage occurs, apparently as a result of either prolonged shock or, occasionally, intracranial hemorrhage. Children in whom profound shock develops rapidly with no detectable diastolic pressure or with unobtainable blood pressure, children in shock with delayed admission to the hospital, or children in shock with gastrointestinal hemorrhage have a poor prognosis. Mortality rates may exceed 50 percent in these groups.

Prevention

Tissue culture–based vaccines for dengue virus types 1, 2, 3, and 4 are immunogenic but not yet licensed for use.[6, 7] Numerous multivalent dengue vaccines using a variety of approaches are in various stages of development.[30, 50, 61, 65] At present, prophylaxis depends on the use of insecticides, repellents, protective body clothing, and screens on houses to avoid mosquito bites. Destruction of *A. aegypti* breeding sites is also effective.[16] If water storage is mandatory, a tight-fitting lid or a thin layer of oil may prevent eggs from being deposited or hatching. A larvicide such as temefos (Abate), which is available as a 1 percent sand granule formulation and effective at a concentration of 1 ppm, may be added safely to drinking water.

EPIDEMIC MEASURES

The WHO recommendations are as follows. On the basis of epidemiologic and entomologic information, the size of the area that requires adult mosquito abatement should be determined. With technical-grade malathion or fenitrothion at 438 mL/hectare, two adulticide treatments at a 10-day interval should be made with the use of a vehicle-mounted or portable ultra-low-volume aerosol generator or mist blower.[71, 120] Cities of moderate size should stockpile at least one vehicle-mounted aerosol generator, five mist blowers, 10 swing fog machines, and 1000 L of ultra-low-volume insecticide to be prepared to perform adulticide operations over a 20-km^2 area rapidly. With limited funds, such equipment and insecticides can be stockpiled centrally for rapid transportation when required. Priority areas for launching ground applications are those that have a concentration of cases. Special attention should be focused on areas where people congregate during daylight hours, such as hospitals and schools. If necessary, ultra-low-volume insecticides may be applied from aircraft. C47 or similar aircraft, smaller agricultural spray planes, and helicopters have been used to make aerial applications.

During the early stages of epidemics, an ultra-low-volume spray of 4 percent malathion in diesel oil or kerosene may be used to spray all houses within a 100-m radius of the residence of DHF patients.

ERADICATION AND CONTROL

A. aegypti was eradicated successfully from countries and whole continents with use of the techniques pioneered by the Rockefeller Foundation in its worldwide program to control urban yellow fever.[106] With time, the species successfully re-established itself in much of its former range. An eradication campaign in the United States was abandoned and replaced by a program of disease surveillance and containment of introduced virus.

Mosquito control or eradication programs require the simultaneous use of two approaches: a reduction in breeding sites and the application of larvicides. Alternatively, a significant reduction in population may be effected by closely spaced applications of adulticide.[82]

Source reduction requires the support of the population, either by legal sanctions or by voluntary actions (see the following section). Source reduction campaigns should be well organized, supervised, and evaluated. Proper disposal of discarded cans, bottles, tires, and other potential breeding sites not used for storage of drinking or bathing water should be performed. Sides of water storage containers should be scrubbed to remove eggs when the water level is low. Water storage containers for drinking and bathing and flower vases should be emptied completely once weekly. Water containers that cannot be emptied should be treated with Abate 1 percent sand granules at a dosage of 1 ppm (e.g., 10 g of sand to 100 L of water). Treatments should be repeated at intervals of 2 to 3 months.

Vehicle-mounted or portable ultra-low-volume aerosol generators or mist blowers can be used to apply technical-grade malathion or fenitrothion at 438 mL/hectare. Three applications made at 1-week intervals can suppress *A. aegypti* populations for about 2 months.

In dengue-endemic countries, little effort has been made to adopt building codes or waste collection methods to reduce mosquito breeding sites.[67] Furthermore, almost no way has been found to use the private sector to effect vector control despite ample evidence of success in the United States.[12, 17]

HEALTH EDUCATION

Control of *A. aegypti* has been maintained effectively in some tropical areas through the simple expedient of emptying water containers once a week. During the yellow fever campaigns, strong sanitary laws made the breeding of mosquitoes on premises a crime punishable by fine or jail.[106] In the modern era, Singapore and Cuba have adopted these measures successfully. Health education through mass media or through the schools has been attempted in Burma, Thailand, Malaysia, and Indonesia, but without spectacular success.[24] The goals of health education and community participation approaches are to make the population aware of the identity of the vector of DHF, describe its biting habits (daytime feeding) and its breeding habits (containers holding clean water), and motivate people to reduce breeding sources by emptying water from containers on a regular basis.[42] The use of piped water rather than water storage should be encouraged. Studies in Malaysia after the 1973 epidemic of DHF indicated a very low level of functional knowledge among the inhabitants of Kuala Lumpur, Malaysia, about the vector of DHF.[24] Discouragingly, persons who were informed correctly, in most instances, took no action to protect themselves against mosquito breeding in their homes. This reaction is in contrast to the present situation in Singapore, where stiff fines and frequent inspections have reduced infestation by *A. aegypti* drastically. Extensive effort is being made to apply social science methods to gain the voluntary participation of the population in sustained mosquito control programs.[70]

REFERENCES

1. Ahmad, K.: Bangladeshi government appeals to WHO. Lancet *356*:409, 2000.
2. Akram, D. S., Igarashi, A., and Takasu, T.: Dengue virus infection among children with undifferentiated fever in Karachi. Indian J. Pediatr. *65*:735–740, 1998.
3. Bethell, D. B., Flobbe, K., Phuong, C. X. T., et al.: Pathophysiologic and prognostic role of cytokines in dengue hemorrhagic fever. J. Infect. Dis. *177*:778–782, 1998.
4. Bethell, D. B., Gamble, J., Pham, P. L., et al.: Noninvasive measurement of microvascular leakage in patients with dengue hemorrhagic fever. Clin. Infect. Dis. *32*:243–253, 2001.
5. Bhamarapravati, N., Toochinda, P., and Boonyapaknavik, V.: Pathology of Thailand hemorrhagic fever: A study of 100 autopsy cases. Ann. Trop. Med. Parasitol. *61*:500–510, 1967.
6. Bhamarapravati, N., and Yoksan, S.: Live attenuated tetravalent dengue vaccine. Vaccine *18*(Suppl. 2):44–47, 2000.
7. Bhamarapravati, N., Yoksan, S., Chayaniyayothin, T., et al.: Immunization with a live attenuated dengue-2-virus candidate vaccine (16681-PDK 53): Clinical, immunological and biological responses in adult volunteers. Bull. World Health Organ. *65*:189–195, 1987.
8. Bokisch, V. A., Top, F. H., Jr., Russell, P. K., et al.: The potential pathogenic role of complement in dengue hemorrhagic shock syndrome. N. Engl. J. Med. *289*:996–1000, 1973.
9. Burke, D. S., Nisalak, A., Johnson, D. E., et al.: A prospective study of dengue infections in Bangkok. Am. J. Trop. Med. Hyg. *38*:172–180, 1988.
10. Carey, D. E., Myers, R. M., and Reuben, R.: Studies on dengue in Vellore, South India. Am J. Trop. Med. Hyg. *15*:580–587, 1966.
11. Carey, S. E.: Chikungunya and dengue: A case of mistaken identity? J. Hist. Med. Allied Sci. *26*:243–262, 1971.
12. Challet, G. L.: Mosquito abatement district programs in the United States. Kaohsiung J. Med. Sci. *10*(Suppl.):67–73, 1994.
13. Chiewsilp, P., Scott, R. M., and Bhamarapravati N.: Histocompatibility antigens and dengue hemorrhagic fever. Am. J. Trop. Med. *30*:1101–1105, 1981.
14. Chuansumrit, A., Pimolthares, V., Tardtong, P., et al.: Transfusion requirements in patients with dengue hemorrhagic fever. Southeast Asian J. Trop. Med. Public Health *31*:10–14, 2000.
15. Chungue, E., Cassar, O., Drouet, M. T., et al.: Molecular epidemiology of dengue-1 and dengue-4 viruses. J. Gen. Virol. *76*:1877–1884, 1995.
16. Chungue, E., Deubel, V., Cassar, O., et al.: Molecular epidemiology of dengue 3 viruses and genetic relatedness among dengue 3 strains isolated from patients with mild or severe form of dengue fever in French Polynesia. J. Gen. Virol. *74*:1765–1770, 1993.
17. Clarke, J. L.: Privatization of mosquito control services in urban areas. Kaohsiung J. Med. Sci. *10*(Suppl.):74–77, 1994.
18. Cohen, S. N., and Halstead, S. B.: Shock associated with dengue infection. I. The clinical and physiologic manifestations of dengue hemorrhagic fever in Thailand, 1964. J. Pediatr. *68*:448–456, 1966.
19. Cuzzubbo, A. J., Vaughn, D. W., Nisalak, A., et al.: Comparison of PanBio dengue duo enzyme-linked immunosorbent assay (ELISA) and MRL dengue fever virus immunoglobulin M capture ELISA for diagnosis of dengue virus infections in Southeast Asia. Clin. Diagn. Lab. Immunol. *6*:705–712, 1999.
20. Deller, J. J., Jr., and Russell, P. K.: Fevers of unknown origin in American soldiers in Vietnam. Ann. Intern. Med. *66*:1129–1143, 1967.
21. DeMadrid, A. T., and Porterfield, J. S.: The flaviviruses (group B arboviruses): A cross neutralization study. J. Gen. Virol. *23*:91–96, 1974.
22. Dengue in the Caribbean, 1977. Proceedings of a Workshop Held in Montego Bay, Jamaica, May 8–11, 1978. Scientific Publication No. 375. Washington, D.C., Pan American Health Organization, 1979, 186 pp.
23. Derrick, E. H., and Bicks, V. A.: The limiting temperature for the transmission of dengue. Aust. Ann. Med. *7*:102, 1958.
24. Dobbins, J. G., and Else, J. G.: Knowledge, attitudes and practices related to control of dengue hemorrhagic fever in an urban Malay kampung. Southeast Asian J. Trop. Med. Public Health *6*:120–126, 1975.
25. Dung, N. M., Day, N. P. J., Tam, D. T. H., et al.: Fluid replacement in dengue shock syndrome: A randomized, double-blind comparison of four intravenous-fluid regimens. Clin. Infect. Dis. *29*:787–794, 1999.
26. Glaziou, P., Chungue, E., Gestas P., et al.: Dengue fever and dengue shock syndrome in French Polynesia. Southeast Asian J. Trop. Med. Public Health *23*:531–532, 1992.
27. Green, S., Vaughn, D. W., Kalayanarooj, S., et al.: Elevated plasma interleukin-10 levels in acute dengue correlate with disease severity. J. Med. Virol. *59*:329–334, 1999.
28. Green, S., Vaughn, D. W., Kalayanarooj, S., et al.: Early immune activation in acute dengue illness is related to development of plasma leakage and disease severity. J. Infect. Dis. *179*:755–762, 1999.
29. Gubler, D. J.: *Aedes aegypti* and *Aedes aegypti*–borne disease control in the 1990's: Top down or bottom up. Am. J. Trop. Med. Hyg. *40*:571–578, 1989.
30. Guirakhoo, F., Weltzin, R., Chambers, T. J., et al.: Recombinant chimeric yellow fever–dengue type 2 virus is immunogenic and protective in nonhuman primates. J. Virol. *74*:5477–5485, 2000.
31. Guzman, M. G., Kouri, G. P., Bravo, J., et al.: Dengue hemorrhagic fever in Cuba, 1981: A retrospective seroepidemiologic study. Am. J. Trop. Med. Hyg. *42*:179–184, 1990.
32. Guzman, M. G., Kouri, G., and Halstead, S. B.: Hypothesis. Do escape mutants explain rapid increase in dengue case-fatality rates within epidemics? Lancet *355*:1902–1903, 2000.
33. Guzman, M. G., Kouri, G., Valdes, L., et al.: Epidemiological studies on dengue, Santiago de Cuba, 1997. Am. J. Epidemiol. *152*:793–799, 2000.
34. Hahn, Y. S., Galler, R., Hunkapiller, T., et al.: Nucleotide sequence of dengue 2 RNA and comparison of the encoded proteins with those of other flaviviruses. Virology *162*:167–180, 1988.
35. Halstead, S. B.: Mosquito-borne haemorrhagic fevers of South and South-east Asia. Bull. World Health Organ. *35*:3–15, 1966.
36. Halstead, S. B.: Etiologies of the experimental dengue of Siler and Simmons. Am. J. Trop. Med. Hyg. *23*:974–982, 1974.
37. Halstead, S. B.: Dengue haemorrhagic fever: A public health problem and a field for research. Bull. World Health Organ. *58*:1–21, 1980.
38. Halstead, S. B.: Immunological parameters of togavirus disease syndromes. *In* Schlesinger, R. W. (ed.): The Togaviruses, Biology, Structure, Replication. New York, Academic Press, 1980, pp. 107–173.
39. Halstead, S. B.: The pathogenesis of dengue: Molecular epidemiology in infectious disease. The Alexander D. Langmuir Lecture. Am. J. Epidemiol. *114*:632–648, 1981.
40. Halstead, S. B.: Dengue: Hematologic aspects. Semin. Hematol. *19*:116–131, 1982.

41. Halstead, S. B.: Immune enhancement of viral infection. Prog. Allergy *31*:301–364, 1982.
42. Halstead, S. B.: Selective primary health care: Strategies for control of disease in the developing world. XI. Dengue. Rev. Infect. Dis. *6*:251–264, 1984.
43. Halstead, S. B.: Pathogenesis of dengue: Challenges of molecular biology. Science *239*:476–481, 1988.
44. Halstead, S. B., Nimmannitya, S., Yamarat, C., et al.: Hemorrhagic fever in Thailand: Newer knowledge regarding etiology. Jpn. J. Med. Sci. Biol. *20*(Suppl.):96–102, 1967.
45. Halstead, S. B., and O'Rourke, E. J.: Dengue viruses and mononuclear phagocytes. I. Infection enhancement by non-neutralizing antibody. J. Exp. Med. *146*:201–217, 1977.
46. Halstead, S. B., and O'Rourke, E. J.: Editorial response: Resuscitation of patients with dengue hemorrhagic fever/dengue shock syndrome. Clin. Infect. Dis. *29*:795–796, 1999.
47. Halstead, S. B., Streit, T. G., Lafontant, J. G., et al.: Haiti: Absence of dengue hemorrhagic fever despite hyperendemic dengue virus transmission. Am. J. Trop. Med. Hyg. *65*:180–183, 2001.
48. Hammon, W. M., Rudnick, A., and Sather, G. E.: Viruses associated with hemorrhagic fevers of the Philippines and Thailand. Science *131*:1102–1103, 1960.
49. He, R. T., Innis, B. L., Nisalak, A., et al.: Antibodies that block virus attachment to Vero cells are a major component of the human neutralizing antibody response against dengue virus type 2. J. Med. Virol. *45*:452–461, 1995.
50. Huang, C. Y., Burapet, S., Pierro, D. J., et al.: Chimeric dengue type 2 (vaccine strain PDK-53)/dengue type 1 virus as a potential candidate dengue type virus vaccine. J. Virol. *74*:3020–3028, 2000.
51. Huerre, M. R., Lan, N. T., Marianneau, P., et al.: Liver histopathology and biological correlates in five cases of fatal dengue fever in Vietnamese children. Virchows Arch. *43*:107–115, 2001.
52. Innis, B. L., Nisalak, A., Nimmannitya, S., et al.: An enzyme-linked immunosorbent assay to characterize dengue infections where dengue and Japanese encephalitis co-circulate. Am. J. Trop. Med. Hyg. *40*:418–427, 1989.
53. Isolation of dengue type 3 virus prompts concern and action. Bull. Pan Am. Health Org. *29*:184–185, 1995.
54. Johnson, K. M., Halstead, S. B., and Cohen, S. N.: Hemorrhagic fevers of Southeast Asia and South America: A comparative appraisal. Prog. Med. Virol. *9*:105–158, 1967.
55. Kalyanarooj, S., Vaughn, D. W., Nimmannitya, S., et al.: Early clinical and laboratory indicators of acute dengue illness. J. Infect. Dis. *176*:313–326, 1997.
56. Karabatsos, N. (ed.): International Catalog of Arbovirus 1985. Ft. Collins, CO, American Society of Tropical Medicine and Hygiene, 1985.
57. Kimura, R., and Hotta, S.: On the inoculation of dengue virus into mice. Nippon Igaku *3379*:629–633, 1944.
58. King, A. D., Nisalak, A., Kalyanarooj, S., et al.: B cells are the principal circulating mononuclear cells infected by dengue virus. Southeast Asian J. Trop. Med. Public Health *30*:718–728, 1999.
59. Kliks, S., Nisalak, A., Brandt, W. E., et al.: Evidence that maternal dengue antibodies are important in the development of dengue hemorrhagic fever in infants. Am. J. Trop. Med. Hyg. *38*:411–419, 1988.
60. Kliks, S. C., Nisalak, A., Brandt, W. E., et al.: Antibody dependent enhancement of dengue virus growth in human monocytes as a risk factor for dengue hemorrhagic fever. Am. J. Trop. Med. Hyg. *40*:444–451, 1989.
61. Kochel, T. J., Raviprakash, K., Hayes, C. G., et al.: A dengue virus serotype-1 DNA vaccine induces virus neutralizing antibodies and provides protection from viral challenge in Aotus monkeys. Vaccine *18*:3166–3173, 2000.
62. Kochel, T. J., Watts, D. M., Halstead, S. B., et al.: Effect of dengue-1 antibodies on American dengue-2 viral infection and dengue haemorrhagic fever. Lancet *360*:310–312, 2002.
63. Kouri, G. P., Guzman, M. G., Bravo, J. R., et al.: Dengue haemorrhagic fever/dengue shock syndrome: Lessons from the Cuban epidemic. Bull. World Health Organ. *67*:375–380, 1989.
64. Kurane, I., and Ennis, F. A.: Cytokines in dengue virus infections: Role of cytokines in the pathogenesis of dengue hemorrhagic fever. Semin. Virol. *5*:443–448, 1994.
65. Lai, C. J., Bray, M., Men, R., et al.: Evaluation of molecular strategies to develop a live dengue vaccine. Clin. Diagn. Virol. *10*:173–179, 1998.
66. La Russa, V. F., and Innis, B. L.: Mechanisms of dengue virus–induced bone marrow suppression. Baillieres Clin. Haematol. *8*:249–270, 1995.
67. Lee, Y. S.: Urban planning and vector control in Southeast Asian cities. Kaohsiung J. Med. Sci. *10*(Suppl.):39–51, 1994.
68. Leitmeyer, K. C., Vaughn, D. W., Watts D. M., et al.: Dengue virus structural differences that correlate with pathogenesis. J. Virol. *73*:4738–4747, 1999.
69. Lewis, J. G., Chang, G. J., Lanciotti, R. S., et al.: Phylogenic relationships of dengue-2 viruses. Virology *197*:216–224, 1993.
70. Lloyd, L. S., Winch, P., Ortega-Canto, J., et al.: The design of a community-based health education intervention for the control of *Aedes aegypti*. Am. J. Trop. Med. Hyg. *50*:401–411, 1994.
71. Lofgren, C. S., Ford, H. R., Tonn, R. J., et al.: The effectiveness of ultra-low volume applications of malathion at a rate of 6 fluid ounces per acre in controlling *Aedes aegypti* in a large-scale test at Nakohn Sawan, Thailand. Bull. World Health Organ. *42*:15–25, 1970.
72. Lumley, G. F., and Taylor, F. H.: Dengue. School of Public Health and Tropical Medicine Service Publication Number 3. Glebe, N. S. W., Australasian Medical Publishing Company, 1943, p. 74.
73. Marchette, N. J., Halstead, S. B., Falkler, W. A., Jr., et al.: Studies on the pathogenesis of dengue infection in monkeys. III. Sequential distribution of virus in primary and heterologous infections. J. Infect. Dis. *128*:23–30, 1973.
74. Mathew, A., Kurane, I., Green, S., et al.: Impaired T cell proliferation in acute dengue infection. J. Immunol. *162*:5609–5615, 1999.
75. Mattingly, P. F.: Symposium on the evolution of arbovirus diseases. II. Ecological aspects of the evolution of mosquito-borne virus diseases. Trans. Soc. Trop. Med. Hyg. *54*:97–112, 1960.
76. Nimmannitya, S.: Clinical spectrum and management of dengue hemorrhagic fever. Southeast Asian J. Trop. Med. Public Health *3*:392–397, 1987.
77. Nimmannitya, S., Halstead, S. B., Cohen, S. N., et al.: Dengue and chikungunya virus infections in man in Thailand, 1962–1964. I. Observations on hospitalized patients with hemorrhagic fever. Am. J. Trop. Med. Hyg. *18*:954–971, 1969.
78. Nisalak, A., Halstead, S. B., Singharaj, P., et al.: Observations related to pathogenesis of dengue hemorrhagic fever. III. Virologic studies of fatal disease. Yale J. Biol. Med. *42*:293–310, 1970.
79. Nogueira, R. M., Zagner, S. M., Martins, I. S., et al.: Dengue haemorrhagic fever/dengue shock syndrome (DHF/DSS) caused by serotype 2 in Brazil. Mem. Inst. Oswaldo Cruz *86*:269, 1991.
80. Qui, F. X., Gubler, D. J., Liu, D. J., et al.: Dengue in China: A clinical review. Bull. World Health Organ. *71*:349–359, 1993.
81. Pathogenetic mechanisms in dengue haemorrhagic fever: Report of an international collaborative study. Bull. World Health Organ. *48*:117–133, 1973.
82. Programma de eliminacion del dengue y erradicacion del Aedes aegypti en Cuba. Bol. Epidemiol. P. A. H. O. *3*:7–10, 1982.
83. Ramirez-Ronda, C. H., and Garcia, C. D.: Dengue in the Western Hemisphere. Infect. Dis. Clin. North Am. *8*:107–128, 1994.
84. Reynes, J. M., Laurent, A., Deubel, V., et al.: The first epidemic of dengue hemorrhagic fever in French Guiana. Am. J. Trop. Med. Hyg. *51*:545–553, 1994.
85. Rice, L.: Dengue fever: A clinical report of the Galveston epidemic of 1922. Am. J. Trop. Med. *3*:73–90, 1923.
86. Rico-Hesse, R.: Molecular evolution and distribution of dengue viruses type 1 and 2 in nature. Virology *174*:479–493, 1990.
87. Rico-Hesse, R., Harrison, R. L., Nisalak, A., et al.: Molecular evolution of dengue type 2 virus in Thailand. Am. J. Trop. Med. Hyg. *58*:96–101, 1998.
88. Roche, J. C., Cordellier, R., Hervey, J. P., et al.: Isolement de 96 souches de virus dengue 2: A partier de moustique captures en Cote-D'Ivoire et Haute-Volta. Ann. Virol. (Inst. Pasteur) *134E*:233–244, 1983.
89. Rosen, L.: The use of Toxorhynchites mosquitoes to detect and propagate dengue and other arboviruses. Am. J. Trop. Med. Hyg. *30*:177–183, 1981.
90. Rosen, L., and Gubler, D.: The use of mosquitoes to detect and propagate dengue viruses. Am. J. Trop. Med. Hyg. *23*:1153–1160, 1974.
91. Rosen, L., Shroyer, D. A., Tesh, R. B., et al.: Transovarial transmission of dengue viruses by mosquitoes *Aedes albopictus* and *Aedes aegypti*. Am. J. Trop. Med. Hyg. *32*:1108–1119, 1983.
92. Rothman, A. L., and Ennis, F. A.: Immunopathogenesis of dengue hemorrhagic fever. Virology *257*:1–6, 1999.
93. Rudnick, A.: Ecology of dengue virus. Conference on DHF. Oct. 24–28, 1977, Singapore. Asian J. Infect. Dis. *2*:156–160, 1978.
94. Russell, P. K., and Nisalak, A.: Dengue virus identification by the plaque reduction neutralization test. J. Immunol. *99*:285–290, 1967.
95. Russell, P. K., Yuill, T. M., Nisalak, A., et al.: An insular outbreak of dengue hemorrhagic fever. II. Virologic and serologic studies. Am. J. Trop. Med. Hyg. *17*:600–608, 1968.
96. Sabin, A. B.: The dengue group of viruses and its family relationships. Bacteriol. Rev. *14*:225–232, 1950.
97. Sabin, A. B.: Research on dengue during World War II. Am. J. Trop. Med. Hyg. *1*:30–50, 1952.
98. Sabin, A. B., and Schlesinger, R. W.: Production of immunity to dengue with virus modified by propagation in mice. Science *101*:640–642, 1945.
99. Sangkawibha, N., Rojansuphot, S., Ahandrik, S., et al.: Risk factors in dengue shock syndrome: A prospective epidemiologic study in Rayong, Thailand. Am. J. Epidemiol. *120*:653–669, 1984.
100. Sariol, C. A., Pelegrino, J. L., Martinez, A., et al.: Detection and genetic relationship of dengue virus sequences in seventeen year-old paraffin-embedded samples from Cuba. Am. J. Trop. Med. Hyg. *61*:994–1000, 1999.
101. Schlesinger, R. W.: Dengue Viruses. Virology Monograph 16. Vienna, Springer, 1977.
102. Sheppard, P. M., MacDonald, W. W., Tonn, R. J., et al.: The dynamics of an adult population of *Aedes aegypti* in relation to dengue haemorrhagic fever in Bangkok. J. Anim. Ecol. *38*:661–702, 1969.

103. Siler, J. F., Hall, M. W., and Hitchens, A. P.: Dengue: Its history, epidemiology, mechanisms of transmission, etiology, clinical manifestations, immunity and prevention. Philippine J. Sci. *29*:1–304, 1926.
104. Simmons, J. S., St. John, J. H., and Reynolds, F. H. K.: Experimental studies of dengue. Philippine J. Sci. *44*:1–247, 1931.
105. Srivastava, V. K., Suri, S., Bhasin, A., et al.: An epidemic of dengue haemorrhagic fever and dengue shock syndrome in Delhi: A clinical study. Ann. Trop. Paediatr. *10*:329–334, 1990.
106. Strode, G. K. (ed.): Yellow Fever. New York, McGraw-Hill, 1951.
107. Sumarmo, Wulur, H., Jahja, E., et al.: Clinical observations on virologically confirmed fatal dengue infections in Jakarta, Indonesia. Bull. World Health Organ. *61*:693–701, 1983.
108. Tassniyom, S., Vasanawathana, V., Chirawatkul, A., et al.: Failure of high-dose methylprednisolone in established dengue shock syndrome: A placebo-controlled, double-blind study. Pediatrics *92*:111–115, 1993.
109. Thisyakorn, U., and Nimmannitya, S.: Nutritional status of children with dengue hemorrhagic fever. Clin. Infect. Dis. *16*:295–297, 1993.
110. Trent, D. W., Grant, J. A., Monath, T. P., et al.: Genetic variation and microevolution of dengue 2 virus in Southeast Asia. Virology *172*:523–535, 1989.
111. Tsai, J. C., Kuo, C. H., and Chen, P. C.: Upper gastrointestinal bleeding in dengue fever. Am. J. Gastroenterol. *86*:33–35, 1991.
112. Vaughn, D. W.: Invited commentary: Dengue lessons from Cuba. Am. J. Epidemiol. *152*:800–803, 2000.
113. Vaughn, D. W., Green, S., Kalayanarooj, S., et al.: Dengue viremia titer, antibody response pattern, and virus serotype correlate with disease severity. J. Infect. Dis. *181*:2–9, 2000.
114. Vitarana, T., and Jayasekara, N.: Dengue haemorrhagic fever outbreak in Sri Lanka. Southeast Asian J. Trop. Med. Public Health *21*:682, 1990.
115. Wang, E., Ni, H., Xu, R., et al.: Evolutionary relationships of endemic/epidemic and sylvatic dengue viruses. J. Virol. *74*:3227–3234, 2000.
116. Watts, D. M., Porter, K., Putvatana, R., et al.: Failure of secondary infections with American genotype dengue 2 viruses to cause dengue haemorrhagic fever. Lancet *354*:1431–1434, 1999.
117. Wen, K. H., Sheu, M. M., Chung, C. B., et al.: The ocular fundus findings in dengue fever. Kaohsiung. J. Med. Sci. *5*:24–30, 1989.
118. Westaway, E. G., Brinton, M. A., Gaidamovich, S. Y. A., et al.: Flaviviridae. Intervirology *24*:183–192, 1985.
119. Western Pacific Regional Officer, WHO: Personal communication, 1995.
120. World Health Organization: Dengue Haemorrhagic Fever: Diagnosis, Treatment Prevention and Control. Geneva, World Health Organization, 1994.
121. Wu, S. J. L., Grouard-Vogel, G., Sun, W., et al.: Human skin Langerhans cells are targets of dengue virus infection. Nat. Med. *6*:816–820, 2000.

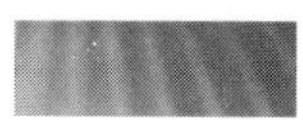

CHAPTER **179D**

Japanese Encephalitis

THEODORE F. TSAI

Japanese encephalitis (JE), a mosquito-borne flaviviral infection, is the leading cause of childhood viral encephalitis in Asia.

History

JE first was recognized after an outbreak in Japan in 1924 led to 6125 cases. The disease was differentiated from von Economo encephalitis, which had a different seasonality and clinical features, by being designated Japanese "B" encephalitis; the "B" subsequently has fallen into disuse. In retrospect, similar summer-autumn outbreaks were recognized as early as 1871 to 1873. In 1933, Hayashi recovered the virus from monkeys and the brain of a patient, and in 1938, Mitamura confirmed its mosquito-borne mode of transmission by isolating the virus from *Culex tritaeniorhychnus*.[31] Inactivated vaccine prepared from infected mouse brain was licensed in Japan in 1956, and its use has led to control of the disease in developed Asian countries.[58, 84, 86] As poliomyelitis has been brought under control in Asia, JE has become the leading viral central nervous system (CNS) infection on that continent.

Etiologic Agent

JE virus is the prototypic member of an antigenic complex that includes St. Louis, Murray Valley, Kunjin encephalitis, and West Nile viruses. Molecular taxonomic studies based on nucleotide sequences of the E protein gene or the pre-M region have segregated JE strains into five genotypes that can be mapped roughly to regions of epidemic and endemic transmission in temperate Asia and India or Southeast Asia (four types, including one limited to Indonesia).[11] However, the virus exists as a single serotype, and correspondence of genotype to human virulence has not been demonstrated epidemiologically.[87] Sequence analysis has been helpful in tracing the potential origins of epidemic strains and has suggested the emergence of ancestral JE virus within the last 300 years.[87]

Strains isolated from nature exhibit a range of virulence in mice. With repeated cell culture passage, biologically derived neuroattenuated strains have been produced for use as vaccines. Combinations of mutations in genes of the E glycoprotein, nonstructural proteins, and noncoding regions have been identified with attenuation of the live vaccine strain SA 14-14-2.[4, 53, 85] Comparisons of neurovirulent and attenuated viruses and manipulations of infectious clones have identified specific codon changes (resulting in amino acid changes principally in the E protein) that make fully replicative viruses avirulent.

As with other flaviviruses, important biologic functions such as viral neutralization are associated with the E glycoprotein. Its proper processing in conjunction with other viral proteins is necessary for authentic expression of disease. Canarypox, yellow fever 17D, and vaccinia recombinant viruses containing various JE viral sequences protect mice from challenge, thus demonstrating the biologic importance of specific genes and their mutations. Some of the recombinants may have utility as synthetic antigens in diagnostic assays or as human or animal vaccines.[53]

Ecology

In its basic transmission cycle, JE virus is transmitted between birds, especially certain egrets and herons, and *Culex* mosquitoes.[6, 71, 86] However, pigs, when present, are the most important source of viral amplification (Fig. 179–7). Pigs maintain a high sustained viremia and may be hosts to thousands of mosquitoes in a single night, thereby providing an abundant source of infected vectors that can transmit the infection further. In the typical setting in rural Asia, the onset of human cases each summer occurs shortly after pigs become infected.[60, 71, 86] The importance of pigs to epidemic

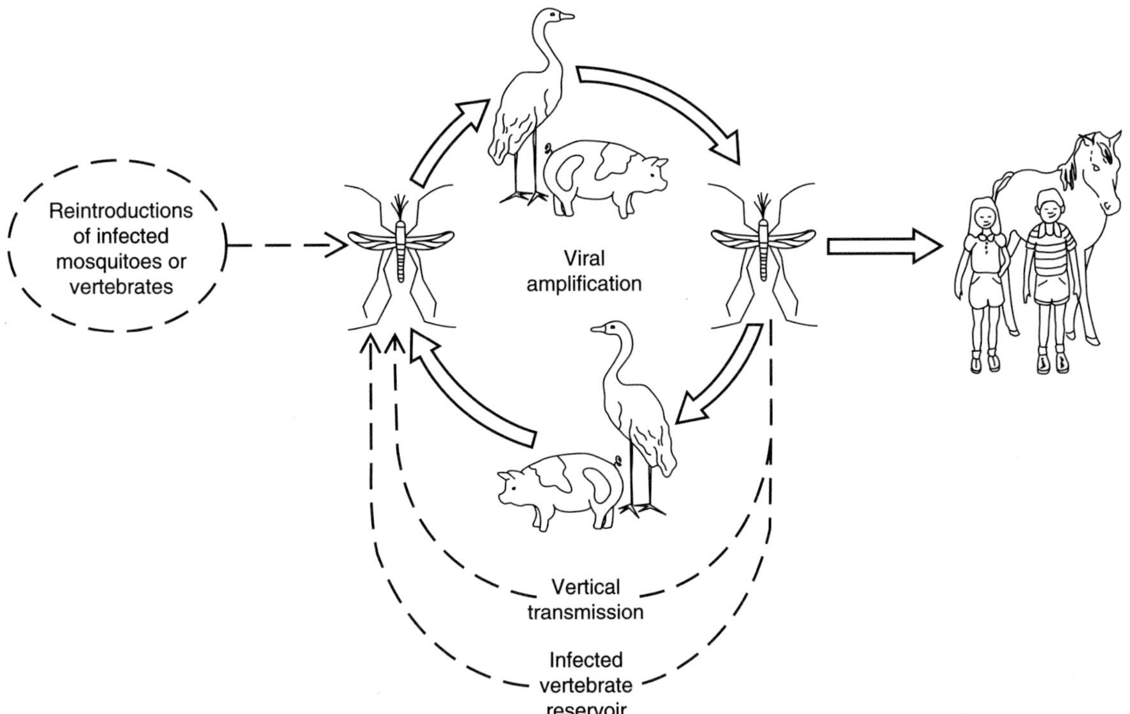

FIGURE 179–7 ■ Transmission cycle of Japanese encephalitis virus. Speculative portions of the cycle are shown in *broken lines.*

transmission can be seen in countries such as Bangladesh, Malaysia, and Indonesia, where JE occurs principally in the non-Moslem population, which does not eschew pigs. However, outbreaks of JE have occurred in areas devoid of pigs, where birds, including ducklings, pigeons, sparrows, and possibly other small birds found near human residences, have been the principal amplifying hosts and other sylvatic cycles have been proposed.[3, 21, 69]

C. tritaeniorhychnus is the major mosquito vector in most areas of Asia, although in various regions, related species *(Culex pseudovishnui, Culex vishnui, Culex gelidus, Culex fuscocephalus,* and *Culex bitaeniorhychnus)* are important locally.[71, 86] *Culex annulirostris* is the principal vector in northern Australia and the Pacific. Certain anopheline mosquitoes may contribute to the transmission of JE in northeastern India. The primary *Culex* vectors use ground pools and especially rice paddies in their pre-adult stages. Immense numbers are produced from the flooded rice paddies that frequently surround individual residences and villages. With the custom of keeping pigs near or inside houses, all elements of the viral transmission cycle are found in close proximity to human activity. The mosquito *C. tritaeniorhychnus* is most active in the evening and night and feeds outdoors. The vector is zoophilic and prefers to feed on large animals rather than humans.

Domestic animals such as dogs and cattle can be infected, but sufficient viremia does not develop to support further transmission. Because they are attractive to JE vectors, their presence may divert mosquitoes from humans (zooprophylaxis). Clinical illness develops in horses after infection and results in periodic outbreaks and economically significant loss of prize horses. Equine vaccines are administered in China, Mongolia, and Japan to prevent disease. Adult pigs remain asymptomatic after infection; however, sows infected during pregnancy abort or deliver piglets with lethal congenital malformations.

The overwintering mechanism for JE virus has not been defined clearly, although considerable evidence suggests a carryover of virus in mosquito eggs, with re-establishment of the transmission cycle by vertically infected mosquitoes.[18, 71] Viral persistence in local mammalian reservoirs such as bats and reintroduction from external sources by migrating birds or windblown mosquitoes also has been proposed.[24, 59]

Epidemiology

The disease occurs mainly in rural areas, where high levels of virus transmission lead to infection at an early age. Nearly all cases occur in children younger than 10 years, with a slight preponderance in boys.[86] More than 99 percent of infections are subclinical, and cumulative exposure with age leads to seroprevalence rates of 80 percent or more by adulthood.[22] In Japan and other developed Asian countries, where children are protected by mass vaccination, adult cases occur principally in the elderly. Waning immunity or other biologic factors associated with aging have been speculated to be risk factors.[39, 84]

Transmission is seasonal: late summer and early fall in temperate regions (July to September) and a longer interval in southern China and Southeast Asia (April to November).[84, 86] The seasonality is more complex in tropical areas, where mosquitoes proliferate after monsoon rains, and two epidemic seasons or year-round transmission is possible in some tropical locations. Although an abundance of mosquitoes usually corresponds to the rainy season, in many locations, vector populations now follow irrigation-controlled schedules of rice field flooding.[57]

JE occurs in nearly every country in Asia[84, 86] (Fig. 179–8), with 30,000 to 50,000 cases reported annually from the region. Transmission is endemic; annual incidence rates of 1 to 10 per 100,000 population are observed in China and most

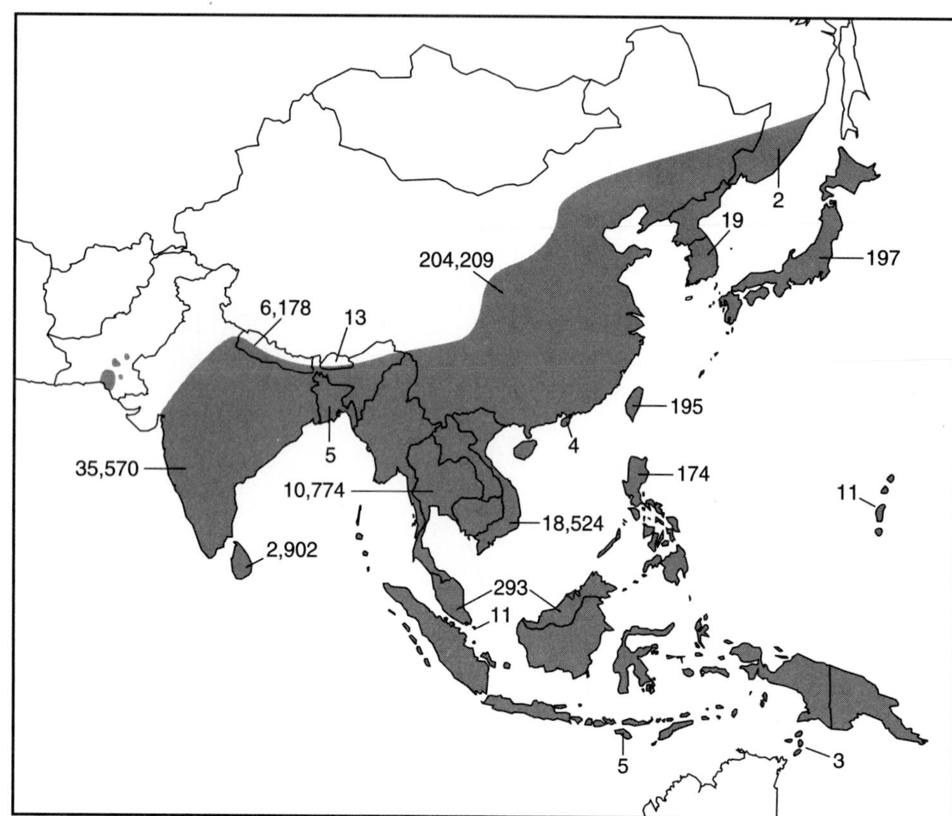

FIGURE 179–8 ■ Geographic distribution of Japanese encephalitis and reported cases from 1985 to 1994. Torres Strait cases are from 1995.

areas of Southeast Asia, but epidemic attack rates as high as 100 per 100,000 population have been described. Only sporadic cases are reported from Indonesia, Malaysia, and the Philippines, whereas periodic, often sizable outbreaks typify transmission in India. Rare outbreaks have occurred in Oceania, on Guam and Saipan in 1949 and 1989, respectively, and in far northern Australia in 1995 and 1998.[24, 59] These outbreaks appeared to have occurred after introduction of the virus by migrating birds or other mechanisms, coupled with unusual conditions of human activity or weather patterns. Establishment of JE virus on the Australian mainland appears to have been limited by immunity in the vertebrate host population as a result of infection by other flaviviruses.[89] Few cases are reported from countries where vaccination rates are high (e.g., Japan, Korea, Taiwan) and where development through urbanization, decreased land under cultivation, and an improved standard of living have reduced human exposure. The use of agricultural pesticides and centralized pig rearing also may have contributed to a decline in infected vectors in these countries.[84, 86] The significant reduction in human cases belies the persistence of enzootic viral transmission in rural areas of these countries, however.

Although economic development has paralleled a decline in JE in some countries, in other areas, development in the form of deforestation, construction of dams, and irrigation schemes has led to increases in transmission of JE virus or its emergence in areas where the disease had not occurred previously. Examples include development projects in the Terai in southern Nepal and the Mahaweli Valley in Sri Lanka, where JE and malaria have become hyperendemic after large-scale programs of deforestation and agricultural development.

Travelers to areas where JE is endemic may be at risk for acquiring the illness.[30, 85] However, risk in the general traveling public is low: fewer than 30 cases have been reported in travelers from North America, Europe, and Australia in the last 20 years, many of them in military personnel and their family members. The risk has been estimated to be in the range of 1 per 15,000 to 1 per 150,000 person-months of exposure. This low rate can be understood by factoring the probability of an illness developing after a single mosquito bite: only certain vector species transmit the virus, typically less than 3 percent of vector mosquitoes are infected, and only one in several hundred infections leads to clinical illness. Because the principal vector species are found in rural areas and they feed mainly outdoors and in the evening and night, the risk is low in the great majority of travelers who can avoid these circumstances of exposure.

Clinical Manifestations

Only one in several hundred infections leads to clinical illness, and the overwhelming majority of infections are inapparent or manifested as mild self-limited illnesses. Patients who come to medical attention may have aseptic meningitis or encephalitis, and 5 to 25 percent die. After an incubation period of 4 to 14 days, the earliest symptoms are lethargy, nausea or abdominal pain, headache, and feverishness (Fig. 179–9). During a period of 2 to 3 days, lethargy increases and the child may exhibit uncharacteristic patterns of behavior and motor abnormalities.[2, 37, 40, 43, 63, 66, 82, 86] In other cases, a long prodrome of a week or more may occur. Vomiting is a common event, and periods of confusion or agitation and unsteadiness may occur. A sudden convulsion is frequently

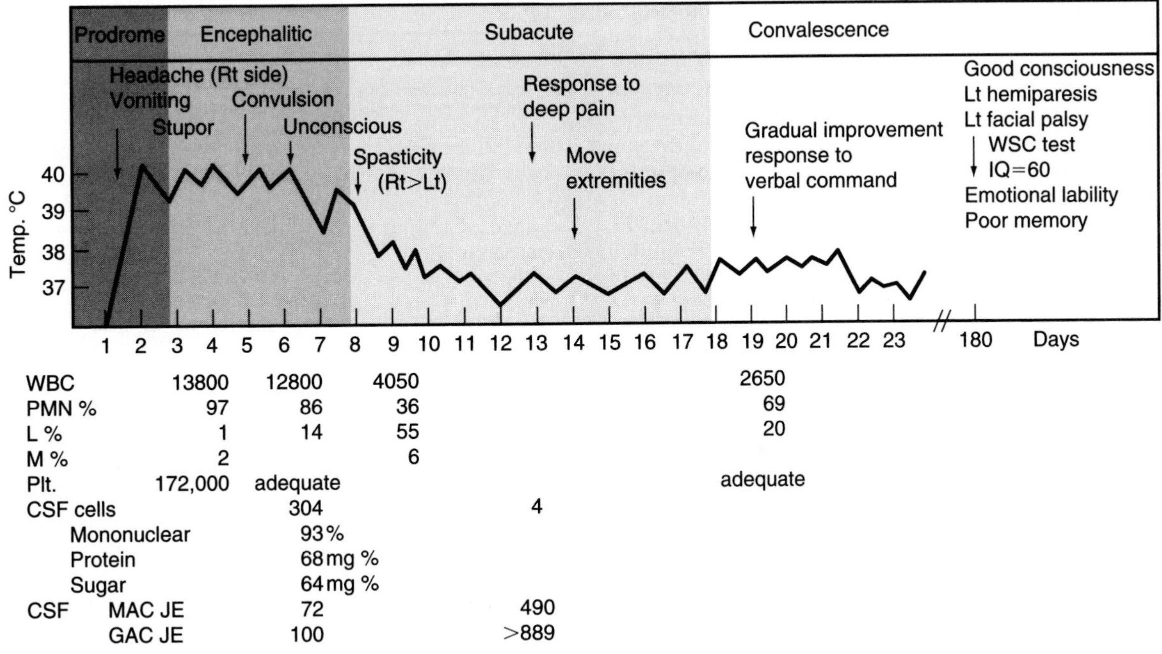

FIGURE 179–9 ■ Clinical stages of a typical Japanese encephalitis case.

the initial symptom. Unusual manifestations, such as acute psychosis and Guillain-Barré syndrome, also have been reported; the latter may lead to a misdiagnosis of acute poliomyelitis in areas of Asia where that disease has not been eradicated.[68, 81]

The principal physical findings are high fever and obvious alterations in consciousness ranging from mild mental clouding, frank disorientation and delirium, to coma. Some children exhibit bizarre behavior, including shouting, spitting, and other personality changes. Mutism is an initial feature in some cases. Signs of meningeal irritation can be elicited in a third to two thirds of cases. Cranial nerve palsies, mainly disconjugate gaze and central facial paralysis, are observed in a third of cases. Muscular weakness, either flaccid or spastic, is a usual symptom. Weakness may be generalized or in many cases is asymmetric, with hemiparesis or an unusual distribution of flaccid and spastic paralysis. Muscular tone generally is increased, with hyperreflexia and ankle clonus; the Babinski sign and other abnormal reflexes are variable. Some patients exhibit erratic flailing movements. Tremor, rigidity, expressionless facies, or thick slurred speech may be initial features, but more frequently, choreoathetosis and other extrapyramidal signs become evident in the second week of illness.[36, 65] Focal or generalized convulsions develop in 50 to 75 percent of patients.[51] Papilledema is seen in 10 percent of cases, and patients occasionally may be hypertensive. Patients with fulminant infections often die during the first 5 days of illness.

In most other cases, fever abates during the next week and neurologic function gradually improves over the course of several weeks. Further recovery of motor function occurs during the next several months to years. In more than a third of patients, coma and respiratory failure necessitate institution of ventilatory support. During this prolonged period of recovery from coma and paralysis, stasis ulcers, urinary tract infections, pneumonia, and bacteremia are frequent complications and may be secondary causes of death. A biphasic pattern of illness has been described in anecdotal cases, with a recurrence of motor and behavioral abnormalities 2 to 5 weeks after initial improvement and larger and more numerous associated magnetic resonance imaging (MRI) lesions.[64]

Routine laboratory studies initially show a peripheral leukocytosis, often with a left shift and a total leukocyte count as high as 30,000/mm^3. Opening pressures on lumbar puncture usually are normal or slightly elevated. Cerebrospinal fluid (CSF) pleocytosis ranges from fewer than 10 cells to several thousand, with a median of several hundred per cubic millimeter. Lymphocytic pleocytosis is a typical finding, but some patients have an initial predominance of polymorphonuclear cells. CSF sugar and protein levels are generally normal (80% of cases); when elevated, protein levels rarely exceed 100 mg/dL.

Electroencephalograms typically show diffuse theta to delta wave slowing, whereas spike and seizure discharges are relatively uncommon findings. Computed tomograms show diffuse white matter edema and nonenhancing low-density areas, mainly in the thalamus, basal ganglia, and pons.[51, 52] Thalamic lesions frequently are associated with unilateral or bilateral hemorrhage. A thalamic location of involvement is consistent with the electroencephalogram's pattern of slowing. MRI shows a similar distribution of abnormalities but is more sensitive with lesions of high or mixed signal intensity on T2 studies in the thalamus, midbrain, basal ganglia, substantia nigra, cerebellum, pons, and spinal cord.[35, 45, 52] JE-associated abnormalities have been reported to appear more frequently in the ipsilateral hemisphere affected by neurocysticercosis-related changes.[79] Electromyograms show a neurogenic pattern consistent with anterior horn cell involvement. Central motor conduction times are prolonged, indicative of diffuse subcortical damage.[52]

Pathology

Pathologic changes are found in the lungs and viscera, in addition to the brain.[17, 27, 33, 34, 44, 76, 90] Grossly, the brain appears swollen, and the meninges may be congested. Punctate hemorrhages may be visible macroscopically. Microscopic examination discloses a moderate inflammatory response in the meninges. Foci of neuronal degeneration with parenchymal and perivascular inflammatory responses are found principally in the thalamus and brain stem, as well as in the hippocampus, temporal cortex, cerebellum, and spinal cord. Areas of neuronophagia may be surrounded by microglial nodules, but sharply defined round areas of softening or necrolysis without an inflammatory response also are seen. Purkinje cells and cerebellar glial shrubs also may be lost.

Pathophysiology

After virus is introduced by a mosquito bite, replication locally and within regional lymphatic tissue leads to a secondary amplified viremia and infection of various organs and the brain. Neuroinvasion is thought to occur through cerebral capillaries; infection crosses from the vascular side of the endothelial cell to the perivascular space, with subsequent neuronal infection.[19] Neurons show evidence of viral antigen in the cell body, axons, and dendrites, and virus spreads within the brain from cell to cell.[17, 34] Infiltrating T cells elicit a broad inflammatory response, with B and T cells and macrophages found in perivascular cuffs and macrophages and T cells in the parenchyma. Neuronophagia proceeds with the formation of microglial nodules and the eventual disappearance of neurons; ghost-like remnants are left, and antigen is accumulated within macrophages.[34]

The rapidity of the neutralizing antibody response is thought to be a principal determinant of outcome.[34, 55, 85] Most fatal cases occurring within approximately 5 days after the onset of illness have no detectable CSF antibody response while virus is recoverable from the CSF, a finding indicative of unimpeded viral replication. In experimentally infected animals, passive immunization reduces mortality, even when it is given 4 to 5 days after inoculation.[55] However, other studies have found that antigen persists in neurons for extensive periods in the presence of intrathecal antibody and immune complexes, thus suggesting a failure of antibody-mediated viral clearance.[17] A role for immunopathologic mechanisms, including the development of antineurofilament antibodies, has been proposed as an alternative correlate of outcome.[16] CSF interleukin-8 levels remain elevated for a longer interval in patients with severe prolonged illness.[78]

Why most JE virus infections are subclinical or lead to no signs of infection in the CNS is unclear. Epidemiologic observations indicate an elevated risk for JE in the elderly and increased severity in young children, but the biologic basis for this increased susceptibility has not been defined. Cross-reactive flaviviral immunity as a result of previous dengue virus infection may modulate the severity of JE in some cases.[17] Pathologic observations have shown a higher prevalence of neurocysticercosis in fatal JE cases than in deaths from other causes, which suggests that physical or physiologic disruption of the brain architecture by infection or other mechanisms could facilitate neuroinvasion (see earlier).[14, 79] Experimental dual infection of animals with JE virus and other agents supports this hypothesis.[48] Other host factors associated with a risk of acquiring illness and having a poor outcome in experimental animals include a specific gene-defining resistance, age, sex hormones, and cold and stress responses.[38]

Complications

The principal complication is secondary bacterial infection occurring in the acute and subacute phases of illness. Stress-induced gastrointestinal hemorrhage and hyponatremia caused by inappropriate antidiuretic hormone secretion also can occur. Concurrent malaria and other parasitic or bacterial infections may complicate management. Although JE occurs in areas of Asia where human immunodeficiency virus (HIV) infection may be prevalent, reports of their interaction have been limited, with no conclusion on differences in outcome.

Cases of clinical relapse with seizures, coma, and weakness, several occurring 6 to 9 months after recovery from the acute illness, have been reported. These patients and other asymptomatic recovered patients had evidence of persistent JE virus infection in peripheral blood mononuclear cells.[77] A study of 253 patients found laboratory evidence of subacute CNS infection in 5 percent of cases, with persistent intrathecal production of JE virus–specific IgM beyond 50 to 180 days or CSF containing JE virus antigen or virus more than 3 weeks after recovery.[67] Further studies are needed to confirm and characterize the persistence of JE virus and its clinical significance.

JE acquired during the first two trimesters of pregnancy may lead to fetal infection and miscarriage. JE virus has been isolated from products of conception in a few cases. Infections acquired during the third trimester have not been associated with adverse outcomes to the pregnancy.[11, 50] Whether congenital JE virus infections are associated with sublethal malformations in humans or whether congenital infections follow subclinical JE virus infection remains unknown. The virus is an important abortifacient in pigs and produces CNS and other lethal in utero malformations.

Laboratory Diagnosis

A specific diagnosis can be confirmed serologically by identifying JE virus–specific IgM antibody in serum or CSF by enzyme-linked immunosorbent assay (ELISA) or by demonstrating fourfold titer changes in neutralization, hemagglutination-inhibition, complement-fixation, or immunofluorescent antibodies between acute- and convalescent-phase serum samples.[9] Serologic cross-reactions with dengue virus and other flaviviruses are a common problem that sometimes can be resolved with cross-neutralization. Some laboratories have established empiric ELISA absorbance cutoffs that can differentiate dengue and JE virus infection.[32] IgM can be detected in serum or CSF (or in both) in nearly all cases by 1 week after the onset of illness.[9] ELISA kits are available commercially, as well as rapid, point-of-care immunoblot assays.[13] Patients who are moribund or severely ill on admission may be seronegative and are most likely to yield viral isolates from CSF.[8] The limited experience with polymerase chain reaction (PCR) suggests poor sensitivity with CSF samples. However, real-time PCR and T-7 promoter-based assays have proved to be sensitive in related West Nile and St. Louis encephalitis cases, and their application to JE should be examined. Immunofluorescent staining of CSF mononuclear cells can provide a specific diagnosis within several hours after a lumbar puncture is performed, but this procedure has a reported sensitivity of only 60 percent.[49]

JE virus occasionally can be isolated from the blood of patients in the pre-neuroinvasive phase of illness, usually no later than 6 to 7 days after onset. Virus can be recovered from brain biopsy and autopsy material by intracerebral inoculation of baby mice and various cell cultures, such as primary chick or duck embryo cells, and in Vero, LLCMK-2, C6-36, and AP-61 cell lines.

Differential Diagnosis

In rural Asia, the principal considerations include tuberculous and pyogenic meningitis; typhoid fever manifested as tremors and ataxia[83]; cerebral malaria; dengue virus infection with encephalopathy[10, 80]; and herpes simplex and measles viruses, enterovirus (especially EV71), HIV, and other causes of viral encephalitis. West Nile virus (and its Kunjin subtype) and Murray Valley encephalitis virus overlap JE virus in their distributions in Asia and Australia, have similar clinical findings, and because of their antigenic relatedness, pose a laboratory diagnostic challenge as well. Nipah virus, a newly described bat-associated paramyxovirus that led to large outbreaks of encephalitis in Malaysia in persons exposed to infected pigs, occurs in the same rural circumstances as does JE virus and may have similar clinical features. The absence of thalamic and basal ganglia involvement and multiple white matter lesions on T2-weighted MRI scans are important differentiating features.[45] In areas of Asia where poliomyelitis still has not been eradicated, JE should be included among the possible causes of acute flaccid paralysis. In a series from Lucknow, India, in which 394 children 6 months to 12 years of age with an acute encephalopathic illness underwent virologic studies, 23 percent had JE. In addition, JE and dengue accounted for 35 percent of defined viral encephalitis cases in Thailand.[12, 41] Meningitis or encephalitis develops in some scrub typhus patients; rash, adenopathy, and an eschar, if present, are helpful diagnostic signs. Acute encephalitis with convulsions is encountered in two thirds of patients with neurocysticercosis, which may be detected by brain imaging. Neurocysticercosis itself may increase the risk for acquiring JE (see "Pathophysiology"). In some developing countries, because aspirin continues to be used in febrile children, individual cases and even outbreaks of Reye syndrome have been mistaken initially as JE.

Noninfectious causes of acute encephalopathy to consider include heat stroke, vascular occlusion and intracranial hemorrhage, acute electrolyte disturbances, lead encephalopathy and other poisonings (especially caused by insect repellents), and inherited metabolic disorders.

Treatment

No specific antiviral therapy is available. A few patients have been treated with interferon-α, but its efficacy has not been evaluated in wider trials.[8, 25, 26] Supportive care and control of intracranial pressure are critical for a good outcome. Mannitol is used routinely in many areas of Asia, but early high-dose dexamethasone therapy was shown to have no clinical efficacy in a prospective controlled clinical trial.[29] Corticosteroids also have been given, without apparent benefit, in the late stages of illness as empiric therapy for late neurologic changes that were presumed to have an immunopathologic basis.[16] Other supportive measures, including control of fever and convulsions, attention to fluid balance, respiratory support, and prevention and treatment of secondary infections, have contributed to increased survival and improved outcomes.

Prognosis

The case-fatality ratio varies from 10 to 35 percent, depending on the accessibility and quality of supportive care. Younger children (<10 years of age) are more likely to die of the infection and to have more serious neurologic complications acutely and as sequelae. Gross neurologic impairment, such as paralysis, weakness, abnormal muscular tone, seizures, ataxia, and extrapyramidal movement disorders, are found in approximately a third to a half of recovered patients several months to a year after onset.[42, 54, 75] Electroencephalographic abnormalities have been detected in more than 50 percent of surviving children 1 year after recovery. Behavioral disorders and subnormal performance on psychologic testing may be found in as many as 75 percent of surviving patients 5 years after onset. Thus, in areas where the disease is prevalent, JE may account for substantial disability in the resident population.

Prevention

In areas of Asia where JE is endemic, universal childhood immunization is recommended.[85] Three JE vaccines are used, the most widely distributed of which is an inactivated vaccine produced from infected mouse brain.[28, 58] The others, a killed primary hamster kidney cell–derived vaccine and a live vaccine made from the attenuated SA 14-14-2 strain, are available exclusively in the People's Republic of China.[85, 88] A single dose of the latter was 99.3 percent effective (94.9 to 100%, 95% confidence interval) when delivered to children days to weeks before exposure to infection.[4] Inactivated mouse brain–derived JE vaccine is distributed in the United States and internationally for use in travelers. Two doses, the schedule recommended in Asia, have a protective efficacy of 91 percent.[28] However, three subcutaneous doses of 1.0 mL (days 0, 7, and 30 or 0, 7, and 14) are needed to produce adequate neutralizing antibody levels in persons from developed countries.[15, 30] The additional dose appears to be necessary because previous flaviviral immunity, generally lacking in residents of developed countries, primes the immune response to vaccination. High antibody titers are sustained for at least 3 years, after which a booster dose may be given.[23] The dose for children 1 to 3 years of age is 0.5 mL; the vaccine is not approved for use in children younger than 1 year. Children vertically infected with HIV in Asia have demonstrated a diminished response to vaccination.[70] JE vaccine has been given concurrently with hepatitis A, diphtheria-tetanus-pertussis, and mumps-measles-rubella vaccines without interference.[5, 85]

Local reactions and mild systemic reactions such as fever, headache, and myalgia occur in 10 to 25 percent of vaccinees.[30] Allergic reactions consisting of generalized urticaria and facial and peripheral angioedema have been a cause of concern because of the potential for respiratory obstruction and anaphylaxis and because the onset of reactions may be delayed for 12 to 72 hours after vaccine administration.[1, 30, 62, 72, 85] Among Japanese vaccinees, immediate reactions (within 1 hour of vaccination) have been associated strongly with IgE specifically reactive to gelatin (a vaccine stabilizer), whereas children with delayed reactions exhibited gelatin-specific IgG. Gelatin hypersensitivity may not underlie all cases with these adverse events. However, an allergic

TABLE 179–4 ■ RISK OF JAPANESE ENCEPHALITIS (JE) BY COUNTRY, REGION, AND SEASON

Country	Affected Areas/Jurisdictions	Transmission Season	Comments
Bangladesh	Few data, probably widespread	Possibly July–December as in northern India	Outbreak reported from Tangail district, Dacca division; sporadic cases in Rajshahi division
Bhutan	No data	No data, presumed to be similar to Nepal	Not applicable
Brunei	Presumed to be sporadic—endemic as in Malaysia	Presumed year-round transmission	
Cambodia	Endemic-hyperendemic countrywide	Presumed to be May–October	Highly prevalent in rural areas near Phnom Penh; confirmed cases in large epidemics October–December 1993–1998
Democratic Republic of Korea	Presumed to be countrywide in rural areas <800 m	July–October	Epidemics in 1970s; few recent data
Hong Kong	Rare cases in new territories	April–October	Vaccine not routinely recommended
India	Reported cases from all states except Arunachal, Dadra, Daman, Diu, Gujarat, Himachal, Jammu, Kashmir, Lakshadweep, Meghalaya, Nagar Haveli, Orissa, Punjab, Rajasthan, and Sikkim	*South India:* May–October in Goa; October– January in Tamil Nadu; August–December in Karnataka; second peak April–June in Mandya district *Andhra Pradesh:* September–December *North India:* July–December	Outbreaks in West Bengal, Bihar, Karnataka, Tamil Nadu, Andhra Pradesh, Kerala, Assam, Uttar Pradesh, Manipure, and Goa Urban cases reported, e.g., Lucknow
Indonesia	Kalimantan, Bali, Nusa Tenggara, Sulawesi, Mollucas, West Irian Java, and Lombok	Probably year-round risk; varies by island; peak risks associated with rainfall, rice cultivation, and presence of pigs Peak periods of risk: November–March; June–July in some years	Endemic on Bali; sporadic cases recognized elsewhere. Vaccine not recommended if travel to urban areas only
Japan*	Rare—sporadic cases on all islands except Hokkaido	June–September except Ryukyu Islands (Okinawa): April–October	Vaccine not routinely recommended for travel to Tokyo and other major cities; enzootic transmission without human cases observed on Hokkaido
Laos	Presumed to be endemic-hyperendemic countrywide	Presumed to be May–October	No data available
Malaysia	Sporadic—endemic in all states of Peninsula, Sarawak, and probably Sabah	November–January peak on Peninsula	Most cases from Penang, Perak, Salangor, Johore, and Sarawak; differentiate from Nipah encephalitis
Myanmar	Presumed to be endemic—hyperendemic countrywide	Presumed to be May–October	Repeated outbreaks in Shan State in Chiang Mai Valley
Nepal	Hyperendemic in southern lowlands (Terai); sporadic cases in Katmandu valley	July–December	Vaccine not recommended for travelers to high-altitude areas only
Pakistan	May be transmitted in central deltas	Presumed to be June–January	Cases reported near Karachi; endemic areas overlap those for West Nile virus
Papua New Guinea	Sporadic cases from Dintrecasteaux islands, Gulf, Milne Bay, South Highland, West Sepik, and Western provinces	Unknown	Vaccine not routinely recommended
People's Republic of China	Cases in all provinces except Xizang (Tibet), Xinjiang, and Qinghai	*Northern China:* May–September *Southern China:* April–October (Guangshi, Yunnan, Gwangdong, southern Fujian, Szechuan, Guizhou, Hunan, and Jiangsi provinces)	Vaccine not routinely recommended for travelers to urban areas only
Philippines	Presumed to be endemic on all islands	Uncertain, speculations based on locations and agro-ecosystems: *West Luzon, Mindoro, Negro Palowan:* April–November; *Elsewhere:* year-round; greatest risk April–January	Outbreaks described in Nueva Ecija, Luzon, and Manila
Republic of Korea	Rare sporadic cases	July–October	Last major outbreaks in 1982–1983
Russia	Far eastern maritime areas south of Khabarousk	Peak period July–September	Sporadic transmission in both rural and sylvatic cycles
Singapore	Rare cases; last in 1992	Year-round transmission no longer detected	Vaccine not routinely recommended. Local transmission on adjacent islands

Continued

TABLE 179–4 ■ RISK OF JAPANESE ENCEPHALITIS (JE) BY COUNTRY, REGION, AND SEASON—cont'd

Country	Affected Areas/Jurisdictions	Transmission Season	Comments
Sri Lanka	Endemic in all but mountainous areas; periodically epidemic in northern and central provinces	October–January; secondary peak of enzootic transmission May–June	Outbreaks in central (Anuradhapura) and northwestern provinces
Taiwan*	Endemic, sporadic cases; island-wide	April–October; June peak	Cases reported in and around Taipei
Thailand	Hyperendemic in north; sporadic-endemic in south. Reduced incidence due to vaccination	May–October	Annual outbreaks in Chiang Mai Valley; sporadic cases in Bangkok suburbs
Vietnam	Endemic, hyperendemic in all provinces	May–October	Highest rates in and near Hanoi
Western Pacific and Australia	Epidemics reported in Guam, Saipan (Northern Mariana Islands), and Torres Strait Islands and Cape York (Australia)	September–January in the Pacific; February–April in northern Australia	Enzootic cycle may not be sustainable; epidemics only follow introduction of virus

*Local JE incidence rates may not reflect risks to nonimmune visitors accurately because of high immunization rates in local populations. Humans are incidental to the transmission cycle. High levels of viral transmission may occur in the absence of human disease.
Note: Assessments are based on publications, surveillance reports, and personal correspondence. Extrapolations have been made from available data. Transmission patterns may change.
From Tsai, T. F., and Yu, Y. X.: Japanese vaccines. *In* Plotkin, S., and Orenstein, W. (eds.): Vaccines. 3rd ed. Philadelphia, W. B. Saunders, 1999, p. 700.

history, including atopy, is a risk factor.[62, 73, 74] In addition to antihistamines, parenteral corticosteroid therapy often has been needed. Allergic side effects are estimated to occur in 0.5 percent of vaccinees, a sufficiently high rate of a potentially serious adverse event that the vaccine has not been recommended as a routine immunization for travel to Asia.[30, 85] In addition, anecdotal cases of temporally associated acute disseminated encephalomyelitis have been reported, with a frequency as high as 1 in 50 to 1 in 75,000 vaccinees.[61] Current recommendations specify that the vaccine be reserved for expatriates, for persons spending 30 days or more in an endemic area during the transmission season, and for persons with briefer itineraries if they have a high risk of exposure (Table 179–4). The course of immunization should be completed 7 to 10 days before the onset of travel.[30]

Inactivated equine vaccines are used widely in some Asian countries, and a DNA equine vaccine recently has been shown to be highly efficacious. Inactivated cell culture–derived and recombinant vaccines for human use are being developed.[53]

Avoidance of outdoor activities during the evening hours, staying in screened or air-conditioned quarters, and sleeping under a bed net will reduce the risk of exposure to vector mosquitoes. Wearing long-sleeved shirts and long pants and using mosquito repellents applied to clothing and exposed skin are recommended for outdoor activities.

The production of vector mosquitoes in rice fields has been controlled by scheduled changes in water levels, application of larvicides and larval predators, and nontargeted effects of agricultural pesticides.

REFERENCES

1. Andersen, M. M., and Ronne, T.: Side effects with Japanese encephalitis vaccine. Lancet *337*:1044, 1991.
2. Benakappa, D. G., Anvekar, G. A., Viswanath, D., et al.: Japanese encephalitis. Indian J. Pediatr. *21*:811–815, 1994.
3. Bhattacharya, S., Chakraborty, S. K., Chakraborty, S., et al.: Density of *Culex vishnui* and appearance of JE antibody in sentinel chicks and wild birds in relation to Japanese encephalitis cases. Trop. Geogr. Med. *38*:46–50, 1986.
4. Bista, M. B., Bannerjee, M. K., Shin, S. H., et al.: Efficacy of single-dose SA 14-14-2 vaccine against Japanese encephalitis: A case control study. Lancet *358*:791–795, 2001.
5. Bock, H. L., Kruppenbacher, J. P., Bienzle, U., et al.: Does the concurrent administration of an inactivated hepatitis A vaccine influence the immune response to other travelers vaccines? J. Travel Med. *7*:74–78, 2000.
6. Buescher, E. L., and Scherer, W. F.: Ecologic studies of Japanese encephalitis virus in Japan. Am. J. Trop. Med. Hyg. *8*:719–722, 1959.
7. Burke, D. S., Lorsomrudee, W., Leake, C. J., et al.: Fatal outcome in Japanese encephalitis. Am. J. Trop. Med. Hyg. *34*:1203–1210, 1985.
8. Burke, D. S., and Morrill, J. C.: Levels of interferon in the plasma and cerebrospinal fluid of patients with acute Japanese encephalitis. J. Infect. Dis. *155*:797–799, 1987.
9. Burke, D. S., Nisalak, A., Ussery, M. A., et al.: Kinetics of IgM and IgG responses to Japanese encephalitis virus in human serum and cerebrospinal fluid. J. Infect. Dis. *151*:1093–1099, 1985.
10. Cam, B. V., Fonsmark, L., Hue, N. B., et al.: Prospective case-control study of encephalopathy in children with dengue hemorrhagic fever. Am. J. Trop. Med. Hyg. *65*:848–851, 2001.
11. Chaturvedi, U. C., Mathur, A., Chandra, A., et al.: Transplacental infection with Japanese encephalitis virus. J. Infect. Dis. *141*:712–715, 1980.
12. Chokephaibulkit, K., Kankirawatana, P., Apintanapong, S., et al.: Viral etiologies of encephalitis in Thai children. Pediatr. Infect. Dis. J. *20*:216–218, 2001.
13. Cuzzubbo, A. J., Vaughn, D. W., Nisalak, A., et al.: Comparison of PanBio dengue duo enzyme-linked immunosorbent assay (ELISA) and MRL dengue fever virus immunoglobulin M capture ELISA for diagnosis of dengue virus infections in Southeast Asia. Clin. Diagn. Lab. Immunol. *6*:705–712, 1999.
14. Das, S. K., Nityanand, S., Sood, K., et al.: Japanese B encephalitis with neurocysticercosis. J. Assoc. Physicians India *39*:643–644, 1991.
15. Defraites, R. F., Gambel, J. M., Hoke, C. H., Jr., et al.: Japanese encephalitis vaccine (inactivated, BIKEN) in U.S. soldiers: Immunogenicity and safety of vaccine administered in two dosing regimens. Am. J. Trop. Med. Hyg. *61*:288–293, 1999.
16. Desai, A., Ravi, V., Guru, S. C., et al.: Detection of autoantibodies to neural antigens in the CSF of Japanese encephalitis patients and correlation of findings with the outcome. J. Neurol. Sci. *122*:109–116, 1994.
17. Desai, A., Shankar, S. K., Ravi, V., et al.: Japanese encephalitis virus antigen in the human brain and its topographic distribution. Acta Neuropathol. *89*:368–373, 1995.
18. Dhanda, V., Mourya, D. T., Mishra, A. C., et al.: Japanese encephalitis virus infection in mosquito reared from field-collected immatures and in wild-caught males. Am. J. Trop. Med. Hyg. *41*:732–736, 1989.
19. Dropulic, B., and Masters, C. L.: Entry of neurotropic arboviruses into the central nervous system: An in vitro study using brain endothelium. J. Infect. Dis. *161*:685–691, 1990.
20. Edelman, R., Schneider, R. J., Chieowanich, P., et al.: The effect of dengue virus infection on the clinical sequelae of Japanese encephalitis: A one-year follow-up study in Thailand. Southeast Asian J. Trop. Med. Public Health *6*:308–315, 1975.
21. Fang, R., Hus, D. R., and Lim, T. W.: Investigation of a suspected outbreak of Japanese encephalitis in Pulau Langkawi. Malaysia J. Pathol. *3*:23–30, 1980.

22. Gajanana, A., Thenmozhi, V., Samuel, P. P., et al.: A community-based study of subclinical flavivirus infections in children in an area of Tamil Nadu, India, where Japanese encephalitis is endemic. Bull. World Health Organ. *73*:237–244, 1995.
23. Gambel, J. M., DeFraites, R., Hoke, C., Jr., et al.: Japanese encephalitis vaccine: Persistence of antibody up to 3 years after a three-dose primary series. J. Infect. Dis. *171*:1074, 1995.
24. Hanna, J. N., Ritchie, S. A., Phillips, D. A., et al.: Japanese encephalitis in north Queensland, Australia, 1998. Med. J. Aust. *170*:533–536, 1999.
25. Harinasuta, C., Nimmanitya, S., and Titsyakorn, U.: The effect of interferon-alpha A on two cases of Japanese encephalitis in Thailand. Southeast Asian J. Trop. Med. Public Health *16*:332–336, 1985.
26. Harrington, D. G., Hilmas, D. E., Elwell, M. L., et al.: Intranasal infection of monkeys with Japanese encephalitis virus: Clinical response and treatment with a nuclease-resistant derivative of poly (I)-poly (C). Am. J. Trop. Med. Hyg. *25*:1191–1198, 1977.
27. Hiyake, M.: The pathology of Japanese encephalitis. Bull. World Health Organ. *30*:153–160, 1964.
28. Hoke, C. H., Nisalak, A., Sangawhipa, N, et al.: Protection against Japanese encephalitis by inactivated vaccines. N. Engl. J. Med. *319*:609–614, 1989.
29. Hoke, C. H., Vaughn, D. W., Nisalak, A., et al.: Effect of high-dose dexamethasone on the outcome of acute encephalitis due to Japanese encephalitis virus. J. Infect. Dis. *165*:631–637, 1992.
30. Immunization Practices Advisory Committee (ACIP): Inactivated Japanese encephalitis virus vaccine: Recommendations of the ACIP. M. M. W. R. Recomm. Rep. *42*(RR-1):1–15, 1993.
31. Inada, R.: Compte rendu des recherches sur l'encephalite epidemique au Japon. Offic. Int. D'Hyg Pub. Bull. Mens. *29*:1389–1401, 1937.
32. Innis, B. L., Nisalak, A., Nimmannitya, S., et al.: An enzyme-linked immunosorbent assay to characterize dengue infections where dengue and Japanese encephalitis cocirculate. Am. J. Trop. Med. Hyg. *40*:418–427, 1989.
33. Ishii, T., Matsushita, M., and Hamada, S.: Characteristic residual neuropathological features of Japanese B encephalitis. Acta Neuropathol. *38*:181–186, 1977.
34. Johnson, R. T., Burke, D. S., Elwell, M., et al.: Japanese encephalitis: Immunocytochemical studies of viral antigen and inflammatory cells in fatal cases. Ann. Neurol. *18*:567–573, 1985.
35. Kalita, J., and Misra, U. K.: Comparison of CT scan and MRI findings in the diagnosis of Japanese encephalitis. J. Neurol. Sci. *174*:3–8, 2000.
36. Kalita, J., and Misra, U. K.: Markedly severe dystonia in Japanese encephalitis. Mov. Disord. *15*:1168–1172, 2000.
37. Kamala, C. S., Venkatwshwara, R. M., George, S., et al.: Japanese encephalitis in children in Bellary Karnataka. Indian Pediatr. *26*:445–452, 1989.
38. Kimura-Kuroda, J., Ichikawa, M., Ogata, A., et al.: Specific tropism of Japanese encephalitis virus for developing neurons in primary rat brain culture. Arch. Virol. *130*:477–484, 1993.
39. Kitaoka, M.: Shift of age distribution of cases of Japanese encephalitis in Japan during the period 1950 to 1967. *In* Hammon, M. W., Kitaoka, M., and Downs, W. G. (eds.): Immunization for Japanese Encephalitis. Amsterdam, Excerpta Medica, 1972, pp. 285–291.
40. Kumar, R., Mathur, A., Kumar, A., et al.: Clinical features and prognostic indicators of Japanese encephalitis in children in Lucknow (India). Indian J. Med. Res. *91*:321–327, 1990.
41. Kumar, R., Mathur, A., Kumar, A., et al.: Virological investigations of acute encephalopathy in India. Indian Council Med. Res. 1228–1230, 1990.
42. Kumar, R., Mathur, A., Singh, K. B., et al.: Clinical sequelae of Japanese encephalitis in children. Indian J. Med. Res. *97*:9–13, 1993.
43. Kumar, R., Selvan, A. S., Sharma, S., et al.: Clinical predictors of Japanese encephalitis. Neuroepidemiology *13*:97–102, 1994.
44. Li, Z. S., Hong, S. F., and Gong, N. L.: Immunohistochemical study of Japanese B encephalitis. Chin. Med. J. (Engl.) *101*:768–771, 1988.
45. Lim, C. C., Sitoh, Y. Y., Hui, F., et al.: Nipah viral encephalitis or Japanese encephalitis? MR findings in a new zoonotic disease. A. J. N. R. Am. J. Neuroradiol. *21*:455–461, 2000.
46. Lincoln, A. F., and Sivertson, S. E.: Acute phase of Japanese B encephalitis: Two hundred and one cases in American soldiers, Korea, 1960. J. Med. Assoc. *150*:268–273, 1952.
47. Liu, Y. F., Teng, C. L., and Liu, K.: Cerebral cysticercosis as a factor aggravating Japanese B encephalitis. Chin. Med. J. (Engl.) *75*:1010, 1957.
48. Lubinieski, A. S., Cypress, C. H., and Lucas, J. P.: Synergistic interaction of two agents in mice: Japanese B encephalitis virus and *Trichinella spiralis*. Am. J. Trop. Med. Hyg. *23*:235–241, 1974.
49. Mathur, A., Kumar, R., Sharma, S., et al.: Rapid diagnosis of Japanese encephalitis by immunofluorescent examination of cerebrospinal fluid. Indian J. Med. Res. *91*:1–4, 1990.
50. Mathur, A., Tandon, H. O., Mathur, K. R., et al.: Japanese encephalitis infection during pregnancy. Indian J. Med. Res. *81*:9–12, 1985.
51. Misra, U. K., and Kalita, J.: Seizures in Japanese encephalitis. J. Neurol. Sci. *190*:57–60, 2001.
52. Misra, U. K., Kalita, J., Jain, S. K., et al.: Radiological and neurophysiological changes in Japanese encephalitis. J. Neurol. Neurosurg. Psychiatry *57*:1484–1487, 1994.
53. Monath, T. P., McCarthy, K., Bedford, P., et al.: Clinical proof of principle of ChimeriVax: Recombinant live, attenuated vaccines against flavivirus infections. Vaccine *20*:1004–1018, 2002.
54. Murgod, U. A., Muthane, U. B., Ravi, V., et al.: Persistent movement disorders following Japanese encephalitis. Neurology *57*:2313–2315, 2001.
55. Nathanson, N., and Cole, G. A.: Fatal Japanese encephalitis virus infection in immunosuppressed spider monkeys. Clin. Exp. Immunol. *6*:161–166, 1970.
56. Ohyama, A., Ishiga, A., Fujita, N., et al.: Effect of human gamma globulin upon encephalitis viruses. Jpn. J. Microbiol. *3*:159–169, 1959.
57. Olson, J. G., Ksiazek, T. G., Tan, R., et al.: Correlation of population indices of female *Culex tritaeniorhynchus* with Japanese encephalitis viral activity in Kapuk, Indonesia. Southeast Asian J. Trop. Med. Public Health *16*:337–340, 1985.
58. Oya, A.: Japanese encephalitis vaccine. Acta Paediatr. Jpn. *30*:175–184, 1988.
59. Paul, W. S., Moore, P. S., Karabatsos, N., et al.: Outbreak of Japanese encephalitis on the island of Saipan, 1990. J. Infect. Dis. *167*:1053–1058, 1993.
60. Peiris, J. S. M., Amerasinghe, F. P., Amerasinghe, P. H., et al.: Japanese encephalitis in Sri Lanka. I. The study of an epidemic-vector incrimination, porcine infection and human disease. Trans. R. Soc. Trop. Med. Hyg. *86*:307–323, 1992.
61. Plesner, A. M., Arlien-Soborg, P. and Herning, M.: Neurological complications to vaccination against Japanese encephalitis. Eur. J. Neurol. *5*:479–485, 1998.
62. Plesner, A. M., Ronne, T., and Wachmann, H.: Case-control study of allergic reactions to Japanese encephalitis vaccine. Vaccine *18*:1830–1836, 2000.
63. Poneprasert, B.: Japanese encephalitis in children in northern Thailand. Southeast J. Trop. Med. Public Health *20*:599–603, 1989.
64. Pradhan, S., Gupta, R. K., Singh, M. B., and Mathur, A.: Biphasic illness pattern due to early relapse in Japanese-B virus encephalitis. J. Neurol. Sci. *183*:13–18, 2001.
65. Pradhan, S., Pandey, N., Shashank, S., et al.: Parkinsonism due to predominant involvement of substantia nigra in Japanese encephalitis. Neurology *53*:1781–1786, 1999.
66. Rathi, A. K., Kushwaha, K. P., Singh, Y. D., et al.: JE virus encephalitis: 1988 epidemic at Gorakhpur. Indian Pediatr. *30*:325–333, 1993.
67. Ravi, V., Desai, A. S., Shenoy, P. K., et al.: Persistence of Japanese encephalitis virus in the human nervous system. J. Med. Virol. *40*:326–329, 1993.
68. Ravi, V., Taly, A. B., Shankar, S. K., et al.: Association of Japanese encephalitis virus infection with Guillain-Barré syndrome in endemic areas of South India. Acta Neurol. Scand. *90*:67–72, 1994.
69. Rodrigues, F. M., Guttikar, S. N., and Pinto, B. D.: Prevalence of antibodies to Japanese encephalitis and West Nile viruses among wild birds in the Krishna-Godavari Delta, Andhra Pradesh, India. Trans. R. Soc. Trop. Med. Hyg. *75*:258–262, 1981.
70. Rojanasuphot, S., Shaffer, N., Chotpitayasunondh, T., et al.: Response to JE vaccine among HIV-infected children, Bangkok, Thailand. Southeast Asian J. Trop. Med. Public Health *29*:443–450, 1998.
71. Rosen, L.: The natural history of Japanese encephalitis virus. Annu. Rev. Microbiol. *40*:395–414, 1986.
72. Ruff, T. A., Eisen, D., Fuller, A., et al.: Adverse reactions to Japanese encephalitis vaccine. Lancet *338*:881–882, 1991.
73. Sakaguchi, M., Miyazawa, H., and Inouye, S.: Specific IgE and IgG to gelatin in children with systemic cutaneous reactions to Japanese encephalitis vaccines. Allergy *56*:536–539, 2001.
74. Sakaguchi, M., Nakashima, K., Takahashi, H., et al.: Anaphylaxis to Japanese encephalitis vaccine. Allergy *56*:804–805, 2001.
75. Schneider, R. J., Firestone, M. H., Edelman, R., et al.: Japanese encephalitis: A one-year follow-up study in Thailand. Southeast Asian J. Trop. Med. Public Health *5*:560–568, 1974.
76. Shankar, S. K., Rao, T. V., Mruthyunjayanna, B. P., et al.: Autopsy study of brains during an epidemic of Japanese encephalitis in Karnataka. Indian J. Med. Res. *78*:431–440, 1983.
77. Sharma, S., Mathur, A., Prakash, R., et al.: Japanese encephalitis virus latency in peripheral blood lymphocytes and recurrence of infection in children. Clin. Exp. Immunol. *85*:85–89, 1991.
78. Singh, A., Kulshreshtha, R., and Mathur, A.: Secretion of the chemokine interleukin-8 during Japanese encephalitis virus infection. J. Med. Microbiol. *49*:607–612, 2000.
79. Singh, P., Kalra, N., Ratho, R. K., et al.: Coexistent neurocysticercosis and Japanese B encephalitis: MR imaging correlation. A. J. N. R. Am. J. Neuroradiol. *22*:1131–1136, 2001.
80. Solomon, T., Dung, N. M., Vaughn, D. W., et al.: Neurological manifestations of dengue infection. Lancet *355*:1053–1059, 2000.
81. Srikanth, S., Ravi, V., Poornima, S., et al.: Viral antibodies in recent onset, nonorganic psychoses: Correspondence with symptomatic severity. Soc. Biol. Psychiatry *36*:517–521, 1994.
82. Thisyakorn, U. S. A., and Nimmannitya, S.: Japanese encephalitis in Thai children, Bangkok, Thailand. Southeast Asian J. Trop. Med. Public Health *16*:93–97, 1985.

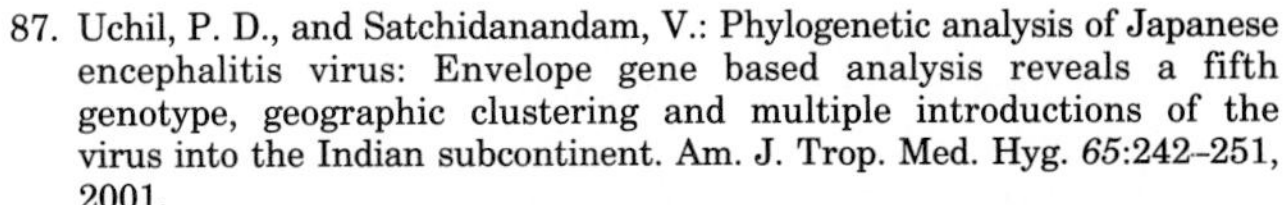

83. Trevett, A. J., Nwokolo, N., Lightfoot, D., et al.: Ataxia in patients infected with *Salmonella typhi* phage type D2: Clinical, biochemical and immunohistochemical studies. Trans. R. Soc. Trop. Med. Hyg. *88*:565–568, 1994.
84. Tsai, T. F.: New initiatives for the control of Japanese encephalitis by vaccination: Minutes of a WHO/CVI meeting, Bangkok, Thailand, 13–15 October, 1998. Vaccine *18*(Suppl. 2):1–25, 2000.
85. Tsai, T. F., Chang, G. J., and Yu, Y. X.: Japanese encephalitis vaccines. *In* Plotkin, S., and Orenstein, W. (eds.): Vaccines. 3rd ed. Philadelphia, W. B. Saunders, 1999, p. 672.
86. Tsai, T. F., Nadhirat, S., and Rojanasuphot, S.: Regional workshop on control strategies for Japanese encephalitis. Southeast Asian J. Trop. Med. Public Health *26*(Suppl. 3):1–59, 1995.
87. Uchil, P. D., and Satchidanandam, V.: Phylogenetic analysis of Japanese encephalitis virus: Envelope gene based analysis reveals a fifth genotype, geographic clustering and multiple introductions of the virus into the Indian subcontinent. Am. J. Trop. Med. Hyg. *65*:242–251, 2001.
88. Yu, Y. X., Ming, A. G., Pen, G. Y., et al.: Safety of a live-attenuated Japanese encephalitis virus vaccine (SA14-14-2) for children. Am. J. Trop. Med. Hyg. *39*:214–217, 1988.
89. Williams, D. T., Daniels, P. W., Lunt, R. A., et al.: Experimental infections of pigs with Japanese encephalitis virus and closely related Australian flaviviruses. Am. J. Trop. Med. Hyg. *65*:379–387, 2001.
90. Zimmerman, H. M.: The pathology of Japanese B encephalitis. Am. J. Pathol. *22*:965–991, 1946.

CHAPTER **179E**

Murray Valley Encephalitis

JOHN G. AASKOV

Outbreaks of an acute, severe encephalitic illness clinically similar to Japanese and St. Louis encephalitis occurred in rural areas of southeastern Australia in 1917, 1918, 1922, 1925, 1951, 1956, 1971, and 1974[1, 9, 16, 17] and in northwestern Australia in 1978, 1981, 1993, and 2000.[8, 13, 34] They are believed to represent a single entity for which various names (Australian X disease, Murray Valley encephalitis, Australian encephalitis) have been used. Approximately 380 cases were reported in the 12 outbreaks, and sporadic cases have occurred each year since 1978 when no outbreaks have taken place.[34]

Case-fatality rates, as high as 60 percent in the early years, declined to 20 percent in the 1974 outbreak and have remained at about this level since then.[10, 13] However, significant residual neurologic disability occurs in as many as 50 percent of survivors.[10, 13]

The presence of this disease in Papua New Guinea was confirmed in 1956.[21] The causative virus was transmitted to experimental animals as early as 1918,[6, 11] although those strains could not be maintained. The definitive isolation and characterization of Murray Valley encephalitis virus in 1951[20] led to epidemiologic studies that suggested its survival in bird-mosquito cycles in northern Australia but not in the area of epidemic occurrence in southern Australia.[1]

In an effort to dissociate a regional disease from a specific locality, the term Australian encephalitis was proposed by residents of Murray Valley for the disease caused by Murray Valley encephalitis virus. Some researchers subsequently have attempted to expand the term Australian encephalitis to include encephalitis caused by any Australian arbovirus. Because the term Australian encephalitis has no scientific validity and is ambiguous, it should not be used.

Etiologic Agent

Murray Valley encephalitis virus was isolated post mortem from the brains of patients in 1951[20] and 1974[23] and shown to be related antigenically to Japanese encephalitis virus.[20, 23]

A partial nucleotide sequence of Murray Valley encephalitis virus[14] has confirmed the previous classification of this virus on serologic grounds as being a member of the Japanese encephalitis, St. Louis encephalitis, West Nile fever subgroup of flaviviruses.[31] Distinguishing Australian strains of Murray Valley encephalitis virus from those isolated in Papua New Guinea has been possible on the basis of limited nucleotide sequencing.[12, 24]

Transmission and Epidemiology

The mosquito *Culex annulirostris* is believed to be the major vector of Murray Valley encephalitis virus,[17, 18, 26] although other mosquitoes such as *Aedes normanensis, Aedes tremulus,* and *Culex quinquefasciatus* also may be involved.[7]

Murray Valley encephalitis virus is believed to survive in cycles of infection between birds and mosquitoes in northern Australia and Papua New Guinea,[1] where regular infection of humans and other animals is indicated by seroconversion in the summer-autumn "wet" season,[15] as well as by clinical disease.[7, 34] Epidemics that occurred in more populous areas of southeastern Australia are believed to have followed the introduction of virus when abnormal spring rainfall allowed chains of bird-mosquito transmission through northern Australia.[2]

However, several studies have suggested interepidemic survival of virus in southern Australia.[22] Isolation of Murray Valley encephalitis virus from wild-caught male *A. tremulus* mosquitoes at the end of the "dry season" in western Australia[7] suggests that vertical transmission may be one mechanism by which it is achieved.

Although disease occurs most commonly in children, clinical infection has developed in individuals of all ages.[1, 4, 8, 10, 13, 17, 25] Data are insufficient to determine whether the lower incidence of disease in adults is due to immunity acquired from previous subclinical infections.

Clinical Manifestations[5, 9, 10, 13, 33]

An initial period of nonspecific prodromal symptoms and signs such as fever, headache, nausea, vomiting, muscle pain, and photophobia is followed within 2 to 5 days by drowsiness, mental obtundation, confusion, disorientation, incongruous behavior, ataxia, speech disturbance, or convulsions, sometimes with a grand mal character. Neurologic signs were present in most cases on admission to the hospital, and additional signs appeared as the disease progressed. In some cases, the signs fluctuated from hour to hour. Bennett[5] recognized three groups of patients according to eventual clinical outcome:

1. Patients with mild cases commonly had disturbed mentation short of coma, incoherent or slurred speech, aphasia, speech perseveration, incontinence, neck stiffness, intention tremor, and limb hypertonicity but rarely required

assistance for respiration. The neurologic changes stabilized in 5 to 10 days, and the patients improved.

2. Patients with severe disease showed more profound central nervous system (CNS) involvement consisting of impairment of consciousness to coma, more marked signs of upper motor neuron involvement, and pharyngeal or respiratory paralysis requiring artificial respiration.

3. In fatal cases, patients had either spastic quadriplegia progressing to almost complete loss of nervous function or severe disease with superimposed infection.

The differential diagnosis of Murray Valley encephalitis has been suggested to be assisted by attention to signs attributable to spinal cord involvement and to cranial nerve palsies, tremor, and the frequency of seizures (seizures rarely develop in adults with Murray Valley encephalitis, whereas they may occur in up to 90 percent of children). Computed tomographic scans in these patients are normal, and electroencephalograms do not show focal features.[10]

Pathology

A period of viremia probably precedes infection of the CNS, but it has not been demonstrated. Pathologic changes in fatal cases were restricted to the CNS and included extensive perivascular cuffing, especially in the cortex, lymphocytic infiltration of the meninges, neuron degeneration and neuronophagia in the cerebellum and spinal cord, and thalamic necrosis. Evidence of repair, including calcification, was described in patients who died late in the disease.[6, 10, 11, 30, 32] These pathologic changes do not distinguish Murray Valley encephalitis from other arthropod-borne encephalitides.

In rodents infected peripherally with Murray Valley encephalitis virus, the virus enters the CNS via the olfactory pathway after replicating in regional lymph nodes. From the olfactory lobe, it spreads via interconnected neural circuits to the cortex, hippocampus, thalamus, cerebellum, medulla oblongata, and spinal cord. Extensive neuronal necrosis was observed in the olfactory bulb and hippocampus. The severity of the subsequent encephalitis correlated with the magnitude of mononuclear and polymorphonuclear cell infiltrates. Infiltration of neutrophils was preceded by increased expression of tumor necrosis factor–α and the chemokine N51/KC in the CNS. Previous depletion of neutrophils or inhibition of inducible nitric oxide synthetase resulted in prolonged survival and decreased mortality in Murray Valley encephalitis virus–infected mice.[3, 27] However, the pronounced mononuclear cell content of cerebrospinal fluid in patients with Murray Valley encephalitis[10] contrasts with the picture in rodents.[27]

Diagnosis

Clinical and epidemiologic features may suggest the diagnosis of Murray Valley encephalitis, especially during recognized epidemics, but individual cases may be difficult to distinguish from cases of encephalitis or encephalopathy of other cause (e.g., herpesvirus).[5, 29] A specific diagnosis depends on serologic evidence of infection concurrent with disease. Detection of IgM antibody that reacts with Murray Valley encephalitis virus in hemagglutination-inhibition[19, 35] or in enzyme-linked immunosorbent assays is the most useful indication of recent infection. Other flaviviruses, especially Kunjin virus, may cause encephalitis, subclinical infection, or minor illness during epidemics of Murray Valley encephalitis, and interpretation of serologic cross-reactions between Kunjin and Murray Valley encephalitis viruses[28] may require specific tests (e.g., neutralization) with several viruses.[17]

Virus isolation has not been successful for antemortem diagnosis. However, a single report[28] has described the use of reverse transcription–polymerase chain reaction (RT-PCR) to detect Murray Valley encephalitis virus RNA in the serum of a child with encephalitis. Subsequent serology confirmed the RT-PCR data. Given the need for rapid clinical intervention in this disease, RT-PCR warrants more extensive use in a diagnostic setting.

Treatment and Prognosis

No specific antiviral therapy is available. Administration of corticosteroids is recommended during the acute phase of the illness to reduce brain edema. Artificial respiration has been lifesaving, and all patients should be transported to base hospitals with facilities for the management of patients with respiratory paralysis.[5] Most patients also require parenteral nutrition or nasogastric feeding.[10]

The early epidemics left some neurologic and psychiatric sequelae, but the lower case-fatality rate in recent outbreaks, presumably because of modern intensive care techniques, has been associated with a high rate of residual disability.[10, 13] Bennett[5] reviewed 18 patients up to 16 months after infection. Four of 11 patients with mild disease had emotional problems and mild degrees of impaired motor coordination and mental acuity. All seven patients with severe disease had serious defects, including paraplegia or quadriplegia and mental disturbance.

This pattern of high residual disability has continued to the present.[10, 13]

Prevention

The irregularity of outbreaks and the large areas in which they occur render preventive measures difficult to institute. However, both government and personal programs for restriction of exposure of humans to the common mosquito vector *C. annulirostris* are likely to minimize disease.

No vaccine is available, and although the killed Japanese encephalitis vaccine elicits antibodies that neutralize Murray Valley encephalitis virus in vitro, whether a Japanese encephalitis vaccine would offer any cross-protection in humans infected with Murray Valley encephalitis virus is not known.

REFERENCES

1. Anderson, S. G.: Murray Valley encephalitis and Australian X disease. J. Hyg. (Camb.) *52*:447–468, 1954.
2. Anderson, S. G., and Eagle, M.: Murray Valley encephalitis: The contrasting epidemiological picture in 1951 and 1952. Med. J. Aust. *1*:478–481, 1953.
3. Andrews, D. M., Matthews, V. B., Sammels, L. M., et al.: The severity of Murray Valley encephalitis in mice is linked to neutrophil infiltration and inducible nitric oxide synthetase activity in the central nervous system. J. Virol. *73*:8781–8790, 1999.
4. Annual report of the National Notifiable Diseases Surveillance System, 1993. Comm. Dis. Int. Bull. *18*:518–547, 1994.
5. Bennett, N. M.: Murray Valley encephalitis, 1974: Clinical features. Med. J. Aust. *2*:446–450, 1976.
6. Breinl, A.: Clinical, pathological, and experimental observations on the "mysterious disease," a clinically aberrant form of acute poliomyelitis. Med. J. Aust. *1*:209–213, 1918.
7. Broom, A. K., Lindsay, M. D. A., Johansen, C. A., et al.: Two possible mechanisms for survival and initiation of Murray Valley encephalitis virus activity in the Kimberley region of Western Australia. Am. J. Trop. Med. Hyg. *53*:95–99, 1995.

8. Bucens, M.: Arbovirus infections diagnosed in Perth, 1981. *In* St. George, T. D., and Kay, B. H. (eds.): Arbovirus Research in Australia. Proceedings, 3rd Symposium, February 15–17, 1982. Commonwealth Scientific and Industrial Research Organisation and Queensland Institute of Medical Research, 1982, p. 171.
9. Burnell, G. H.: The Broken Hill epidemic. Med. J. Aust. *2*:157–161, 1917.
10. Burrow, J. N. C., Whelan, P. I., Kilburn, C. J., et al.: Australian encephalitis in the Northern Territory: Clinical and epidemiological features, 1987–1996. Aust. N. Z. J. Med. *28*:590–596, 1998.
11. Cleland, J. B., Campbell, A. W., and Bradley, B.: Rep. Dir. Gen. Public Health N. S. W., 1917. 1918, pp. 150–280.
12. Coelen, R. J., and MacKenzie, J. S.: The 5′-terminal non-coding region of Murray Valley encephalitis virus RNA is highly conserved. J. Gen. Virol. *71*:241–245, 1990.
13. Cordova, S. P., Smith, D. W., Broom, A. K., et al.: Murray Valley encephalitis in Western Australia in 2000, with evidence of southerly spread. Commun. Dis. Intell. *24*:368–372, 2000.
14. Dalgarno, L., Trent, D. W., Strauss, J. H., et al.: Partial nucleotide sequence of the Murray Valley encephalitis virus genome: Comparison of the encoded polypeptides with yellow fever virus structural and non-structural proteins. J. Mol. Biol. *187*:309–329, 1986.
15. Doherty, R. L.: Arthropod-borne viruses in Australia and their relation to infection and disease. Prog. Med. Virol. *17*:136–192, 1974.
16. Doherty, R. L., Carley, J. G., Cremer, M. R., et al.: Murray Valley encephalitis in eastern Australia, 1971. Med. J. Aust. *2*:1170–1173, 1972.
17. Doherty, R. L., Carley, J. G., Filippich, C., et al.: Murray Valley encephalitis in Australia, 1974: Antibody response in cases and community. Aust. N. Z. J. Med. *6*:446–453, 1976.
18. Doherty, R. L., Carley, J. G., Kay, B. H., et al.: Murray Valley encephalitis virus infection in mosquitoes and domestic fowls in Queensland, 1974. Aust. J. Exp. Biol. Med. Sci. *54*:237–243, 1976.
19. Field, P. R., and Murphy, A. M.: The role of specific IgM globulin estimations in the diagnosis of acquired rubella. Med. J. Aust. *2*:1244–1248, 1972.
20. French, E. L.: Murray Valley encephalitis: Isolation and characterisation of aetiological agent. Med. J. Aust. *1*:100–103, 1952.
21. French, E. L., Anderson, S. G., Price, A. V. G., et al.: Murray Valley encephalitis in New Guinea. 1. Isolation of Murray Valley encephalitis virus from the brain of a fatal case of encephalitis occurring in a Papuan native. Am. J. Trop. Med. Hyg. *6*:827–834, 1957.
22. Gard, G. P., Giles, J. R., Dwyer-Gray, R. J., et al.: Serological evidence of interepidemic infection of feral pigs in New South Wales with Murray Valley encephalitis virus. Aust. J. Exp. Biol. Med. Sci. *54*:297–302, 1976.
23. Lehmann, N. I., Gust, I. D., and Doherty, R.: Isolation of Murray Valley encephalitis virus from the brains of three patients with encephalitis. Med. J. Aust. *2*:450–454, 1976.
24. Lobigs, M., Marshall, I. D., Weir, R. C., et al.: Murray Valley encephalitis virus field strains from Australia and Papua New Guinea: Studies on the sequence of the major envelope protein gene and virulence for mice. Virology *165*:245–255, 1988.
25. Mackenzie, J. S., Smith, D. W., Broom, A. K., et al.: Australian encephalitis in Western Australia, 1979–1991. Med. J. Aust. *158*:591–595, 1993.
26. Marshall, I. D., Woodroofe, G. M., and Hirsch, S.: Viruses recovered from mosquitoes and wildlife serum collected in the Murray Valley of south-eastern Australia, February, 1974, during an epidemic of encephalitis. Aust. J. Exp. Biol. Med. Sci. *60*:457–470, 1982.
27. Matthews, V., Robertson, T., Kendrick, T., et al.: Morphological features of Murray Valley encephalitis virus infection in the central nervous system of Swiss mice. Int. J. Exp. Pathol. *81*:31–40, 2000.
28. McMinn, P. C., Carman, P. G., and Smith, D. W.: Early diagnosis of Murray Valley encephalitis by reverse transcriptase–polymerase chain reaction. Pathology *32*:49–51, 2000.
29. Merritt, A., Phillips, D. A., Carney, I., et al.: A presumptive case of fatal Murray Valley encephalitis acquired in Alice Springs. Commun. Dis. Intell. *22*:103–104, 1998.
30. Pedrau, J. R.: The Australian epidemics of encephalomyelitis (X-disease). J. Pathol. Bacteriol. *42*:59–65, 1936.
31. Pond, W. L., Russ, S. B., Rogers, N. G., et al.: Murray Valley encephalitis virus: Its serological relationship to the Japanese–West Nile–St. Louis encephalitis group of viruses. J. Immunol. *75*:78–84, 1955.
32. Robertson, E. G.: Murray Valley encephalitis: Pathological aspects. Med. J. Aust. *1*:107–110, 1952.
33. Robertson, E. G., and McLorinan, H.: Murray Valley encephalitis: Clinical aspects. Med. J. Aust. *1*:103–107, 1952.
34. Russell, R. C., and Dwyer, D. E.: Arboviruses associated with human disease in Australia. Microbes Infect. *2*:1693–1704, 2000.
35. Wiemers, M. A., and Stallman, N. D.: Immunoglobulin M in Murray Valley encephalitis. Pathology *7*:187–191, 1975.

CHAPTER **179F**

Tick-Borne Encephalitis

CHRISTOPH AEBI ■ THEODORE F. TSAI

Tick-borne encephalitis (TBE) refers here to the neurotropic tick-transmitted flaviviral infections that occur across the Eurasian land mass from the Far East to western Europe. The Far Eastern form of the disease frequently is called Russian spring-summer encephalitis (RSSE); in Europe, where the disease is distinctly milder and often biphasic, it is called simply tick-borne encephalitis, spring-summer meningoencephalitis (Frühsommer Meningoenzephalitis), biphasic meningoencephalitis, central European encephalitis, or because sometimes it is transmitted by raw infected milk, biphasic milk fever.[18, 25, 58, 90]

History

After an outbreak of encephalitis in the Far Eastern region of Russia in 1932, Zilber isolated the virus from viremic humans and from *Ixodes persulcatus* ticks. A milder form of the disease with a similar seasonality had been described previously in Sweden and Austria, but its etiology was not defined until 1948, when the virus was isolated in the Czech Republic and Slovakia. Milk-borne transmission of TBE virus (TBEV) from infected livestock animals first was recognized in an outbreak in 1951 and 1952.

Etiologic Agent

TBEV and the closely related viruses of RSSE and Powassan encephalitis are flaviviruses placed antigenically within a complex of tick-borne flaviviruses that also includes the agents of Kyasanur Forest disease; Omsk hemorrhagic fever; and an encephalomyelitis syndrome in sheep variously called louping ill in the British Isles and Spanish, Greek, or Turkish sheep encephalomyelitis in their respective countries.[33] Molecular taxonomic studies based on nucleotide sequence differences in the virus' E protein gene show the early divergence of a mammal-associated clade from seabird-associated agents. Viruses in the former exhibit a continuous east-to-west cline consistent with an evolutionary origin of TBEV in the Far East and dispersion westward to Europe and the British Isles[21] (Fig. 179–10).

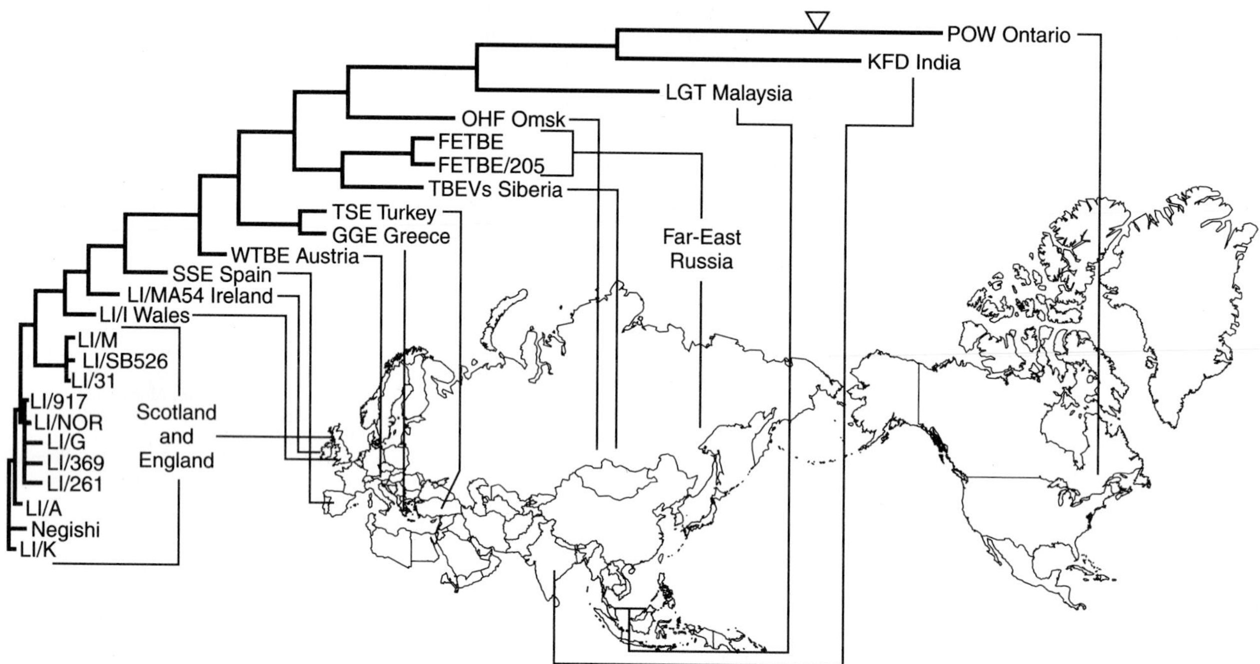

FIGURE 179–10 ■ Cladogram of tick-borne encephalitis complex viruses based on E gene sequences presented from west to east with respect to louping ill (LI) virus. FETBE, Far Eastern tick-borne encephalitis; GGE, Greek goat encephalitis; KFD, Kyasanur Forest disease; LGT, Langat; OHF, Omsk hemorrhagic fever; POW, Powassan encephalitis. SSE, Spanish sheep encephalitis; TSE, Turkish sheep encephalitis; WTBE, western tick-borne encephalitis. The phylogenetics of these and other mosquito-borne flaviviruses are rooted in the Powassan branch indicated by the *triangle.* (From Zanotto, P. M., Gao, G. F., Gritsun, T., et al.: An arbovirus cline across the Northern Hemisphere. Virology *210*:152–159, 1995.)

Ecology

The viruses of RSSE and TBE are transmitted principally by hard ticks in the *Ixodes ricinus* complex: *I. ricinus* in Europe and *I. persulcatus* in the Far East.[18, 25, 58, 90] Other tick vectors include *Ixodes arbicola, Ixodes hexagonus, Haemaphysalis punctata, Haemaphysalis concinna, Dermacentor marginatus,* and *Dermacentor reticulatus.* Viral circulation is maintained by continuous horizontal infection between ticks and animals and through the winter by vertical transmission in vector ticks and by latent infection in hibernating animals. The viruses are transmitted transtadially from larval to nymphal to adult tick stages and transovarially. All stages of the tick and both male and female ticks transmit infection to animals and humans. Ixodid ticks feed on three hosts, one for each of the stages, during the typical 3-year life cycle. Larval and nymphal ticks feed preferentially on birds and small mammals such as wild mice, voles, and dormice, and adult ticks feed on larger mammals such as roe deer, hedgehogs, foxes, hares, badgers, deer, domestic livestock (pigs, goats, sheep, and cows), dogs, cats, and humans. Infections in animals, except occasionally in dogs, are asymptomatic, and the viremia is of brief duration. Therefore, a large population of susceptible vertebrate hosts is needed to maintain viral transmission. Human infections are incidental to the natural cycle of transmission. Birds and large mammals contribute to the spread of vector ticks and viral foci.

Ticks in the *I. ricinus* complex require high soil and ambient humidity (>80–90% relative humidity) and moderate temperature, within the 8° C isotherm. They typically are found in the transitional vegetation zone from the forest edge to fields or meadows or in areas where dense brush or ground vegetation provides a sheltered microenvironment. Vector ticks are absent from mountainous areas with an elevation greater than 1000 m. Foci of TBE transmission are restricted geographically and ecologically to these biotopes and have tended to be highly stable from year to year. However, global warming has been speculated to underlie the changes, both expansion and contraction of transmission foci, in northern and central-southern Europe, respectively (see later).[66, 90]

Tick activity varies with seasonal temperature and humidity. In central Europe, activity begins in March and April, reaches a peak in May, and declines during the summer in July and August. With the return of cooler temperatures, a second peak of activity occurs in September. In temperate regions, tick activity begins later and is greatest in the summer months. In Mediterranean climates, ticks are most active from November to January.

In foci with hyperendemic transmission, tick density may exceed one per square meter. Viral infection rates in ticks are generally in the range of 0.1 to 5 percent. These rates are typically 10-fold lower than *Borrelia burgdorferi* (sensu lato) infection rates in *I. ricinus* in the same areas, although *I. persulcatus* infection rates greater than 10 percent have been reported.[49] The mechanisms underlying this difference are unclear but may include the variable infectiousness of the agents and their interactions with modulatory factors in tick saliva; the relatively brief duration of TBE viremia in animals, which lasts only a few days and thus results in a reduced chance of transmission of virus to feeding ticks, as opposed to the persistent *B. burgdorferi* infections in rodents, with tick feeding more likely to result in infection; and potential differences in the principal reservoir hosts for the respective infectious agents, with a more limited and focal distribution of important hosts for TBEV, such as goats.[84] The two agents evidently do not interfere with each other in their infection of *I. persulcatus* ticks; dually infected ticks and singly TBE-infected and *Borrelia*-infected ticks stand in a ratio of approximately 1:4:14.[49] *I. ricinus* also can be infected with and transmit *Francisella tularensis* and *Ehrlichia*.[114]

The geographic distribution of RSSE and European TBE corresponds to the ranges of their principal tick vectors; however, transmission is highly focal within this range because of the locations of biotopes that support viral circulation (Fig. 179–11). New foci are reported periodically as a result of better recognition of the disease, its natural spread, human modifications of the landscape, and environmental and climate changes (e.g., global warming).[66, 90]

Epidemiology

TBE has been recognized in all countries of Europe except Portugal and the Benelux countries, but endemic transmission is most intense in central Europe.[18, 58] The incidence of TBE previously ranged as high as 50 per 100,000 population in Austria, Poland, Hungary, Russia, the Czech Republic, Slovakia, and the former Yugoslavia, and in certain areas, similar levels of transmission still may prevail. Vaccination has reduced the incidence of disease locally, especially in Austria, where a national program of immunization in effect for 15 years has reduced the incidence to less than 1 per 100,000 population. Currently, isolated cases are reported from France, Greece, and Lichtenstein, and fewer than 100

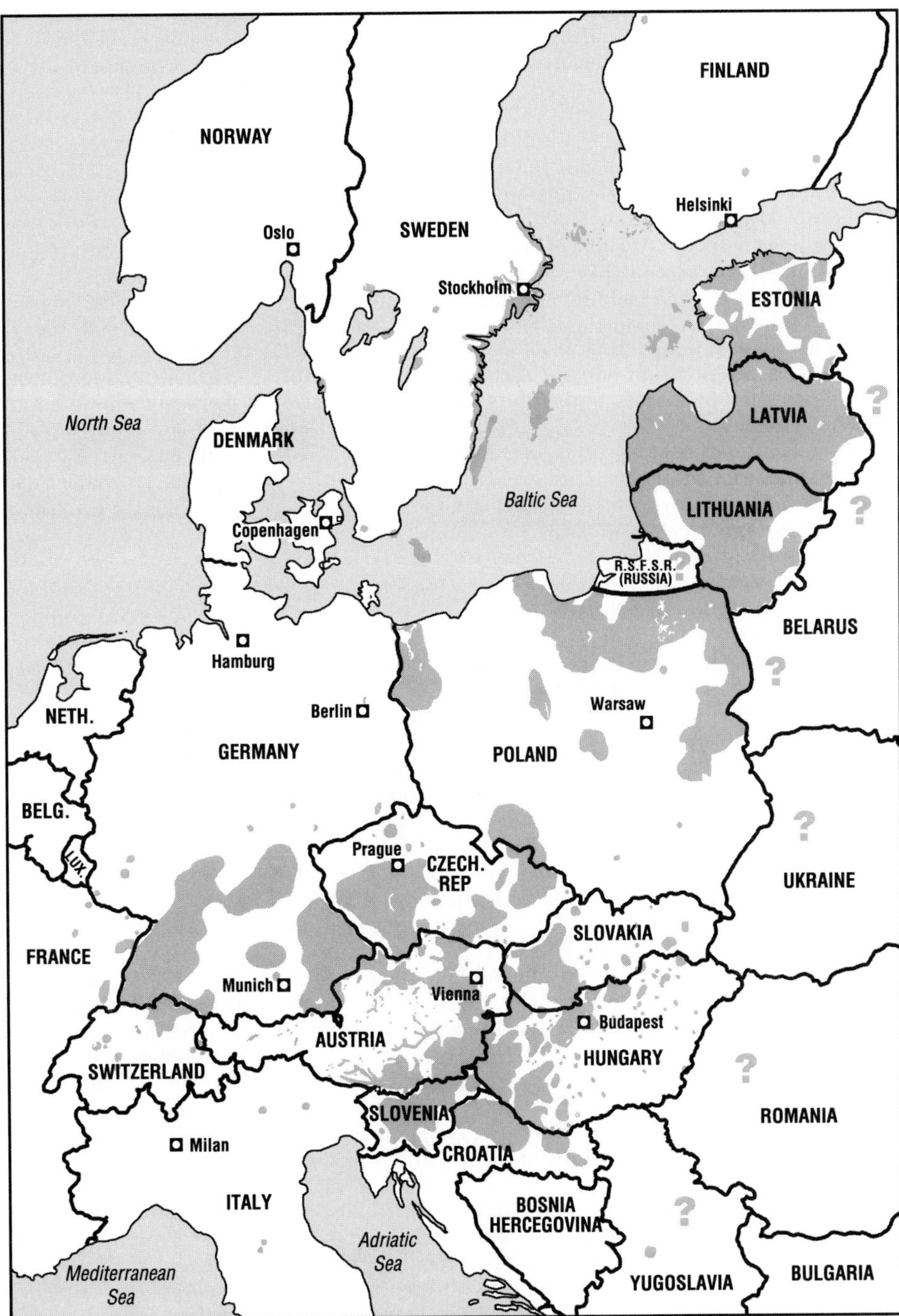

FIGURE 179–11 ■ The geographic distributions of Russian spring-summer encephalitis and European tick-borne encephalitis correspond to the ranges of their principal tick vectors; however, transmission is highly focal within this range because of the locations of biotopes that support viral circulation.

sporadic cases are reported annually in Sweden, Germany, Switzerland, Italy, and Austria. Reporting has increased from other countries of eastern and central Europe (e.g., Slovenia and the Baltic states). In the Far East, cases of RSSE occur principally in forest workers. The disease is recognized in Russia and China, and the first cases acquired in Japan (transmitted by *Ixodes ovatus)* were reported recently.

Within each country, the distribution of cases is highly focal in certain cantons or districts; local seroprevalence may exceed 20 percent, but the general seroprevalence is usually less than 1 per 100,000 population. Frequent exposure during long-term residence leads to a general trend of increasing seroprevalence with age. Seroprevalence rates as high as 50 percent have been observed in groups at high risk of exposure, such as farmers and forestry workers. Although in general, rates are lower (1–5%) and in certain groups are similar to the seroprevalence of hantaviruses, lymphocytic choriomeningitis virus, and *Ehrlichia* spp., *Borrelia* seroprevalence rates are 10-fold higher or more.[76, 82] The frequency of clinical cases of TBE, borreliosis, and dual infection closely approximates the relative frequency of tick infection, singly and dually. Adults 20 to 50 years of age characteristically have made up the majority of cases. In some studies, cases in males (adults and children) predominate by a ratio of 2:1.[19, 31]

Cases have occurred in children as young as 3 months of age, but generally, risk in children increases with age as a result of their increased mobility and activity in the sylvatic environment. These epidemiologic patterns are changing in areas with high immunization coverage. Vaccination effort has focused principally on hyperendemic areas and on high-risk occupational groups such as forestry workers. The low number of cases currently reported from areas where vaccination coverage is high belies the continued transmission of virus in these locations.

Cases may be acquired during outdoor activities, such as berry picking and mushroom gathering, and infection occasionally has been acquired from ticks brought from endemic areas on Christmas trees and other objects. One study found that the seroprevalence in Swedish orienteers (1%) was not substantially different from the general seroprevalence in residents of Stockholm County (5%), an area where TBE is endemic. The absence of a higher risk of acquiring TBE in persons with occasional sylvatic exposure reflects the low infection rate of ticks and the generally low risk to persons with sporadic or short-term exposure. Neither of two studies of American soldiers stationed in central Europe found a clinical case, although one seroconversion in 3297 person-months of exposure, an infection rate of 0.9 per 1000 person-months, and four seroconversions in 959 persons (0.4%) were detected, respectively.[73, 98] With the dissolution of the former Soviet Union and increasing commerce with eastern Europe, interest in the risk of TBE in travelers to Europe and Russia has increased. The available data suggest that the risk is low for most travelers and that vaccination is not indicated except for unusual circumstances of prolonged stay in an endemic area.

The seasonal distribution of cases lags roughly 1 month behind that of tick activity and extends from April until November. The peak incidence in Sweden is in August, and in Austria, the peak occurs in June and July, with a secondary rise in October.

Milk-borne TBE previously accounted for 10 to 20 percent of all cases in central Europe. Infections frequently were acquired from consuming unpasteurized milk or cheese from infected goats, sheep, and cows, and outbreaks resulting in thousands of cases have been reported. Transmission from infected milk is now a rare occurrence, but as recently as 1994, an outbreak in Slovakia led to seven cases in a group that regularly drank raw milk from a family goat.[49] Contact infection, acquired during slaughter of an infected goat, also has been reported.

Clinical Manifestations

Seroepidemiologic studies indicate that greater than 90 percent of human infections with TBEV remain asymptomatic or result in a nonspecific illness.[2, 29, 45] The classic manifestation of the European form of TBE is an acute febrile illness characterized by a biphasic course consisting of a nonspecific prodromal syndrome followed by central nervous system (CNS) disease[24, 106] (Fig. 179–12). Whether infection with TBEV can occur solely as the primary, nonspecific phase without the secondary CNS phase is a matter of controversy.[19, 70] Infection with Far Eastern strains of TBEV results in a more severe, monophasic illness that progresses directly to neurologic involvement with a poorer prognosis for survival and full recovery. TBE has been observed in all age groups, with the exception of neonates. The median age in pediatric case series is 8 to 10 years (range, 3 to 17 years).[13, 31, 67, 110] The youngest patient with serologically documented TBE described in the literature was a 3-month-old infant.[26] Congenital infection has not been reported.

The clinical features of TBE in children are summarized in Table 179–5. The diagnosis of TBE should be considered in all acutely ill patients with fever, CNS abnormalities, and a history of potential tick exposure or ingestion of raw milk in an area endemic for TBE. A high degree of diagnostic awareness is required because the clinical presentation of TBE itself is nonspecific. After an incubation period of 2 to 28 days, in most cases 7 to 14 days,[20, 31, 67, 112] the patient may have a prodromal illness consisting of fever, malaise, nausea and vomiting, headache, myalgia, and occasionally, upper respiratory tract symptoms.[20, 31, 51, 112] Defervescence occurs after 2 to 7 days, and the patient subsequently remains asymptomatic for 1 to 20 days, usually 2 to 8 days.[20, 31, 51, 110] This prodromal illness may be absent. In various case series, a biphasic course was reported in 30 to 90 percent of children with TBE.[31, 43, 67, 110] An abrupt onset of fever, headache, emesis, and symptoms of meningeal irritation heralds the beginning of the second phase of disease.[66] In adults, no association exists between the length of the incubation period and the severity of clinical illness.[43] The typical evolution of fever in a child with TBE is shown in Fig. 179–12.

In this second phase of illness, most children (50–90%) have meningitis without clinical evidence of parenchymal CNS involvement.[31, 50, 55, 67, 79, 93, 110] In adult patients, by contrast, meningitis without encephalitis or myelitis occurs in 20 to 60 percent of cases.[2, 43, 51, 91, 105] On physical examination, fever, signs of meningeal irritation, and photophobia are the most common features.[67, 110] In uncomplicated cases, patients defervesce within 7 days.[31, 67, 110] Meningoencephalitis or meningoencephalomyelitis (or both) manifested by impaired consciousness, seizures, and focal neurologic signs, including limb paresis, occurs in 0 to 34 percent of children.[13, 31, 43, 66, 104] In 13 pediatric patients with parenchymal CNS disease (34% of the case series), Harasek[31] observed ataxia in 10, somnolence in 4, paresthesias and seizures in 2 each, and central facial palsy and nystagmus in 1 each. In two of these patients, transient unilateral shoulder girdle weakness that occurred during the second week of CNS disease suggested involvement of the cervical

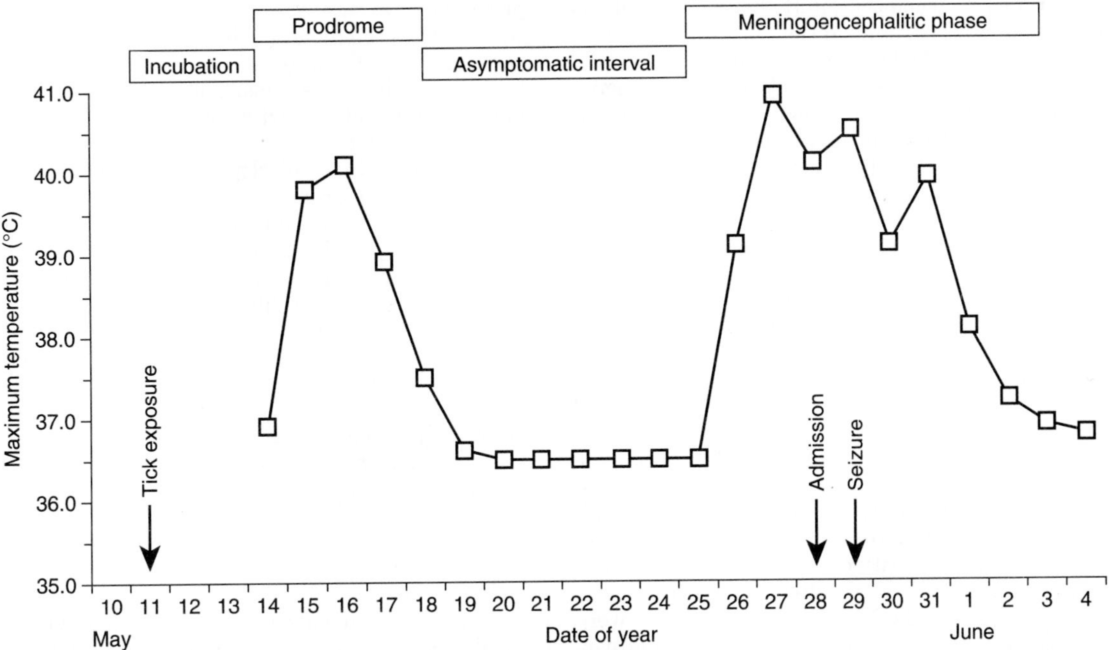

FIGURE 179–12 ■ Clinical course of tick-borne encephalitis (TBE) in a 5-year-old boy exposed to a tick bite in a known endemic area for TBE in the pre-alpine region of central Switzerland. Lumbar puncture on admission revealed mild cerebrospinal fluid (CSF) pleocytosis (14×10^6/L, 50% polymorphonuclear cells). Serum anti-TBE virus IgM and IgG were positive, serum and CSF antibodies against *Borrelia burgdorferi* were negative. CSF enteroviral polymerase chain reaction was negative. Recovery was uneventful.

TABLE 179–5 ■ CLINICAL FEATURES OF SEROLOGICALLY DOCUMENTED TICK-BORNE ENCEPHALITIS IN FIVE PEDIATRIC CASE SERIES (333 CHILDREN)

	Rate (%)
History	
Tick exposure	47–78
Biphasic illness	77–90
Major Symptoms at Initial Evaluation	
Temperature >38.0°C	100
Headache	99–100
Vomiting	60–90
Central Nervous System Signs	
Nuchal rigidity	74–90
Photophobia	10–25
Impaired consciousness	9–11
Ataxia and/or tremor	5–26
Seizures	0–5
Paresis	0–5
Extent of Central Nervous System Involvement	
Meningitis alone	49–89
Meningoencephalitis	9–48
Meningoencephalomyelitis	0–5
Fatal outcome	0
Cerebrospinal Fluid Parameters	
Pleocytosis $>15 \times 10^6$/L	98–100
Glucose normal	100
Protein elevated	9–55
Abnormal electroencephalogram	80–87

Data from references 13, 31, 43, 66, 104

anterior horn or radiculitis. Limb or cranial nerve pareses occur in 0 to 5 percent of children with TBE (see Table 179–5). In a series of 133 children with TBE, Cizman[13] reported transient pareses in 5 patients and irreversible hemiparesis in 1.

In large case series of predominantly adult patients, a paralytic course secondary to bulbar, spinal, or radicular injury was observed in 5 to 25 percent of cases.[43, 47, 74, 105, 112, 115] Unilateral, flaccid paresis of an upper extremity is the most common manifestation of such lower motor neuron disease complicating TBE.[74, 112, 115] Involvement of the cranial nerves occurs somewhat less frequently and is revealed most commonly by external ocular muscle paralysis (usually cranial nerve VI), peripheral facial palsy (VII), otovestibular manifestations (VIII), or involvement of the pharyngeal muscles (IX, X, XI).[20, 43, 74, 106] Lower extremity weakness and, occasionally, autonomic nervous system affliction manifested as bladder dysfunction also may occur.[20, 43, 106] Whereas most manifestations of parenchymal CNS involvement evolve during the acute stage of TBE, paralysis resulting from radiculitis may develop up to 14 days after the onset of CNS disease.[31, 58]

As many as 5 percent of children with TBE experience seizures during the acute stage of TBE.[13, 31, 110] Because most patients are older than 6 years and, thus, are unlikely to suffer from febrile seizures, these episodes probably reflect encephalitis. In adults, seizures have been observed in less than 2 percent of patients.[20, 43]

Extracerebral manifestations of TBE seldom are reported and are of minor clinical relevance. Mild hepatitis[35, 43] and electrocardiographic abnormalities have been described in adults.[108] A single case of myopericarditis in a child with TBE has been reported.[21]

The peripheral white blood cell count characteristically is not altered. Although it is usually in the normal range, both leukopenia and moderate leukocytosis may be found.[31, 66, 106] In adult patients, several investigators observed leukopenia during the viremic prodrome and normal or moderately elevated white blood cell counts during the second phase of illness.[43, 51, 66, 69] In a recent report describing hematologic values during the prodromal phase of TBE, 23 of 28 (82%) patients had mild to moderate thrombocytopenia (60 to 130 × 10^9/L), with values returning to normal during the second phase of illness.[69] Cerebrospinal fluid (CSF) analysis in children with serologically proven TBE reveals predominantly mononuclear pleocytosis in all patients. However, as with enteroviral meningitis, neutrophils may predominate during the first 1 to 3 days of illness.[41] Typically, the CSF white blood cell count is 100 to 1000 × 10^6/L.[31, 54, 66, 106, 110] Occasionally, lower values occur, as reported by Krausler,[50] who found less than 100 × 10^6/L in 24 of 75 (32%) pediatric cases. Wahlberg and colleagues[112] reported an absence of pleocytosis in 18 percent of 94 adult patients examined. Harasek[31] could not find any correlation between the CSF leukocyte count and the severity of clinical disease. In contrast, some investigators[43, 44, 47] reported that adult patients with a high CSF white blood cell count (>300 × 10^6/L) were more likely to experience a severe course of TBE and persistent neurologic sequelae. CSF pleocytosis disappears within 4 to 5 weeks of the onset of acute CNS disease. The CSF glucose concentration is normal,[66] and the protein concentration is normal or moderately elevated (<1000 mg/L),[31, 51, 66, 106] with evidence of blood-brain barrier dysfunction in most patients.[44]

Electroencephalographic (EEG) examination during acute TBE usually is abnormal and characterized by a nonspecific reduction in rhythmic background activity, bilateral periodic slowing, and rarely, focal abnormalities.[31, 42, 43] Attenuation of background activity with periodic delta groups has been shown to correlate with parenchymal CNS involvement in adult TBE patients.[42] Reorganization of EEG activity commonly lags behind clinical improvement, and abnormalities may persist for months to years.[31, 42, 110]

The limited information available on magnetic resonance imaging (MRI) in children with severe TBE indicates that parenchymal lesions characteristically are located in the thalamus[13, 43, 46, 113] (Fig. 179–13). The diagnostic and prognostic value of neuroimaging studies in pediatric TBE has not been established. In adults, MRI studies may be abnormal in approximately 20 percent of patients.[43] Focal lesions are more likely to be found in those with severe neurologic abnormalities[43] and are confined mainly to the thalamus.[5, 8, 43, 68, 88, 111, 113] Less frequently, lesions are located in the basal ganglia,[5, 43, 68, 88] cerebellum,[8, 43] brain stem,[13, 43] and anterior portions of the cervical spine.[8, 13]

Pathology

CNS findings are mainly those of acute meningeal inflammation and focal gray matter encephalomyelitis. The white matter rarely is involved. Macroscopic findings include congestion of the leptomeninges and swelling and hyperemia of the cerebral parenchyma, particularly in the brain stem and cervical region of the spinal cord.[25, 81] Petechial hemorrhages are seen in the brain stem, the anterior horns of the spinal cord, and less consistently, in the cerebellum and the anterior central region of the cortex. Histologic changes are dominated by infiltration and ganglion cell damage in the gray matter of these same areas. Changes are particularly pronounced in the anterior horns of the cervical spine,[101] the medulla oblongata, the cranial nerve nuclei of the pons, and the Purkinje cell layer of the cerebellum.[25] The former locations are consistent with the poliomyelitis-like manifestations of paralytic courses of TBE.[101] Inflammatory foci are characterized by lymphocytic perivascular infiltration and various stages of degenerative changes in neuronal cells. Areas of neuronal necrosis are characterized by perifocal edema, lymphocytic and neutrophilic infiltration, and at a later stage, nodular microglial proliferation at sites of complete neuronophagia. Rarely, the spinal nerve roots, spinal ganglia, and peripheral nerves are involved. Spongiform changes, particularly after protracted illness, appear as sharply defined areas of softening with minimal inflammatory reaction. In the Far Eastern form of the disease, extensive poliomyelitis of the spinal cord with destruction of anterior horn cells, particularly in the upper cervical and lower lumbar areas, and poliomyelitis of the brain stem are noted.

Pathogenesis

Tick-mediated inoculation of TBEV and viral replication within local dermal cells are followed by lymphatic spread to regional lymph nodes, where further replication occurs.[44] Subsequently, viremia leads to generalized infection, especially of reticuloendothelial cells, followed by secondary rounds of viremia that result in neuroinvasion. Viral penetration of the CNS occurs via capillary endothelia and by TBEV-infected, infiltrating mononuclear cells. Envelope glycoprotein E, the immunodominant TBEV-encoded surface protein, mediates attachment to and fusion with the host cellular membrane.[72] The molecular mechanisms of neural invasion by TBEV have not been elucidated in detail. Current knowledge on the molecular pathogenesis of TBEV has been reviewed elsewhere.[32, 33]

Laboratory Diagnosis

Because neither clinical nor CSF findings differentiate TBE from other causes of meningitis or meningoencephalitis, the diagnosis of TBE rests on demonstration of specific antibody by serologic testing. The presence of specific serum IgM or a significant rise in titer of specific IgG antibody in paired sera (or both) is diagnostic of TBE.[38, 44] Enzyme-linked immunosorbent assay (ELISA) has replaced complement-fixation, hemagglutination-inhibition, and neutralization assays in the routine laboratory diagnosis of TBE.[37] ELISA technology offers increased sensitivity, reliably differentiates between IgM and IgG antibodies, and, in contrast to neutralization, uses nonviable viral antigens.[34, 88] For the detection of specific anti-TBEV IgM, an IgM capture ELISA system has proved to be more sensitive and specific than the conventional three-layer ELISA system because high titers of specific IgG and rheumatoid factor do not interfere with IgM binding.[34, 93] With this method, specific IgM virtually always can be demonstrated during the acute illness and thereafter may persist for as long as 9 months.[39, 44, 93] The highly sensitive capture ELISA format allows a determination of anti-TBEV IgM, even in serum samples obtained late during the acute illness, when high titers of specific IgG are already present. A potential problem of TBEV IgG ELISA systems is cross-reactivity with other flaviviruses, notably yellow fever virus and dengue virus.[17, 18, 83] This limitation should be considered in the interpretation of seroprevalence studies

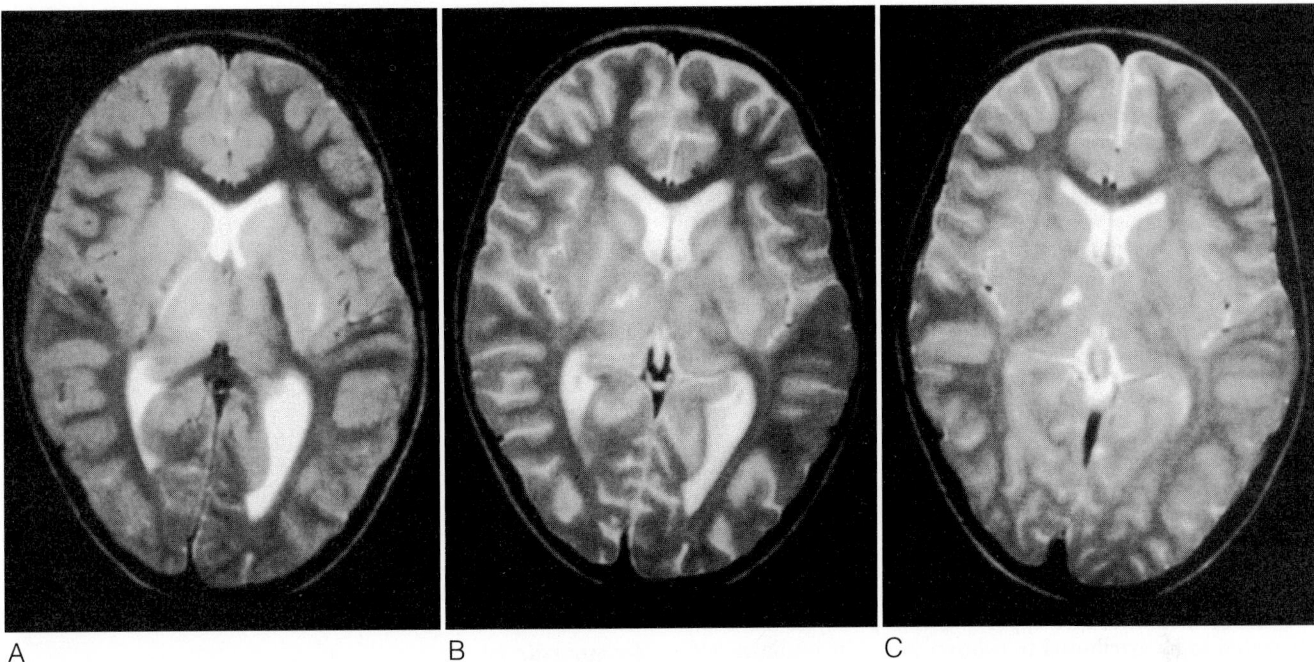

FIGURE 179–13 ■ T2-weighted magnetic resonance imaging series of a 5-year-old girl with a severe course of tick-borne encephalitis. *A*, Acute phase. Note the T2 hyperintensity in the right side of the thalamus, basal ganglia, and diencephalon. *B*, One month later, partial recovery of T2 hyperintensity and enlargement of cerebrospinal fluid (CSF) spaces can be seen. *C*, Three months later, normal T2 intensity and a CSF-filled cavity in the right side of the thalamus are apparent. (Courtesy of Professor David Nadal, M.D., University Children's Hospital, Zurich, Switzerland).

and in patients with a relevant travel or immunization history.

Specific IgM and IgG also can be measured in CSF.[34, 93] Detection of TBEV-specific intrathecal antibody production by ELISA is highly specific for the diagnosis of TBE but somewhat less sensitive than determination of serum IgM during the first several days of CNS disease.[44] Intrathecal TBEV antibody assays are not used widely in clinical practice.

Detection of virus or viral RNA is technically feasible, but it is not used routinely in clinical practice. TBEV can be recovered from blood by viral culture, but because detectable viremia occurs during the prodromal stage (when the diagnosis of TBE seldom is considered), culture is not useful in clinical practice. TBEV may be recovered from the brain tissue of patients who died at an early stage of disease.[14] Amplification of TBEV-specific RNA by reverse transcriptase-polymerase chain reaction (RT-PCR) has been established for detection of TBEV in ticks.[89] Primers that amplify the highly conserved 5′ noncoding region of the TBEV genome have been shown to be sensitive and specific.[104] Successful amplification of TBEV-specific RNA from CSF or brain tissue has been reported in humans.[15, 109, 113] but its diagnostic usefulness in clinical medicine has not been established.

Differential Diagnosis

The clinical course of TBE is nonspecific in most cases, and a history of exposure to ticks in an endemic area can be elicited in 50 to 75 percent of pediatric patients.[31, 43, 67, 79, 103, 110] Because serologic confirmation of the diagnosis is not immediately available in most cases, the differential diagnosis includes a wide spectrum of diseases causing fever and CNS manifestations.

Enteroviruses are the most common etiology of symptomatic CNS infection in children during the warm seasons in regions where TBE is prevalent. Fever in enteroviral infection may be biphasic,[77] although the duration of both the first phase and the asymptomatic interval is usually shorter than noted in TBE.[11] Routine tests of CSF do not differentiate between the two entities. The presence of skin and mucosal manifestations is indicative of enteroviral infection rather than TBE, whereas encephalitis and myelitis can occur in both. Enteroviral meningitis is diagnosed most readily by PCR of CSF[99] or by culture of virus from CSF and mucosal surfaces. *Mumps* meningitis is a major component of the differential diagnosis in cases without parotid enlargement, particularly in areas with low rates of mumps immunization.[107] The diagnosis of mumps meningitis is made by viral culture of CSF or by detection of specific serum IgM antibody. Though a rare occurrence in childhood, *herpes simplex virus (HSV)* encephalitis always should be considered in the differential diagnosis. Because its case-fatality rate is greater than 90 percent if left untreated, therapy with intravenous acyclovir should be initiated without delay if HSV encephalitis is thought possible. The combination of fever, which may be biphasic,[94] and localizing signs observed by neurologic examination, EEG studies, or MRI[40] suggests HSV encephalitis and rarely occurs in pediatric TBE, particularly if the temporal lobe or the orbital portion of the frontal lobe is affected. Meningeal irritation is usually absent in HSV encephalitis. The diagnosis of HSV encephalitis is confirmed by PCR of CSF or by brain biopsy.[7, 64] *Epstein-Barr virus* encephalitis can occur in immunocompetent children and shares with TBEV a preference for causing thalamic and basal ganglia lesions.[43, 86] Other viral etiologies include common respiratory tract viruses such as influenza, parainfluenza, and adenovirus.

Among bacterial infections, partially treated pyogenic meningitis, encephalitis in association with *Mycoplasma pneumoniae* infection,[96] and encephalopathy caused by *Bartonella henselae* may resemble TBE. Tuberculous meningitis runs a subacute course, and although near-normal CSF chemistry may be recorded very early in the disease, hypoglycorrhachia invariably develops and CSF protein rises to high levels. CNS infection by *B. burgdorferi* is particularly important in the differential diagnosis because in Europe, this pathogen and TBEV are transmitted by the same tick vectors, *I. ricinus* and *I. persulcatus*, and because one of the most prevalent European genospecies, *Borrelia garinii,* is more neurotropic than *B. burgdorferi* sensu stricto is.[95] In contrast to TBE, the incubation period for early neuroborreliosis in children is generally 4 to 10 weeks, high-grade fever is unusual, and most patients have cranial nerve paresis. However, several cases of concomitant infection with TBEV and *B. burgdorferi* have been reported in the literature,[1, 12, 53, 85] and coexistence of TBEV and *B. burgdorferi* in ticks has been documented.[49] In some cases of TBE, persistent or late-appearing limb paralysis has been suggested to be attributed to concomitant, but undiagnosed borrelial radiculoneuritis rather than TBE-related myelitis with anterior horn involvement.[53] In this situation, diagnostic evidence of Lyme borreliosis should be sought because this condition requires antimicrobial therapy. Seroepidemiologic evidence suggests that concomitant infection with TBEV and *Ehrlichia phagocytophila,* the agent of human granulocytic ehrlichiosis, also may occur,[49] but no such human cases have been reported.

Treatment

No specific antiviral therapy is available to treat TBE. Specific hyperimmune globulin is indicated exclusively for passive immunization within 96 hours of exposure to ticks. Clinical evidence suggests that the administration of TBE hyperimmune globulin thereafter may have a detrimental effect on the course of disease.[3, 62] In severe cases, supportive therapy is aimed at preventing the development of sequelae related to increased intracranial pressure, seizures, and bulbar dysfunction. After the acute stage, neurorehabilitation may be necessary for patients with motor, cognitive, or emotional disturbances. Because TBE rarely causes a chronic seizure disorder, prolonged anticonvulsive therapy seldom is indicated in patients who had convulsions during acute disease.

Prognosis

The main risk factor for neurologic residua and a fatal outcome of TBE is advanced age.[2, 43, 105] Persistent sequelae appear to be exceedingly rare in children,[31, 43, 55, 67, 110] although no prospective long-term follow-up studies of pediatric TBE patients have been performed to date. Individual cases of children with persistent neurologic damage, including hemiparesis,[13, 46, 113] unilateral arm paresis,[112] epilepsy,[46, 92] and extrapyramidal movement disorder, have been reported.[46] In adult patients, long-term neurologic defects are observed in 2 to 10 percent of patients with clinical evidence of parenchymal CNS involvement during the acute illness.[2, 24, 43, 47, 112] Risk factors for persistent sequelae have been assessed by Kaiser[43] and, by univariate analysis, include impaired consciousness (i.e., Glasgow Coma Scale score <7), ataxia, paresis, abnormal findings on MRI, CSF pleocytosis greater than 300 $\times$ 10^6/L, and CSF protein greater than 600 mg/L. Gunther reported that encephalitic symptoms were associated with low levels of intrathecal IgM in early TBE.[28] Paresis of the extremities and ataxia are the most common persistent findings on neurologic examination.[2, 20, 43, 47, 71, 105] Much more common, however, are ill-defined manifestations such as chronic fatigue, headache, sleep disorders, memory dysfunction, and emotional disturbances, which are reported by most adults recovering from TBE and persist from months to years.[20, 65, 105] In some patients, EEG findings may remain abnormal for prolonged periods, with seizure activity occasionally demonstrated.[31] Most of these patients are asymptomatic, although epilepsy secondary to TBE has been described infrequently.[31, 80] The reported case-fatality rate in adult TBE patients is approximately 1 percent in large series,[2, 20, 24, 43, 47, 71] with most deaths being attributed to severe bulbar encephalitis or related to underlying cardiovascular disease in elderly patients.[20] To date, a single fatal outcome of TBE has been reported in a child.[75]

Prevention

General preventive principles include avoidance of known endemic areas of TBE, the use of protective clothing, and rapid removal of ticks attached to the skin. The topical repellent DEET (*N,N*-diethyl-*m*-toluamide) has a definite, albeit moderate effect against ticks.[97] Because of its potential neurotoxicity, the content of DEET in products used for children should not exceed 15 percent.[10, 87] These measures are effective in reducing tick exposure and transmission of TBEV to some degree. Pasteurization of raw milk prevents enteric transmission of TBEV.[4, 48]

Reliable protection, however, requires active immunization against TBE. Inactivated whole-virus vaccines are produced in Austria (Baxter), Germany (Behring), and Russia. The vaccines are made from different central European TBEV strains and are produced by concentrating and purifying cell culture fluid from infected chick embryo cells. Adjuvants (aluminum hydroxide) are added to the formalin-inactivated cell culture fluid. The Russian vaccine is an inactivated, unconcentrated cell culture fluid from infected African green monkey kidney cells. TBE vaccine is available in the United States under investigational drug exemption to military personnel deployed in endemic areas.[9, 16]

The only vaccine currently approved for children 12 months and older is FSME-Immun Inject (Baxter). Basic immunization consists of three doses given at 0, 1 to 3, and 9 to 12 months. The vaccine is immunogenic and safe.[23, 24, 27, 102] Seroconversion rates for neutralizing antibodies after the first, second, and third dose are 70, 95, and 99 percent, respectively.[57, 61] Reliable protection is achieved 2 weeks after the second dose. Data on the kinetics of vaccine-induced neutralizing serum antibodies led to the recommendation for booster doses every 3 years.[56, 57] Minor adverse events (fever and local reactions) are reported by 4 to 10 percent of vaccinees after receiving the first dose and less frequently after subsequent exposure.[59] Mostly transient neurologic adverse events temporally associated with the administration of TBE vaccine have been reported rarely.[23, 24, 100, 102] Their true incidence has not been established. Based on passive notification of adverse events, an incidence of one neurologic illness in 1 million doses of TBE vaccine has been calculated.[36] Placebo-controlled trials of vaccine

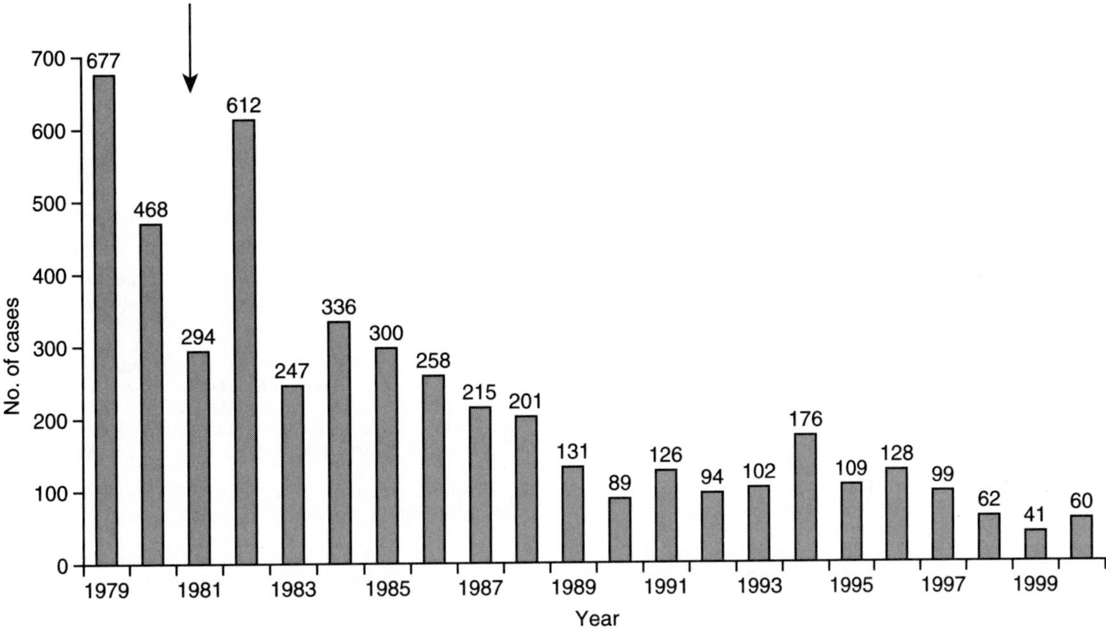

FIGURE 179–14 ■ Annual number of cases of tick-borne encephalitis in Austria before and after the introduction of mass immunization in 1981 *(arrow)*. (Data obtained from the International Scientific Working Group On Tick-Borne-Encephalitis, www.tbe-info.com/report.)

efficacy have not been conducted. Observational studies in Austria using historical controls indicate that the effectiveness of the vaccine is greater than 90 percent.[60, 63] A similar vaccine (Encepur, Behring) is available for both a standard immunization series and an abbreviated three-dose regimen administered on days 0, 7, and 21.[30] In clinical trials, this vaccine was found to be highly reactogenic in children.[22] Currently, it is approved for individuals 12 years and older. A new, preservative-free vaccine (TicoVac, Baxter) introduced in the European Union in 1999 was withdrawn from the market in April 2001 because of an excessive rate of febrile reactions, notably in children younger than 36 months.

In Austria, the TBE vaccine is recommended for mass immunization of all potentially exposed individuals. Since the beginning of the vaccination campaign in 1981, a dramatic reduction in nationally notified cases has been observed[63] (Fig. 179–14). Mass immunization is the probable cause of this decrease because neighboring countries (e.g., Switzerland, Southern Germany, Slowenia) reported stable or increasing numbers of cases of TBE during the same period. In these and other endemic countries of central and eastern Europe, authorities recommend immunization of school-age children and adults who live in endemic areas and have an increased risk of exposure to ticks (e.g., forest workers, orienteers, scouts).[13, 82] In younger children, TBE vaccination usually is not indicated because neurologic complications are exceedingly rare.[13]

A commercial TBE hyperimmune globulin for pre-exposure and postexposure immunoprophylaxis is available in Europe.[3] In several countries, however, this product is not approved for use in children younger than 14 years because numerous breakthrough TBEV infections have been observed in recipients of postexposure prophylaxis.[43, 46, 68, 111] Among these recipients, some unusually severe cases raised concern about a causative role of TBE immunoglobulin in enhancement of disease.[6, 67, 113] Antibody-dependent enhancement, an accepted mechanism of pathogenicity in dengue hemorrhagic fever,[78] was discussed as a possible explanation,[46] but in vivo experimental data in support of this hypothesis in TBE are lacking.[52]

REFERENCES

1. Abshagen, R., and Bahr, J.: Doppelinfektion *Borrelia burgdorferi*–FSME-virus. Kinderaerztliche Praxis *60*:103–104, 1992.
2. Ackermann, R., Krueger, K., Roggendorf, M., et al.: Die Verbreitung der Fruehsommer-Meningoenzephalitis in der Bundesrepublik Deutschland. Dtsch. Med. Wochenschr. *111*:927–933, 1986.
3. Aebi, C., and Schaad, U. B.: FSME-Immunglobulin—eine kritische Beurteilung der Wirksamkeit. Schweiz. Med. Wochenschr. *124*:1837–1840, 1994.
4. Aendekerk, R. P., Schrivers, A. N., and Koehler, P. J.: Tick-borne encephalitis complicated by a polio-like syndrome following a holiday in central Europe. Clin. Neurol. Neurosurg. *98*:262–264, 1996.
5. Alkadhi, H., and Kollias, S. S.: MRI in tick-borne encephalitis. Neuroradiology *42*:753–755, 2000.
6. Arras, C., Fescharek, R., and Gregersen, J. P.: Do specific hyperimmunoglobulins aggravate clinical course of tick-borne encephalitis? Lancet *347*:1331, 1996.
7. Atkins, J. T.: HSV PCR for CNS infections: Pearls and pitfalls. Pediatr. Infect. Dis. J. *18*:823–824, 1999.
8. Beer, S., Brune, N., and Kesselring, J.: Detection of anterior horn lesions by MRI in central European tick-borne encephalitis. J. Neurol. *246*:1169–1171, 1999.
9. Birmingham, K.: Pentagon breaks FDA rules. Nat. Med. *4*:255, 1998.
10. Briassoulis, G., Narlioglu, M., and Hatzis, T.: Toxic encephalopathy associated with use of DEET insect repellents: A case analysis of its toxicity in children. Hum. Exp. Toxicol. *20*:8–14, 2001.
11. Cherry, J. D.: Enteroviruses: Coxsackieviruses, echoviruses, and polioviruses. *In* Feigin, R. D., and Cherry, J. D. (eds.): Textbook of Pediatric Infectious Diseases. 4th ed. Philadelphia, W. B. Saunders, 1998, pp. 1787–1839.
12. Cimperman, J., Maraspin, V., Lotric-Furlan, S., et al.: Concomitant infection with tick-borne encephalitis virus and *Borrelia burgdorferi* sensu lato in patients with acute meningitis and meningoencephalitis. Infection *26*:160–164, 1998.
13. Cizman, M., Rakar, R., Zakotnik, B., et al.: Severe forms of tick-borne encephalitis in children. Wien. Klin. Wochenschr. *111*:484–487, 1999.

14. Clement, J., and Heyman, P.: PCR for diagnosis of viral infections of the central nervous system. Lancet *349*:1256, 1997.
15. Craig, S. C., Pittman, P. R., Lewis, T. E., et al.: An accelerated schedule for tick borne encephalitis vaccine: The American Military experience in Bosnia. Am. J. Trop. Med. Hyg. *61*:874–878, 1999.
16. Dobler, G., Jelinek, T., Frosner, G., et al.: Cross reactions of patients with acute dengue fever to tick-borne encephalitis. Wien. Klin. Wochenschr. *147*:463–464, 1997.
17. Dobler, G., Treib, J., Kiessig, S. T., et al.: Diagnosis of tick-borne encephalitis: Evaluation of sera with borderline titers with the TBE ELISA. Infection *24*:405–406, 1996.
18. Dumpis, U., Crook, D., and Oksi, J.: Tick-borne encephalitis. Clin. Infect. Dis. *28*:882–890, 1999.
19. Duniewicz, M.: Klinisches Bild der Zentraleuropaeischen Zeckenenzephalitis. Munch. Med. Wochenschr. *118*:1609–1613, 1976.
20. Duppenthaler, A., Pfammatter, J. P., and Aebi, C.: Myopericarditis associated with central European tick-borne encephalitis. Eur. J. Pediatr. *159*:854–856, 2000.
21. Gaunt, M. W., Sall, A. A., deLamballerie, X., et al.: Phylogenetic relationships of flaviviruses correlate with their epidemiology, disease association and biogeography. J. Gen. Virol. *82*:1867–1876, 2001.
22. Girgsdies, O. E., and Rosenkranz, G.: Tick-borne encephalitis: Development of a pediatric vaccine. A controlled, randomized, double-blind and multicentre study. Vaccine *14*:1421–1428, 1996.
23. Goerre, S., Kesselring, J., Hartmann, K., et al.: Neurologische Nebenwirkungen nach Impfung gegen die Fruehsommermeningoenzephalitis. Fallbericht und Erfahrungen der Schweizerischen Arzneimittel Nebenwirkungszentrale (SANZ). Schweiz. Med. Wochenschr. *123*:654–657, 1993.
24. Gold, R., Wiethoelter, H., Rihs, I., et al.: Fruehsommer Meningoencephalitis-Impfung. Dtsch. Med. Wochenschr. *117*:112–116, 1992.
25. Grinschgl, G.: Virus meningo-encephalitis in Austria. Bull. World Health Organ. *12*:535–564, 1955.
26. Grubbauer, H. M., Dornbusch, H. J., Spork, D., et al.: Tick borne encephalitis in a 3-month-old child. Eur. J. Pediatr. *151*:743–744, 1992.
27. Grzeszcuk, A., Sokolewicz-Bobrowska, E., and Prokopowicz, D.: Adverse reactions to tick-borne encephalitis vaccine FSME-Immun. Infection *26*:385–388, 1998.
28. Gunther, G., Haglund, M., Lindquist, L., et al.: Intrathecal IgM, IgA and IgG antibody response in tick-borne encephalitis. Long-term follow-up related to clinical course and outcome. Clin. Diagn. Virol. *8*:17–29, 1997.
29. Gustafson, R., Forsgren, M., Gardulf, A., et al.: Clinical manifestations and antibody prevalence of Lyme borreliosis and tick-borne encephalitis in Sweden: A study in five endemic areas close to Stockholm. Scand. J. Infect. Dis. *25*:598–603, 1993.
30. Harabacz, I., Bock, H., Jungst, C., et al.: A randomized phase II study of a new tick-borne encephalitis vaccine using three different doses and two immunization regimens. Vaccine *10*:145–150, 1992.
31. Harasek, G.: Zeckenenzephalitis im Kindesalter. Dtsch. Med. Wochenschr. *99*:1965–1970, 1974.
32. Heinz, F. X.: Tick-borne encephalitis virus: Advances in molecular biology and vaccination strategy in the next century. Zentralbl. Bakteriol. *289*:506–510, 1999.
33. Heinz, F. X., and Mandl, C. W.: The molecular biology of tick-borne encephalitis virus. A. P. M. I. S. *101*:735–745, 1993.
34. Heinz, F. X., Roggendorf, M., Hormann, H., et al.: Comparison of two different enzyme immunoassays of detection of immunoglobulin M antibodies against tick-borne encephalitis virus in serum and cerebrospinal fluid. J. Clin. Microbiol. *14*:141–146, 1981.
35. Hofbauer, K.: Ueber einen Fall mit Fruehsommermeningoenzephalitis mit Leberbeteiligung. Wien. Klin. Wochenschr. *78*:514–517, 1966.
36. Hofmann, H.: Muss nach FSME-Impfung mit dem Auftreten neurologischer Stoerungen gerechnet werden? Wien. Klin. Wochenschr. *107*:509–515, 1995.
37. Hofmann, H., Frisch-Niggemeyer, W., and Heinz, F.: Rapid diagnosis of tick-borne encephalitis by means of enzyme linked immunosorbent assay. J. Gen. Virol. *42*:505–511, 1979.
38. Hofmann, H., Kunz, C., and Heinz, F. X.: Laboratory diagnosis of tick-borne encephalitis. Arch. Virol. *65*:153–159, 1984.
39. Hofmann, H., Kunz, C., Heinz, F. X., and Dippe, H.: Detectability of IgM antibodies against TBE virus after natural infection and after vaccination. Infection *11*:164–166, 1983.
40. Ito, Y., Ando, Y., Kimura, H., et al.: Polymerase chain reaction–proved herpes simplex encephalitis in children. Pediatr. Infect. Dis. J. *17*:29–32, 1998.
41. Jeren, T., and Vince, A.: Cytologic and immunoenzymatic findings in CSF from patients with tick-borne encephalitis. Acta Cytol. *42*:330–334, 1998.
42. Juhasz, C., and Szirmai, I.: Spectral EEG parameters in patients with tick-borne encephalitis: A follow-up study. Clin. Electroencephalogr. *24*:53–58, 1993.
43. Kaiser, R.: The clinical and epidemiological profile of tick-borne encephalitis in southern Germany 1994–98: A prospective study of 656 patients. Brain *122*:2067–2078, 1999.
44. Kaiser, R., and Holzmann, H.: Laboratory findings in tick-borne encephalitis—correlation with clinical outcome. Infection *28*:78–84, 2000.
45. Kaiser, R., Kern, A., Kampa, D., and Neumann-Haefelin, D.: Prevalence of antibodies to *Borrelia burgdorferi* and tick-borne encephalitis virus in an endemic region in southern Germany. Zentralbl. Bakteriol. *286*:534–541, 1997.
46. Kluger, G., Schottler, A., Waldvogel, K., et al.: Tickborne encephalitis despite specific immunoglobulin prophylaxis. Lancet *346*:1502, 1995.
47. Koeck, T., Stuenzner, D., Freidl, W., and Pierer, K.: Zur Klinik der Fruehsommermeningoenzephalitis (FSME) in der Steiermark. Nervenarzt *63*:205–208, 1992.
48. Kohl, I., Kozuch, O., Eleckova, E., et al.: Family outbreak of alimentary tick-borne encephalitis in Slovakia associated with a natural focus of infection. Eur. J. Epidemiol. *12*:373–375, 1996.
49. Korenberg, E. I., Gorban, L. Y., Kovalevskii, Y. V., et al.: Risk for human tick-borne encephalitis, borrelioses, and double infection in the pre-Ural region of Russia. Emerg. Infect. Dis. *7*:459–462, 2001.
50. Krausler, J., Kraus, P., and Moritsch, H.: Klinische und virologisch-serologische Untersuchungsergebnisse bei FSME und anderen Virusinfektionen des Zentralnervensystems. Wien. Klin. Wochenschr. *70*:634–640, 1958.
51. Krech, U., Jung, F., and Jung, M.: Zentraleuropaeische Zeckenenzephalitis in der Schweiz. Schweiz. Med. Wochenschr. *99*:282–285, 1969.
52. Kreil, T. R., and Eibl, M. M.: Pre- and postexposure protection by passive immunization but no enhancement of infection with a flavivirus in a mouse model. J. Virol. *71*:2921–2927, 1997.
53. Kristoferitsch, W., Stanek, G., and Kunz, C.: Doppelinfektion mit Fruehsommermeningoenzephalitis- (FSME-) Virus und *Borrelia burgdorferi*. Dtsch. Med. Wochenschr. *111*:861–864, 1986.
54. Kunz, C.: Arbovirus B-Infektionen. *In* Grumbach, A., and Bonin, O. (eds.): Die Infektionskrankheiten des Menschen und ihre Erreger. 1st ed. Stuttgart, Thieme Verlag, 1969.
55. Kunz, C.: Die Fruehsommer-Meningoenzephalitis. Paediatr. Prax. *14*:189–192, 1974.
56. Kunz, C.: Immunoprophylaxis of encephalitis. *In* Kunz, C. (ed.): Tick-Borne Encephalitis. 1st ed. Vienna, Facultas Verlag, 1980, pp. 1–21.
57. Kunz, C.: Vaccination against tick-borne encephalitis (TBE). Ther. Umsch. *40*:236–238, 1983.
58. Kunz, C.: Tick-borne encephalitis in Europe. Acta Leiden *60*:1–14, 1992.
59. Kunz, C., Heinz, F. X., and Hofmann, H.: Immunogenicity and reactogenicity of a highly purified vaccine against tick-borne encephalitis. J. Med. Virol. *6*:103–109, 1980.
60. Kunz, C., Hofmann, H., and Dippe, H.: TBE vaccination, a prophylactic measure with wide acceptance in Austria. Wien. Med. Wochenschr. *12*:273–276, 1991.
61. Kunz, C., Hofmann, H., Heinz, F., and Dippe, H.: Die Wirksamkeit der Schutzimpfung gegen die Fruehsommermeningoenzephalitis. Wien. Klin. Wochenschr. *92*:809–813, 1980.
62. Kunz, C., Hofmann, H., Kundi, M., and Mayer, K.: Zur Wirksamkeit von FSME-Immunglobulin. Wien. Klin. Wochenschr. *93*:665–667, 1981.
63. Kunze, U., Bernhard, G., Bohm, G., and Groman, E.: Early-summer meningo-encephalitis (ESME) and ESME-vaccination: Status 2000. Wien. Med. Wochenschr. *150*:103–108, 2000.
64. Lakeman, F. D., and Whitley, R. J.: Diagnosis of herpes simplex encephalitis: Application of polymerase chain reaction to cerebrospinal fluid from brain-biopsied patients and correlation with disease. J. Infect. Dis. *171*:857–863, 1995.
65. Lammli, B., Muller, A., and Ballmer, P. E.: Late sequelae of tick-borne encephalitis. Schweiz. Med. Wochenschr. *130*:909–915, 2000.
66. Lindgren, E., and Gustafson, R.: Tick-borne encephalitis in Sweden and climate change. Lancet *358*:16–18, 2001.
67. Logar, M., Arnez, M., Kolbl, J., et al.: Comparison of the epidemiological and clinical features of tick-borne encephalitis in children and adults. Infection *28*:74–77, 2000.
68. Lorenzl, S., Pfister, H. W., Padovan, C., and Yousry, T.: MRI abnormalities in tick-borne encephalitis. Lancet *347*:698–699, 1996.
69. Lotric-Furlan, S., Avsic-Zupanc, T., and Strle, F.: Is an isolated initial phase of a tick-borne encephalitis a common event? Clin. Infect. Dis. *30*:987, 2000.
70. Lotric-Furlan, S., and Strle, F.: Thrombocytopenia—a common finding in the initial phase of tick-borne encephalitis. Infection *23*:203–206, 1995.
71. Mamoli, B., and Pelzl, G.: Residualschaeden nach FSME. Oesterr. Aerzteztg. *45*:45–51, 1990.
72. Mandl, C. W., Kroschewski, H., Allision, S. L., et al.: Adaptation of tick-borne encephalitis virus to BHK-21 cells results in the formation of multiple heparan sulfate binding sites in the envelope protein and attenuation in vivo. J. Virol. *75*:5627–5637, 2001.
73. McNair, A. N. B., and Brown, J. L.: Tick-borne encephalitis complicated by monoplegia and sensorineural deafness. J. Infect. *22*:81–86, 1991.

74. McNeil, J. G., Lednar, W. M., Stansfield, S. K., et al.: Central European tickborne encephalitis: Assessment of risk for persons in the Armed Forces and vacationers. J. Infect. Dis. *152*:650–651, 1985.
75. Messner, H.: Pediatric problems of TBE. *In* Kunz, C. (ed.): Tick-Borne Encephalitis. 1st ed. Vienna, Facultas Verlag, 1981, pp. 25–27.
76. Moll van Charante, A. W., Goren, J., Mulder, P. G., et al.: Occupational risks of zoonotic infections in Dutch forestry workers and muskrat catchers. Eur. J. Epidemiol. *14*:109–116, 1998.
77. Moore, M., Kaplan, M. H., McPhee, J., et al.: Epidemiologic, clinical, and laboratory features of Coxsackie B1–B5 infections in the United States, 1970–79. Public Health Rep. *99*:515–522, 1984.
78. Morens, D. M.: Antibody-dependent enhancement of infection and the pathogenesis of viral disease. Clin. Infect. Dis. *19*:500–512, 1994.
79. Moritsch, H.: Durch Arthropoden uebertragene Virusinfektionen des Zentralnervensystems in Europa. Ergebn. Inn. Med. Kinderheil. *17*:1–57, 1962.
80. Moritsch, H.: Die Arboviren. *In* Haas, R., and Vivell, O. (eds.): Die Virus- und Rickettsieninfektionen des Menschen. 1st ed. Munich, J. F. Lehmanns Verlag, 1965.
81. Moritsch, H., and Krausler, J.: Die endemische Fruehsommer-Meningo-Encephalo-Myelitis im Wiener Becken (Schneider'sche Krankheit). Wien. Klin. Wochenschr. *69*:921–926, 1957.
82. Muller, A.: Active vaccination against tick-borne encephalitis (FSME). Schweiz. Med. Wochenschr. *128*:1110–1116, 1998.
83. Niedrig, M., Vaisviliene, D., Teichmann, A., et al.: Comparison of six different commercial IgG-ELISA kits for the detection of TBEV-antibodies. J. Clin. Virol. *20*:179–182, 2001.
84. Nuttall, P. A.: Pathogen-tick-host interactions: *Borrelia burgdorferi* and TBE virus. Zentralbl. Bakteriol. *289*:492–505, 1999.
85. Oksi, J., Viljanen, M. K., Kalimo, H., et al.: Fatal encephalitis caused by concomitant infection with tick-borne encephalitis virus and *Borrelia burgdorferi*. Clin. Infect. Dis. *16*:392–396, 1993.
86. Ono, J., Shimizu, K., Harada, K., et al.: Characteristic MR features of encephalitis caused by Epstein-Barr virus: A case report. Pediatr. Radiol. *28*:569–570, 1998.
87. Osimitz, T. G., and Murphy, J. V.: Neurological effects associated with use of the insect repellent *N,N*-diethyl-*m*-toluamide. J. Toxicol. Clin. Toxicol. *35*:443–445, 1997.
88. Pfister, H. W., Lorenzl, S., and Yousry, T.: Neuroradiographic manifestations of encephalitis. N. Engl. J. Med. *337*:1393–1394, 1997.
89. Ramelow, C., Suss, J., Berndt, D., et al.: Detection of tick-borne encephalitis virus RNA in ticks *(Ixodes ricinus)* by the polymerase chain reaction. J. Virol. Methods *45*:115–119, 1993.
90. Randolph, S. E.: The shifting landscape of tick-borne zoonoses: Tick-borne encephalitis and Lyme borreliosis in Europe. Philos. Trans. R. Soc. Lond. B. Biol. Sci. *356*:1045–1056, 2001.
91. Rehse-Kuepper, B., Danielova, V., Klenk, W., et al.: Epidemiologie der Zentraleuropaeischen Enzephalitis. Munch. Med. Wochenschr. *118*: 1615–1616, 1976.
92. Roggendorf, M.: Epidemiology of tick-borne encephalitis in Germany. Infection *24*:465–466, 1996.
93. Roggendorf, M., Heinz, F., Deinhardt, F., and Kunz, C.: Serological diagnosis of acute tick-borne encephalitis by demonstration of antibodies of the IgM class. J. Gen. Virol. *7*:41–50, 1981.
94. Rosenfeld, E. A., Radkowski, M. A., and Rowley, A. H.: Biphasic course of illness with disparate outcomes in herpes simplex encephalitis in children. Abstract. Pediatr. Res. *35*:193, 1994.
95. Ryffel, K., Peter, O., Rutti, B., et al.: Scored antibody reactivity determined by immunoblotting shows an association between clinical manifestations and presence of *Borrelia burgdorferi* sensu stricto, *B. garinii, B. afzelii,* and *B. valaisiana* in humans. J. Clin. Microbiol. *37*:4086–4092, 1999.
96. Sakoulas, G.: Brainstem and striatal encephalitis complicating *Mycoplasma pneumonia:* Possible benefit of intravenous immunoglobulin. Pediatr. Infect. Dis. J. *20*:543–545, 2001.
97. Salafsky, B., He, Y. X., Li, J., et al.: Short report: Study on the efficacy of a new long-acting formulation of *N,N*-diethyl-*m*-toluamide (DEET) for the prevention of tick attachment. Am. J. Trop. Med. Hyg. *62*:169–172, 2000.
98. Sanchez, J. L., Craig, S. C., Kohlhase, K., et al.: Health assessment of US military personnel deployed to Bosnia-Herzegovina for operation Joint Endeavor. Mil. Med. *166*:470–474, 2001.
99. Sawyer, M. H.: Enterovirus infections: Diagnosis and treatment. Curr. Opin. Pediatr. *13*:65–69, 2001.
100. Schabet, M., Wietholter, H., Grodd, W., et al.: Neurological complications after simultaneous immunisation against tick-borne encephalitis and tetanus. Lancet *1*:959–960, 1989.
101. Schellinger, P. D., Schmutzhard, E., Fiebach, J. B., et al.: Poliomyelitic-like illness in central European tick-borne encephalitis. Neurology *55*:299–302, 2000.
102. Scholz, E., and Wiethoelter, H.: Postvakzinale Schwerpunktneuritis nach prophylaktischer FSME-Impfung. Dtsch. Med. Wochenschr. *112*:544, 1987.
103. Scholz, H., and Summer, K.: Tick-borne encephalitis 1970 in Styria. In XIII. Symposium de l'Association Europeenne contre la poliomyelite, Helsinki 1971, 1st ed. Bruxelles, Imprimerie des Sciences, 1972.
104. Schrader, C., and Suss, J.: A nested RT-PCR for the detection of tick-borne encephalitis (TBEV) in ticks in natural foci. Zentralbl. Bakteriol. *289*:319–328, 1999.
105. Schwanda, M., Oertli, S., Frauchiger, B., and Krause, M.: Tick-borne meningoencephalitis in Canton Thurgau: A clinical and epidemiological analysis. Schweiz. Med. Wochenschr. *130*:1447–1455, 2000.
106. Spiess, H., Mumenthaler, M., Burkhardt, S., and Keller, H.: Zentraleuropaeische Enzephalitis (Zeckenenzephalitis) in der Schweiz. Schweiz. Med. Wochenschr. *99*:277–282, 1969.
107. Stohrer-Draxl, P., Amstad, H., Grize, L., et al.: Measles, mumps and rubella: Vaccination rates and seroprevalence in 8th grade students of 8 different sites in Switzerland 1995/96. Schweiz. Rundsch. Med. Prax. *319*:352, 1999.
108. Tesarova-Magrova, J., and Kroo, A. H.: Cardiac disease in patients with tick-borne encephalitis. G. Mal. Infett. Parassit. *18*:803–806, 1966.
109. Tomazic, J., Poljak, M., Popovic, P., et al.: Tick-borne encephalitis: Possibly a fatal disease in its acute stage. PCR amplification of TBE RNA from postmortem brain tissue. Infection *25*:41–43, 1997.
110. Torm, S., Zilmer, K., Jaago, K., et al.: Clinical features of tick-borne encephalitis in children in Estonia. Abstract. Presented at a meeting of the European Society of Pediatric Infectious Diseases, 1996, Copenhagen.
111. Valdueza, J. M., Weber, J. R., Harms, L., and Bock, A.: Severe tick borne encephalomyelitis after tick bite and passive immunization. J. Neurol. Neurosurg. Psychiatry *60*:593–594, 1996.
112. Wahlberg, P., Saikku, G., and Grummer-Korvenkontio, M.: Tick-borne viral encephalitis in Finland. The clinical features of Kumlinge disease during 1959–1987. J. Intern. Med. *225*:173–177, 1989.
113. Waldvogel, K., Bossart, W., Huisman, T., et al.: Severe tick-borne encephalitis following passive immunization. Eur. J. Pediatr. *155*: 775–779, 1996.
114. Wicki, R., Sauter, P., Mettler, C., et al.: Swiss Army survey in Switzerland to determine the prevalence of *Francisella tularensis,* members of the *Ehrlichia phagocytophila* genogroup, *Borrelia burgdorferi* sensu lato, and tick-borne encephalitis virus in ticks. Eur. J. Clin. Microbiol. Infect. Dis. *19*:427–432, 2000.
115. Zeipel, G. V., Svedmyr, A., Holmgren, B., and Lindahl, J.: Tick-borne meningoencephalomyelitis in Sweden. Lancet *2*:104, 1959.

CHAPTER **179G**

Other Flaviviral Infections

THEODORE F. TSAI

Powassan Encephalitis

Powassan virus was isolated from a fatally infected patient and named after the patient's Ontario town of residence. The virus is classified within the antigenic complex of tick-borne flaviviruses. Two viral lineages in North America may represent genotypes circulating in separate enzootic cycles. Clinical and pathologic signs of encephalitis have been produced in experimentally infected horses.

EPIDEMIOLOGY AND ECOLOGY

Thirty-two cases of naturally acquired Powassan encephalitis have been reported from North America and others from Russia. Two cases of laboratory-acquired Powassan infection have been reported as well. Half the cases from North America have occurred in children younger than 15 years, and the preponderance of cases have been in males. With one exception, infections have occurred in the summer or early fall; one patient had an onset in December.[19, 34]

The probable sites of exposure of cases have been confined to the eastern states and Canadian provinces: New York, Pennsylvania, and Massachusetts and Ontario and Quebec.* However, the known and suspected geographic distribution of the virus is wider, with isolation of virus recorded from Connecticut, Massachusetts, West Virginia, Colorado, South Dakota, and California, and serologic evidence of infection in humans or animals has been reported from Maine, Wyoming, North Dakota, and British Columbia and Alberta, and Sonora, Mexico. Viral isolates also have been recovered from ticks, mosquitoes, and birds from southeastern Russia, and evidence of viral transmission in China and Southeast Asia has been reported.[26]

In North America, the virus is transmitted by *Ixodes cookei, Ixodes marxi, Ixodes spinipalpus*, and *Dermacentor andersoni* to small mammals (ground hogs, *Marmota monax*; red squirrels, *Tamiasciurus hudsonicus*; weasels, *Mustela*; skunks, *Mephitis*; foxes, *Vulpes*; chipmunks, *Tamias straiatus*; mice, *Peromyscus*; snowshoe hares, *Lepus americanus*; voles, *Microtus*; and gray squirrels, *Scurius carolensis*). In Russia, the virus is transmitted by *Ixodes persulcatus* and various *Haemaphysalis* ticks; *Apodemus* mice and *Microtus* voles are the principal vertebrate hosts. Powassan virus is transmitted transtadially in *D. andersoni* and *Ixodes pacificus*, and transovarial transmission has been shown in other species. Powassan virus infection in humans is probably rare because the implicated ixodid ticks infrequently bite people. Human infections are associated with outdoor activities and subsequent exposure to infected ticks. In one case involving a 13-month-old infant, however, the infecting tick was brought into the home by a domestic cat.[47] Animal serosurveys indicate that infections occur in dogs, and exposure to ticks on domestic animals may be an alternative source of infection. In a human serosurvey from Ontario, 3 percent had Powassan antibody; however, in other areas, the prevalence of antibody has been less than 1 percent. Experimental studies have shown that *Ixodes scapularis*, the vector of Lyme disease, can transmit Powassan virus, and a field isolate has been reported.[9] The absence of a Powassan epidemic paralleling that of Lyme disease suggests differences in the agents' transmission cycles.

Although no Powassan cases have been attributed to milk-borne transmission, experimental studies have shown that domestic goats can be infected with Powassan virus and can shed virus into milk. In a survey of New York goats, 2 percent had serologic evidence of past Powassan virus infection, which indicates the possibility of milk-borne Powassan virus infection in the United States.[49]

CLINICAL MANIFESTATIONS

The incubation period may be several weeks after known exposure to a tick. Fever, headache, lethargy, retro-orbital pain, and photophobia are early symptoms that may be followed abruptly by changes in sensorium, generalized or focal seizures, paresis, and paralysis. Focal neurologic signs have been observed in most patients in whom clinical descriptions have been reported. In one patient, olfactory hallucinations, focal seizures, and localizing electroencephalographic irregularities were concordant and thus suggested a temporal lobe focus.[13, 19]

Three deaths have been reported, and significant neurologic sequelae (hemiplegia, quadriplegia, aphasia), including residual shoulder girdle atrophy and weakness analogous to sequelae that occur after European and Far Eastern tick-borne encephalitis, are common occurrences. In another patient, wasting and weakness of a leg consistent with lumbosacral poliomyelitis were reported.[8, 23]

Clinical and experimental observations of tick-borne encephalitis suggest that chronic central nervous system (CNS) infection characterized by a convulsive disorder (epilepsia partialis continua), weakness, and dementia may occur after recovery from the acute phase of illness. A retrospective study of 22 Canadian patients with a similar clinical syndrome and in whom histologic changes in the brain resembled those of chronic tick-borne encephalitis showed no evidence of Powassan virus infection. However, none of these patients had a history of acute encephalitis.

LABORATORY DIAGNOSIS

Virus has been recovered from the brains of patients with fatal cases of the disease. A serologic diagnosis can be achieved more rapidly by detecting specific IgM antibody in acute-phase serum or spinal fluid. A serologic diagnosis by hemagglutination inhibition and complement fixation is specific in most instances, but heterologous antibodies from other flavivirus infections (e.g., dengue, St. Louis encephalitis) or vaccinations (yellow fever) may obscure the results.

DIFFERENTIAL DIAGNOSIS

The clinical findings of encephalitis in a patient with a history of a tick bite acquired in an endemic area should

*See references 6, 8, 11, 13, 19, 20, 23, 27, 34, 39, 40, 47, 49.

suggest the possibility of Powassan encephalitis. However, because ixodid tick bites may be inconspicuous, a negative history does not exclude the diagnosis. Other viral agents of encephalitis, especially eastern equine encephalitis virus and California group viruses, which are prevalent in New York state and eastern Canada, should be considered in the differential diagnosis. Lyme disease, because of its known geographic distribution and association with a tick vector, also may be associated with neurologic complications; however, a history of having a typical rash and arthritis should differentiate the conditions. In a series of 145 clinical encephalitis cases at a Canadian tertiary pediatric hospital, 1 was attributed to Powassan virus. An imported case of tick-borne encephalitis, encountered in Ohio but acquired in Austria, underscores the value of obtaining a travel history.

TREATMENT AND PREVENTION

No specific therapy for Powassan encephalitis is available. Personal protective measures to avoid tick bites are advised (see the Colorado tick fever section in Chapter 175). Consumption of unpasteurized goat milk should be avoided because of the theoretic risk of contracting Powassan virus infection and the well-documented risk of acquiring other infections associated with raw milk. Commercial inactivated tick-borne encephalitis vaccine does not cross-protect against Powassan virus infection.

West Nile Fever

West Nile fever virus was isolated from an ill viremic person in the West Nile district of Uganda in 1937 and later classified antigenically with viruses in the Japanese encephalitis complex of flaviviruses. Six viral subtypes representing two principal lineages have been proposed, one of which includes strains that have been associated with neurologic infections in humans.[24] The virus' geographic distribution is among the most extensive of all arboviruses in that it encompasses southern, central, eastern, and western Africa, areas of Europe and Russia, the Middle East, Pakistan, India, Southeast Asia, Australia, and with the emergence of outbreaks in the northeastern United States in 1999 to 2001, the Western Hemisphere—including the United States, Canada, and the Carribean.[22, 28] Strains from various geographic regions have been differentiated antigenically and genetically and correlated in a novel application of cluster analysis to patterns of human virulence.[22] U.S. strains are most closely related genetically to strains that circulated as early as 1997 in Israel, where they also were implicated in human outbreaks and epornitic diseases involving principally geese and cranes. Natural infections have been described in a wide variety of birds and mammals, notably including encephalitis outbreaks in horses; mild febrile illness with myopathy in dogs; and widespread epornitic episodes of fatal disseminated viscerotropic and neurotropic infection in North American crows, cranes, geese, and various passerines, columbiformes, and raptors.[12, 42]

The virus is transmitted principally in an avian–*Culex* mosquito cycle, including *Culex univittatus* in Africa; *Culex modestus* and *Culex pipiens* in the Middle East, Europe, and North America; *Culex tritaeniorhychnus* and *Culex vishnui* complex mosquitoes in Asia; and the Kunjin viral subtype by *Culex annulirostris* in Australia.[23] In the United States, a wide range of more than 75 avian species may participate in viral transmission and amplification, but unlike typical arboviral transmission cycles, many avian species die of the infection, possibly reflecting the exotic relationship of the virus to domestic hosts.[12, 28, 38] Transmission between birds and their mites or ticks also has been demonstrated and provides a potential viral overwintering mechanism, but in the United States, evidence of infection in adult overwintering mosquitoes suggests a more likely mechanism that also has been observed for related flaviviruses (St. Louis encephalitis and Japanese encephalitis). Migrating birds appear to be responsible for transferring the virus over long distances, including intercontinental spread between Africa and Europe.[38] The mechanism by which West Nile virus was introduced into the United States, whether by a viremic traveler, an airplane-borne infected mosquito (as occurs in "airport malaria"), a smuggled or wayward viremic bird, or other means, is a matter of speculation.[38] However, the record-breaking high temperatures and drought in New York in the summer of 1999 very conceivably contributed to a receptive environment for introduction of the virus because *C. pipiens*, the virus' principal mosquito vector, paradoxically is more abundant during hot dry years when normally clean water sources become concentrated and polluted and thus favor the mosquito's larval stages. Moreover, the extrinsic incubation period of the virus (the interval required for a mosquito to become infectious after acquiring the virus in a blood meal) is most likely shortened at high ambient temperatures, thereby facilitating viral amplification in the enzootic cycle. The first recognized outbreak of St. Louis encephalitis in 1933 also occurred in the midst of a severe drought. Sindbis virus, an alphavirus, is transmitted in identical avian-mosquito cycles in overlapping geographic areas where combined epidemics have occurred, especially in South Africa.

Seroprevalence rates vary widely according to location and ecologic conditions. For example, seroprevalence rates higher than 80 percent, indicative of a high level of endemic infection, were found in residents near Lake Chad (with an extensive avian population), but 300 km south, seroprevalence rates declined to less than 30 percent, and in Bucharest and New York City, they decreased a further 10-fold lower.[31, 46] Epidemics or equine epizootics have been reported from South Africa, Israel, Algeria, Bulgaria, France, Congo, Morocco, Tunisia, Italy, Czech Republic, Russia, and Romania. The latter outbreak, in 1996, led to nearly 400 neurologic cases, principally in elderly residents of Bucharest. Conditions that resulted in epidemic transmission in South Africa included heavy early season rainfall and warm temperatures, which led to an expanded mosquito breeding habitat, accelerated extrinsic viral incubation in infected vectors, and, consequently, high vector infection rates.

Subclinical infections occur commonly.[31, 46] The incubation period is 1 to 6 days, after which an abrupt onset of fever, headache, muscle aches, conjunctivitis, pharyngitis, and gastrointestinal symptoms occur. Headache often is severe and may be accompanied by ocular pain. Grippe symptoms are followed by a morbilliform rash affecting the trunk and extremities in approximately 50 percent of cases. Lymphadenopathy may be prominent. Arthralgias have been an important component of the illness in some outbreaks. Defervescence usually occurs within 5 days, but like dengue, it may be followed by a recrudescence of fever and symptoms in some cases. Treatment is symptomatic.

Meningoencephalitis is the most common complication.[16, 17, 22, 27, 28, 29, 32, 43, 46] Neurologic signs may be the initial manifestation of illness, or they may develop after the initial grippe prodrome. Neurologic infection has resulted in aseptic meningitis; an encephalitis syndrome with mental status changes, cranial nerve and bulbar palsies, motor weakness, and abnormal reflexes; and myelitis. Optic neuritis and polyradiculitis and polyneuropathy with elements of axonal degeneration also have been reported.[3, 21] During outbreaks in Israel and Romania, CNS infection occurred most frequently in the elderly; however, encephalitis cases have been reported in children in Asia. The case-fatality ratio in neurologic cases is approximately 10 percent, with higher rates in the elderly. Myocarditis, pancreatitis, and fatal hepatitis also have been reported as complications.[4, 18, 36] Peripheral leukopenia and lymphocytosis are usual findings. In patients with CNS infection, pleocytosis and elevated protein are found in cerebrospinal fluid (CSF).

Uncomplicated illness cannot be differentiated clinically from dengue and other febrile illnesses with nonspecific symptoms. The diagnosis also should be suspected in patients with illnesses featuring hepatitis or encephalitis. Because of their overlapping seasonality and similar epidemiologic and clinical features, St. Louis encephalitis always must be excluded in the United States.[29] Virus can be isolated from blood taken early in the illness; it can be recovered from three quarters of samples taken on the first day of onset, whereas only 25 percent of samples from the second or third post-illness day are positive. Virus also has been isolated from the CSF, from liver biopsy specimens, and from the brain and other organs at autopsy. Vero cells and continuous mosquito cell lines generally are used. Intracerebral inoculation of suckling mice is a sensitive system used in reference laboratories for isolation of virus. Direct detection of viral genomic sequences from CSF is highly sensitive, but serologic procedures provide a diagnosis in most cases. Detection of viral-specific IgM in serum is presumptive evidence of recent infection; the presence of IgM in CSF indicates intrathecal production and confirms a recent infection.[45] Cases also can be confirmed by demonstrating four-fold or greater changes in antibody titer by hemagglutination, complement fixation, immunofluorescence, or neutralization. Cross-reactions with dengue and other flaviviruses (Banzi, yellow fever, Wesselsbron, and others in Africa; Japanese encephalitis, Zika, and others in Asia; St. Louis encephalitis and dengue in the United States) can complicate the interpretation of serologic results. Neutralizing antibody assays are most specific and in most cases must be performed to secure the diagnosis.

An inactivated vaccine is licensed for horses, and human vaccines are under development. Personal protection consists of avoiding outdoor activity during the crepuscular periods (when vector mosquitoes are most active) and applying mosquito repellents.

Rocio Encephalitis

Rocio encephalitis virus was isolated from the brain of a fatal encephalitis patient during an outbreak in 1975.[15, 25] The virus is related peripherally to viruses in the Japanese encephalitis viral antigenic complex. The disease has occurred exclusively in the coastal São Paulo State and adjacent Parana State, Brazil, principally in the Ribiera Valley and Santista lowlands. More than 1000 cases were documented in outbreaks between 1975 and 1977; only 1 symptomatic case (in an infant) has been recognized subsequently, although recent infections (IgM in asymptomatic individuals) were documented in serosurveys between 1983 and 1987. Thus, the virus may be transmitted undetected in the Ribiera Valley. The viral transmission cycle has not been elucidated; however, field and laboratory observations suggest transmission between birds and *Psorophora* or *Aedes* mosquitoes. Humans are dead-end hosts. Human cases have occurred principally in men with outdoor occupations, especially fishermen.

The incubation period is estimated to be 7 to 14 days. Prodromal symptoms of fever, headache, malaise, vomiting, and conjunctivitis are followed by mental status changes, meningismus, and motor impairment. Cerebellar signs occur commonly. Signs of bulbar involvement also are seen. Coma and a fatal outcome occur most commonly in children (30%) and in the elderly; overall, 10 percent of cases are fatal and 20 percent of patients have neuropsychiatric sequelae. Pathologic findings of encephalitis principally involve the thalamus, cerebellar dentate nucleus, brain nuclei, brain stem, and spinal cord.

The diagnosis should be suspected in patients with acute encephalitis and a consistent history of exposure. Virus has been isolated from autopsy brain specimens. The presence of viral-specific IgM in CSF or a fourfold change in serum antibody titer confirms a case. IgM in serum is presumptive evidence of recent infection. Treatment is supportive. Emergency application of adulticides and larvicides has been used to control epidemics.

Louping Ill Virus

Louping ill virus derives its name from an old Scottish term describing the leaping motions of encephalitic sheep. Historical accounts of the disease in sheep date from 1795, and the virus was isolated from ill sheep in 1931. Louping ill virus, a member of the antigenic complex of tick-borne flaviviruses, is transmitted by *Ixodes ricinus* to sheep, deer, small mammals, and grouse. The disease is enzootic in pasturelands of Scotland, England, Wales, and Ireland. Naturally acquired human infections have occurred mainly in sheep farmers, veterinarians, and abattoir workers or butchers who had direct contact with animals. Antibody prevalence is 10 percent in abattoir workers in enzootic areas. Laboratory-acquired infections are common and account for half of all reported human cases. These observations suggest that infections are transmitted easily by direct mucous membrane or respiratory infection. Tick-transmitted cases also have been reported. Hospital surveillance in an enzootic area found louping ill virus to be a rare occurrence that was responsible for less than 0.5 percent of encephalitis cases. Related tick-borne viruses in Spain, Greece, Norway, and Turkey have not been associated with human disease. The virus is shed in sheep and goat milk, but unlike tick-borne encephalitis, milk-transmitted cases have not been reported.

The incubation period can be as short as 3 days. Three clinical syndromes have been described.[10] Approximately a third of patients have a self-limited flulike illness with fever, headache, dizziness, and myalgias. The febrile illness is followed by clinical improvement and a second encephalitic phase in more than half the cases. Neurologic symptoms include meningismus, severe headache, vomiting, drowsiness, and tremor; one fatal case was reported. A poliomyelitis syndrome with muscular weakness or paralysis has been described in a few cases. Hemorrhagic fever also was reported in one atypical laboratory-acquired case.

The diagnosis should be suspected in febrile patients with occupational or other exposure, especially if CNS symptoms are present. The diagnosis is confirmed serologically by demonstrating viral-specific IgM in CSF or serum or by a fourfold rise in antibody titer by other techniques. Treatment is symptomatic. The use of unpasteurized milk products should be avoided. Persons with outdoor exposure in enzootic areas are advised to use repellents and other protective measures against tick bites.

Kyasanur Forest Disease

Kyasanur Forest virus was isolated in 1957 after an outbreak of hemorrhagic fever, initially suspected to be the first outbreak of yellow fever in Asia, appeared in India in the Kyasanur Forest of Mysore (now Karnataka).[2] The virus is a member of the tick-borne flaviviral antigenic complex. It is transmitted by *Haemaphysalis spinigera* (among numerous other ixodid ticks) to forest rodents, insectivores, and possibly bats; cattle and other large animals are important tick hosts but do not appear to amplify the virus. Langur monkeys sicken in epizootics and die of the infection. Human cases occur in dry-season epidemics, chiefly in persons who have contact with forests. The disease has spread contiguously as villagers clear forests for pastureland. Between 1982 and 1988, 1847 cases were reported, 254 of which were fatal.

After an incubation period of 3 to 8 days, illness begins abruptly with fever, headache, myalgias, chills, and gastrointestinal symptoms.[35, 37, 41] Facial hyperemia, conjunctival suffusion, lymphadenopathy, hepatomegaly, papulovesicular enanthem, and petechiae are the principal physical findings. Bradycardia and hypotension are present and may progress to become life-threatening. Epistaxis, hemoptysis, and gastrointestinal bleeding may be prominent. Bronchopneumonia and hemorrhagic pulmonary edema complicate the illness in 40 percent of cases. Renal failure may develop. After the resolution of symptoms and an afebrile interval of 1 to 3 weeks, fever, recurrence of symptoms, and meningoencephalitis develop in 15 to 50 percent of cases, as occurs in tick-borne encephalitis. Leukopenia with a left shift, thrombocytopenia, and an elevated hematocrit reflecting hemoconcentration are seen. Elevations in liver enzymes occur commonly. The case-fatality ratio is 3 to 15 percent; keratitis and iritis occur as sequelae. The virus frequently can be isolated from acute-phase blood specimens (<12 days after onset), or the diagnosis can be confirmed serologically. A formalin-inactivated chick embryo cell culture vaccine is distributed in epidemic areas.

Omsk Hemorrhagic Fever

Omsk hemorrhagic fever virus was isolated from a viremic human during a series of outbreaks in the Omsk region of western Siberia from 1945 to 1949.[26, 41] Between 1945 and 1958, approximately 1500 cases were reported in the forest-steppe zones within the Omsk, Novosibirsk, Kurgan, and Tjumen regions. The virus is related antigenically and genetically to other tick-borne flaviviruses. It circulates among microtine rodents and *Dermacentor* ticks, which results in a spring–early summer peak of infected ticks with a smaller peak in early autumn. The disease epidemiology changed after muskrats were introduced into the region; extensive muskrat epizootics occurred and led to an increase in human cases and geographic spread of the disease. Muskrat trappers, who may be infected by direct contact with infected tissue or blood, continue to account for most cases, but tick-borne infections also occur in other local residents, including children. Seroprevalence rates range to higher than 30 percent in some locations. Laboratory-associated cases frequently have occurred in workers not immunized with tick-borne encephalitis vaccine.

The incubation period may be as brief as 2 to 4 days. The illness is similar to Kyasanur Forest disease, but with an earlier onset of hemorrhagic phenomena (e.g., epistaxis). Hemorrhages tend to be less severe, neurologic complications are less frequent, and the overall mortality is lower (less than 3%). Neuropsychiatric sequelae, however, occur commonly. Uncomplicated cases usually resolve within 7 to 10 days. The diagnosis is made serologically. Vaccine produced against tick-borne encephalitis virus is reported to provide some degree of cross-protection.

Other Flaviviral Infections

Flaviviral infections of lesser public health importance or that are recognized less frequently are listed in Table 179-6.

TABLE 179–6 ■ LESS COMMONLY RECOGNIZED FLAVIVIRAL INFECTIONS

Virus	Clinical Syndrome	Geographic Distribution	Transmission Cycle	Mode of Transmission
Alkhurma	Hemorrhagic fever encephalitis	Saudi Arabia	Unknown	Z, DC, ?V
Alma-Arasan	Febrile illness, meningitis	Kazakhstan	*Ixodes persulcatus*—?	V
Apoi	Encephalitis	Japan	Rodent—?	L
Banzi	Nonspecific febrile illness	South, East Africa	*Culex rubinotus*—rodent	V
Bussuquara	Fever, arthralgias	Brazil, Colombia, Panama	*Culex melaconion*—rodent	V
Edge Hill	Fever, polyarthritis	Australia	*Aedes vigilax*—marsupial	V
Ilheus	Fever, myalgia, encephalitis	Argentina, Brazil, Colombia, Guatemala, Panama, Trinidad	*Psorophora ferox*—bird	V, E
Karshi	Nonspecific febrile illness	Uzbekistan	Various ticks—rodent	V
Kokobera	Fever, polyarthralgia	Australia, Papua New Guinea	*Culex annulirostris*—? marsupial	V
Koutango	Fever, rash, arthralgia	Western and central Africa	Tick—rodent	L
Langat	Fever, encephalitis	Malaysia, Thailand, Russia	*Ixodes* tick—rodent	L
Modoc	Aseptic meningitis	Western United States, Canada	Rodent—rodent	Z
Negishi	Encephalitis	Japan, China, Russia	Tick—unknown	L, V
Rio Bravo	Nonspecific febrile illness, meningitis	Western United States, Canada	Bat—bat	Z, L
Sepik	Nonspecific febrile illness	Papua New Guinea	*Mansonia* species—?	V
Spondweni	Fever, arthralgia, rash	Southern and western Africa	*Aedes* species—?	L, V
Usutu	Fever, rash	Southern and central Africa	*Culex* species—bird	V
Wesselsbron	Fever, arthralgia, rash, encephalitis	Sub-Saharan Africa, Thailand	*Aedes* species—?	V, L, DC?
Zika	Fever, rash, arthralgia	Western, eastern, and central Africa; Indonesia, Malaysia	*Aedes* species—monkey	V

DC, direct contact with infected sheep; E, experimental infection; L, laboratory-acquired infection; V, vector-borne infection; Z, zoonotic infection.

Several of the viruses are known to cause human illness only after laboratory exposure. The clinical manifestations of these infections may differ from naturally acquired infection because of their mode of transmission by respiratory, mucosal, or other routes of infection. Other viruses that cause nonspecific syndromes of febrile illness were discovered through fever surveys; although few cases may have been reported, their prevalence may be underestimated because few cases are recognized. Of the zoonotic flaviviruses (transmitted from animal to animal without an arthropod vector), only Rio Bravo and Modoc viruses are known to cause human illness.

REFERENCES

1. Aaskov, J. G., Phillips, D. A., and Wiemers, M. A.: Possible clinical infection with Edge Hill virus. Trans. R. Soc. Trop. Med. Hyg. *87*:452–453, 1993.
2. Adhikari Prabha, M. R., Prabhu, M. G., Raghuveer, C. V., et al.: Clinical study of 100 cases of Kyasanur Forest disease with clinicopathological correlation. Indian J. Med. Sci. *47*:124–130, 1993.
3. Ahmed, S., Libman, R., Wesson, K., et al.: Guillain-Barré syndrome: An unusual presentation of West Nile virus infection. Neurology *55*:144–146, 2000.
4. Albagali, C., and Chaimoff, R.: A case of West Nile myocarditis. Harefuah *57*:274–275, 1959.
5. Boughton, C. R., Hawkes, R. A., and Naim, H. M.: Illness caused by a kokobera-like virus in southeastern Australia. Med. J. Aust. *145*:90–97, 1986.
6. Centers for Disease Control and Prevention: Outbreak of Powassan encephalitis—Maine and Vermont, 1999–2001. J. A. M. A. *286*: 1962–1963, 2001.
7. Charrel, R. N., Zaki, A. M., Attoui, H., et al.: Complete coding sequence of the Alkhurma virus, a tick-borne flavivirus causing severe hemorrhagic fever in humans in Saudi Arabia. Biochem. Biophys. Res. Commun. *287*:455–461, 2001.
8. Conway, D., Rossier, E., Spence, L., et al.: A case report: Powassan virus encephalitis with shoulder girdle involvement. Can. Dis. Wkly. Rep. *2(22):85–87, 1976.*
9. Costero, A., and Grayson, M. A.: Experimental transmission of Powassan virus *(Flaviviridae)* by *Ixodes scapularis* ticks *(Acari: Ixodidae)*. Am. J. Trop. Med. Hyg. *55*:536–546, 1996.
10. Davidson, M. M., Williams, H., and MacLeod, A. J.: Louping ill in man: A forgotten disease. J. Infect. *23*:241–249, 1991.
11. Deibel, R., Srihongse, S., and Woodall, J. P.: Arboviruses in New York State. Am. J. Trop. Med. Hyg. *28*:577–582, 1979.
12. Eidson, M., Kramer, L., Stone, W., et al.: Dead bird surveillance as an early warning system for West Nile virus. Emerg. Infect. Dis. *7*:631–635, 2001.
13. Embil, J., Camfield, P., Artsob, H., et al.: Powassan virus encephalitis resembling herpes simplex encephalitis. Arch. Intern. Med. *143*:341–343, 1983.
14. Essed, W. C. A. H., Van, T., and Ongeran, H. A. E.: Arthropod-borne virus infections in New Guinea. 1. Report of a case of Murray Valley encephalitis in a Papvan woman. Trop. Geogr. Med. *1*:52–55, 1965.
15. Figueiredo, L. T. M.: The Brazilian flaviviruses. Microbes Infect. *2*:1643–1649, 2000.
16. Flatau, E., Kohr, D., Daker, O., et al.: West Nile fever encephalitis. Isr. J. Med. Sci. *17*:1057–1059, 1981.
17. George, S., Prasad, S. R., Rao, J. A., et al.: Isolation of Japanese encephalitis and West Nile viruses from fatal cases of encephalitis. Indian J. Med. Res. *86*:131, 1987.
18. Georges, A. J., Lesbordes, J. L., Georges-Courbot, M. C., et al.: Fatal hepatitis from West Nile virus. Ann. Inst. Pasteur. Virol. *138*:234–237, 1988.
19. Gholam, B. I., Puksa, S., and Provias, J. P.: Powassan encephalitis: A case report with neuropathology and literature review. C. M. A. J. *161*:1419–1422, 1999.
20. Goldfield, M., Austin, S. M., Black, H. C., et al.: A nonfatal human case of Powassan virus encephalitis. Am. J. Trop. Med. Hyg. *22*:78–81, 1973.
21. Gradoth, N., Weitzman, S., and Lehmann, E. E.: Acute anterior myelitis complicating West Nile fever. Arch. Neurol. *36*:172–173, 1979.
22. Hubálek, Z.: Comparative symptomatology of West Nile fever. Lancet *358*:254–255, 2000.
23. Jackson, A. C.: [Leg weakness associated with Powassan virus infection—Ontario.] Can. Dis. Wkly. Rep. *15*(24):123, 1989.
24. Jia, X. Y., Briese, T., Jordan, I., et al.: Genetic analysis of West Nile New York 1999 encephalitis virus. Lancet *354*:1971–1972, 1999.
25. Lopes, O., Sacchetta, L. de A., Coimbra, T. L. M., et al.: Emergence of a new arbovirus disease in Brazil. II. Epidemiologic studies on 1975 epidemic. Am. J. Epidemiol. *108*:394–401, 1978.
26. Lvov, D. K.: Arboviral zoonoses of northern Eurasia (Eastern Europe and The Commonwealth of Independent States). *In* Beran, G. W. (ed.): Handbook of Zoonoses. 2nd ed. Boca Raton, FL, CRC Press, 1994, pp. 237–260.
27. Marberg, K., Golblum, N., Sterk, V. V., et al.: The natural history of West Nile fever. I. Clinical observations during an epidemic in Israel. Am. J. Hyg. *64*:259–265, 1956.
28. Marfin, A. A., and Gubler, D. J.: West Nile encephalitis: An emerging disease in the United States. Clin. Infect. Dis. *33*:1713–1719, 2001.
29. McCarthy, M.: St. Louis encephalitis and West Nile virus encephalitis. Curr. Treat. Options Neurol. *3*:433–438, 2001.
30. McIntosh, B. M., Jupp, P. G., Dos Santos I., et al.: Epidemics of West Nile and Sindbis viruses in South Africa with *Culex univittatus* Theobald as a vector. S. Afr. J. Sci. *72*:295, 1976.
31. Mostashari, F., Bunning, M. L., Kitsutani, P. T., et al.: Epidemic West Nile encephalitis, New York, 1999: Results of a household-based seroepidemiological survey. Lancet *358*:261–264, 2001.
32. Nash, D., Mostashari, F., Fine, A., et al.: The outbreak of West Nile virus infection in the New York City area in 1999. N. Engl. J. Med. *14*:1807–1814, 2001.
33. Nassar, E. S., Coimbra, T. L., Rocco, I. M., et al.: Human disease caused by an arbovirus closely related to Ilheus virus: Report of 5 cases. Intervirology *40*:249–252, 1997.
34. Partington, M. W., Thomson, V., and O'Shaughnessy, M. V.: Powassan virus encephalitis in southeastern Ontario. Can. Med. Assoc. J. *123*:603–604, 1980.
35. Pavri, K.: Clinical, clinicopathologic, and hematologic features of Kyasanur Forest disease. Rev. Infect. Dis. *4*(Suppl. 4):854–859, 1989.
36. Perelman, A., and Stern, J.: Acute pancreatitis in West Nile fever. Am. J. Trop. Med. Hyg. *23*:1150–1152, 1974.
37. Prabha, A., Prabhu, M. G., Raghuvcer, C. V., et al.: Clinical study of 100 cases of Kyasanur Forest disease with clinicopathological correlation. Indian J. Med. Sci. *47*:124–130, 1993.
38. Rappole, J. H., Derrickson, S. R., and Hubalek, Z.: Migratory birds and spread of West Nile virus in the Western Hemisphere. Emerg. Infect. Dis. *6*:319–328, 2000.
39. Rossier, E., Harrison, R. J., and Lemieux, B.: A case of Powassan virus encephalitis. Can. Med. Assoc. J. *110*:1173–1180, 1974.
40. Smith, R., Woodall, J. P., Whitney, E., et al.: Powassan virus infection: A report of three human cases of encephalitis. Am. J. Dis. Child. *127*:691–693, 1974.
41. Smorodintsev, A. A., Kazbintsev, and Chudakov, V. G.: Virus Hemorrhagic Fevers: Israel Program for Scientific Translations. Jerusalem, 1964, pp. 175–192.
42. Snook, C. S., Hyman, S. S., Del Piero, F., et al.: West Nile virus encephalomyelitis in eight horses. J. Am. Vet. Med. Assoc. *218*:1576–1579, 2001.
43. Southam, C. M., and Moore, A. E.: Induced virus infections in man by the Egypt isolates of West Nile virus. Am. J. Trop. Med. Hyg. *3*:19–50, 1954.
44. Sulkin, S. E., Burns, K. F., Shelton, D. F., et al.: Bal salivary gland virus: Infections of man. Tx. Rep. Biol. Med. *20*:113–127, 1962.
45. Tardei, G., Ruta, S., Chitu, V., et al.: Evaluation of immunoglobulin M (IgM) and IgG enzyme immunoassays in serologic diagnosis of West Nile virus infection. J. Clin. Microbiol. *38*:2232–2239, 2000.
46. Tsai, T. F., Popovici, F., Cernescu, C., et al.: West Nile encephalitis epidemic in southeastern Romania. Lancet *352*:767–771, 1998.
47. Wilson, M. S., Wherrett, B. A., and Mahdy, M. S.: Powassan virus meningoencephalitis: A case report. Can. Med. Assoc. J. *121*:320–323, 1979.
48. Wolff, M. S., Calishan, C. H., and McGuire, K.: Spondweni virus infection in a foreign resident of Upper Volta. Lancet *2*:1306–1307, 1982.
49. Woodall, J. P., and Roz, A.: Experimental milk-borne transmission of Powassan virus in the goat. Am. J. Trop. Med. Hyg. *26*:190–192, 1977.
50. Zaki, A. M.: Isolation of a flavivirus related to the tick-borne encephalitis complex from human cases in Saudi Arabia. Trans. R. Soc. Trop. Med. Hyg. *91*:179–181, 1997.

CHAPTER 180

Hepatitis C Virus

ALAN N. MAYER ■ MAUREEN M. JONAS

Since recognition in 1990 that hepatitis C virus (HCV) is the primary cause of non-A, non-B hepatitis, this infection has assumed a prominent role in the field of hepatology and infectious disease. During the last 12 years, substantial progress has been made in understanding the virology, epidemiology, and natural history of HCV infection. An estimated 4 million people in the United States have been infected with this virus, which has become the most common cause of hepatitis, cirrhosis, and end-stage liver disease in this country. On the other hand, HCV does not always cause significant morbidity, at least in the first 2 or 3 decades after infection. HCV remains the subject of numerous studies around the world, in laboratory and clinical settings, and significant advances in definition of molecular virology, viral-host interactions, and effective therapy are expected in the next several years.

Virology

Before the discovery of HCV, the agent responsible for most transfusion-associated non-A, non-B hepatitis was presumed to be a small, enveloped virus. This conclusion was based on the ability to pass the infectious agent through an 80-nm filter and to inactivate it with organic solvents. In 1989, a group at the Chiron Corporation identified a cDNA derived from human plasma[42] that shares sequence similarities with flaviviruses and pestiviruses. Intrahepatic inoculation of the full-length RNA transcribed from this clone was subsequently shown to induce hepatitis in chimpanzees.[100, 192] To date, several technologic obstacles to the study of pathogenesis and replication of HCV remain, including the absence of either a small animal model or an in vitro system in which to propagate the virus.[67] In spite of these difficulties, much has been learned about the molecular virology and physical properties of the viral particles.

HCV VIRION

HCV is approximately 30 to 60 nm in diameter on the basis of filtration studies[100, 192] and electron microscopy.[18, 170] The capsid is thought to be enveloped by a lipid bilayer because infectivity is inactivated by chloroform.[73] The envelope contains two viral glycoproteins, E1 and E2, and the nucleocapsid contained within is composed of core protein and the viral RNA genome.

HCV GENOME

The HCV genome is a 9.6-kb positive, single-stranded RNA (Fig. 180–1). A single open reading frame encodes a 3000–amino acid polyprotein that undergoes proteolytic processing to yield at least 10 individual gene products. Structural proteins (core and envelope) are encoded in the 5′ quarter of the genome, and nonstructural proteins (proteases, helicase, and RNA polymerase) are encoded in the remaining portion. The flanking 5′ and 3′ untranslated regions (UTRs) contain conserved sequences that regulate both genome replication and open reading frame translation.

The HCV 5′ UTR is approximately 340 nucleotides long and is homologous to the 5′ UTRs of the related pestiviruses and GB virus B (GBVB).[34] Translation of the pestivirus and GBVB viral genomes is controlled by a 5′ internal ribosome entry site that bypasses the requirement for a 5′ methyl-G cap. HCV is probably translated by a similar mechanism because computer modeling and cleavage protection studies

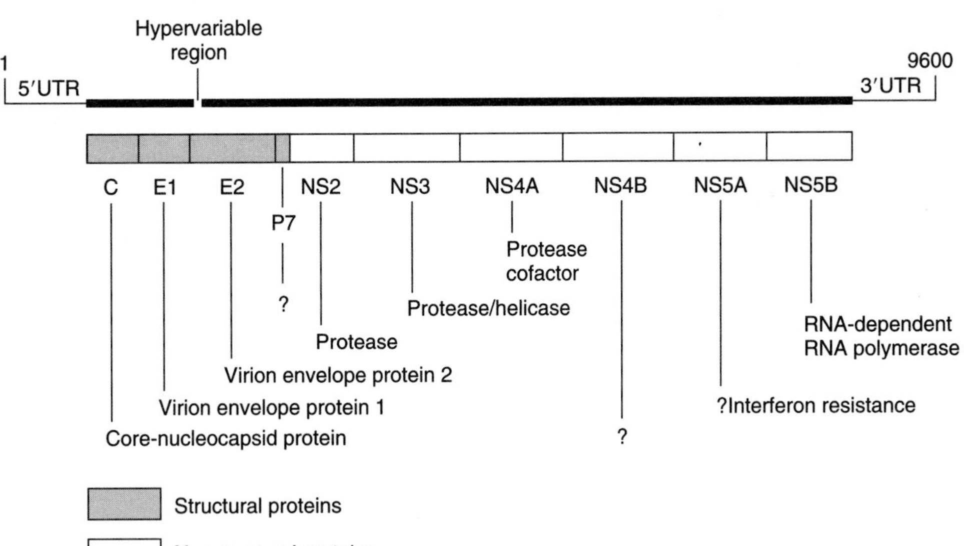

FIGURE 180–1 ■ Schematic of the HCV genome and encoded proteins.

of the HCV 5′ UTR predict the formation of a similar internal ribosome entry site–like structure that includes the canonical four stem-loops.[183] Furthermore, in vitro expression[160] and mutational analysis of the HCV 5′ UTR support this conclusion. Deletion analysis reveals both positive and negative regulatory elements in the 5′ UTR. Deletion of stem-loop I increases translation efficiency, whereas domains II and III are essential for internal ribosome entry site activity. Stem-loop IV contains the initiator AUG, and its destabilization leads to more efficient initiation of translation.[77, 78, 81] Both viral and host-derived factors can bind to the internal ribosome entry site region and alter its activity in vitro,[3, 61, 71] but in vivo roles remain to be defined.

The 3′ UTR contains sequences required for viral replication. The 3′ terminal 98 nucleotides are strongly conserved and are predicted to form a stable stem-loop structure at the 3′ end of the HCV genome. Deleting this structure impairs infectivity in chimpanzees.[193] A polypyrimidine tract in the 3′ UTR unique to HCV and GBVB also is required for infectivity. The sequence conservation and functional importance of the 5′ and 3′ UTRs support their potential utility as targets for novel anti-HCV therapies based on antisense,[35, 72] ribozyme,[121, 122] and small-molecule approaches that are currently in development.[110]

Translation of the single open reading frame results in a single polyprotein precursor that is cleaved by both host and viral proteases. The structural proteins (core, E1 and E2) are processed by host signal peptidase, and the nonstructural proteins are subsequently cleaved by virally encoded NS2–3 and NS3 proteases. The core protein is at the polyprotein N-terminus and together with the viral RNA genome composes the HCV nucleocapsid. The core protein is highly conserved[36] and may be involved in other processes, such as apoptosis,[79] intracellular signaling,[95] transcription,[172] and modulation of the host immune response.[97] The envelope proteins E1 and E2 are N-glycosylated with hydrophobic C-termini that anchor the proteins to the lipid envelope. E2 binds specifically to the host protein CD81,[151, 152] suggesting that it mediates viral entry into the cell. Unlike the core protein, E1 and E2 demonstrate considerable sequence heterogeneity from different isolates. In particular, the N-terminal of E2 contains a "hypervariable" region (HVR1) that is an important viral neutralization determinant.[171] HVR1 also is a T-cell determinant, able to activate helper T-cell responses during HCV infection. The sequence variability of E2 may account, at least in part, for the ability of HCV to elude the host immune system and to establish persistent infection.

The 3′ region of the genome encodes seven nonstructural proteins that participate in post-translational proteolytic processing and replication of HCV genetic material. The HCV polyprotein undergoes processing through a sequence of successive cleavage steps.[191] Initially, host protease generates the NS2–NS3 fusion protein precursor. This intermediate species autoproteolyzes to liberate the individual NS2 and NS3 proteins. NS3, which encodes a multifunctional serine protease, then cleaves the remaining junctions of the HCV polyprotein. NS4A complexes with NS3 and serves as a cofactor for the cleavage of the NS3/4A and NS4B/5A junctions. Whereas the N-terminal domain of NS3 contains the proteolytic domain, its C-terminal contains an RNA helicase that may function during viral replication. Proteins NS4B and NS5A do not yet have defined roles, but NS5A may be a phosphoprotein that is involved in transcriptional activation and cell cycle regulation[14] and may help regulate the viral replication cycle.[22]

Some investigators have designated amino acid residues 2209 to 2248 of the NS5A protein the interferon sensitivity–determining region because mutations within the region are thought to be associated with variation in responsiveness to interferon therapy.[55, 138, 188, 190] However, this designation remains somewhat controversial[143, 166] and is being actively investigated. Additional variables, such as virus genotype (see later) and synergistic mutations (in the NS2 gene), may play roles in modulating interferon responsiveness.

The NS5B protein is the RNA-dependent RNA polymerase thought to be the replicative polymerase for HCV.[114] The enzyme lacks proofreading activity, which may account for the high error rate and consequent sequence divergence.[145] NS5B activity requires a primer for initiation of polymerization, which is thought to occur in vivo by self-priming at the 3′ terminal UTR hairpin.[17] The crystal structure of the NS5B apoenzyme reveals a globular shape unique among polymerases and implicates new structural features important for binding the RNA template and cognate ribonucleotide substrates.[119] These crystallographic results also provide a structure-based framework for biochemical analyses and drug design efforts. In vitro inhibitors of HCV RNA-dependent RNA polymerase have been reported.[2] Yet to be elucidated are the exact steps by which the polymerase replicates the HCV genome, such as in vivo primer requirements, replicative intermediates, and postreplication processing, all of which may provide targets for antiviral agents.

HCV exhibits extensive genetic heterogeneity. Isolates from around the world have been divided into six major genotypes, designated 1 through 6, and more than 100 subtypes. The genomes of the most different HCV isolates differ by up to 35 percent. The impact of HCV genotypes on clinical factors, such as viremia level and severity of liver disease, is controversial. However, clear differences in response to antiviral therapy have been demonstrated.[75, 93, 124, 131]

Within infected individuals, HCV circulates as quasi-species, a mixture of closely related but distinct genomes. Viral genomes of quasi-species typically differ by 1 to 2 percent. In an infected person, quasi-species either may be present from the onset, because of simultaneous transmission, or may develop over time because of accumulation of mutations. Such mutations may enable more efficient HCV replication or evasion of host immune responses. Certain regions of the genome are hypervariable, responsible for most but not all of the genomic differences in quasi-species. HVR1 is found at the N-terminus of the envelope E2 protein, at amino acids 384 to 410. This site is probably on the surface of the folded envelope protein and represents a neutralization epitope for humoral immunity. Although the mutation rate at this site is rapid, it may be even further accelerated in patients subjected to immunostimulation. On the other hand, the rate is decreased in individuals with agammaglobulinemia. Appearance of antibodies against HVR1 in infected subjects is followed by emergence of new variants in the region. For these reasons, HVR1 is believed to play a role in HCV persistence and chronic infection. HVR2 is a second hypervariable region in the E2 protein, identified in genotype 1b isolates.

REPLICATION CYCLE

HCV–host cell interaction and the mechanics of viral replication are not well understood; most information is inferred from conserved mechanisms common to flaviviruses and in vitro studies.[161] Entry of HCV into a cell is mediated by a specific interaction between viral envelope proteins and a host cell surface receptor, and this interaction may underlie host specificity and cellular tropism. The HCV envelope protein E2 has been shown to bind the host cell surface protein CD81,[152] and using an in vitro cell fusion assay, researchers have shown that both E1 and E2 proteins are required for fusion.[177] Additional host proteins other than CD81 may be required for entry of the virus, such as the LDL receptor.[169] Evidence from study of other flaviviruses supports a model in which entry through receptor-mediated endocytosis is followed by envelope fusion with the endosomal membrane to release the nucleocapsid into the cytoplasm. There, ribosome binding to the viral genome enables translation of the encoded polyprotein, with the formation of a replicative ribonucleoprotein complex. The resulting negative-strand intermediate then serves as a template for the production of positive-strand RNA. Virion assembly begins with interaction between the noncoding region of the RNA genome and the capsid proteins to assemble the nucleocapsid. Like other flaviviruses, HCV probably buds into intracellular vesicles, which release free virus from the cell by exocytosis. How HCV acquires its envelope or specifically excludes cellular proteins and RNAs during virion assembly is not known.

Immunopathogenesis

Antibodies to several HCV proteins can be detected by 7 to 30 weeks after infection. However, the extraordinarily high rates of chronic disease and persistent viremia observed in humans suggest that HCV fails to induce an effective neutralizing antibody response. After having a primary HCV infection, convalescent chimpanzees rechallenged with the same or different strains of HCV had reappearance of viremia caused by infection with the subsequent challenge virus.[57] This reappearance of viremia is associated with mild alanine aminotransferase (ALT) elevations and histopathologic signs of acute hepatitis.

Although antibodies to the E2 region of the HCV genome have been identified as potential neutralizing antibodies, their effectiveness is extremely limited and their role in protection has not been demonstrated.[58, 171] Recovery from HCV infection may occur in the absence of any antibody response to the envelope proteins.[125]

Individuals with acute, self-limited HCV infection have both early, vigorous T-helper lymphocyte and cytotoxic T-cell responses.[47, 112] The sequences that are recognized by HCV-specific T-helper cells are immunodominant and conserved among HCV genotypes.[52] Individuals with various major histocompatibility complex haplotypes demonstrate efficient presentation and recognition of a set of common viral epitopes,[107] suggesting that these antigens may be important in development of immune reactivity and might be considered in vaccine development. HCV-specific T-helper ($CD4^+$) and T-suppressor ($CD8^+$) lymphocytes become detectable in blood 3 to 4 weeks after infection. T-cell infiltration of the liver correlates with increase in ALT activity as cytotoxic lymphocytes lyse HCV-infected cells. Effector functions of the $CD4^+$ and $CD8^+$ cells include synthesis of a series of proinflammatory and anti-inflammatory cytokines. After recovery from HCV infection, circulating HCV-specific T-helper and cytotoxic lymphocytes may be present for decades, even when the humoral response declines and HCV antibodies become undetectable.[176]

Although the exact mechanism for viral persistence and the frequent development of chronic infection is not known, HCV-specific cytotoxic T lymphocytes are found at only very low levels in the blood of chronically infected individuals.[74] Patients with stronger polyclonal cytotoxic T-lymphocyte responses in blood and liver have lower levels of HCV viremia.[74] Both HCV-specific and nonspecific $CD8^+$ T cells are found in the liver of infected persons; immune-mediated liver disease is thought to be initiated by the HCV-specific cells but amplified by the nonspecific cytotoxic cells. Several mechanisms have been postulated to explain HCV persistence. They include escape of innate immune response by upregulation of major histocompatibility complex expression on infected cells, viral sequence variations and mutations that eliminate humoral and cellular target epitopes, and lack of susceptibility of HCV to T-cell cytokines. Viral variant sequences are seen more commonly in the presence of cytotoxic T lymphocytes than in their absence.[40] HCV may actively interfere with the host immune response; inhibition of activation of the interferon-inducible protein kinase has been demonstrated by sequences in the HCV E2 and NS5A proteins.[102, 179]

Epidemiology

An estimated 3 percent (170 million) of the world's population has been infected with HCV.[10] It is the most common cause of non-A, non-B hepatitis. In the United States, approximately 2.7 million individuals are chronically infected with HCV,[7] and approximately 28,000 new infections occur each year.[4] This figure represents a substantial decline in incidence compared with 12 years ago (Fig. 180–2), before the first-generation anti-HCV test was used for screening donated blood.

Young adults are at highest risk for acquiring HCV. In the United States, a wide variation in prevalence exists among different subgroups. As risk of acquiring HCV from transfusion has diminished, the proportion of cases associated with intravenous drug abuse has increased rapidly, up to more than 40 percent. Heterosexual contact was reported in 6 percent of infected individuals, household contact in 3 percent, and occupational exposure in only 2 percent. In those with repeated percutaneous exposures, such as injecting drug users, the prevalence is 60 to 90 percent, whereas it is 1 percent in health care workers. Volunteer blood donors, who represent the lowest risk group, have a seroprevalence of less than 0.5 percent. In several early studies, the proportion of cases of HCV infection with no identifiable risk factor had been consistently 35 to 40 percent.[5] However, although high-risk behavior may not be documented within months of diagnosis of HCV, a history of more remote risk factors can be obtained in most of these cases. Thus, more than 90 percent of new cases can be attributed to parenteral or sexual behaviors.[4]

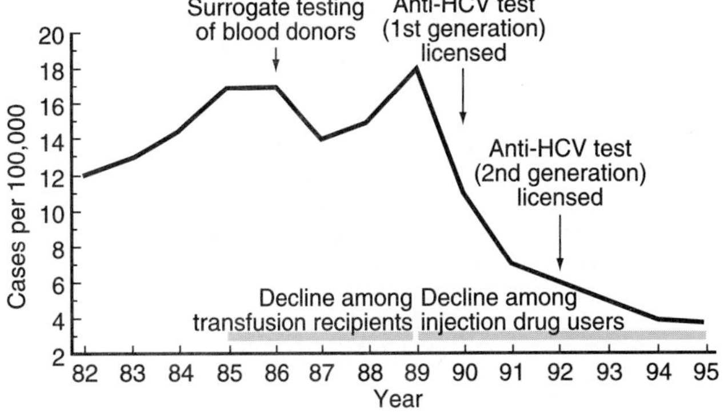

FIGURE 180–2 ■ Estimated incidence of acute hepatitis C in the United States. Incidence has not changed substantially from 1995 to 1999.[11]

The distribution of the different genotypes of HCV varies geographically.[53, 135] Genotypes 1 and 2 are distributed widely throughout the world. Genotype 1 is predominant in North and South America, Europe, and Asia, although the relative frequencies of the different subtypes vary. Genotypes 1a and 1b are common in North and South America and Europe, but only 1b is predominant in Asia. In the United States, genotypes 1a and 1b each account for more than 40 percent of isolates. Type 3 also is distributed widely, and subtype 3a has been seen with increasing frequency among persons who acquired their infection recently. However, subtype 3b has been identified only in Japan, Nepal, Thailand, India, Bangladesh, and Indonesia. Type 4 is predominant in northern and central African countries, and type 5 in southern Africa. Type 6 has been found in 20 to 30 percent of isolates in Hong Kong and Vietnam.

INCIDENCE AND PREVALENCE IN CHILDREN

Infection with HCV occurs throughout the world, in children as well as in adults. The prevalence in pediatric groups varies by risk factors and geographical location. No large seroprevalence studies have been performed in the general pediatric population in the United States, but one survey in an adolescent population revealed very low seroprevalence.[90] Data from other countries disclose widely varying frequencies of HCV infection. A Japanese study of 1442 healthy children found a prevalence of 0 percent anti-HCV positivity.[178] At the other end of the spectrum, 14.5 percent of 696 children randomly sampled in Cameroon were anti-HCV seropositive.[141] Studies looking at household contacts of known HCV-infected individuals found intermediate seroprevalence rates, which increased proportionally to the age of the contact,[1, 154, 162] indicating that duration of contact was an important risk. Mechanism of transmission in these settings has not been clearly defined, but the association with low socioeconomic status indicates the role of crowding and hygiene.

In the United States, the HCV antibody seroprevalence is 0.2 percent in children younger than 12 years and 0.4 percent in those 12 to 19 years of age.[7] Children at risk for HCV infection are listed in Table 180–1. Before 1990, the predominant risk for acquisition of HCV infection by children was through blood or blood product transfusion. Although this mode of transmission is responsible for many current cases of pediatric HCV infection, new infections in children are caused primarily by perinatal (vertical) transmission, as has been demonstrated in Italy.[28] The incidence of new infections in children through this mechanism is not known but could be estimated from the prevalence of HCV infection in women of child-bearing age and the risk of transmission with each pregnancy.

TABLE 180–1 ■ CHILDREN AT RISK FOR HCV INFECTION

- Children repeatedly transfused with blood or blood products for
  - Thalassemia
  - Sickle-cell anemia
  - Other congenital anemias
  - Hemophilia
  - Hemodialysis
  - Hypogammaglobulinemia or other immunodeficiency (IVIG)
- Children with a history of transfusion before 1992 for
  - Childhood malignant disease, especially leukemia
  - Major surgery—cardiac, orthopedic
  - Prematurity, neonatal intensive care
  - Conditions requiring extracorporeal membrane oxygenation
- Adolescents with high-risk behaviors, such as:
  - Intravenous drug use
  - Intranasal drug use
  - Body piercing and tattooing
- Infants of HCV-infected mothers

TRANSFUSION-ASSOCIATED HCV IN CHILDREN

Until recently, receipt of blood or blood products has been the major mode of transmission of HCV to children.[26, 142] In addition to erythrocyte and platelet transfusions, implicated products have included clotting factors,[21, 94] plasma, and intravenous immune globulin.[33] Transmission to children also has been demonstrated by transplanted organs or tissues.[69, 150] In general, as has been described for adults, risk of acquisition of HCV increases with the number or units of blood or blood products received.[91, 96, 140] Children from all parts of the world who have been multiply transfused with either blood or acellular blood products, such as those with thalassemia[105, 159] or hemophilia,[21] have infection rates from 50 to 95 percent. Children with moderate but not ongoing transfusion exposure, such as those who had been treated for childhood malignant neoplasms,[116, 163] those who have been treated with hemodialysis[69, 91] or extracorporeal membrane oxygenation,[140] or those who have undergone surgery for congenital heart disease,[142] have intermediate seroprevalence rates of 10 to 20 percent. Screening of donated blood for anti-HCV, the use of recombinant and heat-inactivated clotting factors, and the addition of virus-inactivating physicochemical processes in the production of immune globulin had drastically reduced the incidence of transmission of HCV by these means. However, these are relatively recent advances instituted within the last 10 years; many children infected with HCV by these products are observed in clinical practices, whereas others are yet to be identified.

PERINATAL TRANSMISSION OF HCV

The frequency of anti-HCV seropositivity in newborns of HCV-infected women was shown to be 14 to 100 percent; in most instances, this antibody was present only transiently, indicating that it had been acquired passively through placental transfer.[59, 64, 157, 181] A more accurate estimate of the frequency of perinatal transmission required the use of the polymerase chain reaction (PCR) technique to detect viral genome in the sera of exposed infants, which then clearly showed that vertical transmission of the virus does occur, albeit at a low rate.[106, 127, 164, 181, 189] Early studies suggested a rate of transmission from anti-HCV seropositive women of 5 to 6 percent, which increased to approximately 10 percent if only women who have HCV RNA in serum at the time of delivery were included. Although a rate of 33 percent was reported in one Italian study,[165] large studies in the United States and Europe suggest a 4 to 5 percent perinatal transmission rate from viremic mothers.[46, 65, 130] This rate compares with a frequency of 40 to 90 percent for the perinatal transmission of hepatitis B virus. Maternal co-infection with human immunodeficiency virus (HIV) increases the rate of perinatal transmission of HCV,[66, 144, 148, 182, 194, 195] even without concomitant transmission of HIV. However, aggressive treatment of HIV-infected pregnant women that results in low or undetectable HIV levels at delivery may mitigate this increase in transmission of HCV.[46] In the absence of co-infection with HIV, the likelihood of transmission of HCV increases with higher levels of maternal HCV viremia. In several studies, no women with less than 10^6 copies/mL of serum HCV RNA transmitted the infection to their newborns,[64, 68, 115, 146] although such was not the case in one report from Italy.[158] The possibility of in utero transmission in at least some cases was suggested by the detection of viremia in six infants on the day of birth.[158] However, in a prospective study, infection documented at birth by detection of HCV RNA in cord blood was often transient and not always predictive of eventual infection of the newborn.[46] If infection is not detected at birth, as is most often the case,[46, 65] transmission around the time of delivery may be more important. The role of peripartum factors, such as prolonged rupture of amniotic membranes and fetal infection by the use of scalp monitors, has been examined.[65, 130] One suggestion is that these factors may increase the likelihood of HCV transmission to neonates.[130] Whether vaginal delivery is a risk factor versus cesarean delivery is not clear,[68] but cases of transmission of HCV after cesarean births have been reported.[148] In one report, transmission frequency was 4 percent after vaginal delivery and 6 percent after cesarean delivery.[158] When this topic was examined by taking into account duration of ruptured membranes, by comparing emergency with elective cesarean deliveries, once again the likelihood of transmission seemed to correlate with this factor rather than the mode of delivery.[65] These studies are somewhat preliminary and need to be confirmed before obstetric practices regarding HCV-infected women are changed, but they provide insight into possible mechanisms of transmission and possible strategies to prevent many new pediatric HCV infections.

Transmission of HCV has been documented in women who have acute infection during the last trimester of pregnancy.[123] Once again, in some instances, viremia in the neonates was transient and not associated with the development of liver disease.[64]

Results regarding the role of breast feeding in the risk of transmission of HCV to infants have been conflicting. When breast feeding was reported in perinatal transmission studies, the frequency of breast feeding overall in the study populations was not discussed, rendering data difficult to interpret. Differences in the duration of breast feeding were noted between uninfected and infected infants in a Japanese study.[146] However, two studies from Italy suggest a lack of additional risk from breast feeding. In the first study, none of 17 breast-fed infants born to HCV-positive HIV-negative mothers was infected after follow-up of 12 to 27 months.[126] In the second study, the perinatal transmission of HCV in breast-fed infants was 7 percent compared with 4 percent in formula-fed infants, but this difference was not statistically significant.[158] None of 76 samples of breast milk from 73 anti-HCV–positive German women contained HCV RNA, even though 62 were HCV RNA seropositive.[153] Only one child had evidence of HCV infection detected 1 month after birth. On the basis of these limited data, currently no recommendation is made to avoid breast feeding by HCV-infected women.

INTRAFAMILIAL AND OTHER HORIZONTAL TRANSMISSION OF HCV

Horizontal transmission refers to transmission to children after the perinatal period or to transmission from infected children to others, such as family members or schoolmates. Studies of household transmission from Europe, South America, and Asia have been accomplished by screening household contacts of index cases for anti-HCV; in some studies, further testing of seropositive contacts with PCR for HCV RNA and even comparative genotype analysis[80] was performed. Prevalence of anti-HCV seropositivity in household contacts varied from 0 to 14.8 percent.[1, 13, 37, 41, 48, 139, 154, 175] Nonspouse seroprevalence rates were 0 to 6.5 percent. Risk of having anti-HCV positivity increased with age and duration of exposure.[41, 154] Rates were particularly low in households of HCV-infected hemophiliacs.[32] The risk to children in the households of chronically HCV-infected individuals separate from perinatal risk was difficult to ascertain, but prevalence rates were very low (approaching zero) in the youngest children and increased steadily with increasing age.[1, 50, 139] Because the mechanism of nonsexual, non-perinatal infection of children in these families is not known, counseling to prevent this transmission is limited to avoidance of sharing household items such as razors, toothbrushes, and fingernail clippers. No justification for having family members avoid sharing of eating utensils or bathrooms exists at this time. HCV-infected adults should be educated about the extremely low likelihood of spreading HCV to their children by routine family contact, including kissing and day-to-day care.

Few data exist regarding the transmission of HCV from infected children to others. In a Spanish study, 80 household contacts (without independent risk factors for infection) of 27 HCV-infected children were tested. None of the parents was found to be infected, but one infected sibling (1 of 32) was identified.[38] In an Italian study of 44 index children, one parent was infected through an accidental needle-stick, and no transmission to other children was demonstrated.[185] Thus, horizontal transmission of HCV between children appears to be rare. Restriction in school or daycare attendance or participation in any routine activity including contact sports is not required for HCV-infected children.[9] In addition, notification of school personnel of a child's HCV infection is not required because routine universal precautions already recommended are adequate for children with HCV.[8]

OTHER MODES OF TRANSMISSION OF HCV IN CHILDREN

The most frequent mode of transmission of HCV in adults is sharing of needles for the purpose of injecting intravenous illicit drugs. To the extent that older children and teenagers participate in this activity, they are at risk for acquiring infection. In fact, in most individuals, infections with HCV occur within 6 to 12 months after beginning intravenous drug use.[62] Other percutaneous exposures that may be more common than intravenous drug use in children and adolescents, such as body piercing and tattooing, have been implicated as a risk in Italy[134] but not in the United States.[45] Studies to evaluate these risks in this country are ongoing. Intranasal administration of cocaine also is considered a risk.[7] Sexual transmission of HCV is thought to occur by both homosexual and heterosexual activities,[6, 180] but their importance to the overall prevalence of infection with HCV is controversial.[147] The prevalence and causes of sporadic or community-acquired HCV infection in children, in the absence of risk factor, are not known.

Diagnosis

The use and significance of methods for diagnosis of HCV infection are summarized in Table 180–2. Direct tests for the viral antigens of HCV in serum are not available. Assays for antibodies directed against several viral antigens have been facilitated by the genomic sequencing of HCV. The first

TABLE 180–2 ■ SEROLOGIC DIAGNOSIS OF HEPATITIS C INFECTION

	Acute HCV	Resolved HCV	Chronic HCV
anti-HCV ELISA-3	+/−	+/−	+*†
anti-HCV IgM (experimental)	+	−	−
anti-HCV RIBA-2 or 3	+/−/indeterminate	+/−	+†
HCV RNA by PCR	+	−	+

*Should be confirmed with another test.
†May be negative in immunosuppressed individuals.

diagnostic test, which became available in 1990, was an enzyme-linked immunosorbent assay (ELISA), which detected antibody to the c100-3 antigen of HCV.[103] Although this important advance quickly resulted in a significant decrease in the incidence of post-transfusion non-A, non-B hepatitis, a high false-positive rate was demonstrated, and delayed development of this antibody in infected individuals did not allow early diagnosis of infection. Currently, the third-generation ELISA-3 is used most widely. It is based on several antigens from both the core (c22-3 antigen) and non-structural (c200 antigen) regions, the latter including the c100-3 antigen used previously. Seropositivity for anti-HCV by the ELISA indicates current or past infection with HCV. A nonreactive test result does not exclude completely either current or past infection because levels of anti-HCV may be undetectable in early infection or may remain undetectable in individuals with altered immunity.

Early problems with sensitivity and specificity of the ELISA led to the development of recombinant immunoblot assay (RIBA) testing for antibodies to the c100-3 antigen as well as another viral antigen, 5-1-1, and superoxide dismutase.[54] Further refinement of this test led to the RIBA-2 assay, which incorporates recombinant antigens c33-C and c22-3.[184] Sera found "positive" for anti-HCV by ELISA are "confirmed" by RIBA-2 if a response of 1+ or greater is observed to any two or more HCV antigens.

Detection of HCV genomes in serum and tissue through the use of PCR currently is the principal method used to detect active infection. This technique has been useful in the identification of seronegative carriers and perinatally transmitted HCV. HCV RNA can be quantified by a variety of methods that differ in sensitivity, linear range, precision, and reproducibility. The quantitative PCR test most widely used can detect levels of virus down to 100 copies/mL of serum. A less cumbersome assay that uses branched DNA and alkaline phosphatase–labeled probes to detect and quantify viral nucleic acid (Quantiplex HCV RNA Assay, Chiron Diagnostics, Emeryville, CA) has been applied to the detection and quantification of HCV RNA.[111] The Quantiplex bDNA 2.0 is as sensitive as some quantitative PCR tests, with great accuracy at high viremia levels.[86] Real-time PCR based on the TaqMan chemistry system (Roche Molecular Diagnostic Systems) promises increased sensitivity, to less than 100 copies/mL, as well as high precision, good reproducibility, and broad linear range. At this point, caution must be used because the values obtained by the different tests are not interchangeable. However, changes in viral load over time with use of the same assay are meaningful. In addition, mathematical equations can be formulated to describe the relationship of one test result to the other.

In summary, the diagnosis of HCV infection in an individual with chronic hepatitis, defined as infection persisting for more than 6 months, includes the detection of anti-HCV in serum and, in low-prevalence populations, confirmation with a positive RIBA-2 result (Fig. 180–3). If this test result is positive, HCV RNA should be determined by a qualitative assay. In a high-prevalence population or an individual with a known risk factor for infection with HCV, a positive anti-HCV test result with use of the standard ELISA should be followed directly with HCV RNA testing to document either active viremia or resolved past infection. The diagnosis of acute HCV infection is more of a problem because anti-HCV may not appear in serum for up to 2 months. In addition, immunocompromised individuals, including patients with hypogammaglobulinemia and immunosuppressed transplant recipients, may not mount an anti-HCV response. For these situations, the diagnosis is made by detection of HCV RNA in serum by either the PCR or bDNA amplification technique. Quantitative HCV RNA testing is reserved for determination of therapeutic response.

Clinical Features

In adults, acute HCV infection is typically mild and most often subclinical. No reports of the clinical manifestations of acute HCV infection in children infected either perinatally or by blood transfusion exist. Acute, severe hepatitis, with atypically high ALT values, jaundice, malaise, anorexia, and hepatomegaly, was seen in some of the children who were infected during the outbreak associated with intravenous

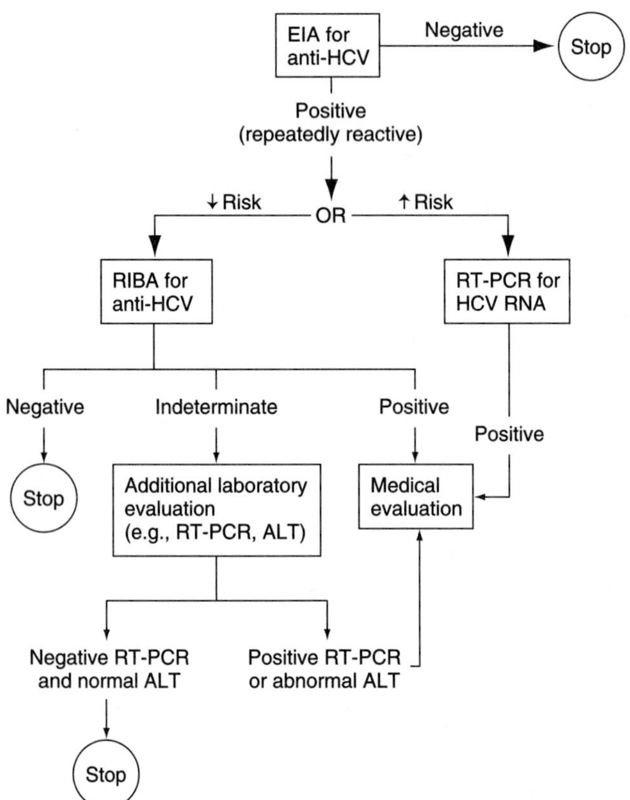

FIGURE 180–3 ■ General algorithm for diagnosis of chronic hepatitis C virus (HCV) in children older than 1 year and adults. ALT, alanine aminotransferase; anti-HCV, antibody to HCV; EIA, enzyme immunoassay; RIBA, recombinant immunobolt assay; RT-PCR, reverse transcriptase polymerase chain reaction. (Source: CDC website at http://www.cdc.gov.)

immune globulin.[88] The reasons for this unusually severe presentation are not clear, but possibilities include greater amounts of virus inoculated, repeated inoculations, and the underlying immunodeficiencies in the hosts. Anecdotally, when chronically infected children are identified, they usually have no history of recognized acute hepatitis. Fulminant hepatitis caused by HCV has not been reported in children.

No reports specifically focusing on clinical features of chronic HCV infection in children exist. Studies of epidemiology, natural history, and treatment often describe the children as being asymptomatic or having nonspecific fatigue or abdominal pain.[26, 27, 30, 31, 82, 89, 116, 142] Most cases are identified by testing of asymptomatic children who are recognized to have a risk for acquiring infection with HCV, such as receipt of transfusion before 1992 or HCV-infected mothers. Once infection is identified and serial ALT values followed, most children are found to have modest elevations in the first years of infection, with normal or nearly normal values for many subsequent years (Fig. 180–4). Nonorgan-specific autoantibodies are occasionally found; antinuclear antibodies have been described in 7.5 to 11 percent, smooth muscle antibodies in 9 to 17.5 percent, and type 1 liver-kidney microsomal antibodies in 10 to 13 percent of European cases.[29, 109] However, clinically apparent autoimmune manifestations are rare. One of the authors has cared for a 13-year-old girl with HCV-associated cirrhosis who also had membranoproliferative glomerulonephritis with nephrotic syndrome, a 6-year-old boy with chronic HCV and lichen planus, and a 17-year-old girl with HCV infection and cutaneous vasculitis that disappeared with antiviral therapy (unpublished data). HCV-associated cryoglobulinemia and porphyria cutanea tarda have not been reported in children. This low frequency of clinical signs or symptoms and the fact that "routine" serum ALT determinations are not performed as part of pediatric medical care indicate that chronic infection with HCV in children is probably under-recognized.

Natural History

Studies of the natural history of infection with HCV in children are smaller and less definitive than those in adults. Factors that influence this natural history in adults include age at infection, mode of acquisition, co-morbid disease, ethanol ingestion, and possibly viral genotype. In children, age and mode of acquisition are often difficult to separate because most infections acquired in infancy are perinatal.

Children treated for leukemia typically receive many blood transfusions, and those treated before 1990 have a very high rate of infection with HCV.[12] Children with thalassemia requiring chronic transfusions also have a very high prevalence of infection with HCV. Many individuals with hemophilia contracted HCV during childhood, before the availability of heat-inactivated and recombinant clotting factors. The natural history of transfusion-associated infection with HCV may differ according to the underlying disease for which the transfusion is required. In one cohort of children transfused during leukemia treatment, many had a delay in development of anti-HCV for several years, and prolonged follow-up of 13 to 27 years did not reveal serious liver disease.[117] Researchers suspected that HCV acquired during a period of immunosuppression from chemotherapy may have prevented or blunted the immune response that plays a role in the pathogenesis of this disease. However, in a small series of 45 American children, cirrhosis developed within 2 years in one child treated for leukemia.[137] Secondary hemochromatosis in thalassemic patients may contribute to the hepatic injury as well as affect the response to therapy for infection with HCV.[43, 105]

Two studies have addressed the natural history of infection with HCV acquired early in life at the time of surgery for congenital heart disease. In a Japanese study, 29 children were observed for at least 4 years, and only 50 percent had persistent viremia. Although they had histologic chronic hepatitis, none had cirrhosis in this period.[133] A study from Germany had similar findings after a longer follow-up period. Of children who were transfused at the time of cardiac surgery, 14.6 percent were positive for anti-HCV 20 years later, but only 55 percent of these subjects were viremic at follow-up.[186] Only one of these HCV RNA–positive patients had an abnormal ALT value, which was possibly explained by the fact that the patient was also in congestive heart failure. Only 17 of the children underwent liver biopsy, and one child (5.9%), who had been co-infected previously with hepatitis B, had cirrhosis. Overall, the clinical course of these children seemed more benign than would be expected if they had been infected as adults. The frequency

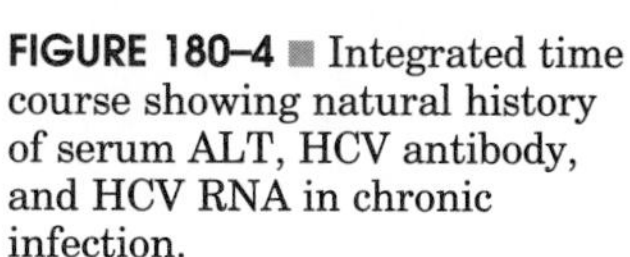

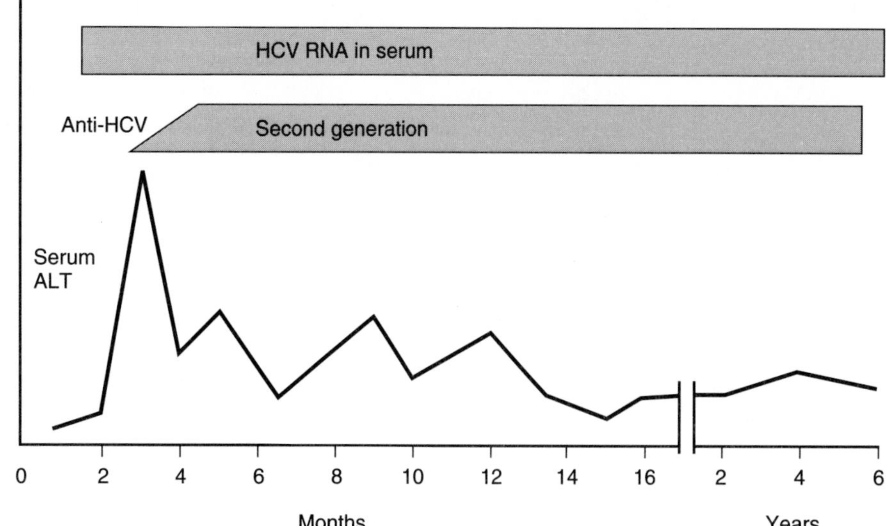

FIGURE 180–4 ■ Integrated time course showing natural history of serum ALT, HCV antibody, and HCV RNA in chronic infection.

of viral persistence is lower than that reported in adults who were infected through transfusion. The reason for this relatively high spontaneous clearance rate is not clear. On the other hand, few of the patients underwent liver biopsy, so the frequency of occult chronic liver disease is not known.

Understanding the natural history of perinatally acquired infection with HCV has become increasingly important because it has become the major route of infection for pediatric patients. Several small reports from Japan and Italy regarding this issue have been published.[27, 149, 167] HCV infection acquired vertically frequently is associated with biochemical evidence of hepatic injury early in life. Spontaneous resolution of infection in some of these infants, even those with active hepatitis as suggested by abnormal ALT values, increasingly is being recognized. However, in most children, perinatally acquired HCV persists for many years. In most cases, it causes only mild chronic hepatitis in the first 1 or 2 decades. The natural history into the third decade and beyond is completely unknown, but infection with HCV acquired at or near the time of birth may cause significant morbidity and mortality later in life. Factors that may predict or alter this course have not been identified.

Histopathologic Features of the Liver in HCV Infection

Histologic features of the liver associated with HCV infection in adults have been described in several series.[19, 99, 113, 168] The major features are portal inflammation with lymphoid aggregates, varying degrees of steatosis, and bile duct injury (Fig. 180–5). In HCV-infected adults, severity of histologic abnormalities does not correlate with biochemical parameters of hepatic dysfunction, such as ALT levels. The implication is that patients may have progressive liver disease in the absence of clinical signs. Thus, histopathologic examination of the liver is an important tool in the understanding of childhood infection with HCV.

Although histologic features in small numbers of HCV-infected children have been described in several reports,[26, 84, 105, 133] most were not systematically examined and scored by conventionally accepted scoring systems.[19, 98, 168] Varying degrees of necroinflammatory activity were noted, but fibrosis was not uniformly described; cirrhosis was reported in 0 to 11 percent of cases. Three papers have focused primarily on histologic findings, with scoring, in

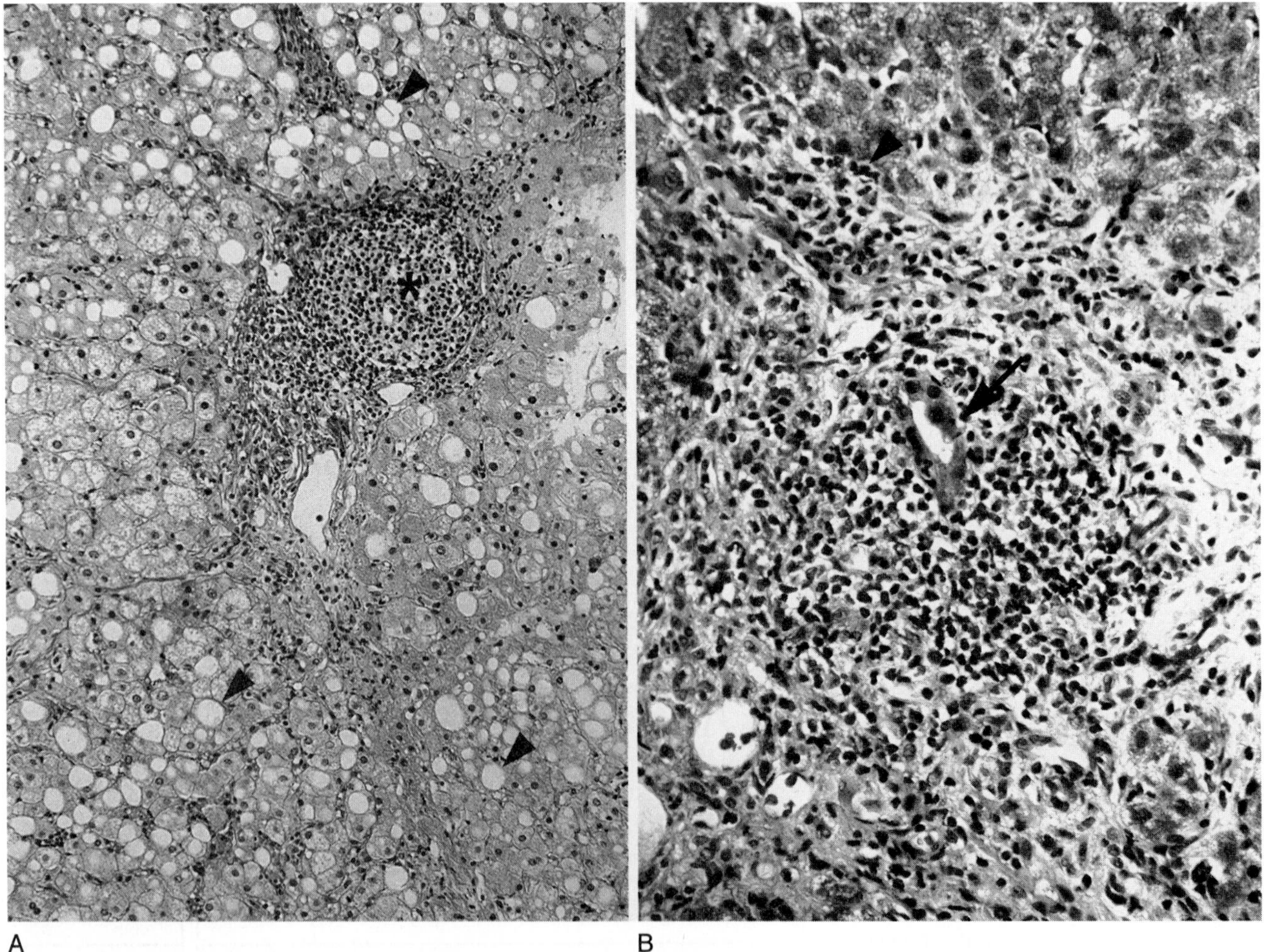

FIGURE 180–5 ■ Photomicrograph of the liver in pediatric patients with chronic hepatitis C. *A* demonstrates portal lymphoid aggregate (*) and moderate steatosis (*arrowheads*) (hematoxylin and eosin). *B* depicts bile duct injury (*arrow*) and interface hepatitis (*arrowhead*) (trichrome). These features are typical of chronic HCV infection in children and adults.

large series of children.[15, 70, 92] In all series, the characteristic histopathologic lesions of infection with HCV (see Fig. 180–5), including portal lymphoid aggregates or follicles, sinusoidal lymphocytes, and steatosis, were seen with approximately the same frequency as in adults. In 109 Japanese children primarily infected through transfusion,[92] the average histologic activity was 3.8 by the Scheuer system.[168] No cases of cirrhosis were encountered, and only 3.6 percent of the children had bridging fibrosis with architectural distortion. Viral genotypes were not reported, and the mean duration of infection was only 2.6 years. In contrast, although histologic activity (Scheuer[168] and METAVIR[19] schemes) was generally mild in a series of children in the United States, portal fibrosis was seen more frequently in 78 percent of specimens from 40 children.[15] Fibrosis was mild in 26 percent, moderate in 22 percent, and severe in 22 percent, and cirrhosis was found in 8 percent. Two of the children with cirrhosis were young adolescents who had acquired HCV infection perinatally. A newly described finding was pericellular fibrosis, typically around the central veins, in 52 percent of specimens; whether this abnormality is unique to pediatric HCV infection has yet to be determined, and this fibrosis was not included in the histologic grading. In this series, 60 percent of children had HCV of genotype 1a, and 32 percent had genotype 1b. The mean duration of infection, in those children in whom it could be determined accurately, was 6.8 ± 5.3 years. In a series of 80 children from Italy and Spain,[70] most of whom were infected with HCV genotype 1a or 1b, with a mean duration of infection of 3.5 ± 4.3 years, inflammatory scores were generally low. The frequency and severity of the bile duct damage and lymphoid follicles increased with the patient's age. Fibrosis was present in 72.5 percent of cases and increased with duration of disease and age of the patient, just as in the American series. Only 1 (1.25%) child had cirrhosis.

These studies demonstrate that histologic features of chronic infection with HCV in childhood are similar to those reported in adults. Necrosis and inflammation are usually mild, but fibrosis commonly is seen and, most important, progresses with increasing age and duration of infection. Thus, the natural history of HCV infection acquired in childhood may in some instances be associated with significant morbidity as the children progress into young adulthood.

Management

Current recommendations for prevention of perinatal transmission of HCV are listed in Table 180–3. Because the rate of perinatal transmission of HCV is low, the risk factors that increase this rate are not fully defined, and because no intervention for the neonate exists at this time, routine screening of all pregnant women is not warranted. Pregnant women, or those considering pregnancy, with risk factors such as intravenous drug use, blood transfusions before 1992, or unexplained ALT elevations, should be offered screening for anti-HCV. However, in a study that screened more than 4000 pregnant women for HCV, a majority (16 of 22) of newly identified cases were without prior identifiable risk factors.[187] Women found to be anti-HCV seropositive should undergo testing with PCR to confirm current infection. At present, no specific recommendations are made to physicians caring for HCV-infected pregnant women in an attempt to reduce the frequency of perinatal transmission.[83] On the basis of preliminary data, avoidance of prolonged amniotic membrane rupture and fetal scalp monitors may prove to be prudent, but confirmatory studies are needed. Post-exposure prophylaxis with immune globulin does not appear to be effective in preventing infection with HCV and is not recommended for infants born to HCV-infected women. Infants born to mothers infected with HCV during pregnancy or at delivery should be tested after 12 to 15 months of age for anti-HCV; a positive test result at that time is likely to correlate with true infection because maternal antibody will have disappeared by that age. The algorithm for identification of women at risk and for detection of perinatally acquired infection is depicted in Figure 180–6.

TABLE 180–3 ■ GUIDELINES FOR PREVENTION OF PERINATAL HCV INFECTION

Recommended (supported by current data)
Targeted testing of pregnant women who have risk factors for HCV
Aggressive treatment of HIV in co-infected pregnant women
Testing of infants for anti-HCV when they are 12 to 15 months of age
Considered (suggested by current data)
Avoid internal fetal scalp monitoring during labor
Deliver infant within 6 hours of rupture of membranes
Not recommended (no current data to support)
Universal testing of pregnant women
Elective cesarean delivery
Avoidance of breast feeding
Immune globulin administration to newborns

Acute infection, which may be acquired from a transfusion, by other parenteral exposure, or at the time of birth, rarely causes symptoms recognizable as acute hepatitis. For this reason, no reports of treatment of acute HCV infection in children exist. Several small studies report the use of interferon in adults with acute HCV infection, with mixed results.[39] Fulminant hepatitis attributed to HCV is extremely rare in children, as it is in adults.

When chronic infection with HCV is diagnosed in children, the duration of infection is likely to be shorter than that in many adult patients who present for treatment. Liver disease is typically mild, with low necroinflammatory and fibrosis scores. Children are less likely to have serious co-morbid conditions, such as HIV infection, chronic alcohol use, and autoimmune disorders, although some will have iron overload secondary to chronic transfusion therapy. This constellation of factors may confer a higher likelihood of having a therapeutic response. Children have a longer life expectancy, with the expectation that progressive hepatic injury and scarring will develop in time. These considerations provide some compelling reasons to examine the role of treatment in children.

No large, multicenter, randomized, controlled therapeutic trials have been performed in children with chronic infection with HCV. Numerous reports of treatment in children have been published, but the studies are usually uncontrolled, include small numbers of patients, and sometimes include only select patient groups, such as hemophiliacs or individuals with thalassemia. Details of the interferon monotherapy trials in children with chronic infection with HCV were reviewed.[87] Only two small controlled trials have been reported; both were performed in Italy. In the first,[25] 5 MU/m^2 recombinant interferon alfa-2b was given to 14 children thrice weekly, and 13 children were left untreated. In the 10 treated children who had at least 50 percent decrease in ALT after 4 months, the interferon was continued for a full 12 months. After a 24-month follow-up, six (43%) of the treated children and none of the untreated children were HCV RNA seronegative. In the second study,[85] 11 children were treated with 3 MU/m^2 of lymphoblastoid interferon alfa three times a week for 12 months, and 10 children received no treatment.

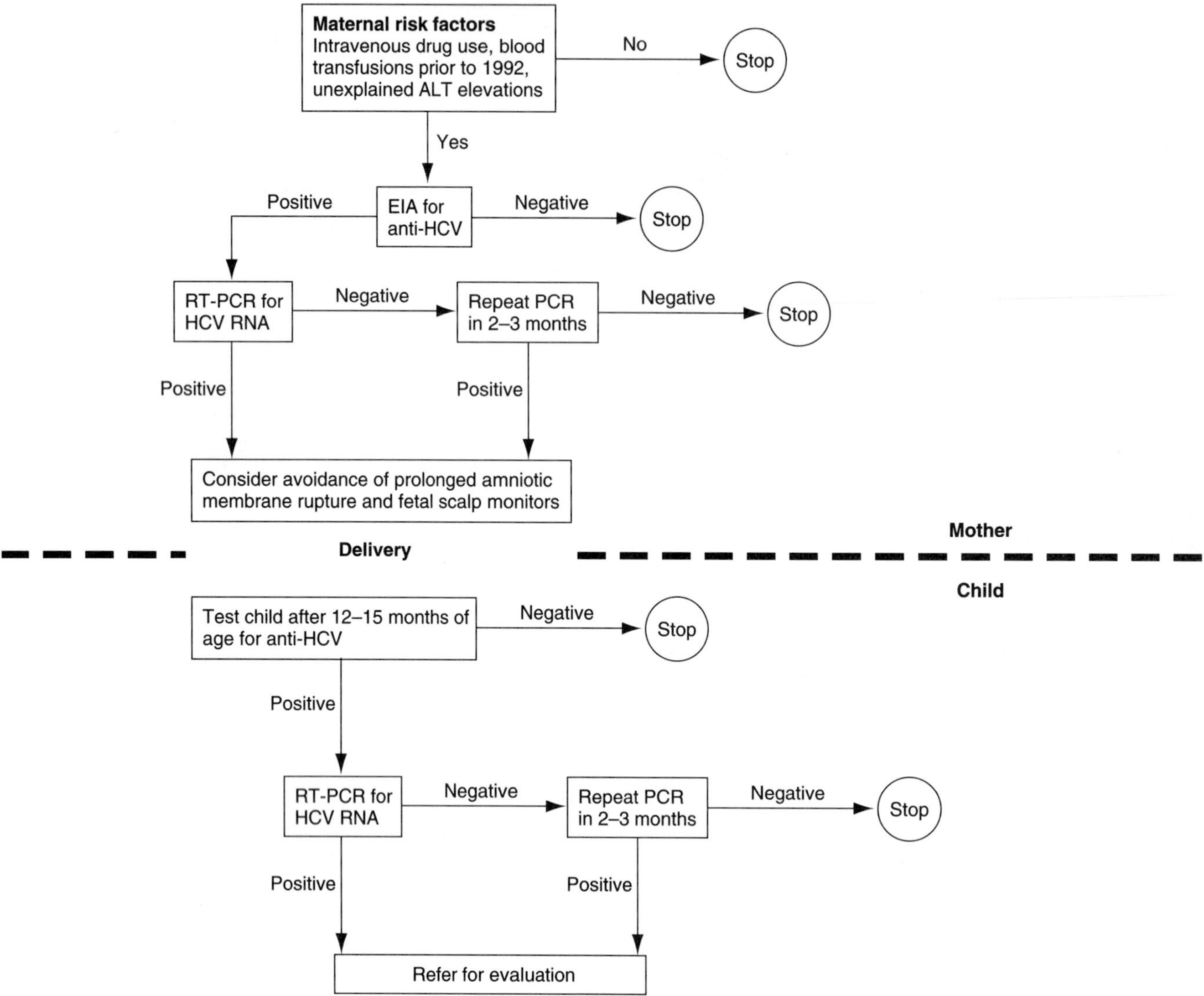

FIGURE 180–6 ■ Algorithm for identification of women at risk and detection of perinatally acquired infection. ALT, alanine aminotransferase; anti-HCV, antibody to HCV; EIA, enzyme immunoassay; HCV, hepatitis C virus; PCR, polymerase chain reaction; RT-PCR, reverse transcriptase polymerase chain reaction.

A sustained virologic response was demo strated in five treated children (45%) and one control subject (10%).

Only two therapeutic trials using interferon monotherapy have been reported from the United States. In the first study, six boys with hemophilia and chronic HCV infection were treated with recombinant interferon alfa-2b at either 3 MU/m^2 or 1.75 MU/m^2 thrice weekly for 24 weeks (one patient received treatment for only 3 weeks).[196] Although two boys became HCV RNA seronegative during therapy, none of these patients had a sustained virologic response. In the second trial, 21 children received interferon alfa-2a at 3 MU/m^2 three times per week for 6 to 12 months.[89] Sustained virologic response was achieved in seven (33%). These responses have been durable, with up to 3 years of post-treatment follow-up in some cases (unpublished data). In general, biochemical responses paralleled virologic responses, and histologic findings in liver biopsy specimens improved in treated patients irrespective of complete virologic response, as has been noted in adult studies.

Even though various small studies have included several types of patients and used different dosages, schedules, and types of interferon, the sustained virologic response rate, when reported, in general was remarkably similar in most studies, ranging from 33 to 45 percent.[25, 49, 60, 85, 89, 101, 128, 132] This rate is significantly higher than the sustained virologic response rates reported in large trials of interferon monotherapy in adult patients. Meta-analysis has proved difficult, given the heterogeneous studies and lack of data in control subjects. Overall, a higher rate of sustained virologic response to interferon alfa monotherapy appears to occur in children with chronic HCV infection compared with adults. This difference may be artifactual because of the small numbers of patients studied. Alternatively, these results may represent true differences in host factors such as younger age, earlier stage of liver disease, different mode of viral acquisition, higher dose of interferon relative to body weight or surface area, or lack of cofactors such as alcohol ingestion or co-morbid diseases. Unfortunately, even with these higher response rates, most children remain infected after treatment. Given the superiority of combination therapy with interferon and ribavirin in adults, a large, randomized, controlled trial of interferon monotherapy is not likely to be undertaken in children with chronic HCV infection.

Although interferon is discontinued because of side effects in a smaller proportion of children compared with adults, this medication is associated with important adverse effects. The influenza-like illness described in adults commonly is seen in children but typically resolves after one or two doses. Dosage reductions commonly are required because of neutropenia, although serious infectious complications have not been described. Although coexisting autoimmune diseases are less common occurrences in children, type II autoimmune hepatitis, associated with liver-kidney microsomal antibody, can be mistaken for or coexist with HCV infection and may be exacerbated with administration of interferon.[29, 70] A frequent side effect of interferon is weight loss with or without anorexia. Children may lose up to 10 percent of their body weight, with serious implications for growth if not promptly addressed.[89] A study of children treated for chronic hepatitis B virus infection suggests that this weight loss and accompanying decrease in linear growth velocity may be transient and improves rapidly once the interferon is discontinued.[44] Significant depression has been described in adults receiving interferon for chronic hepatitis; although no reports of serious mental illness in children treated with interferon alfa have been published, irritability, decreased school performance, and other behavioral disturbances may be precipitated by this medication. One child developed seizures while receiving interferon alfa for HCV infection.[136] Infants treated with interferon alfa for life-threatening hemangiomas were noted to have an increased incidence of spastic diplegia.[16] Judicious use of this drug and careful monitoring are required in young patients. These concerns and others, including the expense of interferon alfa, the potential for serious side effects, and the necessity for parenteral administration, have led some physicians to conclude that treatment with interferon is not warranted in children. No cost-benefit analysis has been performed in this group of patients.

Combination therapy with interferon alfa and ribavirin has proved to be of greater efficacy than is interferon alone in adults. However, ribavirin has the potential to cause serious toxicity, including hemolytic anemia, mutagenicity, and teratogenicity. The use of combination therapy with standard interferon and ribavirin has recently undergone evaluation in a pediatric trial. Recommendations regarding use of this combination in children are not yet standardized. The use of pegylated interferon preparations is not recommended in children except in the context of clinical trials.

Important differences in HCV infection exist between adults and children that may have significant impact on therapy. They are listed in Table 180–4. As transfusion-associated infection declines, the most prevalent means of acquisition of HCV by children will be perinatal transmission. If, as seems probable from small preliminary studies, more of these infections are likely to resolve without treatment or to cause less severe liver disease, treatment of the youngest children may not be necessary. On the other hand, young adolescents with cirrhosis and end-stage liver disease caused by vertically acquired HCV have been encountered. More data are needed about the factors that cause rapid evolution of this disease in pediatric patients so that cogent decisions about selection of patients and timing of treatment can be made.

TABLE 180–4 ■ SPECIAL CONSIDERATIONS FOR TREATMENT OF CHILDREN WITH HCV INFECTION

Differences in Natural History
Mode of acquisition—perinatal
Shorter duration of infection
Co-morbid diseases
Longer anticipated life expectancy
Differences in Liver Disease
Milder grades of necroinflammation
Less frequent severe fibrosis or cirrhosis
Differences in Response to Interferon alfa Treatment
Higher frequency of response*
Lower frequency of relapse*
Less correlation of ultimate response with HCV RNA at 12 weeks*
Fewer instances of drug discontinuation due to side effects
Unknown long-term side effects
No cost-benefit data

*Studies leading to these conclusions include relatively small numbers of patients.

HCV AND HIV CO-INFECTION

HCV and HIV share route of acquisition and risk factors for infection, so co-infection with both viruses is not uncommon. The prevalence of infection with HCV in HIV-infected adults is 33 percent.[174] In the highest risk groups, hemophiliacs and injection drug users, 66 to 100 percent of HIV-infected patients also are infected with HCV.[23] Although sexual transmission of HCV occurs uncommonly, the rate is substantially higher in the presence of HIV co-infection.[51] The same is true for perinatal transmission of HCV.[148, 194, 195]

HCV infection has a more aggressive course in the presence of HIV co-infection. The progression of chronic liver disease is accelerated in co-infection; advanced fibrosis and disease activity correlate with a low CD4 count.[20] A significantly higher fraction of patients infected with HCV and HIV develop liver failure and hepatocellular carcinoma.[24, 56, 129] The presence of HCV infection does not seem to exacerbate HIV infection.[156]

The pathogenic mechanism of this accelerated HCV liver disease is not known, but it is thought to stem from direct cytopathic effects of the virus on hepatocytes, perhaps more so than in immunocompetent individuals. Lower CD4 counts are associated with HCV RNA levels in the blood 10 to 100 times higher than in control subjects, but no correlation has been found between HCV RNA and ALT levels or severity of disease.[63] Additional mechanisms, such as drug toxicity, are likely to play a role in hepatic injury in HIV-infected patients.

Antibody-based tests such as the enzyme immunoassay and RIBA have a higher incidence of false-negative results in immunosuppressed individuals, including those with HIV infection.[120] If the result of anti-HCV testing is negative, direct testing for HCV RNA by use of PCR should be performed to exclude infection with HCV in the HIV-infected patient.

The treatment of patients co-infected with HCV and HIV has been studied only in adults. In a study of 90 patients co-infected with HCV and HIV, the response rate to interferon therapy was similar to that of the non-HIV group (29% vs. 34%), but the relapse rate was higher in the HIV-infected group (31% vs. 12.5%).[173] One study of 20 patients co-infected with HCV and HIV reported the use of ribavirin in combination with interferon, showing viral clearance rates comparable to singly infected patients (50%).[108] However, the toxic side effects of drugs, such as hemolysis induced by ribavirin and myelosuppression by interferon, may be more severe in combination with the anti-retroviral medications used to treat HIV,[104] and these patients should be monitored closely.

Prevention of Hepatitis C

Given the extensive heterogeneity of the HCV envelope proteins, the apparent lack of immunity after a resolved infection, and the lack of a practical cell culture system, no immediate prospects for the development of an effective HCV vaccine exist. However, neutralizing antibodies do exist; they most likely target one or both of the envelope proteins. On the other hand, neutralization may be a short-lived phenomenon given the rapid development of HCV quasi-species in infected individuals. In both humans and chimpanzees, acute self-limited infection with HCV does not confer protection against either heterologous or homologous strains of the virus.[57, 155] Autonomous replication of subgenomic HCV RNA has been demonstrated in a human hepatoma cell line after transfection of constructs composed of nonstructural HCV genes and the neomycin phosphotransferase gene.[118] In addition, purified HCV-like particles have been synthesized in insect cells from a recombinant baculovirus expressing C, E1, and E2 proteins.[18] They are being evaluated as potential immunogens. Synthetic vaccines that include peptides corresponding to cytotoxic T-lymphocyte and helper T-cell epitopes of the HCV core are being used experimentally to induce cytotoxic T-lymphocyte responses and memory in an attempt to stimulate cell-mediated immunity,[76] which may be the more important protective mechanism.

The incidence of new infections with HCV in the United States has decreased markedly during the last several years.[7] The cause of this decrease is not entirely clear because prevention of transfusion-associated infections is responsible for only a small proportion of this dramatic change in incidence. However, no clear indication as yet exists that the incidence of new infections in children is decreasing, especially considering that many currently infected individuals are women of child-bearing age. Although pediatric cases represent a minority of HCV infections and commonly may not progress to serious liver disease during the childhood years, instances of significant morbidity and even mortality from this disease certainly exist. Available therapy is cumbersome, uncomfortable, not without risk, and ineffective in many cases. For these reasons, consideration must be given to measures that might be instituted to prevent new pediatric HCV infections. With recognition of the predominant role of perinatal transmission as the source of most new pediatric infections, this process is the logical target for development of prevention strategies.

REFERENCES

1. Al Nasser, M. N.: Intrafamilial transmission of hepatitis C virus (HCV): A major mode of spread in the Saudi Arabia population. Ann. Trop. Pediatr. *12*:211–215, 1992.
2. Alaoui-Ismaili, M. H., Hamel, M., L'Heureux, L., et al.: The hepatitis C virus NS5B RNA-dependent RNA polymerase activity and susceptibility to inhibitors is modulated by metal cations. J. Hum. Virol. *3*:306–316, 2000.
3. Ali, N., and Siddiqui, A.: The La antigen binds 5′ noncoding region of the hepatitis C virus RNA in the context of the initiator AUG codon and stimulates internal ribosome entry site-mediated translation. Proc. Natl. Acad. Sci. U. S. A. *94*:2249–2254, 1997.
4. Alter, M. J.: Epidemiology of hepatitis C. Hepatology *26*:62S–65S, 1997.
5. Alter, M. J.: Hepatitis C: A sleeping giant? Am. J. Med. *91*:112S–115S, 1991.
6. Alter, M. J., Coleman, P. J., Alexander, J., et al.: Importance of heterosexual activity in the transmission of hepatitis B and non-A, non-B hepatitis. J. A. M. A. *262*:1201–1205, 1989.
7. Alter, M. J., Kruszon-Moran, D., Nainan, O. V., et al.: The prevalence of hepatitis C virus infection in the United States, 1988 through 1994. N. Engl. J. Med. *341*:556–562, 1999.
8. American Academy of Pediatrics: School health. *In* Pickering, L. K. (ed.): 2000 Red Book: Report of the Committee on Infectious Diseases. Elk Grove Village, IL, American Academy of Pediatrics, 2000, pp. 124–127.
9. American Academy of Pediatrics Committee on Sports Medicine and Fitness: Human immunodeficiency virus and other blood-borne viral pathogens in the athletic setting. Pediatrics *104*:1400–1403, 1999.
10. Anonymous: Global surveillance and control of hepatitis C. Report of a WHO Consultation organized in collaboration with the Viral Hepatitis Prevention Board, Antwerp, Belgium. J. Viral Hepat. *6*:35–47, 1999.
11. Anonymous: Summary of notifiable diseases, United States, 1999. M. M. W. R. Morb. Mortal. Wkly. Rep. *48*:1–104, 2001.
12. Aric, M., Maggiore, G., Silini, E., et al.: Hepatitis C virus infection in children treated for acute lymphoblastic leukemia. Blood *84*:2919–2921, 1994.
13. Arif, M., al-Swayeh, M., al-Faleh, F. Z., and Ramia, S: Risk of hepatitis C virus infection among household contacts of Saudi patients with chronic liver disease. J. Viral Hepat. *3*:97–101, 1996.
14. Arima, N., Kao, C. Y., Licht, T., et al.: Modulation of cell growth by the hepatitis C virus nonstructural protein NS5A. J. Biol. Chem. *276*:12675–12684, 2001.
15. Badizadegan, K., Jonas, M. M., Ott, M. J., et al.: Histopathology of the liver in children with chronic hepatitis C viral infection. Hepatology *28*:1416–1423, 1998.
16. Barlow, C. F., Priebe, C. J., Mulliken, J. B., et al.: Spastic diplegia as a complication of interferon alfa-2a treatment of hemangiomas of infancy. J. Pediatr. *132*:527–530, 1998.
17. Bartenschlager, R., and Lohmann, V.: Replication of the hepatitis C virus. Baillieres Best Pract. Res. Clin. Gastroenterol. *14*:241–254, 2000.
18. Baumert, T. F., Ito, S., Wong, D. T., and Liang, T. J.: Hepatitis C virus structural proteins assemble into viruslike particles in insect cells. J. Virol. *72*:3827–3836, 1998.
19. Bedossa, P., and Poynard, T.: An algorithm for the grading of activity in chronic hepatitis C. Hepatology *24*:289–293, 1996.
20. Benhamou, Y., Bochet, M., Di Martino, V., et al.: Liver fibrosis progression in human immunodeficiency virus and hepatitis C virus coinfected patients. The Multivirc Group. Hepatology *30*:1054–1058, 1999.
21. Blanchette, V. S., Vorstmann, E., Shore, A., et al.: Hepatitis C infection in children with hemophilia A and B. Blood *78*:285–289, 1991.
22. Blight, K. J., Kolykhalov, A. A., and Rice, C. M.: Efficient initiation of HCV RNA replication in cell culture. Science *290*:1972–1974, 2000.
23. Bolumar, F., Hernandez-Aguado, I., Ferrer, L., et al.: Prevalence of antibodies to hepatitis C in a population of intravenous drug users in Valencia, Spain, 1990–1992. Int. J. Epidemiol. *25*:204–209, 1996.
24. Bonacini, M., and Puoti, M.: Hepatitis C in patients with human immunodeficiency virus infection: Diagnosis, natural history, meta-analysis of sexual and vertical transmission, and therapeutic issues. Arch. Intern. Med. *160*:3365–3373, 2000.
25. Bortolotti, F., Giacchino, R., Vajro, P., et al.: Recombinant interferon-alfa therapy in children with chronic hepatitis C. Hepatology *22*:1623–1627, 1995.
26. Bortolotti, F., Jara, P., Diaz, C., et al.: Posttransfusion and community-acquired hepatitis C in childhood. J. Pediatr. Gastroenterol. Nutr. *18*:279–283, 1994.
27. Bortolotti, F., Resti, M., Giacchino, R., et al.: Hepatitis C virus infection and related liver disease in children of mothers with antibodies to the virus. J. Pediatr. *130*:990–993, 1997.
28. Bortolotti, F., Resti, M., Giacchino, R., et al.: Changing epidemiologic pattern of chronic hepatitis C virus infection in Italian children. J. Pediatr. *133*:378–381, 1998.
29. Bortolotti, F., Vajro, P., Balli, F., et al.: Non-organ specific autoantibodies in children with chronic hepatitis C. J. Hepatol. *25*:614–620, 1996.
30. Bortolotti, F., Vajro, P., Barbera, C., et al.: Hepatitis C in childhood: Epidemiological and clinical aspects. Bone Marrow Transplant. *12*(Suppl):S21–S23, 1993.
31. Bortolotti, F., Vajro, P., Cadrobbi, P., et al.: Cryptogenic chronic liver disease and hepatitis C virus infection in children. J. Hepatol. *15*:73–76, 1992.
32. Brackmann, S. A., Gerritzen, A., and Oldenburg, J.: Search for intrafamilial transmission of hepatitis C virus in hemophilia patients. Blood *81*:1077–1082, 1993.
33. Bresee, J. S., Mast, E. E., Coleman, P. J., et al.: Hepatitis C virus infection associated with administration of intravenous immunoglobulin. J. A. M. A. *276*:1563–1567, 1996.
34. Brown, E. A., Zhang H., Ping L. H., and Lemon, S. M.: Secondary structure of the 5′ nontranslated regions of hepatitis C virus and pestivirus genomic RNAs. Nucleic Acids Res. *20*:5041–5045, 1992.
35. Brown-Driver, V., Eto, T., Lesnik, E., et al.: Inhibition of translation of hepatitis C virus RNA by 2-modified antisense oligonucleotides. Antisense Nucleic Acid Drug Dev. *9*:145–154, 1999.
36. Bukh, J., Purcell, R. H., and Miller, R. H.: Sequence analysis of the core gene of 14 hepatitis C virus genotypes. Proc. Natl. Acad. Sci. U. S. A. *91*:8239–8243, 1994.
37. Buscarini, E., Tanzi, E., Zanetti, A. R., et al.: High prevalence of antibodies to hepatitis C virus among family members of patients with anti-HCV-positive chronic liver disease. Scand. J. Gastroenterol. *28*:343–346, 1993.
38. Camarero, C., Martos, I., Delgado, R., et al.: Horizontal transmission of hepatitis C virus in households of infected children. J. Pediatr. *123*:98–99, 1993.

39. Camma, C., Almasio, P., and Craxi, A.: Interferon as treatment for acute hepatitis C. A meta-analysis. Dig. Dis. Sci. *41*:1248–1255, 1996.
40. Chang, K. M., Rehermann, B., McHutchison, J. G., et al.: Immunological significance of cytotoxic T lymphocyte epitope variants in patients chronically infected by the hepatitis C virus. J. Clin. Invest. *100*:2376–2385, 1997.
41. Chang, T. T., Liou, T. C., Young, K. C., et al.: Intrafamilial transmission of hepatitis C virus: The important role of inapparent transmission. J. Med. Virol. *42*:91–96, 1994.
42. Choo, Q.-L., Kuo, G., Weiner, A. J., et al.: Isolation of a cDNA derived from a blood-borne non-A, non-B viral hepatitis genome. Science *244*:359–362, 1989.
43. Clemente, M. G., Congia, M., Lai, M. E., et al.: Effect of iron overload on the response to recombinant interferon alpha treatment in transfusion-dependent patients with thalassemia major and chronic hepatitis C. J. Pediatr. *125*:123–128, 1994.
44. Comanor, L., Minor, J., Conjeevaram, H. S., et al.: Impact of chronic hepatitis B and interferon-alpha therapy on growth of children. J. Viral Hepat. *8*:139–147, 2001.
45. Conroy-Cantilena, C., VanRaden, M., Gibble, J., et al.: Routes of infection, viremia, and liver disease in blood donors found to have hepatitis C virus infection. N. Engl. J. Med. *334*:1691–1696, 1996.
46. Conte, D., Fraquelli, M., Prati, D., et al.: Prevalence and clinical course of chronic hepatitis C virus (HCV) infection and rate of HCV vertical transmission in a cohort of 15,250 pregnant women. Hepatology *31*:751–755, 2000.
47. Cooper, S., Erickson, A. L., Adams, E. J., et al.: Analysis of a successful immune response against hepatitis C virus. Immunity *10*:439–449, 1999.
48. Demelia, L., Vallebona, E., Poma, R., et al.: HCV transmission in family members of subjects with HCV related chronic liver disease. Eur. J. Epidemiol. *12*:45–50, 1996.
49. Di Marco, V., Lo Iacono, O., Almasio, P., et al.: Long-term efficacy of alpha-interferon in beta-thalassemics with chronic hepatitis C. Blood *90*:2207–2212, 1997.
50. Diago, M., Zapater, R., Tuset, C., et al.: Intrafamily transmission of hepatitis C virus: Sexual and non-sexual contacts. J. Hepatol. *25*:125–128, 1996.
51. Dienstag, J. L.: Sexual and perinatal transmission of hepatitis C. Hepatology *26*(Suppl 1):66S–70S, 1997.
52. Diepolder, H. M., Gerlach, J. T., Zachoval, R., et al.: Immunodominant CD4+ T-cell epitope within nonstructural protein 3 in acute hepatitis C virus infection. J. Virol. *71*:6011–6019, 1997.
53. Dusheiko, G., Schmilovitz-Weiss, H., Brown, D., et al.: Hepatitis C genotypes: An investigation of type-specific differences in geographic origin and disease. Hepatology *19*:13–18, 1994.
54. Ebeling, F., Naukkarinen, R., and Leikola, J.: Recombinant immunoblot assay for hepatitis C antibody as a predictor of infectivity. Lancet *335*:982–983, 1990.
55. Enomoto, N., Sakuma, I., Asahina, Y., et al.: Mutations in the nonstructural protein 5A gene and response to interferon in patients with chronic hepatitis C virus 1b infection. N. Engl. J. Med. *334*:77–81, 1996.
56. Eyster, M. E., Diamondstone, L. S., Lien, J. M., et al.: Natural history of hepatitis C virus infection in multitransfused hemophiliacs: Effect of coinfection with human immunodeficiency virus. The Multicenter Hemophilia Cohort Study. J. Acquir. Immune Defic. Syndr. *6*:602–610, 1993.
57. Farci, P., Alter, H. J., Govindarajan, S., et al.: Lack of protective immunity against reinfection with hepatitis C virus. Science *258*:135–140, 1992.
58. Farci, P., Alter, H. J., Wong, D. C., et al.: Prevention of hepatitis C virus infection in chimpanzees after antibody-mediated in vitro neutralization. Proc. Natl. Acad. Sci. U. S. A. *91*:7792–7796, 1994.
59. Fortuny, C., Ercilla, M. G., Barrera, J. M., et al.: HCV vertical transmission: Prospective study in infants born to HCV seropositive mothers. *In* Hollinger, F. B., Lemon, S. M., and Margolis, H. S. (eds.): Viral Hepatitis and Liver Disease. Baltimore, Williams & Wilkins, 1991, pp. 418–419.
60. Fujisawa, T., Inui, A., and Ohkawa, T.: Response to interferon therapy in children with chronic hepatitis C. J. Pediatr. *127*:660–662, 1995.
61. Fukushi, S., Kurihara, C., Ishiyama, N., et al.: The sequence element of the internal ribosome entry site and a 25-kilodalton cellular protein contribute to efficient internal initiation of translation of hepatitis C virus RNA. J. Virol. *71*:1662–1666, 1997.
62. Garfein, R. S., Vlahov, D., Galai, N., et al.: Viral infections in short-term injection drug users: The prevalence of the hepatitis C, hepatitis B, human immunodeficiency, and human T-lymphotropic viruses. Am. J. Public Health *86*:655–661, 1996.
63. Ghany, M. G., Chan, T. M., Sanchez-Pescador, R., et al.: Correlation between serum HCV RNA and aminotransferase levels in patients with chronic HCV infection. Dig. Dis. Sci. *41*:2213–2218, 1996.
64. Giacchino, R., Tasso, L., Timitilli, A., et al.: Vertical transmission of hepatitis C virus infection: Usefulness of viremia detection in HIV-seronegative hepatitis C virus–seropositive mothers. J. Pediatr. *132*:167–169, 1998.
65. Gibb, D. M., Goodall, R. L., Dunn, D. T., et al.: Mother-to-child transmission of hepatitis C virus: Evidence for preventable peripartum transmission. Lancet *356*:904–907, 2000.
66. Giovanninni, M., Tagger, A., Ribero, M. L., et al.: Maternal-infant transmission of hepatitis C virus and HIV infections: A possible interaction. Lancet *335*:1166, 1990.
67. Grakoui, A., Hanson, H. L., and Rice, C. M.: Bad time for Bonzo? Experimental models of hepatitis C virus infection, replication, and pathogenesis. Hepatology *33*:489–495, 2001.
68. Granovsky, M. O., Minkoff, H. L., Tess, B. H., et al.: Hepatitis C virus infection in the mothers and infants cohort study. Pediatrics *102*:355–359, 1998.
69. Greco, M., Cristiano, K., Leozappa, G., et al.: Hepatitis C infection in children and adolescents on haemodialysis and after renal transplant. Pediatr. Nephrol. *7*:424–427, 1993.
70. Guido, M., Rugge, M., Jara, P., et al.: Chronic hepatitis C in children: The pathological and clinical spectrum. Gastroenterology *115*:1525–1529, 1998.
71. Hahm, B., Kim, Y. K., Kim, J. H., et al.: Heterogeneous nuclear ribonucleoprotein L interacts with the 3′ border of the internal ribosomal entry site of hepatitis C virus. J. Virol. *27*:8782–8788, 1998.
72. Hanecak, R., Brown-Driver, V., Fox, M. C., et al.: Antisense oligonucleotide inhibition of hepatitis C virus gene expression in transformed hepatocytes. J. Virol. *70*:5203–5212, 1996.
73. He, L. F., Alling, D., Popkin, T., et al.: Determining the size of non-A, non-B hepatitis virus by filtration. J. Infect. Dis. *156*:636–640, 1987.
74. He, X. S., Rehermann, B., Lopez-Labrador, F. X., et al.: Quantitative analysis of hepatitis C virus–specific CD8+ T cells in peripheral blood and liver using peptide-MHC tetramers. Proc. Natl. Acad. Sci. U. S. A. *96*:5692–5697, 1999.
75. Hino, K., Sainokami, S., Shimoda, K., et al.: Genotypes and titers of hepatitis C virus for predicting response to interferon in patients with chronic hepatitis C. J. Med. Virol. *42*:299–305, 1994.
76. Hiranuma, K., Tamaki, S., Nishimura, Y., et al.: Helper T cell determinant peptide contributes to induction of cellular immune responses by peptide vaccines against hepatitis C virus. J. Gen. Virol. *80*:187–193, 1999.
77. Honda, M., Beard, M. R., Ping, L. H., and Lemon, S. M.: A phylogenetically conserved stem-loop structure at the 5′ border of the internal ribosome entry site of hepatitis C virus is required for cap-independent viral translation. J. Virol. *73*:1165–1174, 1999.
78. Honda, M., Brown, E. A., and Lemon, S. M.: Stability of a stem-loop involving the initiator AUG controls the efficiency of internal initiation of translation on hepatitis C virus RNA. RNA *2*:955–968, 1996.
79. Honda, M., Kaneko, S., Shimazaki, T., et al.: Hepatitis C virus core protein induces apoptosis and impairs cell-cycle regulation in stably transformed Chinese hamster ovary cells. Hepatology *31*:1351–1359, 2000.
80. Honda, M., Kaneko, S., Unoura, M., et al.: Risk of hepatitis C virus infection through household contact with chronic carriers: Analysis of nucleotide sequences. Hepatology *17*:971–976, 1993.
81. Honda, M., Ping, L. H., Rijnbrand, R. C., et al.: Structural requirements for initiation of translation by internal ribosome entry within genome-length hepatitis C virus RNA. Virology *222*:31–42, 1996.
82. Hsu, S.-C., Chang, M.-H., Chen, D.-S., et al.: Non-A, non-B hepatitis in children: A clinical, histologic, and serologic study. J. Med. Virol. *35*:1–6, 1991.
83. Hunt, C. M., Carson, K. L., and Sharara, A. I.: Hepatitis C in pregnancy. Obstet. Gynecol. *89*:883–890, 1997.
84. Inui, A., Fujisawa, T., Miyagawa, Y., et al.: Histologic activity of the liver in children with transfusion-associated chronic hepatitis C. J. Hepatol. *21*:748–753, 1994.
85. Iorio, R., Pensati, P., Porzio, S., et al.: Lymphoblastoid interferon alfa treatment in chronic hepatitis C. Arch. Dis. Child. *74*:152–156, 1996.
86. Jacob, S., Baudy, D., Jones, E., et al.: Comparison of quantitative HCV RNA assays in chronic hepatitis C. Am. J. Clin. Pathol. *107*:362–367, 1997.
87. Jonas, M. M.: Treatment of chronic hepatitis C in pediatric patients. *In* Keeffe, E. B. (ed.): Treatment of Chronic Hepatitis C. Philadelphia, W. B. Saunders, 1999, pp. 855–867.
88. Jonas, M. M., Baron, M. J., Bresee, J. S., and Schneider, L. C.: Clinical and virologic features of hepatitis C virus infection associated with intravenous immunoglobulin. Pediatrics *98*:211–215, 1996.
89. Jonas, M. M., Ott, M. J., Nelson, S. P., et al.: Interferon-alpha treatment of chronic hepatitis C virus infection in children. Pediatr. Infect. Dis. J. *17*:241–246, 1998.
90. Jonas, M. M., Robertson, L. M., and Middleman, A. B.: Low prevalence of antibody to hepatitis C virus in an urban adolescent population. J. Pediatr. *131*:314–316, 1997.
91. Jonas, M. M., Zilleruelo, G. E., LaRue, S. I., et al.: Hepatitis C in a pediatric dialysis population. Pediatrics *89*:707–709, 1992.
92. Kage, M., Fujisawa, T., Shiraki, K., et al.: Pathology of chronic hepatitis C in children. Hepatology *26*:771–775, 1997.
93. Kanai, K., Kako, M., and Okamato, H.: HCV genotypes in chronic hepatitis C and response to interferon. Lancet *339*:1543, 1992.
94. Kanesaki, T., Kinoshita, S., Tsujino, G., et al.: Hepatitis C virus infection in children with hemophilia: Characterization of antibody response to four different antigens and relationship of antibody response, viremia, and hepatic dysfunction. J. Pediatr. *123*:381–387, 1993.

95. Kato, N., Yoshida, H., Ono-Nita, S. K., et al.: Activation of intracellular signaling by hepatitis B and C viruses: C-viral core is the most potent signal inducer. Hepatology *32*:405–412, 2000.
96. Khalifa, A. S., Mitchell, B. S., Watts, D. M., et al.: Prevalence of hepatitis C viral antibody in transfused and nontransfused Egyptian children. Am. J. Trop. Med. Hyg. *49*:316–321, 1993.
97. Kittlesen, D. J., Chianese-Bullock, K. A., Yao, Z., et al.: Interaction between complement receptor gC1qR and hepatitis C virus core protein inhibits T-lymphocyte proliferation. J. Clin. Invest. *106*:1239–1249, 2000.
98. Knodell, R. G., Ishak, K. G., Black, W. C., et al.: Formulation and application of a numerical scoring system for assessing histological activity in asymptomatic chronic active hepatitis. Hepatology *1*:431–435, 1981.
99. Kodama, T., Tamaki, T., Katabami, S., et al.: Histological findings in asymptomatic hepatitis C virus carriers. J. Gastroenterol. Hepatol. *8*:403–405, 1993.
100. Kolykhalov, A. A., Agapov, E. V., Blight, K. J., et al.: Transmission of hepatitis C by intrahepatic inoculation with transcribed RNA. Science *277*:570–574, 1997.
101. Komatsu, H., Fujisawa, T., Inui, A., et al.: Efficacy of interferon in treating chronic hepatitis C in children with a history of acute leukemia. Blood *87*:4072–4075, 1996.
102. Korth, M. J., and Katze, M. G.: Evading the interferon response: Hepatitis C virus and the interferon-induced protein kinase, PKR. Curr. Top. Microbiol. Immunol. *242*:197–224, 2000.
103. Kuo, G., Choo, Q.-L., Alter, H. J., et al.: An assay for circulating antibodies to a major etiologic virus of human non-A, non-B hepatitis. Science *244*:362–364, 1989.
104. Lafeuillade, A., Hittinger, G., and Chadapaud, S.: Increased mitochondrial toxicity with ribavirin in HIV/HCV coinfection. Lancet *357*:280–281, 2001.
105. Lai, M. E., DeVirgilis, S., Argiolu, F., et al.: Evaluation of antibodies to hepatitis C virus in a long-term prospective study of posttransfusion hepatitis among thalassemic children: Comparison between first- and second-generation assay. J. Pediatr. Gastroenterol. Nutr. *16*:458–464, 1993.
106. Lam, J. P. H., McOmish, F., Burns, S. M., et al.: Infrequent vertical transmission of hepatitis C virus. J. Infect. Dis. *167*:572–576, 1993.
107. Lamonaca, V., Missale, G., Urbani, S., et al.: Conserved hepatitis C virus sequences are highly immunogenic for $CD4^+$ T cells: Implications for vaccine development. Hepatology *30*:1088–1098, 1999.
108. Landau, A., Batisse, D., Van Huyen, J. P., et al.: Efficacy and safety of combination therapy with interferon-alpha-2b and ribavirin for chronic hepatitis C in HIV-infected patients. AIDS *14*:839–844, 2000.
109. Lang, T., Vogt, M., Schön, C., et al.: Prevalence, autoimmune phenomena, and clinical outcome of posttransfusion HCV infection after cardiac surgery in pediatric patients: A study on 45 patients. Hepatology *26*:463A, 1997.
110. Lau, G. K.: Development of novel therapies for hepatitis C. *In* Liang, T. J., and Hoofnagle, J. H. (eds.): Hepatitis C. San Diego, Academic Press, 2000.
111. Lau, J. Y. N., Davis, G. L., Kniffen, J., et al.: Significance of serum hepatitis C virus RNA levels in chronic hepatitis C. Lancet *341*:1501–1504, 1993.
112. Lechner, F., Wong, D. K., and Dunbar, P. R.: Analysis of successful immune responses in persons infected with hepatitis C virus. J. Exp. Med. *191*:1499–1512, 2000.
113. Lefkowitch, J. H., Schiff, E. R., Davis, G. L., et al.: Pathological diagnosis of chronic hepatitis C: A multicenter comparative study with chronic hepatitis B. Gastroenterology *104*:595–603, 1993.
114. Lesburg, C. A., Radfar, R., and Weber, P. C.: Recent advances in the analysis of HCV NS5B RNA-dependent RNA polymerase. Curr. Opin. Investig. Drugs. *1*:289–296, 2000.
115. Lin, H. H., Kao, J. H., Hsu, H. Y., et al.: Possible role of high-titer maternal viremia in perinatal transmission of hepatitis C virus. J. Infect. Dis. *169*:638–641, 1994.
116. Locasciulli, A., Gornati, G., Tagger, A., et al.: Hepatitis C virus infection and chronic liver disease in children with leukemia in long-term remission. Blood *78*:1619–1622, 1991.
117. Locasciulli, A., Testa, M., Pontisso, P., et al.: Prevalence and natural history of hepatitis C infection in patients cured of childhood leukemia. Blood *90*:4628–4633, 1997.
118. Lohmann, V., Körner, F., Koch, J.-O., et al.: Replication of subgenomic hepatitis C virus RNAs in a hepatoma cell line. Science *285*:110–113, 1999.
119. Lohmann, V., Roos, A., Korner, F., et al.: Biochemical and structural analysis of the NS5B RNA-dependent RNA polymerase of the hepatitis C virus. J. Viral Hepat. *7*:167–174, 2000.
120. Lok, A. S., Chien, D., Choo, Q. L., et al.: Antibody response to core, envelope and nonstructural hepatitis C virus antigens: Comparison of immunocompetent and immunosuppressed patients. Hepatology *18*:497–502, 1993.
121. Macejak, D. G., Jensen, K. L., Jamison, S. F., et al.: Inhibition of hepatitis C virus (HCV)–RNA-dependent translation and replication of a chimeric HCV poliovirus using synthetic stabilized ribozymes. Hepatology *31*:769–776, 2000.
122. Macejak, D. J., Jensen, K. L., Bellon, L., et al.: Inhibition of viral replication by nuclease resistance hammerhead ribozymes directed against hepatitis C virus RNA. Abstract. Hepatology *30*:409A, 1999.
123. Maggiore, G., Ventura, A., De Giacomo, C. C., et al.: Vertical transmission of hepatitis C. Lancet *345*:1122–1123, 1995.
124. Mahaney, K., Tedeschi, V., Maertens, G., et al.: Genotypic analysis of hepatitis C virus in American patients. Hepatology *20*:1405–1411, 1994.
125. Major, M. E., Mihalik, K., Fernandez, J., et al.: Long-term follow-up of chimpanzees inoculated with the first infectious clone for hepatitis C virus. J. Virol. *73*:3317–3325, 1999.
126. Manzini, P., Saracco, G., Cerchier, A., et al.: Human immunodeficiency virus infection as a risk factor for mother-to-child hepatitis C virus transmission; persistence of anti–hepatitis C virus in children is associated with the mother's anti–hepatitis C virus immunoblotting pattern. Hepatology *21*:328–332, 1995.
127. Marcellin, P., Bernuau, J., Martinot-Peignoux, M., et al.: Prevalence of hepatitis C virus infection in asymptomatic anti-HIV1 negative pregnant women and their children. Dig. Dis. Sci. *38*:2151–2155, 1993.
128. Marcellini, M., Kondili, L. A., Comparcola, D., et al.: High dosage alpha-interferon for treatment of children and young adults with chronic hepatitis C disease. Pediatr. Infect. Dis. J. *16*:1049–1053, 1997.
129. Martin, P., Di Bisceglie, A. M., Kassianides, C., et al.: Rapidly progressive non-A, non-B hepatitis in patients with human immunodeficiency virus infection. Gastroenterology *97*:1559–1561, 1989.
130. Mast, E. E., Hwang, L.-Y., Seto, D., et al.: Perinatal hepatitis C virus transmission: Maternal risk factors and optimal timing of diagnosis. Abstract. Hepatology *30*:499A, 1999.
131. Matsumoto, A., Tanaka, E., Suzuki, T., et al.: Viral and host factors that contribute to efficacy of interferon-alpha 2a therapy in patients with chronic hepatitis C. Dig. Dis. Sci. *39*:1273–1280, 1994.
132. Matsuoka, S., Mori, K., and Nakano, O.: Efficacy of interferons in treating children with chronic hepatitis C. Eur. J. Pediatr. *156*:704–708, 1997.
133. Matsuoka, S., Tatara, K., Hayabuchi, Y., et al.: Serologic, virologic, and histologic characteristics of chronic phase hepatitis C virus disease in children infected by transfusion. Pediatrics *94*:919–922, 1994.
134. Mele, A., Corona, R., Tosti, M. E., et al.: Beauty treatments and risk of parenterally transmitted hepatitis: Results from the hepatitis surveillance system in Italy. Scand. J. Infect. Dis. *27*:441–444, 1995.
135. Mellor, J., Holmes, E. C., Jarvis, L. M., et al.: Investigation of the pattern of hepatitis C virus sequence diversity in different geographical regions: Implications for virus classification. The International HCV Collaborative Study Group. J. Gen. Virol. *76*:2493–2507, 1995.
136. Miller, V. S., Zweiner, R. J., and Fielman, B. A.: Interferon-associated refractory status epilepticus. Pediatrics *93*:511–512, 1994.
137. Monteleone, P. M., Andrzejewski, C., and Kelleher, J. F.: Prevalence of antibodies to hepatitis C virus in transfused children with cancer. Am. J. Pediatr. Hematol. Oncol. *16*:309–313, 1994.
138. Murakami, T., Enomoto, N., Kurosaki, M., et al.: Mutations in nonstructural protein 5A gene and response to interferon in hepatitis C virus genotype 2 infection. Hepatology *30*:1045–1053, 1999.
139. Nakashima, K., Ikematsu, H., Hayashi, J., et al.: Intrafamilial transmission of hepatitis C virus among the population of an endemic area of Japan. J. A. M. A. *274*:1459–1461, 1995.
140. Nelson, S. P., and Jonas, M. M.: Hepatitis C infection in children who received extracorporeal membrane oxygenation. J. Pediatr. Surg. *31*:644–648, 1996.
141. Ngatchu, T., Stroffolini, T., Rapicetta, M., et al.: Seroprevalence of anti-HCV in an urban child population: A pilot survey in a developing area, Cameroon. J. Trop. Med. Hyg. *95*:57–61, 1992.
142. Ni, Y.-H., Chang, M.-H., Lue, H.-C., et al.: Posttransfusion hepatitis C virus infection in children. J. Pediatr. *124*:709–713, 1994.
143. Nousbaum, J., Polyak, S. J., Ray, S. C., et al.: Prospective characterization of full-length hepatitis C virus NS5A quasi-species during induction and combination antiviral therapy. J. Virol. *74*:9028–9038, 2000.
144. Novati, R., Theirs, V., Monforte, A. A., et al.: Mother-to-child transmission of hepatitis C virus detected by nested polymerase chain reaction. J. Infect. Dis. *165*:720–723, 1992.
145. Ogata, N., Alter, H. J., Miller, R. H., and Purcell, R. H.: Nucleotide sequence and mutation rate of the H strain of hepatitis C virus. Proc. Natl. Acad. Sci. U. S. A. *88*:3392–3396, 1991.
146. Ohto, H., Terazawa, S., Sasaki, N., et al.: Transmission of hepatitis C virus from mothers to infants. N. Engl. J. Med. *330*:744–750, 1994.
147. Osmond, D. H., Padian, N. S., Sheppard, H. W., et al.: Risk factors for hepatitis C virus seropositivity in heterosexual couples. J. A. M. A. *269*:361–365, 1993.
148. Paccagnini, S., Principi, N., Massironi, E., et al.: Perinatal transmission and manifestation of hepatitis C virus infection in a high risk population. Pediatr. Infect. Dis. J. *14*:195–199, 1995.
149. Palomba, E., Manzini, P., Fiammengo, P., et al.: Natural history of perinatal hepatitis C virus infection. Clin. Infect. Dis. *23*:47–50, 1996.
150. Pastore, M., Willems, M., Cornu, C., et al.: Role of hepatitis C virus in chronic liver disease occurring after orthotopic liver transplantation. Arch. Dis. Child. *75*:363–365, 1995.

151. Petracca, R., Falugi, F., Galli, G., et al.: Structure-function analysis of hepatitis C virus envelope–CD81 binding. J. Virol. *74*:4824–4830, 2000.
152. Pileri, P., Uematsu, Y., Campagnoli, S., et al.: Binding of hepatitis C virus to CD81. Science *282*:938–941, 1998.
153. Polywka, S., Feucht, H., Zollner, B., and Laufs, R.: Hepatitis C virus infection in pregnancy and the risk of mother-to-child transmission. Eur. J. Clin. Microbiol. Infect. Dis. *16*:121–124, 1997.
154. Pramoolsinsap, C., Kurathong, S., and Lerdverasirikul, P.: Prevalence of anti-HCV antibody in family members of anti-HCV-positive patients with acute and chronic liver disease. Southeast Asian J. Trop. Med. Public Health *23*:12–16, 1992.
155. Prince, A. M., Brotman, B., Huima, T., et al.: Immunity in hepatitis C infection. J. Infect. Dis. *165*:438–443, 1992.
156. Quan, C. M., Krajden, M., Grigoriew, G. A., et al.: Hepatitis C virus infection in patients infected with the human immunodeficiency virus. Clin. Infect. Dis. *17*:117–119, 1993.
157. Reinus, J. F., Leikin, E. L., Alter, H, J., et al.: Failure to detect vertical transmission of hepatitis C virus. Ann. Intern. Med. *117*:881–886, 1992.
158. Resti, M., Azzari, C., Mannelli, F., et al.: Mother to child transmission of hepatitis C virus: Prospective study of risk factors and timing of infection in children born to women seronegative for HIV-1. Br. Med. J. *317*:437–441, 1998.
159. Resti, M., Azzari, C., Rossi, M. E., et al.: Hepatitis C virus antibodies in a long-term follow-up of beta-thalassaemic children with acute and chronic non-A, non-B hepatitis. Eur. J. Pediatr. *151*:573–576, 1992.
160. Reynolds, J. E., Kaminski, A., Kettinen, H. J., et al.: Unique features of internal initiation of hepatitis C virus RNA translation. EMBO J. *14*:6010–6020, 1995.
161. Rice, C. M.: The viruses and their replication. *In* Fields, B., Knippe, D., and Howley, P. (eds.): Fields Virology. Philadelphia, Lippincott-Raven, 1996, p. 931.
162. Riestra-Menendez, S., Rodriguez-Garcia, M., Sanchez-SanRoman, F., et al.: Intrafamilial spread of hepatitis C virus. Infection *19*:431–433, 1991.
163. Rossetti, F., Cesaro, S., Pizzocchero, P., et al.: Chronic hepatitis B surface antigen–negative hepatitis after treatment of malignancy. J. Pediatr. *121*:39–43, 1992.
164. Roudot-Thoraval, F., Pawlotsky, J.-M., Thiers, V., et al.: Lack of mother-to-infant transmission of hepatitis C virus in human immunodeficiency virus–seronegative women: A prospective study with hepatitis C virus RNA testing. Hepatology *17*:772–777, 1993.
165. Sabatino, G., Ramenghi, L. A., di Marzio, M., and Pizzigallo, E.: Vertical transmission of hepatitis C virus: An epidemiological study on 2,980 pregnant women in Italy. Eur. J. Epidemiol. *12*:443–447, 1996.
166. Sarrazin, C., Kornetzky, I., Ruster, B., et al.: Mutations within the E2 and NS5A protein in patients infected with hepatitis C virus type 3a and correlation with treatment response. Hepatology *31*:1360–1370, 2000.
167. Sasaki, N., Matsui, A., Momoi, M., et al.: Loss of circulating hepatitis C virus in children who developed a persistent carrier state after mother-to-baby transmission. Pediatr. Res. *42*:263–267, 1997.
168. Scheuer, P. J., Ashrafzadeh, P., Sherlock, S., et al.: The pathology of hepatitis C. Hepatology *15*:567–571, 1992.
169. Seipp, S., Mueller, H. M., Pfaff, E., et al.: Establishment of persistent hepatitis C virus infection and replication in vitro. J. Gen. Virol. *78*(pt 10): 2467–2476, 1997.
170. Shimizu, Y. K., Feinstone, S. M., Kohara, M., et al.: Hepatitis C virus: Detection of intracellular virus particles by electron microscopy. Hepatology *23*:205–209, 1996.
171. Shimizu, Y. K., Hijikata, M., Iwamoto, A., et al.: Neutralizing antibodies against hepatitis C virus and the emergence of neutralization escape mutant viruses. J Virol. *68*:1494–1500, 1994.
172. Shrivastava, A., Manna, S. K., Ray, R., and Aggarwal, B. B.: Ectopic expression of hepatitis C virus core protein differentially regulates nuclear transcription factors. J. Virol. *72*:9722–9728, 1998.
173. Soriano, V., Garcia-Samaniego, J., Bravo, R., et al.: Interferon alpha for the treatment of chronic hepatitis C in patients infected with human immunodeficiency virus. Hepatitis-HIV Spanish Study Group. Clin. Infect. Dis. *23*:585–591, 1996.
174. Staples, C. T., Jr., Rimland, D., and Dudas, D.: Hepatitis C in the HIV (human immunodeficiency virus) Atlanta V.A. (Veterans Affairs Medical Center) Cohort Study (HAVACS): The effect of coinfection on survival. Clin. Infect. Dis. *29*:150–154, 1999.
175. Takahashi, M., Yamada, G., and Tsuji, T.: Intrafamilial transmission of hepatitis C. Gastroenterol. Jpn. *26*:483–488, 1991.
176. Takaki, A., Wiese, M., Maertens, G., et al.: Cellular immune responses persist and humoral responses decrease two decades after recovery from a single-source outbreak of hepatitis C. Nat. Med. *6*:578–582, 2000.
177. Takikawa, S., Ishii, K., Aizaki, H., et al.: Cell fusion activity of hepatitis C virus envelope proteins. J. Virol. *74*:5066–5074, 2000.
178. Tanaka, E., Kiyosawa, K., Soeyama, T., et al.: Prevalence of antibody to hepatitis C virus in Japanese schoolchildren: Comparison with adult blood donors. Am. J. Trop. Med. Hyg. *46*:460–464, 1992.
179. Taylor, D. R., Shi, S. T., Romano, P. R., et al.: Inhibition of the interferon-inducible protein kinase PKR by HCV E2 protein. Science *285*:107–110, 1999.
180. Tedder, R. S., Gilson, R. J. C., Briggs, M., et al.: Hepatitis C virus: Evidence for sexual transmission. Br. Med. J. *302*:1299–1302, 1991.
181. Thaler, M. M., Park, C. K., Landers, D. V., et al.: Vertical transmission of hepatitis C virus. Lancet *338*:17–18, 1991.
182. Tovo, P. A., Palomba, E., Ferraris, G., et al.: Increased risk of maternal-infant hepatitis C virus transmission for women coinfected with human immunodeficiency virus type 1. Italian Study Group for HCV Infection in Children. Clin. Infect. Dis. *25*:1121–1124, 1997.
183. Tsukiyama-Kohara, K., Iizuka, N., Kohara, M., and Nomoto, A.: Internal ribosome entry site within hepatitis C virus RNA. J. Virol. *66*:1476–1483, 1992.
184. Van der Poel, C. L., Cuypers, H. T. M., Reesink, H. W., et al.: Confirmation of hepatitis C virus infection by new four-antigen recombinant immunoblot assay. Lancet *337*:317–319, 1991.
185. Vegnente, A., Iorio, R., Saviano, A., et al.: Lack of intrafamilial transmission of hepatitis C virus in family members of children with chronic hepatitis C infection. Pediatr. Infect. Dis. J. *13*:886–889, 1994.
186. Vogt, M., Lang, T., Hess, J., et al.: Prevalence and clinical outcome of hepatitis C infection in children undergoing cardiac surgery before blood donor screening. N. Engl. J. Med. *341*:866–870, 1999.
187. Ward, C., Tudor-Williams, G., Cotzias, T., et al.: Prevalence of hepatitis C among pregnant women attending an inner London obstetric department: Uptake and acceptability of named antenatal testing. Gut *47*:277–280, 2000.
188. Watanabe, H., Enomoto, N., Nagayama, K., et al.: Number and position of mutations in the interferon (IFN) sensitivity-determining region of the gene for nonstructural protein 5A correlate with IFN efficacy in hepatitis C virus genotype 1b infection. J. Infect. Dis. *183*:1195–1203, 2001.
189. Wejstal, R., Widell, A., Mansson, A.-S., et al.: Mother to infant transmission of hepatitis C virus. Ann. Intern. Med. *117*:887–890, 1992.
190. Witherell, G. W., and Beineke, P.: Statistical analysis of combined substitutions in nonstructural 5A region of hepatitis C virus and interferon response. J. Med. Virol. *63*:8–16, 2001.
191. Wu, Z., Yao, N., Le, H. V., and Weber, P. C.: Mechanism of autoproteolysis at the NS2-NS3 junction of the hepatitis C virus polyprotein. Trends Biochem. Sci. *23*:92–94, 1998.
192. Yanagi, M., Purcell, R. H., Emerson, S. U., and Bukh, J.: Transcripts from a single full-length cDNA clone of hepatitis C virus are infectious when directly transfected into the liver of a chimpanzee. Proc. Natl. Acad. Sci. U. S. A. *94*:8738–8743, 1997.
193. Yanagi, M., St. Claire, M., Emerson, S. U., et al.: In vivo analysis of the 3′ untranslated region of the hepatitis C virus after in vitro mutagenesis of an infectious cDNA clone. Proc. Natl. Acad. Sci. U. S. A. *96*:2291–2295, 1999.
194. Zanetti, A. R., Tanzi, E., Paccagnini, S., et al.: Mother-to-infant transmission of hepatitis C virus. Lombardy Study Group on Vertical HCV Transmission. Lancet *345*:289–291, 1995.
195. Zuccotti, G. V., Ribero, M. L., Giovannini, M., et al.: Effect of hepatitis C genotype on mother-to-infant transmission of virus. J. Pediatr. *127*:278–280, 1995.
196. Zwiener, R. J., Fielman, B. A., Cochran, C., et al.: Interferon-alpha-2b treatment of chronic hepatitis C in children with hemophilia. Pediatr. Infect. Dis. J. *15*:906–908, 1996.

ORTHOMYXOVIRIDAE

CHAPTER 181 Influenza Viruses

W. PAUL GLEZEN

Influenza is an acute respiratory infection caused by strains of the orthomyxoviruses. The first of the human respiratory viruses to be isolated and characterized,[254] influenza viruses also have been studied the most extensively and are the best understood of these agents from a biologic, epidemiologic, and clinical standpoint.[91, 145] Yet, despite great sophistication in our understanding of it as a disease, influenza remains "the last great plague of man."[145]

Despite improvements in living standards and the introduction of antibiotics, the overall impact of influenza on mortality rates has not diminished. In fact, the average number of excess deaths has increased since 1984–1985 to at least 38,000 per year,[87] and the number of hospitalizations attributable to influenza is approximately 300,000 annually.[249, 250] Population dynamics—increasing population density and aging of the world's population—dictate that these numbers will continue to increase. The possibility of a recurrence of the catastrophic 1918–1919 epidemic, in which an estimated 550,000 deaths occurred in the United States alone,[46] seems remote. Nevertheless, an estimated 47,500 excess deaths and $3.8 billion in economic losses[140] were ascribed to the U.S. pandemic of 1968–1969. Annual epidemics have continued unabated. Each year, the peak of influenza virus activity coincides with the peak of health care visits and hospitalizations for acute respiratory tract disease.[43] Despite the decline in overall mortality, an average of 38,000 excess deaths are attributed to influenza each year.[87, 246–248]

As other agents capable of causing respiratory tract infection in children have been identified, influenza has received relatively less attention. Yet the morbidity and mortality rates of influenza in children can be considerable, and the spectrum of clinical manifestations resulting from influenza viral infections is broad.

History

Although the authenticity of influenza in medical antiquity is difficult to establish, apparently the disease has existed for 2000 years. The epidemic in 412 BC described by Hippocrates and Livy probably was influenza.[263] Epidemic influenza-like disease occurred in Europe in the 6th and 10th centuries, but the first generally accepted influenza epidemic occurred in December 1173.[121] Hirsch[121] noted 299 epidemics of influenza between 1173 and 1875. The first pandemic involving Europe, Asia, and North Africa occurred in 1580, and the first epidemic in the Western Hemisphere occurred in 1647. From 1580 until 1918, at least eight influenza pandemics occurred.

In recent times, pandemics of influenza caused by different influenza A subtypes occurred in 1874, 1889, 1900, 1918, 1957, 1968, and 1977. The most noteworthy of all influenza pandemics occurred in 1918. This event has the dubious distinction of producing the greatest morbidity and mortality of all time; more than 20 million deaths occurred in the world.[151]

The term *influenza* may have come from the Latin word *influo,* "to flow in," perhaps indicating its airborne transmission. It may be Italian, relating to an "influence," such as the weather, or mystical astrologic causes.[151]

Properties of the Virus

CLASSIFICATION

Classified taxonomically as orthomyxoviruses, the influenza viruses are negative-sense, single-stranded RNA viruses of three major types—A, B, and C—and multiple subtypes of influenza A viruses.[145] Influenza A and B viruses are most important in human disease and have been studied far more extensively than have influenza C viruses. All have the property of hemagglutination and, with the exception of influenza C, possess the enzyme neuraminidase. For types A and B, these properties reside on a pair of surface glycoproteins, hemagglutinin (HA) and neuraminidase (NA), but influenza C has a single glycoprotein with HA, esterase, and fusion activity.[155] The current World Health Organization system of nomenclature for influenza virus strains specifies type, host (for strains of animal origin), geographic source, strain number, and year of isolation, to which code designations of HA and NA subtypes are appended.[198] Thus, the "Russian" influenza A strain was designated A/USSR/90/77 (H1N1); the "Philippines" influenza A strain was designated A/Philippines/2/82 (H3N2). Strains are characterized and named at the World Health Organization influenza reference centers in Atlanta, Georgia (Centers for Disease Control and Prevention); London, England; Melbourne, Australia; and Tokyo, Japan.

PHYSICAL PROPERTIES

In electron-microscopic preparations, influenza viruses are irregular spherical particles 80 to 120 nm in diameter that also may exhibit filamentous or icosahedral structures[198] (Fig. 181–1). Numerous HA and NA "spikes" bristle from their surfaces. The virion proteins all are specified by the segmented viral genome, but the lipid bilayer and the carbohydrate constituents of glycoproteins and glycolipids in the viral envelope are derived from the host cell (Fig. 181–2). Besides the HA and NA, eight other virus-coded proteins

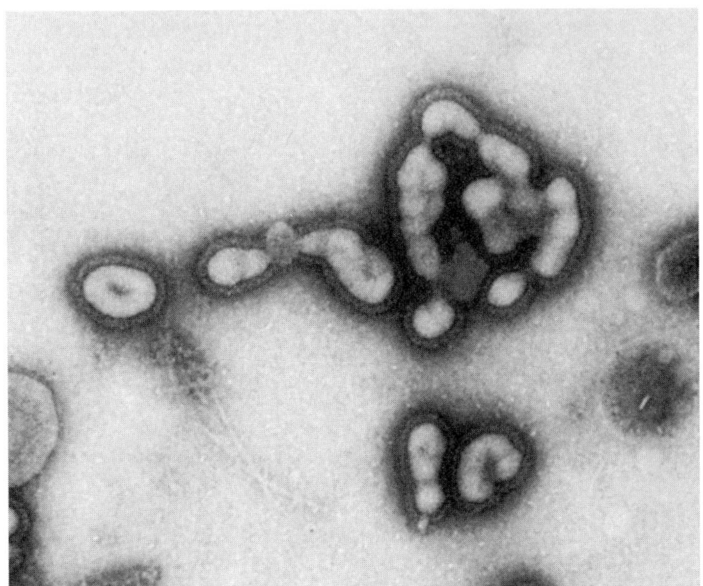

FIGURE 181–1 ■ Influenza A/USSR/90/77 (H1N1). Note hemagglutinin and neuraminidase "spikes" and occasional filamentous forms. (Courtesy of G. R. Noble, M.D., Centers for Disease Control and Prevention.)

have been characterized (Table 181–1). Matrix or membrane protein (M1) is the most abundant protein and the major structural component of the viral envelope. The M2 protein of influenza A virus is a smaller tetrameric protein that acts as an ion channel extending through the viral envelope. M2 has an important role in the penetration and release of viral RNA into the host cell.[259] The function of the comparable polypeptide of influenza B virus, BM2, is unknown.[155] Nucleoprotein is associated with the RNA genome of the virus in ribonucleoprotein complexes in which multiple nucleoprotein molecules are associated with eight segments of the single-stranded RNA. Proteins PB2, PB1, and PA, the largest proteins of the virus, are so designated because two are basic proteins and one is an acidic protein. They are involved with the synthesis of three different kinds of virus-specific RNAs. Evidence suggests that the PB2 protein is the cap-recognizing protein and that PB1 and PA are involved in chain initiation or in chain elongation.[17, 18, 154, 214, 265] Nonstructural proteins, although not incorporated into viral progeny, are virus-coded proteins, NS1 and NS2. NS1 has an anti-interferon effect,[81] and NS2 promotes nuclear export of the viral ribonucleoprotein.[207]

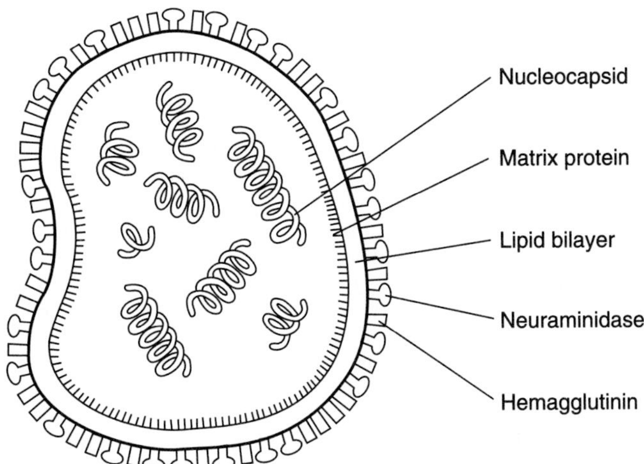

FIGURE 181–2 ■ An influenza virion. Nucleocapsid structures consist of segmented RNA complexed with nucleoprotein and P proteins.

The biologic and antigenic diversity of influenza viruses is attributable in part to their unique, segmented RNA genome. Interchange of corresponding segments of a linear genome, in the traditional sense of genetic recombination, did not account for this extraordinarily high frequency. Hirst,[122] in 1962, proposed the hypothesis that the influenza genome consists of subgenomic pieces capable of semiautonomous replication and random "reassortment" during the process of assembly. This theory accounted for observed recombination frequencies and subsequently was supported by the finding that the RNA of influenza virions was indeed segmented on analysis by polyacrylamide gel electrophoresis.[220] More refined electrophoretic studies in urea-polyacrylamide gels have established that the influenza A genome consists of eight segments (Fig. 181–3). Reassortment in nature has been documented for the 1957 and 1968 pandemic viruses as well as for other A viruses.[198]

ANTIGENIC COMPOSITION

Of the protein constituents of influenza viruses, four are known antigens. The "internal" nucleoprotein and matrix protein are antigenically type specific and stable. Nucleoprotein is the antigenic basis for typing strains as A, B, or C

TABLE 181–1 ■ VIRUS-CODED PROTEINS OF INFLUENZA VIRUS

Gene Segment	Protein Designation	Function	Antigenicity
1	PB2	RNA synthesis	?
2	PB1	RNA synthesis	?
3	PA	RNA synthesis	?
4	HA	Hemagglutinin	Subtype specific
5	NA	Neuraminidase	Subtype specific
6	NP	RNA synthesis	Type specific
7	M1, M2	Matrix	Type specific
8	NS1, NS2	Nonstructural	?

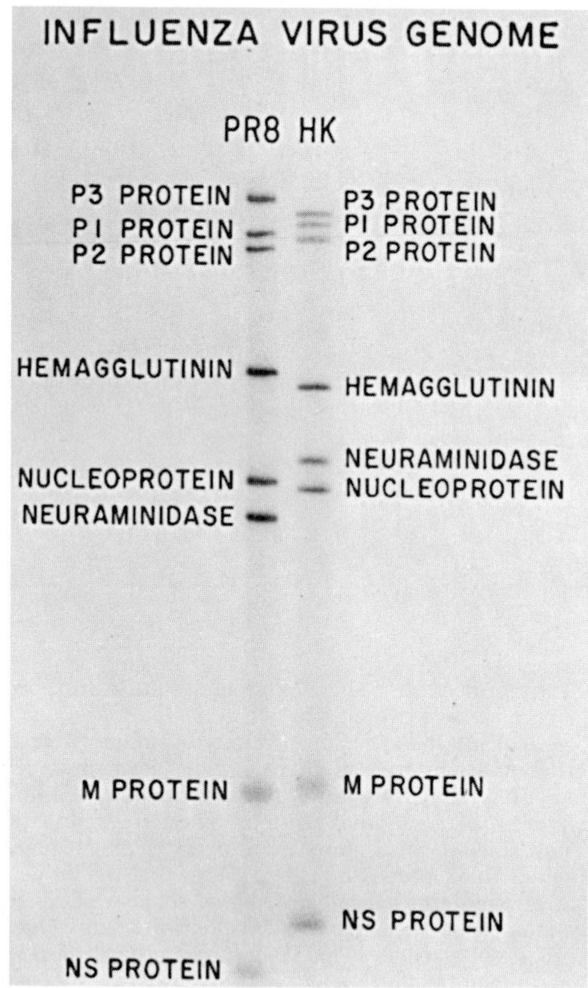

FIGURE 181–3 ■ Polyacrylamide-urea gel electrophoretic maps of the RNA genome of influenza A/PR/8/34 (H0N1) and A/HK/68 (H3N2). (From Ritchey, M. B., Palese, P., and Schulman, J. L.: Mapping of the influenza virus genome. III. Identification of genes coding for nucleoprotein, membrane protein, and nonstructural protein. J. Virol. *20*:307–313, 1976.)

and the predominant constituent of the "soluble" antigen employed for complement-fixation serologic testing. Although antibody against nucleoprotein is formed regularly after natural infection and antibody against matrix protein has been detected after severe illness, these antibodies are short-lived and appear to have no protective value.

In contrast, HA and NA antigens are subtype specific and variable. HA is required for attachment of infecting virus to host-cell membranes. HA-inhibiting antibodies neutralize viral infectivity and are the most important index of immunity against influenza in humans.[123] NA appears to be required for release of virus from infected cells. Specific antineuraminidase antibodies reduce plaque size, mitigate the pathogenic effects of influenza in experimentally infected mice, and correlate inversely with viral shedding and severity of illness.[194] Thus far, three HAs, H1, H2, and H3, and two NAs, N1 and N2, have been recognized in influenza A viruses that spread readily in human populations.

Variation in HA and NA specificity is the basis for antigenic "drift" and "shift" in prevalent viruses. Drift implies a minor change in either antigen, without a change in subtype; shift implies a major change in either or both antigens, with a change in subtype. Antigenic drift occurs in influenza A and B viruses; antigenic shift occurs only in influenza A.

Antigenic drift is the result of point mutations. Selective pressure in an immune population results in selection of mutant viruses with altered antigenic determinants that allow a growth advantage in the presence of prevalent antibody. Supporting this concept are the in vitro studies of Laver and Webster,[158] in which antigenic mutants isolated by serial egg passage in the presence of low-avidity antiserum develop changes in the peptide make-up of their HA subunits.

Antigenic shift occurs when an influenza A virus acquires HA or NA components that differ from antecedent strains by a quantum jump. The phenomenon has been well studied in influenza A viruses. The H3 HA, by chromatographic analysis of peptide composition, is sufficiently distinctive to make highly improbable its emergence by point mutation from the H2 HA of a preceding Asian strain.[159]

Considerable evidence indicates that antigenic shift strains arise by reassortment of gene segments between human and animal influenza viruses during chance simultaneous infection. The 1957 Asian H2N2 virus derived the HA, NA, and PB1 gene segments from an avian virus and the remaining five gene segments from the circulating A (H1N1) strain. The so-called Hong Kong influenza that appeared in 1968, A (H3N2), had avian HA and PB1 gene segments combined with six gene segments from the preceding A (H2N2) virus.[198]

An analogous event initially was suspected as the origin of the swinelike A/New Jersey/8/76 (H1N1) virus recovered from infections in Fort Dix military recruits in 1976. However, the RNA genome of A/NJ now has been shown by polyacrylamide gel chromatography to be virtually identical to other strains of influenza virus isolated from swine.[210] It shows no RNA homology to human strains. The spread of virulent avian viruses with the H5 HA to humans in Hong Kong in 1997 is another alarming event that supports the possibility of emergence of pandemic strains by direct infection of humans with an avian virus possessing surface antigens not previously prevalent in the human population.[126] Thus, the emergence from animal reservoirs of influenza strains with sufficient virulence to cause widespread human epidemics remains a valid hypothesis.

TISSUE CULTURE AND CHICKEN EMBRYO GROWTH

Influenza viruses grow well in a variety of culture systems, although embryonated chicken eggs and the Madin-Darby canine kidney cell line are used most widely. Primary rhesus monkey kidney tissue culture and other monkey cell lines are alternative choices for influenza virus isolation. Intra-amniotic and intra-allantoic inoculation of 10- to 11-day-old eggs is followed by incubation for 3 to 4 days at 33° C. Fluid samples are harvested and tested for the presence of hemagglutinating virus by addition of guinea pig or chicken red blood cells. Monkey kidney cells have maximum sensitivity to influenza viruses when they are maintained after inoculation in a serum-free medium. Subtle cytopathic effects may appear but are variable. Detection of virus is carried out best after 3 to 5 days of incubation at 34° C in the Madin-Darby canine kidney cells or after 7 to 10 days of incubation at 33° C with use of the rhesus kidney cell line, then hemadsorbing with guinea pig red blood cells. Influenza C viruses grow best in eggs; Madin-Darby canine kidney and monkey kidney cells generally give higher yields of influenza A and B viruses. "Blind" repassages may result in an isolation in either system when the initial passage is negative, but the yield drops off sharply. Although parainfluenza viruses also may be isolated in these tissue culture lines, they can be distinguished from influenza viruses by their characteristic syncytial cytopathogenicity and their poor growth in embryonated eggs.[73, 74] Definitive identification of virus isolates is performed by indirect immunofluorescence or hemagglutination inhibition with use of specific antisera. Antigen detection and identification of influenza viruses by use of enzyme-linked immunosorbent assays have been valuable additions to the diagnostic laboratory.[14, 55, 114, 236, 271] Reverse transcription–polymerase chain reaction (PCR) techniques have the possibility of revolutionizing diagnosis of respiratory virus infections.[3, 64]

ANIMAL SUSCEPTIBILITY

Influenza virus types readily grow and produce disease in ferrets.[228] This animal commonly is used for experimental studies. Influenza viruses also can be adapted to grow in mice for research purposes. Other animals, including hamsters, guinea pigs, monkeys, squirrels, chipmunks, chinchillas, and mink, have varying degrees of susceptibility to influenza viruses.

Horses, swine, and birds are infected naturally by type A influenza viruses. In most instances, these animal strains are different from those of human origin; however, the avian strains are the most important reservoir for viruses with pandemic potential.[198]

Epidemiology

INCIDENCE AND PREVALENCE

Influenza is the most important etiology of acute respiratory illnesses that cause patients to seek medical care.[85, 88] Population dynamics that include increasing population and increased population density resulting from urbanization throughout the world facilitates spread of these viruses. Rapid movement of persons throughout the world allows new variants or subtypes to spread readily in a short time. Unless new control measures are added, the impact of epidemics will increase steadily as the population ages. Studies have demonstrated that the hospitalization rates for preschool-age children equal those of the elderly.[134, 200] Furthermore, influenza viruses are the most important causes of acute respiratory tract illnesses leading to hospitalization of schoolchildren.[93, 95, 215]

Although local outbreaks and individual cases of influenza are optionally reportable in all states, information about disease activity as it varies from year to year derives mainly from ongoing surveillance in public health departments and university medical centers.[167] Longitudinal studies of viral respiratory tract illnesses in families,[71, 109, 135, 262] in hospitalized children,[95, 98] in private pediatric practices,[94, 97, 107] and in public clinics[90] have provided useful data about the community impact of influenza infections. Detection of new influenza variants and their spread is facilitated by reporting of virus isolations and serologic responses in specimens submitted to an international network of World Health Organization laboratories.[28]

Weekly tabulations of deaths from "pneumonia" and "influenza" from larger cities in the United States provide a valuable index of mortality from influenza.[247] Several methods have been used to estimate the expected number of deaths in the absence of influenza so that excess mortality can be derived from the observed number during epidemics. Reported deaths in excess of an epidemic threshold usually correlate well with the occurrence of widespread influenza activity (Fig. 181–4).[99, 156, 247]

The highest attack rates of influenza occur in children and tend to proceed to secondary peaks of illness in adult populations.[90, 91] Although case-fatality has been considered to occur most frequently at both extremes of age, increases in pneumonia-influenza deaths in recent years have been most

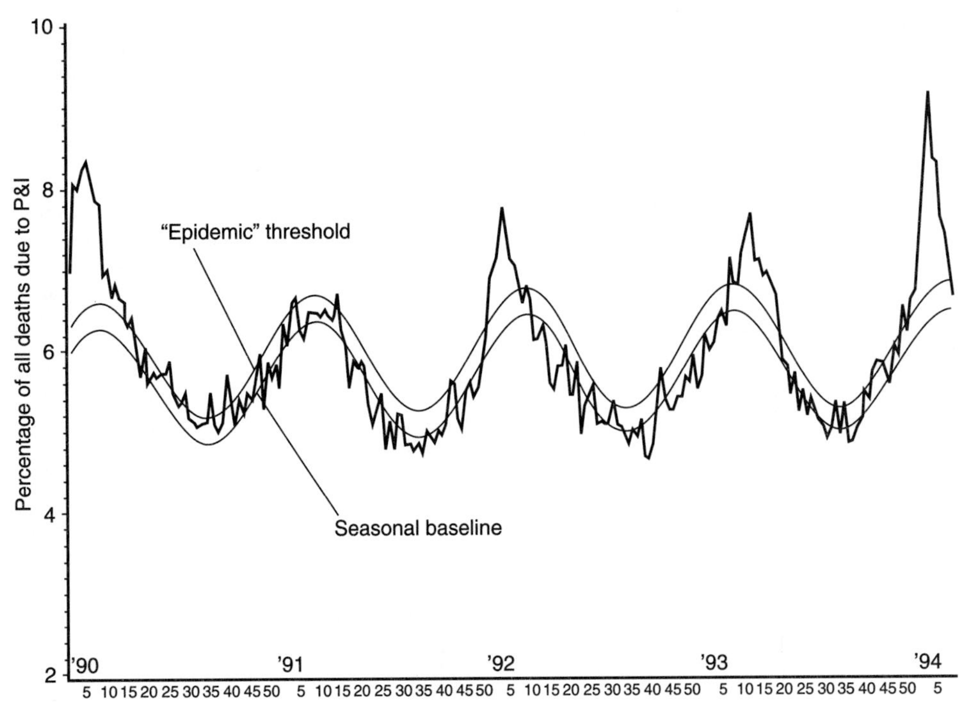

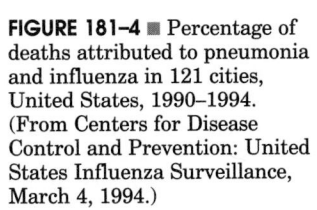

FIGURE 181–4 ■ Percentage of deaths attributed to pneumonia and influenza in 121 cities, United States, 1990–1994. (From Centers for Disease Control and Prevention: United States Influenza Surveillance, March 4, 1994.)

clear-cut in the elderly.[70, 246–248] Regardless of age, influenza is fatal more frequently in persons with preexisting heart disease, chronic pulmonary disorders, diabetes mellitus, chronic renal disease, neuromuscular disorders, and neoplasms.

A remarkable ecologic feature of influenza viruses has been the tendency of one particular virus subtype to achieve worldwide distribution at the same time its predecessor disappears from human circulation.[145] Since their first isolation in the 1930s, three major subtypes of influenza A viruses have circulated widely. At the transition years of these "influenza eras," a major antigenic drift or shift has occurred. The prototypic strains for these time intervals are 1933 to 1957, influenza A/Puerto Rico/8/34 (H1N1); 1957 to 1967, influenza A/Japan/305/57 (H2N2); and 1968 to 1977, influenza A/Hong Kong/8/68 (H3N2). In 1977, influenza A/USSR/90/77 (H1N1) made its appearance; since then, both H1N1 and H3N2 strains have been prevalent.

The antigenic make-up of viruses prevalent before the 1930s has been inferred by seroepidemiologic studies. By this means, researchers have determined that persons born before 1924 have a high prevalence of antibodies against the swinelike H1 HA.[245] Similarly, in serum specimens collected before the emergence of H2N2 and H3N2 strains, high prevalences of antibody against the H3 HA were found in persons born before 1889.[173] Thus, the number of influenza A viruses may be finite and the major subtypes may recycle periodically. This concept is supported by the re-emergence of A/USSR/90/77 (H1N1). Antigenically and genetically, this strain of influenza A was found to be identical to influenza A/Fort Warren/1/50 (H1N1), the H1N1 variant prevalent between 1950 and 1953.[96, 199, 289]

SEASONAL AND GEOGRAPHIC PATTERNS

Influenza infections have marked seasonality.[91] In temperate climates, epidemics occur almost exclusively in winter months. Off-season infections are documented infrequently. Winter circulation in the Southern Hemisphere probably maintains influenza viruses during northern summer months. Occurrence of influenza is less predictable in tropical areas. Some regions may have two annual outbreaks, whereas others may have outbreaks in the rainy season. Geographic variations in the incidence of influenza also may reflect global patterns of spread of new virus strains. Isolated populations may escape the dispersion of new viruses. When outbreaks do occur in such highly susceptible populations, explosive spread and high attack rates in all age groups have been observed.[24, 85]

TRANSMISSION

Droplet spread, with inhalation of airborne particles produced by coughing and sneezing, generally is accepted as the most common mode of natural influenza transmission. Spread also may occur by direct contact, indirect contact, and fine-particle aerosols. Small-particle aerosol, by which virus particles are deposited directly into the lower respiratory tract, is the most efficient means of inducing influenza in volunteer studies. In one such study, a human infectious dose (HID_{50}) of influenza A/Bethesda/10/63 (H2N2) by aerosol was equivalent to 0.6 to 3.0 tissue culture infectious doses ($TCID_{50}$).[1] In contrast, studies in which influenza A/Aichi/2/68 (H3N2) was given by direct instillation or coarse spray into the nose revealed a range of HID_{50} of 127 to 320 $TCID_{50}$.[41, 47] The contribution of small-particle aerosol to transmission of influenza under natural conditions remains uncertain but could be important in the pathogenesis of primary influenza pneumonia.[91]

Once infection is established, peak virus shedding coincides with clinical symptoms. Virus may be recovered for a day before the onset of symptoms with influenza B and up to 6 days in the case of influenza A. Virus shedding is detected for a variable period in children but usually exists for a week or less for influenza A and up to 2 weeks after influenza B infection.[77] At the height of illness, respiratory tract secretions commonly contain 10^6 or more infectious viral particles per milliliter.[193]

The incubation period of influenza ranges from 1 to 7 days but commonly is 2 to 3 days. This brief incubation period, coupled with the large amounts of infectious virus in secretions and the relatively small dose necessary for infection of susceptibles, accounts for the intensity of influenza outbreaks. Spread is most rapid in institutions, such as schools, colleges, military barracks, and nursing homes. In community outbreaks, school-age children usually have the highest attack rates, with secondary spread to their parents and younger siblings (Fig. 181–5).[49, 88, 91, 100]

Nosocomial infection may occur during community epidemics of influenza and has been documented in hospitalized adults,[19] infants,[106] and premature infants.[178, 191] In hospital settings, separating highly susceptible patients from other patients and personnel with acute respiratory tract illness is a reasonable measure.

Pathogenesis and Immunity

VIRAL INFECTION AND PATHOGENESIS

To establish infection, influenza viruses must penetrate the mucous blanket lining the respiratory tract and escape inactivation by nonspecific inhibitors as well as specific local antibodies. The major site of infection is the ciliated columnar epithelial cell.[91, 119] Necrosis of ciliated epithelial cells occurs as early as the first day after the onset of symptoms. Many of the symptoms may be attributed to the release of proinflammatory cytokines and chemokines from the infected epithelial cells.[116, 253] The levels of cytokines and chemokines in nasal secretions coincide with the intensity of symptoms.[79] Local edema and cellular infiltration by lymphocytes, histiocytes, plasma cells, and polymorphonuclear cells follow. Repair of the epithelium begins between the third and fifth days, as indicated by mitoses in the surviving basal cells. A pseudometaplastic response of undifferentiated epithelium reaches its maximum 9 to 15 days after the onset of the infection. After 15 days, cilia and mucus production reappear. With secondary bacterial infection, more extensive inflammatory cell infiltration and destruction of the basal cell layer and basement membrane are seen, with consequent delay in regeneration of the ciliated epithelium.

Pneumonia associated with influenza virus infection may result from primary viral infection, bacterial superinfection, or combined bacterial-viral infection.[168] Fatal primary influenza pneumonia, fortunately a rare occurrence in children, is characterized at autopsy by diffuse hemorrhagic alveolar exudates, necrosis of bronchiolar epithelium, peribronchial lymphocytic infiltration, and marked lymphocytic infiltration of the alveolar walls and interstitial lung tissue.[190]

Although the major pathologic process in influenza is in the respiratory tract, focal and diffuse myocarditis, mediastinal lymph node disorganization and necrosis, and diffuse cerebral edema also have been noted in fatal cases. In recent years, the pathologic entity of diffuse encephalopathy and fatty degeneration of the liver (Reye syndrome) has been

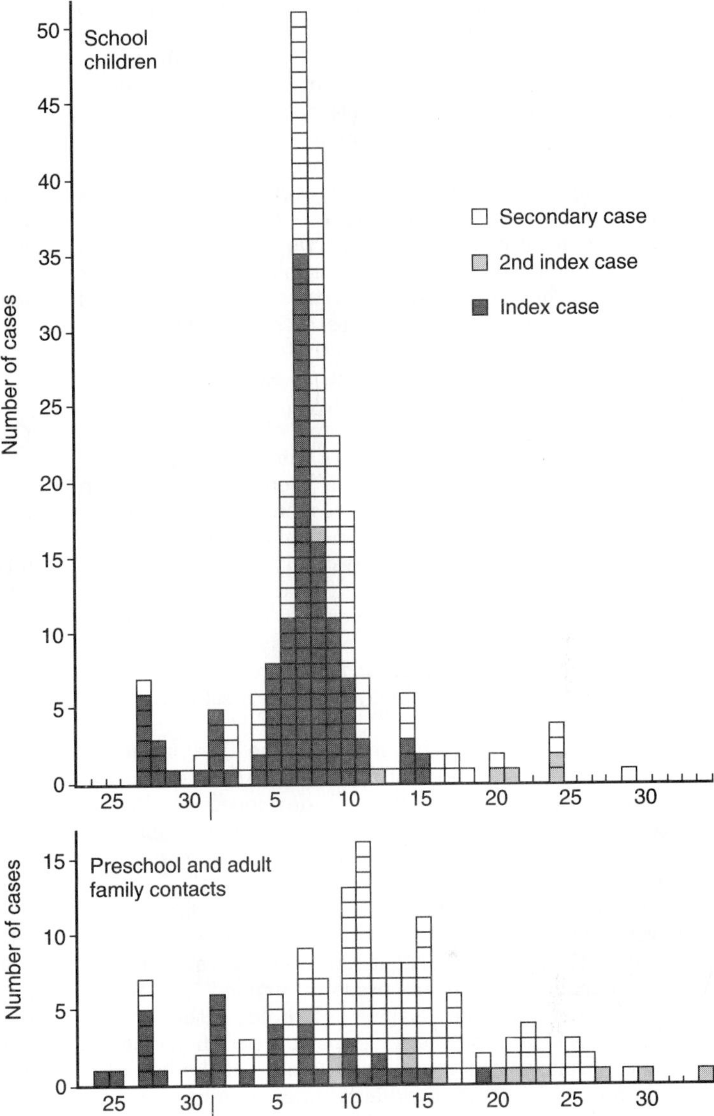

FIGURE 181–5 ■ Epidemic curve of infections by influenza B in Hazleton, Iowa, 1961–1962. Note that the epidemic wave in school-age children precedes the epidemic wave in household contacts. (From Chin, T. D. Y., Mosley, W. H., Poland, J. D., et al.: Epidemiologic studies of type B influenza in 1961–1962. Am. J. Public Health *53*:1068–1074, 1963.)

established as a potential complication of influenza, particularly type B, in children.[161] Reye syndrome was associated with administration of salicylate-containing products to children with influenza or varicella and has declined in incidence as the use of salicylates has decreased.[130] Encephalopathy and encephalitis associated with influenza have been reported frequently in Japan, where an estimated 100 children die each year.[244] The hypotheses for pathogenesis include direct viral invasion of the central nervous system and inflammation secondary to high levels of proinflammatory cytokines.[133]

IMMUNOLOGIC EVENTS

Immunity against influenza results from a complex interplay of humoral, secretory, and cell-mediated mechanisms. Because of the brief incubation period of the disease, anamnestic stimulation of antibody affords little protection. Thus, some degree of preexisting antibody appears to be essential to prevent infection. The sequential antigenic changes that occur in the virus in the course of antigenic drift afford each new variant a selective advantage in establishing infection; the major antigenic changes that accompany antigenic shifts render larger populations susceptible and account for pandemic spread.

After natural influenza infection, both local and humoral antibodies are elicited against HA, NA, nucleocapsid, and matrix protein antigens. Antibodies to the HA are critical for neutralization of virus. Antibodies against NA are associated with diminished severity of illness and reduced rates of person-to-person transmission. Antibodies against NA and matrix protein do not appear to provide protection or to modify transmission. Because influenza is a respiratory epithelial surface infection rather than a systemic infection, some uncertainty exists about the relative degree of protection afforded by local and humoral antibodies. Studies in human volunteers demonstrated good protection against experimental challenge by influenza A/HK/1/68 in subjects who possessed serum antibodies but lacked detectable nasal antibodies.[42] Subjects challenged by influenza B/Eng/65 also demonstrated a better correlation of protection with serum antibody levels than with nasal antibodies.[59] Moreover, in a large experience with volunteers summarized by Hobson and associates,[123] an impressive linear correlation between serum hemagglutination-inhibiting antibody titers and protection was evident. Thus, although an important role for local antibodies as a "first line of defense" against influenza is accepted, serum antibodies clearly contribute to resistance.

Waldman and colleagues[269] have demonstrated that the predominant influenza-neutralizing antibody in nasal secretions is secretory IgA, whereas the predominant neutralizing antibody in tracheobronchial secretions is IgG. A synthesis of the available data suggests that local secretory IgA in nasal secretions may be important in the prevention of infection that is transmitted by droplet spread and that originates in the upper respiratory tract. Serum and local IgG antibodies appear to be of greater importance in neutralizing infection transmitted directly to the lower respiratory tract by aerosol or in preventing extension of upper respiratory tract infection to the lungs.

Cell-mediated immune mechanisms of several varieties have been demonstrated in influenza infection and vaccination. A T-cell "helper" function has been demonstrated in strain-specific humoral antibody response against HA.[268] Both nonspecific and specific mechanisms of lymphocyte cytotoxicity have been found in model systems,[63, 291] but only type-specific cytotoxic T cells have been found in humans.[15, 20, 61] Cytotoxic T lymphocytes are important for recovery from infection in susceptible hosts. Antibody-dependent cell-mediated cytotoxicity has been shown to correlate with the titer of serum anti-HA antibody.[101] This mechanism also may play a role in recovery.[53, 241]

The immunologic imprint made by the first influenza infection of childhood has lasting effects. According to the "doctrine of original antigenic sin," developed by Francis and colleagues[72] from seroepidemiologic data, hemagglutination-inhibiting antibody against the strain of first infection is recapitulated with each subsequent infection by an antigenically distinctive strain of influenza A. Since 1957, however, researchers have found that infections or immunizations with H2N2 or H3N2 strains do not recall antibody against earlier strains in persons primed by H1N1 viruses.[171] Therefore, the doctrine only holds within groups of influenza A strains possessing some degree of homology of antigens. Virelizier and associates[267] analyzed the basis for the phenomenon using irradiated mice immunologically reconstituted with bone marrow from immune donors. Their studies indicate that antigenic "original sin" derives from cross-stimulation of a population of committed memory B lymphocytes that persist after primary infection.

After natural infection, the duration of immunity and the degree of protection against challenge by heterologous variants appear to be variable. On the basis of clinical experience in a Yorkshire general practice, Pickles and associates[216] concluded that natural immunity against influenza A strains lasted at least 4 years. On the other hand, serologic reinfection rates of 2 percent and 12 percent against influenza A and influenza B, respectively, were noted by Hall and colleagues[109] during a 3-year observation period in Seattle children. Some protection against the re-emerged influenza A (H1N1) virus of 1977 was noted for persons who had been infected with a similar virus in the 1950s.[96] The cross-immunity was lost gradually as new H1N1 variants appeared since 1977, demonstrating a divergence in antigenic properties of variants that appeared after 1950 and 1977.

Frank and colleagues[75, 78] reported that variations in reinfection among young children may be multifactorial but, most important, may be related to the age at first infection and the antigenic differences of virus variants in subsequent challenges. Thus, protection against clinical disease appears to persist for many years after influenza infection in older children but may be of much shorter duration in infants and very young children; subclinical reinfection probably occurs after much shorter intervals. A gradual increase in duration and breadth of immunity against related virus strains probably occurs during a period of years. Frank and associates[76] found that unlike the findings for influenza A (H3N2) infections, infection with influenza B virus provided consistent protection for most persons against infection with the next influenza B variant. The protection decreased somewhat for subsequent variants and longer intervals. This decrease may account for the relative infrequency of influenza B infections in adults because only antigenic drift has been documented for this virus. The major antigenic changes occurring in antigenic shifts, however, have the potential to circumvent cumulative immunity in all age groups.

Clinical Manifestations

Disease caused by epidemic influenza A virus has the unique feature that persons of all ages in a population become ill with febrile respiratory tract complaints. In contrast, although other respiratory tract viral agents (respiratory syncytial virus, rhinoviruses, parainfluenza viruses) also may cause community epidemics that involve both children and adults, the illness is different in the two age groups; young children with primary viral infections with noninfluenzal agents have febrile illnesses, whereas older children and adults with similar infections most commonly have common colds and other upper respiratory tract involvement with little or no fever.[83]

The symptoms and signs in children and adults of type A influenza caused by the Asian subtype (H2N2) are compared in Table 181–2.[135] The following findings have occurred significantly more frequently in children: sudden onset, anorexia, abdominal pain, vomiting, nausea, cervical adenopathy, and temperature higher than 38.9° C. Influenza C viruses cause illnesses similar to influenza A infection, but the severity of disease usually is less and the duration shorter. In addition, because antigenic changes in influenza B viruses are less pronounced, frequently a greater difference in illness occurs between children and adults. Influenza B may cause an epidemic in which children will have typical influenza with fever, but many adults in the population will have only upper respiratory tract[92] illnesses without significant fever. In other outbreaks caused by antigenically variant influenza B virus, significant illness has been identified in adults.[93, 111]

OLDER CHILDREN AND ADOLESCENTS (CLASSIC INFLUENZA)

The symptoms and signs of classic influenza in older children and adolescents are presented in Table 181–3. The onset of illness is abrupt, with fever and associated flushed face, chills, headache, myalgia, and malaise.[25, 218, 225, 242] The temperature ranges between 39° C and 41° C (102° F to 106° F), with a general inverse correlation with age. The systemic symptoms are reported to be more severe in older patients, probably because of their ability to describe them. Although a dry cough and coryza also are early manifestations of influenza, these symptoms go unobserved by the patients because of the severity of the systemic manifestations. Sore throat occurs in more than half of the cases and usually is associated with a not otherwise remarkable nonexudative pharyngitis. Ocular symptoms include tearing, photophobia, burning, and pain with eye movement.

In uncomplicated illness, the fever usually persists for 2 to 3 days but may last up to 5 days. A biphasic temperature

TABLE 181–2 ■ FREQUENCY OF SYMPTOMS AND SIGNS OF PROVEN INFLUENZA A (H2N2) IN CHILDREN (0–14 YEARS OF AGE) AND ADULTS*

	Percentage with Symptoms or Signs	
	Children (N = 95)	Adults (N = 30)
Symptoms		
Sudden onset	66*	46
Systemic symptoms		
Feverishness	93	71
Headache	81	72
Anorexia	69*	37
Malaise	68	67
Chilliness	37	64†
Myalgia	33	62†
Respiratory symptoms		
Cough	86	90
Nasal discharge	67	82
Sore throat	62	62
Nasal obstruction	54	52
Sneezing	38	67†
Hoarseness	22	37
Sputum production	19	41†
Other symptoms		
Abdominal pain	31*	0
Vomiting	26*	7
Nausea	23*	4
Diarrhea	2	0
Signs		
Maximum temperature		
≤37.7° C	11	13
37.8° C to 38.8° C	29	58†
≤38.9° C	60*	29
Conjunctival abnormalities	61	56
Pharyngeal injection	60	68
Nasal injection/edema	50	64
Nasal discharge	38	20
Cervical adenopathy	38*	8
Rhonchi or rales	2	0
Pharyngeal exudates	1	0

*Significantly more frequent in children ($p < .05$, Fisher exact test).
†Significantly more frequent in adults ($p < .05$, Fisher exact test).
Data from Jordan, W. S., Denny, F. W., Badger, G. F., et al.: A study of illness in a group of Cleveland families. XVII. The occurrence of Asian influenza. Am. J. Hyg. *68*:190–212, 1958.

pattern may occur, even without apparent secondary bacterial complications. By the second to the fourth day, respiratory tract symptoms become more prominent and the systemic complaints begin to subside. The cough is dry and hacking and usually persists for 4 to 7 days; cough, in association with some degree of general malaise, occasionally persists for 1 or 2 weeks after the rest of the illness has subsided. Illness caused by influenza B virus generally is associated with more prominent nasal and eye complaints and fewer systemic findings, such as dizziness and prostration, than is influenza A illness. In a study in which both influenza A (H1N1) and influenza C were noted in a population of young adults, the illnesses could not be differentiated by clinical findings.[60]

In uncomplicated classic influenza, the leukocyte count most often is normal, but leukopenia (<4500 cells/mm^3) has been noted in approximately 25 percent of cases. The differential cell count is of no diagnostic value, for approximately one third of patients will have normal values, one third will have relative lymphopenia, and one third will have relative neutropenia. The relative proportion of each white blood cell type may depend on the time during the course of infection

TABLE 181–3 ■ RELATIVE FREQUENCY OF SYMPTOMS AND SIGNS DURING CLASSIC INFLUENZA IN OLDER CHILDREN AND ADOLESCENTS

Symptoms	Occurrence*
Chilly sensation	+ + + +
Cough	+ + +
Headache	+ + +
Sore throat	+ + +
Prostration	+ +
Nasal stuffiness	+ +
Dizziness	+
Eye irritation or pain	+
Vomiting	+
Myalgia	+
Signs	
Fever	+ + + +
Pharyngitis	+ + +
Conjunctivitis (mild)	+ +
Rhinitis	+ +
Cervical adenitis	+
Pulmonary rales; wheezes or rhonchi	

*++++, 76 to 100 percent; +++, 51 to 75 percent; ++, 26 to 50 percent; and +, 1 to 25 percent.
From Cherry, J. D.: Influenza viral infections. *In* Vaughan, V., McKay, R., and Behrman, R. (eds.): Nelson Textbook of Pediatrics. 14th ed. Philadelphia W. B. Saunders, 1987, pp. 675–678.

that the differential count is determined.[150] Approximately 10 percent of older children and adolescents will have clinical signs and radiographic evidence of pulmonary involvement.

YOUNGER CHILDREN

GENERAL. Clinical expression of influenza in younger children and infants has been studied intensively, a reflection of increasingly sensitive and specific respiratory tract viral diagnosis. With some exceptions,* most studies have contained disproportionate numbers of hospitalized patients† and thus may tend to exaggerate the more severe end of the influenza spectrum.

In younger children, the manifestations of influenza viral infections frequently are similar to those resulting from other respiratory tract viruses (parainfluenza, respiratory syncytial, rhinovirus, and adenovirus) (Table 181–4). Laryngotracheitis, bronchitis, bronchiolitis, pneumonia, and the common cold all occur. Clinical descriptions of these illnesses are presented in Chapters 161, 171, 182, and 185. The overall rate of hospitalization of children with lower respiratory tract involvement is the same for influenza virus infections as for other viruses, but influenza tends to affect older children.

Primary infection with influenza A in these age categories typically is seen as an undifferentiated febrile upper respiratory tract illness.[280] Infants younger than 2 months frequently are hospitalized for ruling out bacterial sepsis, particularly when influenza A (H3N2) viruses are epidemic.[98] Fever tends to be high, and temperature will exceed 39.5°C in most patients. Affected children appear moderately toxic, with clear nasal discharge, cough, and irritability as almost constant findings. Pharyngitis usually is present, with diffuse erythema and boggy, enlarged tonsillar tissue. Between 5 and 10 percent of those infected will have some degree of pulmonary involvement; in hospitalized children, this percentage may be as high as 50 percent. Vomiting,

*See references 68, 69, 71, 75, 78, 93, 128, 149, 165, 238.
†See references 23, 27, 125, 164, 169, 189, 201, 211, 219, 266, 285.

TABLE 181–4 ■ RELATIVE FREQUENCY OF CLINICAL MANIFESTATIONS OF INFLUENZA VIRAL INFECTIONS IN CHILDREN YOUNGER THAN 5 YEARS

Major Clinical Category	Occurrence*
Upper respiratory tract illness	+ + + +
Laryngotracheitis	+
Bronchitis	+
Bronchiolitis	+
Pneumonia	+
Symptoms	
Cough	+ + + +
Anorexia	+ +
Coryza	+ +
Vomiting	+ +
Diarrhea	+
Sore throat	+
Signs	
Fever	+ + + +
Pharyngitis	+ + +
Cervical adenitis	+ +
Otitis media	+ +
Convulsions	+
Exanthem	+
Generalized adenitis	+

*++++, 76 to 100 percent; +++, 51 to 75 percent; ++, 26 to 50 percent; and +, 1 to 25 percent.

From Cherry, J. D.: Influenza viral infections. *In* Vaughan, V., McKay, R., and Behrman, R. (eds.): Nelson Textbook of Pediatrics. 14th ed. Philadelphia, W. B. Saunders, 1987, pp. 675–678.

diarrhea, otitis media, pneumonitis, and croup frequently are associated findings, and fleeting erythematous, macular or maculopapular discrete rashes occasionally are observed.

GASTROINTESTINAL SYMPTOMS. In contrast to illness symptoms in older children and adults, gastrointestinal symptoms have been noted in several studies of influenza infection in young children. Among 68 children admitted to hospital during a community epidemic of influenza B/Hong Kong/72 in 1974, Kerr and colleagues[143] encountered acute abdominal pain, with minimal associated respiratory tract symptoms, as the presenting complaint in 37 patients. This symptom was noted most frequently in children 4 to 10 years of age and led to unnecessary laparotomy in two patients. In infants, infection by influenza A virus may elicit diarrhea and vomiting. Of 18 infants 6 months of age or younger with proven influenza A/HK/68 infections, Price and associates[221] noted prominent anorexia, diarrhea, or vomiting in 13 (72%), and only 5 (23%) had respiratory tract symptoms alone. Five of the infants with gastrointestinal disturbance had moderate to severe dehydration. Similarly, among 53 hospitalized infants younger than 1 year with infections of influenza A, Paisley and associates[208] found diarrhea to be a prominent symptom in 18 patients (34%). Thus, unlike adults with influenza, infants and young children indeed may display "gastric flu."

FEBRILE CONVULSIONS. Febrile convulsions precipitated by fever of abrupt onset have been cited as common presenting complaints in several studies of hospitalized children with influenza. Among 75 children with infections by influenza A/Hong Kong/68 (H3N2), 26 (35%) of the patients described by Price and associates[221] presented with a febrile convulsion. Of the 77 hospitalized children described by Brocklebank and colleagues,[23] 31 (40%) had convulsions at onset; 27 of the children in this series were 3 years of age or younger, a distribution consistent with the usual age-specific susceptibility pattern of febrile seizures.

CROUP. Acute laryngotracheobronchitis (croup) has been noted as a prominent feature of influenza A in young children during the H3N2 era. Illness tends to be more severe than is the rule for the croup syndrome induced by parainfluenza viruses, and tenacious tracheal secretions may necessitate tracheostomy or endotracheal intubation in a higher proportion of hospitalized patients. During the peak month of a composite of 13 consecutive influenza A outbreaks, influenza A virus was demonstrated in 68 percent of croup patients hospitalized in Washington, D.C.[147] Severe croup caused by influenza virus infection may occur in children at an older age than that of those usually infected with parainfluenza viruses.[62, 129, 219]

NEONATES

In neonates, influenza infection may suggest bacterial sepsis: lethargy, poor feeding, petechiae, poor peripheral circulation with mottling of the skin, and apneic spells. Nosocomial influenza A outbreaks have occurred in neonatal nurseries in association with symptomatic illnesses among nursery staff and parents.[6, 178, 191] Six of the eight infants in one study had apneic spells.[178] Two infants required mechanical ventilation for frequent apneic spells for a period of 6 to 8 days.

HIGH-RISK CHILDREN

Other host characteristics generally considered to influence the clinical expression of influenza include preexisting chronic pulmonary, cardiac, and neuromuscular disease. Most deaths occur in these vulnerable patients.[264] The basis for this doctrine, however, derives almost exclusively from pathologic and epidemiologic analysis of influenza in adult patients.[120] In children with chronic illness, the available data are surprisingly meager. Among the 77 hospitalized children with influenza A described by Brocklebank and colleagues,[23] 13 of 23 (56%) with chronic diseases or congenital malformations developed lower respiratory tract infection, compared with 10 of 54 (19%) without preexisting chronic conditions. Kempe and colleagues[142] studied influenza virus infection in children with malignant neoplasms and found that affected children had both more frequent and more severe influenza-related illnesses than did their healthy contacts or age-matched controls.

The few comprehensive virologic studies conducted in asthmatic children have yielded conflicting results. In a longitudinal study of young children (younger than 3 years) hospitalized for prolonged periods because of severe extrinsic asthma, McIntosh and associates[176] serologically documented 11 episodes of infection by influenza A/Hong Kong/68, all of which were mild and none of which was associated with exacerbations of wheezing. Studies of pediatric outpatients older than 3 years with intrinsic asthma have found that influenza virus infections play important roles in triggering asthma attacks. A population-based study in Houston found that influenza was the most common infection triggering hospitalization of schoolchildren with asthma; 21 percent of all hospitalizations during a 4-year period were associated with influenza virus infection.[95] Other investigators have documented influenza virus infections with exacerbations of asthma in children.[182, 183, 230] A retrospective cohort study has shown that influenza vaccine protects against severe exacerbations in asthmatic children after adjustment for asthma severity.[153] Therefore, the preponderance of evidence from clinical studies incriminates influenza as an important instigator of asthma attacks in children.[89]

Diagnosis

Infection with influenza virus often can be deduced more accurately from epidemiologic features than from clinical presentation. Epidemics occur each winter and usually begin with a sudden increase in presentation to primary care facilities of school-age children with febrile respiratory tract illnesses.[88] Routine laboratory studies provide little help in the differentiation of influenza from other viral respiratory tract diseases. Serial monitoring of induced infections in adults has revealed a characteristic moderate increase in total white blood cell count, with relative lymphopenia, during the height of symptoms and low serum iron values.[54, 56, 65] In children, however, hematologic manifestations are variable, with marked leukocytosis frequently observed in infants.[106] Chest radiographs are useful primarily for determining the presence of complicating interstitial or lobar pneumonia. Transient alterations in tests of pulmonary function have been documented in a high percentage of normal adults with uncomplicated influenza.[110] Thus, oxygen saturation determinations may be useful in children with influenza and clinical evidence of lower respiratory tract involvement, even if chest radiographs do not show infiltrates.

Definite diagnosis of influenza depends on antigen detection or virus isolation from respiratory tract secretions or a significant rise in serum antibody during convalescence. In contrast to shedding of adenoviruses or herpes simplex virus from the respiratory tract, asymptomatic carriage of influenza viruses is a rare occurrence. Thus, virus detection alone is considered conclusive evidence for etiology of an illness. Hemagglutinating agents often can be detected in embryonated eggs, Madin-Darby canine kidney, or primary monkey kidney tissue culture within 72 hours of inoculation. However, longer incubation and serial passage are required before cultures can be regarded as negative.[57] Rapid detection of influenza antigens in nasopharyngeal epithelial cells with specific fluorescent antibody conjugates has been successful in many studies.[163, 206] A combined approach employs short-term incubation of clinical specimens in tissue culture, followed by rapid identification of hemadsorbing agents with fluorescent antibody.[7] Enzyme immunoassay can be used for early detection of influenza A antigen.[55, 271] When this information is available to the clinician in a timely fashion, the use of antibiotics is curtailed and the use of specific antiviral treatment is enhanced.[203] Tests that detect both influenza A and B are now available in primary care settings.[202–204] Further advances in diagnosis of influenza result from incorporation of techniques for reverse transcription–PCR. PCR provides greater sensitivity (95%) than do other antigen detection methods (usually 60–75%).[3] Multiplex quantitative reverse transcription–PCR may allow identification of all of the important respiratory viruses of children—influenza, parainfluenza, and respiratory syncytial virus.[64]

Serologic diagnosis may be accomplished by use of either complement-fixation or hemagglutination-inhibition techniques.[57] The complement-fixation test detects antibody against the "soluble" nucleoprotein antigens that are common to all strains of influenza A or influenza B. Reagents are commercially available, and the test is provided by most clinical laboratories. Complement-fixing antibodies are of relatively brief duration; titers wane within 6 months of infection. Hemagglutination-inhibiting antibodies, which are subtype specific, provide more definitive evidence of infection. However, subtype-specific reagents are required and are less widely available in clinical laboratories. Titers persist for years and are boosted by infection with related strains. The hemagglutination-inhibition test has the added advantage of greater sensitivity. Neutralizing antibodies correlate best with protection against reinfection and are more sensitive indicators. Rises in neuraminidase-inhibiting antibody also may be detected after infection, but such studies are technically cumbersome and restricted to specialized applications. A versatile method for measuring antibodies against influenza antigens employs the enzyme-linked immunosorbent assay.[16, 196] This system is technically simple and has the advantage of permitting specific identification of IgA and IgM antibodies as well as IgG subclasses. It is particularly useful for measurement of antibodies in respiratory secretions that reflect mucosal immunity.

Complications

BACTERIAL INFECTIONS

The most frequent complications of influenza are bacterial infections of the respiratory tract—particularly pneumonia, otitis media, and sinusitis.[66, 118, 168, 184, 208, 243, 251, 257] Characteristically, these complications arise in early convalescence, with bacterial invasion of portions of the respiratory tract resulting in denuded ciliated epithelium and defective mucociliary transport. In 37 young infants experiencing their first infections by influenza A viruses, Wright and colleagues[280] noted otitis media in 10 and pneumonia in 7. Hall and Douglas[106] documented complicating bacterial pneumonia in 5 of 12 patients who developed nosocomial infection by influenza A on an infant ward, most with underlying chronic cardiorespiratory disease. The incidence of complicating bacterial infections in community studies, including children of all ages, is approximately 10 percent, with otitis media being the most frequent finding.[135] A 14-year longitudinal study of young children demonstrated a 28 percent incidence of otitis media after influenza A and B virus infections and an increased risk of recurrent disease.[118] Studies of vaccine effectiveness support reports of influenza-associated acute otitis media of 30 to 40 percent for children in daycare during the respiratory disease season.[86]

Although most cases of bacterial pneumonia complicating influenza are pneumococcal,[243] the two most feared pulmonary complications are progressive primary viral pneumonia and staphylococcal pneumonia.[168] Progressive primary viral pneumonia has been observed most frequently in adult patients with preexisting rheumatic heart disease, but it may occur in previously healthy children as well.[134, 136, 200, 208] It is characterized radiographically by diffuse bronchopneumonic infiltrates and clinically by intense dyspnea and a relentless downhill course, despite antimicrobial and supportive therapy. Staphylococcal pneumonia may occur as a postinfluenzal lobar pneumonia progressing to pneumatoceles and empyema. More characteristically, staphylococcal pneumonia in association with influenza occurs as a fulminant, synergistic, viral-bacterial process with diffuse involvement on radiographs, leukopenia, intense dyspnea, blood-tinged sputum, and rapid death. Necrotizing pneumonitis with microabscesses and positive lung cultures for both influenza A virus and *Staphylococcus aureus* are characteristic.[168]

ACUTE MYOSITIS

Acute myositis occurs in the setting of early convalescence from a typical influenzal illness.[5, 52, 181] Severe pain and tenderness in the calves of both legs come on suddenly, often with the patient refusing to walk. Other muscle groups may be involved as well, but the gastrocnemius and soleus muscles are affected in virtually all cases. Elevated levels of serum creatine kinase and aspartate aminotransferase are characteristic. Influenza B virus has been isolated in 20 of 26 such cases by Middleton and associates[181] and in 11 of 17 cases by Dietzman and colleagues.[52] Infection by influenza A has been documented in one case of the former series. The condition generally is self-limited, but rhabdomyolysis with myoglobinuria and acute renal failure has been described in severe cases occurring in association with influenza A.[31, 51, 141]

ENCEPHALOPATHY AND REYE SYNDROME

Reye syndrome is a condition of obscure pathogenesis characterized by fatty degeneration of the liver and diffuse cerebral edema.[38, 227] Although the condition has been recognized under varying nomenclatures since its partial description by Brain and colleagues[21] in 1929, only somewhat recently has influenza infection been implicated as an inciting factor. Of 85 patients treated at Cincinnati Children's Hospital, 74 (87%) had a respiratory tract prodrome clinically indistinguishable from influenza and 11 patients (13%) had varicella.[212] During the 1974 outbreak in Cincinnati, influenza B/HK/8/73 was isolated from the nasopharyngeal secretions of 9 of 23 affected children, with serologic evidence of influenza B in an additional 3 children.[161] Numerous other reports have demonstrated similar associations of influenza A (H1N1 and H3N2) as well as influenza B with subsequent outbreaks of Reye syndrome.[37, 113, 132, 260, 278] Surveillance data indicate a significant decline in both the incidence and mortality ratio.[2, 4] In a survivor of Reye syndrome, who was studied intensively by Partin and colleagues,[212] influenza A/Vic/3/75 (H3N2) virus was recovered from nasotracheal secretions, cerebrospinal fluid, liver, and skeletal (gastrocnemius) muscle, which led the investigators to postulate visceral dissemination of virus as an element in the pathogenesis of this condition. Clinically, Reye syndrome, most common in white male school-age children, is marked by nausea, vomiting, and stupor during convalescence from a viral illness, most commonly characterized by respiratory tract symptoms.[2, 4] In this setting, the finding of elevated serum transaminase and blood ammonia levels, with unremarkable cerebrospinal fluid, is sufficient for diagnosis.[38] During the 1974 outbreak, Reye syndrome was estimated to have occurred at a rate of 31 to 58 cases per 100,000 infections with influenza B in children,[37–39] although a lower incidence was reported among Colorado children in association with the 1978–1979 H1N1 outbreak.[113] The case-fatality ratio is 26 percent.

An ever-increasing body of data has revealed a strong association between the use of salicylates or salicylate-containing medications and Reye syndrome, with resultant strict warnings against the use of salicylates in children with influenza.[112, 130, 256, 270, 287] The decreased use of aspirin for children with influenza and varicella has paralleled the decline in reporting of cases of Reye syndrome.[2]

Encephalopathy may occur without fatty degeneration of the liver. An encephalitis-like picture is not an uncommon finding among children hospitalized with influenza virus infection.[50, 175] An outbreak associated with influenza B virus infection was reported in Chicago in 1971.[124] Alarming reports of the occurrence of encephalopathy and encephalitis in young children have come from Japan since 1995.[244, 258] More than 200 cases per year have been reported, and more than 100 have been fatal or with permanent neurologic sequelae.[139] Evidence of influenza virus infection has come from virus isolation or PCR detection from the cerebrospinal fluid.[80, 133] The pathogenesis of these illnesses is unknown but may result from direct viral invasion of the central nervous system or from high levels of proinflammatory cytokines that breech the blood-brain barrier.[133, 187]

OTHER COMPLICATIONS

NEUROLOGIC DISEASE. Apart from encephalopathy or Reye syndrome, other severe neurologic illnesses have been noted rarely in association with influenza viral infections.[179, 237] As noted, the most common manifestation is an encephalitis in association with a respiratory tract illness. In most instances, no evidence of a concomitant meningitis is present. Guillain-Barré syndrome and a transverse myelitis also have been associated with influenza.[273]

CARDIAC DISEASE. Pericarditis and myocarditis have been noted rarely in association with influenza viral infections.[34, 44, 184, 257] This cardiac involvement has occurred in normal children and adults as well as in those with preexisting heart disease.

SUDDEN DEATHS. During influenza epidemics, sudden unexpected deaths are observed occasionally. They occur in persons of all ages, and postmortem examination most frequently indicates respiratory tract involvement. Cases of sudden infant death syndrome have been associated with influenza viral infection.[58, 261]

OTHER OBSERVATIONS. Glomerulonephritis and renal failure have been associated with influenza viral infections.[274, 276] In two instances, acute parotitis has occurred with influenza A infection.[19] Although evidence of the transplacental passage of influenza virus to a 30-week-old male fetus has been reported,[286] no epidemiologic evidence of influenza virus teratogenicity is known.[170, 277]

Treatment

SUPPORTIVE THERAPY

Because most influenza infections are unpleasant but uncomplicated illnesses, symptomatic treatment is the cornerstone of management. Bed rest, adequate hydration with oral fluids, control of fever and myalgia with acetaminophen, and maintenance of comfortable breathing by means of nasal decongestants and humidified air suffice in most cases. Prophylactic administration of antibiotics should be discouraged. Persistent irritative cough during convalescence often can be relieved with dextromethorphan or codeine.

Complicated illnesses demand the physician's clinical judgment in the use of other therapeutic modalities. Bacterial infections, suggested by a prolonged febrile course or recrudescence of fever during early convalescence, should be identified as to site, and appropriate cultures should be obtained. Antibiotic therapy then is indicated and should be guided and modified by Gram stain findings and the results of cultures. Because most infections are caused by *Streptococcus pneumoniae, Haemophilus influenzae,* and *Streptococcus pyogenes,* therapy with ampicillin or amoxicillin is adequate for most cases of otitis media or lobar pneumonia. The possibility of penicillin-resistant pneumococci, methicillin-resistant *S. aureus,* and opportunistic gram-negative pathogens should be entertained in fulminant or protracted pneumonias.

Inhalation therapy is an integral part of the management of patients with illnesses complicated by airway compromise (croup), apneic spells, or diffuse pneumonia. Such patients should be monitored carefully. Humidified air is the most important element in management of croup, but nasotracheal intubation or tracheostomy has been required in a high proportion of patients with croup caused by influenza.[129] Provision of supplemental oxygen and, as indicated by oxygen saturation, continuous positive airway pressure or mechanical ventilation may be required in infants and children with apnea or significant alveolar-capillary block due to pneumonia.

SPECIFIC THERAPY

The antiviral agents amantadine and rimantadine are active in vitro against influenza A viruses and have been shown to provide prophylactic and therapeutic benefit in adults.[40] Amantadine acts by blocking the function of the M2 protein, the ion channel that functions to facilitate fusion of viral and cell membranes permitting entry of viral RNA into the host cell.[272] Amantadine lacks activity against influenza B viruses. Numerous pediatric studies also have documented the prophylactic effect of amantadine or its analogue, rimantadine, against community-acquired influenza A.[34, 45, 213, 231, 232] Few pediatric treatment trials have been performed.[67, 148] Rimantadine treatment of young children with limited prior experience with the infecting subtype has resulted in emergence of resistant viruses.[13, 105] Amantadine-rimantadine resistance of influenza A virus results from point mutations of the M2 protein.[10, 13] In some instances, the resistant viruses have been noted to infect susceptible contacts.[115] Despite these observations, less than 1 percent of field isolates of influenza A were found to be resistant to rimantadine.[290] Recommendations for the use of amantadine for prophylaxis have not changed; precautions should be taken to limit contact between patients being treated with amantadine and subjects receiving prophylaxis.[185]

The armamentarium of antiviral drugs for influenza has been supplemented by the addition of NA inhibitors. The inhaled inhibitor zanamivir is approved for use in children 7 years of age and older.[117] Early treatment with zanamivir twice daily shortened the course of illness by 1.25 days compared with placebo. Zanamivir-treated children resumed normal activities 1 day sooner than did placebo recipients and used less relief medication than did placebo recipients. Adverse events occurred with comparable frequency in treated patients and controls. The drug is effective against both influenza A and B, and no resistant viruses were detected with treatment. The inhaled route of administration results in delivery of drug to the site of infection but limits utility in young children unable to use the inhaler and may not be tolerated by persons with reactive airway disease.

An oral NA inhibitor, oseltamivir, is efficacious for treatment of both influenza A and B in children down to age 1 year.[275] In children given a dose of 2 mg/kg twice daily for 5 days starting early in the illness, the resolution of influenza was accelerated by 1.5 days compared with controls. The duration of viral shedding and the quantity of virus in respiratory secretions were significantly decreased in treated children. The incidence of acute otitis media was reduced by 44 percent in the treated children, a medically significant benefit that was reflected in decreased use of antibiotics. The frequency of vomiting in treated children was 5 percent in excess of that in placebo recipients but usually did not result in cessation of therapy. Nausea was reduced by administration with food. Viral isolates with higher than pretreatment values for 50 percent inhibitory concentration for NA inhibition were detected in 5.5 percent of oseltamivir-treated children with influenza A infection; no increased resistance was found for influenza B isolates. The clinical significance of this observation is unknown; resistant strains have been less virulent and less transmissible in laboratory studies.

The broad-spectrum antiviral agent ribavirin has been used successfully in the treatment of both influenza A and B in adult patients when it was administered as an aerosol.[150, 152, 174, 279] Experience with this treatment modality in children is mainly limited to other viruses but has resulted in no significant adverse reactions.[82, 108, 177, 229]

Prognosis

The prognosis for clinical recovery from uncomplicated influenza generally is considered to be excellent. Of the complications of influenza, primary influenza pneumonia, staphylococcal pneumonia, and Reye syndrome have a guarded prognosis. However, a bewildering array of chronic pulmonary conditions has been noted to begin with undifferentiated childhood respiratory tract infections, among which "influenza" often is cited but infrequently proved.[157, 239] These conditions include lobar atelectasis; localized and generalized bronchiectasis; and such clinicopathologic entities as Swyer-James syndrome (unilateral hyperlucent lung), bronchiolitis obliterans, Hamman-Rich syndrome (diffuse interstitial pneumonia), and desquamative interstitial pneumonitis. Only precise virologic diagnosis of acute respiratory tract disease, especially viral pneumonia, will delineate the long-term complications that may occur in a small proportion of cases.

Prevention

Immunization offers the best hope for prevention of influenza. Yet epidemiologic, technologic, pharmacologic, logistic, and political difficulties have hampered widespread implementation of such programs, as witnessed by the storm of controversy that greeted the A/New Jersey/76 "swine flu" vaccine campaign of 1976.[233] Prediction of the epidemic potential of new influenza virus variants is a major difficulty. To be effective, vaccines must contain antigens similar to those of the prevalent influenza viruses. In years when a new variant arises and causes widespread outbreaks, the available vaccine may contain an earlier variant with only modest heterologous immunizing potential. Conversely, in years in which new variants do not arise, vaccines may be formulated ideally but the epidemic potential of virus strains that have already circulated may be diminished, although this is not always true. The A/Sydney (H3N2) variant that predominated from 1997 to 2000 produced severe epidemics for three consecutive seasons. Thus, prevention of epidemics through the use of inactivated vaccines has been difficult.

Only inactivated (formalin-treated) influenza vaccines currently are licensed for use in the United States. Many improvements have been made in these vaccines since their introduction in the late 1930s.[180, 235] These innovations have included enhanced vaccine production by use of high-yield reassortant viruses that grow rapidly in eggs,[209] exclusion of host antigens and other toxic impurities by zonal ultracentrifugation (current "whole-virus" vaccines),[188] disruption of viral particles with ether or detergents (current "split-product" vaccines),[47] and, most recently, physical purification of HA and NA (HANA or "subunit" vaccines).[160]

The antigenicity and reactogenicity of whole-virus and split-product vaccines were studied extensively in children during the trials of A/New Jersey/76 (H1N1) monovalent and A/New Jersey/76 (H1N1)–A/Victoria/75 (H3N2) bivalent vaccines in 1976.[282] Whole-virus vaccines were more immunogenic and, at the same time, more reactogenic than were split-product vaccines because they contained a greater concentration of antigens. In two-dose regimens, the split-product vaccines produced adequate antibody levels without acute reactions. The A/Victoria/75 component of the bivalent vaccines had significantly greater immunogenicity than did the A/New Jersey/76 component in children, which reflects previous priming by H3N2 viral strains but a lack of previous exposure to H1N1-like viruses. The consensus of these studies was that split-product vaccines, by virtue of their minimal reactogenicity, should be preferred for vaccination of children. Similar large-scale trials evaluating monovalent A/USSR/77 (H1N1) and trivalent A/USSR/77 (H1N1), A/Texas/77 (H3N2), and B/Hong Kong/72 inactivated influenza virus vaccines were in agreement with previous results.[284] However, proof of protective efficacy, which with whole-virus vaccines has ranged from 50 to 95 percent after homologous challenge,[146] is comparable for split-product vaccines,[41, 102, 217, 223] even against antigenic drift virus strains.[35, 217] Gruber and associates[104] have reported a protective rate of 60 percent with B/USSR/83 vaccine against the next variant, B/Ann Arbor/86.

The side effects of vaccination with inactivated vaccines in children deserve further comment. Reactions to whole-virus vaccines, when they occur, include fever, "flu-like" symptoms of malaise and myalgia, and local tenderness at the site of inoculation.[282] In the past, febrile convulsions were cited as a particular risk of vaccination in the very young.[172, 281] In the large trials cited, however, 813 children aged 6 months to 5 years received varying doses of whole-virus and split-product vaccines.[102, 282] None of these children had febrile convulsions. During the 1978 trials with subunit vaccines, standardized for HA content, local and systemic reactions were minimal in high-risk children.[284] Therefore, current subunit inactivated influenza vaccines are minimally reactogenic and well tolerated.

Guillain-Barré syndrome occurred in roughly 1 in 100,000 older adult recipients of the A/New Jersey/76 vaccine in the National Influenza Immunization Program.[234, 240] The incidence of this complication among pediatric vaccine recipients as well as among members of the military services who were younger than 25 years was not increased. Surveillance of subsequent years has revealed no excess occurrence of Guillain-Barré syndrome among pediatric influenza vaccine recipients.[28, 131, 137, 138] The risk of developing Guillain-Barré syndrome after acquiring natural influenza virus infection is unknown; although sporadic cases have been reported, influenza infection is not an important triggering agent for this syndrome.[273]

Other influenza vaccines remain experimental in the United States. NA-specific inactivated vaccines offer some degree of protection against severe illness, diminish virus shedding and subsequent transmission, and would be expected to be outdated less frequently by antigenic drift.[205] Addition of adjuvants to inactivated vaccines enhances the height, duration, and breadth of the antibody response they elicit.[235] Candidate live virus vaccines have employed strains spontaneously attenuated after serial passage ("spontaneous" mutants),[255] strains incapable of replication at 37°C ("temperature-sensitive" mutants),[192] and strains adapted to incubation temperatures of 25°C ("cold-adapted" mutants).[48] Live vaccines, administered intranasally, correspond most closely to natural infection in their capacity to produce both secretory and humoral immunity. The most promising ones are the cold-adapted reassortment influenza virus vaccines.[11, 12, 48] These vaccines have been administered to adults and children; both local and systemic antibody responses resulted with no significant side effects.[26, 32, 195, 283, 288] They also have been shown to be safe and nontransmissible in both of these populations and result in protection against challenge with wild influenza virus.[26, 29, 33, 197, 283]

Live attenuated, cold-adapted vaccines administered by nasal spray appear to be the most promising new approach.[166] Trivalent preparations administered to children 15 months to 6 years of age have produced 93 percent protection against culture-positive illness.[12] In the follow-up year, the A/Wuhan (H3N2) vaccine strain provided 86 percent protection against the new variant, A/Sydney (H3N2).[11] The vaccine is well tolerated and accepted by children. Attributable reactions were limited to a mild rhinitis for 9 percent and low-grade fever for 5 percent on day 2 for first-time recipients. No reactions were discernible with subsequent doses.

Vaccination of normal children, who have the highest attack rates during epidemics, has not been advocated routinely in the United States, except for household contacts of high-risk patients.[84] The risk of hospitalization for children younger than 3 years is as high as that for elderly persons,[134, 200] and unlike the elderly, less than 20 percent of young hospitalized children have a chronic underlying condition.[215] Because children are the most important population group in the propagation of epidemics, a vaccine strategy aimed at epidemic prevention would necessarily be focused on this age group. Supporting this concept, mass vaccination of schoolchildren had a measurable effect on the overall incidence of A/HK/68 in Tecumseh, Michigan, during the 1968 epidemic.[186] The protective effect was most evident in adults 20 to 30 years of age, which suggests that immunization of children lowered the incidence of influenza in their parents.

Proof of the concept of indirect protection afforded by childhood immunization is the Japanese program for universal vaccination of schoolchildren.[226] Japanese schoolchildren were required to have two doses of inactivated influenza vaccine for school attendance for many years—particularly during the decade between 1977 and 1987. As many as 80 percent of children aged 9 to 15 years were immunized annually. The program declined when the requirement was relaxed in 1987, and the program was stopped in 1994. Subsequently, total excess mortality has increased remarkably. In retrospect, definite flattening of the mortality curve during the program occurred in contrast to sharp seasonal peaks of mortality rates coinciding with influenza epidemics before and after the program. The only exception was seen in 1975–1976, when a new variant, A/Victoria (H3N2), appeared unexpectedly and produced a severe epidemic; the previous variant, A/Port Chalmers (H3N2), provided no cross-protection against A/Victoria. The immunization of schoolchildren in Japan is estimated to have saved 37,000 to 45,000 lives each year. Vaccine was not recommended for elderly or high-risk persons whose lives were spared; the reduction in mortality rates resulted from the indirect effect of immunizing schoolchildren.

Universal immunization of children in school or daycare not only would reduce significantly serious morbidity in this age group but also would have the potential for dampening epidemics and reducing risk of exposure to virus for vulnerable high-risk patients.[85] The cold-adapted attenuated vaccine developed by Maassab has broader and longer lasting immunity for children younger than 10 years.[35, 217] The administration by nasal spray is accepted better by children and easier to administer than is the inactivated vaccine given by injection. The cold-adapted vaccine is being tested in children as an approach to epidemic control.[166]

Universal immunization of children in the United States would not replace but supplement the current vaccination strategy, focused on the prevention of complicated illness in population groups at highest risk of dying or requiring hospitalization during epidemics. Also given priority for vaccine are women in the later stages of pregnancy as well as health care providers and household contacts (including children) of high-risk patients.[28] In addition, vaccination of children with various illnesses requiring long-term salicylate therapy (e.g., Kawasaki disease, juvenile rheumatoid arthritis) is recommended. Experience has proved that appropriate doses of inactivated vaccines in children older than 6 months can produce acceptable levels of antibody with minimal side effects. Furthermore, vaccination of pregnant women in the second or third trimester of pregnancy will not only reduce their risk of needing hospitalization for pneumonia but will boost the amount of protective antibodies transmitted to their newborn infants and reduce the occurrence of serious infections in the first 6 months of life.[100, 222] Early specific treatment of influenza-infected children with appropriate antiviral drugs will not only shorten the course of illness but also reduce virus in respiratory secretions.[275] This effect should allow reduction in transmission of virus to contacts—another effort to contain this venerable foe.

REFERENCES

1. Alford, R. M., Kasel, J. A., Gerone, P. J., et al.: Human influenza resulting from aerosol inhalation. Proc. Soc. Exp. Biol. Med. *122*:800–804, 1966.
2. Arrowsmith, J. B., Kennedy, D. L., Kuritsky, J. N., et al.: National patterns of aspirin use and Reye syndrome reporting, United States, 1980 to 1985. Pediatrics *79*:858–863, 1987.
3. Atmar, R. L., Baxter B. D., Dominguez, E. A., et al.: Comparison of reverse transcription–PCR with tissue culture and other rapid diagnostic assays for detection of type A influenza virus. J. Clin. Microbiol. *34*:2604–2606, 1996.
4. Barrett, M. J., Hurwitz, E. S., Schonberger, L. B., et al.: Changing epidemiology of Reye syndrome in the United States. Pediatrics *77*:598–602, 1986.
5. Barton, L. L., and Chalhub, E. G.: Myositis associated with influenza A infection. J. Pediatr. *87*:1003–1004, 1975.
6. Bauer, C. K., Elie, K., Spence, L., et al.: Hong Kong influenza in a neonatal unit. J. A. M. A. *223*:1233–1235, 1973.
7. Baxter, B. D., Couch, R. B., Greenberg, S. B., et al.: Maintenance of viability and comparison of identification methods for influenza and other respiratory viruses of humans. J. Clin. Microbiol. *6*:19–22, 1977.
8. Bell, W. E., McKee, A. P., and Utterback, R. A.: Asian influenza virus as the cause of acute encephalitis. Neurology *8*:500–502, 1958.
9. Belshe, R. B.: A review of attenuation of influenza viruses by genetic manipulation. Am. J. Respir. Crit. Care Med. *152*:S72–S75, 1995.
10. Belshe, R. B., Burk, B., Newman, F., et al.: Resistance of influenza A virus to amantadine and rimantadine: Results of one decade of surveillance. J. Infect. Dis. *159*:430–435, 1989.
11. Belshe, R. B., Gruber, W. C., Mendelman, P. M., et al.: Efficacy of vaccination with live attenuated, cold-adapted, trivalent, intranasal influenza virus vaccine against a variant (A/Sydney) not contained in the vaccine. J. Pediatr. *136*:168–175, 2000.
12. Belshe, R. B., Mendelman, P. M., Treanor, J., et al.: The efficacy of live attenuated, cold-adapted, trivalent, intranasal influenzavirus vaccine in children. N. Engl. J. Med. *338*:1405–1412, 1998.
13. Belshe, R. B., Smith, M. H., Hall, C. B., et al.: Genetic basis of resistance to rimantadine emerging during treatment of influenza virus infection. J. Virol. *62*:1508–1512, 1988.
14. Berg, R. A., Yolken, R. H., Rennard, S. I., et al.: New enzyme immunoassays for measurement of influenza A/Victoria/3/75 virus in nasal washes. Lancet *2*:851–853, 1980.
15. Biddison, W. E., Shaw, S., and Nelson, D. L.: Virus specificity of human influenza virus immune cytotoxic T cells. J. Immunol. *122*:660–664, 1979.
16. Bishai, F. R., and Galli, R.: Enzyme-linked immunosorbent assay for detection of antibodies to influenza A and B and parainfluenza type 1 in sera of patients. J. Clin. Microbiol. *8*:648–656, 1978.
17. Blass, D., Patzelt, E., and Kuechler, E.: Identification of the cap binding protein of influenza virus. Nucleic Acids Res. *10*:4803–4812, 1982.
18. Blass, D., Patzelt, E., and Kuechler, E.: Cap recognizing protein of influenza virus. Virology *116*:339–348, 1982.
19. Blumenfeld, L., II, Kilbourne, E. D., Louria, D. B., et al.: Studies on influenza in the pandemic of 1957–1958. I. An investigation of an intrahospital epidemic, with a note on vaccine efficacy. J. Clin. Invest. *38*:199–212, 1959.
20. Braciale, T. J.: Immunologic recognition of influenza-infected cells. 1. Generation of virus strain specific and cross-reactive subpopulations of cytotoxic T cells in response to type A influenza virus infection of different subtypes. Cell. Immunol. *33*:423–426, 1977.
21. Brain, W. R., Hunter, D., and Turnball, H. M.: Acute meningoencephalitis of childhood. Lancet *1*:221–227, 1929.
22. Brill, S. J., and Gilfillan, R. F.: Acute parotitis associated with influenza type A. N. Engl. J. Med. *296*:1391–1392, 1977.
23. Brocklebank, J. T., Coust, S. D. M., McQuillan, J., et al.: Influenza A infections in children. Lancet *2*:497–500, 1972.
24. Brown, P., Gajdusek, D. C., and Morris, J. A.: Epidemic A_2 influenza in isolated Pacific Island populations without pre-epidemic antibody to influenza types A and B, and the discovery of other still unexposed populations. Am. J. Epidemiol. *83*:176–188, 1966.
25. Carey, D. E., Dunn, F. L., Robinson, R. Q., et al.: Community-wide epidemic of Asian strain influenza: Clinical and subclinical illnesses among school children. J. A. M. A. *167*:1459–1463, 1958.
26. Cate, T. R., and Couch, R. B.: Live influenza A/Victoria/75 (H3N2) virus vaccines: Reactogenicity, immunogenicity, and protection against wild-type virus challenge. Infect. Immun. *38*:141–146, 1982.
27. Caul, E. O., Waller, D. K., Clarke, S. K. R., et al.: A comparison of influenza and respiratory syncytial virus infections among infants admitted to hospital with acute respiratory infections. J. Hyg. (Camb.) *77*:383–392, 1976.
28. Centers for Disease Control and Prevention: Prevention and Control of Influenza. M. M. W. R. *49*(RR-3):1–38, 2000.
29. Chanock, R. M., and Murphy, B. R.: Use of temperature-sensitive and cold-adapted mutant viruses in immunoprophylaxis of acute respiratory tract disease. Rev. Infect. Dis. *2*:421–432, 1980.
30. Chin, T. D. Y., Mosley, W. H., Poland, J. D., et al.: Epidemiologic studies of type B influenza in 1961–1962. Am. J. Public Health *53*:1068–1074, 1963.
31. Christenson, J. C., and San Joaquin, V. H.: Influenza-associated rhabdomyolysis in a child. Pediatr. Infect. Dis. J. *9*:60–61, 1990.
32. Clements, M. L., O'Donnell, S., Levine, M. M., et al.: Dose response of A/Alaska/6/77 (H3N2) cold-adapted reassortant vaccine virus in adult volunteers: Role of local antibody in resistance to infection with vaccine. Infect. Immun. *40*:1044–1051, 1983.
33. Clements, M. L., Betts, R. F., and Murphy, B. R.: Advantage of live attenuated cold-adapted influenza A virus over inactivated vaccine for A/Washington/80 (H3N2) wild-type virus infection. Lancet *1*:705–708, 1984.
34. Clover, R. D., Crawford, S. A., Abell, T. D., et al.: Effectiveness of rimantadine prophylaxis of children in families. Am. J. Dis. Child. *140*:706–709, 1986.
35. Clover, R. D., Crawford, S., Glezen, W. P., et al.: Comparison of heterotypic protection against influenza A/Taiwan/86 (H1N1) by attenuated and inactivated vaccines to A/Chile/83-like viruses. J. Infect. Dis. *163*:300–304, 1991.
36. Coltman, C. A., Jr.: Influenza myocarditis. Report of a case with observations on serum glutamic oxaloacetic transaminase. J. A. M. A. *180*:204–208, 1962.
37. Corey, L., Rubin, R. J., and Hattwick, M.: A nationwide outbreak of Reye's syndrome: Its epidemiologic relationship to influenza B. Am. J. Med. *61*:615–626, 1976.
38. Corey, L., Rubin, R. J., Bregman, D., et al.: Diagnostic criteria for influenza B–associated Reye's syndrome: Clinical vs. pathologic criteria. Pediatrics *60*:702–714, 1977.
39. Corey, L., Rubin, R. J., Thompson, T. R., et al.: Influenza B–associated Reye's syndrome: Incidence in Michigan and potential for prevention. J. Infect. Dis. *135*:398–407, 1977.
40. Couch, R. B.: Prevention and treatment of influenza. N. Engl. J. Med. *343*:1778–1787, 2000.
41. Couch, R. B., Douglas, R. G., Fedson, D. S., et al.: Correlated studies of a recombinant influenza-virus vaccine. III. Protection against experimental influenza in man. J. Infect. Dis. *124*:473–480, 1971.
42. Couch, R. B., Douglas, R. G., Rossen, R., et al.: Role of secretory antibody in influenza. *In* The Secretory Immunologic System. Washington, D.C., U.S. Department of Health, Education and Welfare, 1969, pp. 93–112.
43. Couch, R. B., Kasel, J. A., Glezen, W. P., et al.: Influenza: Its control in persons and populations. J. Infect. Dis. *153*:431–440, 1986.
44. Craver, R. D., Sorrells, K., and Gohd, R.: Myocarditis with influenza B infection. Pediatr. Infect. Dis. J. *16*:629–630, 1997.
45. Crawford, S. A., Clover, R. D., Abell, T. D., et al.: Rimantadine prophylaxis in children: A follow-up study. Pediatr. Infect. Dis. J. *7*:379–383, 1988.
46. Crosby, A. W.: Epidemic and Peace, 1918. Westport, CT, Greenwood Press, 1976.
47. Davenport, F. M., Hennessy, A. V., Brandon, F. M., et al.: Comparisons of serologic and febrile responses in humans to vaccination with influenza A viruses or their hemagglutinins. J. Lab. Clin. Med. *63*:5–13, 1964.
48. Davenport, F. M., Hennessy, A. V., Maassab, H. F., et al.: Pilot studies on recombinant cold-adapted live type A and B influenza virus vaccines. J. Infect. Dis. *136*:17–25, 1977.
49. Davis, L. E., Caldwell, G. G., Lynch, R. E., et al.: Hong Kong influenza: The epidemiologic features of a high school family study analyzed and compared with a similar study during the 1957 Asian influenza epidemic. Am. J. Epidemiol. *92*:240–247, 1970.
50. Delorme, L., and Middleton, P. J.: Influenza A virus associated with acute encephalopathy. Am. J. Dis. Child. *133*:822–824, 1979.
51. DiBona, F. J., and Morens, D. M.: Rhabdomyolysis associated with influenza A: Report of a case with unusual fluid and electrolyte abnormalities. J. Pediatr. *91*:943–945, 1977.
52. Dietzman, D. E., Schaller, J. G., Ray, C. G., et al.: Acute myositis associated with influenza B infection. Pediatrics *57*:255–258, 1976.
53. Dolin, R., Murphy, B. R., and Caplan, E. A.: Lymphocyte blastogenic responses to influenza virus antigens after influenza infection and vaccination in humans. Infect. Immun. *19*:867–874, 1978.
54. Dolin, R., Richman, D. D., Murphy, B. R., et al.: Cell-mediated immune responses following induced influenza in humans. J. Infect. Dis. *177*:714–719, 1977.

55. Dominguez, E. A., Taber, L. H., and Couch, R. B.: Comparison of rapid diagnostic techniques for respiratory syncytial and influenza A virus respiratory infections in young children. J. Clin. Microbiol. *31*:2286–2290, 1993.
56. Douglas, R. G., Jr., Alford, R. H., Cate, T. K., et al.: The leukocyte response during viral respiratory illness in man. Ann. Intern. Med. *64*:521–530, 1966.
57. Dowdle, W. A., Kendal, A. P., and Noble, G. R.: Influenza viruses. *In* Lennette, E. H., and Schmidt, N. J. (eds.): Diagnostic Procedures for Viral, Rickettsial and Chlamydial Infections. Washington, D.C., American Public Health Association, 1979, p. 593.
58. Downham, M. A. P. S., Gardner, P. S., McQuillin, J., et al.: Role of respiratory viruses in childhood mortality. Br. Med. J. *1*:235–239, 1975.
59. Downie, J. C., and Stuart-Harris, C. H.: The production of neutralizing activity in serum and nasal secretion following immunization with influenza B virus. J. Hyg. *68*:233–244, 1970.
60. Dykes, A. C., Cherry, J. D., and Nolan, C. E.: A clinical, epidemiologic, serologic, and virologic study of influenza C virus infection. Arch. Intern. Med. *140*:1295–1298, 1980.
61. Effros, R. B., Doherty, P. C., Gerhard, W. E., et al.: Generation of both cross-reactive and virus specific cytotoxic T cell population after immunization with serologically distinct influenza A viruses. J. Exp. Med. *145*:557–558, 1977.
62. Eller, J. J., Fulginiti, V. A., Plunket, D. C., et al.: Attack rates for hospitalized croup in children in a military population: Importance of A_2 influenza infection. Pediatr. Res. *6*:386, 1972.
63. Ennis, F. A., Martin, W. J., Verbonitz, M. W., et al.: Specificity studies on cytotoxic thymus-derived lymphocytes reactive with influenza virus–infected cells: Evidence for dual recognition of H-2 and viral hemagglutinin antigens. Proc. Natl. Acad. Sci. U. S. A. *74*:3006–3010, 1977.
64. Fan, J., Hendrickson, K. J., and Savatski, L. L.: Rapid simultaneous diagnosis of infection with respiratory syncytial viruses A and B, influenza viruses A and B, and human parainfluenza virus types 1, 2, and 3 by multiplex quantitative reverse transcription–polymerase chain reaction–enzyme hybridization assay (Hexaplex). Clin. Infect. Dis. *26*:1397–1402, 1998.
65. Fernandez, H.: Low serum iron in influenza. N. Engl. J. Med. *302*:865, 1980.
66. Finland, M., Strauss, E., and Peterson, O. L.: Staphylococcal pneumonia occurring during an epidemic of clinical influenza. Trans. Assoc. Am. Physicians *56*:139–146, 1941.
67. Fishaut, M., and Mostow, S. R.: Amantadine for severe influenza A pneumonia in infancy. Am. J. Dis. Child. *134*:321–322, 1980.
68. Foy, H. M., Cooney, M. K., Maletzky, A. J., et al.: Incidence and etiology of pneumonia, croup and bronchiolitis in preschool children belonging to a prepaid medical care group over a four-year period. Am. J. Epidemiol. *97*:80–92, 1973.
69. Foy, H. M., Cooney, M. K., McMahan, R., et al.: Viral and mycoplasmal pneumonia in a prepaid medical care group during an eight-year period. Am. J. Epidemiol. *97*:93–102, 1973.
70. Foy, H. M., Cooney, M. K., Allan, I., et al.: Rates of pneumonia during influenza epidemics in Seattle, 1964–1975. J. A. M. A. *241*:253–258, 1979.
71. Fox, J. P., Hall, C. E., Cooney, M. K., et al.: Influenza virus infections in Seattle families, 1975–1979. Am. J. Epidemiol. *116*:212–227, 1982.
72. Francis, T., Davenport, F. M., and Hennessy, A. V.: A serological recapitulation of human infection with different strains of influenza virus. Trans. Assoc. Am. Physicians *66*:231–239, 1953.
73. Frank, A. L., Couch, R. B., Griffis, C. A., et al.: Comparison of different tissue cultures for isolation and quantitation of influenza and parainfluenza viruses. J. Clin. Microbiol. *10*:32–36, 1979.
74. Frank, A. L., Puck, J., Hughes, B. J., et al.: Microneutralization test for influenza A and B and parainfluenza 1 and 2 viruses that uses continuous cell lines and fresh serum enhancement. J. Clin. Microbiol. *12*:426–432, 1980.
75. Frank, A. L., Taber, L. H., Glezen, W. P., et al.: Reinfection with influenza A (H3N2) virus in young children and their families. J. Infect. Dis. *140*:829–836, 1979.
76. Frank, A. L., Taber, L. H., and Porter, C. M.: Influenza B virus reinfection. Am J. Epidemiol. *125*:576–586, 1987.
77. Frank, A. L., Taber, L. H., Wells, C. R., et al.: Patterns of shedding of myxoviruses and paramyxoviruses in children. J. Infect. Dis. *144*:433–441, 1981.
78. Frank, A. L., and Taber, L. H.: Variation in frequency of natural reinfection with influenza A viruses. J. Med. Virol. *12*:17–23, 1983.
79. Fritz, R. S., Hayden, F. G., Calfee, D. P., et al.: Nasal cytokine and chemokine responses in experimental influenza A virus infection: Results of a placebo-controlled trial of intravenous zanamivir treatment. J. Infect. Dis. *180*:586–593, 1999.
80. Fujimoto, Y., Shibata, M., Tsuyuki, M., et al.: Influenza A virus encephalopathy with symmetrical thalamic lesions. Eur. J. Pediatr. *159*:319–321, 2000.
81. Garcia-Sastre, A., Egorov, A., Matassov, D., et al.: Influenza A virus lacking the NS1 gene replicates in interferon-deficient systems. Virology *252*:324–330, 1998.
82. Gelfand, E. W., McCurdy, D., Rao, C. R., et al.: Treatment of viral pneumonitis with ribavirin in severe-combined immunodeficiency disease. Lancet *2*:732–733, 1983.
83. Glezen, W. P.: The common cold. *In* Gorbach, S. L., Bartlett, J. G., and Blacklow, N. R. (eds.): Infectious Diseases. 2nd ed. Philadelphia, W. B. Saunders, 1998, pp. 548–553.
84. Glezen, W. P.: Consideration of the risk of influenza in children and indications for prophylaxis. Rev. Infect. Dis. *2*:408–420, 1980.
85. Glezen, W. P.: Emerging infections: Pandemic influenza. Epidemiol. Rev. *18*:64–76, 1996.
86. Glezen, W. P.: Prevention of acute otitis media by prophylaxis and treatment of influenza virus infections. Vaccine *19*:S56–S58, 2001.
87. Glezen, W. P.: Influenza control—unfinished business. J. A. M. A. *281*:944–945, 1999.
88. Glezen, W. P.: Serious morbidity and mortality associated with influenza epidemics. Epidemiol. Rev. *4*:25–44, 1982.
89. Glezen, W. P.: Reactive airway disorders in children: Role of respiratory viruses. Clin. Chest Med. *5*:635–643, 1984.
90. Glezen, W. P., and Couch, R. B.: Interpandemic influenza in the Houston area, 1974–76. N. Engl. J. Med. *298*:587–592, 1978.
91. Glezen, W. P., and Couch, R. B.: Influenza viruses. *In* Evans, A. S., and Kaslow, R. A. (eds.): Viral Infections of Humans: Epidemiology and Control. 4th ed. New York, Plenum Medical, 1997, pp. 473–505.
92. Glezen, W. P., Couch, R. B., Taber, L. H., et al.: Epidemiologic observations of influenza B virus infections in Houston, Texas, 1976–1977. Am. J. Epidemiol. *111*:13–22, 1980.
93. Glezen, W. P., Decker, M., Joseph, S. W., et al.: Acute respiratory disease associated with influenza epidemics in Houston, 1982–1983. J. Infect. Dis. *155*:1119–1126, 1987.
94. Glezen, W. P., and Denny, F. W.: Epidemiology of acute lower respiratory disease in children. N. Engl. J. Med. *288*:498–505, 1973.
95. Glezen, W. P., Greenberg, S. B., Atmar, R. L., et al.: Impact of respiratory virus infections on persons with chronic underlying conditions. J. A. M. A. *283*:499–505, 2000.
96. Glezen, W. P., Keitel, W. A., Taber, L. H., et al.: Age distribution of patients with medically-attended illnesses caused by sequential variants of influenza A/H1N1: Comparison of age-specific infection rates, 1978–1989. Am. J. Epidemiol. *133*:296–304, 1991.
97. Glezen, W. P., Loda, F. A., Clyde, W. A., Jr., et al.: Epidemiologic patterns of acute lower respiratory disease of children in a pediatric group practice. J. Pediatr. *78*:397–406, 1971.
98. Glezen, W. P., Paredes, A., and Taber, L. H.: Influenza in children related to other respiratory agents. J. A. M. A. *243*:1345–1349, 1980.
99. Glezen, W. P., Payne, A. A., Snyder, D. N., et al.: Mortality and influenza. J. Infect. Dis. *146*:313–321, 1982.
100. Glezen, W. P., Taber, L. H., Frank, A. L., et al.: Influenza virus infections in infants. Pediatr. Infect. Dis. J. *16*:1065–1068, 1997.
101. Greenberg, S. B., Criswell, B. S., and Couch, R. B.: Lymphocyte cytotoxicity to influenza virus–infected cells: Response to vaccination and virus infection. Infect. Immun. *20*:640–645, 1978.
102. Gross, P. A.: Reactogenicity and immunogenicity of bivalent influenza vaccine in one- and two-dose trials in children: A summary. J. Infect. Dis. *136*:S616–S625, 1977.
103. Gross, P. A., Quinnan, G. V., Gaerlaw, P. F., et al.: Influenza vaccines in children: Comparison of a new cetrimonium bromide and standard ether-treated vaccines. Am. J. Dis. Child. *137*:26–28, 1983.
104. Gruber, W. C., Taber, L. H., Glezen, W. P., et al.: Live attenuated and inactivated influenza vaccine in school-age children. Am. J. Dis. Child. *144*:595–600, 1990.
105. Hall, C. G., Dolin, R., Gala, C. L., et al.: Children with influenza A infection: Treatment with rimantadine. Pediatrics *80*:275–282, 1987.
106. Hall, C. B., and Douglas, R. G., Jr.: Nosocomial influenza infection as a cause of intercurrent fevers in infants. Pediatrics *55*:673–677, 1975.
107. Hall, C. B., and Douglas, R. S.: Respiratory syncytial virus and influenza: Practical community surveillance. Am. J. Dis. Child. *130*:615–620, 1976.
108. Hall, C. B., McBride, J. T., Walsh, E. E., et al.: Aerosolized ribavirin treatment of infants with respiratory syncytial viral infections. N. Engl. J. Med. *308*:1443–1447, 1983.
109. Hall, C. E., Cooney, M. K., and Fox, J. P.: The Seattle virus watch. IV. Comparative epidemiologic observations of infections with influenza A and B viruses, 1965–69, in families with young children. Am. J. Epidemiol. *98*:365–380, 1973.
110. Hall, W. J., Douglas, R. G., Jr., Hyde, R. W., et al.: Pulmonary mechanics during uncomplicated influenza A infection. Am. Rev. Respir. Dis. *113*:141–153, 1976.
111. Hall, W. N., Goodman, R. A., Noble, G. R., et al.: An outbreak of influenza B in an elderly population. J. Infect. Dis. *144*:297–302, 1981.
112. Halpin, T. J., Holtzhauer, F. J., Campbell, R. J., et al.: Reye's syndrome and medication use. J. A. M. A. *248*:687–691, 1982.
113. Halsey, N. A., Hurwitz, E. S., Meiklejohn, G., et al.: An epidemic of Reye syndrome associated with influenza A (H1N1) in Colorado. J. Pediatr. *97*:535–539, 1980.
114. Harmon, M. W., and Pawlik, K. M.: Enzyme immunoassay for direct detection of influenza type A and adenovirus antigens in clinical specimens. J. Clin. Microbiol. *15*:5–11, 1982.

115. Hayden, F. G., Belshe, R. B., Clover, R. D., et al.: Emergence and apparent transmission of rimantadine-resistant influenza A virus in families. N. Engl. J. Med. *321*:1696–1702, 1989.
116. Hayden, F. G., Fritz, R. S., Lobo, M. C., et al.: Local and systemic cytokine responses during experimental human influenza A virus infection. J. Clin. Invest. *101*:643–649, 1998.
117. Hedrick, J. A., Barzilai, A., Behre, U., et al.: Zanamivir for treatment of symptomatic influenza A and B infection in children five to twelve years of age: A randomized controlled trial. Pediatr. Infect. Dis. J. *19*:410–417, 2000.
118. Henderson, F. W., Collier, A. M., Sanyal, M. A., et al.: A longitudinal study of respiratory viruses and bacteria in the etiology of acute otitis media with effusion. N. Engl. J. Med. *306*:1377–1383, 1982.
119. Hers, J. F. P.: Disturbances of the ciliated epithelium due to influenza virus. Am. Rev. Respir. Dis. *93*:162–171, 1966.
120. Hers, J. F. P., Masurel, N., and Mulder, J.: Bacteriology and histopathology of the respiratory tract and lungs in fatal Asian influenza. Lancet *2*:1141–1143, 1958.
121. Hirsch, A.: *In* Creighton, C. (ed.): Handbook of Geographical and Historical Pathology. Vol. 1. London, New Sydenham Society, 1883, pp. 7–17.
122. Hirst, G. K.: Genetic recombination with Newcastle disease virus, polioviruses, and influenza. Cold Spring Harbor Symp. Quant. Biol. *27*:303–308, 1962.
123. Hobson, D., Curry, R. L., Beare, A. S., et al.: The role of serum hemagglutination-inhibiting antibody in protection against challenge infection with influenza A2 and B viruses. J. Hyg. *70*:767–777, 1972.
124. Hochberg, F. H., Nelson, K., and Janzen, W.: Influenza type B–related encephalopathy. The 1971 outbreak of Reye syndrome in Chicago. J. A. M. A. *231*:817–821, 1975.
125. Holzel, A., Parker, L., Patterson, W. H., et al.: Virus isolations from throats of children admitted to hospital with respiratory and other diseases, Manchester 1962–4. B. M. J. *1*:614–619, 1965.
126. Horimoto, T., and Kawaoka, Y.: Pandemic threat posed by avian influenza A viruses. Clin. Microbiol. Rev. *14*:129–149, 2001.
127. Horisberger, M. A.: The large P proteins of influenza A viruses are composed of one acidic and two basic polypeptides. Virology *107*:302–305, 1980.
128. Horn, M. E. C., Brain, E., Gregg, I., et al.: Respiratory viral infection in childhood: A survey in general practice, Roehampton 1967–1972. J. Hyg. (Camb.) *74*:157–168, 1975.
129. Howard, J. B., McCracken, G. H., and Luby, J. P.: Influenza A_2 virus as a cause of croup requiring tracheostomy. J. Pediatr. *81*:1148–1149, 1972.
130. Hurwitz, E. S., Barrett, M. J., and Bregman, D.: Public Health Service study of Reye's syndrome and medication: Report of the main study. J. A. M. A. *257*:1905–1911, 1987.
131. Hurwitz, E. S., Holman, R. C., Nelson, D. B., et al.: National surveillance for Guillain-Barré syndrome, January 1978–March 1979. Neurology *33*:150–157, 1983.
132. Hurwitz, E. S., Nelson, D. B., Davis, C., et al.: National surveillance for Reye syndrome: A five year review. Pediatrics *70*:895–900, 1982.
133. Ito, Y., Ichiyama, T., Kimura, H., et al.: Detection of influenza virus RNA by reverse transcription–PCR and proinflammatory cytokines in influenza-virus-associated encephalopathy. J. Med. Virol. *58*:420–425, 1999.
134. Izurieta, H. S., Thompson, W. W., Kramarz, P., et al.: Influenza and the rates of hospitalization for respiratory disease among infants and young children. N. Engl. J. Med. *342*:232–239, 2000.
135. Jordan, W. S., Denny, F. W., Badger, G. F., et al.: A study of illness in a group of Cleveland families. XVII. The occurrence of Asian influenza. Am. J. Hyg. *68*:190–212, 1958.
136. Joshi, V. V., Escobar, M. R., Stewart, L., et al.: Fatal influenza A_2 viral pneumonia in a newborn infant. Am. J. Dis. Child. *126*:839–840, 1973.
137. Kaplan, J. E., Katona, P., Hurwitz, E. S., et al.: Guillain-Barré syndrome in the United States, 1979–80 and 1980–81: Lack of an association with influenza vaccination. J. A. M. A. *248*:698–700, 1982.
138. Kaplan, J. E., Schonberger, L. B., Hurwitz, E. S., et al.: Guillain-Barré syndrome in the United States, 1978–1981: Additional observations from the national surveillance system. Neurology *33*:633–637, 1983.
139. Kasai, T., Togashi, T., and Morishima, T.: Encephalopathy associated with influenza epidemics. Lancet *355*:1558–1559, 2000.
140. Kavet, J.: Influenza and Public Policy [doctoral thesis]. Boston, Harvard School of Public Health, 1973, p. 369.
141. Kelly, K. J., Garland, J. S., Tang, T. T., et al.: Fatal rhabdomyolysis following influenza infection in a girl with familial carnitine palmityl transferase deficiency. Pediatrics *84*:312–316, 1989.
142. Kempe, A., Hall, C. B., MacDonald, N. E., et al.: Influenza in children with cancer. J. Pediatr. *115*:33–39, 1989.
143. Kerr, A. A., Downham, M. A. P. S., McQuillin, J., et al.: Gastric flu: Influenza B causing abdominal symptoms in children. Lancet *1*:291–295, 1975.
144. Khamapirad, T., and Glezen, W. P.: Clinical and radiographic assessment of acute lower respiratory tract disease in infants and children. Semin. Respir. Infect. *2*:130–144, 1987.
145. Kilbourne, E. D.: Influenza. New York, Plenum, 1987.
146. Kilbourne, E. D., Chanock, R. M., Choppin, P. W., et al.: Influenza vaccine: Summary of influenza workshop. V. J. Infect. Dis. *129*:750–771, 1974.
147. Kim, H. W., Brandt, C. D., Arrobio, J. O., et al.: Influenza A and B virus infection in infants and young children during the years 1957–1976. Am. J. Epidemiol. *109*:464–479, 1979.
148. Kitamoto, O.: Therapeutic effectiveness of amantadine hydrochloride in influenza A2: Double blind studies. Jpn. J. Tuberc. Chest Dis. *15*:1–7, 1968.
149. Klein, J. D., Collier, A. M., and Glezen, W. P.: An influenza B epidemic among children in day care. Pediatrics *58*:340–345, 1976.
150. Knight, V., and Gilbert, B. E.: Ribavirin aerosol treatment of influenza. Infect. Dis. Clin. North Am. *1*:441–457, 1987.
151. Knight, V., and Kasel, J. A.: Influenza viruses. *In* Knight, V. (ed.): Viral and Mycoplasmal Infections of the Respiratory Tract. Philadelphia, Lea & Febiger, 1973, pp. 87–123.
152. Knight, V., McClung, H. W., Wilson, S. Z., et al.: Ribavirin small-particle aerosol treatment of influenza. Lancet *2*:945–949, 1981.
153. Kramarz, P., DeStefano, F., Gargiullo, P. M., et al.: Does influenza vaccination prevent asthma exacerbations in children? J. Pediatr. *138*:306–310, 2001.
154. Krug, R. M.: Priming of influenza viral RNA transcription by capped heterologous RNAs. Curr. Top. Microbiol. Immunol. *93*:125–150, 1981.
155. Lamb, R. A., and Krug, R. M.: *Orthomyxoviridae:* The viruses and their replication. *In* Fields, B. N., Knipe, D. M., and Howley, P. M. (eds.): Virology. 3rd ed. Philadelphia, Lippincott-Raven, 1996, pp. 1353–1395.
156. Langmuir, A. D., and Housworth, J.: A critical evaluation of influenza surveillance. Bull. World Health Organ. *41*:393–398, 1969.
157. Laraya-Cuasay, L. R., DeForest, A., Huff, D., et al.: Chronic pulmonary complications of early influenza virus infection in children. Am. Rev. Respir. Dis. *116*:617–625, 1977.
158. Laver, W. G., and Webster, R. G.: Selection of antigenic mutants of influenza viruses: Isolation and peptide mapping of their hemagglutinating proteins. Virology *34*:193–202, 1968.
159. Laver, W. G., and Webster, R. G.: Studies on the origin of pandemic influenza. II. Peptide maps of the light and heavy polypeptide chains from the hemagglutinin subunits of A2 influenza viruses isolated before and after the appearance of Hong Kong influenza. Virology *48*:445–455, 1972.
160. Laver, W. G., and Webster, R. G.: Preparation and immunogenicity of an influenza virus hemagglutinin and neuraminidase subunit vaccine. Virology *69*:511–522, 1976.
161. Linnemann, C. C., Shea, L., Kauffman, C. A., et al.: Association of Reye's syndrome with viral infection. Lancet *2*:179–182, 1974.
162. Little, J. W., Hall, W. J., Douglas, R. G., Jr., et al.: Airway hyperreactivity and peripheral airway dysfunction in influenza A infection. Am. Rev. Respir. Dis. *118*:295–303, 1978.
163. Liu, C.: Diagnosis of influenzal infection by means of fluorescent antibody staining. International Conference on Asian Influenza. Am. Rev. Respir. Dis. *83*(Suppl.):130–138, 1960.
164. Loda, F. A., Clyde, W. A., Jr., Glezen, W. P., et al.: Studies on the role of viruses, bacteria, and *M. pneumoniae* as causes of lower respiratory tract infections in children. J. Pediatr. *72*:161–176, 1968.
165. Loda, F. A., Glezen, W. P., and Clyde, W. A., Jr.: Respiratory disease in group day care. Pediatrics *49*:428–437, 1972.
166. Longini, I. M., Halloran, M. E., Nizam, A., et al.: Estimation of the efficacy of live, attenuated influenza vaccine from a two-year, multi-center vaccine trial: Implications for influenza epidemic control. Vaccine *18*:1902–1909, 2000.
167. Longini, I. M., Koopman, J. S., Monto, A. S., et al.: Estimating household and community transmission parameters for influenza. Am. J. Epidemiol. *115*:736–751, 1982.
168. Louria, D. B., Blumenfeld, H. L., Ellis, J. T., et al.: Studies on influenza in the pandemic of 1957–58. II. Pulmonary complications of influenza. J. Clin. Invest. *38*:213–265, 1959.
169. Macasaet, F. F., Kidd, P. A., Bolano, C. R., et al.: The etiology of acute respiratory infections. III. The role of viruses and bacteria. J. Pediatr. *72*:829–839, 1968.
170. MacKenzie, J. S., and Houghton, M.: Influenza infections during pregnancy: Association with congenital malformations and with subsequent neoplasms in children, and potential hazards of live virus vaccines. Bacteriol. Rev. *38*:356–370, 1974.
171. Maito, M., Soto, T., and Ischida, N.: Antigenic memory in man in response to sequential infections with influenza A viruses. J. Infect. Dis. *126*:61–68, 1972.
172. Marine, W. M., and Stuart-Harris, C.: Reactions and serologic responses in young children and infants after administration of inactivated monovalent influenza A vaccine. J. Pediatr. *88*:26–30, 1976.
173. Masurel, N., and Marine, W. M.: Recycling of Asian and Hong Kong influenza A virus hemagglutinins in man. Am. J. Epidemiol. *97*:44–49, 1973.
174. McClung, H. W., Knight, V., Gilbert, B. E., et al.: Ribavirin aerosol treatment of influenza virus B infection. J. A. M. A. *249*:2671–2674, 1983.

175. McCullers, J. A., Facchini, S., Chesney, P. J., et al.: Influenza B virus encephalitis. Clin. Infect. Dis. *28*:898–900, 1999.
176. McIntosh, K., Ellis, E. F., Hoffman, L. S., et al.: The association of viral and bacterial respiratory infections with exacerbations of wheezing in young asthmatic children. J. Pediatr. *82*:578–590, 1973.
177. McIntosh, K., Kurachek, S. C., Cairns, L. M., et al.: Treatment of respiratory syncytial viral infection in an immunodeficient infant with ribavirin aerosol. Am. J. Dis. Child. *138*:305–308, 1984.
178. Meibalane, R., Sedinak, G. V., Sasidharan, P., et al.: Outbreak of influenza in a neonatal intensive care unit. J. Pediatr. *91*:974–976, 1977.
179. Mellman, W. J.: Influenza encephalitis. J. Pediatr. *53*:292, 1958.
180. Meyer, H. M., Hopps, H. E., Parkman, P. D., et al.: Review of existing vaccines for influenza. Am. J. Clin. Pathol. *70*:146–151, 1978.
181. Middleton, P. J., Alexander, R. M., and Szymonski, M. T.: Severe myositis during recovery from influenza. Lancet *2*:533–535, 1970.
182. Minor, T. E., Dick, E. C., Baker, J. W., et al.: Rhinovirus and influenza type A infections as precipitants of asthma. Am. Rev. Respir. Dis. *113*:149–153, 1976.
183. Minor, T. E., Dick, E. C., DeMeo, A. N., et al.: Virus as precipitants of asthmatic attacks in children. J. A. M. A. *227*:292–298, 1974.
184. Mogabgab, W. J.: The complications of influenza. Med. Clin. North Am. *47*:1191–1199, 1963.
185. Monto, A. S., and Arden, N. H.: Implications of viral resistance to amantadine in control of influenza A. Clin. Infect. Dis. *15*:362–367, 1992.
186. Monto, A. S., Davenport, F. M., Napier, S. A., et al.: Effect of vaccination of a school age population upon the course of an A2/Hong Kong influenza epidemic. Bull. World Health Organ. *41*:537–542, 1969.
187. Mori, S.-I., Nagashima, M., Sasaki, Y., et al.: A novel amino acid substitution at the receptor-binding site on the hemagglutinin of H3N2 influenza A viruses isolated from 6 cases with acute encephalopathy during the 1997–1998 season in Tokyo. Arch. Virol. *144*:147–155, 1999.
188. Mostow, S. R., Schoenbaum, S. C., Dowdle, W. R., et al.: Studies with inactivated influenza vaccine purified by zonal ultracentrifugation. I. Adverse reactions and serological responses. Bull. World Health Organ. *41*:525–530, 1969.
189. Mufson, M. A., Krause, H. E., Mocega, H. E., et al.: Viruses, *Mycoplasma pneumoniae* and bacteria associated with lower respiratory tract disease among infants. Am. J. Epidemiol. *91*:192–202, 1970.
190. Mulder, J., and Hers, J. F. P.: Influenza. Leiden, The Netherlands, Walters-Noordhoff, International School Book Service, 1972.
191. Munoz, F. M., Campbell, J. R., Atmar, R. L., et al.: Influenza A virus outbreak in a neonatal intensive care unit. Pediatr. Infect. Dis. J. *18*:811–815, 1999.
192. Murphy, B. R., Chalhub, E. G., Nusinoff, S. R., et al.: Temperature-sensitive mutants of influenza virus. II. Attenuation of its recombinants for man. J. Infect. Dis. *126*:170–178, 1972.
193. Murphy, B. R., Chalhub, E. G., Nusinoff, S. R., et al.: Temperature-sensitive mutants of influenza virus. III. Further characterization of the ts-1 (E) influenza A recombinant (H3N2) virus in man. J. Infect. Dis. *128*:479–487, 1973.
194. Murphy, B. R., Kasel, J. A., and Chanock, R. M.: Association of serum antineuraminidase antibody with resistance to influenza in man. N. Engl. J. Med. *286*:1329–1332, 1972.
195. Murphy, B. R., Rennels, M. B., Douglas, R. G., Jr., et al.: Evaluation of influenza A/Hong Kong/123/77 (H1N1) ts-1A2 and cold-adapted recombinant viruses in sero-negative adult volunteers. Infect. Immun. *29*:348–355, 1980.
196. Murphy, B. R., Phelan, M. A., Nelson, D. L., et al.: Hemagglutinin-specific enzyme-linked immunosorbent assay for antibodies to influenza A and B viruses. J. Clin. Microbiol. *13*:554–560, 1981.
197. Murphy, B. R., Clements, M. L., Madore, H. P., et al.: Dose response of cold-adapted, reassortant influenza A/California/10/78 virus. J. Infect. Dis. *149*:816, 1984.
198. Murphy, B. R., and Webster, R. G.: Orthomyxoviruses. *In* Fields, B. N., Knipe, D. M., and Howley, P. M. (eds.): Virology. 3rd ed. Philadelphia, Lippincott-Raven, 1996, pp. 1397–1445.
199. Nakajima, K., Desselberger, U., and Palese, P.: Recent human influenza A (H1N1) viruses are closely related genetically to strains isolated in 1950. Nature *274*:334–339, 1978.
200. Neuzil, K. M., Mellen, B. G., Wright, P. F., et al.: The effect of influenza on hospitalizations, outpatient visits, and courses of antibiotics in children. N. Engl. J. Med. *342*:225–231, 2000.
201. Nichol, K. P., and Cherry, J. D.: Bacterial-viral interrelations in respiratory infections of children. N. Engl. J. Med. *277*:667–672, 1967.
202. Noyola, D. E., Clark, B., O'Donnell, F. T., et al.: Comparison of a new neuraminidase detection assay with an enzyme immunoassay, immunofluorescence, and culture for rapid detection of influenza A and B viruses in nasal wash specimens. J. Clin. Microbiol. *38*:1161–1165, 2000.
203. Noyola, D. E., and Demmler, G. J.: Effect of rapid diagnosis on management of influenza A infections. Pediatr. Infect. Dis. J. *19*:303–307, 2000.
204. Noyola, D. E., Paredes, A. J., Clark, B., et al.: Evaluation of a neuraminidase detection assay for the rapid detection of influenza A and B virus in children. Pediatr. Dev. Pathol. *3*:162–167, 2000.
205. Ogra, P. L., Chow, T., Beutner, K. R., et al.: Clinical and immunologic evaluation of neuraminidase-specific influenza A virus vaccine in humans. J. Infect. Dis. *135*:499–506, 1977.
206. Olding-Stenkvist, E., and Grandhen, M.: Rapid diagnosis of influenza A infection by immunofluorescence. Acta Pathol. Microbiol. Scand. B *85*:296–302, 1977.
207. O'Neill, R. E., Talon, J., and Palese, P.: The influenza virus NEP (NS2 protein) mediates the nuclear export of viral ribonucleoproteins. EMBO J. *17*:288–296, 1998.
208. Paisley, J. W., Bruker, F. W., Laner, B. A., et al.: Type A2 influenza viral infections in children. Am. J. Dis. Child. *132*:34–36, 1978.
209. Palese, P., Ritchey, M. B., Schulman, J. L., et al.: Genetic composition of a high-yielding influenza virus recombinant: A vaccine strain against "swine" influenza. Science *194*:334–335, 1976.
210. Palese, P., and Schulman, J. L.: RNA pattern of "swine" influenza virus isolated from man is similar to those of other swine influenza viruses. Nature *263*:528–530, 1976.
211. Parrott, R. H., Kim, H. W., Vargosko, A. J., et al.: Serious respiratory tract illness as a result of Asian influenza and influenza B infections in children. J. Pediatr. *61*:205–213, 1962.
212. Partin, J. C., Schubert, J. C., Partin, J. S., et al.: Isolation of influenza virus from liver and muscle biopsy specimens from a surviving case of Reye's syndrome. Lancet *2*:599–602, 1976.
213. Payler, D. K., and Purdham, P. A.: Influenza A prophylaxis with amantadine in a boarding school. Lancet *1*:502–504, 1984.
214. Penn, C. R., Blaas, D., Kuechler, E., et al.: Identification of the cap-binding protein of two strains of influenza A/FPV. J. Gen. Virol. *62*:177–180, 1982.
215. Perrotta, D. M., Decker, M., and Glezen, W. P.: Acute respiratory disease hospitalizations as a measure of impact of epidemic influenza. Am. J. Epidemiol. *122*:468–476, 1985.
216. Pickles, W. N., Burnet, F. M., and McArthur, M.: Epidemic respiratory infection in a rural population with special reference to the influenza A epidemics of 1933, 1936–37, and 1943–44. J. Hyg. *45*:469–473, 1947.
217. Piedra, P. A., and Glezen, W. P.: Influenza in children: Epidemiology, immunity, and vaccines. Semin. Pediatr. Infect. Dis. *2*:140–146, 1991.
218. Podosin, R. L., and Felton, W. L.: The clinical picture of Far East influenza occurring at the fourth National Boy Scout Jamboree. N. Engl. J. Med. *258*:778–782, 1958.
219. Poland, J. D., Welton, E. R., and Chin, T. D. Y.: Influenza virus B as cause of acute croup syndrome. Am. J. Dis. Child. *107*:54–57, 1964.
220. Pons, U. W., and Hirst, G. K.: Polyacrylamide gel electrophoresis of influenza virus RNA. Virology *34*:385–388, 1968.
221. Price, D. A., Postlethwaite, R. J., and Longson, M.: Influenza virus A2 infections presenting with febrile convulsions and gastrointestinal symptoms in young children. Clin. Pediatr. *15*:361–367, 1976.
222. Puck, J. M., Glezen, W. P., Frank, A. L., et al.: Protection of infants from infection with influenza A virus by transplacentally acquired antibody. J. Infect. Dis. *142*:844–849, 1980.
223. Pyrhonen, S., Suni, J., and Romo, M.: Clinical trial of a subunit influenza vaccine. Scand. J. Infect. Dis. *13*:95–99, 1981.
224. Rebelo-de-Andrade, H., and Zambon, M. C.: Different diagnostic methods for detection of influenza epidemics. Epidemiol. Infect. *124*:515–522, 2000.
225. Rebhan, A. W.: An outbreak of Asian influenza in a girl's camp. Can. Med. Assoc. J. *77*:797–799, 1957.
226. Reichert, T. A., Sugaya, N., Fedson, D. S., et al.: The Japanese experience with vaccinating schoolchildren against influenza. N. Engl. J. Med. *344*:889–896, 2001.
227. Reye, R. D. K., Morgan, G., and Baral, J.: Encephalopathy and fatty degeneration of the viscera. A disease entity in childhood. Lancet *1*:749–752, 1963.
228. Robinson, R. Q., and Dowdle, W. R.: Influenza viruses. *In* Lennette, E. H., and Schmidt, N. J. (eds.): Diagnostic Procedures for Viral and Rickettsial Infections. New York, American Public Health Association, 1969, pp. 414–433.
229. Rodriguez, W. J., Hall, C. B., Welliver, R., et al.: Efficacy and safety of aerosolized ribavirin in young children hospitalized with influenza: A double-blind, multicenter, placebo-controlled trial. J. Pediatr. *125*:129–135, 1994.
230. Roldaan, A. C., and Masurel, N.: Viral respiratory infections in asthmatic children staying in a mountain resort. Eur. J. Respir. Dis. *63*:140–150, 1982.
231. Rose, H. J.: The use of amantadine and influenza vaccine in a type A influenza epidemic in a boarding school. J. R. Coll. Gen. Pract. *30*:619–621, 1980.
232. Rose, H. J.: Use of amantadine in influenza: A second report. J. R. Coll. Gen. Pract. *33*:651–653, 1983.
233. Rubin, D. M., and Hendy, V.: Swine influenza and the news media. Ann. Intern. Med. *87*:769–774, 1977.
234. Safranek, T. J., Lawrence, D. N., Kurland, L. T., et al.: Reassessment of the association between Guillain-Barré syndrome and receipt of swine influenza vaccine in 1976–1977: Results of a two-state study. Am. J. Epidemiol. *133*:940–951, 1991.

235. Salk, J. E., and Salk, D.: Control of influenza and poliomyelitis with killed virus vaccines. Science *195*:834–847, 1977.
236. Sarkkinen, H. K., Halonen, P. E., and Salmi, A. A.: Detection of influenza A virus by radioimmunoassay and enzyme-immunoassay from nasopharyngeal specimens. J. Med. Virol. *7*:213–220, 1981.
237. Schambelan, M., and Sussman, S.: Encephalitis and purpura with influenza infection. Am. J. Dis. Child. *111*:302–303, 1966.
238. Schmidt, J. P., Metcalf, T. G., and Miltenberger, F. W.: An epidemic of Asian influenza in children at Ladd Air Force Base, Alaska, 1960. J. Pediatr. *61*:214–220, 1962.
239. Schneider, R. M., Nevins, D. B., and Brown, H. Z.: Desquamative interstitial pneumonia in a four year old child. N. Engl. J. Med. *277*:1056–1058, 1967.
240. Schonberger, L. B., Bregman, D. J., Sullivan-Bolyai, J. Z., et al.: Guillain-Barré syndrome following vaccination in the national influenza immunization program, United States, 1976–1977. Am. J. Epidemiol. *110*:105–123, 1979.
241. Schulman, J. L., Petigrow, C., and Woodruff, J.: Effects of cell-mediated immunity in influenza virus infection in mice. Dev. Biol. Stand. *39*:385–395, 1977.
242. Schultz, I., Gundelfinger, B., Rosenbaum, M., et al.: Comparison of clinical manifestations of respiratory illness due to Asian strain influenza, adenovirus, and unknown cause. J. Lab. Clin. Med. *55*:497–509, 1960.
243. Schwarzmann, S. W., Adler, J. L., Sullivan, R. L., Jr., et al.: Bacterial pneumonia during the Hong Kong influenza epidemic of 1968–69. Arch. Intern. Med. *127*:1037–1041, 1971.
244. Shinjoh, M., Bamba, M., Jozaki, K., et al.: Influenza A–associated encephalopathy with bilateral thalamic necrosis in Japan. Clin. Infect. Dis. *31*:611–613, 2000.
245. Shope, R. E.: The incidence of neutralizing antibodies for swine influenza virus in the sera of human beings of different ages. J. Exp. Med. *63*:669–684, 1936.
246. Simonsen, L., Clarke, M. J., Schonberger, L. B., et al.: Pandemic influenza mortality: A pattern of changing age distribution. J. Infect. Dis. *178*:53–60, 1998.
247. Simonsen, L., Clarke, M. J., Stroup, D. F., et al.: A method for timely assessment of influenza-associated mortality in the United States. Epidemiology *8*:390–395, 1997.
248. Simonsen, L., Clarke, M. J., Williamson, G. D., et al.: The impact of influenza epidemics on mortality: Introducing a severity index. Am. J. Public Health *87*:1944–1950, 1997.
249. Simonsen, L., Conn, L. A., Pinner, R. W., et al.: Trends in infectious disease hospitalizations in the United States, 1980–1994. Arch. Intern. Med. *158*:1923–1928, 1998.
250. Simonsen, L., Fukuda, K., Schonberger, L. B., et al.: The impact of influenza epidemics on hospitalizations. J. Infect. Dis. *181*:831–837, 2000.
251. Sinclair, D. J., Stuart, F. G., and Ritchie, G. W.: Pulmonary complications of influenza: A radiological review of 30 cases. Can. Med. Assoc. J. *101*:780–784, 1969.
252. Six, H. R., Glezen, W. P., Kasel, J. A., et al.: Heterogeneity of influenza viruses isolated from the Houston community during defined epidemic periods. *In* Nayack, D., and Cox, C. F. (eds.): Genetic Variation among Influenza Viruses. New York, Academic Press, 1981, pp. 505–513.
253. Skoner, D. P., Gentile, D. A., Patel, A., et al.: Evidence for cytokine mediation of disease expression in adults experimentally infected with influenza A virus. J. Infect. Dis. *180*:10–14, 1999.
254. Smith, W., Andrewes, C. H., and Laidlaw, P. P.: A virus obtained from influenza patients. Lancet *2*:66–68, 1933.
255. Smorodintsev, A. A.: The efficacy of live influenza vaccines. Bull. World Health Organ. *41*:585–588, 1969.
256. Starko, K. M., Ray, C.G., Dominguez, L. B., et al.: Reye's syndrome and salicylate use. Pediatrics *66*:859–864, 1980.
257. Stuart-Harris, C. H.: Influenza and its complications. Br. Med. J. *1*:149–150, 1966.
258. Sugaya, N., and Miura, M.: Amantadine therapy for influenza type A–associated encephalopathy. Pediatr. Infect. Dis. J. *18*:734, 1999.
259. Sugrue, R. J., and Hay, A. J.: Structural characteristics of the M2 protein of influenza A viruses: Evidence that it forms a tetrameric channel. Virology *180*:617–624, 1991.
260. Sullivan-Bolyai, J. Z., Mark, J., Johnson, D., et al.: Reye syndrome in Ohio 1973–77. Am. J. Epidemiol. *112*:629, 1980.
261. Sutton, R. N. P., and Emery, J. L.: Sudden death in infancy: A microbiological and epidemiological study. Arch. Dis. Child. *41*:674–677, 1966.
262. Taber, L. H., Paredes, A., Glezen, W. P., et al.: Infection with influenza A/Victoria virus in Houston families, 1976. J. Hyg. (Lond.) *86*:303–313, 1981.
263. Thomson, D.: Influenza (Part I): With special reference to the part played by Pfeiffer's bacillus, streptococci, pneumococci, etc. and the virus theory. Ann. Picket-Thomson Res. Lab. *9*:142, 1933.
264. Troendle, J. F., Demmler, G. J., Glezen, W. P., et al.: Fatal influenza B virus pneumonia in pediatric patients. Pediatr. Infect. Dis. J. *11*:117–121, 1992.
265. Ulmanen, I., Broni, B. A., and Krug, R. M.: Role of two of the influenza virus core P proteins in recognizing cap 1 structure (m^7GpppNm) on RNAs and in initiating viral RNA transcription. Proc. Natl. Acad. Sci. U. S. A. *78*:7355–7359, 1981.
266. Vargosko, A. J., Chanock, R. M., Huebner, R. J., et al.: Association of type 2 hemadsorption (parainfluenza 1) virus and Asian influenza A virus with infectious croup. N. Engl. J. Med. *261*:1–10, 1959.
267. Virelizier, J. L., Allison, A. C., and Schild, G. C.: Antibody responses to antigenic determinants of influenza virus hemagglutinin. II. Original antigenic sin is a bone marrow–derived lymphocyte memory phenomenon modulated by thymus-derived lymphocytes. J. Exp. Med. *140*:1571–1578, 1974.
268. Virelizier, J. L., Postlethwaite, R., Schild, G. C., et al.: Antibody responses to antigenic determinants of influenza virus hemagglutinin. I. Thymus dependence of antibody formation and thymus independence of immunologic memory. J. Exp. Med. *140*:1559–1570, 1974.
269. Waldman, R. H., Gadal, N., Olsen, G. N., et al.: Respiratory tract cell-mediated immunity to influenza. Symp. Ser. Immunobiol. Stand. *20*:222–231, 1973.
270. Waldman, R. J., Hall, W. N., McGee, H., et al.: Aspirin as a risk factor in Reye's syndrome. J. A. M. A. *247*:3089–3094, 1982.
271. Waner, J. L., Todd, S. J., Shalaby, H., et al.: Comparison of Directogen FLU-A with viral isolation and direct immunofluorescence for the rapid detection and identification of influenza A virus. J. Clin. Microbiol. *29*:479–482, 1991.
272. Wang, C., Takeuchi, K., Pinto, L. H., et al.: Ion channel activity of influenza A virus M2 protein: Characterization of the amantadine block. J. Virol. *67*:5585–5594, 1993.
273. Wells, C. E. C., James, W. K. L., and Evans, A. D.: Guillain-Barré syndrome and virus of influenza A (Asian strain). Arch. Neurol. Psychiatry *81*:699–705, 1959.
274. Whitaker, A. N., and Bunce, I.: Disseminated intravascular coagulation and acute renal failure in influenza A2 infection. Med. J. Aust. *2*:196–201, 1974.
275. Whitley, R. J., Hayden, F. G., Reisinger, K. S., et al.: Oral oseltamivir treatment of influenza in children. Pediatr. Infect. Dis. J. *20*:127–133, 2001.
276. Wilson, C. B., and Smith, R. C.: Goodpasture's syndrome associated with influenza A2 virus infection. Ann. Intern. Med. *76*:91–94, 1972.
277. Wilson, M. G., and Stein, A. M.: Teratogenic effects of Asian influenza. An extended study. J. A. M. A. *210*:336–337, 1969.
278. Wilson, R., Miller, J., Greene, H., et al.: Reye's syndrome in three siblings. Am. J. Dis. Child. *134*:1032–1034, 1980.
279. Wilson, S. Z., Gilbert, B. E., Quarles, J. M., et al.: Treatment of influenza A (H1N1) virus infection with ribavirin aerosol. Antimicrob. Agents Chemother. *26*:200–203, 1984.
280. Wright, P. F., Rose, K. B., Thompson, J., et al.: Influenza A infections in young children: Primary natural infection and protective efficacy of live-vaccine-induced or naturally acquired immunity. N. Engl. J. Med. *296*:829–834, 1977.
281. Wright, P. F., Sell, S. H. W., Thompson, J., et al.: Clinical reactions and serologic response following inactivated monovalent influenza type B vaccine in young children and infants. J. Pediatr. *88*:31–35, 1976.
282. Wright, P. F., Thompson, J., Vaughn, W. K., et al.: Trials of influenza A/New Jersey/76 virus vaccine in normal children: An overview of age-related antigenicity and reactogenicity. J. Infect. Dis. *136*:S731–S741, 1977.
283. Wright, P. F., Okabe, N., McKee, K. T., Jr., et al.: Cold-adapted recombinant influenza A virus vaccines in seronegative young children. J. Infect. Dis. *146*:71–79, 1982.
284. Wright, P. F., Cherry, J. D., Foy, H. M., et al.: Antigenicity and reactogenicity of influenza A/USSR/77 virus vaccine in children: A multicentered evaluation of dosage and safety. Rev. Infect. Dis. *5*:758–764, 1983.
285. Wulff, H., Kidd, P., and Wenner, H. A.: Etiology of respiratory infections: Further studies during infancy and childhood. Pediatrics *33*:30–44, 1964.
286. Yawn, D. H., Pyeatte, J. C., Joseph, M., et al.: Transplacental transfer of influenza virus. J. A. M. A. *216*:1022–1023, 1971.
287. Young, R. S., Torretti, D., Williams, R. H., et al.: Reye's syndrome associated with long-term aspirin therapy. J. A. M. A. *251*:754–756, 1984.
288. Zahradnik, J. M., Kasel, J. A., Martin, R. R., et al.: Immune responses in serum and respiratory secretions following vaccination with a live cold-recombinant (CR35) and inactivated A/USSR/77 (H1N1) influenza virus vaccine. J. Med. Virol. *11*:277–285, 1983.
289. Zhdanov, V. M., Lvov, D. K., Zakstelskaya, L. Y., et al.: Return of epidemic A1 (H1N1) influenza virus. Lancet *1*:294–295, 1978.
290. Ziegler, T., Hemphill, M. L., Siegler, M.-L., et al.: Low incidence of rimantadine resistance in field isolates of influenza A viruses. J. Infect. Dis. *180*:935–939, 1999.
291. Zwernick, H. S., Courtneidge, S. A., Skekel, J. J., et al.: Cytotoxic T cells kill influenza virus infected cells but do not distinguish between serologically distinct type A viruses. Nature *267*:354–356, 1977.

PARAMYXOVIRIDAE

CHAPTER 182 Parainfluenza Viruses

CAROLINE BREESE HALL

Physical ills are the taxes laid upon this wretched life;
some are taxed higher, and some lower,
but all pay something.

Philip Stanhope, Lord Chesterfield
Letter to the Bishop of Waterford, 1757

The parainfluenza viruses (PIVs) are ubiquitous agents with well-earned recognition as being among the most important viral respiratory pathogens of humans. The impact of PIV-1 and PIV-2 infections alone is illustrated in the estimates of their causing in young children an annual one-quarter million emergency visits, 70,000 hospitalizations, and a cost of $190 million.[72] The taxes imposed by the burden of all the human PIVs, types 1 to 4, and at all ages are unestimated. Respiratory tract illnesses from the PIVs may occur and recur throughout life, and they are subordinate only to respiratory syncytial virus in the morbidity caused by acute lower respiratory tract disease in infants and young children. Among the agents of acute laryngotracheobronchitis, the PIVs are second to none. The frequently epidemic nature of PIV types 1 and 2, the prolonged seasonal occurrence of type 3, and the ability of all types to cause repeated infections indicate why their import has not been diminished despite the technologic advances available toward control of viral diseases.

History

The historical delineation of the parainfluenza viral family is intertwined with the discovery of the related animal viruses and marked by the colorful names descriptive of their origin (Table 182–1). The first strain of PIV was discovered in Japan and named Sendai, or the hemagglutinating virus of Japan (HVJ).[97] This agent was recovered from mice that had been inoculated with postmortem lung tissue of infants with pneumonia. The first PIV from human sources was recovered several years later by Chanock[17] from infants with croup, and thus it became known as the croup-associated (CA) virus. Subsequently, three additional PIVs that were distinct antigenically were isolated from children with acute respiratory illness.[20, 84] In contrast to the CA virus, which was recognized by its ability to produce syncytia in tissue culture, the strains of the next two types of PIVs produced little or no cytopathic effect but were recognized by their ability to cause hemadsorption of guinea pig erythrocytes to infected tissue culture. These viruses thus were called hemadsorption type 1 (HA-1) and hemadsorption type 2 (HA-2) viruses.

Once the similarity of the familial characteristics of the CA virus with those of the other three viruses was

TABLE 182–1 ■ PARAINFLUENZA VIRUSES

Parainfluenza Virus Type/ Related Animal Virus	Natural Host	Experimental Infection	Preferred Tissue Culture for Initial Isolation	Cytopathic Effect	
				Initial Isolation	*Passage*
Parainfluenza type 1, hemadsorption type 2 (HA-2)	Human, guinea pig, rabbit, monkey, marmoset	Hamster, ferret	Primary monkey kidney, LLC human diploid, human embryonic kidney	+ −	Rounding, cell destruction
Sendai, hemagglutinating virus of Japan (HVJ)	Mouse, pig				
Parainfluenza type 2	Human, monkey, rabbit, guinea pig	Hamster, dog	Primary monkey kidney, human embryonic kidney	+ (syncytial on monkey and human cells)	Syncytial, "Swiss cheese"
Simian virus 5 (SV 5)	Monkey				
Simian virus 41 (SV 41)	Monkey				
Parainfluenza type 3, hemadsorption type 1 (HA-1)	Human, guinea pig, monkey	Hamster, ferret, cotton rat, mouse, lamb	Primary monkey kidney, human embryonic kidney, LLC	±	In monkey cells—elongated, detachment of cell sheet In human cells—syncytial
Shipping fever (SF-4)	Cow				
Parainfluenza type 4	Human	Hamster, guinea pig	Primary monkey kidney	±	Rounding granular, vacuolated

recognized, the viruses were renamed as the human PIVs, type 1 (HA-2), type 2 (CA), and type 3 (HA-1).[4] The fourth human PIV, discovered subsequent to this reclassification, is without a sobriquet and simply is termed PIV-4, with two subtypes, A and B. The first type 4 strain was recovered in monkey kidney cell culture from a college student afflicted with a common cold.[84]

Several animal species appear to be natural hosts to the PIVs (see Table 182–1), with the exception of PIV-4, which has been found only in humans. In animals, PIVs may be important pathogens. Bovine PIV, similar to human PIV-3, often in combination with infection by *Pasteurella* organisms, causes the illness of considerable morbidity and cost in cattle called *shipping fever*.[1] Naturally acquired antibodies to the PIVs are found not only in cows but also in rodents, monkeys, rabbits, and other mammals. A variety of rodents, along with ferrets, dogs, and lambs, have been used for experimental infection. The virus previously called equine morbillivirus has been demonstrated to be in the *Paramyxoviridae* family and named Hendra virus. This virus, which causes lethal illness in horses, was recognized to cause illness in humans also. Individuals in close contact with the horses in Australia contracted the virus, and two died.[5, 6, 61, 135] Subsequently, in 1998, an outbreak of severe, often fatal encephalitis occurred in Malaysia and Singapore in individuals who had close contact with pigs.[24, 40, 61] This virus, called Nipah virus, is phenotypically and antigenically similar to Hendra virus and has a genomic homology of 80 percent.

Characterization of the Viruses

CLASSIFICATION

Human PIVs belong to the genus *Paramyxovirus* and to the *Paramyxoviridae* family. They are distinct from the orthomyxoviruses in size, nucleocapsid structure (nonsegmented), antigenic composition, and laboratory growth characteristics.

COMPOSITION AND PROPERTIES

Human PIVs are single, negative-stranded RNA viruses appearing as pleomorphic enveloped particles with an average diameter of 150 to 300 nm.[27] The genome of all the human PIVs, which consists of an average of 15,000 nucleotides, codes for at least one nonstructural and six structural proteins (Fig. 182–1). Enclosed within the spherical virion is the helical nucleocapsid with its herringbone core tightly wrapped by the nucleocapsid protein (NP). It is surrounded by the host-cell–derived lipid envelope, which is studded with spikes of surface glycoproteins, the hemagglutinin-neuraminidase (HN) and fusion (F) proteins that are the major protective antigens. The large (L) polymerase protein and the phosphorylated nucleocapsid-associated protein (P) also form clusters within the nucleocapsid structure. The sixth structural protein is the nonglycosylated matrix (M) protein, located between the nucleocapsid and the envelope.

The NP along with P and L proteins is responsible for the primary transcription that produces the messenger RNA from which the proteins of the virus are translated. The genome also is replicated from the formation of a full-length antigenome with positive-sense RNA. The assembly of the virion occurs within the host-cell cytoplasm. The NP and the genomic RNA compose the helical structure, and with the subsequent addition of the P and L protein complexes, the nucleocapsid is formed. The envelope proteins are assembled

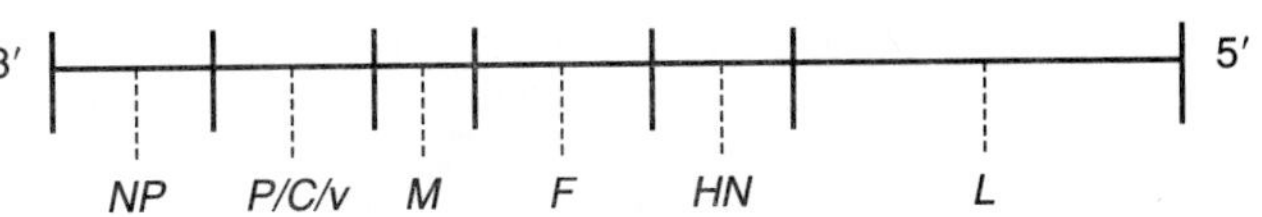

FIGURE 182–1 ■ Schematic representation of the genomic RNA structure of PIV-3.[69] NP, nucleocapsid protein; P, phosphoprotein; C, nonstructural protein (not contained in virion but found in infected cells); v, nonstructural protein encoded by human PIV-2; M, matrix protein; F, fusion protein; HN, hemagglutinin-neuraminidase protein; L, large protein.

at the cell surface. The M protein facilitates the interaction between the nucleocapsid and the surface glycoprotein by the attachment and the insertion of the surface glycoproteins to the host cell and recruitment of the completed nucleocapsid to the budding site of new virions, which are released from the cell surface by evagination of the plasma membrane.

The HN protein is a dimer of two polypeptide portions held together by a disulfide link in the hydrophilic region and at the bases by hydrophobic bonds. The HN mediates the attachment of the virus to the host cell and also is necessary for complete fusion with the host cell.[38] The hemagglutinin component of the HN protein mediates hemagglutination of mammalian erythrocytes through their attachment to mucoprotein receptors on the cellular membranes that contain sialic acid. However, the neuraminidase component of the HN protein subsequently may dislodge this bond by cleaving the sialic acid residues that may serve to aid in the release of the budding viral particles by preventing their reattaching to the cell surface.

The F protein affects the entry of virus by fusing the host and viral cellular membranes. Once adsorption of the virus occurs, the F protein precursor, F0, is cleaved by host proteases into the active F1 and F2 protein fragments, which mediate penetration of the virus into the cell, with subsequent fusion of the viral and cell membranes and hemolysis. Sequences of oligopeptides that mimic the N-terminus of the F1 protein inhibit the penetration of the virus and membrane fusion. A nonstructural protein (C protein), found in infected cells, is encoded by the human PIV-1, PIV-2, and PIV-3 genomes, and a v protein is encoded by the human PIV-2 genome.

Human PIVs share common antigens but also may be differentiated into two antigenic groups, with human PIV-1 and human PIV-3 in one group and human PIV-2, human PIV-4, and mumps virus in the other.[27, 71] Their common antigenicity is illustrated by serologic heterotypic antibody responses to infection with human PIV-1, PIV-2, and PIV-3 and mumps virus. Although the human PIVs do not undergo the major antigenic alterations in their surface antigens, similar to influenza virus, genetic and antigenic variations within all four types have been detected, and their evolution can be determined by analysis of strains obtained over time.[27, 71, 73, 75, 95, 141, 188]

ISOLATION AND IDENTIFICATION

The PIVs are inactivated rapidly by acid at a pH of 3.0 and by exposure to lipid solvents, such as ether and chloroform, which destroy the envelope of the virus. They also are relatively labile to temperatures higher than 37° C.[33, 35] Media containing protein, however, tend to protect against loss of infectivity when the virus is exposed to heat and when it is frozen at −70° C.[33, 79]

Isolation of the human PIVs occurs in permissive cell cultures after an incubation period of 3 to 7 days at 35° C to 37° C. The preferred cell cultures for the growth of PIV are primary or continuous monkey kidney cells, such as LLC-MK; a continuous line of mucoepidermoid human lung carcinoma cells, NCI-H292; and human embryonic kidney cells.[47, 69] PIV-1 also will grow well in human embryonic lung and less well in diploid fibroblastic lines. In other types of kidney tissue, the growth of the PIVs is more variable. PIV-3 replicates in bovine and canine kidney cells and PIV-4 in bovine and hamster kidney cells. After passage, PIV can be propagated in a variety of other cell lines. Persistent infection of some cell lines has been observed with PIV-1, PIV-2, and PIV-3.[48, 119] Cells persistently infected with PIV-3 have little or no cytopathic effect, which is related to the lack of cell fusion, despite the production of large amounts of the cleaved active form of the F1 protein.[175] The growth of the PIVs in embryonated eggs is poor or variable, according to the type and strain. PIV-1, PIV-2, and PIV-3, but not PIV-4, have been adapted to grow in the amniotic cavity of embryonated chicken eggs, although some strains appear resistant to such adaptation.

The production and type of cytopathic effect in tissue culture are variable with PIV (see Table 182–1). PIV-1 and PIV-3 on initial isolation are unlikely to demonstrate distinctive cytopathic effect. On passage, cytopathic effect may be observed, depending on the cell line. PIV-4 is the most difficult PIV to grow in tissue culture. It produces no cytopathic effect and may require 2 to 4 weeks before identification by hemadsorption is possible. Isolation and identification of the PIVs may be accelerated by use of shell viral cultures and rapid antigen identification techniques, as noted later.

The ability of the PIVs to hemadsorb erythrocytes has been the traditional mode of recognizing these viruses in tissue culture. Guinea pig, human group O, or chicken erythrocytes at 4° C or 25° C are used most commonly. PIV-4 hemagglutinates guinea pig and human erythrocytes but not chicken erythrocytes. Staining of infected tissue demonstrates eosinophilic intracytoplasmic inclusions that are the excess nucleocapsids. Specific identification of PIV in tissue culture may be accomplished by testing the hemadsorbing isolates by hemadsorption inhibition, hemagglutination inhibition, or complement-fixation assays. More rapid identification on tissue culture and directly on specimens from patients may be made by antigen detection with assays using immunologic reagents and polymerase chain reaction (PCR) assays.[14, 41, 43, 49, 99] Reverse transcription–PCR (RT-PCR) with differential hybridization techniques, such as hybridization with enzyme immunoassays, has increased the sensitivity of identification of the PIVs in specimens from patients. RT-PCR assays have been developed to detect a single respiratory virus or multiple viruses simultaneously.[2]

Epidemiology

GEOGRAPHIC DISTRIBUTION

The ubiquitous nature of the PIVs has been illustrated by many serologic and viral isolation studies in varied populations, in many parts of the world and in differing climates.* Despite the wide variation in climate and geography, experience with the PIVs is similar in most countries.

*See references 3, 56, 59, 66, 76, 101, 111, 113, 118, 157.

PREVALENCE AND AGE AT INFECTION

The frequency and impact of PIV infections are greatest in preschool-age children and are estimated to account for approximately one third of the lower respiratory tract infections in this age group.[34, 56, 72, 94, 107, 143] Acquisition of PIV-3 usually occurs first, followed by PIV-1 and PIV-2 (Fig. 182–2). The epidemiology of PIV-4 is understood less well, and clinical illness appears to be uncommon or mild. Identifying PIV-4 infection is difficult, however, and the prevalence may be underestimated.[2] Older serologic studies suggest that infection with PIV-4A and PIV-4B is a relatively common occurrence in the preschool years, with 50 percent or more of 5-year-old children possessing antibodies.[52, 92] Infections with PIV-4B may occur less commonly, however; one third or more of adults are seronegative.[52, 92]

Infection with PIV-3 occurs early in life. One half to two thirds of infants have acquired infection by 12 months of age.[55, 56, 76, 134] Experience with PIV-1 and PIV-2 is more gradual. In Washington, D.C., neutralizing antibody was present in less than 10 percent of infants 6 to 12 months of age, in one third of children 4 years of age, and in approximately three fourths of school-age children.[134] By adulthood, virtually everyone has hemagglutination-inhibition antibody to PIV-1 and PIV-3, but acquisition of antibody to PIV-2 is more variable, ranging from 50 to 90 percent.[134, 136, 143]

The frequency of PIV infection in the young child has been illustrated clearly by the Houston Family Studies, in which infections were detected by both viral isolation and serology in children observed from birth.[55, 56, 58] By 2 years of age, 92 percent of the children had experienced at least one infection with PIV-3, and 32 percent had been infected more than once. Serious illness occurs most frequently with primary infection. PIV-3 causes the majority of hospital admissions for lower respiratory tract illness in infants, whereas PIV-1 and PIV-2 are primarily associated with hospitalizations for children 2 to 6 years of age. The age distribution of children with PIV-1 and PIV-3 viral infections seen in private pediatric practice, however, may overlap substantially (see Fig. 182–2). In outpatients in Rochester, New York, approximately half of the PIV-3 viral infections have occurred in children younger than 24 months, compared with approximately one third of the PIV-1 infections.[94] In children 2 to 5 years of age, the reverse was true, with half of the PIV-1 infections and approximately one third of the PIV-3 infections occurring in this older age group (see Fig. 182–2).

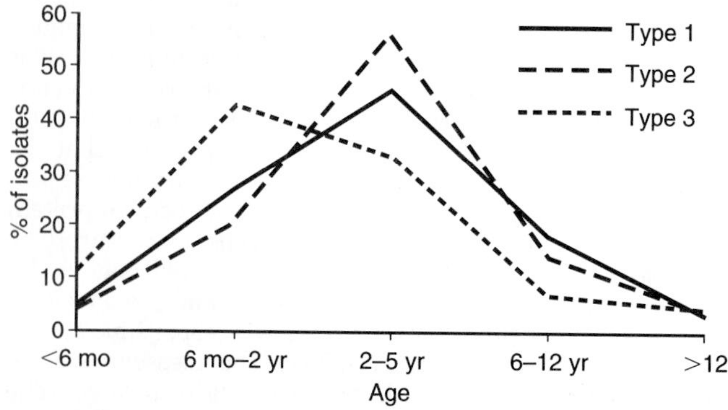

FIGURE 182–2 ■ Age distribution of PIV-1, PIV-2, and PIV-3 infections in outpatient children in Rochester, New York, from 1976 to 1992. (From Knott, A., Long, C. E., and Hall, C. B.: Parainfluenza viral infections in pediatric outpatients: Seasonal patterns and clinical characteristics. Pediatr. Infect. Dis. J. *13*:269–273, 1994.)

SEASONAL OCCURRENCE

The seasonal patterns of the PIVs vary somewhat with the location and the year but in general are distinctive in their predictable and repetitive behavior. Before the early 1960s, the PIVs were mostly endemic.[19] Since the mid-1960s, however, PIV-1 changed its profile by preferentially appearing in the fall. Subsequently, sizable outbreaks of PIV-1 infection were observed to occur every other year, in the even-numbered years, until the 1970s. Then, for unknown reasons, PIV-1 developed temporarily a sporadic nature for a couple of years before settling into its current pattern of causing outbreaks in the autumns of the odd-numbered years.[3, 56–59, 94]

PIV-2 has been even more erratic in its behavior than has PIV-1.[56, 94] During 20 years of surveillance in Rochester, New York, PIV-2 has appeared sporadically in low numbers, usually at the end of PIV-1 fall outbreaks in the odd-numbered years (Fig. 182–3).[67, 94] PIV-3 predominantly has been endemic but has become more epidemic in nature, with swells of activity in the spring to fall.[56, 67, 94] Although 75 percent of PIV-3 isolates obtained during 2 decades of surveillance were recovered in the spring and summer, close to one fourth of the PIV-3 isolates occurred in the fall, primarily in the autumns of the even-numbered years when PIV-1 was absent.

Pathogenesis

TRANSMISSION

Clinical and experimental observations indicate that the PIVs spread readily and effectively.[5, 12, 55, 65, 89, 115, 117, 123, 152] Person-to-person contact appears necessary, allowing direct exposure to infected secretions through large droplets or through self-inoculation. The contagiousness, therefore, will depend on (1) the quantities of virus contained in the nasal secretions[12, 65]; (2) how effectively the infected secretions are propelled into the environment, such as through sneezing and coughing[115, 152]; and (3) how well the infectious virus can survive in the environment.[5, 12, 115, 117] The PIVs are relatively hardy survivors on various surfaces found in hospitals, workplaces, and homes and on skin. The PIVs remain infectious on nonporous surfaces for as long as 10 hours and

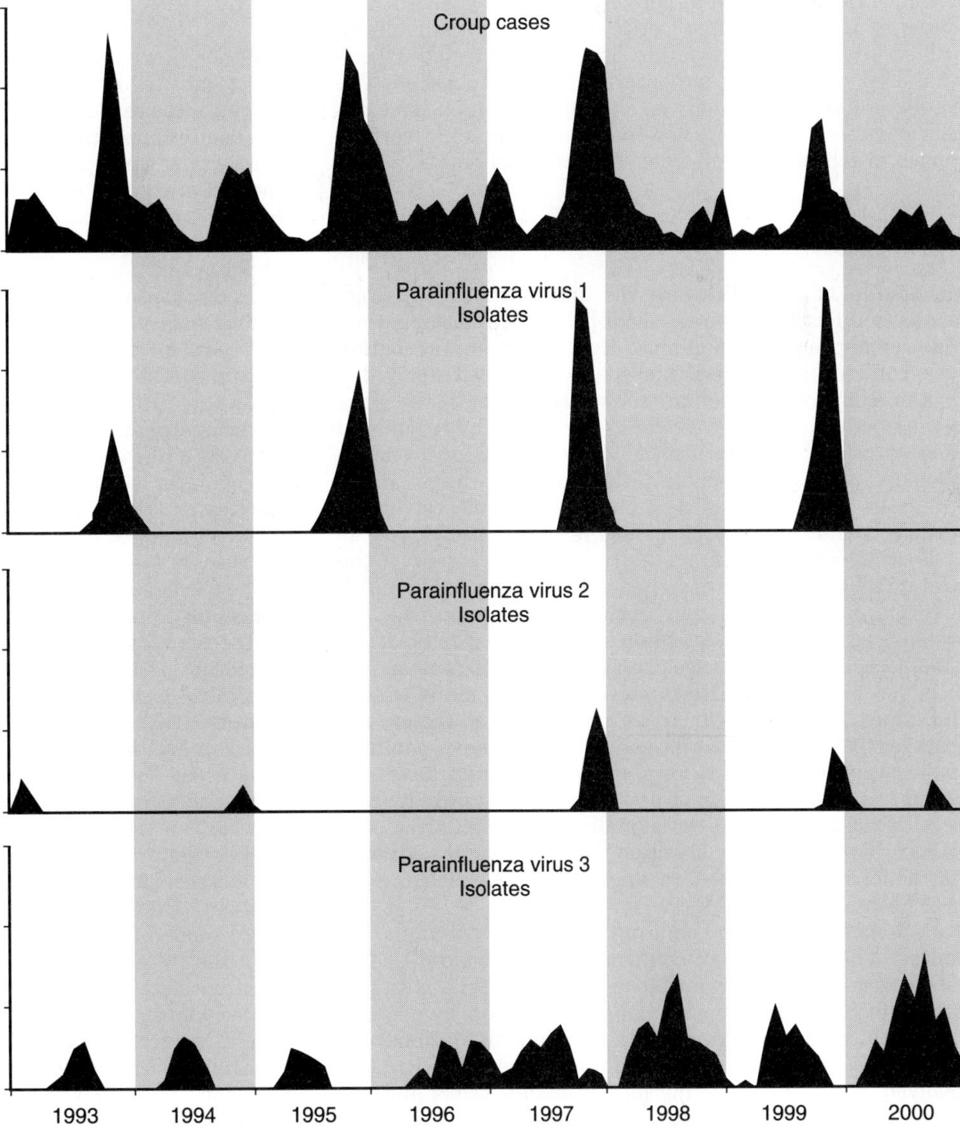

FIGURE 182–3 ■ Number of cases of croup reported by the primary care physicians in Rochester and Monroe County, New York, from 1993 through 2000 to the Community Infectious Disease Surveillance Program of the University of Rochester School of Medicine, Rochester, New York, shown in relation to the periods of isolation of the parainfluenza viruses.

on porous surfaces for as long as 4 hours, but survival may be diminished by drying.[12] PIVs may be transferred to hands from environmental surfaces, suggesting that fomites may play a role in dissemination.[5, 12] A curious conundrum is the survival and persistence of PIV-1 and PIV-3 infections in a group of individuals isolated in the frigid environs of the South Pole for 8.5 months.[122, 132, 133] Despite no outside contacts, infection with PIV-1 and PIV-3 occurred repetitively in the quarantined individuals, raising the possibility that persistent infection may be engendered not only in tissue culture but in humans under certain circumstances, such as extreme environmental conditions.

Children with primary infection caused by PIV-1 have considerable quantities of infectious virus in their nasal secretions, an average of approximately 1000 tissue culture infective doses ($TCID_{50}$) per milliliter.[65] With the tendency of PIVs to cause illnesses associated with frequent sneezing, coughing, and profuse nasal discharge, contamination of the environment from infected individuals is inevitable and probably the primary means of spread of PIV infection. Although PIV-3 has been shown to remain viable for 1 hour in a small-particle aerosol experimentally produced,[115] the secretions disseminated through coughs and sneezes primarily are in the form of large-particle aerosols, which are greater than 15 μm in diameter. For particles of this size to be inhaled, close person-to-person contact is required. The routes of inoculation that occur naturally have not been studied adequately, but adults have been infected experimentally by intranasal and oropharyngeal inoculation. The eye and anterior oral cavity as sites of inoculation have not been examined similarly, however; they may be important portals in self-inoculation from contaminated hands.[88, 166]

PATHOLOGY

Inoculation of the PIVs into the upper respiratory tract results in infection of the nasal epithelium and nasopharynx and the appearance of clinical signs after an incubation period of 2 to 4 days. Specific receptors on the cell membrane of the respiratory epithelium allow attachment of the virus to the host cell, with subsequent penetration by fusion and phagocytosis.[184] After production of the nucleocapsid in the cytoplasm and final assembly of the virus near the cell membrane, the virus is extruded by budding without destruction of the cell, thus allowing continued release of the virus.

The factors determining the tropism and extent of the viral infection are incompletely defined and probably multifactorial. Such factors may include host immunity, the protease activity of various tissues, and virus-specific determinants, such as the cleavage phenotype of the F0 protein.[27, 120] Viral receptors for the PIVs are available on many tissues and, thus, do not appear to be an important factor; the observed pathologic changes generally have been confined to the respiratory tract. Several reports, however, have suggested that spread of the virus may occur not only by cell-to-cell transfer but also occasionally by viremia after both primary and secondary infection.[62, 146] In rodents, viremia and penetration of PIV-1 in migratory mononuclear cells have been observed.[83, 184]

Pathologic studies of children with PIV infections are limited. The few cases of confirmed PIV infection studied pathologically have shown that in the young child with primary infection, inflammation (marked primarily by necrosis of the epithelium) is evident throughout the respiratory tract. The subglottic tissues may appear particularly involved, but the conducting airways at all levels and the alveoli may be affected.[18, 191]

Viral shedding is most abundant and prolonged in young children with primary and severe disease.[65] Children with PIV-1 infections may shed the virus for an average of 4 to 7 days but as long as 12 days. With PIV-3 infections, shedding tends to be longer, occasionally 2 to 3 weeks, and in adults with chronic lung disease, shedding may be both prolonged and intermittent.[62]

Experimental infection of animals with the PIVs has provided a model for the study of the pathophysiology of these infections.[131] Inoculation of rodents with PIV-3 has produced histologically evident, but usually asymptomatic, interstitial pneumonitis or bronchiolitis.[27, 54, 69, 131, 139] In newborn ferrets, PIV infection is progressive and often fatal.[116] Pathologic changes involve the bronchi and peribronchial areas with hyperplasia of the epithelium and surrounding infiltration with pneumocytes and macrophages, causing obliteration of the alveolar spaces. A canine model of PIV-2 into the respiratory tract has produced clinical signs of cough and rhinitis accompanied by histologic changes of denudation of the ciliated epithelium and peribronchial and peribronchiolar lymphocytic infiltrates affecting airways of all sizes.[174]

IMMUNE RESPONSE: ROLE IN PATHOGENESIS AND PROTECTION

Whether illness in PIV infections is related mostly to the direct effects of viral replication or compounded by an immunologic reaction is not clear. Although clinical severity has been related to the degree of viral replication, cellular destruction and pathology also may be engendered by antigen-antibody complexes, IgE antibody, augmented delayed-type hypersensitivity, cytotoxic cellular responses, and release of cytokines and a cascade of other inflammatory mediators.[27, 65]

In contrast to infection from PIV-1 and PIV-2, the most serious form of illness with PIV-3 infection occurs in the first year of life, when infants may possess maternally derived specific antibody, suggesting that the interactions of maternal antibody and virus may be detrimental.[111] In experimental animals, however, passively administered PIV antibody and monoclonal antibodies against F and HN proteins appear protective. Furthermore, the trials with an inactivated trivalent PIV vaccine in the 1960s did not suggest a pathogenic role for antibody. Although not protective, the vaccine was immunogenic and produced serum antibody in the vaccinees. Subsequently, however, they did not experience augmented disease, as observed with the simultaneously tested formalin-inactivated respiratory syncytial virus vaccine.[51]

Clinical observations, furthermore, show that lower respiratory tract infection is confined primarily to primary infection and to young children. Although recurrent infections occur throughout life, they usually are milder, suggesting that naturally acquired immunity is not complete or durable, but nevertheless, protection against severe disease does develop during the first few years of life. For all the PIVs, therefore, the immune response, including serum antibody, that results from natural infection appears to afford some, but not complete, benefit.[27, 134, 156, 177]

In the Houston Family Studies,[55, 58] the level of passively acquired maternal antibody to PIV-3 in the cord blood correlated inversely with the risk of acquiring primary infection. However, recurrent infection occurred frequently in children in several successive years after their primary infection, but the risk of lower respiratory tract disease diminished.

Antigenic variation in the PIVs is not sufficient to explain the lack of complete or durable immunity.[75, 169] More likely, the humoral and cellular immune responses diminish with time. In experimental and natural infection in humans, measurements of the level of immunity have been correlated with the susceptibility to infection and inversely correlated with the degree of viral shedding.[88, 90]

Serum hemagglutination-inhibition antibody and neutralizing antibody are detectable within 1 to 2 weeks.[91] Neutralizing antibody is directed to epitopes on the HN and F proteins. Both of these proteins have important roles in the immunologic and protective responses. In experimental animals, some evidence exists that antibody against the HN protein is more protective than is that formed against the F protein.[142, 159] With repeated infections, an anamnestic antibody response occurs, and antibodies that cross-neutralize the different PIV types develop. In most young children with primary PIV-3 infection, the antibody response to HN protein has been shown to be directed at four of six antigenic sites examined on the HN protein, three of which were neutralizing sites.[169] The response to the F protein, whether with primary or recurrent infection, generally was more variable in magnitude and restricted in terms of antigenic sites. The presence of maternal antibody, however, appeared inhibitory to the infant's ability to produce specific humoral antibody.[169] Previous infection with a heterotypic strain does not produce significant protection against the development of lower respiratory tract disease in young children, but prior homotypic infection has appeared to provide a brief period of such immunity.[177]

The role of mucosal immunity in protection against infection has been demonstrated to be pivotal in PIV infections in numerous animal and human studies. Primary and secondary infections with a heterotypic strain result in low and transient levels of secretory IgA antibody, whereas homotypic reinfection produces an enhanced response.[177] In experimental models, passive administration or induction of mucosal IgA antibody has been demonstrated to be more protective than have serum IgG antibodies.[27, 109, 110, 154, 156, 164] In experimental infection in volunteers, infectivity with PIV was correlated with the neutralizing activity in the secretions rather than in serum.[156, 164]

Even less well defined than the humoral antibody response is the cell-mediated immune response to the PIVs. Genetic and immunologic factors have been suggested as being particularly integral in children who manifest their PIV infections as croup. An abnormal cell-mediated response to PIV in children developing croup has been suggested by their increased lymphoproliferative responses and decreased histamine-induced suppression of lymphocyte transformation responses to PIV compared with children with PIV infection that is manifested as an upper respiratory tract infection.[176] Furthermore, an atopic state, as well as diminished serum IgA levels, has been correlated with a propensity to recurrent croup.[189, 190] The increased severity and prolonged period of viral shedding in immunocompromised hosts, such as those receiving organ transplants, indicate the importance of intact cellular immunity in the control of disease and recovery from PIV infection.[102, 104] In animal models, cell-mediated immunity, which is mediated primarily by CD8 cells, has been demonstrated as being central to recovery and clearance of PIV infections.[27, 78] The presence of histamine and inflammatory mediators, such as the leukotrienes C_4 and D_4, and eosinophilic cationic protein, which are important in bronchoconstriction and in the pathogenesis of inflammation, has been demonstrated during acute PIV infections.[171, 176–180] In children with PIV-3 bronchiolitis, the presence of histamine and leukotrienes in their secretions has been correlated with more severe disease and wheezing.

Clinical Manifestations

The types of illnesses caused by PIV infections have characteristic associations with the age of the child, season, and PIV serotype (Table 182–2 and Fig. 182–4; see also Fig. 182–2).[55–59, 94, 100, 143] In general, most primary infections are symptomatic, and a high proportion of them affect the lower respiratory tract, particularly when the initial infection occurs in the second year of life.[58, 94] Of the primary infections that involve only the upper respiratory tract, fever and laryngeal or tracheal involvement are common occurrences. Reinfections frequently occur at all ages and primarily are mild, involving the upper respiratory tract, or sometimes they even are asymptomatic.[58] In a general practice in Britain, the attack rate of PIV infections in the first 4 years of life was 43.2 per thousand people; at 5 to 14 years of age, the rate was 12 per thousand; and in patients 40 years of age or older, the rate fell to 3.7 per thousand.[8] In the Tecumseh

TABLE 182–2 ■ PROPORTION OF RESPIRATORY SYNDROMES CAUSED BY THE PARAINFLUENZA VIRUSES IN VARIOUS STUDIES

		Percentage of Cases Caused by Parainfluenza Viruses		
Syndrome	**Patient Source**	*Type 1*	*Type 2*	*Type 3*
Croup[15, 21, 25, 32, 59, 94]	Inpatient	10-31	0.5–8	3–8
	Outpatient	7-31	2–4	2–9
Bronchiolitis[21, 25, 59]	Inpatient	1-3	0.4–4	1–13
	Outpatient	2-11	0–2	3–11
Pneumonia[21, 25, 59]	Inpatient	1-3	0.4–4	1–13
	Outpatient	2-11	0–2	3–11
Tracheobronchitis[21, 25, 59]	Inpatient	1-4	0.2–2	2–12
	Outpatient	1-5	0.2–3	4–5
Upper respiratory tract infections[21, 25, 145, 150]	Inpatient	4-12	1–2	5–12
	Outpatient	2-10	0–2	0.4–4
Total upper and lower respiratory tract illnesses[21, 25]	Inpatient	2-5	0.7–2	2–13
	Outpatient	5	2	13

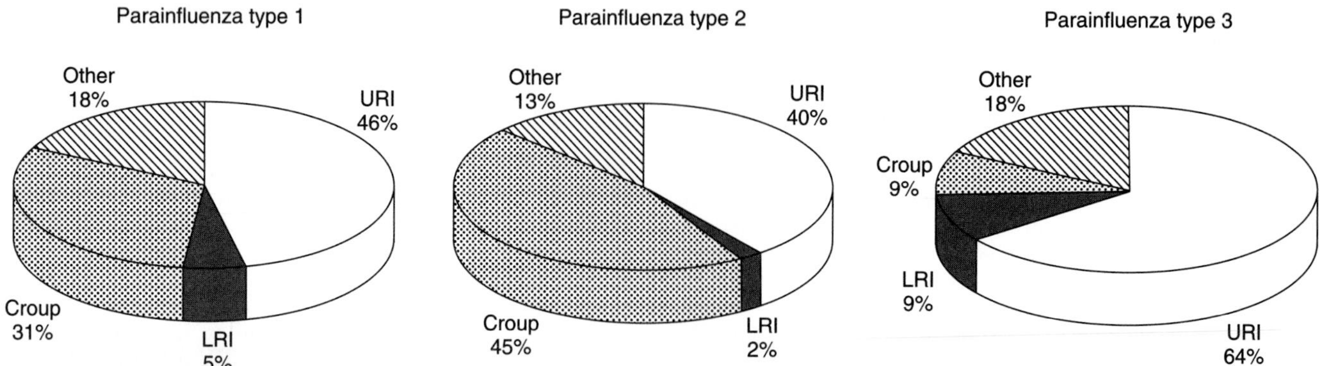

FIGURE 182–4 ■ Clinical manifestations of parainfluenza virus infections according to serotype in pediatric outpatients in Rochester, New York (1976–1992). URI, upper respiratory tract infection (including otitis, colds, pharyngitis); LRI, lower respiratory tract infection other than croup. (From Knott, A., Long, C. E., and Hall, C. B.: Parainfluenza viral infections in pediatric outpatients: Seasonal patterns and clinical characteristics. Pediatr. Infect. Dis. J. *13*:269–273, 1994.)

study, PIVs ranked second only to the rhinoviruses as the most frequently identified agents of upper respiratory tract infections.[118] In persons 20 to 50 years of age, 16 to 28 percent were shown to be infected each year.

The PIVs cause a greater proportion of respiratory illnesses in outpatients than of the respiratory illnesses in hospitalized children.[94, 100] Of all the viral respiratory illnesses examined in a pediatric practice, the PIVs caused approximately two thirds of the croup cases, one fourth of the tracheobronchitis cases, and approximately one half of the upper respiratory tract illnesses, including colds, laryngitis, pharyngitis, and otitis media.

The proportion of hospitalized cases of lower respiratory tract illnesses caused by the PIVs varies according to the year and the age of the children, with infants representing approximately two thirds of the PIV admissions.[56, 100] The risk of needing hospitalization for PIV lower respiratory tract disease is greatest during the fall outbreaks from PIV-1 and PIV-2 in the odd-numbered years and from PIV-3 during the spring.[56] Infants hospitalized with PIV infection, especially those with bronchiolitis or pneumonia, are most likely to be infected by PIV-3. Hospitalization of children beyond 1 year of age through 5 years of age mainly results from PIV-1 and, to a lesser extent, from PIV-2 infections.[55–59, 100]

The various respiratory syndromes associated with PIV-1, PIV-2, and PIV-3 are shown in Table 182–2 and Figures 182–4 and 182–5. Although variation occurs according to the population and type and number of diagnostic methods used for identification of infection, all studies indicate that PIVs are the major cause of croup and an important but less frequent cause of the other lower respiratory tract syndromes in children (see Figs. 182–3 and 182–5). PIV-1 and PIV-2 are associated primarily with croup, especially in hospitalized patients (see Table 182–2).[56, 94, 143] PIV-3 is manifested most frequently in hospitalized patients as pneumonia or bronchiolitis and in outpatients as upper respiratory tract illness.[56, 94] In outpatients, upper respiratory tract infections are produced by all three types of PIV in approximately 40 to 66 percent of cases (see Figs. 182–4 and 182–5).[94, 143]

PIVs have been identified in middle ear aspirates and may play a primary or secondary role of predisposing these patients to bacterial middle ear infection.[23, 70, 94, 121, 148] Otitis media has been shown to complicate upper respiratory tract infections in approximately 10 percent of patients, most frequently infants younger than 6 months. Otitis media from PIV-1 has accounted for approximately one fifth of cases, approximately twice as many as from PIV-3. Of the children 6 years of age or older seen in pediatric practice in Rochester, New York, with a PIV infection, 60 percent had an upper respiratory tract infection (half of these infections primarily were pharyngitis), 14 percent had croup, 9 percent had laryngitis, and 4 percent had tracheobronchitis. Infection with PIV-1, PIV-2, and PIV-3 also may result in an undifferentiated febrile illness without noticeable respiratory signs in 5 to 7 percent of cases.

In the 11-year study of croup in a pediatric practice in Chapel Hill, North Carolina, the PIVs constituted three fourths of the agents isolated. The majority (65%) were type 1.[32] Fifty-eight percent of the lower respiratory tract infections from PIV-1 and 60 percent of those from PIV-2 were manifested as croup, compared with 29 percent of the PIV-3 lower respiratory tract infections.[32] The type and proportion of illnesses associated with PIV-2 are similar to those seen with PIV-1. PIV-2 infections, however, occur about five times less frequently; thus, their impact on health care is less noticeable.[32, 59, 94, 100]

The clinical manifestations associated with PIV-4 are much less well described. This in part may be due to the technical difficulty of isolating PIV-4. According to one study, however, PIV-4 may account for 3 percent of respiratory disease.[16] However, with use of multiplex RT-PCR, PIV-4 accounted for 10 of 64 PIVs identified in nasopharyngeal aspirates.[2] Most PIV-4 isolates have been associated with a mild, usually afebrile, upper respiratory tract infection.[16, 74] However, lower respiratory tract illness associated with PIV-4 has been reported.[103]

The onset of the typical primary PIV infection generally is acute and associated with upper respiratory signs, such as rhinitis and sore throat. Cough and hoarseness frequently are prominent features.[8, 65, 74] Most children with PIV-1 infection during a community outbreak who were seen in a practice setting had fever, upper respiratory tract signs, and tracheobronchial or tracheolaryngeal signs of croup.[65] Fever occurred in 75 percent and frequently was high. Only 12 percent had an afebrile upper respiratory tract illness.

The onset of croup usually is preceded by upper respiratory tract signs. Subsequently, a harsh, barking cough develops, followed by stridor, retractions of the chest wall, and dyspnea. The course of croup characteristically is variable, with an unpredictable waxing and waning in the intensity of the stridor and dyspnea. The acute symptoms usually last

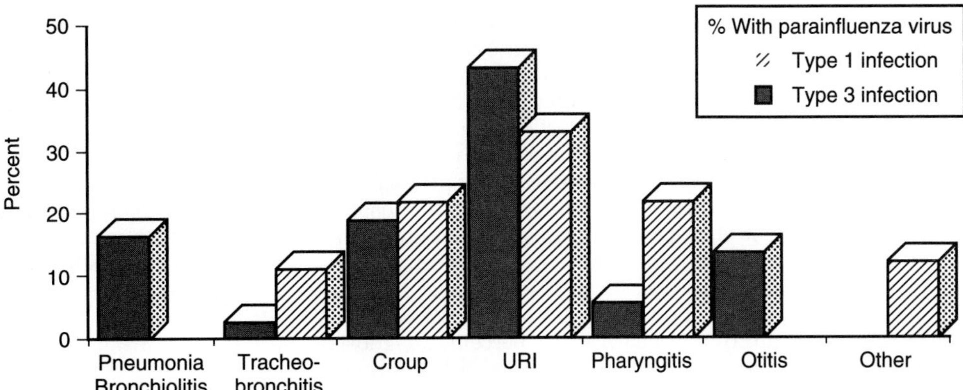

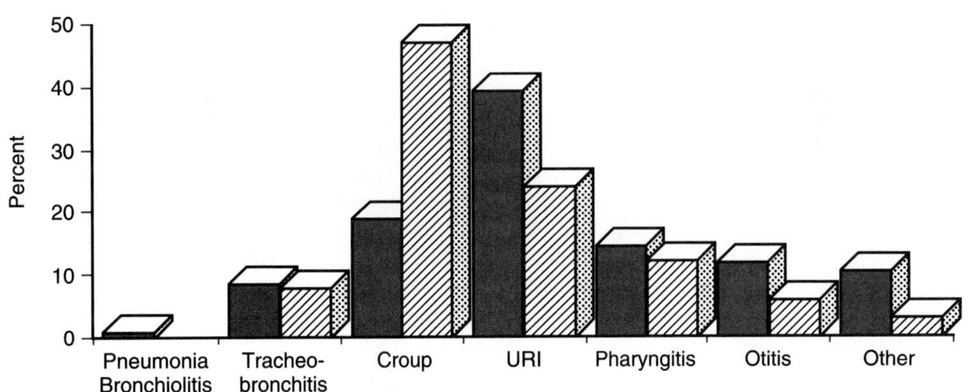

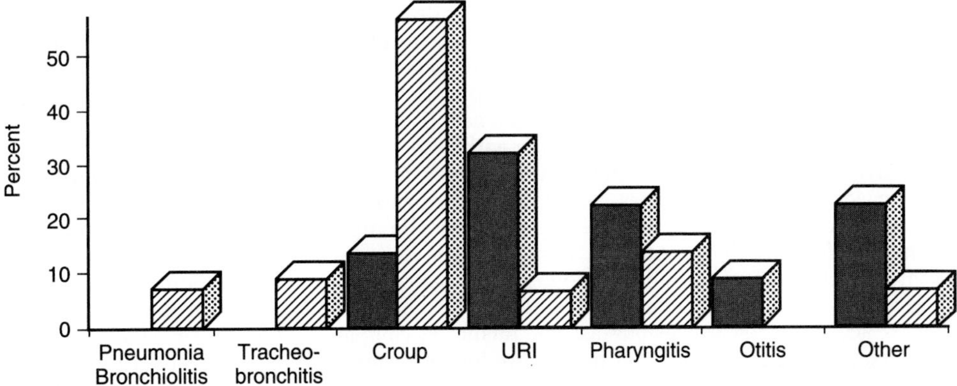

FIGURE 182–5 ■ Type of illness with PIV-1 compared with PIV-3 according to age in outpatients from private pediatric practices presenting with acute respiratory or febrile illnesses. URI, upper respiratory tract infection. (Data obtained 1984 through 1988 from the Community Infectious Disease Surveillance Program of the University of Rochester School of Medicine, Rochester, New York.)

for 3 to 4 days. In the more severely ill, hypoxemia may occur from viral involvement of the lung parenchyma,[125] which, although important in management, may not be recognized because of the focus on the apparent major site of inflammation, the subglottic area.

Reinfections occur commonly in patients with PIV infections and usually are milder, often a common cold. In adults, PIV-1, PIV-2, and PIV-3 constitute approximately 2 to 5 percent of the upper respiratory tract infections, but one fifth or more may be asymptomatic.[11, 36, 74] Of those with clinical illness, approximately 30 to 92 percent develop fever commonly associated with malaise, sore throat, and cough.[11, 36, 74] Rhinorrhea is less common in adults than in children, occurring in less than 25 percent of the adult infections.

PIV infection may cause more severe disease in the elderly and also exacerbations of symptoms in both children and adults with chronic lung disease, including chronic bronchitis, asthma, and cystic fibrosis.* On occasion, as in military recruits, pneumonia has been described with adult

*See references 28, 37, 45, 60, 68, 85, 108, 112, 126, 127, 163.

PIV infections but is rare in a normal, previously healthy population.[42, 182]

PIV infections may result in serious morbidity in immunocompromised hosts. Both children and adults with compromised immunity, especially cellular immunity, are at high risk for development of severe, often fatal, disease, with prolonged periods of viral shedding.[39, 82, 102, 104, 106, 149, 181] At autopsy, multinucleated giant cells have been found in the lung. PIV infection in these high-risk patients is particularly hazardous in transplant units and often is acquired nosocomially. In a study of bone marrow transplant patients conducted from 1974 to 1990, PIV infections were documented in 2.2 percent (15 children and 12 adults).[181] Lower respiratory tract disease occurred in 70 percent of these 27 patients and respiratory failure and death in 22 percent. Diagnosis often was difficult because only in about one third of those with lower respiratory tract involvement was PIV isolated from the upper respiratory tract. Bronchoalveolar lavage was required to obtain a culture that was positive for PIV in 20 percent.

The association of acute PIV infection with a nonrespiratory illness rarely occurs, as does the isolation of PIV from sites other than the respiratory tract. Many case reports have associated PIV infections with a variety of diseases, including adult respiratory distress syndrome, parotitis, myopericarditis, and diseases of the central nervous system.* Anecdotal reports also have associated PIV infection with collagen vascular diseases and a sporadic severe hepatitis, characterized histologically by syncytial giant hepatocytes.[137, 138]

Diagnosis

The diagnosis of PIV infections often may be surmised on clinical and epidemiologic grounds, such as the patient's age, the type of illness, and the seasonal patterns of PIV in the community. Specific diagnosis may be made during the acute phase of the illness by viral isolation, by identification of the viral antigen in specimens from the patient or in culture, and during the patient's convalescence by serologic assays. PIVs, as noted previously, usually are detected in tissue culture by their ability to hemadsorb erythrocytes. Most PIV-1 and PIV-3 strains obtained from acutely ill children may be recognized by hemadsorption within the first 3 to 7 days. PIV-2 and PIV-4 may require longer periods. Specific identification requires subsequent confirmation with use of type-specific serologic assays or one of the rapid techniques for identifying specific viral antigen in tissue culture (see the subsection on isolation and identification).

Serologic diagnosis requiring acute and convalescent sera may be accomplished by various assays, including complement fixation, hemagglutination inhibition, hemadsorption inhibition, neutralizing and enzyme immunoassay, and immunofluorescence.[44] Most of these assays are relatively sensitive, but heterotypic antibody rises may be detected, depending in part on the assay. During reinfection, both homotypic and heterotypic antibody rises may occur, or sometimes little antibody response is detected, despite virus being shed from the nasopharynx.[27, 132] Less is known about the antibody response to PIV-4 infection, but in primary infection, a homotypic response is usual.[92] Detection of specific IgM antibodies, which usually persist for 2 to 11 weeks after infection, has been of limited success as a diagnostic technique.[167, 173]

*See references 6, 7, 31, 77, 80, 81, 147, 151, 172, 183, 185, 192.

Differential Diagnosis

Most of the other major respiratory viral pathogens at times can mimic the illnesses from PIV infections. Differentiation clinically rarely is possible; more helpful are epidemiologic clues, such as the differing seasonal patterns of the respiratory viruses.[64]

Croup from PIVs or any other virus must be differentiated from bacterial tracheitis and epiglottitis, which have rapidly progressive courses and a potentially fatal outcome. With the widespread use of the *Haemophilus influenzae* type b vaccine, epiglottitis now rarely occurs. In contrast, PIV croup usually has a more gradual onset, with a preceding upper respiratory tract infection. Its fluctuating course and prominent "seal's bark" cough without drooling help differentiate it from epiglottitis and bacterial tracheitis. In PIV croup, the peripheral white blood cell count may be normal or initially show a slight elevation and left shift, whereas in these bacterial causes of stridor, the left shift usually is marked. In view of the recent outbreaks of diphtheria in some countries, laryngeal diphtheria may be a consideration in an unimmunized child. In contrast to bacterial tracheitis and epiglottitis, however, laryngeal diphtheria usually is gradual in onset and presents with the characteristic membranous pharyngitis. Stridor and other signs of croup also may be present in children with aspiration of a foreign body, tracheomalacia, and acute angioneurotic edema.

Treatment

Most PIV infections are self-limited and require no treatment. Specific therapy is not available yet for PIV infections. The antiviral drug ribavirin inhibits PIV replication in tissue culture and has appeared beneficial in controlling PIV infection in a limited number of immunocompromised patients.[13, 26, 53, 114, 158]

Therapeutic approaches using immunomodulators, protease inhibitors, synthetic peptides inhibiting viral fusion, and antivirals inhibiting *S*-adenosyl-L-homocysteine hydrolase are being explored.[10, 87, 98, 129, 187] Passive topical administration of IgG, which contains neutralizing antibody to PIV, with and without glucocorticosteroids, also has appeared beneficial against PIV-3 infection in the cotton rat.[130, 140]

Most croup is treated at home, and the armamentarium used during the past century has been varied and usually anecdotal, ranging from cold night air to steam to antiemetics. Yet no such home therapies have proved to be beneficial. After several days of a fluctuating course, most children with croup will improve spontaneously. The more severely affected require hospitalization and may require monitoring for oxygenation and hypercapnia.[29] The hypoxemia usually is responsive to relatively low concentrations of oxygen.

Rapid improvement in the airway obstruction and respiratory distress for the child who is hospitalized or being monitored in the emergency department may be achieved with aerosolized bronchodilators, such as racemic epinephrine.[29, 46] The relief is transient, however, and the hypoxemia, if present, is not affected.[155] Children who continue to have respiratory distress are candidates for treatment with corticosteroids. The dose of corticosteroids is important and probably explains the conflicting results of previous studies using varied doses.[86, 165] In hospitalized patients, high doses of parenteral dexamethasone (>0.3 mg/kg) or its equivalent or oral dexamethasone (0.15 to 0.6 mg/kg) appear necessary to produce the beneficial effect.[29, 86] A single dose of 0.6 mg/kg intramuscularly or intravenously has been recommended to be given in the emergency department to patients requiring hospital admission for croup.[9] For therapy of outpatient croup, a single dose of 0.6 mg/kg of dexamethasone intramuscularly and oral dexamethasone at doses of 0.15 mg/kg or a single oral dose of dexamethasone at 0.6 mg/kg have been shown to be effective.[30, 144] The treatment of croup is discussed more thoroughly in Chapter 22.

Antibiotic therapy should be reserved for documented episodes of secondary bacterial infection, which is an infrequent occurrence in PIV infections.

Prognosis

Most children who previously were healthy recover completely and without complication from PIV infections. The acute complications, morbidity, and mortality relate to the presence of an underlying condition, especially a cardiopulmonary or immunodeficiency disease. Of children hospitalized with PIV infection studied during a 4-year period, 35 percent had preexisting pulmonary or cardiac abnormalities, prematurity, or asthma.[68] Compared with the children who previously were normal, the children with underlying conditions had significantly more severe disease and more complicated courses requiring longer hospitalization. Immunodeficient patients, as described previously, have particular difficulty in controlling and clearing PIV infections, resulting in complicated, prolonged, and recurrent respiratory infections. Follow-up of children with PIV infections supports their generally good prognosis. Some children who have had croup have had pulmonary function abnormalities detected subsequently, but proof that these abnormalities were caused by PIV is lacking.[63, 105]

Prolonged or persistent infection with PIVs also has been noted in some patients with chronic bronchitis, possibly related to the lack of sufficient response of specific antibody in the sputum.[62] The possibility that PIV-like viruses also may be latent in the human central nervous system has been suggested by the occasional detection of such viruses in the central nervous system of patients with chronic neurologic conditions, such as multiple sclerosis, and PIVs may establish persistent infection.[96, 119, 128, 132, 162, 175, 186]

Prevention

For decades, attempts to prevent PIV infections have focused on the development of effective vaccines. A variety of formalin-inactivated, parenteral PIV vaccines have been developed and evaluated in clinical trials.[22, 50, 51, 93, 160, 170] Most of these vaccines have been grown in embryonated hens' eggs and prepared as an aqueous suspension. One vaccine was grown in monkey kidney cell cultures and prepared in alum formulation.[170] The vaccines, whether monovalent, trivalent, or combined with other respiratory vaccines, were able to induce an excellent humoral antibody response but were not protective.[22, 51] Subsequent natural PIV infection in the vaccinees did not result in more severe disease, however, as occurred with the alum-precipitated respiratory syncytial viral vaccine.[22, 51]

Alternative means of immunization have been sought.[27, 69, 87] Live attenuated vaccines compared with inactivated or subunit vaccines have the potential advantages of inducing immunity more closely mimicking natural infection with the production of both humoral and mucosal immunity and a longer duration of protection. Furthermore, because significant antigenic change does not occur yearly with PIVs as with influenza viruses, a single monovalent or polyvalent vaccine may suffice. The potential disadvantages of a live vaccine are the adverse or symptomatic reactions, the possible transmission of the vaccine virus, and its stability (i.e., whether reversion from its attenuated to a more virulent state is possible). Cold-adapted mutant PIV-3 strains have been produced that appear stable and grow well at the lower temperatures of the nasal passages but not at the higher temperatures of the lower respiratory tract.[87, 124] These cold-adapted human strains have been developed into PIV-3 candidate vaccines, one of which appears promising in both seropositive and seronegative young children, including infants.[87, 124, 153]

A second approach has been the use of a strain of virus from another species that is related to the human PIV. Focus has been on the bovine PIV-3 because of its close antigenic relationship to human PIV. The F and HN proteins of the two viruses show more than 75 percent amino acid homology and, more important, have high levels of antigenic relatedness.[27, 69, 87, 124, 168] Immunization with the bovine PIV-3 protects against challenge with human PIV-3, and it has diminished replication in humans.[124] Clinical evaluation of attenuated bovine PIV-3 intranasal vaccine in seronegative children has appeared safe and immunogenic and is undergoing further evaluation. Attenuated chimeric PIV-1 candidate vaccines have been developed with use of reverse genetics by replacement of the HN and F glycoproteins of a live attenuated strain of PIV-3 with the HN and F proteins of PIV-1. These candidate vaccines are immunogenic in animal models and are being investigated further.[87, 154, 161]

Subunit vaccines containing HN and F proteins are being explored concurrently. These glycoproteins have been produced through viral purification procedures and by expression of recombinant viruses with use of vaccinia and baculovirus vectors.[27, 124] Neutralizing antibodies are produced by vaccination with either the HN or the F protein, but protection against infection may require immunization with both glycoproteins. On the basis of the encouraging studies with these subunit vaccines in rodents and in primates, their evaluation is ongoing.

Multiple unique approaches combined with these creative techniques, such as novel adjuvants, immunomodulators, and vehicles for incorporation and administration of the vaccine, are evolving and may enhance further the immune response from PIV immunization.

REFERENCES

1. Abinanti, F. R., Chanock, R. M., Cook, M. K., et al.: Relationship of human and bovine strains of myxovirus parainfluenza 3 (26371). Proc. Soc. Exp. Biol. Med. *106*:466–469, 1961.
2. Aguilar, J., Pérez-Breña, M., Garcí, M., et al.: Detection and identification of human parainfluenza viruses 1, 2, 3, and 4 in clinical samples of pediatric patients by multiplex reverse transcription–PCR. J. Clin. Microbiol. *38*:1191–1195, 2000.
3. Anderson, L. J., Parker, R. A., and Strikas, R. L.: Association between respiratory syncytial virus outbreaks and lower respiratory tract deaths of infants and young children. J. Infect. Dis. *161*:640–646, 1990.
4. Andrewes, C. H., Bang, F. B., Chanock, R. M., et al.: Parainfluenza viruses 1, 2, and 3: Suggested names for recently described myxoviruses. Biology *8*:129–130, 1959.
5. Ansari, S. A., Springthorpe, V. S., Sattar, S. A., et al.: Potential role of hands in the spread of respiratory viral infections: Studies with human parainfluenza virus 3 and rhinovirus 14. J. Clin. Microbiol. *29*:2115–2119, 1991.
6. Arguedas, A., Stutman, H., and Blanding, J. G.: Parainfluenza type 3 meningitis: Report of two cases and review of the literature. Clin. Pediatr. *29*:175–178, 1990.
7. Arisoy, E. S., Demmler, G. J., Thakar, S., et al.: Meningitis due to parainfluenza virus type 3: Report of two cases and review. Clin. Infect. Dis. *17*:995–997, 1993.
8. Banatavala, J. E.: Parainfluenza infections in the community. Br. Med. J. *1*:537–540, 1964.
9. Barkin, R. M.: Pediatric emergency medicine. *In* Concepts and Clinical Practice. St. Louis, C. V. Mosby, 1992, p. 1002.

10. Beppu, Y., Imamura, Y., Tashiro, M., et al.: Human mucus protease inhibitor in airway fluids is a potential defensive compound against infection with influenza A and Sendai viruses. J. Biochem. *121*:309–316, 1997.
11. Bloom, H. H., Johnson, K. M., Jacobsen, R., et al.: Recovery of parainfluenza viruses from adults with upper respiratory illness. Am. J. Hyg. *74*:50–59, 1961.
12. Brady, M. T., Evans, J., and Cuartas, J.: Survival and disinfection of parainfluenza viruses on environmental surfaces. Am. J. Infect. Control *18*:18–23, 1990.
13. Browne, M. J.: Comparative inhibition of influenza and parainfluenza virus replication by ribavirin in MDCK cells. Antimicrob. Agents Chemother. *19*:712–715, 1981.
14. Brumback, B. G., and Wade, C. D.: Simultaneous rapid culture for four respiratory viruses in the same cell monolayer using a differential multicolored fluorescent confirmatory stain. J. Clin. Microbiol. *34*:798–801, 1996.
15. Buchan, K. A., Marten, K. W., and Kennedy, D. H.: Aetiology and epidemiology of viral croup in Glasgow, 1966–1972. J. Hyg. *73*:143–150, 1974.
16. Canchola, J., Vargosko, A. J., Kim, H. W., et al.: Antigenic variation among newly isolated strains of parainfluenza type 4 virus. Am. J. Hyg. *79*:357–364, 1964.
17. Chanock, R. M.: Association of a new type of cytopathogenic myxovirus with infantile croup. J. Exp. Med. *104*:555–576, 1965.
18. Chanock, R. M., Bell, J. A., and Parrott, R. H.: Natural history of parainfluenza infection. Perspect. Virol. *2*:126–139, 1961.
19. Chanock, R. M., and Parrott, R. H.: Acute respiratory disease in infancy and childhood: Present understanding and prospects for prevention. Pediatrics *36*:21–39, 1965.
20. Chanock, R. M., Parrott, R. H., Cook, K., et al.: Newly recognized myxoviruses from children with respiratory disease. N. Engl. J. Med. *258*:207–213, 1958.
21. Chanock, R. M., Parrott, R. H., Johnson, K. M., et al.: Myxoviruses: Parainfluenza. Am. Rev. Respir. Dis. *88*:152–166, 1963.
22. Chin, J., Magoffin, R. L., Shearer, L. A., et al.: Field evaluation of a respiratory syncytial virus vaccine and a trivalent parainfluenza virus vaccine in a pediatric population. Am. J. Epidemiol. *89*:449–463, 1969.
23. Chonmaitree, T., and Henrickson, K.: Detection of respiratory viruses in the middle ear fluids of children with acute otitis media by multiplex reverse transcription:polymerase chain reaction assay. Pediatr. Infect. Dis. J. *19*:258–260, 2000.
24. Chua, K., Bellini, W., Rota, P., et al.: Nipah virus: A recently emergent deadly paramyxovirus. Science *288*:1432–1435, 2000.
25. Clarke, S. K. R.: Parainfluenza virus infections. Postgrad. Med. J. *49*:792–797, 1973.
26. Cobian, L., Houston, S., Greene, J., et al.: Parainfluenza virus respiratory infection after heart transplantation: Successful treatment with ribavirin. Clin. Infect. Dis. *21*:1040–1041, 1995.
27. Collins, P. L., Chanock, R. M., and McIntosh, K.: Parainfluenza viruses. *In* Fields, B. N., Knipe, D. M., and Howley, P. M. (eds.): Fields Virology. Philadelphia, Lippincott-Raven, 1996, pp. 1205–1241.
28. Collinson, J., Nicholson, K., Cancio, E., et al.: Effects of upper respiratory tract infections in patients with cystic fibrosis. Thorax *51*:1115–1122, 1996.
29. Cressman, W. R., and Myer, C. C., III: Diagnosis and management of croup and epiglottitis. Pediatr. Clin. North Am. *41*:265–276, 1994.
30. Cruz, M. N., Stewart, G., and Rosenberg, N.: Use of dexamethasone in the outpatient management of acute laryngotracheitis. Pediatrics *96*:220–223, 1995.
31. Cullen, S. J., and Baublis, J. V.: Parainfluenza parotitis in two immunodeficient children. J. Pediatr. *96*:437–438, 1980.
32. Denny, F. W.: Croup: An 11-year study in a pediatric practice. Pediatrics *71*:871–876, 1983.
33. Denny, F. W.: Certain biologic characteristics of myxovirus parainfluenza 3. Fed. Proc. *19*:409, 1960.
34. Denny, F. W., and Clyde, W. A.: Acute lower respiratory infections in nonhospitalized children. J. Pediatr. *108*:635–646, 1986.
35. Dick, E. C., and Mogabgab, W. J.: Characteristics of parainfluenza 1 (HA-2) virus. III. Antigenic relationships, growth, interaction with erythrocytes and physical properties. J. Bacteriol. *85*:561–571, 1962.
36. Dick, E. C., Mogabgab, W. J., and Holmes, B.: Characteristics of parainfluenza 1 (HA-2) virus 1. Incidence of infection and clinical features in adults. Am. J. Hyg. *73*:263–272, 1961.
37. Drinka, P., Gravenstein, S., Langer, E., et al.: Mortality following isolation of various respiratory viruses in nursing home residents. Infect. Control Hosp. Epidemiol. *20*:812–815, 1999.
38. Ebata, S. N., Cote, M. J., Kang, C. Y., et al: The fusion and hemagglutinin-neuraminidase glycoproteins of human parainfluenza virus 3 are both required for fusion. Virology *183*:437–441, 1991.
39. Englund, J., Piedra, P., and Whimbey, E.: Prevention and treatment of respiratory syncytial virus and parainfluenza viruses in immunocompromised patient. Am. J. Med. *102*:61–70, 1997.
40. Enserink, M.: New virus fingered in Malaysian epidemic. Science *284*:407–410, 1999.
41. Eugene-Ruellan, G., Freymuth, F., Bahloul, C., et al.: Detection of respiratory syncytial virus A and B and parainfluenzavirus 3 sequences in respiratory tracts of infants by a single PCR with primers targeted to the L-polymerase gene and differential hybridization. J. Clin. Microbiol. *36*:796–801, 1998.
42. Evans, A. S., and Brobst, M.: Bronchitis, pneumonitis and pneumonia in University of Wisconsin students. N. Engl. J. Med. *265*:401–409, 1961.
43. Fan, J., Henrickson, K., and Savatski, L.: Rapid simultaneous diagnosis of infections with respiratory syncytial virus A and B, influenza viruses A and B, and human parainfluenza virus types 1, 2, and 3 by multiplex quantitative reverse transcription–polymerase chain reaction–enzyme hybridization assay (Hexaplex). Clin. Infect. Dis. *26*:1397–1402, 1998.
44. Fedova, D., Novotny, J., and Kubinova, I.: Serological diagnosis of parainfluenza virus infections: Verification of the sensitivity and specificity of the hemagglutination-inhibition (HI), complement-fixation (CF), immunofluorescence (IFA) tests and enzyme immunoassay (ELISA). Acta Virol. *36*:304–312, 1992.
45. Fiore, A., Iverson, C., Messmer, T., et al.: Outbreak of pneumonia in a long-term care facility: Antecedent human parainfluenza virus 1 infection may predispose to bacterial pneumonia. J. Am. Geriatr. Soc. *46*:1112–1117, 1998.
46. Fitzgerald, D., Mellis, C., Johnson, M., et al.: Nebulized budesonide is as effective as nebulized adrenaline in moderately severe croup. Pediatrics *97*:722–725, 1996.
47. Frank, A., Couch, R., Griffis, C., et al.: Comparison of different tissue cultures for isolation and quantitation of influenza and parainfluenza viruses. J. Clin. Microbiol. *10*:32–36, 1979.
48. Fraser, K. B., and Anderson, J.: Persistent non-cytocidal infection in BHK 21 cells by human parainfluenza type 2 virus. J. Gen. Microbiol. *44*:47–58, 1966.
49. Freymuth, F., Vabret, A., Galateau-Salle, F., et al.: Detection of respiratory syncytial virus, parainfluenzavirus 3, adenovirus and rhinovirus sequences in respiratory tract of infants by polymerase chain reaction and hybridization. Clin. Diagn. Virol. *8*:31–40, 1997.
50. Fulginiti, V. A., Amer, J., Eller, J. J., et al.: Parainfluenza virus immunization. IV. Simultaneous immunization with parainfluenza types 1, 2, and 3 aqueous vaccines. Am. J. Dis. Child. *114*:26–28, 1967.
51. Fulginiti, V. A., Eller, J. J., Sieber, O. F., et al.: Respiratory virus immunization. I. A field trial of two inactivated respiratory vaccines; an aqueous trivalent parainfluenza virus vaccine and an alum-precipitated respiratory syncytial virus vaccine. Am. J. Epidemiol. *89*:435–448, 1969.
52. Gardner, S. D.: The isolation of parainfluenza 4 subtypes A and B in England and serological studies of their prevalence. J. Hyg. *67*:545–550, 1969.
53. Gelfand, E. W., McCurdy, D., Rao, C. P., et al.: Ribavirin treatment of viral pneumonitis in severe combined immunodeficiency disease. Lancet *2*:732–733, 1983.
54. Giddens, W. E., Van Hoosier, G. L., and Garlinghouse, L. E.: Experimental Sendai virus infection in laboratory rats. II. Pathology and immunohistochemistry. Lab. Anim. Sci. *37*:442–448, 1987.
55. Glezen, W. P.: Incidence of respiratory syncytial and parainfluenza type 3 viruses in an urban setting. Pediatr. Virol. *2*:1–4, 1987.
56. Glezen, W. P.: Serious morbidity associated with the major respiratory viruses. Pediatr. Ann. *19*:535–542, 1990.
57. Glezen, W. P., and Denny, F. W.: Epidemiology of acute lower respiratory disease in children. N. Engl. J. Med. *288*:498–505, 1973.
58. Glezen, W. P., Frank, A. L., Taber, L. H., et al.: Parainfluenza virus type 3: Seasonality and risk of infection in young children. J. Infect. Dis. *150*:851–857, 1984.
59. Glezen, W. P., Loda, F. A., Clyde, W. A., et al.: Epidemiologic patterns of acute lower respiratory disease of children in pediatric group practice. J. Pediatr. *78*:397–406, 1971.
60. Glezen, W., Greenberg, S., Atmar, R., et al: Impact of respiratory virus infections on persons with chronic underlying conditions. J. A. M. A. *283*:499–505, 2000.
61. Goh, K., Tan, C., Chew, N., et al.: Clinical features of Nipah virus encephalitis among pig farmers in Malaysia. N. Engl. J. Med. *342*:1229–1235, 2000.
62. Gross, P. A., Green, R. H., and Curnen, M. G. M.: Persistent infection with parainfluenza type 3 virus in man. Am. Rev. Respir. Dis. *108*:894–898, 1973.
63. Gurwitz, D., Corey, M., and Levison, H.: Pulmonary function and bronchial reactivity in children after croup. Am. Rev. Respir. Dis. *122*:95–99, 1980.
64. Hall, C. B., and Douglas, R. G.: Respiratory syncytial virus and influenza: Practical community surveillance. Am. J. Dis. Child. *130*:615–620, 1976.
65. Hall, C. B., Geiman, J. M., Breese, B. B., et al.: Parainfluenza viral infections in children: Correlation of shedding with clinical manifestations. J. Pediatr. *91*:194–198, 1977.
66. Hall, C. E., Brandt, C. D., Frothingham, T. E., et al.: The virus watch program: A continuing surveillance of viral infections in metropolitan New York families. IX. A comparison of infections with several respiratory pathogens in New York and New Orleans families. Am. J. Epidemiol. *94*:367–385, 1971.
67. Hall, C.: Respiratory syncytial virus and the parainfluenza viruses. N. Engl. J. Med. *344*:1917–1918, 2001.

68. Heidemann, S. M.: Clinical characteristics of parainfluenza virus infection in hospital children. Pediatr. Pulmonol. *13*:86–89, 1992.
69. Heilman, C. A.: Respiratory syncytial and parainfluenza viruses. J. Infect. Dis. *161*:402–406, 1990.
70. Henderson, F. W., Collier, A. M., Sanyal, M. A., et al.: A longitudinal study of respiratory viruses and bacteria in the etiology of acute otitis media. N. Engl. J. Med. *306*:1377–1383, 1982.
71. Henrickson, K. J.: Monoclonal antibodies to human parainfluenza virus type 1 detect major antigenic changes in clinical isolates. J. Infect. Dis. *164*:1128–1134, 1991.
72. Henrickson, K. J., Kuhn, S. M., and Savatski, L.: Epidemiology and cost of human parainfluenza virus type one and two infections in young children. Clin. Infect. Dis. *18*:770–779, 1994.
73. Henrickson, K. J., and Savatski, L. L.: Genetic variation and evolution of human parainfluenza virus type 1 hemagglutinin neuraminidase: Analysis of 12 clinical isolates. J. Infect. Dis. *166*:995–1005, 1992.
74. Herrmann, E. C., and Hable, K. A.: Experiences in laboratory diagnosis of parainfluenza viruses in routine medical practice. Mayo Clin. Proc. *45*:177–188, 1970.
75. Hetherinton, S., Watson, A., Scroggs, R., et al.: Human parainfluenza virus type 1 evolution combines cocirculation of strains and development of geographically restricted lineages. J. Infect. Dis. *169*:248–252, 1994.
76. Hope-Simpson, R. E.: Parainfluenza virus infections in the Cirencester survey: Seasonal and other characteristics. J. Hyg. *87*:393–406, 1981.
77. Hotez, P. J., Goldstein, B., Ziegler, J., et al.: Adult respiratory distress syndrome associated with parainfluenza virus type 1 in children. Pediatr. Infect. Dis. J. *9*:750–752, 1990.
78. Hou, S., and Doherty, P.: Clearance of Sendai virus by $CD8^{+}$ T cells requires direct targeting to virus-infected epithelium. Eur. J. Immunol. *25*:111–116, 1995.
79. Hurrell, J. M.: Methods of storing viruses at low temperatures with particular reference to the myxovirus group. J. Med. Lab. Technol. *24*:30–41, 1967.
80. Jackson, M. A., Olson, L. C., Burry, V. F., et al.: Parainfluenza virus and neurologic signs. Pediatr. Infect. Dis. J. *13*:759–760, 1994.
81. Jantausch, B. A., Wiedermann, B. L., and Jeffries, B.: Parainfluenza virus type 2 meningitis and parotitis in an 11-year-old child. South. Med. J. *88*:230–231, 1995.
82. Jarvis, W. R., Middleton, P. J., and Gelfand, E. W.: Parainfluenza pneumonia in severe combined immunodeficiency disease. J. Pediatr. *94*:423–425, 1979.
83. Johnson, D. P., and Green, R. H.: Viremia during parainfluenza type 3 virus infection of hamsters. Proc. Soc. Exp. Biol. Med. *144*:745–748, 1973.
84. Johnson, K. M., Chanock, R. M., Cook, M. K., et al.: Studies of a new human hemadsorption virus. I. Isolation, properties, and characterization. Am. J. Hyg. *71*:81–92, 1960.
85. Johnston, S., Pattemore, P., Sanderson, G., et al.: Community study of role of viral infections in exacerbations of asthma in 9–11 year old children. Br. Med. J. *310*:1225–1229, 1995.
86. Kairys, S. W., Olmstead, E. M., and O'Connor, G. T.: Steroid treatment of laryngotracheitis: A meta-analysis of the evidence from randomized trials. Pediatrics *83*:683–693, 1989.
87. Kaiser, L., Couch, R., Galasso, G., et al.: First International Symposium on Influenza and Other Respiratory Viruses: Summary and overview: Kapalua, Maui, Hawaii, December 4–6, 1998. Antiviral Res. *42*:149–176, 1999.
88. Kapikian, A. Z., Chanock, R. M., Reichelderfer, T. E., et al.: Inoculation of human volunteers with parainfluenza virus type 3. J. A. M. A. *178*:537–541, 1961.
89. Karron, R. A., O'Brien, K. L., Froehlich, J. L., et al.: Molecular epidemiology of a parainfluenza type 3 virus outbreak on a pediatric ward. J. Infect. Dis. *167*:1441–1445, 1993.
90. Karron, R. A., Wright, P. F., Newman, F. K., et al.: A live human parainfluenza type 3 virus vaccine is attenuated and immunogenic in healthy infants and children. J. Infect. Dis. *172*:1445–1450, 1995.
91. Kasel, J. A., Frank, A. L., Keitel, W. A., et al.: Acquisition of serum antibodies to specific viral glycoproteins of parainfluenza virus 3 in children. J. Virol. *52*:828–832, 1984.
92. Killgore, G. E., and Dowdle, W. R.: Antigenic characterization of parainfluenza 4A and 4B by the hemagglutination-inhibition test and distribution of HI antibody in human sera. Am. J. Epidemiol. *91*:308–316, 1970.
93. Kim, H., Canchola, J. G., Vargosko, A. J., et al.: Immunogenicity of inactivated parainfluenza type 1, type 2, and type 3 vaccines in infants. J. A. M. A. *196*:819–824, 1966.
94. Knott, A., Long, C. E., and Hall, C. B.: Parainfluenza viral infections in pediatric outpatients: Seasonal patterns and clinical characteristics. Pediatr. Infect. Dis. J. *13*:269–273, 1994.
95. Komada, H., Kusagawa, S., Orvell, C., et al.: Antigenic diversity of human parainfluenza virus type 1 isolates and their immunological relationship with Sendai virus revealed by monoclonal antibodies. J. Gen. Virol. *73*:875–884, 1992.
96. Koprowski, H., and ter Meulen, V.: Multiple sclerosis and parainfluenza 1 virus: History of the isolation of the virus and expression of phenotypic differences between the isolated virus and Sendai virus. J. Neurol. *208*:175–190, 1975.
97. Kuroya, M., Ishida, N., and Shirator, T.: New born virus pneumonitis (type Sendai). II. The isolation of a new virus possessing hemagglutination activity. Yokohama M. Bull. *4*:217–233, 1953.
98. Lambert, D., Barney, S., Lambert, A., et al.: Peptides from conserved regions of paramyxovirus fusion (F) proteins are potent inhibitors of viral infusion. Proc. Natl. Acad. Sci. U. S. A. *93*:2186–2191, 1996.
99. Landry, M., and Ferguson, D.: SimulFluor respiratory screen for rapid detection of multiple respiratory viruses in clinical specimens by immunofluorescence staining. J. Clin. Microbiol. *38*:708–711, 2000.
100. Laurichesse, H., Dedman, D., Watson, J., et al.: Epidemiological features of parainfluenza virus infections: Laboratory surveillance in England and Wales, 1975–1997. Eur. J. Epidemiol. *15*:475–484, 1999.
101. Leogrande, G.: Studies on the epidemiology of child infections. 3. Parainfluenza viruses (types 1–4) and respiratory syncytial virus infections. Microbios *72*:55–63, 1992.
102. Lewis, V., Champlin, R., Englund, J., et al.: Respiratory disease due to parainfluenza virus in adult bone marrow transplant recipients. Clin. Infect. Dis. *23*:1033–1037, 1996.
103. Lindquist, S., Darnule, A., Istas, A., et al.: Parainfluenza virus type 4 infections in pediatric patients. Pediatr. Infect. Dis. J. *16*:34–38, 1997.
104. Ljungman, P.: Respiratory virus infections in bone marrow transplant recipients: The European perspective. Am. J. Med. *102*:44–47, 1997.
105. Loughlin, G., and Taussig, L. M.: Pulmonary function in children with a history of laryngotracheobronchitis. J. Pediatr. *94*:365–369, 1979.
106. Madhi, S., Schoub, B., Simmank, K., et al.: Increased burden of respiratory viral associated severe lower respiratory tract infections in children infected with human immunodeficiency virus type-1. J. Pediatr. *137*:78–84, 2000.
107. Marx, A., Török, T., Holman, C., et al.: Pediatric hospitalizations for croup (laryngotracheobronchitis): Biennial increases associated with human parainfluenza virus 1 epidemics. J. Infect. Dis. *176*:1423–1427, 1997.
108. Marx, A., Gary, H., Marston, B., et al.: Parainfluenza virus infection among adults hospitalized for lower respiratory tract infection. Clin. Infect. Dis. *29*:134–140, 1999.
109. Mazanec, M., Kaetzel, C., Lamm, M., et al.: Intracellular neutralization of virus by immunoglobulin A antibodies. Proc. Natl. Acad. Sci. U. S. A. *89*:6901–6905, 1992.
110. Mazanec, M., Lamm, M., Lyn, D., et al.: Comparison of IgA versus IgG monoclonal antibodies for passive immunization of murine respiratory tract. Virus Res. *23*:1–12, 1992.
111. McIntosh, K.: Pathogenesis of severe acute respiratory infections in the developing world: Respiratory syncytial virus and parainfluenza virus. Rev. Infect. Dis. *13*(Suppl.):S492–S500, 1991.
112. McIntosh, K., Ellis, E. F., Hoffman, L. S., et al.: The association of viral and bacterial respiratory infections with exacerbations of wheezing in young asthmatic children. J. Pediatr. *82*:578–590, 1973.
113. McIntosh, K., Halonen, P., and Ruuskanen, O.: Report of a workshop on respiratory viral infections: Epidemiology, diagnosis, treatment, and prevention. Clin. Infect. Dis. *16*:151–164, 1993.
114. McIntosh, K., Kurachek, S. C., Cairns, L. M., et al.: Treatment of respiratory viral infection in an immunodeficient infant with ribavirin aerosol. Am. J. Dis. Child. *138*:305–308, 1984.
115. McLean, D. M., Bannatyne, R. M., and Givan, K. F.: Myxovirus dissemination by air. Can. Med. Assoc. J. *96*:1449–1453, 1967.
116. Metzgar, D. P., Gower, T. A., Larson, E. J., et al.: The effect of parainfluenza virus type 3 on newborn ferrets. J. Biol. Stand. *2*:273–282, 1974.
117. Miller, W. S., and Artenstein, M. S.: Aerosol stability of three acute respiratory disease viruses. Proc. Soc. Exp. Biol. Med. *125*:222–227, 1967.
118. Monto, A. S.: The Tecumseh study of respiratory illness. V. Patterns of infection with the parainfluenza viruses. Am. J. Epidemiol. *97*:338–348, 1973.
119. Moscona, A., and Galinski, M.: Characterization of human parainfluenza virus type 3 persistent infection in cell cultures. J. Virol. *67*:3212–3218, 1990.
120. Moscona, A.: Interaction of human parainfluenza virus type 3 with the host cell surface. Pediatr. Infect. Dis. J. *16*:917–924, 1997.
121. Moyse, E., Lyon, M., Cordier, G., et al.: Viral RNA in middle ear mucosa and exudates in patients with chronic otitis media with effusion. Arch. Otolaryngol. Head Neck Surg. *126*:1105–1110, 2000.
122. Muchmore, H. C., Parkinson, A. J., Humphries, J. E., et al.: Persistent parainfluenza viruses shedding during isolation at the South Pole. Nature *289*:187–189, 1981.
123. Mufson, M. A., Mocega, H. E., and Krause, H. E.: Acquisition of parainfluenza 3 virus infection by hospitalized children. I. Frequencies, rates, and temporal data. J. Infect. Dis. *128*:141–147, 1973.
124. Murphy, B., and Collins, P.: Current status of respiratory syncytial virus (RSV) and parainfluenza virus type 3 (PIV3) vaccine development: Memorandum from a joint WHO/NIAID meeting. Bull. World Health Organ. *75*:307–313, 1997.
125. Newth, C. J., Levinson, H., and Byron, A. C.: The respiratory status of children with croup. J. Pediatr. *81*:1068–1073, 1972.
126. Nicholson, K. G., Kent, J., and Ireland, D. C.: Respiratory viruses and exacerbations of asthma in adults. Br. Med. J. *307*:982–986, 1993.

127. Nicholson, K., Kent, J., Hammersley, V., et al.: Acute viral infections of upper respiratory tract in elderly people living in the community: Comparative, prospective, population based study of disease burden. Br. Med. J. *315*:1060–1064, 1997.
128. Norrby, E., Link, H., Olsson, J. E., et al.: Comparison of antibodies against different viruses in cerebrospinal fluid and serum samples from patients with multiple sclerosis. Infect. Immun. *10*:688–694, 1974.
129. Obara, T., Shuto, S., Saito, Y., et al.: New neplanocin analogues. 7. Synthesis and antiviral activity of 2-halo derivatives of neplanocin A. J. Med. Chem. *39*:3847–3852, 1996.
130. Ottolini, M. G., Hemming, V. G., Piazza, F. M., et al.: Topical immunoglobulin is an effective therapy for parainfluenza type 3 in a cotton rat model. J. Infect. Dis. *172*:243–245, 1995.
131. Ottolini, M., Porter, D., Hemming, V., et al.: Semi-permissive replication and functional aspects of the immune response in a cotton rat model of human parainfluenza virus type 3 infection. J. Gen. Virol. *77*: 1739–1743, 1996.
132. Parkinson, A. J., Muchmore, H. G., Scott, L. V., et al.: Parainfluenza virus upper respiratory tract illness in partially immune adult human subjects: A study at an Antarctic station. Am. J. Epidemiol. *110*:753–763, 1979.
133. Parkinson, A. J., Muchmore, H. G., Scott, E. N., et al.: Survival of human parainfluenza viruses in the South Polar environment. Appl. Environ. Microbiol. *46*:901–905, 1983.
134. Parrott, R. H., Vargosko, A. J., Kim, H. W., et al.: Acute respiratory diseases of viral etiology. III. Myxoviruses: Parainfluenza. Am. J. Public Health *52*:907–917, 1962.
135. Patterson, D., Murray, P., and McCormack, J.: Zoonotic disease in Australia caused by a novel member of the paramyxoviridae. Clin. Infect. Dis. *27*:112–118, 1998.
136. Pereira, M. S., and Fisher, O. D.: An outbreak of acute laryngotracheobronchitis associated with parainfluenza 2 virus. Lancet *2*:790–791, 1960.
137. Phillips, M. J., Blendis, L. M., Poucell, S., et al.: Sporadic hepatitis with distinctive pathological features, a severe clinical course, and paramyxoviral features. N. Engl. J. Med. *324*:455–460, 1991.
138. Phillips, P. E., and Christian, C. L.: Myxovirus antibody increases in human connective tissue disease. Science *168*:982–984, 1970.
139. Porter, D. D., Prince, G. A., Hemming, V. G., et al.: Pathogenesis of human parainfluenza virus 3 infection in two species of cotton rats: *Sigmodon hispidus* develops bronchiolitis, while *Sigmodon fulviventer* develops interstitial pneumonia. J. Virol. *65*:103–111, 1991.
140. Prince, G. A., and Porter, D. D.: Treatment of parainfluenza virus type 3 bronchiolitis and pneumonia in a cotton rat model using topical antibody and glucocorticosteroid. J. Infect. Dis. *173*:598–608, 1996.
141. Prinoski, K., Cote, M. J., Kang, C. Y., et al.: Evolution of the fusion protein gene of human parainfluenza virus 3. Virus Res. *22*:55–69, 1992.
142. Ray, R., Glaze, B. J., and Compans, R. W.: Role of individual glycoproteins of human parainfluenza virus type 3 in the induction of a protective immune response. J. Virol. *62*:783–787, 1988.
143. Reed, G., Jewett, P., Thompson, J., et al.: Epidemiology and clinical impact of parainfluenza virus infections in otherwise healthy infants and young children <5 years old. J. Infect. Dis. *175*:807–813, 1997.
144. Rittichier, K., and Ledwith, C.: Outpatient treatment of moderate croup with dexamethasone: Intramuscular versus oral dosing. Pediatrics *106*:1344–1348, 2000.
145. Robinson, R. Q., Hoshiwara, I., Schaeffer, M., et al.: A survey of respiratory illnesses in a population. I. Viral studies. Am. J. Hyg. *75*:18–27, 1962.
146. Rocchi, G., Arangio-Ruiz, G., Giannini, V., et al.: Detection of viraemia in acute respiratory disease of man. Acta Virol. *14*:405–407, 1970.
147. Roman, G., Phillips, C. A., and Poser, C. M.: Parainfluenza viruses type 3: Isolation from CSF of a patient with Guillain-Barré syndrome. J. A. M. A. *240*:1613–1615, 1978.
148. Ruuskanen, O., Arola, M., Heikkinen, T., et al.: Viruses in acute otitis media: Increasing evidence for clinical significance. Pediatr. Infect. Dis. J. *10*:425–427, 1991.
149. Sable, C., and Hayden, F.: Orthomyxoviral and paramyxoviral infections in transplant patients. Infect. Dis. Clin. North Am. *9*:987–1003, 1995.
150. Sarkkihen, H. C., Haloren, P. E., Arstita, P. P., et al.: Detection of respiratory syncytial, parainfluenza type 3, and adenovirus antigens by radioimmunoassay and enzyme immunoassay in nasopharyngeal specimens from children with acute respiratory disease. J. Clin. Microbiol. *13*:258–265, 1981.
151. Seidman, D., Nass, D., Mendelson, E., et al.: Prenatal ultrasonographic diagnosis of fetal hydrocephalus due to infection with parainfluenza virus type 3. Ultrasound Obstet. Gynecol. *7*:52–54, 1996.
152. Singh-Naz, N., Willy, M., and Riggs, N.: Outbreak of parainfluenza virus type 3 in a neonatal nursery. Pediatr. Infect. Dis. J. *9*:31–33, 1990.
153. Skiadopoulos, M., Surman, S., St. Claire, M., et al.: Attenuation of the recombinant human parainfluenza virus type 3 *cp*45 candidate vaccine virus is augmented by importation of the respiratory syncytial virus *cpts*530 L polymerase mutation. Virology *260*:125–135, 1999.
154. Skiadopoulos, M., Tao, T., Surman, S., et al.: Generation of a parainfluenza virus type 1 vaccine candidate by replacing the HN and F glycoproteins of the live-attenuated PIV3 cp45 vaccine virus with their PIV1 counterparts. Vaccine *18*:503–510, 1999.
155. Skolnik, N. S.: Treatment of croup: A critical review. Am. J. Dis. Child. *143*:1045–1049, 1989.
156. Smith, C. B., Purcell, R. H., Bellanti, J. A., et al.: Protective effect of antibody to parainfluenza type 1 virus. N. Engl. J. Med. *275*:1145–1152, 1966.
157. Sonoda, S., Gotoh, Y., Bann, F., et al.: Acute lower respiratory infections in hospitalized children over a 6 year period in Tokyo. Pediatr. Int. *41*:519–524, 1999.
158. Sparrelid, E., Ljungman, P., Ekelof-Andstrom, E., et al.: Ribavirin therapy in bone marrow transplant recipients with viral respiratory tract infections. Bone Marrow Transplant. *19*:905–908, 1997.
159. Spiggs, M., Murphy, B., Prince, G., et al.: Expression of the F and HN glycoproteins of human parainfluenza virus type 3 recombinant vaccinia viruses: Contributions of the individual to host immunity. J. Virol. *61*:3416–3423, 1987.
160. Sweet, B. H., Tyrell, A. A., Potash, L., et al.: Respiratory virus vaccine. III. Pentavalent respiratory syncytial–parainfluenza–*Mycoplasma pneumoniae* vaccine. Am. Rev. Respir. Dis. *94*:340–349, 1966.
161. Tao, T., Davoodi, F., Cho, C., et al.: A live attenuated recombinant chimeric parainfluenza virus (PIV) candidate vaccine containing the hemagglutinin-neuraminidase and fusion glycoproteins of PIV1 and the remaining proteins from PIV3 induces resistance to PIV1 even in animals immune to PIV3. Vaccine *18*:1359–1366, 2000.
162. ter Meulen, V., Koprowski, H., Iwasaki, Y., et al.: Fusion of cultured multiple sclerosis brain cells with indicator cells: Presence of nucleocapsids and virions and isolation of parainfluenza-type virus. Lancet *2*:1–5, 1972.
163. Treanor, J., and Falsey, A.: Respiratory viral infections in the elderly. Antiviral Res. *44*:79–102, 1999.
164. Tremonti, L. P., Lin, J. S., and Jackson, G. G.: Neutralizing activity in nasal secretions and serum in resistance of volunteers to parainfluenza virus type 2. J. Immunol. *101*:572–577, 1968.
165. Tunnessen, W. W., and Feinstein, A. R.: The steroid-croup controversy: An analytic review of methodologic problems. J. Pediatr. *96*:751–756, 1980.
166. Tyrrell, D. A. J., Bynoe, M. L., Birkum, K., et al.: Inoculation of human volunteers with parainfluenza viruses 1 and 3 (HA2 and HA1). Br. Med. J. *2*:909–911, 1959.
167. van der Logt, J. T., van Loon, A. M., Heessen, F. W., et al.: Diagnosis of parainfluenza virus infection in children and older patients by detection of specific IgM antibody. J. Med. Virol. *16*:191–199, 1985.
168. van Wyke Coelingh, K. L., Winter, C. C., Tierney, E. L., et al.: Attenuation of bovine parainfluenza virus type 3 in nonhuman primates and its ability to confer immunity to human parainfluenza virus type 3 challenge. J. Infect. Dis. *157*:655–662, 1988.
169. van Wyke Coelingh, K. L., Winter, C. C., Tierney, E. L., et al.: Antibody responses of humans and nonhuman primates to individual antigenic sites of the hemagglutinin-neuraminidase and fusion glycoproteins after primary infection or reinfection with parainfluenza type 3 virus. J. Virol. *64*:3833–3843, 1990.
170. Vella, P. P., Weibel, R. E., Woodhour, A. F., et al.: Respiratory virus vaccines. VIII. Field evaluation of trivalent parainfluenza virus vaccine among preschool children in families, 1967–1968. Am. Rev. Respir. Dis. *99*:526–541, 1969.
171. Volovitz, B., Faden, H., and Ogra, P. L.: Release of leukotriene C_4 in respiratory tract during acute viral infection. J. Pediatr. *112*:218–222, 1988.
172. Vreede, R. W., Schellekens, H., and Zuijderwijk, M.: Isolation of parainfluenza virus type 3 from cerebrospinal fluid. J. Infect. Dis. *165*:1166, 1992.
173. Vuorinen, T., and Meurman, O.: Enzyme immunoassays for detection of IgG and IgM antibodies to parainfluenza types 1, 2, and 3. J. Virol. Methods *23*:63–70, 1989.
174. Wagener, J. S., Minnich, L., Sobonya, R., et al.: Parainfluenza type II infection in dogs: A model of viral respiratory tract infection in humans. Am. Rev. Respir. Dis. *127*:771–775, 1983.
175. Wechsler, S. L., Lambert, D. M., Galinski, M. S., et al.: Immediate persistent infection by human parainfluenza virus 3: Unique fusion properties of the persistently infected cells. J. Gen. Virol. *68*:1737–1748, 1987.
176. Welliver, R. C., Sun, M., and Rinaldo, D.: Defective regulation of immune response in croup due to parainfluenza virus. Pediatr. Res. *19*:716–720, 1985.
177. Welliver, R., Wong, D. T., Choi, T. S., et al.: Natural history of parainfluenza virus infection in childhood. J. Pediatr. *101*:180–187, 1982.
178. Welliver, R. C., Wong, D. T., Middleton, E., et al.: Role of parainfluenza virus–specific IgE in pathogenesis of croup and wheezing subsequent to infection. J. Pediatr. *101*:889–896, 1982.
179. Welliver, R. C., Wong, D. T., Sun, M., et al.: Parainfluenza virus bronchiolitis: Epidemiology and pathogenesis. Am. J. Dis. Child. *140*:34–40, 1986.
180. Welliver, R., Wong, D., Sun, M., et al.: The development of respiratory syncytial virus–specific IgE and the release of histamine in nasopharyngeal secretions after infection. N. Engl. J. Med. *305*:841–846, 1981.

181. Wendt, C. H., Weisdorf, D. J., Jordan, M. C., et al.: Parainfluenza virus respiratory infection after bone marrow transplantation. N. Engl. J. Med. *326*:921–926, 1992.
182. Wenzel, R. P., McCormick, D. P., and Beam, W. E.: Parainfluenza pneumonia in adults. J. A. M. A. *221*:294–295, 1972.
183. Wilks, D., and Burns, S.: Myopericarditis associated with parainfluenza virus type 3 infection. Eur. J. Clin. Microbiol. *17*:363–365, 1998.
184. Wolinsky, J. S., and Gilden, D. H.: In vivo studies of parainfluenza I (6/94) virus: Mononuclear cell interactions. Arch. Virol. *49*:25–31, 1975.
185. Wong, V. K., Steinberg, E., and Warford, A.: Parainfluenza virus type 3 meningitis in an 11-month-old infant. Pediatr. Infect. Dis. J. *7*:300–301, 1988.
186. Wroblewska, Z., Santoli, D., Gilden, D., et al.: Persistent parainfluenza type 1 (6/94) infection of brain cells in tissue culture. Arch. Virol. *50*:287–303, 1976.
187. Yao, Q., and Compans, R.: Peptides corresponding to the heptad sequence of human parainfluenza virus fusion protein are potent inhibitors of virus infection. Virology *223*:103–112, 1996.
188. Yurlova, T. I., Sverkunova, M. V., Furaeva, V. A., et al.: Studies of natural population variability of parainfluenza viruses during their epidemic circulation. Acta Virol. *25*:64–70, 1991.
189. Zach, M., Erban, A., and Olinsky, A.: Croup, recurrent croup, allergy, and airways hyperreactivity. Arch. Dis. Child. *56*:336–341, 1981.
190. Zach, M., and Messner, H.: Serum IgA in recurrent croup. Am. J. Dis. Child. *137*:184–185, 1983.
191. Zinserling, A.: Peculiarities of lesions in viral and mycoplasma infections of the respiratory tract. Virchows Arch. Pathol. Anat. *356*:259–273, 1972.
192. Zollar, L. M., and Mufson, M. A.: Acute parotitis associated with parainfluenza 3 virus infection. Am. J. Dis. Child. *119*:147–148, 1970.

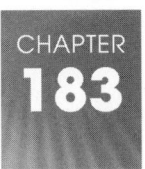

CHAPTER 183 Measles Virus

JAMES D. CHERRY

Measles virus is a singular agent that causes a relatively distinct, exanthematous disease characterized by fever, cough, coryza, conjunctivitis, an erythematous maculopapular confluent rash, and a pathognomonic enanthem. Clinical measles is an epidemic disease, the incidence of which in the United States has been reduced from 315 reported cases per 100,000 population in the prevaccine era to less than 1 per 100,000 since 1992 by the use of attenuated vaccines. However, measles is still a major problem because of its worldwide prevalence, associated morbidity and mortality, and changing epidemiologic pattern in the United States and countries where vaccine use has been widespread.

History

In antiquity, measles and smallpox frequently were confused with each other, as well as with other exanthematous diseases.[25, 292] Major epidemics of both measles and smallpox occurred 1800 years ago in the Roman Empire and China.[39, 248] The first written record of measles generally is credited to Rhazes, a 10th-century Persian physician[25, 39, 193, 390]; however, Rhazes quoted writers, including El Yahudi, a famous Hebrew physician, who lived 300 years earlier.[39] Rhazes identified measles as an entity distinct from smallpox.

During the Middle Ages in Europe, smallpox and measles continued to be confused. By the beginning of the 17th century, however, differentiation between the two diseases was relatively clear; death reports by London parish clerks in 1629 listed measles and smallpox separately.[390] Repeated epidemics of measles were described in the English medical literature during the 17th and 18th centuries.[193]

The first account of measles in America was given by John Hall, who described epidemic disease in Boston in fall 1657.[54] The next epidemic in colonial America was reported in 1687. During the next 150 years, the epidemic interval in Boston gradually decreased from 30 years to about 3 years. Epidemics during the 17th and 18th centuries involved persons of all ages, including neonates; coincident with a reduction in the epidemic interval was a reduction in the age-specific incidence of measles. The reduction in epidemic interval can be attributed to the increased importation of measles as a result of more and faster ships crossing the Atlantic and the gradual increase in population density in North America. By the turn of the 19th century, both Boston and Philadelphia had sufficient population for measles to propagate itself.

The first recognition of the contagiousness of measles is unclear. Shakespeare in *Coriolanus* was aware of its human-to-human transmission.[390] Home[172] in 1758 attempted to immunize against measles by applying a technique similar to the variolation used in smallpox.[313] In 1911, Goldberger and Anderson[137] produced clinical measles in monkeys by injecting filtered material from acute cases of human disease.

The classic epidemiologic study of measles was the account by Panum of the 1846 Faroe Islands epidemic.[302] In this study, Panum confirmed that spread was solely through human-to-human contagion via the respiratory route, the incubation period was 14 days, and infection conveyed lifelong immunity.

The enanthem of measles, which is pathognomonic, was described carefully and presented by Koplik in 1896, 1898, and 1899.[35, 207–209] However, Koplik spots clearly were recognized specifically about a century earlier by John Quier, a physician in Jamaica,[35, 135] and by Richard Hazeltine, a general practitioner in rural Maine.[54]

Although Plotz[314] reported cultivation of measles virus in 1938 and Rake and Shaffer[319] noted similar findings in 1940, reliable tissue culture methods were not available until approximately 10 years later. In 1954, Enders and Peebles[104] isolated eight agents (from cases of measles) in human or simian renal cell cultures. They also demonstrated the ability of convalescent-phase serum from a measles patient to neutralize the viral cytopathogenic effect. The stage for vaccine development was set by tissue culture recovery of the virus,[104] adaptation of viral growth in chicken embryos,[255] and finally, cultivation of the virus in chicken embryo tissue culture cells.[195]

After extensive trials were conducted from 1958 through 1962, tissue culture–grown, inactivated ("killed") and attenuated ("live") measles viral vaccines became available for general use in 1963.[74, 192, 212] In the United States, a nationwide immunization effort instituted in 1965 and 1966 led to a dramatic reduction in epidemic measles for several years. Epidemic measles recurred in 1971, 1977, and 1989, but at lesser overall levels than those in the prevaccine era.[21, 55, 56, 62, 74, 213] After initiation of the Childhood Immunization Initiative in 1977 and the Measles Elimination Program in 1978, the incidence of measles in the United States fell in 1981 to fewer than 1.5 cases per 100,000 population and remained at this low level until 1986.[21, 60, 61] In 1990, the rate was 11.2 cases per 100,000 population, which was the highest it had been since 1977. Since 1990, a substantial decline in measles has occurred in the United States, to a low of 86 confirmed cases in 2000.[63] However, approximately 1 million children worldwide die of measles each year.[132, 299]

Properties

CLASSIFICATION

Measles virus is a relatively large virus with helical capsid symmetry and an RNA genome.[32, 109, 220, 251] It is a singular virus, but antigenically it is related closely to canine distemper. These agents, as well as peste des petits ruminants virus, dolphin morbillivirus, phocine distemper virus, and rinderpest virus, presently are included in the genus *Morbillivirus*; they are members of the family *Paramyxoviridae*. Measles virus differs from the other paramyxoviruses in that it does not possess specific neuraminidase activity and does not adsorb to neuraminic acid–containing cellular receptors.[264, 283, 311, 379] Measles virus hemagglutinates, whereas the other members of its genus do not.

PHYSICAL PROPERTIES

Measles virus is a roughly spherical but pleomorphic virus that ranges from 100 to 300 nm in diameter.[32, 109, 149, 251, 275, 292, 379, 380] The virion is composed of an outer lipoprotein envelope and an internal helical nucleocapsid. The virion contains eight proteins. The outer viral envelope is 10 to 22 nm thick, has short surface projections (peplomers), and contains three virus-coded proteins (F, H, and M).[77, 264, 292] F protein is a dumbbell-shaped peplomer that causes membrane fusion of the virus and host cell and enables penetration of the virus into the host cell. H protein is the hemagglutinin and is a conical peplomer. In infection, H protein reacts with a host cellular receptor. CD46 appears to be the cellular receptor for attenuated measles vaccine strains but not wild-type viral strains.[46, 96, 234, 235, 277, 297] Recent data suggest that the signaling lymphocyte activation molecule (CDw150) is the cellular receptor for wild-type virus.[297] M (matrix) protein is nonglycosylated and associated with the inner lipid bilayer of the envelope. It plays an important role in virus maturation.

The nucleocapsid (N) protein (Fig. 183–1) is a coiled rod with a diameter of 18 nm and a length of 1 μm that contains the viral genomic RNA.[287, 290, 292, 377, 379] N protein has a molecular weight of about 60 kd. Approximately 5 percent of the nucleocapsid is RNA.[160, 372, 378] The other internal proteins of the virus are the L (large), P (phospho), C, and V proteins.

The virus genome has a molecular weight of 4.5×10^6 d; it is a linear, single strand of RNA that contains approximately 15,900 nucleotides.

Measles virus is labile.[193, 194, 270] It is inactivated rapidly by heat, ultraviolet light, lipid solvents such as ether and chloroform, and extreme degrees of acidity and alkalinity (i.e., pH <5 and >10). Longevity is prolonged when protein is present in the viral suspending medium and when the virus is lyophilized with a protein stabilizer. Protein specifically protects against the adverse effects of heat and light. Protein-stabilized measles virus can be stored at −70° C for 5 or more years without significant loss of infectivity. At room temperature, a 60 percent loss in titer occurs in 3 to 5 days; at 56° C, the virus is inactivated within 30 minutes.[36, 270]

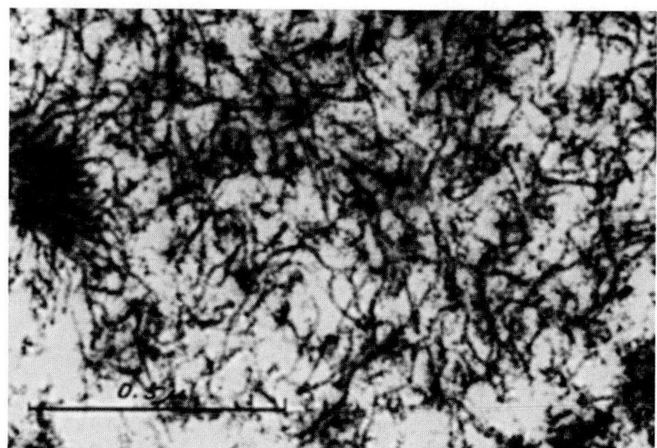

FIGURE 183–1 ■ Nucleocapsid fragments. Electron micrograph. (Courtesy of Dr. John M. Adams.)

ANTIGENIC COMPOSITION

Clinical and epidemiologic data and early laboratory study suggested antigenic homogeneity of all measles strains.[194] Recent nucleotide sequence analysis has identified distinct lineages among wild-type measles virus isolates.[32, 365] The following properties have been associated with measles virus: a hemagglutinin (for simian cells), complement-fixing antigens, hemolytic activity, and a giant-cell–inducing factor.[48, 161, 193, 194, 285, 286, 291, 311, 340] Human measles virus infection results in serum antibodies that are capable of neutralizing viral infectivity, fixing complement with viral antigen, and inhibiting viral hemagglutination and hemolysis.

Cross-seroreactivity occurs among members of the genus *Morbillivirus* but not with other members of the family *Paramyxoviridae*.[40, 52, 179] Measles virus serum antibody in humans reacts with distemper virus, but canine serum after distemper does not react with measles virus. A two-way cross between measles and rinderpest viruses has been demonstrated.

TISSUE CULTURE GROWTH

Measles virus can be propagated in many different primary and cell line tissue cultures.[40, 194, 242] However, for isolation of virus from patient specimens, primary human and monkey kidney cultures have been most successful over the years. In one study, an Epstein-Barr virus–transformed marmoset lymphocytic line (B95-8) was found to be superior to primary monkey kidney cell culture for isolation of virus from nasopharyngeal specimens.[204] In tissue culture, measles virus has two distinct cytopathogenic effects. With initial isolation, syncytial formation occurs as a result of cell fusion, and the resulting giant cells may contain 10 to 50 or more nuclei (Fig. 183–2). On stained preparations, both the nuclei and cytoplasm contain eosinophilic inclusions. The second type of cytopathogenic effect is characterized by the alteration of single cells into spindle shapes or stellate forms. In general, tissue culture–adapted measles viral

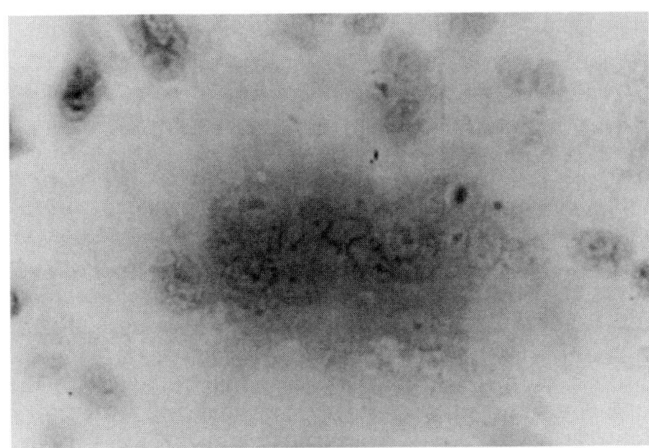

FIGURE 183–2 ■ Measles virus cytopathogenic effect in monkey kidney tissue culture. Giant cell with approximately 20 nuclei.

strains are more likely to cause this cytopathogenic effect than giant-cell formation is. In most cultures, both forms of cytopathogenic effect are evident, and changes in medium composition make one or the other type predominate.

Infection in tissue culture is associated with an attachment-adsorption phase lasting approximately 1 hour and an eclipse period of 6 to 12 hours.[242, 264] Antigen first is noted in the cytoplasm perinuclearly at 12 hours; by 24 hours, it is distributed throughout the cytoplasm. By 30 hours, most antigen is detected at the cell surface. In mature cultures, more cell-associated virus is present than is found free within the medium.

ANIMAL SUSCEPTIBILITY

Humans are the natural hosts of measles virus, but with human contact, monkeys also are infected easily.[253] Laboratory strains of measles virus have been adapted to suckling mice and hamsters.[47, 51, 180, 375]

Epidemiology

PREVALENCE

The prevalence of measles throughout history has been affected markedly by population density and, during the last 40 years, by the use of measles vaccine. Reported cases of measles in the United States from 1963 to 1998, analyzed by year, are presented in Figure 183–3. After the universal use of measles vaccine began in 1965, the number of cases in the United States fell to 22,231 in 1968.[62] In 1971 and 1977, modest epidemics occurred; then, after a national commitment to measles immunization, the number of cases of measles fell to an all-time low of 1497 cases reported in 1983. Beginning in 1986, the number of measles cases again increased, with 27,786 cases reported in 1990. Since 1990, measles in the United States has declined, with an all-time low of 100 cases in 1998.[63] In the 20th century, before the widespread use of measles vaccine, between 200,000 and 600,000 cases of measles were reported annually in the United States.[82, 222] Careful survey has suggested that in the past, reported cases accounted for only approximately 15 percent of the actual number of cases of measles.[74]

In the prevaccine era in the United States and other concentrated populations throughout the world, measles epidemics occurred regularly. In the United States, urban-centered measles epidemics took place every 2 to 5 years, with each epidemic lasting 3 to 4 months.[25, 39, 158, 166, 230, 385, 398] In general, the larger the community, the shorter the interval between epidemics. In the vaccine era, the epidemic pattern has been changed. As noted in Figure 183–3, the total number of cases has been reduced, and the cycle between peaks has lengthened.

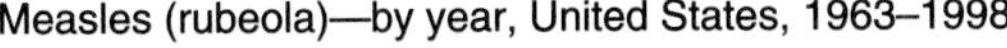

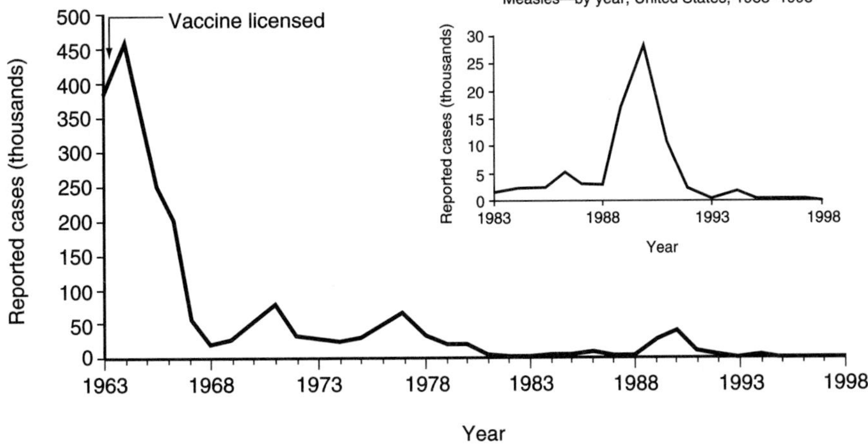

With a record low of 100 measles cases reported in 1998, measles incidence remained at <1 case per million population for the second consecutive year. Of the 100 cases reported, 71% were associated with international importation, suggesting measles is no longer an indigenous disease in the United States.

FIGURE 183–3 ■ Reported measles cases by year in the United States, 1963 to 1998. (From Summary of notifiable diseases—United States, 1998. M. M. W. R. Morb. Mortal. Wkly. Rep. *47* [53]:48, 1999.)

AGE INCIDENCE AND PREVALENCE

In modern times in populous areas, measles has been a disease of children. The age-specific incidence in the United States for selected years is presented in Table 183–1. In the prevaccine era during the 20th century, the highest measles attack rate occurred in children 5 to 9 years of age.[25, 39, 166, 389] In the period 1960 to 1964, data from five reporting areas showed that more than half of all measles cases occurred in this age group.[162] Before the present vaccine era, infections and epidemic loci centered in elementary schools. Younger children acquired measles as secondary cases from their school-attending older siblings. In rural areas, the interval between measles epidemics tended to be greater; therefore, a greater age spread occurred in the percentage of measles cases. In a nationwide serum survey of U.S. military recruits in 1962, Black[38] found that 99 percent had measles antibody.

As noted in Table 183–1, the age incidence and percentage of measles cases by age group have changed markedly since 1964. In 1991, more than 40 percent of measles cases occurred in persons older than 10 years; in the period from 1960 to 1964, less than 10 percent of the patients were older than 10 years. About a third of the cases in 1991 were in adolescents and young adults. Evidence also indicates high primary measles attack rates in newborns to 4-year-old children in areas of suboptimal vaccine utilization.[21, 63, 74, 122, 164] In 2000, a provisional total of 86 confirmed cases of measles were reported.[63] Ten cases (12%) were in infants, 27 (31%) in children 1 to 4 years of age, 17 (20%) in persons aged 5 to 19 years, 20 (23%) in persons aged 20 to 34 years, and 12 (14%) in adults 35 years or older. Most measles cases in the United States since 1994 have been imported or importation associated.[63, 332, 333]

Measles in heavily populated but underdeveloped countries has its greatest incidence in children younger than 2 years.[79, 115, 165, 265, 293]

GEOGRAPHIC DISTRIBUTION

In the 20th century, measles occurred regularly throughout the world in all but the most remote areas.[25, 39] In island and other isolated populations, interepidemic periods can be 10 years or more, and disease occurrence depends on introduction of the disease from outside.

SEASONAL PATTERNS

Epidemic measles is a winter-spring disease in temperate climates, with peak activity in the Northern Hemisphere occurring in March or April. In equatorial regions, epidemics of measles are less marked but tend to occur in the hot, dry seasons.[25, 267, 327, 364]

HOST AND SOCIAL FACTORS

No difference is found in the incidence of measles in males and females. One suggestion, however, is that complication rates are higher in males than females. Tidstrom[368] found that acute laryngitis was more than twice as common in males as females. In other studies, otitis media, pneumonia, and deaths occurred slightly more often in males.[25, 294] Miller,[254] in a large survey in England in 1963, found no difference in the incidence of complications in males and females. Christensen and associates,[78] in studies of an epidemic in Greenland, noted a greater number of complications in female patients older than 15 years, attributable primarily to an increased incidence of pneumonia. In a review of 375 confirmed cases of subacute sclerosing panencephalitis, the male-to-female ratio was 2.4:1.[260] According to Black,[39] antibody titers are slightly higher in women than men. Our studies involving young adults failed to reveal a similar sex difference in antibody levels, however.[352]

Green and associates[144] noted that a group of adult women had a higher postimmunization geometric mean antibody titer than vaccinated men did.

Although the severity of disease in certain populations appears to suggest differences based on race, this difference may be the result of nutritional and other environmental factors. Deseda-Tous and associates[95] were unable to demonstrate any differences in measles antibody by HLA or ABO blood types.

In the prevaccine era, the age of patients at the time of measles infection was related inversely to the number of siblings in the family.[25, 39, 394] In general, measles occurred at an earlier age in city dwellers and those of lower socioeconomic classes than in rural families and well-educated upper income groups.

In the present era of antibiotics and other medical modalities, the greatest factors in measles morbidity and mortality are age and nutritional status. Measles mortality is highest in children younger than 2 years and adults.[25, 39] The severity of measles and rates of mortality correlate in general with the severity of malnutrition.[39, 293] However, extensive investigations by Aaby and others[1, 3, 131] during the last 25 years suggest that overcrowding and intensive exposure may be more important determinants of measles mortality than nutritional status alone is.

Studies of measles early in the 20th century and in developing countries indicated that secondary cases in households are likely to be more severe than primary cases.[1–3, 131]

TABLE 183–1 ■ INCIDENCE AND PERCENT DISTRIBUTION OF REPORTED MEASLES CASES BY AGE GROUP IN SELECTED YEARS, UNITED STATES

	1960–1964*			1974			1979			1991		
Age Group	Cases	%	Incidence†	Cases	%	Incidence†	Cases	%	Incidence†	Cases	%	Incidence†
<1–4	93,653	37.2	766	5,899	26.7	36	2,331	20.7	18.0	4,756	49.3	24.7
5–9	132,956	52.8	1,237	5,391	24.4	30	2,473	21.9	18.1	991	10.2	5.5
10–14	16,403	6.5	169	7,799	35.3	38	3,054	27.1	20.4	905	9.4	5.3
15–19	8,635	3.4	10	2,475	11.2	12	2,633	23.3	15.2	1,102	11.4	6.2
20+				552	2.5	>1	786	7.0	0.6	1,890	19.6	1.8
Totals	251,647			22,094			11,277			9,643		

*Data from four reporting areas: Washington, DC, New York City, Illinois (including Chicago), and Massachusetts.[21, 55, 59, 162]
†Incidence, cases per 100,000 population, extrapolated from the age distribution of known cases.

However, more recent studies in the United States have found no difference in severity between primary and secondary cases in families.[50, 384]

SPREAD OF INFECTION

Measles is a highly contagious disease in nonimmune persons. It is spread from an infected ill person to a new host by the respiratory route.[25, 39, 325, 326, 328] Although monkeys can acquire measles from humans, practically speaking, no animal reservoir exists.[253] Available evidence suggests that infection is spread by persons ill with measles. Asymptomatic contagious carriers are unknown, and persons with acute asymptomatic infection are probably not contagious or only minimally so. The period of greatest contagion occurs during the prodromal period.[137]

Transmission of measles is thought to occur mainly by aerosolized droplets of respiratory secretions. Acquisition of infection by a new host is by the nose and possibly the conjunctivae.[303] Infection can be initiated by small-droplet nuclei, which stay suspended in air for considerable periods, or by direct hits of large droplets at close range.[43, 323] Also possible is that spread involves close person-to-person contact in young children, with large virus-containing droplets of nasal secretions being picked up on the hands of the future host and then applied to the nose.

Pathogenesis and Pathology

VIRAL INFECTION

The sequence of viral events in uncomplicated measles is presented in Table 183–2. Although much is known about measles virus infection in humans, considerable gaps exist regarding specific events. Experimental studies in other primates have been performed in an attempt to fill in the gaps and, therefore, give a more complete picture.[190, 243, 282, 296, 343, 396] The primary site of infection appears to be the respiratory epithelium of the nasopharynx. Measles vaccine virus instilled into the nose or by aerosol results in infection.[41, 211] Papp[303] reported studies suggesting that infection resulted from conjunctival contact and proposed that this means was the primary portal of entry. However, experiments with vaccine virus generally have been unsuccessful when conjunctival inoculation has been performed.[41] Initial infection of the respiratory epithelium appears to be minimal; a more important event is the early spread of virus to regional lymphatics. A presumption based on data derived from Fenner's ectromelia-mouse experimental model[108] is that after such spread, primary viremia occurs. After the initial viremia, extensive multiplication of virus occurs in the reticuloendothelial system at both regional and distant sites. Multiplication of virus also continues at the site of initial infection.

During the fifth to seventh days of infection, extensive secondary viremia takes place and results in the establishment of generalized measles viral infection. The skin, conjunctivae, and respiratory tract are obvious sites of infection, but other organs may be involved as well. From the 11th to the 14th days, the viral content of the blood, respiratory tract, and other organs peaks and then rapidly diminishes over the ensuing 2- to 3-day period.

In immunologically compromised patients with defects in cell-mediated factors, measles virus is not cleared from the secondary infection sites, and progressive, frequently fatal illnesses occur.[8, 103, 257, 259, 268]

TABLE 183–2 ■ SEQUENCE OF MEASLES VIRUS INFECTION IN UNCOMPLICATED PRIMARY DISEASE

Day	Event
0	Measles virus in droplet nuclei or large droplet comes in contact with the epithelial surface of the nasopharynx or possibly the conjunctiva
	Infection of epithelial cells and virus multiplication
1–2	Extension of infection to regional lymphoid tissue
2–3	Primary viremia
3–5	Multiplication of measles virus in respiratory epithelium at site of initial infection and in the reticuloendothelial system regionally and at distant sites
5–7	Secondary viremia
7–11	Establishment of infection in the skin and other viremic sites, including the respiratory tract
11–14	Virus in blood, respiratory tract, skin, and other organs
15–17	Viremia decreases and then ceases
	Viral content in organs rapidly diminishes

From references 147–149, 152, 156, 190, 196, 201, 226, 282, 296, 310, 328, 335, 343, 396.

During infection, measles virus replicates in endothelial cells, epithelial cells, and monocytes and macrophages.[152, 261]

PATHOLOGY

The characteristic pathologic feature of measles is the widespread distribution of multinucleated giant cells, which are the result of cell fusion.* Two main types of giant cells occur in measles: (1) Warthin-Finkeldey cells, which are found in the reticuloendothelium, and (2) epithelial giant cells (Fig. 183–4), which occur principally in the respiratory epithelium but also on other epithelial surfaces.[226]

Warthin-Finkeldey giant cells are found throughout the reticuloendothelial system in the adenoids, tonsils, Peyer

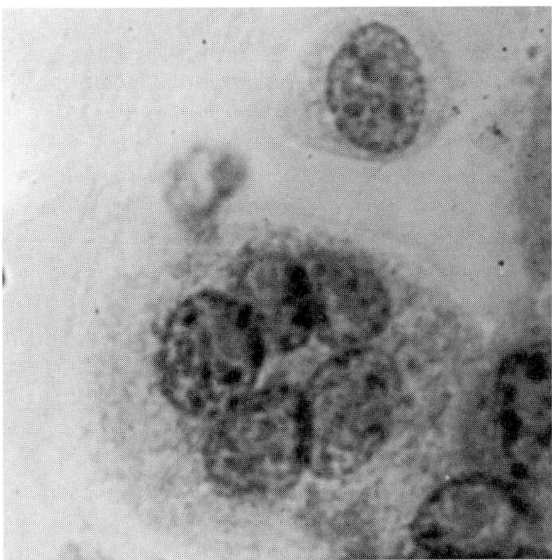

FIGURE 183–4 ■ Epithelial giant cell with five nuclei. Pharyngeal smear. (Courtesy of Dr. John M. Adams.)

*See references 40, 190, 193, 226, 242, 282, 296, 329, 343, 396.

patches, appendix, lymph nodes, spleen, and thymus. They vary in size and contain up to 100 or more nuclei. The cells contain both cytoplasmic and intranuclear eosinophilic inclusions, with cytoplasmic inclusions being more common than intranuclear lesions.

During the prodromal stage of measles, epithelial giant cells regularly are present on respiratory surfaces and frequently are sloughed free (see Fig. 183–4).

Measles Exanthem

Hematoxylin and eosin–stained sections of skin biopsy specimens have revealed typical epithelial syncytial giant cells with nuclear and cytoplasmic inclusions.[201, 361] The giant cells contain 3 to 26 nuclei. Other findings include the following: focal parakeratosis, dyskeratosis, spongiosis, and intracellular edema. The superficial blood vessels are dilated with a sparse, surrounding lymphohistiocytic infiltrate.

Koplik Spots

Suringa and colleagues[361] observed that the histopathologic features of Koplik spots were similar to those of the rash. They noted more giant cells with more nuclei, a greater degree of edema, and a lessened inflammatory response in the enanthem biopsy sample, however.

Respiratory Tract

The extent of respiratory involvement in uncomplicated measles is not known. However, clinical symptoms and the extensive radiographic studies of Kohn and Koiransky[206] suggest that pharyngitis, tracheitis, bronchitis, and pulmonary infiltration are the rule rather than the exception. Unfortunately, the human pathologic data available have been obtained mainly from complicated cases, so the findings cannot be considered representative.[93, 329] In a study in monkeys, Nii and colleagues[282] noted giant cells in the mucosal epithelium of the trachea, bronchi, and bronchioli. The lumina of these airways contained sloughed syncytial cells. Warthin-Finkeldey cells were found in the adjacent lymphatics.

In the lungs of experimentally infected monkeys, interstitial pneumonitis was observed with giant-cell formation.[282] Infiltration of neutrophils, eosinophils, and mononuclear cells also was noted.

IMMUNOLOGIC EVENTS

After natural or attenuated measles virus infection, a large number of specific and nonspecific immunologic responses occur. Many questions relating to immunity in measles remain unanswered, but on the other hand, a considerable body of knowledge has been gathered during the last 50 years.

Antibody

After measles viral infection, an antibody response regularly occurs. Serum antibodies to the N, F, H, and M proteins of measles virus can be demonstrated by hemagglutination-inhibition (HI), complement-fixation (CF), neutralization, immune precipitation, hemolysin inhibition, enzyme-linked immunosorbent assay (ELISA), and fluorescent antibody (FA) methods.[129, 142, 202, 214, 278, 284, 285] Antibody-dependent cellular cytotoxicity and antibody-dependent complement-mediated lysis also can be demonstrated by chromium release assays.[120, 121, 199] In natural infection, HI and neutralizing antibodies appear at approximately the 14th day, peak at around 4 to 6 weeks, and decrease about fourfold from the peak over the course of a year. The vast majority of naturally infected persons have demonstrable HI and neutralizing antibodies for life. Krugman[213] noted an average 16-fold reduction in HI antibody titer 15 years after natural infection in a group of children who had no measles exposure during the observation period.

After immunization, both HI and neutralizing antibodies are present by the 14th day.[129, 214] CF antibody appears slightly later than HI antibody and in general does not persist as long as either HI or neutralizing antibody. Primary infection is characterized by the initial appearance of antibody in the IgM and IgG serum components.[118, 167, 341, 342, 370] The IgM-specific response is short lived, and rarely can measles antibody in this fraction be demonstrated more than 9 weeks after infection.

IgA secretory antibody also occurs regularly after vaccine viral infection and after natural infection.[31, 125]

IgG antibody appearing after infection is primarily subclasses IgG1 and IgG4.[240] Antibody detected by neutralization and by HI is mainly to H protein and correlates with clinical protection against illness.[152, 285] Antibody to N protein is the main antibody detected by CF.[285] Antibody to F protein is demonstrated by inhibition of hemolysis of monkey erythrocytes by measles virus or by immunoprecipitation.[284, 286] Antibody to F protein may contribute to neutralization by disrupting the fusion of virus membrane with host-cell membranes. Only small amounts of antibody to M protein are elicited after infection with wild virus or vaccine virus.[142]

Specific Cell-Mediated Responses

Investigators recognized over 35 years ago that patients with defective cellular resistance factors frequently died of progressive measles virus infections.[274] Approximately 25 years ago, techniques became available that demonstrated measles-specific lymphocyte sensitization.[130, 143, 145, 210, 219, 334] Graziano and colleagues[143] found that lymphocytes from persons who previously had measles had a blastogenic response in vitro when incubated with measles antigen. Labowskie and associates,[219] using an in vitro lymphocyte-mediated cytotoxicity assay, noted that lymphocytes from persons who previously had measles caused cell destruction in a tissue culture chronically infected with measles virus. Ruckdeschel and colleagues[334] observed that two physicians without detectable measles antibody who had experienced repeated recent exposure to measles without illness had strong in vitro cellular responsiveness to measles virus. Krause and associates[210] demonstrated excessive measles-specific lymphocyte blastogenic responses in some persons previously immunized with killed measles vaccine.

Today, T cells are appreciated to be important both in B-cell antiviral antibody responses and as effector cells for the clearance of virus-infected cells from tissues.[152] Both helper ($CD4^+$) and suppressor ($CD8^+$) cells participate in the cellular response.[376] During infection, $CD8^+$ T cells eliminate virus-infected cells by major histocompatibility complex class I–restricted cytotoxic mechanisms.[152] $CD4^+$ T cells respond to measles virus infection by the secretion of cytokines. After initial virus exposure, $CD4^+$ T cells mount a T_H1 response. Before the rash develops, plasma interferon-γ (INF-γ) levels are increased, and with the rash, interleukin-2 (IL-2) appears. With clinical recovery, plasma levels of IL-4 increase (a T_H2 response) and stay elevated for several weeks, whereas the initial T_H1 response subsides.

On reexposure, T_H1 and T_H2 responses occur as indicated by the production of INF-γ, IL-2 and tumor necrosis factor–β (TNF-β), IL-4, IL-5, and IL-10. The T_H1 cytokine response is important for macrophage activation (through the action of INF-γ), lymphocyte proliferation (through IL-2), and major histocompatibility complex class II–restricted cytotoxicity (via TNF-β). The T_H2 cytokine response is important for macrophage deactivation (through the action of IL-4 and IL-10) and B-cell help (via IL-4, IL-5, and IL-10).

Other Responses

Listed in Table 183–3 are nonspecific, immunologically related responses that can be demonstrated during natural or vaccine measles virus infection. Anderson and colleagues[16] demonstrated a temporary defect in neutrophil motility during acute measles that resolved by the 11th day after the onset of rash. Leukopenia has been observed in natural measles[33] and after immunization.[42] With immunization, both neutrophil and lymphocyte numbers are reduced; this reduction lasts approximately 1 week, with an onset approximately 7 days after vaccination. Coovadia and colleagues[83, 85] have shown that the numbers of T, B, and null cells in the lymphocyte population are reduced. With a reduction in the number of T lymphocytes, no change occurs in the ratio of helper and suppressor-cytotoxic cell phenotypes.[10, 18, 186]

Thrombocytopenia occasionally has been associated with natural measles[177] and vaccination.[11, 387] Oski and Naiman[300] noted a mild reduction in the peripheral platelet count during routine measles immunization. Transitory complement defects vary in measles; Charlesworth and associates[66] found evidence of pathologic complement activation in 20 of 50 patents studied. Coovadia and colleagues[85] noted slight but significant reductions in serum IgA levels and elevated IgM values in acute measles virus infections. They found the IgG concentrations to be normal. Increased levels of serum or plasma IgE have been noted in two studies.[150, 344] Delayed hypersensitivity responses in skin are suppressed in both natural and vaccine measles virus infection[112, 353]; similarly, in vitro lymphocyte blastogenic responses to common antigens are suppressed.[386]

MECHANISMS IN RECOVERY FROM MEASLES VIRAL INFECTION

Acute clinical measles is characterized by viral multiplication in many organs of the body and then rapid subsidence of the infection by the 17th day. As noted earlier, measles virus infection is associated with both serum and secretory antibody responses and specific cell-mediated responses that coincide with clinical recovery. All three factors would seem to be important in recovery from acute measles virus infection, but confusing bits of information cloud the issue. For example, researchers have noted that children with simple agammaglobulinemia in whom measurable measles antibodies do not develop after measles virus infection recover from the disease normally.[139] This finding suggests that development of measles antibody is not important for recovery from acute infection. However, by using a sensitive plaque-reduction measles neutralizing antibody technique, Black[37] found small amounts of antibody in the sera of three agammaglobulinemic patients.

In contrast to antibody data, patients with defects in the cell-mediated immune system clearly do poorly with measles virus infection and frequently succumb to progressive infection despite the administration of large doses of measles antibody–containing immunoglobulin. T cells (both $CD4^+$ and $CD8^+$) clear virus-infected cells from tissues by cytotoxicity. INF-α, which is released by a variety of cells, including T cells, inhibits the spread of virus infection.

MECHANISMS IN PREVENTION OF REPEAT ILLNESS IN PERSONS PREVIOUSLY INFECTED WITH MEASLES VIRUS

In contrast to mechanisms of recovery in acute measles, the role of serum antibody in protection against recurrent disease is solid. Before the present vaccine era, researchers repeatedly demonstrated that the administration of measles antibody-containing immunoglobulin could prevent clinical measles.[182, 359] Similarly, infants with transplacentally acquired measles antibody are immune.[214] Whether other

TABLE 183–3 ■ NONSPECIFIC, IMMUNOLOGICALLY RELATED RESPONSES DURING MEASLES VIRUS INFECTION

Category	Findings	Reference
Leukocytes	Defective neutrophil motility	16
	Leukopenia (both lymphocytes and neutrophils)	33, 39
	Decreased T, B, and null lymphocytes	10, 18, 83, 85, 186
	Decreased natural killer cell activity	154
	Decreased helper T cells	89, 200
	Prolonged suppression of interleukin-12 production	20
	Prolonged depression of virus-specific interferon-α production	276
Interferon-α	Elevated plasma levels	155
Neopterin	Elevated plasma levels	155
Interleukin-2 receptor (soluble)	Elevated plasma levels	153
Platelets	Reduction in peripheral count	300
Complement	Frequent pathologic activation of the complement system; reduction of C1q, C4, C3, and C5	66
Serum immunoglobulins	IgA reduced and IgE and IgM elevated	85, 150, 344
In vitro lymphocyte response to phytohemagglutinin	Suppressed In presence of autologous serum; normal in presence of calf serum	386
In vitro lymphocyte response to *Candida*	Suppressed	386
Cutaneous delayed hypersensitivity	Depressed	112
C-reactive protein	Elevated at onset of rash	151
Circulating immune complexes	Noted in 25% of patients 7 to 13 days after rash onset	402

factors are also important in protection against reinfection is not clear. Often cited is that patients with agammaglobulinemia do not have repeated measles virus infections, so other factors must be involved.[139] Ruckdeschel and colleagues[334] reported two physicians who frequently were exposed to measles but in whom no serum antibody could be demonstrated. Both these subjects had measles-specific cell-mediated responses.

Of interest is that patients have been described in whom antibody did not prevent atypical measles after immunization with killed measles vaccine.[228] The data of Krause and associates[210] suggest that persons in whom the capacity for exaggerated measles-specific lymphocyte activity persists (some previous killed vaccine recipients) may be subject to illness in spite of the presence of antibody. However, the antibody produced after killed measles vaccine was incomplete; it lacked specific antibody to F protein.[77] Black[37] noted one child with a low measles neutralizing antibody titer, presumably from natural measles virus infection, in whom measles later developed. Chen and coinvestigators[68] found that some students with measurable but low neutralizing antibody titers were not protected from clinical measles on exposure.

Clinical Manifestations

Before the present vaccine era, measles was an inevitable disease of childhood that was recognized readily by parents and other laypersons, as well as by physicians. Despite the occasional confusion with other exanthematous diseases,[70] the epidemic character of measles usually resulted in an accurate diagnosis. Currently in North America, the epidemiologic pattern of measles has changed, as has general knowledge of the disease by a new generation of parents, physicians, and other medical personnel.

TYPICAL ILLNESS[25, 71, 74, 193, 217, 328, 358]

Incubation Period

The incubation period of measles is approximately 10 (8 to 12) days. Although extensive virologic and immunologic events are occurring during this period, the individual has virtually no outward sign of illness. Goodall[140] suggested (and Partington and Quinton[305] have presented supporting data) that some patients have mild transient respiratory symptoms and fever shortly after initial acquisition of the virus.

Prodromal Period

The prodrome of measles lasts approximately 3 (2 to 4) days. Initial symptoms are respiratory and suggest the possibility of a cold, except for the fact that fever is an early sign. In fact, in situations of close observation, slight temperature elevation has occurred and then subsided for a day or two before the appearance of typical respiratory symptoms.[358]

The onset of clinical measles is characterized by general malaise, fever, coryza, conjunctivitis, and cough. These symptoms worsen over a 2- to 4-day period. Early in the prodromal phase, a transitory rash occasionally has been observed. It has been urticarial or macular, has occurred with the initial onset of fever, and has disappeared before onset of the typical exanthem.

During the prodromal period, the temperature increases gradually to a value of 39.5° ± 1.1° C (103° ± 2° F) over a 4-day period. The nasal symptoms resemble those of other respiratory viral infections and are similar to those of the common cold or acute nasopharyngitis. Sneezing, rhinitis, and congestion are common symptoms. The degree of prodromal conjunctivitis varies considerably. Initially, the conjunctival injection is divided by a transverse marginal line across the lower lids.[357] The conjunctivitis is associated with considerable lacrimation, and older patients in particular are bothered by photophobia, which is frequently severe. Slit-lamp examination reveals both corneal and conjunctival lesions.[24, 114]

The cough in prodromal measles is frequently troublesome. It worsens throughout the period and often has a brassy quality suggesting laryngeal and tracheal involvement. On approximately day 10 ± 1, Koplik spots, the pathognomonic enanthem of measles, first appear (see Fig. 65–1). Koplik[207–209] originally described the lesions as bluish-white specks on a bright red mucosal surface. In my experience, the lesions always have appeared white, and a blue component has not been observed. Koplik spots first arise on the buccal mucosa opposite the lower molars but usually spread quickly to involve most of the buccal and lower labial mucosa. The lesions are about 1 mm in size at first but occasionally seem to coalesce into larger lesions. Initially, only a few lesions appear, but within 12 hours the number is usually uncountable. Of equal importance in diagnosis is the appearance of the background mucosal surface, which is always bright red and granular. Frequently, 1-mm lesions (Fordyce aphthae), which commonly occur normally in adolescents and adults, are confused with Koplik spots.[69] These lesions, however, can be differentiated easily because they appear on a normal pale mucosal surface rather than the bright red background of measles.

During the prodromal period, erythematous maculopapular lesions also are observed occasionally on the palate. At the end of the prodromal period, the posterior pharyngeal wall is usually erythematous and injected, and the patient may complain of a sore throat.

Exanthem Period

In typical measles, the exanthem appears on about the 14th day after exposure. The exanthem occurs at approximately the peak of the respiratory symptoms and when the temperature is usually around 39.5° C (103° F). At this time, the Koplik spots have peaked, and during the next 3 days they disappear. However, after the specific white spots have disappeared, the red, sandpapery mucosal background is still present for a day or two.

The measles exanthem first appears behind the ears and on the forehead at the hair line. Spread of the rash is centrifugal from the head to the feet. By the third day, the rash has involved the face, neck, trunk, upper extremities, buttocks, and lower extremities sequentially. The rash is initially erythematous and maculopapular but progresses to confluence in the same centrifugal manner as it is spread. Confluence is always more prominent on the face; frequently, the lesions on the lower extremities remain discrete. At the height of the rash, the appearance suggests microvesicles on top of a generalized erythematous confluent base (see Fig. 65–2).

The exanthem begins to clear on the third to fourth day, again following the centrifugal course of progression. During the initial stages of the rash, its color is red and it readily blanches on pressure. As the rash fades, it takes on a coppery appearance, after which a brownish discoloration is seen that does not clear with pressure. With healing, a fine desquamation frequently occurs in confluent areas with brownish discoloration. The duration of the exanthem is usually 6 to 7 days.

During the exanthem period, the fever generally peaks on approximately the second or third day of the rash and then falls by lysis during a 24-hour period. Fever that persists after the third or fourth day of exanthem is usually an indication of a complication. Conjunctivitis and nasal symptoms generally subside at about the time of defervescence. Continued nasal discharge, whether purulent or not, suggests bacterial secondary infection. With appearance of the rash, the cough loosens up, and in older persons it frequently becomes productive. The cough may persist for 10 days or more.

Pharyngitis is common during the exanthem period, as is cervical lymph node enlargement. Generalized lymphadenopathy with suboccipital and postauricular involvement is not an uncommon finding, nor is splenomegaly. Young children occasionally have diarrhea, vomiting, laryngitis, and croup. Abdominal pain also can be troublesome.

Laboratory Findings

Laboratory studies rarely are indicated for acute uncomplicated typical measles because the diagnosis can be established on a clinical and epidemiologic basis and the results of studies rarely affect management of the patient. During the periods of prodrome and rash, the total leukocyte count is low. Numbers of neutrophils and lymphocytes are reduced, but the most marked reduction, when absolute counts are considered, is in the number of lymphocytes.[33] In difficult cases, such as the first apparent case in a particular locality, a specific diagnosis can be made by serologic study, most easily by measles CF or HI antibody studies. If an acute serum sample is obtained during the prodrome and a second serum sample is obtained 7 to 10 days later, a fourfold rise in antibody titer usually is demonstrated. At the time of the rash, identification of measles antibody in the IgM fraction is also a useful test.

MODIFIED ILLNESS*

Modified measles is an infection that occurs in a partially immune person. It is characterized by a generally mild illness that usually follows the regular sequence of events in measles. The prodromal period is shorter; cough, coryza, and fever are minimal. Koplik spots are few and transient, and they frequently do not occur. The exanthem follows the progression pattern of regular measles, but confluence of the lesions does not occur. Because serologic studies reveal some children with measles antibody who had never had clinical disease suggestive of measles, some modified infections probably occur without exanthem and perhaps without overt symptoms at all.[37, 215]

Modified measles develops under a variety of circumstances, the most important of which historically was the result of intentional disease alteration by the administration of immune serum globulin to an exposed susceptible child. Naturally occurring modified measles is seen occasionally in infants younger than 9 months because of the presence of transplacentally acquired maternal measles antibody.

Although the magnitude of the problem is unknown, modified measles also occurs as an occasional manifestation of live vaccine failure. In these instances, patients have had modified illness but demonstrated a secondary measles serum antibody response (only IgG antibody).[74, 76, 350] With increasing time from immunization, this response possibly will occur more frequently.[94] However, few data currently support this possibility.

Recurrent measles also rarely results in modified illness. The frequency of recurrent measles is unknown. In general, most authorities have discounted recurrent measles and suggested that the recorded experiences were the result of confusion with infection by other exanthem-producing agents.[70, 212] However, Cherry and colleagues,[74] Schaffner and associates,[338] and Schluederberg[341] have described children with modified illnesses, secondary immunologic responses, and well-documented instances of previous measles.

*See references 25, 28, 68, 74, 76, 101, 128, 169, 182, 217, 307, 324, 338.

ATYPICAL MEASLES

Atypical measles is a clearly defined clinical syndrome that occurs in some previously immunized persons after exposure to natural measles. The overwhelming majority of cases have occurred in persons who initially received inactivated (killed) measles viral vaccines, but some cases also have been noted in children who received only live measles vaccines.[75, 228, 279]

Historical Aspects

The initial studies with inactivated measles vaccines in the early 1960s demonstrated that multiple doses were necessary for stimulation of an antibody response and that measurable serum antibody levels were short lived.[128, 157, 191, 214, 391] In the initial trials, it soon became apparent that some killed vaccine study participants were still susceptible to measles. On exposure to natural measles, typical measles developed in some children and a mild, modified illness in others.[128] As a result, regimens were developed in which children were immunized with two or three doses of killed vaccine at monthly intervals, followed in a month or more by a single dose of Edmonston B live measles vaccine (KKL or KKKL). Studies at the time demonstrated good antibody levels after both regimens. After measles vaccine was licensed in 1963, killed-live measles vaccine regimens enjoyed modest popularity in the United States (as well as in other countries) because live Edmonston B strain vaccine frequently was associated with alarming febrile responses and occasional febrile convulsions.

In 1965, Rauh and Schmidt[321] reported an unusual illness after exposure to natural measles in some children who had received killed vaccine 2 years previously. The significance of their findings became more apparent during the following 2 years when Fulginiti and colleagues[126] and Nader and coworkers[272] noted many instances of "atypical measles" in previous recipients of KKK and KKL vaccination regimens. In these two instances, original immunization had taken place 4 to 6 years before the occurrence of atypical illness.

In 1968, killed measles vaccine was taken off the market in the United States after the distribution of approximately 1.8 million doses in the period from 1963 to 1968.[298] During the 12-year period from 1968 to 1980, atypical measles was reported frequently.* I am unaware of reports since 1980 of further cases of atypical measles. However, I observed one 26-year-old physician and a 28-year-old nurse with the syndrome in the 1980s. Sporadic cases in adults probably still

*See references 17, 45, 67, 127, 136, 159, 170, 176, 223, 246, 256, 279, 281, 289, 383, 384, 399, 400.

are occurring but are misdiagnosed because physicians caring for adults are unaware of the syndrome and, therefore, the history of killed measles vaccine is not uncovered and specific antibody studies are not performed.

In 1971, during study of an extensive measles epidemic, Cherry and colleagues[75] observed six children who had relatively mild, atypical measles-like illnesses but had received only live measles vaccine. Linnemann and colleagues[228] likewise noted two children with atypical measles-like illnesses who had received only live measles vaccine. Nichols[279] and St. Geme and associates[356] also have reported bizarre measles illnesses in former live vaccine recipients.

Clinical Characteristics*

Atypical measles was a common illness from 1967 to 1978. Because killed measles vaccines have not been available in the United States for the last 25 years, two obvious facts need to be mentioned: with each passing year, potential patients and actual patients with atypical measles will be 1 year older and also 1 year farther from the time of the primary killed measles vaccine immunization series. Both these aspects raise concern about whether the clinical manifestations of the syndrome will remain the same today as when the illness first was described. It was my opinion in 1981 that the syndrome had changed slightly but still was recognizable from original descriptions of the illness.[71]

The incubation period of atypical measles is similar to that of typical measles—between 7 and 14 days in duration. The prodromal period is characterized by the sudden onset of high fever (39.5° C to 40.6° C, 103° F to 105° F) and usually headache. Abdominal pain and myalgia are also common complaints. Dry, nonproductive cough is noted in most patients and vomiting in approximately a third of those afflicted. Pleuritic chest pain and weakness are also common complaints. Although few reports to the contrary exist, Koplik spots appear to be rare in atypical measles.

Two to 3 days after onset of the illness, the rash appears. It is unique in that it first develops on the distal ends of the extremities and progresses in a cephalad direction. Usually, the rash is initially erythematous and maculopapular. I have been impressed by a slight yellowish hue of the exanthem when compared with that of typical measles. The rash is particularly prominent on the wrists and ankles; it involves the palms and soles. Spread of the rash varies considerably. In some patients, only the wrists and ankles are involved, whereas in others, the entire extremities as well as the lower part of the trunk are affected. In a peculiar fashion, the rash frequently seems to end its cephalad progression in a line at the level of the nipples. Occasionally, a few erythematous, maculopapular, but discrete lesions are found on the face. In some cases, the rash becomes vesicular, with the lesions being approximately 2 to 3 mm in diameter; they do not proceed to scab formation as in varicella, but occasionally pruritus is a problem, and excoriation occurs from scratching. The exanthem often has a petechial or purpuric component, and urticaria also occurs frequently. Edema of the extremities has been a common finding.

Although coryza has been noted in a few reports, it is not a prominent feature, nor is conjunctivitis. Respiratory distress with dyspnea and rales occurs commonly, and radiographic examination reveals pulmonary involvement in virtually all cases. Most patients have hilar adenopathy and pneumonia. Pleural effusion also occurs frequently. The pneumonia in atypical measles is usually lobular or segmental, with the lesions often appearing nodular (Fig. 183–5). Although initial descriptions of the syndrome suggested an illness of approximately a week's duration, later observations indicated illnesses of 2 weeks or more. In one case, fatigue and other symptoms persisted for more than 1½ years.

In the original description by Rauh and Schmidt,[321] one patient had an exanthem that was biphasic; initially, a transitory rash suggested modified measles. Two weeks later, the more characteristic atypical exanthem developed. The same observers also noted a second case with a biphasic exanthem in which the first lesions were vesicular and occurred when the child had little fever. The second exanthem was maculopapular and associated with a febrile response. Zahradnik and colleagues[400] also noted a similar sequence in two young adults. Two patients who had received killed measles vaccine in the past have had radiographic evidence of characteristic pulmonary findings, but the typical exanthem did not develop.[289, 399]

Other findings in atypical measles include marked hepatosplenomegaly,[321] marked hyperesthesia,[272] weakness,[223] and numbness and paresthesia.[246] Personal observations of cases in adolescents and young adults suggest that the exanthem is less prominent than in past cases and the fever and overall morbidity are of greater duration.[71] Follow-up radiographic studies have demonstrated the persistence of nodular pulmonary lesions for more than 1 year in several patients and up to 6 years in one patient.[223, 256, 399]

Measles antibody studies in atypical measles are remarkably diagnostic. If an initial serum sample is obtained before or at onset of the exanthem, CF and HI titers are usually less than 1:5. By the 10th day of illness, both titers are elevated markedly, with most being 1:1280 or greater. In contrast, in typical natural measles at the 10th day of illness, the titer rarely is greater than 1:160.

Measles virus was not recovered from a patient with atypical measles, but only a few adequately performed studies were carried out. The epidemiologic data presently available suggest that patients with atypical measles are not contagious. Other laboratory studies are not particularly useful in

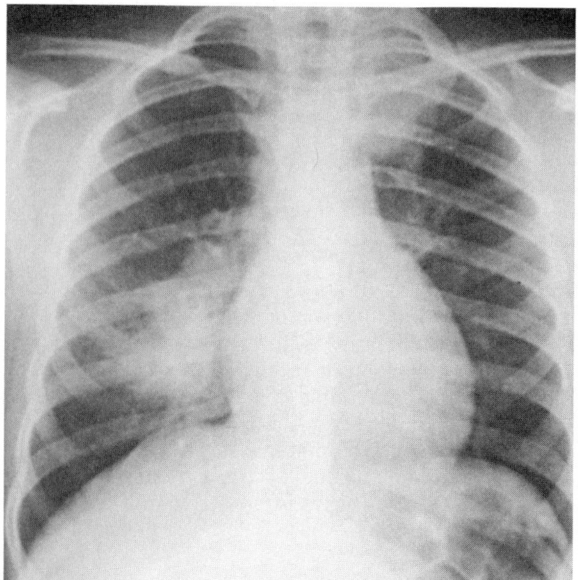

FIGURE 183–5 ■ Nodular pulmonary infiltrates in a child with atypical measles.

*See references 45, 67, 71, 75, 126, 127, 136, 159, 170, 176, 223, 246, 256, 272, 279, 281, 288, 289, 321, 383, 384, 399, 400.

atypical measles. The erythrocyte sedimentation rate is elevated. When serial blood counts have been performed, slight early leukopenia and late eosinophilia have been noted.[126]

The pathogenesis of atypical measles was studied by several investigators, and several possible mechanisms were suggested,[315] including a generalized Arthus reaction, induction of abnormal measles virus–specific delayed-type hypersensitivity, and an imbalance in antibody responses to H and F proteins caused by denaturation of F protein during formalin inactivation of the vaccine virus. In a recent study in monkeys, Polack and associates[315] found that atypical measles resulted from previous priming for a nonproductive type 2 $CD4^+$ T-cell response and not from the lack of functional antibody against F protein.

In revaccination studies performed by our group over 25 years ago, we found that vaccinees with severe local reactions had marked lymphocyte reactivity to inactivated measles virus and absent or minimal HI antibody.[210]

UNUSUAL MANIFESTATIONS AND COMPLICATIONS OF MEASLES

In addition to typical measles, modified measles, and atypical measles, many other clinical manifestations and complications occur at a broad range of frequency. By definition, unusual manifestations are a direct result of the primary viral infection, whereas complications are a result of damage by a secondary infection with another microorganism. In many instances, determining whether a particular manifestation is just viral or involves a second agent is difficult. Combinations of infections are common.

In general, complications resulting from secondary infection are not as common today as they were before the antibiotic era; however, no evidence suggests that unusual manifestations of illness occur less frequently today than formerly. To demonstrate the magnitude of the problem today, the findings in a 1970 to 1971 hospital survey in St. Louis are revealing.[73, 74] In this period, an extensive epidemic occurred, with 10,000 cases of measles. In eight area hospitals, 130 children (1.3%) were admitted; 66 cases of pneumonia and 6 fatalities occurred, and 6 children had encephalitis.

The records of measles patients in three hospitals were reviewed carefully. Of this group of 71 patients, 53 had pneumonia; 37 of the patients with pneumonia had either previous cardiorespiratory or other chronic systemic disorders. Two children had mediastinal and subcutaneous emphysema. All six deaths were caused by fulminant pneumonia. Of the six children with encephalitis, severe residual neurologic damage developed in three. One child had acute measles appendicitis with perforation and peritonitis, and another patient had mesenteric lymphadenitis.

Pneumonia

Pulmonary involvement in measles, as a result of the viral infection, is probably the rule rather than the exception. Kohn and Koiransky[206] performed careful radiographic studies in 130 children with measles and noted that 55 percent had pneumonic infiltration and 74 percent had hilar adenopathy. In most instances, the pneumonia was observed early in the course of the illness, which suggested primary viral involvement rather than secondary bacterial infection. In the 1970 to 1971 St. Louis measles epidemic, approximately 1 in every 150 patients with measles was hospitalized because of pneumonia.

Pneumonia in measles has varied radiographic manifestations.[6, 73, 146, 206, 229, 233, 239, 294, 363] Clearly, viral pneumonia is characterized by bilateral hyperinflation with diffuse fluffy infiltrates that are more confluent at the hilum. Unilateral, segmental, and lobar pneumonias also are observed. Gremillion and Crawford[146] reviewed 106 cases of pneumonia that occurred in 3220 Air Force recruits with measles between 1976 and 1979. Illnesses were severe, but no deaths occurred. Bacterial superinfection was documented in 30.3 percent of the cases; bronchospasm occurred in 17 percent of the recruits with pneumonia. In one study, seven children with massive and bilateral lung consolidation had clinical findings consistent with adult respiratory distress syndrome.[6]

Clinically, young infants have a picture of bronchiolitis with expiratory distress. In severe cases at all ages, a marked ventilation-perfusion deficit is noted.[229, 306] Patients with defects in the cell-mediated immune system are particularly prone to progressive fatal bilateral infection.[103, 205, 257, 259, 349, 351]

Secondary bacterial pneumonia is the result of common respiratory pathogens, particularly *Streptococcus pneumoniae, Haemophilus influenzae, Streptococcus pyogenes,* and *Staphylococcus aureus.* Co-infection with other viruses also was noted in an extensive study of measles-associated pneumonia in the Philippines.[318] In this study, parainfluenza virus and adenoviruses were isolated most commonly.

Other Respiratory Manifestations

Otitis media is the most common complication and is age related. In the immediate prevaccine era in the United States, otitis media developed in approximately 5 to 15 percent of patients with measles. Now it is a less of a problem because of the change in age incidence of measles. The bacterial pathogens in otitis media associated with measles are similar to those in otitis media in children without measles. Mastoiditis was a common complication of measles in the era before antibiotics, but fortunately, today it is rare.

Laryngitis and mild laryngotracheitis occur commonly. Occasionally, frank, severe laryngotracheobronchitis occurs and may require a tracheotomy.[330] Measles-associated bacterial tracheitis is not an uncommon finding.[80] Secondary bacterial infection of the cervical lymph nodes and secondary bacterial pharyngitis are also rather frequent complications of measles. Field[110] attributed 3.2 percent of cases of childhood bronchiectasis to former measles virus infection.[110] Measles also has a deleterious effect on the course of tuberculosis.[354]

Cardiac Manifestations

Myocarditis and pericarditis occasionally occur in measles.[93, 111] Nonspecific, transient electrocardiographic abnormalities were noted in more than half of 71 children with measles in one study.[331] In another study, 19 percent of patients had transient, but clear-cut abnormalities, including T wave changes, atrioventricular conduction defects, and premature auricular contractions.[138] Although cardiac involvement appears to occur commonly in measles, clinical consequences from such involvement are rare.

Neurologic Manifestations

Neurologic involvement is not uncommon in measles.* Gibbs and associates[134] noted that 51 percent of 680 measles

*See references 5, 25, 34, 102, 105, 134, 141, 218, 231, 245, 301, 316, 371, 401.

patients without clinical evidence of encephalitis had abnormal electroencephalographic results during acute or immediate postacute illness. Although the incidence varies, clinically evident encephalitis occurs in approximately 0.5 to 1 of every 1000 measles cases.[25, 57, 74, 102, 192] From 1962 to 1979, the average measles encephalitis-to-case ratio was 0.73:1000.[57] Both mortality and the incidence of sequelae have varied in the reports available. LaBoccetta and Tornay[218] noted a mortality rate of 32 percent in 50 patients in a group seen before 1947 and a rate of 11.5 percent in a group seen between 1947 and 1957. Ziegra[401] reported only 2 deaths in a group of 38 cases. Long-term morbidity data also vary considerably. In general, between 20 and 40 percent of patients who recover from measles encephalitis have manifestations of brain damage. Douglas[97] could find no evidence of later subnormal school performance in a group of children who had uncomplicated measles.

Symptoms of encephalitis usually develop during the period of measles exanthem and within 8 days of the onset of illness.[5, 218, 329] Occasionally, the onset of central nervous system (CNS) signs and symptoms occurs during the prodromal period. LaBoccetta and Tornay[218] noted the following frequencies of signs and symptoms at the onset of measles encephalitis: convulsions, 56 percent; lethargy, 46 percent; coma, 28 percent; and irritability, 26 percent. Patients with encephalitis frequently have multiple findings: headache, abnormalities in respiratory rate and rhythm, twitching and other involuntary movements, and disorientation. Cerebellar ataxia, myelitis, retrobulbar neuritis, transient mental disorders, and hemiplegia are findings noted during the subacute stages of illness. Long-term sequelae include various degrees of retardation and selective brain damage, recurrent seizures, deafness, and hemiplegia and paraplegia.

Examination of cerebrospinal fluid (CSF) in measles encephalitis usually reveals mild pleocytosis with a predominance of mononuclear cells, mildly elevated protein values, and a normal glucose level.[218, 245, 295, 371] In one study, 15 percent of the cases did not have CSF pleocytosis.[218]

Considerable controversy relates to the mechanisms in measles encephalitis.* Some investigators have failed to isolate measles virus or to demonstrate measles virus RNA or other viral antigens in the brains of affected patients.[133, 189, 197, 261] These findings have led to the widespread belief that the illness is autoimmune (acute disseminated encephalomyelitis) and that viral invasion of the CSF is unnecessary. However, other investigators have recovered measles virus from the CSF and brain of affected patients, which indicates that the virus is involved directly in the process.[105, 117, 245, 252] In the hamster model of measles virus encephalitis, virus can be cultured directly from the brain.[304]

Other Manifestations

Measles has been associated with many other manifestations and complications. Of historical interest was the occurrence of a severe, often fatal form of measles called black measles that was characterized by a confluent hemorrhagic skin eruption.[217] Patients with this illness had signs of both encephalitis or encephalopathy and pneumonia. Extensive bleeding from the mouth, nose, and bowel occurred commonly. Severe hemorrhagic measles rarely is seen today, and little is known about its pathogenesis. Disseminated intravascular coagulation would appear to play a role.

*See references 7, 113, 117, 133, 152, 153, 155, 187–189, 197, 245, 252, 261, 273, 308, 312.

Another measles complication involving bleeding is thrombocytopenic purpura.[6, 177] It is a postinfectious illness and different from hemorrhagic measles. Although bleeding is extensive on occasion, the ultimate prognosis is usually good. Stevens-Johnson syndrome has been noted occasionally in measles[236]; other manifestations include pneumomediastinum, subcutaneous emphysema, hepatitis, appendicitis, ileocolitis, mesenteric lymphadenitis, cervicitis, acute glomerulonephritis, corneal ulceration, and gangrene of the extremities.*

Measles in pregnancy results in significant maternal and fetal morbidity and mortality.[23, 100, 185, 268, 355] Jespersen and associates[185] retrospectively reviewed 10 epidemics of measles in Greenland; they obtained adequate data on 327 women infected during pregnancy, and they also were able to examine 252 of the offspring. Thirty-two percent of women infected during the first trimester had spontaneous abortions, and 9 percent of these pregnancies that continued to term resulted in stillbirths. Congenital malformations occurred in 8 of 300 live-born infants.[185] Pneumonia is a common maternal complication of measles during pregnancy.[23, 100]

SUBACUTE SCLEROSING PANENCEPHALITIS

Subacute sclerosing panencephalitis (SSPE) is a rare degenerative CNS disease of children and adolescents caused by persistent measles virus infection. It was described first by Dawson[92] in 1933; he proposed a viral etiologic agent because of the occurrence of inclusion bodies in the neurons of patients dying of the disease. In 1967, Connolly and colleagues[81] reported the observation of measles viral antigen in the brain of a patient with SSPE. They also noted high measles HI and CF titers in the sera and spinal fluid of three afflicted patients. Shortly thereafter, cultures of brain cells from patients with SSPE resulted in syncytial formation and the presence of measles antigen.[29] By cocultivation, measles virus was recovered from the brains of patients with SSPE.[173, 174, 308]

The risk of SSPE developing in children who previously had natural measles is between 0.6 and 2.2 per 100,000 infections.[59, 260] However, the risk is greater in patients who acquire measles at an early age. The mean incubation period from measles illness to the onset of SSPE is 7 years. In contrast to natural measles, the risk of SSPE developing after measles immunization is approximately one per million. In vaccinees in whom SSPE developed, the mean incubation period was 3.3 years.

SSPE has an insidious onset,[65, 366] with progressive behavioral and intellectual deterioration. Symptoms are frequently bizarre and complex and include psychic difficulties, motor incoordination, seizures of various types but most often myoclonic jerks, visual impairment, and difficulties with speech. Progression of the disease leads to stupor, dementia, mutism, central blindness, and finally, decorticate rigidity.

Electroencephalography shows a periodic suppression burst pattern with synchronous myoclonic jerks. Laboratory studies reveal a markedly elevated CSF globulin that is predominantly IgG. Serum measles HI and CF antibody titers are exceptionally high (>1:1280), although demonstration occasionally requires serial determination.[175] Measles antibody (HI and CF) can be detected in CSF.

*See references 123, 168, 192, 198, 217, 227, 247, 262, 280, 348, 369, 395.

At present, no effective treatment exists for SSPE. The average duration of illness from onset to death is approximately 6 to 9 months. A variety of antiviral and immunomodulatory agents have been tried in the treatment of individual patients. Inosiplex and intrathecal INF-α seem to elicit transient improvement in some patients.[98, 99, 232] The incidence of SSPE in the United States decreased dramatically after the extensive use of measles vaccine.[260]

MEASLES IN DEVELOPING COUNTRIES

Measles has been and continues to be a staggering problem in developing countries. The mortality rate in much of Africa is approximately 10 percent,[293] and a reasonable assumption is that the rate is similar in much of Central and South America and Asia.[263, 327, 364] In developing countries, measles is a disease of young children. For example, in Kenya, 25 to 30 percent of children contract measles before their first birthday and 55 to 60 percent before they are 2 years of age; virtually all children have had measles by the time that they are 4 years old.[165] In Kenyan children, mortality peaked in the 17- to 20-month-old age group, and the median age for hospital admission was 14 months.

Although many factors, such as the age at infection, suboptimal medical facilities, and failure to seek medical care, contribute to the excessive morbidity and mortality in children of developing countries, the single overriding factor generally has been thought to be the nutritional status of the infected children.[266, 267, 293] The data of O'Donovan[293] clearly indicate a direct relationship between malnutrition and hospital admissions for measles and deaths. Studies by Coovadia and colleagues[84] and by Carney and associates[53] indicate both humoral and cell-mediated defects in protein-calorie malnutrition. The clinical picture of measles in children with malnutrition is frequently similar to that in patients with known defects in cell-mediated functions.

Low serum retinol concentrations are nearly always present in children with measles in developing countries.[27, 86, 178, 181, 237, 322, 373] Low retinol levels correlate directly with measles mortality, and treatment with vitamin A reduces this mortality rate.[27, 178, 237]

Studies performed during the last decade indicate that the intensive exposure that occurs in children in developing countries is a major factor in measles mortality.[1, 4, 131]

Clinical Manifestations

Measles in children in developing countries is characterized by two different types of severe disease. One type of illness is a fulminant, toxic illness without apparent localizing complications. The other is a more prolonged illness with obvious complications; the complications may be caused by infection with secondary bacterial or other infectious agents, persistent measles virus infection, or a combination of both.

In a group of 507 hospitalized children, O'Donovan[293] noted that 301 had pneumonia; 96, gastroenteritis; 36, croup; 11, convulsions; 67, two or more complications; and 140, nonlocalized systemic toxic effects. The measles rash in malnourished children tends to result in greater confluence and progresses to a dark red and then a violet color.[267] Desquamation is marked and occurs in large scales.[339] After desquamation, patchy depigmentation lasts for some weeks. Another common problem is stomatitis and a resultant sore mouth, which leads to further loss of nutritional intake. Acute corneal ulceration, which occurs after measles in malnourished children, is a common cause of blindness.[336] Multiple skin abscesses and noma (cancrum oris) are rare secondary infectious problems.[192]

MEASLES IN IMMUNOCOMPROMISED HOSTS

Today, because of the extensive use of immunosuppressive therapeutic modalities and greater duration of survival in a number of rapidly fatal diseases, a sizable population of children and adults are immunologically compromised. Measles virus infection in a patient with disease-induced or iatrogenically caused immune deficiency is usually severe and protracted and frequently fatal.

The most common severe measles virus infection in an immunocompromised host is giant-cell pneumonia.[103, 205, 249, 257, 258, 320, 349] The mode of manifestation of this illness varies. Some patients initially have severe but otherwise typical measles after a normal incubation period. Clinical findings at the time of the exanthem indicate pulmonary involvement and respiratory distress, and radiographic findings become rapidly worse over a period of approximately a week or less. Other patients initially have rather vague illness, frequently without rash. In these cases, the pulmonary process may progress over a month or longer. Siegel and associates[349] reported a child with leukemia who recovered from typical measles and then died the following year of diffuse interstitial pneumonia in which characteristic measles giant cells were seen.

A unique form of measles encephalitis also is manifested in immunosuppressed patients.[8, 163, 250, 269, 271, 317, 392] Although the symptoms in different described cases varied, the illness appears to be intermediate between the acute encephalitis occurring in patients without known immunodefects and the chronic picture of SSPE. The incubation period has varied between 5 weeks and 6 months.[8] Convulsions are frequently the initial symptom, and they are a prominent aspect of the illness. The seizures have been focal, unilateral, or permanent localized twitching. Other findings include hemiplegia, stupor, coma, hypertonia, and slurred speech. Most cases have been fatal, and the duration of illness has been from 1 week to 2 months.

Diagnosis

DIFFERENTIAL DIAGNOSIS

The differential diagnosis of typical measles must include all illnesses in which an erythematous maculopapular rash occurs (see also Chapter 65). Of most importance in establishing the diagnosis of measles is a consideration of possible exposure; the duration of the incubation period; the presence of Koplik spots; the presence of the typical febrile prodrome with cough, coryza, and conjunctivitis; and progression of the rash in a caudal direction. The brown discoloration and the intensity of the measles rash are such that the illness usually should not be confused with rubella, erythema infectiosum, roseola infantum, or enteroviral infection. Of greatest differential difficulty are the exanthems of infectious mononucleosis, *Mycoplasma pneumoniae* infection, and drug eruptions.

In the past, atypical measles caused great difficulty in diagnosis. Today, this disease occurs only in adults 35 years or older. The key to diagnosis of this illness is careful elicitation of an accurate vaccination history. Even if it is not known whether the vaccination that the patient received as a child was live or killed vaccine, it usually can be determined by the number of doses given; if a child received more than one dose of vaccine in a short interval, killed vaccine almost certainly was administered. Differential considerations in atypical measles include Rocky Mountain spotted fever, anaphylactoid purpura, *M. pneumoniae* infection, and drug eruptions.

SPECIFIC DIAGNOSIS

Measles virus infection can be diagnosed specifically by isolation of virus in an appropriate tissue culture system; by demonstration of measles antigen in exfoliated cells and tissues by FA techniques or polymerase chain reaction[241]; or by the demonstration of a rise in HI, CF, ELISA, FA, or neutralizing antibody titer in two sequential serum samples or specific measles IgM antibody in a single serum sample (see Chapters 249 and 250). For practical purposes, most measles cases can be diagnosed by the demonstration of specific IgM antibody in an acute-phase serum specimen. False-positive IgM ELISA results may occur.[184]

Treatment

UNCOMPLICATED MEASLES

No specific therapy for uncomplicated measles exists. During the febrile period of illness, activity should be discouraged, and fluid status should be maintained by the liberal provision of soft drinks and ice. Fever may be controlled with acetaminophen. Cough is frequently distressing and can be managed by the judicious use of common antitussives. Room humidification is also useful in controlling the cough and generally can be expected to make the patient more comfortable. As the fever disappears, a gradual return to normal activity is indicated. However, measles virus infection is associated with considerable damage to the ciliated epithelium of the respiratory tract; therefore, resumption of normal activities too soon and exposure to other children and their bacterial pathogens can be associated with severe secondary infection.

Children in developing countries frequently have vitamin A deficiency. Measles morbidity correlates with this deficiency, and treatment with vitamin A is beneficial.[27, 86, 178, 181, 237, 322, 373] Studies in the United States indicate that vitamin A levels are low in a substantial number of measles cases and that morbidity is increased in these deficient children.[14, 19, 49, 124] Vitamin A supplementation also has been shown to enhance IgG antibody levels and total lymphocyte numbers.[87] In 1993, the Committee on Infectious Diseases of the American Academy of Pediatrics recommended vitamin A supplementation in children with measles in selected circumstances.[14] Vitamin A was recommended for children 6 months to 2 years of age who require hospitalization and all patients 6 months or older with immune deficiencies or possible vitamin A deficiency. The dose of vitamin A is 100,000 IU for children 6 months to 1 year of age and 200,000 IU for children 1 year or older. The dose should be repeated 24 hours and 4 weeks after the first dose in children with ophthalmologic evidence of vitamin A deficiency.

ATYPICAL MEASLES

The most important aspect of therapy for atypical measles is proper diagnosis. In patients with atypical measles, Rocky Mountain spotted fever, other septic conditions, lymphoma, or collagen vascular disease frequently is diagnosed erroneously, and their work-up is associated with extensive blood cultures, other diagnostic procedures, and vigorous antibiotic therapy. Careful attention to a history of previous administration of killed measles vaccine should clarify the diagnosis and preclude the unnecessary trauma associated with extensive diagnostic and therapeutic procedures.

In atypical measles, chest radiographs always should be obtained because the pneumonia that usually develops in these patients is frequently much more extensive than the clinical findings would indicate. Activity should be discouraged in acutely ill patients, and follow-up chest radiographs should be used as a guide to resumption of normal activity. In some patients, pulmonary abnormalities have persisted for a considerable period.

COMPLICATIONS OF MEASLES

Otitis Media

Otitis media is the most frequent complication of measles. The infectious agent of otitis media in measles is no different from that in other children without measles of comparable age, so conventional antibiotic therapy is all that is necessary (see Chapter 19).

Laryngotracheitis

Management of the laryngotracheitis caused by measles virus infection is similar to that in other patients with croup caused by other viral etiologic agents. The mainstay of therapy is the administration of humidified air and a concerted effort to relieve the apprehension of the patient. Administration of corticosteroids is contraindicated in measles, and antibiotics are indicated only in patients with laboratory or clinical evidence of secondary bacterial infection (see Chapter 22).

Pneumonia

Pneumonia is a common complication of measles, and it is the leading cause of death. Pneumonia may be a manifestation of primary viral infection, or it may result from a superimposed bacterial infection. The differential diagnosis between primary viral and superimposed bacterial disease cannot be made with certainty. Because the diagnosis of viral pneumonia is often uncertain, most cases should be treated with antibiotics (see Chapters 26 and 27). In primary viral pneumonia, treatment with aerosolized ribavirin should be considered.

In one uncontrolled study in adult patients, intravenous ribavirin was found to be well tolerated, and its use was associated with clinical improvement.[119] In a study in pregnant women, Atmar and associates[23] were unable to demonstrate clear clinical benefit with the administration of aerosolized ribavirin.

Encephalitis

The course of measles encephalitis is unpredictable, and treatment is symptomatic and supportive. Trained nursing care is essential. Careful attention to fluid and electrolyte balance is necessary. In prolonged states of coma, parenteral hyperalimentation is indicated. Status epilepticus should be treated vigorously with the use of a structured protocol for ensuring optimal control (see Chapter 43).

Numerous review papers indicate that measles encephalitis is a postinfectious encephalitis and is predominantly a disease of white matter (acute disseminated encephalomyelitis [ADEM]).[149, 187, 188] This concept resulted from a study of 19 patients with measles encephalitis published in 1984 by Johnson and associates.[189] I am aware of only two patients subsequent to this paper who had ADEM associated with measles virus infection. Clinical evidence supports the fact that ADEM not related to measles virus infection is responsive to corticosteroid therapy.[116, 244]

Considerable evidence indicates that measles encephalitis is not an ADEM and that active direct CNS infection is involved in the process.[105, 117, 245, 252] A controlled trial of 32 children with measles encephalitis failed to find benefit in the steroid-treated group.[401] These data suggest to me that corticosteroids should not be used to treat measles encephalitis unless evidence of ADEM is clear and active measles virus infection has subsided. In patients with severe intractable seizures or other evidence of cerebral edema, the use of intravenous mannitol therapy (0.25 to 1 g/kg of a 20% solution administered over a 30- to 60-minute period) is indicated. In occasional circumstances, respiratory arrest is a problem, and artificial ventilators should be used to tide patients over until respiration becomes normal. Mustafa and coworkers[271] noted improvement in an immunocompromised child with subacute measles encephalitis who was treated with intravenously administered ribavirin.

Appendicitis

Acute abdominal pain occurs occasionally in primary measles, and it can be caused by a generalized mesenteric adenitis secondary to measles virus appendicitis. In appendicitis, evidence of measles virus involvement of the appendix is present. However, therapy should be similar to that in other cases of appendicitis; removal of the appendix is indicated because measles appendicitis perforates with a frequency equal to that in non–measles virus infection.

PROPHYLACTIC ANTIBIOTICS

In the developing world, secondary bacterial infections in measles are a major cause of mortality. Accordingly, recent interest has arisen in the use of antibiotics prophylactically.[64, 345] A meta-analysis in 1997 of studies involving the use of prophylactic antibiotics noted that the available data were poor and provided only weak evidence for giving antibiotics to all children with measles.[345] The recommendation from this study was that antibiotics should be given only if a child has clinical signs of pneumonia or other evidence of sepsis. Chalmers[64] has pointed out the necessity and urgency for performing controlled prophylactic trials.

Prevention

ACTIVE IMMUNIZATION: LIVE ATTENUATED MEASLES VIRUS VACCINE

Attenuated measles vaccines are prepared in chicken embryo tissue cultures. Vaccination produces a mild or inapparent noncommunicable infection that induces active immunity in more than 95 percent of recipients. Vaccine-induced antibodies persist for many years, and although reinfection with illness has been noted on occasion in apparently successfully immunized children, it does not appear that waning immunity is of significant epidemiologic importance.[15, 74, 76, 94, 213] Symptoms associated with measles immunization are minimal and limited to fever, mild malaise, and occasionally a faint rash occurring approximately 1 week after immunization. For complete information and recommendations related to measles immunization, the reader is referred to the most recent recommendations of the Advisory Committee on Immunization Practices,[22, 60, 381] the Committee on Infectious Diseases of the American Academy of Pediatrics,[13] and the manufacturer's package insert. Only a summary of recommendations is presented here.

Recommendations for Use

The widespread epidemics of measles in the United States in 1989 to 1991 were the result of a failure to immunize children at the appropriate age and the increased number of susceptible older children and adults because of vaccine failure.[21, 60, 61, 224, 238] Therefore, eradication of measles in the United States depends on ongoing programs that (1) enroll all children of initial vaccination age and (2) allow revaccination of all persons whose primary vaccine failed. Because routine immunity testing is not a viable public health option, revaccination of primary vaccine failures can be accomplished only by universal reimmunization.

Presently, live measles vaccine is recommended in a two-dose schedule.[13, 60, 381] In general, live measles vaccine should be administered at 12 to 15 months of age and the second dose at school entry.[9, 13, 22, 58, 216, 346, 381, 388, 397] However, the second dose can be given at any time longer than 1 month after administration of the first dose.[22] Children who have not received vaccine during infancy may be immunized at any age, and adults who have not had natural measles also should be immunized. When measles is endemic or epidemic in a community, all children 6 months or older should be immunized. In children who initially were vaccinated before they were 12 months of age, a second vaccination should be administered at 12 to 15 months of age, and a third dose at school entry is necessary to complete the schedule.

Precautions

Measles vaccination should be deferred at times of febrile illness or when interference from another viral infection might cause failure of measles vaccine. Measles immunization also should be postponed for 3 to 11 months in persons who have received whole blood, blood plasma, or immunoglobulin because these products may contain sufficient measles antibody to neutralize the vaccine virus. The duration of postponement depends on the product administered and the dose.[13, 22] Children treated with intravenous immunoglobulin for Kawasaki disease should not receive measles vaccine until 11 months after receiving the immunoglobulin, whereas 3 months' time is adequate for children given immunoglobulin for hepatitis A prophylaxis.

Contraindications

Live measles vaccine should not be administered to pregnant women or to some persons with diseases or therapeutic programs associated with impaired cell-mediated immunity. These conditions in general include leukemia, lymphoma or other generalized malignancies, primary and secondary immunologic disorders, and therapy with steroids, radiation, antimetabolites, or alkylating agents. Measles immunization is recommended for children and adults with asymptomatic human immunodeficiency infection and for symptomatic patients who are not severely immunocompromised.[12, 13]

Complications

Serious complications associated with measles vaccine administration are exceedingly rare. Serious neurologic disease (encephalitis, Reye syndrome, cranial nerve palsy, cerebellar ataxia, and Guillain-Barré syndrome) occurring within 30 days of immunization occurs at a rate of approximately one case per million doses of vaccine administered.[55, 221] This rate is below the rate of occurrence of encephalitis of unknown cause in children for any 30-day period. However, the clustering of cases on days 8 and 9 after immunization noted from claims submitted to the National Vaccine Injury Compensation Program suggests that a causal relationship between measles vaccine and encephalopathy may be a rare complication of immunization.[382] In addition, recovery of measles virus from the CSF of a vaccinated child with encephalitis also suggests that rare vaccine-induced neurologic disease may occur.[117]

Thrombocytopenic purpura, anaphylaxis, hearing loss, and toxic epidermal necrolysis also have been associated with measles immunization.[11, 26, 30, 183, 337, 347, 360, 387]

In developing countries, high-titer measles vaccines were used to induce seroconversion at a young age.[393] However, follow-up studies in some countries noted that mortality was increased in female recipients of these high-titer vaccines over a 3-year period when compared with children who received conventional doses of vaccine.[171, 203] Nonetheless, follow-up studies in other countries showed no increased mortality rates in recipients of high-titer measles vaccine.[3, 225]

Studies by Wakefield and colleagues[367, 374] suggested that measles, mumps, and rubella (MMR) vaccine might have a causal role in inflammatory bowel disease and autism. However, subsequent epidemiologic studies did not support an association between MMR vaccine and either inflammatory bowel disease or autism.[90, 91, 106, 107]

QUARANTINE AND DISEASE CONTAINMENT

Before the widespread use of measles vaccines, quarantine measures were practiced widely but were largely ineffective in preventing the spread of measles. However, disease containment is practical today because the widespread use of measles vaccine has reduced the general number of susceptible young children, which in turn has decreased the rapidity of epidemic development. Epidemic measles now generally involves a greater age range of the population (cases in adolescents and young adults occur frequently), and progression of disease from one age group to another is slower than in epidemics that involve one uniform, largely susceptible population.

Containment is a vital part of the measles prevention policy in the United States. Measles is a reportable disease throughout the United States, and compliance is the obligation of all physicians. After receiving early reports of sporadic measles, health department workers can organize local immunization clinics so that the disease often can be contained in a small geographic area rather than developing into a widespread epidemic.

PASSIVE IMMUNIZATION: IMMUNOGLOBULIN

In the present vaccine era, little need for passive immunization exists. However, when a known susceptible child has had definite exposure to measles, immunoglobulin should be administered in a dose of 0.25 mg/kg (maximal dose, 15 mL). If this treatment is administered within 5 days of exposure, prevention of infection and disease can be expected. Administration of immunoglobulin later in the incubation period may modify the illness but does not prevent it. The use of immunoglobulin is particularly important in children who have not been immunized because of the contraindications to vaccination mentioned previously. In these children, immunoglobulin (0.5 mL/kg; maximal dose, 15 mL) should be administered when measles is epidemic in the community in which they reside. The dosage should be repeated every 4 weeks until the epidemic subsides. Intravenous immunoglobulin may be used (400 mg/kg).

REFERENCES

1. Aaby, P., Bukh, J., Lisse, I. M., et al.: Overcrowding and intensive exposure as determinants of measles mortality. Am. J. Epidemiol. *120*:49–63, 1984.
2. Aaby, P.: Patterns of exposure and severity of measles infection: Copenhagen 1915–1925. Ann. Epidemiol. *2*:257–262, 1992.
3. Aaby, P., Samb, B., Simondon, F., et al.: A comparison of vaccine efficacy and mortality during routine use of high-titre Edmonston-Zagreb and Schwarz standard measles vaccines in rural Senegal. Trans. R. Soc. Trop. Med. Hyg. *90*:326–330, 1996.
4. Aaby, P.: Malnutrition and overcrowding/intensive exposure in severe measles infection: Review of community studies. Rev. Infect. Dis. *10*:478–491, 1988.
5. Aarli, J. A.: Nervous complications of measles: Clinical manifestations and prognosis. Eur. Neurol. *12*:79–93, 1974.
6. Abramson, O., Dagan, R., Tal, A., et al.: Severe complications of measles requiring intensive care in infants and young children. Arch. Pediatr. Adolesc. Med. *149*:1237–1240, 1995.
7. Adams, J. M., Baird, C., and Filloy, L.: Inclusion bodies in measles encephalitis. J. A. M. A. *195*:290–298, 1966.
8. Aicardi, J., Goutieres, F., Arsenio-Nunes, M. L., et al.: Acute measles encephalitis in children with immunosuppression. Pediatrics *59*:232–239, 1977.
9. Albrecht, P., Ennis, F. A., Saltzman, E. J., et al.: Persistence of maternal antibody in infants beyond 12 months: Mechanism of measles vaccine failure. J. Pediatr. *91*:715–718, 1977.
10. Alpert, G., Liebovitz, L., and Danon, Y. L.: Analysis of T-lymphocyte subsets in measles. J. Infect. Dis. *149*:1018, 1984.
11. Alter, H. J., Scanlon, R. T., and Schechter, G. P.: Thrombocytopenic purpura following vaccination with attenuated measles virus. Am. J. Dis. Child. *115*:111–113, 1968.
12. American Academy of Pediatrics, Committee on Infectious Diseases and Committee on Pediatric AIDS: Measles immunization in HIV-infected children. American Academy of Pediatrics. Committee on Infectious Diseases and Committee on Pediatric AIDS. Pediatrics *103*:1057–1060, 1999.
13. American Academy of Pediatrics: Measles. *In* Pickering, L. K. (ed.): 2000 Red Book: Report of the Committee on Infectious Diseases. 25th ed. Elk Grove Village, IL, American Academy of Pediatrics, 2000, pp. 385–396.
14. American Academy of Pediatrics Committee on Infectious Diseases: Vitamin A treatment of measles. Pediatrics *91*:1014–1015, 1993.
15. Anders, J. F., Jacobson, R. M., Poland, G. A., et al.: Secondary failure rates of measles vaccines: A metaanalysis of published studies. Pediatr. Infect. Dis. J. *15*:62–66, 1996.
16. Anderson, R., Rabson, A. R., Sher, R., et al.: Defective neutrophil motility in children with measles. J. Pediatr. *89*:27–32, 1976.
17. Annunziato, D., Kaplan, M. H., Hall, W. W., et al.: Atypical measles syndrome: Pathologic and serologic findings. Pediatrics *70*:203–209, 1982.
18. Arneborn, P., and Biberfeld, G.: T-lymphocyte subpopulations in relation to immunosuppression in measles and varicella. Infect. Immun. *39*:29–37, 1983.
19. Arrieta, A. C., Zaleska, M., Stutman, H. R., et al.: Vitamin A levels in children with measles in Long Beach, California. J. Pediatr. *121*:75–78, 1992.
20. Atabani, S. F., Byrnes, A. A., Jaye, A., et al.: Natural measles causes prolonged suppression of interleukin-12 production. J. Infect. Dis. *184*:1–9, 2001.
21. Atkinson, W. L., Hadler, S. C., Redd, S. B., and Orenstein, W. A.: Measles surveillance: United States, 1991. M. M. W. R. CDC Surveill. Summ. *41*(No. SS-6):1–12, 1992.
22. Atkinson, W. L., Pickering, L. K., Schwartz, B., et al.: General recommendations on immunization. Recommendations of the Advisory Committee on Immunization Practices (ACIP) and the American Academy of Family Physicians (AAFP). M. M. W. R. Recomm. Rep. *51*(RR-2):1–35, 2002.
23. Atmar, R. L., Englund J. A., and Hammill, H.: Complications of measles during pregnancy. Clin. Infect. Dis. *14*:217–226, 1992.
24. Azizi, A., and Krakovsky, D.: Keratoconjunctivitis as a constant sign of measles. Ann. Pediatr. *204*:397–405, 1965.

25. Babbott, F. L., Jr., and Gordon, J. E.: Modern measles. Am. J. Med. Sci. *228*:334–361, 1954.
26. Bachard, A. J., Rubenstein, J., and Morrison, A. N.: Thrombocytopenic purpura following live measles vaccine. Am. J. Dis. Child. *118*:283–285, 1967.
27. Barclay, A. J. G., Foster, A., and Sommer, A.: Retinol supplements and mortality related to measles: A randomised clinical trial. B. M. J. *294*:294–296, 1987.
28. Barsegar, B., Hofmann, H., and Zweymuller, E.: The diagnosis of measles in the newborn and infant age groups. Z. Kinderheilk. *113*:175–184, 1972.
29. Baublis, J. V., and Payne, F. E.: Measles antigen and syncytium formation in brain cell cultures from subacute sclerosing panencephalitis (SSPE). Proc. Soc. Exp. Biol. Med. *129*:593–597, 1968.
30. Beeler, J., Varricchio, F. and Wise, R.: Thrombocytopenia after immunization with measles vaccines: Review of the vaccine adverse events reporting system (1990 to 1994). Pediatr. Infect. Dis. J. *15*:88–90, 1996.
31. Bellanti, J. A., Sanga, R. L., Klutinis, B., et al.: Antibody responses in serum and nasal secretions of children immunized with inactivated and attenuated measles-virus vaccines. N. Engl. J. Med. *280*:628–633, 666–667, 1969.
32. Bellini, W. J., Rota, J. S., and Rota, P. A.: Virology of measles virus. J. Infect. Dis. *170*(Suppl. 1):15–23, 1994.
33. Benjamin, B., and Ward, S. M.: Leukocytic response to measles. Am. J. Dis. Child. *44*:921–963, 1932.
34. Berkovich, S., and Schneck, L.: Ascending paralysis associated with measles. J. Pediatr. *64*:88–93, 1964.
35. Berm, J.: Koplik spots for the record: An illustrated historical note. Clin. Pediatr. (Phila.) *11*:161–163, 1972.
36. Black, F. L.: Growth and stability of measles virus. Virology *7*:184–192, 1959.
37. Black, F. L.: Discussion of paper by Karelitz, S.: Measles vaccine and immunity. N. Y. J. Med. *63*:519–528, 1963.
38. Black, F. L.: A nationwide serum survey of U.S. military recruits, 1962, III. Measles and mumps antibodies. Am. J. Hyg. *80*:304–307, 1964.
39. Black, F. L.: *In* Evans, A. S. (ed.): Viral Infections of Humans: Epidemiology and Control. 3rd ed. New York, Plenum Medical, 1989, pp. 451–469.
40. Black, F. L., Reissig, M., and Melnick, J. L.: Measles virus. Adv. Virus Res. *6*:205–277, 1959.
41. Black, F. L., and Sheridan, S. R.: Studies on an attenuated measles-virus vaccine. IV. Administration of vaccine by several routes. N. Engl. J. Med. *263*:165–169, 1960.
42. Black, F. L., and Sheridan, S. R.: Blood leukocyte response to live measles vaccine. Am. J. Dis. Child. *113*:301–304, 1967.
43. Bloch, A. B., Orenstein, W. A., Ewing, W. M., et al.: Measles outbreak in a pediatric practice: Airborne transmission in an office setting. Pediatrics *75*:676–683, 1985.
44. Boteler, W. L., Luipersbeck, P. M., Fuccillo, D. A., et al.: Enzyme-linked immunosorbent assay for detection of measles antibody. J. Clin. Microbiol. *17*:814–818, 1983.
45. Brodsky, A. L.: Atypical measles: Severe illness in recipients of killed measles virus vaccine upon exposure to natural infection. J. A. M. A. *222*:1415–1416, 1972.
46. Buckland, R., and Wild, T. F.: Is CD46 the cellular receptor for measles virus? Virus Res. *48*:1–9, 1997.
47. Burnstein, T., Frankel, J. W., and Jensen, J. H.: Adaptation of measles virus to suckling hamsters. Fed. Proc. *17*:507, 1958.
48. Bussell, R. H., and Karzon, D. T.: Measles-canine distemper-rinderpest group. *In* Prier, J. E. (ed.): Basic Medical Virology. Baltimore, Williams & Wilkins, 1966, pp. 313–336.
49. Butler, J. C., Havens, P. L., Sowell, A. L., et al.: Measles severity and serum retinol (vitamin A) concentration among children in the U.S. Pediatrics *91*:1176–1181, 1993.
50. Butler, J. C., Proctor, M. E., Fessler, K., et al.: Household-acquisition of measles and illness severity in an urban community in the U.S. Epidemiol. Infect. *112*:569–577, 1994.
51. Carlstrom, G.: Comparative studies on measles and distemper viruses in suckling mice. Arch. Virusforsch. *8*:527–538, 1958.
52. Carlstrom, G.: Relation of measles to other viruses. Am. J. Dis. Child. *103*:287–291, 1962.
53. Carney, J., Stiehm, E. R., Cherry, J. D., et al.: Unpublished data, 1978.
54. Caulfield, E.: Early measles epidemics in America. Yale J. Biol. Med. *15*:531–536, 1943.
55. Centers for Disease Control: Measles Surveillance Report No. 10, 1973–1976. July 1977.
56. Centers for Disease Control: Measles prevention. M. M. W. R. Morb. Mortal. Wkly. Rep. *27*:427–437, 1978.
57. Centers for Disease Control: Measles encephalitis: United States, 1962–1979. M. M. W. R. Morb. Mortal. Wkly. Rep. *30*(29):362–364, 1981.
58. Centers for Disease Control: Measles surveillance, 1977–1981. Issued September 1982.
59. Centers for Disease Control: Recommendations of the Immunization Practices Advisory Committee (ACIP). Measles prevention. M. M. W. R. Morb. Mortal. Wkly. Rep. *31*(17):217–224, 229–231, 1982.
60. Centers for Disease Control: Measles prevention. M. M. W. R. Morb. Mortal. Wkly. Rep. *38*(Suppl. 9):1–18, 1989.
61. Centers for Disease Control and Prevention: Summary of notifiable diseases, United States, 1994. M. M. W. R. Morb. Mortal. Wkly. Rep. *43*(53):1–80, 1995.
62. Centers for Disease Control and Prevention: Summary of Notifiable Diseases, United States, 1998. M. M. W. R. Morb. Mortal. Wkly. Rep. *47*(53):ii–92, 1999.
63. Centers for Disease Control and Prevention: Measles—United States, 2000. M. M. W. R. Morb. Mortal. Wkly. Rep. *51*(6):120–123, 2002.
64. Chalmers, I.: Why we need to know whether prophylactic antibiotics can reduce measles-related morbidity. Pediatrics *109*:312–315, 2002.
65. Chao, D.: Subacute inclusion body encephalitis. J. Pediatr. *61*:501–510, 1962.
66. Charlesworth, J. A., Pussell, B. A., Roy, L. P., et al.: Measles infection: Involvement of the complement system. Clin. Exp. Immunol. *24*:401–406, 1976.
67. Chatterji, M., and Mankad, V.: Failure of attenuated viral vaccine in prevention of atypical measles. J. A. M. A. *238*:2635, 1977.
68. Chen, R. T., Markowitz, L. E., Albrecht, P., et al.: Measles antibody: Reevaluation of protective titers. J. Infect. Dis. *162*:1036–1041, 1990.
69. Cherry, J. D.: Lesions of the lips and mouth. *In* Gellis, S. S., and Kagan, B. M. (eds.): Current Pediatric Therapy: 3. Philadelphia, W. B. Saunders, 1968, pp. 257–260.
70. Cherry, J. D.: Newer viral exanthems. Adv. Pediatr. *16*:233–286, 1969.
71. Cherry, J. D.: Personal observations, 1978.
72. Cherry, J. D.: The "new" epidemiology of measles and rubella. Hosp. Pract. *115*:49–57, 1980.
73. Cherry, J. D., Feigin, R. D., Lobes, L. A., Jr., et al.: Unpublished data, 1971.
74. Cherry, J. D., Feigin, R. D., Lobes, L. A., Jr., et al.: Urban measles in the vaccine era: A clinical, epidemiologic, and serologic study. J. Pediatr. *81*:217–230, 1972.
75. Cherry, J. D., Feigin, R. D., Lobes, L. A., Jr., et al.: Atypical measles in children previously immunized with attenuated measles virus vaccines. Pediatrics *50*:712–717, 1972.
76. Cherry, J. D., Feigin, R. D., Shackelford, P. G., et al.: A clinical and serologic study of 103 children with measles vaccine failure. J. Pediatr. *82*:802–808, 1973.
77. Choppin, P. W., Richardson, C. D., Merz, D. C., et al.: The functions and inhibition of the membrane glycoproteins of paramyxoviruses and myxoviruses and the role of the measles virus M protein in subacute sclerosing panencephalitis. J. Infect. Dis. *143*:352–363, 1981.
78. Christensen, P. E., Schmidt, H., Bang, H. O., et al.: An epidemic of measles in southern Greenland, 1951: Measles in virgin soil. II. The epidemic proper. Acta Med. Scand. *144*:430–449, 1953.
79. Cobban, K.: Measles in Nigerian children. West Afr. Med. J. *12*:18–23, 1963.
80. Conley, S. F., Beste, D. J., and Hoffmann, R. G.: Measles-associated bacterial tracheitis. Pediatr. Infect. Dis. J. *12*:414–415, 1993.
81. Connolly, J. H., Allen, I. V., Hurwitz, L. J., et al.: Measles-virus antibody and antigen in subacute sclerosing panencephalitis. Lancet *1*:542–544, 1967.
82. Conrad, J. L., Wallace, R., and Witte, J. J.: The epidemiologic rationale for the failure to eradicate measles in the U.S. Am. J. Public Health *61*:2304–2310, 1971.
83. Coovadia, H. M., Brain, P., Hallett, A. F., et al.: Immunoparesis and outcome in measles. Lancet *1*:619–621, 1977.
83. Coovadia, H. M., Parent, M. A., Loening, W. E. K., et al.: An evaluation of factors associated with the depression of immunity in malnutrition and in measles. Am. J. Clin. Nutr. *27*:665–669, 1974.
85. Coovadia, H. M., Wesley, A., Henderson, L. G., et al.: Alterations in immune responsiveness in acute measles and chronic post-measles chest disease. Int. Arch. Allergy Appl. Immunol. *56*:14–23, 1978.
86. Coutsoudis, A., Broughton, M., and Coovadia, H. M.: Retinol supplementation reduces morbidity in young African children: A randomised placebo-controlled, double-blind trial. Am. J. Clin. Nutr. *54*:890–895, 1991.
87. Coutsoudis, A., Kiepiela, P., Coovadia, H. M., et al.: Vitamin A supplementation enhances specific IgG antibody levels and total lymphocyte numbers while improving morbidity in measles. Pediatr. Infect. Dis. J. *11*:203–209, 1992.
88. Cremer, N. E., Cossen, C. K., Shell, G., et al.: Enzyme immunoassay versus plaque neutralization and other methods for determination of immune status to measles and varicella-zoster viruses versus complement fixation for serodiagnosis of infections with those viruses. J. Clin. Microbiol. *21*:869–874, 1985.
89. Dagan, R., Phillip, M., Sarov, I., et al.: Cellular immunity and T-lymphocyte subsets in young children with acute measles. J. Med. Virol. *22*:175–182, 1987.
90. Dales, L., Hammer, S. J., and Smith, N. J.: Time trends in autism and in MMR immunization coverage in California. J. A. M. A. *285*:1183–1185, 2001.
91. Davis, R. L., Kramarz, P., Bohlke, K., et al.: Measles-mumps-rubella and other measles-containing vaccines do not increase the risk for inflammatory bowel disease: A case-control study from the Vaccine Safety Datalink project. Arch. Pediatr. Adolesc. Med. *155*:354–359, 2001.

92. Dawson, J. R., Jr.: Cellular inclusions in cerebral lesions of lethargic encephalitis. Am. J. Pathol. *9*:7–16, 1933.
93. Degen, J. A., Jr.: Visceral pathology in measles: A clinicopathologic study of 100 fatal cases. Am. J. Med. Sci. *194*:104–111, 1937.
94. Deseda-Tous, J., Cherry, J. D., Spencer, M. J., et al.: Measles revaccination: Persistence and degree of antibody titer by type of immune response. Am. J. Dis. Child. *132*:287–290, 1978.
95. Deseda-Tous, J. E., Spencer, M. J., Cherry, J. D., et al.: Measles antibody in healthy adults analyzed by HLA and ABO blood types. Abstract. Paper presented at the 16th Interscience Conference on Antimicrobial Agents and Chemotherapy, October 1976, Chicago.
96. Döring, R. E. A., Marcil, A., Chopra, A., et al.: The human CD46 molecule is a receptor for measles virus (Edmonson strain). Cell *75*:295–305, 1993.
97. Douglas, J. W. B.: Ability and adjustment of children who have had measles. B. M. J. *2*:1301–1303, 1964.
98. Dunn, R. A.: Subacute sclerosing panencephalitis. Pediatr. Infect. Dis. J. *10*:68–72, 1991.
99. Durant, R. H., Dyken, P. R., and Swift, A. V.: The influence of inosiplex treatment on the neurological disability of patients with subacute sclerosing panencephalitis. J. Pediatr. *101*:288–293, 1982.
100. Eberhart-Phillips, J. E., Frederick, P. D., Baron, R. C., et al.: Measles in pregnancy: A descriptive study of 58 cases. Obstet. Gynecol. *82*:797–801, 1993.
101. Edmonson, M. B., Addiss, D. G., McPherson, T., et al.: Mild measles and secondary vaccine failure during a sustained outbreak in a highly vaccinated population. J. A. M. A. *263*:2467–2471, 1990.
102. Ehrengut, W.: Measles encephalitis: Age disposition and vaccination. Arch. Virusforsch. *16*:1–5, 1965.
103. Enders, J. F., McCarthy, K., Mitus, A., et al.: Isolation of measles virus at autopsy in cases of giant-cell pneumonia without rash. N. Engl. J. Med. *261*:875–896, 1959.
104. Enders, J. F., and Peebles, T. C.: Propagation in tissue cultures of cytopathogenic agents from patients with measles. Proc. Soc. Exp. Biol. Med. *86*:277–286, 1954.
105. Esolen, L. M., Takahashi, K., Johnson, R. T., et al.: Brain endothelial cell infection in children with acute fatal measles. J. Clin. Invest. *96*:2478–2481, 1995.
106. Farrington, C. P., Miller, E., and Taylor, B.: MMR and autism: Further evidence against a causal association. Vaccine *19*:3632–3635, 2001.
107. Feeney, M., Clegg, A., Winwood, P., et al.: A case-control study of measles vaccination and inflammatory bowel disease. The East Dorset Gastroenterology Group. Lancet *350*:764–766, 1997.
108. Fenner, F.: The pathogenesis of the acute exanthems. Lancet *2*:915–920, 1948.
109. Fenner, F.: Classification and nomenclature of viruses: Second report of the International Committee on Taxonomy of Viruses. Intervirology *7*:1–115, 1976.
110. Field, C. E.: Bronchiectasis in childhood. I. Clinical survey of 160 cases. Pediatrics *4*:21–46, 1949.
111. Finkel, H. E.: Measles myocarditis. Am. Heart J. *67*:679–683, 1964.
112. Fireman, P., Friday, G., and Kumate, J.: Effect of measles vaccine on immunologic responsiveness. Pediatrics *43*:264–272, 1969.
113. Fleischer, B., and Kreth, H. W.: Clonal expansion and functional analysis of virus-specific T lymphocytes from cerebrospinal fluid in measles encephalitis. Hum. Immunol. *7*:239–248, 1983.
114. Florman, A. L., and Agatston, H. J.: Keratoconjunctivitis as a diagnostic aid in measles. J. A. M. A. *179*:192–194, 1962.
115. Foege, W. H.: Measles control in West and Central Africa. Paper presented at the Eighth Annual Immunology Conference, March 1971, Kansas City, MO.
116. Ford-Jones, E. L., MacGregor, D., Richardson, S., et al.: Acute childhood encephalitis and meningoencephalitis: Diagnosis and management. Paediatr. Child Health. *3*:33–40, 1998.
117. Foreman, M. L., and Cherry, J. D.: Isolation of measles virus from the cerebrospinal fluid of a child with encephalitis following measles vaccination. Abstract. Program for the American Pediatric Society, 1967.
118. Forghani, B., Myoraku, C. K., and Schmidt, N. J.: Use of monoclonal antibodies to human immunoglobulin M in "capture" assays for measles and rubella immunoglobulin M. J. Clin. Microbiol. *18*:652–657, 1983.
119. Forni, A. L., Schluger, N. W., and Roberts, R. B.: Severe measles pneumonitis in adults: Evaluation of clinical characteristics and therapy with intravenous ribavirin. Clin. Infect. Dis. *19*:454–462, 1994.
120. Forthal, D. N., Landucci, G., Habis, A., et al.: Measles virus–specific functional antibody responses and viremia during acute measles. J. Infect. Dis. *169*:1377–1380, 1994.
121. Forthal, D. N., Landucci, G., Katz, J., et al.: Comparison of measles virus–specific antibodies with antibody-dependent cellular cytotoxicity and neutralizing functions. J. Infect. Dis. *168*:1020–1023, 1993.
122. Frank, J. A., Jr., Orenstein, W. A., Bart, K. J., et al.: Major impediments to measles elimination: The modern epidemiology of an ancient disease. Am. J. Dis. Child. *139*:881–888, 1985.
123. Frederique, G., Howard, R. O., and Boniuk, V.: Corneal ulcers in rubeola. Am. J. Ophthalmol. *68*:996–1003, 1969.
124. Frieden, T. R., Sowell, A. L., Henning, K. J., et al.: Vitamin A levels and severity of measles: New York City. Am. J. Dis. Child. *146*:182–186, 1992.
125. Friedman, M. G., Phillip, M., and Dagan, R.: Virus-specific IgA in serum, saliva, and tears of children with measles. Clin. Exp. Immunol. *75*:58–63, 1989.
126. Fulginiti, V. A., Eller, J. J., Downie, A. W., et al.: Altered reactivity to measles virus: Atypical measles in children previously immunized with inactivated measles virus vaccines. J. A. M. A. *202*:1075–1080, 1967.
127. Fulginiti, V. A., and Helfer, R. E.: Atypical measles in adolescent siblings 16 years after killed measles virus vaccine. J. A. M. A. *244*:804–806, 1980.
128. Fulginiti, V. A., and Kempe, C. H.: Measles exposure among vaccine recipients: Response to measles exposure and antibody persistence among recipients of measles vaccines. Am. J. Dis. Child. *106*:450–461, 1963.
129. Fulginiti, V. A., and Kempe, C. H.: A comparison of measles neutralizing and hemagglutination-inhibition antibody titers in individual sera. Am. J. Epidemiol. *82*:135–142, 1965.
130. Gallagher, M. R., Welliver, R., Yamanaka, T., et al.: Cell-mediated immune responsiveness to measles: Its occurrence as a result of naturally acquired or vaccine-induced infection and in infants of immune mothers. Am. J. Dis. Child. *135*:48–51, 1981.
131. Garenne, M., and Aaby, P.: Pattern of exposure and measles mortality in Senegal. J. Infect. Dis. *161*:1088–1094, 1990.
132. Gellin, B. G., and Katz, S. L.: Putting a stop to a serial killer: Measles. J. Infect. Dis. *170*(Suppl. 1):1–2, 1994.
133. Gendelman, H. E., Wolinsky, J. S., Johnson, R. T., et al.: Measles encephalomyelitis: Lack of evidence of viral invasion of the central nervous system and quantitative study of the nature of demyelination. Ann. Neurol. *15*:353–360, 1984.
134. Gibbs, F. A., Gibbs, E. L., Carpenter, P. R., et al.: Electroencephalographic abnormality in "uncomplicated" childhood diseases. J. A. M. A. *72*:1050–1055, 1959.
135. Goerka, H.: The life and scientific works of Mr. John Quier. West Indian Med. J. *5*:23, 1956.
136. Gokiert, J. G., and Beamish, W. E.: Altered reactivity to measles virus in previously vaccinated children. Can. Med. Assoc. J. *103*:724–727, 1970.
137. Goldberger, J., and Anderson, J. F.: An experimental demonstration of the presence of the virus of measles in the mixed buccal and nasal secretions. J. A. M. A. *57*:476–478, 1911.
138. Goldfield, M., Boyer, N. H., and Weinstein, L.: Electrocardiographic changes during the course of measles. J. Pediatr. *46*:30–35, 1955.
139. Good, R. A., and Zak, S. J.: Disturbances in gamma globulin synthesis as "experiments of nature." Pediatrics *18*:109–149, 1956.
140. Goodall, E. W.: Measles with an "illness of infection." Clin. J. *54*:69, 1925.
141. Grattan-Smith, P. J., Procopis, P. G., Wise, G. A., et al.: Serious neurological complications of measles: A continuing preventable problem. Med. J. Aust. *143*:385–387, 1985.
142. Graves, M., Griffin, D. E., Johnson, R. T., et al.: Development of antibody to measles virus polypeptides during complicated and uncomplicated measles virus infections. J. Virol. *49*:409–412, 1984.
143. Graziano, K. D., Ruckdeschel, J. C., and Mardiney, M. R., Jr.: Cell-associated immunity to measles (rubeola): The demonstration of in vitro lymphocyte tritiated thymidine incorporation in response to measles complement fixation antigen. Cell. Immunol. *15*:347–359, 1975.
144. Green, M. S., Shohat, T., and Lerman, Y.: Sex differences in the humoral antibody response to live measles vaccine in young adults. Int. J. Epidemiol. *23*:1078–1081, 1994.
145. Greenstein, J. I., and McFarland, H. F.: Response of human lymphocytes to measles virus after natural infection. Infect. Immun. *40*:198–204, 1983.
146. Gremillion, D. H., and Crawford, G. E.: Measles pneumonia in young adults: An analysis of 106 cases. Am. J. Med. *71*:539–542, 1981.
147. Gresser, I., and Chany, C.: Isolation of measles virus from the washed leucocytic fraction of blood. Proc. Soc. Exp. Biol. Med. *113*:695–698, 1963.
148. Gresser, I., and Katz, S. L.: Isolation of measles virus from urine. N. Engl. J. Med. *263*:452–454, 1960.
149. Griffin, D. E.: Measles virus. *In* Knipe, D. M., and Howley, P. M. (eds): Fields Virology. Vol. 1. Philadelphia, Lippincott Williams & Wilkins, 2001, pp. 1401–1441.
150. Griffin, D. E., Cooper, S. J., Hirsch, R. L., et al.: Changes in plasma IgE levels during complicated and uncomplicated measles virus infections. J. Allergy Clin. Immunol. *76*:206–213, 1985.
151. Griffin, D. E., Hirsch, R. L., Johnson, R. T., et al.: Changes in serum C-reactive protein during complicated and uncomplicated measles virus infections. Infect. Immun. *41*:861–864, 1983.
152. Griffin, D. E., Ward, B. J., and Esolen, L. M.: Pathogenesis of measles virus infection: An hypothesis for altered immune responses. J. Infect. Dis. *170*(Suppl. 1):24–31, 1994.
153. Griffin, D. E., Ward, B. J., Jauregui, E., et al.: Immune activation in measles. N. Engl. J. Med. *320*:1667–1672, 1989.
154. Griffin, D. E., Ward, B. J., Jauregui, E., et al.: Natural killer cell activity during measles. Clin. Exp. Immunol. *81*:218–224, 1990.
155. Griffin, D. E., Ward, B. J., Jauregui, E., et al.: Immune activation during measles: Interferon-α and neopterin in plasma and cerebrospinal fluid in

complicated and uncomplicated disease. J. Infect. Dis. *161*:449–453, 1990.
156. Grist, N. R.: The pathogenesis of measles: Review of the literature and discussion of the problem. Glasgow Med. J. *31*:431–441, 1950.
157. Guinee, V. F., Henderson, D. A., Casey, H. L., et al.: Cooperative measles vaccine field trial. I. Clinical efficacy. II. Serologic studies. Pediatrics *37*:649–657, 657–665, 1966.
158. Gunn, W.: Control of common fevers: Measles. Lancet *1*:795–799, 1938.
159. Haas, E. J., and Wendt, V. E.: Atypical measles 14 years after immunization. J. A. M. A. *236*:1050, 1976.
160. Hall, W. W., and Martin, S. J.: Purification and characterization of measles virus. J. Gen. Virol. *19*:175–188, 1973.
161. Hall, W. W., and Martin, S. J.: Structure and function relationships of the envelope of measles virus. Med. Microbiol. Immunol. *160*:143–154, 1974.
162. Halsey, N. A., Nieburg, P. I., Preblud, S. R., et al.: Recent trends in reported measles cases and deaths. Effectiveness of measles vaccine administered at 12 months of age. Simultaneous administration of measles vaccine and DPT antigens. Prepared for the American Academy of Pediatrics Committee on Infectious Diseases, Red Book Committee and Advisory Committee on Immunization Practices. Atlanta, U.S. DHEW, Public Health Service, Centers for Disease Control, 1978.
163. Haltia, M., Tarkkanen, A., Vaheri, A., et al.: Measles retinopathy during immunosuppression. Br. J. Ophthalmol. *62*:356–360, 1978.
164. Hardy, G. E., Jr., Kassanoff, I., Orbach, H. G., et al.: The failure of a school immunization campaign to terminate an urban epidemic of measles. Am. J. Epidemiol. *91*:286–293, 1970.
165. Hayden, R. J.: The epidemiology and nature of measles in Nairobi before the impact of measles immunization. East Afr. Med. J. *51*:199–205, 1974.
166. Hedrich, A. W.: The corrected average attack rate from measles among city children. Am. J. Hyg. *11*:576–600, 1930.
167. Heffner, R. R., Jr., and Schluederberg, A.: Specificity of the primary and secondary antibody responses to myxoviruses. J. Immunol. *98*:668–672, 1967.
168. Heimann, A., Scanlon, R., Gentile, J., et al.: Measles cervicitis: Report of a case with cytologic and molecular biologic analysis. Acta Cytol. *36*:727–730, 1992.
169. Helfand, R. F., Kim, D. K., Gary, H. E., et al.: Nonclassic measles infections in an immune population exposed to measles during a college bus trip. J. Med. Virol. *56*:337–341, 1998.
170. Henderson, J. A. M., and Hammond, D. I.: Delayed diagnosis in atypical measles syndrome. Can. Med. Assoc. J. *133*:211–213, 1985.
171. Holt, E. A., Moulton, L. H., Siberry, G. K., et al.: Differential mortality by measles vaccine titer and sex. J. Infect. Dis. *168*:1087–1096, 1993.
172. Home, F.: Medical Facts and Experiments. London, A. Millar, 1759.
173. Horta-Barbosa, L., Fuccillo, D. A., London, W. T., et al.: Isolation of measles virus from brain cell cultures of two patients with subacute sclerosing panencephalitis. Proc. Soc. Exp. Biol. Med. *132*:272–277, 1969.
174. Horta-Barbosa, L., Fuccillo, D. A., and Sever, J. L.: Subacute sclerosing panencephalitis: Isolation of measles virus from a brain biopsy. Nature *221*:974, 1969.
175. Horta-Barbosa, L., Krebs, H., Ley, A., et al.: Progressive increase in cerebrospinal fluid measles antibody levels in subacute sclerosing panencephalitis. Pediatrics *47*:782–783, 1971.
176. Horwitz, M. S., Grose, C., and Fisher, M.: Atypical measles rash mimicking Rocky Mountain spotted fever. N. Engl. J. Med. *289*:1203–1204, 1973.
177. Hudson, J. B., Weinstein, L., and Chang, T. W.: Thrombocytopenic purpura in measles. J. Pediatr. *48*:48–56, 1956.
178. Hussey, G. D., and Klein, M.: A randomized, controlled trial of vitamin A in children with severe measles. N. Engl. J. Med. *323*:160–164, 1990.
179. Imagawa, D. T.: Relationships among measles, canine distemper and rinderpest viruses. Prog. Med. Virol. *10*:160–193, 1968.
180. Imagawa, D. T., and Adams, J. M.: Propagation of measles virus in suckling mice. Proc. Soc. Exp. Biol. *98*:567–569, 1958.
181. Inua, M., Duggan, M. B., West, C. E., et al.: Postmeasles corneal ulceration in children in northern Nigeria: The role of retinol, malnutrition, and measles. Ann. Trop. Pediatr. *3*:181–191, 1983.
182. Janeway, C. A.: Use of concentrated human serum γ-globulin in the prevention and attenuation of measles. Bull. N. Y. Acad. Med. *21*:202–222, 1945.
183. Jayarajan, V., and Sedler, P. A.: Hearing loss following measles vaccination. J. Infect. *30*:184–185, 1995.
184. Jenkerson, S. A., Beller, M., Middaugh, J. P., et al.: False-positive rubeola IgM tests. N. Engl. J. Med. *332*:1103–1104, 1995.
185. Jespersen, C. S., Littauer, J., and Sagild, U.: Measles as a cause of fetal defects: A retrospective study of ten measles epidemics in Greenland. Acta Pediatr. Scand. *66*:367–372, 1977.
186. Joffe, M. I., Sukha, N. R., and Rabson, A. R.: Lymphocyte subsets in measles: Depressed helper/inducer subpopulation reversed by in vitro treatment with levamisole and ascorbic acid. J. Clin. Invest. *72*:971–980, 1983.
187. Johnson, R. T.: The pathogenesis of acute viral encephalitis and postinfectious encephalomyelitis. J. Infect. Dis. *155*:359–364, 1987.
188. Johnson, R. T.: Acute encephalitis. Clin. Infect. Dis. *23*:219–224, quiz 225–226, 1996.
189. Johnson, R. T., Griffin, D. E., Hirsch, R. L., et al.: Measles encephalomyelitis: Clinical and immunologic studies. N. Engl. J. Med. *310*:137–141, 1984.
190. Kamahora, J., and Nii, S.: Pathological and immunological studies of monkeys infected with measles virus. Arch. Virusforsch. *16*:161–167, 1965.
191. Karzon, D. T., Rush, D., and Winkelstein, W., Jr.: Immunization with inactivated measles virus vaccine: Effect of booster dose and response to natural challenge. Pediatrics *36*:40–50, 1965.
192. Katz, S. L.: Measles: Its complications, treatment and prophylaxis. Med. Clin. North Am. *46*:1163–1175, 1962.
193. Katz, S. L., and Enders, J. F.: Measles virus. *In* Horsfall, F. L., Jr., and Tamm, T. (eds.): Viral and Rickettsial Infections of Man. Philadelphia, J. B. Lippincott, 1965, pp. 784–801.
194. Katz, S. L., and Enders, J. F.: Measles virus. *In* Lennette, E. H., and Schmidt, N. J. (eds.): Diagnostic Procedures for Viral and Rickettsial Infections. Washington, D.C., American Public Health Association, 1969, pp. 504–528.
195. Katz, S. L., Milovanovic, M. V., and Enders, J. F.: Propagation of measles virus in cultures of chick embryo cells. Proc. Soc. Exp. Biol. Med. *97*:23–29, 1958.
196. Kempe, C. H., and Fulginiti, V. A.: The pathogenesis of measles virus infection. Arch. Virusforsch. *16*:103–128, 1965.
197. Kennedy, C. R., and Webster, A. D. B.: Measles encephalitis. N. Engl. J. Med. *311*:330–331, 1984.
198. Khatib, R., Siddique, M., and Abbas, M.: Measles-associated hepatobiliary disease: An overview. Infection *21*:112–114, 1993.
199. Kibler, R., and TerMeulen, V.: Antibody-mediated cytotoxicity after measles virus infection. J. Immunol. *114*:93–98, 1975.
200. Kiepiela, P., Coovadia, H. M., and Coward, P.: T helper cell defect related to severity in measles. Scand. J. Infect. Dis. *19*:185–192, 1987.
201. Kimura, A., Tosaka, K., and Nakao, T.: Measles rash. I. Light and electron microscopic study of skin eruptions. Arch. Virol. *47*:295–307, 1975.
202. Kleiman, M. B., Blackburn, C. K. L., Zimmerman, S. E., et al.: Comparison of enzyme-linked immunosorbent assay for acute measles with hemagglutination inhibition, complement fixation, and fluorescent antibody methods. J. Clin. Microbiol. *14*:147–152, 1981.
203. Knudsen, K. M., Aaby, P., Whittle, H., et al.: Child mortality following standard, medium or high titre measles immunization in West Africa. Int. J. Epidemiol. *25*:665–673, 1996.
204. Kobune, F., Sakata, H., and Sugiura, A.: Marmoset lymphoblastoid cells as a sensitive host for isolation of measles virus. J. Virol. *64*:700–705, 1990.
205. Koffler, D.: Giant cell pneumonia: Fluorescent antibody and histochemical studies on alveolar giant cells. Arch. Pathol. *78*:267–273, 1964.
206. Kohn, J. L., and Koiransky, H.: Successive roentgenograms of the chest of children during measles. Am. J. Dis. Child. *38*:258–270, 1929.
207. Koplik, H.: The diagnosis of the invasion of measles from a study of the exanthema as it appears on the buccal mucous membrane. Arch. Pediatr. *13*:918, 1896.
208. Koplik, H.: A new diagnostic sign of measles. Med. Rec. *53*:505, 1898.
209. Koplik, H.: The new diagnostic spots of measles on the buccal and labial mucous membrane. Med. News *74*:673, 1899.
210. Krause, P. J., Cherry, J. D., Naiditch, M. J., et al.: Revaccination of previous recipients of killed measles vaccine: Clinical and immunologic studies. J. Pediatr. *93*:565–571, 1978.
211. Kress, S., Schluederberg, A. E., Hornick, R. B., et al.: Studies with live attenuated measles-virus vaccine. II. Clinical and immunologic response of children in an open community. Am. J. Dis. Child. *101*:701–707, 1961.
212. Krugman, S.: Present status of measles and rubella immunization in the U.S.: A medical progress report. J. Pediatr. *78*:1–16, 1971.
213. Krugman, S.: Present status of measles and rubella immunization in the U.S.: A medical progress report. J. Pediatr. *90*:1–12, 1977.
214. Krugman, S., Giles, J. P., Friedman, H., et al.: Studies on immunity to measles. J. Pediatr. *66*:471–488, 1965.
215. Krugman, S., Giles, J. P., Jacobs, A. M., et al.: Studies with live attenuated measles-virus vaccine. Am. J. Dis. Child. *103*:353–363, 1962.
216. Krugman, R. D., Rosenberg, R., McIntosh, K., et al.: Further attenuated live measles vaccines: The need for revised recommendations. J. Pediatr. *91*:766–767, 1977.
217. Krugman, S., Ward, R., and Katz, S. L.: Measles (rubeola). *In* Krugman, S., Ward, R., and Katz, S. L. (eds.): Infectious Diseases of Children. 6th ed. St. Louis, C. V. Mosby, 1977, pp. 132–148.
218. LaBoccetta, A. C., and Tornay, A. S.: Measles encephalitis: Report of 61 cases. Am. J. Dis. Child. *107*:247–255, 1964.
219. Labowskie, R. J., Edelman, R., Rustigian, R., et al.: Studies of cell-mediated immunity to measles virus by in vitro lymphocyte-mediated cytotoxicity. J. Infect. Dis. *129*:233–239, 1974.
220. Lamb, R. A., and Kolakofsky, D.: *Paramyxoviridae:* the viruses and their replication. *In* Knipe, D. M., and Howley, P. M. (eds.): Fields Virology, Vol. 1. Philadelphia, Lippincott Williams & Wilkins, 2001, pp. 1305–1339.

221. Landrigan, P. J., and Witte, J. J.: Neurologic disorders following live measles-virus vaccination. J. A. M. A. *223*:1459–1462, 1973.
222. Langmuir, A. D.: Medical importance of measles. Am. J. Dis. Child. *103*:224–226, 1962.
223. Laptook, A., Wind, E., Nussbaum, M., et al.: Pulmonary lesions in atypical measles. Pediatrics *62*:42–46, 1978.
224. Levy, D. L.: The future of measles in highly immunized populations. Am. J. Epidemiol. *120*:39–48, 1984.
225. Libman, M. D., Inrahim, S. A., Omer, M. I. A., et al.: No evidence for short or long term morbidity after increased titer measles vaccination in Sudan. Pediatr. Infect. Dis. J. *21*:112–119, 2002.
226. Lightwood, R., Nolan, R., Franco, M., et al.: Epithelial giant cells in measles as an aid in diagnosis. J. Pediatr. *77*:59–64, 1970.
227. Lin, C.-Y., and Hsu, H.-C.: Measles and acute glomerulonephritis. Pediatrics *71*:398–401, 1983.
228. Linnemann, C. C., Jr., Rotte, T. C., Schiff, G. M., et al.: A seroepidemiologic study of a measles epidemic in a highly immunized population. Am. J. Epidemiol. *95*:238–246, 1972.
229. Lobes, L. A., Jr., and Cherry, J. D.: Fatal measles pneumonia in a child with chickenpox pneumonia. J. A. M. A. *223*:1143–1144, 1973.
230. London, W. P., and Yorke, J. A.: Recurrent outbreaks of measles, chickenpox and mumps. I. Seasonal variation in contact rates. Am. J. Epidemiol. *98*:453–468, 1973.
231. Lyon, G., Ponsot, G., and Lebon, P.: Acute measles encephalitis of the delayed type. Ann. Neurol. *2*:322–327, 1977.
232. Maimone, D., Grimaldi, L. M. E., Incorpora, G., et al.: Intrathecal interferon in subacute sclerosing panencephalitis. Acta Neurol. Scand. *78*:161–166, 1988.
233. Makhene, M. K., and Diaz, P. S.: Clinical presentations and complications of suspected measles in hospitalized children. Pediatr. Infect. Dis. J. *12*:836–840, 1993.
234. Manchester, M., Lisszewski, M. K., Atkinson, J. P., et al.: Multiple isoforms of CD46 (membrane cofactor protein) serve as receptors for measles virus. Proc. Natl. Acad. Sci. U. S. A. *91*:2161–2165, 1994.
235. Manchester, M., Valsamakis, A., Kaufman, R., et al.: Measles virus and C3 binding sites are distinct on membrane cofactor protein (CD46). Proc. Natl. Acad. Sci. U. S. A. *92*:2303–2307, 1995.
236. Maretic, Z., Stihovic, L. J., Ogrizek, M., et al.: Stevens-Johnson syndrome in the course of measles. J. Trop. Med. Hyg. *68*:50–52, 1965.
237. Markowitz, L. E., Nzilambi, N., Driskell, W. H., et al.: Retinol concentration and mortality among hospitalized measles patients, Kinshasa, Zaire. J. Trop. Pediatr. *35*:109–112, 1989.
238. Markowitz, L. E., Preblud, S. R., Orenstein, W. A., et al.: Patterns of transmission in measles outbreaks in the U.S., 1985–1986. N. Engl. J. Med. *320*:75–81, 1989.
239. Mason, W. H., Ross, L. A., Lanson, J., et al.: Epidemic measles in the postvaccine era: Evaluation of epidemiology, clinical presentation and complications during an urban outbreak. Pediatr. Infect. Dis. J. *12*:42–48, 1993.
240. Mathiesen, T., Hammarstrom, L., Fridell, E., et al.: Aberrant IgG subclass distribution to measles in healthy seropositive individuals, in patients with SSPE and in immunoglobulin-deficient patients. Clin. Exp. Immunol. *80*:202–205, 1990.
241. Matszuzono, Y., Narita, M., Ishiguro, N., et al.: Detection of measles virus from clinical samples using the polymerase chain reaction. Arch. Pediatr. Adolesc. Med. *148*:289–293, 1994.
242. Matumoto, M.: Multiplication of measles virus in cell cultures. Bacteriol. Rev. *30*:152–176, 1966.
243. McChesney, M. B., Miller, C. J., Rota, P. A., et al.: Experimental measles. I. Pathogenesis in the normal and the immunized host. Virology *233*:74–84, 1997.
244. McHugh, K. and McMenamin, J. B.: Acute disseminated encephalomyelitis in childhood. Ir. Med. J. *80*:412–414, 1987.
245. McLean, D. M., Best, J. M., Smith, P. A., et al.: Viral infections of Toronto children during 1965. II. Measles encephalitis and other complications. Can. Med. Assoc. J. *94*:905–910, 1966.
246. McLean, D. M., Kettyls, G. D. M., Hingston, J., et al.: Atypical measles following immunization with killed measles vaccine. Can. Med. Assoc. J. *103*:743–744, 1970.
247. McLellan, R. K., and Gleiner, J. A.: Acute hepatitis in an adult with rubeola. J. A. M. A. *247*:2000–2001, 1982.
248. McNeill, W. H.: Plagues and Peoples. Garden City, NY, Anchor Press-Doubleday, 1976, pp. 105, 119.
249. Meadow, S. R., Weller, R. O., and Archibald, R. W. R.: Fatal systemic measles in a child receiving cyclophosphamide for nephrotic syndrome. Lancet *2*:876–878, 1969.
250. Mellor, D. H., and Purcell, M.: Unusual encephalitic illnesses in a child with acute leukaemia in remission: Possible role of measles virus and *Toxoplasma gondii*. Neuropaediatrie *7*:423–430, 1976.
251. Melnick, J. L.: Taxonomy of viruses, 1976. Prog. Med. Virol. *22*:211–221, 1976.
252. Meulen, V. T., Kackell, Y., Muller, D., et al.: Isolation of infectious measles virus in measles encephalitis. Lancet *2*:1172–1175, 1972.
253. Meyer, H. M., Jr., Brooks, B. E., Douglas, R. D., et al.: Ecology of measles in monkeys. Am. J. Dis. Child. *103*:307–313, 1962.
254. Miller, D. L.: Frequency of complications of measles, 1963. B. M. J. *2*:75–78, 1964.
255. Milovanovic, M. V., Enders, J. F., and Mitus, A.: Cultivation of measles virus in human amnion cells and in developing chick embryo. Proc. Soc. Exp. Biol. Med. *95*:120–127, 1957.
256. Mitnick, J., Becker, M. H., Rothberg, M., et al.: Nodular residua of atypical measles pneumonia. A. J. R. Am. J. Roentgenol. *134*:257–260, 1980.
257. Mitus, A., Enders, J. F., Craig, J. M., et al.: Persistence of measles virus and depression of antibody formation in patients with giant-cell pneumonia after measles. N. Engl. J. Med. *261*:882–889, 1959.
258. Mitus, A., Enders, J. F., Edsall, G., et al.: Measles in children with malignancy problems and prevention. Arch. Virusforsch. *16*:331–337, 1965.
259. Mitus, A., Holloway, A., Evans, A. E., et al.: Attenuated measles vaccine in children with acute leukemia. Am. J. Dis. Child. *103*:413–418, 1962.
260. Modlin, J. F., Jabbour, J. T., Witte, J. J., et al.: Epidemiologic studies of measles, measles vaccine, and subacute sclerosing panencephalitis. Pediatrics *59*:505–512, 1977.
261. Moench, T. R., Griffin, D. E., Obriecht, C. R., et al.: Acute measles in patients with and without neurological involvement: Distribution of measles virus antigen and RNA. J. Infect. Dis. *158*:433–442, 1988.
262. Monif, G. R. G., and Hood, G. I.: Ileocolitis associated with measles (rubeola). Am. J. Dis. Child. *120*:245–247, 1970.
263. Moraes, N. D. A.: Medical importance of measles in Brazil. Am. J. Dis. Child. *103*:233–236, 1962.
264. Morgan, E. M., and Rapp, F.: Measles virus and its associated diseases. Bacteriol. Rev. *41*:636–666, 1977.
265. Morley, D. C.: Measles in Nigeria. Am. J. Dis. Child. *103*:230–233, 1962.
266. Morley, D. C., Martin, W. J., and Allen, I.: Measles in East and Central Africa. East Afr. Med. J. *44*:497–508, 1967.
267. Morley, D., Woodland, M., and Martin, W. J.: Measles in Nigerian children: A study of the disease in West Africa, and its manifestations in England and other countries during different epochs. J. Hyg. (Camb.) *61*:115–134, 1963.
268. Moroi, K., Saito, S., Kurata, T., et al.: Fetal death associated with measles virus infection of the placenta. Am. J. Obstet. Gynecol. *164*:1107–1108, 1991.
269. Murphy, J. V., and Yunis, E. J.: Encephalopathy following measles infection in children with chronic illness. J. Pediatr. *88*:937–942, 1976.
270. Musser, S. J., and Underwood, G. E.: Studies on measles virus. II. Physical properties and inactivation studies of measles virus. J. Immunol. *85*:292–297, 1960.
271. Mustafa, M. M., Weitman, S. D., Winick, N. J., et al.: Subacute measles encephalitis in the young immunocompromised host: Report of two cases diagnosed by polymerase chain reaction and treated with ribavirin and review of the literature. Clin. Infect. Dis. *16*:654–660, 1993.
272. Nader, P. R., Horwitz, M. S., and Rousseau, J.: Atypical exanthem following exposure to natural measles: Eleven cases in children previously inoculated with killed vaccine. J. Pediatr. *72*:22–28, 1968.
273. Nagai, K. and Mori, T.: Acute disseminated encephalomyelitis with probable measles vaccine failure. Pediatr. Neurol. *20*:399–402, 1999.
274. Nahmias, A. J., Griffith, D., Salsbury, C., et al.: Thymic aplasia with lymphopenia, plasma cells, and normal immunoglobulins. J. A. M. A. *201*:729–734, 1967.
275. Nakai, M., and Imagawa, D. T.: Electron microscopy of measles virus replication. J. Virol. *3*:187–197, 1969.
276. Nakayama, T., Urano, T., Osano, M., et al.: Long-term regulation of interferon production by lymphocytes from children inoculated with live measles virus vaccine. J. Infect. Dis. *158*:1386–1390, 1988.
277. Naniche, D., Varior-Krisnan, G., Cervoni, F., et al.: Human membrane cofactor protein (CD46) acts as a cellular receptor for measles virus. J. Virol. *67*:6025–6032, 1993.
278. Neumann, P. W., Weber, J. M., Jessamine, A. G., et al.: Comparison of measles antihemolysin test, enzyme-linked immunosorbent assay, and hemagglutination inhibition test with neutralization test for determination of immune status. J. Clin. Microbiol. *22*:296–298, 1985.
279. Nichols, E. M.: Atypical measles syndrome: A continuing problem. Am. J. Public Health *69*:160–164, 1979.
280. Nickell, M. D., Cannady, P. B., Jr., and Schwitzer, G. A.: Subclinical hepatitis in rubeola infections in young adults. Ann. Intern. Med. *90*:354–355, 1979.
281. Nieburg, P. I., D'Angelo, L. J., and Herrmann, K. L.: Measles in patients suspected of having Rocky Mountain spotted fever. J. A. M. A. *244*:808–809, 1980.
282. Nii, S., Kamahora, J., Mori, Y., et al.: Experimental pathology of measles in monkeys. Biken J. *6*:271–297, 1964.
283. Norrby, E.: Hemagglutination by measles virus. II. Properties of the hemagglutinin and of the receptors on the erythrocytes. Arch. Virusforsch. *12*:164–172, 1962.
284. Norrby, E., Enders-Ruckle, G., and ter Meulen, V.: The significance of hemolysing-inhibiting antibodies in protection against measles. Med. Microbiol. Immunol. *160*:232, 1974.
285. Norrby, E., and Gollmar, Y.: Appearance and persistence of antibodies against different virus components after regular measles infections. Infect. Immun. *6*:240–247, 1972.

286. Norrby, E., and Gollmar, Y.: Identification of measles virus–specific hemolysis-inhibiting antibodies separate from hemagglutination-inhibiting antibodies. Infect. Immun. *11*:231–239, 1975.
287. Norrby, E., and Hammarskjold, B.: Structural components of measles virus. Microbios *5*:17–29, 1972.
288. Norrby, E., Lagercrantz, R., and Gard, S.: Measles vaccination. IV. Responses to two different types of preparations given as a fourth dose of vaccine. B. M. J. *1*:813–817, 1965.
289. Norrby, E., Lagercrantz, R., and Gard, S.: Measles vaccination. VII. Followup studies in children immunized with four doses of inactivated vaccine. Acta Paediatr. *58*:261–267, 1969.
290. Norrby, E. C. J., and Magnusson, P.: Some morphological characteristics of the internal component of measles virus. Arch. Virusforsch. *17*:443–447, 1965.
291. Norrby, E. C. J., Magnusson, P., Falksveden, L. G., et al.: Separation of measles virus components by equilibrium centrifugation in CsCI gradients. II. Studies on the large and the small hemagglutinin. Arch. Virusforsch. *14*:462–473, 1964.
292. Norrby, L., and Oxman, M. N.: Measles virus. *In* Fields, B. N., Knipe, D. M., Chanock, R., M., et al. (eds.): Virology. 2nd ed. New York, Raven Press, 1990, pp. 1013–1044.
293. O'Donovan, C.: Measles in Kenyan children. East Afr. Med. J. *48*:526–532, 1971.
294. O'Donovan, C., and Barua, K. N.: Measles pneumonia. Am. J. Trop. Med. Hyg. *22*:73–77, 1973.
295. Ojala, A.: On changes in the cerebrospinal fluid during measles. Ann. Med. Fenn. *36*:321–331, 1947.
296. Ono, K., Iwa, N., Kato, S., et al.: Demonstration of viral antigen in giant cells formed in monkeys experimentally infected with measles virus. Biken J. *13*:329–337, 1970.
297. Ono, N., Tatsuo, H., Hadaka, Y., et al. Measles viruses on throat swabs from measles patients use signaling lymphocytic activation molecule (CDw150) but not CD46 as a cellular receptor. J. Virol. *75*:4399–4401, 2001.
298. Orenstein, W. A., Halsey, N. A., Hayden, G. F., et al.: Current status of measles in the U.S., 1973–1977. J. Infect. Dis. *137*:847–853, 1978.
299. Orenstein, W. A., Markowitz, L. E., Atkinson, W. L., et al.: Worldwide measles prevention. Isr. J. Med. Sci. *30*:469–481, 1994.
300. Oski, F. A., and Naiman, J. L.: Effect of live measles vaccine on the platelet count. N. Engl. J. Med. *275*:352–356, 1966.
301. Pampiglione, G.: Prodromal phase of measles: Some neurophysiological studies. B. M. J. *2*:1296–1300, 1964.
302. Panum, P. L.: Observations made during the epidemic of measles on the Faroe Islands in the year 1846. Med. Classics *3*:829–886, 1939.
303. Papp, K.: Experiences prouvant que la voie d'infection de la rougeole est la contamination de la muqueuse conjonctivale. Rev. Immunol. Ther. Anti-Microb. *20*:27–36, 1956.
304. Parhad, I. M., Johnson, K. P., Wolinsky, J. S., et al.: Encephalitis after inhalation of measles virus: A pathogenetic study in hamsters. Ann. Neurol. *9*:21–27, 1981.
305. Partington, M. W., and Quinton, J. F. P.: The preeruptive illness of measles. Arch. Dis. Child. *34*:149–153, 1959.
306. Pather, M., Wesley, A. G., Schonland, M., et al.: Severe measles-associated pneumonia treated with assisted ventilation. S. Afr. Med. J. *50*:1600–1603, 1976.
307. Paunio, M., Hedman, K., Davidkin, I., et al.: Secondary measles vaccine failures identified by measurement of IgG avidity: High occurrence among teenagers vaccinated at a young age. Epidemiol. Infect. *124*:263–271, 2000.
308. Payne, F. E., Baublis, J. V., and Itabashi, H. H.: Isolation of measles virus from cell cultures of brain from a patient with subacute sclerosing panencephalitis. N. Engl. J. Med. *281*:585–589, 1969.
309. Pearl, P. L., Abu-Farshak, H., Starke, J. R., et al.: Neuropathology of two fatal cases of measles in the 1988–1989 Houston epidemic. Pediatr. Neurol. *6*:126–130, 1990.
310. Peebles, T. C.: Distribution of virus in blood components during the viremia of measles. Arch. Virusforsch. *22*:43–47, 1967.
311. Peries, J. R., and Chany, C.: Studies on measles viral hemagglutination. Proc. Soc. Exp. Biol. Med. *110*:477–482, 1962.
312. Phillips, C. A.: Inclusion bodies in measles encephalitis. J. A. M. A. *195*:167–168, 1966.
313. Plotkin, S. A.: Vaccination against measles in the 18th century. Clin. Pediatr. (Phila.) *6*:312–315, 1967.
314. Plotz, H.: Culture "in vitro" du virus de la rougeole. Bull. Acad. Med. Paris *119*:598, 1938.
315. Polack, F. P., Auwaerter, P. G., Lee, S.-H., et al.: Production of atypical measles in rhesus macaques: Evidence for disease mediated by immune complex formation and eosinophils in the presence of fusion-inhibiting antibody. Nat. Med. *5*:629–634, 1999.
316. Pollack, M. A., Grose, C., and Friend, H.: Measles associated with Bell palsy. Am. J. Dis. Child. *129*:747, 1975.
317. Pullan, C., Noble, T. C., Scott, D. J., et al.: Atypical measles infections in leukaemic children on immunosuppressive treatment. B. M. J. *1*:1562–1565, 1976.
318. Quiambao, B. P., Gatchalian, S. R., Halonen, P., et al.: Coinfection is common in measles-associated pneumonia. Pediatr. Infect. Dis. J. *17*:89–93, 1998.
319. Rake, G., and Shaffer, M. F.: Studies on measles. I. The use of the chorio-allantois of the developing chicken embryo. J. Immunol. *38*:177–200, 1940.
320. Rand, K. H., Emmons, R. W., and Merigan, T. C.: Measles in adults: An unforeseen consequence of immunization? J. A. M. A. *236*:1028–1031, 1976.
321. Rauh, L. W., and Schmidt, R.: Measles immunization with killed virus vaccine: Serum antibody titers and experience with exposure to measles epidemic. Am. J. Dis. Child. *109*:232–237, 1965.
322. Reddy, V., Bhaskaram, P., Raghuramulu, N., et al.: Relationship between measles, malnutrition, and blindness: A prospective study in Indian children. Am. J. Clin. Nutr. *44*:924–930, 1986.
323. Remington, P. L., Hall, W. N., Davis, I. H., et al.: Airborne transmission of measles in a physician's office. J. A. M. A. *253*:1574–1577, 1985.
324. Reyes, M. A., DeBorrero, M. F., Roa, J., et al.: Measles vaccine failure after documented seroconversion. Pediatr. Infect. Dis. J. *6*:848–851, 1987.
325. Riley, E. C., Murphy, G., and Riley, R. L.: Airborne spread of measles in a suburban elementary school. Am. J. Epidemiol. *107*:421–432, 1978.
326. Riley, R. L.: Airborne infection. Am. J. Med. *57*:466–475, 1974.
327. Ristori, C., Boccardo, H., Borgono, J. M., et al.: Medical importance of measles in Chile. Am. J. Dis. Child. *103*:236–241, 1962.
328. Robbins, F. C.: Measles: Clinical features. Pathogenesis, pathology and complications. Am. J. Dis. Child. *103*:266–273, 1962.
329. Roberts, G. B. S., and Bain, A. D.: The pathology of measles. J. Pathol. Immunol. *76*:111–118, 1958.
330. Ross, L. A., Mason, W. H., Lanson, J., et al.: Laryngotracheobronchitis as a complication of measles during an urban epidemic. J. Pediatr. *121*:511–515, 1992.
331. Ross, L. J.: Electrocardiographic findings in measles. Am. J. Dis. Child. *83*:282–291, 1952.
332. Rota, J. S., Rota, P. A., Redd, S. B., et al.: Genetic analysis of measles viruses isolated in the U.S., 1995–1996. J. Infect. Dis. *177*:204–208, 1998.
333. Rota, P. A., Rota, J. S., and Bellini, W. J.: Molecular epidemiology of measles virus. Virology *6*:379–386, 1995.
334. Ruckdeschel, J. C., Graziano, K. D., and Mardiney, M. R., Jr.: Additional evidence that the cell-associated immune system is the primary host defense against measles (rubeola). Cell. Immunol. *17*:11–18, 1975.
335. Ruckle, G., and Rogers, K. D.: Studies with measles virus. II. Isolation of virus and immunologic studies in persons who have had the natural disease. J. Immunol. *78*:341–355, 1957.
336. Sandford-Smith, J. H., and Whittle, H. C.: Corneal ulceration following measles in Nigerian children. Br. J. Ophthalmol. *63*:720–724, 1979.
337. Saxton, N. L.: Thrombocytopenic purpura following the administration of attenuated live measles vaccine. J. Iowa Med. Soc. *57*:1017–1018, 1967.
338. Schaffner, W., Schluederberg, A. E. S., and Byrne, E. B.: Clinical epidemiology of sporadic measles in a highly immunized population. N. Engl. J. Med. *279*:783–789, 1968.
339. Scheifele, D. W., and Forbes, C. E.: Prolonged giant cell excretion in severe African measles. Pediatrics *50*:867–873, 1972.
340. Schluederberg, A.: Separation of measles virus particles in density gradients. Am. J. Dis. Child. *103*:291–296, 1962.
341. Schluederberg, A.: Modification of immune response by previous experience with measles. Arch. Ges. Virusforsch. *16*:347–350, 1965.
342. Schluederberg, A.: Immune globulins in human viral infections. Nature *205*:1232, 1965.
343. Sergiev, P. G., Ryazantseva, N. E., and Shroit, I. G.: The dynamics of pathological processes in experimental measles in monkeys. Acta Virol. *4*:265–273, 1960.
344. Shalit, M., Ackerman, Z., Wollner, S., et al.: Immunoglobulin E response during measles. Int. Arch. Allergy Immunol. *75*:84–86, 1984.
345. Shann, F.: Meta-analysis of trials of prophylactic antibiotics for children with measles: Inadequate evidence. B. M. J. *314*:334–336, 1997.
346. Shasby, D. M., Shope, T. C., Downs, H., et al.: Epidemic measles in a highly vaccinated population. N. Engl. J. Med. *296*:585–589, 1977.
347. Shoss, R. G., and Rayhanzadeh, S.: Toxic epidermal necrolysis following measles vaccination. Arch. Dermatol. *110*:766–770, 1974.
348. Siegel, D., and Hirschman, S. Z.: Hepatic dysfunction in acute measles infection of adults. Arch. Intern. Med. *137*:1178–1179, 1977.
349. Siegel, M. M., Walter, T. K., and Ablin, A. R.: Measles pneumonia in childhood leukemia. Pediatrics *60*:38–40, 1977.
350. Smith, F. R., Curran, A. S., Raciti, K. A., et al.: Reported measles in persons immunologically primed by prior vaccination. J. Pediatr. *101*:391–393, 1982.
351. Sobonya, R. E., Hiller, F. C., Pingleton, W., et al.: Fatal measles (rubeola) pneumonia in adults. Arch. Pathol. Lab. Med. *102*:366–371, 1978.
352. Spencer, M. J., and Cherry, J. D.: Unpublished data, 1976.
353. Starr, S., and Berkovich, S.: Effects of measles, gamma-globulin–modified measles and vaccine measles on the tuberculin test. N. Engl. J. Med. *270*:386–391, 1964.

354. Starr, S., and Berkovich, S.: The effect of measles, gamma globulin modified measles, and attenuated measles vaccine on the course of treated tuberculosis in children. Pediatrics *35*:97–102, 1965.
355. Stein, S. J., and Greenspoon, J. S.: Rubeola during pregnancy. Obstet. Gynecol. *78*:925–929, 1991.
356. St. Geme, J. W., Jr., George, B. L., and Bush, B. M.: Exaggerated natural measles following attenuated virus immunization. Pediatrics *57*:148–150, 1976.
357. Stimson, P. M.: The earlier diagnosis of measles. J. A. M. A. *90*:660–663, 1928.
358. Stokes, J., Jr.: Viral infections, including those presumed to be caused by viruses: Measles (rubeola). *In* Nelson, W. E. (ed.): Textbook of Pediatrics. 6th ed. Philadelphia, W. B. Saunders, 1954, pp. 466–471.
359. Stokes, J., Jr., Maris, E. P., and Gellis, S. S.: Chemical, clinical, and immunological studies on the products of human plasma fractionation. XI. The use of concentrated normal human serum gamma globulin (human immune serum globulin) in the prophylaxis and treatment of measles. J. Clin. Invest. *23*:531–540, 1944.
360. Stratton, K. R., Howe, C. J., and Johnston, R. B., Jr.: Adverse events associated with childhood vaccines other than pertussis and rubella: Summary of a report from the Institute of Medicine. J. A. M. A. *271*:1602–1605, 1994.
361. Suringa, D. W. R., Bank, L. J., and Ackerman, A. B.: Role of measles virus in skin lesions and Koplik's spots. N. Engl. J. Med. *283*:1139–1142, 1970.
362. Sutter, R. W., Markowitz, L. E., Bennetch, J. M., et al.: Measles among the Amish: A comparative study of measles severity in primary and secondary cases in households. J. Infect. Dis. *163*:12–16, 1991.
363. Swift, J. D., Barruga, M. C., Perkin, R. M., et al.: Respiratory failure complicating rubeola. Chest *104*:1786–1787, 1993.
364. Taneja, P. N., Ghal, O. P., and Bhakoo, O. N.: Importance of measles in India. Am. J. Dis. Child. *103*:226–229, 1962.
365. Taylor, M. J., Godfrey, E., Baczko, K., et al.: Identification of several different lineages of measles virus. J. Gen. Virol. *72*:83–88, 1991.
366. Tellez-Nagel, I., and Harter, D. H.: Subacute sclerosing leukoencephalitis. I. Clinico-pathological, electron microscopic and virological observations. J. Neuropathol. Exp. Neurol. *25*:560–581, 1966.
367. Thompson, N. P., Montgomery, S. M., Pounder, R. E., et al.: Is measles vaccination a risk factor for inflammatory bowel disease? Lancet *345*:1071–1074, 1995.
368. Tidstrom, B.: Complications in measles with special reference to encephalitis. Acta Med. Scand. *184*:411–415, 1968.
369. Tishler, M., and Abramov, A. L.: Liver involvement in measles infection of young adults. Isr. J. Med. Sci. *19*:791–793, 1983.
370. Tuokko, H., and Salmi, A.: Detection of IgM antibodies to measles virus by enzyme-immunoassay. Med. Microbiol. Immunol. *171*:187–198, 1983.
371. Tyler, H. R.: Neurological complications of rubeola (measles). Medicine (Baltimore) *36*:147–167, 1957.
372. Udem, S. A., and Cook, K. A.: Isolation and characterization of measles virus intracellular nucleocapsid RNA. J. Virol. *49*:57–65, 1984.
373. Varavithya, W., Stoecker, B., Chaiyaratana, W., et al.: Retinol status of Thai children with measles. Trop. Geogr. Med. *38*:359–361, 1986.
374. Wakefield, A. J., Murch, S. H., Anthony, A., et al.: Ileal-lymphoid-nodular hyperplasia, non-specific colitis, and pervasive developmental disorder in children. Lancet *351*:637–641, 1998.
375. Waksman, B. H., Burnstein, T., and Adams, R. D.: Histologic study of the encephalomyelitis produced in hamsters by a neurotropic strain of measles. J. Neuropathol. Exp. Neurol. *21*:25, 1962.
376. Ward, B. J., Johnson, R. T., Vaisberg, A., et al.: Spontaneous proliferation of peripheral mononuclear cells in natural measles virus infection: Identification of dividing cells and correlation with mitogen responsiveness. Clin. Immunol. Immunopathol. *55*:315–326, 1990.
377. Waters, D. J., and Bussell, R. H.: Isolation and comparative study of the nucleocapsids of measles and canine distemper viruses from infected cells. Virology *61*:64–79, 1974.
378. Waters, D. J., Hersh, R. T., and Bussell, R. H.: Isolation and characterization of measles nucleocapsid from infected cells. Virology *48*:278–281, 1972.
379. Waterson, A. P.: Measles virus. Arch. Ges. Virusforsch. *16*:57–80, 1965.
380. Waterson, A. P., Cruickshank, J. G., Lawrence, G. D., et al.: The nature of measles virus. Virology *15*:379–382, 1961.
381. Watson, J. C., Hadler, S. C., Dykewicz, C. A., et al.: Measles, mumps, and rubella—vaccine use and strategies for elimination of measles, rubella, and congenital rubella syndrome and control of mumps: recommendations of the Advisory Committee on Immunization Practice (ACIP). M. M. W. R. Recomm. Rep. *47*(RR-8):1–57, 1998.
382. Weibel, R. E., Caseta, V., Benor, D. E., et al.: Acute encephalopathy followed by permanent brain injury or death associated with further attenuated measles vaccines: A review of claims submitted to the National Vaccine Injury Compensation Program. Pediatrics *101*:383–387, 1998.
383. Weiner, L. B., Corwin, R. M., Nieburg, P. I., et al.: A measles outbreak among adolescents. J. Pediatr. *90*:17–20, 1977.
384. Welliver, R. C., Cherry, J. D., and Holtzman, A. E.: Typical, modified, and atypical measles. Arch. Intern. Med. *137*:39–41, 1977.
385. Wells, M. W.: The seasonal patterns of measles and chicken pox. Am. J. Hyg. *40*:279–317, 1944.
386. Whittle, H. C., Dossetor, J., Oduloju, A., et al.: Cell-mediated immunity during natural measles infection. J. Clin. Invest. *62*:678–685, 1978.
387. Wilhelm, D. J., and Paegle, R. D.: Thrombocytopenic purpura and pneumonia following measles vaccination. Am. J. Dis. Child. *113*:534–537, 1967.
388. Wilkins, J., and Wehrle, P. F.: Evidence for reinstatement of infants 12 to 14 months of age into routine measles immunization programs. Am. J. Dis. Child. *132*:164–166, 1978.
389. Wilson, E. B., and Worcester, J.: Contact with measles. Proc. Natl. Acad. Sci. U. S. A. *27*:7–13, 1941.
390. Wilson, G. S.: Measles as a universal disease. Am. J. Dis. Child. *103*:219–223, 1962.
391. Winkelstein, W., Jr., Karzon, D. T., Rush, D., et al.: A field trial of inactivated measles virus vaccine in young school children. J. A. M. A. *194*:106–110, 1965.
392. Wolinsky, J. S., Swoveland, P., Johnson, K. P., et al.: Subacute measles encephalitis complicating Hodgkin's disease in an adult. Ann. Neurol. *1*:452–457, 1977.
393. World Health Organization: [Expanded Programme on Immunization. Global Advisory Group. Part I.] Wkly. Epidemiol. Rec. *65*(2):5–12, 1990.
394. Wright, G. P., and Wright, H. P.: The influence of social conditions upon diphtheria, measles, tuberculosis and whooping cough in early childhood in London. J. Hyg. *42*:451–473, 1942.
395. Wynne, J. M., Williams, G. L., and Ellman, B. A. H.: Gangrene of the extremities in measles. S. Afr. Med. J. *52*:117–121, 1977.
396. Yamanouchi, K., Egashira, Y., Uchida, N., et al.: Giant cell formation in lymphoid tissues of monkeys inoculated with various strains of measles virus. Jpn. J. Med. Sci. Biol. *23*:131–145, 1970.
397. Yeager, A. S., Davis, J. H., Ross, L. A., et al.: Measles immunization: Successes and failures. J. A. M. A. *237*:347–351, 1977.
398. Yorke, J. A., and London, W. P.: Recurrent outbreaks of measles, chickenpox, and mumps. II. Systematic differences in contact rates and stochastic effects. Am. J. Epidemiol. *98*:469–482, 1973.
399. Young, L. W., Smith, D. I., and Glasgow, L. A.: Pneumonia of atypical measles: Residual nodular lesions. A. J. R. Am. J. Roentgenol. *110*:439–448, 1970.
400. Zahradnik, J. M., Cherry, J. D., and Rachelefsky, G.: Atypical measles acquired abroad: Foreign travel and pseudoexotic disease. J. A. M. A. *241*:1711–1712, 1979.
401. Ziegra, S. R.: Corticosteroid treatment for measles encephalitis. J. Pediatr. *59*:322–323, 1961.
402. Ziola, B., Lund, G., Muerman, O., et al.: Circulating immune complexes in patients with acute measles and rubella virus infections. Infect. Immun. *41*:578–583, 1983.

CHAPTER

184 Mumps Virus

JAMES D. CHERRY

Mumps (epidemic parotitis) is an acute communicable disease caused by the mumps virus, a member of the genus Rubulavirus. As a result of universal childhood immunization, mumps is an uncommon disease in the United States today.

History[65, 122]

In the fifth century BC, Hippocrates described an outbreak on the island of Thasus.[65] He noted that most patients had bilateral swelling near the ears and that the others had unilateral swelling. He also noted that some patients had bilateral or unilateral pain and swelling of the testicles. The origin of the name *mumps* is not known. It may be from the English noun *mump,* which means "a lump," or the English verb *mump,* one of whose definitions is "mumble." This latter possible origin is based on the mumbling speech that patients with significant parotitis may have.

In 1790, Robert Hamilton presented an extensive study of mumps in which he noted orchitis, associated the illness with neurologic involvement, and described the neuropathology of a fatal case.[50, 51] In 1886, Hirsch[58] noted that mumps occurred throughout the world and that it was a major cause of morbidity in Confederate troops during the American Civil War. In the first half of the 20th century, investigators recognized that mumps virus infection involved multiple organs, and the causative agent was shown to be a filterable virus by Johnson and Goodpasture in 1934.[31, 61]

The growth of mumps virus in embryonated eggs was reported in 1945, and 10 years later its propagation in tissue culture was noted.[48, 53] This latter development led to the development and licensure of a live attenuated mumps vaccine in 1967.[113]

Properties

CLASSIFICATION

Mumps virus is a member of the genus Rubulavirus, subfamily *Paramyxovirinae,* and family *Paramyxoviridae.*[76] It contains a single-stranded, nonsegmented, negative-sense RNA genome that is surrounded by a helical nucleocapsid and a surface envelope.

PHYSICAL PROPERTIES[13, 68, 76]

The virus is generally spherical, but marked pleomorphism occurs. Its size varies from 100 to 600 nm. Seven major proteins exist: a nucleocapsid-associated protein (NP), a phosphoprotein (P), a membrane or matrix protein (M), a fusion protein (F), a hydrophobic membrane-associated protein (SH), a hemagglutinin-neuraminidase (HN), and a polymerase protein (L). The genes for these proteins have been sequenced, and the gene order is 3-NP-P-M-F-SH-HN-L-5. The viral envelope is studded with 12- to 15-nm projections that contain either of the two structural glycoproteins (HN or F).

The P structural protein is associated with the nucleocapsid, and an RNA-dependent RNA polymerase is located within the nucleocapsid structure. The envelope has a high lipid content, and it contains the M protein.

The SH protein gene is the most variable region of the genome and, therefore, can be used to differentiate viral strains.[1, 13, 72, 86, 105] Analysis of the variations in SH gene nucleotide sequences has been used to study outbreaks, identify vaccine viruses, study vaccine adverse events, and identify new viral strains.

Mumps virus infectivity is destroyed by heat (56° C for 20 minutes), and its infectivity is reduced by ultraviolet light, Tween 80, ether, and formalin. The virus is stable at 4° C for several days, and when placed in a buffered salt solution (such as Hanks) with 1 to 2 percent inactivated fetal calf serum, it can be stored indefinitely at −70° C.

ANTIGENIC COMPOSITION[68]

The three major antigenic components of mumps virus are the two glycoproteins (HN or V antigen and F protein) and the nucleocapsid protein (NP or S antigen). The glycoproteins that project from the viral surface are the antigenic target for specific antibodies. Host antibodies to HN and F proteins confer protective immunity against the virus. Mumps viral particles agglutinate erythrocytes of several mammalian and avian species (human, avian, rodent, and simian); at 37° C, the virus causes partial hemolysis of susceptible erythrocytes when it is attached to cellular surface receptors. Specific antibody blocks hemagglutination, hemadsorption, and hemolysis.

Mumps virus is considered to have a single immunotype. However, polyclonal antibodies to parainfluenza and Newcastle disease viral antigens cross-react with antibodies to mumps virus in complement-fixation and hemagglutination-inhibition assays. With monoclonal antibodies, an antigenic relationship between the NH and NP proteins of Sendai virus (a murine parainfluenza type 1 virus) and mumps virus has been demonstrated.[87]

TISSUE CULTURE GROWTH AND ANIMAL SUSCEPTIBILITY[68]

Mumps virus can be propagated in many different primary and cell line tissue cultures. For virus isolation, primary monkey kidney cells generally are used. Its cytopathic effect is similar to that of other paramyxoviruses. When stained, multinucleated giant cells and cytoplasmic eosinophilic inclusions may be observed. In culture, the addition of erythrocytes results in hemadsorption to surface virus.

Mumps virus infects monkeys, rabbits, dogs, cats, and rodents. The virus is isolated readily after inoculation of the amniotic sac of 7- to 8-day-old chicken embryos.

Epidemiology

INCIDENCE

In the United States, mumps was a reportable disease from 1922 to 1950 and has been again since 1967.[21] Between 1950 and 1967, incidence data were gathered from voluntary reporting by cooperating states. Incidence data from 1922 to 1982 are presented in Figure 184–1, and vaccine-era data are presented in Figure 184–2.[21, 113] In the prevaccine era, mumps was a yearly disease, with epidemic peaks occurring approximately every 4 years. The peak epidemic year was 1944, when the rate was 250 per 100,000 population.

In the prevaccine era, mumps was a disease predominantly of young children.[21] However, outbreaks of mumps were a significant problem in young adults in the military.[43, 79] The age distribution of mumps in the United States during selected years is presented in Table 184–1. After the licensure of mumps vaccine in 1967, mumps remained a disease of predominantly young children from 1967 to 1971. However, by 1981, most reported patients were 10 years or older. In 1987, 76 percent of the cases occurred in persons 10 years or older (see Table 184–1). In 1994, 1537 cases were reported, and of those with age noted, 21.8 percent were in patients 20 years or older. The increase in reported cases that occurred in 1987 (see Fig. 184–2) was due to a marked increase in cases in unimmunized persons 10 to 19 years of age. This group had been protected for a time by herd immunity because of the rapidly declining incidence of mumps as a result of routine vaccine use beginning in 1977.[26] In 1998, only 666 cases of mumps were reported in the United States.[14] Nineteen percent of the patients were younger than 5 years, and 36 percent were 15 years or older.

In the prevaccine era, the peak incidence of mumps occurred in the winter and spring months, and this peak continued well into the vaccine era.[21] Since 1989, little seasonal variation in cases has been noted.[14, 113]

MORBIDITY AND MORTALITY

The most common clinical manifestations of mumps virus infection are fever and parotitis. However, approximately 30 percent of infections do not involve parotitis and are not recognized.[71] Epididymo-orchitis occurs in 20 to 30 percent of clinical cases in postpubertal males. Approximately 60 percent of clinical mumps cases involve cerebrospinal fluid (CSF) pleocytosis, but only one sixth of these patients have meningeal symptoms.[4] In 1966, 628 cases of encephalitis (0.5%) were reported, and of these, 10 (1.6%) had a fatal outcome.[21] Encephalitis occurs more commonly in males (61%), and the rate of occurrence is greatest in adults. Deafness after a case of mumps has been estimated to occur in 0.5 to 5.0 per 100,000 cases.[33, 115]

From 1966 to 1975, 200 mumps-associated deaths were reported.[21] Of these, 44 (22%) were in patients with encephalitis; in the others, the causes of death were not identified. Forty-one percent of the deaths occurred in adults 40 years or older. During the 10-year period from 1988 through 1997, only eight deaths caused by mumps were reported.[14]

SPREAD OF INFECTION

Mumps virus is contagious in nonimmune persons. It is spread from an infected person to a new host by the respiratory route. The virus can be isolated from the saliva of infected patients from 7 days before the onset of parotitis to 9 days after onset.[68] Transmission is greatest during a 7-day period beginning 2 days before the onset of parotitis. Asymptomatically infected persons also can transmit the virus. The fact that outbreaks of mumps occurred in young adult populations in the prevaccine era suggests that mumps virus is less contagious than measles; a significant number of persons passed through childhood without being infected with

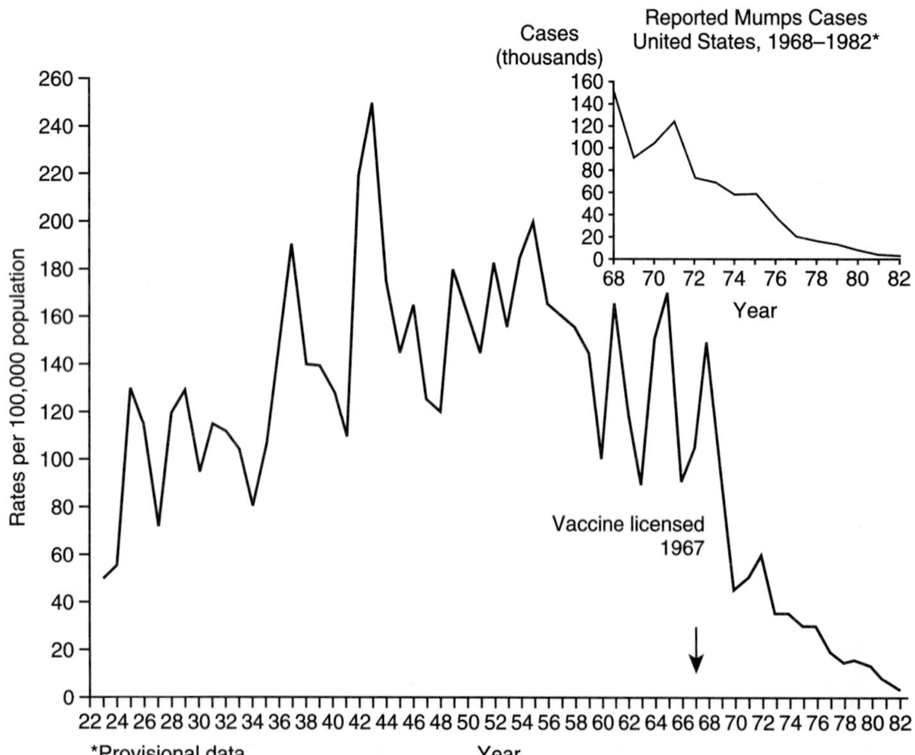

FIGURE 184–1 ■ Incidence of reported mumps in the United States from 1922 to 1982 and the number of reported cases from 1968 to 1982. (From Centers for Disease Control: Mumps surveillance, January 1977–December 1982. Issued September 1984.)

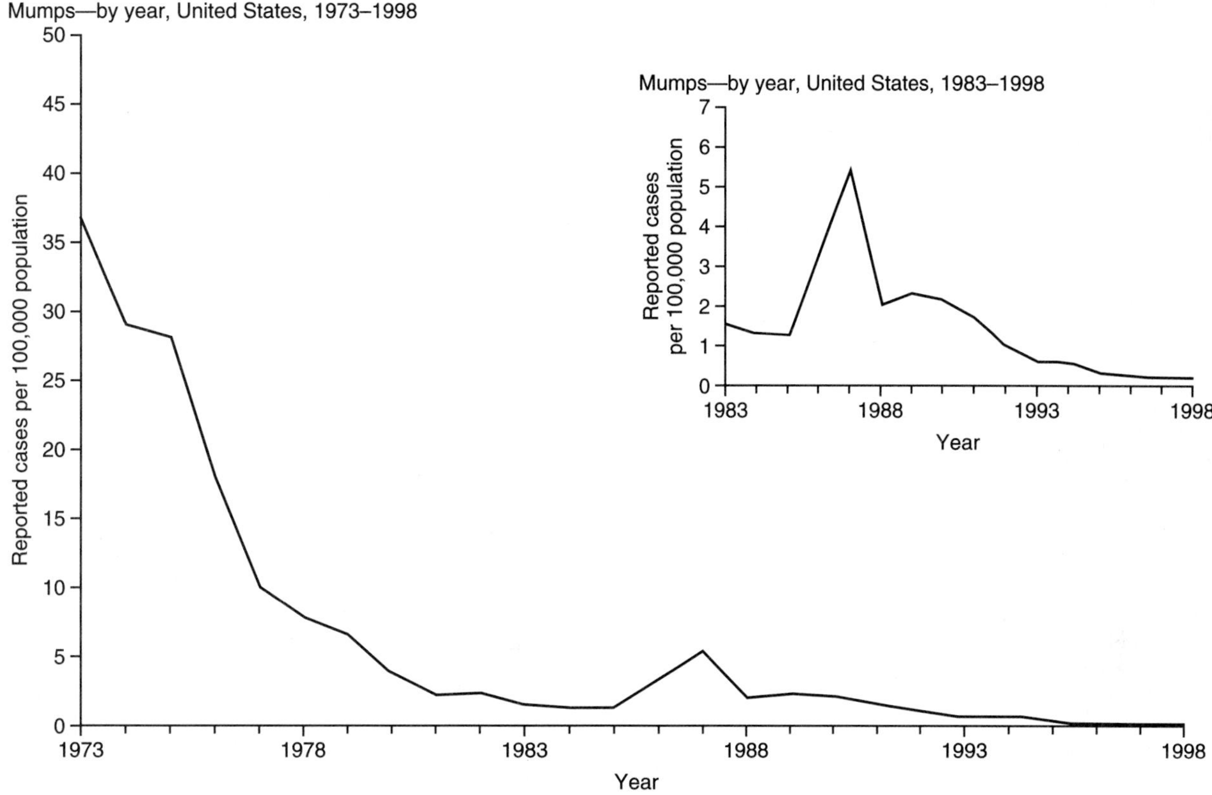

FIGURE 184–2 ■ Incidence of reported mumps in the United States from 1973 to 1998. (From Summary of notifiable diseases, United States, 1998. M. M. W. R. Morb. Mortal. Wkly. Rep. *47*[53]:50, 1999.)

mumps virus. A serologic study reported by Black[7] in 1964 noted that 24 percent of army recruits lacked hemagglutination-inhibition antibody to mumps whereas only 1 percent lacked measles antibody.

The incubation period is most often 16 to 18 days, although it can vary from 12 to 25 days.[68]

Pathogenesis and Pathology

VIRAL INFECTION[34, 68, 122]

After respiratory or perhaps oral acquisition of the virus, primary viral replication occurs in the upper respiratory mucosal epithelium.[122] Virus multiplies and is spread via drainage to local lymph nodes.[34] Subsequently, viremia develops.[63, 88] As a result of viremia, infection occurs in multiple secondary infection sites. Most prominent is infection of the salivary glands resulting in inflammation and swelling. This infection causes virus shedding for 1 to 2 weeks. Other secondary infection sites include the inner ear (cochlea), pancreas, heart, nervous system (meninges and brain), joints, kidneys, liver, gonads, and thyroid.

PATHOLOGY[122]

In the salivary glands, virus infects the ductal epithelium and causes periductal interstitial edema and a local inflammatory reaction involving lymphocytes and macrophages.[120] Tissue damage ensues, and the involved cells desquamate. Virus enters the central nervous system (CNS) by the choroid plexus via infected mononuclear cells. Virus multiplies in choroid and ependymal cells on the ventricular

TABLE 184–1 ■ AGE DISTRIBUTION OF MUMPS CASES IN THE UNITED STATES DURING SELECTED YEARS

	1967–1971*		1987		1994	
Age Group (yr)	*Cases*	%	*Cases*	%	*Cases*	%
<5	2932	17.1	804	6.5	250	17.4
5–9	10413	60.8	2196	17.9	473	33.0
10–14	2372	13.8	4567	37.3	271	18.9
15–19	1418†	8.3	3455	28.2	128	8.9
≥20			1235	10.1	312	20.8

*Average annual reported cases for California, Massachusetts, and New York City.
†Includes all reported cases in patients 15 years or older.
Data from references 18, 21, and 113.

surfaces, and these cells desquamate into the CSF and result in meningitis. In encephalitis, perivascular infiltration with mononuclear cells, scattered foci of neuronophagia, and microglial rod-cell proliferation occur.[10] Periventricular demyelination also takes place.

In the male gonad, the primary site of viral replication is the seminiferous tubules, where infection results in lymphocytic infiltration and edema of interstitial tissue.

IMMUNOLOGIC EVENTS

Infection gives rise to serum antibodies to the HN glycoprotein (V antigen), the F antigen, and the NP protein (S antigen).[68] Antibody to NP protein develops first, 3 to 7 days after the onset of symptoms. Antibodies to NP protein are short lived and are usually absent after 6 months; they cross-react with parainfluenza viruses. Antibodies to HN glycoprotein develop 2 to 4 weeks after the onset of illness and persist for long periods after infection.

IgG and IgM antibody responses (determined by enzyme-linked immunosorbent assay [ELISA]) regularly occur after infection.[111] IgG antibody levels measured by ELISA correlate best with those derived by complement-fixation and hemolysis-in-gel assays. ELISA results are less specific than those achieved with the plaque reduction neutralization assay because of the high rate of cross-reacting antibodies against parainfluenza viruses detected by ELISA.[13, 92] IgM antibodies develop early in infection (second day of illness), peak within the first week of illness, and are usually undetectable 3 months after the onset of illness; occasionally, mumps-specific IgM antibody persists for 5 to 6 months.[68, 111] Mumps-specific IgG antibody appears at the end of the first week of illness, peaks 3 weeks later, and persists throughout life. The IgG response is mainly the IgG1 subclass; a minor IgG3 subclass response also occurs.[13, 96] Salivary IgA antibodies to mumps virus regularly appear after infection.[38]

During infection with vaccine virus, the cell-mediated response to tuberculin is diminished for up to 4 weeks.[73] During the same period, a mumps-specific, cell-mediated immune response develops.[68, 122] It has been demonstrated by skin test hypersensitivity, in vitro lymphocyte proliferative responses, and cytotoxic T-lymphocyte studies.[9, 11, 70]

In general, immunity against recurrent disease has been thought to be lifelong. However, Gut and associates[47] noted 26 patients with mumps who had a previous history of mumps and antibody response patterns suggestive of reinfection and not primary infection. Specifically, they had IgG but not IgM titer rises.

Clinical Manifestations

In epidemics of mumps, cases can be separated into five groups: (1) those with a short course whose signs and symptoms are nonspecific, (2) those in whom the disease is full-blown with salivary swelling but no complications, (3) those with severe mumps and complications (epididymo-orchitis or meningoencephalitis, or both, or other complications), (4) those with no apparent symptoms but with typical antibody responses, and (5) those with meningoencephalitis or orchitis but without involvement of the salivary glands.[104] Approximately 75 percent of all cases of apparent mumps in children belong to the full-blown type without complications. Involvement of the gonads rarely occurs before puberty.

TYPICAL MUMPS WITHOUT COMPLICATIONS[104]

The average case in children has a prodromal period of 1 to 2 days that consists of fever, anorexia, headache, vomiting, and generalized aches and pains. The headache often is particularly marked and probably is caused by mild meningoencephalitis.[36] The temperature usually rises slowly to 102 or 103°F (38.9 or 39.4°C) as the disease becomes full-blown, but at times fever is only slight or absent.

After the prodromal period, one or both parotid glands begin to enlarge (Fig. 184–3). Mumps is bilateral in approximately 70 to 80 percent of cases. A few days to a week or more may intervene between the swelling of the two sides. A distinctive "puckering" sensation is experienced at the angle of the jaw in the early stage, and it may be increased by the application of sour liquids to the tongue, such as lemon juice or vinegar. This sign, when present, may be useful for early diagnosis. The swelling of the gland is also distinctive in that a brawny type of edema occurs about the parotid gland, the borders of which are not discrete, in contrast to the discrete swelling typical of lymphadenitis, in which the node generally is outlined easily. The lobe of the ear is in the center of the swelling, which usually cannot be separated by palpation from the angle of the mandible. Pressure is painful, and opening the jaw is often difficult.

The swelling of an individual gland reaches its maximum in approximately 3 days, remains at its peak for approximately 2 days, and then slowly recedes. The extent of the swelling varies considerably but at times is sufficient to completely distort the outline of the face and head. The submaxillary and sublingual glands may be involved separately or with the parotids in any combination.

During the prodromal phase, slight redness of the orifices of the Stensen or Wharton ducts, when present, has diagnostic significance. The amount of saliva is usually unchanged, although the mouth may be dry or salivation may be extreme. Gellis and Peters[42] described a few cases

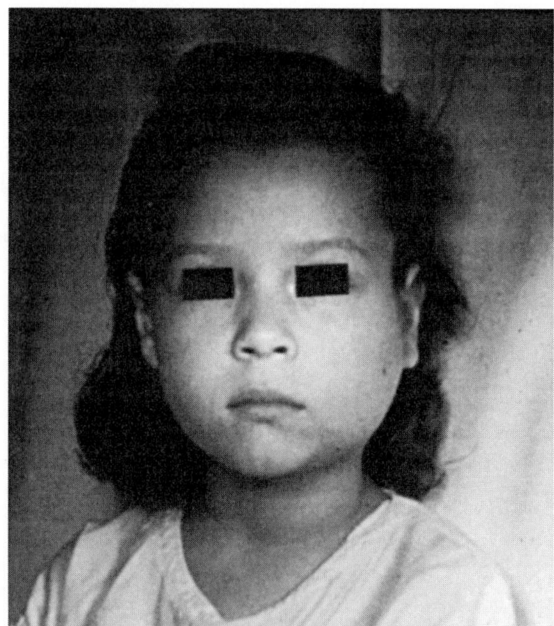

FIGURE 184–3 ■ Note the swelling on the left side of the face related to parotitis secondary to mumps virus infection. The left ear protrudes from the side of the head.

with edema over the upper part of the sternum, apparently caused by pressure on the lymphatics in the neck.

In uncomplicated mumps, the white blood cell count is usually low, with a slight relative lymphocytosis. Serum amylase typically is elevated.

MENINGITIS, MENINGOENCEPHALITIS, AND ENCEPHALITIS

Meningitis and mild meningoencephalitis are the most frequent complications of mumps in children. Azimi and Cramblett[3] reviewed 51 children with mumps meningoencephalitis admitted to Columbus Children's Hospital between July 1964 and December 1967. Of this group of patients, fever occurred in 94 percent, vomiting in 84 percent, nuchal rigidity in 71 percent, lethargy in 69 percent, parotid swelling in 47 percent, headache in 47 percent, convulsions in 18 percent, abdominal pain in 14 percent, sore throat in 8 percent, diarrhea in 8 percent, and delirium in 6 percent.

Clinical findings in neurologic illness caused by mumps virus infection differ by patient age. Meningeal signs are recognized more readily in older children, adolescents, and adults, whereas nonspecific findings such as drowsiness and lethargy occur more commonly in young children.[122] Although seizures develop in 20 to 30 percent of hospitalized patients, electroencephalogram results are usually normal. Even in patients with severe obtundation, the electroencephalogram reveals only diffuse slowing with increased voltage. Focal findings are rare. The outlook in mumps meningoencephalitis is generally good and usually is better than in encephalitis of other viral causes (see Chapter 43). Even patients with profound obtundation generally recover without residual damage. Rarely, deaths do occur, however.[21]

In the typical case, CSF has normal glucose and elevated protein levels and pleocytosis. Glucose is slightly low in approximately 20 percent of cases. At the onset of symptoms, a modest mononuclear pleocytosis is present. The CSF cell count peaks on the third day of illness; counts average 250/mm^3, but counts greater than 1000/mm^3 are not uncommon.

Mumps meningitis usually develops in patients with parotitis approximately 5 days after the onset of illness, but CNS findings can precede the parotid findings and can develop without any salivary gland involvement.

Herndon and colleagues[55] noted that ependymitis regularly occurs in mumps meningitis. A rare complication of mumps appears to be acquired aqueductal stenosis, and researchers have suggested that it may be caused by the preceding ependymitis.[55, 84, 103, 110] In one reported fatal case, hydrocephalus developed within 5 days of disease onset.[85]

A 3-year old boy with mumps cerebellitis, nystagmus, and focal localization of brain lesions noted by electroencephalography was described recently.[77] Also recently reported are facial palsy in a 3-year-old Japanese boy and transverse myelitis in an adult.[32, 114] Haginoya and associates[49] reported a 14-year-old Japanese girl who had chronic progressive mumps virus encephalitis. This child had an illness similar to subacute sclerosing panencephalitis, and her antibody titers suggested that the infecting virus may have had a defect in the HN protein.

GONADAL INFECTION (EPIDIDYMO-ORCHITIS AND OOPHORITIS)

Epididymo-orchitis and oophoritis almost never occur before puberty.[104] However, in adolescent and adult males, epididymo-orchitis is second only to parotitis as a manifestation of mumps virus infection.[71] Cases of orchitis have been reported in children as young as 3 years.[94] In postpubertal males, orchitis develops in 30 to 38 percent with mumps.[5, 91] The rate of orchitis is highest in those 15 to 29 years of age. The greatest number of cases occur during the second, third, and fourth decades of life. Approximately 80 percent of cases of epididymo-orchitis appear during the first 8 days of involvement of the salivary gland, but a few cases occur a considerable time after the parotitis has subsided.[104]

The onset of testicular involvement usually is manifested as chills, recurrence of fever, and swelling of the testes. Pain over the renal area or in the lower part of the abdomen, bilateral or unilateral, may precede or accompany the orchitis. Occasionally, this pain, if on the right side, may suggest appendicitis.

The orchitis is most often unilateral, but bilateral involvement has been reported in 17 to 38 percent of cases.[5, 91] Although atrophy may develop after orchitis, in those with unilateral involvement, sterility is not a concern. Sterility has resulted after some cases of bilateral orchitis, however. The development of malignancies in affected testes has been reported.[5, 62]

Oophoritis occurs in approximately 7 percent of postpubertal females. Pelvic pain and tenderness are noted.[97]

PANCREATITIS

In a retrospective survey of 2482 hospitalized mumps patients, pancreatitis was noted in 75 (3%).[2] Cases occurred in children and adults, and pancreatitis was 1.6 times more common in males than females. Severe involvement of the pancreas is rare, but mild or subclinical infection may occur more commonly than recognized.[97] It may be unassociated with salivary gland manifestations and be misdiagnosed as gastroenteritis. Epigastric pain and tenderness are suggestive; they may be accompanied by fever, chills, vomiting, and prostration. A child with acute hemorrhagic pancreatitis and a pseudocyst caused by mumps virus infection has been reported.[35]

DIABETES MELLITUS[21]

Diabetes mellitus long has been suspected to be associated with antecedent mumps.[52] In experimental animals, mumps virus infection has been linked to hyperglycemia and histologic lesions of the pancreatic islets. Mumps virus can invade the human pancreas and can infect and destroy human and rhesus beta cells in vitro,[93] but pancreatic damage has never been documented in reported cases of diabetes after mumps or mumps vaccination.[102]

In humans, many cases of temporal association have been described both in individuals and in siblings,[28, 29, 67, 81, 83] and outbreaks of diabetes mellitus a few months or years after outbreaks of mumps have been reported.[46, 80, 108] Although evidence has not established a causal association in these cases, a study in Surrey, England, suggested that a small proportion, if any, of diabetes cases that start in childhood (only 15 of the 1663 patients in the study, or <1%) may have resulted from a recent mumps virus infection.[40] Antibody studies have shown fewer positive titers for mumps in diabetics than in normal subjects, even in children.[95] Infection might contribute to the development of diabetes either by specifically damaging islet cells or by precipitating diabetes in patients whose disease is latent.

Teng and colleagues[109] reported an 11-year-old girl with mumps infection complicated by transient hyperinsulinemic hypoglycemia.

NEPHRITIS

Viruria is a common occurrence in uncomplicated mumps, and mild abnormalities in renal function occur.[112] Severe and fatal nephritis has been reported as a rare complication of mumps occurring 10 to 14 days after parotitis.[97] Fujieda and associates[39] reported the demonstration of mumps virus genomic RNA by polymerase chain reaction in a renal biopsy specimen from a 5-year-old girl with IgA nephropathy.

DEAFNESS

Deafness is an important but rare complication of mumps virus infection.[21] Its incidence has been estimated at 0.5 to 5.0 per 100,000 cases of mumps.[33, 115] However, the incidence rate of minor degrees of hearing impairment, such as high-tone hearing loss, is probably much higher.[24]

Mumps-associated deafness occurs with or without meningoencephalitis and may develop after asymptomatic infection.[21, 33, 82] The deafness is usually unilateral and often permanent. Twenty-two of 103 cases (21%) reviewed by Everberg[33] were bilateral. Mumps virus has been isolated from perilymph fluid in a case of sudden-onset, unilateral, complete deafness that began 2 days after the onset of mumps.[121] Vertigo also is noted occasionally in patients with mumps; it occurs most commonly in those in whom deafness develops.[60]

MUMPS AND PREGNANCY[21]

The incidence of mumps during pregnancy was estimated at 0.8 to 10 cases per 10,000 pregnancies[98] before vaccine licensure. No vaccine-era data are available for comparison. Maternal complications such as mastitis,[91] aseptic meningitis,[8] and fatal glomerulonephritis[30] have been reported. Mumps virus has been isolated from human breast milk.[64]

Increased fetal mortality was reported in women who contracted mumps during the first trimester. In a large prospective case-control study, a 27.3 percent rate of fetal wastage was noted in women with mumps during the first trimester versus a 13.0 percent rate in matched, non-ill controls during the first trimester.[101] No significant differences in birth weight were noted among the live births.[100] Because fetal loss usually occurs in such cases within 2 weeks of maternal infection, investigators postulated that factors related to maternal gonadal infection with resulting hormonal changes might be responsible. A histopathologic study of the products of conception in mothers with gestational mumps revealed severe proliferative necrotic villitis and vasculitis in the placenta and viral inclusions, as seen in mumps infection, in fetal tissues.[41] Mumps virus has been isolated from a spontaneously aborted 10-week-old human fetus.[74]

No evidence has shown that gestational mumps in humans increases the risk of fetal malformations,[99] although a few cases of various congenital malformations with no consistent pattern have been reported.[59]

OTHER MANIFESTATIONS

Other rare clinical manifestations include exanthem and enanthem,[23] arthritis,[44] myocarditis,[6] thrombocytopenia,[75] lower respiratory tract infection,[37] and other glandular involvement (thyroiditis, mastitis, dacryoadenitis, and bartholinitis).[71, 89]

Diagnosis

DIFFERENTIAL DIAGNOSIS

Not all patients with mumps have parotid swelling, and mumps virus is not the only cause of parotitis. Mumps virus infection must be considered in all children with aseptic meningitis, meningoencephalitis, and encephalitis (see Chapters 42 and 43). In addition to mumps virus infection, many other infectious agents and noninfectious conditions are associated with parotitis or parotid swelling (see Chapter 16). Other viruses that can cause parotitis include Epstein-Barr virus, coxsackieviruses and echoviruses, influenza A virus, parainfluenza viruses, cytomegalovirus, and lymphocytic choriomeningitis virus.[12] Purulent parotitis can be differentiated from mumps by the exquisite tenderness of the region, an elevated white blood cell count, and the observation of pus coming from the Stensen duct. Other viral causes of parotitis can be differentiated by the respective epidemiologic and clinical characteristics of specific agents and appropriate culture, serologic study, or both.

Enlargement of lymph nodes in proximity to the parotid gland must be differentiated from parotid enlargement (see Chapter 15). The cervical lymph nodes are below the ramus of the mandible. The preparotid nodes are generally anterior to the parotid, and their enlargement usually is associated with conjunctivitis. Occasionally, an enlarged lymph node within the parotid gland may cause some confusion.

Lesions of the ramus of the mandible, such as osteomyelitis, occasionally have been mistaken for parotid enlargement. In this case, the enlargement is usually persistent.

SPECIFIC DIAGNOSIS

In an epidemic situation, the diagnosis of mumps is clinically straightforward, and performing laboratory tests is unnecessary. The critical points are a history of exposure, an incubation period of 2 to 3 weeks, and a typical clinical picture consisting of fever and parotitis. In a sporadic case or in a previously vaccinated child, confirming the etiology by laboratory study is important. Mumps virus as well as most other viruses that cause parotitis can be isolated readily from saliva, throat swabs, or mouth washings during acute illness. In patients with meningoencephalitis, virus also can be recovered from CSF. Virus is isolated in primary monkey kidney tissue culture (see Chapter 249).

Mumps virus infection also can be confirmed by demonstrating a significant antibody titer rise in paired serum specimens by complement fixation, hemagglutination inhibition, or ELISA. However, because mumps cross-reacts with parainfluenza viruses, these methods are not ideal.[92] Mumps-specific IgM antibody also can be determined by ELISA; its presence indicates a recent infection.

In unusual cases in which the source of facial swelling is obscure, determination of a serum amylase level may be helpful; a high value would indicate parotid involvement.

Treatment

Conservative therapy is indicated in the treatment of mumps. Adequate attention to hydration and alimentation of patients is important. Patients may have difficulty with acidic foods such as orange juice. In addition, orange juice may cause vomiting in an already nauseated patient. The diet should be light, with a generous offering of fluids.

Occasionally, analgesics are necessary for severe headache or discomfort caused by parotitis. Stronger analgesics such as codeine or meperidine (Demerol) rarely are required for headache but may be useful for orchitis. Vomiting seldom is sufficiently severe to require intravenous fluids. In these instances, however, electrolytes lost by vomiting should be replaced.

Although lumbar puncture is not often necessary for diagnosis in patients with meningoencephalitis accompanying mumps, patients often indicate that they have experienced relief of headache after this procedure.

No antiviral agent is appropriate or indicated for the treatment of mumps, which is a self-limited illness.

Prognosis

The overall prognosis in uncomplicated mumps is excellent. The outlook in meningoencephalitis is also generally favorable, but death and neurologic damage can occur. Deafness and sterility are rare complications.

Prevention

IMMUNIZATION

A summary of the recommendations of the Advisory Committee on Immunization Practices (ACIP) for the use of mumps vaccine follows.[18, 116] For more complete information, the reader should consult the most recent ACIP statement or the Report of the Committee on Infectious Diseases of the American Academy of Pediatrics.

The mumps virus vaccine available in the United States (official name: mumps virus vaccine, live) is the Jeryl Lynn strain and is prepared in chick embryo cell culture. More than 150 million doses have been distributed in the United States since its introduction in December 1967 through 2002. The vaccine produces a subclinical, noncommunicable infection with few side effects. Mumps vaccine is available in both a monovalent (mumps only) form and combinations: mumps-rubella and measles-mumps-rubella (MMR) vaccines.

The vaccine is approximately 95 percent efficacious in preventing mumps disease,[57, 106] and after vaccination, measurable antibody develops in more than 97 percent of persons known to be susceptible to mumps.[119] Vaccine-induced antibody is protective and long lasting,[117, 118] although it is of considerably lower titer than antibody resulting from natural infection.[119] The duration of vaccine-induced immunity is unknown, but serologic and epidemiologic data collected during 30 years of live vaccine use indicate both persistence of antibody and continuing protection against infection. Estimates of clinical vaccine efficacy ranging from 75 to 95 percent have been calculated from data collected in outbreak settings with the use of different epidemiologic study designs.[22]

In Finland, a two-dose MMR vaccination program with the Jeryl Lynn mumps vaccine strain was launched in 1982.[90] This program has been highly successful, and Finland is the first country documented to be free of indigenous mumps as well as rubella and measles.

General Recommendations

Susceptible children, adolescents, and adults should be vaccinated against mumps unless vaccination is contraindicated. Mumps vaccine is of particular value for children approaching puberty and for adolescents and adults who have not had mumps. MMR is the vaccine of choice for routine administration and should be used in all situations in which recipients are also likely to be susceptible to measles, rubella, or both. The favorable benefit-cost ratio for routine mumps immunization is more marked when vaccine is administered as MMR.[69, 116] Persons should be considered susceptible to mumps unless they have documentation of (1) physician-diagnosed mumps, (2) adequate immunization with live mumps virus vaccine on or after their first birthday, or (3) laboratory evidence of immunity.

Persons who are unsure of their history of mumps disease or mumps vaccination should be vaccinated. No evidence has shown that persons who previously either received mumps vaccine or had mumps are at any increased risk for local or systemic reactions from receiving live mumps vaccine. Testing for susceptibility before vaccination, especially in adolescents and young adults, is not necessary. In addition to the expense, some tests (e.g., mumps skin test, complement-fixation antibody test) may be unreliable, and tests with established reliability (e.g., neutralization, enzyme immunoassay, radial hemolysis antibody test) are not readily available.

Dosage

Two doses of MMR vaccine separated by at least 1 month in the volume specified by the manufacturer should be administered subcutaneously.

Age

Live mumps virus vaccine is recommended at any age on or after the first birthday for all susceptible persons, unless a contraindication exists. In routine circumstances, mumps vaccine should be given in combination with measles and rubella vaccines as MMR, and the currently recommended schedule for administration of measles vaccine should be followed. It should not be administered to infants younger than 12 months because persisting maternal antibody might interfere with seroconversion. To ensure immunity, all persons vaccinated before their first birthday should be revaccinated on or after their first birthday.

PERSONS EXPOSED TO MUMPS

Use of Vaccine

When given after exposure to mumps, live mumps virus vaccine may not provide protection. However, if the exposure did not result in infection, vaccine should induce protection against infection from subsequent exposure. No evidence has indicated that the risk of vaccine-associated adverse events increases if vaccine is administered to persons incubating disease.

Use of Immunoglobulin

Immunoglobulin has not been demonstrated to be of established value in postexposure prophylaxis and is not recommended.

ADVERSE EFFECTS OF VACCINE USE

In field trials before licensure, illnesses did not occur more often in vaccinees than in unvaccinated controls.[56] Reports of illnesses occurring after mumps vaccination mainly have been episodes of parotitis and low-grade fever. Allergic reactions, including rash, pruritus, and purpura, have been associated temporally with mumps vaccination but are uncommon and usually mild and of brief duration. The reported development of encephalitis within 30 days of receiving a mumps-containing vaccine in the United States (0.4 per million doses) is not greater than the observed background incidence rate of CNS dysfunction in the normal population. Other manifestations of CNS involvement in the United States, such as febrile seizures and deafness, also have been reported infrequently. Complete recovery is usual. Reports of nervous system illness occurring after mumps vaccination do not necessarily denote an etiologic relationship between the illness and the vaccine.

In parts of Europe, Canada, and Japan, where different mumps vaccines (Leningrad 3 strain and Urabe Am 9 strain) have been used, rates of vaccine-induced aseptic meningitis have been high.[25, 27, 78, 107]

CONTRAINDICATIONS TO VACCINE USE

Pregnancy

Although mumps vaccine virus has been shown to infect the placenta and fetus,[123] no evidence has indicated that it causes congenital malformations in humans. However, because of the theoretic risk of fetal damage, a prudent approach is to avoid giving live virus vaccine to pregnant women. Vaccinated women should avoid pregnancy for 3 months after vaccination. Routine precautions for vaccinating postpubertal women include asking whether they are or may be pregnant, excluding those who say that they are, and explaining the theoretic risk to those who plan to receive the vaccine. Vaccination during pregnancy should not be considered an indication for termination of pregnancy. However, the final decision about interruption of pregnancy must rest with the individual patient and her physician.

Severe Febrile Illness

Vaccine administration should not be postponed because of minor or intercurrent febrile illnesses such as mild upper respiratory infections. However, vaccination of persons with severe febrile illnesses generally should be deferred until they have recovered.

Allergies

Because live mumps vaccine is produced in chick embryo cell culture, persons with a history of anaphylactic reactions (e.g., hives, swelling of the mouth and throat, difficulty breathing, hypotension, shock) after egg ingestion should be vaccinated only with caution and according to published protocols.[45, 54] Known allergic children should not leave the vaccination site for 20 minutes. Evidence indicates that persons are not at increased risk if they have egg allergies that are not anaphylactic. Such persons may be vaccinated in the usual manner. No evidence has demonstrated that persons with allergies to chickens or feathers are at increased risk of having a reaction to the vaccine.

Because mumps vaccine contains trace amounts of neomycin (25 μg), persons who have experienced anaphylactic reactions to topically or systemically administered neomycin should not receive mumps vaccine. Most often, neomycin allergy is manifested as contact dermatitis, which is a delayed-type (cell-mediated) immune response rather than anaphylaxis. In such persons, the adverse reaction, if any, to 25 μg of neomycin in the vaccine would be an erythematous, pruritic nodule or papule at 48 to 96 hours. A history of contact dermatitis to neomycin is not a contraindication to receiving mumps vaccine. Live mumps virus vaccine does not contain penicillin.

Recent Immunoglobulin Injection

Passively acquired antibody can interfere with the response to live attenuated virus vaccines. Therefore, mumps vaccine should be given at least 2 weeks before the administration of immunoglobulin or be deferred for 3 to 11 months after the administration of immunoglobulin. The duration of deferral depends on the dose of immunoglobulin administered.[116]

Altered Immunity

In theory, replication of the mumps vaccine virus may be potentiated in patients with immune deficiency disease and by the suppressed immune responses that occur with leukemia, lymphoma, or generalized malignancy or with therapy with corticosteroids, alkylating drugs, antimetabolites, or radiation. In general, patients with such conditions should not be given live mumps virus vaccine. Because vaccinated persons do not transmit mumps vaccine virus, the risk of mumps exposure in these patients may be reduced by vaccinating their close susceptible contacts.

An exception to these general recommendations is in children infected with human immunodeficiency virus (HIV): all asymptomatic HIV-infected children should receive MMR vaccine at 12 months of age.[20, 116] If measles vaccine is administered to symptomatic HIV-infected children, the combination MMR vaccine generally is preferred.[19]

Patients with leukemia in remission whose chemotherapy has been terminated for at least 3 months also may receive live mumps virus vaccine. Short-term (less than 2 weeks' duration) corticosteroid therapy, topical steroid therapy (e.g., nasal, skin), and intra-articular, bursal, or tendon injection with corticosteroids are not contraindications to the administration of mumps vaccine. However, mumps vaccine should be avoided if systemic immunosuppressive levels are reached by prolonged, extensive, topical application.

CONTAINMENT OF DISEASE

Containment is important in prevention of mumps in the United States. Mumps is a reportable disease, and compliance is the obligation of all physicians. After early reports of sporadic mumps cases, health department workers can organize local immunization clinics and exclude susceptible students from school so that disease can be contained in a small geographic area.

REFERENCES

1. Afzal, M. A., Buchanan, J., Heath, A. B., et al.: Clustering of mumps virus isolates by SH gene sequence only partially reflects geographical origin. Arch. Virol. *142*:227–238, 1997.
2. A retrospective survey of the complications of mumps. J. R. Coll. Gen. Pract. *24*(145):552–556, 1974.
3. Azimi, P. H., and Cramblett, H. G.: Mumps meningoencephalitis in children. J. A. M. A. *207*:509–512, 1969.
4. Bang, H. O., and Bang, J.: Involvement of the central nervous system in mumps. Bull. Hyg. *19*:503–504, 1944.
5. Beard, C. M., Benson, R. C., Jr., Kelalis, P. P., et al.: The incidence and outcome of mumps orchitis in Rochester, Minnesota, 1935 to 1974. Mayo Clin. Proc. *52*:3–7, 1977.

6. Bengtsson, E., and Orndahl, G.: Complications of mumps with special reference to the incidence of myocarditis. Acta Med. Scand. *149*:381–389, 1954.
7. Black, F. L.: A nationwide serum survey of United States military recruits, 1962. III. Measles and mumps antibodies. Am. J. Hyg. *80*:304–307, 1964.
8. Bowers, D.: Mumps during pregnancy. West. J. Surg. Obstet. Gynecol. *61*:72, 1953.
9. Bruserud, O., and Thorsby, E.: HLA control of the proliferative T lymphocyte response to antigenic determinants on mumps virus: Studies of healthy individuals and patients with type 1 diabetes. Scand. J. Immunol. *22*:509–518, 1985.
10. Bruyn, H. B., Sexton, H. M., and Brainerd, H. D.: Mumps meningoencephalitis: A clinical review of 119 cases with one death. Calif. Med. *86*:155–160, 1957.
11. Callaghan, J. T., Petersen, B. H., Smith, W. C., et al.: Delayed hypersensitivity to mumps antigen in humans. Clin. Immunol. Immunopathol. *26*:102–110, 1983.
12. Caplan, C. E.: Mumps in the era of vaccines. C. M. A. J. *160*:865–866, 1999.
13. Carbone, K. M., and Wolinsky, J. S.: Mumps virus. *In* Knipe, D. M., and Howley, P. M. (eds.): Fields Virology. 4th ed., Vol. 1. Philadelphia, Lippincott Williams & Wilkins, 2001, pp. 1381–1400.
14. Centers for Disease Control and Prevention: Summary of notifiable diseases, United States, 1998. M. M. W. R. Morb. Mortal. Wkly. Rep. *47*(53):ii–92, 1999.
15. Centers for Disease Control and Prevention: Summary of notifiable diseases, United States, 1994. M. M. W. R. Morb. Mortal. Wkly. Rep. *43*(53):1–80, 1995.
16. Centers for Disease Control: Summary of notifiable diseases, United States, 1989. M. M. W. R. Morb. Mortal. Wkly. Rep. *38*(54):1–59, 1990.
17. Centers for Disease Control: Mumps—United States, 1985–1988. M. M. W. R. Morb. Mortal. Wkly. Rep. *38*(7):101–105, 1989.
18. Centers for Disease Control: Mumps prevention. M. M. W. R. Morb. Mortal. Wkly. Rep. *38*(22):388–392, 397–400, 1989.
19. Centers for Disease Control: Immunization of children infected with human immunodeficiency virus: Supplementary ACIP statement. Immunization Practices Advisory Committee. M. M. W. R. Morb. Mortal. Wkly. Rep. *37*(12):181–183, 1988.
20. Centers for Disease Control: Immunization of children infected with human T-lymphotrophic virus type III/lymphadenopathy-associated virus. M. M. W. R. Morb. Mortal. Wkly. Rep. *35*(38):595–596, 603–606, 1986.
21. Centers for Disease Control: Mumps surveillance, January 1977–December 1982. Issued September 1984.
22. Chalken, B. P., Williams, N. M., Preblud, S. R., et al.: The effect of a school entry law on mumps activity in a school district. J. A. M. A. *257*:2455–2456, 1987.
23. Cherry, J. D., and Jahn, C. L.: Exanthem and enanthem associated with mumps virus infection. Arch. Environ. Health *12*:518–521, 1966.
24. Chuden, H. G., Michtl, W., and Stehr, K.: Hearing loss due to mumps. Laryngol. Rhinol. Otol. *57*:745–750, 1978.
25. Cizman, M., Mozetic, M., Radescek-Rakar, R., et al.: Aseptic meningitis after vaccination against measles and mumps. Pediatr. Infect. Dis. J. *8*:302–308, 1989.
26. Cochi, S. L., Preblud, S. R., and Orenstein, W. A.: Perspectives on the relative resurgence of mumps in the United States. Am. J. Dis. Child. *142*:499–507, 1988.
27. Colville, A., and Pugh, S.: Mumps meningitis and measles, mumps and rubella vaccine. Lancet *340*:876, 1992.
28. Craighead, J. E.: The role of viruses in the pathogenesis of pancreatic disease and diabetes mellitus. Prog. Med. Virol. *19*:162–214, 1975.
29. Dacau-Voutetakis, C., Constantinidis, M., Moschos, A., et al.: Diabetes mellitus following mumps. Am. J. Dis. Child. *127*:890–891, 1974.
30. Dutta, P. C.: A fatal case of pregnancy complicated with mumps. J. Obstet. Gynaecol. Br. Emp. *42*:869, 1935.
31. Enders, J. F.: Mumps. *In* Rivers, T. M., and Horsfall, F. L., Jr. (eds.): Viral and Rickettsial Infections of Man. 3rd ed. Philadelphia, J. B. Lippincott, 1959, pp. 780–789.
32. Endo, A., Izumi, H., Miyashita, M., et al.: Facial palsy associated with mumps parotitis. Pediatr. Infect. Dis. J. *20*:815, 2001.
33. Everberg, G.: Deafness following mumps. Acta Otolaryngol. *48*:397–403, 1957.
34. Feldman, H. A.: Mumps. *In* Evans, A. S. (ed.): Viral Infections of Humans: Epidemiology and Control. 3rd ed. New York, Plenum, 1989, pp. 471–491.
35. Feldstein, J. D., Johnson, F. R., Kallick, C. A., and Doolas, A.: Acute hemorrhagic pancreatitis and pseudocyst due to mumps. Ann. Surg. *180*:85–88, 1974.
36. Finkelstein, H.: Meningo-encephalitis in mumps. J. A. M. A. *3*:17–19, 1938.
37. Foy, H. M., Cooney, M. K., Hall, C. E., et al.: Isolation of mumps virus from children with acute lower respiratory tract disease. Am. J. Epidemiol. *94*:467–471, 1971.
38. Friedman, M. G.: Salivary IgA antibodies to mumps virus during and after mumps. J. Infect. Dis. *143*:617, 1981.
39. Fujieda, M., Kinoshita, A., Naruse, K., et al.: Mumps associated with immunoglobulin A nephropathy. Pediatr. Infect. Dis. J. *19*:669–671, 2000.
40. Gamble, D. R.: Relationship of antecedent illness to development of diabetes in children. B. M. J. *12*:99–101, 1980.
41. Garcia, A. G., Pereira, J. M., Vidigal, N., et al.: Intrauterine infection with mumps virus. Obstet. Gynecol. *56*:756–759, 1980.
42. Gellis, S. S., and Peters, M.: Mumps with presternal edema. Bull. Johns Hopkins Hosp. *75*:241, 1944.
43. Gordon, J. E.: The epidemiology of mumps. Am. J. Med. Sci. *200*:412–428, 1940.
44. Gordon, S. C., and Lauter, C. B.: Mumps arthritis: A review of the literature. Rev. Infect. Dis. *6*:338–344, 1984.
45. Greenberg, M. A., and Birx, D. L.: Safe administration of mumps-measles-rubella vaccine in egg-allergic children. J. Pediatr. *113*:504–506, 1988.
46. Gundersen, E.: Is diabetes of infectious origin? J. Infect. Dis. *41*:198–202, 1927.
47. Gut, J. P., Lablache, C., Behr, S., et al.: Symptomatic mumps virus reinfections. J. Med. Virol. *45*:17–23, 1995.
48. Habel, K.: Cultivation of mumps virus in the developing chick embryo and its application to studies of immunity to mumps in man. Public Health Rep. *60*:201–212, 1945.
49. Haginoya, K., Ike, K., Iinuma, K., et al.: Chronic progressive mumps virus encephalitis in a child. Lancet. *346*:50, 1995.
50. Hamilton, R.: An account of a distemper, by the common people in England vulgarly called the mumps. Trans. R. Soc. Edinburgh *2*:59–72, 1790.
51. Hamilton, R.: An account of distemper by the common people of England vulgarly called the mumps. London Med. J. *11*:190–211, 1790.
52. Hams, H. F.: A case of diabetes quickly following mumps. Boston Med. Surg. J. *140*:465–469, 1899.
53. Henle, G., and Deinhardt, F.: Propagation and primary isolation of mumps virus in tissue culture. Proc. Soc. Exp. Biol. Med. *89*:556–560, 1955.
54. Herman, J. J., Radin, R., and Schneiderman, R.: Allergic reactions to measles (rubeola) vaccine in patients hypersensitive to egg protein. J. Pediatr. *102*:196–199, 1983.
55. Herndon, R. M., Johnson, R. T., Davis, L. E., and Descalzi, L. R.: Ependymitis in mumps virus meningitis. Arch. Neurol. *30*:475–479, 1974.
56. Hilleman, M. R., Buynak, E. B., Weibel, R. E., and Stokes, J., Jr.: Live, attenuated mumps-virus vaccine. N. Engl. J. Med. *278*:227–232, 1968.
57. Hilleman, M. R., Weibel, R. E., Buynak, E. B., et al.: Live, attenuated mumps-virus vaccine. 4. Protective efficacy as measured in a field evaluation. N. Engl. J. Med. *276*:252–258, 1967.
58. Hirsch, A.: Handbook of Historical and Geographical Pathology. Translated by Charles Creighton. London, 1886.
59. Holowach, J., Thurston, D. L., and Becker, B.: Congenital defects in infants following mumps during pregnancy: A review of the literature and a report of chorioretinitis due to fetal infection. J. Pediatr. *50*:689–694, 1957.
60. Hyden, D., Odkvist, L. M., and Kylen, P.: Vestibular symptoms in mumps deafness. Acta Otolaryngol. *360*(Suppl.):182–183, 1979.
61. Johnson, C. D., and Goodpasture, E. W.: The etiology of mumps. Am. J. Hyg. *21*:46–57, 1935.
62. Kaufman, J. J., and Bruce, P. T.: Testicular atrophy following mumps: A cause of testis tumor? Br. J. Urol. *35*:67–69, 1963.
63. Kilham, L.: Isolation of mumps virus from the blood of a patient. Proc. Soc. Exp. Biol. Med. *69*:99–100, 1948.
64. Kilham, L.: Mumps virus in human milk and in milk of infected monkey. J. A. M. A. *146*:1231, 1951.
65. Kim-Farley, R. J.: Mumps. *In* Kiple, K. F. (ed.): The Cambridge World History of Human Disease. Cambridge, England, Cambridge University Press, 1993, pp. 887–889.
66. Kim-Farley, R., Bart, S., Stetler, H., et al.: Clinical mumps vaccine efficacy. Am. J. Epidemiol. *121*:593–597, 1985.
67. King, R. C.: Mumps followed by diabetes. Lancet *2*:1055, 1962.
68. Kleiman, M. B., and Leland, D. S.: Mumps virus and Newcastle disease virus. *In* Lennette, E. H., Lennette, D. A., and Lennette, E. T. (eds.): Diagnostic Procedures for Viral, Rickettsial, and Chlamydial Infections. 7th ed. Washington, D. C., American Public Health Association, 1995, pp. 455–463.
69. Koplan, J. P., and Preblud, S. R.: A benefit-cost analysis of mumps vaccine. Am. J. Dis. Child. *136*:362–364, 1982.
70. Kress, H. G., and Kreth, H. W.: HLA restriction of secondary mumps-specific cytotoxic T lymphocytes. J. Immunol. *129*:844–849, 1982.
71. Krugman, S.: Mumps (epidemic parotitis). *In* Krugman, S. (ed.): Infectious Diseases of Children. 7th ed. St. Louis, C. V. Mosby, 1981, pp. 195–207.
72. Kunkel, U., Driesel, G., Henning, U., et al.: Differentiation of vaccine and wild mumps viruses by polymerase chain reaction and nucleotide sequencing of the SH gene: Brief report. J. Med. Virol. *45*:121–126, 1995.
73. Kupers, T. A., Petrich, J. M., Holloway, A. W., and St. Geme, J. W., Jr.: Depression of tuberculin delayed hypersensitivity by live attenuated mumps virus. J. Pediatr. *76*:716–721, 1970.
74. Kurtz, J. B., Tomlinson, A. H., and Pearson, J.: Mumps virus isolated from a fetus. B. M. J. *394*:471, 1982.

75. Lacour, M., Mahyerzi, M., Vienny, H., and Suter, S.: Thrombocytopenia in a case of neonatal mumps infection: Evidence for further clinical presentations. Eur. J. Pediatr. *152*:739–741, 1993.
76. Lamb, R. A., and Kolakofsky, D.: *Paramyxoviridae*: The viruses and their replication. *In* Knipe, and D. M., Howley, P. M. (eds.): Fields Virology. 4th ed., Vol. 1. Philadelphia, Lippincott Williams & Wilkins, 2001, pp. 1305–1340.
77. Majda-Stanislawska, E.: Mumps cerebellitis. Eur. Neurol. *43*:117, 2000.
78. McDonald, J. C., Moore, D. L., and Quennec, P.: Clinical and epidemiologic features of mumps meningoencephalitis and possible vaccine-related disease. Pediatr. Infect. Dis. J. *8*:751–755, 1989.
79. McGuinness, A. C., and Gall, E. A.: Mumps at army camps in 1943. War Med. *5*:95–104, 1944.
80. Melin, K., and Ursung, B.: Diabetes mellitus som komplikation till parotitis: Epidemia. Nord. Med. *60*:1715–1717, 1958.
81. Messaritikas, J., Kalantari, C., Kattamis, C., and Matsaniotis, N.: Diabetes following mumps in sibs. Arch. Dis. Child. *46*:561–562, 1971.
82. Nomura, Y., Harada, T., Sakata, H., and Sugiura, A.: Sudden deafness and asymptomatic mumps. Acta Otolaryngol. (Stockh.) *456*(Suppl.): 9–11, 1988.
83. Notkins, A. L.: Virus-induced diabetes mellitus: Brief review. Arch. Virol. *54*:1–17, 1977.
84. Ogata, H., Oka, K., and Mitsudome, A.: Hydrocephalus due to acute aqueductal stenosis following mumps infection: Report of a case and review of the literature. Brain Dev. *14*:417–419, 1992.
85. Oran, B., Çeri, A., Yilmaz, H., et al.: Hydrocephalus in mumps meningoencephalitis: Case report. Pediatr. Infect. Dis. J. *14*:724–725, 1995.
86. Örvell, C., Kalantari, M., and Johansson, B.: Characterization of five conserved genotypes of the mumps virus small hydrophobic (SH) protein gene. J. Gen. Virol. *78*:91–95, 1997.
87. Örvell, C., Rydbeck, R., and Löve, A.: Immunological relationships between mumps virus and parainfluenza viruses studied with monoclonal antibodies. J. Gen. Virol. *67*:1929–1939, 1986.
88. Overman, J. R.: Viremia in human mumps virus infections. Arch. Intern. Med. *102*:354–356, 1958.
89. Parmar, R. C., Bavdekar, S. B., Sahu, D. R., et al.: Thyroiditis as a presenting feature of mumps. Pediatr. Infect. Dis. J. *20*:637–638, 2001.
90. Peltola, H., Davidkin, I., Paunio, M., et al.: Mumps and rubella eliminated from Finland. J. A. M. A. *284*:2643–2647, 2000.
91. Philip, R. N., Reinhard, K. R., and Lackman, D. B.: Observations on a mumps epidemic in a "virgin" population. Am. J. Hyg. *69*:91–111, 1959.
92. Pipkin, P. A., Afzal, M. A., and Heath, A. B.: Assay of humoral immunity to mumps virus. J. Virol. Methods *79*:219–225, 1999.
93. Prince, G. A., Henson, A. B., Billiups, L. C., and Notkins, A. L.: Infection of human pancreatic beta cell cultures with mumps virus. Nature *271*:158–161, 1978.
94. Reed, D., Brown, G., Merrick, R., et al.: A mumps epidemic on St. George Island, Alaska. J. A. M. A. *199*:967–971, 1967.
95. Samantray, S. K., Christopher, S., Mukundan, P., and Jonson, S. C.: Lack of relationship between viruses and human diabetes mellitus. Aust. N. Z. Med. 7:139, 1977.
96. Sarnesto, A., Julkunen, I., and Makela, O.: Proportion of Ig classes and subclasses in mumps antibodies. Scand. J. Immunol. *22*:345–350, 1985.
97. Scott, T. F. M.: Mumps (epidemic parotitis). *In* Nelson, W. E., Vaughan, V. C., and McKay, R. J. (eds.): Textbook of Pediatrics. 9th ed. Philadelphia, W. B. Saunders, 1969, pp. 647–651.
98. Sever, J., and White, L. R.: Intrauterine viral infections. Annu. Rev. Med. *19*:471, 1968.
99. Siegel, M.: Congenital malformations following chickenpox, measles, mumps, and hepatitis: Results of a cohort study. J. A. M. A. *226*:1521–1524, 1973.
100. Siegel, M., and Fuerst, H. T.: Low birth weight and maternal virus diseases: A prospective study of rubella, measles, mumps, chickenpox, and hepatitis. J. A. M. A. *197*:88, 1966.
101. Siegel, M., Fuerst, H. T., and Peress, N. S.: Comparative fetal mortality in maternal virus diseases: A prospective study on rubella, measles, mumps and chickenpox and hepatitis. N. Engl. J. Med. *274*:768–771, 1966.
102. Sinaniotos, C. A., Daskalopoulou, E., Lapatsanis, P., and Doxiadis, S.: Diabetes mellitus after mumps vaccination. Arch. Dis. Child. *50*:749, 1975.
103. Spartaro, R. F., Lin, S.-R., Horner, F. A., et al.: Aqueductal stenosis and hydrocephalus: Rare sequelae of mumps virus infection. Neuroradiology *12*:11–13, 1976.
104. Stokes, J., Jr.: Mumps (epidemic parotitis). *In* Nelson, W. E. (ed.): Textbook of Pediatrics. 7th ed. Philadelphia, W. B. Saunders, 1959, pp. 505–508.
105. Ströhle, A., Bernasconi, C., and Germann, D.: A new mumps virus lineage found in the 1995 mumps outbreak in western Switzerland identified by nucleotide sequence analysis of the SH gene: Brief report. Arch. Virol. *141*:733–741, 1996.
106. Sugg, W. C., Finger, J. A., Levine, R. H., and Pagano, J. S.: Field evaluation of live virus mumps vaccine. J. Pediatr. *72*:461–466, 1968.
107. Sugiura, A., and Yamada, A.: Aseptic meningitis as a complication of mumps vaccination. Pediatr. Infect. Dis. J. *10*:209–213, 1991.
108. Sultz, H. A., Hart, B. A., Zielezny, M., and Schlesinger, E. R.: Is mumps virus an etiological factor in juvenile diabetes mellitus? Preliminary report. J. Pediatr. *86*:654–656, 1975.
109. Teng, R. J., Wu, T. J., and Ho, M. M.: Mumps infection complicated by transient hyperinsulinemic hypoglycemia. Pediatr. Infect. Dis. J. *16*:416–417, 1997.
110. Thompson, J. A.: Mumps: A cause of acquired aqueductal stenosis. J. Pediatr. *94*:923–924, 1979.
111. Ukkonen, P., Granström, M. L., and Penttinen, K.: Mumps-specific immunoglobulin M and G antibodies in natural mumps infection as measured by enzyme-linked immunosorbent assay. J. Med. Virol. *8*:131–142, 1981.
112. Utz, J. P., and Alling, D.: Clinical and laboratory studies of mumps. IV. Viruria and abnormal renal function. N. Engl. J. Med. *270*:1283–1286, 1964.
113. van Loon, F. P., Holmes, S. J., Sirotkin, B. I., et al.: Mumps surveillance, United States, 1988–1993. M. M. W. R. CDC Surveill. Summ. *44*(SS-3): 1–14, 1995.
114. Venketasubramanian, M.: Transverse myelitis following mumps in an adult—a case report with MRI correlation. Acta Neurol. Scand. *96*:328–331, 1997.
115. Vuori, M., Lahikainen, E. A., and Peltonen, T.: Perceptive deafness in connection with mumps: A study of 298 servicemen suffering from mumps. Acta Otolaryngol. *55*:231–236, 1962.
116. Watson, J. C., Hadler, S. C., Dykewicz, C. A., et al.: Measles, mumps, and rubella—vaccine use and strategies for elimination of measles, rubella, and congenital rubella syndrome and control of mumps: Recommendations of the Advisory Committee on Immunization Practices (ACIP). M. M. W. R. Recomm. Rep. *47*(RR-8):1–57, 1998.
117. Weibel, R. E., Buynak, E. B., McLean, A. A., et al.: Follow-up surveillance for antibody in human subjects following live attenuated measles, mumps and rubella virus vaccines. Proc. Soc. Exp. Biol. Med. *162*:328–332, 1979.
118. Weibel, R. E., Buynak, E. B., McLean, A. A., et al.: Persistence of antibody in human subjects for 7 to 10 years following administration of combined live attenuated measles, mumps and rubella virus vaccines. Proc. Soc. Exp. Biol. Med. *165*:260–263, 1980.
119. Weibel, R. E., Stokes, J., Jr., Buynak, E. B., et al.: Live, attenuated mumps-virus vaccine. 3. Clinical and serologic aspects in a field evaluation. N. Engl. J. Med. *276*:245–251, 1967.
120. Weller, T. H., and Craig, J. R.: Isolation of mumps virus at autopsy. Am. J. Pathol. *25*:1105–1125, 1949.
121. Westmore, G. A., Pickard, B. H., and Stern, H.: Isolation of mumps virus from the inner ear after sudden deafness. B. M. J. *1*:14–15, 1979.
122. Wolinsky, J. S.: Mumps virus. *In* Fields, B. N., and Howley, P. M. (eds.): Fields Virology. 3rd ed. Philadelphia, Lippincott-Raven, 1996, pp. 1243–1265.
123. Yamauchi, T., Wilson, C., and St. Geme, J. W., Jr.: Transmission of live, attenuated mumps virus to the human placenta. N. Engl. J. Med. *290*:710–712, 1974.

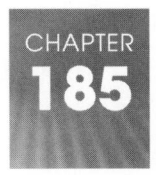

CHAPTER 185 Respiratory Syncytial Virus and Human Metapneumovirus

CHAPTER 185A

Respiratory Syncytial Virus

CAROLINE BREESE HALL

As by one bow on varied strings, the tune is played,
By both the microbe and the host, disease is made.
C. B. H.

Respiratory syncytial virus (RSV) is the most important respiratory pathogen of infancy and early childhood and the major cause of hospitalization for bronchiolitis and pneumonia in infants.[54, 76, 153, 254, 347] According to estimates of the Institute of Medicine, each year approximately 91,000 infants are hospitalized with RSV infection in the United States at a cost of $300 million.[204] Recent studies suggest that these figures currently underestimate the number of hospitalizations for RSV infections. Significant rises in the number of admissions for RSV bronchiolitis have been documented recently in both the United States and Canada.[275, 396] Currently in the United States, 62,500 to 100,000 hospitalizations for RSV bronchiolitis alone are estimated to occur annually in children younger than 5 years. This virus is unique in its ability to produce its most severe disease in the first few weeks to months of life, when specific maternal antibody is uniformly present in the infant's serum. It circulates with an incompletely understood efficiency and causes sizable outbreaks each year such that it infects almost all children in their first years of life. Nearly all of these first infections are symptomatic, and an appreciable proportion involve the lower respiratory tract. RSV does not respect age; symptomatic infections continue throughout life.

History

In 1956, Morris and associates[317] noted a cropping of colds with coryza in a colony of chimpanzees that had been under observation for the previous 3 to 24 weeks. A new virus was recovered from 1 of the 14 afflicted chimpanzees and appropriately named "chimpanzee coryza agent" (CCA). Specific antibody to the CCA agent developed in the remaining 13 animals during convalescence; thus, the attack rate was 100 percent. An upper respiratory tract infection and convalescent antibody to CCA also developed in a person working with these chimpanzees. Isolation of virus, however, was not accomplished. Subsequently, a coryzal illness developed after 3 days in susceptible chimpanzees inoculated with the new agent grown in tissue culture.

A human origin of the chimpanzees' agent was suspected; it was confirmed when Chanock and Finberg[73] recovered two agents indistinguishable from the CCA virus from the throat swabs of an infant with bronchopneumonia (Long strain) and a child with laryngotracheobronchitis (Snyder strain). They studied the increase in antibody to these viruses in patients with respiratory disease and noted that by 4 years of age, 80 percent of children had neutralizing antibody for the Long virus. Nevertheless, they could not determine a definite etiologic association between the virus and the lower respiratory tract disease in their young patients. They proposed to call this group of viruses (Long, Snyder, and CCA) "respiratory syncytial virus" because of their manifestations clinically and in tissue culture. Confirmation of RSV as a major agent in respiratory disease soon accumulated from studies throughout the United States.[75, 242, 375] Subsequently, investigators from many countries have confirmed and further delineated RSV's importance.*

Properties

A tiny thistle—
Of coiled spine
and outer quill. . .
C. B. H.

CLASSIFICATION

The original classification of RSV with the Newcastle disease and parainfluenza group of viruses was based on their similar internal particle structure, eosinophilic inclusions, and syncytial appearance in tissue cultures. However, RSV is antigenically distinct and does not hemagglutinate erythrocytes.[455] Subsequently, the diameter of the nucleocapsid of RSV was determined to be between that of the larger paramyxoviruses and the smaller influenza viruses. Further study of RSV's structure has resulted in its current classification in the order Mononegavirales, which contains the nonsegmented negative-strand RNA viruses, and in the family *Paramyxoviridae* and genus Pneumovirus.[90, 368] Classified with RSV in Pneumovirus are the closely related bovine RSV, ovine RSV, caprine RSV, turkey rhinotracheitis virus, and pneumonia virus of mice.

STRUCTURAL AND ANTIGENIC PROPERTIES

The virion of RSV consists of a nucleocapsid enclosed within a bilayer lipid envelope. The genome of RSV is composed of 15,222 nucleotides (strain A2). It is a nonsegmented, single-stranded, negative-sense RNA genome that is transcribed into 10 major mRNA molecules (Table 185–1), each encoding for one of the major proteins, except for M2 mRNA, which possesses two overlapping open-reading frames that

*See references 47, 76, 144, 145, 153, 253, 301, 332, 347, 401.

TABLE 185–1 ■ RESPIRATORY SYNCYTIAL VIRUS: CHARACTERISTICS AND DIFFERENCES ACCORDING TO STRAIN GROUP

Viral Protein	Gene Length (Nucleotides)	Percent Difference in Strain Groups A vs. B*		Protein Induces
		Nucleotides	*Amino Acids*	
Structural				
Surface				
F	1903	79	89	Viral penetration, major protection, NA, FIA, CTL
G	923	67	53	Viral attachment, strain group protection, NA, no CTL
SH (1A)	410	78	76	Unknown function, CTL, no NA
Matrix				
M	958	—	—†	?Nucleocapsid to envelope, CTL, no NA
M2 (22k)	961	78	92	Unique to pneumoviruses, CTL, no NA
Nucleocapsid Associated				
N	1203	86	96	Major RNA-binding nucleocapsid protein, CTL, no NA
P	914	80	90	Major phosphoprotein, CTL, no NA
L	6578	—	—†	Major polymerase subunit, immune response unknown
Nonstructural				
NS1 (1C)	532	78	92	Unique to pneumoviruses, unknown function, CTL
NS2 (1B)	503	78	87	Unique to pneumoviruses, unknown function, no CTL

*Percent difference between strain A2 (group A) and strain 18537 (group B).
†Dash (—) = difference between strain groups not yet determined.
CTL, cytotoxic lymphocyte response (in humans); FIA, fusion-inhibiting antibody; NA, neutralizing antibody.

encode for two separate proteins (M2–1 and M2–2).[88–90, 219, 420, 456] Eight of them, including the seven largest (L, G, F, N, P, M, and SH), are structural proteins, and two (NS1 and NS2) are nonstructural proteins.[219] Three of the structural proteins, the glycosylated F (fusion) and G (attachment) proteins and the small, nonglycosylated hydrophobic SH (or 1A) protein, are transmembrane surface proteins. Three proteins associated with the genomic mRNA form the viral capsid proteins, N (nucleoprotein), P (phosphoprotein), and L (polymerase). Two matrix proteins, the nonglycosylated M and M2 (membrane-associated proteins), in contrast to the other paramyxoviruses, are also present in RSV. The complete sequence of the genes of the A2 strain now has been determined (Fig. 185–1).

Significant strain variation among RSV isolates has resulted in strains being divided into two major groups.[19, 21] These two major groups, A and B, have intergroup and intragroup variations in several proteins, including F, G, P,

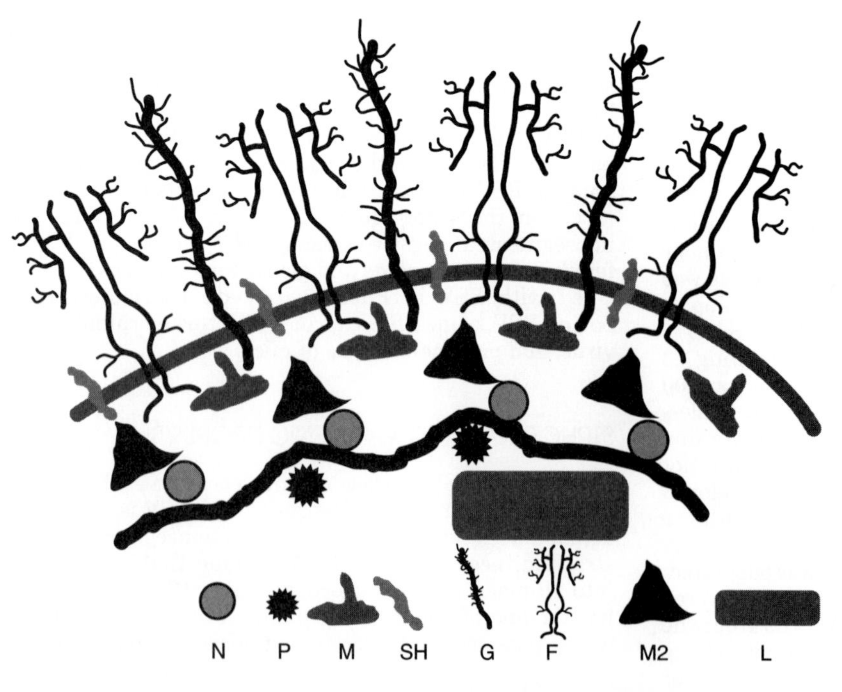

FIGURE 185–1 ■ Schematic representation of the genomic structure of respiratory syncytial virus (RSV). The 10 proteins of RSV are F, G, and SH (surface glycoproteins); M and M2 (matrix proteins); N, P, and L (nucleocapsid-associated proteins); and NS1 and NS2 (nonstructural proteins). (Adapted from Walsh, E. E., and Hall, C. B.: Approaches to the respiratory syncytial virus vaccine. *In* Meyers, R. A., Beaubien, M. P., and Kraus, H.-J. [eds.]: Encyclopedia of Molecular Biology and Molecular Medicine. New York, VCH Publisher, 1996.)

and N (see Table 185–1). The primary difference is in the largest surface glycoprotein, the G protein. The F protein, along with the N, P, M2, NS1, and NS2 proteins, is conserved relatively well, and antibody to F protein is cross-reactive between the two groups.[236, 237, 453] The F proteins of prototype strains from groups A and B have greater than 90 percent amino acid homology and a high degree of antigenic relatedness. In comparison, the amino acid homology between the G proteins of the two groups is 55 percent, and antigenic relatedness is only about 3 to 7 percent.[236, 237, 453] Amino acid diversity for G protein within a group has varied from about 12 percent for group B to about 20 percent for group A.[62]

LABORATORY GROWTH

RSV is relatively labile, which has hampered its purification. At 55° C, it is destroyed rapidly; at 37° C for 24 hours, only 10 percent of infectivity remains; and at 4° C for 1 week, 1 percent remains.[199]

The viability of RSV depends in part on the salt and protein content of the media. At 4° C, the addition of 1 mol/L of magnesium sulfate maintains viral stability for 5 weeks.[127] The virus withstands freezing and thawing poorly.[199, 455] Preservation is enhanced by rapid freezing in a dry ice and alcohol bath and by the addition of sucrose or glycerin to the storage media.[455] Infectivity also is influenced by the pH of the medium; at values less than 5, infectivity rapidly diminishes. The optimal pH for preservation is 7.5.[199] RSV is inactivated rapidly by detergents such as 0.1 percent sodium deoxycholate, sodium dodecyl sulfate, and Triton-X 100, as well as by chloroform and ether. On sucrose gradients, RSV has a density of 1.18 g/cm^3.[127]

RSV generally grows best in cultures of human heteroploid cells such as HEp-2 and HeLa cells. However, the sensitivity of these cell lines is variable, especially with passage, and must be monitored constantly. Other suitable but generally less sensitive cell lines include the primary monkey kidney and human embryonic fibroblast and A549 cell lines. The characteristic cytopathic effect of RSV in continuous cell lines is syncytial formation with eosinophilic cytoplasmic inclusions. The syncytia are usually evident 2 to 7 days after inoculation and progress to complete degeneration within about 4 days.[178] The cytopathic effect, however, depends on the strain of virus, the medium, the sensitivity and thickness of the cell cultures, and the number of passages.[240, 455] In HEp-2 cultures, syncytia formation and the amount of fusion protein produced appear to depend on the presence of calcium and glutamine in the medium.[395] Syncytia tend to be less evident in fibroblast cell lines, and in some primary cell cultures, RSV may produce rounded, refractile cells. In human and animal infections, syncytia may be evident in epithelial cells of the respiratory tract, although they appear to be unnecessary for the pathologic process because most infected cells are not syncytial but contain only one nucleus.

The growth cycle of RSV has been shown to consist of a period of adsorption, with 50 percent of the inoculum being adsorbed in 2 hours, followed by an eclipse period of 12 hours. New virus appears shortly thereafter and enters a log phase of replication lasting for approximately 10 hours.[284] Viral antigen can be documented by fluorescent antibody staining 7 to 10 hours after inoculation into cytoplasm. Shortly thereafter, cell-free virus may be demonstrated in the culture medium, but 50 to 90 percent of the virus remains associated with the cell surface at the time when maximal titers of the virus are obtained.[240, 284] Most of the cell-associated virus consists of incomplete virions that failed to bud entirely and may be released by agitation and sonication. An appreciable portion of the cell-free virus consists of noninfectious, empty virions and aggregated virus, as demonstrated by the 99 percent diminished infectivity after processing through a 0.45-μm filter.[30] With the laboratory Long strain (group A), peak titers usually are reached in 48 hours. For each infected cell, approximately 10 plaque-forming units generally result. Titers of virus are enhanced by inoculation of cell monolayers that are not yet confluent.[255] With continued high passage or propagation of temperature-sensitive mutants of RSV at nonpermissive temperatures, persistent infection may occur, but with loss of cytopathic effect and the amount of cell-free virus.[126, 369]

ANIMAL SUSCEPTIBILITY

The natural hosts for symptomatic RSV infection are primarily humans, chimpanzees, and cows. RSV also has been recovered from asymptomatic goats and sheep. Closely related bovine strains have been isolated from cattle with respiratory disease and, when reinoculated into cattle, sometimes have produced fever and rhinitis.[56, 222, 418, 439, 444] Susceptible animals that could serve as a model for the lower respiratory tract disease of infants have been sought for some time.[59] Although RSV grows in animals such as baboons, guinea pigs, mice, ferrets, mink, chinchillas, marmosets, and hamsters, direct inoculation into their respiratory tract generally produces infection that is clinically and pathologically silent. Other domestic animals such as dogs and cats have been found to possess antibody to RSV, the significance of which is unclear.[290, 380] Several animals have been used as models for studying different aspects of RSV disease, but all have limitations, most frequently diminished replication of RSV and lack of symptomatic infection. Chimpanzees most closely resemble humans in their clinical response to RSV.[43] However, lung pathology and some degree of clinical disease have been induced in numerous other nonhuman primates.[29, 59, 367, 380, 402] Infection in ferrets is age-dependent, with a limited histopathology of the nasal turbinates and trachea developing in adults. In infant ferrets, however, the virus replicates in the lung.[365]

The cotton rat has been the animal model used most widely.[59, 362, 364, 366] With intranasal inoculation, viral titers peak in the lung and nasal turbinates after 4 to 5 days. Histologic changes in the lung are generally minimal and inconsistent, and only a small proportion of cells appear to have productive infection. Inoculation of inbred mice similarly results in the replication of virus in the lung, although the quantity and consistency of the infection may vary with the type and age of the mouse.[160–162, 165, 361, 428] Marked pulmonary pathology may occur in BALB/c mice after high-titer, large-volume inocula, and in older mice it is accompanied by evidence of clinical illness.[165, 443] A lamb model also has been developed, which after challenge with ovine, bovine, or human RSV results in pathologic changes in the lung.[277] Intrathecal or intranasal inoculation of human RSV in the lamb model in one study produced fever and tachypnea more frequently in lambs receiving RSV than in control lambs.[277] The lack of a suitable animal model for human RSV infection has resulted in increased interest in the natural model of bovine RSV in cattle. Despite the appreciable morbidity that naturally occurs with bovine RSV, experimental infection in cattle has been difficult to achieve and is variable.[258]

Epidemiology

What occult power pries loose the lid
to give you winter flight,
But with the lengthening light of spring
gives cloak and leaden wing?

C. B. H.

GEOGRAPHIC DISTRIBUTION

Experience with RSV infection is ecumenical, as is its predominate pathogenicity for the very young and those with underlying high-risk conditions.[49, 301, 316, 401] The timing, length, and intensity of RSV outbreaks, however, vary geographically. Outbreaks in warm and tropical climates tend to be more prolonged, with less distinctive peaks of activity.

SEASONAL PATTERNS

RSV has the distinction of being the only viral respiratory pathogen that regularly produces an important outbreak of infection each year in urban areas.[254, 347] In the United States, RSV activity usually lasts for 20 or more weeks, from November to May.[377] The peak of activity for most areas is January and February, but it is usually slightly earlier in the Southeast. Epidemiologic patterns tend to be the same for other countries with similar temperate climates, whereas in warmer countries, RSV activity may correlate with the rainy seasons.

For 11 consecutive years, the annual arrival of RSV in Washington, D.C., has been associated with a regular increase in the number of children admitted to the hospital with acute lower respiratory tract disease. The yearly number of admissions did not vary by more than 2.7 times.[254] The consistent ramifications of this pathogen in a community have been used to detect its presence. The peak period of admissions each year for children with lower respiratory tract disease is associated mainly with RSV activity.[150, 179, 254] A rise in the number of cases of bronchiolitis or pediatric pneumonia reported from the outpatient offices in a community is also predictive of RSV's arrival[179] (Fig. 185–2). Similar to RSV, influenza A virus and sometimes parainfluenza virus may cause an increase in the number of respiratory tract infections in children in the community, but they do not cause a rise in the number of hospital admissions for respiratory disease consistently.

Usually, during RSV's peak activity in a community, the other major respiratory pathogens are absent or quiescant.[23, 153, 179] Even though outbreaks of RSV and influenza A infection may overlap, the peaks of the epidemics uncommonly coincide.

STRAIN VARIATION

Although RSV consistently causes an annual outbreak of respiratory illness, the severity of the outbreaks may vary from year to year.[197, 397] Variation in circulating strains has been suggested as partly accounting for the fluctuating clinical impact of RSV epidemics. The two major strain groups, A and B, circulate simultaneously during an outbreak, but the proportion of strains from each group may vary by season and geography, as does predominance of the subgroups of A and B strains.* In Rochester during a 20-year period, group A strains predominated in 11 of the years, and group A and B strains were relatively equal in another 5 years[197] (Fig. 185–3). In only four seasons did group B strains account for more than 75 percent of the year's isolates. In Cain, France, however, B strains predominated in 4 of 8 years and accounted for 64 percent of the isolates overall.[134] The strains from 14 cities across the United States over two consecutive seasons were shown to vary greatly, thus suggesting the influence of local rather than national factors.[19] Several distinct but varying genotypes within these strain groups predominate each year in a community, which suggests that homotypic immunity to previous strains may play a role.[18, 61, 319, 352, 420, 463]

The relationship between the circulating strain group and the size of an RSV outbreak does not appear to be strong or consistent, and correlation of strain groups with clinical severity requires further study[61, 197, 300, 341] (see Prognosis and Complications).

*See references 61, 82, 87, 197, 210, 351, 352, 420, 437, 459.

INCIDENCE AND PREVALENCE

RSV is the major cause of inpatient and outpatient pneumonia and bronchiolitis in infancy and early childhood. In young infants, RSV infection produces the greatest morbidity. RSV accounts for approximately 50 percent of all pneumonia in infancy and 50 to 90 percent of cases of bronchiolitis.[54, 76, 155, 205, 299, 326, 348] It also has been associated with 10 to 30 percent of cases of pediatric bronchitis.[254] In contrast, only a relatively small proportion, less than 10 percent, of croup cases have been associated with RSV infection.[155, 254] RSV is isolated rarely from patients (<1%) without respiratory disease.[75, 254]

Specific neutralizing antibody passively received from the mother is present in the sera of all newborns.[156, 347] The level of antibody in a term newborn is similar to the maternal level, with gradual decline in passive antibody during the first 6 months of life. In patients older than 7 months, detectable specific serum antibody is usually the result of natural infection. During the first year of life, approximately 50 to 70 percent or more of infants acquire RSV infection, most during the subsequent season.[151, 156, 157] Essentially all children by 3 years of age and all adults possess specific serum antibody.

Three generalizations may be made about the relationship of age and the incidence and type of RSV disease: (1) lower respiratory tract disease (pneumonia and bronchiolitis) is almost entirely confined to children younger than 3 years, (2) the occurrence of RSV lower respiratory tract disease during the first few weeks of life is relatively uncommon in comparison to the subsequent 6 to 9 months, and (3) reinfections are frequent in both older children and adults.[156, 157, 176, 196, 206, 254, 347]

In infants, the proportion of RSV infections that involve the lower respiratory tract is strikingly high but greatest during the first few months of life. The peak incidence of hospitalized cases of RSV bronchiolitis and pneumonia occurs in children 2 to 5 months of age.[150, 205, 206, 347] In Washington, D.C., approximately 40 percent of primary infections involved the lower respiratory tract, and of every 100 primary RSV infections, 1 resulted in hospital admission for bronchiolitis. In the Houston family studies, lower respiratory tract disease was the manifestation of 33 percent of infections in the first year of life and 16 to 23 percent in the subsequent 3 years[157] (Table 185–2). The risk of hospitalization for an infant infected with RSV during the first 12 months of life was 1.6 percent.

Infants from better socioeconomic environments tend to be older when they first acquire lower respiratory tract

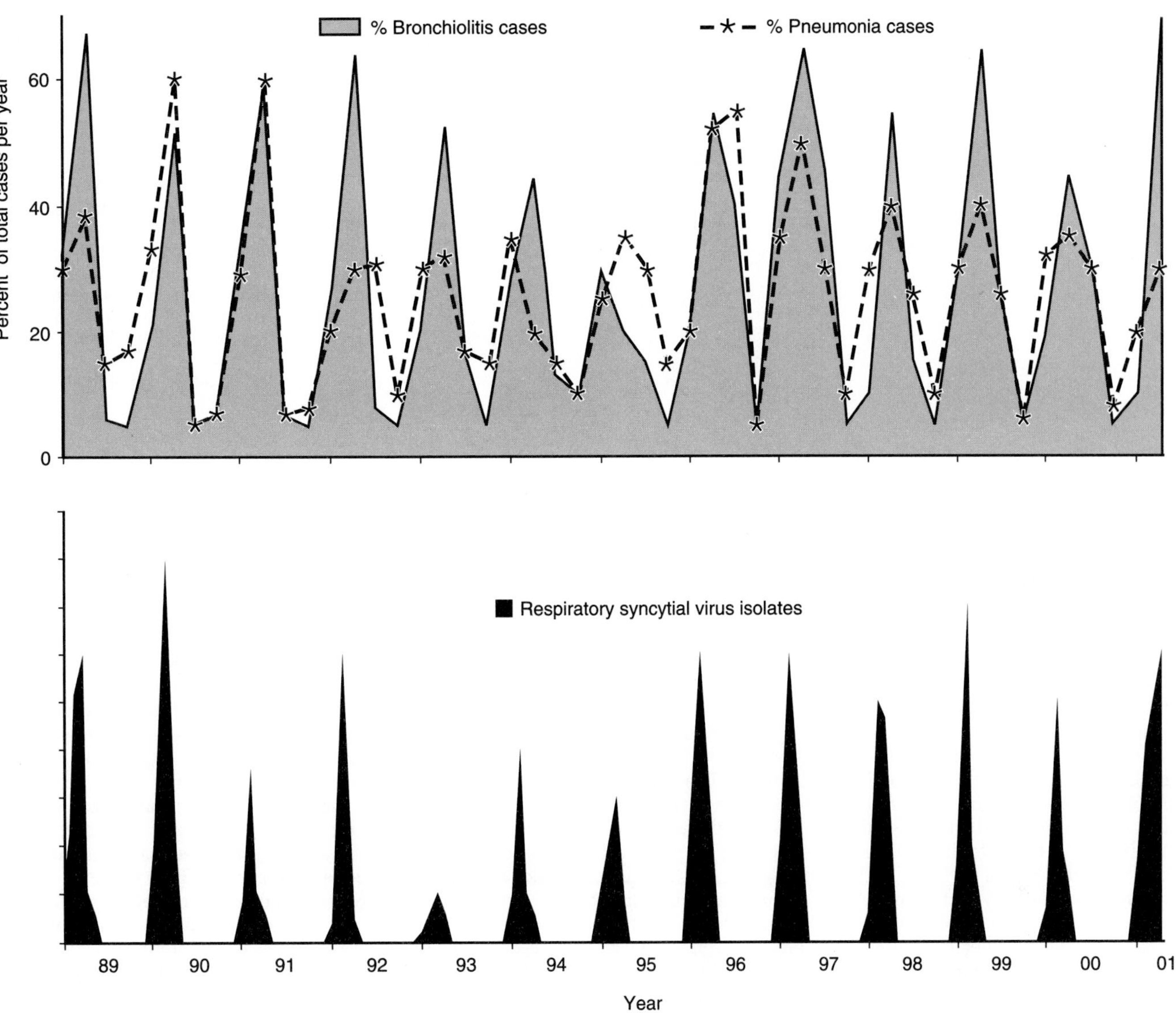

FIGURE 185–2 ■ The proportion of cases of pediatric bronchiolitis and pneumonia in children younger than 2 years reported in Rochester, New York, from 1989 through 2001 is shown in relation to the annual outbreaks of respiratory syncytial virus. The cases are reported weekly by private offices and clinics to the Community Infectious Diseases Surveillance system. The major peaks of bronchiolitis and pneumonia occurred simultaneously and in association with periods of isolation of respiratory syncytial virus.

disease from RSV, and they less frequently have severe disease.[299] In a private practice in Chapel Hill, North Carolina, only 13 percent of bronchiolitis patients were younger than 6 months, as compared with 40 percent in a daycare center and 56 percent of hospitalized cases.[103] The risk of hospitalization for RSV disease in infants from middle-income families in Chapel Hill was less than 1 in 1000, as opposed to a 5- to 10-fold greater risk for infants of low-income families in Houston and Washington, D.C.[156, 157] Similarly, rates of hospitalization for RSV disease have been lower in children from middle-income families in Seattle and a less urban area in Michigan.[131, 315] However, in Huntington, West Virginia, the risk of hospitalization for RSV during the first year of life was 1 per 88 live births.[44] In England, crowding and unemployment also seem to augment the risk of hospital admission.[376, 404] In the urban environs of Tyneside, 1 of every 50 infants required hospital admission during the first year of life for RSV infection.

In most studies of children hospitalized with RSV disease, males predominate in a ratio of approximately 2:1.[178, 347] However, in children with milder RSV illness, boys and girls are affected about equally, thus suggesting that gender influences the expression rather than the rate of illness, with more severe disease developing in boys.[103]

RSV infection in older age groups is a common occurrence. In Tecumseh, RSV infection detected by the relatively insensitive complement-fixation antibody test occurred most frequently in school-age children.[315] Twenty percent of children 5 to 9 years of age were shown to be infected within 1 year. The rate fell to 10 percent in family members 15 to 19 years of age and to 3 to 6 percent in those 20 to 50 years of age. When infection is assessed by viral isolation, the attack rate in family members exposed to young children with RSV infection is appreciable at all ages[157, 186] (Table 185–3). In school-age children and adult family members, the attack rate during an RSV epidemic varied between 38 and 43 percent.

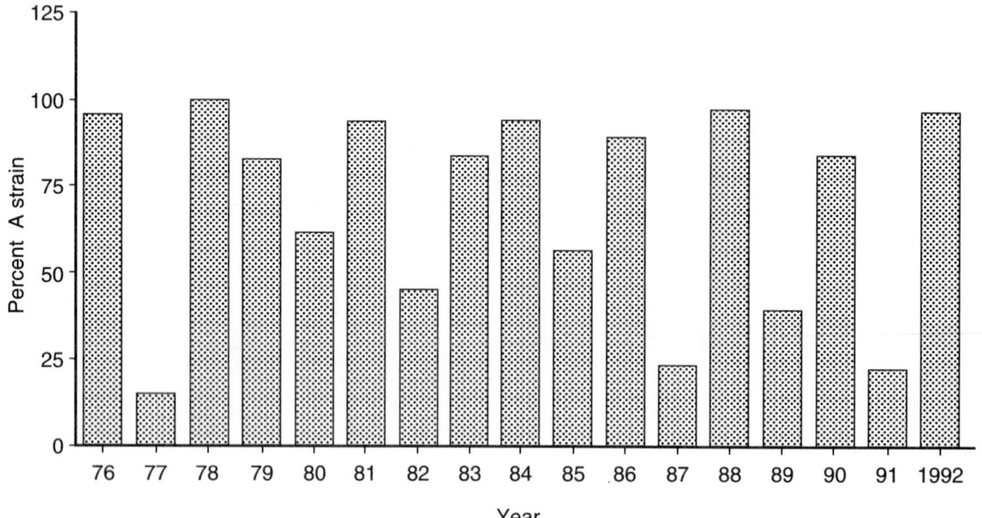

FIGURE 185–3 ■ Proportion of yearly (1976–1992) isolates of respiratory syncytial virus from the Rochester, New York, area that were group A strains. Data were obtained from 1619 respiratory syncytial virus isolates from hospitalized children and from outpatient children included in the Community Surveillance Program of the University of Rochester School of Medicine.

SPREAD OF INFECTION

Each breath's toll is virus spread and shed.[171]

C. B. H.

RSV spreads effectively through exposed families, and introduction of the virus into the family appears to occur most commonly through a school-age child.[47, 186, 315] Serious disease in infancy is, therefore, likely to follow a mild "cold" in an older sibling.[186] In a prospective study of families with an infant and one or more older siblings, 44 percent of the families became infected with RSV during a 3-month epidemic. In almost all these families, older siblings (2 to 16 years of age) introduced the virus into the family, and the infants became secondarily infected. Furthermore, intrafamilial spread of the virus, according to the Tecumseh study, was related to the number of family members.[315] Families with six members had approximately three times the rate of infection observed in families with three members.

The conundrum of how this labile virus can spread so effectively has not been solved. Transmission primarily by small-particle aerosol seems unlikely according to epidemiologic observations.[180, 184] Small-particle aerosols of RSV are unstable at the low relative humidity of 20 to 30 percent usually encountered indoors during the winter months.[372] At 30 and 80 percent relative humidity, RSV in aerosol was maximally inactivated. Maximal stability occurred at 60 percent relative humidity.

Spread may occur, however, through large droplets of secretions or through contact with contaminated secretions.[172, 180] RSV in the nasal secretions of infants with acute infection remains infectious on countertops for longer than 6 hours and on cloth and tissue paper for 30 minutes.[187] Furthermore, these nasal secretions remain infectious after transfer from objects or hands to the hands of another person, thus suggesting that contact with clothing, furniture, or tissue contaminated by the secretions of infected children may be one means of spread. This mode of spread has been supported by studies demonstrating that infection may occur in volunteers who touch surfaces contaminated by secretions and then their eyes or nasal mucosa.[180] In contrast, no infections developed in volunteers exposed to infected infants at a distance of greater than 6 feet, thus suggesting that small-particle aerosol spread of RSV was not a major mode of transmission. Spread of RSV therefore most frequently results from close contact with infected people or their infectious secretions, which tend to be profuse and prolonged in the young; spread is less dependent on the long-distance travel of small-particle aerosols.

TABLE 185–2 ■ FREQUENCY OF RESPIRATORY SYNCYTIAL VIRUS INFECTION IN CHILDREN STUDIED FROM BIRTH*

		No. with Respiratory Syncytial Virus				
Age (mo)	**No. of Child-Years**	*Primary*	*Reinfection*	*Total (Rate/100 Child-Years)*	*LRD (Rate/100 Child-Years)*	*LRD (Rate/100 Infections)*
0–12	125	85	1	86 (68.8)	28 (22.4)	32.6
13–24	92	33	43	76 (82.6)	12 (13.0)	15.8
25–36	65	1	29	30 (46.2)	7 (10.8)	23.3
37–48	39	0	13	13 (33.3)	3 (7.7)	23.1
49–60	24	0	12	12 (50.0)	0 (0)	—
Total	**345**	**119**	**98**	**217 (62.9)**	**50 (14.5)**	**23.0**

*Houston Family Study, 1975 through 1980.
LRD, lower respiratory tract disease.
From Glezen, W. P., Taber, L. H., Frank, A. L., et al.: Risk of primary infection and reinfection with respiratory syncytial virus. Am. J. Dis. Child. *140*:543–546, 1986.

TABLE 185–3 ■ ATTACK RATE OF RESPIRATORY SYNCYTIAL VIRUS IN FAMILIES ACCORDING TO AGE

	Attack Rate*					
	Crude Rate		*In RSV-Positive Families*		*Secondary Rate*	
Age (yr)	**No.†**	**%**	**No.†**	**%**	**No.†**	**%**
<1	10/34	29.4	10/16	62.5	5/11	45.4
1–<2	2/7	28.6	2/5	40.0	0/3	0.0
2–<5	9/34	26.4	9/19	47.0	2/12	16.6
5–<17	9/48	18.7	9/24	38.0	4/19	21.0
17–45	9/55	16.8	9/21	43.0	6/18	33.3
Total	39/178	21.9	39/85	45.9	17/63	27.0

*The crude attack rate according to age is shown for all family members studied and for members of RSV-positive families. The secondary attack rate is also shown for members of RSV-positive families, excluding all primary and co-primary cases.
†Number of persons infected with RSV/total number of persons exposed.
Reprinted, by permission, from Hall, C. B., Geiman, J. M., Biggar, R., et al.: Respiratory syncytial virus infection within families. N. Engl. J. Med. *294*:414–419, 1976.

Pathology and Pathogenesis

The newly born
from mother shorn,
A seed unsown
and shield unknown. . .

C. B. H.

The incubation period of illness from RSV has been reported as being variable, between 2 and 8 days, with 4 to 6 days being the most common.[242, 282, 414] Experimental infection in adult volunteers produced an average incubation period of 5 days.[235, 266] Inoculation is through the upper respiratory tract, and infection occurs in the respiratory epithelium. Both the eye and the nose appear to be equally sensitive routes of inoculation.[185] In contrast, inoculation by mouth much less frequently results in infection. Spread along the respiratory tract occurs mainly by cell-to-cell transfer of the virus along intracytoplasmic bridges. Spread from the upper to the lower respiratory tract may involve the conducting airways at all levels.

The major pathologic findings as shown in infants dying of RSV bronchiolitis are (1) peribronchiolar mononuclear infiltration, (2) necrosis of the epithelium of the small airways, (3) plugging of the lumina, and (4) hyperinflation and atelectasis (Fig. 185–4).[5, 8, 112, 144, 145, 174, 238, 441] The initial lesions in bronchiolitis occur in the small airways (75 to 300 μm).[8] Lymphocytic peribronchiolar infiltration develops along with edema of the walls, the submucosa, and adventitial tissue. Subsequently, the epithelium of the bronchioles undergoes striking necrosis, sometimes with proliferation of the epithelium into the lumen. The necrotic material is sloughed into the lumen of these small airways, thereby impeding the flow of air. In addition, the virus stimulates increased mucus secretion, which compounds the obstruction. The small lumina of an infant's airways are especially vulnerable to obstruction by the edema and exudate.

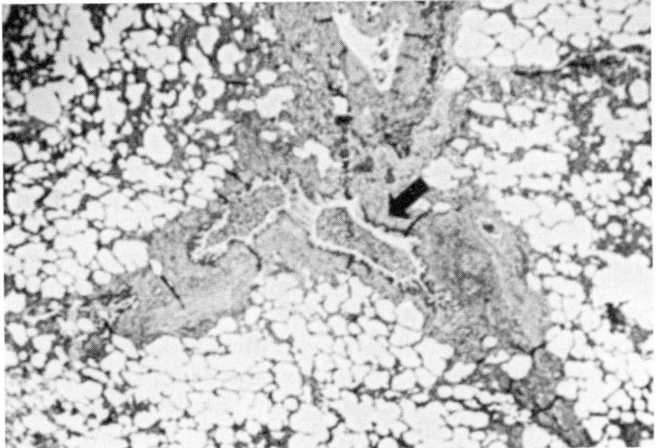

FIGURE 185–4 ■ Histologic examination of an infant dying of respiratory syncytial virus bronchiolitis. The *arrow* denotes a bronchiole filled with inflammatory exudate and comparatively normal alveoli.

Peripheral to the sites of partial occlusion, air trapping occurs similar to a ball-and-valve mechanism. During the negative intrapleural pressure of inspiration, air can flow past the site of partial obstruction. On expiration, however, the positive pressure narrows the lumen, and more complete obstruction and hyperinflation result. In areas where the bronchiolar lumina become completely obstructed, the trapped air may be absorbed and result in multiple areas of focal atelectasis. These pathologic changes adversely affect the mechanics of the infant's respiration by causing markedly increased lung volume and higher expiratory resistance.[477, 478]

Recovery from acute bronchiolitis may be noted histologically within a few days, but complete restoration may take weeks, and some morphologic changes remain.[8, 374] Regeneration of the bronchiolar epithelium may begin in 3 to 4 days, but ciliated cells are rarely present before 2 weeks.[8] The enlarged submucosal glands, augmented numbers of goblet cells, and muscular hypertrophy that often accompany acute bronchiolitis may persist.[374, 477, 478] Although complete clinical recovery is the rule, bronchiolitis may leave a rowen of subtle pathologic changes.

In RSV pneumonia, the characteristic finding is interstitial infiltration of mononuclear cells.[8, 145] In some cases, lymphocytic infiltration of the bronchiolar walls is also present. The lung parenchyma appears edematous, with areas of necrosis leading to alveolar filling, consolidation, and collapse.[8]

ROLE OF THE IMMUNE RESPONSE IN PATHOGENESIS

The characteristics of the immune response of an infant with RSV disease have evoked numerous theories of pathogenesis. Several observations have suggested that immunologic mechanisms may be the key to the severity of RSV lower respiratory tract disease in infancy. First, the most severe disease occurs during the period when the infant possesses specific maternal antibody. Second, this period is also the stage when the infant is immunologically immature. Third, children with high levels of circulating antibody induced by inactivated RSV vaccine had more severe disease than did their unvaccinated counterparts when naturally infected with RSV.[137, 243, 255] In addition, clinical expression of their disease, though exaggerated, was typical of the natural lower respiratory tract disease of infancy. Fourth, shedding of virus is frequently abundant and prolonged in the youngest and most severely affected infants.[182, 183] Immunologic reaction and injury may be more likely in infections in which the antigen persists for prolonged periods.[41]

From such observations, hypotheses that evolved to explain the severity of RSV lower respiratory tract disease in the first few months of life involved one or more immunologic processes, including an immune complex reaction occurring in the lung with viral antigen and maternally acquired IgG antibody, compounded by a lack of IgA secretory antibody; a cell-mediated immune reaction; and an IgE-mediated response in infants with bronchiolitis or wheezing.[74, 256, 467, 469, 470, 472] Alternatively or additionally, the immature development of the immune system and the airway in a young infant may be important in the disease's severity in early life.

The anatomy of a small infant's airway engenders more severe physiologic consequences from the inflammation and obstruction of infection because the proportion of total pulmonary flow resistance derived from the small peripheral airways is much greater than in older children.[214] Anatomic differences in the developing lung also may render it more susceptible to the pathologic sequelae of a viral infection.[374, 477] The submucosal glands of an infant are relatively larger and the collateral ventilation poorer. Hypoxemia, characteristic of RSV infection, tends to produce pulmonary vasoconstriction, which may interfere with normal development of the arterial wall during the first several months of life. The infantile lung may be not only more vulnerable but also less able to compensate for the insult of RSV inflammation.

These hypotheses thus emphasize the imbalance in components of the immune response from numerous potential factors engendered by the singular characteristics of RSV infection—its ubiquity and early age of acquisition. Adding credence to theories suggesting an integral role of the immunologic response in young infants are observations derived from field trials of the initial RSV vaccine.[74, 80, 137, 243, 255, 256, 323] Infants who received this formalin-inactivated vaccine had more severe lower respiratory tract disease than did their RSV-unvaccinated counterparts when they experienced subsequent natural infection with wild RSV. The inactivated vaccine produced little secretory antibody, and although serum antibody levels were high, not all antibody was functional, with some showing diminished neutralizing and fusion-inhibiting capacity.[323, 324] Furthermore, these vaccinated children exhibited an augmented cell-mediated immune response.[256]

More recent studies have suggested a protective role for specific passive or maternal antibody.[156, 169, 175, 338, 345, 359, 373, 462] Furthermore, complement cannot be detected in the lungs of infants dying of RSV disease, nor do the levels of complement fall during the acute phase of illness, as may be expected in an immune complex process.[14] If antibody has a detrimental role, however, it may not be enacted via an immune complex mechanism but rather by enhancement of viral replication.[267]

Multiple immunologic and host factors probably contribute in varying degrees to the pathogenicity of RSV in individual infants. Factors known to be associated with potentially severe RSV disease, however, may be summarized as (1) young age; (2) immunologic immaturity or deficiency; (3) preexisting maternal antibody, which is most likely just a marker of young age; (4) certain underlying diseases, especially prematurity and functionally significant cardiopulmonary disease; (5) abundant and prolonged viral shedding; and (6) administration of the formalin-inactivated vaccine. Whether these factors are intertwining correlates or causes remains a conundrum.

Immune Response

The focus of much recent investigation to delineate the nature of the immune response to RSV has revealed pivotal new pieces of the mosaic of immunity. This information is likely to aid in the development of an effective vaccine and control of RSV infection.

Immunity to RSV infection is variable, incomplete, and not durable. Infections occur throughout life and sometimes even within the same season. Infants may have repetitive lower respiratory tract infections, but the infections that subsequently occur are rarely as severe as the primary infection. This factor, plus the observation that RSV infection after the first several years of life primarily involves the upper respiratory tract, indicates that immunity, though not perfect, does develop.

SERUM ANTIBODY

Maternal antibody is present in essentially all newborns of at least 32 weeks' gestation when appreciable amounts of IgG antibodies are acquired transplacentally. The potentially protective role of maternal antibody has been supported by the correlation of higher levels with older age of the infant at the time of primary infection.[156, 338] Maternal antibody usually declines to undetectable levels by 6 months of age, but it may sometimes remain detectable up to 9 to 12 months of age.[74] Infants with primary infection produce specific serum IgM antibody within several days that is detectable for only a few weeks.[217, 468] Immunoglobulin antibody subsequently appears in the second week, peaks in the fourth week, and declines after 1 to 2 months. The IgA serum antibody response in infants tends to be limited and may not be detectable, depending on the assay.[98, 217, 322, 468] After reinfection, the serum antibody response in all three immunoglobulin classes is enhanced, and antibody titers reach levels similar to those of adults after approximately three infections. Although high levels of IgG antibody to RSV tend to be associated with protection against infection, correlation of the level of specific humoral antibody to susceptibility and clinical severity is relatively poor and not consistently predictive.[99, 196] In animal models, the level of RSV neutralizing antibody correlates well with protection against infection of the lower respiratory tract, but not the upper respiratory tract.[100, 360, 362, 363, 460]

The benefits afforded by specific antibody depend on numerous factors other than titer, including the type, function, and specificity of the protein. The two surface glycoproteins F and G are clearly integral in the immune response. Neutralizing epitopes are present on both F and G, and a fusion epitope is also present on F.[274, 453, 457, 458] Monoclonal antibodies to the F and G proteins but not to the internal proteins N, P, and M, when passively transferred to rodents, afford protection against subsequent RSV challenge.[363, 426, 457, 460]

Immunization with the F, G, and N proteins in experimental animals also produces lower respiratory tract resistance, but the degree of protection varies according to the animal model.[90, 91] The rodent model has verified the broader, heterologous immunity induced by the F protein, whereas antibody induced by the G protein has provided little protection against challenge with a heterologous strain.[90, 236, 409, 457, 473, 474] Immunization with the G but not the F protein also can result in eosinophilic pathology in the mouse lung.[343]

In humans, the roles of F and G proteins also appear integral to the development of immunity to RSV. The response to these proteins in infants, however, is affected by several factors. The quantitative and qualitative humoral response of infants is influenced by the presence of preexisting maternal antibody, by age, and by the particular viral antigens. After infection, young children are able to produce antibodies against both the major surface glycoproteins, F and G, but in the youngest infants the responses are inconsistent, especially to the G protein.[99, 209, 322, 432, 462, 470] The heavily glycosylated G protein is a poorer immunogen in the young, and preexisting serum antibody appears to have a greater dampening effect on response to the G than to the F protein.[209, 321, 322] The effect of young age, however, is greater on the F and IgG antibody responses than on the development of IgM antibody.[321, 432]

The subclass of antibody formed to the F and G proteins is mainly IgG1 and IgG3, the subclasses primarily associated with antibodies to proteins, rather than IgG2, the subclass associated with antibody to carbohydrates.[99] Because the F and G proteins are heavily glycosylated, the lack of an IgG2 response is notable.[318, 448] Adults experimentally infected with RSV responded to the G protein with both IgG1 and IgG2 subclass antibodies, whereas the response to F protein is predominantly IgG1.[449] In addition, the avidity of antibody formed after primary infection versus reinfection differs. In infants with primary infection, the antibody to G protein is of low avidity, whereas the G antibody of adults and in passively derived maternal antibody is of high avidity.[311]

The role of antibodies to the F and G proteins in protection against infection, reinfection, or illness is not entirely delineated. In adults who were challenged with RSV after natural infection, levels of antibody to the F and homologous G proteins and levels of neutralizing antibody to the homologous strain correlated with resistance to reinfection.[196] Protection against symptomatic infection correlated more with antibody to the homologous G protein. The infecting strain also is likely to be a factor in determining the immune and possibly the clinical response. During primary infection, the homologous and heterologous antibody responses to the F proteins of both major subgroups appear to be similar, but there is little heterologous response to the G proteins.[209] Limited data suggest that previous infection with group A strains provides more resistance to reinfection with the homologous or heterologous strain.[209, 318, 319]

LOCAL HUMORAL RESPONSE

Because RSV spreads from cell to cell, it may mostly escape the net of serum neutralizing antibody, thus emphasizing the possible importance of local humoral and cell-mediated immune responses. In animal models, circulating specific antibody has not generally ablated viral replication in the upper respiratory tract, although the administration of high titers of IgG antibody has diminished nasal RSV levels and afforded lower respiratory tract protection.[363, 391, 460] Viral replication has been diminished more effectively in the rodent respiratory tract by local IgA antibody than by serum IgG antibody, but the IgA response and any associated protection are relatively short lived, less than 8 months, whereas IgG antibody in the lower respiratory tract is more durable.[161, 363] Although the neutralizing activity of nasal secretions in children with RSV infection has been examined, correlation with protection from infection or severe disease has not been consistent.[72, 304, 312, 393] In many infants, neutralizing activity was present in the nasal secretions at the time of the infant's admission. The neutralizing activity also appeared to be nonspecific, not related to susceptibility to infection but to diminished viral shedding.[72, 304, 312] Specific IgA antibody, however, can be detected in the nasal secretions of infants of all ages in response to RSV infection, but it may not be neutralizing and does not appear to have a clear role in recovery or in protection against reinfection.[196, 248, 302, 304]

Specific IgA, IgG, IgM, and transient IgE antibodies are present in the secretions of most infected infants.[143, 304, 465] With primary infection, specific IgA, IgG, and IgM antibodies are present in nasal secretions by 3 days in half or more of infants.[217, 248] IgA antibody appears early, with IgM and IgG antibodies peaking in the second week; all three usually disappear within 1 to 3 months. These secretory antibodies are directed to the F, G, and N proteins in both the IgG and IgA isotypes in the nasal washes of infants with primary infection, but IgA tends to dominate.[322] In younger infants, nasal antibody is present less often and in lower quantities. After secondary infection, levels are boosted and more persistent.[217, 248] Small amounts of specific IgE antibody also are produced frequently in the secretions of infants in the early days of acute primary infection.[57, 467, 472] Higher and more persistent titers of IgE and histamine, however, appear to be pathogenic and associated with wheezing and more severe disease acutely and with subsequent airway hyperreactivity.[467, 471, 472] Specific IgE antibody may stimulate a cascade of inflammatory mediators and produce the clinical manifestations of wheezing and hyperreactivity.[146, 398, 429, 446, 447, 469, 470] In vitro and clinical findings suggest that the production of specific antibody results in the release of bronchoactive leukotrienes such as leukotriene C_4 and eosinophil cationic protein, and they may be present in elevated quantities in bronchiolitis.[15, 146, 335, 400, 446, 447, 469, 479]

CELLULAR IMMUNITY

Cellular immunity appears to be most important in recovery and viral clearance. Patients with compromised cell-mediated immunity have more severe and prolonged disease and viral shedding, which suggests that $CD4^+$ and $CD8^+$ T lymphocytes are pivotal in controlling infection. Most of our knowledge of the components and contributions of the cellular response to immunity has come from carefully designed studies in experimental animals, some of which were stimulated by the desire to explain the unfortunate outcome of trials with the formalin-inactivated vaccine.

Active viral infections, including natural RSV infection, usually stimulate helper T cells with a T_H1 cytokine profile (interleukin-2, interferon-γ). In contrast, inactivated or nonreplicating antigens characteristically evoke a T_H2 cytokine pattern (interleukin-4 to interleukin-6). A T_H1-type response usually requires the antigen to be processed in context with class I histocompatibility proteins, which results in the production of IgG2a neutralizing antibody and $CD8^+$

cytotoxic T lymphocytes (CTLs). T_H2 responses, on the other hand, process antigens in association with class II histocompatibility proteins, with the subsequent synthesis of IgG1 but without CTLs. Rodent models have demonstrated that T_H1 responses are evoked by live RSV infection.[109, 159, 164] Specific CTLs have been identified in the liver and spleen of mice after RSV challenge.[34, 427]

The T_H1 response has been demonstrated in vitro to occur in both adults and children, and specific CTLs have been identified in the peripheral blood of adults previously infected with RSV.[22, 35] The pattern of T-cell and cytokine responses evoked in humans is less well delineated.[466] In vitro infection of human peripheral blood mononuclear cells with RSV produces not only interleukin-1 but also inhibitors to interleukin-1.[381] The impaired lymphoproliferative response is evoked only by live, replicating RSV and consists of cell cycle arrest and no proliferative response to mitogens or nonviral antigens. Inactivated virus or live influenza does not result in similar inhibition.[358, 381, 389, 390] These findings may be hypothesized as partly explaining the susceptibility to repetitive RSV infection. Such a cellular inhibitory response may not only be detrimental to recovery from acute RSV but also may dampen the secondary immune response on reinfection.

The clinical effects of these cell-mediated responses in humans are not well defined, but experimental infection in volunteers has suggested that the specific CTL responses are associated with diminished symptoms.[224, 466] Limited data in infants with primary infection suggest that a cell-mediated response with specific CTLs is variably evoked within the first 10 days of infection and that depressed lymphocyte function and several T-cell subsets, along with depressed IL-12 levels and elevated IL-8 levels, are associated with more severe disease.[2, 50, 51, 79, 104, 224]

The N, F, and M2 proteins are targets for CTLs in both rodents and humans.[78, 331, 342] SH, M, and NS2 proteins additionally have been shown to be recognized by human CTLs. CTL responses to G, F, N, and M2 have been associated with resistance to infection in mice, but the protective effect to the N and M2 proteins tends to be transient.[93]

The contribution of the various T-cell subsets to clearance and convalescence from RSV infection has been shown to be complicated and confusing.[164] The type of antigen used for primary immunization is important. In mice, helper T-cell cytokine mRNA expression in the lungs has been shown to differ in animals immunized with live and with inactivated virus; the former stimulates a T_H1-type response with the production of CD4 cells, the characteristic T_H1 cytokines, IgG2a, and CTLs, in contrast to the T_H2 pattern resulting from challenge with the inactivated virus.[33, 64, 163–165, 320] These specific helper T-cell responses, however, are affected by the specific RSV proteins. Immunization with F protein stimulates a T_H1 cytokine response and $CD4^+$ and $CD8^+$ cells. On the other hand, immunization with one G protein produces a T_H2 cytokine pattern with only $CD4^+$ cells.[11, 13] After M2 inoculation, only $CD8^+$ cells are produced.

Graham and colleagues[160–163, 165] have characterized the evoked T-cell subsets in mice and their functional contributions after infection with live and inactivated RSV further. With live RSV infection, mice depleted of $CD4^+$ or $CD8^+$ cells demonstrated prolonged viral shedding but were able to clear the virus. If both subsets were depleted, viral shedding remained high and prolonged. In immune mice depleted of $CD4^+$ cells, $CD8^+$ cells, or both, rechallenge with live RSV resulted in little effect on the ability to clear the infection. Experiments that passively transferred RSV-specific $CD4^+$ or $CD8^+$ cells diminished viral replication in the lung, but in some studies they have been associated with an increase in both morbidity and pathology.[12, 63, 320] The variable degree of pathologic findings in these studies in the murine model may relate to the quantity, timing, specificity, and types of T cells infused or evoked.[45, 90, 159, 164, 226, 238, 412, 434]

These studies in experimental animals offer a possible and piquant explanation for the exaggerated disease observed in infants who had received the formalin-inactivated vaccine. The vaccine, altered from live virus by formalin inactivation, produced an abnormal and unbalanced primary immunization in infants that possibly entailed multiple components of the immune response. As noted earlier, little secretory antibody was produced, and the serum antibody was deficient in neutralizing and fusion-inhibiting activity. However, humoral antibody does not appear to be the major factor in producing the pathologic response because in mice, passive transfer of antibody induced by the formalin-inactivated vaccine did not result in a similar pathologic pulmonary picture. The most widely held explanation currently is that the altered antigens of the formalin-inactivated vaccine, rather than producing the predominant T_H1-type response usually seen with live viral infections, resulted in an imbalance in T_H1 and T_H2 lymphocyte responses. The rodent studies depicting the involved discrete lymphocytic subsets showed that the formalin-inactivated vaccine produced abundant virus-specific memory T cells, $CD4^+$ cells of the T_H2 phenotype, which could be visualized as the predominant cell type in the pulmonary pathology. The plethora of $CD4^+$ cells, however, was not accompanied by an RSV-specific $CD8^+$ CTL response.[160–163, 165] On reinfection with wild RSV, therefore, the memory cells present and able to respond were $CD4^+$ cells. Their rapid proliferation and characteristic inflammatory effects would be unchecked by $CD8^+$ cells, important in the clearance of infection, and also would be unmodified by the presence of local secretory antibody or adequate function of serum antibodies.

These rodent studies further indicated that RSV-specific $CD8^+$ cells also may contribute to the pathologic response to RSV disease. In both immunodeficient and normal mice, clearance of RSV was augmented by CTLs, but so was the lung pathology.[63, 164] Further studies, such as those described previously,[160–163, 165] have indicated that both $CD4^+$ and $CD8^+$ cell subsets are probably involved in the pathologic response, as well as in recovery and protection. This finding supports the hypothesis that a finely tuned and complicated balance among the T-cell subsets and other components of the immune response must be achieved for a beneficial response after natural infection or immunization.[220]

Clinical Manifestations

We view their chests ballooning, with the fears
that they're "pink puffers" of more tender years.[171]

PRIMARY INFECTION

An infant's first encounter with RSV almost always is apparent, but the symptoms may range from those of a mild cold to severe bronchiolitis or pneumonia.[75, 254, 347] RSV rarely is isolated from children with no signs of respiratory illness.[75, 254] The risk of lower respiratory tract disease occurring during this initial experience is high but varies with the setting. Parrott and associates[347] have estimated that 40 percent of primary infections result in febrile pneumonitis, but only a small proportion require hospital admission. According to their estimates, 1 percent of all primary RSV infections led to hospital admission for bronchiolitis.[254] In view of the universal nature of RSV infection, even a small percentage is magnified into the appreciable health and economic problem of an estimated 91,000 infants hospitalized for RSV infection each year in the United States alone.[204]

Certain populations of children are at particularly high risk for lower respiratory tract involvement with primary as well as secondary RSV infection. Higher rates of lower respiratory tract disease have been documented to occur in closed populations and in children from certain geographic areas or with particular ethnic backgrounds or underlying conditions.[242, 245, 282, 289, 301, 405, 414, 464] In daycare centers, the rate of infection is particularly high, not only for primary infection but also in each of the subsequent years for recurrent infection.[206]

In the longitudinal Houston family studies, 69 percent of children in their first year of life acquired RSV infection, and one third of these infections were lower respiratory tract illnesses[157] (see Table 185–2). By 24 months of age, essentially all children had been infected at least once, and half had experienced two infections, such that the rate of infections during the second year of life was 83 percent. The proportion of RSV infections involving the lower respiratory tract remains appreciable during the second, third, and fourth years of life, but the severity decreases (see Tables 185–2 and 185–3). Pneumonia and bronchiolitis occur with diminishing frequency and are replaced by tracheobronchitis and reactive airway disease.[157]

Pneumonia and bronchiolitis are the most common manifestations of RSV lower respiratory tract disease. Croup occurs least commonly, usually accounting for less than 5 percent of cases.[347] In different locations, the ratio of pneumonia to bronchiolitis generally has ranged from 1:1 to 7:1. This variability may stem partly from the difficulty and lack of standard criteria to clinically differentiate bronchiolitis from pneumonia. Wheezing may occur in both syndromes, as may infiltrates on chest radiographs.[141, 253, 379] In bronchiolitis, these shadows are mostly the result of atelectasis rather than the interstitial inflammation and alveolar filling of pneumonia. Radiographic differentiation of the pathogenesis of the observed infiltrates often cannot be achieved. Bronchiolitis is usually clinically defined by the presence of the two cardinal signs: wheezing and hyperinflation of the lung. In pneumonia, the infiltrates on chest radiographs may be accompanied by rales and rhonchi, with or without wheezing. The two syndromes often are combined, and pneumonia appears to be a continuum of bronchiolitis.

The signs associated with lower respiratory tract illness caused by RSV are shown in Table 185–4. Upper respiratory tract symptoms commonly precede lower respiratory tract involvement by several days. Fever occurs commonly in the initial phase of the illness, but by the time of hospitalization, it may be low grade or have disappeared. In a study of 565 hospitalized children with RSV infection, less than half had temperatures higher than 38°C at the time of admission.[194] The duration of fever is usually 2 to 7 days and tends to be milder in infants younger than 6 months than in those 6 to 12 months of age. Although fever occurs more commonly in primary infections, approximately 20 to 40 percent of children with their second, third, or fourth infections are febrile.[206]

Cough also becomes a consistent and prominent finding. Increased coughing may herald lower respiratory tract involvement, which with progression is commonly accompanied by retractions of the chest wall and dyspnea, especially in bronchiolitis. Crackles commonly accompany the wheezing and hyperinflation of bronchiolitis, and wheezes sometimes

TABLE 185–4 ■ SIGNS IN CHILDREN WITH RESPIRATORY SYNCYTIAL VIRAL INFECTIONS

	Percentage of Hospitalized Infants*	Percentage of Ambulatory Infants and Young Children†
Fever	45–65	74–100
Cough	97–100	83–100
Rhinitis	56–82	45–73
Pharyngitis	45–54	20–30
Hoarseness	—	6–20
Dyspnea	50–78	70–90
Retractions	36–68	40–100
Cyanosis	11–25	—
Wheezing	45–76	17–34
Rales	27–72	60–75
Rhonchi	59–78	15–90
Otitis	31	10–34
Conjunctivitis	9	15–30
Vomiting	45–52	20–27

*Data from reference 46 (93% of infants had lower respiratory tract disease), reference 140 (87% of infants had lower respiratory tract disease), and Hall, C. B. (unpublished data on 637 hospitalized infants with lower respiratory tract disease).

†Data from reference 375 (outpatients with bronchiolitis and pneumonia), reference 439 (patients from a British practice survey, two thirds with lower respiratory tract disease), and Hall, C. B. (unpublished data on 434 outpatient children, one third with lower respiratory tract disease).

accompany the crackles in pneumonia.[189, 205, 375] The duration of illness is usually 7 to 12 days.[46, 183] Most infants hospitalized with RSV bronchiolitis or pneumonia show clinical improvement after 3 to 4 days, and most previously normal infants are discharged within 3 to 7 days[182, 189, 305] (Fig. 185–5).

The clinical appearance of improvement, however, often belies the continued inflammation and prolonged physiologic abnormalities in a young infant.[182, 183, 305] In infants hospitalized with RSV lower respiratory tract disease, viral shedding commonly continues despite clinical improvement, and it may be accompanied by continued abnormalities in arterial oxygen saturation, which most likely arise from an abnormally low ratio of ventilation to perfusion rather than from shunting.[182, 183, 189, 194, 378, 477] During hospitalization, the degree of hypoxemia may fluctuate throughout the day, thus necessitating repetitive measurements and monitoring in

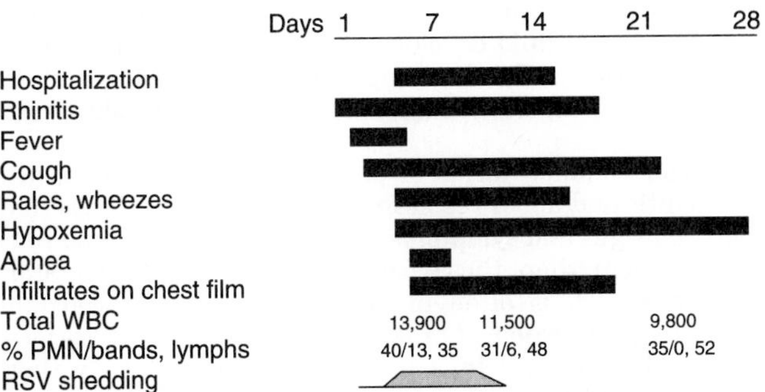

FIGURE 185–5 ■ The course of this 8-week-old infant with pneumonia caused by respiratory syncytial virus (RSV) is characteristic of the course of young infants hospitalized with RSV lower respiratory tract disease. WBC, total white blood cell count per cubic millimeter; % PMN/bands, lymphs, percentage of polymorphonuclear cells, bands, and lymphocytes in the peripheral white blood cell count.

the more severely ill. At discharge, infants may continue to have some degree of hypoxemia. Full recovery from the pathologic processes in the lung may take weeks, the time required for regeneration of the bronchiolar epithelium (see Pathology and Pathogenesis).

Numerous findings have been associated with an increased risk for severe disease and hospitalization.[341, 350, 397] Most of these findings, however, have relatively poor predictive value for individual patients. Among the more consistent and helpful findings are oxygen saturation and global assessment of the degree of illness (i.e., the overall picture of how sick, toxic, or compromised the infant appears to an experienced clinician). Fever does not correlate with severity. Cyanosis is not always present, even in the face of moderate degrees of hypoxemia. The often rapid fluctuations in manifestations, such as retractions and the respiratory rate, are characteristic of moderate to severe RSV lower respiratory disease and further compound the ability to accurately determine the severity of an infant's illness. Making repetitive assessments is often necessary.

The radiographic picture is variable and correlates poorly with severity or outcome. Chest radiographs are not usually necessary for the diagnosis and management of RSV lower respiratory tract disease. Measurements of arterial oxygen saturation, usually by oximetry, physical examination, and the clinical course are frequently more useful and sensitive.

The radiographic findings in infants hospitalized with RSV lower respiratory tract disease include a variety of patterns.[136, 141, 253, 379, 403] The most typical finding is a diffuse interstitial pneumonitis, commonly accompanied by hyperinflation of the lung.[379] In nearly 66 percent of cases, interstitial infiltrates are present in all lobes, and in approximately 20 percent of cases, they are present in only one lobe.[379] In Newcastle-upon-Tyne, hyperaeration was observed in more than 50 percent and peribronchial thickening in 39 percent of children hospitalized with RSV bronchiolitis, pneumonia, or both.[141, 403] Air trapping is particularly indicative of RSV infection and may be the only abnormality. Peribronchial thickening also may be the only finding, but its presence in the Newcastle studies did not correlate more with RSV than with other infections. Alveolar pneumonia, which appears as lobar or segmental consolidation, is evident in about one fourth of children with RSV lower respiratory tract disease, especially in infants younger than 6 months.[136, 141, 403] Lobar or segmental consolidation was noted in about one fifth of the children hospitalized in Chapel Hill, and the right upper lobe was involved in all cases.[379] Consolidated-appearing areas may be caused by pneumonia or atelectasis. Collapse of the lung or demonstrable pleural fluid development is rare. The radiographic abnormalities tend to last longer than the clinical symptoms and signs, with consolidated areas being the slowest to clear.[379]

Other common forms of primary infection are tracheobronchitis and upper respiratory tract infection. The accompanying signs and symptoms in primary infection tend to be more severe than those from other common respiratory agents. Cough is often predominant and prolonged, and fever may be present. Otitis media is frequently associated with RSV infection in young children, particularly those younger than 1 year.[27, 28, 46, 83, 84, 186, 207, 208, 440] RSV has been detected in middle ear aspirates, alone or simultaneously with a bacterial pathogen, thus suggesting that RSV may play both a primary and a secondary role in the pathogenesis of otitis media.[27, 28, 83, 203, 207, 340, 349, 440] RSV-induced otitis media also has been associated with prolonged symptoms and apparent failure of therapy.[27, 28]

REPEATED INFECTION

In Children

Repeated RSV infections are common.[39, 103, 157, 186, 206, 315] Between 6 and 83 percent of children monitored longitudinally have been reinfected each year.[103, 157, 206] The intervals between infections may be no longer than the period between successive outbreaks of RSV infection or even less.[39, 157, 206] Repeated RSV infections are usually but not always milder and consist of tracheobronchitis or an upper respiratory tract infection.[103, 157, 206, 438] Children nevertheless may experience repeated bouts of RSV lower respiratory tract disease. In preschool children, 20 to more than 50 percent of repeated infections involve the lower respiratory tract.[157, 206]

In the longitudinal study of children in a Chapel Hill daycare center, the attack rate for the first infection was 98 percent and, for the second and third infections, 75 and 65 percent, respectively.[206] Of note was the finding that immunity resulting from a single infection appeared to have no ameliorating effect on illness associated with reinfection 1 year later. Not until the third infection was severity reduced appreciably, thus suggesting that both age and immune factors are important. However, the initial illnesses in these children in daycare were relatively mild. In contrast, infants with first infections severe enough to require hospitalization rarely appear to have second or repeated infections of equal severity unless they have an underlying disease that places them at high risk for complications.

In the Houston longitudinal studies, infants in families had similarly high rates of reinfection.[157] Of those experiencing primary infection during the first year of life, 76 percent were reinfected by 24 months of age. One fourth of these second infections involved the lower respiratory tract, but they tended to be mild. Most children had lower respiratory tract illness only once, and those with repetitive lower respiratory tract infections tended to have reactive airway disease.

In Adults

RSV most commonly produces upper respiratory tract illness in adults.[173, 176] In the 1960s, Beem[39] isolated RSV from adults, and Hamre and Procknow[200] recovered the virus from 15 medical students with naturally acquired upper respiratory infection. RSV accounted for more than one fourth of the viruses recovered from these students with colds. In approximately two thirds of military recruits, RSV infection was manifested as a mild upper respiratory tract infection, whereas the rest were asymptomatic.[234] These older studies and those of experimental infection in adult volunteers therefore suggested that in a healthy adult, RSV infection is either asymptomatic or limited to upper respiratory tract manifestations.[235, 266]

Subsequently, however, RSV has been shown in some previously healthy adults to produce more severe illness such as bronchitis, wheezing, and an influenza-like illness.[173, 176, 177] Individuals in contact with young children, such as parents and pediatric hospital staff, frequently acquire infection.[173, 175–177, 184, 186, 196, 198] In these groups, most infections appear to be symptomatic and consist of upper respiratory tract infection with or without fever and tracheobronchitis. Approximately 70 percent of these patients have had an illness more severe and prolonged than the usual "cold" from other causes. Malaise, nasal congestion, and cough may persist for an average of 10 to 14 or more days.[186, 198] Studies by Smith and colleagues[406] from the Cambridge Health Psychology Research Unit have indicated by visual perception tests in experimentally infected volunteers that susceptibility to more symptomatic illness from RSV, but not from other viruses, may be related to behavioral measures. Lower respiratory tract abnormalities, predominantly hyperreactivity of the airway to cholinergic stimuli, also have been detected by pulmonary function studies in young, previously healthy adults.[176, 198] The more severe disease sometimes seen in these groups of adults may relate partly to a high challenge dose from intimate exposure to infants with primary infection because such infants shed high titers of virus abundantly. More severe illness, however, also has been described in both institutionalized and previously normal, community-dwelling adults.[111, 129]

Interest in RSV's role in illness in the elderly has expanded recently. Early in RSV's clinical career, a few reports noted that RSV could cause acute exacerbations of illness in patients with chronic bronchitis.[68, 314, 408] RSV was subsequently recognized in the elderly as a cause of acute and often severe lower respiratory tract disease requiring hospitalization.[133, 257, 445] With the recent increase in recognition and investigation of RSV infection in older populations, researchers have found that RSV clearly possesses potential pathogenicity for multiple groups of older individuals—from those healthy and living in the community to those institutionalized.* Various manifestations of RSV ranging from mostly asymptomatic and mild upper respiratory infection to severe, even fatal lower respiratory tract infection may occur in this population. RSV infection in this population may be commonly manifested as an exacerbation of an underlying condition, particularly cardiac and pulmonary disease, and the viral etiology may not be suspected.[17, 122, 454] The lower respiratory tract disease in this older population also may be combined with concurrent bacterial infection.

Between 2 and 9 percent of all lower respiratory tract hospitalizations in the elderly (14,000 to 62,000 pneumonia hospitalizations) have been estimated to be caused by RSV, with a cost of $150 million to $680 million annually.[17, 201] Not included in these estimates are the additional hospitalizations and cost associated with exacerbations of underlying chronic conditions.

With the increasing numbers of immunocompromised patients, the pathogenicity of RSV in high-risk adult patients has been a growing concern, and the hazard of its nosocomial transmission has been emphasized.[52, 96, 118, 175, 288, 424, 476] Outbreaks in bone marrow transplant units may be devastating, difficult to control, and often not recognized because the manifestations may mimic those seen with other agents more commonly associated with an immunocompromised host. The reported mortality from RSV outbreaks in bone marrow transplant units has ranged from 20 to 100 percent.

INFECTION IN NEONATES

Infection with RSV in the first 4 weeks of life appears to be relatively infrequent.[254, 347, 348] In Washington, D.C., the incidence of RSV infection during the first month of life was noted to be only one third of that during the second month of life. The protected environment of newborns with diminished exposure to others, as well as the high levels of maternal antibody or other early immune factors, may explain in part the generally lower incidence of illness in the newborn period. RSV infection nevertheless may occur during this period, and its clinical expression may be variable, with few or no respiratory signs of severe infection.[190, 354, 385, 407] The atypical clinical features often have resulted in the diagnosis being unsuspected or delayed.[190, 309] In a Newcastle nursery, eight babies were infected and all became symptomatic, usually in the second week of life. The illness was generally mild in these infants and consisted of upper respiratory tract symptoms and cough. Only one infant had radiographic evidence of pneumonia, although three had mild wheezing.[105, 142] In Rochester, 25 percent of infants in a neonatal special care unit for more than 6 days acquired RSV infection during the 3 months that RSV was prevalent in the community.[190] Premature infants were particularly susceptible, the illness was often atypical, and the manifestations appeared to be related to age. Infants older than 3 weeks tended to have the classic lower respiratory tract disease and apnea, whereas babies in the first 3 weeks of life uncommonly had clinical evidence of lower respiratory tract involvement at initial evaluation. Less than half of these younger neonates had upper respiratory tract signs. Most of them had nonspecific signs such as poor feeding, lethargy, and irritability. Nevertheless, four (17%) died, and death was sudden and unexpected in two.

NOSOCOMIAL INFECTION

More than a half a century ago, in 1941, Adams[3] described an epidemic of pneumonitis that occurred in January through February in the nurseries of two Minneapolis hospitals. Thirty-two infants, mostly in the second and third months of life, were affected, and 29 percent died. Cytoplasmic inclusions in bronchial epithelium were observed in all fatal cases. The distinctive epidemiology, clinical syndrome, and pathology of these cases led Adams to propose a viral etiology. Twenty years later, he and his colleagues described a markedly similar epidemic of respiratory illness in infants during which they identified RSV as the cause.[4, 5] RSV was thus indicted as the agent of the earlier, first described nosocomial outbreak.

Nosocomial infection with RSV has become recognized now as a problem of increasing magnitude, especially in immunocompromised patients.* During RSV epidemics, the risk of nosocomial infection spreading from infants hospitalized with RSV lower respiratory tract disease to other infants on the ward admitted with compromising illnesses is high. If RSV is not recognized as a potential nosocomial hazard and specific infection control procedures are not ready to be initiated at the start of the RSV season, the morbidity and mortality may be appreciable. Lower respiratory tract disease has developed in one third or more of infants nosocomially infected and has prolonged their hospital stay significantly.[141, 184] The risk of acquiring nosocomial infection is related to the child's age, underlying disease, length of hospitalization, and clearly, adherence to proper infection control procedures. As many as 45 percent of infants hospitalized for 1 week or more have become infected, and open wards with infants younger than 1 year are particularly fertile ground for frequent cross-infections.[105, 142, 184]

Nosocomial infections in immunocompromised children and adults tend to be serious and difficult to control.[52, 96, 118, 175, 288, 424, 476] As previously noted, outbreaks in transplant units in particular have been associated with a high mortality rate and prolonged transmission. Frequently, the infection is brought into the ward by hospital staff, families, and

*See references 6, 17, 111, 122, 123, 125, 272, 283, 333, 334, 433.

*See references 52, 96, 105, 110, 118, 139, 142, 158, 171, 175, 184, 239, 276, 288, 309, 424, 476.

visitors who may have only a mild cold. Multiple strains of RSV may be introduced during a single outbreak or season.[297] Infection rates in staff members may be high and often require absence from work.[195] However, infection of staff is not necessary for them to spread RSV and may be less important than their transmission of infection via fomites. Staff and others on the ward who come in contact with infectious secretions on environmental surfaces may carry contaminated secretions from patient to patient on their hands and clothing and on objects such as toys.*

Prevention of Nosocomial Infection

Nosocomial acquisition of RSV requires close contact with an infected person or with surfaces contaminated by secretions.[180] Spread occurs by direct inoculation of large particles (droplets) or by self-inoculation after touching contaminated secretions.[175] The risk of acquiring nosocomial infection in an infants' ward has been diminished by a variety of infection control procedures, but most important is careful handwashing by all persons entering and leaving an infant's room and, second, education of the staff with frequent reminders throughout the RSV season.[95, 110, 155, 175, 225, 281] The success of additional barrier precautions such as gowns, gloves, and masks has varied in different settings.[175] When handwashing cannot be strictly enforced, gloves may be effective. In two controlled studies, the routine use of gowns and masks did not add further benefit to conscientious handwashing and other infection control procedures.[181, 325] Other groups have reduced the nosocomial infection rate with procedures that include the use of gowns, gloves, and masks while emphasizing the importance of staff compliance.[281] Because RSV seems to infect mostly via the eyes and nose, regular nose-mouth masks are of limited benefit because touching or rubbing the eyes appears to be the major mode of self-inoculation.[139, 180, 185] Thus, eye-nose goggles or goggles plus a mask appear to be more effective in diminishing nosocomial infection in both staff and infants.[139]

As facilities allow, infants with respiratory signs of unknown etiology should be isolated. With the use of techniques permitting rapid viral diagnosis, infants with RSV infection may be cohorted.[106] Staff with any respiratory signs should preferably not care for patients at high risk for complicated or severe RSV infection.

UNUSUAL MANIFESTATIONS OF DISEASE

RSV infection has been associated with a variety of neurologic, cardiac, and other conditions, generally in case reports. However, in most of these reports, the causal role of RSV is tenuous and unproven. Because of the ubiquitous character of RSV, the concurrent development of RSV infection and other unusual conditions is likely. Acute RSV infection has been demonstrated in case reports of children with various central nervous system disorders, including meningitis, myelitis, ataxia, hemiplegia, and facial palsy.[65, 252, 451] In several of these children with central nervous system disorders, antibody to RSV has been demonstrated in cerebrospinal fluid, thus suggesting local production, and the neurotropism of the virus has been suggested by the production of a neuropathic strain of RSV by intracerebral inoculation of suckling mice.[70]

*See references 139, 158, 171, 172, 175, 179, 180, 181, 184, 188, 337.

Isolated case reports describe an association between RSV infection and cardiac disease, including myocarditis and complete heart block occurring in previously normal children.[31, 149] Exanthems also have been reported occasionally in association with RSV infection,[48, 86] but a causal relationship to RSV is lacking.

Diagnosis

Though minuscule
of micron measure,
It leaves its scent
and prints precise;
A fleeing hare
for hunt and snare. . .

C. B. H.

CLINICAL AND EPIDEMIOLOGIC DIAGNOSIS

Because RSV has a repetitive and distinctive behavior, the diagnosis often may be determined with reasonable accuracy by knowing three factors: (1) the age of the infected child, (2) the clinical syndrome, and (3) the local seasonal patterns of RSV. An infant acquiring lower respiratory tract disease, especially bronchiolitis, in the winter would have a high chance of having RSV infection. Recognition of the historical habits and arrival of RSV in a community, such as by surveillance programs monitoring RSV's activity and the number of bronchiolitis cases or hospital admissions for respiratory illness in young children, may be helpful.[179, 377]

SPECIFIC DIAGNOSIS

A specific diagnosis of RSV infection may be made by isolation of the virus or by a number of rapid antigen detection assays that are clinically useful.* The lability and technical difficulties associated with isolation of RSV in tissue culture render the sensitivity of isolation highly dependent on the quality of the specimen and particularly the expertise of the laboratory.[479] Transported specimens require proper media and cannot be subject to freezing, thawing, and temperature and pH changes.[230, 417] By quantitative assay, a nasal wash is more sensitive than a nasopharyngeal swab specimen for the recovery of RSV.[178, 417] Nasal wash specimens may be obtained with a suction apparatus or simply by the use of a tapered rubber bulb[178] (Fig. 185–6). Specimens thus obtained and inoculated onto sensitive cell lines such as HEp-2 cells have allowed identification of the characteristic cytopathic effect of RSV in an average of 3 to 4 days. The use of cell cultures that are relatively insensitive or too dense, thereby masking the characteristic syncytial appearance, will diminish the chance of detecting the virus. Identification may be expedited by the use of shell vials and detection of antigen in cell culture by rapid techniques such as enzyme-linked immunosorbent assay (ELISA) and immunofluorescence assay (IFA).[107, 116, 293]

Many assays and commercial kits, including IFA, ELISA, radioimmunoassays, DNA-RNA hybridization, and RNA polymerase chain reaction (PCR), are available for rapid diagnosis by antigen detection.† Most involve IFA or ELISA

*See references 107, 116, 211, 231, 250, 251, 286, 293, 416, 417, 425, 455.

†See references 107, 116, 211, 231, 250, 251, 286, 293, 416, 417, 425, 455.

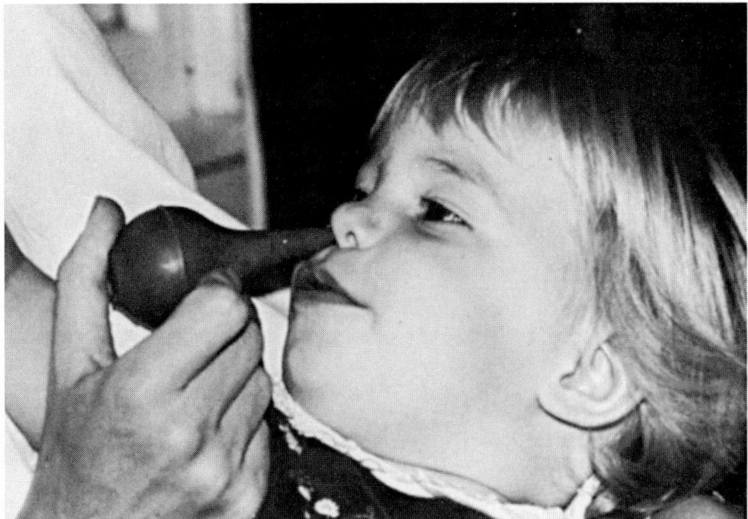

FIGURE 185–6 ■ Simple method for obtaining nasal wash specimens from young children. A 1-oz tapered rubber bulb is used to inject and collect 5 to 10 mL of saline with one squeeze. (From Hall, C. B., and Douglas, R. G., Jr.: Clinically useful method for the isolation of respiratory syncytial virus. J. Infect. Dis. *131*:1–5, 1975.)

on either nasopharyngeal swab or wash specimens and entail the use of polyclonal or monoclonal antibodies. The sensitivity of IFA and ELISA is generally equivalent but has ranged from 32 to 98 percent (most in the range of 70–90%), with IFA tending to be more sensitive and specific. The reported sensitivity of these antigen tests may be falsely high if compared with the sensitivity of tissue culture techniques that are less than optimal, and the specificity may be diminished if the tests are performed during times when RSV is not prevalent in the community.

Serologic diagnosis rarely aids in the clinical management of patients, but it is useful in epidemiologic research. A serologic response may be measured by the complement-fixation, ELISA, neutralization, indirect IFA, fusion inhibition, immunoprecipitation, and Western blot assays.[417, 455] Several of these tests may be used to detect class-specific antibodies directed at the purified viral proteins in both serum and secretions.[121, 231, 306, 417, 454, 470] The complement-fixation test is generally less sensitive than the ELISA or neutralization tests, especially in infants. Solid-phase ELISA is preferable for young infants.[90] A neutralization test combined with an ELISA in microtiter plates has simplified the assay for neutralizing antibodies and appears to be as sensitive as the standard neutralization and plaque reduction assays.[20]

Treatment

Treatment of RSV lower respiratory tract disease is mainly supportive, and the outcome of a severely affected infant has been related directly to the quality of this supportive care.[328, 461] The diminished mortality rate in high-risk infants over the past decade has resulted primarily from technical and physiologic advancements in supportive care for these infants. Because most of these infants are hypoxemic, administering supplemental oxygen is integral to their therapy.[189, 382] Most of the infants respond to relatively low concentrations of oxygen because the physiologic abnormality is primarily one of an unequal ratio of ventilation to perfusion.[477] In those who are more severely ill, arterial blood gas monitoring may need to be performed to detect hypercarbia. Progressive hypercarbia, hypoxemia unresponsive to oxygen administration, and recurrent apnea are potential indications for airway intervention.

Therapy with such agents as bronchodilating agents, corticosteroids, or antibiotics has been highly variable.[40, 259, 279, 461] These agents have been evaluated in infants with RSV infection and generally have been shown to be of limited or no benefit. Nonetheless, a study of Canadian hospitals showed that therapy for RSV infection included bronchodilators in 68 to 93 percent of cases, corticosteroids in 3 to 69 percent of low-risk infants, and antibiotics in 69 percent of high-risk infants and 58 percent of low-risk infants.[279]

The benefit of using bronchodilating agents in infants with bronchiolitis is controversial. The many studies using bronchodilators parenterally, orally, or by nebulization have had conflicting results.[138, 261, 298, 357, 392, 394, 477] A meta-analysis of the efficacy of bronchodilators for the treatment of infants with bronchiolitis, performed on 15 young children who met the selection criteria of the 89 publications identified, indicated that bronchodilators generally resulted in modest clinical improvement in infants who were mildly to moderately ill.[249] The benefit, however, was short lived and did not diminish the risk of needing hospitalization. Most studies have indicated that a minority of all patients with bronchiolitis or wheezing exhibit a discernible benefit. Some studies have indicated that younger infants are least likely to respond to bronchodilators, and some have documented no change in pulmonary resistance with bronchodilators or even have noted a detrimental paradoxical response; others suggest a beneficial effect on airway obstruction.[36, 69, 357, 477] Some researchers have suggested a better response if both alpha and beta receptor agonists are combined in the therapy.[298, 310, 392, 477] Because a subgroup of infants may respond to these agents, many experts advise a carefully monitored trial of bronchodilators, usually aerosolized, in more severely affected infants older than 6 months.

The use of corticosteroids in the treatment of bronchiolitis has been shown to be of no benefit in controlled studies.[58, 60, 102, 262, 386, 411, 413] Although no adverse effect of such therapy has been demonstrated for RSV infection, evidence in children receiving immunosuppressive therapy suggests that it is a possibility.[193]

The only specific treatment currently approved for children hospitalized with RSV infection is ribavirin (1-β-D-ribofuranosyl-1,2,4-triazole-3-carboxamide). This synthetic nucleoside has been administered as a small-particle aerosol for 12 to 22 hours per day for 3 or more days, usually about 3 days. The end-point is clinical improvement. Much shorter, intermittent courses of higher doses also appear to be an acceptable mode of administration.[120] Use of the nucleoside has been associated in various studies with significant improvement in arterial oxygen saturation and lung function; diminished clinical severity, need for mechanical ventilation, and length of hospitalization; and decreased levels of secretory inflammatory mediators associated with severe wheezing and disease.* Some other studies in infants with severe RSV lower respiratory tract disease showed no significant benefit with ribavirin therapy.[228, 280, 308, 371, 475] The total number of patients in these controlled studies is small, however, and the degree of benefit in clinical outcome is unclear. This factor plus the expense of this drug indicates that it should be reserved primarily for infants at high risk for severe disease, as suggested by the American Academy of Pediatrics.[371]

Viral resistance to ribavirin has not been demonstrated. Clinical trials testing additional antiviral therapy for RSV are currently lacking. Vitamin A supplementation has been suggested as adjunctive therapy in severely ill infants.[329] In controlled studies, interferon alpha-2a has been administered intramuscularly to infants with RSV bronchiolitis[81] and intranasally to volunteers without measurable benefit.[213]

Many novel therapeutic agents for RSV are being investigated, including nucleosides other than ribavirin, sulfated polysaccharide compounds, and proteins and peptides that inhibit the replication of RSV.[9, 108, 221, 227, 271, 330, 481]

Prognosis and Complications

Thus, if infected at this tender stage
will they become "blue bloaters" as they age?[171]

Information on the mortality caused by RSV infection is limited. In hospitalized patients with RSV infection or with bronchiolitis, the recent mortality rate has been reported as 1 to 3 percent. However, mortality and morbidity rates from RSV infection vary greatly with the population: they increase in those with certain ethnic backgrounds and underlying diseases, especially infants who are premature, and those with cardiac, pulmonary, and immunodeficient conditions.† Among infants dying of acute respiratory infection, RSV remains the major cause in developed countries. In 1978 and 1979, newspaper headlines described an outbreak of a "mystery disease" ("il male oscuro") in Naples, Italy, where more than 60 young children died in the fall and winter months from an outbreak of respiratory illness. Limited virologic studies implicated RSV as the major cause, and bacterial infection did not appear to play a role.[294, 295] However, in less developed areas, RSV remains a major cause of mortality, in part from complicating bacterial infections.[112, 145, 301, 404]

The risk of acquiring severe or fatal RSV infection has varied appreciably among countries and to some extent from year to year within a community, but the major risk factors for an individual infant are prematurity and young age, in addition to the presence of underlying disease.‡ Approximately 30 to 70 percent of infants hospitalized with RSV infection in large medical centers have an underlying disease.[193, 279, 328] In more than 1200 infants hospitalized in Rochester with RSV infection, 63 percent had one or more underlying conditions, 21 percent of which were prematurity and 11 percent were cardiac abnormalities. Environmental factors, including lower socioeconomic status, passive smoking, crowding, lack of breast-feeding, attendance in daycare, and possibly also variations in the virus itself, have been associated with a poorer prognosis.[197, 215, 218, 300, 328] The proportion of children hospitalized in Rochester with RSV infection who have required intensive care each season has varied between 5 and 25 percent during a 15-year period.[197] Although the reasons for this wide annual variation are not entirely clear, the strain of virus circulating in the community may play a role. Children hospitalized with group A infections had a significantly increased risk of being admitted to the intensive care unit, and during the years in which group A strains strongly predominated in the community, the rate of intensive care admission for RSV was significantly greater than that during the years when B strains were highly dominant.[197] Whether this relationship is causal is unclear. Variations in the proteins of the RSV strains have not shown an effect on clinical severity, and more importantly, an association between the type and severity of clinical disease with either A or B strains has not been consistent.[53, 67, 130, 218, 420, 422, 459]

Infants in the first few months of life with functionally important cardiac disease, lung disease, or both are at the greatest risk, and an appreciable proportion acquire RSV infection nosocomially.* In a prospective study in the early 1980s of hospitalized infants with cardiac lesions, the mortality rate was 37 percent.[291] If the infant's cardiac lesion was complicated by pulmonary hypertension, the mortality rate doubled. Since then, the mortality rate has diminished in infants with cardiac disease, partly because of early surgical correction, advanced techniques, and recognition of the risk associated with RSV infection and the possibility of acquiring it nosocomially. The risk for severe infection nevertheless remains appreciable in these infants.[313, 328] One Canadian study estimated the mortality rate in infants with cardiac disease to be 3 to 4 percent.[328]

Premature infants with lung disease and a complicated neonatal course have a propensity for not only complicated primary infection but also severe reinfections extending into subsequent seasons if their pulmonary function remains compromised.[101, 167, 307] In one prospective study of 30 children younger than 2 years with bronchopulmonary dysplasia, RSV infection was documented in 59 percent during a single season, and two thirds of these children required hospitalization.[167] The chance of development of more severe disease requiring hospitalization was increased in children who were receiving home oxygen therapy or had required oxygen therapy within the last 3 months. The risk of low-birth-weight infants requiring rehospitalization for RSV is considerable.[101, 327, 415] This risk, ranging from approximately 3 to 36 percent, correlates inversely with birth weight and gestational age.

The risk of severe or complicated RSV infection in children with immunocompromising conditions varies with the degree of immunosuppression. Patients with severe forms of congenital immunodeficiency and those with transplants are at particular risk.[52, 96, 193, 229, 288, 355, 476] These patients acquire severe lower respiratory tract disease at any age and have prolonged viral shedding, thus indicating the importance of cellular immunity and $CD4^+$ and $CD8^+$ T lymphocytes in controlling RSV infection.

*See references 37, 66, 94, 147, 170, 191, 192, 195, 264, 265, 287, 303, 382–384, 387, 407, 410, 423, 446, 466.
†See references 154, 173, 232, 245, 279, 289, 313, 328, 397, 405, 418.
‡See references 101, 154, 173, 232, 245, 279, 289, 305, 307, 313, 328, 341, 397, 405, 419.

*See references 1, 101, 167, 193, 279, 291, 292, 305, 307, 328, 404.

Limited information on the effect of human immunodeficiency virus (HIV) infection on RSV infection indicates that the severity of RSV infection is generally less than that in patients with transplants but greater than that in patients with normal immune function, and it may correlate with the degree of immune suppression exerted by the HIV infection. These patients have prolonged shedding and appear to be at increased risk for RSV lower respiratory tract disease and hospitalization, but a fatal outcome is uncommon.[71, 260]

Of increasing recognition and interest is RSV's expanded role in the aggravation of disease in patients with a spectrum of underlying chronic conditions, such as exacerbations and increased severity of illness in patients with pulmonary, cardiac, neurologic, and renal disease.[1, 25, 26, 194, 212, 292] Children with cystic fibrosis have been shown to be at particular risk for exacerbations from RSV infection; these children have reduced lung function and a greater rate of hospitalization (43%) than from any other viral infection.[25, 212]

A major complication of RSV infection in young infants, especially preterm infants, is apnea.[16, 55, 85, 189, 263] Approximately 20 percent of infants hospitalized with RSV infection have demonstrated apnea.[55, 263] It is most likely to occur in the youngest infants, those born prematurely, those with a young postnatal age, especially infants who have not yet reached a postconceptional age of 44 weeks, and those with a history of apnea of prematurity.[85] The apnea usually develops at the beginning of the RSV infection and is short lived and nonobstructive.[16] The prognosis in infants in whom apnea develops in conjunction with RSV infection is not well defined. Although apnea may recur during the acute RSV infection, the prognosis after discharge is generally good.[85] Most infants do not have apnea subsequently, even with later respiratory infections. Infants with apnea or periodic breathing associated with RSV infection require monitoring during the acute phase of their illness, but the subsequent prognosis for normal infants is good.

Secondary bacterial infection is an unusual complication of RSV infection in the United States, and most clinical and pathologic studies indicate that RSV infection rarely predisposes to bacterial infection.[24, 166, 194, 268, 285, 375] In a 9-year prospective study of 565 children hospitalized with RSV lower respiratory tract disease, the rate of subsequent bacterial infection was 1.2 percent in the total group of children infected with RSV and 0.6 percent in the 352 children who received no antibiotics.[194] The highest rate (11%) of subsequent bacterial infection occurred in infants who received broad-spectrum parenteral antibiotics for 5 or more days. Controlled studies with randomized antibiotic treatment of bronchiolitis and pneumonia mostly caused by RSV have shown no difference in the severity or duration of illness or in outcome.[128, 135]

DEVELOPMENT OF CHRONIC LUNG DISEASE

RSV has been suggested as having a role in promoting or exacerbating numerous chronic diseases, especially pulmonary conditions, in later childhood and even in adulthood.

Most prominent among these exacerbations is the possible connection between RSV infection and asthma. Infants with bronchiolitis and particularly those hospitalized with lower respiratory tract disease documented to be from RSV have been shown to be at high risk for subsequent recurrent wheezing or other lower respiratory tract disease.[247] Recurrent respiratory problems have been noted on follow-up to occur in half or more of such infants and tend to be most frequent in the first couple years of life. The development and frequency of recurrent wheezing episodes do not appear to be atopic, nor do they appear to result from direct damage to the lung from RSV infection.[296, 336] The link between RSV and asthma has been suggested by several observations. First, both in the United States and in many other countries, an increase in the number of children with asthma has been documented, as well as an increase in the morbidity associated with asthma.[7, 97] The severity of the illnesses associated with asthma also has increased and disproportionately so in many of the same populations that are at particular risk for the most severe manifestations of RSV.[7, 97, 388] Second, the immunologic response associated with RSV infection is characterized mainly by a T_H2 cytokine phenotype, a pattern also observed during asthmatic attacks.[344, 466] Furthermore, the likelihood of wheezing and the severity of wheezing in children with RSV lower respiratory tract disease have been correlated with increased levels of RSV IgE in secretions, thus suggesting that the inflammatory mediators that play a role in reactive airway disease may be engendered by RSV-induced antibodies as well.[466]

RSV also may affect lung function by altering neural pathways.[278] In animal models, RSV infection has been demonstrated to augment the contractile response of cholinergic pathways and the excitatory nonadrenergic, noncholinergic excitatory (NANCe) system. Additionally, RSV has been shown in the same animal models to diminish the nonadrenargic, noncholinergic inhibitory (NANCi) response. Nevertheless, RSV's role in causing hyperreactivity of the lung is far from clear. Other recent studies have indicated that the theoretic link between RSV infection and asthma is reversed.[32, 296] These studies suggest that the normal inflammatory response at birth is not T_H1, but T_H2, which subsequently shifts to a T_H1 pattern via the stimulus of multiple viral infections and antigenic stimuli early in life. These early infections thus result in T_H1 cells being preferentially selected and provide protection against the development of subsequent wheezing. This area continues to attract much interest and investigation that is likely to show that the development of hyperreactivity of the lung is multifactorial in cause and may well include a genetic predisposition.[115, 273]

Prevention

With perseverance and
the dreamer's scanning scope,
Reality is made of distant hope...

C. B. H.

Control of RSV must await a successful means of immunization. In the interim, alternative methods of prevention are being sought that may offer at least temporary protection during the most vulnerable periods of an infant's life. Because high levels of maternal antibody appear to be protective, the antibodies in pregnant women could be boosted by immunization.[119, 152]

Breast-feeding may offer some protection against RSV infection, but the degree and type of such protection remain unclear.[112, 132, 215, 370, 404] Both in England and in the United States, the proportion of breast-fed infants has been noted to be lower in those hospitalized with RSV infection than in controls. Specific IgA antibodies and, to a lesser extent, IgG and IgM antibodies to RSV have been identified in human colostrum and milk.[112, 269, 431] IgA-specific antibody may persist for prolonged periods in the products of lactation and may be boosted by maternal reinfection.[430] Neutralization of RSV by breast milk appears to be mediated by both immunoglobulin and nonimmunoglobulin components.[269] Direct evidence for the protective effect of breast-feeding on RSV disease is nevertheless lacking.

Licensure in 1996 of high-titer intravenous polyclonal RSV immunoglobulin offered the first mode of prophylaxis for RSV.[359] Monthly administration during the RSV season to high-risk infants who were premature or had chronic lung or congenital heart disease resulted in a significant 63 percent reduction in subsequent hospitalization for RSV infection in those who were premature or had chronic lung disease. However, no benefit, with possibly an adverse outcome, was observed in infants with congenital heart disease.[169, 359] A subsequent placebo-controlled study in premature infants showed a significant 41 percent reduction in hospitalization for RSV infection.[373] Hence, the product was approved for children younger than 24 months with a gestational age of less than 36 weeks or with chronic lung disease but not for infants with congenital heart disease.

The subsequent licensure of an RSV humanized monoclonal antibody (palivizumab) circumvented many of the difficulties and adverse effects of administering a large intravenous dose to small infants. Palivizumab was developed from a mouse monoclonal antibody that recognizes a protective epitope of the surface glycoprotein, the F protein. Only the antigen recognition site from the mouse monoclonal antibody was inserted into the spine of a human antibody, thus diminishing the chance of allergic reactions to the mouse-raised antibody.[359]

Palivizumab, administered intramuscularly, was evaluated in high-risk infants with prematurity and chronic lung disease who still required medical therapy. In a multicenter, placebo-controlled trial, the rate of hospitalization for RSV illness was reduced from 10.6 percent in the placebo group to 4.8 percent in the infants given prophylaxis.[345] The product was approved in 1998 for use in the same group of premature infants as previously approved for the polyclonal RSV antibody. The American Academy of Pediatrics has recommended that prophylaxis be considered for infants and children younger than 2 years who have chronic lung disease and have required medical therapy within 6 months of the beginning of the RSV infection and for premature infants born at 32 weeks' gestation or earlier, even if they do not have chronic lung disease.

Concern has been raised about the estimated cost relative to the benefit of prophylaxis in these infants and whether mutations in the surface of the glycoprotein of the virus could result in resistant strains of RSV.[421]

VACCINES

Control of RSV has long lured but eluded investigators. Although the outcome of infants with RSV infection has improved greatly in recent years, with a marked decrease in the mortality rate, the burden on health care that RSV imposes yearly remains notable not only in children but also in adults.[125, 148] This burden may be alleviated only through immunization. Certain characteristics of RSV infection, however, have posed barriers to the successful development of a vaccine during the 4 decades of effort.

The shroud of past experience with the formalin-inactivated vaccine has conferred caution and concern regarding the development of candidate vaccines. The unfortunate outcome of trials with the formalin-inactivated vaccine nevertheless stimulated research that has divulged information integral to the development of future vaccines. The information derived from rodent models of the exaggerated disease and lung pathology illustrated the importance of the type of immunizing agent in determining whether a beneficial or detrimental humoral and cellular immune response results; these models have suggested that a successful vaccine should produce a balanced T_H1 response with both $CD4^+$ and CTL cells.[90, 109, 164] Furthermore, the specific antigens to be included in a vaccine potentially will alter the immune response, as demonstrated in mice by the greater lung pathology associated with immunization with the G protein than with the F protein.[10, 13] Despite the wealth of information derived from these animal experiments, the lack of an adequate and reliable model to test candidate vaccines remains a significant barrier.

An RSV vaccine also would have to both reflect and improve the variable and nondurable immunity afforded by natural infection. The vaccine would in addition need to be administered in the first few weeks of life, when the most severe disease usually occurs. Little experience exists regarding immunization with live viruses within the neonatal period, and it is likely to be appreciably influenced by the immature and variably developed immune system of the neonate. Maternal antibody also would be most abundant at this period, which has been shown to be potentially inhibitory to the infant's antibody response. Furthermore, the effect of the multiple antigens from other vaccines that are administered within the first few months of life must be considered.

Subsequent to the performance of formalin-inactivated vaccine trials, research focused on the development of an attenuated live vaccine.[90, 114, 117, 241] The initial candidate vaccines were derived from cold-passaged (*cp*) mutants propagated from strains grown at progressively lower temperatures, and strains were selected by growth at low temperatures, below 37°C, after chemical mutagenesis. Trials with these candidate (*cp* and *ts* [temperature-sensitive]) vaccines generally produced promising results in adult volunteers and seropositive children but proved to be unsuitable for infants and young, seronegative children.[77, 90] These vaccines produced unacceptable degrees of illness, were overattenuated, and were not protective, or they were genetically unstable and resulted in the shedding of wild-type virus. Research has progressed toward the development of more suitable candidate strains and vaccines from purified surface glycoproteins, DNA, and synthetic peptides.[90, 92, 99, 117, 241, 244]

Subunit vaccines are being investigated also.[90, 114, 117, 241] Candidate vaccines have consisted of the two major surface glycoproteins, F and G, which have been produced from purified viruses, recombinant vectors, and plasmids containing cDNA of the F and G genes. Two F protein vaccines, PFP-1 and PFP-2, that consist of immunoaffinity-purified, alum-absorbed F glycoprotein have been tested in both adults and children.[42, 124, 168, 346, 353, 435] The PFP-2 vaccine has been evaluated in several high-risk groups: infants with chronic lung disease, children with cystic fibrosis, and elderly institutionalized individuals.[124, 353, 399] In these groups and in normal children and adults, the vaccines have been safe and immunogenic, with good levels of neutralizing antibody produced. However, the vaccinees generally have been seropositive, and the highest risk group—seronegative, young infants—has yet to be evaluated adequately. Also being investigated is immunization with the protective F and G epitopes by using synthetic peptides that mimic the immunogenic regions.[38, 399] They appear promising in rodents and are being developed further.

Immunization with live attenuated vaccine has the potential advantage of intranasal administration and induction of a balanced immune response similar to that gained from natural infection and the acquisition of both systemic and mucosal immunity. Recent candidates have been derived from previously combined *cp* and *ts (cpts)* mutants by repetitive rounds of chemical mutagenesis to induce mutations that have further stability, attenuation, and immunogenicity.[117, 241, 244] Several *cpts* candidates have been evaluated in seronegative children. One candidate, *cpts* 248/404, was immunogenic in seropositive and seronegative children older than 6 months, but upper respiratory tract illness with appreciable nasal congestion developed in younger infants 1 and 2 months old.[480]

New recombinants have been generated from *cpts* 248/404 by reverse genetics. One has the *SH* gene deleted. A second one has the *SH* gene deleted and another attenuating missense mutation in the polymerase.[241, 245] Initial clinical evaluation appears promising.

Recombinant genetic engineering allows novel and more precise designing of new vaccines by constructing full-length RSV cDNA that generates infectious RNA transcripts.[92, 114] The viral genome can be meticulously manipulated to produce optimal mutations for immunogenicity and attenuation and to eliminate detrimental ones.

Successful control of RSV morbidity through immunization will probably require creative and combined approaches. In recognition of the beneficial effect of passive specific antibody, maternal immunization has been suggested as one approach.[152] Novel adjuvants are being investigated; some of them can shift the immune response evoked by subunit vaccines from a T_H2- to a T_H1-type response in experimental animals. Some candidates induce mucosal as well as systemic immunity and potentially allow routes of administration that are preferable to the parenteral route.[339, 452] Enhanced immunogenicity appears possible with enterically active adjuvants and carriers, such as liposomes and biodegradable microspheres, and with adjuvants in vesicles of immunostimulating complexes.[202, 436, 450] The novel development of individual vaccines and approaches is reducing the number of hurdles and detours on the road toward successful control of RSV. In view of the number of different populations from infants to elders who would benefit from protection against RSV infection, multiple approaches and vaccines may be required to achieve effective control of RSV infection and diminish the associated human and financial cost of RSV.

REFERENCES

1. Abman, S. H., Ogle, J. N., Butler-Simon, N., et al.: Role of respiratory syncytial virus in early hospitalization for respiratory distress of young infants with cystic fibrosis. J Pediatr. *113*:826–830, 1988.
2. Abu-Harb, M., Bell, F., Rao, W., et al.: IL-8 and neutrophil elastase levels in the respiratory tract of infants with RSV bronchiolitis. Eur. Respir. J. *14*:139–143, 1999.
3. Adams, J. M.: Primary virus pneumonitis with cytoplasmic inclusion bodies: A study of an epidemic involving thirty-two infants with nine deaths. J. A. M. A. *116*:925–933, 1941.
4. Adams, J. M., Imagawa, D. T., and Zike, K.: Relationship of pneumonitis in infants to respiratory syncytial virus. Lancet *81*:502–506, 1961.
5. Adams, J. M., Imagawa, D. T., and Zike, K.: Epidemic bronchiolitis and pneumonitis related to respiratory syncytial virus. J. A. M. A. *176*:1037–1039, 1961.
6. Agius, G., Dindinaud, G., Biggar, R. J., et al.: An epidemic of respiratory syncytial virus in elderly people: Clinical and serological findings. J. Med. Virol. *30*:117–127, 1990.
7. Aguinaga, O., Arendo, P., Bellido, J., et al.: The prevalence of asthma-related symptoms in 13–14 year old children from 9 Spanish populations. Med. Clin. *112*:171–175 1999.
8. Aherne, W., Bird, T., Court, S. D. M., et al.: Pathological changes in virus infections of the lower respiratory tract in children. J. Clin. Pathol. *23*:7–18, 1970.
9. Ahmad, A., Davies, J., Randall, S., et al.: Antiviral properties of extract of *Opuntia streptacantha*. Antiviral Res. *30*:75–85, 1996.
10. Alwan, W. H., Kozlowska, W. J., and Openshaw, P. J.: Distinct types of lung disease caused by functional subsets of antiviral T cells. J. Exp. Med. *179*:81–89, 1994.
11. Alwan, W. H., and Openshaw, P. J.: Distinct patterns of T- and B-cell immunity to respiratory syncytial virus induced by individual viral proteins. Vaccine *11*:431–437, 1993.
12. Alwan, W. H., Record, F. M., and Openshaw, P. J.: $CD4^+$ T cells clear virus but augment disease in mice infected with respiratory syncytial virus: Comparison with the effects of $CD8^+$ T cells. Clin. Exp. Immunol. *88*:527–536, 1992.
13. Alwan, W. H., Record, F. M., and Openshaw, P. J.: Phenotypic and functional characterization of T cell lines specific for individual respiratory syncytial virus proteins. J. Immunol. *150*:5211–5218, 1993.
14. Ana, P. P. S., Arrobio, J. O., and Kim, H. W.: Serum complement in acute bronchiolitis. Proc. Soc. Exp. Biol. Med. *134*:499–503, 1970.
15. Ananaba, G. A., and Anderson, L. J.: Antibody enhancement of respiratory syncytial virus stimulation of leukotriene production by a macrophagelike cell line. J. Virol. *65*:5052–5060, 1991.
16. Anas, N., Boettrich, C., Hall, C. B., et al.: The association of apnea and respiratory syncytial virus in infants. J. Pediatr. *101*:65–68, 1982.
17. Anderson, L.: Burden of RSV disease in the elderly. Paper presented at the Aventis Pasteur/ICAAC Symposium Respiratory Syncytial Virus in the Elderly, September 17, 2000, Toronto.
18. Anderson, L. J., and Heilman, C. A.: Protective and disease-enhancing immune responses to respiratory syncytial virus. J. Infect. Dis. *171*:1–7, 1995.
19. Anderson, L. J., Hendry, R. M., Pierik, L. T., et al.: Multicenter study of strains of respiratory syncytial virus. J. Infect. Dis. *163*:687–692, 1991.
20. Anderson, L. J., Hierholzer, J. C., Bingham, P. G., et al.: Microneutralization test for respiratory syncytial virus based on an enzyme immunoassay. J. Clin. Microbiol. *22*:1050–1052, 1985.
21. Anderson, L. J., Hierholzer, J. C., Tsou, C., et al.: Antigenic characterization of respiratory syncytial virus strains with monoclonal antibodies. J. Infect. Dis. *151*:626–632, 1985.
22. Anderson, L. J., Tsou, C., Potter, C., et. al.: Cytokine response to respiratory syncytial virus stimulation of human peripheral blood mononuclear cells. J. Infect. Dis. *170*:1201–1208, 1994.
23. Anestad, G.: Interference between outbreaks of respiratory syncytial virus and influenza virus infection. Lancet *2*:502, 1982.
24. Antonow, J., Hansen, K., McKinstry, C., et al.: Sepsis evaluations in hospitalized infants with bronchiolitis. Pediatr. Infect. Dis. J. *17*:231–236, 1998.
25. Armstrong, D., Grimwood, K., Carlin, J., et al.: Severe viral respiratory infections in infants with cystic fibrosis. Pediatr. Pulmonol. *26*:371–379, 1998.
26. Arnold, S., Wang, E., Law, B., et al.:Variable morbidity of respiratory syncytial virus infection in patients with underlying lung disease: A review of the PICNIC RSV database. Pediatr. Infect. Dis. J. *18*:866–869, 1999.
27. Arola, M., Ruuskanen, O., Ziegler, T., et al.: Clinical role of respiratory virus infection in acute otitis media. Pediatrics *86*:848–855, 1990.
28. Arola, M., Ziegler, T., and Ruuskanen, O.: Respiratory virus infection as a cause of prolonged symptoms in acute otitis media. J. Pediatr. *116*:697–701, 1990.
29. Babu, P., Selan, A., Christuraj, S., et al.: A primate model of respiratory syncytial virus infection. Indian J. Exp. Biol. *36*:758–762, 1998.
30. Bachi, T.: Direct observation of the budding and fusion of an enveloped virus by video microscopy. J. Cell Biol. *197*:1689–1695, 1973.
31. Bairan, A. C., Cherry, J. D., Fagan, L. F., et al.: Complete heart block and respiratory syncytial virus. Am. J. Dis. Child. *127*:264–265, 1974.
32. Ball, T., Castro-Rodriguez, J., Griffith, K., et al.: Siblings, day-care attendance, and the risk of asthma and wheezing during childhood. N. Engl. J. Med. *343*:538–543, 2000.
33. Bangham, C. R. M., and Askonas, B. A.: Murine cytotoxic T cells specific to respiratory syncytial virus recognize different antigenic subtypes of the virus. J. Gen. Virol. *67*:623–629, 1986.
34. Bangham, C. R. M., Cannon, M. J., Karzon, D. T., et. al.: Cytotoxic T-cell response to respiratory syncytial virus in mice. J. Virol. *56*:55–59, 1985.
35. Bangham, C., Openshaw, P., Ball, L., et al.:. Human and murine cytotoxic T cells specific to respiratory syncytial virus recognize the viral nucleoprotein (N), but not the major glycoprotein (G), expressed by vaccinia virus recombinants. J. Immunol. *137*:3973–3977, 1986.
36. Barr, F., Patel, N., and Newth, C.: The pharmacologic mechanism by which inhaled epinephrine reduces airway obstruction in respiratory syncytial virus–associated bronchiolitis. J. Pediatr. *136*:699–700, 2000.
37. Barry, W., Cockburn, F., Cornall, R., et al.: Ribavirin aerosol for acute bronchiolitis. Arch. Dis. Child. *61*:593–594, 1986.
38. Bastien, N., Trudel, M., and Simard, C.: Complete protection of mice from respiratory syncytial virus infection following mucosal delivery of synthetic peptide vaccines. Vaccine *17*:832–836, 1999.
39. Beem, M.: Repeated infections with respiratory syncytial virus. J. Immunol. *98*:1115–1122, 1967.
40. Behrendt, C., Decker, M., Burch, D., et al.: International variation in the management of infants hospitalized with respiratory syncytial virus. Eur. J. Pediatr. *157*:215–220, 1998.
41. Bellanti, J. A.: Development of nonimmunologic, nonspecific mechanisms and specific immunologic mechanisms in resistance to airways and pulmonary infections in infants and children. Pediatr. Res. *11*:224–227, 1977.
42. Belshe, R. B., Anderson, E. L., and Walsh, E. E.: Immunogenicity of purified F glycoprotein of respiratory syncytial virus: Clinical and immune responses to subsequent natural infection in children. J. Infect. Dis. *168*:1024–1029, 1993.

43. Belshe, R. B., Richardson, L. S., London, W. T., et al.: Experimental respiratory syncytial virus infection of four species of primates. J. Med. Virol. *1*:157–162, 1977.
44. Belshe, R. B., VanVoris, L. P., Mufson, M. A., et al.: Epidemiology of severe respiratory syncytial virus infections in Huntington, West Virginia. W. V. Med. J. *77*:49–52, 1981.
45. Bembridge, G., Garcia-Beato, R., Lopez, J., et al.: Subcellular site of expression and route of vaccination influence pulmonary eosinophilia following respiratory syncytial virus challenge in BALB/c mice sensitized to the attachment G protein. J. Immunol. *161*:2473–2480, 1998.
46. Berglund, B.: Studies on respiratory syncytial virus infection. Acta Paediatr. Scand. *176*(Suppl.):1–40, 1967.
47. Berglund, B.: Respiratory syncytial virus infection in families: A study of family members of children hospitalized for acute respiratory disease. Acta Paediatr. Scand. *56*:395–404, 1967.
48. Berkovich, S., and Kibrick, S.: Exanthem associated with respiratory syncytial virus infection. J. Pediatr. *65*:368–370, 1964.
49. Berman, S.: Epidemiology of acute respiratory infections in children of developing countries. Rev. Infect. Dis. *13*(Suppl. 6):454–462, 1991.
50. Bont, L., Heijnen, C., Kavalaars, A., et al. Peripheral blood cytokine responses and disease severity in respiratory syncytial virus bronchiolitis. Eur. Respir. J. *14*:144–149, 1999.
51. Bont, L., Kavelaars, A., Heijnen, C., et al.: Monocyte interleukin-12 production is inversely related to duration of respiratory failure in respiratory syncytial virus bronchiolitis. J. Infect. Dis. *181*:1772–1775, 2000.
52. Bowden, R.: Respiratory virus infection after marrow transplant: The Fred Hutchinson Cancer Research Center experience. Am. J. Med. *102*:27–30, 1997.
53. Brandenburg, A., van Beek, R., Moll, H., et al.: G protein variation in respiratory syncytial virus group A does not correlate with clinical severity. J. Clin. Microbiol. *38*:2849–2852, 2000.
54. Brandt, C. D., Kim, H. W., Arrobio, J. O., et al.: Epidemiology of respiratory syncytial virus infection in Washington, D.C. III. Composite analysis of eleven consecutive yearly epidemics. Am. J. Epidemiol. *98*:355–364, 1973.
55. Bruhn, F. W., Mokrohisky, S. T., and McIntosh, K.: Apnea associated with respiratory syncytial virus infection in young infants. J. Pediatr. *90*:382–386, 1977.
56. Bryson, D. G., McNulty, M. S., Logan, E. F., et al.: Respiratory syncytial virus pneumonia in young calves: Clinical pathologic findings. Am. J. Vet. Res. *44*:1648–1655, 1983.
57. Bui, R. H. D., Molinaro, G. A., Kettering, J. D., et al.: Virus-specific IgE and IgG4 antibodies in serum of children infected with respiratory syncytial virus. J. Pediatr. *110*:87–90, 1987.
58. Bülow, S., Nir, M., Levin, E., et al.: Prednisolone treatment of respiratory syncytial virus infection: A randomized controlled trial of 147 infants. Pediatrics *104*:e77, 1999.
59. Byrd, L., and Prince, G.: Animal models of respiratory syncytial virus infection. Clin. Infect. Dis. *25*:1363–1368, 1997.
60. Cade, A., Brownlee, K., Conway, S., et al.: Randomized placebo controlled trial of nebulized corticosteroids in acute respiratory syncytial viral bronchiolitis. Arch. Dis. Child. *82*:126–130, 2000.
61. Cane, P.: Molecular epidemiology of respiratory syncytial virus. Rev. Med. Virol. *11*:103–116, 2001.
62. Cane, P. A., and Pringle, C. R.: Evolution of subgroup A respiratory syncytial virus: Evidence for progressive accumulation of amino acid changes in the attachment protein. J. Virol. *69*:2918–2925, 1995.
63. Cannon, M. J., Openshaw, P. J. M., and Askonas, B. A.: Cytotoxic T cells clear virus but augment lung pathology in mice infected with respiratory syncytial virus. J. Exp. Med. *163*:1163–1168, 1988.
64. Cannon, M. J., Stott, E. J., Taylor, G., et al.: Clearance of persistent respiratory syncytial virus infections in immunodeficient mice following transfer of primed T cells. Immunology *62*:133–138, 1987.
65. Cappel, R., Thiry, L., and Clinet, G.: Viral antibodies in the CSF after acute CNS infections. Arch. Neurol. *32*:629–631, 1975.
66. Caramia, G., and Palazzini, E.: Efficacy of ribavirin aerosol treatment for respiratory syncytial virus bronchiolitis in infants. J. Int. Med. Res. *15*:227–233, 1987.
67. Carballal, G., Videla, C., Sequeira, M., et al.: Respiratory syncytial virus: Changes in prevalence of subgroups A and B among Argentinian children, 1990–1996. J. Med. Virol. *61*:275–279, 2000.
68. Carilli, A. D., Gohd, R. S., and Gordon, W.: A virologic study of chronic bronchitis. N. Engl. J. Med. *270*:123–127, 1964.
69. Carlsen, K.: Inhaled nebulized adrenaline improves lung function in infants with acute bronchiolitis. Respir. Med. *94*:709–714, 2000.
70. Cavallaro, J. J., Maassab, H. F., and Abrams, G. D.: An immunofluorescent and histopathological study of respiratory syncytial (RS) virus encephalitis in suckling mice. Proc. Soc. Exp. Biol. Med. *124*:1059–1064, 1967.
71. Chandwani, S., Borkowsky, W., Krasinski, K., et. al.: Respiratory syncytial virus infection in human immunodeficiency virus–infected children. J. Pediatr. *117*:251–254, 1990.
72. Chanock, R. M.: Control of acute mycoplasmal and viral respiratory tract disease. Science *169*:248–256, 1970.
73. Chanock, R. M., and Finberg, L.: Recovery from infants with respiratory illness of a virus related to chimpanzee coryza agent (CCA). II. Epidemiologic aspects of infection in infants and young children. Am. J. Hyg. *66*:291–300, 1957.
74. Chanock, R. M., Kapikian, A. Z., Mills, J., et al.: Influence of immunological factors in respiratory syncytial virus disease of the lower respiratory tract. Arch. Environ. Health *21*:347–355, 1970.
75. Chanock, R. M., Kim, H. W., Vargosko, A. J., et al.: Respiratory syncytial virus. I. Virus recovery and other observations during 1960 outbreak of bronchiolitis, pneumonia, and minor respiratory diseases in children. J. A. M. A. *176*:647–653, 1961.
76. Chanock, R. M., and Parrott, R. H.: Acute respiratory disease in infancy and childhood: Present understanding and prospects for prevention. Pediatrics *36*:21–39, 1965.
77. Chanock, R. M., Parrott, R. H., Connors, M., et al.: Serious respiratory tract disease caused by respiratory syncytial virus: Prospects for improved therapy and effective immunization. Pediatrics *90*:137–143, 1992.
78. Cherrie, A. H., Anderson, K., and Wertz, G. W.: Human cytotoxic T cells stimulated by antigen on dendritic cells recognize the N, SH, F, M, 22K, and 1b proteins of respiratory syncytial virus. J. Virol. *66*:2102–2110, 1992.
79. Chiba, Y., Higashidato, Y., Suga, K., et al.: Development of cell-mediated cytotoxic immunity to respiratory syncytial virus in human infants following naturally acquired infection. J. Med. Virol. *28*:133–139, 1989.
80. Chin, J., Magoffin, R. L., Shearer, L. A., et al.: Field evaluation of a respiratory syncytial virus vaccine and a trivalent parainfluenza virus vaccine in a pediatric population. Am. J. Epidemiol. *89*:449–463, 1969.
81. Chipps, B. E., Sullivan, W. F., and Portnoy, J. M.: Alpha-2a-interferon for treatment of bronchiolitis caused by respiratory syncytial virus. Pediatr. Infect. Dis. J. *12*:653–658, 1993.
82. Choi, E., and Lee, H.: Genetic diversity and molecular epidemiology of the G protein of subgroups A and B of respiratory syncytial virus isolated over 9 consecutive epidemics in Korea. J. Infect. Dis. *181*:1547–1556, 2000.
83. Chonmaitree, T., and Henrickson, K.: Detection of respiratory viruses in the middle ear fluids of children with acute otitis media by multiplex reverse transcription:polymerase chain reaction assay. Pediatr. Infect. Dis. J. *19*:258–260, 2000.
84. Chonmaitree, T., Owen, M. J., Patel, J. A., et al.: Effect of viral respiratory tract infection on outcome of acute otitis media. J. Pediatr. *120*:856–862, 1992.
85. Church, N. R., Anas, N. G., Hall, C. B., et al.: Respiratory syncytial virus–related apnea in infants: Demographics and outcome. Am. J. Dis. Child. *138*:247–250, 1984.
86. Coffin, S., Gest, K., and Shimamura, A.: Respiratory syncytial virus as a cause of fever and petechiae in infants. Clin. Pediatr. (Phila.) *32*:355–356, 1993.
87. Coggins, W., Lefkowitz, E., and Sullender, W.: Genetic variability among group A and group B respiratory syncytial viruses in a children's hospital. J. Clin. Microbiol. *36*:3552–3557, 1998.
88. Collins, P. L., Dickens, L. E., Buckler-White, A., et al.: Nucleotide sequences for the gene functions of human respiratory syncytial virus reveal distinctive features of intergenic structure and gene order. Proc. Natl. Acad. Sci. U. S. A. *83*:4594–4598, 1986.
89. Collins, P., Hill, M., Cristina, J., et al.: Transcription elongation factor of respiratory syncytial virus, a nonsegmented negative-strand RNA virus. Proc. Natl. Acad. Sci. U. S. A. *93*:81–85, 1996.
90. Collins, P. L., McIntosh, K., and Chanock, R. M.: Respiratory syncytial virus. *In* Fields, B. N., Knipe, D. M., and Howley, P. M. (eds.): Fields Virology. Philadelphia, Lippincott-Raven, 1996, pp. 1313–1351.
91. Collins, P. L., Purcell, R. H., London, W. T., et al.: Evaluation in chimpanzees of vaccinia virus recombinants that express the surface glycoproteins of human respiratory syncytial virus. Vaccine *8*:164–168, 1990.
92. Collins, P., Whitehead, S., Bukreyev, A., et al.: Rational design of live-attenuated recombinant vaccine virus for human respiratory syncytial virus by reverse genetics. Adv. Virus Res. *54*:423–451, 1999.
93. Connors, M., Collins, P. L., Firestone, C. Y., et al.: Respiratory syncytial virus (RSV) F, G, M2 (22K), and N proteins each induce resistance to RSV challenge, but resistance induced by M2 and N proteins is relatively short-lived. J. Virol. *65*:1634–1637, 1991.
94. Conrad, D. A., Christenson, J. C., Waner, J. L., et al.: Aerosolized ribavirin treatment of respiratory syncytial virus infection in infants hospitalized during an epidemic. Pediatr. Infect. Dis. J. *6*:152–158, 1987.
95. Contreras, P., Sami, I., Darnell, M., et al.: Inactivation of respiratory syncytial virus by generic hand dishwashing detergents and antibacterial hand soaps. Infect. Control Hosp. Epidemiol. *20*:57–58, 1999.
96. Couch, R., Englund, J., and Whimbey, E.: Respiratory viral infections in immunocompetent and immunocompromised persons. Am. J. Med. *102*:2–9, 1997.
97. Crain, E. F., Weiss, K. B., Bijur, P. E., et al.: An estimate of the prevalence of asthma and wheezing among inner-city children. Pediatrics *96*:388–389, 1995.
98. Cranage, M. P., and Gardner, P. S.: Systemic cell-mediated and antibody responses in infants with respiratory syncytial virus infections. J. Med. Virol. *5*:161–170, 1980.

99. Crowe, J., Jr.: Immune response of infants to infection with respiratory viruses and live attenuated respiratory virus candidate vaccines. Vaccine *16*:1423–1432, 1998.
100. Crowe, J., Jr., Bui, P., Siber, G., et al.: Cold-passaged, temperature-sensitive mutants of human respiratory syncytial virus (RSV) are highly attenuated, immunogenic, and protective in seronegative chimpanzees, even when RSV antibodies are infused shortly before immunization. Vaccine *13*:847–855, 1995.
101. Cunningham, C. K., McMillan, J. A., and Gross, S. J.: Rehospitalization for respiratory illness in infants of less than 32 weeks' gestation. Pediatrics *88*:527–532, 1991.
102. DeBoeck, K., Van der Aaa, N., Van Lierde, S., et al.: Respiratory syncytial virus bronchiolitis: A double-blind dexamethasone efficacy study. J. Pediatr. *131*:919–921, 1997.
103. Denny, F. W., Collier, A. M., Henderson, F. W., et al.: The epidemiology of bronchiolitis. Pediatr. Res. *11*:234–236, 1977.
104. DeWeerd, W., Twilhaar, W., and Kimpen, J.: T cell subset analysis in peripheral blood of children with RSV bronchiolitis. Scand. J. Infect. Dis. *30*:77–80, 1998.
105. Ditchburn, R. K., McQuillin, J., Gardner, P. S., et al.: Respiratory syncytial virus in hospital cross-infection. B. M. J. *3*:671–673, 1971.
106. Doherty, J., Brookfield, D., Gray, J., et al.: Cohorting of infants with respiratory syncytial virus. J. Hosp. Infect. *38*:203–206, 1998.
107. Doing, K., Jerkofsky, M., Dow, E., et al.: Use of fluorescent-antibody staining of cytocentrifuge-prepared smears in combination with cell culture for direct detection of respiratory viruses. J. Clin. Microbiol. *36*:2112–2114, 1998.
108. Domachowske, J., Dyer, K., Bonville, C., et al.: Recombinant human eosinophil-derived neurotoxin/RNase 2 functions as an effective antiviral agent against respiratory syncytial virus. J. Infect. Dis. *177*:1458–1464, 1998.
109. Domachowske, J., and Rosenberg, H.: Respiratory syncytial virus infection: Immune response, immunopathogenesis, and treatment. Clin. Microbiol. Rev. *12*:298–309, 1999.
110. Donowitz, L. G.: Hospital-acquired infections in children. N. Engl. J. Med. *323*:1836–1837, 1990.
111. Dowell, S., Anderson, L., Gary, J., et al. Respiratory syncytial virus is an important cause of community-acquired lower respiratory infection among hospitalized adults. J. Infect. Dis. *174*:456–462, 1996.
112. Downham, M. A., Gardner, P. S., McQuillin, J., et al.: Role of respiratory viruses in childhood mortality. B. M. J. *1*:235–239, 1975.
113. Downham, M. A., Scott, R., Sims, D. G., et al.: Breast-feeding protects against respiratory syncytial virus infections. B. M. J. *2*:274–276, 1976.
114. Dudas, R., and Karron, R.: Respiratory syncytial virus vaccines. Clin. Microbiol. Rev. *11*:430–439, 1998.
115. Eigen, H.: The RSV-asthma link: The emerging story. J. Pediatr. *135*(Suppl.):1–50, 1999.
116. Engler, H., and Preuss, J.: Laboratory diagnosis of respiratory virus infections in 24 hours of utilizing shell vial cultures. J. Clin. Microbiol. *35*:2165–2167, 1997.
117. Englund, J.: Prevention strategies for respiratory syncytial virus: Passive and active immunization. J. Pediatr. *135*(Suppl.):38–44, 1999.
118. Englund, J. A., Anderson, L. J., and Rhame, F. S.: Nosocomial transmission of respiratory syncytial virus in immunocompromised adults. J. Clin. Microbiol. *29*:115–119, 1991.
119. Englund, J., Glezen, W., and Piedra, P.: Maternal immunization against viral disease. Vaccine *16*:1456–1463, 1998.
120. Englund, J., Piedra, P., Jefferson, L., et al.: High-dose, short-duration ribavirin aerosol therapy in children with suspected respiratory syncytial virus infection. J. Pediatr. *117*:313–320, 1990.
121. Erdman, D. D., and Anderson, L. J.: Monoclonal antibody–based capture enzyme immunoassays for specific serum immunoglobulin G (IgG), IgA, and IgM antibodies to respiratory syncytial virus. J. Clin. Microbiol. *28*:2744–2749, 1990.
122. Falsey, A.: Respiratory syncytial virus infection in older persons. Vaccine *16*:1775–1778, 1998.
123. Falsey, A. R., Cunningham, C. K., Barker, W. H., et al.: Respiratory syncytial virus and influenza A infections in the hospitalized elderly. J. Infect. Dis. *172*:389–394, 1995.
124. Falsey, A., and Walsh, E.: Safety and immunogenicity of a respiratory syncytial virus subunit vaccine (PFP-2) in the institutionalized elderly. Vaccine *15*:1130–1132, 1997.
125. Falsey, A., and Walsh, E.: Respiratory syncytial virus infections in adults. Clin. Microbiol. Rev. *13*:371–384, 2000.
126. Fernie, B. F., Ford E. C., and Gerin, J. L.: The development of BALB/c cells persistently infected with respiratory syncytial virus: Presence of ribonucleoprotein on the cell surface. Proc. Soc. Exp. Biol. Med. *167*:83–86, 1981.
127. Fernie, B. F., and Gerin, J. L.: The stabilization and purification of respiratory syncytial virus using $MgSO_4$. Virology *106*:141–144, 1980.
128. Field, C. M. B., Connolly, J. H., Murtagh, G., et al.: Antibiotic treatment of epidemic bronchiolitis: A double-blind trial. B. M. J. *1*:83–85, 1966.
129. Finger, R., Anderson, L., Dicker, R., et al.: Epidemic infections caused by respiratory syncytial virus in institutionalized young adults. J. Infect. Dis. *155*:1335–1339, 1987.
130. Fletcher, J., Smyth, R., Thomas, H., et al.: Respiratory syncytial virus genotypes and disease severity among children in hospital. Arch. Dis. Child. *77*:508–511, 1997.
131. Foy, H. M., Cooney, M. K., Maletzky, A. J., et al.: Incidence and etiology of pneumonia, croup, and bronchiolitis in preschool children belonging to a prepaid medical care group over a four-year period. Am. J. Epidemiol. *97*:80–92, 1973.
132. Frank, A. L., Taber, L. H., Glezen, W. P., et al.: Breast feeding and respiratory virus infections. Pediatrics *70*:239–245, 1982.
133. Fransen, H., Sterner, G., Forsgren, M., et al.: Acute lower respiratory illness in elderly patients with respiratory syncytial virus infection. Acta Med. Scand. *182*:323–330, 1967.
134. Freymuth, F., Petitjean, J., Pothier, P., et al.: Prevalence of respiratory syncytial virus subgroups A and B in France from 1982 to 1990. J. Clin. Microbiol. *29*:653–655, 1991.
135. Friis, B., Anderson, P., Brenoe, E., et al.: Antibiotic treatment of pneumonia and bronchiolitis: A prospective randomized study. Arch. Dis. Child. *59*:1038–1045, 1984.
136. Friis, B., Eiken, M., Hornsleth, A., et al.: Chest x-ray appearances in pneumonia and bronchiolitis. Acta Paediatr. Scand. *79*:219–225, 1990.
137. Fulginiti, V. A., Eller, J. J., Sieber, O. F., et al.: Respiratory virus immunization. I. A field trial of two inactivated respiratory virus vaccines: An aqueous trivalent parainfluenza virus vaccine, and an alum-precipitated respiratory syncytial virus vaccine. Am. J. Epidemiol. *89*:435–448, 1969.
138. Gadomski, A. M., Lichenstein, R., Horton, L., et al.: Efficacy of albuterol in the management of bronchiolitis. Pediatrics *93*:907–912, 1994.
139. Gala, C. L., Hall, C. B., Schnabel, K. C., et al.: The use of eye-nose goggles to control nosocomial respiratory syncytial virus infection. J. A. M. A. *256*:2706–2708, 1986.
140. Gardner, P. S.: Respiratory syncytial virus infections. Postgrad. Med. J. *49*:788–791, 1973.
141. Gardner, P. S.: How etiologic, pathologic, and clinical diagnoses can be made in a correlated fashion. Pediatr. Res. *11*:254–261, 1977.
142. Gardner, P. S., Court, S. D. M., Brocklebank, J. T., et al.: Virus cross-infection in paediatric wards. B. M. J. *2*:571–575, 1973.
143. Gardner, P. S., and McQuillin, J.: The coating of respiratory syncytial (RS) virus–infected cells in the respiratory tract by immunoglobulins. J. Med. Virol. *2*:165–173, 1978.
144. Gardner, P., McQuillin, J., and Court, S. D. M.: Speculation on pathogenesis in death from respiratory syncytial virus infection. B. M. J. *1*:327–330, 1970.
145. Gardner, P. S., Turk, D. C., Aherne, W. A., et al.: Deaths associated with respiratory tract infection in childhood. B. M. J. *4*:316–320, 1967.
146. Garofalo, R., Kimpen, J. L. L., Welliver, R. C., et al.: Eosinophil degranulation in the respiratory tract during naturally acquired respiratory syncytial virus infection. J. Pediatr. *120*:28–32, 1992.
147. Gelfand, E. W., McCurdy, D., Rao, P., et al.: Ribavirin treatment of viral pneumonitis in severe combined immunodeficiency disease. Lancet *2*:732–733, 1983.
148. Gessner, B.: The cost-effectiveness of a hypothetical respiratory syncytial virus vaccine in the elderly. Vaccine *18*:1485–1494, 2000.
149. Giles, T. D., and Gohd, R. S.: Respiratory syncytial virus and heart disease. J. A. M. A. *236*:1128–1130, 1976.
150. Glezen, W. P.: Viral pneumonia as a cause and result of hospitalization. J. Infect. Dis. *4*:765–770, 1983.
151. Glezen, W.: Incidence of respiratory syncytial and parainfluenza type 3 viruses in an urban setting. Pediatr. Virol. *2*:1–4, 1987.
152. Glezen, W., and Alpers, M.: Maternal immunization. Clin. Infect. Dis. *28*:219–224, 1999.
153. Glezen, W. P., and Denny, F. W.: Epidemiology of acute lower respiratory disease in children. N. Engl. J. Med. *288*:498–505, 1973.
154. Glezen, W., Greenberg, S., Atmar, R., et al.: Impact of respiratory virus infections on persons with chronic underlying conditions. J. A. M. A. *283*:499–505, 2000.
155. Glezen, W. P., Loda, F. A., Clyde, W. A., et al.: Epidemiologic patterns of acute lower respiratory disease of children in the pediatric group practice. J. Pediatr. *78*:397–406, 1971.
156. Glezen, W. P., Paredes, A., Allison, J. E., et al.: Risk of respiratory syncytial virus infection from low-income families in relationship to age, sex, ethnic group and maternal antibody group. J. Pediatr. *98*:708–715, 1981.
157. Glezen, W. P., Taber, L. H., Frank, A. L., et al.: Risk of primary infection and reinfection with respiratory syncytial virus. Am. J. Dis. Child. *140*:543–546, 1986.
158. Goldmann, D. A.: Transmission of infectious diseases in children. Pediatr. Rev. *13*:283–294, 1992.
159. Graham, B.: Pathogenesis of respiratory syncytial virus vaccine–augmented pathology. Am. J. Respir. Crit. Care Med. *152*(Suppl.):63–66, 1995.
160. Graham, B., Bunton, L., Rowland, J., et al.: Respiratory syncytial virus infection in anti-m treated mice. J. Virol. *65*:4936–4942, 1991.
161. Graham, B. S., Bunton, L. A., Wright, P. F., et al.: Reinfection of mice with respiratory syncytial virus. J. Med. Virol. *34*:7–13, 1991.

162. Graham, B. S., Bunton, L. A., Wright, P. F., et al.: The role of T lymphocyte subsets in the pathogenesis of primary RSV infection and rechallenge in mice. J. Clin. Invest. *88*:1026–1033, 1991.
163. Graham, B. S., Henderson, G. S., Tang, Y.-W., et al.: Priming immunization determines T helper cytokine mRNA expression patterns in lungs of mice challenged with respiratory syncytial virus. J. Immunol. *151*:2032–2040, 1993.
164. Graham, B., Johnson, T., and Peebles, R.: Immune-mediated disease pathogenesis in respiratory syncytial virus infection. Immunopharmacology *48*:237–247, 2000.
165. Graham, B. S., Perkins, M. D., Wright, P. F., et al.: Primary respiratory syncytial virus infection in mice. J. Med. Virol. *26*:153–162, 1988.
166. Greenes, D., and Harper, M.: Low risk of bacteremia in febrile children with recognizable viral syndromes. Pediatr. Infect. Dis. J. *18*:258–261, 1999.
167. Groothuis, J. R., Gutierrez, K. M., and Lauer, B. A.: Respiratory syncytial virus infection in children with bronchopulmonary dysplasia. Pediatrics *82*:199–203, 1988.
168. Groothuis, J., King, S., Hogerman, D., et al.: Safety and immunogenicity of a purified F protein respiratory syncytial virus (PFP-2) vaccine in seropositive children with bronchopulmonary dysplasia. J. Infect. Dis. *177*:467–469, 1998.
169. Groothuis, J. R., Simoes, E. A. F., Levin, M. J., et al.: Prophylactic administration of respiratory syncytial virus immune globulin to high-risk infants and young children. N. Engl. J. Med. *329*:1524–1530, 1993.
170. Groothuis, J. R., Woodin, K. A., Katz, R., et al.: Early ribavirin treatment of respiratory syncytial viral infection in high-risk children. J. Pediatr. *117*:792–798, 1990.
171. Hall, C. B.: The shedding and spreading of respiratory syncytial virus. Pediatr. Res. *11*:236–239, 1977.
172. Hall, C. B.: The nosocomial spread of respiratory syncytial virus infections. Annu. Rev. Med. *34*:311–319, 1983.
173. Hall, C. B.: Respiratory syncytial virus: microbe for all ages, mimic of maladies many. *In* Scheld, W., Craig, W., Hughes, J. (eds.): Emerging Infections 4. Washington, DC, ASM Press, 2000, pp. 1–15.
174. Hall, C.: Respiratory syncytial viral infections: Pathology and pathogenicity. *In* Weisman, L., and Groothuis, J. (eds.): Contemporary Diagnosis and Management of Respiratory Syncytial Virus Infection. Newtown, PA, Handbooks in Health Care Company, 2000, pp. 72–93.
175. Hall, C.: Nosocomial respiratory syncytial virus infections: The "cold war" has not ended. Clin. Infect. Dis. *31*:590–596, 2000.
176. Hall, C. B.: Respiratory syncytial virus infections in previously healthy working adults. Clin. Infect. Dis. *33*:792–796, 2001.
177. Hall, C.: Respiratory syncytial virus and the parainfluenza viruses. N. Engl. J. Med. *344*:1917–1923, 2001.
178. Hall, C. B., and Douglas, R. G., Jr.: Clinically useful method for the isolation of respiratory syncytial virus. J. Infect. Dis. *131*:1–5, 1975.
179. Hall, C. B., and Douglas, R. G., Jr.: Respiratory syncytial virus and influenza: Practical community surveillance. Am. J. Dis. Child. *130*:615–620, 1976.
180. Hall, C. B., and Douglas, R. G., Jr.: Modes of transmission of respiratory syncytial virus. J. Pediatr. *99*:100–103, 1981.
181. Hall, C., and Douglas, R. J.: Nosocomial respiratory syncytial virus infections: The role of gowns and masks on prevention. Am. J. Dis. Child. *135*:512–516, 1981.
182. Hall, C. B., Douglas, R. G., Jr., and Geiman, J. M.: Quantitative shedding patterns of respiratory syncytial virus in infants. J. Infect. Dis. *132*:151–156, 1975.
183. Hall, C. B., Douglas, R. G., Jr., and Geiman, J. M.: Respiratory syncytial virus infection in infants: Quantitation and duration of shedding. J. Pediatr. *89*:11–15, 1976.
184. Hall, C. B., Douglas, R. G., Jr., Geiman, J. M., et al.: Nosocomial respiratory syncytial virus infections. N. Engl. J. Med. *293*:1343–1346, 1975.
185. Hall, C. B., Douglas, R. G., Jr., Schnabel, K. C., et al.: Infectivity of respiratory syncytial virus by various routes of inoculation. Infect. Immun. *33*:779–783, 1981.
186. Hall, C. B., Geiman, J. M., Biggar, R., et al.: Respiratory syncytial virus infection within families. N. Engl. J. Med. *294*:414–419, 1976.
187. Hall, C. B., Geiman, J. M., and Douglas, R. G., Jr.: Possible transmission by fomites of respiratory syncytial virus. J. Infect. Dis. *141*:98–102, 1980.
188. Hall, C. B., Geiman, J. M., Douglas, R. G., Jr., et al.: Control of nosocomial respiratory syncytial viral infection. Pediatrics *62*:728–731, 1978.
189. Hall, C. B., Hall, W. J., and Speers, D. M.: Clinical and physiological manifestations of bronchiolitis and pneumonia: Outcome of respiratory syncytial virus. Am. J. Dis. Child. *133*:798–802, 1979.
190. Hall, C. B., Kopelman, A. E., Douglas, R. G., Jr., et al.: Neonatal respiratory syncytial virus infection. N. Engl. J. Med. *300*:393–396, 1979.
191. Hall, C. B., McBride, J. T., Gala, C. L., et al.: Ribavirin aerosol treatment of respiratory syncytial viral infection in infants with underlying cardiac and pulmonary disease. J. A. M. A. *254*:3047–3051, 1985.
192. Hall, C. B., McBride, J. T., Walsh, E. E., et al.: Aerosolized ribavirin treatment of infants with respiratory syncytial viral infection. N. Engl. J. Med. *308*:1443–1447, 1983.
193. Hall, C. B., Powell, K. R., MacDonald, N. E., et al.: Respiratory syncytial viral infection in children with compromised immune function. N. Engl. J. Med. *315*:77–80, 1986.
194. Hall, C. B., Powell, K. R., Schnabel, K. C., et al.: Risk of secondary bacterial infection in infants hospitalized with respiratory syncytial viral infection. J. Pediatr. *113*:266–271, 1988.
195. Hall, C. B., Walsh, E. E., Hruska, J. F., et al.: Ribavirin aerosol treatment of experimental respiratory syncytial viral infection in young adults: A controlled double blind study. J. A. M. A. *249*:2666–2670, 1983.
196. Hall, C. B., Walsh, E. E., Long, C. G., et al.: Immunity and frequency of reinfection with respiratory syncytial virus. J. Infect. Dis. *163*:693–698, 1991.
197. Hall, C. B., Walsh, E. E., Schnabel, K. C., et al.: The occurrence of groups A and B of respiratory syncytial virus over 15 years: The associated epidemiologic and clinical characteristics in hospitalized and ambulatory children. J. Infect. Dis. *162*:1283–1290, 1990.
198. Hall, W. J., Hall, C. B., and Speers, D. M.: Respiratory syncytial virus infections in adults: Clinical, virologic, and serial pulmonary function studies. Ann. Intern. Med. *88*:203–205, 1978.
199. Hambling, M. H.: Survival of the respiratory syncytial virus during storage under various conditions. Br. J. Exp. Pathol. *45*:647–655, 1964.
200. Hamre, D., and Procknow, J. J.: Viruses isolated from natural common colds in the U.S.A. B. M. J. *2*:1382–1385, 1961.
201. Han, L., Alexander, J., and Anderson, L.: Respiratory syncytial virus pneumonia among the elderly: An assessment of disease burden. J. Infect. Dis. *179*:25–30, 1999.
202. Hancock, G. E., Speelman, D. J., Frenchick, P. J., et al.: Formulation of the purified fusion protein of respiratory syncytial virus with the saponin QS-21 induces protective immune responses in BALB/c mice that are similar to those generated by experimental infection. Vaccine *13*:391–400, 1995.
203. Heikkinen, T., Waris, M., Ruuskanen, O., et al.: Incidence of acute otitis media associated with group A and B respiratory syncytial virus infections. Acta Paediatr. *84*:419–423, 1995.
204. Heilman, C. A.: Respiratory syncytial and parainfluenza viruses. J. Infect. Dis. *161*:402–406, 1990.
205. Henderson, F. W., Clyde, W. A., Jr., Collier, A. M., et al.: The etiologic and epidemiologic spectrum of bronchiolitis in pediatric practice. J. Pediatr. *95*:183–190, 1979.
206. Henderson, F. W., Collier, A. M., Clyde, W. A., Jr., et al.: Respiratory syncytial virus infections, reinfections and immunity: A prospective longitudinal study in young children. N. Engl. J. Med. *300*:530–534, 1979.
207. Henderson, F. W., Collier, A. M., Sanyal, M. A., et al.: A longitudinal study of respiratory viruses and bacteria in the etiology of acute otitis media with effusion. N. Engl. J. Med. *306*:1377–1383, 1982.
208. Henderson, F. W., and Giebink, G. S.: Otitis media among children in day care: Epidemiology and pathogenesis. Rev. Infect. Dis. *8*:533–538, 1986.
209. Hendry, R. M., Burns, J. C., Walsh, E. E., et al.: Strain-specific serum antibody responses in infants undergoing primary infection with respiratory syncytial virus. J. Infect. Dis. *157*:640–647, 1988.
210. Hendry, R. M., Pierik, L. T., and McIntosh, K.: Prevalence of respiratory syncytial virus subgroups over six consecutive outbreaks: 1981–1987. J. Infect. Dis. *160*:185–190, 1989.
211. Henkel, J., Aberle, S., Kunde, M., et al.: Improved detection of respiratory syncytial virus in nasal aspirates by seminested RT-PCR. J. Med. Virol. *53*:366–371, 1997.
212. Hiatt, P., Grace, S., Kozinetz, C., et al.: Effects of viral lower respiratory tract infection on lung function in infants with cystic fibrosis. Pediatrics *103*:619–626, 1999.
213. Higgins, P. G., Barrow, G. I., Tyrrell, D. A., et al.: The efficacy of intranasal interferon alpha-2a in respiratory syncytial virus infection in volunteers. Antiviral Res. *14*:3–10, 1990.
214. Hogg, J. C., Williams, J., Richardson, J. B., et al.: Age as a factor in the distribution of lower-airway conductance and in the pathologic anatomy of obstructive lung disease. N. Engl. J. Med. *282*:1283–1287, 1970.
215. Holberg, C. J., Wright, A. L., Martinez, F. D., et al.: Risk factors for respiratory syncytial virus–associated lower respiratory illnesses in the first year of life. Am. J. Epidemiol. *133*:1135–1151, 1991.
216. Holberg, C. J., Wright, A. L., Martinez, F. D., et al.: Child day care, smoking by caregivers, and lower respiratory tract illness in the first 3 years of life. Pediatrics *91*:885–892, 1993.
217. Hornsleth, A., Friis, B., Grauballe, P. C., et al.: Detection by ELISA of IgA and IgM antibodies in secretion and IgM antibodies in serum in primary lower respiratory syncytial virus infection. J. Med. Virol. *13*:149–161, 1984.
218. Hornsleth, A., Klug, B., Nir, M., et al.: Severity of respiratory syncytial virus disease related to type and genotype of virus and to cytokine values in nasopharyngeal secretions. Pediatr. Infect. Dis. J. *17*:1114–1121, 1998.
219. Huang, Y. T., Collins, P. L., and Wertz, G. W.: Characterization of the 10 proteins of human respiratory syncytial virus: Identification of a fourth envelope-associated protein. Virus Res. *2*:157–173, 1985.
220. Hussell, T., Georgiou, A., Sparer, T., et al.: Host genetic determinants of vaccine-induced eosinophilia during respiratory syncytial virus infection. J. Immunol. *161*:6215–6222, 1998.

221. Ikeda, S., Neyts, J., Verma, S., et al.: In vitro and in vivo inhibition of ortho- and paramyxovirus infections by a new class of sulfonic acid polymers interacting with virus-cell binding and/or fusion. Antimicrob. Agents Chemother. *38*:256–259, 1994.
222. Inabu, Y., Tanaka, Y., Sato, K., et al.: Bovine respiratory syncytial virus: Studies on an outbreak in Japan, 1968–1969. Jpn. J. Microbiol. *16*:373–383, 1972.
223. Isaacs, D.: Viral subunit vaccines. Lancet *337*:1223–1224, 1991.
224. Isaacs, D., Bangham, C. R. M., and McMichael, A. J.: Cell-mediated cytotoxic response to respiratory syncytial virus in infants with bronchiolitis. Lancet *2*:769–771, 1987.
225. Isaacs, D., Dickson, H., O'Callaghan, C., et al.: Handwashing and cohorting in prevention of hospital acquired infections with respiratory syncytial virus. Arch. Dis. Child. *66*:227–231, 1991.
226. Jackson, M., and Scott, R.: Different patterns of cytokine induction in cultures of respiratory syncytial (RS) virus–specific human Th cell lines following stimulation with RS virus and RS virus proteins. J. Med. Virol. *49*:161–169, 1996.
227. Jairath, S., Vargas, P., Hamlin, H., et al.: Inhibition of respiratory syncytial virus replication by antisense oligodeoxyribonucleotides. Antiviral Res. *33*:201–213, 1997.
228. Janai, H. K., Stutman, H. R., Zaleska, M., et al. Ribavirin effect on pulmonary function in young infants with respiratory syncytial virus bronchiolitis. Pediatr. Infect. Dis. J. *12*:214–218, 1993.
229. Jarvis, W. R., Middleton, P. J., and Gelfand, E. W.: Significance of viral infections in severe combined immunodeficiency disease. Pediatr. Infect. Dis. *2*:187–192, 1983.
230. Jensen, C., and Johnson, F. B.: Comparison of various transport media for viability maintenance of herpes simplex virus, respiratory syncytial virus, and adenovirus. Diagn. Microbiol. Infect. Dis. *19*:137–142, 1994.
231. Jensen, I., Thisted, E., Glikmann, G., et al. Secretory IgM and IgA antibodies to respiratory syncytial virus in nasopharyngeal aspirates: A diagnostic supplement to antigen detection. Clin. Diagn. Virol. *8*:219–226, 1997.
232. Joffe, S., Escobar, G., Black, S., et al.: Rehospitalization for respiratory syncytial virus among premature infants. Pediatrics *104*:894–899, 1999.
233. Johnson, J., and Graham, B.: The histopathology of fatal untreated human RSV infection: An archival study of autopsy material, 1925–1959. Paper presented at the RSV after 43 Years Symposium, November 8–11, 1999, Stuart, FL.
234. Johnson, K. M., Bloom, H. H., Mufson, M. A., et al.: Natural reinfection of adults by respiratory syncytial virus: Possible relation to mild upper respiratory disease. N. Engl. J. Med. *267*:68–72, 1962.
235. Johnson, K. M., Chanock, R. M., Rifkind, D., et al.: Respiratory syncytial virus. IV. Correlation of virus shedding, serologic response, and illness in adult volunteers. J. A. M. A. *176*:663–667, 1961.
236. Johnson, P. R., Olmsted, R. A., Prince, G. A., et al.: Antigenic relatedness between glycoproteins of human respiratory syncytial virus subgroups A and B: Evaluation of the contributions of F and G glycoproteins to immunity. J. Virol. *10*:3163–3166, 1987.
237. Johnson, P. R., Spriggs, M. K., Olmsted, R. A., et al.: The G glycoprotein of human respiratory syncytial viruses of subgroups A and B: Extensive sequence divergence between antigenically related proteins. Proc. Natl. Acad. Sci. U. S. A. *84*:5625–5629, 1987.
238. Johnson, T., and Graham, B.: Secreted respiratory syncytial virus G glycoprotein induces interleukin-5 (IL-5) IL-13, and eosinophilia by an IL-4 independent mechanism. J. Virol. *73*:8485–8495, 1999.
239. Jones, B., Clark, S., Curran, E., et al.: Control of an outbreak of respiratory syncytial virus infection in immunocompromised adults. J. Hosp. Infect. *44*:53–57, 2000.
240. Jordan, W. S., Jr.: Growth characteristics of respiratory syncytial virus. J. Immunol. *88*:581–590, 1962.
241. Kahn, J.: Respiratory syncytial virus vaccine development. Curr. Opin. Pediatr. *12*:257–262, 2000.
242. Kapikian, A. Z., Bell, J. A., Mastrota, F. M., et al.: An outbreak of febrile illness and pneumonia associated with respiratory syncytial virus infection. Am. J. Hyg. *74*:234–248, 1961.
243. Kapikian, A. Z., Mitchell, R. H., Chanock, R. M., et al.: An epidemiologic study of altered clinical reactivity to respiratory syncytial (RS) virus infection in children previously vaccinated with an inactivated RSV virus vaccine. Am. J. Epidemiol. *89*:405–421, 1969.
244. Karron, R., and Ambrosino, D.: Respiratory syncytial virus vaccines. Pediatr. Infect. Dis. J. *17*:919–920, 1998.
245. Karron, R., Singleton, R., Bulkow, L., et al. Severe respiratory syncytial virus disease in Alaska Native children. J. Infect. Dis. *180*:41–49, 1999.
246. Karron, R., Wright, P., Belshe, R., et al. Evaluation of live recombinant RSV A2 vaccines in children over 6 months of age. Paper presented at the RSV after 43 Years Symposium, November 8–11, 1999, Stuart, FL.
247. Kattan, M.: Epidemiologic evidence of increased airway reactivity in children with a history of bronchiolitis. J. Pediatr. *135*(Suppl.):8–13, 1999.
248. Kaul, T. N., Welliver, R. C., Wong, D. T., et al.: Secretory and antibody response to respiratory syncytial virus infection. Am. J. Dis. Child. *135*:1013–1016, 1981.
249. Kellner, J., Ohlsson, A., Gadomski, A., et al.: Efficacy of bronchodilator therapy in bronchiolitis. Arch. Pediatr. Adolesc. Med. *150*:1166–1172, 1996.
250. Kellogg, J. A.: Culture vs direct antigen assay for the detection of respiratory syncytial virus (RSV). Pan. Am. Group Rapid Viral Diagn. *17*:1–4, 1991.
251. Kellogg, J. A.: Culture vs direct antigen assays for detection of microbial pathogens from lower respiratory tract specimens suspected of containing the respiratory syncytial virus. Arch. Pathol. Lab. Med. *115*:451–458, 1991.
252. Kennedy, C. R., Chrzanowska, K., Robinson, R. O., et al.: A major role for viruses in acute childhood encephalopathy. Lancet *1*:989–991, 1986.
253. Khamapirad, T., and Glezen, W. P.: Clinical and radiographic assessment of acute lower respiratory tract disease in infants and children. Semin. Respir. Infect. *2*:130–144, 1987.
254. Kim, H. W., Arrobio, J. O., Brandt, C. D., et al.: Epidemiology of respiratory syncytial virus infection in Washington, D.C. I. Importance of the virus in different respiratory disease syndromes and temporal distribution of infection. Am. J. Epidemiol. *98*:216–225, 1973.
255. Kim, H. W., Canchola, J. G., Brandt, C. D., et al.: Respiratory syncytial virus disease in infants despite prior administration of antigenic inactivated vaccine. Am. J. Epidemiol. *89*:422–434, 1969.
256. Kim, H. W., Leikin, S. L., Arrobio, J., et al.: Cell-mediated immunity to respiratory syncytial virus induced by inactivated vaccine or by infection. Pediatr. Res. *10*:75–78, 1976.
257. Kimball, A. M., Foy, H. M., Cooney, M. K., et al.: Isolation of respiratory syncytial and influenza viruses from the sputum of patients hospitalized with pneumonia. J. Infect. Dis. *147*:181–184, 1983.
258. Kimman, T. G., Westenbrink, F., Schreuder, B. E. C., et al.: Local and systemic antibody response to bovine respiratory syncytial virus infection and reinfection in calves with and without maternal antibodies. J. Clin. Microbiol. *25*:1097–1106, 1987.
259. Kimpen, J., and Schaad, U.: Treatment of respiratory syncytial virus bronchiolitis: 1995 poll of members of the European Society for Paediatric Infectious Diseases. Pediatr. Infect. Dis. J. *16*:479–481, 1997.
260. King, J., Jr.: Community respiratory viruses in individuals with human immunodeficiency virus infection. Am. J. Med. *102*:19–26, 1997.
261. Klassen, T. P., Rowe, P. C., Sutcliffe, T., et al.: Randomized trial of salbutamol in acute bronchiolitis. J. Pediatr. *118*:807–811, 1991.
262. Klassen, T., Stucliffe, T., Watters, L., et al.: Dexamethasone in salbutamol-treated inpatients with acute bronchiolitis: A randomized, controlled trial. J. Pediatr. *130*:191–196, 1997.
263. Kneyber, M., Brandenburg, A., de Groot, R., et al.: Risk factors for respiratory syncytial virus associated apnoea. Eur. J. Pediatr. *157*:331–335, 1998.
264. Knight, V., and Gilbert, B. E.: Chemotherapy of respiratory viruses. Adv. Intern. Med. *31*:95–118, 1986.
265. Knight, V., Yu, C. P., Gilbert, B. E., et al.: Ribavirin Aerosol Treatment: Emerging Technical and Clinical Summary. Royal Society of Medicine Services Limited. International Congress and Symposium Series, No. 145, London 1988, pp. 69–84.
266. Kravetz, H. M., Knight, V., Chanock, R. M., et al.: Respiratory syncytial virus. III. Production of illness and clinical observations in adult volunteers. J. A. M. A. *176*:657–667, 1961.
267. Krilov, L. R., Anderson, L. J., Marcoux, L., et al.: Antibody-mediated enhancement of respiratory syncytial virus infection in two monocyte/macrophage cell lines. J. Infect. Dis. *160*:777–782, 1989.
268. Kuppermann, N., Bank, D., Walton, E., et al.: Risks for bacteremia and urinary tract infections in young febrile children with bronchiolitis. Arch. Pediatr. Adolesc. Med. *151*:1207–1214, 1997.
269. Laegreid, A., Kolsto Otnaess, A. B., Orstavik, I., et al.: Neutralizing activity in human milk fractions against respiratory syncytial virus. Acta Paediatr. Scand. *75*:696–701, 1986.
270. Laing, I., Riedel, F., Yap, P. L., et al.: Atopy predisposing to acute bronchiolitis during an epidemic of respiratory syncytial virus. B. M. J. *284*:1070–1072, 1982.
271. Lambert, D., Barney, S., Lambert, A., et al.: Peptides from conserved regions of paramyxovirus fusion (F) proteins are potent inhibitors of viral infusion. Proc. Natl. Acad. Sci. U. S. A. *93*:2186–2191, 1996.
272. LaMontagne, J.: RSV pneumonia, a community-acquired infection in adults. Lancet *349*:149–150, 1997.
273. Landau, L. I.: Bronchiolitis and asthma: Are they related? Thorax *49*:293–296, 1994.
274. Langedijk, J., Meloen, R., and van Oirschot, J.: Identification of a conserved neutralization site in the first heptad repeat of the fusion protein of respiratory syncytial virus. Arch. Virol. 143:313–320, 1998.
275. Langley, J., LeBlanc, J., and Wang, E.: Temporal trends in hospitalization for bronchiolitis in Canadian children 1980–97. Paper presented at the RSV after 43 Years Symposium, November 8–11, 1999, Stuart, FL.
276. Langley, J., LeBlanc, J., Wang, E., et al.: Nosocomial respiratory syncytial virus infection in Canadian pediatric hospitals: A Pediatric Investigators Collaborative Network on Infections in Canada Study. Pediatrics *100*:943–946, 1997.

277. Lapin, C. D., Hiatt, P. W., Langston, C., et al.: A lamb model for human respiratory syncytial virus infection. Pediatr. Pulmonol. *15*:151–156, 1993.
278. Larsen, G., and Colasurdo, G.: Neural control mechanisms within airways: Disruption by respiratory syncytial virus. J. Pediatr. *135*(Suppl.):21–27, 1999.
279. Law, B., and Carvalho, V. D.: Respiratory syncytial virus infections in hospitalized Canadian children: Regional differences in patient populations and management practices. Pediatr. Infect. Dis. J. *12*:659–663, 1993.
280. Law, B., Wang, E., MacDonald, N., et al.: Does ribavirin impact on the hospital course of children with respiratory syncytial virus (RSV) infection? An analysis using the Pediatric Investigators Collaborative Network on Infections in Canada (PICNIC) RSV Database. Pediatrics *99*:e7, 1997.
281. LeClair, J. M., Freeman, J., Sullivan, B. F., et al.: Prevention of nosocomial respiratory syncytial virus infections through compliance with glove and gown isolation precautions. N. Engl. J. Med. *317*:329–334, 1987.
282. Lee, G. C.-Y., Funk, G. A., Chen, S. T., et al.: An outbreak of respiratory syncytial virus infection in an infant nursery. J. Formos. Med. Assoc. *72*:39–46, 1973.
283. LeSaux, N.: Canadian experience with RSV in the elderly; Results of an epidemiological study. Paper presented at the Aventis Pasteur/ICAAC Symposium Respiratory Syncytial Virus in the Elderly, September 17, 2000, Toronto.
284. Levine, S., and Hamilton, R.: Kinetics of the respiratory syncytial virus growth cycle in HeLa cells. Arch. Ges. Virusforsch *28*:122–132, 1969.
285. Liebelt, E., Qi, K., and Harvey, K.: Diagnostic testing for serious bacterial infections in infants aged 90 days or younger with bronchiolitis. Arch. Pediatr. Adolesc. Med. *153*:525–530, 1999.
296. Lipson, S., Popiolek, D., Hu, Q., et al.: Efficacy of Directigen RSV testing in patient management following admission from a paediatric emergency department. J. Hosp. Infect. *41*:323–329, 1999.
287. Liss, H. P., and Bernstein, J.: Ribavirin aerosol in the elderly. Chest *93*:1239–1241, 1988.
288. Ljungman, P.: Respiratory virus infections in bone marrow transplant recipients: The European perspective. Am. J. Med. *102*:44–47, 1997.
289. Lowther, S., Shay, D., Holman, R., et al.: Bronchiolitis-associated hospitalizations among American Indian and Alaska Native children. Pediatr. Infect. Dis. *19*:11–17, 2000.
290. Lundgren, D. L., Magnuson, M. G., and Clapper, W. E.: A serologic survey in dogs for antibody to human respiratory viruses. Lab. Anim. Care *19*:352–359, 1969.
291. MacDonald, N. E., Hall, C. B., Suffin, S. C., et al.: Respiratory syncytial viral infection in infants with congenital heart disease. N. Engl. J. Med. *307*:397–400, 1982.
292. MacDonald, N. E., Wolfish, N., McLaine, P., et al.: Role of respiratory viruses in exacerbations of primary nephrotic syndrome. J. Pediatr. *108*:378–382, 1986.
293. Maitreyi, R., Broor, S., Kabra, S., et al. Rapid detection of respiratory viruses by centrifugation enhanced cultures from children with acute lower respiratory tract infections. J. Clin. Virol. *16*:41–47, 2000.
294. Male oscuro—R.S.V.? Lancet *1*:651–652, 1979.
295. Marshall, E.: Visiting experts find the "mystery disease" of Naples is a common virus. Science *203*:908–981, 1979.
296. Martinez, F., Wright, A., Taussig, L., et al.: Asthma and wheezing in the first six years of life. N. Engl. J. Med. *332*:133–138, 1995.
297. Mazzulli, T., Peret, T., McGeer, A., et al.: Molecular characterization of a nosocomial outbreak of human respiratory syncytial virus on an adult leukemia/lymphoma ward. J. Infect. Dis. *180*:1686–1689, 1999.
298. McBride, J., and McConnochie, D.: RSV, recurrent wheezing, and ribavirin. Pediatr. Pulmonol. *25*:145–146, 1998.
299. McConnochie, K. M., Hall, C. B., and Barker, W. H.: Lower respiratory tract illness in the first 2 years of life: Epidemiologic patterns and costs in a suburban pediatric practice. Am. J. Public Health *78*:34–39, 1988.
300. McConnochie, K. M., Hall, C. B., Walsh, E. E., et al.: Variation in severity of respiratory syncytial virus infection with subtype. J. Pediatr. *117*:52–62, 1990.
301. McIntosh, K.: Pathogenesis of severe acute respiratory infections in the developing world: Respiratory syncytial virus and parainfluenza virus. Rev. Infect. Dis. *13*(Suppl.):492–500, 1991.
302. McIntosh, K., Hendry, R. M., Fahnestock, M. L., et al.: Enzyme-linked immunosorbent assay for detection of respiratory syncytial virus infection: Application to clinical samples. J. Clin. Microbiol. *16*:329–333, 1982.
303. McIntosh, K., Kurachek, S. C., Cairns, L. M., et al.: Treatment of respiratory viral infection in an immunodeficient infant with ribavirin aerosol. Am. J. Dis. Child. *138*:305–308, 1984.
304. McIntosh, K., Masters, H. B., Orr, I., et al.: The immunologic response to infection with respiratory syncytial virus in infants. J. Infect. Dis. *138*:24–32, 1978.
305. McMillan, J. A., Tristram, D. A., Weiner, L. B., et al.: Prediction of the duration of hospitalization in patients with respiratory syncytial virus: Use of clinical parameters. Pediatrics *81*:22–26, 1988.
306. Meddens, M. J. M., Herbrink, P., Lindeman, J., et al.: Serodiagnosis of respiratory syncytial virus (RSV) infection in children as measured by detection of RSV-specific immunoglobulins G, M, and A, with enzyme-linked immunosorbent assay. J. Clin. Microbiol. *28*:152–155, 1990.
307. Meert, K., Heidemann, S., Lieh-Lai, M., et al.: Clinical characteristics of respiratory syncytial virus infections in healthy versus previously compromised host. Pediatr. Pulmonol. *7*:167–170, 1989.
308. Meert, K. L., Sarnaik, A. P., Gelmini, M. J., et al.: Aerosolized ribavirin in mechanically ventilated children with respiratory syncytial virus lower respiratory tract diseases: A prospective, double-blind, randomized trial. Crit. Care Med. *22*:566–572, 1994.
309. Meissner, H. C., Murray, S. A., Kiernan, M. A., et al.: A simultaneous outbreak of respiratory syncytial virus and parainfluenza virus type 3 in a newborn nursery. J. Pediatr. *104*:680–684, 1984.
310. Menon, K., Sutcliffe, T., and Klassen, T. P.: A randomized trial comparing the efficacy of epinephrine with salbutamol in the treatment of acute bronchiolitis. J. Pediatr. *126*:1004–1007, 1995.
311. Meurman, O., Waris, M., and Hedman, K.: Immunoglobulin G antibody avidity in patients with respiratory syncytial virus infection. J. Clin. Microbiol. *30*:1479–1484, 1992.
312. Mills, J. V., VanKirk, J. E., Wright, P. F., et al.: Experimental respiratory syncytial virus infection of adults: Possible mechanisms of resistance to infection and illness. J. Immunol. *107*:123–130, 1971.
313. Moler, F. W., Khan, A. S., Meliones, J. N., et al.: Respiratory syncytial virus morbidity and mortality estimates in congenital heart disease patients: A recent experience. Crit. Care Med. *20*:1406–1413, 1992.
314. Monto, A. S., Higgins, M. W., and Ross, H. W.: The Tecumseh study of respiratory illness. VIII. Acute infection in chronic respiratory disease and comparison groups. Am. Rev. Respir. Dis. *111*:27–36, 1975.
315. Monto, A. S., and Lim, S. K.: The Tecumseh study of respiratory illness. III. Incidence and periodicity of respiratory syncytial virus and *Mycoplasma pneumoniae* infections. Am. J. Epidemiol. *94*:290–301, 1971.
316. Morrell, R. E., Marks, M. I., Champlin, R., et al.: An outbreak of severe pneumonia due to respiratory syncytial virus in isolated arctic population. Am. J. Epidemiol. *101*:231–237, 1975.
317. Morris, J. A., Blount, R. E., and Savage, R. E.: Recovery of cytopathogenic agent from chimpanzees with coryza. Proc. Soc. Exp. Biol. Med. *92*:544–549, 1956.
318. Muelenaer, P. M., Henderson, F. W., Hemming, V. G., et al.: Group-specific serum antibody responses in children with primary and recurrent respiratory syncytial virus infections. J. Infect. Dis. *164*:15–21, 1991.
319. Mufson, M. A., Belshe, R. B., Örvell, C., et al.: Subgroup characteristics of respiratory syncytial virus strains recovered from children with two consecutive infections. J. Clin. Microbiol. *25*:1535–1539, 1987.
320. Munoz, J. L., McCarthy, C. A., Clark, M. E., et al.: Respiratory syncytial virus infection in C57BL/6 mice: Clearance of virus from the lungs with virus-specific cytotoxic T cells. J. Virol. *65*:4494–4497, 1991.
321. Murphy, B. R., Alling, D. W., Snyder, M. H., et al.: Effect of age and preexisting antibody on serum antibody response of infants and children to the F and G glycoproteins during respiratory syncytial virus infection. J. Clin. Microbiol. *24*:894–898, 1986.
322. Murphy, B. R., Graham, B. S., Prince, G. A., et al.: Serum and nasal-wash immunoglobulin G and A antibody response of infants and children to respiratory syncytial virus F and G glycoproteins following primary infection. J. Clin. Microbiol. *23*:1009–1014, 1986.
323. Murphy, B. R., Prince, G. A., Walsh, E. E., et al.: Dissociation between serum neutralizing and glycoprotein antibody responses of infants and children who received inactivated respiratory syncytial virus vaccine. J. Clin. Microbiol. *24*:197–202, 1986.
324. Murphy, B. R., and Walsh, E. E.: Formalin-inactivated respiratory syncytial virus vaccine induces antibodies to the fusion glycoproteins that are deficient in fusion-inhibiting activity. J. Clin. Microbiol. *26*:1595–1597, 1988.
325. Murphy, D., Todd, J. R., Chao, R. R., et al.: The use of gowns and masks to control respiratory illness in pediatric hospital personnel. J. Pediatr. *99*:746–750, 1981.
326. Murphy, T. F., Henderson, F. W., Clyde, W. C., Jr., et al.: Pneumonia: An eleven-year study in a pediatric practice. Am. J. Epidemiol. *113*:12–21, 1981.
327. Nachman, S., Navaie-Waliser, M., and Qureshi, M.: Rehospitalization with respiratory syncytial virus after neonatal intensive care unit discharge: a 3-year follow-up. Pediatrics *100*:e8, 1997.
328. Navas, L., Wang, E., de Carvalho, V., et al.: Improved outcome of respiratory syncytial virus infection in a high-risk hospitalized population of Canadian children. J. Pediatr. *121*:348–354, 1992.
329. Neuzil, K. M., Gruber, W. C., Chytil, F., et al.: Serum vitamin A levels in respiratory syncytial virus infection. J. Pediatr. *124*:433–436, 1994.
330. Neyts, J., Reymen, D., Letourneur, D., et al.: Differential antiviral activity of derivatized dextrans. Biochem. Pharmacol. *50*:743–751, 1995.
331. Nicholas, J. A., Rubino, K. L., Levely, M. E., et al.: Cytolytic T-lymphocyte responses to respiratory syncytial virus: Effector cell phenotype and target proteins. J. Virol. *64*:4232–4241, 1990.
332. Nicholson, K.: Impact of influenza and respiratory syncytial virus on mortality in England and Wales from January 1975 to December 1990. Epidemiol. Infect. *116*:51–63, 1996.

333. Nicholson, K.: RSV in community-dwelling elderly. Paper presented at the Aventis Pasteur/ICAAC Symposium Respiratory Syncytial Virus in the Elderly, September 17, 2000, Toronto.
334. Nicholson, K., Kent, J., Hammersley, V., et al.: Acute viral infections of upper respiratory tract in elderly people living in the community: Comparative, prospective, population based study of disease burden. B. M. J. *315*:1060–1064, 1997.
335. Noah, T., and Becker, S.: Chemokines in nasal secretions of normal adults experimentally infected with respiratory syncytial virus. Clin. Immunol. *97*:43–49, 2000.
336. Noble, V., Murray, M., Webb, M., et al.: Respiratory status and allergy nine to 10 years after acute bronchiolitis. Arch. Dis. Child. *76*:315–319, 1997.
337. Nosocomial infection with respiratory syncytial virus. Lancet *340*:1071–1072, 1992.
338. Ogilivie, M. M., Vatheneo, S., Radford, M., et al.: Maternal antibody and respiratory syncytial virus infection in infancy. J. Med. Virol. *7*:263–271, 1981.
339. Oien, N. L., Brideau, R. J., Walsh, E., et al.: Induction of local and systemic immunity against human respiratory syncytial virus using a chimeric FG glycoprotein and cholera toxin B subunit. Vaccine *12*:731–735, 1994.
340. Okamoto, Y., Kudo, K., Shirotori, K., et al.: Detection of genomic sequences of respiratory syncytial virus in otitis media with effusion in children. Ann. Otol. Rhinol. Laryngol. *157*:(Suppl.)7–10, 1992.
341. Opavsky, M. A., Stephens, D., Wang, E. E.-L., et al.: Testing models predicting severity of respiratory syncytial virus infection on the PICNIC RSV database. Arch. Pediatr. Adolesc. Med. *149*:1217–1220, 1995.
342. Openshaw, P. J. M., Anderson, K., Wertz, G. W., et al.: The 22,000-kilodalton protein of respiratory syncytial virus is a major target for Kd-restricted cytotoxic T lymphocytes from mice primed by infection. J. Virol. *64*:1683–1689, 1990.
343. Openshaw, P. J., Clarke, S. L., and Record, F. M.: Pulmonary eosinophilic response to respiratory syncytial virus infection in mice sensitized to the major surface glycoprotein G. Int. Immunol. *4*:493–500, 1992.
344. Openshaw, P., and Walzl, G.: Infections prevent the development of asthma—true, false, or both? J. R. Soc. Med. *92*:495–499, 1999.
345. Palivizumab, a humanized respiratory syncytial virus monoclonal antibody, reduces hospitalization from respiratory syncytial virus infection in high-risk infants. The IMpact-RSV Study Group. Pediatrics *102*:531–537, 1998.
346. Paradiso, P. R., Hildreth, S. W., Hogerman, D. A., et al. Safety and immunogenicity of a subunit respiratory syncytial virus vaccine in children 24 to 48 months old. Pediatr. Infect. Dis. J. *13*:792–798, 1994.
347. Parrott, R. H., Kim, H. W., Arrobio, J. O., et al.: Epidemiology of respiratory syncytial virus infection in Washington, D.C. II. Infection and disease with respect to age, immunologic status, race, and sex. Am. J. Epidemiol. *98*:289–300, 1973.
348. Parrott, R. H., Kim, H. W., Brandt, C. D., et al.: Respiratory syncytial virus in infants and children. Prev. Med. *3*:473–480, 1974.
349. Patel, J., Faden, H., Sharma, S., et al.: Effect of respiratory syncytial virus on adherence, colonization and immunity of non-typable *Haemophilus influenzae*: Implications for otitis media. Int. J. Pediatr. Otorhinolaryngol. *23*:15–23, 1992.
350. Pavon, D., Castro-Rodriguez, J., Rubilar, L. et al.: Relation between pulse oximetry and clinical score in children with acute wheezing less than 24 months of age. Pediatr. Pulmonol. *27*:423–427, 1999.
351. Peret, T., Hall, C., Hammond, G., et al. Circulation patterns of group A and B human respiratory syncytial virus genotypes in 5 communities in North America. J. Infect. Dis. *181*:1891–1896, 2000.
352. Peret, T., Hall, C., Schnabel, K., et al.: Circulation patterns of genetically distinct group A and B strains of human respiratory syncytial virus in a community. J. Gen. Virol. *79*:2221–2229, 1998.
353. Piedra, P., Grace, S., Jewell, A., et al. Purified fusion protein vaccine protects against lower respiratory tract illness during respiratory syncytial virus season in children with cystic fibrosis. Pediatr. Infect. Dis. J. *15*:23–31, 1996.
354. Piedra, P., Wells, J., Cron, S., et al.: Immune responses to respiratory syncytial virus (RSV) in infants and their mothers. Abstract. Pediatr. Res. *45*:171, 1999.
355. Pohl, C., Green, M., Wald, E. R., et al.: Respiratory syncytial virus infections in pediatric liver transplant recipients. J. Infect. Dis. *165*:166–169, 1992.
356. Pons, M. W., Lambert, A. L., Lambert, D. M., et al.: Improvement of espiratory syncytial virus replication in actively growing HEp-2 cells. J. Virol. Methods *7*:217–221, 1983.
357. Prendiville, A., Green, S., and Silverman, M.: Paradoxical response to nebulized salbutamol in wheezy infants, assessed by partial expiratory flow-volume curves. Thorax *42*:86–91, 1987.
358. Preston, F. M., Beier, P. L., and Pope, J. H.: Infectious respiratory syncytial virus (RSV) effectively inhibits the proliferative T cell response to inactivated RSV *in vitro*. J. Infect. Dis. *165*:819–825, 1992.
359. Prevention of respiratory syncytial virus infections: indications for use of palivizumab and update on the use of RSV-IVIG. American Academy of Pediatrics Committee on Infectious Diseases and Committee on Fetus and Newborn. Pediatrics *102*:1211–1216, 1998.
360. Prince, G. A., Hemming, V. G., Horswood, R. L., et al.: Effectiveness of topically administered neutralizing antibodies in experimental immunotherapy of respiratory syncytial virus infection in cotton rats. J. Virol. *61*:1851–1854, 1987.
361. Prince, G. A., Horswood, R. L., Berndt, J., et al.: Respiratory syncytial virus infection in inbred mice. Infect. Immun. *26*:764, 1979.
362. Prince, G. A., Horswood, R. L., Camargo, E., et al.: Mechanisms of immunology to respiratory syncytial virus in cotton rats. Infect. Immun. *42*:81–87, 1983.
363. Prince, G. A., Horswood, R. L., and Chanock, R. M.: Quantitative aspects of passive immunity to respiratory syncytial virus infection in infant cotton rats. J. Virol. *55*:517, 1985.
364. Prince, G. A., Jenson, A. B., Horswood, R. L., et al.: The pathogenesis of respiratory syncytial virus infection in cotton rats. Am. J. Pathol. *93*:771–792, 1978.
365. Prince, G. A., Porter, D. D.: The pathogenesis of respiratory syncytial virus infection in infant ferrets. Am. J. Pathol. *82*:339–352, 1976.
366. Prince, G., Prieels, J., Slaoui, M., et al.: Pulmonary lesions in primary respiratory syncytial virus infection, reinfection, and vaccine-enhanced disease in the cotton rat (*Sigmodon hispidus*). Lab. Invest. 79:1385–1392, 1999.
367. Prince, G. A., Suffin, S. C., Prevar, D. A., et al.: Respiratory syncytial viral infection in owl monkeys: Viral shedding, immunological response, and associated illness caused by wild-type virus and two temperature-sensitive mutants. Infect. Immun. *26*:1009–1013, 1979.
368. Pringle, C. R.: The order Mononegavirales. Arch. Virol. *117*:137–140, 1991.
369. Pringle, C. R., Shirodaria, P. V., Cash, P., et al.: Initiation and maintenance of persistent infection by respiratory syncytial virus. J. Virol. *28*:199–211, 1978.
370. Pullan, C. R., Toms, G. L., Martin, A. J., et al.: Breast feeding and respiratory syncytial virus infection. B. M. J. *281*:1034–1036, 1980.
371. Reassessment of the indications for ribavirin therapy in respiratory syncytial virus infections. American Academy of Pediatrics Committee on Infectious Diseases. Pediatrics *97*:137–140, 1996.
372. Rechsteiner, J., and Winkler, K. C.: Inactivation of respiratory syncytial virus in aerosol. J. Gen. Virol. *5*:405–410, 1969.
373. Reduction of respiratory syncytial virus hospitalization among premature infants and infants with bronchopulmonary dysplasia using respiratory syncytial virus immune globulin prophylaxis. The PREVENT Study Group. Pediatrics *99*:93–99, 1997.
374. Reid, L.: Influence of the pattern of structural growth of lung on susceptibility to specific infectious diseases in infants and children. Pediatr. Res. *11*:210–215, 1977.
375. Reilly, C. M., Stokes, J., Jr., McClelland, L., et al.: Studies of acute respiratory illness caused by respiratory syncytial virus. 3. Clinical and laboratory findings. N. Engl. J. Med. *264*:1176–1182, 1961.
376. Respiratory syncytial virus infection: Admissions to hospitals in industrial, urban and rural areas. Report to the Medical Research Council Subcommittee on Respiratory Syncytial Virus Vaccines. B. M. J. *2*:796–798, 1978.
377. Respiratory syncytial virus activity—United States, 1999–2000 season. M. M. W. R. Morb. Mortal. Wkly. Rep. *49*:1091–1093, 2000.
378. Reynolds, E. O. R.: Arterial blood gas tensions in acute disease of lower respiratory tract in infancy. B. M. J. *1*:1192–1195, 1963.
379. Rice, R. P., and Loda, F.: A roentgenographic analysis of respiratory syncytial virus pneumonia in infants. Radiology *87*:1021–1027, 1966.
380. Richardson, L. S., Belshe, R. B., London, W. T., et al.: Respiratory syncytial virus antibodies in nonhuman primates and domestic animals. Lab. Anim. Sci. *31*:413–415, 1981.
381. Roberts, N. J., Jr., Prill, A. H., and Mann, T. N.: Interleukin 1 and interleukin 1 inhibitor production by human macrophages exposed to influenza virus or respiratory syncytial virus: Respiratory syncytial virus is a potent inducer of inhibitor activity. J. Exp. Med. *163*:511–519, 1986.
382. Rodriguez, W.: Management strategies for respiratory syncytial virus infections in infants. J. Pediatr. *135*(Suppl.):45–50, 1999.
383. Rodriguez, W. J., Kim, H. W., Brandt, C. D., et al.: Aerosolized ribavirin in the treatment of patients with respiratory syncytial virus disease. Pediatr. Infect. Dis. J. *6*:159–163, 1987.
384. Rodriguez, W. J., and Parrott, R. H.: Ribavirin aerosol treatment of serious respiratory syncytial virus infection in infants. Infect. Dis. Clin. North Am. *1*:425–439, 1987.
385. Rohwedder, A., Keminer, O., Forster, J., et al.: Detection of respiratory syncytial virus RNA in blood of neonates by polymerase chain reaction. J. Med. Virol. *54*:320–327, 1998.
386. Roosevelt, G., Sheehan, K., Grupp-Phelan, J., et al.: Dexamethasone in bronchiolitis: A randomized controlled trial. Lancet *348*:292–295, 1996.
387. Rosner, I. K., Welliver, R. C., Edelson, P. J., et al.: Effect of ribavirin therapy on respiratory syncytial virus–specific IgE and IgA responses after infection. J. Infect. Dis. *155*:1043–1047, 1987.
388. Russo, M., McConnochie, K., McBride, J., et al.: Increase in admission threshold explains stable asthma hospitalization rates. Pediatrics *104*:454–462, 1999.

389. Salkind, A. R., McCarthy, D. O., Nichols, J. E., et al.: Interleukin-1-inhibitor activity induced by respiratory syncytial virus: Abrogation of virus-specific and alternate human lymphocyte proliferative responses. J. Infect. Dis. *163*:71–77, 1991.
390. Salkind, A. R., Nichols, J. E., and Roberts, N. J., Jr.: Suppressed expression of ICAM-1 and LFA-1 and abrogation of leukocyte collaboration after exposure of human mononuclear leukocytes to respiratory syncytial virus in vitro. Comparison with exposure to influenza virus. J. Clin. Invest. *88*:505–511, 1991.
391. Sami, I. R., Piazza, F. M., Johnson, S. A., et al.: Systemic immunoprophylaxis of nasal respiratory syncytial virus infection in cotton rats. J. Infect. Dis. *171*:440–443, 1995.
392. Sanchez, I., DeKoster, J., Powell, R. E., et al.: Effect of racemic epinephrine and salbutamol on clinical score and pulmonary mechanics in infants with bronchiolitis. J. Pediatr. *122*:145–151, 1993.
393. Scott, R., and Gardner, P. S.: Respiratory syncytial virus neutralizing activity in nasopharyngeal secretions. J. Hyg. *68*:581–588, 1970.
394. Serwint, J.: Efficacy of albuterol in the management of bronchiolitis. Pediatrics *95*:320, 1995.
395. Shahrabadi, M. S., and Lee, P. W. K.: Calcium requirement for syncytium formation in HEp-2 cells by respiratory syncytial virus. J. Clin. Microbiol. *26*:139–141, 1988.
396. Shay, D., Holman, R., Newman, R., et al.: Bronchiolitis-associated hospitalizations among US children, 1980–1996. J. A. M. A. *282:*1440–1446, 1999.
397. Shay, D., Holman, R., Roosevelt, G., et al.: Bronchiolitis-associated mortality and estimates of respiratory syncytial virus–associated deaths among US children, 1979–1997. J. Infec. Dis. *183*:16–22, 2001.
398. Sheeran, P., Jafri, H., Carubelli, C., et al.: Elevated cytokine concentrations in the nasopharyngeal and tracheal secretions of children with respiratory syncytial virus disease. Pediatr. Infect. Dis. J. *18*:115–122, 1999.
399. Siegrist, C., Plotnicky-Gilquin, H., Cordova, M., et al. Protective efficacy against respiratory syncytial virus following murine neonatal immunization with BBG2Na vaccine: Influence of adjuvants and maternal antibodies. J. Infect. Dis. *179*:1326–1333, 1999.
400. Sigurs, N., Bjarnason, R., and Sigurbergsson, F.: Eosinophil cationic protein in nasal secretion and in serum and myeloperoxidase in serum in respiratory syncytial virus bronchiolitis: Relation to asthma and atopy. Acta Pediatr. *83*:1151–1155, 1994.
401. Simoes, E.: Respiratory syncytial virus infection. Lancet *354*:847–852, 1999.
402. Simoes, E., Hayward, A., Ponnuraj, E., et al.: Respiratory syncytial virus infects the bonnet monkey, *Macaca radiata*. Pediatr. Dev. Pathol. *2*:316–326, 1999.
403. Simpson, W., Hacking, P. M., Court, S. D. M., et al.: The radiological findings in respiratory syncytial virus infection in children. Part II. The correlation of radiological categories with clinical and virological findings. Pediatr. Radiol. *2*:155–160, 1974.
404. Sims, D. G., Downham, M. A. P. S., McQuillin, J., et al.: Respiratory syncytial virus infection in north-east England. B. M. J. *2*:1095–1098, 1976.
405. Singleton, R., Karron, R., Kruse, D., et al. RSV-associated hospitalizations in Alaska Native infants. Int. J. Circumpolar Health *57*:255–259, 1998.
406. Smith, A. P., Tyrrell, D. A. J., Barrow, G. I., et al.: The common cold, pattern sensitivity and contrast sensitivity. Psychol. Med. *22*:487–494, 1992.
407. Smith, D. W., Frankel, L. R., Mathers, L. H., et al.: A controlled trial of aerosolized ribavirin in infants receiving mechanical ventilation for severe respiratory syncytial virus infection. N. Engl. J. Med. *325*:24–29, 1991.
408. Sommerville, R. G.: Respiratory syncytial virus in acute exacerbations of chronic bronchitis. Lancet *2*:1247–1248, 1963.
408. Sparer, T., Matthews, S., Hussell, T., et al. Eliminating a region of respiratory syncytial virus attachment protein allows induction of protective immunity without vaccine-enhanced lung eosinophilia. J. Exp. Med. *187*:1921–1926, 1998.
410. Spinelli, M., Geraci-Ciardullo, K., Palumbo, P. E., et al.: Efficacy of ribavirin for treating respiratory syncytial virus (RSV) pneumonia in high risk infants. Abstract. Pediatr. Res. *19*:304, 1985.
411. Springer, C., Bar-Yishay, E., Uwayyed, K., et al.: Corticosteroids do not affect the clinical or physiological status of infants with bronchiolitis. Pediatr. Pulmonol. *9*:181–185, 1990.
412. Srikiatkachorn, A., and Braciale, T.: Virus-specific memory and effector T lymphocytes exhibit different cytokine responses to antigens during experimental murine respiratory syncytial virus infection. J. Virol. *71*:678–685, 1997.
413. Stecenko, A. A.: Treatment of viral bronchiolitis: Do steroids make sense? Contemp. Pediatr. *4*:121–130, 1987.
414. Sterner, G., Wolontis, S., Bloth, B., et al.: Respiratory syncytial virus: An outbreak of acute respiratory illness in a home for infants. Acta Paediatr. Scand. *55*:273–279, 1966.
415. Stevens, T., Sinkin, R., Hall, C., et al.: Respiratory syncytial virus and premature infants born at 32 weeks' gestation or earlier. Arch. Pediatr. Adoles. Med. *154*:55–61, 2000.
416. Stockton, J., Ellis, J., Saville, M., et al.: Multiplex PCR for typing and subtyping influenza and respiratory syncytial viruses. J. Clin. Microbiol. *36*:2990–2995, 1998.
417. Storch, G.: Respiratory infections. *In* Storch, G. (ed.): Essentials of Diagnostic Virology. St. Louis, Churchill Livingstone, 2000, pp. 59–78.
418. Stott, E. J., Thomas, L. H., Collins, A. P., et al.: A survey of virus infections of the respiratory tract of cattle and their association with disease. J. Hyg. *85*:257–270, 1980.
419. Stretton, M., Ajizian, S. J., Mitchell, I., et al.: Intensive care course and outcome of patients infected with respiratory syncytial virus. Pediatr. Pulmonol. *13*:143–150, 1992.
420. Sullender, W.: Respiratory syncytial virus genetic and antigenic diversity. Clin. Microbiol. Rev. *13*:1–15, 2000.
421. Sullender, W., and Edwards, K.: Mutations of respiratory syncytial virus attachment glycoprotein G associated with resistance to neutralization by primate polyclonal antibodies. Virology *264*:230–236, 1999.
422. Sullender, W., Mufson, M., Prince, G. A., et al.: Antigenic and genetic diversity among the attachment proteins of group A respiratory syncytial viruses that have caused repeat infections in children. J. Infect. Dis. *178*:925–932, 1998.
423. Taber, L. H., Knight, V., Gilbert, B. E., et al.: Ribavirin aerosol treatment of bronchiolitis due to respiratory syncytial virus infection in infants. Pediatrics *72*:613–618, 1983.
424. Takimoto, C. H., Cram, D. L., and Root, R. K.: Respiratory syncytial virus infections on an adult medical ward. Arch. Intern. Med. *151*:706–708, 1991.
425. Tang, Y., Heimgartner, P., Tollefson, S., et al.: A colorimetric microtiter plate PCR system detects respiratory syncytial virus in nasal aspirates and discriminates subtypes A and B. Diagn. Microbiol. Infect. Dis. *34*:333–337, 1999.
426. Taylor, G., Stott, E. J., Bew, M., et al.: Monoclonal antibodies protect mice against respiratory syncytial virus infection in mice. Immunology *52*:137–142, 1984.
427. Taylor, G., Stott, E. J., and Hayle, A. J.: Cytotoxic lymphocytes in the lungs of mice infected with respiratory syncytial virus. J. Gen. Virol. *66*:2533–2538, 1985.
428. Taylor, G., Stott, E. J., Hughes, M., et al.: Respiratory syncytial virus infection in mice. Infect. Immun. *43*:649–655, 1984.
429. Teran, L., Seminario, C., Shute, J., et al.: RANTES, macrophage-inhibitory protein 1a, and the eosinophil product major basic protein are released into upper respiratory secretions during virus-induced asthma exacerbations in children. J. Infect. Dis. *179*:677–681, 1999.
430. Toms, G. L.: Respiratory syncytial virus: Virology, diagnosis, and vaccination. Lung *168*(Suppl.):388–395, 1990.
431. Toms, G. L., Gardner, P. S., Pullan, C. R., et al.: Secretion of RSV inhibitors and antibody in human milk throughout lactation. J. Med. Virol. *5*:351–360, 1980.
432. Toms, G. L., Webb, M. S. C., Milner, P. D., et al.: IgG and IgM antibodies of viral glycoproteins in respiratory syncytial virus infections of graded severity. Arch. Dis. Child. *64*:1661–1665, 1989.
433. Treanor, J., and Falsey, A.: Respiratory viral infections in the elderly. Antiviral Res. *44*:79–102, 1999.
434. Tripp, R., Moore, D., Winter, J., et al.: Respiratory syncytial virus infection and G and/or SH protein expression contribute to substance P, which mediates inflammation and enhanced pulmonary disease in BALB/c mice. J. Virol. *74*:1614–1622, 2000.
435. Tristram, D. A., Welliver, R. C., Mohar, C. K., et al.: Immunogenicity and safety of respiratory syncytial virus subunit vaccine in seropositive children 18–36 months old. J. Infect. Dis. *167*:191–195, 1993.
436. Trudel, M., Nadon, F., Seguin, C., et al.: Initiation of cytotoxic T-cell response and protection of BALB/c mice by vaccination with an experimental ISCOMs respiratory syncytial virus subunit vaccine. Vaccine *10*:107–112, 1992.
437. Tsutsumi, H., Onuma, M., Suga, K., et al.: Occurrence of respiratory syncytial virus subgroup A and B strains in Japan, 1980 to 1987. J. Clin. Microbiol. *26*:1171–1174, 1988.
438. Tsutsumi, H., Sone, S., Takeuchi, R., et al.: Systemic and local immune responses of four cases with lower respiratory tract illness due to reinfection with respiratory syncytial virus. J. Infect. *35*:189–192, 1997.
439. Tyrrell, D. A. J.: Discovering and defining the etiology of acute respiratory disease. Am. Rev. Respir. Dis. *88*:77–84, 1963.
440. Uhari, M., Hietala, J., and Tuokko, H.: Risk of acute otitis media in relation to the viral etiology of infections in children. Clin. Infect. Dis. *20*:521–524, 1995.
441. Urquhart, G. E. D., and Gibson, A. A. M.: RSV infections and infant deaths. B. M. J. *3*:110, 1970.
442. vanDenIngh, T., Averhoeff, I., and VanNieuwstadt, A.: Clinical and pathological observations on spontaneous bovine respiratory syncytial virus infections in calves. Res. Vet. Sci. *33*:152–158, 1982.
443. vanSchaik, S., Enhorning, G., Vargas, I., and Welliver, R.: Respiratory syncytial virus affects pulmonary function in BALB/c mice. J. Infect. Dis. *177*:269–276, 1998.
444. Verhoeff, J., Wierda, A., and Boon, J. H.: Clinical signs following experimental lungworm infection and natural bovine respiratory syncytial virus infection in calves. Vet. Rec. *123*:346–350, 1988.

445. Vikerfors, T., Grandien, M., and Olcen, P.: Respiratory syncytial viral infection in adults. Am. Rev. Respir. Dis. *136*:561–564, 1987.
446. Volovitz, B., Faden, H., and Ogra, P. L.: Releases of leukotriene C4 in respiratory tract during acute viral infection. J. Pediatr. *112*:218–222, 1988.
447. Volovitz, B., Welliver, R. C., de Castro, G., et al.: The release of leukotrienes in the respiratory tract during infection with respiratory syncytial virus: Role in obstructive airway disease. Pediatr. Res. *24*:504–507, 1988.
448. Wagner, D. K., Graham, B. S., Wright, P. F., et al.: Serum immunoglobulin G antibody subclass responses to respiratory syncytial virus F and G glycoproteins after primary infection. J. Clin. Microbiol. *24*:304–306, 1986.
449. Wagner, D., Nelson, D., Walsh, E., et al.: Differential immunoglobulin G subclass antibody titers to respiratory syncytial virus F and G glycoproteins in adults. J. Clin. Microbiol. *25*:748–750, 1987.
450. Walker, R. I.: New strategies for using mucosal vaccination to achieve more effective immunization. Vaccine *12*:387–400, 1994.
451. Wallace, S. J., and Zealley, H.: Neurological, electroencephalographic, and virological findings in febrile children. Arch. Dis. Child. *45*:611–623, 1970.
452. Walsh, E. E.: Mucosal immunization with a subunit respiratory syncytial virus vaccine in mice. Vaccine *11*:1135–1138, 1993.
453. Walsh, E. E., Brandriss, M. W., and Schlesinger, J. J.: Immunological differences between the envelope glycoproteins of two strains of human respiratory syncytial virus. J. Gen. Virol. *68*:2169–2176, 1987.
454. Walsh, E., Falsey, A., and Hennessey, P.: Respiratory syncytial virus and other virus infections in persons with chronic cardiopulmonary disease. Am. J. Respir. Crit. Care Med. *160*:791–795, 1999.
455. Walsh, E. E., and Hall, C. B.: Respiratory syncytial virus. *In* Schmidt, N. J., and Emmons, R. W. (eds.): Diagnostic Procedures for Viral and Rickettsial Infections. New York, American Public Health Association, 1989, pp. 693–712.
456. Walsh, E., and Hall, C.: Approaches to a vaccine for respiratory syncytial virus. *In* Meyers, R. A. (ed.): Encyclopedia of Molecular Biology and Molecular Medicine. Weinheim, Germany, VCH Verlagsgesellschaft, 1996, pp. 286–296.
457. Walsh, E. E., Hall, C. B., Briselli, M., et al.: Protection from respiratory syncytial viral infection in cotton rats by viral glycoprotein subunit immunization. J. Infect. Dis. *55*:1198–1204, 1987.
458. Walsh, E. E., and Hruska, J. F.: Monoclonal antibodies to respiratory syncytial virus proteins: Identification of the fusion protein. J. Virol. *47*:171–177, 1983.
459. Walsh, E., McConnochie, K., Long, C., et al.: Severity of respiratory syncytial virus infection is related to virus strain. J. Infect. Dis. *175*: 14–820, 1997.
460. Walsh, E. E., Schlesinger, J. J., and Brandriss, M. W.: Protection from respiratory syncytial virus infection in cotton rats by passive transfer of monoclonal antibodies. Infect. Immun. *43*:756–758, 1984.
461. Wang, E., Law, B., Boucher, F., et al.: Pediatric Investigators Collaborative Network on Infections in Canada (PICNIC) Study of admission and management variation in patients hospitalized with respiratory syncytial viral lower respiratory tract infection. J. Pediatr. *129*:390–395, 1996.
462. Ward, K. A., Lambden, P. R., Ogilivie, M. M., et al.: Antibodies to RSV polypeptides and their significance in human infection. J. Gen. Virol. *64*:1867–1876, 1983.
463. Waris, M.: Pattern of respiratory syncytial virus epidemics in Finland: Two-year cycles with alternating prevalence of groups A and B. J. Infect. Dis. *163*:464–469, 1991.
464. Weber, M., Dackour, R., Usen, S., et al. The clinical spectrum of respiratory syncytial virus disease in The Gambia. Pediatr. Infect. Dis. J. *17*:224–230, 1998.
465. Welliver, R. C.: Detection, pathogenesis, and therapy of respiratory syncytial virus infections. Clin. Microbiol. Rev. *1*:27–39, 1988.
466. Welliver, R.: Immunologic mechanisms of virus-induced wheezing and asthma. J. Pediatr. *135*(Suppl.):14–20, 1999.
467. Welliver, R. C., Kaul, T. N., and Ogra, P. L.: The appearance of cell-bound IgE in respiratory-tract epithelium after respiratory syncytial virus infection. N. Engl. J. Med. *303*:1198–1202, 1980.
467. Welliver, R. C., Kaul, T. N., Putnam, T. I., et al.: The antibody response to primary and secondary infection with respiratory syncytial virus: Kinetics of class specific response. J. Pediatr. *96*:808–813, 1980.
469. Welliver, R. C., Kaul, T. N., Sun, M., et al.: Defective regulation of immune response in respiratory syncytial virus infection. J. Immunol. *133*:1925–1930, 1984.
470. Welliver, R. C., Sun, M., Hildreth, S. W., et al.: Respiratory syncytial virus–specific antibody responses in immunoglobulin A and E isotypes to the F and G proteins and to intact virus after natural infection. J. Clin. Microbiol. *27*:295–299, 1989.
471. Welliver, R. C., Sun, M., Rinaldo, D., et al.: Predictive value of respiratory syncytial virus specific IgE responses for recurrent wheezing following bronchiolitis. J. Pediatr. *109*:776–790, 1986.
472. Welliver, R. C., Wong, D. T., Sun, M., et al.: The development of respiratory syncytial virus–specific IgE and the release of histamine in nasopharyngeal secretions after infection. N. Engl. J. Med. *305*:841–846, 1981.
473. Wertz, G. W., Stott, E. J., Young, K. K. Y., et al.: Expression of the fusion protein of human respiratory syncytial virus from recombinant vaccinia virus vectors and protection of vaccinated mice. J. Virol. *61*:293–301, 1987.
474. Wertz, G. W., and Sullender, W. M.: Approaches to immunization against respiratory syncytial virus. Biotechnology *20*:151–176, 1992.
475. Wheeler, J. G., Wofford, J., and Turner, R. B.: Historical cohort evaluation of ribavirin efficacy in respiratory syncytial virus infection. Pediatr. Infect. Dis. J. *12*:209–213, 1993.
476. Whimbey, E., Englund, J., and Ljungman, P.: Community respiratory viral infections in the immunocompromised host. Am. J. Med. *102*:1–80, 1997.
477. Wohl, M. E. B.: Bronchiolitis. Pediatr. Ann. *15*:307–313, 1986.
478. Wohl, M., and Chernick, B.: Bronchiolitis. Am. Rev. Respir. Dis. *118*:759–781, 1978.
479. Woodin, K. A., Hall, C. B., Leibenguth, K. C., et al.: Variables affecting the rapid diagnosis of respiratory syncytial virus (RSV). Abstract No. 204. Paper presented at the 28th Interscience Conference on Antimicrobial Agents and Chemotherapy, Los Angeles, 1988, p. 145.
480. Wright, P., Karron, R., Belshe, R., et al.: Evaluation of a live, cold-passaged, temperature-sensitive, respiratory syncytial virus vaccine candidate in infancy. J. Infect. Dis. *182*:1331–1342, 2000.
481. Wyde, P., Moore, D., Pimentel, D., et al.: Recombinant superoxide dismutase (SOD) administered by aerosol inhibits respiratory syncytial virus infection in cotton rats. Antiviral Res. *31*:173–184, 1996.

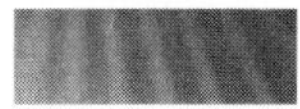

CHAPTER **185B**

Human Metapneumovirus: *Paramyxoviridae*

MICHAEL D. NISSEN

Human metapneumovirus (hMPV) is a novel respiratory tract pathogen first described in 2001.[27] It is the first known mammalian metapneumovirus associated with disease.[26, 27] Avian pneumovirus (APV) is the only other known metapneumovirus.[28] hMPV is considered ubiquitous in humans on the basis of detection of the virus by polymerase chain reaction (PCR) of the respiratory specimens of symptomatic children and adults,[1, 2, 11, 13–24, 28] as well as the presence of a high rate of hMPV-specific antibodies in diverse populations.[14, 27] The features of hMPV infection in children and adults are not yet fully characterized, although the illness is thought to be clinically indistinguishable from human respiratory syncytial virus (hRSV) in many respects.[17, 18, 27]

History

hMPV was isolated initially during a 20-year period from a group of 28 epidemiologically unrelated patients with respiratory tract disease in the Netherlands.[27] All viral isolates were from nasopharyngeal specimens collected in the winter months. The unidentified isolates replicated predominantly in tertiary monkey kidney (tMK) cells. The cytopathic effects of replicating virus were difficult to distinguish from those caused by hRSV, except that the onset of features was delayed by several days. Electron microscopy revealed typical paramyxovirus-like pleomorphic particles and short envelope projections, with nucleocapsids rarely being

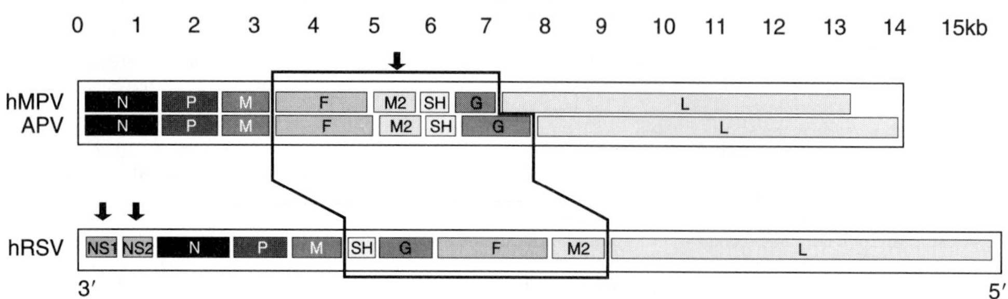

FIGURE 185–7 ■ Genomic map of human metapneumovirus (hMPV) compared with avian metapneumovirus (APV) and human respiratory syncytial virus (hRSV). The putative open-reading frames (ORFs) and the approximate nucleotide (nt) positions within the genome are indicated. *Arrows* signify areas of difference in gene constellation among hMPV, APV, and hRSV.

observed. Reports of hMPV infection from Australia, Canada, England/Wales, Finland, and the United States soon followed.* The virus has been circulating within the Dutch population since at least 1958 based on the universal presence of antibodies to hMPV in sera collected from subjects who were 8 to 99 years old at that time.[27] Researchers have speculated that because APV is the closest relative of hMPV, a possible zoonotic event must have occurred before this time.[27] The late recognition of hMPV as a respiratory pathogen is the result of its unique growth requirements and kinetics in vitro.[27]

Properties

CLASSIFICATION

hMPV has been classified provisionally as a member of the *Metapneumovirus* genus of paramyxoviruses because of its biologic properties, sequence homology, and gene constellation in relation to APV.[26, 27] The metapneumoviruses and pneumoviruses constitute the *Pneumovirinae* subfamily within the *Paramyxoviridae* family.[28] The pneumoviruses contain the RSVs of mammals (bovine, human, ovine RSV) and pneumovirus of mice (PVM).

STRUCTURAL AND ANTIGENIC PROPERTIES

The hMPV virion, like all paramyxoviruses, contains a nucleocapsid of single-stranded, negative-sense RNA within a lipid bilayer envelope derived from the plasma membrane of the host cell.[12] The virion, however, does not contain hemagglutinin or neuraminidase, which distinguishes it as a member of the *Pneumovirinae* subfamily.

Ultrastructural analysis of the hMPV virion by electron microscopy also is typical of paramyxoviruses and demonstrates spherical, pleomorphic, and filamentous particles with short envelope projections.[22, 27] The spherical particles vary from 150 to 600 nm in diameter, with a mean of 209 nm,[22, 27] whereas the envelope projections are 13 to 17 nm in size.[27] The nucleocapsid's diameter is 17 nm with lengths from less than 200 to more than 1000 nm.[22] Filamentous particles average 282 × 62 nm in size.[22]

The entire genomic sequence of hMPV has been determined.[26] The hMPV genome is approximately 13.4 kb in length and consists of eight identifiable open-reading frames (ORFs) that are transcribed into eight viral proteins.[26, 27] All are distinct structural proteins and have been identified as transmembrane surface glycoproteins (fusion [F], attachment [G], and small nonglycoslated hydrophobic [SH]), matrix proteins (M and M2), and nucleocapsid-associated proteins (nucleocapsid [N], phosphoprotein [P], and polymerase [L]). Two structural features principally determine the distinction between the genera *Metapneumovirus* and *Pneumovirus* (Fig. 185–7). Metapneumoviruses lack the nonstructural (NS) proteins NS1 and NS2, and the gene order differs between the two genera. The genetic alignment of the M and L ORFs of metapneumoviruses (3′-N-P-M-F-M2-SH-G-L-5′) is different from that of pneumoviruses (3′-NS1-NS2-N-P-M-SH-G-F-M2-L-5′). However, the location of hMPV viral structural proteins within the virion is similar to that described for hRSV (see Fig. 185–1).

Sequence analysis of the hMPV genome reveals the highest degree of identity with APV.[27] Of the four known serotypes of APV, hMPV most closely resembles APV serotype C, the type most commonly described in birds in the United States[3, 27] (Table 185–5). Sequence information on APV serotype D for comparison with hMPV is limited.[27]

Similar to hRSV, significant genomic sequence or strain variation also exists for hMPV isolates. Phylogenetic analysis of isolates has confirmed the existence of at least two distinct clusters or lineages of hMPV worldwide based on limited sequence analysis of the N, M, F, and L ORFs.[1, 14, 25, 27] In separate studies, overall nucleotide comparison reveals 80 to 88 percent genetic similarity between the two clusters and 93 to 100 percent within each cluster. At the amino acid level, the differences are less distinct, with 94 to 97 percent similarity existing between groups and 97 to 100 percent shared identity found within each group. hMPV genetic strains from both clusters have been noted to co-circulate in the same year.[1] Strains from different years also have been identified in the same subcluster.[1, 27] These genetic clusters may represent subgroups or different serotypes of hMPV,[10] similar to that described for hRSV (i.e., hRSV A and hRSV B). More detailed sequence analysis of hMPV isolates from different geographic regions of the world and definitive serologic studies are required to support this hypothesis.

LABORATORY GROWTH

hMPV is a labile RNA virus like hRSV based on the relatively low yield of positive cell cultures (approximately 16%) in comparison to positive detection by PCR after freezing and thawing of respiratory samples for testing.[14]

The use of tMK or LLC-MK2 (Rhesus monkey kidney) cells has shown the greatest success in culture of hMPV from clinical respiratory samples obtained by nasopharyngeal aspiration, nasopharyngeal swabs, endotracheal aspiration, or bronchoalveolar lavage.[1, 22, 27] The virus replicates poorly in Vero or A549 cells, with no growth detected in chick embryo fibroblast (CEF), Madin-Darby canine kidney (MDCK), or human lung mucoepidermoid carcinoma

*See references 1, 2, 7, 8, 10, 11, 14, 16–18, 21–23, 25, 29.

TABLE 185–5 ■ AMINO ACID SEQUENCE HOMOLOGY OF HUMAN METAPNEUMOVIRUS (hMPV) PROTEINS COMPARED WITH AVIAN METAPNEUMOVIRUS (APV), HUMAN RESPIRATORY SYNCYTIAL VIRUS (hRSV), AND OTHER PARAMYXOVIRUSES*

	Putative ORFs and Genes of hMPV, APV, hRSV, and Other Paramyxoviruses						
	N	P	M	F	M2-1	M2-2	L
APV†	69–88	51–68	76–87	67–81	71–84	26–56	64‡
hRSV§	41	23–24	37–38	33	35–36	18–19	44
Others‖	7–11	4-9	7–10	10–18	—¶	—¶	13–15

*Amino acid sequence homology expressed as a percentage of the known hMPV sequence.
†Range of APV sequence homology for serotypes A, B, and C is listed. APV serotype C exhibited highest sequence homology of the four known serotypes of APV (A, B, C, and D) for all ORFs and genes, except L gene. Sequence data for APV serotype D are incomplete and not included in the data analysis.
‡Sequence data are not available for APV serotypes B and C.
§A range of hRSV sequence homology for serotypes A and B is listed.
‖Other paramyxoviruses include human parainfluenza viruses 2 and 3, Sendai virus, measles virus, Nipah virus, phocine distemper virus, and Newcastle disease virus.
¶ORF absent in the viral genome.
F, fusion protein; L, polymerase genes; M, M2-1, M2-2, matrix proteins; N, nucleocapsid; ORF, open-reading frame; P, phosphoprotein.
Adapted from van den Hoogen, B. G., de Jong, J. C., Groen, J., et al.: A newly discovered human pneumovirus isolated from young children with respiratory tract disease. Nat. Med. 7:719–724, 2001.

(NCI-H292) cells.[1, 14, 22, 27] The characteristic cytopathic effect in cell culture is focal small round, granular, and refringent cells, without large syncytial formation in most cases.[1, 22] The appearance of the cytopathic effect ranges from 3 to 23 days with a mean of 17.3 days.[1, 27]

Other biologic properties of the *Paramyxoviridae* are detected with hMPV culture. Standard chloroform treatment results in a significant reduction in the median tissue culture infective dose ($TCID_{50}$) for tMK cells.[27] Virus-infected cell culture supernatants do not adsorb the erythrocytes (negative hemagglutinating activity) of chickens, guinea pigs, or turkeys.[22, 27] Viral replication in vitro is dependent on the addition of trypsin to the cell culture medium.[27] This last feature of hMPV may have been what contributed to a delay in recognition of the virus as a respiratory pathogen because seminal research performed to identify respiratory agents failed to use trypsin as a culture supplement.[27] Other practices that also would have contributed to this delay include the poor replication of hMPV in the continuous cell culture lines routinely used in diagnostic virology laboratories for viral isolation, slow viral replication in vitro leading to discarding of potential positive isolates before detection, an apparent lack of serologic cross-reactivity to other paramyxoviruses (e.g., hRSV, influenza and parainfluenza viruses), and finally, low nucleotide sequence homology to other known viral pathogens.[27]

ANIMAL SUSCEPTIBILITY

hMPV reproduces efficiently in the respiratory tract of cynomolgus macaques *(Macaca fascicularis)* and causes clinical infection.[27] Virus replication appears to peak between 2 and 8 days after inoculation into either the respiratory tract or conjunctivae.[27] The clinical features of primate infection are consistent with those of mild upper respiratory tract disease and suppurative rhinitis on histologic examination.[27] A similar attempt at experimental infection of turkeys and chickens has been unsuccessful, thus providing further supportive evidence that hMPV is a primate pathogen associated with respiratory tract disease.[27] Intranasal inoculation of guinea pigs and ferrets does lead to the production of virus-specific antisera but no clinically obvious infection.[27]

Epidemiology

GEOGRAPHIC DISTRIBUTION

hMPV is considered to be prevalent worldwide based on reports of infection from three continents and universal seroprevalence in both the Northern and Southern Hemispheres.* Comparison with hRSV is, again, obvious in the global similarities of the age of infected subjects.

SEASONAL PATTERNS

The seasonality of hMPV infection has yet to be determined precisely. In the original description, hMPV was detected and isolated only in respiratory samples collected in the Dutch winter.[27] Subsequent reports in both hemispheres have indicated a seasonal preference from winter to spring, depending on the geographic locale. In North America, most hMPV activity has been recorded by PCR detection in respiratory specimens collected from December until May.[1, 16, 29] In Quebec, Canada, 88 percent of hMPV isolations also were made in this 6-month period,[1] whereas in Rochester, New York, hMPV was active from February to May, with peak activity in April.[16] Further south, in Nashville, Tennessee, infections were noted to begin in March and peak in May, with some disease activity in June and September.[16, 29] Detection of hMPV in Finland was confined to January until April.[11] In Australia, in the Southern Hemisphere, hMPV cases have been noted predominantly in September or the early spring.[14]

Based on these preliminary data, the appearance of hMPV infection tends to follow that of hRSV and influenza, which occur in early to mid-winter, but precedes that of parainfluenza 3 disease activity, which occurs in late spring to early summer.

STRAIN VARIATION

Although hMPV appears to clearly circulate in annual outbreaks of infection, whether the scope or severity of disease

*See references 1, 7, 8, 14, 16, 18, 23, 25, 27, 29.

varies from year to year remains unknown. Whether a clinically recognizable difference in disease severity exists between the two known genetic clusters of hMPV also is unknown. More detailed molecular epidemiologic analysis of community-based hMPV isolates and serologic responses to infection is required to address this question.

INCIDENCE AND PREVALENCE

The true seasonal incidence and prevalence of hMPV disease in children has not been defined. Most reports to date have concentrated on children taken to the hospital for acute respiratory symptoms.[16, 18, 27]

Prospective observation for hMPV disease in the Netherlands and Finland during the winter of 2000 detected the virus in 9 and 10 percent, respectively, of respiratory samples from children with unexplained respiratory tract infection or acute wheezing.[11, 27] In the United States, hMPV was detected retrospectively in 4 percent of hospitalized children younger than 5 years with an acute respiratory illness in which a viral agent could not be identified.[16] In contrast, a community-based retrospective analysis of children in Tennessee during a 25-year period confirmed the presence of hMPV in 20 percent of nasal wash specimens collected from children with an undiagnosed lower respiratory tract illness.[29] In Australia, the annual detection rate of hMPV in respiratory specimens from children was 4.5 percent, although the incidence increased to 13 percent during the months of peak disease activity.[14]

hMPV infection in children, like hRSV, inflicts its burden on children younger than 2 years, particularly those younger than 12 months.[16–18, 27] In children hospitalized for acute respiratory infection in the United States, hMPV affected predominantly children 0 to 12 months of age (50%), followed by those 1 to 2 years of age (42%).[16] Of these infants, infection occurred more commonly in the 7- to 12-month age group (31%) than in those 0 to 6 months of age (19%).[16] Children of white descent were overrepresented when compared with children of all other races (65% versus 35%) in this series of patients.[16]

hMPV is assumed to be widely prevalent based on the high level of hMPV-specific antisera in the community. In the Netherlands, 70 percent of children demonstrated hMPV antibodies on immunofluorescent antigen assay by the time that they reached 5 years of age; by the age of 10 years, 100 percent had these antibodies.[27] Similar work in Australia has confirmed the ubiquitous presence of seropositivity to hMPV, with 90 percent of the population positive at 5 years of age and 98 percent positive by 10 years.[14] Both groups have observed that total antibody titers are higher for those older than 2 years,[14, 27] which may be due to serologic boosting and secondary infection in the second year of life after a primary infection when the child was an infant.

Where stated, most reports of hMPV infection in children treated at hospitals have found a preponderance of affected males to females (1.2 to 2.3:1).[16, 18, 27] hMPV infections in older children have been noted, particularly in those who are immunocompromised or have a preexisting chronic lung condition.[1, 17, 19, 21] hMPV has been touted as a potentially significant pathogen in immunocompromised transplant patients, similar to hRSV.[9, 19] No information is available on the impact of differing socioeconomic environments on the age at initial infection with hMPV or disease severity.

The spread of infection to nonimmune children also has yet to be determined, although it probably follows a pattern similar to that described for hRSV, for which infection is introduced by an older family member.[5] Dissemination of the virus probably occurs via large respiratory droplets, as shown for rhinovirus and hRSV.[4, 6]

Clinical Manifestations

The spectrum of clinical disease associated with hMPV infection is still being delineated. In the original report, the clinical symptoms were said to be largely similar to those caused by hRSV,[27] which included a range of features from mild respiratory problems to bronchiolitis, severe cough, high fever, myalgia, pneumonia, and vomiting. Some patients required hospitalization and mechanical ventilation. Several other studies worldwide have verified this initial description and thus have confirmed the role of hMPV as a major lower respiratory tract pathogen in children.[1, 16–18, 19, 22, 23, 25, 29] Infection with hMPV also has been associated with severe pneumonitis, in some cases leading to death.[1, 18, 19, 21]

The known features of hMPV disease in comparison to those of hRSV in hospitalized children are listed in Table 185–6. Fever, cough, respiratory distress, rhinitis/rhinorrhea, respiratory crackles (rales), wheezing (rhonchi), pharyngitis, otitis media, and conjunctivitis are the signs commonly associated with hMPV infection.[16–18, 23] The symptoms and signs of pediatric hMPV infection in a community-based setting have been described in only a single study to date, although cough (90%), coryza (88%), and fever (52%) remain predominant features.[29]

The most frequent diagnoses given for hMPV infection after medical assessment were bronchiolitis (27 to 59%), pneumonia (8 to 27%), virus-associated exacerbation of asthma (5 to 27%), laryngotracheobronchitis (croup) (3 to 18%), apnea (12%), and otitis media (12%).[16, 17, 29]

When chest radiographs were performed, abnormalities, most frequently bilateral pneumonic infiltrates and hyperinflation, were noted in 39 to 84 percent of cases.[16, 17, 23, 29] A typical chest radiograph of a child infected with hMPV is shown in Figure 185–8.

Severe episodes of pneumonitis have been noted in the two largest case series of hospitalized children with hMPV infection reported to date. Severe complications of infection in these cases included oxygen therapy (32 to 54%), intensive care admission (8 to 15%), and mechanical ventilation (5 to 8%).[16, 17]

TABLE 185–6 ■ SYMPTOMS AND SIGNS OF HUMAN METAPNEUMOVIRUS (hMPV) INFECTION COMPARED WITH HUMAN RESPIRATORY SYNCYTIAL VIRUS (hRSV) INFECTION IN HOSPITALIZED CHILDREN

Symptom/Sign	Percentage of hMPV cases*	Percentage of hRSV cases†
Cough	46–92	97–100
Fever	50–92	45–65
Respiratory distress	43–83	36–78
Rhinitis/rhinorrhea	57–83	56–82
Respiratory crackles/rales	57	27–72
Wheezing/rhonchi	45–50	45–78
Pharyngitis	19–43	45–54
Otitis media	16	31
Conjunctivitis	14	9

*Data from references 16, 17, 23, 29.
†Data adapted from Hall, C. B.: Respiratory syncytial virus. *In* Feigin, R. D., and Cherry, J. D. (eds.): Textbook of Pediatric Infectious Disease, 4th ed. Philadelphia, W. B. Saunders, 1998.

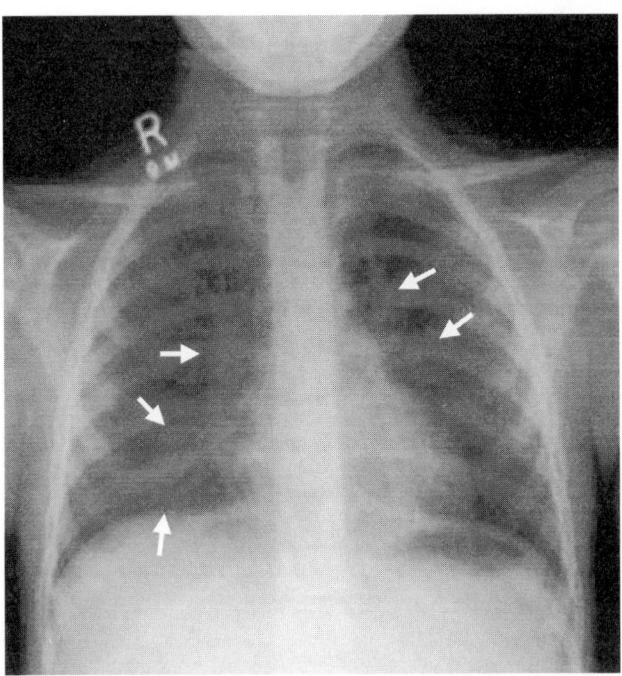

FIGURE 185–8 ■ Chest radiograph of a child infected with human metapneumovirus demonstrating bilateral pneumonic infiltrates *(arrows)* and hyperinflated lung fields.

A single case of reinfection with hMPV has been reported.[21] In a 7-month-old girl undergoing treatment for acute lymphoblastic leukemia with involvement of the central nervous system, pneumonia developed on two occasions 10 months apart with two genetically unrelated lineages of hMPV. The second infection ultimately led to the child's death. Interestingly, the source of the second infection was the child's father, in whom hMPV was isolated by culture after 14 days' incubation.

No clear or significant risk factors for hMPV infection thus far have been recognized. Factors that have been examined include premature birth, breast-feeding, parents who smoke, and daycare attendance.[16, 20] Children who have a positive family history of asthma may be at increased risk for the development of postinfectious bronchial hyperreactivity or asthma.[17, 20, 23] Finnish children with acute wheezing episodes associated with hMPV infection had high levels of interleukin-8 (IL-8) and low levels of RANTES (regulated by activation, normal T cell expressed and secreted).[11] This finding is in contrast to that noted for hRSV infections in vitro, in which RANTES concentrations (chemotactic factor for eosinophils) are high and IL-8 concentrations (chemotactic factor for neutrophils) are variable.[24] Whether the agent or the resultant disease leads to asthma or chronic lung disease is currently debatable, with conflicting reports in two small series of patients infected with hMPV.[11, 23]

hMPV infections in neonates and in hospital settings similar to those caused by hRSV also have been recognized.[17, 20] Therefore, infection control practices identical to those for other diagnosable respiratory virus infections (e.g., hRSV and influenza) should be instituted for known cases of hMPV infection in health care settings. Such practices include strict observance of handwashing by health care workers before and after contact with infected patients or those suspected of being infected and isolation or cohorting of infected cases to decrease transmission to susceptible, particularly immunocompromised patients.

hMPV does not appear to be associated with asymptomatic carriage in the nasopharynx. Van den Hoogen and colleagues noted that no hMPV was found in respiratory samples taken from 400 asymptomatic children younger than 2 years.[27] Co-infections with other known respiratory pathogens do occur. Boivin stated that 24 percent (9 of 38) of their hMPV-positive isolates were co-infected with other viruses. Other viral agents recognized in the respiratory secretions of symptomatic individuals thus far include adenovirus, hRSV, influenza A and B, and measles.[1, 17] Significant clinical bacterial respiratory infections associated with hMPV detection also have been reported, including infection with *Staphylococcus aureus, Streptococcus pneumoniae,* and *Stenotrophomonas maltophilia,* though less frequently than co-infection with other viruses.[1, 17]

Diagnosis

At present, hMPV infection can be diagnosed reliably only by viral culture or reverse transcriptase PCR (RT-PCR) of the respiratory secretions of affected individuals. In contrast to the situation with hRSV, no immunofluorescence test is available yet to inexpensively and rapidly screen respiratory specimens. Such a diagnostic assay is an urgent priority to assist in the widespread epidemiologic and community surveillance for hMPV and determine the true impact of the disease on children and adults.

Viral culture for hMPV is hampered by the long duration until a typical cytopathic effect is noted and requires the use of expensive and noncontinuous cell cultures and trypsin supplementation of culture media. Diagnostic RT-PCR also is expensive, technically demanding, and available only in laboratories with molecular detection capabilities. RT-PCR appears to be superior in sensitivity and turnaround time to viral culture in general. However, no study has examined the sensitivity and specificity of RT-PCR in comparison to viral culture for the diagnosis of hMPV in clinical specimens. RT-PCR can be performed with either a conventional thermocycler or a real-time platform such as the LightCycler (Roche Diagnostics).

Diagnostic RT-PCR assays that have been successful to date have used primer pairs directed at detection of conserved genomic regions of the M, N, F, and L ORFs of the hMPV genome.[1, 11, 13–18, 22, 23, 25, 29] Most of these studies are limited in determination of the true incidence of hMPV in the populations studied because the sensitivity of the RT-PCR assay used is unknown. Targeting diagnostic PCRs to the proximal ORFs (i.e., the 3′ end of the genome) of hMPV has been suggested to possibly be a more sensitive approach because of the differential gene transcription of *Paramyxoviridae.*[25] Only one study thus far has optimized its PCR assay when used as the sole clinical diagnostic assay for hMPV.[13] This study described a LightCycler diagnostic assay that provided faster results and improved the overall sensitivity of detection of hMPV by 10 percent over conventional RT-PCR while maintaining a reproducible and specific testing platform.[13] The authors also reported significant improvement in the sensitivity of their conventional RT-PCR protocol when an enzyme-linked amplicon hybridization assay (ELAHA) was used rather than gel electrophoresis for detection of RT-PCR products and when the concentration of antisense primer was increased over that used for the sense primer (asymmetric primer mixes).[153]

An IgG enzyme immunoassay to assess the incidence and impact of acute hMPV infection in adults has been described recently.[7] A fourfold or greater rise in IgG titer to hMPV was considered significant and indicative of recent infection.

Treatment

To date, no antiviral medications are known to inhibit the growth of hMPV either in vivo or in vitro. Treatment that has been supportive in all hospitalized cases described has included regular nasal suctioning, intravenous fluids, oxygen therapy, and occasionally, mechanical ventilation when necessary.[16, 17, 27]

Prevention

Good infection control practices in health care environments appear to be the only known preventive measures for hMPV infection. No data on viral targets or epitopes for a potential hMPV vaccine have been published. In contrast, attenuated live and inactivated APV vaccines based on the fusion (F) protein of the virus have been created and are used to prevent APV infection in poultry in Europe. These vaccines may offer clues to the future development of a successful vaccine for hMPV.

REFERENCES

1. Boivin, G., Abed, Y., Pelletier, G., et al.: Virological features and clinical manifestations associated with human metapneumovirus: A new paramyxovirus responsible for acute respiratory-tract infections in all age groups. J. Infect. Dis. *186*:1330–1334, 2002.
2. Chan, E. L., Brandt, K., Horsman, G. B., et al.: Human metapneumovirus infection in Saskatchewan. Abstract V-475. Presented at the 42nd Interscience Conference on Antimicrobial Agents and Chemotherapy, September 27–30, 2002, San Diego, California.
3. Cook, J. K. A., and Cavavagh, D.: Detection and differentiation of avian pneumoviruses (metapneuomoviruses). Avian Pathol. *31*:117–132, 2002.
4. Hall, C. B.: The nosocomial spread of respiratory syncytial virus infections. Annu. Rev. Med. *34*:311–319, 1983.
5. Hall, C. B., Geiman, J. M., Biggar, R., et al.: Respiratory syncytial virus infection within families. N. Engl. J. Med. *294*:414–419, 1976.
6. Hendley, J. O., Wenzel, R. P., and Gwaltney, J. M., Jr.: Transmission of rhinovirus colds by self-inoculation. N. Engl. J. Med. *288*:1361–1364, 1973.
7. Falsey, A. R., Erdman, D., Anderson L. J., et al.: Human metapneumovirus (hMPV) infection in elderly and young adults during two winter seasons. Abstract 775. Presented at the 40th Annual Meeting of the Infectious Disease Society of America, October 24–27, 2002, Chicago, Illinois.
8. Howe, M.: Australian find suggests worldwide reach for metapneumovirus. Lancet Infect. Dis. *2*:202, 2002.
9. Ison, M. G., and Hayden, F. G.: Viral infections in immunocompromised patients: What's new with respiratory viruses? Curr. Opin. Infect. Dis. *15*:355–367, 2002.
10. Ison, M. G., Mills, J., and Openshaw, P.: Current research on respiratory viral infections: Fourth International Symposium. Antiviral Res. *55*:227–278, 2002.
11. Jartti, T., van den Hoogen, B., Garofalo, R. P., et al.: Metapneumovirus and acute wheezing in children. Lancet *360*:1393–1394, 2002.
12. Lamb, R. A., and Kolakofsky, D.: *Paramyxoviridae:* The viruses and their replication. *In* Fields, B. N., Knipe, D. M., Howley, P. M., et al. (eds.).: Fields Virology. 3rd ed. Philadelphia, Lippincott-Raven, 1996, pp. 1177–1204.
13. Mackay, I. M., Jacob, K. C., Woolhouse, D., et al.: Molecular assays for detection of human metapneumovirus. J. Clin. Microbiol. *41*:100–105, 2003.
14. Mackay, I. M., Nissen, M. D., Siebert, D. J., et al.: First isolation of human metapneumovirus in Australia. Abstract PP36.1. Presented at the Annual Meeting of the Australian Society for Microbiology, September 29–October 3, 2002, Melbourne.
15. Mackay, I. M., Nissen, M. D., Siebert, D. J, et al.: Human metapneumovirus: From detection to dissection. Abstract PP36.3. Presented at the Annual Meeting of the Australian Society for Microbiology, September 29–October 3, 2002, Melbourne.
16. Mullins, J. A., Erdman, D., Weinberg, G. A., et al.: Human metapneumovirus infection in children hospitalized for respiratory disease. Abstract 774. Presented at the 40th Annual Meeting of the Infectious Disease Society of America, October 24–27, 2002, Chicago, Illinois.
17. Nissen, M. D., Mackay, I. M., Siebert, D. J., et al.: Epidemiological and clinical features of human metapneumovirus in Australian children. Abstract 33. Presented at the 40th Annual Meeting of the Infectious Disease Society of America, October 24–27, 2002, Chicago, Illinois.
18. Nissen, M. D., Siebert, D. J., Mackay I. M., et al.: Evidence of human metapneumovirus in Australian children. Med. J. Aust. *176*:188, 2002.
19. Osterhaus, A. D. M. E.: Myco- and paramyxovirus infections: What's new? Presented at the 5th International Conference on Antiviral Research, 2002, Prague, Czech Republic.
20. Osterhaus, A. D. M. E.: Human metapneumovirus: A new respiratory pathogen. Abstract S84. Presented at the 40th Annual Meeting of the Infectious Disease Society of America, October 24–27, 2002, Chicago, Illinois.
21. Pelletier, G., Dery, P., Abed, Y., et al.: Respiratory tract reinfections by the new human metapneumovirus in an immunocompromised child. Emerg. Infect. Dis. *8*:976–978, 2002.
22. Peret, T. C., Boivin, G., Li, Y., et al.: Characterization of human metapneumoviruses isolated from patients in North America. J. Infect. Dis. *185*:1660–1663, 2002.
23. Rawlinson, W. D., Waliuzzaman, Z., Carter, I. W., et al.: Asthma exacerabations in children are associated with rhinovirus but not human metapneumovirus infection. J. Infect. Dis. *187*:1314–1318, 2003.
24. Saito, T., Deskin, R. W., Casola, A., et al.: Respiratory syncytial virus induces selective production of the chemokine RANTES by upper airway epithelial cells. J. Infect. Dis. *175*:497–504, 1997.
25. Stockton, J., Stephenson, I., Fleming, D., et al.: Human metapneumovirus as a cause of community-acquired respiratory illness. Emerg. Infect. Dis. *8*:897–901, 2002.
26. van den Hoogen, B. G., Bestebroer, T. M., Osterhaus, A. D. M. E., et al.: Analysis of the genomic sequence of a human metapneumovirus. Virology *295*:119–132, 2002.
27. van den Hoogen, B. G., de Jong, J. C., Groen, J., et al.: A newly discovered human pneumovirus isolated from young children with respiratory tract disease. Nat. Med. *7*:719–724, 2001.
28. van Regenmortel, M. H., Fauquet, C. M., Bishop, D. H., et al. (eds.): *Paramxyoviridae. In* Viral Taxonomy: Classification and Nomenclature of Viruses. Seventh Report of the International Committee on Taxonomy of Viruses. San Diego, CA, Academic Press, 2000, pp. 549–561.
29. Williams, J. V.: Clinical manifestations of human metapneumovirus lower respiratory infections in children. Presented at the St. Jude/PIDS Pediatric Microbial Research Conference, February 22–23, 2002, Memphis, Tennessee.

RHABDOVIRIDAE

CHAPTER 186 Rabies Virus

STANLEY A. PLOTKIN ■ H. FRED CLARK

Rabies is a viral infection of the central nervous system (CNS) transmitted from animals to people. Introduction of the agent by bite, scratch, or aerosol enables it to attach to and travel up the nerves to the brain. The encephalitis so caused is characterized by hydrophobia and almost always is fatal.

History[77, 134]

Rabies has a long and colorful history. The Greeks called it *lyssa,* and Democritus is thought to have made the first description of rabies in the dog in 500 BC. The ultimate derivation of the English word *rabies* is from the Sanskrit word *rabhas,* which means "to do violence." Early writers believed that rabies followed the rising of the star Sirius, and the disease became associated with the dog days of summer.

Celsus, the Roman physician, writing in AD 100, displayed an accurate understanding of the disease by attributing infection to a "virus" (i.e., a poison) in the saliva. He advocated cauterization of the wounds produced by rabid animals. Galen, writing a century later, advised surgical resection as the method for preventing rabies.

Rabies was well known in Europe during medieval times, and the great Mohammedan physicians also mention it in their writings. Epizootics, however, were not recorded until 1271, when rabid wolves attacked people in Franconia. Epizootics associated with wolves then occurred frequently in various areas of Europe until early in the 18th century, when epizootics of rabies in domestic dogs began in cities. Rabies probably was transmitted from Europe to the New World, where it became common in North America and the West Indies by the 18th century and spread to South America early in the 19th century. The history of the disease in Asia is not as well known, but rabies clearly has been present since ancient times in China and India, although the current genotype may be from a relatively recent crossover.[94a]

The scientific study of rabies began with the demonstration by Zinke in 1803 that saliva transmitted the disease. The modern prevention of rabies was made possible by the work of Louis Pasteur in the 1880s. He showed that rabies could be transmitted by intracerebral inoculation of a preparation made from the brain of a rabid dog into uninfected rabbits or dogs and then serially transmitted by the same route. He thus demonstrated that rabies is a disease of the CNS. Among Pasteur's other discoveries were the differentiation of furious and dumb rabies, the production of rabies by the intravenous route, and the attenuation of rabies virus in the dried spinal cords of infected rabbits. The famous episode of Joseph Meister, the French boy who received rabies vaccine in 1885, demonstrated that serial inoculations of dried infected rabbit spinal cord, proceeding from most attenuated to least attenuated, in principle could protect against rabies.

Vaccination with nerve tissue vaccines quickly became standard, with important modifications being introduced by Roux, Fermi, and Semple. Semple vaccines, composed of infected sheep or goat brain tissue suspensions in which virus is completely inactivated by phenol, became the standard vaccine in the 1920s and remain in use today in most developing nations.[86]

The Virus

The rabies virus apparently can infect all species of mammals, although wide variations in the sensitivity of different species have been observed. Laboratory propagation may be accomplished readily in mice or other standard laboratory animals; in vitro in neuroblastoma or certain hamster cell cultures; or, after adaptation, in certain other cell lines of human or other mammalian origin.[159]

Electron-microscopic studies reveal that rabies is a bullet-shaped virus typically maturing at cytoplasmic plasma membranes and intracellular membranes of the endoplasmic reticulum in infected cultured cells (Fig. 186–1).[96] Standard virions are approximately 75 nm in diameter and 160 to 180 nm in length. Regular arrays of standard-sized virions maturing from plasma membranes are observed in infected salivary glands. Budding of virus from plasma membrane is much less pronounced in neurons of the CNS than in cell culture or salivary gland cells. However, meticulous electron-microscopic examination of experimentally and naturally infected brains has revealed that budding from membranes of perikarya and dendrites, as well as presence of virus in intracellular spaces of brain (especially at synaptic junctions), occurs regularly.[97] In addition, CNS neurons often exhibit both typical and bizarre morphologic forms of virus maturing in cytoplasm. Cytoplasmic forms often develop in proximity to nucleocapsid matrix inclusions (Negri bodies).[88]

The gross morphologic characteristics and biochemical composition of rabies virus place it within the rhabdovirus group. Until recently, no other rhabdoviruses bearing related antigens were known. However, lyssaviruses of Old World or Australian origin isolated more recently exhibit relationships to rabies, predominantly on the basis of similarities of the nucleoprotein detected by fluorescent antibody and complement-fixation tests, reactions with monoclonal antibodies, and sequencing studies of the N protein gene. Thus, seven types (often designated genotypes) are now recognized.[79]

Rabies virus is lyssavirus type 1 and continues to account for the vast preponderance of isolates. Type 2 (Lagos bat

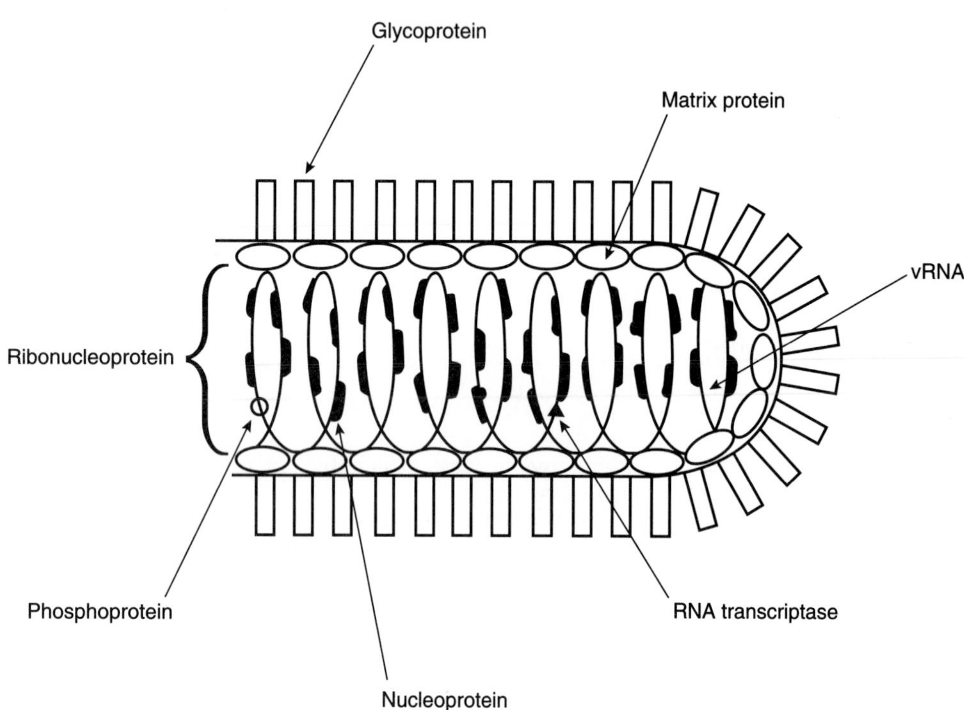

FIGURE 186–1 ■ Drawing of the rabies virus. (Courtesy of Dr. William Wunner, Wistar Institute, Philadelphia.)

virus), type 3 (Mokola virus), and type 4 (Duvenhage) were isolated exclusively in Africa, where they have predominantly bat reservoirs, but only Mokola and Duvenhage viruses have been associated with rare human infections. Lyssaviruses associated with European bat reservoirs have been separated into lyssavirus type 5 (European bat lyssavirus 1, rarely associated with human disease)[38] and type 6 (European bat lyssavirus 2). Lyssavirus type 7 has been identified in Australia (Australian bat lyssavirus) and has a primary reservoir in fruit-eating bats but has caused fatal human infection, thereby ending Australia's previous rabies-free status.[185] Cats in South Africa have been infected frequently with Mokola virus and have died of the infection despite prior vaccination.[221]

The rabies virion now is recognized to be of a molecular composition similar to that of the rhabdovirus prototype virus, vesicular stomatitis virus. It is composed of a helical nucleocapsid core, which contains the RNA genome coupled to nucleoprotein, the transcriptase-associated protein, and a large protein presumably representing the RNA transcriptase replicase.[48] The core is surrounded by a lipoprotein envelope, which contains two matrix proteins, a single glycoprotein, and lipids (primarily phospholipids and cholesterol).[23, 196] The genome is a single-stranded RNA molecule containing 11,932 nucleotides with a molecular mass of approximately 4.0×10^6 daltons.[22] It is a negative-stranded genome, that is, it must be transcribed to produce messenger RNA necessary for replication. However, attempts to demonstrate a virion-bound transcriptase have met with only limited success. Defective virions containing characteristic (for a given strain) sizes of incomplete RNA molecules have been demonstrated in cell culture–propagated virus populations, but their occurrence or role in natural infections has not been determined.

Important surface antigenic properties are associated primarily with the single glycoprotein,[196] a polypeptide containing three major oligosaccharide side chains.[58] Intact rabies virus hemagglutinates goose red blood cells in a medium of pH 6.4 at a temperature of 4° C.[81] Soluble hemagglutinin cannot be recovered from disrupted virions, but viral subunits containing glycoprotein can inhibit the hemagglutination reaction. The glycoprotein is the sole antigen responsible for induction of and reaction with virus-neutralizing antibody. Antibody to nucleoprotein administered passively has no virus-neutralizing or protective capacity but is the essential antibody for the diagnostic detection of intracellular rabies virus antigens (including Negri bodies) by immunofluorescent staining.[238] Active immunization with rabies nucleocapsid may contribute to immune protection, especially to heterotropic lyssaviruses, apparently by induction of a lyssavirus-specific T-cell immune response.[30, 62]

Historically, only a single antigenic type of the rabies type 1 lyssavirus had been identified. Understanding of the past and current epidemiology of rabies has received significant help from genomic sequence analysis[143] and strain differentiation by monoclonal antibodies. By these means, animal-specific strains and geographic distribution of strains can be discerned, and strains from human cases can be traced to the animal and place of origin.[194]

Researchers have demonstrated that rabies virus, like some other RNA viruses, occurs as a quasi-species. The presence of viral subpopulations permits rapid adaptation to new species, although a low level of mutation of nucleotides prevents major changes in the rabies virus.[114, 146]

Antigenic differences between both strains of fixed virus and different field isolates of diverse origin have been detected with use of monoclonal antibodies[236] directed against glycoprotein or nucleoprotein antigens of the virus.[61] The use of monoclonal antibodies also allows easy distinction of rabies from rabies-related viruses.[180] Studies with monoclonal antibodies have revealed that, worldwide, clustering of certain rabies antigenic subtypes is geographic and species specific.[202] As shown in Figure 186–2, six genetic groups of rabies viruses with relatively specific geographic localizations exist.[193] Within those areas, the virus may be transmitted by different species, such as dogs and foxes. Strains recovered from urban dogs fall into the six genotypes according to the location of the city. In the United States,

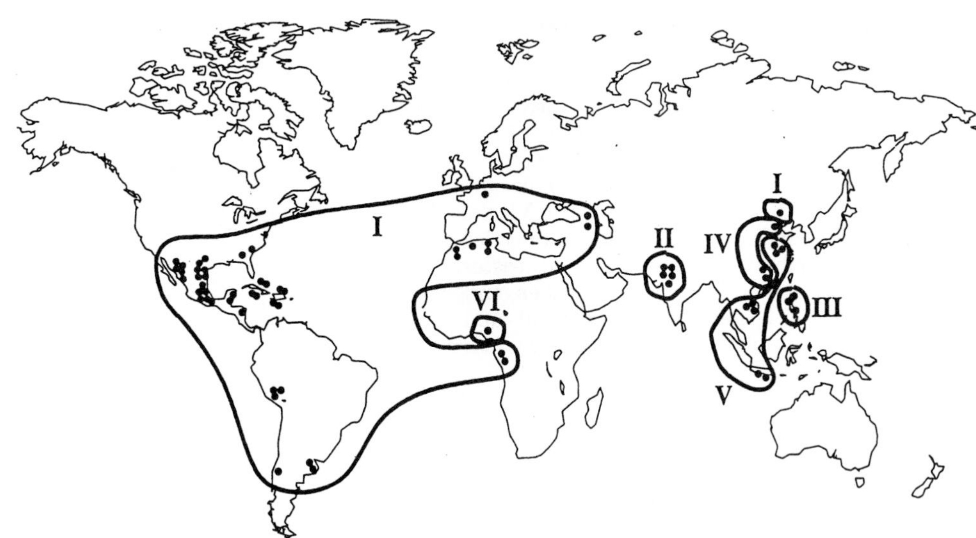

FIGURE 186–2 ■ Distribution of genotypes of rabies virus. (From Smith, J. S., Orciari, L. A., Yager, P. A., et al.: Epidemiologic and historical relationships among 87 rabies virus isolates are determined by limited sequence analysis. J. Infect. Dis. *166*:296–307, 1992. Courtesy of Dr. J. S. Smith, Centers for Disease Control and Prevention, Atlanta.)

readily distinguishable subtypes of rabies virus have been determined to circulate in each of the major terrestrial wild mammal vector species (primarily skunks and raccoons) and in bats.[181] Bat viruses rarely occur in terrestrial animals in North America, whereas in South America, viruses isolated from cows frequently originate from vampire bats.[61] In all well-studied rabies enzootic areas, researchers have determined that rabies circulates predominantly in a limited number of mammalian species characteristic of that area, and a single antigenic phenotype is characteristic of that transmission cycle.[61] However, distinct bat-adapted rabies virus strains may circulate independently in these areas or in areas where terrestrial animals are free of rabies. Different geographic subtypes of street rabies virus share varying proportions of the immunologically critically important glycoprotein epitopes with the vaccine strain (Pasteur) virus. Rabies viruses isolated from human cases of rabies in the United States have been shown to differ quantitatively in their glycoprotein antigenic composition from vaccine strain virus.[235] Despite intense investigation, however, no evidence supports the contention that cross-protection between the Pasteur strain rabies virus vaccine and antigenically distinguishable street strains or non-rabies lyssaviruses is reduced to a degree justifying inclusion of new virus strains in human vaccines. Physicians have every reason to believe that present vaccine strains protect against all feral strains, provided the vaccine is sufficiently potent.

Transmission and Epidemiology[32, 33, 215]

Infection with rabies may be induced readily in experimental animals through the oral, the respiratory, or a variety of parenteral routes. Epidemiologic evidence suggests that the vast preponderance of natural infections of humans and animals is caused by physical inoculation into subcutaneous and muscle tissue by a bite wound and rarely by exposure of mucosal surfaces; saliva is the body fluid that serves as the vehicle for virus to infect other animals or humans. Exceptional infections through the respiratory route have been noted in animals and people exposed to certain caves heavily infested with bats and in persons exposed to virus aerosols experimentally produced in the laboratory.

Domestic animals constitute the largest source of human exposure to rabies in most parts of the world. Dogs and cats are the principal transmitters of rabies to people in Asian countries, such as India, Indonesia, China, and the Philippines. The magnitude of the problem is illustrated by the fact that approximately 12,000 to 20,000 deaths are attributed to rabies annually in India alone,[246] and as many as 50,000 may occur throughout the world.[138] The incidence in India of 2 to 4 rabies deaths per 100,000 population is exceeded only by that of Ethiopia, where the rate is 18 per 100,000.[86] The total number of people given postexposure vaccination probably is 4 million annually. On the other hand, many areas, including the United Kingdom, Japan, Italy, Spain, Scandinavia (except Denmark and Finland), and others, are rabies free.[24]

In a single year of an urban epizootic of dog rabies in one city in Mexico, an estimated 2.5 percent of the population received dog bites and 2.7 percent were given postexposure immunoprophylactic treatment for rabies.[66] In Africa, the dog still is the most important vector, although in the south, jackals, cats, and mongooses also are common sources of rabies exposures.[21, 50] In much of Africa, the incidence of rabies in people and dogs has increased in recent years because of social and political disruptions.[236]

Rabies in wildlife, predominantly foxes, now is enzootic in much of continental Europe, having spread from Poland during the last 60 years.[24] This outbreak gradually has moved westward to involve most of eastern and western Europe, excluding Great Britain and Scandinavia. However, vaccination of wildlife has reduced sharply the incidence in the West, and rabies now rarely occurs in France.[105, 161] The raccoon, dog, and arctic fox are important vectors in eastern Europe and Siberia.[24, 113] Bat rabies exists throughout continental Europe, especially in Denmark, the Netherlands, and coastal areas.[148]

Rabies in Central and South America is related predominantly to dogs, but vampire bats also have considerable importance. The problem caused by bats mostly is indirect; although humans sometimes are bitten, more often they are exposed to cattle infected by bat bites. However, despite common exposure, transmission of rabies from cattle to humans occurs extremely rarely, perhaps because the virus usually is not found in cattle saliva.[55]

In the United States and Canada, the skunk was the rabid animal that most commonly attacks humans. In recent years, the raccoon has replaced the skunk as the most important potential source of infection among terrestrial mammals because of a rapid extension of raccoon rabies northward and southward from Virginia, in a range now continuous from Canada to Florida and west to Ohio.[37, 63] This outbreak stems from human introduction of raccoons into Virginia for hunting from a long-standing nidus of raccoon infection previously restricted to northern Florida and southeastern Georgia. Despite massive spread of raccoon rabies engendering great costs in terms of postexposure treatment and efforts at wildlife control, actual human cases of rabies attributable to raccoons have been rare.[38]

The significance of the bat to rabies epidemiology varies. In the United States, a redoubtable reservoir of rabies in insectivorous bats is present in every state except Hawaii. This bat reservoir probably is responsible for a high proportion of all U.S. cases, including those that have no antecedent history of animal bite.[142, 192] Between 1981 and 1998, an average of two human rabies cases occurred per year; 12 imported cases resulted from dog bite. However, between 1981 and 2000, 26 of 29 domestic cases have been caused by bat strains of rabies, predominantly strains from the silver-haired and Eastern pipistrelle bats.[36, 39, 119] The same trend has been observed in Canada.[5]

Strains isolated from the silver-haired bats are better able to grow in non-neuronal cells, and although prophylactic vaccination is effective, the infectiousness of these strains apparently is high.[146a] In Colorado, 15 percent of tested bats were positive for rabies,[159] which may be a relatively silent infection in that mammal.[173]

Bats may bite sleeping humans but leave little trace behind. Therefore, vaccination always is indicated if a rabid bat is found in the chamber of a sleeping person and may be indicated if a bat entered the chamber but escaped. In Europe, bats have been responsible for transmission of rabies-related lyssaviruses. Despite the rarity of this event, bats and vampirism are linked inextricably in legend with Dracula, the 15th-century despot who lived in current-day Romania.[88] In contrast, true vampire bats in Central and South America are responsible for considerable losses of domestic animals as well as human cases.[11]

Vaccination has curtailed the incidence of rabies in dogs and cats in the United States so greatly that many cities and other areas may be considered free of rabies in terrestrial animals, although the new spread of raccoon rabies has reversed this trend in certain cities of the Middle Atlantic states. The importance of this fact is discussed under Postexposure Prevention.

On the average, only one or two cases of human rabies are reported in the United States each year (a number that has increased slightly in recent years),[38] but thousands of animals still are infected. The distribution of infection among animals is shown in Table 186–1. The cat now is a more important host of domestic rabies than is the dog.

As a result of the rarity of human rabies in the United States, many cases have not been diagnosed until autopsy. Transmission of rabies by corneal transplant to a new host from fatal cases of undiagnosed encephalitis has been reported.[96]

TABLE 186–1 ■ CASES OF ANIMAL RABIES IN THE UNITED STATES, 2001

	Number	Percent
	Wild	
Raccoons	2787	37
Skunks	2282	31
Bats	1281	17
Foxes	432	6
Rodents/lagomorphs	56	0.8
Other	116	1.6
TOTAL	6939	93
	Domestic	
Cats	270	7.6
Dogs	89	1.2
Cattle	82	1.1
Horses/mules	51	0.9
Sheep/goats	3	0.04
Swine	2	0.03
Other	0	0.0
TOTAL	497	7

From Krebs, J. W., Noll, H. R., Rupprecht, C. E., and Childs, J. E.: Rabies surveillance in the United States during 2001. J Am Vet Med Assoc *221*:1690–1701, 2002, with permission.

Pathogenesis

The initial stages of the infectious process are the least understood. Disease certainly depends on the entry of the virus into peripheral nerves, after which centripetal spread occurs rapidly. Replication of virus in muscle cells at a peripheral inoculation site has been demonstrated experimentally and has been shown to persist in myocytes at least 60 days after inoculation[43] but has not been proved to occur in nonexperimental situations.[44, 150] Nevertheless, replication at a low level in myocytes, followed by subsequent infection of nerve cells, would explain the occasionally extended incubation periods of disease. Entry of virus into the peripheral nerve endings probably is mediated by attachment to the nicotinic acetylcholine receptor. However, rabies virus can enter the cell by use of other ganglioside receptors, and once it is in the nervous tissue, cell-to-cell spread can occur by cell-to-cell contact without the requirement of other receptors.[42, 213] In any case, virus is thought to enter peripheral nerves at an extremely variable time after exposure, presumably at the site of neuromuscular or neurotendinal spindles, at motor end-plates, or (in the case of aerosol exposure) at olfactory end-organs.[151] Viremia apparently is an inconstant occurrence and of little import in the dissemination of infection.

The fact that virus transits along nervous pathways has been demonstrated by repeated experimental observations that the progress of disease may be interrupted by surgical excision or chemical destruction of nerves at sites central to the inoculation site.[13] Central progression of virus along neuronal pathways also has been demonstrated by electron-microscopic, immunofluorescent, and serial infectivity studies.[118] Virus appears to be sequestered truly within neuronal cells during the apparently largely passive transmission (by axoplasmic flow) through peripheral nerves, and the virus can therefore be used experimentally to trace synaptic circuits.[110] Intra-axonal retrograde transport appears to be aided by interaction of the rabies P protein with the cytoplasmic protein dynein light chains.[100, 172] Minimal numbers of virions are observed within neurons, and connective tissue elements of nerve sheaths never are infected. Because little maturation and release of virus from nerve plasmalemmal membranes occur during transit, little or no virus is presented to the immune system, which explains the absence of detectable humoral antibody that is characteristic of even prolonged incubation periods with rabies.

Virus enters the CNS at the spinal cord and thereafter travels rapidly to the brain. Early selective infection of the limbic system in the brain may cause disease characterized by extreme excitability and agitation (furious rabies); the more common encephalitic depression symptom is associated with early, widespread infection in the brain. In either case, infection rapidly spreads to infect nearly all brain neurons within a few days of the onset of brain infection and CNS symptoms. Brain infection leads rapidly to death by mechanisms that are poorly understood. Fatal cases of encephalitis reveal little damage of neuronal cells, despite the ubiquitous neuronal infection. On the other hand, persons kept alive by vigorous supportive therapy for lengthy periods after onset of disease may develop severe histopathologic encephalitic lesions. Studies in mice have shown that apoptotic mechanisms may be turned on by rabies virus[98, 217] and that more virulent rabies virus strains may induce less apoptosis by expressing less G protein in neurons[37, 147] or alternatively that the rabies G protein expression may contribute to pathogenesis by down-regulating apoptosis.[147] Although ascending infection is specific to neurons, once the brain is infected, rabies virus spreads centrifugally to peripheral nerve plexuses, salivary glands, muscle fibers, and hair follicles.[99]

The entire manner of progression of the infecting virus, particularly those points in its transit vulnerable to immune intervention, remains to be determined fully. Clearly, preexisting humoral antibody protects, apparently by inactivating virus before it gains entry into the nervous system. After an immunized person is exposed to rabies, disease can be delayed or prevented in some cases by passive antibody, interferon treatment, or both,[104] but protection becomes efficient only when active immunization with potent vaccine accompanies such treatment.

That neutralizing antibodies are key to protection against rabies has been obvious for many years. However, studies have demonstrated the complexity of the immune response.[152] Although some experimental evidence argues for the importance of cytotoxic T lymphocytes in protection against rabies, Hooper and colleagues[95] infected mice that were unable to mount a cellular response and found no difference in disease with respect to normal mice. Nevertheless, early inflammatory responses, as well as rapid production of antibody, correlated with recovery from rabies. Thus, interferon and other mediators may supplement antibody in the prevention of rabies. Although the importance of cellular immunity is unclear, the induction of cytotoxic activity against virus-infected cells by vaccination was shown to correlate with protection. Interestingly, rabies-specific cytotoxic T lymphocytes do not develop during the disease, and wild rabies virus may act as an immunosuppressor. Moreover, chemical immunosuppression enhances the development of experimental rabies. Interferon[14] and interleukin-2,[156] both important immunomodulators produced by cells, enhance protection against rabies. More sophisticated understanding of rabies pathogenesis is required before ideal combinations of immunotherapeutic procedures, possibly including interferon, finally can be formulated.

The reverse side of the coin is shown by the "early death" phenomenon, in which exposed animals or humans developed earlier onset of rabies if previously they had been immunized only partly. Sugamata and associates[199] have shown that early death depends on the presence of T cells, indicating that it is mediated by an immunopathologic cellular response. In addition, some authors have argued that cytotoxic T lymphocytes actually may contribute to rabies neuritic paralysis.[199, 231]

Clinical Manifestations

IN ANIMALS

Rabies encephalitis in animals is expressed in either a paralytic (dumb) or furious syndrome. Typical infections are characterized by behavioral changes and a rapid clinical course leading to coma and death, but occasionally encephalitis can be nonfatal.[9] Because literally millions of animal bites of humans occur annually in the United States, the identification of aberrant behavior is a critical factor in many decisions to treat or not to treat immunoprophylactically for rabies.

The prodromal stage of disease is marked by nonspecific signs, such as restlessness and malaise. Subsequently, placid dogs, cats, cattle, or horses may become vicious. Fear of humans and of areas frequented by them may be lost by wild animals. Thus, rabid foxes, normally nocturnal, may be seen wandering abroad in daylight, even in populous areas. Similarly, rabid bats often have been encountered flying in daytime hours. Early behavioral changes are not accompanied by paralysis.

The clinical course rapidly progresses to either dumb or furious disease. Dumb rabies typically is a depressed encephalitic disease. In addition to lethargy, selectively severe paralysis of throat muscles may be observed, which causes drooling of saliva because of difficulty in swallowing. Hydrophobia is not noted in animals.

Furious rabies is characterized by an unusual state of alertness in which any visual or sound stimulation may incite an attack. Animals may roam indiscriminately, frequently feeding on stones, twigs, and other inanimate objects. Pets alternatively may exhibit unusually affectionate and playful behavior and then viciously bite those playing with them. Biting behavior may be noted by herbivores such as horses, mules, and cattle as well as by normally carnivorous pets and wild animals.

Both dumb and furious rabies have a rapid clinical course in domestic and wild animals. The period between onset of prodromal signs and death caused by respiratory paralysis rarely exceeds 7 to 10 days. Although 10 days usually is given as the limit of virus excretion in the saliva of dogs before death supervenes, rare exceptions involving prolonged or chronic excretion have been reported experimentally and in animals observed in both Africa and Asia.[68, 218]

The diagnosis of rabies in an animal depends on the demonstration of rabies antigens in the brain by fluorescent antibody stains or of rabies RNA by reverse transcriptase–polymerase chain reaction (RT-PCR). However, a test for detection of rabies antigen in the saliva of dogs was developed in Thailand and may be useful for diagnosis in an animal that is being held for observation of symptoms.[109]

Control of Animal Rabies

Aside from large-scale removal of potentially rabid animal species such as stray dogs, the most potent control method is vaccination. In domestic animals, immunization is accomplished readily by a variety of veterinary vaccines, although boosters must be given annually or after other stated intervals depending on the vaccine.[37]

In wild animals, primarily raccoons in the United States and foxes in Europe, oral vaccination with use of baits containing vaccinia-vectored rabies glycoprotein or attenuated live virus has been successful. It is expensive and seems to work better in Europe than in the United States.[63, 161]

IN HUMANS[141, 143, 149, 160]

The incubation period of rabies in some cases may be so long as to qualify it as a slow virus disease. Well-documented cases have occurred as long as 6 years after the bite.[224] However, most cases occur within 20 to 90 days after exposure. The shortest incubation period appears to be 10 days.

That incubation periods are longer after bites on the legs than after bites on the face is well known. The reason for this duration appears to be related not to the length of the nerve that the virus must traverse, because it travels rapidly even from the farthest site, but to the extent of innervation of different parts of the body. Bites on the tips of the fingers or on the genitalia have relatively short incubation periods for this reason. Children in general tend to have shorter incubation periods. Curiously, cases of vaccination failure tend to have shorter incubation periods, a fact that also is observed in experimental trials in animals. This early death effect is discussed under Pathogenesis.

The first symptoms of rabies usually are vague and insidious. The patient simply may feel unwell or have anxiety or depression. Some fever or nausea may be present. The most striking prodromal symptom is itching, pain, or tingling at the site of the bite. This paresthesia is not present always and may take various forms, but its localization is a definite harbinger of rabies. The prodrome lasts 2 to 10 days, when the acute neurologic phase begins. The symptoms of this second phase must be divided into furious versus paralytic rabies, most cases being in the furious category.

In furious rabies, the emphasis is on agitation, hyperactivity, fluctuating consciousness, bizarre behavior, and perhaps nuchal rigidity. Sore throat and hypersalivation are prominent complaints, and laryngospasm may cause hoarseness.

The legendary, but all too real, pathognomonic sign of furious rabies is hydrophobia. Initial attempts to swallow liquid result in painful spasms of the pharyngeal and laryngeal muscles, with aspiration of the liquid into the trachea. A conditioned response appears to be created, in which fear exacerbates the actual spasms. Warrell and associates[225] have hypothesized that brain stem encephalitis leads to destruction of inhibitors of inspiratory motor neurons. Respiratory tract instant reflexes are exaggerated, leading to inspiratory spasms. The hydrophobia has an important psychologic element. In an extreme case, spasms occur if the patient merely is approached with water. Also frequently present is aerophobia, in which spasms occur when a current of air is fanned across the face.

The neurologic examination findings in rabies are not uniform. Meningismus is a commonly occurring abnormality. Even more common occurrences are cranial nerve signs, particularly paralysis of the palate and vocal cords. The voice may develop a hoarse, barking quality. The reflexes may vary from hyperactive to absent, and involuntary movements are prominent.

A distinct pattern of neurologic involvement is shown by approximately 20 to 30 percent of rabies patients, particularly those bitten by vampire bats. Flaccid paralysis may start in the limb that was bitten originally and spread to other limbs. The cranial nerves become involved, and the face, rather than showing agitation, becomes expressionless. Hydrophobia is not a feature. Paralytic rabies is confused easily with Guillain-Barré syndrome. Hemachuda and colleagues[91] emphasize the importance of fever, intact sensation, urinary incontinence, and percussion myoedema in paralytic rabies.

The cerebrospinal fluid (CSF) is abnormal in a minority of patients, particularly those in whom meningismus is present clinically. When abnormal, the CSF shows a mild pleocytosis, mainly mononuclear. The peripheral white blood cell count shows increased polymorphonuclear cells.

Death caused by rabies in the acute stage occurs because of cardiac or respiratory problems. Cardiac arrhythmias with circulatory collapse are common occurrences, and virus may be recovered at autopsy from the heart, which shows pathologic evidence of myocarditis. Respiration becomes increasingly labored, and death may occur during a laryngeal spasm or aspiration.

The acute neurologic phase lasts 2 to 10 days, with eventual deterioration of the patient's mental status into coma. The patient may survive in this state for 2 weeks, particularly in dumb rabies. Before the final deterioration, the patient may have alternating periods of wild agitation and alert cooperation. During the alert state, patients may be able to discuss their illnesses and express fear of impending death. However, most often, death rapidly follows onset of coma, unless intubation and ventilatory assistance are offered, in which case survival may be prolonged for months. During the comatose state, a variety of problems may be present, including cerebral edema, inappropriate antidiuretic hormone secretion, diabetes insipidus, and other manifestations of hypothalamic dysfunction, hypotension or arrhythmia, and pneumonia.

Diagnosis

The diagnosis of rabies in humans begins with its diagnosis in the animal. The technique now most commonly used is to stain the brain of the previously apprehended animal with a fluorescein-labeled antibody to rabies. More recently, enzyme-coupled antibodies have been introduced, allowing the colored product to be seen under the light microscope. Rabies RNA also can be detected by dot hybridization or by PCR amplification.[107] Virus isolation is used for confirmation, either by the classic procedure of intracerebral inoculation in mice or by inoculation of neuroblastoma cells followed by fluorescent antibody staining for rabies antigen.

Unfortunately, no methods for the identification of rabies virus infection before the onset of clinical signs are known. Although the clinical expression of the disease often is characteristic and diagnosis is simplified by history of known exposure to an animal bite, encephalitic illness may occur, in which rabies virus involvement cannot be diagnosed with certainty without laboratory assistance.

When a patient has a history of being bitten by an animal, paresthesia at the wound site, and hydrophobia, determining a clinical diagnosis of rabies is not difficult. Other diseases in which encephalitis occurs, such as those caused by arboviruses, enteroviruses, and herpes simplex virus, occasionally may cause confusion. However, if one finds signs of brain stem involvement in a patient whose sensorium basically is clear and who has no signs of a space-occupying lesion, the other diagnoses usually can be set aside.

Paralytic rabies may be misdiagnosed as Guillain-Barré syndrome, poliomyelitis, or post–rabies vaccine encephalomyelitis. Careful neurologic examination and analysis of the CSF often help to rule out these diagnoses.

The spasms of tetanus can cause momentary confusion, but trismus is not part of rabies, and hydrophobia is not part of tetanus. Botulism (wound or ingestion) will cause paralysis, but the absence of sensory changes should exclude rabies.

Postvaccination encephalitis after nerve tissue vaccine poses a diagnostic problem in countries in which it still is used. It may require the performance of laboratory tests described later.[60]

Perhaps the most confusing differential problem is hysteria in a person who thinks he or she has rabies. Normal blood gas analyses and the absence of variation in bizarre behavior suggest pseudorabies. Psychiatric and drug-induced reactions also may cause transient diagnostic problems.

Laboratory diagnosis now is possible before death. The virus may be demonstrated by fluorescent antibody stain of smears of corneal epithelial cells[116, 187] or sections of skin from the neck at the hairline.[27, 195] These test results are positive because virus migrates down the nerves from the brain, and both the cornea and hair follicles are richly innervated.

Serologic diagnosis also can be obtained if the patient survives beyond the acute period. In persons not given postexposure immunoprophylactic treatment, only low levels of antibodies appear.[90] In contrast, patients who have received vaccine show a rapid rise in titer of virus-neutralizing antibodies between 6 and 10 days after the onset of symptoms.[83] Such antibodies are detected most rapidly by an in vitro rapid fluorescent focus inhibition test or by mouse or plaque-reduction neutralization tests. Rabies may be diagnosed in immunized persons by a rise in titer after the onset of clinical symptoms and is suggested by any antibody titer greater than or equal to 1:5000, a level not usually achieved by vaccines. High antibody levels in CSF are characteristic late in the course of rabies encephalitis; CSF antibody is not induced efficiently by vaccination.[83, 227]

Rabies virus has been isolated from human saliva between days 4 and 24 after onset of disease.[83] Virus also may be isolated in some cases from CSF, brain tissue, or urine sediment during the first 2 weeks of illness. In persons surviving longer than 2 weeks, isolation of virus from body tissues or fluids (or from postmortem brain) may be impossible, presumably because of virus neutralization by humoral antibody.

Postmortem diagnosis can be confirmed by the presence of pathognomonic cytoplasmic inclusions (Negri bodies) in brain tissue, but they are present in less than 80 percent of cases. Rabies antigen may be detected by fluorescent antibody examination, with higher frequency in brain tissues of persons dying after a brief, acute course of disease. In postmortem tissues, histochemical staining with monoclonal antibody to rabies virus ribonucleoprotein especially may be useful because ribonucleoprotein possesses epitopes resistant to the formalin fixation and the paraffin-embedding process.[139] In studies of paraffin-embedded brain tissues (samples up to 40 years old), digestion of sections with proteinase K followed by immunofluorescence or RT-PCR assay gave 100 percent (300 of 300) positive results.[223] However, as in the case of virus isolation attempts, identification of virus antigen in brains of persons kept alive for prolonged periods after onset of disease may be extremely difficult.

Noah and coworkers[155] have summarized the results of attempts to diagnose rabies in humans pre mortem. Their data are summarized in Table 186–2,[166] which shows that RT-PCR analysis of saliva and brain biopsy are the most accurate methods of diagnosis, although even they may not be positive until the fifth day of illness.

Crepin and associates[53] had 100 percent success (9 of 9) in diagnosing rabies using RT-PCR assay of saliva accompanied by immunofluorescent examination of skin biopsy specimens. Most of these patients were diagnosed with specimens collected less than 5 days after onset of symptoms.

Rabies now has been recognized post mortem in patients whose history included transplantation of corneas from donors dying of encephalitis. All cases of undiagnosed fatal encephalitis, therefore, should be studied for rabies, and tissue from such patients should not be used for transplantation.[165]

TABLE 186–2 ■ ANTEMORTEM DIAGNOSTIC TEST RESULTS FOR 20 HUMAN PATIENTS WITH RABIES IN THE UNITED STATES, 1980–1996

Test	No. of Patients Positive for Rabies Virus/ Total No. Tested (%)	Earliest Positive (Day of Illness)
RT-PCR of saliva for rabies virus RNA	10/10 (100)	5
Brain biopsy for rabies virus antigen	3/3 (100)	8
Nuchal skin biopsy for rabies virus antigen	10/15* (67)	5
Virus isolation from saliva	9/15† (60)	5
Antibody to rabies virus in serum	10/18 (56)	5‡
Rabies virus antigen in touch impression from cornea	2/8 (25)	14
Antibody to rabies virus in cerebrospinal fluid	2/13 (15)	15§

*Two patients had earlier skin biopsy findings that were negative but became positive on subsequent biopsy.
†One patient had an earlier test result that was negative.
‡Latest negative 24 days, median to positive 10 days.
§Latest negative 24 days.
Data from Noah, D. L., Drenzek, C. L., Smith, J. S., et al.: Epidemiology of human rabies in the United States, 1980 to 1996. Ann. Intern. Med. *128*:922–930; 1998.

Prognosis

The recovery of a 6-year-old boy from Ohio who developed rabies after a bat bite fueled optimism that survival in rabies might be possible with intensive care.[170] Other rare survivals have been reported,[1, 31, 174] but the optimism seems to be unjustified. Many other patients now have been treated intensively and nevertheless have died after a prolonged clinical course.[17, 56] Antirabies antibodies, interferon and its inducers, and various antivirals have been used without evident success. However, the fact that all survivors have had vaccine administered before or after the bite suggests that some immune mechanism may operate to reduce rabies virus replication or to inhibit virus-induced pathophysiologic changes.

Postexposure Prevention[164]

LOCAL TREATMENT

Removal of saliva containing rabies virus is a crucial part of treatment and should be undertaken urgently. The wound should be flushed copiously with soap and water. Some authors, including us, would follow flushing with a local application of povidone-iodine or ethyl alcohol in whatever form is available immediately. The concentration of ethanol is important; 43 percent (86 proof) or higher gives the best results.[234]

Experimental data suggest that regardless of the solution used, adequate flushing is important, particularly in puncture wounds. Catheters should be inserted into puncture wounds and fluid instilled by means of an attached syringe.[54, 190] If this procedure proves to be too painful, the area can be anesthetized safely with local procaine-type anesthetics.[108, 234] Suturing should be done in line with good surgical practice but avoided when unnecessary.

EQUINE RABIES IMMUNE GLOBULIN

An experimental basis for the desirability of combining antiserum with vaccine was established in 1954.[117] A field test of combined vaccine-serum protection was made possible by a natural disaster, the attack of a rabid wolf on 29 Iranian villagers, 18 of whom were bitten on the head and neck.[16] Rabies developed in 3 of 5 persons who were treated with nerve tissue vaccine only but in only 1 of 13 persons who were given antiserum with nerve tissue vaccine.

Animal rabies serum is no longer available in the United States. However, an immune globulin has been prepared from the serum of rabies-immunized horses (equine rabies immune globulin) and now is used extensively outside of the United States because of its lower price and greater availability (compared with human rabies immune globulin).[241] To reduce allergic reactions, pepsin digestion is used to convert the equine globulin to a $F(ab')_2$ preparation. The product is dispensed at a concentration of 200 IU/mL, and the dose that should be administered is 40 IU/kg, as much as possible infiltrated into the wound. Administration of higher doses dampens the active immune response. The manufacturers recommend an intradermal skin test with the equine rabies immune globulin, but the sensitivity and specificity of the test for prediction of subsequent allergic reactions are poor, and abandonment of the skin test has been proposed.[243] At least one preparation of equine rabies immune globulin was purified sufficiently so that the allergic reaction rate was less than 1 percent,[241] whereas another yielded a 6 percent reaction rate.[242]

A new equine rabies immune globulin is now available, heat treated to reduce the risk of viral contamination.[124]

HUMAN RABIES IMMUNE GLOBULIN

To avoid possible reactions to animal proteins, gamma globulin was prepared from the plasma of volunteers hyperimmunized with rabies vaccine. Although expensive, human rabies immune globulin is preferable to equine rabies immune globulin for use in postexposure treatment in the United States. Because the gamma globulin is homologous in humans, human rabies immune globulin persists longer in the circulation of inoculated persons but, for this reason, may have an even greater dampening effect on active immunization. Thus, Hattwick and associates[84] found that 23 doses of duck embryo vaccine were needed to overcome the suppressive effect on antibody production of 15 to 40 units of human rabies immune globulin per kilogram.

Pharmacokinetic measurements[89, 133, 137, 178] resulted in a recommendation to give 20 IU of human rabies immune globulin per kilogram immediately, with as much as possible being injected locally. Local injection is important because serum levels of antibody after intramuscular injection are not high.[45] Although intravenous administration of human rabies immune globulin produces higher serum titers,[6] local injection still is preferred. No further dose is necessary or desirable because excessive antibody diminishes the active response to vaccine. Moreover, if neither equine nor human rabies immune globulin is available, vaccination should be started immediately, followed by administration of human rabies immune globulin if it arrives within a week.[112] Because of the expense and occasional difficulty in obtaining adequate supplies of human rabies immune globulin, as well as substantial variability of immunoglobin products tested in an animal model,[82] the World Health Organization now is exploring the possibility of using instead "cocktail" mixtures of neutralizing monoclonal antibodies to rabies virus prepared in either murine[189] or human[60] hybridoma cell cultures, but efforts to produce such a product have involved significant technical difficulties.[41]

NERVE TISSUE VACCINE

Most of the rabies vaccine produced in the world today is of nervous tissue origin. Vaccines made in sheep brain or goat brain are used throughout Asia and Africa but are associated with a definite incidence of postvaccinal encephalitis.[8] The susceptibility to rabies vaccine–induced encephalomyelitis has been suggested to vary according to the genetic pattern of major histocompatibility class II alleles in the vaccinated host.[163] Suckling mouse brain vaccines are used in South America and Russia to decrease sensitization to myelinated adult nerve tissue, which is the cause of autoimmune allergic encephalitis.[75]

However, a study from Tunisia found no evidence for humoral response to myelin in patients with encephalitis after nerve tissue vaccine. Instead, antibodies to GM_1 and GD_{1a} gangliosides present on human cells were demonstrated.[127] Thus, the mechanism of encephalitis remains uncertain, beyond the conclusion that it results from non-rabies antigens in the nervous systems of animals, including sheep, lambs, and mice.

The efficacy of nerve tissue vaccine in humans has not been evaluated by controlled studies. The Pasteur Institute of Southern India analyzed the incidence of disease in vaccinated and unvaccinated people bitten by animals that were proved rabid by the transmission of rabies to other animals or humans. Fifty-six percent of untreated persons developed rabies, compared with only 7 percent of vaccinated persons, for an efficacy of approximately 88 percent.[218]

On the other hand, vaccination with nerve tissue vaccine of persons bitten on the head or neck by rabid wolves in Iran still was followed by a 40 percent overall mortality rate. In comparison, 15 of 32 villagers (47%) who failed to seek treatment after being attacked by a rabid wolf developed rabies.[94]

Nerve tissue vaccines are not used in the United States.

DUCK EMBRYO VACCINE

Duck embryo vaccine was developed to overcome the problem of encephalitic reactions to nerve tissue vaccine. In this respect, it was successful; the incidence of neuroparalytic reactions fell from 1 in 1000 with nerve tissue vaccine to 1 in 25,000 with duck embryo vaccine.[164, 177, 186] Unfortunately, a high price was paid in immunogenicity. In postexposure treatment of Americans, Corey and associates[51] found that 8 percent of those given courses of duck embryo vaccine failed to respond with the production of measurable antibody. Even more disturbing was the fact that 23 percent of recipients of duck embryo vaccine plus rabies antiserum did not develop antibody. Duck embryo vaccine contained enough duck protein to produce a significant number of allergic reactions.[177]

CELL CULTURE VACCINES[167]

The ideal solution to the problems of antigenicity and the safety of rabies vaccine clearly lie in the development of vaccines prepared from rabies virus grown in cell culture free of neural tissue. For avoiding inclusion of foreign host proteins in the vaccine, the optimal tissue culture would be of human cells.

The basic ingredients for the production of human diploid-cell vaccine (HDCV), the first cell culture vaccine widely used, were the development of the WI-38 normal human fibroblast cell line by Hayflick and Moorhead[87] and the adaptation of the Pitman-Moore strain of rabies virus to growth in WI-38 by Wiktor and associates.[237] Virus grown in WI-38 or other human fibroblasts is concentrated by ultrafiltration to increase antigen content and then inactivated by beta-propiolactone.

After various schedules of HDCV were tried, researchers found that three properly spaced intramuscular doses invariably produced an immune response. A similar schedule of duck embryo vaccine resulted in titers 10 to 20 times lower. The excellent immunogenicity of HDCV has been confirmed amply,[7, 28, 52, 77, 169, 171, 214, 239] and it has become the "gold standard" against which other vaccines are measured.

Table 186–3 shows the serologic data of three persons who received postexposure immunization from one of the authors.[168]

The crucial test of a rabies vaccine is protection of those actually exposed to the virus. In Europe, the HDCV has been used to treat thousands of people exposed to possible rabies. However, those situations in which rabies was confirmed in the biting animal are particularly important to consider. Kuwert and associates,[120, 121] in Essen, vaccinated 68 persons after exposure to dogs, cats, cows, or wild animals with laboratory-confirmed rabies virus infection or exposed as a result of laboratory accident. The schedule used was 1 mL intramuscularly on days 0, 3, 7, 14, 30, and 90. They had no failures of protection, no significant reactions, and excellent neutralizing and complement-fixing antibody responses.

Bahmanyar and associates in Iran[15] conducted another test of HDCV. Forty-five persons who were bitten by rabid wolves or dogs were given rabies antiserum, followed by the same schedule of vaccine as that used in Germany. Once again, no rabies was seen in vaccinees, despite a 40 percent risk (estimated from previous experience) if they had remained unvaccinated. Antibody measurements showed mean titers as follows: 7 days, 1.1 IU; 14 days, 10.7 IU; 30 days, 49 IU; and 100 days, 312 IU.

The Centers for Disease Control and Prevention (CDC) distributed HDCV of American manufacture after exposure to persons whose exposure to rabies was established.[2] No vaccine failure occurred, and all who received the full schedule of five 1-mL doses intramuscularly responded with antibodies.

Although a small number of vaccine failures have been reported in other countries after administration of the HDCV, ancillary treatment recommendations were not followed scrupulously in each case.[4] The failure rate is estimated to be at most 1 in 12,000 courses of vaccination given in countries with high risk for rabies, such as Thailand.[154] General anesthetics given while the wound is repairing may increase the risk of vaccine failure.[70]

ALTERNATIVE VACCINES TO HUMAN DIPLOID-CELL VACCINE

An effort has been made to produce vaccines with the desirable properties of HDCV at a lower cost that would make them broadly available in the developing nations, where the risk of human rabies is most severe. The products have been produced in Europe and used primarily in Europe or Asia.

Purified Vero rabies vaccine (PVRV) is the Pasteur strain of rabies (as used in HDCV) grown in the Vero cell line in industrial fermenters. The virus is concentrated, inactivated, and purified. PVRV has an immunogenic potency similar to that of HDCV. Successful postexposure experience has been reported in Tunisia,[40] China,[222] and Thailand, even after severe exposure.[101, 201, 207] The Vero cell vaccine has been further purified by chromatography.[124]

Purified chick embryo-cell (PCEC) rabies vaccine is produced in primary chick embryo-cell culture with use of the Flury low egg passage (LEP) strain of rabies virus. It is inactivated, concentrated, and purified, yielding a vaccine preparation of antigenic potency similar to those of PVRV and HDCV.[17] PCEC rabies vaccine was uniformly successful in preventing rabies in postexposure trials in the former Yugoslavia, including subjects who were exposed by wolf bite.[49, 219] PCEC rabies vaccine also was shown to be equivalent to HDCV for boosting previously immunized subjects[26] and for protection of mice against bat strains of rabies.[57]

Purified duck embryo-cell rabies vaccine is produced in embryonated duck eggs. The Pitman-Moore virus harvested from the eggs is purified, concentrated, and inactivated.[111]

Regrettably, although the new vaccines are considerably less expensive than are HDCVs, their costs still place them out of reach of many poorer countries. Therefore, because of expensive purification procedures, these less affluent nations often continue to use predominantly nerve tissue vaccines of high reactogenic potential and variable antigenic potency. However, primary hamster cell kidney vaccine has been produced in China and was demonstrated to be immunogenic and to provide postexposure protection.[67] It now has completely replaced Semple vaccine in China.[67]

An argument has been made that a potent rabies virus might be made at low cost in BHK-21 cells, and if it were inactivated with beta-propiolactone, the beta-propiolactone would so damage the cell DNA that the theoretic danger posed by cell DNA in vaccine would be eliminated totally.[145]

TABLE 186–3 ■ ANTIBODY RESPONSE IN THREE CHILDREN TO POSTEXPOSURE RABIES VACCINATION WITH HUMAN DIPLOID-CELL VACCINE

	Antibody Titers (IU) by Rapid Fluorescent Focus Inhibition Test					
Time after Vaccination	Inoculation Schedule	Case 1	Inoculation Schedule	Case 2	Inoculation Schedule	Case 3
0 day*	V (+ 1 day)†	<0.5	V (+ 3 days)†	<0.4	V (+ 5 days)†	<0.3
3 days	V				V	
7 days	V	<0.1	V	0.6	V	<0.3
14 days	V	13.5	V	1.1	V	0.4
21 days			V			
28 days				17	V	27
30 days	V	20				
38 days		30				
42 days				90		30
3 months		35				
4 months				22		7
7 months						
18 months				2.4		

*Day of first vaccination is day 0.
†Number of days after bite on which human diploid-cell vaccine first was administered.

TABLE 186–4 ■ SCHEDULE OF CELL CULTURE VACCINES FOR IMMUNIZATION AGAINST RABIES

	Vaccine Dosage		
Situation	**Route**	**Volume**	**Schedule (days)**
Postexposure			
United States	IM	1.0 mL	0, 3, 7, 14, 28
WHO	IM	1.0 mL	0, 3, 7, 14, 30, 90
Rapid*	IM	1.0 mL	0 (2 doses), 7, 21
Rapid*	ID	0.1 mL	0 (8 doses), 7 (4 doses), 28, 91
Rapid*	ID	0.1 mL	0 (2 doses), 3 (2 doses), 7 (2 doses), 30, 90
Previously vaccinated	IM	1.0 mL	0, 3
Previously vaccinated*	ID	0.1 mL	0, 3
Pre-exposure			
Primary	IM	1.0 mL	0, 7, 21 or 28
	ID	0.1 mL	0, 7, 21 or 28
Booster	IM	1.0 mL	0
	ID	0.1 mL	0

*Used outside the United States.

Numerous regimens have been developed for rapid immunization of exposed patients in poor countries who may seek medical help late or who may not return for subsequent doses.[200, 220] To reduce costs, advantage is taken of the smaller volume needed for intradermal administration. However, no intradermal vaccine is licensed in the United States (see below). These regimens are listed in Table 186–4 and have the advantage of being less expensive. Note that if the 2-1-1 regimen is chosen, immune globulins will interfere with the response to the vaccine.[124, 246]

Three types of rabies vaccine are available in the United States: HDCV, PCEC, and a tissue culture vaccine made in fetal rhesus diploid cells by the Michigan State Department of Health, called rabies vaccine adsorbed (RVA).*[18] HDCV or RVA is recommended for postexposure immunization when given by the intramuscular route according to the regimens listed in Table 186–4. Note that only five doses are recommended in the United States, although the World Health Organization recommends six.[80] The dose should not be reduced for children.[6] Decreased immune responses have been noted in vaccinees given injections in the gluteal area,[73] and therefore all intramuscular injections of rabies vaccine should be given in the deltoids. Although rabies never has been reported in persons with any prior history of vaccination, in the event of reexposure, they should be given two intramuscular booster doses, as also stated in Table 186–4.

The effectiveness of current rabies vaccines to protect against rabies-related lyssaviruses appears to be good.[79, 148]

DECISIONS TO VACCINATE

The physician must take into account numerous human and zoologic factors in deciding when to vaccinate, although reluctance to use vaccine now is based more on cost than on the pain of injections. A study performed in the United States[144] revealed that administration of rabies prophylaxis was inappropriate in 40 percent of cases in which it was given. However, the study also showed that 6 percent of those not receiving prophylaxis should have received it. Thus, physician judgment needs improvement, not only for medical reasons but also because some incidents of exposure to rabies result in vaccination of many persons, with high cost.[176] Among the factors to be considered are the following.

Pregnancy

Pregnant women tolerate rabies vaccination without problem.[46, 198]

Geography

Terrestrial animal bites in most large urban areas in the developed world are unlikely to be from rabid animals, although Philadelphia, Baltimore, and Washington, D.C., have become part of the raccoon epizootic, with transfer of disease to urban cats.

Type of Animal

Cats always are suspect if they go out of their way to bite. Dogs near the Mexican border are more suspect than are those farther north. Skunks, foxes, and raccoons involved in biting incidents must be considered rabid until proven otherwise. With the exception of woodchucks, rodents such as squirrels are unlikely to be rabid.

Bat Exposures

As stated before, rabies transmission from bats has become a threat to humans in the United States owing to an apparent increase in exposures to silver-haired and Eastern pipistrelle bats. The in vitro characteristics of the bat rabies strains, which may allow them to replicate better in non-neural tissues, plus the small and sometimes imperceptible bites these species inflict, led to the recommendation that vaccination is appropriate when bats are handled without gloves and when sleeping individuals awake to find a bat in the room.[34]

Circumstances of Bite

The attempt to feed an undomesticated animal always must be considered provocative behavior. Invasion of an animal's territory may result in an attack, which is less suggestive of rabies than is an attack by an animal that invades human environments. However, judgment as to whether a bite was provoked is poorly predictive of rabies in enzootic areas.[117] If an animal appears clinically rabid, it should be sacrificed immediately for confirmation of rabies by examination of the brain. If a dog, cat, or ferret appears normal, it may be kept for 10 days to see if it develops rabies.[141] Meanwhile, exposed humans should or should not be started on treatment, depending on the known prevalence of rabies in the particular region.

Animal Vaccination

Rabies is an extremely rare occurrence in properly vaccinated animals.

Table 186–5 summarizes recommendations by the Advisory Committee on Immunization Practices on vaccination against rabies.[28] Advice can be sought from state and local health departments (particularly with regard to the occurrence of rabies in animals) and from the CDC directly.

FAILURE OF RABIES PROPHYLAXIS

The most common cause of vaccine failure is that immune globulin was not used simultaneously.[56, 76, 240] Active immunization will not regularly produce antibodies until

*RVA is temporarily unavailable as of April 1, 2003.

TABLE 186–5 ■ RABIES PRE-EXPOSURE PROPHYLAXIS GUIDE—UNITED STATES[34]

Risk Category	Nature of Risk	Typical Populations	Pre-exposure Recommendations
Continuous	Virus present continuously, often in high concentrations Specific exposure likely to go unrecognized Bite, nonbite, or aerosol exposure	Rabies research laboratory workers* Rabies biologics production workers	Primary course Serologic testing every 6 months; booster vaccination if antibody titer is below acceptable level†
Frequent	Exposure usually episodic with source recognized, but exposure also might be unrecognized Bite, nonbite, or aerosol exposure	Rabies diagnostic laboratory workers* Spelunkers Veterinarians and staff Animal-control and wildlife workers in rabies-enzootic areas	Primary course Serologic testing every 2 years; booster vaccination if antibody titer is below acceptable level†
Infrequent (greater than population at large)	Exposure nearly always episodic with source recognized Bite or nonbite exposure	Veterinarians and animal-control and wildlife workers in areas with low rabies rates Veterinary students Travelers visiting areas where rabies is enzootic and immediate access to appropriate medical care including biologics is limited	Primary course No serologic testing or booster vaccination
Rare (population at large)	Exposure always episodic with source recognized Bite or nonbite exposure	U.S. population at large, including persons in rabies-epizootic areas	No vaccination necessary

*Judgment of relative risk and extra monitoring of vaccination status of laboratory workers are responsibilities of the laboratory supervisor.
†Minimum acceptable antibody level is complete virus neutralization at a 1:5 serum dilution by the rapid fluorescent focus inhibition test. A booster dose should be administered if the titer falls below this level.

10 to 14 days after the first dose. Lack of local infiltration of immune globulins and the immunosuppressive effect of chloroquine account for other failures. The presence of B-cell immunodeficiency in a patient requires measurement of antibodies after vaccination. Patients infected with human immunodeficiency virus (HIV) are likely to respond if their $CD4^+$ lymphocytes are higher than 300/μL. If not, their postvaccination antibodies should also be measured.[102] In HIV-infected children, a standard postexposure course of HDCV had no effect on the level of $CD4^+$ lymphocytes or the HIV viral load.[205] However, even with correct prophylactic treatment, failures may occur, perhaps because virus is deposited directly onto nerve endings[92] or because of inadequate monitoring of vaccine and rabies immune globulin potency in developing countries.[12]

Pre-exposure Immunization

The development of HDCV has made effective immunization of persons at risk of coming into contact with rabies virus possible before the actual exposure. Veterinarians, animal handlers, laboratory workers, and spelunkers need pre-exposure immunization. Large numbers of veterinary students have been vaccinated with HDCV under a three-dose schedule at 0, 7, and 21 or 28 days. Rabies antibody titers were determined on the serum of each veterinary student. Nearly 100 percent developed antibodies, with geometric mean titers of 10 IU or greater, which is equivalent to a neutralizing antibody titer of at least 1:400.[118, 174] The three-dose regimen listed in Table 186–4 induces antibodies in 100 percent of recipients. Pre-exposure immunization may be given with use of HDCV, PCEC, or RVA by intramuscular administration (see Table 186–5). Outside the United States, any one of the alternative cell culture vaccines can be used on the same schedule.[183] Alternatively, and more cheaply, immunization may be performed intradermally according to the same schedule. Intradermal vaccine should not be used for postexposure immunization in the United States; in poor countries, however, considerations of cost may force its use, and alternative schedules have been developed (discussed later).

Although antibody responses are sufficiently regular that postimmunization testing usually is unnecessary, if a test is obtained, neutralizing antibody titers of 1:25 or 0.5 IU are considered protective.

Because rabies in developing countries is primarily a disease of children, exploratory studies have been performed to determine if pre-exposure vaccination could be incorporated into routine pediatric schedules. Preliminary results from Vietnam show that cost aside, routine rabies vaccination in infancy is feasible[123] and could even be performed by low-dose intradermal administration.[205]

Children infected with HIV can be immunized successfully if their $CD4^+$ cells exceed 15 percent of lymphocytes. Those with fewer $CD4^+$ cells will need double doses of rabies vaccine.[205]

Missionaries and Peace Corps personnel operating in rabies-endemic countries should receive pre-exposure vaccination.[10]

INTRADERMAL VACCINATION

For pre-exposure use, the intradermal route is considered an acceptable alternative to intramuscular injection, with the important proviso that persons receiving antimalarial or other immunosuppressive agents and perhaps older persons should have their titers checked after vaccination or receive the injections by the intramuscular route. Trimarchi and Safford[212] reported that about 7 percent of persons failed to develop rabies neutralizing antibodies after intradermal vaccination.

The success of intradermal vaccination depends on a technique that ensures intradermal rather than subcutaneous injection, but a margin of error exists.[19, 72]

To reduce the costs of vaccination, intradermal vaccination for postexposure use has become popular in developing countries, but it no longer is approved in the United States. Although single-dose preparations are not available for the intradermal route, extensive experience in Thailand and elsewhere has validated the successful prevention of rabies with vaccine extracted from vials intended for intramuscular use.[65, 216, 228, 229] However, attention must be paid to the correct administration of the dose into the skin, the sterility of unused portions of the vial, the volume of vaccine in the ampule, and the antigenic content of the vaccine used. The antigenic content should be at least 0.25 IU per 0.1 mL. If it is lower, a 0.2-mL dose may be necessary.[191]

Poor responses to intradermal vaccine have been noted in those concurrently receiving chloroquine or immunosuppressives, such as corticosteroids.[34, 160] Therefore, persons who must be vaccinated while they are taking chloroquine or related antimalarials should be given injections into the deltoid muscle, and postvaccination rabies serologic studies should be obtained on those patients and others who are immunosuppressed.

ALTERNATIVE SCHEDULES

Although the American and World Health Organization (sometimes called Essen) schedules firmly are established for the induction of optimal immune responses, other schedules have been tested extensively to reduce the number of vaccination visits, particularly in the developing world. The most popular of these are the 2-1-1 schedule, in which a double dose is given intramuscularly at day 0, followed by single doses on days 7 and 21,[47, 140] and the regimen developed by Warrell and associates,[228] consisting of eight intradermal doses on day 0, four intradermal doses on day 7, and single doses on days 28 and 91.

The 2-1-1 schedule is not reliable if immune globulins also are administered.[122, 124]

BOOSTER DOSES

Once an immune response to rabies vaccine has developed, a person probably is sensitized forever. Nevertheless, even with administration of HDCV, antibodies fall off rapidly after initial immunization, although most HDCV recipients have some detectable antibody at 2 years after initial vaccination. One booster of HDCV given to previously vaccinated persons results in a dramatic anamnestic response, with titers in one study rising from 2.8 IU to 94 IU at 14 days and more than 100 IU in 35 days.[167] As mentioned, with exposure to rabies in a previously vaccinated person, two intramuscular booster doses are recommended to provide a margin of safety. Single intramuscular or intradermal boosters are given to maintain immunity in individuals chronically exposed to rabies according to the recommendations made by the CDC in Table 186–6.

In persons who have received pre-exposure immunization to rabies, the necessity of boosters is an important issue. Persons who definitely are exposed to a rabid animal should receive two booster doses of vaccine by the intramuscular route. Individuals who are likely to be exposed, such as rabies laboratory workers, are boosted to maintain their antibody titers above 0.5 IU. Booster vaccination is not recommended for others who encounter less exposure, but a follow-up study by Briggs and Schwenke[25] is interesting. They found maintenance of an adequate titer (>0.5 IU) at 1.5 to 2 years after vaccination in 99 percent of subjects who received vaccine by the intramuscular route and in 93 percent who received vaccine by the intradermal route. In Thailand, researchers demonstrated that persons who received pre-exposure rabies vaccination by the intradermal route mounted a slow response to boosters, and the authors suggested that in severe exposures, rabies immune globulin should be given despite the prior immunization.[102] However, the intradermal route can be used successfully to boost prior immunity.[204] On the other hand, Thraenhart and associates[208] observed 100 percent positive antibodies in 18 subjects studied between 2 and 14 years after vaccination.

ADVERSE REACTIONS

The available tissue culture vaccines are well tolerated. In more than 1770 human volunteers receiving pre-exposure immunization with HDCV administered intramuscularly, sore arm was noted in approximately 20 percent, headache in about 8 percent, malaise in 5 percent, and allergic edema

TABLE 186–6 ■ RABIES POSTEXPOSURE PROPHYLAXIS GUIDE—UNITED STATES[34]

Animal Type	Evaluation and Disposition of Animal	Postexposure Prophylaxis Recommendations
Dogs, cats, and ferrets	Healthy and available for 10 days of observation	Persons should not begin prophylaxis unless animal develops clinical signs of rabies*
	Rabid or suspected rabid	Immediately vaccinate
	Unknown (e. g., escaped)	Consult public health officials
Skunks, raccoons, foxes, and most other carnivores; bats	Regarded as rabid unless animal proven negative by laboratory tests†	Consider immediate vaccination
Livestock, small rodents, lagomorphs (rabbits and hares), large rodents (woodchucks and beavers), and other mammals	Consider individually	Consult public health officials Bites of squirrels, hamsters, guinea pigs, gerbils, chipmunks, rats, mice, other small rodents, rabbits, and hares almost never require antirabies postexposure prophylaxis

*During the 10-day observation period, begin postexposure prophylaxis at the first sign of rabies in a dog, cat, or ferret that has bitten someone. If the animal exhibits clinical signs of rabies, it should be euthanized immediately and tested.
†The animal should be euthanized and tested as soon as possible. Holding for observation is not recommended. Discontinue vaccine if immunofluorescence test results of the animal are negative.

in 0.1 percent.[167] During incidents involving mass postexposure treatment, pain, swelling, and other local symptoms occurred in 30 to 74 percent of individuals.[39] Pregnancy is not a contraindication to receiving modern rabies vaccines.[46] Guillain-Barré syndrome and other neurologic problems have been rare, and their relationship to HDCV is uncertain.[115] Guillain-Barré syndrome that occurs after administration of nerve tissue vaccine is associated with antibodies to myelin basic protein.[91]

In contrast, booster vaccinations with HDCV have been associated with allergic reactions in approximately 6 percent of subjects.[35] These reactions are caused by the presence in the vaccine of human albumin that has been altered by the beta-propiolactone used to inactivate the virus.[3, 203, 230] The reactions are of the immune complex type (type III), with urticaria, edema, joint manifestations, fever, and malaise. CDC data suggest that when primary vaccination is given intramuscularly and booster intradermally or vice versa, reactions are more common than if all vaccination is by the same route.[74] Because the reaction is associated with the particular formulation of HDCV rather than with the rabies antigen itself, additional boosters may be given if necessary with PCEC, PVRVg, or HDCV manufactured in Canada (Connaught).[71]

Future Developments

The world of rabies is far from static. Table 186–7 shows the progress of rabies vaccine development for humans. Perhaps the most dramatic future prospect is the development of vaccines in which the gene for rabies glycoprotein has been inserted into a viral vector, such as vaccinia.[182] These vaccines are safe and highly immunogenic when fed to a large variety of animal species.[180] In field studies, raccoons and other wild animals have been immunized successfully with baits containing rabies recombinant vaccine. Other avenues being pursued include the use of potent adjuvants to enhance the immunogenicity of subunit vaccine,[69] the addition of the internal ribonucleoprotein to enhance protection through induction of cellular immune responses and higher antibody responses,[210] animal poxvirus vectors in which the rabies glycoprotein gene has been inserted,[29] synthetic peptides constructed from epitopes of the single glycoprotein and nucleoprotein,[59] and plasmid vectors containing cDNA of the single glycoprotein genes.[248]

Particular effort has been directed toward the development of DNA vaccines. They are alleged to be potentially cheap and particularly thermostable, but to date most have required an unsatisfactory interval to produce virus-neutralizing antibodies (VNA) or have induced VNA of inadequate titer.[130–132] Dogs given two doses of Pasteur strain G protein DNA, administered intramuscularly, were shown to develop VNA to rabies and to European bat lyssaviruses 1 and 2 and to have protection against strict virus challenge.[162] Other investigators reported that rabies G DNA was immunogenic only by the intradermal route in cats.[157] Jallet and colleagues[103] produced chimeric G DNAs of rabies and EBL1, or rabies and Mokola virus, to generate vaccines designed to induce VNA in dogs to either all European lyssaviruses or all African lyssaviruses, respectively. Lodmell and Ewalt[132] showed that rabies G DNA could induce protection after exposure in mice only if the DNA vaccine was inoculated into the pinna of the mouse's ear! In primates, rabies G DNA induced VNA only if it was administered by gene gun.[131] Addition of the adjuvant monophosphoryl lipid A to rabies DNA did not effectively enhance the immunogenic or protective potential of rabies G DNA administered by the intramuscular or intradermal route to mice.

Other approaches have included efforts to express rabies G protein in yeast cells, which failed,[206] and in baculovirus in insect cells, which was successful. Although it is less glycosylated than the virion G protein, the baculovirus-expressed G induced VNA efficiently in mice; its immunogenicity was not improved by adding baculovirus-expressed rabies N protein.[64] In approaches using the rabies G protein cloned into adenovirus, researchers have shown that a replication-defective recombinant elicited enzyme-linked immunosorbent assay antibodies in mice inoculated onto mucosal surfaces[247] and that an adenovirus incorporating a special promoted-intron expression cassette efficiently induced rabies G protein in cell culture that induced VNA in intraperitoneally inoculated mice.[135] The rabies G protein gene was cloned into canine herpesvirus; this recombinant induced VNA efficiently in dogs inoculated by the intranasal route, suggesting that it might be useful as an oral product to control canine rabies.[249]

Molecular biologic approaches have not produced an ideal vaccine, especially for human use. In the near future, the most cost-effective and protective vaccines may be virion products propagated to high titer in an easily managed cell culture system, for example, the BHK-21 continuous cell line or transgenic plants.

TABLE 186–7 ■ SOME RABIES VACCINES DEVELOPED FOR HUMANS

Vaccine Types	Remarks
Pasteur: dried rabbit spinal cord	Residual live virus
Fermi: phenolized sheep or goat brain	Residual live virus
Semple: phenol-inactivated sheep or goat brain	Contains nerve tissue
Fuenzalida: phenol-inactivated suckling mouse brain	Contains less myelin
Duck embryo: beta-propiolactone (BPL) inactivated	Allergy to duck proteins
Human diploid (HDCV): BPL-inactivated fetal human cell culture vaccine	Current standard Booster allergic reactions
Rhesus diploid (RVA): fetal rhesus cell culture BPL-inactivated	Fewer allergic reactions
Vero cell (PVRV): BPL-inactivated virus grown in Vero monkey kidney cell line	Purified by density gradient centrifugation
PCEC rabies vaccine: inactivated virus grown in chick embryo cells	Purified as with PVRV
Vaccine recombinant (VRG): genetic construct expressing rabies glycoprotein	Probably will be used only in animals (see text)

REFERENCES

1. Alvarez, L., Fajardo, R., Lopez, E., et al.: Partial recovery from rabies in a nine-year-old boy. Pediatr. Infect. Dis. J. *13*:1154–1155, 1994.
2. Anderson, L. J., Sikes, R. K., Langkop, C. W., et al.: Postexposure trial of a human diploid cell strain rabies vaccine. J. Infect. Dis. *142*:133–137, 1980.
3. Anderson, M. C., Baer, H., Frazier, D. J., et al.: The role of specific IgE and beta-propiolactone in reactions resulting from booster doses of human diploid cell rabies vaccine. J. Allergy Clin. Immunol. *80*:861–868, 1987.
4. Anonymous: Rabies vaccine failures. Lancet *1*:912, 1988.
5. Anonymous: Human rabies in Canada—1994–2000. Can. Commun. Dis. Rep. *26*:210–211, 2000.
6. Aoki, F. Y., Rubin, M. E., and Fast, M. V.: Rabies neutralizing antibody in serum of children compared to adults following post-exposure prophylaxis. Biologicals *20*:283–287, 1992.

7. Aoki, F. Y., Tyrrell, D. A. J., Hill, L. E., et al.: Immunogenicity and acceptability of a human diploid-cell culture rabies vaccine in volunteers. Lancet *1*:660–662, 1975.
8. Applebaum, E., Greenberg, M., and Nelson, J.: Neurological complications following antirabies vaccine. J. A. M. A. *151*:188–191, 1953.
9. Arko, R. J., Schneider, L. G., and Baer, G. M.: Nonfatal canine rabies. Am. J. Vet. Res. *34*:937–938, 1973.
10. Arguin, P. M., Krebs, J. W., Mandel, E., et al.: Survey of rabies preexposure and postexposure prophylaxis among missionary personnel stationed outside the United States. J. Travel Med. *7*:10–14, 2000.
11. Arrellano-Sota, C.: Biology, ecology, and control of the vampire bat. Rev. Infect. Dis. *10*(Suppl. 4):S615–S619, 1988.
12. Arya, S. C.: Therapeutic failures with rabies vaccine and rabies immunoglobulin. Clin. Infect. Dis. *29*:1605, 1999.
13. Baer, G. M., and Cleary, V. F.: A model in mice for the pathogenesis and treatment of rabies. J. Infect. Dis. *125*:520–527, 1972.
14. Baer, G. M., Moore, S. A., Shaddock, J. H., et al.: An effective rabies treatment in exposed rabies monkeys. Bull. World Health Organ. *57*:807–813, 1979.
15. Bahmanyar, M., Fayaz, A., Nour-Salehi, S., et al.: Successful protection of humans exposed to rabies infection: Postexposure treatment with the new human diploid cell rabies vaccine and antirabies serum. J. A. M. A. *236*:2751–2754, 1976.
16. Baltazard, M., Bahmanyar, M., Ghodssi, M., et al.: Essai pratique du serum antirabique les mordus par loups enrage. Bull. World Health Organ. *13*:747–772, 1955.
17. Barth, R., Gruschkau, H., Bijok, U., et al.: A new inactivated tissue culture rabies vaccine for use in man: Evaluation of PCEC-vaccine by laboratory test. J. Biol. Stand. *12*:29–46, 1984.
18. Berlin, B. S., Mitchell, J. R., Burgoyne, G. H., et al.: Rhesus diploid rabies vaccine (adsorbed): A new rabies vaccine. J. A. M. A. *249*:2663–2665, 1983.
19. Bernard, K. W., Mallonee, J., Wright, J. C., et al.: Preexposure immunization with intradermal human diploid cell rabies vaccine. J. A. M. A. *257*:1059–1063, 1987.
20. Bhatt, D. R., Hattwick, M. A. W., Gerdsen, R., et al.: Human rabies: Diagnosis, complications, and management. Am. J. Dis. Child. *127*:862–869, 1974.
21. Bingham, J., Foggin, C.M., Wandeler, A.I., et al.: The epidemiology of rabies in Zimbabwe. 2. Rabies in jackals (*Canis adustus* and *Canis mesomelas*). Onderstepoort J. Vet. Res. *66*:11–23, 1999.
22. Bishop, D. H. L., Aaslestad, H. G., Clark, H. F., et al.: Evidence for the sequence homology and genome size of rhabdovirus RNA's. *In* Mahy, B. W. J., and Barry, R. D. (eds.): Negative Strand Viruses. Vol. 1. New York, Academic Press, 1975, pp. 259–292.
23. Blough, H. A., Tiffany, J. M., and Aaslestad, H. G.: Lipids of rabies virus and BHK-21 cell membranes. J. Virol. *21*:950–955, 1977.
24. Bourhy, H., Kissi, B., Audry, L., et al.: Ecology and evolution of rabies virus in Europe. J. Gen. Virol. *80*(pt 10):2545–2557, 1999.
25. Briggs, D. J., and Schwenke, J. R.: Longevity of rabies antibody titre in recipients of human diploid cell rabies vaccine. Vaccine *10*:125–129, 1992.
26. Briggs, D. J., Dreesen, D. W., Nicolay, U., et al.: Purified chick embryo cell culture rabies vaccine: Interchangeability with human diploid cell culture rabies vaccine and comparison of one- versus two-dose post-exposure booster regimen for previously immunized persons. Vaccine *19*:1055–1060, 2000.
27. Bryceson, A. D. M., Breenwood, B. M., Warrell, D. A., et al.: Demonstration during life of rabies antigen in humans. J. Infect. Dis. *131*:71–74, 1975.
28. Cabasso, V. J., Dobkin, M. B., Roby, R. E., et al.: Antibody response to a human diploid cell rabies vaccine. Appl. Microbiol. *27*:553–561, 1974.
29. Cadoz, M., Strady, A., Meignier, B., et al.: Immunisation with canarypox virus expressing rabies glycoprotein. Lancet *339*:1429–1432, 1992.
30. Celis, E., Ou, D., Dietzschold, B., et al.: Recognition of rabies and rabies-related viruses by T cells derived from human vaccine recipients. J. Virol. *62*:3128–3134, 1988.
31. Centers for Disease Control: Rabies in a laboratory worker: New York. M. M. W. R. Morb. Mortal. Wkly. Rep. *26*:183, 1977.
32. Centers for Disease Control: Rabies Surveillance: Annual Summary, 1975. Issued August 1976.
33. Centers for Disease Control: Rabies Surveillance: Annual Summary, 1976. Issued October 1977.
34. Centers for Disease Control: Recommendation of the Immunization Practices Advisory Committee, Rabies Prevention—United States. M. M. W. R. *48*(RR-1):1–21, 1999.
35. Centers for Disease Control: Systemic allergic reactions following immunization with human diploid cell rabies vaccine. M. M. W. R. *33*:185–187, 1984.
36. Centers for Disease Control: Update: Raccoon rabies epizootic—United States and Canada, 1999. M. M. W. R. *49*:31–35, 2000.
37. Centers for Disease Control: Compendium of animal rabies prevention and control, 2000. National Association of State Public Health Veterinarians, Inc. M. M. W. R. *49*(RR-8):21–30, 2000.
38. Centers for Disease Control and Prevention. Human rabies—California, Georgia, Minnesota, New York and Wisconsin, 2000. M. M. W. R. *49*:1111–1114, 2000.
39. Centers for Disease Control: Human rabies prevention—United States, 1999. Recommendations of the Advisory Committee on Immunization Practices (ACIP). M. M. W. R. *48*(RR-1):1–21, 1999.
40. Chadli, A., Merieux, C., Arrouji, A., et al.: Study on the efficacy of a vaccine produced from rabies virus cultivated on Vero cells. *In* Vodopija, I., Nicholson, K. G., Smerdel, S., et al. (eds.): Improvements in Rabies Post-Exposure Treatment. Zagreb, Zagreb Institute of Public Health, 1985, pp. 120–136.
41. Champion, J. M., Kean, R. B., Rupprecht, C. E., et al.: The development of monoclonal human rabies virus–neutralizing antibodies as a substitute for pooled human immune globulin in the prophylactic treatment of rabies virus exposure. J. Immunol. Methods *235*:81–90, 2000.
42. Charlton, K. M.: The pathogenesis of rabies and other lyssaviral infections: Recent studies. Curr. Top. Microbiol. Immunol. *187*:95–119, 1994.
43. Charlton, K. M., Nadin-Davis, S., Casey, G. A., and Wandeler, A. I.: The long incubation period in rabies: Delayed progression of infection in muscle at the site of exposure. Acta Neuropathol. (Berl.) *94*:73–77, 1997.
44. Charlton, K. M., and Casey, G. A.: Experimental rabies in skunks: Immunofluorescence light and electron microscopic studies. Lab. Invest. *41*:36–44, 1979.
45. Chomchay, P., Khawplod, P., and Wilde, H.: Neutralizing antibodies to rabies following injection of rabies immune globulin into gluteal fat or deltoid muscle. J. Travel Med. *7–8*:187–188, 2000.
46. Chutivongse, S., Wilde, H., Benjavongkulchai, M., et al.: Postexposure rabies vaccination during pregnancy: Effect on 202 women and their infants. Clin. Infect. Dis. *20*:818–820, 1995.
47. Chutivongse, S., Wilde, H., Fishbein, D. B., et al.: One-year study of the 2-1-1 intramuscular postexposure rabies vaccine regimen in 100 severely exposed Thai patients using rabies immune globulin and Vero cell rabies vaccine. Vaccine *9*:573–576, 1991.
48. Clark, H. F., and Prabhakar, B. S.: Rabies. *In* Olsen, R. G., Krakowka, G. S., and Blakesle, J. R. (eds.): Comparative Pathobiology of Viral Disease. Vol. 2. Boca Raton, CRC Press, 1985, pp. 165–214.
49. Clark, H. F., and Vodopija, I.: Human vaccination against rabies. *In* Baer, G. (ed.): Natural History of Rabies. 2nd ed., Vol. 2. Boca Raton, FL, CRC Press, 1991, pp. 571–595.
50. Cleaveland, S.: Royal Society of Tropical Medicine and Hygiene meeting at Manson House, London, 20 March 1997. Epidemiology and control of rabies. The growing problem of rabies in Africa. Trans. R. Soc. Trop. Med. Hyg. *92*:131–134, 1998, pp. 571–595.
51. Corey, L., Hattwick, M. A. W., Baer, G. W., et al.: Serum neutralizing antibody after rabies postexposure prophylaxis. Ann. Intern. Med. *85*:170–176, 1976.
52. Cox, J. H., and Schneider, L. G.: Prophylactic immunization of humans against rabies by intradermal inoculation of human diploid cell culture vaccine. J. Clin. Microbiol. *3*:96–101, 1976.
53. Crepin, P., Audry, L., Rotivel, Y., et al.: Intravitam diagnosis of human rabies by PCR using saliva and cerebrospinal fluid. J. Clin. Microbiol. *36*:1117–1121, 1998.
54. Dean, D. J., Baer, G. M., and Thompson, W. R.: Studies on the local treatment of rabies-infected wounds. Bull. World Health Organ. *28*:477–486, 1963.
55. Delpietro, H. A., Larghi, O. P., and Russo, R. G.: Virus isolation from saliva and salivary glands of cattle naturally infected with paralytic rabies. Prev. Vet. Med. *48*:223–228, 2001.
56. Deshmukh, R. A., and Yemul, V. L.: Fatal rabies encephalitis despite post-exposure vaccination in a diabetic patient: A need for use of rabies immune globulin in all post-exposure cases. J. Assoc. Physicians India *47*:546–547, 1999.
57. Dietzschold, B., and Hooper, D. C.: Human diploid cell culture rabies vaccine (HDCV) and purified chick embryo cell culture rabies vaccine (PCECV) both confer protective immunity against infection with the silver-haired bat rabies virus strain (SHBRV). Vaccine *16*:1656–1659, 1998.
58. Dietzschold, B.: Oligosaccharides of the glycoprotein of rabies virus. J. Virol. *23*:293–296, 1977.
59. Dietzschold, B., and Ertl, H. C. J.: New developments in the pre-exposure and post-exposure treatment of rabies. Crit. Rev. Immunol. *10*:427–440, 1991.
60. Dietzschold, B., Gore, M., Casali, P., et al.: Biological characterization of human monoclonal antibodies to rabies virus. J. Virol. *64*:3087–3090, 1990.
61. Dietzschold, B., Rupprecht, C. E., Tollis, M., et al.: Antigenic diversity of the glycoprotein and nucleocapsid proteins of rabies and rabies-related viruses: Implications for epidemiology and control of rabies. Rev. Infect. Dis. *10*:S785–S798, 1988.
62. Dietzschold, B., Wang, H., Rupprecht, C. E., et al.: Induction of protective immunity against rabies by immunization with rabies virus ribonucleoprotein. Proc. Natl. Acad. Sci. U. S. A. *84*:9165–9169, 1987.
63. Dobson, A.: Raccoon rabies in space and time. Proc. Natl. Acad. Sci. U. S. A. *97*:14041–14043, 2000.

64. Drings, A., Jallet, C., and Chambert, B.: Is there an advantage to including the nucleoprotein in a rabies glycoprotein subunit vaccine? Vaccine *17*:1549–1557, 1999.
65. Dutta, J. K., Warrell, M. J., and Dutta, T. K.: Intradermal rabies immunization for pre- and post-exposure prophylaxis. Natl. Med. J. India 7:119–122, 1994.
66. Eng, T. R., Fishbein, D. B., Talamante, H. E., et al.: Urban epizootic of rabies in Mexico: Epidemiology and impact of animal bite injuries. Bull. World Health Organ. *71*:615–624, 1993.
67. Fang-Tao, L., and Na, L.: Developments in the production and application of rabies vaccine for human use in China. Trop. Doct. *30*:14–16, 2000.
68. Fekadu, M.: Pathogenesis of rabies virus infection in dogs. Rev. Infect. Dis. *10*:S678–S683, 1988.
69. Fekadu, M., Shaddock, J. H., Ekstrom, J., et al.: An immune stimulating complex (ISCOM) subunit rabies vaccine protects dogs and mice against street rabies challenge. Vaccine *10*:192–197, 1992.
70. Fescharek, R., Franke, V., and Samuel, M. R.: Do anaesthetics and surgical stress increase the risk of post-exposure rabies treatment failure? Vaccine *12*:12–13, 1994.
71. Fishbein, D. B., Dreesen, D. W., Holmes, D. F., et al.: Human diploid cell rabies vaccine purified by zonal centrifugation: A controlled study of antibody response and side effects following primary and booster pre-exposure immunizations. Vaccine 7:437–442, 1988.
72. Fishbein, D. B., Pacer, R. E., Holmes, D. F., et al.: Rabies preexposure prophylaxis with human diploid cell rabies vaccine: A dose-response study. J. Infect. Dis. *156*:50–55, 1987.
73. Fishbein, D. B., Sawyer, L. A., Reid-Sanden, F. L., et al.: Administration of human diploid-cell rabies vaccine in the gluteal area. N. Engl. J. Med. *318*:124–125, 1988.
74. Fishbein, D. B., Yenne, K. M., Dreesen, D. W., et al.: Risk factors for systemic hypersensitivity reactions after booster vaccinations with human diploid cell rabies vaccine: A nationwide prospective study. Vaccine *11*:1390–1394, 1993.
75. Fuenzalida, E., Palacios, R., and Borgono, J. M.: Antirabies antibody response in man to vaccine made from infected suckling-mouse brains. Bull. W. H. O. *30*:431–436, 1964.
76. Gacouin, A., Bourhy, H., Renaud, J. C., et al.: Human rabies despite post-exposure vaccination. Eur. J. Clin. Microbiol. Infect. Dis. *18*:233–235, 1999.
77. Garner, W. O., Jones, D. O., and Pratt, E.: Problems associated with rabies pre-exposure prophylaxis. J. A. M. A. *235*:1131–1132, 1976.
78. Gode, G. R., Jayalakshami, T. S., Raju, A. V., et al.: Intensive care in rabies therapy: Clinical observations. Lancet *2*:6–8, 1976.
79. Gould, A. R., Hyatt, A. D., Lunt, R., et al.: Characterisation of a novel lyssavirus isolated from pteropid bats in Australia. Virus Res. *54*:165–187, 1998.
80. Gross, E. M., Belmaker, I., and Torok, V.: Diploid cell rabies vaccine, six doses or five? Lancet *2*:1339, 1987.
81. Halonen, P. E., Murphy, F. A., Fields, B. N., et al.: Hemagglutinin of rabies and some other bullet-shaped viruses. Proc. Soc. Exp. Biol. Med. *127*:1037–1042, 1968.
82. Hanlon, C. A., Niezgoda, M., Morrill, P. A., and Rupprecht, C. E.: The incurable wound revisited: Progress in human rabies prevention? Vaccine *19*:2273–2279, 2001.
83. Hattwick, M. A. W., and Gregg, M. B.: The disease in man. *In* Baer, G. M. (ed.): The Natural History of Rabies. New York, Academic Press, 1975, pp. 281–304.
84. Hattwick, M. A. W., Rubin, R. H., Music, S., et al.: Postexposure rabies prophylaxis with human rabies immune globulin. J. A. M. A. *227*:407–410, 1974.
85. Hattwick, M. A. W., Weis, T. T., Stechaschulte, C. J., et al.: Recovery from rabies in man. Ann. Intern. Med. *76*:931–942, 1972.
86. Haupt, W.: Rabies—risk of exposure and current trends in prevention of human cases. Vaccine *17*:1742–1749, 1999.
87. Hayflick, L., and Moorhead, P. S.: The serial cultivation of human diploid cell strains. Exp. Cell Res. *25*:585–621, 1961.
88. Heick, A.: Prince Dracula, rabies, and the vampire legend. Ann. Intern. Med. *117*:172–173, 1920.
89. Helmick, C., Johnstone, C., Sumner, J., et al.: A clinical study of Merieux human rabies immune globulin. J. Biol. Stand. *10*:357–367, 1982.
90. Hemachuda, T.: Human rabies: Clinical aspects, pathogenesis, and potential therapy. Curr. Top. Microbiol. Immunol. *187*:121–143, 1994.
91. Hemachuda, T., Griffin, D. E., Chen, W. W., et al.: Immunologic studies of rabies vaccination–induced Guillain-Barré syndrome. Neurology *38*:375–378, 1988.
92. Hemachudha, T., Mitrabhakdi, E., Wilde, H., et al: Additional reports of failure to respond to treatment after rabies exposure in Thailand [in process citation]. Clin. Infect. Dis. *28*:143–144, 1999.
93. Hertzog, M., Fritzell, C., Lafage, M., et al.: T and B cell human responses to European bat lyssaviruses after postexposure rabies vaccination. Clin. Exp. Immunol. *85*:224–230, 1991.
94. Hildreth, E. A.: Prevention of rabies, or the decline of Sirius. Ann. Intern. Med. *58*:833–896, 1963.
94a. Holmes, E. C., Woelk, C. H., Kassis, R., and Bourhy, H.: Genetic constraints and the adaptive evolution of rabies virus in nature. Virology *292*:247–257, 2002.
95. Hooper, D. C., Morimoto, K., Bette, M., et al.: Collaboration of antibody and inflammation in clearance of rabies virus from the central nervous system. J. Virol. *72*:3711–3719, 1998.
96. Houff, S. A., Burton, R. C., Wilson, R. W., et al.: Human-to-human transmission of rabies virus by corneal transplant. N. Engl. J. Med. *300*:603–604, 1979.
97. Iwasaki, Y., Liu, D. S., Yamamoto, T., et al.: The replication and spread of rabies virus in the human central nervous system. J. Neuropathol. Exp. Neurol. *44*:185–195, 1985.
98. Jackson, A. C., and Park, H.: Apoptotic cell death in experimental rabies in suckling mice. Acta Neuropathol. *95*:159–164, 1998.
99. Jackson, A. C., Ye, H., Phelan, C. C., et al.: Extraneural organ involvement in human rabies. Lab. Invest. *79*:945–951, 1999.
100. Jacob, Y., Badrane, H., Ceccaldi, P. E., and Tordo, N.: Cytoplasmic dynein LC8 interacts with lyssavirus phosphoprotein. J. Virol. *74*:10217–10222, 2000.
101. Jaijaroensup, W., Lang, J., Thipkong, P., et al.: Safety and efficacy of purified Vero cell rabies vaccine given intramuscularly and intradermally. (Results of a prospective randomized trial). Vaccine *16*:1559–1562, 1998.
102. Jaijaroensup, W., Limusanno, S., Khawplod, P., et al.: Immunogenicity of rabies postexposure booster injections in subjects who had previously received intradermal preexposure vaccination. J. Travel Med. *6*:234–237, 1999.
103. Jallet, C., Jacob, Y., Bahloul, C., et al.: Chimeric lyssavirus glycoproteins with increased immunological potential. J. Virol. *73*:225–233, 1999.
104. Janis, B., and Habel, K.: Rabies in rabbits and mice: Protective effect of polyribosinic-polyribocytidylic acid. J. Infect. Dis. *125*:345–352, 1972.
105. Jaussaud, R., Strady, C., Lienard, M., and Strady, A.: Rabies in France: An update [in French]. Rev. Med. Interne *21*:679–683, 2000.
106. Johnson, H. N.: Rabies virus. *In* Horsfall, F., and Tamm, I. (eds.): Viral and Rickettsial Diseases of Man. Philadelphia, J. B. Lippincott, 1965.
107. Kamolvarin, N., Tirawatnpong, T., Rattanasiwamoke, R., et al.: Diagnosis of rabies by polymerase chain reaction with nested primers. J. Infect. Dis. *167*:207–210, 1993.
108. Kaplan, M. M., Cohen, D., Koprowski, H., et al.: Studies on the local treatment of wounds for the prevention of rabies. Bull. World Health Organ. *26*:765–775, 1962.
109. Kasempimolporn, S., Saengseesom, W., Lumlertdacha, B., et al.: Detection of rabies virus antigen in dog saliva using a latex agglutination test. J. Clin. Microbiol. *38*:3098–3099, 2000.
110. Kelly, R. M., and Strick, P. L.: Rabies as a transneuronal tracer of circuits in the central nervous system. J. Neurosci. Methods *103*:63–71, 2000.
111. Khawplod, P., Glueck, R., Wilde, H., et al.: Immunogenicity of purified duck embryo rabies vaccine (Lyssavac-N) with use of the WHO-approved intradermal postexposure regimen. Clin. Infect. Dis. *20*:646–651, 1995.
112. Khawplod, P., Wilde, H., Chomchey, P., et al.: What is an acceptable delay in rabies immune globulin administration when vaccine alone had been given previously? Vaccine *14*:389–391, 1996.
113. King, A. A., and Turner, G. S.: Rabies: A review. J. Comp. Pathol. *108*:1–39, 1993.
114. Kissi, B., Badrane, H., Audry, L., et al.: Dynamics of rabies virus quasispecies during serial passages in heterologous hosts. J. Gen. Virol. *80*(pt 8):2041–2050, 1999.
115. Knittel, T., Ramadori, G., Mayet, W. J., et al.: Guillain-Barré syndrome and human diploid cell rabies vaccine. Lancet *1*:1334–1335, 1989.
116. Koch, F. J., Sagartz, J. W., Davidson, D. E., et al.: Diagnosis of human rabies by the cornea test. Am. J. Clin. Pathol. *63*:509–515, 1975.
117. Koprowski, H., and Black, J.: Studies on chick-embryo–adapted rabies virus. V. Protection of animals with antiserum and living attenuated virus after exposure to street strain of rabies virus. J. Immunol. *72*:84–93, 1954.
118. Kramer, T. T.: Personal communication, 1978.
119. Krebs, J. W., Smith, J. S., Rupprecht, C. E., and Childs, J. E.: Mammalian reservoirs and epidemiology of rabies diagnosed in human beings in the United States, 1981–1998. Ann. N. Y. Acad. Sci. *916*:345–353, 2000.
120. Kuwert, E. K., Marcus, I., and Hoher, P. G.: Neutralizing and complement-fixing antibody responses on pre- and postexposure vaccines to a rabies vaccine produced in human diploid cells. J. Biol. Stand. *4*:249–262, 1976.
121. Kuwert, E. K., Werner, J., Marcus, I., et al.: Immunization against rabies with rabies immune globulin, human (RIGH) and a human diploid cell strain (HDCS) rabies vaccine. J. Biol. Stand. *6*:211–219, 1978.
122. Landry, P., Lazzaro, M., and Darioli, R.: Comparative immunogenicity of 2 antirabies vaccines in a 2-1 exposure vaccination schedule [in French]. Schweiz. Rundsch. Med. Prax. *87*:1177–1179, 1998.
123. Lang, J., Duong, G. H., Nguyen, V. G., et al.: Randomised feasibility trial of pre-exposure rabies vaccination with DTP-IPV in infants. Lancet *349*:1663–1665, 1997.
124. Lang, J., Cetre, J. C., Picot, N., et al.: Immunogenicity and safety in adults of a new chromatographically purified Vero-cell rabies vaccine

(PCRV): A randomised, double-blind trial with purified Vero-cell rabies vaccine (PVRV). Biologicals *26*:299–308, 1998.
125. Lang, J., Simanjuntak, G. H., Soerjosembodo, S., and Koesharyono, C.: Suppressant effect of human or equine rabies immunoglobulins on the immunogenicity of post-exposure rabies vaccination under the 2-1-1 regimen: A field trial in Indonesia. MAS054 Clinical Investigator Group. Bull. World Health Organ. *76*:491–495, 1998.
126. Lang, J., Hoa, D. Q., Gioi, N. V., et al.: Immunogenicity and safety of low-dose intradermal rabies vaccination given during an Expanded Programme on immunization session in Viet Nam: Results of a comparative randomized trial. Trans. R. Soc. Trop. Med. Hyg. *93*:208–213, 1999.
127. Laouini, D., Kennou, M. F., Khoufi, S., and Dellagi, K.: Antibodies to human myelin proteins and gangliosides in patients with acute neuroparalytic accidents induced by brain-derived rabies vaccine. J. Neuroimmunol. *91*:63–72, 1998.
128. Lin, F. T., and Lina, N.: Developments in the production and application of rabies vaccine for human use in China. Trop. Doct. *30*:14–16, 2000.
129. Lodmell, D. L., Ray, N. B., Parnell, M. J., et al.: DNA immunization protects nonhuman primates against rabies virus. Nat. Med. *4*:949–952, 1998.
130. Lodmell, D. L., and Ewalt, L. C.: Rabies vaccination: Comparison of neutralizing antibody responses after priming and boosting with different combinations of DNA, inactivated virus, or recombinant vaccinia virus vaccines. Vaccine *18*:2394–2398, 2000.
131. Lodmell, D. L., Ray, N. B., Ulrich, J. T., and Ewalt, L. C.: DNA vaccination of mice against rabies virus: Effects of the route of vaccination and the adjuvant monophosphoryl lipid A (MPL). Vaccine *18*:1059–1066, 2000.
132. Lodmell, D. L., and Ewalt, L. C.: Post-exposure DNA vaccination protects mice against rabies virus. Vaccine *19*:2468–2473, 2001.
133. Loofbourow, J., Cabasso, V., Roby, R., et al.: Human rabies immune globulin: Clinical trials and dose determination. J. A. M. A. *217*:1825–1831, 1971.
134. Matsumoto, S.: Electron microscopy of central nervous system infection. *In* Baer, G. M. (ed.): The Natural History of Rabies. New York, Academic Press, 1975, pp. 33–61.
135. Matthews, D. A., Cummings, D., Evelegh, C., et al.: Development and use of a 293 cell line expressing lac repressor for the rescue of recombinant adenoviruses expressing high levels of rabies virus glycoprotein. J. Gen. Virol. *80*(pt 2):345–353, 1999.
136. Mebatsion, T., Cox, J. H., and Frost, J. W.: Isolation and characterization of 115 street rabies virus isolates from Ethiopia by using monoclonal antibodies: Identification of two isolates as Mokola and Lagos bat virus. J. Infect. Dis. *166*:972–977, 1992.
137. Mertz, G. J., Nelson, K. E., Vithayasai, V., et al.: Antibody responses to human diploid cell vaccine for rabies with and without human rabies immune globulin. J. Infect. Dis. *145*:720–727, 1982.
138. Meslin, F. X., Fishbein, D. B., and Matter, H. C.: Rationale and prospects for rabies elimination in developing countries. Curr. Top. Cell Regul. *187*:1–26, 1994.
139. Metze, K., and Feiden, W.: Demonstration of rabies virus antigen at autopsy. Hum. Pathol. *24*:930, 1993.
140. Meyer, J. P., Tissot, J., Estavoyer, J. M., et al.: Efficacy and immunogenicity of reduced anti-rabies vaccination schedule in subjects in contact with rabies-infected animals. Presse Med. *21*:319, 1992.
141. Mitmoonpitak, C., Tepsumethanon, V., and Wilde, H.: Rabies in Thailand. Epidemiol. Infect. *120*:165–169, 1998.
142. Mlot, C.: Public health. Bat researchers dispute rabies policy. Science *287*:2391–2392, 2000.
143. Modelska, A., Dietzschold, B., Sleysh, N., et al.: Immunization against rabies with plant-derived antigen. Proc. Natl. Acad. Sci. U. S. A. *95*:2481–2485, 1998.
144. Moran, G. J., Talan, D. A., Mower, W., et al.: Appropriateness of rabies postexposure prophylaxis treatment for animal exposures. Emergency ID Net Study Group. J. A. M. A. *284*:1001–1007, 2000.
145. Morgeaux, S., Tordo, N., Gonteur, C., et al.: Propiolactone treatment impairs the biological activity of residual DNA from BHK-21 cells infected with rabies virus. Vaccine *11*:82–90, 1993.
146. Morimoto, K., Hooper, D. C., Carbaugh, H., et al.: Rabies virus quasispecies: Implications for pathogenesis. Proc. Natl. Acad. Sci. U. S. A. *95*:3152–3156, 1998.
146a. Morimoto, K., Patel, M., Corisdeo, S., et al.: Characterization of a unique variant of bat rabies virus responsible for newly emerging human cases in North America. Proc. Natl. Acad. Sci. U. S. A. *93*:5653–5658, 1996.
147. Morimoto, K., Hooper, D. C., and Spitsin, S.: Pathogenicity of different rabies virus variants inversely correlates with apoptosis and rabies virus glycoprotein expression in infected primary neuron cultures. J. Virol. *73*:510–518, 1999.
148. Muller, W. W.: Review of rabies in Europe. Med. Pregl. *51*(Suppl. 1):9–15, 1998.
149. Murphy, F. A.: Morphology and morphogenesis. *In* Baer, G. M. (ed.): The Natural History of Rabies. New York, Academic Press, 1975, pp. 33–61.
150. Murphy, F. A.: Rabies pathogenesis: A brief review. Arch. Virol. *54*:279–297, 1977.
151. Murphy, F. A., and Bauer, S. P.: Early street rabies virus infection in striated muscle and later progression to the central nervous system. Intervirology *3*:256–268, 1974.
152. Nathanson, N., and Gonzalez, S. F.: Immune response to rabies virus. *In* Baer, G. M. (ed.): The Natural History of Rabies. 2nd ed. Boca Raton, FL, CRC Press, 1991, pp. 145–161.
153. Naraporn, N., Khawplod, P., Limsuwan, K., et al.: Immune response to rabies booster vaccination in subjects who had postexposure treatment more than 5 years previously. J. Travel Med. *6*:134–136, 1999.
154. Nicholson, K. G.: Modern vaccines. Lancet *335*:1201–1205, 1990.
155. Noah, D. L., Drenzek, C. L., Smith, J. S., et al.: Epidemiology of human rabies in the United States, 1980 to 1996. Ann. Intern. Med. *128*:922–930, 1998.
156. Numberg, J., II, Doyle, M. U., York, S. M., et al.: Interleukin-2 acts as an adjuvant to increase the potency of inactivated rabies virus vaccines. Proc. Natl. Acad. Sci. U. S. A. *86*:4240–4243, 1989.
157. Osorio, J. E., Tomlinson, C. C., Frank, R. S., et al.: Immunization of dogs and cats with a DNA vaccine against rabies virus. Vaccine *17*:1109–1116, 1999.
158. Paolazzi, C. C., Perez, O., and DeFilippo, J.: Rabies vaccine. Mol. Biotechnol. *11*:137–147, 1999.
159. Pape, W. J., Fitzsimmons, T. D., and Hoffman, R. E.: Risk for rabies transmission from encounters with bats, Colorado, 1977–1996. Emerg. Infect. Dis. *5*:433–437, 1999.
160. Pappaioanou, M., Fishbein, D. B., Dreesen, D. W., et al.: Antibody response to preexposure human diploid-cell rabies vaccine given concurrently with chloroquine. N. Engl. J. Med. *314*:280–284, 1986.
161. Pastoret, P. P., and Brochier, B.: Epidemiology and elimination of rabies in western Europe. Vet. J. *156*:83–90, 1998.
162. Perrin, P., Jacob, Y., Aguilar-Setien, A., et al.: Immunization of dogs with a DNA vaccine induces protection against rabies virus. Vaccine *18*:479–486, 1999.
163. Piyasirisilp, S., Schmeckpeper, B. J., Chandanayingyong, D., et al.: Association of HLA and T-cell receptor gene polymorphisms with Semple rabies vaccine–induced autoimmune encephalomyelitis. Ann. Neurol. *45*:595–600, 1999.
164. Plotkin, S. A., and Clark, H. F.: Committee on immunization: Prevention of rabies in man. J. Infect. Dis. *123*:227–240, 1971.
165. Plotkin, S. A., and Koprowski, H.: Phobia of hydrophobia justified. N. Engl. J. Med. *300*:620–622, 1979.
166. Plotkin, S. A.: Rabies. Clin. Infect. Dis. *30*:4–12, 2000.
167. Plotkin, S. A., and Wiktor, T. J.: Rabies vaccination. Annu. Rev. Med. *29*:583–591, 1978.
168. Plotkin, S. A., and Wiktor, T. J.: Vaccination of children with human cell culture rabies vaccine. Pediatrics *63*:219–221, 1979.
169. Plotkin, S. A., Wiktor, T. J., Koprowski, H., et al.: Immunization schedules for the new human diploid cell vaccine against rabies. Am. J. Epidemiol. *103*:75–80, 1976.
170. Porras, C., Barboza, J. J., Fuenzalida, E., et al.: Recovery from rabies: A case report. Ann. Intern. Med. *85*:44–48, 1976.
171. Public Health Service Advisory Committee on Immunization Practices, Atlanta, Georgia: Rabies: Prevention—United States. M. M. W. R. *33*:393–402, 1984.
172. Raux, H., Flamand, A., and Blondel, D.: Interaction of the rabies virus P protein with the LC8 dynein light chain. J. Virol. *74*:10212–10216, 2000.
173. Ronsholt, L., Sorensen, K. J., Bruschke, C. J., et al.: Clinically silent rabies infection in (zoo) bats [see comments]. Vet. Rec. *142*:519–520, 1998.
174. Rosanoff, E., and Tint, H.: Responses to human diploid cell rabies vaccine: Neutralizing antibody responses of vaccinees receiving booster doses of human diploid cell rabies vaccine. Am. J. Epidemiol. *110*:322–327, 1978.
175. Roscoe, D. E., Holste, W. C., Sorhage, F. E., et al.: Efficacy of an oral vaccinia-rabies glycoprotein recombinant vaccine in controlling epidemic raccoon rabies in New Jersey. J. Wildl. Dis. *34*:752–763, 1998.
176. Rotz, L. D., Hensley, J. A., Rupprecht, C. E., and Childs, J. E.: Large-scale human exposures to rabid or presumed rabid animals in the United States: 22 cases (1990–1996). J. Am. Vet. Med. Assoc. *212*:1198–1200, 1998.
177. Rubin, R. H., Hattwick, M. A. W., Jones, S., et al.: Adverse reactions to duck embryo rabies vaccine. Ann. Intern. Med. *78*:643–649, 1973.
178. Rubin, R., Kikes, K., and Gregg, M.: Human rabies immune globulin: Clinical trials and effects on serum anti-globulins. J. A. M. A. *224*:871–874, 1973.
179. Rupprecht, C. E., Dietzschold, B., Wunner, W. H., et al.: Antigenic relationship of lyssaviruses. *In* Baer, G. (ed.): Natural History of Rabies. 2nd ed., Vol. 1. Boca Raton, FL, CRC Press, 1991.
180. Rupprecht, C. E., Hamir, A. N., Johnston, D. H., et al.: Efficacy of a vaccinia-rabies glycoprotein recombinant virus vaccine in raccoons *(Procyon lotor)*. Rev. Infect. Dis. *10*:S803–S809, 1988.
181. Rupprecht, C. E., and Wiktor, T. J.: Personal communication.
182. Rupprecht, C. E., Wiktor, T. J., Johnston, D. H., et al.: Oral immunization and protection of raccoons *(Procyon lotor)* with a vaccinia-rabies glycoprotein recombinant virus vaccine. Proc. Natl. Acad. Sci. U. S. A. *83*:7947–7950, 1986.

183. Sabchareon, A., Lang, J., Attanath, P., et al.: A new Vero cell rabies vaccine: Results of a comparative trial with HDCV in children. Clin. Infect. Dis. *29*:141–149, 1999.
184. Sakamoto, S., Ide, T., Tokiyoshi, S., et al.: Studies on the structures and antigenic properties of rabies virus glycoprotein analogues produced in yeast cells. Vaccine *17*:205–218, 1999.
185. Samaratunga, H., Searle, J. W., and Hudson, N.: Non-rabies lyssavirus human encephalitis from fruit bats: Australian bat lyssavirus (pteropid lyssavirus) infection. Neuropathol. Appl. Neurobiol. *24*:331–335, 1998.
186. Schlenska, G. K.: Neurological complications following rabies duck embryo vaccination. J. Neurol. *214*:71–74, 1976.
187. Schneider, L. G.: Spread of virus from the central nervous system. *In* Baer, G. M. (ed.): The Natural History of Rabies. New York, Academic Press, 1975, pp. 273–301.
188. Schneider, L. G.: Spread of virus within the central nervous system. *In* Baer, G. M. (ed.): The Natural History of Rabies. New York, Academic Press, 1975, pp. 199–216.
189. Schumacher, C. L., Dietzschold, B., Ertl, H. C. J., et al.: Use of mouse anti-rabies monoclonal antibodies in postexposure treatment of rabies. J. Clin. Invest. *84*:971–975, 1989.
190. Shaughnessy, J. K., and Zichis, J.: Treatment of wounds inflicted by rabid animals. Bull. World Health Organ. *10*:805–813, 1954.
191. Siwasontiwat, D., Lumlertdacha, B., Polsuwan, C., et al.: Rabies: Is provocation of the biting dog relevant for risk assessment? Trans. R. Soc. Trop. Med. Hyg. *86*:443, 1992.
192. Smith, J. S., Fishbein, D. B., Rupprecht, C. E., et al.: Unexplained rabies in three immigrants in the United States. N. Engl. J. Med. *324*:205–211, 1991.
193. Smith, J. S., Orciari, L. A., Yager, P. A., et al.: Epidemiologic and historical relationships among 87 rabies virus isolates as determined by limited sequence analysis. J. Infect. Dis. *166*:296–307, 1992.
194. Smith, J. S., and Seidel, H. D.: Rabies: A new look at an old disease. Prog. Med. Virol. *40*:82–106, 1993.
195. Smith, W. B., Blenden, D. C., Fuh, T., et al.: Diagnosis of rabies by immunofluorescent staining of frozen sections of skin. J. Am. Vet. Med. Assoc. *161*:1495–1501, 1972.
196. Sokol, F.: Recent advances in microbiology. *In* Perez-Miravete, A., and Pelez, D. (eds.): Xth International Congress of Microbiology. Association Mexicana de Microbiologia, Mexico City, 1971, pp. 551–562.
197. Steele, J. H.: History of rabies. *In* Baer, G. M. (ed.): The Natural History of Rabies. New York, Academic Press, 1975, pp. 1–29.
198. Sudarshan, M. K., Madhusudana, S. N., and Mahendra, B. J.: Post-exposure prophylaxis with purified Vero cell rabies vaccine during pregnancy—safety and immunogenicity. J. Commun. Dis. *31*:229–236, 1999.
199. Sugamata, M., Miyazawa, M., Mori, S., et al.: Paralysis of street rabies virus–infected mice is dependent on T lymphocytes. J. Virol. *66*:1252–1260, 1992.
200. Suntharasamai, P., Warrell, M. J., Warrell, D. A., et al.: Early antibody responses to rabies post-exposure vaccine regimens. Am. J. Trop. Med. *36*:160–165, 1987.
201. Suntharasamai, P., Warrell, M. J., Warrell, D. A., et al.: New purified Vero-cell vaccine prevents rabies in patients bitten by rabid animals. Lancet *2*:129–131, 1986.
202. Sureau, P., Rollin, P., and Wiktor, T. J.: Epidemiologic analysis of antigenic variations of street rabies virus: Detection by monoclonal antibodies. Am. J. Epidemiol. *117*:605–609, 1983.
203. Swanson, M. C., Rosanoff, E., Gurwith, M., et al.: IgE and IgG antibodies to β-propiolactone and human serum albumin associated with urticarial reactions to rabies vaccine. J. Infect. Dis. *155*:909–913, 1987.
204. Tantawichien, T., Benjavongkulchai, M., Limsuwan, K., et al.: Antibody response after a four-site intradermal booster vaccination with cell-culture rabies vaccine. Clin. Infect. Dis. *28*:1100–1103, 1999.
205. Thisyakorn, U., Pancharoen, C., Ruxrungtham, K., et al.: Safety and immunogenicity of preexposure rabies vaccination in children infected with human immunodeficiency virus type 1. Clin. Infect. Dis. *30*:218, 2000.
206. Thisyakorn, U., Pancharoen, C., and Wilde, H.: Immunologic and virologic evaluation of HIV-1–infected children after rabies vaccination. Vaccine *19*:1534–1537, 2001.
207. Thongcharoen, P., Wasi, C., Chaitprasithikul, P., et al.: Immunogenicity of a purified Vero cell rabies vaccine. Virus Info Exchange Newsletter for SE Asia *3*:80, 1986.
208. Thraenhart, O., Kreuzfelder, E., Hillebrandt, M., et al.: Long-term humoral and cellular immunity after vaccination with cell culture rabies vaccines in man. Clin. Immunol. Immunopathol. *71*:287–292, 1994.
209. Tims, T., Briggs, D. J., Davis, R. D., et al.: Adult dogs receiving a rabies booster dose with a recombinant adenovirus expressing rabies virus glycoprotein develop high titers of neutralizing antibodies. Vaccine *18*: 2804–2807, 2000.
210. Tollis, M., Dietzschold, B., Volia, C. B., et al.: Immunization of monkeys with rabies ribonucleoprotein (RNP) confers protective immunity against rabies. Vaccine *9*:134–136, 1991.
211. Tordo, N., Poch, O., Ermine, A., et al.: Completion of the rabies virus genome sequence determination: Highly conserved domains among the L (polymerase) proteins of unsegmented negative-strand RNA viruses. Virology *165*:565–576, 1988.
212. Trimarchi, C. V., and Safford, M., Jr.: Poor response to rabies vaccination by the intradermal route. J. A. M. A. *268*:874, 1992.
213. Tsiang, H.: Pathophysiology of rabies virus infection of the nervous system. Adv. Virus Res. *42*:375–412, 1993.
214. Turner, G. S., Aoki, F. Y., Nicholson, K. G., et al.: Human diploid cell strain rabies vaccines: Rapid prophylactic immunization of volunteers with small doses. Lancet *1*:1379–1381, 1976.
215. Turner, G. S.: A review of the world epidemiology of rabies. Trans. R. Soc. Trop. Med. Hyg. *70*:175–178, 1976.
216. Turner, G. S., Aoki, F. Y., Nicholson, K. G., et al.: Human diploid cell strain rabies vaccine: Rapid prophylactic immunisation of volunteers with small doses. Lancet *1*:1379–1381, 1976.
217. Ubol, S., Sukwattanapan, C., and Utaisincharoen, P.: Rabies virus replication induces Bax-related, caspase dependent apoptosis in mouse neuroblastoma cells. Virus Res. *56*:207–215, 1998.
218. Veeraraghavan, N., Ganajana, A., Rangasami, R., et al.: Studies on the salivary excretion of rabies virus by the dog from Surandai. *In* Pasteur Institute Annual Report of the Director 1968, and Science Report 1969. Coonoor, Pasteur Institute, 1970, pp. 68–70.
219. Vodopija, I., Baklaic, Z., and Vodopija, R.: A reliable vaccine for rabies protection. Vaccine *17*:1739–1741, 1999.
220. Vodopija, I., Sureau, P., Lafon, M., et al.: An evaluation of second generation tissue culture rabies vaccines for use in man: A four-vaccine comparative immunogenicity study using a pre-exposure vaccination schedule and an abbreviated 2-1-1 postexposure schedule. Vaccine *4*:245–248, 1986.
221. von Teichman, B. F., de Koker, W. C., Bosch, S. J., et al.: Mokola virus infection: Description of recent South African cases and a review of the virus epidemiology. J. S. Afr. Vet. Assoc. *69*:169–171, 1998.
222. Wang, X. J., Lang, J., Tao, X. R., et al.: Immunogenicity and safety of purified Vero-cell rabies vaccine in severely rabies-exposed patients in China. Southeast Asian J. Trop. Med. Public Health *31*:287–294, 2000.
223. Warner, C. K., Whitfield, S. G., Fekadu, M., and Ho, H.: Procedures for reproducible detection of rabies virus antigen mRNA and genome in situ in formalin-fixed tissues. J. Virol. Methods *67*:5–12, 1997.
224. Warrell, D. A.: The clinical picture of rabies in man. Trans. R. Soc. Trop. Med. Hyg. *70*:175–178, 1976.
225. Warrell, D. A., Davidson, N. M., Pope, H. M., et al.: Pathophysiologic studies in human rabies. Am. J. Med. *60*:180–190, 1976.
226. Warrell, D. A., and Warrell, M. J.: Human rabies and its prevention: An overview. Rev. Infect. Dis. *10*:S726–S731, 1988.
227. Warrell, M. J., Looareesuwan, S., Manatsathit, S., et al.: Rapid diagnosis of rabies and post-vaccinal encephalitides. Clin. Exp. Immunol. *71*:229–234, 1988.
228. Warrell, M. J., Nicholson, K. G., Warrell, D. A., et al.: Economical multiple-site intradermal immunisation with human diploid-cell strain vaccine is effective for post-exposure rabies prophylaxis. Lancet *1*:1059–1062, 1985.
229. Warrell, M. J., Warrell, D. A., Svatbarasamai, P., et al.: An economical regimen of human diploid cell strain anti-rabies vaccine for post-exposure prophylaxis. Lancet *2*:301–304, 1983.
230. Warrington, R. J., Martens, C. J., Rubin, M., et al.: Immunologic studies in subjects with a serum sickness–like illness after immunization with human diploid cell rabies vaccine. J. Allergy Clin. Immunol. *79*:605–610, 1987.
231. Weiland, F., Cox, J. H., Meyer, S., et al.: Rabies virus neuritic paralysis: Immunopathogenesis of nonfatal paralytic rabies. J. Virol. *66*:5096–5099, 1992.
232. Wiktor, T. J., and Clark, H. F.: Growth of rabies virus in cell culture. *In* Baer, G. M. (ed.): The Natural History of Rabies. New York, Academic Press, 1975, pp. 155–179.
233. Wiktor, T. J., and Hattwick, M. A. W.: Rhabdoviruses: Rabies and rabies-related viruses. *In* Kurstak, E., and Kurstak, C. (eds.): Comparative Diagnosis of Viral Diseases. New York, Academic Press, 1977.
234. Wiktor, T. J., and Koprowski, H.: Action locale de certains medicaments sur l'infection rabique de la souris. Bull. World Health Organ. *28*:487–494, 1963.
235. Wiktor, T. J., and Koprowski, H.: Antigenic variants of rabies virus. J. Exp. Med. *152*:99–112, 1980.
236. Wiktor, T. J., and Koprowski, H.: Monoclonal antibodies against rabies virus produced by somatic cell hybridization: Detection of antigenic variants. Proc. Natl. Acad. Sci. U. S. A. *75*:3938–3942, 1978.
237. Wiktor, T. J., Fernandes, M. V., and Koprowski, H.: Cultivation of rabies virus in human diploid cell strain WI-38. J. Immunol. *93*:353–366, 1964.
238. Wiktor, T. J., Gyorgy, E., Schlumberger, H. D., et al.: Antigenic properties of rabies virus components. J. Immunol. *110*:269–276, 1973.
239. Wiktor, T. J., Plotkin, S. A., and Grella, D. W.: Human cell culture rabies vaccine. J. A. M. A. *224*:1170–1171, 1973.
240. Wilde, H., Sirikawin, S., Sabcharoen, A., et al.: Failure of postexposure treatment of rabies in children. Clin. Infect. Dis. *22*:228–232, 1996.
241. Wilde, H., Chomchey, P., Prakongsri, S., et al.: Adverse effects of equine rabies immune globulin. Vaccine 7:10–11, 1989.
242. Wilde, H., Chomkasien, P., Prakongsri, S., et al.: Safety of equine rabies immune globulin. Lancet *2*:1275, 1987.

243. Wilde, H., and Chutivongse, P.: Equine rabies immune globulin: A product with an undeserved poor reputation. Am. J. Trop. Med. Hyg. *42*:175–178, 1990.
244. Wilde, H., Chomchey, P., Punyaratabandhu, P., et al.: Purified equine rabies immune globulin: A safe and affordable alternative to human rabies immune globulin (experience with 3156 patients). Bull. World Health Organ. *67*:731–736, 1989.
245. Wilson, J. M., Hettiarachchi, J., and Wijesuriya, L. M.: Presenting features and diagnosis of rabies. Lancet *2*:1139–1140, 1975.
246. World Health Organization: Guidelines for Dog Rabies Control. Geneva, March 1984.
247. Xiang, Z., and Ertl, H. C.: Induction of mucosal immunity with a replication-defective adenoviral recombinant. Vaccine *17*:2003–2008, 1999.
248. Xiang, Z. Q., Spitalnik, S., Tran, M., et al.: Vaccination with a plasmid vector carrying the rabies virus glycoprotein gene induces protective immunity against rabies virus. Virology *199*:132–140, 1994.
249. Xuan, X., Tuchiya, K., Sato, I., et al.: Biological and immunogenic properties of rabies virus glycoprotein expressed by canine herpesvirus vector. Vaccine *16*:969–976, 1998.

SUBSECTION 9

ARENAVIRIDAE

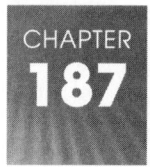

CHAPTER 187 Arenaviral Hemorrhagic Fevers

RÉMI N. CHARREL

History

In the 1950s, a new disease emerged in the Buenos Aires province of Argentina, a rich farming region. The causative agent of Argentine hemorrhagic fever (AHF), named *Junín virus*, was isolated in 1958.[65] Junín virus is hosted by rodents widely distributed in the region, and human infection occurs through contact with infected excreta, usually by the respiratory pathway. AHF is a severe disease that is fatal in approximately 20 percent of cases in the absence of specific treatment. Intensive deforestation and extensive agricultural practices in this region have increased contact between humans and rodents considerably and thereby fueled the emergence of severe annual outbreaks. Cases were expanding progressively into north central Argentina until finally controlled by the availability of a live attenuated vaccine developed in the early 1980s. Junín virus is estimated to have caused approximately 30,000 cases of symptomatic disease since its discovery.

Bolivian hemorrhagic fever (BHF) was described first in 1959 in the El Beni department of eastern Bolivia. The causative agent, named *Machupo virus*, was isolated in 1963 and found to be antigenically and genetically distinct from but related to Junín virus.[41] Machupo virus was responsible for large outbreaks with a high incidence (up to 21% of the population) and a case-fatality rate of approximately 20 percent during the 1960s. Effective rodent control efforts interrupted these epidemics, and since the mid-1970s, no cases of BHF have been reported. After 20 years of silence, a total of 19 additional cases were reported in the same region from 1993 to 1999.[1]

An outbreak of severe hemorrhagic fever began in 1989 in the state of Portuguesa, located in the central plains of Venezuela. Initially thought to be dengue hemorrhagic fever, the causative agent was isolated in 1990, identified as a new arenavirus, and named *Guanarito* after the municipality where the first epidemic occurred.[70] Venezuelan hemorrhagic fever (VHF) has a seasonal occurrence clearly related to intensive agricultural activity and to human contact with the soil and the rodents hosting Guanarito virus.

Little is known about *Sabiá virus,* which was responsible for one fatal case of hemorrhagic fever near São Paulo (Brazil) in 1994.[10] Subsequently, two other cases were reported in laboratory workers. The epidemiology and the natural reservoir of Sabiá virus remain unknown.

In 1999 and 2000, three fatal illnesses were reported in female patients aged 14, 30, and 52 years, two of whom resided in northern California and one in southern California.[19] These cases were associated with *Whitewater Arroyo virus* infection, a recently described arenavirus indigenous to the southwestern United States and hosted by *Neotoma* rodents.[23]

In the Old World, *Lassa fever* initially was described in Nigeria in 1969, and the causative virus was identified during that same year.[5] This disease also occurs in Sierra Leone, Guinea, Liberia, and more sparsely in other countries of West Africa.

Etiologic Agents

Arenaviruses are enveloped single-stranded RNA viruses with a genome consisting of two RNA segments designated large (L) and small (S). The L genomic segment (≈7.2 kb) encodes the viral RNA-dependent RNA polymerase and a zinc-binding protein. The S genomic segment (≈3.5 kb) encodes the nucleocapsid protein (N) and glycoprotein precursor (GPC, secondarily cleaved into the G1 and G2 envelope glycoproteins) in nonoverlapping open-reading frames of opposite polarity.[73] Nucleocapsid antigens are shared by most arenaviruses, and quantitative relationships show the basic split between viruses of Africa and those of the Western Hemisphere. Individual viruses are distinct immunologically by the neutralization test, which depends on the specificity of epitopes contained in the envelope glycoproteins.[66]

At the time that this chapter was written, at least 23 arenaviruses were recognized. They have been classified according to their immunologic characteristics, and two groups are recognized: the Tacaribe serocomplex (including the New World viruses) (Fig. 187–1) and the Lassa–lymphocytic choriomeningitis (LCM) serocomplex (including the ubiquitous LCM virus and all recognized Old World viruses) (Fig. 187–2). Genetic studies are congruent with serologic analyses. They also indicate that the 23 arenaviruses represent four phylogenetic lineages. The Old World (Lassa-LCM serocomplex) lineage comprises five viruses (LCM, Lassa, Mopeia, Mobala, and Ippy) and is deeply rooted to the three New World (Tacaribe serocomplex) lineages designated A, B, and C. Lineage A includes three North American viruses (Whitewater Arroyo, Tamiami, and Bear Canyon) and five South American viruses (Pirital, Pichindé, Flexal, Paraná, and Allpahuayo). Lineage B includes seven South American viruses (Sabiá, Junín, Machupo, Guanarito, Amapari, Tacaribe, and Cupixi), and lineage C consists of three South American viruses (Oliveros, Latino, and Pampa) (Fig. 187–3).

Lassa virus is the only Old World arenavirus that causes human hemorrhagic fever, whereas four New World

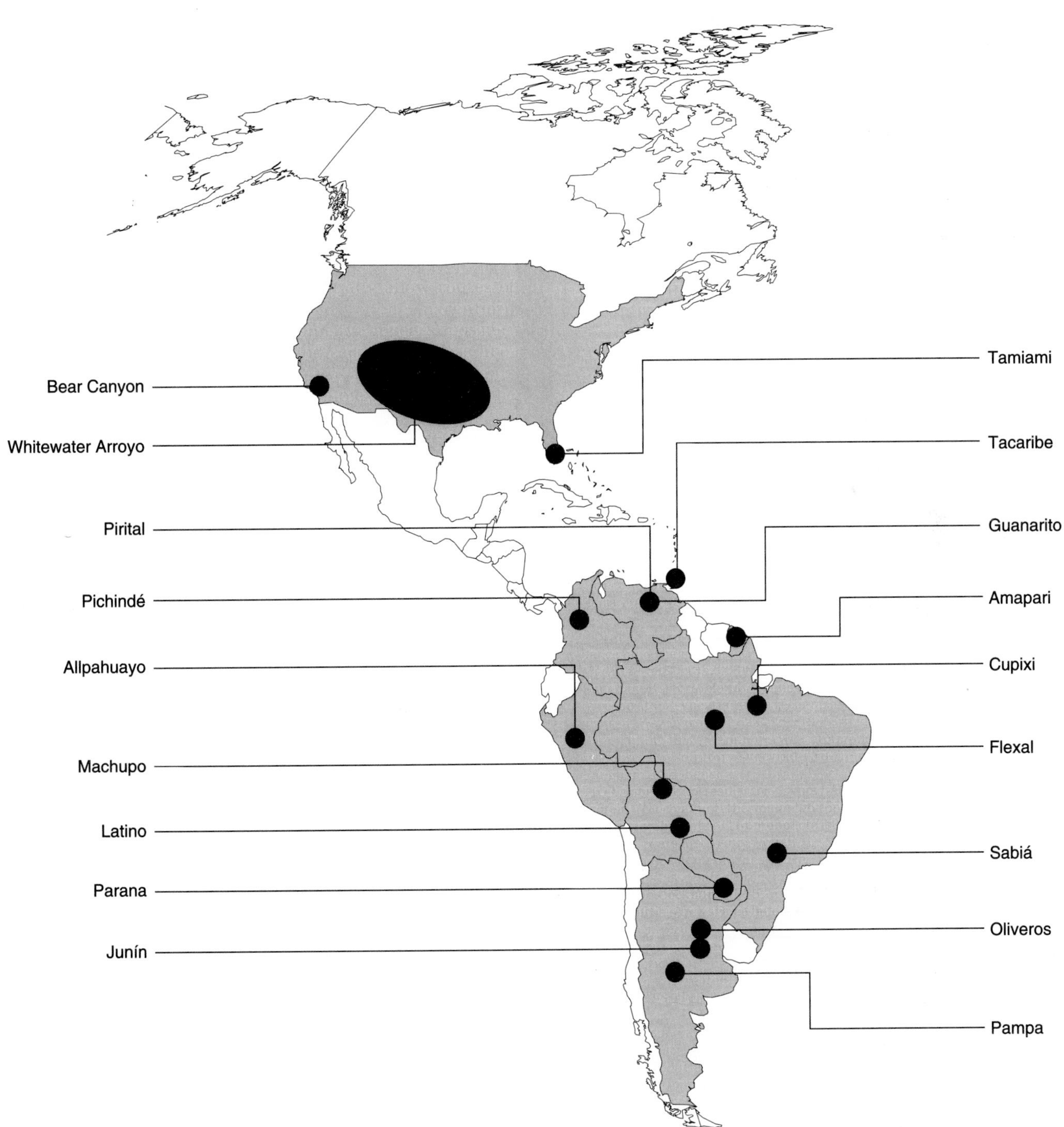

FIGURE 187–1 ■ Geographic distribution of Old World arenaviruses. Lymphocytic choriomeningitis virus is distributed worldwide and is not presented specifically on the map.

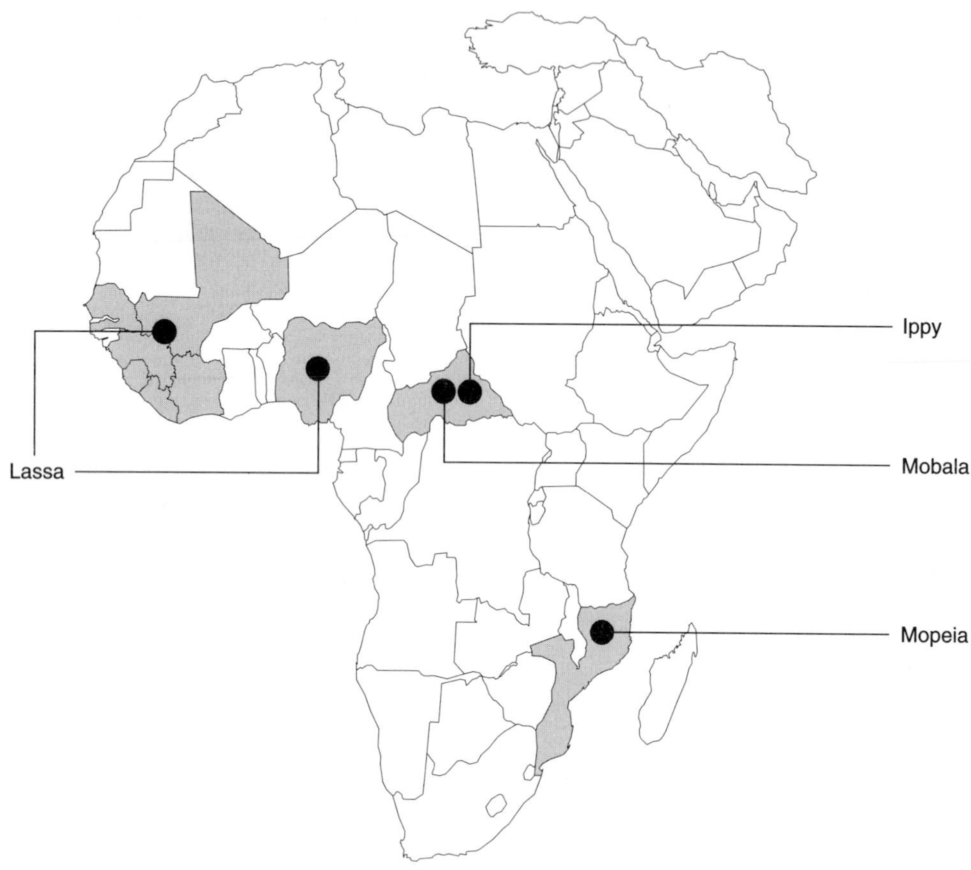

FIGURE 187–2 ■ Geographic distribution of New World arenaviruses. Lymphocytic choriomeningitis virus is distributed worldwide and is not presented specifically on the map.

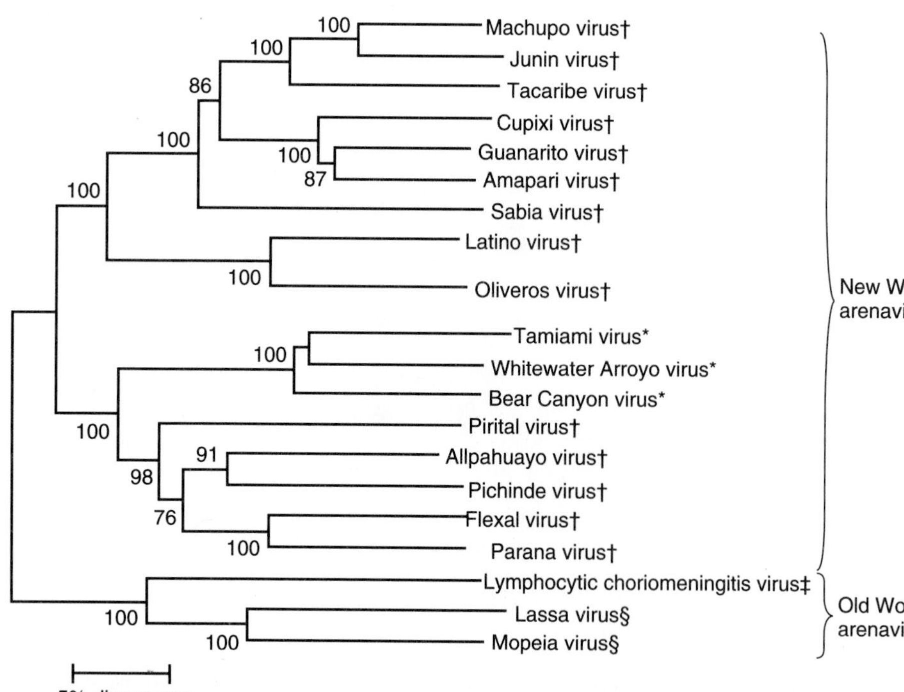

FIGURE 187–3 ■ Phylogenetic relationships of the arenaviruses based on the complete amino acid sequence of the nucleocapsid gene. Genetic distances and groupings were determined by the pairwise-distance algorithm and neighbor-joining method. Bootstrap values corresponding to 500 replications are indicated. The sign after the virus name indicates the geographic distribution: *, North America; †, Central and South America; ‡, worldwide; §, Africa.

members of lineage B (Junín, Machupo, Guanarito, and Sabiá) have been associated with hemorrhagic fever in South America. Whitewater Arroyo virus recently has been associated with fatal human cases in North America.

Epidemiology

Specific rodents (usually one or two closely related species) are the principal hosts of the arenaviruses for which natural host relationships have been characterized (the only exception is Tacaribe virus, associated with bats) (Table 187–1). Now widely recognized is that the diversity of arenaviruses is the result of a long-term, shared evolutionary relationship (termed *co-evolution* or *co-speciation*) between viruses members of the family *Arenaviridae* and rodents of the family Muridae.[2] Chronic infection of the host appears to be crucial to the long-term persistence of arenaviruses in nature. The infection in rodents is accompanied by a chronic viremia or viruria, or both. Because of this specific association, the geographic area where each arenaviral disease is diagnosed is limited by the geographic distribution of the corresponding rodent host.

The rodent host of Junín virus is *Calomys musculinus*, a small field rodent. Since its initial isolation in 1959, the endemic area has expanded from a region of 16,000 km^2 in the north of Buenos Aires province to a region that now is 150,000 km^2 (reaching north of Buenos Aires, south of Santa Fé, southeast of Cordoba, and northeast of La Pampa province). The human population at risk now is estimated at almost 5 million.[18] AHF typically is a seasonal disease, the peak frequency for which occurs during the corn-harvesting season from March to June; during this period, 75 percent of infected people are male agricultural workers who are contaminated by the inhalation of infected aerosol produced from rodent excreta or from rodents caught in mechanical harvesters.[50] Since 1958, cases have been recorded annually, with a range that varies from several hundred to 3500. The mortality rate for patients with confirmed AHF was 14 to 17 percent before immune plasma was used routinely.[51] Evidence has been presented that the number of human cases reflects the proportion of infected *C. musculinus* in a particular area.[62]

Machupo virus, the causative agent of BHF, is hosted by *Calomys laucha* rodents. As for Junín virus, the dynamics of the rodent population determines the epidemiologic features in humans.[60] By contrast to *Calomys callosus*, *C. laucha* invades houses during inundation at the rainy season, with the result that the attack rate in human cases is identical in men, women, and children. The disease has been recorded only from a sparsely populated region in northeast Bolivia, the El Beni province. From 1962 to 1964, a series of outbreaks involved more than 1000 patients, 180 of whom died. Nosocomial transmission of Machupo virus was demonstrated clearly,[67] although most of the recorded infections were acquired by direct contact with *C. laucha* or by aerosolization of infected excreta.

In 1990, new cases of hemorrhagic fever were investigated in Venezuela; the culprit was found to be a new arenavirus designated Guanarito virus after the region where the outbreak occurred.[70] Natural and experimental data suggest that two different rodent species are involved in the transmission cycle of Guanarito virus in nature: the cane rat *Zygodontomys brevicauda* and the cotton rat *Sigmodon alstoni*.[24, 26, 76] Since its discovery, Guanarito virus has been responsible for at least 200 cases of VHF. For unknown reasons, the number of reported human cases has dropped spontaneously since 1992, although rodent infection still can be demonstrated easily inside and even outside the original endemic zone.[81]

In California, three fatal cases recently were associated with Whitewater Arroyo virus, initially isolated from a wood rat (*Neotoma* spp.).[19, 23] The present-day geographic range of rodents of the genus *Neotoma* extends from western Canada southward to Guatemala, Honduras, and Nicaragua. Of the 20 recognized *Neotoma* spp., 9 occur in the United States, and evidence of arenavirus infection has been reported for 5 of them. Recent field studies have provided strong evidence that Whitewater Arroyo virus circulates in the states of New Mexico, Utah, Texas, Oklahoma, Arizona, and Colorado.[6, 25] The abundance and habits of wood rats suggest that potential contact between *Neotoma* rodents and humans is limited.

Lassa virus is associated with rodents belonging to the *Mastomys* genus, and these rodents are distributed widely in sub-Saharan Africa. Documented cases of Lassa fever have been reported in different countries of West Africa, including Nigeria, Liberia, Sierra Leone, Burkina Faso, Guinea, Ivory Coast, Ghana, Senegal, Gambia, and Mali.[7, 27, 29, 35, 59, 71, 77] Between 1985 and 1987, studies of 5000 randomly selected persons living in six central African countries (Cameroon, Central African Republic, Chad, Congo, Equatorial Guinea, and Gabon) tested for serologic evidence of Lassa virus infection found antibody in 3 (0.06%).[31] In contrast, a second study conducted with individuals living in different parts of Nigeria found that 21.3 percent of the 1677 tested were antibody-positive.[77]

Lassa fever is a disease of major public health importance in West Africa because it is responsible for an estimated 5000 deaths and as many as 300,000 infections annually. The first epidemic was described in 1969 in Nigeria,[5] soon followed by several other epidemics in nearby countries. In hospitalized patients, the mortality rate is estimated at 15 to 20 percent.[82] In hospitals located within the endemic area, 10 to 16 percent of the admissions are attributable to Lassa fever. However, serologic surveys suggest that subclinical cases do occur and result in lower overall mortality rates (less than 1%).[59] The overall incidence of Lassa fever in West Africa may be tens of thousands to hundreds of thousands annually.

The main characteristic of Lassa fever is that it is highly transmissible from human to human through direct contact with blood, secretions from infected patients, and aerosol exposure.[43] Many nosocomial outbreaks have been described. Another characteristic of Lassa fever is that numerous cases consist of local residents who seek out rodents for consumption.[75] Because of the prevalence of virus transmission, Lassa fever poses a prominent threat of imported hemorrhagic fever; such cases have been reported in England,[11] Germany,[32] Japan,[36] the Netherlands,[80] Israel,[72] and the United States.[37]

PERSON-TO-PERSON TRANSMISSION

Although human-to-human transmission of BHF has been seen only rarely and then only after intimate contact, Machupo virus clearly was responsible for severe nosocomial outbreaks in which all cases were associated with a single index case who had returned from the endemic region. The only recognized hospital-based outbreak resulted in four secondary cases followed by a tertiary case acquired from a necropsy incident; all but one resulted in death. An epidemic in which seven members of the same family were infected, with a fatal outcome for six, was reported in 1994.[1]

Nosocomial transmission is a common feature of Lassa fever, and many nosocomial outbreaks have been described.[22, 43] However, this aspect of Lassa fever apparently

TABLE 187–1 ■ SOME EPIDEMIOLOGIC FEATURES OF ARENAVIRAL HEMORRHAGIC FEVERS

Fever	Virus	Case, Season, Place, Pattern	Annual Incidence	Geographic Distribution	Ecology	Rodent Reservoir	Comment
Argentine hemorrhagic fever	Junin	Males; corn harvest; March–June	20–200	North central Argentina	Temperate pampa	*Calomys musculinus*	3- to 4-year rodent-disease cycle
Bolivian hemorrhagic fever	Machupo	All ages, both sexes; villages; February–July	<10	Northeast Bolivia	Tropical savanna	*Calomys callosus*	Rodent control successful
Venezuelan hemorrhagic fever	Guanarito	All ages, both sexes equally; house, gardens; no seasonality	0–100	Central Venezuela	Tropical mixed savanna	*Zygodontomys brevicauda, Sigmodon alstoni*	Recently described
Lassa fever	Lassa	All ages, both sexes; villages; no seasonality	10,000	West Africa	Tropical forest savanna	*Mastomys natalensis*	No long-term cycle; nosocomial infections

has been overestimated in reports based on infections in hospitals. The additional risk to hospital workers within the endemic zone is not as great as judged by serosurveys, provided that basic hygiene measures are respected in hospitals when dealing with suspected cases.[34] Good barrier nursing and protection of personnel by the use of gloves, gowns, and eye shields have reduced the incidence of such infection in recent years. Broader surveys of community infections have revealed Lassa fever to be an important community-acquired disease with a wide spectrum of clinical manifestations. Because Lassa virus has been isolated from milk, it clearly poses a risk to nursing children.

In conclusion, data demonstrating nosocomial and human-to-human transmission of several arenaviral diseases reinforce the necessity of implementing biocontainment precautions when dealing with arenavirus-infected patients and materials.

Clinical Manifestations

The clinical picture of South American arenaviral hemorrhagic fever is almost identical regardless of the virus responsible for the disease. The incubation period usually is 7 to 14 days, with extremes extending to 21 days. Infection with a very high inoculum may result in reduction of the incubation period to 2 days. The onset is gradual and consists of fever and malaise, secondarily accompanied by myalgia, back pain, headache, and dizziness. Hyperesthesia of the skin is a common occurrence. Petechiae of the skin and hemorrhage from the gums, vagina, and gastrointestinal tract beginning about the fourth day of illness herald the advent of hypovolemic clinical shock. Blood loss usually is minor, so the hematocrit generally increases as the capillary leak syndrome, the hallmark of the disease, becomes more severe (Table 187–2). Bleeding and the prothrombin time may be prolonged, and a reduction in factors II and VII of the coagulation cascade has been noted. Renal function generally is preserved until shock occurs, but urinary protein may be high. Neurologic manifestations are prominent; intention tremor of the hands and an inability to swallow or to speak clearly may develop and progress to grand mal convulsions, coma, and death in the absence of significant capillary leak or hemorrhagic signs. Death usually occurs 7 to 12 days after onset. Those who survive generally recover completely without permanent sequelae, although transient loss of scalp hair and Beau lines in digital nails are a common consequence of the high and sustained fever.

Symptoms that appear to be more distinctively associated with specific viruses have been reported.[79] Although the frequency of clinical and laboratory findings is identical with Junín and Machupo virus infections, clear differences exist with Guanarito virus infection: pharyngitis, vomiting, and diarrhea are observed more frequently with Guanarito virus; in contrast, petechiae, erythema, facial edema, hyperesthesia of the skin, and shock are observed more frequently in cases of Junín or Machupo infection. A fatal outcome of Junín virus infection is observed more often in pregnant women in the last trimester, and high fetal mortality is associated with infections with Junín and Machupo viruses.[3, 15, 39]

Patients infected with Whitewater Arroyo virus were healthy before the viral infection. In one case, the virus probably was acquired by the aerosol pathway while cleaning rodent droppings in the home. In all cases, no history of travel outside California during the 4 weeks preceding the illness was elicited. The onset was characterized by nonspecific febrile symptoms, including fever, headache, and myalgia. All patients had acute respiratory distress syndrome, and liver failure and hemorrhagic manifestations developed in two. Death occurred within 8 weeks after onset.[19]

Regarding Lassa fever, the clinical description is based on signs observed in hospitalized patients.[28, 42, 66] After an incubation period ranging from 7 to 14 days, patients have an insidious onset characterized by progressive fever, malaise, and generalized myalgia. Retrosternal pain frequently is present in this phase. These symptoms increase in severity during the following week and are accompanied by nausea, vomiting, diarrhea, chest pain, abdominal pain, headache, sore throat, cough, and dizziness. Patients complain of sore throat, pharyngeal inflammation, and chest pain. As the disease progresses, vomiting, diarrhea, hemorrhagic manifestations, encephalopathy, and evidence of vascular permeability may be noted.

During the second week, recovery may begin or the disease progressively worsens until harbingers of a fatal outcome are evident: severe edema, mucosal hemorrhage, pulmonary involvement, encephalopathy (with seizures and coma), or shock; at this stage, pleural and pericardial effusions and ascites are not rare findings. The liver is involved frequently, but icterus is not a usual finding. Death occurs in 15 to 20 percent of hospitalized patients, usually in the second or third week of the course, and is associated with sudden cardiovascular collapse caused by hepatic, pulmonary, and myocardial damage. Few patients have severe central nervous system (CNS) signs, and disturbances in consciousness and convulsions are markers of a poor prognosis. Deafness is an important sequela of Lassa fever; it may be unilateral or bilateral and is a consequence of eighth cranial nerve dysfunction. It can be observed in as many as 30 percent of patients.

Clinical disease in children generally is similar to that in adults. Systematic data are available only for patients with Lassa fever.[64, 82] Fever, vomiting, diarrhea, and cough are common initial symptoms. Pulmonary signs, including rales and pleural effusion, occur more commonly in children than in adults. In very young children, especially those infected antepartum, an unusual condition called "swollen baby

TABLE 187–2 ■ SOME LABORATORY FINDINGS IN ARENAVIRAL HEMORRHAGIC FEVERS

Disease	Viremia	RBC Increase	WBC	Urine Protein	AST/ALT
Argentine hemorrhagic fever	+	++	↓↓	+	N–200
Bolivian hemorrhagic fever	+/–	++	↓↓	+	N–200
Venezuelan hemorrhagic fever	++	++	↓↓	+	??
Lassa fever	++++	++	N–↑	++	100–1500

ALT, alanine aminotransferase; AST, aspartate aminotransferase; RBC, red blood cell; WBC, white blood cell.

syndrome" has been described. It is marked by abdominal distention, widespread edema, and spontaneous bleeding.

Lassa virus replicates at a very high level in the placenta of pregnant women, which might be a reason for the high mortality observed in these patients. The risk of death in pregnant women is estimated to vary from 7 percent in the first two trimesters to 30 percent in the third trimester, in contrast to a 13 percent mortality in nonpregnant women. High fetal mortality varying from 92 percent in early pregnancy to 75 percent in the last trimester is observed.[61, 63, 69]

Very little is known about the health consequences of infection with the other arenaviruses. Aerosol infections are common occurrences in workers at laboratories where arenaviruses are manipulated. Pichindé virus has resulted in numerous seroconversions without any notable clinical significance.[4] Flexal virus was responsible for two symptomatic laboratory infections and should be regarded as potentially dangerous (Pinheiro, F., personal data). Tacaribe virus has resulted in a single case of febrile disease with mild CNS symptomatology (Casals, J., personal data).

Pathogenesis and Pathology

Human and nonhuman primate infection initially involves virus replication at the site of infection, usually in the lung after the deposition of infected aerosol. Replication occurs in the hilar lymph nodes, and despite interstitial infiltration, pneumonic foci usually are not observed. Regardless of the route of infection, the macrophage is a site of important viral replication. With the exception of the hepatitis peculiar to Lassa fever, the pathology of arenaviral hemorrhagic fever is notable for a general lack of parenchymal histologic damage. Edema of tissues and focal hemorrhage of the mucosal surfaces and fascia of many organs are common findings. Rarely are blood clots found that are large enough to be of clinical significance per se. Thus, the crucial and life-threatening lesion in these diseases appears to be capillary leak, in which plasma protein and fluid escape the circulation at a much higher rate than erythrocytes do. How this lesion is produced is not clear, however.[66]

Hemorrhage occurs commonly with the New World arenaviruses that cause hemorrhagic fever. The prominent thrombopenia has a central origin possibly linked to the high levels of interferon observed in these patients.[45] Minor foci of necrosis with acidophilic inclusions (Councilman bodies) have been reported in patients with BHF,[9] and erythroid hypoplasia of bone marrow, as well as lymphoid depletion of nodes and the spleen, may be present. Histologic evidence of disseminated intravascular coagulation generally is absent, and inflammatory lesions of the CNS are lacking. Mild inflammation of the myocardium has been noted in patients with BHF. The Argentine and Bolivian fevers may be marked by encephalopathy. Virus is not recovered from the cerebrospinal fluid (CSF) of patients with such CNS symptoms caused by the South American agents. Macrophages and lymphocytes or their precursors are targets for infection, and the complex cytokine cascade is activated, which can cause the endothelial cells of small capillaries to lose the tight continuity that keeps protein and red cells inside the circulation. As part of this cascade, levels of interferon are elevated. Analysis of serum levels of hematopoietic growth factors suggested a link between granulocyte colony-stimulating factor (G-CSF) serum levels and the severity of the illness in humans.[54] Similarly, interleukin-8 is thought to play an essential role in the activation of neutrophils.[55] Specific antibodies may not appear until 3 to 4 weeks after onset of the disease.

However, New World arenaviruses causing hemorrhagic fever are neutralized more readily, and therapy based on immune serum has been successful in humans. Preliminary studies of VHF suggest that this disease resembles that caused by its other South American relatives.[13, 70] Genetic analysis of the Junín and Guanarito virus sequences amplified from human cases in Argentina and Venezuela, respectively, failed to identify any genetic marker correlating with human pathogenicity or with the severity of the clinical forms.[30, 81]

Although only three cases have been reported to date, Whitewater Arroyo virus infection seems to be associated with profound lymphopenia and thrombocytopenia.[19] To date, no studies have been performed to investigate the pathogenesis of Whitewater Arroyo virus infection. An interesting note is that Whitewater Arroyo virus belongs to lineage A (based on genetic analysis of the nucleocapsid gene), in which no other members have been recognized thus far as human pathogens. However, the small genomic segment of Whitewater Arroyo virus recently has been shown to have a dual origin: the gene encoding the nucleocapsid is inherited from an ancestor belonging to lineage A, whereas the glycoprotein precursor gene is inherited from an ancestor belonging to lineage B.[8] Further investigation is needed to clarify whether the lineage B–inherited GPC gene is responsible for the human pathogenicity of Whitewater Arroyo virus.

The hepatitis of Lassa fever is represented by different stages successively characterized by hepatocellular injury, necrosis, and regeneration, any or all of which may be present at death. In no instance is the degree of hepatic damage sufficient to be responsible for hepatic failure; consequently, the hepatitis of Lassa fever is not the primary cause of death.[40, 58] For cases characterized by encephalopathy, no correlation could be established with the presence of Lassa virus in CSF or with virus antibodies in CSF, serum, or both; no evidence supports the notion that the encephalopathy observed in Lassa fever is a consequence of either direct cytopathic or immune-mediated mechanisms.[12] Direct damage to circulating leukocytes has not been demonstrated, and profound thrombocytopenia does not occur.

In human cases of Lassa fever, no correlation exists between antibody levels and outcome of the disease.[20] More than one third of patients have antibodies to the nucleocapsid of the virus on admission to the hospital. These antibodies do not neutralize the virus, which is found in blood in concentrations much higher in severe infection than in any of the other arenaviral diseases. During convalescence, viral neutralizing antibodies evolve for months and rarely reach levels even a tenth of those that develop after infection with the other viruses in this group. Thus, a reasonable speculation is that compromised cell-mediated immunity is responsible for uncontrolled virus replication and functional capillary collapse. Primates challenged with Lassa virus or naturally infected patients who have recovered from acute Lassa fever usually do not exhibit a measurable neutralizing antibody response. Individuals who are seropositive mount a very strong memory $CD4^+$ T-cell response against the nucleocapsid protein of Lassa virus.[74] Experiments based on inactivated vaccines have shown that in spite of the resulting high titers of antibodies, vaccination does not prevent virus replication and death in nonhuman primates.[20] An obvious conclusion seems to be that control of human Lassa fever mostly involves T cells through a T_H1-type immune response. In addition, an immune response requires epitopes located on both the G1 and G2 glycoproteins to efficiently protect primates challenged with Lassa virus.[20]

Several animals have provided reasonable models for the clinical disease seen in humans. Junín virus causes fatal hemorrhagic disease in guinea pigs, rhesus monkeys are good models for Lassa[38] and Machupo virus infection, and marmosets *(Callithrix jacchus)* reproduce the pathogenesis of Junín virus. Indeed, rhesus monkeys were used to predict the effectiveness of the antiviral drug ribavirin to treat Lassa fever, and guinea pigs were instrumental in the development of an attenuated vaccine for AHF.

Diagnosis and Differential Diagnosis

DIRECT DIAGNOSIS

Serum or heparinized plasma should be collected during the acute febrile stages of the disease; the samples need to be frozen on dry ice or in liquid nitrogen. Storage at a temperature higher than –40° C will result in progressive loss of infectivity. Classically achieved by isolation of virus, a direct diagnosis now may be made by a reverse transcriptase–polymerase chain reaction (RT-PCR)-based assay. Isolation of virus is achieved readily in cell culture, and Vero cells are a sensitive substrate for such direct diagnosis. Because a cytopathic effect not always is observed, cells infected with arenavirus are detected by an immunofluorescence test.

For South American arenaviruses causing hemorrhagic fever, the delay in diagnosis with isolation on Vero cells is 1 to 5 days, much faster than animal inoculation, which requires 7 to 20 days before illness develops. Serum and throat washings collected 3 to 10 days after onset usually yield virus. Virus is isolated less frequently from urine. Specifically, Machupo virus is recovered from only 20 percent of acute-phase sera and even less frequently from throat washings or urine. When serum or throat samples are collected within 2 weeks of clinical onset, success in isolating Lassa virus is very high.

Viral RNA can be purified from serum, plasma, urine, throat washings, and tissues and used as a target for cDNA synthesis with a reverse transcriptase. This cDNA can be amplified by a PCR assay using consensus primers or specific primers, or with both types of primers. The amplified region is sequenced for diagnostic confirmation. RT PCR–based diagnosis offers the advantage of reducing the delay in response, and it has greater sensitivity than possible with cell culture. This technique has been applied successfully to the diagnosis of Lassa fever. Specific primers designed to amplify certain arenaviruses have been proposed but still are not used for diagnostic purpose in epidemic conditions. Molecular tests based on the RT-PCR methodology increasingly are being developed for the diagnosis of arenaviral infections.[48] For Junín and Machupo virus infections specifically, this technique is the only one that is early and sensitive enough to detect the low viremia encountered during the period in which immune plasma therapy can be used effectively.[47] At the time of admission to the hospital, RT-PCR detected Lassa virus RNA in 79 percent of the patients; for comparison, immunofluorescence assay detected antibodies in only 21 percent of these patients. By the third day of admission, 100 percent of the patients tested positive by the RT-PCR test, whereas only 52 percent tested positive by immunofluorescence.[14] The drawback of molecular methods is mostly the need for sophisticated equipment for these methods to be fully applicable in field conditions when an outbreak occurs.

Additional techniques for direct detection of virus in tissues are being developed actively and include in situ nucleic acid hybridization techniques. Antigen-detection enzyme-linked immunosorbent assay (ELISA) has been a sensitive tool in many patients.

INDIRECT DIAGNOSIS

A serologic diagnosis is made by demonstration of a fourfold rise in the titer of specific antibody. A high IgG antibody titer or the presence of specific IgM is indicative of a probable case. Nucleocapsid antigens are shared by most of these viruses, and quantitative relationships show the basic split between the viruses of Africa and those of the Western Hemisphere. Individual viruses are immunologically distinct by the neutralization test, which depends on the specificity of the epitopes contained in the envelope glycoproteins G1 and G2. Samples collected for serologic diagnosis can be kept at –20° C. Blood obtained in early convalescence may be infectious despite the presence of antibodies and, therefore, should be handled accordingly. Antibodies often are detected by the indirect immunofluorescence test because it is an inexpensive, rapid, and sensitive test. An alternative is the ELISA test, which has greater specificity and a sensitivity equal to that of the neutralization test. The latter is the test of choice for differentiating viral strains of arenaviruses, for confirmation of unexpected results, and for detection of infection from the distant past. All these tests have been tested in the conditions of an outbreak and have been shown to be effective.

Antibodies specific to South American arenaviruses appear 12 to 30 days after the onset of infection, and their appearance often correlates with clinical improvement.[68]

In the case of Lassa fever, antibodies detectable by immunofluorescence appear early and often are present during the acute illness with no apparent relationship to viremia or clinical status; IgM or IgG antibodies (or both) develop in 50 percent of patients with Lassa fever during the first week and in more than 66 percent during the next week. Antigen-detection ELISA in conjunction with IgM-capture ELISA has shown promise in the rapid and sensitive diagnosis of Lassa fever. Neutralizing antibodies usually develop only after 4 to 6 months of convalescence.

PREDICTIVE VALUE

In West Africa, the association of fever, pharyngitis, retrosternal pain, and proteinuria resulted in a predictive value of 81 percent. In the endemic area of Argentina, the constellation of asthenia and dizziness accompanied by petechiae and conjunctival congestion has been shown to be indicative of the diagnosis of AHF; the presence of leukopenia, thrombocytopenia, and proteinuria further reinforces a diagnosis suspected on clinical findings. The association of a platelet count less than 100,000/mm^3 and a white blood cell count less than 2500/mm^3 or less than 4000/mm^3 was reported to have a sensitivity of 87 and 100 percent and a specificity of 88 and 71 percent, respectively.[33]

DIFFERENTIAL DIAGNOSIS

The differential diagnosis of Lassa fever should include malaria, typhoid, shigellosis, and dengue and yellow fever. For South American viruses causing hemorrhagic fever, the differential diagnosis includes yellow fever, dengue hemorrhagic fever, hepatitis, leptospirosis, hemorrhagic fever with renal syndrome caused by hantaviruses, rickettsial diseases, typhoid, sepsis with disseminated intravascular coagulation, and in the case of CNS involvement, viral encephalitis.

Suspected cases encountered in the United States should be reported to the local and state health departments or to the Special Pathogen Branch, MS G-14, Centers for Disease

Control and Prevention, 1600 Clifton Road, Atlanta, GA 30333; telephone, (404) 639-1118; FAX, (404) 639-1115; e-mail, dvd1spath@cdc.gov. In Europe, suspected cases should be reported to the Bernhard-Nocht-Institut of Tropical Medicine, Department of Virology, Bernhard-Nocht-Str. 74, 20359 Hamburg, Germany; telephone, (49) 40 42818-0; FAX, (49) 40 42818-378; e-mail, schmitz@bni.uni-hamburg.de, or to the Centre National de Référence des Fièvres Hemorragiques Virales, Institut Pasteur, 21 Av. Tony Garnier, 69365 Lyon cedex 07; telephone (33) 437282421; e-mail, zelles@cervi-lyon.inserm.fr.

Prognosis and Treatment

PROGNOSIS

The case-fatality rate of AHF, which is higher than 15 percent without specific treatment, spectacularly drops to less than 1 percent when specific treatment is available.[33] G-CSF serum level seems to be a marker of severity of the illness.[54]

For Lassa fever, no correlation exists between antibody levels and outcome. Viremia levels in Lassa fever are, however, important in term of prognosis; basically, the higher the viremia, the higher the mortality. The serum aspartate transaminase level also is an accurate prognostic marker: values above 150 IU/mL are associated with 55 percent mortality, whereas the overall mortality rate is approximately 15 percent.[40]

TREATMENT

Arenaviral hemorrhagic fever should be managed by monitoring and correction of fluid, electrolyte, and osmotic imbalances and metabolic acidosis. Hydration should be provided cautiously because of the generalized capillary leak and the possibility of precipitating pulmonary edema. If possible, bleeding should be treated with clotting factor and platelet replacement as guided by laboratory tests.

For Junín virus infection, immune serum therapy is effective in reducing mortality when given within the first 8 days of illness.[16, 51] Experimental evidence suggests that plasma may work by attacking infected cells, as well as by neutralizing virus. An important note is that cerebellar signs such as headache and tremor secondarily developed in 10 percent of the patients who received this treatment. These clinical signs are transient; they are thought to be related to the immunopathologic mechanisms induced by treatment with convalescent plasma.

Despite the recognized efficacy of convalescent plasma for the treatment of Machupo virus infection, the paucity of survivors and the lack of programs for collection and storage of BHF immune plasma may lead to shortages in the event of a new outbreak. In recent cases, ribavirin was offered to two patients with life-threatening infection. Both recovered without sequelae; this promising result suggests that more extensive clinical studies are needed to assess the usefulness of ribavirin in treating BHF.[44]

Junín and Guanarito viruses showed very high in vitro sensitivity to ribavirin and also had an antiviral effect in patients.[17] One of the Sabiá virus infections acquired in the laboratory was treated successfully with ribavirin; treatment was started early after onset of the infection, and no neutralizing antibodies were produced.

The late evolution and low titers of Lassa virus–neutralizing antibodies render immune serum–based therapy less efficient than in treatment of South American arenaviral fever.[56] In contrast, clinical studies have shown ribavirin to be of benefit in severe cases, and, therefore, it should be used as early as possible in the course of the disease. The recommended intravenous regimen is as is follows:

- A loading dose of 30 mg/kg, then
- 15 mg/kg every 6 hours for 4 days, then
- 7.5 mg/kg every 8 hours for 6 days

A recognized side effect of ribavirin is hemolytic anemia, which is reversible when drug administration is interrupted.

Prevention and Control

Prevention of arenavirus disease is achieved by preventing transmission from rodents to humans, from humans to humans, and from infected specimens to laboratory personnel. Strategies for avoiding contact between rodents and humans have been effective in BHF.[49] Simple trapping of *C. callosus* in towns was successful in reducing human contact and thus the incidence of disease to essentially zero. This strategy is more difficult to achieve with AHF because the conditions under which human exposure occurs are different from those of BHF. The distribution of *C. musculinus* (reservoir of Junín virus) is much wider than that of *C. callosus* (reservoir *of* Machupo virus), and Argentine agricultural practices continue to place workers at risk for exposure to reservoir hosts.

A collaborative effort by the U.S. and Argentine governments led to the production of a live attenuated Junín virus vaccine named Candid #1, which has passed safety and immunogenicity tests in U.S. volunteers. Its efficacy was documented in a double-blind trial consisting of 15,000 agricultural workers at risk for acquiring natural infection in Argentina. Subsequently, more than 100,000 persons were immunized with Junín virus vaccine in Argentina. Recent animal protection studies suggest that the Junín virus vaccine could be protective against Machupo virus infections as well. A prospective study of 6500 male agricultural workers in Argentina performed during the course of two epidemic seasons showed that the efficacy of Candid #1 vaccine was 84 percent or higher and that no serious adverse effects could be expected.[52]

For VHF, no preventive measures have been developed. Attenuated Junín virus strains do not protect experimental animals against challenge with Guanarito virus. In VHF, evidence suggests that transmission occurs around houses and in fields, as with BHF, so measures to avoid contact between rodents and humans should be effective, as shown for BHF.

For Lassa fever, reducing contact with *Mastomys natalensis* is a formidable task in West Africa, and this option does not seem to have a promising future. Because person-to-person transmission has been reported in Lassa fever, precautions should be taken to place patients in single rooms. The health care team should be small and adequately trained; they should wear gloves, gowns, and filter masks.[53, 78] All secretions should be decontaminated.[46] Laboratory procedures should be performed with care and inactivating methods used, either heat, chemicals, or irradiation.

In African green monkeys, or vervets *(Cercopithecus aethiops),* the humoral antibody response measured after challenge with purified inactivated Lassa virus was insufficient to protect the animals from a fatal outcome, although it was as high as in humans who recovered from Lassa fever.[57] A naturally attenuated strain (Mopeia virus from Mozambique) protects rhesus monkeys against Lassa virus challenge, but field studies are required to establish the extent and nature of natural human infection with this virus before it can be considered seriously as a candidate for human vaccine development. Alternative approaches, including the use of vaccinia virus vectors bearing the Lassa virus GPC or N genes, are being investigated actively and have shown promising preliminary results.[20, 21]

REFERENCES

1. Bolivian hemorrhagic fever—El Beni department, Bolivia, 1994. M. M. W. R. Morb. Mortal. Wkly. Rep. *43*:943–946, 1994.
2. Bowen, M. D., Peters, C. J., and Nichol, S. T.: Phylogenetic analysis of the Arenaviridae: Patterns of virus evolution and evidence for cospeciation between arenaviruses and their rodent hosts. Mol. Phylogenet. Evol. *8*:301–316, 1997.
3. Briggiler, A. M., Levis, S., Enria, D., et al.: Argentine hemorrhagic fever in pregnant women. Medicina (B. Aires) *50*:443, 1990.
4. Buchmeier, M., Adam, E., and Rawls, W. E.: Serologic evidence of infection by Pichinde virus among laboratory workers. Infect. Immun. *9*:821–823, 1974.
5. Buckley, S. M., and Casals, J.: Lassa fever, a new virus of man from West Africa. III. Isolation and characterization of the virus. Am. J. Trop. Med. Hyg. *19*:680–691, 1970.
6. Calisher, C. H., Nabity, S., Root, J. J., et al.: Transmission of an arenavirus in white-throated woodrats *(Neotoma albigula)*, southeastern Colorado, 1995–1999. Emerg. Infect. Dis. *7*:397–402, 2001.
7. Carey, D. C., Kemp, G. E., White, H. A., et al.: Lassa fever: Epidemiological aspects of the 1970 epidemic, Jos, Nigeria. Trans. R. Soc. Trop. Med. Hyg. *66*:402–408, 1972.
8. Charrel, R. N., de Lamballerie, X., and Fulhorst, C. F.: The Whitewater Arroyo virus: Natural evidence for genetic recombination among Tacaribe serocomplex viruses (family *Arenaviridae)*. Virology *283*:161–166, 2001.
9. Child, P. L., Mackenzie, R. B., Valverde, L. R., et al.: Bolivian haemorrhagic fever: A pathologic description. Arch. Pathol. *83*:434–445, 1967.
10. Coimbra, T. L. M., Nassar, E. S., Burattini, M. N., et al. New arenavirus isolated in Brazil. Lancet *343*:391–392, 1994.
11. Cummins, D.: Lassa fever. Br. J. Hosp. Med. *43*:186–192, 1990.
12. Cummins, D., Benet, D., Fisher-Hoch, S. P., et al.: Lassa fever encephalopathy: Clinical and laboratory findings. J. Trop. Med. Hyg. *95*:197–201, 1992.
13. de Manzione, N., Salas, R. A., Paredes, H., et al.: Venezuelan hemorrhagic fever: Clinical and epidemiological studies of 165 cases. Clin. Infect. Dis. *26*:308–313, 1998.
14. Demby, A. H., Chamberlain, J., Brown, D. W., et al.: Early diagnosis of Lassa fever by reverse transcription-PCR. J. Clin. Microbiol. *32*: 2898–2903, 1994.
15. Douglas, R. G., Wiebenga, N. H., Couch, R. B., et al.: Bolivian hemorrhagic fever probably transmitted by personal contact. Am. J. Epidemiol. *82*:85–91, 1965.
16. Enria, D. A., Briggiler, A. M., Fernandez, N. J., et al.: Dose of neutralising antibodies for Argentine hemorrhagic fever. Lancet *2*:255–256, 1984.
17. Enria, D. A., Briggiler, A. M., Levis, S., et al.: Tolerance and antiviral effects of ribavirin in patients with Argentine hemorrhagic fever. Antiviral Res. *7*:353–359, 1987.
18. Enria, D., and Feuillade, M. R.: Argentine haemorrhagic fever (Junin virus—Arenaviridae): A review on clinical, epidemiological, ecological, treatment and preventive aspects of the disease. *In* Travassos da Rosa, A. P. A., Vasconcelos, P. F. C., and Travassos da Rosa, J. F. S. (eds.): An Overview of Arbovirology in Brazil and Neighboring Countries. Belem, Brazil, Instituto Evandro Chaggas, 1998, pp. 219–232.
19. Fatal illnesses associated with a New World arenavirus—California, 1999–2000. M. M. W. R. Morb. Mortal. Wkly. Rep. *49*:709–711, 2000.
20. Fisher-Hoch, S. P., Hutwagner, L., Brown, B., et al.: Effective vaccine for Lassa fever. J. Virol. *74*:6777–6783, 2000.
21. Fisher-Hoch, S. P., McCormick, J. B., Auperin, D., et al.: Protection of rhesus monkeys from fatal Lassa fever by vaccination with a recombinant vaccinia virus containing the Lassa virus glycoprotein gene. Proc. Natl. Acad. Sci. U. S. A. *85*:1–6, 1988.
22. Fisher-Hoch, S. P., Tomori, O., Nasidi, A., et al.: Review of cases of nosocomial Lassa fever in Nigeria: The high price of poor medical practice. B. M. J. *311*:857–859, 1995.
23. Fulhorst, C. F., Bowen, M. D., Ksiazek, T. G., et al.: Isolation and characterization of Whitewater Arroyo virus, a novel North American arenavirus. Virology *224*:114–120, 1996.
24. Fulhorst, C. F., Bowen, M. D., Salas, R. A., et al.: Natural rodent host associations of Guanarito and Pirital viruses (family *Arenaviridae)* in central Venezuela. Am. J. Trop. Med. Hyg. *61*:325–330, 1999.
25. Fulhorst, C. F., Charrel, R. N., Weaver, S. C., et al.: Geographic distribution and genetic diversity of Whitewater Arroyo virus in the southwestern United States. Emerg. Infect. Dis. *7*:403–407, 2001.
26. Fulhorst, C. F., Ksiazek, T. G., Peters, C. J., et al.: Experimental infection of the cane mouse *Zygodontomys brevicauda* (family Muridae) with Guanarito virus *(Arenaviridae)*, the etiologic agent of Venezuelan hemorrhagic fever. J. Infect. Dis. *180*:966–969, 1999.
27. Frame, J. D.: Surveillance of Lassa fever in missionaries stationed in West Africa. Bull. World Health Organ. *52*:593–598, 1975.
28. Frame, J. D., Baldwin, J. M., Jr., Gocke, D. J., et al.: Lassa fever, a new virus disease of man from West Africa: Clinical description and pathological findings. Am. J. Trop. Med. Hyg. *19*:670–676, 1970.
29. Frame, J. D., Jahrling, P. B., Yalley-Ogunro, J. E., et al.: Endemic Lassa fever in Liberia. II. Serological and virological findings in hospital patients. Trans. R. Soc. Trop. Med. Hyg. *78*:656–660, 1984.
30. Garcia, J. B., Morzunov, S. P., Levis, S., et al.: Genetic diversity of the Junin virus in Argentina: Geographic and temporal patterns. Virology *272*:127–136, 2000.
31. Gonzalez, J. P., Josse, R., Johnson, E. D., et al.: Antibody prevalence against haemorrhagic fever viruses in randomized representative Central African populations. Res. Virol. *140*:319–331, 1989.
32. Gunther, S., Emmerich, P., Laue, T., et al.: Imported Lassa fever in Germany: Molecular characterization of a new Lassa virus strain. Emerg. Infect. Dis. *6*:466–476, 2000.
33. Harrison, L. H., Halsey, N. A., McKee, K. T., Jr., et al.: Clinical case definitions for Argentine hemorrhagic fever. Clin. Infect. Dis. *28*:1091–1094, 1999.
34. Helmick, C. G., Webb, P. A., Scribner, C. L., et al.: No evidence for increased risk of Lassa fever infection in hospital staff. Lancet *2*:1202–1205, 1986.
35. Henderson, B. E., Gary, G. W., Kissling, R. E., et al.: Lassa fever. Virological and serological studies. Trans. R. Soc. Trop. Med. Hyg. *66*:409–416, 1972.
36. Hirabayashi, Y., Oka, S., Goto, H., et al.: An imported case of Lassa fever with late appearance of polyserositis. J. Infect. Dis. *158*:872–875, 1988.
37. Holmes, G. P., McCormick, J. B., Trock, S. C., et al.: Lassa fever in the United States: Investigation of a case and new guidelines for management. N. Engl. J. Med. *323*:1120–1123, 1990.
38. Jahrling, P. B., and Peters, C. J.: Passive antibody therapy of Lassa fever in cynomolgus monkeys: Importance of neutralizing antibody and Lassa virus strain. Infect. Immun. *44*:528–533, 1984.
39. Johnson, K. M., Halstead, S. B., and Cohen, S. N.: Hemorrhagic fevers of Southeast Asia and South America: A comparative appraisal. Prog. Med. Virol. *9*:105–158, 1967.
40. Johnson, K. M., McCormick, J. B., Webb, P. A., et al.: Clinical virology of Lassa fever in hospitalized patients. J. Infect. Dis. *155*:456–464, 1987.
41. Johnson, K. M., Wiebenga, N. H., Mackenzie, R. B., et al.: Virus isolations from human cases of hemorrhagic fever in Bolivia. Proc. Soc. Exp. Biol. Med. *118*:113–118, 1965.
42. Keane, E., and Gilles, H. M.: Lassa fever in Panguma Hospital, Sierra Leone, 1973–1976. B. M. J. *1*:1399–1402, 1977.
43. Keenlyside, R. A., McCormick, J. B., Webb, P. A., et al.: Case-control study of *Mastomys natalensis* and humans in Lassa virus–infected households in Sierra Leone. Am. J. Trop. Med. Hyg. *32*:829–837, 1983.
44. Kilgore, P. E., Ksiazek, T. G., Rollin, P. E., et al.: Treatment of Bolivian hemorrhagic fever with intravenous ribavirin. Clin. Infect. Dis. *24*:718–722, 1997.
45. Levis, S. C., Saavedra, M. C., Ceccoli, C., et al.: Correlation between endogenous interferon and the clinical evolution of patients with Argentine hemorrhagic fever. J. Interferon Res. *5*:383–389, 1985.
46. Lloyd, G., Bowen, E. T. W., and Slade, J. H. R.: Physical and chemical methods of inactivating Lassa virus. Lancet *1*:1046–1048, 1982.
47. Lozano, M. E., Enria, D., Maiztegui, J. I., et al.: Rapid diagnosis of Argentine hemorrhagic fever by reverse transcriptase PCR–based assay. J. Clin. Microbiol. *33*:1327–1332, 1995.
48. Lunkenheimer, K., Hufert, F. T., and Schmitz, H.: Detection of Lassa virus RNA in specimens from patients with Lassa fever by using the polymerase chain reaction. J. Clin. Microbiol. *28*:2689–2692, 1990.
49. Mackenzie, R. B.: Epidemiology of Machupo virus infection. I. Pattern of human infection, San Joaquin, Bolivia, 1962–1964. Am. J. Trop. Med. Hyg. *14*:808–813, 1965.
50. Maiztegui, J. I.: Clinical and epidemiological patterns of Argentine haemorrhagic fever. Bull. World Health Organ. *52*:567–576, 1975.
51. Maiztegui, J. I., Fernandez, N. J., and de Damilano, A. J.: Efficacy of immune plasma in treatment of Argentine hemorrhagic fever and association between treatment and a late neurological syndrome. Lancet *2*:1216–1217, 1979.
52. Maiztegui, J. I., McKee, K. T., Jr., Barrera Oro, J. G., et al.: Protective efficacy of a live attenuated vaccine against Argentine hemorrhagic fever. AHF Study Group. J. Infect. Dis. *177*:277–283, 1998.
53. Management of patients with suspected viral hemorrhagic fever. M. M. W. R. Morb. Mortal. Wkly. Rep. *37*:1–16, 1988.
54. Marta, R. F., Enria, D., and Molinas, F. C.: Relationship between hematopoietic growth factors levels and hematological parameters in Argentine hemorrhagic fever. Am. J. Hematol. *64*:1–6, 2000.
55. Marta, R. F., Montero, V. S., Hack, C. E., et al.: Proinflammatory cytokines and elastase-alpha-1-antitrypsin in Argentine hemorrhagic fever. Am. J. Trop. Med. Hyg. *60*:85–89, 1999.
56. McCormick, J. B., King, I. J., Webb, P. A., et al.: Lassa fever: Effective therapy with ribavirin. N. Engl. J. Med. *314*:20–26, 1986.

57. McCormick, J. B., Mitchell, S. W., Kiley, M. P., et al.: Inactivated Lassa virus elicits a non protective immune response in rhesus monkeys. J. Med. Virol. *37*:1–7, 1992.
58. McCormick, J. B., Walker, D. H., King, I. J., et al.: Lassa virus hepatitis: A study of fatal Lassa fever in humans. Am. J. Trop. Med. Hyg. *35*:401–407, 1986.
59. McCormick, J. B., Webb, P. A., Krebs, J. W., et al.: A prospective study of the epidemiology and ecology of Lassa fever. J. Infect. Dis. *155*:437–444, 1987.
60. Mercado, R.: Rodent control programmes in areas affected by Bolivian haemorrhagic fever. Bull. World Health Organ. *52*:691–695, 1975.
61. Mertens, P. E., Patton, R., Baum, J. J., et al.: Clinical presentation of Lassa fever during the hospital epidemic of Zorzor, Liberia, March–April 1972. Am. J. Trop. Med. Hyg. *22*:780–784, 1973.
62. Mills, J. N., Ellis, B. A., McKee, K. T., et al.: Junin virus activity in rodents from endemic and nonendemic loci in central Argentina. Am. J. Trop. Med. Hyg. *44*:589–597, 1991.
63. Monath, T. P., Maher, M., Casals, J., et al.: Lassa fever in the Eastern Province of Sierra Leone, 1970–1972. II. Clinical observations and virological studies on selected hospital cases. Am. J. Trop. Med. Hyg. *23*:1140–1149, 1974.
64. Monson, M. H., Cole, A. K., Frame, J. D., et al.: Pediatric Lassa fever: A review of 33 Liberian cases. Am. J. Trop. Med. Hyg. *36*:408–415, 1987.
65. Parodi, A. S., Greenway, D. J., Rugiero, H. R., et al.: Sobre la étiologia del brote epidemico de Junin. Diagn. Med. *30*:2300–2301, 1958.
66. Peters, C. J., Buchmeier, M., Rollin, P. E., and Ksiazek, T. G.: Arenaviruses. *In* Fields, B. N., Knipe, D. M., Howley, P. M., et al. (eds.): Fields Virology. 3rd ed. Philadelphia, Lippincott-Raven, 1996, pp. 1521–1551.
67. Peters, C. J., Kuehne, R. W., Mercado, R. R., et al.: Hemorrhagic fever in Cochabamba, Bolivia, 1971. Am. J. Epidemiol. *99*:425–433, 1974.
68. Peters, C. J., and Webb, P. A.: Measurement of antibodies to Machupo virus by the indirect fluorescent technique. Proc. Soc. Exp. Biol. Med. *142*:526–531, 1973.
69. Price, M. E., Fisher-Hoch, S. P., Craven, R. B., et al.: A prospective study of maternal and fetal outcome in acute Lassa fever infection during pregnancy. B. M. J. *297*:584–587, 1988.
70. Salas, R., de Manzione, N., Tesh, R. B., et al.: Venezuelan haemorrhagic fever. Lancet *338*:1033–1036, 1991.
71. Saluzzo, J. F., Adam, F., McCormick, J. B., et al.: Lassa fever in Senegal. J. Infect. Dis. *157*:605, 1988.
72. Schlaeffer, F., Bar-Lavie, Y., Sikuler, E., et al.: Evidence against the high contagiousness of Lassa fever. Trans. R. Soc. Trop. Med. Hyg. *82*:31, 1988.
73. Southern, P. J.: Arenaviridae: The viruses and their replication. *In* Fields, B. N., Knipe, D. M., Howley, P. M., et al. (eds.): Fields Virology. 3rd ed. Philadelphia, Lippincott-Raven, 1996, pp. 1505–1519.
74. Ter Meulen, J., Badusche, M., Kuhnt, K., et al.: Characterization of human CD4(+) T-cell clones recognizing conserved and variable epitopes of the Lassa virus nucleoprotein. J. Virol. *74*:2186–2192, 2000.
75. Ter Meulen, J., Lukashevitch, I., Sidibe, K., et al.: Hunting of peridomestic rodents and consumption of their meat as possible risk factors for rodent-to-human transmission of Lassa virus in the Republic of Guinea. Am. J. Trop. Med. Hyg. *55*:661–666, 1996.
76. Tesh, R. B., Wilson, M. L., Salas, R., et al.: Field studies on the epidemiology of Venezuelan hemorrhagic fever: Implication of the cotton rat *Sigmodon alstoni* as the probable rodent reservoir. Am. J. Trop. Med. Hyg. *49*:227–235, 1993.
77. Tomori, O., Fabiyi, A., Sorungbe, A., et al.: Viral hemorrhagic fever antibodies in Nigerian populations. Am. J. Trop. Med. Hyg. *38*:407–410, 1988.
78. Update: Management of patients with suspected viral hemorrhagic fever. M. M. W. R. Morb. Mortal. Wkly. Rep. *44*:475–479, 1995.
79. Vainrub, B., and Salas, R. A.: Latin American hemorrhagic fever. Infect. Dis. Clin. North Am. *8*:47–59, 1994.
80. Van der Heide, R. M.: A patient with Lassa fever from Burkina Faso (formerly Upper Volta), diagnosed in the Netherlands. Ned. Tijdschr. Geneeskd. *126*:1–7, 1982.
81. Weaver, S. C., Salas, R. A., de Manzione, N., et al.: Guanarito virus (Arenaviridae) isolates from endemic and outlying localities in Venezuela: Sequence comparisons among and within strains isolated from Venezuelan hemorrhagic fever patients and rodents. Virology *266*:189–195, 2000.
82. Webb, P. A., McCormick, J. B., King, I. J., et al.: Lassa fever in children in Sierra Leone, West Africa. Trans. R. Soc. Trop. Med. Hyg. *80*:577–582, 1986.

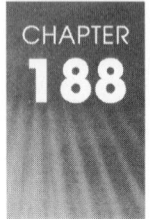

Filoviral Hemorrhagic Fever: Marburg and Ebola Virus Fevers

RÉMI N. CHARREL

Ebola and Marburg viruses are the only members of the family *Filoviridae*. They are maintained in nature through unknown mechanisms and are capable of inducing a severe and highly lethal hemorrhagic fever syndrome in humans. The mortality rates of Ebola and Marburg virus hemorrhagic fever may be as high as 90 and 70 percent, respectively. Recent outbreaks of Ebola virus disease in nonhuman primates from the Philippines and serologic data have provided evidence that filoviruses (at least Ebola virus) are not restricted to Africa.

History

MARBURG VIRUS

In 1967, simultaneous outbreaks of a previously unknown hemorrhagic fever occurred in Marburg and Frankfurt (Germany) and in Belgrade (Serbia, formerly Yugoslavia) (Table 188–1). Infection was traced to contact with African green monkeys *(Cercopithecus aethiops)* from a primate export facility in Entebbe, Uganda. Thirty-one cases developed, including 6 by secondary transmission. Seven deaths occurred in primary cases.[18, 31] An infectious agent unlike any previously seen was recovered from the blood and organs of these persons and was named *Marburg virus* after the name of the German city where the first cases occurred.[14, 29] Since that time, sporadic cases of this disease have been recognized in southern Africa and in Kenya.[8, 12, 30] A more recent outbreak took place during the years 1998 to 2000 at Durba in the east region of the Democratic Republic of Congo (formerly Zaire) (Fig. 188–1). Most of the patients were young gold miners. A total of approximately 130 cases were identified, and the fatality rate reached 71 percent.[38]

EBOLA VIRUS

In 1976, two nearly simultaneous and explosive outbreaks of a similar illness occurred in northwestern Zaire and southern Sudan (see Table 188–1). Viruses morphologically similar to but antigenically distinct from Marburg virus were recovered from patient blood specimens. This agent was named *Ebola virus* after a small river near the epicenter of the epidemic in Zaire.[1, 13] More than 600 persons were affected, and the mortality rate was high: 88 percent in Zaire

TABLE 188–1 ■ YEAR AND LOCATION OF FILOVIRAL HEMORRHAGIC FEVER CASES AND OUTBREAKS

Year	Virus Species	Country	Number of Human Cases	Fatality Rate (%)
1967	*Marburg*	Germany/Serbia	37	19
1975	*Marburg*	South Africa	3	33
1976	*Zaire Ebola*	Zaire	318	88
1976	*Sudan Ebola*	Sudan	284	53
1976	*Sudan Ebola*	England	1	0
1979	*Sudan Ebola*	Sudan	34	65
1980	*Marburg*	Kenya	2	50
1987	*Marburg*	Kenya	1	100
1989	*Reston Ebola**	USA	0	0
1990	*Reston Ebola**	USA	0	0
1992	*Reston Ebola**	Italy	0	0
1994	*Marburg*	Zaire	11	Unknown
1994	*Zaire Ebola*	Gabon	44	63
1994	*Cote d'Ivoire Ebola*	Ivory Coast	1	0
1995	*Zaire Ebola*	Zaire	315	81
1996	*Zaire Ebola*	Gabon	37	57
1996	*Zaire Ebola*	Gabon	60	75
1996	*Zaire Ebola*	South Africa	2	50
1996	*Reston Ebola**	USA	0	0
1996	*Reston Eboal**	Philippines	0	0
1998–2000	*Marburg*	DRC†	130	71
2000	*Sudan Ebola*	Uganda	425	53

*Symptomatic infections and fatal cases were observed in nonhuman primates only.
†The Democratic Republic of the Congo (DRC) formerly was known as Zaire.

and 53 percent in Sudan.[4, 5] A single case of fatal infection was documented in Tandala, Zaire, in 1977,[10] and another outbreak in which 22 of 34 illnesses were fatal occurred in the same area of Sudan in 1979.[39] In 1995, a major epidemic with a mortality rate of more than 80 percent in 315 patients was recorded in the Kikwit region of Zaire, approximately 600 miles southwest of the original site in the Bumba province of Zaire.[35] An isolated and nonfatal Ebola virus infection occurred in 1994 in an anthropologist observing chimpanzees in an Ivory Coast national park.[17] This researcher noted that some of these animals were suffering from a hemorrhagic illness; her infection most likely was acquired in the course of performing an autopsy on one of the chimpanzees.

In 1989, that Ebola virus was not restricted to the African continent became apparent. A group of cynomolgus monkeys *(Macaca fascicularis)* from the Philippines quarantined in a

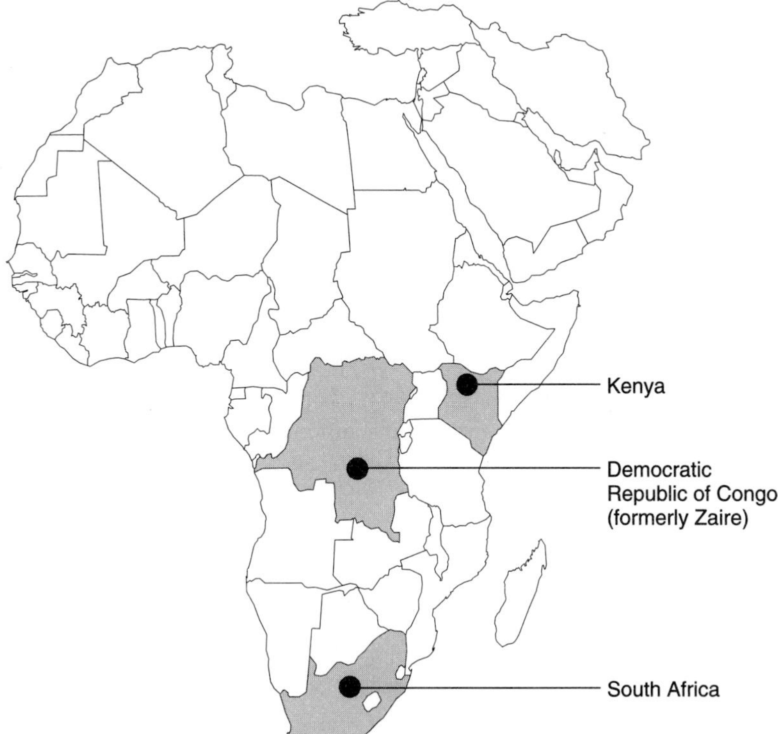

FIGURE 188–1 ■ Geographic distribution of human outbreaks of Marburg virus fever in Africa.

Reston, Virginia, laboratory experienced lethal hemorrhagic disease.[9] Virions antigenically similar to those of Ebola virus were observed in tissues and confirmed by culture in Vero cells.[11] During the next several weeks, the further introduction of new monkeys and the spread of infection to several rooms in the facility necessitated euthanizing the entire cohort of more than 400 animals. The building was fumigated and abandoned. The virus was recovered from another macaque in Philadelphia and later in a laboratory in Italy.[37] Although no human disease was associated with these episodes, several monkey handlers in the United States were infected, as confirmed by serologic conversion from negative to positive for Ebola antibodies.[9] In 1996, a cynomolgus monkey imported from the Philippines died in an animal facility in Texas; two additional cases were recorded in the same facility, with the strain again belonging to the Reston subtype.[28]

A recent epidemic of Ebola hemorrhagic fever occurred in the year 2000 in Uganda and started in the Gulu district. When the outbreak ended in January 2001, a total of 425 cases had been recorded, and 224 lives had been claimed (Fig. 188–2). As reported in a previous outbreak, numerous nosocomially acquired cases developed in health care staff members because of a lack of implementation of infection control measures. The strain of the latter outbreak was closely related to the Sudan subtype.[24]

Etiologic Agents

Filoviridae viruses have a similar morphology. Long filamentous particles often have bizarre configurations (Fig. 188–3) and may be as long as 14,000 nm. They always are 80 nm in width and contain a single negative-sense genome that codes for seven polypeptides. An excellent review of the molecular organization and replication strategy of this virus group and comparison with other related families has been published recently.[26] Filoviruses replicate readily in Vero, MA-104, or SW-13 cell cultures, although specific subtypes seem to prefer individual cell lines, all of which were derived from primates. The viruses also are highly pathogenic for macaques and produce a hemorrhagic disease that usually is more than 75 percent fatal; this hemorrhagic disease is the only useful pathophysiologic model for human infection.

The *Filoviridae* family now comprises two genera.[23] The "Marburg-like viruses" genus has Marburg virus as a unique species. The "Ebola-like viruses" genus includes four antigenically and genetically related species: Zaire Ebola virus (the type species), Reston Ebola virus, Sudan Ebola virus, and Côte d'Ivoire Ebola virus.

With the possible exception of the Ebola virus subtype Reston, filoviruses are highly pathogenic organisms that must be handled only in special laboratories (biosafety level 4) under maximal biologic containment. Recommendations regarding the management of patients and specimens suspected of having these viruses have been published.[34] Further detail is available from the Centers for Disease Control and Prevention (CDC) in Atlanta and can be obtained from their website at *http://www.cdc.gov/ncidod/dvrd/spb*.

Virtually no antigenic relationship exists between Marburg virus and any of the Ebola virus species. The latter, however, exhibit extensive immunologic cross-reactivity, as detected by immunofluorescence or enzyme-linked immunosorbent assay (ELISA). Virus neutralization, in contrast, virtually has been impossible to measure for any of the filoviruses, and this difficulty has proved to be an important obstacle to understanding the epidemiology and ecology of these agents. Unlike the three other species, the Reston Ebola virus strains are not circulating in Africa but in the Philippines. To date, only the Ebola virus strains originating from Africa appear to be human pathogens.

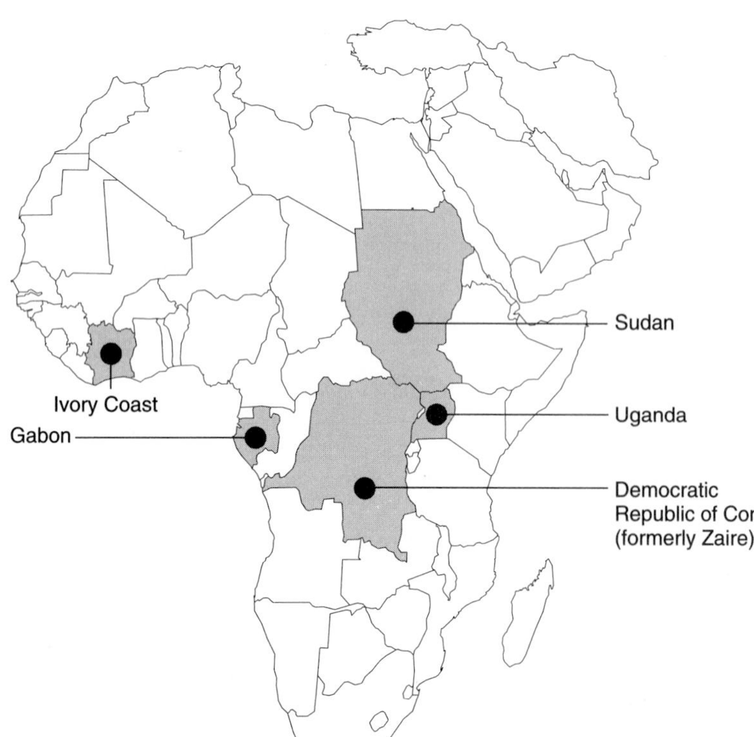

FIGURE 188–2 ■ Geographic distribution of human outbreaks of Ebola virus fever in Africa.

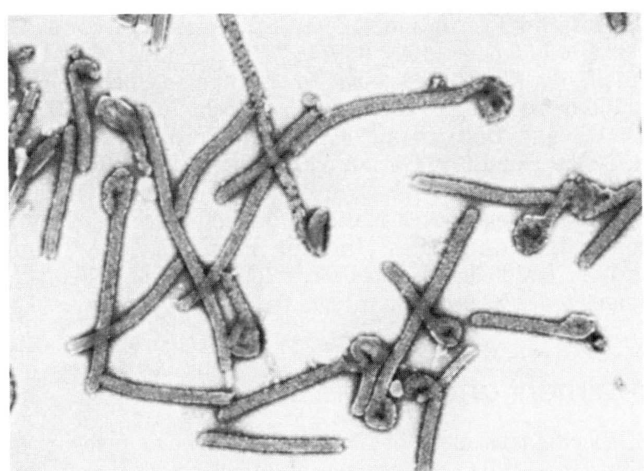

FIGURE 188–3 ■ Electron micrograph of Ebola virus (×38,750). (Courtesy of T. W. Geisbert.)

Epidemiology

Partly because of the infrequent and unpredictable occurrence of filoviruses in humans, the natural reservoirs and vectors (if any) of filoviruses remain a mystery 30 years after initially being recognized. Nonhuman primates cannot be the reservoir host because they become severely ill when infected and die rapidly, as do humans.[2, 21] Limited surveys of vertebrates and certain arthropods at or near sites of human outbreaks have failed to yield even a first clue.[27] The inability to develop a serologic method to search for infection with uniform sensitivity in diverse species is a continuing problem. Studies involving thousands of vertebrates and ten of thousands of invertebrates have been unable to detect any species in which filoviruses can replicate steadily. A recent study reported that only specific species of bats were capable of withstanding Ebola virus replication at high titer without any overt sign of illness, thus rendering bats the most probable reservoir candidate to date.[33]

Much has been published to indicate that humans may be infected without serious disease at prevalence levels of up to 40 percent. Work with ELISA involving the use of purified recombinant antigen suggests that such infection actually is rare.[15] The origin of every index case of human Filovirus disease is unknown. Thus, all outbreaks thus far identified are based on person-to-person transmission. Such transmission is fueled by the high and persistent viremia that marks the syndrome and by the presence of virus in other body fluids, especially when contaminated by blood.

Tissues of monkeys used to prepare cell culture for the manufacture of poliovirus vaccine were the source of the original Marburg outbreak, and secondary infection largely was limited to medical workers who initially failed to take precautions designed to prevent direct skin contact with body fluids. The 1976 Ebola outbreaks were spread primarily by the use of contaminated needles, and the recent Kikwit, Bandundu, epidemic was fomented by ill-advised surgical procedures performed without any protection whatsoever. In the case of the three outbreaks that occurred in Gabon, the index case of each episode was traced back to hunters or inhabitants infected while butchering dead primates; however, the route by which the monkeys became infected remains unknown.

Intimate family contact is also an important factor in the spread of infection, and such infection occurs primarily in persons providing direct care to patients in the home and those preparing corpses for burial. As many as 17 percent of infections in Zaire were thus documented, and this fraction was even higher in the 1995 outbreak. Although these factors mitigate against pediatric disease, of interest is that 20 percent of patients in the 1976 Zaire epidemic were younger than 15 years of age.[5] Aerosol has not been implicated frequently in human infection. However, aerosols have been shown to be infectious for primates, and one anecdotal case from the original Marburg epidemic has been reported.[19] In addition, strong evidence suggests that dissemination of the Reston Ebola virus among monkeys and to monkey handlers was attributable at least partially to respiratory infection.

Epidemiologic investigations have identified the three most important means of transmission as attendance at funerals of presumptive Ebola virus–infected patients where ritual contact with the deceased occurred, intrafamilial transmission, and nosocomial transmission.

Clinical Manifestations

After an incubation period varying from 2 to 21 days (more often 4 to 9 days), the onset of Ebola virus fever is abrupt and, in most patients, characterized by high fever, headache, muscle aches, stomach pain, fatigue, and diarrhea; in some patients, additional signs such as sore throat, hiccups, rash, red and itchy eyes, vomiting of blood, and bloody diarrhea are noted. Within a week, a negative outcome of the disease is manifested as chest pain and shock, sometimes blindness and bleeding, and finally death.[3]

Marburg virus fever is marked by an incubation period almost identical to that of Ebola virus fever, after which the onset also is brutal and characterized by fever, chills, headache, and myalgia. A week after the initiation of clinical signs, a maculopapular rash, nausea, vomiting, chest pain, abdominal pain, diarrhea, and a sore throat may appear. Symptoms increase progressively and may include jaundice, delirium, shock, liver failure, massive hemorrhaging, and multiorgan dysfunction.

Mild leukopenia is a common occurrence early in Filovirus disease, but leukocytosis may appear later as a reflection of secondary bacterial infection, which usually is pulmonary. Thrombocytopenia below 100,000 platelets/mm^3 is uniform, and as bleeding begins, coagulation studies are abnormal. Fibrin split products indicative of disseminated intravascular coagulation have been observed in human and experimentally infected primates. Serum transaminases are elevated markedly, but increased bilirubin and clinical jaundice rarely are noted. Serum protein levels are depressed, the hematocrit is increased, and proteinuria is a common finding.[25]

Pathogenesis and Pathology

Researchers do not understand why some people are able to recover from filoviral fever and others are not. However, what is known is that in patients who die, a significant immune response to the virus usually has not developed at the time of death. Endothelial cells, macrophages, monocytes, and hepatocytes are the main targets of viral infection, with resulting cytopathic effect.[40] A marked elevation in interleukin-2, interleukin-10, tumor necrosis factor–α (TNF-α), interferon-α, and interferon-γ was noted in fatal filoviral hemorrhagic fever cases.[36] TNF-α could trigger the activation of pathways responsible for deleterious effects. Pathologic examination reveals diffuse hemorrhage involving most organ systems, and histologic findings compatible with those of disseminated intravascular coagulation are present.[7] Lymph nodes and the spleen show mild enlargement, edema, and areas of lymphoid necrosis. Diffuse hepatitis with focal necrosis, virtually no inflammatory response, and many Councilman-like bodies are invariably present. Electron microscopy shows that hepatocyte inclusions consist of massive arrays of virus particles.

Diagnosis and Differential Diagnosis

Marburg and Ebola virus fevers must be differentiated from other viral hemorrhagic diseases in Africa, as well as from the many bacterial, rickettsial, and protozoal diseases that may be manifested in a similar manner early in clinical disease. The absence of jaundice helps eliminate yellow fever and Rift Valley fever. For patients seen outside Africa, a travel history is the single most important diagnostic tool available to physicians. Early in the course of the disease, laboratory diagnosis of Ebola virus infection currently is based on antigen-capture ELISA, reverse transcription–polymerase chain reaction (RT-PCR), and virus isolation. These tools are the most accurate for diagnosing acute Ebola virus fever. Later in the course of the disease or after recovery, the diagnosis relies on IgM-capture ELISA or IgG antibody detection; of interest, however, is that specific antibodies do not develop in a significant proportion of patients with a fatal outcome. Because large quantities of Ebola virus are present in dermal tissue, skin biopsies have been proposed for postmortem confirmation of Ebola virus fever by immunohistochemical analysis. Specimens are easy to collect, and formalin fixation renders them safe for transport; nonetheless, the sensitivity of the skin biopsy test does not permit its use for early diagnosis, and it should be reserved for use on dead or dying patients.[41]

For instance, during the Uganda outbreak of Ebola virus fever in the year 2000, patients were classified into three categories depending on the clinical manifestations and epidemiologic data[24]:

- Suspect: Person with fever and contact with a potential case—a patient, a person with unexplained bleeding, an individual with fever and three or more specified symptoms (headache, vomiting, anorexia, diarrhea, weakness or severe fatigue, abdominal pain, body aches or joint pains, difficulty swallowing, difficulty breathing, and hiccups); all unexplained deaths.
- Probable: Person who met these criteria and was assessed and reported by a physician.
- Confirmed: Laboratory-confirmed case—person defined as a patient who met the surveillance case definitions and was positive for either Ebola virus antigen, Ebola virus IgG antibody, or Ebola virus RT-PCR.

Technologic advances have permitted for the first time the performance of confirmatory laboratory tests on the epidemic site in Gulu during the Uganda outbreak. Confirmation was achieved with the RT-PCR assay and antigen detection by ELISA in a local hospital under the supervision of CDC laboratory teams (Rollin, P. E., personal communication).

Marburg virus infection can be diagnosed early in the course of the disease by antigen-capture ELISA, IgM-capture ELISA, RT-PCR, and isolation of virus. IgG-capture ELISA is appropriate for testing persons later in the course of the disease or after recovery.

Suspected cases encountered in the United States should be reported to local and state health departments or to the Special Pathogen Branch, MS G-14, Centers for Disease Control and Prevention, 1600 Clifton Road, Atlanta, GA 30333; telephone, (404) 639–1118; FAX, (404) 639–1115; e-mail, dvd1spath@cdc.gov. In Europe, suspected cases should be reported to the Bernhard-Nocht-Institut of Tropical Medicine, Department of Virology, Bernhard-Nocht-Str. 74, 20359 Hamburg, Germany; telephone, (49) 40 42818–0; FAX, (49) 40 42818–378; e-mail, schmitz@bni.uni-hamburg.de, or Centre National de Référence des Fièvres Hemorragiques Virales, Institut Pasteur, 21 Av. Tony Garnier, 69365 Lyon cedex 07; telephone (33) 437282421; e-mail, zelles@cervi-lyon.inserm.fr.

Treatment and Prevention

No specific treatment of filoviral hemorrhagic fever exists. Ribavirin and interferon have no effect on filoviruses, and the search for other antiviral compounds has not been successful.[25] Treatment relies on symptomatic measures to maintain hydration and nutritional support and to prevent and cure bacterial and parasitic infections. Convalescent plasma has been used on occasion without proven effect. A study conducted during the 1995 Kikwit Ebola epidemic showed that seven of eight patients who received blood collected from convalescent donors recovered; this finding pleads for a thorough evaluation of passive immune therapy.[22] One person infected with Sudan Ebola virus after a laboratory accident survived after receiving such plasma from Zaire Ebola virus survivors.[6] Several patients are thought to have had milder Marburg virus disease after receiving early treatment with plasma.[19] Recent reports also demonstrate that hyperimmune globulin prepared in horses protected baboons in experimental studies.[20] Goat immune globulin was tested in preclinical trials on laboratory animals and was given to researchers suspected of becoming infected with Ebola virus during their laboratory experiments. One researcher highly suspected of having ongoing infection recovered completely after the administration of goat anti-Ebola immune globulin.[16] Attempts to develop a vaccine against Ebola virus currently remain under active investigation. Promising results were obtained recently when vaccinated nonhuman primates survived a challenge with Ebola virus.[32]

REFERENCES

1. Bowen, E. T. W., Lloyd, G., Harris, W. J., et al.: Viral haemorrhagic fever in southern Sudan and northern Zaire. Lancet *1*:571–573, 1977.
2. Breman, J. G., Johnson, K. M., van der Groen, G., et al.: A search for Ebola virus in animals in the Democratic Republic of the Congo and Cameroon: Ecologic, virologic, and serologic surveys, 1979–1980. J. Infect. Dis. *179*(Suppl. 1):139–147, 1999.
3. Colebunders, R., and Borchert, M.: Ebola haemorrhagic fever—a review. J. Infect. Dis. *40*:16–20, 2000.
4. Ebola haemorrhagic fever in Sudan, 1976. Report of a WHO/International Study Team. Bull. World Health Organ. *56*:247–270, 1978.
5. Ebola haemorrhagic fever in Zaire, 1976. Bull. World Health Organ. *56*:271–293, 1978.
6. Edmond, R. T. D., Evans, B., Bowen, E. T., et al.: A case of Ebola virus infection. B. M. J. *2*:541–544, 1977.
7. Fisher-Hoch, S. P., Platt, G. S., Neild, G. H., et al.: Pathophysiology of shock and hemorrhage in a fulminant viral infection (Ebola). J. Infect. Dis. *152*:887–894, 1985.
8. Gear, J. S. S., Cassell, G. A., Gear, A. J., et al.: Outbreak of Marburg virus disease in Johannesburg. B. M. J. *4*:489–493, 1975.
9. Hayes, C. G., Burans, J. P., Ksiazek, T. G., et al.: Outbreak of fatal illness among captive macaques in the Philippines caused by an Ebola-related filovirus. Am. J. Trop. Med. Hyg. *46*:664–671, 1992.
10. Heymann, D. C., Weisfeld, J. S., Webb, P. A., et al.: Ebola hemorrhagic fever, Tandala, Zaire, 1977–1978. J. Infect. Dis. *142*:372–376, 1980.
11. Jahrling, P. B., Geisbert, T. W., Dalgard, D. W., et al.: Preliminary report: Isolation of Ebola virus from monkeys imported to USA. Lancet *335*:502–505, 1990.

12. Johnson, E. D., Roimet, E., Gitau, L. G., et al.: Marburg virus disease: An environmental health threat in Kenya. *In* Kinoti, S. H., Waiyoki, P. G., and Were, B. D. (eds.): Proceedings of the 11th Annual Medical Scientific Conference. Nairobi, Kenya, African Medical Research Foundation, 1990.
13. Johnson, K. M., Webb, P. A., Lange, J., et al.: Isolation and partial characterization of a new virus causing acute haemorrhagic fever in Zaire. Lancet *1*:569–571, 1977.
14. Kissling, R. E., Robinson, R. Q., Murphy, F. A., et al.: Agent of disease contracted from green monkeys. Science *160*:888–890, 1968.
15. Ksiazek, T. G., Rollin, P. E., Jahrling, P. B., et al.: Enzyme immunosorbent assay for Ebola virus antigens in tissues of infected primates. J. Clin. Microbiol. *30*:947–950, 1992.
16. Kudoyarova-Zubavichene, N. M., Sergeyev, N. N., Chepurnov, A. A., et al.: Preparation and use of hyperimmune serum for prophylaxis and therapy of Ebola virus infections. J. Infect. Dis. *179*(Suppl. 1):218–223, 1999.
17. Le Guenno, B., Formentry, P., Wyers, M., et al.: Isolation and partial characterization of a new strain of Ebola virus. Lancet *345*:1271–1274.
18. Martini, G. A., Knauff, H. G., Schmidt, H. A., et al.: A previously unknown infectious disease contracted from monkeys: Marburg virus disease. Dtsch. Med. Wochenschr. *93*:559–571, 1968.
19. Martini, G. A., and Siegert, R. (ed.): Marburg Virus Disease. New York, Springer-Verlag, 1971.
20. Mikhailov, V. V., Borisevich, I. V., Chernikov, N. K., et al.: The evaluation in hamadryas baboons of the possibility for the specific prevention of Ebola fever. Vopr. Virusol. *39*:82–84, 1994.
21. Monath, T. P.: Ecology of Marburg and Ebola viruses: Speculations and directions for future research. J. Infect. Dis. *179*(Suppl. 1):127–138, 1999.
22. Mupapa, K., Massamba, M., Kibadi, K., et al.: Treatment of Ebola hemorrhagic fever with blood transfusions from convalescent patients. J. Infect. Dis. *179*(Suppl.):18–23, 1999.
23. Netesov, S. V., Feldmann, H., Jahrling, P. B., et al.: Family *Filoviridae*. *Reoviridae*. *In* Van Regenmortel, M. H. V., Fauquet, C. M., Bishop, D. H. L., et al. (eds.): Virus Taxonomy. Seventh Report of the International Committee for the Taxonomy of Viruses. New York, Academic, 2000, pp. 539–548.
24. Outbreak of Ebola hemorrhagic fever—Uganda, August 2000–January 2001. M. M. W. R. Morb. Mortal. Wkly. Rep.*50*:73–77, 2001.
25. Peters, C. J., Buchmeier, M., Rollin, P. E., and Ksiazek, T. G.: Filoviridae: Marburg and Ebola viruses. *In* Fields, B. N., Knipe, D. M., Howley, P. M., et al. (eds.): Fields Virology. 3rd ed. Philadelphia, Lippincott-Raven, 1996, pp. 1161–1176.
26. Peters, C. J., Sanchez, A., Rollin, P. E., et al.: *Filoviridae:* Marburg and Ebola viruses. *In* Belshe, B. (ed.): Textbook of Human Virology. 4th ed. St. Louis, Mosby-Year Book, 1996, p. 699.
27. Reiter, P., Turell, M., Coleman, R., et al.: Field investigations of an outbreak of Ebola hemorrhagic fever, Kikwit, Democratic Republic of the Congo, 1995: Arthropod studies. J. Infect. Dis. *179*(Suppl. 1):148–154, 1999.
28. Rollin, P. E., Williams, R. J., Bressler, D. S., et al.: Ebola (subtype Reston) virus among quarantined nonhuman primates recently imported from the Philippines to the United States. J. Infect. Dis. *179*(Suppl. 1):108–114, 1999.
29. Smith, C. E. G., Simpson, D. I. H., Bowen, E. T. W., et al.: Fatal human disease from vervet monkeys. Lancet *2*:1119–1121, 1967.
30. Smith, D. H., Johnson, B. K., Isaacson, M., et al.: Marburg virus disease in Kenya. Lancet *1*:816–820, 1982.
31. Stille, W., Boehle, E., Heim, E., et al.: An infectious disease transmitted by *Cercopthecus aethiops*. Dtsch. Med. Wochenschr. *93*:572–582, 1968.
32. Sullivan, N. J., Sanchez, A., Rollin, P. E., et al.: Development of a preventive vaccine for Ebola virus infection in primates. Nature *408*:605–609, 2000.
33. Swanepoel, R., Leman, P. A., Burt, F. J., et al.: Experimental inoculation of plants and animals with Ebola virus. Emerg. Infect. Dis. *2*:321–325, 1996.
34. Update: Management of patients with suspected viral hemorrhagic fever. M. M. W. R. Morb. Mortal. Wkly. Rep. *44*:475–479, 1995.
35. Update: Outbreak of Ebola virus hemorrhagic fever—Zaire, 1995. M. M. W. R. Morb. Mortal. Wkly. Rep. *44*:399, 1995.
36. Villinger, F., Rollin, P. E., Brar, S. S. et al.: Markedly elevated levels of interferon (IFN)-α, IFN-γ, interleukin (IL)-2, IL-10, and tumor necrosis factor-α associated with fatal Ebola virus infection. J. Infect. Dis. *179*(Suppl. 1):188–191, 1999.
37. Viral haemorrhagic fever in imported monkeys. Wkly. Epidemiol. Rec. *67*:142–143, 1992.
38. Viral haemorrhagic fever/Marburg, Democratic Republic of the Congo. Wkly. Epidemiol. Rec. *74*:157–158, 1999.
39. Viral haemorrhagic fever surveillance. Wkly. Epidemiol. Rec. *44*:2, 1979.
40. Zaki, S. R., and Goldsmith, C. S.: Pathologic features of filovirus infections in humans. Curr. Top. Microbiol. Immunol. *235*:97–116, 1999.
41. Zaki, S. R., Shieh, W.-J., Greer, P. W., et al.: A novel immunohistochemical assay for the detection of Ebola virus in skin: Implications for diagnosis, spread, and surveillance of Ebola hemorrhagic fever. J. Infect. Dis. *179*(Suppl. 1):36–47, 1999.

SUBSECTION **10**

CORONAVIRIDAE

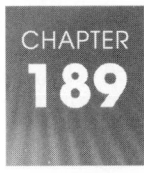

CHAPTER 189 Coronaviruses and Toroviruses, Including Severe Acute Respiratory Syndrome (SARS)

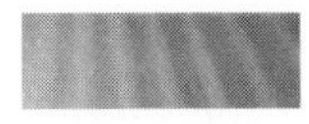

CHAPTER 189A

Coronaviruses and Toroviruses

KENNETH McINTOSH

The family *Coronaviridae* is composed of two genera, Coronavirus and Torovirus. The two genera are related in that they appear quite similar on electron microscopy and they share similar strategies of replication (along with other members of the order Nidovirales, the arteriviruses). They differ, however, in the size of their RNA genome and structural proteins, as well as in the morphology of their nucleocapsids. Coronaviruses are primarily respiratory pathogens in humans, although they cause a wide variety of important diseases in animals, including infectious bronchitis and nephrosis in chickens; gastroenteritis and encephalitis in young piglets; enteritis in turkeys, dogs, and calves; hepatitis and encephalitis in mice; pneumonitis and sialodacryoadenitis in rats; and infectious peritonitis in cats.[48] Toroviruses are, at least as presently known, exclusively enteric pathogens, both in animals and humans.

Since the first report of human coronavirus (HCoV) isolation in 1965,[104] the HCoV group of RNA viruses has been confirmed as a frequent cause of the common cold in children and adults. They also have been implicated as possible contributors in lower respiratory infections in children and adults, and more recently, they have been shown to be important causes of respiratory disease in the elderly.[24, 107] Their role in acute or chronic gastroenteritis is less clear.

The first HCoV was cultivated by Tyrrell and Bynoe at the Common Cold Unit in Salisbury, England, with the use of human embryonic tracheal and nasal epithelial mucosal organ cultures.[104] The authors were able to produce colds regularly in volunteers inoculated with organ culture fluid from the first and later passages of an agent, B814, obtained from a boy with a cold.[8]

Working independently, Hamre and Procknow in 1966 described the isolation of five viruses, including the prototype strain HCoV-229E, in primary human embryonic kidney cell cultures.[31] Four of these agents were obtained from medical students with upper respiratory illnesses and one from a healthy student. These viruses produced a cytopathic effect in human embryonic kidney cells after an initial blind passage and could be adapted to grow and produce a cytopathic effect in the human diploid cell strain WI-38. The growth of six additional HCoVs, including the second human prototype HCoV-OC43, was reported in 1967 by McIntosh and associates, who used human embryonic tracheal organ cultures inoculated with secretions from adults with upper respiratory infections.[62, 64]

That the HCoVs were related to similar agents known to infect animals soon became evident. By electron microscopy, 229E and B814 were demonstrated to be morphologically identical to each other and to avian infectious bronchitis virus.[2] Subsequently, mouse hepatitis virus was demonstrated to be very similar morphologically and to be antigenically related to HCoV-OC43.[62, 66] Shortly thereafter, these and similar agents were placed in the genus Coronavirus of the family *Coronaviridae*, named for the crown-like appearance of their surface projections on electron microscopy.[103]

Poor growth and a lack of cytopathic effect in cell culture have been major deterrents to research on HcoV, which must be isolated (if it can be grown at all) in either human organ culture or human embryonic tissue culture. Because of this handicap, probably fewer than 60 HCoVs have been isolated to date.[31, 38, 49, 66, 87] When sufficient virus has been recovered for characterization, most isolates have proved to be similar, either HCoV-229E–like or HCoV-OC43–like,[57] although several HCoVs, including the very first isolate HCoV-B814, remain antigenically uncharacterized.[7, 9, 66]

Both HCoV-OC43 and HCoV-229E have been adapted to host systems capable of supporting good growth and allowing the production of antigens for serologic tests. HCoV-OC43 has been propagated in suckling mouse brain[62] and was shown to agglutinate and hemadsorb erythrocytes,[39, 40] and both viruses have been adapted to cell lines producing sufficient virus for biochemical studies.

Toroviruses were, like coronaviruses, first described in animals. They were detected in the 1970s and 1980s in the feces of cattle (Breda virus) and horses (Berne virus).[109, 113] Shortly thereafter, Beards and colleagues reported finding particles with a similar appearance in feces of adults and children with gastroenteritis. These particles aggregated in the presence of antiserum to the bovine and equine viruses.[5] Neither the human nor the bovine viruses have been grown in tissue culture.

Etiologic Agents

CORONAVIRUSES

Coronaviruses are medium to large (80 to 220 nm) pleomorphic, spherical, or elliptical enveloped RNA viruses with widely spaced, petal-shaped, 20-nm-long surface projections giving the virus the appearance of a solar corona.[61] They are labile to heat, lipid solvents, and acid pH. The RNA genome is 27 to 32 kb (large for an RNA virus), single stranded, positive sense, and infectious.[48] The genomes of four coronaviruses have been sequenced completely, including those of HCoV-229E and murine hepatitis virus, which resembles HCoV-OC43 antigenically and biologically.[34, 50] The genome and its surrounding capsid are arranged in helical symmetry and enclosed within a lipoprotein envelope.

Within the coronavirus particle, a nucleoprotein (N) surrounds the RNA genome, and together they appear as a coiled tubular helix within the bilayer lipid-containing envelope. The envelope contains two or three glycoproteins: (1) a matrix protein M, which is embedded in the envelope; (2) a surface component S, which is the structural protein of the petal-shaped spikes; and (3) a hemagglutinin esterase HE, which is found in several of the group II viruses, including HCoV-OC43, and which contains sequences closely related to influenza C hemagglutinin. The antigenic interrelationships of these four proteins have permitted arrangement of both the animal coronaviruses and HCoVs into three groups. The two known HCoV serotypes, each along with several other mammalian coronaviruses, have been placed in group I (HCoV-229E) or II (HCoV-OC43), and avian infectious bronchitis virus is the single member of group III. Evidence from RNA base sequencing strengthens the logic of these relationships.[48]

In coronavirus replication, as with other single-stranded, positive-sense viruses, all processes take place in the cytoplasm. In the first step, the virus attaches to the cell membrane by using its HE or S protein in the petal-shaped spike. HCoV-229E uses aminopeptidase N as a cellular receptor,[114] whereas the receptor for HCoV-OC43 still has not been identified definitively. Penetration occurs as a result of S protein–mediated fusion of the viral envelope with the plasma membrane. The genome then codes for the formation of an RNA-dependent RNA polymerase, which initiates the transcription of subgenomic mRNA through a negative-stranded intermediary. The mRNA molecules, as in other members of the virus order Nidovirales, form a nested set, with the sequences of the first open-reading frame at the 5′ end (after a leader sequence) containing the coding region and subsequent sequences through to the polyadenylated 3′ end being untranslated. Virions then are assembled by budding into cytoplasmic vesicles in the rough endoplasmic reticulum and Golgi region. Virus particles are released by cell lysis or fusion of post-Golgi, virion-containing vesicles with the plasma membrane.

TOROVIRUSES

Toroviruses are morphologically very similar to coronaviruses in that they are pleomorphic, membrane-coated viruses, 100 to 120 nm in largest diameter, and bear club-shaped surface projections.[108] A photomicrograph of a torovirus particle is shown in Figure 189–1, juxtaposed to an intestinal coronavirus at the same magnification. The nucleic acid–containing core of the virus has a unique appearance on electron microscopy: it assumes a doughnut shape (i.e., a torus) if viewed from the right angle.[4, 22, 109] Berne virus, first isolated in the 1970s from horses with diarrhea, grows in equine cell tissue culture and has been characterized most thoroughly. The human toroviruses, like the bovine toroviruses, do not grow in tissue culture.

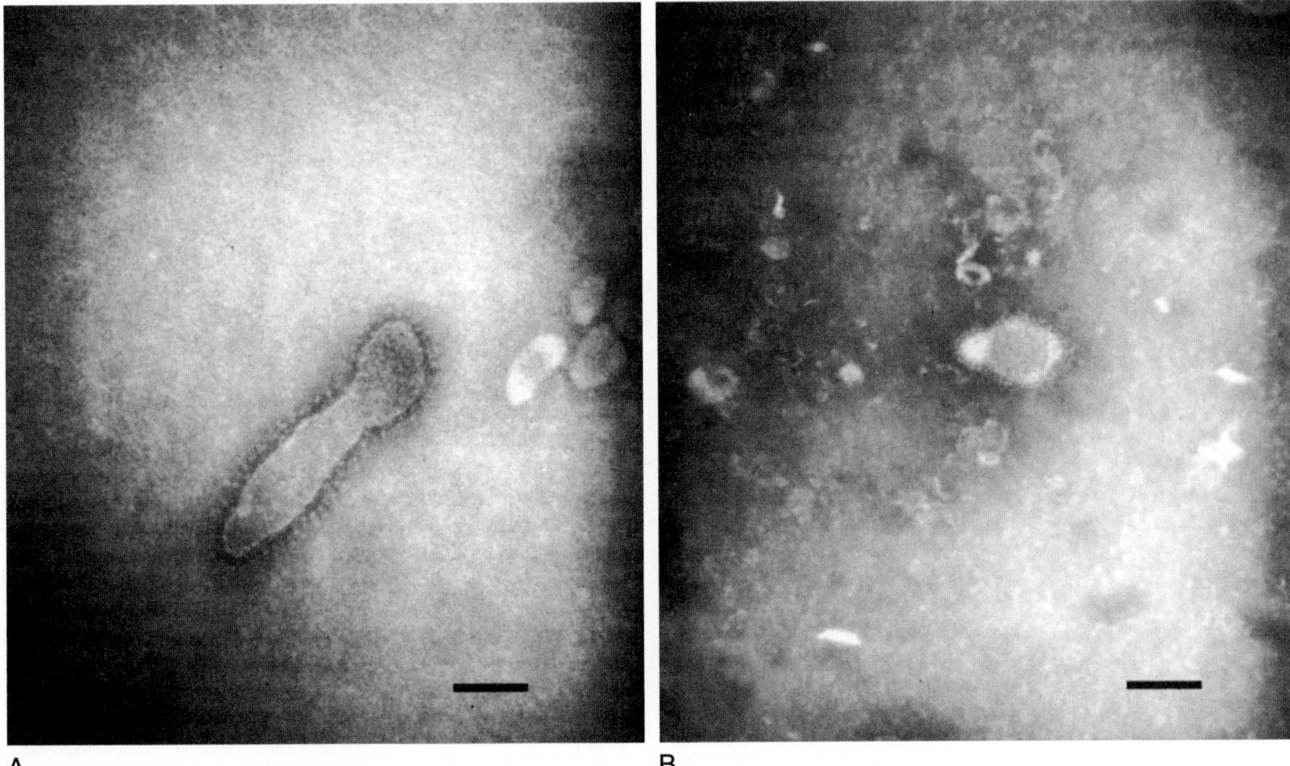

FIGURE 189–1 ■ Negatively stained virus particles in stool samples representing a typical intestinal coronavirus *(A)* and torovirus *(B)*. The *bar* represents 100 nm. The particles both show the typical petal-shaped projections, but those of the coronaviruses are more finely formed and distinct than those of the toroviruses. (Photomicrograph kindly provided by Dr. Martin Petric, Department of Laboratory Medicine, Hospital for Sick Children, Toronto, Canada.)

Toroviruses differ from enteric coronaviruses in being somewhat smaller and more pleomorphic and in having somewhat less distinct surface projections.[22]

Toroviruses contain S glycoproteins on their surface, but no significant sequence homology seems to exist between them and the S proteins of coronaviruses.[98] A second surface protein with HE activity and sequence homology to the HE proteins of both influenza C virus and mouse hepatitis virus has been found on Breda virus, the bovine torovirus, but not on the equine Berne virus.[19] Whether this molecule exists on human toroviruses is not known, although human toroviruses do hemagglutinate rabbit erythrocytes.[22] Toroviruses contain membranes and nucleoproteins similar to those of coronaviruses but with no sequence homology. On the other hand, the replicase contains sequence similarity to that of coronaviruses, and their replication strategy appears to be very similar.[98] Greater than 90 percent identity in the 3′ end of the genome exists between human and animal toroviruses.[22, 98]

The replication strategy of toroviruses probably is very similar to that of coronaviruses in view of the similar organization of the genome and the sequence similarity of their replicase genes.

Epidemiology

Because of the difficulty in isolating respiratory HCoV, most epidemiologic data are derived from serologic surveillance, usually complement fixation, hemagglutination inhibition, neutralization, or enzyme-linked immunosorbent assay (ELISA), with HCoV-229E or HCoV-OC43 viruses used as antigens.[13, 46, 54] Complement-fixation antibody titers frequently are transient, whereas hemagglutination inhibition, neutralization, and ELISA often reflect infection months or years in the past. Because enteric HCoVs rarely have been propagated in culture, epidemiologic study of these agents has been hindered by lack of antigens for serology. Likewise, the epidemiology of human toroviruses has not been well delineated. What information is available about the epidemiology of both enteric coronaviruses and toroviruses is outlined in the later section on clinical manifestations.

GEOGRAPHIC PREVALENCE

Coronavirus infections occur worldwide. Seroprevalence studies of HCoV-229E and HCoV-OC43 infection have been conducted in the United States, Europe, Brazil, and Iraq.[9, 17, 32, 33, 41, 42, 67] With ELISA, antibody prevalence in adults from all areas where they have been examined approaches 90 to 100 percent.

SEASONAL INCIDENCE AND ANNUAL RECYCLING PATTERN

Although HCoV infection may occur at any time of the year, most are seen in midwinter to early spring. Individual serotypes typically predominate in one year, and this pattern then is followed by one or more years of low activity. In healthy children in Atlanta, Georgia, prospectively examined for HCoV-229E and HCoV-OC43 infection from 1960 through 1968 (Fig. 189–2), the incidence of autumn infections approached that of spring infections, and a few infections usually occurred in the summer. In addition, although a very considerable HCoV-229E outbreak occurred in 1961 to 1962, followed by 2 years with a low incidence, in the subsequent 4 years the incidence was quite similar from year to year.[41, 42]

Whatever the season, a single HCoV serotype can cause, at least locally, a high incidence of infection, such as that caused by HCoV-229E in Atlanta children in 1961 to 1962 (see Fig. 189–2). HCoV-229E also was associated with a very significant outbreak in medical students at the University of Chicago in 1966 and 1967.[30] Very substantial proportions of the population can be infected during these intervals. Among the Chicago medical students, 66 (35%) of 191 were infected. In Tecumseh, Michigan, a large HCoV-229E outbreak that occurred between January and April 1967 affected 68 percent of 38 families and 34 percent of 159 individuals tested. Sharp outbreaks also can occur in certain hospitalized infants: at National Jewish Hospital in Denver, 16 of 20 hospitalized asthmatic infants were infected with HCoV-OC43 in December 1968.[65]

RATIO OF CLINICAL TO SUBCLINICAL ILLNESS

In healthy children and adults, HCoVs often are shed asymptomatically. In the 8.5-year surveillance of healthy older children in Atlanta (see Fig. 189–2), only 38 and 47 percent of HCoV-229E and HCoV-OC43 seroconversions, respectively, were associated with respiratory illness. In a group of infants and young children in metropolitan Washington, D.C., tested for HCoV-OC43 seroconversion, at least 50 percent of the infections were subclinical.[67] Susceptibility to HCoV-induced disease may be much greater in certain populations. In the Denver children hospitalized with atopic asthma, 19 were infected with either HCoV-229E or HCoV-OC43 and 17 were symptomatic.[65]

AGE SPECIFICITY OF INFECTION

Antibody to both HCoV-229E and HCoV-OC43 appears in early childhood, and the prevalence increases rapidly with age. On the other hand, asymptomatic and symptomatic infection occurs at all ages, including the elderly, possibly because of small variations in antigenic specificity or the transient nature of immunity. In the Tecumseh families

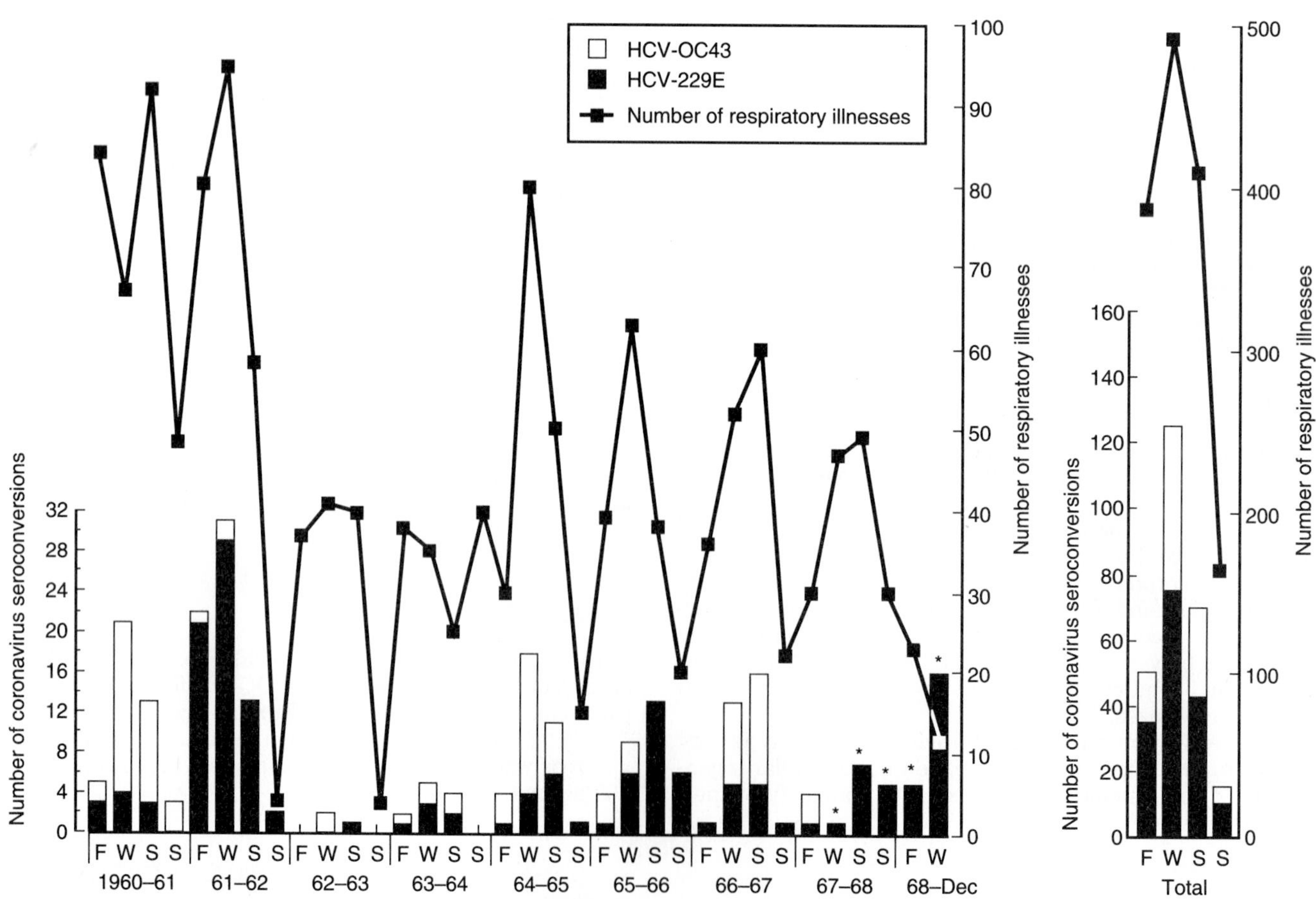

FIGURE 189–2 ■ Seasonal distribution of seroconversion to human coronaviruses OC43 and 229E, 1960 through 1968, in a group of children's cottages in Atlanta, Georgia (120 to 175 children 5 to 19 years of age). Forty-one percent of the seroconversions were associated with respiratory illness. (Adapted from Kaye, H. S., Marsh, H. B., and Dowdle, W. R.: Seroepidemiologic survey of coronavirus [strain OC43] related infections in a children's population. Am. J. Epidemiol. *94*:43–49, 1971; and Kaye, H. S., and Dowdle, W. R.: Seroepidemiologic survey of coronavirus [strain 229E] infections in a population of children. Am. J. Epidemiol. *101*:238–244, 1975.)

studied during a community-wide HCoV-229E epidemic in 1967, only 3 of 54 infections occurred in children younger than 4 years of age. The attack rate then rose to a peak of 14 percent in individuals 15 to 29 years of age and subsequently fell with increasing age.[17] The results were different in an outbreak of HCoV-OC43 infection. With this virus, the highest rate, 29 percent, occurred in children 4 years of age or younger, and rates decreased very little even into adult years, when the incidence was 22 percent.[71]

Several recent studies have emphasized the importance of coronavirus infection in the elderly and the burden of infection, particularly in individuals in chronic care facilities and those with underlying cardiopulmonary disease.[78]

TRANSMISSION

Human volunteers can be infected readily via nosedrops, and a typical cold can develop 2 to 3 days later; therefore, natural infections are assumed to occur through the respiratory route. Monto favors aerosol transmission of HCoV because like influenza viruses, HCoVs often cause sharp and widespread outbreaks.[70] Whatever the means of transmission, HCoVs do not spread easily, at least within families.[17]

Nosocomial transmission of coronavirus respiratory infection has been reported. The study took place in a neonatal intensive care unit, where prospective surveillance by immunofluorescence testing of nasal aspirates performed for 15 months detected 10 infections with coronavirus OC43, all of them nosocomially acquired.[95] All infants had apnea, bradycardia, or abdominal distention, or a combination of these pathologic effects, at the time of infection. Stool samples were not examined. The mode of transmission was not demonstrated in this study.

Infection and Immunity

PATHOGENESIS, INCUBATION PERIOD, AND SEROLOGIC RESPONSE

In healthy adults, HCoVs seem to replicate only in the upper respiratory tract and to produce little direct cytopathology. In human embryonic tracheal organ culture, a decline in ciliary activity after serial passage was the only cytopathic effect observed.[64, 104] In contrast to influenza virus and adenovirus infections, which destroy cells in this system, HCoV-229E and rhinoviruses had no effect, even though these viruses were replicating.[112] Very similar events appear to take place in vivo. Electron microscopy of nasal epithelial biopsy specimens from a young girl with chronic rhinitis and bronchitis showed preservation of cellular structures and cilia despite replication of coronavirus particles.[1]

HCoVs have been detected in nasopharyngeal cells,[68, 77] and HCoV-229E virus titers from 10 to more than 1000 $TCID_{50}$ (median tissue culture infective dose) were found for a week or more in nasopharyngeal washings.[75] Bende and associates studied the course of HCoV-229E colds in 24 volunteers and delineated the typical signs, symptoms, and virus shedding patterns; 8 volunteers were asymptomatic.[6] The incubation period of HCoV colds is, on average, 2 days, and they usually last approximately 1 week.[8]

Little is known about the pathogenesis or immunity of HCoV or torovirus infection of the gastrointestinal tract.

REINFECTION

Repeated infection with HCoVs is a very common occurrence. Among Atlanta children who seroconverted to HCoV-229E, 35 percent had pre-infection antibody titers of 1:10 or higher, and 8 percent had titers of 1:20 or higher.[41] Antibody against HCoV-OC43 also is a common finding in acute sera.[42] No evidence has shown, however, that antibody ameliorates the clinical illness.[71]

Nonetheless, evidence from human volunteer experiments demonstrates that strain-specific antibody can be protective. Reed infected volunteers with one of several HCoV-229E–like viruses. She found that immunity to homotypic challenge endured for at least 1 year, but that immunity to heterotypic HCoV-229E strains in these same volunteers was much lower.[87] IgA antibody may play an important protective role.[12]

Little is known about the role of cell-mediated immunity in resistance to infection with HCoV. In mice, cytotoxic T cells are generated to the mouse hepatitis virus N protein, and immunoreactive lymphocytes probably play a role in both virus clearance and the pathogenesis of neurologic disease.[101] HCoV-229E will replicate in human macrophages,[80] but the role of these cells and cell-mediated immunity in limiting infection is not understood at present.

Clinical Manifestations of Respiratory Tract Infections

THE COMMON COLD AND OTHER UPPER RESPIRATORY TRACT ILLNESSES

A significant association of HCoVs with respiratory illnesses —most of them cold-like—has been demonstrated in prospective studies of adults and families with children. In the Chicago medical students described earlier, HCoV-229E attack rates were 31 percent during "illness periods" and only 9 percent in "wellness periods" ($p < .001$); the illnesses did not differ significantly from undifferentiated acute respiratory tract infections caused by respiratory syncytial virus, parainfluenza viruses, or rhinoviruses.[30] These findings have been confirmed in several other epidemiologic studies.[17, 41, 42]

Symptoms in the adults in the two investigations cited earlier were much like those in human volunteers inoculated with HCoV.[6, 8, 12, 13, 87] Infected volunteers contracted typical common colds, with perhaps more rhinorrhea than occurs in rhinovirus colds; sore throat, cough, malaise, and headache were noted in approximately 50 percent of volunteers. Twenty percent had fever.

The proportion of total respiratory disease or colds attributable to HCoV varies markedly by season and from year to year. In the 8.5-year-long Atlanta study (see Fig. 189–2 and Table 189–1), 7 percent of all respiratory disease was associated with HCoV seroconversion, but in the winter of the epidemic year 1961 to 1962, approximately 16 percent of respiratory illness was associated with HCoV. Most surveys conclude that approximately 8 to 10 percent of all colds are associated with serologically detectable coronavirus infection.[58]

The possible role of coronaviruses in the etiology of otitis media with effusion has been the subject of several recent studies using polymerase chain reaction (PCR) to detect viral nucleic acid in both nasal secretions and middle ear fluid. In one study, 92 children with acute otitis media were investigated. Coronavirus sequences were found in 16 children (17%), in the nasopharynx in 14 and in middle ear fluid in 7. This prevalence was less than that of both respiratory syncytial virus (26%) and rhinoviruses (32%).[83] In another study of middle ear fluid at the time of tube placement, coronavirus sequences rarely were found (only 3 of 100).[82]

TABLE 189–1 ■ CLINICAL FINDINGS IN 61 AND 43 ATLANTA, GEORGIA, CHILDREN* WHO SEROCONVERTED† TO HCV-229E AND HCV-OC43, RESPECTIVELY, 1960 TO 1968

	Virus (%)			Virus (%)	
Initial Complaints	**229E**	**OC43**	**Physical Findings**	**229E**	**OC43**
Sore throat	66	30	Pharyngeal injection	82	72
Coryza	52	19	Coryza	64	49
Cough	43	30	Fever, 37.6° C (99.6° F) and higher	34	40
Fever	21	9			
Headache	15	NR	Fever, 39° C (102.2° F) and higher	8	21
			Cervical adenitis	30	35
			Pulmonary rales (or dullness)	NR	5
			Rash	NR	2

*A changing population of 120 to 175 white children 5 to 19 years of age (median, 9 to 11 years of age) in a church-sponsored home, 1960 to 1968. The children were housed in cottages of 8 to 12 persons, assigned on the basis of age and gender.
†Paired acute and convalescent sera (2 to 3 weeks) showing fourfold or greater antibody rises by indirect hemagglutination (HCV-229E) or hemagglutination inhibition (HCV-OC43).
NR, not reported.
Adapted from Kaye, H.S., Marsh, H.B., and Dowdle, W.R.: Seroepidemiologic survey of coronavirus (strain OC43) related infections in a children's population. Am. J. Epidemiol. *94*:43–49, 1971; and Kaye, H.S., and Dowdle, W.R.: Seroepidemiologic survey of coronavirus (strain 229E) infections in a population of children. Am. J. Epidemiol. *101*:238–244, 1975.

LOWER RESPIRATORY TRACT DISEASE

Asthma and Recurrent Wheezing

Substantial evidence indicates that HCoVs can precipitate asthma attacks.[35, 37, 65, 69, 79, 86] In a 2-year surveillance (1967 to 1969) of 32 mostly atopic children 1 to 5 years of age hospitalized in Denver for severe, recurrent bouts of wheezing, 19 HCoV infections were diagnosed, 16 of them in a typical sharp HCoV epidemic.[65] Six children were infected simultaneously with either parainfluenza virus or respiratory syncytial virus. Of the remaining 13 patients, all were symptomatic: 3 had mild wheezing, and 7 had acute asthma attacks, 2 of which required intravenous therapy. Three patients had pneumonia accompanied by radiographic changes, and four were febrile (>38° C). HCoVs were not as likely to cause wheezing as respiratory syncytial virus was and were more likely to cause only cold-like illnesses and fewer fevers. These findings have been confirmed in several other studies.[69]

Pneumonia and Other Severe Lower Respiratory Tract Infections

Evidence of the etiologic involvement of HCoVs in children hospitalized for lower respiratory tract disease has been more difficult to obtain. For example, among pediatric patients with lower respiratory tract disease at Children's Hospital, Washington, D.C., the incidence of HCoV in ill children, 3.5 percent, was actually lower than that in control patients with nonrespiratory disease, 8.2 percent.[67] In a more recent study of hospitalized patients with acute respiratory disease, HCoV infection was found in only 2 of 83 infants younger than 5 years of age in whom paired sera were available.[23] Better evidence of causation was found in a study of infants hospitalized for lower respiratory tract disease during 1967 to 1970.[63] Infections with both HCoV-229E and HCoV-OC43 were noted, and HCoV was the third most frequently occurring virus (behind respiratory syncytial virus and parainfluenza virus 3), both in incidence and in specific association with pneumonia and bronchiolitis (Table 189–2). Many of these infants required oxygen. HCoV-229E was cultivated from oropharyngeal swabs from two of the infants with pneumonia. In newborns, apnea and bradycardia have been described during coronavirus infection.[94, 95]

HCoV-associated lower respiratory tract disease has been detected in adults. A sharp outbreak of acute respiratory disease sufficient to cause hospitalization of U.S. Marine recruits was attributed at least partially to HCoV-OC43.[111] The clearest association is seen in the elderly with cardiac or chronic obstructive pulmonary disease, in whom infection commonly is associated with lower respiratory tract symptoms, although they rarely lead to hospitalization or death.[11, 25, 29, 96, 107]

TABLE 189–2 ■ RELATIVE INCIDENCE OF VARIOUS RESPIRATORY VIRUS INFECTIONS IN INFANTS WITH PNEUMONIA OR BRONCHIOLITIS, COOK COUNTY HOSPITAL, CHICAGO, ILLINOIS, 1967 TO 1970

	Number of Infants with Indicated Condition Who Were Positive for Virus (%)		
Virus	**Pneumonia**	**Bronchiolitis**	**Total**
Respiratory syncytial	58 (25.1)	48 (32.2)	106 (27.9)
Parainfluenza 3	54 (23.4)	28 (18.8)	82 (21.6)
Coronavirus*	20 (8.7)	10 (6.7)	30 (7.9)
Adenovirus	11 (4.8)	15 (10.1)	26 (6.8)
Parainfluenza 1	11 (4.8)	9 (6.0)	20 (5.3)
Influenza A	10 (4.3)	5 (3.4)	15 (4.0)
Rhinovirus	6 (2.6)	2 (1.3)	8 (2.1)
Parainfluenza 2	3 (1.3)	3 (2.0)	6 (1.6)
Total	126 (55.0)	83 (55.7)	209

Note: Infants were considered positive if virus was recovered or if they had serologic evidence of infection; 231 infants with pneumonia and 149 infants with bronchiolitis were tested. Some infants were positive for more than one virus.
*Both HCV-229E and HCV-OC43.
From McIntosh, K., Chao, R.K., Krause, H.E., et al.: Coronavirus infection in acute lower respiratory tract disease of infants. J. Infect. Dis. *130*:502–507, 1974.

Enteric Human Coronavirus and Torovirus Infections

CORONAVIRUSES

From the earliest descriptions of HCoVs, because of the prominence of coronaviruses as a cause of diarrhea in young calves and pigs, attempts have been made to find coronaviruses in the stool and associate them with enteric disease. The particles that have been seen, often called coronavirus-like particles (CVLPs), have appeared as frequently in stools from well subjects as in those with diarrhea in many studies, and at times they have been difficult to distinguish from cellular membrane fragments. Indeed, their authenticity as viruses has been called into doubt on occasion.[21, 55, 72, 81]

This situation has been confused further by the more recent separation of toroviruses from enteric coronaviruses, although this separation probably will lead ultimately to clarification of this murky field. Many of the specimens that were considered to contain CVLPs in earlier papers may very well have contained toroviruses. At present, electron microscopists think that these virus genera can be distinguished in most instances on the basis of morphology alone,[22] and in many cases the presence of human toroviruses can be confirmed by serologic testing for stool antigens with bovine antisera containing bovine torovirus (Breda virus) antibody.[4, 44, 47]

The first reports of HCoV as a possible cause of human gastroenteritis appeared in 1975; CVLPs were found by electron microscopy in the stools of English adults in three sharp outbreaks of nonbacterial gastroenteritis.[14, 16] In the same year, CVLPs were reported in the stools of healthy adults in India.[60] These rather contrasting publications from England and India heralded the beginning of a continuing controversy on the etiologic importance of these agents as enteric pathogens.[55, 72]

The firmest link of CVLPs to human enteric disease is with gastroenteritis in the very young, especially neonatal necrotizing enterocolitis (NEC). A controlled epidemiologic investigation of NEC was conducted in two hospitals in France, one with and one without an NEC outbreak.[18] Within each hospital, newborns with "no pathologic occurrence" were used as controls. In the NEC-free hospital, no CVLPs were found in the stools of 21 controls, but 2 patients with mild diarrhea had CVLPs. In the NEC hospital, 23 of the 32 (72%) NEC patients had fecal CVLPs, whereas only 3 of 26 (11.5%) controls were positive ($p < .02$). Similarly, CVLPs were observed in infants who were part of a NEC outbreak in a special care nursery in Texas.[88] This outbreak yielded a virus that subsequently has been adapted to growth in tissue culture and to some extent characterized.[53]

In September 1979, an episode of acute, severe (bloody stools, bilious gastric aspirates, abdominal distention) gastroenteritis occurred in a neonatal intensive care unit in Arizona, and several clinical signs were associated significantly with CVLPs in patients' stools.[106] Two children died in this outbreak, and another infant death, with careful electron-microscopic description of coronavirus infection in the distal end of the small bowel, occurred in Oklahoma.[89] In Italy, a case-control study of infants and young children with enteritis found a significant difference in fecal CVLP presence between the ill and control groups: 16.3 percent in ill children and 1.6 percent in controls ($p < .01$).[27]

Despite the foregoing evidence for a causal relationship between CVLPs and gastrointestinal disease, reservation about the role of CVLPs in children's enteric disease still remains, chiefly because CVLPs are found so often in the feces of healthy children, particularly, though not exclusively, in the developing world.[43, 59, 60, 85, 91, 92]

CVLP shedding seems to have little seasonality, even in the endemic southwestern U.S. area.[81]

Attempts have been made to cultivate CVLPs in cell and organ culture and to compare the resultant virus suspensions antigenically with other HCoVs or animal coronaviruses. CVLPs from adults with gastroenteritis were grown in human fetal organ cultures, but no further description of these agents has been reported.[14, 15] As mentioned earlier, another possible enteric HCoV was cultured from a child with NEC, and this virus has been adapted further to growth in a mouse macrophage cell line and mosquito cells.[53] This virus is antigenically unrelated to HCoV-229E and HCoV-OC43. A hemagglutinating coronavirus antigenically and genetically related to a bovine coronavirus, BCV-LY138, has been isolated from a 6-year-old child with severe diarrhea.[115]

TOROVIRUSES

Studies of the clinical manifestations of human torovirus infection are still in their infancy, and certainty of the details is difficult to ascertain. Their pathogenicity still should be considered a matter of some doubt, although the few controlled studies that have been performed have been more consistent than have those of enteric coronaviruses: even though torovirus particles are found in the feces of both symptomatic and asymptomatic individuals, an excess in the former clearly occurs.[36, 45] These studies have included children from Canada and Brazil.

In the study from Brazil, 20 of 91 fecal samples from children in the community with diarrhea contained torovirus antigen detectable by ELISA, and toroviruses were associated significantly with both acute and chronic diarrhea ($p = .02$ in both instances).[45] In the study from Canada, symptomatic and asymptomatic hospitalized children were sampled for fecal viruses: toroviruses were found in 35.0 percent of the former and 14.5 percent of the latter. In comparison to those with stools containing either rotaviruses or astroviruses, torovirus-infected children were older (mean age of 4.0 versus 2.0 years), and their infections more often were acquired nosocomially (57.6% versus 31.3%). Vomiting occurred less commonly with torovirus infection, but occult blood was noted more frequently. A large proportion of symptomatic torovirus infections occurred in immunocompromised children.[36] One case of torovirus found in the feces of a child with acute abdomen has been described.[105]

NEUROLOGIC DISEASES

As described earlier, coronaviruses are the cause of some animal neurologic disorders, including a murine demyelinating disease with some features resembling multiple sclerosis. In humans, a serosurvey of HCoV infection in southern Finland discovered evidence of HCoV-OC43 infection in six patients with acute neurologic episodes, including one with polyradiculitis.[90] Several observations have suggested a possible role of coronavirus infection in multiple sclerosis: (1) isolation of coronaviruses (SK + SD) from the central nervous system tissue of two patients with multiple sclerosis,[10] (2) the demonstration that coronavirus SD can cause demyelination in a primate model,[74] (3) direct visualization of CVLPs in the brain of a patient with multiple sclerosis,[102] and (4) identification by in situ hybridization or PCR of coronavirus RNA in the brains of patients with multiple sclerosis.[3, 73, 100] However, coronaviruses SK and SD are antigenically[26] and genetically[110] very similar to mouse hepatitis virus and were isolated with the use of mouse tissues; the possibility that these isolates were of mouse origin has not been excluded. In addition, other studies have failed to demonstrate coronavirus RNA in the central nervous system tissue of patients with multiple sclerosis[99] or have found such RNA in the same proportion of patients with demyelinating diseases as in controls.[20] Further investigation will be needed to establish whether HCoVs are related causally to any neurologic disease in humans.

Laboratory Diagnosis

VIRUS ISOLATION

Respiratory Coronaviruses

Isolation of HCoVs from clinical material has been limited to a few research laboratories. On primary isolation, some HCoV-229E–type strains will replicate and produce a cytopathic effect in secondary human embryo kidney[31] or certain diploid cell lines: WI-38, MRC-5, and MA-177.[30, 38] The cells become "stringy" after several days' incubation in a roller drum at 33° C or on subsequent passage. However, some HCoV-229E–like strains require organ culture.[49, 57, 87] In contrast, all HCoV-OC43–like strains seem to require organ culture for primary isolation, usually human embryonic trachea or nasal mucosa.

Enteric Coronavirus-like Particles

Growth of these agents in cell or organ culture has been reported,[15, 88, 115] and one isolate has been adapted to growth in tissue culture.[53]

Toroviruses

Human toroviruses have not been grown in any culture system.

VIRUS DETECTION TECHNIQUES

Respiratory Coronaviruses

Respiratory coronaviruses can be sought successfully in clinical samples by direct antigen-detection techniques or by nucleic acid detection. Some evidence that antigens in HCoV-229E and HCoV-OC43 may be representative of the respiratory HCoV group as a whole exists,[57] although this suggestion is not accepted universally. Both immunofluorescence[68, 95] and ELISA have been used successfully for the diagnosis of HCoV infection.[35, 56, 69]

The HCoV genome has been detected successfully both by RNA-RNA hybridization and by reverse transcription PCR. Hybridization has been reported to detect as little as 10 $TCID_{50}$ of virus in nasal washes from volunteers infected with HCoV-229E and to have high specificity as well.[77] PCR amplification of both HCoV-229E and HCoV-OC43 from respiratory secretions also has been described and applied successfully to both nasal washings and middle ear fluid.[76, 82, 83, 93] Few researchers question that these methods will be useful because they are sensitive and specific. In addition, the PCR methodology can use primers that are specific to the HCoV group, but it may pick up infections caused by strains that might be related only distantly to the two prototype strains.[64, 66]

Enteric Coronaviruses

Enteric coronaviruses have been detected primarily by electron microscopy of negatively stained preparations from clarified stool specimens. The possible confusion of coronaviruses and toroviruses in such preparations has been discussed earlier. Immune electron microscopy has been helpful in identifying such viruses in purified preparations, but not directly in stool samples.

An antigen-detection ELISA for enteric coronavirus has been described and applied to fecal specimens from healthy and diarrheal subjects in Thailand.[51, 52] Findings were similar to those of the electron-microscopic stool studies from India: coronavirus excretion was higher in healthy subjects, and excretion of viral antigen was observed occasionally to persist for months. With the adaptation of an antigenically distinct strain of human enteric coronavirus (HEC) to cell culture, constructing antigen-detection systems for further epidemiologic and clinical study of this virus should be possible.[53]

Toroviruses

As with enteric coronaviruses, the primary detection method for toroviruses is electron microscopy of clarified fecal specimens. Torovirus identity can be specified further by either immune electron microscopy or antigen-detection ELISA with the use of antisera prepared against the Breda virus of calves.[4, 44, 45] With increasing experience, electron microscopists can differentiate toroviruses from enteric coronaviruses on the basis of morphology alone.[22, 36]

SERODIAGNOSIS

For respiratory coronaviruses, antigens can be prepared with the use of tissue culture–grown virus or suckling mouse brain preparations. Complement fixation,[17, 63, 67, 71, 90] hemagglutination inhibition (for HCoV-OC43 only),[42] neutralization,[23] ELISA,[13, 28, 46, 56] indirect hemagglutination,[41] and Western blot[84] all have been used.

Serodiagnostic techniques specific for enteric coronaviruses have not been described. Serodiagnosis of torovirus infections has been performed both by immune electron microscopy and by hemagglutination inhibition.[22]

Prevention and Treatment

Even if preparing sufficient antigen for vaccine preparation were possible, the high reinfection rate with these viruses suggests that a vaccine may be ineffective in preventing HCoV-caused respiratory illness. Ribavirin has some in vitro activity against coronavirus and has been shown to reduce hepatitis in mice infected with mouse hepatitis virus, a coronavirus antigenically related to HCoV-OC43.[97]

Acknowledgment

Dr. McIntosh gratefully acknowledges the support of The Bruce R. and Jolene M. McCraw Fund.

REFERENCES

1. Afzelius, B. A.: Ultrastructure of human nasal epithelium during an episode of coronavirus infection. Virchows Arch. *424*:295–300, 1994.
2. Almeida, J. D., and Tyrrell, D. A. J.: The morphology of three previously uncharacterized human respiratory viruses that grow in organ culture. J. Gen. Virol. *1*:175–178, 1967.
3. Arbour, N., Day, R., Newcombe, J., and Talbot, P. J.: Neuroinvasion by human respiratory coronaviruses. J. Virol. *74*:8913–8921, 2000.
4. Beards, G. M., Brown, D. W., Green, J., and Flewett, T. H.: Preliminary characterisation of torovirus-like particles of humans: Comparison with Berne virus of horses and Breda virus of calves. J. Med. Virol. *20*:67–78, 1986.

5. Beards, G. M., Hall, C., Green, J., et al.: An enveloped virus in stools of children and adults with gastroenteritis that resembles the Breda virus of calves. Lancet *1*:1050–1052, 1984.
6. Bende, M., Barrow, I., Heptonstall, J., et al.: Changes in human nasal mucosa during experimental coronavirus common colds. Acta Otolaryngol. *107*:262–269, 1989.
7. Bradburne, A. F.: Antigenic relationships amongst coronaviruses. Arch. Gesamte Virusforsch. *31*:352–364, 1970.
8. Bradburne, A. F., Bynoe, M. L., and Tyrrell, D. A.: Effects of a "new" human respiratory virus in volunteers. B. M. J. *3*:767–769, 1967.
9. Bradburne, A. F., and Somerset, B. A.: Coronavirus antibody titres in sera of healthy adults and experimentally infected volunteers. J. Hyg. (Lond.) *70*:235–244, 1972.
10. Burks, J. S., DeVald, B. L., Jankovsky, L. D., and Gerdes, J. C.: Two coronaviruses isolated from central nervous system tissue of two multiple sclerosis patients. Science *209*:933–934, 1980.
11. Buscho, R. O., Saxtan, D., Shultz, P. S., et al.: Infections with viruses and *Mycoplasma pneumoniae* during exacerbations of chronic bronchitis. J. Infect. Dis. *137*:377–383, 1978.
12. Callow, K. A.: Effect of specific humoral immunity and some non-specific factors on resistance of volunteers to respiratory coronavirus infection. J. Hyg. (Lond.) *95*:173–189, 1985.
13. Callow, K. A., Parry, H. F., Sergeant, M., and Tyrrell, D. A.: The time course of the immune response to experimental coronavirus infection of man. Epidemiol. Infect. *105*:435–446, 1990.
14. Caul, E. O., and Clarke, S. K.: Coronavirus propagated from patient with non-bacterial gastroenteritis. Lancet *2*:953–954, 1975.
15. Caul, E. O. and Egglestone, S. I.: Further studies on human enteric coronaviruses. Arch. Virol. *54*:107–117, 1977.
16. Caul, E. O., Paver, W. K., and Clarke, S. K.: Coronavirus particles in faeces from patients with gastroenteritis. Letter. Lancet. *1*:1192, 1975.
17. Cavallaro, J. J., and Monto, A. S.: Community-wide outbreak of infection with a 229E-like coronavirus in Tecumseh, Michigan. J. Infect. Dis. *122*:272–279, 1970.
18. Chany, C., Moscovici, O., Lebon, P., and Rousset, S.: Association of coronavirus infection with neonatal necrotizing enterocolitis. Pediatrics *69*:209–214, 1982.
19. Cornelissen, L. A., Wierda, C. M., van der Meer, F. J., et al.: Hemagglutinin-esterase, a novel structural protein of torovirus. J. Virol. *71*:5277–5286, 1997.
20. Dessau, R. B., Lisby, G., and Frederiksen, J. L.: Coronaviruses in spinal fluid of patients with acute monosymptomatic optic neuritis. Acta Neurol. Scand. *100*:88–91, 1999.
21. Dourmashkin, R. R., Davies, H. A., Smith, H., and Bird, R. G.: Are coronavirus-like particles seen in diarrhoea stools really viruses? Lancet *2*:971–972, 1980.
22. Duckmanton, L., Luan, B., Devenish, J., et al.: Characterization of torovirus from human fecal specimens. Virology *239*:158–168, 1997.
23. El-Sahly, H. M., Atmar, R. L., Glezen, W. P., and Greenberg, S. B.: Spectrum of clinical illness in hospitalized patients with "common cold" virus infections. Clin. Infect. Dis. *31*:96–100, 2000.
24. Falsey, A. R., McCann, R. M., Hall, W. J., et al.: The "common cold" in frail older persons: Impact of rhinovirus and coronavirus in a senior daycare center. J. Am. Geriatr. Soc. *45*:706–711, 1997.
25. Falsey, A. R., McCann, R. M., Hall, W. J., et al.: Acute respiratory tract infection in daycare centers for older persons. J. Am. Geriatr. Soc. *43*:30–36, 1995.
26. Gerdes, J. C., Klein, I., DeVald, B. L., and Burks, J. S.: Coronavirus isolates SK and SD from multiple sclerosis patients are serologically related to murine coronaviruses A59 and JHM and human coronavirus OC43, but not to human coronavirus 229E. J. Virol. *38*:231–238, 1981.
27. Gerna, G., Passarani, N., Battaglia, M., and Rondanelli, E. G.: Human enteric coronaviruses: Antigenic relatedness to human coronavirus OC43 and possible etiologic role in viral gastroenteritis. J. Infect. Dis. *151*: 796–803, 1985.
28. Gill, E. P., Dominguez, E. A., Greenberg, S. B., et al.: Development and application of an enzyme immunoassay for coronavirus OC43 antibody in acute respiratory illness. J. Clin. Microbiol. *32*:2372–2376, 1994.
29. Gump, D. W., Phillips, C. A., Forsyth, B. R., et al.: Role of infection in chronic bronchitis. Am. Rev. Respir. Dis. *113*:465–474, 1976.
30. Hamre, D., and Beem, M.: Virologic studies of acute respiratory disease in young adults. V. Coronavirus 229E infections during six years of surveillance. Am. J. Epidemiol. *96*:94–106, 1972.
31. Hamre, D., and Procknow, J. J.: A new virus isolated from the human respiratory tract. Proc. Soc. Exp. Biol. Med. *121*:190–193, 1966.
32. Hasony, H. J., and Macnaughton, M. R.: Prevalence of human coronavirus antibody in the population of southern Iraq. J. Med. Virol. *9*:209–216, 1982.
33. Hendley, J. O., Fishburne, H. B., and Gwaltney, J. M.: Coronavirus infections in working adults. Eight-year study with 229 E and OC 43. Am. Rev. Respir. Dis. *105*:805–811, 1972.
34. Herold, J., Raabe, T., and Siddell, S.: Molecular analysis of the human coronavirus (strain 229E) genome. Arch. Virol. Suppl. 7:63–74, 1993.
35. Isaacs, D., Flowers, D., Clarke, J. R., et al.: Epidemiology of coronavirus respiratory infections. Arch. Dis. Child. *58*:500–503, 1983.
36. Jamieson, F. B., Wang, E. E., Bain, C., et al.: Human torovirus: A new nosocomial gastrointestinal pathogen. J. Infect. Dis. *178*:1263–1269, 1998.
37. Johnston, S. L., Pattemore, P. K., Sanderson, G., et al.: Community study of role of viral infections in exacerbations of asthma in 9–11 year old children. B. M. J. *310*:1225–1229, 1995.
38. Kapikian, A. Z., James, H. D., Kelly, S. J., et al.: Isolation from man of "avian infectious bronchitis virus–like" viruses (coronaviruses) similar to 229E virus, with some epidemiological observations. J. Infect. Dis. *119*: 282–290, 1969.
39. Kapikian, A. Z., James, H. D., Jr., Kelly, S. J., et al.: Hemadsorption by coronavirus strain OC43. Proc. Soc. Exp. Biol. Med. *139*:179–186, 1972.
40. Kaye, H. S., and Dowdle, W. R.: Some characteristics of hemagglutination of certain strains of "IBV-like" virus. J. Infect. Dis. *120*:576–581, 1969.
41. Kaye, H. S., and Dowdle, W. R.: Seroepidemiologic survey of coronavirus (strain 229E) infections in a population of children. Am. J. Epidemiol. *101*:238–244, 1975.
42. Kaye, H. S., Marsh, H. B., and Dowdle, W. R.: Seroepidemiologic survey of coronavirus (strain OC 43) related infections in a children's population. Am. J. Epidemiol. *94*:43–49, 1971.
43. Kidd, A. H., Esrey, S. A., and Ujfalusi, M. J.: Shedding of coronavirus-like particles by children in Lesotho. J. Med. Virol. *27*:164–169, 1989.
44. Koopmans, M., Petric, M., Glass, R. I., and Monroe, S. S.: Enzyme-linked immunosorbent assay reactivity of torovirus-like particles in fecal specimens from humans with diarrhea. J. Clin. Microbiol. *31*:2738–2744, 1993.
45. Koopmans, M. P., Goosen, E. S., Lima, A. A., et al.: Association of torovirus with acute and persistent diarrhea in children. Pediatr. Infect. Dis. J. *16*:504–507, 1997.
46. Kraaijeveld, C. A., Reed, S. E., and Macnaughton, M. R.: Enzyme-linked immunosorbent assay for detection of antibody in volunteers experimentally infected with human coronavirus strain 229 E. J. Clin. Microbiol. *12*:493–497, 1980.
47. Krishnan, T., and Naik, T. N.: Electron-microscopic evidence of torovirus like particles in children with diarrhoea. Indian J. Med. Res. *105*:108–110, 1997.
48. Lai, M. M., and Holmes, K. V.: Coronaviridae: The viruses and their replication. *In* Knipe, D. M., Howley, P. M., Griffin, D. E., et al. (eds.): Fields Virology. Philadelphia, Lippincott-Raven, 2001.
49. Larson, H. E., Reed, S. E., and Tyrrell, D. A.: Isolation of rhinoviruses and coronaviruses from 38 colds in adults. J. Med. Virol. *5*:221–229, 1980.
50. Lee, H. J., Shieh, C. K., Gorbalenya, A. E., et al.: The complete sequence (22 kilobases) of murine coronavirus gene 1 encoding the putative proteases and RNA polymerase. Virology *180*:567–582, 1991.
51. Leechanachai, P., Yoosook, C., and Matangkasombut, P.: Epidemiological study of enteric coronavirus excretion by an enzyme-linked immunosorbent assay. J. Med. Assoc. Thai. *72*:452–457, 1989.
52. Leechanachai, P., Yoosook, C., Saguanwongse, S., and Matangkasombut, P.: Comparison of a modified enzyme-linked immunosorbent assay with immunosorbent electron microscopy to detect coronavirus in human faecal specimens. J. Diarrhoeal Dis. Res. *5*:24–29, 1987.
53. Luby, J. P., Clinton, R., and Kurtz, S.: Adaptation of human enteric coronavirus to growth in cell lines. J. Clin. Virol. *12*:43–51, 1999.
54. Macnaughton, M. R.: Occurrence and frequency of coronavirus infections in humans as determined by enzyme-linked immunosorbent assay. Infect. Immun. *38*:419–423, 1982.
55. Macnaughton, M. R., and Davies, H. A.: Human enteric coronaviruses. Brief review. Arch. Virol. *70*:301–313, 1981.
56. Macnaughton, M. R., Flowers, D., and Isaacs, D.: Diagnosis of human coronavirus infections in children using enzyme-linked immunosorbent assay. J. Med. Virol. *11*:319–325, 1983.
57. Macnaughton, M. R., Madge, M. H., and Reed, S. E.: Two antigenic groups of human coronaviruses detected by using enzyme-linked immunosorbent assay. Infect. Immun. *33*:734–737, 1981.
58. Makela, M. J., Puhakka, T., Ruuskanen, O., et al.: Viruses and bacteria in the etiology of the common cold. J. Clin. Microbiol. *36*:539–542, 1998.
59. Marshall, J. A., Birch, C. J., Williamson, H. G., et al.: Coronavirus-like particles and other agents in the faeces of children in Efate, Vanuatu. J. Trop. Med. Hyg. *85*:213–215, 1982.
60. Mathan, M., Mathan, V. I., Swaminathan, S. P., and Yesudoss, S.: Pleomorphic virus-like particles in human faeces. Lancet *1*:1068–1069, 1975.
61. McIntosh, K.: Coronaviruses: A comparative review. Curr. Top. Microbiol. Immunol. *63*:83–129, 1974.
62. McIntosh, K., Becker, W. B., and Chanock, R. M.: Growth in suckling-mouse brain of "IBV-like" viruses from patients with upper respiratory tract disease. Proc. Natl. Acad. Sci. U.S.A. *58*:2268–2273, 1967.
63. McIntosh, K., Chao, R. K., Krause, H. E., et al.: Coronavirus infection in acute lower respiratory tract disease of infants. J. Infect. Dis. *130*:502–507, 1974.
64. McIntosh, K., Dees, J. H., Becker, W. B., et al.: Recovery in tracheal organ cultures of novel viruses from patients with respiratory disease. Proc. Natl. Acad. Sci. U.S.A. *57*:933–940, 1967.
65. McIntosh, K., Ellis, E. F., Hoffman, L. S., et al.: Association of viral and bacterial respiratory infection with exacerbations of wheezing in young asthmatic children. Chest *63*(Suppl.):43, 1973.

66. McIntosh, K., Kapikian, A. Z., Hardison, K. A., et al.: Antigenic relationships among the coronaviruses of man and between human and animal coronaviruses. J. Immunol. *102*:1109–1118, 1969.
67. McIntosh, K., Kapikian, A. Z., Turner, H. C., et al.: Seroepidemiologic studies of coronavirus infection in adults and children. Am. J. Epidemiol. *91*:585–592, 1970.
68. McIntosh, K., McQuillin, J., Reed, S. E., and Gardner, P. S.: Diagnosis of human coronavirus infection by immunofluorescence: Method and application to respiratory disease in hospitalized children. J. Med. Virol. *2*:341–346, 1978.
69. Mertsola, J., Ziegler, T., Ruuskanen, O., et al.: Recurrent wheezy bronchitis and viral respiratory infections. Arch. Dis. Child. *66*:124–129, 1991.
70. Monto, A. S.: Medical reviews. Coronaviruses. Yale J. Biol. Med. *47*:234–251, 1974.
71. Monto, A. S., and Lim, S. K.: The Tecumseh study of respiratory illness. VI. Frequency of and relationship between outbreaks of coronavirus infection. J. Infect. Dis. *129*:271–276, 1974.
72. Mortensen, M. L., Ray, C. G., Payne, C. M., et al.: Coronaviruslike particles in human gastrointestinal disease. Epidemiologic, clinical, and laboratory observations. Am. J. Dis. Child. *139*:928–934, 1985.
73. Murray, R. S., Brown, B., Brian, D., and Cabirac, G. F.: Detection of coronavirus RNA and antigen in multiple sclerosis brain. Ann. Neurol. *31*:525–533, 1992.
74. Murray, R. S., Cai, G. Y., Hoel, K., et al.: Coronavirus infects and causes demyelination in primate central nervous system. Virology *188*:274–284, 1992.
75. Myint, S., Harmsen, D., Raabe, T., and Siddell, S. G.: Characterization of a nucleic acid probe for the diagnosis of human coronavirus 229E infections. J. Med. Virol. *31*:165–172, 1990.
76. Myint, S., Johnston, S., Sanderson, G., and Simpson, H.: Evaluation of nested polymerase chain methods for the detection of human coronaviruses 229E and OC43. Mol. Cell. Probes *8*:357–364, 1994.
77. Myint, S., Siddell, S., and Tyrrell, D.: Detection of human coronavirus 229E in nasal washings using RNA:RNA hybridisation. J. Med. Virol. *29*:70–73, 1989.
78. Nicholson, K. G., Kent, J., Hammersley, V., and Cancio, E.: Acute viral infections of upper respiratory tract in elderly people living in the community: Comparative, prospective, population based study of disease burden. B. M. J. *315*:1060–1064, 1997.
79. Pattemore, P. K., Johnston, S. L., and Bardin, P. G.: Viruses as precipitants of asthma symptoms. I. Epidemiology. Clin. Exp. Allergy *22*:325–336, 1992.
80. Patterson, S., and Macnaughton, M. R.: Replication of human respiratory coronavirus strain 229E in human macrophages. J. Gen. Virol. *60*:307–314, 1982.
81. Payne, C. M., Ray, C. G., Borduin, V., et al.: An eight-year study of the viral agents of acute gastroenteritis in humans: Ultrastructural observations and seasonal distribution with a major emphasis on coronavirus-like particles. Diagn. Microbiol. Infect. Dis. *5*:39–54, 1986.
82. Pitkaranta, A., Jero, J., Arruda, E., et al.: Polymerase chain reaction–based detection of rhinovirus, respiratory syncytial virus, and coronavirus in otitis media with effusion. J. Pediatr. *133*:390–394, 1998.
83. Pitkaranta, A., Virolainen, A., Jero, J., et al.: Detection of rhinovirus, respiratory syncytial virus, and coronavirus infections in acute otitis media by reverse transcriptase polymerase chain reaction. Pediatrics *102*:291–295, 1998.
84. Pohl-Koppe, A., Raabe, T., Siddell, S. G., and ter Meulen, V.: Detection of human coronavirus 229E–specific antibodies using recombinant fusion proteins. J. Virol. Methods *55*:175–183, 1995.
85. Puel, J. M., Orillac, M. S., Bauriaud, R. M., et al.: Occurrence of viruses in human stools in the Ahaggar (Alberia). J. Hyg. (Lond.) *89*:171–174, 1982.
86. Rakes, G. P., Arruda, E., Ingram, J. M., et al.: Rhinovirus and respiratory syncytial virus in wheezing children requiring emergency care. IgE and eosinophil analyses. Am. J. Respir. Crit. Care. Med. *159*:785–790, 1999.
87. Reed, S. E.: The behaviour of recent isolates of human respiratory coronavirus in vitro and in volunteers: Evidence of heterogeneity among 229E-related strains. J. Med. Virol. *13*:179–192, 1984.
88. Resta, S., Luby, J. P., Rosenfeld, C. R., and Siegel, J. D.: Isolation and propagation of a human enteric coronavirus. Science *229*:978–981, 1985.
89. Rettig, P. J., and Altshuler, G. P.: Fatal gastroenteritis associated with coronaviruslike particles. Am. J. Dis. Child. *139*:245–248, 1985.
90. Riski, H., and Hovi, T.: Coronavirus infections of man associated with diseases other than the common cold. J. Med. Virol. *6*:259–265, 1980.
91. Schnagl, R. D., Holmes, I. H., and Mackay-Scollay, E. M.: Coronavirus-like particles in Aboriginals and non-Aboriginals in Western Australia. Med. J. Aust. *1*:307–309, 1978.
92. Sitbon, M.: Human-enteric-coronaviruslike particles (CVLP) with different epidemiological characteristics. J. Med. Virol. *16*:67–76, 1985.
93. Sizun, J., Arbour, N., and Talbot, P. J.: Comparison of immunofluorescence with monoclonal antibodies and RT-PCR for the detection of human coronaviruses 229E and OC43 in cell culture. J. Virol. Methods *72*:145–152, 1998.
94. Sizun, J., Soupre, D., Giroux, J. D., et al.: Nasal colonization with coronavirus and apnea of the premature newborn. Acta Paediatr. *82*:238, 1993.
95. Sizun, J., Soupre, D., Legrand, M. C., et al.: Neonatal nosocomial respiratory infection with coronavirus: A prospective study in a neonatal intensive care unit. Acta Paediatr. *84*:617–620, 1995.
96. Smith, C. B., Golden, C. A., Kanner, R. E., and Renzetti, A. D.: Association of viral and *Mycoplasma pneumoniae* infections with acute respiratory illness in patients with chronic obstructive pulmonary diseases. Am. Rev. Respir. Dis. *121*:225–232, 1980.
97. Smith, R. A., and Kirkpatrick, W.: Ribavirin, Broad Spectrum Antiviral Agent. New York, Academic, 1980.
98. Snijder, E. J., and Horzinek, M. C.: Toroviruses: Replication, evolution and comparison with other members of the coronavirus-like superfamily. J. Gen. Virol. *74*:2305–2316, 1993.
99. Sorensen, O., Collins, A., Flintoff, W., et al.: Probing for the human coronavirus OC43 in multiple sclerosis. Neurology *36*:1604–1606, 1986.
100. Stewart, J. N., Mounir, S., and Talbot, P. J.: Human coronavirus gene expression in the brains of multiple sclerosis patients. Virology *191*:502–505, 1992.
101. Stohlman, S. A., and Hinton, D. R.: Viral induced demyelination. Brain Pathol. *11*:92–106, 2001.
102. Tanaka, R., Iwasaki, Y., and Koprowski, H.: Intracisternal virus-like particles in brain of a multiple sclerosis patient. J. Neurol. Sci. *28*:121–126, 1976.
103. Tyrrell, D. A., Almeida, J. D., Cunningham, C. H., et al.: Coronaviridae. Intervirology *5*:76–82, 1975.
104. Tyrrell, D. A. J., and Bynoe, M. L.: Cultivation of a novel type of common-cold virus in organ cultures. B. M. J. *1*:1467–1470, 1965.
105. Uziel, Y., Laxer, R. M., and Petric, M.: Torovirus gastroenteritis presenting as acute abdomen. Clin. Infect. Dis. *28*:925–926, 1999.
106. Vaucher, Y. E., Ray, C. G., Minnich, L. L., et al.: Pleomorphic, enveloped, virus-like particles associated with gastrointestinal illness in neonates. J. Infect. Dis. *145*:27–36, 1982.
107. Walsh, E. E., Falsey, A. R., and Hennessey, P. A.: Respiratory syncytial and other virus infections in persons with chronic cardiopulmonary disease. Am. J. Respir. Crit. Care Med. *160*:791–795, 1999.
108. Weiss, M., and Horzinek, M. C.: The proposed family Toroviridae: Agents of enteric infections. Brief review. Arch. Virol. *92*:1–15, 1987.
109. Weiss, M., Steck, F., and Horzinek, M. C.: Purification and partial characterization of a new enveloped RNA virus (Berne virus). J. Gen. Virol. *64*:1849–1858, 1983.
110. Weiss, S. R.: Coronaviruses SD and SK share extensive nucleotide homology with murine coronavirus MHV-A59, more than that shared between human and murine coronaviruses. Virology *126*:669–677, 1983.
111. Wenzel, R. P., Hendley, J. O., Davies, J. A., and Gwaltney, J. M.: Coronavirus infections in military recruits. Three-year study with coronavirus strains OC43 and 229E. Am. Rev. Respir. Dis. *109*:621–624, 1974.
112. Winther, B., Gwaltney, J. M., and Hendley, J. O.: Respiratory virus infection of monolayer cultures of human nasal epithelial cells. Am. Rev. Respir. Dis. *141*:839–845, 1990.
113. Woode, G. N., Reed, D. E., Runnels, P. L., et al.: Studies with an unclassified virus isolated from diarrheic calves. Vet. Microbiol. *7*:221–240, 1982.
114. Yeager, C. L., Ashmun, R. A., Williams, R. K., et al.: Human aminopeptidase N is a receptor for human coronavirus 229E. Nature *357*:420–422, 1992.
115. Zhang, X. M., Herbst, W., Kousoulas, K. G., and Storz, J.: Biological and genetic characterization of a hemagglutinating coronavirus isolated from a diarrhoeic child. J. Med. Virol. *44*:152–161, 1994.

CHAPTER **189B**

Severe Acute Respiratory Syndrome (SARS)

ELLIS K. L. HON ■ ALBERT M. LI ■ EDMUND A. S. NELSON ■ CHI WAI LEUNG ■ JAMES D. CHERRY

Severe acute respiratory syndrome (SARS) is a new infectious disease that had its origin in Guangdong Province, China, in the fall of 2002. New information about the epidemiology, etiology, clinical manifestations, and treatment of SARS has been and is being gathered at an unprecedented rate; hence, this chapter, which was written in April 2003 and edited in June 2003, will be incomplete in many areas at the time this book is published. However, the pediatric clinical data reflect the first-hand experience of four of the authors.

The syndrome is associated with considerable morbidity and mortality, and its severity appears to be more marked in adults than in young children.

History

The disease first appeared as an apparent outbreak of atypical pneumonia in Guangdong Province in southern China.[20] The first case of SARS occurred in mid-November 2002 in Foshan City. The Chinese Ministry of Health reported 305 cases, which included 105 health care workers and 5 deaths, occurring between mid-November 2002 and February 9, 2003, in six municipalities in Guangdong Province.

SARS then spread to Hong Kong, where the first recognized case was admitted to a hospital on February 22, 2003. The patient was a 64-year-old male physician from Zhongshan University in Guangdong Province, who, before he was hospitalized, stayed in a Hong Kong hotel for 1 day. Eight guests who stayed on the same floor and two others who stayed on different floors of the hotel acquired the disease, which led to outbreaks of SARS in other countries when they returned home or traveled to other countries. Specifically, secondary cases occurred in two Hong Kong hospitals, and outbreaks in Singapore, Toronto, and Hanoi were observed. As of June 4, 2003, 8402 cases of SARS and 772 deaths from SARS had been reported to the World Health Organization (WHO) from 30 countries and two special administrative regions of China.[22]

Etiology

Poutanen and associates[16] published the results from a study of 10 adult patients with SARS seen in Toronto, Canada, in March 2003. They carried out an extensive search for virus, mycoplasma, chlamydia, rickettsia, bacteria, and fungi. Human metapneumovirus was found by nested polymerase chain reaction (PCR) in bronchoalveolar lavage fluid and nasopharyngeal swabs from five patients. A novel coronavirus was isolated in Vero cell cultures of respiratory specimens from five patients; four of the five patients with coronavirus isolations also had positive PCR results for human metapneumovirus. Subsequently, a novel coronavirus was identified in respiratory specimens from patients with SARS in several countries in WHO network and other laboratories.[4, 8, 12, 21] The coronavirus has a cytopathic effect (CPE) in Vero and FRnK-4 cells, and it can be identified by a reverse transcriptase PCR (RT-PCR) in respiratory specimens. Antibody to this coronavirus can be detected in sera from patients by indirect fluorescent antibody (IFA) testing and enzyme-linked immunosorbent assays (ELISA).[4, 16] Hyperimmune sera against numerous animal coronaviruses and the human 229E coronavirus inhibit the growth of this new coronavirus in tissue culture.

This newly discovered coronavirus is the causative agent of SARS. However, the role of other agents as cofactors is not clear at the present time. Of interest with regard to coronaviruses is that they have a high frequency of recombination.[10, 13] Hence, this new coronavirus possibly has arisen by a reassortment of genes between human and animal coronaviruses during a chance simultaneous infection. The genome of this novel coronavirus (SARS-CoV) has been sequenced.[15, 17] It is approximately 29,750 nucleotides in length, and it has 11 open reading frames. It is similar to other coronaviruses, but it is not closely related to any of the previously characterized human, mammalian, or avian coronaviruses.

Epidemiology

As of June 2003, providing an accurate and complete description of the epidemiology of SARS is impossible. SARS is, however, the first severe and relatively easily transmissible new disease to emerge in the 21st century.[9] In the last century, major influenza A pandemics occurred in 1918, 1957, and 1968, although with the possible exception of the 1918 experience none of these pandemics occurred in totally immunologically virgin human populations.[2] In the mid-1950s, pandemic infection and disease caused by echovirus 9 occurred.[6] Because echovirus 9 apparently was a new virus at that time, the entire world population was susceptible, and over a period of approximately 4 years everyone became infected. Fortunately, in that pandemic disease, mortality and residual morbidity were rare occurrences.

At present, SARS is of major concern because it has a high case-fatality rate of approximately 9 percent, and the entire world population lacks immunity to the coronavirus that is the causative agent.

The incubation period of SARS is 2 to 10 days, with most cases occurring 2 to 7 days after exposure. Most transmissions have been person-to-person through respiratory secretions. Because the coronavirus also has been isolated from feces, fecal-oral or fecal-nasal routes of transmission seem possible as well. In addition, large clusters of cases have suggested the possibility of environmental contamination via sewage or ventilation systems.[9]

A cluster of more than 300 cases linked to a single building in an estate of high-rise apartment buildings in Hong Kong has been noted. Transmission occurred in this building not only among persons living on the same floor but also among persons living on different floors.

Another interesting observation has been the finding of "super spreaders." A super spreader is a patient who apparently has infected a large number of persons. For example, a large cluster of cases in health care workers in Singapore may have been related to contact with a single patient with kidney disease and diabetes. Another possible super spreader in Guangdong, China, may have infected as many as 100 other persons.

As of April 2003, most of the reported cases in the WHO database had occurred in adults, and a large number of secondary cases had occurred in health care workers. The experience of four of the authors from Hong Kong indicates that pediatric cases may play a significant role in the epidemiology of SARS. However, because infection in young children appears to be less severe, these cases may be overlooked, as they could blend with other common respiratory infectious illnesses.

Apparent death rates have varied considerably among geographic areas. These differences may relate to medical care issues, host factors, or perhaps the role of cofactors in disease. In Toronto, the death rate was particularly high, and four of nine patients were found to be infected with both the novel coronavirus and metapneumovirus.[16]

The progression of the present outbreak depends on several factors that affect the epidemic potential of specific infectious agents and includes season, geography, climate, routes of transmission, infectious dose, and effectiveness of preventive measures.

Pathophysiology

From available studies involving adults and some children, the primary site of pathology clearly is the respiratory tract, with bilateral and patchy airspace consolidation in the lungs.[1, 14, 16, 18] In addition, viremia or toxemia is suggested by the presence of lymphopenia and elevated serum enzyme values (ALT, aspartate transaminase [AST], creatine phosphokinase [CPK], and lactate dehydrogenase [LDH]).

Postmortem findings in two cases showed gross consolidation of the lungs and diffuse alveolar damage with pulmonary edema and hyaline membrane formation.[14] Other areas had cellular fibromyxoid organizing exudates in the airspaces. Interstitial spaces had only mild lymphocytic infiltrates. Vacuolated and multinucleated pneumocytes also were noted. In another study, similar findings were noted.[18]

Clinical Presentation

This analysis is based on observations of the first 10 pediatric patients, 5 children and 5 adolescents, hospitalized in two Hong Kong hospitals in March 2003.[11] All cases had histories of contact: household contact in five, contact with health care workers in three, and exposure to a widespread community outbreak in a densely populated residential estate in two. Three children and two adolescents had direct contact with index adult family members with SARS. Five adult index patients had very severe SARS and required intensive care. Two patterns of illness were apparent. In adolescents, SARS is similar to the illness in adults. In contrast, the illness in children has a less severe presentation with no or minimal systemic manifestations except fever, although evidence of pneumonia is present on chest radiographs.

CHILDREN

All five children had fever and were febrile for 1 to 4 days before hospital admission. Other features present on admission included coryza in three patients and cough in four patients. One child had a febrile convulsion, and one child had dizziness. None of the five children had sore throat, chills/rigor, myalgia, or headache.

All children had evidence of pneumonia on initial chest radiographs. In four of the children, focal segmental consolidations were seen on initial radiographs, and one child had an ill-defined patchy consolidation. Computed tomography (CT) of the thorax performed on this patient showed multifocal airspace consolidations, and the features of peripheral and alveolar opacities had the radiologic appearance of bronchiolitis obliterans organizing pneumonia (Fig. 189–3). All five patients had mild progressive consolidative changes on serial chest radiographs, but complete resolution occurred within 14 days. The typical radiographic changes in one of the patients are illustrated in Figure 189–4. None of the children had abnormal interstitial patterns, bronchial dilatation, pleural effusion, cavitation, or mediastinal lymphadenopathy.

In spite of the radiographic findings, wheezing and inspiratory rales were absent or not prominent on physical examination. None of the five patients developed evidence of severe respiratory distress throughout the course of their illnesses, and none was administered supplemental oxygen. The duration of fever was 3 to 7 days. The most impressive laboratory finding was leukopenia with an absolute lymphopenia. The median lowest lymphocyte count was 1.1×10^9/L. Lymphopenia occurred 3 to 4 days after the onset of fever. Two children had modestly low platelet counts. LDH levels were mildly elevated in all five children, but only one child had an elevated CPK value and the ALT values were normal in all five children.

RT-PCR for the novel coronavirus was performed on a nasopharyngeal aspirate specimen from one child and was positive. Thus, although all these children had appropriate contact history and met the clinical case definition of SARS, they possibly might not all have had disease caused by the coronavirus.

ADOLESCENTS

In contrast with the children, all five of the adolescents presented with chills and rigor as well as fever. Four of the five also had cough, myalgia, and headache, and three had coryza. Other complaints included nausea in two patients and abdominal pain in one patient.

Three patients had bilateral lower lobe opacifications on radiographs at the time of admission. These consolidative changes progressed rapidly within days. Despite clinical improvement, the consolidative changes persisted into the second week of the illness. One patient had mild focal airspace consolidation similar to that seen in the CT scan of the 2-year-old boy shown in Figure 189–3. Complete resolution occurred within 14 days in this adolescent. Another patient did not have any radiographic changes at presentation, but high-resolution CT confirmed the presence of focal consolidation in the right lower lobe. This patient did not have any signs of airspace consolidation in the subsequent serial radiographs.

The hematologic manifestations in the teenagers were more marked than those in the children. The lowest total

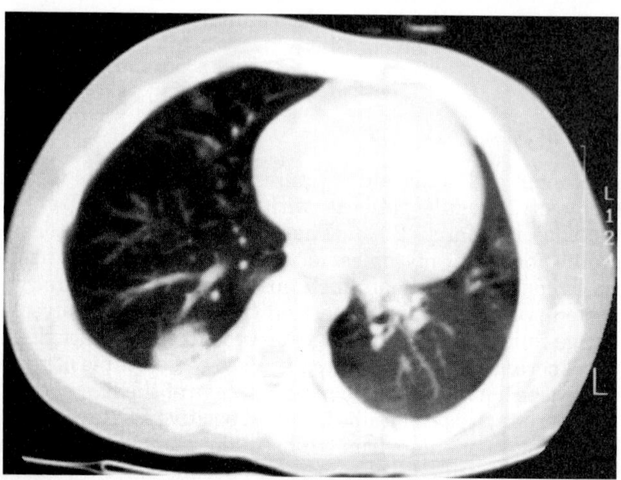

FIGURE 189–3 ■ One frame of a CT scan in a 2-year-old boy. The CT study showed multiple areas of consolidation in the perihilar and subpleural regions and a ground glass opacification that was prominent in the posterior aspects of the lungs.

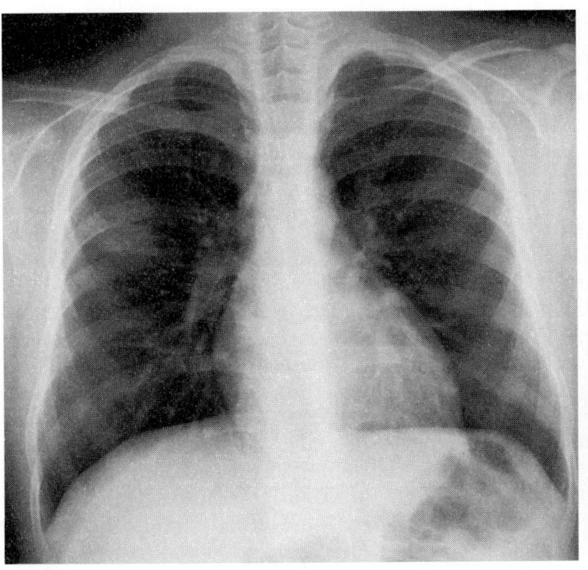
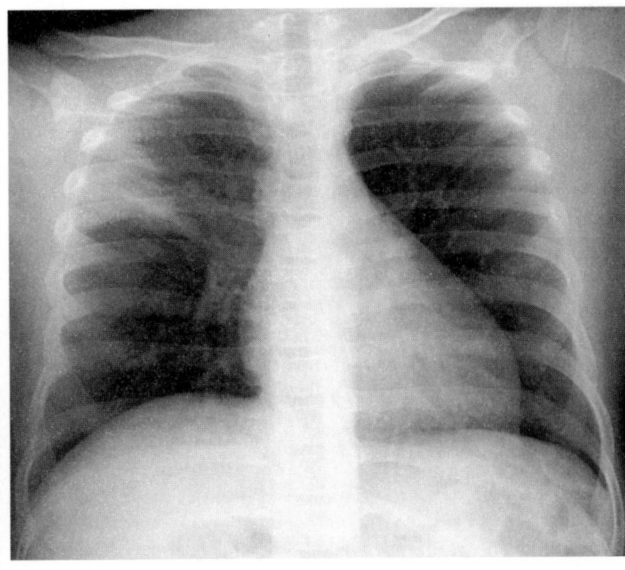

A B

FIGURE 189–4 ■ Serial chest radiographs in a 7½-year-old boy who presented with fever and cough. *A,* Radiograph at presentation shows an ill-defined airspace consolidation in the periphery of the right upper lobe that abuts the horizontal fissure. *B,* This finding was followed by an increased consolidation in the right upper lung field on day 5. Complete resolution of the airspace consolidation occurred by day 14 (not shown). (From Hon, K. L. E., Leung, C. W., Cheng, W. T. F., et al.: Clinical presentations and outcome of severe acute respiratory syndrome in children. Lancet *361*:1701, 2003.)

leukocyte count varied between 1.7 and 4.7 × 10^9/L, and the lymphocyte counts were between 0.3 and 0.8 × 10^9/L. Two of the five had modestly low platelet counts. All adolescents had mildly elevated ALT values, and four had mildly elevated LDH values. Only one patient had a slightly elevated CPK value. RT-PCR for the novel coronavirus was positive in three of five nasopharyngeal aspirate specimens. Four of the five teenagers developed respiratory distress and oxygen desaturation between days 4 and 7 after the onset of fever. Two patients required oxygen supplementation through nasal cannula (2–3 L/min). One patient required bilevel positive airway pressure (BiPAP) support for 5 days. Another patient required intubation and mechanical ventilatory support for 4 days. The highest oxygen requirement for the latter two patients was 50 percent. All patients recovered.

Differential Diagnosis

The differential diagnosis of SARS in children includes the many viral, bacterial, mycoplasmal, and chlamydial agents that cause acute febrile respiratory illnesses in children (see Chapters 23, 25, 26, 27, 161, 181, 182, 185, 189, 194, and 196). Particularly important to consider are agents that cause acute febrile respiratory illnesses in both adults and children. These agents include influenza viruses A and B, several adenoviral types, *Chlamydia pneumoniae, Chlamydia psittaci, Mycoplasma pneumoniae,* and *Legionella pneumophila.*

Specific Diagnosis

For surveillance purposes, both the WHO and the Centers for Disease Control and Prevention (CDC) have developed case definitions.[5, 19] The CDC definition of a suspected case as of March 22, 2003, was as follows:

Respiratory illness of unknown etiology with onset since February 1, 2003, and the following criteria:

- Measured temperature greater than 100.4° F (> 38.0° C)
- One or more clinical findings of respiratory illness (e.g., cough, shortness of breath, difficulty breathing, hypoxia, or radiographic findings of either pneumonia or acute respiratory distress syndrome)
- Travel within 10 days of onset of symptoms to an area with suspected or documented community transmission of SARS (Hong Kong Special Administrative Region and Guangdong Province, China; Hanoi, Vietnam; and Singapore) (excluding areas with secondary cases limited to health care workers or direct household contacts)

or

- Close contact (close contact is defined as having cared for, having lived with, or having had direct contact with respiratory secretions and/or body fluids of a patient suspected of having SARS) within 10 days of onset of symptoms with either a person with a respiratory illness and travel to a SARS area or a person under investigation or suspected of having SARS

Suspected cases with either radiographic evidence of pneumonia or respiratory distress syndrome or evidence of unexplained respiratory distress syndrome by autopsy were designated “probable” cases by the WHO case definition.

Definitive etiologic diagnosis can be established by the identification of the coronavirus in respiratory specimens by RT-PCR or the isolation of the organism in tissue culture. The identification of infection also can be determined by demonstrating specific antibody in sera by IFA or ELISA.[4, 8, 12, 21] Most convincing is the demonstration of seroconversion by studied paired acute-phase and convalescent-phase sera.

SARS should be suspected strongly in a previously healthy patient who has pneumonia and marked lymphopenia.

Treatment

As of April 2003, three case series of adult patients with SARS in which treatment data are presented have been published.[14, 16, 18] Two series are from Hong Kong,[14, 18] and one is from

Canada.[16] In the two series from Hong Kong, all patients were treated with broad-spectrum antibacterial agents, oseltamivir, ribavirin, and corticosteroids. In the series from Canada, the patients received similar therapy except that they were not administered corticosteroids. The 10 pediatric cases noted here all received treatment programs similar to the programs of the adults in Hong Kong except that oseltamivir was not used. Intravenous cefotaxime (25–50 mg/kg/dose, every 6 or 8 hours), oral clarithromycin (15 mg/kg/day, to a maximum dose of 250 mg twice daily), and oral ribavirin (40 mg/kg/day, in 2 or 3 divided doses) were started if a clinical diagnosis of SARS was suspected on admission. Oral prednisolone (0.5 mg/kg/day at one hospital and 2 mg/kg/day at the other hospital) was added if no decrease in fever or improvement in the general well-being of the patient had occurred within 48 hours. If the child was admitted with moderately severe symptoms of high swinging fever and marked malaise, intravenous ribavirin (20 mg/kg/day, in 3 divided doses) and intravenous hydrocortisone (2 mg/kg/dose, every 6 hours) in addition to antibacterial therapy was administered immediately after admission. For patients with persistent fever and progressive clinical or radiologic deterioration, pulse intravenous methylprednisolone (10 to 20 mg/kg/dose) was administered. The decision to provide further pulsed treatment was based on clinical response. Antibacterial agents were discontinued 5 days after defervescence. Ribavirin was administered for 1 to 2 weeks, and corticosteroid was tapered over the course of 2 to 4 weeks, depending on clinical response and radiologic resolution.

Legitimate concerns exist with regard to the use of corticosteroids in the treatment of SARS. Corticosteroid treatment increases the severity of illness and rate of death in many primary viral illnesses such as measles and varicella. As SARS appears to be a primary viral infection caused by a new coronavirus, one might expect that corticosteroids would increase viral load early in infection. The indication for corticosteroid use in severe infectious diseases is the need to decrease inflammation caused by excessive cytokine responses by the host; the rationale for the use of steroids for SARS patients in Hong Kong has been the belief that the severe lung damage is the result of a "cytokine storm" similar to that observed in influenza A subtype H5N1 infection.[7] However, the severe lymphopenia commonly noted in SARS suggests that the inflammatory response already is suppressed. If the above speculation were correct, one would expect a worsening of disease due to the corticosteroid treatment. At present, no evidence shows that worsening has occurred, but this may be explained by an antiviral effect of ribavirin, which has been administered concurrently in all cases.

Because all patients with SARS have pneumonia, one might assume that ribavirin treatment would be more effective if administered by small particle aerosol generator, as this method has been recommended previously for the treatment of respiratory syncytial viral infections in infants and young children (see Chapters 25 and 185). However, this method of administration was not considered in Hong Kong because the first major outbreak of SARS appeared to have been accentuated by the use of a nebulizer on a general ward.[14]

Prognosis

The overall prognosis in children with SARS appears to be good. However, a small number of children have required time in the intensive care unit and mechanical ventilation. The extent of lung damage in recovered children is not known.

Prevention

The mainstay of prevention of SARS is effective hospital infection control practices and quarantine procedures outside hospitals. In retrospect, many secondary cases of SARS in health care personnel were preventable. Unfortunately, the vast majority of hospitals today have not been designed to handle epidemic diseases that are transmitted by the respiratory route. Patients with respiratory illnesses consistent with SARS should be isolated at triage and placed in a negative air pressure room for treatment. Because SARS is spread by the respiratory route and because the nose, mouth, and eyes are sites for primary infection, health care workers should wear masks and goggles while tending patients. Because fomites appear to be important factors in the transmission of other respiratory viruses, medical equipment should be restricted to patient rooms or adequately disinfected after patient contact. Finally, adequate hand-washing before and after patient contact is essential.

Throughout history, quarantines (restraining the movement of people to prevent the spread of infectious disease) have been used successfully to prevent the spread of infectious diseases.[3] In the 1930s and 1940s, quarantine measures were used effectively in reducing exposure during periods of epidemic poliomyelitis. However, during the last 50 years, quarantine has fallen into disfavor because of opinions that it is unworkable and ineffective, which have been fostered by beliefs that modern medicine, civil rights, and technology have made quarantine obsolete. However, quarantine measures have been used appropriately, and should continue to be used, in the present SARS epidemic. Restrictions relating to travel clearly are appropriate, as in the quarantining of exposed symptomatic persons who have traveled to disease-free geographic areas.

REFERENCES

1. Ahuja, A. T., and Wong, J. K. T.: Radiological appearances of recent cases of atypical pneumonia in Hong Kong. www.droid.cunk.edu.ki/we/atypical_pneumonia/atypical_pneumonia.htm, 2003.
2. Boyer, K. M., and Cherry, J. D.: Influenza. *In* Feigin, R. D., Cherry, J. D. (eds.): Textbook of Pediatric Infectious Diseases. 1st ed. Philadelphia, W. B. Saunders, 1981, pp. 1298–1316.
3. Bromberg, J. S., and Vidich, C.: Twenty-first century role for quarantines. Los Angeles Times, April 9, 2003; B13.
4. Centers for Disease Control and Prevention: Severe acute respiratory syndrome (SARS) and coronavirus testing—United States, 2003. M. M. W. R. Morb. Mortal. Wkly. Rep. *52*(14):297–302, 2003.
5. Centers for Disease Control and Prevention: Update: Outbreak of severe acute respiratory syndrome—worldwide, 2003. M. M. W. R. Morb. Mortal. Wkly. Rep. *52*(15):332–336, 2003.
6. Cherry, J. D.: Enteroviruses: Coxsackieviruses, echoviruses, and polioviruses. *In* Feigin, R. D., and Cherry, J. D. (eds.): Textbook of Pediatric Infectious Diseases. 4th ed. Philadelphia, W. B. Saunders, 1998, pp. 1787–1839.
7. Cheung, C., Poon, L., Lau, A., et al.: Induction of proinflammatory cytokines in human macrophages by influenza A (H5N1) viruses: A mechanism for the unusual severity of human disease? Lancet *360*:1831–1837, 2002.
8. Drosten, C., Gunther, S., Preiser, W., et al.: Identification of a novel coronavirus in patients with severe acute respiratory syndrome. N. Engl. J. Med. *348*:1967–1976, 2003.
9. Heymann, D. L.: Status of the global SARS outbreak and lessons for the immediate future. www.who.int/csr/sarsarchive/2003_04_11/en/print.html, 2003.
10. Holmes, K. V.: Coronaviruses. *In* Knipe, D. M., and Howley, P. M. (eds.): Fields Virology. Vol 1. Philadelphia, Lippincott Williams & Wilkins, 2001, pp. 1187–1203.
11. Hon, K. L., Leung, C. W., Cheng, W. T., et al.: Clinical presentations and outcome of severe acute respiratory syndrome in children. Lancet *361*:1701–1703, 2003.
12. Ksiazek, T. G., Erdman, D., Goldsmith, C. S., et al.: A novel coronavirus associated with severe acute respiratory syndrome. N. Engl. J. Med. *348*:1953–1966, 2003.

13. Lai, M. M. C., and Holmes, K. V.: *Coronaviridae*: The viruses and their replication. *In* Knipe, D. M., and Howley, P. M. (eds.): Fields Virology. Vol. 1. Philadelphia, Lippincott Williams & Wilkins, 2001, pp. 685–722.
14. Lee, N., Hui, D., Wu, A., et al.: A major outbreak of severe acute respiratory syndrome in Hong Kong. N. Engl. J. Med. www.nejm.org, 2003.
15. Marra, M. A., Jones, S. J. M., Astell, C. R., et al.: The genome sequence of the SARS-associated coronavirus. Science *300*:1399–1403, 2003.
16. Poutanen, S. M., Low, D. E., Henry, B., et al.: Identification of severe acute respiratory syndrome in Canada. N. Engl. J. Med. www.nejm.org, 2003.
17. Rota, P. A., Oberste, M. S., Monroe, W. A., et al.: Characterization of a novel coronavirus associated with severe acute respiratory syndrome. Science *300*:1394–1398, 2003.
18. Tsang, K. W., Ho, P. L., Ooi, G. C., et al.: A cluster of cases of severe acute respiratory syndrome in Hong Kong. N. Engl. J. Med. www.nejm.org, 2003.
19. World Health Organization: Case definitions for surveillance of severe acute respiratory syndrome (SARS). www.who.int/csr/sars/casedefinition/en/print.html, April 1, 2003.
20. World Health Organization: Severe acute respiratory syndrome (SARS): Multi-country outbreak—Update 24. www.who.int/csr/dom/2003_04_08/en/print.html, April 8, 2003.
21. World Health Organization: Summary on major findings in relation to coronavirus by members of the WHO multi-centre collaborative network on SARS aetiology and diagnosis. www.who.int/csr/sars/findings/en/print.html, April 4, 2003.
22. World Health Organization: Cumulative number of reported probable cases of SARS. *www.who.int/csr/sars/country/2003_06_04/en/print.html.* 2003.

SUBSECTION **11**

BUNYAVIRIDAE

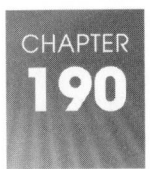

CHAPTER 190

Hantaviruses

C. J. PETERS ■ LOUISA E. CHAPMAN ■ KELLY T. McKEE, Jr.

Historical Perspective

Hantaviruses are the etiologic agents of a diverse group of rodent-borne hemorrhagic fevers that are responsible for considerable morbidity and mortality worldwide. Though recognized by so-called modern medicine only relatively recently, clinical syndromes now known to be associated with these viruses have been described by traditional practitioners across the globe from antiquity.[11, 62, 76] In the 20th century, Soviet scientists reported sporadic outbreaks of febrile renal failure with hemorrhage in the eastern Soviet Union between 1913 and 1930,[8] and Japanese and Soviet scientists recognized annual outbreaks of a similar syndrome in Manchuria and Siberia between 1932 and 1935.[29, 75, 103, 109] In 1934, Swedish scientists described a novel disorder characterized by fever, abdominal and back pain, and renal abnormalities[80, 124]; epidemic disease with these features occurred among German and Finnish troops stationed in Lapland during World War II.[44, 106]

North American medical practitioners initially became acquainted with a similar syndrome in the early 1950s, when a previously unrecognized febrile illness characterized by shock, hemorrhage, and renal failure developed in thousands of soldiers serving with United Nation forces during the Korean War. Physicians called this syndrome, which had a mortality rate of 5 to 15 percent, epidemic hemorrhagic fever.[23, 77]

In 1953, Gajdusek[28] noted similarities among epidemic hemorrhagic fever, the severe and frequently fatal Far Eastern diseases described by Soviet and Japanese scientists, and the Scandinavian disorder and proposed a common etiology. Subsequent validation of this hypothesis (see "The Organism") ultimately prompted adoption of the collective term hemorrhagic fever with renal syndrome (HFRS) to describe this clinical entity characterized by varying degrees of renal dysfunction and hemorrhage with fever.

In June 1993, investigation of a cluster of unexplained respiratory deaths in previously healthy young adult residents of rural areas in the southwestern United States led to recognition of a "new" hemorrhagic fever in North America. Application of sophisticated serologic and virologic tools to diagnostic specimens from patients with this mysterious disease quickly pointed to a hantavirus related to, but distinct from, those causing HFRS.[57, 82] This disorder, now called hantavirus pulmonary syndrome (HPS), proved to be different clinically from classic HFRS, but as virologic and epidemiologic studies of the etiologic agent and its reservoirs were completed, similarities to other hantaviruses became apparent.

The Organism

CLASSIFICATION AND ANTIGENIC COMPOSITION

The genus *Hantavirus* of the family *Bunyaviridae* was defined in 1985.[96, 98] The members of the *Hantavirus* genus are classified among the bunyaviruses because of their shared morphologic, physicochemical, and molecular properties. Like other members of the family *Bunyaviridae,* hantaviruses are negative-stranded, lipid-enveloped RNA viruses with tripartite genomes; genomic segments are designated as large (L), medium (M), and small (S). Also like other bunyaviruses, they display Golgi-associated morphogenesis and usually acquire their envelopes by budding into intracytoplasmic vacuoles.[99] However, they are serologically distinct from other family members and possess unique terminal genomic sequences.[96] The *Hantavirus* genus contains the only members of *Bunyaviridae* that lack arthropod vectors. Each hantavirus is highly adapted to a specific rodent species and depends on persistent asymptomatic infection in wild rodents for maintenance in nature.

TABLE 190–1 ■ SOME CURRENTLY RECOGNIZED HANTAVIRUSES

Virus Strain	Principal Reservoir	Distribution	Disease Association
Hantaan	*Apodemus agrarius*	Far East Northern Asia	HFRS (severe)
Seoul	*Rattus norvegicus*	Worldwide	HFRS (mild/moderate)
Dobrava	*Apodemus flavicollis*	Balkans	HFRS (severe)
Puumala	*Clethrionomys glareolus*	Scandinavia Northern Europe Balkans	HFRS (mild) (nephropathia epidemica)
Sin Nombre	*Peromyscus maniculatus*	North America	HPS
New York	*Peromyscus leucopus*	United States	HPS
Monongohela	*P. maniculatus nubiterrae*	Eastern United States	HPS
Black Creek Canal	*Sigmodon hispidus*	Florida	HPS
Bayou	*Oryzomys palustris*	Southeastern United States	HPS
Prospect Hill	*Microtus pennsylvanicus*	United States	None recognized
Andes	*Oligoryzomys longicaudatus**	South America	HPS
Oran	*Oligoryzomys longicaudatus**	Northern Argentina	HPS
Laguna Negra	*Calomys laucha*	South America	HPS
Choclo	*Oligoryzomys fulvescers*	Panama	HPS
Thottapalayam	*Suncus marinus*	India	None recognized

*The reservoirs of the Andes and Oran viruses are two cryptic species formerly both called *O. longicaudatus* and with exact taxonomy now under study. (D. Enria, personal communication).
HFRS, hemorrhagic fever with renal syndrome; HPS, hantavirus pulmonary syndrome. Additional hantaviruses have been associated with occasional human disease in Europe, Asia, and the Americas.

PHYSICAL PROPERTIES

Morphologically, hantaviruses are spherical, measure 80 to 120 nm in diameter, and have surface glycoprotein projections embedded in a lipid bilayer envelope. Elongated particles (110 to 120 nm long) often are observed, and they display a characteristic grid-like pattern on their surfaces.[35, 99]

SUSCEPTIBILITY

Hantaviruses are inactivated readily by lipid solvents and most disinfectants, including dilute hypochlorite solutions, detergents, ethyl alcohol (70%), most general-purpose household disinfectants, and beta-propiolactone (0.1% at 4° C for 3 days).[36, 56, 93] Limited studies with Hantaan virus have shown sensitivity to a pH of 5 or less and to temperatures of 56° C or higher.[36, 64] The survival time in the environment in the absence of disinfection is not known, but limited studies have shown persistent infectivity in dried cell culture medium for as long as 2 days and in neutral solutions for several hours at 37° C or several days at lower temperatures.[58]

LABORATORY PROPAGATION AND TISSUE CULTURE GROWTH

Hantaviruses are fastidious but can be grown in culture through serial blind passage. They routinely establish persistent, noncytolytic infections and generally do not replicate to high titer.[36, 99] The prototype member of the group, Hantaan virus, was isolated in 1978[69] and propagated successfully in cell culture in the A-549 cell line in 1981.[27] However, Vero E-6 cells subsequently were found to be a better cell culture system for this and other hantaviruses.[36] Hantaviruses have been isolated and propagated successfully through direct inoculation of homogenates of infected tissue from wild-caught rodent hosts onto cell lines or after amplification through serially infected, colonized rodent hosts.[24, 27, 34, 36, 69, 84, 95, 120] Recovering hantaviruses from human specimens has been difficult and infrequent. More than 20 hantaviruses currently are recognized as causing human disease, although many of them have not been fully characterized and their reservoirs have not been determined. The major viruses are listed in Table 190–1. Some hantaviruses have been isolated in cell culture, but many are known only from generic material amplified from human or rodent tissue. This list will be expanded and modified as our knowledge of classification and new viruses expands. Laboratory infection of persons working with cell culture–adapted Hantaan virus has occurred occasionally, but laboratory transmission of hantaviruses from infected rodents to humans is a particularly common occurrence.[20, 21, 49, 65, 66, 73, 111, 112] Consequently, attempts to propagate the virus should be performed only when using biosafety level 3 or 4 facilities and practices.[9, 58]

TRANSMISSION

Hantaviruses are zoonotic; each hantavirus is associated with a distinct rodent species in which it establishes a chronic, inapparent infection. Hantavirus infection of rodents produces a short viremia that results in dissemination of virus to the lungs, salivary glands, and kidneys. Once infected, the rodent sheds virus in urine, saliva, and (to a lesser extent) feces throughout its life, despite the development of neutralizing antibodies.[67] Infection does not diminish the longevity or the reproductive potential of the infected rodent; vertical transmission has not been demonstrated. Enzootic infection appears to be maintained by exposure to nesting materials contaminated with infectious secretions, by grooming behavior, and by intraspecies biting.[65, 67]

Generally accepted is that humans become infected with hantaviruses after contact with contaminated secreta or excreta from infected rodents via inhalation of small-particle aerosols or, rarely, via percutaneous inoculation of infected materials. The primacy of respiratory droplets or airborne particles as the mode of transmission to humans is supported by evidence from outbreaks of disease among laboratory workers and sporadic cases resulting from brief exposure to rodent-infected habitats.*

The risk of human hantavirus infection occurring is a function of the density of the local rodent reservoir population, the

*See references 9, 20, 21, 49, 65–67, 73, 111, 112, 118, 123.

prevalence of infection among rodents, and the frequency of activities that result in contact between humans and rodent excreta. Individual hantavirus infections usually occur when humans disturb rodent habitats or rodents enter human housing. Epidemics generally are associated with either changes in the behavior of human populations that result in large-scale exposure of persons to rodent-infected areas (e.g., military maneuvers, agricultural or forestry activities) or environmental changes that result in rapid increases in the density of the rodent population (e.g., proliferation of food sources). Person-to-person transmission of hantaviruses associated with HFRS has not been demonstrated. The experience to date with HPS has been similar,[114] although interpersonal spread clearly occurred during a single outbreak in South America and may be an occasional feature of the causative agent Andes virus.[25, 116] If subsequent investigations support this observation, a reappraisal of transmission risks associated with this South American hantavirus may be necessary.

Epidemiology

GEOGRAPHIC DISTRIBUTION

Hantaviruses have been found on every continent except Antarctica. With the exception of HFRS caused by Seoul virus, hantavirus diseases occur almost exclusively in rural areas. Hantaan virus, the cause of classic HFRS, is carried by the striped field mouse *Apodemus agrarius.* This rodent is distributed across eastern Russia, China, and the Korean peninsula.[118] The principal reservoir for Puumala virus, the etiologic agent of a milder HFRS variant found in Scandinavia, northern Europe, and Russia west of the Ural Mountains, is the bank vole *Clethrionomys glareolus.*[68, 100]

In the Balkans, at least two viruses have been linked etiologically with HFRS: Puumala and Dobrava; the latter agent is associated with *Apodemus flavicollis,* the yellow-necked field mouse.[2, 4, 5, 34] *Rattus* spp. (primarily *Rattus norvegicus)* serve as reservoirs for the Seoul-like viruses identified worldwide; human infections have been seen most frequently in eastern Asia. Outbreaks of severe and occasionally fatal HFRS among animal handlers and laboratory scientists have been caused by inapparent infection of laboratory rats with Seoul-like viruses.[63]

Numerous hantaviruses associated with native rodents are known to exist in the Americas, and several are of medical importance in the United States.[90] The deer mouse *Peromyscus maniculatus* is the reservoir rodent for Sin Nombre virus, the agent associated most frequently with human disease in North America.[15] This rodent is distributed widely over the United States, Canada, and parts of Mexico. Additionally, HPS cases in the eastern United States have been associated with viruses called New York and Monongahela, which are closely related to Sin Nombre virus and are found in *P. leucopus* (white-footed mouse) and *Peromyscus maniculatus nubiterrae,* respectively.[41, 104] Clinical HPS has been recognized in areas outside the known ranges of *P. maniculatus* and *P. leucopus,* however, and a search for other virus-rodent pairings has yielded at least two additional U.S. hantaviruses, Black Creek Canal virus from *Sigmodon hispidus* (cotton rat) and Bayou virus from *Oryzomys palustris* (rice rat).[40, 51, 54, 81, 94, 108] Prospect Hill virus has been recovered from meadow voles *(Microtus pennsylvanicus)* in Maryland, and related but distinct hantaviruses are inferred to be present in other voles by detection of genetic sequences via reverse transcriptase–polymerase chain reaction (RT-PCR). Another hantavirus, El Moro Canyon virus, has been identified in the harvest mouse *(Reithrodontomys megalotis),* also by RT-PCR. No human infections have been documented with these viruses, and their potential for causing disease, if any, is unknown.[39, 118, 119] Seoul virus from introduced *Rattus* has been associated with human infections in several large cities, but acute (HFRS-like) disease has not been confirmed.[32, 33, 61]

The recognition of clinical HPS in Canada and Central and South America clearly has established HPS as a panhemispheric rather than a geographically circumscribed disease.* However, all HPS agents identified or suspected to date belong to a single genetic group of hantaviruses and are associated with rodents of the family *Muridae,* subfamily *Sigmodontinae.* These rodent species are restricted to the Americas, in accordance with the findings that HPS has been an exclusively Western Hemisphere disease.[90]

SEASONAL PATTERNS

The natural population cycles of rodents and the seasonal nature of certain human behavior result in a pattern of human hantavirus disease that varies both seasonally and annually.[8, 9, 11, 29, 62, 76, 109] Although the incidence of disease varies by season, cases of hantavirus-associated human disease are recognized year-round in all disease-endemic areas.[38, 52, 63, 100]

In eastern Asia and Russia east of the Ural Mountains, HFRS occurs primarily during the late fall and early winter, with smaller peaks during the spring and summer. Most Scandinavian HFRS occurs between the late summer and early spring, whereas European HFRS in warmer regions (e.g., France, Belgium) tends to peak in the spring.[113] In the Balkans, the presence of multiple viral strains results in a more diffuse seasonal distribution of human disease. Persons whose occupations or avocations bring them to rural settings, such as agricultural workers, foresters, biologists, hunters, campers, and soldiers stationed in the field, are at greatest risk for contracting HFRS.

HFRS caused by Seoul virus tends to occur throughout the year, and descriptions of a seasonal occurrence of Seoul virus infection have conflicted.[13, 70] Cases of Seoul virus disease also have a more even age and sex distribution than rural hantavirus infections do, presumably because of the peridomestic nature of the agent's reservoir.

The temporal distribution of HPS cases identified through national surveillance conducted at the Centers for Disease Control and Prevention (CDC) suggests a mild spring-summer seasonality of human disease. Approximately one half of all U.S. cases that have occurred since 1993 have been recognized during May through July. However, these surveillance data are influenced by epidemics of human disease associated with an ecologically circumscribed rapid increase in the population density of infected deer mice in the southwestern United States in relation to El Nino–southern oscillation events.[31, 87] Spring-summer seasonality has been less evident in subsequent years.[38] Additional surveillance is necessary to confirm a consistently seasonal nature of hantavirus infection in the United States.

PREVALENCE

Worldwide, human hantavirus infections may number in the hundreds of thousands of cases annually.[118] Because of the predominantly rural nature of the disease and its prevalence in developing regions of the Eurasian land mass (e.g., rural China), accurate case reporting (and statistical data) for HFRS is limited. Researchers have estimated that more than 100,000 cases of HFRS occur each year in China[118];

*See references 5a, 39, 43, 74, 81, 86, 105, 113a, 113b, 115, 117.

one report suggested an incidence of 1.6 to 29.6 per 100,000 population during 1980.[48] In the former Soviet Union, more than 4000 cases per year were recorded between 1978 and 1989, 96 percent of which occurred in "European" republics. Rates in western regions near the Ural Mountains were higher (20 to 40 per 100,000 population) than were those in eastern districts (2 to 5 per 100,000 population).[107] In Korea, approximately 500 persons with HFRS, around half of whom are soldiers, are hospitalized annually.[107] In central and northern Sweden, a mean annual incidence of 4.3 per 100,000 population has been reported, although northern locales have rates of more than 20 per 100,000 population.[100]

DEMOGRAPHIC FEATURES

Hantavirus infections are recognized infrequently in the pediatric age group.[3, 30, 52, 53, 100, 107, 121] The disease occurs principally in adults, with less than 10 percent of cases being diagnosed in children. A slight male preponderance has been noted in reported cases.

The peak incidence of HFRS in Europe, the Balkans, and the Far East occurs in individuals who are 20 to 50 years of age.[59, 63, 88, 109] Few cases have been reported in children younger than 10 years. Both HFRS and HPS cases in young children often are recognized in association with cases in other family members.[3, 30, 59, 79, 86] A male preponderance of cases has been observed for both the severe (Korean) and milder (European) forms of HFRS in children.[1, 55, 79, 121] Although this pattern, also seen in adults with HFRS, suggests differential susceptibility or risk of exposure by gender, the number of recorded cases, particularly in the youngest age groups, is too small to draw firm conclusions.

The underrepresentation of children recognized to have HFRS and HPS may not be explained by age-related avoidance of activities resulting in exposure. The limited data available (see Clinical Manifestations) suggest that hantavirus infections in children may induce milder disease than that seen in adults, although typical (even fatal) HPS has been described. Comprehensive population-based serosurveys are few in number and have been inadequate to define age-associated infection rates. The apparently immune-mediated pathology of this disease (see Pathogenesis and Pathology) is possibly more evident in persons experiencing infection in adulthood.

Clinical Manifestations

HEMORRHAGIC FEVER WITH RENAL SYNDROME

Two major clinical variants of HFRS have been recognized traditionally. Severe disease associated with high morbidity and mortality occurs primarily in areas of the world where Hantaan and Dobrava viruses are endemic: across the northern half of Asia, China, the Korean Peninsula, and the Balkan nations. Milder illness with little mortality occurs in areas where Puumala virus has been recovered; this latter disease, known also as nephropathia epidemica, is found throughout northern Europe, Scandinavia, and western areas of the former Soviet Union. In the Balkans, the coexistence of Puumala virus–like strains with viruses causing more serious disease has resulted in a mixture of clinical findings in the former Yugoslavia and neighboring countries. Benign manifestations of HFRS are well recognized in many regions where Hantaan virus is found, however, and clinically severe disease occasionally results from Puumala virus infection.[91] Hence, it is important to appreciate the protean nature of this disorder and recognize the potential for disease of any severity whenever and wherever human infection with hantavirus occurs.

Severe HFRS, such as that associated with Hantaan or Dobrava virus, is a complex, multiphasic disorder that presents a substantial challenge in patient management. The clinical course of HFRS caused by Hantaan virus in adults spans a wide spectrum from mildly symptomatic disease to severe hemorrhagic fever and death. Subclinical infections probably occur infrequently.[92, 121] In most cases, the clinical course is relatively benign, with severe disease developing in approximately 20 to 30 percent of patients. Modern-day case-fatality rates range from 2 to 7 percent. In Korea, approximately a third of recognized Hantaan virus infections follow a clinical course consisting of progression through five clinically and pathophysiologically defined stages: febrile, hypotensive, oliguric, diuretic, and convalescent.[70, 101] Phases often blur, however, and in milder cases, one or more phases may not be discernible. After having an incubation period of 2 to 3 weeks (range, 4 to 42 days), most patients report the abrupt onset of high fever, headache, chills, dizziness, myalgia, anorexia, and backache. Approximately a third of patients experience prodromal mild respiratory or gastrointestinal symptoms. Nausea, vomiting, abdominal pain, and intense thirst may be evident at initial evaluation but increase in severity in succeeding days. Photophobia, blurred vision, and eyeball pain are reported frequently. Physical examination reveals a restless, acutely ill patient with flushing of the face, neck, and upper thoracic region. Relative bradycardia is present. Conjunctival and pharyngeal injection, together with facial puffiness, is characteristic. In more than 90 percent of patients, petechiae develop on the soft palate, axillae, lateral aspect of the thorax, conjunctivae, or face, generally between the third and sixth days of illness. Tenderness occurs commonly over the costovertebral angles and diffusely throughout the abdomen. Hematologic studies in the first 3 to 4 days of illness reveal leukocytosis with a left shift in more than 90 percent and thrombocytopenia almost universally; the hematocrit at this stage is generally normal or slightly increased. Proteinuria develops by the third to fourth day, and microscopic hematuria, hyposthenuria, and mild pyuria are reported in most patients; fibrin clots in urine are a characteristic finding.

This febrile phase generally lasts approximately 1 week, followed by abrupt defervescence. Approximately 40 percent of patients then become hypotensive; in most cases, the drop in blood pressure is mild and brief, but in severely ill persons (30–50% of hypotensive patients), clinical shock develops. Tachycardia replaces bradycardia, the pulse pressure narrows, and cyanosis and mental confusion may be seen. The hypotensive phase may last from a few hours to 3 days, and 30 to 40 percent of deaths occur during this period.

As patients recover from hypotension, they enter a period of oliguria. This phase occurs in approximately 60 percent of patients and generally lasts for several days. Anuria develops in approximately 10 percent of patients. Blood pressure normalizes, and hypertension often develops. Clinical manifestations of uremia, including protracted vomiting and hiccups, may be seen. More extensive hemorrhagic manifestations such as ecchymoses, hemoptysis, hematemesis, melena, gross hematuria, and rarely, bleeding in the central nervous system become evident during the oliguric phase. Striking elevations in blood urea nitrogen and creatinine levels are common findings. Biochemical disturbances (electrolyte derangements, metabolic acidosis, uremia) may be severe, and in such cases, dialysis may be lifesaving.

Approximately half of fatalities occur during the oliguric phase.

Between 10 and 14 days into the illness, renal function is restored spontaneously in most patients, and a period of diuresis follows. Polyuria may be substantial, and urine output frequently exceeds 3 to 6 L/day. With the onset of diuresis, clinical recovery is initiated; however, the rapid change in fluid status may precipitate further electrolyte disturbances, so close monitoring remains necessary.

Convalescence typically lasts from 3 to 6 weeks, but in many cases, a longer period passes before health is restored completely. Weight gain and strength are recovered slowly. Proteinuria resolves, but hyposthenuria persists for months. Most patients recover completely, although permanent sequelae may result from such complications as anterior pituitary or other central nervous system hemorrhage.

The disease has been reported infrequently in children.[30, 55, 121] However, the data available indicate that clinical manifestations are similar to and perhaps somewhat less severe than those observed in adults. In a series of 63 children identified retrospectively over a 15-year period in Korea, fever was universal, whereas abdominal pain, headache, and vomiting were present in 73 percent or more of patients[121] (Table 190–2). Proteinuria (100%), leukocytosis (71%), thrombocytopenia (80%), hypocholesterolemia (87%), and elevations in creatinine (94%), blood urea nitrogen (94%), and alanine transaminase (80%) were the laboratory abnormalities found most commonly. Petechiae and hypotension occurred infrequently (38% and 11%, respectively), and frank hemorrhage did so rarely. Eleven patients (18%) required dialysis. The mortality rate was 5 percent, and the remaining patients recovered without sequelae.

HFRS occurring in adults after infection with Seoul virus resembles that described for Hantaan virus infection, but the clinical manifestations are generally much milder.[70] Fever and constitutional symptoms are similar in the two types of infection, but hypotension occurs infrequently in persons infected with Seoul virus (10 percent of cases), and clinical shock is a rare event. The frequency and severity of thrombocytopenia are less with Seoul virus infection, whereas elevations of transaminases occur commonly (more than 60% of cases). The mortality rate for HFRS caused by Seoul virus is 1 percent or less.

The Scandinavian or European form of HFRS (nephropathia epidemica) is generally a much more benign disease than that attributed to Hantaan virus; fatal outcomes are observed, but the case-fatality rate is less than 1 percent. In contrast to the findings with Hantaan virus, subclinical infection apparently occurs commonly with Puumala virus; one report suggests a case-to-infection ratio of 1:10.[85]

In adults, nephropathia epidemica is typically a biphasic disease of 1 to 3 weeks' duration.[18, 88, 113] The onset is usually abrupt, with no apparent prodrome. High fever is the initial symptom in 95 percent of patients. On examination, a facial flush is a usual finding. This febrile phase lasts from 3 to 6 days. The development of nausea, vomiting, abdominal pain, back pain, somnolence, and occasionally, joint pain heralds the onset of the second, or renal, phase. The abdominal pain may be of such severity and character that an acute abdomen is suspected, and many patients have undergone surgery for suspected appendicitis before nephropathia epidemica is diagnosed. Visual disturbances are common, and hypotension, if it develops, is usually mild. Petechiae are relatively infrequent. The renal stage generally lasts 1 to 2 weeks and is characterized by the development of oliguria, proteinuria, hematuria, and hyposthenuria. Modest elevations in blood urea nitrogen and creatinine accompany the oliguria, which typically lasts for no more than a few days before

TABLE 190–2 ■ PROMINENT CLINICAL AND LABORATORY FEATURES OF HEMORRHAGIC FEVER WITH RENAL SYNDROME IN CHILDREN

Features	Korea[121] (%)	Sweden[1] (%)	Finland[79] (%)
Fever	100	100	100
Headache	76	100	59
Anorexia	33	100	NR
Nausea	62	86	81
Vomiting	73	91	72
Abdominal pain	91	93	59
Back/costovertebral angle pain	35	76	63
Dizziness	21	73	9
Thirst	NR	75	NR
Polyuria	NR	57	NR
Diarrhea	NR	57	9
Petechiae	38	NR	NR
Conjunctival hemorrhage	35	NR	3
Proteinuria	100	100	97
Hematuria	67	80	73
Pyuria	8	43	44
Glucosuria	NR	26	12
Casts	NR	33	NR
Leukocytosis	71	22	41
Thrombocytopenia	80	68	87
Elevated hemoglobin	39	NR	28
Elevated C-reactive protein	NR	28	89
Elevated erythrocyte sedimentation rate	NR	58	74
Elevated alanine transaminase	80	NR	53
Elevated creatinine	94	76	84

NR, not recorded.

diuresis begins. Mild leukocytosis and thrombocytopenia occur during the renal phase, whereas electrolyte disturbances sufficient to require dialysis are infrequent events. As with other forms of HFRS, convalescence may be prolonged, and hyposthenuria may persist for many months. Recovery is typically complete, although minor abnormalities in renal function and blood pressure have been described.[60, 83]

As with Hantaan virus–associated HFRS, nephropathia epidemica in children is recognized infrequently. Clinically, the disease also appears to be similar to and, in most cases, milder than that seen in adults. Among 32 Swedish cases reported (18 identified retrospectively and 14 prospectively), fever (100%), headache (100%), anorexia (100%), abdominal pain (93%), vomiting (91%), nausea (86%), and back pain (76%) were the most prevalent symptoms[1] (see Table 190–2). Proteinuria (100%), microscopic hematuria (80%), elevated serum creatinine (76%), and thrombocytopenia (68%) were the laboratory abnormalities most frequently found. Leukocytosis was a relatively uncommon finding (22%) in this series. Six children (19%) had hemorrhagic manifestations, and one complained of blurred vision. In a separate 32-patient series from Finland, fever (100%), nausea (81%), vomiting (72%), and back pain (63%) again were prevalent, but headache and abdominal pain (59%) were reported less frequently[79] (see Table 190–2). Proteinuria (97%), hematuria (73%), and elevated serum creatinine (84%) were common findings. Thrombocytopenia (87%) was reported more prominently among Finnish than Swedish children. Approximately a quarter of Finnish children displayed hemorrhagic manifestations. The proportion of transient visual blurring was identical to that seen in adults (25%). No children in these series required dialysis.

HANTAVIRUS PULMONARY SYNDROME

Classic HPS in adults is a biphasic illness that challenges the diagnostic acumen and clinical management skills of physicians. The clinical features of the prodrome phase are not pathognomonic, and the diagnosis rarely is suspected before the abrupt clinical deterioration that heralds onset of the cardiopulmonary phase. HPS characteristically begins with a prodrome that lasts on average 3 to 4 days but may extend as long as a week or more.[10, 22, 72, 90, 113a] This phase is typified by fever and myalgia, particularly of the back or lower extremities. Although a cough may develop as the prodrome progresses, illnesses initially characterized predominantly by upper respiratory symptoms, such as cough and coryza, are unlikely to be HPS.[10, 22, 72, 78] More than half of HPS patients also have gastrointestinal symptoms (e.g., nausea, vomiting, diarrhea) that are usually mild.[10, 22] Occasionally, HPS-associated gastrointestinal symptoms have been mistaken for an acute surgical abdomen or another intra-abdominal process. The presence of thrombocytopenia in the context of a compatible prodrome is highly suggestive of HPS.[10, 22, 56a, 78, 102]

The onset of the cardiopulmonary phase is abrupt and often life-threatening. Patients usually are hospitalized within 12 to 24 hours of initial medical evaluation, and most deaths occur during the first 24 to 48 hours in the hospital.[10, 12, 22, 72] Clear chest radiographs have progressed to diffuse bilateral pulmonary involvement during the course of several hours. Interstitial edema, present in only 5 percent of patients with adult respiratory distress syndrome, is present in most HPS patients on initial radiography, and alveolar flooding that is usually indistinguishable from the peripheral pattern seen in the acute phase of adult respiratory distress syndrome develops in most patients.[50] This noncardiogenic pulmonary edema, resulting from a diffuse pulmonary capillary leak, can be differentiated from cardiac (hydrostatic) pulmonary edema by the presence of low pulmonary artery occlusion pressure and an increased protein content in edema fluid.[37] Secretions recovered when HPS patients are intubated are generally acellular, resemble plasma or pulmonary edema fluid, and have been observed to clot in severe cases.[22, 37] The presence of significant numbers of polymorphonuclear leukocytes in pulmonary secretions suggests an alternative etiology.

The pulmonary decline usually is accompanied by the onset of shock caused by myocardial dysfunction and relative hypovolemia.[10, 37, 72] In severe cases, hemodynamic measurements show high systemic vascular resistance combined with low cardiac and stroke volume indices. Progression to death is associated with worsening cardiac dysfunction unresponsive to treatment, even despite adequate oxygenation.[37]

Thrombocytopenia may be present in the late prodrome and is almost always found during the cardiopulmonary phase. Additional laboratory abnormalities in hospitalized patients include hemoconcentration, prolonged prothrombin and partial thromboplastin times, elevated serum lactate dehydrogenase concentration, decreased serum protein concentration, mild leukocytosis with a marked left shift, and the frequent presence of myeloid precursors on the peripheral smear.[10, 22, 56a, 72, 90] Proteinuria is a common occurrence. Serum creatinine often is elevated modestly in severe cases, although renal failure is not characteristic of infection with Sin Nombre virus despite episodes of hypotension and other predisposing conditions in many patients. Among patients who survive, recovery may be as dramatic as the decline; survivors may be extubated within 3 to 7 days after admission to the intensive care unit and may be discharged from the hospital within 2 weeks.[90]

Renal failure has been more prominent in two reported cases of HPS caused by infection with Black Creek Canal virus and Bayou virus.[22, 54] The hantavirus disease associated with Andes virus[74] in Argentina and Chile and that from other related virus infections in Brazil[81] and Paraguay[117] closely resembles Sin Nombre virus disease. Renal failure has accompanied some cases in a focus in northern Argentina.[86]

Subclinical or mild disease rarely follows Sin Nombre virus infection.[102] However, although initial case-fatality rates of 70 to 80 percent were reported in 1993, a wider clinical spectrum has been recognized as clinicians have developed a heightened suspicion and diagnostic assays have become more readily available. As of May 2003, the overall case-fatality rate for HPS cases identified in the United States is 35 percent. This apparent decline in the incidence of mortality may reflect improvement in survival attributed to improved clinical management. However, it undoubtedly also reflects a decrease in the tendency to suspect this diagnosis only with the fatal and near-fatal disease that existed early in the clinical understanding of this syndrome.

HPS has been recognized infrequently in children younger than 17 years. Several case reports and reviews of pediatric HPS patients (identified through CDC surveillance and a university database) indicate that the geographic distribution, clinical course, and mortality rates in children and adolescents are similar to those described for adults.[3, 7, 53, 61a, 93a] Fever, headache, dyspnea or cough, gastrointestinal disturbances, and myalgia are common in the prodromal phase. Tachypnea and fever are frequent on hospital admission; in one case series, however, hypotension at presentation was uncommon (33%).[93a] In one patient, dizziness with an apparent vestibular component was described.[53] Thrombocytopenia, a "left shift" in the leukocyte differential, elevated levels of hepatic transaminases and lactate dehydrogenase, and hypoalbuminemia are typically seen on admission. Although leukocytosis and hemoconcentration are not found early reliably, they may appear later in the course of illness. There have been suggestions that mortality among prepubertal children may be somewhat lower than that seen in older individuals,[7] but as patient numbers have accumulated over time, overall case-fatality rates in pediatric and adolescent patients seem to be similar to those seen in adults (30–40%). In one series, hypotension and absence of fever at admission were found to be predictive of respiratory failure, whereas elevated prothrombin time (≥14 seconds) at admission was predictive of mortality.[93a]

Complications

In general, human infection with HFRS-associated hantaviruses results in an acute illness with prolonged incapacitation followed by complete recovery. Unless complicated by organ hemorrhage (e.g., central nervous system bleeding), residua have not been observed. However, epidemiologic associations between hypertensive renal disease and evidence of previous U.S. hantavirus infection have been reported.[32, 33] These data require further study to determine their significance.

Although prolonged prothrombin and partial thromboplastin times occur commonly in hospitalized HPS patients, overt disseminated intravascular coagulation and overt hemorrhage are infrequent.[10, 122] Patients in whom disseminated intravascular coagulation is established rarely survive longer than 48 hours. One patient who did survive a cardiopulmonary phase accompanied by overt disseminated intravascular coagulation died 3 weeks later of gangrenous complications.

The South American viruses have been associated with more extrapulmonary manifestations than have the Sin Nombre infections in the United States. Evidence of bleeding is found more commonly, and other complications are reported with greater frequency.

Pathogenesis and Pathology

Serum antibodies develop within 3 to 7 days of the onset of illness in patients infected with hantaviruses. Early clinical events are presumed to be accompanied by viremia; however, significant signs and symptoms develop in temporal association with the onset of a measurable antibody response. Pathologic studies of fatal HFRS cases indicate that multiple organ systems are involved, but a triad of lesions consisting of hemorrhagic necrosis of the renal medulla, anterior pituitary, and cardiac right atrium is described as characteristic.[46] In HPS, multiple organ involvement with variable degrees of vascular congestion is noted in all fatal cases. However, the predominant findings at autopsy have involved the lungs, with pulmonary edema and serous effusions seen grossly and interstitial pneumonitis with a mononuclear cell infiltrate, intra-alveolar edema, and focal hyaline membrane formation described microscopically. Immunohistochemical studies demonstrate the widespread presence of hantavirus antigens in endothelial cells of the microvasculature, particularly in the lungs but also in the kidneys, heart, spleen, pancreas, lymph nodes, skeletal muscle, intestine, adrenal gland, adipose tissue, urinary bladder, and brain. However, few histologic changes have been noted in the kidney, brain, and heart of autopsied patients with HPS.[122]

The underlying pathologic lesion leading to hemodynamic alterations in hantavirus infection is damage to the vascular endothelium. The cause of the injury is unknown, but both cellular and humoral immune-mediated mechanisms have been implicated.[19, 23, 46, 110, 122] Soluble factors acting on the hematologic and immunologic systems also are released. The abrupt onset of noncardiogenic pulmonary edema in HPS occurs after the development of an immune response directed against viral antigen present throughout the endothelial cells lining the pulmonary capillaries, and such edema leads to a pulmonary capillary leak syndrome.[89]

Diagnosis and Differential Diagnosis

A high index of suspicion is essential for recognition of hantavirus infection in persons living or traveling in disease-endemic areas. The protean nature of the disease in children is such that almost any ill-defined febrile disease associated with abdominal or back pain in an appropriate geographic setting should stimulate consideration of the diagnosis, particularly if the clinical syndrome is accompanied by myalgia, if thrombocytopenia or proteinuria is present, or if a history of exposure to rodents or rural environments in disease-endemic areas is elicited.[102]

The differential diagnosis of HFRS includes rickettsial disease, leptospirosis, meningococcemia, other viral diseases, post-streptococcal syndromes, pyelonephritis, leukemia, and hemolytic-uremic syndrome. Differentiation from an acute intra-abdominal or pelvic process, such as appendicitis, may be extremely difficult on clinical grounds.

The differential diagnosis of HPS includes rickettsial diseases, legionellosis, *Yersinia pestis* infection (plague), meningococcemia, brucellosis, mycoplasmal and fungal pneumonias (including *Coccidioides immitis* and *Histoplasma* pneumonias), tularemia, psittacosis, pancreatitis accompanied by adult respiratory distress syndrome, and autoimmune disorders (including thrombotic thrombocytopenia purpura). A prominent cough or sore throat or a localized infiltrate on a chest radiograph that does not generalize within hours argues for a non-hantaviral etiology.[10, 78] A constellation of the absence of a cough in the presence of dizziness, nausea or vomiting, a low platelet count, a low serum bicarbonate level, and an elevated hematocrit discriminated HPS from similar patients with unexplained adult respiratory distress syndrome in two studies.[10, 78] Thrombocytopenia or a falling platelet count provides a valuable clue late in the prodrome. After onset of pulmonary edema, the presence of four of five findings (thrombocytopenia, myelocytosis, hemoconcentration, lack of significant toxic granulations in neutrophils, and more than 10 percent of lymphocytes with immunoblastic morphologic findings) has sensitivity for HPS of 96 percent and specificity of 99 percent.[56a] Frequent use of pulse oximetry also is of assistance.

Laboratory diagnosis of HFRS or HPS is made by demonstration of specific anti-hantavirus IgM antibodies in acute-phase serum by enzyme immunoassay in the IgM capture format. A fourfold or greater rise in specific IgG antibodies by enzyme immunoassay or immunofluorescence[57, 71] in sequential sera (ideally obtained 2 or more weeks apart) also is useful. The availability of purified recombinant hantavirus antigens has enhanced diagnostic specificity in both the enzyme immunoassay and Western blot assay systems.[26, 47, 125] Enzyme-linked immunosorbent assay and indirect fluorescent antibody tests are broadly cross-reactive, particularly among viruses from rodents of the same subfamily.[16, 17] For example, a recombinant Sin Nombre virus antigen detects antibodies against Bayou, Black Creek Canal, Andes, and several other viruses from sigmodontine rodents, and it maintains reactivity with antibodies directed against arvicolid rodent–associated viruses (e.g., Puumala and Prospect Hill). Neutralizing antibody assays are more specific, but technical requirements preclude their routine use. Immunohistochemical techniques have been applied to tissue samples from patients infected with hantaviruses.[122] Nucleic acid primers from several hantavirus strains have been generated, which has enabled nucleotide sequences from fresh or frozen tissues to be amplified by RT-PCR. RT-PCR is usually successful on whole blood or blood clots obtained within the first 7 to 10 days of illness. However, the expense and effort of performing the method are not justified unless the resulting genetic sequence information is needed for definition of the viral strain or for epidemiologic studies.[2, 82] Attempts to isolate hantaviruses from human specimens are generally unrewarding.

Treatment

Cautious fluid management and hemodynamic and intensive care unit support are the most important aspects of the clinical management of any hantavirus disease.[37, 72] Early hospitalization and avoidance of even minor trauma are essential to maintain the integrity of damaged vascular beds in these patients. Transport of patients should be minimized; the barotrauma associated with transport in underpressurized aircraft may be particularly hazardous.[6] Attention to fluid management and metabolic status is especially critical. In patients with HFRS, restriction of fluids may be necessary early in the course of disease as renal function diminishes, but large input may be required later during diuresis to cover massive losses. Electrolyte abnormalities and metabolic acidosis occur commonly. Peritoneal dialysis or hemodialysis may be lifesaving in severe cases.[6] In HPS, the nature of the pulmonary pathology predisposes to iatrogenic pulmonary edema; careful attention must be paid to maintaining appropriate central venous and pulmonary arterial pressure to avoid such complications. Tissue perfusion and adequate oxygenation are the goals of supportive therapy with this syndrome. Oxygen supplementation and mechanical ventilation are required nearly always. Inotropic agents may be necessary to maintain tissue perfusion.[37, 72]

Hantaan and Sin Nombre viruses exhibit similar in vitro sensitivity to ribavirin. One prospective, placebo-controlled trial suggested that intravenous ribavirin was effective in reducing the mortality and morbidity rates associated with HFRS in China.[45] In contrast, although 30 patients with HPS who received investigational, open-label intravenous ribavirin generally tolerated it well, treatment was accompanied by a low frequency of early drug-associated adverse events, most significantly, anemia and resulting transfusion, and no clear evidence of benefit was obtained.[10, 12] This contrast in clinical experience is not explained by differences in dosing schedules; patients in both protocols received identical doses.[12, 45] All hantaviruses have been sensitive to the antiviral effects of ribavirin in vitro. The lack of any dramatic effect by intravenous ribavirin in HPS is probably due to the rapid progression of disease; HPS-associated deaths usually occur within the first 48 hours after admission and therapeutic intervention.[10–12, 22, 37, 45, 72]

Ribavirin is not licensed for intravenous use in the United States. Teratogenic concerns mandate careful informed consent if the use of this drug is considered in children, pregnant women, or nursing mothers. A randomized placebo-controlled trial to ascertain whether intravenous ribavirin has efficacy for HPS was stopped short of a definitive endpoint because of slow enrollment.[12]

Prevention

PRIMARY PREVENTION

The most effective preventive measure available for hantavirus infection is the avoidance of rodents and their habitats. However, eradication of the rodent reservoir hosts in disease-endemic areas is not feasible. Prevention efforts are directed more appropriately toward reducing the frequency of rodent-human interactions through environmental hygiene practices that minimize rodent density in home and work environments and avoidance of known rodent-infested areas and activities that increase the risk of human exposure to aerosolized infectious rodent excreta. Such avoidance may be particularly important during times of high rodent populations and in various ecologic zones for specific reasons. In fact, in the southwestern United States, remote sensing patterns from the year before can predict local areas of disease, thus allowing precisely targeted public health messages and interventions.[31]

Detailed guidelines on measures appropriate to eliminate rodents from homes in disease-endemic areas, to clean rodent-contaminated areas safely, and to minimize the risk for workers occupationally exposed to rodents and participants in outdoor recreational activities have been published.[14] Although rodent ectoparasites do not transmit hantaviruses, in the southwestern United States, several rodent species are also hosts to fleas that transmit *Y. pestis*. In such areas, insecticides should be used in conjunction with rodent extermination measures because eradication of rodents without concurrent control of the associated fleas may increase the risk of human plague occurring.[14]

VACCINE PROSPECTS

Inactivated vaccines to Hantaan and Seoul viruses have been developed in South Korea and China. Some of these vaccines induce neutralizing antibody responses in humans and are being tested in field studies. A recombinant vaccinia strain expressing Hantaan antigens has been tested in human volunteers in the United States and has been shown to induce a serum neutralizing antibody response.[97] An immediate need exists for a vaccine effective against Hantaan virus, but several obstacles to accepting the aforementioned candidates remain. No realistic animal model of human disease permits full preclinical evaluation, the disease process is immunopathologic, and some monoclonal antibodies can enhance macrophage infection. Thus, even more than with other viral vaccines, double-blinded, placebo-controlled trials are needed urgently to provide definitive evidence of protection and to exclude adverse effects.

HOSPITAL INFECTION CONTROL

The use of universal precautions in handling the blood and body fluids of all patients is prudent practice. In addition, a certified biologic safety cabinet should be used for all handling of human body fluids in situations in which splatter or aerosolization is possible.[58] Viral antigens can be detected in necropsy specimens, and RT-PCR readily detects viral genetic material in necropsy tissue and in blood and plasma obtained from hantavirus-infected persons early in the course of the disease.[42, 122] However, secondary transmission of hantaviruses associated with HFRS has not been documented after contact with acutely ill persons or exposure to their clinical laboratory specimens. The experience with American hantaviruses linked to HPS has been similar.[58, 114] A single well-documented episode of person-to-person spread during an Andes virus outbreak in South America and subsequent anecdotal experience with this agent suggest that it may be an exception.[25, 116] This latter incident notwithstanding, the many years of experience with HFRS and HPS indicate that once the diagnosis has been confirmed, isolation of hospitalized patients to prevent nosocomial transmission generally is not required. Sera and other specimens from hantavirus-infected persons can be handled safely by using biosafety level 2 facilities and practices. Higher biosafety levels are recommended for attempts to propagate hantaviruses.[11, 58]

REFERENCES

1. Ahlm, C., Settergren, B., Gothefors L., et al.: Nephropathia epidemica (hemorrhagic fever with renal syndrome) in children: Clinical characteristics. Pediatr. Infect. Dis. J. *13*:45, 1994.
2. Antoniadis, A., Stylianakis, A., Papa, A., et al.: Direct genetic detection of Dobrava virus in Greek and Albanian haemorrhagic fever with renal syndrome (HFRS) patients. J. Infect. Dis. *174*:407, 1996.
3. Armstrong, L. R., Bryan, R. T., Sarisky, J., et al.: Mild hantaviral disease caused by Sin Nombre virus in a four-year-old child. Pediatr. Infect. Dis. J. *14*:1108, 1995.
4. Avsic-Zupnac, T., Likar, M., Novakovic, S., et al.: Evidence of the presence of two hantaviruses in Slovenia. Arch. Virol. *115*(Suppl. 1):87, 1990.
5. Avsic-Zupanc, T., Xiao, S.-Y., Stojanovic, R., et al.: Characterization of Dobrava virus: A hantavirus from Slovenia. J. Med. Virol. *38*:132, 1992.
5a. Bohlman, M. C., Morzumor, S. P., Meissner, J., et al.: Analysis of hantavirus genetic diversity in Argentina: S segment–derived phylogeny. J. Virol. 76:3765, 2002.
6. Bruno, P., Hassell, L. H., Brown, J., et al.: The protean manifestations of hemorrhagic fever with renal syndrome: A retrospective review of 26 cases from Korea. Ann. Intern. Med. *113*:385, 1990.
7. Bryan, R. T., Doyle, T. J., Moolenaar, R. L., et al.: Hantavirus pulmonary syndrome in children. Semin. Pediatr. Infect. Dis. *8*:1–7, 1997.
8. Casals, J., Henderson, B. E., Hoogstraal, H., et al.: A review of Soviet viral hemorrhagic fevers, 1969. J. Infect. Dis. *122*:437–453, 1970.
9. Centers for Disease Control and Prevention/National Institutes of Health: Biosafety in Microbiological and Biomedical Laboratories. 3rd ed. Washington, DC, U.S. Department of Health and Human Services, Public Health Service, 1993, HHS Publication No. (CDC) 93–8395.

10. Chapman, L. E., Ellis, B. A., Koster, F. T., et al.: Discriminators between hantavirus-infected and uninfected persons enrolled in a trial of intravenous ribavirin for presumptive hantavirus pulmonary syndrome. Clin. Infect. Dis. *34*:293–304, 2002.
11. Chapman, L. E., and Khabbaz, R. F.: Review: Etiology and epidemiology of the Four Corners hantavirus outbreak. Infect. Agents Dis. *3*:234, 1994.
12. Chapman, L. E., Mertz, G. J., Peters, C. J., et al.: Safety and tolerance during one year of open label experience. Antiviral Ther. *4*:211–219, 1999.
13. Chen, H.-X., Qiu, F.-X., Dong, B.-J., et al.: Epidemiological studies on hemorrhagic fever with renal syndrome in China. J. Infect. Dis. *154*:394, 1986.
14. Childs, J. E., Kaufmann, A. F., Petere, C. J., and Ehrenberg, R. L.: Hantavirus infection—southwestern United States: Interim recommendations for risk reduction. Centers for Disease Control and Prevention. M. M. W. R. Recomm. Rep. *42*(RR-11):1–13, 1993.
15. Childs, J. E., Ksiazek, T. G., Spiropoulou, C. F., et al.: Serologic and genetic identification of *Peromyscus maniculatus* as the primary rodent reservoir for a new hantavirus in the southwestern United States. J. Infect. Dis. *169*:1271, 1994.
16. Chu, Y. K., Jennings, G., Schmaljohn, A., et al.: Cross-neutralization of hantaviruses with immune sera from experimentally infected animals and from hemorrhagic fever with renal syndrome and hantavirus pulmonary syndrome patients. J. Infect. Dis. *172*:1581, 1995.
17. Chu, Y. K., Rossi, C., LeDuc, J. W., et al.: Serological relationships among viruses in the *Hantavirus* genus, family *Bunyaviridae*. Virology *198*:196, 1994.
18. Collan, Y., Mihatsch, M. J., Lahdevirta, J., et al.: Nephropathia epidemica: Mild variant of hemorrhagic fever with renal syndrome. Kidney Int. *40*(Suppl. 35):62, 1991.
19. Cosgriff, T. M.: Mechanisms of disease in hantavirus infection: Pathophysiology of hemorrhagic fever with renal syndrome. Rev. Infect. Dis. *13*:97, 1991.
20. Desmyter, J., LeDuc, J. W., Johnson, K. M., et al.: Laboratory rat associated outbreak of haemorrhagic fever with renal syndrome due to Hantaan-like virus in Belgium. Lancet *2*:445, 1983.
21. Dournon, E., Moriniere, B., Matheron, S., et al.: HFRS after a wild rodent bite in the Haute-Savoie and risk of exposure to Hantaan-like virus in a Paris laboratory. Lancet *1*:676, 1984.
22. Duchin, J. S., Koster, F. T., Peters, C. J., et al.: Hantavirus pulmonary syndrome: A clinical description of 17 patients with a newly recognized disease. N. Engl. J. Med. *330*:949, 1994.
23. Earle, D. P.: Symposium on epidemic hemorrhagic fever. Am. J. Med. *16*:619, 1954.
24. Elliott, L., Ksiazek T. G., Rollin P. E., et al.: Isolation of the causative agent of hantavirus pulmonary syndrome. Am. J. Trop. Med. Hyg. *51*:102, 1994.
25. Enria, D., Padula, P., Segura, E. L., et al.: Hantavirus pulmonary syndrome in Argentina: Possibility of person-to-person transmission. Medicina *56*:709–711, 1996.
26. Feldmann, H., Sanchez, A., Morzunov, S., et al.: Utilization of autopsy RNA for the synthesis of the nucleocapsid antigen of a newly recognized virus associated with hantavirus pulmonary syndrome. Virus Res. *30*:351, 1993.
27. French, G. R., Foulke, R. S., Brand, O. A., et al.: Korean hemorrhagic fever: Propagation of the etiologic agent in a cell line of human origin. Science *211*:1046, 1981.
28. Gajdusek, D. C.: Acute infectious hemorrhagic fevers and mycotoxicoses in the Union of Soviet Socialist Republics. Medical Science Publication No. 2. Washington, D.C., Army Medical Service Graduate School, Walter Reed Army Medical Center, 1953.
29. Gajdusek, D. C.: Hemorrhagic fevers in Asia: A problem in medical ecology. Geogr. Rev. *41*:20, 1956.
30. Gajdusek, D. C.: Virus hemorrhagic fevers: Special reference to hemorrhagic fever with renal syndrome (epidemic hemorrhagic fever). J. Pediatr. *60*:841, 1962.
31. Glass, G. E., Cheek, J. E., Patz, J. A., et al.: Using remotely sensed data to identify areas at risk for hantavirus pulmonary syndrome. Emerg. Infect. Dis. *6*:238–247, 2000.
32. Glass, G. E., Watson, A. J., LeDuc, J. W., et al.: Infection with rat borne hantavirus in U.S. residents is consistently associated with hypertensive renal disease. J. Infect. Dis. *167*:614, 1993.
33. Glass, G. E., Watson, A. J., LeDuc, J. W., et al.: Domestic cases of hemorrhagic fever with renal syndrome in the United States. Nephron *68*:48, 1994.
34. Gligic, A., Dimkovic, N., Xiao, S.-Y., et al.: Belgrade virus: A new hantavirus causing severe hemorrhagic fever with renal syndrome in Yugoslavia. J. Infect. Dis. *166*:113, 1992.
35. Goldsmith, C. S., Elliot, L. H., Peters, C. J., et al.: Ultrastructural characteristics of Sin Nombre virus, causative agent of hantavirus pulmonary syndrome. Arch. Virol. *140*:2107, 1995.
36. Gonzalez-Scarano, F., and Nathanson, N.: *Bunyaviridae*. *In* Fields, B. N., Knipe, D. M., Howley, P. M., et al. (eds.): Fields' Virology. 3rd ed. Philadelphia, Lippincott-Raven, 1996, pp. 1473–1504.
37. Hallin, G. W., Simpson, S. Q., Crowell, R. E., et al.: Cardiopulmonary manifestations of hantavirus pulmonary syndrome. Crit. Care Med. *24*:252, 1996.
38. Hantavirus pulmonary syndrome—United States, 1995 and 1996. M. M. W. R. Morb. Mortal. Wkly. Rep. *45*(14):291–295, 1996.
39. Hjelle, B., Chavez-Giles, F., Torrez-Martinez, N., et al.: Genetic identification of a novel hantavirus of the harvest mouse *Reithrodontomys megalotis*. J. Virol. *68*:6751, 1994.
40. Hjelle, B., Goade, D., Torrez-Martinez, N., et al.: Hantavirus pulmonary syndrome, renal insufficiency and myositis associated with infection by Bayou hantavirus. Clin. Infect. Dis. *23*:495–500, 1996.
41. Hjelle, B., Krolikowski, J., Torrez-Martinez, N., et al.: Phylogenetically distinct hantavirus implicated in a case of hantavirus pulmonary syndrome in the northeastern United States. J. Med. Virol. *46*:21, 1995.
42. Hjelle, B., Spiropoulou, C. F., Torrez-Martinez, N., et al.: Detection of Muerto Canyon virus RNA in peripheral blood mononuclear cells from patients with hantavirus pulmonary syndrome. J. Infect. Dis. *170*:1013, 1994.
43. Hjelle, B., Torrez-Martinez, N., and Koster, F. T.: Hantavirus pulmonary syndrome–related virus from Bolivia. Lancet *347*:57, 1996.
44. Hortling, H.: En epidemi av falteben in finska Lappland. Nord. Med. *30*:1001, 1946.
45. Huggins, J. W., Hsiang, C. M., Cosgriff, T. M., et al.: Prospective, double-blind, concurrent, placebo-controlled clinical trial of intravenous ribavirin therapy of hemorrhagic fever with renal syndrome. J. Infect. Dis. *164*:1119, 1991.
46. Hullinghorst, R. L., and Steer, A.: Pathology of epidemic hemorrhagic fever. Ann. Intern. Med. *38*:77, 1953.
47. Jenison, S., Yamada, T., Morris, C., et al.: Characterization of human antibody responses to Four Corners hantavirus infections among patients with hantavirus pulmonary syndrome. J. Virol. *68*:3000, 1994.
48. Jiang, Y.-T.: A preliminary report on hemorrhagic fever with renal syndrome in China. Chin. Med. J. *96*:265, 1983.
49. Kawamata, J., Yamanouchi, T., Dohmae, K., et al.: Control of laboratory acquired hemorrhagic fever with renal syndrome (HFRS) in Japan. Lab. Anim. Sci. *37*:431, 1987.
50. Ketai, L. H., Williamson, M. R., Telepak, R. J., et al.: Hantavirus pulmonary syndrome: Radiographic findings in 16 patients. Radiology *191*:665, 1994.
51. Khan, A. S., Gaviria, M., Rollin, P. E., et al.: Hantavirus pulmonary syndrome in Florida: Association with the newly identified Black Creek Canal virus. Am. J. Med. *100*:46, 1996.
52. Khan, A. S., Khabbaz, R. F., Armstrong, L. R., et al.: Hantavirus pulmonary syndrome: The first 100 U.S. cases. J. Infect. Dis. *173*:1297, 1996.
53. Khan, A. S., Ksiazek, T. G., Zaki, S. R., et al.: Fatal hantavirus pulmonary syndrome in an adolescent. Pediatrics *95*:276, 1995.
54. Khan, A. S., Spiropoulou, C. F., Morzunov, S., et al.: Fatal illness associated with a new hantavirus in Louisiana. J. Med. Virol. *46*:281, 1995.
55. Ko, K. W.: Korean hemorrhagic fever in Korean children. *In* Murakami, K., and Sakai, Y. (eds.): Recent Advances in Pediatric Nephrology. Amsterdam, Elsevier, 1987, pp. 643–646.
56. Kolman, J.: Some physical and chemical properties of Uukuniemi virus, strain Potepli-63. Acta Virol. *14*:159, 1970.
56a. Koster, F., Foucar, K., Hjelle, B., et al.: Rapid presumptive diagnosis of hantavirus cardiopulmonary syndrome by peripheral blood smear review. Am. J. Clin. Pathol. *116*:665, 2001.
57. Ksiazek, T. G., Peters, C. J., Rollin, P. E., et al.: Identification of a new North American hantavirus that causes acute pulmonary insufficiency. Am. J. Trop. Med. Hyg. *52*:117, 1995.
58. Laboratory management of agents associated with hantavirus pulmonary syndrome: Interim biosafety guidelines. Centers for Disease Control and Prevention. M. M. W. R. Recomm. Rep. *43*(RR-7):1–7, 1994.
59. Lahdevirta, J.: Nephropathia epidemica in Finland: A clinical, histological and epidemiological study. Ann. Clin. Res. *3*(Suppl. 8):1, 1971.
60. Lahdevirta, J., Collan, Y. K., Jokinen, E. J., et al.: Renal sequelae to nephropathia epidemica. Acta Pathol. Microbiol. Scand. *86*:265, 1978.
61. LeDuc, J. W., Childs, J. E., and Glass, G. E.: The hantaviruses, etiologic agents of hemorrhagic fever with renal syndrome: A possible cause of hypertension and chronic renal disease in the United States. Annu. Rev. Public Health *13*:79, 1992.
61a. Lee, B. E., Joffe, A. R., and Vaudry, W.: Hantavirus pulmonary syndrome: Report of the first Canadian pediatric case. Can. J. Infect. Dis. 9:319, 1998.
62. Lee, H. W.: Epidemiologic features of Korean hemorrhagic fever and research activities on this disease in the Republic of Korea. Paper presented by the WHO Working Group on Hemorrhagic Fever with Renal Syndrome, February 1982, Tokyo.
63. Lee, H. W.: Epidemiology. *In* Lee, H. W., and Dalrymple, J. M. (eds.): Manual of Hemorrhagic Fever with Renal Syndrome. Seoul, Korea University, World Health Organization Collaborating Center for Virus Reference and Research Institute for Viral Diseases, 1989, pp. 39–48.
64. Lee, H. W., Baek, L. J., Seong, I. W., et al.: Physico-chemical properties of Hantaan virus. II. The effect of temperature and pH on infectivity of Hantaan virus. J. Korean Soc. Virol. *13*:23, 1983.
65. Lee, H. W., French, G. R., Lee, P. W., et al.: Observations on natural and laboratory infection of rodents with the etiologic agent of Korean hemorrhagic fever. Am. J. Trop. Med. Hyg. *30*:477, 1981.
66. Lee, H. W., and Johnson, K. M.: Laboratory-acquired infections with Hantaan virus, the etiologic agent of Korean hemorrhagic fever. J. Infect. Dis. *146*:645, 1982.

67. Lee, H. W., Lee, P. W., Baek, L. J., et al.: Intraspecific transmission of Hantaan virus, etiologic agent of Korean hemorrhagic fever, in the rodent *Apodemus agrarius*. Am. J. Trop. Med. Hyg. *30*:1106, 1981.
68. Lee, H. W., Lee, P. W., Baek, L. J., et al.: Geographical distribution of hemorrhagic fever with renal syndrome and hantaviruses. Arch. Virol. *115*(Suppl. 1):5, 1990.
69. Lee, H. W., Lee, P. W., and Johnson, K. M.: Isolation of the etiologic agent of Korean hemorrhagic fever. J. Infect. Dis. *137*:298, 1978.
70. Lee, J. S.: Clinical features of hemorrhagic fever with renal syndrome in Korea. Kidney Int. *40*(Suppl. 35):88, 1991.
71. Lee, P. W., Meegan, J. M., LeDuc, J. W., et al.: Serologic techniques for detection of Hantaan virus infection, related antigens and antibodies. *In* Lee, H. W., and Dalrymple, J. M. (eds.): Manual of Hemorrhagic Fever with Renal Syndrome. Seoul, Korea University, World Health Organization Collaborating Center for Virus Reference and Research Institute for Viral Diseases, 1989, pp. 36–38.
72. Levy, H., and Simpson, S. Q.: Hantavirus pulmonary syndrome. Am. J. Respir. Crit. Care Med. *149*:1710, 1994.
73. Lloyd, G., Bowen, E. T. W., Jones N., et al.: HFRS outbreak associated with laboratory rats in UK. Lancet *1*:175, 1984.
74. Lopez, N., Padula, P., Rossi, C., et al.: Genetic identification of a new hantavirus causing severe pulmonary syndrome in Argentina. Virology *220*:223, 1996.
75. Mayer, C. F.: Epidemic hemorrhagic fever of the Far East, or endemic hemorrhagic nephroso-nephritis, a short outline of the disease, with supplemental data on the results of experimental inoculation of human volunteers. Mil. Surg. *110*:276, 1952.
76. McKee, K. T., Jr., LeDuc, J. W., and Peters, C. J.: Hantaviruses. *In* Belshe, R. B. (ed.): Textbook of Human Virology. 2nd ed. Littleton, MA, PSG Publishing, 1991, pp. 615–632.
77. McNinch, J. H.: Far East command conference on epidemic hemorrhagic fever. Ann. Intern. Med. *38*:53, 1953.
78. Moolenaar, R. L., Dalton, C., Lipman, H. B., et al.: Clinical features that differentiate hantavirus pulmonary syndrome from three other acute respiratory illnesses. Clin. Infect. Dis. *21*:643, 1995.
79. Mustonen, J., Huttunen, N.-P., Brummer-Korvenkontio, M., et al.: Clinical picture of nephropathia epidemica in children. Acta Pediatr. *83*:526, 1994.
80. Myhrman, G.: En njursjukdorn med egenartad symptombild. Nord. Med. Tidsskr. 7:793, 1934.
81. Nichol, S. T., Rollin, P. E., Ksiazek, T. G., et al.: Hantavirus pulmonary syndrome and newly described hantaviruses in the United States. *In* Elliott, R. H. (ed.): *Bunyaviridae*. New York, Plenum, 1996, pp. 269–280.
82. Nichol, S. T., Spiropoulou, C. F., Morzunov, S., et al.: Genetic identification of a hantavirus associated with an outbreak of acute respiratory illness. Science *262*:914, 1993.
83. Niklasson, B., Hellsten, G., and LeDuc, J.: Hemorrhagic fever with renal syndrome: A study of sequelae following nephropathia epidemica. Arch. Virol. *137*:241, 1994.
84. Niklasson, B., and LeDuc, J. W.: Isolation of the nephropathia epidemica agent in Sweden. Lancet *1*:1012, 1984.
85. Niklasson, B., LeDuc, J., Nystrom, K., et al.: Nephropathia epidemica: Incidence of clinical cases and antibody prevalence in an endemic area of Sweden. Epidemiol. Infect. *99*:559, 1987.
86. Parisi, M. D. N., Enria, D. A., Piri, N. C., et al.: Retrospective detection of clinical infection caused by hantavirus in Argentina. Medicina *56*:1, 1996.
87. Parmenter, R. R., Brunt, J. W., Moore, D. I., et al.: The hantavirus epidemic in the Southwest: Rodent population dynamics and the implications for transmission of hantavirus-associated adult respiratory distress syndrome (HARDS) in the Four Corners region. Sevilleta LTER Publications Nos. 41 and 45. Albuquerque, University of New Mexico, 1993.
88. Peco-Antic, A., Popovic-Rolovic, M., Gligic, A., et al.: Clinical characteristics of haemorrhagic fever with renal syndrome in children. Pediatr. Nephrol. *6*:335, 1992.
89. Peters, C. J.: Pathogenesis of viral hemorrhagic fevers. *In* Nathanson, N., Ahmed, R., Gonzalez-Scarano, F., et al. (eds.): Viral Pathogenesis. Philadelphia, Lippincott-Raven, 1996, pp. 779–800.
90. Peters, C. J., and Khan, A. S.: Hantavirus pulmonary syndrome: The new American hemorrhagic fever. Clin. Infect. Dis. *34*:1224–1231, 2002.
91. Pilaski, J., Feldman, H., Morzunov, S., et al.: Genetic identification of a new Puumala virus strain causing severe hemorrhagic fever with renal syndrome in Germany. J. Infect. Dis. *170*:1456, 1994.
92. Pon, E., McKee, K. T., Jr., Diniega, B. M., et al.: Outbreak of hemorrhagic fever with renal syndrome among U.S. Marines in Korea. Am. J. Trop. Med. Hyg. *42*:612, 1990.
93. Prince, H. N., Prince, D. L., and Prince, R. N.: Principles of viral control and transmission. *In* Block, S. S. (ed.): Disinfection, Sterilization, and Preservation. 4th ed. Philadelphia, Lea & Febiger, 1991, pp. 411–444.
93a. Ramos, M. M., Overturf, G. D., Crowley, M. R., et al.: Infection with Sin Nombre hantavirus: Clinical presentation and outcome in children and adolescents. Pediatrics *108*:E27, 2001.
94. Rollin, P. E., Ksiazek, T. G., Elliot, L. H., et al.: Isolation of Black Creek Canal virus, a new hantavirus from *Sigmodon hispidus* in Florida. J. Med. Virol. *46*:35, 1995.
95. Schmaljohn, A., Li, D., Negley, D. L., et al.: Isolation and initial characterization of a new found hantavirus from California. Virology *206*:963, 1995.
96. Schmaljohn, C. S., and Dalrymple, J. M.: Analysis of Hantaan virus RNA: Evidence for a new genus of *Bunyaviridae*. Virology *131*:482, 1983.
97. Schmaljohn, C. S., Hasty, S. E., and Dalrymple, J. M.: Preparation of candidate vaccinia-vectored vaccines for haemorrhagic fever with renal syndrome. Vaccine *10*:10, 1992.
98. Schmaljohn, C. S., Hasty, S. E., Dalrymple, J. M., et al.: Antigenic and genetic properties of viruses linked to hemorrhagic fever with renal syndrome. Science *227*:1041, 1985.
99. Schmaljohn, C. S., and Hooper, J. W.: *Bunyaviridae:* The viruses and their replication. *In* Knipe, D. M., Howley, P. M., Griffin, D. E. (eds.): Fields' Virology. 4th ed. Philadelphia, Lippincott, Williams, & Wilkins, 2001, pp. 1635–1668.
100. Settergren, B.: Nephropathia epidemica (hemorrhagic fever with renal syndrome) in Scandinavia. Rev. Infect. Dis. *13*:736, 1991.
101. Sheedy, J. A., Froed, B. F., Batson, H. A., et al.: The clinical course of epidemic hemorrhagic fever. Am. J. Med. *16*:619, 1954.
102. Simonsen, L., Dalton, M. J., Breiman, R. F., et al.: Evaluation of the magnitude of the 1993 hantavirus outbreak in the southwestern United States. J. Infect. Dis. *172*:729, 1995.
103. Smorodintsev, A. A., Kazbintsev, L. I., and Chudakov, V. G.: Viral Hemorrhagic Fevers. Washington, DC, Office of Technical Services, U.S. Department of Commerce, 1964, p. 1.
104. Song, J. W., Back, L. J., Gajdusek, D. C., et al.: Isolation of pathogenic hantavirus from white-footed mouse *(Peromyscus leucopus)*. Lancet *344*:1637, 1994.
105. Stevens, C., Johnson, M., and Bell, A.: First reported cases of hantavirus pulmonary syndrome in Canada. Can. Commun. Dis. Rep. *20*:121, 1994.
106. Stuhlfauth, K.: Bericht über ein neues schlammtieberahnliches Krankheitsbild bei deutschen Truppen in Lappland. Dtsch. Med. Wochenschr. *69*:439, 1973.
107. Tkachenko, E. A., and Lee, H. W.: Etiology and epidemiology of hemorrhagic fever with renal syndrome. Kidney Int. *40*(Suppl. 35):54, 1991.
108. Torrez-Martinez, N., and Hjelle, B.: Enzootic of Bayou hantavirus in rice rats *(Oryzomys palustris)* in 1983. Lancet *346*:780, 1995.
109. Trencseni, T., and Keleti, B.: Clinical Aspects and Epidemiology of Haemorrhagic Fever with Renal Syndrome. Budapest, Akademiai Kiado, 1971.
110. Tsai, T. F.: Hemorrhagic fever with renal syndrome: Clinical aspects. Lab. Anim. Sci. *37*:419, 1987.
111. Tsai, T. F.: Hemorrhagic fever with renal syndrome: Mode of transmission to humans. Lab. Anim. Sci. *37*:428, 1987.
112. Umenai, T., Lee, H. W., Lee, P. W., et al.: Korean haemorrhagic fever in staff in an animal laboratory. Lancet *1*:314, 1979.
113. van Ypersele de Strihou, C.: Clinical features of hemorrhagic fever with renal syndrome in Europe. Kidney Int. *40*(Suppl. 35):80, 1991.
113a. Verity, R., Prasad, E., Grimsrud, K., et al.: Hantavirus pulmonary syndrome in northern Alberta, Canada: Clinical and laboratory findings for 19 cases. Clinical Infectious Diseases *31*:942, 2000.
113b. Vincent, M. J., Quiroz, E., Gracia, F., et al: Hantavirus pulmonary syndrome in Panama: Identification of novel hantaviruses and their likely reservoirs. Virology *277*:14, 2000.
114. Vitek, C. R., Breiman, R. F., Ksiazek, T. G., et al.: Evidence against person-to-person transmission of hantavirus to health-care workers. Clin. Infect. Dis. *22*:824, 1996.
115. Weissenbacher, M. C., Cura, E., Segura, E. L., et al.: Serological evidence of human hantavirus infection in Argentina, Bolivia, and Uruguay. Medicina *56*:17, 1996.
116. Wells, R. M., Sosa Estani, S., Yadon, Z. E., et al.: An unusual hantavirus outbreak in southern Argentina: Person-to-person transmission? Emerg. Infect. Dis. *3*:171–174, 1997.
117. Williams, R. J., Bryan, R. T., Mills, J. N., et al.: An outbreak of hantavirus pulmonary syndrome among Mennonite colonies in western Paraguay. Am. J. Trop. Med. Hyg. *57*:274–282, 1997.
118. Yanagihara, R.: Hantavirus infection in the United States: Epizootiology and epidemiology. Rev. Infect. Dis. *12*:449, 1990.
119. Yanagihara, R., Gajdusek, D. C., Gibbs, C. J., Jr., et al.: Prospect Hill virus: Serological evidence for infection in mammologists. N. Engl. J. Med. *310*:1325, 1984.
120. Yanagihara, R., Goldgaber, D., Lee, P. W., et al.: Propagation of nephropathia epidemica in cell culture. Lancet *1*:1013, 1984.
121. Yoo, K. H., and Choi, Y.: Haemorrhagic fever with renal syndrome in Korean children. Korean Society of Pediatric Nephrology. Pediatr. Nephrol. *8*:540–544, 1994.
122. Zaki, S. R., Greer, P. W., Coffield, L. M. et al.: Hantavirus pulmonary syndrome: Pathogenesis of an emerging infectious disease. Am. J. Pathol. *146*:552, 1995.
123. Zeitz, P. S., Butler, J. C., Cheek, J. E., et al.: A case-control study of hantavirus pulmonary syndrome during an outbreak in the southwestern United States. J. Infect. Dis. *171*:864, 1995.
124. Zetterholm, S. G.: Akuta mefriter simulerande akuta bukfall. Svenska Lakartidningen *31*:425, 1934.
125. Zoller, L., Yang, S., Gott, P., et al.: Use of recombinant nucleocapsid proteins of the Hantaan and nephropathia epidemica serotypes of hantaviruses as immunodiagnostic antigens. J. Med. Virol. *39*:200, 1993.

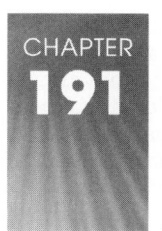

La Crosse Encephalitis and Other California Serogroup Viruses

JAMES E. McJUNKIN ■ LINDA L. MINNICH ■ THEODORE F. TSAI

Terminology

The term *California serogroup* does not describe the widespread geographic distribution of viruses in the serogroup but simply reflects the name of the prototype virus initially discovered in California in 1943. In fact, La Crosse (LAC) virus, the most prevalent and pathogenic member of the serogroup, produces disease in the Midwest and eastern United States but not in the West Coast region.[1, 13, 40, 44, 74, 106, 107] LAC virus is estimated to cause 8 to 30 percent of all cases of encephalitis in the United States annually and is the most common arboviral infection of children in North America.[93] The other members of the California serogroup also are addressed briefly.

Clinical information of greatest relevance to practitioners is contained in the following sections: Clinical Manifestations, Diagnosis, Differential Diagnosis, and Treatment.

Etiologic Agent

In 1960, a 4-year-old girl died of "rural encephalitis" in a hospital in La Crosse County, Wisconsin. Four years later, Dr. Wayne Thompson and colleagues isolated a novel virus from frozen homogenates of the child's brain by intracerebral inoculation of suckling mice.[103, 105] Soon after its discovery, LAC virus was identified as a member of the California serogroup and is one of five (prototype California encephalitis [CE], LAC, snowshoe hare, Jamestown Canyon [JC], and trivittatus) viruses causing human disease in North America. Inkoo and Tahyna viruses are members of the California serogroup distributed in Europe.

The California serogroup is 1 of 16 in the Bunyavirus genus. Bunyaviruses are spherical particles 75 to 115 nm in diameter with nucleocapsid cores 60 to 70 nm in diameter enveloped by a membrane bilayer 4 nm thick.[101] Virions bud directly by vesicular fusion from the cisternae of Golgi or the endoplasmic reticulum. The genome is composed of three pieces of negative-sense, single-stranded circularized RNA. Each of the three RNA segments (L, M, and S) is associated with a nucleoprotein encoded by the S segment and small quantities of L protein (a viral polymerase), and these proteins form the three nucleocapsids.[39, 42, 49] The circular, helical nucleocapsids are enclosed in a lipid envelope in which the G1 and G2 glycoproteins are located on 5- to 10-nm-long spikes.

The M segment that encodes the G1 and G2 glycoproteins is a major determinant of viral neuro-invasiveness in mice and susceptibility of *Aedes triseriatus* mosquitoes to oral and intrathoracic infection.[5, 37, 40, 95] Neuro-invasiveness may be linked to the cell receptor and fusion functions associated with glycoproteins.[37, 39] The G1 protein of LAC virus is involved in viral attachment to mammalian cell receptors, hemagglutination, and viral neutralization.[37, 40, 67, 68, 95] Group- and LAC virus–specific epitopes are present on G1. The G2 glycoprotein mediates viral attachment to insect cells,[73] but recent work emphasizes that G1 also is required for infection of mosquito cells (in vitro and in vivo).[50] Antibodies to the nucleocapsid protein neither hemagglutinate nor neutralize.

Although the M segment genome largely determines *neuro-invasiveness* (i.e., the ability to invade the central nervous system [CNS] from an extraneural site) via its glycoprotein products (especially G1), recent evidence using viral reassortants of different virulence implicates the L segment as a major factor in determining *neurovirulence* (i.e., the ability to infect CNS tissue after direct cerebral injection).[34] Recent work has shown that a truncated G1 protein preparation induces a protective immune response in the suckling mouse model via neutralizing antibody (see "Prevention").[88] Apparently, neutralizing antibody can prevent neuro-invasion by interruption of the transient viremia, which occurs just after virus inoculation.

Oligonucleotide maps of LAC viral isolates from various areas of the United States have grouped the viruses into three types. Upper Midwest viral strains are of two types, A and B; type C varieties are found in scattered areas of the eastern part of the United States.[32, 70] Strain variation indicates that changes in the viral genome occur by genetic drift. Genetic reassortment through exchange of RNA segments also has been demonstrated in nature. Study of the genome of viral isolates from three fatal cases indicated a high degree of conservation of nucleotide sequences among these isolates.[18, 55]

Ecology

Ochlerotatus triseriatus (formerly known as *A. triseriatus*), the eastern tree hole mosquito, is the reservoir of LAC virus in nature and the vector for transmission of infection to humans.[44, 109, 110] Humans do not maintain prolonged viremia and, therefore, are dead-end hosts. The mosquito is distributed principally in eastern hardwood deciduous forests, where it breeds in tree holes; however, it also is adapted to breeding in small artificial containers that hold rainwater, such as discarded cans, bottles, and tires. The mosquito is diurnal and feeds actively during the day. Although they disperse over a wide area, fairly permanent foci of infected mosquitoes are observed in sharply delimited areas, and virus isolation and human cases recur each summer in established foci.[44, 69, 100]

The most important mechanism for maintenance of LAC virus in nature is vertical (transovarial) transmission in *O. triseriatus*. The virus overwinters in infected eggs, which give rise to infected mosquito progeny the following year, thereby providing the mechanism of recurrent disease each summer in endemic areas.[80, 99, 110] Recent work has indicated that transovarial transmission of LAC virus in *O. triseriatus* is controlled by a single gene locus.[43] The LAC virus also is maintained in nature via horizontal transmission by venereal propagation in *O. triseriatus* and through amplification of the virus in the vertebrate hosts on which vector mosquitoes feed.[80, 109, 110] Vector competence, related in part to the ability of the female mosquito to become infected in the first place, may be associated with malnutrition of the mosquito, which compromises her mesenteric barrier and might then allow infection to occur after taking a LAC virus–infected blood meal.[43, 87] The principal amplifying hosts involved in horizontal transmission are chipmunks and squirrels.[115] Other wild vertebrates such as foxes and woodchucks also may contribute to amplification. Although domestic livestock and pets do not contribute to horizontal amplification of the virus, certain species do show seroconversion to California serogroup viruses, and these species may prove to be useful markers of viral presence in a given area.[36] For example, outbreaks of fatal encephalitis have occurred in puppies, and dogs have been used in an animal model of CNS infection.[11]

Aedes canadensis is an important secondary vector found in Ohio and West Virginia.[9, 84] LAC virus varieties with a type C oligonucleotide pattern are found in this species in Ohio and New York. Concern that *Aedes albopictus,* the Asian tiger mosquito, could enter the transmission cycle for LAC[23, 24, 46] was confirmed recently when LAC virus–infected *A. albopictus* mosquitos were isolated in nature in areas proximate to human cases.[35] This species, which is dispersed widely in the southeastern region of the United States, has significant potential to expand the geographic range and circumstances in which LAC virus (and possibly other California serogroup viruses) might be transmitted.

Although JC virus first was isolated in Colorado and is distributed widely in the West and Midwest, most cases of human illness have been reported in New York, New England, Ontario, and the upper Midwest. Recently, seroconversion for JC virus also was found frequently (18%) in native Alaskans.[108] Various *Aedes* mosquitoes (e.g., *Aedes communis* in the West, *Aedes stimulans* in the upper Midwest, *Aedes abserratus* in Connecticut) function as vectors.[26, 44, 45, 47] As opposed to LAC virus, in which large mammals do not play a role in viral propagation in nature, JC virus has deer as the primary amplifying host, with up to 80 percent seroconversion found in adult deer populations in endemic areas.[85, 86, 116] The overwintering mechanism of JC virus has not been elucidated, although transovarial transmission in *Aedes provocans* has been demonstrated.[10]

Snowshoe hare virus is distributed throughout Canada, including the Yukon and Northwest Territories, in adjacent northern states, and in Russia and China. *Culiseta inorata* and various *Aedes* spp. transmit the virus to snowshoe hares *(Lepus americanus),* ground squirrels *(Citellus undulatus),* and other mammals. Transovarial transmission in vector mosquitoes has been demonstrated.[52]

Trivittatus virus is transmitted and maintained through vertical transmission by *A. trivittatus* in the Midwest and is vectored in the South by *Aedes infirmatus.* CE virus is distributed in the western part of the United States, where *Aedes melanimon* and *Aedes dorsalis* are the principal vectors.[43, 51, 91, 104] Inkoo and Tahyna viruses cause a febrile illness with CNS and respiratory tract infection, respectively, in Scandinavia, Central Europe, and western Russia. Viral recombinants have been demonstrated.[29] Inkoo also has been found recently in native Alaskans.[108]

Epidemiology

LAC encephalitis principally is a disease of children. Among reported cases in the United States from 1972 to 1981, 75 percent were in children younger than 10 years, and only 3 percent occurred in persons 20 years or older.[65, 113] The majority of cases are seen in males, with a ratio of approximately 2:1 in most series, probably related to a higher exposure rate of males to sylvan vectors.[82, 103] The annual incidence of CNS LAC virus infection in individuals younger than 15 years in endemic regions is approximately 10 to 30 per 100,000.[66, 112] LAC virus infections are endemic in the United States, with infections typically occurring from July through October, chiefly in rural areas of the east-central states.[65, 106] The geographic distribution of LAC virus infection corresponds to natural divisions where beech, oak, and maple woodlots are prevalent.[44] Although LAC encephalitis has been considered a disease of the Midwestern and mid-Atlantic states (with highly endemic zones in Minnesota, Wisconsin, Illinois, Iowa, Ohio, and West Virginia), cases have been found in 28 states, mostly east of the Mississippi. One highly endemic focus has been recognized in western North Carolina for many years,[99] and sporadic cases have been found as far south as Louisiana and as far east as Connecticut (Fig. 191–1). Although the appearance is that certain foci of infection tend to remain well localized,[81, 99] recent work in eastern Tennessee showing a low seroprevalence in the general population (only 0.5%), despite a recent marked increase in the number of pediatric cases in that region, suggests that true increases in the prevalence of LAC infection (indicating a newly established endemic focus) are occurring in some areas as well.[62, 63] Active surveillance efforts can increase case-finding markedly, as seen in West Virginia,[66] where after the death of a child from LAC encephalitis in 1987, more than 150 cases were diagnosed during the next 8 years (versus only 15 cases ever previously reported in West Virginia).[78] Centers for Disease Control and Prevention (CDC) records further showed that from 1987 to 1997, West Virginia became the most highly endemic state in the United States, often accounting for roughly half or more of the cases reported to the CDC annually. Therefore, the public health importance of LAC encephalitis nationally is not known fully because the virus is distributed discontinuously in the eastern part of the United States, where the disease could be endemic but under-recognized.[8, 58, 112] Improved recognition will require a high index of suspicion by clinicians because the virus typically is not recoverable on culture of cerebrospinal fluid (CSF) and therefore requires specific serologic testing (see Diagnosis).

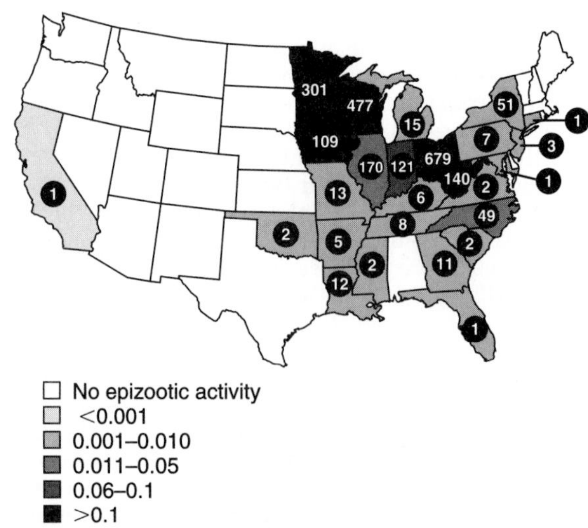

FIGURE 191–1 ■ Reported cases of encephalitis attributable to California serogroup virus by state and incidence per 10,000 population, 1964 to 1995.

Further confounding efforts to understand the true prevalence of disease is the fact that inapparent infections are far more prevalent than clinically evident disease is (see Clinical Manifestations).[65] Seroprevalence rises with age in endemic areas.[99, 100] Serosurveys have shown that point-prevalence rates vary in endemic locations from 30 percent in rural areas to 15 percent in urban locations.[82] Although the risk appears to be highest in rural areas, many cases occur in suburban residential locations, and travel to forested recreational areas in endemic regions is reported by other patients.[27, 58, 104] A case-control study performed in a highly endemic county found several characteristics of the peridomestic environment to be associated with a risk of acquiring LAC encephalitis: tree holes on the residential premise, proximity of the house to the forest edge, and the presence of artificial containers and large numbers of discarded tires. Various types of behavior (e.g., time spent outdoors, use of air conditioners) were not risk factors.[112] This study supports other work pointing to the proximity and abundance of natural and artificial mosquito breeding sites as the principal risk factor from an environmental perspective.[81, 84]

Serosurveys indicate JC virus seroprevalence rates of 5 to 40 percent in the upper Midwest. The preponderance of reported cases (21 of 29 in one series) occur in males.[97] Unlike LAC encephalitis, cases are found in all age groups. Human infections with snowshoe hare virus have been documented by serosurvey in Alaska and throughout Canada.[44] Antibody prevalence rates were more than 30 percent in some areas; seroprevalence in males was double the rate in females. Sporadic infection with CE viruses is probably frequent in the western part of the United States.[91] The prevalence of seroreactors was approximately one third in a study of the residents of Kern County, California. However, symptomatic cases rarely occur.

Pathogenesis

LAC virus, which infects the salivary glands of the mosquito vector, is introduced into the host's skin and subcutaneous tissue during feeding. Probing alone is infectious. Completion of a blood meal is not necessary for transmission. Local viral replication in adjacent muscle tissue leads to a systemic viremia that seeds the reticuloendothelial system, muscle, and chondrocytes; such seeding results in further amplification of the viremia and allows invasion of the CNS.[38, 39, 59, 61] Entrance to the CNS probably is gained via infection of vascular endothelial cells initially, followed by infection of neurons and glial cells.[59, 61] Recent case reports suggest that vascular involvement in human LAC encephalitis may be important in the pathogenesis of focal deficits (from stroke) and more generalized cerebral edema (possibly from vasogenic edema).[72, 77] Polymerase chain reaction (PCR) studies of the location of LAC virus within the CNS found evidence of viral RNA within the cortex but not in other tissues of the CNS.[18] The latter is consistent with the results of magnetic resonance imaging (MRI) in a recent study, which showed findings predominantly consistent with lesions in cortical areas.[76]

Studies indicate that the extraneural phase of viral replication and neuro-invasiveness are mediated largely by the M segment of the genome primarily via G1 glycoprotein, which has cell receptor and fusion functions.[37, 39, 40, 95] A more recent study in adult mice has indicated that once the virus has gained access to the CNS, replication in CNS tissue, that is, neurovirulence, is mediated largely by the L RNA segment, probably via viral polymerase.[33, 40] Previous work had implicated the M segment in neurovirulence as well, but in that study neurovirulence was defined as time to death after intracutaneous inoculation.[95] The host immune response involves neutralizing antibody, which mediates viral aggregation, inhibition of viral attachment to cells, and inhibition of viral penetration and uncoating.[68] Other aspects of the immune response recently shown to play a role in protection against CNS LAC virus infection in animal models are $CD4^+$ T cells and MxA protein, the latter of which is induced by the interferon-α/β system.[53, 94] Susceptibility and complications of LAC encephalitis may have an immunogenic component, as indicated by an association of illness and seizures with certain human leukocyte antigens.[15] Neuronal cell death may be mediated largely by apoptosis (programmed cell death), as determined by studies in mice.[89]

Clinical Manifestations

The clinical spectrum of illness in LAC virus infections ranges from inapparent infection or a mild febrile illness to aseptic meningitis and fatal encephalitis.[3, 4, 19, 20, 22, 48, 54, 102, 114] The ratio of inapparent to clinical infection has ranged from 26:1 to 322:1.[65] Most clinically apparent infections are associated with signs and symptoms of meningoencephalitis. Severe cases tend to mimic herpes simplex encephalitis at initial evaluation, whereas mild cases may be manifested as aseptic meningitis. Although the case-fatality rate is less than 1 percent, a recent series of 127 hospitalized patients included 3 with the near-lethal complication of cerebral herniation, and a high percentage (25%) of patients required intensive support, such as mechanical ventilation.[76]

Children typically have a 3- to 4-day prodrome of fever, headache, and vomiting; diarrhea is usually absent. The illness further evolves such that disorientation (42%) or seizures (46%), or both, are seen frequently on the day of admission. Most seizures are partial or partial with secondary generalization (58%), with the remainder being generalized. Status epilepticus develops in approximately one fourth of children with seizures. Rare patients may have a sudden onset of seizures with little or no preceding fever or headache.[76]

On examination, signs of meningeal irritation and mental status changes are found in approximately one quarter and one third of patients, respectively.[76] Focal neurologic signs, principally focal seizures, paresis, aphasia, and abnormal reflexes, are seen in 16 to 25 percent of cases of LAC encephalitis. Focal and generalized seizures occur in 42 to 62 percent of cases, and status epilepticus develops in 10 to 15 percent. Focal neurologic signs, whether found on physical examination or on electroencephalographic (EEG) or imaging studies, generally should be taken as evidence of presumptive herpes simplex encephalitis until a diagnosis of LAC encephalitis can be confirmed.[113]

In the largest and most recent series studied (n = 127),[76] the hospital course was complicated by hyponatremia (21%) generally consistent with the syndrome of inappropriate antidiuretic hormone (SIADH) secretion, recurrent or de novo seizures (13%), signs of increased intracranial pressure (13%), and cerebral herniation (2.3%). Approximately 1 in 10 patients (including the 3 with herniation and 10 others with recurrent seizures, coma, or both) experienced significant neurologic deterioration usually between 36 and 72 hours of admission. Possible risk factors associated with deterioration were the presence of disorientation or vomiting at admission and a trend toward seizures at admission. Such neurologic deterioration appeared to be related temporally to a decrease in serum sodium or an increase in body temperature in some cases.

Clinical findings in patients infected with other members of the California serogroup deserve brief mention. JC virus infections often are associated with prodromal respiratory symptoms in conjunction with aseptic meningitis or clinical encephalitis. Among 39 patients with proven or suspected CNS infection with JC virus, 10 had encephalitis and 7 reported upper respiratory symptoms or pneumonia.[44, 97]

The few reported cases of snowshoe hare virus infection have had manifestations ranging from an influenza-like illness to aseptic meningitis and fatal encephalitis. One fatality was reported in a 14-year-old girl who had symptoms and signs that suggested Reye syndrome.[30] In a 59-year-old man, radiologic and EEG findings showed a temporal lobe focus, which led to brain biopsy and a clinical and pathologic diagnosis of herpes encephalitis, although herpes virus was not isolated. Serologic examination later confirmed the diagnosis of snowshoe hare virus infection. Mild febrile illness attributed to infection with trivittatus virus has been described in some patients, and CNS infections have been identified in others.[82] Three cases of infection caused by prototype CE virus have been reported. All three patients had signs and symptoms of encephalitis.[51]

Laboratory examinations for LAC virus infection have been well outlined in a recent series.[76] The total CSF leukocyte count typically is elevated only moderately (in this series, the median white blood cell [WBC] count in CSF was 75), and 25 percent of patients had red blood cells in CSF.[76] Elevated protein levels are observed in less than a third of cases.[3, 20, 22, 54, 76] Approximately 10 percent of children will have negative or equivocal findings on initial CSF analysis, only to have numerous WBCs within 24 to 48 hours on repeat lumbar puncture. The peripheral leukocyte count was elevated in half the cases (>15,000 WBCs/mm^3), and neutrophilia was often present.[76]

Brain imaging techniques are usually negative, but they have a higher yield in more advanced disease. In 127 children in a recent study, 92 had computed tomography (CT) scans. Only 11 were positive, 8 showing generalized edema and 3 with focal findings, all in supratentorial locations. In three children whose courses were complicated by cerebral herniation, CT scans became positive only after the herniation event (i.e., admission CT scans were negative [Fig. 191–2]). From this same series *(n* = 127), 10 children had MRI of the brain, 4 of which were abnormal and showed focal areas of gadolinium enhancement, predominantly in cortical areas[76] (see Fig. 191–2). Recent case reports suggest that MRI may reveal lesions not detected by CT in LAC encephalitis. In a 20-month-old infant with right hemiparesis, CT on admission was negative, but MRI on day 1 showed evidence of acute infarction of the left basal ganglia.[72] In another 12-month-old child with clinical evidence of neurodegeneration, MRI showed areas of increased signal intensity in the periventricular white matter, even though the initial CT scan had been negative.[34] *It must be emphasized, however, that the technical difficulties in performing MRI in children (especially nonintubated children) still favor CT as the initial imaging study.*

EEG abnormalities have been found in 71 to 90 percent of patients tested. Focal EEG findings, usually slowing, may appear in as many as 44 percent of abnormal EEGs. Recent evidence indicates that periodic lateralizing epileptiform discharges (PLEDs), previously thought to be virtually pathognomonic of herpes simplex encephalitis, also are seen in LAC encephalitis, with 8 of 90 EEGs in one recent series positive for PLEDs.[28, 76] In four of these eight cases, patients required continuous EEG surveillance to monitor treatment of nonconvulsive status epilepticus.[76]

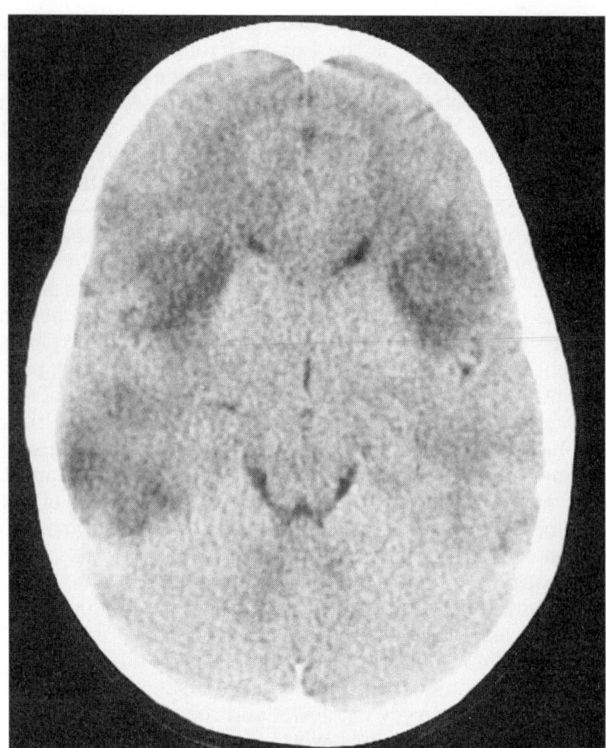

FIGURE 191–2 ■ A computed tomographic scan of an unusually severe case of La Crosse encephalitis shows small ventricles and multifocal hypodense lesions with loss of gray-white differentiation in the right frontotemporoparietal and left temporal regions. Computed tomographic scans are usually negative in La Crosse encephalitis (see text).

Diagnosis

Of importance is that clinicians communicate with virology laboratory colleagues when choosing diagnostic tests for encephalitis so that the limitations of these tests are understood. To select appropriate laboratory tests, information about the clinical findings and travel history must be combined with knowledge of the local epidemiology and natural history of viral infections.

Although the preferred approach to the diagnosis of viral encephalitis is to identify the viral agent by isolation or detection of antigen or nucleic acid in CSF, limitations of these procedures for LAC virus require the diagnosis to be made by serologic methods. Despite one report of isolation of LAC virus from CSF, culture still is not a reliable means of diagnosis or documentation of infection. LAC virus has been isolated from the brain on three occasions (two postmortem and one via brain biopsy in a surviving patient).[64, 81] No isolation from CSF was reported in a series of 34 LAC encephalitis patients.[84] Identification of viral antigen in infected mosquitoes or in brain autopsy or biopsy specimens can be accomplished by immunohistochemical techniques such as immunofluorescence (IF) and immunoperoxidase staining.[16] Viral genome components can be identified by hybridization.[17] PCR assays have been developed but have not been evaluated clinically.[14, 71] The additional inherent problems of processing and transport of specimens for RNA isolation render the challenges of reverse transcriptase PCR for LAC virus greater than those encountered with the more stable DNA of herpes simplex.

Given the limitations for identification of virus in CSF, serologic methods continue to be the primary method of diagnosis. IgM-specific antibody to LAC virus can be detected by an IgM capture enzyme immunoassay (EIA) or by IF in CSF and serum specimens. IgM capture EIA is a sensitive serologic test that detects virus-specific IgM in 83 to 100 percent of cases.[6, 7, 11, 12, 29, 31] Absorbance values are usually higher in CSF than in serum, but serum may be positive for IgM-specific antibody earlier in the course of infection. Even though serum IgM can persist for as long as 9 months after primary infection, the seasonal occurrence of LAC infection renders IgM-specific serologic study a useful tool in diagnosing acute infection. IgM has been reported to persist for 1 to 7 years after acute infection in patients with postencephalitic seizures, but whether this presence is due to the persistence of viral infection in patients with CNS sequelae is not clear. Standardized procedures and reagents are not available commercially. Reagents must be produced by the laboratory or obtained from the CDC and then cross-titrated by the end user. Procedures for titration of reagents and their utilization also lack standardization. Microtiter plates must be prepared with the capture antibody for human IgM, and the usual procedure requires overnight incubation. The time and technical expertise required for this procedure restrict its routine use. In addition, the overnight incubation needed for maximal sensitivity of the IgM capture assay renders its use as a "rapid" diagnostic test much less practical than use of the IF test, which can be completed in 2 to 3 hours.

The only diagnostic serologic kit approved by the Food and Drug Administration (FDA) is an indirect IF test for LAC, eastern equine, western equine, and St. Louis encephalitis viruses (Focus Technologies, Inc.). Despite the cost of reagents, this technique is better suited for rapid (same-day) results and processing of single specimens. Although the procedure is not difficult technically for individuals familiar with IF procedures, experience and observation of strict criteria for positive readings are critical to ensure the specificity of IgM-specific tests. Pretreatment of serum to remove or inactivate IgG, comparison of reactivity among the four viral antigens, and a requirement for intracytoplasmic inclusions are essential to maintain specificity of the test. The sensitivity of 60 to 80 percent of cases positive for IgM at the time of hospital admission can be enhanced further (to more than 90%) by repeat serologic testing 3 to 7 days later in cases in which the initial testing is negative but clinical suspicion has not been allayed. (Note that a similar relationship between the timing of testing and sensitivity applies to IgM capture EIA as well.) Specificity is related directly to observation of the reading criteria but approaches 100 percent in a laboratory with experienced technologists. A presumptive diagnosis of recent LAC virus infection can be made with an elevated IgM titer (10 or greater) or a single highly elevated IgG titer (160 or greater).

Fourfold or greater rises in IgM or IgG (or both) may be used to confirm infection determined by either indirect IF or IgM capture (see earlier). Fourfold or greater changes in hemagglutination-inhibition and neutralization antibody titers also may be used to confirm infection. A stable or single elevated serum IgG titer of 64/80 or higher by hemagglutination or neutralization is presumptive evidence of recent infection. Complement fixation, though less expensive to perform and frequently offered by commercial laboratories, never should be used alone because of lack of sensitivity.

In all diagnostic tests for LAC encephalitis, false-positive results (compromised specificity) remain the key clinical issue. A false-positive test could result in serious consequences if, for example, antiviral therapy for herpes simplex virus infection were discontinued erroneously or if antibiotic therapy for partially treated bacterial meningitis were discontinued. Therefore, clinicians should be in direct communication with laboratory colleagues concerning specificity data for their laboratory, particularly in cases in which treatable alternative diagnoses, such as herpes simplex encephalitis or partially treated meningitis, remain in the differential diagnosis on clinical grounds.

From a practical standpoint, the use of rapid diagnostic techniques for LAC virus (such as detection of IgM by indirect IF) in highly endemic areas may benefit patients by reducing unnecessary antibiotic or antiviral therapy, provided that the positive IgM test for LAC virus (indicative of a provisional diagnosis) also is combined with negative tests for other bacterial and viral agents (especially a negative PCR test for herpes simplex virus DNA in patients with severe disease or focal encephalitis). In centers studying investigational antiviral therapy in highly endemic areas, the need for rapid diagnosis is more compelling, but the same caveats of ruling out other organisms apply. In such a center in West Virginia, the IF test has proven sensitive (>80%) and virtually 100 percent specific, and it has excellent turnaround time (<24 hours) to facilitate expeditious assignment to the investigational therapeutic protocol. The same IF serologic test then is used for convalescent titers (in 2 to 6 weeks), which if positive, will be consistent with a confirmed case of LAC infection. In areas where LAC virus is not endemic and such testing is not available, rapid diagnostic testing still might be sought in severe, deteriorating cases of encephalitis in which no diagnosis is yet confirmed. In milder cases, such as those with signs of a mild, resolving aseptic meningitis, the diagnosis is primarily of epidemiologic importance, and acute and convalescent titers may be determined reasonably in reference laboratories with less rapid techniques.

Differential Diagnosis

The principal consideration in the differential diagnosis is herpes simplex encephalitis (HSE). Clinical descriptions consistently disclose a high rate of focal neurologic findings or focal seizures, or both, in LAC encephalitis (approximately 30%). The frontal and temporal lobe locations of abnormalities detected by EEG (including PLEDs in some cases) and by brain imaging studies in some cases of LAC encephalitis also may point to a presumptive diagnosis of herpes simplex encephalitis.[3, 76] Because late institution of therapy in herpes simplex encephalitis is associated with a poor outcome, a reasonable approach is to make an early diagnosis of presumptive herpes simplex encephalitis in cases of encephalitis with focal findings, pending definitive diagnosis.[111]

In patients with less fulminant signs of CNS infection, enteroviral aseptic meningitis is a common consideration, especially because it can occur in summer and early fall. The presence of rash, pharyngitis, myocarditis, or conjunctivitis is a clue to enterovirus and is not characteristic of LAC virus infection. In areas where immunizations might be eschewed for religious reasons, poliomyelitis remains an important diagnostic consideration. Mumps encephalitis is another consideration, even in the absence of parotid swelling, and low CSF glucose levels may be a clue to this diagnosis.[83]

Zoonotic infections that cause meningitis or encephalitis should be considered carefully in the differential diagnosis because of the rural distribution of LAC virus infections. Patients with Rocky Mountain spotted fever exhibit signs of CNS disturbance, but the disorder usually is characterized by rash or evidence of viscerotropic infection (or both). Leptospirosis can be differentiated by the presence of rash, conjunctivitis, and pulmonary and cardiac involvement. In non-immunocompromised patients, *Listeria* encephalitis occurs principally at the extremes of age. Encephalomyocarditis virus infections of the CNS have been reported in Europe; in the United States, antibody to the virus has been found in human serosurveys, but clinical evidence of disease has not been documented. Cat-scratch encephalopathy should be brought into the differential diagnosis, especially in southeastern states, where the disease is most prevalent. Rabies should be considered in the differential diagnosis because patients may have signs of encephalitis in the absence of hydrophobia and without a history of an animal bite. *Mycoplasma pneumoniae* can be complicated by encephalitis in rare instances.

Treatment

A reasonable general strategy is to assess these patients as one would assess a child with closed head injury because in both instances, (1) changes in the level of consciousness cannot be assumed to be caused by a normal need to sleep and therefore need to be monitored serially and (2) changes in the level of consciousness are generally the best and earliest indicator of evolving intracranial pathology, as opposed to brain stem signs (e.g., pupillary abnormalities, bradycardia with hypertension). *Therefore, serial monitoring of the level of consciousness is the most important aspect of neurologic monitoring (using the Glasgow Coma Scale [GCS]), even if the child has minimal change in level of consciousness at the time of admission.*

Three particularly important decision points in management depend on the presence or absence of (1) *disorientation,* (2) *further deterioration in GCS scores,* and (3) *focal findings.* Children who remain lethargic but do not progress to disorientation may be observed carefully on the general pediatric floor. Once the child becomes *disoriented* (GCS score typically <13), as shown by mental status changes in an older child or a lack of recognition of parents in an infant, the child might best be monitored in an intensive care setting. *Further deterioration in the GCS* to a score of 8 or less generally indicates that the patient is no longer able to adequately protect the airway, and appropriate intervention is needed. Cases that suggest herpes simplex encephalitis because of *focal findings* or deep coma, or both, warrant presumptive treatment with acyclovir.

Many of the same strategies that apply in treating children at risk for increased intracranial pressure are used in treating those with LAC encephalitis. A reasonable approach is to perform funduscopy and consider CT of the brain before performing lumbar puncture and to note the opening pressure of the latter. General treatment strategies include airway and ventilatory management designed to avoid hypercapnia; hemodynamic management to optimize mean arterial pressure (and presumably cerebral perfusion pressure); neurologic strategies to optimize seizure control and measures to avoid an excessive cerebral metabolic rate; and strategies designed to avoid hypo-osmolality, hyperthermia, and other factors that may exacerbate intracranial hypertension. Intubated patients should be adequately sedated and may need additional analgesia/sedation before noxious procedures such as endotracheal suctioning are performed.

Recent data suggest that hyponatremia and hyperthermia might be related temporally to clinical deterioration in some patients with LAC encephalitis. In general, physicians no longer recommend restriction of fluids for patients with CNS infection but instead use *isotonic fluids* (normal saline or 5% dextrose in normal saline) *at maintenance rates (plus deficit replacement)* to minimize the tendency for the development of hyponatremia while maintaining intravascular volume.[76] Serum sodium should be monitored approximately every 8 hours during the acute phase of the illness. If evidence of SIADH is documented (and cerebral salt wasting is ruled out) by careful monitoring of fluid status and urine and serum sodium and osmolality, careful restriction of fluids might be considered. Maintaining intravascular volume in such a situation may be aided by monitoring central venous pressure.

Because of data suggesting that hyperthermia may be associated with neurologic deterioration in some patients, having a low threshold for treatment of fever with antipyretics is recommended. Cooling blankets may be indicated for persistent fever, especially in critically ill patients with evidence of increased intracranial pressure, provided that shivering and discomfort are controlled.

Patients suffering neurologic deterioration in spite of implementation of the aforementioned measures may need repeat EEG or brain imaging studies (or both) because nonconvulsive status epilepticus can occur and the initial brain imaging results may be normal but later imaging may show evidence of cerebral edema. Recently, some experience has been gained in the monitoring of intracranial pressure in LAC encephalitis.[64] High intracranial pressure was documented in three of six patients in whom monitors were placed, and such monitoring was found to be a useful adjunct in managing elevated intracranial pressure.[76]

Currently, no specific antiviral therapy is approved by the FDA for the treatment of LAC encephalitis, but intravenous ribavirin has been used on a compassionate-use basis in a few cases. Ribavirin can inhibit the replication of LAC virus in vitro (primarily by a direct effect on viral polymerase activity) at levels potentially achievable in CSF. Also relevant to the potential use of ribavirin in LAC encephalitis is that other bunyaviruses have been shown to be sensitive to ribavirin in vitro or in animal studies, or in both.[21, 56, 57, 77, 79, 90, 96, 98] Hantaan virus, for example, which causes lethal encephalitis in the suckling mouse model (as does LAC virus), produces less viremia and mortality in mice treated with ribavirin.[57] Intravenous ribavirin initially was used on a compassionate-use basis in a human case of severe LAC encephalitis in 1994,[79] and subsequently it has been used similarly in six severe cases without serious adverse effects (unpublished data of the author). Recently, a randomized, double-blind, placebo-controlled clinical trial of intravenous ribavirin was started in the highly endemic region of southern West Virginia by McJunkin and coworkers, where its use has been limited to severe cases.

Outcome

LAC and JC virus infections are associated with a case-fatality rate of less than 1 percent. However, a recent series (n = 127) indicated near-lethal disease from cerebral herniation in 3 cases and a sizable proportion of patients who required mechanical ventilation (25%) and/or intensive care (50%).[76]

Six to 15 percent of patients who have recovered from LAC encephalitis have recurrent seizures.[20, 25] The risk of a recurrent convulsive disorder was approximately 25 percent in patients who experienced a seizure during the acute phase of illness.[25, 41] The interval between the onset of recurrent seizures and recovery from acute infection ranged from a few days to years (mean, 4 years).[25] Persistent hemiparesis was a residual abnormality in 2 of 151 patients monitored for up to 6 years after recovery, but 1 patient had a brain biopsy performed on the opposite hemisphere.[20] Unilateral infarction of the basal ganglia and hemiparesis were described recently in the case of an infant.[72] Another infant with a presumed LAC infection initially had an apparent neurodegenerative disease secondary to acute disseminated encephalomyelitis.[34]

Until recently, psychometric evaluation of recovered patients has failed to show significant differences in standard tests of cognitive ability when compared with controls or normative data in the general population.[75, 92] However, a recent study of 28 recovered patients showed a mean full-scale intelligence quotient (IQ) of 87.8 (95% confidence interval, 82.2 to 93.2), with 35 percent of these patients having an IQ less than 80 and 46 percent demonstrating significant disparities between verbal and performance IQ scores. In addition, 60 percent of this group had positive testing for attention-deficit/hyperactivity disorder.[76] Previous data indicating changes in performance on tests administered before and after illness suggested effects in children who were more seriously ill.[75] In another small series, abnormalities in visual-motor function and intellectual impairment were observed more often in patients who had focal abnormalities in the acute illness.[92]

Pathology

Pathologic descriptions of two fatal cases have been reported.[64] In gross appearance, the brain is swollen and the meninges are congested. The principal brain lesions are neuronal degeneration, patchy inflammatory lesions, and vasculitis. The cerebrum and basal ganglia are the principal sites of involvement, but petechial hemorrhages and edema were noted in the spinal cord of one patient. In both cases, lesions in the cerebrum were confined to the frontal, parietal, and temporal lobes, and the cerebellum was not involved.

The focal inflammatory lesions and perivascular reactions are composed primarily of mononuclear cells. Neuronolysis and neuronophagia are observed in foci of inflammation and necrosis, along with reactive polymorphonuclear, mononuclear, and microglial responses. Small extravasations of erythrocytes may appear as well. Lymphocytic perivascular cuffs are seen, but inclusion bodies are not. In one case, a focal area of necrosis, hemorrhage, and hematoma formation was present in the temporal lobe, which corresponded to a mass lesion seen on CT.

In a recent case, brain biopsy material examined by indirect IF demonstrated LAC viral antigen in neurons and perhaps in endothelial cells. The same biopsy material from this patient showed minimal necrosis and perivascular cuffing on light microscopy.[77] The finding of minimal necrosis despite abnormal CT findings and deep coma is interesting in view of the relatively benign outcome of LAC encephalitis (vs. HSE), even in patients who experience deep coma or exhibit CT abnormalities. This finding is in marked contradistinction to herpes simplex encephalitis, in which the presence of either deep coma or CT lesions would be a very poor prognostic factor consistent with the extensive necrosis seen pathologically.[111] Recent findings in a mouse model indicate that neuronal cell death in LAC encephalitis may be mediated largely by apoptosis (as opposed to necrosis).[89]

Prevention

Large-scale spraying of insecticides is not an effective intervention for elimination of *O. triseriatus* because this tree-dwelling mosquito tends to be protected by the leaf canopy of its habitat. Public health prevention has focused on elimination of breeding sites of *O. triseriatus*. Such efforts in endemic areas have included removal of used tires and other containers that hold small pools of water and (less commonly) sealing tree holes with cement or gypsum wool insulation.[104] The sheer number of such potential breeding sites necessitates intervention on a community-wide basis.[80] Public health education has been directed at communities at risk and at children through magazines such as *Ranger Rick*[2] and more recently via a CDC educational program called *Neato Mosquito* (available at www.CDC.gov). In La Crosse, Wisconsin, in 1979, measures to decrease breeding sites were implemented in a community-wide mosquito control program, in addition to ovitraps and adulticides when adult mosquito populations reached critical levels. After the program's inception in 1978, a gradual reduction in the number of cases was observed. However, surrounding untreated counties experienced a similar decline in incidence (W. Thompson, personal communication). The proper use of repellents (see Table 178–2), playing in open sunny fields, and avoidance of tree-shaded areas may confer a reduction in risk by minimizing exposure to the vector. Insect repellents for use in children should contain less than 10 percent DEET and can be applied to the child's clothing and then in lesser amounts to areas of exposed skin.

The potential for development of a vaccine comes from recent work with a truncated G1 protein preparation that induces a protective immune response in suckling mice via neutralizing antibody.[88] Protection against neuro-invasion was achieved by interruption of the transient viremia, which occurs just after inoculation of the virus. More recently, a DNA-based vaccine that encodes for viral glycoproteins (G1 and G2) also induced a protective neutralizing antibody response in mice.[94] Should ecologic preventive measures fail to lower disease rates in endemic areas, development of a vaccine for use in persons living in these areas may prove worthwhile.

REFERENCES

1. Artsob, H., and Spence, L.: California encephalitis: Quebec. Can. Dis. Wkly. Rep. *7*:194–195, 1981.
2. Athey, E., and Thomas, N.: Fight that bite! Ranger Rick *18*:13–15, 1984.
3. Balfour, H. H., Jr., Siem, R. A., Bauer, H., and Quie, P. G.: California arbovirus (La Crosse) infections. I. Clinical and laboratory findings in 66 children with meningoencephalitis. Pediatrics *52*:680–691, 1973.
4. Balkhy, H. H., and Schreiber, J. R.: Severe La Crosse encephalitis with significant neurologic sequelae. Pediatr. Infect. Dis. J. *19*:77–80, 2000.
5. Beaty, B., and Bishop, D. H. L.: Bunyavirus-vector interactions. Virus Res. *10*:289–302, 1988.
6. Beaty, B. J., Casals, J., Brown, K. L., et al.: Indirect fluorescent-antibody technique for serological diagnosis of La Crosse (California) virus infections. J. Clin. Microbiol. *15*:429–434, 1982.
7. Beaty, B. J., Jamnback T. L., Hildreth, S. W., et al.: Rapid diagnosis of La Crosse virus infections: Evaluation of serologic and antigen detection techniques for the clinically relevant diagnosis of La Crosse encephalitis. *In* Thompson, W. H., and Calisher, C. H. (eds.): California Serogroup Viruses. New York, Alan R. Liss, 1983, pp. 293–302.
8. Beghi, E., Nicolosi, A., Kurland, L. T., et al.: Encephalitis and aseptic meningitis, Olmsted County, Minnesota, 1950–1981. I. Epidemiology. Ann. Neurol. *16*:283–294, 1984.
9. Berry, R. L., Parsons, M. A., LaLonde-Weigert, B. J., et al.: *Aedes canadensis*, a vector of La Crosse virus (California serogroup) in Ohio. J. Am. Mosq. Control Assoc. *2*:73, 1986.
10. Berry, R. L., Weigert, J. L., Calisher, C. H., et al.: Evidence for transovarial transmission of Jamestown Canyon virus in Ohio. Mosq. News *37*:494–496, 1977.

11. Black, S. S., Harrison, L. R., Purcell, A. R., et al.: Necrotizing panencephalitis in puppies infected with LaCrosse virus. J. Vet. Diagn. Invest. *6*:250–254, 1994.
12. Calisher, C. H., Pretzman, C. I., Muth, D. J., et al.: Serodiagnosis of La Crosse virus infections in humans by detection of immunoglobulin M class antibodies. J. Clin. Microbiol. *23*:667–671, 1976.
13. Campbell, G. L., Reeves, W. D, Hardy, J. L., et al.: Seroepidemiology of California and Bunyamwera serogroup bunyavirus infections in humans in California. Am. J. Epidemiol. *136*:308–319, 1992.
14. Campbell, W. P., and Huang, C.: Detection of California serogroup viruses using universal primers and reverse transcription–polymerase chain reaction. J. Virol. Methods *53*:55–61, 1995.
15. Case, K. L, West, R. M., and Smith, M. J.: Histocompatibility antigens and La Crosse encephalitis. J. Infect. Dis. *168*:358–360, 1993.
16. Cassidy, L. F., and Patterson, J. L.: Mechanism of La Crosse virus inhibition by ribavirin. Antimicrob. Agents Chemother. *33*:2009–2011, 1989.
17. Chandler, L. J., Beaty, B. J., Bishop, D. H. L., et al.: Detection of La Crosse and snowshoe hare viral nucleic acids by in situ hybridization. Am. J. Trop. Med. Hyg. *40*:561–568, 1989.
18. Chandler L. J., Borucki M. K., Dobie D. K., et al.: Characterization of La Crosse virus RNA in autopsied central nervous system tissues. J. Clin. Microbiol. *36*:3332–3336, 1998.
19. Chun, R. W. M.: Clinical aspects of La Crosse encephalitis: Neurological and psychological sequelae. *In* Thompson, W. H., and Calisher, C. H. (eds.): California Serogroup Viruses. New York, Alan R. Liss, 1983, pp. 193–201.
20. Chun, R. W. M., Thompson, W. H., Grabow, J. D., et al.: California arbovirus encephalitis in children. Neurology *18*:369–375, 1968.
21. Connor, E., Morrison, S., Lane, J., et al.: Safety tolerance and pharmacokinetics of systemic ribavirin in children with human immunodeficiency virus infection. Antimicrob. Agents Chemother. *37*:532–539, 1993.
22. Cramblett, H. G., Stegmiller, H., and Spencer, C.: California encephalitis virus infections in children: Clinical and laboratory studies. J. A. M. A. *198*:128–132, 1966.
23. Craven, R. B., Eliason, D. A., Francy, D. B., et al.: Importation of *Aedes albopictus* and other exotic mosquito species into the United States in used tires from Asia. J. Am. Mosq. Control Assoc. *4*:138–142, 1988.
24. Cully, J. F., and Streit, T. G.: Transmission of La Crosse virus by four strains of *Aedes albopictus* to and from the eastern chipmunk *(Tamias striatus)*. J. Am. Mosq. Control Assoc. *8*:237–240, 1992.
25. Deering, W. M.: Neurologic aspects and treatment of La Crosse encephalitis. *In* Thompson, W. H., and Calisher, C. H. (eds.): California Serogroup Viruses. New York, Alan R. Liss, 1983, pp. 187–191.
26. Deibel, R., Srihongse, S., and Grayson, M. A.: Jamestown Canyon virus: The etiologic agent of an emerging human disease? *In* Thompson, W. H., and Calisher, C. H. (eds.): California Serogroup Viruses. New York, Alan R. Liss, 1983, pp. 313–325.
27. Deibel, R., Srihongse, S., and Woodall, J. P.: Arboviruses in New York State: An attempt to determine the role of arboviruses in patients with viral encephalitis and meningitis. Am. J. Trop. Med. Hyg. *28*:577–582, 1979.
28. de los Reyes, E., Glauser, T. A., McJunkin, J. E., et al.: Periodic lateralizing epileptiform discharges and La Crosse encephalitis: Diagnostic and public health implications. Neurology *46*:150–151, 1996.
29. Demikhov, V. G., Chaitsev, V. G., Dutenko, A. M., et al.: California serogroup virus infections in the Ryazan region of the USSR. Am. J. Trop. Med. Hyg. *45*:371–376, 1991.
30. Disease Control and Epidemiology Service, Ontario Ministry of Health: Surveillance of arboviruses in Ontario in 1983: The increased detection of seropositive cases to the California group viruses (CGV). Ontario Dis. Surveill. Rep. *5*:394–400, 1984.
31. Dykers, T. I., Brown, K. L., Gundersen, C. B., et al.: Rapid diagnosis of La Crosse encephalitis: Detection of specific immunoglobulin M in cerebrospinal fluid. J. Clin. Microbiol. *22*:740–744, 1985.
32. El Said, L. H., Vorndam, V., Gentsch, J. R., et al.: A comparison of La Crosse virus isolates obtained from different ecological niches and an analysis of the structural components of California encephalitis serogroup viruses and other bunyaviruses. Am. J. Trop. Med. Hyg. *28*:364–386, 1979.
33. Endres, M. J., Griot, C., Gonzalez-Scarano, F., et al.: Neuroattenuation of an avirulent bunyavirus variant maps to the L RNA segment. J. Virol. *65*:5465–5470, 1991.
34. Garg, B. P., and Kleiman, M. B.: Acute disseminated encephalomyelitis presenting as a neurodegenerative disease in infancy. Pediatr. Neurol. *11*:57–58, 1994.
35. Gerhardt, R. R., Gottfried, K. L., Apperson, C. S., et al.: First isolation of La Crosse virus from naturally infected *Aedes albopictus*. Emerg. Infect. Dis. *7*:807–811, 2001.
36. Godsey, M. S., Amoo, F., Yuill, T. M., et al.: California serogroup virus infections in Wisconsin domestic animals. Am. J. Trop. Med. Hyg. *39*:409–416, 1988.
37. Gonzalez-Scarano, F., Beaty, B. J., Sudin D., et al.: Genetic determinants of the virulence and infectivity of La Crosse virus. Microb. Pathog. *4*:1–7, 1988.
38. Gonzalez-Scarano, F., Endres, M. J., and Nathanson, N.: *Bunyaviridae*: Pathogenesis. Curr. Top. Microbiol. Immunol. *169*:217–249, 1991.
39. Gonzalez-Scarano, F., Pobjecky, N., and Nathanson, N.: La Crosse bunyavirus can mediate pH-dependent fusion from without. Virology *132*:222–225, 1984.
40. Gonzalez-Scarano, F., Pobjecky, N., and Nathanson, N.: Bunyaviruses. *In* Fields, B. N., and Knipe, D. M. (eds.): Virology. New York, Raven Press, 1990, pp. 1195–1228.
41. Grabow, J. D., Matthews, C. G., Chun, R. W. M., et al.: The electroencephalogram and clinical sequelae of California arbovirus encephalitis. Neurology *19*:394–404, 1969.
42. Grady, L. J., Sanders, M. L., and Campbell, W. P.: The sequence of the MRNA of an isolate La Crosse virus. J. Gen. Virol. *68*:3057–3071, 1987.
43. Graham, D. H., Holmes, J. L., Higgs, S., et al.: Selection of refractory and permissive strains of *Aedes triseriatus* (Diptera: Culicidae) for transovarial transmission of La Crosse virus. J. Med. Entomol. *36*:671–678, 1999.
44. Grimstad, P. R.: California group virus disease. *In* Monath, T. P. (ed.): The Arbovirus: Epidemiology and Ecology. Vol. 2. Boca Raton, FL, CRC Press, 1988, pp. 99–136.
45. Grimstad, P. R., Haroff, R. N., Wentworth, B. B., et al.: Jamestown Canyon virus (California serogroup) is the etiologic agent of widespread infection in Michigan humans. Am. J. Trop. Med. Hyg. *35*:376–386, 1986.
46. Grimstad, P. R., Kobayashi, J. F., Zhand, M., et al.: Recently introduced *Aedes albopictus* in the United States: Potential vector of La Crosse virus *(Bunyaviridae:* California serogroup). J. Am. Mosq. Control Assoc. *5*:422–426, 1989.
47. Grimstad, P. R., Shabino, C. L., Calisher, C. H., et al.: A case of encephalitis in a human associated with a serologic rise of Jamestown Canyon virus. Am. J. Trop. Med. Hyg. *31*:1238–1244, 1982.
48. Gundersen, C. B., and Brow, K. L.: Clinical aspects of La Crosse encephalitis: Preliminary report. *In* Thompson, W. H., and Calisher, C. H. (eds.): California Serogroup Viruses. New York, Alan R. Liss, 1983, pp. 169–177.
49. Hacker, D., Rochat, S., and Kolakofsky, D.: Anti-mRNAs in La Crosse bunyaviruses-infected cells. J. Virol. *64*:5051–5057, 1990.
50. Hacker, J. K., Volkman, L. E., and Hardy, J. L.: Requirement for the G1 protein of California encephalitis virus in infection in vitro and in vivo. Virology *206*:945–953, 1995.
51. Hammon, W. M., and Reeves, W. C.: California encephalitis virus: A newly described agent. Calif. Med. *77*:303–309, 1952.
52. Heard, P. B., Zhang, M. B., and Grimstad, P. R.: Laboratory transmission of Jamestown Canyon and snowshoe hare viruses *(Bunyaviridae:* California serogroup) by several species of mosquitoes. J. Am. Mosq. Control Assoc. *7*:94–102, 1991.
53. Hefti, H. P., Frese, M., Landis, H., et al.: Human MxA protein protects mice lacking a functional alpha/beta interferon system against La Crosse virus and other lethal viral infections. J. Virol. *73*:698–691, 1999.
54. Hilty, M. D., Haynes, R. E., Azimi, P. H., et al.: California encephalitis in children. Am. J. Dis. Child. *124*:530–533, 1972.
55. Huang, C., Thompson, W. H., and Campbell, W. P.: Comparison of the M RNA genome segments of two human isolates of La Crosse virus. Virus Res. *36*:177–185, 1995.
56. Huggins, J. W., Jahrling, P., Kende, M., et al.: Efficacy of ribavirin against virulent RNA virus infections. *In* Smith, R. A., Knight, V., and Smith, J. A. D. (eds.): Clinical Applications of Ribavirin. Orlando, FL, Academic Press, 1984, pp. 49–63.
57. Huggins, J. W., Kim, G. R., Brand, O. M., et al.: Ribavirin therapy for Hantaan virus infection in suckling mice. J. Infect. Dis. *153*:489–497, 1986.
58. Hurwitz, E. S., Schell, W., Nelson, D., et al.: Surveillance of California encephalitis group virus illness in Wisconsin and Minnesota, 1978. Am. J. Trop. Med. Hyg. *32*:595–601, 1983.
59. Janssen, R., Gonzalez-Scarano, F., and Nathanson, N.: Mechanisms of bunyavirus virulence: Comparative pathogenesis of a virulent strain of La Crosse and an avirulent strain of Tahyna virus. Lab. Invest. *50*:447–455, 1984.
60. Johnson, A. J., Martin, D. A., Karabatsos, N., et al.: Detection of anti-arboviral immunoglobulin G by using a monoclonal antibody–based capture enzyme-linked immunosorbent assay. J. Clin. Microbiol. *38*:1827–1831, 2000.
61. Johnson, K. P., and Johnson, R. T.: California encephalitis. II. Studies of experimental infection in the mouse. J. Neuropathol. Exp. Neurol. *27*:390–400, 1968.
62. Jones, T. F., Craig, A. S., Nasci, R. S., et al.: Newly recognized focus of La Crosse encephalitis in Tennessee. Clin. Infect. Dis. *28*:93–97, 1999.
63. Jones, T. F., Erwin, P. C., Craig, A. S., et al.: Serological survey and active surveillance for La Crosse virus infections among children in Tennessee. Clin. Infect. Dis. *31*:1284–1287, 2000.
64. Kalfayan, B.: Pathology of La Crosse virus infection in humans. *In* Thompson, W. H., and Calisher, C. H. (eds.): California Serogroup Viruses. New York, Alan R. Liss, 1983, pp. 179–186.
65. Kappus, K. D., Monath, T. P., Kaminski, R. M., et al.: Reported encephalitis associated with California serogroup virus infections in the United States, 1963–1981. *In* Thompson, W. H., and Calisher, C. H. (eds.): California Serogroup Viruses. New York, Alan R. Liss, 1983, pp. 31–41.

66. Kindle, A. A., McJunkin, J. E., Meek, J. R., et al.: La Crosse encephalitis in West Virginia. M. M. W. R. Morb. Mortal. Wkly. Rep. *37*:1449–1453, 1988.
67. Kingsford, L., and Boucquey, K. H.: Monoclonal antibodies specific for the G1 glycoprotein of La Crosse virus that react with other California serogroup viruses. J. Gen. Virol. *71*:523–530, 1990.
68. Kingsford, L., Boucquey, K. H., and Cardoso, T. P.: Effects of specific monoclonal antibodies on La Crosse virus neutralization: Aggregation, inactivation by Fab fragments, and inhibition of attachment to baby hamster kidney cells. Virology *181*:591–601, 1991.
69. Kitron, U., Michael, J., Swanson J., et al.: Spatial analysis of the distribution of La Crosse encephalitis in Illinois, using a geographic information system and local and global spatial statistics. Am. J. Trop. Med. Hyg. *57*:469–475, 1997.
70. Klimas, R. A., Thompson, W. H., Calisher, C. H., et al.: Genotypic varieties of La Crosse isolated from different geographic regions of the continental United States and evidence for naturally occurring intertypic recombinant La Crosse virus. Am. J. Epidemiol. *114*:112–131, 1981.
71. Kuno, G., Mitchell, C. J., Chang, G. J., et al.: Detecting bunyaviruses of the Bunyamwera and California serogroups by a PCR technique. J. Clin. Microbiol. *34*:1184–1188, 1996.
72. Leber, S. M., Brunberg, J. A., and Pavkovic, I. M.: Infarction of basal ganglia associated with California encephalitis virus. Pediatr. Neurol. *12*:346–349, 1995.
73. Ludwig, G., Israel, B. A., Christensen, B. M., et al.: Role of La Crosse virus glycoproteins in attachment of virus to host cells. Virology *181*:564–571, 1991.
74. Mancao, M. Y., Law, I. M., and Roberson-Trammell, K.: California encephalitis in Alabama. South. Med. J. *89*:992–993, 1996.
75. Matthews, C. G., Chun, R. W. M., Grabow, J. D., et al.: Psychological sequelae in children following California arbovirus encephalitis. Neurology *18*:1023–1030, 1968.
76. McJunkin, J. E., de los Reyes, E. C., Irazuzta, J. E., et al.: La Crosse encephalitis in children. N. Engl. J. Med. *344*:801–807, 2001.
77. McJunkin, J. E., Minnich, L. L., Huang, E.: Evaluation of the efficacy of ribavirin in treatment of experimentally-induced La Crosse encephalitis in mice. Poster Session, Pediatric Academic Societies Annual Meeting. Baltimore, MD, May 6, 2002.
78. McJunkin, J. E., Khan R. R., and Tsai, T. F.: California–La Crosse encephalitis. Infect. Dis. Clin. North. Am. *12*:83–93, 1998.
79. McJunkin, J. E., Khan, R., de los Reyes, E. C., et al.: Treatment of severe case of La Crosse encephalitis with intravenous ribavirin following diagnosis by brain biopsy. Pediatrics *99*:261–267, 1997.
80. Miller, B. R., DeFoliart, G. R., and Yuill, T. M.: Vertical transmission of La Crosse virus (California encephalitis group): Transovarial and filial infection rates in *Aedes triseriatus* (Diptera: Culicidae). J. Med. Entomol. *14*:437–440, 1977.
81. Mitchell, C. J., Hramis, L. D., Karabatsos, N., et al.: Isolation of La Crosse, Cache Valley, and Potosi viruses from *Aedes* mosquitoes (Diptera: Culicidae) collected at used-tire sites in Illinois during 1994–1995. J. Med. Entomol. *35*:573–577, 1998.
82. Monath, T. P., Nuckolls, J. G., Berall, J., et al.: Studies on California encephalitis in Minnesota. Am. J. Epidemiol. *92*:40–50, 1970.
83. Mumps meningitis and MMR vaccination. Lancet *2*:1015–1016, 1989.
84. Nasci, R. S., Moore, C. G., Biggerstaff, B. J., et al.: La Crosse encephalitis virus habitat associations in Nicholas County, West Virginia. J. Med. Entomol. *37*:559–770, 2000.
85. Neitzel, D. F., and Grimstad, P. R.: Serological evidence of California group and Cache Valley virus infection in Minnesota white-tailed deer. J. Wildl. Dis. *27*:230–237, 1991.
86. Osorio, J. E., Godsey, M. S., Defoliart, G. R., et al.: La Crosse viremia in white-tailed dear and chipmunks exposed by infection of mosquito bite. Am. J. Trop. Med. Hyg. *54*:338–342, 1996.
87. Paulson, S. L., and Hawley, W. A.: Effect of body size on the vector competence of field and laboratory populations of *Aedes triseriatus* for La Crosse virus. J. Am. Mosq. Control Assoc. 7:170–175, 1991.
88. Pekosz, A., Griot, C., Stillmock, K., et al.: Protection from La Crosse virus encephalitis with recombinant glycoproteins: Role of neutralizing anti-G1 antibodies. J. Virol. *69*:3475–3481, 1995.
89. Pekosz, A., Phillips, J., Pleasure, D., et al.: Induction of apoptosis by La Crosse virus infection and role of neuronal differentiation and human bcl-2 expression in its prevention. J. Virol. *70*:5329–5335, 1996.
90. Peters, C. J., Reynolds, J. A., Slone, T. W., et al.: Prophylaxis of Rift Valley fever with antiviral drugs, immune serum, interferon inducer, and a macrophage activator. Antiviral Res. *6*:285–297, 1986.
91. Reeves, W. C., Emmons, R. W., and Hardy, J. L.: Historical perspectives on California encephalitis virus in California. *In* Thompson, W. H., and Calisher, C. H. (eds.): California Serogroup Viruses. New York, Alan R. Liss, 1983, pp. 19–29.
92. Rie, H. E., Hilty, M. D., and Cramblett, H. G.: Intelligence and coordination following California encephalitis. Am. J. Dis. Child. *125*:824–827, 1973.
93. Rust, R. S., Thompson, W. H., Matthews, C. G., et al.: La Crosse and other forms of California encephalitis. J. Child. Neurol. *14*:1–14, 1999.
94. Schuh, T., Schultz, J., Moelling, K., et al.: DNA-based vaccine against La Crosse virus: Protective immune response mediated by neutralizing antibodies and $CD4^+$ T-cells. Hum. Gene Ther. *10*:1649–1658, 1999.
95. Shope, R. E., Rozhon, E. J., and Bishop, D. H. L.: Role of the middle-sized bunyavirus RNA segment in mouse virulence. Virology *114*: 273–276, 1981.
96. Sidwell, R. W., Huffman, J. H., Barnett, B. B., et al.: In vitro and in vivo phlebovirus inhibition by ribavirin. Antimicrob. Agents Chemother. *32*:331–336, 1988.
97. Srihongse, S., Grayson, M. A., and Deibel, R.: California serogroup viruses in New York State: The role of subtypes in human infections. Am. J. Trop. Med. Hyg. *33*:1218–1227, 1984.
98. Stephen, E. L., Jones, D. E., Peters, C. J., et al.: Ribavirin treatment of toga- arena- and bunyavirus infection in subhuman primates and other laboratory animal species. *In* Smith, R. A., and Kirkpatrick, W. (eds.): Ribavirin: A Broad-Spectrum Antiviral Agent. New York, Academic Press, 1980, pp. 169–183.
99. Szumlas, D. E., Apperson, C. S., Hartig, P. C., et al.: Seroepidemiology of La Crosse virus infection in humans in western North Carolina. Am. J. Trop. Med. Hyg. *54*:332–337, 1996.
100. Szumlas, D. E., Apperson, C. S., and Powell E. E.: Seasonal occurrence and abundance of *Aedes triseriatus* and other mosquitoes in a La Crosse virus–endemic area in western North Carolina. J. Am. Mosq. Control Assoc. *12*:184–193, 1996.
101. Talmon, Y., Pradad, B. V. V., Clerx, J. P. M., et al.: Electron microscopy of vitrified-hydrated La Crosse virus. J. Virol. *61*:2319–2321, 1987.
102. Taylor, M. R., Carpenter, D. E., Currier, R. D., et al.: California encephalitis virus causes subacute encephalomyelitis in an adult. Arch. Neurol. *42*:88–89, 1985.
103. Thompson, W. H., and Evans, A. S.: California encephalitis virus studies in Wisconsin. Am. J. Epidemiol. *81*:230–244, 1965.
104. Thompson, W. H., and Gundersen, C. B.: La Crosse encephalitis: Occurrence of disease and control in a suburban area. *In* Thompson, W. H., and Calisher, C. H. (eds.): California Serogroup Viruses. New York, Alan R. Liss, 1983, pp. 225–236.
105. Thompson, W. H., Kalfayan, B., and Anslow, R. O.: Isolation of California encephalitis group virus from a fatal human illness. Am. J. Epidemiol. *81*:245–263, 1965.
106. Tsai, T. F.: Arboviral infection in the United States. Infect. Dis. Clin. North Am. *5*:73–102, 1991.
107. Tsai, T. F.: Arboviruses. *In* Murray, P. R. (ed.): Manual of Clinical Microbiology. 6th ed. Washington, D.C., ASM Press, 1995, pp. 980–993.
108. Walters, L. L., Tirrell, S. J., and Shope, R. E.: Seroepidemiology of California and Bunyamwera serogroup *(Bunyaviridae)* virus infections in native populations of Alaska. Am. J. Trop. Med. Hyg. *60*:806–821, 1999.
109. Watts, D. M., Pantuwatana, S., Yuill, T. M., et al.: Transovarial transmission of La Crosse virus in *Aedes triseriatus*. Ann. N. Y. Acad. Sci. *266*:135–143, 1975.
110. Watts, D. M., Thompson, W. H., Yuill, T. M., et al.: Overwintering of La Crosse virus in *Aedes triseriatus*. Am. J. Trop. Med. Hyg. *23*:694–700, 1974.
111. Whitley, R. J.: Viral encephalitis. N. Engl. J. Med. *323*:242–250, 1990.
112. Woodruff, B. A., Baron, R. C., and Tsai, T. F.: Symptomatic La Crosse viral infections in the central nervous system: A study of risk factors in an endemic area. Am. J. Epidemiol. *136*:320–327, 1992.
113. Wurtz, R., and Paleologos, N.: La Crosse encephalitis presenting like herpes simplex encephalitis in an immunocompromised adult. Clin. Infect. Dis. *31*:1113–1114, 2000.
114. Young, D. J.: California encephalitis virus: Report of three cases and review of the literature. Ann. Intern. Med. *65*:419–428, 1966.
115. Yuill, T. M.: The role of mammals in the maintenance and dissemination of La Crosse virus. *In* Thompson, W. H., and Calisher, C. H. (eds.): California Serogroup Viruses. New York, Alan R. Liss, 1983, pp. 77–87.
116. Zamparo, J. M., Andreadis, T. G., and Shope, R. E.: Serologic evidence of Jamestown Canyon virus infection in white-tailed deer populations from Connecticut. J. Wildl. Dis. *33*:623–627, 1997.

CHAPTER 192 Other Bunyaviruses

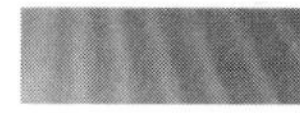

CHAPTER 192A Rift Valley Fever

ROBERT E. SHOPE

Rift Valley fever (RVF) is primarily a disease of sheep and cattle. It is transmitted by mosquitoes and caused by a virus with selective affinity for the parenchymal cells of the liver, which undergo characteristic eosinophilic degeneration. Infection with RVF virus causes a short, but severe disease in sheep and cattle. Most pregnant ewes and cows abort, and more than 90 percent of newborn lambs die. Case-fatality rates in older sheep and cattle are lower, but nonetheless significant. People usually acquire the infection from aerosols generated from the body fluids and tissues of animals dying of the disease and, less commonly, from bites of infected mosquitoes, especially during epidemics. See Swanepoel and Coetzer[10] for a comprehensive review.

History

RVF probably has occurred for many years in Africa and first was recognized at the beginning of the 20th century with the introduction of intensive livestock husbandry. In 1912, large numbers of newborn lambs died of an unknown disease in the Rift Valley of Kenya, and in the following year the clinical features first were described. Daubney and associates[3] proved that the causal agent was a filterable virus, which they suspected was transmitted by mosquitoes because animals protected by screens did not contract the disease. In 1944, the virus was isolated from mosquitoes caught in the Semliki Forest in western Uganda, and it was proved later that *Erethmapodites chrysogaster* was able to transmit the infection under experimental conditions. Between 1950 and 1974, at least 15 major epizootics of RVF occurred in livestock in various areas of sub-Saharan Africa. During 1975, an extensive epizootic of RVF took place in South Africa, with many human cases and several deaths documented.[4]

An extensive epizootic of RVF also occurred in lower Egypt in 1977. Hundreds of thousands of domestic animals were lost, including cattle, buffaloes, goats, and sheep. Associated with this epizootic was the largest human epidemic of the disease ever known, in which 200,000 humans were infected and 600 died.[5] This outbreak emphasized the increasing threat of RVF to humans and domestic animals and showed that RVF virus was an important cause of hemorrhagic fever in Africa. In 1987, an epidemic of RVF occurred in Mauritania after flooding of the Senegal River basin following completion of the Diama dam; at least 1200 human cases and 200 deaths occurred in one affected area alone. Epidemics and epizootics were reported in Madagascar in 1990,[7] Egypt in 1993,[2] eastern Africa in 1997–1998,[1] and Yemen and Saudi Arabia in 2000.[8] The cases in the Arabian peninsula are the first outside Africa and demonstrate the potential of RVF to spread.

Based on virus isolation, RVF probably occurs sporadically throughout most of sub-Saharan Africa. Zinga virus, previously described as a cause of sporadic human disease in central Africa, has been shown to be a strain of RVF virus.

Etiologic Agent

RVF virus is destroyed by solvents such as ether and is inactivated readily by formalin; it is destroyed by heating at 56° C for 40 minutes. When stored at 4° C or −10° C, the virus loses its infectivity in about 3 months. The virus can be preserved indefinitely on dry ice at −70° C or in lyophilized form.

Fully formed virions are spherical and approximately 94 nm in diameter. They mature in the cytoplasm, although intranuclear inclusions occur in vivo and in cell culture. The virus readily multiplies in a variety of cell lines of animal and human origin. RVF virus has been assigned to the Phlebovirus genus of the family *Bunyaviridae*.

The virus is highly pathogenic for mice, young rats, and hamsters, and death occurs in 95 to 100 percent of these animals 36 to 96 hours after inoculation.

Vectors

In studies in South Africa, the virus has been transmitted experimentally by *Culex theileri, Culex zombaensis, Culex neavei, Aedes juppi,* and *Erethmapodites quinquevittatus.* Epizootics of RVF have occurred in years of unusually heavy rains that filled natural depressions in the land (pans or dambos), thereby favoring the proliferation of flood-water mosquitoes. Studies in Kenya have shown that transovarial transmission of the virus in pan-breeding *Aedes* of the subgenus *Neomelanoconion* is the probable mechanism of virus maintenance and periodic recrudescence. *Culex pipiens* was implicated as a vector in Egypt during the 1977–1978 epidemic. During epizootics, domestic livestock serve as viremic, amplifying hosts in the transmission cycle.

Clinical Manifestations

Humans are very susceptible to RVF virus. During the epizootics in South Africa, most veterinarians and many farmers engaged in work with sick sheep and cattle became infected. In most cases, infection was linked to direct contact with the carcasses, tissues, and organs of animals that died of RVF. Transmission was probably by the aerosolized body fluids of the animals. Some patients gave no history of such contact; in these cases, the infection is presumed to have been transmitted by mosquitoes or possibly acquired by drinking infected milk. The virus can be transmitted readily to laboratory personnel by direct contact with infected animals or by the respiratory route from aerosol droplet infection.

The incubation period of RVF is 3 to 7 days; its onset is sudden, with chills, myalgia, joint pain, headache, and a biphasic fever that lasts approximately 1 week. Patients often feel nauseated and may vomit or complain of abdominal fullness and pain. The face is flushed, the conjunctivae are injected, and the tongue is furred. Bradycardia is present, and slight tenderness over the liver, which may be enlarged, can be present. Many patients become delirious, and some have hallucinations. In a small proportion (<1%) of patients, the infection is complicated by retinitis. Late in the course of the illness or early in convalescence, unclear vision may be noted and the patient may have a central blind spot. This visual defect is associated with a cotton-wool exudate on the macula. Both eyes are involved occasionally, and the loss of vision is a severe handicap. These lesions gradually resolve, and the patient's vision returns to normal in most cases. Meningoencephalitis manifested as intense headache, confusion, and stupor may occur as a complication in less than 1 percent of patients during or after the second wave of fever. Lumbar puncture relieves the headache. Cerebrospinal fluid (CSF) shows a slight pleocytosis, mostly of lymphocytes, a normal glucose level, and a slightly increased protein content. Antibody to RVF virus may be demonstrated in the fluid. Few patients with encephalitis die. Recovery is usually complete but may be prolonged. Occasionally, the patient is left with permanent sequelae.

Hemorrhagic fever, a complication with a case-fatality rate of 15 percent, develops in approximately 1 percent of patients with RVF. Mortality was disproportionately less in children than adults during the 1977 Egyptian epidemic. In cases of severe illness, a hemorrhagic diathesis may develop that includes epistaxis, hematemesis, melena, and sometimes, cerebral hemorrhage. Profuse gastrointestinal hemorrhage may be fatal. Jaundice may be evident.

Laboratory Findings

The patient has an initial leukocytosis that is followed by leukopenia. Profound thrombocytopenia and other defects in coagulation may be observed. Disturbance in liver and kidney function also may be documented.

The diagnosis of RVF is suggested when human beings suffer from an acute, severe, but short febrile illness at the same time that an epizootic with high mortality is occurring in sheep.

The diagnosis usually can be confirmed by isolation of the virus in mice or cell culture from blood and, in fatal cases, from the liver. The development of antibodies can be demonstrated by immunofluorescence, IgM enzyme-linked immunosorbent assay, hemagglutination inhibition, complement fixation, and neutralization. In patients with encephalitis, IgM antibodies are detectable in CSF.

Treatment

Treatment is symptomatic. When a hemorrhagic diathesis develops, treatment should be directed toward controlling bleeding. Transfusions of fresh-frozen plasma and platelets may be beneficial. Disseminated intravascular coagulation has been documented in a monkey model, but its role in human disease is uncertain.

Prevention

RVF is mainly a disease of adults and usually is acquired occupationally. It is a serious hazard faced by veterinarians, ranchers, and laboratory personnel in the course of their work. Because RVF usually is acquired by direct contact with the tissues of infected sheep and cattle, the risk of infection can be reduced by wearing gloves, protective masks, and goggles when postmortem examinations are carried out on animals that have died of unknown causes. Because of the value of domestic animals in many economically depressed areas of Africa, sheep and cattle often are housed within family compounds. Sick or dying animals usually are killed to salvage their meat. In this peridomestic environment, children also can be exposed to virus aerosols and readily become infected. Infection from a mosquito bite is possible as well, and for this reason, the use of repellents and bed nets is recommended.

The primary strategy for preventing RVF in both humans and animals relies on vaccination of sheep and cattle, which are the amplifying hosts. Attenuated strains of the virus have been developed and used successfully on a mass scale to immunize livestock. These attenuated vaccines are associated with some abortions in pregnant ewes and cows. An inactivated vaccine is safe and is in widespread use in Africa.

A new, live attenuated vaccine designated MP-12 has been developed by passage of RVF virus in the presence of the mutagen 5-fluorouracil.[6] The vaccine has proved safe for use in domestic livestock, does not produce abortions, and offers considerable promise as a veterinary and human vaccine. Formalin-inactivated vaccines produced in cell culture[9] have been used on an investigational basis in more than 3000 persons with a seroconversion rate greater than 95 percent. A single case of Guillain-Barré syndrome has been reported, but its relationship to vaccination is uncertain. Human vaccination is recommended for high-risk occupational groups. Various genetically engineered vaccine candidates are under development.

REFERENCES

1. An outbreak of Rift Valley fever, eastern Africa, 1997–1998. Wkly. Epidemiol. Rep. *73*:105–109, 1998.
2. Arthur, R. R., el-Sharkawy, M. S., Cope, S. E., et al.: Recurrence of Rift Valley fever in Egypt. Lancet *342*:1149–1150, 1993.
3. Daubney, R., Hudson, J. R., and Garnham, P. C.: Enzootic hepatitis or Rift Valley fever: An undescribed virus disease of sheep, cattle and man from East Africa. J. Pathol. Bacteriol. *34*:545–579, 1931.
4. Gear, J.: Hemorrhagic fevers in South Africa: An account of two recent outbreaks. J. S. Afr. Vet. Assoc. *48*:5–8, 1977.
5. Meegan, J. M.: Rift Valley fever in Egypt: An overview of the epizootics in 1977 and 1978. Contrib. Epidemiol. Biostat. *3*:100–113, 1981.
6. Morrill, J. C., Jennings, G. B., Caplen, H., et al.: Pathogenicity and immunogenicity of a mutagen-attenuated Rift Valley fever virus immunogen in pregnant ewes. Am. J. Vet. Res. *48*:1042–1047, 1987.
7. Morvan, J., Rollin, P. E., Laventure, S., et al.: Rift Valley fever epizootic in the central highlands of Madagascar. Res. Virol. *143*:407–415, 1992.
8. Outbreak of Rift Valley fever, Yemen, August–October 2000. Wkly. Epidemiol. Rec. *75*:392–395, 2000.
9. Randall, R., Gibbs, C. J., Anlisio, C. G., et al.: The development of a formalin-killed Rift Valley fever vaccine for use in man. J. Immunol. *89*:660–671, 1962.
10. Swanepoel, R. and Coetzer, J. A. W.: Rift Valley fever. *In* Coetzer, J. A. W., Thomson, G. R., and Tustin, R. C. (eds.): Infectious Diseases of Livestock. Cape Town, South Africa, Oxford University Press, 1994, pp. 688–717.

CHAPTER **192B**

Crimean-Congo Hemorrhagic Fever

ROBERT B. TESH

Crimean-Congo hemorrhagic fever (CCHF) is an acute febrile viral illness, often with severe hemorrhagic manifestations. The clinical entity and its viral etiology were described first by Chumakov in 1945,[7] but the agent was not propagated or available for study until 1967. Since then, CCHF has been reported from many countries in eastern Europe, central Asia, and Africa. Ticks or contact with the blood of infected livestock is the usual source of infection, but numerous nosocomial outbreaks of CCHF also have been reported.

Etiologic Agent

CCHF virus, the etiologic agent, is a member of the genus Nairovirus, family *Bunyaviridae*. It is lethal to newborn mice and rats after intracerebral inoculation. CCHF virus replicates in many vertebrate cell lines, but it usually does not cause any discernible cytopathogenic effect under fluid overlay. Thus, indirect methods such as immunofluorescence must be used to detect viral infection/antigen in the cells.

A relatively high level of viremia (up to 6.2 $\log_{10}$ median lethal dose per milliliter) develops in persons with CCHF and persists for 8 to 12 days after onset of the illness. Blood from patients with CCHF is quite infectious, and numerous nosocomial infections have occurred in hospital personnel caring for acutely ill patients with hemorrhagic symptoms.[7] CCHF virus is relatively stable in blood and serum and has been recovered from specimens stored as long as 2 or 3 weeks at 4° C.

Epidemiology

CCHF virus is known to occur over a wide geographic area, including eastern Europe, central Asia, and much of Africa. The endemic zone of CCHF has been well delineated in Russia and other states of the former Soviet Union and in South Africa, but in other regions of central Asia and Africa, most cases probably are unrecognized as a result of their sporadic occurrence and largely rural distribution.

The epidemiology of CCHF is complex and not well understood because of the variety of tick and mammalian species that have been found to be infected naturally with the virus. The basic transmission cycle of the virus varies from region to region, depending on the developmental stage and species of ticks involved and their preferred mammalian hosts.[5] In addition, transovarial and trans-stadial transmission of CCHF virus also has been demonstrated in some tick vectors. In general, human cases of CCHF usually are associated with periods of tick abundance and feeding activity. For example, in eastern Europe, cases of CCHF typically occur between May and August, when the tick population is active. Humans usually acquire CCHF from a tick bite or from contact with blood or other tissues of infected livestock.[5] Most patients are adult males engaged in the livestock industry (farmers, slaughterhouse workers, and veterinarians).

Numerous nosocomial outbreaks of CCHF have occurred in hospital workers and laboratory technicians.[1, 3, 7] These persons usually have had direct contact with the blood of patients with CCHF. The mortality rate in reported secondary cases has been high (≈30%). The disease also has been reported in persons slaughtering or performing autopsies on infected and presumably viremic domestic animals.[7]

Clinical Manifestations

The incubation period of CCHF is 1 to 6 days.[5–7] The disease begins suddenly, with fever, nausea, severe headache, dizziness, myalgia, and general toxemia. Vomiting, abdominal pain, diarrhea, and depression also occur commonly. Patients often are flushed, and their conjunctivae are injected. Hepatomegaly is present in approximately 50 percent of cases. In general, hemorrhagic manifestations do not appear before the third or fourth day of the illness, at which point the patient's condition deteriorates markedly. Patients typically become asthenic, apathetic, and occasionally delirious during this stage. Central nervous system changes characterized clinically by loss of consciousness, agitated or myotonic movements, decreased tendon reflexes, and meningeal symptoms occur quite frequently. The appearance of a petechial rash, bruises, and ecchymoses on the skin and mucous membranes indicates onset of the hemorrhagic phase of this disease, which generally lasts 3 to 6 days. Hemorrhages varying in size from petechiae to large hematomas develop on the mucous membranes and skin of the trunk and extremities, especially at the site of injections, trauma, or tight-fitting clothing. Bleeding from the nose, gums, and buccal cavity also occurs commonly. In severe cases of CCHF, gastric, uterine, intestinal, genitourinary, and pulmonary hemorrhage occurs in decreasing frequency. In patients with profuse hemorrhage, tachycardia, shock, and death may ensue. If the patient survives the hemorrhagic phase of the disease, recovery begins by the 9th or 10th day, and a 2- to 6-week period of slow convalescence follows. Viremia is intense and prolonged in CCHF, especially in fatal cases, so blood from these patients should be treated with extreme care.

Leukopenia and thrombocytopenia are a consistent feature of CCHF and occur early in the disease.[2, 6] Other abnormal laboratory findings usually include elevated levels of serum aspartate and alanine aminotransaminase, lactate dehydrogenase, bilirubin, creatinine, and urea. Clinical studies of patients with CCHF in South Africa[6] found markedly elevated values for the prothrombin time, activated partial thromboplastin time, thrombin time, and fibrin degradation products, findings indicative of disseminated intravascular coagulopathy. Many of these abnormal clinical laboratory values were evident early in the disease and had a high predictive value for the outcome.

Pathogenesis

Fluorescent antibody studies on organs in fatal cases of CCHF show a concentration of viral antigen in the reticuloendothelial cells of the liver and spleen, thus suggesting that these cells are a major site of virus replication.[6] Other pathologic changes observed at autopsy include generalized vascular lesions with endothelial damage that give rise to scattered focal hemorrhage and edema in most organs.[5] In severe cases, marked renal involvement and kidney failure may occur.

Diagnosis

A clinical diagnosis of CCHF is difficult to make before the onset of hemorrhagic manifestations because the initial symptoms are nonspecific and cases are usually sporadic in occurrence. As a result of the frequency and severity of the abdominal pain associated with the prodromal phase of CCHF, occasionally it is misdiagnosed as appendicitis or gastric ulcer, and patients are subjected to unnecessary surgery, which can be fatal to both the patient and the attending medical personnel.[1, 3, 7] Once hemorrhagic manifestations appear, the differential diagnosis should include erythema multiforme (Stevens-Johnson syndrome), leptospirosis, hemorrhagic fever with renal syndrome, Ebola virus infection, Lassa fever, Rift Valley fever, Q fever, and yellow fever, depending on the region of the world where the patient was exposed.

A definitive diagnosis of CCHF can be made by isolation of the virus from the patient's blood during the first weeks of illness. IgG and IgM antibodies become demonstrable 7 to 10 days after the onset of symptoms in nonfatal cases.[4]

Treatment

Treatment of CCHF is symptomatic but should include immediate hospitalization and strict bed rest.[7] Because death usually results from acute blood loss and shock, patients may require transfusions of fresh blood, platelets, or plasma (or all three). Administration of immune plasma obtained from convalescent donors also is recommended early in the course of the illness or to persons such as hospital personnel who are exposed to the virus inadvertently. One report[2] indicated that ribavirin was beneficial in the treatment of severe cases.

Prognosis

The mortality rate of CCHF varies from approximately 10 to 50 percent.[2, 6, 7] If the patient survives the hemorrhagic phase of the disease, recovery is complete and permanent immunity results.

Prevention

A killed CCHF virus vaccine prepared in mouse brain has been used experimentally in Russia and Bulgaria.[7] It is recommended for use in laboratory and hospital personnel and in other high-risk populations; however, few data are available on its efficacy.

To protect hospital personnel, strict isolation should be maintained when caring for all CCHF patients.

Other measures designed to prevent CCHF include spraying fields and animals with insecticide for tick control, using personal insect repellents, wearing protective clothing to prevent tick bites, and providing public education about the epidemiology of CCHF.

REFERENCES

1. Burney, M. I., Ghafoor, A., Saleen, M., et al.: Nosocomial outbreak of viral hemorrhagic fever caused by Crimean hemorrhagic fever–Congo virus in Pakistan, January 1976. Am. J. Trop. Med. Hyg. *29*:941–947, 1980.
2. Fisher-Hoch, S. P., Khan, J. A., Rehman, S., et al.: Crimean-Congo haemorrhagic fever treated with oral ribavirin. Lancet *346*:472–475, 1995.
3. Joubert, J. R., King, J. B., Rossouw, D. J., et al.: A nosocomial outbreak of Crimean-Congo hemorrhagic fever at Tygerberg Hospital. Part 3. Clinical pathology and pathogenesis. S. Afr. Med. J. *68*:772–778, 1985.
4. Shepherd, A. J., Swanepoel, R., and Leman, P. A.: Antibody response in Crimean-Congo hemorrhagic fever. Rev. Infect. Dis. *11*(Suppl. 4): 801–806, 1989.
5. Swanepoel, R.: Nairovirus infections. *In* Porterfield, J. S. (ed.): Exotic Viral Infections. London, Chapman & Hall, 1995, pp. 285–293.
6. Swanepoel, R., Gill, D. E., Shepherd, A. J., et al.: The clinical pathology of Crimean-Congo hemorrhagic fever. Rev. Infect. Dis. *11*(Suppl. 4):794–800, 1989.
7. Watts, D. M., Ksiazek, T. G., Linthicum, K. J., et al.: Crimean-Congo hemorrhagic fever. *In* Monath, T. P. (ed.): The Arboviruses: Epidemiology and Ecology. Vol. 2. Boca Raton, FL, C. R. C. Press, 1989, pp. 177–222.

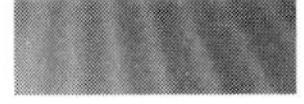

CHAPTER **192C**

Phlebotomus Fever (Sandfly Fever)

ROBERT B. TESH

Phlebotomus fever, an acute, self-limited febrile illness of 2 to 4 days' duration, is acquired from the bite of infected phlebotomine sandflies. Phlebotomus fever is also known as sandfly fever, pappataci fever, and 3-day fever. The disease is endemic in many areas of central Asia, northern Africa, and southern Europe. Historically, phlebotomus fever has been largely of military interest because the introduction of large numbers of susceptible troops into endemic areas often has resulted in epidemics of the disease[7]; more recently, the disease has been reported with increasing frequency in tourists visiting endemic areas.[3, 6]

In 1909, Doerr and associates first demonstrated that the causative agent of the illness was a virus transmitted by *Phlebotomus papatasi*. In 1954, Sabin successfully adapted the agent to mice and described two distinct serologic types designated the Naples and Sicilian strains.[7] Subsequently, 44 additional serotypes have been isolated from various regions of the world; all these agents are included in the genus Phlebovirus, family *Bunyaviridae*. Although most of the phleboviruses are probably capable of producing human illness, the discussion here is limited to the three (Naples, Sicilian, and Toscana) that most commonly are associated with the disease. Rift Valley fever virus is also a member of this genus and frequently causes a phlebotomus fever–like illness in infected persons.[4] However, humans generally acquire Rift Valley fever from the bite of infected mosquitoes or from aerosol, and the sequelae of the latter disease are more severe and occasionally fatal.

Etiologic Agent

The phleboviruses are RNA-containing viruses, spherical in shape and 90 to 100 nm in diameter.[7] The Naples, Sicilian, and Toscana viruses produce a cytopathic effect, as well as plaques in Vero cells. Most laboratory animals are not susceptible to infection with these viruses, although they can be adapted to newborn mice by serial passage intracerebrally. For this reason, tissue culture is recommended for primary isolation of these agents.

Epidemiology

The geographic distribution of the Naples and Sicilian virus types in the Old World closely parallels that of their presumed vector, *Phlebotomus papatasi*[7] (Fig. 192–1). Toscana virus has been isolated in Portugal, Spain, Italy, and Cyprus and has been associated with two other peridomestic sandfly species, *Phlebotomus perniciosus* and *Phlebotomus perfiliewi*.

These phlebotomine species are tiny, sand-colored biting flies about 2 to 3 mm long. Because of their small size, they have little difficulty squeezing through ordinary screens and mosquito netting. They are usually nocturnal in their activity, and only the female bites. Sandflies move in short hops and usually do not travel more than a few hundred meters from their resting and breeding sites. During the day, peridomestic species such as *P. papatasi* and *P. perniciosus* rest in dark corners and crevices, often within houses. The larvae develop in loose soil and organic debris in stone walls, animal sheds, privies, open wells, and gardens. Because of their indoor habits, these peridomestic species are quite vulnerable to residual insecticides.

In central Asia and the Mediterranean region, sandflies are active during the late spring and summer. The incidence of phlebotomus fever follows the same seasonal pattern.

Many phlebotomus fever viruses appear to be maintained in the sandfly population by transovarial (vertical) transmission.[7] Thus, sandflies appear to serve as both vectors and reservoirs of these viruses. Unlike most other arboviruses, whose activity depends on the presence of susceptible and viremic vertebrate hosts, phlebotomus fever viruses are probably active continuously during each sandfly season. Serologic studies of persons living in endemic areas of the disease indicate that most of the residents are infected early in life.[7] In these communities, sporadic cases of phlebotomus fever occur in children because most of the adult population is already immune. However, because of the benign nature of the disease, its sporadic occurrence, and its similarity to many other viral diseases of childhood, most cases are unrecognized. Still, when a large number of susceptible persons (soldiers, tourists, refugees, and so on) enter an endemic area of phlebotomus fever, bite transmission occurs and an epidemic of the disease quickly appears.[6, 7]

Clinical Manifestations

The incubation period for phlebotomus fever averages 3 to 5 days.[1, 7] The illness begins suddenly with fever, severe frontal headache, retro-orbital pain, conjunctival injection, photophobia, malaise, anorexia, nausea, vomiting, myalgia, and lower back pain. The face may be flushed, but a true rash is absent. The disease is self-limited, and symptoms usually disappear within 1 to 3 days; however, a general feeling of weakness and depression is not an uncommon occurrence for a week or more after the illness.

Meningitis and meningoencephalitis also have been described in persons with Toscana virus infection.[2, 6] In addition to the classic symptoms of phlebotomus fever, these patients exhibit nuchal rigidity, a positive Kernig sign, a clouded sensorium, and occasionally, nystagmus and tremor. To date, no deaths have been recorded. Childhood cases of the meningoencephalitic form of Toscana virus infection have been reported,[2] but this form of the infection occurs more commonly in adults.

One attack of phlebotomus fever usually confers lifelong immunity against the infecting virus type but not against heterologous serotypes.[7] For this reason, second cases of the disease have been reported in the same individual in areas where two or more virus serotypes are active.

A marked leukopenia usually is observed with phlebotomus fever.[1] It is characterized by an initial lymphopenia, followed by protracted neutropenia (Fig. 192–2). In patients with central nervous system involvement, pleocytosis and an elevated protein content are observed in the CSF.

Pathology

Fatalities caused by phlebotomus fever have not been reported, and little is known of the pathologic changes produced by these viruses.

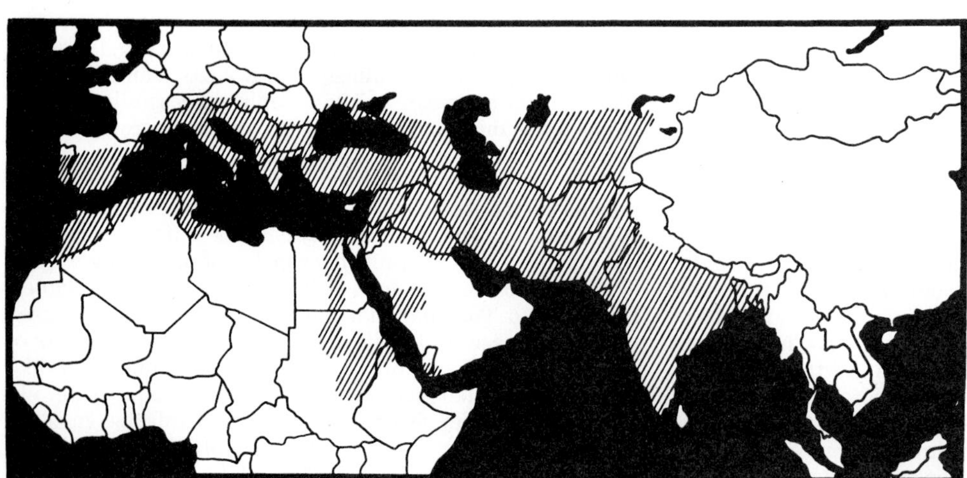

FIGURE 192–1 ■ The known geographic distribution of *Phlebotomus papatasi,* the presumed vector of sandfly fever (Naples and Sicilian types), in central Asia, the Mediterranean region, and adjacent areas of Africa. (Modified from Tesh, R. B., Gajdamovic, S. J., Rodhain, F., et al.: Serological studies on the epidemiology of sandfly fever in the Old World. Bull. World Health Organ. *54*:663–674, 1976.)

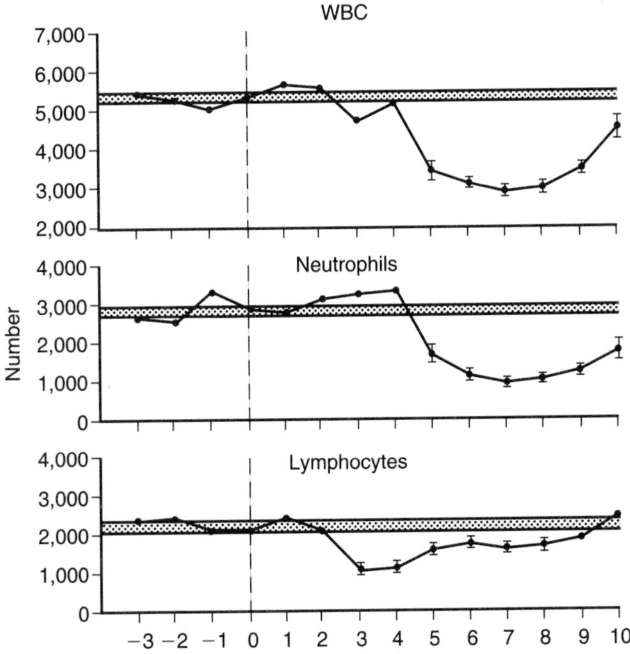

FIGURE 192–2 ■ Mean total leukocyte count as well as absolute neutrophil and lymphocyte counts in 11 adult volunteers inoculated (day 0) with the Sicilian strain of phlebotomus fever virus. The average incubation period in the subjects was about 70 hours. WBC, white blood cells. (Modified from Bartelloni, P. J., and Tesh, R. B.: Clinical and serologic responses of volunteers infected with phlebotomus fever virus [Sicilian type]. Am. J. Trop. Med. Hyg. *25*:456–462, 1976.)

Diagnosis

The diagnosis of phlebotomus fever usually is made on the basis of clinical and epidemiologic evidence. A sudden outbreak during the summer months of a short febrile illness with severe headache in visitors or other newcomers to an endemic area where sandflies are abundant should suggest the disease. Depending on the region, the differential diagnosis might include dengue, West Nile fever, malaria, influenza, and numerous other respiratory and enteroviral infections.

A transient viremia (24 to 36 hours) occurs during this illness, which means that isolation of the virus from blood is unusual. In a few instances, Toscana virus has been isolated directly from the CSF of persons with central nervous system symptoms.[2] Serologic tests offer the simplest method for a specific diagnosis of phlebotomus fever. Antibodies are present in serum 7 to 14 days after infection and can be demonstrated by immunofluorescence,[3] enzyme immunoassay,[4] or neutralization.[1] A fourfold rise in antibody titer from acute to convalescent sera or the presence of specific IgM antibodies provides presumptive evidence of a recent phlebotomus fever virus infection. At present, these serologic tests generally are not available and usually are performed in only a few arbovirus laboratories.

Treatment

Treatment is symptomatic, and hospitalization is not usually necessary. Occasionally, narcotics are required to relieve the severe headache associated with the disease.

Prognosis

Phlebotomus fever is a self-limited, nonfatal disease. Recovery is complete.

Prevention

Control measures are directed primarily against the vector. Household spraying with residual insecticides is quite effective in reducing peridomestic vector populations and controlling the disease. The use of personal insect repellents (e.g., diethyltoluamide) and fine mesh bed nets is also effective in avoiding sandfly bites.

REFERENCES

1. Bartelloni, P. J., and Tesh, R. B.: Clinical and serologic responses of volunteers infected with phlebotomus fever virus (Sicilian type). Am. J. Trop. Med. Hyg. *25*:456–462, 1976.
2. Braito, A., Grazia Ciufolini, M., and Pippi, L.: *Phlebotomus*-transmitted Toscana virus infections of the central nervous system: A seven-year experience in Tuscany. Scand. J. Infect. Dis. *30*:505–508, 1998.
3. Eitrem, R., Niklasson, B., and Weiland, O.: Sandfly fever among Swedish tourists. Scand. J. Infect. Dis. *23*:451–457, 1991.
4. Eitrem, R., Vene, S., and Niklasson, B.: ELISA for detection of IgM and IgG antibodies to sandfly fever Sicilian virus. Res. Virol. *142*:387–394, 1991.
5. Meagan, J. M., and Bailey, C. L.: Rift Valley fever. *In* Monath, T. P. (ed.): The Arboviruses: Epidemiology and Ecology. Vol. 4. Boca Raton, FL, C. R. C. Press, 1989, pp. 51–76.
6. Schwarz, T. F., Gilch, S., and Jager, G.: Aseptic meningitis caused by sandfly fever virus, serotype Toscana. Clin. Infect. Dis. *21*:669, 1995.
7. Tesh, R. B.: Phlebotomus fever. *In* Monath, T. P. (ed.): The Arboviruses: Epidemiology and Ecology. Vol. 4. Boca Raton, FL, C. R. C. Press, 1989, pp. 15–27.
8. Tesh, R. B., Saidi, S., Gajdamovic, S. J., et al.: Serological studies on the epidemiology of sandfly fever in the Old World. Bull. World Health Organ. *54*:663–674, 1976.

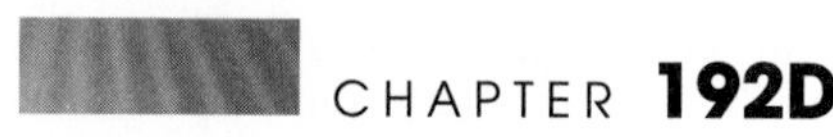

CHAPTER **192D**

Oropouche Fever

FRANCISCO P. PINHEIRO ■
AMELIA P. A. TRAVASSOS DA ROSA ■
PEDRO FERNANDO DA C. VASCONCELOS

Oropouche fever is an arbovirus infection that causes an acute febrile episode accompanied by headache, myalgia, arthralgia, and other systemic symptoms. The symptoms usually recur a few days after the end of the first febrile episode, at which time they are generally less severe. Aseptic meningitis may develop in some patients. Patients make a full recovery, without any apparent aftereffects, even in the most serious cases. No fatalities have been confirmed as being attributable to Oropouche fever. One of the most striking characteristics of Oropouche virus (OROV) is its ability to produce epidemics in urban population centers, most of which reportedly have occurred in the Brazilian Amazon region. Many of these outbreaks have had a major impact on the stricken cities.

The first case of the disease was described in 1955 in a resident of Vega de Oropouche, Trinidad, from whose blood the agent was isolated.[1] The disease was detected again in 1961, this time in the city of Belém, Pará State, northern Brazil, where it caused an epidemic that affected at least 11,000 people.[15] This epidemic was followed by many other epidemics, several of an explosive nature, in urban population centers throughout the Brazilian states of Pará, Amapá, Amazonas, Tocantins, Maranhão, Rondônia, and Acre.[6, 10, 15, 19, 20, 22, 25, 26] Outside Brazil, epidemics of Oropouche fever were reported in Panama in 1989 (Quiroz, E., and associates, Panama, unpublished data, 1989) and in the Amazon region of Peru in 1992[4] and in 1994 (Ministry of Health, Peru, and U.S. Naval Medical Research Institute Detachment [NAMRID], Lima, 1994).

Etiologic Agent

Oropouche fever is caused by OROV, which belongs to the genus Bunyavirus of the family *Bunyaviridae*.[21] The virus has enveloped spherical particles 90 to 100 nm in diameter, the capsid has helical symmetry, and the RNA contains three segments.[11, 21] Phylogenetic analysis has revealed that all OROV strains form a monophylogenetic group consisting of three distinct lineages. Lineage I contains the prototype strain from Trinidad and most of the Brazilian strains, lineage II contains six Peruvian strains isolated between 1992 and 1998 and two strains from western Brazil isolated in 1991, and lineage III comprises four strains isolated from Panama during 1989.[24] Antigenically, it belongs to the Simbu group, which in turn is part of the Bunyamwera supergroup of arboviruses. The virus has a hemagglutinin that is active against geese erythrocytes, and it can be recovered from infected hamster serum treated with acetone (Travassos da Rosa, Belém, unpublished data, 1969). Intracerebral and intraperitoneal inoculation of OROV into baby mice and intracerebral, intraperitoneal, and subcutaneous inoculation of the virus into adult hamsters produce lethal infections. The virus replicates in numerous cell cultures, including Vero, BHK-21, and primary chicken embryo fibroblast, and causes a cytopathic effect.[21] The agent is sensitive to the action of sodium deoxycholate.[9]

Epidemiology

GEOGRAPHIC DISTRIBUTION

Thus far, the only reported cases of Oropouche fever have occurred in Brazil, Panama, Peru, and Trinidad (Fig. 192–3). However, most cases have been limited to the Brazilian Amazon region, with none reported in other areas of Brazil.

With a few exceptions, all episodes of Oropouche fever have been in the form of urban epidemics, including those in Belém and Manaus, the largest cities in the Brazilian Amazon region. The city of Belém, capital of Pará State, was struck by three major epidemics during a 20-year period. The city of Santarém and surrounding villages also were affected by a major epidemic in 1974 and 1975.[19] The first epidemics that occurred outside the State of Pará, those striking the cities of Manaus and Barcelos in the State of Amazonas[3] and the city of Mazagão in what was then the Amapá Territory, were reported early in the 1980s.[13] After a period of quiescence lasting until 1988, new outbreaks of the disease struck the cities of Porto Franco and Tocantinópolis in the states of Maranhão and Tocantins, respectively.[26] The next reported epidemics occurred in 1991, this time in more distant locations, namely, in the cities of Ariquemes and Ouro Preto D'Oeste in the State of Rondônia; the epidemic's impact on these cities was so great that it was reported in the national press. In 1994, another outbreak involving at least 6000 people was recorded in Serra Pelada, Pará State.[25] The last outbreaks were recorded in 1996 and affected at least five urban centers in the states of Pará, Amazonas, and Acre.[22] Thus, during 1961 to 1996, more than 30 epidemics of Oropouche fever have been recorded in Brazil. Serologic surveys[6, 13, 17, 20] have estimated that more than 357,000 people have been infected during this period. However, this estimate is actually quite conservative because the incidence of this viral disease had not been computed in many major outbreaks (Belém, 1968; Porto Franco and Tocantinópolis, 1988). Accordingly, possibly more than a half million people in the Brazilian Amazon region may have been infected with the Oropouche virus since the beginning of the 1960s.

In addition to the aforementioned epidemic areas, countless small villages scattered throughout virtually the entire Amazon region have residents who show hemagglutination-inhibition antibodies against OROV. In general, the prevalence of these antibodies is less than 3 percent, with the exception of Ilha de Gurupá, where it is 10.7 percent.[20]

Outside Brazil, outbreaks were reported in Panama and Peru. The outbreak in Panama occurred in 1989 in the village of Bejuco, which is located approximately 50 km west of the capital (Quiroz, E., and associates, Panama, unpublished data, 1989). The first epidemic in Peru was reported in 1992 in the city of Iquitos in the Peruvian Amazon region[4]; subsequently, an outbreak occurred in Puerto Maldonado, Madre de Dios, also in the Peruvian Amazon region (Ministry of Health, Peru, and NAMRID, Lima, 1994). Studies performed in Peru suggest that transmission of OROV occurs continuously in the population of the city of Iquitos and surrounding villages.[27] Evidence of immunity to OROV was detected in nonhuman primates in Colombia, thus suggesting its presence in that country as well.[9]

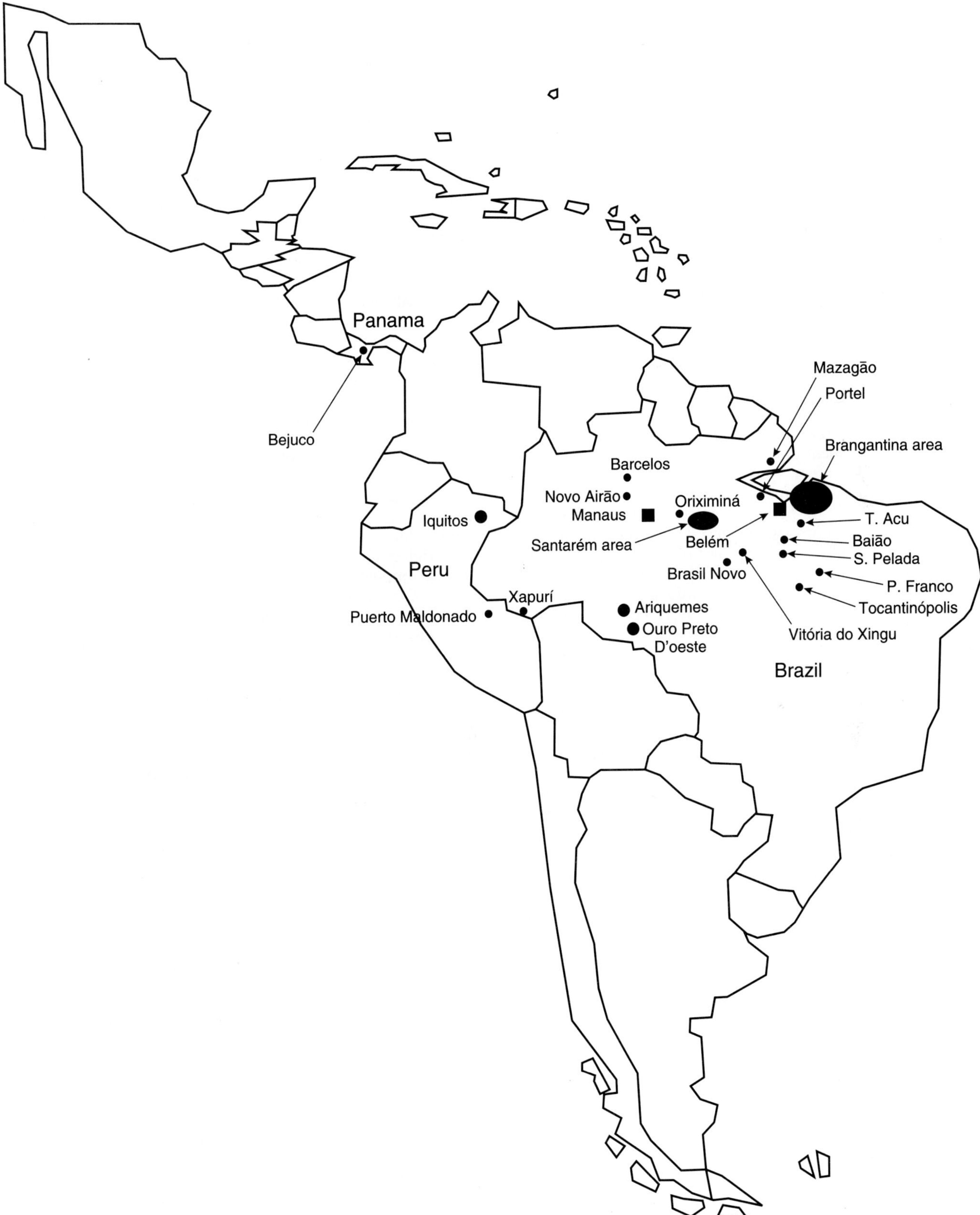

FIGURE 192–3 ■ Outbreaks of Oropouche fever reported in the Americas from 1961 to 2000.

INCIDENCE

A significant characteristic of Oropouche fever has been the exceptionally high attack rates seen during several outbreaks. Although incidence rates have varied in different outbreaks, a rate of 30 percent was quite common. The proportion of those infected who suffer overt disease is not known with certainty, but in one epidemic, clinical disease developed in 63 percent of those infected.[6]

Gender-specific attack rates vary, with rates in females slightly higher than those in males in villages in the Bragantina area, eastern Pará State, struck by the virus in 1979,[6] with the opposite being true in the outbreak in Belém that same year. However, in the reported epidemics in Santarém, the infection struck females twice as often as males.[5] Oropouche fever affects all age groups, although in certain outbreaks its incidence was higher in children and young adults.

DIFFUSION OF EPIDEMICS

As indicated earlier, Oropouche fever epidemics have struck different locations at varying intervals. However, many outbreaks were marked by bona fide epidemic sweeps, with countless numbers of villages within a particular geographic area being affected by the virus. This diffusion phenomenon was observed in Bragança in 1967, in Santarém in 1974 and 1975, and even more so in Belém and in the Bragantina area from 1978 to 1980 (where at least 10 towns were stricken), as well as in Rondônia in 1991. Virus spread is most likely due to the movement of viremic individuals throughout areas in which the virus vector is present.

SEASONAL FLUCTUATION

Most epidemics of Oropouche fever typically occur during the rainy season, which in the case of the state of Pará, corresponds to the period between the months of January and June. However, many epidemics have extended into the dry season, though with less intensity. The seasonal nature of Oropouche fever most likely is linked to the higher density of populations of *Culicoides paraensis*, commonly known as the biting midge, the urban virus vector, in months with higher levels of rainfall, combined with a higher concentration of exposed individuals. Downward trends in epidemics of Oropouche fever generally are associated with arrival of the dry season and the resulting lower density of biting midge populations and smaller numbers of exposed individuals [11, 22]

ENDEMIC TRANSMISSION

During interepidemic periods, isolated cases of Oropouche fever undoubtedly occur in Brazil but remain undiagnosed. Although no systematic studies have been conducted to investigate endemic transmission of OROV in Brazil, seroepidemiologic investigations have indicated that the prevalence of anti-OROV antibodies in humans is 0 to 2 percent in areas where endemic transmission has not been reported[20] but increases to 17 to 44 percent after outbreaks.[5, 11, 21] These data suggest that endemic transmission of OROV is quite low in Brazil.

TRANSMISSION MECHANISM

Laboratory studies and broad-based surveys conducted by the Evandro Chagas Institute during the course of epidemics point to the importance of the insect *C. paraensis* in the *Ceratopogonidae* family as the urban vector for OROV.[14, 18] These tiny insects, commonly known as maruins (biting midges) in the Amazon region, are active during the day, particularly in the late afternoon hours. They crave human blood and bite people inside as well as outside their homes.[8, 19, 23] The disease is transmitted by inoculation of the virus into exposed individuals by bites of infected midges.

TRANSMISSION CYCLES

Studies conducted by the Evandro Chagas Institute[20] suggest that OROV is perpetuated in nature through two different cycles, namely, an urban cycle and a wild cycle.

In the urban or epidemic cycle, the virus is transmitted from person to person by the bite of *C. paraensis*. One of the most conclusive pieces of evidence attesting to this assertion lies in demonstration of the ability of *C. paraensis*, after feeding on the blood of viremic patients, to transmit the virus to hamsters bitten by the midges 5 or more days later.[18] Moreover, these midges typically are found in high densities during periods of epidemics. They breed mostly in the decomposing trunks of felled banana trees, in rotting husks of cocoa beans,[7] and in piles of detritus formed in tree hollows.[12] They are scattered throughout the tropical and subtropical areas of the Americas.[12]

Attempts to transmit the virus from one hamster to another through the bite of the *Culex quinquefasciatus* mosquito (a species commonly found in urban areas throughout the Amazon region) demonstrated that it was transmitted only in the presence of extremely high levels of viremia, which rarely occurs in infected humans.[14] Thus, this finding virtually rules out all likelihood of the epidemic vector being *C. quinquefasciatus*. Curiously, the virus isolation rate from *C. paraensis* during periods of epidemics is only 1:12,500,[11] which suggests that we are dealing with a low-efficiency vector. Apparently, humans are the only vertebrate involved in the urban cycle of OROV because studies of domestic animals conducted during the course of numerous outbreaks have ruled out the possibility of these animals playing an amplifying role.

As far as its wild, silent cycle is concerned, evidence suggests that among vertebrates, the Edentata (sloth), nonhuman primates, and possibly certain species of wild birds serve as hosts. Although to date OROV has been isolated from a single pool of *Aedes serratus* in Brazil and once from *Coquillettidia venezuelensis* in Trinidad,[1, 20] the possible involvement of biting midges in the virus' wild cycle nonetheless should be investigated.

The link between the two cycles is most likely humans themselves, who after contracting the infection in enzootic forested areas and then returning to an urban setting during the viremic phase become a source of infection for biting midges. The virus replicates in the tissues of biting midges, which after the extrinsic incubation period, bite and infect exposed individuals. These individuals in turn serve as a source of infection for other midges, thereby forming a chain of transmission resulting in the unleashing of an epidemic.

INCUBATION PERIOD

Observations conducted during numerous epidemics suggest that the incubation period ranges from 4 to 8 days. A laboratory worker who accidentally was infected orally exhibited symptoms of the viral disease 3 days later, and another technician fell ill 4 days after being infected, probably through the respiratory route.[20]

TRANSMISSIBILITY PERIOD

The blood of infected patients is infectious to *C. paraensis* for the first 3 or 4 days after the onset of symptoms, when the level of viremia is high enough to infect the midges. Experimental studies have shown the length of the extrinsic incubation period to be 5 or more days.[18] The virus is not transmitted directly from one person to another.

RATIO OF SYMPTOMATIC CASES

A prospective study conducted in the city of Santa Izabel in the state of Pará during the course of the epidemic of 1979 showed the ratio of symptomatic to asymptomatic cases to be roughly 2:1.[6] The study was performed during the period from March through June of that year. It involved 274 individuals exposed to the virus who were monitored by clinical examination and laboratory testing on a weekly basis throughout the study. By the end of the study period, 78 (28.5%) of these individuals had serologic evidence of OROV infection, with clinical manifestations of the disease developing in 49 (63%) of the 78.

Clinical Manifestations

In most cases of Oropouche fever, the infection takes the form of an acute febrile episode, which runs its course. However, certain patients may show typical signs and symptoms of aseptic meningitis, which also runs its course without complications.

CLASSIC FEBRILE FORM

This form of the disease is characterized by the sudden onset of symptoms after an incubation period ranging from 4 to 8 days. The first symptoms to appear are fever, headache, chills, dizziness, muscular pain, arthralgia, and photophobia. Retro-ocular pain and conjunctival congestion also may be present. In addition, some patients suffer from nausea, which may be accompanied by episodes of vomiting. Not uncommonly, patients have severe anorexia and insomnia. At times, cough and coryza will be present as well, although these manifestations may be attributable to intercurrent infections. Certain patients complain of fleeting burning or stinging sensations in different parts of their body. The presence of an exanthem is a rare finding. Two laboratory workers who were infected accidentally reported a longer and heavier than usual menstrual flow.[19, 20, 25] The fever can be quite high, 39° C or 40° C, and in some cases it may be higher than 40° C. The headache usually is localized in the front or back part of the head, although it also may be diffuse. It is generally severe and, in some cases, may not respond readily to common analgesics. Generalized myalgia is present and sharpest in the neck, along the vertebral column, and in the area of the sacrum. The pain may be extremely strong and cause the patient a great deal of discomfort. Patients generally describe feeling as though their body had been crushed or they had been beaten. Usually, generalized arthralgia is also present. Certain patients have dizzy spells so severe that in some cases they collapse. Any epigastralgia is generally mild. Patients have no sign of jaundice, hepatomegaly, or splenomegaly. Occasionally, swollen lymph nodes are detected in the submaxillary and occipital regions, which could be totally unrelated to the viral infection.

The intensity of the clinical symptoms varies. In some cases the symptoms are quite severe and even may cause prostration, whereas in others, they can be rather mild. Many patients are bedridden and, in the case of certain epidemics, flood area hospitals, thus causing serious overcrowding.

The acute phase of the disease generally lasts 2 to 5 days but can be as long as a week. The myalgia, on the other hand, may persist for a period of 3 to 5 days after the fever has disappeared. Some patients report having prolonged asthenia for as long as a month. Certain patients complain of a persistent headache lasting up to several weeks. No deaths have been attributed to OROV infection of humans.[11]

Nearly 60 percent of all patients have one or more recurrences in the first or second week after disappearance of the manifestations of the acute phase of the disease.[6, 13, 14] Relapses may take the form of reappearance of all the acute-phase symptoms of the disease, or they may be limited strictly to fever, asthenia, and dizziness. In some patients, relapses were accompanied by a urinary tract infection of bacterial origin. An abscess most likely of bacterial origin developed in the oropharynx of one particular patient approximately 10 days after recovery from the original febrile condition. In some cases, patients may suffer a series of relapses during a period of 2 to 3 weeks.[20] All attempts to isolate OROV during relapses have failed.

Observations made during the course of the 1980 outbreak in Belém revealed that an exanthem developed in approximately 5 percent of all laboratory-confirmed cases.[13] The exanthem appeared between the third and sixth day after onset of the fever, disappeared 2 or 3 days later, and mainly involved the thorax, back, arms, and legs.[13, 17] During the outbreak in Manaus, many patients exhibited a maculopapular exanthem beginning on the torso and subsequently spreading to the upper and lower extremities.[3] In another rare case, a 4-year-old child whose infection was confirmed by serodiagnosis experienced nystagmus, generalized tremors, and somnolence.[6] These symptoms lasted approximately 8 days, with the child apparently making a full recovery.

The effects of Oropouche fever on pregnancy are essentially unknown. The only available data in this regard come from studies conducted in Manaus of nine pregnant patients, two of whom, both in the second month of their pregnancy at the time, suffered miscarriages.[3]

ASEPTIC MENINGITIS

At first, patients exhibit manifestations typical of the initial acute phase of the infection. As the illness progresses, a few days later, the headache and dizziness become increasingly severe, and some patients begin to experience other neurologic symptoms, generally during the second week of the illness, that lead them to seek medical care. The main complaints cited by patients are fever, extremely severe headache in the back of the head, and dizziness. Approximately a third of all patients complain of nausea and vomiting. Some patients suffer from moderate lethargy. They also may have trouble holding themselves in an upright position. Some patients complain of double vision or diplopia. They generally try to keep from moving their heads to avoid aggravating their pain. In most cases, physical examination of these patients reveals varying degrees of stiffness of the neck but no signs of paresis or paralysis. Some patients experience nystagmus. Despite the seriousness of these neurologic symptoms, patients make a full recovery. Encephalograms taken of four patients showed no abnormalities. The incidence of meningitis in patients who seek medical care is less than 5 percent.[16]

Pathogenesis

Little is known about the pathogenesis of Oropouche fever. Apparently, the agent produces a systemic infection in humans that induces a viremic phase, but the organ or organs in which the virus replicates are not known. Virtually all infected patients exhibit viremia during the first 2 days of their illness. By the third day, the rate of viremia drops to 72 percent, and it falls to 44 and 23 percent by the fourth and fifth days, respectively. Viremia titers are generally above 3.0 $\log_{10}$ median lethal dose per 0.02 mL in mice, with approximately 10 percent of patients exhibiting virus titers as high as 5.0 to 5.3 during the course of the first 2 days of their illness. By the third day, virus titers are 1 log lower than in the first 2 days, with titers plummeting by the fourth day.[20]

Likewise, little is known about the pathogenesis of relapses, which occur commonly. That no sign of viremia could be detected in any of the countless patients examined while suffering relapses is noteworthy.

The fact that OROV is capable of causing aseptic meningitis, combined with the fact that it was isolated from the CSF in one case of meningitis,[16] suggests that the virus has the ability to penetrate the blood-brain barrier.

With no known confirmed fatalities attributable to OROV, no data are available on the possible organic lesions caused by this agent in humans.

Laboratory tests on young hamsters inoculated with OROV have shown that it has essentially hepatoviscerotropic properties, with isolated necrosis of hepatocytes or focal necrosis and the involvement of Kupffer cells exhibiting reactive hyperplasia; animals invariably succumb to the infection. In newborn mice the virus exhibits marked neurotropism, with animals showing signs of focal encephalitis within 24 to 48 hours after inoculation.[2]

Laboratory Findings

Leukopenia associated with neutropenia is found commonly, although in certain cases moderate leukocytosis may be present. The leukopenia can be severe, with reports of leukocyte counts as low as 2000/mm^3. No signs of cell abnormalities are present. Aspartate and alanine aminotransferase levels are normal or may show a moderate increase, but in no case do they exceed 135 U/mL of serum. Platelet counts are usually normal but occasionally may be slightly low. The sedimentation rate and levels of urea, creatinine, and glucose in blood are normal, as are urine tests.[20]

The CSF of patients with aseptic meningitis shows pleocytosis and an increased concentration of protein.[16] The cell count varies from 7 to 310 cells/mm^3 of CSF; both segmented and mononuclear cells are present, with a predominance of segmented cells. In one case, the cell count in CSF fell from 130 to 30 in a 1-week period, and another patient's cell count fell from 70 to 10 cells over a 3-week interval. In general, a moderate increase in protein levels occurs in the CSF, although one patient's protein level was more than 100 mg/mL. Sugar levels remain normal.

Laboratory Diagnosis

Specific confirmation of the infection is made by isolating the virus from patients' blood or by performing OROV-specific serologic assays.[21] To isolate the virus, blood samples need to be taken during the first 5 days of the illness, preferably in the first 2 days when viremia is present in virtually all cases. The virus can be isolated by intracerebral or intraperitoneal inoculation of serum from infected patients into baby mice or young hamsters (in this case, subcutaneous inoculation can be used as well). Viral isolates also can be recovered in different cell cultures, such as Vero and BHK-21. The virus is identified by complement fixation or neutralization using OROV-specific ascitic fluid or antisera. Serodiagnosis is accomplished by the demonstration of an increase in antibody in paired serum samples taken during the acute and convalescent phases of the disease by hemagglutination inhibition, complement fixation, or neutralization. A positive IgM antibody-capture enzyme-linked immunosorbent assay (MAC-ELISA) on a single serum sample provides a presumptive diagnosis of recent infection, particularly in the presence of a clinical picture consistent with the disease; the test is usually positive after the fifth day of illness.

Differential Diagnosis

Because of the nonspecific nature of the symptoms, a clinical diagnosis of Oropouche fever is difficult to make, and often the disease is mistaken for other febrile illnesses such as dengue fever and malaria. In fact, malaria and dengue fever initially were suspected as the cause of numerous epidemics of Oropouche fever. Detailed clinical records combined with epidemiologic data can help establish a differential diagnosis, the certainty of which hinges on the absence of plasmodia in blood samples and the lack of laboratory evidence of dengue infection. Other viral and bacterial febrile diseases must be considered in the differential diagnosis. Accordingly, clinical and epidemiologic data and nonspecific tests will need to be taken into account, although making an accurate diagnosis requires specific tests.

Febrile forms of the disease accompanied by an exanthem need to be distinguished from other exanthematous febrile symptoms caused by dengue, measles, enteroviruses, and allergies to medication.

Finally, differentiating cases of aseptic meningitis associated with OROV infection from cases of aseptic meningitis associated with other causative agents requires a specific etiologic diagnosis.

Treatment

Because Oropouche fever has no specific treatment, the only type of management for infection with the virus is symptomatic. Rest is important and should be continued for several days after disappearance of the initial acute manifestations because relapses are thought to occur more often in patients prematurely resuming regular activities, particularly strenuous ones. Aspirin or another antipyretic should be taken to lower the fever, with the use of ordinary analgesics recommended for headache, myalgia, and arthralgia. However, certain patients whose headaches failed to respond to this treatment were treated with morphine derivatives. Also recommended are fruit juices or glucose solutions. Severely dehydrated patients may be treated with intravenous fluids.

Prevention and Control

The most effective way to prevent, avert, or curb the impact of epidemics of Oropouche fever is to combat its vector *C. paraensis*. To be effective, vector control effort needs to focus on the midge's adult and larval forms. Given that *C. paraensis* is habitually active during the day, application of insecticides to its habitats by thermonebulization or ultra-low-volume aerosolization may help reduce populations of adult biting midges. Because this *Culicoides* spp. is most active during the late afternoon hours,[23] ultra-low-volume spraying may be more effective during this period. However, carefully planned studies are needed to assess how to maximize the effectiveness of spraying by determining the type and concentration of insecticide to be used, the necessary volume of insecticide per treatment area, the size of the droplets, the frequency and timing of applications, and other factors. At the same time, making an effort to control its larvae by applying larvicides to corresponding habitats or, better yet, by conducting drives to eliminate or burn breeding sites such as rotting cocoa bean husks and the decomposing trunks of felled banana trees is essential.[7] Obviously, the success of these measures will depend largely on community involvement. Providing proper community education is important. Individuals can protect themselves by applying insecticides directly to the skin. However, these types of products provide only temporary action, and they may be unaffordable to the poor.

No vaccine against Oropouche fever exists at this time. In light of the relatively benign nature of this viral disease, developing a general-purpose vaccine for at-risk populations living in areas where they are exposed to the disease is hard to justify.

REFERENCES

1. Anderson, C. R., Spence, L., Downs, W. G., et al.: Oropouche virus: A new human disease agent from Trinidad, West Indies. Am. J. Trop. Med. Hyg. *10*:574–578, 1961.
2. Araújo, R., Pinheiro, F. P., Araújo, M. T., et al.: Patogenia das lesões hepáticas na infecção experimental com o vírus Oropouche (BeAn 19991): Análise comparativa das curvas virémica e de infectividade com as alterações ultra-estruturais. Hiléia Médica Belém *1*:7–12, 1979.
3. Borborema, C. A. T., Pinheiro, F. P., Albuquerque, B. C., et al.: Primeiro registro de epidemias causadas pelo vírus Oropouche no Estado do Amazonas. Rev. Inst. Med. Trop. Sao Paulo *24*:132–139, 1982.
4. Chavez, R., Colan, E., and Phillips I.: Fiebre de Oropouche en Iquitos: Reporte preliminar de 5 casos. Rev. Farmacol. Terap. *2*:12–14, 1992.
5. Dixon, K. E., Travassos da Rosa, A. P. A., Travassos da Rosa, J. F. S., et al.: Oropouche virus. II. Epidemiological observations during an epidemic in Santarém, Pará, Brazil, in 1975. Am. J. Trop. Med. Hyg. *30*:161–164, 1981.
6. Freitas, R. B., Pinheiro, F. P., Santos, M. A. V., et al.: Epidemia de virus Oropouche no leste do Estado do Pará, 1979. *In* Pinheiro, F. P. (ed.): International Symposium on Tropical Arboviruses and Haemorrhagic Fevers, Rio de Janeiro, Academia Brasileira de Ciências, 1982, pp. 419–439.
7. Hoch, A. L., Roberts, D. R., and Pinheiro, F. D. P.: Breeding sites of *Culicoides paraensis*, and other options for control by environmental management. Bull. Pan Am. Health Organ. *20*:284–293, 1986.
8. Hoch, A. L., Roberts, D. R., and Pinheiro, F. P.: Host-seeking behavior and seasonal abundance of *Culicoides paraensis* (Diptera: Ceratopogonidae) in Brazil. J. Am. Mosq. Control Assoc. *6*:110–114, 1990.
9. Karabatsos, N. (ed.): International Catalogue of Arboviruses, 1985. 3rd ed. San Antonio, TX, American Society of Tropical Medicine and Hygiene, 1985.
10. LeDuc, J. W., Hoch, A. L., Pinheiro, F. P., et al.: Epidemic Oropouche virus disease in northern Brazil. Bull. Pan Am. Health Organ. *15*:97–103, 1981.
11. LeDuc, J. W., and Pinheiro, F. P.: Oropouche fever. *In* Monath, T. P. (ed.): The Arboviruses: Epidemiology and Ecology. Vol. IV. Boca Raton, FL, C. R. C. Press, 1986, pp. 1–14.
12. Linley, J. R., Hoch, A. L., and Pinheiro, F. P.: Biting midges (Diptera: Ceratopogonidae) and human health. J. Med. Entomol. *20*:347–364, 1983.
13. Pinheiro, F. P.: Febre do Oropouche. J. Brasil. Med. *44*:46–62, 1983.
14. Pinheiro, F. P., Hoch, A. L., Gomes, M. L. C., et al.: Oropouche virus. IV. Laboratory transmission by *Culicoides paraensis*. Am. J. Trop. Med. Hyg. *30*:172–176, 1981.
15. Pinheiro, F. P., Pinheiro, M., Bensabath, G., et al.: Epidemia de vírus Oropouche em Belém. Rev. Serv. Esp. Saúde Publ. *12*:15–23, 1962.
16. Pinheiro, F. P., Rocha, A. G., Freitas, R. B., et al.: Meningite associada às infecções por vírus Oropouche. Rev. Inst. Med. Trop. Sao Paulo *24*:246–251, 1982.
17. Pinheiro, F. P., Travassos da Rosa, A. P. A., Freitas, R. B., et al. Arbovírus. Aspectos clínico-epidemiológicos: *In* Instituto Evandro Chagas, 50 Anos de Contribuição às Ciências Biológicas e à Medicina Tropical. Belém, Fundação Serviços de Saúde Pública, 1986, pp. 349–357.
18. Pinheiro, F. P., Travassos da Rosa, A. P. A., Gomes, M. L. C., et al.: Transmission of Oropouche virus from man to hamster by the midge *Culicoides paraensis*. Science *215*:1251–1253, 1982.
19. Pinheiro, F. P., Travassos da Rosa, A. P. A., Travassos da Rosa, J. F., et al.: An outbreak of Oropouche virus disease in the vicinity of Santarém, Pará, Brazil. Tropenmed. Parasitol. *27*:213–223, 1976.
20. Pinheiro, F. P., Travassos da Rosa, A. P. A., Travassos da Rosa, J. F., et al.: Oropouche virus. I. A review of clinical, epidemiological and ecological findings. Am. J. Trop. Med. Hyg. *30*:149–160, 1981.
21. Pinheiro, F. P., Travassos da Rosa, A. P. A. and Vasconcelos, P. F. C.: Arboviral zoonoses of Central and South America. Part G. Oropouche fever. *In* Beran, G. W. (ed.): Handbook of Zoonoses. 2nd ed. Boca Raton, FL, C. R. C. Press, 1994, pp. 214–217.
22. Pinheiro, F. P., Travassos da Rosa, A. P. A., and Vasconcelos, P. F. C.: An overview of Oropouche fever epidemics in Brazil and neighbour countries. *In* Travassos da Rosa, A. P. A., Vasconcelos, P. F. C., and Travassos da Rosa, J. F. S. (eds.): An Overview of Arbovirology in Brazil and Neighbouring Countries. Belém, The Erandro Chagas Institute, 1998, pp. 186–192.
23. Roberts, D. R., Hoch, A. L., Dixon, K. E., et al.: Oropouche virus. III. Entomological observations from three epidemics in Pará, Brazil, 1975. Am. J. Trop. Med. Hyg. *30*:165–171, 1981.
24. Saeed, M. F., Wang, H., Nunes, M., et al.: Nucleotide sequences and phylogeny of the nucleocapsid gene of Oropouche virus. J. Gen. Virol. *81*:743–748, 2000.
25. Travassos da Rosa, A. P. A., Rodrigues, S. G., and Nunes, M. R., et al.: Epidemia de febre do Oropouche em Serra Pelada, Município de Curionópolis, Pará, 1994. Rev. Soc. Bras. Med. Trop. *29*:537–541, 1996.
26. Vasconcelos, P. F. C., Travassos da Rosa, J. F. S., Guerreiro, S. C., et al.: Primeiro registro de epidemias causadas pelo vírus Oropouche nos estados do Maranhão e Goiás, Brasil. Rev. Inst. Med. Trop. Sao Paulo *31*:271–278, 1989.
27. Watts, D. M., Phillips, I., Callahan, J. D., et al. Oropouche virus transmission in the Amazon River basin of Peru. Am. J. Trop. Med. Hyg. *56*:148–152, 1997.

RETROVIRIDAE

CHAPTER

193 Human Retroviruses

CHAPTER **193A**

Oncoviruses (Human T-Cell Lymphotropic Viruses Types I and II) and Lentiviruses (Human Immunodeficiency Virus Type 2)

LYNNE M. MOFENSON

The discovery of human T-cell lymphotropic virus type I (HTLV-I) in 1980 demonstrated for the first time that humans could be infected by retroviruses, which previously were known as animal pathogens that could cause malignancies.[6, 91, 261] HTLV-I subsequently was found to cause adult T-cell leukemia/lymphoma (ATLL) and now is recognized to be associated with a spectrum of disease manifestations, including a chronic degenerative neurologic disease (HTLV-I–associated myelopathy [HAM]/tropical spastic paraparesis [TSP]); a relapsing, severe generalized dermatitis in children (infective dermatitis); and numerous inflammatory or autoimmune conditions, or both, such as uveitis, arthropathy, polymyositis, bronchoalveolitis, and Sjögren syndrome.[42, 190, 205, 298] In 1982, a second antigenically related retrovirus of the oncovirus subfamily, HTLV-II, was identified from a patient with a T-cell variant of hairy-cell leukemia.[146] The pathogenicity of this virus remains unclear, although the virus has been found in some individuals with $CD8^+$ lymphoproliferative diseases and neuromyopathies.[96]

Identification of HTLV played a critical role in advancing virologic science. The research methodology developed to culture T lymphocytes and isolate HTLV-I was fundamental in enabling the identification of human immunodeficiency virus (HIV) type 1, a retrovirus of the lentivirus subfamily, as the cause of acquired immunodeficiency syndrome (AIDS) in 1983. In 1986, a second antigenic variant, HIV-2, was identified in some individuals with AIDS from West Africa.[48]

HTLV-related research also has had important ramifications outside the field of virology.[21] Improved understanding of cellular transcriptional and post-transcriptional events was facilitated by research that demonstrated the functional properties of the HTLV transactivator protein Tax, which serves to increase viral expression and regulate the function of host cell genes, and Rex, a transport protein that ferries between the nucleus and cytoplasm and serves to export unspliced viral mRNA to the cytoplasm for translation into viral proteins. HTLV-I–related research led to discovery of the cytokines interleukin-9 (IL-9) and IL-15 and the IL-2 receptor, as well as identification of chemokine production by $CD8^+$ T lymphocytes. Finally, the study of oncogenesis has been stimulated by research into the mechanism by which HTLV-I induces malignant transformation.

With the explosion of information concerning the molecular, biologic, clinical, and epidemiologic aspects of retroviruses, an important model has been provided for exploring the pathobiology of many human diseases ranging from neoplastic disorders to autoimmune and immunodeficiency syndromes. Given the rapid pace of breakthroughs in retrovirology, new isolations probably will result in the discovery of additional examples of these types of viruses, perhaps unlocking secrets of some human diseases for which the etiology is currently unknown.

The Retroviruses

CLASSIFICATION

Retroviruses form a family of single-stranded RNA viruses that are unusual because they contain a diploid RNA genome that replicates by flow of genetic information through a DNA intermediate, a process known as *reverse transcription;* the name *retrovirus* is derived from this characteristic. This unique capability is due to the presence of a virally encoded, RNA-dependent DNA polymerase, reverse transcriptase, that catalyzes transcription of viral RNA into a double-stranded DNA copy. This viral DNA intermediary becomes integrated into host-cell DNA, where it then resides as a provirus; this process occurs by a specialized recombination mechanism requiring another viral protein, integrase. This capacity for genomic integration correlates with the capability of retroviruses to cause lifelong infection, evade the usual mechanisms of immune clearance, and produce chronic diseases in the host that become manifested only after a long asymptomatic period that may last years to decades.

Retroviruses have been grouped historically into two broad categories, classic/simple and complex, based on the complexity of the viral genome and replication mechanisms[79, 338] (Table 193–1). Simple retroviruses contain only three genes (*env, gag,* and *pol*) that encode for two classes of transcripts, unspliced genomic RNA and spliced RNA; these transcripts code for viral enzymes or structural components. Simple retroviruses cause disease in animals and are not discussed further in this chapter.

Complex retroviruses that can infect humans have a more complicated genome that encodes for numerous regulatory genes involved in modulating viral replication. These retroviruses have been divided historically into three

TABLE 193–1 ■ *RETROVIRIDAE* FAMILY

Type of Retrovirus	Prototype Viruses
Classic (or Simple) Retroviruses	
D-type Retroviruses	Mason-Pfizer monkey virus
B-type Retroviruses	Mouse mammary tumor virus
C-type Retroviruses a	Rous sarcoma virus
C-type Retroviruses b	Murine leukemia virus
Complex Retroviruses	
Oncoretroviruses, human	Human T-cell lymphotropic virus types I and II
Lentiretroviruses, human	Human Immunodeficiency virus types 1 and 2
Spumaretroviruses (foamy viruses)	Human spumaretrovirus

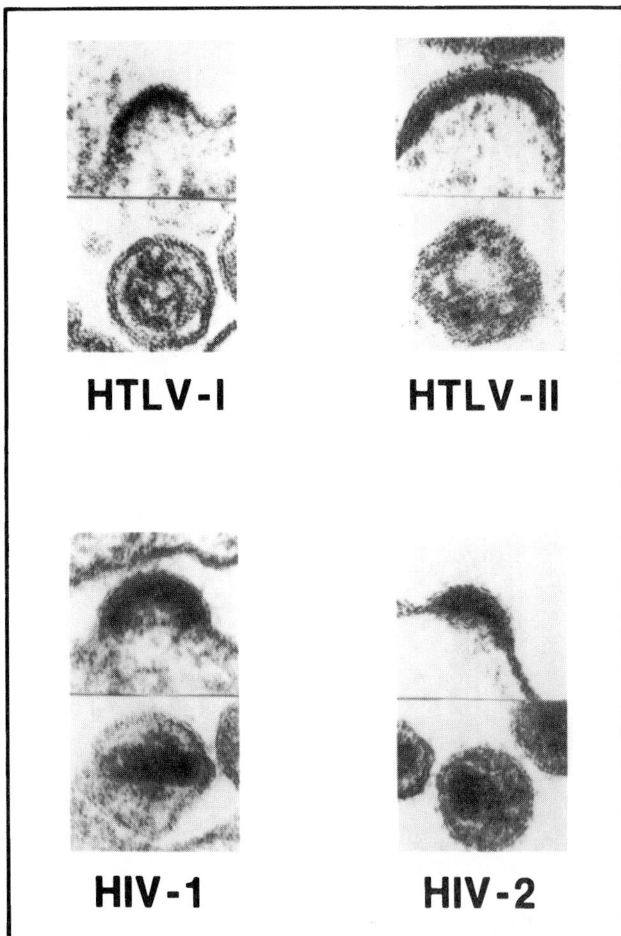

FIGURE 193–1 ■ Electron micrographs of HTLV-I, HTLV-II, HIV-1, and HIV-2. In the *upper panel* for each virus is shown the budding particle; in the *lower panel,* the mature virion. (From Blattner, W. A.: Retroviruses. *In* Evans A. S. [ed.]: Viral Infections of Human Epidemiology and Control. 3rd ed. New York, Plenum, 1989, pp. 545–592.)

subfamilies on the basis of nucleotide sequences and genetic organization. The subfamilies included the *Oncovirinae* (oncogenic or transforming viruses, which include HTLV-I and HTLV-II); the *Lentivirinae* (slow viruses with cytopathic effects, which include HIV-1 and HIV-2); and the *Spumavirinae* (foamy viruses).

Although they share some similarities in genomic structure and life cycle, the different subfamilies of retroviruses have distinct in vitro and in vivo effects and different strategies for evading host immunity. Oncoviruses generally transform cells in culture, stimulate target-cell proliferation, and cause tumors in their hosts. Lentiviruses cause cell fusion and multinucleated giant-cell formation, are cytopathic in cell culture, and cause slow infections characterized by immunodeficiency in their hosts. The spumaviruses also are cytopathic for susceptible cells, and they induce syncytial giant cells and vacuolation in cells in vitro.[79] Transgenic mice carrying the spumavirus *bel* gene were found to express the transgene in the central nervous system (CNS) and smooth muscle and to develop a progressive degenerative encephalopathy and myopathy.[31] However, spumavirus replication in vivo is extremely limited, and unlike the oncoviruses and lentiviruses, no evidence has been found that these viruses are pathogenic in either naturally or accidentally infected animals and humans.[175, 176] Thus, the relevance of spumaviruses as human pathogens is unknown, and they are not discussed further.

MORPHOLOGY/GENOMIC STRUCTURE

Retroviruses have a distinct morphology. They are enveloped RNA viruses that have diameters of 80 to 120 nm, a thin electron-dense outer envelope, and an electron-dense core that is either spherical (HTLV-I and HTLV-II) or cylindric (HIV-1 and HIV-2) (Fig. 193–1). The envelope of all retroviruses is composed of a lipid bilayer derived from the host-cell plasma membrane during budding of the virus from the cell surface, with surface projections consisting of the viral envelope proteins (Fig. 193–2). The retroviral core protein encloses a ribonucleoprotein of genomic RNA complexed with viral reverse transcriptase and integrase.[49] The genome is a messenger-sense, linear, single-stranded RNA composed of two identical subunits held together by hydrogen bonds at their 5′ ends. The 5′ and 3′ ends of the RNA contain repeated sequences that give rise to elements in viral DNA called long terminal repeats (LTRs). The LTRs are composed of nucleic acid sequences that provide signals critical for structural transformation of the viral genome, including initiation and progression of reverse transcription of viral RNA into DNA, integration of viral DNA into the host genome by viral integrase, initiation of viral mRNA transcription from the integrated provirus and binding sites for viral and cellular proteins and that positively and negatively influence mRNA transcription.[269, 323, 335, 366] Between the LTRs are the genes that encode the major structural proteins of the virus, the enzymes found in the viral particles, and additional proteins with specialized intracellular functions.

As noted earlier, all retroviruses contain a minimum of three genes, *gag* (group-specific antigen), *pol* (polymerase), and *env* (envelope). They are arranged in a 5′ to 3′ order, with LTRs at each end[106] (Fig. 193–3). The *gag* gene encodes the structural protein products that form the core particle of the virus, including nucleocapsid, capsid, and matrix proteins. The *pol* gene products include the enzymes required for genome replication (viral RNA-dependent DNA polymerase and ribonuclease H), proviral integration (integrase), and polyprotein processing (protease). The *env* gene encodes the major components of the viral coat, the surface

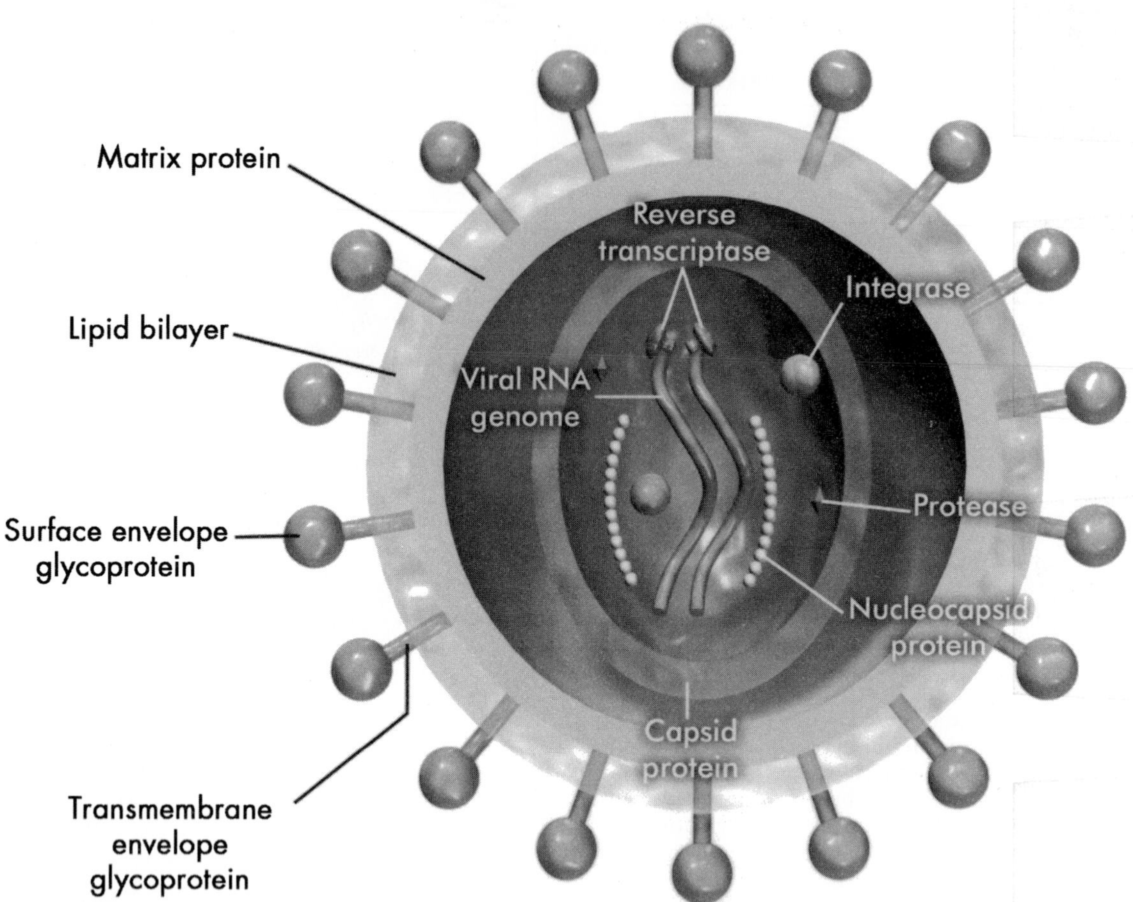

FIGURE 193–2 ■ Retroviral structure. The mature retroviral virion is spherical; the central viral core is spherical in HTLV oncoviruses and cylindric in HIV lentiviruses. The core is surrounded by a lipid bilayer envelope derived from the host-cell membrane during budding, with surface projections consisting of the viral surface and transmembrane envelope proteins. The viral matrix protein surrounds the virion core and is associated with the viral transmembrane envelope glycoproteins. The virion core is a structural shell composed of the viral capsid proteins. Within the shell are two copies of single-stranded viral RNA and multiple copies of the virally encoded reverse transcriptase, protease, and integrase enzymes. The viral nucleocapsid protein is bound to the RNA copies and may serve to condense the viral RNA into the capsid shell during virion assembly.

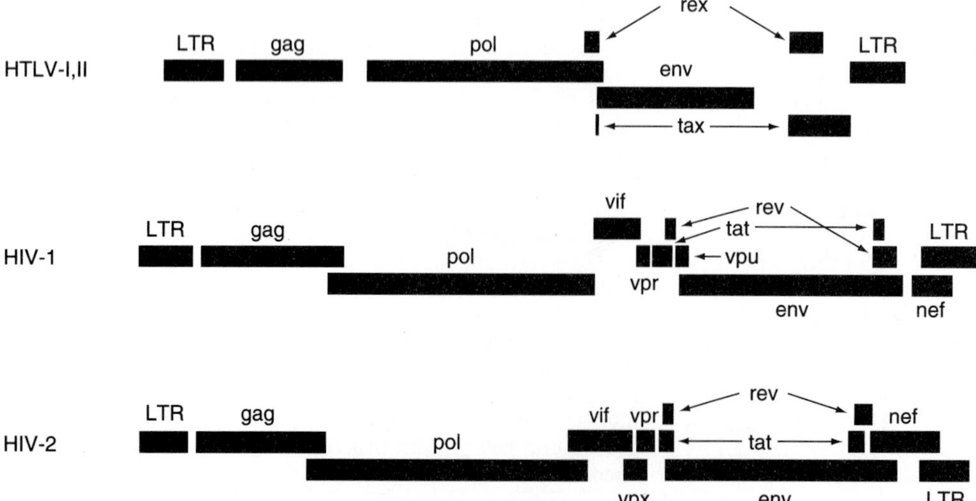

FIGURE 193–3 ■ Retroviral genome. This schematic depiction of the HTLV and HIV genomes shows that HTLV has a more complex genome than most animal retroviruses do and that HIV in turn has additional regulatory genes. Details of the functions of these genes are summarized in text. (Reprinted by permission from Gallo, R. C., Wong-Staal, F., Montagnier, L., et al.: HIV/HTLV gene nomenclature. Nature *333*:504, 1988. Copyright © Macmillan Magazines, Ltd.)

and transmembrane glycoproteins. Retroviral genes generally are expressed first as large overlapping polyproteins that undergo processing into functional peptide products by viral or cellular proteases. A complex array of additional genes with various regulatory functions are also present (Table 193–2).

Oncoviral Regulatory and Accessory Genes

In addition to the standard retroviral genes, the oncoviruses HTLV-I and HTLV-II contain several regulatory and accessory genes important for viral replication and activation of host genes that are encoded in open-reading frames (ORFs) in a unique region at the 3′ end of the genome called the pX region.[5, 134] The HTLV-I pX region contains four ORFs, whereas HTLV-II contains five ORFs. Two of these ORFs common to both viruses (ORF III and ORF IV) encode the regulatory proteins Rex and Tax.

The *rex* (regulator of expression of virion proteins) gene encodes a nucleolus-localizing phosphoprotein that affects mRNA splicing and export from the nucleus to the cytoplasm. For cellular genes, mRNA splicing and export are tightly coupled. After cellular genes are transcribed into mRNA, splicing occurs in the cell nucleus before mRNA can be exported into the cytoplasm for translation into proteins. Incompletely spliced mRNA molecules are retained in the nucleus.[203, 323] However, for retroviral reproduction, the export of full-length, unspliced viral RNA into the cytoplasm is required to serve as genomic RNA for integration into progeny virions and to serve as mRNA for the production of viral structural proteins. Thus, retroviruses had to develop a mechanism to bypass the cellular regulatory process; for HTLV, the Rex protein serves this function. This protein is expressed predominantly at an early stage of viral gene expression and enhances the transport of single-spliced and unspliced viral mRNA coding for structural proteins, as well as transport of the viral genome from the nucleus to the cytoplasm. The Rex protein also exerts a negative effect on the transport of multiply spliced viral mRNA to the cytoplasm. These multiply spliced mRNA molecules code for regulatory proteins, including Rex and Tax.[335]

The *tax* (transactivator) gene encodes a nuclear protein that plays a critical role in the regulation of viral replication and also stimulates a large number of cellular genes involved in activation and proliferation of T cells, including lymphokines, lymphokine receptors, and nuclear proto-oncogenes.[373, 374] The Tax protein does not bind directly to DNA but rather interacts with host-cell transcriptional factors to produce a multifaceted array of molecular effects.[21] The Tax protein activates mRNA transcription by binding to several different host-cell transcription-enhancing factors, including those of the nuclear factor NF-κB family. In addition

TABLE 193–2 ■ RETROVIRAL GENOME TERMINOLOGY AND FUNCTION

Name of Gene	Function of Protein
Major Structural Genes (All Retroviruses)	
gag	Expressed late; proteins form nucleocapsid, capsid, and matrix
pol	Expressed late; proteins form reverse transcriptase, ribonuclease H, protease, and integrase enzymes
env	Expressed late; proteins form envelope surface and transmembrane proteins
Accessory Regulatory Genes (Oncoviruses and Lentiviruses Only)	
Oncoviruses HTLV-I and HTLV-II	
tax	Expressed early; binds to host-cell transcription factors that enhance transcription of viral mRNA from integrated proviral genome, as well as many cellular genes; suppresses expression of tumor suppression genes; suppresses expression of genes for cellular DNA repair enzyme (DNA polymerase-beta); directly binds to and inhibits some cell cycle regulation and tumor suppressor proteins
rex	Expressed early; directs selective transport of unspliced genomic and partially spliced viral structural and enzyme mRNA from nucleus to cytoplasm; down-regulates transport of multiply spliced regulatory viral mRNA
Lentiviruses HIV-1 and HIV-2	
tat	Expressed early; binds to long terminal repeat sequence in integrated provirus (*tat* activation region (*TAR*)) to enhance viral mRNA transcript elongation
rev	Expressed early; directs selective transport of unspliced genomic and partially spliced structural and enzyme viral mRNA from nucleus to cytoplasm; down-regulates transport of multiply spliced regulatory viral mRNAs
nef	Expressed early; enhances cytoplasmic delivery of viral particles from cell membrane (allowing dissociation of pre-integration complex from virion capsid proteins?); down-regulates CD4 and MHC expression on cell surface
vif	Expressed late; stabilizes cytoplasmic nucleoprotein pre-integration complex; prevents premature processing of viral proteins in cytoplasm; ensures that viral peptides needed for viral assembly are available at plasma membrane
vpr	Vpr protein is present in virion itself and associated with nucleoprotein pre-integration complex; interacts with nucleoporins to facilitate transport of pre-integration complex with viral DNA into the nucleus
vpu (HIV-1 only)	Expressed late; induces intracellular degradation of cytoplasmic domain CD4; down-regulates MHC expression; important in virion assembly and release
vpx (HIV-2 only)	Present in the virion itself; affects efficiency of early replication events by unknown mechanism

MHC, major histocompatibility complex.

to activating transcription of the HTLV genome, the "Tax transcription factor complex" acts to stimulate transcription of many cellular genes, including those encoding IL-2, IL-2 receptor-alpha, tumor necrosis factor, cyclooxygenase 2 (a prostaglandin synthetase), and some nuclear oncogenes.[212, 373, 374] Tax also represses transcription of tumor suppression genes and the expression of cellular DNA polymerase-beta, a key enzyme for repair of damaged DNA. Additionally, Tax can bind directly to and inhibit some cell cycle regulation and tumor suppressor proteins, thereby interfering with cell cycle regulation and resulting in abnormal promotion of the cell cycle and enhancement of cellular proliferation.[374] Finally, Tax increases the genetic instability of the cell by impairing cellular DNA repair mechanisms, which leads to an accumulation of mutations and an increase in chromosomal anomalies. In vitro, Tax protein can immortalize human T cells and induce tumors in transgenic mice. However, in vivo, malignancy develops in less than 5 percent of HTLV-I–infected individuals. Thus, although the *tax* gene probably is involved in malignant transformation of infected T cells, it is not sufficient by itself to explain the final development of malignancy.[7, 338, 373, 374]

Less is known about the function of the HTLV accessory proteins that are encoded by the remaining ORFs in the pX region (e.g., p12, p13, and p30 in HTLV-I and p10, p11, p22/20, and p28 in HTLV-II). The best characterized accessory protein is HTLV-I p12 from ORF I, which is a conserved, hydrophobic protein localized to the internal cell plasma membrane and perinuclear regions of the cell.[43] The p12 protein contains amino acid motifs commonly found in proteins involved in intracellular signaling pathways and probably interacts with cellular proteins, perhaps cellular kinases, to modulate intracellular signaling in infected cells. The protein also interacts with the beta and gamma chains of the IL-2 receptor. This protein may be required for activation of host cells during the early stages of infection, for cellular transformation, and for efficient viral infectivity, similar to the function of the *nef* gene of the lentivirus HIV-1.[5] Interestingly, the corresponding ORF I protein in HTLV-II, p10, does not bind the IL-2 receptor and is not associated with the constitutive activation of the IL-2 signaling pathway that is seen with HTLV-I–transformed cells.[43] These differences may be associated with differences in pathogenicity between the two oncoviruses.

Lentiviral Regulatory and Accessory Genes

More detailed data are available about the function of lentiviral genes.[72] The lentiviruses HIV-1 and HIV-2 have more complex genomes containing at least six regulatory genes in addition to *env, gag,* and *pol* (see Table 193–2). The lentiviral genes corresponding to the oncoviral *tax* and *rex* are called *tat* and *rev*; these genes are found in all known human and animal lentiviruses and appear to be essential for replication.[203]

Like the oncoviral *rex* gene, *rev* is expressed early in the viral replication cycle and undergoes splicing in the nucleus; multiply spliced *rev* mRNA transcripts then are exported to produce Rev protein in the cytoplasm. This protein contains a nuclear localization signal that facilitates entry of the protein back into the nucleus. Rev then binds to unspliced viral mRNA at a *cis*-acting Rev response element (RRE) located on the mRNA. A nuclear export signal sequence on the carboxy-terminal domain of Rev next targets the unspliced viral mRNA for export to the cytoplasm by binding to the cellular protein CRM1 (exportin 1) and exiting the nucleus via the host-cell export pathway.[53] The full-length unspliced viral mRNA then serves as a translational template for expression of the Gag, and Pol proteins and also serves as genomic RNA for incorporation into new virions.

In contrast to the oncoviral Tax protein, which binds to host-cell proteins and has multiple effects in addition to promoting initiation of HTLV gene transcription, the lentiviral Tat protein binds to an RNA target, the Tat activation region (TAR), located immediately 3′ to the LTR transcription start site, and plays a primary role in the expression of HIV viral transcripts by enhancing mRNA elongation. At least two host-cell cofactors are involved in this process.[323] Cellular cyclin T binds to the activation domain of Tat, which increases both the affinity and specificity of the resulting complex for TAR. A host-cell encoded kinase then is recruited to the "Tat–cyclin T–TAR" complex and phosphorylates the carboxyl-terminal domain of the host-cell RNA polymerase II, which in turn enhances mRNA transcript elongation.

The remaining lentiviral accessory regulatory genes *nef, vpr,* and *vif* provide fine-tuning by enhancing or, less commonly, by diminishing viral replication. Another accessory gene, *vpu,* is found only in HIV-1, whereas HIV-2 and simian immunodeficiency virus (SIV) lack the *vpu* gene but contain a gene called *vpx*. The *nef* gene, like *tat* and *rev,* is expressed early in the replication cycle. Similar to the HTLV-I p12 protein, *nef* encodes a hydrophobic, membrane-associated protein that probably interacts with and modulates cellular signaling pathways and is required for optimal infectivity in vivo and for activation of infected host cells. Nef protein significantly enhances the cytoplasmic delivery of viral particles entering the cell via fusion at the plasma membrane, possibly by enhancing phosphorylation of the viral matrix protein and thereby allowing dissociation of the matrix and associated pre-integration nucleoprotein complex from the virion capsid proteins.[286, 323] Nef also down-regulates cell surface expression of CD4 by accelerating CD4 receptor endocytosis through interaction with the cytoplasmic tail of CD4 and a protein complex (AP-2 adaptor complex) responsible for recruiting membrane-associated proteins to clathrin-coated pits for endocytosis.[72] This process reduces the potential interference of membrane-associated CD4 with the release of budding virions. Major histocompatibility complex (MHC) class I receptor expression also is down-regulated by Nef.

The Vpr protein is present in the virion itself, may act to regulate cellular events after penetration and uncoating of the virus to facilitate viral replication, and is involved in efficient localization of the nucleoprotein pre-integration complex into the nucleus.[49, 115] Vpr appears to interact with a specific site on nucleoporins in the nuclear pore complex to facilitate nuclear entry.[323] Similar to the Vpr protein, the HIV-2 Vpx protein is found in the virion and appears to affect the efficiency of early replication events, but the precise mechanism is unknown.[49, 174]

The *vif* (virion infectivity factor) accessory gene is expressed late, along with structural and enzymatic proteins. The Vif protein is predominantly cytoplasmic but also exists in a membrane-associated form.[203] Vif protein is phosphorylated by a host-cell protein kinase, which seems to be important for interaction of Vif with cellular and viral proteins or for targeting to certain cellular compartments. Vif appears to stabilize the pre-integration provirus; viral particles that are produced in the absence of Vif are incapable of incorporating the provirus into host-cell chromosomes.[203] Vif also may function to prevent premature processing of Gag precursor proteins by viral protease in the cytoplasm, thereby ensuring that the Gag-derived peptides that form the viral nucleoprotein core are available at the plasma membrane for assembly with other viral components.

The HIV-1 *vpu* gene also is expressed late. The Vpu protein is associated with the endoplasmic reticulum in infected cells, where it binds the CD4 molecule and prevents it from translocating to the plasma membrane; instead, the CD4 molecule is targeted for proteolysis through the cytoplasmic ubiquitin-proteasome pathway.[72, 323] This process prevents trapping and subsequent degradation of HIV envelope proteins by CD4 in the cytoplasm, thus increasing the ability of the viral envelope proteins to reach the cell membrane. Vpu, like Nef, also down-regulates MHC class I receptor expression. In addition, Vpu may be important in virion assembly and particle release.[44, 94, 346]

VIRAL REPLICATION

The lentiviruses can infect and replicate in nondividing, terminally differentiated cells, and transmission can occur by cell-free or cell-associated virus. HIV-1 has high replication rates in vivo, with an average of 10^9 to 10^{10} viral particles produced each day. Free viral particles are estimated to have a half-life of less than 6 hours, and productively infected cells have a half-life of about 1 day.[132, 239, 355] The relentless rounds of reverse transcription rapidly generate extensive viral genetic variation within a single individual, which results in a genetically related "swarm," or quasi-species, of viruses and provides the ability to rapidly escape the host immune response.

In contrast, the oncoviruses require that the host cell undergo division for productive infection to be established, and they replicate in vivo largely via mitosis rather than reverse transcription.[192] Additionally, transmission is predominantly, if not solely, accomplished by means of cell-cell contact.[60] The events that occur during primary HTLV infection are reverse transcription of the viral genome, integration of the provirus into DNA, transcription of mRNA, synthesis of viral proteins, and a burst of viral expression. However, after a period of active replication, viral persistence is facilitated by a prolonged phase of clonal proviral expansion produced by transactivation of host-cell genes by Tax, which results in cellular DNA replication and the production of new cells containing the HTLV proviral genome.[215] Unlike viral nucleic acid replication by the error-prone viral reverse transcriptase, cellular mitosis is much less prone to mutation and generates little viral genetic variation. Moreover, the provirus remains hidden from immune surveillance. Thus, oncoviruses have extraordinary genetic stability in comparison to lentiviruses. The genetic variability of the HIV-1 envelope protein that exists within the viral quasi-species in a single individual 5 years after infection is greater than the genetic variability found in all HTLV-I proteins identified worldwide to date.[352]

These differences are related to divergence among the retroviral subfamilies in genetic organization, transcription, and function of the major regulatory genes (*tax* and *rex* for the HTLVs and *tat* and *rev* for HIVs). The Tax and Tat proteins both are transactivating enhancer proteins. However, the HTLV Tax protein interacts with cellular proteins and activates cellular genes, thereby resulting in disruption of the cell cycle and induction of cell proliferation. In contrast, the HIV Tat protein has more focal effects; it recognizes a small RNA domain in the HIV LTR and serves primarily to transactivate HIV replication. The Rex and Rev proteins have similar functions; both interact with genomic mRNA structures (the Rex responsive element and Rev responsive element) to enhance transport of the unspliced and partly spliced viral mRNA molecules from the nucleus to the cytoplasm, and both also down-regulate the transport of multiply spliced mRNA transcripts that encode for early regulatory proteins, including the mRNA molecules coding for themselves. In the oncoviruses, Tax and Rex are derived from the same mRNA, and therefore down-regulation of Rex mRNA transport results in decreased Tax mRNA transport and protein production. This process leads to diminished transactivation of HTLV genome transcription and prevents massive viral production. In contrast, the HIV Tat protein comes in two functionally equivalent forms, a 72- and an 86-residue protein. The 72-residue Tat protein is derived from a joint Rev/Tat mRNA, but the 86-residue Tat protein comes from a small Rev-independent mRNA. Although Rev, like Rex, has a negative effect on its own expression, as well as that of Tat, this effect is mitigated by the expression of a Tat mRNA that is not dependent on expression of Rev mRNA, thereby resulting in continued production of the Tat transactivating protein and constant and massive transcription of the HIV genome.

Retroviral Life Cycle

All retroviruses have two phases in their life cycle: an infection phase (including viral attachment, entry, reverse transcription, and proviral integration) and an expression phase (including transcription, translation, assembly, and budding of the virion) (Fig. 193–4).[49] In general, more detail is known about replication in lentiviruses than in oncoviruses.

INFECTION PHASE OF RETROVIRAL REPLICATION

Retroviruses attach to cells through recognition and binding of viral outer surface envelope proteins to specific proteins on the surface of the host cell; such cell surface receptor specificity probably accounts for the species and cellular tropism of retroviruses.[144, 235] The surface glycoprotein of the retroviral envelope has three structural and functional domains separated by conserved hinges and is noncovalently linked to the transmembrane protein via disulfide bonds. The envelope transmembrane protein anchors the entire envelope glycoprotein complex on the virion surface and is responsible for the fusogenic capacity of the viral envelope. The transmembrane protein of all retroviruses has several conserved motifs, including a "leucine zipper" coiled motif followed by the N-terminal hydrophobic "fusion peptide" responsible for fusion with the host-cell membrane. After binding of the viral surface protein to the host-cell receptor, conformational changes permit correct exposure of the transmembrane fusion peptide to the host-cell membrane. The interaction of several fusion peptides may serve to destabilize the lipid bilayer of the target-cell membrane by forming a "fusion pore" between the two bilayers[84] to facilitate fusion of the viral and cellular membranes and release of the viral RNA-protein complex into the cytoplasm.[105, 311, 338]

The cell surface receptor for HTLV-I and HTLV-II has not been characterized completely. Oncoviruses transmit infection primarily by fusion of infected cells with uninfected cells and the subsequent formation of syncytia. In HTLV-I, fusion is thought to be mediated by the HTLV envelope proteins expressed on the surface of infected cells and by cell adhesion molecules, such as vascular cell adhesion molecule type 1 (VCAM-1), intracellular adhesion molecule type 1 (ICAM-1), ICAM-3, and the membrane permease CD98, on target-cell surfaces.[21] Although HTLV-I envelope-expressing infected cells can form syncytia with cells from most cell lines, in vivo, HTLV-1 is found only in CD4 lymphocytes.[60] In contrast, HTLV-II displays a preferential tropism for cells of the $CD8^+$ T-lymphocyte phenotype.[138, 168]

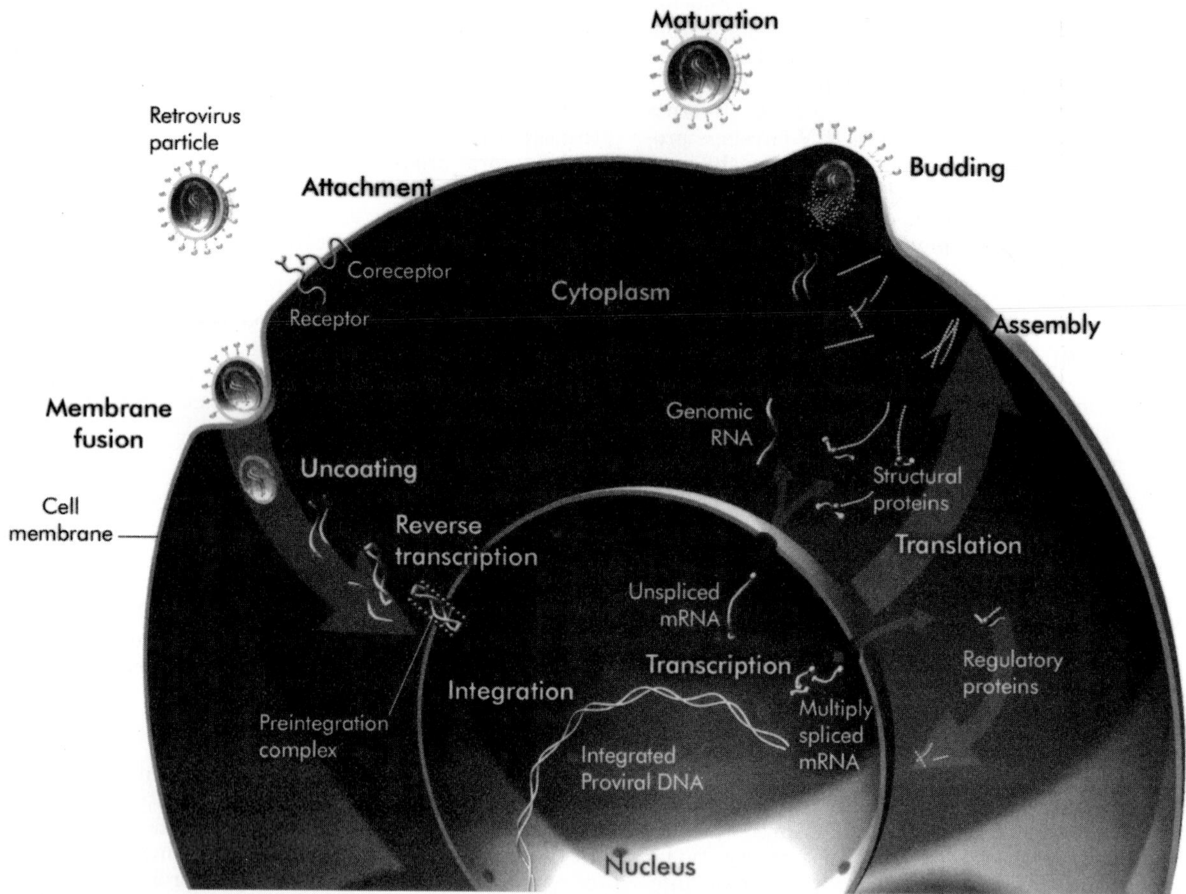

FIGURE 193–4 ■ Life cycle of retroviruses. Details of viral replication are discussed in the text. (Modified from Furtado, M. R., Callaway, D. S., Phair, J. P., et al.: Persistence of HIV-1 transcription in peripheral blood mononuclear cells in patients receiving potent antiretroviral therapy. N. Engl. J. Med. *340*:1620, 1999.)

The lentiviruses HIV-1 and HIV-2 infect cells that express CD4, the HLA class II receptor, on their cell surface.[235] These cells include CD4$^+$ T-lymphocytes, cells of the monocyte/macrophage lineage, and microglia in the brain. A high-affinity interaction between the surface glycoprotein and the CD4 receptor produces a conformational change that results in exposure of another site with high affinity for a secondary co-receptor required for the entry of HIV-1 and some HIV-2 isolates into the cell. The chemokine receptor CCR5 is the co-receptor used by monocyte/macrophage–tropic HIV-1, whereas the CXCR4 chemokine receptor is used by T-lymphocyte–tropic HIV-1; although most HIV-1 strains use only one receptor, some strains of HIV-1 are dually tropic and can use both receptors.[28, 63, 69, 241] Additional co-receptors may support the entry of more restricted types of HIV isolates. For example, the chemokine receptor CCR3 is used by some macrophage-tropic HIV-1 strains and mediates entry of the virus into microglia; CCR2b, CR8, STLR/STRL-22, GPR15, GPR1, and the cytomegalovirus protein US28 also support entry by various HIV-1 and HIV-2 strains.[111, 323] Whereas nearly all strains of HIV-2 can use CD4 together with the chemokine receptor CCR5 or CXCR4 (or both), most HIV-2 isolates also can interact with multiple other co-receptors.[213, 288] Additionally, some HIV-2 isolates can use CXCR4 or other receptors, such as CCR3, as a primary receptor and infect cells lacking the CD4 molecule.[73]

Early postentry events include uncoating of the virus, which appears to require interaction of viral structural proteins with host-cell components that may have been incorporated into the virion during viral assembly. In HIV-1, interaction of the viral capsid protein with the host-cell cyclophilin A that is associated with the virion core during viral assembly may destabilize the multimeric capsid complex.[323] Additionally, a virion-associated host-cell protein kinase phosphorylates the viral matrix protein and thereby allows dissociation of the capsid and nucleocapsid proteins from the rest of the virus at the cell membrane. The HIV-1 Vif protein, which co-localizes with the Gag-derived proteins, is thought to confer enhanced stability to the remaining cytoplasmic viral nucleoprotein complex.

Retroviral RNA-to-DNA transcriptional events are initiated in the cytoplasm through the action of the viral enzymes reverse transcriptase (RNA-directed DNA polymerase) and ribonuclease. Viral single-stranded RNA is transcribed into a viral RNA/DNA hybrid complex by the DNA polymerase; the ribonuclease then destroys the original RNA and permits the DNA polymerase to complete transcription of a second DNA strand to form a linear double-stranded DNA copy of the original viral RNA.[105] Retroviral integration is mediated by a large nucleoprotein complex that forms in the cytoplasm and is called the preintegration complex. This complex includes the viral nucleic acids and a subset of viral proteins, including the matrix protein, reverse transcriptase, integrase, and in the lentiviruses, Vpr.[323] The viral integrase enzyme component of this complex recognizes specific sequences within the viral LTR and cleaves two nucleotides from the 3′ ends as an initial processing step for integration; this process occurs while the pre-integration complex is still in the cytoplasm.[13] In the lentiviruses, which can infect nondividing cells, the pre-integration complex is imported actively into the nucleus during interphase. Nuclear transport is mediated by nuclear localization sequences on the matrix protein and on integrase and by interactions of Vpr with nucleoporins in the nuclear pore complex.

Once nuclear entry has been gained, the integrase joins the recessed 3′ ends to phosphates in the host DNA for insertion of the DNA duplex into the host genome.[13, 50] A final step in integration is thought to involve cellular factors involved in DNA repair, in particular, a DNA-dependent protein kinase. This kinase is hypothesized to repair gaps left by the integrase around the sequence inserted into the host DNA; the result is a fully integrated provirus.[50, 57]

EXPRESSION PHASE OF RETROVIRAL REPLICATION

Once viral DNA is integrated into the host cell, the proviral genome resembles other cellular genes and becomes highly dependent on the host cell for further replication, with the host cell machinery being used for replication, expression, and protein production. Regulation of transcription is a complex process requiring interaction among the integrated proviral LTRs, host-cell DNA transcription factors, and the lentiviral Tat protein or oncoviral Tax protein.

The early phase of viral gene expression is characterized by the presence of spliced and unspliced viral mRNA in the nucleus, but only multiply spliced mRNA in the cytoplasm. In HTLVs, these mRNA molecules serve to direct production of the Tax and Rex regulatory proteins; in HIVs, they direct production of the Tat, Rev, and Nef proteins. The transition from early regulatory to late structural gene expression is characterized by the selective transport of unspliced and partially spliced mRNA into the cytoplasm; as discussed previously, in lentiviruses this process is dependent on sufficient amounts of the Rev protein and, in oncoviruses, the Rex protein.[49, 338] The unspliced/partially spiced mRNA transcripts that enter the cytoplasm encode for structural proteins and are first expressed as large overlapping polyproteins. These polyproteins undergo processing into functional peptide viral structural components by the action of virally encoded and host-cell protease enzymes.

The retroviral Env protein is synthesized as a large precursor protein; it undergoes initial glycosylation in the endoplasmic reticulum, with subsequent disulfide bonding, folding, and oligomerization, and then is transported to the Golgi complex, where it is cleaved by a host-cell protease into surface and transmembrane proteins, which undergo further glycosylation.[60] The two mature glycoproteins are noncovalently associated via disulfide bonds. After cleavage occurs, the complexed proteins are transported and inserted into the plasma cell membrane via the cellular secretory pathway.[82]

The retroviral *gag* and *pol* genes are transcribed into a single mRNA transcript, which subsequently is translated into two separate polyprotein precursors, the Gag and Gag-Pol precursor proteins; the Gag-Pol polyprotein is translated via a ribosomal frame shift between the Gag and Pol mRNA reading frames. The Pol component of the Gag-Pol precursor protein is cleaved to form the viral enzymes reverse transcriptase, ribonuclease, and protease. The Gag precursor encodes the major structural proteins of the virion core, which do not undergo proteolytic processing into mature proteins until after assembly of the immature virion at the plasma membrane.

Virion assembly and budding occur through targeting, accumulation, and association of different domains of the Gag and Gag-Pol precursor proteins at the inner face of the plasma membrane where the envelope proteins are being expressed.[82, 83, 271, 345] The M domain, an amino acid sequence contained in the N-terminal area of the matrix portion of the Gag protein, has a membrane-targeting sequence that directs the Gag and Gag-Pol polyproteins to the cytoplasmic face of the plasma membrane. Myristylation of the N-terminal portion of some (lentiviruses) or all (oncoviruses) of the Gag precursor protein matrix domain is required for membrane targeting to occur and allow Gag protein assembly at the membrane. In lentiviruses, the matrix domain interacts with the long cytoplasmic tail of the viral envelope transmembrane protein inserted into the membrane of the cell.[83] The I domain, an amino acid sequence contained in the nucleocapsid portion of the Gag polyprotein, participates in the Gag-Gag interactions to promote protein polymerization and also appears to be required for incorporation of the Gag-Pol precursor into virions.[82] The nucleocapsid domain of the Gag polyprotein interacts with viral genomic RNA through specific (sequence-specific nucleic acid binding) and nonspecific (interaction of basic residues with RNA) mechanisms and plays an important role in RNA binding, dimerization, and encapsidation and in facilitating Gag protein interactions and packaging into tight complexes.[47, 82]

The interactions of these three domains in the precursor protein thus lead to assembly and emergence (but not release) of the viral "bud" from the cell surface.[256] On electron microscopy, large electron-dense patches of Gag multimers are visualized under the plasma membrane that deform the membrane outward as they grow. More advanced intermediates appear as spheres connected to the cell by a thin stalk. During the process of budding, substantial amounts of cellular surface antigens, such as β_2-microglobulin and HLA-DR, are incorporated into the viral envelope. Additionally, during the process of virion assembly, host-cell proteins may be incorporated into the virion. For example, in HIV-1, a host-cell protein, cyclophilin A, interacts with the Gag polyprotein to form a complex in the virion core.[81, 327] This host factor appears to be required for the formation of infectious virions, and it may play a role in early events after viral entry, as discussed earlier.[54, 323]

In addition to the capsid, nucleocapsid, and matrix protein domains, other polypeptide segments that are required during the late stages of viral assembly are contained in the Gag polyprotein. They are referred to collectively as "late assembly" or "L" domains, and they are found in both lentiviruses and oncoviruses. In lentiviruses, the C-terminal portion of Gag (p6) includes a highly conserved amino acid motif that is needed to recruit the cellular machinery required for efficient release of budding virus from the cell membrane.[256, 290, 306, 345] The Gag protein of oncoviruses also contains a late domain, although it is located in the N-terminal region of the protein.[306] Some investigators have suggested that these domains engage in interactions with host proteins at the plasma membrane that facilitate final release of the budding virus from the cell.

In HIV-1, the late domain is thought to interact with the cellular protein ubiquitin. Ubiquitin is a small protein present in cells that together with cellular proteasomes, is involved in collecting or destroying cellular proteins that are damaged or no longer needed; it exists in cells as a free molecule or is covalently attached to lysines in a variety of proteins. When a protein is linked to multiple ubiquitin molecules (polyubiquitination), the protein becomes targeted for degradation by cellular proteasomes. However, when a protein is linked to a single ubiquitin molecule (mono-ubiquitination), instead of degradation, protein function is modulated; for example, mono-ubiquitination of plasma membrane receptor proteins promotes internalization and down-regulation of the receptor through endocytosis in a nonproteolytic process that has some similarities to virus budding. After protein degradation, the ubiquitin molecule is recycled as a free molecule. HIV-1 particles have been shown to contain ubiquitin, predominantly as a free molecule, but 2 to 5 percent of the Gag-derived, "late assembly domain" protein p6 is mono-ubiquitinated.[306] One hypothesis is that the late domain of Gag contains an amino acid sequence that binds to residues on the ubiquitin ligase enzyme and thereby results in mono-ubiquitination of the Gag protein. The Gag-ubiquitin conjugate may then attract undefined cellular factors, perhaps those normally involved in endocytosis, that trigger release of the retrovirus from the cell membrane.[256] In the absence of the late domain, an infected cell becomes covered with virus that remains tethered to the plasma membrane by narrow stalks.

Maturation of the virion requires cleavage of the Gag precursor by the virally encoded protease and triggers structural changes that produce mature virions with the characteristic spherical oncoviral or cylindrical lentiviral capsid. The Gag polyprotein gives rise to the matrix protein, which lines the inner face of the viral membrane; the capsid protein, which forms a core shell surrounding the viral RNA genome and its associated proteins; and the nucleocapsid protein, which coats and condenses the RNA genome. This step occurs concomitantly with or immediately after the external budding process.

GENERAL METHODS OF DIAGNOSIS OF RETROVIRAL INFECTION

Detection of retroviral antibody has been the test most widely used to diagnose infection in older children and adults. However, because of transplacental passage of maternal antibody, antibody testing during infancy is not diagnostic of infection, and direct viral detection methods are necessary for making the diagnosis. In addition, during primary infection, a window period exists during which ongoing viral replication is detectable by virologic tests, but antibody tests will be negative or indeterminant because a detectable antibody response has not developed.

Antibody testing for retroviruses most frequently involves the use of an initial screening test followed by performance of a more specific confirmatory test. Initial screening generally involves the detection of viral antigens from disrupted whole virus or synthetic or recombinant viral antigens in an enzyme-linked immunosorbent assay (ELISA). A positive ELISA is confirmed by the more specific immunoblot (or Western blot), which measures the presence of antibodies to a number of virus-associated proteins, both structural and nonstructural. Viral antigens (from disrupted whole virus or synthetic or recombinant antigens) undergo electrophoresis through a polyacrylamide gel to separate the antigens by size. The separated antigens then are transferred to nitrocellulose paper, incubated with the patient's serum, and subsequently incubated with enzyme-linked antihuman antibody and chromogenic substrate, which results in visible bands where patient antibodies are bound by antigens. Analysis of band patterns permits more specific identification of the virus. Other techniques used to measure antibodies to retroviruses include indirect immunofluorescence (IFA), radioimmunoprecipitation assay (RIPA), and biologic assays for antibody to envelope glycoproteins (neutralization or syncytium inhibition assays).

Because of antigenic differences between HIV-1 and HIV-2, HIV-1 screening tests are not reliable for the detection of HIV-2. A commercial HIV-1/HIV-2 combination assay is available that has high sensitivity for detection of both viruses; a supplemental immunoblot assay is used to confirm the viral subtype.[40, 193] Serologic diagnosis of HTLV infection is similar to that of HIV and involves the use of a screening enzyme immunoassay (EIA) and confirmatory immunoblot or RIPA. However, these tests do not distinguish between antibodies directed at HTLV-I or HTLV-II.[42] In patients with positive serology, virologic detection tests have been used, such as proviral amplification by polymerase chain reaction (PCR) or viral isolation. Assays containing several synthetic peptides and recombinant proteins have been developed and appear to be capable of differentiating between HTLV-I and HTLV-II.[29, 275]

Direct detection of virus by culture is intensive, expensive, and time consuming, with several weeks often required for results. The ability to isolate HTLV and HIV is dependent on the patient's disease state, immune status, and viral load. The ability to culture retroviruses has been improved by co-cultivation of patient cells with human peripheral blood mononuclear cells that have been stimulated in vitro with mitogens (e.g., phytohemagglutinin) and growth factors (e.g., IL-2), as well as by removal of patient $CD8^+$ (suppressor) cells from the co-culture. In infants and children, the small volume of blood available for culture and the low virus load in some cases may render virus isolation challenging.

Other methods used for detecting virus include (1) antigen capture assays to detect free circulating viral antigens (e.g., p24 HIV-1 core antigen), (2) IFA and immunohistochemistry to detect viral antigens in tissue, (3) detection of viral nucleic acids by Southern blot analysis, (4) in situ hybridization or dot blots, (5) PCR to detect proviral DNA in leukocytes or tissue, and (6) assays to detect viral RNA in plasma or other fluids. DNA PCR can be used to quantitate virus and is highly sensitive because it is capable of amplifying tiny quantities of viral nucleic acids enzymatically to detectable levels with a system of specific nucleotide primers and probes. This technique can be modified to detect viral RNA by using reverse transcription to convert viral RNA to DNA and performing PCR on the DNA product or by using other techniques such as branched-chain amplification or nucleic acid sequence–based amplification.[34, 253, 303]

Oncoviruses: HTLV Types I and II

HTLV-I

HTLV-I was the first human retrovirus identified and was isolated initially from a patient with cutaneous T-cell lymphoma.[261] HTLV-I now is known to be the causative agent of malignancy (ATLL), neurologic disorders (HAM/TSP), infective dermatitis in children, and numerous other disorders that are possibly autoimmune in nature (Table 193–3).

Epidemiology

Evaluation of the global distribution of HTLV-I initially was complicated by the considerable antigenic similarity between HTLV-I and HTLV-II (≈60% homology in nucleotide sequences). The first ELISA and Western blot assays designed to detect HTLV were not able to discriminate

TABLE 193–3 ■ DISEASES ASSOCIATED WITH HUMAN T-LYMPHOTROPIC VIRUS TYPES I AND II

Strength of Association	Human T-Lymphotropic Virus Type I	Human T-Lymphotropic Virus Type II
Strong	Adult T-cell leukemia/lymphoma Myelopathy (HTLV-1-associated myelopathy/tropical spastic paraparesis) Infective dermatitis Uveitis Arthropathy Interstitial pneumonitis Immune deficiency with opportunistic infections	Neurologic disorders (spastic paraparesis/myelopathy to more widespread involvement of central nervous system)
Intermediate	Polymyositis Cutaneous lymphomata such as mycosis fungoides, Sézary syndrome Sjögren syndrome/sicca syndrome	$CD8^+$ cell cancers Immune deficiency with opportunistic infections
Weak	Renal failure B-cell leukemias Small cell lung cancer	

between the presence of antibodies to HTLV-I and those to HTLV-II; DNA PCR was required to distinguish type-specific proviral sequences. Thus, early epidemiologic studies often were unable to distinguish between HTLV-I and HTLV-II infection. Second-generation assays use synthetic type-specific peptides that enable differentiation between HTLV-I and HTLV-II antibodies.[29, 275] More recent studies have been better able to discriminate the epidemiologic distribution of the two viruses.

On a global basis, an estimated 15 to 25 million individuals are infected with HTLV-I. Based on genetic analysis, HTLV-I is classified into three major types.[204, 371] The Melanesian type, which was isolated from Melanesians in Papua New Guinea and the Solomon Islands in the South Pacific and from Australian aborigines, is the most divergent in that it exhibits only 93 percent sequence similarity in the envelope gene with other HTLV-I strains.[16, 372] The other two HTLV-I types exhibit 97 percent sequence similarity. The second distinct genetic type is found in central Africa. The third, the Cosmopolitan type, includes isolates from various areas, and it represents the majority of HTLV-I isolates. The Cosmopolitan group has been further divided into four subtypes based on LTR sequencing: Transcontinental (A), Japanese (B), West African (C), and North African (D). Subtype A, the most widespread, has been isolated from Japan, the Caribbean basin, South America, India, Iran, far-eastern Russia, and South Africa (hence the name "Transcontinental"). Subtypes B and C are more restricted geographically, with subtype B found primarily in Japan and rarely in India and subtype C found in West Africa and the Caribbean basin. Subtype D was identified more recently in Morocco, Algeria, and North Africa.

Because the genetic variability and intra-subtype genetic drift of HTLV-I are limited, the geographic distribution of viral types has been hypothesized to represent the anthropologic movement of virus-carrying populations over time.[371] Most HTLV-I isolates from the same ethnic group in different locations and from different groups inhabiting the same area have phylogenetic similarities. For example, in North and South America and the Caribbean, most HTLV-I isolates belong to subtype A and are thought to have originated from ancestral Mongoloids who migrated from Asia to the American continents. In addition to subtype A, subtype C has been identified in the Caribbean and may reflect forced migration of black slaves from West Africa to the New World. Two HTLV-I subtypes have been found in Japan, with subtype A being predominant in the northern and southern territories and subtype B more predominant in southwestern Japan, which has led to speculation that these differences reflect immigration of different populations to different areas of the Japanese archipelago.

HTLV-I is highly endemic in southwestern Japan, particularly on the islands of Kyushu, Shikoku, and Okinawa, where roughly 30 percent of the adult population is seropositive.[134, 368] Geographic clustering of HTLV-I infection in southwestern Japan is observed, and marked variation may be observed within small geographic areas; such microclustering has been speculated to be due to the limited interchange, particularly intermarriage, between neighboring communities in Japan.[368]

Regions of moderate HTLV-I endemicity include areas of the Caribbean, such as Jamaica, Trinidad, Barbados, and the West Indies, where seroprevalence rates range between 2 to 5 percent in black adults.[17, 186, 220, 353] Parts of Africa also appear to have large reservoirs of HTLV-I infection; possible endemic areas have been identified within Gabon, Chad, Nigeria, Cameroon, Guinea, Democratic Republic of Congo (formerly Zaire), and the Ivory Coast.[42, 65, 341] The seroprevalence rate in the African adult population is approximately 0.5 to 1 percent; however, the distribution of HTLV-I is not uniform and is characterized by clusters of high endemicity. Foci of HTLV-I infection also have been identified in Central and South America, including Panama, Brazil, Colombia, Venezuela, Surinam, Guyana, Ecuador, and Peru.[51, 220] HTLV-I seroprevalence rates in Brazilian blood donors range from 0.08 percent in the south to 1.8 percent in the northeast, although seroprevalence in specific populations such as Brazilian Indians has been as high as 38 percent.[51, 89, 198] The HTLV-I seroprevalence rate in pregnant women in northeastern Brazil was 0.84 percent.[25]

HTLV-I seroprevalence in low-risk populations in the United States and Europe is under 1 percent. Seroprevalence rates in blood donors in the United States in the year after initiation of blood screening were 0.016 to 0.021 percent. Females and blacks, Hispanics, and Asians were more likely to be seropositive than were males and whites.[38] During the same period, seropositivity in applicants for the U.S. Armed Forces was similarly relatively low, but twice that observed in blood donors, 0.41 per 1000.[276] Similar to the demographics observed for seropositive blood donors, the prevalence in black applicants was more than 30 times that in white applicants, and a disproportionate rate of seropositivity in female applicants was observed. Clusters of HTLV-I infection also have been reported in blacks in the southern and southeastern United States and in immigrants from HTLV-I–endemic areas.[64, 68, 133, 356] HTLV-I seroprevalence rates in blood donors in Europe have ranged between 0 and 0.02 percent.[328] In inner-city London, HTLV seroprevalence in pregnant women was 1.1 per 1000 women, with the highest prevalence noted in women from the Caribbean (17.0 per 1000) and western and central Africa (3.2 per 1000); in women born in nonendemic areas and who were not black Caribbean, seroprevalence was 0.06 to 0.12 per 1000.[3]

Factors that influence HTLV-I seropositivity are age, race, sex, and geography. In endemic areas, the prevalence in children is low but starts to increase during the teenage years; this age-related increase is more marked for females than males. By 40 to 50 years of age, women are significantly more likely to be infected than men are. This sex- and age-related pattern may be the result of more efficient male-to-female sexual transmission of HTLV-I among sexually active adults.[27, 318]

With the development of advanced immunoassays, differentiation of the epidemiology of HTLV-II and HTLV-I infection has been possible. In a study of 1.7 million blood donors in the United States, the prevalence of HTLV-I and HTLV-II infection was 9.1 and 22.3 per 100,000 donors, respectively.[225] Thus, approximately 30 percent of volunteer blood donors found to be HTLV-seropositive are infected with HTLV-I and 70 percent with HTLV-II.[150] HTLV-I seroprevalence was associated with older age; female sex; hepatitis C seropositivity; black, Hispanic, or Asian race/ethnicity; and birth outside the United States.[225] These data are consistent with HTLV-I infection in the United States in that it is concentrated primarily in persons born in or having sexual contact with persons from HTLV-I–endemic areas of Africa, the Caribbean, and Japan. In contrast, HTLV-II has been found primarily in injecting drug users and their sexual contacts.[150]

Modes of Transmission

HTLV-I does not replicate efficiently in vivo and is transmitted through infected T cells in breast milk, semen, and blood. Modes of HTLV-I transmission are similar to those of HIV-1: sexual contact, parenteral transmission through blood transfusion of a cellular blood product or through intravenous drug use, and perinatally, most often via breast milk. The efficiency of HTLV transmission appears to be significantly lower than that of HIV because HTLV is highly cell associated whereas HIV can be transmitted in a cell-free and cell-associated manner.

SEXUAL TRANSMISSION

Sexual transmission is a significant source of HTLV-I acquisition in adults. Male-to-female sexual transmission appears to be more efficient than female-to-male transmission.[368] In one study from Japan, the risk of transmission of HTLV-I from an infected husband to his wife over a 10-year period was 61 percent, whereas the risk of transmission from an infected wife to her husband was less than 1 percent.[145] Sexual transmission of HTLV-I from infected men to their wives in Japan increased with older age of the male partner and elevated HTLV-I antibody titer, thus suggesting that a longer duration of infection and an elevated viral load may be associated with increased transmissibility.[307]

Data from studies in the United States are consistent with the findings in Japan. Risk factors for male-to-female HTLV-I sexual transmission were examined in the Retrovirus Epidemiology Donation Study, which since 1988 has enrolled volunteer blood donors from five participating blood centers who have been found to be seropositive for HTLV. The proportion of female sexual partners of infected men who were infected themselves (38%) was nearly twice that of male partners of infected female donors (20%).[150] In addition, ratios of transmitter-to-nontransmitter couples were similar for HTLV-I and HTLV-II, thus suggesting similar transmission efficacy of the two viruses. HTLV-transmitting men had been in their sexual relationships longer (mean of 225 versus 122 months) and had higher proviral loads than nontransmitters did. Transmitting men also tended to have higher antibody titers against various viral proteins than nontransmitters did; in general, antibody titers correlated highly with viral load.

In Japan, rates of seropositivity also have been found to be higher in persons with a history of sexually transmitted diseases, which suggests that disruption of the genital mucosa or an increase in leukocytes in genital secretions and semen, or both, may increase the risk of transmission.[232] In studies from several different countries, HTLV-I prevalence has been found to be elevated in female sex workers[61, 101, 232, 363]; lack of consistent use of condoms, the duration of prostitution, older age, infection with *Chlamydia trachomatis* or syphilis, antibody to herpes simplex virus type 1, and concomitant HIV-1 infection were associated with elevated HTLV-I prevalence.[101, 232] An increased risk for HTLV-I seropositivity also has been observed in persons attending clinics that treat sexually transmitted diseases[77, 155, 232, 359]; in such clinics in the United States, HTLV seropositivity ranged from 0.18 to 2.0 percent.[155] Risk factors for the acquisition of HTLV-I infection by females included multiple sexual partners, bruising during sex, syphilis, and concomitant HIV infection, whereas for men, hepatitis B antigenemia, bruising during sex, older age at onset of sexual activity, married status, and an agricultural occupation were associated with an increased risk.[77]

Homosexual men in endemic areas have an increased risk of HTLV-I acquisition, presumably through anal intercourse. In Trinidad, HTLV-I seropositivity was sixfold higher in homosexual men than the general population, and in Baltimore, Maryland, male-to-male sexual activity was associated with an elevated risk of seropositivity in men seen in clinics for sexually transmitted diseases.[15, 359] The higher rate of HIV than HTLV infection in homosexual men in Trinidad is an indication of the higher efficiency of HIV transmission.

MOTHER-TO-CHILD TRANSMISSION

HTLV-I infection does not appear to interfere with the course of pregnancy and is not associated with congenital abnormalities.[25] However, mother-to-child transmission of HTLV-I is the major source of infection in children. Studies in Japan have shown that more than 90 percent of HTLV-I–seropositive children have mothers who are seropositive themselves; overall, 15 to 25 percent of children born to infected women become infected.[88, 123, 145, 336, 361] Transmission to the infant appears to occur predominantly postpartum, as reflected by infant seroconversion to seropositivity after the loss of passively transferred maternal antibodies. Depending on the study, 11 to 40 percent of breast-fed children of HTLV-I–infected women become infected versus 0 to

13 percent of bottle-fed children.[122, 124, 240, 319, 332, 361, 362, 375] Numerous variables are associated with a risk of HTLV-I transmission, including longer duration of breast-feeding, elevated maternal HTLV-I antibody titer, high maternal HTLV-I proviral load, presence of HTLV-I–bearing cells in breast milk, female gender of the child, older maternal age, long duration of membrane rupture (>4 hours), and lower maternal income.[121, 122, 124, 152, 188, 319, 336, 361, 362]

Substantial evidence supports the conclusion that most HTLV-I transmission occurs through breast-feeding.[123] HTLV-I antigen has been detected in the breast milk of seropositive mothers, and HTLV-I proviral DNA has been identified by PCR in mononuclear cells from the breast milk of HTLV-I carrier women.[156, 229] HTLV-I infection of milk cells may not be restricted to T lymphocytes. Breast-derived luminal epithelial cells, which are present in human milk during early and long-term lactation, can be persistently infected with HTLV-I and undergo transformation in vitro. These cells can transmit HTLV-I infection to epithelial cells in breast milk or the intestines or to T cells derived from milk or blood.[305] In a marmoset animal model, transmission of HTLV-I has been shown to occur by oral feeding of lymphocytes from the breast milk of HTLV-I–infected mothers.[157, 370] Lymphocyte-facilitated infection of gastrointestinal epithelial cells has been hypothesized to be the mechanism for transmission.[376]

The risk of transmission via breast milk is most likely multifactorial and involves the duration of exposure, the amount and activation level of the virus, and the presence of protective or enhancing specific and nonspecific immunity. The median time to infection in a Jamaican cohort was estimated to be 11.9 months.[88] A duration of breast-feeding longer than 6 months appears to be associated with at least a threefold increased risk of transmission.[319, 361, 362] In one study in Japan, no child who breast-fed for less than 6 months became infected, and in a study in Jamaica, children born to mothers with higher titers of HTLV-I antibody had a delayed time to seroconversion, thus suggesting that passive transfer of maternal HTLV-I antibody may affect transmission timing and risk.[188, 317, 319] In an experimental rabbit model, passive immunization with HTLV-I hyperimmunoglobulin prevented milk-borne transmission of HTLV-I.[285] However, in some studies, higher levels of maternal antibody were associated with a higher risk of transmission, presumably because higher antibody levels may reflect a higher viral load.[361] Current recommendations are to provide formula feeding for infants born to HTLV-I–seropositive women.[42, 122] However, in situations in which formula feeding is not possible, cessation of breast-feeding when the child reaches the age of 6 months, or earlier, may reduce the risk of transmission.[320]

Transmission may be possible, albeit infrequently, during the in utero or intrapartum period. Approximately 3 to 4 percent of infants born to carrier mothers are infected despite bottle feeding, which suggests that intrauterine or intrapartum transmission may occur, but with much lower efficiency than with transmission via breast milk.[122, 154, 317] The finding that the duration of membrane rupture is associated with HTLV-I transmission suggests that some percentage of transmission may occur intrapartum. HTLV-I has been shown to infect intestinal and cervical epithelial cell lines in vitro.[376, 377] Thus, theoretically, one possibility is that infected cells in maternal genital secretions are swallowed by the infant during passage through the birth canal and HTLV-I is transmitted to intestinal cells in the infant.

Restricted infection of human trophoblast cells by HTLV-I has been demonstrated in vitro.[177] However, in an in vitro study, infection of trophoblast cells with HTLV-I was found to induce apoptosis in placental villous cells, and in a study of placentas from HTLV-I–seropositive and HTLV-I–seronegative women, the number of apoptosis-positive cells was significantly higher in the placentas from seropositive women.[78, 86] Researchers hypothesized that apoptosis of HTLV-I–infected cells could lead to clearance of infected cells without further proliferation and spread of infection, thereby providing a defense mechanism against transplacental infection. HTLV-I has been identified in the cord blood and placentas from HTLV-I–positive mothers by antigen-detection tests and DNA PCR, although positive findings have not always correlated with the eventual infection status of the infant[85, 154, 283]; in one study, none of seven children with positive cord blood were found to be infected during 2 to 4 years of follow-up.[154]

Genetic susceptibility to HTLV-I infection was suggested in a large genetic epidemiologic survey in an HTLV-I–endemic population in French Guiana.[259] A segregation analysis was consistent with the presence of a yet-unidentified dominant major gene predisposing to HTLV-I infection, in addition to the expected familial correlations caused by sexual and perinatal HTLV-I transmission. Almost all HTLV-I–seropositive children younger than 10 years were predicted to be genetically predisposed to infection, whereas most HTLV-I–seropositive adults were sporadic cases.

PARENTERAL TRANSMISSION

Parenteral transmission by transfusion and intravenous drug use is well documented and appears to be the most efficient mode of transmission, with a 15 to 60 percent chance of infection in those receiving HTLV-I–infected cellular products.[246, 274] Comparative rates of transmission of HTLV-I, HTLV-II, and HIV-1 were evaluated retrospectively in a large repository of U.S. blood donor serum from the Transfusion Safety Study.[67] Consistent with a requirement for cell-cell contact for transmission of HTLV and in contrast to HIV-1, HTLV-I and HTLV-II transmission was observed only with the transfusion of cellular blood components. Infectivity appeared to decrease with an increasing period of blood storage; no apparent transmission occurred after the transfusion of components stored more than 10 days, which suggests that the known decrease in the ability of donor lymphocytes to be activated or proliferate with storage renders the cells noninfectious. In this study, rates of transfusion-related transmission of HTLV-I and HTLV-II were similar, with approximately 27 percent of recipients of blood components from seropositive donors becoming infected. In contrast, 89 percent of the recipients of HIV-1–positive blood became infected, regardless of the blood product component type, and no effect of storage on transmission risk was seen. The median time to seroconversion after the transfusion of HTLV-I–contaminated blood products is 51 days.[45]

In a study of HTLV-infected blood donors, both HTLV-I and HTLV-II infection was associated with low educational attainment, accidental needle-sticks or cuts, previous blood transfusion, seven or more sexual partners, and a sexual partner from an HTLV-I–endemic area.[289] However, injection drug use or sex with injecting drug users was associated with HTLV-II only and not HTLV-I infection.

Screening of blood donors in the United States since 1988, as well as in other countries such as Japan, has reduced transfusion-related transmission markedly. However, in countries in which HTLV-I and HTLV-II screening of blood is not performed, transfusions provide an important source of infection. In a study of hospitalized children in Gabon in Africa, multiple blood transfusions secondary to complications of sickle-cell disease were as predominant a mode of HTLV-I transmission as perinatal transmission was.[62] Similarly, in Martinique, HTLV-I seroprevalence in patients with sickle-cell anemia was 10 percent versus 1 to 3 percent in normal blood donors, and HTLV-I–seropositive patients had received more transfusions than seronegative persons did.[284]

Descriptive studies have suggested that ecologic factors may influence the rate of seropositivity in a population; for example, residence in a lower-altitude, tropical environment was associated with higher rates of seropositivity in some reports.[186, 201] A role for insect vectors, such as mosquitoes, was postulated. However, no evidence has shown that retroviruses can replicate in arthropods, and any hypothesized insect-borne transmission would need to occur mechanically via the mouth parts of biting insects that were contaminated with a significant amount of infected and infectious lymphocytes; such transmission, if it occurs, would be expected to be very unusual.[80] Additionally, the prevalence of antibodies to arboviruses was not significantly greater in HTLV-seropositive than HTLV-seronegative persons.[218]

Disease Associations

After infection with HTLV-I, most infected individuals remain clinically asymptomatic for life. However, persistent viral infection and antigen production elicit a strong humoral and cellular immune response in infected individuals that results in high antibody titers to HTLV-I structural and regulatory proteins and increased circulating activated HTLV-I Tax protein–specific cytotoxic T lymphocytes.[55, 137] Additionally, even in asymptomatic patients, spontaneous in vitro proliferation of lymphocytes is observed.[160]

Early in the course of primary infection, the HTLV-I proviral load is high but becomes rapidly controlled. Within 90 days of primary infection, a narrow range of proviral load is observed in an individual, which generally stays relatively constant over time.[191, 245, 325] Antibody titer is highly correlated with proviral load after the initial set-point is reached. The HTLV-I proviral load in asymptomatic HTLV-I carriers can be as high as 5 percent of all peripheral blood mononuclear cells, and it is particularly high in individuals with HAM/TSP, in whom as many as 20 percent of peripheral blood mononuclear cells can be infected.[191, 214] A high peripheral blood proviral load appears to predate the development of neurologic and ophthalmologic HTLV-I–associated disease entities.

In adults, the diseases associated with HTLV-I infection are malignancies and chronic degenerative neurologic syndromes. Pediatric manifestations of HTLV-I infection have been identified, and researchers now recognize that exposure to HTLV-I early in life may be critical in the development of HTLV-I–associated diseases in adulthood, years to decades later. HTLV-I may be a prototype for other retroviruses yet to be discovered that predispose to the development of active diseases with long latency after exposure at birth or early in life.

Adult T-Cell Leukemia and Other Malignancies

ATLL was the first clinical disease to be linked with HTLV-I infection. This aggressive form of leukemia/lymphoma first was described in Japan in 1977, before the discovery of HTLV-I. Although an infectious etiology was postulated because of geographic clustering of ATLL in southern Japan, only after the discovery of HTLV-I in 1980 was a causal link established between HTLV-I seropositivity and ATLL.[261] ATLL is the most common form of leukemia in Japan, with approximately 700 new cases diagnosed yearly.[315, 316]

ATLL is found primarily in HTLV-I–endemic areas or in migrants from such areas. The incidence of ATLL in the United States is low, with cases seen primarily in immigrants from HTLV-I–endemic areas or in blacks in the southeastern United States, in whom endemic HTLV-I infection has been documented.[270] In a study in central Brooklyn, which has a large Caribbean migrant population, the annual incidence of ATLL in African Americans was approximately 3.1 per 100,000 person-years.[171]

ATLL occurs more commonly in females in Africa and the Caribbean but more commonly in males in Japan (male-to-female ratio of 1.4:1).[126, 257] The mean age at onset is between 40 and 60 years; however, the average age at onset of ATLL is somewhat lower in patients from the Caribbean and Africa (43 years) than in those from Japan (58 years).[368] The disease very rarely occurs in children. The incubation period for ATLL appears to be 20 to 30 years or longer after infection with HTLV-I, and researchers have postulated that ATLL results from HTLV-I infection acquired during the first few years of life.[224] The lifetime risk for development of ATLL is estimated to be 2 to 5 percent in individuals infected before the age of 20 years.[42, 190, 217]

During the long latent period of HTLV-I infection, most infected individuals show polyclonal proliferation of cells harboring integrated HTLV-I provirus. Asymptomatic HTLV-I carriers may experience a pre-ATLL state associated with mild leukocytosis or the presence of abnormal lymphocytes with characteristic lobulated nuclei ("flower cells") that are found to have monoclonal or oligoclonal HTLV-I provirus integrated into the cell genome. More than 50 percent of such persons will experience resolution of the leukocytosis spontaneously. Why ATLL will develop in only a small percentage of HTLV-I–infected individuals is not clear. Because malignant transformation is probably a multistep process, intermediate factors such as the host immune response or oncogenic environmental stimuli, or both, may be involved.[134] Diagnostic criteria for ATLL[299] are shown in Table 193–4.

Clinical manifestations of ATLL include lymphadenopathy in 50 to 80 percent of patients and hepatosplenomegaly in 25 to 67 percent (Table 193–5). Skin lesions, which occur in 40 to 60 percent of patients, include large nodules, plaques, ulcers, a generalized papular rash appearing on the limbs, trunk, or face, or any combination of these lesions. An elevated white blood cell count ranging from 10,000 to 300,000/mm^3 occurs in approximately two thirds of patients, and abnormal T lymphocytes ("flower cells") containing lobulated nuclei may be seen. Hypercalcemia occurs in 32 to 63 percent of patients. In patients with hypercalcemia, ATLL cells have been found to secrete excessive amounts of parathyroid hormone–related peptide, probably because of Tax-mediated transactivation of the gene for this protein.[71] Osteolytic bone lesions occur in 2.5 to 10 percent. The CNS, which is affected in 2.5 to 10 percent of patients, can act as a sanctuary and has been found to be an important site

TABLE 193–4 ■ REQUIREMENTS FOR DIAGNOSIS OF ADULT T-CELL LEUKEMIA/LYMPHOMA

1. HTLV-I seropositivity
2. Histologic or cytologic proven lymphoid malignancy with T-cell surface antigens present
3. Abnormal T lymphocytes ("flower cells") consistently present in peripheral blood (except for the lymphoma subtype of ATLL)
4. Demonstration of clonality of proviral DNA as well as clonal integration of proviral DNA

TABLE 193–5 ■ CLINICAL FINDINGS IN ADULT T-CELL LEUKEMIA/LYMPHOMA

Median age of onset	40–60 yr
Gender	Caribbean, Africa: females > males Japan: males slightly > females (1.4:1)
Clinical/laboratory findings	
Generalized lymphadenopathy	50–80%
Hepatosplenomegaly	25–67%
Skin involvement	40–60%
Elevated white cell count	60–66%
Hypercalcemia	32–63%
Pulmonary involvement	14%
Lytic bone lesions	2–10%
Central nervous system involvement	2–10%

for relapse when chemotherapy is given to treat ATLL.[257] Opportunistic infections occur commonly because of the defective T-cell–mediated immunity observed in ATLL and are a primary cause of mortality. In patients with preexisting infestation with the roundworm *Strongyloides stercoralis,* a hyperinfection syndrome accompanied by gram-negative sepsis may occur and has a mortality rate of over 70 percent. Other common opportunistic infections include bacterial infections, *Pneumocystis* pneumonia, and serious fungal infections. Findings indicative of poor survival include age older than 40 years, increased tumor bulk, poor performance status, high lactate dehydrogenase level, hypercalcemia, and the presence of clones of cells containing multiple or defective copies of the HTLV-I provirus.[180, 272]

Clinical and laboratory criteria have been used to differentiate ATLL into four subtypes: acute, chronic, lymphoma, and smoldering[42, 257, 299, 368] (Table 193–6). The distribution of clinical ATLL subtypes varies geographically. In Japan, most cases are acute ATLL with leukemic manifestations; however, in the Caribbean, most cases are initially of the lymphoma subtype.[171, 172] Acute ATLL is the rapidly aggressive form of leukemia/lymphoma that first was recognized in Japan. It is the most common subtype and has the shortest survival time. Clinical findings include a characteristic cutaneous involvement in 40 percent of patients that ranges from a maculopapular rash to tumorous lesions; leukemia with circulating abnormal lymphocytes; generalized lymphadenopathy, hepatomegaly, splenomegaly, or any combination of these conditions; lytic bone lesions; hypercalcemia; and immunodeficiency leading to opportunistic infections. Chronic and lymphoma-type ATLL each are seen in approximately a fifth of ATLL patients. Chronic ATLL has a more indolent clinical course than acute ATLL does, with a median survival of approximately 24 months. Chronic ATLL overlaps with cases of T-cell chronic lymphocytic leukemia and is associated with moderate leukocytosis, with 0.5 to 3 percent of circulating cells being malignant. Cutaneous manifestations may be observed, but nodal or extranodal involvement occurs rarely and hypercalcemia is absent. Lymphoma-type ATLL has a median survival of approximately 10 months and overlaps with T-cell non-Hodgkin lymphoma, with prominent lymphadenopathy and the presence of monoclonally integrated HTLV-I in the malignant cells and little to no peripheral blood involvement. Smoldering ATLL occurs least commonly, in approximately 5 percent of patients, and is relatively indolent. It is characterized by abnormal cells in the absence of leukocytosis and resembles mycosis fungoides, with slow progression, cutaneous involvement manifested as erythema or infiltrative plaques or tumors, and mild lymphadenopathy or splenomegaly, or both.

The pathogenesis of ATLL is not known. The typical phenotype of ATLL cells is $CD3^+$, $CD4^+$, $CD8^-$, and $CD25^+$ (IL-2 receptor–positive). Monoclonal HTLV-I provirus is found integrated into the DNA of ATLL malignant cells. HTLV-I is known to transform normal CD4 lymphocytes in vitro and result in immortalization, high levels of IL-2 expression, and increased expression of the IL-2 alpha-chain receptor on the cell surface. The presence of excessive receptors for IL-2, a known growth factor for T cells, may be linked to development of the proliferative leukemic process of ATLL.[368] Additionally, the HTLV-I Tax protein activates the promoters of many genes involved in cell growth and differentiation and interferes with DNA repair functions.[215] One hypothesis is that the continuous proliferation observed in HTLV-I–infected cells may render them more susceptible to spontaneous mutagenesis, as well as to the effect of external

TABLE 193–6 ■ CLINICAL SUBTYPES OF ADULT T-CELL LEUKEMIA/LYMPHOMA: CLINICAL AND LABORATORY FINDINGS

	Adult T-Cell Leukemia/Lymphoma Clinical Subtype			
	Acute	Chronic	Lymphoma	Smoldering
Percentage with subtype	57%	19%	19%	5%
Survival				
Median	6 mo	24 mo	10 mo	> 24 mo
Four-year rate	5%	27%	6%	63%
Clinical Findings				
Lymphadenopathy	+/–	+/–	Yes	No
Hepatomegaly/splenomegaly	+/–	+/–	+/–	No
Skin involvement	+/–	+/–	+/–	+/–
Bone lesions	+/–	No	+/–	No
Bone marrow involvement	+/–	No	+/–	No
Laboratory Findings				
Absolute lymphocyte count ($\times 10^9$)	≥4	≥4	<4	<4
Abnormal circulating lymphocytes	≥5%	≥5%	≤1%	≥5%*
Polylobated lymphocytes (flower cells)	Yes	Occasional	No	Occasional
Calcium	Normal or elevated	Normal	Normal or elevated	Normal
Lactate dehydrogenase	Normal or elevated	<2 times normal	Normal or elevated	<1.5 times normal

*If less than 5% of circulating abnormal lymphocytes are present in the smoldering ATLL subtype, at least one histologically proven lesion from the lungs or skin should be present.

carcinogens.[1] Although *tax* does not directly transform cells and has no homology to known proto-oncogenes, the finding that persistent clonal expansion of HTLV-I–infected cells precedes the development of ATLL suggests that tumor cells may originate in clonally expanding nonmalignant cells through a multistep process that may include the acquisition of mutations in genes such as *p53* or *p16*.

The host immune response also may be involved in malignant transformation. An association between progression to ATLL and HTLV-I antibody titer has been reported. In a study of 5 cases of ATLL and 38 matched HTLV-I–infected controls without ATLL, researchers found a 1.6-fold increase in the risk of ATLL with every 2-fold increase in HTLV-I antibody titer.[125] However, despite having higher HTLV-I antibody levels, all patients with ATLL had low or undetectable levels of HTLV-I anti-Tax antibody for up to 10 years preceding the diagnosis of ATLL when compared with HTLV-I carriers without ATLL. Malignant ATLL cells are also less likely to express detectable levels of Tax mRNA and more likely to have partial deletion of the HTLV-I genome. The Tax protein is the major target of cytotoxic T cells in HTLV-I infection, and suppression or defective expression of the Tax protein on the surface of infected cells may permit escape from immune-mediated cell lysis.[125] Indeed, HTLV-I–infected patients with ATLL have poorly detectable Tax-specific cytotoxic T-cell activity,[148, 244] which could permit more unrestrained proliferation of infected cells and lead to increased HTLV-I viral load, higher HTLV-I antibody levels to non-Tax viral proteins, and eventually, malignant transformation.

Treatment regimens for ATLL remain unsatisfactory, with high rates of relapse. Combination chemotherapy with cytotoxic agents results in a complete response in 20 to 45 percent of individuals, but the duration of the response is short, generally lasting only a few months.[257, 314] The combination of zidovudine and interferon-α has been shown to be active in the treatment of ATLL, even in patients in whom conventional multiagent chemotherapy has failed.[99, 119] Because viral replication is not required for malignant transformation to ATLL and the level of viral replication during the leukemic phase of ATLL is barely detectable, clinical response is not likely to be due directly to an antiretroviral effect of these drugs. Zidovudine produces cytostatic effects through termination of DNA replication and may exert direct antitumor effects; this agent has been shown to block HTLV-I–induced cell transformation in vitro. Interferon-α has multiple biologic effects, including an antiproliferative effect through inhibition of protein synthesis and cell growth, and it also may enhance immune recognition of tumor cells by inducing the expression of MHC molecules on the tumor cell surface. However, although survival is prolonged, this therapy is not curative, and relapse occurs. Novel treatments are being investigated. ATLL cells are known to overexpress IL-2 receptor on their surface. Therefore, immunotherapy with toxin-conjugated monoclonal antibodies to the alpha chain of the IL-2 receptor has been studied in clinical trials, with remissions lasting from 9 weeks to 3 years.[348–350] Topoisomerase inhibitors and retinoids also have been evaluated.[257] In vitro, ATLL cells are susceptible to lysis by Tax-specific cytotoxic T cells, which has led to the hypothesis that stimulation of cellular immunity to Tax might inhibit tumor growth.[148, 244] In a rat model, the use of an HTLV-I Tax-directed DNA vaccine induced cytotoxic T-cell activity against Tax-expressing cells, and adoptive transfer of these cells effectively suppressed in vivo growth of HTLV-I–transformed tumor cells.[244]

Other malignancies have been associated with HTLV-I infection, although the supporting evidence for these associations is less clear than that for ATLL. Cutaneous T-cell lymphomata, such as mycosis fungoides and Sézary syndrome, have been described in adults and a child with HTLV-I infection.[17, 108, 347, 380] In one small study of eight patients with Sézary syndrome, HTLV-I mRNA expression was found in four patients.[98] Multiple myeloma and B-cell chronic lymphocytic leukemia also have been described in HTLV-I–infected patients. These malignancies may arise as a result of chronic antigenic stimulation of B cells by HTLV-I–infected T cells, with such stimulation leading to uncontrolled B-cell expansion. In the Caribbean, HTLV-I has been associated with the development of T-cell non-Hodgkin lymphoma.[189] A single case of small cell cancer of the lung with monoclonally integrated HTLV-I in the tumor has been reported. A pulmonary infiltrative syndrome resembling lymphoid pulmonary hyperplasia seen in HIV-1–infected children has been reported in patients with HTLV-I–associated myelopathy.[309]

HTLV-I–Associated Myelopathy

In the 1880s, a "multiple neuritis" syndrome consisting of a predominantly ataxic motor neuropathy was reported in Jamaica. In subsequent years, similar syndromes of unknown etiology were described in other geographic locales and given different names, including "Strachan disease," "central neuritis," "Jamaican neuropathy," "tropical spastic paraplegia," and "tropical spastic paraparesis."[381] The identification of HTLV-I in 1980, the development of antibody tests to diagnose HTLV-I infection, and the recognition that HTLV-I and TSP were endemic in the same geographic locations led to the hypothesis that these entities might be associated. In 1985, Gessain and colleagues performed a case-control study in Martinique in which patients with TSP of unknown cause were compared with a control group of nurses and blood donors without neurologic disease. Sixty percent of the TSP patients versus only 4 percent of controls had HTLV-I serum antibodies detected.[85, 95] In the same year, a report was published on the detection of HTLV-I antibodies in the cerebrospinal fluid (CSF) and serum of individuals afflicted with TSP.[278] In 1986, a series of Japanese patients with a similar clinical syndrome who also had HTLV-I antibodies in their CSF were described, and these investigators proposed that the syndrome be called "HTLV-I–associated myelopathy."[249] At a 1988 meeting of the World Health Organization's Scientific Group on HTLV-I Infections and Its Associated Disease, researchers proposed that HAM and HTLV-I–associated TSP were clinically and pathologically identical and recommended that it be known by the acronym HAM/TSP.[367]

The disease usually occurs in HTLV-I–endemic areas, including the Caribbean, southern Japan, equatorial Africa, Central and South America, Melanesia, and southern Africa.[97] Sporadic cases have been described in nonendemic areas, usually in immigrants from endemic areas or their sexual contacts or in recipients of blood transfusions (before HTLV blood screening). Incidence and prevalence estimates are unreliable because of the insidious nature of the disease and the lack of recognition of early symptoms by clinicians. In HTLV-I–seropositive persons in Japan, the incidence of HAM/TSP is 3.1 per 100,000 HTLV-I–infected persons per year.[97] In contrast, the annual incidence of HAM/TSP in HTLV-I–infected persons in Jamaica and Trinidad was 22.1 per 100,000 persons.[184] This difference in incidence is hypothesized to reflect an association between the time that HTLV-I infection is acquired and the type of disease manifestation that occurs. In the Caribbean, most HTLV-I infection is acquired sexually during adult life, and HAM/TSP is the most common clinical manifestation of the disease; in contrast, in Japan, most infection is acquired by maternal-to-child transmission during infancy, and ATLL is the most common disease manifestation. Case reports of HAM/TSP occurring after blood transfusion and the finding in Japan and Martinique that 13 to 20 percent of HAM/TSP cases had a history of blood transfusion accelerated the decision of blood banks in the United States to screen for HTLV-I antibodies. In Japan, a 16 percent decrease in the number of HAM/TSP cases occurred in the 2 years after initiation of blood screening.[90, 248]

Although the mean onset of disease is in the fourth decade of life, incubation of this disease appears to be shorter than that of ATLL. In patients with HTLV-I infection acquired by transfusion in whom HAM/TSP subsequently developed, the median time to development of symptoms after receiving a transfusion was 3.3 years, and in one report, HAM/TSP occurred 18 weeks after blood transfusion.[102, 248] Onset of symptoms is uncommon in persons younger than 20 or older than 70 years. However, HAM/TSP has been reported in a child as young as 6 years after the development of transfusion-acquired HTLV-I infection.[248] The rate of HAM/TSP increases with age from 20 through 50 years of age and then declines.[184] The lifetime risk of HAM/TSP developing in an HTLV-I–infected person is estimated to be 1.9 percent overall, with a slightly higher incidence in women (1.8%) than men (1.3%).[184]

The clinical features of HAM/TSP include chronic progressive spastic paraparesis and weakness of the limbs, particularly the legs, which results in an insidious onset of gait disturbance (Table 193–7). Mild sensory loss and painful paresthesias may develop and result in complaints of extremity numbness or dysesthesia and low back pain. Bowel and bladder sphincter impairment may occur and cause constipation, urinary frequency/incontinence, and impotence. Neurologic examination shows hyperactive deep tendon reflexes, clonus, extensor plantar reflexes, proximal muscle wasting, and a spastic paraparesis with a slow, scissoring gait; mild sensory changes may be observed. Cognitive function and the cranial nerves usually are spared. Systemic non-neurologic symptoms suggestive of an autoimmune process, such as pulmonary alveolitis, uveitis, arthropathy, Sjögren syndrome, and vasculitis, also may be noted.[134, 135, 309] Progression is variable; 10 years after onset, 30 percent of patients are bedridden and 45 percent require crutches to walk.[97]

Nonspecific lesions of the brain are observed with magnetic resonance imaging in as many as 75 percent of patients, but no clear correlation has been established between the lesions and symptoms. Atrophy of the spinal cord may occur, usually in the thoracic region. Multiple foci of increased T2 signal intensity are found in the periventricular white matter, similar to the findings observed in patients with multiple sclerosis. However, cognitive impairment may be noted in multiple sclerosis but is not found in HAM/TSP, and HTLV-I sequences have not been detected in the peripheral blood or CNS of multiple sclerosis patients.[247]

High HTLV-I antibody levels are found in both peripheral blood and CSF. In CSF, a mild to moderate pleocytosis, increased protein, or oligoclonal immunoglobulin bands (or any combination of these findings) may be observed. Elevated CSF neopterin, an indicator of cellular immune activation, may be present. In approximately 50 percent of patients, atypical "flower" lymphocytes are observed and account for approximately 1 to 15 percent of peripheral blood lymphocytes; these cells also may be seen in CSF.[135] Unlike the monoclonal integration observed in ATLL, polyclonal integration of HTLV-I is noted in cells from patients with HAM/TSP.[97]

TABLE 193–7 ■ CLINICAL FINDINGS IN HUMAN T-LYMPHOTROPIC VIRUS TYPE I-ASSOCIATED MYELOPATHY/TROPICAL SPASTIC PARAPARESIS

Incidence	Primarily sporadic and occurring in adults, rare in childhood; female preponderance (2:1)
Onset	Usually insidious, rarely abrupt
Main neurologic findings	Chronic spastic paraparesis, slowly progressive
	Leg weakness, more marked proximally
	Bladder disturbance with urinary incontinence usually early, constipation later; impotence or decreased libido
	Paresthesias (tingling, pins/needles, burning) more prominent than objective physical signs
	Low lumbar pain with radiation to legs
	Impaired vibration sense, proprioception less often
	Hyperreflexia of lower limbs, often with clonus and Babinski signs
	Hyperreflexia of upper limbs; weakness may be absent
	Exaggerated jaw jerk in some patients
	Normal cognitive function
Less frequent neurologic findings	Cerebellar signs, optic atrophy, deafness,nystagmus, other cranial nerve deficits, hand tremor, absent or depressed ankle jerk
	Rarely, convulsions, cognitive impairment, dementia, impaired consciousness
Other possible neurologic findings	Muscular atrophy, fasciculation (rare), polymyositis, peripheral neuropathy, polyradiculopathy, cranial neuropathy, meningitis, encephalopathy
Possible systemic non-neurologic findings	Pulmonary alveolitis, uveitis, Sjögren syndrome, arthropathy, vasculitis, ichthyoses, cryoglobulinemia, monoclonal gammopathy, adult T-cell leukemia or lymphoma
Laboratory diagnosis	Detection of HTLV-I antibodies or antigens and/or viral isolation in blood and CSF
	Mild lymphocytic pleocytosis in CSF
	Lobulated lymphocytes in blood or CSF
	Mild to moderate increase in protein in CSF

CSF, cerebrospinal fluid.

Pathologically, HAM/TSP is characterized by perivascular demyelination and neuronal lesions. Macroscopic atrophy of the spinal cord occurs, with changes consistent with a chronic inflammatory process characterized by perivascular cuffing of mononuclear cells and lymphocytic infiltration of the brain and spinal cord. Early in the disease, these lymphocytes consist of both $CD8^+$ and $CD4^+$ T cells, along with B lymphocytes and macrophages in areas of parenchymal damage.[139] HTLV-I proviral DNA can be demonstrated in $CD4^+$ cells in the infiltrates by in situ PCR. Evidence suggests that these HTLV-I–infected cells migrate from the peripheral blood and cross the blood-brain barrier to enter the nervous system.[37] Later in the disease, the inflammatory cells are fewer in number and consist primarily of CD8+ cytotoxic T cells. Marked myelin and axonal destruction and astrocytic gliosis are prominent. The lower thoracic cord is particularly affected, and parenchymal damage of both white and gray matter of the cord may be present. In the brain, although perivascular mononuclear cell infiltration may be seen, parenchymal damage is an unusual finding. However, rare patients may have white matter lesions, cerebellar symptoms, amyotrophic lateral sclerosis–like symptoms, or neuropathy.[135]

The pathogenesis of HAM/TSP is not known. An increased HTLV-I viral load and an augmented humoral and cellular immune response to HTLV-I are reported in patients with HAM/TSP. When compared with asymptomatic HTLV-I–seropositive individuals or those with ATLL, patients with HAM/TSP have higher HTLV-I antibody titers, a higher proviral load, and elevated levels of spontaneous lymphocyte proliferation and proinflammatory cytokines, including IL-1, interferon-α, and tumor necrosis factor–α.[191, 227, 228] HTLV-I–specific CD8+ cytotoxic T cells can be found in the CSF as well as peripheral blood of patients with HAM/TSP, and a significant reduction in the naive T-cell population occurs with a concomitant increase in the memory/effector CD8+ cell population.[140, 141, 227] Examination of the T-cell receptor repertoire shows significant expansion of the CD8+ T-cell population in patients with HAM/TSP as opposed to asymptomatic carriers. Many of these CD8+ cells correspond to cytotoxic T lymphocytes directed against epitopes of the immunodominant Tax protein of HTLV-I.[337]

One postulated mechanism for nervous system damage is direct infection of CNS glial cells by HTLV-I; a direct cytotoxic immune response to the glial cell is generated and results in demyelination.[134] However, HTLV-I expression appears to be localized to infiltrating CD4+ lymphocytes within the spinal cord lesions rather than nervous system parenchymal cells, and no clear evidence has established that HTLV-I infects CNS cells.[230] Alternatively, the heightened HTLV-I–specific immune response in patients with HAM/TSP and neuropathologic findings suggests that immune-mediated mechanisms may have a role in the pathogenesis of disease.[170] The activated HTLV-I–specific cytotoxic CD8+ T cells observed in patients with HAM/TSP could secrete cytokines that might induce demyelination as well as increase the transmigration of additional HTLV-I–infected lymphocytes to the inflammatory lesion.[134, 227, 230]

Specific characteristics of the virus also may influence disease manifestations. In one study, a specific *tax* gene phylogenetic subgroup, *tax* A, was found to occur more commonly in patients with HAM/TSP than in healthy HTLV-I carriers, thus suggesting that functional or immunogenic differences in the transactivating Tax protein among HTLV-I viral types may play a role in causing disease.[87] Another hypothesized mechanism is more indirect and involves HTLV-I–associated activation of autoreactive cells, which could lead to an autoimmune process that induces myelin destruction. The finding that numerous autoimmune-like diseases may occur in HTLV-I–infected patients and may coexist with HAM/TSP is consistent with the latter hypothesis.[135] A genetic susceptibility to the development of HAM/TSP also may exist. HTLV-I–infected patients with the class I allele HLA-A*02 had a proviral load one third less than that of HTLV-I carriers who lack this allele, and they had half the odds for development of HAM/TSP.[143] Because the risk for HAM/TSP is related to proviral load, this relationship may be due to a more efficient antiviral cellular immune response in individuals with a particular class I HLA allele.

Similar to ATLL, no curative treatment has been developed. However, prolonged survival may be seen. Mean survival after the onset of symptoms is 10 years, and the major causes of death are infection and cancer.[335] Symptomatic treatment includes measures to maintain muscle function and reduce spasticity. Treatment with systemic or intrathecal corticosteroids may induce a transient benefit in approximately 50 percent of patients, particularly those with early-stage disease, and zidovudine alone or combined with interferon-α therapy has shown some promise.[103, 113, 134]

HTLV-I–Associated Uveitis

An idiopathic, noninfectious uveitis has been reported to occur in HTLV-I–seropositive individuals, usually those who otherwise are asymptomatic.[205, 206, 231, 298] In endemic areas in Japan, 38 percent of patients with idiopathic uveitis were infected with HTLV-I as compared with 19 percent of patients with nonuveitic ocular disease and 10 percent with uveitis of known etiology.[207] In the younger age group (20 to 49 years) with idiopathic uveitis, HTLV-I seroprevalence was 49 percent. Similarly, in Brazil, an area of lower HTLV-I endemicity, HTLV-I seroprevalence also was elevated in patients with idiopathic uveitis; 1.8 percent of patients with idiopathic uveitis were HTLV-I–seropositive versus none of those with uveitis of known etiology.[369] In a survey of 105 asymptomatic Brazilian HTLV-I carriers, uveitis was found in 2.8 percent of infected persons. In epidemiologic surveys in Japan, the prevalence rate of HTLV-I–associated uveitis in HTLV-1 carriers was lower, estimated to be approximately 0.1 percent.[369] The mean age at onset in a series of Japanese patients was 43 years in men and 48 years in women.[207] As noted for HAM/TSP, genetic factors also may be associated with a susceptibility to or the severity of HTLV-I–associated uveitis.[293]

The syndrome is characterized by the abrupt onset of blurred vision, foggy vision, floaters, or any combination of these findings. The predominant finding on ocular examination is an intermediate uveitis with infiltrating cells and lacework-like membranous vitreous opacities. Approximately 14 percent of patients have panuveitis with uveoretinal lesions and mild retinal vasculitis, and 5 percent have iritis alone.[207] The uveitis is generally mild to moderate, and visual acuity is affected only slightly in most patients. Uveitis is unilateral in 57 percent and bilateral in 43 percent. The disease usually responds to topical or systemic steroids within a few weeks, although recurrence may be seen in 25 to 50 percent of cases within 2 months to 2 years after therapy is discontinued.[207, 231] Many patients (≈20%) had hyperthyroidism (Graves disease) that preceded or followed the onset of uveitis. A study of 105 asymptomatic Brazilian HTLV-I–seropositive adults found abnormal results in at least one lacrimal film evaluation test in 40 percent versus 23 percent of uninfected controls,[369] thus suggesting that abnormal early ocular abnormalities may be present in asymptomatic HTLV-1 carriers.

HTLV-I antibody has been detected in the aqueous humor of patients with HTLV-I uveitis.[207] Additionally, proviral HTLV-I DNA has been demonstrated in T cells found in the intraocular fluid of 59 percent or more Japanese patients with HTLV-I uveitis. Production of cytokine by HTLV-I–infected T cells is hypothesized to be the cause of the intraocular inflammation.[207, 282, 335] Significant amounts of cytokines, including tumor necrosis factor–α, are produced by HTLV-I–infected T-cell clones that have been established from the ocular fluid of patients with HTLV-I–associated uveitis and by the retinal glial cells of rats experimentally infected with HTLV-I.[282, 293]

Pediatric Manifestations

INFECTIVE DERMATITIS

A severe, generalized, chronic relapsing dermatitis of childhood called infective dermatitis was described first in Jamaican children in 1966.[312] In 1967, researchers observed that cultures of the nares or skin lesions in children with infective dermatitis often were positive for *Staphylococcus aureus* or beta-hemolytic streptococci.[351] These infections responded well to antibiotic therapy but relapsed once therapy was withdrawn. The refractory nature of the disorder with frequent exacerbations, infections with bacteria that are usually nonvirulent, and resistance to treatment suggested an association with immune dysfunction. After the identification of HTLV-I in 1980, epidemiologic studies demonstrated that HTLV-I was endemic in Jamaica; because HTLV-I infection was known to be associated with immune dysfunction and enhanced susceptibility to infections,[196] an association between infective dermatitis and HTLV-I infection was hypothesized.

In 1990, La Grenade and colleagues first described an association of infective dermatitis and HTLV-I infection in Jamaican children.[163] In a study of 14 children with typical infective dermatitis and 11 with atopic dermatitis, all children with infective dermatitis were found to be HTLV-I–seropositive versus none of those with atopic dermatitis. In a later, expanded report, all of 50 children with infective dermatitis were found to be HTLV-I–seropositive as opposed to only 14 percent of 35 with atopic dermatitis.[164] Subsequently, cases of infective dermatitis were reported in HTLV-I–infected children in Trinidad, Colombia, Brazil, and Japan.[26, 310, 333]

The clinical features of infective dermatitis include the acute onset in early childhood of a severe exudative eczema, typically without preceding infantile eczema. It is characterized by exudation and crusting involving the perinasal skin and nostrils, external ear and retroauricular areas, eyelid margins, scalp, neck, axillae, and groin. The eczema may be accompanied by a generalized fine papular rash on the trunk and back. A dermatopathic lymphadenitis with palpable lymph nodes also may be observed.[164] A chronic watery nasal discharge in the absence of other causes of rhinitis is common, and *S. aureus* or beta-hemolytic streptococci often are cultured from nose and skin lesions. Long-term antibiotic therapy is required to control the disease.

Diagnostic criteria for HTLV-I–associated infective dermatitis are shown in Table 193–8. The age at onset is usually the second to third year of life; 60 percent of patients are female.[190] The dermatitis may become less severe as the child gets older. In a study in Jamaica, the estimated incidence rate for infective dermatitis in HTLV-I–infected children was 552 cases per 100,000 child-years (95% confidence interval, 14 to 3080).[185]

In Jamaican children with infective dermatitis, HTLV-I antibody titers were significantly higher than those in asymptomatic HTLV-I–infected children. Children with infective dermatitis were more likely than those with atopic dermatitis to be anemic and to have lower serum albumin, higher white blood cell counts and erythrocyte sedimentation rates, lymphocytosis with atypical lymphocytes, and elevated serum immunoglobulins.[164] These findings are consistent with chronic inflammation and antigenic stimulation caused by the relapsing bacterial infections characteristic of infective dermatitis. However, elevated levels of T-cell activation also were seen in children with infective dermatitis, along with a higher $CD4^+$ and $CD8^+$ T-lymphocyte number, $CD4^+/CD8^+$ ratio, and percentage of HLA-DR antigen–positive T cells. These findings may be related primarily to HTLV-I infection rather than being secondary to infective dermatitis. In a cross-sectional study of asymptomatic HTLV-I–seropositive and HTLV-I–seronegative Jamaican children 11 to 31 months of age, HTLV-I infection was associated with an increase in $CD4^+$ cells expressing HLA-DR on their surface that was progressive and related to the duration of infection.[187] This finding may be an early marker for HTLV-I infection in children and indicative of an early perturbation in the immune system.

TABLE 193–8 ■ DIAGNOSIS OF HUMAN T-LYMPHOTROPIC VIRUS TYPE I–ASSOCIATED INFECTIVE DERMATITIS

Type of Criteria	Clinical/Laboratory Findings
Major criteria (diagnosis requires the presence of items 1–3, with at least 1 additional item present)	1. Crusting eczema involving the scalp, eyelid margins, perinasal skin, external ear and retroauricular areas, axillae, groin, and/or neck (must include 2 sites or more)
	2. Chronic watery nasal discharge and/or crusting of the anterior nares without other signs of rhinitis
	3. HTLV-I seropositivity
	4. Chronic relapsing dermatitis with prompt response to appropriate antibiotic therapy but prompt recurrence as soon as therapy is stopped
	5. Onset in early childhood
Minor or less specific criteria	1. Positive skin or anterior nares cultures for *Staphylococcus aureus* and/or beta-hemolytic streptococci
	2. Fine, generalized papular rash
	3. Generalized lymphadenopathy (with histologic dermatopathic lymphadenitis on biopsy, if performed)
	4. Anemia
	5. Elevated erythrocyte sedimentation rate
	6. Hyperimmunoglobulinemia (IgD and IgE)
	7. Elevated $CD4^+$ and $CD8^+$ T-cell count and elevated $CD4^+/CD8^+$ ratio

Complications of infective dermatitis occur in 30 to 35 percent of patients. The most common complications are crusted (Norwegian) scabies, corneal opacities, chronic bronchiectasis, and infection with parasitic worms such as *S. stercoralis*.[162] Other reported complications include lymphocytic interstitial pneumonitis and glomerulonephritis, which reflect the systemic complications of HTLV-I infection. Early death caused by severe bacterial infections with sepsis or the development of other later manifestations of HTLV-I infection may occur. Although ATLL and HAM/TSP are only rarely reported in children, a few cases of ATLL or HAM/TSP developing in patients with infective dermatitis after 12 to 25 years have been reported.[109, 165, 333] The class II HLA haplotype DRB1*DQB1* has been found in HTLV-I–infected children with infective dermatitis and also in infected Japanese adults with HAM/TSP.[166] These data suggest a possible genetically increased susceptibility to some HTLV-I disease manifestations, perhaps secondary to an exaggerated host immune response to HTLV-I infection in individuals with this haplotype.[166, 185] Children with HTLV-I–associated infective dermatitis, therefore, may be at risk for more serious HTLV-I–associated disorders later in life.

Histologically, an inflammatory lymphocytic infiltrate is seen within the skin lesions. The HTLV-I genome has been detected by PCR in lymphocytes cultured from biopsy specimens of skin lesions in patients with infectious dermatitis, although cultured fibroblasts were negative, thus suggesting that HTLV-I–infected lymphocytes had infiltrated the skin.[162] Cultured keratinocytes from children with infectious dermatitis have been shown to exhibit overexpression of proinflammatory and anti-inflammatory cytokines, which could be induced directly or indirectly by HTLV-I infection.[340] Secretion of cytokines by HTLV-I–infected cells might amplify or maintain a persistent inflammatory reaction in the skin and, when combined with the enhanced susceptibility to infection induced by HTLV-I–associated immunodysfunction, could result in the clinical manifestations of infective dermatitis. In a rabbit model, infection with HTLV-I by intravenous inoculation was associated with the development of a generalized exfoliative papillary dermatitis characterized by T-cell infiltrates in the epidermis and epithelium of the hair follicle, similar to that seen in cutaneous T-cell lymphoma.[302] HTLV-I envelope sequences were detected by DNA PCR in rabbit skin biopsy samples, and HTLV-I was isolated from cultures of affected skin. Researchers have postulated that infective dermatitis represents an HTLV-I–associated immunodeficiency syndrome resulting from exposure to HTLV-I in early life, primarily through mother-to-child transmission.

Treatment of infective dermatitis is symptomatic and targeted at controlling bacterial superinfection with the use of antibiotic therapy. However, long-term therapy is needed because of the relapsing nature of the illness. Occasionally, mild topical steroids are used for severe dermatitis.

OTHER PEDIATRIC MANIFESTATIONS

Renal manifestations rarely have been reported in association with infective dermatitis in children. Miller and colleagues reported a syndrome of infective dermatitis, glomerulonephritis, renal failure, severe hypertension with hypertensive encephalopathy, microangiopathic hemolytic anemia, and significant glomerulosclerosis with fibrosis on renal biopsy specimens in two Jamaican children infected with HTLV-I.[202] Pulse methylprednisolone was effective in reversing the renal failure in a child who was in the early stage of illness, but steroids were ineffective in a child treated later in the course of illness. In HTLV-I–infected adults, a syndrome of hemolytic-uremic syndrome or thrombotic thrombocytopenic purpura with severe hypertension, or both, has been reported.[66, 334] Chronic renal failure has been reported rarely in adults with ATLL. In one patient with ATLL, HTLV-I antigen with bound immunoglobulin was demonstrated by immunofluorescence in the glomerulus, thus suggesting that glomerular deposition of HTLV-I–associated immune complexes may be the etiology of the renal damage.[226] Alternatively, concomitant infection with group A beta-hemolytic *Streptococcus* during the immunodeficiency associated with HTLV-I could result in streptococcal-associated glomerulonephritis.

Other Disorders

Numerous autoimmune disorders have been associated with HTLV-I. In a study of 113 HTLV-I–infected patients in southern Florida, rheumatologic or autoimmune diseases were not uncommon.[113] An HTLV-I–associated large joint chronic arthropathy has been described. Clinically, the disorder is manifested as an oligoarthritis of the shoulder, wrists, or knees with a chronic course. Some patients may have accompanying myalgia or bronchitis.[234] Proliferative changes are observed in nonlymphocytic mesenchymal and synovial cells, along with synovial overgrowth. HTLV-I antibodies are detected in the synovial fluid of affected joints, and HTLV-I proviral DNA has been found in synovial cells and synovial fluid lymphocytes.[158, 335] A chronic inflammatory arthropathy can develop in HTLV-I transgenic mice.[138] HTLV-I Tax protein may be associated with proliferation of synovial cells leading to erosion of cartilage and bone.

HTLV-I–associated polymyositis has been described in patients with HAM/TSP, as well as those without neurologic impairment.[210, 252, 368] Muscle biopsy is consistent with a myositis with mononuclear interstitial infiltrates, necrosis, and regeneration. HTLV-I provirus has been identified by in situ hybridization in $CD4^+$ cells in the inflammatory cell infiltrate.[120] The mechanism by which HTLV-I produces disease is unknown. It is probably not a direct viral effect because HTLV-I does not appear to infect muscle cells.[252] As hypothesized for HAM/TSP, the pathologic process could be the result of an autoimmune response, or it could be due to the production of cytokines in focal inflammatory infiltrates in muscle by activated HTLV-I–infected $CD4^+$ cells and subsequent bystander damage to the myofibers.

An asymptomatic, subclinical lymphocytic pneumonitis has been described in patients with HAM/TSP. Bronchoalveolar lavage has shown the presence of a T-lymphocyte alveolitis, with high soluble IL-2 receptor levels also found in lavage fluid from these patients.[308, 309] On lung biopsy, a marked lymphocytic infiltration of the lung is seen. The presence of HTLV-I provirus in alveolar lymphocytes obtained by lavage has been described in 7.5 to 30 percent of patients with HAM/TSP and in less than 5 percent of HTLV-I–infected patients without myelopathy.[135]

HTLV-I also has been associated with Sjögren syndrome, a chronic exocrinopathy causing keratoconjunctivitis sicca, xerostomia, and sialadenitis and characterized by a lymphocytic infiltration of the lacrimal and salivary glands; the etiology has been hypothesized to be autoimmune in nature. In a study in Japan, HTLV-I seroprevalence in patients with Sjögren syndrome was 23 percent, significantly higher than the 3 percent HTLV-I seroprevalence in blood donors.[326] HTLV-I antibody titers in HTLV-I–seropositive patients with Sjögren syndrome were significantly higher than those in asymptomatic HTLV-I carriers and similar to those seen in patients with HAM/TSP. However, in contrast to HAM/TSP patients, the HTLV-I proviral load in peripheral blood was not always high. HTLV-I salivary IgA antibodies occurred commonly in HTLV-I–seropositive patients with Sjögren syndrome but very rarely in asymptomatic HTLV-I patients or those with HAM/TSP, thus suggesting potential increased viral activity within the salivary glands.[326] In a study of HTLV-I–infected patients from Guadeloupe, French West Indies, a sicca-like syndrome was found in almost 80 percent of patients, approximately half of whom also had neurologic findings.[18] HTLV-I provirus has been identified by PCR in acini cells and inflammatory infiltrates in the labial salivary glands of HAM/TSP patients, as well as in healthy HTLV-I carriers with the sicca syndrome.[324] In addition, one of the symptoms of Sjögren syndrome is impaired sweating, and HTLV-I pX sequences have been identified in samples of eccrine sweat gland epithelia from HTLV-I–infected individuals.[295] Transgenic animal models have indicated that HTLV-I is tropic for ductal epithelium of the salivary and lacrimal glands.[104]

HTLV-I infection, even in the absence of other disease manifestations, is associated with immune dysfunction. Perturbations in lymphokine and cytokine production have been observed with HTLV-I in vitro, most likely caused by Tax-mediated transactivation of various host-cell pathways. Spontaneous lymphocyte proliferation is seen in asymptomatic seropositive patients, as well as in HAM/TSP patients,[354] and changes in T-cell subsets reflecting an increase in activation markers, such as the IL-2 receptor, also may be observed. Opportunistic infections such as *Pneumocystis* pneumonia and Norwegian scabies can develop in HTLV-I–infected patients without other disease manifestations, and these patients are more likely to experience numerous other infections, including tuberculosis, leprosy, and strongyloidiasis.[221, 222, 277, 342] HTLV-I–infected patients have lower eosinophil counts than uninfected patients do, which may be related to the increased susceptibility of HTLV-I–infected persons to parasitic diseases.[223]

Dual Infection with HIV-1

Because some of the geographic areas endemic for HTLV-I are also endemic for HIV-1, dual infection with both viruses may occur.[15] In a study in the coastal port of Santos, Brazil, concurrent infection with HTLV-I and HTLV-II was seen in 6.0 and 7.4 percent of HIV-1–infected individuals, respectively.[74] Intravenous drug use and seropositivity to hepatitis C virus were correlated with co-infection with either HTLV-I or HTLV-II.

Based on in vitro studies indicating that the HTLV-I *tax* gene product can interact with the Tat response element of the HIV-1 LTR and enhance HIV-1 replication, researchers have proposed that dual infection might increase HIV-1 disease progression or increase the frequency of HTLV-I–associated diseases.[300] However, whether enhanced replication of HIV-1 occurs in dually infected patients in vivo is unclear. In one study in Brazil, no significant difference in HIV-1 plasma RNA levels was observed in 23 patients with HIV-1/HTLV-I co-infection and 92 patients with HIV-1 infection alone.[114]

Several small clinical studies are consistent with the hypothesis of potential enhanced disease progression with co-infection. HTLV-I/HIV-1 co-infection in intravenous drug users was found to be associated with a threefold increase in mortality when compared with drug users who had only HIV-1 infection.[254] In a study in Trinidad, co-infected individuals had more rapid progression to AIDS than did those with HIV-1 infection alone, and in a study from Rio de Janeiro, patients dually infected with HIV-1 and HTLV-I had a more advanced World Health Organization HIV disease stage.[14, 287] Interestingly, those with advanced disease and dual infection had higher $CD4^+$ lymphocyte counts than did those with a similar disease stage but infected with HIV-1 alone; similar findings also were reported in another study.[75, 287] The $CD4^+$ number, therefore, may be an unreliable predictor of immunodeficiency in dually infected patients; HTLV-I may induce an elevated $CD4^+$ number through enhancement of lymphocyte proliferation, but the function of these cells may be abnormal.[35]

In addition, HIV-1 infection possibly increases the likelihood for development of some HTLV-I–associated diseases. HTLV-I and HTLV-II expression appears to be up-regulated in patients co-infected with HIV-1.[19] Several reports have been published of patients with dual infection in whom a typical HAM/TSP syndrome developed, and antibodies to HIV-1 and HTLV-I were present in the blood and CSF of one dually infected patient with neurologic disease.[2, 20, 199]

HTLV-II

HTLV-II first was identified in patients with hairy-cell leukemia.[146, 279, 280] HTLV-II is closely related to HTLV-I, with approximately 60 percent homology in nucleotide sequences.[161] HTLV-II infection is endemic in native American Indian populations and is probably an ancient infection that has been maintained in the population by sexual transmission and mother-to-child transmission through breastfeeding.[107] More recently, HTLV-II has been introduced into urban settings in the United States, Europe, and Asia, where transmission is primarily through intravenous drug use or transfusion of contaminated blood. The role of this virus in causation of disease has not been as definitively established as that for HTLV-I, but a possible association with lymphoproliferative and neurologic disorders has been suggested (see Table 193–3).

Viral Pathogenesis/Molecular Biology

Like HTLV-I, HTLV-II can transform cells in vitro. However, HTLV-II displays a preferential tropism for and induces clonal expansion of cells of the $CD8^+$ T-lymphocyte phenotype.[46, 136, 179] In an evaluation of HTLV-II–infected patients, HTLV-II was detected exclusively within $CD8^+$ lymphocytes in most individuals and less frequently in both $CD4^+$ and $CD8^+$ T cells in some individuals.[136, 168] Whether the difference in cell tropism between HTLV-I and HTLV-II might lead to variations in pathogenicity between the two viruses is unknown.

Based on nucleotide sequencing of the viral envelope and phylogenetic analysis, two major molecular subtypes of HTLV-II have been identified and designated HTLV-IIA and HTLV-IIB; these subtypes have a 4 to 7 percent divergence in the gene encoding the envelope transmembrane protein.[108] Studies focusing on the LTR and pX regions of the provirus have shown additional differences. The Tax protein appears to differ in length between the two subtypes, with the HTLV-IIB Tax protein being 25 amino acids longer than the HTLV-IIA Tax protein.[255] Functionally, the HTLV-IIA Tax protein is a weaker inactivator of the *p53* tumor suppressor gene and a less potent transactivator of the viral LTR in vitro than is the Tax protein from HTLV-I or HTLV-IIB, and limited data suggest that the proviral load may be lower in HTLV-IIA–infected than HTLV-IIB–infected individuals.[70, 181] Based on phylogenetic analysis of nucleotide sequences in the LTR region of the virus, two additional subtypes have been identified in restricted geographic locations, HTLV-IIC and HTLV-IID.[70, 181] The Tax protein of HTLV-IIC is the same length as that of HTLV-IIB, and the length of Tax in HTLV-IID is intermediate between the A and B-C subtypes.

Epidemiology

HTLV-II is endemic in a large number of Native American Indian populations in the United States (Navajo and Pueblo Indians in New Mexico and the Seminole Indians in Florida) and numerous indigenous Amerindian populations in Latin America, including Panama, Colombia, Argentina, Brazil, and Chile.[108, 117, 129, 130, 173, 183, 357] HTLV-II seroprevalence in these Amerindian tribes varies between 2 and 30 percent.[128, 183, 217, 343] Although HTLV-I is endemic in Africa, HTLV-II seroprevalence appears to be relatively low; in one study, the prevalence of HTLV-II was 0.8 percent in the Ivory Coast, 0.05 percent in Guinea, and 0.02 percent in Senegal.[30] However, in a study in Eritrea, 2.1 percent of female sexual workers were found to be HTLV-II–seropositive.[9]

In the United States, Europe, and Southeast Asia, HTLV-II infection is found primarily in intravenous drug users, with seroprevalence rates ranging from 3 to 18 percent.[32, 33, 155] In the United States, HTLV-II accounts for the vast majority of HTLV infections in intravenous drug users.[42] In a study of HTLV-II and HIV seroprevalence in drug users from eight metropolitan areas in the United States, the overall prevalence of HTLV-II alone was 15.1 percent, the prevalence of HIV-1 alone was 9.9 percent, and that of dual HIV-1/HTLV-II infection was 3.3 percent; HTLV-II prevalence was higher in the Southwest and Midwest than the

Northeast, whereas HIV-1 prevalence was highest in the Northeast.[32] HTLV-II seroprevalence in drug users was highest in black and Hispanic persons, increased with age, and was higher in women than men in all age groups. The female preponderance of HTLV-II infection may indicate more efficient sexual transmission of HTLV-II from men to women than vice versa; similar findings have been noted with HTLV-I. In persons attending clinics for sexually transmitted diseases in the United States, nearly two thirds of HTLV infections are caused by HTLV-II.[155] In a study involving blood donors in the United States, HTLV-II prevalence was 22.3 per 100,000 donors and was highest in West Coast blood centers.[225] HTLV-II infection was associated with an age of 40 to 49 years, first-time blood donation, female sex, high-school or lower education, and hepatitis C seropositivity.

The geographic distribution of HTLV-II subtypes varies.[107] HTLV-IIA is the predominant infection in intravenous drug users in North America and Europe and is widespread worldwide. HTLV-IIB predominates in Paleoindian groups, such as the North American Native Indian population, although a mixture of HTLV-IIA and HTLV-IIB also has been reported in some tribes.[131] In South America, HTLV-IIB infection is seen in native populations in Panama, Colombia, and Argentina, but an indigenous Brazilian Indian population in the Amazon appears to be infected with HTLV-IIC, also seen in intravenous drug users in urban areas of Brazil.[70] In Europe, a mixture of infections is noted; for example, HTLV-IIA is primarily found in Sweden, whereas HTLV-IIB is more prevalent in Spain and Italy. HTLV-IID has been detected in central African Pygmies.

Modes of Transmission

HTLV-II, like HTLV-I, is transmitted by transfusion of contaminated cellular blood products, by injection with contaminated needles, sexually, and from mother to child. Whether differences in transmission efficiency exist between the two viruses is unclear.

Sexual transmission is an important mode of HTLV-II acquisition, although data are more limited for HTLV-II than for HTLV-I. Studies in non–drug-using native populations have shown a strong association of HTLV-II infection between spouses.[182, 343] Among Guaymi Indians in Panama, HTLV-II seroprevalence approaches 10 percent. Seropositivity in women is associated with an early age at first sexual intercourse, the number of lifetime sexual partners, and the number of long-term sexual relationships; in males, intercourse with prostitutes is associated with seropositivity.[182] In HTLV-II–seropositive injecting drug users, higher rates of seropositivity are found in individuals with a history of sexually transmitted diseases.[32, 292, 344] Preferential male-to-female transmission has been reported, as with HTLV-I. In HTLV-II–seropositive blood donors, a history of sexual contact with an intravenous drug user or an HTLV-II–infected sexual partner has been associated with increased risk of HTLV-II seropositivity.[289] In addition, a high prevalence of HTLV-II seropositivity in patients who are not intravenous drug users but who have sexually transmitted diseases also supports the role of sexual contact in HTLV-II transmission.[289]

Injecting drug use is the primary mode of HTLV-II acquisition in the United States. In a study of HTLV-infected blood donors (the Retrovirus Epidemiology Donor Study), HTLV-II infection was significantly associated with injection drug use or sexual contact with an injecting drug user, whereas HTLV-I infection was not.[289] Having had an abortion also was an independent risk factor for the acquisition of HTLV-II infection by female blood donors, probably because of abortion being a marker of increased unprotected sexual activity. Other risk factors, such as seven or more sexual partners, were common to both HTLV-I and HTLV-II. Sex with an injecting drug user was a particular risk factor for women; 65 percent of HTLV-II–infected women reported that they had a sexual partner who used injection drugs, and 20 percent of women reported that they also injected drugs themselves. HTLV-II infection in drug users has been associated with nonwhite race, older age, markers of previous hepatitis B virus infection, the use of a specific needle-sharing practice called backloading, a history of herpes simplex virus type 2 infection, and a history of receiving money for sex.[32, 292, 344] In an Italian study of HTLV risk factors in patients seen in a clinic for sexually transmitted diseases, injecting drug use was associated with HTLV-II infection, whereas HTLV-I infection was associated more with sexual behavior.[100] Among injecting drug users, seroprevalence for HTLV-II was 8.2 percent versus 2.1 percent for HTLV-I. HTLV-I infection was associated with exposure to syphilis and non-European nationality.

HTLV-II also has been detected in the breast milk of carrier mothers, and mother-to-child transmission has been described in those who breast-feed.[118, 167, 169, 343] The rate of HTLV-II breast milk transmission described in the few small studies available (≈14%) is slightly lower than that found for HTLV-I. Like HTLV-I, HTLV-II appears to be transmitted infrequently in the absence of breast-feeding.[90, 107, 149, 339] Passive immunization with HTLV-II hyperimmunoglobulin in rabbits prevented blood-borne transmission of HTLV-II–infected cells.[211] Interestingly, only HTLV-II and not HTLV-I immunoglobulin was effective in preventing HTLV-II transmission, thus suggesting that despite some cross-reactivity on conventional ELISAs, cross-neutralization between the viruses is minimal or nonexistent.[211]

Clinical Disease

When compared with HTLV-I, HTLV-II infection appears to be associated with a much lower prevalence of virus-associated neoplasia. Although HTLV-II was isolated initially from the cells of patients with hairy-cell leukemia,[28, 146] subsequent studies have not confirmed this association. In an HTLV-II–endemic population of Native Americans in New Mexico, no apparent increase in the incidence of hairy-cell leukemia, mycosis fungoides, and chronic lymphocytic leukemia was observed over that in other ethnic groups.[129]

When cancers do develop, they are of the $CD8^+$ cell phenotype. Unusual skin disorders resembling cutaneous lymphoma have been reported in a small number of patients co-infected with HIV-1 and HTLV-II. A severe erythroderma with subsequent exfoliation of the skin accompanied by eosinophilia and dermatopathic lymphadenopathy was reported in two intravenous drug users with dual infection.[151] In contrast to most cutaneous lymphomata in the United States, which are of the $CD4^+$ cell phenotype, the infiltrating T cells were of the $CD8^+$ phenotype. In a third HIV-1/HTLV-II co-infected patient with a cutaneous $CD8^+$ T-cell lymphoma, the skin infiltrate was found to contain $CD8^+$ cells with HTLV-II DNA.[260] HTLV-II infection of $CD8^+$ cells has been described in one patient with large granular cell lymphocytosis and one with large granular lymphocytic leukemia.[178, 197] However, HTLV-II was found in only 2 percent of patients with large granular lymphocytic leukemia in a subsequent study of 51 patients.[116] HTLV-II infection also has been described in one patient with mycosis fungoides.[379]

Evidence suggests that HTLV-II may be associated with neurologic disorders ranging from a spastic paraparesis-myelopathy similar to HAM/TSP to more widespread involvement of the CNS.[219] Myeloneuropathies indistinguishable from HAM/TSP have been reported in patients infected with HTLV-II alone or co-infected with HIV-1.[20, 127, 217, 219, 225] In addition, a chronic neurodegenerative disorder with ataxia as a prominent feature has been reported in patients with HTLV-II infection.[112, 297] In patients in whom HTLV-II was subtyped, type A was identified. Most cases occurred in women, similar to the observed female preponderance in patients with HAM/TSP. Patients with HIV-1 infection who have sensory peripheral polyneuropathy have been found to have a higher prevalence of HTLV-II co-infection, as diagnosed by serology and DNA PCR, than have HIV-1–infected patients without neuropathy, thus suggesting that HTLV-II may be involved in the pathogenesis of the neuropathy.[378]

Although immune deficiency and an increased risk of infections have been reported in HTLV-I–infected individuals, the data are less clear for HTLV-II. An initial report from San Francisco described an association of HTLV-II seropositivity and bacterial infections, particularly skin and soft tissue infections and bacterial pneumonia, but the results were confounded by intravenous drug use, which in itself could increase the risk for infections, in nearly all HTLV-II–seropositive patients.[208] In a case-control study of intravenous drug users from Baltimore with an overall HTLV-II seroprevalence of 7 percent, no significant association between HTLV-II seropositivity and the development of bacterial pneumonia, infective endocarditis, and skin abscess was found.[281] However, in a study of blood donors infected with HTLV-I or HTLV-II and also HIV-1–seronegative, HTLV-II infection was associated with an increased incidence of bronchitis, bladder or kidney infection, oral herpes simplex virus infection, and a borderline increase in the incidence of pneumonia.[222] It is clear that the natural history and clinical manifestations of HTLV-II need further delineation in the context of ongoing prospective natural history studies.

Lentiviruses: HIV-2

HIV-1 is discussed in the latter half of this chapter (193B) and is not discussed here. HIV-2 has a morphology and life cycle similar to that of HIV-1, but with significant antigenic, biologic, epidemiologic, and clinical differences (Table 193–9). Both viruses have similar modes of transmission and can result in immune depletion and AIDS. However, whereas HIV-1 has a global distribution, HIV-2 is confined primarily to west Africa and found only sporadically in Europe, the United States, and other countries, and the clinical latency period and rates of perinatal and sexual transmission are lower than those for HIV-1. The basis of such differences in natural history between these two lentiviruses is unknown and may result from characteristics of the virus, the host, or both.

VIRAL GENOME/PATHOGENESIS

Although HIV-1 and HIV-2 share a similar genetic organization, significant divergence in genetic sequence exists, with differences of 58 percent for the *gag* gene, 59 percent for the *pol* gene, and 39 percent for the *env* gene.[48, 242] More

TABLE 193–9 ■ COMPARISON OF HUMAN IMMUNODEFICIENCY VIRUS TYPES 2 AND 1

Characteristic	HIV-2	HIV-1
Viral genome	*vpx* gene, no *vpu* gene *nef* gene longer in HIV-2, defective *nef* gene in 10% Difference in number and identity of transcription enhancers for LTR (less responsive to stimulation?)	*vpu* gene, no *vpx* gene Defective *nef* gene in <1% Greater responsiveness of LTR to transcription enhancers?
Geographic distribution	West Africa Restricted distribution outside Africa, primarily in countries with ties to West Africa Europe: Portugal, France, Germany, Spain South America: Brazil India	Global
Modes of transmission	Sexual, blood-borne, mother-to-child	Sexual, blood-borne, mother-to-child
Risk of sexual transmission	3-fold lower than HIV-1	
Seroconversion in commercial sex workers in Senegal[147,194]	Incidence of seroconversion in commercial sex workers in Senegal, 1% per year	Incidence of seroconversion in commercial sex workers in Senegal, 2–3% per year
Risk of mother-to-child transmission (without antiretroviral prophylaxis)	0–4%	25–35%
Viral load (without therapy)	28- to 30-fold lower than HIV-1	
Viral set point:		
Seroconverters in Guinea-Bissau[8]	Median RNA, 2500 copies/mL	Median RNA, 70,000 copies/mL
Commercial sex workers in Senegal[262, 263]	Median RNA, 263 copies/mL	Median RNA, 7182 copies/mL
Pregnant women in the Gambia[243]	Geometric mean RNA, 410 copies/mL	Geometric mean RNA, 15,100 copies/mL
Rate of $CD4^+$ T-cell decline	1% per year	10% per year
Time to development of AIDS	<0.5% per year	3–5% per year
Increase in mortality above that of HIV-seronegative individuals	2- to 4-fold increase	10-fold increase

LTR, long terminal repeat.

similarity is seen between HIV-2 and primate SIV, in which the nucleic acid sequence homology between HIV-2 and SIV_{SM} and SIV_{MAC} strains is approximately 75 percent.[193] Because of this antigenic variation, HIV-1 antibody screening EIAs may not detect antibody to HIV-2, and thus combination screening tests containing antigens from both viruses have been developed and are in use in the United States for screening of blood donors.[39, 41] Additionally, confirmatory Western blot testing to detect HIV-2 requires the use of HIV-2–specific assays because not all samples from persons infected with HIV-2 will be positive on HIV-1 Western blot; some will test indeterminate or, rarely, negative. Seven genetic groups of HIV-2 (A to G) have been identified. However, current data suggest that only HIV-2 subtypes A and B are established in significant amounts in human populations.[22] No differences in replication potential between the two subtypes appear to exist.[56]

HIV-1 and HIV-2 differ in the number and size of their accessory genes. HIV-2 lacks the genetic equivalent of the HIV-1 *vpu* gene. The HIV-1 Vpu protein plays an important role in intracellular processing of $CD4^+$: down-regulation of $CD4^+$ receptor expression on HIV-1–infected cells. This characteristic could enhance the ability of cytoplasmic HIV-1 envelope proteins to reach the cell membrane and also enhance release of budding virions; no equivalent functional protein exists in HIV-2. HIV-2 contains the *vpx* gene, which is not found in HIV-1 but shares homology with the HIV-1 *vpr* gene and may affect early events in the replication cycle. Additionally, the *nef* ORF in HIV-1 is shorter than that in HIV-2, and the prevalence of defective *nef* genes in patients with HIV-2 infection (≈10%) is significantly higher than previously seen in HIV-1–infected individuals (<1%).[313] In HIV-1, deletions in the *nef* gene have been described in patients with long-term nonprogression.

Whereas both HIV-1 and HIV-2 infect $CD4^+$ T lymphocytes and use the CXCR4 or CCR5 co-receptors for cell entry, HIV-2 can use multiple additional co-receptors.[213] The cytopathicity of HIV-2 appears to be similar to that of HIV-1 and is determined by the type of co-receptor used for cell entry.

In an in vitro study comparing HIV-1 and HIV-2 co-receptor use and cytopathicity in human lymphoid cells, HIV-2 specificity for the CCR5 co-receptor alone or in combination with other co-receptors was associated with restricted cytopathicity, whereas specificity for CXCR4 was linked to a more virulent phenotype, as observed for HIV-1.[288] Thus, the lesser virulence of HIV-2 than HIV-1 does not appear to be due to a restriction in co-receptor use or lower intrinsic cytopathic potential.

Studies indicate that levels of integrated proviral HIV-2 DNA in peripheral blood mononuclear cells are similar to those in comparable groups of HIV-1–infected individuals.[10, 24, 138, 262] However, levels of HIV-2 plasma RNA and proviral DNA do not appear to have a significant correlation.[262] Despite similar proviral levels in HIV-1 and HIV-2, patients infected with HIV-2 have a significantly lower plasma viral load, thus suggesting a lower rate of expression of the HIV-2 proviral DNA template.[23, 58, 262, 263, 296, 301, 322, 329] In a study of sero-incident cases of HIV-1 and HIV-2 infection in Guinea-Bissau, the viral set-point after seroconversion was 28-fold lower in HIV-2 than in HIV-1 recent seroconverters.[8, 238] Other studies have shown a broader-based neutralizing antibody response and higher antibody levels in HIV-2– than HIV-1–infected individuals.[194, 321] These findings suggest that HIV-2 may have low rates of viral replication or a reduced ability to mutate and escape the host immune response, or both.

Productive lentiviral infection is dependent on continued activation of target cells. The lower rate of viral production in HIV-2–infected cells also could reflect a lesser ability of infected cells to respond to activation or could indicate that the cells themselves have lower activation states. The transcriptional enhancer/promoter region of the HIV-2 LTR differs from that of the HIV-1 LTR in the number and identity of enhancer elements, and transcriptional up-regulation of viral production may be disrupted more easily than for HIV-1.[193, 262] This factor could result in lower responsiveness of the HIV-2 LTR to transcription factors in activated T cells. For example, the HIV-2 LTR has been shown to be less responsive to stimulation of viral gene expression by tumor necrosis factor–α than the HIV-1 LTR is.[110]

Lentiviral envelope glycoproteins can induce cytokine production and other immunologic disturbances; differences in the effect of the HIV-1 and HIV-2 envelope glycoprotein also could contribute to differences in the pathogenicity of the viruses. Recombinant HIV-2 envelope glycoprotein is superior to the HIV-1 envelope in stimulating the production of interferon-γ and IL-16, both of which inhibit viral replication, and less effective in producing expression of IL-4, which stimulates viral replication.[233, 294] The HIV-2 envelope glycoprotein inhibits T-cell proliferation more than the glycoprotein of HIV-1 does in vitro, and it also was found to inhibit expression of cell surface activation markers.[36] The presence of an HIV-2 protein that reduces immune system stimulation may decrease replication, result in lower levels of HIV-2 viremia, and also decrease $CD4^+$ cell apoptosis. The rate of total lymphocyte apoptosis has been found to be lower in HIV-2 than HIV-1 infection.[200]

EPIDEMIOLOGY

HIV-2 is endemic in certain areas of western Africa, including Guinea-Bissau, Burkina Faso, the Gambia, Cape Verde, Senegal, and the Ivory Coast, as well as in Angola and Mozambique in southern Africa.[193] Transmission is principally through heterosexual contact. The overall prevalence of HIV-2 in these areas is approximately 1 to 2 percent, although seroprevalence rates of 8 percent in pregnant women in Guinea-Bissau have been observed[329]; in high-risk groups such as urban commercial sex workers, HIV-2 prevalence rates of 15 to 64 percent have been reported.[193] HIV-2 group A infections have been identified predominantly in the western part of West Africa, mainly Guinea-Bissau, Senegal, the Gambia, and Mali.[22] HIV-2 group B infections have been found in central and eastern West African countries such as the Ivory Coast, Ghana, and Nigeria.

When compared with HIV-1, the seroprevalence of HIV-2 is higher in older age groups[364]; in a study in Guinea-Bissau, among individuals older than 50 years, HIV-2 prevalence was 12 percent in men and 16 percent in women.[264] In contrast, HIV-1 infection was more prevalent in younger individuals. The older age of HIV-2–infected persons may be a result of the longer clinical latency period allowing more prolonged survival in HIV-2–infected persons.

HIV-2 has only limited distribution outside West Africa and has been described primarily in regions in Europe, South America, and India with historical socioeconomic ties to West Africa. The greatest numbers of HIV-2 cases have been reported in Portugal, France, and Germany.[268] The cultural and economic ties of Portugal to its former colonies in West Africa probably facilitated the spread of HIV-2 to Europe and possibly Brazil, also a former Portuguese colony. As many as 4.5 percent of AIDS cases in Portugal are caused by HIV-2, and in northern Portugal, HIV-2 accounts for 12 percent of HIV infections.[304] In France, 1 to 2 percent of all pediatric HIV infections are caused by HIV-2.[76] In North

America and most countries in Europe, the majority of reported HIV-2 infections occur in individuals of West African origin or their sexual contacts. However, indigenous HIV-2 transmission also may occur inasmuch as HIV-2 infections not directly linked to West Africa have been reported in Portugal, France, and Spain. HIV-2 infection has been reported in India; some studies suggest that 7 to 8 percent of all HIV infections in Bombay are caused by HIV-2. In the United States, fewer than 100 cases of HIV-2 infection have been reported to the Centers for Disease Control and Prevention (CDC), and since the implementation of combination HIV-1/HIV-2 screening of the blood supply in June 1992, no transfusion-acquired HIV-2 cases have been reported to the CDC.[40,41]

Although some reports have suggested that infection with HIV-2 may be protective against HIV-1 infection, it has not been confirmed in other studies.[12, 236, 330, 331, 360] In two studies, HIV-2–positive subjects actually had a tendency toward a higher risk of acquiring HIV-1 infection than did seronegative individuals.[236, 360] Dual infection with HIV-1 and HIV-2, confirmed by PCR and culture, has been observed in areas that are endemic for both viruses.[93, 258] Susceptibility to dual HIV-1 and HIV-2 infection was studied in a macaque model of HIV infection.[251] Interestingly, the timing of secondary virus exposure was found to be a critical factor in the risk of acquiring infection. Productive mixed infections were established with simultaneous exposure or if viral challenge occurred within 4 weeks after primary infection. However, animals exposed at 8 weeks or more after primary inoculation were resistant to secondary infection. The mechanism of protection is not known. In one study, 50 percent of peripheral blood mononuclear cells from HIV-2–infected commercial sex workers resisted in vitro challenge with CCR5-dependent HIV-1 but not CXCR4-dependent HIV-1.[159] Additionally, high levels of beta-chemokines RANTES (regulated upon activation, normal T-cell expressed and secreted), macrophage inflammatory protein 1-alpha (MIP-1α), and MIP-1β, the natural ligands of the CCR5 receptor, were secreted when these resistant peripheral blood mononuclear cells from HIV-2–infected individuals underwent stimulation. These investigators hypothesized that beta-chemokine–mediated resistance might play a role in the potential protection of some HIV-2–infected individuals from secondary HIV-1 infection.

MODE OF TRANSMISSION

The modes of HIV-2 acquisition appear to be identical to those of HIV-1: heterosexual and homosexual intercourse, intravenous drug use, receipt of contaminated blood products, and perinatally. However, the infectivity of HIV-2 seems to be lower than that of HIV-1, and transmission of HIV-2 via sexual intercourse appears to be less frequent than that observed with HIV-1.[147] One estimate is that the likelihood of sexual transmission of HIV-2 per sexual exposure is threefold less than with HIV-1.[147, 194]

In a study in Guinea-Bissau, the overall prevalence of HIV-2 infection in 1996 was 9.7 percent in police officers and 5.5 percent in pregnant women, as opposed to 0.9 percent in each group for HIV-1.[236] However, during the 7-year period from 1990 to 1996, the incidence of HIV-1 infection increased significantly in both groups whereas the incidence of HIV-2 decreased, thus implying more efficient transmission of HIV-1. In a similar study of commercial sex workers in Senegal, the incidence of HIV-1 infection increased 12-fold despite a prevalence of HIV-2 at baseline that was approximately 2-fold higher than that for HIV-1.[147, 194] The lower likelihood of sexual transmission of HIV-2 may explain its more limited geographic distribution.

Data from most studies of mother-infant pairs indicate that perinatal transmission of HIV-2 appears to be rare, with mother-to-child transmission rates ranging from 0 to 4 percent.[4, 92, 243, 266, 329] In one large prospective study from the Ivory Coast, the risk of perinatal transmission from HIV-1–infected mothers was 21-fold greater than from HIV-2–infected mothers; transmission rates were 1.2 percent from HIV-2–infected mothers versus 24.7 percent from HIV-1–infected mothers.[4] In another large study in the Gambia, the estimated rate of mother-to-child transmission of HIV-2 was 4.0 percent versus 24.4 percent for HIV-1.[243] Interestingly, in this study, three of eight HIV-2–infected infants were infected after 2 months of age, which suggests that HIV-2, like HIV-1, can be transmitted postnatally through breast milk.

The maternal plasma viral load is a significant risk factor for perinatal transmission of both HIV-1 and HIV-2 infection. In the study in the Gambia, for every 1 $\log_{10}$ increase in plasma RNA, the odds of transmission was 2.7 for HIV-1 and 2.8 for HIV-2.[243] However, maternal RNA levels were significantly lower in HIV-2–infected than HIV-1–infected mothers. After adjusting for viral load, the odds of transmitting HIV-1 were similar to those for HIV-2, thus suggesting that the level of viremia, as opposed to the type of virus, was the major determinant of the difference in mother-to-child transmission rates between HIV-1 and HIV-2.

Transmission from women who are dually seropositive for HIV-1 and HIV-2 has been described; HIV-1 appears to be transmitted more efficiently than HIV-2 does, and HIV-1 transmission rates from dually infected women were similar to those from women infected with HIV-1 alone. Transmission of dual infection to the infant, though a rare occurrence, has been described. In the Ivory Coast cohort, 19.0 percent of women with dual HIV-1 and HIV-2 infection transmitted HIV to their infants; of 11 infected infants, 10 were infected with HIV-1 alone and 1 was dually infected.[4] Mortality in infants born to HIV-1–infected or dually infected mothers was 2.6 to 4.2 times higher than that in infants born to HIV-2–infected mothers (mortality rates of 133, 82, and 32 per 1000, respectively).[58]

CLINICAL MANIFESTATIONS

HIV-2 is fully pathogenic in humans, and the clinical spectrum of disease caused by HIV-2 is similar to that of HIV-1. However, the rate of $CD4^+$ T-cell depletion and clinical progression to AIDS is slower, and more favorable survival is observed, although the mortality rate is increased in comparison to seronegative persons.[142, 153, 193, 195, 358] In a cohort study of HIV-2– and HIV-1–infected women in Senegal, the rate of decline in $CD4^+$ T-lymphocyte count was approximately 1 percent per year for women infected with HIV-2 versus 10 percent per year for HIV-1.[195] The median time to development of AIDS in HIV-1–infected women was 10 years; in contrast, HIV-2 AIDS-free survival was so high that a median estimate of the time to a diagnosis of AIDS was not able to be determined.[194] In community-based studies comparing the risk of death in infected versus uninfected adults, the relative risk of dying with HIV-2 infection was increased by 2- to 4-fold, in contrast to a 10-fold increase with HIV-1 infection.[216, 265, 273]

Immunologic findings are similar to those in HIV-1 infection, with polyclonal hypergammaglobulinemia, increased T-cell activation, decreased lymphocyte proliferation, reduced antigen recall, and mildly elevated $CD8^+$ and reduced $CD4^+$ T-lymphocyte counts. However, in most cases, these changes are not as severe as those observed with HIV-1 infection. As for HIV-1, viral load significantly correlates with disease progression as measured by $CD4^+$ T-cell decline or mortality, and differences in viral load throughout most of the natural history of HIV-1 and HIV-2 infection probably account for the differences in disease progression and transmissibility reported between the two viruses.[8, 11, 262, 263, 304] In a comparison of HIV-1– and HIV-2–infected persons with similar $CD4^+$ T-cell counts, the quantitative viral load was significantly lower in those infected with HIV-2.[296] In patients with a $CD4^+$ cell count greater than 500/mm^3, none of the HIV-2–infected individuals had a detectable plasma viral load as compared with 52 percent of HIV-1–infected persons. In a study of seroincident cases of single or dual infection with HIV-1 and HIV-2 in Guinea-Bissau, dually infected individuals had lower plasma RNA levels than singly infected individuals did.[8]

Similar to the clinical outcome of HIV-2 infection in adults, slower rates of disease progression and better survival have been observed in HIV-2– versus HIV-1–infected or dually infected children.[4, 59, 237, 250, 267] In a prospective study in the Gambia, the 18-month mortality rate of children born to HIV-2–infected mothers did not differ significantly from that of children born to HIV-seronegative women (7 versus 6%, respectively).[250] In contrast, the relative risk of death in children born to HIV-1– versus HIV-2–infected or seronegative mothers was increased by 2.3- and 2.6-fold, respectively. The excess deaths in children of HIV-1–infected mothers were primarily caused by HIV-1 infection in the child; the mortality rate was 35 percent in HIV-1–infected children, as opposed to 9 percent in uninfected children born to HIV-1–infected mothers. In contrast, no deaths occurred in HIV-2–infected children. In Guinea-Bissau, overall child mortality was similar in children born to HIV-2–seropositive and HIV-seronegative women (16.3 versus 14.6%, respectively).[237] However, despite generally slower progression in HIV-2–infected children, severe immunodeficiency and AIDS occurring early in life rarely have been reported with HIV-2 infection.[92, 209]

Antiretroviral therapy for HIV-2 infection may be possible, but the drugs available may be less effective against HIV-2 than HIV-1.[291] HIV-2 is inhibited in vitro by nucleoside analogue reverse transcriptase inhibitors such as zidovudine or didanosine, though somewhat less so than HIV-1 is. Non-nucleoside reverse transcriptase inhibitors generally show little to no inhibition of HIV-2 in vitro at nontoxic levels.[365] Preliminary data indicate that HIV-1 protease inhibitors also may inhibit HIV-2.[194]

REFERENCES

1. Aboud, M., Rosner, M., Dombrovsky, A., et al.: Interactions between retroviruses and environmental carcinogens and their role in animal and human leukemogenesis. Leuk. Res. *16*:1061–1069, 1992.
2. Aboulafia, D. M., Saxton, E. H., Koga, H., et al.: A patient with progressive myelopathy and antibodies to human T-cell leukemia virus type 1 and human immunodeficiency virus type 1 in serum and cerebrospinal fluid. Arch. Neurol. *47*:477–479, 1990.
3. Ades, A. E., Parker, S., Walker, J., et al.: Human T cell leukemia/lymphoma virus infection in pregnant women in the United Kingdom: Population study. B. M. J. *320*:1497–1501, 2000.
4. Adjorlolo-Johnson, G., De Cock, K. M., Ekpini, E., et al.: Prospective comparison of mother-to-child transmission of HIV-1 and HIV-2 in Abidjan, Ivory Coast. J. A. M. A. *272*:462–466, 1994.
5. Albrecht, B., Collins, N. D., Burniston, M. T., et al.: Human T-lymphotropic virus type 1 open reading frame I p12^I is required for efficient viral infectivity in primary lymphocytes. J. Virol. *74*:9828–9835, 2000.
6. Anderson, G. A., Guerena, M., and Dixon, C. M.: Human non-HIV retroviral infections. Infect. Med. *11*:545–549, 1994.
7. Anderson, S., Shugars, D., Swanstrom, R., et al.: Nef from primary isolates of human immunodeficiency virus type 1 suppresses surface CD4 expression in human and mouse T cells. J. Virol. *67*:4923–4931, 1993.
8. Andersson, S., Norrgren, H., da Silva, Z., et al.: Plasma viral load in HIV-1 and HIV-2 singly and dually infected individuals in Guinea-Bissau, West Africa. Arch. Intern. Med. *160*:3286–3293, 2000.
9. Andersson, S., Tessema, H. G., and Wahren, B.: Is there a focus of HTLV-II infections in the horn of Africa? J. Acquir. Immune Defic. Syndr. Hum. Retrovirol. *21*:353–354, 1999.
10. Ariyoshi, K., Berry, N., Wilkins, A., et al.: A community-based study of human immunodeficiency virus type 2 provirus load in a rural village in West Africa. J. Infect. Dis. *173*:245–248, 1996.
11. Ariyoshi, K., Jaffar, S., Alabi, A. S., et al.: Plasma viral load predicts the rate of CD4 T cell decline and death in HIV-2–infected patients in West Africa. A. I. D. S. *14*:339–344, 2000.
12. Ariyoshi, K., van der Loeff, M. S., Sabally, S., et al.: Does HIV-2 infection provide cross-protection against HIV-1 infection? A. I. D. S. *1*:1053–1054, 1997.
13. Asante-Appiah, E., and Skalka, A. M.: Molecular mechanisms in retrovirus DNA integration. Antiviral Res. *36*:139–156, 1997.
14. Bartholomew, C., Blattner, W., and Cleghorn, F.: Progression to AIDS in homosexual men coinfected with HIV and HTLV-I in Trinidad. Lancet *2*:1469, 1987.
15. Bartholomew, C., Saxinger, C., Clark, J. W., et al.: Transmission of HTLV-I and HIV among homosexuals in Trinidad. J. A. M. A. *257*:2604–2608, 1987.
16. Bastian, I., Gardner, J., Webb, D., et al.: Isolation of a strain of human T-lymphotropic virus type I from Australian aboriginals. J. Virol. *67*:843–851, 1993.
17. Bazarbachi, A., Saal, F., Laroche, L., et al.: HTLV-I provirus and mycosis fungoides. Science *259*:1470–1471, 1993.
18. Beby-Defaux, A., Frugier, F., Bourgoin, A., et al.: Nucleotide sequence analysis of human T-cell lymphotropic virus type I pX and LTR regions from patients with sicca syndrome. J. Med. Virol. *59*:245–255, 1999.
19. Beilke, M. A., Japa, S., and Vinson, D. G.: HTLV-I and HTLV-II virus expression increase with HIV-1 coinfection. J. Acquir. Immune Defic. Syndr. Hum. Retrovirol. *17*:391–397, 1998.
20. Berger, J. R., Svenningsson, A., Raffanti, S., and Resnick, L.: Tropical spastic paraparesis–like illness occurring in a patient dually infected with HIV-1 and HTLV-II. Neurology *41*:85–87, 1991.
21. Berneman, Z. N.: Meeting report: HTLV molecular biology and pathogenesis: Airlie Center, Warrenton, VA, USA, 17–19 March 2000. Leukemia *15*:647–654, 2001.
22. Berry, N., Ariyoshi, K., Balfe, P., et al.: Sequence specificity of the human immunodeficiency virus type 2 (HIV-2) long terminal repeat U3 region in vivo allows subtyping of the principal HIV-2 viral subtypes A and B. A. I. D. S. Res. Hum. Retroviruses *17*:263–267, 2001.
23. Berry, N., Ariyoshi, K., Jaffar, S., et al.: Low peripheral blood viral HIV-2 RNA in individuals with high CD4 percentage differentiates HIV-2 from HIV-1 infection. J. Hum. Virol. *1*:457–468, 1998.
24. Berry, N., Ariyoshi, K., Jobe, O., et al.: HIV type 1 proviral load measured by quantitative polymerase chain reaction correlates with CD4+ lymphopenia in HIV type 2 infected individuals. A. I. D. S. Res. Hum. Retroviruses *10*:1031–1037, 1994.
25. Bittencourt, A. L., Dourado, I., Filho, P. D., et al.: Human T-cell lymphotropic virus type I infection among pregnant women in northeast Brazil. J. Acquir. Immune Defic. Syndr. Hum. Retrovirol. *26*:490–494, 2001.
26. Blank, A., Herrera, M., Lourido, M. A., et al.: Infective dermatitis in Colombia. Lancet *346*:710, 1996.
27. Blattner, W., Saxinger, C., Riedel, D., et al.: A study of HTLV-I and its associated risk factors in Trinidad and Tobago. J. Acquir. Immune Defic. Syndr. *90*:1102–1108, 1990.
28. Bleul, C. C., Farzan, M., Choe, H., et al.: The lymphocyte chemoattractant SDF-1 is a ligand for LESTR/fusin and blocks HIV-1 entry. Nature *382*:829–833, 1996.
29. Bonis, J., Baillou, A., Barin, F., et al.: Discrimination between human T-cell lymphotropic virus type I and II (HTLV-I and HTLV-II) infections by using synthetic peptides representing an immunodominant region of the core protein (p19) of HTLV-I and HTLV-II. J. Clin. Microbiol. *31*:1481–1485, 1993.
30. Bonis, J., Verdier, M., Dumas, M., et al.: Low human T cell leukemia virus type II seroprevalence in Africa. J. Infect. Dis. *169*:225–227, 1994.
31. Bothe, K., Aguzzi, A., Lassmann, H., et al.: Progressive encephalopathy and myopathy in transgenic mice expressing human foamy virus genes. Science *253*:555–557, 1991.
32. Briggs, N. C., Battjes, R. J., Cantor, K. P., et al.: Seroprevalence of human T cell lymphotropic virus type II infection, with or without human immunodeficiency virus type 1 coinfection, among US drug users. J. Infect. Dis. *172*:51–58, 1995.
33. Calabró, M. L., Luparello, M., Grottola, A., et al.: Detection of human T lymphotropic virus type II/b in human immunodeficiency virus type 1–coinfected persons in southeastern Italy. J. Infect. Dis. *168*:1273–1277, 1993.
34. Caliendo, A. M.: Laboratory methods for quantitating HIV RNA. A. I. D. S. Clin. Care 7:89–93, 1995.
35. Casseb, J.: Is human T-cell lymphotropic virus type I more clever than human immunodeficiency virus type 1? Clin. Infect. Dis. *27*:1309–1310, 1998.

36. Cavaleiro, R., Sousa, A. E., Loureiro, A., and Victorino, R. M. M.: Marked immunosuppressive effects of the HIV-1 envelope protein in spite of lower HIV-2 pathogenicity. A. I. D. S. *14*:2679–2686, 2000.
37. Cavrois, M., Gessain, A., Gout, O., et al.: Common human T cell leukemia virus type 1 (HTLV-I) integration sites in cerebrospinal fluid and blood lymphocytes of patients with HTLV-I–associated myelopathy/tropical spastic paraparesis indicate that HTLV-I crosses the blood-brain barrier via clonal HTLV-I–infected cells. J. Infect. Dis. *182*:1044–1050, 2000.
38. Centers for Disease Control and Prevention: Human T-lymphotropic virus type I screening in volunteer blood donors—United States, 1989. M. M. W. R. Morb. Mortal. Wkly. Rep. *39*(50):915, 921–924, 1990.
39. Centers for Disease Control and Prevention: Testing for antibodies to human immunodeficiency virus type 2 in the United States. M. M. W. R. Recomm. Rep. *41*(RR-12):1–9, 1992.
40. Centers for Disease Control and Prevention: Update: HIV-2 infection among blood and plasma donors—United States, June 1992–June 1995. M. M. W. R. Morb. Mortal. Wkly. Rep. *44*(32):603–606, 1995.
41. Centers for Disease Control and Prevention: CDC update: Human immunodeficiency virus type 2. Atlanta, Centers for Disease Control and Prevention, 1998.
42. Centers for Disease Control and Prevention, U.S.P.H.S. Working Group: Guidelines for counseling persons infected with human T-lymphotropic virus type I (HTLV-I) and type II (HTLV-II). Ann. Intern. Med. *118*:448–454, 1993.
43. Cereseto, A., Mulloy, J.C., Granchini, G.: Insights on the pathogenicity of human T-lymphotropic/leukemia virus types I and II. J. Acquir. Immune Defic. Syndr. Hum. Retrovirol. *13*(Suppl 1):S69–S75, 1996.
44. Chen, M. Y., Maldarelli, F., Karczewski, M., et al.: Human immunodeficiency virus type 1 vpu protein induces degradation of CD4 *in vitro*: The cytoplasmic domain of CD4 contributes to vpu sensitivity. J. Virol. *67*:3877–3884, 1993.
45. Chen, Y.C., Wang, C.H., Su, J.J., et al.: Infection of human T-cell leukemia virus type I and development of human T-cell leukemia/lymphoma in patients with hematologic neoplasms: A possible linkage to blood transfusion. Blood *74*:388–394, 1989.
46. Cimarelli, A., Duclos, C. A., Gessain, A., et al.: Clonal expansion of human T-cell leukemia virus type II in patients with high proviral load. Virology *223*:362–364, 1996.
47. Cimarelli, A., Sandin, S., Hoglund, S., and Luban, J.: Basic residues in human immunodeficiency virus type 1 nucleocapsid promote virion assembly via interaction with RNA. J. Virol. *74*:3046–3057, 2000.
48. Clavel, F., Guyader, M., Guetard, D., et al.: Molecular cloning and polymorphism of the human immunodeficiency virus type 2. Nature *324*:691–695, 1986.
49. Clements, J. E., and Zink, M. C.: Molecular biology and pathogenesis of animal lentivirus infection. Clin. Microbiol. Rev. *9*:100–117, 1996.
50. Coffin, J. M., and Rosenberg, N.: Closing the joint. Nature *399*:413–415, 1999.
51. Cortes, E., Dietels, R., Aboulafia, D. M., et al.: HIV-1, HIV-2 and HTLV-I infection in high-risk groups in Brazil. N. Engl. J. Med. *320*:953–958, 1989.
52. Cox, S. W., Aperia, K., Albert, J., and Wahren, B.: Comparison of the sensitivities of primary isolates of HIV type 2 and HIV type 1 to antiviral drugs and drug combinations. A. I. D. S. Res. Hum. Retroviruses *10*:1725–1729, 1994.
53. Cullen, B. R.: Retroviruses as model systems for the study of nuclear RNA export pathways. Virology *249*:203–210, 1998.
54. Cullen, B. R., and Heitman, J.: Chaperoning a pathogen. Nature *372*:319–320, 1994.
55. Daenke, S., Kermonde, A., Hall, S. E., et al.: High activated and memory cytotoxic T-cell responses to HTLV-I in healthy carriers and patients with tropical spastic paraparesis. Virology *217*:139–146, 1996.
56. Damond, F., Apetrei, C., Robertson, D. L., et al.: Variability of human immunodeficiency virus type 2 (HIV-2) infecting patients living in France. Virology *280*:19–30, 2001.
57. Daniel, R., Katz, R. A., and Skalka, A. M.: A role for DNA-PK in retroviral DNA integration. Science *284*:644–647, 1999.
58. De Cock, K. M., Adjorlolo, G., Ekpini, E., et al.: Epidemiology and transmission of HIV-2: Why there is no HIV-2 pandemic. J. A. M. A. *270*:2083–2086, 1993.
59. De Cock, K. M., Zadi, F., Adjorlolo, G., et al.: Retrospective study of maternal HIV-1 and HIV-2 infections and child survival in Abidjan, Côte d'Ivoire. B. M. J. *308*:441–443, 1994.
60. Delamarre, L., Rosenberg, A. R., Pique, C., et al.: The HTLV-I envelope glycoproteins: Structure and function. J. Acquir. Immune Defic. Syndr. Hum. Retrovirol. *13*(Suppl. 1):85–91, 1996.
61. Delaporte, E., Buve, A., Nzila, N., et al.: HTLV-I infection among prostitutes and pregnant women in Kinshasa, Zaire: How important is high-risk sexual behavior? J. Acquir. Immune Defic. Syndr. Hum. Retrovirol. *8*:511–515, 1995.
62. Delaporte, E., Peeters, M., Bardy, J.-L., et al.: Blood transfusion as a major risk factor for HTLV-I infection among hospitalized children in Gabon (Equatorial Africa). J. Acquir. Immune Defic. Syndr. *6*:424–428, 1993.
63. Deng, H. K., Liu, R., Ellmeier, W., et al.: Identification of a major co-receptor for primary isolates of HIV-1. Nature *381*:661–666, 1996.
64. deShazo, R. D., Chadha, N., Morgan, J. E., et al.: Immunologic assessment of a cluster of asymptomatic HTLV-I–infected individuals in New Orleans. Am. J. Med. *86*:65–69, 1989.
65. de Thé, G., Giordano, C., Gessain, A., et al.: Human retroviruses HTLV-I, HIV-1, and HIV-2 and neurological diseases in some equatorial areas of Africa. J. Acquir. Immune Defic. Syndr. *2*:550–556, 1989.
66. Dixon, A. C., Kwock, D. W., Nakamura, J. M., et al.: Thrombotic thrombocytopenic purpura and human T-lymphotropic virus, type I (HTLV-I). Ann. Intern. Med. *100*:93–94, 1989.
67. Donegan, E., Lee, H., Operskalski, E. A., et al.: Transfusion transmission of retroviruses: Human T-lymphotropic virus types I and II compared with human immunodeficiency virus type 1. Transfusion *34*:478–483, 1994.
68. Dosik, H., Goldstein, M. F., Poiesz, B. J., et al.: Seroprevalence of human T-lymphotropic virus in blacks from a selected central Brooklyn population. Cancer Invest. *12*:289–295, 1994.
69. Dragic, T., Litwin, V., Allaway, G. P., et al.: HIV-1 entry into CD4(+) cells is mediated by the chemokine receptor CC-CKR-5. Nature *381*:667–673, 1996.
70. Eiraku, N., Novoa, P., da Costa Ferreira, M., et al.: Identification and characterization of a new and distinct molecular subtype of human T-cell lymphotropic virus type 2. J. Virol. *70*:1481–1492, 1996.
71. Ejima, E., Rosenblatt, J., Massari, M., et al.: Cell-type specific transactivation of the parathyroid hormone–related protein gene promoter by the human T-cell leukemia virus type I (HTLV-I) tax and HTLV-II tax proteins. Blood *81*:1017–1024, 1993.
72. Emerman, M., and Malim, M. H.: HIV-1 regulatory/accessory genes: Keys to unraveling viral and host biology. Science *280*:1880–1884, 1998.
73. Endres, M. J., Clapham, P. R., Marsh, M., et al.: CD4-independent infection by HIV-2 is mediated by fusin/CXCR-4. Cell *87*:745–756, 1996.
74. Etzel, A., Shibata, G. Y., Rozman, M., et al.: HTLV-1 and HTLV-2 infections in HIV-infected individuals from Santos, Brazil: Seroprevalence and risk factors. J. Acquir. Immune Defic. Syndr. Hum. Retrovirol. *26*:185–190, 2001.
75. Fantry, L., De Jonge, E., Auwaeter, P. G., et al.: Immunodeficiency and elevated CD4 T lymphocyte counts in two patients coinfected with human immunodeficiency virus and human lymphotropic virus type I. Clin. Infect. Dis. *21*:1466–1468, 1995.
76. Faye, A., Burgard, M., Crosnier, H., et al.: Human immunodeficiency virus type 2 infection in children. J. Pediatr. *130*:994–997, 1997.
77. Figueroa, J. P., Morris, J., Brathwaite, A., et al.: Risk factors for HTLV-I among heterosexual STD clinic attenders. J. Acquir. Immune Defic. Syndr. Hum. Retrovirol. *9*:81–88, 1995.
78. Fujino, T., Iwamoto, I., Otsuka, H., et al.: Apoptosis in placentas from human T-lymphotropic virus type I–seropositive pregnant women: A possible defense against transmission from mother to fetus. Obstet. Gynecol. *94*:279–283, 1999.
79. Flugel, R. M.: Spumaviruses: A group of complex retroviruses. J. Acquir. Immune Defic. Syndr. *4*:739–750, 1991.
80. Foil, L. D., and Issel, C. J.: Transmission of retroviruses by arthropods. Annu. Rev. Entomol. *36*:355–381, 1991.
81. Franke, E. K., Yuan, H. E. H., and Luban, J.: Specific incorporation of cyclophilin A into HIV-1 virions. Nature *372*:359–362, 1995.
82. Freed, E. O.: HIV-1 gag proteins: Diverse functions in the virus life cycle. Virology *251*:1–15, 1998.
83. Freed, E. O., and Martin, M. A.: Virion incorporation of envelope glycoproteins with long but not short cytoplasmic tails is blocked by specific, single amino acid substitutions in the human immunodeficiency virus type 1 matrix. J. Virol. *69*:1984–1989, 1995.
84. Freed, E. O., and Martin, M. A.: The role of human immunodeficiency virus type 1 envelope glycoprotein in virus infection. J. Biol. Chem. *270*:23883–23886, 1995.
85. Fujino, T., Fujiyoshi, T., Yashiki, S., et al.: HTLV-I transmission from mother to fetus via placenta. Lancet *340*:1157, 1992.
86. Fujino, T., Iwamoto, I., Otsuka, H., et al.: Apoptosis in placentas from human T-lymphotropic virus type I–seropositive pregnant women: A possible defense mechanism against transmission from mother to fetus. Obstet. Gynecol. *94*:279–283, 1999.
87. Funukawa, Y., Yamashita, M., Usuku, K., et al.: Phylogenetic subgroups of human T cell lymphotropic virus (HTLV) type I in the *tax* gene and their association with different risks for HTLV-I–associated myelopathy/tropical spastic paraparesis. J. Infect. Dis. *182*:1343–1349, 2000.
88. Furnia, A., Lal, R., Maloney, E., et al.: Estimating the time of HTLV-I infection following mother-to-child transmission in a breast-feeding population in Jamaica. J. Med. Virol. *59*:541–546, 1999.
89. Gabbai, A. A., Bordin, J. O., Vieira-Filho, J. B. P., et al.: Selectivity of human T-lymphotropic virus type-I (HTLV-1) and HTLV-2 among different populations in Brazil. Am. J. Trop. Med. Hyg. *49*:664–671, 1993.
90. Gallo, D., Petru, A., Yeh, E. T., et al.: No evidence of perinatal transmission of HTLV-II. J. Acquir. Immune Defic. Syndr. *6*:1168–1170, 1993.
91. Gallo, R. C.: Human retroviruses: A decade of discovery and link with human disease. J. Infect. Dis. *164*:235–243, 1991.

92. Gayle, H. D., Gnaore, E., Adjorlolo, G., et al.: HIV-1 and HIV-2 infection in children in Abidjan, Cote d'Ivoire. J. Acquir. Immune Defic. Syndr. *5*:513–517, 1992.
93. George, J. R., Ou, C.-Y., Parekh, B., et al.: Prevalence of HIV-1 and HIV-2 mixed infections in Cote d'Ivoire. Lancet *340*:337–339, 1992.
94. Geraghty, R., and Panganiban, A.: Human immunodeficiency virus type 1 vpu has a CD4- and an envelope glycoprotein-independent function. J. Virol. *67*:4190–4194, 1993.
95. Gessain, A., Barin, F., Vernant, J. C., et al.: Antibodies to human T-lymphotropic virus type-1 in patients with tropical spastic paraparesis. Lancet *2*:407–410, 1985.
96. Gessain, A., and de Thè, G.: Geographic and molecular epidemiology of primate T lymphotropic retroviruses: HTLV-I, HTLV-II, STLV-PP, and PTLV-L. Adv. Virus Res. *47*:377–426, 1996.
97. Gessain, A., and Gout, O.: Chronic myelopathy associated with human T-lymphotropic virus type I (HTLV-I). Ann. Intern. Med. *117*:933–946, 1992.
98. Ghosh, S. K., Abrams, J. T., Terunuma, H., et al.: Human T-cell leukemia virus type 1 *tax/rex* DNA and RNA in cutaneous T-cell lymphoma. Blood *84*:2663–2671, 1994.
99. Gill, P. S., Harrington, W., Kaplan, M. H., et al.: Treatment of adult T-cell leukemia-lymphoma with a combination of interferon alpha and zidovudine. N. Engl. J. Med. *332*:1744–1748, 1995.
100. Giuliani, M., Rezza, G., Lepri, A. C., et al.: Risk factors for HTLV-I and II in individuals attending a clinic for sexually transmitted diseases. Sex. Transm. Dis. *27*:87–92, 2000.
101. Gottuzzo, E., Sanchez, J., Escamilla, J., et al.: Human T cell lymphotropic virus type 1 infection among female sex workers in Peru. J. Infect. Dis. *169*:754–759, 1994.
102. Gout, O., Baulac, M., Gessain, A., et al.: Rapid development of myelopathy after HTLV-I infection acquired by transfusion during cardiac transplantation. N. Engl. J. Med. *322*:383–388, 1990.
103. Gout, O., Gessain, A., Iba-Zizen, M., et al.: The effect of zidovudine on chronic myelopathy associated with HTLV-1. J. Neurol. *238*:108–109, 1991.
104. Green, J. E., Hinrichs, S. H., Vogel, J., and Jay, G.: Exocrinopathy resembling Sjögren's syndrome in HTLV-I *tax* transgenic mice. Nature *341*:72–74, 1989.
105. Greene, W. C.: The molecular biology of human immunodeficiency virus type 1 infection. N. Engl. J. Med. *324*:308–317, 1991.
106. Hahn, B. H.: Viral genes and their products. *In* Broder, S., Merigan, T. C., Jr., and Bolognesi, D. (eds.): Textbook of AIDS Medicine. Baltimore, Williams & Wilkins, 1994, pp. 21–43.
107. Hall, W. W., Ishak, R., Zhu, S. W., et al.: Human T lymphotropic virus type II (HTLV-II): Epidemiology, molecular properties and clinical features of infection. J. Acquir. Immune Defic. Syndr. Hum. Retrovirol. *13*(Suppl. 1):204–214, 1996.
108. Hall, W. W., Liu, C. R., Schneewind, O., et al.: Deleted HTLV-I provirus in blood and cutaneous lesions of patients with mycosis fungoides. Science *253*:317–320, 1991.
109. Hanchard, B., La Grenade, L., Carberry, C., et al.: Childhood infective dermatitis evolving into adult T-cell leukemia after 17 years. Lancet *338*:1593–1594, 1991.
110. Hannibal, M. C., Markovitz, D. M., Clark, N., and Nabel, G. J.: Differential activation of human immunodeficiency virus type 1 and type 2 transcription by specific T-cell activation signals. J. Virol. *67*:5035–5040, 1993.
111. Harouse, J. M., Bhat, S., Spitalnik, S. L., et al.: Inhibition of entry of HIV-1 into neural cell lines by antibodies against galactosyl ceramide. Science *253*:320–323, 1991.
112. Harrington, W. J., Shermata, W., Hjelle, B., et al.: Spastic ataxia associated with human T-cell lymphotropic virus type II infection. Ann. Neurol. *33*:411–414, 1993.
113. Harrington, W. J., Ucar, A., Gill, P., et al.: Clinical spectrum of HTLV-I in South Florida. J. Acquir. Immune Defic. Syndr. Hum. Retrovirol. *8*:466–473, 1995.
114. Harrison, L. H., Quinn, T. C., and Schechter, M.: Human T cell lymphotropic virus type I does not increase human immunodeficiency virus viral load in vivo. J. Infect. Dis. *175*:438–440, 1997.
115. Heinzinger, N. K., Bukrinsky, M. I., Haggerty, S. A., et al.: The vpr protein of human immunodeficiency virus type 1 influences nuclear localization of viral nucleic acids in nondividing cells. Proc. Natl. Acad. Sci. U. S. A. *91*:7311–7315, 1994.
116. Heneine, W., Chan, W. C., Lust, J. A., et al.: HTLV-II infection is rare in patients with large granular lymphocyte leukemia. J. Acquir. Immune Defic. Syndr. *7*:736–737, 1994.
117. Heneine, W., Kaplan, J. E., Gracia, F., et al.: HTLV-II endemicity among Guyami Indians in Panama. N. Engl. J. Med. *324*:565, 1991.
118. Heneine, W., Woods, T., Green, D., et al.: Detection of HTLV-II in breastmilk of HTLV-II infected mothers. Lancet *340*:1157–1158, 1992.
119. Hermine, O., Bouscary, D., Gessain, A., et al.: Treatment of adult-T-cell leukemia-lymphoma with zidovudine and interferon alfa. N. Engl. J. Med. *332*:1749–1751, 1995.
120. Higuchi, I., Hashimoto, K., Matsuoka, E., et al.: The main HTLV-I–harboring cells in the muscles of viral carriers with polymyositis are not macrophages but CD4+ lymphocytes. Acta Neuropathol. *92*:358–361, 1996.
121. Hino, S., Katamine, S., Miyamoto, T., et al.: Association between maternal antibodies to the external envelope glycoprotein and vertical transmission of human T-lymphotropic virus type I—maternal anti-env antibodies correlate with protection in non–breast-fed children. J. Clin. Invest. *95*:2920–2925, 1995.
122. Hino, S., Katamine, S., Miyata, H., et al.: Primary prevention of HTLV-I in Japan. J. Acquir. Immune Defic. Syndr. Hum. Retrovirol. *13*(Suppl. 1):199–203, 1996.
123. Hino, S., Yamaguchi, K., Katamine, S., et al.: Mother-to-child transmission of human T-cell leukemia virus type-I. Jpn. J. Cancer Res. *76*:474–480, 1985.
124. Hirata, M., Hayashi, J., Noguchi, A., et al.: The effects of breastfeeding and presence of antibody to p40tax protein of human T cell lymphotropic virus type I on mother to child transmission. Int. J. Epidemiol. *21*:989–994, 1992.
125. Hisada, M., Okayama, A., Shiryo, S., et al.: Risk factors for adult T-cell leukemia among carriers of human T-lymphotropic virus type I. Blood *92*:3557–3561, 1998.
126. Hisada, M., Okayama, A., Spiegelman, D., et al.: Sex-specific mortality from adult T-cell leukemia among carriers of human T-lymphotropic virus type I. Int. J. Cancer *91*:497–499, 2001.
127. Hjelle, B., Appenzeller, O., Mills, R., et al.: Chronic neurodegenerative disease associated with HTLV-II infection. Lancet *339*:645–646, 1992.
128. Hjelle, B., Khabbaz, R. F., Conway, G. A., et al.: Prevalence of human T-cell lymphotropic virus type II in American Indian populations of the southwestern United States. Am. J. Trop. Med. Hyg. *51*:11–15, 1994.
129. Hjelle, B., Mills, R., Swenson, S., et al.: Incidence of hairy cell leukemia, mycosis fungoides and chronic lymphocytic leukemia in first known HTLV-II–endemic population. J. Infect. Dis. *163*:435–440, 1991.
130. Hjelle, B., Scalf, R., and Swenson, S.: High frequency of human T-cell leukemia-lymphoma virus type II infection in New Mexico blood donors: Determination by sequence-specific oligonucleotide hybridization. Blood *76*:450–454, 1990.
131. Hjelle, B., Zhu, S. W., Takahashi, H., et al.: Endemic human T cell leukemia virus type II infection in southwestern U.S. Indians involves two prototype variants of virus. J. Infect. Dis. *168*:737–740, 1993.
132. Ho, D. D., Neumann, A. U., Perelson, A. S., et al.: Rapid turnover of plasma virions and CD4 lymphocytes in HIV-1 infection. Nature *373*:123–126, 1995.
133. Ho, G. Y. F., Nomura, A. M. Y., Nelson, K., et al.: Declining seroprevalence and transmission of HTLV-I in Japanese families who immigrated to Hawaii. Am. J. Epidemiol. *134*:981–987, 1991.
134. Höllsberg, P., and Hafler, D. A.: Pathogenesis of diseases induced by human lymphotropic virus type I infection. N. Engl. J. Med. *328*:1173–1182, 1993.
135. Ijichi, S., and Osame, M.: Human T lymphotropic virus type I (HTLV-I)-associated myelopathy/tropical spastic paraparesis (HAM/TSP): Recent perspectives. Intern. Med. *34*:713–721, 1995.
136. Ijichi, S., Ramundo, M. B., Takahashi, H., et al.: In vivo cellular tropism of human T cell leukemia virus type II. J. Exp. Med. *176*:293–296, 1992.
137. Ishihara, S., Okayama, A., Stuver, S., et al.: Association of HTLV-I antibody profile of asymptomatic carriers with proviral DNA levels in peripheral blood mononuclear cells. J. Acquir. Immune Defic. Syndr. *7*:199–203, 1994.
138. Iwakura, Y., Tosu, M., Yoshida, E., et al.: Induction of inflammatory arthropathy resembling rheumatoid arthritis in mice transgenic for HTLV-I. Science *253*:1026–1028, 1991.
139. Izumo, S., Umehara, F., Kashio, N., et al.: Neuropathology of HTLV-I–associated myelopathy (HAM/TSP). Leukemia *22*(Suppl. 3):82–84, 1997.
140. Jacobson, S., McFarlin, D. E., Robinson, S., et al.: HTLV-I–specific cytotoxic T lymphocytes in the cerebrospinal fluid of patients with HTLV-I–associated neurological disease. Ann. Neurol. *32*:651–657, 1992.
141. Jacobson, S., Shida, H., McFarlin, D. E., et al.: Circulating CD8+ cytotoxic T lymphocytes specific for HTLV-I pX in patients with HTLV-I–associated neurological disease. Nature *348*:245–248, 1990.
142. Jaffar, S., Wilkins, A., Ngom, T., et al.: Rate of decline of percentage CD4+ cells is faster in HIV-1 than in HIV-2 infection. J. Acquir. Immune Defic. Syndr. Hum. Retrovirol. *16*:327–332, 1997.
143. Jeffrey, K. J., Usuku, K., Hall, S. E., et al.: HLA alleles determine human T-lymphotropic virus-I (HTLV-I) proviral load and the risk of HTLV-I–associated myelopathy. Proc. Natl. Acad. Sci. U. S. A. *96*:3848–3853, 1999.
144. Johnson, M. A., and Cann, A. J.: Molecular determination of cell tropism of human immunodeficiency virus. Clin. Infect. Dis. *14*:747–755, 1992.
145. Kajiyama, W., Kashiwagi, S., Ikematsu, H., et al.: Intrafamilial transmission of adult T cell leukemia virus. J. Infect. Dis. *154*:851–857, 1986.
146. Kalyanaraman, V. S., Sarngadharan, M. G., Robert-Guroff, M., et al.: A new subtype of human T-cell leukemia virus (HTLV-II) associated with a T-cell variant of hairy cell leukemia. Science *218*:571–573, 1982.

147. Kanki, P. J., Travers, K. U., MBoup, S., et al.: Slower heterosexual spread of HIV-2 than HIV-1. Lancet *343*:943–946, 1994.
148. Kannagi, M., Matsushita, S., Shida, H., and Harada, S.: Cytotoxic T cell response and expression of the target antigen in HTLV-I infection. Leukemia *8*(Suppl.):54–59, 1994.
149. Kaplan, J. E., Abrams, E., Shaffer, N., et al.: Low risk of mother-to-child transmission of human T lymphotropic virus type II in non–breast fed infants. J. Infect. Dis. *166*:892–895, 1992.
150. Kaplan, J. E., Khabbaz, R. F., Murphy, E. L., et al.: Male-to-female transmission of human T-cell lymphotropic virus types I and II: Association with viral load. J. Acquir. Immune Defic. Syndr. Hum. Retrovirol. *12*:193–201, 1996.
151. Kaplan, M. H., Hall, W. W., and Susin, M.: Syndrome of severe skin disease, eosinophilia, and dermatopathic lymphadenopathy in patients with HTLV-II complicating human immunodeficiency virus infection. Am. J. Med. *91*:300–309, 1991.
152. Kashiwagi, S., Kajiyama, W., Hayashi, J., et al.: Antibody to p40tax protein of human T cell leukemia virus I and infectivity. J. Infect. Dis. *161*:426–429, 1990.
153. Kassim, S., Sassan-Morokro, M., Ackah, A., et al.: Two-year follow-up of persons with HIV-1– and HIV-2–associated pulmonary tuberculosis treated with short-course chemotherapy in West Africa. A. I. D. S. *9*:1185–1191, 1995.
154. Katamine, S., Moriuchi, R., Yamamoto, T., et al.: HTLV-I proviral DNA in umbilical cord blood of babies born to carrier mothers. Lancet *343*:1326–1327, 1994.
155. Khabbaz, R. F., Onorato, I. M., Cannon, R. O., et al.: Seroprevalence of HTLV-I and HTLV-II among intravenous drug users and persons in clinics for sexually transmitted diseases. N. Engl. J. Med. *326*:375–380, 1992.
156. Kinoshita, K., Hino, S., Amagasaki, T., et al.: Demonstration of adult T cell leukemia virus antigen in milk from three seropositive mothers. Jpn. J. Cancer Res. *75*:103–105, 1984.
157. Kinoshita, K., Yamanouchi, K., Ikeda, S., et al.: Oral infection of a common marmoset with human T cell leukemia virus type I (HTLV-I) by inoculating fresh human milk of HTLV-I carrier mothers. Jpn. J. Cancer Res. *76*:1147–1153, 1985.
158. Kitajima, I., Yamamoto, K., Sato, K., et al.: Detection of human T cell lymphotropic virus type I proviral DNA and its gene expression in synovial cells in chronic inflammatory arthropathy. J. Clin. Invest. *88*:1315–1322, 1991.
159. Kokkotou, E. G., Sankalé, J.-L., Mani, I., et al.: In vitro correlates of HIV-2–mediated HIV-1 protection. Proc. Natl. Acad. Sci. U. S. A. *97*:6797–6802, 2000.
160. Kramer, A., Jacobsen, S., Reuben, J., et al.: Spontaneous lymphocyte proliferation in symptom-free HTLV-I positive Jamaicans. Lancet *2*:923–924, 1989.
161. Kubota, T., Morishita, N., Tanaka, Y., et al.: Establishment of novel lymphoid cell lines dually infected with human T cell lymphotropic viruses types I and II. J. Infect. Dis. *172*:220–224, 1995.
162. La Grenade, L.: HTLV-I-associated infective dermatitis: Past, present and future. J. Acquir. Immune Defic. Syndr. Hum. Retrovirol. *13*(Suppl. 1):46–49, 1996.
163. La Grenade, L., Hanchard, B., Fletcher, V., et al.: Infective dermatitis of Jamaican children: A marker for HTLV-I infection. Lancet *336*:1345–1347, 1990.
164. La Grenade, L., Manns, A., Fletcher, V., et al.: Clinical, pathologic, and immunologic features of human T-lymphotropic virus type 1–associated infective dermatitis in children. Arch. Dermatol. *134*:439–444, 1998.
165. La Grenade, L., Morgan, C., Carberry, C., et al.: Tropical spastic paraparesis occurring in HTLV-I–associated infective dermatitis: Report of two cases. West Indian Med. J. *44*:34–35, 1995.
166. La Grenade, L., Sonoda, S., Miller, W., et al.: HLA DRB1*DQB1* haplotype in HTLV-I–associated familial infective dermatitis may predict development of HTLV-I–associated myelopathy/tropical spastic paraparesis. Am. J. Med. Genet. *61*:37–41, 1996.
167. Lal, R. B., Gongora-Biachi, R. A., Pardi, D., et al.: Evidence for mother-to-child transmission of human T lymphotropic virus type II. J. Infect. Dis. *168*:586–591, 1993.
168. Lal, R. B., Owen, S. M., Rudolph, D. L., et al.: In vivo cellular tropism of human T lymphotropic virus type II is not restricted to CD8+ cells. Virology *210*:41–47, 1995.
169. Lal, R. B., Owen, S. M., Segurado, A. A. C., et al.: Mother-to-child transmission of human T-lymphotropic virus type II (HTLV-II). Ann. Intern. Med. *120*:300–301, 1994.
170. Levin, M. C., Lehky, T. J., Flerlage, A. N., et al.: Immunologic analysis of a spinal cord-biopsy specimen from a patient with human T-cell lymphotropic virus type I–associated neurologic disease. N. Engl. J. Med. *336*:839–845, 1997.
171. Levine, P. H., Cleghorn, F. R., Manns, A., et al.: Adult T-cell leukemia/lymphoma: A working point-score classification for epidemiologic studies. Int. J. Cancer *59*:491–493, 1994.
172. Levine, P. H., Dosik, H., Joseph, E. M., et al.: A study of adult T-cell leukemia/lymphoma incidence in Central Brooklyn. Int. J. Cancer *80*:662–666, 1999.
173. Levine, P. H., Jacobson, S., Elliott, R., et al.: HTLV-II infection in Florida Indians. A. I. D. S. Res. Hum. Retroviruses *9*:123–127, 1993.
174. Levy, D., Fernandes, L., Williams, W., et al.: Induction of cell differentiation by human immunodeficiency virus 1 vpr. Cell *72*:541–550, 1993.
175. Linial, M.: Foamy viruses are unconventional retroviruses. J. Virol. *73*:1747–1755, 1999.
176. Linial, M.: Why aren't foamy viruses pathogenic? Trends Microbiol. *8*:284–289, 2000.
177. Liu, X. D., and Ebbesen, P.: In vitro HTLV-I transfer to human trophoblast cells: Implications for transplacental passage. Abstract. J. Acquir. Immune Defic. Syndr. Hum. Retrovirol. *10*:263, 1995.
178. Loughran, T. P., Jr., Coyle, T., Sherman, M. P., et al.: Detection of human T-cell leukemia/lymphoma virus type II in a patient with large granular lymphocyte leukemia. Blood *80*:1116–1169, 1992.
179. Love, J. L., Marchioli, C. C., Dube, S., et al.: Expansion of clonotypic T-cell populations in peripheral blood of asymptomatic Gran Chaco Amerindians infected with HTLV-IIB. J. Acquir. Immune Defic. Syndr. Hum. Retrovirol. *18*:178–185, 1998.
180. Lymphoma Study Group: Major prognostic factors of patients with adult T-cell leukemia-lymphoma: A cooperative study. Leuk. Res. *15*:81–90, 1991.
181. Mahieux, R., Pise-Masison, C. A., Lambert, P. F., et al.: Differences in the ability of human T-cell lymphotropic virus type 1 (HTLV-1) and HTLV-2 to inhibit p53 function. J. Virol. *74*:6866–6874, 2000.
182. Maloney, E. M., Armien, B., Gracia, F., et al.: Risk factors for human T cell lymphotropic virus type II infection among the Guaymi Indians of Panama. J. Infect. Dis. *180*:876–879, 1999.
183. Maloney, E. M., Biggar, R. J., Neel, J. V., et al.: Endemic human T cell lymphotropic virus type II infection among isolated Brazilian Amerindians. J. Infect. Dis. *166*:100–107, 1992.
184. Maloney, E. M., Cleghorn, F. R., St. Claire Morgan, O., et al.: Incidence of HTLV-I–associated myelopathy/tropical spastic paraparesis (HAM/TSP) in Jamaica and Trinidad. J. Acquir. Immune Defic. Syndr. Hum. Retrovirol. *17*:167–170, 1998.
185. Maloney, E. M., Hisada, M., Palmer, P., et al.: Human T cell lymphotropic virus type I–associated infective dermatitis in Jamaica: A case report of clinical and biologic correlates. Pediatr. Infect. Dis. J. *19*:560–565, 2000.
186. Maloney, E. M., Murphy, E. L., Figueroa, J. P., et al.: Human T-lymphotropic virus type I (HTLV-I) seroprevalence in Jamaica. II. Geographic and ecologic determinants. Am. J. Epidemiol. *133*:1125–1134, 1991.
187. Maloney, E. M., Pate, E., Wiktor, S. Z., et al.: The relative distribution of T cell subsets is altered in Jamaican children infected with human T cell lymphotropic virus type I. J. Infect. Dis. *172*:867–870, 1995.
188. Maloney, E. M., Wiktor, S. Z., Pate, E. J., et al.: HTLV-I titers in children are associated with maternal titers. Abstract. J. Acquir. Immune Defic. Syndr. Hum. Retrovirol. *10*:259, 1995.
189. Manns, A., Cleghorn, F. R., Falk, R. T., et al.: Role of HTLV-I in development of non-Hodgkin lymphoma in Jamaica and Trinidad and Tobago. Lancet *342*:1447–1450, 1993.
190. Manns, A., Hisada, M., La Grenade, L.: Human T-lymphotropic virus type 1 infection. Lancet *353*:1951–1958, 1999.
191. Manns, A., Miley, W. J., Wilks, R. J., et al.: Quantitative proviral DNA and antibody levels in the natural history of HTLV-I infection. J. Infect. Dis. *180*:1487–1493, 1999.
192. Mansky, L. M.: In vivo analysis of human T-cell leukemia virus type 1 reverse transcription accuracy. J. Virol. *74*:9525–9531, 2000.
193. Markovitz, D. M.: Infection with the human immunodeficiency virus type 2. Ann. Intern. Med. *118*:211–218, 1993.
194. Marlink, R.: Lessons from the second AIDS virus, HIV-2. A. I. D. S. *10*:689–699, 1996.
195. Marlink, R., Kanki, P., Thior, I., et al.: Reduced rate of disease development after HIV-2 infection as compared to HIV-1. Science *265*:1587–1590, 1994.
196. Marsh, B. J.: Infectious complications of human T cell leukemia/lymphoma virus type I infection. J. Infect. Dis. *23*:138–145, 1996.
197. Martin, M. P., Biggar, R. J., Hamlin-Greer, G., et al.: Large granular lymphocytosis in a patient infected with HTLV-II. A. I. D. S. Res. Hum. Retroviruses *9*:715–719, 1993.
198. Matutes, E., Schulz, T., Andrada Serpa, M. J., et al.: Report of the second international symposium on HTLV in Brazil. Leukemia *8*:1092–1094, 1994.
199. McArthur, J. C., Griffen, J. W., Cornblath, D. R., et al.: Steroid responsive myeloneuropathy in a man dually infected with HIV-1 and HTLV-I. Neurology *40*:938–944, 1990.
200. Michel, P., Balde, A. T., Roussilhon, C., et al.: Reduced immune activation and T cell apoptosis in human immunodeficiency virus type 2 compared to type 1: Correlation of T cell apoptosis with beta-2-microglobulin concentration and disease evolution. J. Infect. Dis. *181*:64–75, 2000.
201. Miller, G. J., Lewis, L. L., Colman, S. M., et al.: Clustering of human T lymphotropic virus type I seropositivity in Monserrat, West Indies: Evidence for an environmental factor in transmission of the virus. J. Infect. Dis. *170*:44–50, 1994.

202. Miller, M. E. Y., Shah, D. J., Barton, E. N., et al.: Human T-cell lymphotropic virus-1–associated renal disease in Jamaican children. Pediatr. Nephrol. *16*:51–56, 2001.
203. Miller, R. J., Cairns, J. S., Bridges, S., and Sarver, N.: Human immunodeficiency virus and AIDS: Insights from animal lentiviruses. J. Virol. *74*:7187–7195, 2000.
204. Miura, T., Fukunaga, T., Igarashi, T., et al.: Phylogenetic subtypes of human T-lymphotropic virus type I and their relations to the anthropological background. Proc. Natl. Acad. Sci. U. S. A. *91*:1124–1127, 1994.
205. Mochizuki, M., Tajima, K., Watanabe, T., and Yamaguchi, K.: Human T lymphotropic virus type 1 uveitis. Br. J. Ophthalmol. *78*:149–154, 1994.
206. Mochizuki, M., Watanabe, T., Yamaguchi, K., et al.: Uveitis associated with human T-cell lymphotropic virus type 1. Am. J. Ophthalmol. *114*:123–129, 1992.
207. Mochizuki, M., Watanabe, T., Yamaguchi, K., et al.: Uveitis associated with human T-lymphotropic virus type I: Seroepidemiological, clinical and virological studies. J. Infect. Dis. *166*:943–944, 1992.
208. Modahl, L. E., Young, K. C., Varney, K. F., et al.: Are HTLV-II seropositive injection drug users at increased risk of bacterial pneumonia, abscess, and lymphadenopathy? J. Acquir. Immune Defic. Syndr. Hum. Retrovirol. *16*:169–175, 1997.
209. Morgan, G., Wilkins, H. A., Pepin, J., et al.: AIDS following mother-to-child transmission of HIV-2. AIDS *4*:879–882, 1990.
210. Morgan, O., Rodgers-Johnson, P., Mora, C., and Char, G.: HTLV-I and polymyositis in Jamaica. Lancet *2*:1184–1187, 1989.
211. Morishita, N., Ishii, K., Tanaka, Y., et al.: Immunoglobulin prophylaxis against human T cell lymphotropic virus type II in rabbits. J. Infect. Dis. *169*:620–623, 1994.
212. Moriuchi, M., Inoue, H., and Moriuchi, H.: Reciprocal interactions between human T-lymphotropic virus type 1 and prostaglandins: Implications for viral transmission. J. Virol. *75*:192–198, 2001.
213. Mörner, A., Björndal, A., Albert, J., et al.: Primary human immunodeficiency virus type 2 (HIV-2) isolates, like HIV-1 isolates, frequently use CCR5 but show promiscuity in coreceptor use. J. Virol. *73*:2343–2349, 1999.
214. Mortreux, F., Kazanji, M., Gabet, A.-S., et al.: Two-step nature of human T-cell leukemia virus type 1 replication in experimentally infected squirrel monkeys *(Saimiri sciureus)*. J. Virol. *75*:1083–1089, 2001.
215. Mortreux, F., Leclercq, I., Gabet, A.-S., et al.: Somatic mutation in human T-cell leukemia virus type I provirus and flanking cellular sequences during clonal expansion in vivo. J. Natl. Cancer Inst. *93*:367–377, 2001.
216. Mulder, D. W., Nunn, A. J., Kamabi, A., et al.: Two year HIV-1 associated mortality in a Ugandan rural population. Lancet *343*:1021–1023, 1994.
217. Murphy, E. L.: Clinical epidemiology of human T-lymphotropic virus type II (HTLV-II). J. Acquir. Immune Defic. Syndr. Hum. Retrovirol. *13*(Suppl. 1):215–219, 1996.
218. Murphy, E. L., Calisher, C. H., Figueroa, J. P., et al.: HTLV-I infection and arthropod vectors. N. Engl. J. Med. *320*:1146, 1989.
219. Murphy, E. L., Engstrom, J. W., Miller, K., et al.: HTLV-II associated myelopathy in a 43 year old woman. Lancet *371*:757–758, 1993.
220. Murphy, E. L., Figueroa, J. P., Gibbs, W. N., et al.: Human T-lymphotropic virus type I (HTLV-I) seroprevalence in Jamaica. I. Demographic determinants. Am. J. Epidemiol. *133*:1114–1124, 1991.
221. Murphy, E. L., Glynn, S. A., Fridey, J., et al.: Increased prevalence of infectious diseases and other adverse outcomes in human T-lymphotropic virus types I– and II–infected blood donors. J. Infect. Dis. *176*:1468–1475, 1997.
222. Murphy, E. L., Glynn, S. A., Fridey, J., et al.: Increased incidence of infectious diseases during prospective follow-up of human T-lymphotropic virus type II– and I–infected blood donors. Arch. Intern. Med. *159*:485–491, 1999.
223. Murphy, E. L., Glynn, S., Watanabe, K., et al.: Laboratory test differences associated with HTLV-I and HTLV-II infection. J. Acquir. Immune Defic. Syndr. Hum. Retrovirol. *17*:332–338, 1998.
224. Murphy, E. L., Hanchard, B., Figueroa, J. P., et al.: Modelling the risk of adult T-cell leukemia/lymphoma in persons infected with human T-lymphotropic virus type I. Int. J. Cancer *43*:250–252, 1989.
225. Murphy, E. L., Watanabe, K., Nass, C. C., et al.: Evidence among blood donors for a 30-year-old epidemic of human T lymphotropic virus type II infection in the United States. J. Infect. Dis. *180*:1777–1783, 1999.
226. Myoshi, I., Yoshimoto, S., Ohtsuki, Y., et al.: Adult T-cell leukemia antigen in renal glomerulus. Lancet *1*:768–769, 1983.
227. Nagai, M., Kubota, R., Greten, T. F., et al.: Increased activated human T cell lymphotropic virus type I (HTLV-I) Tax11-19–specific memory and effector CD8+ cells in patients with HTLV-I–associated myelopathy/tropical spastic paraparesis: Correlation with HTLV-I provirus load. J. Infect. Dis. *183*:197–205, 2001.
228. Nagai, M., Usuku, K., Matsumoto, W., et al.: Analysis of HTLV-I proviral load in 202 HAM/TSP patients and 243 asymptomatic HTLV-I carriers: High proviral load strongly predisposes to HAM/TSP. J. Neurovirol. *4*:586–593, 1998.
229. Nagamine, M., Nakashima, Y., Uemura, S., et al.: DNA amplification of human T lymphotropic virus type I (HTLV-I) proviral DNA in breast milk of HTLV-I carriers. J. Infect. Dis. *164*:1024–1025, 1991.
230. Nakamura, T.: Immunopathogenesis of HTLV-I–associated myelopathy/tropical spastic paraparesis. Ann. Med. *32*:600–607, 2000.
231. Nakao, K., and Ohba, N.: Clinical features of HTLV-I–associated uveitis. Br. J. Ophthalmol. *77*:274–279, 1993.
232. Nakashima, K., Kashiwagi, S., Kajiyama, W., et al.: Sexual transmission of human T-lymphotropic virus type I among female prostitutes and among patients with sexually transmitted diseases in Fukuoka, Kyushu, Japan. Am. J. Epidemiol. *141*:305–311, 1995.
233. Neoh, L. P., Akimoto, H., Kaneko, H., et al.: The production of beta-chemokines induced by HIV-2 envelope glycoprotein. A. I. D. S. *11*:1062–1063, 1997.
234. Nishioka, K., Nakajima, T., Hasanama, T., et al.: Rheumatic manifestations of human leukemic virus infection. Rheum. Dis. Clin. North Am. *19*:489–503, 1993.
235. Norkin, L. C.: Virus receptors: Implications for pathogenesis and design of antiviral agents. Clin. Microbiol. Rev. *8*:293–315, 1995.
236. Norrgren, H., Andersson, S., Biague, A. J., et al.: Trends and interaction of HIV-1 and HIV-2 in Guinea-Bissau, West Africa: No protection of HIV-2 against HIV-1 infection. A. I. D. S. *13*:701–707, 1999.
237. Norrgren, H., Fonseca, A., Andersson, S., et al.: Child survival in children born to HIV-2 infected women in Guinea-Bissau, West Africa. Acta Trop. *72*:309–315, 1999.
238. Norrgren, H., Marquina, S., Leitner, T., et al.: HIV-2 genetic variation and DNA load in asymptomatic carriers and AIDS cases in Guinea-Bissau. J. Acquir. Immune Defic. Syndr. Hum. Retrovirol. *16*:31–38, 1997.
239. Nowak, M. A.: AIDS pathogenesis: From models to viral dynamics in patients. J. Acquir. Immune Defic. Syndr. Hum. Retrovirol. *10*(Suppl. 1):1–5, 1995.
240. Nyambi, P. N., Ville, Y., Louwagie, J., et al.: Mother to child transmission of human T-cell lymphotropic virus types I and II (HTLV-I/II) in Gabon: A prospective follow-up of 4 years. J. Acquir. Immune Defic. Syndr. Hum. Retrovirol. *12*:187–192, 1996.
241. Oberlin, E., Amara, A., Bachelerie, F., et al.: The CXC chemokine SDF-1 is the ligand for LESTR/fusin and prevents infection by T-cell-line–adapted HIV-1. Nature *382*:833–835, 1996.
242. O'Brien, T. R., George, J. R., and Holmberg, S. D.: Human immunodeficiency virus type 2 infection in the United States: Epidemiology, diagnosis and public health implications. J. A. M. A. *267*:2775–2779, 1992.
243. O'Donovan, D., Airyoshi, K., Milligan, P., et al.: Maternal plasma viral RNA levels determine marked differences in mother-to-child transmission rates of HIV-1 and HIV-2 in the Gambia. A. I. D. S. *14*:441–448, 2000.
244. Ohashi, T., Hanabuchi, S., Kato, H., et al.: Prevention of adult T-cell leukemia–like lymphoproliferative disease in rats by adoptively transferred T cells from a donor immunized with human T-cell leukemia virus type I Tax-coding DNA vaccine. J. Virol. *74*:9610–9616, 2000.
245. Okayama, A., Stuver, S., Iga, M., et al.: Sequential change of virus markers in seroconverters with community-acquired infection of human T lymphotropic virus type I. J. Infect. Dis. *183*:1031–1037, 2001.
246. Okochi, K., Sato, H., and Hinuma, Y.: A retrospective study on transmission of adult T cell leukemia virus by blood transfusion: Seroconversion in recipients. Vox Sang. *46*:245–253, 1984.
247. Oksenberg, J. R., Mantegazza, R., Kakai, K., et al.: HTLV-I sequences are not detected in peripheral blood genomic DNA or in brain cDNA of multiple sclerosis patients. Ann. Neurol. *28*:574–577, 1990.
248. Osame, M., Janssen, R., Kubota, H., et al.: Nationwide survey of HTLV-I–associated myelopathy in Japan: Association with blood transfusion. Ann. Neurol. *28*:50–56, 1990.
249. Osame, M., Usuku, K., Izumo, S., et al.: HTLV-I– associated myelopathy, a new clinical entity. Lancet *1*:1031–1032, 1986.
250. Ota, M. O. C., O'Donovan, D., Alabi, A., et al.: Maternal HIV-1 and HIV-2 infection and child survival in The Gambia. A. I. D. S. *14*:435–439, 2000.
251. Otten, R. A., Ellenberger, D. L., Adams, D. R., et al.: Identification of a window period for susceptibility to dual infection with two distinct human immunodeficiency virus type 2 isolates in a *Macaca nemestrina* (pig-tailed macaque) model. J. Infect. Dis. *180*:673–684, 1999.
252. Ozden, S., Gessain, A., Gout, O., and Mikol, J.: Sporadic inclusion body myositis in a patient with human T cell leukemia virus type 1–associated myelopathy. Clin. Infect. Dis. *32*:510–514, 2001.
253. Pachl, C., Todd, J. A., and Kern, D. G.: Rapid and precise quantification of HIV-1 RNA in plasma using a branched DNA signal amplification assay. J. Acquir. Immune Defic. Syndr. Hum. Retrovirol. *8*:446–454, 1995.
254. Page, J. B., Lai, S. H., Chitwood, D. D., et al.: HTLV-I/II seropositivity and death from AIDS among HIV-1 seropositive intravenous drug users. Lancet *385*:1439–1441, 1990.
255. Pardi, D., Kaplan, J. E., Coligan, J. E., et al.: Identification and characterization of an extended Tax protein in human T-cell lymphotropic virus type II subtype b isolates. J. Virol. *67*:7663–7667, 1993.

256. Patnaik, A., Chau, V., Wills, J. W.: Ubiquitin is part of the retrovirus budding machinery. Proc. Natl. Acad. Sci. U. S. A. *97*:13069–13074, 2000.
257. Pawson, R., Mufti, G. H., and Pagliuca, A.: Management of adult T-cell leukaemia/lymphoma. Br. J. Hematol. *100*:453–458, 1998.
258. Peeters, M., Gersky-Damet, G.-M., Fransen, K., et al.: Virological and polymerase chain reaction studies of HIV-1/HIV-2 dual infections in Cote d'Ivoire. Lancet *340*:339–340, 1992.
259. Plancoulaine, S., Gessain, A., Joubert, M., et al.: Detection of a major gene predisposing to human T-lymphotropic virus type I infection in children among an endemic population of African origin. J. Infect. Dis. *182*:405–412, 2000.
260. Poiesz, B., Dube, D., Dube, S., et al.: HTLV-II–associated cutaneous T-cell lymphoma in a patient with HIV-1 infection. N. Engl. J. Med. *342*:930–936, 2000.
261. Poiesz, B. J., Ruscetti, F. W., Gazder, A. F., et al.: Detection and isolation of type C retrovirus particles from fresh and cultured lymphocytes of a patient with cutaneous T-cell lymphoma. Proc. Natl. Acad. Sci. U. S. A. *77*:7415–7419, 1980.
262. Popper, S., Dieng Sarr, A., Gueye-Ndiaye, A., et al.: Low plasma human immunodeficiency virus type 2 viral load is independent of proviral load: Low virus production in vivo. J. Virol. *74*:1554–1547, 2000.
263. Popper, S., Dieng-Sarr, A., Travers, K., et al.: Lower human immunodeficiency virus (HIV) type 2 viral load reflects the difference in pathogenicity of HIV-1 and HIV-2. J. Infect. Dis. *180*:1116–1121, 1999.
264. Poulsen, A.-G., Aaby, P., Jensen, H., and Dias, F.: Risk factors for HIV-2 seropositivity among older people in Guinea-Bissau—a search for the early history of HIV-2 infection. Scand. J. Infect. Dis. *32*:169–175, 2000.
265. Poulsen, A.-G., Aaby, P., Larsen, O., et al.: Nine year HIV-2 associated mortality in an urban community in Bissau, West Africa. Lancet *349*:911–919, 1997.
266. Poulson, A. G., Kvinesdal, B. B., Aaby, P., et al.: Lack of evidence of vertical transmission of human immunodeficiency virus type 2 in a sample of the general population in Bissau. J. Acquir. Immune Defic. Syndr. *5*:25–30, 1992.
267. Prazuck, T., Yameogo, J.-M. V., Heylinck, B., et al.: Mother-to-child transmission of human immunodeficiency virus type 1 and type 2 and dual infection: A cohort study in Banfora, Burkino Faso. Pediatr. Infect. Dis. J. *14*:940–947, 1995.
268. Quinn, T. C.: Population migration and the spread of types 1 and 2 human immunodeficiency viruses. Proc. Natl. Acad. Sci. U. S. A. *91*:2407–2414, 1994.
269. Ratner, L.: Molecular biology and pathogenesis of HIV infection. Curr. Opin. Infect. Dis. *6*:181–190, 1993.
270. Ratner, L., and Poiesz, B. J.: Leukemias associated with human T-cell lymphotropic virus type I in a non-endemic region. Medicine (Baltimore) *67*:401–422, 1988.
271. Rayne, F., Bouamr, F., Lalanne, J., and Mamoun, R. Z.: The NH_2-terminal domain of the human T-cell leukemia virus type 1 capsid protein is involved in particle formation. J. Virol. *75*:5277–5287, 2001.
272. Renjifo, B., Chou, K., Ramirez, L. S., et al.: Human T-cell leukemia virus type I (HTLV-I) molecular genotypes and disease outcome. J. Acquir. Immune. Defic. Syndr. Hum. Retrovirol. *13*(Suppl. 1):146–153, 1996.
273. Ricard, D., Wilkins, A., Ngom, P. T., et al.: The effects of HIV-2 infection in a rural area of Guinea-Bissau. A. I. D. S. *8*:977–982, 1994.
274. Rios, M., Khabbaz, R. F., Kaplan, J. E., et al.: Transmission of human T cell lymphotropic (HTLV) type II by transfusion of HTLV-I screened blood products. J. Infect. Dis. *170*:206–210, 1994.
275. Roberts, B. D., Foung, S. K. H., Lipka, J. J., et al.: Evaluation of an immunoblot assay for serological confirmation and differentiation of human T-cell lymphotropic virus types I and II. J. Clin. Microbiol. *31*:260–264, 1993.
276. Roberts, C. R., Fipps, D. R., Brundage, J. F., et al.: Prevalence of human T-lymphotropic virus in civilian applicants for the United States Armed Forces. Am. J. Public Health *82*:70–73, 1992.
277. Robinson, R. D., Lindo, J. F., Neva, F. A., et al.: Immunoepidemiologic studies of *Strongyloides stercoralis* and human T lymphotropic virus type I infections in Jamaica. J. Infect. Dis. *169*:692–696, 1994.
278. Rodgers-Johnson, P., Gajdusek, D. C., Morgan, O. S., et al.: HTLV-I and HTLV-II antibodies and tropical spastic paraparesis. Letter. Lancet *2*:1247–1248, 1985.
279. Rosenblatt, J. D., Giorgi, J. V., Golde, D. W., et al.: Integrated human T-cell leukemia virus II genome in CD8+ cells from a patient with "atypical" hairy cell leukemia: Evidence for distinct T and B cell lymphoproliferative disorders. Blood *71*:363–369, 1988.
280. Rosenblatt, J. D., Golde, D. W., Wachsman, W., et al.: A second isolate of HTLV-II associated with atypical hairy-cell leukemia. N. Engl. J. Med. *315*:372–377, 1986.
281. Safaeian, M., Wilson, L. E., Taylor, E., et al.: HTLV-II and bacterial infections among injection drug users. J. Acquir. Immune Defic. Syndr. Hum. Retrovirol. *24*:483–487, 2000.
282. Sagawa, K., Mochizuki, M., Masuoka, K., et al.: Immunopathological mechanisms of human T cell lymphotropic virus type I (HTLV-I) uveitis: Detection of HTLV-I–infected T cells in the eye and their constitutive cytokine production. J. Clin. Invest. *95*:852–858, 1995.
283. Saito, S., Furuki, K., Ando, Y., et al.: Identification of HTLV-I sequence in cord blood mononuclear cells of neonates born to HTLV-I antigen/antibody positive–mothers by polymerase chain reaction. Jpn. J. Cancer Res. *81*:890–895, 1990.
284. Sanhadji, K., Gessain, A., Chout, R., et al.: HTLV-I antibody and cell-mediated immunity status in sickle cell anemia. Clin. Immunol. Immunopathol. *43*:140–144, 1987.
285. Sawada, T., Iwahara, Y., Ishii, K., et al.: Immunoglobulin prophylaxis against milkborne transmission of human T cell leukemia virus type I in rabbits. J. Infect. Dis. *164*:1193–1196, 1991.
286. Schaeffer, E., Geleziunas, R., and Greene, W. C.: Human immunodeficiency virus type 1 nef functions at the level of virus entry by enhancing cytoplasmic delivery of virions. J. Virol. *75*:2993–3000, 2000.
287. Schechter, M., Harrison, L. H., Halsey, N. A., et al.: Coinfection with human T-cell lymphotropic virus type I and HIV in Brazil. J. A. M. A. *271*:353–357, 1994.
288. Schramm, B., Penn, M. L., Palacios, E. H., et al.: Cytopathicity of human immunodeficiency virus type 2 (HIV-2) in human lymphoid tissue is coreceptor dependent and comparable to that of HIV-1. J. Virol. *74*:9594–9600, 2000.
289. Schreiber, G. B., Murphy, E. L., Horton, J. A., et al.: Factors for human T-cell lymphotropic virus types I and II (HTLV-I and -II) in blood donors: The Retrovirus Epidemiology Donor Study. J. Acquir. Immune Defic. Syndr. Hum. Retrovirol. *14*:263–271, 1997.
290. Schubert, U., Ott, D. E., Chertova, E. N., et al.: Proteasome inhibition interferes with Gag polyprotein processing, release, and maturation of HIV-1 and HIV-2. Proc. Natl. Acad. Sci. U. S. A. *97*:13057–13062, 2000.
291. Schutten, M., van der Ende, M. E., and Osterhaus, A. E. M. E.: Antiretroviral therapy in patients with dual infection with human immunodeficiency virus types 1 and 2. N. Engl. J. Med. *342*:1758–1760, 2000.
292. Schwebke, J., Calsyn, D., Shriver, K., et al.: Prevalence and epidemiologic correlates of human T cell lymphotropic virus infection among intravenous drug users. J. Infect. Dis. *169*:962–967, 1994.
293. Seki, N., Yamaguchi, K., Yamada, A., et al.: Polymorphism of the 5′-flanking region of the tumor necrosis factor (TNF)-alpha gene and susceptibility to human T-cell lymphotropic virus type I (HTLV-I) uveitis. J. Infect. Dis. *180*:880–883, 1999.
294. Sekigawa, I., Kaneko, H., Neoh, L. P., et al.: Differences of the HIV envelope proteins between HIV-1 and HIV-2—possible relation to the lower virulence of HIV-1. Viral Immunol. *11*:1–8, 1998.
295. Setoyama, M., Mizoguchi, S., and Eizuru, Y.: Human T-cell lymphotropic virus type I infects eccrine sweat gland epithelia. Int. J. Cancer *80*:652–655, 1999.
296. Shanmugam, V., Switzer, W. M., Nkengasong, J. N., et al.: Lower HIV-2 plasma viral loads may explain differences between the natural histories of HIV-1 and HIV-2 infections. J. Acquir. Immune Defic. Syndr. Hum. Retrovirol. *24*:257–263, 2000.
297. Sheremata, W. A., Harrington, W. J., Jr., Bradshaw, P. A., et al.: Association of "(tropical) ataxic neuropathy" with HTLV-II. Virus Res. *29*:71–77, 1993.
298. Shibata, K., Shimamoto, Y., Nishimura, T., et al.: Ocular manifestations of adult T-cell leukemia/lymphoma. Ann. Hematol. *74*:163–168, 1997.
299. Shimoyama, M.: Diagnostic criteria and classification of clinical subtypes of adult T-cell leukemia-lymphoma. A report from the Lymphoma Study Group (1984–87). Br. J. Haematol. *79*:428–437, 1991.
300. Siekevitz, M., Josephs, S. F., Dukovich, M., et al.: Activation of the HIV-1 LTR by T-cell mitogens and the trans-activator protein of HTLV-I. Science *238*:1575–1578, 1987.
301. Simon, F., Matheron, S., Tamalet, C., et al.: Cellular and plasma viral load in patients infected with HIV-1. A. I. D. S. *11*:1411–1417, 1993.
302. Simpson, R. M., Leno, M., Hubbard, B. S., et al.: Cutaneous manifestations of human T cell leukemia virus type I infection in an experimental model. J. Infect. Dis. *173*:722–726, 1996.
303. Sison, A. V., and Campos, J. M.: Laboratory methods for early detection of human immunodeficiency virus type 1 in newborns and infants. Clin. Microbiol. Rev. *5*:238–247, 1992.
304. Soriano, V., Gomes, P., Heneine, W., et al.: Human immunodeficiency virus type 2 (HIV-2) in Portugal: Clinical spectrum, circulating subtypes, virus isolation and plasma viral load. J. Med. Virol. *61*:111–116, 2000.
305. Southern, S. O., and Southern, P. J.: Persistent HTLV-I infection of breast luminal epithelial cells: A role in HTLV transmission? Virology *241*:200–214, 1998.
306. Strack, B., Calistri, A., Accola, M. A., et al.: A role for ubiquitin ligase recruitment in retrovirus release. Proc. Natl. Acad. Sci. U. S. A. *97*:13063–13068, 2000.
307. Stuver, S. O., Tachibana, N., Olayama, A., et al.: Heterosexual transmission of human T-cell leukemia/lymphoma virus type I among married couples in southwestern Japan: An initial report from the Miyazaki cohort study. J. Infect. Dis. *167*:57–63, 1993.
308. Sugimoto, M., Nakashima, H., Matsumoto, M., et al.: Pulmonary involvement in patients with HTLV-I–associated myelopathy: Increased soluble IL-2 receptors in bronchoalveolar lavage fluid. Am. Rev. Respir. Dis. *139*:1329–1335, 1989.

309. Sugimoto, M., Nakashima, H., Watanabe, S., et al.: T-lymphocytic alveolitis in HTLV-I–associated myelopathy. Lancet *2*:1220, 1987.
310. Suite, M., Jack, N., Basdeo-Mahuraj, K., et al.: Infective dermatitis in Trinidad and Tobago. A. I. D. S. Res. Hum. Retroviruses *10*:447, 1994.
311. Sullivan, N., Sun, Y., Sattentau, Q., et al.: CD4-induced conformational changes in the human immunodeficiency virus type 1 gp120 glycoprotein: Consequences for virus entry and neutralization. J. Virol. *72*:4694–4703, 1998.
312. Sweet, R. D.: A pattern of eczema in Jamaica. Br. J. Dermatol. *78*:93–100, 1966.
313. Switzer, W. M., Wiktor, S., Soriano, V., et al.: Evidence of Nef truncation in human immunodeficiency virus type 2 infection. J. Infect. Dis. *177*:65–71, 1998.
314. Taguchi, H., Kinoshita, K., Takatsuki, K., et al.: An intensive chemotherapy of adult T-cell leukemia/lymphoma: CHOP followed by etoposide, vindesine, ranimustine, and mitoxantrone with granulocyte colony-stimulating factor support. J. Acquir. Immune Defic. Syndr. Hum. Retrovirol. *12*:182–186, 1996.
315. Tajima, K.: The 4th nation-wide study of adult T-cell leukemia/lymphoma (ATL) in Japan: Estimates of risk of ATL and its geographical and clinical features. The T- and B-Cell Malignancy Study Group. Int. J. Cancer *45*:237–243, 1990.
316. Tajima, K., Fujita, K., Tsukidate, S., et al.: Seroepidemiologic studies on the effects of filarial parasites on infestation of adult T-cell leukemia virus in the Goto Islands, Japan. Gann *74*:188–191, 1983.
317. Tajima, K., Takezaki, T., Ito, M., et al.: Short-term breast feeding may reduce the risk of vertical transmission of HTLV-I. Abstract. J. Acquir. Immune Defic. Syndr. Hum. Retrovirol. *10*:285, 1995.
318. Takahashi, K., Tajima, K., Komoda, H., et al.: Incidence of human T lymphotropic virus type I seroconversion after age 40 among Japanese residents in an area where the virus is endemic. J. Infect. Dis. *171*:559–565, 1995.
319. Takahashi, K., Takezaki, T., Oki, T., et al.: Inhibitory effect of maternal antibody on mother-to-child transmission of human T-lymphotropic virus type I. Int. J. Cancer *49*:673–677, 1991.
320. Takezaki, T., Tajima, K., Ito, M., et al.: Short-term breastfeeding may reduce the risk of vertical transmission of HTLV-I. Leukemia *11*(Suppl. 3):60–62, 1997.
321. Talalet, C., Simon, F., Dhiver, C., et al.: Autologous neutralizing antibodies and viral load in HIV-2–infected individuals. A. I. D. S. *9*:90–91, 1995.
322. Tamalet, C., Lafeuillade, A., Yahi, N., et al.: Comparison of viral burden and phenotype of HIV-1 isolates from lymph nodes and blood. A. I. D. S. *8*:1083–1088, 1994.
323. Tang, H., Kuhen, K. L., and Wong-Staal, F.: Lentivirus replication and regulation. Annu. Rev. Genet. *33*:133–170, 1999.
324. Tangy, F., Ossondo, M., Vernant, J.-C., et al.: Human T cell leukemia virus type I expression in salivary glands of infected patients. J. Infect. Dis. *179*:497–502, 1999.
325. Taylor, G. P., Tosswill, J. H. C., Matutes, E., et al.: Prospective study of HTLV-I infection in an initially asymptomatic cohort. J. Acquir. Immune Defic. Syndr. Hum. Retrovirol. *22*:92–100, 1999.
326. Terada, K., Katamine, S., Eguchi, K., et al.: Prevalence of serum and salivary antibodies to HTLV-I in Sjögren's syndrome. Lancet *344*:1116–1119, 1994.
327. Thali, M., Bukovsky, A., Kondo, E., et al.: Functional association of cyclophilin A with HIV-1 virions. Nature *372*:363–365, 1994.
328. The European HTLV Research Network.: Seroepidemiology of the human T-cell leukemia/lymphoma viruses in Europe. J. Acquir. Immune Defic. Syndr. Hum. Retrovirol. *13*:68–77, 1996.
329. The HIV Infection in Newborns French Collaborative Study Group: Comparison of vertical human immunodeficiency virus type 2 and human immunodeficiency virus type 1 transmission in the French prospective cohort. Pediatr. Infect. Dis. J. *13*:502–506, 1994.
330. Travers, K. U., Eisen, G. E., Marlink, R. G., et al.: Protection from HIV-1 infection by HIV-2. A. I. D. S. *12*:224–225, 1998.
331. Travers, K., Mboup, S., Marklink, R., et al.: Natural protection against HIV-1 infection provided by HIV-2. Science *268*:1612–1615, 1995.
332. Tsuji, Y., Doi, H., Yamabe, T., et al.: Prevention of mother to child transmission of human T-lymphotropic virus type 1. Pediatrics *86*:11–17, 1990.
333. Tsukasaki, K., Yamada, Y., Ikeda, S., and Tomonaa, M.: Infective dermatitis among patients with ATL in Japan. Int. J. Cancer *57*:293, 1994.
334. Ucar, A., Fernandez, H. F., Byrnes, J. J., et al.: Thrombotic microangiopathy and retroviral infections: A 13-year experience. Am. J. Hematol. *45*:304–309, 1994.
335. Uchiyama, T.: Human T cell leukemia virus type I (HTLV-I) and human diseases. Annu. Rev. Immunol. *15*:15–37, 1997.
336. Ureta-Vidal, A., Angelin-Duclos, C., Tortevoye, P., et al.: Mother-to-child transmission of human T-cell leukemia/lymphoma virus type I: Implication of high antiviral titer and high proviral load in carrier mothers. Int. J. Cancer *82*:832–836, 1999.
337. Ureta-Vidal, A., Pique, C., Garcia, Z., et al.: Human T cell leukemia virus type I (HTLV-I) infection induces greater expansions of CD8 T lymphocytes in persons with HTLV-I–associated myelopathy/tropical spastic paraparesis than in asymptomatic carriers. J. Infect. Dis. *183*:857–864, 2001.
338. Urnovitz, H. B., and Murphy, W. H.: Human endogenous retroviruses: Nature, occurrence and clinical implications in human disease. Clin. Microbiol. Rev. *9*:72–99, 1996.
339. Van Dyke, R. B., Heneine, W., Perrin, M. E., et al.: Mother-to-child transmission of human T-lymphotropic virus type II. J. Pediatr. *127*:924–928, 1995.
340. Venkateshan, C. N., La Grenade, L., De, S. K., et al.: Overexpression of pro- and anti-inflammatory cytokines by cultured keratinocytes from HTLV-I associated familial infective dermatitis. A. I. D. S. Res. Hum. Retroviruses *11*(Suppl. 1):143, 1995.
341. Verdier, M., Denis, F., Sangare, A., et al.: Prevalence of antibody to human T cell leukemia virus type 1 (HTLV-1) in populations of Ivory Coast, Africa. J. Infect. Dis. *160*:363–370, 1989.
342. Verdier, M., Denis, F., Sangare, A., et al.: Antibodies to human T lymphotropic virus type I in patients with leprosy in tropical areas. J. Infect. Dis. *161*:1309–1310, 1990.
343. Vitek, C. R., Gracia, F. I., Fiusti, R. A., et al.: Evidence for sexual and mother-to-child transmission of human T lymphotropic virus type II among Guaymi Indians, Panama. J. Infect. Dis. *171*:1022–1026, 1995.
344. Vlahov, D., Khabbaz, R. F., Cohn, S., et al.: Incidence and risk factors for human T-lymphotropic virus type II seroconversion among injecting drug users in Baltimore, Maryland, U.S.A. J. Acquir. Immune Defic. Syndr. Hum. Retrovirol. *9*:89–96, 1995.
345. Vogt, V. M.: Ubiquitin in retrovirus assembly: Actor or bystander? Proc. Natl. Acad. Sci. U. S. A. *97*:12945–12947, 2000.
346. von Schwedler, U., Song, J., Aiken, C., et al.: Vif is crucial for human immunodeficiency virus type 1 proviral DNA synthesis in infected cells. J. Virol. *67*:4945–4955, 1993.
347. Wagner, M., Rose, V. A., Linder, R., et al.: Human pathogenic virus-associated pseudolymphomas and lymphomas with primary cutaneous manifestations in humans and animals. Clin. Infect. Dis. *27*:1299–1308, 1998.
348. Waldmann, T. A.: Human T-cell lymphotropic virus type I–associated adult T-cell leukemia: The Joseph Goldberger Clinical Investigator Lecture. J. A. M. A. *273*:735–737, 1995.
349. Waldmann, T. A., White, J. D., Carrasuillo, J. A., et al.: Radioimmunotherapy of interleukin-2R alpha–expressing adult T-cell leukemia with yttrium-90–labeled anti-Tac. Blood *86*:4063–4075, 1995.
350. Waldmann, T. A., White, J. D., Goldman, C. K., et al.: The interleukin-2 receptor: A target for monoclonal antibody treatment of human T-cell lymphotropic virus I–induced adult T-cell leukemia. Blood *82*:1701–1712, 1993.
351. Walshe, M. M.: Infective dermatitis in Jamaican children. Br. J. Dermatol. *79*:229–236, 1967.
352. Wattel, E., Cavrois, M., Gessain, A., and Wain-Hobson, S.: Clonal expansion of infected cells: A way of life for HTLV-I. J. Acquir. Immune Defic. Syndr. Hum. Retrovirol. *13*(Suppl. 1):92-99, 1996.
353. Wattel, E., Mariotti, M., Agis, F., et al.: Human T lymphotropic virus (HTLV) type I and II DNA amplification in HTLV-I/II–seropositive blood donors of the French West Indies. J. Infect. Dis. *165*:369–372, 1992.
354. Wattel, E., Vartanian, J. P., Pannetier, C., and Wain-Hobson, S.: Clonal expansion of human T-cell leukemia virus type 1–infected cells in asymptomatic and symptomatic carriers without malignancy. J. Virol. *69*:2863–2866, 1995.
355. Wei, Z., Ghosh, S. K., Taylor, M. E., et al.: Viral dynamics in human immunodeficiency virus type 1 infection. Nature *373*:117–122, 1995.
356. Weinberg, J. B., Spiegel, R. A., Blazey, D. L., et al.: Human T-cell lymphotropic virus I and adult T-cell leukemia: Report of a cluster in North Carolina. Am. J. Med. *95*:51–58, 1988.
357. Weiss, S. H.: The evolving epidemiology of human T-lymphotropic virus type II. J. Infect. Dis. *169*:1080–1083, 1994.
358. Whittle, H., Morris, J., Todd, T., et al.: HIV-2–infected patients survive longer than HIV-1–infected patients. A. I. D. S. *8*:1617–1620, 1994.
359. Wiktor, S. Z., Cannon, R. O., Atkinson, W. L., et al.: Infection with human T lymphotropic virus types I and II in sexually transmitted disease clinics in Baltimore and New Orleans. J. Infect. Dis. *165*:920–924, 1992.
360. Wiktor, S. Z., Nkengasong, J. N., Ekpini, E. R., et al.: Lack of protection against HIV-1 infection among women with HIV-2 infection. A. I. D. S. *13*:695–699, 1999.
361. Wiktor, S. Z., Pate, E. J., Murphy, E. L., et al.: Mother-to-child transmission of human T-cell lymphotropic virus type I (HTLV-I) in Jamaica: Association with antibodies to envelope glycoprotein (gp46) epitopes. J. Acquir. Immune Defic. Syndr. *6*:1162–1167, 1993.
362. Wiktor, S. Z., Pate, E. J., Rosenberg, P. S., et al.: Mother-to-child transmission of human T-cell lymphotropic virus type I associated with prolonged breast-feeding. J. Hum. Virol. *1*:37–44, 1997.
363. Wiktor, S. Z., Piot, P., Mann, J. M., et al.: Human T cell lymphotropic virus type I (HTLV-I) among female prostitutes in Kinshasa, Zaire. J. Infect. Dis. *161*:1073–1077, 1990.
364. Wilkens, A., Ricard, D., Todd, J., et al.: The epidemiology of HIV infection in a rural area of Guinea-Bissau. A. I. D. S. *7*:1119–1122, 1993.

365. Witvrouw, M., Pannecouque, C., Van Laethem, K., et al.: Activity of non-nucleoside reverse transcriptase inhibitors against HIV-2 and SIV. A. I. D. S. *13*:1477–1483, 1999.
366. Wolinsky, S. M.: Retrovirology. Curr. Opin. Infect. Dis. *7*:65–71, 1994.
367. World Health Organization: Report of the Scientific Group on HTLV-I and Associated Diseases. Kagoshima, Japan, December 1988: Viral diseases. Wkly. Epidemiol. Rec. *49*:382–383, 1989.
368. Yamaguchi, K.: Human T-lymphotropic virus type I in Japan. Lancet *343*:213–216, 1994.
369. Yamamoto, J. H., Segurado, A. A., Hirata, C. E., et al.: Human T-cell lymphotropic virus type 1 infection and ocular manifestations in Sao Paulo, Brazil. Arch. Ophthalmol. *117*:513–517, 1999.
370. Yamanouchi, K., Kinoshita, K., Moriuchi, R., et al.: Oral transmission of human T cell leukemia virus type I into a common marmoset *(Callithrix jacchus)* as an experimental model for milk-borne transmission. Jpn. J. Cancer Res. *76*:481–487, 1985.
371. Yamashita, M., Ido, E., Miura, T., and Hayami, M.: Molecular epidemiology of HTLV-I in the world. J. Acquir. Immune Defic. Syndr. Hum. Retrovirol. *13*(Suppl. 1):124–131, 1996.
372. Yanagihara, R., Nerurkar, V. R., and Ajdukiewicz, A. B.: Comparison between strains of human T lymphotropic virus type 1 isolated from inhabitants of the Solomon Islands and Papua New Guinea. J. Infect. Dis. *164*:443–449, 1991.
373. Yoshida, M.: Molecular biology of HTLV-I: Recent progress. J. Acquir. Immune Defic. Syndr. Hum. Retrovirol. *13*(Suppl. 1):63–68, 1996.
374. Yoshida, M.: Multiple viral strategies of HTLV-I for dysregulation of cell growth control. Annu. Rev. Immunol. *19*:475–496, 2001.
375. Yoshinaga, M., Yashiki, S., Oki, T., et al.: A maternal risk factor for mother to child HTLV-I transmission: Viral antigen-producing capacities in culture of peripheral blood and breast milk cells. Jpn. J. Cancer Res. *86*:649–654, 1995.
376. Zacharopoulos, V. R., Perotti, M. E., and Phillips, D. M.: Lymphocyte-facilitated infection of epithelia by human T-cell lymphotropic virus type I. J. Virol. *66*:4601–4605, 1992.
377. Zacharopoulos, V. R., and Phillips, D. M.: Infection of a cervix-derived epithelial cell line with HTLV-I. J. Acquir. Immune Defic. Syndr. *10*:249, 1995.
378. Zehender, G., De Maddalena, C., Osio, M., et al.: High prevalence of human T cell lymphotropic virus type II infection in patients affected by human immunodeficiency type 1–associated predominantly sensory polyneuropathy. J. Infect. Dis. *172*:1595–1598, 1995.
379. Zucker-Franklin, D., Hooper, W. C., and Evatt, B. L.: Human lymphotropic retroviruses associated with mycosis fungoides and evidence that human T-cell lymphotropic virus type II (HTLV-II) as well as HTLV-I may play a role in the disease. Blood *80*:1537–1545, 1992.
380. Zucker-Franklin, D., Kosann, M. K., Pancake, B. A., et al.: Hypopigmented mycosis fungoides associated with human T cell lymphotropic virus type 1 Tax in a pediatric patient. Pediatrics *103*:1039–1044, 1999.
381. Zunt, J. R.: Tropical spastic paraparesis: An old disease with a new name. Arch. Neurol. *58*:122–124, 1985.

CHAPTER **193B**

Lentiviruses (Human Immunodeficiency Virus Type 1 and Acquired Immunodeficiency Syndrome)

I. CELINE HANSON ■ WILLIAM T. SHEARER

This half of the chapter provides an overview of human immunodeficiency virus type 1 (HIV-1 or simply HIV) infection and the resultant associated acquired immunodeficiency syndrome (AIDS).

Impact of HIV and AIDS

HIV infection and AIDS have had a significant clinical impact on children worldwide.[66, 191] The World Health Organization has estimated that 40 million people were infected with HIV-1 in 2001.[279] Of these 40 million, 5 million were newly infected and half of these newly infected individuals were young people 15 to 24 years of age. Eight hundred thousand children younger than 15 years were infected in 2001, and more than 90 percent acquired their infection by perinatal transmission.[251] The global specter of HIV infection in women, and subsequently in their children, is presented in Figure 193–5.[57] Despite advances in care, HIV/AIDS continues its worldwide spread, even in developed nations such as the United States.[213]

The few early cases of pediatric HIV infection/AIDS in the United States have been replaced with increasing numbers; 8908 AIDS cases in children younger than 13 years have been reported through December 2000. Although AIDS mortality decreased in 1996 through 1999 with the introduction of newer treatment strategies, young minority women of child-bearing age showed some of the smallest proportional decreases in mortality.[150] HIV infection/AIDS looms, then, as a significant health care threat to infants and children of all nations, including the United States. Because of the wide spectrum of clinical expression, all clinical and health care specialists (including primary caregivers, pediatric subspecialists, nursing personnel, and social service professionals) who provide care to children should familiarize themselves with HIV-1 infection, develop expertise, and anticipate provision of services to this population.

Definition and Staging

Pediatric AIDS first was reported to the Centers for Disease Control and Prevention (CDC) in 1982 and appeared at the same time as an epidemic of adult AIDS.[64] The first definitions of pediatric AIDS, provided in 1985, proved cumbersome, and in 1987, the CDC developed a classification system that more accurately and adequately represented infants; by then, HIV was recognized as the etiologic agent of adult and pediatric AIDS.[46] In 1994, the classification system again was revised to include more advanced viral diagnostic technology and a system for staging pediatric HIV disease that involved both clinical and immunologic axes.[52] This new staging system accommodates the criticisms of many clinicians who thought that the 1987 strict pediatric AIDS definition did not allow for reporting infants and children with significant morbidity from HIV infection but without a diagnosis of AIDS.[45] Table 193–10 outlines the clinical axis of the staging system, which is composed of four clinical categories (N, A, B, C).[52] The clinical axis is intended for unidirectional use in any individual child—that is, disease severity proceeds from N (asymptomatic), to A (mildly symptomatic), to B (moderately symptomatic), to C (severely symptomatic), and then to HIV-associated death. Clinical category C describes children with AIDS-defining characteristics, namely, wasting, encephalopathy, opportunistic infections, and malignancies, but it excludes lymphoid interstitial pneumonitis/pulmonary lymphoid hyperplasia (LIP/PLH). Clinical category B describes children with other specific HIV-associated illnesses (e.g., single episodes of bacteremia, leiomyosarcomas, lymphoproliferative lung disorders, anemia, thrombocytopenia) and excludes children with a clinical category C event. Clinical category A describes children with two or more specific HIV-associated illnesses, namely,

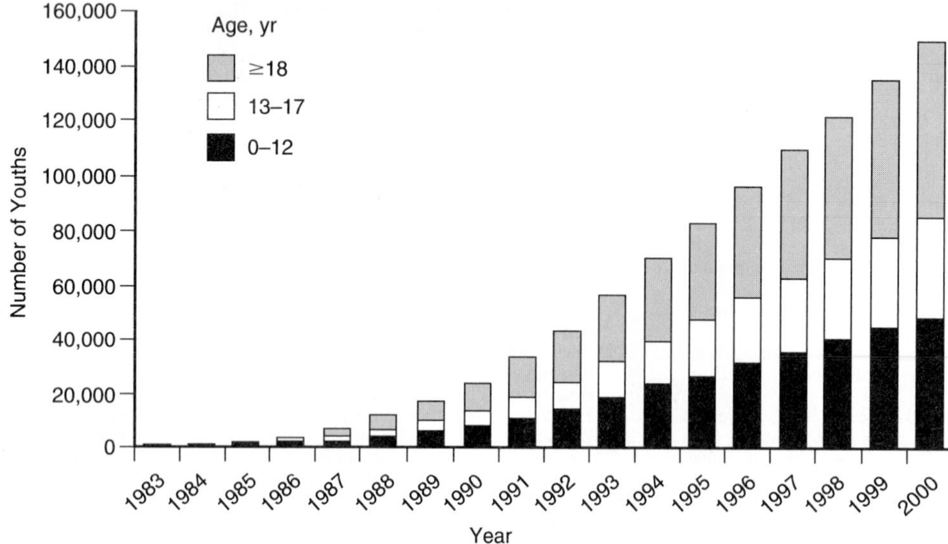

FIGURE 193–5 ■ Estimation of the cumulative number of motherless children, adolescents, and young adults orphaned by the HIV/AIDS epidemic in the United States, 1983 through 2000. (From Michaels, D., and Levine, C.: Estimates of the number of motherless youth orphaned by AIDS in the United States. J. A. M. A. *268*:3456–3461, 1992. Copyright 1992, American Medical Association.)

lymphadenopathy, hepatomegaly, splenomegaly, upper respiratory tract infections/sinusitis/otitis media, parotitis, and dermatitis, and excludes children with a clinical category C or B event. Clinical category N describes children without clinical category C, B, or A events; these children may or may not be completely asymptomatic (single category A events may exist, i.e., lymphadenopathy).

Table 193–11 provides an expanded description of the immunologic axis of the staging system, which includes categories 1 (no evidence of immune suppression), 2 (moderate immunosuppression), and 3 (severe immunosuppression).[52] The immune axis is limited to quantitative assessment (absolute count, percentage, or both) of the peripheral blood helper T-cell (CD4) population. Each category is linked to age-matched CD4 counts and percentages; age groups include 0 to 11 months, 12 to 71 months, and 72 months and older. Age-matched CD4 percentages and count standards for moderate to severe immunosuppression are identical to those provided in the 1995 revised guidelines for pediatric *Pneumocystis* prophylaxis interventions.[54]

Epidemiology and Transmission

TRANSMISSION BY BLOOD PRODUCTS

Pediatric HIV transmission has been documented by blood and blood products, predominantly before the spring of 1985 (transfusion-associated AIDS and hemophilia-associated AIDS), by perinatal transmission from mothers with identified risk factors, by sexual transmission to children and adolescents, and by breast milk.[88, 113, 263] The first case report of transfusion-associated AIDS was linked to a transfusion given in 1977. Investigation of the demographic characteristics of 72 children with neonatal transfusion-associated HIV infection has documented a 54 percent incidence in children of color (Hispanic and black children) and equal gender representation.[105] In the hemophiliac population, the incidence of HIV seropositivity approaches 80 percent for persons born before 1985 (before adaptation of HIV screening techniques to pooled blood products, namely, factor concentrate therapy). The demographic data of hemophiliac patients with AIDS closely resemble the characteristics of the hemophiliac population as a whole (predominance of affected white males).[146] In transfusion-associated pediatric AIDS and hemophiliac-associated AIDS cases, the symptom-free period has been reported to range from a median of 18 months to 5 years and more nearly approximates the adult HIV experience of longer than 10 years.[76, 105]

PERINATAL TRANSMISSION

Perinatal transmission of HIV infection accounts for more than 90 percent of newly reported pediatric AIDS cases.[226] In the United States, 7828 cases of perinatally transmitted AIDS were reported to the CDC through June 1999. This perinatal predominance is mimicked worldwide, especially in countries where adult heterosexual transmission is

TABLE 193–10 ■ PEDIATRIC HIV CLASSIFICATION—CLINICAL CATEGORIES

Immunologic Categories	N: No Signs/Symptoms	A: Mild Signs/Symptoms	B: Moderate Signs/Symptoms	C: Severe Signs/Symptoms
1. No evidence of suppression	N1	A1	B1	C1
2. Evidence of moderate suppression	N2	A2	B2	C2
3. Severe suppression	N3	A3	B3	C3

Adapted from Centers for Disease Control and Prevention: 1994 Revised classification system for human immunodeficiency virus infection in children less than 13 years of age. M. M. W. R. Morb. Mortal. Wkly. Rep. *43*:2, 1994.

TABLE 193–11 ■ IMMUNOLOGIC CATEGORIES BASED ON AGE-SPECIFIC CD4⁺ T-LYMPHOCYTE COUNTS AND PERCENTAGE OF TOTAL LYMPHOCYTES

	Age of Child					
	<12 mo		1–5 yr		6–12 yr	
Immunologic Category	μL	%	μL	%	μL	%
1. No evidence of suppression	≥1500	≥25	≥1000	≥25	≥500	≥25
2. Evidence of moderate suppression	750–1499	15–24	500–999	15–24	200–499	15–24
3. Severe suppression	<750	<15	<500	<15	<200	<15

Adapted from Centers for Disease Control and Prevention: 1994 revised classification system for human immunodeficiency virus infection in children less than 13 years of age. M. M. W. R. Morb. Mortal. Wkly. Rep. *43:4,* 1994.

uniquely prevalent (e.g., in Africa).[39, 88, 232, 255] The transmission rate for perinatally acquired HIV infection without perinatal antiretroviral intervention has been reported to be between 12 and 25 percent in the United States and Europe and is probably higher in Africa.[64, 72, 228, 262, 264] Recent advances in perinatal primary antiretroviral therapy (antepartum, peripartum, and postpartum delivery of zidovudine in HIV-infected women without severe immunosuppression) have led to a decrease in perinatal transmission rates to approximately 8 percent.[72] Implementation of published guidelines promoting the use of zidovudine and highly active antiretroviral therapy (HAART) to suppress the viral load and restore or preserve immune function in pregnant HIV-infected women has resulted in a further reduction in transmission rates in the United States.[73] These guidelines target prevention of perinatal transmission by promoting early testing, counseling, and treatment intervention in women of child-bearing age with newly identified HIV infection.[58] High maternal seroprevalence rates in any given community predict an increased incidence of perinatal transmission unless HIV prevention interventions are implemented actively.[226] Maternal HIV seroprevalence rates vary by site and can be matched to trends documenting increasing rates of sexually transmitted diseases (e.g., syphilis). This association is especially true in urban centers and in the southeastern United States. The perinatal transmission rates reported define transmission only in the context of live infant outcomes. The incidence of spontaneous fetal loss in HIV-infected pregnant women has been suggested to be increased and may represent increased HIV perinatal morbidity.[164]

Maternal risk factors as identified through national surveillance in reported AIDS cases include drug abuse, heterosexual infection by sexual partners with risk factors for acquiring HIV disease, and maternal transfusion before 1985.[226, 238]

Prospective and retrospective evaluations of maternal predictors for perinatal HIV transmission have been the focus of multiple studies. Maternal predictors identified to date include maternal viremia (measured as quantitative RNA or viral load),[93, 110] maternal immunosuppression or an inadequate immune response (measured by the CD4 count, neutralizing antibody production),[79, 80, 93] and viral characteristics (syncytium formation, phenotype and resistance patterns of maternal virus at delivery or infant virus at birth).[29] Pregnancy and placental variables (delivery mode, duration of rupture of membranes, vitamin A deficiency, chorioamnionitis) also may influence the risk of perinatal transmission of HIV.[94, 162, 237, 254, 277, 278] Infant variables under evaluation as predictors of HIV transmission include HLA frequency and the infant cellular immune response (cytokine production, cytotoxic T-cell function).[79, 92, 95, 153, 178] In addition, genetic factors have been suggested to confer protection against progression of disease.[235]

Perinatal HIV transmission has been proposed to take place in the antepartum, peripartum, and postpartum periods.[84, 114, 246] However, the distribution of transmission across these timing periods has not been defined precisely. The timing of the first positive culture in perinatally infected infants—that is, early (the first 7 days of life) versus late (second week of life or later)—has been used to epidemiologically differentiate children potentially infected in utero from those with intrapartum infection.[35] Such distinctions and a need for more precise definition of the timing distribution of perinatal transmission are of paramount importance in defining interventions for interruption of transmission.[16] Such interruption is especially important because investigators have suggested that early HIV-1 infection can have an impact on the rate of neurodevelopmental dysfunction within the first 2 years of life.[196, 245]

The demographics of the perinatally infected pediatric cohort include an enhanced prevalence in black and Hispanic children and no significant distinction between male and female cases.[226] In contrast to transfusion-associated pediatric AIDS, perinatally infected infants exhibit symptoms shortly after birth (6.4 versus 17.8 months), even with treatment intervention.[117] Attempts to assess progression of disease have led to descriptions of subpopulations of HIV-infected children: rapid, usual, and slow progressors.[23, 81, 121, 145, 156, 245, 269] Standardized definitions for rapid or usual progressors are lacking. A stringent definition of slow progressors has been proposed (≤8 years of age without evidence of clinical or immunologic decline).[121, 145] Multicenter studies performed to assess the demographic, virologic, and immunologic characteristics of these rapid, usual, and slow progressors are ongoing. In addition, isolated reports of children with documented HIV infection and evidence of clearance have prompted careful study of perinatally exposed, but uninfected infants with evidence of HIV-indeterminant status as documented by a single positive HIV culture.[36, 128]

SEXUAL TRANSMISSION

In the adult population, sexual acquisition of HIV infection is the predominant transmission pattern. The intersection of pediatric sexual abuse and HIV transmission has been reported increasingly.[113, 123] Sexual abuse in young children and infants may be associated with the transmission of sexual disease (syphilis, gonorrhea, etc.). HIV infection should be considered in the differential diagnosis of possible sexually transmitted diseases in children under assessment for sexual assault. In contrast to the infrequent reports of sexual transmission in infants and children younger than 13 years, adolescents, who account for 1 percent of AIDS cases in the United States, are infected frequently by sexual transmission.[172] Because the symptom-free period for clinical expression of HIV infection in adolescents may approach adult standards (i.e., more than 10 years), many young adults (20 to 29 years of age) with AIDS probably became infected with HIV during adolescence.[172] Adolescents with AIDS, like affected infants and children, are more likely to be poor and black or Hispanic. Reported risks for transmission in adolescents vary by age, sex, and race or ethnicity. The youngest teenage AIDS patients more often are linked to receipt of blood products for hemophilia or coagulopathies and the oldest, to sexual transmission (males who have sex with males and heterosexual contact). Female adolescents with AIDS (all ages) report heterosexual contact or known HIV risk most frequently. The category of heterosexual contact accounted for the largest proportional increase in the reported risk of transmission in both female and male adolescent AIDS cases. The nature of youth (experimentation, search for self and sexual identity, and inability to access health care easily) places adolescents at risk for heterosexual transmission of HIV infection.[32] From 1994 to 2000, surveillance of HIV infection has identified a reduction in the number of persons in whom HIV infection was newly diagnosed; in adolescents, the trend is toward stabilization rather than a reduction in these numbers.[59, 60]

OTHER MODES OF TRANSMISSION

Less frequently reported transmission routes of HIV infection are important for pediatric health care providers to acknowledge and target. The risk of transmission of HIV through breast-feeding has been reported infrequently. In a study of HIV-infected breast-feeding mothers and their exposed infants, Dunn and associates[88] documented a 14 percent risk of HIV transmission through breast-feeding above and beyond the established perinatal transmission risk. These studies have prompted the adoption of guidelines for preventing transmission via this route by avoiding breast-feeding in HIV-seropositive postpartum mothers in the United States.[43] Transmission of HIV to infants by breast-feeding represents approximately a third to a half of all perinatal transmission in underdeveloped countries.[104] Research efforts to evaluate the efficacy of antiretrovirals in reducing transmission by breast-feeding are ongoing.

The pediatric population has undergone careful epidemiologic assessment for casual (household contact) transmission of HIV. Isolated cases of transmission of HIV to children have been reported, but blood exposure has been implicated in these cases and casual transmission has *not* been documented.[102, 241] To date, *no* data suggest that HIV infection is transmitted casually from HIV-infected children to siblings, playmates, or caregivers.[107, 229, 241] In addition, no evidence suggests that exposed, noninfected children would be at greater risk for acquisition of HIV than noninfected, immunologically mature adults are. Documentation of transmission routes and lack of casual transmission have prompted guidelines from the American Academy of Pediatrics and the CDC for appropriate "mainstreaming" of HIV-infected children and families.[42, 218] These guidelines include school, daycare, and foster care placement for HIV-infected children and promote social incorporation of these children.

Etiology

Identification of the etiology of AIDS followed closely behind the clinical description of this complex immunodeficiency. In 1983, investigators worldwide identified a viral etiology for AIDS and described human lymphotropic virus III, lymphadenopathy-associated virus, and a virus associated with persistent generalized lymphadenopathy.[69, 112] These viruses subsequently have been identified as similar and now are called HIV-1, or simply HIV[77] (Fig. 193–6). Two species of HIV are recognized: HIV-1 and HIV-2. HIV-1 has been the more prevalent pathogenic species and, especially in the United States, almost uniformly has been associated with reported AIDS cases.[47, 49]

HIV belongs to the virus family *Retroviridae,* genus *Lentivirus,* first described almost 50 years ago. It is an RNA virus that acts as an infectious agent by penetrating cell membranes and using a pivotal and integral enzyme carried in its core, reverse transcriptase, to become integrated into the host-cell genome.[96] Genetic mapping of HIV has identified genes common to human retroviruses (*gag, pol,* and *env*) and necessary for replication. Considerable heterogeneity of the *env* gene, which codes for viral envelope proteins, has been noted in multiple HIV isolates. The *env* gene produces a glycosylated protein (gp160) that is cleaved into an external component (gp120) and a transmembrane component (gp41). The heterogeneity of the *env* gene and the resulting gp120 structural variability render preparation of an effective vaccine difficult. The group-specific antigen (*gag*) gene codes for a polyprotein that is cleaved by the HIV protease into the matrix, capsid, and nucleocapsid proteins found in virions: The *pol* gene codes for the production of enzymes required for HIV replication, namely, a heterodimeric reverse transcriptase (p66/p51), and the viral integrase (p31) and protease proteins. Five other HIV genes—*tat, rev, nef, vif,* and *vpr*—encode proteins that play crucial roles in HIV replication and pathogenesis. For example, the Tat protein (transactivator of transcription) binds to a specific nucleotide sequence in the viral RNA, and attracts cellular proteins that increase the efficiency of elongation of viral transcripts. The Rev protein blocks the splicing of viral RNA, allowing RNA molecules to reach the cytoplasm that are translated into gp160, or packaged into progeny virions. Further discussion of the other accessory proteins of HIV are found in Chapter 193A.

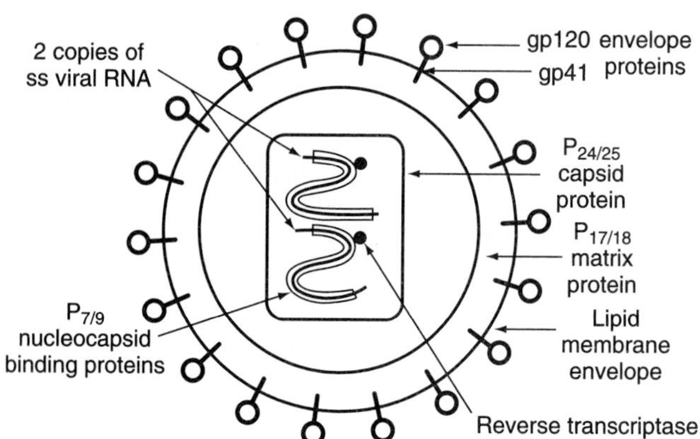

FIGURE 193–6 ■ Diagram of the virion of HIV-1. (From Demmler, G. J., and Taber, L. H.: Virology of HIV-1. Semin. Pediatr. Infect. Dis. *1*:17–20, 1990.)

Many investigators have compared HIV with the animal lentivirus visna, which infects sheep, because both share a tropism for lymphocytes and central nervous system (CNS) tissue. Comparison with simian immunodeficiency virus infection in primates has provided important information about early infection and the potential for interruption of infection.[270] In animal models, the introduction of HIV has led to rapid seroconversion; however, clinical disease with immune defects and opportunistic infection has not been reproduced. Despite these problems, continued exploration of the effects of HIV infection in animal models may yield new insight into the pathogenesis of HIV disease in humans.

Pathogenesis

VULNERABILITY OF THE FETAL AND NEONATAL IMMUNE SYSTEM TO HIV INFECTION

The human fetus and neonate are particularly susceptible to the devastating effects of HIV infection because the normal networking of components of the immune system has not developed.[192] Although B- and T-lymphocyte differentiation can begin as early as 10 weeks of gestational life, transmission of HIV from mother to fetus can occur even earlier.[248] Such early HIV infection in a host characterized by immunologic naiveté possibly leads to rapid and full expression of the fatal illness by the early age of 2 to 3 years.[121, 145, 234] Undoubtedly, the longer survival of HIV-infected adults can be attributed, at least in part, to their fully developed T- and B-cell repertoire; the immune memory of humoral and cellular responses; mature complement components; and an intact phagocytic system of monocytes, macrophages, and polymorphonuclear leukocytes. All these defense mechanisms have been shown to be impaired in normal newborns, and a reasonable conclusion is that this secondary state of immunodeficiency in the newborn lends itself to the early establishment and rapid development of full-blown HIV infection.[8, 192] At every level of the immune response—inflammation, antigen presentation, primary immune response, secondary immune response—the newborn is expected to be unable to protect itself against HIV infection and against the secondary infections that inexorably follow.

THE DEVELOPING IMMUNE SYSTEM AND HIV INFECTION

Perhaps the easiest way to envision the disruption that HIV creates in the newborn immune system is to consider the intricate normal differentiation pathways of the bone marrow stem cell as it creates the many cellular components of the immune system.[272] The T- and B-lymphocyte differentiation pathways present multiple opportunities for genetic defects, such as occurs in states of congenital immunodeficiency (Fig. 193–7). Most certainly, the precise differentiation of lymphocyte subsets and the secretion and interaction of interleukins are disrupted severely by HIV infection. Most important among these lymphocyte subsets is the helper T or CD4 lymphocyte, the central role of which in the production of normal immune responses has been compared with that of a symphony conductor in the production of beautiful music.[96] For some inexplicable reason, this all-important CD4 lymphocyte bears a receptor (the CD4 molecule itself) for the gp120 component of the HIV virion coat, thus rendering it particularly susceptible to attack, paralysis, and destruction by HIV.[96] One can understand the pathogenesis of HIV infection best by considering all the important roles that the CD4 lymphocyte plays in the immune response[96] (Fig. 193–8). In many regards, the immunodeficiency of neonatal HIV infection parallels that of genetically inherited immune disorders.

In addition to its central role in the pathogenesis of pediatric HIV infection, the immune system also seems to contribute directly to perhaps the most devastating aspect of pediatric HIV infection, that of HIV-induced encephalopathy[34, 133] (Fig. 193–9). HIV-induced encephalopathy is also important in adults, but it is particularly devastating in

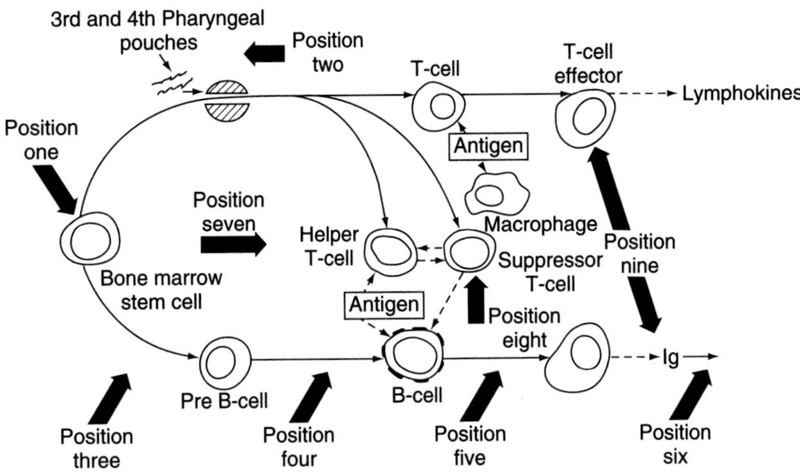

FIGURE 193–7 ■ Model of the events of cellular maturation, cellular interaction, and cellular biosynthesis required for a normal immune response. The *arrows* indicate presumed defects in various immunodeficiency states. Position 1: Failure of B- and T-cell development (e.g., severe combined immunodeficiency disease). Position 2: Failure of development of the thymus (e.g., DiGeorge syndrome). Position 3: Failure of maturation of stem cells into pre-B cells (e.g., thymoma, hypogammaglobulinemia). Position 4: Failure of maturation of pre-B cells into B cells (e.g., X-linked hypogammaglobulinemia). Position 5: Failure of maturation of B cells into plasma cells (e.g., common variable hypogammaglobulinemia). Position 6: Hypercatabolism of immunoglobulin (e.g., myotonic dystrophy). Position 7: Reduced helper T cells (e.g., subset of common variable hypogammaglobulinemia). Position 8: Increase in suppressor T-cell activity (e.g., subset of common variable hypogammaglobulinemia). Position 9: Excessive loss of immunoglobulins and lymphocytes (e.g., intestinal lymphangiectasia). (From Waldmann, T. A.: Immunodeficiency diseases: Primary and acquired. *In* Samter, M., Talmage, D. W., Frank, M. M., et al. [eds.]: Immunological Diseases. 4th ed. Boston, Little, Brown, 1988, pp. 411–465.)

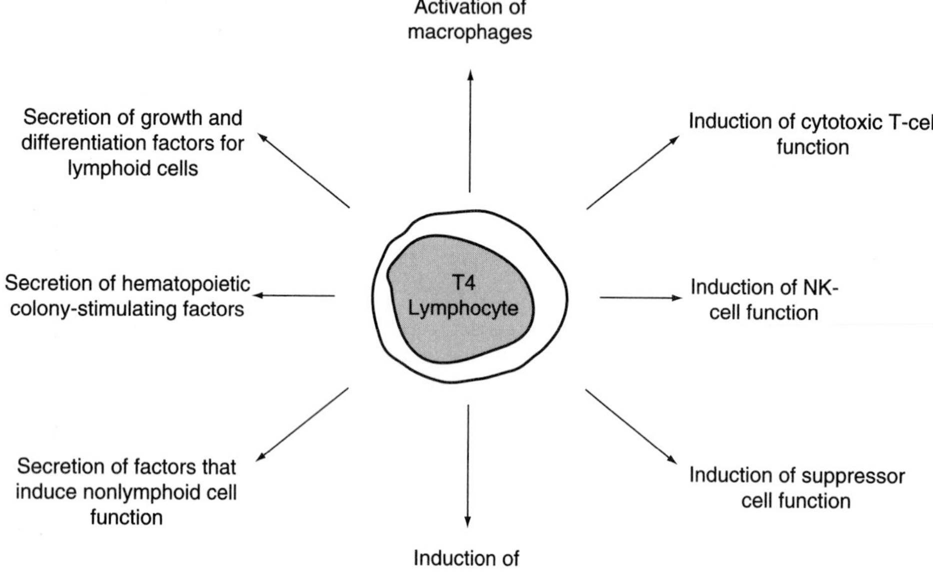

FIGURE 193–8 ■ Critical role of the T4 (CD4) lymphocyte in the human response. The T4 cell is responsible directly or indirectly for the induction of a wide array of functions of multiple limbs of the immune response, as well as for certain nonlymphoid cell functions. This activity is effected for the most part by secretion of a variety of soluble factors that have trophic or inductive effects (or both) on the cells in question. (From Fauci, A. S.: The human immunodeficiency virus: Infectivity and mechanisms of pathogenesis. Science *239*:617–622, 1988. Copyright 1988 by the American Association for the Advancement of Science.)

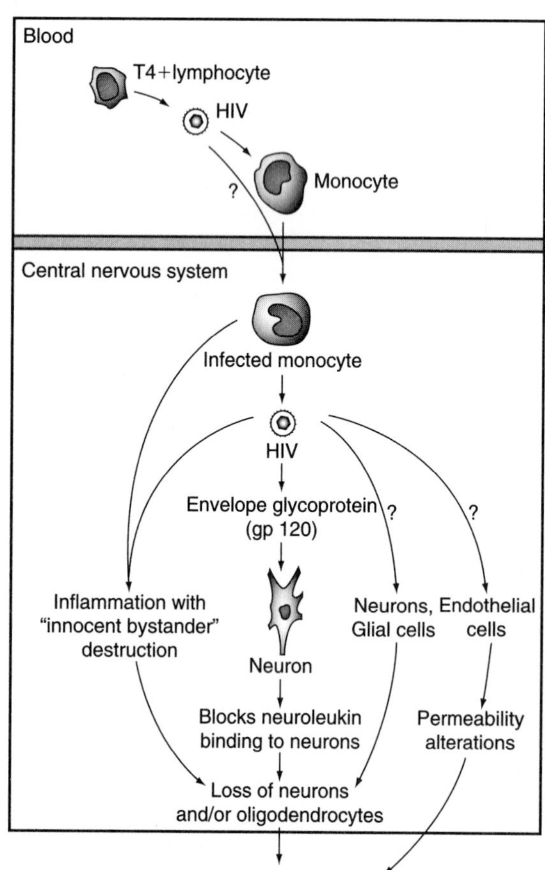

FIGURE 193–9 ■ Role of the immune system in pediatric HIV-induced encephalopathy. HIV-infected CD4 lymphocytes and macrophages enter the central nervous system. HIV may escape from these transport cells and infect nerve cells directly or cause indirect damage to neurons by the release of cytokines such as tumor necrosis factor and interleukin-2. (Reprinted, by permission, from Ho, D., Pomerantz, R. J., and Kaplan, J. C.: Pathogenesis of infection with human immunodeficiency virus. N. Engl. J. Med. *317*:278–286, 1987.)

young infants who fail to reach early motor milestones or, worse, regress from acquired early development. Possibly, the incomplete state of myelination of CNS tissue accounts for this extraordinary susceptibility to the neurologic effects of HIV infection. HIV-infected CD4 lymphocytes and HIV-containing macrophages, which may serve as HIV reservoirs, are thought to transport HIV into the CNS, where the virus appears to be able to infect nerve cells directly.[133] Data implicate cytokines (interleukin-1α [IL-1α] or IL-1β) and reactive oxygen species released by HIV-infected lymphocytes and macrophages in the damage seen in exposed nerve tissue.[270]

IMMUNE DYSFUNCTION IN HIV INFECTION

The immune abnormalities of HIV-infected adult hosts are characterized better than those of HIV-infected pediatric patients. Classically, abnormalities in adult HIV infection include leukopenia, lymphopenia, and decreased CD4 helper-inducer cells with an expanded CD8 cell population, which results in an inverted CD4/CD8 ratio, usually with a number much less than 1.0. Early in infection, T-lymphocyte function has been noted to be diminished (<50%), with decreased in vitro responses to soluble antigens preceding CD4 cell depletion.[130] Although in vitro responses to common mitogens, such as phytohemagglutinin, concanavalin A, and pokeweed, appear to be normal early in HIV infection, these responses begin to decrease with clinical decline; characteristically, pokeweed mitogen responses disappear first. Additionally, in vivo T-lymphocyte function typically reveals cutaneous anergy to *Candida,* tetanus, and mumps antigens.[96] Because of HIV-related paralysis of CD4 cells, IL-2 production is reduced, thereby weakening the immune amplification system.[96] HIV-infected CD4 cells release soluble IL-2 receptors. These elevated serum IL-2 receptor levels produce a blockade of cell-bound IL-2 receptors by competition for IL-2.

Changes in immunologic function in the presence of HIV infection have been observed in infants and children. Children with HIV infection are infrequently lymphopenic in terms of values observed in adults.[64] If lymphopenia is observed in children with HIV infection, it usually is seen in older children with transfusion-associated infection or in children who have progressed to end-stage HIV disease. CD4 cell depletion may be less dramatic in children as a consequence of their relative lymphocytosis. In fact, CD4 cell counts in HIV-infected children commonly exceed 400 cells/mm^3. Moreover, Denny and associates[78] have shown that in infants 12 to 24 months of age, a CD4 value of less than 1000 cells/mm^3 is significant for HIV-related CD4 depletion; in infants younger than 12 months, a value of less than 1500 cells/mm^3 similarly applies. Because of altered relative proportions of CD4 and CD8 cells, the inverted CD4/CD8 ratio observed in children is similar to that in adults. As in adults, lymphoproliferative responses to recall antigens have been documented as relatively normal early in infection; decline is correlated with the onset of clinical symptoms.[28] HIV-1–specific CD8 cytotoxic-suppressor cell function has been documented as nondetectable in infants with primary infection (early perinatal infection).[178] The impact of cytotoxic cell function on progression of disease is currently under analysis.[109] Cutaneous anergy is a usual finding in children with HIV infection; however, interpretation in children younger than 2 years may be difficult because of the relative degree of anergy in very young normal children.

In addition to T-lymphocyte dysfunction in HIV-infected adults, B-cell dysfunction is similarly marked (e.g., hypergammaglobulinemia occurs in adults and can be used to monitor disease progression). HIV-infected adults also demonstrate circulating immune complexes and autoantibody production secondary to polyclonal activation of B cells by HIV itself or concomitant viral infection with cytomegalovirus (CMV) or Epstein-Barr virus.[163] Other host defense cells are affected by HIV infection[26, 244] (e.g., natural killer cells in HIV infection have been shown to be unable to kill target cells normally, despite adequate binding, and cytotoxic T-cell function has been demonstrated to be diminished, although patients have sufficient numbers of precursor cytotoxic T lymphocytes).[151, 179] Monocytes and macrophages most likely play a major role in the pathogenesis of HIV infection by serving as HIV reservoirs that are spared the cytopathic effects of HIV. Defective chemotaxis and bacterial killing have been observed in HIV-infected monocytes and macrophages, as well as defective induction of IL-1, which possibly accounts for the decreased IL-2 response in CD4 cells.[244]

Hypergammaglobulinemia is particularly prominent in infants and children with HIV infection and frequently heralds HIV infection at a time when the HIV enzyme-linked immunosorbent assay (ELISA) and Western blot are nondiagnostic because of the presence of maternal antibody. This evidence of B-cell activation or dysregulation often precedes other evidence of immune dysfunction, namely, CD4 depletion, an inverted CD4/CD8 ratio, or in vitro evidence of T-cell dysfunction. In particular, IgG levels may rise to 2 to 3 SD above the mean of normal values, and serum IgA, IgM, and IgE levels may be elevated as well. This extreme hypergammaglobulinemia in children may be caused by polyclonal stimulation of B cells by HIV or co-infection with CMV or Epstein-Barr virus, or it may be caused by the absence of normal CD4 immunoregulatory cells.[215] Functional activity has been documented as inadequate in children with HIV infection despite elevation of serum immunoglobulin levels.[7, 20, 27, 28]

ORIGIN OF IMMUNODEFICIENCY IN HIV INFECTION

Hypotheses have been proposed to explain the immune aberrations, specifically, CD4 depletion and dysfunction, noted in HIV infection; Table 193–12 lists several of these hypotheses.[212] None of these proposals is entirely satisfactory in explaining the secondary immunodeficiency of HIV infection in adults or children. Probably the first and second of these proposals (CD4 cell depletion and CD4 cell syncytial formation) are the easiest to comprehend because removal of CD4 cells or CD4 function from the immune system would render it progressively weaker and unable to thwart secondary infections. However, more recent data elucidating the immunopathogenesis of HIV infection have documented that HIV-1 replication in vivo is continuous and drives rapid and constant turnover of CD4 lymphocytes, in contrast to the notion that inconstant HIV replication produces a stepwise decline in circulating CD4 lymphocytes.[135, 274] Rabin and associates[222] and Roederer and colleagues[225] noted depletion of CD8-naive T cells and CD4 depletion in children and adults, respectively. CD8 expansion, characteristic of early asymptomatic infection, was noted especially with CD8 memory T cells. CD4 depletion preferentially involved naive T cells. These findings suggest a relationship between depletion of naive CD4 T cells and poor new T-cell–mediated responses. The idea that immunopathogenesis may be related to syncytium formation is provocative because of already existing immunopathologic viral models of infection, such as with respiratory syncytial virus.[240]

TABLE 193–12 ■ POTENTIAL MECHANISMS OF THE FUNCTIONAL AND QUANTITATIVE DEPLETION OF CD4 T LYMPHOCYTES

Direct HIV-mediated cytopathic effects (single-cell killing)
HIV-mediated formation of syncytia
Virus-specific immune responses
  HIV-specific cytolytic T lymphocytes
  Antibody-dependent cellular cytotoxicity
  Natural killer cells
Autoimmune mechanisms
Anergy caused by inappropriate cell signaling through gp120-CD4 interaction
Superantigen-mediated perturbation of T-cell subgroups
Programmed cell death (apoptosis)

Reprinted, by permission, from Pantaleo, G., Grazosi, C., and Fauci, A. S.: The immunopathogenesis of human immunodeficiency virus infection. N. Engl. J. Med. *328*:327–335, 1993.

In most children, the additional complexity of maternal-fetal transmission of HIV is a consideration, and few data define the immunopathogenesis of HIV infection in this transplacental or perinatal event. The maternal immunologic status and the role of the placenta in affording protection or permitting infection should be defined, and potential perinatal cofactors (such as intravenous drug abuse, sexually transmitted diseases, maternal malnutrition) should be understood better. Langston and associates[164] suggest that HIV may be fetotoxic, with impact most notably reported in the thymus, where precocious involution, epithelial injury, and occasionally, severe thymitis are described. Loss of lymphocytes at the corticomedullary junction of the thymus implies a defect induced by HIV in the immunologic selection process. Pediatric virus-specific immune responses (i.e., the roles of CD8$^+$ cytotoxic cells and monocytes and neutralizing antibody production) are being studied. Normal mechanisms of cell death, programmed cell death or apoptosis, may be enhanced by cross-linking of the CD4 molecule with HIV gp120 complexes or circulating immune complexes.[120, 212] Vigano and associates[269] documented the predominant production of type 2 cytokines (IL-4, IL-10) in children with symptomatic infection and proposed that it might increase clinical progression and CD4 depletion by enhancing apoptosis or HIV replication.

Abundant epidemiologic information clearly documents that serious and life-threatening clinical manifestations develop more rapidly in children with perinatally acquired HIV infection and immune dysfunction than in adults, who typically are symptom-free for approximately 10 years after the acquisition of HIV infection.[226, 276] In the case of perinatal HIV infection, symptoms generally occur by 2 years and ultimately lead to death.[228, 234] These epidemiologic data indicate that the immunologically naive, pediatric host defense system is affected more quickly by HIV infection, most likely on the basis of several defects in host defense.[276]

Clinical Manifestations

In children and adults, HIV infection causes a spectrum of clinical abnormalities that affect multiple organ systems and include the symptom constellation of AIDS. Table 193–13 lists many of the presumed or documented opportunistic infections that satisfy the current criteria for a diagnosis of pediatric AIDS.[46] Wasting, encephalopathy, lymphoproliferative lung disorders, and oncologic processes are also diagnostic of AIDS. Infection with HIV, independent of an AIDS diagnosis, may be attended by nonspecific clinical findings, including mild failure to thrive (not sufficient to meet the AIDS wasting definition), hepatosplenomegaly, acquired microcephaly, parotitis, generalized lymphadenopathy, nonspecific intermittent diarrhea, intermittent fever, and chronic skin disease.[207] These clinical symptoms are shared by other pediatric disease processes and can, when manifested singly in an HIV-infected host, cause a delay in diagnosis. However, a careful and detailed history should provide helpful insight into potential HIV risk factors and prompt inclusion of HIV infection in the differential diagnosis. The major clinical features of AIDS are discussed here by broad categories: opportunistic infections, pulmonary complications, CNS complications, and so forth.

OPPORTUNISTIC INFECTIONS

Opportunistic infections plague HIV-infected individuals and are the most prominent cause of morbidity and mortality in this cohort. Of note, the introduction of effective HAART interventions that have provided host immune restoration have significantly modified the expression of certain opportunistic infections in adults and children.[258] The administration of combination HIV therapy, including protease inhibitors in adults and children, has improved the survival of perinatally infected children.[4, 115, 209]

Pneumocystis Pneumonia

P. carinii pneumonia (PCP) ranks second only to lymphoid interstitial pneumonitis as the most common pulmonary disease.[125, 242] PCP has a fulminant course in the pediatric population, with the highest mortality rates occurring in affected children younger than 1 year.[242] In a study of 172 children with perinatal HIV infection, 9 percent had PCP when younger than 1 year, with a median survival of 1 month.[234] Clinical expression of pediatric PCP often can be distinguished from other pulmonary diseases by the severity of the hypoxemia (higher alveolar-arterial oxygen gradients), elevated serum lactate dehydrogenase levels, the rapidity of progression of disease with tachypnea and fever, characteristic diffuse interstitial infiltrates on radiography, and the usual lack of digital clubbing.[127] The more insidious manifestation of PCP characteristic of HIV-infected adults, namely, prolonged fever (>7 weeks), cough, and dyspnea (averaging 3 weeks), is appreciated less commonly in infants and children. Radiographically, pediatric PCP is associated with diffuse interstitial markings progressing to the "white-out" picture of adult respiratory distress syndrome (Fig. 193–10). However, PCP can be seen initially as a unilateral streaky pneumonic infiltrate, as lobar consolidation, or with accompanying pleural effusions.

As in primary immunodeficiency disorders, aggressive diagnostic measures may be indicated to establish a diagnosis of PCP. Lung biopsy remains the gold standard for distinguishing PCP from other lung diseases in AIDS. However, bronchoscopic alveolar lavage has proved to be a useful diagnostic tool in adults and children and should be considered a first diagnostic choice for presumed PCP in children who cannot provide sputum specimens for evaluation.[127] In older children and adults, evaluation of sputum for the presence of *Pneumocystis* with appropriate stains or monoclonal antibodies may preempt the need for invasive diagnostic measures.

TABLE 193–13 ■ OPPORTUNISTIC INFECTIONS THAT ESTABLISH THE DIAGNOSIS OF AIDS

Documented HIV Infection
Presumptive diagnosis
- Esophageal candidiasis
- Cytomegalovirus retinitis
- *Pneumocystis* pneumonia
- Toxoplasmosis of the brain (after 1 mo of age)
- Disseminated atypical mycobacterial infection

Definitive histologically confirmed diagnosis
- Disseminated coccidioidomycosis
- Disseminated histoplasmosis
- Isosporiasis
- Extrapulmonary cryptococcosis
- Extrapulmonary *Mycobacterium tuberculosis*
- Recurrent *Salmonella* septicemia
- Disseminated/persistent herpes simplex

Indeterminate HIV Infection
All opportunists listed above are applicable but must be diagnosed definitively, i.e., histologic confirmation

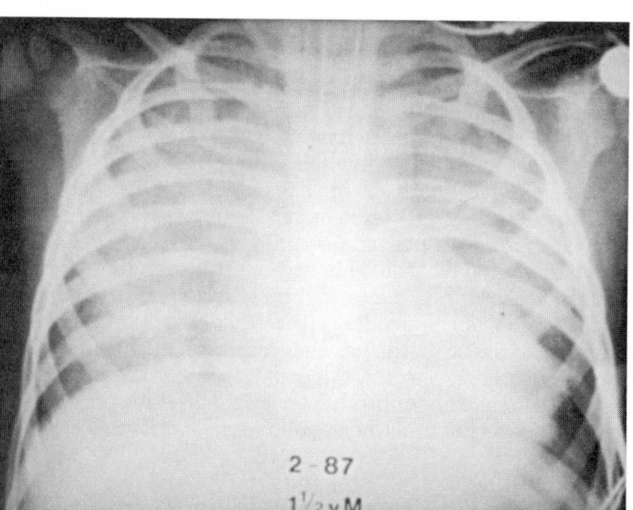

FIGURE 193–10 ■ Classic diffuse interstitial infiltrates of acute and fatal *Pneumocystis carinii* pneumonia in a 15-month-old child with perinatal AIDS. (From Hanson, I. C.: Respiratory infections in HIV-infected children. Immunol. Allergy Clin. North Am. *13*:205–217, 1993.)

Acute PCP is treated traditionally with parenteral trimethoprim-sulfamethoxazole (TMP-SMX) or pentamidine or, for those with hypersensitivity, with atovaquone.[140] Adjunctive corticosteroid therapy given early in moderate to severe PCP provides significant benefit with only limited evidence of concomitant immune suppression and attendant infectious complications.[111, 243, 261]

Secondary PCP prophylaxis (therapy initiated after resolution and complete treatment of acute PCP) for adults and children is accepted as standard care.[48, 50, 54, 139] Proposed pediatric regimens include TMP-SMX at 150 mg/m^2/day and 750 mg/m^2/day, respectively, three times a week (single dose on 3 consecutive days a week, two divided doses on 3 alternate days a week, two divided doses daily), dapsone at 2 mg/kg (single dosing not to exceed 100 mg/day), and pentamidine (aerosolized [300 mg via Respirgard II inhaler monthly]).[54, 141] Although lower doses of TMP-SMX have been reported to be effective in the prevention of PCP in a small cohort of HIV-infected children, no controlled, prospective study of alternative dosing has been conducted.[100] In children younger than 13 years, evidence supporting interruption of secondary prophylaxis based on immune reconstitution is being evaluated. This approach contrasts with recommendations to discontinue secondary PCP prophylaxis in adults and adolescents with evidence of restoration of immunity (CD4$^+$ T- lymphocyte counts that have increased to greater than 200 cells/mm^3 for 3 months or longer as a result of HAART).[62] Primary PCP prophylaxis for adults and children is well defined by the CDC.[54, 65] In 1993, the CDC published the first PCP prophylaxis guidelines for HIV-infected children; these guidelines linked the institution of therapy to the level of immunosuppression as measured by the CD4 count or percentage.[48, 168] After implementation of these guidelines, Simonds and associates[242] reviewed the incidence of reported PCP cases to the CDC and noted no decline in case numbers. Of 300 children with PCP reported to the CDC between January 1991 and June 1993, 66 percent had never received prophylaxis. In addition, 18 percent of infants younger than 1 year experienced PCP with CD4 counts that were above the guideline thresholds for immunosuppression. Based on these data, guidelines for PCP prophylaxis in children were modified in 1995, and Table 193–14 outlines the institution of therapy by age and CD4 monitoring.[54] The most significant changes in the revised guidelines include (1) an emphasis on early detection of HIV infection in infants for optimal implementation of the guidelines, (2) provision of PCP prophylaxis to all HIV-exposed infants in the first months of life, and (3) emphasis on quarterly CD4 monitoring to evaluate immunosuppression thresholds in HIV-infected children. The low potential for associated morbidity from the administration of PCP prophylaxis allows for implementation of therapy to all infants, independent of HIV status, in the first months of life, when their risk has been documented to be highest and is least likely to correlate with CD4 monitoring.[242]

Mycobacterium avium–intracellulare Complex

The *M. avium–intracellulare* complex (MAC), which caused disseminated infections in both adults and children with HIV infection in the early 1980s and 1990s, has waned significantly with increasing and successful use of HAART.[87] In a 1990 review of opportunistic infections in pediatric AIDS patients, 43 of 552 (7.8%) children from birth to 9 years of age were found to have disseminated MAC.[127] Epidemiologically, MAC has been linked with evidence of significant immunosuppression (CD4 counts below 50 cells/mm^3) in adults.[51, 62, 137] Researchers have noted that the development of MAC infection in children may be associated with CD4 counts greater than 50 cells/mm^3, especially in those younger than 6 years.[62, 154, 231] Symptoms of MAC infection include fever, malaise, weight loss, anorexia, and night sweats. Gastrointestinal manifestations are not uncommon and have included abdominal pain, diarrhea, malabsorption, and intestinal perforation. Rarely, MAC has been reported with extrabiliary obstructive jaundice (presumed to be secondary to lymphadenopathy) and endobronchial masses. The diagnosis of disseminated MAC infection relies on identification of these microorganisms from the blood, lymph tissue, bone marrow, liver, lungs, and gastrointestinal tract. Therapy for disseminated MAC infection in the pediatric population includes some combination of clarithromycin or azithromycin (maximal dosing of 500 mg and 250 mg, respectively) and/or rifabutin (maximal dosing of 300 mg).[4, 125, 138] The epidemiologic link with severe immunosuppression and the advent of therapeutic prophylactic interventions (clarithromycin or azithromycin and/or rifabutin) has prompted the implementation of MAC prophylaxis guidelines for adults, adolescents, and older children (6 years and older) with CD4 counts less than 50 cells/mm^3.[51] In adults,

TABLE 193–14 ■ RECOMMENDATIONS FOR *PNEUMOCYSTIS* PNEUMONIA PROPHYLAXIS AND CD4$^+$ MONITORING FOR HIV-EXPOSED INFANTS AND HIV-INFECTED CHILDREN BY AGE AND HIV INFECTION STATUS

Age/HIV Infection Status	PCP Prophylaxis	CD4$^+$ Monitoring
Birth to 4–6 wk, HIV exposed	No prophylaxis	1 mo
4–6 wk to 4 mo, HIV exposed	Prophylaxis	3 mo
4–12 mo		
HIV infected or indeterminate	Prophylaxis	6, 9, and 12 mo
HIV infection reasonably excluded	No prophylaxis	None
1–5 yr, HIV infected	Prophylaxis *if* CD4$^+$ count is <500 cells/μL or CD4$^+$ percentage is <15%	Every 3–4 mo
6–12 yr, HIV infected	Prophylaxis *if* CD4$^+$ count is <200 cells/μL or CD4$^+$ percentage is <15%	Every 3–4 mo

From Centers for Disease Control and Prevention: 1995 Revised guidelines for prophylaxis against *Pneumocystis carinii* pneumonia for children infected with or perinatally exposed to human immunodeficiency virus. National Pediatric and Family HIV Resource Center and National Center for Infectious Diseases, Centers for Disease Control and Prevention: M. M. W. R. Recomm. Rep. *44*(RR-4):6, 1995.

discontinuation of primary MAC prophylaxis has been linked to evidence of sustained immune restoration ($CD4^+$ T-lymphocyte counts that exceed 100 cells/mm^3 for 3 or more months). Such studies have not been conducted with great numbers of HIV-infected children. However, because of issues of compliance (nausea, vomiting) with the drugs available for MAC prophylaxis, many clinicians have elected to discontinue primary and even secondary MAC prophylaxis in children with evidence of sustained age-matched restoration of immunity as a result of HAART.

Mycobacterium tuberculosis

The increasing incidence of tuberculosis globally has affected the HIV-infected population because factors that increase the transmission of tuberculosis also have an impact on HIV transmission.[195] In a cohort of pregnant and nonpregnant HIV-infected women monitored in a multicenter longitudinal study, the prevalence of tuberculosis determined by medical history or positive skin tests was 14 percent.[198] In tuberculosis-positive individuals 25 to 44 years of age in the United States, the incidence of co-infection with HIV ranges from 9.9 to 24.2 percent in low to higher reporting states.[61] Factors associated with the acquisition of pediatric tuberculosis primarily have included family and caregiver risks.[15] In a study of 60 HIV-infected families, the incidence of tuberculosis was approximately 6 percent, with both HIV-infected and HIV-uninfected children affected.[13] The vector for transmission was identified as an infected family member or caregiver. Tuberculosis should be considered in the differential diagnosis of pulmonary disease in HIV-exposed children, and routine testing for tuberculosis should be standard care for this population. Treatment of active tuberculosis in an HIV-infected child includes at least a four-drug regimen, and the duration of treatment is 9 to 12 months, with the longest duration in children with extrapulmonary disease. Careful monitoring of antiretroviral therapy is necessary in HIV-infected children receiving concomitant antituberculosis therapy because interactions can be complex. For example, rifampin induces hepatic cytochrome P-450 and may have an impact on antiretroviral agents metabolized through that same pathway. Each HIV-infected child should be evaluated annually for exposure to tuberculosis.

Cytomegalovirus

In 1987 reports to the CDC, disseminated CMV infection occurred in 19 percent of pediatric patients with AIDS.[228] The adult spectrum of CMV disease, including retinitis, pneumonitis, esophagitis, gastritis, colitis, hepatitis, cholangitis, and encephalitis, is not defined as precisely in the pediatric AIDS literature. CMV clearly can cause primary pneumonitis in children or can be found in association with other pulmonary pathogens, especially *Pneumocystis*. Unusual gastrointestinal manifestations have included pyloric obstruction, enterocolitis, and oral and esophageal ulcers. CMV retinitis in children, in contrast to adults, is described infrequently. This discrepancy may reflect the lack of good subjective complaints in the pediatric population or early demise from other infections such as PCP. Treatment of CMV disease associated with HIV infection focuses on progression of disease and not a curative outcome. Therapeutic intervention includes the use of ganciclovir, valganciclovir, foscarnet, or cidofovir. These drugs have significant side effects, including bone marrow suppression and renal toxicity.[82] Drug dosing with these agents is divided into induction and maintenance dosing. The optimal interval for efficacy has not been determined clearly and usually is chosen on an individual basis. Although many adults report subjective and objective improvement on receiving therapy, discontinuation of therapy is associated with high relapse rates, independent of the affected site. Careful monitoring of children receiving CMV treatment and antiretroviral therapy is imperative because the use of both classes of agents may depress bone marrow function. Guidelines to prevent CMV infection in HIV-infected persons have been published and include the use of oral ganciclovir.[106] Oral ganciclovir may provide primary prophylaxis in HIV- and CMV-infected children with severe immunosuppression ($CD4^+$ T-lymphocyte count <50 cells/mm^3). Prevention of complications of CMV in HIV-infected children with severe immunosuppression should include careful and regular (every 4 to 6 months) retinal monitoring for evidence of eye disease.[55] Once initiated, discontinuation of secondary prophylaxis for disseminated CMV disease should be considered on a case-by-case basis because current data to support discontinuation are limited.

Other Herpesvirus Infections

Infections with the herpesvirus family are not uncommon in HIV-infected children, with chronic herpes simplex virus infection reported in 5 percent of children with AIDS.[228] In general, herpes simplex virus infection in pediatric AIDS has been limited to mild to severe localized infections without reports of dissemination. Varicella-zoster and herpes-zoster virus infections have contributed significant morbidity to HIV-infected persons. Disseminated and chronic herpes-zoster virus infections are reported in pediatric patients with AIDS. The judicious use of acyclovir for chronic infection is warranted to lessen the probability of emergence of resistant strains. Prevention of herpes infections in school-age children is especially important because varicella exposure may be considerable. Administering varicella-zoster immune globulin should be considered for susceptible HIV-infected children with exposure to varicella-zoster virus. Because the varicella vaccine is an attenuated live viral vaccine, its use in HIV-infected children is limited currently to children with asymptomatic or mildly symptomatic HIV disease and evidence of 25 percent $CD4^+$ T lymphocytes or greater.[56]

Fungal Diseases

Chronic *Candida* infection plagues HIV-infected children.[64, 207] Affected mucous membranes or skin often does not respond well to treatment with topical antifungal agents. Fluconazole has been documented in an open multicenter study to be as effective and safe as ketoconazole for the treatment of oropharyngeal candidiasis.[132] In severe fungal infections, amphotericin B should be administered intravenously. Prophylaxis for candidal infections is not recommended because of concern about the development of resistance to azoles such as fluconazole, which could limit their use significantly in the care of disseminated or mucosal disease.[55, 62]

Other disseminated fungal diseases, such as histoplasmosis and cryptococcosis, less commonly affect pediatric patients with AIDS. Histoplasmosis may be prevalent in HIV-infected children who reside in parts of the United States where *Histoplasma capsulatum* is endemic.[275] Symptoms of histoplasmosis include fever, rash, cough, lymphadenopathy, splenomegaly, thrombocytopenia, low-grade disseminated intravascular coagulopathy, adult respiratory distress syndrome, meningoencephalitis, and neurologic abnormalities consistent with intracranial mass lesions. Symptoms of cryptococcosis include fever, headache, pulmonary involvement, and subacute meningitis or meningoencephalitis. Primary prophylaxis for adults and adolescents is suggested for those with immune system compromise. Specifically, itraconazole is suggested as primary cryptococcosis prophylaxis for adults and adolescents with $CD4^+$ lymphocyte counts of less than 50 cells/mm^3 and fluconazole for histoplasmosis prophylaxis in adults and adolescents with $CD4^+$ lymphocyte counts of less than 100 cells/mm^3. Recommendations to discontinue prophylaxis as a result of HAART-related improved immune function have been developed for cryptococcosis and include sustained (6 months or greater) $CD4^+$ lymphocyte counts higher than 100 to 200 cells/mm^3. In contrast, no such recommendations exist for discontinuation of histoplasmosis prophylaxis in HIV-infected adults or adolescents with evidence of HAART-related reconstitution of immunity.

Bacterial Diseases

Pediatric patients have an increased incidence of severe bacterial infections, including *Streptococcus pneumoniae, Staphylococcus aureus,* and various gram-negative organisms.[3] The risk of contracting community-acquired invasive bacterial infections has been estimated to be three times higher than the rate in non–HIV-infected children.[9] In a study of 372 HIV-infected children monitored for a median of 17 months, 14 percent experienced one or more laboratory-proven serious bacterial infections.[260] Clinical infections included bacteremia, pneumonia, osteomyelitis, meningitis, and sinusitis. Therapy is directed against the specific isolated bacterial pathogen, and the dosing and duration of therapy are dependent on the affected site. Prophylaxis against bacterial infections initially should include vaccination with appropriate childhood vaccines, including *Haemophilus influenzae* type b and pneumococcal conjugate vaccines.[14] Other medications available for bacterial prophylaxis include intravenous immunoglobulin (IVIG) and TMP-SMX. In a study that predated the widespread use of antiretroviral agents in children, the use of IVIG (400 mg/kg every 28 days) increased the time free from serious bacterial infections in those with CD4 counts exceeding 199 cells/mm^3 and decreased morbidity as measured by hospitalizations.[197] A subsequent analysis of concomitant IVIG and zidovudine use documented the efficacy of IVIG in children not also receiving TMP-SMX for PCP prophylaxis.[247] Given the expense and cumbersome route of administration, IVIG has been reserved as prophylaxis for HIV-infected children with evidence of hypogammaglobulinemia or those resistant to antibiotic prophylaxis options.

PULMONARY COMPLICATIONS

In addition to PCP and chronic sinopulmonary infection, the noninfectious pulmonary complications of pediatric AIDS are associated with significant morbidity. In a series of more than 150 children with perinatal HIV infection, the lymphoproliferative lung disorders LIP/PLH were reported most frequently, and 17 percent of these children were affected.[234] Histopathologically, LIP and PLH appear to be distinct entities, although whether these disorders represent a continuum of reactive hyperplasia of lymphoid tissue is somewhat controversial.[96] In LIP, small lymphoid infiltrates are dispersed throughout parenchymal lung tissue and often are accompanied by alveolar epithelial hyperplasia and interstitial widening. PLH describes larger, dense nodular aggregates of lymphoid tissue both in distal parenchymal tissue and in the walls of bronchi and bronchioles (Fig. 193–11*A*). Compression of blood and lymphatic vessels by these nodules may contribute to the accompanying clinical interstitial widening. The etiology of LIP/PLH has not been defined. Associations with in situ Epstein-Barr virus and the HIV genome have been noted, and an increase in local nonspecific and HIV-specific IgG and IgA production has been described.[125]

Clinically, LIP/PLH is characterized by a nonproductive cough and the insidious onset of progressive hypoxia. The hypoxemia may be subtle and best appreciated during febrile, upper respiratory tract illnesses. Digital clubbing, generalized lymphadenopathy, chronic parotitis, or failure to thrive may accompany LIP/PLH. Radiographically, LIP/PLH often demonstrates characteristic interstitial infiltrates with a nodular pattern (See Fig. 193–11*B*). This radiographic picture frequently mimics that of miliary tuberculosis and warrants exclusion of this pulmonary infection. In an immunocompromised, anergic, HIV-positive child, simple delayed hypersensitivity skin testing for exclusion of tuberculosis may not suffice, and bronchoalveolar lavage or gastric aspiration for detection of acid-fast microorganisms may be necessary. Lung biopsy is the definitive diagnostic procedure for LIP/PLH. However, in HIV-infected children, a presumed diagnosis of LIP/PLH by the less invasive exclusion of infectious pathogens is preferred.

Therapy for LIP/PLH is not defined clearly because the clinical outcome is variable. HIV-infected children with LIP/PLH have been noted to have spontaneous remissions without therapeutic intervention, whereas other affected children progress to respiratory insufficiency and failure. Therapeutic interventions have included IVIG supplementation; antiretroviral therapy, specifically, zidovudine and corticosteroids (daily or alternate-day dosing ranging from 0.5 to 2.0 mg/kg/day); and observation.[125] No significant associated infectious sequelae (bacteremia, fungemia) of corticosteroid use were reported in treated children. Supportive therapy consisting of oxygen supplementation, chest physiotherapy, and attention to adequate nutritional intake is helpful adjunctive treatment.

In general, children with LIP/PLH have prolonged survival in comparison to those with PCP or other AIDS-defining events. Of note, LIP/PLH is included as a category B event in the 1994 revised pediatric classification and staging system.[52] Scott and associates[234] described a median survival time of 72 months for children with LIP/PLH, in contrast to median survival times of 12 and 11 months for children with *Candida* esophagitis and HIV encephalopathy, respectively.

Other noninfectious pulmonary complications have been reported less frequently in the pediatric HIV-infected population and include bronchiectasis, vasculitis, and diffuse interstitial pneumonitis. Pulmonary B-cell lymphoproliferative disorders (non-Hodgkin lymphoma) have been described in pediatric AIDS cases, often associated with lymphoproliferative lung disorders (LIP/PLH) and detection of Epstein-Barr virus by polymerase chain reaction (PCR), immunochemistry, and Southern blot analysis.[185, 205]

CENTRAL NERVOUS SYSTEM COMPLICATIONS

Neurologic abnormalities have been documented in persons with HIV and can be attributed to opportunistic infections, adverse events of primary treatment, or primary infection with HIV, especially in light of HIV's described tropism for monocytes. Ten percent of adults with AIDS initially have neurologic symptoms, and 40 percent are affected during their clinical course.[183] An appreciation of the neurologic abnormalities in pediatric AIDS lagged behind documentation of immunodeficiency and concomitant opportunistic

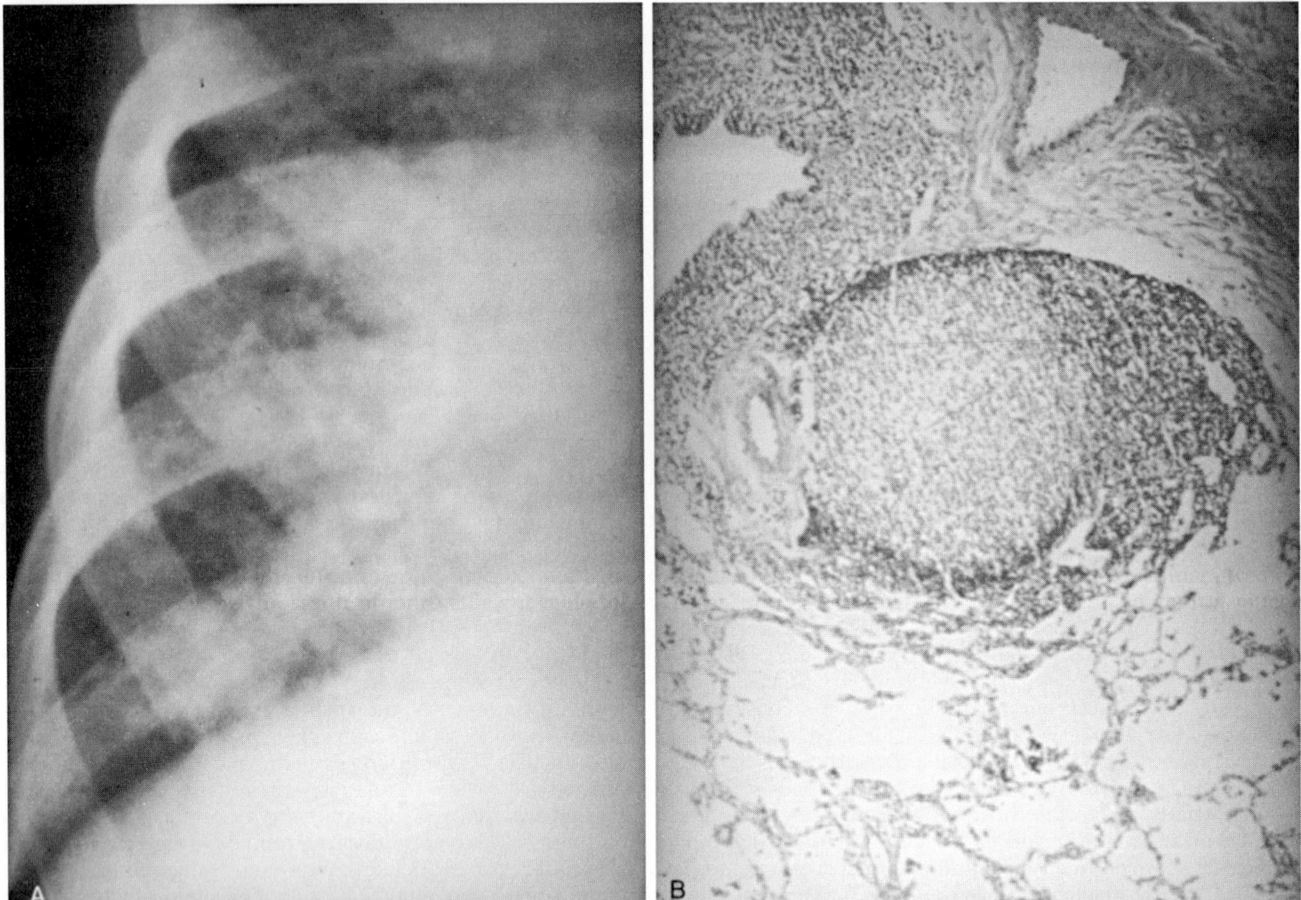

FIGURE 193–11 ■ *A*, Chest radiograph documenting parenchymal nodularity in a 3-year-old child with perinatal AIDS. *B*, Pulmonary lymphoid hyperplasia in the same infant with perinatal AIDS and histologic changes, including interstitial widening and prominent peribronchial lung nodes.

infections and lung disease in the literature. Belman and associates (1988)[18] and Epstein and colleagues (1986)[91] described significant neurologic complications, including seizure disorders, attention-deficit disorders, developmental delay, and acquired microcephaly and encephalopathy, in association with HIV disease. In 1987, expansion of the CDC surveillance criteria for the diagnosis of AIDS incorporated and acknowledged neurologic deficits by defining AIDS dementia or encephalopathy.[46] In adults, *dementia* included "clinical findings of disabling cognitive and/or motor dysfunction interfering with occupation or activities of daily living." In children, this definition incorporated progressive loss of behavioral or developmental milestones. A diagnosis of AIDS dementia in adults and HIV encephalopathy in children requires the exclusion of concurrent illnesses or conditions other than HIV infection, such as infectious agents (congenital or acquired toxoplasmosis or CMV infection) or malignancy. In 1994, the definition of HIV encephalopathy was adapted directly to children and consists of at least one of the following present for at least 2 months: (1) failure to attain or loss of developmental milestones or loss of intellectual ability, verified by a standard developmental scale or neuropsychologic tests; (2) impaired brain growth or acquired microcephaly demonstrated by head circumference measurements or brain atrophy identified by computed tomography (CT) or magnetic resonance imaging (MRI) (serial imaging is required for children younger than 2 years); and (3) acquired symmetric motor deficit manifested by two or more of the following: paresis, pathologic reflexes, ataxia, or gait disturbance.[52] The incidence of HIV encephalopathy in the pediatric AIDS population is high. In an early large multicenter surveillance cohort of perinatal HIV-infected children, 23 percent exhibited clinical symptoms consistent with the diagnosis of HIV encephalopathy.[175] Other neurologic abnormalities described in adult patients with AIDS, including neuropathy, myopathy, radiculopathy, and vacuolar myelopathy, have been reported infrequently in the pediatric AIDS cohort. The onset of encephalopathy has been described in association with profound immune deficiency. Lobato and colleagues[175] reported CD4 counts of less than 500 cells/mm^3 in children younger than 1 year with HIV encephalopathy. Isolated encephalopathy without other AIDS-defining opportunists or characteristics has been reported infrequently in the pediatric literature.

The precise pathogenesis of the encephalopathic changes associated with HIV infection remains elusive, although cellular tropism of HIV has been implicated.[11] Histopathologically, most children with involvement of the CNS (not related to malignancy or opportunistic infection) show significant brain atrophy. Of note, inflammatory lesions are usually sparse and alone cannot account for the significant amount of atrophy observed. Other purported factors potentially contributing to diminished brain size have included the following: (1) direct or indirect interference of HIV with brain growth (HIV toxic effect versus competition with brain growth factors such as neuroleukin), (2) severe malnutrition, (3) severe hypoxia from cardiac and pulmonary compromise, and (4) therapeutic regimens for infectious or noninfectious processes that mandate the prolonged use of medications that may inhibit brain growth.[11, 193] In addition to cortical atrophy, myelin pallor and basal ganglia calcifications are reported at histology and by the use of nuclear imaging techniques (CT or MRI). These latter findings often have no correlation with clinical neurologic abnormality and suggest that further study of CNS involvement in pediatric patients is warranted.

Behavioral abnormalities have been described in the literature in the pediatric HIV-infected cohort. In hemophiliac patients in Pennsylvania, the mean intelligence quotient was higher than the state average, but attention-deficit/hyperactivity disorder, learning disability, and graphomotor weakness were described in higher proportion in the HIV-infected group.[182]

Therapy for noninfectious and nonmalignant encephalopathy in HIV-infected children has included antiretroviral therapy.[187, 217] Behavioral, neurodevelopmental, and occasionally, imaging improvements have been documented with nucleoside analogue intervention. Clearly, antiviral therapy not only must achieve effective serum and plasma concentrations but also must be able to cross the blood-brain barrier and affect HIV-infected CNS monocytes. Children with neurologic or behavioral deficits and HIV infection should be evaluated by a pediatric neurologist, and obtaining developmental, audiologic, and ophthalmologic assessments is warranted.[166] This cohort of children often needs special support systems that may include physical therapy, medications to assist with seizure control or contractures, specialized equipment (braces, splints, wheelchairs, etc.), and as needed, medications or devices to assist with swallowing or food ingestion.

A clinical syndrome of aseptic meningitis, often recurring and presumed to be solely related to HIV infection, has been described in adults.[183] In pediatric AIDS, bacterial pathogens predominate as the most common cause of meningitis, and the aforementioned recurrent aseptic meningitis syndrome appears to be a rare occurrence.[12] Cerebrospinal fluid (CSF) assessments in HIV-infected children without overt clinical CNS involvement are usually normal but occasionally reveal pleocytosis, elevated protein content, and elevated intrathecal antibody synthesis directed toward HIV itself or HIV antigen.[116] HIV rarely is isolated from CSF. Other pathogens reported in the pediatric HIV-infected population include *Candida* spp., CMV, tuberculosis, *Toxoplasma,* and *Cryptococcus.*[194]

GASTROINTESTINAL COMPLICATIONS

Gastrointestinal complications of HIV disease are encountered frequently in both children and adults. Among children with AIDS reported to the CDC in 1988 and 1989, wasting syndrome was described in 16 percent.[226] Wasting has been revised from the 1987 definition to its present definition (1994): (1) persistent weight loss greater than 10 percent of baseline, (2) downward crossing of at least two of the percentile lines on the weight-for-age chart in a child 1 year or older, *or* (3) less than the 5th percentile on a weight-for-height chart on two consecutive measurements at least 30 days apart, *plus* (a) chronic diarrhea (at least two loose stools per day for ≥30 days) *or* (b) documented fever (≥30 days, intermittent or constant).[46, 52] Associated protein and micronutrient (zinc, selenium) deficiencies have been documented in HIV-infected adults and children.[201] Nutritional defects may be related to inadequate caloric intake (anorexia from concomitant infection such as MAC or tuberculosis, neuropsychiatric abnormalities, or dysphagia from infectious etiologies such as chronic oral herpes or *Candida* esophagitis), malabsorption with or without diarrhea, or increased energy expenditure (persistent fever with resultant increased metabolic rates). In a study of 27 adults with HIV wasting, Macallan and associates[180] documented that reduced energy intake and not elevated energy expenditure was the prime determinant in weight loss.

In two separate analyses of HIV-infected children, somatic growth (weight for age and length for age) has been shown to decline by 4 to 6 months of age and to be significantly different from that of HIV-uninfected, but exposed controls.[188, 201] These studies have prompted careful attention to the nutritional needs of HIV-infected children. In addition to provision of optimal caloric and nutritional supplementation, therapies that serve as appetite stimulants have been used increasingly and include cyproheptadine, megestrol acetate (Megace), and dronabinol (Marinol). The documented efficacy of these agents is not usually permanent, especially when concomitant opportunistic infections are evident.[85, 261] The use of treatment regimens that include a protease inhibitor has not always correlated with significant increases in somatic growth for HIV-infected children.[37]

Opportunistic infections commonly affect the length of the gastrointestinal tract. Oral ulcers, diarrhea, malabsorption, intestinal perforation, and colitis have been associated ith herpesvirus, isosporiasis, cryptosporidiosis, *M. avium–intracellulare* infection, CMV infection, *Giardia* infection, and bacterial infections (*Salmonella, Shigella, Campylobacter*). Specific therapeutic intervention should be designed to treat the pathogens that have been isolated.[97] Long-term maintenance therapy often is required to keep the patient as free of infection as possible.

MALIGNANCY

Early in the HIV epidemic, adults were not uncommonly afflicted by oncologic processes. B-cell non-Hodgkin lymphomata occurred in 3 to 4 percent of patients, and Kaposi sarcoma occurs in as many as 40 percent of HIV-infected male homosexuals.[10, 185] With increasing use of HAART in the mid-1990s, the incidence rate of primary CNS lymphomata in HIV-infected adults has declined.[148] Malignancy continues to be reported in HIV-infected children as they live longer (improved antiretroviral and supportive therapy) and their numbers increase. In a study of 4954 children with AIDS in the United States, approximately 2.5 percent had documented malignancies: non-Hodgkin lymphoma (n = 100), Kaposi sarcoma (n = 8), leiomyosarcoma (n = 4), and Hodgkin disease (n = 2); 10 others had unspecified cancers.[21] McClain and Rosenblatt[185] reviewed the literature and documented 26 children (younger than 13 years) with AIDS and lymphomata. The most prevalent symptom complex included fever, weight loss, hepatomegaly, and abdominal distention. Of note, seven patients had initial neurologic complaints. Respiratory complaints were noted in a handful of children with pulmonary lymphomata in association with the lymphoproliferative lung disorders LIP/PLH. Associated in situ infection with HIV, Epstein-Barr virus, or both has been documented, although its precise role in pathogenesis is not defined. Early chemotherapeutic intervention has enhanced the quality of life and longevity and often has been provided in conjunction with antiretroviral therapy.

Kaposi sarcoma clearly occurs much less commonly[180] in HIV-infected children than in their adult counterparts. The pathogenesis of Kaposi sarcoma, both HIV and non–HIV related, has been elucidated more recently, and the novel human herpesvirus–8 has been documented in lesions.[131, 199] Pathogenesis has been linked to oncogenesis and cytokine-induced growth. The clinical manifestations of Kaposi sarcoma associated with AIDS affect multiple organs. The skin, gastrointestinal tract, lungs, and heart have been affected by Kaposi sarcoma proliferations. The prognosis for Kaposi sarcoma in adults has been linked to clinical progression of the underlying HIV disease, with poorer responses in patients with more profound immunodeficiency (lowered CD4 counts) or opportunistic infections. Not surprisingly, management of Kaposi sarcoma has improved with increasing use of HAART to restore immune function in HIV-infected individuals.[41] Treatment of Kaposi sarcoma in adults has included antiretroviral therapy, chemotherapy (vinca alkaloids), radiation therapy, and most recently, interferon-α therapy.[56, 184] New agents being used for more widespread Kaposi sarcoma include anthracyclines, anti-angiogenic agents, and retinoic acids.[41]

Since 1987, more than 13 children with AIDS have been reported with smooth muscle malignancies, specifically, leiomyosarcomas of the gastrointestinal tract.[63, 184] Previously described in small numbers of children in the world's literature, this upsurge in such an uncommon malignancy in pediatric AIDS patients suggests a distinct relationship to HIV or other concomitant infections. McClain and colleagues[184] documented the association of Epstein-Barr virus (by PCR and in situ hybridization techniques) with leiomyosarcoma in children with AIDS.

Such unusual clinical manifestations have prompted pediatric oncologists nationwide to establish a pediatric AIDS cancer registry to define and better understand the oncologic processes in HIV-infected children. Such effort should be helpful in the development of concerted oncologic intervention as the number of children with AIDS who survive beyond childhood increases.

OTHER COMPLICATIONS

Cardiac Abnormalities

Cardiac manifestations of HIV infection in children have been described.[174] In a study of almost 600 HIV-infected infants, progressive left ventricular dysfunction as measured by a diminished shortening fraction was associated with decreased CD4 lymphocyte counts.[30] Clearly, opportunistic infections (cryptococcosis, aspergillosis) and malignancy (Kaposi sarcoma) have had an affect on cardiac disease and AIDS in children and adults. Clinically, HIV-infected children have been described with congestive heart failure and cardiomegaly, cardiac tamponade, nonbacterial thrombotic endocarditis, conduction disturbances, and sudden death, presumably secondary to primary ventricular arrhythmia associated with severe cardiomyopathy. In one study, four of six HIV-infected infants with cardiac abnormalities were found to have focal myocarditis when myocardial histologic studies were performed.[171]

In a study of 81 HIV-infected children, unexpected cardiorespiratory arrest occurred in 9 percent, chronic congestive heart failure in 10 percent, and dysrhythmias in 35 percent of children.[177] Asymptomatic children with HIV infection additionally have been documented to exhibit cardiac abnormalities, including ventricular dysfunction and dilation and pericardial effusions. The routine use of echocardiography increases the documentation of such cardiac abnormalities. No evidence suggests that HIV is directly cardiotoxic, although HIV has been documented within myocardial cells by in situ hybridization.[101] Other factors may have an impact on the development of cardiac abnormalities and include malnutrition and infectious agents such as CMV and Epstein-Barr virus. Decreased left ventricular function associated with pharmacologic therapy (antiretroviral agents, pentamidine, steroids, etc.) has been reported. In one study of HIV-infected children receiving antiretroviral nucleoside analogue therapy (zidovudine or didanosine), the odds for development of cardiomyopathy were 8.4 times greater in children receiving zidovudine but *not* didanosine.[83] Treatment includes traditional cardiac agents such as angiotensin-converting enzyme inhibitors and diuretics.

Increasing use of HAART and, specifically, protease inhibitors in the pediatric HIV-infected population has prompted careful management of associated hypercholesterolemia and hyperlipidemia.[132] Routine evaluation of cholesterol and lipid profiles is suggested with persistent HAART use. Rising or increased levels should prompt consultation with a pediatric cardiologist for the best individual management practice.

Renal Dysfunction

Renal disease is yet another clinical manifestation of HIV infection. In a retrospective evaluation of 155 pediatric AIDS patients, 12 were noted to have significant proteinuria.[256] The renal abnormalities described in this cohort included nephritis (focal glomerulosclerosis and mesangial hyperplasia) and nephrosis. In fact, focal sclerosis and segmental sclerosis have been described in more than half of reported children.[257] The immunopathologic characteristics of HIV-associated nephropathy include inflammatory infiltrations predominantly composed of activated T cells (CD4 cells usually exceeding CD8 cells).[224, 229] Renal disease in HIV-infected children often appears in concert with profound immunodeficiency and end-stage HIV disease. Toxic therapy, concomitant infection, HIV alone, and circulating immune complexes have been implicated in the pathogenesis of this entity. Because most pediatric AIDS patients with renal disease have vertically acquired HIV infection, the importance of congenital or early concomitant infections (e.g., CMV) has been postulated to affect pathogenesis. Lending further credence to this postulate is documentation of concurrent viral illnesses in both primarily immunodeficient and HIV-infected children with renal disease.[103] Of note, renal disease was manifested histologically as focal glomerulosclerosis in both populations. The uniqueness of HIV nephropathy then becomes questionable. The nephrosis of HIV disease can be particularly difficult to treat in an already malnourished, hypoproteinemic, HIV-infected child. Corticosteroid therapy may be attempted but often ameliorates symptoms with variable efficacy. Nutritional supplementation and dietary restriction may be supportive adjunctive therapy.

Bone Marrow Suppression

Hematologic abnormalities associated with HIV infection in children include leukopenia, anemia, and thrombocytopenia. Of note, leukopenia and, in particular, lymphopenia, so characteristic of HIV-infected adults, are uncharacteristic clinical findings early in pediatric HIV infection, especially in perinatally infected infants.[77] Neutropenia often has been described in association with circulating antineutrophil antibodies and may respond to blockade therapy with IVIG. Granulocyte colony-stimulating factor has been used successfully in neutropenia, both drug induced and HIV associated.[118, 202] The anemia of HIV infection may be microcytic, hypochromic as seen in chronic infection, autoimmune with positive Coombs testing, or typical of nutritional deprivation (iron or vitamin B_{12} deficiency). The etiology of anemia in AIDS cases is difficult to sort out and is confounded by multiple cofactors that affect red blood cell counts—that is, poor nutritional status and concomitant use of toxic therapeutic agents (zidovudine). In adults and children, recombinant erythropoietin has been beneficial in treating anemia associated with antiviral therapy.[31, 98, 171]

Immune thrombocytopenia has been reported in 13 percent of children with symptomatic HIV infection and an onset as early as the first year of life.[89] This phenomenon appears to be mediated immunologically, although its pathogenesis is not defined clearly. Two proposed explanations are (1) nonspecific binding of platelets to circulating antibody complexes, which are documented so commonly in HIV-infected adults and children, and (2) production of antibodies specifically targeted to platelets and triggered by the same stimulus that produces almost universal hypergammaglobulinemia in HIV-infected children. The presence of platelet-associated IgG in HIV-infected children has been reported to have a sensitivity of 93 percent; however, its specificity is only 13 percent, thus suggesting that platelet-associated IgG is unlikely to be a cause of thrombocytopenia.[90] Therapy for thrombocytopenia in children and adults has included no intervention, platelet transfusions, systemic corticosteroids, IVIG, antiretroviral therapy, and most recently in adults, interferon-α. Immune thrombocytopenia has resolved spontaneously in some children with simple supportive measures. These therapeutic interventions have produced variable responses in individuals.

Diagnosis of HIV Infection in Infants and Children

EARLY TRANSMISSION OF HIV TO FETUSES

Information is scant on the role of the human placenta in transmitting HIV infection from mother to fetus. Studies have suggested that fetal infection can take place as early as 9 to 11 weeks of gestational age.[33, 65, 181, 248, 266] In one study, 16- to 24-week-old fetal tissue obtained from HIV-infected mothers was examined for the presence of HIV DNA by PCR amplification.[248] HIV DNA was found in 19 of 31 thymic samples and in 22 of 33 spleen samples studied, which indicates that HIV can be transmitted early in gestation. Preliminary examination of birth placental tissue from HIV-infected mothers in another study indicated that HIV core antigens can be detected in approximately 50 percent of the cases studied (23 of 51); furthermore, HIV antigens were localized in the Hofbauer cells.[266] Another group suggests that HIV infection does not cause significant pathology in the placenta and that HIV antigens and RNA synthesis only rarely are detected in placental tissue.[58] Finally, investigators have documented that placental trophoblasts can be infected by CD4-independent isolates of HIV-1 in vitro.[5] Thus, little doubt exists that HIV can be transmitted in utero to the fetus and result in an infected infant,[165, 233] although other modes of HIV transmission from mother to infant, such as by exposure to infected amniotic fluid, mixing of maternal blood with fetal blood at the time of delivery, exposure to infected cervical secretions in the birth canal, and breast milk, have been observed.[84, 204] Because the rate of transmission of HIV from an infected mother to her fetus or infant is estimated to range from 12 to 25 percent,[64, 74, 264] to suspect that some pathologic HIV-related effect on the placenta permits such an extraordinary transmission rate of virus seems reasonable.

An increase in intrauterine fetal demise has been demonstrated in the literature in HIV-infected pregnant women.[86, 164] In HIV-negative fetuses, placental or fetal lesions known to be associated with fetal demise were identified: abruption, infarction, and other infections (CMV). In HIV-positive fetuses, no such placental lesions could be identified, and death was attributed to HIV infection of fetal tissue as detected by in situ hybridization. Two hypotheses for transmission are proposed: (1) direct cell-to-cell spread of HIV from infected maternal mononuclear cells through the placental cells and eventually to fetal tissue itself and (2) infected maternal cells that gain access to the fetal circulation.

METHODS USED TO DIAGNOSE HIV INFECTION IN CHILDREN OLDER THAN 18 MONTHS

In children older than 18 months in whom the presence of maternal anti-HIV antibody is no longer a confounding variable, the conventional tests used to diagnose HIV infection in adults are applicable[129] (Table 193–15). Thus, ELISA, Western blot analysis, indirect fluorescent antibody assay, p24 HIV antigen analysis (p24Ag), HIV culture, and HIV PCR may be used. Of these tests, ELISA and Western blot analysis are the most practical, and two positive ELISAs plus a positive Western blot confirm a diagnosis of HIV infection.

The ELISA for detection of serum antibodies to HIV is a standardized screening test for identifying present or past infection with HIV. It is a test that is overly sensitive because it tends to overpredict the number of positive subjects and must be confirmed by the more specific Western blot test. Many commercial testing kits have been approved by the Food

TABLE 193–15 ■ GUIDELINES FOR THE DIAGNOSIS OF HIV INFECTION IN INFANTS BORN TO HIV-INFECTED MOTHERS

Definitive HIV Diagnosis for Infants 18 mo or Older

Two positive enzyme-linked immunosorbent assays and a positive confirmatory serologic test, e.g., Western blot or immunofluorescence assay

OR

Any 2 positive viral detection assays on separate specimens:
- HIV culture
- HIV polymerase chain reaction
- p24 antigen test

OR

Documentation of a pediatric AIDS-defining illness

Presumptive Diagnosis for Infants Younger Than 18 mo

A single positive viral detection assay (excluding cord blood):
- HIV culture
- HIV polymerase chain reaction
- p24 antigen assay

Definitive Diagnosis for Infants Younger Than 18 mo

Any 2 positive viral detection assays on separate specimens:
- HIV culture
- HIV polymerase chain reaction
- p24 antigen test

OR

Documentation of a pediatric AIDS-defining illness

From Hanson, I.C., and Shearer, W.T.: Diagnosis of HIV infection. Semin. Pediatr. Infect. Dis. 5:266–271, 1994.

and Drug Administration (FDA) and the CDC for screening of individuals, and more recently, combination kits that test for both HIV-1 and HIV-2 are being used.[259] The method consists of adding patient serum to microwells in a plastic plate that have been coated with native or recombinant HIV antigens. After reaction and washing, reagents containing a colored dye are added to the microwells, and the resulting solutions are read at a certain wavelength in a special spectrophotometer.

The Western blot assay is a method in which individual proteins of an HIV lysate are separated according to size by polyacrylamide gel electrophoresis. The viral proteins then are transferred onto nitrocellulose paper and reacted with the patient's serum. Any antibody from the patient's serum is detected by an antihuman IgG antibody conjugated with an enzyme that in the presence of substrate will produce a colored band. Positive and negative control specimens are run simultaneously to allow identification of viral proteins. Western blot results are interpreted as positive, negative, or indeterminate[129, 250] (Table 193–16).

METHODS USED TO MAKE AN EARLY DIAGNOSIS OF HIV INFECTION IN INFANTS AND CHILDREN YOUNGER THAN 18 MONTHS

The clinical manifestations of HIV infection in children are varied and nonspecific and include chronic pneumonitis, failure to thrive, hepatosplenomegaly, thrombocytopenia, and chronic diarrhea. In children younger than 18 months, a positive serologic determination of HIV is not accepted as indicative of HIV infection because passive maternal antibody confuses the serologic picture. Documentation of HIV infection in children younger than 18 months, whether symptomatic or not, requires more thorough investigation of the immune system with CD4 (helper T lymphocyte) determination, exclusion of congenital immunodeficiency, and identification of viral components from serum or CSF—that is, p24 HIV antigen determination (including the immune complex–dissociated p24 antigen), HIV culture (blood or CSF) and the use of reverse transcriptase assay or p24 HIV antigen determination, or HIV PCR.[52]

Table 193–15 outlines the current guidelines for determining positive HIV infection status in infants younger than 18 months who are born to HIV-infected mothers.[52, 129, 186] Diagnostic distinctions are made in accordance with the infant's age and the number and type of positive virologic assays. Note that a single positive diagnostic test does *not* confirm HIV infection, except in the presence of clinical AIDS-defining events. To date, the methods that have been used to make an early diagnosis in high-risk infants include culture of peripheral blood mononuclear cells for HIV[185, 221]; DNA PCR of peripheral blood mononuclear cells for HIV[70, 208, 227]; detection of HIV antigen (p24Ag or immune complex–dissociated p24Ag) in blood or spinal fluid[99, 210, 215]; assays for neonatal IgA, IgM, and IgG and for neonatal IgG3 specific for HIV[40, 221]; and in vitro assays to determine the ability of neonatal peripheral blood mononuclear cells to secrete HIV-specific IgG antibody.[6, 214, 223]

TABLE 193–16 ■ ASSOCIATION OF STATE AND TERRITORIAL PUBLIC HEALTH LABORATORY DIRECTORS/CENTERS FOR DISEASE CONTROL AND PREVENTION CRITERIA FOR POSITIVE INTERPRETATION OF WESTERN BLOT ASSAYS

Any 2 of
p24
gp41
gp120/160*

*Distinction between the 120/160 bands is not required, and these bands may be considered as a single reactant for interpretation of Western blot. From Hanson, I. C., and Shearer, W. T.: Diagnosis of HIV infection. Semin. Pediatr. Infect. Dis. 5:266–271, 1994.

Cord blood determinations for HIV are problematic because of contamination by maternal cells. Experience with the use of PCR or culture technology in neonates born to HIV-infected women has documented HIV infection as early as the first days or month of life.[196] In these earliest settings, DNA PCR is the preferred testing tool. The estimated sensitivity of DNA PCR is 38 percent at birth, 93 percent by 14 days of age, and 96 percent by 28 days of age.[87] The HIV-1 RNA PCR currently used to predict disease progression and manage HIV treatment has not been approved for the diagnosis of HIV-1 in neonates.

In the past, exclusion of HIV infection in infants born to HIV-infected mothers (≈80% of children born to HIV-infected mothers) was delayed temporally to 15 to 18 months, when HIV serology was determined to be negative. Based on evaluation of the specificity and sensitivity of viral diagnostic tests, current pediatric PCP prophylaxis guidelines suggest that infants with two negative virologic assays (HIV culture or HIV PCR), both at 1 month or older and at 4 months or older, most likely are not infected with HIV, and interruption of the therapeutic intervention is warranted.[54] Hence, early diagnosis in HIV-exposed infants has been improved both for identification of HIV-infected children (as early as the first month of life) and for uninfected children labeled as serorevertеrs (as early as the fourth month of life). Schedules for testing of HIV-exposed infants vary nationally. However, advancements in diagnostic technology allow for early testing of HIV-exposed infants, including shortly after birth, every 3 months in the first year of life, and every 6 months until the infant's HIV infection status can be determined.

Although the aforementioned viral diagnostic assays can identify HIV infection early in neonatal life, more imperative is that exposure be identified in utero to interrupt perinatal HIV transmission. Hence, diagnostic tests to quickly identify maternal infection during delivery or the immediate postpartum period are needed. Current studies in the United States are under way to evaluate the potential for implementation of rapid HIV testing in pregnant women.

Treatment

SECONDARY AND SUPPORTIVE TREATMENT

Therapeutic intervention for HIV-infected children includes prompt and aggressive treatment of acute infections, particularly opportunistic infections. Because immunodeficiency often precludes complete eradication of microorganisms, long-term, chronic maintenance therapy often is required. Relapses with and without preventive therapy are not uncommon. With its high morbidity and mortality in children, PCP has focused clinicians on preventive or prophylactic regimens. Of note, other opportunists (herpes zoster, pneumococcosis) can recur frequently and might require prophylactic therapeutic regimens.[190] Other preventive measures applicable to all immunodeficient children are particularly important in an HIV-infected host. Examples include measles, influenza, and varicella prophylaxis after exposure. Additionally, routine childhood health care preventive measures, including adequate nutritional support, age and developmentally appropriate stimulation, dental and skin hygiene, and immunizations, should be offered to

TABLE 193–17 ■ SUGGESTED IMMUNIZATIONS FOR HIV-INFECTED OR HIV-SUSPECTED CHILDREN

TOPV	No
IPV	Yes
DTP	Yes
MMR	Yes
HBV	Yes
Hib	Yes
Pneumococcal	Yes
Influenza	Yes

*Authors' recommendations compiled from guidelines suggested by the Centers for Disease Control and Prevention.[14]

DTP, diphtheria-tetanus-pertussis; HBV, hepatitis B virus; Hib, *Haemophilus influenzae* type b; IPV, inactivated poliovirus vaccine; MMR, measles-mumps-rubella; TOPV, trivalent oral poliovirus vaccine.

All HIV infected children should receive immunization against pneumococcal infection. Pneumococcal conjugate vaccine is recommended for children under 24 months of age. Children older than 24 months may be immunized with 23 valent polysaccharide vaccine alone, or following a dose of conjugate vaccine.

children with HIV infection or AIDS.[44, 55] Table 193–17 outlines suggested immunizations for HIV-infected children. Note that the live viral measles, mumps, and rubella vaccine is recommended for children without evidence of severe immune compromise. Varicella vaccine is recommended for children without significant immune compromise and also limited clinical symptoms; immunization of healthy household infants is recommended. Influenza vaccine should be administered yearly according to general age-related guidelines for HIV-infected children.

The efficacy of IVIG in reducing the development of serious laboratory-proven bacterial and clinically diagnosed infections has been documented in symptomatic HIV-infected children with CD4 counts higher than 200/mm^3.[200, 260] In a study of IVIG therapy in conjunction with zidovudine therapy, IVIG again demonstrated a reduction in morbidity from serious bacterial infections, but only in children not concomitantly receiving TMP-SMX as PCP prophylaxis. For children receiving TMP-SMX, no differences in morbidity from bacterial infections were noted between the immunoglobulin-treated group and placebo (albumin) controls. Current indications for immunoglobulin intervention are limited and include (1) all children with documentation of hypogammaglobulinemia and (2) children with more than two invasive bacterial infections in a 1-year period.[55]

PRIMARY (ANTI-HIV) TREATMENT

Much effort has been expended in rapidly and safely evaluating chemotherapeutic agents with purported antiretroviral activity. Large multicenter studies to assess the effect of antiretroviral agents in adults and children have been the focus of the National Institutes of Health, AIDS Clinical Trial Group (ACTG). Many important collaborative studies documenting the efficacy of antiretroviral and opportunistic therapy are the result of these efforts.[67, 72, 159, 160, 187, 247, 249, 260]

Current antiretroviral intervention has targeted different steps in HIV's replication cycle[17, 157] (Fig. 193–12). Because of the special nature and challenge of pediatric HIV infection, few of the steps in the HIV life cycle have been approached therapeutically, in contrast to the situation in

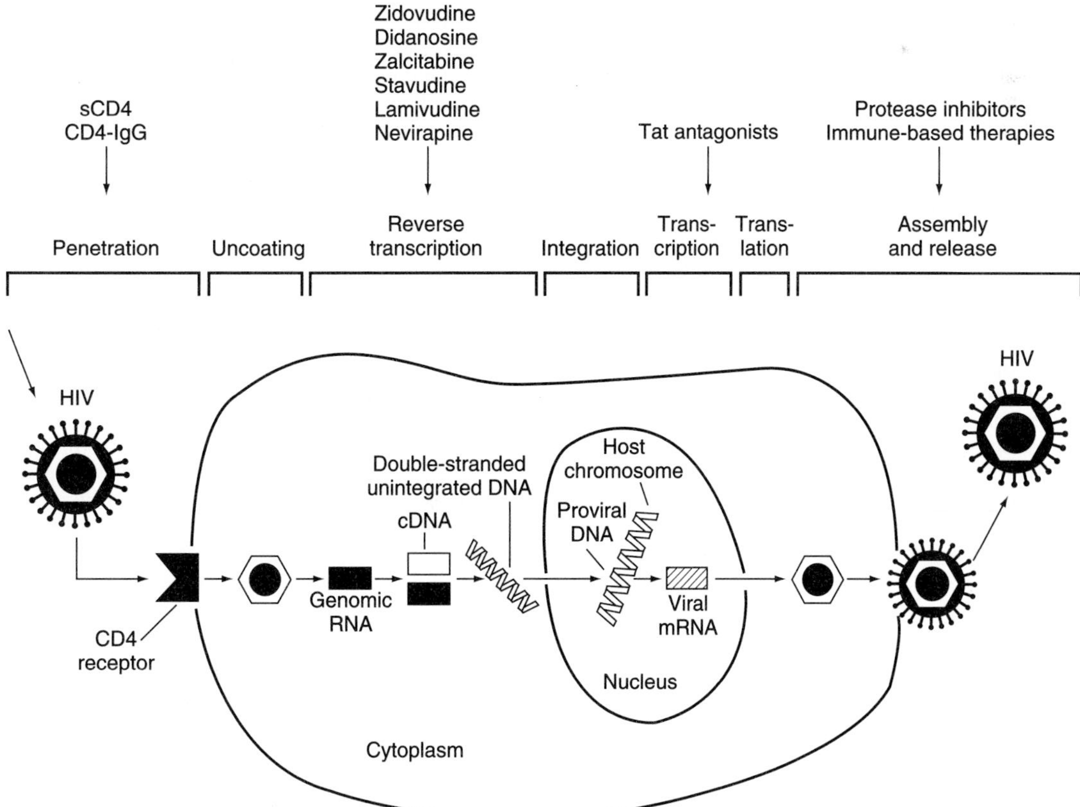

FIGURE 193–12 ■ Life cycle of HIV, with illustration of targets for pharmacologic intervention. (From Kline, M. W., and Shearer, W. T.: HIV infection and AIDS in children. *In* Rich, R. R., Fleischer, T. A., Schwartz, W. T., et al. [eds.]: Clinical Immunology. St. Louis, Mosby, 1996, pp. 739–750.)

adults with HIV infection, in whom many experimental regimens have been attempted. The discussion of therapy should be considered in the context of not only the HIV replication cycle but also the designed impact on the targeted population (i.e., interruption of perinatal transmission or the effect on already established pediatric HIV infection). Selection of treatment options dramatically changed in the mid-1990s with the advent of numerous available agents targeting multiple sites of the viral replication cycle and also with the commercial availability and increasing use of markers such as CD4 and HIV viral load (RNA PCR levels) to predict progression of the disease.[211]

Guidelines for initiation of therapy differ for adults and children. Current pediatric recommendations include initiation of therapy for symptomatic and immunosuppressed HIV-infected children. Many clinicians elect to begin therapy in any child identified as being infected with HIV but delay immediate provision of therapy until issues of compliance and adherence have been investigated thoroughly. Selection of treatment regimens is dependent on multiple factors: (1) patient acceptability and compliance, (2) clinical evidence of progression of disease, (3) evidence of deterioration of immunity (declining CD4 count on two separate measures), and (4) evidence of virologic failure (increasing RNA PCR measures of viral load). In the face of compliance and depending on the resources available, genotypic or phenotypic resistance testing may assist in selecting alternative treatment options for HIV-infected children with treatment failure.

Blockade of HIV by CD4/Co-receptors

Because HIV first attaches by binding its gp120 envelope protein to cellular CD4, antiretroviral therapy has been proposed to block the target binding site, CD4.[142] Recombinant human CD4 (rCD4) molecules have been evaluated in animal models and humans for their safety and pharmacokinetics as target binders[149, 220] but have been hampered by their short half-life. In an effort to prolong the half-life and perhaps enhance efficacy, rCD4 has been constructed to include the Fc region of human IgG1, which produces a chimeric molecule rCD4-IgG.[136] For use in children, rCD4-IgG may cross the placenta in a fashion similar to that of native IgG and offer potential protection to an HIV-exposed fetus. Shearer and associates[239] studied the pharmacokinetics and safety of rCD4-IgG in six mother-infant pairs and documented safety, clear evidence of placental transfer of rCD4-IgG, and appropriate elimination. Studies of rCD4-IgG in adults have demonstrated a potential for modulation of immunity, but no evidence to date for short-term activity in halting the progression of disease.[68] The finding that HIV binds to CD4 cell in tandem with co-receptors (CCR5 or CXCR4) has led to studies evaluating the use of mutant co-receptors known to resist cellular infection.[253] Phase I studies are under way with agents that block CCR5 and impede HIV from fusing to the CD4 cell membrane and infecting the cell.

Blockade of HIV by Fusion Inhibitors

Fusion of the HIV envelope (glycoprotein gp41) with the target cell membrane is an important step in cellular infection. gp41 contains three important regions (fusion peptide [FP] and N- and C-terminal repeats); FP is inserted into the cell membrane, and then, when the N- and C-terminal repeats fold into a six-helix bundle, FP promotes the fusion of cellular and viral membranes. Enfuvirtide (also known as T20) is a synthetic peptide that binds to amino acids in the C-terminal repeat, preventing the formation of this six-helix bundle.[147] Modest decreases in HIV viral load are seen in clinical studies involving both adults[152] and children.[68a] Enfuvirtide is administered twice daily by subcutaneous injection. Adverse effects have included pain and discomfort, induration, erythema, and other skin changes at the injection site. Other adverse events reported in trials included insomnia, myalgia, peripheral neuropathy, and depression, but their relation to the use of this agent is unclear. Resistance to enfuvirtide has already been reported, and this agent will likely need to be used in combination with other retroviral agents.[124] Clinical studies are under way to determine the optimal use of this new drug in children.

Nucleosides (Proviral DNA Reverse Transcriptase Inhibitors)

Several investigational efforts have been directed toward inhibiting the formation of proviral DNA by HIV reverse transcriptase. Although nucleosides have no effect on reverse transcriptase itself but affect the elongation of its proviral DNA product, these drugs are considered reverse transcriptase inhibitors. Because this antiviral approach best inhibits only actively replicating cells, latently infected, resting cells may derive little benefit from reverse transcriptase inhibition alone.[143]

ZIDOVUDINE. Zidovudine (azidothymidine, AZT, Retrovir) was the first nucleoside analogue to be evaluated in adults and children. Early placebo-controlled trials in adults with AIDS documented a significant reduction in mortality rates and prompted licensure of zidovudine for adults in 1987.[99] The initial recommended doses (1200 mg/day) were reassessed in dose-controlled trials in adults with AIDS and in placebo-controlled trials in asymptomatic HIV-infected adults. The current standard of care for adults in the United States includes a lower dose intervention (600 mg/day) at the onset of symptoms or significant immunodeficiency (CD4 count <500/mm^3).[250] Controversy continues to exist regarding the efficacy of zidovudine in adults with asymptomatic disease.[134, 170, 271] In pediatric studies conducted according to the perspective of historical controls and the clinical status of patients before and after receiving drug treatment, zidovudine has been documented to be efficacious both by continuous infusion and by oral intermittent dosing.[187, 217] Parameters defining efficacy in children included an enhanced sense of well-being, improvement in dementia (especially in cognitive abilities), reduced hepatosplenomegaly and lymphadenopathy, and increased appetite and weight gain. Immunologically, zidovudine has been associated in children with a decline in serum immunoglobulin levels and a transient increase in CD4 helper T-lymphocyte numbers. This latter phenomenon was observed best in early trials in children in which therapy was initiated when CD4 cell counts were higher than 100/mm^3. However, the immunologic changes noted with zidovudine treatment alone, particularly changes in CD4 counts, could not be sustained consistently. Most children's CD4 counts drifted back to baseline within several months of undergoing therapy.

Zidovudine pharmacokinetics by oral, intermittent dosing has documented good oral bioavailability (65%) and CNS penetration with a mean serum half-life of 1 to 1.5 hours. Because zidovudine requires phosphorylation to be active against HIV infection, the active metabolite (zidovudine triphosphate) accumulates intracellularly and has a longer half-life. Zidovudine is metabolized hepatically, and 25 percent of its clearance is via renal secretion and glomerular filtration. Hence, primary renal or hepatic compromise or drugs that affect flow or hepatic glucuronidation (acetaminophen) may alter the metabolism of zidovudine and result in accumulation and toxicity.

Zidovudine has documented toxic effects, including prominent macrocytic anemia, leukopenia/neutropenia, and chemical hepatitis. Leukopenia and particularly neutropenia are the most common dose-limiting toxicities. Most clinicians rely on bimonthly blood counts to monitor bone marrow suppression. Human granulocyte colony-stimulating factor has been used in adults and children with AIDS to enhance myelopoiesis and correct both HIV- and zidovudine-induced neutropenia.[119, 206] Transfusion-dependent anemia is not an uncommon event and often responds to dose reduction. Recombinant erythropoietin has proved efficacious in adults and children with zidovudine-induced anemia.[31, 171]

Zidovudine was licensed in the United States for pediatric use in 1990. Licensing closely followed documentation of the efficacy of intermittent oral zidovudine therapy in pediatric clinical trials. Not surprisingly, the recommended dosing for children was the same as that used in these trials, 180 mg/m^2 per dose every 6 hours, not to exceed 500 mg/day.[187] Most clinicians currently use 90 to 180 mg/m^2/day delivered every 6 to 8 hours. For adolescents, adult standards (zidovudine intervention not to exceed 600 mg/day [300 mg two times per day]) often are used.

Early animal model studies that documented the safety and success of zidovudine in limiting transmission of simian virus paved the way for human studies.[268] The remarkable success of ACTG protocol 076 in preventing perinatal HIV transmission with zidovudine has expanded the drug's use to yet another population, the fetus.[72] Early pharmacokinetic and safety trials of zidovudine documented safety with only mild reversible anemia in infants. Pharmacokinetic data suggested that doses of 1.5 mg/kg (intravenously) or 2.0 mg/kg (orally) were safe and associated with minimal toxicity. In ACTG protocol 076, the efficacy of zidovudine delivered during gestation (500 mg/day orally), during labor and delivery (intravenous loading dose of 2 mg/kg, followed by a continuous infusion of 1 mg/kg), and to newborn infants (2.0 mg/kg per dose every 6 hours orally or, for infants not able to tolerate oral dosing, 1.5 mg/kg per dose every 6 hours intravenously) in reducing perinatal transmission was dramatic (Fig. 193–13). The decrease from 25 to 8 percent represented a 66 percent reduction in vertical transmission and has altered the standard of care for HIV-infected pregnant women and their exposed fetuses.[53, 273] The short-term toxicity of therapy was linked to reversible anemia not requiring transfusion.

The toxicity associated with zidovudine and other nucleoside analogues used in drug regimens to prevent perinatal transmission of HIV has been described in small study cohorts and includes significant mitochondrial dysfunction in uninfected children, low birth weight, and premature delivery.[24, 176] Several large studies have refuted some of these findings. Three multicenter studies in the United States of HIV-exposed infants with concomitant exposure to nucleoside analogues did not detect evidence of mitochondrial dysfunction in either infected or uninfected infants exposed in utero or during the intrapartum or postpartum period.[75, 126, 173] A small Swiss study reported a 33 percent rate of premature delivery in HIV-infected pregnant women receiving combination antiviral therapy that included zidovudine.[176] In a study of more than 2000 pregnant HIV-infected women in the United States, more than 500 of whom received combination therapy, the risk of premature delivery, low birth weight, and low Apgar scores did not exceed that noted in women with either no therapy or monotherapy.[265] Concern about the longer-term effects

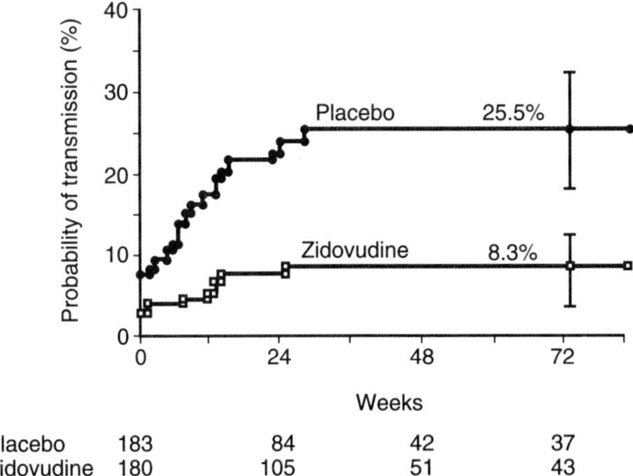

FIGURE 193–13 ■ Analysis demonstrating a 66 percent reduction in perinatal transmission rates from 25 to 8 percent with antepartum, peripartum, and postpartum zidovudine therapy in HIV-infected pregnant women and their infants. (Reprinted, by permission, from Connor, E. M., Sperling, R. S., Gelber, R., et al.: Reduction of maternal-infant transmission of human immunodeficiency virus type 1 with zidovudine treatment: Pediatric AIDS Clinical Trials Group Protocol 076 Study Group. N. Engl. J. Med. 331:1173–1180, 1994.)

related to nucleoside and other antiretroviral agents with potential for mitochondrial toxicity or other complications in the fetus has prompted continued surveillance to monitor the specific potential for adverse outcomes in HIV-exposed infant cohorts who have received antiretroviral therapy.

Resistance to zidovudine has been identified in the HIV-1 isolates of patients receiving long-term therapy. Mutations at codon 215 of the HIV-1 reverse transcriptase have been described as characteristic of resistance to zidovudine in both adults and children.[144] Resistance to didanosine or zalcitabine is reported less frequently, but the clinical significance of this finding is not understood fully. Nielsen and associates[206] examined 34 children for evidence of zidovudine-resistant isolates and documented increased progression of disease (failure to thrive, onset of opportunistic infections) in these children as opposed to those with nonresistant isolates. Evidence of such resistance has fueled the development of combination therapies to reduce not only toxicity but also the potential for development of resistance. With concerns related to drug resistance looming, attention has turned to enhancing compliance with therapy, and protocols to enhance adherence are ongoing.[267]

DIDEOXYINOSINE. Dideoxyinosine (ddI) has been evaluated in phase I/II trials both at the National Cancer Institute by Butler and associates[38] and at the National Institute for Allergy and Infectious Diseases by Lambert and colleagues.[161] Both adults and children have been reported with ddI-associated, dose-limiting neuropathy. Additional toxicity related to ddI includes pancreatitis, lactic acidosis, hypercholesterolemia, and lipodystrophy. ddI is a common alternative or adjunct to zidovudine therapy in combination regimens. A nucleoside analogue, ddI has a prolonged intracellular half-life (approximately 12 hours), which allows for twice- and three-times-daily dosing. Blanche and associates[22] described the efficacy of ddI in an open-label trial in children. In July 1991, the FDA approved the use of ddI in adults and children based on available clinical data and the urgent need for alternative drugs for treating HIV infection. The current recommended dose is 90 to 150 mg/m^2 every 12 hours. For optimal absorption, ddI should be administered on an empty stomach. Periodic assessment of liver function tests and amylase, neurologic examination, and ophthalmologic examination (retinal depigmentation has been described) are warranted.

DIDEOXYCYTIDINE. Dideoxycytidine (ddC), a nucleoside analogue akin to ddI, is a potent in vitro inhibitor of HIV replication. Initially limited by the route of administration (intravenous, subcutaneous) and high-dose toxicity (peripheral neuropathy), ddC has produced palliation of clinical symptoms, decreased virologic parameters (serum p24Ag levels), and improved immunologic status at lower oral doses in adults.[2] The most frequently reported adverse effects of ddC include aphthous ulcers, painful peripheral neuropathy, and rash. Because of poor penetration of the CNS, ddC probably may be limited in use to children with zidovudine or ddI failure or as a component of combination regimens.[216] The current recommended dose is 0.01 mg/kg every 8 hours.

STAVUDINE. Stavudine (d4T) has been evaluated in clinical trials in children with HIV infection. Like zidovudine, ddI, and ddC, d4T is a potent inhibitor of in vitro HIV replication and functions as a nucleoside analogue.[155] Pharmacokinetic studies document that the oral bioavailability of the drug ranges from 61 to 78 percent. d4T crosses the blood-brain barrier, and CSF concentrations range from 16 to 97 percent 2 to 3 hours after administration of an oral dose. In a cohort of 37 children (7 months to 15 years of age), d4T was well tolerated, and no drug-associated adverse events were noted. Efficacy data have shown improvement by an increase in CD4 count, decrease in viral load, and no clinical evidence of progression of disease. The current recommended dose is 1 mg/kg (up to 30 kg) every 12 hours. Adverse events include lactic acidosis, lipodystrophy, pancreatitis, and peripheral neuropathy.

LAMIVUDINE. Lamivudine (3TC) is licensed for use in adults and children. Its antiviral potency is very good, with reductions of 1 log or greater realized in clinical trials. 3TC is tolerated well orally and is used in twice-daily dosing. The recommended dose is 4 mg/kg, and the drug is available both as a solution and as tablets. A combined product (Combivir) provides a preformed tablet formulation of zidovudine (300 mg) and 3TC (150 mg) available for use twice daily. Reported adverse events include pancreatitis and, rarely, lactic acidosis.

ABACAVIR. Abacavir (ABC) also has demonstrated good in vitro and in vivo potency in reducing the HIV viral load, specifically as part of combination therapy. Limitations of ABC therapy are linked to a rare adverse event that can be life-threatening, namely, early idiosyncratic rash. The symptom complex includes fever, vomiting, diarrhea, and fatigue and sometimes can be confused with transient viral or bacterial infections. Known hypersensitivity to ABC should prohibit further use. The recommended dosing is 8 mg/kg twice daily, and the drug is available as an oral solution and as a tablet. A combined product (Trizivir) provides a preformed tablet formulation of zidovudine (300 mg), 3TC (150 mg), and ABC (300 mg) available for use twice daily.

Nucleotide Reverse Transcriptase Inhibitors

Tenofovir is a nucleotide reverse transcriptase inhibitor that contains an intramolecular phosphate. This agent was licensed in 2002 for treatment of HIV infection in adults, and dose finding studies are currently under way in children. Tenofovir has been associated with osteomalacia and reduced bone density in animals when given at very high doses. Renal insufficiency has also developed at high doses in animals, but neither the bone toxicity nor renal dysfunction has been observed in adult subjects. These careful observations of the tect bone or renal toxicities are part of ongoing trials in children.

Non-nucleosides

Non-nucleoside reverse transcriptase inhibitors include nevirapine, efavirenz, and delavirdine. These drugs work by binding directly to the enzymatic site of reverse transcriptase and do not require phosphorylation. Non-nucleosides have proven efficacy in reducing viral load and improving clinical status in both adults and children. However, this group of agents is limited by the ease of development of resistance. Nevirapine was the first of the agents to be approved for use in children, and its use in previously treated HIV-infected children initially showed great promise. The recommended dose is 120 to 200 mg/m^2 every 12 hours, and it is available as both an oral formulation and a tablet. Because of its metabolism, dosing should be graded, with half-dosing in the first week and then full dosing in week 2. Perhaps the most promising use of nevirapine has been documented in the prevention of perinatal HIV transmission. In clinical trials in Uganda (HIVNET 012) in a breast-feeding cohort, a single 200-mg oral dose at the onset of labor combined with a single 2-mg/kg dose to the infant at 48 to 72 hours of life resulted in a 12 percent transmission rate as compared with a 21 per-cent rate with short-course zidovudine use.[122] In a U.S., European, Brazilian, and Caribbean study (PACTG 316), nevirapine was added to traditional combination therapy during pregnancy. In this study of more than 1500 HIV-infected pregnant women, nevirapine (200 mg) or placebo was provided at the onset of labor to the HIV-infected women, and nevirapine or placebo was given to the infant at 48 hours of life and matched to the mothers' randomization. The risk of transmission was not different between combination therapy/nevirapine (1.4%) and combination therapy/ placebo (1.6%).[84] Adverse events related to nevirapine include hepatitis and a Stevens-Johnson–like rash.

Delavirdine is used only rarely in pediatric patients because an oral solution is not available. The recommended adolescent or adult dosing is 400 mg three times daily. In contrast, efavirenz has enjoyed widespread use since its approval by the FDA for both adults and children. This agent is particularly attractive because its use is approved as a single daily dose. Pediatric dosing ranges from 200 to 600 mg each day based on weight, but the drug is limited to a capsule formulation. Adverse events include hepatitis, rash (including a Stevens-Johnson–like syndrome), disassociated CNS symptoms (insomnia, irritability, bad dreams) for the first weeks that the drug is taken, hypercholesterolemia, hyperlipidemia, and lipodystrophy. Warnings for women of reproductive age are warranted because in animal models efavirenz has been associated with anencephaly. Use of the agent can cause a false-positive cannabinoid screening.

Protease Inhibitors

Increased use of protease inhibitors in the mid-1990s heralded significant changes in HIV-related morbidity and mortality. Protease inhibitors share features with viral protease and function by binding to and inhibiting viral protease. They are efficacious in dramatically reducing RNA viral loads. Each shares metabolic activation through the hepatic cytochrome P-450 enzyme system and, hence, is capable of significant drug-drug interactions. The use of protease inhibitors in combination regimens requires careful evaluation of the impact of this therapy on other antiretrovirals, including other protease inhibitors, prophylaxis for opportunistic infection, and any drug that also is activated by cytochrome P-450. Examples of such interactions include oral contraceptives, antituberculosis drugs, antiepileptic drugs, some antihistamines, and methadone.

One of the first approved protease inhibitors was ritonavir. Its use in children was limited initially to previously treated children as part of salvage therapy. The drug is available as a liquid formulation or a powder, and its palatability is affected by accompanying nausea and vomiting. Despite these limitations, ritonavir was used widely after its approval for use in children. The recommended dosing for children is 350 to 400 mg/m^2 every 12 hours. Adverse events include gastrointestinal intolerance, paresthesias, and lipodystrophy. Since its initial use as a primary antiretroviral agent, ritonavir has been more widely used as an enhancer of newer protease inhibitor therapy, namely, indinavir, lopinavir, saquinavir, and amprenavir. Saquinavir is available as a soft gel capsule (Fortovase) and is more potent than the hard gel capsule formulation (Invirase), which realistically should be used only in combination with ritonavir. Current dosing of Fortovase is 50 mg/kg in three daily doses. Adverse events include headache, gastrointestinal intolerance, hepatic toxicity, and lipodystrophy. Indinavir is available as a capsule, and the recommended dosing is 500 mg/m^2 every 8 hours. In adults, dosing may be shifted to twice daily, with the addition of ritonavir. Adverse events include renal stones or proteinuria (or both) without adequate hydration, gastrointestinal intolerance, lipodystrophy, and mucocutaneous symptoms (alopecia, paronychia). Nelfinavir has been used more widely in pediatric populations and is available as a powder formulation and as tablets. The recommended dosing is 30 mg/kg every 8 hours. Children older than 6 years of age can be managed using 55 mg/kg twice daily. Adverse events include gastrointestinal intolerance (i.e., secretory diarrhea) and lipodystrophy. Amprenavir is available as an oral formulation and as capsules. Its recommended dosing is 20 mg/kg twice daily, and adverse events include gastrointestinal intolerance (diarrhea, vomiting), rash (including Stevens-Johnson–like syndrome), mood disorders, and lipodystrophy. Patients with TMP-SMX hypersensitivity usually tolerate the drug even though it is a sulfonamide. The oral formulation contains a high concentration of propylene glycol and should be used with caution in individuals with hepatic or renal failure. Additional new protease inhibitors are currently under study in both adults and children. Among these is atazanavir, which has shown excellent responses in therapy-naïve adults and children. The potential advantage of this new agent is the fact that it has minimal effects on blood lipid profiles.

Inclusion of protease inhibitors in combination therapy should be performed with the assistance of a physician experienced in prescribing HAART and in identifying drug-drug interactions to ensure that appropriate drug levels are maintained and that resistance is not fostered because of subtherapeutic levels. Resistance occurs not infrequently with protease inhibitor therapy, so careful attention to compliance with protocols and selection of agents that do not lower therapeutic levels are warranted. For example, patients with significant diarrhea might best avoid nelfinavir because absorption might be affected and the drug itself carries an intrinsic risk for the development of secretory diarrhea.

Immunomodulators

Because antiretroviral therapy has not been shown to eradicate HIV infection, many investigators have turned their attention to restoration of the secondary immunodeficiency associated with HIV infection in an attempt to augment natural antiretroviral defenses. Immune modulators have been assessed as single therapeutic agents or in combination regimens in adult clinical trials. Kovacs and associates[158] documented increases in CD4 T lymphocytes after intermittent infusions of IL-2 in adults with HIV infection and CD4 counts of 200 cells/mm^3 or higher. In European and U.S. studies, subcutaneous injections of IL-2 resulted in increased circulating CD4$^+$ cells but not in a decrease in RNA viral load.[1, 252] Combination antiretroviral and immunomodulator therapy is promising and the subject of ongoing trials (IL-2 and nucleoside analogues, interferon-α and nucleoside analogues).

Interferons, especially interferon-α, have been documented to produce in vitro antiretroviral activity.[230] Interferons are presumed to inhibit HIV replication by diminishing the assembly and release of mature virus particles (virion budding) from an infected cell surface. Trials to assess the efficacy of interferons in vivo have documented increases in CD4 counts with combination therapy when compared with zidovudine monotherapy.[108] Alternating zidovudine and interferon-α regimens for children have been proposed and approved in principle by the Pediatric Core Committee of the ACTG. The toxicity of interferon-α is not insignificant and includes fever, malaise, myalgia, and suppression of bone marrow. Of note, interferon-α is licensed for use in adults with Kaposi sarcoma,[91] and clinical trials are ongoing to assess its role in ameliorating HIV-induced immune thrombocytopenia.

Vaccines

Significant problems attend the development of vaccines against HIV.[25, 71, 199] Effective viral vaccines afford protection by the production of functional neutralizing antibodies in immunized hosts. Neutralizing antibodies to HIV have been detected in 10 to 80 percent of HIV-infected patients. Currently, no clear method exists to decipher whether these circulating antibodies with in vitro activity afford in vivo protection from HIV and diminish progression of the disease. The current paucity of animals that seroconvert to HIV and become immunodeficient and subject to clinical manifestations renders the process of evaluating antibody function more difficult to approach. Complicating this issue is the heterogeneity of the HIV envelope glycoprotein, which additionally renders development of a vaccine problematic.

Despite obstacles and in the face of a growing HIV epidemic, vaccine development is progressing. Killed or synthetic virus vaccine trials using gp120 candidate vaccines in animal models[19, 203, 219] and more recently in HIV-infected pregnant women and their offspring did not predict the complex nature of CD4 and its chemokine receptor binding sites.[73] Attention recently has been focused on stimulating cellular immune responses, and a prime boost in macaques and humans suggests the potential for DNA and recombinant pox virus vaccines.[189] To meet the needs for both a neutralizing antibody and cellular response, some investigators have proposed that multiple vaccines may be necessary to achieve success. Because the vast majority of children infected with HIV acquire their infection at birth, development of a vaccine or vaccines for perinatal interruption is a high priority.

Prognosis

Before the use of HAART, T-cell immunodeficiency persisted in patients with AIDS.[167, 236] Mortality rates for adult patients with AIDS have been described, with one report documenting the median survival for all patients as 12.5 months.[171] These rates have been modified by the advent of effective antiretroviral therapy for adults and are reflected by a decrease in recent mortality rates in patients with AIDS.

Accelerated research efforts directed toward developing early diagnostic methods for documenting HIV infection have resulted in earlier diagnosis, earlier administration of primary viral therapy, and prompt treatment and prevention of opportunistic infections. This advance has resulted in diminished morbidity and mortality rates in HIV-infected children, particularly those with more rapid onset of symptoms and abrupt clinical and immunologic decline. Pediatric research should continue to emphasize the development of new therapeutic interventions that might reduce perinatal transmission rates even further. For example, effective vaccine development clearly would have a significant worldwide impact on adults and children exposed to HIV.

Research efforts must now be coupled with socioeconomic and political efforts to find the will to have a global impact on HIV transmission and treatment. Duplication of the successes realized in industrialized countries are needed desperately in sub-Saharan Africa, East Asia, and Central America, where competing medical needs limit the available funding for prevention of HIV transmission and HIV treatment. When viewed from this perspective, placing the highest priority on global confrontation of this epidemic that threatens the future of our children is imperative.

REFERENCES

1. Abrams, D. I., Bebchuk, J. D., Denning, E. T., et al.: Randomized, open-label study of the impact of two doses of subcutaneous recombinant interleukin-2 on viral burden in patients with HIV-1 infection and CD4+ cells counts of > or = 300/mm^3: CPCRA 059. J. Acquir. Immune Defic. Syndr. *29*:221–231, 2002.
2. Abrams, D. I., Goldman, A. I., Launer, C., et al.: A comparative trial of didanosine or zalcitabine after treatment with zidovudine in patients with human immunodeficiency virus infection: The Terry Beirn Community Programs for Clinical Research on AIDS. N. Engl. J. Med. *330*:657–662, 1994.
3. Abrams, E. J.: Opportunistic infections and other clinical manifestations of HIV disease in children. Pediatr. Clin. North Am. *47*:79–108, 2000.
4. Abrams, E. J., Weedon, J., Bertolli, J., et al.: Aging cohort of perinatally human immunodeficiency virus–infected children in New York City. New York City Pediatric Surveillance of Disease Consortium. Pediatr. Infect. Dis. J. *20*:511–517, 2002.
5. Al-Harthi, L., Guilbert, L. J., Hoxie, J. A., et al.: Trophoblasts are productively infected by CD4-independent isolate of HIV type 1. A. I. D. S. Res. Hum. Retroviruses *18*:13–17, 2002.
6. Amadori, A., de Rossi, A., Giaquinto, C., et al.: In vitro production of HIV-specific antibody in children at risk of AIDS. Lancet *1*:852–854, 1988.
7. Ammann, A. J., Schiffman, G., Abrams, D., et al.: B cell immunodeficiency in acquired immunodeficiency syndrome. J. A. M. A. *251*:1447–1449, 1984.
8. Anderson, D. C., Hughes, B. J., and Smith, C. W.: Abnormal mobility of neonatal polymorphonuclear leukocytes: Relationship to impaired redistribution of surface adhesion sites by chemotactic factor or colchicine. J. Clin. Invest. *63*:863–874, 1981.
9. Andiman, W. A., Mezger, J., and Shapiro, E.: Invasive bacterial infections in children born to women infected with human immunodeficiency virus type 1. J. Pediatr. *124*:846–852, 1994.
10. Arico, M., Caselli, D., D'Argenio, P., et al.: Malignancies in children with human immunodeficiency virus type 1 infection: The Italian Multicenter Study on Human Immunodeficiency Virus Infection in Children. Cancer *68*:2473–2477, 1991.
11. Armstrong, D. D., and Kirkpatrick, J. B.: Neuropathology of pediatric AIDS. Semin. Pediatr. Infect. Dis. *1*:112–123, 1990.
12. Ashkenazi, S., and Kohl, S.: Central nervous system abnormalities in pediatric HIV infection and AIDS. Semin. Pediatr. Infect. Dis. *1*:94–106, 1990.
13. Association of State and Territorial Public Health Laboratory Directors: Seventh Annual Conference on Human Retrovirus Testing, Chicago, March 1992, pp. 1–26.
14. Atkinson, W. L., Pickering, L. K., Schwartz, B., et al.: General recommendations on immunizations. Recommendations of the Advisory Committee on Immunization Practices (ACIP) and the American Academy of Family Physicians (AAFP). M. M. W. R. Recomm. Rep. *51*(RR-2):1–35, 2002.
15. Bakshi, S. S., Alvarez, D., Hilfer, C. L., et al.: Tuberculosis in human immunodeficiency virus–infected children: A family infection. Am. J. Dis. Child. *147*:320–324, 1993.
16. Balasubranamian, R., and Lagakos, S. W.: Estimation of the timing of perinatal transmission of HIV. Biometrics *57*:1048–1058, 2001.
17. Balis, F. M., and Poplack, D. G.: Drug development and clinical pharmacology. *In* Pizzo, P. A., and Wilfert, C. M. (eds.): Pediatric AIDS: The Challenge of HIV Infection in Infants, Children, and Adolescents. Baltimore, Williams & Wilkins, 1990, pp. 457–477.
18. Belman, A. L., Diamond, G., Dickson, D., et al.: Pediatric acquired immunodeficiency syndrome: Neurologic syndromes. Am. J. Dis. Child. *142*:29–35, 1988.
19. Berman, P. W., Gregory, T. J., Riddle, L., et al.: Protection of chimpanzees from infection by HIV-1 after vaccination with recombinant glycoprotein gp120 but not gp160. Nature *345*:622–625, 1990.
20. Bernstein, L. J., Ochs, H. D., Wedgwood, R. J., et al.: Defective humoral immunity in pediatric acquired immune deficiency syndrome. J. Pediatr. *107*:352–356, 1985.
21. Biggar, R. J., Frisch, M., and Goedert, J. J.: Risk of cancer in children with AIDS. AIDS-Cancer Match Registry Study Group. J. A. M. A. *284*:2593–2594, 2000.
22. Blanche, S., Calvez, T., Rouzioux, C., et al.: Randomized study of two doses of didanosine in children infected with human immunodeficiency virus. J. Pediatr. *122*:966–973, 1993.
23. Blanche, S., Tardieu, M., Duliege, A. M., et al.: Longitudinal study of 94 symptomatic infants with perinatally acquired human immunodeficiency virus infection: Evidence for a bimodal expression of clinical and biological symptoms. Am. J. Dis. Child. *144*:1210–1215, 1990.
24. Blanche, S., Tardieu, M., Rustin, P., et al.: Persistent mitochondrial dysfunction and perinatal exposure to antiretroviral nucleoside analogues. Lancet *354*:1084–1089, 1999.
25. Bolognesi, D. P.: AIDS vaccines: Progress and unmet challenges. Ann. Intern. Med. *114*:161–162, 1991.
26. Bonavida, B., Katy, J., and Gottlieb, M.: Mechanism of defective NK cell activity in patients with acquired immunodeficiency syndrome (AIDS) and AIDS-related complex. I. Defective trigger of NK cells for NKLF production by target cells, and partial restoration by IL-2. J. Immunol. *137*:1157–1163, 1986.
27. Borkowsky, W., Rigaud, M., Krasinski, K., et al.: Cell-mediated and humoral immune responses in children infected with human immunodeficiency virus during the first four years of life. J. Pediatr. *120*:371–375, 1992.
28. Borkowsky, W., Steele, C. J., Grubman, S., et al.: Antibody responses to bacterial toxoids in children infected with human immunodeficiency virus. J. Pediatr. *110*:563–566, 1987.
29. Brenner, T. J., Dahl, K. E., Olson, B., et al.: Relation between HIV-1 syncytium inhibition antibodies and clinical outcome in children. Lancet *337*:1001–1005, 1991.
30. Bricker, J. T., for the P^{2}C^2 HIV Study Group: Transmission, immunodeficiency, and infectious complications. Abstract. Seattle, Presented at a meeting of the American Thoracic Society, Seattle, May 1995.
31. Brigitta, U. M., Jacobsen, F., Butler, K. M., et al.: Combination treatment with azidothymidine and granulocyte colony-stimulating factor in children with human immunodeficiency virus infection. J. Pediatr. *121*:797–802, 1992.
32. Brookmeyer, R.: Reconstruction and future trends of the AIDS epidemic in the United States. Science *253*:37–42, 1991.
33. Brossard, Y., Aubin, J. T., Madnelbrot, L., et al.: Frequency of early in utero HIV-1 infection: A blind DNA polymerase chain reaction study on 100 fetal thymuses. A. I. D. S. *9*:359–366, 1995.
34. Brouwers, P., Belman, A., and Epstein, L. G.: Central nervous system involvement: Manifestations, evaluation and pathogenesis. *In* Pizzo, P. A., and Wilfert, C. M., (eds.): Pediatric AIDS: The Challenge of HIV Infection in Infants, Children, and Adolescents. Baltimore, Williams & Wilkins, 1994, pp. 433–455.
35. Bryson, Y. J., Luzuriaga, K., Sullivan, J. L., et al.: Proposed definitions for in utero versus intrapartum transmission of HIV-1. N. Engl. J. Med. *327*:1246–1247, 1992.
36. Bryson, Y. J., Pang, S., Wei, L. S., et al.: Clearance of HIV infection in a perinatally infected infant. N. Engl. J. Med. *332*:833–838, 1995.
37. Buchacz, K., Cervia, J. S., Lindsey, J. C., et al.: Impact of protease inhibitor–containing combination antiretroviral therapies on height and weight growth in HIV-infected children. Pediatrics *108*:E72, 2001.
38. Butler, K., Husson, R. N., Balis, F. M., et al.: Dideoxyinosine (ddI) in children with symptomatic HIV infection. N. Engl. J. Med. *324*:137–144, 1991.
39. Canosa, C. A.: Epidemiology of HIV infection in children in Europe. Acta Paediatr. *400*:8–14, 1994.

40. Caselli, D., Marconi, M., Maccabruni, A., et al.: HIV-specific IgG3 in cord blood: Predictive value for seroreversion. Ann. N. Y. Acad. Sci. *693*:262–263, 1993.
41. Cattelan, A. M., Tervenzoli, M., and Aversa, S. M.: Recent advances in the treatment of AIDS-related Kaposi's sarcoma. Am. J. Clin. Dermatol. *3*:451–462, 2002.
42. Centers for Disease Control: Education and foster care of children infected with human T-lymphotropic virus type III/lymphadenopathy-associated virus. M. M. W. R. Morb. Mortal. Wkly. Rep. *34*(34):517–521, 1985.
43. Centers for Disease Control: Recommendations for assisting in the prevention of perinatal transmission of human T-lymphotropic virus type III/lymphadenopathy-associated virus and acquired immunodeficiency syndrome. M. M. W. R. Morb. Mortal. Wkly. Rep. *34*(48):721–726, 731–732, 1985.
44. Centers for Disease Control: Immunization of children infected with human T-lymphotropic virus type III/lymphadenopathy-associated virus. M. M. W. R. Morb. Mortal. Wkly. Rep. *35*(38):595–598, 603–606, 1986.
45. Centers for Disease Control: Revision of the CDC surveillance case definition for acquired immunodeficiency syndrome. Council of State and Territorial Epidemiologists; AIDS Program, Center for Infectious Diseases. M. M. W. R. Morb. Mortal. Wkly. Rep. *36*(Suppl. 1):1–15, 1987.
46. Centers for Disease Control: Classification system for human immunodeficiency virus (HIV) infection in children under 13 years of age. M. M. W. R. Morb. Mortal. Wkly. Rep. *36*(15):225–230, 235–236, 1987.
47. Centers for Disease Control: First 100,000 cases of acquired immunodeficiency syndrome—United States. M. M. W. R. Morb. Mortal. Wkly. Rep. *38*(32):561–563, 1989.
48. Centers for Disease Control and Prevention: Guidelines for prophylaxis against *Pneumocystis carinii* pneumonia for children infected with human immunodeficiency virus. M. M. W. R. Recomm. Rep. *40*(RR-2): 1–13, 1991.
49. Centers for Disease Control and Prevention: Summary of notifiable diseases, United States, 1991. M. M. W. R. Morb. Mortal. Wkly. Rep. *40*(53):1–63, 1992.
50. Centers for Disease Control and Prevention: Recommendations for prophylaxis against *Pneumocystis carinii* pneumonia for adults and adolescents infected with human immunodeficiency virus. M. M. W. R. Recomm. Rep. *41*(RR-4):1–11, 1992.
51. Centers for Disease Control and Prevention: Recommendations on prophylaxis and therapy for disseminated *Mycobacterium avium* complex for adults and adolescents infected with human immunodeficiency virus. U.S. Public Health Service Task Force on prophylaxis and therapy for *Mycobacterium avium* complex. M. M. W. R. Recomm. Rep. *42*(RR-9):14–20, 1993.
52. Centers for Disease Control and Prevention: 1994 Revised classification system for human immunodeficiency virus infection in children less than 13 years of age. M. M. W. R. Morb. Mortal. Wkly. Rep. *43*:1–17, 1994.
53. Centers for Disease Control and Prevention: Recommendations of the U.S. Public Health Service Task Force on the use of zidovudine to reduce perinatal transmission of human immunodeficiency virus. M. M. W. R. Recomm. Rep. *43*(RR-11):1–20, 1995.
54. Centers for Disease Control and Prevention: 1995 revised guidelines for prophylaxis against *Pneumocystis carinii* pneumonia for children infected with or perinatally exposed to human immunodeficiency virus. National Pediatric and Family HIV Resource Center and National Center for Infectious Diseases, Centers for Disease Control and Prevention. M. M. W. R. Recomm. Rep. *44*(RR-4):1–11, 1995.
55. Centers for Disease Control and Prevention: USPHS/IDSA guidelines for the prevention of opportunistic infections in persons infected with human immunodeficiency virus: A summary. M. M. W. R. Recomm. Rep. *44*(RR-8):1–34, 1995.
56. Centers for Disease Control and Prevention: Prevention of varicella. Updated recommendations of the Advisory Committee on Immunization Practices (ACIP). M. M. W. R. *48*(RR-6):1–5, 1999.
57. Centers for Disease Control and Prevention: The global HIV and AIDS epidemic, 2001. M. M. W. R. Morb. Mortal. Wkly. Rep. *50*(21):434–439, 2001.
58. Centers for Disease Control and Prevention: Revised recommendations for HIV screening of pregnant women. M. M. W. R. Recomm. Rep. *50*(RR-19):63–85, 2001.
59. Centers for Disease Control and Prevention: Update AIDS—United States, 2000. M. M. W. R. Morb. Mortal. Wkly. Rep. *51*(27):592–595, 2002.
60. Centers for Disease Control and Prevention: Diagnosing and reporting of HIV and AIDS in states with HIV/AIDS surveillance—United States, 1994–2000. M. M. W. R. Recomm. Rep. *51*(27):595–598, 2002.
61. Centers for Disease Control and Prevention: Progressing toward tuberculosis elimination in low-incidence areas of the United States: Recommendations of the advisory council for the elimination of tuberculosis. M. M. W. R. Recomm. Rep. *51*(RR-5):1, 2002.
62. Centers for Disease Control and Prevention: Guidelines for preventing opportunistic infections among HIV-infected persons—2002. Recommendations of the U.S. Public Health Service and the Infectious Diseases Society of America. M. M. W. R. Recomm. Rep. *51*(RR-8):1–52, 2002.
63. Chadwick, E. G., Connor, E. J., Hanson, I. C., et al.: Tumors of smooth muscle origin in pediatric HIV-infected patients: A new association of AIDS and cancer. J. A. M. A. *263*:3182–3184, 1990.
64. Chadwick, E. G., and Yogev, R.: Pediatric AIDS. Pediatr. Clin. North Am. *42*:969–992, 1995.
65. Chandwani, E., Greco, M. A., Mittal, K., et al.: Pathology and HIV expression in term placentas from seropositive women. Abstract MBP 20. Presented at the Fifth International Conference on AIDS, June 1989, Montreal, p. 225.
66. Chin, J.: Current and future dimensions of the HIV/AIDS pandemic in women and children. Lancet *336*:221–224, 1990.
67. Chougnet, C., Jankelevich, S., Fowke, K., et al.: Long-term protease inhibitor–containing therapy results in limited improvement in T cell function but not restoration of interleukin-12 production in pediatric patients with AIDS. J. Infect. Dis. *184*:201–205, 2001.
68. Chowdhury, I. H., Koyanagi, Y., Takamatsu, K., et al.: Evaluation of anti–human immunodeficiency virus effect of recombinant CD4-immunoglobulin in vitro: A good candidate for AIDS treatment. Med. Microbiol. Immunol. *180*:183–192, 1991.
68a. Church, J. A., Cunningham, C., Hughes, M., et al.: Safety and antiretroviral activity of chronic subcutaneous administration of T-20 in human immunodeficiency virus 1–infected children. Pediatr. Infect. Dis. J. *21*: 653–659, 2002.
69. Clavel, F., Guetard, D., Brun-Vezinet, F., et al.: Isolation of a new human retrovirus from West African patients with AIDS. Science *233*:343–346, 1986.
70. Comeau, A. M., Hsu, H.-W., Schwerzier, M., et al.: Identifying human immunodeficiency virus infection at birth: Application of polymerase chain reaction to Guthrie cards. J. Pediatr. *123*:252–258, 1993.
71. Connor, E. M., and McSherry G.: Immune-based interventions in perinatal human immunodeficiency virus infection. Pediatr. Infect. Dis. J. *13*:440–448, 1994.
72. Connor, E. M., Sperling, R. S., Gelber, R., et al.: Reduction of maternal-infant transmission of human immunodeficiency virus type 1 with zidovudine treatment: Pediatric AIDS Clinical Trials Group Protocol 076 Study Group. N. Engl. J. Med. *331*:1173–1180, 1994.
73. Cooper, E. R., Charurat, M., Mofenson, L., et al.: Combination antiretroviral strategies for the treatment of pregnant HIV-1–infected women and prevention of perinatal HIV-1 transmission. J. Acquir. Immune Defic. Syndr. *29*:484–494, 2002.
74. Cowan, M. J., Hellman, D., Chudwin, D., et al.: Maternal transmission of acquired immune deficiency syndrome. Pediatrics *73*:382–386, 1984.
75. Culnane, M., Fowler, M. G., Lee, S. S., et al.: Lack of long-term effects of in utero exposure to zidovudine among uninfected children born to HIV-infected women. J. A. M. A. *281*:151–157, 1999.
76. Curran, J. W., Lawrence, D. N., Jaffe, H., et al.: Acquired immunodeficiency syndrome (AIDS) associated with transfusions. N. Engl. J. Med. *310*:492–497, 1984.
77. Demmler, G. J., and Taber, L. H.: Virology of HIV-1. Semin. Pediatr. Infect. Dis. *1*:17–20, 1990.
78. Denny, T. N., Yogev, R., Gelman, R., et al.: Lymphocyte subsets in healthy children during the first 5 years of life. J. A. M. A. *267*:1484–1488, 1992.
79. DeRossi, A., Zanotto, C., Mammano, F., et al.: Pattern of antibody response against the v3 loop in children with vertically acquired immunodeficiency type-1 (HIV-1) infection. A. I. D. S. Res. Hum. Retroviruses *9*:221–228, 1993.
80. Devash, Y., Calvelli, T. A., Wood, D. G., et al.: Vertical transmission of human immunodeficiency virus is correlated with the absence of high-affinity/avidity maternal antibodies to the gp120 principal neutralizing domain. Proc. Natl. Acad. Sci. U. S. A. *87*:3445–3449, 1990.
81. Dickover, R. E., Dillon, M., Gillete, S. G., et al.: Rapid increases in load of human immunodeficiency virus correlate with early disease progression and loss of CD4 cells in vertically infected infants. J. Infect. Dis. *170*:1279–1284, 1994.
82. Dieterich, D. T., Kotler, D. P., Busch, D. F., et al: Ganciclovir treatment of cytomegalovirus colitis in AIDS: A randomized, double-blind, placebo-controlled multicenter study. J. Infect. Dis. *167*:278–282, 1993.
83. Domanski, M. J., Sloas, M. M., Follmann, D. A., et al.: Effect of zidovudine and didanosine treatment on heart function in children infected with human immunodeficiency virus. J. Pediatr. *127*:137–146, 1995.
84. Dorenbaum, A., Cunningham, C. K., Gelver, R. D., et al.: Two-dose intrapartum/newborn nevirapine and standard antiretroviral therapy to reduce perinatal HIV transmission: A randomized trial. J. A. M. A. *288*:189–198, 2002.
85. Drug approval for weight loss in AIDS news. Am. Fam. Physician *47*:997, 1993.
86. D'Ubalo, C., Pezzotti, P., Rezza, G., et al.: Association between HIV-1 infection and miscarriage: A retrospective study. DIANAIDS Collaborative Study Group. Diagnosi Iniziale Anomalie Neoplastiche AIDS. A. I. D. S. *12*:1087–1093, 1998.

87. Dunn, D. T., Brandt, C. D., and Krivine, A.: The sensitivity of HIV-1 DNA polymerase chain reaction in the neonatal period and the relative contributions of intra-uterine and intra-partum transmission. A. I. D. S. *9*:F7–F11, 1995.
88. Dunn, D. T., Newell, M. L., Ades, A. E., et al.: Risk of human immunodeficiency virus type 1 transmission through breastfeeding. Lancet *340*:585–588, 1992.
89. Ellaurie, M., Burns, E. R., Bernstein, L. J., et al.: Thrombocytopenia and human immunodeficiency virus in children. Pediatrics *82*:905–908, 1988.
90. Ellaurie, M., Burns, E. R., and Rubinstein, A.: Platelet-associated IgG in pediatric HIV infection. Pediatr. Hematol. Oncol. *8*:179–185, 1991.
91. Epstein, L. G., Sharer, L. R., Oleske, J. M., et al.: Neurologic manifestations of HIV infection in children. Pediatrics *78*:678–687, 1986.
92. European Collaborative Study: Children born to women with HIV-1 infection: Natural history and transmission. Lancet *337*:253–260, 1991.
93. European Collaborative Study: Risk factors for mother-to-child transmission of HIV-1. Lancet *339*:1007–1012, 1992.
94. European Collaborative Study: Caesarean section and risk of vertical transmission of HIV-1 infection. Lancet *343*:1464–1467, 1994.
95. Fabio, G., Scorza, R., Lazzarin, A., et al.: HLA-associated susceptibility to HIV-1 infection. Clin. Exp. Immunol. *87*:20–23, 1992.
96. Fauci, A. S.: The human immunodeficiency virus: Infectivity and mechanisms of pathogenesis. Science *239*:617–622, 1988.
97. Fehir, K. M., Decker, W. A., Samo, T., et al.: Immune globulin (GAMMAGARD) prophylaxis of CMV infections in patients undergoing organ transplantation and allogeneic bone marrow transplantation. Transplant. Proc. *21*:3107–3109, 1989.
98. Fischl, M. A., Galpin, J. E., Levine, J. D., et al.: Recombinant human erythropoietin for patient with AIDS treated with zidovudine. N. Engl. J. Med. *322*:488–493, 1990.
99. Fischl, M. A., Richman, D. D., Grieco, M. H., et al.: The efficacy of azidothymidine (AZT) in the treatment of patients with AIDS and AIDS-related complex. N. Engl. J. Med. *313*:192–197, 1987.
100. Fisher, R. G., Nageswaran, S., Valentine, M. E., et al.: Successful prophylaxis against *Pneumocystis carinii* pneumonia in HIV-infected children using smaller than recommended dosages of trimethoprim-sulfamethoxazole. A. I. D. S. Patient Care. *15*:263–269, 2001.
101. Fisher, S., D., and Lipshultz, S. E.: Epidemiology of cardiovascular involvement in HIV disease and AIDS. Ann. N. Y. Acad. Sci. *946*:13–22, 2002.
102. Fitzgibbon, J. E., Gaur, S., Frenkel, L. D., et al.: Transmission from one child to another of human immunodeficiency virus type 1 with a zidovudine-resistance mutation. N. Engl. J. Med. *329*:1835–1841, 1993.
103. Foster, S., Hawkins, E., Hanson, C. G., et al.: Pathology of the kidney in childhood immunodeficiency: Is AIDS-related nephropathy unique? Pediatr. Pathol. *11*:63–74, 1991.
104. Fowler, M. G., and Newell, M. L.: Breast-feeding and HIV-1 transmission in resource-limited settings. J. Acquir. Immune Defic. Syndr. *30*:230–239, 2002.
105. Frederick, T., Mascola, L., Eller, A., et al.: Progression of human immunodeficiency virus disease among infants and children infected perinatally with human immunodeficiency virus or through neonatal blood transfusion. Pediatr. Infect. Dis. J. *13*:1091–1097, 1994.
106. Frenkel, L. M., Capparelli, E. V., Dankner, W. M., et al.: Oral ganciclovir in children: Pharmacokinetics, safety, tolerance, and antiviral effects. The Pediatric AIDS Clinical Trials Group. J. Infect. Dis. *182*:1616–1624, 2000.
107. Friedland, G., Kahl, P., Slatzman, B., et al.: Additional evidence for lack of transmission of HIV infection by close interpersonal (casual) contact. A. I. D. S. *4*:639–644, 1990.
108. Frissen, P. H., Van der Ende, M. E., ten Napel, C. H., et al.: Zidovudine and interferon-alpha combination therapy versus zidovudine monotherapy in subjects with symptomatic human immunodeficiency virus type 1 infection. J. Infect. Dis. *169*:1351–1355, 1994.
109. Froebel, K. S., Aldhous, M. C., Mok, J. Y., et al.: Cytotoxic T lymphocyte activity in children infected with HIV. A. I. D. S. Res. Hum. Retroviruses *10*:83–88, 1994.
110. Gabiano, C., Tovo, P., de Martino, M., et al.: Mother-to-child transmission of human immunodeficiency virus type-1: Risk of infection and correlates of transmission. Pediatrics *90*:369–374, 1992.
111. Gagnon, S., Boota, A. M., Fischl, M. A., et al.: Corticosteroids as adjunctive therapy for severe *Pneumocystis carinii* pneumonia in the acquired immunodeficiency syndrome: A double-blind, placebo-controlled trial. N. Engl. J. Med. *323*:1444–1450, 1990.
112. Gallo, R. C., Salahuddin, S. Z., Shearer, G. M., et al.: Frequent detection and isolation of cytopathic retroviruses (HTLV-III) from patients with AIDS and at risk for AIDS. Science *224*:500–503, 1984.
113. Gellert, G. A., Durfee, M. J., Berkowitz, C. D., et al.: Situational and sociodemographic characteristics of children infected with human immunodeficiency virus from pediatric sexual abuse. Pediatrics *91*:39–44, 1993.
114. Goedert, J. J., Duliege, A., Amos, C. I., et al.: High risk of HIV-1 infection for first-born twins. Lancet *338*:1471–1475, 1991.
115. Gortmaker, S. L., Hughes, M., Cervia J., et al.: Effect of combination therapy including protease inhibitors on mortality among children and adolescents infected with HIV-1. N. Engl. J. Med. *345*:1522–1528, 2001.
116. Goudsmit, J., de Wolf, F., Paul, D. A., et al.: Expression of human immunodeficiency virus antigen (HIV-Ag) in serum and cerebrospinal fluid during acute and chronic infection. Lancet *2*:177–180, 1986.
117. Greene, W. C.: AIDS and the immune system. Sci. Am. *269*:105–117, 1993.
118. Groopman, J. E., Mitsuyasu, R. T., Delco, M. J., et al.: Effect of recombinant human granulocyte-macrophage colony-stimulating factor on myelopoiesis in the acquired immunodeficiency syndrome. N. Engl. J. Med. *317*:593–598, 1987.
119. Groopman, J. E., and Scadden, D. T.: Interferon therapy for Kaposi sarcoma associated with the acquired immunodeficiency syndrome (AIDS). Ann. Intern. Med. *110*:335–337, 1989.
120. Groux, H., Torpier, G., Monte, D., et al.: Activation-induced death by apoptosis in CD4+ T cells from human immunodeficiency virus–infected asymptomatic individuals. J. Exp. Med. *175*:331–340, 1992.
121. Grubman, S., Gross, E., Lerner-Weiss, N., et al.: Older children and adolescents living with perinatally acquired human immunodeficiency virus infection. Pediatrics *95*:657–663, 1995.
122. Guay, L. A., Musoke, P., Fleming, T., et al.: Intrapartum and neonatal single-dose nevirapine compared with zidovudine for prevention of mother-to-child transmission of HIV-1 in Kampala, Uganda: HIVNET 012 randomised trial. Lancet *354*:795–802, 1999.
123. Gutman, L. T., St. Claire, K. K., Weedy, C., et al.: Human immunodeficiency virus transmission by child sexual abuse. Am. J. Dis. Child. *145*:137–141, 1991.
124. Hanna, S. L., Yang, C., Owen, S. M., et al.: Resistance mutation in HIV entry inhibitors. A. I. D. S. *16*:1603–1608, 2002.
125. Hanson, I. C.: Respiratory infections in HIV-infected children. Immunol. Allergy Clin. North Am. *13*:205–217, 1993.
126. Hanson, I. C., Antonelli, T. A., Sperling, R. S., et al.: Lack of tumors in infants with perinatal HIV-1 exposure and fetal/neonatal exposure to zidovudine. J. Acquir. Immune Defic. Syndr. Hum. Retrovirol. *20*:463–467, 1999.
127. Hanson, I. C., and Kaplan, S. L.: Opportunistic infections. Semin. Pediatr. Infect. Dis. *1*:31–39, 1990.
128. Hanson, I. C., Pitt, J., Sherrieb, K., et al.: Followup of single positive or indeterminate HIV cultures among infants in a multisite perinatal HIV study. Abstract. Presented at a meeting of the Infectious Disease Society of America, September 16, 1995, San Francisco.
129. Hanson, I. C., and Shearer, W. T.: Diagnosis of HIV infection. Semin. Pediatr. Infect. Dis. *5*:266–271, 1994.
130. Hay, J. F., Lewis, D. E., and Miller, G. G.: Functional versus phenotypic analysis of T cells in subjects seropositive for the human immunodeficiency virus: A prospective study of in vitro responses to *Cryptococcus neoformans*. J. Infect. Dis. *158*:1071–1078, 1988.
131. Hengge, U. R., Ruzicka, T., Tyring, S. K., et al.: Update on Kaposi's sarcoma and other HHV8 associated diseases. Part 2: pathogenesis, Castleman's disease, and pleural effusion lymphoma. Lancet Infect. Dis. *2*:344–352, 2002.
132. Hernandez-Sampelayo, T.: Fluconazole versus ketoconazole in the treatment of oropharyngeal candidiasis in HIV-infected children: Multicentre study group. Eur. J. Clin. Microbiol. Infect. Dis. *13*:340–344, 1994.
133. Ho, D., Pomerantz, R. J., and Kaplan, J. C.: Pathogenesis of infection with human immunodeficiency virus. N. Engl. J. Med. *317*:278–286, 1987.
134. Ho, D. D.: Time to hit HIV, early and hard. N. Engl. J. Med. *333*:450–451, 1995.
135. Ho, D. D., Neumann, A. U., Perelson, A. S., et al.: Rapid turnover of plasma virions and CD4 lymphocytes in HIV-1 infection. Nature *373*:123–126, 1995.
136. Hodges, T. L., Kahn, J. O., Kaplan, L. D., et al.: Phase 1 study of recombinant CD4–immunoglobulin G therapy of patients with AIDS and AIDS-related complex. Antimicrob. Agents Chemother. *35*:2580–2586, 1991.
137. Horsburgh, C. R.: *Mycobacterium avium* complex infection in the acquired immunodeficiency syndrome. N. Engl. J. Med. *324*:1332–1338, 1991.
138. Horsburgh, C. R., Havlik, J. A., Metchock, B. G., et al.: Oral therapy of disseminated *Mycobacterium avium* complex infection in AIDS relieves symptoms and is well tolerated. Am. Rev. Respir. Dis. *143*:115, 1991.
139. Hughes, W. T.: *Pneumocystis carinii* pneumonia. N. Engl. J. Med. *297*:1381, 1971.
140. Hughes, W. T., Leoung, G., Dramer, F., et al.: Comparison of atovaquone (566C80) with trimethoprim-sulfamethoxazole to PCP in patients with AIDS. N. Engl. J. Med. *328*:1521–1527, 1993.
141. Hughes, W. T., Rivera, G. K., Schell, M. J., et al.: Successful intermittent chemoprophylaxis for *Pneumocystis carinii* pneumonitis. N. Engl. J. Med. *316*:1627–1632, 1987.
142. Hussey, R. E., Richardson, N. E., Kowalski, M., et al.: A soluble CD4 protein selectively inhibits HIV replication and syncytium formation. Nature *331*:78–81, 1988.

143. Husson, R. N., Mueller, B. U., Farley, M., et al.: Zidovudine and didanosine combination therapy in children with human immunodeficiency virus infection. Pediatrics *93*:316–322, 1994.
144. Husson, R. N., Shirasaka, T., Butler, K. M., et al.: High-level resistance to zidovudine but not to zalcitabine or didanosine in human immunodeficiency virus from children receiving antiretroviral therapy. J. Pediatr. *123*:9–16, 1993.
145. Italian Register for HIV Infection in Children: Features of children perinatally infected with HIV-1 surviving longer than 5 years. Lancet *343*:191–195, 1994.
146. Jason, J. M., Stehr-Green, J., Holman, R. C., et al.: Human immunodeficiency virus infection in hemophilic children. Pediatrics *82*:565–570, 1988.
147. Jiang, S., Zhao, Q., and Debnath, A. K.: Peptide and non-peptide HIV fusion inhibitors. Curr. Pharm. Des. *8*:563–580, 2002.
148. Kadan-Lottick, N. S., Skluzacek, M. D., and Gurney, J. G.: Decreasing incidence rates of primary central nervous system lymphoma. Cancer *95*:193–202, 2002.
149. Kahn, J. O., Allan, J. D., Hodges, T. L., et al.: The safety and pharmacokinetics of recombinant soluble CD4 (rCD4) in subjects with the acquired immunodeficiency syndrome (AIDS) and AIDS-related complex: A phase 1 study. Ann. Intern. Med. *112*:254–261, 1990.
150. Karon, J. M., Fleming, P. L., Steketee, R. W., et al.: HIV in the United States at the turn of the century: An epidemic in transition. Am. J. Public Health *91*:1060–1068, 2001.
151. Katzman, M., and Lederman, M. M.: Defective postbinding lysis underlies the impaired natural killer activity in factor VIII–treated human T-lymphotropic virus type III seropositive hemophiliacs. J. Clin. Invest. *77*:1067–1062, 1986.
152. Kilby, J. M., Lalezari, J. P., Eron, J. J., et al.: The safety, plasma pharmacokinetics, and antiviral activity of subcutaneous enfuvirtide (T-20) a peptide inhibitor of gp41-mediated virus fusion, in HIV-infected adults. A. I. D. S. Res. Hum. Retroviruses *18*:685–693, 2002.
153. Kilpatrick, D. C., Hague, R. A., Yap, P. L., et al.: HLA antigen frequencies in children born to HIV-infected mothers. Dis. Markers *9*:21–26, 1991.
154. Kirkpatrick, S., Hanson, I. C., Bohannon, B., et al.: *Mycobacterium avium* complex (MAC) in HIV-infected children less than 13 years of age. Abstract. Presented at a meeting of the Infectious Disease Society of America, September 16, 1995, San Francisco.
155. Kline, M. W., Dunkle, L. M., Church, J. A., et al.: A phase I/II evaluation of stavudine (d4T) in children with human immunodeficiency virus infection. Pediatrics *96*:247–252, 1995.
156. Kline, M. W., Paul, M. E., Bohannon, B., et al.: Characteristics of children surviving to five years of age or older with vertically acquired human immunodeficiency. Pediatr. A. I. D. S. *6*:350–353, 1995.
157. Kline, M. W., and Shearer, W. T.: HIV infection and AIDS in children. *In* Rich, R. R., Fleischer, T. A., Schwartz, W. T., et al. (eds.): Clinical Immunology. St. Louis, Mosby, 1996, pp. 739–750.
158. Kovacs, J. A., Baseler, M., Dewar, R. J., et al.: Increases in CD4 T lymphocytes with intermittent courses of interleukin-2 in patients with human immunodeficiency virus infection. N. Engl. J. Med. *332*:567–575, 1995.
159. Krogstad, P., Lee, S., Johnson, G., et al.: Nucleoside-analogue reverse-transcriptase inhibitors plus nevirapine, nelfinavir, or ritonavir for pretreated children infected with human immunodeficiency virus type 1. Clin. Infect. Dis. *34*:991–1001, 2002.
160. Krown, S. E.: AIDS-associated Kaposi sarcoma: Pathogenesis, clinical course and treatment. A. I. D. S. *2*:71–80, 1980.
161. Lambert, J. S., Seidlin, M., Reichman, R. C., et al.: 2′3′-dideoxyinosine (ddI) in patients with the acquired immunodeficiency syndrome or AIDS-related complex. N. Engl. J. Med. *322*:1333–1340, 1990.
162. Landesman, S. A., Kalish, L. A., Burns, D., et al.: Obstetrical factors in vertical transmission of HIV: Role of duration of ruptured membranes. N. Engl. J. Med. *334*:1617–1623, 1996.
163. Lane, H. C., Depper, J. M., Green, W. C., et al.: Qualitative analysis of immune function in patients with the acquired immunodeficiency syndrome: Evidence for a selective defect in soluble antigen recognition. N. Engl. J. Med. *313*:79–84, 1985.
164. Langston, C., Lewis, D. E., Hammill, H. A., et al.: Excess intrauterine fetal demise associated with maternal HIV infection. J. Infect. Dis. *172*:1451–1460, 1995.
165. Lapointe, N., Michaud, J., Pekovic, D., et al.: Transplacental transmission of HTLV-III virus. N. Engl. J. Med. *312*:1325–1326, 1985.
166. Laufer, M., and Scott, G. B.: Medical management of HIV disease in children. Pediatr. Clin. North Am. *47*:127–153, 2000.
167. Lee, J. W., and Pizzo, P. A.: Management of specific problems in children with leukemias and lymphomas. *In* Patrick, C. C. (ed.): Infections in Immunocompromised Infants and Children. New York, Churchill Livingstone, 1992, pp. 195–214.
168. Leibovitz, E., Rigaud, M., Pollack, H., et al.: *Pneumocystis carinii* pneumonia in infants infected with the human immunodeficiency virus with more than 450 CD4 T-lymphocytes per cubic millimeter. N. Engl. J. Med. *323*:631–633, 1990.
169. Lemp, G. F., Payne, S. F., Neal, D., et al.: Survival trends for patients with AIDS. J. A. M. A. *263*:402–406, 1990.
170. Lenderking, W. R., Gelber, R. D., Cotton, D. J., et al.: Evaluation of the quality of life associated with zidovudine treatment in asymptomatic human immunodeficiency virus infection: The AIDS Clinical Trials Group. N. Engl. J. Med. *330*:738–743, 1994.
171. Levine, R. L., Englard, A., McKinley, G. F., et al.: The efficacy and lack of toxicity of escalating doses of recombinant erythropoietin (rHuEPO) in anemic AIDS patients on zidovudine (AZT). Blood *74*:1–7, 1989.
172. Lindegren, M. L., Hanson, C., Miller, K., et al.: Epidemiology of human immunodeficiency virus infection in adolescents, United States. Pediatr. Infect. Dis. J. *13*:525–535, 1994.
173. Lindegren, M. L., Rhodes, P., Gordon, L., et al.: Drug safety during pregnancy and in infants. Lack of mortality related to mitochondrial dysfunction among perinatally HIV-exposed children in pediatric HIV surveillance. Ann. N. Y. Acad. Sci. *918*:222–235, 2000.
174. Lipshultz, S. E., Chanock, S., Sanders, S. P., et al.: Cardiovascular manifestations of human immunodeficiency virus infection in infants and children. Am. J. Cardiol. *63*:1489–1497, 1989.
175. Lobato, M. N., Caldwell, M. B., and Oxtoby, M. J.: Encephalopathy in children with perinatally acquired human immunodeficiency virus infection: Pediatric spectrum of disease clinical consortium. J. Pediatr. *126*:710–715, 1995.
176. Lorenzi, P., Spicher, V. M., Laubereau, B., et al.: Antiretroviral therapies in pregnancy: Maternal, fetal and neonatal effects. Swiss HIV Cohort Study, the Swiss Collaborative HIV and Pregnancy Study and the Swiss Neonatal HIV Study. A. I. D. S. *12*:F241–F247, 1998.
177. Luginbuhl, L. M., Orav, E., McIntosh, K., et al.: Cardiac morbidity and related mortality in children with HIV infection. J. A. M. A. *269*:2869–2875, 1993.
178. Luzuriaga, K., Koup, R. A., Pikora, C. A., et al.: Deficient human immunodeficiency virus type-1 specific cytotoxic T-cell responses in vertically infected children. Pediatrics *119*:230–236, 1991.
179. Luzuriaga, K., McQuilken, P., Alimenti, A., et al.: Early viremia and immune responses in vertical human immunodeficiency virus type 1 infection. J. Infect. Dis. *167*:1008–1013, 1993.
180. Macallan, D. C., Noble, C., Baldwin, C., et al.: Energy expenditure and wasting in human immunodeficiency virus infection. N. Engl. J. Med. *333*:83–88, 1995.
181. Maury, W., Potts, B. J., and Rabson, A. B.: HIV-1 infection of first trimester and term human placental tissue: A possible mode of maternal-fetal transmission. J. Infect. Dis. *160*:583–588, 1989.
182. Mayes, S. D., Handford, H. A., Schaefer, J. H., et al.: The relationship of HIV status, type of coagulation disorder, and school absenteeism to cognition, educational performance, mood, and behavior of boys with hemophilia. J. Genet. Psychol. *157*:137–151, 1996.
183. McArthur, J. C.: Neurologic manifestations of AIDS. Medicine (Baltimore) *66*:407–437, 1987.
184. McClain, K. L., Leach, C. T., Jenson, H. B., et al.: Association of Epstein-Barr virus with leiomyosarcomas in children with AIDS. N. Engl. J. Med. *332*:12–18, 1995.
185. McClain, K. L., and Rosenblatt, H.: Pediatric HIV infection and AIDS: Clinical expression of malignancy. Semin. Pediatr. Infect. Dis. *1*:124–129, 1990.
186. McIntosh, K., Pitt, J., Brambilla, D., et al.: Blood culture in the first 6 months of life for the diagnosis of vertically transmitted human immunodeficiency virus infection: The Women and Infants Transmission Study Group. J. Infect. Dis. *170*:996–1000, 1994.
187. McKinney, R. E., Pizzo, P. A., Scott, G. B., et al.: Safety and tolerance of intermittent intravenous and oral zidovudine therapy in human immunodeficiency virus–infected pediatric patients. J. Pediatr. *116*:640–647, 1990.
188. McKinney, R. E., and Robertson, J. W.: Effect of human immunodeficiency virus infection on the growth of young children: Duke Pediatric AIDS Clinical Trials Unit. J. Pediatr. *123*:579–582, 1993.
189. McMichael, A., Mwau, M., and Hanke, T.: Design and tests of an HIV vaccine. Br. Med. Bull. *62*:87–98, 2002.
190. Metselaar, H. J., Velzing, J., Rothbarth, P. H., et al.: Prophylactic use of anti-CMV immunoglobulins in heart transplant recipients: A study on its safety. Transplant. Proc. *21*:2504–2505, 1989.
191. Michaels, D., and Levine, C.: Estimates of the number of motherless youth orphaned by AIDS in the United States. J. A. M. A. *268*: 3456–3461, 1992.
192. Miller, M. E.: Immunodeficiencies of immaturity. *In* Stiehm E. R. (ed.): Immunologic Disorders of Infants and Children. 3rd ed. Philadelphia, W. B. Saunders, 1989, pp. 196–225.
193. Mintz, M.: Elevated serum levels of tumor necrosis factor are associated with progressive encephalopathy in children with acquired immunodeficiency syndrome. Am. J. Dis. Child. *143*:771–774, 1989.
194. Mintz, M., and Epstein, L. G.: Neurologic manifestation of pediatric acquired immunodeficiency syndrome: Clinical features and therapeutic approaches. Semin. Neurol. *12*:51–56, 1992.
195. Mitsuya, H., and Broder, S.: Strategies for antiviral therapy in AIDS. Nature *325*:773–778, 1987.

196. Mofenson, L. M., and Committee on Pediatric AIDS: Technical report: Perinatal human immunodeficiency virus testing and prevention of transmission. Pediatrics *106*:e88, 2000.
197. Mofenson, L. M., Moye, J., Korelitz, J., et al.: Crossover of placebo patients to intravenous immunoglobulin confirms efficacy for prophylaxis of bacterial infections and reduction of hospitalizations in human immunodeficiency virus–infected children. Pediatr. Infect. Dis. J. *13*:477–484, 1994.
198. Mofenson, L. M., Rodriguez, E. M., Hershow, R., et al.: *Mycobacterium tuberculosis* infection in pregnant and nonpregnant women infected with HIV in the Women and Infants Transmission Study. Arch. Intern. Med. *155*:1066–1072, 1995.
199. Moore, P. S., and Chang, Y.: Detection of herpesvirus-like DNA sequences in Kaposi sarcoma in patients with and those without HIV infection. N. Engl. J. Med. *332*:1181–1185, 1995.
200. Morgan, E. T., and Smalley, L. A.: Varicella in immunocompromised children: Incidence of abdominal pain and organ involvement. Am. J. Dis. Child. *137*:883, 1983.
201. Moye, J. M., Rich, K. C., Kalish, L. A., et al.: Natural history of somatic growth in pediatric HIV infection. J. Pediatr. *128*:58–69, 1996.
202. Mueller, B. U., Jacobsen, F., Butler, K. M., et al.: Combination treatment with azidothymidine and granulocyte colony-stimulating factor in children with human immunodeficiency virus infection. J. Pediatr. *121*:797–802, 1992.
203. Murphey-Corb, M., Martin, L., Davison-Fairburn, B., et al.: A formalin-inactivated whole SIV vaccine confers protection in macaques. Science *246*:1293–1297, 1989.
204. Mwanyumba, F., Gaillard, P., Inion, I., et al.: Placental inflammation and perinatal transmission of HIV-1. J. Acquir. Immune Defic. Syndr. *1*:29, 2002.
205. Nadal, D., Caduff, R., Frey, E., et al.: Non-Hodgkin lymphoma in four children infected with the human immunodeficiency virus: Association with Epstein-Barr virus and treatment. Cancer *73*:224–230, 1994.
206. Nielsen, K., Wei, L. S., Sim, M. S., et al.: Correlation of clinical progression in human immunodeficiency virus–infected children with in vitro zidovudine resistance measured by a direct quantitative peripheral blood lymphocyte assay. J. Infect. Dis. *172*:359–364, 1995.
207. Oleske, J. M., Minnefor, A. B., Cooper, R., et al.: Immune deficiency syndrome in children. J. A. M. A. *249*:2345–2349, 1983.
208. Ou, C. Y., Kwok, S., Mitchell, S. W., et al.: DNA amplification for direct detection of HIV-1 in DNA of peripheral blood mononuclear cells. Science *239*:295–297, 1988.
209. Palella, F. J., Jr., Delaney, K. M., Moorman, A. C., et al.: Declining morbidity and mortality among patients with advanced human immunodeficiency virus infection. HIV Outpatient Study Investigators. N. Engl. J. Med. *338*:853–860, 1998.
210. Palomba, E., Gay, V., DeMartino, M., et al.: Early diagnosis of human immunodeficiency virus infection in infants by detection of free and complexed p24 antigen. J. Infect. Dis. *165*:394–395, 1992.
211. Palumbo, P. E.: Antiretroviral therapy of HIV infection in children. Pediatr. Clin. North Am. *47*:155–169, 2000.
212. Pantaleo, G., Grazosi, C., and Fauci, A. S.: The immunopathogenesis of human immunodeficiency virus infection. N. Engl. J. Med. *328*:327–335, 1993.
213. Parker, R.: The global HIV/AIDS pandemic, structural inequalities, and the politics of international health. Am. J. Public Health *92*:343–346, 2002.
214. Pawha, S., Chirmule, N., Leombruno, C., et al.: In vitro synthesis of human immunodeficiency virus–specific antibodies in peripheral blood lymphocytes of infants. Proc. Natl. Acad. Sci. U. S. A. *86*:7532–7536, 1989.
215. Pawha, S., Fikrig, S., Mesey, R., et al.: Pediatric acquired immunodeficiency syndrome: Demonstration of B lymphocyte defects in vivo. Diagn. Immunol. *4*:24–30, 1986.
216. Pizzo, P. A., Butler, K., Balis, F., et al.: Dideoxycytidine alone and in an alternating schedule with zidovudine in children with symptomatic human immunodeficiency virus infection. J. Pediatr. *117*:799–808, 1990.
217. Pizzo, P. A., Eddy, J., Falloon, J., et al.: Effect of continuous intravenous infusion of zidovudine (AZT) in children with symptomatic HIV infection. N. Engl. J. Med. *319*:889–896, 1988.
218. Plotkin, S. A., and the Task Force on Pediatric AIDS: Pediatric guidelines for infection control of human immunodeficiency virus infection (acquired immunodeficiency virus) in hospitals, medical offices, schools and other settings. Pediatrics *82*:801–807, 1988.
219. Purcell, R. H.: Animal models for the development of a vaccine for the acquired immunodeficiency syndrome. Ann. Intern. Med. *110*:381–385, 1989.
220. Putkonen, P., Thorstensson, R., Ghavamzadeh, L., et al.: Prevention of HIV-2 and SIVsm infection by passive immunization in cynomolgus monkeys. Nature *352*:436–438, 1991.
221. Quinn, T. C., Kline, R. L., Halsey, N., et al.: Early diagnosis of perinatal HIV infection by detection of viral-specific IgA antibodies. J. A. M. A. *24*:3439–3442, 1991.
222. Rabin, R. L., Roederer, M., Maldonado, Y., et al.: Altered presentation of naive and memory CD8 T cell subsets in HIV-infected children. J. Clin. Invest. *95*:2054–2060, 1995.
223. Report of a consensus workshop. Siena, Italy, January 17–18, 1992: Early diagnosis of HIV infection in infants. J. Acquir. Immune Defic. Syndr. *5*:1169–1178, 1992.
224. Rey, L., Viciana, A., and Ruiz, P.: Immunopathological characteristics of in situ T-cell subpopulations in human immunodeficiency virus–associated nephropathy. Hum. Pathol. *26*:408–415, 1995.
225. Roederer, M., Dubs, J. G., Anderson, M. T., et al.: CD8 naive T cell counts decrease progressively in HIV-infected adults. J. Clin. Invest. *95*:2061–2066, 1995.
226. Rogers, M. F., Caldwell, M. B., Gwinn, M. L., et al.: Epidemiology of pediatric human immunodeficiency virus infection in the United States. Acta Paediatr. *400*:5–7, 1994.
227. Rogers, M. F., Ou, C. Y., Rayfield, M., et al.: Use of the polymerase chain reaction for early detection of the proviral sequences of human immunodeficiency virus in infants born to seropositive mothers. N. Engl. J. Med. *320*:1649–1654, 1989.
228. Rogers, M. F., Thomas, P. A., Starcher, E. T., et al.: Acquired immunodeficiency syndrome in children: Report of the Centers for Disease Control National Surveillance, 1982 to 1985. Pediatrics *79*:1008–1014, 1987.
229. Rogers, M. F., White, C. R., Sanders, R., et al.: Lack of transmission of human immunodeficiency virus from infected children to their household contacts. Pediatrics *85*:210–215, 1990.
230. Rusconi, S., Merrill, D. P., Hirsch, M. S., et al.: Inhibition of human immunodeficiency virus type 1 replication in cytokine-stimulated monocytes/macrophages by combination therapy. J. Infect. Dis. *170*:1361–1366, 1994.
231. Rutstein, R., Cobb, P., McGowan, K., et al.: *Mycobacterium avium-intracellulare* complex in HIV-infected children. A. I. D. S. *7*:507–512, 1993.
232. Ryder, R. W., Nsa, W., Hassig, S. E., et al.: Perinatal transmission of the human immunodeficiency virus type 1 to infants of seropositive women in Zaire. N. Engl. J. Med. *320*:1637–1642, 1989.
233. Scott, G. B., Fischl, M. A., Klimas, N., et al.: Mothers of infants with the acquired immunodeficiency syndrome: Evidence for both symptomatic and asymptomatic carriers. J. A. M. A. *253*:363–365, 1985.
234. Scott, G. B., Hutto, C., McKuch, R. W., et al.: Survival in children with perinatally acquired human immunodeficiency virus type 1 infection. N. Engl. J. Med. *321*:1791–1796, 1989.
235. Sei, S., Boler, A. M., Nguyen, G. T., et al.: Protective effect of CCR5 delta 32 heterozygosity is restricted by SDF-1 genotype in children with HIV-1 infection. A. I. D. S. *27*:1343–1352, 2002.
236. Selik, R. M., Chu, S., and Buehler, J. S.: HIV infection as leading cause of death among young adults in US cities and states. J. A. M. A. *269*:2991–2994, 1993.
237. Semba, R. D., Miotti, P. G., Chiphangwi, J. D., et al.: Maternal vitamin A deficiency and mother-to-child transmission of HIV-1. Lancet *343*:1593–1597, 1994.
238. Semprini, A. E., Vucetich, A., Pardi, G., et al.: HIV infection and AIDS in newborn babies of mothers positive for HIV antibody. B. M. J. *294*:610, 1987.
239. Shearer, W. T., Duliege, A. M., Kline, M. W., et al.: Transport of recombinant human CD4–immunoglobulin G across the human placenta: Pharmacokinetics and safety in six mother-infant pairs in AIDS clinical trial group protocol 146. Clin. Diagn. Lab. Immunol. *2*:281–285, 1995.
240. Shigita, S., Henuima, Y., Suto, T., et al.: The cell to cell infection of respiratory syncytial virus in HEp-2 monolayer cultures. J. Gen. Virol. *3*:129–131, 1968.
241. Simonds, R. J., and Chanock, S.: Medical issues related to caring for human immunodeficiency virus–infected children in and out of the home. Pediatr. Infect. Dis. J. *12*:845–852, 1993.
242. Simonds, R. J., Lindegren, M. L., Thomas, P., et al.: Prophylaxis against *Pneumocystis carinii* pneumonia among children with perinatally acquired human immunodeficiency virus infection in the United States. N. Engl. J. Med. *332*:786–790, 1995.
243. Sleasman, J. W., Hemenway, C., Klein, A. S., et al.: Corticosteroids improve survival of children with AIDS and *Pneumocystis carinii* pneumonia. Am. J. Dis. Child. *147*:30–34, 1993.
244. Smith, P. D., Ohura, K., Masur, H., et al.: Monocyte function in the acquired immunodeficiency syndrome: Defective chemotaxis. J. Clin. Invest. *74*:2121–2128, 1984.
245. Smith, R., Malee, K., Charurat, M., et al.: Timing of perinatal human immunodeficiency virus type 1 infection and rate of neurodevelopment. The Women and Infant Transmission Study Group. Pediatr. Infect. Dis. *19*:862–871, 2000.
246. Soeiro, R., Rubinstein, A., Rashburn, W. K., et al.: Maternofetal transmission of AIDS: Frequency of human immunodeficiency virus type 1 nucleic acid sequences in human fetal DNA. J. Infect. Dis. *166*:699–703, 1992.
247. Spector, S. A., Gelber, R. D., McGrath, N., et al.: A controlled trial of intravenous immune globulin for the prevention of serious bacterial infections in children receiving zidovudine for advanced human immunodeficiency virus infection. N. Engl. J. Med. *331*:1181–1187, 1994.

248. Sprecher, S., Soumenkoff, G., Pussant, F., et al.: Vertical transmission of HIV in 15-week fetus. Lancet *2*:288–289, 1986.
249. Starr, S. E., Fletcher, C. V., Spector, S. A., et al.: Combination therapy with efavirenz, nelfinavir, and nucleoside reverse-transcriptase inhibitors in children infected with human immunodeficiency virus type 1. N. Engl. J. Med. *341*:1874–1881, 1999.
250. State-of-the-art conference on azidothymidine therapy for early HIV infection. Am. J. Med. *89*:335–344, 1990.
251. Steinbrook, R.: Preventing HIV infection in children. N. Engl. J. Med. *346*:1842–1843, 2002.
252. Stellbrink, H. J., VanLunzen, J., Westby, M., et al.: Effects of interleukin-2 plus highly active antiretroviral therapy on HIV-1 replication and proviral DNA (COSMIC trial). A. I. D. S. *16*:1479–1487, 2002.
253. Stephenson, J.: Researchers explore new anti-HIV agents. J. A. M. A. *287*:1635–1637, 2002.
254. St. Louis, M. E., Kamenga, M., Brown, C., et al.: Risk of perinatal transmission according to maternal immunologic, virologic, and placental factors. J. A. M. A. *269*:2853–2859, 1993.
255. Stoneburner, R., Sato, P., Burton, A., et al.: The global HIV pandemic. Acta. Paediatr. *400*(Suppl.):1–4, 1994.
256. Strauss, J., Abitbol, C., Zilleruelo, G., et al.: Renal disease in children with the acquired immunodeficiency syndrome. N. Engl. J. Med. *321*:625–630, 1989.
257. Strauss, J., Zilleruelo, G., Abitbol, C., et al.: Human immunodeficiency virus nephropathy. Pediatr. Nephrol. *7*:220–225, 1993.
258. Sullivan, J. L., and Luzuriaga, K.: The changing face of pediatric HIV-1 infection. N. Engl. J. Med. *345*:1568–1569, 2001.
259. Tchekmedyian, N. S., Hickman, M., and Heber, D.: Treatment of anorexia and weight loss with megestrol acetate in patients with cancer or acquired immunodeficiency syndrome. Semin. Oncol. *18*:35–42, 1991.
260. The National Institute of Child Health and Human Development Intravenous Immunoglobulin Study Group: Intravenous immune globulin for the prevention of bacterial infections in children with symptomatic human immunodeficiency virus infection. N. Engl. J. Med. *325*:73–80, 1991.
261. The National Institutes of Health–University of California Expert Panel for Corticosteroids as Adjunctive Therapy for *Pneumocystis* Pneumonia: Consensus statement on the use of corticosteroids as adjunctive therapy for *Pneumocystis* pneumonia in the acquired immunodeficiency syndrome. N. Engl. J. Med. *323*:1500–1504, 1990.
262. The Working Group on Mother-to-Child Transmission of HIV: Rates of mother-to-child transmission of HIV-1 in Africa, America, and Europe: Results from 13 perinatal studies. J. Acquir. Immune Defic. Syndr. Hum. Retrovirol. *8*:506–510, 1995.
263. Thiry, L., Sprecher-Goldberger, S., Jonckheer, T., et al.: Isolation of AIDS virus from cell free breast milk of three healthy virus carriers. Lancet *2*:891–892, 1985.
264. Thomas, P. A., Weedon, J., Krasinski, K., et al.: Maternal predictors of perinatal human immunodeficiency virus transmission: The New York City Perinatal HIV Transmission Collaborative Study Group. Pediatr. Infect. Dis. J. *13*:489–495, 1994.
265. Tuomala, R. E., Shapiro, D. E., Mofenson, L. M., et al.: Antiretroviral therapy during pregnancy and the risk of an adverse outcome. N. Engl. J. Med. *346*:1863–1870, 2002.
266. Unger, M., Jimenez, E., Backe, E., et al.: Allantoic vasculopathy of the placenta in HIV-exposed pregnancies: Correlation to clinical findings. Abstract FB452. Presented at the Sixth International Conference on AIDS, June 1990, San Francisco, p. 191.
267. VanDyke, R. B., Lee, S., Johnson, G. M., et al.: Reported adherence as a determinant of response to highly active antiretroviral therapy in children who have human immunodeficiency virus infection. Pediatrics *109*:e61, 2002.
268. VanRompay, K. K., Otsyula, M. G., Marthas, M. L., et al.: Immediate zidovudine treatment protects simian immunodeficiency virus–infected newborn macaques against rapid onset of AIDS. Antimicrob. Agents Chemother. *39*:125–131, 1995.
269. Vigano, A., Principi, N., Villa, M. L., et al.: Immunologic characterization of children vertically infected with human immunodeficiency virus, with slow or rapid disease progression. J. Pediatr. *126*:368–374, 1995.
270. Vivani, B., Corsini, E., Binaglia, M., et al.: Reactive oxygen species generated by glia are responsible for neuron death induced by human immunodeficiency virus–glycoprotein 120 in vitro. Neuroscience *107*:51–58, 2001.
271. Volberding, P. A., Lagakos, S. W., Grimes, J. M., et al.: A comparison of immediate with deferred zidovudine therapy for asymptomatic HIV-infected adults with CD4 cell counts of 500 or more per cubic millimeter: AIDS Clinical Trials Group. N. Engl. J. Med. *333*:401–407, 1995.
272. Waldmann, T. A.: Immunodeficiency diseases: Primary and acquired. *In* Samter, M., Talmage, D. W., Frank, M. M., et al. (eds.): Immunological Diseases. 4th ed. Boston, Little, Brown, 1988, pp. 411–465.
273. Watts, D. H.: Management of human immunodeficiency virus infection in pregnancy. N. Engl. J. Med. *346*:1879–1891, 2002.
274. Wei, X., Sajal, K. G., Taylor, M. E., et al.: Viral dynamics in human immunodeficiency virus type 1 infection. Nature *373*:117–122, 1995.
275. Wheat, L. J., Salma, T. G., and Zechkel, M. L.: Histoplasmosis in the acquired immune deficiency syndrome. Am. J. Med. *78*:203–210, 1985.
276. Wilfert, C. M., Wilson, C., Luzuriaga, K., et al.: Pathogenesis of pediatric human immunodeficiency virus type 1 infection. J. Infect. Dis. *170*:286–292, 1994.
277. Wofsy, C. B., Cohen, J. B., Hauer, L. B., et al.: Isolation of AIDS-associated retrovirus from genital secretions of women with antibodies to the virus. Lancet *1*:527–529, 1986.
278. Wolinsky, S. M., Wike, C. M., Korber, B. T., et al.: Selective transmission of human immunodeficiency virus type 1 variants from mothers to infants. Science *5048*:1134–1137, 1992.
279. WHO Report: More than 36 million worldwide have HIV/AIDS. AIDS Policy Law *1*:10, 2001.

SECTION XVIII

Chlamydia

CHAPTER 194

Chlamydia Infections

MARGARET R. HAMMERSCHLAG

Chlamydiae are obligate intracellular pathogens that have established a unique niche within the host cell. They cause a variety of diseases in animal species at virtually all phylogenic levels. Traditionally, the order has contained one genus with four recognized species: *Chlamydia trachomatis, Chlamydia psittaci, Chlamydia pneumoniae*, and *Chlamydia pecorum*.[37, 44, 54] *C. trachomatis* and *C. pneumoniae* are the most significant human pathogens, and *C. psittaci* is an important zoonosis. Recent taxonomic analysis involving the 16S and 23S rRNA genes have found that the order Chlamydiales contains at least four distinct groups at the family level and that within the order Chlamydiaceae are two distinct lineages.[37] This analysis has suggested splitting the genus *Chlamydia* into two genera, *Chlamydia* and *Chlamydophila*. Two new species, *Chlamydia muridarum* (formerly the agent of mouse pneumonitis—MoPn) and *Chlamydia suis,* would join *C. trachomatis*. *Chlamydophila* would contain *C. pecorum, C. pneumoniae,* and *C. psittaci,* and three new species split off from *C. psittaci*: *C. abortus*, *C. caviae* (formerly *C. psittaci* Guinea pig conjunctivitis strain), and *C. felis.* Controversy regarding this reclassification is continuing, but for the purposes of this chapter, we will continue to refer to these organisms as *Chlamydia*.

Chlamydiae are characterized by a unique developmental cycle with morphologically distinct infectious and reproductive forms: the elementary body (EB) and reticulate body (RB). They have a gram-negative envelope without detectable peptidoglycan, although recent genomic analysis has revealed that both *C. trachomatis* and *C. pneumoniae* encode for proteins forming a nearly complete pathway for the synthesis of peptidoglycan, including penicillin-binding proteins.[96, 141] This finding is the basis for the so-called chlamydial peptidoglycan paradox, given that it has been known for decades that chlamydial development is sensitive to β-lactam antibiotics. Chlamydiae also share a group-specific lipopolysaccharide (LPS) antigen and utilize host adenosine triphosphate (ATP) for the synthesis of chlamydial protein.[120] Although chlamydiae are auxotrophic for three of four nucleoside triphosphates, they do encode functional glucose-catabolizing enzymes that can be used for the generation of ATP. As with peptidoglycan synthesis, for some reason these genes are turned off.[141] All chlamydiae also encode an abundant protein, the major outer membrane protein (MOMP or OmpA), that is surface exposed in *C. trachomatis* and *C. psittaci* but apparently not in *C. pneumoniae*.[141] MOMP is the major determinant of the serologic classification of *C. trachomatis* and *C. psittaci* isolates.

After infection, the infectious EBs, which are 200 to 400 μm in diameter, attach to the host cell by a process of electrostatic binding and are taken into the cell by endocytosis that does not depend on the microtubule system. Within the host cell, the EB remains within a membrane-lined phagosome. The phagosome does not fuse with the host cell lysosome. The inclusion membrane is devoid of host cell markers, but lipid markers traffic to the inclusion, which suggests functional interaction with the Golgi apparatus. The EBs then differentiate into RBs that undergo binary fission. After approximately 36 hours, RBs differentiate into EBs. At about 48 hours, release may occur by cytolysis or by a process of exocytosis or extrusion of the whole inclusion, with the host cell left intact. Chlamydiae also may enter a persistent state after treatment with certain cytokines such as interferon gamma, treatment with antibiotics, or restriction of certain nutrients. While in the persistent state, metabolic activity is reduced. The ability to cause prolonged, often subclinical infection is one of the major characteristics of chlamydiae.

Infection Caused by *Chlamydia trachomatis*

EPIDEMIOLOGY

C. trachomatis infection is the most prevalent sexually transmitted infection and infectious disease in the United States today.[56, 57] The Centers for Disease Control and Prevention (CDC) estimates that the number of new *C. trachomatis* infections exceeds 4 million annually.[56] The prevalence of chlamydial infection is more weakly associated with socioeconomic status, urban or rural residence, and race or ethnicity than is the case with gonorrhea and syphilis. The prevalence of *C. trachomatis* infection is consistently higher than 5 percent among sexually active adolescent and young adult women attending outpatient clinics, regardless of the region of the country, location of the clinic (urban or rural), and the race or ethnicity of the population.[45] In sexually active adolescents, the prevalence commonly exceeds 10 percent and may exceed 20 percent.[45] Decreasing age at first intercourse and increasing age at marriage have contributed importantly to the higher prevalence of infection with *C. trachomatis*. Infection with *C. trachomatis* tends to be asymptomatic and of long duration. If a pregnant woman has active infection during delivery, the infant may acquire the infection and, as a consequence, either conjunctivitis or pneumonia. Rarely, children also may acquire chlamydial infection as a result of sexual abuse.

TABLE 194–1 ■ SELECTED STUDIES OF PERINATAL CHLAMYDIAL INFECTION

	Prevalence of Maternal Genital Infection		Proportion of Infants with Chlamydial Infection Born to Infected Mothers				
Author, Year, City	*Total*	*No. Infected (%)*	*Total*	*Conjunctivitis*	*Pneumonia*	*NP*	*Rectum/Vagina*
Frommell et al., 1979, Denver[42]	340	30 (8.8)	67	39%	11%	6%	NS
Schachter et al., 1986, San Francisco[147]	5531	262 (4.7)	131	17.6%	16%	11.5%	14%
Hammerschlag et al., 1989, Brooklyn[66]	4357	341 (7.8)	45	15%	1%	4%	NS

NP, nasopharynx; NS, not studied.

INFECTIONS IN INFANTS

Neonatal conjunctivitis and pneumonia can develop in infants born to mothers with *C. trachomatis* cervical infection. Epidemiologic evidence strongly suggests that the infant acquires chlamydial infection from the mother during vaginal delivery[42, 59, 64, 147] (Table 194–1). Infection after cesarean section occurs rarely, usually after early rupture of the amniotic membrane.[8] No evidence supports postnatal acquisition from the mother or other family members. Approximately 50 to 75 percent of infants born to infected women become infected at one or more anatomic sites, including the conjunctiva, nasopharynx, rectum, and vagina. However, the epidemiology of perinatal *C. trachomatis* infection has changed during the past decade. The introduction of highly sensitive and specific nucleic acid amplification tests (NAATs) for detection of *C. trachomatis,* coupled with systematic screening and treatment of chlamydial infection in pregnant women, has resulted in a marked decrease in perinatally acquired *C. trachomatis* infection.[68]

Inclusion Conjunctivitis

C. trachomatis is the most frequent identifiable infectious cause of neonatal conjunctivitis and the major clinical manifestations of neonatal chlamydial infection. Conjunctivitis develops in approximately 30 to 50 percent of infants born to *Chlamydia*-positive mothers.[42, 59, 64, 147] Studies in the 1980s identified *C. trachomatis* in 14 to 46 percent of infants younger than 1 month of age with conjunctivitis.[72, 73, 135, 140] As stated earlier, chlamydial ophthalmia appears to occur much less frequently now as a result of systematic screening and treatment of pregnant women. The incubation period is 5 to 14 days after delivery or earlier if membranes have ruptured prematurely. At least 50 percent of infants with chlamydial conjunctivitis also have nasopharyngeal infection.[6, 64] The clinical findings vary widely and range from mild conjunctival injection with scant mucoid discharge to severe conjunctivitis with copious purulent discharge, chemosis, and pseudomembrane formation. The conjunctiva can be friable and may bleed when stroked with a swab. Chlamydial conjunctivitis needs to be differentiated from gonococcal ophthalmia in some infants, especially those born to mothers who did not receive any prenatal care, had gonorrhea during pregnancy, or abused drugs. Overlap in both incubation period and clinical expression is possible.

Pneumonia

The nasopharynx is the most frequent site of perinatally acquired chlamydial infection,[60, 64] with approximately 70 percent of infected infants having positive cultures at that site. Most of these nasopharyngeal infections are asymptomatic and may persist for 3 years or more.[9, 88, 147] Chlamydial pneumonia develops in only about 30 percent of infants with nasopharyngeal infection. In those in whom pneumonia does develop, the manifestations and clinical findings are characteristic.[6, 77] *C. trachomatis* pneumonia is usually apparent in infected infants between 4 and 12 weeks of age. A few cases have been reported as early as 2 weeks of age, but no cases have been noted to occur beyond the age of 4 months. Infected infants frequently have a history of cough and congestion with an absence of fever. On physical examination, the infant is tachypneic, and rales are heard on auscultation of the chest; wheezing is a distinctly uncommon occurrence. The only specific radiographic finding is hyperinflation.[6, 77] A review of the chest films of 125 infants with chlamydial pneumonia revealed bilateral hyperinflation; diffuse infiltrates with a variety of radiographic patterns, including interstitial and reticulonodular; atelectasis; and bronchopneumonia.[134] Lobar consolidation and pleural effusions were not seen. Significant laboratory findings include peripheral eosinophilia (>300 cells/cm^3) and elevated serum immunoglobulin levels.[6, 77]

C. trachomatis is rarely isolated from the lungs of infants with chlamydial pneumonia, which led some researchers to suggest that an immune mechanism is involved in its pathogenesis.[41] Histopathologic studies have not revealed any characteristic features. Biopsy material has shown pleural congestion and near-total alveolar and partial bronchiolar mononuclear consolidation with occasional eosinophils, granular pneumocytes, and focal aggregations of neutrophils. In addition, necrotic change in the bronchioles is marked.[41] Follow-up studies have suggested that infantile chlamydial pneumonia may be associated with pulmonary function test abnormalities and respiratory tract symptoms 7 to 8 years after recovery from the acute illness.[45]

Infections at Other Sites

Infants born to *Chlamydia*-positive mothers also may become infected in the rectum and vagina.[147] Although infection at these sites appears to be totally asymptomatic, the infection may cause confusion if detected later. Schachter and associates[147] reported finding subclinical rectal and vaginal infection in 14 percent of infants born to *Chlamydia*-positive women; some of these infants remained culture-positive at 18 months of age. Bell and colleagues[9] monitored 22 infants born to women with culture-proven chlamydial infections and found that positive cultures were detected in these children as late as 28.5 months after birth. The longest duration of perinatally acquired infection occurred in the nasopharynx or oropharynx, 28.5 months as just mentioned. Nine infants had rectal or vaginal infections that persisted for slightly more than 12 months.

INFECTIONS IN OLDER CHILDREN

C. trachomatis has not been associated with any specific clinical syndrome in older infants and children. Most attention to *C. trachomatis* infection in these children has concentrated on its relationship to sexual abuse. Isolation of *C. trachomatis* from a rectal or genital site in children without previous sexual activity may be a marker of sexual abuse; moreover, evidence for other modes of spread, such as through fomites, is lacking for this organism. As previously mentioned, perinatal maternal-to-infant transmission resulting in vaginal or rectal infection has been documented, with prolonged infection lasting for periods of up to 3 years.[9, 147] It is an important confounding variable.

Vaginal infection with *C. trachomatis* was reported uncommonly in prepubertal children before 1980. The possibility of sexual contact frequently was not even discussed. In 1981, Rettig and Nelson[137] reported concurrent or subsequent chlamydial infection in 9 of 33 (27%) episodes of gonorrhea in a group of prepubertal children. However, *C. trachomatis* was not found in any of 31 children with urethritis or vaginitis that was not gonococcal. No information was given about possible sexual activity.

Most studies have identified rectogenital chlamydial infection in 2 to 3 percent of sexually abused children when these children underwent routine culture for the organism. Most of those with chlamydial infection were asymptomatic. In two early studies that had control groups, similar percentages of control patients also were infected.[67, 89] A larger study subsequently conducted by Ingram and colleagues[90] found a stronger association between vaginal chlamydial infection and a history of sexual abuse, but not with pharyngeal infection, which was found in a similar number of controls. Rectal infection was detected in only 1 of 124 abused children.

In the setting of repeated abuse by a family member over the course of a long time, the development of infection would be difficult to demonstrate. The 2001 Guidelines for the Treatment of Sexually Transmitted Diseases from the CDC does not recommend that samples for culture of *C. trachomatis* be routinely obtained from the pharynx and urethra in children who are suspected victims of sexual abuse.[57] The major reasons were the low yield from the urethra, the tendency for longer persistence of perinatally acquired pharyngeal infection, and the potential confusion with *C. pneumoniae.*[5]

Although asymptomatic, perinatally acquired nasopharyngeal infection with *C. trachomatis* may persist for at least 2 years, respiratory tract infection in older children and adults appears to be a distinctly uncommon occurrence, the reasons for which are not clear. Studies of the interaction of *C. trachomatis* and alveolar macrophages from normal healthy adults have demonstrated that these cells efficiently kill *C. trachomatis.*[121] *C. trachomatis* has been isolated from the pharynx of some adults, which is apparently related to certain sexual practices. These infections have been asymptomatic. Two earlier studies based entirely on serology suggested that *C. trachomatis* might be a cause of pharyngitis and community-acquired pneumonia in adults.[99, 100] Subsequent studies using culture methods did not confirm this theory.[49, 85] Possibly, the original studies actually detected cross-reacting antibody to *C. pneumoniae.*

C. trachomatis can cause pneumonia in older children or adults in two specific situations. One is in immunosuppressed persons. Several well-documented cases of *C. trachomatis* pneumonia in persons with leukemia, bone marrow transplant recipients, and those with acquired immunodeficiency syndrome (AIDS) have been reported.[46, 92, 111, 114] In all these cases, *C. trachomatis* was isolated from biopsy specimens of lung tissue or bronchoalveolar lavage fluid. Several patients also had a serologic response that was diagnostic of acute *C. trachomatis* infection. Unfortunately, no clinical findings were characteristic. These adults had none of the features that are distinctive of infantile chlamydial pneumonia.

Several cases of pulmonary infection after exposure to *C. trachomatis* serovars L_1 and L_2 in the laboratory also have been reported.[10] The infections were probably acquired by inhalation of aerosolized organisms. Clinically, these patients had high fever, night sweats, and cough and were found to have mediastinal lymphadenopathy, pneumonitis, or splenomegaly alone or in any combination. In two cases, the diagnosis of lymphoma was seriously considered. These findings are not unexpected given the severity of lymphogranuloma venereum genital infection. Accidental exposure to the aerosolized trachoma biovar of *C. trachomatis* has not been associated with the development of significant illness.

DIAGNOSIS OF *C. TRACHOMATIS* INFECTIONS

The "gold standard" of diagnosis remains isolation by culture of *C. trachomatis* from the conjunctiva, nasopharynx, vagina, or rectum. *Chlamydia* culture has been defined further by the CDC as isolation of the organism in tissue culture and confirmation by microscopic identification of the characteristic inclusions by fluorescent antibody staining.[56, 57] Several nonculture methods have been approved by the Food and Drug Administration (FDA) for the diagnosis of chlamydial conjunctivitis, including enzyme immunoassays (EIAs), specifically, Chlamydiazyme (Abbott Diagnostics, Chicago) and MicroTrak EIA (Genetic Systems, Seattle), and direct fluorescent antibody tests, including Syva MicroTrak (Genetic Systems) and Pathfinder (Sanofi-Pasteur, Chaska, MN). These tests appear to perform well on conjunctival specimens, with 90 percent or greater sensitivity and 95 percent or greater specificity in comparison to culture.[72, 73, 135, 140] Unfortunately, their performance with nasopharyngeal specimens has not been as good, with sensitivity ranging from 33 to more than 90 percent.[72, 73, 125, 140] The commercially available DNA probe Pace II (Gen-Probe, San Diego, CA, has FDA approval only for cervical and urethral sites in adults, in whom its performance has been similar to that of most of the approved EIAs available. It does not have approval for any site in children.

A major advance in the diagnosis of *C. trachomatis* infection during the past decade has been the introduction of NAATs. These tests have high sensitivity, perhaps even detecting 10 to 20 percent more cases than possible with culture, while retaining high specificity.[11] Currently, three commercially available NAATs are FDA approved: polymerase chain reaction (PCR) (Amplicor [Roche Molecular Diagnostics, Nutley, NJ]),* transcription-mediated amplification (TMA) (GenProbe), and strand displacement amplification (SDA) (ProbeTec, Becton Dickson, Sparks, MD). PCR and SDA are DNA amplification tests; both use primers that target gene sequences on the cryptogenic *C. trachomatis* plasmid, which has approximately 10 copies per cell. TMA is an RNA amplification assay. NAATs that are currently commercially available have FDA approval for cervical swabs from women, urethral swabs from men, and urine from men and women. Information on the use of NAATs in children is limited, but preliminary data suggest that PCR is equivalent to culture for the detection of *C. trachomatis* in the conjunctiva and nasopharynx of infants with conjunctivitis.[74] The use of noninvasive specimens such as urine is especially helpful in high-prevalence populations such as sexually active adolescents.[45, 56]

Nonculture tests should never be used for rectal or vaginal sites in children or for any forensic purposes in adolescents or adults.[56, 57] Only culture should be used; isolation of the organism in tissue culture should be confirmed by microscopic identification of the inclusions by staining with a fluorescein-conjugated, *C. trachomatis* spp.–specific monoclonal antibody. EIAs are not acceptable for confirmation of culture results, and their use has led to false-positive reports.[62, 132] Isolates of *C. trachomatis* also should be preserved. The use of nonculture tests for detection of *C. trachomatis* in vaginal and rectal specimens has been associated with a large number of false-positive results.[62, 132] Fecal material can give false-positive reactions with any EIA; none is approved for this site in adults. Common bowel organisms, including *Escherichia coli, Proteus* spp., vaginal organisms such as group B *Streptococcus* and *Gardnerella vaginalis,* and even some respiratory tract flora such as group A *Streptococcus,* can also give positive reactions with EIAs.[132] These types of tests are best for screening for genital infection in adolescents and adults in high-prevalence populations (prevalence of infection >7%).[11] Because all of the available EIAs use genus-specific antibodies, if performed on respiratory tract specimens, these tests will detect *C. pneumoniae* as well.[5] NAATs also are not approved for the detection of *C. trachomatis* in rectogenital specimens from prepubertal children and rectal specimens in adults. The major problem with rectal specimens is the presence of inhibitors of DNA polymerase, which can lead to false-negative results. Data on the use of NAATs for vaginal specimens or urine from children are very limited and insufficient to allow recommendation of their use.[34, 50, 107] The CDC recommended that NAATs be used as an alternative to culture *only* if confirmation is available.[56, 57] Confirmation tests should consist of a second FDA-approved NAAT that targets a gene sequence different from the one used in the initial test.

PREVENTION AND CONTROL

Because *C. trachomatis* infections are transmitted vertically from mother to infant during delivery, several options are possible for intervention. One of the first to be considered was neonatal ocular prophylaxis. The general assumption, based on the results of prospective studies of mother-to-infant transmission of *C. trachomatis*, has been that neonatal ocular prophylaxis with silver nitrate does not prevent the development of chlamydial conjunctivitis. Because erythromycin and tetracycline ophthalmic ointments also were approved and used for ocular prophylaxis, physicians suggested that they also might be effective for prevention of chlamydial conjunctivitis.

In 1980, Hammerschlag and associates[63] in Seattle found that of 60 infants born to *Chlamydia*-positive women, chlamydial conjunctivitis did not develop in the 24 who received erythromycin but did develop in 33 percent (12 of 36) of those who received silver nitrate drops. No effect on the incidence of nasopharyngeal infection or the later development of chlamydial pneumonia was found. Subsequent studies have not confirmed this observation.[7, 23, 66, 91] In 1989, Hammerschlag and associates[66] compared silver nitrate, erythromycin, and tetracycline as neonatal ocular prophylaxis in a large urban hospital in Brooklyn. The prophylaxis preparations were given within 30 minutes of birth. Chlamydial conjunctivitis developed in 20 percent of infants (15 of 76) born to infected mothers who received silver nitrate drops, in 14 percent (13 of 92) of those who received erythromycin, and in 11 percent (7 of 62) of those who received tetracycline. The incidence of nasopharyngeal infection and pneumonia was not affected. A subsequent study from Taiwan compared silver nitrate, the two antibiotics, and no prophylaxis.[23] However, this study, in contrast to previous studies, did not specifically monitor infants born to women with culture-documented chlamydial infection, but included all infants delivered during the period of the study, for 4 weeks or when conjunctivitis developed. Again, no difference was found in the incidence of neonatal chlamydial conjunctivitis among the four groups. The incidence of chlamydial conjunctivitis in the tetracycline, erythromycin, silver nitrate, and no-prophylaxis groups was 1.3, 1.5, 1.7, and 1.6 percent, respectively. *C. trachomatis* was diagnosed by a direct fluorescent antibody test rather than by culture. No data were given regarding the prevalence of maternal infection with *C. trachomatis* or *Neisseria gonorrhoeae*. Respiratory tract infection was not assessed.

Povidone-iodine also has been suggested as an agent for neonatal ocular prophylaxis because it has a broad antibacterial spectrum in vitro; it is also antiviral and inexpensive in comparison to other prophylaxis agents. Data on its use and efficacy are very limited, however. In one study from Kenya, povidone-iodine appeared to result in a 50 percent reduction in the number of cases of *C. trachomatis* conjunctivitis when compared with silver nitrate (5.5% versus 10.5% of infants) and an approximately 30 percent reduction when compared with erythromycin (7.4%).[91] No difference was noted in the proportions of infants in whom gonococcal ophthalmia developed. The pregnant women enrolled were not screened for *C. trachomatis* prenatally, and chlamydial conjunctivitis in the infants was diagnosed by a direct fluorescent antibody test. Mothers were told to bring the infants back if conjunctivitis developed. Because of the structure of the study, one cannot be sure whether every infant with conjunctivitis returned to the clinic. Because the prevalence of chlamydial infection in the pregnant women in the population was unknown, the investigators did not know how many cases of chlamydial ophthalmia to expect. Directing neonatal ocular prophylaxis primarily toward preventing gonococcal ophthalmia would appear to be prudent because it is the agent that poses the greatest risk of eye injury. However, silver nitrate is no longer manufactured in the United States.

The most effective method of controlling perinatal chlamydial infection appears to be screening and treatment of pregnant women. The CDC currently recommends either erythromycin base or amoxicillin as the first-line regimen for treating *C. trachomatis* infection in pregnant women.[29, 57] Single-dose azithromycin is listed as an alternative regimen with the caveat that data on its use are insufficient to recommend the routine use of azithromycin in pregnant women.[57] However, clinical experience and preliminary data suggest that azithromycin is safe and effective.[112] Reasons for failure of maternal treatment to prevent infantile chlamydial infection include poor compliance and reinfection from an untreated sexual partner. Even with effective screening, some infected women will be missed, depending on the diagnostic methods used. In addition, some women do not seek prenatal care.

TREATMENT

Oral erythromycin suspension (ethylsuccinate or stearate) (50 mg/kg/day for 14 days) is the therapy of choice for the treatment of chlamydial conjunctivitis and pneumonia in infants.[57] It provides better and faster resolution of the conjunctivitis, and it treats any concurrent nasopharyngeal infection, which prevents the development of pneumonia. Administration of additional topical therapy is not needed. The efficacy of this regimen has been reported to range from

80 to 90 percent; thus, as many as 20 percent of infants may require another course of therapy.[64, 81, 126, 135] Erythromycin at the same dose for 2 to 3 weeks is the treatment of choice for pneumonia, and it does result in clinical improvement as well as elimination of the organism from the respiratory tract. An association between treatment with oral erythromycin and infantile hypertrophic pyloric stenosis has been reported in infants younger than 6 weeks who were given the drug for prophylaxis after nursery exposure to pertussis.[57] Data on the use of other macrolides (azithromycin or clarithromycin) for the treatment of neonatal chlamydial infection are limited. The results of one small study suggest that a short course of azithromycin, 20 mg/kg/day orally, one dose daily for 3 days, may be effective.[68]

Chlamydial infections in older children may be treated with oral erythromycin (50 mg/kg/day four times a day orally to a maximum of 2 g/day for 7 to 14 days). Children older than 8 years may be treated with tetracycline (25 to 50 mg/kg/day four times a day orally for 7 days). Azithromycin, 1 g orally as a single dose, also may be used in children who weigh at least 45 kg, are 8 years of age or older, or both.

Infection Caused by *Chlamydia psittaci*

Human infection with *C. psittaci* was described first probably by Juergensen in 1874 or Ritter in 1876. Ritter described seven cases of an unusual pneumonia that appeared to be caused by parrots and finches that were caged in the study of his brother's home in Switzerland. After these reports, several outbreaks of a similar disease in Europe established the association with exposure to birds. The term *psittacosis* was coined by Morange in 1892 from the Greek word for parrots, *psittakos*.[2]

THE ORGANISM

C. psittaci is a diverse species that affects nonpsittacine birds and many mammalian species as well. The known host range includes 15 mammalian species and 130 avian species representing 10 orders.[2] *C. psittaci* also can be differentiated from *C. trachomatis* by a lack of glycogen in the inclusions, the morphologic features of the inclusions, and resistance to sulfonamides.[2]

The diversity of *C. psittaci* is probably a reflection of its wide host range; indeed, recent genomic analysis has suggested reorganizing the organism into four separate species in a new genus, *Chlamydophila*.[37] Strains of *C. psittaci* have been analyzed by patterns of pathogenicity, inclusion morphology in tissue culture, DNA restriction endonuclease analysis, and monoclonal antibodies, which indicate that nine mammalian serovars, seven avian serovars, and two koala biovars exist.[2, 82, 156] Mammalian strains differ greatly from avian strains in their antigenic characteristics. Two of the avian serovars, psittacine and turkey, are of major importance in the avian population of the United States. Each is associated with important host preferences and disease characteristics.

All strains of the turkey serovar have been associated with serious disease in either birds or human beings, with major epizootics in turkeys often resulting in disease in humans. The psittacine serovar also has been associated with serious disease in humans; however, human involvement usually is limited to sporadic cases after exposure to pet birds or pigeons. The pathogenicity of each *C. psittaci* strain for humans is unknown.

EPIDEMIOLOGY

According to the most recent report from the CDC, 85 percent of cases of psittacosis in the United States were associated with exposure to birds; 70 percent of these reported cases were the result of exposure to caged pet birds.[27] Individuals at highest risk of acquiring psittacosis included bird owners or fanciers and pet shop employees. Since 1984, several major outbreaks of psittacosis have occurred in the United States in turkey-processing plants, where approximately 300 persons were infected.[80, 133] Workers exposed to turkey viscera were at the highest risk of acquiring infection.[80] In 1995, the CDC investigated an outbreak of avian chlamydiosis in a shipment of more than 700 pet birds from a Florida bird distributor to the Atlanta area.[117] Affected birds included parrots, parakeets, finches, lovebirds, cockatiels, conures, and canaries. Clinical psittacosis or serologic evidence of *C. psittaci* infection was found in 30.7 percent of households with birds from the infected flock. An average of 21 days (range, 1 to 47) elapsed between purchase of the bird and the onset of symptoms. Most of the infected individuals had mild or asymptomatic illnesses. Among persons in exposed households, illness occurred more frequently if the recently purchased bird had become sick or had died. Kissing or nuzzling, handling, and feeding the bird were all significantly associated with the development of clinical psittacosis, but in contrast to earlier studies, cleaning the bird's cage was not. The risk for clinical psittacosis varied significantly by type of bird to which the individual was exposed. The attack rate was highest for individuals exposed to parrots.

Inhalation of infectious aerosols derived from the feces, fecal dust, or secretions of *C. psittaci*–infected animals is believed to be the primary route of infection. The source birds can be infected asymptomatically or can show signs of infection such as anorexia, ruffled feathers, depression, and watery green droppings. Psittacosis is frequently a systemic infection in birds, and the turkey strains can induce severe pericarditis. The gastrointestinal tract also is infected frequently. The psittacine serovar appears to be much less virulent in both turkeys and pigeons than in psittacine birds.[2]

Psittacosis is an uncommon occurrence in children. In a series of 135 cases from Australia observed during a 15-year period, the youngest patient was 17 years of age.[164] Children may be less likely to be exposed to birds. Bird keeping is more commonly a hobby of adults, and the parents are the ones who usually clean the cage of the family's pet bird. An outbreak of psittacosis involving two adolescents was reported from a small village in Scotland. The source of the infection appeared to be the local pet shop, which had taken delivery of four lovebirds, two of which died shortly after arrival.[118] Another report describes a family outbreak during which three members of a family of nine persons contracted severe pneumonia.[17] A newly purchased cockatiel appeared to be the primary source, but person-to-person transmission was likely between 19-year-old twin brothers who shared a bedroom, one of whom had no direct contact with the bird. A retrospective review of the records of the Public Health Laboratory at Leeds, England, for cases with a fourfold rise in *Chlamydia* complement-fixation (CF) titer identified 219 patients during a 24-year period from 1965 to 1989.[30] The ages ranged from 9 months to 87 years; only 5 (2.2%) of the patients were younger than 10 years, but on review, only 34 of the total cases were thought to be psittacosis. All involved antecedent avian exposure, but the ages were not specified.

CLINICAL MANIFESTATIONS

Infection with *C. psittaci* in humans may range from clinically inapparent to severe infection involving multiple organ systems, as well as pneumonia. The mean incubation period is 15 days after exposure (range, 5 to 21 days). The onset is usually abrupt, with complaints of fever, cough, and headache. The fever is high and frequently associated with rigors and sweats. The headache can be so severe that meningitis can be considered a possibility; 33 percent of patients in the Australian series underwent lumbar puncture.[164] The cough is usually nonproductive, and rales may be heard on auscultation. Chest radiographs are generally abnormal, with variable infiltrates. Pleural effusions also may be present. In contrast, most of the individuals in the Atlanta outbreak had very mild disease characterized by fever, headache, and cough.[117]

LABORATORY FINDINGS

The white blood cell count usually is not elevated, but mild leukocytosis may be present. Almost 50 percent of patients in the Australian series had abnormal liver function test results, including elevated levels of aspartate aminotransferase, alkaline phosphatase, and bilirubin.[164]

DIAGNOSIS

Because of the varying clinical findings, making the diagnosis of psittacosis can be difficult. A history of exposure to birds is important, although as many as 20 percent of patients with psittacosis may not have a history of such contact.[159] In the Australian series, 85 percent of patients had a history of recent bird contact, 71 percent of whom described a strong bird contact history.[164] Only five patients had been exposed to poultry. Pneumonia caused by *C. pneumoniae* also can have similar clinical findings.[129, 130] Data from both Sweden and Denmark have suggested that many cases of "psittacosis" caused by *C. pneumoniae* with no history of exposure to birds probably have occurred, and the diagnosis has been established serologically with CF.[43, 116] An outbreak of suspected psittacosis in a boys' boarding school in England was reported in 1984.[129] The outbreak involved 20 children 13 to 18 years of age and 4 adults. The illness was mild and characterized by pharyngitis and flulike symptoms, including headache, fever, and cough. The diagnosis was made on the basis of serology (CF titers). No avian source was identified. Because the cases occurred during a 3-month period, person-to-person spread was suggested. Subsequent analysis of the sera suggested that the outbreak was caused by *C. pneumoniae.*[130] Person-to-person spread rarely occurs in psittacosis; secondary cases tend to be severe, however.

Other infections that can produce the syndrome of pneumonia with high fever, unusually severe headache, and myalgia include *Mycoplasma pneumoniae* infection, tularemia, tuberculosis, fungal infection, legionnaires' disease, and various bacterial infections. The diagnosis of psittacosis in the human population is based primarily on clinical findings, epidemiology, and serology.

The diagnosis of human infection with *C. psittaci* has not changed substantially for many years. The mainstay of diagnosis remains serology with the CF test. According to the 2000 recommendations from the CDC,[27] a confirmed case of psittacosis requires a compatible clinical illness, usually with a good history of avian exposure. Laboratory confirmation can be made by one of the three following methods: (1) culture of *C. psittaci* from respiratory secretions, (2) fourfold or greater increase in CF or microimmunofluorescence (MIF) titer in sera collected at least 2 weeks apart, and (3) an MIF IgM titer of 16 or greater. A probable case should be epidemiologically linked to a confirmed case or have a single CF or MIF antibody titer of 32 or higher in a least one serum sample obtained after the onset of symptoms. As with use of the MIF for the diagnosis of *C. pneumoniae* infection, cross-reactions with other *Chlamydia* spp. and bacteria can occur.[119] Recently, a cross-reaction with *Legionella longbeachae* was described in a patient with fulminant pneumonia caused by *C. psittaci.*[150]

Although *C. psittaci* will grow in the same culture systems used for the isolation of *C. trachomatis* and *C. pneumoniae,* very few laboratories culture for *C. psittaci,* mainly because of the potential biohazard.

CF is a genus-specific test; thus, infection caused by *C. pneumoniae* can give titers of 32 or higher. Early treatment with tetracycline also may suppress the antibody response. Even though many laboratories can isolate *C. psittaci,* it is not a service provided routinely by most clinical microbiology laboratories. The CDC reported using a modification of the MIF test for the serodiagnosis of human psittacosis.[160] In the 78 patients examined, psittacosis was diagnosed on the basis of compatible clinical symptoms after exposure to sick birds. Conventional CF was positive in 36 (46%) of the patients. The MIF test detected diagnostic antibody responses in all the CF-positive patients and in another 12 patients whose sera were negative or anticomplementary according to CF. Seven other patients were thought to have *C. pneumoniae* infection because of their MIF antibody response.

Several reports also have examined the use of nonculture methods, including direct fluorescent antibody, EIA, and PCR, for the direct identification of *C. psittaci* in clinical specimens. Several in-house PCR assays for detection of *C. psittaci* have been reported in the literature.[105, 109, 124, 154] Several of these assays have a multiplex format intended to detect *C. pneumoniae, C. trachomatis,* and *C. psittaci* in a single sample.[105, 109, 154] Most reported studies have assessed only the ability of these assays to amplify laboratory isolates; they have not been evaluated extensively for detection of *C. psittaci* in clinical specimens from humans with suspected psittacosis. Only a small number of human cases of psittacosis documented by PCR have been reported in the literature.[109, 124] In 1997, the CDC reported one of the most extensive evaluations of the use of PCR in the investigation of a psittacosis outbreak.[109] Most of the specimens tested were from birds. The target sequence of the assay was the 16S rRNA gene. The first amplification was genus-specific, and the second was multiplexed and could differentiate among *C. psittaci, C. pneumoniae,* and *C. trachomatis* on the basis of the molecular weight of the amplicon. With the use of this assay, *C. psittaci* was detected in 13 (17.3%) of 75 sick or dead birds involved in three avian psittacosis outbreaks; 5 of the 13 PCR-positive birds were also culture-positive. None of the throat swab specimens from four humans involved in this outbreak were positive by PCR or culture, but one individual had a *C. psittaci*–specific MIF IgG titer of 512. The CDC[27] provides a list of laboratories that test human specimens in its current recommendations for the control of *C. psittaci* infection in humans and pet birds (Table 194–2).

TREATMENT

The recommended treatment of psittacosis in adults and children older than 8 years is 500 mg of tetracycline orally every 6 hours for 7 to 10 days. Erythromycin (50 mg/kg/day,

TABLE 194–2 ■ LABORATORIES THAT TEST HUMAN SPECIMENS FOR *CHLAMYDIA PSITTACI*

Laboratory	Tests Performed	Telephone Number
Respiratory Diseases Laboratory Section, CDC, Atlantia	MIF CF PCR Culture	(404) 639-3563
Focus Technology, Cypress, CA	IFA PCR Culture	(800) 445-4032
Laboratory Corp. of America, Burlington, NC	Culture Polyclonal antibody	(800) 334-5161
Specialty Labs., Santa Monica, CA	MIF	(800) 421-4449

CDC, Centers for Disease Control and Prevention; CF, complement fixation; IFA, immunofluorescent antibody; MIF, microimmunofluorescence; PCR, polymerase chain reaction.
From Compendium of measures to control *Chlamydia psittaci* infection among humans (psittacosis) and pet birds (avian chlamydiosis). M. M. W. R. Morb. Mortal. Wkly. Rep. *49* (RR-8):3–17, 2000.

up to 2 g/day, for 7 to 10 days) also can be used. The experience in the Australian series[164] and anecdotal reports suggest that tetracycline may be more effective than erythromycin. The initial infection does not appear to be followed by long-term immunity. Reinfection and clinical disease can develop within 2 months of treatment; two well-documented cases of reinfection are reported in the literature. A pet shop employee had two episodes of psittacosis 11 months apart. Each episode met the CDC's confirmed case definition.[22]

Infection Caused by *Chlamydia pneumoniae*

THE ORGANISM

The first isolates of *C. pneumoniae* were obtained serendipitously during trachoma studies in the 1960s.[53] After the recovery of a similar isolate from the respiratory tract of a college student with pneumonia in Seattle, Grayston and colleagues[55] applied the designation TWAR after their first two isolates, TW-183 and AR-39. On the basis of inclusion morphology and staining characteristics in cell culture, *C. pneumoniae* initially was considered a *C. psittaci* strain. Subsequent analysis, however, has demonstrated that this organism is distinct from both *C. psittaci* and *C. trachomatis*. Sequencing has revealed that *C. pneumoniae* differs significantly from *C. trachomatis* in several areas. *C. pneumoniae* encodes for 21 polymorphic membrane proteins (PMPs) versus 9 in *C. trachomatis*. PMPs may be surface exposed in *C. pneumoniae*.[96] Ultrastructural studies have demonstrated an EB morphology distinct from that of *C. trachomatis* and *C. psittaci*[24] (Fig. 194–1). However, some isolates of *C. pneumoniae*, including IOL-207, have been found to have round EBs.[21, 131] Thus, it may not be a consistent species characteristic. Restriction endonuclease pattern analysis, nucleic acid hybridization studies, and amplified fragment length polymorphism analysis suggest a high degree of genetic relatedness (>95%) among the *C. pneumoniae* isolates examined thus far and less than 10 percent homology with either *C. trachomatis* or *C. psittaci*.[19, 28, 54, 110] At this point, we do not have a strain typing system for *C. pneumoniae*. Plasmids have not been detected in any human isolate of *C. pneumoniae*.

EPIDEMIOLOGY

C. pneumoniae appears to be a common human pathogen. The organism also has been isolated from nonhuman species, including a horse, koalas, and reptiles and amphibians, although the role that these infections may play in human disease is unknown.[94, 136] The mode of transmission remains uncertain but probably involves infected respiratory tract secretions. Acquisition of infection by droplet aerosol was described during a laboratory accident.[86] *C. pneumoniae* can remain viable on Formica countertops for 30 hours and can survive small-particle aerosolization.[38, 152] Spread of *C. pneumoniae* within families and enclosed populations such as military recruits has been described.[65, 98, 162]

Several serologic surveys have documented rising chlamydial antibody prevalence rates in school-age children that reach 30 to 45 percent in adolescents.[18, 33, 146] This increasing prevalence of chlamydial antibody during childhood is probably attributable to *C. pneumoniae*. The proportion of community-acquired pneumonia associated with *C. pneumoniae* infection has ranged from 2 to 19 percent; it varies with geographic location, the age group examined, and the diagnostic methods used.*

Several studies of the role of *C. pneumoniae* in lower respiratory tract infections in pediatric populations have found evidence of infection in 0 to more than 18 percent (Table 194–3). Most of these studies have relied entirely on serology for diagnosis. Early studies that relied on serology suggested that infection in children younger than 5 years in Seattle and Scandinavia was rare[53]; however, in a study of Filipino children younger than 5 years with lower respiratory tract infection, nearly 10 percent had either acute or chronic antibody to *C. pneumoniae*.[143] In Brooklyn, the proportion of lower respiratory tract infections associated with *C. pneumoniae*, as determined by culture, increased from 9 percent in children younger than 5 years to 19 percent in children and adolescents 5 to 16 years of age.[25]

Studies that have used culture have found a poor correlation between culture and serology, especially in children.[15, 35, 76] Although 7 to 13 percent of children 6 months to 16 years of age enrolled in two multicenter pneumonia treatment studies were culture-positive and 7 to 18 percent met the serologic criteria for acute infection with the MIF test, they were not the same patients.[15, 76] Only 1 to 3 percent of the culture-positive children met the serologic criteria, and approximately 70 percent were seronegative.

In studies to date, acute infection with *C. pneumoniae* does not appear to vary by season. In Seattle and Scandinavia, cycles lasting several years during which the incidence of new infection with *C. pneumoniae* waxed and waned have been described.[53]

Prolonged culture positivity lasting from several weeks to several years after acute infection has been reported.[25, 31, 35, 53, 65] Asymptomatic nasopharyngeal carriage also occurs in 2 to 5 percent of adults and children.[14, 35, 51, 87] The role that asymptomatic carriage plays in the epidemiology of *C. pneumoniae* is not known, but possibly these persons serve as a reservoir for spread of infection.

*See references 15, 25, 39, 47, 53, 76, 95, 143, 144, 153.

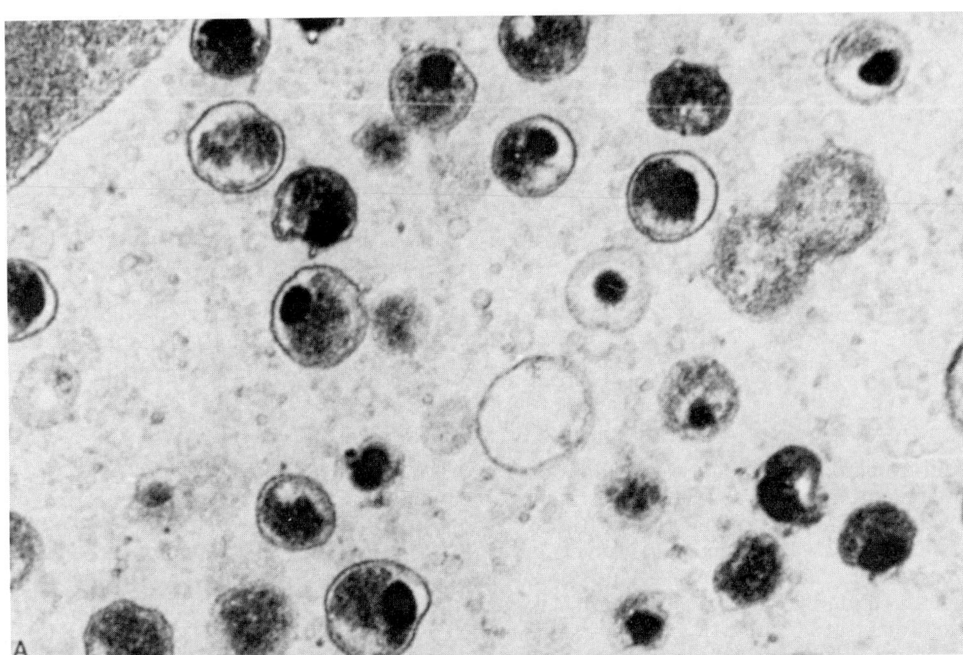

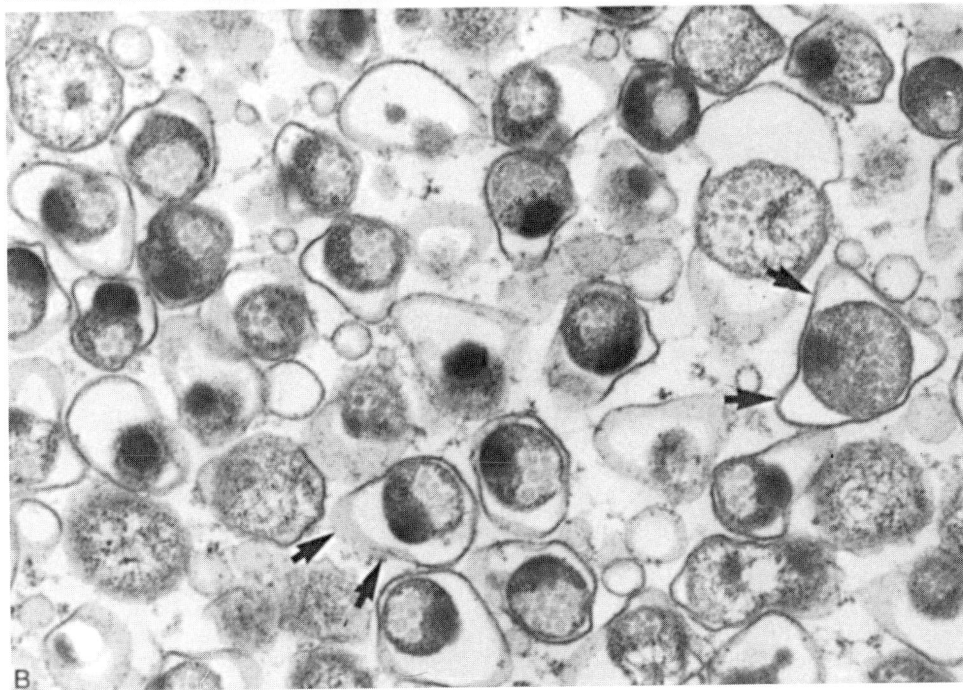

FIGURE 194–1 ■ Electron micrograph of *Chlamydia trachomatis (A)* and *Chlamydia pneumoniae (B)* inclusions demonstrating the morphology of the elementary body (EB). The EBs of *C. pneumoniae* have a pear shape because of a loose periplasmic membrane *(arrows)*, unlike the typically round EBs of *C. trachomatis* and *Chlamydia psittaci.*

CLINICAL MANIFESTATIONS

The spectrum of disease associated with *C. pneumoniae* is expanding. Most infections are probably mild or asymptomatic. Longitudinal serologic data obtained during an epidemic among military recruits in Finland suggest that only about 10 percent of infections result in clinically apparent pneumonia.[98]

Initial reports emphasized mild atypical pneumonia clinically resembling that associated with *M. pneumoniae.*[53, 144] In several subsequent studies, however, pneumonia associated with *C. pneumoniae* has been clinically indistinguishable from other pneumonias.[15, 53, 76] Co-infection with other pathogens, especially *M. pneumoniae* and *Streptococcus pneumoniae,* can be a frequent occurrence.[15, 76] Twenty percent of the children in one multicenter pneumonia treatment study with positive *C. pneumoniae* cultures were co-infected with *M. pneumoniae*; they could not be distinguished from children who were infected with either organism alone.[15] *C. pneumoniae* has been associated with severe illness and even death, although the role of preexisting chronic conditions as contributing factors in many of these patients is difficult to assess. In some cases, however, *C. pneumoniae* clearly appears to be implicated as a serious pathogen, even in the absence of underlying disease. *C. pneumoniae* was isolated from the respiratory tract and the pleural fluid of a previously healthy adolescent boy with severe pneumonia complicated by respiratory tract failure and pleural effusions[4] (Fig. 194–2).

The role of host factors remains to be determined. Although *C. pneumoniae* has been detected in bronchoalveolar lavage

TABLE 194–3 ■ STUDIES OF *CHLAMYDIA PNEUMONIAE* ACUTE LOWER RESPIRATORY TRACT INFECTION IN CHILDREN

Study	Year	Country	Age	No	No. Positive Results/No. Tested (%)		
					Culture	PCR	MIF
Saikku et al.[143]	1988	Philippines	<5 yr	220	ND	ND	14/220 (6.4)
Forgie et. al.[39]	1991	Gambia	1–9 yr	74	ND	ND	9/74 (12.1)
Yeung et al.[163]	1993	Canada	<6 mo	86	ND	ND	0/86 (0)
Herrmann et al.[83]	1994	Sudan	<12 yr	110	3/110 (2.7)	0/110 (0)	4/110 (3.6)
Jantos et al.[95]	1995	Germany	2 days–15 yr	290	1/290 (0.3)	2/290 (0.7)	2/101(2.0)
Block et al.[15]	1995	USA	3–12 yr	260	34/260 (13/1)	ND	48/260 (18.5)
Harris et al.[76]	1998	USA	6 mo–16 yr	456	31/420 (7.3)	ND	37/420 (8.8)

MIF, microimmunofluorescence; ND, not done; PCR, polymerase chain reaction.

fluid from 10 percent of a group of patients with AIDS and pneumonia, its clinical role in these patients is uncertain because most were co-infected with other well-recognized pathogens such as *Pneumocystis carinii* and *Mycobacterium tuberculosis*.[3] Gaydos and colleagues[47] identified *C. pneumoniae* infection by PCR in 11 percent of a group of immunocompromised adults with human immunodeficiency virus infection, malignancies, and other immune disorders, including systemic lupus erythematosus, sarcoidosis, and common variable immunodeficiency. *C. pneumoniae* appeared to be responsible for 6 of 31 (19%) episodes of acute chest syndrome in children with sickle-cell disease.[113] The *C. pneumoniae* infection in these patients seemed to be associated with more severe hypoxia than infection with *M. pneumoniae* did.

C. pneumoniae may act as an inflammatory trigger for asthma. Several cases of culture-documented *C. pneumoniae* infection in patients with significant bronchospasm have been reported.[58, 65] Asthmatic bronchitis was diagnosed in one patient, and she was receiving systemic and topical steroids.[65] This patient did not improve until her chlamydial infection was treated. Hahn and associates[58] reported an association between serologic evidence of acute *C. pneumoniae* infection and wheezing in adults seen for lower respiratory tract illness. However, they were able to isolate the organism from only 1 of 365 patients. As part of a study in children, *C. pneumoniae* was isolated from 13 of 118 children (11%) 5 to 15 years of age who were initially evaluated for either new or acute exacerbations of asthma.[35] Treatment of the infection appeared to result in both clinical improvement and improvement in pulmonary function test scores. Only five of the children with confirmed infection had detectable IgG antibody to *C. pneumoniae*. One child who did not comply with his antibiotic therapy was culture-positive on five occasions during a 3-month period. Anti–*C. pneumoniae* antibody as determined by MIF was never detected. Specific anti–*C. pneumoniae* IgE was, however, detected in 85.7 percent of the culture-positive asthmatics as compared with 9 percent of the children with *C. pneumoniae* pneumonia who were not wheezing.[36] This finding suggests that the bronchial reactivity seen with *C. pneumoniae* infection may be IgE mediated. The potential prolonged, persistent *C. pneumoniae* infection may produce chronic inflammation and trigger bronchospasm in susceptible persons. *C. pneumoniae* has been demonstrated to induce in vitro ciliostasis in ciliated bronchial epithelial cells.[149] Animal studies also suggest that steroids can reactivate *C. pneumoniae* lung infection in mice.[106] In addition, immune-mediated phenomena, including erythema nodosum and iritis, have been described as complicating *C. pneumoniae* infection.[151, 161]

The role of *C. pneumoniae* in upper respiratory infections is less well defined. *C. pneumoniae* has been isolated from the middle ear fluid of children and adults with otitis media.[14, 123] Block and colleagues recovered *C. pneumoniae* from the middle ear fluid of eight children 3 months through 14 years of age with acute otitis media.[14] *C. pneumoniae* was the sole pathogen isolated in two patients. Co-pathogens in the remaining six patients included β-lactamase–positive *Haemophilus influenzae* and *Moraxella catarrhalis,* along

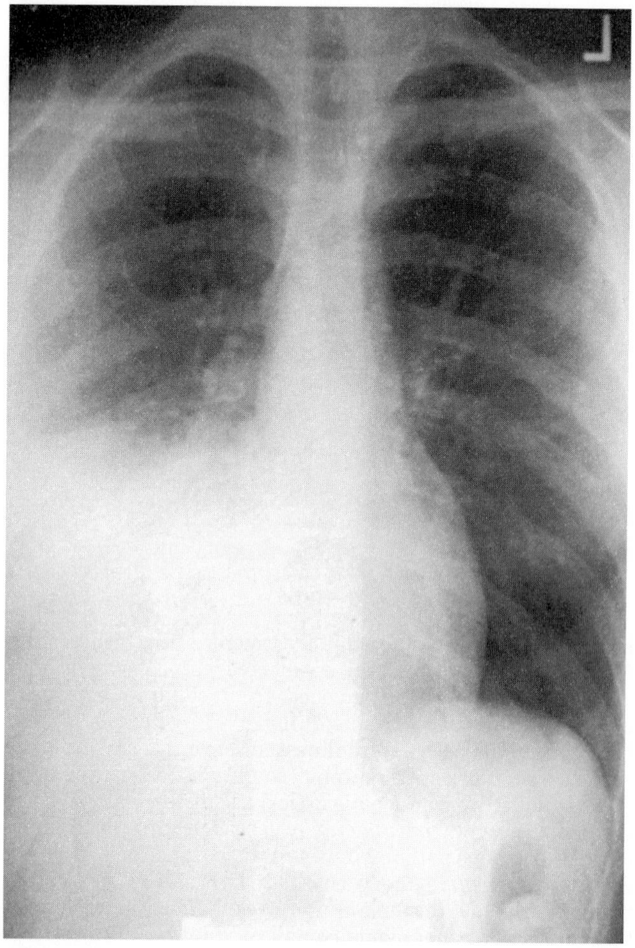

FIGURE 194–2 ■ Chest radiograph of a 19-year-old man with *Chlamydia pneumoniae* pneumonia demonstrating pleural effusion in the right lung. *C. pneumoniae* was isolated from the pleural fluid.

with penicillin-resistant and penicillin-sensitive *S. pneumoniae*. Five of the *C. pneumoniae*–positive children responded favorably despite not being treated with antibiotics active against the organism, either a course of an oral β-lactam or single-dose intramuscular ceftriaxone. Symptoms suggestive of sinus involvement are not uncommon in patients with upper respiratory tract infection associated with *C. pneumoniae,* but only one case of isolation of the organism, from a 47-year-old man with sinusitis, has been reported.[79] Data also are limited on the potential role of *C. pneumoniae* in pharyngitis. Only two studies have been published, and diagnosis was limited to serology. Although one study found serologic evidence of *C. pneumoniae* in 8.5 percent of adult patients with pharyngitis,[84] Hyman and associates[87] reported that 19 percent of asymptomatic adults who were culture- or PCR-negative (or negative by both modalities) fulfilled the serologic criteria for acute *C. pneumoniae* infection.

DIAGNOSIS

A specific laboratory diagnosis of *C. pneumoniae* infection can be made by isolation of the organism from nasopharyngeal or throat swabs, sputa, or pleural fluid, if present. The nasopharynx appears to be the optimal site for isolation of the organism.[15] The relative yield from throat swabs and sputum is not known. Isolation of *C. pneumoniae* requires culture in tissue; the organism cannot be propagated in cell-free media. Initial studies suggested that *C. pneumoniae* was more difficult to isolate in tissue culture than *C. trachomatis* was.[53] Originally, the same methods were used: HeLa or McCoy cells pretreated with dextran diethylaminoethyl. Multiple passages were needed, the inclusions were small and difficult to see, and in general, the yield was poor. *C. pneumoniae* grows more readily in other cell lines derived from respiratory tract tissue, specifically, HEp-2 and HL cells.[26, 138] Omission of pretreatment with dextran diethylaminoethyl results in much larger inclusions, and specimens need only one passage. Culture with an initial inoculation and one passage should take 4 to 7 days.

Nasopharyngeal cultures can be obtained with Dacron-tipped, wire-shafted swabs. Each lot of swabs should be treated in a mock infection system to ensure that no inhibitory effects occur on either the viability of cells or recovery of chlamydiae. Specimens for culture should be placed in appropriate transport media, usually a sucrose phosphate buffer with antibiotics and fetal calf serum, and stored immediately at 4° C for no longer than 24 hours. Viability decreases if specimens are held at room temperature. If the specimen cannot be processed within 24 hours, it should be frozen at −70° C until culture can be performed. After 72 hours of incubation, culture confirmation can be performed by staining with either a *C. pneumoniae* spp.–specific or a *Chlamydia* genus–specific (anti-LPS) fluorescein-conjugated monoclonal antibody.[115] Inclusions of *C. pneumoniae* do not contain glycogen and thus do not stain with iodine. Unfortunately, the availability of commercially produced *C. pneumoniae*–specific reagents is limited. If a genus-specific antibody is used, *C. pneumoniae* should be confirmed by differential staining with a specific *C. trachomatis* antibody; if the latter is negative, the isolate is either *C. pneumoniae* or *C. psittaci*. If the patient has not had avian exposure, psittacosis would be highly likely.

Because isolation of *C. pneumoniae* was initially considered to be difficult and limited, emphasis was placed on serologic diagnosis. However, performance of the MIF test also is limited to a small number of research laboratories. The MIF test was modified from the test used for *C. trachomatis* by using EBs from TW-183 or other *C. pneumoniae* strains as the antigen. With the MIF test, one can detect IgG, IgM, and IgA antibodies. Grayston and colleagues[53] proposed a set of criteria for the serologic diagnosis of *C. pneumoniae* infection with the MIF test that have been used by many laboratories and clinicians. For acute infection, the patient should have a fourfold rise in IgG titer, a single IgM titer of 16 or higher, or a single IgG titer of 512 or higher. Past or preexisting infection is defined as an IgG titer of 16 or higher, but lower than 512. These researchers further proposed that the pattern of antibody response in primary infection differed from that seen in reinfection. In initial infection, the IgM response appears at about 3 weeks after the onset of illness and the IgG response at 6 to 8 weeks. In reinfection, the IgM response may be absent and the IgG response occurs earlier, within 1 to 2 weeks.[53] A fourfold titer rise or a titer of 64 or higher with CF also is considered to be diagnostic. Initially, Grayston and colleagues[52] found that less than one third of hospitalized patients with suspected *C. pneumoniae* infection had detectable CF antibody. However, in a report of a small outbreak of *C. pneumoniae* infection in University of Washington students, all seven patients with pneumonia had CF titers of 64 or higher.[52] CF is genus-specific.

Because of the relatively long period until the development of a serologic response in primary infection, the antibody response may be missed if convalescent sera are obtained too soon (i.e., earlier than 3 weeks after the onset of illness). The use of paired sera also affords only a retrospective diagnosis, which is of little help in terms of deciding how to treat a patient. The criteria for use of a single serum sample have not been correlated with the results of culture and are based primarily on data from adults. The antibody response in acute infection may take longer than 3 months to develop. Acute, culture-documented infection also can occur without seroconversion, especially in children.[15, 25, 36, 76] Only 28 percent of the culture-positive children enrolled in a multicenter pneumonia treatment study had detectable anti–*C. pneumoniae* antibody by MIF, and only 1 percent met the serologic criteria for acute infection.[15] Most had no detectable antibody by the MIF test, even after 3 months of follow-up.[15] However, the results of immunoblotting revealed that these children have antibody to numerous *C. pneumoniae* proteins but that less than 30 percent react with MOMP, which is the antigen presented in the MIF test.[102] Although MOMP has been demonstrated to be immunodominant in *C. trachomatis* infection, it does not appear to be immunodominant for *C. pneumoniae*.[12, 88, 102]

Background rates of seropositivity also can be high in some populations. Hyman and associates,[87] as part of a study of asymptomatic *C. pneumoniae* infection in subjectively healthy adults in Brooklyn, found 81 percent to have IgG or IgM titers of 16 or higher. Seventeen percent had evidence of "acute infection" (IgG titer >512, IgM titer >16, or both). However, none of these persons was culture- or PCR-positive. Similar results were reported by Kern and associates[97] in healthy firefighters and policemen in Rhode Island. The specificity of the MIF IgM assay can be affected by the presence of rheumatoid factor. A study from the Netherlands found an increased probability of false-positive results caused by rheumatoid factor with increasing age.[157] Sera should be routinely absorbed before MIF IgM testing is performed. Hyman and colleagues[87] absorbed all the IgM-positive sera, and the titers did not change. Some IgG antibody may result from a heterotypic response to other chlamydial species because cross-reactions with MOMP occur among the three species, as do cross-reactions caused by the genus LPS antigen. Moss and colleagues[119] reported that antibodies to *C. pneumoniae* and *C. psittaci* were found in as many as half of all chlamydial IgG–positive persons attending a clinic for sexually transmitted diseases. This point is reinforced by the observation that studies from the early 1980s suggesting that *C. trachomatis* was a cause of community-acquired pneumonia and pharyngitis in adults and children were probably detecting antibody to *C. pneumoniae* rather than *C. trachomatis*.[78, 99, 100] Other organisms that have been reported as possibly causing cross-reactions on MIF are *Bartonella*[108] and *Bordetella pertussis*.[93] The latter could be significant because adults with pertussis frequently have a chronic cough or severe bronchitis, which is a clinical feature often ascribed to *C. pneumoniae*. Recent studies have found significant homology between human and *C. pneumoniae* heat shock protein 60 (HSP-60) and *E. coli* GroEL.[122] Picornavirus proteins also have been reported to share antigenic determinants with HSP-60/65, including the HSP-60 of humans and *C. pneumoniae*, which conceivably could lead also to cross-reactions in the MIF assay.[75]

Moreover, the MIF test is not standardized, and reading the slides has a very large subjective component and requires a very experienced microscopist. A recent study by Peeling and coworkers[127] attempted to address the problem of interlaboratory variation in performance of the MIF test by sending a panel of 22 acute and convalescent sera to 14 different laboratories. Nine of the laboratories used an in-house MIF. The antigens in most of the assays were either AR-39 or TW-183. Three laboratories used one of two commercially available kits, which included either AR-39 or Kajaani 6 as the antigen. The remaining two laboratories used the Washington Research Foundation kit, which uses TW-183. The overall agreement in assay results (to get within one twofold dilution of the "gold standard," as read at the University of Washington) was 80 percent. The range was 50 to 100 percent, depending on the isotype. Agreement in serodiagnostic criteria was 69 percent for negative, 68 percent for "chronic," and 87 percent for a fourfold increase in IgG.

Although EIA serology test kits offer the promise of standardized performance and objective end-points, none have been evaluated adequately in comparison to culture or PCR.[32] Most have been compared only with MIF. None have FDA clearance or approval for use in the United States. One commercial assay, the Medac rELISA, uses a recombinant LPS antigen; others are based on LPS-extracted EBs or synthetic peptides.[32, 103, 128, 155] These kits can measure IgG, IgM, and IgA antibodies, but cutoffs vary from kit to kit, and the criteria for a positive result (acute infection, past infection) can be very complex.[32, 103, 155] A study from the United States compared recombinant LPS EIA with culture and found that the sensitivity ranged from 13 percent for IgM antibody in children to 78 percent for either IgA or IgG antibody in adults with respiratory infection.[103] Specificity in comparison to culture ranged from 21 to 91 percent. Recently, Persson and Haidl[128] reported cross-reactions with rEIA and parvovirus, primarily for IgM, but it also was seen to a lesser extent with IgG and IgA. This cross-reaction was not seen with MIF.

The CDC[32] has proposed some modifications of the serologic criteria for diagnosis. Although the MIF test was considered to be the only serologic test currently acceptable, the criteria were made significantly more stringent. Acute infection as determined by MIF was defined as a fourfold rise in IgG or an IgM titer of 16 or greater, and the use of a single elevated IgG titer was discouraged. An IgG titer of 16 or greater was considered to indicate past exposure, but neither elevated IgA titer nor any other serologic marker was thought to be a validated indicator of persistent or chronic infection. The CDC did not recommend the use of any EIA for detection of antibody to *C. pneumoniae*.

Direct detection of *C. pneumoniae* EBs in clinical specimens by fluorescent antibody stains is occasionally possible but is insensitive and frequently nonspecific.[55] No commercially available reagents have been evaluated or approved for this purpose. All the chlamydial EIAs currently available detect *C. pneumoniae* and *C. trachomatis* because they use polyclonal or genus-specific monoclonal antibodies. However, few data exist on the use of these assays in this setting, and the data that are available also suggest that EIAs are insensitive for detection of *C. pneumoniae* in respiratory tract specimens. Chirgwin and associates[25] obtained nasopharyngeal specimens from 91 patients with pneumonia for testing with Chlamydiazyme. Although no false-positive results occurred, the EIA detected only 2 of 15 patients (13.3%) who were culture-positive for *C. pneumoniae*.

The number of *C. pneumoniae* organisms present in the respiratory tract of persons with pneumonia or other respiratory tract diseases is smaller than the number found in genital *C. trachomatis* infection. DNA amplification methods (e.g., PCR) appear to be the most promising technology in the development of a rapid, nonculture method for detection of *C. pneumoniae*. At least 18 in-house PCR assays for detection of *C. pneumoniae* in clinical specimens have been reported in the literature.[16] None of these assays is standardized or extensively validated in comparison to culture for detection of *C. pneumoniae* in respiratory specimens. None is commercially available or has FDA approval. Major variations in these methods include collecting and processing specimens, primer design, nucleic acid extraction, detection and identification of amplification products, and ways to prevent possible false-positive and inhibitory reactions. The primers used most frequently have been those based on the *omp1* gene, the 16S rRNA gene, the 16S and 16S–23S spacer rRNA genes, and a *C. pneumoniae*–specific cloned *Pst* I fragment.[16] Some assays have used single amplification; some have been nested. Methods for detecting the amplification product include agarose gel electrophoresis, Southern blot, EIA, and polyacrylamide gel electrophoresis.[16] Recent studies suggest significant interlaboratory variation in performance of PCR for *C. pneumoniae*.[32] The CDC does not recommend any specific assay because of a lack of comparative data[32] and suggests that more studies need to be conducted with proper controls and larger numbers of clinical specimens from patients. The CDC suggested that any new PCR assay be compared with a sensitive culture system.

TREATMENT

Chlamydia spp. are susceptible to the tetracyclines, macrolides, and quinolones.[61] *C. pneumoniae*, like *C. psittaci*, is resistant to sulfonamides.[61] To date, few published data have described the response of *C. pneumoniae* to antimicrobial therapy. Most of the treatment studies of pneumonia caused by *C. pneumoniae* published thus far have relied entirely on diagnosis by serology; consequently, microbiologic efficacy could not be assessed. Anecdotal reports have suggested that prolonged courses, up to 3 weeks, of either tetracyclines or erythromycin may be needed to eradicate *C. pneumoniae* from the nasopharynx of adults with flulike illness and pharyngitis.[65] The results of two pediatric multicenter pneumonia treatment studies found that 10-day courses of erythromycin and clarithromycin and 5 days of azithromycin suspension were equally efficacious; they eradicated the organism in 79 to 86 percent of children.[15, 76, 139] Quinolones, including levofloxacin and moxifloxacin, also have been demonstrated to have 70 to 80 percent efficacy in eradicating *C. pneumoniae* from adults with community-acquired pneumonia.[70, 71]

Most patients improved clinically despite persistence of the organism. Persistence does not appear to be secondary to the development of antibiotic resistance.[70, 71, 139]

Based on these limited data, the following regimens for respiratory tract infection caused by *C. pneumoniae* can be suggested: in adults, doxycycline, 100 mg twice a day for 14 to 21 days; tetracycline, 250 mg four times a day for 14 to 21 days; azithromycin, 1.5 g over a period of 5 days; levofloxacin, 500 mg/day orally or intravenously for 7 to 14 days; or moxifloxacin, 400 mg/day orally for 10 days. For children, suggested regimens include erythromycin suspension, 50 mg/kg/day for 10 to 14 days; clarithromycin suspension, 15 mg/kg/day for 10 days; or azithromycin suspension, 10 mg/kg on day 1 followed by 5 mg/kg/day once daily on days 2 to 5. Some patients may require re-treatment.

REFERENCES

1. Alary, M., Joly, J. R., Moutquin, J. M., et al.: Randomised comparison of amoxycillin and erythromycin in treatment of genital chlamydial infection in pregnancy. Lancet *344*:1461–1466, 1994.
2. Andersen, A. A., and Tappe, J. P.: Genetic, immunologic, and pathologic characterization of avian chlamydial strains. J. Am. Vet. Med. Assoc. *195*:1512–1526, 1989.
3. Augenbraun, M. H., Roblin, P. M., Chirgwin, K., et al.: Isolation of *Chlamydia pneumoniae* from the lungs of patients infected with the human immunodeficiency virus. J. Clin. Microbiol. *29*:401–402, 1990.
4. Augenbraun, M. H., Roblin, P. M., Mandel, L. J., et al.: *Chlamydia pneumoniae* pneumonia with pleural effusion: Diagnosis by culture. Am. J. Med. *91*:437–438, 1991.
5. Bauwens, J. E., Gibbons, M. S., Hubbard M. M., et al.: *Chlamydia pneumoniae* (strain TWAR) isolated from two symptom-free children during evaluation for possible sexual assault. J. Pediatr. *119*:591–593, 1991.
6. Beem, M. O., and Saxon, E. M.: Respiratory-tract colonization and a distinctive pneumonia syndrome in infants infected with *Chlamydia trachomatis*. N. Engl. J. Med. *296*:306–310, 1977.
7. Bell, T. A., Sandstrom, K. I., Gravett, M. G., et al.: Comparison of ophthalmic silver nitrate solution and erythromycin ointment for prevention of natally acquired *Chlamydia trachomatis*. Sex. Transm. Dis. *14*:195–200, 1987.
8. Bell, T. A., Stamm, W. E., Kuo, C. C., et al.: Risk of perinatal transmission of *Chlamydia trachomatis* by mode of delivery. J. Infect. *29*:165–169, 1994.
9. Bell, T. A., Stamm, W. E., Wang, S. A., et al.: Chronic *Chlamydia trachomatis* infections in infants. J. A. M. A. *267*:400–402, 1992.
10. Bernstein, D. I., Hubbard, T., Wenman, W. M., et al.: Mediastinal and supraclavicular lymphadenitis and pneumonitis due to *Chlamydia trachomatis* serovars L_1 and L_2. N. Engl. J. Med. *311*:1543–1546, 1984.
11. Black, C.M.: Current methods of laboratory diagnosis of *Chlamydia trachomatis* infection. Clin. Microbiol. Rev. *10*:160–184, 1997.
12. Black, C. M., Johnson, J. E., Farshy, C. E., et al.: Antigenic variation among strains of *Chlamydia pneumoniae*. J. Clin. Microbiol. *29*: 1312–1316, 1991.
13. Black, S. B., Grossman, M., Cles, L., et al.: Serologic evidence of chlamydial infection in children. J. Pediatr. *98*:65–67, 1981.
14. Block, S., Hammerschlag, M. R., Hedrick, J., et al.: *Chlamydia pneumoniae* in acute otitis media. Pediatr. Infect. Dis. J. *16*:858–862, 1997.
15. Block, S., Hedrick, J., Hammerschlag, M. R., et al.: *Mycoplasma pneumoniae* and *Chlamydia pneumoniae* in pediatric community-acquired pneumonia: Comparative efficacy and safety of clarithromycin vs. erythromycin ethylsuccinate. J. Pediatr. Infect. Dis. *14*:471–477, 1995.
16. Boman, J., Gaydos, C. A., and Quinn, T. C.: Molecular diagnosis of *Chlamydia pneumoniae* infection. J. Clin. Microbiol. *37*:3791–3799, 1999.
17. Bourke, S. J., Carrington, D., Frew, C. E., et al.: Serological cross-reactivity among chlamydial strains in a family outbreak of psittacosis. J. Infect. *19*:41–45, 1989.
18. Burney, P., Forsey, T., Darougar, S., et al.: The epidemiology of chlamydial infections in childhood: A serological investigation. Int. J. Epidemiol. *13*:491–495, 1984.
19. Campbell, L. A., Kuo, C.-C., and Grayston, J. T.: Characterization of the new *Chlamydia* agent, TWAR, as a unique organism by restriction endonuclease analysis and DNA-DNA hybridization. J. Clin. Microbiol. *25*:1911–1916, 1987.
20. Campbell, L. A., Melgosa, M. P., Hamilton, D. J., et al.: Detection of *Chlamydia pneumoniae* by polymerase chain reaction. J. Clin. Microbiol. *30*:434–439, 1992.
21. Carter, M. W., Sah, A. M., Treharne, J. D., et al.: Nucleotide sequence and taxonomic value of the major outer membrane protein gene of *Chlamydia pneumoniae* IOL-207. J. Gen. Microbiol. *137*:465–475, 1991.
22. Cartwright, K. A. V., Caul, E. O., and Lamb, R. W.: Symptomatic *Chlamydia psittaci* reinfection. Lancet *1*:1004, 1988.
23. Chen, J. Y.: Prophylaxis of ophthalmia neonatorum: Comparison of silver nitrate, tetracycline, erythromycin and no prophylaxis. J. Pediatr. Infect. Dis. *11*:1026–1030, 1992.
24. Chi, E. Y., Kuo, C.-C., and Grayston, J. T.: Unique ultrastructure in the elementary body of *Chlamydia* sp. strain TWAR. J. Bacteriol. *169*: 3757–3763, 1987.
25. Chirgwin, K., Roblin, P. M., Gelling, M., et al.: Infection with *Chlamydia pneumoniae* in Brooklyn. J. Infect. Dis. *163*:757–761, 1991.
26. Cles, L. D., and Stamm, W. E.: Use of HL cells for improved isolation and passage of *Chlamydia pneumoniae*. J. Clin. Microbiol. *28*:938–940, 1990.
27. Compendium of measures to control *Chlamydia psittaci* infection among humans (psittacosis) and pet birds (avian chlamydiosis). M. M. W. R. Recomm. Rep. *49*(RR-8):3–17, 2000.
28. Cox, R. L., Kuo, C.-C., Grayston, J. T., et al.: Deoxyribonucleic acid relatedness of *Chlamydia* sp strain TWAR to *Chlamydia trachomatis* and *Chlamydia psittaci*. Int. J. Syst. Bacteriol. *38*:265–268, 1988.
29. Crombleholme, W. R., Schachter, J., Grossman, M., et al.: Amoxicillin therapy for *Chlamydia trachomatis* in pregnancy. Obstet. Gynecol. *75*: 752–756, 1990.
30. Crosse, B. A.: Psittacosis: A clinical review. J. Infect. *21*:251–259, 1990.
31. Dean, D., Roblin, P. M., Mandel, L., et al.: Molecular evaluation of serial isolates from patients with persistent *Chlamydia pneumoniae* infection. *In* Stephens, R. S., Byrne, G. I., Christiansen, G. I., et al. (eds.): Chlamydial Infections. Proceedings of the Ninth International Symposium on Human Chlamydial Infection. University of California Press, San Francisco, 1998, pp. 219–222.
32. Dowell, S. F., Peeling, R. W., and Boman, J.: Standardizing *Chlamydia pneumoniae* assays: Recommendations from the Centers for Disease Control and Prevention (USA) and the Laboratory Centre for Disease Control (Canada). Clin. Infect. Dis. 33:492–503, 2001.
33. Dwyer, R. S. C., Treharne, J. D., Jones, B. R., et al.: *Chlamydia* infection: Results of micro-immunofluorescence tests for the detection of type-specific antibody in certain chlamydial infections. Br. J. Venereol. Dis. *48*:452–459, 1972.
34. Embree, J. E., Lindsay, D., Williams, T., et al. Acceptability and usefulness of vaginal washes in premenarcheal girls as a diagnostic procedure for sexually transmitted diseases. Pediatr. Infect. Dis. J. *8*:662–667, 1996.
35. Emre, U., Roblin, P. M., Gelling, M., et al.: The association of *Chlamydia pneumoniae* infection and reactive airway disease in children. Arch. Pediatr. Adolesc. Med. *148*:727–732, 1994.
36. Emre, U., Sokolovskaya, N., Roblin, P. M., et al.: Detection of anti-*Chlamydia pneumoniae* IgE in children with reactive airway disease. J. Infect. Dis. *172*:265–267, 1995.
37. Everett, K. D. E., Bush, R. M., and Anderson, A. A.: Emended description of the order Chlamydiales, proposal of Parachlamydiaceae fam. nov. and Simkaniaceae fam. nov., each containing one monotypic genus, revised taxonomy of the family Chlamydiaceae, including a new genus and five new species, and standards for identification of organisms. Int. J. Syst. Bacteriol. *49*:425–440, 1999.
38. Falsey, A. R., and Walsh, E. E. Transmission of *Chlamydia pneumoniae*. J. Infect. Dis. *168*:493–496, 1993.
39. Forgie, I. M., O'Neill, K. P., Lloyd-Evans, N., et al.: Etiology of acute lower respiratory tract infections in Gambian children. II. Acute lower respiratory tract infection in children ages one to nine years presenting at the hospital. J. Pediatr. Infect. Dis. *10*:42–47, 1991.
40. Fransen, L., Nsanze, H., Klauss, V., et al.: Ophthalmia neonatorum in Nairobi, Kenya: The roles of *Neisseria gonorrhoeae* and *Chlamydia trachomatis*. J. Infect. Dis. *153*:862–870, 1986.
41. Frommell, G. T., Bruhn, F. W., and Schwartzman, J. D.: Isolation of *Chlamydia trachomatis* from infant lung tissue. N. Engl. J. Med. *296*: 1150–1152, 1977.
42. Frommell, G. T., Rothenberg, R., Wang, S. P., et al.: Chlamydial infection of mothers and their infants. J. Pediatr. *95*:28–32, 1979.
43. Fryden, A., Kihlstrom, E., Maller, R., et al.: A clinical and epidemiological study of "ornithosis" caused by *Chlamydia psittaci* and *Chlamydia pneumoniae* (strain TWAR). Scand. J. Infect. Dis. *21*:681–691, 1989.
44. Fukushi, H., and Hirai, K.: *Chlamydia pecorum*: The fourth species of genus *Chlamydia*. Microbiol. Immunol. *37*:516–522, 1993.
45. Gaydos, C. A., Crotchfelt, K. A., Howell, M. R., et al.: Molecular amplification assays to detect chlamydial infections from high school female students and to monitor the persistence of chlamydia DNA after therapy. J. Infect. Dis. *177*:417–24, 1998.
46. Gaydos, C. A., Eiden, J. J., Oldach, D., et al.: Diagnosis of *Chlamydia pneumoniae* infection in patients with community-acquired pneumonia by polymerase chain reaction enzyme immunoassay. Clin. Infect. Dis. *19*: 157–160, 1994.
47. Gaydos, C. A., Fowler, C. L., Gill, V. J., et al.: Detection of *Chlamydia pneumoniae* by polymerase-chain reaction–enzyme immunoassay in an immunocompromised population. Clin. Infect. Dis. *17*:718–723, 1993.
48. Gaydos, C. A., Roblin, P. M., Hammerschlag, M. R., et al.: Diagnostic utility of PCR–enzyme immunoassay, culture and serology for detection of *Chlamydia pneumoniae* in symptomatic and asymptomatic patients. J. Clin. Microbiol. *32*:903–905, 1994.

49. Gerber, M. A., Ryan, R. W., Tilton, R. C., et al.: Role of *Chlamydia trachomatis* in acute pharyngitis in young adults. J. Clin. Microbiol. *20*:993–994, 1984.
50. Giradet, R. G., McClain, N., Lahoti, S., et al.: Comparison of the urine-based ligase chain reaction test to culture for detection of *Chlamydia trachomatis* and *Neisseria gonorrhoeae* in pediatric sexual abuse victims. Pediatr. Infect. Dis. J. *20*:144–147, 2001.
51. Gnarpe, J., Gnarpe, H., and Sundelof, B.: Endemic prevalence of *Chlamydia pneumoniae* in subjectively healthy persons. Scand. J. Infect. Dis. *23*: 387–388, 1991.
52. Grayston, J. T., Aldous, M. B., Easton, A., et al.: Evidence that *Chlamydia pneumoniae* causes pneumonia and bronchitis. J. Infect. Dis. *168*: 1231–1235, 1993.
53. Grayston, J. T., Campbell, L. A., Kuo, C.-C., et al.: A new respiratory tract pathogen: *Chlamydia pneumoniae* strain TWAR. J. Infect. Dis. *161*: 618–625, 1990.
54. Grayston, J. T., Kuo, C.-C., Campbell, L. A., et al.: *Chlamydia pneumoniae* sp. nov. for *Chlamydia* sp. strain TWAR. Int. J. Syst. Bacteriol. *39*:88–90, 1989.
55. Grayston, J. T., Kuo, C. C., Wang, S. P., et al.: A new *Chlamydia psittaci* strain, TWAR, isolated in acute respiratory tract infections. N. Engl. J. Med. *315*:161–168, 1986.
56. 2001 Guidelines for the laboratory detection of *Chlamydia trachomatis* and *Neisseria gonorrhoeae* infections. M. M. W. R. Morb. Mortal. Wkly. Rep. *51*(RR-15)1–39, 2002.
57. 2001 Guidelines for the treatment of sexually transmitted diseases. M. M. W. R. Morb. Mortal. Wkly. Rep. *51*(RR-6):1–80, 2002.
58. Hahn, D. L., Dodge, R. W., and Golubjatnikov, R.: Association of *Chlamydia pneumoniae* (strain TWAR) infection with wheezing, asthmatic bronchitis, and adult-onset asthma. J. A. M. A. *266*:225–230, 1991.
59. Hammerschlag, M. R.: *Chlamydia trachomatis* infections and pregnancy. *In* Reeve, P. (ed.): Chlamydial Infections. Heidelberg, Germany, Springer-Verlag, 1987, pp. 56–71.
60. Hammerschlag, M. R.: Chlamydial infections. J. Pediatr. *114*:727–734, 1989.
61. Hammerschlag, M. R.: Antimicrobial susceptibility and therapy of infections caused by *Chlamydia pneumoniae.* Antimicrob. Agents Chemother. *38*:1873–1878, 1994.
62. Hammerschlag, M. R., Ajl, S., and Laraque, D.: Inappropriate use of nonculture tests for the detection of *Chlamydia trachomatis* in suspected victims of child sexual abuse: A continuing problem. Pediatrics *104*: 1137–1139, 1999.
63. Hammerschlag, M. R., Chandler, J. W., Alexander, E. R., et al.: Erythromycin ointment for ocular prophylaxis of neonatal chlamydial infection. J. A. M. A. *244*:2291–2293, 1980.
64. Hammerschlag, M. R., Chandler, J. W., Alexander, E. R., et al.: Longitudinal studies on chlamydial infections in the first year of life. Pediatr. Infect. Dis. J. *1*:395–401, 1982.
65. Hammerschlag, M. R., Chirgwin, K., Roblin, P. M., et al.: Persistent infection with *Chlamydia pneumoniae* following acute respiratory illness. Clin. Infect. Dis. *14*:178–182, 1992.
66. Hammerschlag, M. R., Cummings, C., Roblin, P. M., et al.: Efficacy of neonatal ocular prophylaxis for the prevention of chlamydial and gonococcal conjunctivitis. N. Engl. J. Med. *320*:769–772, 1989.
67. Hammerschlag, M. R., Doraiswamy, B., Alexander, R., et al.: Are rectogenital chlamydial infections a marker of sexual abuse in children? Pediatr. Infect. Dis. J. *3*:100–104, 1984.
68. Hammerschlag, M. R., Gelling, M., Roblin, P. M., et al.: Treatment of neonatal chlamydial conjunctivitis with azithromycin. Pediatr. Infect. Dis. J. *17*:1049–1050, 1998.
69. Hammerschlag, M. R., Golden, N. H., Oh, M. K., et al.: Single dose of azithromycin for the treatment of genital chlamydial infections in adolescents. J. Pediatr. *122*:961–965, 1993.
70. Hammerschlag, M. R., and Roblin, P. M.: Microbiologic efficacy of moxifloxacin for the treatment of community-acquired pneumonia due to *Chlamydia pneumoniae.* Int. J. Antimicrob. Agents *15*:149–152, 2000.
71. Hammerschlag, M. R., and Roblin, P. M.: Microbiologic efficacy of levofloxacin for the treatment of community-acquired pneumonia due to *Chlamydia pneumoniae.* Antimicrob. Agents Chemother. *44*:1409, 2000.
72. Hammerschlag, M. R., Roblin, P. M., Cummings, C., et al.: Comparison of enzyme immunoassay and culture for diagnosis of chlamydial conjunctivitis and respiratory infections in infants. J. Clin. Microbiol. *25*: 2306–2308, 1987.
73. Hammerschlag, M. R., Roblin, P. M., Gelling, M., et al.: Comparison of two enzyme immunoassays to culture for diagnosis of chlamydial conjunctivitis and respiratory infections in infants. J. Clin. Microbiol. *28*: 1725–1727, 1990.
74. Hammerschlag, M. R., Roblin, P. M., Gelling, M., et al.: Use of polymerase chain reaction for the detection of *Chlamydia trachomatis* in ocular and nasopharyngeal specimens from infants with conjunctivitis. Pediatr. Infect. Dis. J. *16*:293–297, 1997.
75. Harkonen, T., Puolakkainen, M., Sarvas, M., et al.: Picornavirus proteins share antigenic determinants with heat shock proteins 60/65. J. Med. Virol. *62*:383–391, 2000.
76. Harris, J.-A., Kolokathis, A., Campbell, M., et al.: Safety and efficacy of azithromycin in the treatment of community acquired pneumonia in children. Pediatr. Infect. Dis. J. *17*:865–871, 1998.
77. Harrison, H. R., English, M. G., Lee, C. K., et al.: *Chlamydia trachomatis* infant pneumonitis: Comparison with matched controls and other infant pneumonitis. N. Engl. J. Med. *298*:702–708, 1978.
78. Harrison, H. R., Magder, L. S., Boyce, W. T., et al.: Acute *Chlamydia trachomatis* respiratory infection in childhood. Am. J. Dis. Child. *140*: 1068–1072, 1986.
79. Hashigucci, K.: Isolation of *Chlamydia pneumoniae* from the maxillary sinus of a patient with purulent sinusitis. Clin. Infect. Dis. *15*:570–571, 1992.
80. Hedberg, K., White, K. E., Forfang, J. C., et al.: An outbreak of psittacosis in Minnesota turkey industry workers: Implications for modes of transmission and control. Am. J. Epidemiol. *130*:569–577, 1989.
81. Heggie, A. D., Jaffe, A. C., Stuard, L. A., et al.: Topical sulfacetamide vs oral erythromycin for neonatal chlamydial conjunctivitis. Am. J. Dis. Child. *139*:564–566, 1985.
82. Herring, A. J.: Typing *Chlamydia psittaci:* A review of methods and recent findings. Br. Vet. J. *149*:455–475, 1993.
83. Herrmann, S. B., Salih, M. A. M., Yousif, B. E., et al.: Chlamydial etiology of acute lower respiratory tract infections in children in the Sudan. Acta Paediatr. *83*:169–172, 1994.
84. Huovinen, P., Lahtonen, R., Zeigler, T., et al.: Pharyngitis in adults: The presence and coexistence of viruses and bacterial organisms. Ann. Intern. Med. *110*:612–616, 1989.
85. Huss, H., Jungkind, D., Amadio, P., et al.: Frequency of *Chlamydia trachomatis* as the cause of pharyngitis. J. Clin. Microbiol. *22*:858–860, 1985.
86. Hyman, C. L., Augenbraun, M. H., Roblin, P. M., et al.: Asymptomatic respiratory tract infection with *Chlamydia pneumoniae.* J. Clin. Microbiol. *29*:2082–2083, 1991.
87. Hyman, C. L., Roblin, P. M., Gaydos, C. A., et al.: Prevalence of asymptomatic nasopharyngeal carriage of *Chlamydia pneumoniae* in subjectively healthy adults: Assessment by polymerase chain reaction–enzyme immunoassay and culture. Clin. Infect. Dis. *20*:1174–1178, 1995.
88. Iijima, Y., Miyashita, N., Kishimoto, T., et al.: Characterization of *Chlamydia pneumoniae* species-specific proteins immunodominant in humans. J. Clin. Microbiol. *32*:583–588, 1994.
89. Ingram, D. L., Runyan, D. K., Collins, A. D., et al.: Vaginal *Chlamydia trachomatis* infection in children with sexual contact. Pediatr. Infect. Dis. *3*:97–99, 1984.
90. Ingram, D. L., White, S. T., Occhiuti, A. R., et al.: Childhood vaginal infections: Association of *Chlamydia trachomatis* with sexual contact. Pediatr. Infect. Dis. *5*:226–229, 1986.
91. Isenberg, S. J., Apt, L., and Wood, M.: A controlled trial of povidone-iodine as prophylaxis against ophthalmia neonatorum. N. Engl. J. Med. *332*:562–566, 1995.
92. Ito, J. I., Comess, K. A., Alexander, E. R., et al.: Pneumonia due to *Chlamydia trachomatis* in an immunocompromised adult. N. Engl. J. Med. *307*:95–98, 1982.
93. Jackson, L. A., Cherry, J. D., Wang, S. P., and Grayston, J. T.: Frequency of serological evidence of *Bordetella* infections and mixed infections with other respiratory pathogens in university students with cough illnesses. Clin. Infect. Dis. *31*:3–6, 2000.
94. Jackson, M., White, N., Giffard, P., and Timms, P.: Epizootiology of *Chlamydia* infections in two free-range koala populations. Vet. Microbiol. *65*:255–264, 1999.
95. Jantos, C. A., Wienpahl, B., Schiefer, H. G., et al.: Infection with *Chlamydia pneumoniae* in infants and children with acute lower respiratory tract disease. Pediatr. Infect. Dis. J. *14*:117–122, 1995.
96. Kalman, S., Mitchell, W., Marathe, R., et al.: Comparative genomes of *Chlamydia pneumoniae* and *C. trachomatis.* Nat Genet *21*:385–389, 1999.
97. Kern, D. G., Neill, M. A., and Schachter, J.: A seroepidemiologic study of *Chlamydia pneumoniae* in Rhode Island. Chest *104*:208–213, 1993.
98. Kleemola, M., Saikku, P., Visakorpi, R., et al.: Epidemics of pneumonia caused by TWAR, a new *Chlamydia* organism, in military trainees in Finland. J. Infect. Dis. *157*:230–236, 1988.
99. Komaroff, A. L., Aronson, M. D., Pass, C. T., et al.: Serologic evidence of chlamydial and mycoplasmal pharyngitis in adults. Science *222*:927–928, 1983.
100. Komaroff, A. L., Aronson, M. D., and Schachter, J.: *Chlamydia trachomatis* infection in adults with community-acquired pneumonia. J. A. M. A. *245*:1319–1322, 1981.
101. Kroon, F. P., van't Wout, J. W., Weiland, H. T., et al.: *Chlamydia trachomatis* pneumonia in an HIV-seropositive patient. N. Engl. J. Med. *320*:806–807, 1989.
102. Kutlin, A., Roblin, P. M., and Hammerschlag, M. R.: Antibody response to *Chlamydia pneumoniae* infection in children with respiratory illness. J. Infect. Dis. *177*:720–724, 1998.
103. Kutlin, A., Tsumura, N., Emre, U., et al.: Evaluation of *Chlamydia* immunoglobulin M (IgM), IgG, and IgA rELISAs Medac for diagnosis of *Chlamydia pneumoniae* infection. Clin. Diagn. Lab. Immunol. *4*:213–216, 1997.

104. Laga, M., Plummer, F. A., Piot, P., et al.: Prophylaxis of gonococcal and chlamydial ophthalmia neonatorum. N. Engl. J. Med. *318*:653–657, 1988.
105. Madico, G., Quinn, T. C., Boman, J., and Gaydos, C. A.: Touchdown enzyme time release–PCR for detection and identification of *Chlamydia trachomatis*, *C. pneumoniae*, and *C. psittaci* using the 16S and 16S–23S spacer rRNA genes. J. Clin. Microbiol. *38*:1085–1093, 2000.
106. Malinverni, R., Kuo, C. C., Campbell, L. A., et al.: Reactivation of *Chlamydia pneumoniae* lung infection in mice by cortisone. J. Infect. Dis. *172*:593–595, 1995.
107. Mathews-Greer, J., Sloop, G., Springer, A., et al.: Comparison of detection methods for *Chlamydia trachomatis* in specimens obtained from pediatric victims of suspected sexual abuse. Pediatr. Infect. Dis. J. *18*:165–167, 1999.
108. Maurin M., Eb, F., Etienne, J., and Raoult, D.: Serologic cross-reactions between *Bartonella* and *Chlamydia* species: Implications for diagnosis. J. Clin. Microbiol. *35*:2283–2287, 1997.
109. Messmer, T. O., Skelton, S. K., Moroney, J. F., et al.: Application of a nested, multiplex PCR to psittacosis outbreaks. J. Clin. Microbiol. *35*: 2043–2046, 1997.
110. Meijer, A., Morrè, S. A., van den Brule, A. J. C., et al.: Genomic relatedness of *Chlamydia* isolates determined by amplified fragment length polymorphism analysis. J. Bacteriol. *181*:4469–4475, 1999.
111. Meyers, J. D., Hackman, R. C., and Stamm, W. E.: *Chlamydia trachomatis* infection as a cause of pneumonia after human marrow transplantation. Transplantation *36*:130–134, 1983.
112. Miller, J. M., and Martin, D. H.: Treatment of *Chlamydia trachomatis* infections in pregnant women. Drugs *60*:597–605, 2000.
113. Miller, S. T., Hammerschlag, M. R., Chirgwin, K., et al.: The role of *Chlamydia pneumoniae* in acute chest syndrome of sickle cell disease. J. Pediatr. *118*:30–33, 1991.
114. Moncada, J. V., Schachter, J., and Wofsy, C.: Prevalence of *Chlamydia trachomatis* lung infection in patients with acquired immune deficiency syndrome. J. Clin. Microbiol. *23*:986, 1986.
115. Montalban, G. S., Roblin, P. M., and Hammerschlag, M. R.: Performance of three commercially available monoclonal reagents for confirmation of *Chlamydia pneumoniae* in cell culture. J. Clin. Microbiol. *32*:1406–1407, 1994.
116. Mordhorst, C. D., Wang, S.-P., Myhra, W., et al.: *Chlamydia pneumonia*, strain TWAR, infections in Denmark 1975–1987. *In* Bowie, W. R., Caldwell, H. R., Jones, R. P., et al. (eds.): Chlamydial Infections. Proceedings of the Seventh International Symposium on Human Chlamydial Infections. Cambridge, Cambridge University Press, 1990, pp. 418–421.
117. Moroney, J. F., Guevara, R., Iverson, C., et al.: Detection of chlamydiosis in a shipment of pet birds, leading to recognition of an outbreak of clinically mild psittacosis in humans. Clin. Infect. Dis. *26*:1425–1429, 1998.
118. Morrison, W. M., Hutchinson, R. B., Thomason, J., et al.: An outbreak of psittacosis. Br. Soc. Study Infect. *91*:71–75, 1991.
119. Moss, T. R., Darougar, S., Woodland, R. M., et al.: Antibodies to chlamydia species in patients attending a genitourinary clinic and the impact of antibodies to *Chlamydia pneumoniae* and *Chlamydia psittaci* on the sensitivity and the specificity of *Chlamydia trachomatis* serology tests. Sex. Transm. Dis. *20*:61–65, 1993.
120. Moulder, J. W.: Interaction of chlamydiae and host cells in vitro. Rev. Clin. Microbiol. *55*:143–190, 1991.
121. Nakajo, M. N., Roblin, P. M., Hammerschlag, M. R., et al.: Chlamydicidal activity of human alveolar macrophages. Infect. Immun. *58*:3640–3644, 1990.
122. Ochiai, Y., Fukushi, H., Yan, C., et al.: Comparative analysis of the putative amino acid sequences of chlamydial heat shock protein 60 and *Escherichia coli* GroEL. J. Vet. Med. Sci. 62:941–945, 2000.
123. Ogawa, H., Hashiguchi, K., and Kazuyama, Y.: Recovery of *Chlamydia pneumoniae* in six patients with otitis media with effusion. J. Laryngol. Otol. *106*:490–492, 1992.
124. Oldach, D. W., Gaydos, C. A., Mundy, L. M., et al.: Rapid diagnosis of *Chlamydia psittaci* pneumonia. Clin. Infect. Dis. *17*:338–343, 1993.
125. Paisley, J. W., Lauer, B. A., Melinkovich, P., et al.: Rapid diagnosis of *Chlamydia trachomatis* pneumonia in infants by direct immunofluorescence microscopy of nasopharyngeal secretions. J. Pediatr. *109*:653–655, 1986.
126. Patamasucon, P., Rettig, P. J., Faust, K. L., et al.: Oral vs topical erythromycin therapies for chlamydial conjunctivitis. Am. J. Dis. Child. *136*:817–821, 1982.
127. Peeling, R., Wang, S., and Grayston, J.: *Chlamydia pneumoniae* serology: Interlaboratory variation in microimmunofluorescence assay results. J. Infect. Dis. *181*(Suppl. 3):426–429, 2000.
128. Persson, K., and Haidl, S.: Evaluation of a commercial test for antibodies to the chlamydial lipopolysaccharide (Medac) for serodiagnosis of acute infections by *Chlamydia pneumoniae* (TWAR) and *Chlamydia psittaci*. A. P. M. I. S. *108*:131–138, 2000.
129. Pether, J. V. S., Noah, N. D., Lau, Y. K., et al.: An outbreak of psittacosis in a boys' boarding school. J. Hyg. (Camb.) *92*:337–343, 1984.
130. Pether, J. V. S., Wang, S. P., and Grayston, J. T.: *Chlamydia pneumoniae*, strain TWAR, as the cause of an outbreak in a boys' school previously called psittacosis. Epidemiol. Infect. *103*:395–400, 1989.
131. Popov, V. L., Shatkin, A. A., Pankratova, V. N., et al.: Ultrastructure of *Chlamydia pneumoniae* in cell culture. FEMS Microbiol. Lett. *84*: 129–134, 1991.
132. Porder, K., Sanchez, N., Roblin, P. M., et al.: Lack of specificity of Chlamydiazyme for detection of vaginal chlamydial infection in prepubertal girls. Pediatr. Infect. Dis. J. *8*:358–360, 1989.
133. Psittacosis at a turkey processing plant—North Carolina, 1989. M. M. W. R. Morb. Mortal. Wkly. Rep. *39*:460–469, 1990.
134. Radkowski, M. A., Kransler, J. K., Beem, M. O., et al.: *Chlamydia* pneumonia in infants: Radiography in 125 cases. A. J. R. Am. J. Roentgenol. *137*:703–706, 1981.
135. Rapoza, P. A., Quinn, T. C., Kiessling, L. A., et al.: Assessment of neonatal conjunctivitis with a direct immunofluorescent monoclonal antibody stain for *Chlamydia*. J. A. M. A. *255*:3369–3373, 1986.
136. Reed, K. D., Ruth, G. R., Meyer, J. A., and Shukla, S. K.: *Chlamydia pneumoniae* infection in a breeding colony of African clawed frogs *(Xenopus tropicalis)*. Emerg. Infect. Dis. *6*:196–199, 2000.
137. Rettig, P. J., and Nelson, J. D.: Genital tract infection with *Chlamydia trachomatis* in prepubertal children. J. Pediatr. *99*:206–210, 1981.
138. Roblin, P. M., Dumornay, W., and Hammerschlag, M. R.: Use of HEp-2 cells for improved isolation and passage of *Chlamydia pneumoniae*. J. Clin. Microbiol. *30*:1968–1971, 1992.
139. Roblin, P. M., and Hammerschlag, M. R.: Microbiologic efficacy of azithromycin and susceptibility to azithromycin of isolates of *Chlamydia pneumoniae* from adults and children with community acquired pneumonia. Antimicrob. Agents Chemother. *42*:194–196, 1998.
140. Roblin, P. M., Hammerschlag, M. R., Cummings, C., et al.: Comparison of two rapid microscopic methods and culture for detection of *Chlamydia trachomatis* in ocular and nasopharyngeal specimens from infants. J. Clin. Microbiol. *27*:968–970, 1989.
141. Rockey, D. D., Lenart, J., and Stephens, R. S.: Genome sequencing and our understanding of chlamydiae. Infect. Immun. *68*:5473–5479, 2000.
142. Rowe, D. S., Aicardi, E. Z., Dawson, C. R., et al.: Purulent ocular discharge in neonates: Significance of *Chlamydia trachomatis*. Pediatrics *63*:628–632, 1979.
143. Saikku, P., Ruutu, P., Leinonen, M., et al.: Acute lower-respiratory-tract infection associated with chlamydial TWAR antibody in Filipino children. J. Infect. Dis. *158*:1095–1097, 1988.
144. Saikku, P., Wang, S. P., Kleemola, M., et al.: An epidemic of mild pneumonia due to an unusual *Chlamydia psittaci* strain. J. Infect. Dis. *151*:832–839, 1985.
145. Sandstrom, K. I., Bell, T. A., Chandler, J. W., et al.: Microbial causes of neonatal conjunctivitis. J. Pediatr. *105*:706–712, 1984.
146. San Joaquin, V. H., Rettig, P. J., Newton, J. Y., et al.: Prevalence of chlamydial antibodies in children. Am. J. Dis. Child. *136*:425–427, 1982.
147. Schachter, J., Grossman, M., Sweet, R. L., et al.: Prospective study of perinatal transmission of *Chlamydia trachomatis*. J. A. M. A. *255*: 3374–3377, 1986.
148. Schachter, J., Sweet, R. L., Grossman, M., et al.: Experience with the routine use of erythromycin for chlamydial infections in pregnancy. N. Engl. J. Med. *314*:276–279, 1986.
149. Shemer, A. Y., and Lieberman, D.: *Chlamydia pneumoniae*–induced ciliostasis in ciliated bronchial epithelial cells. J. Infect. Dis. *171*: 1274–1278, 1995.
150. Soni, R., Seale, J. P., and Young, I. H.: Fulminant psittacosis requiring mechanical ventilation and demonstrating serological cross-reactivity between *Legionella longbeachae* and *Chlamydia psittaci*. Respirology *4*:203–205. 1999.
151. Sundelof, B., Gnarpe, H., and Gnarpe, J.: An unusual manifestation of *Chlamydia pneumoniae* infection: Meningitis, hepatitis, iritis and atypical erythema nodosum. Scand. J. Infect. Dis. *25*:259–261, 1993.
152. Theunissen, H. J. H., Toom, N. A. L., Burggraaf, A., et al.: Influence of temperature and relative humidity on the survival of *Chlamydia pneumoniae* in aerosols. Am. Soc. Microbiol. *59*:2589–2593, 1993.
153. Thom, D. H., Grayston, T., Wang, S. P., et al.: *Chlamydia pneumoniae* strain TWAR, *Mycoplasma pneumoniae* and viral infections in acute respiratory disease in a university study health clinic population. Am. J. Epidemiol. *132*:248–256, 1990.
154. Tong, C. Y. W., and Sillis, M.: Detection of *Chlamydia pneumoniae* and *Chlamydia psittaci* in sputum samples by PCR. J. Clin. Pathol. *46*: 313–317, 1993.
155. Tuuminen, T., Palomaki, P., and Paavonen, J.: The use of serologic tests for the diagnosis of chlamydial infections. J. Microbiol. Methods *42*: 265–279, 2000.
156. Van Buuren, C. E., Dorrestein, G. M., and Van Dijk, J. E.: *Chlamydia psittaci* infections in birds: A review on the pathogenesis and histopathological features. Vet. Q. *16*:38–41, 1994.
157. Verkooyen, R. P., Hazenberg, M. A., Van Haaren, G. H., et al.: Age-related interference with *Chlamydia pneumoniae* microimmunofluorescence serology due to circulating rheumatoid factor. J. Clin. Microbiol. *30*:1287–1289, 1992.
158. Weiss, S. G., Newcomb, R. W., and Beem, M. O.: Pulmonary assessment of children after chlamydial pneumonia of infancy. J. Pediatr. *108*:659–664, 1986.

159. Williams, L. P.: Review of the epidemiology of chlamydiosis in the United States. J. Am. Vet. Med. Assoc. *195*:1518–1521, 1989.
160. Wong, K. H., Skelton, S. K., and Daugharty, H.: Utility of complement fixation and microimmunofluorescence assays for detecting serologic responses in patients with clinically diagnosed psittacosis. J. Clin. Microbiol. *32*:2417–2421, 1994.
161. Yamada, S., Tsumura, N., Nagai, K., et al.: A child with iritis due to *Chlamydia pneumoniae* infection. J. Jpn. Assoc. Infect. Dis. *68*: 1543–1547, 1994.
162. Yamazaki, T., Nakada, H., Sakurai, N., et al.: Transmission of *Chlamydia pneumoniae* in young children in a Japanese family. J. Infect. Dis. *162*: 1390–1392, 1990.
163. Yeung, S. M., McLeod, K., Wang, S. P., et al.: Lack of evidence of *Chlamydia pneumoniae* infection in infants with acute lower respiratory tract disease. Eur. J. Clin. Microbiol. Infect. Dis. *12*:850–853, 1993.
164. Yung, A. P., and Grayson, M. L.: Psittacosis: A review of 135 cases. Med. J. Aust. *148*:228–233, 1988.

SECTION XIX

Rickettsial Diseases

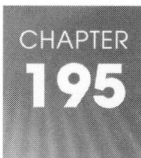

CHAPTER 195

Rickettsial Diseases

MORVEN S. EDWARDS ■ RALPH D. FEIGIN

The rickettsial diseases are caused by a family of microorganisms that have characteristics common to both bacteria and viruses. Rickettsiae depend on the intracellular milieu of animal cells for growth and reproduction; thus, they are considered by some physicians to occupy a position between bacteria and viruses. The following properties, however, indicate their predominantly bacterial character: (1) they multiply by transverse binary fission, (2) they contain both DNA and RNA, (3) at least one species contains muramic acid, (4) they possess enzymes of the Krebs cycle and enzymes for electron transport and protein synthesis, (5) they are retained by a filter, and (6) their growth is inhibited by a variety of antibacterial agents. Their primary resemblance to viruses is that they grow only within living cells.

These microorganisms have been named rickettsiae to honor Dr. H. T. Ricketts, who early in the 20th century discovered and elaborated the cycle of the rickettsia causing Rocky Mountain spotted fever and who in 1910 lost his life in Mexico after contracting typhus fever, which he was investigating.

The rickettsial diseases are grouped together because they possess the following common characteristics: (1) the etiologic agents are similar in size and shape, and all can be seen as coccobacillary forms under the light microscope; (2) they multiply intracellularly within certain cells of susceptible hosts; (3) the characteristic pathologic lesion is widespread vasculitis of the small blood vessels, except in Q fever, in which pneumonitis may be of equal importance; (4) all are acute infectious diseases clinically characterized by fever, headache, and a rash, with the exception of Q fever, which has no rash, and ehrlichiosis, which frequently has no rash; (5) in the early stages of the disease, all infections are susceptible to several of the broad-spectrum antibiotics; (6) all rickettsiae take on a characteristic red color when stained by the Gimenez method; (7) in all rickettsial infections, except Q fever, rickettsialpox, and ehrlichiosis, agglutinins are produced to the OX-19, OX-2, or OX-K strains of the bacillus *Proteus vulgaris* (Weil-Felix reaction); and (8) all rickettsial organisms occur under natural conditions in either insects (lice and fleas) or arachnids (ticks and mites), and these arthropods are, in all cases except Q fever, the primary means by which these diseases are transmitted to humans.

All rickettsial organisms, except the heterogeneic strains of scrub typhus and *Ehrlichia,* produce complement-fixing antibodies. Data from complement fixation and, if available, the Weil-Felix reaction, supplemented with the clinical and epidemiologic features of each individual patient, constitute definitive criteria for diagnosing each of the rickettsial diseases.

The immunity produced by any one of the rickettsial infections is usually of long duration and effective against reinfection by the same etiologic agent. Scrub typhus is an exception.

Four major groups of rickettsial diseases are found within the tribe Rickettsieae.[4] *Ehrlichia* is a genus within a separate rickettsial tribe, Ehrlichieae. With the exception of *Ehrlichia,* an infection by a rickettsia organism belonging to one of these four groups usually confers partial or complete immunity against an infection by any of the other rickettsiae belonging to the same group. In contrast, little or no cross-immunity is conferred for infections caused by rickettsiae belonging to different groups. As an exception, a minor degree of serologic cross-reaction exists between some rickettsiae of the typhus and spotted fever groups. In general, immunity after natural infection is more prolonged than immunity after immunization. Immunization, however, usually prevents mortality and has been used in specific populations.

A final general characteristic is that mammals and arthropods are natural hosts of rickettsiae. However, infection also can occur by an airborne route when infectious microorganisms gain access to the conjunctival or respiratory surfaces. The airborne route appears to be a common mode of laboratory infection.

In all rickettsial infections except louse-borne typhus, humans are only an incidental and accidental blind-end host and do not contribute to survival of the rickettsial species. Rickettsial diseases vary enormously in severity, from benign, self-limited illnesses without mortality to some of the most fulminating infections known. A high index of suspicion leading to prompt diagnosis and institution of appropriate therapy is an important factor in enhancing the survival of patients with rickettsial disease. Table 195–1 summarizes the epidemiologic characteristics of rickettsial diseases.

The Spotted Fevers

The spotted fevers are a group of infectious diseases caused by *Rickettsia rickettsii* and its antigenic variants. Because they are all transmitted by ticks, they are also called tick typhuses.

Rocky Mountain spotted fever (RMSF) is by far the most severe and important disease in the spotted fever group; it occurs throughout the temperate zone of North America. An illness apparently identical to RMSF occurs in South America, where it is called São Paulo disease. Other less severe forms of tick typhus occur in Europe, Asia, Africa, and Australia; they are distinguished from each other by

A portion of the material in this chapter was originally written by Edward S. Murray, now deceased.

TABLE 195–1 ■ IMPORTANT EPIDEMIOLOGIC CHARACTERISTICS OF RICKETTSIAL DISEASES

		Epidemiologic Features		
Disease	**Agent**	*Geographic Occurrence*	*Usual Mode of Human Transmission*	**Mammalian Host**
Typhus group				
Epidemic typhus	*R. prowazekii*	Worldwide	Infected louse feces rubbed into broken skin or as aerosol to membranes	Humans, flying squirrel
Brill-Zinsser disease	*R. prowazekii*	Worldwide	Recrudescence months or years after primary attack of louse-borne typhus	Humans
Murine typhus	*R. typhi*	Scattered pockets, worldwide	Flea bite	Rodents
Murine typhus–like	*R. felis*	United States	Flea bite	Opossums
Spotted fever group				
Rocky Mountain spotted fever	*R. rickettsii*	Western Hemisphere	Tick bite	Wild rodents, dogs
Mediterranean spotted fever (boutonneuse)	*R. conorii**	Mediterranean, Caspian, and Black Sea coastal regions, Africa, Southeast Asia	Tick bite	Wild rodents, dogs
Rickettsialpox	*R. akari*	Worldwide	Mite bite	Mice
Scrub typhus	*Orientia tsutsugamushi*	Japan, Southeast Asia, west and southwest Pacific	Mite bite	Wild rodents
Q fever	*Coxiella burnetii*	Worldwide	Inhalation of infected particles from environment of infected animals	Mammals
Ehrlichiosis group				
Human monocytic erlichiosis	*Ehrlichia chaffeensis*	Worldwide	Tick bite	Deer, dogs, humans
Human granulocytic erlichiosis	HGE agent†	United States, Europe	Tick bite	Deer, humans, other mammals

*In addition, *Rickettsia australis* (Queensland tick typhus) in Australia, *Rickettsia siberica* (Siberian tick typhus) in North Asia, and *Rickettsia japonica* (Oriental spotted fever) in Japan are antigenically and geographically distinct entities.
†*Anaplasma (E.) phagocytophilia*–like agent.

geographic location, as well as by differences in the spotted fever rickettsiae that cause them.[37]

The spotted fever group of rickettsiae multiply not only in the cytoplasm but also fairly frequently in the nucleus of susceptible animal cells,[38] in contradistinction to other rickettsiae that grow exclusively in cytoplasm.

ROCKY MOUNTAIN SPOTTED FEVER

This disease, caused by *R. rickettsii,* was recognized first in parts of Idaho and Montana at the turn of 20th century. For several decades it was thought to be limited to the Rocky Mountain area; however, beginning in the 1930s, the disease began to be recognized in eastern regions of the United States and now has been reported in all geographic areas of the country. For a decade after the discovery of broad-spectrum antibiotics around 1950, the incidence of RMSF declined in both the east and the west, but beginning in the early 1960s, the incidence of RMSF soared exponentially, from fewer than 200 cases in 1960 to a peak of 1192 cases in 1981.[27] Since 1981, however, infection rates have waned considerably (Fig. 195–1), with 812 cases reported to the Centers for Disease Control and Prevention in 1996.[36]

Inexplicably, the incidence of RMSF in the Rocky Mountain area had begun a steady decline even before the era of broad-spectrum antibiotic use in the 1950s; by 1988, fewer than 20 RMSF cases were reported in all the Rocky Mountain and Pacific Coast areas. This trend has continued, and the major endemic regions now include the south Atlantic and the western south-central regions (Fig. 195–2).

Today, RMSF is the most prevalent rickettsial disease in the United States and a growing infectious disease problem. Pediatricians have a special interest in RMSF for several reasons. Nearly two thirds of RMSF patients are younger than 15 years. In addition, although both chloramphenicol and tetracyclines are highly effective against RMSF, the overall case-fatality rate is 3.9 percent. Although this mortality can be attributed to various causes, a considerable number of deaths in children with RMSF can be ascribed to failure to consider and diagnose this disorder at a time when an accurate diagnosis followed by proper therapy would almost certainly have been curative.

Etiology, Morphology, Growth, and Metabolism

R. rickettsii, the etiologic agent of RMSF, consists of small coccobacillary microorganisms measuring 0.3 to 0.5 μm in diameter and 0.3 to 4 μm in length. They usually occur singly but also may appear in strands. The most typical stained form is a diplobacillus with slightly pointed ends and a transparent band between the two bacilli. Electron microscopy reveals a two-layered cell wall and a cytoplasmic membrane. The chemical composition of rickettsiae is similar to that of gram-negative bacteria. Rickettsiae must penetrate into living cells to grow and multiply. They are grown most readily in the yolk sacs of embryonated eggs, but under special conditions, they also grow well in certain tissue culture cells. Once inside, rickettsial cells multiply by transverse binary fission.

Rickettsiae remain viable for several days in blood at +4° C (+39° F). Hence, a sample of blood taken early from a

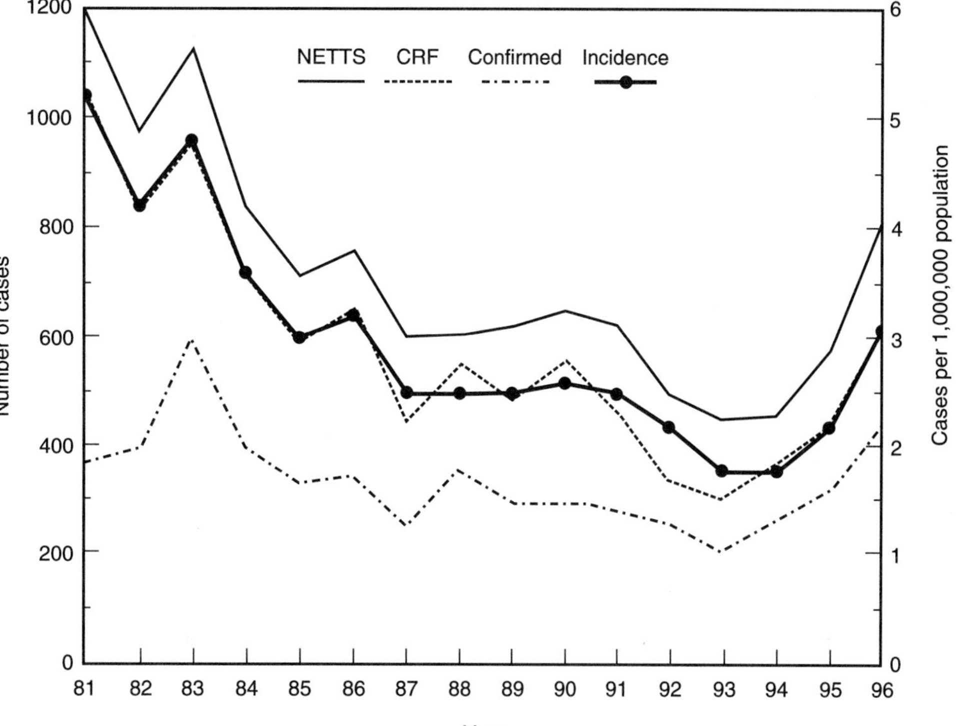

FIGURE 195–1 ■ Number and incidence of Rocky Mountain spotted fever per million population in the United States, 1981 to 1996. (Data from Treadwell, T. A., Holman, R. C., Clarke, M. J., et al.: Rocky Mountain spotted fever in the United States, 1993–1996. Am. J. Trop. Med. Hyg. *63*:21–26, 2000.)

patient with suspected rickettsial disease can be held for a day or more in a refrigerator, pending isolation procedures.

Rickettsiae take on a characteristic red color when stained with Gimenez stain. *R. rickettsii* organisms possess a soluble antigenic moiety that is shared with all their antigenic variants in the spotted fever group, as well as with rickettsialpox. Living *R. rickettsii* organisms contain a toxin; when these organisms are injected intravenously, mice die within 6 to 12 hours, long before significant multiplication has occurred.

Epidemiology and Transmission

Because RMSF rickettsiae are primarily parasites of ticks, the epidemiology of human disease is intimately associated

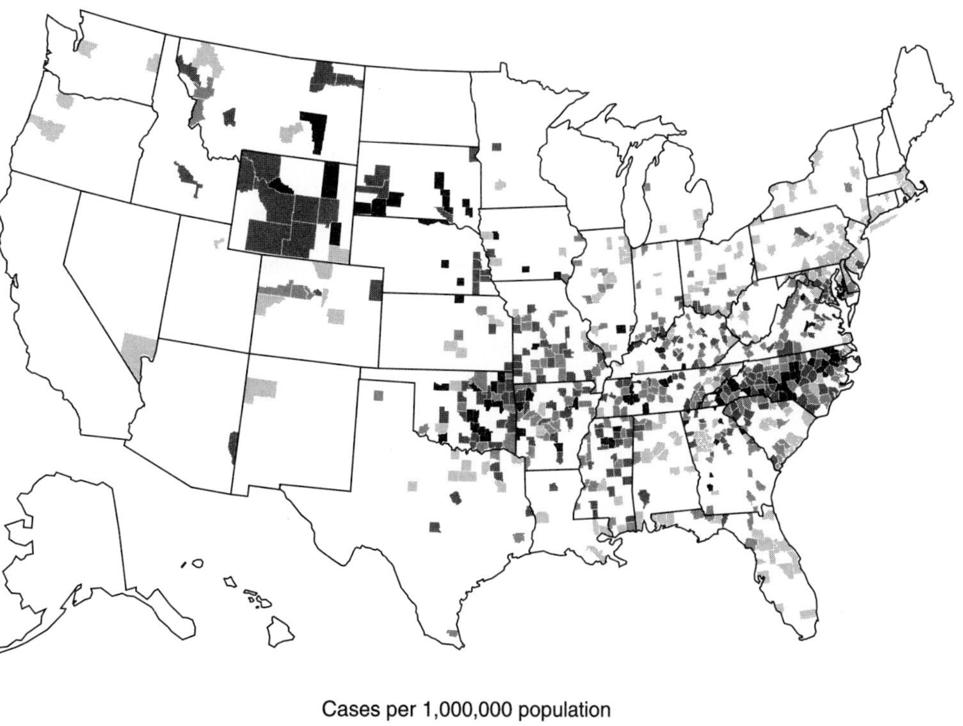

FIGURE 195–2 ■ Average annual incidence of Rocky Mountain spotted fever per million population by county in the United States, 1993–1996, based on reports from the National Electronic Telecommunications System for Surveillance (NETTS) and case report forms (CRF) submitted to the Centers for Disease Control and Prevention. (Data from Treadwell, T. A., Holman, R. C., Clarke, M. J., et al.: Rocky Mountain spotted fever in the United States, 1993–1996. Am. J. Trop. Med. Hyg. *63*:21–26, 2000.)

with the biology of the ticks that transmit it. Disease may be acquired in the laboratory, and workers must comply with protective measures. RMSF has been transmitted by blood transfusion[46] and by the aerosol route.[18, 26]

The wood tick (*Dermacentor andersoni*) in the west, the dog tick (*Dermacentor variabilis*) in the east, and the Lone Star tick (*Amblyomma americanum*) in the southwest are natural carriers and vectors of the disease. RMSF rickettsiae do not kill their arthropod hosts but are passed transovarially through unending generations of ticks. Congenitally acquired rickettsiae in tick eggs can persist through the larval and nymphal stages and finally to the adult stage over a 2-year cycle; infected adults have been shown to survive for as long as 4 years without feeding.

The ticks require only three blood meals during a lifetime: just before molting from larva to nymph, again before molting from nymph to adult, and during copulation as adults before the female lays eggs. The larval and nymphal stages of the tick feed on a small mammal to proceed to the next stage. Adult females generally obtain their blood meal from a large domestic animal, such as a dog, sheep, or horse, and are the only stage of tick that feeds on humans.

A study in Maryland and Virginia in the late 1960s showed that 15 different mammals, including field mice, and 18 types of birds can be intermediate hosts. Many small wild animals as well as dogs possess antibodies to RMSF, which indicates that they may be involved in promoting infection in the tick-mammal-tick cycle. Mammals act as the all-important blood meal source for the ticks during their various metamorphoses. Still, the exact importance of these mammals in maintaining or increasing infection in the RMSF cycle is not clear because ticks themselves are reservoirs of the disease.[38]

Dogs have long been suspected of being an important link in the RMSF cycle in nature. Between 1975 and 1977 on Cape Cod, rickettsial strains were isolated for the first time from the blood of sick or dying dogs; the five rickettsial strains isolated appear to be closely antigenically related to or are identical to *R. rickettsii,* which causes RMSF disease in humans. In addition, rising titers of RMSF antibodies have been demonstrated in more than 30 clinically ill dogs. Dogs appear to be susceptible to virulent *R. rickettsii* organisms.

However, the epidemiology of RMSF in dogs is complicated by the fact that many dogs have residual RMSF antibodies without any history of previous illness and, at least on Cape Cod, less than 1 percent of ticks examined appeared to be infected with rickettsial-like organisms.

Moreover, all but a few of these rickettsiae found in ticks appear to be antigenically distinct from the rickettsiae isolated from both sick dogs and humans. The data presently available do not clarify the role of dogs in the RMSF cycle. Dogs may be accidental hosts of RMSF rickettsiae, much as humans are, they may mechanically transport ticks from infected tick islands to the proximity of humans, or they may play an important role in maintaining or increasing the reservoir of virulent *R. rickettsii* in nature.

The decline of RMSF in the west to fewer than 20 cases a year and its increased incidence in the east have been discussed; neither of these phenomena has been explained satisfactorily, although numerous hypotheses have been proposed.

Three additional prominent epidemiologic features of RMSF are (1) its seasonal character—most cases occur during the period of greatest tick activity, from April to September; (2) the fact that approximately two thirds of cases in the United States occur in children younger than 15 years[38]; and (3) its focal nature—relatively small areas in a state may account for a high percentage of that state's recorded RMSF cases. For example, 89 percent or more of all cases of RMSF occurring in New York State are reported from Long Island, Clermont County in Ohio reports approximately 10 percent of all Ohio cases of RMSF, and Cape Cod and the offshore islands generally account for almost all the cases reported in Massachusetts.

Pathogenesis

The primary pathologic lesion of RMSF is found in the vascular system after the bite of an infected tick. Rickettsiae multiply in the endothelial cells lining small blood vessels and become widely disseminated by way of the bloodstream. They can be demonstrated in both the cytoplasm and the nucleus of cells.[38] Focal areas of endothelial proliferation and perivascular mononuclear cell infiltration lead to thrombosis and leakage of red blood cells into the surrounding tissues. Numerous mechanisms of cellular injury have been postulated, including (1) injury to cell membranes caused by the penetration of multiple rickettsiae, followed by a crescendo of rickettsial release; (2) depletion of adenosine 5′-triphosphate by intracellular rickettsiae, which causes failure of the sodium pump and an influx of water; (3) competition by *R. rickettsii* for crucial metabolic substrates; and (4) damage to the cell by toxic products of rickettsial metabolism.[42, 45, 48]

Vascular lesions appear to account for the more prominent clinical manifestations, such as rash, headache, and mental confusion, as well as terminal heart failure and shock. Vascular lesions can be found everywhere but are most readily appreciated in the skin, gonads, and adrenal glands. Parenchymatous inflammation accompanies vasculitis in the heart and central nervous system. Interstitial myocarditis, patchy in distribution, can be demonstrated regularly in fatal cases. The location of rickettsiae by immunofluorescence coincides with the patchy distribution of the myocarditis. Pathologic examination reveals interstitial edema and inflammation with relative preservation of myocardial fibers.[44] In the neural parenchyma itself, both mononuclear infiltration and focal proliferative glial nodules are usually topographically related to inflamed blood vessels.[11] In the kidney, inflammation involves both vessels and the interstitium in most patients. Acute tubular necrosis occurs. In one study, immunofluorescence failed to demonstrate immune complex deposition, which suggests that the pathologic renal lesions in RMSF are not immune mediated.[5] In the lung, rickettsial involvement of the pulmonary microcirculation results in interstitial pneumonia, as evidenced by alveolar septal congestion and interstitial edema, alveolar edema and hemorrhage with a fibrinous and mononuclear exudate, and interlobular septal edema. Organisms can be demonstrated in the pulmonary microcirculation by direct immunofluorescence, which indicates that the pathologic changes are most likely caused by direct infection rather than a circulating toxin. Hepatic lesions found to be statistically significant, when compared with age- and sex-matched controls, were portal triaditis consisting of polymorphonuclear leukocytes and large mononuclear cells, portal vasculitis, sinusoidal leukocytosis, erythrophagocytosis by Kupffer cells, and increased hepatic weight. Again, via immunofluorescence microscopy, rickettsial organisms were demonstrated in portal blood vessels and sinusoidal lining cells.[17, 28]

More recent data have added significantly to our understanding of the pathophysiology of this disease. Negative nitrogen balance may be extreme. Early in infection, it may be related to excretion of nitrogen in urine, but after several days, it is related to insufficient protein intake. The serum albumin concentration may be depressed as a result of protein loss, hepatic dysfunction related to the disease process itself, and leakage of protein through the damaged endothelium of the blood vessel walls.

Profound hyponatremia occurs commonly, and studies by Liu and associates[23] suggest that it is related to several factors, including (1) a shift in water from the intracellular to the extracellular space, (2) loss of sodium via excretion in urine, and (3) an exchange of sodium for potassium at the cellular level. Intracellular sodium increases slightly. Destruction of some cells results in increased serum concentrations of potassium and massive losses of potassium in urine. Intracellular overhydration of the medulla oblongata also has been suggested as a contributing factor in some patients who suffer a cerebral death. Plasma concentrations of aldosterone and antidiuretic hormone have been increased in some persons with this disease, but they have been normal in others.[20, 32]

Clinical Manifestations

Fever, headache, rash, toxicity, mental confusion, and myalgia are the major clinical features of RMSF.[38]

The onset of the disease in humans, which usually occurs 2 to 8 days after a bite by an infected tick, may be either gradual or abrupt. The temperature rises rapidly to 40° C or 40.6° C (104° F or 105° F). Although the pattern of fever may remain persistently high, a considerable number of patients show dramatic temperature oscillations of 1.8° C to 2.8° C (3° F to 6° F) over a period of a few hours.

The rash associated with RMSF is an important pathognomonic feature of the disease; it appears by the second or third day in most patients, but occasionally it may be delayed until the sixth day or later. Characteristically, the initial lesions are small erythematous macules that blanch on pressure. These lesions rapidly become maculopapular and petechial and later, in untreated patients, may even become confluently hemorrhagic. Rarely, they progress to massive skin necrosis.[14]

Usually, the rash first appears peripherally on the wrists and ankles and, within a few hours, spreads up the extremities to the trunk. An especially diagnostic feature of the rash of RMSF is its regular occurrence on the palms and soles. Eschars, which are characteristic of other rickettsial diseases, have been reported with RMSF rarely.[39] On occasion, RMSF may be "spotless" or "almost spotless."[33] The absence of a rash should not delay the institution of appropriate therapy if the historical and clinical features suggest a diagnosis of RMSF.[13, 29]

The headache in adults and older children is characteristic. It is intense, persistent night and day, and intractable to all efforts at alleviation. However, young children may not complain of headaches. Toxicity is a salient feature of the disease. Signs of meningoencephalitis are common; the patient is restless, irritable, and apprehensive, and this stage may progress rapidly to mental confusion and delirium. Children may become comatose. Meningismus is not always accompanied by abnormalities in cerebrospinal fluid. In fact, cerebrospinal fluid is generally clear, with minor elevations in the lymphocyte count ($<10/mm^3$). A case of eosinophilic meningitis caused by RMSF has been reported.[8] Grand mal or focal seizures may be noted. Cortical blindness and central deafness (transient or persistent) also have been reported.[4] Other forms of neurologic involvement may include ataxia, spastic paralysis, and sixth nerve palsy. These signs and symptoms are usually short lived but may persist beyond the period of hospitalization.[12, 38] RMSF exerts a mild, but consistent effect on intellectual functioning,[14] which in turn suggests a higher probability of learning disability and a corresponding difficulty with school performance in children who previously had RMSF.[50]

Cardiac involvement occurs frequently in RMSF. Close observation and evaluation with an electrocardiogram, echocardiogram, and chest radiograph are indicated. Congestive heart failure and arrhythmias are common.[24]

Pulmonary involvement occurs in 10 to 40 percent of reported cases and is manifested as rales, abnormal chest radiograph, or abnormal arterial blood gas measurements. The chest radiograph may show focal infiltrates or pulmonary edema and cardiomegaly.[9, 25]

Myalgia or muscle tenderness is a common feature. Characteristically, the patient complains bitterly when the calf or thigh muscles are squeezed.

Ocular manifestations occur most commonly in the retina and include venous engorgement, retinal edema, papilledema, cotton-wool spots, retinal hemorrhage, and retinal artery occlusion. One patient has been reported with severe anterior segment uveitis and an iris nodule, presumed to be due to the widespread vasculitic process that occurs in RMSF.[10]

Other signs include edema of the extremities or face, a stiff neck, and conjunctival suffusion. Enlargement of the spleen or liver occurs relatively infrequently, yet gastrointestinal symptoms and signs are common during the early course of RMSF. In one series of 131 patients, 56 percent reported nausea or vomiting, 34 percent reported abdominal pain, and 20 percent reported diarrhea at the initial visit for medical care. Jaundice also has occurred with RMSF.[41]

As noted with other rickettsial diseases but not adequately explained, patients with glucose-6-phosphate dehydrogenase deficiency appear to account for a disproportionate number of those who die of RMSF.[40]

Diagnosis

No laboratory test is available to quickly establish the diagnosis of RMSF early in the course of illness. Specific treatment must be initiated promptly; it is imperative that physicians recognize that they must make a clinical diagnosis based almost solely on symptoms, signs, and epidemiologic considerations. *R. rickettsii* may be identified by fluorescent or peroxidase-tagged antibody testing of a skin specimen obtained by biopsy.[47, 49] Such testing may be a practical means of confirming the diagnosis during the early stages of illness before positive serologic reactions can be obtained. In one series, 9 of 17 cases of RMSF were diagnosed by immunofluorescence, with no false-negative results in these patients. Once should recognize, however, that an experienced rickettsiologist is usually required to interpret the biopsy specimen and that false-negative results may occur. Under optimal conditions, these tests are moderately sensitive (≥70%) and extremely specific (100%).[2, 22] Significant serologic data rarely become available before the 10th to 12th day of illness, by which time most of the 20 percent of patients who will die if untreated are already moribund or dead.

A few laboratory data may give helpful clues to the diagnostician. For example, for the first 4 or 5 days after onset, the white blood cell count is normal or shows leukopenia (an uncommon feature of severe bacterial infection). As the disease progresses, secondary bacterial infections supervene, and leukocyte counts may rise to anywhere between 11,000 and 30,000 cells/mm^3.

Thrombocytopenia of varying severity develops in most cases, as with other severe infections.[30] Studies suggest that the adherence of platelets to the surface of *Rickettsia*-infected endothelial cells contributes to the reduction in the number of circulating platelets. Frequent monitoring for this development is critical because severe and unrecognized thrombocytopenia may lead to a fatal outcome despite adequate specific antibiotic therapy.[34]

An additional hemostatic abnormality is the occurrence of an acquired coagulation inhibitor in association with RMSF. Acquired inhibitors also may accompany other infectious illnesses in children.[31]

The diagnosis can be established by demonstrating a fourfold or greater change in titer between acute and convalescent sera by one of a number of rickettsial group–specific serologic tests. Tests available include enzyme immunoassay (EIA), indirect immunofluorescence antibody (IFA), latex agglutination, indirect hemagglutination (IHA), microagglutination, and complement-fixation tests. The most sensitive and specific of these tests are EIA, IHA, and IFA. An interval of 7 to 10 days after the onset of illness is required before an antibody response is detectable; on occasion, arriving at a probable diagnosis from a single high-titer convalescent serum specimen is necessary. A single serum titer of 1:64 or greater by IFA, 1:128 or greater by IHA, latex agglutination, or microagglutination, or 1:16 by complement fixation in convalescent serum constitutes a probable diagnosis. The Weil-Felix serologic test is insensitive and nonspecific, and it should no longer be used as a diagnostic tool for rickettsial infections.[3]

A microtiter enzyme-linked immunosorbent assay (ELISA) was developed to characterize the IgM and IgG response in RMSF. It is highly sensitive and accurate. However, as with other tests, the value of ELISA in rapid diagnosis is limited because IgG and IgM seroconversion cannot be demonstrated until 6 days after the onset of illness. These tests may be useful in seroepidemiologic studies.[19]

A polymerase chain reaction (PCR) assay has been developed that enables detection of specific sequences of DNA at the theoretic limit of one molecule and, therefore, one organism. A known pair of primers permits the detection of a common sequence found in the genome of *R. rickettsii, Rickettsia prowazekii,* and *Rickettsia typhi.* It is therefore a specific and useful screening and diagnostic tool for the most common rickettsial illnesses in the United States. The test can detect as few as 30 organisms per sample, takes approximately 48 hours to complete, and enables therapeutic intervention during the acute illness.[6]

With use of the specific complement-fixation or IFA tests for diagnosis, extensive cross-reactions are observed between *R. rickettsii* and *Rickettsia conorii.* Differences in titer and less cross-reactivity with the murine typhus group make distinction possible. If the geographic origin of the infection is known or if IFA is used, the disease can be distinguished as RMSF or Mediterranean spotted fever.[15]

Differential Diagnosis

Measles and meningococcemia are the disorders for which RMSF is most frequently mistaken. However, a petechial rash that involves the palms and soles and spreads centripetally is unlike true or modified measles. A centripetally spreading rash, however, may be seen in the atypical measles syndrome. Thus, a careful history of previous measles immunization, particularly with killed vaccine, should be obtained. Meningococcemia can be a more difficult problem; early in both diseases, a normal or low leukocyte count, signs of meningeal irritation, and moderate cerebrospinal fluid pleocytosis may be present. An inability to definitively differentiate RMSF from meningococcemia cannot be allowed to delay antimicrobial therapy because both diseases are potentially fulminating and fatal infections. Treatment should be initiated promptly with one of the tetracyclines or chloramphenicol, as well as with penicillin G (as for meningococcal infection). When the diagnosis is certain, use of the inappropriate drug can be discontinued.

Other febrile illnesses that can be considered in the differential diagnosis include typhoid fever, leptospirosis, rubella, scarlet fever, disseminated gonococcal disease, infectious mononucleosis, secondary syphilis, rheumatic fever, enteroviral infection, immune thrombocytopenic purpura, thrombotic thrombocytopenic purpura, immune complex vasculitis, hypersensitivity reactions to drugs, murine typhus, rickettsialpox, recrudescent typhus, and sylvatic *R. prowazekii* infection, which is enzootic in flying squirrels.[38]

Treatment

GENERAL CONSIDERATIONS FOR THE TREATMENT OF ALL RICKETTSIAL DISEASES

The rickettsial diseases, especially RMSF, louse-borne typhus, and scrub typhus, are potentially fatal infections for which specific therapy is available.

Adequate antibiotic treatment is highly effective, so patients who are treated during the first week of illness almost invariably improve promptly. On the other hand, if the disease is allowed to proceed into the second week untreated, even optimal therapy becomes progressively less effective.

SPECIFIC TREATMENT

Because rickettsial diseases—particularly RMSF—can be fulminant, initiation of prompt and optimal specific therapy is important. Initiation of treatment before the fifth day of illness optimizes the likelihood of a good outcome.

Doxycycline is the drug of choice. Although tetracyclines should not generally be used in children younger than 8 years, the rationale for their use in this setting is severalfold: (1) staining of teeth by tetracycline is dose related and unlikely to occur in association with one or two short courses of therapy; (2) doxycycline is less likely to stain developing teeth than the other tetracyclines are, possibly because it binds less to calcium; (3) doxycycline is also the treatment of choice for ehrlichiosis, which can be confused clinically with RMSF.[1] Chloramphenicol, formerly recommended for the treatment of RMSF, may be less effective than tetracyclines and may not be effective against ehrlichiosis.[3] The fluoroquinolones are a potential therapeutic option for RMSF, but their efficacy in human disease has not been established.[35]

For children weighing less than 45 kg, the dosage of doxycycline is 2 mg/kg orally or intravenously twice daily on the first day of treatment and once or twice daily thereafter. Older children should receive 100 mg twice daily on the first day and once or twice daily thereafter.

Treatment can be terminated 2 or 3 days after the temperature returns to normal for a full 24-hour period. The usual course is 7 to 10 days. (For scrub typhus, sporadic late doses are given to prevent relapse.)

The thrombocytopenia and blood coagulation deficiencies that frequently develop in RMSF often signal the danger of disseminated intravascular coagulation. Initiation of prompt, adequate antimicrobial therapy is the first essential step. Severe thrombocytopenia may be treated with concentrates of platelets prepared from freshly drawn blood.

Because of the widespread endothelial damage that occurs in severe rickettsial infection, a severely ill patient may be even more desperately ill than is apparent. Providing supportive care to the patient is important. Careful sequential evaluation of serum and urine electrolytes, renal function, and body weight is essential for planning and guiding fluid therapy. Hyponatremia is most frequently best managed by providing maintenance fluids (1500 mL/m^2/day) or by instituting modest fluid restriction. Administration of sodium-rich fluids generally precipitates cardiac decompensation and pulmonary edema without substantially raising the serum sodium concentration. Patients who are hypotensive and concomitantly hypoalbuminemic may be helped by the administration of albumin (1 g/kg immediately). When the clotting time is prolonged in patients without disseminated intravascular coagulation, administration of vitamin K may be helpful. Marked anemia may require blood transfusion.

Prognosis

Before the advent of specific therapy, the overall mortality rate from RMSF was approximately 25 percent. Today, if appropriate antimicrobials are provided before the end of the first week of illness, recovery is the rule. Nevertheless, the overall mortality rate from RMSF in the United States still hovers between 5 and 7 percent; death occurs primarily in patients in whom the diagnosis is delayed until the second week of illness. When death occurs (usually between the 9th and 12th day of illness), vascular collapse, thrombocytopenia, and renal or heart failure, alone or in combination, are noted. Central nervous system involvement and disseminated intravascular clotting commonly occur.

Complications are uncommon, especially if patients receive treatment. Bronchopneumonia may develop in seriously ill patients, and overzealous administration of parenteral fluid may precipitate cardiac failure. The disease is usually mild in immunized persons. Solid immunity follows recovery from RMSF, even if therapy is begun as early as a day or two after onset.

Prevention

Two major preventive measures are effective: personal avoidance or reduction in tick contact and the use of killed vaccines.

Personal measures for reducing the amount of contact with ticks when in infected areas can be highly effective. Wearing pants tucked into boots, limiting access to exposed skin around the neck and wrists, and frequent inspection for ticks reaching these areas are important means of reducing contact. Early deticking is particularly valuable because infected ticks must be attached and feeding for 4 to 6 or more hours before they can transmit the disease. These facts should be emphasized in preventive education programs, particularly in geographic areas where the disease is endemic. The application of repellents such as dimethyl phthalate to clothes and exposed parts of the body affords additional protection.

Killed vaccines have proved to be valuable in preventing deaths, although they do not always protect against acquisition of the disease. The original vaccine was prepared in 1924 by Parker and Spence. They crushed ticks in phenol and injected a suspension of this product. Several years later, in 1938, a yolk sac–derived vaccine was developed, commercial distribution of which began in 1948. Neither vaccine conferred immunity in humans, and the latter vaccine was subsequently withdrawn from the market in the United States. A chicken embryo vaccine was then developed.[21] This vaccine was safe in the 52 volunteers vaccinated, and two doses elicited low levels of antibodies to *R. rickettsii* in 50 percent of the vaccinees.[7]

Although this vaccine provided only partial protection against RMSF, it ameliorated the illness when it did occur. Because an attack of RMSF imparts solid immunity, vaccination with attenuated living strains of *R. rickettsii* or other live, but less pathogenic rickettsiae has been suggested as a means to provide broader and more durable immunity than that afforded by killed vaccines.[43] A cell culture vaccine was tested but failed to protect vaccinated volunteers when they were challenged.[38]

Control of ticks in the field with permethrin, a product with little toxicity for humans and other mammals but toxic to tick larvae and nymphs, is costly and not practical on a long-term basis.[16]

MEDITERRANEAN SPOTTED FEVER

This disease was first described by Connor in 1910 and is a tick-borne infection caused by *R. conorii*. In September 1932 at the First International Congress of Mediterranean Hygiene, the name Mediterranean spotted fever was adopted. Other names given to this illness include boutonneuse fever, Kenya tickbite fever, African tick typhus, India tick typhus, Israeli spotted fever, and Marseilles fever. A resurgence of this disease has been reported, especially in Mediterranean countries such as Spain, Italy, and Israel.[57, 60]

Epidemiology

R. conorii is an obligate intracellular parasite of mites, which inoculate the microorganism directly into the dermis during feeding. In the Mediterranean area, the vector is the brown dog tick *Rhipicephalus sanguineus,* but other species of mites (*Hyalomma, Ixodes, Haemaphysalis*) may act as vectors in other geographic areas.[60]

Rickettsiae are widespread in ticks and can parasitize many organs, including the ovaries. The tendency of these parasites to invade not only the cytoplasm but also the nuclei of cells explains why they eventually may be transmitted transovarially. These vectors constitute a reservoir of infection. *R. conorii* can be identified in ticks by use of optical microscopy with Gimenez and Stamp staining or by immunofluorescence.

The epidemiologic pattern of Mediterranean spotted fever is determined by the biology of the tick, and consequently, a consistent seasonal peak occurs from late June to mid-October. The natural cycle of the tick-borne rickettsiae may include dogs, wild rodents, and birds. Humans are introduced into the cycle accidentally and become a dead end in the transmission chain. Habitual contact with dogs appears to be the most common factor in people who acquire the infection. Occasionally, the disease develops after defleaing a dog or from bites by ticks that are found on the ground.[64]

The exact prevalence of the disease is unknown. The incidence seems to be rising, however, perhaps because of an increase in recognition of the infection, an increase in the number of dogs in urban areas, and possibly weather conditions such as the serious droughts that have occurred in the Mediterranean region.[58]

Mediterranean spotted fever occurs in all age groups of both sexes. The incidence in certain occupational subgroups can be reduced through better standards of hygiene.[57]

Clinical Manifestations

The infecting bite passes unnoticed in most cases, and the incubation period varies from 6 to 10 days. The primary lesion, tache noire (black spot), was described and named by Pieri in 1925.[67] It develops at the site of the tick bite, is not painful, and is rarely pruritic. The lesion becomes necrotic at its center, an eschar develops, and enlargement of the regional lymph glands occurs. The initial lesion heals slowly and clears after 10 to 20 days without scarring. Discrete residual pigmentation can remain indefinitely.[52]

The tache noire is pathognomonic but not always present, with reported incidence rates varying from 30 to 90 percent. Instances of multiple ulcers have been reported occasionally. The lesion appears to be the result of a combination of a substance secreted by the tick and another of rickettsial origin; it is not produced by a separate bite of an uninfected tick or by experimental inoculation of *R. conorii*. An inflammatory infiltrate, predominantly mononuclear, accumulates at the site of the tache noire and suggests the importance of T-cell–mediated immunity in local host defense.

The tache noire is localized predominantly on the head of children and on the legs of adults. Rickettsiae may be inoculated by scratching, as well as by the conjunctival route.

The onset of disease is usually abrupt, with severe headache, malaise, and fever that reaches temperatures of 39° C to 40° C (102.2° F to 104° F) within the first 2 or 3 days. The fever continues for 6 to 12 days, but antibiotics can shorten the febrile period. Generalized myalgia, especially of the leg muscles, is a prominent feature. Myositis can be demonstrated by electromyography and muscle biopsy, although performance of these tests is usually unnecessary.[65]

The cutaneous features are almost universally present and are helpful diagnostically. The rash usually develops on the third, fourth, or fifth febrile day. The initial lesions appear on the extremities; after 24 to 36 hours, the rash spreads to the trunk, neck, face, buttocks, palms, and soles. The first lesions are macular, pink, and irregularly defined but become maculopapular after a few hours. They generally measure 1 to 4 mm in diameter. The rash persists for 10 to 20 days after the remission of clinical symptoms. It may become purpuric or intensely pruritic, or it may be absent. Atypical cutaneous manifestations such as nodular lesions or maculoerythematous lesions resembling the rash of murine typhus develop in a few patients.[52, 57]

The cutaneous manifestations are caused by involvement of the vascular structures of the dermis. Rickettsemia during the incubation period probably seeds the endothelial cells of the capillaries, arterioles, and venules. The vasculitis produced is much like that seen in RMSF. It gradually disappears during convalescence, and as the maculopapules fade, a brown discoloration of the skin may be noticed.

Cardiovascular and respiratory changes are transient and nonspecific. Bradycardia is the most consistent finding, but other dysrhythmias have been reported. In more seriously ill patients, pericarditis, heart failure, and myocarditis have developed.

Phlebitis of the lower limbs is the main vascular complication. Venous thrombosis is a recognized complication, and pregnant patients are particularly prone to venous thrombosis. Pneumonitis, pleuritis, pleuropericarditis, and adult respiratory distress syndrome have been described in association with Mediterranean spotted fever.

In addition to the headache that is characteristic of rickettsial illnesses, varying degrees of impaired consciousness may occur. Rarely, stupor, delirium, convulsions, and transient hypoacusis may be noted. Neurologic sequelae have been observed after rickettsial encephalitis.

Renal function is not altered in most cases, although nephritis with acute renal failure has occurred occasionally. The liver is palpable in a third of patients, and the spleen may be enlarged in 20 percent of children. Tests of hepatic function reveal an increase in serum transaminase levels in more than half of cases. Alkaline phosphatase levels are elevated in one third of patients. Needle biopsy of the liver reveals foci of hepatocellular necrosis and a predominantly mononuclear reaction to the necrosis at sites of infection by *R. conorii*. The lesion differs from a true granuloma in that it is not an aggregate of epithelioid macrophages.[68]

A variety of other systemic symptoms may occur. Photophobia and bilateral conjunctivitis have been reported. Severe unilateral conjunctivitis suggests transmission of the disease via the conjunctival route. Uveitis, choroiditis, retinal artery occlusion, and neuroretinitis are uncommon ocular disturbances.[51, 56]

Hematologic abnormalities include isolated cases of autoimmune anemia and mixed cryoglobulinemia associated with Mediterranean spotted fever. Some studies report a high incidence of hypoproteinemia. At least two cases of leukocytoclastic vasculitis secondary to infection with *R. conorii* have been described.[55, 57]

On occasion, Mediterranean spotted fever may take a malignant, rapidly fatal course, even in previously healthy children. The illness is consistent with a widespread vasculitis characterized by irreversible shock, encephalopathy, disseminated intravascular coagulopathy, and renal failure.[70]

Diagnosis

If biopsy is performed early in the course of disease, rickettsial organisms can be detected by immunofluorescence or by restriction fragment length polymorphism analysis of a PCR product from the tache noire.[69] *R. conorii* cannot be isolated from blood cultures by routine laboratory procedures. The clinical findings, geographic location, and epidemiologic considerations help establish the diagnosis. Laboratory diagnosis is an important adjunct and involves serologic identification of serum antibody.[63]

Complement-fixation, microagglutination, Western blot, and indirect IFA tests are available. Identification of specific IgM by immunofluorescence helps differentiate acute infection from a carrier state. Some patients with proven Mediterranean spotted fever treated early with antibiotics have normal IgM levels, however. One latex agglutination test for detection of antibodies to *R. conorii* is both sensitive and specific. It is simpler and more rapid to perform than microimmunofluorescence/immunoglobulin and can be performed in laboratories without specially trained personnel or sophisticated equipment.[54, 57, 61, 66]

Differential Diagnosis

Before the rash appears, differentiating Mediterranean spotted fever from other acute infections is difficult. Even after appearance of the rash, the disease can be confused with measles, meningococcemia, secondary syphilis, and leukocytoclastic angiitis. Other rickettsial diseases should be considered, especially in the absence of a tache noire. Cross-reactions among rickettsiae occur with indirect immunofluorescence. Differentiation from typhoid fever is possible when agglutinins develop against antigens of typhoid or paratyphoid bacilli.

Treatment and Prevention

Mediterranean spotted fever generally runs a benign course, and fatalities are rare. Doxycycline is the drug of choice. Successful treatment also has been achieved with tetracycline, chloramphenicol, and ciprofloxacin.[53] The optimal duration of specific therapy has not been definitively established, and different antibiotic regimens ranging from single doses to treatment for up to 15 days have been reported.[59]

The major effective methods of control involve avoidance of tick bites. Natural immunity occurs after infection, and specific antibodies have been shown to persist for as long as 4 years after acute illness. Effective vaccines are not available.[62]

OTHER TICK TYPHUS FEVERS

Three other antigenically distinct diseases are Siberian tick typhus, Queensland tick typhus, and Oriental spotted fever. The etiologic agents share the same antigen with *R. rickettsii* but have distinguishing type-specific antigens demonstrated by complement-fixation and neutralization tests. Siberian tick typhus has been diagnosed throughout central Asia, Queensland tick typhus occurs in eastern Australia, and Oriental spotted fever is found in Japan.[37]

Dogs are the principal mammalian reservoir; ticks also act as reservoirs by virtue of transovarial transmission. These diseases have similar clinical, pathologic, and epidemiologic patterns. They produce a mild disease, similar to that of Mediterranean spotted fever. As in RMSF, patients with glucose-6-phosphate dehydrogenase deficiency are suggested to be at risk for more severe complications from these diseases. This susceptibility becomes an important factor in areas of the world with a high incidence of glucose-6-phosphate dehydrogenase deficiency.[71]

Treatment is similar to that for RMSF.

Rickettsialpox

First recognized in New York City in 1946, rickettsialpox is a benign rickettsial infection caused by *Rickettsia akari,* an organism that is antigenically related to the spotted fever group.[78, 80, 88] Certain features of the disease that distinguish rickettsialpox include transmission by a mite, an eschar at the site of the infectious mite bite, a vesiculopapular rash, and the absence of Weil-Felix agglutinins.

THE ORGANISM

The etiologic agent, *R. akari,* like that of RMSF, grows in the nucleus as well as in the cytoplasm of cells[75]; its soluble antigen cross-reacts with RMSF and the three other tick typhus rickettsiae, thus rendering it a bona fide member of the spotted fever group of organisms. However, its clinical, epidemiologic, and serologic features clearly set it apart from other diseases of the spotted fever group.

EPIDEMIOLOGY AND TRANSMISSION

Most cases of rickettsialpox in the United States have been reported from New York City. However, cases of rickettsialpox have been observed in many other cities in the northeastern portion of the United States, and what is probably the same disease has been described in Ukrainian and other former Soviet cities. In addition, a disease clinically consistent with rickettsialpox has been described in the Republic of South Africa; a typical strain of *R. akari* also has been isolated from a field mouse in Korea. The number of reported cases has declined. Whether the incidence of the disease is decreasing or the disease is simply underreported is unclear. Sporadic periodic outbreaks of this disease are described.[73]

Whereas house mice are the natural hosts of the mite transmitting rickettsialpox in the United States, commensal rats have been shown to be infected in Russia, and wild rodents are suspected of carrying the disease in South Africa. Rickettsialpox therefore may be much more prevalent worldwide than reported, and its reservoir may extend to many other wild or domestic animals than those that have been implicated thus far.

The disease has a natural cycle between the mite vector (*Liponyssoides sanguineus*) and the house mouse (*Mus musculus*). The mite passes the disease transovarially, so it is both a reservoir and vector. Humans acquire infection when a depleted supply of mouse hosts caused by reduced availability of food, poison, disease, or trapping forces infected mites to seek an alternative host, namely, people. The disease affects persons of all ages. Males and females are equally susceptible.[73, 76, 79, 80, 85]

PATHOLOGY

Because no mortality occurs, no comprehensive pathologic study is available. Biopsy studies demonstrate thrombosis and necrosis of capillaries with mononuclear cell infiltration analogous to the angiitis of the other rickettsial diseases. A skin biopsy is not usually necessary to confirm a diagnosis of rickettsialpox, although the histologic changes are sufficiently characteristic to aid in the diagnosis if a biopsy is performed.[73, 74] Organisms have not been demonstrated in skin biopsy specimens by light or electron microscopy, but they have been detected by direct fluorescent antibody testing of eschars.[82]

CLINICAL MANIFESTATIONS

The incubation period of rickettsialpox is 9 to 14 days, but it is difficult to precisely determine because most patients have continuous exposure to the vector in their home and are usually unaware of the mite bite.[87, 89]

Initially, a red papule develops at the site of the mite bite. This lesion slowly progresses through a papulovesicular stage to become a black scab or eschar at about the time of onset of the fever. Although the lesion is most often solitary, two eschars have been described in many cases.[75] Regional lymph nodes related to the primary eschar are almost invariably enlarged.

The fever is irregular; it fluctuates between 37.8° C and 39.5° C (100° F and 103° F) and rarely lasts longer than 6 or 7 days. Usually, it is accompanied by the headache characteristic of rickettsial disease. Rhinorrhea, cough, sore throat, nausea, vomiting, and abdominal pain have been reported.[75, 77, 83, 86]

The rash is the most remarkable aspect of the disease. It usually develops within several days of the onset of fever as scattered nonpruritic macules, which rapidly become firm maculopapules; within a day or two, vesicles develop on the summits of the papules. The lesions usually appear on the face, trunk, and extremities, with sparing of the palms and soles.[72] The number of lesions ranges from 5 or 6 to more than 100. The haphazard distribution of the characteristic papulovesicles is similar in appearance to chickenpox rash in an adult.

DIAGNOSIS

The diagnosis can be made serologically by either complement-fixation or immunofluorescence tests with use of either RMSF or rickettsialpox antigens. Antibodies to *R. akari* have cross-reactivity with those to *R. rickettsii*. Absorption of serum samples may be performed to distinguish a specific antibody response. Weil-Felix tests are negative because no *Proteus* agglutinins are produced.[81] Immunofluorescence of paraffin-embedded eschar material obtained by skin biopsy may be used to confirm the diagnosis.[82] The major differential diagnostic problem is adult chickenpox. Infectious mononucleosis, gonococcemia, and infection with echovirus (types 9 and 16), coxsackievirus A (types 9 and 16), or coxsackievirus B (type 5) should also be considered.[74, 84, 85] Patients often give a history of having worked in basements, around incinerators, or in similar areas that might be infested by house mice and their mites.

TREATMENT

Deaths have not been reported. Doxycycline is the drug of choice for treatment of the disease; chloramphenicol is an acceptable alternative.[73] A treatment course of 3 to 5 days is sufficient. In infants and young children with mild illness, antibiotics may be withheld because the disease is self-limited.

Typhus Group

Three diseases—louse-borne typhus, Brill-Zinsser disease, and murine flea-borne typhus—make up the typhus group. Clinically and pathologically, these three illnesses are similar; epidemiologically, they are different and are hence described under separate headings.

PRIMARY LOUSE-BORNE TYPHUS FEVER

Primary louse-borne typhus fever is an acute infectious disease transmitted to humans by the body louse. Louse-borne typhus has played a major role in the history of nations for the past 5 centuries. It has undoubtedly been more decisive than military campaigns, as Zinsser[108] has convincingly described in his book *Rats, Lice and History*.

Typhus fever occurs only in the presence of the lice, which multiply to astronomic numbers during periods of war, famine, and social upheaval. During the 19th century, epidemics occurred in Europe, Asia, Africa, and sporadically in the United States; the last recorded American epidemic occurred in Philadelphia in 1893. After World War I, more than 30 million people in eastern Europe were infected with typhus fever, and an estimated 3 million died. During World War II, louse-borne typhus again infected millions of people in prison camps, the eastern European combat zone, and North Africa. In the 1970s, tens of thousands of louse-borne typhus cases occurred in uncontrolled epidemics in Burundi and Rwanda in central Africa. In the 1980s, Ethiopia and Nigeria reported the greatest number of cases worldwide.[100] A small outbreak occurred in Russia in 1997.[102]

Since 1976, at least 30 cases of disease caused by *R. prowazekii* have been documented in the United States. They have occurred sporadically. The presumed source of infection is the flying squirrel (*Glaucomys volans*).[94, 99]

The Organism

The etiologic agent is *R. prowazekii*. Its morphologic features, growth, metabolism, toxin production, and staining characteristics are similar to those described for rickettsiae of the spotted fever group. Antigenically, the organisms of louse-borne and flea-borne (murine) typhus form a separate group, although they show some minor antigenic cross-over with the spotted fever group.

Epidemiology and Transmission

The causative agent of epidemic typhus has been assumed to exist only in the human-louse-human cycle, and patients who recovered from typhus were thought to be the reservoir of *R. prowazekii* in interepidemic periods. If such were the case, eradication of epidemic typhus would theoretically be possible because few patients with Brill-Zinsser disease would be alive after long interepidemic periods. The presence of sporadic *R. prowazekii* infection, however, suggests that perpetuation of epidemic typhus is possible because it may persist in an animal reservoir.

The chain of typhus infection starts when *R. prowazekii* appears in a patient's blood during the acute febrile infection. A louse becomes infected during one of its frequent blood meals. After 5 to 10 days of incubation in the louse, large numbers of rickettsiae appear in the louse feces. Transmission of rickettsiae from an infected louse to a new host can occur by several mechanisms. Because a louse defecates as it feeds, infected feces can be rubbed into the louse bite wound. Additionally, dried louse feces can gain access to the mucous membranes of the eye or respiratory tract. The epidemic spread of typhus throughout a community is related to the temperature preferences of the louse. Lice prefer blood meals on humans with a normal temperature; hence, they tend to leave febrile patients (as well as the dead). Crowding during wars and famine renders transfer to new hosts easy.

Pathology

The pathologic process is similar to that described for the spotted fever group of diseases.

Clinical Manifestations

From 1 to 2 weeks after the bite of an infected louse, illness usually begins abruptly. The major clinical signs and symptoms are fever, headache, and a rash. Body temperature generally rises rapidly to 40° C (104° F) or higher. In untreated patients, it remains at this level with minor fluctuations until death or recovery. The rash usually appears on the trunk by the fourth to seventh day; it spreads peripherally to the extremities and typically spares the face, palms, and soles. At first, the rash consists of macules that fade on pressure; they soon become fixed as maculopapules and later become petechial or hemorrhagic. A severe, intractable headache is a characteristic symptom. Cases of typhus fever manifested as encephalitis, meningitis, or meningoencephalitis have been reported. Severe, untreated cases can progress to prostration, stupor, or delirium with terminal myocardial and renal failure. Complications occur uncommonly but can include gangrene, parotitis, otitis media, acute pericarditis, myocarditis, pericardial effusion, pleurisy, pleural effusion, and pneumonia.[93, 106, 107]

Diagnosis

The various factors concerned with the diagnosis of louse-borne typhus are analogous to those discussed for the diagnosis of RMSF, with a few differences. The rash of louse-borne typhus begins centrally on the trunk and spreads peripherally to the extremities, whereas the reverse is true for RMSF. Moreover, a rash on the palms and soles, a common event in RMSF, is rarely observed in louse-borne typhus. Differentially, typhus usually occurs in epidemics under conditions of crowding and high louse populations.

A definitive diagnosis can be established by demonstrating a fourfold change in antibody titer between serum specimens obtained acutely and during convalescence. Several serologic methods are available, including EIA, microagglutination, and latex agglutination, but the indirect IFA test is the preferred method. Detecting rickettsia by PCR or visualization of rickettsia in tissue also may be performed to establish the diagnosis definitively. As noted in the section The Spotted Fevers, antigenic crossing between any of the members of the typhus and spotted fever groups of organisms is a common occurrence.

Treatment

Tetracycline, chloramphenicol, or a fluoroquinolone is the antimicrobial of choice. Therapy is given until the child is afebrile for 48 to 72 hours. The usual duration of therapy is 7 to 10 days.

Prognosis

Case-fatality rates in untreated cases correlate with age. The rate of mortality, an uncommon occurrence in children, is 10 percent in young adults and may run as high as 60 to 70 percent in those older than 50 years. Recovery from an attack gives rise to enduring immunity. (For exceptions, see Brill-Zinsser Disease.)

Prevention

Two highly effective measures, vaccination and louse control, are available for controlling typhus epidemics. Potent killed vaccines produced from yolk sacs grown in chick embryos have proved highly effective in preventing mortality; these vaccines do not, however, regularly prevent infection. DDT and the newer insecticides lindane and malathion have proved highly effective in reducing louse infestation during typhus epidemics. Dusting insecticides onto the clothes of louse-infested populations is effective in ridding the community of lice and curtailing louse-borne typhus epidemics.

BRILL-ZINSSER DISEASE

Brill-Zinsser disease is a relapse or recrudescence of louse-borne typhus that occurs years after the primary attack.[97] This relapsing form of typhus is in many ways analogous to a relapse of malaria. After a primary attack, the typhus rickettsiae remain dormant somewhere in the body, probably most commonly in cells of the reticuloendothelial system. Years later, they are reactivated by stress or some unknown factor to multiply and cause a second acute infection. Because of partial immunity remaining from the primary typhus attack, the recrudescent infection is almost always a milder, shorter, and less debilitating illness. The causative agent is the same as for primary louse-borne typhus; the symptoms, signs, and pathologic changes are similar to those described in the section Primary Louse-Borne Typhus Fever.

Tetracycline is the drug of choice. A single dose of doxycycline may lead to prompt resolution of clinical symptoms in selected cases.[101]

MURINE TYPHUS

Murine typhus is a disease of rats passed from rat to rat by the rat flea and only occasionally and accidentally transmitted to humans by the bite of an infected rat flea.[104] The disease occurs worldwide, primarily along coastal areas and around granaries where rats abound. During the first half of the 20th century, it was highly prevalent along the Atlantic seaboard and Gulf Coast areas. Unlike other rickettsial infections, murine typhus is often acquired in cities—hence one of its names, urban fever.[92]

The Organism

The causative organism, *R. typhi* (formerly *Rickettsia mooseri*), is similar to *R. prowazekii* in metabolism, growth, toxin production, and staining characteristics, although it is slightly smaller and more uniform in size. Because they possess a large common antigenic moiety, *R. typhi* and *R. prowazekii* are classed together in one group. A new rickettsial agent tentatively designated as the ELB agent also has been identified as a cause of murine typhus.[103]

Epidemiology and Transmission

Murine typhus is usually acquired by humans in the following manner. The rat flea *Xenopsylla cheopis* is the vector and becomes infected when feeding on an acutely ill rat. The rickettsiae multiply in the flea without causing any ill effects, but the feces of the infected flea teem with rickettsiae for the rest of the flea's life. Rat fleas prefer to feed on rats but will feed on people if rats are not available. When an infected flea sucks blood, its dejecta is teeming with rickettsiae. If the flea bites a person, the infected feces may be rubbed into the bite wound or transferred in a dried aerosol to the conjunctivae or respiratory tract. Humans are obviously not related to the maintenance of *R. typhi* in nature. However, serologic and molecular analysis suggests that the cat flea *Ctenocephalides felis*, which has a propensity to feed on humans, also may serve as a vector.[95] In California, sporadic cases have been related to transmission of *R. typhi* by fleas from opossums to humans.[90]

In the early 1940s, 2000 to 5000 cases of murine typhus were reported annually in the United States, primarily in the southeastern and Gulf Coast states. Murine typhus is not reported in many states, and only 60 to 80 cases are presently reported annually. However, the overall seroprevalence of 0.6 percent in childhood and the finding of antibody-positive children residing in Kentucky, Oklahoma, and Missouri suggest that typhus may not be confined to the Gulf Coast region.[98]

Pathology

The pathologic process is analogous to that described for the spotted fever group of organisms.

Clinical Manifestations

The incubation period ranges from 6 to 14 days. The most common clinical features are fever, which is found in all patients, and rash and headache, each observed in three fourths or more of patients. The symptoms and signs are similar to those of louse-borne typhus, the principal differences being that murine typhus is milder and shorter in duration. The classic triad of fever, headache, and rash occurs in only half of affected children.[105] The fever does not rise much above 39° C (102° F). The headache is less severe, and the maculopapular rash is both less extensive and of shorter duration. Children who receive an appropriate antibiotic undergo defervescence in 1 to 3 days; without appropriate treatment, defervescence occurs after 2 to 3 weeks.[96] Complications seldom occur, and the mortality rate is 1 percent or less.

Diagnosis

A fourfold change in titer between acute and convalescent sera by indirect IFA, latex agglutination, complement fixation, or EIA is diagnostic. Differentiating between antibodies produced in response to epidemic typhus is difficult but may be accomplished by using an IgM-specific EIA, if needed. The diagnostic tool used most recently is the PCR assay described in the RMSF section. This test, available only in research laboratories, permits confirmation of rickettsial infection in 48 hours and theoretically allows therapeutic intervention during the acute illness.[6]

Because the flea is the vector for murine typhus, epidemiologic considerations used by the physician to make a tentative diagnosis include studies of the patient's contact with rats, fleas, or both. Because murine typhus is a mild illness and the rash may be evanescent, the disease may be confused with any disease that causes a fever of unknown origin in a patient who does not generally appear to be acutely ill.

Treatment

The treatment of choice is a single dose of doxycycline. Additional effective treatment choices include other tetracyclines, chloramphenicol, or a fluoroquinolone.[91]

Prevention

Limiting the size of rat populations is the principal factor in prevention and control of murine typhus. The first step is to scatter insecticides on rat runs to reduce the flea population. Rat populations then can be reduced by poisoning, trapping, and eliminating rat harborages and by rat-proofing buildings. Such preventive measures initiated in the coastal cities of the southeastern part of the United States have reduced the incidence from more than 5000 cases immediately after World War II to only 60 to 80 cases per year.

Tsutsugamushi Disease (Scrub Typhus)

Scrub typhus is an acute infectious disease of variable severity that is transmitted to humans by certain chiggers. The focus of the disease is restricted almost exclusively to a vast and roughly triangular area in the southwest Pacific and in Southeast Asia. The points of the triangle are Japan, the Solomon Islands, and Pakistan. Patients who are seen with scrub typhus infection elsewhere almost certainly contracted their disease in this restricted triangle.

THE ORGANISM

The causative organism, *Orientia* (formerly *Rickettsia*) *tsutsugamushi,* is distinguished by remarkable antigenic heterogeneity. The marked strain differences in scrub typhus rickettsiae also appear to be related to the striking differences in severity of disease in the same or different localities. This antigenic heterogeneity also has thwarted all effort until the present to develop an effective vaccine or a generally applicable specific serologic test. A slight modification of the Gimenez method is required to stain scrub typhus rickettsiae a bright red.

EPIDEMIOLOGY AND TRANSMISSION

Trombiculid mites serve as both reservoirs and vectors, and they transmit the rickettsiae to their own progeny via infected ova. They also possibly transmit the disease to the small rodents on which they feed. Of the four stages of trombiculid mites in nature, only one, the six-legged larval form, feeds on small mammals—or people who happen to camp on or traverse the soil where the mites breed and live. All other stages of the mite are spent in the soil, where they feed on organic matter.

Because of the prolonged persistence of *O. tsutsugamushi* in the human host, fetal infection acquired transplacentally is a possibility. One examination pairing mother-cord sera in an endemic area found no serologic evidence of transplacental infection.[119] Twenty-nine percent of the mothers demonstrated serologic evidence of past infection; however, no mother was acutely infected at the time of the study. Isolation of *O. tsutsugamushi* from the placenta has not been reported in humans.

PATHOLOGY

The basic pathologic process of scrub typhus is a perivasculitis of the small blood vessels analogous to the other rickettsial diseases. In addition, an eschar or necrotic inflammatory lesion develops at the site of the mite bite, with subsequent regional lymphadenopathy similar to that caused by rickettsialpox. General lymphadenopathy occurs commonly in scrub typhus but rarely or not at all in all other rickettsial diseases.

CLINICAL MANIFESTATIONS

In more than 50 percent of cases, an initial lesion develops into a necrotic eschar. Because mites are frequently acquired when people walk through the brush, the initial lesion is commonly on a lower limb; regional lymphadenopathy almost invariably accompanies the primary lesion. The incubation period is approximately 1 to 2 weeks, and at approximately the same time that the initial mite bite lesion and eschar are noted, the main characteristic features of the disease develop—fever, headache, rash, and general lymphadenopathy. After regression of the eschar, a scar often remains and has been shown to persist for up to 25 years.[114]

A macular rash frequently appears on the trunk for only a short time, between the fifth and eighth day of illness. Less commonly, the rash persists, becomes maculopapular, and extends to the extremities. The general lymphadenopathy is especially prominent in the axilla, neck, and inguinal areas. Hepatosplenomegaly and conjunctival injection are common; deafness and tinnitus occur less commonly but are helpful diagnostic features when they do appear. Atypical pneumonia and overwhelming pneumonia resembling adult respiratory distress syndrome have been described.[110] Myocarditis and disseminated intravascular coagulation also have been reported.[116] The severity of the clinical manifestations varies widely because several different strains of *R. tsutsugamushi* exist.

DIAGNOSIS

The Weil-Felix OX-K strain agglutination reaction may be the only serologic test available in less developed countries. It can aid in confirming (in early convalescence) a tentative diagnosis made during the acute phase of the disease when specific therapy can be lifesaving. However, it is not very sensitive; OX-K agglutinins develop in only a little more than 50 percent of scrub typhus patients. Moreover, OX-K agglutinins are also produced by relapsing fever.

Immunofluorescent tests are much more diagnostic and reliable. Unfortunately, because of the multiplicity of scrub typhus strains, eight or more antigenic strains must be included in the sophisticated immunofluorescent tests for scrub typhus; these tests are available in only a few specialized laboratories.

The antibody to *O. tsutsugamushi* measured by immunofluorescence is short lived[118]; thus, the true incidence of scrub typhus in endemic areas is probably much greater than initially described. Apparently, a high immunofluorescent titer may represent repeated infections. An indirect immunoperoxidase test is now available and is sensitive, specific, and reproducible. No cross-reactivity occurs when testing against diseases other than scrub typhus. The indirect immunoperoxidase test is superior to the Weil-Felix reaction and comparable to the immunofluorescent test in the serodiagnosis of scrub typhus and seems to be a practical substitute for immunfluorescence.[111, 115] A dot immunoassay also has been applied to the serodiagnosis of scrub typhus. The results are easily interpreted by untrained personnel because the naked eye readily distinguishes the differences in intensity of color between positive and negative reactions.[117, 122]

Diagnostic methods have been developed that allow identification of the rickettsial strain in infected patients. One of them uses strain-specific monoclonal antibodies in an inhibition ELISA. In another, PCR with strain-specific primers offers a method suitable for diagnosis in the acute stage of the illness.[112, 113]

Scrub typhus can be suspected when a patient gives a history of recent exposure in a geographic area where scrub typhus occurs. If, in addition, a local eschar, evanescent rash, and general and regional lymphadenopathy along with fever, headache, and conjunctival suffusion are present, the physician should be alerted to suspect scrub typhus; however, it cannot be differentiated with certainty from dengue, leptospirosis, malaria, or typhoid fever.

TREATMENT

Both chloramphenicol and the tetracyclines are highly effective. One study demonstrated that a single 200-mg dose of doxycycline was as effective as a 7-day course of tetracycline in treating patients with scrub typhus.[109] However, in this study, therapy was not instituted until day 10 of the disease. Immunity begins to develop only during the second week of the illness. Because both chloramphenicol and doxycycline are rickettsiostatic, patients with scrub typhus who are treated in the first week of illness may require sporadic short courses of antibiotic therapy for prevention of relapse.[120, 121] Strains with reduced susceptibility to antibiotics have been observed in northern Thailand. Rifampin may offer an alternative for treatment of infection acquired in that locale.[123]

PROGNOSIS

The prognosis varies widely because of significant differences in the severity of disease caused by different strains in different populations and in various geographic areas. Mortality rates in the pre-antibiotic era varied from 1 to 60 percent. With the use of antimicrobials, fatalities rarely occur.

When treatment is begun early in the course of scrub typhus, relapses as well as definite second attacks of the disease are common.[120] The wide heterogeneity of scrub typhus strains is believed to account for the frequent reinfections that occur after scrub typhus infection; reinfections are rarely or never seen after other rickettsial diseases.

PREVENTION

Vector control involves impregnating clothing and smearing exposed skin surfaces with dimethyl or dibutyl phthalate.

Short-term vector control of camping grounds can be accomplished by cutting, burning, or bulldozing vegetation along with heavy spraying with insecticides such as dieldrin or lindane.

Chemoprophylaxis is feasible for persons with high-risk exposure for short periods. Doxycycline given once a week provides effective chemoprophylaxis against naturally transmitted scrub typhus if the prophylaxis is started before exposure to infection and continued for 6 weeks after exposure.[121] No satisfactory vaccine has been produced.

Q Fever

Q fever is an acute rickettsial infection worldwide in distribution that is characterized in humans by fever, headache, and an associated pneumonitis in more than 50 percent of cases.[152] It is unique among the human rickettsial infections in that it is primarily a disease of animals transmitted to humans by inhalation of the agent rather than by an arthropod bite.

THE ORGANISM

The Q-fever rickettsia was discovered in the late 1930s independently by Burnet and Freeman in Australia and by Cox in the United States; the rickettsia has been named *Coxiella burnetii.* The organism is distinctive among rickettsiae in being highly resistant to heat, desiccation, and chemicals. Moreover, like *R. akari,* it fails to stimulate cross-reacting *Proteus* strain agglutinins (Weil-Felix reaction).

EPIDEMIOLOGY AND TRANSMISSION

The epidemiology of Q fever differs markedly from that of the other rickettsiae. Q fever is primarily a zoonosis infecting cattle, sheep, goats, and rodents worldwide, as well as marsupials in Australia and cats in Canada.[150, 162] Humans contract the disease when and where they come in contact with infected animals or material contaminated by them.

In domestic livestock, the infection is usually inapparent and remains latent until some stress or physiologic alteration such as parturition leads to multiplication of the organism in birth tissues and excretion of rickettsiae in milk, urine, and feces.[142] At the time of parturition, the placental tissues and fluids of sheep, cattle, and goats contaminate the ground; dried dust particles containing the markedly resistant organisms can be blown about and remain potential sources of infection for many months.

Epidemics of Q fever occur in abattoirs when infected (especially pregnant) animals are slaughtered; massive contamination of workers takes place, and aerosols are created that may be carried by air-conditioning systems to infect personnel far removed from the slaughtering area.[128] Several outbreaks of Q fever have been reported in research laboratories.[132, 143] Q fever also commonly occurs in textile plants where bales of wool are processed, in tanneries, and in shearing camps, as well as in children in rural areas who are exposed at the annual spring lambing time.[133]

Infection, in most cases, is by inhalation. Ticks are a negligible factor in passing the disease to humans but appear to be an important mode of transmission of the disease to small wild rodents and to some domestic animals. Chronic Q fever in pregnancy may involve the placenta. The use of a suppressive regimen that controls the mother's placentitis may contribute to the delivery of a healthy baby.[125] At least two confirmed cases of *C. burnetii* infection in a human fetus have been reported; however, no teratogenic effects have been described. Human milk can serve as a source of infection in breast-fed babies.[154]

The prevalence of Q fever is probably underestimated. More than 40 percent of persons who have frequent contact with farm animals such as goats, cattle, and sheep were found to be seropositive for Q-fever antibodies. The disease has been diagnosed in an increasing number of children younger than 3 years and should be considered during an evaluation for fever of unknown origin.[154]

PATHOLOGY

Mortality from the disease is rare, but the pathologic process has been well defined with the use of both autopsy and biopsy specimens. *C. burnetii* has been demonstrated in lung macrophages at autopsy[161] and more recently in specimens obtained at transbronchoscopic lung biopsy.[149] Abnormalities in liver function tests, as well as the common hepatosplenomegaly, suggest disease in these organs. Liver biopsy specimens demonstrate granulomatous changes with a dense fibrin ring surrounding a lipid vacuole. Rickettsial organisms are not found in these lesions, which are highly suggestive but not pathognomonic for Q fever.[135, 148] Similar granulomata have been noted in bone marrow.[160] Valvular vegetations are seen when endocarditis complicates Q fever.[137] *Rickettsia* has been isolated from affected valves.[124, 140]

CLINICAL MANIFESTATIONS

After an incubation period of 9 to 20 days, the disease usually begins abruptly with chills, high fever, general malaise, myalgia, chest pain, and an intractable headache of the type characteristic of rickettsial disease; however, no rash is present.[155] Although physical findings in the chest are remarkably few, a radiograph reveals multiple round segmental opacities in more than 50 percent of patients. Other less common findings include pleural effusion, lobar consolidation, and linear atelectasis.[144, 146] Even though pneumonitis is one of the primary characteristics of this disease, Q fever is nonetheless a systemic disease like the other rickettsioses. Hepatitis is another common clinical form of Q fever, especially in younger patients.[152] Other findings include gastroenteritis, pericarditis, rhabdomyelitis, petechial rash, and hemolytic anemia.[129, 134, 141, 159] The disease is usually mild and self-limited and lasts only 1 or 2 weeks. The overall mortality rate is approximately 1 percent. Patients in whom chronic Q fever and endocarditis develop, however, have a mortality rate of 30 to 60 percent.[157] Other reported complications include myocarditis, pericarditis, meningoencephalitis,[131] glomerulonephritis,[158] and inappropriate secretion of antidiuretic hormone.[127]

DIAGNOSIS

EIA, complement fixation, immune adherence hemagglutination antibody tests, and immunofluorescent tests measuring anti–phase I and anti–phase II antibodies are highly efficacious in diagnosing Q fever. Anti–phase II antibody is present in early primary disease. Anti–phase I antibody is present in patients with chronic disease who have endocarditis or granulomatous hepatitis.[147] Reference or research laboratories have the capability of measuring specific IgG, IgA, or IgM antibodies by immunofluorescence or EIA methods.[136, 145]

Attempts to isolate the organism are both unnecessary and dangerous because isolation may predispose laboratory personnel to infection. PCR can be used on paraffin-embedded tissues.[151] Immunoblotting techniques also have been used in research laboratories to diagnose Q fever. Although the clinical features of Q fever are not specific, careful evaluation of epidemiologic data can be valuable in suggesting a possible Q-fever diagnosis.

The often severe and puzzling cases of myocarditis, pericarditis, or endocarditis may develop months after the original infection. In such patients, serologic tests using Q-fever antigens may reveal extremely high Q-fever antibodies, thus providing a clue to the correct diagnosis.[153]

TREATMENT

Tetracycline or doxycycline is the drug of choice for the disease, which responds promptly to the tetracyclines; relapses rarely occur. Chloramphenicol is an alternative drug. The most appropriate drug and duration of therapy for patients with endocarditis caused by Q fever are unclear. Therapy that combines doxycycline or tetracycline with a fluoroquinolone, rifampin, or trimethoprim-sulfamethoxazole has been used with varying degrees of success.[157, 163]

PROGNOSIS

The overall mortality rate from uncomplicated Q fever is approximately 1 percent. Most patients recover completely in a month or two with or without specific therapy, although antimicrobial therapy shortens the symptomatic period. In the rare instances of complications such as myocarditis, pericarditis, and especially endocarditis, permanent disability and even fatal outcomes have been reported in 30 to 60 percent of patients.[157]

IFA quantitative titers have been suggested as an aid in the prognosis of patients with Q fever. Particularly high IgM titers were found in cases of granulomatous hepatitis. IgA antibodies against phase I were found in cases of Q fever endocarditis, although patients with fatal Q fever have been shown to have few or no IgA antibodies despite high IgG and IgM titers.[130]

PREVENTION

Q-fever vaccine candidates are being investigated. Details concerning the phase variation of *C. burnetii,* as well as its genetic and antigenic stability, must be worked out, but the outlook of Q-fever immunoprophylaxis is certainly promising.[138, 139]

Controlling infected herds of economically valuable domestic animals has proved to be difficult. Instituting effective control has been stymied because the mild nature of the disease has failed to arouse public demand for control. Hence, mild Q-fever infection continues to simmer in domestic animals, and epidemics of mild human disease appear sporadically. With the advent of antimicrobial therapy, morbidity from the disease has decreased further. This decreased morbidity, in turn, additionally diminishes public pressure for developing preventive measures.

With the outbreaks of Q fever reported in research laboratories, specific control measures have been formulated. If possible, research laboratories using sheep should be separated from other laboratories. If such separation is not possible, other control measures should be instituted, including the following: (1) sheep should never be transported through a patient care area; ideally, any transport should be contained in a cart specifically designed to protect the environment from fomite and aerosol transmission; (2) all enclosed Q-fever biohazard areas should have an exhaust air ventilation system; (3) every investigator using sheep should register them as biohazards with the designated biosafety officer; (4) protective clothing should be provided for use in and around sheep research and housing areas; and (5) all personnel who come in contact with the sheep or sheep products should be identified and enrolled in a health education and medical surveillance program. The effectiveness of surveillance programs, including serologic monitoring, skin testing, and vaccination in susceptible laboratory personnel, is being investigated.[126, 156]

Ehrlichiosis

Two human tick-borne diseases caused by *Ehrlichia* spp. have been recognized in the United States since 1986. Both human monocytic ehrlichiosis (HME) and human granulocytic ehrlichiosis (HGE) are febrile illnesses characterized by headache, anorexia, and myalgia, often with associated leukopenia. Many patients have experienced tick attachment or a bite within weeks before the onset of illness. Since the initial description of human illness by Maeda and associates in 1987,[191] numerous cases in children have been reported, and the spectrum of infection has broadened considerably.

THE ORGANISMS

Members of the genus *Ehrlichia,* named after Paul Ehrlich, have been classified into three genogroups into which all previously recognized species fit.[164] One group includes *Ehrlichia chaffeensis*, the agent of HME. *Ehrlichia canis* is the most extensively studied *Ehrlichia* organism in this group because it was recognized as a cause of acute febrile illness in dogs in 1935. During the 1960s in Vietnam, the illness came to be known as tropical canine pancytopenia when a large number of trained military working dogs died with symptoms of anorexia, weight loss, and pancytopenia followed by fatal epistaxis.[205] *E. chaffeensis*, a name derived from Fort Chaffee, Arkansas, where the isolate originated, was identified in 1991 as the agent causing HME. The second group is represented by *Ehrlichia sennetsu* and *Ehrlichia risticii*. Sennetsu fever is a mononucleosis-like illness caused by *E. sennetsu* that is geographically limited to Japan and the Far East. The third group is represented by *Anaplasma* (formerly *Ehrlichia*) *phagocytophila*, a veterinary pathogen that infects the neutrophils of sheep, cattle, and deer, and by *Ehrlichia equi*, the agent of canine and equine granulocytic ehrlichiosis. HGE is caused by an *Ehrlichia* organism that is closely related to these two species, but the final species designation for the causative agent of HGE has not been determined.[166, 173] A third species, *Ehrlichia ewingii* can cause human illness also.[172]

EPIDEMIOLOGY AND TRANSMISSION

Since the initial report of human illness, more than 700 cases of HME in adults and at least 20 cases in children have been described.[168–170, 175, 178, 185, 187, 188, 190, 192, 193] Cases of ehrlichiosis have been diagnosed from every state except North Dakota and South Dakota.[194] Reported cases of HME are concentrated in the southeastern and south-central areas of the country. Illness occurs in the months when ticks are prevalent, from March to October,[183] and approximately 80 percent of the children in whom the infection is diagnosed have a history of a tick bite within the 3 weeks before the onset of symptoms.

The Lone Star tick *A. americanum* is the principal vector of HME, although alternative tick vectors such as *Dermacentor* may exist in some geographic regions. The reservoir for HME has not been clarified, but deer and livestock are the preferred hosts of *A. americanum*. Proximity to a wildlife reserve served as a risk factor for acquiring HME in one reported cluster of cases.[203]

The initial reports of HGE were from the upper Midwestern states of Wisconsin and Minnesota. Infections have been reported also from Connecticut, New York, Maryland, California, Florida, and Europe. More than 600 patients have been identified. A tick bite frequently precedes the illness, and the deer tick *Ixodes scapularis* is the principal vector in the northeastern and upper Midwestern states. The black-legged tick *Ixodes pacificus* is the primary vector in the Pacific western states. Because the predominant host of the deer tick, the white-tailed deer, has a wide geographic distribution, HGE may be more prevalent than currently documented.[168, 186, 196, 200] The tick vector for the variant HGE caused by *E. ewingii* is *A. americanum*.

Perinatal transmission of ehrlichiosis has been documented. The mother was apparently infected with the agent of HGE toward the end of her pregnancy and gave birth to a normal infant. Symptoms in both the mother and infant resolved after treatment with doxycycline.[189]

PATHOGENESIS AND PATHOLOGY

The pathogenesis of ehrlichiosis is incompletely elucidated. Though capable of establishing infection in numerous organs and tissues, the primary target cell for HGE is the granulocyte and for HME it is the macrophage. Granulomata of the bone marrow occur frequently in HME, thus suggesting that involvement of the reticuloendothelial system may be important in pathogenesis.[176]

Ehrlichia organisms enter the cytoplasm of host cells and proliferate in phagosomes into elementary bodies. These individual *Ehrlichia* organisms multiply by binary fission into immature inclusions called initial bodies. Mature groups of elementary bodies form morulae, which are released by rupture of the cell to reinitiate the infecting process.[191]

CLINICAL MANIFESTATIONS

The estimated incubation period for HME is 12 to 14 days. Like RMSF, HME is an acute febrile illness manifested as fever, headache, anorexia with or without vomiting, and myalgia.[184, 197, 204] The features of HME are shown in Table 195–2.

Rash, which may be macular, maculopapular, or petechial, seldom develops in adult infections. In pediatric infections, rash appears to be a common symptom, with a distribution often including both the trunk and extremities.

Meningitis as a manifestation of HME has been reported in seven children. Symptoms may range from irritability and meningismus to obtundation with response only to painful stimuli.[168, 171, 174, 185] Initial examination of cerebrospinal fluid has revealed pleocytosis ranging from approximately 50 to 1400 white blood cells, usually with a predominance of mononuclear cells; a range of 5 to 40 red blood cells; mildly elevated protein (85 to 120 mg/dL); and a normal to slightly low glucose value. The patients recovered completely.

Half to two thirds of adults and children have mild leukopenia and thrombocytopenia. One child had a documented decline in the white blood cell count from 13,000 to 1600 over a period of several hours.[179] Usually, thrombocytopenia is not associated with clinical bleeding; however, disseminated intravascular coagulopathy has been reported.[191] Elevations of aspartate aminotransferase, usually modest, peak at approximately 1 week into the illness, with values ranging from twice normal to several thousand. Other uncommon manifestations of illness include protracted fever,[202] elevated renal function test values (occasionally of sufficient severity to require dialysis), hyponatremia, hypoalbuminemia, and toxic shock syndrome.[181] Persistent infection over a 2-month interval and infection complicating human immunodeficiency virus disease have been documented.[177, 195]

The clinical features of HGE are similar to those of HME, with fever, malaise, myalgia, and headache occurring consistently. Rash occurs in less than 10 percent of cases. Morulae may be demonstrated in the cytoplasm of neutrophils but not mononuclear cells. Leukopenia, generally mild, is a feature of the illness in approximately half of the patients, and thrombocytopenia develops in most. As with HME, the level of serum aspartate aminotransferase is elevated in most cases.

DIAGNOSIS AND DIFFERENTIAL DIAGNOSIS

The diagnosis of HME or HGE is confirmed most often by documenting a fourfold change in antibody titer by indirect IFA in acute- and convalescent-phase serum samples. Sera should be collected acutely and 3 to 6 weeks after the onset of illness for analysis. Assays have been developed for the detection of both HME and HGE by PCR.[165, 167, 180] A case also may be confirmed by PCR amplification of ehrlichial DNA from a clinical sample or by detection of intraleukocytic morulae and a single IFA titer of 64 or more. A probable case is defined as a single IFA titer of 64 or more or the presence of morulae within infected leukocytes.[194]

Human ehrlichiosis must be distinguished from other tick-borne diseases, especially RMSF. The illnesses are similar in that both have manifestations of diffuse vasculitis. Clinically, ehrlichiosis is less likely to be accompanied by rash and more likely to have leukopenia or pancytopenia as a laboratory feature. The similarity of ehrlichiosis and RMSF is emphasized by two retrospective serosurveys in which approximately 10 percent of specimens, from patients lacking the serologic criteria for a diagnosis of RMSF, fulfilled the criteria for the diagnosis of ehrlichiosis.[188, 201] Other tick-borne illnesses such as Lyme disease, babesiosis, Colorado tick fever, relapsing fever, and tularemia should be included in the differential diagnosis.

Simultaneous HME and *Borrelia burgdorferi* infection has been described.[168] Whether it represents dual infection or is an instance of antigenic cross-reactivity is unknown. In children, Kawasaki syndrome may have features mimicking ehrlichiosis; paired sera from a group of children with Kawasaki syndrome, however, failed to react with a panel of *Ehrlichia* antigens.[199]

TABLE 195–2 ■ CLINICAL AND LABORATORY FEATURES OF ADULT AND PEDIATRIC MONOCYTIC EHRLICHIOSIS

	Percentage of Cases	
Feature*	*Adult (N = 46)*	*Pediatric (N = 20)*
Fever	96	100
Anorexia	76	78
Headache	80	100
Myalgia	74	67
Rash	20	65
Leukopenia†	61	72
Thrombocytopenia‡	52	78
Elevated aspartate aminotransferase§	76	83

*Some features not specified for all patients.
†Fewer than 4000 white blood cells/mm³.
‡Fewer than 150,000 platelets/mm³.
§More than 55 U/L.

TREATMENT

The drug of choice for treatment of human ehrlichiosis is doxycycline. The recommended dosage is 3 to 4 mg/kg/day in two divided doses (maximum, 200 mg/day). Data concerning the clinical efficacy of chloramphenicol are conflicting. Several children have been treated with chloramphenicol with apparent improvement, but cases of its ineffectiveness also have been reported. Mild clinical illness may resolve without specific antimicrobial treatment, although fever may be protracted.[183, 184, 197] However, human ehrlichiosis may have a fatal outcome, so doxycycline treatment should be initiated when the diagnosis is suspected, without regard for the age of the child.[182, 198]

REFERENCES

General Characteristics

Murray, E. S.: The rickettsial diseases. *In* Conn, H. F., and Conn, R. R., Jr. (eds.): Current Diagnosis 5. Philadelphia, W. B. Saunders, 1977.

Rocky Mountain Spotted Fever

1. Abramson, J. S., and Givner, L. B.: Should tetracycline be contraindicated for therapy of presumed Rocky Mountain spotted fever in children less than 9 years of age? Pediatrics *86*:123–124, 1990.
2. Abramson, J. S., and Givner, L. B.: Rocky Mountain spotted fever. Semin. Pediatr. Infect. Dis. *5*:131–136, 1994.
3. American Academy of Pediatrics: Rocky Mountain spotted fever. *In* Pickering, L. K. (ed.): 2000 Red Book: Report of the Committee on Infectious Diseases. 25th ed. Elk Grove Village, IL, American Academy of Pediatrics, 2000, pp. 491–493.
4. Bell, W. E., and Lascari, A. D.: Rocky Mountain spotted fever. Neurology *20*:841–847, 1970.
5. Bradford, W. D., Croker, B. P., and Tisher, C. C.: Kidney lesion in Rocky Mountain spotted fever. Am. J. Pathol. *97*:381–392, 1979.
6. Carl, M., Tibbs, C. W., Dobson, M. E., et al.: Diagnosis of acute typhus infections using the polymerase chain reaction. J. Infect. Dis. *161*: 791–793, 1990.
7. Clements, M. L., Wisseman, C. L., Woodward, T. E., et al.: Reactogenicity, immunogenicity, and efficacy of a chick embryo cell–derived vaccine for Rocky Mountain spotted fever. J. Infect. Dis. *148*:922–930, 1983.
8. Crennan, J. M., and VanScoy, R. E.: Eosinophilic meningitis caused by Rocky Mountain spotted fever. Am. J. Med. *80*:288–289, 1986.
9. Donohue, J.: Lower respiratory tract involvement in Rocky Mountain spotted fever. Arch. Intern. Med. *140*:223–227, 1980.

10. Duffey, R. J., and Hammer, M. E.: The ocular manifestations of Rocky Mountain spotted fever. Ann. Ophthalmol. *19*:301–306, 1987.
11. Feigin, R. D., Kissane, J. M., Eisenberg, C. S., et al.: Rocky Mountain spotted fever. Clin. Pediatr. (Phila.) *8*:331–343, 1969.
12. Gorman, R. J., Saxon, S., and Snead, O. C.: Neurologic sequelae of Rocky Mountain spotted fever. Pediatrics *67*:354–357, 1981.
13. Green, W. R., Walker, D. H., and Cain, B. G.: Fatal viscerotropic Rocky Mountain spotted fever. Am. J. Med. *64*:523–528, 1978.
14. Griffith, G. L., and Luce, E. A.: Massive skin necrosis in Rocky Mountain spotted fever. South. Med. J. *71*:1337–1340, 1978.
15. Hechemy, K. E., Stevens, R. W., Sasowski, S., et al.: Discrepancies in Weil-Felix and microimmunofluorescence test results for Rocky Mountain spotted fever. J. Clin. Microbiol. *9*:292–293, 1979.
16. Imperato, P. J.: Ticks, Lyme disease, and spotted fever. N. Y. State J. Med. *89*:313–314, 1989.
17. Jackson, M. D., Kirkman, C., Bradford, W. D., et al.: Rocky Mountain spotted fever: Hepatic lesions in childhood cases. Pediatr. Pathol. *5*:379–388, 1986.
18. Johnson, V. E., III, and Kadull, P. J.: Rocky Mountain spotted fever acquired in a laboratory. N. Engl. J. Med. *277*:812, 1967.
19. Jones, D., Anderson, B., Olson, J., et al.: Enzyme-linked immunosorbent assay for detection of human immunoglobulin G to lipopolysaccharide of spotted fever group rickettsiae. J. Clin. Microbiol. *31*:138–141, 1993.
20. Kaplowitz, L. G., and Robertson, G. L.: Hyponatremia in Rocky Mountain spotted fever: Role of antidiuretic hormone. Ann. Intern. Med. *98*: 334–335, 1983.
21. Kenyon, R. H., and Pedersen, C. E., Jr.: Preparation of Rocky Mountain spotted fever vaccine suitable for human immunization. J. Clin. Microbiol. *1*:500–503, 1975.
22. Linneman, C. C.: Skin biopsy in diagnosis of Rocky Mountain spotted fever. J. Pediatr. *96*:781–782, 1980.
23. Liu, C. T., Hilmas, D. E., Griffin, M. J., et al.: Alterations of body fluid compartments and distribution of tissue water and electrolytes in monkeys during Rocky Mountain spotted fever. J. Infect. Dis. *138*:42–48, 1978.
24. Marin-Garcia, J., and Barrett, F. F.: Myocardial function in Rocky Mountain spotted fever: Echocardiographic assessment. Am. J. Cardiol. *51*:341–343, 1983.
25. Martin, W., Chaplin, R. H., and Sheitzer, M. E.: The chest radiograph in Rocky Mountain spotted fever. A. J. R. Am. J. Roentgenol. *139*:889–893, 1982.
26. Oster, C. N., Burke, D. J., Kenyon, R. H., et al.: Laboratory acquired Rocky Mountain spotted fever. N. Engl. J. Med. *297*:859–863, 1977.
27. Rocky Mountain spotted fever: United States, 1990. M. M. W. R. Morb. Mortal. Wkly. Rep. *40*:451–453, 459, 1991.
28. Roggli, V. L., Keener, S., Bradford, W. D., et al.: Pulmonary pathology of Rocky Mountain spotted fever in children. Pediatr. Pathol. *4*:47–57, 1985.
29. Roth, R. M., and Gleckman, R. A.: Human infections derived from dogs. Postgrad. Med. *77*:169–180, 1985.
30. Rubio, T., Riley, H. D., Jr., Nida, J. R., et al.: Thrombocytopenia in Rocky Mountain spotted fever. Am. J. Dis. Child. *116*:88–96, 1968.
31. Scimeca, P. G., Weinblatt, M. E., and Kochen, J. A.: Acquired coagulation inhibitor in association with Rocky Mountain spotted fever. Clin. Pediatr. (Phila.) *26*:459–463, 1987.
32. Sexton, D. J., and Clapp, J.: Inappropriate antidiuretic hormone secretion. Arch. Intern. Med. *137*:362–363, 1977.
33. Sexton, D. J., and Corey, G. R.: Rocky Mountain "spotless" and "almost spotless" fever: A wolf in sheep's clothing. Clin. Infect. Dis. *15*:439–448, 1992.
34. Silverman, D. J.: Adherence of platelets to human endothelial cells infected by *Rickettsia rickettsii*. J. Infect. Dis. *153*:694–700, 1986.
35. Thorner, A. R., Walker, D. H., and Petri, W. A., Jr.: Rocky Mountain spotted fever. Clin. Infect. Dis. *27*:1353–1360, 1998.
36. Treadwell, T. A., Holman, R. C., Clarke, M. J., et al.: Rocky Mountain spotted fever in the United States, 1993–1996. Am. J. Trop. Med. Hyg. *63*:21–26, 2000.
37. Uchida, T.: *Rickettsia japonica*, the etiologic agent of Oriental spotted fever. Microbiol. Immunol. *37*:91–102, 1993.
38. Walker, D. H.: Rocky Mountain spotted fever: A disease in need of microbiological concern. Clin. Microbiol. Rev. *2*:227–240, 1989.
39. Walker, D. H., Gay, R. M., and Valdes-Dapena, M.: The occurrence of eschars in Rocky Mountain spotted fever. J. Am. Acad. Dermatol. *4*:571–576, 1981.
40. Walker, D. H., Hawkins, H. K., and Hudson, P.: Rocky Mountain spotted fever: Idiopathic characteristics associated with glucose-6-phosphate dehydrogenase deficiency. Arch. Pathol. Lab. Med. *107*:121–125, 1983.
41. Walker, D. H., Henderson, F. W., and Hutchins, G. M.: Rocky Mountain spotted fever: Mimicry of appendicitis or acute surgical abdomen? Am. J. Dis. Child. *140*:742–744, 1986.
42. Walker, D. H., and Mattern, W. B.: Acute renal failure in Rocky Mountain spotted fever. Arch. Intern. Med. *139*:443–448, 1979.
43. Walker, D. H., Montenegro, M. R., Hegarty, B. C., et al.: Rocky Mountain spotted fever vaccine. South. Med. J. *77*:447–449, 1984.
44. Walker, D. H., Paletta, C. E., and Cain, B. G.: Pathogenesis of myocarditis in Rocky Mountain spotted fever. Arch. Pathol. Lab. Med. *104*:171–174, 1980.
45. Weiss, E.: Growth and physiology of rickettsiae. Bacterial Dis. *37*:259–283, 1973.
46. Wells, G. M., Woodward, T. E., Fiset, P., et al.: Rocky Mountain spotted fever caused by blood transfusion. J. A. M. A. *239*:2763–2765, 1978.
47. White, W. L., Patrick, J. D., and Miller, L. R.: Evaluation of immunoperoxidase techniques to detect *Rickettsia rickettsii* in fixed tissue specimens. Am. J. Clin. Pathol. *101*:747–752, 1994.
48. Wolbach, S. B.: Studies on Rocky Mountain spotted fever. J. Med. Res. *41*:1–198, 1919.
49. Woodward, T. E., Pedersen, C. E., Jr., Oster, C. N., et al.: Prompt confirmation of Rocky Mountain spotted fever: Identification of rickettsiae in skin tissues. J. Infect. Dis. *134*:297–305, 1976.
50. Wright, L.: Intellectual sequelae of Rocky Mountain spotted fever. J. Abnorm. Psychol. *80*:315–316, 1972.

Mediterranean Spotted Fever

51. Adan, A., Lopez-Soto, A., Moser, C., et al.: Use of steroids and heparin to treat retinal arterial occlusion in Mediterranean spotted fever. J. Infect. Dis. *151*:1139, 1988.
52. Anderson, J. A., Magnarelli, L. A., Burgdorfer, W., et al.: Importation into the United States from Africa of *Rhipicephalus simus* on a boutonneuse fever patient. Am. J. Trop. Med. Hyg. *30*:897–899, 1981.
53. Cascio, A., Colomba, C., Di Rosa, D., et al.: Efficacy and safety of clarithromycin as treatment for Mediterranean spotted fever in children: A randomized controlled trial. Clin. Infect. Dis. *33*:409–411, 2001.
54. De La Fuente, L., Anda, P., Rodriguez, I., et al.: Evaluation of a latex agglutination test for *Rickettsia conorii* antibodies in seropositive patients. J. Med. Microbiol. *28*:69–72, 1989.
55. DeMicco, C., Raoult, D., Benderitter, T., et al.: Immune complex vasculitis associated with Mediterranean spotted fever. J. Infect. *14*:163–165, 1987.
56. Diez Ruiz, A., Ramos Jimenez, A., Lopez Ruz, M. A., et al.: Boutonneuse fever transmitted by conjunctival inoculation. Klin. Wochenschr. *66*:1212–1213, 1988.
57. Font-Creus, B., Bella-Cueto, C., Tringali, G. R., et al.: Mediterranean spotted fever: A cooperative study of 227 cases. Rev. Infect. Dis. *7*: 635–642, 1985.
58. Gross, E. M., Yagupsky, P., Torok, V., et al.: Resurgence of Mediterranean spotted fever. Lancet *2*:1107, 1982.
59. Gudiol, F., Pallares, R., Carratala, J., et al.: Randomized double-blind evaluation of ciprofloxacin and doxycycline for Mediterranean spotted fever. Antimicrob. Agents Chemother. *33*:987–988, 1989.
60. Harris, R. L., Kaplan, S. L., Bradshaw, M. W., et al.: Boutonneuse fever in American travelers. J. Infect. Dis. *153*:126–128, 1986.
61. Hechemy, K. E., Raoult, D., Eisemann, C., et al.: Detection of antibodies to *Rickettsia conorii* with latex agglutination test in patients with Mediterranean spotted fever. J. Infect. Dis. *153*:132–135, 1986.
62. Mansueto, S., Vitale, G., Bentinegna, M., et al.: Persistence of antibodies to *Rickettsia conorii* after an acute attack of boutonneuse fever. J. Infect. Dis. *151*:377, 1985.
63. Montenegro, M. R., Mansueto, S., Hegarty, B. C., et al.: The histology of "taches noires" of boutonneuse fever and demonstration of *Rickettsia conorii* in them by immunofluorescence. Virchows Arch. *900*:309–317, 1983.
64. Moraga, F. A., Martinez-Roig, A., Alonso, J. L., et al.: Boutonneuse fever. Arch. Dis. Child. *57*:149–151, 1982.
65. San Jose, A., Bosch, J. A., Arderiu, A., et al.: Myositis due to *Rickettsia conorii* infection. Trans. R. Soc. Trop. Med. Hyg. *82*:346, 1988.
66. Teysseire, N., and Raoult, D.: Comparison of Western immunoblotting and microimmunofluorescence for diagnosis of Mediterranean spotted fever. J. Clin. Microbiol. *30*:455–460, 1992.
67. Walker, D. H., Occhino, C., Tringali, G. R., et al.: Pathogenesis of rickettsial eschars: The tache noire of boutonneuse fever. Hum. Pathol. *19*:1449–1454, 1988.
68. Walker, D. H., Staiti, A., Mansueto, S., et al.: Frequent occurrence of hepatic lesions in boutonneuse fever. Acta Trop. *43*:175–181, 1986.
69. Williams, W. J., Radulovic, S., Dasch, G. A., et al.: Identification of *Rickettsia conorii* infection by a polymerase chain reaction in a soldier returning from Somalia. Clin. Infect. Dis. *19*:93–99, 1994.
70. Yagupsky, P., and Wolach, B.: Fatal Israeli spotted fever in children. Clin. Infect. Dis. *17*:850–853, 1993.

Other Tick Typhus Fevers

71. Prias, M. A., Calia, G., Saba, F., et al.: Glucose-6-phosphate dehydrogenase deficiency in male patients with Mediterranean spotted fever in Sardinia. J. Infect. Dis. *147*:607–608, 1983.

Rickettsialpox

72. Boyd, A. S.: Rickettsialpox. Dermatol. Clin. *15*:313–318, 1997.
73. Brettman, C. R., Lewin, S., Holymein, R. S., et al.: Rickettsialpox: Report of an outbreak and a contemporary review. Medicine (Baltimore) *60*:363–372, 1981.
74. Dolgopol, V. V.: Histologic changes in rickettsialpox. Am. J. Pathol. *24*:119, 1948.

75. Greenberg, M., and Pellitteri, O. J.: Rickettsialpox. Bull. N. Y. Acad. Med. *23*:338, 1947.
76. Greenberg, M., Pellitteri, O. J., and Jellison, W. L.: Rickettsialpox: A newly recognized rickettsial disease. III. Epidemiology. Am. J. Public Health *37*:860–868, 1947.
77. Greenberg, M., Pellitteri, O. J., Klein, I. F., et al.: Rickettsialpox: A newly recognized rickettsial disease. II. Clinical observation. J. A. M. A. *133*:901, 1947.
78. Huebner, R. J., Jellison, W. L., and Armstrong, C.: Rickettsialpox: A newly recognized rickettsial disease. V. Recovery of *Rickettsia akari* from a house mouse (*Mus musculus*). Public Health Rep. *62*:777–780, 1947.
79. Huebner, R. J., Jellison, W. L., and Pomerantz, C.: Rickettsialpox: A newly recognized rickettsial disease. IV. Isolation of a rickettsia apparently identical with the causative agent of rickettsialpox from *Allodermanyssus sanguineus,* a rodent mite. Public Health Rep. *61*:1677–1682, 1946.
80. Huebner, R. J., Stamps, P., and Armstrong, C.: Rickettsialpox: A newly recognized rickettsial disease. I. Isolation of the etiologic agent. Public Health Rep. *61*:1605–1614, 1946.
81. Jacobson, J. M., Desmond, E. P., Kornblee, L. V., et al.: Positive Weil-Felix reactions in a case of rickettsialpox. Int. J. Dermatol. *28*:271–272, 1989.
82. Kass, E. M., Szaniawski, W. K., Levy, H., et al.: Rickettsialpox in a New York City hospital, 1980 to 1989. N. Engl. J. Med. *331*:1612–1617, 1994.
83. LaBocetta, A. C., Israel, H. L., Perri, A. M., et al.: Rickettsialpox: Report of four apparent cases in Pennsylvania. Am. J. Med. *13*:413, 1952.
84. Lerner, A. M., Klein, J. O., Cherry, J. D., et al.: New viral exanthems. N. Engl. J. Med. *269*:678, 736, 1963.
85. Murray, E. S., and Snyder, J. C.: Brill's disease. II. Etiology. Am. J. Hyg. *53*:22, 1951.
86. Shankman, B.: Report of an outbreak of endemic febrile illness not identified, occurring in NYC. N. Y. State J. Med. *46*:2156, 1946.
87. Sleisinger, M. H., Murray, E. S., and Cohen, S.: Rickettsialpox case due to laboratory infection. Public Health Rep. *66*:311, 1951.
88. Sussman, L. N.: Kew Gardens' spotted fever. N. Y. Med. *2*:27, 1946.
89. Zdrodovskii, P. F., and Golinevich, E. H.: Vesicular and varioliform rickettsioses (rickettsialpox). *In* Zdrodovskii, P. F., and Golinevich, E. H. (eds.): The Rickettsial Diseases. New York, Pergamon, 1960, pp. 340–353.

Typhus Group

90. Adams, W. H., Emmons, R. W., and Brooks, J. E.: The changing ecology of murine (endemic) typhus in southern California. Am. J. Trop. Med. Hyg. *19*:311–318, 1970.
91. American Academy of Pediatrics: Endemic typhus. *In* Pickering, L. K. (ed.): 2000 Red Book: Report of the Committee on Infectious Diseases. 25th ed. Elk Grove Village, IL, American Academy of Pediatrics, 2000, pp. 620–621.
92. Brezina, R.: Diagnosis and control of rickettsial diseases. Acta Virol. *29*:338–349, 1985.
93. Diab, S. M., Araj, G. F., and French, F. F.: Cardiovascular and pulmonary complications of epidemic typhus. Trop. Geogr. Med. *41*:76–79, 1989.
94. Duma, R. J., Soneshine, D. E., Bozeman, F. M., et al.: Epidemic typhus in the United States associated with flying squirrels. J. A. M. A. *245*:2318–2323, 1981.
95. Dumler, J. S.: Murine typhus. Semin. Pediatr. Infect. Dis. *5*:137–142, 1994.
96. Fergie, J. E., Purcell, K., and Wanat, D.: Murine typhus in South Texas children. Pediatr. Infect. Dis. J. *19*:535–538, 2000.
97. Gaon, J. A., and Murray, E. S.: The natural history of recrudescent typhus (Brill-Zinsser disease) in Bosnia. Bull. World Health Organ. *35*:133–141, 1966.
98. Marshall, G. S.: *Rickettsia typhi* seroprevalence among children in the southeast United States. Pediatr. Infect. Dis. J. *19*:1103–1104, 2000.
99. McDade, J. E., Shepard, C. C., Redus, M. A., et al.: Evidence of *Rickettsia prowazekii* infections in the United States. Am. J. Trop. Med. Hyg. *29*:277–284, 1980.
100. Perine, P. L., Chandler, B. P., Krause, D. K., et al.: A clinico-epidemiological study of epidemic typhus in Africa. Clin. Infect. Dis. *14*:1149–1158, 1992.
101. Perine, P. L., Krause, D. W., Awoke, S., et al.: Single-dose doxycycline treatment of louse-borne relapsing fever and epidemic typhus. Lancet *2*:742–744, 1974.
102. Raoult, D., and Roux, V.: The body louse as a vector of reemerging human diseases. Clin. Infect. Dis. *29*:888–911, 1999.
103. Schriefer, M. E., Sacci, J. B., Jr., and Dumler, J. S.: Identification of a novel rickettsial infection in a patient diagnosed with murine typhus. J. Clin. Microbiol. *32*:949–954, 1994.
104. White, P. C., Jr.: A brief historical review of murine typhus in Virginia and the United States. Va. Med. Monthly *94*:16–23, 1970.
105. Whiteford, S. F., Taylor, J. P., and Dumler, J. S.: Clinical, laboratory, and epidemiologic features of murine typhus in 97 Texas children. Arch. Pediatr. Adolesc. Med. *155*:396–400, 2000.
106. Wolfman, D. E., Fenton, W., Jr., and Donald, P. J.: Typhus-induced facial necrosis. Otolaryngol. Head Neck Surg. *94*:390–393, 1986.
107. Woo, M. L., Leung, J. W., and French, G. L.: Rickettsial infection presenting as culture-negative meningitis. Postgrad. Med. J. *64*:614–616, 1988.
108. Zinsser, H.: Rats, Lice and History. New York, Blue Ribbon Books, 1943.

Scrub Typhus

109. Brown, G. W., Saunders, J. P., Singh, S., et al.: Single dose doxycycline therapy in scrub typhus. Trans. R. Soc. Trop. Med. Hyg. *72*:412–416, 1978.
110. Chayakul, P., Panich, V., and Silpapojakul, K.: Scrub typhus pneumonitis: An entity which is frequently missed. Q. J. Med. *68*:595–602, 1988.
111. Crum, J. W., Hanchaley, S., and Eamsila, C.: New paper enzyme-linked immunosorbent technique compared with microimmunofluorescence for detection of human serum antibodies to *Rickettsia tsutsugamushi.* J. Clin. Microbiol. *11*:584–588, 1980.
112. Furuya, Y., Yamamoto, S., Otu, M., et al.: Use of monoclonal antibodies against *Rickettsia tsutsugamushi* Kawasaki for serodiagnosis by enzyme-linked immunosorbent assay. J. Clin. Microbiol. *29*:340–345, 1991.
113. Furuya, Y., Yoshida, Y., Katayama, T., et al.: Serotype-specific amplification of *Rickettsia tsutsugamushi* DNA by nested polymerase chain reaction. J. Clin. Microbiol. *31*:1637–1640, 1993.
114. Jin-ju, W., Gui-zhong, T., and Shi-feng, S.: Study on *Leptotrombidium gaohuensis* sp. nov.: Newly discovered vectors of tsutsugamushi disease. Chin. Med. J. *100*:590–594, 1987.
115. Kelly, D. J., Wong, P. W., Gan, E., et al.: Comparative evaluation of the indirect immunoperoxidase test for the serodiagnosis of rickettsial disease. Am. J. Trop. Med. Hyg. *38*:400–406, 1988.
116. Ognibene, A. J., O'Leary, D. S., Czarnecki, S. W., et al.: Myocarditis and disseminated intravascular coagulation in scrub typhus. Am. J. Med. Sci. *262*:233–239, 1971.
117. Ohashi, N., Tamura, A., and Suto, T.: Immunoblotting analysis of anti-rickettsial antibodies produced in patients of tsutsugamushi disease. Microbiol. Immunol. *32*:1085–1092, 1988.
118. Saunders, J. P., Brown, G. W., Shirai, A., et al.: The longevity of antibody to *Rickettsia tsutsugamushi* in patients with confirmed scrub typhus. Trans. R. Soc. Trop. Med. Hyg. *74*:253–257, 1980.
119. Shirai, A., Brown, G. W., Gan, E., et al.: *Rickettsia tsutsugamushi* antibody in mother cord pairs of sera. Jpn. J. Med. Sci. Biol. *34*:37–39, 1981.
120. Smadel, J. E., Bailey, C. A., and Diercks, F. H.: Chloramphenicol (chloromycetin) in the chemoprophylaxis of scrub typhus (tsutsugamushi disease). IV. Relapses of scrub typhus in treated volunteers and their prevention. Am. J. Hyg. *51*:229–241, 1950.
121. Twartz, J. C., Shirai, A., Selvaraju, G. , et al.: Doxycycline prophylaxis for human scrub typhus. J. Infect. Dis. *146*:811–818, 1982.
122. Urakami, H., Yamamoto, S., Tsuruhar, T., et al.: Serodiagnosis of scrub typhus with antigens immobilized on nitrocellulose sheet. J. Clin. Microbiol. *27*:1841–1846, 1989.
123. Watt, G., Kantipong, P., Jongsakul, K., et al.: Doxycycline and rifampin for mild scrub-typhus infections in northern Thailand: A randomised trial. Lancet *356*:1057–1061, 2000.

Q Fever

124. Andrews, P. S., and Marmion, B. P.: Morbid anatomical and bacteriological findings in a patient with endocarditis. B. M. J. *1*:983, 1959.
125. Bental, T., Fejgin, M., Keysary, A., et al.: Chronic Q fever of pregnancy presenting as *Coxiella burnetii* placentitis: Successful outcome following therapy with erythromycin and rifampin. Clin. Infect. Dis. *21*:1318–1321, 1995.
126. Bernard, K. W., Parham, G. L., Winkler, W. G., et al.: Q fever control measures: Recommendations for research facilities using sheep. Infect. Control *3*:461–464, 1982.
127. Biggs, B. A., Douglas, J. G., Grant, I. W., et al.: Prolonged Q fever associated with inappropriate secretion of antidiuretic hormone. J. Infect. *8*:61–63, 1984.
128. Brown, G. L., Colwell, D. L., and Hooper, W. L.: An outbreak of Q fever in Staffordshire. J. Hyg. (Camb.) *66*:649–655, 1968.
129. Cardellach, F., Font, J., Agusti, A. G., et al.: Q fever and hemolytic anemia. J. Infect. Dis. *148*:769, 1983.
130. Edlinger, E.: Immunofluorescence serology: A tool for prognosis of Q fever. Diagn. Microbiol. Infect. Dis. *3*:343–351, 1985.
131. Ferrante, M. A., and Dolan, M. J.: Q fever meningoencephalitis in a soldier returning from the Persian Gulf War. Clin. Infect. Dis. *16*:489–496, 1993.
132. Hall, C. J., Richmond, S. J., Caul, E. O., et al.: Laboratory outbreak of Q fever acquired from sheep. Lancet *1*:1004–1006, 1982.
133. Henderson, R. J.: Q fever and leptospirosis in the dairy farming community and allied workers of Worcestershire. J. Clin. Pathol. *22*:511–514, 1969.
134. Hervás, J. A., de la Fuente, M. A., García, F., et al.: *Coxiella burnetii* myopericarditis and rhabdomyolysis in a child. Pediatr. Infect. Dis. J. *19*:1104–1106, 2000.
135. Hofmann, C. E., and Heaton, J. W., Jr.: Q fever hepatitis: Clinical manifestations and pathological findings. Gastroenterology *83*:474–479, 1982.
136. Hunt, J. G., Field, P. R., and Murphy, A. M.: Immunoglobulin responses to *Coxiella burnetii* (Q fever): Single-serum diagnosis of acute infection using an immunofluorescence technique. Infect. Immun. *39*:977–981, 1983.

137. Hunter, W. H.: Some problems in Q fever infections in New South Wales. Med. J. Aust. *1*:900–904, 1968.
138. Kazar, J.: Immunity in Q fever. Acta Virol. *32*:358–368, 1988.
139. Kazar, J., and Rehacek, J.: Q fever vaccines: Present status and application in man. Zentralbl Bakteriol *267*:74–78, 1987.
140. Kimbrough, R. C., III, Ormsbee, R. A., and Peacock, M. G.: Q fever endocarditis: A three and one-half year follow-up. *In* Burgdorfer, W., and Anacker, R. L. (eds.): Rickettsiae and Rickettsial Diseases. New York, Academic, 1981, pp. 125–132.
141. Lim, K. C., and Kang, J. Y.: Q fever presenting with gastroenteritis. Med. J. Aust. *1*:327, 1980.
142. Luoto, L., and Huebner, R. J.: Q fever studies in southern California. IX. Isolation of Q fever organisms from parturient placentas of naturally infected dairy cows. Public Health Rep. *65*:541–544, 1950.
143. Meiklejohn, G., Reimer, L. G., Graves, P. S., et al.: Cryptic epidemic of Q fever in a medical school. J. Infect. Dis. *144*:107–113, 1981.
144. Millar, J. K.: The chest film findings in Q fever: A series of 35 cases. Clin. Radiol. *29*:371–375, 1978.
145. Murphy, A. M., and Hunt, J. G.: Retrospective diagnosis of Q fever in a country abattoir by the use of specific IgM globulin estimations. Med. J. Aust. *2*:326–327, 1981.
146. Murphy, P. P., and Richardson, S. G.: Q fever pneumonia presenting as an eosinophilic pleural effusion. Thorax *44*:228–229, 1989.
147. Peacock, M. G., Philip, R. N., Wilhams, J. C., et al.: Serological evaluation of Q fever in humans: Enhanced phase I titers of immunoglobulin G and A are diagnostic for Q fever endocarditis. Infect. Immun. *41*:1089–1098, 1983.
148. Pellegrin, M., Delsol, G., Auvergnat, J. C., et al.: Granulomatous hepatitis in Q fever. Hum. Pathol. *11*:51–57, 1980.
149. Pierce, T. H., Tucht, S. C., Gorin, A. B., et al.: Q fever pneumonitis: Diagnosis by transbronchoscopic lung biopsy. West. J. Med. *130*: 453–455, 1979.
150. Pinsky, R. L., Fishbein, D. B., Greene, C. R., et. al.: An outbreak of cat-associated Q fever in the United States. J. Infect. Dis. *164*:202–204, 1991.
151. Raoult, D., and Marrie, T.: Q fever. Clin. Infect. Dis. *20*:489–496, 1995.
152. Raoult, D., Tissot-Dupont, H., Foucault, C., et al.: Q fever 1985–1998. Clinical and epidemiologic features of 1,383 infections. Medicine (Baltimore) *79*:109–123, 2000.
153. Raoult, D., Urvolgyi, J., Etienne, J., et al.: Diagnosis of endocarditis in acute Q fever by immunofluorescence serology. Acta Virol. *32*:70–74, 1988.
154. Richardus, J. H., Dumas, A. M., Huisman, J., et al.: Q fever in infancy: A review of 18 cases. Pediatr. Infect. Dis. *4*:369–373, 1985.
155. Ruiz-Contreras, J., Montero, R. G., Amador, J. T. R., et al.: Q fever in children. Am. J. Dis. Child. *147*:300–302, 1993.
156. Simor, A. E., Bruntan, J. L., Salit, I. E., et al.: Q fever: Hazard from sheep used in research. Can. Med. Assoc. J. *130*:1013–1016, 1984.
157. Tobin, M. J., Cahill, N., Gearty, G., et al.: Q fever endocarditis. Am. J. Med. *72*:396–400, 1982.
158. Uff, J. S., and Evans, D. J.: Mesangio-capillary glomerulonephritis associated with Q fever endocarditis. Histopathology *1*:463–472, 1977.
159. van Hensbroek, M. B., de Vries, E., Dolan, G., et al.: Rash and petechiae as presenting signs of Q fever. Pediatr. Infect. Dis. J. *19*:358, 2000.
160. Voigt, J. J., Delsol, G., and Fabre, J.: Liver and bone marrow granulomas in Q fever. Gastroenterology *84*:887–888, 1983.
161. Whittick, J. W.: Necropsy findings in a case of Q fever in Britain. B. M. J. *1*:979–980, 1950.
162. Wisniewski, H. J., and Krumbiegel, E. R.: Epidemiological studies of Q fever in humans. Arch. Environ. Health *21*:66–70, 1970.
163. Yeaman, M. R., Roman, M. J., and Baca, O. G.: Antibiotic susceptibilities of two *Coxiella burnetii* isolates implicated in distinct clinical syndromes. Antimicrob. Agents Chemother. *33*:1052–1057, 1989.

Ehrlichiosis

164. Anderson, B. E., Dawson, J. E., Jones, D. C., et al.: *Ehrlichia chaffeensis*, a new species associated with human ehrlichiosis. J. Clin. Microbiol. *29*:2838–2842, 1991.
165. Anderson, B. E., Sumner, J. W., Dawson, J. E., et al.: Detection of the etiologic agent of human ehrlichiosis by polymerase chain reaction. J. Clin. Microbiol. *30*:775–780, 1992.
166. Bakken, J. S., and Dumler, J. S.: Human granulocytic ehrlichiosis. Clin. Infect. Dis. *31*:554–560, 2000.
167. Bakken, J. S., Dumler, J. S., Chen, S.-M., et al.: Human granulocytic ehrlichiosis in the upper Midwest United States: A new species emerging? J. A. M. A. *272*:212–218, 1994.
168. Barton, L. L., Dawson, J. E., Letson, G. W., et al.: Simultaneous ehrlichiosis and Lyme disease. Pediatr. Infect. Dis. J. *9*:127–129, 1990.
169. Barton, L. L., and Foy, T. M.: *Ehrlichia canis* infection in a child. Pediatrics *4*:580–582, 1989.
170. Barton, L. L., Rathore, M. H., and Dawson, J. E.: Infection with *Ehrlichia* in childhood. J. Pediatr. *120*:998–1001, 1992.
171. Berry, D. S., Miller, R. S., Hooke, J. A., et al.: Ehrlichial meningitis with cerebrospinal fluid morulae. Pediatr. Infect. Dis. J. *18*:552–555, 1999.
172. Buller, R. S., Arens, M., Hmiel, S. P., et al.: *Ehrlichia ewingii*, a newly recognized agent of human ehrlichiosis. N. Engl. J. Med. *341*:148–155, 1999.
173. Chen, S.-M., Dumler, J. S., Bakken, J. S., et al.: Identification of a granulocytotropic *Ehrlichia* species as the etiologic agent of human disease. J. Clin. Microbiol. *32*:589–595, 1994.
174. Dimmitt, D. C., Fishbein, D. B., and Dawson, J. E.: Human ehrlichiosis associated with cerebrospinal fluid pleocytosis: A case report. Am. J. Med. *87*:677–678, 1989.
175. Doran, T. I., Parmley, R. T., Logas, P. C., et al.: Infection with *Ehrlichia canis* in a child. J. Pediatr. *114*:809–812, 1989.
176. Dumler, J. S., Dawson, J. E., and Walker, D. H.: Human ehrlichiosis: Hematopathology and immunohistologic detection of *Ehrlichia chaffeensis*. Hum. Pathol. *24*:391–396, 1993.
177. Dumler, J. S., Sutker, W. L., and Walker, D. H.: Persistent infection with *Ehrlichia chaffeensis*. Clin. Infect. Dis. *17*:903–905, 1993.
178. Edwards, M. S.: Ehrlichiosis in children. Semin. Pediatr. Infect. Dis. *5*: 143–147, 1994.
179. Edwards, M. S., Jones, J. E., Leass, D. L., et al.: Childhood infection caused by *Ehrlichia canis* or a closely related organism. Pediatr. Infect. Dis. J. *7*:651–654, 1988.
180. Everett, E. D., Evans, K. A., Henry, R. B., et al.: Human ehrlichiosis in adults after tick exposure: Diagnosis using polymerase chain reaction. Ann. Intern. Med. *120*:730–735, 1994.
181. Fichtenbaum, C. J., Peterson, L. R., and Weil, G. J.: Ehrlichiosis presenting as a life-threatening illness with features of toxic shock syndrome. Am. J. Med. *95*:351–357, 1993.
182. Fishbein, D. B., Dawson, J. E., and Robinson, L. E.: Human ehrlichiosis in the United States, 1985 to 1990. Ann. Intern. Med. *120*:736–743, 1994.
183. Fishbein, D. B., Kemp, A., Dawson, J. E., et al.: Human ehrlichiosis: Prospective active surveillance in febrile hospitalized patients. J. Infect. Dis. *160*:803–809, 1989.
184. Fishbein, D. B., Sawyer, L. A., Holland, C. J., et al.: Unexplained febrile illnesses after exposure to ticks: Infection with an *Ehrlichia?* J. A. M. A. *257*:3100–3104, 1987.
185. Golden, S. E.: Aseptic meningitis associated with *Ehrlichia canis* infection. Pediatr. Infect. Dis. J. *8*:335–337, 1989.
186. Hardalo, C. J., Quagliarello, V., and Dumler, J. S.: Human granulocytic ehrlichiosis in Connecticut: Report of a fatal case. Clin. Infect. Dis. *21*:910–914, 1995.
187. Harkess, J. R., Ewing, S. A., Brumit, T., et al.: Ehrlichiosis in children. Pediatrics *87*:199–203, 1991.
188. Harkess, J. R., Ewing, S. A., Crutcher, J. M., et al.: Human ehrlichiosis in Oklahoma. J. Infect. Dis. *159*:576–579, 1989.
189. Horowitz, H. W., Kilchevsky, E., Haber, S., et al.: Perinatal transmission of the agent of human granulocytic ehrlichiosis. N. Engl. J. Med. *339*: 375–378, 1998.
190. Jacobs, R. F., and Schutze, G. E.: Ehrlichiosis in children. J. Pediatr. *131*:184–192, 1997.
191. Maeda, K., Markowitz, N., Hawley, R. C., et al.: Human infection with *Ehrlichia canis,* a leukocytic rickettsia. N. Engl. J. Med. *316*:853–856, 1987.
192. Malpass, D. G., Heiman, H. S., and Sumaya, C. V.: Childhood ehrlichiosis: A case report and review of the literature. Int. Pediatr. *6*:354–358, 1991.
193. McDade, J. E.: Ehrlichiosis: A disease of animals and humans. J. Infect. Dis. *161*:609–617, 1990.
194. McQuiston, J. H., Paddock, C. D., Holman, R. C., et al.: The human ehrlichioses in the United States. Emerg. Infect. Dis. *5*:635–642,1999.
195. Paddock, C. D., Suchard, D. P., Grumbach, K. L., et al.: Brief report: Fatal seronegative ehrlichiosis in a patient with HIV infection. N. Engl. J. Med. *329*:1164–1167, 1993.
196. Pancholi, P., Kolbert, C. P., Mitchell, P. D., et al.: *Ixodes dammini* as a potential vector of human granulocytic ehrlichiosis. J. Infect. Dis. *172*:1007–1012, 1995.
197. Petersen, L. R., Sawyer, L. A., Fishbein, D. B., et al.: An outbreak of ehrlichiosis in members of an army reserve unit exposed to ticks. J. Infect. Dis. *159*:562–568, 1989.
198. Purvis, J. J., and Edwards, M. S.: Doxycycline use for rickettsial disease in pediatric patients. Pediatr. Infect. Dis. J. *19*:871–874, 2000.
199. Rauch, A. M.: Kawasaki syndrome: Review of new epidemiologic and laboratory developments. Pediatr. Infect. Dis. J. *6*:1016–1021, 1987.
200. Reed, K. D., Mitchell, P. D., Persing, D. H., et al.: Transmission of human granulocytic ehrlichiosis. J. A. M. A. *273*:23, 1995.
201. Rohrbach, B. W., Harkess, J. R., Ewing, S. A., et al.: Epidemiologic and clinical characteristics of persons with serologic evidence of *E. canis* infection. Am. J. Public Health *80*:442–445, 1990.
202. Roland, W. E., McDonald, G., Caldwell, C. W., et al.: Ehrlichiosis: A cause of prolonged fever. Clin. Infect. Dis. *20*:821–825, 1995.
203. Standaert, S. M., Dawson, J. E., Schaffner, W., et al.: Ehrlichiosis in a golf-oriented retirement community. N. Engl. J. Med. *333*:420–425, 1995.
204. Taylor, J. P., Betz, T. G., Fishbein, D. B., et al.: Serological evidence of possible human infection with *Ehrlichia* in Texas. J. Infect. Dis. *158*:217–220, 1988.
205. Walker, J. S., Rundquist, J. D., Taylor, R., et al.: Clinical and clinicopathologic findings in tropical canine pancytopenia. J. Am. Vet. Med. Assoc. *157*:43–55, 1970.

SECTION XX

Mycoplasma

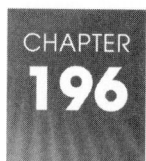

CHAPTER 196 Mycoplasma and Ureaplasma Infections

JAMES D. CHERRY ■ NATASCHA CHING

Mycoplasmas and ureaplasmas, the smallest free-living microorganisms, are ubiquitous in nature. More than 100 species have been recovered from many animals, including human beings.[552, 669] Of this group, 15 have been identified as human pathogens or as part of the "normal" human flora, with *Mycoplasma pneumoniae, Mycoplasma hominis,* and *Ureaplasma urealyticum* found to cause disease frequently in children. A protean array of illnesses in children are caused by infection with these organisms.

The generic name *Mycoplasma* is derived from Greek and Latin. *Myco* refers to the mycelial, or filamentous, characteristic, and *plasma* indicates the plasticity and pleomorphism of the organism.[648] *Urea* in *Ureaplasma* indicates the presence of urease in this genus.[227]

History

In 1898, Nocard and Roux[503] recovered the first *Mycoplasma* organism from cattle with contagious pleuropneumonia. Shortly after the original discovery, many other mycoplasmas were recovered from several different animals.[272] These other mycoplasmas, which frequently were not associated with disease, originally were called pleuropneumonia-like organisms; this designation was abbreviated to PPLO. The term PPLO enjoyed general use until the early 1960s.

The first isolation of a mycoplasma from a human was reported in 1937 by Dienes and Edsall.[157] This organism, now recognized as *M. hominis,* was recovered from an abscessed Bartholin gland. In 1944, Eaton and colleagues[169] reported the recovery of an organism, originally called the Eaton agent, from persons ill with primary atypical pneumonia. For many years, the Eaton agent was considered to be a virus, even though it was inhibited by streptomycin and chlortetracycline.[167, 168] In 1961, Marmion and Goodburn[437] noted that the Eaton agent was morphologically similar to PPLOs. In 1962, the organism now known as *M. pneumoniae* was cultivated on a cell-free agar medium and was shown in human volunteer studies to be the etiologic agent of primary atypical pneumonia.[97, 99, 272]

In 1954, Shepard[592] reported the recovery of PPLOs with a distinctive small-colony characteristic from men with and without nongonococcal urethritis. These T strains (T for tiny), as they were called, now are classified as *U. urealyticum.* More recently, another mycoplasma, *Mycoplasma genitalium,* has been associated with genital tract infections, and three mycoplasma species have been noted to co-infect patients with human immunodeficiency virus (HIV) infection.[469, 654]

Classification

Mycoplasma and *Ureaplasma* are the two genera of the family Mycoplasmataceae, in the order Mycoplasmatales, which belongs to the class Mollicutes.[227, 552] Both *Mycoplasma* and *Ureaplasma* require cholesterol for growth, have a genome with a molecular weight of approximately 4.5×10^8, and have nicotinamide adenine dinucleotide (NADH) oxidase localized in the cytoplasm. These species lack a cell wall, as do all organisms within the class Mollicutes.[305] Members of the genus *Mycoplasma* do not hydrolyze urea, whereas the three species within the genus *Ureaplasma* do.

The "normal" human mollicate flora includes 13 *Mycoplasma,* 1 *Ureaplasma,* and 1 *Acholeplasma* spp.[93, 171, 227, 399, 662, 669] These organisms are listed by site of most common isolation and frequency of occurrence in Table 196–1. *Mycoplasma salivarium* and *Mycoplasma orale* are commonly part of the normal respiratory flora and have not been associated with illness in non-immunocompromised persons. *M. hominis* and *U. urealyticum* also are recovered commonly from humans, and frequently they are related causally to illness.

TABLE 196–1 ■ MOLLICUTES FLORA OF HUMANS LISTED BY SITE OF MOST COMMON ISOLATION AND PREVALENCE

Organism	Prevalence
Respiratory tract	
Mycoplasma salvarium	Very common
Mycoplasma orale	Very common
Mycoplasma buccale	Rare
Mycoplasma faucium	Rare
Mycoplasma lipophilum	Rare
Mycoplasma pneumoniae	Common
Acholeplasma laidlawii	Rare
Genitourinary tract	
Mycoplasma hominis	Very common
Mycoplasma genitalium	Rare
Mycoplasma fermentans	Rare
Mycoplasma primatum	Rare
Mycoplasma spermatophilum	Rare
Mycoplasma penetrans	Rare
Ureaplasma urealyticum	Very common
Blood	
Mycoplasma pirum	Rare

Data from references 399, 435, 619, 662, 668, 672.

Mycoplasma buccale, Mycoplasma faucium, Mycoplasma primatum, Acholeplasma laidlawii, and *Mycoplasma lipophilum* rarely are isolated and are not thought to cause disease in non-immunocompromised humans. *M. genitalium* and *Mycoplasma fermentans* have biologic and morphologic features that suggest they may be pathogenic in people, but their role in human genital disease has not been established.[649, 668] Persistent infections in blood, bones, joints, and kidneys with *M. fermentans, U. urealyticum, Mycoplasma penetrans, Mycoplasma pirum,* and *M. hominis* have occurred in patients with immunodeficiencies.[29, 467, 668] *M. pneumoniae* is a common cause of respiratory and other human illness.

Mycoplasma pneumoniae

PROPERTIES

Morphology

Because mycoplasmas lack a cell wall, they all tend to be pleomorphic. Kammer and colleagues[336] studied the morphologic characteristics of *M. pneumoniae* organisms grown in broth medium by scanning electron microscopy and grouped their observations by days of incubation. From 0.3 to 2 days, the predominant morphologic feature consisted of 0.51 ± 0.011-μm symmetric round forms in tightly packed clusters. During the interval from day 2 to day 6, branched and straight filaments and bulbs were the predominant forms. The bulbous elements had a diameter of 0.25 ± 0.006 μm, and the filamentous forms were 0.19 ± 0.005 μm in diameter. The filaments were intertwined, and occasional round forms were observed. From day 6 to day 10, the organisms had a rounded shape but were asymmetric. Their diameter was 0.72 ± 0.027 μm, and they occurred in groups of three or four cells. Biberfeld and Biberfeld[42] noted that *M. pneumoniae* filamentous forms varied in length from 1 to 5 μm.

The ultrastructure of *M. pneumoniae,* as well as that of all members of the family Mycoplasmataceae, is relatively simple and consists of a cell membrane and cytoplasm.[227, 667] In 7-day *M. pneumoniae* cultures, Domermuth and associates[159] noted the following characteristics: elementary bodies 105 × 120 nm in diameter, mature cells with a maximal diameter of 690 × 750 nm and an average diameter of 440 × 590 nm, asymmetry of the limiting membrane, electron-dense lines outside the limiting membrane, and dense bodies as cytoplasmic inclusions.

Wilson and Collier[713] studied the ultrastructure of *M. pneumoniae* in hamster tracheal organ culture and noted filamentous organisms with trilaminar membranes; the cells were polymorphic, but each had a specialized terminal structure at the site of attachment to the organ culture. This terminal structure had a dense central core containing a denser central filament. Between the organism and the organ culture cell, fusion was not detected, but a loose network of fibrils was noted between the two surfaces. The bodies of the mycoplasmas contained densely staining fibrillar material and cytoplasmic granules, both of which contained nucleic acid.

Motility and Multiplication

Bredt[66] studied *M. pneumoniae* motility and multiplication on a glass surface in liquid medium by phase-contrast microscopy. The organisms were observed to multiply by binary fission; first, short filamentous structures were formed, which then separated into two cells. A growth cycle between two separations lasted approximately 3 hours. After division, the new cells moved by means of a gliding motion. The gliding speed has been noted to be approximately 0.2 to 0.5 μm/sec, but maximal speeds of 1.5 to 2.0 μm/sec have been observed.[547]

Composition

Mycoplasmas are composed of approximately 40 to 60 percent protein, 10 to 20 percent lipid, and a variable amount of carbohydrate. The *M. pneumoniae* genome is circular, double-stranded DNA with a contour length of 4.8×10^8 d.[473] The guanosine plus cytosine content of the DNA is 38.6 to 40.8 percent.[59, 496, 552, 651]

Growth Characteristics and Physical Properties[94, 272, 552, 648, 667]

M. pneumoniae grows in *Mycoplasma* broth medium and on agar enriched with yeast extract and animal serum. *M. pneumoniae* ferments carbohydrates and requires sterol for growth. It grows under both anaerobic and aerobic conditions, but growth is more consistent when it is incubated in nitrogen and 5 percent carbon dioxide. When compared with other mycoplasmas isolated from humans, *M. pneumoniae* grows relatively slowly, with visible formation of colonies rarely occurring in less than 1 week and possibly taking 3 weeks or more. Repeated agar passage results in more rapid growth, and laboratory strains thus treated produce colonies in 3 days.

M. pneumoniae colonies on agar generally appear different from the classic *Mycoplasma* "fried egg" look noted with other types recovered from humans. The *M. pneumoniae* colony is spherical and dense, with a rough ("mulberry") surface.

M. pneumoniae has the following enzyme systems: $NADH_2$ oxidase, nicotinamide adenine dinucleotide phosphate ($NADPH_2$) oxidase, lactate dehydrogenase, probably succinic dehydrogenase, and diaphorases.[272] In liquid medium, the following can be noted: acid color change in medium with added glucose and phenol red as a result of glucose metabolism, reduction of methylene blue in medium as a result of dehydrogenase activity, and reduction of 2-3-5 tetrazolium chloride to red formazan by dehydrogenase activity.[648]

On agar, *M. pneumoniae* hemolyzes erythrocytes in an agar overlay by liberation of peroxide. Erythrocytes and other cells adsorb to *M. pneumoniae* colonies, and organisms in suspension cause hemagglutination.

Mycoplasmas, including *M. pneumoniae*, are heat-sensitive. They have a half-life of less than 2 minutes at 50° C and lose viability within 1 week at room temperature.[667] They can be stored for several years at −20° C, but −70° C is optimal for long-term storage.

Mycoplasmas are resistant to osmotic environmental changes but are sensitive to detergents. They are inhibited by gold salts and antibiotics not directed against cell wall synthesis.

Antigenic Composition

The following immunologic reactions have been noted in association with *M. pneumoniae*–host serum interactions: specific complement fixation; precipitation in gel; growth inhibition; indirect hemagglutination; metabolic inhibition; antigen-antibody union identified by immunofluorescence, enzyme-linked immunosorbent assay (ELISA), and radioimmunoassay; adherence inhibition assay; and nonspecific complement fixation (positive serologic test result for syphilis) and agglutination (cold and *Streptococcus* MG agglutinins).[83, 299, 313, 399, 543, 648] *M. pneumoniae* organisms have both membrane and cytoplasmic antigens.[190, 344] Two membrane antigens can be identified by immunodiffusion,[535] with the major membrane antigen being found in the lipid fraction of the organism.[344] The antigens are glycolipids and are of major importance in complement fixation, metabolic inhibition, and mycoplasmacidal reactions.[77] The cytoplasmic (soluble) antigen, which also contains lipid, can be identified by complement fixation when the antigen is prepared by phenol extraction.

Humans have an IgG immune response to six principal protein antigens.[146, 147, 225, 370, 551, 686] These six polypeptides have the following molecular masses: 170, 130, 90, 45, 35, and 30 kd. The 170-kd antigen is the P1 protein. This protein is localized at the surface of the terminal organelle (terminal structure), is the major adhesin responsible for attachment, and is the cause of the gliding motility of the organism. Antibodies to P1 protein inhibit hemadsorption and adherence to respiratory epithelium.[295, 297, 298, 312, 333, 371, 634] Another important adhesin is the 30-kd protein (P30 adhesin). In addition to the P1 and P30 proteins, at least six accessory proteins are involved in the adherence of *M. pneumoniae* to host cells.[552] These accessory proteins are HMW1, HMW2, HMW3, and A, B, and C.

M. pneumoniae strains can be divided into two types based on sequence variation in the P1 gene.[161,162] Five subtypes of the type 1 strain and three subtypes of the type 2 strain have been noted by restriction fragment length polymorphism (RFLP).

Membrane determinants of *M. pneumoniae* cross-react with the erythrocyte glycoprotein containing the I antigen and the related sugar chain (F1)[278, 316]; with pneumococcal serotypes 23 and 32[13]; with the glycolipids of spinach, parsnips, carrots, and selected strains of *Staphylococcus aureus* and group A streptococci; and with perhaps the filamentous hemagglutinin of *Bordetella pertussis*.[254, 310, 345, 683]

Animal Susceptibility

M. pneumoniae grows and causes pneumonia in hamsters and cotton rats and causes inapparent infection of the bronchial epithelium of chicken embryos.[543]

EPIDEMIOLOGY

Epidemic Pattern

In large urban areas, *M. pneumoniae* is endemic; infection and disease occur throughout the year. Foy and associates[207, 213] noted cultural or serologic evidence of *M. pneumoniae* infection in a Seattle prepaid medical care group during all seasons throughout an 11-year period. Similar endemicity has been reported in other studies.[464, 470, 502] In addition to the background endemic pattern, *M. pneumoniae* enjoys a cyclic epidemic pattern that is specific for a particular urban community. Epidemics have occurred at 3- to 7-year intervals.[176, 213, 331, 402, 502] Epidemics, which develop slowly, usually start in the fall and persist in the community for 12 to 30 months.

As part of an influenza surveillance program, Layani-Milon and associates[382] studied acute respiratory infections in outpatients for six winters in the Rhône-Alpes region of France by using a polymerase chain reaction (PCR) plus hybridization–based detection system. Each year from 1992 to 1997, at least one peak of *M. pneumoniae* infection was noted in the late fall. Overall, they studied 3897 children and adults with acute respiratory illnesses, and 7.3 percent were found to be infected with *M. pneumoniae*. The yearly rate of *M. pneumoniae* cases fell from 10.1 percent in 1992 to 1993 to 2.0 percent in 1995 to 1996; in the subsequent year (1996 to 1997), it rose to 4.2 percent.

Incidence of Infection and Disease

In the past, most pediatricians and other physicians considered *M. pneumoniae* illness to be uncommon in the general population. The initial epidemiologic studies were concerned mainly with the occurrence of pneumonia in closed populations, such as the military and boarding schools.[98, 464, 573, 631, 632, 680] During the last 37 years, however, many large studies in civilian populations, coupled with more sensitive serologic techniques, have indicated that both infection and disease with *M. pneumoniae* occur commonly.*

Hornsleth[292] examined 367 serum samples collected from children hospitalized in Copenhagen from September 1963 to May 1965 for complement-fixing antibodies. He noted that 42 percent of infants 6 to 11 months of age had demonstrable antibody; from 1 to 9 years of age, more than two thirds of the children had antibody. Suhs and Feldman[638] found a similar high prevalence of hemagglutination-inhibiting antibody in the sera of residents of Point Barrow, Alaska, but only 5 percent of the serum samples from a children's home in Syracuse had measurable antibody.

Brunner and associates[78] detected serum antibody by the sensitive radioimmunoprecipitation test in 28 percent of 7- to 12-month-old infants, 55 percent of 13- to 24-month-old children, 67 percent of 25- to 60-month-old children, and 97 percent of persons older than 17 years. The high antibody prevalence noted in this study, as well as the findings in Copenhagen and Alaska, suggests an infection incidence rate of approximately 20 to 30 percent per year in a susceptible population of young children. The prevalent antibody noted at an early age in these studies possibly is not caused specifically by *M. pneumoniae* infection but, instead could be the result of exposure to the many cross-reacting antigens in nature.[13, 235, 345] However, studies by Fernald and colleagues,[194] in which infants and children in a daycare center were monitored systematically, indicated a yearly infection rate of approximately 12 percent.

Monto and colleagues,[470] in a large study involving 3243 persons, investigated the incidence of infection in six yearly cohort groups of children and adults. Infection was determined by significant rises in titer of complement-fixing antibody on three serum specimens collected during a 1-year period from each subject. The overall yearly infection rate was found to be 5.3 percent. The highest rate (8.8%) occurred in the 5- to 9-year-old group. Infants younger than 1 year had a rate of 2.8 percent.

Brunner and associates[78] noted that geometric mean antibody titers tended to increase with increasing age, which suggested that the older children were being reinfected. Fernald and colleagues[194] reported that 5 of 22 children infected with *M. pneumoniae* in their investigation experienced reinfections during the 5-year observation period. In the study of Monto and associates,[470] 24.4 percent of the 172 infections detected in subjects of all ages were reinfections. During a 12-year serologic surveillance period, Foy and coworkers[213] noted great variation in the incidence of

*See references 10, 24, 26, 46, 78, 89, 136, 156, 165, 171, 194, 208–211, 213, 216, 218, 242, 243, 245, 251, 292, 318, 326, 331, 402, 415, 470, 471, 502, 638.

M. pneumoniae infection; in the period from October 1965 to May 1966, only 0.2 percent of 398 children had fourfold rises in complement-fixation antibody titer, whereas during the May 1973 to May 1974 period, 35 percent of 246 subjects 10 to 20 years old had serologic evidence of infection.

The incidence of disease caused by *M. pneumoniae* depends on the endemic or epidemic prevalence of the organism in the community and is age related. The incidence of *M. pneumoniae* by age for two epidemics and the surrounding endemic periods in Seattle was studied by Foy and associates.[213] The highest epidemic attack rate was 14 per 1000 children 5 to 9 years of age, and the highest endemic attack rate (4 per 1000) occurred in the same age group. Ten- to 14-year-old children had the second highest attack rate during both epidemic and endemic periods. The attack rate in children younger than 5 years was about twice that observed in young adults.

The ratio of symptomatic to asymptomatic infection has varied in different studies. In family studies, both Balassanian and Robbins[26] and Foy and associates[211] noted that only 15 percent of infections were asymptomatic, whereas Saliba and associates[573] noted that 55 percent of the residents of a boys' home had asymptomatic infection. Chanock and colleagues[98] observed that only 1 of 30 infections in Marine recruits was manifested as clinically apparent pneumonia.

Incubation Period

The reported incubation period has varied from a mean of approximately 1 week in volunteer studies and point-source epidemics to 3 weeks in community outbreaks.* In a volunteer study, Rifkind and colleagues[557] administered tissue culture–grown *M. pneumoniae* in a concentration of 320 to 1280 EID_{50} (mean egg-infective dose) into the nose and posterior pharyngeal area of 27 men with no demonstrable antibody. In this study, pneumonia occurred 9 to 12 days after inoculation, following 1 to 3 days of upper respiratory illness. In six volunteers, only upper respiratory illness was noted, and the incubation period varied from 4 to 9 days. In a similar study in which volunteers received 10^6 to 10^7 broth-grown organisms, the incubation period was 8 to 10 days.[609]

In an interesting common-source outbreak caused by an intense 8-hour exposure at a party, the peak incubation period was 13 days, and most of the cases occurred between days 11 and 14.[179] In another probable point-source outbreak, which may have resulted from a room aerosol, the incubation period varied from 4 to 9 days.[576] In studies of case-to-case intervals in families, Foy and associates[211] reported a median incubation time of 23 days, with most of the cases occurring between days 16 and 25. In similar studies, Copps and colleagues[136] noted an average interval of 21 days, and Biberfeld and Sterner[46] found a modal value of 20 days. A point-source outbreak in a family unit was described in which all seven family members became ill 10 to 16 days after the onset of symptoms in the index case.[346]

The longer incubation period in the family situation than in the volunteer studies and the point-source outbreaks may be the result of larger inocula in the last instances. An alternative explanation may be that in the community case-to-case situation, the index case may not transmit the organism effectively until symptoms have been manifested for a week or more.

*See references 46, 136, 179, 208, 211, 215, 557, 576, 610, 669.

Communicability

In contrast to other respiratory illnesses such as measles and influenza, the spread of disease caused by *M. pneumoniae* in both closed populations, such as military training units and boarding schools, and open communities is usually slow. For example, the introduction of influenza or measles into a family most often results in infection of all susceptible persons from the primary case. In contrast, the spread of *M. pneumoniae* through a family of six people probably would require three or four passages. Foy and associates[211] noted secondary attack rates in families of 64 percent for children and 17 percent for adults. Biberfeld and Sterner[46] reported secondary infection rates of 41 and 84 percent, respectively, for adults and children in families. In contrast to family groups, the spread of *M. pneumoniae* in schools and other situations of brief exposure is low.[208, 217] In one Seattle elementary school, the infection rate was 18 percent. Foy and Alexander[208] believe that neighborhood spread among playmates is more important than school exposure in community transmission of *M. pneumoniae*.

Transmission in families occurs during the acute phase of illness, and transmission by persons with asymptomatic infection has not been documented.[208]

Geography

The endemic and epidemic presence of *M. pneumoniae* has been demonstrated in the urban areas of developed countries with temperate climates throughout the world.* Serologic investigations in more remote areas, including both arctic and tropical zones, also indicate the presence of *M. pneumoniae* infection. Suhs and Feldman[638] found measurable antibody in the serum of 68 percent of 169 persons in Point Barrow, and Golubjatnikov and associates,[245] in a study of children in a remote Mexican highland community, detected seropositivity in 16 percent of 637 children. Serologic evidence of infection also has been noted in Cairo, Singapore, Hong Kong, the West Indies, and southern Africa.[95, 331] Incidence studies have not been performed in rural areas, but patterns of infection probably would be characterized by epidemic periods of a year or so and then complete absence of *M. pneumoniae* circulation for several years.

Sex

Although the results of studies have varied, the difference in the incidence of *M. pneumoniae* disease by sex is small. During the 11 years of study in Seattle, Foy and associates[213] noted that the rate of *M. pneumoniae* pneumonia was higher in women than in men in the 30- to 39-year age group (1.8 versus 1.2 per 1000); in infants, boys were afflicted more often than girls, but otherwise the rates for children by sex were virtually identical. Jensen and associates[326] found that pneumonia, otitis media, and nasopharyngitis in various combinations occurred more commonly in boys than in girls. Monto and colleagues[470] noted that boys younger than 5 years of age had more infections, but that the reverse was true for children 5 to 14 years of age. In other studies involving all age groups, males have shown a slightly greater frequency of illness than females.[436, 502] In the Seattle family studies, symptoms were more severe in boys than in girls.

*See references 46, 156, 186, 208, 213, 318, 402, 424, 436, 487, 502, 626.

PATHOGENESIS AND PATHOLOGY

Sequence of Events in Infection

M. pneumoniae infection is acquired via the respiratory route from the respiratory secretions of an ill person infected with this agent. Spread can be accomplished by small-particle aerosols or large droplets of secretions coming in contact with the epithelial surface of the nasopharynx and perhaps the surfaces of the lower respiratory tract (trachea, bronchi, and bronchioles) as well. In volunteer studies, Couch[139] observed that the 50 percent human infectious dose by small-particle aerosol was 1 colony-forming unit (nasal instillation required a dose that was 100 times greater).

Because epidemiologic data indicate the need for close and perhaps prolonged personal contact for transmission of infection, transmission by small-particle aerosol probably occurs rarely under natural conditions. After acquisition of the infectious agent, multiplication occurs extracellularly on mucous membrane surfaces. The incubation period, which varies from 4 days to more than 3 weeks, probably depends strongly on the size of the original inoculum. The extent of the respiratory infection increases during the incubation period, and shedding of organisms in respiratory secretions can be observed 2 to 8 days before clinical illness.[139] Initial symptoms of infection include headache, malaise, fever, sore throat, and cough; evidence of lower respiratory tract disease is present within the succeeding 3 days.[156, 557] The method of extension of infection within the respiratory tract is unknown. The extent of disease possibly depends totally on the initial distribution of the infectious agent at the time of acquisition rather than on spread of infection from a primary upper respiratory site.

After the onset of clinical symptoms, the concentration of *M. pneumoniae* in respiratory secretions peaks, remains high for approximately 1 week, and then persists for 4 to 6 weeks or longer.[139, 156] The associated symptoms and signs in disease caused by *M. pneumoniae* (meningitis, arthritis, hemolytic anemia, rash, pericarditis) suggest the possibility of frequent dissemination of the organism from the respiratory tract. Many reviews on the subject tend to discount the possibility of generalized *M. pneumoniae* infection and attribute the associated systemic clinical findings to immunologic events related to respiratory infection.[139, 156] However, little published evidence indicates that the organism has been sought carefully in the blood and other sites of dissemination. In many instances, *M. pneumoniae* has been recovered from or identified by PCR in the blood, pericardial fluid, middle ear fluid, vesicular skin lesions, pleural fluid, kidneys, brain, and cerebrospinal fluid (CSF).* In addition, the observation of low CSF glucose in *M. pneumoniae* meningoencephalitis suggests direct involvement by the organism.[358]

Pathology

Pathologic findings in *M. pneumoniae* disease of children have not been reported, and only minimal data from adults are available. However, a reasonable understanding of the pathologic process of *M. pneumoniae* disease can be constructed from studies in the hamster, various tracheal organ cultures, and human biopsy and postmortem material.[160, 332, 427, 458, 524, 658, 717] The primary damage in *M. pneumoniae* infection is to the epithelial lining of the mucosal surfaces of the respiratory tract. This damage has been observed on the surface of bronchi, bronchioles, and alveoli, and clinical symptoms in children suggest that similar pathologic changes occur in the trachea and upper respiratory tract as well. Specifically conspicuous is destruction of the ciliated epithelium of the bronchi and bronchioles. Because of mucosal desquamation and ulceration, the lumina contain considerable debris; added to this debris is an inflammatory exudate consisting of fibrin, mononuclear cells, and neutrophils. The alveolar spaces contain similar exudate and edema fluid.

The walls of the bronchi and bronchioles are thickened by edema and contain an infiltrate of macrophages, lymphocytes, and plasma cells. The alveolar walls are also thickened and contain lymphocytes, mononuclear cells, and erythrocytes. Dilation of the septal capillaries occurs. Edema and cellular infiltration extend into the interstitial spaces. Gross examination of the lungs reveals areas of hemorrhage and congestion. The pleura may contain patches of fibrinous exudate, and pleural fluid may be present. The pneumonic areas may be discrete or widespread.

A biopsy specimen of a vesiculopustular skin lesion revealed an epidermis with mild acanthosis and marked edema that primarily was intracellular.[658] The papillary and upper reticular dermis contained neutrophils and round cells, and hemorrhagic foci were present within the upper corium and epidermis. The blister fluid contained plasma protein and neutrophils. Findings in other organs include mesenteric lymphadenitis, focal hepatic necrosis, follicular splenitis, acute myocarditis, and hemorrhagic encephalitis.

Immunologic Events

SPECIFIC ANTIBODY. A specific serum antibody response usually occurs after infection with *M. pneumoniae*, and it can be measured by many different serologic techniques: immunofluorescence, complement fixation, indirect hemagglutination, precipitation, growth inhibition, mycoplasmacidal antibody test, ELISA, radioimmunoassay, adherence inhibition assay, and radioimmunoprecipitation test.* Complement-fixing antibodies occur early in *M. pneumoniae* disease, reach a peak titer in approximately 1 month, and then decline slowly over a variable period. Fluorescent-staining antibodies and antibody determined by ELISA have temporal patterns similar to those of complement-fixing antibodies. Growth-inhibiting antibodies appear later (2 to 3 weeks after the onset of illness), peak later, and persist longer than complement-fixing antibodies do. The initial serum immune response includes specific IgM, IgG, and IgA antibodies. After clinical illness and convalescence, specific antibody is located mainly in the IgG serum fraction. Occasionally, significant levels of IgM antibody persist for several months or years after infection.[41, 79, 174, 328] Antibody titer responses in infected children are generally of a lesser magnitude than those in adults.[165] Asymptomatic infections in children may not be associated with a measurable serum antibody response. *M. pneumoniae*–specific IgE antibodies have been detected in the sera of patients with asthma, atopic dermatitis, or both conditions.[664]

After infection, specific antibody is also present in nasal secretions and sputum.[40, 75] In volunteer studies, Brunner and colleagues[75] noted that 42 and 73 percent of subjects had respective IgA nasal and sputum responses. Biberfeld and Sterner[47] found specific antibody in 44 of 55 sputum

*See references 2, 9, 30, 33, 49, 204, 303, 338, 362, 417, 418, 422, 483, 486, 493, 494, 552, 615, 616, 641, 665.

*See references 76–78, 83, 164, 193, 273, 299, 313, 399, 410, 543, 584, 656.

specimens from patients with *M. pneumoniae* infection of the lower respiratory tract. They noted IgA antibody in all specimens tested, IgG antibody in 24 of 31 specimens, and IgM antibody in 13 of 27 specimens.

SPECIFIC CELL-MEDIATED IMMUNITY. Fernald and coworkers[188, 189, 195] have shown that lymphocytes from adults previously infected with *M. pneumoniae* undergo blast transformation when cultured in vitro in the presence of *M. pneumoniae* organisms. In age-related studies, researchers noted that only one of nine children younger than 4 years with documented previous infection had evidence of specific cell-mediated immunity as measured by lymphocyte stimulation.[194] In contrast, 7 of 12 children older than 4 years and 87 percent of an adult group demonstrated specific lymphocyte stimulation. This study suggests that specific cell-mediated immunity increases as a function of age and depends on repeated infection. Koh and colleagues[359] noted high levels of interleukin-4 (IL-4) and a high IL-4/interferon-γ ratio in the bronchoalveolar lavage fluid of children with *M. pneumoniae* pneumonia, thus suggesting a predominant T_H2-like cytokine response.

Martin and colleagues[440] found that leukocytes from volunteers with *M. pneumoniae* infection demonstrated chemotaxis in the presence of the organism whereas leukocytes collected before infection did not. Patients infected with *M. pneumoniae* also respond with interferon-α in their blood and nasopharyngeal secretions early in infection and with interferon-γ during convalescence.[488, 489]

NONSPECIFIC RESPONSES. Antibodies to several diverse antigens develop during human infection with *M. pneumoniae.* The best known of these antibodies are cold agglutinins, and they are useful in the diagnosis of *M. pneumoniae* pneumonia.[138, 185, 273, 318, 612] Cold agglutinins are directed against the I antigen of erythrocytes.[316, 403, 612] Most pneumonias in which serum cold agglutinins are noted are caused by *M. pneumoniae.* Cold agglutinins are detected in the serum of approximately 75 percent of patients with *M. pneumoniae* pneumonia; they are less common in *M. pneumoniae* infection without pneumonia.[94]

Patients with *M. pneumoniae* also frequently develop antibodies to the MG strain of nonhemolytic streptococci[401] and occasionally to *M. genitalium,*[405] *M. hominis,*[579] *Mycoplasma hyorhinis, Mycoplasma orale, Mycoplasma pulmonis, M. salivarium,* and *Mycoplasma mycoides* variety *mycoides,* the etiologic agent of contagious pleuropneumonia of cattle.[391] Other heterologous antibodies found in the serum of patients with *M. pneumoniae* infection include those to smooth muscle, the mitotic spindle apparatus, brain, lung, liver, and Wasserman (WR) cardiolipin antigen.[40, 48, 404] In addition to these findings, Biberfeld and Norberg detected immune complexes by the platelet aggregation technique in the sera of 16 of 39 patients with acute respiratory illness caused by *M. pneumoniae.*[44] Mizutani and Mizutani[461] demonstrated the presence of circulating immune complexes in most patients with pneumonia caused by *M. pneumoniae.* The same investigators also detected rheumatoid factor in the sera of patients with *M. pneumoniae* disease.[462]

Possible Mechanisms of Disease Production

Numerous studies have been performed in an attempt to understand the pathogenesis of respiratory disease caused by mycoplasmas.[78, 109–112, 122–124, 129, 131–134] Of particular interest in human *M. pneumoniae* infection is the apparent high prevalence of infection in infants, children, adolescents, and young adults but the frequently mild nature of disease in infants and young children in comparison to older patients. Some studies suggest that the more severe disease in older patients is associated with reinfection and is mediated somewhat by immunologic responses.

Organ culture and animal studies indicate that damage at the site of primary infection—the respiratory epithelium—is the result of close organism-cell attachment.[109, 132, 134, 296, 407, 408, 481, 540, 675] This attachment of organism to cell uses neuraminic acid receptors on the cell.[614] In an organ culture system with *M. mycoides* variety *capri,* ciliary damage was decreased when the cellular receptor sites were treated with receptor-destroying enzyme.[110] Lipman and associates[407, 408] noted that one attenuated *M. pneumoniae* strain had lost its ability to cytadsorb. The close association of organism and cell allows the transport of specific damaging material to the cell. Although the precise nature of this substance is not known, the data available suggest that it might be hydrogen peroxide. It is liberated by *M. pneumoniae* in vitro; in organ culture studies, hydrogen peroxide has been shown to be the damaging factor in another *Mycoplasma* infection.[109, 408, 409] In cell culture, *M. pneumoniae* inhibits host-cell catalase activity.[15] This inhibition of catalase activity enhances the toxicity of the hydrogen peroxide generated by the microorganism. *M. pneumoniae* also enters host cells and persists intracellularly for at least 7 days.[28]

Fernald and associates[194] noted that specific cell-mediated immunity to *M. pneumoniae* as measured by lymphocyte transformation becomes more prevalent with increasing age, as does specific antibody. Their studies suggest that more than one exposure to antigen may be necessary to elicit both humoral and cellular responses. Fernald and Glezen,[195] in an inactivated *M. pneumoniae* vaccine trial in children, noted that lymphocyte sensitivity developed in many recipients, but not a humoral antibody response. In a trial of an inactivated vaccine in adults, Smith and associates[609] found that on challenge infection, an exaggerated illness occurred in vaccinees who failed to form humoral antibodies after immunization. These findings have led to the consideration that persistent specific cell-mediated responsiveness might contribute to the pulmonary process in *M. pneumoniae* infection. However, the incubation period of illness in adults and children is similar, which argues against the sensitization theory.[119]

Foy and associates[214] noted that complement-fixing antibodies remained elevated for 2 to 9 years after infection with pneumonia but fell quickly after the second year in persons with mild illness. Protection against reinfection was better in those who previously had pneumonia than in those with mild symptoms.

CLINICAL MANIFESTATIONS

Pneumonia

Pneumonia is the most important clinical manifestation of *M. pneumoniae* infection, and this agent is responsible for 10 to 20 percent of all cases of pneumonia.[126, 156, 217, 218, 224, 275, 276, 294, 453] The highest incidence of pneumonia caused by *M. pneumoniae* in Seattle occurred in children 5 to 14 years of age.[213] In a study in Chiba Prefecture, Japan, researchers noted that the peak age of lower respiratory tract illness caused by *M. pneumoniae* was 4 years.[485] In a prospective study of community-acquired pneumonia in Finland, 11 percent of the children with *M. pneumoniae* infection were younger than 5 years of age, 32 percent were between 5 and 9 years of age, and 57 percent were 10 to 14 years of age.[275] Although researchers frequently state that *M. pneumoniae* pneumonia rarely occurs in children younger than 5 years of age, in

TABLE 196–2 ■ FREQUENCY OF CLINICAL FINDINGS IN CHILDREN AND ADULTS WITH *MYCOPLASMA PNEUMONIAE* PNEUMONIA

Finding	Frequency
Symptoms	
Fever	++++
Cough	++++
Malaise	+++
Headache	++
Sputum	++
Chills	++
Hoarseness	+
Earache	+
Coryza	+
Sore throat	+
Diarrhea	+
Nausea and/or vomiting	+
Chest pain	+
Signs	
Rales	+++
Pharyngitis	++
Lymphadenopathy	+
Conjunctivitis	±
Rash	±
Otitis media	±

++++, close to 100 percent; +++, 75 percent; ++, 50 percent; +, 25 percent; ±, 0 to 10 percent.
Compiled from eight studies in which both children and adults were included: references 43, 45, 136, 217, 224, 319, 430, 487.

actuality, the incidence in this group was found to be about twice that noted in young adults in Seattle.[213] Pneumonia caused by *M. pneumoniae* occurs less commonly in children younger than 2 years of age and rarely in infants younger than 6 months of age. The apparent frequency of *M. pneumoniae* pneumonia is influenced by the relative occurrence of pneumonia caused by other pathogens. During the child's first 5 years of life, *M. pneumoniae* is only one of many agents (e.g., respiratory syncytial virus, adenoviruses, parainfluenza viruses, influenza viruses, *Streptococcus pneumoniae, Haemophilus influenzae*) that cause pneumonia. During later childhood and adolescence, pneumonia as a consequence of infection with these other agents is a rare event; therefore, *M. pneumoniae* is the leading cause of pneumonia in these persons.

Because isolation rates of *M. pneumoniae* during both endemic and epidemic periods do not vary greatly by season, as do those of common respiratory viruses, the proportion of patients with *M. pneumoniae* pneumonia increases during the summer months.

SYMPTOMS AND SIGNS. Since 1961, a large number of studies have reported the frequency of signs and symptoms in *M. pneumoniae* infection.* Unfortunately, many studies have included only special populations such as the military, and with few exceptions, community investigations have failed to indicate differences by age. In only three investigations have data regarding children been itemized separately.[72, 210, 633] Table 196–2 presents the relative frequency of symptoms and signs as compiled from eight studies in which both children and adults were included. The hallmark of pneumonia caused by *M. pneumoniae* is fever and cough. The onset of illness usually cannot be demarcated clearly, but malaise, fever, and headache are early complaints. Cough has an onset 3 to 5 days after the beginning of illness and is initially nonproductive. Foy and colleagues[217] and Biberfeld and coworkers[45] noted that 77 and 100 percent, respectively, of the patients that they studied had maximal temperatures greater than 38.9° C (102° F). Copps and associates[136] found that 58 percent of the group that they evaluated had temperatures higher than 39.4° C (103° F) and that 4 percent had temperatures higher than 40.6° C (105° F).

The reporting of headache in association with *M. pneumoniae* pneumonia has varied considerably. Nakao and associates[487] noted this complaint in only 8 percent of subjects, whereas Biberfeld and associates[45] and Foy and colleagues[217] reported it in two thirds of those studied. Chills and the production of sputum are present in about 50 percent of ill patients. Again, great differences among investigations are noted, and they probably are related to the relative ages of the patients.

Coryza is unusual in *M. pneumoniae* pneumonia; therefore, its occurrence should suggest another etiologic agent for illness in a specific patient. In a study involving children exclusively, Stevens and colleagues[633] noted that coryza occurred more commonly in young children; as might be expected, they found productive cough more frequently in their older patients. Hoarseness, earache, sore throat, gastrointestinal complaints, and chest pain occur in approximately 25 percent of patients.

On physical examination, about 75 percent of patients have auscultatory evidence of pneumonia, and approximately half have pharyngitis. Remarkable lymphadenopathy, particularly with cervical involvement, is noted in approximately 25 percent of patients. Twenty-one percent of the patients studied by Foy and associates[217] had otitis media. In other studies, this manifestation was noted in about 5 to 10 percent of cases. Conjunctivitis was reported in almost half the patients reported by Fransen and associates.[224] In contrast, except for Jansson and colleagues,[319] who noted conjunctivitis in 3 percent of their study group, this finding was not mentioned in the other reports. Similarly, rash was reported in 6, 11, and 17 percent, respectively, in the studies in Minnesota, Wisconsin, and Seattle,[136, 218, 430] but it was not mentioned in the other studies.

The most common finding on chest auscultation is dry rales, but musical rales with expiration are noted occasionally. Rales usually persist for 2 weeks, and hearing them a month or more after the onset of disease is not unusual. Occasionally, patients have no auscultatory evidence of pulmonary disease throughout their illness, in spite of the presence of abnormalities on chest radiographs. During illness, cough becomes increasingly prominent; initially it is nonproductive, but later, it may produce a frothy white sputum in older children and adolescents. The sputum also may appear purulent and contain blood. Cough persists for 3 to 4 weeks and longer after nonrespiratory symptoms such as fever and headache have subsided.

In a study of 44 children with lower respiratory illness caused by *M. pneumoniae,* Stevens and associates[633] noted the following frequencies of symptoms and signs: cough, 97 percent; malaise, 82 percent; vomiting, 40 percent; abdominal pain, 35 percent; headache, 32 percent; rash, 20 percent; fever higher than 38° C (>100.4° F), 78 percent; rales, 78 percent; pharyngitis, 32 percent; rhonchi, 30 percent; bronchial breathing, 27 percent; and otitis media, 27 percent. Foy and coworkers[210] found that chills and productive cough were more common in adults than children and that temperatures tended to be higher in children.

In a large study involving 108 children with *M. pneumoniae* infection, wheezing occurred with the acute illness in 40 percent.[570] When the children in this study were evaluated

*See references 43, 45, 72, 104, 114, 126, 136, 176, 177, 186, 210, 224, 235, 266, 277, 306, 319, 430, 464, 477, 487, 570, 633.

3 years after their acute illness, they were found to have three indicators of lung function that had mean values significantly lower than those in control children.

Few reports specifically describe pneumonia caused by *M. pneumoniae* in young children.[25, 103, 127, 211, 258, 485, 605, 633] However, a review of the case descriptions available indicates that illness, when it occurs, can be severe and relatively prolonged when compared with common viral and bacterial infections. Singer and DeVoe[605] reported a 3-year-old severely ill child who had a temperature of 39.4° C, a pulse of 150, and a respiratory rate of 40. Diffuse pulmonary involvement of the right upper lobe and lingular segments of the left lower lobe was observed by radiography, although rales and altered breath sounds could not be heard. The patient's condition worsened over a 6-day period. At this time, specific therapy with erythromycin was instituted, and slow recovery followed. The child had a normal white blood cell count, transiently elevated serum aspartate aminotransferase and alanine aminotransferase values, and microscopic hematuria. Grix and Giammona[258] observed two 5-year-old children with extensive pneumonia, pleural effusions, and febrile periods of 10 and 16 days. Stevens and associates[633] reported a 5-year-old boy with pulmonary consolidation and aseptic meningitis, and Clyde and Denny[127] described an asymptomatic 3-year-old boy with a "feathery infiltrate" in the right upper lung field. In a family study, Foy and colleagues[211] investigated four children younger than 6 years. In a 4-year-old child, the pneumonia persisted for more than 1 month, and in this child's brother, the illness lasted approximately 2 weeks. I have seen a 4.5-year-old girl with scattered infiltrates throughout both lung fields and febrile illness of 14 days' duration.[103]

Severe and extensive pulmonary disease occurs occasionally in *M. pneumoniae* infection.* Massive lobar pneumonia is noted on occasion, and pleural effusions are fairly common findings.† The adult respiratory distress syndrome has been observed, and illness has suggested pulmonary embolism with infarction.[202, 548, 603, 679] Chronic interstitial pulmonary fibrosis and fulminant fatal diffuse interstitial fibrosis have been noted in two adults with *M. pneumoniae* pneumonia, and localized bronchiectasis developed in a 20-year-old man at the site of previous acute lung infection.[116, 247, 333, 642] Children who had a delay in onset or inadequate duration of macrolide treatment were found by Marc and associates[431] to have reduced lung diffusion capacity after contracting *M. pneumoniae* pneumonia. A 5-year-old girl had severe necrotizing pneumonitis, and an adult had bronchiolitis obliterans organizing pneumonia.[411, 508] *M. pneumoniae* pneumonia is generally more severe in patients with preexisting cardiorespiratory problems, immunodeficiencies, and sickle-cell disease.[34, 118, 222, 230, 322, 457, 532, 598, 618]

Four patients—one child, one adolescent, and two adults—have been found to have lung abscesses in association with *M. pneumoniae* infection.[116, 397, 601] The illness in the adolescents and adults was characterized by productive cough and chest pain for 2 to 4 weeks. In one patient, clinical recovery and clearance of the pulmonary lesion were dramatic with tetracycline therapy; two other patients received suboptimal therapy but eventually recovered. The child with a lung abscess was a 6-year-old girl who had a 7-day history of cough and a 4-day history of fever.[116] In addition to the abscess, she had pleural effusion, thrombocytopenia, and disseminated intravascular coagulation. One 18-year-old man with extensive consolidation of the right lower lung field had residual pleural scarring 8 months after the acute illness.[478]

A newborn who contracted congenital pneumonia, probably via vertical transmission of *M. pneumoniae,* has been described.[677]

Clyde[126] reported factors that correlated with *M. pneumoniae* pneumonia in a study of 1139 subjects with community-acquired pneumonia. Positive factors were sore throat, headache, fever of 38.9° C or higher, exanthem, family size of four or more, and ear infection. In the same study, pneumonia did not correlate with coryza, leukocytosis (15×10^9/L or more and 10×10^9/L or more), preexisting disease, recurrent pneumonia, hospitalization for treatment, or cigarette smoking.

Although recovery from *M. pneumoniae* pneumonia is usually complete, two studies suggest that persistent abnormalities in lung function can occur after illness.[468, 570]

RADIOGRAPHY. Because the classic clinical entity, primary atypical pneumonia, has numerous causes but often is used as a synonym for *M. pneumoniae* pneumonia, much confusion has ensued about the spectrum of the radiographic appearance of the specific mycoplasmal infection. The radiographic pattern of primary atypical pneumonia is varied, but bilateral, diffuse, reticular infiltrates are common components.[416, 585, 608] Subsequent study has indicated that the diffuse interstitial pattern is an uncommon finding in *M. pneumoniae* infection and more often is the result of infection with other agents such as viruses, fungi, and *Chlamydia.*[70, 234, 495, 545, 674]

Brolin and Wernstedt[70] carefully evaluated the radiographic findings in 56 patients with significant *M. pneumoniae* pneumonia; 21 of the patients were younger than 20 years. They noted the following distribution of different patterns: typical lobar pneumonia, 8 patients; predominantly alveolar but not total consolidation, 13; interstitial (either reticular or noduloreticular), 20; a combination of lobar pneumonia and other alveolar involvement without total consolidation, 2; a combination of lobar involvement and interstitial, 10; and a combination of alveolar involvement without total consolidation and interstitial, 3. Alveolar patterns were more common in females; interstitial involvement was found more frequently in males. Twenty-two percent of patients had enlargement of the hilar or paratracheal lymph nodes, and 14 percent had pleural effusion.

The persistence of radiographic changes is variable. Brolin and Wernstedt[70] noted that 13 percent of their patients who underwent follow-up studies had abnormal findings more than 4 weeks after the initial study. They observed that persistence tended to be longer in patients with alveolar disease than in those with interstitial patterns. The degree of clinical symptoms and pulmonary physical findings frequently correlates poorly with the apparent degree of involvement noted on radiographs. In many patients with significant symptoms, only minimal interstitial changes are observed. In other instances, patients with lobar pneumonia often have few clinical findings indicating pulmonary disease.

Kim and associates[349] performed high-resolution computed tomography on 38 children who had been hospitalized with *M. pneumoniae* pneumonia 1 to 2.2 years previously. Abnormalities in two or more lobes, which corresponded to the initial chest radiographic infiltrates, were found in 37 percent of the children. Young age (<8 years) at the time of hospitalization and high *M. pneumoniae* antibody titer were found to be risk factors for the subsequent abnormalities.

*See references 105, 108, 116, 118, 135, 199, 202, 208, 258, 261, 341, 397, 411, 428, 431, 457, 477, 486, 504, 508, 524, 548, 558, 598, 601, 603, 605, 618, 625.

†See references 24, 108, 115, 128, 154, 199, 202, 258, 414, 417, 478, 484, 486, 504, 605, 625.

NONSPECIFIC LABORATORY DATA. The total leukocyte count in patients with pneumonia caused by *M. pneumoniae* is most often normal, but variation is considerable.* In a group of more than 250 children younger than 15 years, Foy and associates[210] noted that 30 percent and 6 percent had total leukocyte counts greater than 10,000 and 15,000 cells/mm^3, respectively. In a group of 45 children, Stevens and colleagues[633] observed leukocytosis in 33 percent of patients and leukopenia in one patient. Sixty-seven percent of the children had neutrophilia, and one patient had neutropenia. An increased percentage of band form neutrophils in *M. pneumoniae* pneumonia is an unusual finding.

The erythrocyte sedimentation rate is elevated in all cases,[43, 136, 318] and this elevation is usually marked. Biberfeld and colleagues[43] noted that 16 of 37 patients had erythrocyte sedimentation rates of 50 mm/hr. Serologic tests for syphilis are found to be falsely positive on occasion, and serum cold agglutinins and antibodies to *Streptococcus* MG antigen are common findings.[41, 94, 98, 156] Results of the direct Coombs test are frequently positive, and elevated levels of serum IgM are noted.[41, 185] Urinalysis results are generally normal.

Respiratory Disease Other Than Pneumonia

COMMON COLD AND UNSPECIFIED UPPER RESPIRATORY ILLNESS. By strict definition (significant nasal symptoms, no pharyngitis, and minimal fever), *M. pneumoniae* rarely causes the common cold. However, mild upper respiratory illness is noted frequently as the only manifestation of *M. pneumoniae* infection in children, adolescents, and young adults.† The frequency of unspecified upper respiratory tract illness as a manifestation of *M. pneumoniae* infection, when compared with other manifestations resulting from infection with this agent, varies considerably among studies. Feizi[184] studied patients from a country practice in England and noted that 50 percent of the patients had upper respiratory tract symptoms. Illness in these persons was often prolonged, however, and lasted as long as 7 to 10 weeks. In a review in Scotland, only 3 percent of 596 *M. pneumoniae* infections were classified as upper respiratory tract illness. In studies of common respiratory illnesses in children in which viruses and other agents were sought, *M. pneumoniae* was noted in 2 to 5 percent of patients with upper respiratory tract illness.[95, 156, 415]

PHARYNGITIS AND NASOPHARYNGITIS. As noted in Table 196–2, pharyngitis is observed in approximately half of all patients with *M. pneumoniae* pneumonia. However, pharyngitis as the major manifestation of *M. pneumoniae* infection occurs less commonly. Parrott[526] found that 12 percent of children admitted to the hospital with severe "bronchitis-pharyngitis" had *M. pneumoniae* infection. Jensen and associates[326] noted the frequent occurrence of pharyngitis and otitis media in children infected with *M. pneumoniae.* In a study of 715 children and adolescents with pharyngitis, Glezen and colleagues[241] reported that 36.8 percent had group A streptococcal infection and 3.1 percent were infected with *M. pneumoniae.* When the *M. pneumoniae* infections were grouped by age, the peak (11.4%) occurred in the 12- to 14-year-old group, and none were observed in children younger than 6 years. Five patients with *M. pneumoniae* infection had concomitant group A streptococcal infection, but the illnesses in these cases could not be distinguished clinically from those caused by either agent alone. Cervical lymphadenopathy occurred in approximately 50 percent of those infected, and the pharyngeal lesion was exudative in 43 percent.

In a study involving 131 adult patients with pharyngitis, 10.6 percent were found to have serologic evidence of *M. pneumoniae* infection.[364]

OTITIS MEDIA AND BULLOUS HEMORRHAGIC MYRINGITIS. Although the incidence has varied in different studies, otitis media is noted in approximately 5 percent of children and adolescents with *M. pneumoniae* pneumonia. The role of *M. pneumoniae* as an etiologic agent in common acute otitis media in children is unclear. Halsted and associates[262] noted that 12 percent of children with otitis media had serologic evidence of *M. pneumoniae* infection, but they were unable to recover the agent from middle ear fluid. In a study in which children were selected because of *M. pneumoniae* infection in a family member, 47 of 49 children with otitis media had *M. pneumoniae* infection.[326] Räty and Kleemola[550] used PCR to detect *M. pneumoniae* in 16 of 380 (4%) middle ear fluid samples from 138 children with acute otitis media.

In a volunteer study, myringitis developed in 13 of 52 subjects.[557] Findings were usually bilateral and associated with throbbing pain. The appearance of the tympanic membrane varied from mild injection to severe inflammation with edema. Hemorrhagic areas on the drum were noted in five subjects, and serous-appearing blebs containing blood were observed in two. Bullous myringitis also has been noted only occasionally with natural *M. pneumoniae* infection.[72, 127, 211, 217, 430, 615] However, in one study of 148 children and adults with *M. pneumoniae* pneumonia, 27 (18%) were found to have bullous myringitis.[430]

SINUSITIS. Although clinically recognized sinusitis has been reported rarely in patients with *M. pneumoniae* infection, Griffin and Klein[257] found radiographic evidence of sinusitis in approximately two thirds of a group of Navy recruits with *M. pneumoniae* pneumonia. In general, the patients with sinusitis had more prolonged illness than did recruits without sinusitis. Savolainen and colleagues[581] noted that 11 of 310 patients with acute maxillary sinusitis had fourfold or greater rises in complement-fixing antibody to *M. pneumoniae.* In chronic suppurative maxillary sinusitis, cultures for *M. pneumoniae* have been performed, but no organisms were isolated.[39, 621]

ACUTE BRONCHITIS. Acute bronchitis characterized by fever, cough, and rhonchi, with or without associated pharyngitis, is a frequent manifestation of *M. pneumoniae* infection.* Of 40 patients with *M. pneumoniae* infection, Feizi[184] reported that 6 had bronchitis, 3 had upper respiratory tract illness plus bronchitis, and 1 had sinusitis plus bronchitis. In contrast to these findings, Hornsleth[292] noted that only 1 of 25 patients with *M. pneumoniae* infection had acute bronchitis. In the differential diagnosis of acute bronchitis, *M. pneumoniae* infection accounts for 10 to 20 percent of cases.[96, 100, 156, 177, 535]

CROUP. *M. pneumoniae* infection has been associated only occasionally with croup. Parrott[526] found no instances of *M. pneumoniae* infection in a large number of children with croup, and Chanock and Parrott[100] did not list this agent as an etiologic consideration in croup. In contrast, extensive studies in both Seattle and Chapel Hill have revealed that approximately 2 percent of croup cases are associated with

*See references 43, 136, 176, 210, 217, 224, 318, 464, 633, 674.
†See references 95, 137, 156, 165, 182, 184, 186, 194, 211, 217, 291, 382, 415, 464, 487, 498, 573.

*See references 95, 96, 100, 177, 184, 291, 292, 487, 498, 526, 573.

M. pneumoniae infection.[156, 209, 243, 414] Because no descriptions of clinical illness are available, a reasonable assumption is that croup caused by *M. pneumoniae* infection is generally mild and without distinguishing characteristics.

BRONCHIOLITIS AND INFECTIOUS ASTHMA. Approximately 5 percent of cases of bronchiolitis are caused by infection with *M. pneumoniae,* but the percentage varies among studies.[95, 96, 100, 156, 165, 209, 243, 414, 526] In two large studies, no instances of *M. pneumoniae*–associated bronchiolitis were reported.[291, 292] *M. pneumoniae* also is a relatively common cause of asthmatic bronchitis and recurrent wheezing in asthmatic children.[38, 290, 300] Horn and associates[290] noted that *M. pneumoniae* was isolated from 6.6 percent of children with wheezy bronchitis, and Berkovich and associates[38] found *M. pneumoniae* infection in 7 of 33 episodes of wheezing in asthmatic children. Wheezing also occurs during *M. pneumoniae* pneumonia.[25, 570] Freymuth and colleagues[228] identified *M. pneumoniae* in nasal aspirate samples by PCR in 3 of 132 children (2%) with acute exacerbations of asthma.

OTHER. Exacerbations of chronic obstructive pulmonary disease have been associated with *M. pneumoniae* infection.[113, 378, 454, 611, 707] By culture, Cherry and associates[113] did not obtain any *M. pneumoniae* isolates from the bronchial specimens of adults with chronic bronchitis. However, more recently, Kraft and colleagues,[369] using PCR, detected *M. pneumoniae* in the bronchoalveolar lavage or bronchial biopsy specimens of 9 of 18 adults with chronic asthma. Smith and associates[611] were unable to show that patients with chronic obstructive pulmonary disease had increased susceptibility to infection in comparison to normal subjects. Illness suggestive of pertussis has been described in three children.[379, 633]

Exanthem and Enanthem

Exanthem as a manifestation of *M. pneumoniae* infection is a common occurrence, but its incidence has varied considerably among different studies.* In large studies involving children in which *M. pneumoniae* infection was evaluated in a specific geographic area, the incidence of exanthem has varied from 3 to 33 percent.† Foy and associates[217] noted rash in 17 percent of 319 patients with *M. pneumoniae* pneumonia during a 5-year surveillance period. In a study involving only children, Stevens and colleagues[633] noted exanthem in 9 percent of their patients. Copps and coworkers,[136] in a community outbreak in La Crosse, Wisconsin, found that 11 percent of their patients with pneumonia also had rash.

The cutaneous manifestations in *M. pneumoniae* infection are protean. Most common is an erythematous maculopapular rash that is most prominent on the trunk and back; the lesions may be discrete (rubelliform) or confluent (morbilliform). Though not the most common cutaneous manifestations of *M. pneumoniae* infection, erythema multiforme and Stevens-Johnson syndrome are the most often reported and the most serious.‡

In Table 196–3, the clinical findings in 29 well-documented cases of *M. pneumoniae* infection with exanthem are presented; in Table 196–4, the specific mucocutaneous findings in 20 of the 29 patients are itemized. Of the total group, all but 8 were males, 24 of the 29 were younger than 20 years, and 12 of the 20 were younger than 11 years. The duration of exanthem was longer than 7 days in all but 2 patients; all patients were febrile, and in 17 cases, the rash occurred during fever.

Fourteen patients had generalized ulcerative stomatitis, and seven had tonsillitis or pharyngitis. Severe conjunctivitis was observed in eight patients, and this manifestation was seen only in those with vesicular or bullous cutaneous lesions. All eight patients with severe conjunctivitis also had generalized ulcerative stomatitis. Surprisingly, vesicular or bullous exanthems with oral and eye lesions (Stevens-Johnson syndrome) rarely occur in females.[24, 442, 633]

As noted in Table 196–3, 25 of the 29 patients had pneumonia. The occurrence of rash as the major manifestation of *M. pneumoniae* infection is probably rare. In a study of 112 patients who had suspected infectious exanthems without pneumonia, Cherry and associates[107] could find none with

TABLE 196–3 ■ SELECTED CLINICAL FINDINGS IN 29 PATIENTS WITH *MYCOPLASMA PNEUMONIAE* INFECTION AND EXANTHEM

Clinical Findings	No. of Patients
Predominant components of exanthem	
Erythematous macular	4
Erythematous maculopapular	14
Vesicular	14
Bullous	6
Petechial	1
Urticarial	2
Discrete lesions	11
Confluent lesions	7
Pruritic	6
Predominant distribution of exanthem	
Hands	9
Arms	20
Feet	8
Legs	19
Trunk	19
Face	11
Buttocks	9
Genitals	8
Duration of exanthem (days)	
<7	2
7–14	11
>14	10
Time of onset of exanthem	
Before fever	2
With fever	4
During fever	17
After fever	1
Antibiotics administered before exanthem	
Yes	17
No	10
Enanthem	
Generalized ulcerative stomatitis	14
Tonsillitis of pharyngitis	7
Conjunctivitis	
Severe	8
Mild	3
Pneumonia	
Yes	25
No	4

From Cherry, J. D.: Anemia and mucocutaneous lesions due to *Mycoplasma pneumoniae* infections. Clin. Infect. Dis. *17*(Suppl. 1): 47–51, 1993.

*See references 9, 86, 106, 108, 118, 135, 136, 176, 186, 205, 211, 215, 217, 246, 251, 261, 291, 318, 340, 379, 381, 383, 419, 422, 424, 430, 486, 487, 498, 567, 577, 627, 633, 637, 658, 674.
†See references 136, 186, 211, 217, 291, 318, 379, 424, 430, 487, 498, 627, 633.
‡See references 24, 86, 108, 135, 184, 186, 215, 335, 340, 419, 422, 442, 498, 555, 577, 583, 600, 633, 637, 674, 682.

TABLE 196–4 ■ MUCOCUTANEOUS FINDINGS IN 20 PATIENTS WITH *MYCOPLASMA PNEUMONIAE* INFECTIONS AND EXANTHEM

Case	Reference	Age (yr)	Sex	Distinguishing Characteristic of Exanthem	Generalized Ulcerative Stomatitis	Severe Conjunctivitis
1	108	16	M	Fiery-red confluent maculopapular	0	0
2	108	17	F	Blotchy erythematous	0	0
3	103	4.5	F	Morbilliform	0	0
4	205	9	M	Erythematous maculopapular	+	0
5	205	8	M	Papulovesicular; "target" appearance	+	0
6	215	14	M	Symmetric macular and bullous	+	+
7	340	19	M	Erythematous maculopapular, vesicles; "iris" lesions	+	0
8	379	10	F	Macular and petechial	0	0
9	381	16	M	Varicella-like	+	+
10	674	8	M	Macular	+	0
11	674	6	M	Diagnosed as measles	0	0
12	419	16	M	Scattered vesicular; generalized	+	+
13	419	6	M	Vesicular; generalized	+	0
14	486	7	M	Urticarial	0	0
15	486	9	M	Maculopapular	0	0
16	577	10	M	Vesiculobullous and maculopapular	+	+
17	658	27	M	Vesiculopustular to papular; "pityriasis-like"	0	0
18	208	10	M	Vesiculobullous; generalized	+	0
19	383	5	M	Maculopapular	0	0
20	424	11	F	Papular; most marked on hands and feet	0	0

Modified from Cherry, J.D., Hurwitz, E.S., and Welliver, R.C.: *Mycoplasma pneumoniae* infections and exanthems. J. Pediatr. *87*:369–373, 1975.

M. pneumoniae infection. Foy and colleagues[211] noted a 2-year-old child with only rash, Stutman[637] reported a 15-year-old boy with Stevens-Johnson syndrome but not pneumonia from whom the organism was recovered from a vesicular lesion, and Ruhrmann and Holthusen[567] observed frequent cases of mild erythema multiforme without pneumonia.

In an analysis of 42 cases of erythema multiforme seen during a 20-year period, Villiger and associates[682] noted a presumptive or definite diagnosis of *M. pneumoniae* infection in 14 children. Nine of the children were boys (64%), and eight of the illnesses had mucous membrane involvement.

Many patients with *M. pneumoniae* infection and exanthem have a history of antibiotic administration before development of the rash; this observation suggests the possibility that the rash is drug induced rather than a result of the infectious process. As noted in Table 196–3, 17 patients had received antibiotics before the rash appeared, and the exanthem was present before the administration of antibiotic therapy in 10. Whereas these data incriminate the infection as a cause of exanthem, the large number of cases in association with the administration of antibiotic raises the possibility that the antibiotic intensifies the dermosensitive potential of the infectious agent in a manner similar to that noted between Epstein-Barr virus and ampicillin in infectious mononucleosis. *M. pneumoniae* has been recovered from the blister fluid of two patients with erythema multiforme.[422]

Other unusual cutaneous manifestations include erythema nodosum, pityriasis rosea, varicella-like urticaria, and Cockade purpura.[108, 246, 251, 381, 486, 567, 587, 658]

Cardiac Manifestations

Cardiac involvement during *M. pneumoniae* infection generally is considered to be unusual.* However, studies of Pönkä[538] and Sands and associates[578] and survey data of Noah[502] and Assaad and Borecka[23] indicate that *M. pneumoniae* myocarditis and pericarditis are important causes of both morbidity and mortality. In a study of fatal viral and mycoplasmal infections, Assaad and Borecka[23] noted six cardiovascular deaths related to *M. pneumoniae* infection during a 9-year period. Noah[502] found that 1 percent of 700 patients with *M. pneumoniae* infection had cardiac manifestations as the main clinical feature. Pönkä[538] published findings of a 7-year study involving 560 patients with serologic evidence of *M. pneumoniae* infection. In this group, 69 patients with cardiac manifestations were detected; of these 69 patients, 25 had carditis for which no causal agent other than *M. pneumoniae* could be incriminated. Pönkä[538] also reviewed the world literature and found a total of 33 other cases of carditis.

Of 25 carefully studied patients, 17 had respiratory symptoms before the diagnosis of carditis, and 10 had radiologically confirmed pneumonia. All but four patients had fever. Of the 25 patients, 2 were younger than 10 years and 2 were in the 10- to 19-year age group. Of the 33 cases in the literature, 7 were 20 years or younger. Of this survey group, 25 of the 33 had respiratory illness, and in 19 it was recorded as pneumonia.

Of the 25 patients in Finland reviewed by Pönkä, 6 had pericarditis and the remainder had perimyocarditis. Antibiotic therapy in 11 patients did not appear to shorten the duration of illness or diminish the number of cardiac sequelae. At a 16-month follow-up, 11 patients had persistent cardiac damage. Another interesting aspect of this study was the finding of rises in *M. pneumoniae* complement-fixing antibody titer in five adults with myocardial infarcts.

Chergui and associates[102] described a 45-year-old man with bilateral interstitial infiltrates and second-degree heart block. He was treated with erythromycin, and the heart block, fever, and respiratory distress cleared on hospital day 5.

*See references 101, 102, 114, 180, 183, 229, 251, 343, 347, 379, 396, 483, 501, 641.

Hematologic Manifestations

Severe hemolytic anemia has been reported on several occasions in patients with *M. pneumoniae* infection.* Most cases of *M. pneumoniae* hemolytic anemia have been associated with marked pulmonary involvement. Stevens-Johnson syndrome is a common associated finding, and myocarditis has been noted on two occasions.[135, 183, 184, 347, 633] In general, severity of illness correlates with high titers of cold agglutinins.

The hemolysis may be severe and acute, often with a 50 percent reduction in hemoglobin concentration. In contrast to uncomplicated pulmonary disease, the leukocyte count in patients with hemolytic anemia frequently is elevated markedly with a predominance of neutrophils. Results of the direct Coombs test are usually positive. Clinical experience suggests that administration of steroids in conjunction with proper antibiotic therapy may be beneficial in this illness. Boccardi and associates[57] observed a 7-year-old boy with hemolytic anemia and transitory paroxysmal cold hemoglobinuria.

Feizi[185] has demonstrated that clinically inapparent compensated hemolysis frequently is associated with *M. pneumoniae* pulmonary infection. Fiala and associates[198] noted that bone marrow suppression also contributed to the anemia in a patient whom they studied. Ruhrmann and Holthusen[567] reported a hemorrhagic variant of erythema multiforme (Cockade purpura) similar to Henoch-Schönlein disease in *M. pneumoniae* infection; they also noted severe thrombocytopenia not associated with hemolytic anemia. Gill and Marrie[239] reported a 27-year-old man who had hemophagocytosis with an *M. pneumoniae* infection.

Severe *M. pneumoniae* infection with pneumonia, thrombocytopenia, and disseminated intravascular coagulation has been described.[116, 117]

Gastrointestinal Findings

NONSPECIFIC FINDINGS. Approximately 25 percent of patients with *M. pneumoniae* pneumonia have nausea, vomiting, diarrhea, or some combination thereof (see Table 196–2). Aside from these complaints, gastrointestinal problems in association with *M. pneumoniae* infection are rare events. Stevens and associates[633] found that 15 percent of a group of 44 children with infection had notable abdominal pain. Referred abdominal pain with pneumonia also has been observed.[184]

LIVER INVOLVEMENT. Liver involvement in *M. pneumoniae* infection is a surprisingly rare event. Levine and Lerner[395] reported that mild increases in transaminases occur and that acute and chronic active hepatitis has been noted with respiratory symptoms and proven *M. pneumoniae* infection, but they provided no further information. MacLean[424] reported a 13-year-old girl who initially had a sore throat and then 9 days later had clinical and laboratory evidence of hepatitis. Murray and associates[480] presented a case report of an adult with typical *M. pneumoniae* pneumonia in whom liver function and enzyme studies indicated hepatitis. Helms and colleagues[277] noted that 6 of 17 patients with *M. pneumoniae* pneumonia had elevated aspartate aminotransferase values. Enzyme changes have been observed in other case evaluations,[397, 430, 605] and hepatic necrosis has occurred.[427]

*See references 106, 135, 152, 183, 185, 198, 294, 347, 427, 561, 588, 604, 633, 644.

Simonian and Janner[604] reported a 12-year-old boy who had pleural effusion, hepatitis, and hemolytic anemia. Narita and associates[494] noted two children with lymphadenopathy and liver dysfunction. These two patients are of interest because both had mycoplasmemia and neither had pneumonia.

PANCREATITIS. In 1974, Mårdh and Ursing[435] reported six patients with respiratory illnesses, serologic evidence of *M. pneumoniae* infection, and pancreatitis. In four patients, pancreatic symptoms began 1 to 2 weeks after the onset of respiratory illness; in the other two patients, the pancreatitis was subclinical. Diabetes developed in two patients, one of whom died. At postmortem examination, pneumonitis and pancreatitis were confirmed. In a study of pancreatitis, Leinikki and Pantzar[389] noted that sera from 18 of 56 patients had rises in complement-fixing antibody titer to *M. pneumoniae.* Because none of the patients in this study had respiratory illness suggestive of *M. pneumoniae,* the investigators suggested that perhaps the antibody responses were not specific for *M. pneumoniae* infection but were caused by a cross-reacting infection or were the result of autoantigens from pancreatic damage. Leinikki and associates[390] have conducted further studies; their belief is that the antibody response is nonspecific, but their data neither confirm nor refute this assumption. In another study, Freeman and McMahon[226] also noted serologic evidence of *M. pneumoniae* infection in 33 percent of patients with pancreatitis. Oderda and Kraut[507] reported a 22-month-old girl with pancreatitis and a rise in complement-fixing antibody titer to *M. pneumoniae.* This child had no respiratory symptoms.

Arthritis

Mycoplasmas other than *M. pneumoniae* are a common cause of arthritis in animals other than human beings.[130, 317] In many instances, the animal diseases suggest human rheumatoid arthritis. Consequently, researchers have searched extensively for mycoplasmas in humans with rheumatoid arthritis, but to date, no associations have been established. However, *M. pneumoniae* infection clearly is associated occasionally with joint manifestations.* In a review of 1259 patients with *M. pneumoniae* infection, Pönkä[537] noted transient arthritis in 0.9 percent. Two patients were found to have Reiter syndrome. Hernandez and colleagues[281] reported seven instances of arthritis in 38 persons with *M. pneumoniae* respiratory disease. In one patient, the illness lasted 18 months and was associated with the development of rheumatoid factor.

Eighteen instances of illness suggestive of rheumatic fever have been described.[36, 120, 329, 377, 472, 483, 490, 705] In all 18 patients, large joints were involved; 15 patients had joint swelling or effusion, whereas 3 had only pain. Most patients had a history of preceding respiratory illness with sore throat, and 10 of the 18 had radiographic evidence of pneumonia. The sedimentation rate was elevated in all patients in whom the test was performed. One child had an erythema marginatum–like rash, as well as polyarthritis and fever.[472] Poggio and colleagues[534] reported a child with reactive arthritis 3 weeks after the onset of diarrhea and a respiratory tract infection. Leukocytoclastic vasculitis plus polyarthritis associated with *M. pneumoniae* infection has been described in a young adult.[531]

*See references 36, 151, 230, 235, 281, 329, 377, 379, 435, 481, 490, 537, 569, 705.

Muscular Disease

Berger and Wadowksy[37] reported a 15-year-old girl with right lower lobe pneumonia, hepatitis, and rhabdomyolysis associated with *M. pneumoniae* infection. Polymyositis has been noted in association with *M. pneumoniae* infection on six occasions.[530]

Neurologic Disease

Several large community and military studies of *M. pneumoniae* pneumonia and other respiratory illnesses are notable in that neurologic disease is not described.[98, 136, 176, 217, 318, 464, 477] However, other studies, particularly those performed more recently, indicate a surprising spectrum of neurologic illness associated with *M. pneumoniae* infection.* The failure to find neurologic disease in the initial large studies mentioned was probably due not to its absence but to the orientation of the investigators; neurologic disease was not studied under the respiratory investigation protocols. In three large studies of *M. pneumoniae* illness involving 1856 cases, 2.6 to 4.8 percent had neurologic illness.[498, 502, 539] Assaad and Borecka[23] noted five fatal *M. pneumoniae* infections in which central nervous system (CNS) findings were the major clinical manifestations.

In 1973, Lerer and Kalavsky[394] reported 5 cases of neurologic disease associated with *M. pneumoniae* infection and analyzed 45 cases from the literature. They noted the following frequencies of specific clinical involvement: generalized encephalitis, 30 percent; spinal nerve roots, 30 percent; meningitis, 20 percent; cranial nerves, 20 percent; focal encephalitis, 16 percent; cerebellum, 14 percent; psychosis, 8 percent; and spinal cord, 2 percent. Combined involvement was noted in 36 percent of cases; in 79 percent, a history of antecedent respiratory illness was elicited. Fifty-three percent of the patients were 20 years or younger, and 15 percent were younger than 10 years. Eighty percent of the children and adolescents were males. The onset of neurologic disease occurred 3 to 23 days after the onset of respiratory illness, with a mean value of 10 days. Five deaths were noted, and 22 percent of the survivors had residual neurologic deficits.

In a review of 61 patients with *M. pneumoniae*–associated neurologic disease during a 24-year period in Helsinki, Finland, Koskiniemi[367] noted that 45 of the patients were children and that all these children had encephalitis. Of the total group, 5 patients (8%) died and 14 (23%) had severe sequelae.

In a study of acute childhood encephalitis in Toronto, Canada, 9 of 50 children (18%) with adequate microbiologic study had evidence of *M. pneumoniae* infection.[363] Interesting, four of the nine children also had evidence of concomitant viral infection. In a further study of encephalitis at the same center during a 5-year-period, researchers noted that 50 of 159 children (31%) with encephalitis had evidence of *M. pneumoniae* infection[49]; in this analysis, 30 of the 50 cases (60%) had microbiologic evidence of other concomitant infections. Respiratory prodromal symptoms preceded the encephalitis in approximately 67 percent of the patients in whom the diagnosis was based on culture, PCR, or both. Two children had acute demyelinating encephalomyelitis. Long-term neurologic sequelae occurred in 48 to 64 percent of cases.

In other studies, aseptic meningitis is reported more frequently; other less common findings include poliomyelitis-like syndrome, bilateral sensorineural deafness, Reye syndrome, cerebral infarction, optic disk swelling, brain stem syndrome, transverse myelitis, psychosis, cerebellar syndrome, radiculopathy, brachial plexus neuropathy, Bell palsy, and Guillain-Barré syndrome.* Klimek and associates[358] reported a 13-year-old boy with meningoencephalitis and transverse myelitis in association with low CSF glucose values. Arthur and Margolis[21] noted the appearance of *Mycoplasma*-like structures in granulomatous angiitis of the CNS at postmortem examination of a 35-year-old man.

Mixed Infections

In many studies of *M. pneumoniae* infection, cultural or serologic evidence of concomitant or sequential infection with other infectious agents has been noted.† In a large study of patients hospitalized with acute respiratory illness, Fransen and associates[224] found that 64 percent of patients with rises in complement-fixing antibody titer to *M. pneumoniae* also had antibody titer rises to viral, chlamydial, or bacterial agents. In this group, the most common concomitant infections were with parainfluenza viruses. The occurrence of mixed infection did not appear to have a pronounced effect on clinical manifestations; the only significant difference between patients with mixed infection and those with single *M. pneumoniae* infection was the more common finding of a high erythrocyte sedimentation rate in the former group. In several other large studies of disease caused by *M. pneumoniae,* concomitant infections were common, but no evidence of synergistic or antagonistic roles of one agent for another was noted.[186, 241, 465, 626, 627] Renner and associates[554] found a lower than expected frequency of seropositivity to *M. pneumoniae* in 91 serum pairs with seroconversion to influenza A virus.

The high rate of possible mixed infections in the large encephalitis study in Toronto is of particular interest.[49] In addition to common respiratory viruses and enteroviruses, they noted herpes group viruses, *Bartonella henselae,* and *Mycobacterium tuberculosis.* In studies of *Bordetella pertussis* infection, evidence of mixed infection with *M. pneumoniae* or perhaps serologic cross-reactivity has been found repeatedly.[310, 683]

The observation by Grady and Gilfillan[248] that 81 percent of patients with legionnaires' disease also had serologic evidence of *M. pneumoniae* infection is interesting. In the same study, 29 percent of all patients seropositive for *M. pneumoniae* also were seropositive for the legionnaires' disease antigen. Comparable studies performed by the Centers for Disease Control and Prevention failed to find a similar rate of high co-positivity in sera obtained in other legionnaires' disease epidemics. Another study found no serologic relationship between *M. pneumoniae* and *Legionella pneumophila.*[553] Severe bacterial disease after *M. pneumoniae* infection has been reported occasionally. Stadel and colleagues[622] noted *H. influenzae* pneumonia and bacteremia after a mild *M. pneumoniae* illness; Biberfeld and

---

*See references 2, 5, 6, 8, 16, 19, 21, 23, 26, 30, 32, 33, 43, 46, 49, 73, 125, 160, 166, 175, 178, 184, 196, 203, 224, 244, 284, 285, 294, 309, 338, 342, 348, 351, 358, 363, 365–367, 372, 380, 388, 406, 420, 459, 474, 491, 498, 500, 502, 506, 507, 515, 523, 539, 566, 572, 596, 606, 616, 627, 630, 633, 646, 665, 675, 702, 708.

*See references 2, 16, 19, 32, 160, 166, 244, 271, 284, 309, 348, 351, 358, 366, 380, 406, 474, 500, 505, 523, 525, 566, 572, 596, 627, 633, 675, 702, 708.

†See references 9, 26, 49, 186, 187, 224, 241, 248, 255, 310, 363, 392, 403, 439, 464, 465, 491, 554, 622, 626, 627, 683.

colleagues[45] reported staphylococcal septicemia in two cases of *M. pneumoniae* pneumonia, and Rykner and associates[569] recovered pneumococci from the pleural exudate of a patient with *M. pneumoniae* pneumonia.

Kleemola and Kayhty[356] found fourfold or greater increases in *M. pneumoniae* complement-fixing antibody titer in 40.7 percent of 54 patients with bacterial meningitis. However, they thought that this antibody response was not caused by specific *M. pneumoniae* infection but by cross-reactive glycolipids resulting from the bacterial infection.[355, 356]

Lind and associates[406] reported that 4 of 19 patients with neurologic disease and *M. pneumoniae* infection had serologic evidence of concomitant viral infection.

Other Disease Associations

Foy and colleagues[211] noted that both ear involvement and pneumonia as manifestations of *M. pneumoniae* infection occurred more commonly in children with previous tonsillectomy. Putman and associates[544] found that in all but 3 of 31 patients with sarcoidosis, the serum complement-fixing antibody titer to *M. pneumoniae* was 1:32 or higher, whereas in a similar-sized control group without sarcoidosis, only 2 persons had titers of 1:32 and none had higher titers. Other interesting observations include multiple birth defects in a newborn exposed to *M. pneumoniae* in utero,[65] a tubo-ovarian abscess in a young woman from whom *M. pneumoniae* was isolated in pure culture,[661] fever of unknown origin in a 32-year-old man,[373] glomerulonephritis in a few patients with pneumonia,[536] inappropriate secretion of antidiuretic hormone in a 6-year-old boy,[409] and optic disk swelling and iritis.[574]

Recurrent Disease

The results of several investigations suggest that recurrent *M. pneumoniae* infection is a frequent finding.[75, 195, 631] Repeat infections can be associated with severe disease, such as pneumonia. In the Seattle studies, second attacks of pneumonia have been documented, and similar findings have been observed in England.[207, 219, 221, 291]

DIAGNOSIS

Differential Diagnosis

Because the clinical manifestations of *M. pneumoniae* infection are protean and because infections occur commonly in children and adolescents, this agent should be considered in the differential diagnosis of most infectious illnesses. Most important is its consideration in patients with pulmonary disease, in whom illnesses caused by viruses (particularly adenoviruses, parainfluenza viruses, influenza viruses), *Chlamydia psittaci, Chlamydia pneumoniae, Coxiella burnetii,* bacteria (particularly *S. pneumoniae, B. pertussis, H. influenzae, M. tuberculosis),* and fungi (particularly *Histoplasma capsulatum* and *Coccidioides immitis)* are the main differential possibilities. Because the clinical manifestations, including the radiographic appearance of the lungs, are frequently similar in the various differential possibilities, the following other factors are important: status of the host (normal or immunologically compromised), the environment (human, animal, or inanimate source), the age of the patient, the incubation period, and the season.

In otherwise healthy children, *M. pneumoniae* is a common cause of pneumonia in those older than 3 years and is the leading cause of pneumonia in older children and adolescents. The lack of coryza is sometimes useful in differentiating *M. pneumoniae* pneumonia from that caused by common viral agents, and elevation of the white blood cell count along with an increase in band form neutrophils is evidence against a mycoplasmal etiologic agent, except in patients with concomitant hemolytic anemia. The occurrence of exanthem and, in particular, Stevens-Johnson syndrome should lead the physician to suspect *M. pneumoniae;* similarly, the occurrence of hemolytic anemia, joint manifestations, or neurologic signs and symptoms with pneumonia should lead the physician to strongly suspect *M. pneumoniae* as the etiologic agent. Because the pulmonary manifestations of *M. pneumoniae* infection are not always clinically apparent, a physician investigating an unusual acute or subacute case (aseptic meningitis or other neurologic illness; exanthem; enanthem; hepatitis; pancreatitis; pericarditis, myocarditis, or both; and arthritis) would be wise to consider the possibility of *M. pneumoniae* as the etiologic agent and to obtain appropriate chest radiographs, as well as definitive cultures and serologic studies.

Specific Diagnosis

SERUM COLD AGGLUTININS. Despite the considerable confusion in the literature and by physicians in general regarding the diagnostic value of the serum cold agglutination test for *M. pneumoniae* infection, our opinion is that when it is used appropriately, the test is a simple and useful procedure. One cause for confusion was a report in 1966 in which only 1 of 28 children with positive cold agglutination titers actually had serologic evidence of *M. pneumoniae* infection by complement fixation.[639] However, this report can be criticized because the study population consisted of 444 children younger than 4 years and only 170 of this group had pneumonia. Because cold agglutinins are noted occasionally in the sera of patients of all ages with a variety of illnesses, for useful results, their study should have been restricted to patients likely to have *M. pneumoniae* lower respiratory tract disease.[108, 200, 235, 402] In various studies of pneumonia, serum cold agglutinins at a titer of 1:32 or higher were found in 50 to 90 percent of patients with *M. pneumoniae* infection.[46, 94, 98, 224, 235, 318, 477, 633, 680] In general, the cold agglutinin response correlates directly with the severity of pulmonary involvement; patients with extensive lobar involvement nearly always have positive titers[3] (1:32), whereas those with only minimal findings on radiographic study frequently have equivocal or negative titers. Positive cold agglutination titers have been observed in 18 percent of adenoviral pneumonias in a study involving a military population.[235] In general, the higher the cold agglutinin titer, the more likely that a particular illness is caused by *M. pneumoniae.*

A rapid screening test for cold agglutinins is available and useful.[232, 256] This test is performed by adding 4 drops of blood to a tube containing sodium citrate or another anticoagulant. The tube is placed in ice water (0° to 4° C) in a freezer for approximately 30 seconds and then examined immediately for coarse agglutination by tilting the tube on its side. When the tube is warmed, the agglutination should resolve, and it can be reproduced again by repeating the ice water cooling procedure.

SPECIFIC ANTIBODY DETERMINATIONS. Several specific antibody tests (growth inhibition, immunofluorescence, indirect hemagglutination, precipitation, mycoplasmacidal antibody, complement fixation, ELISA, adherence inhibition assay, radioimmunoassay, and radioimmunoprecipitation) can be used to measure serum antibodies to *M. pneumoniae,* but until relatively recently, only the complement-fixation test was available routinely. A fourfold rise in complement-fixation antibody titer indicates acute *M. pneumoniae* infection. Because complement-fixation antibody in *M. pneumoniae* infection is of relatively short duration, the observation of a fourfold fall in titer also can be useful on occasion in assigning etiologic significance in a particular illness. High single titers (≥1:256) usually indicate recent infection but rarely can be used to relate the cause of an illness specifically to *M. pneumoniae.* Because *M. pneumoniae* infection is associated with a relatively long incubation period, the development of antibodies is significant at the time of acute disease. As a consequence of this development, fourfold changes in titer can occur in a short interval (5 days), and collection of paired sera 5 to 7 days apart usually reveals a significant rise in complement-fixation antibody titer.

In recent years, most diagnostic laboratories have replaced the complement-fixation test with commercial immunofluorescence or ELISA for demonstration of antibodies to *M. pneumoniae* antigens.* These tests, in addition to demonstrating rises in antibody values in paired sera, can identify specific IgM and IgA antibodies in single serum samples. In general, when used by experienced laboratory personnel, both immunofluorescence and ELISA have sensitivities and specificities similar to those of the complement-fixation test for determining significant increases in antibody values in paired serum specimens. In addition, demonstration of specific IgM or IgA antibody in a single serum sample suggests a recent infection. However, the specific IgM and IgA responses after infection may last for several months; therefore, demonstration of these antibodies in a single serum sample may be misleading with regard to the diagnosis of specific illness. Hence, in most instances, paired sera (5 to 14 days apart) should be examined to confirm a clinical diagnosis.

CULTURE. With proper media, experienced personnel have little difficulty isolating *M. pneumoniae* from throat swabs of infected patients.[14, 671] However, because *M. pneumoniae* is relatively slow growing, in most instances requiring more than 1 week of incubation, culture is of less use for diagnosis of routine cases than serologic study is. Cultures should be performed in all unusual situations; specifically, joint fluid, CSF, pericardial fluid, and biopsy material should be cultured. The modified SP-4 medium, which is more sensitive than conventional mycoplasma culture media, coupled with the agar plate immunofluorescence identification procedure, may facilitate the cultural diagnosis of *M. pneumoniae.*[671]

DIRECT ANTIGEN DETECTION. Because *M. pneumoniae* culture is clinically impractical in view of the long time until organisms can be identified, direct detection of antigen in respiratory secretions is an important priority. In 1987, a species-specific probe (Gen-Probe) that uses iodine 125–labeled complementary DNA, homologous to *M. pneumoniae* ribosomal RNA, became available.[268, 270, 354, 663] Clinical results with this probe have been variable. Hata and colleagues,[270] in a study involving throat swabs in a pediatric population, noted a sensitivity of 76.7 percent and a specificity of 91.7 percent when compared with culture. Tilton and colleagues[663] found a sensitivity of 100 percent and a specificity of 98 percent in a study of sputum and throat cultures performed in two hospital clinics in Connecticut. Kleemola and coworkers[354] also noted good sensitivity (95%) and specificity (85%) with sputum specimens in army conscripts. In contrast to these results, Harris and associates[268] identified only 22 percent of culture-positive patients with the Gen-Probe assay. This test is no longer available.[353]

Studies with indirect immunofluorescence and ELISA offer promise for antigen detection in clinical specimens.[283, 361]

DETECTION BY POLYMERASE CHAIN REACTION. A large number of studies have indicated the usefulness of PCR for demonstration of specific *M. pneumoniae* DNA in nasopharyngeal, blood, CSF, urine, and tissue specimens.* Numerous different primers have been used to identify gene sequences of the P1 cytoadhesin protein, the adenosine triphosphatase asperon, or 16S ribosomal RNA gene sequences. Using culture plus serologic criteria as the comparative standard, several studies have shown excellent sensitivity and specificity.

TREATMENT

Antimicrobial Therapy

M. pneumoniae is sensitive in vitro to erythromycin, tetracyclines, chloramphenicol, clarithromycin, azithromycin, several aminoglycosides, and quinolones.[31, 156, 307, 308, 320, 432, 499, 607] It is resistant to all penicillins and for practical purposes to the cephalosporins. In spite of this demonstrated in vitro sensitivity of the organism, plus several studies that have shown clinical therapeutic effectiveness,† a common misconception in many physicians is that antibiotic therapy is of little value in the treatment of illness caused by *M. pneumoniae.* This idea had its origin before the present era, when many patients with viral pneumonia were given a diagnosis of primary atypical pneumonia and treated unsuccessfully with antibiotics.

In 1961, Kingston and associates[350] demonstrated the therapeutic effectiveness of demethylchlortetracycline for pneumonia caused by *M. pneumoniae.* Since then, several other antibiotics have been studied carefully and also have been found to be effective against *M. pneumoniae* pneumonia.[94, 156, 217, 235, 318, 567, 589, 607, 610] The drugs of choice for pneumonia caused by *M. pneumoniae* are either erythromycins or tetracyclines. Because of the adverse effects of tetracyclines on teeth, an erythromycin is the drug of choice in children. In *M. pneumoniae* pneumonia, the dose of erythromycin for children is 40 to 50 mg/kg/24 hr administered every 6 hours for a minimum of 10 days. For adolescents and adults, the dose of erythromycin or tetracycline is 2 g/24 hr administered every 6 hours. In general, the effectiveness of antibiotic therapy correlates directly with the severity of pneumonia and the elapsed time of illness before the initiation of therapy.

Azithromycin and clarithromycin both are approved for the treatment of community-acquired pneumonia in children.[55, 267] Their advantage is less frequent dosing, shorter duration of therapy, and less gastrointestinal disturbance in older patients. The azithromycin dosing schedule is 10 mg/kg/day (maximal dose, 1 g/day) on day 1, followed by 5 mg/kg daily (maximal dose, 500 mg/day) for 4 days. The clarithromycin dose is 15 mg/kg/day administered every 12 hours for 10 days (maximal dose, 1 g/day).

In all other clinical manifestations of *M. pneumoniae* infection except pneumonia (e.g., nonpulmonary respiratory infection, neurologic disease, Stevens-Johnson syndrome),

*See references 11, 87, 170, 181, 201, 311, 360, 385, 475, 549, 602, 613, 659, 660, 676, 701.

*See references 1, 2, 49, 51, 82, 85, 153, 163, 268, 289, 304, 324, 334, 421, 438, 482, 492, 556, 590, 616, 643, 681, 712.

†See references 55, 94, 156, 211, 217, 235, 318, 350, 567, 586, 589, 607, 610.

antibiotic therapy has not been evaluated adequately. In general, otitis media, pharyngitis, croup, and bronchiolitis appear to be mild, self-limited illnesses that require no therapy. In more serious illness, such as Stevens-Johnson syndrome and neurologic disease, individual case studies have indicated little evidence of therapeutic benefit with either erythromycin or tetracycline therapy. However, our opinion is that when diagnosed, most *M. pneumoniae* infections should be treated because there is little to lose and in vitro data suggest the possibility of efficacy. Jensen and colleagues[326] noted that prophylactic administration of oxytetracycline to family contacts prevented disease but not infection. Azithromycin prophylaxis has been used successfully in two hospital outbreaks of *M. pneumoniae* pneumonia.[302, 352]

General Management

Children and adolescents with *M. pneumoniae* pneumonia should be discouraged from engaging in excessive physical activity during the acute illness and for a 2-week period during convalescence because clearance, as observed by radiography, is slow and lags behind apparent clinical well-being. Older children and adolescents should be advised of their contagiousness to others; this risk period exists as long as cough persists, even with successful antibiotic therapy.

Steroids have been used in the management of severe pulmonary disease, Stevens-Johnson syndrome, encephalitis, and hemolytic anemia. Although definitive data are lacking, several case studies suggest associated clinical benefit; steroids seem to be particularly useful in treating severe hemolytic anemia. A 6-year-old girl with brain stem and striatal encephalitis complicating *M. pneumoniae* pneumonia experienced neurologic improvement within 48 hours of administration of intravenous immunoglobulin.[572]

PREVENTION

Because of the marked and prolonged morbidity associated with *M. pneumoniae* infection, which has been particularly troublesome in the military, much effort has been directed toward the development of vaccines. In 1965, Jensen and associates[325] reported encouraging initial trials with an inactivated vaccine. In this study, significant rises in *M. pneumoniae* growth-inhibiting antibody titer developed in 25 of 30 volunteers. Later challenge studies with the same vaccine indicated that 9 of 10 volunteers with serum antibody were protected, but illness more severe than that in the unvaccinated control group occurred in vaccinees who did not have an antibody response after initial immunization.[609] This altered reactivity on challenge suggested a sensitization process perhaps similar to that observed with other inactivated antigen vaccines and indicated the need for caution in further trials.[142, 195] Other trials of inactivated vaccines in both adults and children have had varying degrees of success.[456, 466, 706]

A trial with a live attenuated vaccine (a temperature-sensitive mutant) gave encouraging results.[252] However, because further study of natural *M. pneumoniae* disease indicated that reinfection occurs commonly and because sensitization may play a role in pathogenesis, proceeding slowly in conducting further vaccine trials in children seems prudent.[194]

The degree of contagion of *M. pneumoniae* is relatively low, so isolation methods should be effective in preventing spread of disease. The studies of Jensen and associates[326] and the hospital azithromycin trials[302, 352] indicate that in certain circumstances (in particular, high-risk subjects such as patients with sickle-cell disease and high-risk populations), prophylactic administration of antibiotics may be justified.

Ureaplasma urealyticum

PROPERTIES

Ureaplasmas (formerly T-strain mycoplasmas) are distinguished from all other members of the order Mycoplasmatales by their production of urease and their ability to hydrolyze urea.[594, 595, 653] The genus *Ureaplasma* contains a single species *(U. urealyticum)* with 14 serovars.[400, 560, 704] The morphologic characteristics of *U. urealyticum* in young liquid medium culture are similar to those of other mycoplasmas. Round-ovoid elements approximately 330 nm in diameter with a range of 100 to 850 nm are found; rod-shaped and filamentous structures also occur, and the latter have a length of 2 μm and a width of 50 to 300 nm.[50, 595, 710] In clinical material, short, bacillary forms with monopointed ends are common findings. Organisms are surrounded by a single trilaminar membrane approximately 10 nm thick with pilus-like structures radiating from the surface. Multiplication occurs by a simple budding process and perhaps by binary fission.

On unbuffered standard *Mycoplasma* agar with a pH of 6.0, *U. urealyticum* colonies are small (20 to 30 μm) and circular, with irregular borders, and grow downward into the agar.[595] On buffered agar, *U. urealyticum* colonies are bigger and often have the "fried egg" appearance of typical large colony-forming mycoplasmas.[428]

Isolation of *U. urealyticum* from clinical material is facilitated by the demonstration of urease activity.[197, 593, 655] In liquid medium containing urea and phenol red, growth of *U. urealyticum* results in the production of ammonia, with a resultant increase in pH and a change in color. Subculture from broth to agar medium that contains urea and manganese sulfate yields dark brown ureaplasmal colonies.

EPIDEMIOLOGY

The main reservoirs of human strains of *U. urealyticum* are the genital tracts of adult men and women.[20, 216, 446–448, 655, 669, 675] Infants become colonized with *U. urealyticum* during passage through the birth canal of an infected woman.[220, 357, 386, 640] With ruptured membranes, the infant can be infected in utero.[357] *U. urealyticum* has been recovered from the following sites in newborn infants: throat, nose, genitourinary tract of girls, urine of boys, external auditory canal, umbilicus, and perineum. Not all infants of infected women become colonized, and neonatal colonization tends to not persist. In one study in which *U. urealyticum* was recovered from 38 percent of girls and 6 percent of boys at birth, follow-up during a 2-year period revealed a decreasing prevalence of colonization; at 2 years, none of the children had positive cultures.[216]

During prepubertal childhood, *U. urealyticum* is recovered only rarely from urine or genital specimens.[212, 386] After puberty, colonization is a common occurrence and is primarily the result of sexual contact.[444, 446, 448] Colonization in adults is related directly to sexual activity. In population studies, *U. urealyticum* rarely is isolated from persons with no sexual experience, but it occurs in approximately 50 percent of men and 75 percent of women for whom sexual intercourse with three or more partners is reported.

CLINICAL MANIFESTATIONS

Because *U. urealyticum* can be recovered with considerable frequency from the throat, eyes, and genitourinary tract of babies and from the genitourinary tract of postpubertal males and females who are well, establishing cause-and-effect relationships in disease frequently has been difficult. Studies suggest the following disease associations with *U. urealyticum* in human genitourinary and reproductive disease: good to strong association with nongonococcal urethritis, prostatitis, and urethral syndrome; moderate association with epididymitis, involuntary infertility, repeated spontaneous abortion and stillbirth, chorioamnionitis, and low birth weight; weak association with urinary calculi, pyelonephritis, Reiter disease, and pelvic inflammatory disease; and no association with Bartholin gland abscess, vaginitis, cervicitis, postabortal fever, and postpartum fever.* Most illnesses related to or possibly related to *U. urealyticum* infection are not pediatric problems; only those of direct or indirect importance in pediatric and adolescent medicine are considered here.

Nongonococcal Urethritis

Nongonococcal urethritis occurs more commonly than gonococcal urethritis in men in most developed countries.[269, 315, 443, 687] Approximately 40 percent of cases of nongonococcal urethritis are caused by *Chlamydia trachomatis,* and 20 to 30 percent are the result of *U. urealyticum* infection.[60, 61, 140, 286, 447, 582] Clinical differentiation of disease caused by *C. trachomatis* and *U. urealyticum* has not been studied, but nongonococcal and gonococcal urethritis have been evaluated comparatively.[264, 315, 387, 685]

The incubation period in nongonococcal urethritis is relatively long, with most cases occurring 10 to 20 days after exposure, whereas with gonorrhea, the period is shorter, usually less than 1 week.[264] The onset of symptoms in nongonococcal urethritis is generally more gradual than that associated with gonorrhea. Virtually all men with gonorrhea have a urethral discharge, and most have both discharge and dysuria. In contrast, Jacobs and Kraus[315] found that only 38 percent of men with nongonococcal urethritis had both dysuria and discharge. In the same study, 15 percent of patients with nongonococcal urethritis had only dysuria, whereas only 2 percent of those with gonococcal urethritis had a similar complaint. On examination, Handsfield[264] found the discharge in nongonococcal urethritis to be purulent in 36 percent of his cases, nonpurulent in 9 percent, and of an intermediate character in the remaining 55 percent. In contrast, 73 percent of patients with gonorrhea had a purulent discharge, 27 percent had an intermediate discharge, and none had a nonpurulent discharge. Because of the more gradual onset and the usually less severe symptoms, patients with nongonococcal urethritis are less prompt in seeking medical care than those with gonorrhea are. Jacobs and Kraus[315] found that 76 percent of patients with discharge and gonococcal infection came to the clinic within 4 days of onset whereas only 43 percent of similar nongonococcal urethritis patients visited the clinic within 4 days of disease onset. Without treatment, nongonococcal urethritis symptoms subside gradually in some patients during a 1- to 3-month period.[516]

*See references 80, 91, 93, 173, 374, 376, 452, 628, 636, 655, 657, 666.

After penicillin, ampicillin, or spectinomycin treatment of men with urethral gonorrhea, urethritis recurs (postgonococcal urethritis) in many patients.[288] Studies of postgonococcal urethritis indicate an etiologic role for *C. trachomatis; U. urealyticum* is probably responsible for some cases.[517]

A 7.5-year-old sexually inactive boy with recurrent urethritis associated with *U. urealyticum* infection has been described.[591]

Low Birth Weight

In 1969, Klein and associates[357] found that isolation of *Mycoplasma* was associated with low birth weight in a study of 221 newborns. Colonized babies (mainly with *U. urealyticum)* had a statistically lower mean birth weight (2605 g) than did babies in whom colonization was not detected (2952 g). In a second prospective study at the same center involving 484 pregnant women, researchers noted that 28 percent of babies with a birth weight of 2500 g or less were colonized by *U. urealyticum* whereas only 5 percent of babies weighing more than 2500 g were colonized.[64] In this study, the association of *U. urealyticum* and low birth weight was not related to a shortened gestational period.

Since these early studies, at least 17 investigations involving more than 8000 pregnant women have been conducted to evaluate the role of cervical ureaplasmal infection in prematurity.* In several studies, a correlation between vaginal colonization, cervical colonization, or both and premature birth has been observed. Alfa and coworkers[12] studied 108 full-term mothers and 104 preterm mothers in a tertiary care hospital and noted *U. urealyticum* genital carriage rates of 25 percent and 19.2 percent, respectively. Acquisition of ureaplasmas in the respiratory tract of the infants occurred significantly more frequently in the preterm group (8.5%) than in the term infants (0.9%). Newborns weighing 1500 g or less had a colonization rate of 19 percent (5 of 26). In a case-control study involving 395 women, Abele-Horn and colleagues[4] found that the *U. urealyticum* colonization rate was 41 percent in preterm deliveries versus 10 percent in non-preterm deliveries. Yoon and associates[715] found that the presence of *U. urealyticum* in amniotic fluid correlated with an increased risk of premature delivery. In contrast to these results, neither Paul and coworkers[528] nor Benito and Blusewicz[35] found a direct association between *U. urealyticum* colonization and preterm delivery.

In spite of the possible association between colonization with *U. urealyticum* and premature birth, a specific cause-and-effect relationship seems unlikely.[92, 175]

Chorioamnionitis

In a study of 249 puerperal women and their babies, Shurin and colleagues[599] noted on histologic examination of the placentas that *U. urealyticum* was recovered from 37.5 percent of babies whose placentas showed chorioamnionitis and from only 19 percent of those with normal placentas. In this study, no adverse effects could be attributed to either the placental lesions or colonization of the babies. Some studies suggest that chorioamnionitis caused by *U. urealyticum* is a cause of premature delivery.[4, 92, 175, 282, 715] Caspi and associates[88] reported a 32-year-old woman with amnionitis in whom *U. urealyticum* was recovered from her blood. After delivery, the same organism was recovered from the blood of one of the twin infants. *U. urealyticum* has been recovered

*See references 4, 12, 35, 92, 174, 216, 528, 564, 565, 715.

from fetal tissue after abortion, stillbirth, and neonatal death.[158, 426, 563]

Neonatal Pneumonia

In a study of pneumonitis in early infancy, Stagno and associates[623] isolated *U. urealyticum* from the nasopharynx of 8 of 38 children (21%) with pneumonia but from only 2 of 49 control children (4%). Quinn and colleagues[546] noted fatal neonatal pneumonia resulting from an intrauterine infection with *U. urealyticum,* and Waites and associates[691] reported three neonates with pneumonia caused by *U. urealyticum* associated with persistent pulmonary hypertension. Several other studies indicate that *U. urealyticum* is a cause of acute respiratory distress and pneumonia in newborns.[81, 92, 143, 509, 513, 522, 523, 689]

Chronic Lung Disease

Several large studies have found a significant association between *U. urealyticum* colonization of the respiratory tract in low-birth-weight infants and the development of bronchopulmonary dysplasia.* In contrast to these studies, Heggie and associates,[274] da Silva and co-investigators,[150] and Couroucli and colleagues[141] found no association between *U. urealyticum* and the development of bronchopulmonary dysplasia. Bowman and coworkers[62] treated *U. urealyticum*–colonized, extremely low birth weight infants with erythromycin and found no association between the initial colonization and the development of chronic lung disease. They also called attention to the fact that in the study by Heggie and associates,[274] a substantial proportion of the colonized infants were treated with erythromycin, which might explain the lack of an association between colonization and subsequent chronic lung disease.

One theory suggests that *U. urealyticum* is not the primary cause of bronchopulmonary dysplasia but that the organism might be the cause of an undetected pneumonia.[90] This pneumonia results in an increased requirement for supplemental oxygen. The bronchopulmonary dysplasia is the result of oxygen toxicity caused by the supplemental oxygen therapy.

Ollikainen[511] found that preterm infants who were colonized with *U. urealyticum* had higher leukocyte counts on the first 2 days of life and that they needed oscillatory ventilation more often than noncolonized infants did. Patterson and colleagues[527] found that *U. urealyticum* colonization in preterm infants was associated with an increase in IL-1β and tumor necrosis factor–α relative to IL-6 in tracheal aspirate samples. Manimtim and coworkers[429] speculated that *U. urealyticum* enhances the proinflammatory response to a second infection by blocking IL-6 and IL-10, which would predispose a preterm infant to prolonged inflammation, lung injury, and impaired clearance of secondary infections.

Overall, *U. urealyticum* infection appears to contribute to the development of bronchopulmonary dysplasia in some cases.†

Neonatal Central Nervous System Infections

Garland and Murton[231] reported a 786-g newborn in whom meningitis caused by *U. urealyticum* developed on day 10. The baby recovered after being treated with erythromycin and then chloramphenicol therapy. In a prospective study, Waites and coworkers[694] isolated *U. urealyticum* from the CSF of eight infants who were being treated for meningitis or investigated for hydrocephalus. Six of these culture-positive babies had intraventricular hemorrhage, and hydrocephalus developed in three cases. In a second study, Waites and associates[693] studied an additional 318 infants in four suburban community hospitals and found 5 babies from whom *U. urealyticum* was recovered from the CSF. Three of the five babies did not have pleocytosis, and they recovered without treatment. The fifth baby died as a result of right frontal hemorrhage. In contrast to the findings of Waites and colleagues, Likitnukul and coworkers[398] cultured the CSF and blood of 203 infants with suspected sepsis and failed to isolate *U. urealyticum.* Several additional studies have confirmed the association between *U. urealyticum* infection and meningitis.[92, 280, 512, 624, 689]

Sepsis

U. urealyticum has been recovered from the blood of newborns with pneumonia and meningitis.[85, 689]

Other Infections

U. urealyticum has been isolated from an abscess at the site of an internal fetal heart rate monitor and was determined to be the cause of postoperative mediastinitis in an adult after undergoing coronary artery bypass surgery.[233, 263]

DIAGNOSIS AND TREATMENT

Demonstration of infection by *U. urealyticum* can be established easily by presently available culture techniques. However, assigning causation of disease is more difficult because of its ubiquitous presence in normal persons. In clinical practice, the most important differential consideration is between gonococcal infection and nongonococcal urethritis. Although the symptoms of the two illnesses are frequently different, sufficient overlap exists to render arriving at a specific diagnosis without laboratory aid hazardous. Microscopic examination of a urethral specimen is essential. In most instances, the observation of gram-negative cell-associated diplococci on Gram stain is sufficient for a diagnosis of *Neisseria gonorrhoeae* infection. When smears reveal polymorphonuclear neutrophils without organisms suggestive of gonococci, a specific bacterial culture should be performed. Because infection with multiple agents occurs commonly and postgonococcal urethritis is a frequent problem, one is advised to investigate initial illnesses completely in adolescents with cultures for bacteria, *Chlamydia,* and *Ureaplasma. U. urealyticum* also can be detected by PCR.[52]

Patients with nongonococcal urethritis should be treated with tetracycline (40 mg/kg/24 hr every 6 hours; persons weighing more than 50 kg should receive 500 mg every 6 hours) for 10 days.[264, 287] *Chlamydia* and *Ureaplasma* are also sensitive to erythromycin, so this antibiotic is a useful alternative for patients in whom tetracycline is contraindicated. With adolescent patients, to seek out and treat the sex partners whenever possible is prudent.

After diagnosis, *U. urealyticum* CNS and respiratory infections should be treated with erythromycin.[690, 695] The study by Bowman and associates[62] suggests that consideration should be given to erythromycin treatment of *U. urealyticum* colonization in very low birth weight infants.

*See references 3, 4, 7, 90, 92, 265, 293, 330, 510, 520, 529, 533, 575, 629, 696–698.

†See references 3, 4, 265, 293, 330, 510, 520, 529, 533, 629, 696, 698.

Mycoplasma hominis

PROPERTIES

Three basic morphologic forms of *M. hominis* have been observed by phase-contrast microscopy: coccoidal cells 30 to 80 nm in diameter, diploforms and filamentous forms with a thickness of 30 to 40 nm, and forms with variable lengths reaching 40 µm or more.[56, 67, 69, 159] Bredt[68] studied newly isolated strains and noted that coccoid forms and ring- or disk-shaped cells were predominant; with some strains, filamentous forms of variable length also were noted. Multiplication occurs by binary fission, by fragmentation of filaments and rings, and by budding.[56, 559]

Anderson and Barile[18] studied the ultrastructure of *M. hominis* and noted considerable variability in internal components. In some cells, ribosome-like granules in the cytoplasm and a more central area of net-like strands were present, suggestive of a nucleus. Other cells had only irregular densities within the cytoplasm. In some instances, dense cytoplasmic bodies were observed; in other cells, vacuoles were seen.

On *Mycoplasma* agar, *M. hominis* colonies are approximately 200 to 300 µm in diameter and have the typical mycoplasmal "fried egg" appearance.[655] *M. hominis* grows on ordinary blood agar and produces pinpoint nonhemolytic colonies. *M. hominis* metabolizes arginine to ammonia, so arginine-supplemented liquid medium with a pH indicator (phenol red) can be used for primary isolation. *M. hominis* can be identified specifically and differentiated from other human mycoplasmas that metabolize arginine by growth inhibition by specific antibody.

M. hominis has two cytoadhesins that are membrane proteins; they allow attachment to cells of the urogenital tract.[279] Attachment is to sulfated glycolipids of the host cells.[514]

EPIDEMIOLOGY

Like those of *U. urealyticum,* the main reservoirs of *M. hominis* are the genital tracts of adult men and women.[220, 444, 446, 448–450, 655] Infants become colonized during passage through the birth canal, but such colonization tends to not persist. In a recent study of 208 women at delivery, *M. hominis* was recovered from cervicovaginal specimens in 11 percent and the gastric secretions of 1 percent of newborns.[249] In prepubertal children, *M. hominis* only rarely is recovered from urine or genital specimens. Postpubertal genital tract colonization results primarily from sexual contact.

M. hominis can be recovered from the oral cavity of 1 to 5 percent of normal adults.[619]

CLINICAL MANIFESTATIONS

Studies suggest the following disease associations with *M. hominis* in human genitourinary and reproductive diseases: good to strong association with pyelonephritis, pelvic inflammatory disease, postabortal fever, and postpartum fever; moderate association with prostatitis, vaginitis, and cervicitis; weak association with Bartholin gland abscess and low birth weight; and no association with nongonococcal urethritis, epididymitis, urinary calculi, Reiter disease, urethral syndrome, involuntary infertility, repeated spontaneous abortion and stillbirth, and chorioamnionitis.* With the exception of pelvic inflammatory disease and complications of pregnancy, which occur in adolescents, the other disease associations reported do not involve pediatric patients.

Sacker and colleagues[571] reported a 5-day-old baby who had several abscess lesions in the supraclavicular area from which only *M. hominis* was recovered on incision and drainage. Another newborn had submandibular lymphadenitis caused by *M. hominis.*[541] Wound infections with *M. hominis* have been reported in neonates after cardiac surgery.[71, 393]

In three large studies in which CSF was obtained in the work-up of suspected neonatal sepsis, *M. hominis* was recovered from the fluid in 23 of 387 patients.[678, 693, 694] Of the 23 with isolates, only 1 had CSF findings indicative of meningitis. Several case reports of newborn babies with meningitis caused by *M. hominis* have been reported.[17, 58, 236, 238, 433] Examination of CSF reveals pleocytosis, with most cells being polymorphs, as well as increased protein and decreased glucose concentrations. Appropriate antibiotic therapy usually is delayed because the CSF is not examined routinely for mycoplasmas. *M. hominis* has been recovered on two occasions from the CSF of a 2.5-year-old girl with a ventriculoperitoneal shunt.[692] Because she had no complications from the infection and only minimal CSF inflammation, no treatment was initiated. Three months later, the organism could not be isolated from CSF and the child was doing well.

M. hominis was recovered from the amniotic fluid of a baby who later died of respiratory distress syndrome.[74] Postmortem examination revealed interstitial pneumonia. A stillbirth attributed to an *M. hominis* infection acquired in utero has been reported.[455] Jones and Tobin[327] noted eight *M. hominis* eye infections in 250 newborns studied. In volunteer studies in adults, researchers found that *M. hominis* could produce exudative pharyngitis.[476] Moffet and associates[463] isolated *M. hominis* from the throat of 1 of 174 infants and children with pharyngitis but made no similar isolation from a control group of children without pharyngitis. Neu and Ellner[497] recovered *M. hominis* from the throat of 1 child in a group of 56 with exudative pharyngitis. Other *M. hominis* infections include a scalp abscess as a complication of intrapartum monitoring,[240] massive pericardial effusion in a newborn,[461] septicemia in a 10-month-old burned infant,[149] chronic multifocal osteomyelitis in an 8-year-old,[301] septicemia after heart surgery in a 5-year-old girl,[148] and exudative vaginitis in a 10-year-old girl.[688]

In adult patients, the following clinical manifestations have been caused by *M. hominis:* mediastinitis,[441] wound abscesses in renal and liver transplant recipients,[620, 684] brain abscess,[716] pneumonia in a lung transplant recipient, and bacteremia in a patient with multiple injuries.[259, 423]

DIAGNOSIS AND TREATMENT

Illness caused by *M. hominis* infection rarely occurs in children. This organism should be considered an etiologic possibility in neonates with meningitis and those with abscesses in which routine cultures are negative. The possibility of *M. hominis* as an etiologic agent also should be considered in adolescent girls with pelvic inflammatory disease.

M. hominis is usually sensitive to tetracycline, and this antibiotic is the drug of choice unless it is otherwise contraindicated.[63, 84, 635, 647, 648, 709] During the last decade, resistance of *M. hominis* to tetracyclines has increased.[144, 445] The organism also is usually sensitive to clindamycin, rifampicin, and chloramphenicol. In two cases of neonatal meningitis,

*See references 54, 80, 91, 172, 173, 237, 260, 375, 518, 519, 565, 597, 628, 655, 657, 672.

treatment with chloramphenicol failed to eradicate the organism from the CSF.[238, 451] Eradication was accomplished by doxycycline in one infant and clindamycin in the other. In contrast to *U. urealyticum* and *M. pneumoniae, M. hominis* is markedly resistant to erythromycin.

Mycoplasma fermentans, Mycoplasma genitalium, Mycoplasma penetrans, Mycoplasma pirum, and AIDS-Associated Mycoplasmal Infections

MYCOPLASMA FERMENTANS

M. fermentans originally was isolated from the genital tract of men and women 50 years ago, but it has not been established as a cause of genitourinary disease.[568, 650, 669] This organism has been isolated from the blood of leukemia patients, from the joint fluid of patients with arthritis, and from the blood and urine of patients with acquired immunodeficiency syndrome (AIDS).[28, 53, 434, 469, 479, 703, 711] *M. fermentans* has been identified by PCR in the peripheral blood mononuclear cells and lymph nodes of HIV-infected patients.[271, 339, 370, 580] The organism also has been recovered from the blood of homosexual men without HIV infection.[339, 370, 425] *M. fermentans* has been identified in synovial fluid samples from 15 patients with inflammatory arthritic diseases, including rheumatoid arthritis.[617]

MYCOPLASMA GENITALIUM

M. genitalium first was identified and reported in 1981.[654, 657, 669, 672] It was cultured from the urethral swabs of two men with nongonococcal urethritis. The organism also has been recovered from the respiratory tract of patients with pneumonia who were participating in an *M. pneumoniae* vaccine trial.[27] Although *M. genitalium* has biologic features that indicate its pathogenic potential and it has caused infection and disease in experimentally infected chimpanzees, its role in human disease has not been established clearly.[654, 669, 673] With the use of PCR, Jensen and associates[323] presented evidence suggesting a causative role in some cases of nongonococcal urethritis. The organism also has been recovered in mixed culture with *M. pneumoniae* from the synovial fluid of a patient with pneumonia and subsequent polyarthritis.[670]

MYCOPLASMA PENETRANS

M. penetrans is a relatively newly recognized species isolated from the urogenital tract of patients with AIDS.[412, 413] In a seroprevalence study, Wang and associates[699] found that 35.4 percent of HIV-infected patients had antibody versus only 0.4 percent of HIV-seronegative subjects. They subsequently noted a high prevalence of antibody to *M. penetrans* in the sera of homosexual men but not in the sera of other HIV transmission groups.[700] In a more recent study, Grau and colleagues[250] found that 18.2 percent of HIV-infected patients had antibody to *M. penetrans* whereas only 1.3 percent of HIV-seronegative persons had antibody. *M. penetrans* antibody seroprevalence increased with progression of HIV-associated disease, and it was associated predominantly with homosexual practices in the HIV-infected patients. No pediatric data relating to *M. penetrans* seroprevalence are available.

MYCOPLASMA PIRUM

M. pirum originally was recovered from eukaryotic cell cultures, and its origin was traced to a human tumor cell line.[11, 155, 384] It has been recovered more recently from primary lymphocyte cells in patients with AIDS.[53]

AIDS-ASSOCIATED MYCOPLASMAL INFECTIONS

The frequent identification of *M. fermentans, M. pirum,* and *M. penetrans* infections in HIV-infected patients has led to the consideration that they may function as cofactors in the progression of HIV infection.[53, 368, 469] Although these mycoplasmas have the capacity to invade cells and to be potent immunomodulators, their pathogenic role, if any, in association with HIV has not been determined yet.

Mycoplasma and *Ureaplasma* Infections in Immunocompromised Patients

Patients with hypogammaglobulinemia are susceptible to severe persistent infection with *U. urealyticum, M. hominis, M. pneumoniae,* and *M. orale.*[22, 206, 223, 467, 542, 562] Clinical manifestations include osteomyelitis, arthritis, cellulitis, and chronic respiratory illness. Patients need to be treated for prolonged periods with high-dose intravenous immunoglobulin and antibiotics to which the specific agents are susceptible. Severe and persistent infections also have occurred in liver, kidney, and bone marrow transplant recipients, as well as other immunocompromised patients.[121, 314, 337, 460, 532]

Yechouron and associates[714] reported a 64-year-old man with Hodgkin lymphoma who died of septicemia caused by *Mycoplasma arginini,* an animal pathogen.[714]

REFERENCES

1. Abele-Horn, M., Busch, U., Nitschko, H., et al.: Molecular approaches to diagnosis of pulmonary diseases due to *Mycoplasma pneumoniae.* J. Clin. Microbiol. *36*:548–551, 1998.
2. Abele-Horn, M., Franck, W., Busch, U., et al.: Transverse myelitis associated with *Mycoplasma pneumoniae* infection. Clin. Infect. Dis. *26*:909–912, 1998.
3. Abele-Horn, M., Genzel-Boroviczény, O., Uhlig, T., et al.: *Ureaplasma urealyticum* colonization and bronchopulmonary dysplasia: A comparative prospective multicentre study. Eur. J. Pediatr. *157*:1004–1011, 1998.
4. Abele-Horn, M., Genzel-Boroviczény, O., Wolff, C., et al.: Vaginal *Ureaplasma urealyticum* colonization: Influence on pregnancy outcome and neonatal morbidity. Infection *25*:286–291, 1997.
5. Abramovitz, P., Schvartzman, P., Harel, D., et al.: Direct invasion of the central nervous system by *Mycoplasma pneumoniae:* A report of two cases. J. Infect. Dis. *155:*487, 1987.
6. Acharya, A. B., and Lakhani, P. K.: Hopkins syndrome associated with *Mycoplasma* infection. Pediatr. Neurol. *16*:54–55, 1997.
7. Agarwal, P., Rajadurai, V. S., Pradeepkumar, V. K., et al.: *Ureaplasma urealyticum* and its association with chronic lung disease in Asian neonates. J. Paediatr. Child Health *36*:487–490, 2000.
8. Agustin, E. T., Gill, V., and Cunha, B. A.: *Mycoplasma pneumoniae* meningoencephalitis complicated by diplopia. Heart Lung *23*:436–437, 1994.
9. Aiello, L. F., and Luby, J. P.: Concomitant *Mycoplasma* and adenovirus infection in a family. Am. J. Dis. Child. *128:*874–877, 1974.
10. Alexander, E. R., Foy, H. M., Kenny, G. E., et al.: Pneumonia due to *Mycoplasma pneumoniae:* Its incidence in the membership of a co-operative medical group. N. Engl. J. Med. *275:*131–136, 1966.
11. Alexander, T. S., Gray, L. D., Kraft, J. A., et al.: Performance of meridian immunocard *Mycoplasma* test in a multicenter clinical trial. J. Clin. Microbiol. *34*:1180–1183, 1996.
12. Alfa, M. J., Embree, J. E., Degagne, P., et al.: Transmission of *Ureaplasma urealyticum* from mothers to full and preterm infants. Pediatr. Infect. Dis. J. *14*:341–345, 1995.
13. Allen, P. Z., and Prescott, B.: Immunochemical studies on a *Mycoplasma pneumoniae* polysaccharide fraction: Cross-reactions with types 23 and 32 antipneumococcal rabbit sera. Infect. Immun. *20*:421–429, 1978.

14. Allen, V., Sueltmann, S., and Lawson, C.: Laboratory diagnosis of *Mycoplasma pneumoniae* in a public health laboratory. Health Lab. Sci. *4*:90–95, 1967.
15. Almagor, M., Yatziv, S., and Kahane, I.: Inhibition of host cell catalase by *Mycoplasma pneumoniae:* A possible mechanism for cell injury. Infect. Immun. *41*:251–256, 1983.
16. Al-Mateen, M., Gibbs, M., Dietrich, R., et al.: Encephalitis lethargica–like illness in a girl with mycoplasma infection. Neurology *38*:1155–1158, 1988.
17. Alonso-Vega, C., Wauters, N., Vermeylen, D., et al.: A fatal case of *Mycoplasma hominis* meningoencephalitis in a full-term newborn. J. Clin. Microbiol. *35*:286–287, 1997.
18. Anderson, D. R., and Barile, M. F.: Ultrastructure of *Mycoplasma hominis.* J. Bacteriol. *90*:180–192, 1965.
19. Anikster, Y., Glustein, J. Z., Weill, M., et al.: Extrapulmonary manifestations of *Mycoplasma pneumoniae* infections. Israel J. Med. Sci. *30*:412–413, 1994.
20. Archer, J. F.: "T" strain *Mycoplasma* in the female urogenital tract. Br. J. Vener. Dis. *44*:232–234, 1968.
21. Arthur, G., and Margolis, G.: *Mycoplasma*-like structures in granulomatous angiitis of the central nervous system: Case reports with light and electron microscopic studies. Arch. Pathol. Lab. Med. *101*:382–387, 1977.
22. Asmar, B. I., Andresen, J., and Brown, W. J.: *Ureaplasma urealyticum* arthritis and bacteremia in agammaglobulinemia. Pediatr. Infect. Dis. J. *17*:73–76, 1998.
23. Assaad, F., and Borecka, I.: Nine-year study of WHO virus reports on fatal viral infections. Bull. World Health Organ. *55*:445–453, 1977.
24. Azimi, P. H., Chase, P. A., and Petru, A. M.: Mycoplasmas: Their role in pediatric disease. Curr. Probl. Pediatr. *14*:1–46, 1984.
25. Azimi, P. H., and Koranyi, K. I.: *Mycoplasma pneumoniae* infections in a family. Clin. Pediatr. (Phila.) *16*:1138–1139, 1977.
26. Balassanian, N., and Robbins, F. C.: *Mycoplasma pneumoniae* infection in families. N. Engl. J. Med. *277*:719–725, 1967.
27. Baseman, J. B., Dallo, S. F., Tully, J. G., et al.: Isolation and characterization of *Mycoplasma genitalium* strains from the human respiratory tract. J. Clin. Microbiol. *26*:2266–2269, 1988.
28. Baseman, J. B., Lange, M., Criscimagna, N. L., et al.: Interplay between mycoplasmas and host target cells. Microb. Pathog. *19*:105–116, 1995.
29. Bauer, F. A., Wear, D. J., Angritt, P., and Lo, S.-C.: *Mycoplasma fermentans* (incognitus strain) infection in the kidneys of patients with acquired immunodeficiency syndrome and associated nephropathy: A light microscopic immunohistochemical, and ultrastructural study. Hum. Pathol. *22*:63–69, 1991.
30. Bayer, A. S., Galpin, J. E., Theofilopoulos, A. N., et al.: Neurologic disease associated with *Mycoplasma pneumoniae* pneumonitis: Demonstration of viable *Mycoplasma pneumoniae* in cerebrospinal fluid and blood by radioisotopic and immunofluorescent tissue culture techniques. Ann. Intern. Med. *94*:15–20, 1981.
31. Bébéar, C., Dupon M., Renaudin, H., et al.: Potential improvements in therapeutic options for mycoplasmal respiratory infections. Clin. Infect. Dis. *17*(Suppl. 1):202–207, 1993.
32. Beirne, P., Taylor, P., Choudhury, R. P., et al.: Cerebellar syndrome complicating *Mycoplasma pneumoniae* pneumonia. J. R. Soc. Med. *93*:28–29, 2000.
33. Bencina, D., Dovc, P., Mueller-Premru, M., et al.: Intrathecal synthesis of specific antibodies in patients with invasion of the central nervous system by *Mycoplasma pneumoniae.* Eur. J. Clin. Microbiol. Infect. Dis. *19*:521–530, 2000.
34. Benisch, B. M., Fayemi, A., Gerber, M. A., et al.: Mycoplasmal pneumonia in a patient with rheumatic heart disease. Am. J. Clin. Pathol. *58*:343–348, 1972.
35. Benito, C. W., and Blusewicz, T. A.: The relationship of *Ureaplasma urealyticum* cervical colonization and preterm delivery in high-risk pregnancies. Obstet. Gynecol. *97*:S45–S46, 2001.
36. Berant, M., Cohen, N., and Wagner, Y.: *Mycoplasma pneumoniae* infection presenting as acute rheumatic fever. Helv. Paediatr. Acta *36*:567–572, 1981.
37. Berger, R. P., and Wadowksy, R. M.: Rhabdomyolysis associated with infection by *Mycoplasma pneumoniae:* A case report. Pediatrics *105*:433–436, 2000.
38. Berkovich, S., Millian, S. J., and Snyder, R. D.: The association of viral and *Mycoplasma* infections with recurrence of wheezing in the asthmatic child. Ann. Allergy *28*:43–49, 1970.
39. Bhattacharyya, T. K., Mehra, Y. N., and Agarwal, S. C.: Incidence of bacteria, L-form and mycoplasma in chronic sinusitis. Acta Otolaryngol. *74*:293–296, 1972.
40. Biberfeld, G.: Antibodies to brain and other tissues in cases of *Mycoplasma pneumoniae* infection. Clin. Exp. Immunol. *8*:319–333, 1971.
41. Biberfeld, G.: Antibody responses in *Mycoplasma pneumoniae* infection in relation to serum immunoglobulins, especially IgM. Acta Pathol. Microbiol. Scand. [B] *79*:620–634, 1971.
42. Biberfeld, G., and Biberfeld, P.: Ultrastructural features of *Mycoplasma pneumoniae.* J. Bacteriol. *102*:855–861, 1970.
43. Biberfeld, G., Johnsson, T., and Jonsson, J.: Studies on *Mycoplasma pneumoniae* infection in Sweden. Acta Pathol. Microbiol. Scand. *63*:469–475, 1965.
44. Biberfeld, G., and Norberg, R.: Circulating immune complexes in *Mycoplasma pneumoniae* infection. J. Immunol. *112*:413–415, 1974.
45. Biberfeld, G., Stenbeck, J., and Johnsson, T.: *Mycoplasma pneumoniae* infection in hospitalized patients with acute respiratory illness. Acta Pathol. Microbiol. Scand. *74*:287–300, 1968.
46. Biberfeld, G., and Sterner, G.: A study of *Mycoplasma pneumoniae* infections in families. Scand. J. Infect. Dis. *1*:39–46, 1969.
47. Biberfeld, G., and Sterner, G.: Antibodies in bronchial secretions following natural infection with *Mycoplasma pneumoniae.* Acta Pathol. Microbiol. Scand. [B] *79*:599–605, 1971.
48. Biberfeld, G., and Sterner, G.: Smooth muscle antibodies in *Mycoplasma pneumoniae* infection. Clin. Exp. Immunol. *24*:287–291, 1976.
49. Bitnun, A., Ford-Jones, E. L., Petric, M., et al.: Acute childhood encephalitis and *Mycoplasma pneumoniae.* Clin. Infect. Dis. *32*:1674–1684, 2001.
50. Black, F. T., Birch-Andersen, A., and Freundt, E. A.: Morphology and ultrastructure of human T-mycoplasmas. J. Bacteriol. *111*:254–259, 1972.
51. Blackmore, T. K., Reznikov, M., and Gordon, D. L.: Clinical utility of the polymerase chain reaction to diagnose *Mycoplasma pneumoniae* infection. Pathology *27*:177–181, 1995.
52. Blanchard, A., Hentschel, J., Duffy, L., et al.: Detection of *Ureaplasma urealyticum* by polymerase chain reaction in the urogenital tract of adults, in amniotic fluid, and in the respiratory tract of newborns. Clin. Infect. Dis. *17*(Suppl. 1):148–153, 1993.
53. Blanchard, A., and Montagnier, L.: AIDS-associated mycoplasmas. Annu. Rev. Microbiol. *48*:687–712, 1994.
54. Blanco, J. D., Gibbs, R. S., Malherbe, H., et al.: A controlled study of genital mycoplasmas in amniotic fluid from patients with intra-amniotic infection. J. Infect. Dis. *147*:650–653, 1983.
55. Block, S., Hedrick J., Hammerschlag, M. R., et al.: *Mycoplasma pneumoniae* and *Chlamydia pneumoniae* in pediatric community-acquired pneumonia: Comparative efficacy and safety of clarithromycin vs. erythromycin ethylsuccinate. Pediatr. Infect. Dis. J. *14*:471–477, 1995.
56. Boatman, E. S.: Morphology and ultrastructure of the Mycoplasmatales. *In* Barile, M. F., and Razin, S. (eds.): The Mycoplasmas. Vol. 1. New York, Academic Press, 1979, pp. 63–102.
57. Boccardi, V., D'Annibali, S., DiNatale, G., et al.: *Mycoplasma pneumoniae* infection complicated by paroxysmal cold hemoglobinuria with anti-P specificity of biphasic hemolysin. Blut *34*:211–214, 1977.
58. Boe, O., Diderichsen, J., and Matre, R.: Isolation of *Mycoplasma hominis* from cerebrospinal fluid. Scand. J. Infect. Dis. *5*:285–288, 1973.
59. Bové, J. M.: Molecular features of mollicutes. Clin. Infect. Dis. *17*(Suppl. 1):10–31, 1993.
60. Bowie, W. R., Alexander, E. R., Floyd, J. F., et al.: Differential response of chlamydial and *Ureaplasma*-associated urethritis to sulphafurazole (sulfisoxazole) and aminocyclitols. Lancet *2*:1276–1278, 1976.
61. Bowie, W. R., Wang, S.-P., Alexander, E. R., et al.: Etiology of nongonococcal urethritis: Evidence for *Chlamydia trachomatis* and *Ureaplasma urealyticum.* J. Clin. Invest. *59*:735–742, 1977.
62. Bowman, E. D., Dharmalingam, A., Fan, W.-Q., et al.: Impact of erythromycin on respiratory colonization of *Ureaplasma urealyticum* and the development of chronic lung disease in extremely low birth weight infants. Pediatr. Infect. Dis. J. *17*:615–620, 1998.
63. Braun, P., Klein, J. O., and Kass, E. H.: Susceptibility of genital mycoplasmas to antimicrobial agents. Appl. Microbiol. *19*:62–70, 1970.
64. Braun, P., Lee, Y.-H., Klein, J. O., et al.: Birth weight and genital mycoplasmas in pregnancy. N. Engl. J. Med. *284*:167–171, 1971.
65. Bray, P. F., and Hackett, T. N.: Multiple birth defects in a newborn exposed to *Mycoplasma pneumoniae* in utero. Am. J. Dis. Child. *130*:312–314, 1976.
66. Bredt, W.: Motility and multiplication of *Mycoplasma pneumoniae:* A phase contrast study. Pathol. Microbiol. *32*:321–326, 1968.
67. Bredt, W.: Filamentous growth of some *Mycoplasma* species of man. Experientia *25*:1118–1119, 1969.
68. Bredt, W.: Cellular morphology of newly isolated *Mycoplasma hominis* strains. J. Bacteriol. *105*:449–450, 1971.
69. Bredt, W., Heunert, H. H., Hofling, K. H., et al.: Microcinematographic studies of *Mycoplasma hominis* cells. J. Bacteriol. *113*:1223–1227, 1973.
70. Brolin, I., and Wernstedt, L.: Radiographic appearance of mycoplasmal pneumonia. Scand. J. Respir. Dis. *59*:179–189, 1978.
71. Brooker, R. J., Eason, J. D., and Solimano, A.: *Mycoplasma* surgical wound infection in a neonate. Pediatr. Infect. Dis. J. *13*:751–753, 1994.
72. Broome, C. V., LaVenture, M., Kaye, H. S., et al.: An explosive outbreak of *Mycoplasma pneumoniae* infection in a summer camp. Pediatrics *66*:884–888, 1980.
73. Bruch, L. A., Jefferson, R. J., Pike, M. G., et al.: *Mycoplasma pneumoniae* infection, meningoencephalitis, and hemophagocytosis. Pediatr. Neurol. *25*:67–70, 2001.
74. Brunell, P. A., Dische, R. M., and Walker, M. B.: *Mycoplasma*, amnionitis, and respiratory distress syndrome. J. A. M. A. *207*:2097–2099, 1969.
75. Brunner, H., Greenberg, H. B., James, W. D., et al.: Antibody to *Mycoplasma pneumoniae* in nasal secretions and sputa of experimentally infected human volunteers. Infect. Immun. *8*:612–620, 1973.
76. Brunner, H., Horswood, R. L., and Chanock, R. M.: More sensitive methods for detection of antibody to *Mycoplasma pneumoniae.* J. Infect. Dis. *127*(Suppl.):52–55, 1973.

77. Brunner, H., James, W. D., Horswood, R. L., et al.: Measurement of *Mycoplasma pneumoniae* mycoplasmacidal antibody in human serum. J. Immunol. *108*:1491–1498, 1972.
78. Brunner, H., Prescott, B., Greenberg, H., et al.: Unexpectedly high frequency of antibody to *Mycoplasma pneumoniae* in human sera as measured by sensitive techniques. J. Infect. Dis. *135*:524–530, 1977.
79. Brunner, H., Schaeg, W., Bruck, U., et al.: Determination of IgG, IgM, and IgA antibodies to *Mycoplasma pneumoniae* by an indirect staphylococcal radioimmunoassay. Med. Microbiol. Immunol. *165*:29–41, 1978.
80. Brunner, H., Weidner, W., and Schiefer, H.-G.: Studies on the role of *Ureaplasma urealyticum* and *Mycoplasma hominis* in prostatitis. J. Infect. Dis. *147*:807–813, 1983.
81. Brus, F., van Waarde, W. M., Schoots, C., et al.: Fatal ureaplasmal pneumonia and sepsis in a newborn infant. Eur. J. Pediatr. *150*:782–783, 1991.
82. Buck, G. E., O'Hara, L. C., and Summersgill, J. T.: Rapid, sensitive detection of *Mycoplasma pneumoniae* in simulated clinical specimens by DNA amplification. J. Clin. Microbiol. *30*:3280–3283, 1992.
83. Busolo, F., Tonin, E., and Meloni, G. A.: Enzyme-linked immunosorbent assay for serodiagnosis of *Mycoplasma pneumoniae* infections. J. Clin. Microbiol. *18*:432–435, 1983.
84. Bygdeman, S. M., and Märdh, P. A.: Antimicrobial susceptibility and susceptibility testing of *Mycoplasma hominis:* A review. Sex. Transm. Dis. *10*:366–370, 1983.
85. Cadieux, N., Lebel, P., and Brousseau, R.: Use of a triplex polymerase chain reaction for the detection and differentiation of *Mycoplasma pneumoniae* and *Mycoplasma genitalium* in the presence of human DNA. J. Gen. Microbiol. *139*:2431–2437, 1993.
86. Cannell, H., Churcher, G. M., and Milton-Thompson, G. J.: Stevens-Johnson syndrome associated with *Mycoplasma pneumoniae* infection. Br. J. Dermatol. *81*:196–199, 1969.
87. Carter, J. B.: Serologic diagnosis of *Mycoplasma pneumoniae* infection: Introduction of an indirect fluorescent antibody (IFA) procedure. Immunopathology *8*:1–7, 1984.
88. Caspi, E., Herczeg, E., Solomon, F., et al.: Amnionitis and T strain mycoplasmemia. Am. J. Obstet. Gynecol. *111*:1102–1106, 1971.
89. Cassell, G. H., and Cole, B. C.: Mycoplasmas as agents of human disease. N. Engl. J. Med. *304*:80–89, 1981.
90. Cassell, G. H., Crouse, D. T., Waites, K. B., et al.: Does *Ureaplasma urealyticum* cause respiratory disease in newborns? Pediatr. Infect. Dis. J. *7*:535–541, 1988.
91. Cassell, G. H., Davis, R. O., Waites, K. B., et al.: Isolation of *Mycoplasma hominis* and *Ureaplasma urealyticum* from amniotic fluid at 16–20 weeks of gestation: Potential effect on outcome of pregnancy. Sex. Transm. Dis. *10*:294–302, 1983.
92. Cassell, G. H., Waites, K. B., Watson, H. L., et al.: *Ureaplasma urealyticum* intrauterine infection: Role in prematurity and disease in newborns. Clin. Microbiol. Rev. *6*:69–87, 1993.
93. Cassell, G. H., Younger, J. B., Brown, M. B., et al.: Microbiologic study of infertile women at the time of diagnostic laparoscopy: Association of *Ureaplasma urealyticum* with a defined subpopulation. N. Engl. J. Med. *308*:502–505, 1983.
94. Chanock, R. M.: *Mycoplasma* infections of man. N. Engl. J. Med. *273*:1199–1206, 1257–1264, 1965.
95. Chanock, R., Chambon, L., Chang, W., et al.: WHO respiratory disease survey in children: A serological study. Bull. World Health Organ. *37*:363–369, 1967.
96. Chanock, R. M., Cook, M. K., Fox, H. H., et al.: Serologic evidence of infection with Eaton agent in lower respiratory illness in childhood. N. Engl. J. Med. *262*:648–654, 1960.
97. Chanock, R. M., Hayflick, L., and Barile, M. F.: Growth on artificial medium of an agent associated with atypical pneumonia and its identification as a PPLO. Proc. Natl. Acad. Sci. U. S. A. *48*:41–49, 1962.
98. Chanock, R. M., Mufson, M. A., Bloom, H. H., et al.: Eaton agent pneumonia. J. A. M. A. *175*:213–220, 1961.
99. Chanock, R. M., Mufson, M. A., and Somerson, N. L.: Role of *Mycoplasma* (PPLO) in human respiratory disease. Am. Rev. Respir. Dis. *88*:218–231, 1963.
100. Chanock, R. M., and Parrott, R. H.: Acute respiratory disease in infancy and childhood: Present understanding and prospects for prevention. Pediatrics *36*:21–39, 1965.
101. Chen, S.-C., Tsai, C. C., and Nouri, S.: Carditis associated with *Mycoplasma pneumoniae* infection. Am. J. Dis. Child. *140*:471–472, 1986.
102. Chergui, K., Fourme, T., Veillard-Baron, A., et al.: *Mycoplasma pneumoniae* and second-degree heart block. Clin. Infect. Dis. *27*:1534–1535, 1998.
103. Cherry, J. D.: Newer viral exanthems. Adv. Pediatr. *16*:233–286, 1969.
104. Cherry, J. D.: Newer respiratory viruses: Their role in respiratory illnesses of children. Adv. Pediatr. *20*:225–289, 1973.
105. Cherry, J. D.: *Mycoplasma* infections. *In* Shen, J. T. Y. (ed.): The Clinical Practice of Adolescent Medicine. New York, Appleton-Century-Crofts, 1980, pp. 80–93.
106. Cherry, J. D.: Anemia and mucocutaneous lesions due to *Mycoplasma pneumoniae* infections. Clin. Infect. Dis. *17*(Suppl. 1):47–51, 1993.
107. Cherry, J. D., Allen, V. D., and Sueltmann, S.: Search for *Mycoplasma pneumoniae* infection in patients with exanthem but without pneumonia. Arch. Environ. Health *16*:911–912, 1968.
108. Cherry, J. D., Hurwitz, E. S., and Welliver, R. C.: *Mycoplasma pneumoniae* infections and exanthems. J. Pediatr. *87*:369–373, 1975.
109. Cherry, J. D., and Taylor-Robinson, D.: Growth and pathogenesis of *Mycoplasma mycoides* var. *capri* in chicken embryo tracheal organ cultures. Infect. Immun. *2*:431–438, 1970.
110. Cherry, J. D., and Taylor-Robinson, D.: Peroxide production by mycoplasmas in chicken tracheal organ cultures. Nature *228*:1099–1100, 1970.
111. Cherry, J. D., and Taylor-Robinson, D.: Growth and pathogenicity studies of *Mycoplasma gallisepticum* in chicken tracheal organ cultures. J. Med. Microbiol. *4*:441–449, 1971.
112. Cherry, J. D., and Taylor-Robinson, D.: *Mycoplasma* pathogenicity studies in organ cultures. Ann. N. Y. Acad. Sci. *225*:290–303, 1973.
113. Cherry, J. D., Taylor-Robinson, D., Willers, H., et al.: A search for mycoplasma infections in patients with chronic bronchitis. Thorax *26*:62–67, 1971.
114. Cherry, J. D., and Welliver, R. C.: *Mycoplasma pneumoniae* infections of adults and children. West. J. Med. *125*:47–55, 1976.
115. Chester, A., Kane, J., and Garagusi, V.: *Mycoplasma* pneumonia with bilateral pleural effusions. Am. Rev. Respir. Dis. *112*:451–456, 1975.
116. Chiou, C. C., Liu, Y. C., Lin, H. H., et al.: *Mycoplasma pneumoniae* infection complicated by lung abscess, pleural effusion, thrombocytopenia and disseminated intravascular coagulation. Pediatr. Infect. Dis. J. *16*:327–329, 1997.
117. Chryssanthopoulos, C., Eboriadou, M., Monti, K., et al.: Fatal disseminated intravascular coagulation caused by *Mycoplasma pneumoniae.* Pediatr. Infect. Dis. J. *20*:634-635, 2001.
118. Chusid, M. J., Lachman, B. S., and Lazerson, J.: Severe *Mycoplasma* pneumonia and vesicular eruption in SC hemoglobinopathy. J. Pediatr. *93*:449–451, 1978.
119. Cimolai, N., Mah, D. G., Taylor, G. P., et al.: Bases for the early immune response after rechallenge or component vaccination in an animal model of acute *Mycoplasma pneumoniae* pneumonitis. Vaccine *13*:305–309, 1995.
120. Cimolai, N., Malleson, P., Thomas, E., et al.: *Mycoplasma pneumoniae* associated arthropathy: Confirmation of the association by determination of the antipolypeptide IgM response. J. Rheumatol. *16*:1150–1152, 1989.
121. Clough, W., Cassell, G. H., Duffy, L. B., et al.: Septic arthritis and bacteremia due to *Mycoplasma* resistant to antimicrobial therapy in a patient with systemic lupus erythematosus. Clin. Infect. Dis. *15*:402–407, 1992.
122. Clyde, W. A.: An experimental model for human *Mycoplasma* disease. Yale J. Biol. Med. *40*:436–443, 1968.
123. Clyde, W. A.: Immunopathology of experimental *Mycoplasma pneumoniae* disease. Infect. Immun. *4*:757–763, 1971.
124. Clyde, W. A.: *Mycoplasma pneumoniae* infections of man. *In* Tully, J. G., and Whitcomb, R. F. (eds.): The Mycoplasmas. Vol. II. New York, Academic Press, 1979, pp. 275–306.
125. Clyde, W. A.: Neurological syndromes and mycoplasmal infections. Arch. Neurol. *37*:65–66, 1980.
126. Clyde, W. A., Jr.: Clinical overview of typical *Mycoplasma pneumoniae* infections. Clin. Infect. Dis. *17*(Suppl. 1):32–36, 1993.
127. Clyde, W. A., and Denny, F. W.: *Mycoplasma* infections in childhood. Pediatrics *40*:669–684, 1967.
128. Cockcroft, D. W., and Stilwell, G. A.: Lobar pneumonia caused by *Mycoplasma pneumoniae.* Can. Med. Assoc. J. *124*:1463–1468, 1981.
129. Cohen, G., and Somerson, N. L.: Glucose-dependent secretion and destruction of hydrogen peroxide by *Mycoplasma pneumoniae.* J. Bacteriol. *98*:547–551, 1969.
130. Cole, B. C., and Cassell, G. H.: *Mycoplasma* infections as models of chronic joint inflammation. Arthritis Rheum. *22*:1375–1381, 1979.
131. Collier, A. M., and Baseman, J. B.: Organ culture techniques with mycoplasmas. Ann. N. Y. Acad. Sci. *225*:277–289, 1973.
132. Collier, A. M., and Clyde, W. A.: Relationships between *Mycoplasma pneumoniae* and human respiratory epithelium. Infect. Immun. *3*:694–701, 1971.
133. Collier, A. M., Clyde, W. A., and Denny, F. W.: Biologic effects of *Mycoplasma pneumoniae* and other mycoplasmas from man on hamster tracheal organ culture. Proc. Soc. Exp. Biol. Med. *132*:1153–1158, 1969.
134. Collier, A. M., Clyde, W. A., and Denny, F. W.: *Mycoplasma pneumoniae* in hamster tracheal organ culture: Immunofluorescent and electron microscopic studies. Proc. Soc. Exp. Biol. Med. *136*:569–573, 1971.
135. Copps, S. C.: Primary atypical pneumonia: With hemolytic anemia and erythema multiforme. Clin. Pediatr. (Phila.) *3*:491–495, 1964.
136. Copps, S. C., Allen, V. D., Sueltmann, S., et al.: A community outbreak of *Mycoplasma* pneumonia. J. A. M. A. *204*:123–128, 1968.
137. Cordero, L., Cuadrado, R., Hall, C. B., et al.: Primary atypical pneumonia: An epidemic caused by *Mycoplasma pneumoniae.* J. Pediatr. *71*:1–12, 1967.
138. Costea, N., Yakulis, V. J., and Heller, P.: Inhibition of cold agglutinins (anti-I) by *M. pneumoniae* antigens. Proc. Soc. Exp. Biol. Med. *139*:476–479, 1972.

139. Couch, R. B.: *Mycoplasma pneumoniae* (primary atypical pneumonia). *In* Mandell, G. L., Douglas, R. G., Jr., and Bennett, J. E. (eds.): Principles and Practice of Infectious Diseases. New York, John Wiley & Sons, 1980, pp. 1484–1498.
140. Coufalik, E. D., Taylor-Robinson, D., and Csonka, G. W.: Treatment of nongonococcal urethritis with rifampicin as a means of defining the role of *Ureaplasma urealyticum*. Br. J. Vener. Dis. *55*:36–43, 1979.
141. Couroucli, X. I., Welty, S. E., Ramsay, P. L., et al.: Detection of microorganisms in the tracheal aspirates of preterm infants by polymerase chain reaction: Association of adenovirus infection with bronchopulmonary dysplasia. Pediatr. Res. *47*:225–232, 2000.
142. Craighead, J. E.: Report of a workshop: Disease accentuation after immunization with inactivated microbial vaccines. J. Infect. Dis. *131*:749–753, 1975.
143. Crouse, D. T., Odrezin, G. T., Cutter, G. R., et al.: Radiographic changes associated with tracheal isolation of *Ureaplasma urealyticum* from neonates. Clin. Infect. Dis. *17*(Suppl. 1):122–130, 1993.
144. Cummings, M. C., and McCormack, W. M.: Increase in resistance of *Mycoplasma hominis* to tetracyclines. Antimicrob. Agents Chemother. *34*:2297–2299, 1990.
145. Dajani, A. S., Clyde, W. A., and Denny, F. W.: Experimental infection with *Mycoplasma pneumoniae* (Eaton's agent). J. Exp. Med. *121*:1071–1086, 1965.
146. Dallo, S. F., Chavoya, A., and Baseman, J. B.: Characterization of the gene for a 30-kilodalton adhesin-related protein of *Mycoplasma pneumoniae*. Infect. Immun. *58*:4163–4165, 1990.
147. Dallo, S. F., Lazzell, A. L., Chavoya, A., et al.: Biofunctional domains of the *Mycoplasma pneumoniae* P30 adhesin. Infect. Immun. *64*:2595–601, 1996.
148. Dan, M., and Robertson, J.: *Mycoplasma hominis* septicemia after heart surgery. Am. J. Med. *84*:976–977, 1988.
149. Dan, M., Tyrrell, D. L. J., Stemke, G. W., et al.: *Mycoplasma hominis* septicemia in a burned infant. J. Pediatr. *99*:743–745, 1981.
150. Da Silva, O., Gregson, D., and Hammerberg, O.: Role of *Ureaplasma urealyticum* and *Chlamydia trachomatis* in development of bronchopulmonary dysplasia in very low birth weight infants. Pediatr. Infect. Dis. J. *16*:364–369, 1997.
151. Davis, C. P., Cochran, S., Lisse, J., et al.: Isolation of *Mycoplasma pneumoniae* from synovial fluid samples in a patient with pneumonia and polyarthritis. Arch. Intern. Med. *148*:969–970, 1988.
152. Daxböck, F., Zedtwitz-Liebenstein, K., Burgmann, H., et al.: Severe hemolytic anemia and excessive leukocytosis masking mycoplasma pneumonia. Ann. Hematol. *80*:180–182, 2001.
153. deBarbeyrac, B., Bernet-Poggi, C., Febrer, F., et al.: Detection of *Mycoplasma pneumoniae* and *Mycoplasma genitalium* in clinical samples by polymerase chain reaction. Clin. Infect. Dis. *17*(Suppl. 1):83–89, 1993.
154. Decancq, H. G., Jr., and Lee, F. A.: *Mycoplasma pneumoniae* pneumonia: Massive pulmonary involvement and pleural effusion. J. A. M. A. *194*:1010–1011, 1965.
155. Del Giudice, R. A., Tully, J. G., Rose, D. L., et al.: *Mycoplasma pirum* sp. nov., a terminal structured mollicute from cell cultures. Int. J. Syst. Bacteriol. *35*:285–291, 1985.
156. Denny, F. W., Clyde, W. A., and Glezen, W. P.: *Mycoplasma pneumoniae* disease: Clinical spectrum, pathophysiology, epidemiology, and control. J. Infect. Dis. *123*:74–92, 1971.
157. Dienes, L., and Edsall, J.: Observations on L-organisms of Klieneberger. Proc. Soc. Exp. Biol. Med. *36*:740–744, 1937.
158. Dische, M. R., Quinn, P. A., Czegledy-Nagy, E., et al.: Genital *Mycoplasma* infection. Intrauterine infection: Pathologic study of the fetus and placenta. Am. J. Clin. Pathol. *72*:167–174, 1979.
159. Domermuth, C. H., Nielsen, M. H., Freundt, E. A., et al.: Ultrastructure of *Mycoplasma* species. J. Bacteriol. *88*:727–744, 1964.
160. Dorff, B., and Lind, K.: Two fatal cases of meningoencephalitis associated with *Mycoplasma pneumoniae* infection. Scand. J. Infect. Dis. *8*:49–51, 1976.
161. Dorigo-Zetsma, J. W., Dankert, J., and Zaat, S. A.: Genotyping of *Mycoplasma pneumoniae* clinical isolates reveals eight P1 subtypes within two genomic groups. J. Clin. Microbiol. *38*:965–970, 2000.
162. Dorigo-Zetsma, J. W., Wilbrink, B., Dankert, J., et al.: *Mycoplasma pneumoniae* P1 type 1- and type 2-specific sequences within the P1 cytadhesin gene of individual strains. Infect. Immun. *69*:5612–5618, 2001.
163. Dorigo-Zetsma, J. W., Zaat, S. A., Vriesema, A. J. M., et al.: Demonstration by a nested PCR for *Mycoplasma pneumoniae* that *M. pneumoniae* load in the throat is higher in patients hospitalised for M. pneumoniae infection than in non-hospitalised subjects. J. Med. Microbiol. *48*:1115–1122, 1999.
164. Dowdle, W. R., and Robinson, R. Q.: An indirect hemagglutination test for diagnosis of *Mycoplasma pneumoniae* infections. Proc. Soc. Exp. Biol. Med. *116*:947–950, 1964.
165. Dowdle, W. R., Stewart, J. A., Heyward, J. T., et al.: *Mycoplasma pneumoniae* infections in a children's population: A five-year study. Am. J. Epidemiol. *85*:137–146, 1967.
166. Dowling, P. C., and Cook, S. D.: Role of infection in Guillain-Barré syndrome: Laboratory confirmation of herpesviruses in 41 cases. Ann. Neurol. *9*:44–55, 1981.
167. Eaton, M. D., and Liu, C.: Studies on sensitivity to streptomycin of the atypical pneumonia agent. J. Bacteriol. *74*:784–787, 1957.
168. Eaton, M. D.: Action of aureomycin and chloromycetin on the viruses of primary atypical pneumonia. Proc. Soc. Exp. Biol. Med. *73*:24–26, 1950.
169. Eaton, M. D., Meiklejohn, G., and van Herick, W.: Studies on the etiology of primary atypical pneumonia: A filterable agent transmissible to cotton rats, hamsters, and chick embryos. J. Exp. Med. *79*:649–668, 1944.
170. Echivarria, J. M., Leon, P., Balfagon, P., et al.: Diagnosis of *Mycoplasma pneumoniae* infection by microparticle agglutination and antibody-capture enzyme immunoassay. Eur. J. Clin. Microbiol. Infect. Dis. *9*:217–220, 1990.
171. Embree, J. E., and Embil, J. A.: Mycoplasmas in diseases of humans. Can. Med. Assoc. J. *123*:105–111, 1980.
172. Embree, J. E., Krause, V. W., and Embil, J. A.: *Mycoplasma hominis*: A placental pathogen? Sex. Transm. Dis. *10*:307–310, 1983.
173. Embree, J. E., Krause, V. W., Embil, J. A., et al.: Placental infection with *Mycoplasma hominis* and *Ureplasma urealyticum:* Clinical correlation. Obstet. Gynecol. *56*:475–481, 1980.
174. Emmons, J., Schluenderberg, A., and Cordero, L.: An aid to the rapid diagnosis of *Mycoplasma pneumoniae* infections. J. Infect. Dis. *119*:650–653, 1969.
175. Eschenbach, D. A.: *Ureaplasma urealyticum* and premature birth. Clin. Infect. Dis. *17*(Suppl. 1):100–106, 1993.
176. Evans, A. S., Allen, V., and Sueltmann, S.: *Mycoplasma pneumoniae* infections in University of Wisconsin students. Am. Rev. Respir. Dis. *96*:237–244, 1967.
177. Evans, A. S., and Brobst, M.: Bronchitis, pneumonitis and pneumonia in University of Wisconsin students. N. Engl. J. Med. *265*:401–409, 1961.
178. Evans, M. R. W., and Marshall, A. J.: Recovery from *Mycoplasma* meningoencephalitis, credited to penicillin allergy. Lancet *1*:1100, 1990.
179. Evatt, B. L., Dowdle, W. R., Johnson, M., Jr., et al.: Epidemic *Mycoplasma* pneumonia. N. Engl. J. Med. *285*:374–377, 1971.
180. Farraj, R. S., McCully, R. B., Oh, J. K., et al.: *Mycoplasma*-associated pericarditis. Mayo Clin. Proc. *72*:33–36, 1997.
181. Fedorko, D. P., Emery, D. D., Franklin, S. M., et al.: Evaluation of a rapid enzyme immunoassay system for serologic diagnosis of *Mycoplasma pneumoniae* infection. Diagn. Microbiol. Infect. Dis. *23*:85–88, 1995.
182. Feikin, D. R., Moroney, J. F., Talkington, D. F., et al.: An outbreak of acute respiratory disease caused by *Mycoplasma pneumoniae* and adenovirus at a federal service training academy: New implications from an old scenario. Clin. Infect. Dis. *29*:1545–1550, 1999.
183. Feizi, O., Grubb, C., Skinner, J. I., et al.: Primary atypical pneumoniae due to *Mycoplasma pneumoniae* complicated by haemorrhagic pleural effusion, haemolytic anaemia and myocarditis. Br. J. Clin. Pract. *27*:99–101, 1973.
184. Feizi, T.: Syndromes associated with mycoplasmas. Postgrad. Med. J. *43*:106–108, 1967.
185. Feizi, T.: Cold agglutinins, the direct Coombs' test and serum immunoglobulins in *Mycoplasma pneumoniae* infection. Ann. N. Y. Acad. Sci. *143*:801–812, 1967.
186. Feizi, T., Maclean, H., Sommerville, R. G., et al.: Studies on an epidemic of respiratory disease caused by *Mycoplasma pneumoniae.* B. M. J. *1*:457–460, 1967.
187. Fekety, F. R., Jr., Caldwell, J., Gump, D., et al.: Bacteria, viruses, and mycoplasmas in acute pneumonia in adults. Am. Rev. Respir. Dis. *104*:499–507, 1971.
188. Fernald, G. W.: In vitro response of human lymphocytes to *Mycoplasma pneumoniae*. Infect. Immun. *5*:552–558, 1972.
189. Fernald, G. W.: Role of host response in *Mycoplasma pneumoniae* disease. J. Infect. Dis. *127*(Suppl.):55–58, 1973.
190. Fernald, G. W.: Humoral and cellular immune responses to mycoplasmas. *In* Tully, J. G., and Whitcomb, R. F. (eds.): The Mycoplasmas. Vol. II. New York, Academic Press, 1979, pp. 399–423.
191. Fernald, G. W., and Clyde, W. A., Jr.: Pulmonary immune mechanisms in *Mycoplasma pneumoniae* disease. *In* Kirkpatrick, C. H., and Reynolds, H. Y. (eds.): Immunologic and Infectious Reactions in the Lung. New York, Marcel Dekker, 1976, pp. 101–130.
192. Fernald, G. W., Clyde, W. A., and Bienenstock, J.: Immunoglobulin-containing cells in lungs of hamsters infected with *Mycoplasma pneumoniae.* J. Immunol. *108*:1400–1408, 1972.
193. Fernald, G. W., Clyde, W. A., and Denny, F. W.: Nature of the immune response to *Mycoplasma pneumoniae.* J. Immunol. *98*:1028–1038, 1967.
194. Fernald, G. W., Collier, A. M., and Clyde, W. A.: Respiratory infections due to *Mycoplasma pneumoniae* in infants and children. Pediatrics *55*:327–335, 1975.
195. Fernald, G. W., and Glezen, W. P.: Humoral and cellular immune responses to an inactivated *Mycoplasma pneumoniae* vaccine in children. J. Infect. Dis. *127*:498–504, 1973.

196. Fernandez, C. V., Bortolussi, R., Gordon, K., et al.: *Mycoplasma pneumoniae* infection associated with central nervous system complications. J. Child. Neurol. *8*:27–31, 1993.
197. Fiacco, V., Miller, M. J., Carney, E., et al.: Comparison of media for isolation of *Ureaplasma urealyticum* and genital *Mycoplasma* species. J. Clin. Microbiol. *20*:862–865, 1984.
198. Fiala, M., Myhre, B. A., Chinh, L. T., et al.: Pathogenesis of anemia associated with *Mycoplasma pneumoniae.* Acta Haematol. *51*:297–301, 1974.
199. Fine, N. L., Smith, L. R., and Sheedy, P. F.: Frequency of pleural effusions in *Mycoplasma* and viral pneumonias. N. Engl. J. Med. *283*:790–793, 1970.
200. Finland, M., Peterson, O. L., Allen, H. E., et al.: Cold agglutinins. I. Occurrence of cold isohemagglutinins in various conditions. J. Clin. Invest. *24*:451–457, 1945.
201. Fischer, G. S., Sweimler, W. I., and Kleger, B.: Comparison of MYCOPLASM-ELISA with complement fixation test for measurement of antibodies to *Mycoplasma pneumoniae.* Diagn. Microbiol. Infect. Dis. *4*:139–145, 1986.
202. Fischman, R. A., Marschall, K. E., Kislak, J. W., et al.: Adult respiratory distress syndrome caused by *Mycoplasma pneumoniae.* Chest *74*:471–473, 1978.
203. Fisher, R. S., Clark, A. W., Wolinsky, J. S., et al.: Postinfectious leukoencephalitis complicating *Mycoplasma pneumoniae* infection. Arch. Neurol. *40*:109–113, 1983.
204. Fleischaur, P., Hube, U., Mertens, H., et al.: Nachweis von *Mycoplasma pneumoniae* in Liquor bei akuter Polyneuritis. Dtsch. Med. Wochenschr. *97*:678–682, 1972.
205. Fleming, P. C., Krieger, E., Turner, J. A. P., et al.: Febrile mucocutaneous syndrome with respiratory involvement, associated with isolation of *Mycoplasma pneumoniae.* Can. Med. Assoc. J. *97*:1458–1459, 1967.
206. Forgacs, P., Kundsin, R. B., Margles, S. W., et al.: A case of *Ureaplasma urealyticum* septic arthritis in a patient with hypogammaglobulinemia. Clin. Infect. Dis. *16*:293–294, 1993.
207. Foy, H. M.: Infections caused by *Mycoplasma pneumoniae* and possible carrier state in different populations of patients. Clin. Infect. Dis. *17*(Suppl. 1):37–46, 1993.
208. Foy, H. M., and Alexander, E. R.: *Mycoplasma pneumoniae* infections in childhood. Adv. Pediatr. *16*:301–323, 1969.
209. Foy, H. M., Cooney, M. K., Maletzky, A. J., et al.: Incidence and etiology of pneumonia, croup and bronchiolitis in preschool children belonging to a prepaid medical care group over a four-year period. Am. J. Epidemiol. *97*:80–92, 1973.
210. Foy, H. M., Cooney, M. K., McMahan, R., et al.: Viral and mycoplasmal pneumonia in a prepaid medical care group during an eight-year period. Am. J. Epidemiol. *97*:93–102, 1973.
211. Foy, H. M., Grayston, J. T., Kenny, G. E., et al.: Epidemiology of *Mycoplasma pneumoniae* infection in families. J. A. M. A. *197*:859–866, 1966.
212. Foy, H., Kenny, G., Bor, E., et al.: Prevalence of *Mycoplasma hominis* and *Ureaplasma urealyticum* (T strains) in urine of adolescents. J. Clin. Microbiol. *2*:226–230, 1975.
213. Foy, H. M., Kenny, G. E., Cooney, M. K., et al.: Long-term epidemiology of infections with *Mycoplasma pneumoniae.* J. Infect. Dis. *139*:681–687, 1979.
214. Foy, H. M., Kenny, G. E., Cooney, M. K., et al.: Naturally acquired immunity to pneumonia due to *Mycoplasma pneumoniae.* J. Infect. Dis. *147*:967–973, 1983.
215. Foy, H. M., Kenny, G. E., and Koler, J.: *Mycoplasma pneumoniae* in Stevens-Johnson's syndrome. Lancet *2*:550–551, 1966.
216. Foy, H. M., Kenny, G. E., Levinsohn, E. M., et al.: Acquisition of mycoplasmata and T-strains during infancy. J. Infect. Dis. *121*:579–587, 1970.
217. Foy, H. M., Kenny, G. E., McMahan, R., et al.: *Mycoplasma pneumoniae* in the community. Am. J. Epidemiol. *93*:55–67, 1970.
218. Foy, H. M., Kenny, G. E., McMahan, R., et al.: *Mycoplasma pneumoniae* pneumonia in an urban area: Five years of surveillance. J. A. M. A. *214*:1666–1672, 1970.
219. Foy, H. M., Kenny, G. E., Sefi, R., et al.: Second attacks of pneumonia due to *Mycoplasma pneumoniae.* J. Infect. Dis. *135*:673–677, 1977.
220. Foy, H. M., Kenny, G. E., Wentworth, B. B., et al.: Isolation of *Mycoplasma hominis,* T-strains, and cytomegalovirus from the cervix of pregnant women. Am. J. Obstet. Gynecol. *106*:635–643, 1970.
221. Foy, H. M., Nugent, C. G., Kenny, G. E., et al.: Repeated *Mycoplasma pneumoniae* pneumonia after 4 and one half years. J. A. M. A. *216*:671–672, 1971.
222. Foy, H. M., Ochs, H., and Davis, S. D.: *Mycoplasma pneumoniae* infections in patients with immunodeficiency syndromes: Report of four cases. J. Infect. Dis. *127*:388–393, 1973.
223. Frangogiannis, N. G., and Cate, T. R.: Endocarditis and *Ureaplasma urealyticum* osteomyelitis in a hypogammaglobulinemic patient. A case report and review of the literature. J. Infect. *37*:181–184, 1998.
224. Fransen, H., Forsgren, M., Heigl, Z., et al.: Studies on *Mycoplasma pneumoniae* in patients hospitalized with acute respiratory illness. Scand. J. Infect. Dis. *1*:91–98, 1969.
225. Franzoso, G., Hu, P. C., Meloni, G. A., et al.: The immunodominant 90-kilodalton protein is localized on the terminal tip structure of *Mycoplasma pneumoniae.* Infect. Immun. *61*:1523–1530, 1993.
226. Freeman, R., and McMahon, M. J.: Acute pancreatitis and serological evidence of infection with *Mycoplasma pneumoniae.* Gut *19*:367–370, 1978.
227. Freundt, E. A., and Edward, D. G.: Classification and taxonomy. *In* Barile, M. F., and Razin, S. (eds.): The Mycoplasmas. Vol. I. New York, Academic Press, 1979, pp. 1–41.
228. Freymuth, F., Vabret, A., Brouard, J., et al.: Detection of viral, *Chlamydia pneumoniae* and *Mycoplasma pneumoniae* infections in exacerbations of asthma in children. J. Clin. Virol. *13*:131–139, 1999.
229. Friedli, B., Renebey, F., and Rouge, J. C.: Complete heart block in a young child presumably due to *Mycoplasma pneumoniae* myocarditis. Acta Paediatr. Scand. *66*:385–388, 1977.
230. Ganick, D. J., Wolfson, J., Gilbert, E. F., et al.: *Mycoplasma* infection in the immunosuppressed leukemic patient. Arch. Pathol. Lab. Med. *104*:535–536, 1980.
231. Garland, S. M., and Murton, L. J.: Neonatal meningitis caused by *Ureaplasma urealyticum.* Pediatr. Infect. Dis. J. *6*:868–870, 1987.
232. Garrow, D. H.: A rapid test for the presence of increased cold agglutinins. B. M. J. *2*:206–208, 1958.
233. Geers, T. A., Taege, A. J., Longworth, D. L., et al.: *Ureaplasma urealyticum*: Unusual cause of culture-negative mediastinitis. Clin. Infect. Dis. *29*:949–950, 1999.
234. George, R. B., Weill, H., Rasch, J. R., et al.: Roentgenographic appearance of viral and mycoplasma pneumonias. Am. Rev. Respir. Dis. *96*:1144–1150, 1967.
235. George, R. B., Ziskind, M. M., Rasch, J. R., et al.: *Mycoplasma* and adenovirus pneumonias: Comparison with other atypical pneumonias in a military population. Ann. Intern. Med. *65*:931–942, 1966.
236. Gewitz, M., Dinwiddie, R., Rees, L., et al.: *Mycoplasma hominis:* A cause of neonatal meningitis. Arch. Dis. Child. *54*:231–239, 1979.
237. Gibbs, R. S., Blanco, J. D., St. Clair, P. J., et al.: *Mycoplasma hominis* and intrauterine infection in late pregnancy. Sex. Transm. Dis. *10*:303–306, 1983.
238. Gilbert, G. L., Law, F., and Macinnes, S. J.: Chronic *Mycoplasma hominis* infection complicating severe intraventricular hemorrhage, in a premature neonate. Pediatr. Infect. Dis. J. *7*:817–818, 1988.
239. Gill, K., and Marrie, T. J.: Hemophagocytosis secondary to *Mycoplasma pneumoniae* infection. Am. J. Med. *82*:668–670, 1987.
240. Glaser, J. B., Engelberg, M., and Hammerschlag, M.: Scalp abscess associated with *Mycoplasma hominis* infection complicating intrapartum monitoring. Pediatr. Infect. Dis. *2*:468–470, 1983.
241. Glezen, W. P., Clyde, W. A., Senior, R. J., et al.: Group A streptococci, mycoplasmas, and viruses associated with acute pharyngitis. J. A. M. A. *202*:455–460, 1967.
242. Glezen, W. P., and Denny, F. W.: Epidemiology of acute lower respiratory disease in children. N. Engl. J. Med. *288*:498–504, 1973.
243. Glezen, W. P., Loda, F. A., Clyde, W. A., et al.: Epidemiologic patterns of acute lower respiratory disease of children in a pediatric group practice. J. Pediatr. *78*:397–406, 1971.
244. Goldschmidt, B., Menonna, J., Fortunato, J., et al.: *Mycoplasma* antibody in Guillain-Barré syndrome and other neurological disorders. Ann. Neurol. *7*:108–112, 1980.
245. Golubjatnikov, R., Allen, V. D., Olmos-Blancarte, A. M. P., et al.: Serologic profile of children in a Mexican highland community: Prevalence of complement-fixing antibodies to *Mycoplasma pneumoniae,* respiratory syncytial virus and parainfluenza viruses. Am. J. Epidemiol. *101*: 458–464, 1975.
246. Goodburn, G. M., Marmion, B. P., and Kendall, E. J. C.: Infection with Eaton's primary atypical pneumonia agent in England. Br. J. Med. *1*:1266–1270, 1963.
247. Goudie, B. M., Kerr, M. R., and Johnson, R. N.: *Mycoplasma* pneumonia complicated by bronchiectasis. J. Infect. *7*:151–152, 1983.
248. Grady, G. F., and Gilfillan, R. F.: Relation of *Mycoplasma pneumoniae* sero-reactivity, immunosuppression, and chronic disease to Legionnaires' disease: A twelve-month prospective study of sporadic cases in Massachusetts. Ann. Intern. Med. *90*:607–610, 1979.
249. Grattard, F., Soleihac, B., de Barbeyrac, B., et al.: Epidemiologic and molecular investigations of genital mycoplasmas from women and neonates at delivery. Pediatr. Infect. Dis. J. *14*:853–859, 1995.
250. Grau, O., Slizewicz, B., Tuppin, P., et al.: Association of *Mycoplasma penetrans* with human immunodeficiency virus infection. J. Infect. Dis. *172*:672–681, 1995.
251. Grayston, J. T., Alexander, E. R., Kenny, G. E., et al.: *Mycoplasma pneumoniae* infections: Clinical and epidemiologic studies. J. A. M. A. *191*:369–374, 1965.
252. Greenberg, H., Helms, C. M., Brunner, H., et al.: Asymptomatic infection of adult volunteers with a temperature sensitive mutant of *Mycoplasma pneumoniae.* Proc. Natl. Acad. Sci. U. S. A. *71*:4015–4019, 1974.
253. Greenberg, H., Helms, C. M., Grizzard, M. B., et al.: Immunoprophylaxis of experimental *Mycoplasma pneumoniae* disease: Effect of route of administration on the immunogenicity and protective effect of inactivated *M. pneumoniae* vaccine. Infect. Immun. *16*:88–92, 1977.

254. Greenberg, H., Prescott, B., Brunner, H., et al.: Sharing of glycolipid antigenic determinants by *Mycoplasma pneumoniae* vegetables and certain bacteria. *In* Proceedings of the Symposium on New Approaches for Inducing Natural Immunity to Pyogenic Organisms, Winter Park, Florida, 1973. Washington, D.C., U.S. Department of Health, Education and Welfare, Publication No. (NIH) 74–553, 1973, pp. 151–156.
255. Greenstone, G.: Infectious mononucleosis complicated by pneumonia due to *Mycoplasma pneumoniae:* Report of two cases. J. Pediatr. *90*:492–493, 1977.
256. Griffin, J. P.: Rapid screening for cold agglutinins in pneumonia. Ann. Intern. Med. *70*:701–705, 1969.
257. Griffin, J. P., and Klein, E. W.: Role of sinusitis in primary atypical pneumonia. Clin. Med. *78*:23–27, 1971.
258. Grix, A., and Giammona, S. T.: Pneumonitis with pleural effusion in children due to *Mycoplasma pneumoniae.* Am. Rev. Respir. Dis. *109*:665–671, 1974.
259. Guerrero, M. L. F., Manuel Ramos, J., and Soriano, F.: *Mycoplasma hominis* bacteraemia not associated with genital infections. J. Infect. *39*:91–94, 1999.
260. Gump, D. W., Gibson, M., Ashikaga, T.: Lack of association between genital mycoplasmas and infertility. N. Engl. J. Med. *310*:937–941, 1984.
261. Gump, D. W., and Hawley, H. B.: Severe *Mycoplasma pneumoniae* pneumonia. Respiration *33*:475–486, 1976.
262. Halsted, C., Lepow, M. L., Balassanian, R., et al.: Otitis media: Clinical observations, microbiology and evaluation of therapy. Am. J. Dis. Child. *115*:542–551, 1968.
263. Hamrick, H. J., Mangum, M. E., and Katz, V. L.: *Ureaplasma urealyticum* abscess at site of an internal fetal heart rate monitor. Pediatr. Infect. Dis. J. *12*:410–411, 1993.
264. Handsfield, H. H.: Gonorrhea and nongonococcal urethritis. Med. Clin. North Am. *62*:925–943, 1978.
265. Hannaford, K., Todd, D. A., Jeffery, H., et al.: Role of *Ureaplasma urealyticum* in lung disease of prematurity. Arch. Dis. Child. Fetal Neonatal Ed. *81*:F162–F167, 1999.
266. Hanukoglu, A., Hebroni, S., and Fried, D.: Pulmonary involvement in *Mycoplasma pneumoniae* infection in families. Infection *14*:3–8, 1986.
267. Harris, J. A., Kolokathis, A., Campbell, M., et al.: Safety and efficacy of azithromycin in the treatment of community- acquired pneumonia in children. Pediatr. Infect. Dis. J. *17*:865–871, 1998.
268. Harris, R., Marmion, B. P., Varkanis, G., et al.: Laboratory diagnosis of *Mycoplasma pneumoniae* infection. 2. Comparison of methods for the direct detection of specific antigen or nucleic acid sequences in respiratory exudates. Epidemiol. Infect. *101*:685–694, 1988.
269. Hart, G.: Sexually transmitted diseases. *In* Shen, J. T. Y. (ed.): The Clinical Practice of Adolescent Medicine. New York, Appleton-Century-Crofts, 1980, pp. 101–110.
270. Hata, D., Kuze, F., Mochizuki, Y., et al.: Evaluation of DNA probe test for rapid diagnosis of *Mycoplasma pneumoniae* infections. J. Pediatr. *116*:273–276, 1990.
271. Hawkins, R. E., Rickman, L. S., Vermund, S. H., et al.: Association of *Mycoplasma* and human immunodeficiency virus infection: Detection of amplified *Mycoplasma fermentans* DNA in blood. J. Infect. Dis. *165*:581–585, 1992.
272. Hayflick, L.: Fundamental biology of the class Mollicutes, order Mycoplasmatales. *In* Hayflick, L. (ed.): The Mycoplasmatales and the L-Phase of Bacteria. New York, Appleton-Century-Crofts, 1969, pp. 15–47.
273. Hayflick, L., and Chanock, R. M.: *Mycoplasma* species of man. Bacteriol. Rev. *29*:185–221, 1965.
274. Heggie, A. D., Bar-Shain, D., Boxerbaum, B., et al.: Identification and quantification of ureaplasmas colonizing the respiratory tract and assessment of their role in the development of chronic lung disease in preterm infants. Pediatr. Infect. Dis. J. *20*:854–859, 2001.
275. Heiskanen-Kosma, T., Korppi, M., Jokinen, C., et al.: Etiology of childhood pneumonia: Serologic results of a prospective, population-based study. Pediatr. Infect. Dis. J. *17*:986–991, 1998.
276. Heiskanen-Kosma, T., Korppi, M., Laurila, A., et al. : *Chlamydia pneumoniae* is an important cause of community-acquired pneumonia in school-aged children: Serological results of a prospective, population-based study. Scand. J. Infect. Dis. *31*:255–259, 1999.
277. Helms, C. M., Viner, J. P., Sturm, R. H., et al.: Comparative features of pneumococcal, mycoplasmal, and legionnaires' disease pneumonias. Ann. Intern. Med. *90*:543–547, 1979.
278. Hengge, U. R., Kirschfink, M., Konig, A. L., et al.: Characterization of I/FI glycoprotein as a receptor for *Mycoplasma pneumoniae.* Infect. Immun. *60*:79–83, 1992.
279. Henrich, B., Feldmann, R. C., and Hadding, U.: Cytoadhesins of *Mycoplasma hominis.* Infect. Immun. *61*:2945–2951, 1993.
280. Hentschel, J., Abele-Horn, M., and Peters, J.: *Ureaplasma urealyticum* in the cerebrospinal fluid of a premature infant. Acta Paediatr. *82*:690–693, 1993.
281. Hernandez, L. A., Urquhart, G. E. D., and Dick, W. C.: *Mycoplasma pneumoniae* infection and arthritis in man. B. M. J. *2*:14–16, 1977.
282. Hillier, S. L., Martius, J., Krohn, M., et al.: A case-control study of chorioamnionic infection and histologic chorioamnionitis in prematurity. N. Engl. J. Med. *319*:972–978, 1988.
283. Hirai, Y., Shiode, J., Masayoshi, T., et al.: Application of an indirect immunofluorescence test for detection of *Mycoplasma pneumoniae* in respiratory exudates. J. Clin. Microbiol. *29*:2007–2012, 1991.
284. Hodges, G. R., Fass, R. J., and Saslaw, S.: Central nervous system disease associated with *Mycoplasma pneumoniae* infection. Arch. Intern. Med. *130*:277–282, 1972.
285. Hodges, G. R., and Perkins, R. L.: Landry-Guillain-Barré syndrome associated with *Mycoplasma pneumoniae* infection. J. A. M. A. *210*:2088–2090, 1969.
286. Holmes, K. K., Handsfield, H. H., Wang, S. P., et al.: Etiology of nongonococcal urethritis. N. Engl. J. Med. *292*:1199–1205, 1975.
287. Holmes, K. K., Johnson, D. W., and Floyd, T. M.: Studies of venereal disease. III. Double-blind comparison of tetracycline hydrochloride and placebo in treatment of nongonococcal urethritis. J. A. M. A. *202*:138–140, 1967.
288. Holmes, K. K., Johnson, D. W., Floyd, T. M., et al.: Studies of venereal disease. II. Observations on the incidence, etiology, and treatment of the postgonococcal urethritis syndrome. J. A. M. A. *202*:131–137, 1967.
289. Honda, J., Yano, T., Kusaba, M., et al.: Clinical use of capillary PCR to diagnose *Mycoplasma pneumoniae.* J. Clin. Microbiol. *38*:1382–1384, 2000.
290. Horn, M. E. C., Brain, E. A., Gregg, I., et al.: Respiratory viral infection and wheezy bronchitis in childhood. Thorax *34*:23–28, 1969.
291. Horn, M. E. C., Brain, E., Gregg, I., et al.: Respiratory viral infection in childhood: A survey in general practice, Roehampton 1967–1972. J. Hyg. (Camb.) *74*:157–168, 1975.
292. Hornsleth, A.: *Mycoplasma pneumoniae* infection in infants and children in Copenhagen 1963–65: Incidence of complement-fixing antibodies in age groups 0–9 years. Acta Pathol. Microbiol. Scand. *69*:304–313, 1967.
293. Horowitz, S., Landau, D., Shinwell, E. S., et al.: Respiratory tract colonization with *Ureaplasma urealyticum* and bronchopulmonary dysplasia in neonates in southern Israel. Pediatr. Infect. Dis. J. *11*:847–851, 1992.
294. Hosker, H. S. R., Tam, J. S., Chan, C. H. S., et al.: *Mycoplasma pneumoniae* infection in Hong Kong: Clinical and epidemiological features during an epidemic. Respiration *60*:237–240, 1993.
295. Hu, P. C., Cole, R. M., Huang, Y. S., et al.: *Mycoplasma pneumoniae* infection: Role of a surface protein in the attachment organelle. Science *216*:313–315, 1982.
296. Hu, P., Collier, A. M., and Baseman, J. B.: Interaction of virulent *Mycoplasma pneumoniae* with hamster tracheal organ cultures. Infect. Immun. *14*:217–224, 1976.
297. Hu, P. C., Huang, C. H., Collier, A. M., et al.: Demonstration of antibodies to *Mycoplasma pneumoniae* attachment protein in human sera and respiratory secretions. Infect. Immun. *41*:437–439, 1983.
298. Hu, P. C., Huang, C. H., Huang, Y. S., et al.: Demonstration of multiple antigenic determinants on *Mycoplasma pneumoniae* attachment protein by monoclonal antibodies. Infect. Immun. *50*:292–296, 1985.
299. Hu, P. C., Powell, D. A., Albright, F., et al.: A solid-phase radioimmunoassay for detection of antibodies against *Mycoplasma pneumoniae.* J. Clin. Lab. Immunol. *11*:209–213, 1983.
300. Huhti, E., Mokka, T., Nikoskelainen, J., et al.: Association of viral and mycoplasma infections with exacerbations of asthma. Ann. Allergy *33*:145–149, 1974.
301. Hummell, D. S., Anderson, S. J., Wright, P. F., et al.: Chronic recurrent multifocal osteomyelitis: Are mycoplasmas involved? N. Engl. J. Med. *317*:510–511, 1987.
302. Hyde, T. B., Gilbert, M., Schwartz, S. B., et al.: Azithromycin prophylaxis during a hospital outbreak of *Mycoplasma pneumoniae* pneumonia. J. Infect. Dis. *183*:907–912, 2001.
303. Ieven, M., Demey, H., Ursi, D., et al.: Fatal encephalitis caused by *Mycoplasma pneumoniae* diagnosed by the polymerase chain reaction. Clin. Infect. Dis. *27*:1552–1553, 1998.
304. Ieven, M., Ursi, D., van Bever, H., et al.: Detection of *Mycoplasma pneumoniae* by two polymerase chain reactions and role of *M. pneumoniae* in acute respiratory tract infections in pediatric patients. J. Infect. Dis. *173*:1445–1452, 1996.
305. International Committee on Systematic Bacteriology, Subcommittee on the Taxonomy of Mollicutes: Proposal of minimal standards for descriptions of new species of the class Mollicutes. Int. J. Syst. Bacteriol. *29*:172–180, 1979.
306. Ionno, J. A., and Westfall, R. E.: *Mycoplasma pneumoniae* pneumonia: Clinical course and complications. Mil. Med. *135*:459–463, 1970.
307. Ishida, K., Kaku, M., Irifune, K., et al.: In vitro and in vivo activities of macrolides against *Mycoplasma pneumoniae.* Antimicrob. Agents Chemother. *38*:790–798, 1994.
308. Ishida, K., Kaku, M., Irifune, K., et al.: In vitro and in vivo activity of a new quinolone AM-1155 against *Mycoplasma pneumoniae.* J. Antimicrob. Chemother. *34*:875–883, 1994.
309. Jachuck, S. J., Clark, F., Gardner-Thorpe, C., et al.: A brainstem syndrome associated with *Mycoplasma pneumoniae* infection: A report of two cases. Postgrad. Med. J. *51*:475–477, 1975.
310. Jackson, L. A., Cherry, J. D., Wang, S. P., et al.: Frequency of serological evidence of *Bordetella* infections and mixed infections with other respiratory pathogens in university students with cough illnesses. Clin. Infect. Dis. *31*:3–6, 2000.

311. Jacobs, E.: Serological diagnosis of *Mycoplasma pneumoniae* infections: A critical review of current procedures. Clin. Infect. Dis. *17*(Suppl. 1): 79–82, 1993.
312. Jacobs, E., Rock, R., and Dalehite, L.: A B cell, T cell–linked epitope located on the adhesin of *Mycoplasma pneumoniae.* Infect. Immun. *58*:2464–2469, 1990.
313. Jacobs, E., Schopperle, K., and Bredt, W.: Adherence inhibition assay: A specific serological test for detection of antibodies to *Mycoplasma pneumoniae.* Eur. J. Clin. Microbiol. *4*:113–118, 1985.
314. Jacobs, F., van de Stadt, J., Gelin, M., et al.: *Mycoplasma hominis* infection of perihepatic hematomas in a liver transplant recipient. Surgery *98*:98–100, 1992.
315. Jacobs, N. F., and Kraus, S. J.: Gonococcal and nongonococcal urethritis in men: Clinical and laboratory differentiation. Ann. Intern. Med. *82*:7–12, 1975.
316. Janney, F. A., Lee, L. T., and Howe, C.: Cold hemagglutinin cross-reactivity with *Mycoplasma pneumoniae.* Infect. Immun. *22*:29–33, 1978.
317. Jansson, E.: Mycoplasmas and arthritis. Scand. J. Rheumatol. *4*:39–42, 1975.
318. Jansson, E., von Essen, R., and Tuuri, S.: *Mycoplasma pneumoniae* pneumonia in Helsinki 1962–1970. Scand. J. Infect. Dis. *3*:51–54, 1971.
319. Jansson, E., Wager, O., Stenstrom, R., et al.: Studies on Eaton PPLO pneumonia. B. M. J. *1*:142–145, 1964.
320. Jao, R. L., and Finland, M.: Susceptibility of *Mycoplasma pneumoniae* to 21 antibiotics *in vitro.* Am. J. Med. Sci. *253*:639–650, 1967.
321. Jemski, J. V., Hetsko, C. M., Helms, C. M., et al.: Immunoprophylaxis of experimental *Mycoplasma pneumoniae* disease: Effect of aerosol particle size and site of deposition of *M. pneumoniae* on the pattern of respiratory infection, disease, and immunity in hamsters. Infect. Immun. *16*:93–98, 1977.
322. Jensen, J. S., Heilmann, C., and Valerius, N. H.: *Mycoplasma pneumoniae* infection in a child with AIDS. Clin. Infect. Dis. *19*:207, 1994.
323. Jensen, J. S., Orsum, R., Dohn, B., et al.: *Mycoplasma genitalium:* A cause of male urethritis? Genitourin. Med. *69*:265–269, 1993.
324. Jensen, J. S., Songergard-Andersen, J., Uldum, S. A., et al.: Detection of *Mycoplasma pneumoniae* in simulated clinical samples by polymerase chain reaction. A. P. M. I. S. *97*:1046–1048, 1989.
325. Jensen, K. E., Senterfit, L. B., and Chanock, R. M.: An inactivated *Mycoplasma pneumoniae* vaccine. J. A. M. A. *194*:248–252, 1965.
326. Jensen, K. J., Senterfit, L. B., Scully, W. E., et al.: *Mycoplasma pneumoniae* infections in children: An epidemiologic appraisal in families treated with oxytetracycline. Am. J. Epidemiol. *86*:419–432, 1967.
327. Jones, D. M., and Tobin, B.: Neonatal eye infections due to *Mycoplasma hominis.* B. M. J. *3*:467–468, 1968.
328. Jones, G. R., and Stewart, S. M.: A prospective study of the persistence of *Mycoplasma pneumoniae* antibody levels. Scott. Med. J. *19*:129–133, 1974.
329. Jones, M. C.: Arthritis and arthralgia in infection with *Mycoplasma pneumoniae.* Thorax *25*:748–750, 1970.
330. Jonsson, B., Karell, A.-C., Ringertz, S., et al.: Neonatal *Ureaplasma urealyticum* colonization and chronic lung disease. Acta Paediatr. *83*:927–930, 1994.
331. Joosting, A. C. C., Harwin, R. M., Coppin, A., et al.: A serological investigation of *Mycoplasma pneumoniae* infection on the Witwatersrand. S. Afr. Med. J. *50*:2134–2135, 1976.
332. Jordan, W. S., Jr., and Dingle, J. H.: *Mycoplasma pneumoniae* infections. *In* Dubos, R. J., and Hirsch, J. G. (eds.): Bacterial and Mycotic Infections of Man. Philadelphia, J. B. Lippincott, 1965, pp. 810–824.
333. Kahane, I., Tucker, S., Leith, D. K., et al.: Detection of the major adhesin P1 in triton shells of virulent *Mycoplasma pneumoniae.* Infect. Immun. *50*:944–946, 1985.
334. Kai, M., Kamiya, S., Yabe, H., et al.: Rapid detection of *Mycoplasma pneumoniae* in clinical samples by the polymerase chain reaction. J. Med. Microbiol. *38*:166–170, 1993.
335. Kalb, R. E., Grossman, M. E., and Neu, H. C.: Stevens-Johnson syndrome due to *Mycoplasma pneumoniae* in an adult. Am. J. Med. *79*:541–544, 1985.
336. Kammer, G. M., Pollack, J. D., and Klainer, A. S.: Scanning-beam electron microscopy of *Mycoplasma pneumoniae.* J. Bacteriol. *104*:499–502, 1970.
337. Kane, J. R., Shenep, J. L., Krance, R. A., et al.: Diffuse alveolar hemorrhage associated with *Mycoplasma hominis* respiratory tract infection in a bone marrow transplant recipient. Chest *105*:1891–1892, 1994.
338. Kasahara, I., Otsubo, Y., Yanase, T., et al.: Isolation and characterization of *Mycoplasma pneumoniae* from cerebrospinal fluid of a patient with pneumonia and meningoencephalitis. J. Infect. Dis. *152*:823–825, 1985.
339. Katseni, V. L., Gilroy, C. B., Ryait, B. K., et al.: *Mycoplasma fermentans* in individuals seropositive and seronegative for HIV-1. Lancet *341*:271–272, 1993.
340. Katz, H. I., Wooten, J. W., Davis, R. G., et al.: Stevens-Johnson syndrome: Report of a case associated with culturally proven *Mycoplasma pneumoniae* infection. J. A. M. A. *199*:504–506, 1967.
341. Kaufman, J. M., Cuvelier, C. A., and van der Straeten, M.: *Mycoplasma* pneumonia with fulminant evolution into diffuse interstitial fibrosis. Thorax *35*:140–144, 1980.
342. Keegan, B. M., Lowry, N. J., and Yager, J. Y.: *Mycoplasma pneumoniae*: A cause of coma in the absence of meningoencephalitis. Pediatr. Neurol. *21*:822–825, 1999.
343. Kenney, R. T., Li, J. S., Clyde, W. A., Jr., et al.: Mycoplasmal pericarditis: Evidence of invasive disease. Clin. Infect. Dis. *17*(Suppl. 1):58–62, 1993.
344. Kenny, G. E.: Antigenic determinants. *In* Barile, M. F., and Razin, S. (eds.): The Mycoplasmas. Vol. I. New York, Academic Press, 1979, pp. 351–384.
345. Kenny, G. E., and Newton, R. M.: Close serological relationship between glycolipids of *Mycoplasma pneumoniae* and glycolipids of spinach. Ann. N. Y. Acad. Sci. *225*:54–61, 1973.
346. Khatib, R., and Schnarr, D.: Point-source outbreak of *Mycoplasma pneumoniae* infection in a family unit. J. Infect. Dis. *151*:186–187, 1985.
347. Khatib, R. E., and Lerner, A. M.: Myocarditis in *Mycoplasma pneumoniae* pneumonia: Occurrence with hemolytic anemia and extraordinary titers of cold isohemagglutinins. J. A. M. A. *231*:493–494, 1975.
348. Kidron, D., Barron, S. A., and Mazliah, J.: Mononeuritis multiplex with brachial plexus neuropathy coincident with *Mycoplasma pneumoniae* infection. Eur. Neurol. *29*:90–92, 1989.
349. Kim, C. K., Chung, C. Y., Kim, J. S., et al.: Late abnormal findings on high-resolution computed tomography after *Mycoplasma* pneumonia. Pediatrics *105*:372–378, 2000.
350. Kingston, J. R., Chanock, R. M., Mufson, M. A., et al.: Eaton agent pneumonia. J. A. M. A. *176*:118–123, 1961.
351. Klar, A., Gross-Kieselstein, E., Hurvitz, H., et al.: Bilateral Bell's palsy due to *Mycoplasma pneumoniae* infection. Isr. J. Med. Sci. *21*:692–694, 1985.
352. Klausner, J. D., Passaro, D., Rosenberg, J., et al.: Enhanced control of an outbreak of *Mycoplasma pneumoniae* pneumonia with azithromycin prophylaxis. J. Infect. Dis. *177*:161–166, 1998.
353. Kleemola, M., Heiskanen-Kosma, T., Nohynek, H., et al.: Diagnostic efficacy of a *Mycoplasma pneumoniae* hybridization test in nasopharyngeal aspirates of children. Pediatr. Infect. Dis. J. *12*:344–345, 1993.
354. Kleemola, S. R. M., Karjalainen, J. E., and Raty, R. K. H.: Rapid diagnosis of *Mycoplasma pneumoniae* infection: Clinical evaluation of a commercial probe test. J. Infect. Dis. *162*:70–75, 1990.
355. Kleemola, M., and Kayhty, H.: Increase in titers of antibodies to *Mycoplasma pneumoniae* in patients with purulent meningitis. J. Infect. Dis. *146*:284–288, 1982.
356. Kleemola, M., Kayhty, H., and Raty, R.: Presence of antibodies to *Mycoplasma pneumoniae* in patients with bacterial meningitis: Reply. J. Infect. Dis. *148*:363–365, 1983.
357. Klein, J. O., Buckland, D., and Finland, M.: Colonization of newborn infants by mycoplasmas. N. Engl. J. Med. *280*:1025–1030, 1969.
358. Klimek, J. J., Russman, B. S., and Quintiliani, R.: *Mycoplasma pneumoniae* meningoencephalitis and transverse myelitis in association with low cerebrospinal fluid glucose. Pediatrics *58*:133–135, 1976.
359. Koh, Y. Y., Park, Y., Lee, H. J., et al.: Levels of interleukin-2, interferon-gamma, and interleukin-4 in bronchoalveolar lavage fluid from patients with *Mycoplasma* pneumonia: Implication of tendency toward increased immunoglobulin E production. Pediatrics *107*:E39, 2001.
360. Kok, T. W., Marmion, B. P., Varkanis, G., et al.: Laboratory diagnosis of *Mycoplasma pneumoniae* infection. 3. Detection of IgM antibodies to *M. pneumoniae* by a modified indirect haemagglutination test. Epidemiol. Infect. *103*:613–623, 1989.
361. Kok, T. W., Varkanis, G., Marmion, B. P., et al.: Laboratory diagnosis of *Mycoplasma pneumoniae* infection. 1. Direct detection of antigen in respiratory exudates by enzyme immunoassay. Epidemiol. Infect. *101*:669–684, 1988.
362. Koletsky, R. J., and Weinstein, A. J.: Fulminant *Mycoplasma pneumoniae* infection: Report of a fatal case, and a review of the literature. Am. Rev. Respir. Dis. *122*:491–496, 1980.
363. Kolski, H., Ford-Jones, E. L., Richardson, S., et al.: Etiology of acute childhood encephalitis at The Hospital for Sick Children, Toronto, 1994–1995. Clin. Infect. Dis. *26*:398–409, 1998.
364. Komaroff, A. L., Aronson, M. D., Pass, T. M., et al.: Serologic evidence of chlamydial and mycoplasmas pharyngitis in adults. Science *222*:927–928, 1983.
365. Komatsu, H., Kuroki, S., Shimizu, Y., et al.: *Mycoplasma pneumoniae* meningoencephalitis and cerebellitis with antiganglioside antibodies. Pediatr. Neurol. *18*:160–164, 1998.
366. Kopelman, P.: Raised mean cell volume and meningoencephalitis associated with *Mycoplasma pneumoniae* infection. B. M. J. *1*:881–882, 1977.
367. Koskiniemi, M.: CNS manifestations associated with *Mycoplasma pneumoniae* infections: Summary of cases at the University of Helsinki and review. Clin. Infect. Dis. *17*(Suppl. 1):52–57, 1993.
368. Kovacic, R., Launay, V., Tuppin, P., et al.: Search for the presence of six *Mycoplasma* species in peripheral blood mononuclear cells of subjects seropositive and seronegative for human immunodeficiency virus. J. Clin. Microbiol. *34*:1808–1810, 1996.
369. Kraft, M., Cassell, G. H., Henson, J. E., et al.: Detection of *Mycoplasma pneumoniae* in the airways of adults with chronic asthma. Am. J. Respir. Crit. Care Med. *158*:998–1001, 1998.

370. Krause, D. C.: *Mycoplasma pneumoniae* cytadherence: Unravelling the tie that binds. Mol. Microbiol. *20*:247–253, 1996.
371. Krause, D. C., and Baseman, J. B.: Inhibition of *Mycoplasma pneumoniae* hemadsorption and adherence to respiratory epithelium by antibodies to a membrane protein. Infect. Immun. *39*:1180–1186, 1983.
372. Kumada, S., Kusaka, H., Okaniwa, M., et al.: Encephalomyelitis subsequent to mycoplasma infection with elevated serum anti–Gal C antibody. Pediatr. Neurol. *16*:241–244, 1997.
373. Kundsin, R. B., Driscoll, S. G., Monson, R. R., et al.: Association of *Ureaplasma urealyticum* in the placenta with perinatal morbidity and mortality. N. Engl. J. Med. *310*:941–945, 1984.
374. Kundsin, R. B., Driscoll, S. G., and Pelletier, P. A.: *Ureaplasma urealyticum* incriminated in perinatal morbidity and mortality. Science *213*:474–476, 1981.
375. Ladefoged, S. A.: Molecular dissection of *Mycoplasma hominis.* A. P. M. I. S. *97*(Suppl.):1–45, 2000.
376. Lam, K., and Bayer, A. S.: *Mycoplasma pneumoniae* as a cause of the "fever of unknown origin" syndrome. Arch. Intern. Med. *142*:2312–2313, 1982.
377. Lambert, H. P.: Syndrome with joint manifestations in association with *Mycoplasma pneumoniae* infection. B. M. J. *3*:156–157, 1968.
378. Lambert, H. P.: Antibody to *Mycoplasma pneumoniae* in normal subjects and in patients with chronic bronchitis. J. Hyg. (Camb.) *66*:185–189, 1968.
379. Lambert, H. P.: Infections caused by *Mycoplasma pneumoniae.* Br. J. Dis. Chest *63*:71–82, 1969.
380. Larsen, P. D., and Crisp, D.: Acute bilateral striatal necrosis associated with *Mycoplasma pneumoniae* infection. Pediatr. Infect. Dis. J. *15*:1124–1126, 1996.
381. Lascari, A. D., Garfunkel, J. M., and Mauro, D. J.: Varicella-like rash associated with *Mycoplasma* infection. Am. J. Dis. Child. *128*:254–255, 1974.
382. Layani-Milon, M. P., Gras, I., Valette, M., et al.: Incidence of upper respiratory tract *Mycoplasma pneumoniae* infections among outpatients in Rhone-Alpes, France, during five successive winter periods. J. Clin. Microbiol. *37*:1721–1726, 1999.
383. Leach, A., and Lewis, B. W.: Unusual *Mycoplasma pneumoniae.* B. M. J. *1*:185, 1969.
384. Leach, R. H., Hales, A., Furr, P. M., et al.: Problems in the identification of *Mycoplasma pirum* isolated from human lymphoblastoid cell cultures. F. E. M. S. Microbiol. Lett. *44*:293–297, 1987.
385. Lee, S. H., Charoenying, S., Brennan, T., et al.: Comparative studies of three serologic methods for the measurement of *Mycoplasma pneumoniae* antibodies. Am. J. Clin. Pathol. *92*:342–347, 1989.
386. Lee, Y. H., McCormack, W. M., Marcy, S. M., et al.: The genital mycoplasmas: Their role in disorders of reproduction and in pediatric infections. Pediatr. Clin. North Am. *21*:457–466, 1974.
387. Lee, Y. H., Rosner, B., Alpert, S., et al.: Clinical and microbiological investigation of men with urethritis. J. Infect. Dis. *138*:798–803, 1978.
388. Lehtokoski-Lehtiniemi, E., and Koskiniemi, M.-L.: *Mycoplasma pneumoniae* encephalitis: A severe entity in children. Pediatr. Infect. Dis. J. *8*:651–653, 1989.
389. Leinikki, P., and Pantzar, P.: Acute pancreatitis in *Mycoplasma pneumoniae* infections. B. M. J. *1*:554, 1973.
390. Leinikki, P. O., Pantzar, P., and Tykka, H.: Immunoglobulin M antibody response against *Mycoplasma pneumoniae* lipid antigen in patients with acute pancreatitis. J. Clin. Microbiol. *8*:113–118, 1978.
391. Lemcke, R. M., Shaw, E. J., and Marmion, B. P.: Related antigens in *Mycoplasma pneumoniae* and *Mycoplasma mycoides* var. *mycoides.* Aust. J. Exp. Biol. Med. Sci. *18*:761–770, 1965.
392. Lepow, M. L., Balassanian, N., Emmerich, J., et al.: Interrelationships of viral, mycoplasmal, and bacterial agents in uncomplicated pneumonia. Am. Rev. Respir. Dis. *97*:533–545, 1968.
393. Lequier, L., Robinson, J., and Vaudry, W.: Sternotomy infection with *Mycoplasma hominis* in a neonate. Pediatr. Infect. Dis. J. *14*:1010–1012, 1995.
394. Lerer, R. J., and Kalavsky, S. M.: Central nervous system disease associated with *Mycoplasma pneumoniae* infection: Report of five cases and review of the literature. Pediatrics *52*:658–667, 1973.
395. Levine, D. P., and Lerner, A. M.: The clinical spectrum of *Mycoplasma pneumoniae* infections. Med. Clin. North Am. *62*:961–978, 1978.
396. Lewes, D., Rainford, D. J., and Lane, W. F.: Symptomless myocarditis and myalgia in viral and *Mycoplasma pneumoniae* infections. Br. Heart J. *36*:924–932, 1974.
397. Lewis, J. E., and Sheptin, C.: Mycoplasmal pneumonia associated with abscess of the lung. Calif. Med. *117*:69–72, 1972.
398. Likitnukul, S., Kusmiesz, H., Nelson, J. D., et al.: Role of genital mycoplasmas in young infants with suspected sepsis. J. Pediatr. *109*:971–974, 1986.
399. Lin, J.-S. L.: Human mycoplasmal infections: Serologic observations. Rev. Infect. Dis. *7*:216–231, 1985.
400. Lin, J.-S. L., Kendrick, M. I., and Kass, E. H.: Serologic typing of human genital T-mycoplasmas by a complement-dependent mycoplasmacidal test. J. Infect. Dis. *126*:658–663, 1972.
401. Lind, K.: Immunological relationships between *Mycoplasma pneumoniae* and *Streptococcus* MG. Acta Pathol. Microbiol. Scand. *73*:237–244, 1968.
402. Lind, K.: Incidence of *Mycoplasma pneumoniae* infection in Denmark from 1958 to 1969. Acta Pathol. Microbiol. Scand. [B] *79*:239–247, 1971.
403. Lind, K.: Production of cold agglutinins in rabbits induced by *Mycoplasma pneumoniae, Listeria monocytogenes* or *Streptococcus* MG. Acta Pathol. Microbiol. Scand. [B] *81*:487–496, 1973.
404. Lind, K., Hoier-Madsen, M., and Wiik, S.: Autoantibodies to the mitotic spindle apparatus in *Mycoplasma pneumoniae* disease. Infect. Immun. *56*:714–715, 1988.
405. Lind, K., Lindhardt, B. O., Schutten, H. J., et al.: Serological cross-reactions between *Mycoplasma genitalium* and *Mycoplasma pneumoniae.* J. Clin. Microbiol. *20*:1036–1043, 1984.
406. Lind, K., Zoffmann, H., Larsen, S. O., et al.: *Mycoplasma pneumoniae* infection associated with infection of the central nervous system. Acta Med. Scand. *205*:325–332, 1979.
407. Lipman, R. P., and Clyde, W. A., Jr.: The interrelationship of virulence, cytadsorption, and peroxide formation in *Mycoplasma pneumoniae.* Proc. Soc. Exp. Med. Biol. *131*:1163–1167, 1969.
408. Lipman, R. P., Clyde, W. A., Jr., and Denny, F. W.: Characteristics of virulent, attenuated, and avirulent *Mycoplasma pneumoniae* strains. J. Bacteriol. *100*:1037–1043, 1969.
409. Little, T. M., and Dowdle, R. H.: *Mycoplasma* pneumonia with inappropriate secretion of antidiuretic hormone. B. M. J. *1*:571, 1975.
410. Liu, C., Eaton, M. D., and Heyl, J. T.: Studies on primary atypical pneumonia. II. Observations concerning the development and immunological characteristics of antibody in patients. J. Exp. Med. *109*:545–556, 1959.
411. Llibre, J. M., Urban, A., Garcia, E., et al.: Bronchiolitis obliterans organizing pneumonia associated with acute *Mycoplasma pneumoniae* infection. Clin. Infect. Dis. *25*:1340–1342, 1997.
412. Lo, S. C., Hayes, M. M., Tully, J. G., et al.: *Mycoplasma penetrans* sp. nov., from the urogenital tract of patients with AIDS. Int. J. Syst. Bacteriol. *42*:357–364, 1992.
413. Lo, S. C., Hayes, M. M., Wang, R. Y. H., et al. Newly discovered *Mycoplasma* isolated from patients infected with HIV. Lancet *388*:1415–1418, 1991.
414. Loda, F. A., Clyde, W. A., Jr., Glezen, W. P., et al.: Studies on the role of viruses, bacteria, and *M. pneumoniae* as causes of lower respiratory tract infections in children. J. Pediatr. *72*:161–176, 1968.
415. Loda, F. A., Glezen, W. P., and Clyde, W. A., Jr.: Respiratory disease in group day care. Pediatrics *49*:428–437, 1972.
416. Longcope, W. T.: Bronchopneumonia of an unknown etiology (variety X). Bull. Johns Hopkins Hosp. *67*:268, 1940.
417. Loo, V. G., Richardson, S., and Quinn, P.: Isolation of *Mycoplasma pneumoniae* from pleural fluid. Diagn. Microbiol. Infect. Dis. *14*:443–445, 1991.
418. Lorber, J., Kalhan, S. C., and Mahgrefte, B.: Treatment of ventriculitis with gentamicin and cloxacillin in infants born with spina bifida. Arch. Dis. Child. *45*:178–185, 1970.
419. Ludlam, G. B., Bridges, J. B., and Benn, E. C.: Association of Stevens-Johnson syndrome with antibody for *Mycoplasma pneumoniae.* Lancet *1*:958–959, 1964.
420. Lum, G., and Kulhanjian, J.: Severe encephalitis in a three-year-old girl. Pediatr. Infect. Dis. J. *15*:181, 184–186, 1996.
421. Luneberg, E., Jensen, J. S., and Frosch, M.: Detection of *Mycoplasma pneumoniae* by polymerase chain reaction and nonradioactive hybridization in microtiter plates. J. Clin. Microbiol. *31*:1088–1094, 1993.
422. Lyell, A., Gordon, A. M., Dick, H. M., et al.: Mycoplasmas and erythema multiforme. Lancet *2*:1116–1118, 1967.
423. Lyon, G. M., Alspaugh, A., Meredith, F. T., et al.: *Mycoplasma hominis* pneumonia complicating bilateral lung transplantation: Case report and review of the literature. Chest *112*:1428–1432, 1997.
424. MacLean, D. W.: *Mycoplasma pneumoniae:* One year's experience in an urban practice. Scott. Med. J. *14*:312–320, 1969.
425. Macon, W. R., Lo, S.-C., Poiesz, B. J., et al.: Acquired immunodeficiency syndrome–like illness associated with systemic *Mycoplasma fermentans* infection in a human immunodeficiency-virus–negative homosexual man. Hum. Pathol. *24*:554–558, 1993.
426. Madan, E., Meyer, M. P., and Amortigui, A. J.: Isolation of genital mycoplasmas and *Chlamydia trachomatis* in stillborn and neonatal autopsy material. Arch. Pathol. Lab. Med. *112*:749–751, 1988.
427. Maisel, J. C., Babbitt, L. H., and John, T. J.: Fatal *Mycoplasma pneumoniae* infection with isolation of organisms from lung. J. A. M. A. *202*:287–290, 1967.
428. Manchee, R. J., and Taylor-Robinson, D.: Enhanced growth of T-strain mycoplasmas with *N*-2-hydroxy-ethylpiperazine-*N*¢-2-ethanesulfonic acid buffer. J. Bacteriol. *100*:78–85, 1969.
429. Manimtim, W. M., Hasday, J. D., Hester, L., et al.: *Ureaplasma urealyticum* modulates endotoxin-induced cytokine release by human monocytes derived from preterm and term newborns and adults. Infect. Immun. *69*:3906–3915, 2001.
430. Mansel, J. K., Rosenow, E. C., III, Smith, T. F., et al.: *Mycoplasma pneumoniae* pneumonia. Chest *95*:639–646, 1989.

431. Marc, E., Chaussain, M., Moulin, F., et al.: Reduced lung diffusion capacity after *Mycoplasma pneumoniae* pneumonia. Pediatr. Infect. Dis. J. *19*:706–710, 2000.
432. Mårdh, P.-A.: Human respiratory tract infections with mycoplasmas and their in vitro susceptibility to tetracyclines and some other antibiotics. Chemotherapy *21*(Suppl. 1):27–57, 1975.
433. Mårdh, P.-A.: *Mycoplasma hominis* infection of the central nervous system in newborn infants. Sex. Transm. Dis. *10*:331–334, 1983.
434. Mårdh, P.-A., Nilsson, F. J., and Bjelle, A.: Mycoplasmas and bacteria in synovial fluid from patients with arthritis. Ann. Rheum. Dis. *32*:319–325, 1973.
435. Mårdh, P.-A., and Ursing, B.: The occurrence of acute pancreatitis in *Mycoplasma pneumoniae* infection. Scand. J. Infect. Dis. *6*:167–171, 1974.
436. Markham, J. G.: *Mycoplasma pneumoniae* infection in 1978. N. Z. Med. J. *90*:473–474, 1979.
437. Marmion, B. P., and Goodburn, G. M.: Effect of an organic gold salt on Eaton's primary atypical pneumonia agent and other observations. Nature *189*:247–248, 1961.
438. Marmion, B. P., Williamson, J., Worswick, D. A., et al.: Experience with newer techniques for the laboratory detection of *Mycoplasma pneumoniae* infection: Adelaide, 1978–1992. Clin. Infect. Dis. *17*(Suppl. 1):90–99, 1993.
439. Martelli, A.: Sulla reazione di fissazione del complemento per *Mycoplasma pneumoniae* nella diagnosi sierologica di affezioni respiratorie. G. Batteriol. Virol. Immunol. *65*:43–49, 1972.
440. Martin, E. R., Warr, G., Couch, R., et al.: Chemotaxis of human leukocytes: Responsiveness to *Mycoplasma pneumoniae.* J. Lab. Clin. Med. *81*:520–529, 1973.
441. Mattila, P. S., Carlson, P., Sivonen, A., et al.: Life-threatening *Mycoplasma hominis* mediastinitis. Clin. Infect. Dis. *29*:1529–1537, 1999.
442. McCormack, J. G.: *Mycoplasma pneumoniae* and the erythema multiforme Stevens-Johnson syndrome. J. Infect. *3*:32–36, 1981.
443. McCormack, W. M.: Common sexually transmitted diseases and their treatment. Bull. N. Y. Acad. Med. *54*:216–222, 1978.
444. McCormack, W. M.: Epidemiology of *Mycoplasma hominis.* Sex. Transm. Dis. *10*:261–262, 1983.
445. McCormack, W. M.: Susceptibility of mycoplasmas to antimicrobial agents: Clinical implications. Clin. Infect. Dis. *17*(Suppl. 1):200–201, 1993.
446. McCormack, W. M., Almeida, P. C., Bailey, P. E., et al.: Sexual activity and vaginal colonization with genital mycoplasmas. J. A. M. A. *221*:1375–1377, 1972.
447. McCormack, W. M., Braun, P., Lee, Y.-H., et al.: The genital mycoplasmas. N. Engl. J. Med. *288*:78–89, 1973.
448. McCormack, W. M., Lee, Y.-H., and Zinner, S. H.: Sexual experience and urethral colonization with genital mycoplasmas. Ann. Intern. Med. *78*:696–698, 1973.
449. McCormack, W. M., Rosner, B., Alpert, S., et al.: Vaginal colonization with *Mycoplasma hominis* and *Ureaplasma urealyticum.* Sex. Transm. Dis. *13*:67–70, 1986.
450. McCormack, W. M., Rosner, B., and Lee, Y.-H.: Colonization with genital mycoplasmas in women. Am. J. Epidemiol. *97*:240–245, 1973.
451. McDonald, J. C., and Moore, D. L.: *Mycoplasma hominis* meningitis in a premature infant. Pediatr. Infect. Dis. *7*:795–798, 1988.
452. McDonald, M. I., Lam, M. H., Birch, D. F., et al.: *Ureaplasma urealyticum* in patients with acute symptoms of urinary tract infection. J. Urol. *128*:517–519, 1982.
453. McIntosh, J. C., and Gutierrez, H. H.: Mycoplasmal infections: Epidemiology, immunology, diagnostic techniques, and therapeutic strategies. Immunol. Allergy Clin. North Am. *13*:43–57, 1993.
454. McNamara, M. J., Phillips, I. A., and Williams, O. B.: Viral and *Mycoplasma pneumoniae* infections in exacerbations of chronic lung disease. Am. Rev. Respir. Dis. *100*:19–24, 1969.
455. Meis, J. F., van Kuppeveld, F. J., Kremer, J. A., et al.: Fatal intrauterine infection associated with *Mycoplasma hominis.* Clin. Infect. Dis. *15*:753–754, 1992.
456. Metzgar, D. P., Woodhour, A. F., Vella, P. P., et al.: Respiratory virus vaccines. II. *Mycoplasma pneumoniae* (Eaton agent) vaccines. Am. Rev. Respir. Dis. *94*:1–9, 1966.
457. Meyers, B. R., and Hirschman, S. Z.: Fatal infections associated with *Mycoplasma pneumoniae:* Discussion of three cases with necropsy findings. Mt. Sinai J. Med. *39*:258–264, 1972.
458. Miller, T. C., Baman, S. I., and Albers, W. H.: Massive pericardial effusion due to *Mycoplasma hominis* in a newborn. Am. J. Dis. Child. *136*:271–272, 1982.
459. Mills, R. W., and Schoolfield, L.: Acute transverse myelitis associated with *Mycoplasma pneumoniae* infection: A case report and review of the literature. Pediatr. Infect. Dis. J. *11*:228–231, 1992.
460. Miranda, C., Carazo, C., Bañón, R., et al.: *Mycoplasma hominis* infection in three renal transplant patients. Diagn. Microbiol. Infect. Dis. *13*:329–331, 1990.
461. Mizutani, H., and Mizutani, H.: Immunologic responses in patients with *Mycoplasma pneumoniae* infections. Am. Rev. Respir. Dis. *127*:175–179, 1983.
462. Mizutani, H., and Mizutani, H.: Circulating immune complexes in patients with mycoplasmal pneumonia. Am. Rev. Respir. Dis. *130*:627–629, 1984.
463. Moffet, H. L., Siegel, A. C., and Doyle, H. K.: Nonstreptococcal pharyngitis. J. Pediatr. *73*:51–60, 1968.
464. Mogabgab, W. J.: *Mycoplasma pneumoniae* and adenovirus respiratory illnesses in military and university personnel, 1959–1966. Am. Rev. Respir. Dis. *97*:345–358, 1968.
465. Mogabgab, W. J.: Beta-hemolytic streptococcal and concurrent infections in adults and children with respiratory disease, 1958 to 1969. Am. Rev. Respir. Dis. *102*:23–34, 1970.
466. Mogabgab, W. J.: Protective efficacy of killed *Mycoplasma pneumoniae* vaccine measured in large-scale studies in a military population. Am. Rev. Respir. Dis. *108*:899–908, 1973.
467. Mohiuddin, A. A., Corren, J., Harbeck, R. J., et al.: *Ureaplasma urealyticum* chronic osteomyelitis in a patient with hypogammaglobulinemia. J. Allergy Clin. Immunol. *87*:104–107, 1991.
468. Mok, J. Y., Waugh, P. R., and Simpson, H.: *Mycoplasma pneumoniae* infection: A follow-up study of 50 children with respiratory illness. Arch. Dis. Child. *54*:506–511, 1979.
469. Montagnier, L., and Blanchard, A.: Mycoplasmas as cofactors in infection due to the human immunodeficiency virus. Clin. Infect. Dis. *17*(Suppl. 1):309–315, 1993.
470. Monto, A. S., Bryan, E. R., and Rhodes, L. M.: The Tecumseh study of respiratory illnesses. VII. Further observations on the occurrence of respiratory syncytial virus and *Mycoplasma pneumoniae* infections. Am. J. Epidemiol. *100*:458–468, 1975.
471. Monto, A. S., and Lim, S. K.: The Tecumseh study of respiratory illness. III. Incidence and periodicity of respiratory syncytial virus and *Mycoplasma pneumoniae* infections. Am. J. Epidemiol. *94*:290–301, 1971.
472. Moore, P., and Martland, T.: *Mycoplasma pneumoniae* infection mimicking acute rheumatic fever. Pediatr. Infect. Dis. J. *13*:81–82, 1994.
473. Morowitz, H. J., and Wallace, D. C.: Genome size and life cycle of the mycoplasma. Ann. N. Y. Acad. Sci. *225*:62–73, 1973.
474. Moskal, M. J., Kaylarian, V. H., and Doro, J. M.: Psychosis complicating *Mycoplasma pneumoniae* infection. Pediatr. Infect. Dis. *3*:63–66, 1984.
475. Moule, J. H., Caul, E. O., and Wreghitt, T. G.: The specific IgM response to *Mycoplasma pneumoniae* infection: Interpretation and application to early diagnosis. Epidemiol. Infect. *99*:685–692, 1987.
476. Mufson, M. A., Ludwig, W. M., Purcell, R. H., et al.: Exudative pharyngitis following experimental *Mycoplasma hominis* type 1 infection. J. A. M. A. *192*:1146–1152, 1965.
477. Mufson, M. A., Manko, M. A., Kingston, J. R., et al.: Eaton agent pneumonia: Clinical features. J. A. M. A. *178*:369–374, 1961.
478. Mufson, M. A., Sanders, V., Wood, S. C., et al.: Primary atypical pneumonia due to *Mycoplasma pneumoniae* (Eaton agent): Report of a case with a residual pleural abnormality. N. Engl. J. Med. *268*:1109–1111, 1963.
479. Murphy, W. H., Bullis, C., Dabich, L., et al.: Isolation of *Mycoplasma* from leukemic and nonleukemic patients. J. Natl. Cancer Inst. *45*:243–251, 1970.
480. Murray, H. W., Masur, H., Senterfit, L. B., et al.: The protean manifestations of *Mycoplasma pneumoniae* infection in adults. Am. J. Med. *58*:229–242, 1975.
481. Muse, K. E., Powell, D. A., and Collier, A. M.: *Mycoplasma pneumoniae* in hamster tracheal organ culture studied by scanning electron microscopy. Infect. Immun. *13*:229–237, 1976.
482. Nadal, D., Bossart, W., Zucol, F., et al.: Community-acquired pneumonia in children due to *Mycoplasma pneumoniae*: Diagnostic performance of a seminested 16S rDNA-PCR. Diagn. Microbiol. Infect. Dis. *39*:15–19, 2001.
483. Naftalin, J. M., Wellisch, G., Kahana, Z., et al.: *Mycoplasma pneumoniae* septicemia. J. A. M. A. *228*:565, 1974.
484. Nagayama, Y., Sakurai, N., Tamai, K., et al.: Isolation of *Mycoplasma pneumoniae* from pleural fluid and/or cerebrospinal fluid: Report of four cases. Scand. J. Infect. Dis. *19*:521–524, 1987.
485. Nagayama, Y., Sakurai, N., Yamamoto, K., et al.: Isolation of *Mycoplasma pneumoniae* from children with lower respiratory tract infections. J. Infect. Dis. *157*:911–917, 1988.
486. Nakao, T., Orii, T., and Umetsu, M.: *Mycoplasma pneumoniae* pneumonia with pleural effusion, with special reference to isolation of *Mycoplasma pneumoniae* from pleural fluid. Tohoku J. Exp. Med. *104*:13–18, 1971.
487. Nakao, T., Umetsu, M., Watanabe, N., et al.: An outbreak of *Mycoplasma pneumoniae* infection in a community. Tohoku J. Exp. Med. *102*:23–31, 1970.
488. Nakayama, T., Sonoda, S., Urano, T., et al.: Interferon production during the course of *Mycoplasma pneumoniae* infection. Pediatr. Infect. Dis. J. *11*:72–77, 1992.
489. Nakayama, T., Urano, T., Osano, M., et al.: Alpha interferon in the sera of patients infected with *Mycoplasma pneumoniae.* J. Infect. Dis. *154*:904–906, 1986.
490. Naraqi, S., and Kabins, S. A.: *Mycoplasma pneumoniae* monoarticular arthritis. J. Pediatr. *83*:621–623, 1973.

491. Narita, M., Itakura, O., Matsuzono, Y., et al.: Analysis of mycoplasmal central nervous system involvement by polymerase chain reaction. Pediatr. Infect. Dis. J. *14*:236–237, 1995.
492. Narita, M., Matsuzono, Y., Itakura, O., et al.: Survey of mycoplasmal bacteremia detected in children by polymerase chain reaction. Clin. Infect. Dis. *23*:522–525, 1996.
493. Narita, M., Matsuzono, Y., Itakura, O., et al.: Analysis of mycoplasmal pleural effusion by the polymerase chain reaction. Arch. Dis. Child. *78*:67–69, 1998.
494. Narita, M., Yamada, T., Nakayama, T., et al.: Two cases of lymphadenopathy with liver dysfunction due to *Mycoplasma pneumoniae* infection with mycoplasmal bacteraemia without pneumonia. J. Infect. *42*:154–156, 2001.
495. Nastro, J. A., Littner, M. R., Tashkin, D. P., et al.: Diffuse, pulmonary, interstitial infiltrate and mycoplasmal pneumonia. Am. Rev. Respir. Dis. *110*:659–662, 1974.
496. Neimark, H. C.: Division of mycoplasmas into subgroups. J. Gen. Microbiol. *63*:249–263, 1970.
497. Neu, H. C., and Ellner, P. D.: Role of *Mycoplasma* in exudative pharyngitis. N. Y. State J. Med. *69*:3026–3028, 1969.
498. News and Notes: Epidemiology: *Mycoplasma pneumoniae* 1977. B. M. J. *1*:726, 1978.
499. Niitu, Y., Hasegawa, S., Suetake, T., et al.: Resistance of *Mycoplasma pneumoniae* to erythromycin and other antibiotics. J. Pediatr. *76*:438–443, 1970.
500. Nishioka, K., Fujimoto, M., Date, R., et al.: Bilateral sensorineural deafness associated with *Mycoplasma pneumoniae* infection: The first case report. Hiroshima J. Med. Sci. *33*:585–589, 1984.
501. Nissen, M., McEniery, J., Delbridge, G., et al.: Acute hypertrophic cardiomyopathy possibly associated with *Mycoplasma pneumoniae* infection. Pediatr. Infect. Dis. J. *14*:74–75, 1995.
502. Noah, N. D.: *Mycoplasma pneumoniae* infection in the United Kingdom: 1967–73. B. M. J. *1*:544–546, 1974.
503. Nocard, E., and Roux, E. R.: Le microbe de la pleuro-pneumoniae. Ann. Inst. Pasteur (Paris) *12*:240–262, 1898.
504. Noriega, E. R., Simberkoff, M. S., Gilroy, F. J., et al.: Life-threatening *Mycoplasma pneumoniae* pneumonia. J. A. M. A. *229*:1471–1472, 1974.
505. Novelli, V. M., and Marshall, W. C.: Optic disc swelling and *Mycoplasma pneumoniae*. Pediatr. Infect. Dis. *3*:597, 1985.
506. Novelli, V. M., Matthew, D. J., and Dinwiddie, R. D.: Acute fulminant toxic encephalopathy associated with *Mycoplasma pneumoniae* infection. Pediatr. Infect. Dis. *4*:413–415, 1985.
507. Oderda, G., and Kraut, J. R.: Rising antibody titer to *Mycoplasma pneumoniae* in acute pancreatitis. Pediatrics *66*:305–306, 1980.
508. Oermann, C., Sockrider, M. M., and Langston, C.: Severe necrotizing pneumonitis in a child with *Mycoplasma pneumoniae* infection. Pediatr. Pulmonol. *24*:61–65, 1997.
509. Ohlsson, A., Wang, E., and Vearncombe, M.: Leukocyte counts and colonization with *Ureaplasma urealyticum* in preterm neonates. Clin. Infect. Dis. *17*(Suppl. 1):144–147, 1993.
510. Ollikainen, J.: Perinatal *Ureaplasma urealyticum* infection increases the need for hospital treatment during the first year of life in preterm infants. Pediatr. Pulmonol. *30*:402–405, 2000.
511. Ollikainen, J., Heiskanen-Kosma, T., Korppi, M., et al.: Clinical relevance of *Ureaplasma urealyticum* colonization in preterm infants. Acta Paediatr. *87*:1075–1078, 1998.
512. Ollikainen, J., Hiekkaniemi, H., Korppi, M., et al.: *Ureaplasma urealyticum* cultured from brain tissue of preterm twins who died of intraventricular hemorrhage. Scand. J. Infect. Dis. *25*:529–531, 1993.
513. Ollikainen, J., Hiekkaniemi, H., Korppi, M., et al.: *Ureaplasma urealyticum* infection associated with acute respiratory insufficiency and death in premature infants. J. Pediatr. *122*:756–760, 1993.
514. Olson, L. D., and Gilbert, A. A.: Characteristics of *Mycoplasma hominis* adhesion. J. Bacteriol. *175*:3224–3227, 1993.
515. Ong, E. L. C., Ellis, M. E., and Yuill, G. M.: Neurological complication of *Mycoplasma pneumoniae* infection. Respir. Med. *83*:441–442, 1989.
516. Oriel, J. D.: Treatment of nongonococcal urethritis. *In* Hobson, D., and Holmes, K. K. (eds.): Nongonococcal Urethritis and Related Infections. Washington, D.C., American Society for Microbiology, 1977, pp. 38–42.
517. Oriel, J. D., Ridgway, G. L., Reeve, P., et al.: The lack of effect of ampicillin plus probenecid given for genital infections with *Neisseria gonorrhoeae* on associated infections with *Chlamydia trachomatis*. J. Infect. Dis. *133*:568–571, 1976.
518. Paavonen, J., Miettinen, A., Stevens, C. E., et al.: *Mycoplasma hominis* in nonspecific vaginitis. Sex. Transm. Dis. *10*:271–275, 1983.
519. Paavonen, J., Miettinen, A., Stevens, C. E., et al.: *Mycoplasma hominis* in cervicitis and endometritis. Sex. Transm. Dis. *10*:276–280, 1983.
520. Pacifico, L., Panero, A., Roggini, M., et al.: *Ureaplasma urealyticum* and pulmonary outcome in a neonatal intensive care population. Pediatr. Infect. Dis. J. *16*:579–586, 1997.
521. Panero, A., Pacifico, L., Rossi, N., et al.: Elevated white blood cell counts associated with *Ureaplasma urealyticum* colonization in preterm neonates. Clin. Infect. Dis. *19*:980–981, 1994.
522. Panero, A., Pacifico, L., Rossi, N., et al.: *Ureaplasma urealyticum* as a cause of pneumonia in preterm infants: Analysis of the white cell response. Arch. Dis. Child. *73*:F37–F40, 1995.
523. Papaevangelou, V., Falaina, V., Syriopoulou, V., et al.: Bell's palsy associated with *Mycoplasma pneumoniae* infection. Pediatr. Infect. Dis. J. *18*:1024–1026, 1999.
524. Parker, F., Jolliffe, L. S., and Finland, M.: Primary atypical pneumonia: Report of eight cases with autopsies. Arch. Pathol. *44*:581–608, 1947.
525. Parker, P., Puck, J., and Fernandez, F.: Cerebral infarction associated with *Mycoplasma pneumoniae*. Pediatrics *67*:373–375, 1981.
526. Parrott, R. H.: Viral respiratory tract illnesses in children. Bull. N. Y. Acad. Med. *39*:629–648, 1963.
527. Patterson, A. M., Taciak, V., Lovchik, J., et al.: *Ureaplasma urealyticum* respiratory tract colonization is associated with an increase in interleukin 1-beta and tumor necrosis factor alpha relative to interleukin 6 in tracheal aspirates of preterm infants. Pediatr. Infect. Dis. J. *17*:321–328, 1998.
528. Paul, V. K., Gupta, U., Singh, M., et al.: Association of genital mycoplasma colonization with low birth weight. Int. J. Gynaecol. Obstet. *63*:109–114, 1998.
529. Payne, N. R., Steinberg, S. S., Ackerman, P., et al.: New prospective studies of the association of *Ureaplasma urealyticum* colonization and chronic lung disease. Clin. Infect. Dis. *17*(Suppl. 1):117–121, 1993.
530. Perez, C., Gurtubay, I., Martinez-Ibañez, F., et al.: More on polymyositis associated with *Mycoplasma pneumoniae* infection. Scand. J. Rheumatol. *28*:125, 1999.
531. Perez, C., Mendoza, H., Hernandez, R., et al.: Leukocytoclastic vasculitis and polyarthritis associated with *Mycoplasma pneumoniae* infection. Clin. Infect. Dis. *25*:154–155, 1997.
532. Perez, C. R., and Leigh, M. W.: *Mycoplasma pneumoniae* as the causative agent for pneumonia in the immunocompromised host. Chest *100*:860–861, 1991.
533. Perzigian, R. W., Adams, J. T., Weiner, G. M., et al.: *Ureaplasma urealyticum* and chronic lung disease in very low birth weight infants during the exogenous surfactant era. Pediatr. Infect. Dis. J. *17*:620–625, 1998.
534. Poggio, T. V., Orlando, N., Galanternik, L., et al.: Microbiology of acute arthropathies among children in Argentina: *Mycoplasma pneumoniae* and *hominis* and *Ureaplasma urealyticum*. Pediatr. Infect. Dis. J. *17*:304–308, 1998.
535. Pollack, J. D., Somerson, N. L., and Senterfit, L. B.: Isolation, characterization, and immunogenicity of *Mycoplasma pneumoniae* membranes. Infect. Immun. *2*:326–329, 1970.
536. Pönkä, A.: The occurrence and clinical picture of serologically verified *Mycoplasma pneumoniae* infections with emphasis on central nervous system, cardiac and joint manifestations. Ann. Clin. Res. *11*(Suppl. 24):1–60, 1979.
537. Pönkä, A.: Arthritis associated with *Mycoplasma pneumoniae* infection. Scand. J. Rheumatol. *8*:27–32, 1979.
538. Pönkä, A.: Carditis associated with *Mycoplasma pneumoniae* infection. Acta Med. Scand. *206*:77–86, 1979.
539. Pönkä, A.: Central nervous system manifestations associated with serologically verified *Mycoplasma pneumoniae* infection. Scand. J. Infect. Dis. *12*:175–184, 1980.
540. Powell, D. A., Hu, P. C., Wilson, M., et al.: Attachment of *Mycoplasma pneumoniae* to respiratory epithelium. Infect. Immun. *13*:959–966, 1976.
541. Powell, D. A., Miller, K., and Clyde, W. A., Jr.: Submandibular adenitis in a newborn, caused by *Mycoplasma hominis*. Pediatrics *63*:798–799, 1979.
542. Puéchal, X., Hilliquin, P., Renoux, M., et al.: *Ureaplasma urealyticum* destructive septic polyarthritis revealing a common variable immunodeficiency. Arthritis Rheum. *38*:1524–1526, 1995.
543. Purcell, R. H., and Chanock, R. M.: Mycoplasmas of human origin. *In* Lennette, E. H. (ed.): Diagnostic Procedures for Viral and Rickettsial Infections. New York, American Public Health Association, 1969, pp. 786–825.
544. Putman, C. E., Baumgarten, A., and Gee, J. B. L.: The prevalence of mycoplasmal complement-fixing antibodies in sarcoidosis. Am. Rev. Respir. Dis. *111*:364–365, 1975.
545. Putman, C. E., Curtis, A. M., Simeone, J. F., et al.: *Mycoplasma* pneumonia: Clinical and roentgenographic patterns. A. J. R. Am. J. Roentgenol. *124*:417–422, 1975.
546. Quinn, P. A., Gillan, J. E., Markestad, T., et al.: Intrauterine infection with *Ureaplasma urealyticum* as a cause of fatal neonatal pneumonia. Pediatr. Infect. Dis. *4*:538–543, 1985.
547. Radestock, U., and Bredt, W.: Motility of *Mycoplasma pneumoniae*. J. Bacteriol. *129*:1495–1501, 1977.
548. Radisic, M., Torn, A., Gutierrez, P., et al.: Severe acute lung injury caused by *Mycoplasma pneumoniae:* Potential role for steroid pulses in treatment. Clin. Infect. Dis. *31*:1507–1511, 2000.
549. Rastawicki, W., and Jagielski, M.: Enzyme-linked immunosorbent assay, complement fixation test and immunoelectroprecipitation test in the diagnosis of *Mycoplasma pneumoniae* infections: Comparative analysis. Zentralbl. Bakteriol. *283*:477–484, 1996.

550. Räty, R., and Kleemola, M.: Detection of *Mycoplasma pneumoniae* by polymerase chain reaction in middle ear fluids from infants with acute otitis media. Pediatr. Infect. Dis. J. *19*:666–668, 2000.
551. Razin, S., and Jacobs, E.: *Mycoplasma* adhesion. J. Gen. Microbiol. *138*:407–422, 1992.
552. Razin, S., Yogev, D., and Naot, Y.: Molecular biology and pathogenicity of mycoplasmas. Microbiol. Mol. Biol. Rev. *62*:1094–1156, 1998.
553. Renner, E. D., Helms, C. M., Hall, N. H., et al.: Seroreactivity to *Mycoplasma pneumoniae* and *Legionella pneumophila:* Lack of a statistically significant relationship. J. Clin. Microbiol. *13*:1096–1098, 1981.
554. Renner, E. D., Helms, C. M., Johnson, W., et al.: Coinfections of *Mycoplasma pneumoniae* and *Legionella pneumophila* with influenza A virus. J. Clin. Microbiol. *17*:146–148, 1983.
555. Reichert-Penetrat, S., Barbaud, A., Antunes, A., et al.: An unusual form of Stevens-Johnson syndrome with subcorneal pustules associated with *Mycoplasma pneumoniae* infection. Pediatr. Dermatol. *17*:202–204, 2000.
556. Reznikov, M., Blackmore, T. K., Finlay-Jones, J. J., et al.: Comparison of nasopharyngeal aspirates and throat swab specimens in a polymerase chain reaction–based test for *Mycoplasma pneumoniae*. Eur. J. Clin. Microbiol. Infect. Dis. *14*:58–62, 1995.
557. Rifkind, D., Chanock, R., Kravetz, H., et al.: Ear involvement (myringitis) and primary atypical pneumonia following inoculation of volunteers with Eaton agent. Am. Rev. Respir. Dis. *85*:479–489, 1962.
558. Roberts, J. E., and Isaacs, D.: Neurological and pulmonary complications of *Mycoplasma pneumoniae* infection in a preschool child. J. Infect. *12*:251–252, 1986.
559. Robertson, J., Gonersall, M., and Gill, P.: *Mycoplasma hominis:* Growth, reproduction, and isolation of small viable cells. J. Bacteriol. *124*:1007–1018, 1975.
560. Robertson, J. A., and Stemke, G. W.: Expanded serotyping scheme for *Ureaplasma urealyticum* strains isolated from humans. J. Clin. Microbiol. *5*:873–878, 1982.
561. Roberts-Thomson, I. C., Cottew, G. S., and Fraser, J. R. E.: *Mycoplasma* pneumonia with severe haemolytic anaemia. Med. J. Aust. *2*:1046–1047, 1973.
562. Roifman, C. M., Rao, C. P., Lederman, H. M., et al.: Increased susceptibility to *Mycoplasma* infection in patients with hypogammaglobulinemia. Am. J. Med. *80*:590–594, 1986.
563. Romano, N., Romano, F., and Carollo, F.: T-strains of *Mycoplasma* in bronchopneumonic lungs of an aborted fetus. N. Engl. J. Med. *285*:950–952, 1971.
564. Romero, R., Mazor, M., Oyarzun, E., et al.: Is genital colonization with *Mycoplasma hominis* or *Ureaplasma urealyticum* associated with prematurity/low birth weight? Obstet. Gynecol. *73*:532, 1989.
565. Ross, J. M., Furr, P. M., Taylor-Robinson, D., et al.: The effect of genital mycoplasmas on human fetal growth. Br. J. Obstet. Gynecol. *88*:749–755, 1981.
566. Rothstein, T. L., and Kenny, G. E.: Cranial neuropathy, myeloradiculopathy, and myositis: Complications of *Mycoplasma pneumoniae* infection. Arch. Neurol. *36*:476–477, 1979.
567. Ruhrmann, G., and Holthusen, W.: *Mycoplasma* infection and erythromycin therapy in childhood. Scott. Med. J. *22*:401–403, 1977.
568. Ruiter, M., and Wentholt, H. M. M.: A pleuropneumonia-like organism in primary fusospirochetal gangrene of the penis. J. Invest. Dermatol. *15*:301–304, 1950.
569. Rykner, G., Bonnafous, J., and Manigand, G.: Sérologie des infections B *Mycoplasma pneumoniae* par le test d'inhibition metabolique. Semin. Hop. Paris *47*:1498, 1970.
570. Sabato, A. R., Martin, A. J., Marmion, B. P., et al.: *Mycoplasma pneumoniae:* Acute illness, antibiotics, and subsequent pulmonary function. Arch. Dis. Child. *59*:1034–1037, 1984.
571. Sacker, I., Walker, M., and Brunell, P. A.: Abscess in newborn infants caused by mycoplasma. Pediatrics *46*:303–304, 1970.
572. Sakoulas, G.: Brainstem and striatal encephalitis complicating *Mycoplasma pneumoniae* pneumonia: Possible benefit of intravenous immunoglobulin. Pediatr. Infect. Dis. J. *20*:543–545, 2001.
573. Saliba, G. S., Glezen, W. P., and Chin, T. D. Y.: *Mycoplasma pneumoniae* infection in a resident boys' home. Am. J. Epidemiol. *86*:408–418, 1967.
574. Salzman, M. B., Sood, S. K., Slavin, M. L., et al.: Ocular manifestations of *Mycoplasma pneumoniae* infection. Clin. Infect. Dis. *14*:1137–1139, 1992.
575. Sanchez, P. J., and Regan, J. A.: *Ureaplasma urealyticum* colonization and chronic lung disease in low birth weight infants. Pediatr. Infect. Dis. J. 7:542–546, 1988.
576. Sande, M. A., Gadot, F., and Wenzel, R. P.: Point source epidemic of *Mycoplasma pneumoniae* infection in a prosthodontics laboratory. Am. Rev. Respir. Dis. *112*:213–217, 1975.
577. Sanders, D. Y., and Johnson, H. W.: Stevens-Johnson syndrome associated with *Mycoplasma pneumoniae* infection. Am. J. Dis. Child. *121*:243–245, 1971.
578. Sands, M. J., Jr., Satz, J. E., Turner, W. E., Jr., et al.: Pericarditis and perimyocarditis associated with active *Mycoplasma pneumoniae* infection. Ann. Intern. Med. *86*:544–548, 1977.
579. Sasaki, T., Bonissol, C., and Stoiljkovic, B.: Cross-reactive antibodies to mycoplasmas found in human sera by the enzyme-linked immunosorbent assay (ELISA). Microbiol. Immunol. *31*:521–530, 1987.
580. Sasaki, Y., Honda, M., Naitou, M., et al.: Detection of *Mycoplasma fermentans* DNA from lymph nodes of acquired immunodeficiency syndrome patients. Microb. Pathog. *17*:131–135, 1994.
581. Savolainen, S., Jousimies-Somer, H., Kleemola, M., et al.: Serological evidence of viral or *Mycoplasma pneumoniae* infection in acute maxillary sinusitis. Eur. J. Clin. Microbiol. Infect. Dis. *8*:131–135, 1989.
582. Schachter, J., Hanna, L., Hill, E. C., et al.: Are chlamydial infections the most prevalent venereal disease? J. A. M. A. *231*:1252–1255, 1975.
583. Schamberger, M. S., Goel, J., Braddock, S. R., et al.: Stevens-Johnson syndrome and respiratory failure in a 9-year-old boy. South. Med. J. *90*:755–757, 1997.
584. Schmidt, N. J., Lennette, E. H., Dennis, J., et al.: On the nature of complement-fixing antibodies to *Mycoplasma pneumoniae.* J. Immunol. *97*:95–99, 1966.
585. Schmitz, R. C.: Primary atypical pneumonia of unknown cause. Arch. Intern. Med. *75*:222–232, 1945.
586. Schönwald, S., Barsic, B., Klinar, I., et al.: Three-day azithromycin compared with ten-day roxithromycin treatment of atypical pneumonia. Scand. J. Infect. Dis. *26*:706–710, 1994.
587. Schulman, P., Piemonte, T. C., and Singh, B.: Acute renal failure, hemolytic anemia, and *Mycoplasma pneumoniae.* J. A. M. A. *244*:1823–1824, 1980.
588. Sequeira, W., Jones, E., and Bronson, D. M.: *Mycoplasma pneumoniae* infection with arthritis and a varicella-like eruption. J. A. M. A. *246*:1936–1937, 1981.
589. Shames, J. M., George, R. B., Holliday, W. B., et al.: Comparison of antibiotics in the treatment of mycoplasmal pneumonia. Arch. Intern. Med. *125*:680–684, 1970.
590. Sharma, S., Brousseau, R., and Kasatiya, S.: Detection and confirmation of *Mycoplasma pneumoniae* in urogenital specimens by PCR. J. Clin. Microbiol. *36*:277–280, 1998.
591. Shawn, D. H., Quinn, P. A., Prober, C., et al.: Recurrent urethritis associated with *Ureaplasma urealyticum* in a prepubertal boy. Pediatr. Infect. Dis. J. *6*:687–688, 1987.
592. Shepard, M. C.: The recovery of pleuropneumonia-like organisms from Negro men with and without nongonococcal urethritis. Am. J. Syph. *38*:113–124, 1954.
593. Shepard, M. C., and Lunceford, C. D.: Differential agar medium (A7) for identification of *Ureaplasma urealyticum* (human T mycoplasmas) in primary cultures of clinical material. J. Clin. Microbiol. *3*:613–625, 1976.
594. Shepard, M. C., Lunceford, C. D., Ford, D. K., et al.: *Ureaplasma urealyticum* gen. nov. sp. nov.: Proposed nomenclature for the human T (T-strain) mycoplasmas. Int. J. Syst. Bacteriol. *24*:160–171, 1974.
595. Shepard, M. C., and Masover, G. K.: Special features of ureaplasmas. *In* Barile, M. F., and Razins, S. (eds.): The Mycoplasmas. Vol. I. New York, Academic Press, 1979, pp. 451–494.
596. Sheth, R. D., Goulden, K. J., and Pryse-Phillips, W. E.: The focal encephalopathies associated with *Mycoplasma pneumoniae.* Can. J. Neurol. Sci. *20*:319–323, 1993.
597. Shimada, M., Kotani, T., Sameshima, H., et al.: Two patients with premature labour associated with *Mycoplasma hominis* infection. J. Med. Microbiol. *47*:179–182, 1998.
598. Shulman, S. T., Bartlett, J., Clyde, W. A., Jr., et al.: The unusual severity of mycoplasmal pneumonia in children with sickle-cell disease. N. Engl. J. Med. *287*:164–167, 1972.
599. Shurin, P. A., Alpert, S. Rosner, B., et al.: Chorioamnionitis and colonization of the newborn infant with genital mycoplasmas. N. Engl. J. Med. *293*:5–8, 1975.
600. Sieber, O. F., John, T. J., Fulginiti, V. A., et al.: Stevens-Johnson syndrome associated with *Mycoplasma pneumoniae* infection. J. A. M. A. *200*:79–81, 1967.
601. Siegler, D. I. M.: Lung abscess associated with *Mycoplasma pneumoniae* infection. Br. J. Dis. Chest *67*:123–127, 1973.
602. Sillis, M.: The limitations of IgM assays in the serological diagnosis of *Mycoplasma pneumoniae* infections. J. Med. Microbiol. *33*:253–258, 1990.
603. Simmons, B. P., and Aber, R. C.: *Mycoplasma pneumoniae* pneumonia: Symptoms mimicking pulmonary embolism with infarction. J. A. M. A. *241*:1268–1269, 1979.
604. Simonian, N., and Janner, D.: Pleural effusion, hepatitis and hemolytic anemia in a twelve-year-old male child. Pediatr. Infect. Dis. J. *17*:173–174, 1998.
605. Singer, J. I., and DeVoe, W. M.: Severe *Mycoplasma pneumoniae* infection in otherwise healthy siblings. J. Pediatr. *95*:999–1001, 1979.
606. Skoldenberg, B.: Aseptic meningitis and meningoencephalitis in cold-agglutinin–positive infections. B. M. J. *1*:100–102, 1965.
607. Slotkin, R. I., Clyde, W. A., Jr., and Denny, R. W.: The effect of antibiotics on *Mycoplasma pneumoniae* in vitro and in vivo. Am. J. Epidemiol. *86*:225–237, 1967.
608. Smiley, D. F., Showacre, E., Lee, W., et al.: Acute interstitial pneumonitis: A new disease entity. J. A. M. A. *112*:1901, 1939.

609. Smith, C. B., Friedewald, W. T., and Chanock, R. M.: Inactivated *Mycoplasma pneumoniae* vaccine: Evaluation in volunteers. J. A. M. A. *199*:353–358, 1967.
610. Smith, C. B., Friedewald, W. T., and Chanock, R. M.: Shedding of *Mycoplasma pneumoniae* after tetracycline and erythromycin therapy. N. Engl. J. Med. *276*:1172–1175, 1967.
611. Smith, C. B., Golden, C. A., Kanner, R. E., et al.: Association of viral and *Mycoplasma pneumoniae* infections with acute respiratory illness in patients with chronic obstructive pulmonary disease. Am. Rev. Respir. Dis. *121*:225–232, 1980.
612. Smith, C. B., McGinniss, M. H., and Schmidt, P. J.: Changes in erythrocyte I agglutinogen and anti-I agglutinins during *Mycoplasma pneumoniae* infection in man. J. Immunol. *99*:333–339, 1967.
613. Smith, T. F.: *Mycoplasma pneumoniae* infections: Diagnosis based on immunofluorescence titer of IgG and IgM antibodies. Mayo Clin. Proc. *61*:830–831, 1986.
614. Sobeslavsky, O., Prescott, B., and Chanock, R. M.: Adsorption of *Mycoplasma pneumoniae* to neuraminic acid receptors of various cells and possible role in virulence. J. Bacteriol. *96*:695–705, 1968.
615. Sobeslavsky, O., Syrucek, L., Bruckova, M., et al.: The etiological role of *Mycoplasma pneumoniae* in otitis media in children. Pediatrics *35*:652–657, 1965.
616. Socan, M., Ravnik, I., Bencina, D., et al.: Neurological symptoms in patients whose cerebrospinal fluid is culture- and/or polymerase chain reaction–positive for *Mycoplasma pneumoniae*. Clin. Infect. Dis. *32*:E31–E35, 2001.
617. Sohaeverbeke, T., Gilroy, C. B., Bébéar, C., et al.: *Mycoplasma fermentans* in joints of patients with rheumatoid arthritis and other joint disorders. Lancet *347*:1418, 1996.
618. Solanki, K. L., and Berdoff, R. L.: Severe mycoplasma pneumonia with pleural effusions in a patient with sickle cell–hemoglobin C (SC) disease: Case report and review of the literature. Am. J. Med. *66*:707–710, 1979.
619. Somerson, N. L., and Cole, B. C.: The *Mycoplasma* flora of human and nonhuman primates. *In* Tully, J. G., and Whitcomb, R. F. (eds.): The Mycoplasmas. Vol. II. New York, Academic Press, 1979, pp. 191–216.
620. Souweine, B., Mathevon, T., Bret, L., et al.: Successful treatment of infection due to *Mycoplasma hominis* with streptogramins in a renal transplant patient: Case report and review. Clin. Infect. Dis. *26*:1233–1234, 1998.
621. Sprinkle, P. M.: Current status of Mycoplasmatales and bacterial variants in chronic otolaryngologic disease. Laryngoscope *82*:737–747, 1972.
622. Stadel, B. V., Foy, H. M., Nuckolls, J. W., et al.: *Mycoplasma pneumoniae* infection followed by *Haemophilus influenzae* pneumonia and bacteremia. Am. Rev. Respir. Dis. *112*:131–133, 1975.
623. Stagno, S., Brasfield, D. M., Brown, M. B., et al.: Infant pneumonitis associated with cytomegalovirus, *Chlamydia, Pneumocystis,* and *Ureaplasma:* A prospective study. Pediatrics *68*:322–329, 1981.
624. Stahelin-Massik, J., Levy, F., Friderich, P., et al.: Meningitis caused by *Ureaplasma urealyticum* in a full term neonate. Pediatr. Infect. Dis. J. *13*:419–421, 1994.
625. Stallings, M. W., and Archer, S. B.: Atypical *Mycoplasma* pneumonia. Am. J. Dis. Child. *126*:837–838, 1973.
626. Stallman, N. D., and Allan, B. C.: A survey of antibodies to *Mycoplasma pneumoniae* in Queensland. Med. J. Aust. *1*:800–802, 1970.
627. Stallman, N. D., Allan, B. C., and Wiemers, M. A.: Infection with *Mycoplasma pneumoniae:* Clinical and serological data on 286 patients. Med. J. Aust. *1*:340–343, 1976.
628. Stamm, W. E., Running, K., Hale, J., et al.: Etiologic role of *Mycoplasma hominis* and *Ureaplasma urealyticum* in women with the acute urethral syndrome. Sex. Transm. Dis. *10*:318–322, 1983.
629. Stancombe, B. B., Walsh, W. F., Derdak, S., et al.: Induction of human neonatal pulmonary fibroblast cytokines by hyperoxia and *Ureaplasma urealyticum.* Clin. Infect. Dis. *17*(Suppl. 1):154–157, 1993.
630. Steele, J. C., Gladstone, R. M., Thanasophon, S., et al.: *Mycoplasma pneumoniae* as a determinant of the Guillain-Barré syndrome. Lancet *2*:710–714, 1969.
631. Steinberg, P., White, R. J., Fuld, S. L., et al.: Ecology of *Mycoplasma pneumoniae* infections in marine recruits at Parris Island, South Carolina. Am. J. Epidemiol. *89*:62–73, 1969.
632. Sterner, G., DeHevesy, G., Tunevall, G., et al.: Acute respiratory illness with *Mycoplasma pneumoniae:* An outbreak in a home for children. Acta Paediatr. Scand. *55*:280–286, 1966.
633. Stevens, D., Swift, P. G. F., Johnston, P. G. B., et al.: *Mycoplasma pneumoniae* infections in children. Arch. Dis. Child. *53*:38–42, 1978.
634. Stevens, M. K., and Krause, D. C.: Disulfide-linked protein associated with *Mycoplasma pneumoniae* cytadherence phase variation. Infect. Immun. *58*:3430–3433, 1990.
635. Stewart, S. M., Burnet, M. E., and Young, J. E.: In vitro sensitivity of strains of mycoplasmas from human sources to antibiotics and to sodium aurothiomalate and tylosin tartrate. J. Med. Microbiol. *2*:287–292, 1969.
636. Stray-Pedersen, B., Bruu, A. L., and Molne, K.: Infertility and uterine colonization with *Ureaplasma urealyticum.* Acta Obstet. Gynecol. Scand. *61*:21–24, 1982.
637. Stutman, H. R.: Stevens-Johnson syndrome and *Mycoplasma pneumoniae:* Evidence for cutaneous infection. J. Pediatr. *111*:845–847, 1987.
638. Suhs, R. H., and Feldman, H. A.: Serologic epidemiologic studies with *M. pneumoniae.* II. Prevalence of antibodies in several populations. Am. J. Epidemiol. *83*:357–365, 1966.
639. Sussman, S. J., Magoffin, R. L., Lennette, E. H., et al.: Cold agglutinins, Eaton agent, and respiratory infections of children. Pediatrics *38*:571–577, 1966.
640. Syrogiannopoulos, G. A., Kapatais-Zoumbos, K., Decavalas, G. O., et al.: *Ureaplasma urealyticum* colonization of full term infants: Perinatal acquisition and persistence during early infancy. Pediatr. Infect. Dis. J. *9*:236–240, 1990.
641. Szymanski, M., Petric, M., Saunders, F. E., et al.: *Mycoplasma pneumoniae* pericarditis demonstrated by polymerase chain reaction and electron microscopy. Clin. Infect. Dis. *34*:E16–E17, 2002.
642. Tablan, O. C., and Reyes, M. P.: Chronic interstitial pulmonary fibrosis following *Mycoplasma pneumoniae* pneumonia. Am. J. Med. *79*:268–270, 1985.
643. Talkington, D. F., Thacker, W. L., Keller, D. W., et al.: Diagnosis of *Mycoplasma pneumoniae* infection in autopsy and open-lung biopsy tissues by nested PCR. J. Clin. Microbiol. *36*:1151–1153, 1998.
644. Tanowitz, H. B., Robbins, N., and Leidich, N.: Hemolytic anemia: Associated with severe *Mycoplasma pneumoniae* pneumonia. N. Y. State J. Med. *78*:2231–2232, 1978.
645. Taylor, G., Taylor-Robinson, D., and Fernald, G. W.: Reduction in the severity of *Mycoplasma pneumoniae*–induced pneumonia in hamsters by immunosuppressive treatment with antithymocyte sera. J. Med. Microbiol. *7*:343–348, 1974.
646. Taylor, M. J., Burrow, G. N., Strauch, B., et al.: Meningoencephalitis associated with pneumonitis due to *Mycoplasma pneumoniae.* J. A. M. A. *199*:813–816, 1967.
647. Taylor-Robinson, D.: Mycoplasmas of various hosts and their antibiotic sensitivities. Postgrad. Med. J. *43*(Suppl.):100–104, 1967.
648. Taylor-Robinson, D.: The biology of mycoplasmas: Symposium on acute respiratory diseases. J. Clin. Pathol. *21*(Suppl. 2):38–51, 1968.
649. Taylor-Robinson, D.: *Mycoplasma* infections of the human urogenital tract with particular reference to nongonococcal urethritis. Ann. Microbiol. *135A*:129–134, 1984.
650. Taylor-Robinson, D.: Genital *Mycoplasma* infections. Clin. Lab. Med. *9*:501–523, 1989.
651. Taylor-Robinson, D.: The Mycoplasmatales: *Mycoplasma, Ureaplasma, Acholeplasma, Spiroplasma* and *Anaeroplasma. In* Parker, M. T., and Duerden, B. I. (eds.): Principles of Bacteriology, Virology and Immunity. Vol. 2. Systemic Bacteriology. Philadelphia, B. C. Decker, 1990, pp. 664–681.
652. Taylor-Robinson, D., and Cherry, J. D.: A nonpathogenic mycoplasma inhibiting the effect of a pathogenic mycoplasma in organ culture. J. Med. Microbiol. *5*:291–298, 1972.
653. Taylor-Robinson, D., and Furr, P. M.: The distribution of T-mycoplasmas within and among various animal species. Ann. N. Y. Acad. Sci. *225*:108–117, 1973.
654. Taylor-Robinson, D., Gilroy, C. B., and Hay, P. E.: Occurrence of *Mycoplasma genitalium* in different populations and its clinical significance. Clin. Infect. Dis. *17*(Suppl. 1):66–68, 1993.
655. Taylor-Robinson, D., and McCormack, W. M.: The genital mycoplasmas. N. Engl. J. Med. *302*:1003–1010, 1063–1067, 1980.
656. Taylor-Robinson, D., Shirai, A., Sobeslavsky, O., et al.: Serologic response to *Mycoplasma pneumoniae* infection. II. Significance of antibody measured by different techniques. Am. J. Epidemiol. *84*:301–313, 1966.
657. Taylor-Robinson, D., Tully, J. G., Furr, P. M., et al.: Urogenital *Mycoplasma* infections of man: A review with observations on a recently discovered *Mycoplasma.* Isr. J. Med. Sci. *17*:524–530, 1981.
658. Teisch, J. A., Shapiro, L., and Walzer, R. A.: Vesiculopustular eruption with *Mycoplasma* infection. J. A. M. A. *211*:1694–1697, 1970.
659. Thacker, W. L., and Talkington, D. F.: Comparison of two rapid commercial tests with complement fixation for serologic diagnosis of *Mycoplasma pneumoniae* infections. J. Clin. Microbiol. *33*:1212–1214, 1995.
660. Thacker, W. L., and Talkington, D. F.: Analysis of complement fixation and commercial enzyme immunoassays for detection of antibodies to *Mycoplasma pneumoniae* in human serum. Clin. Diagn. Lab. Immunol. *7*:778–780, 2000.
661. Thomas, M., Jones, M., and Ray, S.: *Mycoplasma pneumoniae* in a tubo-ovarian abscess. Lancet *2*:774–775, 1975.
662. Thomsen, A. C.: Occurrence and pathogenicity of *Mycoplasma hominis* in the upper urinary tract: A review. Sex. Transm. Dis. *10*:323–326, 1983.
663. Tilton, R. C., Dias, F., Kidd, H., et al.: DNA probe versus culture for detection of *Mycoplasma pneumoniae* in clinical specimens. Diagn. Microbiol. Infect. Dis. *10*:109–112, 1988.
664. Tipirneni, P., Moore, B. S., Hyde, J. S., et al.: IgE antibodies to *Mycoplasma pneumoniae* in asthma and other atopic diseases. Ann. Allergy *45*:1–7, 1980.
665. Tjhie, J. H., Van de Putte, E. M., Haasnoot, K., et al.: Fatal encephalitis caused by *Mycoplasma pneumoniae* in a 9-year-old girl. Scand. J. Infect. Dis. *29*:424–425, 1997.

666. Toth, A., Lesser, M. L., Brooks, C., et al.: Subsequent pregnancies among 161 couples treated for T-*Mycoplasma* genital-tract infection. N. Engl. J. Med. *308*:505–508, 1983.
667. Tully, J. G.: Biology of the mycoplasmas. *In* McGarrity, G. J., Murphy, D. G., and Nichols, W. W. (eds.): *Mycoplasma* Infection of Cell Cultures. New York, Plenum, 1978, pp. 1–33.
668. Tully, J. G.: *Mycoplasma* flora of humans. Personal communication. Dec. 1, 1991.
669. Tully, J. G.: Current status of the mollicute flora of humans. Clin. Infect. Dis. *17*(Suppl. 1):2–9, 1993.
670. Tully, J. G., Rose, D. L., Baseman, J. B., et al.: *Mycoplasma pneumoniae* and *Mycoplasma genitalium* mixture in synovial fluid isolate. J. Clin. Microbiol. *33*:1851–1855, 1995.
671. Tully, J. G., Rose, D. L., Whitcomb, R. F., et al.: Enhanced isolation of *Mycoplasma pneumoniae* from throat washings with a newly modified culture medium. J. Infect. Dis. *139*:478–482, 1979.
672. Tully, J. G., Taylor-Robinson, D., Rose, D. L., et al.: *Mycoplasma genitalium,* a new species from the human urogenital tract. Int. J. Syst. Bacteriol. *33*:387–396, 1983.
673. Tully, J. G., Taylor-Robinson, D., Rose, D. L., et al.: Urogenital challenge of primate species with *Mycoplasma genitalium* and characteristics of infection induced in chimpanzees. J. Infect. Dis. *153*:1046–1054, 1986.
674. Turner, J. A. P., Burchak, E. C., Bannatyne, R. M., et al.: The protean manifestations of *Mycoplasma* infections in childhood. Can. Med. Assoc. J. *99*:633–637, 1968.
675. Twomey, J. A., and Espir, M. L. E.: Neurological manifestations and *Mycoplasma pneumoniae* infection. B. M. J. *2*:832–833, 1979.
676. Uldum, S. A., Jensen, J. S., Søndergård-Andersen, J., et al.: Enzyme immunoassay for detection of immunoglobulin M (IgM) and IgG antibodies to *Mycoplasma pneumoniae.* J. Clin. Microbiol. *30*:1198–1204, 1992.
677. Ursi, D., Ursi, J.-P., Ieven, M., et al.: Congenital pneumonia due to *Mycoplasma pneumoniae.* Arch. Dis. Child. *72*:F118–F120, 1995.
678. Valencia, G. B., Banzon, F., Cummings, M., et al.: *Mycoplasma hominis* and *Ureaplasma urealyticum* in neonates with suspected infection. Pediatr. Infect. Dis. J. *12*:571–573, 1993.
679. Van Bever, H. P., Van Doorn, J. W. D., and Demey, H. E.: Adult respiratory distress syndrome associated with *Mycoplasma pneumoniae* infection. Eur. J. Pediatr. *151*:227–228, 1992.
680. Van der Veen, J., and Van Nunen, C. J.: Role of *Mycoplasma pneumoniae* in acute respiratory disease in a military population. Am. J. Hyg. *78*:293–301, 1963.
681. Van Kuppeveld, F. J., Johansson, K. E., Galama, J. M., et al.: 16S rRNA based polymerase chain reaction compared with culture and serological methods for diagnosis of *Mycoplasma pneumoniae* infection. Eur. J. Clin. Microbiol. Infect. Dis. *13*:401–405, 1994.
682. Villiger, R. M., von Vigier, R. O., Ramelli, G. P., et al.: Precipitants in 42 cases of erythema multiforme. Eur. J. Pediatr. *158*:929–932, 1999.
683. Vincent, J. M., Cherry, J. D., Nauschuetz, W. F., et al.: Prolonged afebrile nonproductive cough illnesses in American soldiers in Korea: A serological search for causation. Clin. Infect. Dis. *30*:534–539, 2000.
684. Vogel, U., Lüneberg, E., Kuse, E.-R., et al.: Extragenital *Mycoplasma hominis* infection in two liver transplant recipients. Clin. Infect. Dis. *24*:512–513, 1997.
685. Volk, J., and Kraus, S. J.: Nongonococcal urethritis: A venereal disease as prevalent as epidemic gonorrhea. Arch. Intern. Med. *134*:511–514, 1974.
686. Vu, A. C., Foy, H. M., Cartwright, F. D., et al.: The principal protein antigens of isolates of *Mycoplasma pneumoniae* as measured by levels of immunoglobulin G in human serum are stable in strains collected over a 10-year period. Infect. Immun. *55*:1830–1836, 1987.
687. Vulliemin, J. F.: Nongonococcal urethritis: Therapeutic considerations. Curr. Ther. Res. *26*:719–725, 1979.
688. Waites, K. B., Brown, M. B., Stagno, S., et al.: Association of genital mycoplasmas with exudative vaginitis in a 10-year-old: A case of misdiagnosis. Pediatrics *71*:250–252, 1983.
689. Waites, K. B., Crouse, D. T., and Cassell, G. H.: Systemic neonatal infection due to *Ureaplasma urealyticum.* Clin. Infect. Dis. *17*(Suppl. 1):131–135, 1993.
690. Waites, K. B., Crouse, D. T., and Cassell, G. H.: Therapeutic considerations for *Ureaplasma urealyticum* infections in neonates. Clin. Infect. Dis. *17*(Suppl. 1):208–214, 1993.
691. Waites, K. B., Crouse, D. T., Philips, J. B., III, et al.: Ureaplasmal pneumonia and sepsis associated with persistent pulmonary hypertension of the newborn. Pediatrics *83*:79–85, 1989.
692. Waites, K. B., Duffy, L. B., Baldus, K., et al.: Mycoplasmal infections of cerebrospinal fluid in children undergoing neurosurgery for hydrocephalus. Pediatr. Infect. Dis. J. *10*:952–953, 1991.
693. Waites, K. B., Duffy, L. B., Crouse, D. T., et al.: Mycoplasmal infections of cerebrospinal fluid in newborn infants from a community hospital population. Pediatr. Infect. Dis. J. *9*:241–245, 1990.
694. Waites, K. B., Rudd, P. T., Crouse, D. T., et al.: Chronic *Ureaplasma urealyticum* and *Mycoplasma hominis* infections of central nervous system in preterm infants. Lancet *1*:17–21, 1988.
695. Waites, K. B., Sims, P. J., Crouse, D. T., et al.: Serum concentrations of erythromycin after intravenous infusion in preterm neonates treated for *Ureaplasma urealyticum* infection. Pediatr. Infect. Dis. J. *13*:287–293, 1994.
696. Wang, E. E. L., Cassell, G. H., Sanchez, P. J., et al.: *Ureaplasma urealyticum* and chronic lung disease of prematurity: Critical appraisal of the literature on causation. Clin. Infect. Dis. *17*(Suppl. 1):112–116, 1993.
697. Wang, E. E. L., Frayha, H., Watts, J., et al.: Role of *Ureaplasma urealyticum* and other pathogens in the development of chronic lung disease of prematurity. Pediatr. Infect. Dis. J. *7*:547–551, 1988.
698. Wang, E. E. L., Ohlsson, A., and Kellner, J. D.: Association of *Ureaplasma urealyticum* colonization with chronic lung disease of prematurity: Results of a metaanalysis. J. Pediatr. *127*:640–644, 1995.
699. Wang, R. Y. H., Shih, J. W. K., Grandinetti, T., et al.: High frequency of antibodies to *Mycoplasma penetrans* in HIV-infected patients. Lancet *340*:1312–1316, 1992.
700. Wang, R. Y. H., Shih, J. W. K., Weiss, S. H., et al.: *Mycoplasma penetrans* infection in male homosexuals with AIDS: High seroprevalence and association with Kaposi's sarcoma. Clin. Infect. Dis. *17*:724–729, 1993.
701. Waris, M. E., Toikka, P., Saarinen, T., et al.: Diagnosis of *Mycoplasma pneumoniae* pneumonia in children. J. Clin. Microbiol. *36*:3155–3159, 1998.
702. Warren, P., Fischbein, C., Mascoli, N., et al.: Poliomyelitis-like syndrome caused by *Mycoplasma pneumoniae.* J. Pediatr. *93*:451–452, 1978.
703. Watanabe, T., Shibata, K., Yoshikawa, T., et al.: Detection of *Mycoplasma salivarium* and *Mycoplasma fermentans* in synovial fluids of temporomandibular joints of patients with disorders in the joints. F. E. M. S. Immunol. Med. Microbiol. *22*:241–246, 1998.
704. Watson, H. L., Blalock, D. K., and Cassell, G. H.: Variable antigens of *Ureaplasma urealyticum* containing both serovar-specific and serovar-cross-reactive epitopes. Infect. Immun. *58*:3679–3688, 1990.
705. Weinstein, M. P., and Hall, C. B.: *Mycoplasma pneumoniae* infections associated with migratory polyarthritis. Am. J. Dis. Child. *127*:125–126, 1974.
706. Wenzel, R. P., Craven, R. B., Davies, J. A., et al.: Protective efficacy of an inactivated *Mycoplasma pneumoniae* vaccine. J. Infect. Dis. *136*(Suppl.):204–207, 1977.
707. Westerberg, S. C., Smith, C. B., and Renzetti, A. D.: *Mycoplasma* infections in patients with chronic obstructive pulmonary disease. J. Infect. Dis. *127*:491–497, 1973.
708. Westernfelder, G. O., Akey, T., Corwin, S. J., et al.: Acute transverse myelitis due to *Mycoplasma pneumoniae* infection. Arch. Neurol. *38*:317–318, 1981.
709. Westrom, L., and March, P. A.: The effect of antibiotic therapy on *Mycoplasma* in the female genital tract: In vitro and in vivo studies on the sensitivity of *Mycoplasma hominis* and T-mycoplasmas to tetracyclines and other antibiotics. Acta Obstet. Gynecol. Scand. *50*:25–31, 1971.
710. Whitescarver, J., and Furness, G.: T-mycoplasmas: A study of the morphology, ultrastructure and mode of division of some human strains. J. Med. Microbiol. *8*:349–355, 1975.
711. Williams, M. H., Brostoff, J., and Roitt, I. M.: Possible role of *Mycoplasma fermentans* in pathogenesis of rheumatoid arthritis. Lancet *2*:277–280, 1970.
712. Williamson, J., Marmion, B. P., Kok, T., et al.: Confirmation of fatal *Mycoplasma pneumoniae* infection by polymerase chain reaction detection of the adhesin gene in fixed lung tissue. J. Infect. Dis. *170*:1052–1053, 1994.
713. Wilson, M. H., and Collier, A. M.: Ultrastructural study of *Mycoplasma pneumoniae* in organ culture. J. Bacteriol. *125*:332–339, 1976.
714. Yechouron, A., Lefebvre, J., and Robson, H. G.: Fatal septicemia due to *Mycoplasma arginini:* A new human zoonosis. Clin. Infect. Dis. *15*:434–438, 1992.
715. Yoon, B. H., Chang, J. W., and Romero, R.: Isolation of *Ureaplasma urealyticum* from the amniotic cavity and adverse outcome in preterm labor. Obstet. Gynecol. *92*:77–82, 1998.
716. Zheng, X., Olson, D. A., Tully, J. G., et al.: Isolation of *Mycoplasma hominis* from a brain abscess. J. Clin. Microbiol. *35*:992–994, 1997.
717. Zinserling, A.: Peculiarities of lesions in viral and *Mycoplasma* infections of the respiratory tract. Virchows Arch. Pathol. Anat. *356*:259–273, 1972.

SECTION XXI

Fungal Diseases

CHAPTER 197 Classification of Fungi

DEXTER H. HOWARD ■ HEIDI M. KOKKINOS

The medically important fungi are contained in a biologic kingdom called Fungi.[8] These organisms are divided into two groups on the basis of their basic growth pattern: yeasts and molds. Yeasts are unicellular fungi that reproduce by budding or by fission. Molds are multicellular fungi that grow by means of filamentous threads called *hyphae.* On the hyphae are developed reproductive propagules.[2, 3]

Fungi may reproduce sexually or asexually. The sexual form of growth is called the teleomorph, and the asexual form is called the anamorph.* The sexual means of reproduction forms the basis of the taxonomy of fungi. Each of the products of meiosis that result from sexual reproduction is housed in specialized structures called sexual spores. Among medically important fungi, the three types of sexual spores are zygospores, ascospores, and basidiospores, so named to indicate their particular method of formation.[2, 3, 8] The phyla of medically important fungi within the kingdom Fungi (along with the type of sexual spore formed by members of those phyla) are (1) Zygomycota (zygospores), (2) Ascomycota (ascospores), and (3) Basidiomycota (basidiospores). In addition, another group that is not taxonomically referred to as a phylum contains fungi that do not produce sexual spores. The group is referred to as the Mitosporic Fungi or Fungi Imperfecti.

A group of microorganisms with flagellated asexual spores usually are considered to be fungi.[1] These forms now are contained within three biologic kingdoms: Fungi, Straminipila, and Protoctista. The motile forms in the kingdom Fungi (phylum Chytridiomycota) and in the kingdom Protoctista do not contain human pathogens. One rare human pathogen exists in the kingdom Straminipila: *Pythium insidiosum*. Because of the limited involvement in human disease, the taxonomy of the kingdom Straminipila is not included in this coverage.

The taxonomic scheme depicted is based on various sources,[1, 4, 7, 8, 9] and the original draft of the scheme was published recently.[7]

The basic taxonomic units are the species, and they are grouped into a hierarchical system that includes genera, families, orders, classes, and phyla. The categories may be subdivided (e.g., subphylum, subclass, suborder) to indicate degrees of relationship. Populations within a given species that have some characteristics in common may be set apart as tribes or varieties or some other subset designation. Delineation of the zoopathogen *Ajellomyces capsulatum*, the teleomorph of *Histoplasma capsulatum*, is as follows:

- Kingdom: Fungi
  - Phylum: Ascomycota
    - Class: Ascomycetes
      - Order: Onygenales
        - Family: Onygenaceae
          - Genus: *Ajellomyces*
            - Species: *Ajellomyces capsulatum* (anamorph: *Histoplasma capsulatum)*
              - Variety: The varietal state applies to the anamorph (2): *H. capsulatum* var. *capsulatum, H. capsulatum* var. *duboisii*, and *H. capsulatum* var. *farciminosum*

This consideration includes *only* those taxa known to contain medically important species. Classes, orders, and families not known to contain such pathogens are omitted. More detailed considerations can be obtained by consulting the references indicated.

- Kingdom: Fungi
  - Phylum: Zygomycota: the teleomorph consists of zygospores; the anamorph consists of sporangiospores within a sporangium.
    - Class: Zygomycetes
      - Order: Mucorales
        - Family: Mucoraceae. Agents of mucormycosis are found in this family.
          - Genera: *Apophysomyces, Absidia, Mucor, Rhizomucor, Rhizopus*
        - Family: Cunninghamellaceae
          - Genus: *Cunninghamella*
        - Family: Mortierellaceae
          - Genus: *Mortierella*
        - Family: Saksenaeaceae
          - Genus: *Saksenaea*
        - Family: Syncephalastraceae
          - Genus: *Syncephalastrum*
        - Family: Thamnidiaceae
          - Genus: *Cokeromyces*
      - Order: Entomophthorales—agents of entomophthoromycoses
        - Family: Basidiobolaceae
          - Genus: *Basidiobolus*
        - Family: Ancylistaceae
          - Genus: *Conidiobolus*
  - Phylum: Ascomycota: the teleomorph consists of ascospores borne in an ascus; the anamorph may be unicellular yeasts or multicellular molds. Molecular

*Of note is that teleomorphs and anamorphs have different names, although they are the same fungus; for example, *Filobasidiella neoformans* (teleomorph) and *Cryptococcus neoformans* (anamorph). By common agreement, the anamorph name is the one used in reports from a clinical microbiology laboratory.

phylogeny studies have allowed associations to be realized even when a known teleomorph for a given anamorph has not been revealed. These associations are suggested throughout.

Class: Endomycetes—yeasts (unicellular fungi)
- Order: Saccharomycetales—ascomata absent. Asci formed singly or in chains. Anamorphs: yeast cells that divide by budding or fission
  - Genera: Teleomorphs of *Candida, Geotrichum,* etc.

Class: Ascomycetes—molds. The coverage given here is abbreviated. For a more complete consideration, see elsewhere[4, 9]
- Order: Onygenales. Ascomata are cleistothecia.
  - Family: Arthrodermataceae—agents of tinea (ringworm)
    - Genus: *Arthroderma* (anamorphs *Microsporum, Trichophyton*). The genus *Epidermophyton* is related closely, but no teleomorph has yet been described
  - Family: Onygenaceae—agents of endemic pulmonary mycoses
    - Genus: *Ajellomyces* (anamorphs: *Histoplasma, Blastomyces*, and *Emmonsia*). The asexual genera *Coccidioides* and *Paracoccidioides* are related closely, but no teleomorph has yet been discovered.
- Order: Eurotiales (ascomata are cleistothecia)
  - Family: Trichocomaceae (contains the greatest number of human pathogens and is the only one included here). Agents of aspergillosis, penicilliosis, and related types of infections
    - Genera: Teleomorphs of the anamorphs *Aspergillus* and *Penicillium*. Another familiar anamorph pathogen, *Paecilomyces,* has no teleomorph.
- Order: Ophiostomatales (ascomata are perithecia with long necks)
  - Family: Ophiostomataceae
    - Genus: *Ophiostoma* (anamorph: *Sporothrix*). The agent of sporotrichosis, *S. schenckii*, is related closely to *Ophiostoma.*
- Order: Hypocreales (ascomata mostly perithecia)
  - Family: Hypocreaceae—agents of a wide diversity of mycoses
    - Genera: Teleomorphs of *Fusarium* spp. Other related anamorphs without a teleomorph include *Acremonium, Trichoderma,* and *Verticillium.*
- Order: Microascales (ascomata cleistothecia or perithecia)
  - Family: Microascaceae
    - Genera: *Pseudallescheria* (anamorph: *Scedosporium*), *Microascus* (anamorph: *Scopulariopsis*)
- Order: Sordariales (ascomata cleistothecia or perithecia). Rare human pathogens. Details are not included.
- Order: Dothidiales (ascomata are cleistothecia). Some disagreement about the family contents of this order remains. The synthesis herein is derived from other publications[4, 7, 9]
  - Family: Didymosphaeriaceae
    - Genus: *Neotestudina* (no anamorph)—agent of mycetoma
  - Family: Piedraiaceae
    - Genus: *Piedraia* (no anamorph)—cause of black piedra
  - Family: Herpotrichiellaceae—mainly agents of phaeohyphomycoses and chromoblastomycoses
    - Genera: Human pathogens are manifested only as anamorphs, for example, *Phialophora, Rhinocladiella, Cladophialophora, Exophiala, Fonsecaea.*
- Order: Pleosporales
  - Family: Pleosporaceae
    - Genus: *Cochliobolus* (anamorphs: *Curvularia* and *Bipolaris*)

Phylum: Basidiomycota—the teleomorph is a basidium bearing basidiospores; anamorphs are yeasts or molds. Arthroconidia are reproductive propagules of some of the molds.
- Class: Hymenomycetes
  - Order: Filobasidiales—agent of cryptococcosis
    - Genus: *Filobasidium* (anamorph: *Cryptococcus*)
  - Order: Trichosporonales—agent of trichosporonosis
    - Genus: *Trichosporon* (anamorph)
- Class: Ustilaginomycetes
  - Order: Malasseziales
    - Genus: *Malassezia*—agent of pityriasis versicolor
- Class: Urediniomycetes
  - Order: Sporidiales—species found in clinical materials
    - Genera: *Rhodotorula* and *Sporobolomyces*

MITOSPORIC FUNGI. Mitosporic Fungi, or the Fungi Imperfecti, are fungi with no known teleomorphs. Molecular techniques have allowed these anamorphic fungi to be related to teleomorphic groups, and these relationships have been indicated earlier. Nevertheless, a large number of pathogens exist for which no teleomorph is known, and gathering such forms into a separate category (i.e., the Mitosporic Fungi) is convenient for discussing them as a separate group. At one time, these anamorphic fungi were collected into a phylum, Deuteromycota, but this designation no longer is used commonly in medical mycology. Mitosporic Fungi are divided into subgroups but not given hierarchical names such as orders, families, and so on. The subgroups are Blastomycetes, Hyphomycetes, Coelomycetes, and Agonomycetes.

Blastomycetes. The subgroup Blastomycetes consists of unicellular fungi that reproduce by budding or fission. These yeasts do not have teleomorphs that have been recognized at this time, but they obviously are related to ascomycetes and basidiomycetes. These associations have been indicated in the foregoing scheme. Some representative genera of these yeasts are *Candida, Cryptococcus, Trichosporon,* and *Rhodotorula.*

Hyphomycetes. Hyphomycetes includes molds that produce asexual conidia. Moniliaceous forms have hyaline hyphae and conidia. As with the Blastomycetes, these forms have ascomycete or basidiomycete affinities. Sometimes it is expressed as a teleomorph. Examples have been given in the foregoing material, and some instances of closely related anamorphs for which a teleomorph has not yet been detected have been indicated. Representative genera of moniliaceous hyphomycetes are *Coccidioides, Aspergillus, Penicillium, Acremonium, Fusarium, Sporothrix*, and more. Dematiaceous forms have dark conidia and hyphae and are agents of chromoblastomycosis and phaeohyphomycosis. Genera of dematiaceous hyphomycetes include *Cladosporium, Bipolaris, Curvularia, Phialophora, Cladophialopora,* and others.

Coelomycetes. Coelomycetes includes molds that produce reproductive elements within pycnidia or on acervuli. They are agents of mycetoma and wound infection. Two representative genera are *Phoma* (pycnidium-forming) and *Colletotrichum* (acervulus-forming).

Agonomycetes (Mycelia Sterilia). This subgroup consists of molds that produce no reproductive propagules of any kind. One example is the genus *Rhizoctonia.*

Organisms of Uncertain Position. *Rhinosporidium seeberi* (rhinosporidiosis) and *Pneumocystis carinii* (pneumocystosis) are of uncertain taxonomic position. Rhinosporidiosis causes tumor-like masses, commonly in the nasal mucosa or on the conjunctiva of humans and animals.[8] The taxonomic position of *R. seeberi* always has been uncertain.[6] Recently, studies involving 18S rRNA genes from tissue infected with the fungus have shown a phylogenetic relationship to a novel group of protists that infect fish and amphibians. The fungus is "... the first known human pathogen from the DRIPs clade, a novel clade of aquatic protistan parasites (Icthyasporea)."[6]

P. carinii (recently also referred to as *Pneumocystis jiroveci*)[8a] originally was considered a protozoan, and most of the information about this important opportunistic pathogen is found in the literature on animal parasites. However, studies of ribosomal RNA sequences have established that *P. carinii* is a member of the kingdom Fungi.[5] The systematic position of *P. carinii* within the kingdom Fungi is uncertain, but the best evidence indicates that it is an ascomycete.[10]

Protothecosis is a rare cutaneous disease caused by *Prototheca* spp. The taxonomic position of these microorganisms is not established clearly, but they are thought to be achloric algae. Although they are not, therefore, considered to be fungi, they often are included in texts of medical mycology.[8]

REFERENCES

1. Alexopoulos, C. J., Mims, C. W., and Blackwell, M.: Introductory Mycology. 4th ed. New York, John Wiley & Sons, 1996.
2. Baron, E. J., Chang, R. S., Howard, D. H., et al.: Medical Microbiology: A Short Course. New York, Wiley-Liss, 1984.
3. Crissey, J. T., Lang, H., Parish, L. C.: Manual of Medical Mycology. Cambridge, Blackwell, 1995.
4. deHoog, G. S., and Guarro, J.: Atlas of Clinical Fungi. Baarn and Delft, The Netherlands, Centraalbureau voor Schimmelcultures, 2000.
5. Edman, J. C., Kovacs, J. A., Mansur, H., et al.: Ribosomal RNA sequence shows *Pneumocystis carinii* to be a member of the fungi. Nature *334*:519–522, 1988.
6. Fredricks, D. N., Jolly, J. A., Lepp, P. W., et al.: *Rhinosporidium seeberi*: A human pathogen from a novel group of aquatic protistan parasites. Emerg. Infect. Dis. 6:273–282, 2000.
7. Howard, D. H.: An introduction to the taxonomy of zoopathogenic fungi. *In* Howard, D. H. (ed.): Pathogenic Fungi of Humans and Animals. 2nd ed. New York, Marcel Dekker, 2003.
8. Kwon-Chung, K. J., Bennett, J. E.: Medical Mycology. Philadelphia, Lea & Febiger, 1992.

8a. Stringer, J. R., Beard, C. B., Miller, R. F., et al.: A new name (*Pneumocystis jiroveci*) for pneumocystis from humans. Emerging Int. Dis. *8*: 897–898, 2002.

9. Sutton, D. A., Fothergill, A. W., and Rinaldi, M. G.: Guide to Clinically Significant Fungi. Baltimore, Williams & Wilkins, 1998.
10. Taylor, J. W., Swann, E., and Berbee, M. L. Molecular evolution of ascomycete fungi. *In* Hawksworth, D. E. (ed.): Ascomycete Systematics: Problems and Perspectives in the Nineties. New York, Plenum, 1994.

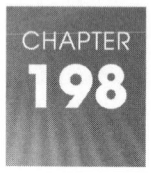

CHAPTER 198 *Aspergillus* Infections

MICHAEL D. BLUM ■ BERNHARD L. WIEDERMANN

The term *Aspergillus* (Latin *aspergere,* "to scatter"), first coined by the Florentine botanist Micheli[124] in his *Nova Plantarum Genera* of 1729, referred to the perforated globe, or aspergillum, used to sprinkle holy water during religious ceremonies. The human disease was described first by Sluyter[181] in 1847 and reviewed by Virchow[201] in his classic paper of 1856. In 1897, Renon[155] reported an association of the disease with certain occupations, such as wig cleaning and pigeon handling. However, not until 1952 were the diverse clinical manifestations of aspergillosis realized,[69] and only recently has the importance of *Aspergillus* infection in immunosuppressed patients been recognized. Systemic disseminated aspergillosis is a product of medical progress and a consequence of the widespread use of antibiotics and immunosuppressive agents in the modern age.

The genus *Aspergillus* includes more than 900 recognized species, only a small number of which have been documented to be pathogenic to the human host. *Aspergillus fumigatus* is the most common cause of human disease worldwide, and *Aspergillus flavus, Aspergillus nidulans, Aspergillus niger,* and *Aspergillus terreus* account for most of the remainder. However, many other species have been reported to cause illness in humans.[42, 154, 161] *Aspergillus* spp. all exhibit thermotolerance, which may enhance pathogenicity in the human host.[161]

Fungi in the genus *Aspergillus* reproduce by means of asexual spores called *conidia.* In tissue preparation of clinical specimens, conidiophores are usually absent. Specimens characteristically show dichotomously branching, septate hyphae, which are suggestive of, but not specific for, this genus. In culture, however, *Aspergillus* spp. are identified by their characteristic colony appearance and by microscopic examination of the conidia and spore-bearing structures. For example, the major pathogenic species, *A. fumigatus,* is characterized by smoky, gray-green colonies; compact, columnar conidia; and phialides, which cover the upper half of flask-shaped vesicles. The mycologic characteristics of other *Aspergillus* spp. and techniques for preparation of fungal material have been well described.[57, 161, 188]

Aspergillus spp. are known to produce a variety of mycotoxins in nonhuman hosts, including aflatoxin, ochratoxin, fungiclavine, and kojic acid. Although these toxins have not been isolated from an infected human host, several cases of acute aflatoxicosis have developed as a result of the consumption of contaminated food.[31] Many putative virulence factors produced by *Aspergillus* spp., particularly *A. fumigatus,* have been studied[42, 100] and ultimately may lead to novel approaches to therapy.

Epidemiology

Aspergillus spp. are ubiquitous worldwide and occur in a variety of natural substrates, including grain, decaying vegetation, soil, and dung.[180] *Aspergillus* is frequently isolated from the air because spores are lightweight, resistant to desiccation, and easily dispersed. The fungus can be recovered from sputum for several days after exposure to a cloud of *Aspergillus* conidia.[161]

Inhalation of spores combined with an immune response has been described in regular smokers of contaminated marijuana.[85] In addition, hospital outbreaks have been associated with airborne contamination secondary to bird droppings in air ducts,[99] road construction adjacent to hospital windows,[103] and hospital renovation.[215] Demolition of ducts and false ceilings close to a neonatal intensive care unit[95] and an adult hematology department[146] resulted in fatal pulmonary aspergillosis in immunocompromised patients. An outbreak of invasive aspergillosis in widely varying areas of one hospital was traced to construction activity in the central radiology suite.[70]

Control of such outbreaks has focused on removing immunosuppressed patients from construction sites, equipping rooms with high-efficiency air filters, and using laminar air flow isolation.[9] Phenotypic methods such as biotyping by the killer system have permitted tracking of nosocomial outbreaks of aspergillosis.[50] However, genotypic methods such as restriction fragment length polymorphism using random amplified polymorphic DNA probes[25] and polymerase chain reaction (PCR) amplification of intergenic spacer regions[152] provide better discrimination among isolates in the outbreak setting. The epidemiology of invasive aspergillosis was reviewed recently.[109, 197]

Pathogenesis

Phagocytic response, rather than production of antibodies, provides the primary host defense against *Aspergillus* infections. Because conidia are the inhaled particles that initiate infection, macrophages form the "front line" of defense by rapidly killing the fungus in the conidial stage. Neutrophils are involved only if the conidia escape the reticuloendothelial system and begin mycelial growth.[170]

Aspergillosis is a relatively uncommon occurrence in patients with acquired immunodeficiency syndrome (AIDS),[42, 84, 177] which implies a relative lack of importance of cell-mediated immunity in defense against this fungus. Invasive aspergillosis usually occurs in patients with advanced AIDS and has been considered to result from independent predisposing factors such as neutropenia, corticosteroid therapy, or intravenous drug use.[179] Human immunodeficiency virus (HIV)–infected children with age-adjusted $CD4^+$ lymphocyte counts less than 25 percent of the normal median for age have been shown to have significant defects in the ability of neutrophils to damage nonopsonized hyphae of *A. fumigatus*.[163] Moreover, HIV-infected children manifested significantly decreased phagocytic activity of peripheral blood monocyte-derived macrophages when compared with normal controls.[164] These host defects may account for the fact that, in some series of invasive aspergillosis in patients with AIDS,[105, 177] predisposing factors independent of HIV infection were present in no more than half of the cases.

Aspergillus accounts for the vast majority of fungal infections in patients with chronic granulomatous disease[32] and on occasion may account for an unusual manifestation of the disease.[173] The predisposition of patients with chronic granulomatous disease[214] or selective defects in phagocytic killing[52, 139] underscores the importance of oxidative killing in human host defense against this disease.

With more severe immunosuppression, invasive aspergillosis can ensue. Predisposing factors include (1) corticosteroid treatment, (2) neutropenia, (3) cytotoxic chemotherapy, (4) broad-spectrum antimicrobial therapy, (5) acute leukemia in relapse, and (6) acute organ rejection.[159] Newer treatments such as infliximab also may predispose to the development of aspergillosis.[213] In addition, invasive aspergillosis in children has been reported after influenza infection,[76, 104] subacute hepatic necrosis,[207] liver transplantation,[166] heart transplantation,[7] and bone marrow transplantation.[148, 202] Invasive aspergillosis occurs in 5 to 11 percent of patients after undergoing bone marrow transplantation[202] and has been associated with delayed engraftment,[129] graft-versus-host disease,[123] and graft rejection.[119] Although aspergillosis after autologous bone marrow transplantation usually occurs before engraftment, with allogeneic transplant it is more likely to occur after engraftment.[202] The attack rate of invasive aspergillosis has been reported to be higher in patients with organ transplants who previously had cytomegalovirus infection and in those requiring antirejection therapy.[67] Despite the absence of neutropenia, invasive aspergillosis was reported to occur in almost 2 percent of one large series of patients with liver transplants and has been associated with the use of OKT3.[98] Aspergillosis in children with cancer has been reviewed recently.[1, 61]

Rare cases of fulminant aspergillosis have been described in normal hosts.[59] Aspergillosis is an uncommon disease in the newborn period and usually is manifested as widely disseminated disease,[157] although primary cutaneous aspergillosis has been reported increasingly in premature infants.[60, 64] Predisposing factors for the development of aspergillosis in newborn infants include the use of broad-spectrum antibiotics or corticosteroids, prematurity, chronic granulomatous disease, and necrotizing enterocolitis.[60, 174]

In immunosuppressed patients, *Aspergillus* tends to invade blood vessels and results in infarction, necrosis, and widespread hematogenous dissemination. Examination of affected organs reveals numerous septate hyphae with dichotomous branching, as well as conidial heads when fungi are present in air-containing tissues.[116] In contrast, widespread dissemination secondary to vascular invasion seldom occurs in patients with chronic granulomatous disease, who typically have isolated pneumonia with or without contiguous spread.[32] The unusual finding of diffuse nodular pneumonia in childhood may provide a clue for the diagnosis of chronic granulomatous disease and aspergillosis.[30]

Allergic reactions to *Aspergillus* may play a role in the pathologic process of this disease, as evidenced by patients with allergic bronchopulmonary aspergillosis. In this condition, patients with chronic respiratory diseases such as asthma[158] and cystic fibrosis[107] trap *A. fumigatus* in tenacious mucus, which results in an immune response and exacerbation of respiratory symptoms. Despite the presence of numerous luminal hyphae in tissues, however, invasion of the bronchial wall and fungal dissemination have been reported rarely in the absence of other risk factors (e.g., indwelling catheters, hyperalimentation, corticosteroid therapy).[22, 29]

An immune response to trapped fungi also may result in allergic fungal sinusitis, a chronic disease that tends to occur in young adults with a history of atopy, asthma, or nasal polyposis. It is caused more commonly by dematiaceous fungi than by *Aspergillus*.[72] Patients often report expelling dark rubbery nasal casts of allergic mucin in which hyphal forms can be found. As many as 30 percent of patients with allergic *Aspergillus* sinusitis may exhibit expansion or bony erosion of the involved sinus; invasion, however, has not been reported.[65]

Clinical Manifestations

A variety of saprophytic and pathologic conditions have been attributed to *Aspergillus* spp. (Table 198–1). Invasiveness appears to depend on the genetic and immune status of the host, as well as the extent and duration of exposure to spores. Disseminated aspergillosis, defined as infection of two or more noncontiguous organs, is the most severe form of clinical aspergillosis. Patients usually have pulmonic disease and widespread organ involvement. The clinical features of invasive *Aspergillus* infection in a large pediatric hospital were reviewed recently.[204] The most common sites of *Aspergillus* infection in children are discussed in the following sections.

TABLE 198–1 ■ CLINICAL SPECTRUM OF ASPERGILLOSIS IN CHILDREN

Ear
- Otitis externa
- Invasive otitis externa

Paranasal sinuses
- Indolent sinus aspergillosis
- Aspergilloma
- Invasive sinus aspergillosis

Eye
- Traumatic keratitis
- Postoperative endophthalmitis
- Contiguous spread from paranasal sinuses

Lungs
- Primary pulmonary aspergillosis
- Hypersensitivity pneumonitis
- Allergic bronchopulmonary aspergillosis
- Mucoid impaction
- Eosinophilic pneumonitis
- Bronchocentric granulomatosis
- Extrinsic allergic alveolitis
- Aspergilloma
- Invasive pulmonary aspergillosis

Central nervous system
- Traumatic inoculation
- Contiguous spread from paranasal sinuses
- Disseminated disease

Bone
- Traumatic osteomyelitis
- Contiguous spread from lung or overlying skin

Skin and nails
- Onychomycosis
- Primary cutaneous aspergillosis
- Contiguous spread from paranasal sinuses
- Disseminated disease

Heart
- Postoperative endocarditis
- Isolated cardiac aspergillosis

Genitourinary tract
- Ascending infection
- Disseminated disease

Other
- Splenic aspergillomas
- Intraperitoneal aspergillosis

EAR AND SINUS

Otomycosis, defined as fungal infection of the external ear canal, more commonly occurs in tropical and subtropical regions and is particularly prevalent in groups that regularly cover their ears with traditional garb.[144] It is predominantly a unilateral disease caused by *Aspergillus* or *Candida* spp. and is found often in association with *Staphylococcus aureus, Pseudomonas, Proteus,* or other bacterial pathogens.[132] *Aspergillus* otomycosis, most commonly secondary to *A. niger*,[48] produces a mass of black spores that start close to the tympanic membrane and spread outward to fill the ear canal. Disease in immunosuppressed patients rarely results in invasive otitis externa,[149] but in general *Aspergillus* otomycosis is a localized, noninfiltrative process. Thorough removal of debris from the external canal and treatment directed against the underlying chronic otitis externa generally result in a good therapeutic response. Topical antifungal agents also have been successful.[144, 185]

Aspergillus is the most common fungal infection of the nose and paranasal sinuses. It may be manifested as an indolent case, aspergilloma, or fulminant disease. Indolent sinus aspergillosis may occur locally in the absence of predisposing factors, most commonly in warm, damp climates[8] or in association with dental disease or dental fillings.[101] Patients have the typical manifestations of chronic sinusitis, including rhinorrhea, nasal obstruction, and sinus fullness. Radiographic studies usually indicate opacification without evidence of bone erosion. Mucosal thickening with necrotic brownish-green material is noted commonly at surgery.[127] On occasion, patients with these symptoms have a mass (aspergilloma) in the maxillary or ethmoid sinuses. Local surgery with drainage usually results in complete resolution in these cases of noninvasive sinus aspergillosis.[185]

In contrast, invasive sinus aspergillosis, which generally occurs in immunosuppressed patients, may be fulminant, with early bone destruction, direct extension to the orbit and anterior cranial fossa, and widespread dissemination.[118] The most common initial symptoms are fever, periorbital swelling, and nasal congestion.[74] Infection usually progresses anteriorly; it spreads from the nose to the facial skin and leaves a path of blackened, necrotic tissue destruction. This progression contrasts with that of the yellow-black, necrotic ulcerations of intraoral aspergillosis, which usually spread from the soft palate posteriorly.[46]

Fulminant aspergillosis caused by primary infection of the paranasal sinuses occurs infrequently in children, generally in the setting of immunosuppression or neutropenia or after the administration of broad-spectrum antimicrobials.[13, 16] These children have facial pain, swelling, and erythema; nasal crusting or ulceration occurs less commonly. The mortality rate is high in this group of patients. Because granulocytopenia may mask the signs and symptoms of sinus aspergillosis, aggressive attempts to diagnose this condition with computed tomography (CT) and early biopsy are necessary to reduce the high mortality rate associated with this entity. Characteristic CT findings include unilateral involvement of several sinuses, normal sinus cells between completely opacified cells, absence of air-fluid levels, and smooth, thickened sinus linings. In contrast with orbital cellulitis, bone destruction may be evident, but periosteal separation from the medial orbital wall typically does not occur.[27]

Invasive *Aspergillus* sinusitis has been reported increasingly in bone marrow transplant[28, 167] and AIDS[121] patients. *Aspergillus* sinusitis was reported to occur in 4 percent of pediatric bone marrow transplant recipients in one series[28]; frequent careful anterior rhinoscopy was considered critical in diagnosing infection in this high-risk group.

EYE

Involvement of the orbit and its contents is manifested most commonly as orbital aspergillosis secondary to local extension from the sinuses,[223] traumatic keratitis,[140, 199] or postoperative endophthalmitis.[108] Mycotic keratitis occurs most frequently in developing countries with humid climates. Trauma is the most common predisposing factor, and *Aspergillus* has been reported to be the most frequently occurring fungal pathogen.[140] Corneal scraping for fungal culture is recommended to guide medical or surgical treatment.

Aspergillus endophthalmitis is typically characterized by the rapid onset of pain and severe visual loss, often with a confluent yellowish macular infiltrate on ophthalmoscopy.[218] A case of *Aspergillus* endophthalmitis without any detectable cause has been described in an immunologically normal 1-month-old infant.[178] Rarely, patients with disseminated disease[40] or an occult focus of *Aspergillus* infection[184] present with endophthalmitis. In postmortem studies, approximately 8 percent of patients with disseminated *Aspergillus* infection had evidence of ocular involvement.[117] Bilateral retinal infarction secondary to disseminated disease has been reported in a 10-month-old infant.[81]

LUNG

Pulmonary involvement occurs in approximately 90 percent of *Aspergillus* infections, and in 70 percent, it is the only site of infection[38] (Fig. 198–1). It is the most common site of invasive *Aspergillus* disease. Noninvasive pulmonary aspergillosis includes primary pulmonary aspergillosis, hypersensitivity reactions, and aspergilloma.

Noninvasive Pulmonary Aspergillosis

Primary pulmonary aspergillosis is believed to occur in normal hosts without preexisting disease, although the existence of this entity has been questioned.[38] This rare disease, usually caused by the inhalation of massive amounts of *A. fumigatus,* may be chronic and indolent or, on occasion, fulminant and fatal. Chest radiographs may show a variety of diffuse or localized cavitary or infiltrative processes.

The symptoms of allergic bronchopulmonary aspergillosis result from a host immune response to the fungus, which becomes trapped within the tenacious mucus of patients with asthma or cystic fibrosis. In addition, mucoid impaction, bronchocentric granulomatosis, or eosinophilic pneumonia may develop in a subset of this population. Extrinsic allergic alveolitis represents a hypersensitivity lung reaction in normal hosts secondary to heavy, primarily occupational exposure to *Aspergillus* spores. Diagnostic criteria have been well described.[158] Administration of corticosteroids is the primary therapy.[185]

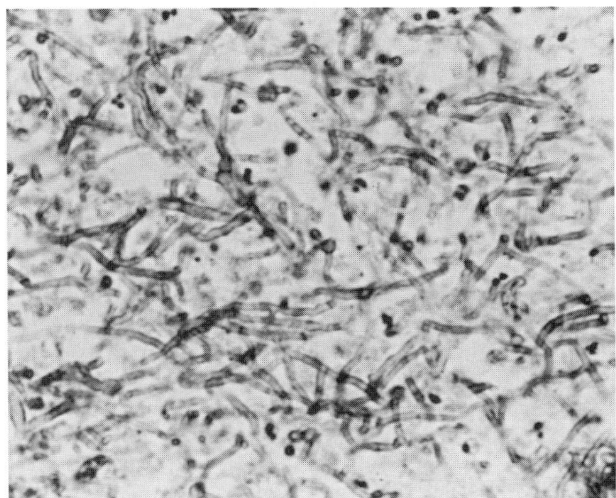

FIGURE 198–1 ■ Pulmonary aspergillosis illustrating septate hyphae and dichotomous branching (hematoxylin and eosin staining, ×64.)

Aspergilloma, usually secondary to *A. fumigatus,* is the most frequent form of pulmonary aspergillosis. The pathologic lesion is a mycetoma, a ball of mycelia growing in a poorly drained lung space that communicates with the bronchial tree. Tuberculosis, especially in patients receiving a long course of antituberculous therapy, is the most common predisposing factor for the development of an aspergilloma, with an incidence ranging from 2 percent of all tuberculosis patients[75] to almost 20 percent of patients with residual cavities larger than 2.5 cm.[39] Other conditions predisposing to aspergilloma in children include bronchiectasis,[113] congenital heart disease,[55] congenital pulmonary cysts,[182] healed abscess cavities,[182] histoplasmosis,[175] sarcoidosis,[225] and invasive aspergillosis in immunosuppressed hosts.[122]

Clinical features of aspergilloma include hemoptysis, productive cough, clubbing, fever, and localizing sounds at the site of the lesion.[38] Hemoptysis on occasion may be massive and fatal.[90] The characteristic radiologic finding is an apical, pulmonary air meniscus sign,[195] that is, crescent-shaped air adjacent to an intracavitary body with surrounding fibrocavitary changes. The diagnosis is confirmed by histologic examination and culture of a biopsy specimen; the presence of serum antibodies to *Aspergillus* and a positive sputum culture provide supportive evidence.[114] Treatment must be individualized,[37] with surgical resection generally recommended only for patients with severe hemoptysis.[79] Spontaneous resolution of pulmonary aspergillomas has been described in a few patients.[39]

Invasive Pulmonary Aspergillosis

Invasive pulmonary aspergillosis (Fig. 198–2) has become an increasingly important cause of morbidity and mortality in immunosuppressed patients with hematologic malignancies.[183] In one series,[227] 90 percent of patients with invasive aspergillosis had underlying hematologic malignancy, with 70 percent having a granulocyte count less than 500/mm^3. Invasive pulmonary aspergillosis after bone marrow transplantation has a particularly high mortality rate.[35]

Neutropenia is of paramount importance in this disease. In persistently febrile, neutropenic children receiving broad-spectrum antibiotics, approximately 50 percent of new pulmonary infiltrates are indicative of fungal pneumonia, usually caused by either *Candida* or *Aspergillus.*[34] Survival in these cases depends largely on recovery of the granulocyte count.

Invasive pulmonary aspergillosis is manifested most commonly as necrotizing bronchopneumonia or hemorrhagic infarction, although single or multiple abscesses, granulomata, or lobar infiltrates are occasionally present. Positive surveillance nasal cultures for *Aspergillus* frequently precede the development of invasive pulmonary aspergillosis.[2]

The propensity for *Aspergillus* to invade blood vessels results in a variety of pulmonary manifestations of invasive disease, such as focal necrosis, pulmonary infarction, and hemorrhagic consolidation. Several unusual variants in children have been reported, including necrotizing bronchitis with pseudomembrane formation,[147] invasive tracheitis,[196] tracheoesophageal fistula,[86] and pleural aspergillosis.[87]

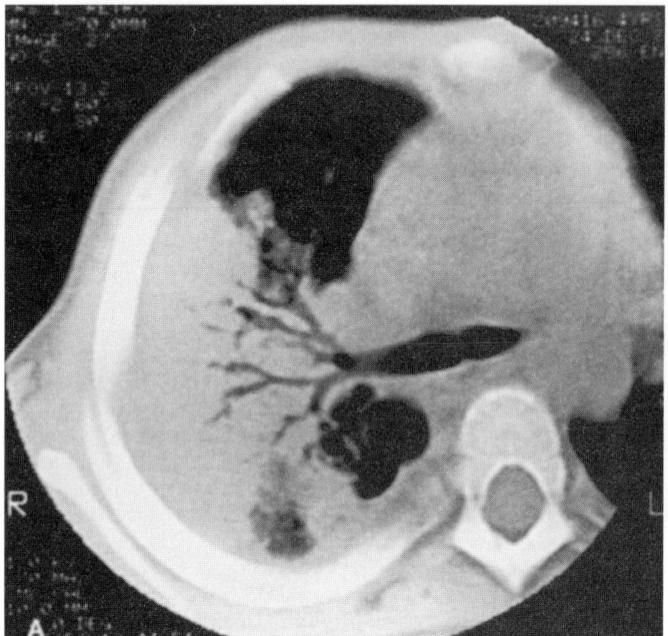

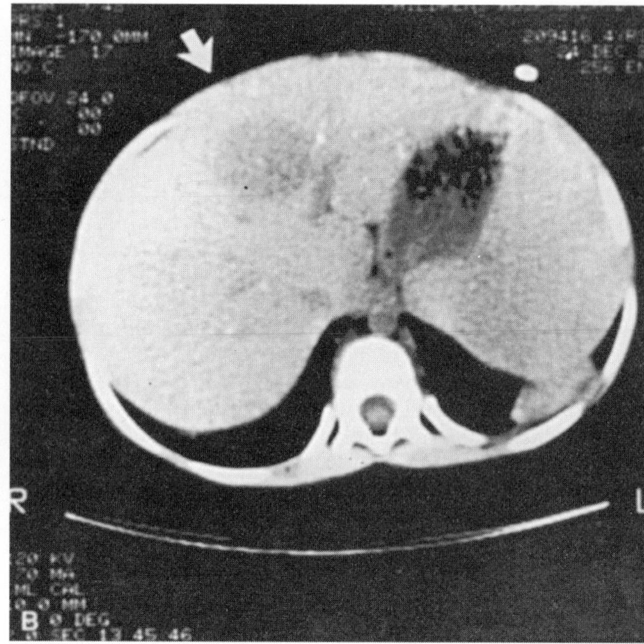

FIGURE 198–2 ■ Invasive aspergillosis in a 4-year-old boy with chronic granulomatous disease of childhood. *A,* A computed tomographic scan of the chest shows consolidation in the right lower lobe, with evidence of bronchiectasis. *B,* A computed tomographic scan of the upper part of the abdomen shows involvement of the right lobe of the liver *(arrow).*

Clinical manifestations consist of fever, dyspnea, nonproductive cough, mild hemoptysis, and pleuritic chest pain, which may be especially prominent in patients with hemorrhagic pulmonary infarction. The diagnostic specificity of isolation of *Aspergillus* from the respiratory tract directly correlates with the degree of immunosuppression. Isolation of *A. fumigatus* or *A. flavus* from the respiratory tract of neutropenic, leukemic patients is highly suggestive of invasive pulmonary disease.[229] The lower specificity and sensitivity of sputum cultures in immunosuppressed, non-neutropenic patients, however, may warrant a more invasive diagnostic procedure. Histologic demonstration of parenchymal invasion of the lung by *Aspergillus* remains the gold standard of diagnosis.

As is the case with patients who do not have HIV, pulmonary aspergillosis in HIV-infected patients usually is manifested as cavitary upper lobe disease, focal alveolar infiltrates, or bilateral alveolar or interstitial infiltrates. However, distinct differences appear to exist.[125] Cavitary upper lobe disease disseminates only rarely regardless of whether patients are infected with HIV; however, hemoptysis is fatal more often in HIV-infected patients. Focal infiltrates can persist for months in HIV-infected patients, but they usually either progress or resolve spontaneously with recovery of granulocytes in patients with leukemia or bone marrow transplants. The clinical manifestations of invasive tracheobronchitis caused by *Aspergillus* in patients with AIDS have been reviewed.[88] This clinical entity also appears to be an evolving concern in lung transplant recipients.[220] Large-airway disease appears to occur less commonly in HIV-infected children than in adults.[177]

CENTRAL NERVOUS SYSTEM

Aspergillosis of the central nervous system (CNS) may result from direct spread from the paranasal sinuses or, more commonly, from widespread dissemination in immunosuppressed patients. Unusual cases of inoculation of the brain through an unsuspected encephalocele[138] or rooster pecking[17] have been reported. Most cases are not recognized before the patient dies. In one study, cerebral aspergillosis was detected at autopsy in 20 percent of liver transplant patients.[23] Symptomatic patients generally have focal neurologic signs secondary to hemorrhagic infarcts.[209] Invasion of the CNS by hyphal forms of *Aspergillus* results in CT findings consistent with those of vascular occlusion, infarction, and abscess formation.[221] Although nodular enhancing lesions secondary to caseating granulomas more commonly result from yeast forms such as *Cryptococcus* or *Histoplasma*, cerebral[142] and cerebellar[169] aspergillomas have been described. Analysis of cerebrospinal fluid is not generally helpful in diagnosing aspergillosis of the CNS because infection of the meninges is relatively infrequent and not usually diffuse.[145, 209]

Aspergillus may invade the brain stem directly,[10] but involvement of the spinal cord usually results from compression caused by direct or hematogenous spread to the adjacent vertebral body.[51, 150] Rarely, myelopathy can be the initial sign of invasive aspergillosis in immunosuppressed children.[94]

BONE AND SKIN

Aspergillus osteomyelitis occurs predominantly in immunosuppressed patients, although traumatic tibial osteomyelitis has been reported in an immunologically normal adolescent.[36] In most cases, bone is invaded from a contiguous preexisting lesion in the lung or overlying skin. Spread from contiguous pneumonia most commonly occurs in patients with chronic granulomatous disease.[189] Because the radiologic findings are generally nonspecific, surgical biopsy and culture are needed for confirmation of the diagnosis.

Aspergillus spp. were the fungi most frequently grown from superficial white onychomycosis in one series.[112] Skin involvement by *Aspergillus* is usually secondary to hematogenous dissemination or local spread in immunosuppressed patients. In fact, painless cutaneous induration and erythema of the face may be the earliest signs of fulminant sinus aspergillosis.[217] Primary cutaneous aspergillosis also occurs in immunosuppressed patients. The usual environmental precipitants include intravenous arm boards[115] or intravenous cannulas.[5] Lesions typically occur at the point of contact, such as the palm or foot for arm boards and the entry site for intravenous catheters. Lesions progress from erythematous or violaceous papules or plaques through a hemorrhagic bullous stage to a purpuric ulcer with central necrosis.[62] Infection occasionally invades the underlying tendons and necessitates widespread débridement.[83] Potassium hydroxide preparation and early skin biopsy may allow prompt diagnosis and treatment.[4] A recent review of cases of invasive aspergillosis in a large pediatric hospital, as well as reported cases in the literature, suggests that children have cutaneous aspergillosis more commonly than previously suspected.[204] Prematurity invariably has been present in reported cases of primary cutaneous aspergillosis in neonates.[141]

HEART

Aspergillus endocarditis, most commonly found in association with open heart surgery, is associated with a high mortality rate in adults and children.[11] Unlike *Candida* endocarditis, inoculation usually is airborne intraoperatively rather than catheter-related. Postmortem studies indicate more invasiveness than in candidal disease, with erosion through synthetic or natural tissue and widespread embolization.[210]

The cardinal features include persistent fever, evidence of embolic phenomena, and consumption coagulopathy after cardiac surgery. Peripheral blood cultures are rarely positive. Echocardiography may be useful for the detection of mycotic aneurysms, intracardiac vegetations, or intra-aortic vegetations.[91] Although the diagnosis usually depends on isolation of *Aspergillus* from surgical specimens, a biopsy specimen of an embolus may grow the fungus or demonstrate characteristic histopathologic features.[11]

Isolated cardiac aspergillosis has been reported in a child who underwent bone marrow transplantation for aplastic anemia.[82] Although *Aspergillus* infections most commonly extend from the endocardium outward, several cases of *Aspergillus* pericarditis from contiguous pleural foci have been described.[206] *Aspergillus* pericarditis almost never is the sole intrathoracic location of aspergillosis.[102] It usually is symptomatic, often occurring with cardiac tamponade.

GENITOURINARY TRACT

Aspergillosis of the genitourinary tract generally results from hematogenous spread or ascending infection. Introduction of the organism via contaminated surgical material also has been reported.[89] The disease generally is more destructive than candidal involvement of the kidney, with resultant large areas of thrombosis and necrosis of cortical and papillary tissue.[153] Clinical manifestations include fever, chills, and microhematuria. Unilateral flank pain may occur with ascending infection.[54] On occasion, an isolated unilateral *Aspergillus* cast of the renal pelvis develops and may be passed through the urethra. Although urinary mycetomas usually are caused by *Candida* spp., an aspergilloma in a child with leukemia has been described during relapse.[110] Urine culture may be negative despite almost total renal destruction.[54]

OTHER

Although they are less common than candidal abscesses, multiple splenic aspergillomas have been described in leukemic patients with no evidence of systemic involvement.[97] Fever may be the only initial sign; left upper quadrant abdominal pain and splenomegaly occur in less than half of affected patients.[80] Intraperitoneal aspergillosis has been reported in children undergoing continuous cycling peritoneal dialysis.[96] Prompt removal of the peritoneal catheter is recommended in such cases.[190] Several children have experienced rupture of a mycotic aortic aneurysm secondary to invasive aspergillosis of the posterior mediastinum.[219] Primary lymph node granulomatous aspergillosis has been described in an adolescent with no apparent risk factors for *Aspergillus* infection.[111] Involvement of the gastrointestinal tract, liver, thyroid, testis, and adrenal has been reported.[227]

Diagnosis

Ideally, the diagnosis of aspergillosis should be based on (1) clinical and radiographic evidence of infection at a given site, (2) isolation and identification of *Aspergillus* in a high-quality specimen from that site, and (3) histologic identification of tissue invasion by a fungus with the same morphologic characteristics as those of the recovered agent. Potential diagnostic pitfalls include contamination of the clinical specimen, colonization of the site with noninvasive *Aspergillus* spp., lack of specificity of fungal morphologic features in histologic samples, and confusion of a pathologic diagnosis with an etiologic diagnosis.[203]

Aspergillus spp. readily grow on almost all laboratory media. Because most species are inhibited by cycloheximide, only antibacterial antibiotics should be present in the isolation medium. Recommended media for primary isolation include Sabouraud dextrose agar, brain-heart infusion agar, 2 percent malt extract agar, and potato flakes agar.[159] Characteristic conidiophores usually are present within 48 hours of incubation at 37° C, the optimal temperature for growth of most pathogenic species of *Aspergillus*.[161] Transfer of purified isolates to Czapek-Dox or malt extract agar solution may facilitate species identification in individual cases.[42, 57] Speciation of *Aspergillus* isolates may increase in importance as variations in antifungal drug susceptibility become better characterized.[42]

Respiratory specimens growing *Aspergillus* spp. may be misleading because uninfected persons may be colonized in the tracheobronchial tree.[122] However, the finding of two or more positive cultures of *A. flavus* or *A. fumigatus* is highly suggestive of pulmonary aspergillosis, particularly if the growth is heavy and free of other *Aspergillus* spp.[192] Adding microscopy to culture of respiratory fluid specimens increases the diagnostic yield over culture alone.[42] The positive predictive value of respiratory culture is highest for bone marrow transplant recipients, followed by those with hematologic malignancies.[71]

Blood cultures rarely are positive in disseminated aspergillosis.[47, 227] The lack of specificity inherent in indirect sampling (e.g., sputum) and the potential morbidity associated with direct sampling have spawned efforts to detect early invasive disease by serologic means. IgG antibody to *Aspergillus* has been detected by immunodiffusion,[53] immunofluorescence,[171] and enzyme-linked immunosorbent assay (ELISA).[172] These techniques often fail to detect early invasive disease because of a delay in antibody response or insufficient antibody production in immunosuppressed patients. In addition, an age-related increase in *Aspergillus* antibodies secondary to widespread environmental exposure limits the specificity of antibody detection.[171]

Significant work is ongoing to develop clinically useful antigen detection methods for *Aspergillus,* and it is a rapidly changing field. Attempts to detect *Aspergillus* antigen by ELISA,[143, 162, 168, 186] radioimmunoassay,[216] or immunoblotting[228] have been more reliable for detecting early invasive disease but are not yet recommended for routine application.[14] A new sensitive sandwich ELISA that recognizes the galactofuran side chain of the galactomannan molecule may have utility in pediatric hematology patients.[162] PCR techniques have not been as promising.[24] Nested PCR on serum may be useful for the detection of invasive pulmonary aspergillosis.[226] Techniques for antigen detection in invasive aspergillosis have been reviewed.[6, 224] With antigen or antibody testing, serial assays may have more utility than isolated tests have.[200]

Treatment

Intravenous amphotericin B remains the drug of choice for treating invasive *Aspergillus* infection.[44] Early diagnosis and treatment with intravenous amphotericin B substantially improve the outcome in this disease.[3] In general, the endpoint of treatment is determined by resolution of neutropenia or improvement after discontinuation of corticosteroids rather than by a total cumulative dose.[58, 185] Ideally, the clinical and radiologic findings of aspergillosis should have resolved and cultures returned to negative when therapy is ceased.[185] The Infectious Diseases Society of America recently published practice guidelines for the treatment of diseases caused by *Aspergillus*.[185]

Oral and intravenous formulations of itraconazole, a triazole, have been approved by the Food and Drug Administration (FDA) for the treatment of pulmonary and extrapulmonary aspergillosis in patients who are intolerant of or refractory to amphotericin B. Although efficacy has been shown in uncontrolled clinical trials,[78] relapse may be a problem in immunocompromised patients despite long courses of therapy.[43] Itraconazole has been anecdotally successful in the treatment of invasive aspergillosis in patients with chronic granulomatous disease,[92, 133] and interferon gamma may be a useful adjunct to therapy in this patient population.[18] Itraconazole treatment has been associated with fewer episodes of allergic bronchopulmonary aspergillosis in cystic fibrosis patients, and it has allowed a reduction in daily steroid use.[134]

New antifungal agents are being developed in an attempt to reduce the toxicity associated with amphotericin B. The FDA has approved new formulations of amphotericin B in lipid vehicles for the treatment of aspergillosis in patients refractory to or intolerant of conventional amphotericin B therapy. Although the number of pediatric patients enrolled in prelicensure studies was limited,[135, 137, 208] experience with the use of these agents in children is growing.[92, 160, 212] Less nephrotoxicity and fewer infusion-related reactions appear to be associated with the lipid formulations than with conventional amphotericin B.[68, 93, 212, 222] Caspofungin acetate, a once-daily intravenous glucan synthesis inhibitor, recently has been approved by the FDA for the treatment of invasive aspergillosis in patients who are refractory to or intolerant of other therapies.[26] Experience is limited in children. Combination polyene-azole antifungal therapy may hold promise for the future.[33, 56, 187] Standards for in vitro susceptibility testing of *Aspergillus* spp. are being revised as more antifungal agents are developed.[49, 128, 130]

Administration of hematopoietic growth factors can play a role in the management of neutropenic patients with aspergillosis.[126] Liposomal amphotericin B and granulocyte colony-stimulating factor, with or without surgery, successfully treated invasive pulmonary aspergillosis in a limited number of children with malignancy.[45] One group has proposed the administration of elutriated monocytes, perhaps in conjunction with hematopoietic growth factors and interferon gamma, as a future form of therapy.[165]

Surgical excision has been successful in the treatment of children with *Aspergillus* sinusitis,[151] cerebral mycetoma,[33, 66] infected prosthetic valves,[11] and localized pulmonic infections.[176] Some physicians have advocated early, complete resection of pulmonary lesions, combined with antifungal therapy, for the treatment of bone marrow transplant patients.[106] Surgical excision of pulmonary aspergillomas usually is restricted to patients with severe hemoptysis and adequate pulmonary function for tolerating the procedure.[12, 79, 198] Performing selective bronchial artery embolization may be necessary before resection.[73] Intracavitary administration of antifungal agents may be an alternative to resection in localized pulmonic infections.[15, 63]

Surgical débridement is the mainstay of therapy for indolent sinus aspergillosis and is used in conjunction with antifungal therapy for invasive sinus aspergillosis. Surgical removal of infected tissue, combined with the administration of amphotericin B, is optimal for the treatment of *Aspergillus* endocarditis.[11] Surgery combined with oral therapy may be sufficient for bone infections.[185] A combined medical and surgical approach was used successfully in a child with leukemia and cerebral and sinus aspergillosis.[66] Performing surgical débridement or resection in conjunction with antifungal therapy may be necessary for locally advanced primary cutaneous aspergillosis.[205] Vitrectomy combined with intravitreous amphotericin B has been considered the preferred treatment of *Aspergillus* endophthalmitis.[218] For most other sites of *Aspergillus* infection, surgical débridement seems to offer little advantage over medical therapy alone.

Prevention

Because the mortality of invasive aspergillosis remains high despite current therapy,[41] attempts to reduce the exposure of immunosuppressed or neutropenic patients to *Aspergillus* spores are of paramount importance for prevention of this disease.[156] Strategies to prevent invasive fungal infections in patients with neoplastic diseases have been reviewed.[21, 109, 211] High-risk patients should be isolated from areas of construction activity and placed in rooms equipped with high-efficiency particulate air filters. Ornamental plants and flowers should be removed from these rooms. Aerosolized copper-8-quinolinolate, a nontoxic antifungal powder, has been used for outbreak control.[136]

Because the toxicity of systemic amphotericin B precludes prophylactic use, several innovative approaches to antifungal prophylaxis have been initiated recently. Amphotericin B nasal spray may be effective in controlling respiratory and sinus colonization in neutropenic patients,[120] as well as the frequency of invasive disease.[77] In one study, fatal aspergillosis occurred less frequently after the prophylactic administration of amphotericin B nasal spray to pediatric bone marrow transplant patients.[194] In addition, aerosolized amphotericin B, delivered by a small-particle aerosol generator, has been studied for prophylactic use.[19, 20] Prophylactic itraconazole, with[191] or without[193] nasal amphotericin B, has been shown in preliminary studies to protect patients with prolonged granulocytopenia from fatal aspergillosis and also may be useful in patients with chronic granulomatous disease.[131] The clinical use of hematopoietic growth factors may provide the best prophylaxis in the future against *Aspergillus* infections.[126]

REFERENCES

1. Abbasi, S., Shenep, J. L., Hughes, W. T., et al.: Aspergillosis in children with cancer: A 34-year experience. Clin. Infect. Dis. *29*:1210, 1999.
2. Aisner, J., Murillo, J., Schimpff, S. C., et al.: Invasive aspergillosis in acute leukemia: Correlation with nose cultures and antibiotic use. Ann. Intern. Med. *90*:4, 1979.
3. Aisner, J., Schimpff, S. C., and Wiernik, P. H.: Treatment of invasive aspergillosis: Relation of early diagnosis and treatment to response. Ann. Intern. Med. *86*:539, 1977.
4. Allen, U., Smith, C. R., and Prober, C. G.: The value of skin biopsies in febrile, neutropenic, immunocompromised children. Am. J. Dis. Child. *140*:459, 1986.
5. Allo, M. D., Miller, J., Townsend, T., et al.: Primary cutaneous aspergillosis associated with Hickman intravenous catheters. N. Engl. J. Med. *317*:1105, 1987.
6. Andriole, V. T.: Infections with *Aspergillus* species. Clin. Infect. Dis. *17*(Suppl. 2):481, 1993.
7. Austin, J. M., Schulman, L. L., and Mastrobattista, J. D.: Pulmonary infection after cardiac transplantation: Clinical and radiologic correlations. Radiology *172*:259, 1989.
8. Bahadur, S., Kacker, S. K., D'Souza, B., et al.: Paranasal sinus aspergillosis. J. Laryngol. Otol. *97*:863, 1983.
9. Barnes, R. A., and Rogers, T. R.: Control of an outbreak of nosocomial aspergillosis by laminar air-flow isolation. J. Hosp. Infect. *14*:89, 1989.
10. Barrios, N., Tebbi, C. K., Rotstein, C., et al.: Brainstem invasion by *Aspergillus fumigatus* in a child with leukemia. N. Y. State J. Med. *88*:656, 1988.
11. Barst, R. J., Prince, A. S., and Neu, H. C.: *Aspergillus* endocarditis in children: Case report and review of the literature. Pediatrics *68*:73, 1981.
12. Battaglini, J. W., Murray, G. F., Keagy, B. A., et al.: Surgical management of symptomatic pulmonary aspergilloma. Ann. Thorac. Surg. *39*:512, 1985.
13. Baydala, L. T., Yanofsky, R., Akabutu, J., et al.: Aspergillosis of the nose and paranasal sinuses in immunocompromised children. Can. Med. Assoc. J. *138*:927, 1988.
14. Bennett, J. E.: Rapid diagnosis of candidiasis and aspergillosis. Rev. Infect. Dis. *9*:398, 1987.
15. Bennett, M. R., Weinbaum, D. L., and Fiehler, P. C.: Chronic necrotizing pulmonary aspergillosis treated by endobronchial amphotericin B. South. Med. J. *83*:829, 1990.
16. Berkow, R. L., Weisman, S. J., Provisor, A. J., et al.: Invasive aspergillosis of paranasal tissues in children with malignancies. J. Pediatr. *103*:49, 1983.
17. Berkowitz, F. E., and Jacobs, D. W.: Fatal case of brain abscess caused by rooster pecking. Pediatr. Infect. Dis. J. *6*:941, 1987.
18. Bernhisel-Broadbent, J., Camargo, E. E., Jaffe, H.-S., et al.: Recombinant human interferon-γ as adjunct therapy for *Aspergillus* infection in a patient with chronic granulomatous disease. J. Infect. Dis. *163*:908, 1991.
19. Beyer, J., Barzen, G., Risse, G., et al.: Aerosol amphotericin B for prevention of invasive pulmonary aspergillosis. Antimicrob. Agents Chemother. *37*:1367, 1993.
20. Beyer, J., Schwartz, S., Barzen, G., et al.: Use of amphotericin B aerosols for the prevention of pulmonary aspergillosis. Infection *22*:143, 1994.
21. Beyer, J., Schwartz, S., Heinemann, V., et al.: Strategies in prevention of invasive pulmonary aspergillosis in immunosuppressed or neutropenic patients. Antimicrob. Agents Chemother. *38*:911, 1994.
22. Bhargava, V., Tomashefski, J. F., Jr., Stern, R. C., et al.: The pathology of fungal infection and colonization in patients with cystic fibrosis. Hum. Pathol. *20*:977, 1989.
23. Boon, A. P., Adams, D. H., and McMaster, P.: Cerebral aspergillosis in liver transplantation. J. Clin. Pathol. *43*:114, 1990.
24. Bretagne, S., Costa, J.-M., Marmorat-Khuong, M., et al.: Detection of *Aspergillus* species DNA in bronchoalveolar lavage samples by competitive PCR. J. Clin. Microbiol. *33*:1164, 1995.
25. Buffington, J., Reporter, R., Lasker, B. A., et al.: Investigation of an epidemic of invasive aspergillosis: Utility of molecular typing with the use of random amplified polymorphic DNA probes. Pediatr. Infect. Dis. J. *13*:386, 1994.
26. Caspofungin (Cancidas) for aspergillosis. Med. Lett. Drugs Ther. *43*:58, 2001.
27. Centeno, R. S., Bentson, J. R., and Mancuso, A. A.: CT scanning in rhinocerebral mucormycosis and aspergillosis. Radiology *140*:383, 1981.
28. Choi, S. S., Milmoe, G. J., Dinndorf, P. A., et al.: Invasive *Aspergillus* sinusitis in pediatric bone marrow transplant patients. Arch. Otolaryngol. Head Neck Surg. *121*:1188, 1995.
29. Chung, Y., Kraut, J. R., Stone, A. M., et al.: Disseminated aspergillosis in a patient with cystic fibrosis and allergic bronchopulmonary aspergillosis. Pediatr. Pulmonol. *17*:131, 1994.
30. Chusid, M. J., Sty, J. R., and Wells, R. G.: Pulmonary aspergillosis appearing as chronic nodular disease in chronic granulomatous disease. Pediatr. Radiol. *18*:232, 1988.
31. Ciegler, A., Burmeister, H. R., and Vesonder, R. F.: Poisonous fungi: Mycotoxins and mycotoxicoses. *In* Howard, D. H. (ed.): Fungi Pathogenic for Humans and Animals. Vol. 3, Part B. New York, Marcel Dekker, 1983, p. 413.
32. Cohen, M. S., Isturiz, R. E., Malech, H. L., et al.: Fungal infection in chronic granulomatous disease. Am. J. Med. *71*:59, 1981.
33. Coleman, J. M., Hogg, G. G., Rosenfeld, J. V., et al.: Invasive central nervous system aspergillosis: Cure with liposomal amphotericin B, itraconazole, and radical surgery—case report and review of the literature. Neurosurgery *36*:858, 1995.
34. Commers, J. R., Robichaud, K. J., and Pizzo, P. A.: New pulmonary infiltrates in granulocytopenic cancer patients being treated with antibiotics. Pediatr. Infect. Dis. *3*:423, 1984.
35. Cordonnier, C., Bernaudin, J. F., Bierling, P., et al.: Pulmonary complications occurring after allogeneic bone marrow transplantation. Cancer *58*:1047, 1986.
36. Corrall, C. J., Merz, W. G., Rekedal, K., et al.: *Aspergillus* osteomyelitis in an immunocompetent adolescent: A case report and review of the literature. Pediatrics *70*:455, 1982.
37. Daly, R. C., Pairolero, P. C., Piehler, J. M., et al.: Pulmonary aspergilloma. J. Thorac. Cardiovasc. Surg. *92*:981, 1986.
38. Dar, M. A., Ahmad, M., Weinstein, A. J., et al.: Thoracic aspergillosis. Cleve. Clin. Q. *51*:615, 1984.
39. Davies, D. (Chairman): Aspergilloma and residual tuberculous cavities: The results of a resurvey. A report of the Research Committee of the British Thoracic and Tuberculosis Association. Tubercle *51*:227, 1970.
40. Demicco, D. D., Reichman, R. C., Violette, E. J., et al.: Disseminated aspergillosis presenting with endophthalmitis. Cancer *53*:1995, 1984.
41. Denning, D. W.: Therapeutic outcome in invasive aspergillosis. Clin. Infect. Dis. *23*:608, 1996.
42. Denning, D. W.: Invasive aspergillosis. Clin. Infect. Dis. *26*:781, 1998.
43. Denning, D. W., Lee, J. Y., Hostetler, J. S., et al.: NIAID mycosis study group multicenter trial of oral itraconazole therapy for invasive aspergillosis. Am. J. Med. *97*:135, 1994.
44. Denning, D. W., and Stevens, D. A.: Antifungal and surgical treatment of invasive aspergillosis: Review of 2121 published cases. Rev. Infect. Dis. *12*:1147, 1990.
45. Dornbusch, H. J., Urban, C. E., Pinter, H., et al.: Treatment of invasive pulmonary aspergillosis in severely neutropenic children with malignant disorders using liposomal amphotericin B (AmBisome), granulocyte colony-stimulating factor, and surgery: Report of five cases. Pediatr. Hematol. Oncol. *12*:577, 1995.
46. Dreizen, S., Bodey, G. P., McCredie, K. B., et al.: Orofacial aspergillosis in acute leukemia. Oral Surg. Oral Med. Oral Pathol. *59*:499, 1985.
47. Duthie, R., and Denning, D. W.: *Aspergillus* fungemia: Report of two cases and review. Clin. Infect. Dis. *20*:598, 1995.
48. Enweani, I. B. and Igumbor, H. Prevalence of otomycosis in malnourished children in Edo State, Nigeria. Mycopathologia *140*:85, 1998.
49. Espinel-Ingroff, A., Bartlett, M., Chaturvedi, V., et al.: Optimal susceptibility testing conditions for detection of azole resistance in *Aspergillus* spp.: NCCLS collaborative evaluation. Antimicrob. Agents Chemother. *45*:1828, 2001.
50. Fanti, F., Conti, S., Campani, L., et al.: Studies on the epidemiology of *Aspergillus fumigatus* infections in a university hospital. Eur. J. Epidemiol. *5*:8, 1989.
51. Ferris, B., and Jones, C.: Paraplegia due to aspergillosis: Successful conservative treatment in two cases. J. Bone Joint Surg. Br. *67*:800, 1985.
52. Fietta, A., Sacchi, F., Mangiarotti, P., et al.: Defective phagocyte *Aspergillus* killing associated with recurrent pulmonary *Aspergillus* infections. Infection *12*:10, 1984.
53. Fisher, B. D., Armstrong, D., Yu, B., et al.: Invasive aspergillosis: Progress in early diagnosis and treatment. Am. J. Med. *71*:571, 1981.
54. Flechner, S. M., and McAninch, J. W.: Aspergillosis of the urinary tract: Ascending route of infection and evolving patterns of disease. J. Urol. *125*:598, 1981.
55. Flye, M. W., and Sealy, W. C.: Pulmonary aspergilloma: A report of its occurrence in two patients with cyanotic congenital heart disease. Ann. Thorac. Surg. *20*:196, 1975.
56. George, D., Kordick, D., Miniter, P., et al.: Combination therapy in experimental invasive aspergillosis. J. Infect. Dis. *168*:692, 1993.
57. Gray, L. D., and Roberts, G. D.: Laboratory diagnosis of systemic fungal diseases. Infect. Dis. Clin. North Am. *2*:779, 1988.
58. Graybill, J. R.: Therapeutic agents. Infect. Dis. Clin. North Am. *2*:805, 1988.
59. Greif, Z., Moscuna, M., Suprun, H., et al.: Fatal childhood pulmonary aspergillosis from contact with pigeons. Clin. Pediatr. (Phila.) *20*:357, 1981.
60. Groll, A. H., Jaeger, G., Allendorf, A., et al.: Invasive pulmonary aspergillosis in a critically ill neonate: Case report and review of invasive

aspergillosis during the first 3 months of life. Clin. Infect. Dis. *27*:437, 1998.
61. Groll, A. H., Kurz, M., Schneider, W., et al.: Five-year-survey of invasive aspergillosis in a paediatric cancer centre. Epidemiology, management, and long-term survival. Mycoses *42*:431, 1999.
62. Grossman, M. E., Fithian, E. C., Behrens, C., et al.: Primary cutaneous aspergillosis in six leukemic children. J. Am. Acad. Dermatol. *12*:313, 1985.
63. Guleria, R., Gupta, D., and Jindal, S. K.: Treatment of pulmonary aspergilloma by endoscopic intracavitary instillation of ketoconazole. Chest *103*:1301, 1993.
64. Gupta, M., Weinberger, B., and Whitley-Williams, P. N.: Cutaneous aspergillosis in a neonate. Pediatr. Infect. Dis. J. *15*:464, 1996.
65. Hartwick, R. W., and Batsakis, J. G.: Sinus aspergillosis and allergic fungal sinusitis. Ann. Otol. Rhinol. Laryngol. *100*:427, 1991.
66. Henze, G., Aldenhoff, P., Stephani, U., et al.: Successful treatment of pulmonary and cerebral aspergillosis in an immunosuppressed child. Eur. J. Pediatr. *138*:263, 1982.
67. Hibberd, P. L., and Rubin, R. H.: Clinical aspects of fungal infection in organ transplant recipients. Clin. Infect. Dis. *19*(Suppl. 1):33, 1994.
68. Hiemenz, J. W., and Walsh, T. J.: Lipid formulations of amphotericin B: Recent progress and future directions. Clin. Infect. Dis. *22*(Suppl. 2):133, 1996.
69. Hinson, K. E., Moon, A. J., and Plummer, N. S.: Bronchopulmonary aspergillosis: A review and report of eight new cases. Thorax *7*:317, 1952.
70. Hopkins, C. C., Weber, D. J., and Rubin, R. H.: Invasive *Aspergillus* infection: Possible non-ward common source within the hospital environment. J. Hosp. Infect. *13*:19, 1989.
71. Horvath, J. A., and Dummer, S.: The use of respiratory-tract cultures in the diagnosis of invasive pulmonary aspergillosis. Am. J. Med. *100*:171, 1996.
72. Houser, S. M., and Corey, J. P.: Allergic fungal rhinosinusitis: Pathophysiology, epidemiology, and diagnosis. Otolaryngol. Clin. North Am. *33*:399, 2000.
73. Hughes, C. F., Waugh, R., and Lindsay, D.: Surgery for pulmonary aspergilloma: Preoperative embolisation of the bronchial circulation. Thorax *41*:324, 1986.
74. Iwen, P. C., Rupp, M. E., and Hinrichs, S. H.: Invasive mold sinusitis: 17 cases in immunocompromised patients and review of the literature. Clin. Infect. Dis. *24*:1178, 1997.
75. Jain, S. K., Agrawal, R. L., and Agrawal, M.: *Aspergillus* infection in pulmonary tuberculosis. Indian J. Med. Sci. *36*:48, 1982.
76. Jariwalla, A. G., Smith, A. P., and Melville-Jones, G.: Necrotising aspergillosis complicating fulminating viral pneumonia. Thorax *35*:215, 1980.
77. Jeffery, G. M., Beard, M. E. J., Ikram, R. B., et al.: Intranasal amphotericin B reduces the frequency of invasive aspergillosis in neutropenic patients. Am. J. Med. *90*:685, 1991.
78. Jennings, T. S., and Hardin, T. C.: Treatment of aspergillosis with itraconazole. Ann. Pharmacol. *27*:1206, 1993.
79. Jewkes, J., Kay, P. H., Paneth, M., et al.: Pulmonary aspergilloma: Analysis of prognosis in relation to haemoptysis and survey of treatment. Thorax *38*:572, 1983.
80. Johnson, J. D., and Raff, M. J.: Fungal splenic abscess. Arch. Intern. Med. *144*:1987, 1984.
81. Johnson, R., and Rootman, J.: Bilateral retinal infarction in disseminated aspergillosis. Can. J. Ophthalmol. *17*:223, 1982.
82. Johnson, R. B., Wing, E. J., Miller, T. R., et al.: Isolated cardiac aspergillosis after bone marrow transplantation. Arch. Intern. Med. *147*:1942, 1987.
83. Jones, N. F., Conklin, W. T., and Albo, V. C.: Primary invasive aspergillosis of the hand. J. Hand Surg. [Am.] *11*:425, 1986.
84. Joshi, V. V., Path, F. R., Oleske, J. M., et al.: Pathology of opportunistic infections in children with acquired immune deficiency syndrome. Pediatr. Pathol. *6*:145, 1986.
85. Kagen, S. L., Kurup, V. P., Sohnle, P. G., et al.: Marijuana smoking and fungal sensitization. J. Allergy Clin. Immunol. *71*:389, 1983.
86. Kapdushnik, J., Springer, C., Naparstek, E., et al.: Tracheoesophageal fistula induced by *Aspergillus* infection following bone marrow transplantation. Pediatr. Pulmonol. *17*:202, 1994.
87. Kearon, M. C., Power, J. T., Wood, A. E., et al.: Pleural aspergillosis in a 14-year-old boy. Thorax *42*:477, 1987.
88. Kemper, C. A., Hostetler, J. S., Follansbee, S. E., et al.: Ulcerative and plaque-like tracheobronchitis due to infection with *Aspergillus* in patients with AIDS. Clin. Infect. Dis. *17*:344, 1993.
89. Khan, Z. U., Gopalakrishnan, G., Al-Awadi, K., et al.: Renal aspergilloma due to *Aspergillus flavus*. Clin. Infect. Dis. *21*:210, 1995.
90. Kibbler, C. C., Milkins, S. R., Bhamra, A., et al.: Apparent pulmonary mycetoma following invasive aspergillosis in neutropenic patients. Thorax *43*:108, 1988.
91. Kleiman, M. B.: Echocardiography in *Aspergillus* endocarditis. Pediatrics *69*:252, 1982.
92. Kline, M. W., Bocobo, F. C., Paul, M. E., et al.: Successful medical therapy of *Aspergillus* osteomyelitis of the spine in an 11-year-old boy with chronic granulomatous disease. Pediatrics *93*:830, 1995.
93. Kline, S., Larsen, T. A., Fieber, L., et al.: Limited toxicity of prolonged therapy with high doses of amphotericin B lipid complex. Clin. Infect. Dis. *21*:1154, 1995.
94. Koh, S., Ross, L. A., Gilles, F. H., et al.: Myelopathy resulting from invasive aspergillosis. Pediatr. Neurol. *19*:135, 1998.
95. Krasinski, K., Holzman, R. S., Hanna, B., et al.: Nosocomial fungal infection during hospital renovation. Infect. Control *6*:278, 1985.
96. Kravitz, S. P., and Berry, P. L.: Successful treatment of *Aspergillus* peritonitis in a child undergoing continuous cycling peritoneal dialysis. Arch. Intern. Med. *146*:2061, 1986.
97. Kulkarni, R., Murray, D. L., Gupta, S., et al.: Multiple splenic aspergillomas in a patient with acute lymphoblastic leukemia. Am. J. Pediatr. Hematol. Oncol. *4*:141, 1982.
98. Kusne, S., Torre-Cisneros, J., Mañez, R., et al.: Factors associated with invasive lung aspergillosis and the significance of positive *Aspergillus* culture after liver transplantation. J. Infect. Dis. *166*:1379, 1992.
99. Kyriakides, G. K., Zinneman, H. H., Hall, W. H., et al.: Immunologic monitoring and aspergillosis in renal transplant patients. Am. J. Surg. *131*:246, 1976.
100. Latgé, J.-P.: *Aspergillus fumigatus* and aspergillosis. Clin. Microbiol. Rev. *12*:310, 1999.
101. Legent, F., Billet, J., Beauvillain, C., et al.: The role of dental canal fillings in the development of *Aspergillus* sinusitis. Arch. Otorhinolaryngol. *246*:318, 1989.
102. Le Moing, V., Lortholary, O., Timsit, J. F., et al.: *Aspergillus* pericarditis with tamponade: Report of a successfully treated case and review. Clin. Infect. Dis. *26*:451, 1998.
103. Lentino, J. R., Rosenkranz, M. A., Michaels, J. A., et al.: Nosocomial aspergillosis: A retrospective review of airborne disease secondary to road construction and contaminated air conditioners. Am. J. Epidemiol. *116*:430, 1982.
104. Lewis, M., Kallenbach, J., Zaltzman, M., et al.: Invasive pulmonary aspergillosis complicating influenza A pneumonia in a previously healthy patient. Chest *87*:691, 1985.
105. Lortholary, O., Meyohas, M.-C., Dupont, B., et al.: Invasive aspergillosis in patients with acquired immunodeficiency syndrome: Report of 33 cases. Am. J. Med. *95*:177, 1993.
106. Lupinetti, F. M., Behrendt, D. M., Giller, R. H., et al.: Pulmonary resection for fungal infection in children undergoing bone marrow transplantation. J. Thorac. Cardiovasc. Surg. *104*:684, 1992.
107. Maguire, S., Moriarty, P., Tempany, E., et al.: Unusual clustering of allergic bronchopulmonary aspergillosis in children with cystic fibrosis. Pediatrics *82*:835, 1988.
108. Mahajan, V. M.: Postoperative ocular infections: An analysis of laboratory data on 750 cases. Ann. Ophthalmol. *16*:847, 1984.
109. Manuel, R. J., and Kibbler, C. C.: The epidemiology and prevention of invasive aspergillosis. J. Hosp. Infect. *39*:95, 1998.
110. Marchand, R., Ahronheim, G. A., Patriquin, H., et al.: Aspergilloma of the renal pelvis in a leukemic child. Pediatr. Infect. Dis. J. *4*:103, 1985.
111. Mazzoni, A., Ferrarese, M., Manfredi, R., et al.: Primary lymph node invasive aspergillosis. Infection *24*:37, 1996.
112. McAleer, R.: Fungal infections of the nails in western Australia. Mycopathologia *73*:115, 1981.
113. McCarthy, D. S., and Pepys, J.: Pulmonary aspergilloma: Clinical immunology. Clin. Allergy *3*:57, 1973.
114. McCarthy, G., FitzGerald, M. X., and Keelan, P.: The spectrum of pulmonary aspergillosis. Ir. J. Med. Sci. *157*:316, 1988.
115. McCarty, J. M., Flam, M. S., Pullen, G., et al.: Outbreak of primary cutaneous aspergillosis related to intravenous arm boards. J. Pediatr. *108*:721, 1986.
116. McDonald, G. S., and Crowe, P.: Clinicopathological patterns of invasive and superficial fungal infection. Ir. J. Med. Sci. *157*:185, 1988.
117. McDonnell, P. J., McDonnell, J. M., Brown, R. H., et al.: Ocular involvement in patients with fungal infections. Ophthalmology *92*:706, 1985.
118. McGill, T. J., Simpson, G., and Healy, G. B.: Fulminant aspergillosis of the nose and paranasal sinuses: A new clinical entity. Laryngoscope *90*:748, 1980.
119. McWhinney, P. H. M., Kibbler, C. C., Hamon, M. D., et al.: Progress in the diagnosis and management of aspergillosis in bone marrow transplantation: 13 years' experience. Clin. Infect. Dis. *17*:397, 1993.
120. Meunier, F.: Prevention of mycoses in immunocompromised patients. Rev. Infect. Dis. *9*:408, 1987.
121. Meyer, R. D., Gaultier, C. R., Yamashita, J. T., et al.: Fungal sinusitis in patients with AIDS: Report of 4 cases and review of the literature. Medicine (Baltimore) *73*:69, 1994.
122. Meyer, R. D., Young, L. S., Armstrong, D., et al.: Aspergillosis complicating neoplastic disease. Am. J. Med. *54*:6, 1973.
123. Meyers, J. D.: Fungal infections in bone marrow transplant patients. Semin. Oncol. *17*(Suppl. 6):10, 1990.
124. Micheli, P.: Nova Plantarum Genera juxta Tournefortii Methodum Disposita. Florentiae, Paperinii, 1729.
125. Miller, W. T., Sais, G. J., Frank, I., et al.: Pulmonary aspergillosis in patients with AIDS. Chest *105*:37, 1994.
126. Milliken, S. T., and Powles, R. L.: Antifungal prophylaxis in bone marrow transplantation. Rev. Infect. Dis. *12*(Suppl.):374, 1990.

127. Min, Y., Kim, H. S., Lee, K., et al.: *Aspergillus* sinusitis: Clinical aspects and treatment outcomes. Otolaryngol. Head Neck Surg. *115*:49, 1996.
128. Moore, C. B., Walls, C. M., and Denning, D. W.: In vitro activities of terbinafine against *Aspergillus* species in comparison with those of itraconazole and amphotericin B. Antimicrob. Agents Chemother. *45*:1882, 2001.
129. Morrison, V. A., Haake, R. J., and Weisdorf, D. J.: Non-candidal fungal infections after bone marrow transplantation: Risk factors and outcome. Am. J. Med. *96*:497, 1994.
130. Mosquera, J., Warn, P. A., Morrissey, J., et al.: Susceptibility testing of *Aspergillus flavus*: Inoculum dependence with itraconazole and lack of correlation between susceptibility to amphotericin B in vitro and outcome in vivo. Antimicrob. Agents Chemother. *45*:1456, 2001.
131. Mouy, R., Veber, F., Blanche, S., et al.: Long-term itraconazole prophylaxis against *Aspergillus* infections in thirty-two patients with chronic granulomatous disease. J. Pediatr. *125*:998, 1994.
132. Mugliston, T., and O'Donoghue, G.: Otomycosis: A continuing problem. J. Laryngol. Otol. *99*:327, 1985.
133. Neijens, H. J., Frenkel, J., de Muinck Keizer-Schrama, S. M., et al.: Invasive *Aspergillus* infection in chronic granulomatous disease: Treatment with itraconazole. J. Pediatr. *115*:1016, 1989.
134. Nepomuceno, I. B., Esrig, S., and Moss, R. B.: Allergic bronchopulmonary aspergillosis in cystic fibrosis. Chest *115*:364, 1999.
135. Ng, T. T., and Denning, D. W.: Liposomal amphotericin B (AmBisome) therapy of invasive fungal infections: Evaluation of United Kingdom compassionate use data. Arch. Intern. Med. *155*:1093, 1995.
136. Opal, S. M., Asp, A. A., Cannady, P. B., Jr., et al.: Efficacy of infection control measures during a nosocomial outbreak of disseminated aspergillosis associated with hospital construction. J. Infect. Dis. *153*:634, 1986.
137. Oppenheim, B. A., Herbrecht, R., and Kusne, S.: The safety and efficacy of amphotericin B colloidal dispersion in the treatment of invasive mycoses. Clin. Infect. Dis. *21*:1145, 1995.
138. Ouammou, A., el Ouanzazi, A., Belghmaidi, M., et al.: Cerebral aspergillosis and encephalomeningocele. Childs Nerv. Syst. *2*:216, 1986.
139. Pagani, A., Spalla, R., Ferrari, F. A., et al.: Defective *Aspergillus* killing by neutrophil leucocytes in a case of systemic aspergillosis. Clin. Exp. Immunol. *43*:201, 1981.
140. Panda, A., Sharma, N., Das, G., et al.: Mycotic keratitis in children: Epidemiologic and microbiologic evaluation. Cornea *16*:295, 1997.
141. Papouli, M., Roilides, E. M., Bibashi, E., et al.: Primary cutaneous aspergillosis in neonates: Case report and review. Clin. Infect. Dis. *22*:1102, 1996.
142. Partridge, B. M., and Chin, A. T.: Cerebral aspergilloma. Postgrad. Med. J. *57*:439, 1981.
143. Patterson, T. F., Miniter, P., Patterson, J. E., et al.: *Aspergillus* antigen detection in the diagnosis of invasive aspergillosis. J. Infect. Dis. *171*:1553, 1995.
144. Paulose, K. O., Al Khalifa, S., Shenoy, P., et al.: Mycotic infection of the ear (otomycosis): A prospective study. J. Laryngol. Otol. *103*:30, 1989.
145. Peacock, J. E., McGinnis, M. R., and Cohen, M. S.: Persistent neutrophilic meningitis: Report of four cases and review of the literature. Medicine (Baltimore) *63*:379, 1984.
146. Perraud, M., Piens, M. A., Nicoloyannis, N., et al.: Invasive nosocomial pulmonary aspergillosis: Risk factors and hospital building works. Epidemiol. Infect. *99*:407, 1987.
147. Pervez, N. K., Kleinerman, J., Kattan, M., et al.: Pseudomembranous necrotizing bronchial aspergillosis. Am. Rev. Respir. Dis. *131*:961, 1985.
148. Peterson, P. K., McGlave, P., Ramsay, N. K., et al.: A prospective study of infectious diseases following bone marrow transplantation: Emergence of *Aspergillus* and cytomegalovirus as the major causes of mortality. Infect. Control *4*:81, 1983.
149. Phillips, P., Bryce, G., Shepherd, J., et al.: Invasive external otitis caused by *Aspergillus*. Rev. Infect. Dis. *12*:277, 1990.
150. Polatty, R. C., Cooper, K. R., and Kerkering, T. M.: Spinal cord compression due to an aspergilloma. South. Med. J. *77*:645, 1984.
151. Quiney, R. E., Rogers, M. J., Davidson, R. N., et al.: Craniofacial resection for extensive paranasal sinus aspergilloma. J. Laryngol. Otol. *102*:1172, 1988.
152. Radford, S. A., Johnson, E. M., Leeming, J. P., et al.: Molecular epidemiological study of *Aspergillus fumigatus* in a bone marrow transplantation unit by PCR amplification of ribosomal intergenic spacer sequences. J. Clin. Microbiol. *36*:1294, 1998.
153. Raghavan, R., Date, A., and Bhaktaviziam, A.: Fungal and nocardial infections of the kidney. Histopathology *11*:9, 1987.
154. Raper, K. B., and Fennell, D. I.: The Genus *Aspergillus*. Baltimore, Williams & Wilkins, 1965.
155. Renon, L.: Etude sur l'Aspergillose chez les Animaux et chez l'Homme. Paris, Masson, 1897.
156. Rhame, F. S., Streifel, A. J., Kersey, J. H., Jr., et al.: Extrinsic risk factors for pneumonia in the patient at high risk of infection. Am. J. Med. *76*(5A):42, 1984.
157. Rhine, W. D., Arvin, A. M., and Stevenson, D. K.: Neonatal aspergillosis. Clin. Pediatr. (Phila.) *25*:400, 1986.
158. Ricketti, A. J., Greenberger, P. A., Mintzer, R. A., et al.: Allergic bronchopulmonary aspergillosis. Chest *86*:773, 1984.
159. Rinaldi, M. G.: Invasive aspergillosis. Rev. Infect. Dis. *5*:1061, 1983.
160. Ringden, O., and Tollemar, J.: Liposomal amphotericin B (AmBisome) treatment of invasive fungal infections in immunocompromised children. Mycoses *36*:187, 1993.
161. Rippon, J. W.: Medical Mycology. 3rd ed. Philadelphia, W. B. Saunders, 1988.
162. Rohrlich, P., Sarfati, J., Mariani, P., et al.: Prospective sandwich enzyme-linked immunosorbent assay for serum galactomannan: Early predictive value and clinical use in invasive aspergillosis. Pediatr. Infect. Dis. J. *15*:232, 1996.
163. Roilides, E., Holmes, A., Blake, C., et al.: Impairment of neutrophil antifungal activity against hyphae of *Aspergillus fumigatus* in children infected with human immunodeficiency virus. J. Infect. Dis. *167*:905, 1993.
164. Roilides, E., Holmes, A., Blake, C., et al.: Defective antifungal activity of monocyte-derived macrophages from human immunodeficiency virus–infected children against *Aspergillus fumigatus*. J. Infect. Dis. *168*:1562, 1993.
165. Roilides, E., Holmes, A., Blake, C., et al.: Antifungal activity of elutriated human monocytes against *Aspergillus fumigatus* hyphae: Enhancement by granulocyte-macrophage colony-stimulating factor and interferon-gamma. J. Infect. Dis. *170*:894, 1994.
166. Rossi, G., Tortorano, A. M., Viviani, M. A., et al.: *Aspergillus fumigatus* infections in liver transplant patients. Transplant. Proc. *21*:2268, 1989.
167. Saah, D., Raverman, E., Drakos, P. E., et al.: Rhinocerebral aspergillosis in patients undergoing bone marrow transplantation. Ann. Otol. Rhinol. Laryngol. *103*:306, 1994.
168. Sabetta, J. R., Miniter, P., and Andriole, V. T.: The diagnosis of invasive aspergillosis by an enzyme-linked immunosorbent assay for circulating antigen. J. Infect. Dis. *152*:946, 1985.
169. Salmon, M. A.: Aspergilloma of the cerebellum. J. R. Soc. Med. *76*:611, 1983.
170. Schaffner, A., Douglas, H., and Braude, A.: Selective protection against conidia by mononuclear and against mycelia by polymorphonuclear phagocytes in resistance to *Aspergillus*. J. Clin. Invest. *69*:617, 1982.
171. Schonheyder, H., and Andersen, P.: An indirect immunofluorescence study of antibodies to *Aspergillus fumigatus* in sera from children and adults without aspergillosis. Sabouraudia *20*:41, 1982.
172. Schonheyder, H., and Andersen, P.: IgG antibodies to purified *Aspergillus fumigatus* determined by enzyme-linked immunosorbent assay. Int. Arch. Allergy Appl. Immunol. *74*:262, 1984.
173. Schoumacher, R. A., Tiller, R. E., and Berkow, R. L.: Invasive pulmonary aspergillosis in an infant: An unusual presentation of chronic granulomatous disease. Pediatr. Infect. Dis. J. *6*:215, 1987.
174. Schwartz, D. A., Jacquette, M., and Chawla, H. S.: Disseminated neonatal aspergillosis: Report of a fatal case and analysis of risk factors. Pediatr. Infect. Dis. J. *7*:349, 1988.
175. Schwartz, J., Baum, G. L., and Straub, M.: Cavitary histoplasmosis complicated by fungus ball. Am. J. Med. *31*:692, 1961.
176. Shamberger, R. C., Weinstein, H. J., Grier, H. E., et al.: The surgical management of fungal pulmonary infections in children with acute myelogenous leukemia. J. Pediatr. Surg. *20*:840, 1985.
177. Shetty, D., Giri, N., Gonzalez, C. E., et al.: Invasive aspergillosis in human immunodeficiency virus–infected children. Pediatr. Infect. Dis. J. *16*:216, 1997.
178. Sihota, R., Agarwal, H. C., Grover, A. K., et al.: *Aspergillus* endophthalmitis. Br. J. Ophthalmol. *71*:611, 1987.
179. Singh, N., Yu, V. L., and Rihs, J. D.: Invasive aspergillosis in AIDS. South. Med. J. *84*:822, 1991.
180. Sinski, J. T.: The epidemiology of aspergillosis. *In* Al-Doory, Y. (ed.): The Epidemiology of Human Mycotic Disease. Springfield, IL, Charles C Thomas, 1975, pp. 210–226.
181. Sluyter, T.: De Vegetabilibus Organismi Animalis Parasitis ac de novo Epiphyto Pityriasi Versicolore Obvio (Diss.). Berlin, G. Schade, 1847.
182. Solit, R. W., McKeown, J. J., and Smullens, S.: The surgical implications of intracavitary mycetomas (fungus balls). J. Thorac. Cardiovasc. Surg. *62*:411, 1971.
183. Spearing, R. L., Pamphilon, D. H., and Prentice, A. G.: Pulmonary aspergillosis in immunosuppressed patients with hematologic malignancies. Q. J. Med. *59*:611, 1986.
184. Stenson, S., Brookner, A., and Rosenthal, S.: Bilateral endogenous necrotizing scleritis due to *Aspergillus oryzae*. Ann. Ophthalmol. *14*:67, 1982.
185. Stevens, D. A., Kan, V. L., Judson, M. A., et al.: Practice guidelines for diseases caused by *Aspergillus*. Clin. Infect. Dis. *30*:696, 2000.
186. Stynen, D., Goris, A., Sarfati, J., et al.: A new sensitive sandwich enzyme-linked immunosorbent assay to detect galactofuran in patients with invasive aspergillosis. J. Clin. Microbiol. *33*:497, 1995.
187. Sugar, A. M.: Use of amphotericin B with azole antifungal drugs: What are we doing? Antimicrob. Agents Chemother. *39*:1907, 1995.
188. Sutton, D. A., Fothergill, A. W., and Rinaldi, M. G.: Guide to Clinically Significant Fungi. Baltimore, Williams & Wilkins, 1998.

189. Tack, K. J., Rhame, F. S., Brown, B., et al.: *Aspergillus* osteomyelitis: Report of four cases and review of the literature. Am. J. Med. *73*:295, 1982.
190. Tanis, B. C., Verburgh, C. A., van't Wout, J. W., et al.: *Aspergillus* peritonitis in peritoneal dialysis: Case report and a review of the literature. Nephrol. Dial. Transplant. *10*:1240, 1995.
191. Todeschini, G., Murari, C., Bonesi, R., et al.: Oral itraconazole plus nasal amphotericin B for prophylaxis of invasive aspergillosis in patients with hematologic malignancies. Eur. J. Clin. Microbiol. Infect. Dis. *12*:614, 1993.
192. Treger, T. R., Visscher, D. W., Bartlett, M. S., et al.: Diagnosis of pulmonary infection caused by *Aspergillus*: Usefulness of respiratory cultures. J. Infect. Dis. *152*:572, 1985.
193. Tricot, G., Joosten, E., Boogaerts, M. A., et al.: Ketoconazole vs. itraconazole for antifungal prophylaxis in patients with severe granulocytopenia: Preliminary results of two nonrandomized studies. Rev. Infect. Dis. *9*(Suppl.):94, 1987.
194. Trigg, M. E., Morgan, D., Burns, T. L., et al.: Successful program to prevent aspergillus infections in children undergoing marrow transplantation: Use of nasal amphotericin. Bone Marrow Transplant. *19*:43, 1997.
195. Tuncel, E.: Pulmonary air meniscus sign. Respiration *46*:139, 1984.
196. Vail, C. M., and Chiles, C.: Invasive pulmonary aspergillosis: Radiologic evidence of tracheal involvement. Radiology *165*:745, 1987.
197. VandenBergh, M. F. Q., Verweij, P. E., and Voss, A.: Epidemiology of nosocomial fungal infections: Invasive aspergillosis and the environment. Diagn. Microbiol. Infect. Dis. *34*:221, 1999.
198. Varkey, B., and Rose, H. D.: Pulmonary aspergilloma: A rational approach to treatment. Am. J. Med. *61*:626, 1976.
199. Venugopal, P. L., Venugopal, T. L., Gomathi, A., et al.: Mycotic keratitis in Madras. Indian J. Pathol. Microbiol. *32*:190, 1989.
200. Verweij, P. E., Brinkman, K., Kremer, H. P. H., et al.: *Aspergillus* meningitis: Diagnosis by non–culture-based microbiological methods and management. J. Clin. Microbiol. *37*:1186, 1999.
201. Virchow, R.: Beitrage zur Lehre von den beim menschen vorkommenden pflanzlichen Parasiten. Arch. Pathol. Anat. Physiol. Klin. Med. *9*:557, 1856.
202. Wald, A., Leisenring, W., van Burik, J., et al.: Epidemiology of *Aspergillus* infections in a large cohort of patients undergoing bone marrow transplantation. J. Infect. Dis. *175*:1459, 1997.
203. Walker, D. H., and McGinnis, M. R.: Opportunistic fungal infection: What the clinician, pathologist, and mycologist can accomplish if they work together. Clin. Lab. Med. *2*:407, 1982.
204. Walmsley, S., Devi, S., King, S., et al.: Invasive *Aspergillus* infections in a pediatric hospital: A ten-year review. Pediatr. Infect. Dis. J. *12*:673, 1993.
205. Walsh, T. J.: Primary cutaneous aspergillosis—an emerging infection among immunocompromised patients. Clin. Infect. Dis. *27*:453, 1998.
206. Walsh, T. J., and Bulkley, B. H.: *Aspergillus* pericarditis: Clinical and pathologic features in the immunocompromised patient. Cancer *49*:48, 1982.
207. Walsh, T. J., and Hamilton, S. R.: Disseminated aspergillosis complicating hepatic failure. Arch. Intern. Med. *143*:1189, 1983.
208. Walsh, T. J., Hiemenz, J. W., Seibel, N. L., et al.: Amphotericin B lipid complex for invasive fungal infections: Analysis of safety and efficacy in 556 cases. Clin. Infect. Dis. *26*:1383, 1998.
209. Walsh, T. J., Hier, D. B., and Caplan, L. R.: Aspergillosis of the central nervous system: Clinicopathological analysis of 17 patients. Ann. Neurol. *18*:574, 1985.
210. Walsh, T. J., Hutchins, G. M., Bulkley, B. H., et al.: Fungal infections of the heart: Analysis of 51 autopsy cases. Am. J. Cardiol. *45*:357, 1980.
211. Walsh, T. J., and Lee, J. W.: Prevention of invasive fungal infections in patients with neoplastic diseases. Clin. Infect. Dis. *17*(Suppl. 2):468, 1993.
212. Walsh, T. J., Seibel, N. L., Arndt, C., et al.: Amphotericin B lipid complex in pediatric patients with invasive fungal infections. Pediatr. Infect. Dis. J. *18*:702, 1999.
213. Warris, A., Bjørneklett, A., and Gaustad, P.: Invasive pulmonary aspergillosis associated with infliximab therapy. N. Engl. J. Med. *344*:1099, 2001.
214. Washburn, R. G., Gallin, J. I., and Bennett, J. E.: Oxidative killing of *Aspergillus fumigatus* proceeds by parallel myeloperoxidase-dependent and -independent pathways. Infect. Immun. *55*:2088, 1987.
215. Weems, J. J., Jr., Davis, B. J., Tablan, O. C., et al.: Construction activity: An independent risk factor for invasive aspergillosis and zygomycosis in patients with hematologic malignancy. Infect. Control *8*:71, 1987.
216. Weiner, M. H., Talbot, G. H., Gerson, S. L., et al.: Antigen detection in the diagnosis of invasive aspergillosis. Ann. Intern. Med. *99*:777, 1983.
217. Weingarten, J. S., Crockett, D. M., and Lusk, R. P.: Fulminant aspergillosis: Early cutaneous manifestations and the disease process in the immunocompromised host. Otolaryngol. Head Neck Surg. *97*:495, 1987.
218. Weishaar, P. D., Flynn, H. W., Jr., Murray, T. G., et al.: Endogenous aspergillus endophthalmitis. Ophthalmology *105*:57, 1998.
219. Wells, W. J., Fox, A. H., Theodore, P. R., et al.: Aspergillosis of the posterior mediastinum. Ann. Thorac. Surg. *57*:1240, 1994.
220. Westney, G. E., Kesten, S., de Hoyos, A., et al.: *Aspergillus* infection in single and double lung transplant recipients. Transplantation *61*:915, 1996.
221. Whelan, M. A., Stern, J., and de Napoli, R. A.: The computed tomographic spectrum of intracranial mycosis: Correlation with histopathology. Radiology *141*:703, 1981.
222. White, M. H., Anaissie, E. J., Kusne, S., et al.: Amphotericin B colloidal dispersion vs. amphotericin B as therapy for invasive aspergillosis. Clin. Infect. Dis. *24*:635, 1997.
223. Whitehurst, F. O., and Liston, T. E.: Orbital aspergillosis: Report of a case in a child. J. Pediatr. Ophthalmol. Strabismus *18*:50, 1981.
224. Williamson, E. C. M., and Leeming, J. P.: Molecular approaches for the diagnosis and epidemiological investigation of *Aspergillus* infection. Mycoses *42*(Suppl. 2):7, 1999.
225. Wollschlager, C., and Khan, F.: Aspergillomas complicating sarcoidosis. Chest *86*:585, 1984.
226. Yamakami, Y., Hashimoto, A., Yamagata, E., et al.: Evaluation of PCR for detection of DNA specific for *Aspergillus* species in sera of patients with various forms of pulmonary aspergillosis. J. Clin. Microbiol. *36*:3619, 1998.
227. Young, R. C., Bennett, J. E., Vogel, C. L., et al.: Aspergillosis: The spectrum of disease in 98 patients. Medicine (Baltimore) *49*:147, 1970.
228. Yu, B., Niki, Y., and Armstrong, D.: Use of immunoblotting to detect *Aspergillus fumigatus* antigen in sera and urines of rats with experimental invasive aspergillosis. J. Clin. Microbiol. *28*:1575, 1990.
229. Yu, V. L., Muder, R. R., and Poorsattar, A.: Significance of isolation of *Aspergillus* from the respiratory tract in diagnosis of invasive pulmonary aspergillosis. Am. J. Med. *81*:249, 1986.

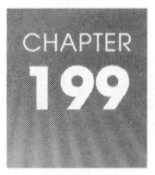

Blastomycosis

GORDON E. SCHUTZE

Blastomyces dermatitidis is a dimorphic fungus that is responsible for a systemic disease characterized by granulomatous and suppurative lesions. Illness occurs when fungal spores are inhaled into the lungs and undergo transition into an invasive yeast phase. Once in the yeast phase, these organisms may not be cleared by bronchopulmonary phagocytes and may proliferate before the development of immunity. The infection may be halted and resolved by the host at this point, or progression of the infection leading to localized pulmonary involvement or extrapulmonary disease may occur. Such dissemination results in the involvement of other organs, most notably the skin and bones. Although the highest prevalence of disease with this organism is observed in North America, blastomycosis has been documented to occur worldwide.

Gilchrist and Stokes[22, 23] were the first to describe blastomycosis in the late 1890s. During the next decade, the heightened awareness of the disease by the medical community produced reports from various regions of the United States, with most cases occurring in the Chicago area.[50] Because of this finding, blastomycosis became known as Chicago disease or Gilchrist disease. A widely accepted concept during these early studies was that two forms of the disease (cutaneous and systemic) existed and that each represented a different portal of entry by the organism. Many years later, Schwarz and Baum[56] established that blastomycosis was a primary pulmonary process and that the cutaneous manifestations were secondary to dissemination from the lung. More recently, blastomycosis became known as North American blastomycosis because of an erroneous belief that the disease was limited to North America, but because this disease now is recognized as having a worldwide distribution, it is known at present as blastomycosis.

The Organism

B. dermatitidis is the causative agent of blastomycosis. The organism has two forms: sexual (the teleomorphic or perfect state) and asexual (the anamorphic or imperfect state). The sexual form of the fungus is named *Ajellomyces dermatitidis*, whereas the asexual form is actually *B. dermatitidis*. The asexual stage exhibits dimorphism, during which the fungus grows as a yeast form at body temperature and as a mycelial form at room temperature. At 37° C, the yeast form appears as a large round organism (6 to 15 µm in diameter) with a thick wall that can produce a single bud (Fig. 199–1). Characteristically, this bud is connected to the parent yeast by a wide base of attachment and usually will equal the size of the parent before detachment. At 25° C to 30° C on laboratory medium, *B. dermatitidis* grows as a white to gray-brown mold (mycelia) with a delicate, silky appearance. Microscopically, the mold is characterized by filamentous colonies composed of thin, uniform septate hyphae (1 to 2 µm in width) that produce conidiophores that branch at right angles to the main hyphal segment. The solitary conidia (spores), which are located at the end of the conidiophores, are small (2 to 10 µm in diameter) and may be oval or pyriform (pear shaped). These conidia are similar to the microconidia of *Histoplasma capsulatum*, but the conidia of *B. dermatitidis* do not form tuberculate macroconidia as do those of *Histoplasma*. The appearance of *B. dermatitidis* mycelia is not pathogenic for the organism, and definitive identification depends on conversion of the organism to the yeast form by culture at 37° C.

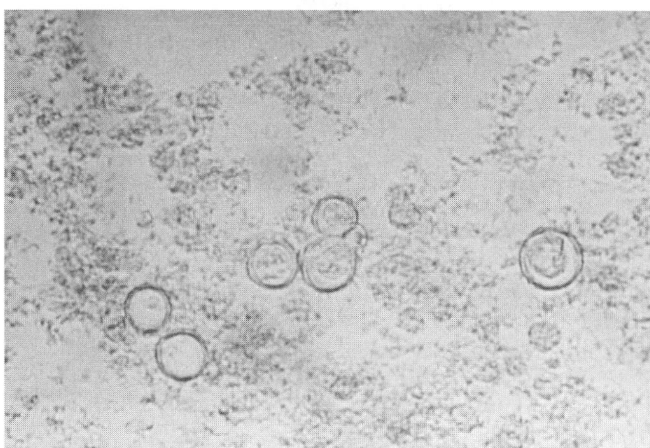

FIGURE 199–1 ■ Wet preparation demonstrating the spherical shape of *Blastomyces dermatitidis*.

Ecology and Epidemiology

Only a paucity of data concerning the ecology and epidemiology of this disease exist. Without data on the ecology of the organism, knowledge about the epidemiology of disease caused by this organism is derived from studies of sporadic cases. Although significant data on the epidemiology of the disease have been gathered with such studies, gaps in our knowledge will become clarified when the ecology of the agent is defined better. Because *B. dermatitidis* cannot be recovered easily from nature and an adequate skin test antigen is not available for conducting population surveys, the present knowledge of this disease is based on case reports of sporadic infections and outbreaks of human and canine disease. The use of new molecular techniques such as polymerase chain reaction may provide fresh insight into the epidemiology of this organism in the coming years.[39]

The natural reservoir of *B. dermatitidis* is not defined as precisely as the reservoirs for other systemic mycoses (e.g., bird droppings, *H. capsulatum*), but this organism is assumed to have its reservoir in a similar habitat as that of the other dimorphic fungi. *B. dermatitidis* appears to be a soil saprophyte and presumably exists in the mycelial form in nature. The organism probably thrives in a location that is high in organic material, is abundant in moisture, has an acid pH, and even may be enriched with animal excreta.[33] The yeast and mycelial phases of the organism appear to disappear rapidly when placed in the soil, whereas conidia can survive for several weeks.[40] Desiccation of such an area with subsequent disturbance of the site results in an infectious aerosol of mycelial fragments and conidia. Conidia also may be released from mycelia on the soil or from decaying material when wetted or disturbed.[29, 31]

Speculation on the natural source of this organism began shortly after it was recognized. Several investigators have noted an association between water and *B. dermatitidis*. Denton and Di Salvo[17] were able to recover the organism in 10 of 356 samples along 1 mile of road by the Savannah River. Furcolow and associates[21] published an extensive review of cases of canine and human blastomycosis that occurred during a prolonged period (1885 to 1968); a high incidence of disease was demonstrated south of the Ohio River and east of the Mississippi River. In addition, at least five human outbreaks of blastomycosis have occurred along river banks.[11, 32, 33, 61] The exact role of the water, however, currently is not understood.

Blastomycosis has been reported to occur worldwide, but many of these reported cases have not withstood scrutiny. Unequivocal cases of blastomycosis from South America have not been described in the last 4 decades. Isolated cases have been reported from England, Switzerland, and Poland, and sporadic infections have been found in the Middle East and India. Most cases, however, are reported from the eastern portion of North America (east of the 100th meridian), with a smaller number scattered throughout Africa.[2]

All age groups are susceptible to blastomycosis. The age distribution varies with each series of cases published because of differences in the populations examined. Most patients, however, are between the ages of 20 and 70 years; only 3 to 11 percent of reported cases occur in patients younger than 20 years.[21, 36, 41] Two patients who were 3 weeks of age or younger have been reported.[38, 63] Exceptions to this age spectrum occur in outbreaks, in which cases in children can predominate. Although some studies in adults have demonstrated a preponderance of males infected with *B. dermatitidis*, previous studies in children and adolescents have not shown such a trend.[35, 49, 59, 66] Case rates for blastomycosis have been described to be highest for African American patients, but the general speculation is that the racial difference in case rates reflects the population in the community of the endemic region. The age, sex, and race distributions of children with blastomycosis therefore appear to be a matter of exposure and not susceptibility of the individual.

Dogs seem to be as susceptible to *B. dermatitidis* as humans. Because of this finding, canine blastomycosis has become a surrogate marker for human blastomycosis. The incidence and prevalence of canine blastomycosis have been studied extensively to supplement our knowledge about the geographic distribution of the disease. Menges and associates[42] were among the first to conclude that humans and dogs acquire their infections from the same source and that no evidence has been found of passive transmission of illness from dog to human or vice versa.

Pathogenesis and Pathology

Five methods of *B. dermatitidis* transmission have been described: inhalation, accidental inoculation, dog bites, conjugal transmission, and intrauterine transmission. By far the most common portal of entry into the body is through the lungs. Not until the work of Schwarz and Baum[56] in the early 1950s did researchers recognize that *B. dermatitidis* was inhaled from the environment and resulted in a subclinical or mild respiratory illness. In most situations, disease at other body sites is a result of hematogenous spread from the lungs, even if not recognized clinically. Primary cutaneous blastomycosis has occurred secondary to accidental needle inoculation, often in a veterinarian or pathologist or via dog bites.[24, 34] Person-to-person spread of blastomycosis does not occur, except in certain situations. One well-recognized case of conjugal transmission and two of intrauterine transmission to neonates have been reported.[13, 38, 63]

Blastomycosis begins with inhalation of the conidia of *B. dermatitidis* into the lungs, followed by an inflammatory response with neutrophils and macrophages. Most conidia are killed easily by these phagocytes, but those that succeed in changing into the yeast form are more resistant to phagocytosis. The large size of the yeast form and resistance to the oxidative mechanisms of killing used by phagocytes render the yeast form more difficult to kill. During the next 4 to 8 weeks, unphagocytosed yeast forms proliferate, and patients may be asymptomatic or complain of an influenza-like illness with fever, arthralgia, myalgia, a productive cough, and pleuritic chest pain.[54] The infection may be halted by the host at this stage, or progression of the infection may lead to localized pulmonary and extrapulmonary disease.

Subclinical cases of blastomycosis probably develop more commonly than symptomatic ones do.[62] The high number of asymptomatic infections supports the theory that healthy individuals are fairly resistant to infection. The exact mechanism of both natural and acquired resistance to infection is not understood. Natural resistance is thought to be mediated by neutrophils, monocytes, and alveolar macrophages. Human neutrophils phagocytize the conidia of *B. dermatitidis* rapidly and effectively, and within 2 hours 90 percent of the conidia are located intracellularly,[20] whereas the yeast forms are moderately resistant to killing by neutrophils. Human alveolar macrophages exhibit phase transition–associated fungicidal and fungistatic activities by irreversibly blocking conidial phase transition to the yeast form or reversibly inhibiting phase transition by causing the accumulation of unusual intermediate forms.[60]

Only recently have we been able to characterize features of acquired resistance in blastomycosis. No relationship between the presence of specific antibody against *B. dermatitidis* and the development of resistance to disease has been found. Specific cellular immunity, however, appears to occur in all patients infected with this organism. Antigen-specific T cells are stimulated to produce lymphokines (e.g., interferon-γ) that activate macrophages, thereby resulting in enhanced fungicidal activity.[4]

Clinical Manifestations

PULMONARY DISEASE

Symptomatic illness develops in approximately 50 percent of infected children, with most of these illnesses initially appearing as an acute or chronic pulmonary process. Patients with acute pulmonary blastomycosis have symptoms similar to those of an acute bacterial process. Cough (which may be productive), fever, malaise, and chest pain are the most common complaints of patients.[49] In many instances, patients may respond initially to routine antimicrobial therapy, only to have their constitutional symptoms return at a later date. Unlike adults, whose disease may take years to progress to a chronic pulmonary process, children's disease rarely progresses longer than 6 months without a return of symptoms.[66]

A mass effect, fibronodular patterns, and consolidation are frequent findings on chest radiography in adults with blastomycosis.[7, 15, 48] Little information exists on the chest radiographic patterns commonly encountered in children, but extensive consolidation of the involved lobes appears to be the most common finding.[9, 35, 49, 55] Consolidation has been described to involve all lobes of the lung and may be multilobar or bilateral. Multiple small cavitary lesions, pleural effusions, hilar adenopathy, and nodular infiltrates also have been described. Mass lesions, which occur commonly in adults, frequently are not demonstrated in children, probably because mass lesions are associated more commonly with chronic disease whereas lobar consolidation is more consistent with acute disease. The consolidation demonstrated on chest radiography may mimic that of an acute bacterial process (Fig. 199–2), whereas the chronic chest abnormalities associated with blastomycosis (e.g., mass lesions, cavitary lesions) may be confused with tuberculosis or neoplasms. Mass lesions, consolidation, air bronchograms, nodular infiltrates, and satellite lesions commonly are found in adults with pulmonary blastomycosis who have undergone computed tomography of the chest.[64] Computed tomographic findings in children have been limited to consolidation, pulmonary abscess, and paratracheal adenopathy[55] (Fig. 199–3). Patients with severe radiographic disease may have slow pulmonary recovery and suffer from long-term sequelae, but most patients with pulmonary blastomycosis have normal pulmonary function testing at follow-up.[1]

DISSEMINATED DISEASE

Even though the numbers are small, disseminated disease appears to be present in 50 to 80 percent of children in whom blastomycosis is diagnosed.[55, 59, 66] The most common site of disseminated disease in children is the bones (Fig. 199–4). Although the long bones (e.g., the tibia, humerus), ribs, and

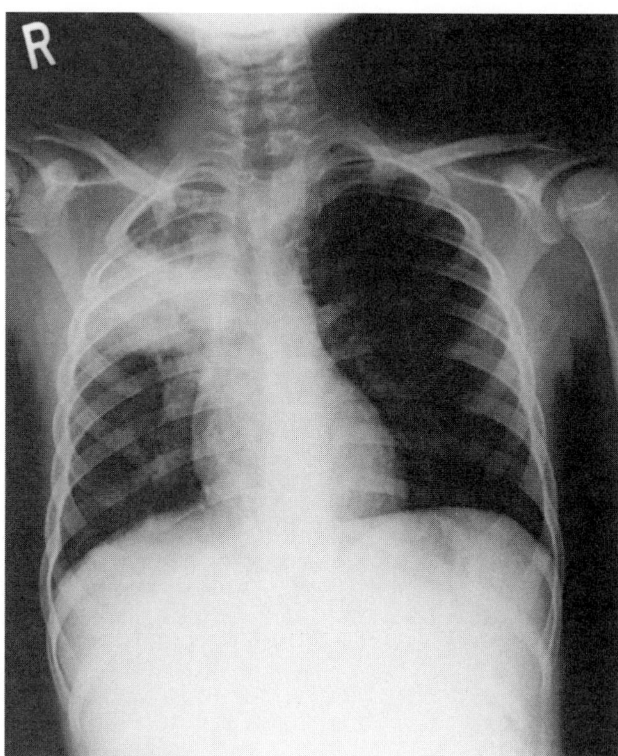

FIGURE 199–2 ■ Chest radiograph of a right upper lobe infiltrate secondary to infection with *Blastomyces dermatitidis*.

vertebrae (Fig. 199–5) are involved most frequently, almost any bone is vulnerable.[51] Skin disease has been described in children, but the classic verrucous lesions seen in adults are uncommon (Fig. 199–6). Pustular or ulcerative lesions may be demonstrated, but they usually occur in children as a result of underlying bony involvement (Figs. 199–7 and 199–8). Skin lesions involving sun-exposed areas of the body (e.g., the nose, ears) also may be seen (Fig. 199–9). Other areas of involvement that have been described include the liver, spleen, heart,

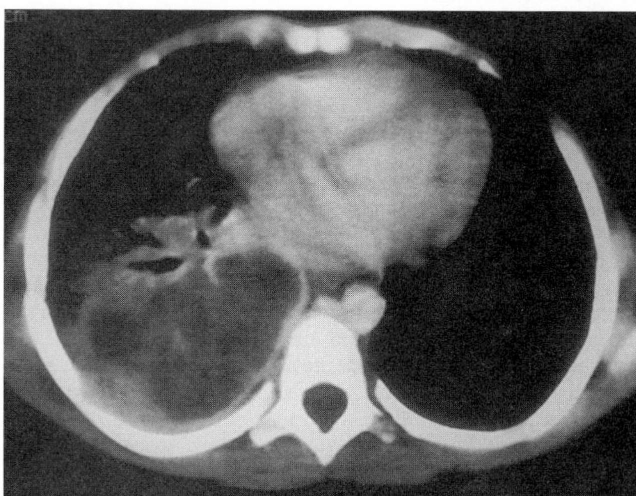

FIGURE 199–3 ■ Computed tomographic scan of the chest revealing consolidation and abscess formation in the right lower lobe of the lung.

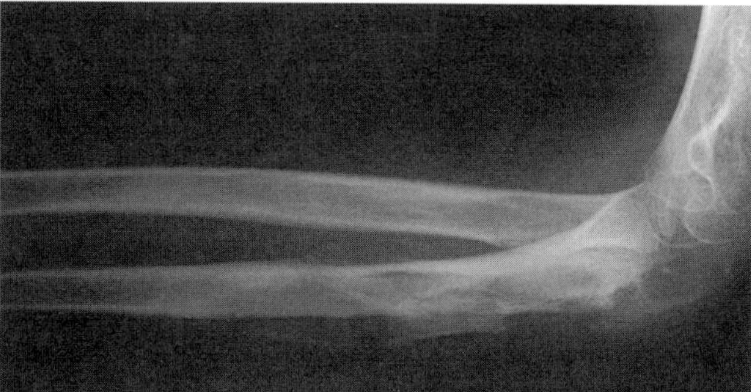

FIGURE 199–4 ■ Bony destruction of the ulna by blastomycosis.

lymph nodes, psoas muscle, kidney, middle ear, and the central nervous system[26, 28, 66] (Fig. 199–10).

DISEASE IN IMMUNOCOMPROMISED PATIENTS

Information concerning infection with *B. dermatitidis* in immunocompromised children is lacking, and only limited data exist on blastomycosis in immunocompromised adults.[47, 57, 65] Unlike other fungi (e.g., *H. capsulatum, Cryptococcus neoformans*), this agent has caused infection in only

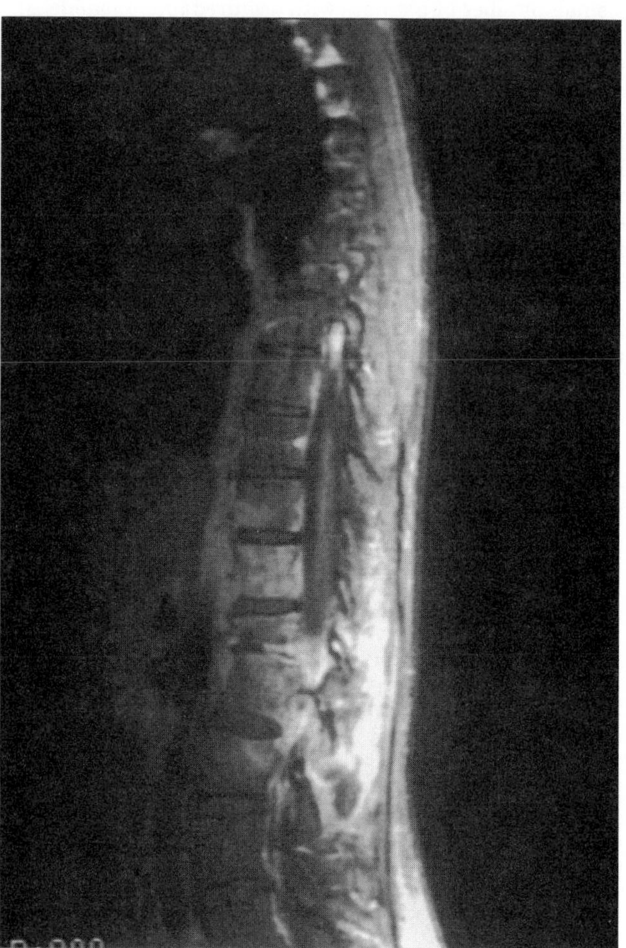

FIGURE 199–5 ■ Magnetic resonance image of the spine demonstrating signal abnormalities at T11 through L3 with a severe compression deformity of the L1 vertebral body and multiple oval lytic lesions caused by blastomycosis.

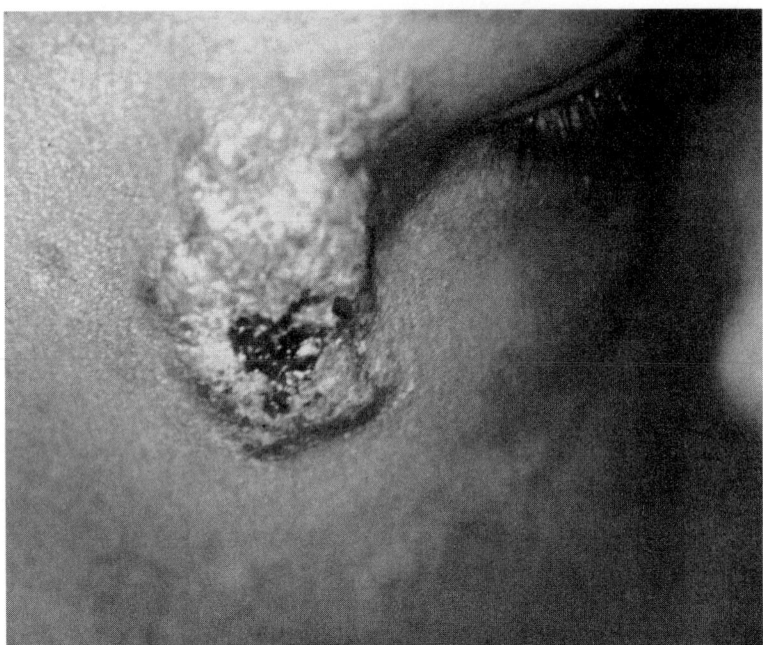

FIGURE 199–6 ■ Verrucous lesion of blastomycosis on the face of a child.

a small number of patients with acquired immunodeficiency syndrome, probably because many of these patients have less exposure to regions endemic for the organism. Pulmonary involvement is the most common manifestation of disease in immunocompromised patients, and adult respiratory distress syndrome is encountered more frequently than in immunologically normal hosts. Multiple organ and central nervous system involvement in these patients is relatively common when compared with normal hosts. Increased mortality rates (30–54%) have been described, with a large proportion of patients who die of other causes having evidence of persistent blastomycosis at the time of death. Many issues regarding therapy for this group of patients are not understood, but lifetime suppressive therapy appears to be indicated.

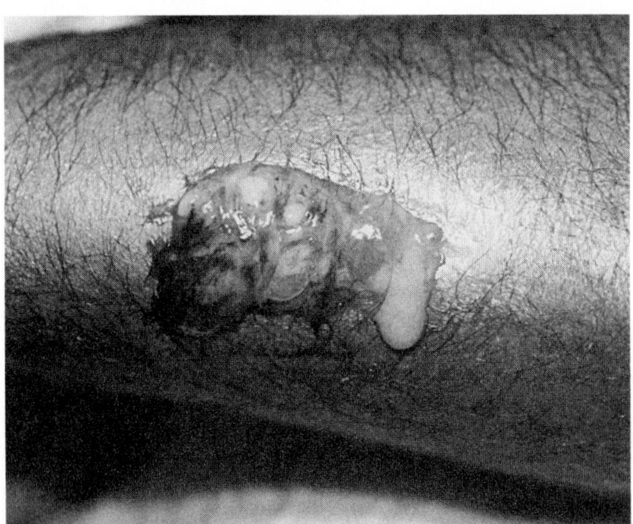

FIGURE 199–7 ■ Purulent wound drainage overlying a region of osteomyelitis with blastomycosis.

DISEASE DURING PREGNANCY

Prenatal diagnosis of blastomycosis in pregnant women has been well documented.[12, 16, 25, 27, 37, 44] Of the seven women described in these reports, evidence of disseminated disease was noted in three, three had pulmonary disease alone, and adult respiratory distress syndrome requiring ventilatory support and early cesarean section developed in the remaining patient. These seven pregnancies culminated in the birth of eight infants (one set of twins). None of the infants was found to be infected at birth, nor did signs or symptoms consistent with blastomycosis develop at a later date. The placentas of the three women with disseminated disease and the woman with adult respiratory distress syndrome were examined for evidence of *B. dermatitidis*. Only the mother with adult respiratory distress syndrome had organisms in the placenta.[37] The organisms were located on the maternal as well as the fetal side of the placenta.

NEONATAL DISEASE

Two neonates who had an acute onset of respiratory distress within 3 weeks of birth and in whom pulmonary blastomycosis was diagnosed have been described.[38, 63] Both infants died of their illness, and abnormalities on autopsy were limited to the lungs. One mother was noted to have lesions consistent with blastomycosis on her face and thigh,[63] whereas the second mother had a lesion on her right lower extremity.[38] Only one mother allowed an extensive physical examination to be performed, and her genital examination was unremarkable. The second mother denied having genital lesions; she refused therapy for blastomycosis and 2.5 years later died of a disseminated illness caused by *B. dermatitidis*. Autopsy findings revealed that her uterus and both ovaries had multiple abscesses, with the left ovary being almost entirely unrecognizable as a result of chronic infection.[67] The pathophysiology of neonatal disease is not understood entirely. Because the pathologic changes caused by *B. dermatitidis* were limited to the lungs in these neonates,

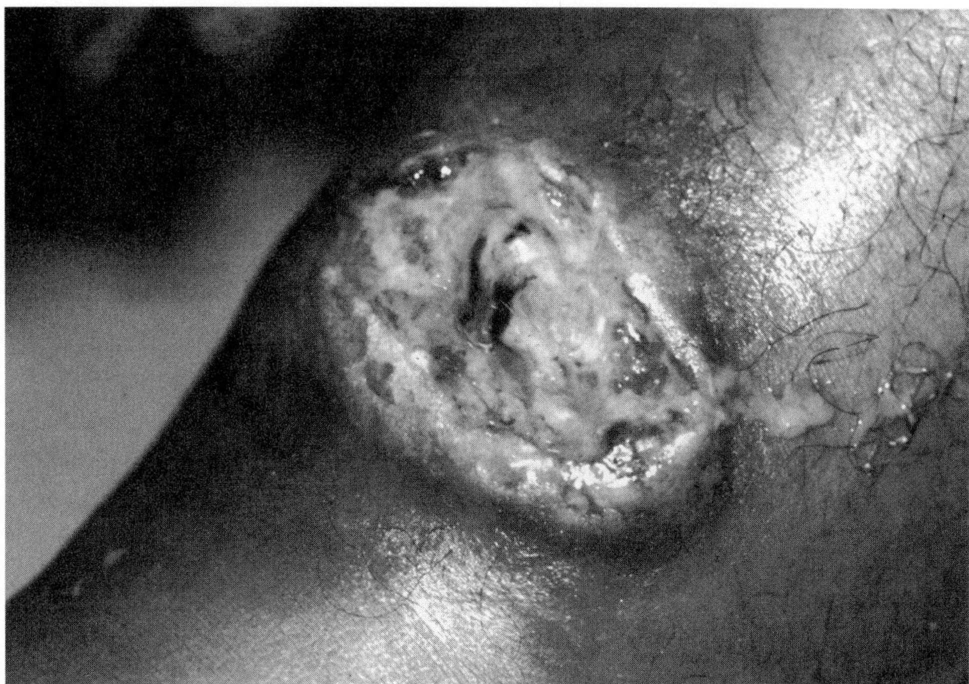

FIGURE 199–8 ■ Ulcerative lesion overlying a region of osteomyelitis secondary to blastomycosis.

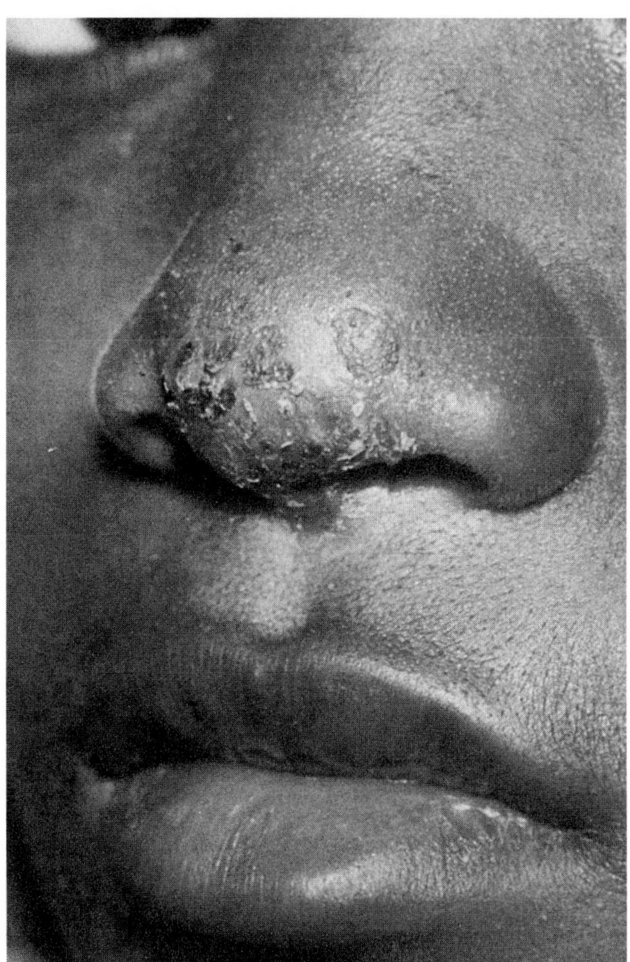

FIGURE 199–9 ■ Crusted skin lesion on the nose caused by *Blastomyces dermatitidis*.

this illness certainly could have been caused by aspiration of vaginal secretions that were colonized with this organism at birth. Autopsy findings in the second mother, however, certainly raise the question of transplacental passage of the organism.

Diagnosis

Because no clinical syndrome is characteristic of blastomycosis, an unequivocal diagnosis requires isolation of the organism from a clinical specimen. A presumptive diagnosis can be made when the characteristic yeast is visualized in respiratory secretions, purulent material, or histopathologic sections. For patients with pulmonary disease, respiratory secretions can be obtained through sputum production, bronchoscopy with bronchoalveolar lavage, or open lung biopsy. Sputum samples are more commonly helpful in older patients; such specimens are difficult to obtain in young children. Likewise, obtaining adequate specimens with the use of bronchoscopy and bronchoalveolar lavage in young children has been shown to be problematic. The need for open lung biopsy in patients with pulmonary blastomycosis after negative results from flexible bronchoscopy and bronchoalveolar lavage demonstrates the technical limitations of this procedure in the pediatric population.[55] Bronchial brushings and bronchoscopically directed biopsy would improve recovery of the organism, but these procedures are technically difficult to perform in younger patients at this time. Because of the difficulty of establishing the diagnosis of pulmonary blastomycosis in young patients, it is recommended that children and adolescents who are suspected of having blastomycosis undergo lung biopsy if sputum and bronchoscopic examination are nondiagnostic.[55]

Respiratory or purulent wound secretions can be examined by light microscopy of wet preparations with or without the use of potassium hydroxide to visualize the characteristic yeast forms. Other staining techniques, such as the calcofluor

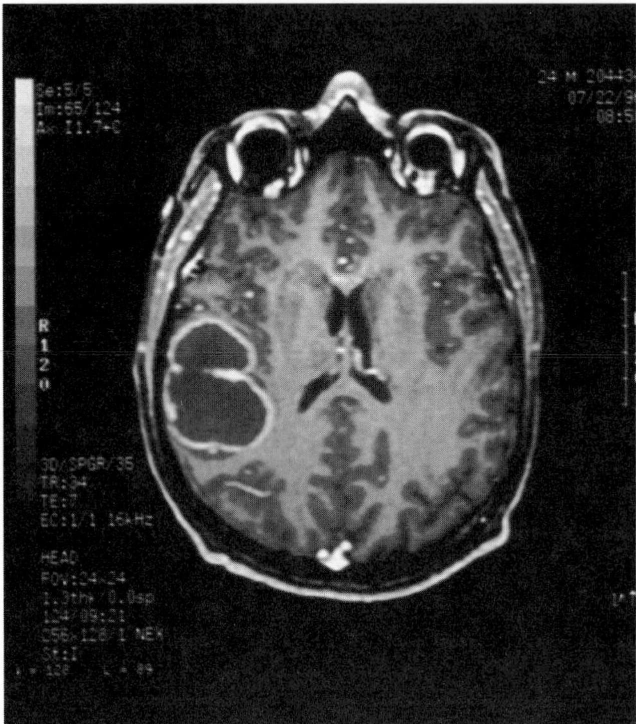

FIGURE 199–10 ■ Computed tomography of the brain demonstrating a multiloculated abscess in the right temporal lobe as a result of infection with *Blastomyces dermatitidis*.

white stain, can be useful for analyzing specimens when the number of organisms in the specimen is limited. Gomori methenamine silver or periodic acid–Schiff stain may be useful for examining histopathologic specimens[36] (Fig. 199–11). The presence of pyogranulomata in a pathologic specimen should alert one to the diagnosis of blastomycosis, but organisms may be difficult to locate with the use of hematoxylin and eosin stains; in such instances, Gomori methenamine silver or periodic acid–Schiff stain may be helpful. Specimens collected for culture should be placed on a culture medium that will ensure recovery of all clinically significant fungi. The use of a more enriched agar, such as Sabouraud agar with brain-heart infusion, is essential for the recovery of such organisms as *B. dermatitidis*. Specimens potentially contaminated with bacteria or other fungal agents should be placed on an additional agar containing antimicrobial agents (e.g., chloramphenicol, cycloheximide) to inhibit the growth of these contaminants.

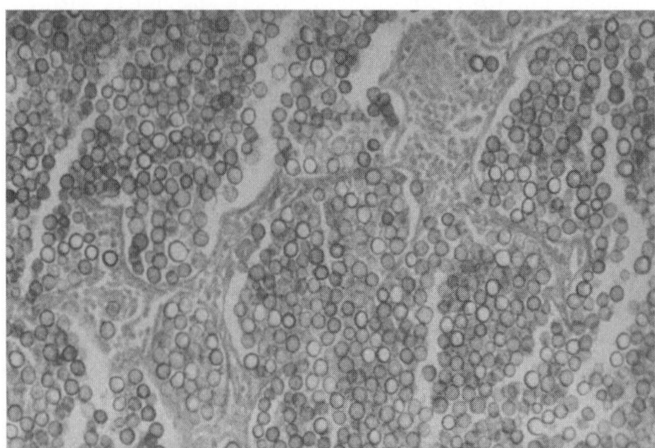

FIGURE 199–11 ■ Overwhelming infection with *Blastomyces dermatitidis* demonstrated in lung tissue with a silver stain.

In some situations, however, isolation attempts are unsuccessful, and alternative laboratory tests may be used. Most currently available serologic tests are performed by complement fixation, immunodiffusion, or enzyme immunoassay with a yeast-phase antigen (A antigen). These assays have been most useful as epidemiologic tools, not for the clinical diagnosis of disease, because of poor sensitivity and specificity resulting from cross-reactivity with the antigens of other fungi (e.g., *H. capsulatum*). The most sensitive of these tests is the commercially available enzyme immunoassay.[5] However, a 120-kDa protein that reacts with antibodies to *Blastomyces* has been identified.[30] This surface protein, designated WI-1, has been demonstrated to be a key antigenic target of humoral and cellular responses during infection. In a study comparing WI-1 and A antigen, WI-1 was found to be more reactive and specific for the binding of serum antibodies to *Blastomyces*.[31] Preliminary testing with WI-1 used as a target in a radioimmunoassay demonstrated that 93 percent of 27 patients with blastomycosis had positive serology within 60 days of diagnosis and that only 5 percent of 84 patients from whom the fungus was not identified were positive.[58] Even though advances have been made, the role of serology remains limited in establishing a diagnosis. If serology is used, the most accurate method of testing is enzyme immunoassay.

Treatment

Before antifungal medications were available, the mortality rate associated with blastomycosis usually exceeded 60 percent. After the introduction of effective medications for the treatment of blastomycosis, all patients received therapy when the diagnosis was established. This concept has been challenged because of the toxicity of amphotericin B and the recognition that self-limited cases of pulmonary blastomycosis exist.[53] Since the advent of safe and effective oral medications for the treatment of blastomycosis in adults, this controversy has lessened.[8] However, for children with blastomycosis, in whom as many as 80 percent have disseminated disease, the decision to withhold therapy for pneumonia secondary to blastomycosis can be dangerous. If a culture diagnosis of blastomycosis is established after the patient has made a spontaneous recovery without therapy, the use of antifungal therapy might be questioned. If therapy is withheld, patients must be monitored carefully for months or even years for evidence of reactivation or dissemination of disease. Accidental introduction of blastomycosis into the skin through needle puncture or bite wounds usually can be treated locally by vigorous cleaning with tincture of iodine, an iodophor, or chlorhexidine.

The use of ketoconazole (400 to 800 mg/day for 6 months) for blastomycosis in adults has achieved cure rates of up to 89 percent.[6] However, little is known about the use of ketoconazole for blastomycosis in children. The recommended dose of ketoconazole in children, as established for the treatment of *Candida* infection, is 5 to 10 mg/kg/day given as a once-daily dose,[14] which would approximate the 400 to 800 mg suggested for blastomycosis in a 70-kg individual. When such a dose was used in five children with blastomycosis, two had relapses (one associated with noncompliance) and two had progression of their disease. The one patient who was cured also underwent a lobectomy, which would have eliminated the area with a large number of organisms.[55] Until more data become available, ketoconazole appears not to be effective for the treatment of blastomycosis in pediatric patients.

Fluconazole has been demonstrated to be effective against blastomycosis in 65 percent of adults at a dose of 200 to 400 mg daily.[46] A treatment failure rate of 30 percent was observed in the high-dose (400 mg/day) group, which included the youngest patient in the study. The investigators concluded that fluconazole was moderately effective against blastomycosis in adults and that its efficacy was similar to that of ketoconazole. No data on the treatment of blastomycosis with fluconazole are available for patients younger than 18 years. Hence, fluconazole does not have a role in the treatment of blastomycosis in pediatric patients.

The recommended therapy of choice for acute non–life-threatening blastomycosis in adults is itraconazole (200 to 400 mg/day) for 6 months.[8, 19, 52] Few data exist on the use of itraconazole in pediatric patients with blastomycosis, but doses of 5 to 10 mg/kg daily have been used safely and effectively in infants and children in other situations.[3, 18, 43, 45] One study used itraconazole (5 to 7 mg/kg/day; maximum, 200 mg/day) to treat four pediatric patients with blastomycosis.[55] Two patients were treated successfully with itraconazole after an initial treatment failure with a previous antifungal regimen. A third patient's initial trial with itraconazole for his pulmonary blastomycosis failed despite directly observed therapy. This patient had undetectable itraconazole levels in his serum, presumably caused by drug-drug interactions between primidone and itraconazole. The fourth patient completed a 6-month course of itraconazole for her pulmonary blastomycosis without relapse. Although data are limited because of the extremely small numbers of patients studied, itraconazole appears to be superior to ketoconazole or fluconazole for the treatment of blastomycosis in children. Because the exact dose has not been established, 5 to 10 mg/kg/day delivered in a single daily or a twice-daily regimen should be used at this time.

The agent with the greatest proven success for the treatment of blastomycosis in pediatric patients remains amphotericin B deoxycholate.[49, 55, 59, 66] A total course of 25 to 30 mg/kg approaches a 100 percent cure rate. Therefore, for patients with life-threatening or central nervous system disease, neonates, and pregnant or immunocompromised patients, amphotericin B deoxycholate is recommended. Lipid preparations of amphotericin B are effective in treating animal models of blastomycosis, but they have not been evaluated adequately for human disease. The limited clinical experience with the lipid preparations, however, does indicate that they may provide an alternative for selected patients who are unable to tolerate amphotericin B deoxycholate.[10]

Specific treatment recommendations are outlined in Table 199–1. In cases of mild to moderate pulmonary disease or mild to moderate non–central nervous system disseminated disease, a combination of amphotericin B and itraconazole may be used. Treatment can be initiated with amphotericin B and changed to itraconazole to complete 6 months of therapy once the patient has been stabilized. In most of instances, this change occurs after approximately 10 to 14 doses of amphotericin B deoxycholate at 1 mg/kg per dose. Caution should be used in patients with osteomyelitis because many experts suggest that these patients should receive a total of 1 year of itraconazole therapy.[8]

Because of the unpredictable nature of drug interactions, any patient receiving itraconazole with other medications that may interact with itraconazole should be monitored closely and have documentation of adequate serum levels. Close follow-up of these patients for identification of those with progression or relapse of their disease is mandatory. If patients do not have a clinical response within 2 to 4 weeks, if adequate serum levels cannot be obtained, or if clinical deterioration is documented, amphotericin B should be substituted for itraconazole for the treatment of blastomycosis.

TABLE 199–1 ▪ TREATMENT RECOMMENDATIONS FOR BLASTOMYCOSIS IN CHILDREN

Type of Disease	Drug of Choice	Alternative
Pulmonary		
Life-threatening	Amphotericin B	May change to itraconazole when patient improves
Mild-moderate	Itraconazole	
Central nervous system	Amphotericin B	
Non-central nervous system		
Life-threatening	Amphotericin B	May change to itraconazole when patient improves
Mild-moderate	Itraconazole	
Immunocompromised host	Amphotericin B	Suppressive therapy should be continued with itraconazole
Neonate	Amphotericin B	

Surgery, other than for establishment of the diagnosis, has a limited role in therapy for blastomycosis. Surgery is indicated for drainage of large abscesses or for removal of devitalized tissue in the occasional patient with osteomyelitis who is responding poorly to therapy. Surgery never should be considered curative and always should be performed in association with appropriate antifungal therapy. The duration of therapy should not be shortened simply because the patient has undergone surgical resection of the involved area.

Isolation of patients with pulmonary disease caused by blastomycosis is not required because the person-to-person spread of this disease has never been attributed to respiratory secretions. Furthermore, no special precautions are required for patients with open wounds caused by blastomycosis.

REFERENCES

1. Alkrinawi, S., and Pianosi, P.: Pulmonary function following blastomycosis in childhood. Clin. Pediatr. (Phila.) *39*:27–31, 2000.
2. Baily, G. G., Robertson, V. J., Neill, P., et al.: Blastomycosis in Africa: Clinical features, diagnosis, and treatment. Rev. Infect. Dis. *13*:1005–1008, 1991.
3. Bhandari, V., and Narang, A.: Oral itraconazole therapy for disseminated candidiasis in low birth weight infants. J. Pediatr. *120*:330, 1992.
4. Bradsher, R. W., Balk, R. A., and Jacobs, R. F.: Growth inhibition of *Blastomyces dermatitidis* in alveolar and peripheral macrophages from patients with blastomycosis. Am. Rev. Respir. Dis. *135*:412–417, 1987.
5. Bradsher, R. W., and Pappas, P. G.: Detection of specific antibodies in human blastomycosis by enzyme immunoassay. South. Med. J. *88*:1256–1259, 1995.
6. Bradsher, R. W., Rice, D. C., and Abernathy, R. S.: Ketoconazole therapy for endemic blastomycosis. Ann. Intern. Med. *103*:872–879, 1985.
7. Brown, L. R., Swenson, S. J., Van Scoy, R. E., et al.: Roentgenologic features of pulmonary blastomycosis. Mayo Clin. Proc. *66*:29–38, 1991.
8. Chapman, S. W., Bradsher, R. W., Jr., Campbell, G. D., Jr., et al.: Practice guidelines for the management of patients with blastomycosis. Clin. Infect. Dis. *30*:679–683, 2000.
9. Chesney, J. C., Gourley, G. R., Peters, M. E., et al.: Pulmonary blastomycosis in children: Amphotericin B therapy and a review. Am. J. Dis. Child. *133*:1134–1139, 1979.
10. Chowfin, A., Tight, R., and Mitchell, S.: Recurrent blastomycosis of the central nervous system: Case report and review. Clin. Infect. Dis. *30*:969–971, 2000.

11. Cockerill, F. R., III, Roberts, G. D., Rosenblatt, J. E., et al.: Epidemic of pulmonary blastomycosis (Namekagon fever) in Wisconsin canoeists. Chest *86*:688–692, 1984.
12. Cohen, I.: Absence of congenital infection and teratogenesis in three children born to mothers with blastomycosis and treated with amphotericin B during pregnancy. Pediatr. Infect. Dis. J. *6*:76–77, 1987.
13. Craig, M. W., Davey, W. N., and Green, R. A.: Conjugal blastomycosis. Am. Rev. Respir. Dis. *102*:86–90, 1970.
14. Cross, J. T., Jr., Hickerson, S. L., and Yamauchi, T.: Antifungal drugs. Pediatr. Rev. *16*:123–129, 1995.
15. Cush, R., Light, R. W., and George, R. B.: Clinical and roentgenographic manifestations of acute and chronic blastomycosis. Chest *69*:345–349, 1976.
16. Daniel, L., and Salit, I. E.: Blastomycosis during pregnancy. Can. Med. Assoc. J. *131*:759–761, 1984.
17. Denton, J. F., and Di Salvo A, F.: Isolation of *Blastomyces dermatitidis* from natural sites at Augusta, Georgia. Am. J. Trop. Med. Hyg. *13*:716–722, 1964.
18. De Repentigny, L., Ratelle, J., Leclerc, J. M., et al.: Repeated-dose pharmacokinetics of an oral solution of itraconazole in infants and children. Antimicrob. Agents Chemother. *42*:404–408, 1998.
19. Dismukes, W. E., Bradsher, R. W., Jr., Cloud, G. C., et al.: Itraconazole therapy for blastomycosis and histoplasmosis. Am. J. Med. *93*:489–497, 1992.
20. Drutz, D. J., and Frey, C. L.: Intracellular and extracellular defenses of human phagocytes against *Blastomyces dermatitidis* conidia and yeasts. J. Lab. Clin. Med. *105*:737–750, 1985.
21. Furcolow, M. L., Chick, E. W., Busey, J. F., et al.: Prevalence and incidence studies of human and canine blastomycosis. I. Cases in the United States, 1885–1968. Am. Rev. Respir. Dis. *102*:60–67, 1970.
22. Gilchrist, T. C.: A case of blastomycetic dermatitis in man. Johns Hopkins Hosp. Rep. *1*:269–283, 1896.
23. Gilchrist, T. C., and Stokes, W. R.: The presence of an *Oidium* in the tissues of a case of pseudo-lupus vulgaris: Preliminary report. Johns Hopkins Hosp. Bull. *7*:129–133, 1896.
24. Gnann, J. W., Jr., Bressler, G. S., Bodet, C. A., et al.: Human blastomycosis after a dog bite. Ann. Intern. Med. *98*:48–49, 1983.
25. Hager, H., Welt, S. I., Cardasis, J. P., et al.: Disseminated blastomycosis in a pregnant woman successfully treated with amphotericin B: A case report. J. Reprod. Med. *33*:485–488, 1988.
26. Hughes, W. T., Franco, S., and Oh, M. H. K.: Systemic blastomycosis in childhood: Case report and review. Clin. Pediatr. (Phila.) *8*:597–601, 1969.
27. Ismail, M. A., and Lerner, S. A.: Disseminated blastomycosis in a pregnant woman: Review of amphotericin B usage during pregnancy. Am. Rev. Respir. Dis. *126*:350–353, 1982.
28. Istorico, L. J., Sanders, M., Jacobs, R. F., et al.: Otitis media due to blastomycosis: Report of two cases. Clin. Infect. Dis. *14*:355–358, 1992.
29. Kitchen, M. S., Reiber, C. D., and Eastin, G. B.: An urban epidemic of North American blastomycosis. Am. Rev. Respir. Dis. *115*:1063–1066, 1977.
30. Klein, B. S., and Jones, J. M.: Isolation, purification, and radiolabeling of a novel 120-kD surface protein on *Blastomyces dermatitidis* yeasts to detect antibody in infected patients. J. Clin. Invest. *85*:152–161, 1990.
31. Klein, B. S., and Jones, J. M.: Purification and characterization of the major antigen WI-1 from *Blastomyces dermatitidis* yeasts and immunological comparison with A antigen. Infect. Immun. *62*:3890–3900, 1994.
32. Klein, B. S., Vergeront, J. M., Di Salvo, A. F., et al.: Two outbreaks of blastomycosis along rivers in Wisconsin: Isolation of *Blastomyces dermatitidis* from riverbank soil and evidence of its transmission along waterways. Am. Rev. Respir. Dis. *136*:1333–1338, 1987.
33. Klein, B. S., Vergeront, J. M., Weeks, R. J., et al.: Isolation of *Blastomyces dermatitidis* in soil associated with a large outbreak of blastomycosis in Wisconsin. N. Engl. J. Med. *314*:529–534, 1986.
34. Larson, D. M., Eckman, M. R., Alber, R. L., et al.: Primary cutaneous (inoculation) blastomycosis: An occupational hazard to pathologists. Am. J. Clin. Pathol. *79*:253–255, 1983.
35. Laskey, W. K., and Sarosi, G. A.: Blastomycosis in children. Pediatrics *65*:111–114, 1980.
36. Lemos, L. B., Guo, M., and Baliga, M.: Blastomycosis: Organ involvement and etiologic diagnosis. A review of 123 patients from Mississippi. Ann. Diagn. Pathol. *4*:391–406, 2000.
37. MacDonald, D., and Alguire, P. C.: Adult respiratory distress syndrome due to blastomycosis during pregnancy. Chest *98*:1527–1528, 1990.
38. Maxson, S., Miller, S. F., Tryka, A. F., et al.: Perinatal blastomycosis: A review. Pediatr. Infect. Dis. J. *11*:760–763, 1992.
39. McCullough, M. J., DiSalvo, A. F., Clemons K. V., et al.: Molecular epidemiology of *Blastomyces dermatitidis*. Clin. Infect. Dis. *30*:328–335, 2000.
40. McDonough, E. S., Van Prooien, R., and Lewis, A. L.: Lysis of *Blastomyces dermatitidis* yeast phase cells in natural soil. Am. J. Epidemiol. *81*:86–94, 1965.
41. Menges, R. W., Doto, I. L., and Weeks, R. J.: Epidemiologic studies of blastomycosis in Arkansas. Arch. Environ. Health *18*:956–971, 1969.
42. Menges, R. W., Furcolow, M. L., Selby, L. A., et al.: Clinical and epidemiologic studies on seventy-nine canine blastomycosis cases in Arkansas. Am. J. Epidemiol. *81*:164–179, 1965.
43. Mouy, R., Veber, F., Blanche, S., et al.: Long-term itraconazole prophylaxis against *Aspergillus* infection in thirty-two patients with chronic granulomatous disease. J. Pediatr. *125*:998–1003, 1994.
44. Neiberg, A. D., Mavromatis, F., Dyke, J., et al.: *Blastomyces dermatitidis* treated during pregnancy: Report of a case. Am. J. Obstet. Gynecol. *128*:911–912, 1977.
45. Neijens, H. J., Frenkel, J., de Muinck Keizer-Schrama, S. M. P. F., et al.: Invasive *Aspergillus* infection in chronic granulomatous disease: Treatment with itraconazole. J. Pediatr. *115*:1016–1019, 1989.
46. Pappas, P. G., Bradsher, R. W., Chapman, S. W., et al.: Treatment of blastomycosis with fluconazole: A pilot study. Clin. Infect. Dis. *20*:267–271, 1995.
47. Pappas, P. G., Threlkeld, M. G., Bedsole, G. D., et al.: Blastomycosis in immunocompromised patients. Medicine (Baltimore) *72*:311–325, 1993.
48. Patel, R. G., Patel, B., Petrini, M. F., et al.: Clinical presentation, radiographic findings, and diagnostic methods of pulmonary blastomycosis: A review of 100 consecutive cases. South. Med. J. *92*:289–295, 1999.
49. Powell, D. A., and Schuit, K. E.: Acute pulmonary blastomycosis in children: Clinical course and follow-up. Pediatrics *63*:736–740, 1979.
50. Ricketts, H. T.: Oidiomycosis (blastomycosis) of the skin and its fungi. J. Med. Res. *6*:373–547, 1901.
51. Saccente, M., Abernathy, R. S., Pappas, P. G., et al.: Vertebral blastomycosis with paravertebral abscess: Report of eight cases and review of the literature. Clin. Infect. Dis. *26*:413–418, 1998.
52. Sarosi, G. A., and Davies, S. F.: Therapy for fungal infections. Mayo Clin. Proc. *69*:1111–1117, 1994.
53. Sarosi, G. A., Davies, S. F., and Phillips, J. R.: Self-limited blastomycosis: A report of 39 cases. Semin. Respir. Infect. *1*:40–44, 1986.
54. Sarosi, G. A., Hammerman, K. J., Tosh, F. E., et al.: Clinical features of acute pulmonary blastomycosis. N. Engl. J. Med. *290*:540–543, 1974.
55. Schutze, G. E., Hickerson, S. L., Fortin, E. M., et al.: Blastomycosis in children. Clin. Infect. Dis. *22*:496–502, 1996.
56. Schwarz, J., and Baum, G. L.: Blastomycosis. Am. J. Clin. Pathol. *21*:999–1029, 1951.
57. Serody, J. S., Mill, M. R., Detterbeck, F. C., et al.: Blastomycosis in transplant recipients: Report of a case and review. Clin. Infect. Dis. *16*:54–58, 1993.
58. Soufleris, A. J., Klein, B. S., Courtney, B. T., et al.: Utility of anti–WI-1 serological testing in the diagnosis of blastomycosis in Wisconsin residents. Clin. Infect. Dis. *19*:87–92, 1994.
59. Steele, R. W., and Abernathy, R. S.: Systemic blastomycosis in children. Pediatr. Infect. Dis. J. *2*:304–307, 1983.
60. Sugar, A. M., Picard, M., Wagner, R., et al.: Interactions between human bronchoalveolar macrophages and *Blastomyces dermatitidis* conidia: Demonstration of fungicidal and fungistatic effects. J. Infect. Dis. *171*:1559–1562, 1995.
61. Tosh, F. E., Hammerman, K. J., Weeks, R. J., et al.: A common source epidemic of North American blastomycosis. Am. Rev. Respir. Dis. *109*:525–529, 1974.
62. Vaaler, A. K., Bradsher, R. W., and Davies, S. F.: Evidence of subclinical blastomycosis in forestry workers in northern Minnesota and northern Wisconsin. Am. J. Med. *89*:470–476, 1990.
63. Watts, E. A., Gard, P. D., and Tuthill, S. W.: First reported case of intrauterine transmission of blastomycosis. Pediatr. Infect. Dis. J. *2*:308–310, 1983.
64. Winer-Muram, H. T., Beals, D. H., and Cole, F. H., Jr.: Blastomycosis of the lung: CT features. Radiology *182*:829–832, 1992.
65. Witzig, R. S., Hoadley, D. J., Greer, D. L., et al.: Blastomycosis and human immunodeficiency virus: Three new cases and review. South. Med. J. *87*:715–719, 1994.
66. Yogev, R., and Davis, T.: Blastomycosis in children: A review of the literature. Mycopathologia *68*:139–143, 1979.
67. Young, L., and Schutze, G. E.: Perinatal blastomycosis: The rest of the story. Pediatr. Infect. Dis. J. *14*:83, 1995.

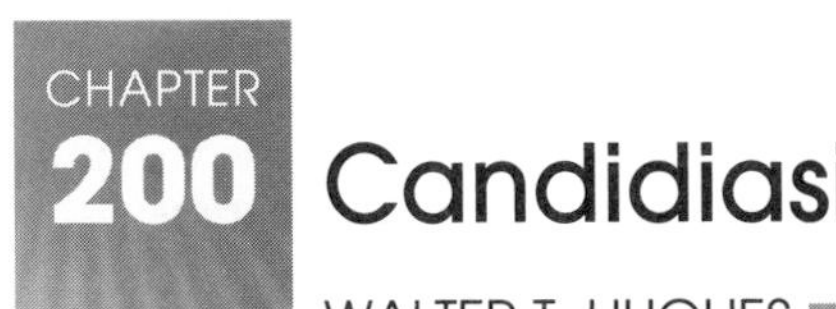

Candidiasis

WALTER T. HUGHES ■ PATRICIA M. FLYNN

Candidiasis is a "white plague" of the immunocompromised host. Clinical expression of the disease implies debility, ranging in magnitude from the weak neonate to the individual with a profound congenital or acquired immunodeficiency disorder. For some 2000 years after Hippocrates described thrush in the mouths of babies, the infection was viewed as an annoying and insignificant superficial disease. Only within the past century has candidiasis of deep organs been recognized. Since the 1960s, certain important therapeutic and diagnostic advances in medicine have affected host defenses and microbial ecology to the extent that these ubiquitous yeasts have gained prominence as pathogens of the first order with capabilities of producing life-threatening disease. Fortunately, in ordinary circumstances, the totally healthy person has little need to fear the malady.

The Organism

Members of the genus *Candida* characteristically are round to oval vegetative cells possessing the ability to produce pseudohyphae (chains of elongated yeast forms) under certain conditions and the inability to develop ascospores (spores within a parent cell). They often are classified as Fungi Imperfecti (Deuteromycetes). The taxonomy of yeasts is far from complete. Organisms of the genus *Torulopsis* have been reclassified as *Candida*. The earlier terms *Monilia* and *Oidium* are obsolete and no longer applied to the genus *Candida*.

The Latin word *candidus* means "dazzling white" and is appropriately applied to the appearance of the thallus (colony). *Candida* spp. form round, well-demarcated, smooth, glistening, and creamy-white colonies on culture media. The yeast form of *Candida* is round to oval, measures 2 to 6 μm in diameter, and reproduces by budding. It does not possess a capsule, a feature that easily differentiates it from species of *Cryptococcus*. It is a dimorphic yeast in that it may, under appropriate conditions, exist as a yeast form (blastospore) or a pseudohyphal form. Some cells may produce septated cylindrical extensions from the blastospore. This phenomenon is called a *germ tube* and can be provoked by the incubation of *Candida* blastospores in human serum. Laboratories have taken advantage of this characteristic to provide quick (tentative) identification of a yeast such as *Candida albicans*. Most *C. albicans* strains undergo chlamydospore formation under controlled stressful conditions. This feature is sufficiently unique to *C. albicans* for use as a diagnostic test. However, a few other yeasts, such as *Candida tropicalis,* may develop chlamydospores. The use of carbohydrate substrates varies sufficiently among *Candida* spp. to serve as a biochemical basis for identification. By determining the use of selected carbohydrates as carbon sources in the presence of oxygen (assimilation) and in the absence of oxygen (fermentation), profiles have been established for the purpose of speciation. Most medically important *Candida* spp. cannot use potassium nitrate as a sole source of nitrogen, although *Candida utilis* is an exception.

Recent application of restriction enzyme analysis of *C. albicans* genomic DNA, using digestion with the restriction endonuclease $E_{CO}RI$, have demonstrated broad genotypic groups (A, B, C, and D) of the species.[120]

More than 150 species of *Candida* have been described, but only a portion of them are considered to be of medical importance; however, a reasonable expectation is that others eventually will be associated with disease in the immunocompromised host. *C. albicans* is by far the most frequent species causing disease in humans. Of considerable concern has been the observation from several sources that disease caused by non-*albicans* species is increasing in prevalence. They include *Candida tropicalis, Candida pseudotropicalis, Candida paratropicalis, Candida krusei, Candida guilliermondi, Candida parapsilosis, Candida lusitaniae, Candida rugosa,* and *Candida stellatoidea.*

HOST SUSCEPTIBILITY

An axiom that most simply expresses the host-parasite relationship of *Candida* spp. and humans can be formulated as follows: extent of disease equals number of organisms times virulence, divided by host resistance. Knowledge accrued to date suggests that little strain-to-strain variation exists in virulence of *C. albicans,* as well as other *Candida* spp., although *C. albicans* usually is more virulent than are other species. Compared with organisms that cause disease in the immunocompetent host, *Candida* spp. possess relatively low virulence factors. Thus, for establishment of a disease state, (1) the host resistance mechanisms must be impaired, (2) the number of organisms to which the host is exposed must be high, or (3) a combination of these characteristics is required.

The importance of the number of organisms to which the host is challenged should not be minimized. For example, a healthy adult volunteer experimentally ingested a suspension of *C. albicans* in the enormous amount of 80 g (more than 10^{12} organisms). Within 3 hours, he was febrile, and *C. albicans* was cultured from blood and urine samples.[100] In practice, the number of organisms to which the patient is exposed usually is not known, and because virulence is rather constant, the predominant determinant for disease is the extent of impairment to normal host defenses. As might be expected, no single defect in the immune response can account for increased susceptibility to infection. However, in one specific form of the disease, chronic mucocutaneous candidiasis, defects in cell-mediated immunity have been well established. Here, the most consistent abnormality involves subnormal production of lymphokines by T cells in response to *Candida* antigens.[92]

Studies of responses of the immunocompetent host to *Candida* spp. suggest that eventually all components of the immune system respond to the microbe. Receptor sites on buccal and vaginal epithelial cells permit adherence of the yeast.[90] Lysozyme (muramidase) causes agglutination and killing of *C. albicans.*[115] Secretory and humoral anti-*Candida* immunoglobulin A (IgA) antibodies are generated.[124] Also, specific anti-*Candida* IgE antibodies are demonstrable.[118] Most normal adults have circulating IgG antibodies to

Candida antigens.[174] Transient IgM antibody response occurs with the infection.[174] IgG antibodies effectively opsonize *C. albicans.* The organism activates the alternative complement pathway.[168] Polymorphonuclear leukocytes,[31] monocytes, and eosinophils[104, 105] ingest and kill *Candida.* A polysaccharide component of *C. albicans* can induce the formation of suppressor lymphocytes,[138] and mitogen-stimulated lymphocytes produce a lymphokine that kills the organism.[37] Unsaturated lactoferrin has antifungal activity that can be reversed with iron, an essential element for growth of *Candida.*[93] The normal skin is resistant to colonization and infection with *Candida* spp. Also, the ecology of the microbial flora of the skin and mucosal surfaces is an important defense system against *Candida* spp.

Using restriction enzyme analysis and hybridization with *C. albicans*–specific DNA probe, genetically distinct strains of *C. albicans* with elevated secretory proteinase production have been associated with diarrhea in hospitalized children, suggesting important virulence factors of the organisms as well as risk for an immunodeficient host.[116]

The underlying diseases and immunocompromising factors that have been associated with increased susceptibility to candidiasis are noted in Table 200–1. A detailed review of disorders that predispose to candidiasis has been prepared by Odds.[132]

Epidemiology

Candida spp. of medical importance have a rather restricted distribution in nature and are found primarily in association with humans and other warm-blooded animals.[132] Even when *C. albicans* has been isolated from soil, foliage, or the atmosphere, it has been at sites where human or animal contamination was probable. *C. stellatoidea* has been isolated only from humans. From 1980 to 1989, the rates of disseminated candidiasis increased 11 times (from 0.013 to 0.15 case per 1000 admissions to United States hospitals).[46] During the 1990s, the rate of fungal liver infection (largely *Candida)* in 731 bone marrow transplantation patients was 9 percent.[150] A recent population-based surveillance for candidemia in Atlanta and San Francisco showed the annual incidence at both sites to be 8 per 100,000 population. The highest incidence (75 per 100,000) occurred among infants 1 year of age and younger. Underlying conditions of those with candidemia were cancer (26%), abdominal surgery (14%), diabetes mellitus (13%), and human immunodeficiency virus (HIV) infection (10%). In one half the cases, species other than *C. albicans* were isolated, especially *C. parapsilosis, Candida glabrata,* and *C. tropicalis.*[88]

In considering colonization rates for *Candida* in people without candidiasis, a distinction must be made between healthy infants and children and those who are hospitalized or suffering from an illness. Also, colonization varies with topographic sites. The frequency of *C. albicans* in isolates as determined in selected studies is given in Table 200–2.

C. albicans organisms, and in some instances other *Candida* spp., have been isolated from monkeys, chimpanzees, baboons, gorillas, cats, dogs, goats, horses, pigs, sheep, cattle, mice, rats, rabbits, chickens, ducks, turkeys, pigeons, parrots, seagulls, sparrows, and other animals.[132]

The transmission of *Candida* under usual circumstances seems to require direct approximation of a colonized site with a susceptible mucous membrane or skin surface. Oral and cutaneous infections in the neonate are acquired from the infected vaginal mucosa during passage of the infant through the birth canal.[98, 126] Transmission between the breast and infant's oral mucosa may result from breast feeding.[61] Intrauterine infection of the fetus is a rare occurrence and has been attributed to ascending infection from the vagina of the mother, although transplacental transmission may be a possible route for infection.[36] Midgley and Clayton[123] were able to culture *C. albicans* readily from the air of rooms housing patients with cutaneous candidiasis. The significance of airborne transmission has not been established. Studies on infant-to-infant transmission of *Candida* in hospital nurseries indicate that cross-infection occurs uncommonly and that segregation of infected infants with thrush has little impact on infection rates.[65, 99] However, recent epidemiologic studies using restriction enzyme analyses have demonstrated that the organism may be acquired from the environment or from staff members in bone marrow transplantation and neonatal intensive care units.[14, 152, 180]

Nosocomial candidiasis has been reported with increased frequency in recent years.[22, 111, 128] Information from the National Nosocomial Infection Surveillance system from 1980 to 1990 noted a fivefold overall increase in the incidence of nosocomial bloodstream infections.[9] A case-control study in nonleukemic, hospitalized patients identified seven risk factors for candidemia: (1) a central line, (2) a bladder catheter, (3) two or more antibiotics, (4) azotemia, (5) transfer from another hospital to a tertiary hospital, (6) diarrhea, and (7) candiduria.[22] An increase in the rate of *C. parapsilosis* has been observed recently in children's hospitals, usually associated with prematurity, presence of central venous catheter, and the use of total parenteral nutrition.[108] New typing procedures for differentiating isolates of *C. albicans* with the use of DNA restriction enzyme fragment analysis offer promise for more powerful epidemiologic studies.[52, 166]

Pathogenesis and Pathology

The initial step in colonization is the adherence of *Candida* blastospores to the mucosal or dermal epithelial cells. Before, during, or after invasion, the filamentous or pseudohyphal form of the organism develops. This transformation may be related to the resistance factors or microenvironmental conditions of the host tissue.[40] As the infection is established, the cascade of events mentioned in the section on host susceptibility ensues, depending on the capabilities and the immunocompetence of the host. Invasion of the mucous membrane results in the formation of an adherent pseudomembrane composed of epithelial cells, leukocytes, keratin, and food debris associated with both blastospore and pseudohyphal forms of *Candida.* Especially in the intestinal tract, mucosal lesions progress to sharply demarcated ulcers, with a base of granulation tissue covered by a fibrinous exudate and granulocytes intermixed with the organisms. Dissemination of *Candida* to deep visceral organs likely is by hematogenous routes. One can deduce that the portal of entry for systemic infection primarily is from mucous membrane lesions. With systemic disease, the kidneys, lungs, liver, brain, and spleen are affected most frequently, although all organs of the body have been involved. With systemic disease, a pyogenic response occurs with formation of microabscesses. Granulomatous reactions can occur but do so infrequently.

Studies have helped to elucidate the pathogenic mechanism of systemic candidiasis. Toxic components of *Candida* have been isolated by Iwata and Yamamoto[80] and others. This "canditoxin" is acutely toxic to mice. Glycoproteins isolated from *C. albicans* by these investigators may act

TABLE 200–1 ■ DISEASES AND COMPROMISING FACTORS THAT PREDISPOSE TO CANDIDIASIS

Category	Selected References	Category	Selected References
Infancy	Baley et al., 1984[7]	Tranquilizers	Pollack et al., 1964[141]
	Baley et al., 1988[8]	Antibiotics	Winner and Hurley, 1964[177]
	Stamos et al.,1995[164]		Odds, 1979[132]
	Botas et al., 1995[20]		Seelig, 1966[155]
	Leibovitz et al., 1992[106]		Smits et al., 1966[159]
	Ward et al., 1983[173]		Caruso, 1964[25];
	Fiax, 1984,[42] 1992[43]		Fitzpatrick and
	Johnson et al., 1984[82]		Topley, 1966[48]
	Odds, 1979[132]		Lehner and Ward, 1970[103]
	Klein et al., 1972[95]		Lehner and Ward, 1970[103]
	Taschdjian and		Toala et al., 1970[169]
	Kozinin, 1957[167]	Corticosteroids	Bernhardt et al., 1972[13]
	Winner and Hurley 1964[177]		Lehner and Ward, 1970[103]
Pregnancy	Stanley et al., 1972[165]		Zegarelli and
	Pederson, 1964[135]		Kutscher, 1964[181]
	Bland et al., 1937[15]		Godfrey et al., 1974[60]
Hypovitaminosis A	Montes et al., 1973[125, 126]	Oral contraceptives	Bourg, 1964[21]
Malnutrition	Barbhaiya, 1966[10]		Walsh et al., 1968[171]
Iron-deficiency anemia	Fletcher et al., 1975[49]		Diddle et al., 1969[32]
		Intravascular catheters	Freeman et al., 1972[55]
Trauma	Mailbach and Kligman,	and hyperalimentation	Glew et al., 1975[59]
	1962[112]		Henderson et al., 1981[66]
	Dixon et al., 1969[33]		Solomon et al., 1984[162]
Diabetes mellitus	Hesseltine, 1955[65]		Michel et al., 1979[122]
	Sonck and Somersalo,1963[163]		Hughes, 1982[72]
Addison disease	Podolsky and		Toala et al., 1970[169]
	Ferguson, 1970[140]	Urinary catheters	Bernhardt et al., 1972[13]
	Hung et al., 1963[76]		Schönebeck 1972[153]
Cushing syndrome	Giombetti et al., 1971[58]		Fisher et al., 1982[45]
Hypothyroidism	Odds, 1979[132]		Toala et al., 1970[169]
Hypoparathyroidism	Odds, 1979[132]	X-irradiation	Chen and Webster, 1974[26]
	Hung et al., 1963[76]	Surgery	Bernhardt et al., 1972[13]
Polyendocrinopathy	Ahonen et al., 1990[1]		Gaines and Remington, 1972[56]
	Anttila, et al., 1994[3]		Richards et al., 1972[146]
Malignancy	Boggs et al., 1961[19]	Organ transplantation	Wingard et al., 1991[176]
	Bodey, 1966[16]		Atkinson et al., 1979[6]
	Schumacher et al., 1964[154]		Goodrich et al., 1991[62]
	Richet et al., 1991[147]		Lipton et al., 1984[110]
	Hughes, 1971[71]		Clift, 1984[28]
	Young et al., 1974[180]	Congenital immune	Edwards et al., 1978[38]
	Robbins et al., 1974[148]	deficiency disorders	
	Kostiala et al., 1982[97]	Acquired immuno-	Gottlieb et al., 1981[63]
	Hughes, 1982[72]	deficiency syndrome	
	Bodey, 1984[17]		
	Maksymiuk et al., 1984[113]		
	Klein et al., 2000[94]		

to release histamine, which accounts for some of the clinical manifestations of the disease.

Clinical Types

Although *Candida* spp. may cause disease at any body site from scalp to toenail, certain areas are affected more frequently than are others. Also, the site and extent of the infection often serve as indicators of the immunocompetence of the host. For example, a healthy-appearing infant with oral thrush or cutaneous candidiasis of the diaper area usually has no underlying immunodeficiency disorder, whereas the patient with chronic mucocutaneous candidiasis or systemic candidiasis likely has a significant underlying abnormality. A topographic classification of candidiasis provides the most useful approach to the clinical features of the disease.

OROPHARYNGEAL CANDIDIASIS

Three patterns of oropharyngeal candidiasis have been described.

Thrush (Acute Pseudomembranous Candidiasis)

Thrush is the most common type of candidiasis in infants and children. The lesions become visible as superficial strands or patches of pearly-white material on the mucosal surface, resembling curds of milk. These lesions may become confluent to form an adherent pseudomembrane composed of desquamated epithelial cells, leukocytes, keratin, necrotic tissue, and food deposits.[35] Blastospore and pseudohyphal forms are abundant, although these organisms rarely penetrate deeper than the stratum corneum. The subepithelial tissues may be involved, with edema and microabscesses. Removal of the pseudomembrane leaves a denuded erythematous lesion. In mild cases, the lesions are not painful. The

TABLE 200–2 ■ COLONIZATION RATES FOR *CANDIDA ALBICANS* IN PATIENTS WITHOUT EVIDENCE OF CANDIDIASIS

Site and Category	Number Studied	Patients with *C. albicans* (%)	Reference
Mouth			
Healthy children (5–18 yr)	503	5.4	Clayton and Noble, 1966[27]
Hospitalized children	200	46.0*	Marks et al., 1975[114]
Normal infants	68	17.6	Dixon et al., 1969[33]
Infants with skin lesions	117	30.6	Dixon et al., 1969[33]
Feces			
Healthy children (school age)	743	12.2	Pan and Pan, 1964[133]
Hospitalized children	86	16.3	Pan and Pan, 1964[133]
Normal infants	69	23.2	Pederson, 1969[136]
Infants with skin lesions	117	41.9	Dixon et al., 1969[33]
Skin			
Normal children	31	0.0	Hughes and Kim, 1973[75]
Fingers, normal children	407	0.6	Clayton and Noble, 1966[27]
Children, chronic leg disorders	86	3.5	Hughes and Kim, 1973[75]
Breast, women in labor	259	0.4	Gillespie et al., 1960[57]
Vagina			
Obstetric patients	1194	27.6	Hurley, 1966[77]
Obstetric patients	6629	21.8	Hurley et al., 1973[78]
Nonpregnant patients	81	24.7	Marks et al., 1971[114]

*Includes all yeast isolates.

sites involved most frequently are the buccal mucosa, dorsum, and lateral areas of the tongue, gingivae, and pharynx. *C. albicans* is by far the most frequent cause of thrush.

Acute Atrophic Candidiasis (Glossitis)

Glossitis occurs as a result of antibiotic therapy and is manifested by erosions of the oral mucosa and depapillation of the dorsum of the tongue. The white pseudomembranous lesions are minimal or absent. The tongue appears smooth and erythematous. Glossodynia (painful tongue) is a frequent complaint. This lesion is believed to evolve from the effects of broad-spectrum, rarely narrow-spectrum, oral antibiotics on the bacterial flora of the mouth. The lesions and symptoms usually resolve after the discontinuation of antibiotics.

Angular Cheilosis (Perlèche)

Perlèche is characterized by fissuring, erythema, and pain at the corners of the mouth. It results from habitual licking at the corners of the mouth, which provides a site for infection with *Candida*. The lesions may become granular, with shiny erythematous erosions and desquamation of the epithelium surrounded by hyperkeratosis.

Two additional *Candida* lesions of the mouth, leukoplakia and chronic atrophic candidiasis, are seen in adults but rarely in children.

ESOPHAGEAL CANDIDIASIS

The most frequent symptom of esophageal candidiasis is dysphagia. Pain may be experienced with swallowing or as a persistent retrosternal, paravertebral, intrascapular, or subscapular annoyance. Nausea and vomiting may occur. Hematemesis and melena rarely occur. About one half of these patients have thrush.[156] Many patients experience no symptoms from esophageal candidiasis. In the immunocompromised host, concomitant infection with herpes simplex virus and bacteria may occur.[37] The site most frequently affected with *Candida* is the inferior one third of the esophagus, although any area may be involved. Endoscopy reveals thrushlike lesions on an erythematous and friable mucosa. An esophagram with barium typically shows ulcerations of the mucosa, which produces a cobblestone-like pattern. In advanced lesions, edema and inflammation may result in tumor-like lesions or strictures. Perforation of the esophagus and fistulas may be found. Often, patients with esophageal candidiasis have no symptoms or signs of oropharyngeal disease.

GASTROINTESTINAL CANDIDIASIS

The true incidence of gastric and intestinal candidiasis is not known. Cases that have been documented adequately have been associated with an underlying abnormality. Gastric lesions have been found predominantly in patients with peptic ulcers or malignancies and after gastric resection. Abdominal pain and weight loss have been noted in such cases.

The association of clinical manifestations and intestinal candidiasis must be approached with caution. Whereas diarrhea and abdominal pain have been reported, substantiation of cause and effect is lacking. Kumar and colleagues[101] attributed the cause of diarrhea to *Candida* in 15 of 592 Indian infants with diarrhea. They were of the opinion that the finding of pseudohyphal forms in fecal specimens was of diagnostic importance. A recent review of the literature concluded that the available data show a strong correlation between cessation of diarrhea in patients with *Candida* spp. in their stools and treatment with an antifungal drug compared with those not so treated.[107]

In 109 children with cancer and systemic candidiasis (deep organ involvement) studied ante mortem and at autopsy, *Candida* lesions were found in the esophagus in 49, stomach in 40, small intestine in 37, and colon in 48. Signs and symptoms could not be attributed accurately to these lesions.[71] More than 30 cases of biliary and gallbladder candidiasis have been reported.[129] *Candida* spp. have been implicated in typhlitis in immunocompromised patients.

PERITONEAL CANDIDIASIS

Peritonitis caused by *Candida* spp. may occur as a complication of peritoneal dialysis or intestinal surgery or with bowel perforation. The typical signs of peritonitis may be absent.[79] Abdominal distention, fever, and vomiting may occur in some cases. Candidal infection of the peritoneal cavity tends to remain localized, and dissemination to other organs is an uncommon occurrence.[12, 81, 161] Clinical features of fungal peritonitis cannot be differentiated from bacterial peritonitis, except by Gram stain and culture of peritoneal fluid.[39] The outcome of fungal peritonitis in children is usually more favorable than in adults undergoing dialysis.[172]

CANDIDIASIS OF THE URINARY TRACT

Candida may cause infections of the kidney, bladder, ureter, and urethra. *Candida* in voided urine is not an uncommon occurrence in the immunocompromised host, in those receiving antibiotics, or in those with an indwelling catheter. Data show that 100,000 or more colonies of *Candida* spp. per milliliter of urine is no more indicative of urinary tract infection than are lower counts.[132] The symptoms of urinary tract candidiasis are similar to those that occur with bacterial infections at respective sites.[45] Lesions similar to oral thrush may be seen by cystoscopy on the bladder mucosa with cystitis. Renal microabscesses, papillary necrosis, calyceal distortion, perinephritic abscesses, and obstructive lesions from a fungus ball may be caused by *Candida*. In 26 cases with candidiasis and candiduria at the Mayo Clinic, 23 (88%) had urinary tract abnormalities.[2]

VAGINAL CANDIDIASIS

Vaginitis caused by *C. albicans* occurs commonly and does not imply necessarily a serious underlying disease. Pruritus and vaginal discharge are the most frequent symptoms. The discharge is white and creamy or watery; the vaginal mucosa is erythematous, with typical lesions of thrush. Skin of the perineum may be involved, with intertriginous papular or ulcerative lesions.

RESPIRATORY TRACT CANDIDIASIS

Candida may affect the respiratory tract in three ways: by colonization of the mucous membrane, by invasive infiltration of deeper tissues, and by an allergic response to the antigens. Any site may be involved. A distinct syndrome of extensive oral candidiasis and hoarseness has been described in patients undergoing immunosuppression therapy for cancer or HIV infection. In these children, discrete plaques can be visualized on the vocal cords by laryngoscopy.[102, 149]

Candidiasis limited to the bronchi rarely occurs and is associated more frequently with pulmonary and systemic disease. Pulmonary candidiasis with invasion of the parenchyma may present as localized or diffuse pneumonia, nodular lesions, abscesses, or empyema.[63, 132, 178] Fever and tachypnea are frequent symptoms, and a definitive diagnosis requires an invasive procedure, such a lung biopsy, to demonstrate the organism in tissue.

Pulmonary allergy is not well defined, but several studies suggest that the entity exists. *C. albicans* has provoked asthmatic attacks in atopic patients.[85] Both polysaccharide and protein extracts of *C. albicans* have induced respiratory reactions.

BONE, JOINT, AND MUSCLE CANDIDIASIS

Candida arthritis has been reported in patients ranging in age from newborns to elderly adults. In most cases, the infection has been associated with systemic candidiasis. The knee has been the joint most frequently affected. Joints may be infected by direct inoculation, in association with osteomyelitis, or from hematogenous spread. Nonsystemic candidal infection occurring after prosthetic arthroplasty has been reported in 10 cases.[30]

Candida osteomyelitis of the spine, wrist, femur, scapula, costochondral junction, humerus, mandible, ribs, and sternum has been reported.[38, 132] More than 22 cases of arthritis and osteomyelitis have been reported in infants younger than 14 weeks of age. Typically, the lesion is a fusiform swelling of the lower extremity and is warm to the touch; radiographs reveal osteolysis and cortical bone erosion.[173] Candidal infection of muscle, in which pain has been the localized symptom, has been described.[5]

CARDIAC CANDIDIASIS

Candida spp. may invade the endocardium, myocardium, and pericardium. The clinical manifestations of *Candida* endocarditis are similar to those found with subacute bacterial endocarditis. Unlike bacterial endocarditis, blood cultures frequently are sterile with the fungal infection. In a review of 319 cases of fungal endocarditis, *Candida* accounted for 67 percent of cases.[120] Of 109 children with systemic candidiasis, 28 had cardiac lesions.[72] Whereas 5 (18%) of the 28 children with carditis had indwelling central venous catheters, only 3 (3.7%) of the 81 without cardiac involvement had catheters. Furthermore, an increase in the incidence of *Candida* carditis was related temporally to the introduction of central venous catheters into the clinical management of cancer patients. The valves involved most commonly are the aortic and mitral; however, infection of all areas of the heart has been described. Lesions of carditis include colonization and invasion of the endocardium with yeast and pseudohyphal forms, emboli occluding major arteries, necrosis, and microabscess formation. Nonspecific electrocardiographic changes with myocarditis include supraventricular arrhythmias, QRS changes, and marked T-wave changes.[54] Rarely, valvular lesions of *Candida* endocarditis may be discernible by two-dimensional echocardiography.

CENTRAL NERVOUS SYSTEM CANDIDIASIS

Primary candidiasis of the brain and meninges is rare, whereas the central nervous system (CNS) frequently is involved in disseminated candidiasis. In a review of 29,659 autopsies, Vorreith[170] found 7 (0.023%) cases with CNS candidiasis; 5 of them also had other organs infected. Nearly a decade later, Parker and associates[134] reported the rate of 0.3 percent of CNS candidiasis in 2040 autopsies. In studies of systemic candidiasis, one fourth[72] to one half[110] have had CNS involvement. Likely, the prevalence of CNS candidiasis is increasing, and in almost all cases, other organs also are involved. In a report of 12 children with candidal meningitis and cancer, the duration of profound neutropenia and fever, antibiotic therapy, and the use of total parenteral nutrition were significant variables compared with the case-matched control subjects. *Candida tropicalis* was the causative species in 11 of the 12 cases. All cases were fatal.[119]

Of 106 premature infants with systemic candidiasis in a large neonatal intensive care unit, 23 had candidal meningitis, most often manifested by respiratory decompensation. Prompt treatment with amphotericin B monotherapy was associated with an excellent outcome.[41]

The neuropathologic lesions include macroabscesses and microabscesses, noncaseating granulomata, diffuse glial nodules, vasculitis, thrombosis, meningitis, ependymitis, mycotic aneurysm, densely packed balls of pseudohyphae, demyelination, and transverse myelitis.[110]

The clinical features are not well defined; they range from signs and symptoms of meningeal inflammation or encephalitis to no discernible CNS abnormality. With meningeal involvement, no more than one half of patients have cerebrospinal fluid pleocytosis or hypoglycorrhachia. If present, the organisms can be visualized with Gram stain. Computed axial tomography and magnetic resonance imaging often help in revealing rather typical, well-demarcated, abscess-like lesions of the brain. The frequent concomitant occurrence of cardiac and CNS candidiasis dictates the need to evaluate patients for both lesions when one is found.

OPHTHALMIC CANDIDIASIS

Candida keratitis may develop after minor trauma but more frequently occurs as a secondary invader of keratitis of other causes when topical antibiotics and corticosteroids are used.[182] In recent years, *Candida* endophthalmitis as a component of systemic candidiasis has been established clearly as a clinical entity—so much so that, in any patient suspected of having systemic candidiasis, a careful examination of the retina is mandatory. The typical lesions are white, cotton-like, chorioretinal abnormalities that may extend to the vitreous. They often resemble a colony of *Candida* growing on blood agar. Color photographs of these lesions are provided in the report by Fishman and colleagues.[47] Pain, blurred vision, "spots before the eyes," scotomata, and photophobia have been associated with the infection.

Candida endophthalmitis has been found frequently in patients receiving intravenous hyperalimentation. In a prospective study, Montgomerie and Edwards[127] found lesions in 5 of 25 such patients, and Henderson and associates[66] reported that 13 (9%) of 131 postoperative patients receiving hyperalimentation developed the lesion. In a careful study of 10 low-birth-weight infants with systemic candidiasis, 4 had retinal lesions.[7] Routinely monitoring patients in these high-risk categories with careful ophthalmoscopic examination seems wise. Retinal infections may occur in other immunocompromised patients with systemic candidiasis. Some experimental evidence suggests that such lesions may not be discernible readily in severely neutropenic patients, possibly because of the lack of inflammatory response.[67]

CUTANEOUS CANDIDIASIS

Candida is a frequent cause of intertrigo or diaper dermatitis in healthy children (see Fig. 65–23). Affected infants often will demonstrate obvious discomfort when urinating onto skin infected with *Candida*. *Candida* paronychia or nail infection is seen most often in healthy children because of thumb sucking or other trauma to the nail or its surrounding tissues. Clinically, profound erythema of the involved tissues is seen. Occasionally, scant purulent discharge may be seen.

Candidal infections of the skin are seen with great frequency in immunocompromised patients. Individuals infected with HIV, patients diagnosed with lymphoproliferative disease, and patients on immunosuppressive medications reperesent a few examples. As a distinct group demonstrating immunodeficiency, neonates have been seen to present with a distinct clinical type of candidal infection. Very premature infants have been noted to have erythema and crusting over dependent or intertriginous areas of skin. This infection has been assumed to be due to a high rate of maternal colonization with *C. albicans*. Although other fungi also have been implicated, *C. albicans* proved to be the cause of most cases reported from our institution. Of great importance was the fact that 69 percent of those children found to have such disease ultimately prove to have disseminated infection. Cheilitis, balanitis, and an interdigital form of cutaneous candidiasis also can be seen. Nystatin is a topical agent for use in cutaneous candidiasis. Ketoconazole, fluconazole, and itraconazole also may be effective.

ACUTE DISSEMINATED (SYSTEMIC) CANDIDIASIS

Disseminated candidiasis may involve any tissue of the body, but in most cases the infection is predominant in two or three organs. The term *disseminated* is used to designate disease in which deep organs of the body are infected with *Candida*. The portals of entry usually are lesions of the gastrointestinal tract or oral mucosa or skin puncture sites, and organisms are disseminated by the hematogenous route to the tissues of one or more organs. Transient candidemia may occur without discernible foci of infection. In severely immunocompromised patients, however, most with candidemia have disseminated disease.[180] The most frequent sites of infection in patients with disseminated candidiasis include the lungs, kidneys, liver, spleen, and brain. The clinical manifestations depend on the sites involved and the extent of involvement. The aforementioned descriptions of topographic infections apply to organs involved with disseminated candidiasis. Infants with the disseminated disease appear clinically similar to those with sepsis caused by other organisms.

Those with underlying conditions who are more likely to have disseminated candidiasis include cancer patients, patients with acquired immunodeficiency syndrome, recipients of organ transplants, debilitated premature infants, patients with indwelling central venous catheters and hyperalimentation lines, and patients with immunodeficiency disorders who have undergone complicated major surgery.

Two clinical manifestations of disseminated candidiasis strongly indicate this infection. One of them is the ocular lesions of *Candida* endophthalmitis described earlier; the other is a maculopapular rash. The skin lesions have been found in patients with hematologic malignancies. In one study, 10 (13%) of 77 patients with disseminated candidiasis and cancer had cutaneous lesions.[18, 86] Typically, the discrete, firm, erythematous papules measure 0.5 to 1 cm in diameter. A nodular center often is surrounded by an erythematous halo. The rash may be generalized, and biopsy specimens show yeast and pseudohyphal forms.

Mycotic cervical lymphadenitis occurring after oral mucositis and neutropenia has been observed in children with cancer and may herald systemic candidiasis.[157] In recent years, disseminated candidiasis has become more prevalent in low-birth-weight infants who require intensive care management. In the study by Baley and associates,[7] the infants had one or more of the following clinical abnormalities: respiratory deterioration, abdominal distention, melena, carbohydrate intolerance, hypotension, candiduria, endophthalmitis, meningitis, skin abscesses, temperature instability, or erythematous rash. The mean age at the time of diagnosis was 1 month. In other cases, carditis, arthritis, and osteomyelitis have occurred.[83] *C. albicans* is the most frequent cause, but other *Candida* spp. also may cause the infection.

Of the organ transplant recipients, those undergoing bone marrow transplantation are at greatest risk for developing disseminated candidiasis. In an autopsy study of 266 bone marrow transplant recipients, 23 had disseminated candidiasis.[28] The incidence was higher in those with aplastic anemia (17.5%) than in those with hematologic malignancies (5.9%).

A study of 109 children with disseminated candidiasis and cancer provides some insight into the clinical features of the infection.[72] These cases were evaluated for 2 months before death, and clinical manifestations were compared with autopsy findings. Fever, granulocytopenia, relapse of the malignancy, and therapy with antibiotics and immunosuppressive drugs made up the clinical profile in about 90 percent of the cases. The major organs involved, in order of highest frequency, were the lungs, spleen, kidney, liver, heart, and brain. In 88 percent of these cases, more than one organ was involved, excluding the gastrointestinal tract; much of this organ involvement was not apparent from clinical evaluation. For example, in one half the patients with *Candida* infection of the pulmonary parenchyma, the lesions were not detectable by radiographs made within the last 10 days of life, whereas 93 percent of the pulmonary lesions were grossly visible at autopsy. Renal and hepatic function tests were normal in one half the patients with candidiasis of these organs. Candiduria was not a dependable indicator of systemic or renal disease. *Candida* carditis occurred more frequently in patients with indwelling central venous catheters.

Despite frequent sampling with antemortem blood cultures (1032 specimens), only 17 percent of pediatric patients yielded the organism. However, 93 percent of these children were colonized at one or more sites with *Candida* spp. Recent studies have shown an increased incidence of hematogenous candidiasis in pediatric patients who are colonized at multiple sites compared with those who are not colonized.[116, 117] Important to note is that candidiasis was the cause of death in only 15 percent of cases. This statistic underscores the need for thorough and repeated evaluation of patients with systemic candidiasis for concomitant infections, especially those of bacterial origin. Other studies have noted similar findings.[113]

Diagnosis

The diagnosis of candidiasis basically requires the association of clinical observations with laboratory tests for the isolation and identification of the organism. In some types of candidiasis, a biopsy may be required to demonstrate the causative organism in diseased tissue.

Direct microscopic examination of materials swabbed or scraped from surface lesions, fluids aspirated from closed lesions, or imprints from biopsy specimens may help to establish a diagnosis quickly. Specimens from surface lesions can be mounted in 10 to 20 percent potassium hydroxide to reveal the ovoid budding yeast cells about 3 to 7 μm in diameter, pseudohyphae, or both. The organisms stain well with periodic acid–Schiff, Gomori methenamine silver nitrate, toluidine blue, or Gram stain. Even typical organisms can be identified only tentatively as *Candida*. In some preparations, differentiating *Aspergillus, Trichosporon,* and *Geotrichum* spp. from *Candida* may be difficult.

In biopsy specimens, the early tissue reaction is acute suppurative inflammation that may progress to granulomatous inflammation. Microabscess formation is frequent. Both yeast and pseudohyphae are found in the diseased tissue.

Candida spp. may be cultured on Sabouraud dextrose media. If specimens are likely to be contaminated with bacteria, chloramphenicol should be incorporated into the media. Cycloheximide, sometimes included in media to prevent saprophytic fungal overgrowth, should not be used because it may inhibit some strains of *Candida*. Blood culture bottles should be vented for optimal growth, although some strains may grow anaerobically. A radiometric blood culture system was found to provide earlier identification of *Candida* and other yeasts than is obtained with the more standard methods.[70] The lysis-centrifugation (Isolator) blood culture method also is reported to improve detection of *Candida* spp. compared with standard methods.[64, 91] On solid media, *Candida* spp. appear as white or cream-colored colonies that are moist and pasty with well-demarcated borders. In contrast to most other species, *C. albicans* produces germ tubes when suspended in human serum, or serum from certain lower animals, for a period of 1 to 4 hours. Biochemical fermentation and assimilation tests serve specifically to identify *Candida* spp.

Many serologic tests for antibody to *Candida* have been studied, but none has proved useful for the specific diagnosis of candidiasis. In recent years, attention has been directed to the detection of antigenic components and metabolic products of *Candida* in blood and other body fluids of patients with systemic forms of candidiasis. Techniques such as precipitation, agglutination, enzyme-linked immunosorbent assay, counterimmunoelectrophoresis, gas-liquid chromatography, and radioimmunoassay have been applied. Techniques for the detection of mannan,[109, 175] cytoplasmic antigen,[4] and D-arabinitol[89] offer promise but have not been perfected for general application in the diagnosis of candidiasis of deep organs. Preliminary studies of polymerase chain reaction have proved successful in identifying clinical specimens with *Candida*.[23, 69, 87]

A definitive diagnosis of deep-organ or disseminated candidiasis is difficult to establish. Cultivation of *Candida* from otherwise sterile body fluids (blood, spinal fluid, bone marrow) with compatible clinical features in an immunocompromised patient, in whom other causes of infection have been excluded, warrants the diagnosis. Computed axial tomography scans are especially helpful in recognizing involvement of the liver, spleen, kidneys, or brain. Lesions at these sites sufficiently are characteristic for a presumptive diagnosis.[11, 51] In patients with hematologic malignancies requiring frequent bone marrow examination, routine cultures of the marrow occasionally reveal *Candida* spp. of clinical significance.[71]

Treatment and Prevention

Several drugs are available for the treatment of candidiasis. Selection of the appropriate drug, or drug combination, depends on the location and extent of infection. Anti-*Candida* drugs in general use include nystatin, clotrimazole, gentian violet, amphotericin B, flucytosine, fluconazole, itraconazole, and ketoconazole.[29] In 2000, an expert panel from the Infectious Diseases Society of America prepared a comprehensive and authoritative set of guidelines for the treatment of candidiasis.[145] These guidelines and the following recommendations for treatment are similar.

Oropharyngeal candidiasis usually responds to the administration of nystatin oral suspension, 200,000 U every 4 to 6 hours for at least 1 week or longer. The suspension is swished in the mouth for 5 minutes or longer and then swallowed. In infants and patients not able to retain the drug in the mouth, the dose should be given at least six times daily. Clotrimazole also is effective and is given as a 10-mg dissolvable troche five or six times daily. The troche is held in the mouth until it dissolves completely.[179] Alternatively, a vaginal suppository of nystatin, 100,000 units every 4 hours, may be held in the mouth until it is dissolved.[35] Gentian violet as a 0.5 or 1.0 percent solution swabbed onto the buccal mucosa twice daily is moderately effective but causes irritation and ulceration of the mucosa with prolonged use. Fluconazole suspension given as a 6-mg/kg dose followed by a single daily dose of 3 mg/kg for 13 days has proved superior to nystatin for the treatment of oropharyngeal candidiasis in immunocompromised children, including those undergoing cancer therapy or with HIV infection.[49] Itraconazole and ketoconazole[74] are also effective but less effective than fluconazole.[145] Severe cases of oral candidiasis, especially in granulocytopenic patients, may benefit from short courses of amphotericin B, 0.5 mg/kg/day intravenously for 3 to 5 days. With bottle- or breast-fed and thumb-sucking infants, these respective sites may be colonized with *Candida;* nystatin cream applied four to six times daily to the skin areas and boiling of bottle nipples (or using disposable nipples) are important techniques in management. Avoidance of antibacterial drugs also is desirable.

Vaginal candidiasis is treated equally well with clotrimazole, miconazole, terconazole, tioconazole, or nystatin suppositories. Butoconazole cream also is effective.[68] Oral fluconazole in a single dose of 150 mg successfully treats vaginal candidiasis in adults.[130, 137]

Esophageal candidiasis is treated with a 2- to 3-week course of fluconazole or itraconazole. Ketoconazole is less effective. Refractory cases may be treated with intravenous amphotericin B (0.3 to 0.7 mg/kg/day) as needed to produce a response.[145] This site is prone to complications of stricture, secondary infection, and perforation.

Candida cystitis, without renal or systemic involvement, can be treated with fluconazole or flucytosine orally, irrigation of the bladder with amphotericin B, or a combination of these drugs.[44, 53, 145, 170] Isolated candiduria has been treated successfully with short courses of intravenous amphotericin B (less than 10 days) in cases in which the therapy mentioned earlier was not successful.[96] Candiduria can be effectively cleared with oral fluconazole for 14 days, but infection recurs after treatment in most cases.[160] With an indwelling catheter, continuous or intermittent irrigation with a solution of 50 μg/mL of amphotericin B in sterile water should be used.[154] The duration of treatment required can be determined by monitoring cultures of urine samples. In patients with renal candidiasis and in those in whom disseminated infection is suspected, intravenous amphotericin B with flucytosine (if the strain is susceptible) provides the most effective treatment, and 4 to 6 weeks of therapy usually is required.

Patients with systemic candidiasis, as well as those with *Candida* ophthalmitis, endocarditis, meningitis, or pneumonitis, should be treated with amphotericin B intravenously initially. When clinically stable and with azole-susceptible strains, fluconazole orally at 6 mg/kg/day may replace amphotericin B for continuation therapy. In mild, uncomplicated systemic candidiasis, some physicians use fluconazole alone for therapy. The studies show that the combination of amphotericin B and flucytosine may be synergistic in the treatment of *Candida* meningitis. Amphotericin B penetrates into the spinal fluid poorly, whereas effective spinal fluid levels of flucytosine are easily achievable. Patients should be maintained on 0.5 to 1 mg/kg/day of amphotericin B as a daily infusion over 4 to 6 hours and 150 mg/kg/day of flucytosine orally in four equally divided doses. A lysosomal preparation of amphotericin B is an option for children who are intolerant of or develop renal dysfunction with conventional amphotericin B. Treatment should be continued for at least 1 month and for longer in complicated cases. Antibiotics and immunosuppressive drugs should be avoided if possible.

Butler and associates[24] treated neonates with systemic candidiasis successfully using amphotericin B alone. If it was associated with a central intravascular catheter, the candidemia was treated with a total course dose of 10 to 15 mg/kg amphotericin B and removal of the device. Similar success with short courses of intravenous amphotericin B (7 to 14 days after sterilization of blood) has been reported after removal of infection-associated devices.[34] For severe, disseminated candidiasis, a total course dose of 25 to 30 mg/kg was used.

Systemic candidiasis treated with intravenous miconazole or ketoconazole is not recommended; it is followed by recovery in only 20[17] to 37 percent of patients.

In febrile, granulocytopenic (less than 500 granulocytes/mm^3) cancer patients with no causative agent identified and infections that fail to respond to broad-spectrum antibiotics within a week or so, the likelihood of systemic fungal infection is sufficient (about 30% of cases) to warrant consideration of empirical amphotericin B therapy.[73, 139] A study of 206 adults with neutropenia and candidemia randomized to receive amphotericin B or fluconazole showed that the treatments were successful in 79 and 70 percent of the patients, respectively ($p = 0.22$).[144] The use of colony-stimulating factors has not been studied adequately in such patients but may offer promise in management.

Of considerable concern is the report by Powderly and associates[142] showing that some *Candida* spp. isolated from severely immunocompromised patients with systemic candidiasis were resistant to the usual concentrations of amphotericin B attainable in vivo. All episodes of candidemia caused by isolates with minimal inhibitory concentrations greater than 0.8 μg/mL of amphotericin B were fatal, whereas one half of those with minimal inhibitory concentrations of 0.8 μg/mL and less recovered. A more recent study by Rex and associates,[143] using the National Committee for Clinical Laboratory Standards method, failed to demonstrate that the results of in vitro susceptibility testing for amphotericin B and fluconazole predicted outcome of therapy for patients with candidemia.

Several studies have evaluated the administration of antifungal drugs prophylactically to patients at high risk for acquiring the infection.[84, 121] Nonabsorbable oral agents are not effective. Fluconazole has been effective in reducing topical and systemic candidiasis in bone marrow transplant recipients.[158, 176] However, an increase in colonization with fluconazole-resistant *Candida* spp. may occur. Double-blind, randomized placebo-controlled studies have shown both fluconazole[151] and itraconazole[131] to be effective in the prevention of invasive systemic fungal infection in profoundly neutropenic patients with cancer. Such approaches must be individualized carefully to specific cases and medical centers.

REFERENCES

1. Ahonen, P., Myllärniemi, S., Sipila, I., et al.: Clinical variation of autoimmune polyendocrinopathy-candidiasis-ectodermal dystrophy (APECED) in a series of 68 patients. N. Engl. J. Med. *322*:1829, 1990.

2. Ang, B. S. P., Telenti, A., King, B., et al.: Candidemia from a urinary tract source: Microbiological aspects and clinical significance. Clin. Infect. Dis. *17*:662, 1993.
3. Anttila, V.J., Ruutu, P., Bondestam, S., et al.: Hepatosplenic yeast infection in patients with acute leukemia: A diagnostic problem. Clin. Infect. Dis. *18*:979, 1994.
4. Araj, G. F., Hopfer, R. L., Chestnut, S., et al.: Diagnostic value of the enzyme-linked immunoadsorbent assay for detection of *Candida albicans* cytoplasmic antigen in sera of cancer patients. J. Clin. Microbiol. *16*:46, 1982.
5. Arena, F. P., Perlin, M., and Brahman, H.: Fever, rash and myalgias of disseminated candidiasis during antifungal therapy. Arch. Intern. Med. *141*:1233, 1981.
6. Atkinson, K., Storb, R., Prentice, R. L., et al.: Analysis of late infections in 89 long-term survivors of bone marrow transplantation. Blood *53*:720, 1979.
7. Baley, J. E., Kliegman, R. M., and Faranoff, A. A.: Disseminated fungal infection in very low-birth-weight infants: Clinical manifestations and epidemiology. Pediatrics *73*:144, 1984.
8. Baley, J. E., and Silverman, R. A.: Systemic candidiasis: Cutaneous manifestations in low birth weight infants. Pediatrics *82*:211, 1988.
9. Banerjee, S. N., Emori, T. G., and Culver, D. H.: Secular trends in nosocomial primary bloodstream infection in the United States, 1980–1989. Am. J. Med. *91*(Suppl. 3B):86S, 1991.
10. Barbhaiya, H. C.: Antifungal prophylaxis during antibiotic therapy. Indian J. Med. Sci. *20*:145, 1966.
11. Bartley, D. L., Hughes, W. T., Parvey, L. S., et al.: Computed tomography of hepatic and splenic fungal abscesses in leukemic children. Pediatr. Infect. Dis. *1*:317, 1982.
12. Bayer, A. S., Blumenkrantz, M. J., Montgomerie, J. Z., et al.: *Candida* peritonitis: Report of 22 cases and review of the English literature. Am. J. Med. *61*:832, 1976.
13. Bernhardt, H. E., Orlando, J. C., Benfield, J. R., et al.: Disseminated candidiasis in surgical patients. Surg. Gynecol. Obstet. *134*:819, 1972.
14. Betremieux, P., Chevrier, S., Quindos, G., et al.: Use of DNA fingerprinting and biotyping methods to study a *Candida albicans* outbreak in a neonatal intensive care unit. Pediatr. Infect. Dis. J. *13*:899, 1994.
15. Bland, P. B., Rakoff, A. E., and Pincus, I. J.: Experimental vaginal and cutaneous moniliasis: Clinical and laboratory study of certain monilias associated with vaginal, oral and cutaneous thrush. Arch. Dermatol. Syph. *36*:760, 1937.
16. Bodey, G. P.: Fungal infections complicating acute leukemia. J. Chronic Dis. *19*:667, 1966.
17. Bodey, G. P.: Candidiasis in cancer patients. Am. J. Med. *77*:13, 1984.
18. Bodey, G. P., and Luna, M.: Skin lesions associated with disseminated candidiasis. J. A. M. A. *229*:1466, 1974.
19. Boggs, D. R., Williams, A. F., and Howell, A.: Thrush in malignant neoplastic disease. Arch. Intern. Med. *107*:354, 1961.
20. Botas, C. M., Kurlat, I., Young, S. M., et al.: Disseminated candidal infections and intravenous hydrocortisone in preterm infants. Pediatrics *95*:883, 1995.
21. Bourg, R.: Les candidiases vaginales ont-elles une incidence hormonale? Bull. Acad. R. Med. Belge *7*:699, 1964.
22. Bross, J., Talbot, G. H., Maislin, G., et al.: Risk factors for nosocomial candidemia: A case-control study in adults without leukemia. Am. J. Med. *87*:614, 1989.
23. Burgener-Kairuz, P., Zuber, J. P., Jaunin, P., et al.: Rapid detection and identification of *Candida albicans* and *Torulopsis (Candida) glabrata* in clinical specimens by species-specific nested PCR amplification of a cytochrome P-450 lanosterol-alpha-demethylase (L1A1) gene fragment. J. Clin. Microbiol. *32*:1902, 1994.
24. Butler, K. M., Rench, M. A., and Baker, C. J.: Amphotericin B as a single agent in the treatment of systemic candidiasis in neonates. Pediatr. Infect. Dis. *9*:51, 1990.
25. Caruso, L. J.: Vaginal moniliasis after tetracycline therapy. Am. J. Obstet. Gynecol. *90*:374, 1964.
26. Chen, T. Y., and Webster, J. H.: Oral monilia study on patients with head and neck cancer during radiotherapy. Cancer *34*:246, 1974.
27. Clayton, Y. M., and Noble, W. C.: Observations on the epidemiology of *Candida albicans*. J. Clin. Pathol. *19*:76, 1966.
28. Clift, R. A.: Candidiasis in the transplant patient. Am. J. Med. *77*:34, 1984.
29. Como, J. A., and Dismukes, W. E.: Oral azole drugs as systemic antifungal therapy. N. Engl. J. Med. *330*:263, 1994.
30. Darouiche, R. O., Hamill, R. J., Musher, D. M., et al.: Periprosthetic candidal infections following arthroplasty. Rev. Infect. Dis. *11*:89, 1989.
31. Diamond, R. D., Krzesicki, R., and Wellington, J.: Damage to pseudohyphal forms of *Candida albicans* by neutrophils in the absence of serum in vitro. J. Clin. Invest. *61*:349, 1978.
32. Diddle, A. W., Gardner, W. H., Williamson, P. J., et al.: Oral contraceptive medication and vulvovaginal candidiasis. Obstet. Gynecol. *34*:373, 1969.
33. Dixon, P. N., Warin, R. P., and English, M. P.: Role of *Candida albicans* infection in napkin rashes. B. M. J. *2*:23, 1969.
34. Donowitz, L. G., and Hendley, J. O.: Short-course amphotericin B therapy for candidemia in pediatric patients. Pediatrics *95*:888, 1995.
35. Dreizen, S.: Oral candidiasis. Am. J. Med. *77*:28, 1984.
36. Dvorak, A. M., and Gavaller, B.: Congenital systemic candidiasis. N. Engl. J. Med. *274*:540, 1966.
37. Edwards, J. E.: *Candida* species. *In* Mandell, G. L., Douglas, R. G., and Bennett, J. E. (eds.): Principles and Practice of Infectious Diseases. 2nd ed. New York, John Wiley & Sons, 1985, pp. 1435–1447.
38. Edwards, J. E., Lehrer, R. I., Stiehm, E. R., et al.: Severe candidal infections: Clinical perspective, immune defense mechanisms, and current concepts of therapy. Am. J. Med. *89*:91, 1978.
39. Eisenberg, E. S., Leviton, I., and Soeiro, R.: Fungal peritonitis in patients receiving peritoneal dialysis: Experience with 11 patients and review of the literature. Rev. Infect. Dis. *8*:309, 1986.
40. Epstein, J. B., Truelove, E. L., and Izutzu, K. T.: Oral candidiasis: Pathogenesis and host defense. Rev. Infect. Dis. *6*:96, 1984.
41. Fernandez, M., Moylett, E. H., Noyola, D. E., Baker, C. J. Candidal meningitis in neonates: a 10-year review. Clin. Infect. Dis. *31*:458, 2000.
42. Fiax, R. G.: Systemic *Candida* infections in infants in intensive care nurseries: High incidence of central nervous system involvement. J. Pediatr. *105*:616, 1984.
43. Fiax, R. G.: Invasive neonatal candidiasis: Comparison of *albicans* and *parapsilosis* infection. Pediatr. Infect. Dis. J. *11*:88, 1992.
44. Fisher, J. F. Candiduria: When and how to treat it. Curr. Infect. Dis. Rep. *2*:523, 2000.
45. Fisher, J. F., Chew, W. H., Shadomy, S., et al.: Urinary tract infection due to *Candida albicans*. Rev. Infect. Dis. *4*:1107, 1982.
46. Fisher-Hoch, S. P., and Hutwagner, L.: Opportunistic candidiases: An epidemic of the 1980s. Clin. Infect. Dis. *21*:897, 1995.
47. Fishman, L. S., Griffin, J. R., Sapico, F. L., et al.: Hematogenous *Candida* endophthalmitis: A complication of candidemia. N. Engl. J. Med. *286*:675, 1972.
48. Fitzpatrick, J. J., and Topley, H. E.: Ampicillin therapy and *Candida* outgrowth. Am. J. Med. Sci. *252*:310, 1966.
49. Fletcher, J., Mather, J., Lewis, M. J., et al.: Mouth lesions in iron-deficiency anemia: Relationship to *Candida albicans* in saliva and the impairment of lymphocyte transformation. J. Infect. Dis. *131*:44, 1975.
50. Flynn, P. M., Cunningham, C. K., Kerkering, T., et al.: Oropharyngeal candidiasis in immunocompromised children: A randomized, multicenter, study of orally administered fluconazole suspension versus nystatin. J. Pediatr. *127*:322, 1995.
51. Flynn, P. M., Shenep, J. L., Crawford, R., Hughes, W. T. Use of abdominal computed tomography for identifying disseminated fungal infection in pediatric cancer patients. Clin. Infect. Dis. *20*:964, 1995.
52. Fox, B. C., Mobley, H. L. T., and Wade, J. C.: The use of a DNA probe for epidemiological studies candidiasis in immunocompromised hosts. J. Infect. Dis. *159*:488, 1989.
53. Fan-Haward, P., O'Donovan, C., Smith, S. M., et al.: Oral fluconazole versus amphotericin B bladder irrigation for treatment of candidal funguria. Clin. Infect. Dis. *21*:960, 1995.
54. Franklin, W. G., Simon, A. B., and Sodeman, T. M.: *Candida* myocarditis without valvulitis. Am. J. Cardiol. *38*:924, 1976.
55. Freeman, J. B., Lemire, A., and Maclean, L. D.: Intravenous alimentation and septicemia. Surg. Gynecol. Obstet. *135*:708, 1972.
56. Gaines, J. D., and Remington, J. S.: Disseminated candidiasis in the surgical patient. Surgery *72*:730, 1972.
57. Gillespie, H. L., Inmon, W. B., and Slater, V.: Incidence of *Candida* in the vagina during pregnancy: Study utilizing the Pagano-Levin culture medium. Obstet. Gynecol. *16*:185, 1960.
58. Giombetti, R., Hagstrom, J. W. C., Landey, S., et al.: Cushing's syndrome in infancy: A case complicated by monilial endocarditis. Am. J. Dis. Child. *122*:264, 1971.
59. Glew, R. H., Buckley, H. R., Rosen, H. M., et al.: Value of prospective *Candida* precipitins in fungemia in patients with hyperalimentation. Surg. Forum *26*:113, 1975.
60. Godfrey, S., Hambleton, G., and König, P.: Steroid aerosols and candidiasis. B. M. J. *2*:387, 1974.
61. Gonzalez-Ochoa, A., and Dominiguez, L.: Algunas observaciones epidimiologicas y patogenicas sobre la moniliasis oral del recien nacido. Rev. Inst. Salub. Enprm. Trop. *17*:1, 1957.
62. Goodrich, J. M., Reed, E. C., Mori, M., et al.: Clinical features and analysis of risk factors for invasive candidal infection after marrow transplantation. J. Infect. Dis. *164*:731, 1991.
63. Gottlieb, M. S., Schroff, R., Schauber, H. M., et al.: *Pneumocystis carinii* pneumonia and mucosal candidiasis in previously healthy homosexual men. N. Engl. J. Med. *305*:1425, 1981.
64. Guerra-Romero, L., Edson, R. S., Cockerill, F. R., III, et al.: Comparison of DuPont Isolator and Roche Septi-Chek for detection of fungemia. J. Clin. Microbiol. *25*:1623, 1987.
65. Harris, L. J.: Further observations on a simple procedure to eliminate thrush from hospital nurseries. Am. J. Obstet. Gynecol. *80*:30, 1959.
66. Henderson, D. K., Edwards, J. E., and Montgomerie, J. Z.: Hematogenous *Candida* endophthalmitis in patients receiving parenteral hyperalimentation fluids. J. Infect. Dis. *143*:655, 1981.
67. Henderson, D. K., Edwards, J. E., Jr., Ishida, K., et al.: Experimental hematogenous *Candida* endophthalmitis diagnostic approaches. Infect. Immun. *23*:858, 1979.

68. Hesseltine, H. C.: Specific therapy for vaginal mycosis. Am. J. Obstet. Gynecol. *70*:403, 1955.
69. Holmes, A. R., Cannon, R. D., Shepherd, M. G., et al.: Detection of *Candida albicans* and other yeasts in blood by PCR. J. Clin. Microbiol. *32*:228, 1994.
70. Hopfer, R. L., Orengo, A., Chestnut, S., et al.: Radiometric detection of yeasts in blood cultures of cancer patients. J. Clin. Microbiol. *12*:329, 1980.
71. Hughes, W. T.: Leukemia monitoring with fungal bone marrow cultures. J. A. M. A. *218*:441, 1971.
72. Hughes, W. T.: Systemic candidiasis: A study of 109 fatal cases. Pediatr. Infect. Dis. *1*:11, 1982.
73. Hughes, W. T., Armstrong, D., Bodey, G. P., et al.: Guidelines for the use of antimicrobial agents in neutropenic patients with unexplained fever. Clin. Infect. Dis. *25*:551, 1997.
74. Hughes, W. T., Bartley, D. L., Patterson, G. G., et al.: Ketoconazole and candidiasis: A controlled study. J. Infect. Dis. *147*:1060, 1983.
75. Hughes, W. T., and Kim, H. K.: Mycoflora in cystic fibrosis: Some ecologic aspects of *Pseudomonas aeruginosa* and *Candida albicans*. Mycopathol. Mycol. Appl. *50*:261, 1973.
76. Hung, W., Migeon, C. J., and Parrott, R. H.: Possible autoimmune basis for Addison's disease in three siblings, one with idiopathic hypoparathyroidism, pernicious anemia and superficial moniliasis. N. Engl. J. Med. *269*:65–68, 1963.
77. Hurley, R.: Pathogenicity of genus *Candida*. *In* Weiner, H. I., and Hurley, R. (eds.): Symposium on *Candida* Infections. London, Livingstone, 1966, pp. 13–25.
78. Hurley, R., Leask, B. G. S., Faktor, J. A., et al.: Incidence and distribution of yeast species and *Trichomonas vaginalis* in the vagina of pregnant women. J. Obstet. Gynaecol. Br. Commonw. *80*:252, 1973.
79. Hurwich, B. J.: Monilial peritonitis. Arch. Intern. Med. *117*:405, 1966.
80. Iwata, K., and Yamamoto, Y.: Glycoprotein toxins produced by *Candida albicans*. *In* The Black and White Yeasts. Proceedings of the Fourth International Conference on the Mycoses, Pan American Health Organizations Scientific Publ. No. 356. Washington, D.C., 1978, pp. 246–257.
81. Jacobs, L. G., Skidmore, E. A., Cardoso, L. A., and Ziv, F.: Bladder irrigation with amphotericin B for treatment of fungal urinary tract infections. Clin. Infect. Dis. *18*:313, 1994.
82. Johnson, D. E., Conroy, M. M., Foker, J. E., et al.: *Candida* peritonitis in the newborn infant. J. Pediatr. *97*:298, 1980.
83. Johnson, D. E., Thompson, T. R., Green, T. P., et al.: Systemic candidiasis in very low-birth-weight infants (1500 grams). Pediatrics *73*:138, 1984.
84. Jones, P. G., Kauffman, C. A., McAuliffe, L., et al.: Ketoconazole vs. nystatin for prevention of fungal infections in neutropenic patients. 23rd Interscience Conference on Antimicrobial Agents and Chemotherapy, 1983, p. 265. Abstract 982.
85. Kabe, J., Aoki, Y., Ishizaki, T., et al.: Relationship of dermal and pulmonary sensitivity to extracts of *Candida albicans*. Am. Rev. Respir. Dis. *104*:348, 1971.
86. Kaidbey, K. H., and Kurban, A. K.: Unusual granuloma of the skin seen in Lebanon. Acta Derm. Venereol. *51*:225, 1971.
87. Kan, V. L.: Polymerase chain reaction for the diagnosis of candidemia. J. Infect. Dis. *168*:779, 1993.
88. Kao, A. S., Brandt, M. E., Pruitt, W. R., et al. The epidemiology of candidemia in two United States cities: Results of a population-based active surveillance. Clin. Infect. Dis. 29:1164, 1999.
89. Kiehn, T. E., Bernard, E. M., Gold, J. W. M., et al.: Candidiasis detection by gas-liquid chromatography of D-arabinitol, a fungal metabolite, in human serum. Science *206*:577, 1979.
90. King, R. D., Lee, J. C., and Morris, A. L.: Adherence of *Candida albicans* and other *Candida* species to mucosal epithelial cells. Infect. Immun. *27*:667, 1980.
91. Kirkley, B. A., Easley, K. A., and Washington, J. A.: Controlled clinical evaluation of Isolator and EXP aerobic blood systems for detection of bloodstream infections. J. Clin. Microbiol. *32*:1547, 1994.
92. Kirkpatrick, C. H.: Host factors in defense against fungal infections. Am. J. Med. *77*:1, 1984.
93. Kirkpatrick, C. H., Green, I., Rich, R. R., et al.: Inhibition of growth of *Candida albicans* by iron-insaturated lactoferrin: Relation to host defense mechanisms in chronic mucocutaneous candidiasis. J. Infect. Dis. *124*:539, 1971.
94. Klein, R. S., Arnsten, J. H., Sobel, J. D. Oropharyngeal *Candida* colonization and human immunodeficiency virus type 1 infection. J. Infect. Dis. 181:812, 2000.
95. Klein, J. D., Yamauchi, T., and Horlick, S. P.: Neonatal candidiasis, meningitis, and arthritis: Observation and a review of the literature. J. Pediatr. *81*:31, 1972.
96. Kohn, D. B., Uehling, D. T., Peters, M. E., et al.: Short-course amphotericin B therapy for isolated candiduria in children. J. Pediatr. *110*:310, 1987.
97. Kostiala, I., Kostiala, A. A., Kahanpää, A., et al.: Acute fungal stomatitis in patients with hematologic malignancies: Quantity and species of fungi. J. Infect. Dis. *146*:101, 1982.
98. Kozinin, P. J., Taschdjian, C. L., and Wiener, H.: Incidence and pathogenesis of neonatal candidiasis. Pediatrics *21*:421, 1958.
99. Kozinin, P. J., Wiener, H., Taschdjian, C. L., et al.: Is isolation of infants with thrush necessary? J. A. M. A. *170*:1172, 1959.
100. Krause, W., Matheis, H., and Wulf, K.: Fungaemia and funguria after oral administration of *Candida albicans*. Lancet *1*:598, 1969.
101. Kumar, V., Chandrasekaran, R., and Kumar, L.: *Candida* diarrhea. Lancet *1*:752, 1976.
102. Lawson, R., Bodey, G., and Luna, M.: Case report: *Candida* infection presenting as laryngitis. Am. J. Med. Sci. *280*:173, 1980.
103. Lehner, T., and Ward, R. G.: Iatrogenic oral candidiasis. Br. J. Dermatol. *83*:161, 1970.
104. Lehrer, R. I.: Measurement of candidal activity of specific leukocyte types in mixed cell population. II. Normal and chronic granulomatous disease eosinophils. Infect. Immun. *3*:800, 1971.
105. Lehrer, R. I.: The fungicidal mechanisms of human monocytes. I. Evidence for myeloperoxidase-linked and myeloperoxidase-independent candidicidal mechanisms. J. Clin. Invest. *53*:338, 1975.
106. Leibovitz, E., Juster-Reicher, A., Amitai, M., et al.: Systemic candidal infections associated with use of peripheral venous catheters in neonates: A 9-year experience. Clin. Infect. Dis. *14*:485, 1992.
107. Levine, J., Dykoski, R. K., and Janoff, E. N.: *Candida*-associated diarrhea: A syndrome in search of credibility. Clin. Infect. Dis. *21*:881, 1995.
108. Levy, I., Rubin, L.G., Vasishtha, S., et al. Emergence of *Candida parapsilosis* as the predominant species causing candidemia in children. Clin. Infect. Dis. *26*:1086, 1998.
109. Lew, M. A., Siber, G. R., Donahue, D. M., et al.: Enhanced detection with enzyme-linked immunosorbent assay of *Candida* marrow in antibody-containing serum after heat extraction. J. Infect. Dis. *145*:45, 1982.
110. Lipton, S. A., Hickey, W. F., Morris, J. H., et al.: Candidal infection in the central nervous system. Am. J. Med. *76*:101, 1984.
111. MacDonald, L., Baker, C., Chenoweth, C. Risk factors for candidemia in a children's hospital. Clin. Infect. Dis. 26:642, 1998.
112. Mailbach, H. I., and Kligman, A. M.: The biology of experimental human cutaneous moniliasis *(Candida albicans)*. Arch. Dermatol. *85*:233, 1962.
113. Maksymiuk, A. W., Thongprasert, S., Hopfer, R., et al.: Systemic candidiasis in cancer patients. Am. J. Med. *77*:20, 1984.
114. Marks, M. I., Marks, S., and Brazean, M.: Yeast colonization in hospitalized and nonhospitalized children. J. Pediatr. *87*:524, 1975.
115. Marquis, G., Montplaisir, S., Gargon, S., et al.: Fungitoxicity of muramidase: Ultrastructural damage to *Candida albicans*. Lab. Invest. *46*:627, 1982.
116. Mathaba, L. T., Paxman, A. E., Ward, P. D., et al. Genetically distinct strains of *Candida albicans* with elevated secretory proteinase production are associated with diarrhoea in hospitalized children. J. Gastroenterol. Hepatol. *15*:53, 2000.
117. Martino, P., Girmenia, C., Micozzi, A., et al.: Prospective study of *Candida* colonization, use of empiric amphotericin B and development of invasive mycosis in neutropenic patients. Eur. J. Clin. Microbiol. Infect. Dis. *13*:797, 1994.
118. Martino, P., Girmenia, C., Vendetti, M., et al.: *Candida* colonization and systemic infection in neutropenic patients: A retrospective study. Cancer *64*:2030, 1989.
119. McCullers, J. A., Vargas, S., Flynn, P. M., et al. Candidal meningitis in children with cancer. Clin. Infect. Dis. *31*:451, 2000.
120. McLeod, R., and Remington, J. S.: Postoperative fungal endocarditis. *In* Duma, R. J. (ed.): Infections of Prosthetic Heart Valves and Vascular Grafts: Prevention, Diagnosis and Treatment. Baltimore, University Park Press, 1977, p. 163.
121. Meunier-Carpentier, F., Cruciani, M., and Klastersky, J.: Oral prophylaxis with miconazole or ketoconazole of invasive fungal disease in neutropenic cancer patients. Eur. J. Cancer Clin. Oncol. *19*:43, 1983.
122. Michel, L., McMichan, J. C., and Bachy, J. L.: Microbial colonization of indwelling central nervous catheter: Statistical evaluation of potential contaminating factors. Am. J. Surg. *137*:745, 1979.
123. Midgley, G., and Clayton, Y. M.: Distribution of dermatophytes and *Candida* spores in the environment. Br. J. Dermatol. *86*:69, 1972.
124. Milne, J. D., and Warnock, D. W.: Antibodies to *Candida albicans* in human cervicovaginal secretions. Br. J. Vener. Dis. *53*:375, 1977.
125. Montes, L. F., Krumdieck, C., and Cornwell, P. E.: Hypovitaminosis A in patients with mucocutaneous candidiasis. J. Infect. Dis. *128*:227, 1973.
126. Montes, L. F., Pittilo, R. F., Hunt, D., et al.: Microbial flora of infant's skin. Arch. Dermatol. *103*:400, 1971.
127. Montgomerie, J. Z., and Edwards, J. E., Jr.: Association of infection due to *Candida albicans* with intravenous hyperalimentation. J. Infect. Dis. *137*:197, 1978.
128. Moro, M. L., Maffei, C., Manso, E., et al.: Nosocomial outbreak of systemic candidiasis associated with parenteral nutrition. Infect. Control Hosp. Epidemiol. *11*:27, 1990.
129. Morris, A. B., Sands, M. L., Shiraki, M., et al.: Gallbladder and biliary tract candidiasis: Nine cases and review. Rev. Infect. Dis. *12*:483, 1990.
130. Multicentre Study Group: Treatment of vaginal candidiasis with a single oral dose of fluconazole. Eur. J. Clin. Microbiol. Infect. Dis. *7*:364, 1988.

131. Nucci, M., Biasoli, I., Akiti, T., et al. A double-blind, randomized, placebo-controlled trial of itraconazole capsules as antifungal prophylaxis for neutropenic patients. Clin. Infect. Dis. *30*:300, 2000.
132. Odds, F. C.: *Candida* and Candidiasis. Baltimore, University Park Press, 1979, p. 382.
133. Pan, N. C., and Pan, I. H.: Prevalence rate of *Candida* species in stool of children in Taipei. J. Formosan Med. Assoc. *63*:396, 1964.
134. Parker, J. C., McClosky, J. J., Solanki, K. V., et al.: Candidiasis: The most common postmortem cerebral mycosis in an endemic fungal area. Surg. Neurol. *6*:123, 1976.
135. Pederson, G. T.: Yeasts isolated from the throat, rectum, and vagina in 60 women examined during pregnancy and 1/2 to 1 year after labour. Acta Obstet. Gynaecol. Scand. *6*[Suppl. 42]:47, 1964.
136. Pederson, G. T.: Yeast flora in mother and child: A mycological-clinical study of women followed up during pregnancy, the puerperium and 5–12 months after delivery, and their children on the 7th day of life and at the age of 5–12 months. Nord. Med. *81*:207, 1969.
137. Perry, C. M., Whittington, R., and McTavish, D.: Fluconazole: An update of its antimicrobial activity, pharmacokinetic properties, and therapeutic use in vaginal candidiasis. Drugs *49*:984, 1995.
138. Piccolella, E., Lombardi, G., and Morelli, R.: Generation of suppressor cells in the response of human lymphocytes to a polysaccharide from *Candida albicans*. J. Immunol. *126*:2151, 1981.
139. Pizzo, P. A., Robichand, K. J., Gill, F. A., et al.: Empiric antibiotics and antifungal therapy for cancer patients with prolonged fever and granulocytopenia. Am. J. Med. *72*:101, 1982.
140. Podolsky, S., and Ferguson, B. D.: Fatal systemic candidiasis following treatment of Addison's crisis in a juvenile diabetic. Diabetes *19*:438, 1970.
141. Pollack, B., Buck, I. F., and Kalmins, L.: An oral syndrome complicating psychopharmacotherapy: Study II. Am. J. Psychiatry *121*:384, 1964.
142. Powderly, W. G., Kobayashi, G. S., Herzig, G. P., et al.: Amphotericin B-resistant yeast infection in severely immunocompromised patients. Am. J. Med. *84*:826, 1988.
143. Rex, J. H., Bennett, J. E., Sugar, A. M., et al.: Intravascular catheter exchange and duration of candidemia. Clin. Infect. Dis. *21*:994, 1995.
144. Rex, J. H., Bennett, J. E., Sugar, A. M., et al.: A randomized trial comparing fluconazole with amphotericin B for the treatment of candidemia in patients without neutropenia. N. Engl. J. Med. *331*:1325, 1994.
145. Rex, J. H., Walsh, T. J., Sobel, J. D., et al. Practice guidelines for the treatment of candidiasis. Clin. Infect. Dis. *30*:662, 2000.
146. Richards, K. E., Pierson, C. L., Bucciarelli, L., et al.: Monilial sepsis in the surgical patient. Surg. Clin. North Am. *52*:1399, 1972.
147. Richet, H. M., Andremont, A., Tancrede, C., et al.: Risk factors for candidemia in patients with acute lymphocytic leukemia. Rev. Infect. Dis. *13*:211, 1991.
148. Robbins, J. S., Mittemeyer, B. T., and Borski, A. A.: Primary renal candidiasis masking transitional-cell carcinoma. Urology *4*:332, 1974.
149. Roig, P., Carrasco, R., Salavert, M., et al.: Laringitis candidiascia e infeccion por VIH: Descripcion de cuatro casos. Rev. Clin. Esp. *191*:261, 1992.
150. Rossetti, F., Brawner, D. L., Bowden, R. et al.: Fungal liver infection in marrow transplant recipients: Prevalence at autopsy, predisposing factors, and clinical features. Clin. Infect. Dis. *20*:8801, 1995.
151. Rotstein, C., Bow, E. J., Laverdiere, M., et al. Randomized placebo-controlled trial of fluconazole prophylaxis for neutropenic cancer patients: benefit based on purpose and intensity of cytotoxic therapy. Clin. Infect. Dis. *28*:311, 1999.
152. Sanchez, V., Vazquez, J. A., Barth-Jones, D., et al.: Nosocomial acquisition of *Candida parapsilosis:* An epidemiologic study. Am. J. Med. *94*:577, 1993.
153. Schönebeck, J.: Asymptomatic candiduria prognosis, complications and some other considerations. Scand. J. Urol. Nephrol. *6*:136, 1972.
154. Schumacher, H. R., Ginns, D. A., and Warren, W.: Fungus infection complicating leukemia. Am. J. Med. Sci. *247*:313, 1964.
155. Seelig, M. S.: Mechanisms by which antibiotics increase the incidence and severity of candidiasis and alter the immunological defense. Bacteriol. Rev. *30*:442, 1966.
156. Sheft, D. J., and Shrago, G.: Esophageal moniliasis, the spectrum of the disease. J. A. M. A. *213*:1859, 1970.
157. Shenep, J. L., Kalwinsky, D. K., Feldman, S., et al.: Mycotic cervical lymphadenitis following oral mucositis in children with leukemia. J. Pediatr. *106*:243, 1985.
158. Slavin, M. A., Osborne, B., Adams, R., et al.: Efficacy and safety of fluconazole prophylaxis for fungal infections after marrow transplantation: A prospective randomized, double-blind study. J. Infect. Dis. *171*:1545, 1995.
159. Smits, B. J., Prior, A. P., and Arablaster, P. G.: Incidence of *Candida* in hospital in-patients and the effects of antibiotic therapy. B. M. J. *1*:208, 1966.
160. Sobel, J. D., Kauffman, C. A., McKinsey, D., et al. Candiduria: A randomized, double-blind study of treatment with fluconazole and placebo. Clin. Infect. Dis. *30*:19, 2000.
161. Solomkin, J. S., Flohr, A. B., Quie, P. G., et al.: The role of *Candida* in intraperitoneal infections. Surgery *88*:524, 1980.
162. Solomon, S. L., Khabbaz, R. F., Parker, R. H., et al.: An outbreak of *Candida parapsilosis* bloodstream infection in patients with parenteral nutrition. J. Infect. Dis. *149*:98, 1984.
163. Sonck, C. E., and Somersalo, O.: The yeast flora of the anogenital region in diabetic girls. Arch. Dermatol. *88*:846, 1963.
164. Stamos, J. K., and Rowley, A. H.: Candidemia in a pediatric population. Clin. Infect. Dis. *20*:571, 1995.
165. Stanley, V. C., Hurley, R., and Carrol, C. J.: Distribution and significance of *Candida* precipitins in sera from pregnant women. J. Med. Microbiol. *5*:313, 1972.
166. Stevens, D. A., Odds, F. C., and Scherer, S.: Application of DNA typing methods to *Candida albicans* epidemiology and correlations with phenotype. Rev. Infect. Dis. *12*:258, 1990.
167. Taschdjian, C. L., and Kozinin, P. J.: Laboratory and clinical studies on candidiasis in the newborn infant. J. Pediatr. *50*:426, 1957.
168. Thong, Y. H., and Ferrante, A.: Alternative pathway of complement activation by *Candida albicans*. Aust. N. Z. J. Med. *8*:620, 1978.
169. Toala, P., Schroeder, S. A., Raly, A. K., et al.: *Candida* at Boston City Hospital. Arch. Intern. Med. *136*:983, 1970.
170. Vorreith, M.: Mycotic encephalitis. Acta Neuropathol. (Berlin) *11*:55, 1968.
171. Walsh, H., Hilderbrandt, R. J., and Prystowsky, H.: Oral progestational agents as a cause of *Candida* vaginitis. Am. J. Obstet. Gynecol. *101*:991, 1968.
172. Warady, B. A., Bashir, M., Donaldson, L. A. Fungal peritonitis in children receiving peritoneal dialysis: a report of the NAPRTCS. Kidney Int. *58*:384, 2000.
173. Ward, R. M., Sattler, F. R., and Dalton, A. S.: Assessment of antifungal therapy in an 800-gram infant with candidal arthritis and osteomyelitis. Pediatrics *72*:234, 1983.
174. Warnock, D. W., Milne, J. D., and Fielding, A. W.: Immunoglobulin classes of human serum antibodies in vaginal candidiasis. Mycopathologia *63*:173, 1978.
175. Wiener, M. H., and Yount, W. J.: Mannan antigenemia in the diagnosis of invasive *Candida* infections. J. Clin. Invest. *58*:1045, 1976.
176. Wingard, J. R., Merz, W. G., Rinaldi, M. G., et al.: Increase in *Candida krusei* infections among patients with bone marrow transplantation and neutropenia treated prophylactically with fluconazole. N. Engl. J. Med. *325*:1274, 1991.
177. Winner, H. I., and Hurley, R.: *Candida albicans*. London, Churchill, 1964, pp. 62–75.
178. Winston, D. J., Chandrasekar, P. H., Lazarus, H. M., et al.: Fluconazole prophylaxis of fungal infections in patients with acute leukemia. Ann. Intern. Med. *118*:495, 1993.
179. Yap, B. S., and Bodey, G. P.: Oropharyngeal candidiasis treated with a troche form of clotrimazole. Arch. Intern. Med. *139*:646, 1979.
180. Young, R. C., Bennett, J. E., Geelhoed, G. W., et al.: Fungemia with compromised host resistance: A survey of 70 cases. Ann. Intern. Med. *80*:605, 1974.
181. Zegarelli, E. V., and Kutscher, A. H.: Oral moniliasis following intraoral topical corticosteroid therapy. J. Oral Ther. *1*:304, 1964.
182. Zimmerman, L. E.: Keratomycosis. Surv. Ophthalmol. *8*:1, 1963.

CHAPTER 201 Coccidioidomycosis

ZIAD M. SHEHAB

Coccidioidomycosis is an infection caused by a dimorphic fungus: *Coccidioides immitis.* The primary pulmonary infection produced by this organism usually is self-limited, but disseminated and fatal disease also may occur. In the United States, coccidioidomycosis is an endemic disease of the southwestern states and results in 100,000 infections per year.[62] In other parts of the United States, it is seen also in individuals who have traveled or lived in the endemic areas of the Southwest or Mexico.[21, 45, 154] The disease is endemic in other areas of the Western Hemisphere, most notably in northern Mexico and in certain countries in South and Central America.[119] With population growth in the endemic areas of the Southwest and increased population mobility, clinicians in nonendemic parts of the country probably will encounter this disease, particularly in its more severe or disseminated forms.

The history[40, 56] of coccidioidomycosis exemplifies the process of chance, insight, and careful scientific study as it applies to the acquisition of medical knowledge. Coccidioidal granuloma, a form of disseminated coccidioidomycosis, first was described by Posadas in 1892 in Argentina. The disease initially was thought to be a form of skin tumor. Rixford and Gilchrist associated it with what they thought was a protozoon resembling coccidia and named it *Coccidioides.* They divided it into two species: *immitis* and *pyogenes.* Ophüls and Moffitt, in 1900, were the first to attribute coccidioidal granuloma to the fungus *C. immitis.* Although investigators earlier had noted fungal growth on cultures from pathologic specimens, they dismissed these organisms as contaminants. Between 1900 and 1936, numerous reports of coccidioidal granuloma appeared in the medical literature, but the association between coccidioidal granuloma and acute pulmonary infection remained unrecognized. In 1936, Gifford and associates[69] and Dickson[47] were responsible for demonstrating the concept that *C. immitis* could cause either a primary or a secondary type of illness. The primary form previously had been known in California as San Joaquin fever or valley fever.

In the period that followed, the epidemiology of the disease[146, 151] and the ecology of the organism[52, 104] were studied carefully by many investigators, led by the effort of Dr. Charles Smith. Many different forms of therapy for the disseminated disease were tried during this era, but none proved satisfactory.[56] In 1957, amphotericin B became available, and the prognosis associated with the disseminated form of the disease improved with the advent of effective antifungal therapy.

As with many pathogenic fungi, the life cycle of *C. immitis* has two distinct phases: a saprophytic, or vegetative, phase and a parasitic phase. In nature and on most laboratory media, the organism grows as a mycelium with branching, septate hyphae. After 5 to 7 days, the aerial mycelia show the development of rectangular spores (arthrospores, arthroconidia) separated by empty nonviable cells[37] (Fig. 201–1). At this stage, the hyphae become fragile, and the arthroconidia, which measure 2 to 8 μm in diameter, easily become airborne. Because of their size, they can reach the alveolar spaces of the lung when inhaled.

On gaining access to the tissues of the mammalian host, the arthroconidia begin the parasitic phase of their life cycle. They enlarge and in approximately 48 hours develop into spherules that undergo internal segmentation and contain endospores 2 to 5 μm in size. The spherules (Fig. 201–2) are round, double-walled structures 20 to 100 μm in diameter. The endospores are released into the surrounding tissues by rupture of the spherule wall. These endospores, in turn, may mature into spherules in vivo, thereby repeating the tissue phase of the life cycle of the organism. Alternatively, when the spherule ruptures and releases endospores into the environment, hyphal formation can occur, and the cycle thus is repeated in nature.[88]

C. immitis grows on laboratory media relatively easily and produces colonies that become visible in 3 to 4 days. They represent the mycelial phase of the fungus and appear as flat, smooth, and gray colonies from which spicules may project in some whereas others have the look of a velvety membrane. The colonies appear as tufts in the second week and then develop cobweb-like aerial hyphae. Pigmentation may be seen after 2 weeks and is observed best as a brownish undersurface. Variability in colony morphology can be significant, but only one species of *C. immitis* is recognized

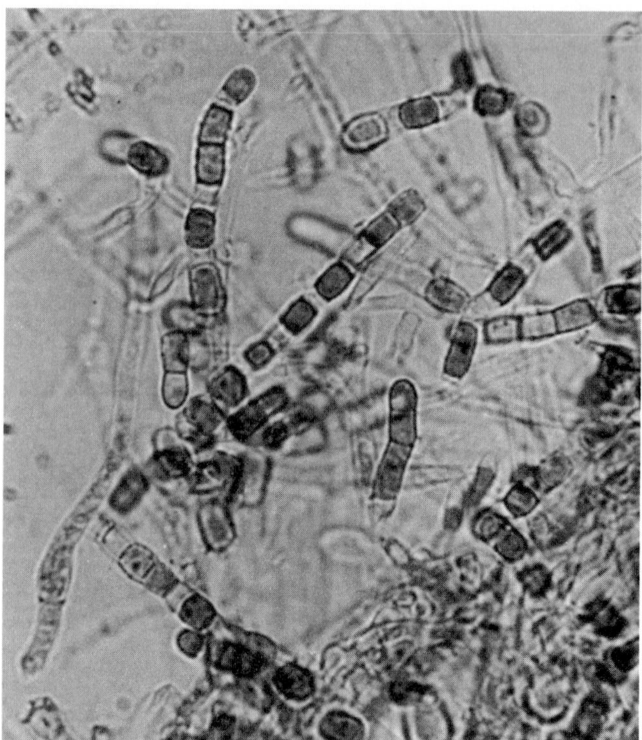

FIGURE 201–1 ■ Mycelial form of *Coccidioides immitis.* Arthroconidia are separated by vacuolated cells. (From Davis, B. D., Delbecco, R., Eisen, H. W., et al.: Microbiology: Including Immunology and Molecular Genetics. 3rd ed. Hagerstown, MD, Harper & Row, 1980.)

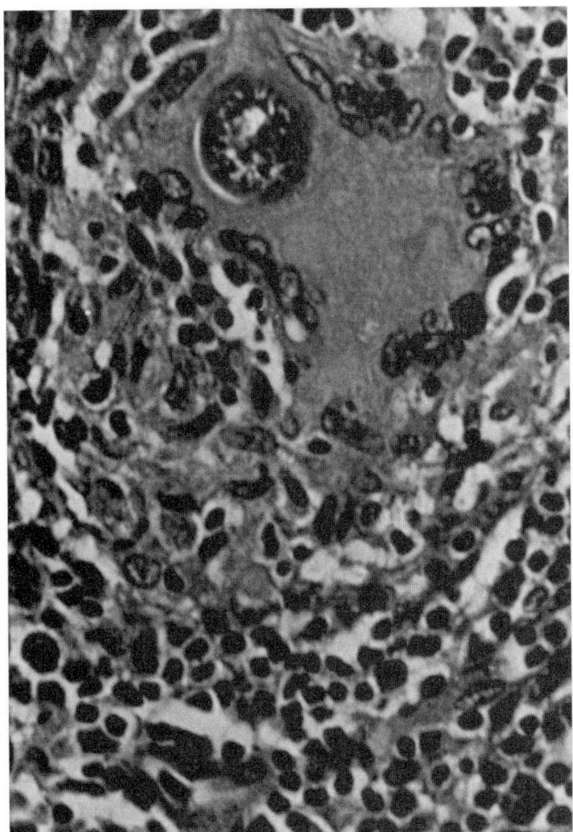

FIGURE 201–2 ■ Coccidioidal granuloma showing a multinucleated giant cell containing a spherule filled with endospores. The adjacent field contains lymphocytes and plasma cells.

currently. Identification is accomplished by inoculating mycelia into laboratory animals and demonstrating conversion of the fungus to the spherule phase. However, reliable techniques showing in vitro conversion to the spherule stage, demonstration of specific exoantigens, and identification of the organism by genetic probes have been developed and obviate the need for animal inoculation.[39, 118, 155, 158]

Epidemiology

Coccidioidomycosis is endemic in the Western Hemisphere between 40 degrees' latitude north and south. In the United States, these areas lie in the southwestern states, especially western Texas, New Mexico, Arizona, and California. The areas in which coccidioidomycosis is prevalent generally correspond to the lower Sonoran life zone.[119] This life zone is characterized by an arid to semiarid climate, hot summers, and relatively short winters with limited rainfall and few freezes. Most of the fungal growth occurs during the rainy season in alkaline soil and at low altitudes, conditions that favor growth of the creosote bush, which often coexists with *C. immitis*.[52] The fungus is found in the soil to a depth of 20 cm, especially in the walls of rodent burrows, and is isolated infrequently from surface soil during hot, dry weather[52] or in soil rich with other organisms.[104] Environmental conditions in endemic regions apparently inhibit the growth of competitive organisms.[52] Naturally acquired infection has been shown to develop in a variety of animals, including rodents, cattle, sheep, and dogs. Arthroconidia become airborne during wind storms[60] or after disruption of soil by construction work and farming. Prolonged droughts followed by heavy rains also have resulted in an increase in cases, such as occurred in California in 1992 and 1993.[29] Archeologic excavations and digging by children in soil containing the organism have been reported to result in local outbreaks.[132, 159, 170, 174] In addition, transmission has been reported to occur by contaminated fomites, such as dusty clothing and farm products.[1, 139] Because of the ease by which arthroconidia become airborne, the organism is dangerous to laboratory personnel. Epidemics have resulted from inadvertent opening of a single culture plate.[92]

Primary coccidioidal infection occurs most frequently in summer and fall, after the rainy seasons. Arthroconidia are more likely to become dispersed because of the dry weather after promotion of greater hyphal growth by the wet environment.[52, 63, 96, 119, 146, 148] Variation in seasonal infection rates also is explained partially by the occurrence of dust storms[119, 148] and earthquake activity, but these factors fail to account for the large increases in cases seen, such as the multiyear epidemic that occurred in central California in the early 1990s.[5, 63]

Susceptibility to primary coccidioidal infection is unaffected by age, sex, or racial background.[56] Estimates of infection rates in endemic areas that are based on the risk of infection developing in children have been declining. For example, infection rates measured by skin test reactivity to skin test antigens have declined from approximately 10 percent between 1937 and 1939 to 2 percent in 1959 and to less than 1 percent thereafter in kindergarten and first-grade students who had lived all of their 5 to 7 years in Kern County, California.[99] Similarly, the annual risk has been estimated to be down to between 2 and 4 percent in college students in Tucson, Arizona.[96] Incidence rates are higher in older male children, in rural areas, during wind storms, and for those with occupational exposure.[135, 137, 146] In contrast to susceptibility to primary infection, the frequency of dissemination varies considerably: it is higher in infants,[28, 31, 89, 144] Filipinos, Hispanics, and blacks.[60, 69, 83] Filipinos have 170 times and blacks 10 times the incidence of dissemination noted in non-Hispanic whites. However, some of this increased risk may reflect environmental exposure to high inocula of *C. immitis*.[7] Immunosuppressed hosts also are at increased risk for dissemination. In particular, patients with active coccidioidomycosis and infection with human immunodeficiency virus (HIV) have a greatly increased risk for severe pulmonary disease and disseminated infection.[59, 64, 176]

The tissue phase of the infection is the spherule, which is not infectious. Although mycelial growth can be found in cavities when searched for carefully, no evidence of person-to-person spread of *C. immitis* exists,[57, 77, 130, 172] except in special situations in which the fungus is allowed to revert to its airborne form, such as growth from wound drainage on a plaster cast.[51] Patients with coccidioidomycosis do not require isolation, even when draining wounds are present. In such circumstances, dressings should be changed frequently to prevent growth of the fungus and the formation of arthroconidia.

Once limited to the lower Sonoran life zone, the disease cannot be ignored throughout the country because more cases are seen everywhere as a result of the ease and frequency of travel, increased population in endemic areas, and reactivation of infection in immunocompromised hosts, including transplant recipients and patients with acquired immunodeficiency syndrome (AIDS). In these patients, delay in diagnosis can be fatal, and rapid recognition of the diagnosis and prompt institution of appropriate therapy mandate timely and accurate diagnosis.

Pathogenesis and Pathology

Acquisition of *C. immitis* infection is usually via the respiratory tract. Most human infections are surmised to result from exposure to only a single spore[62] (Fig. 201–3). Rarely, direct cutaneous inoculation may occur by puncture of the skin with a contaminated object.[72, 82, 114, 117] Growth of the organism stimulates an intense inflammatory response, and in most patients, the infection remains localized to the lungs and hilar nodes. In a minority of patients, clinically significant extrapulmonary dissemination occurs by way of the lymphatics or bloodstream.

The initial inflammatory response of acute pulmonary coccidioidomycosis is predominantly a polymorphonuclear leukocyte reaction, possibly related to a chemotactic effect of endospores or complement activation from other *C. immitis* antigens. Tissue necrosis, spherules, and a few mononuclear cells are present at this stage of the disease, but epithelial giant cells are noted infrequently. This bronchopneumonic process can occur in any lobe of the lung. The inflammatory response, however, is ineffective because neutrophils do not show any killing of coccidioidal forms at any stage of growth of the organism. Although this response may slow progression of the infection temporarily, it ultimately cannot arrest the disease process.[62] Killing has been demonstrated with natural killer cells and mononuclear leukocytes. Numerous studies have shown the importance of T cells in controlling the infection as evidenced by delayed cutaneous hypersensitivity, peripheral lymphocyte transformation, and production of interferon-γ.[62] Dermal hypersensitivity correlates well with other measures of peripheral blood lymphocyte responsiveness such as lymphocyte transformation and cytokine production.[3] As the disease progresses, cell-mediated immune defenses become defective, possibly as a result of antigen overload, suppressor cells, immune complexes, or fungal immunosuppressive substances, and such defects result in an ineffective response by type 2 helper cells.[156]

Disseminated coccidioidomycosis resembles progressive tuberculosis of childhood in its spread, which usually occurs within weeks or months after the initial infection. However, endogenous reactivation of treated primary disease may occur, particularly in individuals receiving immunosuppressive therapy[44, 113] or those with HIV infection.[20, 63, 64] Extrapulmonary spread may occur anywhere in the body, but lesions develop most frequently in bone, soft tissue, lymph nodes, and the meninges.[84] The bone lesions resemble chronic osteomyelitis (Fig. 201–4). Infection of the brain substance is a rare event, but meningitis occurs commonly and frequently localizes in the basilar area.[17, 83]

The pathologic findings of fatal coccidioidomycosis have been reviewed extensively.[84] The tissue reaction in disseminated disease is predominantly granulomatous but can be accompanied by elements of acute inflammation. Typically, the granulomatous lesions contain abundant giant cells and histiocytes. Caseous necrosis occurs commonly, and spherules usually can be identified lying freely and within macrophages (see Fig. 201–2). Fibrous tissue may surround areas of inflammation, but calcification is found infrequently. Autopsy studies in patients with coccidioidomycosis and AIDS show poor granulomatous responses and larger numbers of organisms in lung tissue than in non-AIDS patients.[73]

Most cases of disseminated coccidioidal infection in the first months of life have been associated with heavy exposure to dust, with these infants apparently acquiring their infection by the respiratory route.[32, 89] Nearly all the reported infants in this age group have had severe disease,[28, 31, 89, 161] but primary infection sometimes may go unrecognized.[31] Although women in whom coccidioidomycosis develops late in pregnancy may have an increased risk for disseminated disease,[167] with few exceptions[26, 101] infants nearly always are born free of infection.[32, 33, 145, 165] In several patients with apparent perinatal transmission, the mothers had coccidioidal endometritis, and infected amniotic fluid was the most likely source of their infants' infections.[14, 101, 142, 153]

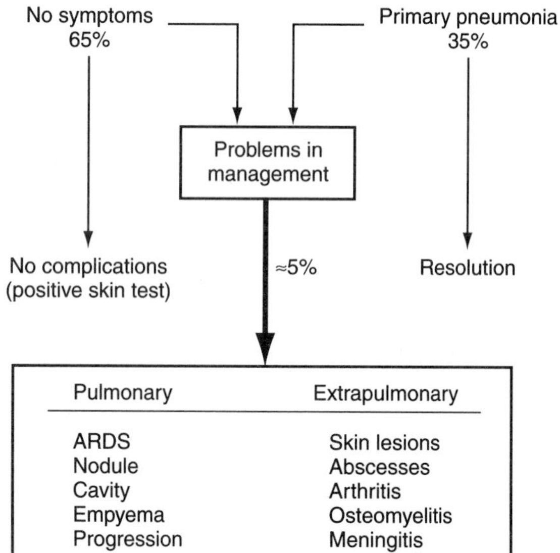

FIGURE 201–3 ■ Clinical spectrum of coccidioidomycosis. ARDS, adult respiratory distress syndrome. (From Galgiani, J. N.: Coccidioidomycosis. West. J. Med. *159*:153–171, 1993.)

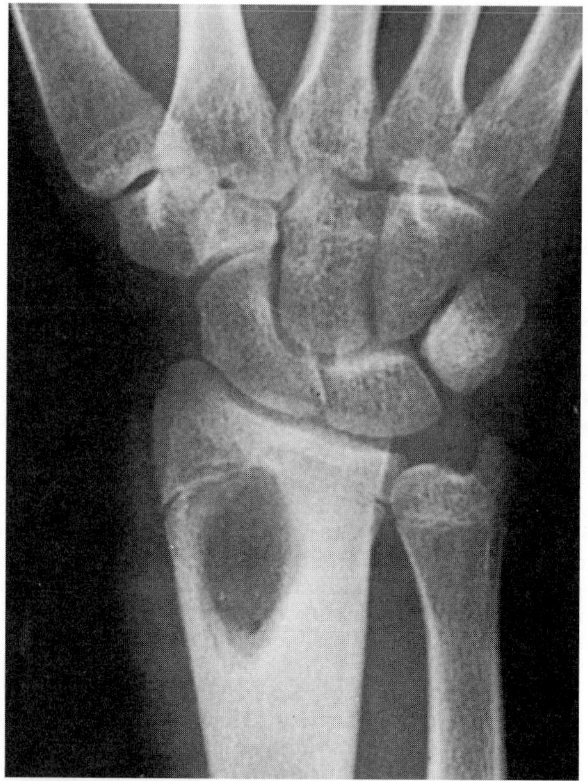

FIGURE 201–4 ■ Osteomyelitis in a 14-year-old boy with disseminated coccidioidomycosis. An osteolytic lesion involves the distal end of the radius.

Dissemination of coccidioidomycosis occurs more frequently in immunosuppressed patients who have resided in an endemic area,[44, 63, 106] but immunologic abnormalities have not been detected in other groups who also are at high risk for disseminated disease, such as Filipinos. Once dissemination occurs, the patient's cell-mediated immunity frequently is impaired,[24, 36, 152] especially if extensive infection is present.[12, 150] Dissemination can occur in patients who have a selective lack of response to coccidioidal antigens, as evidenced by negative skin test results to coccidioidin and spherulin, and who do not have evidence of generalized anergy. In vitro measurements of lymphocyte reactivity (transformation) to phytohemagglutinin or to specific cell wall antigens of *C. immitis* also are depressed.[12, 34–36, 43] In contrast, patients with disseminated disease and positive skin test results usually have normal in vitro lymphocyte responses that are similar to those found in healthy persons who have recovered from primary infection.[36, 42, 116, 179] Furthermore, after recovery from severe disseminated disease, patients may show return of specific and nonspecific cell-mediated immunity.[12, 24, 56, 152] Infected children have immunologic findings similar to those described in adults, but they have not been as well studied.

Clinical Manifestations

PRIMARY INFECTION

The clinical features of acute coccidioidomycosis in children are thought to be similar to those observed in adults.[149] Studies in Air Force personnel indicate that infection is subclinical or indistinguishable from a mild upper respiratory tract infection in 60 percent of non-immunocompromised hosts.[149, 152] In the remaining 40 percent, the severity varies from insignificant flulike illness lasting 1 to 2 days to severe lower respiratory illness with lobar pneumonia, pleural effusions, and occasionally, pericarditis.[56, 62, 126, 147] At times, the disease may mimic bacterial pneumonia and sepsis.[10, 103] The most common form of symptomatic infection is a subacute, self-limited pulmonary illness, but some patients will experience more complicated pulmonary infections or even extrapulmonary disease. The latter patients are those most likely to be seen by physicians outside endemic areas, and these patients may require extensive work-up and experience delays in diagnosis if coccidioidomycosis is not considered.[21, 45] Severe disease is more likely to develop in individuals with diabetes or those with a recent history of cigarette smoking.[138]

The usual incubation period is 10 to 16 days but may range from less than a week to almost a month.[56] In young adults, fatigue (77%), cough (64%), chest pain (53%), and dyspnea (17%) are the most common symptoms. Fever was present in 46 percent, with arthralgia, myalgia, and headaches being reported in 22 percent each.[105, 160] In infants, stridor rarely may be present as a result of primary infection of subglottic tissue.[68, 78] Chest pain is sometimes severe and usually pleuritic.[160] It may be followed by vague chest pain that persists for several months.[50, 56, 62]

Transient rashes probably occur more frequently in children than adults and are observed in slightly more than half of symptomatic children.[82, 135] Two types of rash are seen, depending on the time of initial evaluation and the patient's immune status. Those seen early in the illness are erythematous and maculopapular.[56, 82, 170, 174] They vary in severity from diffuse eruptions resembling measles or scarlet fever to more common and less extensive processes localized to the lower part of the trunk and thighs.[56, 82] In a few patients, urticarial lesions may be present.[170] Erythema nodosum and erythema multiforme appear somewhat later in the course of illness, usually after the third day to as late as 3 weeks.[56, 147] Erythema nodosum correlates with the development of cell-mediated immunity and is associated with a low incidence of dissemination.[50, 56, 146] This symptom complex may occur in other diseases, including tuberculosis, histoplasmosis, and group A beta-hemolytic streptococcal infection. However, its presence in a child residing in some endemic areas, such as the San Joaquin Valley, nearly always signifies acute coccidioidal infection. For unknown reasons, erythema nodosum occurs less frequently in infected children inhabiting other endemic areas, such as Tucson.[135] The condition is self-limited and usually resolves within a few days to several weeks. Erythema nodosum occurs two to four times more frequently in women than men, but this gender difference is not apparent in childhood infection.[146] The rash occurs infrequently in blacks, Hispanics, and Filipinos. Erythema multiforme for some reason occurs more commonly in children.

Acute arthritis or arthralgia is an additional hypersensitivity manifestation, and occasionally one or both accompany primary coccidioidal infection. Because these findings are usually transient and do not signify dissemination, spherules are presumed to not be present in the involved joints at this stage of the disease.[50]

The radiographic appearance of primary coccidioidomycosis is not specific.[13, 27, 76, 135] Bronchopneumonic infiltrates are the most frequent finding and often are associated with hilar lymphadenopathy. Segmental or lobar consolidation and nodular or patchy pulmonary infiltrates also can occur. Small pleural effusions or pleuropericardial reactions occur frequently (Fig. 201–5) and are usually sterile.[102] These radiographic findings resolve in 90 to 95 percent of symptomatic cases, albeit slowly in some, and usually do not necessitate specific therapy.

In a minority of patients, cavitation, nodule formation, bronchiectasis, or calcification may develop at the site of the pulmonic infiltrate.[15, 22] The cavities are usually thin walled and asymptomatic and rarely require surgical therapy. Many resolve spontaneously[97] but nonetheless result in a need for prolonged care and convalescence. Rarely, the cavities lead to the development of empyema or a bronchopleural fistula. These complications are much more

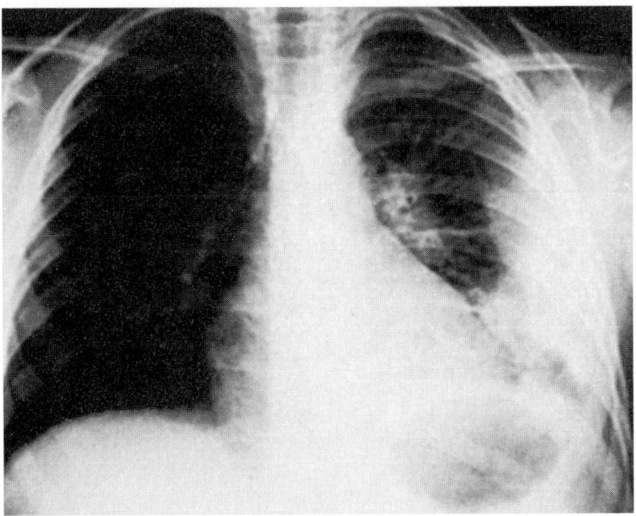

FIGURE 201–5 ■ Chest radiograph of a patient with acute pulmonary coccidioidomycosis showing pulmonary infiltrates, extensive pleural fluid, and enlargement of the left hilum.

likely to develop in patients with immunosuppression or diabetes.[90] Nodules and thin-walled cavities develop in 5 percent of patients with coccidioidal pneumonia.[156] These lesions are well circumscribed, typically single, and less than 6 cm in diameter. In most patients, the lesions are asymptomatic. In adults, these nodules may be confused with carcinoma of the lung, thus requiring excision or diagnostic fine-needle aspiration.[48]

A miliary pattern indicative of hematogenous or lymphatic spread sometimes can be appreciated in immunocompromised hosts and, infrequently, in immunocompetent hosts as well.[11] Rarely, endotracheal or endobronchial lesions can be demonstrated by endoscopy.[127]

In neonates, the constellation of radiographic findings of focal consolidation with diffuse nodular densities associated with nonspecific symptoms and minimal clinical evidence of respiratory tract infection has been described but is not specific for coccidioidomycosis at this age.[14, 27] Chorioretinitis as a manifestation of systemic disease also has been reported.[70]

In contrast to primary pulmonary infection, primary cutaneous coccidioidomycosis is an uncommon finding.[72, 114, 117] Most cases have been reported in laboratory workers,[92] but this form of infection also is recognized in children.[114] The lesion of primary cutaneous disease resembles a chancre and is associated with regional lymphadenitis. In adults, usually only mild constitutional symptoms are present, and the process spontaneously resolves within 2 to 3 months. However, in children, progressive and prolonged infection may occur more commonly; antifungal therapy may be necessary.[114, 173]

The manifestations of primary coccidioidal disease thus are varied, and because no constellation of symptoms and signs is sufficiently pathognomonic, specific laboratory tests are required for diagnosis.

DISSEMINATED COCCIDIOIDOMYCOSIS

Except in very young children, dissemination appears to occur less frequently in pediatric patients than in adults (0.5%), although this view has been questioned.[93, 144, 147] Spread of infection usually becomes apparent within a few weeks to a few months after development of the initial infection and is heralded by persistent fever, toxicity, and the insidious development of lesions outside the chest. Disseminated disease develops in occasional patients after an asymptomatic primary infection[38, 55, 93] and can be manifested as involvement of the larynx.[18]

Skin Disease

The most common cutaneous manifestation of disseminated coccidioidomycosis is verrucous granuloma, which characteristically is located at the nasolabial fold.[56, 82] These lesions may heal or continue to progress. The lesions mimic those caused by other fungi, tuberculosis, actinomycetes, and syphilis. The subcutaneous tissues also may be involved and result in large "cold" abscesses and the development of sinus tracts leading to chronic ulcers.[50]

Bone and Joint Disease

Invasion of bone by *C. immitis* results in chronic osteomyelitis,[16, 41, 91] which may drain into soft tissue (Fig. 201–6) and form fistulas to the overlying skin.[38] The bones most frequently infected are the vertebrae, tibia, metatarsals, skull, and metacarpals. Lesions are present in a single bone in 60 percent of cases; two bones are involved in 20 percent and three in another 10 percent. Radiographically, the lesions are typically lytic (see Fig. 201–4). Vertebral osteomyelitis is characterized by involvement of all parts of the vertebra, with relative sparing of the disk.[50] Meningitis is a serious concern with vertebral osteomyelitis.

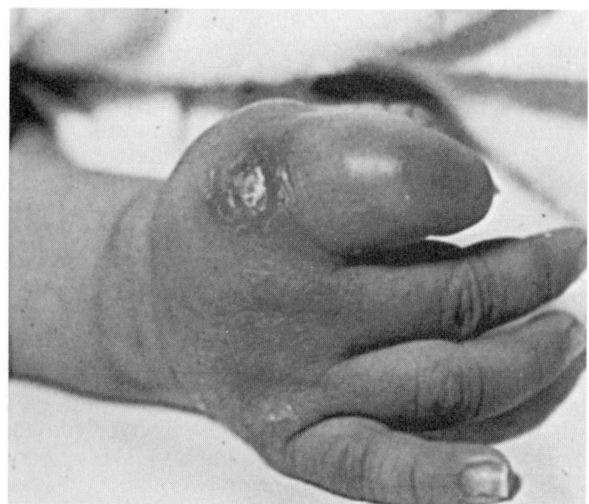

FIGURE 201–6 ■ Swelling and a chronic draining sinus over the proximal phalanx of the index finger. The infant has disseminated coccidioidomycosis with involvement of the underlying bone.

Meningitis

Meningitis may be the sole manifestation of extrapulmonary disease, particularly in whites, but it also occurs as part of widespread dissemination.[17, 81, 95, 143] It may develop acutely with the primary infection or appear up to 6 months later. The most common symptoms are headache, sluggishness, ataxia, and vomiting. The child often lacks signs of meningeal irritation and sometimes has signs of focal neurologic deficits. The pathology is that of granulomatous and suppurative basilar meningitis, with frequent parenchymal involvement and granulomas and abscesses of the spinal cord and brain.[54, 112] Vasculitic complications with infarction and strokelike findings have been described and may be abrupt in onset.[54, 171] Cerebrospinal fluid (CSF) analysis usually reveals moderate pleocytosis with mononuclear cell predominance, low CSF glucose, and an elevated protein level.[25, 81, 143] The presence of eosinophilic pleocytosis in the CSF is a common finding in coccidioidal meningitis but is of no prognostic value.[131] CSF culture is often negative for the fungus, whereas CSF antibody is often detectable.[25] The diagnosis is confirmed by positive CSF culture, serology, or both. These findings are typical for lumbosacral CSF; however, considerable variation exists in the cell count, chemistry, and antibody content of fluid obtained from the ventricles, cisterna magna, or lumbosacral space,[71, 81, 143] with the last exhibiting the more severe changes. Evidence is supported by a positive serum serologic result or culture of *C. immitis* from a nonpulmonary site. Before the availability of amphotericin B, coccidioidal meningitis was uniformly fatal, and the average length of survival in children was 5.5 months. Death from coccidioidal meningitis is now a relatively rare event.

Coccidioidomycosis in Pregnancy

Like tuberculosis, coccidioidomycosis can involve the pelvic organs. Early studies had indicated an alarming risk of dissemination and death in women who acquired coccidioidomycosis, especially during the third trimester of pregnancy.[125] In a population-based study, Wack and colleagues[167] showed that coccidioidomycosis occurs infrequently during pregnancy but remains associated with serious complications when the disease develops in the third trimester or soon after delivery. Coccidioiduria may be a silent manifestation of disseminated disease.[124]

Coccidioidomycosis in Immunocompromised Hosts

Conditions that result in immune suppression, particularly T-lymphocyte dysfunction, such as seen in patients with lymphoma or bone marrow or solid organ transplantation, predispose to more fulminant forms of coccidioidomycosis.[30, 79, 136] Solid organ transplant recipients are at the highest risk in the first year after transplantation, especially during their primary infection. Dissemination also can occur late as a result of reactivation of old infection. Lymphopenia is an important risk factor for dissemination. Cell-mediated immunity probably is the most important host factor in controlling coccidioidal infection. Therefore, one is not surprised that patients infected with HIV have a greatly increased risk for severe forms of pulmonary coccidioidomycosis[59] and extrapulmonary disease, including meningitis.[176] In HIV-infected patients, active coccidioidomycosis may represent recrudescence of old healed disease.[20] However, coccidioidomycosis in most of these patients probably represents a primary infection.[64] A CD4 count less than 250/μL is associated significantly with the development of active disease.[4] The clinical manifestations range from minimal systemic symptoms without a pulmonary focus to severe cough and dyspnea associated with diffuse pulmonary disease and a radiographic pattern showing a discretely nodular appearance resembling *Pneumocystis carinii* infection. The severity of symptoms is correlated inversely with CD4 counts, and severe disease occurs most commonly in patients with CD4 counts less than 200/μL.[64] Black race and a history of pharyngeal or esophageal candidiasis are associated with an increased risk for coccidioidomycosis in HIV-infected individuals living in endemic areas. Protease inhibitor therapy and the use of azoles for at least 3 weeks of the preceding 3 months result in a reduced risk in those with candidiasis.[176] Even with appropriate antifungal therapy, the prognosis of HIV-infected patients with depressed CD4 counts in whom diffuse pulmonary coccidioidomycosis develops is poor, with a mortality rate of 70 percent.[59, 64] HIV-infected patients also may initially have evidence of extrapulmonary dissemination. Patients who have documented extrapulmonary dissemination in association with positive serologic tests for HIV are regarded as sufficiently immuno-incompetent to be classified as having AIDS.[134] An important note is that many HIV-infected patients who have positive serologic results without evidence of active disease eventually contract active coccidioidomycosis[9] and may be candidates for therapy.

Diagnosis

In endemic areas where physicians are aware of the disease, the diagnosis of coccidioidomycosis usually is established readily by appropriate laboratory studies. In other locations, the diagnosis is not considered unless a travel history is obtained. One should remember that cases have occurred even after brief exposure in an endemic area. Primary pulmonary coccidioidomycosis resembles other lower respiratory illnesses, including those caused by viruses, bacteria, *Mycoplasma, Mycobacterium tuberculosis,* and other fungi (e.g., *Histoplasma).*

The hematologic findings in primary coccidioidal infection consist of elevation of the erythrocyte sedimentation rate, leukocytosis, and frequently eosinophilia.[56, 147] Marked eosinophilia may be a clue that dissemination has occurred.[80] Specific diagnosis usually is based on the results of skin tests, serologic reactions, and sputum examination.

CULTURE AND IDENTIFICATION OF THE FUNGUS

The organism is detected readily by direct examination and culture from purulent material. The yield from other sources, such as pleural fluid, blood, and gastric aspirates, is somewhat lower. Only about a third of spinal fluid samples are culture-positive, and direct examination of CSF almost always yields negative results.[81, 143] Detection of the fungus in blood occurs uncommonly and is associated with severe forms of disseminated disease.[6]

In severe pulmonary or disseminated disease, microscopic examination of bronchopulmonary lavage fluid, exudates, or biopsy specimens is diagnostic if typical spherules containing endospores are seen. Hematoxylin and eosin–stained sections can be used to demonstrate spherules but are used mainly to show the inflammatory process. The periodic acid–Schiff stain is useful for demonstrating the spherule contents (Fig. 201–7), whereas methenamine silver stains highlight the wall of the spherule. Cytologic examination of sputa is more sensitive than potassium hydroxide stains.[168] The spherules do not pick up the Gram stain.

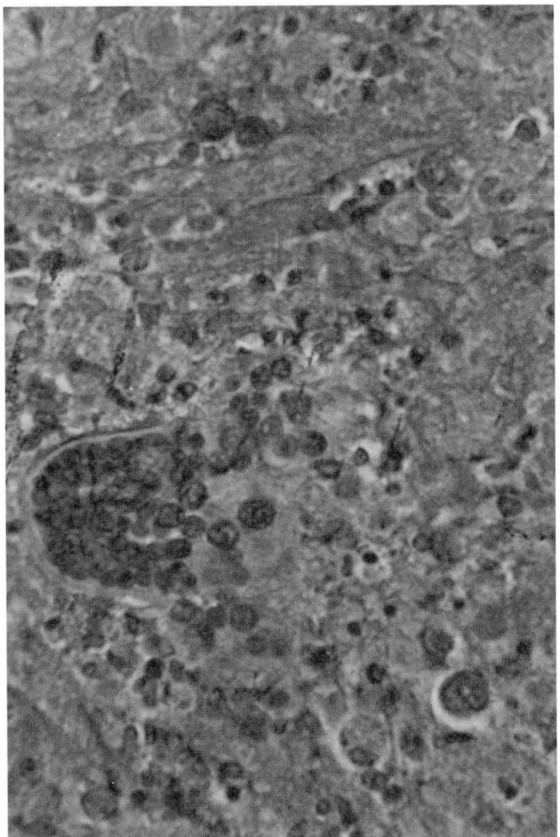

FIGURE 201–7 ■ A spherule that has ruptured recently and is in the process of releasing endospores.

In HIV-infected patients with pulmonary infiltrates, coccidioidal spherules may be identified in bronchopulmonary lavage specimens by the same methenamine silver stain used to identify *P. carinii*. Indeed, in areas endemic for coccidioidomycosis, the possibility of concomitant pulmonary infection with both *C. immitis* and *P. carinii* or other pathogens should be kept in mind in this patient group.[64, 107] Cytologic examination of bronchial washings or bronchoalveolar fluid is diagnostic in only about a third of persons with or without HIV infection and is less sensitive than culture.[48] With the rare exception of persons with primary cutaneous infection, the finding of spherules in tissues outside the thoracic cavity is evidence that the patient has disseminated disease. For this reason, biopsy may be useful for establishing a diagnosis, particularly in patients with borderline or low complement-fixation antibody titers. Culture of *C. immitis* from body fluids, sputum, or exudates can be performed on most laboratory media. If *C. immitis* is suspected, the use of mycologic media containing cycloheximide can be helpful. Handling of the cultures is hazardous and requires special biosafety precautions.[92] Once a nonpigmented mold has grown, final identification requires conversion of the mycelial phase to the spherule stage. Such conversion is accomplished by animal inoculation or by the use of special media.[158] A more rapid confirmation method is the detection of specific exoantigens of the fungus in the culture media[39, 155] or the use of genetic probes, which allow for rapid confirmation, usually within hours.[118]

SKIN TEST

The clinical usefulness of skin testing in patients suspected of having coccidioidomycosis has been reviewed. Two antigenic preparations derived from lysates of either the mycelial phase (coccidioidin) or the spherule phase (spherulin) are used clinically to elicit delayed hypersensitivity.[133, 157] A positive skin test result to either preparation means that the patient has had infection at some time.[82, 140] The skin test results become positive 2 to 21 days after the onset of symptoms, usually before the serologic results have become positive. By the second week of illness, a negative skin test result would be unusual in primary coccidioidomycosis (<10%).[152] However, a negative skin test result 1 month after the onset of symptoms frequently suggests latent dissemination or the potential for later dissemination.[56, 147, 152]

The skin test is applied intradermally, and the presence of 5 mm or more of induration at 48 hours is interpreted as a positive result. The standard dose of coccidioidin is a dilution of 1:100; with spherulin, 0.1 mL of a solution containing 2.8 µg is applied. In patients with erythema nodosum, a wise approach is to initiate skin testing with a 10-fold dilution of these preparations to avoid severe local and systemic reactions. A low level of cross-reactivity exists with antigens from *Histoplasma capsulatum* or *Blastomyces dermatitidis*. However, skin testing does not induce delayed hypersensitivity[133] or serum antibody responses to coccidioidin,[147] but it may induce cross-reacting antibodies to histoplasmin.[123]

The skin test may be unreliable in immunosuppressed patients, in whom a delayed hypersensitivity response may be impossible.

In a child who is a long-time resident of an endemic area, a positive skin test result is not helpful in the diagnosis of acute infection unless one can show that the patient's skin test was previously negative. The greatest usefulness of the skin test is in population surveys for obtaining prevalence data and as a measure of cellular immunity, a factor in prognosis.

SEROLOGIC STUDIES

Figure 201–8 illustrates the serologic and skin test responses of symptomatic patients with primary coccidioidomycosis. The initial antibody response to coccidioidal infection is predominantly in the IgM fraction and is responsible for the positive precipitin test result that accompanies primary infection.[122, 141] These responses can be measured by tube precipitins, latex agglutination, enzyme immunoassay, or immunodiffusion methods.[123] Fifty percent of patients have positive results in the first week, and 90 percent show precipitins within 2 to 3 weeks.[151] Thereafter, antibody reversion occurs, and by 5 months, only 10 percent of patients with uncomplicated infection have positive results.[151] Serum precipitins may persist in some patients with disseminated infection or may reappear with reactivation of infection. Precipitating IgM antibody detected by the tube precipitin assay or by immunodiffusion usually indicates acute infection.[151] In contrast to that seen with complement fixation, the magnitude of the precipitating antibody titer does not correlate with an increased risk of dissemination.[150] Occasionally, IgM antibody has been detected in the cord blood of newborns whose mothers had detectable antibody. These infants did not have any evidence of infection on follow-up.[123] Latex agglutination is sensitive, rapid, and easy to perform but frequently yields false-positive reactions,[123] and positive results should be confirmed by a second method. It also gives false-positive results in spinal fluid and diluted sera and should not be used for these specimens.[121]

Serum IgG antibodies that fix complement usually appear later and last 6 to 8 months.[123] They are found more commonly in more symptomatic infections and are detected in 50 to 90 percent by 3 months after the onset of symptoms. At least 90 percent of persons show a positive IgM or IgG response after having symptomatic primary infection. The main methods of detecting these antibodies are immunodiffusion, immunoassay, and complement fixation.[109, 123, 169, 177] These assays correlate well, and immunodiffusion is particularly useful for detection of antibody in patients whose sera are anticomplementary.[123]

Immunodiffusion yields few false-positive results and can detect early asymptomatic infection in persons infected with HIV.[9] This method seems to be slightly more sensitive than complement fixation in detecting early infection.[94]

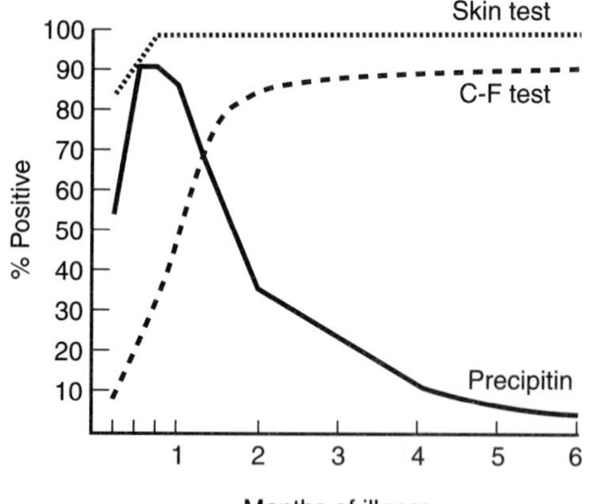

FIGURE 201–8 ■ Immunologic reactions in symptomatic primary coccidioidomycosis, with time of appearance and duration related to the frequency of positive reactions. (Based on Smith, C. E., Beard, R. R., Rosenberger, H. G., et al.: Effect of season and dust control on coccidioidomycosis. J. A. M. A. *132*:833–838, 1946.)

More recently, enzyme immunoassay has become available. This assay compares well with more traditional assays (complement fixation, immunodiffusion, latex agglutination) and does not suffer from the subjectivity required to interpret the other assays.[61, 109] The IgG enzyme immunoassay has a sensitivity of 92 percent, whereas the IgM assay has a sensitivity of 77 percent. When both assays are combined, the sensitivity is excellent,[94, 109] but the test suffers from false-positive results in patients with blastomycosis or suspected noncoccidioidal pulmonary illness.[94]

Antibodies measured by complement fixation are slower to develop and are found primarily in the IgG fraction.[123, 124] Usually, they are not detected in serum samples obtained during the first week of infection, and their rise may occur as late as 3 months after the onset of symptoms.[86, 151]

The magnitude of the complement-fixation antibody response correlates closely with the severity of infection and the likelihood of dissemination.[151] Although antibody titer cannot be used as the sole indicator of dissemination, titers of 1:32 or greater in most laboratories are highly suggestive of extrapulmonary spread of infection[85, 151]; 61 percent of these patients have a titer of at least 1:16, whereas 95 to 100 percent of those without dissemination have a titer lower than 1:16. The titer of complement-fixation antibody parallels disease activity and is useful in monitoring the progress of patients with disseminated disease. In a few patients, especially those with extensive pulmonary involvement and pleural effusion, high titers develop without other clinical evidence of dissemination.[102] Conversely, some patients with dissemination, particularly those with single lesions in skin, bone, or the meninges, have lower titers.

Some patients with immunodeficiency disease, in particular, HIV infection, may have extensive disease with low or undetectable antibody levels[8, 29, 59, 123] and negative skin test results to coccidioidal and other antigens.[64] Bone marrow transplant recipients may have no serologic or skin test response before or shortly after bone marrow transplantation and may require aggressive attempts at culturing the fungus for diagnosis.[136] Some patients with HIV infection may have persistently positive serologic test results in the absence of any clinical disease. These patients are at high risk for active coccidioidomycosis and should be treated early.[9]

Complement-fixation antibody is detectable in the CSF of 70 percent of patients at the time that coccidioidal meningitis is diagnosed and eventually becomes detectable in all patients. The antibody measured is not a reflection of serum levels but rather is thought to indicate specific immunoglobulin biosynthesis by cells residing within or contiguous to the central nervous system. Occasionally, patients with vertebral osteomyelitis or epidural abscesses have low complement-fixation titers in CSF without other evidence of meningeal involvement.

Treatment

PRIMARY INFECTION

In more than 90 percent of children, primary coccidioidomycosis is a self-limited illness, and antifungal therapy is not needed. In some children with severe primary disease, therapy with antifungal antibiotics may be justified to either abbreviate the period of morbidity or lessen the chance of dissemination in those with an elevated complement-fixation titer.

Which patients with primary uncomplicated pulmonary infection should receive therapy remains controversial. In general, evidence of severe infection or concurrent risk factors such as immunosuppression should lead to initiation of therapy. Severe infections usually are heralded by weight loss of more than 10 percent, intense night sweats for longer than 3 weeks, infiltrates involving more than half of one lung or portions of both lungs, prominent or persistent hilar adenopathy, a complement-fixation titer to *C. immitis* greater than 1:16, failure of development of normal skin test hypersensitivity to coccidioidal antigens, inability to work, or symptoms that persist for longer than 2 months.[65] A diagnosis of primary coccidioidomycosis during the third trimester of pregnancy or immediately postpartum should raise consideration of treatment. Persons of African or Filipino ancestry have a higher risk of dissemination, and this risk should be taken into consideration. Therapy typically consists of oral azoles for 3 to 6 months. Amphotericin is recommended for pregnant women because of the teratogenic potential of fluconazole and possibly the other azoles.[65] When reticulonodular or miliary disease is seen, therapy usually is initiated with amphotericin followed by oral azoles after evidence of response. The total course of therapy should last at least 1 year and be followed by oral azole therapy for secondary prophylaxis.[65]

Asymptomatic pulmonary cavities generally do not require therapy, but consideration should be given to excision of some cavities that persist longer than 2 years. In patients with cavities that result in local discomfort, superinfection, or hemoptysis, therapy with oral azoles may alleviate the symptoms. Resection of localized cavities is an option to recurrent courses of antifungal therapy.[65] Pyopneumothorax results from rupture of a cavity into the pleural space. Its treatment is surgical with or without a course of antifungal therapy. Chronic fibrocavitary disease usually is treated with oral azoles for at least a year. In patients with inadequate responses, increasing the dose of azole, switching to a different azole, and administering amphotericin B are options. Surgical resection may be helpful in localized disease or when significant hemoptysis has occurred.[65]

DISSEMINATED DISEASE

Nonmeningeal Dissemination

Patients with disseminated disease who have clinically apparent lesions outside the thoracic cavity almost always should receive antifungal therapy; the agent of choice in fulminant infections is amphotericin B.

Treatment is indicated for patients with extrapulmonary dissemination. The classic therapy consists of amphotericin B administered initially at 1 to 1.5 mg/kg/day and then tapered to 1 to 1.5 mg/kg/day three times a week.[49] The usual total dose in adults is 1 to 2.5 g. In children, the maximal dose has not been defined because children tolerate amphotericin B better than adults do.[178] Local instillation or irrigation of abscesses and cavities with amphotericin B or other antifungal agents may be beneficial but has not been studied systematically.[16, 91] Amphotericin lipid-complexed preparations offer the possibility of administering higher doses with less toxicity; their role in the treatment of coccidioidomycosis remains to be defined and needs further study.

The total dose of amphotericin B depends on the patient's age and the severity of disease. Most patients respond to between 15 and 45 mg/kg, with the total dose and duration of therapy determined by the patient's response. The azoles have been tested extensively in this form of the disease. The main agents used for this purpose are itraconazole and fluconazole. In a randomized, double-blind study of progressive nonmeningeal coccidioidomycosis, a trend toward better efficacy with itraconazole was demonstrated, especially in the subgroup of patients with skeletal infections.[67] In children, such treatment has to be weighed against the need for more frequent drug administration and diet limitations related to the absorption of itraconazole. Ketoconazole has the advantage of being significantly less costly than the other two azoles; it is associated, however, with more gastrointestinal discomfort and may impair testosterone secretion and adrenal steroid synthesis without causing an adrenal crisis.[19, 129] Itraconazole and ketoconazole have important drug interactions, most notably with cyclosporine and diphenylhydantoin.[74] In general, the azoles are used for a few months after the resolution of symptoms or for at least a year of therapy. Caution should be exercised with the use of fluconazole in pregnancy because four infants with multiple congenital malformations somewhat reminiscent of the Antley-Bixler syndrome have been described.[2] The role of echinocandins is unclear at present.

Surgical therapy seldom is required in patients with primary disease, but therapeutic thoracentesis may be indicated rarely when pneumonitis is complicated by large pleural effusions.[102] Surgery is also necessary when pericardial involvement is complicated by tamponade. Patients with persistent coccidioidal cavities (>1 year) may require lobectomy, especially if the lesions are symptomatic.[108] Coccidioidal lymphadenopathy occasionally requires excision. In general, bone and joint disease requires a combined surgical and medical approach. Coccidioidal arthritis typically responds poorly to systemic therapy, and synovectomy may aid in the control of symptoms.[16, 128, 175] When surgical procedures are performed, a course of systemic therapy in the perioperative period is advisable to prevent further spread of disease.[58] Osteomyelitis is treated optimally by curettage and draining of the involved bone along with the addition of amphotericin B, itraconazole, or fluconazole therapy.[16, 23, 41, 67] Within endemic areas, a useful approach may be to screen HIV-infected patients serologically by immunodiffusion or complement fixation at a frequency of once every 6 months to identify active cases early. Consideration should be given to offering antifungal prophylaxis to these persons.[110] Whether such prophylaxis is effective is unclear, and the potential for development of drug resistance should be weighed. In a retrospective cohort study, clinical response, the lowest complement-fixation titer, the end-of-therapy complement-fixation titer, or a fourfold drop in complement-fixation titer was not predictive of relapse in nonmeningeal forms of disseminated coccidioidomycosis, whereas a peak complement-fixation titer of more than 1:256 or a persistently negative coccidioidin skin test was independently associated with increased risk.[115]

Meningeal Disease

Amphotericin treatment of coccidioidal meningitis has been associated with a marked improvement in survival.[53, 95, 98] However, such treatment needs to include prolonged intrathecal therapy via lumbar, ventricular, or cisternal administration. This therapy is associated with significant side effects that include headache, nausea, vomiting, chills and fever, arachnoiditis, and occasionally, paralysis, seizures, and coma. The symptoms of arachnoiditis may be indistinguishable from those of microbiologic relapse.[81] Ketoconazole has been used with some success in meningitis but also is associated with a high relapse rate[46]; in high doses (1200 mg daily in adults, 15 to 23 mg/kg/day in children), therapy has been successful, but such doses tend to be tolerated poorly in adults.[62, 75, 81, 143]

Studies using 400 mg of fluconazole or itraconazole in the treatment of meningitis without the concurrent use of amphotericin B show good results, with response rates of approximately 80 percent.[66, 162–164] Many patients who do not show improvement with this regimen demonstrate clinical improvement when the dose is increased up to 800 mg of fluconazole or 600 mg of itraconazole. Fluconazole is the preferred drug.[65] Based on limited data, the pediatric dose of fluconazole would be approximately 12 mg/kg/day. Patients generally respond clinically within 1 to 2 months, although abnormalities in CSF may persist in some patients for a prolonged period. When therapy has been stopped, increases in CSF cell count or complement-fixation antibody titer may be the only indication of reactivation of meningeal disease and signify a need to intensify therapy.[50]

Significant attention should be paid to CSF flow dynamics, because in almost all children with coccidioidal meningitis obstructive hydrocephalus develops and requires ventriculoperitoneal shunting and rarely a second shunt to drain a "trapped" fourth ventricle.[81, 143] Hence, the advantage of such a drug as fluconazole, which can be given systemically, obviates the problems of impaired CSF flow that are encountered when intrathecal or intraventricular therapy is used.

Recent studies have indicated that the relapse rate after discontinuation of azole therapy is high. Eleven of 14 (78%) persons treated with azoles (ketoconazole, itraconazole, or fluconazole) for periods ranging from 8 to 101 months for coccidioidal meningitis had a relapse of disseminated coccidioidomycosis within 0.5 to 30 months after therapy was stopped. No clinical or laboratory findings can be used to predict which patients are at risk for relapse. The data thus indicate that moderately prolonged azole therapy for coccidioidal meningitis suppresses but does not eradicate the infection, and therefore prolonged, if not lifelong, therapy might be necessary.[46, 156]

Prognosis

Primary pulmonary coccidioidal infection usually is self-limited, with complete recovery occurring in 1 to 3 weeks. In a small proportion of cases, localized complications of the primary infection, such as pleural effusion or pericarditis, prolong the clinical course. Dissemination is rare in whites and is less likely to occur in patients with positive skin test results. Until the late 1950s, no effective therapy was available for the more severe forms of coccidioidomycosis, and the mortality rate of patients with disseminated disease was approximately 50 percent.[56] The mortality rate of patients with multiple sites of dissemination and those with coccidioidal meningitis approached 100 percent.[53, 166] Presently, therapy with amphotericin B or azoles may cure some of these patients and in many others prolongs useful life. Certain forms of disseminated infection, such as joint involvement, are particularly resistant to systemic therapy and may persist for many years without other signs of dissemination. For patients with HIV infection, therapy for disseminated coccidioidomycosis is not usually curative, and lifelong suppressive therapy with intermittent doses of amphotericin B or oral azoles may be required to prevent relapses.[111] Some experts even advise the use of lifelong suppressive therapy for HIV-infected patients with uncomplicated pulmonary coccidioidomycosis.

Prevention

A killed vaccine has been prepared from spherules and is efficacious in experimental animals.[87, 100] In trials conducted in adult humans, the vaccine was tolerated reasonably well but did not result in significant decreases in attack rates or severity of disease.[120] Live attenuated strains of *C. immitis* are also highly immunogenic in experimental animals, but viable organisms tend to persist in immunized hosts. Furthermore, the strains are unstable and revert to their virulent form after several passages in animals. For these reasons, no effective means is currently available for prevention of human coccidioidomycosis.

Other efforts at prevention have been aimed at dust control and eradication of the organisms from soil.[148] Whether these measures are effective is unproved, and in rural areas they are costly and impractical. Immunosuppressed children with negative skin test results should be advised to not engage in field activities or organized excursions into areas highly endemic for coccidioidomycosis.[159, 170]

REFERENCES

1. Albert, B. L., and Sellers, T. F., Jr.: Coccidioidomycosis from fomites. Arch. Intern. Med. *112*:253–261, 1963.
2. Aleck, K. A., and Bartley, D. L.: Multiple malformations syndrome following fluconazole use in pregnancy: Report of an additional patient. Am. J. Med. Genet. *72*:253–256, 1997.
3. Ampel, N. M., Bejarano, G. C., Salas, S. D., et al.: In vitro assessment of cellular immunity in human coccidioidomycosis: Relationship between dermal hypersensitivity, lymphocyte transformation, and lymphokine production by peripheral blood mononuclear cells from healthy adults. J. Infect. Dis. *165*:710–715, 1992.
4. Ampel, N. M., Dols, C. L., and Galgiani, J. N.: Coccidioidomycosis during human immunodeficiency virus infection: Results of a prospective study in a coccidioidal endemic area. Am. J. Med. *94*:235–240, 1993.
5. Ampel, N. M., Mosley, D. G., England, B., et al.: Coccidioidomycosis in Arizona: Increase in incidence from 1990 to 1995. Clin. Infect. Dis. *27*:1528–1530, 1998.
6. Ampel, N. M., Ryan, K. J., Carry, P. J., et al.: Fungemia due to *Coccidioides immitis:* An analysis of 16 episodes in 15 patients and a review of the literature. Medicine (Baltimore) *65*:312–321, 1986.
7. Ampel, N. M., Wieden, M. A., and Galgiani, J. N.: Coccidioidomycosis: Clinical update. Rev. Infect. Dis. *11*:897–911, 1989.
8. Antoniskis, D., Larsen, R. A., Akil, B., et al.: Seronegative disseminated coccidioidomycosis in patients with HIV infection. AIDS *4*:691–693, 1990.
9. Arguinchona, H. L., Ampel, N. M., Dols, C. L., et al.: Persistent coccidioidal seropositivity without clinical evidence of active coccidioidomycosis in patients with human immunodeficiency virus. Clin. Infect. Dis. *20*:1281–1285, 1995.
10. Arsura, A. L., Bellinghausen, P. L., Kilgore, W. B., et al.: Septic shock in coccidioidomycosis. Crit. Care Med. *26*:62–65, 1998.
11. Arsura, E. L., and Kilgore, W. B.: Miliary coccidioidomycosis in the immunocompetent. Chest *117*:404–409, 2000.
12. Barbee, R. A., and Hicks, M. J.: Clinical usefulness of lymphocyte transformation in patients with coccidioidomycosis. Chest *93*:1003–1007, 1988.
13. Batra, P.: Pulmonary coccidioidomycosis. J. Thorac. Imaging *7*:29–38, 1992.
14. Bernstein, D. I., Tipton, J. R., Schott, S. F., et al.: Coccidioidomycosis in a neonate: Maternal-infant transmission. J. Pediatr. *99*:752–754, 1981.
15. Birsner, J. W.: The roentgen aspects of five hundred cases of pulmonary coccidioidomycosis. A. J. R. Am. J. Roentgenol. *72*:556–573, 1954.
16. Bisla, R. S., and Taber, T. H., Jr.: Coccidioidomycosis of bone and joints. Clin. Orthop. *121*:196–204, 1976.
17. Bouza, E., Dreyer, J. S., Hewitt, W. L., et al.: Coccidioidal meningitis: An analysis of thirty-one cases and review of the literature. Medicine (Baltimore) *60*:139–172, 1981.
18. Boyle, J. O., Coulthard, S. W., and Mandel, R. M.: Laryngeal involvement in disseminated coccidioidomycosis. Arch. Otolaryngol. Head Neck Surg. *117*:433–438, 1991.
19. Britton, H., Shehab, Z., Lightner, E., et al.: Adrenal response in children receiving high doses of ketoconazole for coccidioidomycosis. J. Pediatr. *112*:488–492, 1988.
20. Bronnimann, D. A., Adam, R. D., Galgiani, J. N., et al.: Coccidioidomycosis in acquired immune deficiency syndrome. Ann. Intern. Med. *106*:372–379, 1987.
21. Cairns, L., Blythe, D., Kao, A., et al.: Outbreak of coccidioidomycosis in Washington State residents returning from Mexico. Clin. Infect. Dis. *30*:61–64, 2000.
22. Castellino, R. A., and Blank, N.: Pulmonary coccidioidomycosis: The wide spectrum of roentgenographic manifestations. Calif. Med. *109*:41–49, 1969.
23. Catanzaro, A., Galgiani, J. N., Levine, B. E., et al.: Fluconazole in the treatment of chronic pulmonary and nonmeningeal disseminated coccidioidomycosis: NIAID Mycoses Study Group. Am. J. Med. *98*: 249–256, 1995.
24. Catanzaro, A., Spitler, L. E., and Moser, K. M.: Cellular immune response in coccidioidomycosis. Cell. Immunol. *15*:360–371, 1975.
25. Caudill, R. G., Smith, C. E., and Reinarz, J. A.: Coccidioidal meningitis: A diagnostic challenge. Am. J. Med. *49*:360–365, 1970.
26. Charlton, V., Ramsdell, K., and Sehring, S.: Intrauterine transmission of coccidioidomycosis. Pediatr. Infect. Dis. J. *18*:561–563, 1999.
27. Child, D. C., Newell, J. D., Bjelland, J. C., et al.: Radiographic findings of pulmonary coccidioidomycosis in neonates and infants. A. J. R. Am. J. Roentgenol. *145*:261–263, 1985.
28. Christian, J. R., Sarre, S. G., Peers, J. H., et al.: Pulmonary coccidioidomycosis in a twenty-one-day-old infant. Am. J. Dis. Child. *92*:66–73, 1956.
29. Coccidioidomycosis—United States, 1991–1992. M. M. W. R. Morb. Mortal. Wkly. Rep. *42*(2):21–24, 1993.
30. Cohen, I. M., Galgiani, J. N., Potter, D., et al.: Coccidioidomycosis in renal replacement therapy. Arch. Intern. Med. *142*:489–494, 1982.
31. Cohen, R.: Coccidioidomycosis: Case studies in children. Arch. Pediatr. *66*:241–265, 1949.
32. Cohen, R.: Placental *Coccidioides*: Proof that congenital *Coccidioides* is nonexistent. Arch. Pediatr. *68*:59–66, 1951.
33. Cohen, R., and Burnip, R.: Coccidioidin skin testing during pregnancy and in infants and children. Calif. Med. *72*:31–33, 1950.
34. Cox, R. A.: Cross-reactivity between antigens of *Coccidioides immitis, Histoplasma capsulatum,* and *Blastomyces dermatitidis* in lymphocyte transformation assays. Infect. Immun. *25*:932–938, 1979.
35. Cox, R. A., Brummer, E., and Lecara, G.: In vitro lymphocyte responses of coccidioidin skin test–positive and –negative persons to coccidioidin, spherulin, and a *Coccidioides* cell wall antigen. Infect. Immun. *15*:751–755, 1977.
36. Cox, R. A., Vivas, J. R., Gross, A., et al.: In vivo and in vitro cell-mediated responses in coccidioidomycosis: Immunologic responses of persons with primary, asymptomatic infections. Am. Rev. Respir. Dis. *114*:937–943, 1976.
37. Davis, B. D., Delbecco, R., Eisen, H. W., et al.: Microbiology: Including Immunology and Molecular Genetics. 3rd ed. Hagerstown, MD, Harper & Row, 1980.
38. Dennis, J. L., and Hansen, A. E.: Coccidioidomycosis in children. Pediatrics *14*:481–494, 1954.
39. Denys, G. A., Newman, M. A., and Standard, P. G.: Evaluation of a commercial exoantigen test system for the rapid identification of systemic fungal pathogens. Am. J. Clin. Pathol. *79*:379–381, 1983.
40. Deresinski, S. C.: History of coccidioidomycosis: Dust to dust. *In* Stevens, D. A. (ed.): Coccidioidomycosis: A Text. New York, Plenum Medical, 1980, pp. 1–20.
41. Deresinski, S. C.: Coccidioidomycosis of bone and joints. *In* Stevens, D. A. (ed.): Coccidioidomycosis: A Text. New York, Plenum Medical, 1980, pp. 195–224.
42. Deresinski, S. C., Applegate, R. J., Levine, H. B., et al.: Cellular immunity to *Coccidioides immitis:* In vitro lymphocyte response to spherules, arthrospores, and endospores. Cell. Immunol. *32*:110–119, 1977.
43. Deresinski, S. C., Levine, H. B., and Stevens, D. A.: Soluble antigens of mycelia and spherules in the in vitro detection of immunity to *Coccidioides immitis.* Infect. Immun. *10*:700–704, 1974.
44. Deresinski, S. C., and Stevens, D. A.: Coccidioidomycosis in compromised hosts. Medicine (Baltimore) *54*:377–395, 1974.
45. Desai, S. A., Minai, O. A., Gordon, S. M., et al.: Coccidioidomycosis in non-endemic areas: A case series. Respir. Med. *95*:305–309, 2001.
46. Dewsnup, D. H., Galgiani, J. N., Graybill, J. R., et al.: Is it ever safe to stop azole therapy for *Coccidioides immitis* meningitis? Ann. Intern. Med. *124*:305–310, 1996.
47. Dickson, E. C.: "Valley fever" of the San Joaquin Valley and fungus. Calif. West. Med. *47*:151–155, 1937.
48. DiTomasso, J. P., Ampel, N. M., Sobonya, R. E., et al.: Bronchoscopic diagnosis of pulmonary coccidioidomycosis: Comparison of cytology, culture, and transbronchial biopsy. Diagn. Microbiol. Infect. Dis. *18*:83–87, 1994.
49. Drutz, D. J.: Amphotericin B in the treatment of coccidioidomycosis. Drugs *26*:337–346, 1983.
50. Drutz, D. J., and Catanzaro, A.: Coccidioidomycosis. Am. Rev. Respir. Dis. *117*:559–585, 727–771, 1978.
51. Eckmann, B. H., Schaefer, G. L., and Huppert, M.: Bedside interhuman transmission of coccidioidomycosis via growth on fomites: An epidemic involving six persons. Am. Rev. Respir. Dis. *89*:175–185, 1964.
52. Egeberg, R. O., and Ely, A. F.: *Coccidioides immitis* in the soil of the southern San Joaquin Valley. Am. J. Med. Sci. *23*:151–154, 1956.
53. Einstein, H. E., Holemann, C. W., Sandidge, L. L., et al.: Coccidioidal meningitis: The use of amphotericin B in treatment. Calif. Med. *94*:339–343, 1961.
54. Erly, W. K., Bellon, R. J., Seeger, J. F., et al.: MR imaging of acute coccidioidal meningitis. A. J. N. R. Am. J. Neuroradiol. *20*:509–514, 1999.
55. Feigin, R. D., Shackelford, P. G., Lins, R. D., et al.: Subcutaneous abscess due to *Coccidioides immitis.* Am. J. Dis. Child. *124*:734–735, 1972.
56. Fiese, M. J.: Coccidioidomycosis. Springfield, IL, Charles C Thomas, 1958.
57. Fiese, M. J., Cheu, S., and Sorensen, R. H.: Mycelial forms of *Coccidioides immitis* in sputum and tissues of the human host. Ann. Intern. Med. *43*:255–270, 1955.

58. Findlay, F. M., and Melick, D. W.: Treatment of cavitary coccidioidomycosis. *In* Ajello, L. (ed.): Coccidioidomycosis. Tucson, University of Arizona Press, 1967, pp. 79–83.
59. Fish, D. G., Ampel, N. M., Galgiani, J. N., et al.: Coccidioidomycosis during human immunodeficiency virus infection: A review of 77 patients. Medicine (Baltimore) *69*:384–391, 1990.
60. Flynn, N. M., Hoeprich, P. D., Kawachi, M. M., et al.: An unusual outbreak of windborne coccidioidomycosis. N. Engl. J. Med. *301*:358–361, 1979.
61. Gade, W., Ledman, D. W., Wethington, R., et al.: Serological responses to various *Coccidioides* antigen preparations in a new enzyme immunoassay. J. Clin. Microbiol. *30*:1907–1912, 1992.
62. Galgiani, J. N.: Coccidioidomycosis. West. J. Med. *159*:153–171, 1993.
63. Galgiani, J. N.: Coccidioidomycosis: A regional disease of national importance. Rethinking approaches for control. Ann. Intern. Med. *130*:293–300, 1999.
64. Galgiani, J. N., and Ampel, N. M.: Coccidioidomycosis in human immunodeficiency virus–infected patients. J. Infect. Dis. *162*:1165–1169, 1990.
65. Galgiani, J. N., Ampel, N. M., Catanzaro, A., et al.: Practice guidelines for the treatment of coccidioidomycosis. Clin. Infect. Dis. *30*:658–661, 2000.
66. Galgiani, J. N., Catanzaro, A., Cloud, G. A., et al.: Fluconazole therapy for coccidioidal meningitis: The NIAID-Mycoses Study Group. Ann. Intern. Med. *119*:28–35, 1993.
67. Galgiani, J. N., Catanzaro, A., Cloud, G. A., et al.: Comparison of oral fluconazole and itraconazole for progressive, nonmeningeal coccidioidomycosis. A randomized, double-blind trial. Ann. Intern. Med. *133*:676–686, 2000.
68. Gardner, S., Seilheimer, D., Catlin, F., et al.: Subglottic coccidioidomycosis presenting with persistent stridor. Pediatrics *66*:623–625, 1980.
69. Gifford, M. A., Buss, W. I. C., and Duds, R. J.: Data on *Coccidioides* fungus infection, Kern County, 1900–1936. *In* Kern County Health Department Annual Report. 1936–1937, pp. 39–54.
70. Golden, S. E., Morgan, C. M., Bartley, D. L., et al.: Disseminated coccidioidomycosis with chorioretinitis in early infancy. Pediatr. Infect. Dis. *5*:272–274, 1986.
71. Goldstein, E., Winship, M. J., Pappagianis, D.: Ventricular fluid and the management of coccidioidal meningitis. Ann. Intern. Med. *77*:243–246, 1972.
72. Goodman, D. H., and Schabarum, B.: Primary cutaneous coccidioidomycosis: Visible classic demonstration of delayed hypersensitivity. Ann. Intern. Med. *59*:84–90, 1963.
73. Graham, A. R., Sobonya, R. E., Bronnimann, D. A., et al.: Quantitative pathology of coccidioidomycosis in acquired immunodeficiency syndrome. Hum. Pathol. *19*:800–806, 1988.
74. Graybill, J. R.: Treatment of coccidioidomycosis. Curr. Top. Med. Mycol. *5*:151–179, 1993.
75. Graybill, J. R., Stevens, D. A., Galgiani, J. N., et al.: Ketoconazole treatment of coccidioidal meningitis. Ann. N. Y. Acad. Sci. *544*:488–496, 1988.
76. Greendyke, W. H., Resnick, D. L., and Harvey, W. C.: The varied roentgen manifestations of primary coccidioidomycosis. A. J. R. Am. J. Roentgenol. *109*:491–499, 1970.
77. Hagman, H. M., Madnick, E. G., D'Agostino, A. N., et al.: Hyphal forms of the central nervous system of patients with coccidioidomycosis. Clin. Infect. Dis. *30*:349–355, 2000.
78. Hajare, S., Rakusan, T. A., Kalia, A., et al.: Laryngeal coccidioidomycosis causing airway obstruction. Pediatr. Infect. Dis. *8*:54–56, 1989.
79. Hall, K. A., Sethi, G. K., Rosado, L. J., et al.: Coccidioidomycosis and heart transplantation. J. Heart Lung Transplant. *12*:525–526, 1993.
80. Harley, W. B., and Blaser, M. J.: Disseminated coccidioidomycosis associated with extreme eosinophilia. Clin. Infect. Dis. *18*:627–629, 1994.
81. Harrison, H. R., Galgiani, J. N., Sprunger, L., et al.: Amphotericin B and imidazole therapy for coccidioidal meningitis in children. Pediatr. Infect. Dis. *2*:216–221, 1983.
82. Hobbs, E. R.: Coccidioidomycosis. Dermatol. Clin. *7*:227–239, 1989.
83. Huntington, R. W., Jr.: Morphology and racial distribution of fatal coccidioidomycosis: Report of a 10-year autopsy series in an endemic area. J. A. M. A. *169*:115–118, 1959.
84. Huntington, R. W.: Pathology of coccidioidomycosis. *In* Stevens, D. A. (ed.): Coccidioidomycosis: A Text. New York, Plenum Medical, 1980, pp. 113–132.
85. Huppert, M.: Serology of coccidioidomycosis. Mycopathol. Mycol. Appl. *41*:107–113, 1970.
86. Huppert, M., and Bailey, J. W.: The use of immunodiffusion tests in coccidioidomycosis. I. The accuracy and reproducibility of the immunodiffusion test which correlates with complement fixation. Am. J. Clin. Pathol. *44*:364–373, 1965.
87. Huppert, M., Levine, H. B., Sun, S. H., et al.: Resistance of vaccinated mice to typical and atypical strains of *Coccidioides immitis*. J. Bacteriol. *94*:924–927, 1967.
88. Huppert, M., and Sun, S. H.: Overview of mycology, and the mycology of *Coccidioides immitis*. *In* Stevens, D. A. (ed.): Coccidioidomycosis: A Text. New York, Plenum Medical, 1980, pp. 21–46.
89. Hyatt, H. W., Sr.: Coccidioidomycosis in a 3-week-old infant. Am. J. Dis. Child. *105*:93–98, 1963.
90. Hyde, L.: Coccidioidal pulmonary cavitation. Dis. Chest *54*(Suppl. 1): 273–277, 1968.
91. Iger, M.: Coccidioidal osteomyelitis. *In* Ajello, L. (ed.): Coccidioidomycosis. Miami, Symposia Specialists, 1977, pp. 177–190.
92. Johnson, J. E., III, Perry, J. E., Fekety, F. R., et al.: Laboratory-acquired coccidioidomycosis: A report of 210 cases. Ann. Intern. Med. *60*:941–956, 1964.
93. Kafka, J. A., and Catanzaro, A. T.: Disseminated coccidioidomycosis in children. J. Pediatr. *98*:355–361, 1981.
94. Kaufman, L., Sekhon, A. S., Moledina, N., et al.: Comparative evaluation of commercial Premier EIA and microimmunodiffusion and complement fixation tests for *Coccidioides immitis* antibodies. J. Clin. Microbiol. *33*:618–619, 1995.
95. Kelly, P. C.: Coccidioidal meningitis. *In* Stevens, D. A. (ed.): Coccidioidomycosis: A Text. New York, Plenum Medical, 1980, pp. 163–193.
96. Kerrick, S. S., Lundergan, L. L., and Galgiani, J. N.: Coccidioidomycosis at a university health service. Am. Rev. Respir. Dis. *131*:100–102, 1985.
97. Knoper, S. R., and Galgiani, J. N.: Coccidioidomycosis. Infect. Dis. Clin. North Am. *2*:861–875, 1988.
98. Labadie, E. L., and Hamilton, R. H.: Survival improvement in coccidioidal meningitis by high-dose intrathecal amphotericin B. Arch. Intern. Med. *146*:2013–2018, 1986.
99. Larwood, T. R.: Coccidioidin skin testing in Kern County, California: Decrease in infection rate over 58 years. Clin. Infect. Dis. *30*:612–613, 2000.
100. Levine, H. B., Pappagianis, D., and Cobb, J. M.: Development of vaccines for coccidioidomycosis. Mycopathol. Mycol. Appl. *41*:177–185, 1970.
101. Linsangan, L. C., and Ross, L. A.: *Coccidioides immitis* infection of the neonate: Two routes of infection. Pediatr. Infect. Dis. J. *18*:171–173, 1999.
102. Lonky, S. A., Catanzaro, A., Moser, K. M., et al.: Acute coccidioidal pleural effusion. Am. Rev. Respir. Dis. *114*:681–688, 1976.
103. Lopez, A. M., Williams, P. L., and Ampel, N. M.: Acute pulmonary coccidioidomycosis mimicking bacterial pneumonia and septic shock: A report of two cases. Am. J. Med. *95*:236–239, 1993.
104. Lubarsky, R., and Plunkett, O. A.: Some ecologic studies of *Coccidioides immitis* in soil. *In* Sternberg, T. H., Newcomer, V. D. (eds.): Therapy of Fungus Diseases, an International Symposium. Boston, Little, Brown, 1955, pp. 308–310.
105. Lundergan, L. L., Kerrick, S. S., and Galgiani, J. N.: Coccidioidomycosis at a university outpatient clinic: A clinical description. *In* Einstein, H. E., and Catanzaro, A. (eds.): Coccidioidomycosis. Proceedings of the Fourth International Conference. Washington D.C., National Foundation for Infectious Diseases, 1985, pp. 47–54.
106. MacDonald, N., Steinhoff, M. C., and Powell, K. R.: Review of coccidioidomycosis in immunocompromised children. Am. J. Dis. Child. *135*:553–556, 1981.
107. Mahaffey, K. W., Hippenmeyer, C. L., Mandel, R., et al.: Unrecognized coccidioidomycosis complicating *Pneumocystis carinii* pneumonia in patients infected with the human immunodeficiency virus and treated with corticosteroids: A report of two cases. Arch. Intern. Med. *153*:1496–1498, 1993.
108. Marks, T. S., Spence, W. F., and Baisch, B. F.: Limited resection for pulmonary coccidioidomycosis. *In* Ajello, L. (ed.): Coccidioidomycosis. Tucson, University of Arizona Press, 1967, pp. 73–78.
109. Martins, T. B., Jaskowski, T. D., Mouritsen, C. L., et al.: Comparison of commercially available enzyme immunoassay with traditional serological tests for detection of antibodies to *Coccidioides immitis*. J. Clin. Microbiol. *33*:940–943, 1995.
110. McNeil, M. M., and Ampel, N. M.: Coccidioidomycosis in patients infected with human immunodeficiency virus: Prevention issues and priorities. Clin. Infect. Dis. *21*(Suppl.):111–113, 1995.
111. Minamoto, G., and Armstrong, D.: Fungal infections in AIDS: Histoplasmosis and coccidioidomycosis. Infect. Dis. Clin. North Am. *2*:447–456, 1988.
112. Mischel, P. S., and Vinters, H. V.: Coccidioidomycosis of the central nervous system: Neuropathological and vasculopathic manifestations and clinical correlates. Clin. Infect. Dis. *20*:400–405, 1995.
113. Murphy, S. M., Drash, A. L., and Donnelly, W. H.: Disseminated coccidioidomycosis associated with immunosuppressive therapy following renal transplantation. Pediatrics *48*:144–145, 1971.
114. O'Brien, J. J., and Gilsdorf, J. R.: Primary cutaneous coccidioidomycosis in childhood. Pediatr. Infect. Dis. *5*:485–486, 1986.
115. Oldfield, E. C., III, Bone, W. D., Martin, C. R., et al.: Prediction of relapse after treatment of coccidioidomycosis. Clin. Infect. Dis. *25*:1205–1211, 1997.
116. Opelz, G., and Scheer, M. I.: Cutaneous sensitivity and in vitro responsiveness of lymphocytes in patients with disseminated coccidioidomycosis. J. Infect. Dis. *132*:250–255, 1975.
117. Overholt, E. L., and Hornick, R. B.: Primary cutaneous coccidioidomycosis. Arch. Intern. Med. *114*:149–153, 1964.
118. Padhye, A. A., Smith, G., Standard, P. G., et al.: Comparative evaluation of chemiluminescent DNA probe assays and exoantigen tests for rapid identification of *Blastomyces dermatitidis* and *Coccidioides immitis*. J. Clin. Microbiol. *32*:867–870, 1994.
119. Pappagianis, D.: Epidemiology of coccidioidomycosis. Curr. Top. Med. Mycol. *2*:199–238, 1988.

120. Pappagianis, D.: Evaluation of the protective efficacy of the killed *Coccidioides immitis* spherule vaccine in humans: The Valley Fever Vaccine Study Group. Am. Rev. Respir. Dis. *148*:656–660, 1993.
121. Pappagianis, D., Krasnow, R. I., and Beall, S.: False-positive reactions of cerebrospinal fluid and diluted sera with the coccidioidal latex agglutination test. Am. J. Clin. Pathol. *66*:916–921, 1976.
122. Pappagianis, D., Lindsey, N. J., Smith, C. E., et al.: Antibodies in human coccidioidomycosis: Immunoelectrophoretic properties. Proc. Soc. Exp. Biol. Med. *118*:118–122, 1965.
123. Pappagianis, D., and Zimmer, D. L.: Serology of coccidioidomycosis. Clin. Microbiol. Rev. *3*:247–268, 1990.
124. Petersen, E. A., Friedman, B. A., Crowder, E. D., et al.: Coccidioiduria: Clinical significance. Ann. Intern. Med. *85*:34–38, 1976.
125. Peterson, C. M., Schuppert, K., Kelly, P. C., et al.: Coccidioidomycosis and pregnancy. Obstet. Gynecol. Surv. *48*:149–156, 1993.
126. Pinckney, L., and Parker, B. R.: Primary coccidioidomycosis in children presenting with massive pleural effusion. A. J. R. Am. J. Roentgenol. *130*:247–249, 1978.
127. Polesky, A., Kirsch, C. M., Snyder, L. S., et al.: Airway coccidioidomycosis—report of cases and review. Clin. Infect. Dis. *28*:1273–1280, 1999.
128. Pollock, S. F., Morris, J. M., and Murray, W. R.: Coccidioidal synovitis of the knee. J. Bone Joint Surg. Am. *49*:1397–1407, 1967.
129. Pont, A., Williams, P. L., Azhar, S., et al.: Ketoconazole blocks testosterone synthesis. Arch. Intern. Med. *142*:2137–2140, 1982.
130. Puckett, T. F.: Hyphae of *Coccidioides immitis* in tissues of the human host. Am. Rev. Tuberc. *70*:320–327, 1954.
131. Ragland, A. S., Arsura, E., Ismail, Y., et al.: Eosinophilic pleocytosis in coccidioidal meningitis: Frequency and significance. Am. J. Med. *95*:254–257, 1993.
132. Ramras, D. G., Walch, H. A., Murray, J. P., et al.: An epidemic of coccidioidomycosis in the Pacific Beach area of San Diego. Am. Rev. Respir. Dis. *101*:975–978, 1970.
133. Rapaport, F. T., Lawrence, H. S., Millar, J. W., et al.: The immunologic properties of coccidioidin as a skin test reagent in man. J. Immunol. *84*:368–373, 1960.
134. 1993 Revised classification system of HIV infection and expanded surveillance case definition for AIDS among adolescents and adults. M. M. W. R. Recomm. Rep. *41*(RR-17):1–19, 1992.
135. Richardson, H. B., Jr., Anderson, J. A., and McKay, B. M.: Acute pulmonary coccidioidomycosis in children. J. Pediatr. *70*:376–382, 1967.
136. Riley, D. K., Galgiani, J. N., O'Donnell, M., et al.: Coccidioidomycosis in bone marrow transplant recipients. Transplantation *56*:1531–1533, 1993.
137. Roberts, P. L., and Lisciandro, R. C.: A community epidemic of coccidioidomycosis. Am. Rev. Respir. Dis. *96*:766–772, 1967.
138. Rosenstein, N. E., Emery, K. W., Werner, S. B., et al.: Risk factors for severe pulmonary and disseminated coccidioidomycosis: Kern County, California, 1995–1996. Clin. Infect. Dis. *32*:708–715, 2001.
139. Rothman, P. E., Graw, R. G., and Harris, J. C.: Coccidioidomycosis: Possible fomite transmission: A review and report of a case. Am. J. Dis. Child. *118*:792–801, 1969.
140. Sarosi, G. A., Catanzaro, A., Daniel, T. M., et al.: Clinical usefulness of skin testing in histoplasmosis, coccidioidomycosis, and blastomycosis. Am. Rev. Respir. Dis. *138*:1081–1082, 1988.
141. Sawaki, Y., Huppert, M., Bailey, J. W., et al.: Patterns of human antibody reactions in coccidioidomycosis. J. Bacteriol. *91*:422–427, 1966.
142. Shafai, T.: Neonatal coccidioidomycosis in premature twins. Am. J. Dis. Child. *132*:634, 1978.
143. Shehab, Z. M., Britton, H., and Dunn, J. H.: Imidazole therapy of coccidioidal meningitis in children. Pediatr. Infect. Dis. J. 7:40–44, 1988.
144. Sievers, M. L.: Disseminated coccidioidomycosis among southwestern American Indians. Am. Rev. Respir. Dis. *109*:602–612, 1974.
145. Smale, L. E., and Waechter, K. G.: Dissemination of coccidioidomycosis in pregnancy. Am. J. Obstet. Gynecol. *107*:356–361, 1970.
146. Smith, C. E.: Epidemiology of acute coccidioidomycosis with erythema nodosum ("San Joaquin" or "Valley Fever"). Am. J. Public Health *30*:600–611, 1940.
147. Smith, C. E.: Coccidioidomycosis. Pediatr. Clin. North Am. *2*:109–125, 1955.
148. Smith, C. E., Beard, R. R., Rosenberger, H. G., et al.: Effect of season and dust control on coccidioidomycosis. J. A. M. A. *132*:833–838, 1946.
149. Smith, C. E., Beard, R. R., Whiting, E. G., et al.: Varieties of coccidioidal infection in relation to the epidemiology and control of the diseases. Am. J. Public Health *36*:1394–1402, 1946.
150. Smith, C. E., Saito, M. T., Beard, R. R., et al.: Serological tests in the diagnosis and prognosis of coccidioidomycosis. Am. J. Hyg. *52*:1–21, 1950.
151. Smith, C. E., Saito, M. T., and Simons, S. A.: Pattern of 39,500 serologic tests in coccidioidomycosis. J. A. M. A. *160*:546–552, 1956.
152. Smith, C. E., Whiting, E. G., Baker, E. E., et al.: The use of coccidioidin. Am. Rev. Tuberc. *57*:330–360, 1948.
153. Spark, R. P.: Does transplacental spread of coccidioidomycosis occur? Arch. Pathol. Lab. Med. *105*:347–350, 1981.
154. Standaert, S. M., Schaffner, W., Galgiani, J. N., et al.: Coccidioidomycosis among visitors to a *Coccidioides immitis*–endemic area: An outbreak in a military reserve unit. J. Infect. Dis. *171*:1672–1675, 1995.
155. Standard, P. G., and Kaufman, L.: Immunological procedure for the rapid and specific identification of *Coccidioides immitis* cultures. J. Clin. Microbiol. *5*:149–153, 1977.
156. Stevens, D. A.: Coccidioidomycosis. N. Engl. J. Med. *332*:1077–1082, 1995.
157. Stevens, D. A., Levine, H. B., Ten Eyck, D. R., et al.: Dermal sensitivity to different doses of spherulin and coccidioidin. Chest *65*:530–533, 1974.
158. Sun, S. H., Huppert, M., and Vukovich, K. R.: Rapid in vitro conversion and identification of *Coccidioides immitis*. J. Clin. Microbiol. *3*:186–190, 1976.
159. Teel, K. W., Yow, M. D., and Williams, T. W., Jr.: A localized outbreak of coccidioidomycosis in southern Texas. J. Pediatr. *77*:65–73, 1970.
160. Tom, P. F., Long, T. J., and Fitzpatrick, S. B.: Coccidioidomycosis in adolescents presenting as chest pain. J. Adolesc. Health Care *8*:365–371, 1987.
161. Townsend, T. E., and McKey, R. W.: Coccidioidomycosis in infants. Am. J. Dis. Child. *86*:51–53, 1953.
162. Tucker, R. M., Denning, D. W., Dupont, B., et al.: Itraconazole therapy for chronic coccidioidal meningitis. Ann. Intern. Med. *112*:108–112, 1990.
163. Tucker, R. M., Galgiani, J. N., Denning, D. W., et al.: Treatment of coccidioidal meningitis with fluconazole. Rev. Infect. Dis. *12*(Suppl.): 380–389, 1990.
164. Tucker, R. M., Williams, P. L., Arathoon, E. G., et al.: Pharmacokinetics of fluconazole in cerebrospinal fluid and serum in human coccidioidal meningitis. Antimicrob. Agents Chemother. *32*:369–373, 1988.
165. Vaughan, J. E., and Ramirez, H.: Coccidioidomycosis as a complication of pregnancy. Calif. Med. *74*:121–125, 1951.
166. Vincent, T., Galgiani, J. N., Huppert, M., et al.: The natural history of coccidioidal meningitis: VA-Armed Forces cooperative studies, 1955–1958. Clin. Infect. Dis. *16*:247–254, 1993.
167. Wack, E. E., Ampel, N. M., Galgiani, J. N., et al.: Coccidioidomycosis during pregnancy: An analysis of ten cases among 47,120 pregnancies. Chest *94*:376–379, 1988.
168. Warlick, M. A., Quan, S. F., and Sobonya, R. E.: Rapid diagnosis of pulmonary coccidioidomycosis: Cytologic v. potassium hydroxide preparations. Arch. Intern. Med. *143*:723–725, 1983.
169. Weiden, M. A., Galgiani, J. N., and Pappagianis, D.: Comparison of immunodiffusion techniques with standard complement fixation assay for quantitation of coccidioidal antibodies. J. Clin. Microbiol. *18*:529–534, 1983.
170. Werner, S. B., Pappagianis, D., Heindl, I., et al.: An epidemic of coccidioidomycosis among archeology students in northern California. N. Engl. J. Med. *28*:507–512, 1972.
171. Williams, P. L., Johnson, R., Pappagianis, D., et al.: Vasculitic and encephalitic complications associated with *Coccidioides immitis* infection of the central nervous system in humans: Report of 10 cases and review. Clin. Infect. Dis. *14*:673–682, 1992.
172. Winn, R. E., Johnson, R., Galgiani, J. N., et al.: Cavitary coccidioidomycosis with fungus ball formation: Diagnosis by fiberoptic bronchoscopy with coexistence of hyphae and spherules. Chest *105*:412–416, 1994.
173. Winn, W. A.: Primary cutaneous coccidioidomycosis. Arch. Dermatol. *9*:221–228, 1965.
174. Winn, W. A., Levine, H. B., Broderick, J. E., et al.: A localized epidemic of coccidioidal infection: Primary coccidioidomycosis occurring in a group of ten children infected in a backyard playground in the San Joaquin Valley of California. N. Engl. J. Med. *268*:867–870, 1963.
175. Winter, W. G., Jr., Larson, R. K., Honeggar, M. M., et al.: Coccidioidal arthritis and its treatment: 1975. J. Bone Joint Surg. Am. *57*:1152–1157, 1975.
176. Woods, C. W., McRill, C., Plikaytis, B. D., et al.: Coccidioidomycosis in human immunodeficiency virus–infected persons in Arizona, 1994–1997: Incidence, risk factors, and prevention. J. Infect. Dis. *181*:1428–1434, 2000.
177. Zartarian, M., Petersen, E. M., and de la Maza, L. M.: Detection of antibodies to *Coccidioides immitis* by enzyme immunoassay. Am. J. Clin. Pathol. *107*:148–153, 1997.
178. Ziering, W. H., and Rockas, H. R.: Coccidioidomycosis: Long-term treatment with amphotericin B of disseminated disease in a three-month-old baby. Am. J. Dis. Child. *108*:454–459, 1964.
179. Zweiman, B., Pappagianis, D., Mailbach, H., et al.: Coccidioidin delayed hypersensitivity: Skin test and in vitro lymphocyte reactivities. J. Immunol. *102*:1284–1289, 1969.

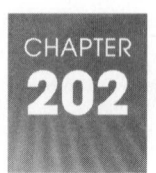

CHAPTER 202 Paracoccidioidomycosis

ANGELA RESTREPO-MORENO ■ GIL BENARD

Paracoccidioidomycosis, formerly known as South American blastomycosis, usually is a progressive chronic disease that preferentially affects the lungs, skin, mucous membranes, adrenals, and reticuloendothelial system. Benign, self-limited infections also have been documented occasionally. Two types of clinical presentations are described: the acute-subacute (juvenile) and the chronic (adult) forms of the disease. Children generally present with the acute form, which affects predominantly the reticuloendothelial system organs. The mycosis is limited geographically to various Latin American countries.[3, 14, 17, 20, 44, 55, 56, 59, 80]

The disease was described originally by Lutz[55] in Brazil in 1908 and initially observed in children in 1911 by Montenegro.[58]

The Organism

Paracoccidioides brasiliensis is the etiologic agent of this disease. It is an imperfect, dimorphic fungus that grows as a mold at room temperature (14° to 24° C) and as a yeast at 37° C. In the mycelial phase, growth is slow, about 3 to 4 weeks; the colony is white to tan and compact, with short aerial mycelia. Microscopically thin, septated hyphae and chlamydospores are seen, but under special conditions (natural substrates, media with reduced carbohydrate content), arthroconidia and aleurioconidia also are produced.[20] The small size of these conidia (less than 5 μm) renders them compatible with alveolar deposition; furthermore, such conidia have been shown to be infectious when inhaled.[69]

The mycelial phase is not distinctive, and subcultures at 37° C are required for complete identification. At this temperature, *P. brasiliensis* produces soft, wrinkled, cream-colored colonies that develop in about 6 to 10 days. Microscopically, the most characteristic feature is the presence of multiple budding yeast cells; the parent cell produces various peripheral buds and acquires the appearance of a pilot's wheel. Single buds and short chains also are produced, but they are not diagnostic. Cells are quite variable in size (2 to 40 μm) and have a thick cell wall and internal vacuoles. This phase of growth is identical to the one observed in tissue and pathologic materials.[3, 20, 44, 55, 75, 80, 86] The organism does not readily take most bacterial or hematologic stains. *P. brasiliensis* is aerobic and, in its mycelial phase, grows well in the regular mycologic media to which antibiotics and cycloheximide have been added in order to reduce growth of bacteria and saprophytic fungi.[20, 55]

Transmission

Paracoccidioidomycosis is not a contagious disease.[20, 44, 55, 80, 92, 110] Although a single case of placental involvement that did not result in fetal infection has been reported,[16] Epidemic outbreaks have not been reported, and only a few cases in family members have been documented,[3, 55–57, 80, 110] which could be attributed to the long periods of mycosis latency between the moment of infection and the appearance of overt clinical manifestations.[3, 59, 93] Consequently, the memory of the activity conducive to the infection of the patient or of the accompanying individuals usually has been forgotten,[19] which prompted Borelli to coin the name "reservarea" for those places in the endemic areas where the fungus has its habitat and humans acquire the infection. This concept differs from that of an "endemic area," which implicates the place where the disease is diagnosed.[19]

P. brasiliensis infection in animals as proved by culture or histology has been shown consistently only in armadillos, mammals that probably acquire the infection when disturbing the terrestrial habitat of the fungus.[5, 22, 94, 104] Unfortunately, the microniche of *P. brasiliensis* has not been identified properly; soil has been incriminated, but the number of isolates from this source is small.[45] Recently, the role played by deforestation in increasing both exposure and incidence rates has been documented in Brazil in Amerindians and in children.[32, 42, 96] The ecological factors that prevail in the reservarea also have been characterized, with the following being significantly associated with the disease: altitude from 1000 to 1499 meters above sea level, rainfall from 2000 to 2999 mm, and presence of humid forests and of coffee and tobacco crops.[24] In Colombia, the fertile Andean regions have the highest incidence rates of paracoccidioidomycosis.[107]

Paracoccidioidomycosis was thought, and still is by some, to be acquired by trauma; however, clinical and experimental data indicate that infection is acquired most commonly by inhalation.[20, 47, 57, 75, 81]

Epidemiology

AGE

More than 70 percent of the patients are 30 years of age or older. Until recently, the number of childhood cases was shown to be only 2.1 percent in the first decade of life.[7, 8, 27, 55, 58, 110] In 1976, Castro and del Negro[27] published one of the largest series of children with paracoccidioidomycosis diagnosed in a 30-year period. They found that among 1899 patients with this disease seen at the Hospital das Clinicas in São Paulo, Brazil, only 70 (3.6%) of the patients were 14 years of age or younger. However, in 1999 and in the same state, Blotta and colleagues[17] found that 5.6 percent of the paracoccidioidomycosis patients diagnosed between 1988 and 1996 were younger than 14 years of age, thus showing an increase over the 1976 figure. In 1998, Rios-Gonçalves and associates[96] analyzed the records of 36 children who had been diagnosed in the state of Rio de Janeiro during a period of 25 years. In a similar lapse, Fonseca's group[42] described 13 children, 12.7 percent of all cases, who had been diagnosed in the Amazonian states of Pará and Tocantins, forest areas that have been colonized since the 1970s and where paracoccidioidomycosis formerly had been regarded as rare.

In certain places, the infection rates measured by a positive skin test reaction also are high. In 1976, Pedrosa[85] conducted a skin testing survey among rural children (6 to 11 years of age) in a particular county of Rio de Janeiro where

TABLE 202–1 ■ AGE AND GENDER DISTRIBUTION IN 235 CHILDREN WITH PARACOCCIDIOIDOMYCOSIS

Gender*	Age		Total by gender (%)
	3–9 yr	10–14 yr	
Males	55	86	141 (60)
Females	45	49	94 (40)
Totals by age (%)	100 (43.0)	135 (57.8)	235 (100)

*Male-to-female=1.5:1.
Data taken from references 17, 23, 30, 31, 42, 73, 85, 95, and 96.

paracoccidioidomycosis had been previously diagnosed in a 3-year-old boy. He found that 34 percent of the children tested positive for paracoccidioidin, a figure indicative of early exposure to *P. brasiliensis*.

In 1996, Londero and colleagues[58] compiled the records of 106 children with the mycosis, including those formerly analyzed by Castro and del Negro.[27] This series, a recent compilation,[8] several individual reports, and a thesis* have revealed that the disease occurs more frequently in individuals 12 to 15 years of age than in younger children (Table 202–1). More than 250 reports of paracoccidioidomycosis in children aged 3 to 14 years, including those analyzed by Londero and colleagues,[58] have been found in a literature search.[†]

The relative paucity of children with this mycosis in comparison with the figures reported in adults, close to 10,000 cases,[3, 14, 17, 37, 45, 55–57, 62, 100, 109] may be explained, in part, by the effective control exerted by most hosts on the progression of the primary infection, by the long incubation period characteristic of the mycosis, and by the establishment of latent foci that may become apparent clinically many years after initial exposure.[3, 12, 20, 29, 43, 47, 57, 59, 93] Benard and associates[10] consider that the association with different age groups is related to the epidemiology of paracoccidioidomycosis because in the endemic areas, as previously shown, children become exposed to the fungus at an early age. In healthy children, appropriate defenses usually curtail development of the mycosis, but in infants of low socioeconomic conditions, the transition from infection to overt disease may be accelerated and aggravated by the mycosis itself, by malnutrition, or by other associated conditions.[8, 10, 17, 27, 42, 96] In addition, unknown susceptibility factors, the intensity of exposure to the infectious source, the virulence of certain *P. brasiliensis* isolates, and other factors may well contribute to the development of the disease in children.[8, 9, 12, 31, 42, 58, 110]

GENDER

Adult males are afflicted with much greater frequency than are females (male-to-female ratio of 14:1).[3, 14, 17, 20, 42, 55, 57, 80, 110] In children, however, the disease affects males and females in about equal proportions.[14, 17, 27, 42, 58, 96, 110] In the review published by Londero and associates,[58] which included children up to 14 years of age, a slight predominance of male patients was noted in the older group (see Table 202–1). These findings suggest that the sex hormones, the hormone-dependent immunologic factors, or both play a role in determining the outcome of the host-parasite interaction.[4, 12, 20, 91] Researchers have shown that *in vitro* estrogens inhibit *P. brasiliensis* mycelium-to-yeast transition, thereby hindering the progression of the infection.[4, 20, 91]

*See references 7, 17, 22, 23, 30, 31, 42, 85, 95, 96.
†See references 2, 7, 8, 17, 22, 23, 30, 31, 39, 42, 58, 73, 85, 95, 96.

OCCUPATION AND RACE

Almost one half of the reported cases in adults occur in individuals whose occupations require extensive exposure to the soil.* Adult residents of areas in which paracoccidioidomycosis is endemic generally develop disease that is less severe than that seen in immigrants or in people who migrate to highly endemic settings. These people often develop disseminated infection, much like the juvenile cases do.[3, 10, 12, 29, 55–58, 71, 80, 88, 110] The influence of genetic traits on the mycosis has not been elucidated.[35]

GEOGRAPHIC DISTRIBUTION

Paracoccidioidomycosis is restricted to Latin America, from Mexico to Argentina; some countries within this area (Chile and some of the Caribbean Islands), however, are free of the disorder. In endemic countries, the disease's distribution is uneven, and most cases occur in individuals living in regions corresponding to the humid tropical and subtropical forests.[†] The endemic area is centered in Brazil; 7000 of the about 10,000 patients reported to date were natives of this country.[14, 17, 44, 55–57, 62, 80, 96, 110] Although paracoccidioidomycosis has been reported in patients not living in endemic areas, prior residence in Latin America has been documented in every case.[59, 93] In some of these patients, the interval between residence in the endemic area and clinical manifestations of the disease has been 10 to 40 years.[3, 55, 93] Within endemic areas, 10 to 50 percent of healthy adult individuals react to the intradermal administration of paracoccidioidin, suggesting previous contact or subclinical infection with *P. brasiliensis*.[18, 20, 22, 32, 58, 85] Recent molecular biology studies have indicated the existence of at least five different groups of *P. brasiliensis* strains and their close correspondence with the borders of the various endemic countries.[82] Despite its apparently restricted ecological niche, the habitat of the etiologic agent has not been determined precisely.[90, 94]

Pathogenesis and Pathology

The initial stages of the host-parasite interaction are unknown because of our inability to detect the precise moment when infection does occur.[43] In the past, traumatic implantation of the fungal propagules into skin and mucosa was thought to cause primary lesions, whereas other manifestations were regarded as secondary. However, through the study of many cases, including autopsies, what has become apparent is that pulmonary lesions are primary, with the infection taking place by inhalation of fungal propagules.[20, 47] In experimental animals, the inhalatory route has been shown to give rise to disseminated disease.[69] In most cases, the initial pulmonary infection does not cause undue symptoms.[43, 56] Once the conidia reach the terminal bronchi or the alveolar spaces, yeast transformation ensues.[69] In some cases, the fungus promptly disseminates by the lymphohematogeneous route, producing distant

*See references 3, 14, 17, 20, 44, 55, 56, 80, 92, 110.
†See references 14, 17, 19, 22, 23, 24, 32, 42, 62, 90, 94, 107.

subclinical and quiescent foci. Apparently, the local defenses are capable of controlling fungal spread, but some viable yeast cells may remain dormant in such foci in the pulmonary and mediastinal lymph nodes. Rarely, the initial pulmonary infection outweighs the host's immune defenses, causing an acute-subacute disease, the juvenile type, with predominant involvement of the reticuloendothelial system.[44] The disease in children falls into this category. Often, the quiescent foci remain so throughout life, as demonstrated by the high number of subclinical infections compared with the low disease incidence of this mycosis in the endemic regions.[110] Nevertheless, the most common clinical presentation of the disease is the chronic form, or adult-type disease, believed to result from fungal reactivation in these foci. This reactivation frequently occurs when the patient has left the endemic area, as demonstrated by the cases reported outside Latin America, in countries where paracoccidioidomycosis is considered an imported pathology.[29, 59, 93]

Thus, in the acute or subacute form, the initial lung infection may pass unnoticed but is followed by prompt dissemination to other organs and tissues. In the chronic form, lung pathology frequently occurs. Pathology is restricted to the lungs in some of these patients, but in most, other organs also are afflicted. This may be caused by lymphohematogeneous dissemination from reactivated pulmonary foci or directly from foci at virtually any organ. Actually, paracoccidioidomycosis, in the acute, subacute, or chronic forms, is more frequently a disseminated disease, even though clinical manifestations appear to be restricted to a sole organ.[44, 71, 80] However, determination of the degree of dissemination certainly is influenced by the availability of diagnostic procedures. After appropriate therapy, residual lesions, mostly fibrotic, become established.[43, 71]

As already mentioned, the disease in children is acute or subacute and progressive (the juvenile form).[8, 27, 58] The time that elapses between infection and the onset of symptoms is not known precisely but has been estimated to be short, a few months.[43, 44] In such patients, paracoccidioidomycosis is a severe, systemic disorder that involves preferentially the reticuloendothelial system to such an extent that it is the hallmark of the process.[7, 8, 58]

In adults, pulmonary lesions may be micronodular or miliary, nodular, infiltrative or interstitial, cavitary, fibrotic, and mixed types.[71, 109] Emphysematous areas, pleural thickening, and enlarged hilar and mediastinal lymph nodes also can be observed. Right ventricular hypertrophy may be found in cases of long duration.[109] Lung involvement probably is secondary to a chronic lymphangitic process caused by the fungus itself and to the host's response represented by formation of granulomata and fibrosis, the latter of which predominates at the perihilar region. This aspect correlates with the butterfly-like (perihilar) micronodular and interstitial infiltration observed on plain films.[108] Obstruction and reversal of lymphatic flow lead to the spread of the inflammatory process throughout the lungs.

In children and adolescents, the pulmonary component tends to pass unnoticed, and neither clinical examination nor radiologic studies reflect the real damage.[47] Actually, only a minor proportion of the cases reported have had lung symptomatology[58] (Fig. 202–1). However, lack of notification may be more apparent than actual because the weight of the extrapulmonary lesions tends to minimize the less intense respiratory manifestations. Frequently, the mycosis is misdiagnosed, especially with tuberculosis and certain lymphomatous disorders.[58] Nonetheless, a careful search of pulmonary samples, including induced sputum, may reveal the characteristic multiple-budding *P. brasiliensis* yeast cells.[58, 89] New imaging methods, such as gallium and computed tomography, have allowed detection of incipient or discrete interstitial pulmonary lesions not revealed by plain radiographs.[23, 46, 111]

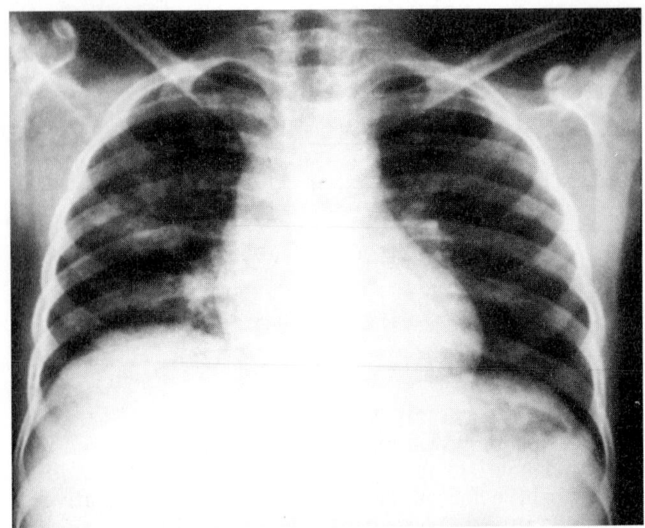

FIGURE 202–1 ■ Lung radiographs showing bilateral fluffy infiltrates mainly in the central and lower fields of the right lung, with tendency to coalesce. The patient is a 12-year-old child with extensive lymph node and skin involvement.

Lesions in the oropharyngeal and laryngeal mucosa occur frequently in the chronic form. They may be infiltrative, ulcerated, nodular, or vegetative and usually have a granulomatous aspect.[71, 99] The base of the ulcerated lesions usually is covered by small abscesses (the mulberry-like lesions) that probably represent fungal dissemination through the lymphatic system because they usually are accompanied by regional lymph node involvement.[28]

In children, such mucosal lesions are rather exceptional, but skin involvement occurs more commonly and tends to be multiple, in contrast with the adult chronic form.[64] In the latter, lesions are represented mostly by contiguous involvement of the periorificial mucosal lesions or draining lymph nodes. In children or young adults, and eventually in adults with the chronic severe disseminated disease, they represent hematogenous spread of the fungus. In this case, the lesions may appear as ulcerated or ulcerovegetative lesions, papules, or crust-covered ulcers, usually at the same stage of development. Reports of septic shock caused by septicemia by *P. brasiliensis* show that the fungus can be blood-borne.[71]

The reticuloendothelial system is the target organ in both children and young adults.[7] Almost every child with paracoccidioidomycosis exhibits involvement of the superficial or deep lymph node chains. Lymph nodes vary in size, number, consistency, and location; with time, they liquefy, forming abscesses or fistulas (Fig. 202–2). The spleen and liver frequently are involved in these same groups. Abdominal lymph node involvement also is a common occurrence in children.[7, 58] Hypertrophied lymph nodes, usually generalized but particularly periaortic, around the hepatic hilum and retroperitoneally can be detected by ultrasonography, computed tomography, or magnetic resonance imaging.[66] Coalescent masses may become palpable and may result in pathology caused by extrinsic compression of adjacent structures, such as jaundice by compression of the biliary duct,[18] pancreatitis,[18] or an intestinal obstruction.[67]

Splenic lesions are nodular or miliary. Gross hepatic lesions may not be apparent, but histopathologic examination regularly reveals fungal invasion of this organ.[7, 8, 58, 75]

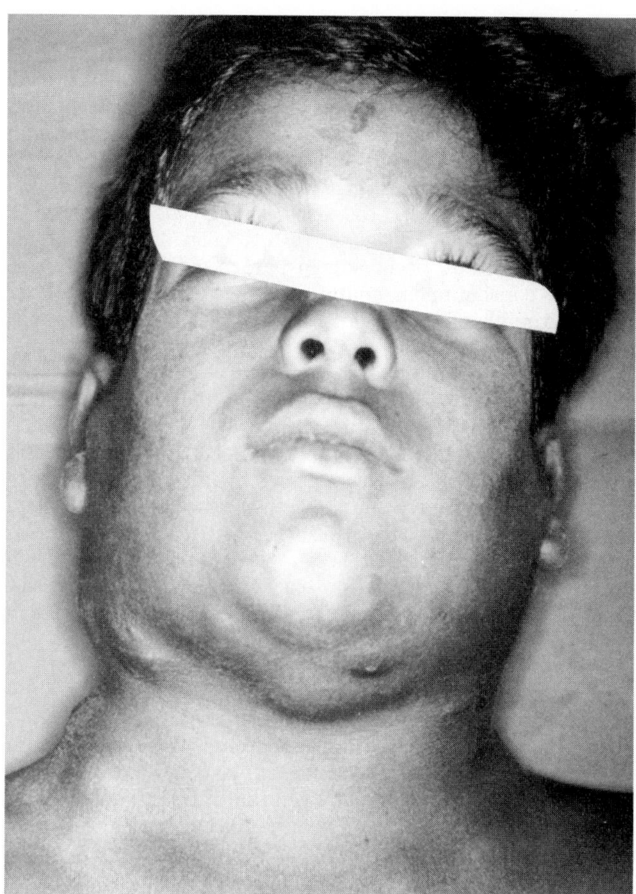

FIGURE 202–2 ■ Hypertrophied lymph nodes of the cervical and maxillary regions in a 10-year-old child.

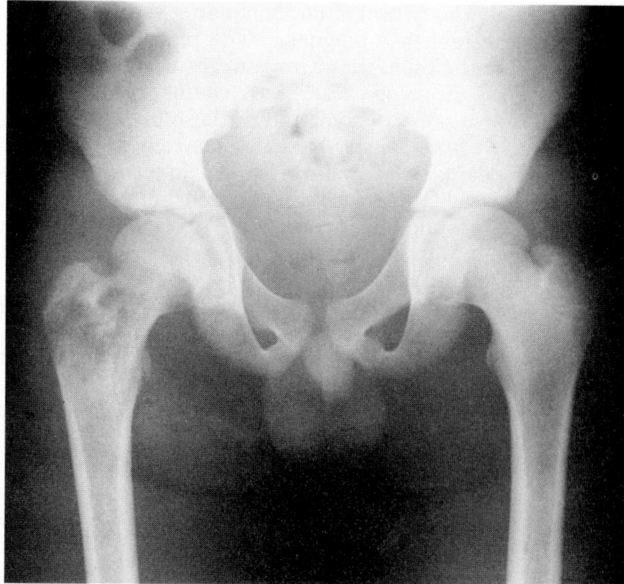

FIGURE 202–3 ■ Osteolytic lesions of the femur in a 9-year-old boy with subacute disseminated paracoccidioidomycosis.

In a series of fatal cases of paracoccidioidomycosis, 56.7 percent revealed the presence of yeast cells in the liver, associated with a granulomatous tissue response. Thirty percent of the cases had only widening of the portal tracts by fibrosis (31.6%), whereas 11.6 percent had an essentially normal liver.[105]

The intestinal mucosa may be affected, but similar to the lungs, its involvement is secondary to blockade of the regional lymphatic flow, with retrograde progression of *P. brasiliensis* to the mucosa, a process resulting in mycotic enteritis.[18, 41, 67] In this case, the submucosal inflammatory process is granulomatous; fungal cells are visualized; and the intestinal changes may vary from dilated loops, edema, congestion, and nodule formation to multiple mucosal ulcers.[41, 67]

Recent studies also have shown bone marrow infiltration mainly, but not exclusively, in the acute-subacute form of the disease: 25.7 percent of the patients examined during active disease and 36.4 percent of those who died of paracoccidioidomycosis revealed this type of involvement.[87] The histologic pattern was variable, but appropriate staining always displayed fungal cells. Bone marrow invasion frequently is associated with marked eosinophilia.[87, 102] In addition, bone (Fig. 202–3) and joint lesions are frequent occurrences in the acute-subacute form of the disease[2, 8, 39, 58] and appear closely related to bone marrow infiltration.[87]

The adrenals often are involved in patients with the chronic form of the mycoses, many of whom suffer from adrenal hypofunction or insufficiency (Addison disease). The glands contain multiple granulomatous foci, and diffuse necrosis may be seen in the most severe cases. Hyperplasia of the adrenal glands also occurs commonly.[71]

Histologically, formation of granulomata is the rule, except in patients with severe disseminated disease such as those with the acute-subacute form.[44] The granulomatous inflammation is associated with a mixed pyogenic component, especially in the case of ulcerated skin lesions or ruptured lymph nodes. Caseation and central necrosis may be present. In compact granulomata, abundant epithelial cells, Langerhans or foreign-body giant cells, plasmacytes, and lymphocytes are seen; often, phagocytosis of the yeast cells can be observed. $CD4^+$ lymphocytes dominate over $CD8^+$ lymphocytes and appear as peripheral mantles around aggregates of macrophages and histiocytes.[76] In the juvenile disseminated disease, the inflammatory reaction is diffuse, with abundance of both mononuclear and yeast cells but sparse formation of compact granulomas.[10, 27, 88] Loose granulomata appear unable to circumscribe fungal antigens, and at their periphery, *P. brasiliensis* antigens may permeate throughout the intercellular space.[98] Skin and mucous membrane lesions usually exhibit pseudoepitheliomatous hyperplasia and intraepithelial microabscesses.[3, 75, 98]

An interesting aspect drawn from the previously described histologic studies is the frequent description of areas of extremely active disease characterized by pyogenic reaction and loose granulomata, rich in budding fungal cells, intermingled with areas with compact granulomata, rare fungal cells, and variable degrees of fibrosis. This mixed aspect can be observed in lymph nodes, skin, or pulmonary lesions, suggesting that the disease evolves through localized new bouts of fungal multiplication and tissue invasion, whereas the adjacent older lesions are in their way to fibrotic resolution. Computed tomographic imaging of the lung confirmed this aspect by depicting areas with alveolar condensation along with fibrotic and emphysematous zones.[46]

Tissue reactions are nonspecific; thus, diagnosis depends on finding *P. brasiliensis*. If the parasite is abundant, it may be identified by hematoxylin and eosin stains. Special fungal stains (e.g., Grocott silver methenamine), however, always should be employed, especially when granulomata are examined. The typical multiple budding yeast cells must be found to establish a diagnosis. The presence of fungal cells of different sizes (2 to 40 μm) suggests the presence of *P. brasiliensis*. In some cases, short chains and cells with single buds also are observed, and in these patients, differentiation of *P. brasiliensis* from *Cryptococcus neoformans*, *Blastomyces dermatitidis*, and even *Histoplasma capsulatum* must be made. When the disease is chronic, most of the fungal cells are found inside the macrophages, but free yeast cells predominate in disseminated cases. Internalized yeast cells exhibit altered morphology.[3, 75, 93]

Interestingly, in old apparently inactive lesions, the remaining fungi have aberrant morphology and low viability indices, and they require a long time to multiply in microaerophilic conditions, which could explain the long latency period needed for the mycosis to become manifested in the chronic form patients.[93]

In paracoccidioidomycosis, the host-parasite interaction is complex, and both arms of the immune system participate in the immune response.[8, 10, 20] Patients with the mycosis have no deficiency in antibody production; on the other hand, a polyclonal activation of the humoral system, with high serum concentrations of specific immunoglobulin A (IgA), IgG isotypes, and IgE, is present.[8, 10, 15, 112] However, a protective role for antibodies has not been clearly demonstrated. In this mycosis, the patient has a depression of T-cell–mediated immunity characterized by lymphocyte proliferation and hypersensitivity skin tests hyporesponsiveness, the intensity of which parallels the severity of the infectious process and correlates inversely with the amount of anti–*P. brasiliensis*–specific antibodies produced.[77, 78] Patients with localized disease may have normal or nearly normal cell-mediated immune parameters and low or undetectable specific antibody responses, whereas in those with disseminated disease, cell-mediated immunity is depressed but the antibody titers are very high. This imbalance was particularly noted when antigen-specific responses were analyzed.[11, 13, 38, 78] Several studies showed that a particular cytokine pattern underlies this imbalance: low production of T_H1 cytokines such as interleukins-2 (IL-2) and interferon-γ (IFN-γ) and normal or increased production of helper T-cell subtype 2 (T_H2) cytokines such as IL-10, IL-5, and IL-4.[13, 52, 53, 60] That T_H2-type responses dominated more than T_H1 types in severe paracoccidioidomycosis was anticipated by elegant studies on mice models mimicking the progressive forms of the disease.[26, 51] In these models, both the T-cell–mediated and the antibody response were suggestive of a T_H2 control of the immune response.

In humans, researchers showed that, in the acute-subacute form of the disease, as well as in chronic cases with severely disseminated disease, the specific antibody isotypes also were under the influence of a T_H2 control. High levels of IgE and IgG4 (switch dependent on IL-4) were present, whereas these same isotypes were either low or undetectable in patients with the chronic form or less severe disease.[6, 60] Another aspect in favor of a T_H2 control was the observation of peripheral and bone marrow eosinophilia in severe cases, an abnormality linked to increased production of IL-5.[82a, 102] Apparently, in the acute-subacute disease, which usually is more severe and disseminated, the immune response fails to control the fungus from the beginning of the infectious process. Possibly, a consequence of the high antigen challenge or the participation of particular antigen-presenting cell subsets[1] is that the immune response is driven to a T_H2 pattern. This pattern would not be counteracted by T_H1 responses because the latter are profoundly down-modulated.[11, 60, 83a] In chronic, less severe cases, the initial infection was apparently controlled, which may allow a better balance of the immune responses, lower antigenic challenges, and a less marked T_H2 immune response. These clinical and experimental studies also indicated that such imbalance tended to disappear with response to treatment and resolution of the disease.[11, 51, 52, 60] Patients who were apparently cured demonstrated high lymphocyte proliferative responses as well as positive skin tests, and reestablishment of the capacity to secrete T_H1-type cytokines in response to fungal antigens. It has been shown that the immunodepression occurring in paracoccidioidomycosis has yet other consequences, manifested by the apparition of certain microbial infections with further decline of the health status of the patient.[9, 101]

Macrophages activated by cytokines represent the most important single host defense mechanism against *P. brasiliensis*. Intracellular killing of *P. brasiliensis* yeast cells and conidia has been shown to occur only when previous activation has taken place.[50] Studies with patients' monocytes have shown the important and synergistic role of tumor necrosis factor-α and IFN-γ in the arming of macrophages for efficient anti–*P. brasiliensis* activity.[25] In general, adequate correlation exists between active cellular immune responses and restriction of fungal growth in tissues.[20, 77]

Polymorphonuclear leukocytes (PMNs) also can be seen permeating some paracoccidioidodal lesions, especially those representing acute inflammation or microabscesses[98, 105, 108]; in experimental models, they appear early in the inflammatory process and likely play a role in the control of the initial infection.[21] Recent studies showed that human PMNs can be activated by cytokines to have enhanced anti–*P. brasiliensis* activity.[54]

Clinical Manifestations

Paracoccidioidomycosis is a polymorphic disorder that at a particular time may involve more than one organ system. Thus, making a topographic classification is unrealistic, and the classification of the mycosis currently accepted takes into consideration not only the organs involved but also the host's immune condition and the disease's natural history.[43] The infection is categorized as a *subclinical form*, and the overt process is subdivided into *acute-subacute* or *chronic disease*. The acute-subacute pattern predominates in children and young adults who are at greater risk than are patients exhibiting the chronic disease. According to the severity of the process, juvenile patients are assigned to two subgroups: severe and moderate. The adult type, which is the chronic progressive form of paracoccidioidomycosis, may be localized to pulmonary lesions, the unifocal disease, or disseminated from its primary foci, the multifocal process. Disseminated disease is characterized by involvement of the skin; mucosa; reticuloendothelial system; adrenal glands; and, less frequently, the gastrointestinal or the genitourinary tract; bones; and central nervous system.[7, 16, 47, 64, 71, 75, 88] The chronic form can be mild, moderate, or severe.[43]

Patients with acute or subacute disease develop signs and symptoms of a wasting process. Fever, malaise, listlessness, weight loss, and emaciation are recorded frequently. The severity of these symptoms is proportional to the degree of the organic involvement. Londero and associates[58] gathered the information published up to 1994 and found 269 cases in children younger than 14 years of age; however, sufficient clinical data for analysis of the prominent organic involvement were provided for only 77 children. The clinical characteristics exhibited by these children and by other patients reported more recently are shown in Table 202–2.

TABLE 202–2 ■ CLINICAL FINDINGS AT THE MOMENT OF DIAGNOSIS IN 98 CHILDREN WITH PARACOCCIDIOIDOMYCOSIS

Clinical Findings	No. of Children (%)
Lymph node enlargement	
Superficial	74 (75.5)
Thoracic	17 (17.3)
Abdominal	12 (12.2)
Abdominal masses	15 (15.3)
Hepatomegaly and/or splenomegaly	56 (57.1)
Ascites	13 (13.3)
Jaundice	5 (5.1)
Diarrhea, vomiting, abdominal pain, or distention	25 (25.5)
Joint or bone lesions	35 (35.7)
Skin lesions	34 (34.7)
Respiratory symptoms	16 (15.3)
Pulmonary consolidations or infiltrates	9 (9.2)
Pleural effusion	5 (5.1)
Oral and upper respiratory tract mucosal lesions	9 (9.2)

Data from references 2, 23, 31, 39, 42, 58, 73, and 87.

These findings support the notion that juvenile paracoccidioidomycosis is a disease of the reticuloendothelial system resulting in damage of the corresponding organs caused by severe macrophage dysfunction, as suggested previously.[44] Superficial lymph node enlargement was the predominant sign (75%) in these cases. Cervical and submandibular lymph node chains were involved most commonly, followed by those of the supraclavicular and axillary regions; however, any chain can be affected. Lymph nodes may vary in size from slightly enlarged to large, painful, coalescent masses; they may be mobile and of elastic consistency or fixed to the adjacent tissues; hypertrophied nodes may progress to fistulization and discharge purulent material rich in *P. brasiliensis* yeast cells.

The next most important finding in Londero's series[58] was hepatomegaly or splenomegaly (57.1%), which usually was asymptomatic. Jaundice was an infrequent occurrence and more closely related to extrinsic compression of the biliary tree.[18] Liver enzymes, especially alkaline phosphatase, were abnormal in some cases, but not markedly increased. Portal hypertension also was a rare occurrence. Findings and complaints relating to the abdomen and digestive tract, such as presence of abdominal masses, lymph node enlargement, diarrhea, vomiting, abdominal distention or pain, and ascites also were recorded (see Table 202–2). Signs and symptoms of an acute abdomen, caused by masses formed by hypertrophied lymph nodes, also have been reported; this problem leads to intestinal occlusion, blockage of lymphatic drainage, and later, ascites.[7, 8, 58]

In a series comprising predominantly patients with the juvenile form of the disease, abdominal radiographic studies (double-contrast barium) revealed ileal and jejunal alterations in 42 to 51 percent.[41, 67] The main findings were distortion and coarsening of the mucosal pattern and loop dilation. However, part of these alterations was probably nonspecific because jejunal biopsies performed in a small number of patients revealed neither granulomatous response nor *P. brasiliensis* yeast cells.[67] On the other hand, histopathologic examination of autopsies (probably the more severe cases) showed a specific granulomatous enteritis in 80 percent.[41] Additionally, in a magnetic resonance imaging study of patients, mostly with the juvenile form, 48 percent had abdominal lymph node enlargement, even if no abdominal signs and symptoms had been recorded.[66] This lymph node involvement causes mesenteric lymphatic stasis and enteric mucosal edema that may progress to fungal enteritis accompanied by abnormal intestinal function such as reduced absorption of fat.[68] The newer imaging procedures (computed tomography, magnetic resonance imaging) are helpful in determining the extent and nature of abdominal involvement.[66] These consequences of the primary fungal process adversely affect the health status of the patient.[9, 101]

Bone damage and articular problems also were important components (29.6%) of disseminated disease, especially in younger children. In these patients, the long bones frequently were affected, with the lytic lesions located at the diaphyseal or metaphyseal-epiphyseal regions,[2] probably because of their higher vascularization, emphasizing the hematogenous dissemination that typically occurs in this form of the disease. Ribs, skull, phalanges, and vertebral lytic lesions also have been documented. Differently from the painful, motion-restriction joint lesions, the bone lesions usually were silent.[2, 8, 39, 74] A pathologic fracture occasionally may occur.[74]

Skin lesions were noted in 34.7 percent of the juvenile cases, with a tendency toward higher frequency with increasing patient age. Distribution of cutaneous lesions was variable, but face and trunk were involved more frequently.[64] Lung abnormalities were recorded in a smaller proportion of cases. However, even in the absence of clinical and radiologic involvement, colonization of the lung by *P. brasiliensis* can be demonstrated by direct examination and by culture.[89] When chest radiographs were abnormal, enlarged hilar lymph nodes and miliary infiltrates predominated.[47, 58, 89]

Anemia, an increased erythrocyte sedimentation rate, severe hypoalbuminemia, and hypergammaglobulinemia with high IgG serum concentrations are found regularly.[7, 8, 44] Nonetheless, anti–*P. brasiliensis* antibodies may prove undetectable in some patients.[34, 49] Eosinophilia, as well as elevated IgE antibody titers, has been detected in severely compromised patients.[102, 112]

A recently review analyzed the association between human immunodeficiency virus (HIV) infection and paracoccidioidomycosis.[12] The youngest patient reported was a 15-year-old boy who had enlargement of superficial and mediastinal lymph nodes, skin nodules, and pulmonary infiltrates.[30] The mycosis also was diagnosed occasionally in other patients whose immune function was depressed by certain conditions or medications.[65] Of interest, however, is that the incidence of this mycosis has not increased in HIV-infected patients as might be expected.[12]

In the chronic, progressive, adult form of paracoccidioidomycosis, signs and symptoms differ substantially from those found in children. Descriptions of the disease in adults are beyond the scope of this text but are referenced.[3, 44, 71, 80, 92, 99]

Diagnosis

Disseminated or pulmonary paracoccidioidomycosis both can be confused with tuberculosis, histoplasmosis, leukemia, malignancies, or Hodgkin disease. When the skin or mucous membranes are affected, paracoccidioidomycosis must be differentiated from histoplasmosis, leishmaniasis, leprosy, syphilis, lupus erythematosus, and a variety of malignancies. In children, tuberculosis, acute abdominal syndrome, intestinal obstruction, osteomyelitis, and rheumatic fever also are important considerations in the differential diagnoses of this disorder.*

Specific diagnosis depends solely on laboratory confirmation. Histopathologic study of biopsy materials is one of the best methods for establishing the diagnosis. Although the hematoxylin and eosin stain is acceptable, precise identification is facilitated by the special fungal stain (Grocott silver methenamine).[3, 75] Experimental studies indicate that immunohistochemical detection of specific glycoproteins by means of monoclonal antibodies also is a valuable procedure.[40]

In the mycology laboratory, *P. brasiliensis* can be observed by direct (potassium hydroxide) preparations. When multiple samples of carefully collected specimens are examined, diagnosis can be made by direct examination in 85 to 95 percent of cases.[20, 55] The characteristic multiple budding yeast cells (pilot's wheel), the various sizes of the blastoconidia, and the walls' refractivity establish the diagnosis. *P. brasiliensis* blastoconidia may be confused with *B. dermatitidis*, *C. neoformans*, large *H. capsulatum* yeast cells,[3, 20, 55] or even *Pneumocystis carinii*.[103] This is why the multiple budding structure should always be found for specific diagnosis.

Recently, several molecular biology diagnostic tests based on polymerase chain reaction assays have been implemented. As an example, *P. brasiliensis gp43* gene was amplified in sputum samples, and the results indicated that 10 yeast cells/mL was the lower limit of detection, providing great accuracy to the diagnosis.[48]

Cultures should be obtained to support the diagnosis and to establish the viability of the fungus. However, they are not always positive because the presence of other, more rapidly growing microorganisms in the samples renders isolation difficult. At room temperature, *P. brasiliensis* is a slow-growing fungus that can be overgrown readily by bacteria, yeasts (especially *Candida*), and contaminant molds. Isolation should be attempted by the concomitant use of modified Sabouraud agar and yeast extract agar plus antibiotics and cycloheximide. In noncontaminated samples, the use of brain-heart infusion agar plus blood and antibiotics (without cycloheximide), a hemoglobin-containing agar incubated at 37° C, or both also is advisable. Cultures should be observed for 4 to 6 weeks depending on temperature of incubation, with a definitive classification being accomplished only in the yeast phase.[20, 55, 80, 92]

Serologic procedures are extremely valuable for both diagnosis and therapy follow-up of patients. Agar gel immunodiffusion (ID) and complement fixation (CF) tests have been employed most often. Nonetheless, such techniques as immunoelectrophoresis, indirect immunofluorescence, enzyme-linked immunosorbent assays (ELISA), and the newer dot-blot immunobinding and Western blotting all have been used.[15, 34, 55, 57, 72] Some of the newer tests have employed purified antigens, such as glycoprotein 43, which are well characterized and more specific.[34] ID and CF that employ crude antigens derived from the yeast phase can detect between 85 and 95 percent of active cases. Titers are highest and the number of precipitin bands greatest in the most severe cases. Cross-reactions between patient sera and *Histoplasma* spp. antigens occur but with insufficient frequency to invalidate the test.[15, 20, 34] ID is very simple and specific. Three precipitin bands, two of which are specific for *P. brasiliensis*, have been identified.[20, 34]

CF also has prognostic value. When CF and ID are nonreactive on two successive occasions at least 3 months apart, treatment can be discontinued. If positive CF titers persist at a low level, prognosis also appears to be good.[15, 20, 34, 71, 72, 80, 92]

Counterimmunoelectrophoresis (CIF) and ELISA also are capable of showing a decline in antibody levels in parallel with clinical improvement. Antibodies thus measured are cleared 1 to 2 years after cessation of therapy, depending on the clinical form. Relapses are accompanied by increased antibody levels.[34]

The use of purified versus crude antigens has resulted in improvement of the serologic tests presently available. Antibodies against the dominant *P. brasiliensis gp43* glycoprotein can be detected by several techniques in almost all patients with paracoccidioidomycosis.[34] On the same token, a recombinant antigen (pb27) has been tested in Western and ELISA tests, with important increases in specificity.[84]

Developments in the detection in patients' sera of specific fungal antigens have been introduced recently.[49] They allow a more precise diagnosis in patients with disseminated childhood and adult multifocal disease, in whom antibodies are undetectable because of their coupling to excess antigen or incapacity to rise antibodies. Antigenemia follow-up studies permit a more precise determination of improvement as antigen load decreases with treatment response.[49]

The skin test with paracoccidioidin is not considered a diagnostic test because 30 to 50 percent of the patients prove nonreactive when tested initially.[20, 22, 80, 85] Conversely, a positive skin test indicates previous contact with the fungus but not necessarily active disease. When histoplasmin skin test material is used, cross-reactions have been verified.[20, 32, 80, 85] When the skin test with paracoccidioidin is negative and the patient is treated, the skin test may become positive, in which case the patient's prognosis is considered satisfactory.[20, 80]

Treatment

The treatment of paracoccidioidomycosis is divided in two phases: attack and maintenance. Two different drugs can be used for each phase, or the same drug can be used for the two phases but at different dosages. Among the reasons for this two-phase prolonged treatment are the chronic progressive nature of the disease and the knowledge that all currently available drugs, albeit with apparently different efficacies, are only fungistatic. Thus, an adequate humoral and cellular immune response is required to control the mycosis. Cellular immunity, however, may be impaired in a large number of patients because of malnutrition or the disease process itself.[7, 8, 77] Providing supportive therapy, therefore, is imperative. Bed rest, adequate nutrition, correction of anemia, and treatment of other concomitant infections are essential.[72] Paracoccidioidomycosis is the only fungal disease that can be treated successfully with sulfa drugs. Until 1958, when amphotericin B was introduced, no other treatment was available. In children, sulfadiazine can be provided orally at daily doses of 60 to 100 mg/kg divided in four to six equal parts; in adults, a maximum daily dose of 6 g can be used. Water intake and urine alkalinization (usually by bicarbonated water intake) should be encouraged during therapy to prevent crystalluria and tubular deposits of sulfadiazine.[72, 100] Duration of the attack treatment is dictated by the patient's response after clinical and serologic improvement have been attained; in the chronic form, 2 to 6 months are required. A slow-acting sulfa

*See references 2, 10, 18, 27, 29, 41, 44, 46, 57, 58, 64, 71, 80, 99.

drug (sulfamethoxypyridazine or sulfadimethoxine) can be provided as maintenance treatment, at a maximum daily dosage of 1 g.

In children, the precise total duration of therapy is variable according to the severity of the disease, and as such should also be dictated by the clinical and serologic responses of the patient to treatment. The importance of continuous treatment must be emphasized because relapses occur if the drug is not taken regularly. Moreover, if the drug is interrupted prematurely, the patient's isolate may become resistant to sulfonamides.[72, 92] Sulfonamides can be used by patients with mild or moderately severe disease. They also can be used for patients who have been treated initially with amphotericin B.[72] Brazilian physicians frequently employ trimethoprim-sulfamethoxazole (80 mg of trimethoprim and 400 mg of sulfamethoxazole per tablet) given at a dose of two tablets and administered orally at 12-hour intervals. In general, children should be given one half the dose given to adults.[7, 72] The Redbook recommends 8 to 10 mg/kg of trimethoprim daily. This combination has the advantage of permitting alternative parenteral administration whenever necessary. Serum concentrations of sulfonamides should be obtained when this drug is used and should not be less than 50 μm/mL. Duration of the acute treatment with this drug varies in each case, but it usually lasts for 6 months. Maintenance treatment in these cases can be achieved by using one half the dose of the attack treatment or by using a slow-acting sulfa. The advent of the imidazole drugs has decreased the use of sulfa drugs by patients with adequate economical resources.[72, 79]

Amphotericin B is effective but should be reserved for severely disseminated cases.[8, 72] It also can be used by patients who relapse during the course of or after treatment with sulfonamide or any orally administered drug because gastrointestinal involvement may impair drug absorption in these cases. The effectiveness of therapy with azoles has curtailed the need for more aggressive regimens. Amphotericin B should be provided as described in other chapters of this book. More than one course of therapy may be required in some patients.

Some investigators have suggested the use of a combined amphotericin B–sulfonamide treatment. In adults, a total cumulative dose of amphotericin B of 1 to 2 g followed by sulfa drugs, given as indicated previously, usually is sufficient.[63] With this drug combination, clinical improvement can be achieved in about 75 percent of patients; about 10 percent do not respond as well, and the remainder die during treatment. Relapses are expected in about 10 to 15 percent of optimally treated patients.[72] Data regarding effectiveness of the new amphotericin B lipid formulations in paracoccidioidomycosis are insufficient.[36]

The use of oral ketoconazole has improved greatly the prognosis of patients with the progressive forms of this disease.[33, 37, 63, 66, 79] Lesions clear at the same rate with ketoconazole and with amphotericin B, but compared with sulfonamide therapy, less time is required to ensure a sustained remission (6 months in some patients). Ketoconazole is not as toxic as is amphotericin B and does not require parenteral administration. Adults have been treated with 200 to 400 mg once daily for periods of 6 to 12 months with no problems and have shown a lower relapse rate (10%).[72, 92] However, other studies have indicated that patients may need 18 months or more of treatment to achieve good results.[34, 37, 61, 63]

The role of ketoconazole in treating childhood paracoccidioidomycosis remains controversial because relatively few children have been treated. The results available to date suggest that the drug is effective. When careful observation during therapy is possible, children may be treated with ketoconazole administered at doses varying from 5 to 8 mg/kg/day, in accordance with the manufacturer's indications. Children treated with ketoconazole should be monitored for changes in liver enzymes.[63, 71, 80] In adults, liver toxicity and gonadal changes also should be evaluated, especially during prolonged therapy.[72]

Ketoconazole no longer is considered the therapy of choice because of its side effects and numerous drug interactions. When the new triazole derivatives for oral administration (itraconazole, fluconazole) became available, they were tested in patients with paracoccidioidomycosis. Today, more experience has been gained with itraconazole, albeit the number of juvenile patients treated thus far still is small.[72, 79, 92] This triazole is more potent and less toxic than is ketoconazole and is equally or even more effective than is the parent compound. It is administered in 100-mg capsules that should be given with a meal.

One to two capsules, depending on the severity of the fungal process, taken daily for 6 months have been shown to be effective in reducing all active lesions. Most (98%) of the patients, including children and young adults, respond.[72, 79] Posttherapy observations indicate a low proportion of relapses (2.1%).[106] Side effects have been few and include transient elevation of hepatic enzymes.[72, 79, 80, 106] At present, several well-conducted trials have been reported favoring this new triazole, which appears to be the preferred drug for the treatment of paracoccidioidomycosis in most patients. This drug is costly and may be unaffordable by patients of low socioeconomic status.[72, 80] Recently, a randomized trial with sulfadiazine, ketoconazole, and itraconazole for the treatment of patients with disease of moderate severity failed to show higher efficacy of a particular regimen over the others.[100] However, long-term follow-up was not evaluated in this study.

A liquid formulation of itraconazole in cyclodextrin solution recently has become available, and it appears to be preferable to the original capsule formulation for children and infants because it is easily administered. It can be given at a dose of 5 mg/kg/day for variable periods according to clinical and laboratory responses. Absorption is enhanced by cyclodextrin, with serum levels higher than those with the capsules. Although we have no experience with this liquid formulation in treating children with paracoccidioidomycosis, the medication has proved to be of value in immunocompromised children with opportunistic mycoses.[106a] Itraconazole maintenance therapy is recommended at a dose of 4 to 10 mg/kg daily, with a maximum dosage of 200 mg twice daily.

Fluconazole is not as effective in this disorder; higher doses, up to 600 mg/day, and longer treatment periods are required. Recrudescence and relapse of disease occur more frequently than when itraconazole is used.[8, 72, 80] Fluconazole may be useful in severely ill patients who must be treated intravenously.[72] The literature has only one report of the successful use of terbinafine in an adult patient.[83]

Many questions remain to be answered regarding optimal treatment of paracoccidioidomycosis. The role of adjunct therapy with immunomodulators, such as cytokines, for cases refractory to conventional therapy remains to be investigated. Alpha glucan obtained from *Saccharomyces cerevisiae* has been investigated.[70] The clinical and laboratory criteria that allow the transition from the attack to the maintenance treatment phases have not been standardized, nor have the parameters that could be used to end treatment with the assurance that the patient is cured. Progressive decrease in the titers of the serologic tests currently available is one of the laboratory parameters used most frequently; restoration of some cellular immunity responses, such as reactivity to the paracoccidioidin skin test, also are used. Newer methods (e.g., antigenemia detection and molecular biology approaches) are being standardized.[48, 49] Meanwhile, most specialists agree that treatment decisions need to be tailored according to the patient.

Prognosis

Paracoccidioidomycosis is considered to be progressive in most cases and fatal if left untreated. However, residual lesions have been observed in a few patients with no known history of active mycotic infection.[43, 47, 71] Prognosis depends on the status of the patient at the time of diagnosis. Children and young adults in whom fungemia has taken place and who have multiple organ involvement do not respond well to therapy. In less disseminated cases, the response to treatment depends on the severity of disease at the time of diagnosis. The fatality rate in young patients at one time was reported to be 31 percent,[27] but it now is much lower as a result of earlier diagnoses and better treatments. In the adult group, patients have a greater chance of survival because of the usually less severely disseminated nature of the chronic form. Once specific treatment is instituted, lesions regress promptly; skin lesions may heal completely in 2 to 4 weeks.[64, 72] Complete remission is possible in most patients with the acute-subacute and chronic form of the disease. Prognosis has improved as a result of earlier diagnosis, new antifungal drugs that facilitated compliance, and better knowledge of the disease. The latter has provided better clinical and laboratory follow-up and the notion that the disease needs prolonged surveillance, as shown by the decrease in positive mycologic tests during and after therapy.[72, 80, 106] Some investigators consider the term *cure* inappropriate because of the inability to confirm complete eradication of the organism; the term *apparent cure* should instead be used.[72]

Paracoccidioidomycosis persists as a disease with low mortality but high morbidity. Complications vary and, like prognosis, their occurrence depends on the extent of fungal invasion. In the juvenile form, early complications that may lead to surgical intervention are intestinal obstruction and jaundice, both of which result from enlarged mesenteric lymph nodes. Disabsorptive syndromes may be associated, aggravating the nutritional status of the patients.[9, 101] Patients also may present with ascites or chylothorax. Lymph nodes may suppurate, and fistulas can develop. A late complication that has been described recently is abdominal malakoplakia.[97] In the adult form, acute complications of mucosal involvement are dysphagia and dysphonia, edema of the glottis, respiratory insufficiency, and Addison disease, among others. Sequelae are not as common in children as in adults. In general, fibrosis is the cause of serious problems in patients who respond to therapy. Despite the newer, very effective therapies, these sequelae preclude, in many cases, the complete restoration of the patients' previous health status.[71, 72, 79, 80, 92, 106] In the former group, scarring and fibrosis of the affected nodes and residual pulmonary fibrosis have been noted.[3, 58] Malabsorption syndrome probably is the most serious sequela in the juvenile form because of the enteric loss of proteins and inflammatory cells that results in immunodeficiency and opportunistic infections.[9, 101] In adults, the sequelae described most frequently are microstomia, laryngeal stenosis leading to permanent tracheostomy, adrenal insufficiency, pulmonary fibrosis, and emphysema.[3, 75, 109]

REFERENCES

1. Almeida, S. R., Moraes, J. Z., Camargo, Z. P., et al.: Pattern of immune response to GP43 from *Paracoccidioides brasiliensis* in susceptible and resistant mice is influenced by antigen-presenting cells. Cell. Immunol. *190*:68–76, 1998.
2. Amstalden, E. M. I., Xavier, R., Kattapuran, S. V., et al.: Paracoccidioidomycosis of bone and joints. Medicine *75*:212–225, 1996.
3. Angulo, A., and Pollak, L.: Paracoccidioidomycosis. *In* Baker, R. D. (ed.): The Pathologic Anatomy of the Mycoses: Human Infections with Fungi, Actinomycetes and Algae. Berlin, Springer Verlag, 1971, pp. 507–576.
4. Aristizábal, B. H., Clemons, K. V., Stevens, D. A., et al.: Morphological transition of *Paracoccidioides brasiliensis* conidia to yeast cells: In vivo inhibition in females. Infect. Immun. *66*:5587–5591, 1998.
5. Bagagli E., Sano A., Coelho K. I., et al.: Isolation of *Paracoccidioides brasiliensis* from armadillos (*Dasypus noveminctus*) captured in an endemic area of paracoccidioidomycosis. Am. J. Trop. Med. Hyg. *58*:505–512, 1998.
6. Baida, H., Biselli, P. J., Juvenale, M., et al.: Differential antibody isotype expression to the major *Paracoccidioides brasiliensis* antigen in juvenile and adult form paracoccidioidomycosis. Microb. Infect. *1*: 273–278, 1999.
7. Barbosa, G. L. Paracoccidioidimicose na criança. Rev. Pat. Trop. (Brazil) *21*:269–383, 1992.
8. Benard, G., Ori, N. W., Marques, H. H. S., et al.: Severe acute paracoccidioidomycosis in children. Pediatr. Infect. Dis. *13*:510–515, 1994.
9. Benard, G., Gryschek, R. C., Duarte, A. J., et al.: Cryptococcosis as an opportunistic infection in immunodeficiency secondary to paracoccidioidomycosis. Mycopathologia *133*:65–69, 1996.
10. Benard, G., Neves, C. P., Gryschek, R. C. B., et al.: Severe juvenile type paracoccidioidomycosis in an adult. J. Med. Vet. Mycol. *33*:67–71, 1995.
11. Benard, G., Mendes-Giannini, M. J., Juvenale, M., et al.: Immunosuppression in paracoccidioidomycosis: T cell hyporesponsiveness to two *Paracoccidioides brasiliensis* glycoproteins that elicit strong humoral immune response. J. Infect. Dis. *175*:1263–1267, 1997.
12. Benard, G., and Duarte, A. J. S.: Paracoccidioidomycosis: A model for evaluation of the effects of human immunodeficiency virus infection on the natural history of endemic tropical diseases. Clin. Infect. Dis. *31*:1032–1039, 2000.
13. Benard, G., Romano, C. C., Cacere, C. R., et al.: Imbalance of IL-2, IFN-gamma and IL-10 secretion in the immunosuppression associated with human paracoccidioidomycosis. Cytokine *13*:248–252, 2001.
14. Bethlem, E. P., Capone, D., Maranhao B., et al.: Paracoccidoidiomycosis. Curr. Opin. Pulm. Med. *5*:319–325, 1999.
15. Biagioni, L., Souza, M. J., Chamma, L. G., et al.: Serology of paracoccidioidomycosis. II. Correlation between class-specific antibodies and clinical forms of the disease. Trans. R. Soc. Trop. Med. Hyg. *78*:617–621, 1984.
16. Blotta, M. H. S., Altermani, A. M., Amaral, E., et al.: Placental involvement in paracoccidioidomycosis. J. Med. Vet. Mycol. *31*:249–257, 1993.
17. Blotta, M. H., Mamoni, R. L., Oliveira, S. J., et al.: Endemic regions of paracoccidioidomycosis in Brazil: A clinical and epidemiologic study of 584 cases in the southeast region. Am. J. Trop. Med. Hyg. *61*:390–394, 1999.
18. Boccalandro, I., and Albuquerque, F. J. M.: Icterícia e comprometimento hepático na blastomicose sulamericana. A propósito de 10 casos e revisão bibliográfica. Rev. Paul. Med. *56*:350–366, 1960.
19. Borelli, D. Some ecological aspects of paracoccidioidomycosis. In: Proc. Panam. Symp. Paracoccidioidomycosis. Washington DC, Pan American Health Organization, Scientific Publication. *254*:59–64, 1972.
20. Brummer, E., Castañeda, E., and Restrepo, A.: Paracoccidioidomycosis: An update. Clin. Microbiol. Rev. *6*:89–117, 1993.
21. Burger, E., Miyaji, M., Sano, A., et al.: Histopathology of paracoccidioidomycotic infection in athymic and euthymic mice: a sequential study. Am. J. Trop. Med. Hyg. *55*:235–242, 1996.
22. Cadavid, D., and Restrepo, A.: Factors associated with *Paracoccidiodes brasiliensis* infection among permanent residents of 3 endemic areas in Colombia. Epidemiol. Infect. *111*:121–133, 1993.
23. Calegaro, J. U., Gomes, E. F., and Rodah, J. E.: Paracoccidioidomicose infantil. Relato de dos casos estudados por galio[67] (^{67}Ga). Radiol. Bras. *30*:343–346, 1997.
24. Calle, D., Rosero, D. S., Orozco, L. C., et al.: Paracoccidioidomycosis in Colombia: An ecological study. Epidemiol Infect. *126*:309–315, 2001.
25. Calvi, S. A., Peraçoli, M. T., Mendes, R. P., et al.: Effect of cytokines on the in vitro fungicidal activity of monocytes from paracoccidioidomycosis patients. Microbes Infect. *5*:107–113, 2003.
26. Cano, L. E., Kashino, S. S., Arruda, C., et al.: Protective role of gamma interferon in experimental pulmonary paracoccidioidomycosis. Infect. Immun. *66*:800–806, 1998.
27. Castro, R. M., and del Negro, G.: Particularidades clinicas da paracoccidioidomicose na crianca. Rev. Hosp. Clin. Fac. Med. São Paulo *31*:194–198, 1976.
28. Castro, C. C., Benard, G., Ygaki, et al.: MRI of head and neck paracoccidioidomycosis. Br. J. Radiol. *72*:717–722, 1999.

29. Chikamori, T., Saka, S., Nagano, H., et al.: Paracoccidioidomycosis in Japan. Report of a case. Ver. Inst. Med. Trop. São Paulo *26*:267–271, 1984.
30. Cimerman, S., Bacha, H. A., Ladeira, M. C. T., et al.: Paracoccidioidomycosis in a boy infected with HIV. Mycoses *40*:434–444, 1997.
31. Colares, S. M., Marcantônio, S., Zambonato, S., et al.: Paracoccidioidomicose aguda/subaguda disseminada. Primeiro caso no Rio Grande do Sul. Rev. Soc. Bras. Med. Trop. *31*:563–576, 1998.
32. Coimbra, C. E. A., Wanke, B., Santos, R. V., et al.: Paracoccidioidin and histoplasmin sensitivity in the Tupí-Mondé Amerindian populations from Brazilian Amazonia. Ann. Trop. Med. Parasitol. *88*:197–207, 1994.
33. Del Negro, G.: Ketoconazole in paracoccidioidomycosis. A long-term therapy study with prolonged folllow-up. Rev. Inst. Med. Trop. São Paulo *24*: 27–39, 1982.
34. Del Negro, G. M. B., Pereira, C. N., Andrade, H. F., et al.: Evaluation of tests for antibody response in the follow-up of patients with acute and chronic forms of paracoccidioidomycosis. J. Med. Microbiol. *49*:37–46, 2000.
35. Dias, M. F., Pereira, A. C., Pereira, A., et al.: The role of HLA antigens in the development of paracoccidioidomycosis. Eur. Acad. Dermatol. Venereol. *14*:166–171, 2000.
36. Dietze, R., Fowler, V. G., Steiner, T. S., et al.: Failure of amphotericin B colloidal dispersion in the treatment of paracoccidioidomycosis. Am. J. Trop. Med. Hyg. *60*:837–839, 1999.
37. Dillon, N. L., Habermann, M. C., Marques, S. A., et al.: Ketoconazole. Tratamento da paracoccidioidomicose no período de 2 anos. An. Bras. Dermatol. *60*:45–48, 1985.
38. Diniz, S. N., Cisalpino, P. S., Koury, M. C. et al.: In vitro human immune reactivity of fast protein liquid chromatography fractionated *Paracoccidioides brasiliensis* soluble antigens. Microb. Infect. *1*:353–360, 1999.
39. Doria, A. S., and Taylor, G. A. Bony involvement in paracoccidioidomycosis. Pediatr. Radiol. *27*:67–69, 1997.
40. Figueroa, J. L., Hamilton, A., Allen, M., et al.: Immunohistochemical detection of a novel 22- to 25-Da glycoprotein of *Paracoccidioides brasiliensis* in biopsy materials and partial characterization by using species-specific monoclonal antibodies. J. Clin. Microbiol. *32:*1566–1574, 1994.
41. Fonseca, L. C., and Mignone, C.: Paracoccidioidomicose do intestino delgado, aspectos anatomo-clínicos e radiológicos de 125 casos. Rev. Hosp. Clin. Fac. Med. São Paulo *31*:199–207, 1976.
42. Fonseca, E. R., Pardal, P. P., and Severo L. C.: Paracoccidioidomicose em crianças em Belém do Pará. Rev. Soc. bras. Med. Trop. *32*:31–33, 1999.
43. Franco, M., Mendes, R. P., Dillon, N. L., and Mota, N. G. S.: Paracoccidioidomycosis, a recently proposed classification of its clinical forms. Rev. Soc. Bras. Med. Trop. *20*:129–132, 1987.
44. Franco, M., Mendes, R. P., Moscardi-Bacchi, M. M., et al.: Paracoccidioidomycosis. Bailliere's Clin. Trop. Med. Comm. Dis. *4:*185–220, 1989.
45. Franco, M., Bagagli, E., Scapolio, S., and da Silva Lacaz, C.: A critical analysis of isolation of *Paracoccidioides brasiliensis* from soil. Med. Mycol. *38:*185–191, 2000.
46. Funari, M., Kavakama, J., Shikanai-Yasuda, M. A., et al.: Chronic pulmonary paracoccidioidomycosis (South American blastomycosis): High-resolution CT findings in 41 patients. A. J. R. Am. J. Roentgenol. *173*:59–64, 1999.
47. Giraldo, R., Restrepo, A., Gutierrez, F., et al.: Pathogenesis of paracoccidioidomycosis: A model based on the study of 46 patients. Mycopathologia *58:*63–70, 1976.
48. Gomes, G. M., Cisalpino, P. S., Taborda, C. P., et al.: PCR for diagnosis of paracoccidioidomycosis. J. Clin. Microbiol. *38*:3478–3480, 2000.
49. Gómez, B. L., Figueroa, J. I., Hamilton, A. J., et al.: Antigenemia in patients with paracoccidioidomycosis: Detection of the 87 kDa determinant during and after antifungal therapy, J. Clin. Microbiol. *36*:3309–3316, 1998.
50. Gonzalez, A., de Gregory, W., Velez, D., et al.: Nitric oxide participation in the fungicidal mechanism of gamma interferon-activated murine macrophages against P. *brasiliensis* conidia. Infect. Immun. *68:* 2546–2552, 2000.
51. Hostetler, J. S., Brummer, E., Coffman, R. L., et al.: Effect of anti-IL4, interferon gamma and an antifungal triazole (Sch-42427) in paracoccidioidomycosis: Correlation of IgE levels with outcome. Clin. Exp. Immunol. *94:*11-16, 1993.
52. Karhawi, A. S., Colombo, A. L., Salomao, R.: Production of IFN-gamma is impaired in patients with paracoccidioidomycosis during active disease and is restored after clinical remission. Med. Mycol. *38*:225–229, 2000.
53. Kashino, S. S., Fazioli, R. A., Cafalli-Favati, C., et al.: Resistance to *Paracoccidioides brasiliensis* infection is linked to a preferential Th1 immune response, whereas susceptibility is associated with absence of IFN-gamma production. J. Interf. Cytok. Res. *20*:89–97, 2000.
54. Kurita, N., Oarada, M., Miyaji, M., et al.: Effect of cytokines on antifungal activity of human polymorphonuclear leucocytes against yeast cells of *Paracoccidioides brasiliensis*. Med. Mycol. *38*:177–182, 2000.
55. Lacaz, C. S., Porto, E., and Martins, J. E. C.: Paracoccidioidomicose. *In* Lacaz, C. S, Porto, E., and Martins, J. E. C. (eds.): Micologia Medica. 4th ed. São Paulo, Sarvier Publishers, 1991, pp. 248–261.
56. Londero, A. T., and Melo, I. S.: Paracoccidioidomicose. J. Brasil. Med. *55*:96–111, 1988.
57. Londero, A. T.: Paracoccidioidomicose: Patogenia, formas clinicas, manifestacões pulmonares e diagnostico. J. Pneumol. (Brazil) *12*:41–57, 1986.
58. Londero, T. A., Rios-Gonçalves, A. J., Terra, G. M., et al.: Paracoccidioidomycosis in Brazilian children. A critical review (1911–1994). Arq. Bras. Med. *70*:197–203, 1996.
59. Manns, B. J., Baylis, B. W., Urbanski, S. J., et al.: Paracoccidioidomycosis: case report and review. Clin. Infect. Dis., *23:*1026–1032, 1996.
60. Mamoni, R. L., Nouér, S. A., Oliveira, S. J., et al.: Enhanced production of specific IgG4, IgE, IgA, and TGF-beta in sera from patients with the juvenile form of paracoccidioidomycosis. Med. Mycol. *40*:153–159, 2002.
61. Marcondes, J., Meira, D. A., Mendes, R. P., et al.: Avaliação do tratamento da paracoccidioidomicose com o ketoconazole. Rev. Inst. Med. Trop. São Paulo *26*:113–121, 1984.
62. Marques, S. A., Franco, M. F., Mendes, R. P., et al.: Some epidemiological aspects of paracoccidioidomycosis in Botucatú endemic area, State of São Paulo, Brazil. Rev. Inst. Med. Trop. São Paulo *25:*87–92, 1983.
63. Marques, S. A., Dillon, N. L., Franco, M. F., et al.: Paracoccidioidomycosis: A comparative study of the evolutionary serologic, clinical and radiologic results for patients treated with ketoconazole or amphotericin B plus sulfonamides. Mycopathologia *89:*19–25, 1985.
64. Marques, S. A.: Cutaneous lesions. *In* Franco, M., Lacaz, C. S., Restrepo, A., et al. (eds.): Paracoccidioidomycosis. Boca Raton, FL, CRC Press, 1994, pp. 259–266.
65. Marques, S. A., and Shikanai-Yasuda, M. A.: Paracoccidioidomycosis associated to immunosuppression, AIDS, and Cancer. *In* Franco, M., Lacaz, C. S., Restrepo, A., et al. (eds.): Paracoccidioidomycosis. Boca Raton, FL, CRC Press, 1994, pp. 393–405.
66. Martinez, R., Belluci, A. D., Fiorillo, A. M.: A tomografia computadorizada na avaliação do comprometimento abdominal na paracoccidiodomicose. Rev. Soc. Bras. Med. Trop. *21*:47, 1988.
67. Martinez, R., Meneghelli, U. G., Dantas, R. O., et al.: O comprometimento gastrintestinal na blastomicose sul-americana (paracoccidioidomicose). I. Estudo clínico, radiológico e histopatológico. Rev. Ass. Med. Bras. *25*:31–34, 1979.
68. Martinez, R., Meneghelli, U. G., Dantas, R. O., et al.: O comprometimento gastrintestinal na blastomicose sul-americana (paracoccidioidomicose) II. Estudo funcional do intestino delgado. Rev. Ass. Med. Bras. *25*:70–73, 1979.
69. McEwen, J. G., Bedoya, V., Patiño, M. M., et al.: Experimental paracoccidioidomycosis induced by the inhalation of conidia. J. Med. Vet. Mycol. *25*:165–175, 1987.
70. Meira, D. A., Pereira, P. C., Marcondes-Machado, J., et al.: The use of glucan as immunostimulant in the treatment of paracoccidioidomycosis. Am. J. Trop. Med. Hyg. *55*:496–503, 1996.
71. Mendes, R. P. M. The gamut of clinical manifestations. *In* Franco, M., Lacaz, C. S., Restrepo, A., et al. (eds.): Paracoccidioidomycosis. Boca Raton, FL, CRC Press, 1994, pp. 233–258.
72. Mendes, R. P., Negroni, R., Arachevala, A.: Treatment and control of cure. *In* Franco, M., Lacaz, C. S., Restrepo, A., et al. (eds.): Paracoccidioidomycosis. Boca Raton, FL, CRC Press, 1994, pp. 373–392.
73. Migliari D. A., Sugaya N. N., Mimura, M. A. et al.: Periodontal aspects of the juvenile form of paraccoccidioidomycosis. Rev. Inst. Med. Trop. São Paulo *40*:15–18, 1998.
74. Miranda-Aires, E., Costa Alves, C. A., Ferreira, A. V., et al.: Bone paracoccidioidomycosis in an HIV-positive patient. Braz. J. Infect. Dis. *1*:260–265, 1997.
75. Montenegro, M. R., and Franco, M.: Pathology. *In* Franco, M., Lacaz, C. S., Restrepo, A., et al. (eds.): Paracoccidioidomycosis. Boca Raton, FL, CRC Press, 1994, pp. 131–150.
76. Moscardi-Bacchi, M., Mendes, R. P., Marques, S. A. et al.: In situ localization of T lymphocyte subsets in human paracoccidioidomycosis. J. Med. Vet. Mycol. *27*:149–158, 1989.
77. Mota, N. G. S., Rezkallah-Iwasso, M. T., Peraçoli, M. T., et al.: Correlation between cell-mediated immunity and clinical forms of paracoccidioidomycosis. Trans. R. Soc. Trop. Med. Hyg. *79*:765–771, 1985.
78. Musatti, C. C., Rezkallah, M. T., Mendes, E., et al.: In vivo and in vitro evaluation of cell-mediated immunity in patients with paracoccidioidomycosis. Cell. Immunol. *24*:365–378, 1976.
79. Naranjo, M. S. Trujillo, M., Munera, M. I., et al.: Treatment of paracoccidioidomycosis with itraconazole. J. Med. Vet. Mycol. *28*:67–76, 1990.
80. Negroni, R. Paracoccidioidomycosis (South American blastomycosis, Lutz mycosis). Int. J. Dermatol. *12*:847–859, 1993.
81. Negroni, R.: Pathogenesis. *In* Franco, M., Lacaz, C. S., Restrepo, A., et al. (eds.): Paracoccidioidomycosis. Boca Raton, FL, CRC Press, 1994, pp. 203–212.
82. Niño-Vega, G. A., Calgagno, A. M., San Blas, G., et al.: RFLP analysis reveals marked geographical isolation between strains of *Paracoccidioides brasiliensis*. Med. Mycol. *38*:437–441, 2000.

82a. Oliveira, S. J., Mamoni, R. L., Musatti, C. C., et al.: Cytokines and lymphocyte proliferation in juvenile and adult forms of paracoccidioidomycosis: Comparison with infected and non-infected controls. Microbes Infect. *4*:139–144, 2002.

83. Ollague, J. M., de Zurita, A. M., and Calero, G.: Paracoccidioidomycosis (South American blastomycosis) successfully treated with terbinafine: first case report. Br. J. Dermatol. *143*:188–191, 2000.

84. Ortiz, B., Díez, S., Urán, M. E., et al.: Use of the 27 kDa recombinant protein from *Paracoccidioides brasiliensis* and its use in the serodiagnosis of paracoccidioidomycosis. Clin. Diagn. Immunol. *5*:826–830, 1998.
85. Pedrosa, P. N. Paracoccidioidomicose. Inquérito intradérmico com paracoccidioidina em zona rural do Estado do Rio de Janeiro. MSc thesis, Universidade Federal do Rio de Janeiro, Rio de Janeiro, Brazil, 1976.
86. Queiroz-Telles, F.: *Paracoccidioides brasiliensis:* Ultrastructural findings. *In* Franco, M., Lacaz, C. S., Restrepo, A., et al. (eds.): Paracoccidioidomycosis. Boca Raton, FL, CRC Press, 1994, pp. 27–48.
87. Resende, L. S. R.: Mielopatia infiltrativa por paracoccidioidomicose. Ph.D. thesis, Faculdade de Medicina de Botucatu, UNESP, São Paulo State, Brazil, 2000.
88. Restrepo, A., Robledo, M., Giraldo, R., et al.: The gamut of paracoccidioidomycosis. Am. J. Med. *61*:33–42, 1976.
89. Restrepo, A., Trujillo, M., and Gómez, I.: Inapparent lung involvement in patients with the subacute juvenile type of paracoccidioidomycosis. Rev. Inst. Med. Trop. São Paulo *31*:18–22, 1989.
90. Restrepo, A.: Ecology of *Paracoccidioides brasiliensis*. *In* Franco, M., Lacaz, C. S., Restrepo, A., et al. (eds.): Paracoccidioidomycosis. Boca Raton, FL, CRC Press, 1994, pp. 121–130.
91. Restrepo, A., Salazar, M. E., Clemons, K. V., et al.: Hormonal influences in the host-interplay with *Paracoccidioides brasiliensis*. In: Stevens, D. A., Vanden Bosche, H., Odds, F. (eds.): Topics on Fungal Infections. Bethesda, MD, National Foundation for Infectious Diseases. 1997, pp. 125–133.
92. Restrepo, A.: *Paracoccidioides brasiliensis*. *In* Mandell, G. L., Dollin, R., and Bennett, J. E. (eds.): Principles and Practice of Infectious Diseases. 5th ed. Philadelphia, W. B. Saunders, 2000, pp. 2768–2772.
93. Restrepo, A.: Morphological aspects of *Paracoccidioides brasiliensis* in lymph nodes: Implications for the prolonged latency of paracoccidioidomycosis? Med. Mycol. *38*:317–322, 2000.
94. Restrepo A., McEwen, J. G., and Castañeda, E.: The habitat of *Paracoccidioides brasiliensis*: How far from solving the riddle? Med. Mycol. 40:213–216, 2001.
95. Rios-Gonçalves, A. J., Terra, G. M. F., Rosembaum, R., et al.: Paracoccidioidomicose disseminada “tipo juvenil.” Arq. Brasil. Med. *66*:335–337, 1992.
96. Rios-Gonçalves, A. J., Londero, A. T., Terra, G. M. F., et al: Paracoccidioidomycosis in children in the state of Rio de Janeiro (Brazil). Geographic distribution and the study of a “reservarea.” Rev. Inst. Med. Trop. São Paulo *40*:11–13, 1998.
97. Rocha, N., Suguiama, E. H., Maia, D., et al.: Intestinal malakoplakia associated with paracoccidiodomycosis: A new association. Histopathology *30*:79–83, 1997.
98. Sandoval, M., De Brito, T., Sotto, M. N., et al.: Antigen distribution in mucocutaneous biopsies of human paracoccidioidomycosis. Int. J. Surg. Pathol. *3*:181–188, 1996.
99. Sant’Anna, G. D., Mauri, M., Arrarte, H., Jr., et al.: Laryngeal manifestations of paracoccidioidomycosis (South American blastomycosis). Arch. Otolaryngol. Head Neck Surg. *125*:1375–1378, 1999.
100. Shikanai-Yasuda, M. A., Benard, G., Higaki, Y., et al.: Randomized trial with itraconazole, ketoconazole and sulfadiazine in paracoccidioidomycosis. Med. Mycol. *40*:411–417, 2002.
101. Shikanai-Yasuda, M. A., Segurado, A. A. C., Pinto, W. P., et al.: Immunodeficiency secondary to juvenile paracoccidioidomycosis. Mycopathologia *120*:23–28, 1992.
102. Shikanai-Yasuda, M. A., Higaki, Y., Uip, D. E., et al.: Comprometimiento da medula ossea e eosinofilia na paracoccidiodiomicose. Rev. Inst. Med. Trop. São Paulo *34*:85–90, 1992.
103. Silletti, R. P., Glezerov, V., Schwartz, I. S., et al.: Pulmonary paracoccidioidomycosis misdiagnosed as *Pneumocystis* pneumonia in an immunocompromised host. J. Clin. Microbiol. *34*:2328–2330, 1996.
104. Silva-Vergara, M. L., and Martinez, R.: Role of the armadillo *Dasypus novemcinctus* in the epidemiology of paracoccidioidomycosis. Mycopathologia *144*:131–133, 1999.
105. Teixeira, F., Gayotto, L. C., and De Brito, T.: Morphological patterns of the liver in South American blastomycosis. Histopathology *2*:231–237, 1978.
106. Tobón, A. M., Gómez, I., Franco, L., et al.: Seguimiento post-terapia en pacientes con paracoccidioidomicosis tratados con itraconazol. Rev. Colombiana Neumol. *7*:74–78, 1995.
106a. Tobón, A. M., Franco, L., Espinal, D., et al.: Disseminated histoplasmosis in children: The role of itraconazol therapy. Pediatr. Infect. Dis. J. *15*:1002–1008, 1996.
107. Torrado, E., Castañeda, E., de la Hoz, F., et al.: Paracoccidioidomicosis: Definición de las áreas endémicas de Colombia. *Biomédica* *20*:327–334, 2000.
108. Tuder, R. M., El Ibrahim, R., Godoy, C. E., et al.: Pathology of the pulmonary paracoccidioidomycosis. Mycopathologia *92*:179–188, 1985.
109. Valle, A. C. F, Guimarães, R. R., Lopes, D. J., et al.: Aspectos radiológicos torácicos na paracoccidioidomicose. Rev. Inst. Med. Trop. São Paulo *34*:107–115, 1992.
110. Wanke, B., and Londero, A. T.: Epidemiology and paracoccidioidomycosis infection. *In* Franco, M., Lacaz, C. S., Restrepo, A., et al. (eds.): Paracoccidioidomycosis. Boca Raton, FL, CRC Press, 1994, pp. 109–120.
111. Yamaga, L. Y., Benard, G. Hironaka, F. H., et al.: The role of gallium-67 scan in defining the extent of disease in an endemic deep mycosis, paracoccidioidomycosis: A predominantly multifocal disease. Eur. J. Nucl. Med. Mol. Imaging *30*:888–894, 2003.
112. Yarzábal, L., Dessaint, J. P., Arango, M., et al.: Demonstration and qualification of IgE antibodies against *Paracoccidioides brasiliensis* in paracoccidioidomycosis. Int. Arch. Allergy Immunol. *62*:346–351, 1980.

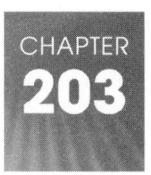

CHAPTER 203 Cryptococcosis

WALTER T. HUGHES

Cryptococcosis is a life-threatening systemic fungal infection caused by the monomorphic yeast *Cryptococcus neoformans*. Historically, the disease has been referred to as torulosis, European blastomycosis, and Busse-Buschke disease. Both the organism and the disease that it causes were discovered independently more than a century ago. In 1894, Busse, a German pathologist, found the yeast in the tibial lesion of a 31-year-old woman who later died of systemic infection under the medical care of Buschke, her physician. Meanwhile, in 1895, Sanfelice, an Italian, had cultured for the first time the encapsulated yeast *Saccharomyces* (later *Cryptococcus*) *neoformans* from peach juice. Sanfelice pointed out the similarity between the isolates from Busse's case and the yeast from the peach juice. The first case in which *C. neoformans* was recognized as the cause of meningitis was reported in 1914 by Verse, although in retrospect other cases had been described earlier.

Cryptococcosis involves predominantly the central nervous system (CNS), lungs, skin, and bones, but other organs also have been affected. Although most cases are in immunocompromised patients, the systemic disease also may occur in seemingly immunocompetent individuals.

The Organism

Cryptococcosis is caused by *C. neoformans*, 1 of 19 species of the genus *Cryptococcus*. Only rarely do other species of *Cryptococcus*, such as *Cryptococcus laurentii*, cause disease. *C. neoformans* is an encapsulated yeast varying in size from 4 to 8 μm or more in diameter. Two varieties of *neoformans* have been identified. Variety *neoformans* in the telemorphic state is designated *Filobasidiella neoformans* variety *neoformans* and has two serotypes, A and D. Variety *gattii*, also *F. neoformans* variety *gattii*, has two serotypes, B and C.

C. neoformans replicates by budding. As budding occurs, a long, slender neck between the parent and daughter cells may be seen. A feature of all *C. neoformans* strains is the mucopolysaccharide capsule surrounding the cell wall. This capsule may vary in size from twice the diameter of the yeast to a barely detectable thickness. The presence of this capsule is useful for identification of the genus and may be recognized with the use of a mucicarmine stain or with negative staining using India ink. The Fontana-Masson stain is useful in the identification of *C. neoformans* in fixed tissues. This stain detects melanin precursors in the cell wall and differentiates *C. neoformans* from other yeasts.[27]

C. neoformans forms smooth, mucoid colonies on solid media. Initially cream colored, the colonies become dry and tan, pinkish, or yellow with aging. The fungus produces urease, is nonfermative, and uses several carbohydrates. Species of the genus are separated with carbohydrate assimilation tests and potassium nitrate. The organism grows at 37° C, is lactose negative, and does not produce pseudomycelia on cornmeal agar. It does not grow well at room temperature (25° C). The development of DNA probes for hybridization with RNA of organisms appears promising for rapid and sensitive methods for the identification of *C. neoformans*.[15] Growth on agar containing L-canavanine, glycine, and thymol-blue indicator serves to differentiate serotypes B and C from A and D. Color change occurs with B and C but not with A and D serotypes.[23]

Epidemiology

Cryptococcosis occurs worldwide as a sporadic infection but not in epidemics. *C. neoformans* is found in soil, especially in sites enriched with avian guano. Although pigeons have been associated with cryptococcosis, the organism resides in the feces, and the birds are not infected. Serotypes A and D of *C. neoformans* are found worldwide and usually associated with pigeon excreta, whereas serotypes B and C more often are located in tropical and subtropical countries. *C. neoformans* variety *gattii* (serotype B) has been found to flourish in the environment of the river red gum tree (*Eucalyptus camaldulensis*).[8, 20] Naturally acquired infections occur in lower mammals, especially cats. Neither animal-to-human nor human-to-human infections have been reported.[9] However, a recent study provided convincing data to associate isolates of *C. neoformans* from feces of a pet cockatoo with cryptococcal meningitis in an adult.[30] Another study showed a higher rate of delayed hypersensitivity skin test reactions to cryptococcal antigen in normal people with heavy exposure to pigeons than in those without such exposure.[29]

Cryptococcal infection is thought to be acquired by inhalation of the yeast into the lungs from a soil reservoir. From the lungs, hematogenous dissemination may occur. Systemic infection may occur in otherwise normal individuals, but most cases of cryptococcosis occur in immunosuppressed individuals. Some of the underlying immunosuppressive conditions include leukemia, lymphoma, Hodgkin disease, lupus erythematosus, Cushing syndrome, sarcoidosis, organ transplantation, chronic mucocutaneous candidiasis, congenital immunodeficiency disorders, and acquired immunodeficiency syndrome (AIDS). The AIDS epidemic has become a major factor in the increased prevalence of cryptococcosis since 1980.[7] Cryptococcosis occurs in an estimated 8 percent of AIDS patients in the United States.[17] An active, population-based surveillance from 1992 to 1994 in four U. S. cities showed the incidence of cryptococcosis to be 1.8 to 6.7 cases per 100,000 population and up to 0.9 cases per 100,000 in the population not infected with human immunodeficiency virus (HIV). Eighty-six percent of the 1083 cases occurred in patients with AIDS. Only four of the patients with cryptococcosis were younger than 18 years of age.[14] In adults with AIDS, cryptococcal meningitis occurs most frequently in blacks, Haitians, and intravenous drug users.

No explanation has been found for the higher rate of cryptococcosis in males than in females.

Cryptococcosis seems to occur less frequently in children than in adults. A Brazilian study[39] found 4 cases of cryptococcosis among 170 HIV-infected children. Of 100 adult patients studied post mortem, 8 had cryptococcal infection.[5]

Pathophysiology

Considerable evidence suggests that *C. neoformans* becomes airborne from soil or dried pigeon excreta. These organisms, or fomites, usually measure less than 2 µm in diameter and, therefore, are of a size that easily can reach the lung parenchyma through the airways of the lower respiratory tract.[28, 33–35] After inhalation, the yeast becomes deposited in the alveolar spaces, where replication may or may not occur and where alveolar macrophages and the primary immune response attempt to protect the host from invasion.

The variety of *C. neoformans* may be a factor in the pathology of the infection. Some studies show that infection with *C. neoformans* variety *gattii* (serotypes B and C) more often is associated with immunocompetent individuals with cerebral mass lesions (with or without hydrocephalus) and pulmonary lesions than is infection with *C. neoformans* variety *neoformans*.[25] However, the histopathologic features are indistinguishable.

After inhalation of the yeast, localized pulmonary infection may occur, although it may not be evident clinically at the time of and after hematogenous dissemination. Early lesions are characterized by collections of encapsulated yeasts surrounded by a gelatinous-like material. Granulomatous and chronic inflammatory reactions occur after the acute infection. Four basic patterns of reaction are seen in the lung: one or more peripheral granulomata, granulomatous pneumonia with intra-alveolar organisms and varying degrees of inflammatory response, diffuse invasion of organisms within alveolar capillaries and interstitial tissues with little or no inflammation, and massive intra-alveolar and intravascular organisms.[22]

Studies in the experimental rat show that *C. neoformans* penetrates the lung parenchyma shortly after infection (2 hours), immunocompetent rats control the infection effectively with minimal extrapulmonary spread and low levels of the capsular glucuronoxylomannan, and macrophage activation plays a key role in limiting infection to the lung.[13]

The lesions of the brain and meninges are different from those of the lung. Typically, cystlike lesions, especially of the cerebral cortex, are seen. They represent masses of yeast forms and little, if any, inflammatory reaction. When an inflammatory response is seen, macrophages predominate, and *C. neoformans* may be found in the cytoplasm of these cells. Granulomatous lesions are uncommon occurrences in the brain. The meninges may be thickened with the gelatinous polysaccharide of the yeast capsule.[11]

Bone lesions may be found in 5 percent or more of cases of extrapulmonary cryptococcosis. Here, acute and chronic inflammation occurs, often associated with giant cells and granulomata.[2] Other sites of dissemination include skin, joints, eye, urinary tract, adrenal, liver, lymph nodes, sinuses, gastrointestinal tract, and the female reproductive system.

The capsular polysaccharide of *C. neoformans* is predominantly glucuronoxylomannan. This material elicits an antibody and is the determinant for the yeast's serotype. It does not, in the purified state, elicit a delayed hypersensitivity reaction. Whole-cell organisms, as well as protein-containing fractions, will elicit a delayed hypersensitivity reaction.

Impaired cell-mediated immunity of the host is a major determinant in the infection and progression of this infection. Furthermore, evidence suggests that, during the infection, cryptococcosis affects some specific components of cell-mediated immunity.[6] Athymic (nude) mice and T-cell–depleted mice are highly susceptible to cryptococcal infection. When normal mice are inoculated with *C. neoformans,* a response of $CD4^+$ and $CD8^+$ T lymphocytes limits the infection and prevents dissemination.[24] *C. neoformans* undergoes attachment, ingestion, and digestion by phagocytes when provided antibody and complement. As a facultative intracellular pathogen, the yeast survives in phagocytic cells with intracellular polysaccharide production.[10] Some evidence suggests that the organism's polysaccharide capsule may impair phagocytosis and killing and that administration of monoclonal antibodies to the capsular polysaccharide may be protective.[26]

Clinical Manifestations

One of the most comprehensive studies of the clinical features of cryptococcosis is the publication of 171 well-documented cases of both immunocompromised and immunocompetent patients.[34] This report studied all cases from 24 health care institutions in Brazil during a period of 30 years. Of the 171 cases, only 3 patients (1.8 percent) were 10 years of age or younger and only 10 patients (5.8 percent) were younger than 20 years of age. Of these 10 patients, 2 had AIDS, 2 had other causes of immunocompromise, and 6 were not immunocompromised. The CNS was involved in 76 percent of the 171 patients, with similar rates for the immunocompetent and immunosuppressed patients with or without AIDS. Disseminated cryptococcosis occurred in 92 percent of patients and pulmonary cryptococcosis in 8 percent.

CENTRAL NERVOUS SYSTEM INVOLVEMENT

Headache and fever are the most common symptoms. Nausea and vomiting occur in one half of the cases. Stiff neck is seen in 75 percent of those who are not immunocompromised and in only 33 percent of those with AIDS. Other, less frequent manifestations include alteration of consciousness, impaired mental function, cranial nerve lesions, visual deficits, papilledema, seizures, diplopia, focal neurologic deficits, photophobia, and abnormal cerebellar signs.[34] The duration of symptoms before diagnosis varies from less than 1 week to as long as 18 months.

PULMONARY INVOLVEMENT

Primary pulmonary cryptococcosis has not been well described in children because most cases of this infection are disseminated at the time of diagnosis. Based on studies in adults,[4] about one third of the cases are asymptomatic in the immunocompetent host. About one half the patients have cough or chest pain, and lower percentages have sputum production (32%), weight loss (26%), fever (26%), and hemoptysis (18%). In the immunocompromised host, the onset may be more severe and the course more rapid.[24]

CUTANEOUS LESIONS

A variety of skin lesions caused by *C. neoformans,* including ulcers, nodules, vesicles, abscesses, papules, cellulitis, acneiform plaques, and purpuric and sinus tracts, have been described (see Fig. 65–24). Thus, histologic examination and culture are essential to identify specifically the cryptococcal skin lesion.

EXTRAPULMONARY CRYPTOCOCCOSIS IN IMMUNOCOMPROMISED INFANTS AND CHILDREN

The extent of knowledge about cryptococcosis in infants and children is reflected by reports and reviews.[1, 18, 19] From 1966 to 1997, only 22 non-AIDS immunosuppressed children and 30 children with AIDS and extrapulmonary cryptococcosis have been reported. Aspects of these cases are summarized in Table 203–1.

Diagnosis

The diagnosis is established by the demonstration of *C. neoformans* during the disease state. This demonstration may be done by direct examination using India ink preparations for cerebrospinal fluid (CSF), urine, or sputum

TABLE 203–1 ■ EXTRAPULMONARY CRYPTOCOCCOSIS IN IMMUNOSUPPRESSED INFANTS AND CHILDREN REPORTED SINCE 1966

Clinical Type	Chronic Cutaneous Candidiasis n=4	Systemic Lupus Erythematosis n=6	Acute Lymphoblastic Leukemia n=9	AIDS* n=30	Other† n=3
Years of Age: Range (Mean)	3-4 (10)	8-7 (12)	3-17 (13)	5 mo–16 yr (9)	1/2-10 (5)
Meningitis	3	3	4	14	
Meningitis +cutaneous			1		
Disseminated + meningitis					1
Disseminated	1	1	1	11	
Cryptococcemia			1		2
Cryptococcemia + meningitis		1			
Peritonitis		1			
Cutaneous only			2		

*Clinical data incomplete on patients with acquired immunodeficiency syndrome (AIDS).
†Hyperimmunoglobulin E, severe combined immunodeficiency syndrome, renal transplantation.
Data from Leggiadro, R. J., Barrett, F. F., and Hughes, W. T.: Extrapulmonary cryptococcosis in immunosuppressed infants and children. Pediatr. Infect. Dis. J. *11*:43–47, 1992; Leggiadro, R. J., Kline, M. W., and Hughes, W. T.: Extrapulmonary cryptococcosis in children with acquired immunodeficiency syndrome. Pediatr. Infect. Dis. J. *10*:658–662, 1991; and Abadi, J., Nachman, S., Kressel, A. B., Pirofski, L. A. Cryptococcosis in children with AIDS. Clin. Infect. Dis. *28*:309–313, 1999.

specimens, or using mucicarmine and Masson-Fontana silver stains for histologic examinations; by isolation in culture; and by the detection of cryptococcal antigen. With cryptococcal meningitis, the India ink preparation reveals the yeast in 77 to 94 percent of cases; the culture yields the organism in 87 to 100 percent, and the cryptococcal antigen test is positive in 83 to 100 percent of cases. The leukocyte count of the CSF may be normal or increased to low levels rarely exceeding 100 cells/mm^3, and the glucose is less than 50 mg/dL in 65 to 75 percent of the patients.[34]

A high yield from cultures is influenced by the collection and processing of specimens. The methods suggested by Kwon-Chung and Bennett[17] are optional. For the initial culture, Sabouraud agar and Niger seed agar medium are used, and cultures are maintained at 30° to 32° C (not 37° or 25° C). The sediment from centrifuged CSF or urine specimens is spread on several plates or slants. Alternatively, 2 to 5 mL of CSF can be inoculated into Sabouraud broth and incubated on a shaker. Cycloheximide should not be used because it may inhibit the growth of *C. neoformans*. Blood should be cultured by the lysis-centrifugation procedure (Isolator tube) (Dupont, Wilmington, DE.).[38] Evidence of growth may be seen as early as 3 days, but cultures should be held for 3 to 4 weeks before being considered sterile.

Detection of cryptococcal antigen in CSF, serum, and urine offers a highly sensitive and specific diagnostic tool. Latex agglutination uses hyperimmune rabbit immunoglobulin anti–*C. neoformans* antibodies bound to latex particles. Titers of 1:4 and greater suggest cryptococcal infection. Commercial kits detect as little as 10 ng of cryptococcal antigen and have a sensitivity rate of about 95 percent in experienced hands. Enzyme immunoassays use monoclonal or polyclonal antibody to detect antigen. Comparison studies show close agreement between latex agglutination and enzyme immunoassays.[12] Both latex agglutination and enzyme immunoassay kits are available commercially.

The antigen-detection test (CALAS, Meridian Diagnostics, Cincinnati, OH) has been applied to the diagnosis of pulmonary cryptococcosis.[21] In 41 patients suspected of having pulmonary cryptococcosis, 8 were proved to have *C. neoformans* infection by culture and histology. The transthoracic needle aspirate was positive for cryptococcal antigen in all 8 cases, and only 1 of the 33 patients without cryptococcosis had a false-positive test. The CALAS test also is highly sensitive and specific for detection of antigen in CSF and serum.[16]

Polymerase chain reaction amplification of *C. neoformans* DNA is being developed, but this technique probably will have the greatest application to epidemiologic investigations because the antigen tests are adequate for diagnostic purposes and can be done quickly in most hospital laboratories.

Treatment

Three factors must be considered in guiding the treatment of cryptococcosis: (1) the underlying disease (none or immunocompromised); (2) extent of infection (pulmonary or extrapulmonary with and without neural involvement); and (3) choice of drugs.

Most investigators agree that a 6- to 10-week course of treatment usually is adequate for treating systemic cryptococcosis in immunocompetent individuals and in some patients who are immunocompromised for a limited period. However, AIDS patients require continuation of antifungal drugs indefinitely because of the high recurrence rate of cryptococcosis. As for the extent of infection, some immunocompetent patients with pulmonary cryptococcosis have recovered without antifungal therapy. However, cases must be evaluated individually as to the wisdom of this approach. Several years ago, the choice of a drug for treatment was simple because amphotericin B was the only drug with efficacy. Now several drugs with therapeutic efficacy, including flucytosine, fluconazole, and itraconazole, are available.

Reliable in vitro susceptibility tests to predict the in vivo efficacy are desirable, but such tests are not sufficiently standardized and applicable to general hospital laboratories at this time. However, of all the fungi causing serious human infection, *C. neoformans* seems to hold great promise for such testing. Velez and associates[40] found a positive correlation between the minimum inhibitory concentration determined in vitro for *C. neoformans* and in vivo responses of murine cryptococcal meningitis treated with fluconazole.

Experts from the National Institute of Allergy and Infectious Disease Mycoses Study Group and the Infectious Diseases Society of America established year 2000 guidelines for the management of cryptococcal infections.[36] A summary of these recommendations follows. The main determinants for treatment are the status of the host immune system and the topographic location of the disease.

TREATMENT OF CRYPTOCOCCOSIS IN THE IMMUNOCOMPETENT HOST

Pulmonary and Non–Central Nervous System Disease

Some patients with normal immunocompetence and cryptococcosis of limited extent and nonprogressive disease may recover without treatment. However, in most infants and children, exclusion of extrapulmonary dissemination is difficult, and treatment is warranted. Performing a lumbar tap is essential in all cases of pulmonary disease. Immunocompetent patients with asymptomatic and mild-to-moderate symptoms should be treated with 3 to 6 mg/kg/day of fluconazole for 6 to 12 weeks. An alternative drug for those unable to take fluconazole is itraconazole (Table 203–2). If oral azoles cannot be taken or progression of the disease occurs, amphotericin B, 0.4 to 0.7 mg/kg/day, is recommended. Severe pulmonary disease is treated like CNS disease.

Central Nervous System Disease in the Immunocompetent Host

The combination of amphotericin B, 0.7 to 1.0 mg/kg/day, and flucytosine, 100 mg/kg/day, is used as induction therapy for 2 weeks, then fluconazole, 100 mg/kg/day, is used as induction therapy for 2 weeks; then fluconazole, 100 mg/kg/day, may be used for a minimum of 10 weeks.[3, 32, 37] Alternatively, the amphotericin B and flucytosine combination may be continued for 6 to 10 weeks. A spinal tap should be done after 2 weeks of therapy, at which time 60 to 70 percent of cases will have sterile spinal fluid. Patients with positive cultures at 2 weeks require a more prolonged course of treatment. Intraventricular and intrathecal amphotericin B may be needed for refractory cases.

Lipid formulations of amphotericin B should be used in place of amphotericin B in patients with renal dysfunction.

TREATMENT OF CRYPTOCOCCOSIS IN THE IMMUNOCOMPROMISED HOST WITH ACQUIRED IMMUNODEFICIENCY SYNDROME

Cryptococcal Pneumonia

All HIV-infected patients with pulmonary cryptococcal infection must be treated because they are at high risk for

TABLE 203–2 ■ AZOLE ALTERNATIVES FOR THE TREATMENT OF CRYPTOCOCCOSIS

Category	Fluconazole	Itraconazole*
Dose	3–6 mg/kg/day† Adults = 200–400 mg/day	Child† 3–16 years of age = 100 mg/day Adults = 200–400 mg/day
Route	Intravenous or oral; once daily	Oral: once or twice daily
Peak plasma concentration	4.5 to 8 μg/mL	0.234 μg/mL
Protein binding	11%	99%
Volume of distribution (Vol_D)	0.7 to 1.0 L/kg	796 L (adult)
Central nervous system distribution	54%–85% serum level	<10% of serum level
Half-life (normal renal function)	14–20 hrs	64 hours (steady state)
Elimination: renal excretion	>80%	0.03%
biliary excretion	Small	3%–18%
Major adverse effects	Nausea, vomiting, diarrhea, rash, increase in serum aminotransferase levels	Nausea, vomiting, rash, hypertension, increase in serum aminotransferase levels

*No Food and Drug Administration approval for pediatric use in cryptococcosis.
†No pediatric dose has been established; dose estimate.

disseminated infection. Treatment of developing mild and moderately severe pneumonia is fluconazole, 100 mg/kg/day for life. Some evidence suggests that AIDS patients responding with immune reconstitution after effective highly active antiretroviral therapy (HAART) may not require lifelong maintenance therapy. An alternative to fluconazole is itraconazole. For patients with severe pneumonia, amphotericin B should be used until the patient is asymptomatic, at which time fluconazole can be substituted for maintenance therapy.

Cryptococcal Meningitis

The initial induction and consolidation phases of treatment are identical to the treatment of CNS cryptococcosis in the immunocompetent patient as described earlier.[31, 37] Amphotericin B plus flucytosine is given for 2 weeks, followed by fluconazole for a minimum of 10 weeks (Table 203–3). However, in the immunocompromised host with AIDS, maintenance with an anticryptococcal drug is required for lifelong coverage. Fluconazole daily is the preferred drug for maintenance, but oral itraconazole daily or intravenous amphotericin B one to three times a week is a reasonable alternative.

Other therapy includes the occasional need for a ventricular shunt for hydrocephalus or corticosteroids for cerebral edema.

Prognosis

Based on the reports of extrapulmonary cryptococcosis in immunosuppressed infants and children, the prognosis for severe systemic cryptococcosis is reasonably good. Of the 13 children with AIDS and cryptococcosis,[19] 2 untreated patients died, and 10 of the 11 treated patients had a clinical response to amphotericin B with or without flucytosine, although 7 of the 10 had died of HIV infection at the time of the report. Of the 15 non-AIDS but immunosuppressed patients reviewed by Leggiadro and associates,[18] responses also were favorable but difficult to evaluate clearly because of other diseases and complications.

The cryptococcal antigen titer in CSF and serum has been used as a guide to therapeutic response in patients with meningitis caused by *C. neoformans*. In non-AIDS patients, high titers of cryptococcal antigen in serum and CSF at baseline were correlated with higher mortality rate

TABLE 203–3 ■ BASIC INFORMATION FOR AMPHOTERICIN B AND FLUCYTOSINE TREATMENT FOR CRYPTOCOCCAL MENINGITIS

Category	Amphotericin	Flucytosine
Dose	0.5–0.7 mg kg/day or 1 mg/kg every other day	100 mg/kg/day
Route	Intravenous, single dose over 2–6 hours	Oral, in four divided doses
Peak plasma concentration	0.5–2.0 μg/mL (dose of 0.5 mg/kg/day)	30–40 μg/mL (2-g dose)
Protein binding	≥90%	2%–4%
Volume of distribution	Neonate = 1.5–9.4 L per kg Child = 0.4–8.3 L per kg Adult = 4.0 L per kg	Approximates total body water
Central nervous system distribution	Poor	60%–90% of serum level
Elimination	Renal = 40% over 7 days Biliary = minimal Dialysis = poorly dialyzable	Renal = >90%
Major adverse effects	Hypokalemia, renal impairment, anemia, thrombophlebitis, cardiac arrhythmias	Anemia, leukopenia, thrombocytopenia, rash, confusion; greatest when serum levels >100 μg/mL

during therapy.[2, 6] A study of AIDS-associated meningitis showed no correlation between outcome and antigen titer.[31] However, during therapy for acute meningitis, an unchanged or increased titer of antigen in CSF correlated with clinical and microbiologic failure to respond to treatment.

REFERENCES

1. Abadi, J., Nachman, S., Kressel, A. B., and Pirofski, L. A.: Cryptococcosis in children with AIDS. Clin. Infect. Dis. *28*:309–313, 1999.
2. Behrman, R. E., Masci, J. R., and Nicholas, P.: Cryptococcal skeletal infections: Case report and review. Rev. Infect. Dis. *12*:181–190, 1990.
3. Bennett, J. E., Dismukes, W. E., Duma, R. J., et al.: A comparison of amphotericin B alone and combined with flucytosine in the treatment of cryptococcal meningitis. N. Engl. J. Med. *301*:126–131, 1979.
4. Campbell, G. D.: Primary pulmonary cryptococcosis. Am. Rev. Respir. Dis. *94*:236–243, 1966.
5. Climent, C., DeVinatea, M. L., Lasala, G., et al.: Geographical pathology profile of AIDS in Puerto Rico: The first decade. Mod. Pathol. *7*:647–651, 1994.
6. Diamond, R. D., and Bennett, J. E.: Prognostic factors in cryptococcal meningitis: A study in 111 cases. Ann. Intern. Med. *80*:176–181, 1974.
7. Dismukes, W. E.: Cryptococcal meningitis in patients with AIDS. J. Infect. Dis. *157*:624–628, 1988.
8. Ellis, D. H., and Pfeiffer, T. J.: Natural habitat of *Cryptococcus neoformans gattii*. J. Clin. Microbiol. *28*:1642–1644, 1990.
9. Faggi, E., Gargani, G., Pizzirani, C., et al.: Cryptococcosis in domestic mammals. Mycoses *36*:165–170, 1993.
10. Feldmesser, M., Kress, Y., Novikoff, P., et al.: *Cryptococcus neoformans* is a faculative intracellular pathogen in murine pulmonary infection. Infect. Immun. *68*:4225–4237, 2000.
11. Fetter, B. F., Klintworth, G. K., and Henry, W. S.: Mycoses of the Central Nervous System. Baltimore, Williams & Wilkins, 1976, p. 100.
12. Frank, U. K., Nishimura, S. L., Li, N. C., et al.: Evaluation of an enzyme immunoassay for detection of cryptococcal capsular polysaccharide antigen in serum and cerebrospinal fluid. J. Clin. Microbiol. *31*:97–101, 1993.
13. Goldman, D., Lee, S. C., and Casadevall, A.: Pathogenesis of pulmonary *Cryptococcus neoformans* infection in the rat. Infect. Immun. *62*: 4755–4761, 1994.
14. Hajjeh, R. A., Conn, L. A., Stephens, D. S., et al.: Cryptococcosis: Population-based, multisite, active surveillance and risk factors in human immunodeficiency virus-infected persons. J. Infect. Dis. *179*:449–454, 1999.
15. Huffnagle, K. E., and Gander, R. M.: Evaluation of Gen-Probe's *Histoplasma capsulatum* and *Cryptococcus neoformans* AccuProbes. J. Clin. Microbiol. *31*:419–421, 1993.
16. Jaye, D. L., Waites, K. B., Parker, B., et al.: Comparison of two rapid latex agglutination tests for detection of cryptococcal capsular polysaccharide. Am. J. Clin. Pathol. *109*:634–641, 1998.
17. Kwon-Chung, K. J., and Bennett, J. E.: Medical Mycology. Philadelphia, Lea & Febiger, 1992.
18. Leggiadro, R. J., Barrett, F. F., and Hughes, W. T.: Extrapulmonary cryptococcosis in immunosuppressed infants and children. Pediatr. Infect. Dis. J. *11*:43–47, 1992.
19. Leggiadro, R. J., Kline, M. W., and Hughes, W. T.: Extrapulmonary cryptococcosis in children with acquired immunodeficiency syndrome. Pediatr. Infect. Dis. J. *10*:658–662, 1991.
20. Levitz, S. M.: The ecology of *Cryptococcus neoformans* and the epidemiology of cryptococcosis. J. Infect. Dis. *13*:1163–1169, 1991.
21. Liaw, Y. S., Yang, P. C., Yu, C. V., et al.: Direct determination of cryptococcal antigen in transthoracic needle aspirates for diagnosis of pulmonary cryptococcosis. J. Clin. Microbiol. *33*:1588–1591, 1995.
22. McDonnell, J. M., and Hutchins, G. M.: Pulmonary cryptococcosis. Hum. Pathol. *16*:121–128, 1985.
23. Min, K. H., and Kwon-Chung, K. J.: The biochemical basis for the distribution between the two *Cryptococcus neoformans* varieties with CGB medium. Centralbl. Bakteriol. *261*:481, 1986.
24. Mitchell, T. G., and Perfect, J. R.: Cryptococcosis in the era of AIDS: 100 years after the discovery of *Cryptococcus neoformans*. Clin. Microbiol. Rev. *8*:515, 1995.
25. Mitchell, D. H., Sorrell, T. C., Allworth, A. M., et al.: Cryptococcal disease of the CNS in immunocompromised hosts: Influence of cryptococcal variety on clinical manifestations and outcome. Clin. Infect. Dis. *20*:611–616, 1995.
26. Mukherjee, S., Lee, S., Mukherjee, J., et al.: Monoclonal antibodies to *Cryptococcus neoformans* capsular polysaccharide modify the course of intravenous infection in mice. Infect. Immun. *62*:1079–1088, 1994.
27. Murray, P. R., Baron, E. J., Pfaller, M. A., et al.: Manual of Clinical Microbiology. 6th ed. Washington, D.C., ASM Press, 1995.
28. Neilson, J. B., Fromtling, R. A., and Bulmer, G. S.: *Cryptococcus neoformans*: Size range of infectious particles from aerosolized soil. Infect. Immun. *17*:634–638, 1977.
29. Newberry, W. M., Walter, J. E., Chandler, J. W., et al.: Epidemiologic study *Cryptococcus neoformans*. Ann. Intern. Med. *67*:724–732, 1967.
30. Nosanchuk, J. D., Shoham, S., Fries, B. C., et al.: Evidence of zoonitic transmission of *Cryptococcus neoformans* from a pet cockatoo to an immunocompromised host. Ann. Intern. Med. *132*:205–208, 2000.
31. Powderly, W. G.: Therapy for cryptococcal meningitis in patients with AIDS. Clin. Infect. Dis. *140*(Suppl. 1):554–559, 1992.
32. Powderly, W. G., Cloud, G. A., Dismukes, W. E., et al.: Measurement of cryptococcal antigen in serum and cerebrospinal fluid: Value in the management of AIDS-associated cryptococcal meningitis. Clin. Infect. Dis. *18*:789–792, 1994.
33. Powell, K. E., Dahl, B. A., Weeks, R. J., et al.: Airborne *Cryptococcus neoformans*: Particles from pigeon excreta compatible with alveolar deposition. J. Infect. Dis. *125*:412, 1972.
34. Rosenbaum, R., and Goncalves, A. J. R.: Clinical epidemiological study of 171 cases of cryptococcosis. Clin. Infect. Dis. *18*:369–380, 1994.
35. Ruiz, A., and Blumer, G. S.: Particle size of airborne *Cryptococcus neoformans* in a tower. Appl. Environ. Microbiol. *41*:1225, 1981.
36. Saag, M. S., Graybill, R. J., Larsen, R. A., et al.: Practice guidelines for the management of cryptococcal disease. Clin. Infect. Dis. *30*:710–718, 2000.
37. Saag, M. S., Powderly, W. G., Cloud, G. A., et al.: Comparison of amphotericin B with fluconazole in the treatment of acute AIDS-associated cryptococcal meningitis. N. Engl. J. Med. *326*:83–89, 1992.
38. Tarrand, J. J., Guillot, C., Wenglar, M., et al.: Clinical comparison of the resin-containing BACTEC 26 Plus and the Isolator 10 blood culturing systems. J. Clin. Microbiol. *29*:2245–2249, 1991.
39. Valada, M. G., Nunes, C., Jacob, C. M., et al.: Cryptococcosis in HIV-infected children. International Conference on AIDS *10*:254 (Abstract No. PB0446). Aug. 7–12, 1994.
40. Velez, J. D., Allendoefer, R., Luther, M., et al.: Correlation of in vitro azole susceptibility with in vivo response in a murine model of cryptococcal meningitis. J. Infect. Dis. *168*:508–510, 1993.

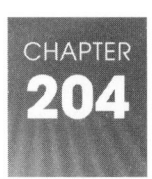

Histoplasmosis

MARTIN B. KLEIMAN

Histoplasmosis is the most common pulmonary and systemic mycosis in humans and affects millions of people. Although infections occur worldwide, a substantial proportion occur in the United States, where approximately 500,000 persons are infected annually.[283] Of these, an estimated 55,000 to 200,000 infected individuals become symptomatic and 1500 to 4000 require hospitalization.[180] Its public health significance as an opportunistic infection is escalating in proportion to the increasing numbers of persons who are immunosuppressed.[173]

Histoplasma capsulatum, the etiologic agent of histoplasmosis, first was described[238] in 1906 by Samuel Darling, a pathologist in the Panama Canal Zone,[50] while examining autopsy specimens of a man from Martinique who had died of a chronic, wasting illness. He observed an organism within histiocytes and thought it to be an encapsulated plasmodium; the illness caused by this new pathogen was named reticuloendothelial cytomycosis.[176] In 1932, Dodd and Tompkins[64] demonstrated intracellular *H. capsulatum* in the peripheral blood smear of a febrile child, and DeMonbreum[60] subsequently grew the organism from this same child and correctly classified it as a fungus. In 1944, Christie and Peterson[42] developed histoplasmin and, after subcutaneous inoculation, demonstrated a positive cutaneous reaction in a child with histoplasmosis.

In 1945, Parson and Zarafonetis[198] characterized the disease as rare and usually fatal after studying 71 patients with disseminated histoplasmosis. However, with the use of histoplasmin skin testing, Christie and Peterson[42] soon demonstrated histoplasmosis to be a common and usually a mild disease. They correctly recognized that histoplasmosis was the etiology of pulmonary calcifications in large numbers of patients who were presumed to have tuberculosis but in whom tuberculin skin tests were negative. Further characterization of the natural habitat and transmission of the fungus occurred in the late 1940s and early 1950s with demonstration of the organism in soil and air samples.[2, 75, 220, 284]

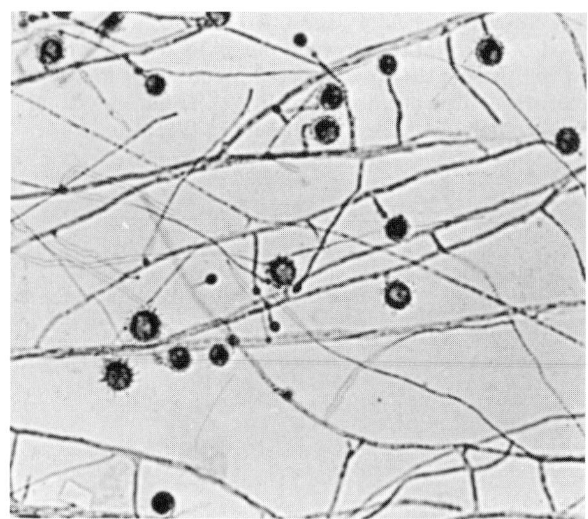

FIGURE 204–1 ■ Culture of *Histoplasma capsulatum* from sputum illustrating tuberculate macroaleuriospores and microaleuriospores (lactophenol cotton blue, ×52).

The Organism

H. capsulatum variety *capsulatum,* the anamorphic (asexual) form of the organism, is a thermally dimorphic, saprophytic fungus of the class Ascomycetes, family Gymnoascaceae, subdivision Ascomycotina. The mold form displays heterothallic sexual reproduction with plus (+) and minus (-) mating types. Ninety percent of infections are caused by the minus type. The ascomycetous teleomorph produced by mating opposite types was isolated in 1972 and termed *Emmonsiella capsulata*[142]; the current taxonomy of this perfect (sexual) form is *Ajellomyces capsulatus.*[168, 221] Because the fungus is isolated in the laboratory as the anamorph, the more common name *Histoplasma capsulatum* is used in this text.

At temperatures of 25° to 30° C, the fungus grows as a fluffy colony with an aerial mycelium that varies from white to buff brown. Mycelia, microconidia (3 to 5 μm), and tuberculate and nontuberculate macroconidia (8 to 16 μm) are seen microscopically[147] (Fig. 204–1). The organism grows slowly, with 1 to 2 weeks required for laboratory strains and as long as 8 to 12 weeks for growth from clinical specimens. When cultured at 37° C on enriched media containing cysteine, the mold transforms to the yeast form in 7 to 10 days.[180] The small, heaped, pasty colonies appear microscopically as ovoid, budding yeasts (1 to 3 μm × 3 to 5 μm) with rare pseudohyphae.[180, 193]

In its natural habitat, the soil, *H. capsulatum* exists as mycelia and spores. It survives best in moist (95–100% humidity), nitrogen-rich soil at temperatures of 37° C or higher and can be found as deep as 1 mile below the soil surface.[275, 283] The droppings in roosting sites of chickens, blackbirds, and starlings contain nutrients that promote fungal growth and, at least in the case of chickens, may contain substances that discourage the growth of competitive organisms in the soil.[245] Many species of colonial New World bats become infected and excrete the fungus in their guano; bat guano also contains substances that encourage growth of the fungus.[74, 159, 258, 259] Although birds excrete the fungus in droppings, they remain uninfected, probably because of their high body temperature. *H. capsulatum* can remain viable in droppings or other contaminated sites for many years.[318]

Early techniques used to differentiate strains of *H. capsulatum* included serotyping and chemotyping.[65] Current techniques involve restriction fragment length polymorphisms of DNA. Three broad classes that show geographic and possibly clinical differences have been delineated.[134, 277] Class 2 strains are found most frequently in North America, and class 3 strains are found in Central and South America. Class 1 strains are isolated almost exclusively from immunocompromised patients. Individual strains within each class have been examined further with additional nucleic acid–based and genome-wide approaches to reveal considerable genetic diversity. Such strain differences are useful for molecular epidemiologic investigations.[120, 218] Studies have suggested that patients with acquired immunodeficiency syndrome (AIDS) may be infected with less virulent, temperature-sensitive variants of *H. capsulatum.*[249]

Histoplasma duboisii, the etiology of African histoplasmosis, was reclassified as a variant of *H. capsulatum* when it was shown that mating of isolates from each type produced cleistothecia and ascospores identical to those of *E. capsulata* (now termed *A. capsulatus).*[143, 220] *H. capsulatum* variety *duboisii* is indistinguishable from *H. capsulatum* variety *capsulatum* in its mycelial stage, but its tissue phase is much larger and consists of thick-walled oval yeast forms that are 10 to 15 μm in diameter. Infections caused by *H. capsulatum* variety *duboisii* have been described across central and western Africa and occur along with histoplasmosis caused by *H. capsulatum.*[193]

Epidemiology

Histoplasmosis is acquired almost exclusively when environmental sites that are contaminated with *H. capsulatum* are disturbed and spores become aerosolized and then are inhaled. Early understanding of its epidemiology was heavily influenced by findings in sudden outbreaks of acute infection among small groups of people exposed to relatively large inocula. However, because most infections are asymptomatic or self-limited, such investigations skewed the true epidemiology. A more accurate understanding was achieved when the results of skin test epidemiology, cultures of environmental sources, birds, and other animals, and careful analysis of the history of exposure also were considered.[32]

Histoplasmosis has been reported worldwide in tropical, subtropical, and most frequently, temperate areas.[78] Regions with a relatively high incidence of infection are termed endemic, and the majority of infections occur in these areas. Most infections occur sporadically and cannot be associated with exposure to a specific site or activity. They are presumed to result when environmental conditions are conducive to growth of the fungus, and dry windy weather or other events or activities facilitate the airborne transmission of spores. Although early reports emphasized that the infection usually was associated with occupational exposure in primarily rural environments, infection is recognized commonly in urban areas,[230] where it may affect large numbers of people.[311] Infections occur commonly in children and frequently remain unrecognized because as investigations of outbreaks have shown, children often remain asymptomatic.[24, 106] In a skin test survey of a highly endemic area in Tennessee, skin test reactivity was found in 80 percent of children 10 years of age.[329]

The incidence of human infection varies widely in endemic regions. Within short distances of areas in which residents demonstrate only a moderate incidence of skin test reactivity may be hyperendemic areas in which the incidence of infection is considerably higher. Still more localized and very heavily contaminated sites, termed microfoci, may be found in which localized, sometimes severe outbreaks occur. Because the droppings of birds and bats[62] accelerate growth of the fungus in the environment, sites that have been implicated in localized outbreaks have included blackbird and pigeon roosting areas, chicken houses, bat-infested caves, attics, chimneys, old buildings, and decaying woodpiles and trees. Activities that disturb these types of sites have been implicated in localized outbreaks.[209, 283] Infections in children have been associated with exploring caves; playing in barns or hollow trees; cleaning abandoned buildings; cutting firewood or tree stumps; renovating the walls, attics, or basements of older homes; digging in contaminated sites; being downwind of the excavation/demolition of buildings; cleaning seldom-used fireplaces; and being in indoor environments contaminated by fungal aerosols gaining access to air intakes.

Edwards and colleagues[71, 72] described the geographic distribution of *H. capsulatum* in the United States by performing histoplasmin skin testing on 275,558 Navy recruits between 1958 and 1965. The highest incidence of reactivity was found in residents of the Ohio-Mississippi-Missouri, the St. Lawrence, and the Rio Grande River valleys.[180] In four states (Arkansas, Kentucky, Missouri, and Tennessee) the percentage of positive adult reactors ranged from 57 to 68 percent. In the adjacent states (Illinois, Indiana, Ohio, and Oklahoma), skin test reactivity ranged from 50 to 73 percent among adults in farm areas. Of the other seven states in the endemic area, lifetime prevalence rates exceeding 50 percent were demonstrated in one or more counties.[1] Epidemiologic studies of this scale have not been repeated, and as has been demonstrated with other endemic mycoses,[149] population shifts and changes in land use may alter these patterns.

Numerous histoplasmosis outbreaks have been documented and offer some means of assessing the epidemiology and clinical spectrum of infections acquired in point-source and sustained outbreaks. The largest sustained outbreak was reported to occur in Indianapolis, Indiana, involved an estimated 100,000 persons within a 400-square-mile area, and lasted nearly 1 year.[311] Symptomatic cases were identified in 435 individuals (including 49 younger than 15 years), and disseminated disease developed in 46 of them. Persons 15 to 34 years of age were more likely to become infected than were other age groups. An equal sex distribution of cases occurred before puberty; males predominated in a 3:1 ratio in older individuals. Localized outbreaks related to high-risk sites and activities noted previously are well documented. Isolated cases may not be associated readily with such activities. Infections acquired during travel to endemic regions may go unrecognized, particularly in persons without a history of contact with a site commonly associated with histoplasmosis, such as occurred in a large group of college students whose only known common exposure was vacationing at a hotel in Mexico.[38]

Although a variety of wild and domestic animals may become infected, transmission to humans does not occur.[177] Infection of an infant after exposure to a pillow that contained contaminated feathers has been reported.[31] Even though a case of sexual transmission that resulted from exposure to the mucosal lesions of a patient with disseminated histoplasmosis has been reported,[243] human-to-human transmission is an extremely rare occurrence. Transmission has been confirmed, with the use of molecular typing methodology, in the recipients of two cadaveric organs transplanted from a donor who had resided in an endemic area.[155] Infections caused by direct inoculation of contaminated material in the environment or from laboratory accidents occur rarely.

Pathophysiology

H. capsulatum has unique biologic capabilities that contribute to its success as a human pathogen. Key among them are its ability to infect and gain access to macrophages; to alter the intracellular environment, thereby allowing it to survive, replicate, and disseminate; to remain viable during clinically inapparent infection; and to become reactivated when host immune factors permit.[29, 323] The onset of infection results in a brisk innate immune response that is followed by an acquired immune response. During these events, the fungus induces an orderly modulation of the host inflammatory and cytokine responses. Production of cytokine begins within 24 hours of primary infection and continues for approximately 3 weeks, thus bridging the innate and acquired immune reactions. Successful clearance of the infection is highly dependent on the integrity of the cellular immune response. The clinical manifestations and outcome are determined by this complex interplay of events.

The incubation period of histoplasmosis is variable and depends on the size of the inoculum, the integrity of the host immune response, the presence of immunity from previous infection, and strain-to-strain differences in fungal virulence.[94, 139] Although the range of incubation periods is reported to be 1 to 3 weeks in nonimmune hosts, it is largely based on data gathered from point-source outbreaks in which the time of exposure is readily determined. However, in these settings, the size of the infecting inoculum probably is larger than that resulting in sporadic infections.[32] Because the overwhelming majority of infections occur sporadically and are either asymptomatic or result in nonspecific flulike illnesses that are not diagnosed, the upper range may be longer. In patients who retain specific cellular immunity from previous infection, re-exposure results in less severe symptoms and shorter incubation periods, usually approximately 4 to 7 days.[32] Normal infants and individuals with a primary or acquired deficiency in cellular immune function are more likely to experience symptomatic illness after exposure.[94]

In experimental animals, acute pneumonitis develops after inhalation of *H. capsulatum* microconidia or mycelial fragments.[14] Because of their smaller size, microconidia gain access to the smaller airways more readily than macroconidia do. Within 2 to 3 days after being inhaled, spores germinate within alveoli and convert to the yeast form of the fungus. This step appears to be a critical determinant of virulence because chemical blockage of conversion from the mycelial to the yeast phase impairs virulence in a murine model.[175] Additional determinants of fungal virulence have been described, and newly developed molecular techniques have been used to identify two genes *(URA5, CBPI)* that have a role in pathogenesis.[323] In the first week, a neutrophil response occurs at the site of the infection; it is followed in about 2 weeks by the accumulation of helper T lymphocytes and macrophages.[211] The yeast forms attach to integrins of the CD11/CD18 group of cell surface receptors and enter neutrophils[234] and macrophages.[27] This process may be an adaptive microbe entry mechanism that enables the organism to evade the host oxidative burst response associated with host-directed opsonophagocytosis.[323] Human neutrophils possess fungistatic activity that resides within azurophil granules.[25, 189] Neutrophils have been shown to play a role in the primary immune response in a murine model[332]; however, depletion of neutrophils in a systemic model of secondary infection did not alter the course. Traditional opsonophagocytosis facilitated by binding to complement or to immunoglobulin after the development of humoral immunity also occurs.[323]

Yeasts appear to have a competitive advantage within the membrane-bound vacuoles of macrophages.[186, 187] In mouse models, strategies used by the organism to survive and replicate in this ordinarily hostile environment include increasing the alkalinity, tolerating nutrient starvation, and resisting the toxic effects of host reactive oxygen and nitrogen intermediates, degradative enzymes, and antimicrobial peptides.[323] Lysis of infected cells results in the release of additional yeasts and infection of additional macrophages. During this period of fungal sequestration and replication, lymphohematogenous dissemination distributes yeast from the lungs to the reticuloendothelial system and to other organs.[186]

The cellular immune system plays the pivotal role in a host's successful response to infection with *H. capsulatum.*[187, 211] Although infection usually results in a brisk antibody response, humoral immunity does not contribute substantially to primary or secondary immunity.[227] Human dendritic cells that reside in the lung link the innate and adaptive immune responses. More efficient antigen-presenting cells than alveolar macrophages, dendritic cells phagocytose and rapidly degrade the organism, present *H. capsulatum* antigen for lymphocyte proliferation, and facilitate the induction of cell-mediated immunity.[102, 187] Some of the strategies used by the fungus that facilitate its survival and replication within macrophages, such as prevention of phagolysosomal fusion, do not take place in dendritic cells. The resultant rapid destruction of yeast within dendritic cells may represent an important role for these cells in the innate immune response.[187] After their participation in the innate immune response, several endogenous cytokines induced by the development of acquired cellular immunity[187] activate macrophages, which then act as the primary cellular effectors that control the infection.[186] Cytokines that play key roles in the resolution of primary or secondary infection (protective immunity) in animal models include tumor necrosis factor-α (TNF-α),[5, 7, 8, 326, 332] interferon-γ (IFN-γ),[5, 6, 46, 146, 276] interleukin-12 (IL-12),[6, 30, 333, 334] and granulocyte-macrophage colony-stimulating-factor (GM-CSF).[4, 6, 7, 56, 58, 246] IL-12's effect results from its induction of IFN-γ; it is active in primary infection but not in reinfection.[6] Cytokines that activate human macrophages and induce them to become fungistatic are GM-CSF, macrophage-stimulating factor, and IL-3[188]; the mechanisms by which the colony-stimulating factors stimulate fungistatic activity are not clear. Human macrophages also express antifungal activity that is not cytokine-dependent. The latter mechanism is stimulated by attachment of macrophages to type 1 collagen matrices and is mediated, at least in part, by overcoming the ability of yeasts to inhibit phagolysosomal fusion.[190]

In addition to macrophages, specific T-cell subpopulations are also capable of killing *H. capsulatum.* $CD4^+$ cells have been shown to be essential for fungal clearance in mouse models.[55, 92] The importance of these cells in human infection is supported by observations showing that the risk of severe histoplasmosis developing in adults with human immunodeficiency virus (HIV) infection increases when the $CD4^+$ count falls below 200/μL.[294] $CD8^+$ cells also mediate immunity in mice, but their contribution is not as significant as that of $CD4^+$ cells. $CD8^+$ cell clearance of *H. capsulatum* involves both perforin-dependent and -independent mechanisms.[331] Perforin also plays an independent and essential role in primary immunity in a mouse model.[331] Cytokines such as IFN-γ and TNF-α also work in concert with cytolytic mechanisms to provide protective immunity against *H. capsulatum.*[331] The role of natural killer (NK) cells has been studied in murine models.[200] NK cells participate to a limited degree in the immune response in immunocompetent animals and play a more substantial role in animals depleted of T cells.[187]

In immunocompetent hosts, cellular immunity is suppressed[204] early in the course of histoplasmosis, especially in disseminated histoplasmosis of infancy.[44, 192] Cellular immune function returns to normal after 4 to 6 weeks of treatment. In the mouse model, *H. capsulatum* infection is associated with the generation of suppressor T-cell activity; this activity depresses the production of T-cell–dependent, delayed-type hypersensitivity, mitogen-induced lymphocyte transformation, and cytotoxic activity.[13] T-cell immunity develops approximately 10 to 21 days after exposure, and splenic suppressor T-cell numbers decrease while helper T-cells increase.

In a study of the cellular immune response of HIV-1–infected patients with recent histoplasmosis, all had nonreactive skin tests. Lymphoproliferative responses and IFN-γ production were depressed in those with $CD4^+$ counts between 200 and 500 cells/mm^3; lymphoproliferative responses approached normal in patients with $CD4^+$ counts above 500 cells/mm^3.[273] In addition to having defective cellular immunity resulting from decreased numbers of $CD4^+$ cells, persons with HIV infection have macrophages that show a diminished ability to control *H. capsulatum.* These macrophages have a profound defect in their ability to recognize and bind to yeast and also demonstrate permissiveness for intracellular growth of the fungus.[39] The HIV envelope glycoprotein gp120 appears to play a role in inhibiting phagocytosis of *H. capsulatum* by macrophages, but it is not responsible for the capacity for accelerated growth of yeast within macrophages.[40]

Pathology

With the exception of patients who have progressive disseminated infection, particularly those with preexisting congenital or acquired cellular immune dysfunction, histopathologic findings in histoplasmosis are characterized by granulomatous inflammation, usually in association with caseating and noncaseating granulomata. Granulomata appear after the development of an effective acquired immune response; the cellular elements in these lesions consist primarily of mononuclear phagocytes and lymphocytes, largely T cells. Langerhans giant cells are often present, and typical yeast forms occasionally, but not consistently, are visible within macrophages. Inflammation progresses to fibrosis and often is accompanied by calcification.[94] The rate of calcification is age-dependent, and it may occur within months in children and for up to several years in adults.[94, 252] Exuberant granulomatous inflammation or fibrosis, or both, can result in obstruction or dysfunction of adjacent mediastinal or biliary tract structures. Although viable yeasts remain in quiescent granulomata, they are few in number and infrequently seen. In areas endemic for histoplasmosis, old granulomata in the lung, bone marrow, or other sites may be seen as incidental findings, the significance of which is dependent on clinical assessment. Yeasts almost never are observed in histologic sections of extensive fibrosis in late histoplasmosis.

In patients with acutely progressive manifestations of histoplasmosis, especially those with preexisting cellular immune dysfunction or infants, the inflammatory response is impaired and granuloma formation is poor.[96] In these instances, extensive parasitization of macrophages by yeasts occurs, and organisms may be seen readily in a variety of reticuloendothelial structures, especially the bone marrow, and sometimes within leukocytes in the peripheral blood. Many other organ systems are involved. The histopathologic findings in central nervous system (CNS) infection consist of granulomatous basilar meningeal and vascular inflammation, perineural inflammatory changes in cranial nerves, and many organisms at the periphery of mass lesions.[289] The adrenals and gastrointestinal tract commonly are affected in disseminated infection.

Clinical Manifestations

Approximately 95 percent of infections caused by *H. capsulatum* occur in normal persons and either are asymptomatic or cause brief, self-limited illness with no sequelae. The only residual findings are the incidental radiographic demonstration of typical granulomata in the lung parenchyma or calcifications in the hilar/mediastinal lymph nodes or the spleen. In immunocompetent hosts, the size of the inoculum is the single most important determinant of whether infection will be accompanied by clinical symptoms. After exposure to small inocula, symptoms will develop in only 1 percent of individuals, but after heavy exposure, 50 to 100 percent will become ill.[283] Similarly, the symptoms that develop are more severe in individuals who are exposed to large inocula. Severity may be reduced by preexisting immunity derived from previous infection. However, protection is not complete, and severe disease can occur after re-exposure to a heavy inoculum. A critical determinant of susceptibility and severity also is host-dependent. Individuals with cell-mediated immune deficiency and normal infants younger than 1 year are at a disproportionately high risk for the development of symptoms after exposure and are at far greater risk for progression of early fungal dissemination.

As with the other endemic mycoses, histoplasmosis begins as an acute inflammatory pneumonitis, undergoes self-limited or progressive dissemination, and requires an effective host immune response for its control. Clinical manifestations (Table 204–1) are varied because they result from any or all of the following: the nonspecific systemic effects caused by the infection, symptoms resulting from either the primary inflammatory focus or perturbation of function of anatomic structures adjacent to primary sites of inflammation, hypersensitivity phenomena resulting from the acquired immune response, symptoms caused by hematogenously infected sites, life-threatening multisystem symptoms resulting from progressive parasitization of the reticuloendothelial and other organ systems, symptoms caused by chronically progressive forms of pneumonitis or dissemination, or exacerbation of quiescent disease. Recognition, confirmation of the diagnosis, and selection of prudent therapeutic options require understanding of these diverse clinical manifestations.

TABLE 204–1 ■ CLINICAL MANIFESTATIONS OF PEDIATRIC HISTOPLASMOSIS

Manifestation
Asymptomatic infection
Pulmonary disease
Acute (mild, moderate, severe forms)
Mediastinal adenopathy (granuloma)
Obstruction (mediastinal structures)
Mediastinal fibrosis
Pericarditis
Chronic disease with cavitation*
Progressive disseminated infection
Acute
Infancy (PDH of infancy)
Immunocompromised (non-HIV)
HIV
Subacute*
Chronic*
Presumed ocular histoplasmosis†
Primary cutaneous infection

*Infrequent manifestation during childhood.
†Rare in children.
HIV, human immunodeficiency virus; PDH, progressive disseminated histoplasmosis.

PULMONARY HISTOPLASMOSIS

The most common symptoms of acute primary histoplasmosis encompass a spectrum of respiratory and systemic complaints of varying severity. Eighty percent of infections are mild, undifferentiated, flulike illnesses with cough, myalgia, headache, and variable low-grade fever; symptoms are self-limited and resolve in 3 to 5 days.[283] In more significant fungal exposure, fever is present and often accompanied by headache, myalgia, chills, more persistent cough, and more significant chest pain.[94] These symptoms may persist for as long as 2 weeks and be associated with nausea, vomiting, diarrhea, asthenia, weight loss, or fatigue. This manifestation also is self-limited, although fatigue and weight loss improve slowly after the fever resolves. In primary infections that last longer than 2 weeks, fever is higher and often accompanied by greater weight loss, chills, night sweats, fatigue, and chest pain. In general, the chest pain that occurs in histoplasmosis is typically nonpleuritic, may be substernal or lateralized, usually is brief in duration, and recurs frequently; this pattern may last from a week to a few months.[94] Wheezing is a common initial symptom.[28, 282] Hepatosplenomegaly occasionally is present, although its occurrence should raise suspicion of early dissemination. In these prolonged illnesses, resolution without treatment may occur, but with the safe and effective oral antifungal agents available, most experts recommend treatment with antifungal therapy. Finally, in acute primary infections that occur after intense exposure to large numbers of spores, the resulting diffuse pneumonitis may be associated with dyspnea or adult respiratory distress syndrome early in the infection. In these instances, the ordinarily self-limited early dissemination has a high risk of becoming progressive, and treatment is required. After development of the respiratory complaints that accompany primary infection, rheumatologic syndromes may be seen within several months of infection. They usually consist of erythema multiforme,[174] erythema nodosum,[94, 158, 197, 239] acute migratory polyarthritis, or any combination of these conditions.[45, 224] The rheumatologic symptoms are immune mediated and usually self-limited or respond to anti-inflammatory therapy.

A variety of symptoms may result from complications arising from intrathoracic or, less commonly, intra-abdominal lymphadenitis caused by *H. capsulatum*. One of the most problematic is acute primary infection accompanied by fever, weight loss, and a mediastinal mass demonstrated by chest radiography. This scenario, as well as the presence of mediastinal lymphadenopathy in the absence of any recognized clinical symptoms, often requires definitive diagnosis to exclude malignancy, especially lymphoma.[84, 301, 325] Pediatric series that have examined the definitive diagnosis of such manifestations have found rates of histoplasmosis to vary from 1 to 57 percent,[21, 84, 281, 325] a discrepancy best explained by considering whether the study population lived in an endemic region. In endemic regions, the etiology of a mass within the middle mediastinum was histoplasmosis if the histoplasmal complement-fixation (CF) titer was greater than 1:16.[84]

Complications of acute primary histoplasmosis may be seen when granulomatous lymphadenitis results in inflammation, compression, or obstruction of contiguous structures within the thorax; this manifestation occasionally is termed mediastinal granuloma. Structures most commonly affected are, in decreasing order of frequency, the bronchi, trachea, pericardium, pulmonary vasculature and great vessels, lymphatics,[267] esophagus, and nerves.[69, 199, 219, 324] Symptoms include bronchial compression/obstruction with distal pneumonitis; pericarditis; pulmonary infarction; esophageal diverticula, fistula formation, or dysmotility, alone or in combination; tracheoesophageal fistula formation; and phrenic or recurrent laryngeal nerve palsy. Children are more susceptible than adults to tracheobronchial compression as a result of encroachment by enlarged lymph nodes.[86] The risk of involvement of contiguous structures by such mediastinal granulomata is related to the thickness of the capsule rather than the overall size of the node.[94] In highly endemic regions, histoplasmosis is the etiology of up to 25 percent of acute pericarditis cases; approximately one fourth of patients have symptoms of tamponade.[284] In almost all instances it is caused by pericardial inflammation resulting from an infected lymph node adjacent to the pericardium and not by frank fungal pericarditis.[328] The pericardial fluid is exudative and bloody. Most patients with histoplasmal pericarditis improve with nonsteroidal anti-inflammatory agents. Rarely, contiguous adenitis or broncholiths erode through the pericardium and cause fungal contamination of the pericardial space.[94, 328] Pleural effusions occur very infrequently in children with histoplasmosis and, similar to pericarditis, appear to result from pleural inflammatory reactions to adjacent granulomata; cultures of pleural fluid are negative.[214] Broncholithiasis may result from calcifications that erode through bronchi,[18] but they rarely occur in children. Lower cervical[284] or supraclavicular adenitis is a rare manifestation of histoplasmosis and usually is seen in association with mediastinal involvement. Lymphadenitis occasionally affects the intra-abdominal lymph nodes and has been reported to cause biliary tract obstruction[201, 217] in children.

Subacute or chronic manifestations of intrathoracic histoplasmosis may occur in children, although they most commonly affect older adults. Of these entities, mediastinal fibrosis may affect adolescents. In these instances, granulomatous inflammation progresses to dense fibrosis, which in turn causes stenosis, obstruction, or malfunction of contiguous critical mediastinal structures. Although symptoms are similar to those caused by active granulomatous inflammation that impairs the function of these structures, the fibrosis is progressive and irreversible and responds to neither antifungal therapy nor anti-inflammatory agents. Common complications include the superior vena cava syndrome and stenosis or obstruction of the trachea, bronchi, pulmonary artery, or esophagus.[161] Late constrictive pericarditis was reported[94] to develop in 14 percent of adults with histoplasmal pericarditis, but data have been descriptive. Long-term data in children are lacking. Additional late complications of intrathoracic histoplasmosis seen primarily in adults include pulmonary histoplasmomas, which are granulomata in the peripheral lung fields that become encased in dense fibrous tissue, often with calcification, enlarge slowly over a period of several years, and may cause symptoms of a mass lesion.[97] Cavitary (also termed chronic) pulmonary histoplasmosis has been reported in a child[17] but typically is seen in adults with underlying chronic obstructive pulmonary disease.[315] Early symptoms include episodes of low-grade fever, productive cough, weakness, weight loss, and fatigue.[99] Early pulmonary findings consist of interstitial pneumonitis that eventually progresses to fibrosis, cavitation, and gradual spread to uninvolved areas of the lung. If chronic plasmosis is untreated, disseminated infection eventually develops in approximately 80 percent of patients with this disorder.[82, 226]

PRIMARY CUTANEOUS HISTOPLASMOSIS

Primary cutaneous histoplasmosis can develop after accidental inoculation of skin or mucocutaneous structures,[88] such as the conjunctiva[264] or vulva.[243] The infection is characterized by a chancriform ulcer that often is associated with regional adenopathy. Lesions involute and heal spontaneously in several months. Spread to contiguous structures and dissemination can occur in hosts who are immunocompromised.[49]

PROGRESSIVE DISSEMINATED HISTOPLASMOSIS

The clinical entity of progressive disseminated histoplasmosis (PDH) is defined as an illness that occurs in association with continuing replication of *H. capsulatum* in multiple organ systems. This definition excludes the transient fungal dissemination that uniformly occurs in early primary infection and is aborted by the acquired cellular immune response. However, it does include the rare instance in which intense exposure results in severe primary infection that overwhelms the host's ability to mount an effective cellular immune response and dissemination progresses. Relatively distinct clinical manifestations of PDH in adults permit subclassification into acute, subacute, and chronic forms. In contrast to adult infection, PDH in children occurs exclusively as an acute, progressive, life-threatening infection.[122] Most of these infections develop in immunocompetent infants or in children with acquired or congenital cellular immune deficiency. Rarely, PDH occurs in an immunocompetent child.[51]

PDH may result from exogenous exposure of a susceptible or immune host or from reactivation of endogenous quiescent foci of infection. Precise differentiation of these mechanisms of pathogenesis is complicated by the risk for re-exposure in endemic areas and the unavailability of methodology that easily distinguishes strain differences in isolates. Although reactivation of infection may occur in an immunosuppressed host, epidemiologic data in immunosuppressed individuals who reside in areas highly endemic for histoplasmosis favor exogenous exposure as the most likely mechanism. Supporting evidence consists of observations showing that rates of PDH in immunocompromised patients increase only during periods in which infection rates increase in the general population and do not increase in interepidemic periods.[206, 233, 272, 314] Using the results of histoplasmin skin testing obtained at the time of diagnosis of malignancy in a large cohort of children, Hughes[118] found that skin test reactivity was absent in all children in whom PDH subsequently developed and that in none of those known to be skin test–positive at the time of diagnosis of their neoplastic diseases did PDH develop later.

PROGRESSIVE DISSEMINATED HISTOPLASMOSIS OF INFANCY. PDH of infancy usually affects children younger than 1 year and has been reported to occur in a 6-week-old infant.[151, 192] It is usually a subacute illness in which symptoms often are reported to have been present for 1 to 12 weeks before initial evaluation; as the disease progresses, patients eventually become profoundly ill and usually die unless treated. Early symptoms include fever, failure to thrive,[250] and hepatosplenomegaly in almost all instances. Pallor, cough, tachypnea, oropharyngeal ulcerations, lymphadenopathy, gastrointestinal bleeding, or hemorrhagic skin lesions may develop. Abnormalities that are seen in laboratory studies and inexorably worsen include anemia, thrombocytopenia, leukopenia,[96, 151] disseminated intravascular coagulopathy, and marked depression of immunoregulatory cells[44, 192]; these abnormalities reflect the overwhelming fungal parasitization of the reticuloendothelial system and often suggest the diagnosis of a lymphoreticular malignancy. The chest radiograph may show signs of focal pneumonitis, mediastinal adenopathy, or miliary disease, but more than 50 percent of chest radiographs are normal at the time of diagnosis. Organs commonly affected are the spleen, liver, bone marrow, lymph nodes, gastrointestinal tract, and adrenal glands.[34] CNS abnormalities were reported in 62 percent of a large series of PDH cases in Costa Rican infants.[192]

PDH of infancy was uniformly fatal before the availability of effective antifungal agents[151]; survival rates are now excellent. In a series of Costa Rican children that included some infants with malnutrition, 90 percent of patients treated with amphotericin B survived; of the four who died, two had received amphotericin B for either 33 or 35 days and were treated with ketoconazole orally thereafter. Both families declined further treatment and were lost to follow-up (C. Odio, personal communication); each returned, within 5 weeks of discharge, with massive gastrointestinal hemorrhage and recurrent dissemination. The other two were gravely ill and died after having received only either two or three doses. Survival was 100 percent in an Indiana series of PDH of infancy (M. Kleiman, unpublished data).

PROGRESSIVE DISSEMINATED HISTOPLASMOSIS IN IMMUNOCOMPROMISED HOSTS. Immunosuppressed individuals, especially those in whom the primary medical condition or therapy has depressed cellular immunity, are at risk for dissemination if they acquire histoplasmosis.[118] Common predisposing conditions include AIDS, immunosuppressive therapy for reticuloendothelial malignancies,[118] organ transplantation, and dialysis.* In children who are receiving chemotherapy for malignancies, disseminated histoplasmosis can occur during either remission or relapse.[118] The most common initial symptom is persistent fever, often without localizing symptoms and unassociated with toxicity. As the illness evolves, fever continues, and liver and spleen enlargement may occur. Laboratory abnormalities include progressively worsening anemia, leukopenia, and thrombocytopenia; disseminated intravascular coagulopathy also occurs commonly. The chest radiograph may be normal.[118] *Histoplasma* antibody assays are usually negative, and the diagnosis can be confirmed most easily by histoplasmal antigen assay of urine or serum. Another common symptom complex consists of respiratory complaints and tachypnea. In these instances, fever is present and followed in several days by dyspnea. The chest radiograph, though occasionally normal at the onset of symptoms, demonstrates diffuse interstitial infiltrates that progressively worsen. Hypoxemia usually accompanies the symptoms and also is progressive. The clinical findings are not specific for histoplasmosis and are identical to those caused by *Pneumocystis carinii,* cytomegalovirus, various viral respiratory pathogens, other opportunistic fungi, and bacterial septicemia.[104] The diagnosis may be made noninvasively with the urine antigen assay; if negative, lung biopsy is the most sensitive and specific diagnostic method and may provide important information about other potential etiologies. Examination of bronchoalveolar lavage fluid for histoplasmal antigen is useful in adults but has not been studied adequately in children. Treatment with antifungal agents is needed for immunocompromised children with PDH (see Table 204–3). Outcome has been excellent, with survival of all 29 children given amphotericin B; 3 children who relapsed responded to re-treatment.[118]

A subacute form of PDH is seen primarily in adults, although in one report of 19 cases, it was found in seven infants and one child.[96] The principal clinical features that distinguish the subacute from the acute form of PDH are more prolonged symptoms at initial evaluation, a higher frequency of focal lesions, and less pronounced fever and fewer hematologic abnormalities in subacute infection. Early complaints are nonspecific and may be present for 1 to 6 months; fever, malaise, and weight loss occur frequently. Hepatosplenomegaly is seen almost uniformly, and intestinal ulceration, sometimes with perforation, occurs commonly. The terminal ileum often is involved.[33] Oropharyngeal ulcerations occur and are large and deep and can mimic neoplasms.[96] Seventy-five percent of patients demonstrate adrenal involvement, sometimes unilateral[257]; adrenal insufficiency occurs less commonly but is reported in 15 percent of adults.[96, 100, 247] CNS infections are seen occasionally and may be manifested as chronic meningitis, focal mass lesions, or focal areas of cerebritis. Endovascular infections occur and may involve abnormal or normal native valves, most commonly the aortic or mitral valves or prosthetic valves.[3, 41, 89] Cardiac disease generally is typical of fungal endocarditis, with large valvular vegetations and a high rate of embolic phenomena.[89] Vaginal and penile ulcers, soft tissue nodules, recurrent panniculitis, carpal tunnel syndrome, osteomyelitis and arthritis, enteropathies, immune hemolytic anemia, and epididymitis all have occurred.[124, 129, 136, 196, 212, 224, 243, 253, 282] Although the progression of subacute PDH is slower than that seen in acute PDH, it is a progressive infection that is fatal in 2 to 24 months if untreated.[96]

*See references 78, 117, 128, 163, 179, 180, 216, 261, 283, 284, 313.

Chronic disseminated histoplasmosis is seen almost exclusively in adults.[96] Oropharyngeal ulcers are accompanied by chronic, mild, intermittent constitutional symptoms. A chronic relapsing disseminated form of the disease has been described in two younger patients, 9 and 20 years of age, with chronic mucocutaneous candidiasis.[78, 202]

PROGRESSIVE DISSEMINATED HISTOPLASMOSIS IN HIV-INFECTED PATIENTS. Histoplasmosis is an AIDS-defining opportunistic infection[36] and commonly occurs in HIV-infected persons residing in endemic areas. Disseminated infection develops in more than 90 percent of HIV-infected adults with histoplasmosis.[294] In 1988, less than 0.5 percent of adult patients with AIDS had disseminated disease.[98] In endemic areas, it has been reported in approximately 5 percent of patients[108, 166, 171] and in as many as 21 to 53 percent during epidemic periods.[20, 294, 312, 313] In a multivariate analysis of risk factors for the development of histoplasmosis in HIV-infected adults residing in endemic areas, receipt of antiretroviral therapy and triazole drugs was independently associated with decreased risk[109, 172]; one study found the risk to be increased with positive baseline serology, $CD4^+$ cell counts below 150/µL, and exposure to chicken coops.[171] Comparable studies have not been performed in children. In Arkansas, a highly endemic area, histoplasmosis was the AIDS-defining illness in 8 percent of 40 children who acquired HIV in the perinatal period.[237] Histoplasmosis occasionally is seen in nonendemic regions, perhaps because of reactivation of quiescent foci of infection.[228, 229]

In HIV-infected adults with disseminated histoplasmosis, symptoms are often nonspecific; prolonged unexplained fever and weight loss are seen almost uniformly, and respiratory complaints occur in about half of patients.[229, 294] Gastrointestinal symptoms are reported commonly and are usually nonspecific; abdominal pain, weight loss, and diarrhea occur in 50 to 70 percent of patients.[107, 110, 145, 254] Liver and spleen enlargement is found in approximately 25 percent. Ten percent of patients are initially gravely ill with signs of a septic shock–like syndrome.[294] Clinical and laboratory abnormalities associated with shock, respiratory failure, or death have been reported.[291] Mucocutaneous lesions occur in approximately 10 percent of adult patients and include nonspecific maculopapular rash, papules, nodules, pustules, ulcerative lesions, acneiform lesions, mucosal ulcers, and vegetative plaques[105]; histopathologic examination of skin biopsy specimens is often diagnostic. CNS involvement, including meningitis, encephalitis, and focal brain lesions, occurs in approximately 18 percent of patients.[11, 12, 20, 121, 165, 229, 289] Symptoms include headache, encephalopathy, or complaints arising from focal neurologic abnormalities.[289] Published reports of histoplasmosis complicating HIV infection in children are few; in four HIV-infected children in Indiana, fever was present in all and cutaneous lesions were absent; hepatosplenomegaly was found in one, and an abdominal mass caused by an infected abdominal lymph node was seen in one. In adults, initial chest radiographs are normal in approximately 40 percent and show diffuse interstitial or reticulonodular infiltrates in about 50 percent and localized lesions in approximately 5 percent. Diffuse abnormalities commonly appear during treatment of individuals whose chest radiographs initially were normal.[229]

CENTRAL NERVOUS SYSTEM INFECTION. CNS manifestations occur in 10 to 20 percent of adults with disseminated histoplasmosis, but they also may occur as chronic meningitis without any other manifestations of dissemination.[226, 231, 247, 289] Meningitis occurs in 60 percent of CNS infections; single or multiple mass lesions affecting the brain or spinal cord and encephalitis account for the balance of infections. Symptoms of meningitis are usually present 1 to 6 months before diagnosis, but they have been reported to be present for 7 years.[90] Symptoms include headache, decreased level of consciousness, confusion, and cranial nerve deficits in 28 to 56 percent of cases.[289] Diagnosis is most problematic in patients with meningitis but without disseminated infection. It is suspected ante mortem in only 40 percent of cases; symptoms and findings mimic those caused by other granulomatous infections, sarcoidosis,[289] cerebral vasculitis,[251] or neoplasms.[125] The diagnosis is confirmed either by isolating *H. capsulatum* from cerebrospinal fluid (CSF), detecting histoplasmal antigen or antibody in CSF, or identifying the organism in non-CNS sites. CSF findings are nonspecific and include mild pleocytosis, elevated protein, and depressed glucose. CNS infection in children usually is reported in association with dissemination[236, 240]; meningitis was found in 62 percent of cases of PDH of infancy in one series.[192] A chronic, progressive infection of the CNS has been reported in a child.[222] Other reports describe isolated meningitis with focal neurologic abnormalities occurring after an acute respiratory illness,[16] cerebellar ataxia that was diagnosed only presumptively as histoplasmosis,[241] and cerebellar and medullar lesions.[278] One child with a symptom complex of cervical lymphadenopathy, CSF pleocytosis, arthritis, and interstitial nephritis has been described.[282]

PRESUMED OCULAR HISTOPLASMOSIS SYNDROME. The entity termed presumed ocular histoplasmosis syndrome consists of a triad of findings, including discrete atrophic choroidal scars in the macula or midperiphery (histo spots), peripapillary atrophy, and choroidal neovascularization that can lead to loss of central vision.[43, 232] The peripapillary atrophy occurs in the absence of inflammatory changes in the vitreous or anterior chambers. Presumed ocular histoplasmosis primarily affects histoplasmin skin test–positive adults who reside in endemic areas. Because the clinical syndrome also occurs in individuals residing in nonendemic regions,[195, 256, 280] a cause-effect relationship with *H. capsulatum* has not been established firmly. Presumed ocular histoplasmosis does not appear to occur in children younger than 10 years, although among patients included in a review of the operative management of this entity were 11 children from 12 to 18 years old and one 7-year-old.[268]

ILLNESS CAUSED BY INFECTION WITH *HISTOPLASMA CAPSULATUM* VARIETY *DUBOISII*

In patients infected with *Histoplasma capsulatum* variety *duboisii,* focal lesions are seen more commonly in bones (usually the femur, ribs, or skull) and skin (cutaneous or subcutaneous). The lungs, gastrointestinal tract, liver, spleen, and lymph nodes rarely are involved. A progressive disseminated form of infection with *H. capsulatum* variety *duboisii* occurs and is associated with pyogranulomatous inflammation involving multiple organs.[47, 162, 319]

RADIOGRAPHIC FINDINGS

The radiographic findings seen most commonly in patients with histoplasmosis are not pathognomonic[137] and may mimic those seen in other granulomatous processes and, in some cases, neoplastic conditions, especially lymphoma. After small or moderate degrees of fungal exposure, the plain chest radiograph is normal in approximately 75 percent of skin test converters.[317] Computed tomography (CT) is more sensitive and likely to reveal parenchymal infiltrates that are not seen on plain radiography. The most common pulmonary parenchymal changes are "soft" interstitial infiltrates 2 to 15 mm in diameter, often found in the basilar portions of the lungs (Fig. 204–2). They may either fully resolve or consolidate into granulomata that persist, with or without calcification, as common findings in residents or visitors to endemic areas.[194]

The appearance of enlarged hilar/mediastinal nodes, either in association with pulmonary infiltrates or as isolated findings, is also a common radiographic finding of acute pulmonary infection. With CT, low-signal intensity within nodes sometimes is demonstrated, although frank suppuration is unusual. Infected nodes may enlarge sufficiently to compress or obstruct adjacent mediastinal structures. Nodes usually have reached their peak at the time of diagnosis and decrease in size or return to normal in several months; calcification may, but does not consistently, occur. In infants and young children, clusters of small infiltrates occasionally coalesce into a larger bronchopneumonic lesion.[94] Although small pleural effusions are present in 10 percent of adults with acute histoplasmosis,[311] they occur infrequently in children.[213, 267] Isolated calcifications may be seen in the spleen or liver (or both) months to years after infection. They result from the self-limited fungal dissemination that takes place during primary infection and often are appreciated as incidental findings in individuals who have lived in endemic regions.

After intense fungal exposure, three distinct chest radiographic patterns have been described.[94] Individuals from nonendemic areas initially may have scattered infiltrates that later evolve into "buckshot" calcifications. The second and most common pattern is the presence of smaller, nodular lesions as shown in Figure 204–3. This form is seen in individuals from endemic and nonendemic areas. Finally, a diffuse miliary pattern may occur, often in a patient with protective immunity.

In PDH, the chest radiograph may show abnormalities in only 25 to 50 percent of patients. In immunocompromised children, diffuse interstitial infiltrates are the most common radiographic findings; they worsen rapidly and in concert with progressive hypoxia, especially in patients with HIV infection or those receiving immunosuppressive therapy. The presence of interstitial infiltrates at admission has been reported in 62 percent of children with PDH of infancy[192] in a Costa Rican series, but chest radiographs were uniformly normal in a series of Indiana patients (M. Kleiman, unpublished data). Abdominal sonography or CT, or both, may show evidence of adrenal enlargement in chronic disseminated disease in adults.[160, 322]

Fibrosing mediastinitis caused by histoplasmosis is seen radiographically as pronounced thickening of the mediastinum that often compresses or obstructs the superior

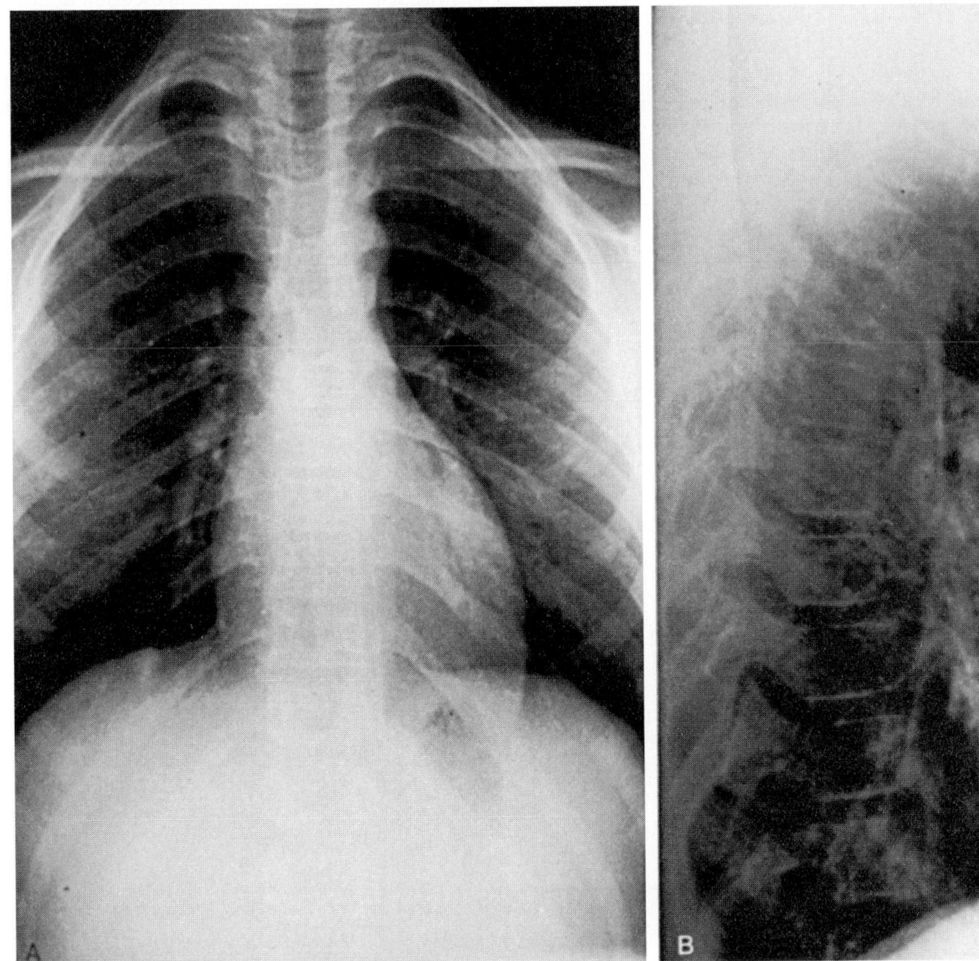

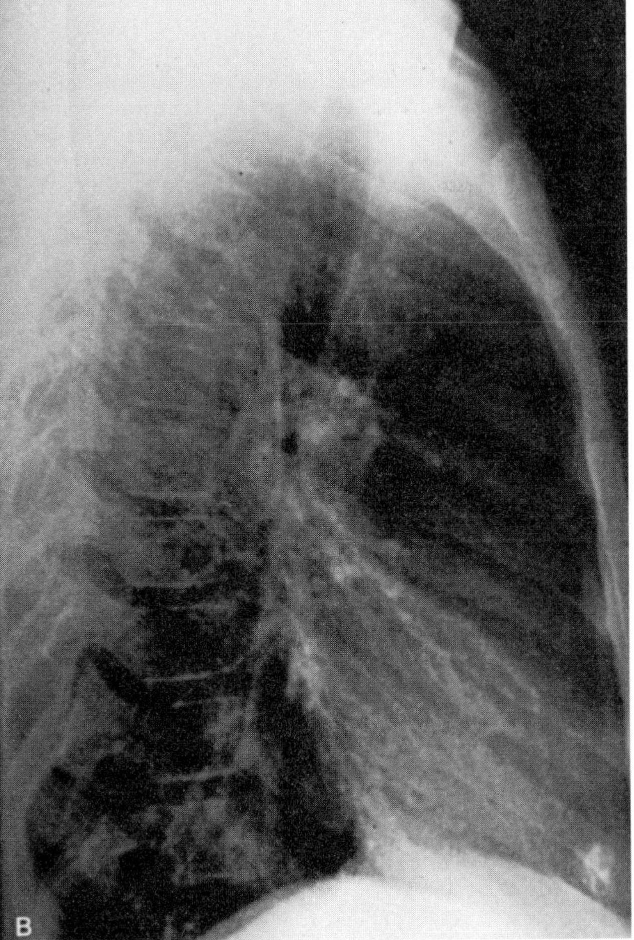

FIGURE 204–2 ■ Chest radiograph of an asymptomatic boy showing in the right lower lobe a calcification overlying the diaphragm between ribs 10 and 11 in the posteroanterior view *(A)* and overlying the apex of the heart in the lateral view *(B)*. These films also demonstrated punctate calcifications overlying the spleen and right axilla (not shown).

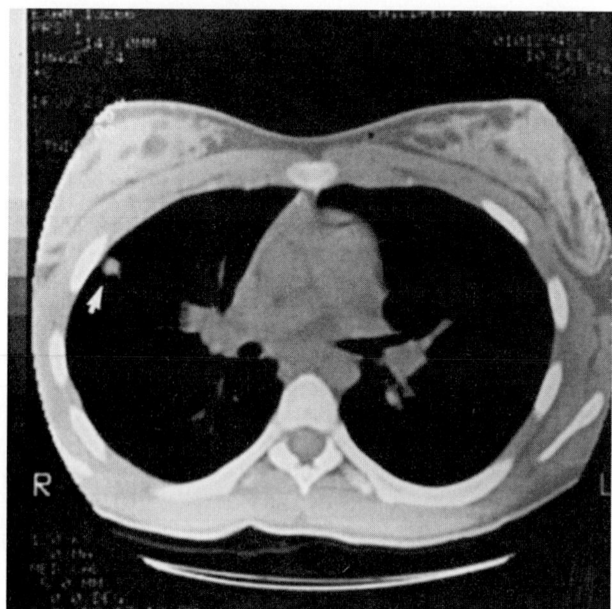

FIGURE 204–3 ■ Computed tomographic view of the chest of a teenage girl from Tennessee complaining of right arm pain when swimming. A nodular density is seen in the periphery of the right lung field *(arrow),* and the right hilum is enlarged slightly. Serologic tests and needle biopsy of the lesion were nondiagnostic, but excisional biopsy showed necrotizing granulomata with numerous histoplasmal yeast forms.

vena cava, major bronchi, esophagus, or other critical structures. It can be found in a localized pattern that frequently contains calcification, but it must be carefully differentiated from idiopathic fibrosis or non–infection-induced fibrosis, which may cause similar symptoms.[242] CT and magnetic resonance imaging (MRI) help differentiate active inflammation from fibrosis and aid in monitoring progression.[223, 225]

Diagnosis

Several laboratory tests play key roles in the diagnosis of histoplasmosis. Although each has value, their optimal use depends on an understanding of their differing sensitivities and specificities in various clinical settings. Table 204–2 provides general guidelines for their interpretation.

HISTOLOGIC DEMONSTRATION OF ORGANISMS

In clinical and epidemiologic settings compatible with histoplasmosis, observation of 2- to 4-μm typical yeast forms in histopathologic specimens is strong supportive evidence of histoplasmosis (Fig. 204–4). Care must be taken to differentiate *H. capsulatum* from the intracellular pathogens *Leishmania donovani* and *Toxoplasma gondii,* as well as small variants of *Blastomyces dermatitidis,* endospores and young spherules of *Coccidioides immitis, Penicillium marneffei,* and the yeast forms of *Cryptococcus neoformans.* Giemsa and hematoxylin and eosin stains demonstrate intracellular yeasts in sputum, blood smears, bone aspirates, and biopsy specimens. The Gomori methenamine silver stain is the most sensitive reagent and also has the advantage that calcification artifacts dissolve during the staining procedure[193]; its disadvantage is that it does not provide adequate cellular detail.

Although observation of yeast forms in specimens provides important diagnostic information, the disadvantage of this method is that it requires either a body fluid with a large fungal load or tissue that must be obtained by biopsy. The yield is excellent in disseminated forms of histoplasmosis,

TABLE 204–2 ■ INTERPRETIVE GUIDELINES FOR LABORATORY TESTS IN CHILDREN WITH ACUTE HISTOPLASMOSIS

Test	Result	Interpretation*	
		Normal Host	Immunocomprised Host
Complement-fixation antibody assay†	≤1:8	–	(–)
	1:16	+	+
	≥1:32	++	++
Immunodiffusion antibody assay†	M bands and H bands negative	–	(–)
	M present only	+	+
	H present only	++	++
	M and H present	++‡	++‡
Urine antigen	<5 U	(–)	(–)
	≥ 5 U	++§	++§
Histologic findings			
Node/mass	Negative	–	–
Infected organ	Granulomata, no yeast form	++	++
	Granulomata, yeast forms	+++	+++
Bone marrow/blood	No yeast forms	(–)	(–)
	Yeast forms seen	+++§	+++§
Culture any site	Negative	(–)	(–)
Any site	Positive	+++	+++
Bone marrow/blood	Positive	+++§	+++§

*(–), does not exclude infection; –, recent infection unlikely (≤5% probability); +, recent infection possible; ++, strongly suggestive of acute or recent infection; +++, confirms current infection.
†Seroconversion confirms acute/recent infection.
‡Progressive disseminated infection unlikely.
§Strongly suggestive of progressive disseminated infection or acute primary infection.
Excerpted from Long, S., Pickering, L. K., and Prober, C. G. (eds.): Principles and Practice of Pediatric Infectious Diseases. New York, Churchill Livingstone. 1997, p. 1347.

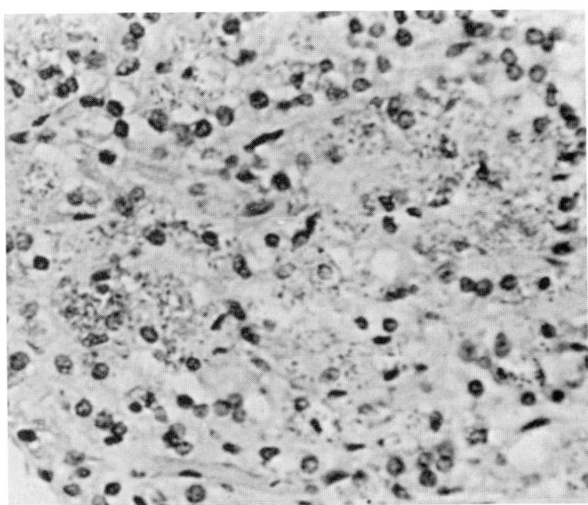

FIGURE 204–4 ■ Histoplasmosis of the adrenal gland illustrating the histiocytic response with numerous cells of *Histoplasma capsulatum* within the cytoplasm (hematoxylin and eosin, ×52).

in which yeasts are demonstrated easily in bone marrow, in tissue, and often in blood smears.[121] It is less sensitive in self-limited primary infections[320] because few organisms may be present in granulomata. The technique is usually unrewarding in patients with calcified and fibrotic lesions.[164, 166, 320] Limited experience exists with an immunoperoxidase *Histoplasma* antibody stain that can be used on tissue specimens.[138] In one study of patients with mediastinal fibrosis or mediastinal granuloma, antigen staining showed the presence of yeasts in 4 of 22 (18.2%) patients.[61] Sensitive and specific oligonucleotide probes for yeastlike fungi have been developed and hold promise for application to clinical specimens.[156]

CULTURE

Normally sterile specimens and minced or homogenized tissue can be inoculated onto suitable media such as brain-heart infusion agar, inhibitory mold agar, Sabourad's glucose (dextrose) agar (SGA), and enriched broth such as brain-heart infusion broth. The optimal method for recovery of *H. capsulatum* from blood is the lysis-centrifugation technique, which lyses white blood cells, inhibits complement, and prevents coagulation; after processing, the resulting concentrate is transferred to culture media. Specimens from nonsterile sites should be cultured on media that inhibit bacteria and saprophytic fungi; non–cycloheximide-containing media also should be used to permit the growth of other opportunistic pathogens.[147] Cultures are incubated aerobically at 25° to 30° C and held for at least 12 weeks before being considered negative. Most isolates grow in 3 to 4 weeks.[301] Use of the lysis-centrifugation system for blood culture has shortened the time for identification of a positive culture from approximately 16 days to 9 days.[19, 203] The fungus is recovered in its mycelial form, and confirmation of identification requires that it be converted to the yeast form, be shown to produce the H or M exoantigen, or react positively with a specific nucleic acid probe[251] (AccuProbe; Gen-Probe, Inc., San Diego, CA).

Recovery of *H. capsulatum* from a clinical specimen obtained from a symptomatic patient confirms the diagnosis of active histoplasmosis. The only exception is the infrequent event in which an incidental granuloma is found to be culture-positive but histoplasmosis is not a likely cause of the clinical symptoms. The sensitivity of culture depends heavily on the severity of the infection and the fungal burden. In primary acute, self-limited histoplasmosis, less than 15 percent of patients have a positive culture from any site. In contrast, cultures are positive in 82 to 90 percent of adults with PDH, including those who are immunocompetent or immunosuppressed or have HIV infection. In these patients, sites from which *H. capsulatum* commonly is recovered include the lower respiratory tract, blood, bone marrow, CSF, liver, spleen, skin lesions, and synovium.[9, 181] The highest yield in PDH is from bone marrow, which is positive in 75 percent of instances.[231, 284] Urine is positive in 40 to 70 percent and sputum in 60 percent.[247] In adults with PDH, rates of positive lysis-centrifugation cultures of peripheral blood are 90 to 100 percent in acute, 50 percent in subacute, and very rarely seen in chronic manifestations.[160] Radiometric mycobacterial broth blood cultures also may yield *H. capsulatum,* particularly in patients with AIDS.[178]

In forms of pulmonary histoplasmosis other than low-inoculum infection, sputum may be a reliable site for recovery of the organism in culture but not the best choice of diagnostic methods. High-inoculum infection after exposure to heavily contaminated sites usually results in moderate to severe infection in which patients seek medical attention within 2 weeks of inhaling spores. In these instances, the fungal burden is high, and respiratory secretions or lung tissue may demonstrate the organism, thus allowing prompt diagnosis; culture also may be positive, but the 2- to 4-week delay in achieving growth renders culture less desirable than other diagnostic methods, especially antigen detection. In adults with chronic cavitary pulmonary infection, sputum culture is positive in 50 to 85 percent of instances.[95, 288] The sensitivity of sputum culture may be increased with multiple sampling.[299] Cultures of extrapulmonary sites rarely are positive in chronic pulmonary disease.[315] Bronchoscopy with bronchoalveolar lavage may be helpful in patients with pulmonary disease. In a study of bronchoscopy in 71 adults, bronchoalveolar lavage was positive in only 4 percent of individuals with a single pulmonary nodule, but it increased to 55 percent in the remainder of the patient group. The highest yield of 88 percent (seven of eight) was in patients with infiltrates or cavitary disease.[213] Bronchoscopy did not appear to be helpful in evaluating patients with adenopathy, chronic pleural effusion, or bronchopleural fistulas. In children, culture plus staining of bronchoalveolar lavage fluid has been rewarding in diagnosing high–fungal burden infection in patients with HIV, but it is less sensitive than lung biopsy in other immunocompromised patients, especially those receiving chemotherapy for reticuloendothelial malignancy. In patients with mediastinal granuloma and fibrosis, cultures were positive in only 3.8 to 10 percent.[61, 161]

Cultures are usually negative in rheumatologic manifestations of histoplasmosis such as arthritis, erythema nodosum, erythema multiforme, and pericarditis because these manifestations generally occur months after low-burden infection in patients whose acquired cellular immune response has controlled fungal replication. CNS infection is an uncommon finding in children, although it was reported to occur in 62 percent of 40 cases in one series of PDH of infancy, and yeasts were observed in the CSF of 5 patients.[192] Recognizing CNS infection in adults is difficult unless concurrent dissemination, which occurs in approximately 20 to 40 percent of cases, is present.[288, 289] Invasive procedures sometimes are needed to confirm the diagnosis. Culture is positive in 20 to 60 percent of CSF specimens and in 50 percent of cultures obtained from other sites in adults.[288] Because the number of organisms in CSF is small, the yield of culture is improved substantially by using large volumes (10 to 20 mL in adults) on at least two occasions.

ANTIBODY AND ANTIGEN DETECTION

The serologic methods that are used most commonly for the diagnosis of histoplasmosis are immunodiffusion (ID) and CF. Each has equal sensitivity (75–85%); however, ID is slightly more specific (>95% versus 85–90%).[284, 285] In immunocompetent patients, either or both tests are positive in 95 percent of patients with acute primary pulmonary infection. CF titers often become positive 2 to 4 weeks earlier, usually by 4 to 6 weeks after infection.[284] In patients with CF antibody, 25 percent have a negative ID result; only 1 percent of those reactive by ID are CF-negative.[52] However, when the ID test is reactive, it remains positive longer after the symptoms have resolved than CF does. An extremely important limitation of both serologic assays is their reduced sensitivity in immunosuppressed patients; only 50 percent of immunosuppressed children and adults with disseminated histoplasmosis are seropositive.[53, 118]

Cross-reactivity with other fungal antigens affects both CF and ID assays. It occurs most commonly with blastomycosis, coccidioidomycosis, and paracoccidioidomycosis,[301] but cross-reactions also occur with candidiasis, tuberculosis, aspergillosis, and cryptococcosis.[164, 301] Cross-reactions with blastomycosis are especially common findings in the histoplasmosis CF assay, in which titers of 1:8 to 1:16 frequently are observed[132]; comparison of results of a single serum sample performed in the same assay often reveals CF antibody concentrations to be higher for the homologous infection. In these instances, ID tests are sometimes corroborative because the blastomycosis ID method is more specific and less likely to cross-react in histoplasmosis. However, ID has been noted to show false positivity in 25 to 50 percent of other fungal infections.[301] Cross-reactivity also is seen occasionally in patients with chronic cavitary tuberculosis, although simultaneous infection with tuberculosis and fungal pathogens can occur.[83] Variability in the specificity of commercial reagents has been reported to cause false-negative results.[152]

Complement Fixation

CF uses sensitized sheep red blood cells, killed whole *H. capsulatum* yeast cells, and histoplasmin, a soluble mycelium-form filtrate antigen.[180] After exposure in acute primary pulmonary histoplasmosis, the titer becomes positive in as many as 6 percent of individuals at 3 weeks, 73 percent at 4 weeks, and 77 percent at 6 weeks.[52, 301] With resolution of infection, titers decrease to 1:8 to 1:16 within 4 to 6 months and become undetectable (less than 1:8) by 9 months in most instances. Reported sensitivities for a single titer vary from 70 to 95 percent and depend on the threshold for considering a result positive. Single titers of 1:32 performed by an experienced laboratory are strong supportive evidence of acute or recent infection, especially when the accompanying clinical symptoms are compatible. One report[263] showed that 12 of 28 patients with non-*Histoplasma* febrile pneumonia had falsely positive CF titers of 1:32 or greater, so other laboratory and clinical data need to be considered. The presence of a fourfold rise between acute and convalescent sera is the best serologic evidence of recent infection. Both the individual yeast (CF-Y) and mycelial (CF-M) phases can be measured. CF-Y is more sensitive than CF-M for recent or active infection. In a series of 11 children with acute pulmonary histoplasmosis, CF-Y was 1:32 or greater in 9, but CF-M was 1:32 or greater in only 3 children.[325] In endemic regions, background low-titer CF serologic reactions may be present in 5 to 15 percent of adults,[283] but they have been reported to occur in as many as 30 percent.[91, 94, 160, 302]

The serologic response appears to correlate with the severity of disease in immunocompetent individuals with acute infection.[283] In an outbreak of histoplasmosis, seropositivity was 90 to 100 percent in severe acute histoplasmosis, 86 percent in moderate, 75 percent in mild, and 18 percent in asymptomatic infections.[148] Twenty-five percent of patients with acute histoplasmosis have CF titers that could be termed borderline positive, between 1:8 and 1:16.[52] Although they may result from previous infection, these titers should not be disregarded if clinical symptoms are suggestive of acute infection. In adults with chronic pulmonary histoplasmosis, the CF titer is greater than 1:32 in almost all patients.[127] In children with mediastinal masses caused by histoplasmosis, 67 percent have CF titers of 1:32 or greater.[84] Serologic responses do not differ sufficiently to use them as criteria for therapeutic decisions.[302]

The serologic diagnosis of meningitis caused by *H. capsulatum* often is problematic. Both CF and ID can be positive in CSF, but as many as half of patients with other chronic fungal meningeal infections may show falsely positive results.[210, 300] CF-M antibody appears to be the most sensitive and specific test for the diagnosis of meningitis caused by histoplasmosis. In one study, no false-positive CSF CF-M titers occurred in patients with cryptococcal meningitis, but CF-Y was falsely positive in 5 of 18 patients.[300] Individuals with fibrosing mediastinitis or mediastinal granuloma generally have negative or very low levels of CF antibody.[283]

Immunodiffusion

The micro-ID method[131] detects precipitins (reported as bands) against the H and M glycoprotein antigens of *H. capsulatum*.[180, 302] The M band is present in 25 percent of infections by the fourth week of infection and in 50 to 86 percent by the sixth week.[15, 52, 207] It can persist for 18 to 36 months after recovery but eventually becomes nonreactive. In endemic areas, in which serologic surveys show that 24 percent of healthy adult blood donors have CF-Y titers of 1:8 or 1:16, ID serology is positive in less than 1 percent.[91] Because it is more specific, ID can be of value to confirm the diagnosis of histoplasmosis in patients with *Histoplasma* CF titers in the borderline 1:8 to 1:16 range.[279]

The H band is present infrequently in patients with histoplasmosis; when seen, it is transient and its presence is suggestive of active infection.[94] In patients with active pulmonary histoplasmosis, between half and three fourths have an M band alone. The H band is present in only 10 to 20 percent of acute infections,[9, 99, 132, 302] and only 10 percent of individuals have both M and H bands present.[9] The latter finding is highly suggestive of active histoplasmosis.[131] The H band is detected less consistently in children with histoplasmosis.[282] In adults with disseminated disease, both bands are present in 25 percent of individuals.[9] The M band has been detected in 52 and 57 percent of patients with chronic pulmonary and disseminated disease, respectively.[99]

Antibody Detection by Radioimmunoassay and Enzyme Immunoassay

Antibody detection methods that use radioimmunoassay (RIA) and enzyme immunoassay have been developed. They can detect antibody slightly earlier than possible with ID and CF, can detect antibody to histoplasmin and yeast antigens, and can measure IgG- and IgM-specific histoplasmal antibodies.[52, 144, 207, 302, 305, 335] The disadvantages of cross-reactivity,[301] complexity and cost of the methodology, poor reproducibility, and negligible clinically relevant superiority over standard serologic methods have restricted their commercial availability. Neither RIA nor enzyme immunoassay is recommended for diagnosis.

Antigen Detection

The semiquantitative histoplasmal antigen assay fills an important gap in laboratory diagnosis. When performed on serum, urine, or other selected body fluids, it provides rapid diagnostic information for the most serious manifestations of disease, especially in immunocompromised patients, in whom serologic methods are often negative.[306] Although antigen assay has been studied almost exclusively in adults, it also provides important diagnostic information in childhood infections.

Antigen detection is most sensitive in manifestations that are associated with high fungal burdens, especially in immunosuppressed patients, in whom antibody responses occur in less than 50 percent. It is also useful in primary infection before cellular immunity has cleared the hematogenous dissemination and seroconversion has occurred. In addition to its use as a diagnostic test, antigen assay also provides a measure of the adequacy of response to therapy and, after treatment, a convenient laboratory monitor that can predict relapse in patients who are at high risk for recurrence.[293, 295–297] Measurement of antigen was developed with the use of RIA technology, but an enzyme-linked immunoassay yields rapid and reliable results[70]; an inhibition assay is less precise in the lower end of the detection range.[87]

The sensitivity of antigen detection in urine specimens is high in patients with acute primary pulmonary infection. The range of sensitivity is 25 to 75 percent, with the highest rates occurring in those seen within a few weeks of exposure and in patients with heavy fungal inhalation and extensive pulmonary involvement.[288, 320] Other pulmonary manifestations such as subacute and chronic cavitary infection in adults have lower fungal burdens and are positive in only 25 percent and 10 percent, respectively. The sensitivity of antigen detection is very high in progressive forms of histoplasmosis. In adults with disseminated histoplasmosis, antigen is found in blood or urine, or in both, in 82 percent of immunosuppressed and non-immunosuppressed patients and in 95 percent of patients with AIDS.[288] In 22 children with PDH, urinary antigen testing was positive in 100 percent.[79] From 1991 through 2001 at Riley Hospital for Children in Indianapolis, urine antigen testing was positive in all instances of disseminated histoplasmosis (M. Kleiman, unpublished data).

Although histoplasmal antigen may be detected in serum, the sensitivity is less than that of urine. Of immunosuppressed adult patients with disseminated histoplasmosis, antigen was found in 50 percent of serum samples and 92 percent of urine specimens. Similarly, in patients with disseminated histoplasmosis complicating AIDS, antigenuria was seen in 95 percent versus 85 percent in serum.[306, 320] Antigen often is found in the bronchoalveolar lavage fluid of patients after intense exposure and in immunocompromised patients with hematogenous dissemination and lung involvement.[294, 298] In adults with isolated meningitis, antigen detection in CSF may be the sole basis for confirming the diagnosis.[302, 307] The range of antigen positivity in all cases of meningitis is 40 to 66 percent; the highest rates are found in severe infections with heavy fungal burdens, especially those that occur in immunosuppressed patients. In patients with clinical findings suggestive of meningitis but in whom antigen is not present in CSF, antigen found in extrameningeal sites sometimes can confirm the diagnosis.

Antigen levels in blood or urine decline during treatment and should clear completely in infections that are treated adequately.[304] Conversely, the persistence of moderate antigenuria has been associated with a risk of recrudescence. This risk has been demonstrated best in patients with AIDS and histoplasmosis, in whom significant antigenuria often persists after cessation of therapy.[295, 296, 309] Monitoring urine antigen in such patients has shown that increasing urine antigen concentrations foretell recurrence.[295] However, the sensitivity of the antigen assay is high, and the pattern of antigen clearance has not been established firmly in other clinical settings. For example, infants with PDH who have been treated adequately have had a good clinical response, and those in whom urine antigen levels have substantially decreased during therapy often have persistence of low levels of urine antigen after completion of amphotericin B therapy. In these infants, no relapse has been observed after treatment with a total dose of 30 mg/kg of amphotericin B (M. Kleiman, unpublished data). Residual excretion of urine antigen continues to decrease and eventually ceases; monitoring is recommended to confirm resolution.[79] To demonstrate significant changes in concentration, specimens should be collected at intervals of at least 2 weeks; monitoring of urine samples for recurrence should be performed at 3- to 6-month intervals and at times of suspected relapse.

Cross-reactions in the histoplasmal antigen assay occur in paracoccidioidomycosis, African histoplasmosis, blastomycosis, and infections caused by *P. marneffei.*[316] Because these infections have distinguishing epidemiologic and clinical features and supportive diagnostic tests may further aid in differentiating them from histoplasmosis, cross-reactions usually create little disadvantage in interpretation of positive test results. Furthermore, treatment is similar for these endemic mycoses, so appropriate therapy may be given while confirmatory data are sought. Blood, urine, bronchoalveolar lavage fluid, and CSF are specimens that yield reliable results in the antigen assay. False-positive results may occur with pleural fluid and other high-protein–containing body fluids such as peritoneal, synovial, and pericardial fluid; these fluids and tissue specimens are not suitable specimens. The test is commercially available at the Histoplasmosis Reference Laboratory, Indianapolis, IN (1-800-HISTODGN).

SKIN TESTING

A skin test for histoplasmosis has been a valuable epidemiologic and investigational tool but has little diagnostic usefulness[94]; it is no longer commercially available. Skin testing is performed with standardized histoplasmin antigen prepared from mycelial-phase culture filtrate. After intradermal administration, an area of induration of 5 mm or larger at 48 hours is considered positive.[180] Skin test reactivity usually develops within 2 to 4 weeks after infection.[81] In chronic pulmonary disease, including cavitary disease, the skin test is positive in three fourths of patients.[81] In contrast, individuals with disseminated disease seldom have positive results.[10] Eighty percent of children who are older than 12 years and reside in an endemic area may be reactive.[283] Cutaneous reactivity may diminish, wax, or wane with re-exposure,[94, 283, 329] but it usually persists indefinitely in most individuals. The problem of serologic boosting by skin testing also has limited its diagnostic use.[9, 10, 26, 115, 130, 133, 180] Cross-reactions occur in patients with blastomycosis and coccidioidomycosis.[71–73]

MOLECULAR METHODS

Molecular methods designed to detect *H. capsulatum* in clinical samples are not available.[41] Epidemiologic studies have used restriction fragment length polymorphisms of DNA. Nucleic acid–based and genome-wide approaches have been used to explore the genetic diversity of the pathogen.[134, 277] Molecular methods also have been used to examine strains recovered from patients who have failed therapy[308] and to identify relatedness in isolates recovered after organ transplantation.[155]

Treatment

A substantial majority of individuals with histoplasmosis recover without treatment and do not require specific antifungal therapy.[94] Bed rest often is recommended for symptomatic acute histoplasmosis.[116] Treatment almost always is required for patients with severe illness or evidence suggestive of progressive dissemination. Consensus practice guidelines have been developed for adults and were based on controlled trials in patients with disseminated infection and those with chronic pulmonary infection; descriptive studies of other manifestations of histoplasmosis, as well as the clinical experience of experts, were also considered. No controlled therapeutic trials have been conducted in children, and the entities of chronic pulmonary infection and subacute and chronic dissemination syndromes rarely occur in children. Table 204–3 summarizes recommendations for treating the clinical manifestations of histoplasmosis seen most frequently in children. They have been derived from clinical experience, the few available descriptive reports, and results of adult data. Surgical management of histoplasmosis rarely is indicated.

MEDICAL MANAGEMENT FOR MANIFESTATIONS REQUIRING ANTIFUNGAL THERAPY

Because most patients with light or moderate exposure to fungal spores recover without treatment, the first decision is to determine whether to carefully observe the patient or to begin administering an antifungal agent. The two criteria that are key to making this decision are clinical assessment of the severity or duration of the symptoms (or both) and an assessment of the adequacy of the patient's cellular immunity. Once treatment with antifungals has been elected, a regimen is selected that is appropriate for the initial findings. Manifestations of histoplasmosis in children that most often require antifungal treatment are severe or protracted symptoms resulting from acute primary pulmonary infection, mediastinal granuloma that is causing compression of adjacent structures, disseminated infection, and active infection in immunocompromised hosts.[255]

Amphotericin B and itraconazole are the antifungal agents that play primary roles in medical management. Amphotericin B is fungicidal for *H. capsulatum,* whereas itraconazole is fungistatic. Based largely on the results of its superiority in animal studies[48] and its faster clearance of fungemia in patients with AIDS,[123] amphotericin B is more effective for severe disease than itraconazole is.[303] Amphotericin B is used most commonly as "induction" therapy, and after substantial improvement has occurred, it is stopped and itraconazole then is used to complete treatment. Itraconazole is preferred for the treatment of patients who have mild or moderate symptoms. In addition to regimens that are used to treat acute infections, suppressive (secondary prophylactic) regimens are used for patients with AIDS because they have a high risk of recurrence when treatment is stopped.[294] Finally, primary prophylactic regimens have been developed for use by patients with AIDS who live in highly endemic areas.[172]

A detailed discussion of the antifungal agents used to treat histoplasmosis is found in Chapter 239. Amphotericin B generally is well tolerated and effective in children. Its lipid formulations, though less nephrotoxic, are substantially more expensive.[260] A comparative trial of amphotericin B deoxycholate and liposomal amphotericin B in adults with disseminated histoplasmosis and AIDS showed improved survival with the liposomal preparation.[123] If the newer formulations are used, doses should be adjusted. Both liposomal and standard amphotericin B formulations clear fungemia faster than itraconazole does.[292] If amphotericin B is used as monotherapy for severe or disseminated infection

TABLE 204–3 ■ SUMMARY OF TREATMENT RECOMMENDATIONS FOR CHILDREN WITH HISTOPLASMOSIS

	Treatment	
Manifestation	Severe Illness	Moderate of Mild Illness
Acute pulmonary	AmB,* then Itr for 12 wk	Symptoms <4 wk, none; persistent symptoms for >4 wk, Itr for 6–12 wk
Disseminated (non-HIV)	AmB,† or AmB followed by Itr for 6 mo	Itr for 6–8 mo‡ or same as for severe
Disseminated (with HIV)	AmB,†,§ or AmB followed by Itr	Itr, then Itr suppression for life
Meningitis	AmB for 3 mo, then Flu for 12 mo	Same as for severe because of poor outcome
Granulomatous mediastinitis	AmB, then Itr for 6 mo	Itr for 6 mo
Fibrosing mediastinitis	Itr for 3 mo‖	Same as for severe
Pericarditis	Pericardial drainage for severe tamponade + NSAID for 2–12 wk	NSAID for 2–12 wk
Rheumatologic	NSAID for 2–12 wk	Same as for severe
Compression of contiguous structures by granulomatous adenitis		Corticosteroids, concurrent Itr

*The effectiveness of concomitant corticosteroids is controversial.
†If amphotericin B is used for the entire course of treatment, 30 mg/kg should be given over a 4-week period.
‡Therapy should continue until *Histoplasma* antigen concentrations are less than 4 U in urine.
§Liposomal amphotericin B may be superior to amphotericin B deoxycholate in patients with HIV (see text).
‖Probably ineffective if fibrotic; when granulomatous mediastinitis could be present, it may be considered.
AmB, amphotericin B; Flu, fluconazole; Itr, itraconazole; NSAID, nonsteroidal anti-inflammatory drug.
Modified from Wheat, J., Sarosi, G., McKinsey, D., et al.: Practice guidelines for the management of patients with histoplasmosis. Clin. Infect. Dis. *30*:688–695, 2000.

in a normal or immunocompromised host, a total dose of at least 30 mg/kg administered for 4 to 6 weeks is recommended. Failures of 30 and 35 mg/kg total dose have been reported in PDH of infancy,[192] and because recurrences have been observed in immunosuppressed patients,[118] close follow-up, preferably with monitoring of urine antigen, is required after completion. When amphotericin B is used as induction therapy, it should be continued until substantial improvement in clinical and laboratory findings is achieved; in adults, improvement usually takes 3 to 10 days.[181] Success with shorter courses of therapy for PDH of infancy has been reported.[80, 151, 157] One such study reported cure in five infants[80] (only two with microbiologic confirmation and another in which PDH was highly probable) with an initial dose of 0.25 mg/kg, 0.5 mg/kg given on the second day, and 1 mg/kg/day administered for 7 to 11 days thereafter. Not enough data are available to recommend short courses of amphotericin B for treatment, and because of the availability of itraconazole, such treatment seldom is needed.

Itraconazole generally is well tolerated by children and, in adults, is more effective than the other azoles[76, 85, 111, 113, 184, 208, 248, 274]; trials with itraconazole have not been performed in children. Nonetheless, itraconazole is the azole of choice for the treatment of histoplasmosis when an oral agent is used. The erratic bioavailability of the capsule form can be improved when it is taken with liquids with low pH and caloric content. Coca-Cola Classic aids in absorption,[119] but serum levels should be monitored, particularly if symptoms persist. The liquid suspension of itraconazole is better absorbed but may have adverse gastrointestinal effects. As with the other azoles, important drug interactions need to be considered in patients receiving agents known to affect excretion of the azole or whose excretion is affected by the antifungal. The 90 percent minimal inhibitory concentration (MIC_{90}) of itraconazole for *H. capsulatum* is 0.02 µg/mL; the optimal therapeutic level has not been determined, but serum concentrations in excess of 1 µg/mL should be effective, and levels in excess of this amount are easily achieved, well tolerated, and effective.[112] Itraconazole is quite expensive.

Fluconazole was less effective than itraconazole in treating adults with chronic pulmonary histoplasmosis[170] or disseminated histoplasmosis.[308] It also has been associated with relapse in disseminated infection,[309] is less effective than itraconazole for secondary prophylaxis in adults with disseminated infection,[172] and clears fungemia more slowly in adults with disseminated infection than itraconazole does.[293] Fluconazole is recommended for use in patients who either do not tolerate itraconazole or fail to absorb it. When used, careful follow-up with urine antigen monitoring is needed to detect relapse. Because itraconazole does not enter the CSF easily, fluconazole may be considered in patients with CNS infection. However, the relationship between CSF concentrations and outcome has not been determined.[310] Antagonism is a concern when fluconazole is used in conjunction with amphotericin B for the treatment of meningitis.[153]

Ketoconazole is less well tolerated than either itraconazole or fluconazole.[23, 59, 114, 154, 266] It is reasonably effective in adults with chronic pulmonary infection[63, 154, 183, 244] and in those with disseminated infection, although relapse is a common occurrence.[181, 215] In histoplasmosis complicating AIDS, the response to ketoconazole was only 9 percent versus 74 to 88 percent with amphotericin B and 85 percent with itraconazole.[185, 271, 287]

PRIMARY PULMONARY INFECTION. Primary pulmonary histoplasmosis that occurs after intense exposure to spores may result in life-threatening illness with high fever, diffuse pulmonary infiltrates, hypoxemia, and the adult respiratory distress syndrome.[67, 94, 96, 181, 286, 310] Infection of this severity should be treated promptly, and induction with amphotericin B is recommended until substantial clinical improvement occurs. Thereafter, itraconazole should be continued for at least 3 months. In patients who may not appear as ill but in whom laboratory or clinical evidence is suggestive of progressive primary dissemination, empiric therapy should be initiated.

Patients without respiratory distress but in whom severe systemic complaints such as high fever, chills, mild chest pain, and weight loss persist for 2 to 4 weeks or longer are also candidates for antifungal therapy. In these instances, firm criteria have not been established to guide the timing of this decision, and treatment must be individualized. Still, as observed when amphotericin B was the only effective treatment and its toxicity and inconvenience resulted in deferring therapy for longer than currently practiced, a significant proportion of these symptoms could be expected to undergo spontaneous resolution. The convenience of oral antifungal agents renders the decision less problematic because these protracted, but mild to moderately severe symptoms may be treated with itraconazole. Itraconazole should be used for at least 6 weeks in these instances (see Table 204–3). No clinical studies have been conducted to show whether treatment shortens the duration of symptoms or prevents later complications.[181] Only anecdotal evidence indicates that corticosteroids are of benefit in treating patients with severe inhalation and adult respiratory distress syndrome.[101, 126, 262, 327]

MEDIASTINAL GRANULOMA. One of the most common initial complaints in children is mediastinal granuloma in which an infected node compresses or obstructs adjacent structures. Most often affected are bronchi and the trachea and, less commonly, the superior vena cava, esophagus,[182] and the phrenic or recurrent laryngeal nerves. Symptoms usually associated with airway compression are mild tachypnea, exertion with activity, asthma, and mild chest pain; the superior vena cava syndrome may accompany obstruction of the superior vena cava. Fever is an unusual occurrence unless secondary bacterial pneumonitis caused by obstruction is present. The illness is generally self-limited but may persist for several weeks. Although only anecdotal evidence supports the benefit of treatment, itraconazole may be helpful in patients with active inflammation. The presence of an elevated erythrocyte sedimentation rate and CF titer could be considered markers compatible with active inflammation. As also demonstrated in a study involving dogs with mediastinal granuloma,[235] adjunctive treatment with steroids is sometimes beneficial[101, 262] and, if effective, results in prompt improvement (M. Kleiman, unpublished data). If steroids are used, they should be given with an antifungal agent because of the risk of dissemination resulting from steroid-induced depression of cellular immunity. Itraconazole should be continued for 6 to 12 months. Although fibrosing mediastinitis is a late complication of histoplasmosis, no evidence has shown that mediastinal granuloma is its precursor and that antifungal therapy will prevent its occurrence.

DISSEMINATED INFECTION. Progressive disseminated infections in children occur in several settings, and all require antifungal therapy. Among immunocompetent children, they occur in infants younger than 1 year and, though very infrequently, in children at any age after intense exposure. In immunocompromised children, dissemination is seen most often in patients who are receiving immunosuppressive agents that impair the cellular immune system, in patients with AIDS, and rarely in patients with inherited disorders of cellular immunity. Table 204–3 reviews treatment recommendations.

Immunocompetent Patients and Immunosuppressed Patients without HIV Infection. The mortality rate of acute progressive disseminated histoplasmosis approaches 100 percent.[96, 151] In adults with acute, subacute, and chronic disseminated manifestations of histoplasmosis, the mortality rate without treatment is 80 percent[226]; therapy with antifungal agents reduces the rate to under 25 percent.[181] Treatment with amphotericin B results in survival of more than 90 percent of infants with PDH.[151, 192] In a report[117] describing 31 immunocompromised children with disseminated histoplasmosis, 19 of 20 recovered after receiving treatment with amphotericin B. Three experienced late recurrences that responded to re-treatment. One patient died after receiving only one dose. Four patients also responded to a 3- to 5-month course of ketoconazole, and three responded to sulfa regimens. All four untreated patients died. Little reported experience using itraconazole for the treatment of disseminated infection in children exists. Only one report has described the outcome of itraconazole monotherapy in children with disseminated histoplasmosis. Seven children 2 to 14 years of age were treated.[265] One died shortly after treatment was stopped at 1 month. "Marked improvement" was noted in patients treated for 3 months (four patients) and 6 months (one patient), and complete resolution was reported in one patient after 12 months of therapy with itraconazole. In spite of the paucity of published data in children, itraconazole is recommended, although initial induction with amphotericin B is used for severe infections. Itraconazole's recommendation is based largely on its demonstrated effectiveness in clinical trials in adults and its ease of administration and tolerability in children. Absorption should be confirmed and urine antigen monitored during therapy to ensure that the fungal burden is decreasing. If amphotericin B is elected as monotherapy, a total dose of 30 to 35 mg/kg over 4 weeks is recommended.

Disseminated Infection in Patients with AIDS. The severity of the initial signs of illness heavily influences the outcome and recommended treatment regimens for patients with disseminated histoplasmosis complicating HIV infection (see Table 204–3). Regimens are based on trials conducted in adults. Amphotericin B was effective in 74 to 88 percent of all cases,[287, 294] whereas patients treated for infections that were sufficiently severe to require hospitalization had a 50 percent mortality rate.[287] In those with moderate to severe disseminated histoplasmosis, liposomal amphotericin B provided a survival benefit in comparison to amphotericin B deoxycholate.[123] Patients with only mild or moderate symptoms were treated successfully with itraconazole monotherapy in 85 percent of instances.[303] Fungemia is cleared more rapidly by amphotericin B deoxycholate and liposomal amphotericin B than by itraconazole or fluconazole.[293]

Because of a high rate of recurrence of infection after cessation of therapy in patients with AIDS, chronic maintenance therapy (secondary prophylaxis) is needed.[122, 290, 294, 312] In adults, amphotericin B (50 mg weekly or biweekly) is effective in 81 to 97 percent,[169, 294] itraconazole in 90 percent,[112, 304] and fluconazole in 90 percent of those who were treated with amphotericin B induction.[191] Fluconazole was not as effective for secondary prophylaxis when it was used also as induction therapy; among the third of patients who experienced relapses, 50 percent of the isolates were resistant.[309] Itraconazole is the azole of choice for mildly or moderately ill patients, in whom it may be used as induction therapy and secondary prophylaxis. Fluconazole should be reserved for use as secondary prophylaxis only if patients received amphotericin B as induction therapy or if itraconazole is poorly tolerated or its high cost renders it unavailable. Whether withdrawal of secondary prophylaxis is appropriate when the patient's $CD4^+$ count increases above 150 while receiving retroviral therapy remains unclear. Primary prophylaxis with itraconazole is effective for patients with AIDS who live in highly endemic areas[172] and have absolute $CD4^+$ counts below 150; the selection of drug-resistant *Candida* is a potential disadvantage of this approach.

The antigen assay is a convenient and effective laboratory monitoring test that can be used during treatment and maintenance. In patients with HIV infection complicated by disseminated histoplasmosis, it can document reduction in fungal burden during induction and is predictive of clinical relapse if antigen levels rise during treatment.[191, 295] Although antigen levels become normal in successfully treated immunocompetent patients and in most whose immunosuppression is caused by etiologies other than AIDS, patients with HIV infection often continue to excrete antigen in urine. In this setting, monitoring of urine antigen should be performed at 3- to 6-month intervals. Levels should be measured when clinical or other laboratory data are suggestive of relapse.

CENTRAL NERVOUS SYSTEM INFECTION. CNS infections occur infrequently in children. In adults, manifestations include meningitis, focal infection of the brain or spinal cord, thrombotic events caused by focal vasculitis or emboli, and diffuse encephalitis. Mortality is almost uniformly invariable if untreated. Response rates are low; treatment is effective in only 20 to 40 percent of patients with meningitis, and 50 percent of responders relapse after cessation of treatment.[289] Amphotericin B at a total dose of 35 mg/kg administered for a 3- to 4-month period has been used most often to treat adults with meningitis. Although both amphotericin B deoxycholate and liposomal amphotericin B enter the CSF poorly,[68, 103, 150] liposomal amphotericin B reaches higher concentrations in brain tissue.[103] Comparative studies of these agents for the treatment of CNS infections caused by histoplasmosis have not been performed. Although fluconazole probably should not be used concurrently with amphotericin B because of its potential for antagonism,[153] its ability to enter CSF renders it more attractive than itraconazole for long-term treatment after induction therapy with amphotericin B. Serum concentrations of fluconazole should be monitored to ensure that they are optimal (80 to 150 μg/mL).[181] Focal cerebral or spinal cord lesions that are not associated with meningitis should be treated with liposomal amphotericin B induction; itraconazole may be used thereafter because achieving adequate CSF levels may not be needed for cure.[289]

MEDICAL MANAGEMENT OF MANIFESTATIONS THAT DO NOT REQUIRE ANTIFUNGAL THERAPY

Several common and uncommon manifestations of histoplasmosis do not require antifungal treatment. Apart from mild primary pulmonary infection, one of the most common is pericarditis. Because it is rarely associated with frank fungal infection of the pericardium, it often resolves spontaneously or with nonsteroidal anti-inflammatory agents. Indomethacin is often effective[328] in rapidly reducing inflammation, can reverse signs of impending tamponade, and is preferred. Steroids have been reported to be effective but, if used, should be accompanied by antifungal therapy. Rheumatologic symptoms of arthritis, with or without erythema multiforme or erythema nodosum, also respond to nonsteroidal anti-inflammatory agents.[239] Fibrosing mediastinitis is a late complication of histoplasmosis, but it occurs occasionally in children. Once granulomatous lesions evolve to become densely fibrotic, antifungal and anti-inflammatory therapy is ineffective. However, the clinical and laboratory criteria that are used to assess whether active inflammation is present are inexact, and a trial of antifungal therapy usually is warranted upon diagnosis. Treatment with antifungals is generally unsuccessful,[181] but improvement has been reported.[269]

Presumed ocular histoplasmosis is seen almost exclusively in adults and does not improve with antifungal therapy; its management has been extensively reviewed.[43]

SURGICAL

Operative intervention rarely is needed to manage patients with histoplasmosis. In a review of 94 patients 10 to 40 years of age, the most common reason for evaluation was obstruction of thoracic structures by mediastinal masses.[86] Seventy-five underwent surgery or endoscopy to relieve obstruction of the pulmonary artery, superior vena cava, bronchus, or esophagus. Recurrent pneumonia, tracheoesophageal fistula, hemoptysis, and broncholithiasis were other indications for surgical procedures.[86, 140, 330] Because attempts to completely excise caseous nodes sometimes can damage contiguous structures, the preferable approach is to incise and evacuate debris from such lesions and leave the adherent portion of the capsule intact.[77, 86, 205, 321]

Surgery has little place in the management of post-histoplasmosis fibrosing mediastinitis. The dense fibrous consolidation of mediastinal structures coupled with the hypervascularity of mediastinal tissues renders the risk for development of serious hemorrhage and other life-threatening surgical complications high[167]; excisional biopsy carries a prohibitive risk.[54] Once calcification has occurred in fibrosing mediastinitis, surgical repair is not feasible,[164] and the fibrosis continues after surgery. Some success has been achieved with relief of vascular obstruction by percutaneous placement of intravascular stents.[66] Prophylactic excision of large mediastinal nodes has not been shown to prevent fibrosis, and patients with large mediastinal lymph nodes who are otherwise asymptomatic rarely progress to mediastinal fibrosis.[283]

Prognosis

Histoplasmosis is either unrecognized or self-limited in the vast majority of individuals who sustain this most common of the endemic mycoses. Histoplasmosis results in serious illness in infants, immunocompromised patients, and older individuals, particularly those with emphysematous pulmonary disease.[22, 180] The cure rate for children who receive therapy for serious acute manifestations is high. Little prospective information is available about the long-term outcome in acute pulmonary histoplasmosis. A study that examined pulmonary function in six children and their parents after intense exposure found restrictive (three patients) and obstructive (two patients) patterns and a reduction in CO diffusing capacity in five of six tested. At 2 years, a diffusing capacity abnormality remained in three, and hypoxemia persisted in the most severely affected patient.[141] No data that can be used to predict the occurrence of long-term complications such as mediastinal fibrosis are available. When it does occur, mediastinal fibrosis is progressive and therapeutic options are few; because by definition mediastinal fibrosis invades the airways and pulmonary vasculature, its prognosis is influenced heavily by whether it affects one or both lungs.[54] The prognosis is poor in the latter instance. Although lifelong secondary prophylaxis is recommended for HIV-infected patients with histoplasmosis, ongoing clinical trials are examining the risk of recurrence in those who demonstrate immunologic reconstitution after effective antiretroviral therapy.

Prevention

Complete prevention of histoplasmosis is not possible currently, but reasonable precautions can greatly decrease the risk to individuals who are highly likely to suffer serious complications if they become infected. Individuals who reside in endemic regions (or planning travel to endemic areas) and have impaired cellular immunity caused by inherited disorders, immunosuppressive agents, or HIV infection should be counseled about the potentially serious consequences of infection. Counseling should include education about the sites likely to be contaminated with *H. capsulatum* and the activities that may potentially expose them to spores; primary prophylactic regimens using itraconazole may be considered for HIV-infected patients with exposure to soil mixed with bird or bat droppings[109] (see "Epidemiology"). If such activities are unavoidable, the use of National Institute for Occupational Safety and Health (NIOSH)-certified high-efficiency mask filtration devices[270] should be encouraged; however, devices appropriate for use by small children may not be available. Attempts to sterilize sites by formaldehyde spray[35, 270] have been made, but the toxicity of this agent renders its use undesirable and, in some settings, ineffective.[37] When potentially contaminated sites are disturbed, aerosols containing spores can be substantially reduced by thoroughly dampening the material with water before it is manipulated. Although education and counseling of high-risk patients affords some protection against acquiring infection from microfoci, some of which can result in intense exposure, it does not protect against "sporadic" infections. For the general population, education in endemic areas is also beneficial, particularly for protecting individuals whose occupational and recreational activities may expose them to *H. capsulatum*.

No vaccine for prevention of histoplasmosis exists, although active investigation is under way to identify potential vaccine targets[57, 323] in animal models. A recombinant protein vaccine has been made from cloned sequences of DNA coding for the cell wall glycoprotein heat shock protein 60, which has been found to be protective in mice against a lethal intravenous inoculum of *H. capsulatum*.[93] This vaccine protected mice in a model of pulmonary infection. In contrast to the failure of H antigen to protect mice against an intravenous challenge with yeasts, mice immunized with H antigen and challenged intranasally were protected at 1 month and had some limited protection 3 months after immunization.

REFERENCES

1. Ajello, L.: Distribution of *Histoplasma capsulatum* in the United States. *In* Histoplasmosis. Proceedings of the Second National Conference. Springfield, IL, Charles C Thomas, 1971.
2. Ajello, L., and Zeidberg, L. D.: Isolation of *Histoplasma capsulatum* and *Allescheria boydii* from soil. Science *113*:662, 1951.
3. Alexander, W. J., Mowry, R. W., Cobb, C. G., and Dismukes, W. E.: Prosthetic valve endocarditis caused by *Histoplasma capsulatum*. J. A. M. A. *242*:1399–1400, 1979.
4. Allendoerfer, R., Biovin, G. P., and Deepe, G. S., Jr.: Modulation of immune response in murine pulmonary histoplasmosis. J. Infect. Dis. *175*:905–914, 1997.
5. Allendorfer, R., Brunner, G. D., and Deepe, G. S., Jr.: Complex requirements for nascent and memory immunity in pulmonary histoplasmosis. J. Immunol. *162*:7389–7396, 1999.

6. Allendoerfer, R., and Deepe, G. S., Jr.: Intrapulmonary response to *Histoplasma capsulatum* in gamma interferon knockout mice. Infect. Immun. *65*:2564–2669, 1997.
7. Allendoerfer, R., and Deepe, G. S., Jr.: Blockade of endogenous TNF-alpha exacerbates primary and secondary pulmonary histoplasmosis by differential mechanisms. J. Immunol. *160*:6072–6082, 1998.
8. Allendoerfer, R., and Deepe, G. S., Jr.: Regulation of infection with *Histoplasma capsulatum* by TNFR1 and 2. J. Immunol. *165*:2657–2664, 2000.
9. American Thoracic Society: Medical Section of the American Lung Association: Laboratory diagnosis of mycotic and specific fungal infections. Am. Rev. Respir. Dis. *132*:1373–1379, 1985.
10. American Thoracic Society: Clinical usefulness of skin testing in histoplasmosis, coccidioidomycosis and blastomycosis. Am. Rev. Respir. Dis. *138*:1081–1082, 1988.
11. Anaissie, E., Fainstein, V., Samo, T., et al.: Central nervous system histoplasmosis. An unappreciated complication of the acquired immunodeficiency syndrome. Am. J. Med. *84*:215–217, 1988.
12. Anders, K. H., Guerra, W. F., Tomiyasu, U., et al.: The neuropathology of AIDS: UCLA experience and review. Am. J. Pathol. *124*:537–558, 1986.
13. Artz, R. P, and Bullock, W. E.: Immunoregulatory responses in experimental disseminated histoplasmosis: Depression of T-cell–dependent and T-cell–effector responses by activation of splenic suppressor cells. Infect. Immun. *23*:893–902, 1979.
14. Baughman, R. P., Kim, C. K., Vinegar, A., et al.: The pathogenesis of experimental pulmonary histoplasmosis: Correlative studies of histopathology, bronchoalveolar lavage, and respiratory function. Am. Rev. Respir. Dis. *134*:771–776, 1986.
15. Bauman, D. S., and Smith, C. D.: Comparison of immunodiffusion and complement fixation tests in the diagnosis of histoplasmosis. J. Clin. Microbiol. *2*:77–80, 1975.
16. Bellin, E. L., Silva, M., and Lawyer, T.: Central nervous system histoplasmosis in a Puerto Rican. Neurology *12*:148–152, 1962.
17. Bennish, M., Radkowski, M. A., and Rippon, J. W.: Cavitation in acute histoplasmosis. Chest *84*:496–497, 1983.
18. Bhagavan, B. S., Rao, D. R. G., and Weinberg, T.: Histoplasmosis producing broncholithiasis. Arch. Pathol. *91*:577–579, 1971.
19. Bille, J., Stockman, L., Roberts, G. D., et al.: Evaluation of a lysis-centrifugation system for recovery of yeasts and filamentous fungi from blood. J. Clin. Microbiol. *18*:469–471, 1983.
20. Bonner, J. R., Alexander, W. J., Dismukes, W. E., et al.: Disseminated histoplasmosis in patients with the acquired immune deficiency syndrome. Arch. Intern. Med. *144*:2178–2181, 1984.
21. Bower, R. J., and Kiesewetter, W. B.: Mediastinal masses in infants and children. Arch. Surg. *112*:1003–1009, 1977.
22. Bradsher, R. W., Alford, R. H., Hawkins, S. S., et al.: Conditions associated with relapse of amphotericin B–treated disseminated histoplasmosis. Johns Hopkins Med. J. *150*:127–131, 1982.
23. Brass, C., Galgiani, J. N., Blaschke, T. F., et al.: Disposition of ketoconazole, an oral antifungal, in humans. Antimicrob. Agents Chemother. *21*:151–158, 1982.
24. Brodskey, A. L., Gregg, M. B., Loewenstein, M. S., et al.: Outbreak of histoplasmosis associated with the 1970 Earth Day activities. Am. J. Med. *54*:333–342, 1973.
25. Brummer, E., Kurita, N., Yosihida, S., et al.: Fungistatic activity of human neutrophils against *Histoplasma capsulatum:* Correlation with phagocytosis. J. Infect. Dis. *164*:158–162, 1991.
26. Buechner, H. A., Seabury, J. H., Campbell, C. C., et al.: The current status of serologic, immunologic and skin tests in the diagnosis of pulmonary mycoses. Chest *63*:259, 1973.
27. Bullock, W. E., and Wright, S. D.: Role of the adherence-promoting receptors, CR3, LFA-1, and pl50,95 in binding of *Histoplasma capsulatum* by human macrophages. J. Exp. Med. *165*:195–210, 1987.
28. Butler, J. C., Heller, R., and Wright, P. F.: Histoplasmosis during childhood. South. Med. J. *87*:476–480, 1994.
29. Cain, J. A., and Deepe, G. S., Jr.: Evolution of the primary immune response to *Histoplasma capsulatum* in murine lung. Infect. Immun. *66*:1473–1481, 1998.
30. Cain, J. A., and Deepe, G. S., Jr.: Interleukin-12 neutralization alters lung inflammation and leukocyte expression of CD80, CD86, and major histocompatibility complex class II in mice infected with *Histoplasma capsulatum*. Infect. Immun. *68*:2069–2076, 2000.
31. Campbell, C. C., Hill, G. B., and Falgout, B. T.: *Histoplasma capsulatum* isolated from feather pillow associated with histoplasmosis in an infant. Science *136*:1050, 1962.
32. Cano, M. V. C., and Hajjeh, R. A: The epidemiology of histoplasmosis: A review. Semin. Respir. Dis. *16*:109–118, 2001.
33. Cappell, M. S., Mandell, W., Grimes, M. M., et al.: Gastrointestinal histoplasmosis. Dig. Dis. Sci. *33*:353–360, 1988.
34. Case records of the Massachusetts General Hospital: Weekly clinicopathological exercises. Case 24-1984. Pancytopenia and fever in a renal-transplant recipient. N. Engl. J. Med. *310*:1584–1594, 1984.
35. Centers for Disease Control and Prevention: Histoplasmosis control: Decontamination of bird roosts, chicken houses, and other point sources. Atlanta, U. S. Department of Health, Education, and Welfare, Public Health Service, 1979, HEW Publication No. (CDC) 80–8380.
36. Centers for Disease Control and Prevention: Revision of the CDC surveillance case definition for the acquired immunodeficiency syndrome. Council of State and Territorial Epidemiologists; AIDS Program, Centers for Infectious Diseases. M. M. W. R. Morb. Mortal. Wkly. Rep. *36*(Suppl. 1):1–15, 1987.
37. Centers for Disease Control and Prevention: Cave-associated histoplasmosis: Costa Rica. M. M. W. R. Morb. Mortal. Wkly. Rep. *37*(29):312–313, 1988.
38. Centers for Disease Control and Prevention: Update: Outbreak of acute febrile respiratory illness among college students—Acapulco, Mexico, March 2001. M. M. W. R. Morb. Mortal. Wkly. Rep. *50*(18):359–360, 2001.
39. Chaturvedi, S., Frame, P., and Newman, S. L.: Macrophages from human immunodeficiency virus–positive persons are defective in host defense against *Histoplasma capsulatum*. J. Infect. Dis. *171*:320–327, 1995.
40. Chaturvedi, S., and Newman, S. L.: Modulation of the effector function of human macrophages for *Histoplasma capsulatum* by HIV-1. Role of the envelope glycoprotein gp120. J. Clin. Invest. *100*:1465–1474, 1997.
41. Chemaly, R. F., Tomford, J. W., Hall, G. S., et al.: Rapid diagnosis of *Histoplasma capsulatum* endocarditis using the AccuProbe on the excised valve. J. Clin. Microbiol. *39*:2640–2641, 2001.
42. Christie, A., and Peterson, J. C.: Pulmonary calcification in negative reactors to tuberculin. Am. J. Public Health *35*:1131, 1945.
43. Ciulla, T. A., Piper, H. C., and Wheat, L. J.: Presumed ocular histoplasmosis syndrome: Update on epidemiology, pathogenesis, and photodynamic, antiangiogenic, and surgical therapies. Curr. Opin. Ophthalmol. *6*:442–449, 2001.
44. Clapp, D. W., Kleiman, M. B., and Brahmi, Z.: Immunoregulatory lymphocyte populations in disseminated histoplasmosis of infancy. J. Infect. Dis. *156*:687–688, 1997.
45. Class, R. N., and Cascio, F. S.: Histoplasmosis presenting as acute polyarthritis. N. Engl. J. Med. *287*:1133–1134, 1972.
46. Clemons, K. V., Darbonne, W. C., Curnutte, J. T., et al.: Experimental histoplasmosis in mice treated with anti–murine interferon-gamma antibody and in interferon-gamma gene knockout mice. Microbes Infect. *2*:997–1001, 2000.
47. Cockshott, W. P., and Lucas, A. O.: Histoplasmosis duboisii. Q. J. Med. *133*:223, 1964.
48. Connolly, P., Wheat, J., Schnizlein-Bick, C., et al.: Comparison of a new triazole antifungal agent, Schering 56592, with itraconazole and amphotericin B for treatment of histoplasmosis in immunocompetent mice. Antimicrob. Agents Chemother. *43*:322–328, 1999.
49. Cott, G. R., Smith, T. W., Hinthorn, D. R., and Liu, C.: Primary cutaneous histoplasmosis in immunosuppressed patient. J. A. M. A. *242*:456–457, 1979.
50. Darling, S. T.: A protozoan general infection producing pseudo tubercles in the lungs and focal necrosis in the liver, spleen, and lymph nodes. J. A. M. A. *46*:1283, 1906.
51. Daubenton, J. D., and Beatty, D. W.: Disseminated histoplasmosis in an "immunocompetent child." S. Afr. Med. J. *88*:270–271, 1998.
52. Davies, S. F.: Serodiagnosis of histoplasmosis. Semin. Respir. Infect. *1*:9–15, 1986.
53. Davies, S. F., Khan, M., and Sarosi, G. A.: Disseminated histoplasmosis in immunologically suppressed patients: Occurrence in a non-endemic area. Am. J. Med. *64*:98–100, 1978.
54. Davis, A. M., Pierson, R. N., and Loyd, J. E.: Mediastinal Fibrosis. Semin. Respir. Infect. *16*:119–130, 2001.
55. Deepe, G. S., Jr.: Protective immunity in murine histoplasmosis: Functional comparison of adoptively transferred T-cell clones and splenic T cells. Infect. Immun. *56*:2350–2355, 1988.
56. Deepe, G. S., Jr., and Gibbons, R.: Recombinant murine granulocyte-macrophage colony-stimulating factor modulates the course of pulmonary histoplasmosis in immunocompetent and immunodeficient mice. Antimicrob. Agents Chemother. *44*:3328–3336, 2000.
57. Deepe, G. S., Jr., and Gibbons, R.: Protective efficacy of H antigen from *Histoplasma capsulatum* in a murine model of pulmonary histoplasmosis. Infect. Immun. *69*:3128–3134, 2001.
58. Deepe, G. S., Gibbons, R., and Woodward, E.: Neutralization of endogenous granulocyte-macrophage colony-stimulating factor subverts the protective immune response to *Histoplasma capsulatum*. J. Immunol. *163*:4985–4993, 1999.
59. DeFelice, R., Johnson, D. G., and Galgiani, J. N.: Gynecomastia with ketoconazole. Antimicrob. Agents Chemother. *19*:1073–1074, 1981.
60. DeMonbreum, W. A.: The cultivation and cultural characteristics of Darling's *H. capsulatum*. Am. J. Trop. Med. *14*:93, 1934.
61. Dines, D. E., Payne, W. S., Bernatz, P. E., et al.: Mediastinal granuloma and fibrosing mediastinitis. Chest *75*:320–324, 1979.
62. DiSalvo, A. F.: The role of bats in the ecology of *Histoplasma capsulatum*. *In* Histoplasmosis: Proceedings of the Second National Conference. Springfield, IL, Charles C Thomas, 1971.
63. Dismukes, W. E., Cloud, G., Bowles, C., et al.: Treatment of blastomycosis and histoplasmosis with ketoconazole: Results of a prospective randomized clinical trial. Ann. Intern. Med. *103*:861–872, 1985.
64. Dodd, K., and Tompkins, E.: Case of histoplasmosis of Darling in an infant. Am. J. Trop. Med. *14*:127, 1934.

65. Domer, J. E.: Monosaccharide and chitin content of cell walls of *Histoplasma capsulatum* and *Blastomyces dermatitidis*. J. Bacteriol. *107*:870–877, 1971.
66. Doyle, T. P., Loyd, J. E., and Robbins, I. M.: Percutaneous pulmonary artery and vein stenting. A novel treatment for mediastinal fibrosis. Am. J. Respir. Crit. Care Med. *164*:657–660, 2001.
67. Drutz, D. J., Spickard, A., Rogers, D. E., et al.: Treatment of disseminated mycotic infections. Am. J. Med. *45*:405–418, 1968.
68. Dugoni, B., Guglielmo, B. J., and Hollander, H.: Amphotericin B concentration in cerebrospinal fluid of patients with AIDS and cryptococcal meningitis. Clin. Pharm. *8*:220–221, 1989.
69. Dukes, R. J., Strimian, V., Dines, D. E., et al.: Esophageal involvement with mediastinal granuloma. J. A. M. A. *236*:2313–2315, 1976.
70. Durkin, M. M., Connolly, P. A., and Wheat, L. J.: Comparison of radioimmunoassay and enzyme-linked immunoassay methods for detection of *Histoplasma capsulatum* var *capsulatum* antigen. J. Clin. Microbiol. *35*:2252–2255, 1997.
71. Edwards, L. B., Acquaviva, F. A., and Livesay, V. T.: Further observations on histoplasmin sensitivity in the United States. Am. J. Epidemiol. *98*:315–325, 1973.
72. Edwards, L. B., Acquaviva, F. A., Livesay, V. T., et al.: An atlas of sensitivity to tuberculin, PPD-B, and histoplasmin in the United States. Am. Rev. Respir. Dis. *99*(Suppl.):1–132, 1969.
73. Edwards, P. Q.: Histoplasmin sensitivity patterns around the world. *In* Histoplasmosis. Proceedings of the Second National Conference. Springfield, IL, Charles C Thomas, 1971.
74. Emmons, C. W., Klite, P. D., Baer, G. M., et al.: Isolation of *Histoplasma capsulatum* from bats in the United States. Am. J. Epidemiol. *84*:103–109, 1966.
75. Emmons, C. W., Morlan, H. B., and Hill, E. L.: Isolation of *Histoplasma capsulatum* from soil. Public Health Rep. *64*:892, 1949.
76. Epsinel-Ingroff, A., Shadomy, S., and Gebhardt, R. J.: In vitro studies with R 51,211. Antimicrob. Agents Chemother. *26*:5–9, 1984.
77. Ferguson, T. B., and Burford, T. H.: Mediastinal granuloma: A 15-year experience. Ann. Thorac. Surg. *1*:125, 1965.
78. Flynn, P. M., Barrett, F. F., and Herrod, H. G.: Disseminated histoplasmosis in two patients with chronic mucocutaneous candidiasis. Pediatr. Infect. Dis. *6*:691–693, 1987.
79. Fojtasek, M. F., Kleiman, M. B., Connolly-Stringfield, P., et al.: The *Histoplasma capsulatum* antigen assay in disseminated histoplasmosis in children. Pediatr. Infect. Dis. J. *13*:801–805, 1994.
80. Fosson, A. R., and Wheeler, W. E.: Short-term amphotericin B treatment of severe childhood histoplasmosis. J. Pediatr. *86*:32–36, 1975.
81. Furcolow, M. L.: Tests of immunity in histoplasmosis. N. Engl. J. Med. *268*:357, 1963.
82. Furcolow, M. L.: Course and prognosis of untreated histoplasmosis. J. A. M. A. *177*:292–296, 1977.
83. Furcolow, M. L., Schubert, J., Tosh, F. E., et al.: Serologic evidence of histoplasmosis in sanatoriums in the U. S. J. A. M. A. *180*:109, 1962.
84. Gaebler, J. W., Kleiman, M. B., Cohen, M., et al.: Differentiation of lymphoma from histoplasmosis in children with mediastinal masses. J. Pediatr. *104*:706–709, 1984.
85. Ganer, A., Arathoon E., and Stevens, D. A.: Initial experience in therapy for progressive mycoses with itraconazole, the first clinically studied triazole. Rev. Infect. Dis. *9*(Suppl. 1):77–86, 1987.
86. Garrett, H. E., Jr., and Roper, C. L.: Surgical intervention in histoplasmosis. Ann. Thorac. Surg. *42*:711–722, 1986.
87. Garringer, A. T. O., Wheat, L. F., and Brisendine, E. J.: Comparison of an established antibody sandwich method with an inhibition method of *Histoplasma capsulatum* antigen detection. J. Clin. Microbiol. *38*:2909–2913, 2000.
88. Gass, M., and Kobayashi, G. S.: Histoplasmosis: An illustrative case with unusual vaginal and joint involvement. Arch. Dermatol. *100*:724–727, 1969.
89. Gaynes, R. P., Gardner, P., and Causey, W.: Prosthetic valve endocarditis caused by *Histoplasma capsulatum*. Arch. Intern. Med. *141*:1533–1537, 1981.
90. Gelfand, J. A., and Bennett, J. E.: Active *Histoplasma* meningitis of 22 years' duration. J. A. M. A. *233*:1294–1295, 1975.
91. George, R. B., and Lambert, R. S.: Significance of serum antibodies to *Histoplasma capsulatum* in endemic areas. South. Med. J. *77*:161–163, 1984.
92. Gomez, A. M., Bullock, W. E., Taylor, C. L., and Deepe, G. S., Jr.: Role of L3T4+ T cells in host defense against *Histoplasma capsulatum*. Infect. Immun. *56*:1685–1691, 1988.
93. Gomez, F. J., Allendoerfer, R., and Deepe, G. S., Jr.: Vaccination with recombinant heat shock protein 60 from *Histoplasma capsulatum* protects mice against pulmonary histoplasmosis. Infect. Immun. *63*:2587–2595, 1995.
94. Goodwin, R. A., Loyd, J. E., and Des Prez, R. M.: Histoplasmosis in normal hosts. Medicine (Baltimore) *60*:231–266, 1981.
95. Goodwin, R. A., Owens, F. T., Snell, J. D., et al.: Chronic pulmonary histoplasmosis. Medicine (Baltimore) *55*:413–452, 1976.
96. Goodwin, R. A., Shapiro, J. L., Thurman, G. H., et al.: Disseminated histoplasmosis: Clinical and pathologic correlation. Medicine (Baltimore) *59*:1–33, 1980.
97. Goodwin, R. A., and Snell, J. D., Jr.: The enlarging histoplasmoma: Concept of tumor-like phenomenon encompassing the tuberculoma and coccidioidoma. Am. Rev. Respir. Dis. *100*:1–12, 1969.
98. Graybill, J. R.: Histoplasmosis and AIDS. J. Infect. Dis. *158*:623–626, 1988.
99. Graybill, J. R., Patino, M. M., Gomez, A. M., et al.: Detection of histoplasmal antigens in mice undergoing experimental pulmonary histoplasmosis. Am. Rev. Respir. Dis. *132*:752–756, 1985.
100. Greene, L. W., Cole, W., Greene, J. B., et al.: Adrenal insufficiency as a complication of the acquired immunodeficiency syndrome. Ann. Intern. Med. *101*:497–498, 1984.
101. Greenwood, M. F., and Holland, P.: Tracheal obstruction secondary to *Histoplasma* mediastinal granuloma. Chest *62*:642–643, 1972.
102. Gildea, L. A., Morris, R. E., and Newman, S. L.: *Histoplasma capsulatum* yeasts are phagocytosed via very late antigen-5, killed, and processed for antigen presentation by human dendritic cells. J. Immunol. *166*:1049–1056, 2001.
103. Groll, A., Giri, N., Petratitis, V., et al.: Comparative efficacy and distribution of lipid formulations of amphotericin B in experimental *Candida albicans* infection of the central nervous system. J. Infect. Dis. *182*:274–282, 2000.
104. Groll, A. H., Irwin, R. S., Patrick, C. C., et al.: Management of specific infectious complications in children with leukemias and lymphomas. *In* Clinical Management of Infections of Immunocompromised Infants and Children. Philadelphia, Lippincott Williams & Wilkins, 2001, pp. 111–143.
105. Grossman, M. E.: Cutaneous Manifestations of Infection in the Immunocompromised Host. Baltimore, Wilkins & Wilkins, 1995, pp. 22–28.
106. Gustafson, T. L., Kaufman, L., Weeks, R., et al.: Outbreak of acute pulmonary histoplasmosis in members of a wagon train. Am. J. 71:759–765, 1981.
107. Haggerty, C. M., Britton, M. C., Dorman, J. M., et al.: Gastrointestinal histoplasmosis in the acquired immune deficiency syndrome. West. J. Med. *143*:244–246, 1985.
108. Hajjeh, R. A.: Disseminated histoplasmosis in persons infected with human immunodeficiency virus. Clin. Infect. Dis. *21*(Suppl. 1):108–110, 1985.
109. Hajjeh, R. A., Pappas, P. G., Henderson, H., et al.: Multicenter case-control study of risk factors for histoplasmosis in human immunodeficiency virus–infected persons. Clin. Infect. Dis. *32*:1215–1220, 2001.
110. Halline, A. G., Madlonado-Lutomirsky, M., Ryoo, J. W., et al.: Colonic histoplasmosis in AIDS: Unusual endoscopic findings in two cases. Gastrointest. Endosc. *45*:199–204, 1997.
111. Hay, R. J., Dupont, B., and Graybill, J. R.: First international symposium on itraconazole: A summary. Rev. Infect. Dis. *9*(Suppl. 1):1–152, 1987.
112. Hecht, F. M., Wheat, J., Korzun, A. H., et al.: Itraconazole maintenance treatment for histoplasmosis in AIDS: A prospective, multicenter trial. J. Acquir. Immune Defic. Syndr. Hum. Retrovirol. *16*:100–107, 1997.
113. Heeres, J., Backx, L. J. J., and Van Custem, J.: Antimycotic azoles. 7. Synthesis and antifungal properties of a series of novel triazol-3-ones. J. Med. Chem. *27*:894–900, 1984.
114. Heiberg, J. K., and Svejaard, E.: Toxic hepatitis during ketoconazole therapy. B. M. J. *283*:825–826, 1981.
115. Heusinkveld, R., Tosh, F., and Newberry, W.: Antibody response to the histoplasmin skin test. Am. Rev. Respir. Dis. *96*:1069–1071, 1967.
116. Horton, G. E., Larkin, J. C., and Phillips, S.: Acute pulmonary histoplasmosis. South. Med. J. *52*:912, 1959.
117. Hostoffer, R. W., Berger, M., Clark, H. T., et al.: Disseminated *Histoplasma capsulatum* in a patient with hyper IgM immunodeficiency. Pediatrics *94*:234–236, 1994.
118. Hughes, W. T.: Hematogenous histoplasmosis in the immunocompromised child. J. Pediatr. *105*:569–575, 1984.
119. Jaruratanasirikul, S., and Kleepkaew, A.: Influence of an acidic beverage (Coca-Cola) on the absorption of itraconazole. Eur. J. Clin. Pharmacol. *52*:235–237, 1997.
120. Jiang, B., Bartlett, M. S., Allen, S. D., et al.: Typing of *Histoplasma capsulatum* isolates based on nucleotide sequence variation in the internal transcribed spacer regions of rRNA genes. J. Clin. Microbiol. *38*:241–245, 2000.
121. Johnson, P. C., Khardori, N., Butt, F., et al.: Progressive disseminated histoplasmosis in patients with acquired immunodeficiency syndrome. Am. J. Med. *85*:152–158, 1988.
122. Johnson, P. C., Sarosi, G. A., and Septimus, E. J.: Progressive disseminated histoplasmosis in patients with the acquired immunodeficiency syndrome: A report of 12 cases and a literature review. Semin. Respir. Infect. *1*:1–8, 1986.
123. Johnson, P. C., Wheat, L. J., Cloud, G. A., et al.: Safety and efficacy of liposomal amphotericin B compared with conventional amphotericin B for induction therapy of histoplasmosis in patients with AIDS. Ann. Intern. Med. *137*:105–109, 2002.
124. Jones, R. C., and Goodwin, R. A.: Histoplasmosis of the bone. Am. J. Med. *70*:864–866, 1981.
125. Karalakulasingam, R., Arora, K. K., Adams, G., et al.: Meningoencephalitis caused by *Histoplasma capsulatum*. Arch. Intern. Med. *136*:217–220, 1983.

126. Kataria, Y. P., Campbell, P. B., and Burlingham, B. T.: Acute pulmonary histoplasmosis presenting as adult respiratory distress syndrome: Effect of therapy on clinical and laboratory features. South. Med. J. *74*:534–537, 1981.
127. Kauffman, C. A.: Pulmonary histoplasmosis. Curr. Infect. Dis. Rep. *3*:279–285, 2001.
128. Kauffman, C. A., Israel, M. S., Smith, J. W., et al.: Histoplasmosis in immunosuppressed patients. Am. J. Med. *64*:923–932, 1978.
129. Kauffman, C. A., Slama, T. G., and Wheat, L. J.: *Histoplasma capsulatum* epididymitis. J. Urol. *125*:434–435, 1981.
130. Kaufman, L.: Serological tests for histoplasmosis: Their use and interpretation. *In* Ajello, L., Chick, E. W., and Furcolow, M. L. (eds.): *In* Histoplasmosis. Proceedings of the Second National Conference. Springfield, IL, Charles C Thomas, 1971, p. 321.
131. Kaufman, L., Kovacs, J. A., and Reiss, E.: Clinical immunomycology. *In* Rose, N. R. (ed.): Manual of Clinical Laboratory Immunology. Washington, D.C., American Society of Microbiology Press, 1997, pp. 595–596.
132. Kaufman, L., and Reiss, E.: Serodiagnosis of fungal diseases. *In* Lennette, E. H., Balows, A., Hausler, W. J., Jr., et al.: (eds.): Manual of Clinical Microbiology. 4th ed. Washington, D.C., American Society of Microbiology, 1985, p. 924.
133. Kaufman, L., Terry, R. T., Schubert, J. H., et al.: Effect of a single histoplasmin skin test on the serological diagnosis of histoplasmosis. J. Bacteriol. *94*:798, 1967.
134. Keath, E. J., Kobayashi, G. S., and Medoff, G.: Typing of *Histoplasma capsulatum* by restriction fragment length polymorphisms in a nuclear gene. J. Clin. Microbiol. *30*:2104–2107, 1992.
135. Keller, F. G., and Kurtzberg, J.: Disseminated histoplasmosis: A cause of infection-associated hemophagocytic syndrome. Am. J. Pediatr. Hematol. Oncol. *16*:368–371, 1994.
136. King, R. W., and Kraikitpanitch, S.: Subcutaneous nodules caused by *Histoplasma capsulatum*. Ann. Intern. Med. *86*:586–587, 1977.
137. Kirchner, S. G., Hernanz-Schulman, M., Stein, S. M., et al.: Imaging of pediatric mediastinal histoplasmosis. Radiographics *3*:365–381, 1991.
138. Klatt, E. C., Cosgrove, M., and Meyer, P. R.: Rapid diagnosis of disseminated histoplasmosis in tissues. Arch. Pathol. Lab. Med. *110*:1173–1175, 1986.
139. Klimpel, K. R., and Goldman, W. E.: Isolation and characterization of spontaneous avirulent variants of *Histoplasma capsulatum*. Infect. Immun. *55*:528–533, 1987.
140. Knight, P. J., Mulne, A. F., and Vassay, L. E.: When is lymph node biopsy indicated in children with enlarged peripheral nodes? Pediatrics *69*:391–396, 1982.
141. Kritski, A. L., Lemle, A., de Souza, G. R. M., et al.: Pulmonary function changes in the acute stage of histoplasmosis, with follow-up: An analysis of eight cases. Chest *97*:1244–1245, 1990.
142. Kwong-Chung, K. J.: Sexual stage of *Histoplasma capsulatum*. Science *175*:326, 1972.
143. Kwon-Chung, K. J.: Perfect state *(Emmonsiella capatalata)* of the fungus using large-form African histoplasmosis. Mycologia *67*:980, 1975.
144. Lambert, R. S., and George, R. B.: Evaluation of enzyme immunoassay as a rapid screening test for histoplasmosis and blastomycosis. Am. Rev. Respir. Dis. *136*:316–319, 1987.
145. Lamps, L. W., Molina, C. P., West, A. B., et al.: The pathologic spectrum of gastrointestinal and hepatic. Am. J. Clin. Pathol. *113*:64–72, 2000.
146. Lane, T. E., Wu-Hsieh, B. A., and Howard, D. H.: Gamma interferon cooperates with lipopolysaccharide to activate mouse splenic macrophages to an antihistoplasma state. Infect. Immun. *61*:1468–1473, 1993.
147. Larone, D. H., Mitchell, T. G., Walsh, T. J.: *Histoplasma, Blastomyces, Coccidioides,* and other dimorphic fungi causing systemic mycoses. *In* Murray, P. R., Baron, E. J., Pfaller, M. A., et al.: (eds.): Manual of Clinical Microbiology. 7th ed. Washington, D.C., American Society of Microbiology, 1999, pp. 1259–1268.
148. Larrabee, W. F., Ajello, L., and Kaufman, L.: An epidemic of histoplasmosis on the isthmus of Panama. Am. J. Trop. Med. Hyg. *27*:281–283, 1977.
149. Larwood, T. R.: Coccidioidin skin testing in Kern County, California: Decrease in infection rate over 58 years. Clin. Infect. Dis. *30*:612–613, 2000.
150. Leender, A., Reiss, P., Portegies, P.., et al.: Liposomal amphotericin B (AmBisome) compared with amphotericin B both followed by oral fluconazole in the treatment of AIDS-associated cryptococcal meningitis. A. I. D. S. *11*:1463–1471, 1997.
151. Leggiadro, R. J., Barrett, F. F., and Hughes, W. T.: Disseminated histoplasmosis of infancy. Pediatr. Infect. Dis. *7*:799–805, 1988.
152. Leland, D. S., Zimmerman, S. E., Cunningham, E. B., et al.: Variability in commercial *Histoplasma* complement fixation antigens. J. Clin. Microbiol. *29*:1723–1724, 1991.
153. LeMonte, A. M., Washum, K. E., Smedema, M. L., et al.: Amphotericin B combined with itraconazole or fluconazole for treatment of histoplasmosis. J. Infect. Dis. *182*:545–550, 2000.
154. Lewis, J. H., Zimmerman, H. J., Benson, G. D., et al.: Hepatic injury associated with ketoconazole therapy: Analysis of 33 cases. Gastroenterology *86*:503–513, 1984.
155. Limaye, A. P., Connolly, P. A., Manish, S., et al.: Brief Report: Transmission of *Histoplasma capsulatum* by organ transplantation. N. Engl. J. Med. *343*:1163–1166, 2000.
156. Lindsley, M. D., Hurst, S. F., Iqbal, N. J., et al.: Rapid identification of dimorphic and yeast-like fungal pathogens using specific DNA probes. J. Clin. Microbiol. *39*:3505–3511, 2001.
157. Little, J., Bruce, J., Andrews, H., et al.: Treatment of disseminated infantile histoplasmosis with amphotericin B. Pediatrics *24*:1, 1959.
158. Little, J. A., and Steigman, A. J.: Erythema nodosum in primary histoplasmosis. J. A. M. A. *173*:875, 1960.
159. Lockwood, G. F., and Garrison, R. G.: The possible role of uric acid in the ecology of *Histoplasma capsulatum*. Mycopathologia *35*:377–388, 1968.
160. Loyd, J. E., Des Prez, R. M., and Goodwin, R. A., Jr.: *Histoplasma capsulatum. In* Mandell, G. L., Douglas, R. G., Jr., and Bennett, J. E. (eds.): Principles and Practice of Infectious Diseases. 3rd ed. New York, Churchill Livingstone, 1990, p. 1989.
161. Loyd, J. E., Tillman, B. F., Atkinson, J. B., et al.: Mediastinal fibrosis complicating histoplasmosis. Medicine (Baltimore) *67*:295–310, 1988.
162. Lucas, A. O.: Cutaneous manifestations of African histoplasmosis. Br. J. Dermatol. *82*:435–447, 1970.
163. Ma, K. W.: Disseminated histoplasmosis in dialysis patients. Clin. Nephrol. *24*:155–157, 1985.
164. Macher, A.: Histoplasmosis and blastomycosis. Med. Clin. North Am. *64*:447–459, 1980.
165. Macher, A., Rodrigues, M. M., Kaplan, W., et al.: Disseminated bilateral chorioretinitis due to *Histoplasma capsulatum* in a patient with acquired immunodeficiency syndrome. Ophthalmology *92*:1159–1164, 1985.
166. Mashburn, J. D., Dawson, D. F., and Young, J. M.: Pulmonary calcifications and histoplasmosis. Am. Rev. Respir. Dis. *84*:208, 1961.
167. Mathisen, D. J., and Grillo, H. C.: Clinical manifestation of mediastinal fibrosis and histoplasmosis. Am. Thorac. Surg. *54*:1053–1058, 1992.
168. McGinnis, M. R., and Katz, B.: *Ajellomyces* and its synonym *Emmonsiella*. Mycotaxonomy *8*:157–164, 1979.
169. McKinsey, D. S., Gupta, M. R., Riddler, S. A., et al.: Long-term amphotericin B therapy for disseminated histoplasmosis in patients with the acquired immune deficiency syndrome. Ann. Intern. Med. *111*:655–659, 1989.
170. McKinsey, D. S., Kauffman, C. A., Pappas, P. G., et al.: Fluconazole therapy for histoplasmosis. Clin. Infect. Dis. *23*:996–1001, 1996.
171. McKinsey, D. S., Spiegel, R. A., Hutwagner, L., et al.: Prospective study of histoplasmosis in patients infected with human immunodeficiency virus: Incidence, risk factors, and pathophysiology. Clin. Infect. Dis. *24*:1995–2003, 1997.
172. McKinsey, D. S., Wheat, L. J., Cloud, G. A., et al.: Itraconazole prophylaxis for fungal infections in patients with advanced human immunodeficiency virus infection: Randomized, placebo-controlled, double-blind study. Clin. Infect. Dis. *28*:1049–1056, 1999.
173. McNeil, M. M., Nash, S. L., Hajjeh, R. A., et al.: Trends in mortality due to invasive mycotic diseases in the United States, 1990–1997. Clin. Infect. Dis. *33*:641–647, 2001.
174. Medeiros, A. A., Marty, S. D., Tosh, F. E., et al.: Erythema nodosum and erythema multiforme as clinical manifestations of histoplasmosis in a community outbreak. N. Engl. J. Med. *274*:415–420, 1966.
175. Medoff, G., Kobayashi, G. S., Painter, A., et al.: Morphogenesis and pathogenicity of *Histoplasma capsulatum*. Infect. Immun. *55*:1355–1358, 1987.
176. Meleney, H. E.: Histoplasmosis (reticulo-endothelial cytomycosis): A review with mention of 13 unpublished cases. Am. J. Trop. Med. *20*:603, 1940.
177. Menges, R. W.: Clinical manifestations of animal histoplasmosis. *In* Histoplasmosis. Proceedings of the Second National Conference. Springfield, IL, Charles C Thomas, 1971.
178. Merz, W. G., Kodsy, S., and Merz, C. S.: Recovery of *Histoplasma capsulatum* from blood in a commercial radiometric mycobacterium medium. J. Clin. Microbiol. *30*:237–239, 1992.
179. Miller, C. R., and Grossmann, H.: Disseminated histoplasmosis in chronic mucocutaneous candidiasis. Pediatr. Radiol. *23*:104–105, 1993.
180. Mitchell, T. G.: Systemic mycoses. *In* Joklik, W. K., Willett, H. P., and Amos, D. B. (eds.): Zinsser Microbiology. 14th ed. Norwalk, CT, Appleton-Century-Crofts, 1984, p. 1138.
181. Mocheria, S., and Wheat, L. J.: Treatment of histoplasmosis. Semin. Respir. Infect. *16*:141–148, 2001.
182. Monzon, C. M., Cooperstock, M. S., Singsen, B. H., et al.: Meningitis and multiple cerebral abscesses in a ten year old boy. J. Pediatr. *112*:830–835, 1988.
183. National Institute of Allergy and Infectious Diseases Mycoses Study Group, Birmingham, Alabama, and Bethesda, Maryland: Treatment of blastomycosis and histoplasmosis with ketoconazole. Ann. Intern. Med. *103*:861–872, 1985.
184. Negroni, R., Palmieri, O., Koren, F., et al.: Oral treatment of paracoccidioidomycosis and histoplasmosis with itraconazole in humans. Rev. Infect. Dis. *9*(Suppl. 1):47–50, 1987.

185. Negroni, R., Robles, A. M., Arechavala, A., et al.: Ketoconazole in the treatment of paracoccidioidomycosis and histoplasmosis. Rev. Infect. Dis. *2*:643–649, 1980.
186. Newman, S. L.: Macrophages in host defense against *Histoplasma capsulatum.* Trends Microbiol. 7:67–71, 1999.
187. Newman, S. L.: Cell-mediated immunity to *Histoplasma capsulatum.* Semin. Respir. Infect. *162*:102–108, 2001.
188. Newman, S. L., and Gootee, L.: Colony-stimulating factors activate human macrophages to inhibit intracellular growth of *Histoplasma capsulatum* yeasts. Infect. Immun. *60*:4593–4597, 1992.
189. Newman, S. L., Gootee, L., and Gabay, J. E.: Human neutrophil-mediated fungistasis against *Histoplasma capsulatum:* Localization of fungistatic activity to the azurophil granules. J. Clin. Invest. *92*:624–631, 1993.
190. Newman, S. L., Gootee, L., Kidd, C., et al.: Activation of human macrophage fungistatic activity against *Histoplasma capsulatum* upon adherence to type 1 collagen matrices. J. Immunol. *158*:1779–1786, 1997.
191. Norris, S., Wheat, J., McKinsey, D., et al.: Prevention of relapse of histoplasmosis with fluconazole in patients with the acquired immunodeficiency syndrome. Am. J. Med. *96*:504–508, 1994.
192. Odio, C. M., Navarrete, M., Carrillo, J. M., et al.: Disseminated histoplasmosis in infants. Pediatr. Infect. Dis. J. *18*:1065–1068, 1999.
193. O'Hara, M.: Histopathologic diagnosis of fungal diseases. Infect. Control *7*:78–84, 1986.
194. Okudiara, M., Straub, M., and Schwarz, J.: The etiology of discrete splenic and hepatic calcifications in an endemic area of histoplasmosis. Am. J. Pathol. *39*:599, 1961.
195. Ongkosuwito, J. V., Kortbeek, L. M., Van der Lelij, A., et al.: Aetiological study of the presumed ocular histoplasmosis syndrome in the Netherlands. Br. J. Ophthalmol. *83*:535–539, 1999.
196. Orchard, J. L., Luparello, F., and Brunskill, D.: Malabsorption syndrome occurring in the course of disseminated histoplasmosis. Am. J. Med. *66*:331–336, 1979.
197. Ozols, I. I., and Wheat, L. J.: Erythema nodosum in an epidemic of histoplasmosis in Indianapolis. Arch. Dermatol. *117*:1709–1712, 1981.
198. Parsons, R. J., and Zarafonetis, C. J. D.: Histoplasmosis in man: Report of 7 cases and a review of 71 cases. Arch. Intern. Med. *75*:1, 1945.
199. Pate, J. W., and Hammon, J.: Superior vena cava syndrome due to histoplasmosis in children. Ann. Surg. *166*:778, 1965.
200. Patino, M. M., Williams, D. M., Ahrens, J., et al.: Experimental histoplasmosis in the beige mouse. J. Leukoc. Biol. *41*:228–235, 1987.
201. Patrick, C. C., Flynn, P. M., Henwick, S., et al.: Disseminated histoplasmosis presenting as a cystic duct obstruction. Pediatr. Infect. Dis. J. *11*:593–594, 1992.
202. Paya, C. V., Hermans, P. E., Van Scoy, R. E., et al.: Repeatedly relapsing disseminated histoplasmosis: Clinical observations during long-term follow-up. J. Infect. Dis. *156*:308–312, 1987.
203. Paya, C. V., Roberts, G. D., and Cockerill, F. R.: Transient fungemia in acute pulmonary histoplasmosis: Detection by new blood-culturing techniques. J. Infect. Dis. *156*:313–315, 1987.
204. Payan, D. G., Wheat, L. J., Brahmi, Z., et al.: Changes in immunoregulatory lymphocyte populations in patients with histoplasmosis. J. Clin. Immunol. *4*:98–107, 1984.
205. Peabody, J. W., Jr., Brown, R. B., Davis, E. W., et al.: Surgical implications of mediastinal granulomas. Am. Surg. *25*:357, 1959.
206. Peddi, V. R., Hariharan, S., and First, M. R.: Disseminated histoplasmosis in renal allograft recipients. Clin. Transplant. *10*:160–165, 1996.
207. Penn, R. L., Lambert, R. S., and George, R. B.: Invasive fungal infections: The use of serologic tests in diagnosis and management. Arch. Intern. Med. *143*:1215–1220, 1983.
208. Phillips, P., Fetchick, R., Weisman, I., et al.: Tolerance to and efficacy of itraconazole in treatment of systemic mycoses: Preliminary results. Rev. Infect. Dis. *9*(Suppl. 1):87–93, 1987.
209. Pladson, T. R., Stiles, M. A., and Kuritsky, J. N.: Pulmonary histoplasmosis: A possible risk in people who cut decayed wood. Chest *86*:435–438, 1984.
210. Plouffe, J. F., and Fass, R. J.: *Histoplasma* meningitis: Diagnostic value of cerebrospinal fluid serology. Ann. Intern. Med. *92*:189–191, 1980.
211. Porta, A., and Maresca, B.: Host response and *Histoplasma capsulatum*/macrophage molecular interactions. Med. Mycol. *38*:399–406, 2000.
212. Pottage, J. C., Trenholme, G. M., Aronson, I. K., et al.: Panniculitis with histoplasmosis and alpha-1-antitrypsin deficiency. Am. J. Med. *75*:150–153, 1983.
213. Prechter, G. C., and Prakash, U. B.: Bronchoscopy in the diagnosis of pulmonary histoplasmosis. Chest *95*:1033–1036, 1989.
214. Quasney, M. W., and Leggiadro, R. J.: Pleural effusion associated with histoplasmosis. J. Pediatr. Infect. Dis. *12*:415–418, 1993.
215. Quinones, C. A., Reuben, A. G., Hamill, R. J., et al.: Chronic cavitary histoplasmosis: Failure of oral treatment with ketoconazole. Chest *95*:914–916, 1989.
216. Racela, L. S., Papasian, C. J., Watanabe, I., et al.: Systemic talc granulomatosis associated with disseminated histoplasmosis in a drug abuser. Arch. Pathol. Lab. Med. *112*:557–560, 1988.
217. Rescorla, F. J., Kleiman, M. B., and Grosfeld, J. L.: Obstruction of the common bile duct in histoplasmosis. Pediatr. Infect. Dis. J. *13*:1017–1019, 1994.
218. Retallack, D. M., and Woods, J. P.: Molecular epidemiology, pathogenesis, and genetics of the dimorphic fungus *Histoplasma capsulatum.* Microbes Infect. *1*:817–824, 1999.
219. Riggs, W., and Nelson, P.: The roentgenographic findings in infantile and childhood histoplasmosis. A. J. R. Am. J. Roentgenol. *97*:181, 1966.
220. Riley, H. D.: The history of histoplasmosis. S. Okla. State Med. Assoc. *76*:31–40, 1983.
221. Rippon, J. W.: The pathogenic fungi and the pathogenic actinomycetes. *In* Medical Mycology: The Pathogenic Fungi and the Pathogenic Actinomycetes. 3rd ed. Philadelphia, W. B. Saunders, 1988, p. 424.
222. Rivera, I. V., Curless, R. G., Indacochea, F. J., et al.: Chronic progressive CNS histoplasmosis presenting in childhood: Response to fluconazole therapy. Pediatr. Neurol. *8*:151–153, 1992.
223. Rodriquez, E., Soler, R., Pombo, F., et al.: Fibrosing mediastinitis: CT and MR findings. Clin. Radiol. *53*:907–910, 1998.
224. Rosenthal, J., Brandt, K. D., Wheat, L. J., et al.: Rheumatologic manifestations of histoplasmosis in the recent Indianapolis epidemic. Arthritis Rheum. *26*:1065–1070, 1983.
225. Rossi, S. E., McAdams, H. P., Rosado-de-Christenson, M. L., et al.: Fibrosing mediastinitis. Radiographics 21:737–757, 2001.
226. Rubin, H., Furcolow, M. L., and Yates, J. L.: The course and prognosis of histoplasmosis. Am. J. Med. *27*:278, 1959.
227. Salvin, S. B.: Acquired resistance in experimental histoplasmosis. Trans. N. Y. Acad. Sci. *18*:462–468, 1955.
228. Salzman, S. H., Smith, R. L., and Aranda, C. P.: Histoplasmosis in patients at risk for the acquired immunodeficiency syndrome in a nonendemic setting. Chest *93*:916–921, 1988.
229. Sarosi, G. A., and Johnson, P. C.: Disseminated histoplasmosis in patients infected with human immunodeficiency virus. Clin. Infect. Dis. *14*(Suppl. 1):60–67, 1992.
230. Sarosi, G. A., Parker, J. D., and Rosh, F. E.: Histoplasmosis outbreaks: Their patterns. *In* Histoplasmosis Proceedings of the Second National Conference. Springfield, IL, Charles C Thomas, 1971.
231. Sathapatayavongs, B., Batteiger, B. E., Wheat, L. J., et al.: Clinical and laboratory features of disseminated histoplasmosis during two large urban outbreaks. Medicine (Baltimore) *62*:263–270, 1983.
232. Schlaegel, T. F.: Update on ocular histoplasmosis. Ophthalmol. Clin. *23*:1, 1983.
233. Schlech, W. F., 3rd, Wheat, L. J., Ho, J. L., et al.: Recurrent urban histoplasmosis, Indianapolis, Indiana, 1980–1981. Am. J. Epidemiol. *118*:301–312, 1983.
234. Schnur, R. A., and Newman, S. L.: The respiratory burst response to *Histoplasma capsulatum* by human neutrophils. Evidence for intracellular trapping of superoxide anion. J. Immunol. *144*:4765–4772, 1990.
235. Schulman, R. L., McKiernan, B. C., and Schaeffer, D. J.: Use of corticosteroids for testing dogs with airway obstruction secondary to hilar lymphadenopathy caused by chronic histoplasmosis: 16 cases (1979–1997). J. Am. Vet. Med. Assoc. *214*:1345–1348, 1999.
236. Schulz, D. M.: Histoplasmosis of the central nervous system. J. A. M. A. *151*:549–551, 1953.
237. Schutze, G. E., Tucker, N. C., and Jacobs, R. F.: Histoplasmosis and perinatal human immunodeficiency virus. Pediatr. Infect. Dis. J. *11*:501–502, 1992.
238. Schwarz, J., and Baum, G. L.: The history of histoplasmosis, 1906 to 1956. N. Engl. J. Med. *256*:255–258, 1957.
239. Sellers, T. F., Jr., Price, W. N., Jr., and Newberry, W. M., Jr.: An epidemic of erythema multiforme and erythema nodosum caused by histoplasmosis. Ann. Intern. Med. *62*:1244–1262, 1965.
240. Shapiro, J. L., Lux, J. J., and Sprofkin, B. E.: Histoplasmosis of the central nervous system. Am. J. Pathol. *31*:319–330, 1955.
241. Shearer, W. T.: Presumptive histoplasmosis presenting as cerebellar ataxia with spontaneous recovery. Pediatrics *57*:150–152, 1976.
242. Sherrick, A. D., Brown, L. R., Harms, G. F., et al.: The radiographics findings of fibrosing mediastinitis. Chest *106*:484–489, 1994.
243. Sills, M., Schwartz, A., and Weg, J. G.: Conjugal histoplasmosis: A consequence of progressive dissemination in the index case after steroid therapy. Ann. Intern. Med. *79*:221–224, 1973.
244. Slama, T. G.: Treatment of disseminated and progressive cavitary histoplasmosis with ketoconazole. Am. J. Med. *74*(1B):70–73, 1983.
245. Smith, C. D.: The role of birds in the ecology of *Histoplasma capsulatum. In* Histoplasmosis. Proceedings of the Second National Conference. Springfield, IL, Charles C Thomas, 1971.
246. Smith, J. G., Magee, D. M., Williams, D. M., et al.: Tumor necrosis factor-alpha plays a role in host defense against *Histoplasma capsulatum.* J. Infect. Dis. *162*:1349–1353, 1990.
247. Smith, J. W., and Utz, J. P.: Progressive disseminated histoplasmosis. Ann. Intern. Med. *76*:557–565, 1972.
248. Sobel, J. D., and Muller, G.: Comparison of itraconazole and ketoconazole in the treatment of experimental candidal vaginitis. Antimicrob. Agents Chemother. *26*:266–267, 1984.

249. Spitzer, E. D., Keath, E. J., Travis, S. J., et al.: Temperature-sensitive variants of *Histoplasma capsulatum* isolated from patients with acquired immunodeficiency syndrome. J. Infect. Dis. *162*:258–261, 1990.
250. Steele, C. J., and Kleiman, M. B.: Disseminated histoplasmosis, hypercalcemia and failure to thrive. Pediatr. Infect. Dis. J. *13*:421–422, 1994.
251. Stone, J. H., Pomper, M. G., and Hellmann, D. B.: Histoplasmosis mimicking vasculitis of the central nervous system. J. Rheumatol. *25*:1644–1648, 1998.
252. Straub, M., and Schwarz, J.: Healed primary complex in histoplasmosis. Am. J. Clin. Pathol. *25*:727, 1955.
253. Strayer, D. S., Gutwein, M. B., Herbold, D., et al.: Histoplasmosis presenting as the carpal tunnel syndrome. Am. J. Surg. *141*:286–288, 1981.
254. Suh, K. N., Anekthannaon, T., and Mariuz, P. R.: Gastrointestinal histoplasmosis in patients with AIDS: Case report and review. Clin. Infect. Dis. *32*:485–491, 2001.
255. Sutliff, W. D.: Histoplasmosis cooperative study 4. Amphotericin B dosage for chronic pulmonary histoplasmosis. Am. Rev. Respir. Dis. *105*:60–67, 1972.
256. Suttorp-Schulten, M. S., Bollemeijer, J. G., Box, P. J., et al.: Presumed ocular histoplasmosis in the Netherlands—an area without histoplasmosis. Br. J. Ophthalmol. *81*:1, 1997.
257. Swartz, M. A., Scofield, R. H., Dickey, W. D., et al.: Unilateral adrenal enlargement due to *Histoplasma capsulatum*. Clin. Infect. Dis. *23*:813–815, 1996.
258. Taylor, M. I., Chavez-Tapia, C. B., Vargas-Yanez, R., et al.: Environmental conditions favoring bat infection with *Histoplasma capsulatum* in Mexican shelters. Am. J. Trop. Med. Hyg. *61*:914–919, 1999.
259. Taylor, M. L., Diaz, S., Gonzalez, P. A., et al.: Relationship between pathogenesis and immune regulation mechanisms in histoplasmosis: A hypothetical approach. Rev. Infect. Dis. *6*:775–782, 1984.
260. Taylor, R. L., Williams, D. M., Craven, P. C., et al.: Amphotericin B in liposomes: A novel therapy for histoplasmosis. Am. Rev. Respir. Dis. *125*:610–611, 1982.
261. Tebib, J. G., Piens, M. A., Guillaux, M., et al.: Sarcoidosis possibly predisposing to disseminated histoplasmosis. Thorax *43*:73–74, 1988.
262. Tegeris, A. S., and Smith, D. T.: Acute disseminated pulmonary histoplasmosis treated with cortisone and MRID-112. Ann. Intern. Med. *48*:1414, 1958.
263. Terry, P. B., Rosenow, E. C., and Roberts, G. D.: False-positive complement fixation serology in histoplasmosis. J. A. M. A. *238*:2453–2456, 1978.
264. Tesh, R. B., and Schneidau, J. C., Jr.: Primary cutaneous histoplasmosis. N. Engl. J. Med. *275*:597, 1966.
265. Tobon, A. M., Franco, L., Espinal, D., et al.: Disseminated histoplasmosis in children: The role of itraconazole therapy. Pediatr. Infect. Dis. J. *15*:1002–1008, 1996.
266. Tucker, W. S., Jr., Snell, B. B., Island, D. P., et al.: Reversible adrenal insufficiency induced by ketoconazole. J. A. M. A. *253*: 2413–2414, 1985.
267. Tutor, J. D., Schoumacher, R. A., and Chesney, P. J.: Chylothorax associated with histoplasmosis in a child. Pediatr. Infect. Dis. J. *19*:262–263, 2000.
268. Uemura, A., and Thomas, M. A.: Visual outcome after surgical removal of choroidal neovascularization in pediatric patients. Arch. Ophthalmol. *118*:1373–1378, 2000.
269. Urschel, H. C., Jr., Razzuk, M. A., Netto, G. J., et al.: Sclerosing mediastinitis: Improved management with histoplasmosis titer and ketoconazole. Ann. Thorac. Surg. *50*:215–221, 1990.
270. U. S. Department of Health and Human Services: Histoplasmosis: Protecting Workers at Risk. Washington, D.C., National Institute of Occupational Safety and Health, 1997, DHHS (NIOSH) Publication 97-146.
271. Utz, J. P.: Chemotherapy of the systemic mycoses. Med. Clin. North Am. *66*:221–233, 1982.
272. Vail, G. M., Filo, R. S., Cornetta, K., et al.: Incidence of histoplasmosis following allogeneic bone marrow transplant or solid organ transplant in a hyperendemic area, Abstract #346, Program and Abstracts of the Infectious Disease Society of American 36th Annual Meeting, Denver CO, November 12–15. Clin. Infect. Dis. *27*:986, 1998.
273. Vail, G. M., Mocherla, S., Wheat, L. F., et al.: Cellular immune response in HIV-infected patients with histoplasmosis. J. Acquir. Immune Defic. Syndr. *29*:49–53, 2002.
274. Van Cauteren, H., Heykants, J., De Coster, R., et al.: Itraconazole: Pharmacologic studies in animals and humans. Rev. Infect. Dis. *9*(Suppl. 1):43–46, 1987.
275. Vandiviere, H. M., Goodman, N. L., Melvin, I. G., et al.: Histoplasmosis in Kentucky: Can it be prevented? J. Ky. Med. Assoc. *79*:719–726, 1981.
276. Villaret, L., Fries, R., Kolhekar, S., et al.: Impaired responsiveness to gamma interferon of macrophages infected with lymphocytic choriomeningitis virus clone 13: Susceptibility to histoplasmosis. Infect. Immun. *63*:1468–1472, 1995.
277. Vincent, R., Goewert, R., Goldman, W. E., et al.: Classification of *Histoplasma capsulatum* isolates by restriction fragment polymorphisms. J. Bacteriol. *165*:813–818, 1986.
278. Vos, M. J., Debets-Ossenkopp, Y. J., Claessenn, F. A. P., et al.: Cerebellar and medullar histoplasmosis. Neurology *54*:141, 2000.
279. Ward, J. I., Weeks, M., Allen, D., et al.: Acute histoplasmosis: Clinical, epidemiologic and serologic findings of an outbreak associated with exposure to a fallen tree. Am. J. Med. *66*:587–595, 1979.
280. Watzke, R. C., Kleiman, M. L., and Wener, M. H.: Histoplasmosis-like choroiditis in a nonendemic area: The northwest United States. Retina *18*:204–212, 1998.
281. Weber, T. R., Grosfeld, J. L., Kleiman, M. B., et al.: Surgical implications of endemic histoplasmosis in children. J. Pediatr. Surg. *18*:486–491, 1983.
282. Weinberg, G. A., Kleiman, M. B., Grosfeld, J. L., et al.: Unusual manifestations of histoplasmosis in childhood. Pediatrics *72*:99–105, 1983.
283. Wheat, L. J.: Histoplasmosis. Infect. Dis. Clin. North Am. *2*:841, 1988.
284. Wheat, L. J.: Diagnosis and management of histoplasmosis. Eur. J. Clin. Microbiol. Infect. Dis. *8*:480, 1989.
285. Wheat, J.: Histoplasmosis in Indianapolis. Clin. Infect. Dis. *14*(Suppl.):91–99, 1992.
286. Wheat, J.: Histoplasmosis: Recognition and treatment. Clin. Infect. Dis. *19*(Suppl.):19–27, 1994.
287. Wheat, L. J: Histoplasmosis in the acquired immunodeficiency syndrome. Curr. Top. Med. Mycol. *7*:7–18, 1996.
288. Wheat, L. J.: Laboratory diagnosis of histoplasmosis: Update 2000. Semin. Respir. Infect. *16*:131–140, 2001.
289. Wheat, L. J., Batteiger, B. E., and Sathapatayavongs, B.: *Histoplasma capsulatum* infections of the central nervous system. A clinical review. Medicine (Baltimore) *69*:244–260, 1990.
290. Wheat, L. J., and Butkus-Small, C.: Disseminated histoplasmosis in the acquired immune deficiency syndrome. Arch. Intern. Med. *144*:2147–2149, 1984.
291. Wheat, L. J., Chetchotisakd, P., Williams, B., et al.: Factors associated with severe manifestations of histoplasmosis in AIDS. Clin. Infect. Dis. *30*:877–881, 2000.
292. Wheat, L. J., Cloud, G., Johnson, P. C., et al.: Clearance of fungal burden during treatment of disseminated histoplasmosis in liposomal amphotericin B verus itraconazole. Antimicrob. Agents Chemother. *45*:2354–2357, 2001.
293. Wheat, L. J., Connolly, P., Haddad, N., et al.: Antigen clearance during treatment of disseminated histoplasmosis with itraconazole versus fluconazole in patients with AIDS. Antimicrob. Agents Chemother. *46*:248–250, 2002.
294. Wheat, L. J., Connolly-Stringfield, P. A., Baker, R. I., et al.: Disseminated histoplasmosis in the acquired immune deficiency syndrome. Clinical findings, diagnosis and treatment, and review of the literature. Medicine (Baltimore) *69*:361–374, 1990.
295. Wheat, L. J., Connolly-Stringfield, P., Blair, R., et al.: Histoplasmosis relapse in patients with AIDS: Detection using *Histoplasma capsulatum* variety *capsulatum* antigen levels. Ann. Intern. Med. *115*:936–941, 1991.
296. Wheat, L. J., Connolly-Stringfield, P., Blair, R., et al.: Effect of successful treatment with amphotericin B on *Histoplasma capsulatum* variety *capsulatum* polysaccharide antigen levels in patients with AIDS and histoplasmosis. Am. J. Med. *92*:153–160, 1992.
297. Wheat, L. J., Connolly-Stringfield, P., Kohler, R. B., et al.: *Histoplasma capsulatum* polysaccharide antigen detection in diagnosis and management of disseminated histoplasmosis in patients with acquired immunodeficiency syndrome. Am. J. Med. *87*:396–400, 1989.
298. Wheat, L. J., Connolly-Stringfield, P., Williams, B., et al.: Diagnosis of histoplasmosis in patients with the acquired immunodeficiency syndrome by detection of *Histoplasma capsulatum* polysaccharide antigen in bronchoalveolar lavage fluid. Am. Rev. Respir. Dis. *145*:1421–1424, 1992.
299. Wheat, L. J., and French, M. L. V.: Diagnosis of histoplasmosis (in response to letter). Ann. Intern. Med. *98*:260, 1983.
300. Wheat, L. J., French, M. L., Batteiger, B., et al.: Cerebrospinal fluid *Histoplasma* antibodies in central nervous system histoplasmosis. Arch. Intern. Med. *145*:1237, 1985.
301. Wheat, L. J., French, M. L. V., Kamel, S., et al.: Evaluation of cross-reactions in *Histoplasma capsulatum* serologic tests. J. Clin. Microbiol. *23*:493–499, 1986.
302. Wheat, L. J., French, M. L. V., Kohler, R. B., et al.: The diagnostic laboratory tests for histoplasmosis. Ann. Intern. Med. *97*:680–685, 1982.
303. Wheat, J., Hafner, R., Korzun, A. H., et al.: Itraconazole treatment of disseminated histoplasmosis in patients with the acquired immunodeficiency syndrome. Am. J. Med. *98*:336–342, 1995.
304. Wheat, L. J., Hafner, R., Wulfsohn, M., et al.: Prevention of relapse of histoplasmosis with itraconazole in patients with the acquired immunodeficiency syndrome. Ann. Intern. Med. *118*:610–616, 1993.
305. Wheat, L. J., Kohler, R. B., French, M. L. V., et al.: Immunoglobulin M and G *Histoplasma* antibody response in histoplasmosis. Am. Rev. Respir. Dis. *128*:65–70, 1982.
306. Wheat, L. J., Kohler, R. B., and Tewari, R. P.: Diagnosis of disseminated histoplasmosis by detection of *Histoplasma capsulatum* in serum and urine specimens. N. Engl. J. Med. *314*:83–88, 1986.
307. Wheat, L. J., Kohler, R. B., Tewari, R. P., et al.: Significance of *Histoplasma* antigen in the cerebrospinal fluid of patients with meningitis. Arch. Intern. Med. *149*:302–304, 1989.
308. Wheat, J., Marichal, P., Vanden Bossche, H., et al.: Hypothesis on the mechanism of resistance to fluconazole in *Histoplasma capsulatum*. Antimicrob. Agents Chemother. *41*:410–414, 1997.

309. Wheat, J., MaWhinney, S., Hafner, R., et al.: Treatment of histoplasmosis with fluconazole in patients with acquired immunodeficiency syndrome. National Institute of Allergy and Infectious Disease Acquired Immunodeficiency Syndrome Clinical Trials Group and Mycoses Study Group. Am. J. Med. *103*:223–232, 1997.
310. Wheat, J., Sarosi, G., McKinsey, D., et al.: Practice guidelines for the management of patients with histoplasmosis. Clin. Infect. Dis. *30*:688–695, 2000.
311. Wheat, L. J., Slama, T. G., Eitzen, H. E., et al.: A large urban outbreak of histoplasmosis: Clinical features. Ann. Intern. Med. *94*:331–337, 1981.
312. Wheat, L. J., Slama, T. G., and Zeckel, M. L.: Histoplasmosis in the acquired immune deficiency syndrome. Am. J. Med. *78*:203–210, 1985.
313. Wheat, L. J., and Small, C. B.: Disseminated histoplasmosis in the acquired immunodeficiency syndrome. Arch. Intern. Med. *144*:2147–2149, 1984.
314. Wheat, L. J., Smith, E. J., Sathapatayavongs, B., et al.: Histoplasmosis in renal allograft recipients. Two large urban outbreaks. Arch. Intern. Med. *143*:703–707, 1983.
315. Wheat, L. J., Wass, J., Norton, J., et al.: Cavitary histoplasmosis occurring during two large urban outbreaks: Analysis of clinical, epidemiologic, roentgenographic, and laboratory features. Medicine (Baltimore) *63*:201–209, 1984.
316. Wheat, J., Wheat, H., Connolly, P., et al.: Cross-reactivity in *Histoplasma capsulatum* variety *capsulatum* antigen assays of urine samples from patients with endemic mycoses. Clin. Infect. Dis. *24*:1169–1171, 1997.
317. Whitehouse, W. M., Davey, W. M., Engelke, O. K., et al.: Roentgen findings in histoplasmin-positive school children. J. Mich. Med. Soc. *58*:1266, 1959.
318. Wilcox, K. R., Waisbren, B. A., and Martin, J.: The Walworth, Wisconsin, epidemic of histoplasmosis. Ann. Intern. Med. *49*:338, 1958.
319. Williams, A. O., Lawson, E. A., and Lucas, A. O.: African histoplasmosis due to *Histoplasma duboisii*. Arch. Pathol. *87*:306–318, 1969.
320. Williams, B., Fojtasek, M., Connolly-Stringfield, P., et al.: Diagnosis of histoplasmosis by antigen detection during an outbreak in Indianapolis, Ind. Arch. Pathol. Lab. Med. *118*:1205–1208, 1994.
321. Williams, K. R., and Burford, T. H.: Surgical treatment of granulomatous paratracheal lymphadenopathy. J. Thorac. Cardiovasc. Surg. *48*:13, 1964.
322. Wilson, D. A., Nguyen, C. L., and Tytle T. L., et al.: Sonography of the adrenal glands in chronic disseminated histoplasmosis. J. Ultrasound Med. *5*:69–73, 1986.
323. Woods, J. P., Heinecke, E. L., Luecke, J. W., et al.: Pathogenesis of *Histoplasma capsulatum*. Semin. Respir Infect. *16*:91–101, 2001.
324. Woods, L. P.: Mediastinal granuloma causing tracheal compression in a 4-year-old child. Surgery *58*:448, 1965.
325. Woods, W. G., Singher, L. J., Krivit, W., et al.: Histoplasmosis simulating lymphoma in children. J. Pediatr. Surg. *14*:423–425, 1979.
326. Wu-Hsieh, B. A., Lee, G. S., Franco, M., et al.: Early activation of splenic macrophages by tumor necrosis factor alpha is important in determining the outcome of experimental histoplasmosis in mice. Infect. Immun. *60*:4230–4238, 1992.
327. Wynne, J. W., and Olsen, G. N.: Acute histoplasmosis presenting as the adult respiratory distress syndrome. Chest *66*:158–161, 1974.
328. Young, E. J., Vainrub, B., and Musher, D. M.: Pericarditis due to histoplasmosis. J. A. M. A. *240*:1750–1751, 1978.
329. Zeidberg, L. D., Dillon, A., and Gass, R. S.: Some factors in the epidemiology of histoplasmin sensitivity in Williamson County, Tennessee. Am. J. Public Health *41*:80, 1951.
330. Zeiss, J., Woldenberg, L. S., Morgan, R., et al.: Pulmonary histoplasmoma presenting as massive hemoptysis. Pediatr. Infect. Dis. *6*:689–691, 1987.
331. Zhou, P., Freidag, B. L., Caldwell, C. C., et al.: Perforin is required for primary immunity to *Histoplasma capsulatum*. J. Immunol. *166*:1968–1974, 2001.
332. Zhou, P., Miller, G., and Seder, R. A.: Factors involved in regulating primary and secondary immunity to infection with *Histoplasma capsulatum:* TNF-alpha plays a critical role in maintaining secondary immunity in the absence of IFN-gamma. J. Immunol. *160*:1359–1368, 1998.
333. Zhou, P., Sieve, M. C., Bennett, J., et al.: IL-12 prevents mortality in mice infected with *Histoplasma capsulatum* through induction of IFN-gamma. J. Immunol. *155*:785–795, 1995.
334. Zhou, P., Sieve, M. C., Tewari, R. P., et al.: Interleukin-12 modulates the protective immune response in SCID mice infected with *Histoplasma capsulatum*. Infect. Immun. *65*:936–942, 1997.
335. Zimmerman, S. E., Stringfield, P. C., Wheat, L. J., et al.: Comparison of sandwich solid-phase radioimmunoassay and two enzyme-linked immunosorbent assays for detection of *Histoplasma capsulatum* polysaccharide antigen. J. Infect. Dis. *160*:678–685, 1989.

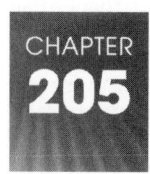

Sporotrichosis

BERNHARD L. WIEDERMANN

Sporotrichosis is an infection caused by the fungus *Sporothrix schenckii* that is manifested most commonly as an ulcerating nodule at a site of local trauma, with spread along regional lymphatic channels. Infection of other tissues or widespread dissemination is a rare occurrence. It is a relatively uncommon problem in children, but young adults appear to be infected more frequently, presumably owing to more frequent exposure to soil, plants, and decaying vegetable matter that harbor the organism. The disease first was described by a medical student, Benjamin Schenck, in 1898, and most of what is known about the clinical syndrome has been learned from study of large outbreaks, particularly one occurring in gold miners near Johannesburg, South Africa, in the early 1940s.[67, 76]

The Organism

S. schenckii is a dimorphic fungus found principally in decaying vegetable matter or plant debris, even though it does not appear to be a plant pathogen. It grows well on most culture media and is resistant to cycloheximide. Preferred culture media are Sabouraud glucose agar and blood agar, incubated at 25° to 27° C. Most isolates grow readily from clinical material within 3 to 5 days, although occasional instances of slow growth have been reported, and cultures should be held at least 4 weeks before being called negative. Incubation on blood agar at higher temperatures (37° C) allows growth of the yeast phase, which is necessary for specific identification of the organism in culture.[63]

Epidemiology

Most cases of sporotrichosis are reported from Central and South America, especially from Mexico and Brazil, and cases in the United States appear to cluster in the Midwest, particularly along the Mississippi and Missouri River areas.[31, 58] Disease in humans usually results from inoculation of minor wounds by debris containing *S. schenckii*, and thus gardeners and nursery workers, forestry workers, miners, and other people exposed to contaminated plant materials are at higher risk for acquiring the disease.[11, 15] Disseminated disease has been the initial presentation of some human immunodeficiency virus–infected individuals.[2] Laboratory personnel working with the organism have become infected after incurring needle-stick injuries.[75] The large South African epidemic in the gold mines of Transvaal probably resulted from the miners' brushing against rotting timbers in the mines, and a cluster of cases after a brick-throwing incident in Florida was traced to *S. schenckii* in the packing straw of the bricks.[65, 76] Contaminated hay was the source of one outbreak linked to a Halloween haunted house.[21] Pulmonary disease may result from inhalation of spores.[58] Uncommonly, transmission of disease from animals, particularly domestic cats with cutaneous disease, or from family members occurs.[23, 27, 28, 61] One adult acquired the disease after being bitten by a squirrel.[66] In South America, armadillo hunters are at risk for developing sporotrichosis, but it has been shown to be acquired from the decaying plant debris in armadillo nests rather than from the animals themselves.[51] DNA typing of isolates can be useful in investigations of outbreaks.[14]

Pathogenesis and Pathology

As indicated, the most common mode of acquisition of sporotrichosis is by inoculation of the organism into skin structures, although disease also may develop from inhalation of spores of the organism. The incubation period varies considerably, commonly ranging from 7 to 30 days after cutaneous inoculation, but possibly as long as 6 months.[63] The disease usually remains relatively localized: of the 2825 cases of sporotrichosis in the Transvaal mine epidemic, none had systemic spread.[76]

S. schenckii, like other yeasts, appears to bind specifically to the glycosphingolipid lactosylceramide, which is present on the cell surface of animal cells.[39] This mechanism may be one by which the organism establishes a foothold in the host. Cell-mediated immune responses probably are important for containment of infection. One study documented intact responses in patients with cutaneous forms of the disease, whereas patients with systemic sporotrichosis had impaired cell-mediated immunity.[57] This study is supported by the observation that systemic disease tends to occur in people with underlying diseases that alter cell-mediated immunity.

Histopathologic examination of primary cutaneous lesions usually reveals changes in the epithelium, with hyperkeratosis, parakeratosis, and pseudoepitheliomatous hyperplasia. Intraepidermal microabscesses may be seen as well. In more established lesions, the pathologic process involves the dermis and below, with inflammatory infiltrate extending perivascularly.[49] The classic lesion on microscopic examination is a granuloma with an asteroid body at the center, although this picture is not pathognomonic for sporotrichosis. The asteroid body is an antigen-antibody complex deposited on the surface of the organism.[48] Unfortunately, demonstrating fungi in tissue sections often is difficult, even with special staining techniques, because of the paucity of organisms in tissue. They may be seen on Gram stain as gram-positive but irregularly staining bodies, sometimes as cigar-shaped 3- to 5-μm yeast forms. Periodic acid–Schiff and silver stains probably are better suited for detection of fungi in tissue sections.[49, 63] Immunohistochemical staining techniques may prove superior to standard methods.[52, 55]

Clinical Manifestations

Sporotrichosis can occur in both cutaneous and extracutaneous forms, with the cutaneous varieties accounting for about 80 percent of all cases.[63] These categories can be broken down further into the organ system involved (Table 205–1).

TABLE 205–1 ■ CLINICAL FORMS OF SPOROTRICHOSIS

Cutaneous	Extracutaneous
Lymphocutaneous	Osteoarticular
Fixed cutaneous	Pulmonary
	Muscular
	Ocular
	Genitourinary
	Central nervous system

Data from references 1, 33, 34, 45, 58, 64.

CUTANEOUS SPOROTRICHOSIS

Cutaneous disease with *S. schenckii* can be either lymphocutaneous or fixed cutaneous, with the fixed cutaneous form occurring less frequently. In lymphocutaneous cases, the initial lesion appears as a firm, slightly tender subcutaneous nodule. It progresses along local lymphatic channels, with multiple nodules appearing. The lesions typically enlarge and then may ulcerate and suppurate (Fig. 205–1). Untreated, they may heal slowly over months or persist, and recurrences are frequent. Differential diagnosis includes cutaneous nocardiosis, atypical mycobacterial disease, leishmaniasis, rosacea, syphilis, and pyoderma gangrenosum as well as cutaneous manifestations of other fungal diseases.[19, 43, 74, 82]

The fixed cutaneous form of the disease is just as the name implies, with no evidence of lymphatic spread. The primary lesions are identical to those seen in the lymphocutaneous form. Although some researchers have suggested that sporotrichosis in childhood is more likely to appear in the fixed cutaneous form, compared with adults, this theory has not been borne out in prior studies. Table 205–2 shows results from six reports of series of cases of sporotrichosis in childhood. The 60 percent rate for the lymphocutaneous form may not differ much from the 90 percent figure quoted

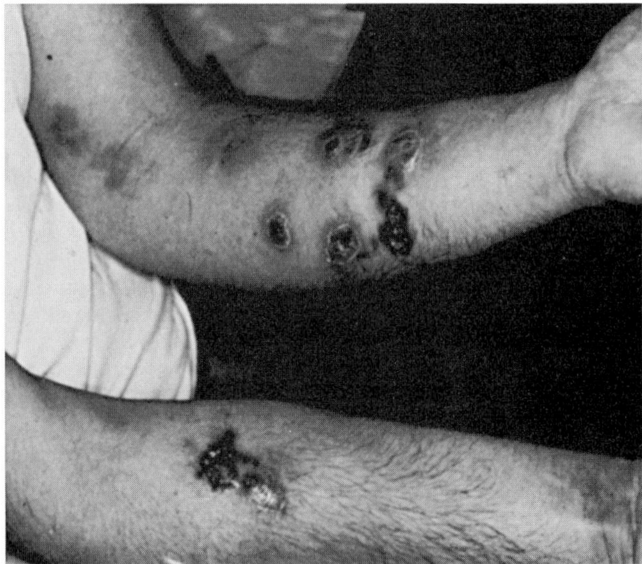

FIGURE 205–1 ■ Cutaneous lymphatic sporotrichosis of both arms. Note the characteristic involvement of lymphatics that drain the sites of the primary lesions. (Courtesy of G. Medoff and G. S. Kobayashi.)

TABLE 205–2 ■ SUMMARY OF 42 CASES OF PEDIATRIC SPOROTRICHOSIS

Duration of symptoms before diagnosis	3–10 weeks
Lymphatic involvement	28/47*
Culture-positive	39/44
Relapse after therapy	1/21

*Numerator is number of patients positive; denominator is number of patients tested.
Data from references 9, 12, 17, 30, 50, and 53.

for adults when one takes into account that many pediatric studies are reports of small numbers of cases and may have resulted from selection bias. A large series of patients from Peru documented a disproportionate number of children with facial lesions (86 of 143 children versus 23 of 95 adults) but did not classify fixed versus lymphocutaneous forms by age.[56] Fixed cutaneous disease in children has been confused with impetigo.[9] A recent study from Peru also documented a predilection of children to develop lymphocutaneous lesions on the face and neck.[50a] Risk factors for disease in children in this study included playing in fields, ownership of a cat, and residence in a house with dirt floors.

EXTRACUTANEOUS SPOROTRICHOSIS

Sporotrichosis occurring in extracutaneous sites may either be localized (related to an unusual area of trauma) or represent disseminated disease. In the absence of trauma, the presence of extracutaneous sporotrichosis should raise suspicion of disseminated disease and consideration of immunodeficiency states. Overall, infection of bones and joints is the most common form of extracutaneous disease.[80] Sporotrichal arthritis usually is an indolent and slowly progressive disease that may occur with or without cutaneous or lymphatic disease, which suggests a hematogenous route of infection for most cases. Diagnosis generally requires synovial biopsy with culture for demonstrating the organism.[68, 80] Two studies showed diagnostic delays averaging 17 and 25 months, respectively, from the onset of symptoms.[5, 16] Sporotrichal osteomyelitis usually occurs with concomitant arthritis, but isolated bone involvement has been recorded. Lytic lesions and periosteal changes are noted most frequently.[32, 80]

Pulmonary sporotrichosis seldom occurs with cases of disseminated disease and probably develops after inhalation of spores, as with primary pulmonary histoplasmosis.[58] The presence of cavitary lesions in the upper lobes often leads to a diagnosis of tuberculosis, and fungal culture of sputum, bronchoscopic specimens, lung tissue, or gastric aspirate usually is needed for diagnosis.[24, 58, 78] Pleural involvement is an uncommon occurrence (3 of 47 cases in one review), and complications such as massive hemoptysis rarely occur.[25, 35, 58]

Sporotrichosis has been found to involve virtually every organ system in the body as part of disseminated disease.[80] Most commonly, underlying immunodeficiency states, such as diabetes, prolonged steroid therapy, alcoholism, and acquired immunodeficiency syndrome, are present.[1, 26, 33, 36, 45, 73, 80] Fungemia in the absence of disseminated disease has been documented in one otherwise healthy adult with a lysis-centrifugation blood culture system.[44] Interestingly, dissemination in patients with neoplasia seldom occurs.

Diagnosis

A high index of suspicion is necessary to make the diagnosis of sporotrichosis. In the largest outbreak in the United States, which occurred in 1988 among horticulturists and forestry workers, only 15 percent of cases were diagnosed at the time of initial presentation to a physician.[13] Culture is the gold standard for diagnosing sporotrichosis. Although organisms occasionally are seen on pathologic specimens, the yield is low enough to render biopsy unnecessary. If the diagnosis is suspected, scrapings of cutaneous lesions for culture should be sufficient to establish the diagnosis.[63]

Serodiagnosis has been explored in recent years. A skin test antigen has been available for many years, but, as with the histoplasmin skin test for histoplasmosis, it is useful mainly as an epidemiologic tool. Immunoprecipitation or commercially available slide latex agglutination can be useful when material for culture is difficult to obtain or cultures are negative, such as with sporotrichal meningitis.[20, 69] Similarly, an enzyme-linked immunosorbent assay has been used for diagnosis. Antibody titers in cerebrospinal fluid tend to fall with successful therapy, and such tests might prove useful for monitoring response to therapy.[69] Western blotting has been used to detect sporotrichal antibody.[70] Using a crude antigen preparation, Scott and Muchmore[70] determined that detection of antibody to three antigens, 32, 40 and 70 kd, appears to be both sensitive and specific for diagnosis of active sporotrichosis. Furthermore, patients with extracutaneous disease appeared to form antibody to a greater number of *S. schenckii* organisms than did those with cutaneous disease. Further studies of the immune response in sporotrichosis should enable development of better serodiagnostic tests than those that now are routinely available.

Treatment and Prognosis

Sporotrichosis may resolve spontaneously, but treatment is indicated in most circumstances.[4, 59] The Mycoses Study Group of the Infectious Diseases Society of America has published practice guidelines for management of patients with sporotrichosis.[42]

Heat applied to the site of cutaneous disease has been reported anecdotally to cause resolution of lesions in patients in whom medical therapy was contraindicated.[29, 64, 77] One prospective study demonstrated good results using benzene pocket warmers for heat therapy of facial lesions in children.[37] Surgical removal of infected skin and soft tissue has been used, but skin grafting may be required.[8] This form of treatment usually is unnecessary with the availability of medical management, except possibly for some cases of pulmonary infection (particularly if it is confined to one lobe) and other extracutaneous disease.[16, 32, 58] Hyperthermia remains an option for treating sporotrichosis in pregnancy, for which other agents may be contraindicated.[42]

A saturated solution of potassium iodide (SSKI), a proteolytic agent for which the mechanism of action in sporotrichosis is unclear,[47] can be used for uncomplicated sporotrichosis. The in vitro growth of *S. schenckii* is not inhibited appreciably by iodide, but free iodine has a marked inhibitory effect on growth.[79] The small amount of free iodine in a saturated solution of potassium iodide may be sufficient to cause resolution of disease. The pediatric dosage of a saturated solution of potassium iodide is somewhat empiric, but it usually is given three times daily in juice or milk, starting at a low dose (e.g., 1 to 2 drops per year of age) and increasing the dose over the course of several days to a maximum of 30 to 40 drops per dose.[12, 50, 53] For younger children, lower dosages may be acceptable.[50, 60] Treatment is continued until a few weeks after all lesions have resolved. Adverse reactions, such as salivary gland swelling, excessive lacrimation or salivation, nausea, vomiting, and abdominal pain, may resolve with temporary cessation of therapy followed by reinstitution at a lower dosage. SSKI currently is only an alternative treatment for lymphocutaneous and cutaneous forms of the disease.[42]

Itraconazole, an oral azole derivative, is the drug of choice for treatment of cutaneous, lymphocutaneous, and osteoarticular forms of sporotrichosis.[7, 40, 41, 42, 72] Restrepo and colleagues[62] showed clinical cures in all 17 patients with cutaneous forms of sporotrichosis treated with itraconazole (100 mg/day), with no major side effects. However, Borelli[6] reported a treatment failure in a patient treated with 100 mg/day who subsequently responded when the dose was increased to 200 mg/day. Systemic disease also has been treated with itraconazole with favorable clinical responses, although all information is from cases in adults.[3, 46, 54, 72, 81]

Intravenous amphotericin B remains the drug of choice for treating patients with disseminated or severe sporotrichosis.[42, 80] Duration of therapy in children has not been studied but probably should require 30 mg/kg as a total dose. Occasionally, intra-articular amphotericin B is used for treating sporotrichal arthritis if response to other therapy is poor.[22] Amphotericin B therapy in patients with pulmonary sporotrichosis is less effective than with other forms of sporotrichosis, which has prompted many clinicians to use a combined medical-surgical approach.[42, 58] Itraconazole is an alternative therapy and may be useful for long-term suppression.[42] Amphotericin B appears to be effective in treating sporotrichal meningitis when it is given early in the course of the disease, but adjunctive therapy with flucytosine or rifampin might be helpful.[68] Itraconazole and fluconazole also may have roles in treating meningitis.[40, 42]

S. schenckii does not appear to be particularly susceptible to ketoconazole in vitro, and clinical experience with ketoconazole treatment of sporotrichosis has been mixed.[10, 18, 71] Possibly, relatively large doses of ketoconazole are needed to produce a good clinical response. Terbinafine, an allylamine, cured five adults with cutaneous sporotrichosis, but further experience with this agent is needed.[38]

Prognosis for cutaneous forms of disease is excellent, but the extracutaneous forms are associated with significant morbidity and mortality, in part related to the underlying conditions predisposing these patients to disseminated disease. Many cases of osteoarticular disease result in permanent disability.[16]

Prevention

The key to prevention of sporotrichosis is the elimination of exposure to the organism, particularly with regard to skin surfaces and mucous membranes. Usually, it can be accomplished by the use of protective clothing during high-risk procedures, such as working with sphagnum moss or other decaying, moist plant material.[11, 13] Nursery workers should be educated about the hazards and early signs of sporotrichosis, and physicians and veterinarians should be aware of the uncommon circumstances of spread of the infection from family members and domestic cats. The epidemic in the Transvaal gold mines was stopped when timbers in the mine shafts were sprayed with a fungicide.[76] Although reporting of individual cases of sporotrichosis is not required in the United States, reporting of clusters of cases can aid epidemiologic investigations and stop the spread of the disease.

REFERENCES

1. Agger, W. A., Caplan, R. H., and Maki, D. G.: Ocular sporotrichosis mimicking mucormycosis in a diabetic. Ann. Ophthalmol. *10*:767, 1978.
2. al-Tawfiq J. A., and Wools, K. K. Disseminated sporotrichosis and *Sporothrix schenckii* fungemia as the initial presentation of human immunodeficiency virus infection. Clin. Infect. Dis. *26*:1403, 1998.
3. Baker, J. H., Goodpasture, H. C., Kuhns, H. R., Jr., et al.: Fungemia caused by an amphotericin B—resistant isolate of *Sporothrix schenckii*: Successful treatment with itraconazole. Arch. Pathol. Lab. Med. *113*:1279, 1989.
4. Bargman, H. B.: Sporotrichosis of the nose with spontaneous cure. Can. Med. Assoc. J. *124*:1027, 1981.
5. Bayer, A. S., Scott, V. J., and Guz, C. B.: Fungal arthritis. III. Sporotrichal arthritis. Semin. Arthritis Rheum. *9*:66, 1979.
6. Borelli, D.: A clinical trial of itraconazole in the treatment of deep mycoses and leishmaniasis. Rev. Infect. Dis. *9*(Suppl. 1):S57, 1987.
7. Breeling, J. L., and Weinstein, L.: Pulmonary sporotrichosis treated with itraconazole. Chest 103:313, 1993.
8. Bullpitt, P., and Weedon, D.: Sporotrichosis: A review of 39 cases. Pathology *10*:249, 1978.
9. Burch, J. M., Morelli, J. G., and Weston, W. L.: Unsuspected sporotrichosis in childhood. Pediatr. Infect. Dis. J. 20:442, 2001.
10. Calhoun, D. L., Waskin, H., White, M. P., et al.: Treatment of systemic sporotrichosis with ketoconazole. Rev. Infect. Dis. 13:47, 1991.
11. Centers for Disease Control: Multistate outbreak of sporotrichosis in seedling handlers, 1988. M. M. W. R. Morb. Mortal. Wkly. Rep. *37*:652, 1988.
12. Chandler, J. W., Jr., Kriel, R. L., and Tosh, F. E.: Childhood sporotrichosis. Am. J. Dis. Child. *115*:368, 1968.
13. Coles, F. B., Schuchat, A., Hibbs, J. R., et al.: A multistate outbreak of sporotrichosis associated with sphagnum moss. Am. J. Epidemiol. *136*:475, 1992.
14. Cooper, C. R., Jr., Breslin, B. J., Dixon, D. M., et al.: DNA typing of isolates associated with the 1988 sporotrichosis epidemic. J. Clin. Microbiol. *30*:1631, 1992.
15. Cote, T. R., Kasten, M. J., and England, A. C., III: Sporotrichosis in association with Arbor Day activities. N. Engl. J. Med. *319*:1290, 1988.
16. Crout, J. E., Brewer, N. S., and Tompkins, R. B.: Sporotrichosis arthritis: Clinical features in seven patients. Ann. Intern. Med. *86*:294, 1977.
17. Dahl, B. A., Silberfarb, P. M., Sarosi, G. A., et al.: Sporotrichosis in children: Report of an epidemic. J. A. M. A. *215*:1980, 1971.
18. Dall, L., and Salzman, G.: Treatment of pulmonary sporotrichosis with ketoconazole. Rev. Infect. Dis. *9*:795, 1987.
19. Day, T. W., Gibson, G. H., and Guin, J. D.: Rosacea-like sporotrichosis. Cutis *33*:549, 1984.
20. de Albornoz, M. B., Villanueva, E., and de Torres, E. D.: Application of immunoprecipitation techniques to the diagnosis of cutaneous and extracutaneous forms of sporotrichosis. Mycopathologia *85*:177, 1984.
21. Dooley, D. P., Bostic, P. S., and Beckius, M. L.: Spook house sporotrichosis. A point-source outbreak of sporotrichosis associated with hay bale props in a Halloween haunted-house. Arch. Intern. Med. *157*:1885, 1997.
22. Downs, N. J., Hinthorn, D. R., Mhatre, V. R., et al.: Intra-articular amphotericin B treatment of *Sporothrix schenckii* arthritis. Arch. Intern. Med. *149*:954, 1989.
23. Dunstan, R. W., Langham, R. F., Reimann, K. A., et al.: Feline sporotrichosis: A report of five cases with transmission to humans. J. Am. Acad. Dermatol. *15*:37, 1986.
24. England, D. M., and Hochholzer, L.: *Sporothrix* infection of the lung without cutaneous disease: Primary pulmonary sporotrichosis. Arch. Pathol. Lab. Med. *111*:298, 1987.
25. Fields, C. L., Ossorio, M. A., and Roy, T. M.: Empyema associated with pulmonary sporotrichosis. South. Med. J. 82:910, 1989.
26. Fitzpatrick, J. E., and Eubanks, S.: Acquired immunodeficiency syndrome presenting as disseminated cutaneous sporotrichosis. Int. J. Dermatol. *27*:406, 1988.
27. Frean, J. A., Isaacson, M., Miller, G. B., et al.: Sporotrichosis following a rodent bite: A case report. Mycopathologia *116*:5, 1991.
28. Frumkin, A., and Tesserand, M. E.: Sporotrichosis in a father and son. J. Am. Acad. Dermatol. 20:964, 1989.
29. Galiana, J., and Conti-Diaz, I. A.: Healing effects of heat and a rubefacient on nine cases of sporotrichosis. Sabouraudia *3*:64, 1963.
30. Gluckman, I.: Sporotrichosis in children. S. Afr. Med. J. 39:991, 1965.
31. Goncalves, A. P.: Geopathology of sporotrichosis. Int. J. Dermatol. *12*:115, 1973.
32. Govender, S., Rasool, M. N., and Ngcelwane, M.: Osseous sporotrichosis. J. Infect. *19*:273, 1989.
33. Gullberg, R. M., Quintanilla, A., Levin, M. L., et al.: Sporotrichosis: Recurrent cutaneous, articular, and central nervous system infection in a renal transplant recipient. Rev. Infect. Dis. *9*:369, 1987.
34. Halverson, P. B., Lahiri, S., Wojno, W. C., et al.: Sporotrichal arthritis presenting as granulomatous myositis. Arthritis Rheum. *28*:1425, 1985.
35. Haponik, E. F., Hill, M. K., and Craighead, C. C.: Case report: Pulmonary sporotrichosis with massive hemoptysis. Am. J. Med. Sci. *297*:251, 1989.

36. Heller, H. M., and Fuhrer, J.: Disseminated sporotrichosis in patients with AIDS: Case report and review of the literature. AIDS 5:1243, 1991.
37. Hiruma, M., Kawada, A., Noguchi, H., et al.: Hyperthermic treatment of sporotrichosis: Experimental use of infrared and far infrared rays. Mycoses *35*:293, 1992.
38. Hull, P. R., and Vismer, H. F.: Treatment of cutaneous sporotrichosis with terbinafine. Br. J. Dermatol. *126*(Suppl. 39):51, 1992.
39. Jimenez-Lucho, V., Ginsburg, V., and Krivan, H. C.: Cryptococcus neoformans, Candida albicans, and other fungi bind specifically to the glycosphingolipid lactosylceramide (GalB1—4GlcB1—1Cer), a possible adhesion receptor for yeasts. Infect. Immun. *58*:2085, 1990.
40. Kauffman, C. A.: Old and new therapies for sporotrichosis. Clin. Infect. Dis. *21*:981, 1995.
41. Kauffman, C. A.: Sporotrichosis. Clin. Infect. Dis. *29*:231, 1999.
42. Kauffman, C. A., Hajjeh, R., Chapman, S. W., et al.: Practice guidelines for the management of patients with sporotrichosis. Clin. Infect. Dis. *30*:684, 2000.
43. Kibbi, A. G., Karam, P. G., and Kurban, A. K.: Sporotrichoid leishmaniasis in patients from Saudi Arabia: Clinical and histologic features. J. Am. Acad. Dermatol. *17*:759, 1987.
44. Kosinski, R. M., Axelrod, P., Rex, J. H., et al.: Sporothrix schenckii fungemia without disseminated sporotrichosis. J. Clin. Microbiol. *30*:501, 1992.
45. Kurosawa, A., Pollock, S. C., Collins, M. P., et al.: Sporothrix schenckii endophthalmitis in a patient with human immunodeficiency virus infection. Arch. Ophthalmol. *106*:376, 1988.
46. Lavalle, P., Suchil, P., De Ovando, F., et al.: Itraconazole for deep mycoses: Preliminary experience in Mexico. Rev. Infect. Dis. *9*(Suppl. 1): S64, 1987.
47. Lieberman, J., and Kurnick, N. B.: Induction of proteolysis within purulent sputum by iodides. Clin. Res. *11*:81, 1963.
48. Lurie, H. I.: Histopathology of sporotrichosis: Notes on the nature of the asteroid body. Arch. Pathol. *75*:93, 1963.
49. Lurie, H. I., and Still, W. J. S.: The "capsule" of Sporotrichum schenckii and the evolution of the asteroid body: A light and electron microscopic study. Sabouraudia 7:64—70, 1969.
50. Lynch, P. J., and Botero, F.: Sporotrichosis in children. Am. J. Dis. Child. *122*:325, 1971.
50a. Lyon, G. M., Zurita, S., Casquero, I., et al.: Population-based surveillance and a case-control study of risk factors for endemic lymphocutaneous sporotrichosis in Peru. Clin. Infect. Dis. *36*:34, 2003.
51. Mackinnon, J. E., Conti-Diaz, I. A., Gezuele, E., et al.: Isolation of Sporothrix schenckii from nature and considerations on its pathogenicity and ecology. Sabouraudia 7:38, 1969.
52. Marques, M. E. A., Coelho, K. I. R., Sotto, M. N., et al.: Comparison between histochemical and immunohistochemical methods for diagnosis of sporotrichosis. J. Clin. Pathol. *45*:1089, 1992.
53. Orr, E. R., and Riley, H. D., Jr.: Sporotrichosis in childhood: Report of ten cases. J. Pediatr. 78:951, 1971.
54. Oscherwitz, S. L., and Rinaldi, M. G.: Disseminated sporotrichosis in a patient infected with human immunodeficiency virus. Clin. Infect. Dis. *15*:568, 1992.
55. Padhye, A. A., Kaufman, L., Durry, E., et al.: Fatal pulmonary sporotrichosis caused by Sporothrix schenckii var. luriei in India. J. Clin. Microbiol. *30*:2492, 1992.
56. Pappas, P. G., Tellez, I., Deep, A. E., et al.: Sporotrichosis in Peru: Description of an area of hyperendemicity. Clin. Infect. Dis. 30:65, 2000.
57. Plourre, J. F., Jr., Silva, J., Jr., Fekety, R., et al.: Cell-mediated immune responses in sporotrichosis. J. Infect. Dis. *139*:152, 1979.
58. Pluss, J. L., and Opal, S. M.: Pulmonary sporotrichosis: Review of treatment and outcome. Medicine *65*:143:1986.
59. Pueringer, R. J., Iber, C., Deike, M. A., et al.: Spontaneous remission of extensive pulmonary sporotrichosis. Ann. Intern. Med. 104:366, 1986.
60. Rafal, E. S., and Rasmussen, J. E.: An unusual presentation of fixed cutaneous sporotrichosis: A case report and review of the literature. J. Am. Acad. Dermatol. *25*(5 Pt. 2):928, 1991.
61. Reed, K. D., Moore, F. M., Geiger, G. E., et al.: Zoonotic transmission of sporotrichosis: Case report and review. Clin. Infect. Dis. *16*:384, 1993.
62. Restrepo, A., Robledo, J., Gomez, I., et al.: Itraconazole therapy in lymphangitic and cutaneous sporotrichosis. Arch. Dermatol. *122*:413, 1986.
63. Rippon, J. W.: Medical Mycology: The Pathogenic Fungi and the Pathogenic Actinomycetes. 3rd ed. Philadelphia, W. B. Saunders, 1988.
64. Romig, D. A., Voth, D. W., and Liu, C.: Facial sporotrichosis during pregnancy: A therapeutic dilemma. Arch. Intern. Med. *130*:910, 1972.
65. Sanders, E.: Cutaneous sporotrichosis: Beer, bricks, and bumps. Arch. Intern. Med. *127*:482, 1971.
66. Saravanakumar, P. S., Eslami, P., and Zar, F. A.: Lymphocutaneous sporotrichosis associated with a squirrel bite: Case report and review. Clin. Infect. Dis. *23*:647, 1996.
67. Schenck, R. B.: On refractory subcutaneous abscesses caused by a fungus possibly related to sporotricha. Bull. Johns Hopkins Hosp. *9*:286, 1898.
68. Schwartz, D. A.: Sporothrix tenosynovitis: Differential diagnosis of granulomatous inflammatory disease of the joints. J. Rheumatol. *16*:550, 1989.
69. Scott, E. N., Kaufman, L., Brown, A. C., et al.: Serologic studies in the diagnosis and management of meningitis due to Sporothrix schenckii. N. Engl. J. Med. *317*:935, 1987.
70. Scott, E. N., and Muchmore, H. G.: Immunoblot analysis of antibody responses to Sporothrix schenckii. J. Clin. Microbiol. *27*:300, 1989.
71. Shadomy, S., White, S. C., Yu, H. P., et al.: Treatment of systemic mycoses with ketoconazole: In vitro susceptibilities of clinical isolates of systemic and pathogenic fungi to ketoconazole. J. Infect. Dis. *152*:1249, 1985.
72. Sharkey-Mathis, P. K., Kauffman, C. A., Graybill, J. R., et al.: Treatment of sporotrichosis with itraconazole. Am. J. Med. *95*:279, 1993.
73. Shaw, J. C., Levinson, W., and Montanaro, A.: Sporotrichosis in the acquired immunodeficiency syndrome. J. Am. Acad. Dermatol. *21*:1145, 1989.
74. Spiers, E. M., Hendrick, S. J., Jorizzo, J. L., et al.: Sporotrichosis masquerading as pyoderma gangrenosum. Arch. Dermatol. *122*:691, 1988.
75. Thompson, D. W., and Kaplan, W.: Laboratory-acquired sporotrichosis. Sabouraudia *15*:167, 1977.
76. Transvaal Mine Medical Officers' Association: Sporotrichosis infection in mines of the Witwatersrand: A symposium. Johannesburg, Transvaal Chamber of Mines, 1947.
77. Trejos, A., and Ramirez, O.: Local heat in the treatment of sporotrichosis. Mycopathol. Mycol. Appl. *30*:47, 1966.
78. Velji, A. M., Hoeprich, P. D., and Slovak, R.: Multifocal systemic sporotrichosis with lobar pulmonary involvement. Scand. J. Infect. Dis. *20*:565, 1988.
79. Wada, R.: Studies on mode of action of potassium iodide upon sporotrichosis. Mycopathol. Mycol. Appl. *34*:97, 1968.
80. Wilson, D. E., Mann, J. J., Bennett, J. E., et al.: Clinical features of extracutaneous sporotrichosis. Medicine *46*:265, 1967.
81. Winn, R. E., Anderson, J., Piper, J., et al.: Systemic sporotrichosis treated with itraconazole. Clin. Infect. Dis. *17*:210, 1993.
82. Wlodaver, C. G., Tolomeo, T., and Benear, J. B., II: Primary cutaneous nocardiosis mimicking sporotrichosis. Arch. Dermatol. *124*:659, 1988.

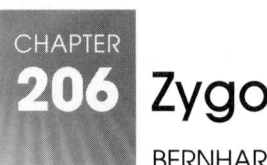

Zygomycosis

BERNHARD L. WIEDERMANN

Zygomycosis is the preferred nomenclature for infectious syndromes, previously called phycomycosis or mucormycosis, caused by fungi of the class Zygomycetes. The designation phycomycosis refers to a now outdated taxonomic scheme, but references to mucormycosis still occur in the literature and probably still are useful. However, this term could be misleading because the clinical syndromes caused by members of Zygomycetes include organisms in the order Entomophthorales as well as those in the order Mucorales. Although members of Entomophthorales tend to produce disease in normal hosts that is markedly different from the classic mucormycosis seen in immunocompromised patients, this distinction is becoming blurred and has resulted in adoption of the taxonomically proper term zygomycosis. Some authors use the term entomophthoromycosis for the more indolent clinical syndromes caused by members of this order. In this chapter, zygomycosis refers to infections caused by any of the organisms in the class Zygomycetes; mucormycosis and entomophthoromycosis are used to describe disease caused by members of the two pathogenic orders of the Zygomycetes.

Human disease consistent with zygomycosis probably was described initially by Kurchenmeister in 1855, but the first English-language description of the disease did not appear until Gregory and associates[33] described rhinocerebral disease in three diabetic patients in 1943. Since then, zygomycosis has been recognized as clearly encompassing a relatively uncommon but frequently fatal group of diseases occurring predominantly in immunocompromised hosts, particularly those with diabetes mellitus or impairment of neutrophil function, as well as a syndrome of relatively limited infection of skin and soft tissue caused by fungi in the order Entomophthorales in healthy people.[47, 85, 86]

The Organisms

Members of Zygomycetes are ubiquitous in nature and perhaps have a wider impact on humans as plant pathogens causing fruit decay than as human and animal pathogens.[8, 86] A detailed review of clinical microbiologic aspects of the Zygomycetes was published recently.[83] The class consists of two orders, Mucorales and Entomophthorales, each containing several species reported to cause disease in humans (Table 206–1). They grow readily on common laboratory media but are inhibited by cycloheximide.[3] With members of Mucorales, on solid agar plates one sees rapid growth of woolly colonies, often with spores seen as tiny dark dots to the naked eye. Hyphae characteristically are large (10 to 30 μm in diameter), nonseptate, and, often, twisted or ribbonlike. The lack of septation and the tendency of hyphae to branch at right angles usually serve to distinguish them from *Aspergillus* spp., which are septate and smaller and branch at acute angles.[3] Genera usually are differentiated from one another by examination of mycelia. Speciating the members of Zygomycetes often is difficult.

For members of Entomophthorales, growth also occurs readily on solid media but appears as flat, gray, or pale yellow waxy colonies with velvety white mycelia on the surface.[3, 86] The hyphae often are septate, and differentiation between genera and among species is based on morphologic characteristics of cultured organisms.

TABLE 206–1 ■ FUNGI CAUSING ZYGOMYCOSIS IN HUMANS

Order Mucorales
Family Mucoraceae
Absidia corymbifera, Absidia ramosa[55, 99]
Actinomucor elegans[20]
Apophysomyces elegans[17, 113]
Mucor indicus, M. ranosissimus, M. circinelloides, M. hiemalis[46, 77, 105]
Rhizomucor pusillus[112]
Rhizopus arrhizus, R. oryzae, R. rhizopodiformis (*is. 4*)[21, 30, 111]
Family Cunninghamellaceae
Cunninghamella bertholletiae[64, 80, 82, 84, 104]
Family Choanophoraceae
Cokermyces recurvatus[6, 79]
Family Saksenaeaceae
Saksenaea vasiformis[31, 75, 78]

Order Entomophthorales
Family Entomophthoraceae
Conidiobolus coronatus, C. incongruus[2, 35, 63, 65, 98]
Family Basidiobolaceae
Basidiobolus ranarum[23, 54, 93]

Epidemiology

All members of Zygomycetes are ubiquitous in nature and are found in all parts of the world, regardless of climate or other factors. Many of them are animal pathogens. Members of Mucorales are present in soil and occasionally are isolated from the hospital environment.[46, 108, 110] Studies have suggested a relationship between activities involved in hospital construction and development of zygomycosis in immunocompromised hosts.[46, 88, 110] *Rhizopus* spp. frequently are found in moldy bread and fruits.[86] Members of Entomophthorales commonly are found in feces of reptiles and other animals as well as in decaying vegetable matter, and some are insect pathogens.[86]

The ubiquitous nature of these organisms, coupled with the paucity of human disease associated with them, is strong evidence for their relatively saprophytic characteristics. Most human disease caused by members of Mucorales is concentrated in North America, perhaps because of a concentration of seriously immunocompromised hosts.[8] *Rhizopus, Rhizomucor,* and *Absidia* are the most common genera encountered in clinical medicine. On the other hand, infections caused by the Entomophthorales genera *Basidiobolus* and *Conidiobolus* occur predominantly in Africa, India, and the Far East, although a few cases have been acquired in North and South America.[86] Typically, *Basidiobolus* spp. infections are seen in young children and adolescents with superficial infections of the trunk or extremities, whereas *Conidiobolus* tends to infect rhinofacial areas of young adult males.[58]

Mucormycosis

PATHOGENESIS AND PATHOLOGY

Mucormycosis usually is acquired by humans after inhalation of spores, and the organisms may colonize the sinuses and nasopharynx of some patients.[86] Occasionally, mucormycosis results from cutaneous inoculation of spores, as has occurred with contaminated elastic adhesive tape, and disseminates from the cutaneous or subcutaneous site.[21, 30] Person-to-person transmission has not been documented. The key to production of disease, however, is the immune status of the host. The neutrophil appears to be the primary component of the immune response against these organisms and may serve to prevent germination of inhaled spores.[22] Diabetes mellitus, in particular diabetic ketoacidosis, is the most common underlying disease in patients with mucormycosis.[44, 85] Other underlying diseases accompanied by acidosis, such as uremia or sepsis, also may predispose to mucormycosis.[53, 85] Other predisposing illnesses, some of which are accompanied by acidosis, are listed in Table 206–2. Important by its absence is acquired immunodeficiency syndrome (AIDS), which, of course, predominantly is a lymphocytic disorder. Zygomycosis reported in patients with AIDS tends to occur in intravenous drug users and may reflect this risk factor more than does the immunodeficiency itself.[64, 95] Disease may follow a less fulminant course in patients with AIDS compared with other immunocompromised populations.[9] Perhaps further evidence of the low virulence of these organisms is that mucormycosis still is an uncommon disease, even though many of the illnesses listed in Table 206–2 are common.

TABLE 206–2 ■ UNDERLYING DISEASES COMMONLY ASSOCIATED WITH INCREASED RISK FOR MUCORMYCOSIS

Diabetes mellitus[12, 44, 74]
Neutropenia or neutrophil dysfunction[44]
Malignancy[44, 60, 74]
Malnutrition[66]
Deferoxamine therapy[34, 82, 92, 114]
Intravenous drug use[64]
Organ transplantation[34, 99, 105, 116]
Trauma or surgery[4, 24, 32, 55, 75]
Burns[17, 56]
Corticosteroid therapy[60]
Methylmalonicaciduria[50]

Serum from patients with diabetic ketoacidosis does not inhibit the growth of *Rhizopus* spp., but serum from those same patients after treatment of the ketoacidosis does show inhibitory properties similar to those of normal human serum.[13, 28] Furthermore, iron may play a key role in lowering host defenses, as demonstrated by the tendency for deferoxamine therapy to result in progression of both natural and experimental mucormycosis.[19, 34, 82, 92] This phenomenon appears to occur commonly, particularly in patients undergoing hemodialysis.[10, 114] Studies in experimental animals suggest that deferoxamine may serve as a siderophore for *Rhizopus* spp., with resultant increased fungal growth and increased mortality in a guinea pig model.[18] However, in vitro data conflict on the exact effects of iron or deferoxamine on promoting the growth of members of Mucorales.[68] Much remains to be understood about the pathogenesis of mucormycosis, and a unifying concept will have to incorporate the effects of steroids, acidosis, and iron on host neutrophils and macrophages in failing to suppress fungal replication.

The hallmark of histologic examination of mucormycosis is vascular invasion with resultant thrombosis and tissue necrosis and accompanying acute and chronic inflammation.[66, 74, 86] Most of the clinical findings of progressive disease can be related to these effects on blood vessels. Septic emboli may affect all parts of the body. Perineural invasion also occurs commonly.[27] In the rhinocerebral form, the disease may progress along nerve roots during intracranial spread. Although relatively sparse, hyphal forms may be seen in tissue on routine hematoxylin and eosin staining more than with silver or other special fungal stains[86] (Fig. 206–1).

CLINICAL MANIFESTATIONS

The clinical forms of mucormycosis are considered best by type of organ system involvement (Table 206–3).

Acute Rhinocerebral Mucormycosis

The acute rhinocerebral form of mucormycosis occurs most commonly in the setting of diabetic ketoacidosis and has a high mortality rate.[47, 57, 94] Initially, the patient may have a history of pain, swelling, or tenderness of the face, with proptosis, headache, and altered mental status appearing as the infection progresses. Bloody or necrotic lesions may appear at the nasal turbinates or palate, but soon, symptoms of central nervous system involvement predominate. The functions of cranial nerves II, III, IV, and VI become impaired, and cranial nerves I, V, and VII also are involved commonly.

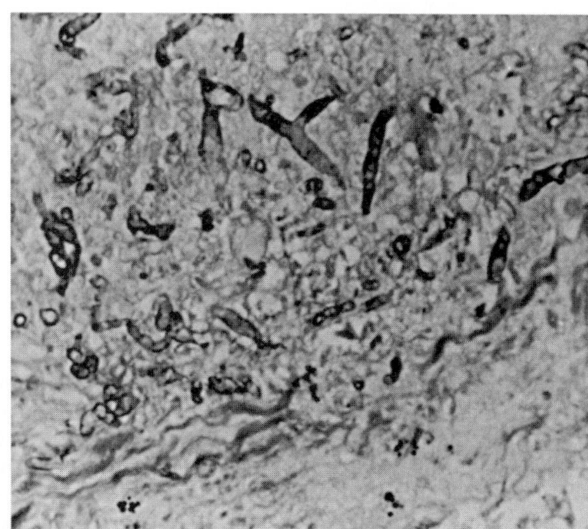

FIGURE 206–1 ■ Zygomycosis caused by *Rhizopus* species. Observe the varied morphologic features of the coenocytic hyphae and large size. (Hematoxylin and eosin, original magnification ×64.)

Thrombosis of the cavernous sinus or internal carotid artery is a feared complication.

Cutaneous Mucormycosis

Cutaneous mucormycosis occurs occasionally, usually at the site of trauma, burns, or invasive procedures in immunocompromised hosts.[17, 43, 100, 112] Of 25 patients with mucormycosis treated during a recent 14-year period, 10 had cutaneous infections.[1] Several cases of mucormycotic cellulitis caused by contaminated elastic adhesive bandages occurred in the 1970s, and later, other dressings were implicated.[30, 111] Some affected patients have developed locally aggressive or disseminated disease. In general, the lesions varied morphologically initially, but local progression was devastating in some cases. Overall, cutaneous mucormycosis either may appear as a relatively indolent, local infection with ulceration or may cause gangrenous cellulitis with local and distant extension.[90] This latter complication appears to occur more commonly with burn wound infections and in immunocompromised hosts, including newborn infants.[4, 56]

Neonatal zygomycosis occurs rarely, with only 33 cases well described in the English-language literature.[51, 69, 87] Skin is the most common point of entry for these patients, with adhesive tape, monitor leads, or central venous access sites predominating. Premature infants represented 72 percent of cases, and the overall mortality rate was 75 percent.

In addition to primary inoculation of zygomycosis in cutaneous or subcutaneous sites, nodular skin lesions resulting from hematogenous spread also may occur.[43] Often, making a diagnosis of disseminated disease is rendered possible by the appearance of skin lesions that then undergo biopsy.

TABLE 206–3 ■ CLINICAL FORMS OF MUCORMYCOSIS

Rhinocerebral
Cutaneous
Pulmonary
Gastrointestinal
Disseminated
Miscellaneous

Blood cultures generally are negative, but this form of cutaneous disease is an indication of widespread dissemination and is associated with poor outcome, regardless of therapy.[85, 86]

Pulmonary Mucormycosis

Pulmonary disease caused by mucormycosis occurs most commonly in the setting of disseminated infection, but it also is well described as an isolated phenomenon.[59, 60, 74, 80, 99, 116] Mucormycotic pneumonia typically develops in severely immunocompromised patients, such as those with malignancy and neutropenia, but also has occurred in patients with juvenile diabetes and in a normal host.[15, 40, 85] Affected patients usually are febrile and have hemoptysis. Massive pulmonary hemorrhage may result from vascular erosion. Radiographic appearance may vary from a nonspecific infiltrate to formation of a cavity. Pleural involvement rarely occurs. Rarely, fungus balls have been noted.[74] The disease usually is fulminant but may be milder in hosts with less severe immune compromise.

Gastrointestinal Mucormycosis

Gastrointestinal involvement probably results from ingestion of fungal spores, either from the environment or from colonized upper airways. Occasionally, hematogenous or direct extension routes result in intestinal tract involvement. Malnutrition, prematurity, uremia, and underlying gastrointestinal disease such as typhoid fever or amebiasis are predisposing factors.[48, 61, 62, 66] All sites along the intestinal tract can be involved, with the stomach and colon being most common ones.[66] Nonspecific abdominal pain with hematemesis, hematochezia, or melena may occur. Premature infants may experience necrotizing enterocolitis, with or without pneumatosis intestinalis.[101, 115] Dissemination to other sites may occur by hematogenous routes. Perforation after bowel wall necrosis is a common occurrence. Diagnosis usually is made at autopsy.

Disseminated Mucormycosis

Disseminated mucormycosis not surprisingly occurs in the most severely immunocompromised patients and most commonly is an autopsy diagnosis.[38, 103] Clinical findings are nonspecific, and a high index of suspicion and readily accessible tissue for biopsy are needed for diagnosis. The pulmonary system is affected most commonly, followed by the central nervous system, but virtually any organ can be involved. A subacute form of disseminated disease with a protracted but fatal course has been reported.[70] The combination of severe immune compromise and subtle clinical findings renders this form of mucormycosis the most difficult to treat.

Miscellaneous Forms of Mucormycosis

A variety of case reports of mucormycosis involving isolated areas of the body are found in the literature. Thus, mucormycotic endocarditis, myocarditis, meningitis, brain abscess, peritonitis, Budd-Chiari syndrome, osteomyelitis, arthritis, myositis, endophthalmitis, pyelonephritis, and cystitis all have been reported.* Common to these disease manifestations is some type of local trauma, either accidental or surgical, that results in a ready access site for invasion of fungal organisms. Outcome varies highly and depends on the underlying condition of the host as well as the extent of disease.

*See references 6, 11, 12, 24, 26, 55, 73, 75, 76, 96, 102.

DIAGNOSIS

Diagnosing mucormycosis can be difficult. As mentioned previously, blood cultures usually are negative, even in the presence of hematogenous dissemination. Growth of an organism from the respiratory tract or wound also is not proof of infection because these fungi may colonize body surfaces.[86] The gold standard of diagnosis is tissue biopsy showing characteristic hyphal forms invading tissue. Specimens obtained through skinny needle biopsy or bronchoalveolar lavage also likely reflect mucormycosis accurately.[49, 89] Although this type of information alone does not permit absolute identification of the organism involved (growth in culture is needed for speciation), it is sufficient to diagnose infection by a member of Mucorales.

Work continues on other methods of diagnosis. Although many members of Mucorales have antigenic cross-reactivity, ability to detect specific antibodies in patients with mucormycosis has been somewhat disappointing. A comparison of immunodiffusion with enzyme-linked immunosorbent assays for antibody to antigens of *Rhizopus arrhizus* and *Rhizomucor pusillus* in 46 patients with zygomycosis (43 with infections caused by members of Mucorales) showed relatively poor sensitivity and specificity. With 43 control cases of aspergillosis, candidiasis, cryptococcosis, and pseudallescheriasis, sensitivities were only 66 percent and 81 percent for immunodiffusion and enzyme immunoassay, respectively.[42] False positivity in patients with aspergillosis and candidiasis was encountered. Part of the problem with antibody detection may result from the poor immune responses seen in patients with mucormycosis, and antigen detection methods may be more rewarding for diagnosis.

TREATMENT

Mucormycosis occurs too rarely to allow accurate assessment of the effects of specific therapeutic regimens. Therefore, most treatment recommendations have resulted from anecdotal experiences rather than controlled trials. In an infectious syndrome occurring predominantly in immunocompromised hosts, attempting to correct or improve the underlying disease as much as possible is essential. In the case of mucormycosis, it would include aggressive correction of hyperglycemia and acidosis in diabetic patients; discontinuation of deferoxamine therapy in those receiving this drug; and decreasing doses of or discontinuing immunosuppressive therapy, such as cancer chemotherapy, corticosteroids, and cyclosporine. The role of white blood cell transfusions or colony-stimulating factors in ameliorating the neutropenic state has not been addressed critically in mucormycosis.

Standard medical therapy is amphotericin B, given at maximal dosages of 1 to 1.5 mg/kg/day, based on the individual's tolerance of side effects.[5] The most seriously diseased patients are given a total of at least 30 mg/kg. Some cases have been reported of cure with shorter duration of therapy, which should be reserved for well-localized disease in relatively normal hosts, in combination with surgical débridement.[91] Amphotericin B lipid complex has been used successfully in at least two pediatric patients.[107] Whether lipid formulations of amphotericin B confer any advantage over conventional amphotericin B for mucormycosis is unclear.[45]

Christenson and colleagues[14] reported on a diabetic child with mucormycotic pneumonia treated with a combination of amphotericin B and rifampin in whom clinical improvement appeared to coincide with addition of the rifampin. In vitro susceptibility testing of the clinical isolate *(Rhizopus oryzae)* and other strains suggested evidence of synergy. The child's serum fungistatic activity increased when rifampin was added to the amphotericin B therapy. Flucytosine occasionally has been used in combination with amphotericin B.[16, 67] Ketoconazole was used, perhaps successfully, to treat one patient with mucormycosis, but in general, these organisms are resistant to the azole compounds.[7, 29] Azole drugs in combination with fluoroquinolones showed some efficacy in a mouse model of *R. oryzae* pulmonary disease.[97] These studies certainly suggest the need for further work on combination drug therapy for these situations.

Most authorities agree that aggressive surgical débridement, when possible, is a necessary complement to medical therapy.[32, 36, 71] All necrotic-appearing tissue should be removed, and often patients require repeated surgical procedures for removal of devitalized tissue. Surgical débridement alone may be sufficient to cure localized cutaneous disease.[78]

Hyperbaric oxygen therapy has been used for some of these patients in an attempt to limit the extent of gangrene and tissue necrosis.[25, 32] In one retrospective study, two of six patients receiving hyperbaric oxygen, along with standard medical and surgical therapy, died, compared with four deaths in seven patients not receiving hyperbaric oxygen.[25] Hyperbaric oxygen therapy in combination with administration of liposomal amphotericin B and interferon-γ was successful in one patient with trauma-associated mucormycosis.[72] Although this regimen might appear promising, the number of patients evaluated with this form of treatment is much too small to permit any firm conclusions on benefit.

In summary, no specific treatment regimens for mucormycosis have proved effective. In a retrospective study of adult cancer patients, high-dose amphotericin B (total, 2 g), combined with surgical débridement and immune reconstitution therapy, was associated with improved outcome.[45] Well-organized prospective clinical trials are needed to refine treatment of this rare but serious condition.

PROGNOSIS AND PREVENTION

As indicated throughout this section, mucormycosis is a serious disease that occurs largely in immunocompromised hosts and results in a high mortality rate. However, some evidence exists for improved prognosis. In one study of 33 cases over the course of a 44-year period, a shift in the 1970s from a predominantly postmortem diagnosis to a predominantly premortem diagnosis occurred.[74] Furthermore, survival increased from 6 to 73 percent during this time. More aggressive means of diagnosis and treatment plus the availability of amphotericin B likely accounted for this shift. Still, survival is tied most closely to the extent of the infection and the severity of the underlying immunocompromised state, and not all reports suggest improvement in outcome. In Kline's[44] review of mucormycosis at one large children's center, only 1 of 15 confirmed patients survived, but mucormycosis was diagnosed in only 3 of the 15 before death. An overall survival rate of about 50 percent in cases diagnosed before death seems reasonably accurate.[85] Any improvement in prognosis during the next few years likely will result from a heightened index of suspicion of the disease in the appropriate clinical settings, combined with continued aggressive means of diagnosis and medical and surgical treatment.

Prevention of mucormycosis can be addressed in three areas. First, control of underlying disease such as diabetes can limit the risk for developing disease. Second, use of less immunosuppressive drugs for transplantations and other conditions will help, as will lessening the degree of neutropenia during treatment of malignancies. Finally, patients at risk should be shielded from situations in which they are likely to encounter the organisms (e.g., at construction sites, around decaying plant matter) and from the use of nonsterile dressings over wound sites. Hospitals can exercise caution in exposure of immunocompromised patients to construction activity within the hospital and use filtering systems to prevent transmission of spores by the airborne route.

Entomophthoromycosis

PATHOGENESIS AND PATHOLOGY

Entomophthoromycosis presumably develops through inhalation of spores to cause sinus disease or cutaneous inoculation to cause cutaneous or subcutaneous infection. However, the exact mechanisms are unclear, and no specific animal model has been developed. The organisms are of extremely low virulence, as manifested by the rare occurrence of these infections even though the fungi are ubiquitous. Although discrete clinical syndromes have been assigned to the two genera causing disease, this distinction is artificial, and one should recognize that either group could cause either form of entomophthoromycosis or even a syndrome more suggestive of mucormycosis.[93, 106, 109]

Histopathologic examination of affected tissues shows some similarities to mucormycosis. Areas of acute and chronic inflammation are found in association with broad hyphal elements that may or may not display septations. The hyphae are more visible with hematoxylin and eosin staining than with more specific fungal stains.[86] However, the tendency for vascular invasion typical of mucormycosis does not occur with entomophthoromycosis, and necrosis is an uncommon occurrence. Instead, a so-called Splendore-Hoeppli phenomenon, likely consisting of hyphae surrounded by eosinophilic material in a stellate pattern, occurs.[86] However, this feature is not pathognomonic of entomophthoromycosis and has been seen in cases of mucormycosis.

CLINICAL MANIFESTATIONS

Chronic Rhinofacial Zygomycosis

Chronic rhinofacial zygomycosis, also called entomophthoromycosis conidiobolae because most infections are caused by *Conidiobolus coronatus,* is an indolent subcutaneous infection involving the face.[35, 63, 65] Typically, bilateral intranasal swelling eventually progresses to invasion of the sinuses and soft tissue swelling of the face, unaccompanied by fever or pain. One infant developed orbital involvement from *C. coronatus* dacryocystitis.[52] Symptoms commonly persist for weeks or months, but deep-tissue progression is unlikely to occur.

Chronic Subcutaneous Zygomycosis

Chronic subcutaneous zygomycosis, also known as entomophthoromycosis basidiobolae, is similar to chronic rhinofacial disease with the exception that the lesions usually are on the trunk or extremities. The etiologic agent is

Basidiobolus ranarum. Painless subcutaneous nodules may progress to invade deeper soft tissues, and massive soft tissue swelling may develop. Facial infection similar to that of chronic rhinofacial zygomycosis also may occur.[23] *Conidiobolus incongruus* has caused orbitofascial disease in a child residing in the Middle East.[2] With rare exceptions, most cases of subcutaneous zygomycosis are slowly progressive.[39, 86]

Gastrointestinal Basidiobolomycosis

Gastrointestinal basidiobolomycosis is an extremely rare condition resulting from *B. ranarum* infection of the gastrointestinal tract. A cluster of cases was identified in Arizona in the late 1990s, suggesting a possible emerging infection in the region. In a case-control study including 7 adult patients in Arizona, infected patients tended to be more likely to use ranitidine and to have resided in Arizona for a longer period of time compared with controls.[54] Clinical features included abdominal pain, leukocytosis, and eosinophilia. Combined surgical resection and itraconazole appeared to be effective treatment.

DIAGNOSIS

Entomophthoromycosis often can be diagnosed presumptively on the basis of clinical presentation and geographic origin of the patient, but usually biopsy is required.[58, 86] Recent work on serodiagnosis by immunodiffusion has had promising results.[37, 41] Onchocerciasis, filariasis, and Burkitt lymphoma sometimes are in the differential diagnosis.[39, 58]

TREATMENT

Evaluation of therapy for this group of diseases is difficult to make because of occasional reports of spontaneous resolution. Many agents have been tried with varying success. Taylor and colleagues[98] treated a young man with rhinofacial disease with amphotericin B, corticosteroids, miconazole, and multiple surgical procedures before noting resolution some months after any therapy had been given. They performed susceptibility testing, which showed minimal inhibitory effects of amphotericin B and no benefit of adding flucytosine or rifampin. Miconazole, ketoconazole, and potassium iodide did not have impressive in vitro activity in their assay. Restrepo[81] recommends potassium iodide therapy, with trimethoprim-sulfamethoxazole as an alternative.

Other anecdotal reports of efficacy of trimethoprim-sulfamethoxazole, ketoconazole, or itraconazole raise hopes for effective therapy but must be tempered by the fact that small numbers of patients have been treated.[35, 54, 98] Currently, no "drug of choice" has been determined for this condition, although some type of medical therapy seems indicated for all cases. The role of surgery is less for this group of disorders than for mucormycosis, but patients with well-circumscribed areas, such as nodular lesions, may benefit from surgical excision. Even so, recurrence of disease after surgery is not uncommon in such patients.[98]

PROGNOSIS AND PREVENTION

Mortality caused by the entomophthoromycoses is unlikely to occur, but morbidity and disfigurement are common occurrences. The efficacy of medical and surgical therapy is unclear, but probably all patients should receive attempts at treatment because the natural history of the disease is one of slow progression. Specific means for disease prevention are not available because so little is known about factors predisposing to these chronic zygomycotic syndromes.

REFERENCES

1. Adam, R. D., Hunter G., DiTomasso, J., et al.: Mucormycosis: Emerging prominence of cutaneous infections. Clin. Infect. Dis. *19*:67, 1994.
2. Al-Hajjar, S., Perfect, J., Hashem, F., et al.: Orbitofascial conidiobolomycosis in a child. Pediatr. Infect. Dis. J. *15*:1130, 1996.
3. American Thoracic Society: Laboratory diagnosis of mycotic and specific fungal infections. Am. Rev. Respir. Dis. *132*:1373, 1985.
4. Arisoy, A. E., Arisoy, E. S., Correa-Calderon, A., et al.: *Rhizopus* necrotizing cellulitis in a preterm infant: A case report and review of the literature. Pediatr. Infect. Dis. J. *12*:1029, 1993.
5. Armstrong, D.: Problems in management of opportunistic fungal diseases. Rev. Infect. Dis. *11*(Suppl. 7):S1591, 1989.
6. Axelrod, P., Kwon-Chung, K. J., Frawley, P., et al.: Chronic cystitis due to *Cokermyces recurvatus:* A case report. J. Infect. Dis. *155*:1062, 1987.
7. Barnert, J., Behr, W., and Reich, H.: An amphotericin B–resistant case of rhinocerebral mucormycosis. Infection *13*:134, 1985.
8. Benbow, E. W., and Stoddart, R. W.: Systemic zygomycosis. Postgrad. Med. J. *62*:985, 1986.
9. Blatt, S. P., Lucey, D. R., DeHoff, D., et al.: Rhinocerebral zygomycosis in a patient with AIDS. J. Infect. Dis. *164*:215, 1991.
10. Boelaert, J. R., Fenves, A. Z., and Coburn, J. W.: Mucormycosis among patients on dialysis. N. Engl. J. Med. *321*:190, 1989.
11. Branton, M. H., Johnson, S. C., Brooke, J. D., et al.: Peritonitis due to *Rhizopus* in a patient undergoing continuous ambulatory peritoneal dialysis. Rev. Infect. Dis. *13*:19, 1990.
12. Case Records of the Massachusetts General Hospital (Case 36–1988). N. Engl. J. Med. *319*:629, 1988.
13. Chinn, R. Y. W., and Diamond, R. D.: Generation of chemotactic factors by *Rhizopus oryzae* in the presence and absence of serum: Relationship to hyphal damage mediated by human neutrophils and effects of hyperglycemia and ketoacidosis. Infect. Immun. *38*:1123, 1982.
14. Christenson, J. C., Shalit, I., Welch, D. F., et al.: Synergistic action of amphotericin B and rifampin against *Rhizopus* species. Antimicrob. Agents Chemother. *31*:1775, 1987.
15. Cohen-Abbo, A., Bozeman, P. M., and Patrick, C. C.: *Cunninghamella* infections: Review and report of two cases of *Cunninghamella* pneumonia in immunocompromised children. Clin. Infect. Dis. *17*:173, 1993.
16. Cook, B. A., White, C. B., Blaney, S. M., et al.: Survival after isolated cerebral mucormycosis. Am. J. Pediatr. Hematol. Oncol. *11*:330, 1989.
17. Cooter, R. D., Lim, I. S., Ellis, D. H., et al.: Burn wound zygomycosis caused by *Apophysomyces elegans*. J. Clin. Microbiol. *28*:2151, 1990.
18. Cutsem, J. V., and Boelaert, J. R.: Effects of deferoxamine, feroxamine and iron on experimental mucormycosis (zygomycosis). Kidney Int. *36*:1061, 1989.
19. Daly, A. L., Velazquez, L. A., Bradley, S. F., et al.: Mucormycosis: Association with deferoxamine therapy. Am. J. Med. *87*:468, 1989.
20. Davel, G., Featherston, P., Fernandez, A., et al.: Maxillary sinusitis caused by *Actinomucor elegans*. J. Clin. Microbiol. *39*:740, 2001.
21. Dennis, J. E., Rhodes, K. H., Cooney, D. R., et al.: Nosocomial *Rhizopus* infection (zygomycosis) in children. J. Pediatr. *96*:824, 1980.
22. Diamond, R. D., Krzesicki, R., Epstein, B., et al.: Damage to hyphal forms of fungi by human leukocytes in vitro: A possible host defense mechanism against aspergillosis and mucormycosis. Am. J. Pathol. *91*:313, 1978.
23. Dworzack, D. L., Pollock, A. S., Hodges, G. R., et al.: Zygomycosis of the maxillary sinus and palate caused by *Basidiobolus haptosporus*. Arch. Intern. Med. *138*:1274, 1978.
24. Fergie, J. E., Fitzwater, D. S., Einstein, P., et al.: *Mucor* peritonitis associated with acute periotoneal dialysis. Pediatr. Infect. Dis. J. *11*:498, 1992.
25. Ferguson, B. J., Mitchell, T. G., Moon, R., et al.: Adjunctive hyperbaric oxygen for treatment of rhinocerebral mucormycosis. Rev. Infect. Dis. *10*:551, 1988.
26. Fong, K. M., Seneviratne, E. M. E., and McCormack, J. G.: Mucor cerebral abscess associated with intravenous drug use. Aust. N. Z. J. Med. *20*:74, 1990.
27. Frater, J. L., Hall, G. S., and Procop, G. W.: Histologic features of zygomycosis: Emphasis on perineural invasion and fungal morphology. Arch. Pathol. Lab. Med. *125*:375, 2001.
28. Gale, G. R., and Welch, A.: Studies of opportunistic fungi. I. Inhibition of *R. oryzae* by human serum. Am. J. Med. Sci. *45*:604, 1971.
29. Galgiani, J. N.: Fluconazole, a new antifungal agent. Ann. Intern. Med. *113*:177, 1990.
30. Gartenberg, G., Bottone, E. J., Keusch, G. T., et al.: Hospital-acquired mucormycosis *(Rhizopus rhizopodiformis)* of skin and subcutaneous tissue: Epidemiology, mycology and treatment. N. Engl. J. Med. *299*:1115, 1978.
31. Gonis, G., and Starr, M.: Fatal rhinoorbital mucormycosis caused by *Saksenaea vasiformis* in an immunocompromised child. Pediatr. Infect. Dis. J. *16*:714, 1997.

32. Gordon, G., Indeck, M., Bross, J., et al.: Injury from silage wagon accident complicated by mucormycosis. J. Trauma *28*:866, 1988.
33. Gregory, J. E., Golden, A., and Haymaker, W.: Mucormycosis of the central nervous system: A report of three cases. Bull. Johns Hopkins Hosp. *73*:405, 1943.
34. Hamdy, N. A. T., Andrew, S. M., Shortland, J. R., et al.: Fatal cardiac zygomycosis in a renal transplant patient treated with desferrioxamine. Nephrol. Dial. Transplant. *4*:911, 1989.
35. Herstoff, J. K., Bogaars, H., and McDonald, C. J.: Rhinophycomycosis entomophthorae. Arch. Dermatol. *114*:1674, 1978.
36. Hsu, J., Clayman, J. A., and Geha, A. S.: Survival of a recipient of renal transplantation after pulmonary phycomycosis. Ann. Thorac. Surg. *47*:617, 1989.
37. Imwidthaya, P., and Srimuang, S.: Immunodiffusion test for diagnosing basidiobolomycosis. Mycopathologia *118*:127, 1992.
38. Ingram, C. W., Sennesh, J., Cooper, J. N., et al.: Disseminated zygomycosis: Report of four cases and review. Rev. Infect. Dis. *11*:741, 1989.
39. Jelliffe, D. B., Burkitt, D., O'Conor, G. T., et al.: Subcutaneous phycomycosis in an East African child. J. Pediatr. *59*:124, 1961.
40. Johnson, G. M., and Baldwin, J. J.: Pulmonary mucormycosis and juvenile diabetes. Am. J. Dis. Child. *135*:567, 1981.
41. Kaufman, L., Mendoza, L., and Standard, P. G.: Immunodiffusion test for serodiagnosing subcutaneous zygomycosis. J. Clin. Microbiol. *28*:1887, 1990.
42. Kaufman, L., Turner, L. F., and McLaughlin, D. W.: Indirect enzyme-linked immunosorbent assay for zygomycosis. J. Clin. Microbiol. *27*:1979, 1989.
43. Khardori, N., Hayat, S., Rolston, K., et al.: Cutaneous *Rhizopus* and *Aspergillus* infections in five patients with cancer. Arch. Dermatol. *125*:952, 1989.
44. Kline, M. W.: Mucormycosis in children: Review of the literature and report of cases. Pediatr. Infect. Dis. *4*:672, 1985.
45. Kontoyiannis, D. P., Wessel, V. C., Boday, G. P., et al.: Zygomycosis in the 1990s in a tertiary-care center. Clin. Infect. Dis. *30*:851, 2000.
46. Krasinski, E., Holzman, R. S., Hanna, B., et al.: Nosocomial fungal infection during hospital renovation. Infect. Control *6*:278, 1985.
47. Lehrer, R. I., Howard, D. H., Sypherd, P. S., et al.: Mucormycosis. Ann. Intern. Med. *93*:93, 1980.
48. Levinson, S. E., and Isaacson, C.: Spontaneous perforation of the colon in the newborn infant. Arch. Dis. Child. *35*:378, 1960.
49. Levy, S. A., Schmitt, K. W., and Kaufman, L.: Systemic zygomycosis diagnosed by fine needle aspiration and confirmed with enzyme immunoassay. Chest *90*:146, 1986.
50. Lewis, L. L., Hawkins, H. K., and Edwards, M. S.: Disseminated mucormycosis in an infant with methylmalonicaciduria. Pediatr. Infect. Dis. J. *9*:851, 1990.
51. Linder, N., Keller, N., Huri, C., et al.: Primary cutaneous mucormycosis in a premature infant: Case report and review of the literature. Am. J. Perinatol. *15*:35, 1998.
52. Lithander, J., Louon, A., Scrimgeour, E., et al.: Orbital entomophthormycosis in an infant: Recovery following surgical debridement, combination antifungal therapy and use of hyperbaric oxygen. Br. J. Ophthalmol. *85*:374, 2001.
53. Lloyd, T. R., and Bolte, R. G.: Rhinocerebral mucormycosis in an infant with streptococcal sepsis and purpura fulminans. Pediatr. Infect. Dis. *5*:575, 1986.
54. Lyon, G. M., Smilack, J. D., Komatsu, K. K., et al.: Gastrointestinal basidiobolomycosis in Arizona: Clinical and epidemiological characteristics and review of the literature. Clin. Infect. Dis. *32*:1448, 2001.
55. Mackenzie, D. W. R., Soothill, J. F., and Millar, J. H. D.: Meningitis caused by *Absidia corymbifera*. J. Infect. *17*:241, 1988.
56. Majeski, J. A., and MacMillan, B. G.: Fatal systemic mycotic infections in the burned child. J. Trauma *17*:320, 1977.
57. Maniglia, A. J., Mintz, D. H., and Novak, S.: Cephalic phycomycosis: A report of eight cases. Laryngoscope *92*:755, 1982.
58. Manson-Bahr, P. E. C., and Bell, D. R.: Manson's Tropical Diseases. 19th ed. London, Ballière Tindall, 1987.
59. Medoff, G., and Kobayashi, G. S.: Pulmonary mucormycosis. N. Engl. J. Med. *286*:86, 1972.
60. Meyer, R. D., Rosen, P., and Armstrong, D.: Phycomycosis complicating leukemia and lymphoma. Ann. Intern. Med. *77*:871, 1972.
61. Michalak, D. M., Cooney, D. R., Rhodes, K. H., et al.: Gastrointestinal mucormycoses in infants and children: A cause of gangrenous intestinal cellulitis and perforation. J. Pediatr. Surg. *15*:320, 1980.
62. Mooney, J. E., and Wanger, A.: Mucormycosis of the gastrointestinal tract in children: Report of a case and review of the literature. Pediatr. Infect. Dis. J. *12*:872, 1993.
63. Moretz, M. L., Grist, W. J., and Sewell, C. W.: Zygomycosis presenting as nasal polyps in a healthy child. Arch. Otolaryngol. Head Neck Surg. *113*:550, 1987.
64. Mostaza, J. M., Barbado, F. J., Fernandez-Martin, J., et al.: Cutaneoarticular mucormycosis due to *Cunninghamella bertholletiae* in a patient with AIDS. Rev. Infect. Dis. *11*:316, 1989.
65. Nathan, M. D., Keller, A. P., Jr., Lerner, C. J., et al.: Entomophthorales infection of the maxillofacial region. Laryngoscope *92*:767, 1982.
66. Neame, P., and Raynor, D.: Mucormycosis: A report of twenty-two cases. Arch. Pathol. *70*:261, 1960.
67. Ng, P. C., and Dear, P. R. F.: Phycomycotic abscesses in a preterm infant. Arch. Dis. Child. *64*:862, 1989.
68. Niimi, O., Kokan, A., and Kashiwagi, N.: Effect of deferoxamine mesylate on the growth of Mucorales. Nephron *53*:281, 1989.
69. Nissen, M. D., Jana, A. K., Cole, M. J., et al.: Neonatal gastrointestinal mucormycosis mimicking necrotizing enterocolitis. Acta Paediatr. *88*:1290, 1999.
70. Nolan, R. L., Carter, R. R., III, Griffith, J. E., et al.: Case report: Subacute disseminated mucormycosis in a diabetic male. Am. J. Med. Sci. *298*:252, 1989.
71. Ochi, J. W., Harris, J. P., Feldman, J. I., et al.: Rhinocerebral mucormycosis: Results of aggressive surgical debridement and amphotericin B. Laryngoscope *98*:1339, 1988.
72. Okhuysen, P. C., Rex, J. H., Kapusta, M., et al.: Successful treatment of extensive posttraumatic soft-tissue and renal infections due to *Apophysomyces elegans*. Clin. Infect. Dis. *19*:329, 1994.
73. Orgel, I. K., and Cohen, K. L.: Postoperative zygomycetes endophthalmitis. Ophthalmic Surg. *20*:584, 1989.
74. Parfrey, N. A.: Improved diagnosis and prognosis of mucormycosis: A clinicopathologic study of 33 cases. Medicine *65*:113, 1986.
75. Pierce, P. F., Wood, M. B., Roberts, G. D., et al.: *Saksenaea vasiformis* osteomyelitis. J. Clin. Microbiol. *25*:933, 1987.
76. Polo, J. R., Luno, J., Menarguez, C., et al.: Peritoneal mucormycosis in a patient receiving continuous ambulatory peritoneal dialysis. Am. J. Kidney Dis. *13*:237, 1989.
77. Prevoo, R. L., Starink, T. M., and de Haan, P.: Primary cutaneous mucormycosis in a healthy young girl: Report of a case caused by *Mucor hiemalis* Wehmer. J. Am. Acad. Dermatol. *24*(5 Pt. 2):882, 1991.
78. Pritchard, R. C., Muir, D. B., Archer, K. H., et al.: Subcutaneous zygomycosis due to *Saksenaea vasiformis* in an infant. Med. J. Aust. *145*:630, 1986.
79. Ramani, R., Newman, R., Salkin, I. F., et al.: *Cokermyces recurvatus* as a human pathogenic fungus: Case report and critical review of the published literature. Pediatr. Infect. Dis. J. *19*:155, 2000.
80. Reed, A. E., Body, B. A., Austin, M. B., et al.: *Cunninghamella bertholletiae* and *Pneumocystis carinii* pneumonia as a fatal complication of chronic lymphocytic leukemia. Hum. Pathol. *19*:1470, 1988.
81. Restrepo, A.: Treatment of tropical mycoses. J. Am. Acad. Dermatol. *31(Suppl.)*:S91, 1994.
82. Rex, J. H., Ginsberg, A. M., Fries, L. F., et al.: *Cunninghamella bertholletiae* infection associated with deferoxamine therapy. Rev. Infect. Dis. *10*:1187, 1988.
83. Ribes, J. A., Vanover-Sams, C. L., and Baker, D. J.: Zygomycetes in human disease. Clin. Microbiol. Rev. *13*:236, 2000.
84. Rickerts, V., Böhme, A., Viertel, A., et al.: Cluster of pulmonary infections caused by *Cunninghamella bertholletiae* in immunocompromised patients. Clin. Infect. Dis. *31*:910, 2000.
85. Rinaldi, M. G.: Zygomycosis. Infect. Dis. Clin. North Am. *3*:19, 1989.
86. Rippon, J. W.: Medical Mycology: The Pathogenic Fungi and the Pathogenic Actinomycetes. 3rd ed. Philadelphia, W. B. Saunders, 1988.
87. Robertson, A. F., Joshi, V. V., Ellison, D. A., et al.: Zygomycosis in neonates. Pediatr. Infect. Dis. J. *16*:812, 1997.
88. Rosen, P. P., and Sternberg, S. S.: Decreased frequency of aspergillosis and mucormycosis. N. Engl. J. Med. *295*:1319, 1976.
89. Rozich, J., Oxendine, D., Heffner, J., et al.: Pulmonary zygomycosis: A cause of positive lung scan diagnosed by bronchoalveolar lavage. Chest *95*:238, 1989.
90. Ryan, M. E., and Ochs, J.: Primary cutaneous mucormycosis: Superficial and gangrenous infections. Pediatr. Infect. Dis. *1*:110, 1982.
91. Ryan-Poirier, K., Eiseman, R. M., Beaty, J. H., et al.: Post-traumatic cutaneous mucormycosis in diabetes mellitus: Short-term antifungal therapy. Clin. Pediatr. *27*:609, 1988.
92. Sane, A., Manzi, S., Perfect, J., et al.: Deferoxamine treatment as a risk factor for zygomycete infection. J. Infect. Dis. *159*:151, 1989.
93. Schmidt, J. H., Howard, R. J., Chen, J. L., et al.: First culture proven gastrointestinal entomophthoromycosis in the United States: A case report and review of the literature. Mycopathologia *95*:101, 1986.
94. Schwartz, J. N., Donnelly, E. H., and Klintworth, G. K.: Ocular and orbital phycomycosis. Surv. Ophthalmol. *22*:3, 1977.
95. Smith, A. G., Bustamante, C. I., and Gilmor, G. D.: Zygomycosis (absidiomycosis) in an AIDS patient. Mycopathologia *105*:7, 1989.
96. Stave, G. M., Heimberger, T., and Kerkering, T. M.: Zygomycosis of the basal ganglia in intravenous drug users. Am. J. Med. *86*:115, 1989.
97. Sugar, A. M., and Liu, X. P.: Combination antifungal therapy in treatment of murine pulmonary mucormycosis: Roles of quinolones and azoles. Antimicrob. Agents Chemother. *44*:2004, 2000.
98. Taylor, G. D., Sekhon, A. S., Tyrrell, D. L. J., et al.: Rhinofacial zygomycosis caused by *Conidiobolus coronatus:* A case report including in vitro sensitivity to antimycotic agents. Am. J. Trop. Med. Hyg. *36*:398, 1982.
99. Tazelaar, H. D., Baird, A. M., Mill, M., et al.: Bronchocentric mycosis occurring in transplant recipients. Chest *96*:92, 1989.

100. Umbert, I. J., and Su, W. P. D.: Cutaneous mucormycosis. J. Am. Acad. Dermatol. *21*:1232, 1989.
101. Vadeboncoeur, C., Walton, J. M., Raisen, J., et al.: Gastrointestinal mucormycosis causing an acute abdomen in the immunocompromised pediatric patient: Three cases. J. Pediatr. Surg. *29*:1248, 1994.
102. Vallaeys, J. H., Praet, M. M., Roels, H. J., et al.: The Budd-Chiari syndrome caused by a zygomycete: A new pathogenesis of hepatic vein thrombosis. Arch. Pathol. Lab. Med. *113*:1171, 1989.
103. Varricchio, F., Reyes, M. G., and Wilks, A.: Undiagnosed mucormycosis in infants. Pediatr. Infect. Dis. J. *8*:660, 1989.
104. Ventura, G. J., Kantarjian, H. M., Anaissie, E., et al.: Pneumonia with *Cunninghamella* species in patients with hematologic malignancies: A case report and review of the literature. Cancer *58*:1534, 1986.
105. Wajszczuk, C. P., Dummer, J. S., Ho, M., et al.: Fungal infections in liver transplant recipients. Transplantation *40*:347, 1985.
106. Walker, S. D., Clark, R. V., King, C. T., et al: Fatal disseminated *Conidiobolus coronatus* infection in a renal transplant patient. Am. J. Clin. Pathol. *98*:559, 1992.
107. Walsh, T. J., Hiemenz, J. W., Seibel, N., et al.: Amphotericin B lipid complex in the treatment of 228 cases of invasive mycosis. 34th ICAAC, Orlando, 1994, poster M69.
108. Walsh, T. J., and Pizzo, P. A.: Nosocomial fungal infections: A classification for hospital-acquired fungal infections and mycoses arising from endogenous flora or reactivation. Ann. Rev. Microbiol. *42*:517, 1988.
109. Walsh, T. J., Renshaw, G., Andrews, J., et al: Invasive zygomycosis due to *Conidiobolus incongruus*. Clin. Infect. Dis. *19*:423, 1994.
110. Weems, J. J., Jr., Davis, B. J., Tablan, O. C., et al.: Construction activity: An independent risk factor for invasive aspergillosis and zygomycosis in patients with hematologic malignancy. Infect. Control *8*:71–75, 1987.
111. White, C. B., Barcia, P. J., and Bass, J. W.: Neonatal zygomycotic necrotizing cellulitis. Pediatrics *78*:100, 1986.
112. Wickline, C. L., Cornitius, T. G., and Butler, T.: Cellulitis caused by *Rhizomucor pusillus* in a diabetic patient receiving continuous insulin infusion pump therapy. South. Med. J. *82*:1432, 1989.
113. Wieden, M. A., Steinbronn, K. K., Padhye, A. A., et al.: Zygomycosis caused by *Apophysomyces elegans*. J. Clin. Microbiol. *22*:522, 1985.
114. Windus, D. W., Stokes, T. J., Julian, B. A., et al.: Fatal *Rhizopus* infections in hemodialysis patients receiving deferoxamine. Ann. Intern. Med. *107*:678, 1987.
115. Woodward, A., McTigue, C., Hogg, G., et al.: Mucormycosis of the neonatal gut: A "new" disease or a variant of necrotizing enterocolitis? J. Pediatr. Surg. *27*:737, 1992.
116. Zeluff, B. J.: Fungal pneumonia in transplant recipients. Semin. Respir. Infect. *5*:80, 1990.

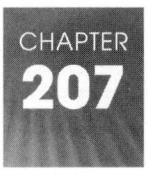

CHAPTER 207 Miscellaneous Mycoses

JUDITH L. ROWEN

Entities

Fungi other than the classic mycoses generally cause disease in two distinct ways: first, organisms present in the environment are inoculated accidentally into the host, and second, immunocompromised hosts cannot defend against the ubiquitous fungi and acquire systemic infection with organisms that rarely are seen as pathogens in a normal host. When the infection is due to inoculation, several distinct entities occur that may be caused by many different fungi. Table 207–1 lists etiologies reported for these clinical syndromes.

MYCOTIC KERATITIS. In a review of 51 cases of microbial keratitis in children, 18 percent were attributed to fungal pathogens.[40] Corneal infection with fungi often occurs after trauma to the eye, frequently with contamination of the injury by organic matter.[36, 139] Thus, nearly any fungus normally found in such organic matter can invade injured tissue. After *Aspergillus,* the most common fungi implicated are *Fusarium, Alternaria,* and *Curvularia.*[139] The diagnosis often is delayed because the child has been presumptively treated with antibacterial, antiviral, or corticosteroid drops before the acquisition of corneal scrapings.[139] Gram staining or potassium hydroxide wet-mount examination frequently results in a proper diagnosis.[179] Appropriate therapy with topical or oral antifungal agents, or both, is successful in most cases; surgical therapy is required for patients with large areas of infiltrate or after failure of medical treatment.[65, 71] Natamycin, a topical polyene, is used most frequently.

SOFT TISSUE INFECTION, INCLUDING MYCETOMA. Smoldering infection may occur when environmental fungi are inoculated directly into normal tissue. The classic manifestation of this process is mycetoma, a chronic granulomatous disorder affecting all the soft tissues in the area of inoculation, occasionally also involving bone and distant organs.[189] The condition is characterized by abscesses, nodules, and sinuses that may drain characteristic granules. Figure 207–1 depicts a characteristic granule. Approximately two thirds of mycetomata actually are caused by bacteria such as *Nocardia,* whereas the remaining third (also referred to as "eumycetoma") are caused by fungi.[30] In the United States, the pathogen found most frequently is *Scedosporium apiospermum* (sexual phase, *Pseudallescheria boydii*),[30] but in the subtropics, where the condition is more prevalent, the organism isolated most frequently is *Madurella mycetomatis.*[189] The disease occurs more commonly in men than women and is more likely to affect adults than children.[189] In one case series, however, 15 percent of cases occurred in children. The lower extremity, especially the foot, is the body part most commonly involved, followed by the thorax, but cases have been reported that involve all body areas.[30, 189] The differential diagnosis includes cutaneous tuberculosis, tumor, osteomyelitis, and sporotrichosis.[189] Examination of exudates from draining sinuses may reveal the diagnosis, but surgical biopsy might be required.[30, 189] Therapy should be directed at the pathogen isolated; itraconazole has shown some promise in selected cases.[24, 189]

FUNGAL PERITONITIS. Patients undergoing peritoneal dialysis are actually compromised hosts because of both direct violation of the mucocutaneous barrier by the dialysis catheter and the immunosuppressive effect of the underlying renal disease.[15] Fungal peritonitis occurs after contamination of the dialysis system. *Candida* spp. are the most common causative agent,[186] but several other yeasts and filamentous fungi have been reported as the etiology (see Table 207–1). Fungi are responsible for 2.9 percent of

TABLE 207–1 ■ SELECTED MISCELLANEOUS FUNGI IMPLICATED IN COMMON CLINICAL SYNDROMES

Clinical Syndrome	Genus	Reference(s)
Keratitis	*Acremonium*	60, 75
	Alternaria	139
	Aureobasidium	71
	Bipolaris	71
	Curvularia	139
	Exophiala	4
	Fusarium	139
	Metarhizium	41
	Paecilomyces	139
	Penicillium	139
Mycetoma/soft tissue infection	*Acremonium*	60, 75, 189
	Alternaria	27
	Exophiala jeanselmei	189
	Fusarium	189
	Madurella grisea	24, 30
	Madurella mycetomatis	30, 189
	Pseudallescheria boydii/ Scedosporium apiospermum	30, 189
Peritonitis	*Acremonium*	60, 185
	Alternaria	152
	Bipolaris	1, 91, 138
	Exophiala	91
	Fusarium	64, 91
	Paecilomyces	39, 109, 150, 185
	Penicillium	185
	Pichia	125
	Rhodotorula	19, 51, 185
	Saccharomyces	119
	Scedosporium	159
	Trichosporon	33, 44, 117, 185
Sinusitis	*Acremonium*	60
	Alternaria	48, 123
	Bipolaris	48, 187
	Curvularia	48, 86, 127
	Exserohilum	1, 48
	Fusarium	48
	Pseudallescheria	185
	Scopulariopsis	53, 95

Note: The fungi listed are those within the purview of this section on "miscellaneous mycoses." Many of these syndromes are commonly caused by *Candida, Aspergillus,* and the zygomycetes as well.

episodes of peritonitis that occur in children undergoing peritoneal dialysis.[186] Treatment includes removal of the dialysis catheter and antifungal therapy, but the ideal timing for removal of the catheter is not clear.[22, 186] Amphotericin has very poor penetration into the dialysate when given intravenously[22] and is irritating when given intraperitoneally.[58] Penetration of fluconazole into dialysate is rapid and efficient.[22] Both fluconazole and itraconazole have been used successfully as therapy.[22, 31, 68, 120, 185] The outcome of fungal peritonitis may be better in children than adults, with a larger percentage successfully continuing peritoneal dialysis.[186]

FUNGAL SINUSITIS. Fungal sinusitis appears to be a spectrum of diseases ranging from a purely allergic condition through invasive forms that may progress to brain abscess as erosion through the sinus walls continues.[45] Noninvasive sinusitis takes two forms: allergic fungal sinusitis and sinus mycetoma. In allergic fungal sinusitis, the sinus (most commonly a maxillary sinus) fills with a gelatinous material often described as having the consistency of peanut butter or cottage cheese.[45] This material consists of mucin, eosinophils, Charcot-Leyden crystals, and sparse fungal hyphae.[48] Patients have signs and symptoms of chronic sinusitis, and proptosis and distortion of facial features may develop.[48, 127] Most case series include pediatric patients, with the youngest patients being in the early elementary school years.[48, 96, 156] The disease is more common in humid, coastal areas.[45] The fungi implicated most commonly include *Curvularia* and *Bipolaris* spp.[38, 48, 156]; *Aspergillus, Exserohilum,* and *Alternaria* spp. also have been reported.[38, 45]

The diagnosis of allergic fungal sinusitis should be suspected in patients with chronic sinusitis, especially those with a history of atopy. Nasal polyps are found frequently, and many patients may recall production of nasal casts.[48, 156] Computed tomography (CT) and magnetic resonance imaging (MRI) may highly suggest the diagnosis; on non–contrast-enhanced CT, the sinuses contain areas of high attenuation, and by MRI, areas of T2-weighted signal void are seen.[103] Figure 207–2 presents a typical CT scan from a patient with allergic fungal sinusitis. Many patients will show loss of bony margins; this loss is not from invasive destruction but from bone compression caused by a mass effect.[48] The diagnosis is confirmed by histopathology; to meet

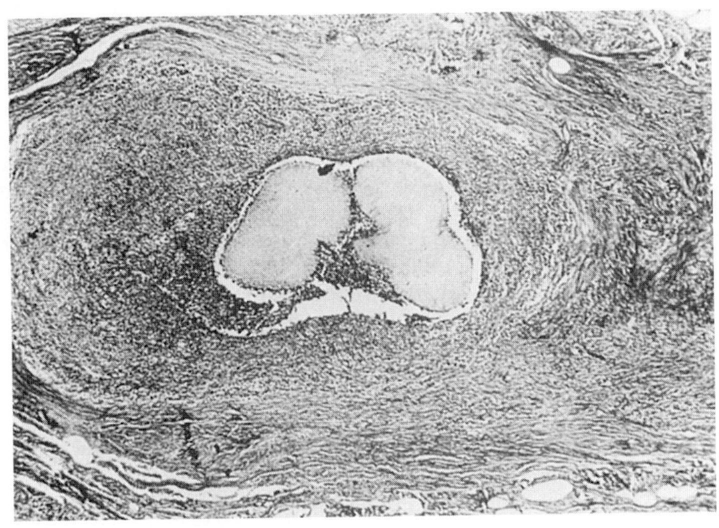

FIGURE 207–1 ■ Large granule of *Pseudallescheria boydii* in the sinus tract of a mycetoma. Extensive fibrosis is seen in the periphery of the tract, and the tract is filled with a mixed granulomatous and pyogenic infiltrate (hematoxylin and eosin, ×100). (Courtesy of Centers for Disease Control and Prevention.)

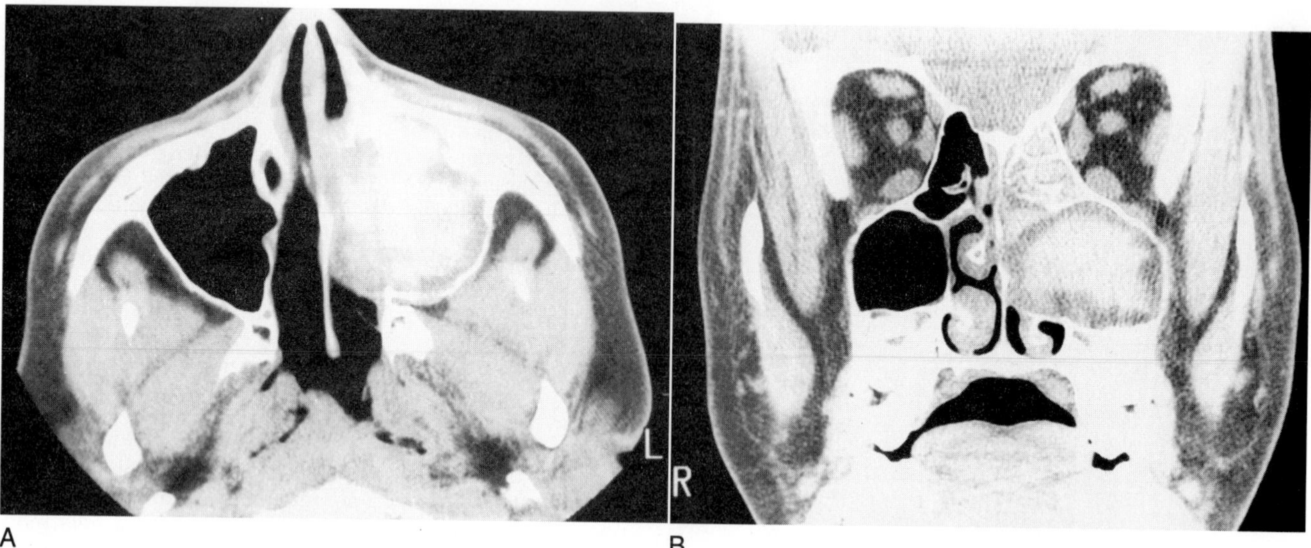

FIGURE 207–2 ■ Allergic *Curvularia* sinusitis in a 12-year-old girl. *A,* Axial computed tomographic image demonstrating a large space-occupying mass involving the left maxillary sinus with expansion of its medial and lateral posterior walls. The mass has high density centrally with a peripheral zone of decreased density. *B,* Coronal image, again showing the mass with centrally increased density and low density in the periphery. Additionally, the ethmoid air cells are involved. (Photos courtesy of Eric Hendrick, M.D.)

the criteria for allergic fungal sinusitis, the patient must be immunocompetent, have radiographic evidence of sinusitis, and have histologic specimens with eosinophil-rich allergic mucin, positive fungal stain, or culture and no evidence of invasion.[48]

Treatment predominantly is surgical, usually endoscopic removal of the allergic mucin and improvement in aeration and drainage.[45, 48, 96, 106] The pathophysiology is assumed to be very similar to that of allergic bronchopulmonary aspergillosis in that the disease is the result of the host's response to inhaled fungi that lodge in the sinuses rather than the result of true infection.[38] Elevated IgE is noted frequently.[48, 156] Thus, corticosteroids, both systemic and nasally inhaled, are administered after surgical drainage.[45, 106, 157] Immunotherapy with fungal allergens also has been used by some clinicians.[106] Recurrences are common, especially if corticosteroid use is stopped prematurely.[157] Itraconazole has been reported to be helpful in allergic bronchopulmonary aspergillosis[168]; it has been used in some cases of allergic fungal sinusitis, but its utility is yet unproven.[11]

The other form of noninvasive fungal sinusitis is sinus mycetoma, which essentially is a fungus ball in the sinuses, usually the maxillary sinuses.[46, 94] The patient initially has nasal obstruction, facial pain, and a fetid odor (cacosmia).[45, 46] Similar to allergic fungal sinusitis, distortion of the bony margins may occur,[46] although one large series noted this finding in only 4% of patients.[94] Although *Aspergillus fumigatus* is the fungus most frequently implicated, *Pseudallescheria* and *Alternaria* also are reported.[46, 94] Clay-like, cheesy material, similar in appearance to the material present in allergic fungal sinusitis but without the findings of allergic mucin on histopathology, is seen at surgery.[45] However, although hyphae are sparse in allergic fungal sinusitis, they are abundant in mycetoma but frequently fail to grow on culture.[45] Treatment is surgical, with wide opening of the sinuses and removal of the mycetoma; recurrences are relatively rare.[94]

Acute, fulminant invasive fungal sinusitis is associated most frequently with Zygomycetes or *Aspergillus* in immunocompromised individuals.[45] However, increasing reports of this entity implicate other fungi such as *Pseudallescheria, Fusarium, Alternaria,* and *Scopulariopsis.*[45, 53, 95, 123] Affected patients are usually immunocompromised as a result of cancer, transplantation, or poorly controlled diabetes mellitus.[47] Initial signs and symptoms may be limited to fever with headache and epistaxis; careful physical examination may reveal nasal mucosal ulcers or eschars.[45] The hallmark of this entity is histopathologic evidence of invasion into the mucosa or other tissues.[45, 47] The disease may progress rapidly and lead to orbital apex syndrome and further intracranial involvement.[45] Therapy includes wide surgical excision and amphotericin B; lipid formulations of amphotericin B may be useful in this syndrome.[45]

Etiologies

The taxonomy of fungi has undergone significant revision with the addition of molecular techniques to the classic morphologic methods. When presented with a patient with a fungal infection, the clinician rarely can identify the taxonomic group of the invading organism until final culture results are available. Instead, the appearance of the organism in tissue specimens is what is appreciated first. Thus, in the following discussion of infection caused by specific pathogens, the organisms will be grouped by their appearance in tissue. For detailed review of fungal taxonomy, the reader is referred to several excellent resources.[172, 193]

YEASTS

In contrast to the filamentous fungi, which tend to invade locally at the site of initial inoculation, with later dissemination if at all, yeasts tend to cause disease after hematogenous dissemination without significant local disease. End-organ deposition, however, may lead to focal disease after hematogenous spread. In addition to *Candida* and the classic dimorphic fungi of endemic infections, several yeast-like pathogens have emerged as significant pathogens.

Malassezia Species

Also known by the obsolete term *Pityrosporum,* these fungi are most familiar as the cause of a minor skin infection, tinea versicolor. However, *Malassezia furfur* and *Malassezia pachydermatis* also cause bloodstream infection, usually in association with central venous catheters. *M. furfur* is obligatorily lipophilic, which probably explains the concordance of systemic disease with the use of intravenous lipid emulsions. Systemic infection with *Malassezia* was described first in 1981 by Redline and Dahms; the patient was an extremely low-birth-weight infant, which is typical for this disease.[148] Catheter-related *Malassezia* fungemia also has been described in older children and adults with immunocompromising conditions.[16] In a review of 55 cases in neonates, the most common underlying condition was prematurity, followed by short-gut syndrome; all infants were receiving lipid supplementation.[105] In contrast, *M. pachydermatis* does not require lipids for growth. This organism is most familiar as a causative agent of otitis externa in dogs, and at least one nursery outbreak has been associated with colonized pets of health care workers.[32]

Adults are colonized nearly universally with *Malassezia* organisms.[105] Colonization in neonates varies from 30 to 100 percent of those sampled and occurs early in life.[3, 98, 145, 161] Factors correlated with colonization include length of hospitalization, lower gestational age, time in an isolette, and use of occlusive dressings.[105] The organisms resist superficial cleaning and may persist on plastic surfaces for prolonged periods of at least 3 months, which may facilitate outbreaks within an intensive care nursery.[180]

Clinically, infected infants have fever (53%), respiratory distress (53%), lethargy, poor feeding, bradycardia, and hepatosplenomegaly.[105] Thrombocytopenia occurs in 48 percent. Frequently, blood drawn directly from the central catheter will be culture-positive, with negative peripheral blood cultures. The laboratory should be alerted that *Malassezia* is suspected because lipid supplementation may enhance recovery of the organism.[134] The 2.5- to 6.0-μm yeasts may be seen on a smear of blood drawn through the catheter.[74, 104] Treatment should include removal of the implicated central catheter. Antifungal therapy usually is provided, although testing suggests only moderate susceptibility to amphotericin B.[104] Even though most infants recover, those succumbing to infection frequently have heavy involvement of the lungs and heart at autopsy.[104, 105]

Trichosporon Species

Most infections caused by *Trichosporon* are attributed to *Trichosporon beigelii* in the literature; however, revision of the genus has suggested that most invasive disease is caused by *Trichosporon asahii,* with other species predominantly implicated in superficial disease such as white piedra.[172] White piedra affects the shafts of terminal hairs and results in nodules or coalescent concretions; one epidemiologic survey found it in 40 percent of men and 14 percent of women tested.[90] Invasive disease usually affects neutropenic cancer patients or neonates.[8, 62, 77, 80, 82] Table 207–2 summarizes other reports of *Trichosporon* infection causing unusual manifestations of disease or affecting patients with other underlying conditions.

Trichosporon is isolated from blood cultures as a yeast that is germ tube–negative and urease-positive. In tissue sections, hyaline hyphae with septations and rectangular arthroconidia (2 to 4 by 3 to 7 μm) are seen, with pseudohyphae and blastoconidia noted occasionally.[172] The organism may be found in soil, water, vegetation, and animal excreta.[82, 172] *Trichosporon* shares a heat-stable antigen with *Cryptococcus neoformans,* which may cause the latex agglutination test for cryptococcal capsular polysaccharide to be positive in the setting of disseminated *Trichosporon* infection.[115] The results of the cryptococcal antigen test have been followed in an experimental model and in patients to document response to therapy; however, the initial antigen testing may be negative despite disseminated disease.[76, 171, 183]

Most affected neonates have been below 1000 g birth weight and born between 23 and 25 weeks' gestational age.[62, 173, 195] Disease was identified most frequently in the second week of life, with the bloodstream and skin being the sites most commonly involved. Most of these infants succumbed to their infection.

Immunocompromised hosts frequently have fever during periods of neutropenia. Skin involvement occurs in the setting of disseminated disease and is described as papular, purpuric, or necrotic lesions.[54, 88] The organism is recovered from blood cultures, skin lesions, urine, sputum, and liver and kidney biopsy specimens, thus indicating the organism's widespread involvement.[54, 82] Isolated fungemia and infection limited to the lungs also have been reported.[7, 121] Mortality rates are high.[54, 82]

TABLE 207–2 ■ SUMMARY OF REPORTED *TRICHOSPORON* INFECTIONS

Type of Infection	Underlying Condition	Reference
Bloodstream	Burns	76
Disseminated	Hemophagocytic syndrome	42, 81
Endocarditis	Repaired congenital heart disease	13
Invasive fungal dermatitis	Prematurity	153
Lung abscess	Chronic granulomatous disease	142
Meningitis	Acute lymphocytic leukemia	171
Oral mucositis	Acute myelogenous leukemia	83
Parvertebral abscess	Acute lymphoblastic leukemia	17
Peritonitis	Continuous ambulatory peritoneal dialysis for renal failure	117
Pneumonia	Trauma	118
Sepsis with shock	Diabetes mellitus	50
Septic arthritis	Acute myelogenous leukemia	116
Shunt infection	Arachnoid cyst	14
Urinary tract infection	Renal transplant	100

Although amphotericin B often is used, some experts recommend therapy with one of the newer azoles. The organism has been described as tolerant to amphotericin B,[184] but animal models have shown good efficacy with fluconazole.[8, 183] A new triazole, voriconazole, has good activity in vitro, but clinical data are lacking.[113] Successful therapy with lipid-based amphotericin B has been reported.[173]

Penicillium marneffei

Occasional reports describe opportunistic infection with *Penicillium* molds, but the major pathogen in this genus is *P. marneffei,* which is the only species that is a dimorphic fungus. At 25° C, it grows as a filamentous mold and produces a diffusible red pigment, whereas at 37° C, it grows as a yeast form that reproduces by fission rather than budding.[37] The hyphae are septate and hyaline, and the yeast forms are 3 to 5 μm in size, similar to the size of *Histoplasma.*[172] Initial reports confused the organism with *Histoplasma*; one histopathologic feature that may be helpful is that the yeasts of *P. marneffei* frequently have visible cross walls that form during fission.[37, 43] Adding to the potential confusion, infection with *P. marneffei* may lead to a false-positive *Histoplasma* antigen test.[37]

The fungus was isolated first from bamboo rats captured in Vietnam, and the disease is endemic to Southeast Asia, including areas of Myanmar, Cambodia, southern China, Indonesia, Laos, Malaysia, Thailand, and Vietnam.[132] Disease caused by *P. marneffei* was listed as an acquired immunodeficiency syndrome (AIDS)–defining condition in 1992, and it is the third most common opportunistic infection in the Chiang Mai region of Thailand, with 16 percent of all patients infected with human immunodeficiency virus (HIV).[37] The exact mode of transmission is unclear; bamboo rats and humans are thought to be infected from a common source rather than transmission being from rats to humans.[49] An inhalational route of infection is supported by an infection in a physician from Africa who was HIV-positive and whose only possible exposure was during a visit to the Pasteur Institute, where other laboratory workers were handling the fungus.[132] The incubation period may be as short as 2 weeks to very prolonged; the first recognized human case was in a U.S. missionary with Hodgkin disease who had traveled in Southeast Asia 2 years before the discovery of his infection.[132]

In most cases, the disease is disseminated, with prominent involvement of the skin by umbilicated papules reminiscent of molluscum contagiosum, as shown in Figure 207–3.[37] In a review of 21 children with HIV and penicilliosis, the initial signs and symptoms included generalized lymphadenopathy (90%), hepatomegaly (90%), fever (81%), skin lesions (67%), splenomegaly (67%), failure to thrive (52%), severe anemia (43%), and thrombocytopenia (21%).[166] The infection was manifested at a later age than most opportunistic infections in this population (32 versus 7 months of age). In adults, fever, weight loss, and anemia are also prominent, and a painful cough is noted frequently.[49] The organism usually is isolated from blood cultures, and skin biopsy cultures also frequently yield the organism.[49, 166]

More focal involvement of lymph nodes may occur. In children with HIV, mesenteric adenitis with prolonged fever and abdominal pain may mimic acute appendicitis.[178] Chronic lymphadenopathy resembling scrofula has been reported in a previously healthy child.[196] This child and another without underlying disease had transient lymphocyte abnormalities that resolved after treatment of the infection.[97, 196]

The diagnosis is dependent primarily on isolation of the organism from cultures or characteristic findings on histopathologic examination with a consistent clinical history. Serologic and DNA amplification tests have been devised but remain experimental.[49, 132] Amphotericin B followed by itraconazole is the usual mode of therapy. As with many fungal infections in HIV patients, relapse occurs frequently once therapy is halted.[169] In a placebo-controlled trial of itraconazole maintenance therapy, relapse did not occur in the treatment arm, whereas 20 of 35 placebo recipients relapsed at a mean of 24 weeks after therapy.[170]

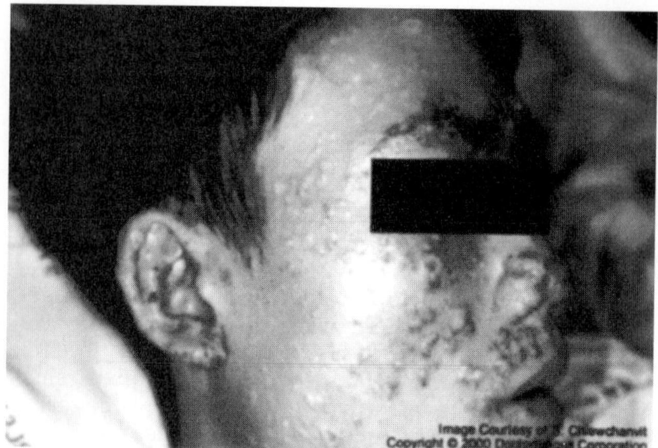

FIGURE 207–3 ■ Skin lesions from *Penicillium marneffei.* (Photograph courtesy of S. Chiewchanvit, provided by *www.doctorfungus.org.*)

Pichia Species

Pichia anomala (formerly known as *Hansenula anomala)* and *Pichia angusta* (formerly known as *Hansenula polymorpha)* are rare causes of human disease. *P. anomala* is the teleomorph, or sexual stage, of *Candida pelliculosa.* It characteristically has one to four hat-shaped ascospores when asci are produced.[172] It may colonize the human gastrointestinal tract and also is found in pigeon excreta, plants, and fruit.[12]

Human infection has been reported primarily in immunocompromised hosts and premature neonates.[6, 12, 114, 125, 128, 158, 164, 175, 194] Nursery outbreaks with high levels of colonization have been described.[12, 128, 164] Neonates with fungemia are lethargic and have mottling, apnea, bradycardia, and an increased need for ventilatory support.[128] Abscesses may occur at the site of insertion of peripheral intravenous catheters.[128] Jaundice and fever also have been described.[12] Almost every patient reported had recently received broad-spectrum antibiotics and had a central catheter in place, frequently for parenteral nutrition.[12] The organism often is isolated from blood cultures and the catheter tip.[6, 194] Other infections have included ventriculitis, lymphadenitis, and necrotizing enteritis.[114, 125, 128]

Despite the fragile nature of the patients affected, disease caused by *Pichia* rarely is fatal. Most reported cases have been treated with amphotericin B plus 5-flucytosine and removal of central venous catheters. Although many isolates are susceptible to fluconazole, elevated minimal inhibitory concentrations (MICs) have been found in patient isolates associated with poor clinical response to this drug.[6, 194]

Rhodotorula Species

Rhodotorula grows as glistening pink to red colonies. Usually, no pseudohyphae are formed; the yeast cells are ovoid or elongate, 2 to 5.5 by 2.5 to 14 μm.[172] The organism is urease-positive and does not ferment carbohydrates.[172] It can be found colonizing normal human skin, mucous membranes, shower curtains, bathtubs, and toothbrushes and can be isolated from cheese, milk, air, soil, and water.[93, 162, 172] Most human infections have been associated with catheters in patients with cancer or HIV.[93, 162, 182] Endocarditis in a child with presumed underlying rheumatic heart disease also has been described.[131] The pathogen appears to be of low virulence, with few deaths attributable to infection. Resistance to fluconazole occurs commonly, whereas in vitro testing suggests that most strains are susceptible to voriconazole, itraconazole, and amphotericin B.[55, 93] Clinical cases have been treated successfully with amphotericin B or 5-flucytosine monotherapy and by removal of catheters, without antifungal therapy.[93, 131]

Saccharomyces cerevisiae

This yeast is best known as baker's yeast or brewer's yeast. Strains (often called *Saccharomyces boulardii*) also have been used as a biotherapeutic agent for severe diarrhea, especially *Clostridium difficile*–associated diarrhea.[78] The yeast is distributed ubiquitously in the environment and may be found as a commensal in the human gastrointestinal tract.[176] Clinical isolates have enhanced virulence in comparison to environmental strains when evaluated in animal models.[144] *Saccharomyces* is responsible for 3 percent of cases of fungal vaginitis, especially in women with a history of recurrent or chronic vaginitis.[144, 167] Invasive infection develops in patients with multiple medical problems, usually with a central venous catheter in place.[7, 61, 120, 176] The source of infection is presumed to be via translocation from the gastrointestinal tract or from indwelling venous lines.[176] Mortality rates with these infections are high, near 50 percent.[61] Organisms have been isolated from the blood, peritoneum, kidneys, lungs, liver, and spleen.[61] Infections associated with the use of *S. boulardii* (actually not a separate species) seem to be less clinically devastating, although septic shock developed in one patient, who later recovered.[78, 143] Environmental sampling has indicated that the organisms can be isolated from the air, environmental surfaces, and the hands of caretakers opening packets for administration to the patient, so direct contamination of central venous catheters may be the source, although gut translocation also has been postulated.[78, 143] Therapy includes removal of implicated catheters and administration of antifungal agents. MICs are low for amphotericin B and 5-flucytosine, and itraconazole and voriconazole seem to have better activity than fluconazole does.[55, 176]

Blastoschizomyces capitatus

This pathogen was formerly known as *Trichosporon capitatum* and *Geotrichum capitatum*. It may be found in soil and beach sand and as part of the normal human flora of the gastrointestinal tract.[172] Infection has been seen predominantly in immunocompromised hosts, especially those with hematologic malignancies. In a review of 12 patients with *Blastoschizomyces* infection, blood cultures were positive in 11.[108] Eight of the patients had lesions comparable to those seen with hepatosplenic candidiasis, and the fungus did grow from liver specimens.[108] Five patients had neurologic findings, and focal lesions were seen on CT scans of the brain.[108] Chronic meningitis in a patient after bone marrow transplantation has been described.[73] Organisms have been isolated from the blood, heart, lungs, liver, spleen, cerebrospinal fluid (CSF), skin, stomach, urine, kidneys, and intracerebral lesions.[13, 73, 108] The lung lesions may resemble those of an aspergilloma, with cavitation and a typical crescent sign.[108] In tissue, pleomorphic yeasts 3 to 8 μm in diameter and septate hyphae are seen. Successful therapy generally requires recovery from neutropenia. Amphotericin B with and without 5-flucytosine and fluconazole have been used. A patient with chronic meningitis responded clinically to a prolonged course of fluconazole, but fungi were noted in the meninges at autopsy, so the infection was not eradicated.[73] Voriconazole has better activity in vitro than the other azoles do; clinical correlation has not been reported.[55]

MOLDS

In contrast to the pathogens found in tissues as yeasts, molds are rarely part of the normal human flora and instead have arisen from the environment. A portal of entry, be it a minor wound, a central catheter, or the lungs, is often recognizable. With increasing numbers of immunocompromised hosts, the variety of fungi assuming greater clinical importance has expanded similarly. In tissue specimens, making a definitive diagnosis of the particular mold involved is rarely possible. One useful differentiation is between the "black molds," or dematiaceous fungi, which lead to clinical infections collectively known as phaeohyphomycoses, and the hyaline molds, which cause hyalohyphomycoses. Dematiaceous fungi contain melanin in their cell walls, which can be seen in tissue sections, especially with Masson-Fontana staining. Table 207–3 lists the genera included in this group. In addition to phaeohyphomycosis, other clinical syndromes associated with the dematiaceous fungi, such as mycetoma (discussed previously) and chromoblastomycosis, are sufficiently unique to be discussed separately.

Agents of hyalohyphomycosis are listed in Table 207–4. In tissue section, the hyaline molds may be presumed to be *Aspergillus* or *Candida*. Although the distinction is difficult to make, a few characteristics may allow differentiation of these molds from the more common *Aspergillus*. The hyphae are septate, frequently with marked variation in diameter.[99] Whereas *Aspergillus* nearly uniformly branches at 45 degrees, the hyaline molds may exhibit both 45- and

TABLE 207–3 ■ DEMATIACEOUS FUNGI

Alternaria*	*Gamsia*	***Phialophora***
Aureobasidium	*Gliomastix*	*Phoma*
Bipolaris	*Hannebertia*	*Pithomyces*
Botrymyces	*Helminthosporium*	*Pleurophragmium*
Byssoascus	*Hormonema*	*Ramichloridium*
Cephalotrichum	*Humicola*	*Rhinocladiella*
Chaetomium	*Hypoxylon*	*Rosellinia*
Chloridium	*Khuskia*	***Scedosporium prolificans***
Cladophialophora	*Lecythophora*	*Scolecobasidium*
Cladosporium	*Leptodontium*	*Scytalidium*
Coniothyrium	*Leptosphaeria*	*Sporidesmium*
Curvularia	***Madurella***	*Stachybotrys*
Dactylaria	*Microascus*	*Stemphylium*
Doratomyces	*Mycocentrospora*	*Stephanosporium*
Drechstera	*Nigrospora*	*Taeniolella*
Echinobotryum	*Ochroconus*	*Torula*
Epicoccum	*Oidiodendron*	*Ulocladium*
Exophiala	*Periconia*	*Wangiella*
Exserohilum	*Phaeoacremonium*	*Wardomyces*
Fonsecaea	*Phialemonium*	*Xylar*

*Genera in bold type are most frequently implicated in human disease.

TABLE 207–4 ■ AGENTS OF HYALOHYPHOMYCOSIS

Acremonium*
Aphanoascus (anamorph = *Chrysosporium*)
Arthrographis
Beauveria
Chrysosporium
Coprinus (actually a mushroom)
Cylindrocarpon
Fusarium
Myriodontium
Paecilomyces
Penicillium
Schizophyllum commune (actually a bracket fungus)
Trichoderma
Tritrachium
Volutella

*The most frequently implicated genera are presented in bold type.

90-degree branching.[99] Careful investigation frequently reveals evidence of adventitious sporulation through the presence of phialoconidia and phialides; *Aspergillus* generally only undergoes in vivo sporulation in aerated spaces such as lung cavities.[99] Confusion with Zygomycetes occurs less commonly, but the hyphae of hyaline molds are narrower and more frequently septate than those of Zygomycetes and thus less likely to twist in a ribbon-like pattern.[99]

Phaeohyphomycosis

The range of clinical diseases attributed to the phaeoid, or dematiaceous, fungi is broad. The term *phaeohyphomycosis* literally means "condition of fungi with dark hyphae" and thus does not reflect the disease produced but the pathogen producing the disease. The presence of melanin in the cell wall may act as a virulence factor, as has been shown for *Wangiella dermatitidis* in animal models.[110] Focal diseases attributed to this group of fungi include bone and joint infection after local trauma, sinusitis, peritonitis associated with dialysis, and keratitis. Implicated genera include *Alternaria, Curvularia, Bipolaris, Exserohilum,* and *Exophiala*.[1, 27, 59, 110] Allergic bronchopulmonary pneumonitis also has been described.[1]

Phaeomycotic brain abscess often is caused by *Cladophialophora bantiana* (formerly named *Xylohypha bantiana)* or *Ochroconus gallopavum* (formerly named *Dactylaria gallopavum)*.[110, 165] *Bipolaris* also has been reported as a cause of brain abscess and granulomatous meningoencephalitis.[1, 124] Many of these patients are immunocompetent, without underlying disease. Brain abscess caused by *C. bantiana* is manifested as chronic headache, fever, and hemiparesis.[110] Young males are affected predominantly, and the frontal lobes are involved most commonly. Lumbar puncture reveals elevated opening pressure, high protein and depressed glucose levels, and negative cultures. Abscess cultures must be obtained.[110]

Disseminated disease usually occurs in the setting of altered host immunity. Most patients have hematologic malignancies with resultant neutropenia. In a review of 72 cases of disseminated phaeohyphomycosis, the mortality rate was 79 percent.[149] Fever was present in 76 percent, with skin manifestations in 33 percent, central nervous system (CNS) symptoms in 31 percent, gastrointestinal symptoms in 31 percent, and apparent sepsis in 11 percent.[149] Blood cultures were positive in more than half the patients.[149] Fungemia with *Exophiala jeanselmei* has been described in association with central venous catheters.[137] Eosinophilia may be a hint that disseminated phaeomycosis is the cause of fever in an immunocompromised host, although it was noted in only 11 percent of such patients.[149]

Infection in organ transplant recipients is manifested somewhat differently than in those with hematologic malignancies. The length of time post-transplant until the development of symptomatic disease is prolonged, with a median time of 22 months.[165] Skin, soft tissue, or joint infection develops in most organ transplant patients, with *Exophiala* being the pathogen most frequently implicated.[165] The second most common manifestation is brain abscess, which occurs much earlier in the course, at a mean of 3 months post-transplant.[165]

Premature neonates are another population of immunocompromised hosts susceptible to unusual pathogens. Infection caused by the agents of phaeohyphomycosis in premature infants predominantly have been in the form of invasive fungal dermatitis with necrotic ulcers. Two cases caused by *Curvularia* and one by *Bipolaris* have been described.[29, 59, 152]

Skin lesions attributed to phaeohyphomycosis may take many forms, including papules, plaques, pustules, nodules, and nonhealing ulcers, most commonly on the extremities.[165] In a review of 89 cases of cutaneous alternariosis, the lesions were noted to be shallow-based, nonhealing ulcers that evolved from nodules, subcutaneous noninflammatory cysts, verrucous lesions, and confluent scaly patches.[101] In the setting of disseminated disease, skin manifestations may take the form of a rash rather than discreet lesions.[149]

Therapy for phaeohyphomycosis depends on the site of infection. If surgical resection is feasible, it should be pursued. Generally, amphotericin B does not have good activity, whereas itraconazole has more consistent activity.[149] In vitro results of 15 species of dematiaceous fungi demonstrated low MICs for both itraconazole and terbinafine.[112] Itraconazole led to clinical improvement, remission, or stabilization in 11 of 17 patients.[160]

STACHYBOTRYS

A cluster of 10 cases of pulmonary hemorrhage and hemosiderosis in infants in Cleveland, Ohio, initially was attributed to environmental exposure to *Stachybotrys chartarum* (also referred to as *Stachybotrys atra*).[52, 57] This mold produces trichothecene mycotoxins, so researchers postulated that the disease in infants was caused by exposure to mycotoxins from fungi growing in water-damaged households. However, further evaluation by the Centers for Disease Control and Prevention found that the association was not substantiated.[67] If similar outbreaks recur, more careful analysis of the role of fungi and mycotoxins is warranted.

CHROMOBLASTOMYCOSIS

Chromoblastomycosis is a chronic infection of skin and subcutaneous tissue; the agent most commonly isolated is *Fonsecaea pedrosoi,* but other implicated fungi are *Cladophialophora carrionii* and *Phialophora verrucosa.* The disease is limited to the tropical and subtropical regions of the world, usually in warm, humid areas.[23] Infection begins with inoculation of the organism, typically through minor trauma. Most affected patients are men, frequently farmers.[23] The median age of affected patients is 35 years, but pediatric patients have been reported.[23] The mean duration of illness before initial medical evaluation is 3 years, thus attesting to the slow-growing nature of this process.[23] The lesions are markedly hyperkeratotic and may be nodular, verrucous, or psoriaform[23] (Fig. 207–4). Common symptoms include pruritus and pain.[23] Scratching the lesions may be the mode of spread for the frequent development of satellite lesions.[111] Bacterial superinfection is a common complication; the fungi do not usually disseminate to deeper tissues, although brain involvement has been reported.[23, 111] A late complication is fibrosis leading to lymphatic obstruction and a clinical picture similar to that of elephantiasis.[111] Most cases can be diagnosed by direct potassium hydroxide smears, which reveal the pathognomonic sclerotic bodies.[23] Sclerotic bodies also have been referred to as muriform cells and Medlar bodies. They are round to polyhedral, chestnut brown, thick-walled cells 5 to 12 μm in diameter with horizontal or vertical septae.[111] If biopsy is performed, the sclerotic bodies once again will be noted, and the dermis will reveal granulomata.[23, 111] The fungi readily grow in culture, but a few weeks may be necessary for colonies to be evident. The differential diagnosis includes verrucous cutaneous tuberculosis, sporotrichosis, mycetoma, leishmaniasis, coccidioidomycosis, psoriasis, hyperkeratotic tinea, blastomycosis, leprosy, and tertiary syphilis.[23, 111] Differentiating features include the distinct margins and frequent satellite lesions of chromoblastomycosis.[111] Treatment has included local excision when feasible, with some practitioners using either cryosurgery or the application of heat.[23, 111] Antifungal therapy with itraconazole or terbinafine has shown promising results.[23, 56]

SCEDOSPORIUM/PSEUDALLESCHERIA

Classification of these organisms as agents of phaeohyphomycosis versus hyalohyphomycosis has been controversial.[110] *Scedosporium prolificans* is listed more commonly as dematiaceous, and *S. apiospermum* infection is listed most commonly as a hyalohyphomycosis. *S. apiospermum* is the asexual anamorph of *P. boydii*; other obsolete names for this fungus include *Petriellidium boydii, Monosporium apiospermum,* and *Allescheria boydii. S. prolificans* was referred to previously as *Scedosporium inflatum* but was found to be conspecific with a fungus named *Lomentospora prolificans* isolated from the soil of potted plants in a Belgian greenhouse; thus, the previously assigned specific nomenclature was adopted.[20] The two species differ morphologically, with *S. prolificans* having annellides with a distinctive, swollen base.[192] In addition, *P. boydii* will grow on Sabouraud agar containing cycloheximide whereas *S. prolificans* will not.[192] Both species of *Scedosporium* cause disseminated disease in

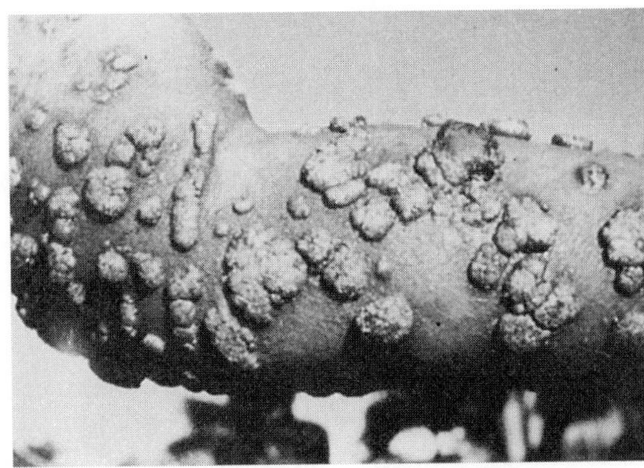

FIGURE 207–4 ■ Chromoblastomycosis. The warty-like growth of epidermis and dermis is a result of traumatic implantation of the etiologic agent and subsequent autoinoculation from scratching. The agent was *Fonsecaea pedrosoi.*

immunocompromised hosts, but differences in the form of localized disease most associated with the species do occur. In the United States, *P. boydii* is the causative agent most commonly isolated from mycetoma.[30] *P. boydii* is widely distributed in soil, sewage, and contaminated water.[172] Its presence in polluted water is most likely responsible for the unique occurrence of brain abscess caused by this fungus in patients who have survived near-drowning. In a review of 38 cases of CNS infection, most of the patients had immunocompromising conditions, but 28 percent had sustained near-drowning.[135] Abscesses may be single or multiple.[135] Although the fungus may be isolated from CSF, direct inspection of brain tissue usually is required to make the diagnosis.[92]

P. boydii may be isolated from respiratory secretions in the absence of disease.[177] In patients with cystic fibrosis, 8.6 percent had *S. apiospermum* isolated from sputum cultures, the most frequent filamentous fungus after *A. fumigatus.*[34] Two of the patients had signs and symptoms compatible with allergic bronchopulmonary disease occurring after chronic colonization with *S. apiospermum.*[34] Invasive pulmonary disease also develops in both immunocompetent and immunocompromised hosts.[89, 126, 177] Clinically, it may resemble aspergillosis. In addition to pulmonary infection, other focal forms of the disease have included endocarditis related to an indwelling catheter, osteomyelitis, surgical wound infection, sinusitis, and olecranon bursitis.[64, 177, 190]

S. prolificans initially was recognized as a cause of focally invasive disease, especially musculoskeletal infections occurring after penetrating trauma or surgery.[192] However, recently the organism has been recognized as an emerging pathogen of immunocompromised hosts.[141, 144] Some clusters of cases have occurred in association with hospital renovation, thus suggesting a possible environmental source, but such an etiology has not been conclusively demonstrated.[20] Because many of the cases have been reported from Spain, Australia, and California, it has been suggested that climactic factors may influence the likelihood of infection. Cases in California have been suspected to be coccidioidomycosis.[136]

The usual finding of disseminated *S. prolificans* infection is fever unresponsive to broad-spectrum antibiotics, followed by pulmonary involvement and later neurologic manifestations, skin lesions, and finally, widespread involvement with frequent renal failure.[144, 146] In a review of 16 cases of disseminated infection, chest radiographs were abnormal in 12 patients, with bilateral focal infiltrates in 6, diffuse infiltrates in 5, and a solitary pulmonary nodule in a single patient.[20] The skin lesions are usually multiple and may be erythematous or nodular or have necrotic centers.[20, 136] One patient had intense myalgias preceding the eruption of skin lesions.[136] Meningoencephalitis may occur; one case was attributed to direct inoculation during lumbar puncture for intrathecal chemotherapy.[102] At autopsy, the fungus is found most commonly in the kidney, lung, brain, and spleen.[20] The mortality rate is very high, 87.5 percent in one series.[20] Blood cultures are frequently positive, with the organism growing in 9 to 15 days in routine blood culture detection systems but much more rapidly in fungal isolator tubes.[20]

Both clinically important species of *Scedosporium* are resistant to amphotericin B.[20, 55] Therapy usually includes wide surgical débridement whenever possible. Some joint infections apparently have responded to débridement plus intra-articular amphotericin B; the high local concentration may improve its effectiveness.[192] As with most mold infections, recovery of neutrophil counts in immunocompromised hosts is critical for improvement. *P. boydii* is susceptible to some of the newer triazoles such as posaconazole, ravuconazole, and voriconazole, none of which are available commercially.[144] Some strains of *S. prolificans* were also susceptible, and a triazole, as yet unnamed, also showed some activity.[144] Successful treatment of *P. boydii* with voriconazole has been reported.[126, 135] Itraconazole has some activity and has proved effective in localized disease, but decreased concentrations in brain tissue may limit its effectiveness.[65, 135]

Hyalohyphomycosis

FUSARIUM SPECIES

Fusarium initially was recognized as a plant pathogen that caused crown rot on cereal grains.[133] The organisms are distributed widely in soil and vegetation and in all climates, and they may be airborne.[133] Pathogenic species also have been isolated from hospital water systems, thus suggesting the possibility of nosocomial acquisition.[10] The species most commonly associated with invasive human disease are *Fusarium solani, Fusarium oxysporum,* and *Fusarium verticilloides* (also known as *Fusarium moniliforme*).[79]

The first human disease states attributed to *Fusarium* were secondary not to invasion but to elaboration of mycotoxins. Alimentary toxic aleukia was responsible for epidemics in the Soviet Union during World War II.[133] This disease results from the consumption of grains colonized with *Fusarium sporotrichioides* after overwintering. The fungus elaborates a toxin designated T-2, which is a potent protein synthesis inhibitor. The disease begins with a burning sensation from the mouth to the stomach, followed by vomiting and diarrhea, abdominal pain, headache, and fatigue. Progressive leukopenia develops, and hemorrhage and necrosis eventually may lead to death. A similar disease known as scabby grain intoxication, or akakabi-byo, has occurred in Japan.[133] Mycotoxins have never been demonstrated conclusively during invasive fusariosis, but they have been postulated to contribute to virulence through further suppression of the host's immune system.[133] Other possible virulence factors include production of enzymes and adherence and invasion of prosthetic materials.[133]

In immunocompetent hosts, *Fusarium* may cause localized disease such as onychomycosis and fungal keratitis. Onychomycosis from *Fusarium* may result in a characteristic milky discoloration of the nail.[133] *Fusarium* is the most common fungal etiology of keratitis in the United States.[133] Corneal injury accompanied by contamination with fungal material may progress to keratitis, possibly aided by the elaboration of proteases by *F. solani.*[133, 139] The organism can survive on contact lenses, thus affording another possible mode of entry.[133] Burn wounds also are colonized frequently with *Fusarium.*[141] In central Africa, *Fusarium* is a frequent cause of mycotic external otitis.[133] Bone and joint infections have been reported after traumatic inoculation,[25, 133] and hematogenous osteomyelitis has been described in an adolescent with leukemia.[28] Peritonitis associated with continuous ambulatory peritoneal dialysis catheters also may occur.[63, 91, 133]

The incidence of infection caused by *Fusarium* has been increasing, most probably in concert with the increased use of immunosuppressive regimens. Most cases are described in patients with hematologic malignancies, but other underlying conditions include aplastic anemia, AIDS, solid tumors, and burns.[107] Eight percent of all non-*Candida* fungal infections occurring after bone marrow transplantation are caused by *Fusarium.*[122] The vast majority of patients are neutropenic at the time of infection. In a review of 81 cases, the infection was disseminated in 88 percent.[107] Common sites of infection were the skin (79%), lungs (42%), and the upper respiratory tract, including the sinuses (22%).[107] Localized disease, specifically onychomycosis, precedes disseminated infection in a substantial number of cases, thus underscoring the need for careful inspection and treatment of local infection before the institution of immunosuppressive therapy.[107, 133] Infection in patients after receiving solid organ transplants usually is localized and occurs at a median of 9 months post-transplant.[155]

In immunocompromised hosts, skin involvement is characteristic (Fig. 207–5 provides an example). The lesions are found predominantly on the extremities and begin as tender,

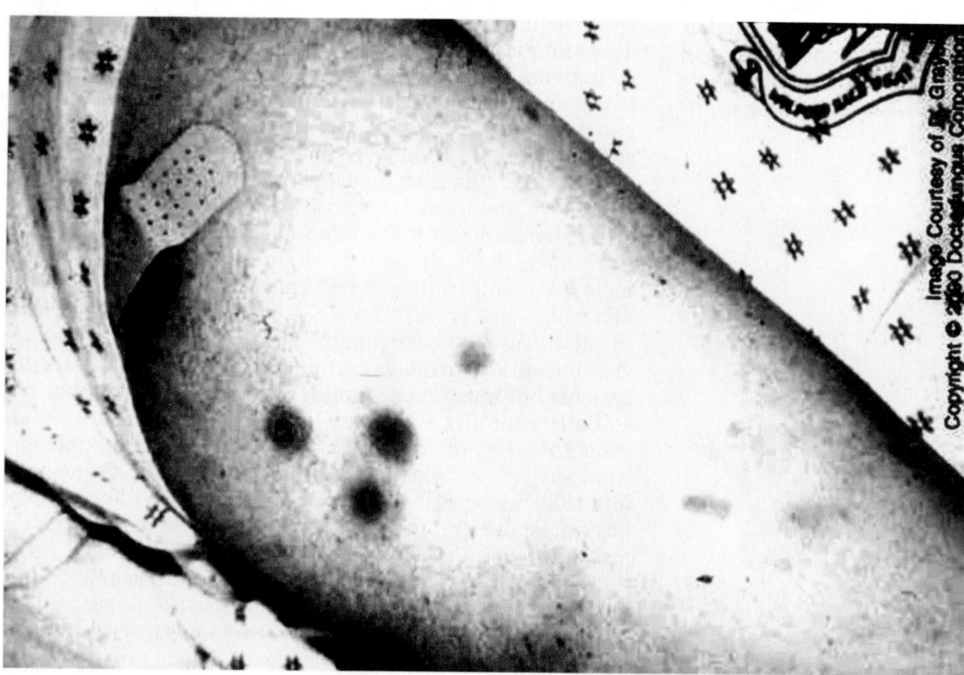

FIGURE 207–5 ■ Skin lesions of disseminated fusariosis in an immunocompromised host. The lesions often resemble ecthyma gangrenosum. (Photograph courtesy of D. Graybill, provided by *www.doctorfungus.org.*)

erythematous papules that may become vesicular and later develop a necrotic center very reminiscent of ecthyma gangrenosum.[70, 129, 133, 155] The lesions usually occur in the setting of disseminated disease with hematogenous spread, but they also may follow direct inoculation. Nasal lesions may resemble those of zygomycosis or aspergillosis, with painless, black necrotic eschars.[70]

Infection has been reported in neonates as well. One 28-week-gestation infant has been described with a fungal mass in the renal pelvis akin to renal fungus balls after candidiasis; the infant recovered after resection of the mass.[130] Endocarditis, most likely related to a central venous catheter, has been described in a term neonate.[84]

In a large case series, histopathology or blood cultures, or both, were positive in 80 percent of cases; blood cultures were positive in 47 percent.[107] This prevalence is in contrast to aspergillosis, in which positive blood cultures are distinctly unusual. The high rate of positive blood cultures in fusariosis most likely is related to the production of adventitious unicellular propagules and the vaso-invasive nature of the fungus.[141, 144] In tissue sections, the fungi often have a perivascular distribution, with frank vascular invasion leading to thrombosis and necrosis.[70, 133] The fungus grows rapidly in culture, and mature colonies develop by 4 to 5 days.[70] Sickle- or banana-shaped macroconidia are noted, and the reverse is deeply pigmented.[70]

Mortality rates from *Fusarium* infection are high—76 percent in one case series, 57 percent in another, and 26 percent in a third report.[79, 107, 147] The outcome appears to be better in patients with solid organ transplants than in those with bone marrow transplants, with resolution in five of six patients in one series.[155] Therapy generally has been disappointing in neutropenic patients, and recovery of neutrophil counts appears to be mandatory for clinical resolution.[70] Catheter-related infections respond fairly well with removal of the catheter and administration of antifungal therapy; however, most reported cases also had normal neutrophil counts.[181] In burn patients, very high-dose topical nystatin therapy has been reported to be effective.[18] Whenever feasible, wide surgical resection is necessary. Antifungal therapy for disseminated infection has been disappointing. The organisms are resistant to amphotericin in animal models.[9] The activity of amphotericin B may be enhanced, however, by the addition of agents providing synergy; a recent report describes encouraging in vitro results with the combination of amphotericin B plus azithromycin.[35] Amphotericin B lipid complex has been used to achieve levels above the MIC.[26, 140] Because neutrophils are clearly critical to recovery, granulocyte transfusions and colony-stimulating factors have been used.[21, 26, 72, 140, 144, 147] In vitro testing shows the activity of voriconazole to be fairly similar to that of amphotericin B and itraconazole against *Fusarium*.[55]

PAECILOMYCES SPECIES

Paecilomyces lilacinus and *Paecilomyces variotii* both have been reported as human pathogens. The organisms are widely distributed in soil and decomposing vegetation. They were previously classified with *Penicillium* and bear some resemblance microscopically but never have the blue-green coloration frequently seen in *Penicillium* colonies. *P. lilacinus* has a faint violet, mauve, or reddish-gray tint, whereas *P. variotii* has powdery colonies that initially are buff but eventually turn yellowish-brown.[172] Localized infection, such as peritonitis, complicating continuous ambulatory peritoneal dialysis and keratitis has been described.[39, 109, 139, 150, 185] Resistance to commonly used disinfectants has contributed to outbreaks from contaminated solutions and topical agents; an outbreak occurring after intraocular lens implantation was traced to contaminated bicarbonate solution, and skin infection in immunocompromised patients was linked to contaminated moisturizing lotion.[87, 188] Cases of sinusitis, endophthalmitis, endocarditis after placement of cardiac grafts, orbital cellulitis, pulmonary infection, and cutaneous and subcutaneous infection have been reported.[141, 174] Infection has been noted in patients with underlying hematologic malignancies, chronic granulomatous disease, and diabetes mellitus and after receiving bone marrow transplants.[87, 154, 163, 174, 191] Even in immunocompromised hosts, the infection usually remains localized, but dissemination has been described.[87, 141] Skin lesions may resemble those seen in fusariosis, and they range from erythematous macules to nodules, pustules, vesicular lesions, and necrotic crusts.[87] Blood cultures may be positive, especially in infection related to indwelling vascular access devices.[141, 164] Skin biopsy samples frequently yield positive cultures.[87] Clinical outcome was poor in 30 of 47 cases reviewed.[174] Removal of vascular devices and surgical débridement are recommended.[141, 176] Speciation is important when devising optimal therapy because *P. lilacinus* is frankly resistant to amphotericin B and fluconazole whereas *P. variotii* is generally susceptible to both amphotericin B and the azoles.[2]

ACREMONIUM SPECIES

Acremonium previously was named *Cephalosporium,* and this name for the genus is the one most familiar to clinicians; cephalosporin first was isolated from *Acremonium chrysogenium*.[75] The organisms are widely distributed in soil, plant debris, and rotting mushrooms.[75] The most common form of infection caused by *Acremonium* is focally invasive disease after trauma, with mycetoma and keratitis predominating.[60, 75] Other reported manifestations include hypersensitivity pneumonitis, fungus balls, sinusitis, bone and joint infection, arteriovenous fistula infection, peritonitis, empyema, meningitis, and endocarditis.[60] Many patients have had recent surgery, injury, intravenous drug injection, or immunosuppressive therapy as predisposing factors.[60] In immunocompromised hosts, fungemia, including catheter-related fungemia, and papular rashes have been reported.[75, 151] Recovery is usually dependent on restoration of normal neutrophil function. *Acremonium* is resistant to most antifungals when tested in vitro; amphotericin B has the best activity.[75] Many different therapeutic regimens have been attempted, with variable success.[75] Catheter-related fungemia has responded to removal of the catheter followed by liposomal amphotericin B.[151]

"MYCOSES" CAUSED BY ORGANISMS OTHER THAN FUNGI

Two diseases, protothecosis and rhinosporidiosis, generally were considered mycoses until molecular genetic techniques revealed the true nature of the pathogens. Protothecosis is caused by an achlorophyllic alga, and rhinosporidiosis recently has been attributed to a protistan parasite.

Rhinosporidiosis

The disease consists of warty, vegetative growths, usually found in the nose or eyes (Fig. 207–6 provides an example). The growths do not cause pain and grow very slowly. Epidemiologically, the disease is associated with exposure to stagnant pools or fresh water. Eighty-eight percent of cases

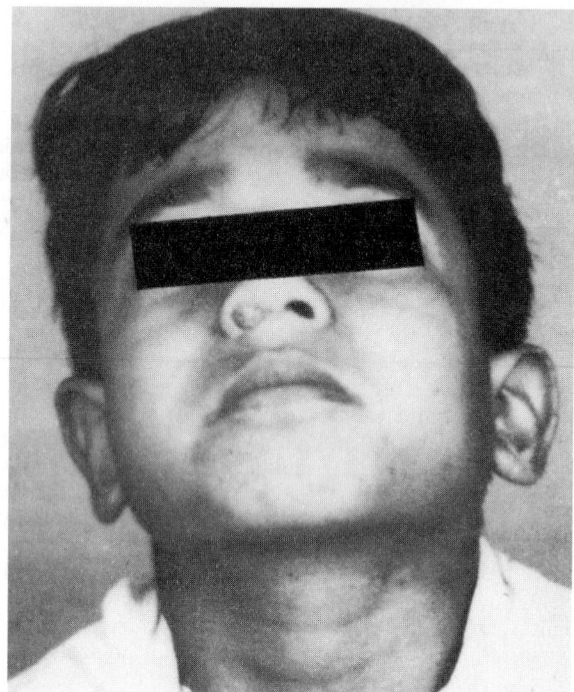

FIGURE 207–6 ■ Rhinosporidiosis. Polyps are developing in the nose. (Courtesy of S. Banerjee.)

are reported from India; however, cases also are reported from South America and the United States.[5, 69] The lesions may resemble nasal polyps, but mucous cysts are absent, and histopathology reveals the characteristic "sporangia." The spherules of *Rhinosporidium seeberi* are visible with most commonly used tissue stains. The spherules also stain with mucicarmine, which stains *C. neoformans* as well. The only known therapy to date is surgical removal, which may lead to copious bleeding and secondary infection. The organism never has been grown in culture, but recent evaluation of 18S ribosomal RNA has revealed that *R. seeberi* is most closely related to the DRIPs clade of aquatic protistan parasites; close phylogenetic relatives include known fish parasites.[66] Further evaluation of these related parasites may result in better understanding of the natural history of infection and the ideal approach to therapy.

Protothecosis

The algae responsible for protothecosis grow readily on Sabouraud agar unless cycloheximide is incorporated.[172] The species most commonly implicated is *Prototheca wickerhamii,* but *Prototheca zopfii* and *Prototheca stagnora* also have been reported.[85] Forms of infection include cutaneous or subcutaneous infection, olecranon bursitis, catheter-related infection, and systemic disease.[85] Half the reported patients have an underlying immunocompromising condition.[85] Infection frequently occurs after local trauma. Histologically, granulomata often are noted.[86] Disseminated disease usually involves the abdominal cavity with the development of multiple nodular lesions.[85] The organisms are usually susceptible to amphotericin B, so treatment is generally surgical excision (if feasible), followed by amphotericin B, although olecranon bursitis frequently is treated with bursectomy alone.[85, 173]

REFERENCES

1. Adam, R. D., Paquin, M. L., Petersen, E. A., et al.: Phaeohyphomycosis caused by the fungal genera *Bipolaris* and *Exserohilum.* A report of 9 cases and review of the literature. Medicine (Baltimore) *65*:203–217, 1986.
2. Aguilar, C., Pujol, I., Sala, J., and Guarro, J.: Antifungal susceptibilities of *Paecilomyces* species. Antimicrob. Agents Chemother. *42*:1601–1604, 1998.
3. Ahtonen, P., Lehtonen, O. P., Kero, P., et al.: *Malassezia furfur* colonization of neonates in an intensive care unit. Mycoses *33*:543–547, 1990.
4. al Hedaithy, S. S., and al Kaff, A. S.: *Exophiala jeanselmei* keratitis. Mycoses *36*:97–100, 1993.
5. Allen, F. R., and Dave, M.: Treatment of rhinosporidiosis in man based on sixty cases. Indian Med. Gaz. *71*:376–395, 1936.
6. Alter, S. J., and Farley, J.: Development of *Hansenula anomala* infection in a child receiving fluconazole therapy. Pediatr. Infect. Dis. J. *13*:158–159, 1994.
7. Anaissie, E., Bodey, G. P., Kantarjian, H., et al.: New spectrum of fungal infections in patients with cancer. Rev. Infect. Dis. *11*:369–378, 1989.
8. Anaissie, E., Gokaslan, A., Hachem, R., et al.: Azole therapy for trichosporonosis: Clinical evaluation of eight patients, experimental therapy for murine infection, and review. Clin. Infect. Dis. *15*:781–787, 1992.
9. Anaissie, E., Hachem, R., Legrand, C., et al.: Lack of activity of amphotericin B in systemic murine fusarial infection. J. Infect. Dis. *165*:1155–1157, 1992.
10. Anaissie, E. J., Kuchar, R. T., Rex, J. H., et al.: Fusariosis associated with pathogenic fusarium species colonization of a hospital water system: A new paradigm for the epidemiology of opportunistic mold infections. Clin. Infect. Dis. *33*:1871–1878, 2001.
11. Andes, D., Proctor, R., Bush, R. K., and Pasic, T. R.: Report of successful prolonged antifungal therapy for refractory allergic fungal sinusitis. Clin. Infect. Dis. *31*:202–204, 2000.
12. Aragao, P. A., Oshiro, I. C., Manrique, E. I., et al.: *Pichia anomala* outbreak in a nursery: Exogenous source? Pediatr. Infect. Dis. J. *20*:843–848, 2001.
13. Arnold, A. G., Gribbin, B., De Leval, M., et al.: *Trichosporon capitatum* causing recurrent fungal endocarditis. Thorax *36*:478–480, 1981.
14. Ashpole, R. D., Jacobson, K., King, A. T., and Holmes, A. E.: Cysto-peritoneal shunt infection with *Trichosporon beigelii.* Br. J. Neurosurg. *5*:515–517, 1991.
15. Ault, B. H., Jones, D. P., and Wyatt, R. J.: Infections in children with renal disease. *In* Patrick, C. C. (ed.): Clinical Management of Infections in Immunocompromised Infants and Children. Philadelphia, Lippincott Williams & Wilkins, 2000, pp. 242–258.
16. Barber, G. R., Brown, A. E., Kiehn, T. E., et al.: Catheter-related *Malassezia furfur* fungemia in immunocompromised patients. Am. J. Med. *95*:365–370, 1993.
17. Barbor, P. R., Rotimi, V. O., and Fatani, H.: Paravertebral abscess caused by *Trichosporon capitatum* in a child with acute lymphoblastic leukaemia. Letter. J. Infect. *31*:251–252, 1995.
18. Barret. J. P., Ramzy, P. I., Heggers, J. P., et al.: Topical nystatin powder in severe burns: A new treatment for angioinvasive fungal infections refractory to other topical and systemic agents. Burns *25*:505–508, 1999.
19. Benevent, D., Peyronnet, P., Lagarde, C., and Leroux-Robert, C.: Fungal peritonitis in patients on continuous ambulatory peritoneal dialysis. Three recoveries in 5 cases without catheter removal. Nephron *41*:203–206, 1985.
20. Berenguer, J., Rodriguez-Tudela, J. L., Richard, C., et al.: Deep infections caused by *Scedosporium prolificans.* A report on 16 cases in Spain and a review of the literature. Scedosporium Prolificans Spanish Study Group. Medicine (Baltimore) *76*:256–265, 1997.
21. Blazar, B. R., Hurd, D. D., Snover, D. C., et al.: Invasive *Fusarium* infections in bone marrow transplant recipients. Am. J. Med. *77*:645–651, 1984.
22. Blowey, D. L., Garg, U. C., Kearns, G. L., and Warady, B. A.: Peritoneal penetration of amphotericin B lipid complex and fluconazole in a pediatric patient with fungal peritonitis. Adv. Perit. Dial. *14*:247–250, 1998.
23. Bonifaz, A., Carrasco-Gerard, E., and Saúl, A.: Chromoblastomycosis: Clinical and mycologic experience of 51 cases. Mycoses *44*:1–7, 2001.
24. Borelli, D.: A clinical trial of itraconazole in the treatment of deep mycoses and leishmaniasis. Rev. Infect. Dis. *9*(Suppl.):57–63, 1987.
25. Bourguignon, R. L., Walsh, A. F., Flynn, J. C., et al.: *Fusarium* species osteomyelitis. Case report. J. Bone Joint Surg. Am. *58*:722–723, 1976.
26. Boutati, E. I., and Anaissie, E. J.: *Fusarium,* a significant emerging pathogen in patients with hematologic malignancy: Ten years' experience at a cancer center and implications for management. Blood *90*:999–1008, 1997.
27. Brady, R. C., and Sommerkamp, T. G.: Thorn-induced *Alternaria* flexor tenosynovitis of the hand. Pediatr. Infect. Dis. *20*:1097–1098, 2001.
28. Brint, J. M., Flynn, P. M., Pearson, T. A., and Pui, C. H.: Disseminated fusariosis involving bone in an adolescent with leukemia. Pediatr. Infect. Dis. J. *11*:965–968, 1992.
29. Bryan, M. G., Elston, D. M., Hivnor, C., and Honl, B. A.: Phaeohyphomycosis in a premature infant. Cutis *65*:137–140, 2000.

30. Castro, L. G., Belda, J. W., Salebian, A., and Cuce, L. C.: Mycetoma: A retrospective study of 41 cases seen in Sao Paulo, Brazil, from 1978 to 1989. Mycoses *36*:89–95, 1993.
31. Chan, T. H., Koehler, A., and Li, P. K.: *Paecilomyces varioti* peritonitis in patients on continuous ambulatory peritoneal dialysis. Am. J. Kidney Dis. *27*:138–142, 1996.
32. Chang, H. J., Miller, H. L., Watkins, N., et al.: An epidemic of *Malassezia pachydermatis* in an intensive care nursery associated with colonization of health care workers' pet dogs. N. Engl. J. Med. *338*:706–711, 1998.
33. Cheng, I. K., Fang, G. X., Chan, T. M., et al.: Fungal peritonitis complicating peritoneal dialysis: Report of 27 cases and review of treatment. Q. J. Med. *71*:407–416, 1989.
34. Cimon, B., Carrere, J., Vinatier, J. F., et al.: Clinical significance of *Scedosporium apiospermum* in patients with cystic fibrosis. Eur. J. Clin. Microbiol. Infect. Dis. *19*:53–56, 2000.
35. Clancy, C. J., and Nguyen, M. H.: The combination of amphotericin B and azithromycin as a potential new therapeutic approach to fusariosis. J. Antimicrob. Chemother. *41*:127–130, 1998.
36. Clinch, T. E., Robinson, M. J., Barron, B. A., et al.: Fungal keratitis from nylon line lawn trimmers. Am. J. Ophthalmol. *114*:437–440, 1992.
37. Cooper, C. R., Jr.: From bamboo rats to humans: The odyssey of *Penicillium marneffei*. A. S. M. News *64*:390–397, 1998.
38. Corey, J. P., Delsupehe, K. G., and Ferguson, B. J.: Allergic fungal sinusitis: Allergic, infectious, or both? Otolaryngol. Head Neck Surg. *113*:110–119, 1995.
39. Crompton, C. H., Balfe, J. W., Summerbell, R. C., and Silver, M. M.: Peritonitis with *Paecilomyces* complicating peritoneal dialysis. Pediatr. Infect. Dis. J. *10*:869–871, 1991.
40. Cruz, O. A., Sabir, S. M., Capo, H., and Alfonso, E. C.: Microbial keratitis in childhood. Ophthalmology *100*:192–196, 1993.
41. De Garcia, M. C., Arboleda, M. L., Barraquer, F., and Grose, E.: Fungal keratitis caused by *Metarhizium anisopliae* var. *anisopliae*. J. Med. Vet. Mycol. *35*:361–363, 1997.
42. del Palacio, A., Perez-Revilla, A., Albanil, R., et al.: Disseminated neonatal trichosporosis associated with the hemophagocytic syndrome. Pediatr. Infect. Dis. J. *9*:520–522, 1990.
43. Deng, Z. L., and Connor, D. H.: Progressive disseminated penicilliosis caused by *Penicillium marneffei*. Report of eight cases and differentiation of the causative organism from *Histoplasma capsulatum*. Am. J. Clin. Pathol. *84*:323–327, 1985.
44. De Saedeleer, B., Sennesael, J., Van der Niepen, P., and Verbeelen, D.: Intraperitoneal fluconazole therapy for *Trichosporon cutaneum* peritonitis in continuous ambulatory peritoneal dialysis. Nephrol. Dial. Transplant. *9*:1658–1659, 1994.
45. deShazo, R. D., Chapin, K., and Swain, R. E.: Fungal sinusitis. N. Engl. J. Med. *337*:254–259, 1997.
46. deShazo, R. D., O'Brien, M., Chapin, K., et al.: Criteria for the diagnosis of sinus mycetoma. J. Allergy Clin. Immunol. *99*:475–485, 1997.
47. deShazo, R. D., O'Brien, M., Chapin, K., et al.: A new classification and diagnostic criteria for invasive fungal sinusitis. Arch. Otolaryngol. Head Neck Surg. *123*:1181–1188, 1997.
48. deShazo, R. D., and Swain, R. E.: Diagnostic criteria for allergic fungal sinusitis. J. Allergy Clin. Immunol. *96*:24–35, 1995.
49. Duong, T. A.: Infection due to *Penicillium marneffei,* an emerging pathogen: Review of 155 reported cases. Clin. Infect. Dis. *23*:125–130, 1996.
50. Ebright, J. R., Fairfax, M. R., and Vazquez, J. A.: *Trichosporon asahii,* a non-*Candida* yeast that caused fatal septic shock in a patient without cancer or neutropenia. Clin. Infect. Dis. *33*:E28–E30, 2001.
51. Eisenberg, E. S., Leviton, I., and Soeiro, R.: Fungal peritonitis in patients receiving peritoneal dialysis: Experience with 11 patients and review of the literature. Rev. Infect. Dis. *8*:309–321, 1986.
52. Elidemir, O., Colasurdo, G. N., Rossmann, S. N., and Fan, L. L.: Isolation of *Stachybotrys* from the lung of a child with pulmonary hemosiderosis. Pediatrics *104*:964–966, 1999.
53. Ellison, M. D., Hung, R. T., Harris, K., and Campbell, B. H.: Report of the first case of invasive fungal sinusitis caused by *Scopulariopsis acremonium:* Review of scopulariopsis infections. Arch. Otolaryngol. Head Neck Surg. *124*:1014–1016, 1998.
54. Erer, B., Galimberti, M., Lucarelli, G., et al.: *Trichosporon beigelii:* A life-threatening pathogen in immunocompromised hosts. Bone Marrow Transplant. *25*:745–749, 2000.
55. Espinel-Ingroff, A.: In vitro activity of the new triazole voriconazole (UK-109,496) against opportunistic filamentous and dimorphic fungi and common and emerging yeast pathogens. J. Clin. Microbiol. *36*:198–202, 1998.
56. Esterre, P., Inzan, C. K., Ramarcel, E. R., et al.: Treatment of chromomycosis with terbinafine: Preliminary results of an open pilot study. Br. J. Dermatol. *134*:33–36, 1996.
57. Etzel, R. A., Montana, E., Sorenson, W. G., et al.: Acute pulmonary hemorrhage in infants associated with exposure to *Stachybotrys atra* and other fungi. Arch. Pediatr. Adolesc. Med. *152*:757–762, 1998.
58. Fabris, A., Pellanda, M. V., Gardin, C., et al.: Pharmacokinetics of antifungal agents. Perit. Dial. Int. *13*(Suppl.):380–382, 1993.
59. Fernandez, M., Noyola, D. E., Rossmann, S. N., and Edwards, M. S.: Cutaneous phaeohyphomycosis caused by *Curvularia lunata* and a review of *Curvularia* infections in pediatrics. Pediatr. Infect. Dis. J. *18*:727–731, 1999.
60. Fincher, R. M., Fisher, J. F., Lovell, R. D., et al.: Infection due to the fungus *Acremonium (Cephalosporium).* Medicine (Baltimore) *70*:398–409, 1991.
61. Fiore, N. F., Conway, J. H., West, K. W., and Kleiman, M. B.: *Saccharomyces cerevisiae* infections in children. Pediatr. Infect. Dis. J. *17*:1177–1179, 1998.
62. Fisher, D. J., Christy, C., Spafford, P., et al.: Neonatal *Trichosporon beigelii* infection: Report of a cluster of cases in a neonatal intensive care unit. Pediatr. Infect. Dis. J. *12*:149–155, 1993.
63. Flynn, J. T., Meislich, D., Kaiser, B. A., et al.: *Fusarium* peritonitis in a child on peritoneal dialysis: Case report and review of the literature. Perit. Dial. Int. *16*:52–57, 1996.
64. Forrest, G., and Redfield, R.: Photo quiz. A 40-year-old man with chronic elbow swelling after minor trauma. Clin. Infect. Dis. *34*:354, 398–399, 2002.
65. Forsterm R. K., Rebellm, G., and Wilson, L. A.: Dematiaceous fungal keratitis. Clinical isolates and management. Br. J. Ophthalmol. *59*:372–376, 1975.
66. Fredricks, D. N., Jolley, J. A., Lepp, P. W., et al.: *Rhinosporidium seeberi:* A human pathogen from a novel group of aquatic protistan parasites. Emerg. Infect. Dis. *6*:273–282, 2000.
67. From the Centers for Disease Control and Prevention. Update: Pulmonary hemorrhage/hemosiderosis among infants—Cleveland, Ohio, 1993–1996. J. A. M. A. *283*:1951–1953, 2000.
68. Gadallah, M. F., White, R., el Shahawy, M. A., et al.: Peritoneal dialysis complicated by *Bipolaris hawaiiensis* peritonitis: Successful therapy with catheter removal and oral itraconazole without the use of amphotericin-B. Am. J. Nephrol. *15*:348–352, 1995.
69. Gaines, J. J., Clay, J. R., Chandler, F. W., et al.: Rhinosporidiosis: Three domestic cases. South. Med. J. *89*:65–67, 1996.
70. Gamis, A. S., Gudnason, T., Giebink, G. S., and Ramsay, N. K.: Disseminated infection with *Fusarium* in recipients of bone marrow transplants. Rev. Infect. Dis. *13*:1077–1088, 1991.
71. Garg, P., Gopinathan, U., Choudhary, K., and Rao, G. N.: Keratomycosis: Clinical and microbiologic experience with dematiaceous fungi. Ophthalmology *107*:574–580, 2000.
72. Girmenia, C., Iori, A. P., Boecklin, F., et al.: *Fusarium* infections in patients with severe aplastic anemia: Review and implications for management. Haematologica *84*:114–118, 1999.
73. Girmenia, C., Micozzi, A., Venditti, M., et al.: Fluconazole treatment of *Blastoschizomyces capitatus* meningitis in an allogeneic bone marrow recipient. Eur. J. Clin. Microbiol. Infect. Dis. *10*:752–756, 1991.
74. Glaser, C. A., and Atwater, S. K.: Febrile infant with a percutaneous vascular catheter. Pediatr. Infect. Dis. J. *14*:163, 165–166, 1995.
75. Guarro, J., Gams, W., Pujol, I., and Gene, J.: *Acremonium* species: New emerging fungal opportunists—in vitro antifungal susceptibilities and review. Clin. Infect. Dis. *25*:1222–1229, 1997.
76. Hajjeh, R. A., and Blumberg, H. M.: Bloodstream infection due to *Trichosporon beigelii* in a burn patient: Case report and review of therapy. Clin. Infect. Dis. *20*:913–916, 1995.
77. Haupt, H. M., Merz, W. G., Beschorner, W. E., et al.: Colonization and infection with *Trichosporon* species in the immunosuppressed host. J. Infect. Dis. *147*:199–203, 1983.
78. Hennequin, C., Kauffmann-Lacroix, C., Jobert, A., et al.: Possible role of catheters in *Saccharomyces boulardii* fungemia. Eur. J. Clin. Microbiol. Infect. Dis. *19*:16–20, 2000.
79. Hennequin, C., Lavarde, V., Poirot, J. L., et al.: Invasive *Fusarium* infections: A retrospective survey of 31 cases. The French Groupe d'Etudes des Mycoses Opportunistes GEMO. J. Med. Vet. Mycol. *35*:107–114, 1997.
80. Henwick, S., Henrickson, K., Storgion, S. A., and Leggiadro, R. J.: Disseminated neonatal *Trichosporon beigelii.* Pediatr. Infect. Dis. J. *11*:50–52, 1992.
81. Higgins, E. M., Layton, D. M., Arya, R., et al.: Disseminated *Trichosporon beigelii* infection in an immunosuppressed child. J. R. Soc. Med. *87*:292–293, 1994.
82. Hoy, J., Hsu, K. C., Rolston, K., et al.: *Trichosporon beigelii* infection: A review. Rev. Infect. Dis. *8*:959–967, 1986.
83. Hsu, C. F., Wang, C. C., Hung, C. S., et al.: *Trichosporon beigelii* causing oral mucositis and fungemia: Report of one case. Chung Hua Min Kuo Hsiao Erh Ko I Hsueh Hui Tsa Chih *39*:191–194, 1998.
84. Hsu, C. M., Lee, P. I., Chen, J. M., et al.: Fatal *Fusarium* endocarditis complicated by hemolytic anemia and thrombocytopenia in an infant. Pediatr. Infect. Dis. J. *13*:1146–1148, 1994.
85. Iacoviello, V. R., DeGirolami, P. C., Lucarini, J., et al.: Protothecosis complicating prolonged endotracheal intubation: Case report and literature review. Clin. Infect. Dis. *15*:959–967, 1992.
86. Ismail, Y., Johnson, R. H., Wells, M. V., et al.: Invasive sinusitis with intracranial extension caused by *Curvularia lunata.* Arch. Intern. Med. *153*:1604–1606, 1993.
87. Itin, P. H., Frei, R., Lautenschlager, S., et al.: Cutaneous manifestations of *Paecilomyces lilacinus* infection induced by a contaminated skin lotion in patients who are severely immunosuppressed. J. Am. Acad. Dermatol. *39*:401–409, 1998.

88. Itoh, T., Hosokawa, H., Kohdera, U., et al.: Disseminated infection with *Trichosporon asahii.* Mycoses *39*:195–199, 1996.
89. Jabado, N., Casanova, J. L., Haddad, E., et al.: Invasive pulmonary infection due to *Scedosporium apiospermum* in two children with chronic granulomatous disease. Clin. Infect. Dis. *27*:1437–1441, 1998.
90. Kalter, D. C., Tschen, J. A., Cernoch, P. L., et al.: Genital white piedra: Epidemiology, microbiology, and therapy. J. Am. Acad. Dermatol. *14*:982–993, 1986.
91. Kerr, C. M., Perfect, J. R., Craven, P. C., et al.: Fungal peritonitis in patients on continuous ambulatory peritoneal dialysis. Ann. Intern. Med. *99*:334–336, 1983.
92. Kershaw, P., Freeman, R., Templeton, D., et al.: *Pseudallescheria boydii* infection of the central nervous system. Arch. Neurol. *47*:468–472, 1990.
93. Kiehn, T. E., Gorey, E., Brown, A. E., et al.: Sepsis due to *Rhodotorula* related to use of indwelling central venous catheters. Clin. Infect. Dis. *14*:841–846, 1992.
94. Klossek, J. M., Serrano, E., Peloquin, L., et al.: Functional endoscopic sinus surgery and 109 mycetomas of paranasal sinuses. Laryngoscope *107*:112–117, 1997.
95. Kriesel, J. D., Adderson, E. E., Gooch, W. M., III, and Pavia, A. T.: Invasive sinonasal disease due to *Scopulariopsis candida:* Case report and review of scopulariopsosis. Clin. Infect. Dis. *19*:317–319, 1994.
96. Kupferberg, S. B., and Bent, J. P.: Allergic fungal sinusitis in the pediatric population. Arch. Otolaryngol. Head Neck Surg. *122*:1381–1384, 1996.
97. Kwan, E. Y., Lau, Y. L., Yuen, K. Y., et al.: *Penicillium marneffei* infection in a non–HIV infected child. J. Paediatr. Child. Health *33*:267–271, 1997.
98. Leeming, J. P., Sutton, T. M., and Fleming, P. J.: Neonatal skin as a reservoir of *Malassezia* species. Pediatr. Infect. Dis. J. *14*:719–721, 1995.
99. Liu, K., Howell, D. N., Perfect, J. R., and Schell, W. A.: Morphologic criteria for the preliminary identification of *Fusarium, Paecilomyces,* and *Acremonium* species by histopathology. Am. J. Clin. Pathol. *109*:45–54, 1998.
100. Lussier, N., Laverdiere, M., Delorme, J., et al.: *Trichosporon beigelii* funguria in renal transplant recipients. Clin. Infect. Dis. *31*:1299–1301, 2000.
101. Lyke, K. E., Miller, N. S., Towne, L., and Merz, W. G.: A case of cutaneous ulcerative alternariosis: Rare association with diabetes mellitus and unusual failure of itraconazole treatment. Clin. Infect. Dis. *32*:1178–1187, 2001.
102. Madrigal, V., Alonso, J., Bureo, E., et al.: Fatal meningoencephalitis caused by *Scedosporium inflatum (Scedosporium prolificans)* in a child with lymphoblastic leukemia. Eur. J. Clin. Microbiol. Infect. Dis. *14*:601–603, 1995.
103. Manning, S. C., Merkel, M., Kriesel, K., et al.: Computed tomography and magnetic resonance diagnosis of allergic fungal sinusitis. Laryngoscope *107*:170–176, 1997.
104. Marcon, M. J., and Powell, D. A.: Epidemiology, diagnosis, and management of *Malassezia furfur* systemic infection. Diagn. Microbiol. Infect. Dis. *7*:161–175, 1987.
105. Marcon, M. J., and Powell, D. A.: Human infections due to *Malassezia* spp. Clin. Microbiol. Rev. *5*:101–119, 1992.
106. Marple, B. F., and Mabry, R. L.: Comprehensive management of allergic fungal sinusitis. Am. J. Rhinol. *12*:263–268, 1998.
107. Martino, P., Gastaldi, R., Raccah, R., and Girmenia, C.: Clinical patterns of *Fusarium* infections in immunocompromised patients. J. Infect. *28*:7–15, 1994.
108. Martino, P., Venditti, M., Micozzi, A., et al.: *Blastoschizomyces capitatus:* An emerging cause of invasive fungal disease in leukemia patients. Rev. Infect. Dis. *12*:570–582, 1990.
109. Marzec, A., Heron, L. G., Pritchard, R. C., et al.: *Paecilomyces variotii* in peritoneal dialysate. J. Clin. Microbiol. *31*:2392–2395, 1993.
110. Matsumoto, T., Ajello, L., Matsuda, T., et al.: Developments in hyalohyphomycosis and phaeohyphomycosis. J. Med. Vet. Mycol. *32*:329–349, 1994.
111. McGinnis, M. R.: Chromoblastomycosis and phaeohyphomycosis: New concepts, diagnosis, and mycology. J. Am. Acad. Dermatol. *8*:1–16, 1983.
112. McGinnis, M. R., and Pasarell, L.: *In vitro* evaluation of terbinafine and itraconazole against dematiaceous fungi. Med. Mycol. *36*:243–246, 1998.
113. McGinnis, M. R, Pasarell, L., Sutton, D. A., et al.: In vitro evaluation of voriconazole against some clinically important fungi. Antimicrob. Agents Chemother. *41*:1832–1834, 1997.
114. McGinnis, M. R., Walker, D. H., and Folds, J. D.: *Hansenula polymorpha* infection in a child with chronic granulomatous disease. Arch. Pathol. Lab. Med. *104*:290–292, 1980.
115. McManus, E. J., Jones, J. M.: Detection of a *Trichosporon beigelii* antigen cross-reactive with *Cryptococcus neoformans* capsular polysaccharide in serum from a patient with disseminated *Trichosporon* infection. J. Clin. Microbiol. *21*:681–685, 1985.
116. McWhinney, P. H., Madgwick, J. C., Hoffbrand, A. V., et al.: Successful surgical management of septic arthritis due to *Trichosporon beigelii* in a patient with acute myeloid leukaemia. Scand. J. Infect. Dis. *24*:245–247, 1992.
117. Melez, K. A., Cherry, J., Sanchez, C., et al.: Successful outpatient treatment of *Trichosporon beigelii* peritonitis with oral fluconazole. Pediatr. Infect. Dis. J. *14*:1110–1113, 1995.
118. Miro, O., Sacanella, E., Nadal, P., et al.: *Trichosporon beigelii* fungemia and metastatic pneumonia in a trauma patient. Eur. J. Clin. Microbiol. Infect. Dis. *13*:604–606, 1994.
119. Mocan, H., Murphy, A. V., Beattie, T. J., and McAllister, T. A.: Fungal peritonitis in children on continuous ambulatory peritoneal dialysis. Scott. Med. J. *34*:494–496, 1989.
120. Montane, B. S., Mazza, I., Abitbol, C., et al.: Fungal peritonitis in pediatric patients. Adv. Perit. Dial. *14*:251–254, 1998.
121. Morrison, V. A., Haake, R. J., and Weisdorf, D. J.: The spectrum of non-*Candida* fungal infections following bone marrow transplantation. Medicine (Baltimore) *72*:78–89, 1993.
122. Morrison, V. A., Haake, R. J., and Weisdorf, D. J.: Non-*Candida* fungal infections after bone marrow transplantation: Risk factors and outcome. Am. J. Med. *96*:497–503, 1994.
123. Morrison, V. A., and Weisdorf, D. J.: *Alternaria:* A sinonasal pathogen of immunocompromised hosts. Clin. Infect. Dis. *16*:265–270, 1993.
124. Morton, S. J., Midthun, K., and Merz, W. G.: Granulomatous encephalitis caused by *Bipolaris hawaiiensis.* Arch. Pathol. Lab. Med. *110*:1183–1185, 1986.
125. Moses, A., Maayan, S., Shvil, Y., et al.: *Hansenula anomala* infections in children: From asymptomatic colonization to tissue invasion. Pediatr. Infect. Dis. J. *10*:400–402, 1991.
126. Munoz, P., Marin, M., Tornero, P., et al.: Successful outcome of *Scedosporium apiospermum* disseminated infection treated with voriconazole in a patient receiving corticosteroid therapy. Clin. Infect. Dis. *31*:1499–1501, 2000.
127. Muntz, H. R.: Allergic fungal sinusitis in children. Otolaryngol. Clin. North Am. *29*:185–222, 1996.
128. Murphy, N., Buchanan, C. R., Damjanovic, V., et al.: Infection and colonisation of neonates by *Hansenula anomala.* Lancet *1*:291–293, 1986.
129. Musa, M. O., Al Eisa, A., Halim, M., et al.: The spectrum of *Fusarium* infection in immunocompromised patients with haematological malignancies and in non-immunocompromised patients: A single institution experience over 10 years. Br. J. Haematol. *108*:544–548, 2000.
130. Nakar, C., Livny, G., Levy, I., et al.: Mycetoma of the renal pelvis caused by *Fusarium* species. Pediatr. Infect. Dis. J. *20*:1182–1183, 2001.
131. Naveh, Y., Friedman, A., Merzbach, D., and Hashman, N.: Endocarditis caused by *Rhodotorula* successfully treated with 5-fluorocytosine. Br. Heart J. *37*:101–104, 1975.
132. Nelson, K. E., Kaufman, L., Cooper, C. R., Jr., and Merz, W. G.: *Penicillium marneffei:* An AIDS-related illness from Southeast Asia. Infect. Med. *16*:118–128, 1999.
133. Nelson, P. E., Dignani, M. C., and Anaissie, E. J.: Taxonomy, biology, and clinical aspects of *Fusarium* species. Clin. Microbiol. Rev. *7*:479–504, 1994.
134. Nelson, S. C., Yau, Y. C., Richardson, S. E., and Matlow, A. G.: Improved detection of *Malassezia* species in lipid-supplemented Peds Plus blood culture bottles. J. Clin. Microbiol. *33*:1005–1007, 1995.
135. Nesky, M. A., McDougal, E. C., and Peacock, J. E., Jr.: *Pseudallescheria boydii* brain abscess successfully treated with voriconazole and surgical drainage: Case report and literature review of central nervous system pseudallescheriasis. Clin. Infect. Dis. *31*:673–677, 2000.
136. Nielsen, K., Lang, H., Shum, A. C., et al.: Disseminated *Scedosporium prolificans* infection in an immunocompromised adolescent. Pediatr. Infect. Dis. J. *12*:882–884, 1993.
137. Nucci, M., Akiti, T., Barreiros, G., et al.: Nosocomial fungemia due to *Exophiala jeanselmei* var. *jeanselmei* and a *Rhinocladiella* species: Newly described causes of bloodstream infection. J. Clin. Microbiol. *39*:514–518, 2001.
138. Oh, S. H., Conley, S. B., Rose, G. M., et al.: Fungal peritonitis in children undergoing peritoneal dialysis. Pediatr. Infect. Dis. *4*:62–66, 1985.
139. Panda, A., Sharma, N., Das, G., et al.: Mycotic keratitis in children: Epidemiologic and microbiologic evaluation. Cornea *16*:295–299, 1997.
140. Patterson, T. S., Barton, L. L., Shehab, Z. M., and Hutter, J. J.: Amphotericin B lipid complex treatment of a leukemic child with disseminated *Fusarium solani* infection. Clin. Pediatr. (Phila.) *35*:257–260, 1996.
141. Perfect, J. R., and Schell, W. A.: The new fungal opportunists are coming. Clin. Infect. Dis. *22*(Suppl.):112–118, 1996.
142. Piwoz, J. A., Stadtmauer, G. J., Bottone, E. J., et al.: *Trichosporon inkin* lung abscesses presenting as a penetrating chest wall mass. Pediatr. Infect. Dis. J. 19:1025–1027, 2000.
143. Pletincx, M., Legein, J., and Vandenplas, Y.: Fungemia with *Saccharomyces boulardii* in a 1-year-old girl with protracted diarrhea. J. Pediatr. Gastroenterol. Nutr. *21*:113–115, 1995.
144. Ponton, J., Ruchel, R., Clemons, K. V., et al.: Emerging pathogens. Med. Mycol. *38*:225–236, 2000.
145. Powell, D. A., Hayes, J., Durrell, D. E., et al.: *Malassezia furfur* skin colonization of infants hospitalized in intensive care units. J. Pediatr. *111*:217–220, 1987.

146. Rabodonirina, M., Paulus, S., Thevenet, F., et al.: Disseminated *Scedosporium prolificans (S. inflatum)* infection after single-lung transplantation. Clin. Infect. Dis. *19*:138–142, 1994.
147. Rabodonirina, M., Piens, M. A., Monier, M. F., et al.: *Fusarium* infections in immunocompromised patients: Case reports and literature review. Eur. J. Clin. Microbiol. Infect. Dis. *13*:152–161, 1994.
148. Redline, R. W., and Dahms, B. B.: *Malassezia* pulmonary vasculitis in an infant on long-term Intralipid therapy. N. Engl. J. Med. *305*:1395–1398, 1981.
149. Revankar, S. G., Patterson, J. E., Sutton, D. A., et al.: Disseminated phaeohyphomycosis: Review of an emerging mycosis. Clin. Infect. Dis. *34*:467–476, 2002.
150. Rinaldi, S., Fiscarelli, E., and Rizzoni, G.: *Paecilomyces variotii* peritonitis in an infant on automated peritoneal dialysis. Pediatr. Nephrol. *14*:365–366, 2000.
151. Roilides, E., Bibashi, E., Acritidou, E., et al.: *Acremonium* fungemia in two immunocompromised children. Pediatr. Infect. Dis. J. *14*:548–550, 1995.
152. Rossmann, S. N., Cernoch, P. L., and Davis, J. R.: Dematiaceous fungi are an increasing cause of human disease. Clin. Infect. Dis. *22*:73–80, 1996.
153. Rowen, J. L., Atkins, J. T., Levy, M. L., et al.: Invasive fungal dermatitis in the < or = 1000-gram neonate. Pediatrics *95*:682–687, 1995.
154. Saberhagen, C., Klotz, S. A., Bartholomew, W., et al.: Infection due to *Paecilomyces lilacinus:* A challenging clinical identification. Clin. Infect. Dis. *25*:1411–1413, 1997.
155. Sampathkumar, P., and Paya, C. V.: *Fusarium* infection after solid-organ transplantation. Clin. Infect. Dis. *32*:1237–1240, 2001.
156. Schubert, M. S., and Goetz, D. W.: Evaluation and treatment of allergic fungal sinusitis. I. Demographics and diagnosis. J. Allergy Clin. Immunol. *102*:387–394, 1998.
157. Schubert, M. S., and Goetz, D. W.: Evaluation and treatment of allergic fungal sinusitis. II. Treatment and follow-up. J. Allergy Clin. Immunol. *102*:395–402, 1998.
158. Sekhon, A. S., Kowalewska-Grochowska, K., Garg, A. K., and Vaudry, W.: *Hansenula anomala* fungemia in an infant with gastric and cardiac complications with a review of the literature. Eur. J. Epidemiol. *8*:305–308, 1992.
159. Severo, L. C., Oliveira, F., Garcia, C. D., et al.: Peritonitis by *Scedosporium apiospermum* in a patient undergoing continuous ambulatory peritoneal dialysis. Rev. Inst. Med. Trop. Sao Paulo *41*:263–264, 1999.
160. Sharkey, P. K., Graybill, J. R., Rinaldi, M. G., et al.: Itraconazole treatment of phaeohyphomycosis. J. Am. Acad. Dermatol. *23*:577–586, 1990.
161. Shattuck, K. E., Cochran, C. K., Zabransky, R. J., et al.: Colonization and infection associated with *Malassezia* and *Candida* species in a neonatal unit. J. Hosp. Infect. *34*:123–129, 1996.
162. Sheu, M. J., Wang, C. C., Wang, C. C., et al.: *Rhodotorula* septicemia: Report of a case. J. Formos. Med. Assoc. *93*:645–647, 1994.
163. Shing, M. M., Ip, M., Li, C. K., et al.: *Paecilomyces varioti* fungemia in a bone marrow transplant patient. Bone Marrow Transplant. *17*:281–283, 1996.
164. Singh, K., Chakrabarti, A., Narang, A., and Gopalan, S.: Yeast colonisation & fungaemia in preterm neonates in a tertiary care centre. Indian J. Med. Res. *110*:169–173, 1999.
165. Singh, N., Chang, F. Y., Gayowski, T., and Marino I. R.: Infections due to dematiaceous fungi in organ transplant recipients: Case report and review. Clin. Infect. Dis. *24*:369–374, 1997.
166. Sirisanthana, V., and Sirisanthana, T.: Disseminated *Penicillium marneffei* infection in human immunodeficiency virus–infected children. Pediatr. Infect. Dis. J. *14*:935–940, 1995.
167. Sobel, J. D., Vazquez, J., Lynch, M., et al.: Vaginitis due to *Saccharomyces cerevisiae*: Epidemiology, clinical aspects, and therapy. Clin. Infect. Dis. *16*:93–99, 1993.
168. Stevens, D. A., Schwartz, H. J., Lee, J. Y., et al.: A randomized trial of itraconazole in allergic bronchopulmonary aspergillosis. N. Engl. J. Med. *342*:756–762, 2000.
169. Supparatpinyo, K., Chiewchanvit, S., Hirunsri, P., et al.: An efficacy study of itraconazole in the treatment of *Penicillium marneffei* infection. J. Med. Assoc. Thai. *75*:688–691, 1992.
170. Supparatpinyo, K., Perriens, J., Nelson, K. E., and Sirisanthana, T.: A controlled trial of itraconazole to prevent relapse of *Penicillium marneffei* infection in patients infected with the human immunodeficiency virus. N. Engl. J. Med. *339*:1739–1743, 1998.
171. Surmont, I., Vergauwen, B., Marcelis, L., et al.: First report of chronic meningitis caused by *Trichosporon beigelii*. Eur. J. Clin. Microbiol. Infect. Dis. *9*:226–229, 1990.
172. Sutton, D. A., Fothergill, A. W., and Rinaldi, M. G.: Guide to Clinically Significant Fungi. Baltimore, Williams & Wilkins, 1998.
173. Sweet, D., and Reid, M.: Disseminated neonatal *Trichosporon beigelii* infection: Successful treatment with liposomal amphotericin B. J. Infect. *36*:120–121, 1998.
174. Tan, T. Q., Ogden, A. K., Tillman, J., et al.: *Paecilomyces lilacinus* catheter-related fungemia in an immunocompromised pediatric patient. J. Clin. Microbiol. *30*:2479–2483, 1992.
175. Thuler, L. C., Faivichenco, S., Velasco, E., et al.: Fungaemia caused by *Hansenula anomala*—an outbreak in a cancer hospital. Mycoses *40*:193–196, 1997.
176. Tiballi, R. N., Spiegel, J. E., Zarins, L. T., and Kauffman, C. A.: *Saccharomyces cerevisiae* infections and antifungal susceptibility studies by colorimetric and broth macrodilution methods. Diagn. Microbiol. Infect. Dis. *23*:135–140, 1995.
177. Travis, L. B., Roberts, G. D., and Wilson, W. R.: Clinical significance of *Pseudallescheria boydii*: A review of 10 years' experience. Mayo Clin. Proc. *60*:531–537, 1985.
178. Ukarapol, N., Sirisanthana, V., and Wongsawasdi, L.: *Penicillium marneffei* mesenteric lymphadenitis in human immunodeficiency virus–infected children. J. Med. Assoc. Thai. *81*:637–640, 1998.
179. Vajpayee, R. B., Angra, S. K., Sandramouli, S., et al.: Laboratory diagnosis of keratomycosis: Comparative evaluation of direct microscopy and culture results. Ann. Ophthalmol. *25*:68–71, 1993.
180. van Belkum, A., Boekhout, T., and Bosboom, R.: Monitoring spread of *Malassezia* infections in a neonatal intensive care unit by PCR-mediated genetic typing. J. Clin. Microbiol. *32*:2528–2532, 1994.
181. Velasco, E., Martins, C. A., and Nucci, M.: Successful treatment of catheter-related fusarial infection in immunocompromised children. Eur. J. Clin. Microbiol. Infect. Dis. *14*:697–699, 1995.
182. Walsh, T. J., Gonzalez, C., Roilides, E., et al.: Fungemia in children infected with the human immunodeficiency virus: New epidemiologic patterns, emerging pathogens, and improved outcome with antifungal therapy. Clin. Infect. Dis. *20*:900–906, 1995.
183. Walsh, T. J., Lee, J. W., Melcher, G. P., et al.: Experimental *Trichosporon* infection in persistently granulocytopenic rabbits: Implications for pathogenesis, diagnosis, and treatment of an emerging opportunistic mycosis. J. Infect. Dis. *166*:121–133, 1992.
184. Walsh, T. J., Melcher, G. P., Rinaldi, M. G., et al.: *Trichosporon beigelii*, an emerging pathogen resistant to amphotericin B. J. Clin. Microbiol. *28*:1616–1622, 1990.
185. Wang, A. Y., Yu, A. W., Li, P. K., et al.: Factors predicting outcome of fungal peritonitis in peritoneal dialysis: Analysis of a 9-year experience of fungal peritonitis in a single center. Am. J. Kidney Dis. *36*:1183–1192, 2000.
186. Warady, B. A., Bashir, M., and Donaldson, L. A.: Fungal peritonitis in children receiving peritoneal dialysis: A report of the NAPRTCS. Kidney Int. *58*:384–389, 2000.
187. Washburn, R. G., Kennedy, D. W., Begley, M. G., et al.: Chronic fungal sinusitis in apparently normal hosts. Medicine (Baltimore) *67*:231–247, 1988.
188. Webster, R. G., Jr., Martin, W. J., Pettit, T. J., et al.: Eye infection after plastic lens implantation. M. M. W. R. Morb. Mortal. Wkly. Rep. *24*:437–438, 1975.
189. Welsh, O.: Mycetoma: Current concepts in treatment. Int. J. Dermatol. *30*:387–398, 1991.
190. Welty, F. K., McLeod, G. X., Ezratty, C., et al.: *Pseudallescheria boydii* endocarditis of the pulmonic valve in a liver transplant recipient. Clin. Infect. Dis. *15*:858–860, 1992.
191. Williamson, P. R., Kwon-Chung, K. J., and Gallin, J. I.: Successful treatment of *Paecilomyces varioti* infection in a patient with chronic granulomatous disease and a review of *Paecilomyces* species infections. Clin. Infect. Dis. *14*:1023–1026, 1992.
192. Wilson, C. M., O'Rourke, E. J., McGinnis, M. R., and Salkin, I. F.: *Scedosporium inflatum:* Clinical spectrum of a newly recognized pathogen. J. Infect. Dis. *161*:102–107, 1990.
193. www.doctorfungus.org.
194. Yamada, S., Maruoka, T., Nagai, K., et al.: Catheter-related infections by *Hansenula anomala* in children. Scand. J. Infect. Dis. *27*:85–87, 1995.
195. Yoss, B. S., Sautter, R. L., and Brenker, H. J.: *Trichosporon beigelii,* a new neonatal pathogen. Am. J. Perinatol. *14*:113–117, 1997.
196. Yuen, W. C., Chan, Y. F., Loke, S. L., et al.: Chronic lymphadenopathy caused by *Penicillium marneffei:* A condition mimicking tuberculous lymphadenopathy. Br. J. Surg. *3*:1007–1008, 1986.

Parasitic Diseases

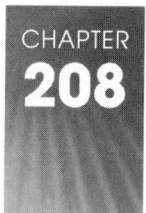

CHAPTER 208

Classification and Nomenclature of Human Parasites

LYNNE S. GARCIA

Although common names frequently are used to describe parasitic organisms, these names may represent different parasites in different parts of the world. In order to eliminate these problems, a binomial system of nomenclature in which the scientific name consists of the genus and species is used. These names generally are of Greek or Latin origin. In certain publications, the scientific name often is followed by the name of the individual who originally named the parasite. The date of naming also may be provided. If the name of the individual is in parentheses, it means that the person used a generic name no longer considered to be correct.

On the basis of life histories and morphologic characteristics, systems of classification have been developed to indicate the relationship among the various parasite species. Closely related species are placed in the same genus, related genera in the same family, related families in the same order, related orders in the same class, and related classes in the same phylum, one of the major categories in the animal kingdom. As one progresses up the classification schema, each category becomes more broad; however, each category still has characteristics in common.

Parasites of humans are classified in five major divisions. They include the Protozoa (amebae, flagellates, ciliates, sporozoans, coccidia, microsporidia), the Platyhelminthes or flatworms (cestodes, trematodes), the Acanthocephala or thorny-headed worms, the Nematoda or roundworms, and the Arthropoda (insects, spiders, mites, ticks, and so on). Although these categories appear to be well defined, often considerable confusion occurs in attempting to classify parasitic organisms. One of the primary reasons is the lack of known specimens. Some organisms recovered from humans are very rare; thus, difficulty arises in determining morphologic and physiologic variation among such groups. Type specimens must be deposited for study before a legitimate species name can be given. Even when certain parasites are numerous, they may represent strains or races of the same species with slightly different characteristics.

Generally, reproductive mechanisms are a valid concept in determining definitions of species, but so many exceptions exist within parasite groups that taking into consideration properties such as sexual reproduction, parthenogenesis, and asexual reproduction is difficult. Another difficulty in recognition of species is the ability and tendency of the organisms to alter their morphologic forms according to age, host, or nutrition, which often results in several names being given to the same organism. An additional problem involves alternation of parasitic and free-living phases in the life cycle. These organisms may be very different and difficult to recognize as belonging to the same species. Despite these difficulties, newer, more sophisticated molecular methods of grouping

TABLE 208–1 ■ HUMAN VECTOR-BORNE INFECTIONS

Infection (Disease)	Causative Agent	Vector (Common Name)
Protozoal		
Malaria	*Plasmodium* species	Mosquitoes
Leishmaniasis	*Leishmania* species	Sandflies
Chagas disease	*Trypanosoma cruzi*	Triatomid bugs
East African trypanosomiasis	*T. brucei rhodesiense*	Tsetse flies
West African trypanosomiasis	*T. brucei gambiense*	Tsetse files
Babesiosis	*Babesia* species	Ticks
Helminthic		
Filariasis	*Wuchereria bancrofti*	Mosquitoes
Filariasis	*Brugia malayi*	Mosquitoes
Filariasis	*Dirofilaria* species	Mosquitoes
Filariasis	*Mansonella perstans*	Biting midges
Filariasis	*M. streptocerca*	Biting midges
Filariasis	*M. ozzardi*	Biting midges
Onchocerciasis	*Onchocerca volvulus*	Black flies
Loiasis	*Loa loa*	Deer flies
Dog tapeworm infection	*Dipylidium caninum*	Dog lice and fleas, human fleas
Rat tapeworm infection	*Hymenolepis diminuta*	Rat fleas, beetles, grain beetles
Dwarf tapeworm	*H. nana*	Grain beetles (rare)

TABLE 208–2 ■ MEDICALLY IMPORTANT ARTHROPODS

Local or Systemic Problems	Vector (Common Name)	Local or Systemic Problems	Vector (Common Name)
Skin reaction to bites	Sucking lice Bedbugs Kissing bugs Biting midges Sandflies Black flies Mosquitoes Deer flies Tsetse flies Soft ticks Hard ticks	Painful sting, potential anaphylaxis	Honeybees Bumblebees Wasps, hornets, yellowjackets Fire ants Scorpions
		Dermatitis, ulcerations	Fleas
		Nodular ulceration with subsequent secondary infection	Chigoe flea
		Blistering of skin after contact with adult beetles	Blister beetles
Painful bite	Horseflies Fire ants Centipedes	Bite, usually painless, delayed systemic reaction	Black widow spiders
Intense itching	Human itch mites Chiggers	Initial blister followed by extensive necrosis and slow healing	Brown recluse spiders South American brown spiders

organisms often have confirmed taxonomic conclusions reached hundreds of years earlier by experienced taxonomists.

As investigations continue in parasitic genetics, immunology, and biochemistry, the species designation will be defined more clearly. Originally, these species designations were determined primarily by morphologic differences, resulting in a phenotypic approach. With the use of highly sophisticated molecular techniques, the approach will continue to be more genotypic. Benefits of these studies also include the development of highly specific and sensitive diagnostic tests and the ability to diagnose parasitic infections based on molecular parameters, rather than merely phenotypic characteristics.

Although gaps in our knowledge concerning classification of all human parasites remain, the binomial system has allowed the classification of 1.5 million species of organisms in the animal kingdom such that all published information can be retrieved, regardless of the language spoken. The difficulty for the clinician arises when one considers the rapid increase in information concerning microbiology during the past few years and changing considerations such as the role of immunosuppression in the host-parasite interaction and the modified definitions of "normal flora" and "nonpathogenic" in this patient population.

The classification of parasites is presented in tabular form. Although certain designations of species may be somewhat controversial, this classification scheme is designed to provide some order and meaning to a widely divergent group of organisms. No attempt has been made to include every possible organism, and only those considered clinically relevant in the context of human parasitology are included. The main groups that are presented include protozoa, nematodes (roundworms), cestodes (tapeworms), and trematodes (flukes). Some relevant information on arthropods is presented in Tables 208–1 and 208–2. The hope is that this information will provide some insight into the parasite groupings, thus leading to a better understanding of parasitic infections and the appropriate diagnostic and clinical approach.

I. PROTOZOA

1. (Amebae)— Intestinal

These organisms are characterized by having pseudopods (motility) and trophozoite and cyst stages in the life cycle and include some exceptions in which a cyst form has not been identified. Amebae usually are acquired by humans through fecal-oral transmission or mouth-to-mouth contact (*Entamoeba gingivalis*).

Current Name	
*Entamoeba histolytica**	*Entamoeba gingivalis*
*Entamoeba dispar**	*Endolimax nana*
Entamoeba hartmanni†	*Iodamoeba bütschlii*
Entamoeba coli	*Blastocystis hominis*
Entamoeba polecki	

**Entamoeba histolytica* is being used to designate true pathogens, whereas *Entamoeba dispar* now is being used to designate nonpathogens. Unless trophozoites containing ingested red blood cells (*E. histolytica*) are seen, the two organisms cannot be differentiated on the basis of morphology seen in permanent stained smears of fecal specimens and will be reported as *E. histolytica/E. dispar*. Immunoassays are available commercially for identifying the *E. histolytica/E. dispar* group and for differentiating *E. hisolytica* from *E. dispar*. Because the differences in pathogenicity are genetic and not just phenotypic, the decision to treat is one that must be determined by the physician. Reports of finding organisms in the *E. histolytica/E. dispar* group in patient specimens must continue to be reported to state and county Departments of Public Health (follow your particular state reporting regulations).

†*Entamoeba hartmanni* is non-pathogenic and is totally different from *E. histolytica*. "Small race *E. hisolytica*" is incorrect and should not be used at any time to designate *E. hartmanni*.

2. (Flagellates)—Intestinal

These organisms move by means of flagella and are acquired by fecal-oral transmission. With exception of *Dientamoeba fragilis* (internal flagella) and those in the genera *Trichomonas* and *Pentatrichomonas,* they have the trophozoite and cyst stages in the life cycle. *D. fragilis, Trichomonas,* and *Pentatrichomonas* species do not have a cyst state.

Current Name

*Giardia lamblia**
Chilomastix mesnili
Dientamoeba fragilis
Pentatrichomonas hominis
Trichomonas tenax
Enteromonas hominis
Retortamonas intestinalis

*Although some individuals have changed the species designation for the genus *Giardia* to *G. intestinalis* or *G. duodenalis,* no consensus exists. Therefore, for this listing, we retain the name *Giardia lamblia.*

3. (Ciliates)—Intestinal

These organisms, which move by means of cilia, are acquired by humans through fecal-oral transmission. They have both the trophozoite and cyst forms in the life cycle.

Current Name

Balantidium coli

4. (Coccidia, Microsporidia)—Intestinal

These organisms are acquired by humans by ingestion of various meats or through fecal-oral transmission through contaminated food or water.

Current Name

Coccidia

Cryptosporidium parvum
Cyclospora cayetanensis
Isospora belli
Sarcocystis hominis
Sarcocystis suihominis
Sarcocystis bovihominis
Sarcocystis "lindemanni"

Microsporidia

Enterocytozoon bieneusi
Encephalitozoon (Septata) intestinalis†

†Formerly called *Septata intestinalis.*

5. (Amebae, Flagellates)—Other Body Sites

The amebae are pathogenic, free-living organisms that may be associated with warm, fresh-water areas. They have been found in the central nervous system, the eye, and other sites. *Trichomonas vaginalis* usually is acquired by sexual transmission. This particular flagellate is found in the genitourinary system.

Current Name

Amebae

Naegleria fowleri
Acanthamoeba species
Hartmanella species
Balamuthia mandrillaris

Flagellates

Trichomonas vaginalis

6. (Coccidia, Microsporidia, Undecided Classification)—Other Body Sites

These organisms are particularly important in the compromised patient. They also may infect many individuals who have no apparent symptoms. On the basis of several RNA studies, *Pneumocystis carinii* is linked more closely to the fungi and has been reclassified with those organisms. However, for the present, it will be listed here.

Current Name

Coccidia

Toxoplasma gondii

Sarcocystis "lindemanni"

Microsporidia

Nosema connori
Vittaforma corneae (Nosema corneum)
Pleistophora
Trachipleistophora hominis
Trachipleistophora anthropophthera
Brachiola vesicularum
Encephalitozoon hellem
Encephalitozoon cuniculi
*Encephalitozoon (Septata) intestinalis**
Enterocytozoon bieneusi[†]
"Microsporidium"[‡]

*Formerly called *Sepata intestinalis.*
[†]*Enterocytozoon bieneusi* has been recovered from sites other than the intestinal tract (findings confirmed in 1996 and 1997).
[‡]This designation is not a true genus, but a "catch-all" for those organisms that have not been (or may never be) identified to the genus or species levels.

Undecided Classification

*Pneumocystis carinii**

**Pneumocystis carinii* now has been reclassified with the fungi and renamed *Pneumocystis jiroveci* in human intestines.

7. (Sporozoa, Flagellates)—Blood and Tissues

All of these organisms are arthropod borne. Diagnosis may be somewhat more difficult to make than is that of the intestinal protozoa, particularly if automated blood differential systems are used. The *leishmania* have undergone extensive revisions in classification. However, from a clinical perspective, recovery and identification of the organisms still are related to body site. Recovery of the organisms is limited to the site of the lesion in infections other than those caused by the *Leishmania donovani* complex (visceral leishmaniasis).

Current Name

Sporozoa (Malaria, Babesiosis)

Malaria
- *Plasmodium vivax*
- *Plasmodium ovale*
- *Plasmodium malariae*
- *Plasmodium falciparum*

Babesiosis
- *Babesia* species

Flagellates (Leishmaniasis, Trypanosomiasis)

Leishmaniasis
- *Leishmania tropica* complex (cutaneous leishmaniasis)
- *Leishmania mexicana* complex (cutaneous leishmaniasis)
- *Leishmania braziliensis* complex (mucocutaneous leishmaniasis)
- *Leishmania donovani* complex (visceral leishmaniasis)

Trypanosomiasis
- *Trypanosoma brucei gambiense* (West African trypanosomiasis)
- *Trypanosoma brucei rhodesiense* (East African trypanosomiasis)
- *Trypanosoma cruzi* (American trypanosomiasis)
- *Trypanosoma rangeli*

II. NEMATODES

1. Intestinal

These organisms normally are acquired by ingestion of eggs or penetration of the skin by larval forms from the soil.

Current Name	
Ascaris lumbricoides	*Trichostrongylus* species
Enterobius vermicularis (pinworm)	*Trichuris trichiura* (whipworm)
Ancylostoma duodenale (Old World hookworm)	*Capillaria philippinensis*
Necator americanus (New World hookworm)	*Oesophagostomum* species (*O. bifurcum* most common in humans—West Africa)
Strongyloides stercoralis	*Ternidens diminutus* (as high as 80% in Zimbabwe)

2. Tissue

For the most part, these organisms rarely are seen within the United States; however, the first three are more important.

Current Name	
Trichinella spiralis	*Angiostrongylus costaricensis*
Trichinella species	*Gnathostoma spinigerum*
Toxocara canis or *T. cati* (visceral or ocular larva migrans)	*Gnathostoma* species
Ancylostoma braziliense or *A. caninum* (cutaneous larva migrans)	Anisakiasis (larvae from salt-water fish)
Baylisascaris procyonis (severe systemic visceral larva migrans)	*Anisakis* species
Dracunculus medinensis	*Phocanema* species
Angiostrongylus cantonensis	*Contracaecum* species
	Pseudoterranova species
	Capillaria hepatica
	Thelazia species

3. (Filarial Worms)—Blood, Other Body Fluids, Skin

These organisms also are arthropod borne. The adult worms tend to live in the tissues of lymphatics. Diagnosis is made on the basis of the recovery and identification of the larval worms (microfilariae) in the blood, other body fluids, or skin. Elephantiasis may be associated with some of the organisms listed.

Current Name	
Wuchereria bancrofti	*Mansonella streptocerca*
Brugia malayi	*Mansonella perstans*
Brugia timori	*Dirofilaria immitis* ("coin" lesion in the lung) (dog heartworm)
Loa loa	*Dirofilaria* species (may be found in subcutaneous nodules)
Onchocerca volvulus	
Mansonella ozzardi	

III. CESTODES

1. Intestinal

The adult form of these organisms is acquired by humans through ingestion of the larval forms contained in poorly cooked or raw meats or fresh-water fish. In the case of *Dipylidium caninum*, infection is acquired by the accidental ingestion of dog fleas. Both *Hymenolepis nana* and *H. diminuta* are transmitted by ingestion of certain arthropods (fleas, beetles). Also, *H. nana* can be transmitted through egg ingestion (life cycle can bypass the intermediate beetle host). Humans can serve as both the intermediate and definitive hosts in *H. nana* and *Taenia solium* infections.

Current Name

Diphyllobothrium latum (broad, fish tapeworm)
Dipylidium caninum (dog tapeworm)
Hymenolepis nana (dwarf tapeworm)
Hymenolepis diminuta (rat tapeworm)
Taenia solium (pork tapeworm)
Taenia saginata (beef tapeworm)
Taenia asiatica (Taiwanese variant of *T. saginata*)

2. (Larval Forms)—Tissue

The ingestion of certain tapeworm eggs or accidental contact with certain larval forms can lead to the diseases shown in parantheses.

Current Name

Taenia solium (cysticercosis)
Echinococcus granulosus (hydatid disease)
Echinococcus multilocularis (alveolar hydatid disease)
Echinococcus oligarthrus (polycystic hydatid disease)
Multiceps multiceps (coenurosis)
Diphyllobothrium species (sparganosis)
Spirometra mansonoides (sparganosis)

IV. TREMATODES

1. Intestinal

These organisms are uncommon within the United States, except for four species of *Alaria,* which are endemic within North America.

Current Name

Fasciolopsis buski (giant intestinal fluke)
Echinostoma ilocanum
Eurytrema pancreaticum
Heterophyes heterophyes
Metagonimus yokogawai
Alaria species

2. Liver, Lung

These organisms are not seen commonly within the United States; however, some Southeast Asian refugees do harbor some of these parasites.

Current Name

Clonorchis (Opisthorchis) sinensis (Chinese liver fluke)
Paragonimus westermani (lung fluke)
Paragonimus species
Opisthorchis viverrini
Fasciola hepatica (sheep liver fluke)
Metorchis conjunctus (North American liver fluke)

3. Blood

The schistosomes are acquired by penetration of the skin by the cercarial forms that are released from fresh-water snails. Although they are not endemic within the United States, occasionally patients are seen who may have these infections.

Current Name

Schistosoma mansoni
Schistosoma haematobium
Schistosoma japonicum
Schistosoma intercalatum
Schistosoma mekongi

V. ARTHROPODS

See Tables 208–1 and 208–2.

REFERENCES

1. Beaver, C. B., Jung, R. C., and Cupp, E. W.: Clinical Parasitology. Philadelphia, Lea & Febiger, 1984, 825 pp.
2. Edman, J. C., Kovacs, J. A., Masur, H., et al.: Ribosomal RNA sequence shows *Pneumocystis carinii* to be a member of the fungi. Nature *334*:519–522, 1988.
3. Fayer, R.: *Cryptosporidium* and Cryptosporidiosis. Boca Raton, FL, CRC Press, 1997, 251 pp.
4. Garcia, L. S.: Diagnostic Medical Parasitology. 4th ed. Washington, D.C., ASM Press, 2001, 1092 pp.
5. Hartskeerl, R. A., Van Gool, T., Schuitema, A. R. J., et al.: Genetic and immunological characterization of the microsporidian *Septata intestinalis* Cali, Kotler, and Orenstein, 1993: Reclassification to *Encephalitozoon intestinalis*. Parasitology *110*:277–285, 1995.
6. Levine, N. D.: Veterinary Parasitology. Minneapolis, Burgess Publishing, 1978, 236 pp.
7. Molina, J. M., Oksenhendler, E., Beauvais, B., et al.: Disseminated microsporidiosis due to *Septata intestinalis* in patients with AIDS: Clinical features and response to albendazole therapy. J. Infect. Dis. *171*:245–249, 1995.
8. Meyers, W. M., Neafie, R. C., Marty, A. M., et al. (eds.): Pathology of Infectious Diseases. Vol. 1. Helminthiases. Washington, D.C., Armed Forces Institute of Pathology, 2000, 561 pp.
9. Murray, P. R., Baron, E. J., Pfaller, M. A., et al. (eds.): Manual of Clinical Microbiology. 8th ed. Washington, D.C., ASM Press, 2003, 2113 pp.
10. Ortega, Y., Sterling, C. R., Gilman, R. H., et al.: *Cyclospora* species: A new protozoan pathogen of humans. N. Engl. J. Med. *328*:1308–1312, 1993.
11. Pape, J. W., Verdier, R. I., Boncy, M., et al.: *Cyclospora* infection in adults infected with HIV: Clinical manifestations, treatment, and prophylaxis. Ann. Intern. Med. *121*:654–657, 1994.
12. Stringer, S. L., Hudson, K., Blase, M. A., et al.: Sequence from ribosomal RNA of *Pneumocystis carinii* compared to those of four fungi suggests an ascomycetous affinity. J. Protozool. *36*:14S–16S, 1989.
13. Wittner, M., and Weiss, L. M.: The Microsporidia and Microsporidiosis. Washington, D.C., ASM Press, 1999, 553 pp.
14. Zierdt, C. H.: *Blastocystis hominis*: Past and future. Clin. Microbiol. Rev. *4*:61–79, 1991.

SUBSECTION 1

PROTOZOA

A. AMEBAE

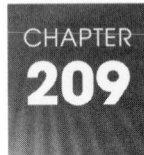

Amebiasis

PETER J. HOTEZ ■ ALAN D. STRICKLAND

Amebiasis is a major infectious diarrheal disease among children living in the developing countries of the tropics as well as those who emigrate from these areas to the United States. The frequency of amebiasis in less developed countries is high. For instance, about 10 to 20 percent of Mexican children harbor amebae, and as many as 5 percent of their episodes of acute diarrhea are caused by amebiasis.[70] More than one half of all patients treated for amebiasis in a hospital in Lagos, Nigeria, were children younger than 10 years of age.[70] As in many other parasitic diseases, infants and toddlers with amebiasis often present with clinical features of their disease that usually are not found in adults, including a fulminating variant of amebic colitis.[30, 38, 65]

Amebiasis is caused by either *Entamoeba histolytica,* a protozoan named for the pathologic evidence of "lysis" of tissues, or *Entamoeba dispar,* which is identical morphologically but so far has been implicated only as a cause of an asymptomatic carrier state.[87] The first demonstration of the organism in human tissues was made by V. D. Lambl in 1859 in the postmortem examination of the colon of a child who died as a result of having excessive diarrhea.[15, 71] No correlation of the organism with the disease was made until 1875, when Losch, in St. Petersburg, Russia, found the organism at autopsy in the colon of a woodcutter. Losch induced diarrhea and ulcerations in a dog given feces from the patient.[56] He did not, however, think that a connection existed between the organism and the disease. The first patient described in the United States was a physician treated by William Osler for an amebic liver abscess in 1890.[71] Councilman and Lafleur[22, 40] described the organism and the disease in 1891. Further investigation of the disease was delayed until a better understanding of the life cycle of *E. histolytica* could be obtained.[26] In recent years, the application of modern molecular biology techniques to the study of *E. histolytica* and *E. dispar* has resulted in an explosion of information about the mechanisms of virulence, pathogenicity, and immune responses to these organisms.[87, 92]

Etiology

Studies using molecular (DNA and RNA) and immunologic (monoclonal antibodies) probes demonstrated the existence of two distinct species of the genus *Entamoeba*, which are identical morphologically.[13, 16, 20, 24, 66, 75, 114] *E. histolytica* is the pathogenic species having the capacity to invade tissue and cause symptomatic disease, whereas *E. dispar* (as well as *E. histolytica*) is associated with the asymptomatic carrier state.[87] In the research laboratory, specific DNA probes have been used in a polymerase chain reaction and specific monoclonal antibodies have been used in immunoassays in order to distinguish the two different species.[39, 118, 122] Diagnostically useful assays with these molecular probes are under clinical development. Morphologically distinct members of the genus *Entamoeba*, such as *Entamoeba coli* and *Entamoeba hartmanni,* also are nonpathogenic.

Members of the genus *Entamoeba* (protozoan organisms belonging to the subphylum Sarcodina) have both trophozoite and cyst forms. The cysts of *E. histolytica* and *E. dispar* are almost spherical, being surrounded by a cell wall composed of chitin. The cysts may have one to four nuclei, although quadrinucleate cysts are most typical. This feature allows differentiation from *Escherichia coli,* which usually has six to eight nuclei in the cysts and may have as many as 32 nuclei.[72] Cysts of *E. histolytica* are 5 to 20 μm in diameter (average, 12 μm) and have a greenish tint in the unstained condition.[59] Young cysts contain chromatoid bodies, which are composed of ribosome particles in crystalline arrays.[12] The cysts of *E. hartmanni* appear identical to those of *E. histolytica* except for having a smaller size of 4 to 10 μm. *E. histolytica* cysts can survive for days in the dried state at 30° C or for months at 0° to 4° C. They can be killed by temperatures above 50° C for 5 minutes.[40] They are completely resistant to the concentrations of chlorine used in water supplies but may be killed with hyperchlorination or with iodine solutions.[59, 72] They are filtered out of water supplies that pass through a sand filtration phase. They resist acids well.

When these quadrinucleate cysts are ingested, they resist the acid pH of the stomach and ultimately excyst in the alkaline environment of the bowel. The process of excystation results in the release of four trophozoites that divide by binary fission to produce eight trophozoites. The usual trophozoites have a diameter of 25 μm, with a range between 10 and 60 μm.[26, 87] They have a single nucleus that is 3 to 5 μm in diameter and contains fine peripheral chromatin with a slightly eccentric karyosome. There is a granular endoplasm that typically contains vacuoles in which bacteria and debris can be seen. Some glycogen is present and can be stained with periodic acid–Schiff stain. Mitochondria, Golgi membranes, and rough endoplasmic reticulum are absent.[36] The presence of ingested erythrocytes is a characteristic feature of *E. histolytica* but not *E. dispar*.[87] Movement is accomplished by extension of clear pseudopodia. Replication is by binary fission. These protozoa live in the colon of humans and other mammals. Trophozoites die quickly outside the body and are quite sensitive to acid—they generally are not considered to be infective.[36] When cooled (as when feces are expelled and gradually cool from body temperature) or stimulated by as yet undefined luminal conditions, the trophozoites form cysts that can remain viable for weeks to months upon excretion.[87]

Trophozoites of *E. coli* are 15 to 50 μm in diameter, have much more sluggish motility than *E. histolytica,* and have blunt pseudopodia rather than the sharp, finger-like pseudopodia of *E. histolytica.* Trophozoites of *E. hartmanni* are 4 to 14 μm in diameter and have much less glycogen than do those of *E. histolytica*.[26]

Epidemiology

Amebiasis is worldwide in distribution. Estimates indicate that about 500 million people are carrying either *E. dispar* or *E. histolytica,* that 50 million people each year will have active disease, and that between 50,000 and 100,000 deaths per year are caused by the organism.[80, 86, 123] Generally speaking, asymptomatic *E. dispar* infection is about 10-fold more common than is *E. histolytica* infection, and symptomatic invasive amebiasis develops in only about 10 percent of individuals infected with *E. histolytica*.[87] Thus, only about 1 percent of patients found to harbor *Entamoeba* by stool microscopy develop clinically apparent amebiasis.

The prevalence of *Entamoeba* infection varies from an estimated 5 percent of the population of the United States to as high as 50 percent of the population of certain underdeveloped parts of Africa and Indochina and of areas of South and Central America.[15, 26, 86] High rates of invasive disease occur among Mexican Americans who are recent immigrants to the United States. Most immigrants who develop amebic liver abscess from *E. histolytica* infection usually present within 5 months from the time of entry into their new country.[50] Other high-risk groups in the United States include institutionalized populations[74] and, at one time, the homosexual male populations of New York City and San Francisco.[63, 106, 113] The prevalence of *Entamoeba* infection among these men has decreased in recent years as a consequence of the implementation of safer sex practices.[25] Small children serve as sources of infection for entire families. Cases of severe disease and fatality have been recorded in contacts of humans who have asymptomatic infections.[26] The age distribution is reported as a bimodal one, with a peak incidence between 2 and 3 years of age (with a case-fatality rate of 20%) and another peak after 40 years of age (with a case-fatality rate of 69%).[53]

Pathogenesis and Pathology

Clinical amebiasis occurs when trophozoites invade the colonic tissue. This process is initiated when the trophozoite adheres to the mucins lining the surface of the large bowel,[40, 72, 86] followed by enzymatic destruction of the basement membrane of the mucosa and its underlying tissue. Host inflammatory responses also contribute to the destruction of tissue.

In the relatively anaerobic environment of the colon, the 10- to 20-μm trophozoites of *E. histolytica* to attach themselves to bacteria actively through a surface receptor that can be blocked by mannose.[68] *Entamoeba coli* is highly favored for attack by *E. histolytica,* which rapidly lyses the bacteria and ingests them. These trophozoites also may attach to the interglandular region of the intestinal mucosa[36, 40, 72, 86] or to colonic mucus.[18] The adherence to the mucus and the intestinal wall is associated with two amebic adherence lectins of 260 kd and 220 kd; the former comprise 170-kd and 35-kd subunits.[77, 88] The 170-kd subunit is the functional component that binds to galactose and consists of a short cytoplasmic domain, a transmembrane domain, and a large extracellular portion that is cysteine-rich.[9, 18, 19, 23, 76, 77, 90, 115] The 170-kd subunit of the amebic lectin protects the parasite by blocking the assembly of host complement components onto its surface.[14] The cysteine-rich component of the 170-kd lectin is immunogenic and has been shown to be effective in animals as a potential subunit vaccine target.[19]

Lectin-mediated adherence by the trophozoite is a prerequisite for the subsequent lysis of target interglandular intestinal cells. Target cell lysis is a complex process requiring the presence of calcium[91] and several parasite-derived virulence factors, including a calcium-dependent phospholipase,[55, 89] a target cell ionophore,[52] a hemolysin,[43] and a neuraminidase. Thus, cytolysis of the target cell is completed extracellularly by the trophozoite. The killed cells then can be engulfed with intact cell membrane, or the cytoplasm and the nucleus can be ingested through a broken membrane.[36, 62] The nucleus of the target cell loses its membrane even before ingestion and no longer stains in the usual electron-dense manner.

Invasion of the mucosa then may occur, but many factors are involved in instituting this invasion. The presence and adherence of bacteria often are required for invasiveness.[53, 62, 68] Parasite-derived hydrolytic enzymes greatly contribute to the destruction of cells and the surrounding extracellular matrix. They include several types of proteases[47, 70, 93, 95, 107] and glycosidases.[118, 125] The former has been shown to participate in parasite-mediated immune evasion by degrading immunoglobulin A (IgA) molecules and mimicking the activity of certain complement components.[48]

A vigorous infiltration by neutrophils and other inflammatory cells occurs in response to invasion by trophozoite.[36, 62, 86, 87, 96] Host cell recruitment occurs in part by the parasite-induced stimulation of host interleukin 8.[128] The host polymorphonuclear response greatly contributes to the destruction of host tissues. The 170-kd lectin of *E. histolytica* attaches the trophozoite to polymorphonuclear neutrophils, peripheral blood mononuclear cells, monocytes, and monocyte-derived macrophages.[86, 117] Neutrophils are killed and lysed similarly to intestinal cells. However, cytolysis of neutrophils releases some substance or substances that are locally effective in augmenting the cytolytic efficacy of virulent *E. histolytica,* thus causing the inflammatory response to increase the damage rather than contain the infection.[103] Invading trophozoites release substances that have not been characterized but strongly attract more neutrophils to the invading *E. histolytica* and allow these neutrophils to be killed as well.[98] Thus, the immune response to the initial infection with *E. histolytica* often is not effective, and few viable neutrophils are found in the material left behind the active infection. Nevertheless, cell-mediated immunity has an important role in limiting the extent of invasive amebiasis and in protecting the host from a recurrence.[87, 92] The major cell-mediated effector mechanisms include killing of trophozoite by activated macrophages and $CD8^+$ cytotoxic lymphocytes.[98–103] Cytokines such as tumor necrosis factor and interferon-γ contribute to immunocompetent cell activation, whereas nitric oxide also has a prominent effector role. Humoral antibodies produced during a primary infection have been shown to protect against further infection and cause further damage to the host. One IgG antibody was found to be cytotoxic to *E. histolytica* in a manner independent of the complement system.[105] Another antibody has been found to be a liver autoantibody.[27] Numerous other antibodies have been noted, but their significance in most cases awaits further study.[44, 49, 112, 116]

The initial lesions of clinical amebiasis often are small interglandular ulcers with a diameter of about 1 mm. They extend only to the muscularis mucosa.[15, 62] The margins may be hyperemic, and there is slight edema of the surrounding mucosa. *E. histolytica* organisms seen in these ulcers will stain quite well with periodic acid–Schiff stain.[79] Bleeding and friability are not prominent at this stage, although proctoscopic examination may find mucus coming from these ulcers with abundant amebae present.

The next stage of intestinal disease is the production of deeper ulcers. These "buttonhole" ulcers may be as large as 1 cm in diameter and may extend into the submucosa.[15, 79] The ulcer often extends laterally under normal-appearing mucosa, forming a characteristic flask shape. Occasional perforation through the serosa with resultant peritonitis or pneumoperitoneum is found.[111] Extensive necrosis may be present, but usually only very little inflammation is present. Rarely, a pseudomembranous colitis may develop.[29] The edema is more intense, but the mucosa between ulcers is relatively normal in contrast to the marked inflammatory response seen in bacterial enteritis. When ulceration is more extensive, the edema surrounding the ulcers becomes confluent, and the mucosa appears gelatinous. In young children, this condition can progress to a fulminant necrotizing colitis associated with transmural necrosis. The pathologic events associated with this phenomenon are not understood. Rarely, an inflammatory response is present, resulting in granulation tissue with a fibrous outer wall.[72] It is given the name *ameboma.* Occasionally, an ameboma fills a significant portion of the lumen, which causes stricture or obstruction. Other complications of intestinal amebiasis result from direct extension of the ulcers. This extension may result in cutaneous involvement of the perianal area or lesions of the penis, vulva, vagina, or cervix.[3, 72] Cutaneous and ophthalmologic amebiasis also is caused by fecal contamination of the face.[64]

Amebas disseminate to the liver in as many as 50 percent of patients with fulminant amebiasis.[3, 4] Dissemination to other organs directly from the intestine probably does not occur, but dissemination from the liver to lung, heart, brain, spleen, scapula, larynx, stomach, and aorta has been described.[15] Amebic abscess of the liver occurs more often in adult males than in females by a ratio of 16:1 but occurs equally often in prepubertal children of both sexes.[4, 15] Abscesses occur more commonly in adults but occur in children as young as 4 months of age.[69] These abscesses vary from microscopic lesions to massive necrosis of as much as 90 percent of the liver. Fever, right upper quadrant pain, and the presence of serum antibodies to amebae point to hepatic amebic abscess.[86] The abscesses usually are free of bacterial contamination and have little inflammatory component. Examination of the fluid from such an abscess frequently reveals a reddish "anchovy paste" fluid that rarely may appear white or green. The fluid is acidic, with a pH ranging from 5.2 to 6.7.[85] Amebas are found in the walls of the abscess and only rarely in the fluid of the abscess. The walls are composed of a thin connective-tissue capsule. The right lobe of the liver is involved with amebic liver abscess about six times as often as is the left lobe. Abscesses in the right lobe can perforate and cause disease below the diaphragm or in the thoracic cavity. Abscesses in the left lobe can lead to pericardial effusions, which are less common than pleural effusions.[37, 42]

Pleural effusions can remain loculated or lead to cutaneous fistulas or to bronchopleural fistulas. Drainage from these fistulas is acidic, in contrast to the neutral secretions in the normal lung. Seeding of the cardiac valves and of the brain has been described.[15] Cerebral abscesses have the same microscopic findings as do liver abscesses, with a thin capsule of connective tissue surrounding a fluid with little or no associated inflammatory response.

Clinical Manifestations

INTESTINAL AMEBIASIS

Asymptomatic Intraluminal Amebiasis

The most common type of amebic infestation is an asymptomatic cyst-passing carrier state. All *E. dispar* infections and as many as 90 percent of *E. histolytica* infections are asymptomatic, presenting only with *Entamoeba* cysts in the feces.[34, 80] Some investigators have suggested that stools of these individuals generally are more liquid than in individuals without trophozoites.[26] Furthermore, no longitudinal studies have been conducted to determine whether *E. dispar* or asymptomatic *E. histolytica* infections cause intermittent episodes of diarrhea or contribute to malnutrition and physical growth impairment of children.

Acute Amebic Colitis

Amebic dysentery is the most common form of symptomatic invasive amebiasis. Seventy percent of patients have a gradual onset of symptoms over 3 or 4 weeks after infestation, with increasingly severe diarrhea as the primary complaint, accompanied by general abdominal tenderness. Occasionally, the onset may be acute or may be delayed for several months after infestation. The diarrhea is associated with pain in virtually 100 percent of children. Pain may be of such severity that an acute abdomen is suspected.[3, 10, 45, 79] The stools contain blood and mucus in virtually all cases.[3, 78, 79] Fever occurs in fewer than one half of the patients. Abdominal distention and dehydration occur in fewer than 10 percent of patients. In young children, intussusception, perforation, and peritonitis, or necrotizing colitis may develop rapidly.[10, 45, 111]

Ameboma

Ameboma is an unusual presentation of intestinal amebiasis occurring in fewer than 1 percent of patients with amebic colitis. These patients present with an abdominal mass that gives an apple-core appearance on radiographs, which can mimic colonic carcinoma.

EXTRAINTESTINAL AMEBIASIS

Amebic Liver Abscess

The second most frequent presentation of invasive amebiasis is an amebic liver abscess, which occurs in 1 to 7 percent of children with invasive amebiasis[15, 69, 97] and in 10 to 50 percent of adults with invasive intestinal amebiasis.[4, 15] However, fewer than 30 percent of patients with amebic liver abscess have active diarrhea at any time before presentation. Symptoms of amebic liver abscess in adults include upper abdominal pain in 77 percent of patients, fever in 90 percent, hepatomegaly with tenderness in 93 percent, and poor right diaphragmatic excursion in 58 percent. Jaundice occurs in 12 percent of patients.[51, 84, 97] Occasionally, pain is reported in the right shoulder or the right side of the chest.

In children, abdominal pain is reported infrequently with amebic liver abscess.[38, 65] More commonly, high fever, abdominal distention, irritability, and tachypnea are noted. Some of these children are admitted to the hospital with a fever of unknown origin. Hepatomegaly occurs frequently, but elicitation of hepatic tenderness is not well documented. In one report, four of five children younger than 5 years of age died with amebic liver abscesses because the diagnosis was not suspected.[51] Death usually results from rupture of the liver abscess into the peritoneum, thorax, or pericardium but may follow extensive hepatic damage and liver failure.[4, 84]

Metastatic Amebiasis

Extra-abdominal amebiasis presumably follows direct extension from liver abscesses rather than direct dissemination from the intestine.[4, 15] Thoracic amebiasis is the most common type of extra-abdominal amebiasis and occurs in about 10 percent of patients with amebic liver abscess.[15, 42] Symptoms depend on the type of involvement. Empyema, bronchohepatic fistulas, or extension of a pleuropulmonary abscess into the pericardium may occur. Pericardial amebiasis is the next most common form of extraintestinal involvement and may result from rupture of a liver abscess in the left lobe of the liver into the pericardium or through extension of the right-sided pleural amebiasis.[15, 28, 32, 37] It is estimated to occur in 3 percent of patients with hepatic abscesses.[32] It presents as acute pericarditis with tamponade and, occasionally, as pneumopericardium.[28] Amebic liver abscess in the left lobe also may rupture directly into the left chest.[61]

Cerebral amebic abscesses were found in 8 percent of patients with amebic infections discovered at autopsy in one study.[54] In other studies, lower rates of only 0.66 to 4.7 percent of patients with amebic liver abscess having brain abscesses were reported.[41] Patients with cerebral amebiasis frequently are so ill from the intestinal, liver, and possibly lung involvement that neurologic signs are not always assessed easily. However, in 18 patients with proven cerebral amebiasis, initial neurologic examination was normal in 13, and only 1 later developed seizures.

Other foci of infection are rare, but amebic rectovesical fistula formation and involvement of pharynx, heart, aorta, and scapula have been reported. Cutaneous extension after the adherence of perforated, inflamed bowel to the skin is an extremely painful and rare complication.[15, 72] This situation also may arise after invasion of the skin by trophozoites emerging out from the rectum.

Diagnosis

As many as 40 percent of adults with amebiasis and an even greater percentage of children escape diagnosis because this disease is not included as a diagnostic consideration. The diagnosis of amebiasis should be considered in any child who is passing bloody stools or stools with mucus; any child with a hepatic abscess; and any febrile child with right upper quadrant pain, abdominal distention, or tachypnea.[51, 65]

MICROSCOPIC DIAGNOSIS

The investigation of a child for amebiasis should include examination of three stools by wet mount (within 1 to 2 hours of stool passage) and by fixation in formalin and polyvinyl alcohol for permanent stains and concentration.[40, 72, 110] Multiple examinations often are necessary because the cysts are shed only intermittently. The stools should not be contaminated with water and urine (because these destroy trophozoites) or with interfering substances such as barium, laxatives, antibiotics, and soapsuds enemas.[72, 87] Saline does not destroy the trophozoites. A single, formed stool reveals amebic cysts by these techniques in 30 to 50 percent of infected individuals.[40, 72] Examination of three stools, taken at daily intervals, diagnoses 60 to 70 percent of patients with amebic colitis and 40 to 50 percent of patients with amebic hepatic abscesses. The polyvinyl alcohol preserves trophozoites well, and the formalin allows good preservation and concentration of the cysts.[72] Staining with periodic acid–Schiff stain highlights the trophozoite forms, and the trichrome stain provides definition of intracellular characteristics of both trophozoites and cysts. Being certain that any organisms seen are *E. histolytica* (or *E. dispar*) rather than the nonpathogenic *E. coli* or *E. hartmanni* is important. A negative stool examination should not preclude further work-up if no other explanation of the patient's symptoms has been found by this stage.

LABORATORY, SEROLOGIC, AND MOLECULAR DIAGNOSTIC TESTS

Most patients with amebic colitis have occult blood in their feces, often a useful and inexpensive screening test.[87] Most patients with amebic liver abscess have a leukocytosis and an elevated alkaline phosphatase. In contrast, liver transaminases often are not elevated. The erythrocyte sedimentation rate typically is increased.

Serologic studies also can be helpful in the diagnosis of invasive amebiasis, whereas asymptomatic infections with *E. dispar* usually do not elicit a measurable serologic response. Moreover, the absence of serum antibodies to *E. histolytica* after 1 week of symptoms is evidence against the diagnosis of invasive amebiasis.[1, 87, 109] Gel diffusion (both agar gel diffusion and cellulose acetate diffusion), counterimmunoelectrophoresis, indirect hemagglutination, indirect immunofluorescent test, and enzyme-linked immunosorbent assay (ELISA) are tests that are currently available.[6, 31, 72, 104, 110, 127] Indirect immunofluorescent and indirect hemagglutination titers persist for years after an infection, rendering them less useful in endemic areas.[72, 110] Counterimmunoelectrophoresis and gel diffusion results often revert to negative within months. Purified recombinant parasite antigens have been used in serologic tests for amebic liver abscesses and to distinguish between acute and convalescent infections.[1, 87] ELISA using genetically engineered polypeptides likely will become an important new tool for the diagnosis of invasive amebiasis.[112]

Newer molecular diagnostic tools ultimately may allow the clinician to distinguish the nonpathogenic *E. dispar* spp. from *E. histolytica*. They include ELISAs, which employ monoclonal antibodies developed against pathogen-specific epitopes,[1, 39, 94, 112] and the polymerase chain reaction, which uses species-specific oligonucleotides to differentiate *E. histolytica* from *E. dispar* in stool samples.[1, 2, 33, 39, 94, 112, 118, 122]

RADIOGRAPHIC STUDIES

Radiologic imaging has become helpful in the diagnosis of extraintestinal amebiasis. Ultrasonography, computed tomography (CT), and magnetic resonance imaging (MRI) all have been shown to be helpful in demonstrating extracolonic amebiasis in the liver, paracecal masses, brain, and other sites.[81–83, 121, 122] These modalities also improve the precision with which needle aspirations of these abscesses can be done.[122] At present, CT and MRI appear to have no advantage over ultrasonography of the liver. Most patients with amebic liver abscess have a single abscess in the right lobe of the liver, although multiple lesions also can occur.[5] Chest radiographs show elevation of the right diaphragm in 56 percent of patients with hepatic abscess.[4] The diagnosis of cerebral amebiasis requires careful neurologic evaluation and radiographic evaluation with either CT or MRI.[15, 41, 54] Because of the risk for perforation, barium studies are relatively contraindicated in patients with amebic colitis.

BIOPSY STUDIES

The colonic and rectal mucosa in amebic colitis usually reveals ulcerations with a diameter of 1 to 10 mm. Amebic trophozoites often are at the periphery of these necrotic areas, which can be sampled through a biopsy specimen taken during sigmoidoscopy or colonoscopy.[35, 40] Because of the potential for perforation, colonoscopy should be undertaken with caution.

Amebic trophozoites are found near the capsule of amebic liver abscesses. In instances when a clinical diagnosis of amebic liver abscess is in doubt, needle aspiration of the liver abscess under CT or ultrasound guidance can be performed. This procedure has associated risks, including bleeding, peritoneal spillage of trophozoites, secondary superinfection, and accidental rupture of an echinococcal cyst.[87, 92]

Differential Diagnosis

Invasive amebic colitis may resemble ulcerative colitis, Crohn disease of the colon (inflammatory bowel disease), bacillary dysentery, or tuberculous colitis.[11, 17, 29, 40] Stool examinations, colonoscopic examination with biopsies, and serologic examination should be able to differentiate amebic colitis from these diseases. Histologic examination of involved colonic mucosa should differentiate amebic colitis, with its relative lack of inflammation and rare granulation tissue, from the inflammatory responses seen in ulcerative colitis, bacillary dysentery, and Crohn disease of the colon. Tuberculous colitis and Crohn disease are more likely to show granuloma formation than is amebiasis. Ileocecal or small bowel involvement as seen on barium studies would suggest Crohn disease or tuberculosis of the gastrointestinal tract rather than amebiasis. Tuberculous colitis usually is associated with pulmonary tuberculosis and with a strong reaction to tuberculin skin testing. In some cases, differentiating between invasive amebic colitis and inflammatory bowel disease may not be possible. If a patient with this differential diagnosis is placed on corticosteroids and deteriorates, the corticosteroids should be stopped and repeat investigation for amebiasis performed.[17, 65, 72]

Amebic liver abscess must be differentiated from pyogenic abscesses and neoplastic lesions. Total leukocyte counts and cultures of blood may help to differentiate pyogenic and amebic abscesses. However, many children with pyogenic liver abscesses have negative blood cultures. Often, amebic and pyogenic liver abscesses show similar features on CT and MRI. Occasionally, nuclear imaging with gallium is helpful because, unlike a pyogenic abscess, very few neutrophils are contained within the amebic liver abscess (in this instance, the term *amebic liver abscess* is a misnomer).[87, 92] Hence, gallium scanning of an amebic liver abscess may reveal a cold spot, possibly with a bright rim. Several investigators recommend a trial with an appropriate drug for amebic abscess for 3 or 4 days while serologic and culture results are awaited.[65, 126] Patients with amebic liver abscess should respond to treatment in this length of time by becoming afebrile. No change in size of the liver or size of the abscess should be noted at this time because resolution of the abscess usually takes 2 months to several years.[5, 81, 82, 108, 124] Neoplastic lesions frequently can be proved by ultrasound examination to be solid masses. A history of weight loss without symptoms of dysentery or presence of *E. histolytica* in the stool suggests neoplastic disease.

Complications

Complications of amebiasis may be prevented by early diagnosis and treatment with appropriate agents.[41, 65] When complications occur, the prognosis generally is poor.

Invasive intestinal amebiasis has been associated most commonly with perforation and peritonitis,[7, 10, 45, 65, 111, 120] which apparently are an end result of "necrotizing" or "toxic" amebic colitis. In children, perforation may be heralded by the appearance of an acute abdomen or pneumoperitoneum, with rapid progression to death, presumably from sepsis.[7, 65, 120] Surgical resection and therapy for endotoxic shock improve the prognosis.[120] This complication is not rare and accounts for more than 30 percent of the deaths from amebiasis in childhood.[11, 46] Massive intestinal hemorrhage causes about 3 percent of deaths from amebiasis. Intussusception occasionally occurs and can be reduced with gentle barium enema. Multiple colonic strictures also can occur and cause obstructive symptoms. Fistulas to other organs or to the skin may develop.

Liver abscesses and their resultant complications account for about 40 percent of the deaths from amebiasis.[46] Liver abscess also was found in 13 percent of patients with amebiasis who had postmortem examinations. Liver abscess with rupture into the abdomen was present in 8 percent of patients who died with amebiasis, and rupture of a liver abscess into the right pleural space was found in 12 percent.[46] Bacterial superinfection was found in 10 percent of cases of pleural amebiasis.[42] In cases free of bacterial contamination, the fluid has few inflammatory cells and an acidic pH. Amebic pericarditis or pneumopericardium occurs rarely and is found in only 1 percent of patients whose deaths were caused by amebiasis.[28, 32, 37, 46] The fluid is similar to that found in the pleural space. A cerebral abscess was found in 4 percent of patients with amebiasis who died.[46] It has been reported in fewer than 10 children, only 1 of whom survived.[8, 15, 41, 54] Other complications include infections of the retroperitoneal space, stomach, spleen, esophagus, and duodenum.[54]

Prevention

Prevention of amebiasis requires sanitation, health education, early treatment of cases, and adequate surveillance and control programs.[87, 92] Because the only known mode of infection is ingestion of matter contaminated with cysts of *E. histolytica*, their removal through the disposal of human feces and water sterilization is essential. The cysts can be removed adequately from drinking water by sand filtration, hyperchlorination, or boiling.[59, 72] However, spread through raw fruits or vegetables contaminated with cysts still can occur. Infected food handlers are a major source of transmission. Travelers can avoid infection by avoiding eating unpeeled fruits and vegetables and by drinking only boiled, bottled, or disinfected (iodination with tetraglycine hydroperiodide) water.[92] Early treatment of patients with intraluminal amebiasis also is important because asymptomatic individuals excrete up to 15 million cysts per day, which can survive in water for several weeks and often are resistant to the levels of chlorination used commonly for water purification.[67]

Therapy that targets individuals with *E. histolytica* but not *E. dispar* infections may become possible during the next few years as molecular diagnostic techniques improve.

Recombinant vaccines that employ derivatives of either the major amebic lectin or a serine-rich amebic protein are under development.[41]

Treatment

INTESTINAL AMEBIASIS

Asymptomatic Intraluminal Amebiasis

Treatment of asymptomatic cyst passers is controversial. Many authors suggest that such treatment is mandatory because these individuals serve as a source of infection for other individuals and themselves may become symptomatic with a change in the intracolonic environment.[63, 67, 113] Other authors suggest that asymptomatic individuals not be treated because the medications have severe toxicities, amebiasis is so widespread, and some individuals rid themselves of the disease with no therapy.[113] This controversy most likely will disappear once diagnostic methods that distinguish between *E. histolytica* and *E. dispar* infections become more widely available to clinicians. Until that time, treating all children is most prudent. Controversies surrounding the treatment of amebiasis during pregnancy are not addressed here.

The three intraluminal agents most widely used to treat asymptomatic intraluminal amebiasis are iodoquinol, diloxanide furoate, and paromomycin. Each one has a high rate of success for eradication of cyst passage.[57, 58]

Iodoquinol, or diiodohydroxyquin, is a poorly absorbed amebicidal agent with side effects of abdominal pain, nausea, vomiting, and diarrhea in the usual doses.[3, 57–60, 126] A small fraction is absorbed and can cause skin rashes or, through deiodination, thyroid function test abnormalities. In very large doses for prolonged periods, it has been reported to cause optic neuritis, optic atrophy, and peripheral neuropathy. It is not useful for extraintestinal amebiasis. The dosage of iodoquinol (Yodoxin) is 30 to 40 mg/kg/day to a maximum of 2 g in three divided oral doses for 20 days.

Diloxanide furoate (Furamide) is a poorly absorbed agent that is quite active against only intraluminal amebiasis but treats symptomatic as well as asymptomatic disease.[31, 60, 126] Cure rates have been more than 90 percent with a 10-day oral course of diloxanide furoate at 20 mg/kg/day in three divided doses (maximum dose of 1500 mg/day).[57, 58, 73] It has few side effects; marked flatulence is the main problem. It is available through the Centers for Disease Control and Prevention (CDC) by calling the CDC Drug Service (telephone: 404-639-3670).

Paromomycin is a nonabsorbable aminoglycoside that is active against both the cyst and trophozoite stages. High cure rates have been reported with a 7-day oral dose of paromomycin at 25 to 35 mg/kg/day in three divided doses.

Acute Amebic Colitis

Metronidazole is an imidazole compound that is available as a well-absorbed oral agent or as an intravenous medication.[3, 4, 21, 60, 79, 87, 92, 126] It is the most effective amebicide for treatment of amebic colitis and works by exploiting the anaerobic metabolism of the organism. By undergoing reduction and reacting with nucleic acids, metronidazole causes some mutagenicity and carcinogenicity in mice and hamsters, but no genetic disturbances have been found in humans.[60] Other side effects include nausea, headaches, a metallic taste of the saliva, dizziness, abdominal pain, glossitis, stomatitis, and diarrhea. Rarely, seizures or neuropathy occurs. It has an effect similar to that of disulfiram if taken when the patient consumes ethanol.[60] The oral dosage is 35 to 50 mg/kg/day (to a maximum of 2250 mg/day) in three divided doses for 7 to 10 days for severe intestinal or extraintestinal amebiasis. Cure rates for extraintestinal amebiasis are excellent, but one third of patients with intraluminal amebiasis treated with metronidazole alone will have a relapse.[126] Therefore, treatment should be followed by administration of an intraluminal agent, usually iodoquinol. Related imidazoles such as tinidazole (60 mg/kg/day [maximum, 2 g] for 5 days) and ornidazole may prove to be tolerated better than metronidazole.

Emetine and its derivative dehydroemetine are tissue-active amebicides derived from an ipecac alkaloid that inhibits protein synthesis.[60, 126] They have many side effects. Very common problems include diarrhea, vomiting, precordial chest pain, arrhythmias, electrocardiographic changes of inverted T waves and prolonged Q-T intervals, and tachycardia (especially if the patient is ambulatory). Emetine is cleared by renal excretion and still can be detected in urine up to 2 months after cessation of treatment; therefore, side effects may continue after stopping the emetine. Given the apparent success of the imidazoles for the treatment of amebiasis, the use of emetine and dehydroemetine for intestinal amebiasis likely will continue to decrease.

Agents such as metronidazole that are active against invasive and extraintestinal amebiasis are well absorbed and do not necessarily stay in the lumen long enough to have an effect on intestinal amebiasis. Thus, these agents should be used in conjunction with a luminal agent either simultaneously or with the luminal agent used after the tissue-active-agent.

EXTRAINTESTINAL AMEBIASIS

Amebic Liver Abscess and Metastatic Amebiasis

Extraintestinal and severe intestinal amebiasis must be treated with the tissue-active agents. Metronidazole (35 to 50 mg/kg/day in three divided doses for 10 days) is the preferred drug because it is both effective and relatively free of serious side effects.[3, 4, 60, 87, 92, 126] It is effective for extraintestinal amebiasis in any location, although amebic brain abscesses usually are not treated successfully with any medications. Most patients with amebic liver abscess respond to metronidazole within 72 hours. As for amebic colitis, follow-up therapy with a luminal agent is very important because of the high rates of asymptomatic intestinal colonization in patients with amebic liver abscess.

If metronidazole cannot be used, a combination of chloroquine with either emetine or dehydroemetine has been used in the past, but side effects are a problem.

Because extraintestinal amebiasis begins most commonly with a hepatic abscess that ruptures into the abdomen, the right side of the chest, the pericardium, or the left side of the chest (from the left lobe of the liver), the issue of draining the hepatic abscess or the site of rupture must be considered.[46] Draining is indicated for (1) cysts larger than 12 cm that are in danger of rupture, (2) failure to respond to medical therapy, (3) a left lobe abscess that might predispose to pericardial rupture, (4) initial diagnosis to exclude pyogenic liver abscess, or (5) a ruptured abscess.[87, 119]

Prognosis

Available statistics suggest that, worldwide, 500 million people are infected with *E. histolytica*. Invasive disease develops in 50 million people each year, and 50,000 to 100,000 deaths per year are caused by the invasive disease.[80, 86, 87] Hence, the case-fatality ratio is between 1 in 500 and 1 in 1000 diagnosed cases. However, among patients with illness severe enough to require hospitalization, the case-fatality ratio is higher. One small study in children reported a 9 percent mortality rate and a 27 percent morbidity rate.[65]

Bowel necrosis or perforation is the cause of death from purely intestinal amebiasis, and early surgical intervention can lower the mortality rate from these complications from 100 to 28 percent.[120] Amebic liver abscess has a case-fatality rate of 10 to 15 percent in combined figures of adults and children.[51, 69, 84] The mortality rate when pleural involvement is noted is 14 percent.[42, 51] Amebic pericarditis has a case-fatality rate of 40 percent.[37] Cerebral amebiasis has a case-fatality rate of 96 percent.

REFERENCES

1. Abd-Alla, M., Jackson, T. F. H. G., Gathirim, V., et al.: Differentiation of pathogenic from nonpathogenic *Entamoeba histolytica* infection by detection of galactose-inhibitable adherence protein antigen in sera and feces. J. Clin. Microbiol. *31*:2845–2850, 1993.
2. Acuna-Soto, R., Samuelson, J., De Girolami, P., et al.: Application of the polymerase chain reaction to the epidemiology of pathogenic and nonpathogenic *Entamoeba histolytica*. Am. J. Trop. Med. Hyg. *48*:58–70, 1993.
3. Adams, E. B., and MacLeod, I. N.: Invasive amebiasis. I. Amebic dysentery and its complications. Medicine *56*:315–323, 1977.
4. Adams, E. B., and MacLeod, I. N.: Invasive amebiasis. II. Amebic liver abscess and its complications. Medicine *56*:325–334, 1977.
5. Ahmed, L., Salama, Z. A., El Rooby, A., et al.: Ultrasonographic resolution time for amebic liver abscess. Am. J. Trop. Med. Hyg. *41*:406–410, 1989.
6. Ambroise-Thomas, P., and Truong, T. K.: Fluorescent antibody test in amebiasis: Clinical applications. Am. J. Trop. Med. Hyg. *21*:907–911, 1972.
7. Azar, H., Nazarian, I., and Sadrieh, M.: A study of cause of death in patients with fulminant amebic colitis. Am. J. Proctol. *28*:80–84, 1977.
8. Bachy, A.: Cerebral abscesses in amebiasis. J. Pediatr. *88*:364–365, 1976.
9. Bailey, G. B., Nudelman, E. D., Day, D. B., et al.: Specificity of glycosphingolipid recognition by *Entamoeba histolytica* trophozoites. Infect. Immun. *58*:43–47, 1990.
10. Balikian, J. P., Bitar, J. G., Rishani, K. K., et al.: Fulminant necrotizing amebic colitis in children. Am. J. Proctol. *28*:69–73, 1977.
11. Balikian, J. P., Uthman, S. M., and Kabakian, H. A.: Tuberculous colitis. Am. J. Proctol. *28*:75–79, 1977.
12. Barker, D. C.: Differentiation of *Entamoeba*. Patterns of nucleic acids and ribosomes during encystation and excystation. *In* Van den Bossche H. (ed.): Biochemistry of Parasites and Host-Parasite Relationships. Amsterdam, Elsevier Biomedical, 1976, p. 253.
13. Bhattacharya, S., Bhattacharya, A., Diamond, L. S., et al.: Circular DNA of *Entamoeba histolytica* encodes ribosomal RNA. J. Protozool. *36*:455–458, 1989.
14. Braga, L. L., Ninomiya, H., McCoy, J. J., et al. Inhibition of the complement membrane attack complex by the galactose-specific adhesion of *Entamoeba histolytica*. J. Clin. Invest. *90*:1131–1137, 1992.
15. Brandt, H., and Tamayo, R. P.: Pathology of human amebiasis. Hum. Pathol. *1*:351–385, 1970.
16. Burch D. J., Li, E., Reed, S., et al.: Isolation of a strain-specific *Entamoeba histolytica* cDNA clone. J. Clin. Microbiol. *29*:297–302, 1991.
17. Case records of the Massachusetts General Hospital: Weekly clinicopathological exercises: Case 32-1977. N. Engl. J. Med. *297*:322–330, 1977.
18. Chadee, K., Petri, W. A., Jr., Innes, D. J., et al.: Rat and human colonic mucins bind and inhibit adherence lectin of *Entamoeba histolytica*. J. Clin. Invest. *80*:1245–1254, 1987.
19. Chu-Jing, G. S., Kain, K. C., Abd-Alla, M., et al.: A recombinant cysteine-rich section of the *Entamoeba histolytica* galactose-inhibitable lectin is efficacious as a subunit vaccine in the gerbil model of amebic liver abscess. J. Infect. Dis. *171*:645–651, 1995.
20. Clark, C. G., and Diamond, L. S.: Ribosomal RNA genes of "pathogenic" *Entamoeba histolytica* are distinct. Mol. Biochem. Parasitol. *49*:297–302, 1991.
21. Cohen, H. G., and Reynolds, T. B.: Comparison of metronidazole and chloroquine for the treatment of amoebic liver abscess. Gastroenterology *69*:35–41, 1975.
22. Councilman, W. T., and Lafleur, H. A.: Amoebic dysentery. Johns Hopkins Hosp. Rep. *2*:395–548, 1891.
23. DeMeester, F., Shaw, E., Scholze, H., et al.: Specific labeling of cysteine proteinases in pathogenic and nonpathogenic *Entamoeba histolytica*. Infect. Immun. *58*:1396–1401, 1990.
24. Diamond, L. S., and Clark, C. G.: A redescription of *Entamoeba histolytica* Schaudinn. 1903 (Emended Walker, 1911) separating it from *Entamoeba dispar* (Brumpt, 1925). J. Eukaryotic Microbiol. *40*:340–344, 1993.
25. Druckman, D. A., and Quinn, T. C.: *Entamoeba histolytica* infection in homosexual men. *In* Ravdin, J. I. (ed.): Amebiasis: Human Infection by *Entamoeba histolytica*. New York, Churchill Livingstone, 1988, pp. 563–571.
26. Elsdon-Dew, R.: The epidemiology of amoebiasis. Adv. Parasitol. *6*:1–62, 1968.

27. Faubert, G. M., Meerovitch, E., and McLaughlin, J.: The presence of liver auto-antibodies induced by *Entamoeba histolytica* in the sera from both naturally infected humans and immunized rabbits. Am. J. Trop. Med. Hyg. *27*:892–895, 1978.
28. Freeman, A. L., and Bhoola, K. D.: Pneumopericardium complicating amoebic liver abscess: A case report. S. Afr. Med. J. *50*:551–553, 1976.
29. Friedrich, I. A., Korsten, M. A., and Gottfried, E. B.: Necrotizing amebic colitis with pseudomembrane formation. Am. J. Gastroenterol. *74*:529–531, 1980.
30. Fuchs, G., Ruiz-Palacios, G., and Pickering, L. K.: Amebiasis in the pediatric population. *In* Ravdin J. I. (ed.): Amebiasis: Human Infection by *Entamoeba histolytica*. New York, Churchill Livingstone, 1988, pp. 594–613.
31. Gandhi, B. M., Irshad, M., Acharya, S. K., et al.: Amebic liver abscess and circulating immune complexes of *Entamoeba histolytica* proteins. Am. J. Trop. Med. Hyg. *39*:440–444, 1988.
32. Ganesan, T. K., and Kandaswamy, S.: Amebic pericarditis. Chest *67*:112–113, 1975.
33. Garfinkel, L. I., Giladi, M., Huber, M., et al.: DNA probes specific for *Entamoeba histolytica* possessing pathogenic and nonpathogenic zymodemes. Infect. Immun. *57*:926–931, 1989.
34. Gathiram, V., and Jackson, T. F. H. G.: A longitudinal study of asymptomatic carriers of pathogenic zymodemes of *Entamoeba histolytica*. S. Afr. Med. J. 72:669–672, 1987.
35. Gilman, R., Islam, M., Paschi, S., et al.: Comparison of conventional and immunofluorescent techniques for the detection of *Entamoeba histolytica* in rectal biopsies. Gastroenterology *78*:435–439, 1980.
36. Griffin, J. L.: Human amebic dysentery: Electron microscopy of *Entamoeba histolytica* contacting, ingesting, and digesting inflammatory cells. Am. J. Trop. Med. Hyg. *21*:895–906, 1972.
37. Guimaraes, A. C., Vinhaes, L. A., Filho, A. S., et al.: Acute suppurative amebic pericarditis. Am. J. Cardiol. *34*:103–106, 1974.
38. Haffar, A., Boland, J., and Edwards, M. S.: Amebic liver abscess in children. Pediatr. Infect. Dis. *1*:322–327, 1982.
39. Haque, R., Ali, I.K., Akther, S., and Petri, W. A. Jr.: Comparison of PCR isoenzyme analysis, and antigen detection for diagnosis of *Entamoeba histolytica* infection. J. Clin. Microbiol. 36:449–452, 1998.
40. Harries, J.: Amoebiasis: A review. J. R. Soc. Med. *75*:190–197, 1982.
41. Huston, C.D. and Petri W.A. Jr.: Host-pathogen interaction in amebiasis and progress in vaccine development. Eur. J. Clin. Microbiol. Infect. Dis. 17:601–614, 1998.
42. Ibarra-Perez, C., and Selman-Lama, M.: Diagnosis and treatment of amebic "empyema": Report of eighty-eight cases. Am. J. Surg. *134*:283–287, 1977.
43. Jansson, A., Gillin, F., Kagardt, U., et al.: Coding of hemolysins within the ribosomal RNA repeat on a plasmid in *Entamoeba histolytica*. Science *263*:144–1443, 1994.
44. Joyce, M. P., and Ravdin, J. I.: Antigens of *Entamoeba histolytica* recognized by immune sera from liver abscess patients. Am. J. Trop. Med. Hyg. *38*:74–80, 1988.
45. Kala, P. C., Sharma, G. C., and Haldia, K. N.: Fulminating amoebic colitis with multiple perforations. Am. J. Proctol. *28*:31–34, 1977.
46. Kean, B. H., Gilmore, H. R., Jr., and Van Stone, W. W.: Fatal amebiasis: Report of 148 fatal cases from the Armed Forces Institutes of Pathology. Ann. Intern. Med. *44*:831–843, 1956.
47. Keene, W. E., Petitt, M. G., Allen, S., et al.: The major neutral proteinase of *Entamoeba histolytica*. J. Exp. Med. *163*:536–549, 1986.
48. Kelsall, B. L., and Ravdin, J. I.: Proteolytic degradation of human IgA by *Entamoeba histolytica*. J. Infect. Dis. *168*:1319–1322, 1993.
49. Kettis, A. A., Thorstensson, R., and Utter, G.: Antigenicity of *Entamoeba histolytica* strain NIH 200: A survey of clinically relevant antigenic components. Am. J. Trop. Med. Hyg. *32*:512–522, 1983.
50. Knobloch J., and Mannweiler D.: Development and persistence of antibodies to *Entamoeba histolytica* in patients with amebic liver abscess: analysis of 216 cases. Am. J. Trop. Med. Hyg. *32*:727–732, 1983.
51. Lamont, A. C., and Wicks, A. C. B.: Amoebic liver abscess in Rhodesian Africans. Trans. R. Soc. Trop. Med. Hyg. *70*:302–305, 1976.
52. Leippe, M., Tannich, E., Nickel, R., et al.: Primary and secondary structure of the pore-forming protein produced by *Entamoeba histolytica*. EMBO J. *11*:3501–3506, 1992.
53. Leitch, G. J.: Intestinal lumen and mucosal microclimate H+ and NH3 concentrations as factors in the etiology of experimental amebiasis. Am. J. Trop. Med. Hyg. *38*:480–486, 1988.
54. Lombardo, L., Alonso, P., Arroyo, L. S., et al.: Cerebral amebiasis: Report of 17 cases. J. Neurosurg. *21*:704–709, 1964.
55. Long-Krug, S. A., Hysmith, R. M., Fischer, K. J., et al.: The phospholipase A enzymes of *Entamoeba histolytica*: Description and subcellular localization. J. Infect. Dis. *152*:536–541, 1985.
56. Losch, F.: Massenhafte entwicklung von amoben in dickdarm. Virchows Arch. [A] *65*:196–211, 1975.
57. McAuley, J. B., Herwaldt, B. L., Stokes, S. L., et al.: Diloxanide furoate for treating asymptomatic *Entamoeba histolytica* cyst passers: 14 years' experience in the United States. Clin. Infect. Dis. *15*:464–468, 1992.
58. McAuley, J. B., and Juranek, D. D.: Luminal agents in the treatment of amebiasis. Clin. Infect. Dis. *14*:1161–1162, 1992.
59. Mahmoud, A. A. F., and Warren, K. S.: Algorithms in the diagnosis and management of exotic diseases. XVII. Amebiasis. J. Infect. Dis. *134*:639–643, 1976.
60. Mandell, W. F., and Neu, H. C.: Parasitic infections: Therapeutic considerations. Med. Clin. North Am. *72*:669–690, 1988.
61. Markwalder, K.: Left-side pleuropulmonary amoebiasis: A case report from Chad. Trans. R. Soc. Trop. Med. Hyg. *75*:308–309, 1981.

61. Markwalder, K.: Left-side pleuropulmonary amoebiasis: A case report from Chad. Trans. R. Soc. Trop. Med. Hyg. *75*:308–309, 1981.

62. Martinez-Palomo, A., Tsutsumi, V., Anaya-Velazquez, F., et al.: Ultrastructure of experimental intestinal invasive amebiasis. Am. J. Trop. Med. Hyg. *41*:273–279, 1989.
63. Mathews, H. M., Moss, D. M., Healy, G. R., et al.: Isoenzyme analysis of *Entamoeba histolytica* isolated from homosexual men. J. Infect. Dis. *153*:793–795, 1986.
64. Mendoza, J. B., and Barba, E. J. R.: Cutaneous amebiasis of the face: A case report. Am. J. Trop. Med. Hyg. *35*:69–71, 1986.
65. Merritt, R. J., Coughlin, E., Thomas, D. W., et al.: Spectrum of amebiasis in children. Am. J. Dis. Child. *136*:785–789, 1982.
66. Mirelman, D., Bracha, R., Rozenblatt, S., et al.: Repetitive DNA elements characteristic of pathogenic *Entamoeba histolytica* strains can also be detected after polymerase chain reaction in a cloned nonpathogenic strain. Infect. Immun. *58*:1660–1663, 1990.
67. Mirelman, D., DeMeester, F., Stolarsky, T., et al.: Effects of covalently bound silica-nitroimidazole drug particles on *Entamoeba histolytica*. J. Infect. Dis. *159*:303–309, 1989.
68. Mirelman, D., Feingold, C., Wexler, A., et al.: Interactions between *Entamoeba histolytica,* bacteria and intestinal cells. Ciba Found. Symp. *99*:2–30, 1983.
69. Moorthy, B., Mehta, S., Mitra, S. K., et al.: Amoebic liver abscess in a four-month-old infant. Aust. Paediatr. J. *13*:53–55, 1977.
70. Munoz, O.: Clinical spectrum of amebiasis in children. *In* Kretschmer, R. R. (ed.): Amebiasis: Infection and Disease by *Entamoeba histolytica*. Boca Raton, CRC Press, 1990, pp. 209–220.
71. Osler, W.: On the *Amoeba coli* in dysentery and in dysenteric liver abscess. Johns Hopkins Hosp. Bull. *1*:53–54, 1890.
72. Patterson, M., and Schoppe, L. E.: The presentation of amoebiasis. Med. Clin. North Am. *66*:689–705, 1982.
73. Pehrson, P., and Bengtsson, E.: Treatment of non-invasive amoebiasis: A comparison between tinidazole alone and in combination with diloxanide furoate. Trans. R. Soc. Trop. Med. Hyg. *77*:845–846, 1983.
74. Petri, W. A., and Ravdin, J. I.: Amebiasis in institutionalized populations. *In* Ravdin, J. I. (ed.): Amebiasis: Human Infection by *Entamoeba histolytica*. New York, Churchill Livingstone, 1988.
75. Petri, W. A., Jr., Jackson, T. F. H. G., Gathiram, V., et al.: Pathogenic and nonpathogenic strains of *Entamoeba histolytica* can be differentiated by monoclonal antibodies to the galactose-specific adherence lectin. Infect. Immun. *58*:1802–1806, 1990.
76. Petri, W. A., Jr., Smith, R. D., Schlesinger, P. H., et al.: Isolation of the galactose-binding lectin that mediates the in vitro adherence of *Entamoeba histolytica*. J. Clin. Invest. *80*:1238–1244, 1987.
77. Petri, W. A., Jr., Chapman, M. D., Snodgrass, T., et al.: Subunit structure of the galactose and *N*-acetyl galactosamine-inhibitable adherence lectin of *Entamoeba histolytica*. J. Biol. Chem. *264*:3007–3012, 1989.
78. Pittman, F. E., El-Hashimi, W. K., and Pittman, J. C.: Studies of human amebiasis. I. Clinical and laboratory findings in eight cases of acute amebic colitis. Gastroenterology *65*:581–587, 1973.
79. Pittman, F. E., El-Hashimi, W. K., and Pittman, J. C.: Studies of human amebiasis. II. Light and electron microscopic observations of colonic mucosa and exudate in acute amebic colitis. Gastroenterology *65*:588–603, 1973.
80. Prevention and Control of Intestinal Parasitic Infections. World Health Organization Technical Report *749*:1–80, 1987.
81. Radin, D. R, Ralls, P. W., Colletti, P. M., et al.: CT of amebic liver abscess. A. J. R. Am. J. Roentgenol. *150*:1297–1301, 1988.
82. Ralls, P. W., Henley, D. S., Colletti, P. M., et al.: Amebic liver abscess: MR imaging. Radiology *165*:801–804, 1987.
83. Ralls, P. W., Quinn, M. F., Boswell, W. D., et al.: Patterns of resolution in successfully treated hepatic amebic abscess: Sonographic evaluation. Radiology *149*:541–543, 1983.
84. Ramachandran, S., Goonatillake, H. D., and Induruwa, P. A. C.: Syndromes in amoebic liver abscess. Br. J. Surg. *63*:220–225, 1976.
85. Ramachandran, S., Induruwa, P. A. C., and Perera, M. V. F.: pH of amoebic liver pus. Trans. R. Soc. Trop. Med. Hyg. *70*:159–160, 1976.
86. Ravdin, J. I.: *Entamoeba histolytica:* From adherence to enteropathy. J. Infect. Dis. *159*:420–429, 1989.
87. Ravdin, J. I.: Amebiasis. Clin. Infect. Dis. 20:1453–1466, 1995.
88. Ravdin, J. I., and Guerrant, R. L.: Role of adherence in cytopathogenic mechanisms of *Entamoeba histolytica*. J. Clin. Invest. *68*:1305–1313, 1981.
89. Ravdin, J. I., Murphy, C. F., Guerrant, R. L., et al.: Effect of calcium and phospholipase A antagonists on the cytopathogenicity of *Entamoeba histolytica*. J. Infect. Dis. *152*:542–549, 1985.
90. Ravdin, J. I., Murphy, C. F., Salata, R. A., et al.: *N*-acetyl-D-galactosamine-inhibitable adherence lectin of *Entamoeba histolytica*. I.

Partial purification and relation to amoebic virulence in vitro. J. Infect. Dis. *151*:804–815, 1985.
91. Ravdin, J. I., Moreau, F., Sullivan, J. A., et al.: The relationship of free intracellular calcium ions to the cytolytic activity of *Entamoeba histolytica*. Infect. Immun. *56*:1505–1512, 1988.
92. Reed, S. L., and Ravdin J. I.: Amebiasis. *In* Blaser, M. J., Smith P. D., Ravdin, J. I., et al. (eds.): Infections of the Gastrointestinal Tract. New York, Raven Press, 1995, pp. 1065–1080.
93. Reed, S. L., Keene, W. E., McKerrow, J. H., et al.: Cleavage of C3 by a neutral cysteine proteinase of *Entamoeba histolytica*. J. Immunol. *143*:189–195, 1989.
94. Reed, S. L., Flores, B. M., Batzer, M. A., et al: Molecular and cellular characterization of the 29-kDa peripheral membrane protein of *Entamoeba histolytica*: Differentiation between pathogenic and nonpathogenic isolates. Infect. Immun. *60*:542–549, 1992.
95. Reed, S., Bouvier, J., Pollack, A. S., et al.: Cloning of a virulence factor of *Entamoeba histolytica*. J. Clin. Invest. *91*:1532–1540, 1993.
96. Rodriguez, M. A., and Orozco, E.: Isolation and characterization of phagocytosis- and virulence-deficient mutants of *Entamoeba histolytica*. J. Infect. Dis. *154*:27–32, 1986.
97. Rustgi, A. K., and Richter, J. M.: Pyogenic and amebic liver abscess. Med. Clin. North Am. *73*:847–858, 1989.
98. Salata, R. A., Ahmed, P., and Ravdin, J. I.: Chemoattractant activity of *Entamoeba histolytica* for human polymorphonuclear neutrophils. J. Parasitol. *75*:644–646, 1989.
99. Salata, R. A., Martinez-Palomo, A., Murray, H. W., et al.: Patients treated for amebic liver abscess develop cell-mediated immune responses effective in vitro against *Entamoeba histolytica*. J. Immunol. *136*:2633–2639, 1986.
100. Salata, R. A., Murray, H. W., Rubin, B. Y., et al.: The role of gamma interferon in the generation of human macrophages and T lymphocytes cytotoxic for *Entamoeba histolytica*. Am. J. Trop. Med. Hyg. *37*:72–78, 1987.
101. Salata, R. A., Pearson, R. D., and Ravdin, J. I.: Interaction of human leukocytes and *Entamoeba histolytica*. Killing of virulent amebae by the activated macrophage. J. Clin. Invest. *76*:491–499, 1985.
102. Salata, R. A., and Ravdin, J. I.: N-acetyl-D-galactosamine-inhibitable adherence lectin of *Entamoeba histolytica*. II. Mitogenic activity for human lymphocytes. J. Infect. Dis. *151*:816–822, 1985.
103. Salata, R. A., and Ravdin, J. I.: The interaction of human neutrophils and *Entamoeba histolytica* increases cytopathogenicity for liver cell monolayers. J. Infect. Dis. *154*:19–26, 1986.
104. Sathar, M. A., Bredenkamp, B. L., Gathiram, V., et al.: Detection of *Entamoeba histolytica* immunoglobulins G and M to plasma membrane antigen by enzyme-linked immunosorbent assay. J. Clin. Microbiol. *28*:332–335, 1990.
105. Saxena, A., Chugh, S., and Vinayak, V. K.: Elucidation of cellular population and nature of anti-amoebic antibodies in cytotoxicity to *Entamoeba histolytica* (NIH:200). J. Parasitol. *72*:434–438, 1986.
106. Schmerin, M. J., Gelstron, A., and Jones, T. C.: Amebiasis: An increasing problem among homosexuals in New York City. J. A. M. A. *238*:1386–1387, 1977.
107. Schulte, W., and Scholze, H.: Action of the major protease from *Entamoeba histolytica* on proteins of the extracellular matrix. J. Protozool. *36*:538–543, 1989.
108. Sheen, I. S., Chien, C. S. C., Lin, D. Y., et al.: Resolution of liver abscesses: Comparison of pyogenic and amebic liver abscesses. Am. J. Trop. Med. Hyg. *40*:384–389, 1989.
109. Shetty, N., Das, P., Pal, S. C., et al.: Observations on the interpretation of amoebic serology in endemic areas. J. Trop. Med. Hyg. *91*:222–227, 1988.
110. Shetty, N., and Prabhu, T.: Evaluation of faecal preservation and staining methods in the diagnosis of acute amoebiasis and giardiasis. J. Clin. Pathol. *41*:694–699, 1988.
111. Sotela-Avila, C., Kline, M., Silberstein, M. J., et al.: Bloody diarrhea and pneumoperitoneum in a 10-month-old girl. J. Pediatr. *113*:1098–1104, 1988.
112. Stanley S. L., Jackson, T. F. H. G., Reed, S. L., et al.: Serodiagnosis of invasive amebiasis using a recombinant *Entamoeba histolytica* protein. J. A. M. A. *266*:1984–1986, 1991.
113. Takeuchi, T., Okuzawa, E., Nozaki, T., et al.: High seropositivity of Japanese homosexual men for amebic infection. J. Infect. Dis. *159*:808, 1989.
114. Tannich, E., Horstmann, R. D., Knobloch, J., et al.: Genomic DNA differences between pathogenic and nonpathogenic *Entamoeba histolytica*. Proc. Natl. Acad. Sci. U. S. A. *86*:5118–5122, 1989.
115. Tannich, E., Ebert, F., and Horstmann, R. D.: Primary structure of the 170-kDa surface lectin of pathogenic *Entamoeba histolytica*. Proc. Natl. Acad. Sci. U. S. A. *88*:1849–1853, 1991.
116. Torian, B. E., Reed, S. L., Flores, B. M., et al.: Serologic response to the 96,000-Da surface antigen of pathogenic *Entamoeba histolytica*. J. Infect. Dis. *159*:794–797, 1989.
117. Torian, B. E., Reed, S. L., Flores, B. M., et al.: The 96-kilodalton antigen as an integral membrane protein in pathogenic *Entamoeba histolytica*: Potential differences in pathogenic and nonpathogenic isolates. Infect. Immun. *58*:753–760, 1990.
118. Troll, H., Marti, H., Weiss, N.: Simple differential detection of Entamoeba histolytica and Entamoeba dispar in fresh stool specimens by sodium acetate-acetic acid-formalin concentration and PCR. J. Clin. Microbiol. *35*:1701–1705, 1997.
119. vanSonnenberg, E., Mueller, P. R., Schiffman, H. R., et al.: Intrahepatic amebic abscess: Indications for and results of percutaneous catheter drainage. Radiology *156*:631–635, 1985.
120. Vargas, M., and Pena, A.: Toxic amoebic colitis and amoebic colon perforation in children: An improved prognosis. J. Pediatr. Surg. *11*:223–225, 1976.
121. Vicary, F. R., Cusick, G., Shirley, I. M., et al.: Ultrasound and amoebic liver abscess. Br. J. Surg. *64*:113–114, 1977.
122. Walderich, B. Development of monoclonal antibodies specifically recognizing the cyst stage of Entamoeba histolytica. Am. J. Trop. Med. Hyg. *59*:347–351, 1998.
123. Wanke, C., Butler, T., and Islam, M.: Epidemiologic and clinical features of invasive amebiasis in Bangladesh: A case-control comparison with other diarrheal diseases and postmortem findings. Am. J. Trop. Med. Hyg. *38*:335–341, 1988.
124. Watt, G., Padre, L. P., Adapon, B., et al.: Nonresolution of an amebic liver abscess after parasitologic cure. Am. J. Trop. Med. Hyg. *35*:501–504, 1986.
125. Werries, E., Nebinger, P., and Franz, A.: Degradation of biogene oligosaccharides by beta-N-acetylglucosaminidase secreted by *Entamoeba histolytica*. Mol. Biochem. Parasitol. *7*:127–140, 1983.
126. Wolfe, M. S.: The treatment of intestinal protozoan infections. Med. Clin. North Am. *66*:707–720, 1982.
127. Yang, J., and Kennedy, M. T.: Evaluation of enzyme-linked immunosorbent assay for the serodiagnosis of amebiasis. J. Clin. Microbiol. *10*:778–785, 1979.
128. Yu, Y and Chadee, K. Secreted Entamoeba histolytica proteins stimulate interleukin-8 mRNA expression and protein production in human colonic epithelial cells. Arch. Med. Res. *28*:223–224, 1997.

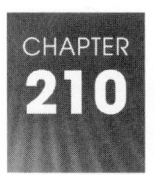

CHAPTER 210 *Blastocystis hominis* Infection

PETER J. HOTEZ

Blastocystis hominis is a protist that inhabits the gastrointestinal tract of humans and possibly other animals. Although new information about the molecular and cell biology of this organism has been acquired in recent years, considerable controversy regarding its true taxonomy and life cycle remains.[4, 26] The pathogenicity of *B. hominis* and its ability to cause gastrointestinal illness in humans are equally controversial.[10, 11, 13, 16, 23, 24]

Etiology and Pathogenesis

Since its discovery in the early part of the 20th century by Alexeieff[1] and then Brumpt,[6] *B. hominis* has been assigned to many different phyla in both animal and plant kingdoms. Early on, it was identified by various workers as vegetable material, a yeast, a fungus, or a protozoan. Although the organism was identified as a protozoan parasite in 1967, its subphylum status bounced between the Sporozoa and the Sarcodina.[4] Nucleic acid sequencing data now suggest that *B. hominis* does not belong to either category but instead probably constitutes its own group more closely related to the ameboflagellates belonging to a new proposed subphylum called Blastocysta.[4, 13, 14] Additional molecular taxonomic data suggest that the intraspecific variation among stocks of *B. hominis* is sufficiently different to warrant at least two separate species assignments for the organism.[5] This observation ultimately may have a bearing on the current controversies surrounding the pathogenicity of the organism.

Ultrastructural information gathered from light and electron microscopy on organisms obtained from in vitro culture and from fresh fecal material indicates the existence of several different parasite forms, including cyst forms, ameboid forms, and the so-called granular, avacuolar, and vacuolar forms.[4] The *B. hominis* vacuolar cell is the most distinctive and appears as a thin peripheral band of cytoplasm surrounding a large membrane-enclosed central vacuole.[4] The central vacuole may have a storage function. Although *B. hominis* is believed to have predominantly anaerobic metabolism, structures that look like mitochondria have been identified on transmission electron microscopy. *Blastocystis* mitochondria may function only in lipid biosynthesis and not oxidative phosphorylation.[4, 28] Alternatively, what appears to be a *Blastocystis* mitochondrion on electron microscopy actually may be a hydrogenosome.[4]

Several highly speculative life cycles of *B. hominis* have been proposed.[4, 14] The infective stage probably is a dormant cyst form that undergoes excystation in response to host gastric acid and intestinal enzymes. Excystation may result in the release of avacuolar forms that can undergo facultative transformation to either an ameboid or a multivacuolar form. The multivacuolar form, in turn, may either encyst to an infective stage or coalesce to the vacuolar form.[4] These stages are believed to predominate in the large intestine, although organisms also have been recovered from duodenal aspirates. Which, if any, of these life cycle stages invade tissue or cause disease is not known. Acquisition of knowledge in this area has been hampered by lack of a suitable animal model, although infection of gnotobiotic guinea pigs with this organism was reported to result in mild intestinal hyperemia and superficial invasion of *B. hominis* into the mucosa of the cecum. Nonspecific inflammation (infiltration of lymphocytes and plasmocytes) and edema of the colonic mucosa have been seen during sigmoidoscopy with biopsy in some patients.[4] Thus far, no serologic antibody response to the organism has been demonstrated.[7] The possibility remains that *B. hominis* is entirely commensal in humans. The epidemiologic association between infection and disease is reviewed next.

Epidemiology and Clinical Manifestations

B. hominis has a worldwide distribution in both tropical and temperate regions, with up to 54 percent infection rates among some populations.[2–4, 8, 9, 20, 21, 24, 27] High rates of infection also have been reported in individuals with a recent history of travel,[23] with exposure to pets or farm animals,[8] and living in institutionalized settings.[4] In many of these individuals, however, *B. hominis* probably is a commensal parasite. Although *B. hominis* is found commonly in preschool-age and school-age children,[20–22] children overall do not appear to be at increased risk for infection.[4]

Most studies investigating the association between *B. hominis* infection and disease are based primarily on clinical laboratory isolates of the organism in patients exhibiting gastrointestinal symptoms. Common clinical complaints include abdominal discomfort, bloating, cramping, diarrhea, and vomiting.[2] Immunoglobulin G2 seroconversion to *B. hominis* has been linked to irritable bowel syndrome.[12] Weight loss associated with a protein-losing enteropathy also has been described. Infective arthritis also has been reported.[16] Because *B. hominis* commonly is found in both symptomatic and asymptomatic individuals, some investigators have proposed that only very heavy infections result in disease.[17, 19, 25] Many of these studies were not controlled, however. Shlim and colleagues[25] conducted a large prospective controlled study among a population of expatriates and tourists in Katmandu, Nepal, who were at high risk for traveler's diarrhea. They concluded that *B. hominis* in high concentrations was not associated with diarrhea and the presence of higher concentrations of the organism in stool was not associated with more severe symptoms.[25] In a subsequent editorial, several design features were cited that may "weaken the authors' conclusions."[15] At least four other prospective trials have been conducted, with one supporting *B. hominis* as a cause of diarrhea, one arguing against it, and two others that were inconclusive.[23] The confusion may be resolved partly by the identification of separate human "demes" of *Blastocystis*,[5, 14] which might lead to improved molecular diagnostic techniques for distinguishing pathogenic from nonpathogenic species. This situation is somewhat analogous to the morphologically identical species of

Entamoeba (*Entamoeba histolytica* and *Entamoeba dispar*), only the former of which causes colitis.

Diagnosis

Light microscopy of wet preparations of fresh or concentrated stool usually identify *B. hominis*. Staining of preparations with iodine or trichome also is of some benefit. Many laboratories attempt to identify the characteristic vacuolar forms, which actually may be under-represented in clinical material.[4] Under these circumstances, the services of an experienced technologist are required to identify the less distinctive multivacuolar forms in the feces. Organisms also can be recovered from biopsy material obtained during sigmoidoscopy and colonoscopy.

Treatment

Given the controversy surrounding the pathogenicity of *B. hominis*, a prudent approach is to refrain from treating asymptomatic immunocompetent individuals.[18] In individuals who have gastrointestinal illness and in whom other pathogens have been excluded, administering a course of antiprotozoal chemotherapy may be reasonable. Some investigators have reported symptomatic improvement in patients receiving either metronidazole or tinidazole.[4, 9] Using an in vitro assay that employed metabolic labeling, researchers found that the drugs emetine, satranidazole, furazolidone, and quinacrine were superior in activity to either metronidazole or tinidazole.[4] The authors caution, however, that the in vitro assay does not take into account the pharmacokinetic properties of the drugs. Furazolidone is available in suspension and, therefore, may be suitable for pediatric use.[11] Trimethoprim-sulfamethoxazole has also been reported as an alternative regimen.

REFERENCES

1. Alexeieff, A.: Sur la nutre des formations dites "kystes de *Trichomonas intestinalis*." Comptes Rendus des Seances de la Societe de Biologies *71*:296–298, 1911.
2. Al-Tawil, Y. S., Gilger, M. A., Gopalakrishna, G. S., et al.: Invasive *Blastocystis hominis* infection in a child. Arch. Pediatr. Adolesc. Med. *148*:882–885, 1994.
3. Ashford, R. W., and Atkinson, E. A.: Epidemiology of *Blastocystis hominis* infection in Papua New Guinea: Age-prevalence and associations with other parasites. Ann. Trop. Med. Parasitol. *86*:129–136, 1992.
4. Boreham, P. F. L., and Stenzel, D. J.: Blastocystis in humans and animals: Morphology, biology, and epizootiology. Adv. Parasitol. *32*:1–70, 1993.
5. Boreham, P. F., Upcroft, J. A., and Dunn, L. A.: Protein and DNA evidence for two demes of *Blastocystis hominis* from humans. Int. J. Parasitol. *22*:49–53, 1992.
6. Brumpt, E.: *Blastocystis hominis* n. sp. et formes voisines. Bull. Soc. Pathol. Exot. Filiales *5*:725–730, 1912.
7. Chen, J., Vaudry, W. L., Kowalewska, K., and Wenman, W.: Lack of serum immune response to *Blastocystis hominis*. Lancet *1*:1021, 1987.
8. Doyle, P. W., Helgason, M. M., Mathias, R. G., and Proctor, E. M.: Epidemiology and pathogenicity of *Blastocystis hominis*. J. Clin. Microbiol. *28*:116–121, 1990.
9. El Masry, N. A., Bassily, S., and Farid, Z.: *Blastocystis hominis*: Clinical and therapeutic aspects. Trans. R. Soc. Trop. Med. Hyg. *82*:173, 1988.
10. Garcia, L. S., Bruckner, D. A., and Clancy, M. N.: Clinical relevance of *Blastocystis hominis*. Lancet *1*:1233–1234, 1984.
11. Hotez, P.: The other intestinal protozoa: enteric infections caused by *Blastocystis hominis*, *Entamoeba coli*, and *Dientamoeba fragilis*. Semin. Pediatr. Infect. Dis. *11*:178–181, 2000.
12. Hussain, R., Jaferi, W., Zuberi, S., et al.: Significantly increased IgG2 subclass antibody levels to *Blastocystis hominis* in patients with irritable bowel syndrome. Am. J. Trop. Med. Hyg. *56*:301–306, 1997.
13. Jiang, J. H., and He, J. G.: Taxonomic status of *Blastocystis hominis*. Parasitol. Today *9*:2–3, 1993.
14. Johnson, A. M., Thanous, A., Boreham, P. F. L., and Baverstock, P. R.: *Blastocystis hominis*: Phylogenetic affinities determined by rRNA sequence comparison. Exp. Parasitol. *68*:283–288, 1989.
15. Keystone, J. S.: Editorial: *Blastocystis hominis* and traveler's diarrhea. Clin. Infect. Dis. *21*:102–103, 1995.
16. Lee, M. G., Rawlins, S. C., Didier, M., et al.: Infective arthritis due to *Blastocystis hominis*. Ann. Rheum. Dis. *49*:192–193, 1990.
17. Logar, J., Andlovic, A., and Poljsak-Prijatel, M.: Incidence of *Blastocystis hominis* in patients with diarrhoea. J. Infect. *28*:151–154, 1994.
18. Markell, E. K.: Editorial: Is there any reason to continue treating *Blastocystis* infections? Clin. Infect. Dis. *21*:104–105, 1995.
19. Markell, E. K., and Udkow, M. P.: *Blastocystis hominis*: Pathogen or fellow traveler? Am. J. Trop. Med. Hyg. *35*:1023–1026, 1986.
20. Nimri, L. F.: Evidence of an epidemic of *Blastocystis hominis* infections in preschool children in northern Jordan. J. Clin. Microbiol. *31*:2706–2708, 1993.
21. Nimri, L. F., and Batchoun, R.: Intestinal colonization of symptomatic and asymptomatic schoolchildren with *Blastocystis hominis*. J. Clin. Microbiol. *32*:2865–2866, 1994.
22. O'Gorman, M. A., Orenstein, S. R., Proujansky, R., et al.: Prevalence and characteristics of *Blastocystis hominis* infection in children. Clin. Pediatr. *32*:91–96, 1993.
23. Patterson, J. E., Patterson, T. F., Edberg, S. C., et al.: The traveler with *Blastocystis hominis*: Experience from a traveler's clinic and review. Infect. Dis. Clin. Pract. *1*:28–32, 1992.
24. Senay, H., and MacPherson, D.: *Blastocystis hominis*: Epidemiology and natural history. J. Infect. Dis. *162*:987–990, 1990.
25. Shlim, D. R., Hoge, C. W., Rajah, R., et al.: Is *Blastocystis hominis* a cause of diarrhea in travelers? A prospective controlled study in Nepal. Clin. Infect. Dis. *21*:97–101, 1995.
26. Udkow, M. P., and Markell, E. K.: *Blastocystis hominis*: Prevalence in asymptomatic versus symptomatic hosts. J. Infect. Dis. *168*:242–244, 1993.
27. Zierdt, C. H.: *Blastocystis hominis*, a protozoan parasite and intestinal pathogen of human beings. Clin. Microbiol. Newslett. *5*:57–59, 1983.
28. Zierdt, C. H.: *Blastocystis hominis*: Past and future. Clin. Microbiol. Rev. *4*:61–79, 1992.

CHAPTER 211

Entamoeba coli Infection

PETER J. HOTEZ

Until recently, *Entamoeba coli* was considered to be entirely nonpathogenic and was of interest to the clinician only because of its morphologic similarities to *Entamoeba histolytica* that might result in misdiagnosis. In 1991, however, several case reports from northern Europe appeared that implicated *Entamoeba coli* as a possible cause of infectious diarrhea.[2, 5, 7] Two cases of diarrhea associated with *Entamoeba coli* have been described in children.[2]

Etiology and Pathogenesis

Entamoeba coli, like other members of the genus *Entamoeba*, has both trophozoite and cyst forms. The trophozoite is similar in size to *E. histolytica* (15 to 50 μm) but has a more sluggish motility with short pseudopodia.[4] The cytoplasm is described as granular, coarse, or frothy and contains numerous bacteria, yeasts, and other food materials.[4, 6] Occasionally, red blood cells are seen in the cytoplasm, but their occurrence is not nearly as common as in pathogenic strains of *E. histolytica*. During passage through the colon, the trophozoite will round up and synthesize a chitin-containing cyst wall. *Entamoeba coli* cysts measure 10 to 35 μm and usually contain 8 to 16 nuclei, although 32 nuclei are seen on occasion.

Transmission of *Entamoeba coli* infection occurs through the fecal-oral route in the same manner as does *E. histolytica* infection. Upon cyst ingestion, the total number of excysting trophozoites usually is less than eight.[4] The *Entamoeba coli* trophozoites colonize the lumen of the large intestine. Very little is known about the events by which *Entamoeba coli* trophozoites occasionally cause human gastrointestinal illness. Even with a pathogenic *Entamoeba coli* strain, the invasive potential of this organism is presumed not to be nearly as great as is that of *E. histolytica* because diarrheal disease in patients infected with *Entamoeba coli* is not associated with dysentery or accompanied by a leukocytosis or elevated serum immunoglobulin A.[7]

Epidemiology and Clinical Manifestations

Entamoeba coli is worldwide in distribution, although it occurs more commonly in warmer climates and in some populations of homosexual men.[4] In 1991, Wahlgren[7] described eight patients from Sweden with mild or persistent diarrhea who harbored *Entamoeba coli*. Before receiving specific antiamebic chemotherapy, all eight patients had their stools examined repeatedly by (1) light microscopy, to exclude other protozoa and helminths; (2) electron microscopy, to exclude the presence of some pathogenic viruses; and (3) both aerobic and anaerobic culture, to exclude pathogenic bacteria. These patients typically complained of a long history of loose but not watery stools (without blood or mucus), flatulence, and colicky pain. One patient was a parasitology laboratory technician who had symptoms for more than 15 years. Every patient responded to specific antiamebic chemotherapy.[7] Two children with similar symptoms who also responded to antiamebic chemotherapy subsequently were described in Ireland.[2]

Diagnosis and Treatment

Entamoeba coli sometimes is difficult to distinguish from *E. histolytica*, particularly because the nuclear structures of their trophozoite stages are similar.[3] Some differences, however, including the karyosome, which is eccentric in *Entamoeba coli* but central in *E. histolytica*, and the cytoplasm, which is coarse and seldom contains red blood cells in *Entamoeba coli*, in contrast to *E. histolytica*, exist.[3] The differences between the cyst stages of *Entamoeba coli* and *E. histolytica* (and *Entamoeba dispar*) are more apparent. For example, the *Entamoeba coli* cyst typically has two to four times more nuclei than do those in *E. histolytica*. The *Entamoeba coli* cyst has been reported to become more refractive during fixation, so that it often is visualized better in a wet preparation.[4]

Generally speaking, *Entamoeba coli* still is regarded by most investigators as a commensal organism. However, in patients with persistent diarrhea whose diagnostic fecal evaluation reveals only the presence of *Entamoeba coli*, administering a course of specific antiamebic therapy is reasonable.[1] All of the Swedish patients were reported to respond to a 10-day course of diloxanide furoate in a dose of 500 mg three times daily.[7] Children also may respond to an equivalent pediatric dose of 20 mg/kg/day in three divided doses for 10 days. As of 1994, diloxanide furoate was available in the United States from the Centers for Disease Control and Prevention Drug Service. Alternatively, two children from Ireland (where diloxanide furoate was not available) were treated successfully for *Entamoeba coli*–associated diarrhea with metronidazole.[2]

REFERENCES

1. Cooperstock, M., DuPont, H. L., Corrado, M. L., et al.: Evaluation of new anti-infective drugs for the treatment of diarrhea caused by *Entamoeba histolytica*. Clin. Infect. Dis. *15*(Suppl. 1):S254–S258, 1992.
2. Corcoran, G. D., O'Connell, B., Gilleece, A., and Mulvihill, T. E.: *Entamoeba coli* as possible cause of diarrhea. Lancet *338*:254, 1991.
3. Despommier, D. D., Gwadz, R. W., and Hotez, P. J.: Parasitic Diseases. 3rd ed. New York, Springer-Verlag, 1995, pp. 232–233.
4. Garcia, L. S., and Bruckner, D. A.: Diagnostic Medical Parasitology. 2nd ed. Washington, D.C., American Society for Microbiology, 1992, pp. 18–20.
5. Hotez, P. The other intestinal protozoa: Enteric infections caused by *Blastocystis hominis*, *Entamoeba coli*, and *Dientamoeba fragilis*. Semin. Pediatr. Infect. Dis. *11*:178–181, 2000.
6. Proctor, E. M.: Laboratory diagnosis of amebiasis. Clin. Lab. Med. *11*:829–859, 1991.
7. Wahlgren, M.: *Entamoeba coli* as cause of diarrhoea? Lancet *337*:675, 1991.

B. FLAGELLATES (INTESTINAL)

CHAPTER

212 Giardiasis

JAMES S. SEIDEL*

Giardiasis is caused by an infection with the protozoan parasite *Giardia lamblia* (also known as *Giardia duodenalis* or *Giardia intestinalis*). Anton van Leeuwnhoek first described the parasite when examining his own stool under a microscope. Vilem Lambl described the trophozoite in 1859 and Grassi the cyst in 1879.[32] This flagellate parasite, which belongs to the family Hexamititadae, is one of the most primitive eukaryotes and lacks many organelles, including Golgi apparatus and mitochondria.[11] The two morphologic forms are the infectious cyst, which is relatively resistant to chemicals and environmental stresses, and the trophozoite, which is responsible for the disease. The trophozoite lives in the small intestine and divides by binary fission. The species that infects humans is morphologically indistinguishable from that of other mammals. Isoenzyme and genetic analyses indicate that isolates from infected individuals are heterogeneous and can be placed in four groups.[3] The different isolates within groups demonstrate some specificity for infection in various mammals versus humans.

Epidemiology

Giardia infections are ubiquitous, and outbreaks occur in developed and underdeveloped countries throughout the world. Many species exist (e.g., *G. duodenalis, Giardia bovis, Giardia catti, Giardia muris*) that are somewhat host specific. Cross-transmission occurs between animals and humans.[6] Transmission involves the fecal-oral, water-borne, and food-borne transmission of cysts; thus, the level of sanitation is directly related to the prevalence of infection.[2, 8, 19, 23, 30, 34, 47] It is one of the most common parasites in the United States and is found in 4.2 to 7 percent of specimens submitted to the laboratory for examination.[22] Data from the National Giardiasis Surveillance System of the Centers for Disease Control and Prevention estimate that 2.5 million cases occur each year in the United States.[9] Cases per 100,000 population range from 0.9 to 42.3, with 10 states reporting more than 20 cases per 100,000 population. In 1997, New York State had the highest number of cases, with 42.3 cases per 100,000 population, accounting for 14.5 percent of cases nationally. Cases have equal sex distribution, and rates are highest in children 0 to 5 years of age, followed closely by adults 31 to 40 years of age. Most cases are reported in the late summer and early fall. Giardia is a frequent cause of diarrhea in daycare centers around the world, with infection rates of 1 to 50 percent.[1, 25, 35, 38, 40] Most children have symptoms. Chronic passage of cysts in some preschool-aged children in daycare centers is for as long as 5 to 6 months after the initial diagnosis. Transmission from these infants and children to adult family members is not an uncommon occurrence. Prevalence rates decline after children are toilet trained. Sexual transmission may occur in heterosexual and homosexual contact.[24, 29] Campers in national parks and wilderness areas are at risk because of vertical transmission from animals and water-borne outbreaks.[53] In addition, many outbreaks have been reported in municipal water supplies that have not been treated with flocculation or filtration. From 1985 to 1994, *Giardia* was responsible for 44 percent of the outbreaks of water-borne diarrheal illness in which an etiology could be determined. Sixty-four percent of these outbreaks were associated with unfiltered water. According to a sample survey of 66 reservoir sites in Canada and the United States, 81 percent contained Giardia cysts at a concentration of 3 cysts per liter before treatment and 1.7 cysts per liter after treatment.[26, 27] Treatment of water with iodine preparations kills most cysts, but they are relatively resistant to chlorination. Swimming pools may be another source of infection when used by diapered infants and developmentally delayed individuals.[41] Another mode of transmission is through food, in which as few as 10 cysts may be required to establish infection.[33, 43] Travelers to high areas of endemicity are at risk for infection. Patients who were infected during travel had longer exposures times in countries where the prevalence was high.[21]

Pathogenesis

Humans are infected by coming in contact with as few as 10 to 25 cysts.[43] Excystation occurs in the stomach and small intestine, and the trophozoites are found in large numbers in the upper part of the small intestine, where they closely apply their sucking disks to the mucosa (Fig. 212–1). They may penetrate into the secretory tubules of the mucosa and, at times, are found in the gallbladder and in the biliary drainage. Scanning electron micrographs of the intestinal mucosa (Fig. 212–2) demonstrate the mechanical damage caused by the presence of the organisms on the mucosal surface. The histologic changes seen in the tissues do not always correlate with the presence or absence of symptoms. Biopsies of the small intestine in children and adults show normal histology despite the presence of diarrhea and other symptoms.[46] On the other hand, flattening of the brush border, damage to epithelial cells, and slight flattening of the villi with increased mitotic index, increased goblet cells, and infiltration with inflammatory cells also may be present.[5, 36, 44, 54] The causes of symptoms are not well understood and include (1) the parasite as a physical barrier to absorption, (2) disruption of the brush border with loss of enzymatic activity, (3) elaboration of toxins by the parasite, (4) changes in fat absorption in the small intestine, and (5) activation of cytokines after damage to enterocytes. Persistence of infection in nude mice suggests a role for T-cell activity.[45, 51] Immune responses involve both humeral and cellular mechanisms. Humans produce serum immunoglobulin G (IgG), IgM, IgA, and IgE in response to

*Deceased

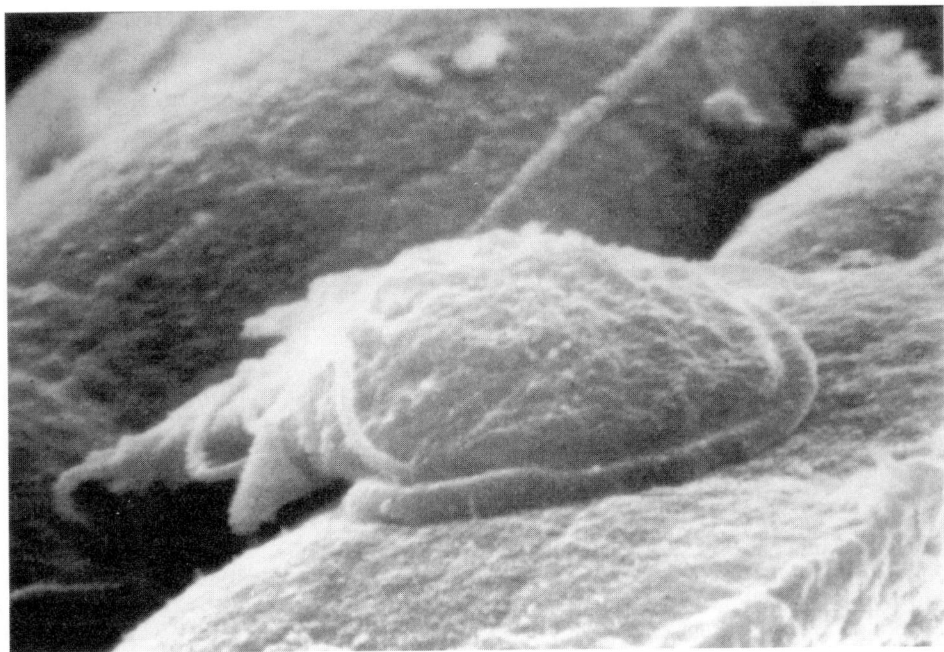

FIGURE 212–1 ■ Trophozoite of *Giardia lamblia* adhering to the intestinal surface.

infection.[12, 14, 39, 49, 52] IgA response appears to play a role in the modulation of infection, as does migration of infiltrating lymphocytes in the intestinal mucosa. Eighty-four percent of human volunteers self-cured in 18.4 days, whereas the remainder became chronically infected.[43] Human milk has been shown to kill the trophozoites of *G. lamblia* by generating toxic lipolytic products.[11, 12, 42] Infection may be severe and difficult to eradicate in immunodeficient individuals. In severe cases, damage to the mucosal surface may lead to disaccharide deficiency. Disruption of digestion by bile and proteases may produce malabsorption, diarrhea, and resulting malnutrition.

Giardiasis long has been associated with hypogammaglobulinemia, nodular lymphoid hyperplasia of the small intestine, and chronic diarrhea.[17] Patients with hypogammaglobulinemia, absence of plasma cells in the intestinal lamina propria, and human immunodeficiency virus (or acquired immunodeficiency syndrome) are susceptible to chronic giardiasis.[20] Individuals with X-linked hypogammaglobulinemia, selective IgA deficiency, and Wiskott-Aldrich or Nezelof syndrome are less susceptible.[37, 48]

Clinical Manifestations

Many patients carrying the parasite are asymptomatic. Symptoms may vary from mild abdominal discomfort and diarrhea to severe cramping, bloating, and severe diarrhea

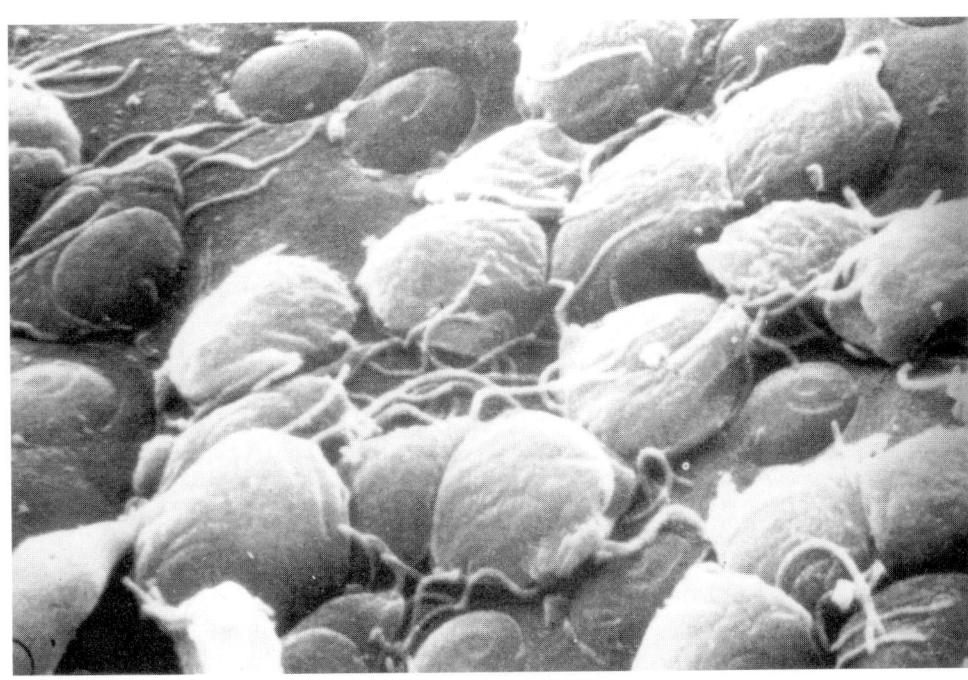

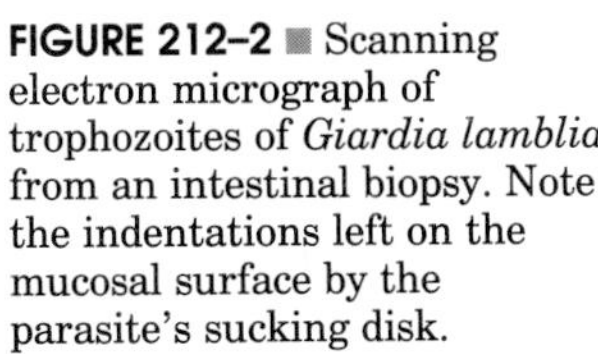

FIGURE 212–2 ■ Scanning electron micrograph of trophozoites of *Giardia lamblia* from an intestinal biopsy. Note the indentations left on the mucosal surface by the parasite's sucking disk.

TABLE 212–1 ■ SYMPTOMS IN PATIENTS WITH GIARDIASIS

Symptom	Frequency (%)
Flatulence	56
Anorexia	56
Cramps	53
Foul-smelling stool	52
Abdominal distention	31
Belching	30
Weight loss	18

TABLE 212–2 ■ STOOL CHARACTERISTICS IN PATIENTS WITH GIARDIASIS

Stool Characteristic	Frequency (%)
Mushy	52
Formed	33
Watery	12
Mucous	3
Blood	0

(Table 212–1). Patients and caretakers describe a constellation of signs and symptoms, including abdominal bloating, flatulence, and frequent foul-smelling diarrhea. Young infants may exhibit anorexia, weight loss, or a malabsorption syndrome that resembles sprue. Lactose intolerance may develop and persist after the infection has been eradicated.[48] Anecdotal reports have attributed a variety of other symptoms, including rash, arthralgia, arthritis, and fever, to giardiasis, but no data support *G. lamblia* as the cause of these symptoms. Stooling patterns vary from normal to mushy, foul-smelling diarrhea (Table 212–2). Signs of inflammatory diarrhea, such as tenesmus and bloody diarrhea, do not occur. Cyst passers may be asymptomatic and may serve as a reservoir of infection for others. This fact is particularly important for food handler and daycare center outbreaks. Severe prolonged illness that requires hospitalization is found in 2 per 100,000 cases, which is similar to that for shigellosis.[28] Hospital admission usually is of young children and pregnant women because of volume depletion and failure to thrive.[50]

Parasitic infection, including giardiasis, should be considered in the evaluation of the child who fails to thrive and in immunocompromised infants and children who have diarrhea or gastrointestinal complaints. It also should be considered in the differential diagnosis of any child who is in daycare or who has traveled outside of the United States and has gastrointestinal symptoms.[16, 35]

Diagnosis

Obtaining a thorough travel history is important in making the diagnosis of giardiasis. Recent travel to the wilderness or a national park and travel to St. Petersburg or other endemic areas are important parts of the history in any patient with persistent diarrhea. Examination of preserved fecal specimens reveals cysts or trophozoites in most infections. Organisms are excreted in a highly variable pattern; therefore, because examination of only a single stool sample may miss from 10 to 50 percent of infections, multiple samples taken on different days are required.[4] Recently, commercially available tests to detect antigen by an enzyme-linked immunosorbent assay (ELISA) have been shown to be highly sensitive and specific. The ELISA may be particularly useful in screening mass outbreaks. Monoclonal antibodies usually are employed to detect antigen either by an ELISA or immunofluorescence assay. Some of these assays have a sensitivity of 91 to 95 percent.[7, 31] Antigen may be best detected when the stool is preserved in formalin.[7] These tests do not replace microscopic examination of the stool because of the possibility of infection with multiple organisms in travelers. Infections may be missed in some patients, and in cases with a high index of suspicion, the organism may be recovered by duodenal biopsy or duodenal aspiration. Invasive techniques may be important in immunosuppressed individuals and in those with sprue, for whom histology of the bowel also may be important in planning therapy.

Treatment

All patients with either cysts or trophozoites in the stool should be treated. Drugs that are used throughout the world are shown on Table 212–3. Only metronidazole, albendazole, paromomycin, and furazolidone are available in the United States. Although albendazole has been shown to be curative either in single doses or a 5-day course, it is not approved for use in giardiasis in the United States.[15, 55] Quinacrine, which is inexpensive and has excellent efficacy, also is no longer available in the United States.[10] It may cause hemolysis in children with glucose-6-phosphate dehydrogenase deficiency. Furazolidone is an effective alternative and is available in a liquid form. However, it is administered four

TABLE 212–3 ■ DRUGS FOR THE TREATMENT OF GIARDIASIS

Drug	Dose	Efficacy (%)	Side Effects
Metronidazole	15 mg/kg/day tid × 5–7 days (max, 750 mg/day)	80–95	Metallic taste, nausea, vomiting, headache, disulfiram effects, rash, neuropathy
Tinidazole	50 mg/kg × 1 (max, 2 g)	90–98	Metallic taste, nausea, vomiting, headache, disulfiram effects
Albendazole	10 mg/kg/day (max, 400 mg/day) for 3–5 days	81–95	Gastrointestinal upset
Secnidazole	30 mg/kg/day in three doses × 1 (max, 2 g)	92–100	Nausea, vomiting, abdominal pain
Furazolidone	6 mg/kg/day in four doses × 7–10 days (max, 400 mg/day)	80	Allergic reactions, gastrointestinal upset, headache, hemolysis, neuropathy
Paromomycin	25–30 mg/kg/day in three doses (max, 1.5 g/day)	60–70	Gastrointestinal upset
Quinacrine	6 mg/kg/day × 5–7 days (max, 300 mg/day)	90–95	Nausea, vomiting, gastrointestinal upset, yellow skin, toxic psychosis, hemolysis
Nitazoxanide	12–47 mo, 200 mg/day in two doses × 3 days; 4–11 yr, 400 mg/day in two doses × 3 days. Taken with food	85	Nausea, anorexia, flatulence, appetite increase, enlarged salivary glands, increased creatinine and serum glutamic-pyruvic transaminase, yellow eyes, discolored urine

times a day for 7 to 10 days and is associated with side effects that include rash, nausea, and vomiting. Tinidazole has been shown to eliminate the parasite after single-dose therapy.[18] It is not available in the United States. A new member of the 5-nitromidazoles, which include metronidazole and tinidazole, secnidazole has been shown to be well tolerated as a 30-mg/kg/day (maximum, 2 g) and may become an option for therapy.[13] Paromomycin, an aminoglycoside that is not well absorbed, is the only drug that can be used in pregnancy. It is not as effective as other medications in eradicating the parasite but may induce clinical improvement. A 3-day course of a new drug recently released by the U.S. Food and Drug Administration, nitazoxanide (Alinia), has been shown to treat successfully 85 percent of children with diarrhea caused by *Giardia*.[46a]

Although outbreaks in daycare centers are common, treating all children in the daycare center is not efficacious because recurrence rates are high and a chance of a drug reaction always exists. Treatment is reserved for symptomatic children.

REFERENCES

1. Addis, D. G., Stewart, J. M., Finton, R. J., et al.: *Giardia lamblia* and cryptosporidium infections in child day-care centers in Fulton County, Georgia. Pediatr. Infect. Dis. *10*:907–911, 1991.
2. Anonymous: Waterborne giardiasis—California, Colorado, Oregon, Pennsylvania. M. M. W. R. Morb. Mortal. Wkly. Rep. *29*:121, 1980.
3. Chadhuri, P., De, A., Bhattacharya, A., and Pal, S. C.: Isolation and heterogeneity in human isolates of by isoenzyme studies. Int. J. Med. Microbiol. *274*:490–495, 2001.
4. Danciger, M., and Lopez, M.: Numbers of *Giardia* in the feces of infected children. Am. J. Trop. Med. *24*:237–241, 1975.
5. Duncombe, V. M., Bolin, T. D., Davis, A. E., et al.: Histopathology in giardiasis. A correlation with diarrhea. Aust. N. Z. J. Med. 8:392–396, 1978.
6. Dykes, A. C., Juranekl, D. D., Lorenz, R. A., et al.: Municipal waterborne giardiasis. An epidemiological investigation. Beavers implicated as a possible reservoir. Ann. Intern. Med. *92*:165–170, 1980.
7. Fedorko, D. P., Williams, E. C., Nelson, N. A., et al.: Performance of three enzyme immunoassays and two different fluorescence assays for detection of *Giardia lamblia* in stool specimens preserved in ECOFIX. J. Clin. Microbiol. *38*:2781–2783, 2000.
8. Fraser, C. T., and Cooke, K.: Epidemic giardiasis and municipal water supply. Am. J. Public Health. *81*:760–762, 1991.
9. Furness, B. W., Beach, M. J., and Roberts, J. M.: Giardiasis surveillance—United States 1992–1997. M. M. W. R. Morb. Mortal. Wkly. Rep. *49*:1–13, 2000.
10. Gardner, T. B., and Hill, D. R.: Treatment of giardiasis. Clin. Microbiol. Rev. *14*:114–128, 2001.
11. Gillin, F. D., Reiner, D. S., and McCaffery, J. M.: Cell biology of the primative eucaryote *Giardia lamblia*. Annu. Rev. Microbiol. *50*:679, 1996.
12. Gillin, F. E., Reiner, D. S., and Wang, C. S.: Killing of *Giardia lamblia* trophozoites by normal human milk. J. Cell Biochem. *23*:47–56, 1983.
13. Gillis, J. C., and Wiseman, L. R. Secnidazole: A review of its antimicrobial activity, pharmacokinetic properties and therapeutic use in the management of protozoal infections and bacterial vaginosis. Drugs *51*:621–628, 1996.
14. Goka, J. A. K., Mathan, V. I., Rolston, D. D. K., et al.: Diagnosis of giardiasis by specific IgM antibody enzyme-linked immunosorbent assay. Lancet *2*:184–186, 1989.
15. Hall, A., and Nahar, Q.: Albendazole as a treatment for infections with *Giardia duodendalis* in children in Bangladesh. Trans. R. Soc. Trop. Med. Hyg. *87*:84–86, 1993.
16. Hardie, R. M., Wall, P. G., Gott, P., et al.: Infectious diarrhea in tourists staying in a resort hotel. Emerg. Infect. Dis. *5*:168–171, 1999.
17. Hermans, P. E., Huizemnga, K. A., Hoffman, H. N., et al.: Dysgammaglobinemia associated with nodular hyperplasia of the small intestine. Am. J. Med. *40*:78–89, 1965.
18. Hill, D. R.: Giardiasis. Issues in diagnosis and management. Infect. Dis. Clin. North Am. 7:503–525, 1993.
19. Issac-Renton, J. L., Cordiero, C., Sarafis, K., et al.: Characteristics of *Giardia duodenalis* isolates from a waterborne outbreak. J. Infect. Dis. *167*:431–440, 1993.
20. Janoff, E. N., Smith, P. D., and Blaser, M. J.: Acute antibody responses to *Giardia lamblia* are depressed in patients with AIDS. J. Infect. Dis. *157*:798–804, 1988.
21. Jellinek, T., and Loscher, T.: Epidemiology of giardiasis in German travelers. J. Trav. Med. 7:70–73, 2000.
22. Kappus, K. D., Lundgren, R. G. J., Juranek, D. D., et al.: Intestinal parasitism in the United States: Update on a continuing problem. Am. J. Trop. Med. Hyg. *50*:705–713, 1994.
23. Kent, G. P., Greenspan, J. R., Hendon, J. L., et al.: Epidemic giardiasis caused by a contaminated public water supply. Am. J. Public Health *78*:139–143, 1988.
24. Keystone, J. S., Keystone, D. L., and Proctor, E. M.: Intestinal parasitic infections in homosexual men: Prevalence, symptoms and factors in tansmission. Can. Med. Assoc. J. *123*:512–514, 1980.
25. Keystone, J. S., Krajden, S., and Warren, M. R.: Person-to-person transmission of *Giardia lamblia* in day-care nurseries. Can. Med. Assoc. J. *12*:241–242, 1978.
26. LeChevallier, M. W., Norton, W. E., and Lee, R. G.: *Giardia* and *Cryptosporidium* in filtered drinking water supplies. Appl. Environ. Microbiol. *57*:2617–2621, 1991.
27. LeChevallier, M. W., Norton, W. E., and Lee, R. G.: Occurrence of *Giardia* and *Cryptosporidium* spp in surface water supplies. Appl. Environ. Microbiol. *57*:2610–2616, 1991.
28. Lengerich, E. J., Addiss, D. G., and Juranek, D. D.: Severe giardiasis in the United States. Clin. Infect. Dis. *18*:760–763, 1994.
29. Levine, G. I.: Sexually transmitted parasitic diseases. Prim. Care Clin. Office Practice *18*:101–128, 1991.
30. Lopez, C. E., Dykes, A. C., Juranek, D. D., et al.: Waterborne giardiasis: A communitywide outbreak of disease and a high rate of asymptomatic infection. Am. J. Epidemiol. *112*:495–507, 1980.
31. Maraha, B., and Buiting, A. G.: Evaluation of four enzyme immunoassays for detection of Giardia lamblia antigen in stool specimens. Eur. J. Clin. Microbiol. Infect. Dis. *19*:485–487, 2000.
32. Meyer, E. A. (ed.): Giardiasis. Amsterdam, Elsevier Science 1990, p. 51.
33. Mintz, E. D., Hudson Wragg, M., Mshar, P., et al.: Foodborne giardiasis in a corporate office setting. J. Infect. Dis. *167*:250–253, 1993.
34. Moore, G. T., Cross, W. M., McGuire, D., et al.: Epidemic giardiasis at a ski resort. N. Engl. J. Med. *282*:402–407, 1969.
35. Nunez, F. A., Hernandez, M., and Finlay, C. M.: Longitudinal study of giardiasis in three day care centers of Havana City. Acta Trop. *73*:237–242, 1999.
36. Oberhuber, G., Kastner, N., and Stolte, M.: Giardiasis. A histologic analysis of 567 cases. Scand. J. Infect. Dis. *32*:48–58, 1997.
37. Ochs, H. D., Ament, M. E., and Davis, S. D.: Giardiasis with malabsorption in X-linked agammaglobulinemia. N. Engl. J. Med. *287*:341–342, 1972.
38. Overturf, G. D.: Endemic giardiasis in the United States: Role of the day care center [Editorial]. Clin. Infect. Dis. *18*:764, 1994.
39. Perez, O., Lastre, M., Bandera, F., et al.: Evaluation of the immune response to symptomatic and asymptomatic human giardiasis. Arch. Med. Res. *25*:171–177, 1994.
40. Pickering, L. K., Woodward, W. E., DuPont, H. L., et al.: Occurrence of *Giardia lamblia* in children in day care centers. J. Pediatr. *104*:522–526, 1984.
41. Porter, J. D., Ragassoni, H. P., Buchanin, J. D., et al.: *Giardia* transmission in a swimming pool. Am. J. Public Health *78*:659–662, 1988.
42. Reiner, D. S., Wang, C. S., and Gillin, F. D.: Human mold kills *Giardia lamblia* by generating toxic lipolytic products. J. Infect. Dis. *154*:825–832, 1986.
43. Rendtorff, R. C.: The experimental transmission of human intestional protozoan parasites II. *Giardia lamblia* cysts given in capsules. Am. J. Hyg. *59*:209–212, 1954.
44. Ridley, M. J., and Ridley, D. S.: Serum antibiodies and jejunal histology in giardiasis. J. Clin. Pathol. *29*:30–34, 1976.
45. Roberts-Thomson, I. C., and Mitchel, G. F.: Giardiasis in mice. I. Prolonged infection in certain mouse strains and hypothymic (nude) mice. Gastroenterology *75*:42–46, 1978.
46. Rodrigyez-da-Silva, J., Coutinho, S. G., Dias, L., et al.: Histopathologic changes in giardiasis: A biopsy study. Am. J. Dig. Dis. *9*:355–365, 1964.

46a. Rossignol J. F., Ayoub, A., and Ayers, M. S. D.: Treatment of diarrhea caused by *Giardia intestinalis* and *Entamoeba histolytica* or *E. dispar*: A randomized double-blind, placebo-controlled study of nitazoxanide. J. Infect. Dis. *184*:381–384, 2001.

47. Shaw, P. K., Brodsky, R. E., Lyman, D. O., et al.: A community-wide outbreak of giardiasis with evidence of tranmission by a municipal water supply. Ann. Intern. Med. *87*:426, 1977.
48. Singh, K. D., Bhasin, D. K., Rana, S. V., et al.: Effect of *Giardia lamblia* on dudonenal disaccharisase levels in humans. Trop. Gastroenterol. *21*:174–176, 2000.
49. Smith, P. D., Gillin, F. D., Brown, W. R., et al.: IgG antibody to *Giardia lamblia* detected by enzyme-linked immunosorbent assay. Gastroenterology *80*:1476–1480, 1982.
50. Solomons, N. W.: Giardiaisis nutritional implications. Rev. Infect. Dis. *4*:859–869, 1982.
51. Stevens, D. P., Frank, D. M., and Mahmoud, A. A. F.: Thymus dependency of host resistance to *Giardia muris* infection: Studies in nude mice. J. Immunol. *120*:680–682, 1978.

52. Visvesvera, G. S., Smith, P. D., Healy, G. R., et al.: An immunofluorescence test to detect serum antibody to *Giardia lamblia.* Ann. Intern. Med. *93*:802–805, 1980.
53. Welch, T. P.: Risk of giardiasis from consumption of wilderness water in North America: A systematic review of the epidemiologic data. Int. J. Infect. Dis. *4*:100–103, 2000.
54. Yardley, J. H., Takano, J., and Hendrix, T. R.: Epithelial and other mucosal lesions of the jejunum in giardiasis. Jejunal biopsy studies. Bull. Johns Hopkins Hosp. *115*:389–406, 1964.
55. Zaat, J. O., Mank, T. H., and Assendelft, W. J.: Drugs for treating giardiasis. Cochrane Database Syst Rev 71:CD000217, 2000.

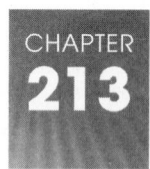

CHAPTER 213 *Dientamoeba fragilis* Infections

LISA M. FRENKEL

Dientamoeba fragilis is a protozoan that may inhabit the human gastrointestinal tract. In 1918, *D. fragilis* was recognized as a distinct species by Jepps and Dobell, who believed it to be a rare intestinal commensal.[31] In unpreserved feces, the morphologic characteristics of *D. fragilis* do not persist, which most likely accounts for its perceived rarity in some surveys. Careful studies using preserved and stained fecal specimens have found an association between *D. fragilis* infection and acute and chronic gastrointestinal symptoms, which has led to acceptance of its role as a pathogen.

The Organism

D. fragilis, unlike most other intestinal protozoa, has no known cyst form. The trophozoite initially was classified in the genus *Endamoeba.* However, the similarity of *D. fragilis* to flagellates, specifically to *Histomonas meleagridis,* the cause of "blackhead" enterohepatitis in fowl, was noted on careful examination under the light microscope.[16] *H. meleagridis* is a flagellate when it is found in the cecum of fowl; however, its flagella are lost when it invades tissue.[16] *D. fragilis* in the binucleate form resembles the tissue form of *Histomonas.*[16] Nonetheless, despite this resemblance, *D. fragilis* has not been found to invade tissues. Its antigenic and ultrastructural relatedness to *Histomonas* has been based on fluorescent antibody and electron-microscopic studies, respectively.[12, 17] *D. fragilis* was reclassified in 1974 by Honigberg as a nonflagellate trichomonad of the order Trichomonadida, family Monocercomonadidae, subfamily Dientamoebinae, and genus *Dientamoeba.*[8, 19]

D. fragilis infects the mucosal crypts of the large intestine in close proximity to mucosal epithelium from the cecum to the rectum. The organism varies in size from 3 to 18 μm in diameter, but it is usually 7 to 12 μm. The pseudopodia of *D. fragilis* have a delicate, leaf-like appearance and serrated margins.[30] This protozoan is seen to move actively in fresh feces but quickly becomes rounded after standing. *D. fragilis* is relatively easy to isolate and grow in vitro in media containing solid rice starch.[16] Cultures should be maintained at 37° to 38° C (98.6° to 100.4° F) because the organism rounds up and stops moving and feeding at lower temperatures. *D. fragilis* will thrive in temperatures up to 41° C (105.8° F). This organism feeds on bacteria and starch grains and will ingest human red blood cells. *D. fragilis* reproduces by binary fission.[16] Although the organisms are found most commonly in the binucleate form, approximately 20 percent are in the uninucleate form, and a few are multinucleate.[30, 31, 34, 63, 66] Each nucleus contains a large, fragmented (four to eight granules) karyosome surrounded by a clear zone with no peripheral chromatin and a fine nuclear membrane.[31, 65] Occasionally, some aberrant forms may be found. These forms usually are uninucleate and may be as large as 20 μm; they do not reproduce. Humans appear to be the natural host of *D. fragilis,* but *D. fragilis* infection has been reported in two simian species.[16] Multiple attempts to infect other animals have been unsuccessful.

Epidemiology and Transmission

D. fragilis was thought to be uncommon until improved techniques for preserving the organism were used.[22, 25, 54] The trophozoites of *D. fragilis* have been noted to be quite sensitive to an aerobic environment.[12] The organisms die and disintegrate within 1 hour in an isotonic salt solution at room temperature; when smeared on slides, they round up and become granular within 15 minutes during microscopic examination at room temperature and low humidity.[12]

D. fragilis has been reported worldwide, with a prevalence of 1.4 to 38 percent in selected populations.* Higher prevalence rates, from 19 to 69 percent, have been reported in various crowded living situations such as institutions and communal groups[5, 38, 40, 41, 60] and in persons traveling outside the United States.[35, 50, 57] A serologic survey in Canada using indirect immunofluorescence techniques detected antibodies to *D. fragilis* in 87 to 100 percent of healthy children between 1 and 19 years of age,[11] thus suggesting infection of most children in infancy. Although the antibodies detected in this survey did not absorb when incubated with *Klebsiella pneumoniae* or *Bacteroides vulgatus,* which are known to contaminate the antigen source of *D. fragilis,* additional studies are needed to confirm the specificity of the assay and define the seroprevalence in other populations.

The mode of transmission of *D. fragilis* is unknown; however, two mechanisms have been postulated. One hypothesis is that *D. fragilis* is transmitted in the eggs of

*See references 3–5, 9, 12, 18, 35, 37–39, 42, 45, 46, 49, 51, 58–60, 63, 64, 67, 70.

Enterobius vermicularis (pinworm) in a manner similar to the transmission of *H. meleagridis* in the eggs of the avian nematode *Heterakis gallinae*.[6, 16, 61, 64] In support of this theory, numerous investigators have noted a high frequency of concomitant infection with *D. fragilis* and *E. vermicularis*.[6, 16, 26, 61] Ockert provided the most convincing support for this theory when after ingesting the eggs of *E. vermicularis,* which he had washed with water and exposed to pepsin and hydrochloric acid, he became infected with both *E. vermicularis* and *D. fragilis*.[43] Other researchers, noting a high rate of concomitant infection of *D. fragilis* and organisms transmitted by the fecal-oral route, suggest this mode of transmission.[37, 38, 40, 64]

Clinical Manifestations

Gastrointestinal and, less frequently, systemic symptoms have been reported to occur in association with *D. fragilis* in the fecal specimens of children and adults.* Symptomatic infections develop in 15 to 85 percent of infected individuals.[32, 36, 37, 41, 45, 50, 55–57, 68, 70] Both acute watery diarrhea and a chronic recurrent abdominal pain syndrome have been associated with *D. fragilis* in children and adults.†

Persons with acute diarrhea also have reported abdominal pain, anorexia, nausea, vomiting, and less frequently, fever, weight loss, headache, malaise, fatigue, irritability, and weakness.[13–15, 27, 32, 33, 47, 55, 56, 66, 71] The stools have been described as greenish-brown, mushy or sticky with a foul odor, and at times bloody and with mucus.[32, 33] Abdominal tenderness has been found commonly on physical examination.[13, 32, 56]

D. fragilis infection, when symptomatic, is associated most frequently with chronic abdominal pain,[13, 39, 55, 56] which may persist for months to years.[27, 66] The pain frequently is described as dull, achy, crampy, or colicky and usually is located in the lower abdominal quadrants.[54, 56, 66] Complaints of flatulence, fatigue, and alternating diarrhea and constipation are not uncommon in persons with *D. fragilis* infection.[31, 56] Laboratory and radiologic studies are usually normal. Eosinophilia, not generally seen with protozoal infections, has been reported in infected children and adults, most commonly in association with chronic symptoms.[13, 55, 56] However, eosinophilia has not been observed by others.[32] The high prevalence of *D. fragilis* in fecal surveys, typically without symptoms, and the nonserious nature of symptomatic infections should steer clinicians to look for an alternative diagnosis in seriously ill children.

Diagnosis

Infection with *D. fragilis* should be considered when abdominal pain or diarrhea, or both, persists beyond 1 week, particularly if the child lives in an institution, has lived or traveled to a location where sanitary practices are poor, or is infected with pinworms.

Investigation for *D. fragilis* infection should include the collection of at least three stool specimens immediately placed in a stool preservative such as polyvinyl alcohol to retain the morphologic characteristics of the delicate trophozoite.[54] The diagnosis also can be made by examination of a permanently stained smear of a fresh or purged fecal specimen.[6, 25, 63] Detection of the organism does not appear to be compromised by the use of "environmentally friendly" mercury-free stool preservative and stain (EcoFix and EcoStain).[23] Three fecal specimens properly collected and stained will lead to identification of this intestinal protozoan in 70 to 93 percent of infected individuals.[29, 53] Stool specimens should be collected on alternate days because excretion of *D. fragilis* appears to occur in a cyclic pattern.[14] Stool samples should be collected before radiologic studies with barium are performed because barium interferes with detection of the protozoa.[21] Other medications interfering with identification of the parasite include antibiotics, mineral oil, antimalarials, antiprotozoan agents, nonabsorbable diarrheal preparations, and bismuth.[21] These substances may interfere with the detection of parasites for as long as 3 weeks.[21]

After arrival in the laboratory, stool specimens are processed with the use of a formalin-ether sedimentation concentration technique, stained with either iron hematoxylin or trichrome, and examined by qualified and experienced individuals for the proper identification of *D. fragilis*.[20, 23] Garcia and associates[21, 22] reported that 92.2 percent of *D. fragilis* trophozoites were determined solely on the basis of trichrome-stained smears, and subsequent studies indicated a comparable sensitivity with the use of EcoStain.[23] Diagnostic characteristics of *D. fragilis* on a permanently stained smear include a high percentage of binucleate trophozoites and nuclei without peripheral chromatin but with four to eight chromatin granules in a central mass.[19] Detection of *D. fragilis* by indirect immunofluorescence[10] or by culture[52] appears promising in limited investigations. One serologic test has been developed; however, the high seroprevalence of *D. fragilis* precludes its use as a diagnostic tool.[11]

Treatment

Several different agents have been used for the treatment of *D. fragilis* infection. At present, one of four drugs is recommended for the treatment of *D. fragilis* infection: iodoquinol, tetracycline, paromomycin, and metronidazole.[1, 2, 10, 36, 56] However, because of the lack of clinical studies, tetracycline and paromomycin are considered investigational by the U.S. Food and Drug Administration.[1] Iodoquinol, 650 mg three times a day for 20 days, is recommended for adults and 40 mg/kg/day divided three times a day for children. The tablets should be taken with meals. Side effects include abdominal discomfort, diarrhea, anal irritation and pruritus, headache, and dysesthesias of the hands and feet. Paromomycin in a dosage of 500 mg three times a day for adults and 25 to 35 mg/kg/day in three divided doses in children for 7 days may be more effective than iodoquinol.[69] Adverse reactions to paromomycin include nausea, abdominal cramps, and diarrhea. It is absorbed poorly after oral administration and, unfortunately, is no longer available in syrup form in the United States. Alternative therapy is tetracycline hydrochloride or metronidazole. Tetracycline is recommended at a dosage of 500 mg four times a day for adults or 40 mg/kg/day in four divided doses in children for 10 days. Tetracycline should be given on an empty stomach because food and dairy products may interfere with absorption of the drug. Tetracycline may cause gastrointestinal and central nervous system symptoms. It should not be given to children younger than 9 years because it may cause discoloration of teeth. Metronidazole treatment is recommended at a dosage of 500 to 750 mg three times daily for 10 days in adults or 20 to 40 mg/kg/day

*See references 7, 10, 13, 15, 24, 26–33, 40, 41, 44, 45, 47, 48, 50, 56, 57, 59, 62, 63, 66, 68, 71.

†See references 13, 15, 25–31, 38, 39, 40, 44–47, 52–55, 58, 59, 66.

divided into three doses for children. Treatment with metronidazole may cause gastrointestinal and central nervous system symptoms. Because of the adverse reactions associated with these drugs, the clinician should evaluate the need for therapy in each case carefully and discuss treatment options with the child's family.

REFERENCES

1. Abromowicz, M. (ed.): Drugs for parasite infections. Med. Lett. Drugs Ther. April:1–12, 2002.
2. American Academy of Pediatrics. *In* Pickering, L. K., (ed.): 2000 Red Book: Report of the Committee on Infectious Diseases. 25th ed. Elk Grove Village, IL, American Academy of Pediatrics, 2000, pp. 693, 698, 720.
3. Boe, J.: The occurrence of human intestinal protozoa in Norway. Acta Med. Scand. *113*:321–328, 1943.
4. Bruckner, D. A., Garcia, L. S., and Voge, M.: Intestinal parasites in Los Angeles, California. Am. J. Med. Technol. *45*:1020–1022, 1979.
5. Brug, S. L.: Observation on *Dientamoeba fragilis.* Ann. Trop. Med. Parasitol. *30*:441–452, 1936.
6. Burrows, R. B., and Swerdlow, H. A.: *Enterobius vermicularis:* A probable vector of *Dientamoeba fragilis.* Am. J. Trop. Med. Hyg. *5*:256–264, 1956.
7. Butler, W. P.: *Dientamoeba fragilis:* An unusual intestinal pathogen. Dig. Dis Sci. *41*:1811–1813, 1996.
8. Camp, R. R., Mattern, C. F. T., and Honigberg, B. M.: Study of *Dientamoeba fragilis,* Jepps and Dobell. I. Electron microscopic observations of the binucleate stages. II. Taxonomic position and revision of genus. J. Protozool. *21*:69–82, 1974.
9. Centers for Disease Control: Intestinal parasite surveillance. Annual summary 1978. Georgia, U.S. Public Health Service, 1979.
10. Chan, F. T. H., Guan, M. X., Mackinzie, A. M. R., and Diaz-Mitoma, F.: Susceptibility testing of *Dientamoeba fragilis* ATCC 30948 with iodoquinol, paromomycin, tetracycline, and metronidazole. Antimicrob. Agents Chemotherapy. *38*:1157–1160, 1994.
11. Chan, F., Stewart, N., Guan, M., et al.: Prevalence of *Dientamoeba fragilis* antibodies in children and recognition of a 39 kDa immunodominant protein antigen of the organism. Eur. J. Microbiol. Infect. Dis. *15*:950–954, 1996.
12. Chang, M.: Parasitization of the parasite. J. A. M. A. *223*:1510, 1973.
13. Cuffari, C., Oligny, L., and Seidman, E. G: *Dientamoeba fragilis* masquerading as allergic colitis. J. Pediatr. Gastroenterol. Nutr. *26*:16–20, 1998.
14. Desser, S. S., and Yang, Y. J.: *Dientamoeba fragilis* in idiopathic gastrointestinal disorders. Can. Med. Assoc. J. *114*:290–293, 1976.
15. Dickinson, E. C., Cohen, M. A., and Schlenker, M. K: *Dientamoeba fragilis:* A significant pathogen. Am. J. Emerg. Med. *20*:62–63, 2002.
16. Dobell, C: Researches on the intestinal protozoa of monkeys and man. X. The life-history of *Dientamoeba fragilis.* Observations, experiments, and speculations. Parasitology *32*:417–461, 1940.
17. Dwyer, D. M.: *Trichomonas, Histomonas, Dientamoeba* and *Entamoeba.* I. Quantitative fluorescent antibody methods. J. Protozool. *19*:316–325, 1972.
18. Fantham, H. B., and Porter, A.: Some entozoa of man as seen in Canada and South Africa. Can. Med. Assoc. J. *34*:414–421, 1936.
19. Faust, E. C., Beaver, P. C., and Jung R. C.: Animal Agents and Vectors of Human Disease. 4th ed. Philadelphia, Lea & Febiger, 1975.
20. Forbes, B. A., Sahm, D. F., Weissfeld, A. S. (eds.): Bailey and Scott's Diagnostic Microbiology. 11th ed. St. Louis, C. V. Mosby, 2002.
21. Garcia, L. S., and Ash, L. R.: Diagnostic Parasitology. St. Louis, C. V. Mosby, 1975, pp. 9–20.
22. Garcia, L. S., Brewer, T. C., and Bruckner, D. A.: A comparison of the formalin-ether concentration and trichrome-stained smear methods for the recovery and identification of intestinal protozoa. Am. J. Med. Technol. *45*:932–935, 1979.
23. Garcia, L. S., and Shumuzu, R. Y.: Evaluation of intestinal protozoan morphology in human fecal specimens preserved in EcoFix: Comparison of Wheatley's trichrome stain and EcoStain. J. Clin. Microbiol. *36*:1974–1976, 1998.
24. Gittings, J. C., and Waltz, A. D.: *Dientamoeba fragilis.* Am. J. Dis. Child. *34*:543–546, 1927.
25. Goldman, M., and Brooke, M. M.: Protozoans in stools unpreserved and preserved in PVA-fixative. Public Health Rep. *68*:703, 1953.
26. Grendon, J. H., Di Giacomo, R. F., and Frost, F. J.: Descriptive features of *Dientamoeba fragilis* infections. J. Trop. Med. Hyg. *98*:309–315, 1995.
27. Hakansson, E. G.: *Dientamoeba fragilis,* some further observations. Am J. Trop. Med. Hyg. *16*:175–183, 1936.
28. Hakansson, E. G.: *Dientamoeba fragilis,* some further observations. Am. J. Trop. Med. Hyg. *17*:349–352, 1937.
29. Hiatt, R. A., Markell, E. K., and Ng, E.: How many stool examinations are necessary to detect pathogenic intestinal protozoa? Am. J. Trop. Med. Hyg. *53*:36–39, 1995.
30. Hood, M.: Diarrhea caused by *Dientamoeba fragilis.* J. Lab. Clin. Med. *25*:914–918, 1940.
31. Jepps, M. W., and Dobell, C.: *Dientamoeba fragilis,* N. G., N.. Sp., a new intestinal amoeba from man. Parasitology *10*:352–367, 1918.
32. Kean, B. H., and Malloch, C. L.: The neglected amoeba: *Dientamoeba fragilis.* A report of 100 pure infections. Am. J. Dig. Dis. *11*:735–744, 1966.
33. Knoll, E. W., and Howell, K. M.: Studies on *Dientamoeba fragilis:* Its incidence and possible pathogenicity. Am. J. Clin. Pathol. *15*:178–183, 1945.
34. Kudo, R.: Observation on *Dientamoeba fragilis.* Am. J. Trop. Med. Hyg. *6*:299–305, 1926.
35. Mackie, T. T., Larsh, J. E., Jr., and Mackie, J. W.: A survey of intestinal parasitic infections in the Dominican Republic. Am. J. Trop. Med. *31*:825–832, 1951.
36. Markell, E. K., John, D., and Krotoski, W.: Medical Parasitology. 8th ed. Philadelphia, W. B. Saunders, 1999, pp. 68–70.
37. McQuay, R. M.: Parasitologic studies in a group of furloughed missionaries. I. Intestinal protozoa. Am. J. Trop. Med. Hyg. *16*:154–160, 1967.
38. Melvin, D. M., and Brooke, M. M.: Parasitologic surveys on Indian reservations in Montana, South Dakota, New Mexico, Arizona and Wisconsin. Am. J. Trop. Med. Hyg. *11*:765–772, 1962.
39. Miller, M. J.: The intestinal protozoa of man in midwestern Canada. J. Parasitol. *25*:355–357, 1939.
40. Millet, V. E., Spencer, M. J., Chapin, M. R., et al.: Intestinal protozoan infection in a semicommunal group. Am. J. Trop. Med. Hyg. *32*:54–60, 1983.
41. Millet, V. E., Spencer, M. J., Chapin, M. R., et al.: Intestinal protozoan infection in a semicommunal group. Dig. Dis. Sci. *28*:335–339, 1983.
42. Naimen, H. L., Sekla, L., and Albritton, W. L.: Giardiasis and other parasitic infections in a Manitoba residential school for the mentally retarded. Can. Med. Assoc. J. *122*:185–188, 1980.
43. Ockert, G.: Zur Epidemiologie von *Dientamoeba fragilis.* II. Mitteilung: Versuche über die Übertragung der Art mit Enterobius-Eiern. J. Hyg. Epidemiol. Immunol. *16*:222–225, 1972.
44. Oxner, R. B., Paltridge, G. P., Chapman, B. A., et al.: *Dientamoeba fragilis:* A bowel pathogen? N. Z. Med. J. *100*:64–65, 1987.
45. Oyofo, B. A., Persuski, L. F. Ismail, T. F., et al: Enteropathogens associated with diarrhoea among military personnel during operation bright star 96, in Alexandria, Egypt. Mil. Med. *162*:396–400, 1997.
46. Porter, A.: Remarks on intestinal parasites in Montreal and the relation of *Entamoeba histolytica* to colitis. Can. Med. Assoc. J. *30*:134–137, 1934.
47. Robertson, A.: Note on a case infected with *Dientamoeba fragilis.* Jepps and Dobell. Am. J. Trop. Med. Hyg. *1923*:26–243, 1917.
48. Rothman, M. D., and Epstein, H. J.: Clinical symptoms associated with the so-called nonpathogenic amoeba. J. A. M. A. *116*:694–700, 1941.
49. Ruebush, T. K., Juranek, D. D., and Brodsky, R. E.: Diagnoses of intestinal parasites by state and territorial public health laboratories, 1976. J. Infect. Dis. *138*:114–117, 1978.
50. Sapero, J. J.: Clinical studies in nondysenteric intestinal amebiasis. Am. J. Trop. Med. Hyg. *19*:497–514, 1939.
51. Saunders, L. G.: A survey of helminth and protozoan incidence in man and dogs at Fort Chipewyan, Alberta. J. Parasitol. *35*:31–34, 1949.
52. Sawangjaroen, N., Luke, R., and Prociv, P.: Diagnosis by faecal culture of Dientamoeba fragilis infections in Australian patients with diarrhoea. Trans. R. Soc. Trop. Med. Hyg. *87*:163–165, 1993.
53. Sawitz, W. G., and Faust, E. C.: The probability of detecting intestinal protozoa by successive stool examinations. Am. J. Trop. Hyg. *22*:131–136, 1942.
54. Scholten, T. H., and Yang, J.: Evaluation of unpreserved and preserved stools for the detection of intestinal parasites. Am. J. Clin. Pathol. *62*:563–567, 1974.
55. Spencer, M. J., Chapin, M. R., and Garcia, L. S.: *Dientamoeba fragilis,* a gastrointestinal protozoan parasite in adults. Am. J. Gastroenterol. *70*:565–569, 1982.
56. Spencer, M. J., Garcia, L. S., and Chapin, M. R.: *Dientamoeba fragilis,* an intestinal pathogen in children? Am. J. Dis. Child. *133*:390–393, 1979.
57. Spencer, M. J., Millet, V. E., and Garcia, L. S.: Parasitic infections in a pediatric population. Pediatr. Infect. Dis. *2*:110–113, 1983.
58. Stein, B., and Talis, B.: The prevalence of *Dientamoeba fragilis* in Tel Aviv and its surroundings. Res. Council Israel *8E*:55, 1959.
59. Steinitz, H., Talis, B., and Stein, B.: *Entamoeba histolytica* and *Dientamoeba fragilis* and the syndrome of chronic recurrent intestinal amoebiasis in Israel. Digestion *3*:146–153, 1970.
60. Svennson, R. M.: A survey of human intestinal protozoa in Sweden and Finland. Parasitology *20*:237–249, 1928.
61. Swerdlow, M. A., and Burrows, R. B.: *Dientamoeba fragilis.* An intestinal pathogen. J. A. M. A. *158*:176–178, 1955.
62. Taliafero, W. H., and Becker, E. R.: A note on the human intestinal amoeba, *Dientamoeba fragilis.* Am. J. Hyg. *4*:71–74, 1924.
63. Thompson, J. G.: *Dientamoeba fragilis,* Jepps and Dobell, 1917: A case of human infection in England. J. Trop. Med. Hyg. *26*:135–136, 1923.

64. Weiner, D., Brooke, M. M., and Witkow, A.: Investigation of parasitic infections in the central area of Philadelphia. Am. J. Trop. Med. Hyg. *8*:625–629, 1959.
65. Wenrich, D. H.: Studies on *Dientamoeba fragilis* (protozoa) I. Observations with special reference to nuclear structure. J. Parasitol. *22*:76–83, 1936.
66. Wenrich, D. H.: Studies on *Dientamoeba fragilis* (protozoa) II. Report on unusual morphology in one case with suggestions as to pathogenicity. J. Parasitol. *23*:183–196, 1937.
67. Wenrich, D. H., Stabler, R. M., and Arnett, J. H.: *Entamoeba histolytica* and other intestinal protozoa in 1,060 college freshmen. Am. J. Trop. Med. Hyg. *15*:331–345, 1935.
68. Windsor, J. J., Rafay, A. M., Shenoy, A. K., and Johnson, E. H: Incidence of *Dientamoeba fragilis* in faecal samples submitted for routine microbiological analysis. Br. J. Biomed. Sci. *55*:172–175, 1998.
69. Wolfe, M. S.: In Strickland, G. (ed.): Hunter's Tropical Medicine. Philadelphia, W. B. Saunders, 1991, p. 580.
70. Yang, J., and Scholten, T.: *Dientamoeba fragilis*. A review with notes on its epidemiology, pathogenicity, mode of transmission and diagnosis. Am. J. Trop. Med. Hyg. *26*:16–22, 1977.
71. Yoeli, M.: A report on intestinal disorders accompanied by large number of *Dientamoeba fragilis*. Trop. Med. Hyg. *58*:38–41, 1955.

CHAPTER 214 *Trichomonas* Infections

JOAN S. PURCELL ■ MARIAM R. CHACKO

Trichomonas spp. are found in both animals and humans. The most widely studied member of this species is *Trichomonas vaginalis* because it is the trichomonad most relevant to human disease. Donne first described *T. vaginalis* in 1836 as motile microorganisms in the purulent frothy leukorrhea of women with vaginal discharge and genital irritation.[14] Epidemiologic information concerning *Trichomonas* infection is most detailed in the adult population; nevertheless, studies that document the epidemiology of *T. vaginalis* in children and adolescents are available.*

Bacteriology

Trichomonads are acellular flagellated protozoans. The Trichomonadidae family is characterized as mononucleate with an axial organelle that has an undulating membrane.[60] The *Trichomonas* genus includes protozoans that have organelles with three to four anterior flagella and an undulating membrane composed of the posterior flagellum.[60] Five and three *Trichomonas* spp. infect humans and animals, respectively. In humans, the five species of *Trichomonas* include *Trichomonas tenax, Trichomonas ardin delteili, Trichomonas faecalis, Trichomonas hominis,* and *T. vaginalis*.[60]

T. vaginalis is the most clinically relevant human trichomonad; the other four species are nonpathogenic. The structure of *T. vaginalis* consists of four anterior flagella and a posterior flagellum incorporated into the undulating membrane. *T. vaginalis* can survive but cannot multiply at room temperature. In contrast, *T. hominis* has five anterior flagella and a trailing posterior flagellum and can survive and multiply at room temperature. Only *T. hominis* can survive in media without serum and in feces for up to 24 hours.[60]

Pathogenesis

Virulence factors associated with *T. vaginalis* infection have been defined and include adherence, contact-independent factors, hemolysis, and host macromolecule acquisition. Epithelial cell adherence is dependent on an intact cytoskeleton and *Trichomonas* protein ligands and proteases, which are necessary to activate adherence molecules.[10, 17] Cell contact–independent factors include pH variability and cell-detaching factor, which in vitro inhibit reorganization of cells infected with *T. vaginalis*. *T. vaginalis* produces lactic and acetic acid as a byproduct of glucose metabolism.[10] These acids lower the pH, which is cytotoxic to epithelial cells. Another metabolic byproduct of *T. vaginalis* is cell-detaching factor, which has a cytopathic effect on epithelial cells and increases subepithelial vascularity, thereby producing the clinical sign of "strawberry cervix."[10] The activity of cell-detaching factor is optimal at pH 5.0 or greater. Hemolysis is seen only in the presence of live trichomonads. Cysteine proteases appear to be important for hemolysis because introduction of their inhibitors in vitro eliminates hemolysis by *T. vaginalis*.[10, 25] The addition of metronidazole reduces levels of hemolysis by 50 percent.[10] The hemolytic activity of *T. vaginalis* is temperature-dependent, with maximal hemolysis at 37° C. Hemolysis is inhibited via separation of trichomonads from erythrocytes by a 3-μm filter, thus suggesting a contact-dependent mechanism.[10] As a parasite, *T. vaginalis* is also dependent on host macromolecules for nutrition, including plasma proteins and lactoferrin.

The host responds to *T. vaginalis* infection at the cellular level with polymorphonuclear cells and lymphocyte activity. *T. vaginalis* secretes proteases that are chemotactic to polymorphonuclear leukocytes, with resultant phagocytosis and killing of the trichomonad by oxidative mechanisms.[10] *T. vaginalis* secretions are mitogenic to lymphocytes; they enhance phagocytosis by polymorphonuclear cells and may suppress the host immune response if large numbers of suppressor lymphocytes are activated. Clinically, *T. vaginalis* infection has gender differences. Women are largely symptomatic, whereas only a small minority of men have symptoms with *T. vaginalis* infection, many of which undergo spontaneous cure. Estrogen levels in females directly correlate with infection at peak estradiol levels. In an early study of premenarchal vaginitis in children 3 months to 9 years of age, *T. vaginalis* infection accounted

*See references 8, 9, 15, 18, 20–22, 24, 31, 33, 34, 43, 48, 56.

for only 2.8 to 4.4 percent of cases of vaginitis in unestrogenized vaginas, as compared with 50 percent of infections in the fully estrogenized vaginas of patients nearing puberty.[18] In asymptomatic males infected with *T. vaginalis,* the prostate gland serves as a reservoir. Men may remain asymptomatic because of the concentration of zinc salts in prostatic fluid, which is cytocidal for trichomonads.[29] In vitro, testosterone decreases the growth of *T. vaginalis* as well.[16]

In the host, trichomonads may serve as a vector for bacteria and viruses, as demonstrated by the high coinfection rate with *T. vaginalis* and human papillomavirus. Whereas bacteria contaminate trichomonads externally, trichomonads are thought to ingest virus-infected cells and destroy them, with the active virus left intact.[20] *T. vaginalis* has been implicated in the etiology of pelvic inflammatory disease via ascension from the vagina to the fallopian tubes. Studies in vitro have demonstrated *Escherichia coli* strains, a part of the normal vaginal flora, intimately attached to trichomonads by glycoprotein strands.[25] Trichomonads contaminated with bacteria serve as a vector for the bacteria to produce pelvic infection on reaching the uterus, fallopian tubes, or peritoneum.[25] In contrast, vaginal colonization with *Lactobacillus* spp. was thought to inhibit trichomonal invasion by lowering vaginal pH. In a study of 336 African women 15 to 49 years of age, 199 of whom were pregnant, 31 percent were culture-positive for *T. vaginalis,* whereas only 40 percent of the patients tested positive for *Lactobacillus.* Although the rate of *Lactobacillus* colonization in these African women was low, the high rate of *T. vaginalis* infection was not related to the absence of *Lactobacillus.* Thus, trichomonads may not alter the vaginal flora substantially.[39]

A spectrum of severity of disease exists in patients infected with *T. vaginalis.* Some patients are asymptomatic, whereas others experience severe symptomatic inflammation and discomfort. The virulence of *T. vaginalis* isolates varies; whether this variance is caused by the host response or inherent properties of the parasite is unknown. The Golgi apparatus in *T. vaginalis* is a prominent structure and seems to be a key station in the production of adhesins.[6] However, evidence indicates that the dramatic heterogeneity that exists on the surface of the parasite leads to antigenic diversity among different isolates of *T. vaginalis.* In one study, prominent immunogens absent on the surface of *T. vaginalis* isolates led to an enhanced ability of the parasite to cause cytoadherence-dependent killing of HeLa cells in monolayer culture. In addition, only the adherent parasites possessed adhesins, which directly affected the parasites' cytoadherence and cytotoxicity.[1] The cysteine proteases of *T. vaginalis* may be responsible for the cytoadherence, nutrient acquisition, and cytotoxicity of *T. vaginalis.* These proteinases are shed during the life cycle and growth of *T. vaginalis.* One hundred percent of sera from women infected with *T. vaginalis* but none from normal uninfected women possessed IgG to numerous trichomonad cysteine proteinases. This serum antiproteinase antibody disappeared after the women received effective therapy for the infection.[3]

Immunology

The interaction between *T. vaginalis* and host immunoglobulins is not clear. In women infected with *T. vaginalis,* specific local antibodies, IgG and IgA, are seen in vaginal secretions. IgA may serve to increase opsonization of the parasite by IgG and thus result in enhanced phagocytosis. IgG specific for *Trichomonas* cysteine proteases and surface proteins is seen, but it does not help rid the host of infection.[3] *T. vaginalis* synthesizes high-molecular-weight proteins with variable surface expression.[2] Of samples obtained from women infected with *T. vaginalis,* 70 percent of vaginal washes and 80 percent of vaginal mucus samples had IgG to a specific *T. vaginalis* surface protein immunogen with a molecular mass of 230,000 d (P230). In contrast, no antibody to P230 was detected in uninfected women or in detergent extract depleted of P230, thus suggesting a highly specific antibody.[2] Clinically, this finding may account for the lack of resistance to repeated *Trichomonas* infections and variable host antibody titers in infected persons.

Epidemiology

In humans, five species of *Trichomonas* have been identified; the most clinically important one is *T. vaginalis. T. vaginalis* is not part of the normal flora but is found in the human vagina, urethra, and prostate. Inoculation experiments with *T. vaginalis* in the mouth and intestines failed to establish infection in these sites.[60] *T. tenax* is found in the mouth, whereas *T. hominis, T. ardin delteili,* and *T. faecalis* are found in the bowel. *T. tenax* is detected in approximately 5 percent of patients with *T. vaginalis.*[60] *T. tenax, T. ardin delteili,* and *T. faecalis* are part of the normal flora and are nonpathogenic.[60] *T. hominis* can infect humans and is associated with gastroenteric dysentery.[60] The incidence of *T. hominis* in humans is between 0.4 and 3.5 percent. *T. hominis* is found only rarely in the stools of patients who concomitantly have *T. vaginalis.*[60]

T. vaginalis infection may be the sexually transmitted disease most commonly encountered. The prevalence of *T. vaginalis* urogenital infection varies from 5 to 65 percent in different studies conducted predominantly in adults. Many of the studies of urogenital trichomoniasis are biased because of lack of random sampling, variance in the sensitivity and specificity of the diagnostic tests used, and sample selection, often from sexually transmitted disease clinics.[37] One of the reasons for the high prevalence of *T. vaginalis* infection is its rate of asymptomatic carriage; accordingly, reliance on clinical symptoms alone will cause a practitioner to miss as many as 80 percent of infections.[42]

Trichomonal infection is found in all age groups, from neonates to adults. It has been detected in newborns and infants, presumably from contamination on passage through an infected birth canal.[48] Most of the cases reported have involved premature infant girls. Vertical transmission of the organism occurs as the infant passes through the infected maternal birth canal.

T. vaginalis is seen most commonly in postmenarchal sexually active females; however, *T. vaginalis* vaginitis is noted occasionally in children.[20] *T. vaginalis* in a prepubertal or non–sexually active female must raise suspicion of sexual abuse and prompt an evaluation for other sexually transmitted diseases.[15, 43, 60] In a study of 409 children suspected of having been sexually abused, *T. vaginalis* was diagnosed in 4 children 10 to 12 years of age by wet-mount examination of vaginal secretions. This study may have underrepresented cases of *T. vaginalis* in patients suspected of having been sexually abused because a saline wet-mount preparation was available in only 18 of the 409 children.[59] One study of 54 premenarchal girls (median age, 5.8 years) with vulvovaginitis failed to identify *T. vaginalis.*[42] Lang[34] found *T. vaginalis* in 3.6 percent of 9- to 12-year-old girls. In adolescents, the prevalence of *T. vaginalis* is between 5.5 and 34 percent.[21]

Trichomonal infections can be found in both males and females, although the incidence is greater in females. The incidence of *T. vaginalis* infection is between 10 and 25 percent in sexually active females worldwide. In males attending a sexually transmitted disease clinic, the prevalence of *T. vaginalis* was 22 percent in sexual contacts of females with trichomoniasis and 6 percent in homosexual males attending the same clinic.[27] *T. vaginalis* was found in 58 percent of 85 black males 16 to 22 years of age who currently were sexually active.[47] Sixty-nine percent previously had a sexually transmitted disease.

The rate of infection with *T. vaginalis* is increased in black females, as well as in females with other sexually transmitted diseases. In addition, it is increased in females who have gonococcal cervicitis with a vaginal pH shift above 4.5 and in those who are pregnant, and it may be increased around the time of menarche and after menopause.[13, 41, 60] Trichomoniasis does not appear to have a seasonal pattern of infection.[37] Urogenital trichomoniasis is seen more commonly in inner-city patients and those in the 20- to 30-year-old age group.[37] Infection with *T. vaginalis* increases in direct relation to the number of sexual partners. Oral contraceptives diminish the rate of infection with *T. vaginalis* when compared with an intrauterine device or tubal ligation.[37] The use of nonoxinol 9 spermicidal cream was not related significantly to a decrease in *Trichomonas* infection.[4] In another study of 226 women attending a sexually transmitted disease clinic, trichomonal infection was noted in 44 percent of the patients.[41] No association was found among patient age, frequency of coitus, date of most recent coitus, day of the menstrual cycle, antibiotic use, contraceptive methods, or symptoms of discharge or pruritus.[41] Other risk factors for females may involve a change in the normal vaginal flora, such as overgrowth of *Gardnerella vaginalis, Bacteroides,* or *Peptostreptococcus.* These bacteria may serve as sources of nutrients for trichomonads and allow them to thrive. In males, sexual contact with a female infected with *T. vaginalis,* nongonococcal urethritis, or nongonococcal nonchlamydial urethritis was associated with an increased risk for infection with *T. vaginalis.*[30] In trichomoniasis, lactobacilli are absent from the vagina. This absence promotes alkalinity of the vaginal pH, thereby enhancing the overgrowth of anaerobes and trichomonads.[54] Another study performed in Africa failed to demonstrate a significant role for *Lactobacillus* in patients with *T. vaginalis* infection.[12, 39]

T. vaginalis usually is transmitted sexually in adolescents and adults. Large numbers of trichomonads are found in the prostatic secretions of husbands of women with recurrent *T. vaginalis* infection. In a clinic for patients with sexually transmitted diseases, 60 percent of husbands of women who were suffering from chronic, repeated *T. vaginitis* infection were culture-positive for *T. vaginalis,* in contrast to 8 percent in a control group of male patients attending the same clinic.[57] These data support the concept of sexual transmission of *T. vaginalis.*

Nonsexual transmission of *T. vaginalis* has been reported. In rural India, a point prevalence survey of random samples from juvenile and adolescent females complaining of leukorrhea revealed that 76 percent were infected with *T. vaginalis.* Of those who were infected, 38 percent were younger than 12 years. In this study, poor genital hygiene and underwear use were correlated with a higher incidence of infection. In addition, a significantly higher risk occurred in females who washed or bathed in tanks or rivers versus those who used pipe or well water. Thus, in the tropics, nonsexual transmission may account for infection with *T. vaginalis* in juvenile and adolescent females.[9] *T. vaginalis* can survive on toilet seats for up to 1 hour, on wet clothes for 3 hours, in fresh water for 30 minutes, in warm mineral water for 2 or 3 days, and in urine for hours. Thus, according to the literature, transmission of *Trichomonas* may occur via fomites (washcloths, towels), particularly when people are living together in crowded, confined spaces.[43]

Clinical Manifestations

The vagina of an infant may serve as a reservoir of infection that goes unnoticed until the infant is initially evaluated 5 to 6 weeks after birth for fever. Motile trichomonads and pyuria are seen on examination of the urine. Symptoms resolve after treatment with metronidazole.[48] Premenarchal children have diffuse bubbly leukorrhea and pruritus.[34] Vaginitis with a purulent foul-smelling discharge is the most common manifestation of infection with *T. vaginalis* in females; in some patients, trichomonads may be found in the urine initially, with the development of frank signs of vaginitis 7 to 28 days later.[24]

As many as 50 percent of females and 90 percent of males infected with *T. vaginalis* will be asymptomatic.[56] When one controls for co-infection with other organisms, *T. vaginalis* infection is associated significantly with purulent discharge, vulvar itching, colpitis macularis ("strawberry cervix"), and vaginal and vulvar erythema. The sensitivity of the other signs and symptoms of *Trichomonas* vaginitis, including vaginal burning, dysuria, urinary frequency, dyspareunia, frothy discharge, and cervical friability, is low.[59] Although frothy leukorrhea was associated most frequently with *Trichomonas* infection, 29 percent of the patients with frothy discharge in one study did not have *Trichomonas* infection.[59] Strawberry cervix was pathognomonic of *T. vaginalis* infection, but it was noted in only 2 to 3 percent of patients. Thus, one cannot depend on this finding to establish a clinical diagnosis of *T. vaginalis* vaginitis in most patients.[13] Accordingly, the diagnosis of *Trichomonas* infection should be entertained in any female with a vaginal discharge.

Trichomonads may ascend the fallopian tubes and, if contaminated with bacteria, can produce the syndrome of pelvic inflammatory disease.[8, 25] In males, *T. vaginalis* may be manifested as symptomatic urethritis with dysuria secondary to urethral inflammation and discharge. On examination, the discharge often is not visualized. When a discharge is present, it is clear to cloudy but not grossly purulent. On microscopy, numerous inflammatory cells are seen.[27, 32] *T. vaginalis* also may be a cause of chronic nonbacterial prostatitis and be manifested as chronic prostatitis resistant to standard therapy.[23, 32] In addition, *T. vaginalis* has been reported to be an etiologic agent of epididymitis in males, with purulent urethral discharge, scrotal swelling, and enlargement of the epididymis.[13] Though rare, *T. vaginalis* has been reported to infect the median raphe of the penis.[53]

Diagnosis

CLINICAL EXAMINATION

In females, the presence of a frothy purulent discharge, vulvar/vaginal erythema, and a strawberry cervix should suggest *Trichomonas* infection. Males tend to be asymptomatic or, if symptomatic, have a purulent urethral discharge and urethral inflammation. Eighty percent of infections will be missed if the physician relies on clinical examination alone.[14, 54]

WET-MOUNT EXAMINATION

The diagnosis of trichomoniasis in women usually is made by wet-mount examination of vaginal secretions. Wet-mount preparations are obtained by swabbing the lateral and anterior vaginal fornices to obtain discharge material with vaginal epithelial cells; the secretions are placed in a tube with normal saline and then mounted on a slide. This method also may be used to obtain urethral specimens in males. These preparations are easy to prepare, and the method is cost-effective, but its sensitivity is low (51%).[14] In addition, the validity of the result is dependent on the technical skill of the examiner and the rapidity with which the specimen is examined; cooling greatly affects the motility of trichomonads, which may hinder identification.[31]

PAPANICOLAOU SMEAR

Papanicolaou smears can detect trichomonads. However, this method is considered unreliable for the diagnosis of trichomoniasis. *T. vaginalis* does not always appear in its typical pear-shaped morphology after fixation on the slide. Rather, it may appear to be more rounded, similar to a polymorphonuclear leukocyte. Cytopathologic diagnostic criteria for *Trichomonas* infection include the presence of perinuclear halos and a dirty granular background. However, these features are nonspecific, and a similar background and halos can be found with certain other conditions. Therefore, the sensitivity of Papanicolaou smears for diagnosing *Trichomonas* in culture-proven infection is as low as 56 percent.[29] In a study of 1199 women, *T. vaginalis* infection would have been diagnosed falsely in 37 percent based on Papanicolaou smear results. In a second study, *T. vaginalis* infection would not have been diagnosed in 44 percent of patients with culture-proven infection because of negative Papanicolaou smear findings.[45]

STAINING TECHNIQUES

Acridine orange is a compound that differentially stains DNA (yellow-green) and RNA (bright red). *T. vaginalis* stains brick-red with an oval, yellow-green nucleus. The flagella do not stain. Unfixed smears are kept at room temperature for as long as 24 hours; fixed slides may be kept as long as 5 days. Acridine orange stains may permit a rapid, accurate diagnosis of *T. vaginalis* infection. The diagnosis can be confirmed by other diagnostic methods in 93 percent of cases.[40] Acridine orange staining appears to be at least as sensitive as wet-mount examination.[7, 49]

CULTURE

Diagnosis of *T. vaginalis* by culture has been considered the gold standard. However, this diagnostic method generally is used in clinical research. Secretions are collected from the vagina or urethra with a cotton-tipped swab and placed directly on culture media. The reformulated media currently prepared commercially are Diamond, Kupferberg, and Lash media.[50] These media contain antibiotics to inhibit bacterial overgrowth and may contain yeast extract, horse or sheep serum, or both.[50] Cultures are incubated for 7 days, and a drop of sediment from the culture tube is placed on a slide and a wet-mount examination performed. Culture of *T. vaginalis* on these media detected fewer than 10 trichomonads, and cultures were not affected by douching in the previous 24 hours. In contrast, the sensitivity of wet-mount preparations decreased from 57 to 22 percent after douching.[14] Limitations of culture include the failure of culture media to support the growth of trichomonads in some cases by culture day 7. Growth in culture media is also inoculum-dependent; less sensitive media require higher inocula of trichomonads.[50] In males, the combination of prostatic massage before collection of the specimen and culture of both urethral samples and urinary sediment has a sensitivity of 94 to 98 percent.[30, 47]

The plastic envelope or pouch method is a simplified and now standard method of culture that is selective for *T. vaginalis*. Vaginal secretions are placed in a dry medium that is reconstituted with distilled water. The solution then is placed in pouches with separate chambers that are mixed easily for culture. Subsequently, the upper chamber is placed on a slide mount and viewed for motile trichomonads. Both wet-mount and immediate examinations of the envelope for motile trichomonads are reported to have a sensitivity of 66 percent versus traditional culture (sensitivity, 89–91%) and the envelope or pouch culture (sensitivity, 89–97%). In another recent study, the sensitivity plus specificity of culture via the pouch method was 94 and 96 percent, that for vaginal wet-mount examination was 58 and 100 percent, and that for vaginal polymerase chain reaction was 89 and 97 percent.[35] The pouch or envelope method is more convenient to use than the wet-mount preparation and traditional culture. In addition, these methods have equivalent sensitivity for diagnosing *T. vaginalis* infection and are relatively inexpensive.[5, 11] Furthermore, the pouch culture method allows direct daily visualization without sampling or opening the pouches.[12]

DIRECT FLUORESCENT ANTIBODY STAINING

The sensitivity of direct fluorescent antibody (DFA) staining approaches 86 percent when compared with culture and is not related to the number of trichomonads seen on wet-mount examination. The sensitivity of DFA staining is superior to that of wet-mount examination or acridine orange staining in females who have *T. vaginalis* infection and is comparable to the sensitivity of these techniques in females infected with multiple organisms.[6, 27, 49] Interpretation of DFA staining may be accomplished in less than 1 hour.[27] In a study of high-risk males who underwent prostatic massage before collection of the specimen, DFA staining on urethral samples had a sensitivity of 63 percent.[47]

A monoclonal-based enzyme-linked immunosorbent assay (ELISA) was developed for use with a monoclonal antibody specific for a 65-kd surface polypeptide of *T. vaginalis*. Polyclonal rabbit anti–*T. vaginalis* antibody labeled with horseradish peroxidase was used as the probe. In a limited study of 36 females, this ELISA had a sensitivity of 89 percent and a specificity of 97 percent.[36]

OTHER RAPID DIAGNOSTIC TESTS

Rapid diagnostic tests such as DNA amplification techniques are being used for clinical research purposes to diagnose trichomoniasis. They are being made available for clinical use. Several primer sets have been described, and sensitivities using vaginal swabs have ranged from 8.5 to 100 percent.[35] In contrast, the sensitivity of using a urine specimen to detect trichomoniasis is 64 percent.[35]

Treatment

Metronidazole is the treatment of choice for *T. vaginalis* infection and is currently the only drug available for treatment of trichomoniasis in the United States. Worldwide, other drugs used for trichomoniasis include nifuratel, nimorazole, tinidazole, ornidazole, secnidazole, and carnidazole. Despite the availability of these other drugs, metronidazole remains the standard therapy for trichomoniasis. Metronidazole enters the trichomonad via passive diffusion, and its nitro group is reduced to a cytotoxic intermediate that reacts with DNA and causes cell death. Metronidazole is 93 to 95 percent bioavailable, and after oral administration, peak serum levels are attained in 1 to 3 hours and a steady state in 2 to 3 days. Metronidazole is metabolized by the liver, with only 20 percent being protein-bound; thus, the drug is distributed well in the body.[38] Side effects reported with the use of metronidazole include nausea, vomiting, anorexia, a metallic taste, headache, dizziness, diarrhea, and darkening of the urine. Urticaria, reversible peripheral neuropathy, seizures, and ataxia have been reported with intravenous use. The side effects tend to be dose related and self-limited.[38] In a study of 1199 females with *T. vaginalis* infection treated with metronidazole, only 4 to 5 percent experienced symptoms of nausea, coated tongue, dryness of the mouth, anorexia, or diarrhea. All symptoms disappeared within a few days of completion of treatment, and in only one case was treatment discontinued because of side effects. In addition, relative and absolute leukopenia was not observed in these subjects. Of note, metronidazole enhances or reactivates the growth of *Candida albicans* in the vagina.[45] Metronidazole may potentiate the actions of anticonvulsants and warfarin. Because a significant disulfiram-like effect is produced when the drug is combined with moderate intake of alcohol,[38] alcohol should be avoided during and for 48 hours after completion of a course of therapy with metronidazole.

T. vaginalis infection should be treated to relieve symptoms, prevent further transmission of disease, and prevent chronic inflammation of the Bartholin and Skene glands.[56] In males, chronic infection may lead to prostatitis or urethral stricture.[56] Adolescent and adult males who are asymptomatic may harbor *T. vaginalis* in their prostatic secretions and thereby reinfect their partners. Therefore, male partners of females infected with *T. vaginalis* should be treated.[57]

Treatment of *T. vaginalis* is metronidazole, 2 g orally in a single dose or 500 mg twice daily for 7 days in adolescents and adults. Each regimen is 95 percent effective.[19] Metronidazole vaginal suppositories are not recommended for the treatment of trichomoniasis. Some strains of *T. vaginalis* have reduced susceptibility to metronidazole, with low-level metronidazole-resistant strains reported in 2.9 percent of infected cases. Though rare, higher-level resistance also has been reported.[36, 51, 52] Treatment options for metronidazole-resistant cases are limited. If the infection fails to respond to either of the aforementioned regimens, it should be retreated with metronidazole, 500 mg twice daily for 7 days.[19] If treatment failure continues, the patient can be treated with 2 g of metronidazole once daily for 3 to 5 days.[19] Metronidazole is contraindicated in the first trimester of pregnancy because of possible teratogenic effects on the fetus, but it may be used safely after the first trimester.[19]

TABLE 214–1 ■ DOSING OF METRONIDAZOLE IN CHILDREN

Age (yr)	Weight (kg)	Metronidazole Administered (mg) Orally*	Metronidazole Administered (mg) Locally†
0–1	10	150	10
1–6	20.5	250	50
7–12	40	500	150
>12	>40	500–1000	250–500

*Oral dose = one third of the total dose administered every 8 hours for 5 to 10 days.
†Local dose = total dose administered intravaginally once daily or half the total dose administered twice daily for 5 to 10 days.
Adapted from Kurnatowska, A., and Komorowska, A.: Urogenital trichomoniasis in children. *In* Honigberg, B. M. (ed.): Trichomonads Parasitic in Humans. New York, Springer-Verlag, 1989, p. 268.

However, a recent study of asymptomatic pregnant women (16 to 23 weeks) treated with single-dose metronidazole found that significantly more women were likely to go into premature labor.[26] A breast-fed infant consumes approximately 1 percent of a single 2-g oral dose of metronidazole; therefore, infants of mothers who are breast-feeding and who are treated with a single dose of metronidazole for trichomoniasis should be removed from the breast for at least 24 hours after treatment.[38]

In children with infections of the genital organs, local therapy with metronidazole is preferred because it has fewer systemic side effects. Cotton-tipped swabs saturated with metronidazole are introduced into the hymen and applied locally. In multifocal infections, genital infections that fail to respond to local therapy, and infections in newborn or infant boys, oral therapy with metronidazole is given[33] (Table 214–1). Before the administration of oral or intravenous metronidazole to children, baseline hematologic, renal, and liver function tests should be obtained to monitor changes as therapy continues. Resolution of the signs and symptoms of infection indicates a response to treatment. Eradication of *T. vaginalis* should be confirmed by wet-mount examination or culture (if available) 3 to 5 days after completion of treatment in children.[33]

Prognosis

If untreated, *T. vaginalis* can lead to chronic inflammation of the Bartholin and Skene glands in females and to prostatitis and urethritis with urethral stricture formation in males.[52] Complete resolution of symptoms plus eradication of *T. vaginalis* usually is noted when treatment is provided promptly.

REFERENCES

1. Alderete, J. F.: Alternating phenotypic expression of two classes of *Trichomonas vaginalis* surface markers. Rev. Infect. Dis. *10*(Suppl.): 408–412, 1988.
2. Alderete, J. F., Newton, E., Dennis, C., et al.: Vaginal antibody of patients with trichomoniasis is to a prominent surface immunogen of *Trichomonas vaginalis*. Genitourin. Med. *67*:220–225, 1991.
3. Alderete, J. F., Newton, E., Dennis, C., et al.: Antibody in sera of patients infected with *Trichomonas vaginalis* is to trichomonad proteinases. Genitourin. Med. *67*:331–334, 1991.
4. Barbone, F., Austin, H., Louv, W. C., et al.: A follow-up study of methods of contraception, sexual activity, and rates of trichomoniasis, candidiasis, and bacterial vaginosis. Am. J. Obstet. Gynecol. *163*:510–514, 1990.
5. Beal, C., Goldsmith, R., Kotby, M., et al.: The plastic envelope method: A simplified technique for culture diagnosis of trichomoniasis. J. Clin. Microbiol. *30*:2265–2268, 1992.

6. Benchimol, M., Ribeiro, K. C., Mariante, R. M., and Alderete, J. F.: Structure and division of the Golgi complex in *Trichomonas vaginalis* and *Trichomonas fetus*. Eur. J. Cell. Biol. *80*:593–607, 2001.
7. Bickley, L. S., Krisher, K. K., Punsalang, A., Jr., et al.: Comparison of direct fluorescent antibody, acridine orange, wet mount, and culture for detection of *Trichomonas vaginalis* in women attending a public sexually transmitted diseases clinic. Sex. Transm. Dis. *16*:127–131, 1989.
8. Cates, W., Jr., and Rauh, J. L.: Adolescents and sexually transmitted diseases: An expanding problem. J. Adolesc. Health Care *6*:257–261, 1985.
9. Charles, S. X.: Epidemiology of *Trichomonas vaginalis* in rural adolescent and juvenile children. J. Trop. Pediatr. *37*:90, 1991.
10. Dailey, D. C., Chang, T., and Alderete, J. F.: Characterization of *Trichomonas vaginalis* hemolysis. Parasitology *101*:171–175, 1990.
11. Draper, D., Parker, R., Patterson, E., et al.: Detection of *Trichomonas vaginalis* in pregnant women with the In Pouch TV Culture System. J. Clin. Microbiol. *31*:1016–1018, 1993.
12. Ekwempu, C. C., Lawande, R. V., and Egler, L. J.: Microbial flora of the lower genital tract of women in labour in Zaria, Nigeria. J. Clin. Pathol. *34*:82–83, 1981.
13. Fisher, I., and Morton, R. S.: Epididymitis due to *Trichomonas vaginalis*. Br. J. Vener. Dis. *45*:252–253, 1969.
14. Fouts, A. C., and Kraus, S. J.: *Trichomonas vaginalis:* Reevaluation of its clinical presentation and laboratory diagnosis. J. Infect. Dis. *141*:137–143, 1980.
15. Frau, L. M., and Alexander, E. R.: Public health implications of sexually transmitted diseases in pediatric practice. Pediatr. Infect. Dis. *4*:453–467, 1985.
16. Garber, G. E., Lemchuk-Favel, L. T., and Rousseau, G.: Effect of estradiol on cell detaching factor of *Trichomonas vaginalis*. Clin. Microbiol. *29*:1847–1849, 1991.
17. Graves, A., and Gardner, W. A., Jr.: Pathogenicity of *Trichomonas vaginalis*. Clin. Obstet. Gynecol. *36*:145–152, 1993.
18. Gray, L. A., and Kotcher, E.: Vulvovaginitis in childhood. Clin. Obstet. Gynecol. *3*:165–174, 1960.
19. 2002 Guidelines for treatment of sexually transmitted disease. Centers for Disease Control and Prevention. M. M. W. R. Recomm. Rep. *51*(RR-6), 2002.
20. Hammerschlag, M. R., Alpert, S., Rosner, I., et al.: Microbiology of the vagina in children: Normal and potentially pathogenic organisms. Pediatrics *62*:57–62, 1978.
21. Hardy, P. H., Hardy, J. B., Nell, E. E., et al.: Prevalence of six sexually transmitted disease agents among pregnant inner-city adolescents and pregnancy outcome. Lancet *2*:333–337, 1984.
22. Honigberg, B. M.: Trichomonads Parasitic in Humans. New York, Springer-Verlag, 1989.
23. Ireton, R. C., and Berger, R. E.: Prostatitis and epididymitis. Urol. Clin. North Am. *11*:87–88, 1984.
24. Jones, J. G., Yamauchi, T., and Lambert, B.: *Trichomonas vaginalis* infestation in sexually abused girls. Am. J. Dis. Child. *139*:846–847, 1985.
25. Keith, L. G., Berger, G. S., Edelman, D. A., et al.: On the causation of pelvic inflammatory disease. Am. J. Obstet. Gynecol. *149*:215–224, 1983.
26. Klebanoff, M. A., Carey, J. C., Hauth, J. C., et al.: Failure of metronidazole to prevent preterm delivery among pregnant women with asymptomatic *Trichomonas vaginalis* infection. N. Engl. J. Med. *16*:487–493, 2001.
27. Krieger, J. N., Jenny, C., Verdon, M., et al.: Clinical manifestations of trichomoniasis in men. Ann. Intern. Med. *118*:844–849, 1993.
28. Krieger, J. N., and Rein, M. F.: Zinc sensitivity of *Trichomonas vaginalis:* In vitro studies and clinical implications. J. Infect. Dis. *146*:341–345, 1982.
29. Krieger, J. N., Tam, M. R., Stevens, C. E., et al.: Diagnosis of trichomoniasis: Comparison of conventional wet-mount examination with cytologic studies, cultures, and monoclonal antibody staining of direct specimens. J. A. M. A. *259*:1223–1227, 1988.
30. Krieger, J. N., Verdon, M., Siegel, N., et al.: Risk assessment and laboratory diagnosis of *Trichomoniasis* in men. J. Infect. Dis. *166*:1362–1366, 1992.
31. Krowchuk, D. P., Anglin, T. M., and Kumar, M. L.: Rapid diagnosis of common sexually transmitted diseases in adolescents: A review. Pediatr. Dermatol. *6*:278–279, 1989.
32. Kuberski, T.: *Trichomonas vaginalis* associated with nongonococcal urethritis and prostatitis. Sex. Transm. Dis. 7:135–136, 1980.
33. Kurnatowska, A., and Komorowska, A.: Urogenital trichomoniasis in children. *In* Honigberg, B. M. (ed.): Trichomonads Parasitic in Humans. New York, Springer-Verlag, 1989, pp. 246–273.
34. Lang, W. R.: Premenarchal vaginitis. Obstet. Gynecol. *13*:723–729, 1959.
35. Lawing, L. F., Hedges, S. R., and Schwebke, J. R.: Detection of trichomoniasis in vaginal and urine specimens from women by culture and PCR. J. Clin. Microbiol. *38*:3585–3588, 2000.
36. Lisi, P. J., Dondero, R. S., Kwiatkoski, D., et al.: Monoclonal-antibody–based enzyme-linked immunosorbent assay for *Trichomonas vaginalis*. J. Clin. Microbiol. *26*:1684–1686, 1988.
37. Lossick, J.: Epidemiology of urogenital trichomoniasis. *In* Honigberg, B. M. (ed.): Trichomonads Parasitic in Humans. New York, Springer-Verlag, 1989, pp. 311–323.
38. Lossick, J.: Therapy of urogenital trichomoniasis. *In* Honigberg, B. M. (ed.): Trichomonads Parasitic in Humans. New York, Springer-Verlag, 1989, pp. 324–341.
39. Mason, P. R., MacCallum, M. J., and Poynter, B.: Association of *Trichomonas vaginalis* with other microorganisms. Lancet *1*:1067, 1982.
40. Mason, P. R., Super, H., and Fripp, P. J.: Comparison of four techniques for the routine diagnosis of *Trichomonas vaginalis* infection. J. Clin. Pathol. *29*:154–157, 1976.
41. McLellan, R., Spence, M. R., Brockman, M., et al.: The clinical diagnosis of trichomoniasis. Obstet. Gynecol. *60*:30–34, 1982.
42. Moldwin, R. M.: Sexually transmitted protozoal infections. Urol. Clin. North Am. *19*:93–96, 1992.
43. Neinstein, L. S., Goldenring, J., and Carpenter, S.: Nonsexual transmission of sexually transmitted diseases: An infrequent occurrence. Pediatrics *74*:71–72, 1984.
44. Paradise, J. E., Campos, J. M., Friedman, H. M., et al.: Vulvovaginitis in premenarchal girls: Clinical features and diagnostic evaluation. Pediatrics *70*:193–198, 1982.
45. Perl, G. A.: Errors in the diagnosis of *Trichomonas vaginalis* infection as observed among 1199 patients. Obstet. Gynecol. *39*:7–9, 1972.
46. Rubino, S., Muresu, R., Rappelli, P., et al.: Molecular probe for identification of *Trichomona vaginalis*. J. Clin. Microbiol. *29*:702, 1991.
47. Saxena, S. B., and Jenkins, R. R.: Prevalence of *Trichomonas vaginalis* in men at high risk for sexually transmitted diseases. Sex. Transm. Dis. *18*:138–142, 1991.
48. Schares, T., Machtinger, S., D'Harlingue, A. E., et al.: *Trichomonas vaginalis* urinary tract infection in an infant. Pediatr. Infect. Dis. *1*:340–341, 1982.
49. van der Schee, C., van Belkum, A, Zwijgers, L., et al.: Improved diagnosis of *Trichomonas vaginalis* infection by PCR using vaginal swabs and urine specimens compared to diagnosis by wet-mount microscopy, culture, and fluorescent staining. J. Clin. Microbiol. *37*:4127–4130, 1999.
50. Schmid, G. P., Matheny, L. C., Zaidi, A. A., et al.: Evaluation of six media for the growth of *Trichomonas vaginalis* from vaginal secretions. J. Clin. Microbiol. *6*:1230–1233, 1989.
51. Schmid, G., Narcisi, E., Mosure, D., et al.: Prevalence of metronidazole-resistant *Trichomonas vaginalis* in a gynecology clinic. J. Reprod. Med. *46*:545–549, 2001.
52. Sobel, J. D., Nagappan, V., and Nyirjesy, P.: Metronidazole-resistant vaginal trichomoniasis: An emerging problem. N. Engl. J. Med. *341*:292–293, 1999.
53. Sowmini, C. N., Vijayalakshmi, K., Chellamuthiah, C., et al.: Infections of the median raphe of the penis: Report of three cases. Br. J. Vener. Dis. *49*:469–474, 1972.
54. Spence, M. R., Hollander, D. H., Smith, J., et al.: The clinical and laboratory diagnosis of *Trichomonas vaginalis* infection. Sex. Transm. Dis. 7:168–171, 1980.
55. Spiegel, C: Microflora associated with *Trichomonas vaginalis* and vaccination against vaginal trichomoniasis. *In* Honigberg, B. M. (ed.): Trichomonads Parasitic in Humans. New York, Springer-Verlag, 1989, pp. 213–224.
56. Thomason, J. L., and Gelbart, S. M.: *Trichomonas vaginalis*. Obstet. Gynecol. *74*:536–540, 1989.
57. Watt, L., and Jennison, R. F.: Incidence of *Trichomonas vaginalis* in marital partners. Br. J. Vener. Dis. *36*:163–166, 1960.
58. White, S. T., Loda, F. A., Ingram, D. L., et al.: Sexually transmitted diseases in sexually abused children. Pediatrics *72*:16–21, 1983.
59. Wolner-Hanssen, P. W., Krieger, J. N., Stevens, C. E., et al.: Clinical manifestations of vaginal trichomoniasis. J. A. M. A. *261*:571–576, 1989.
60. Wilcox, R. R.: Epidemiological aspects of human trichomoniasis. Br. J. Vener. Dis. *36*:167–174, 1960.

C. CILIATES (INTESTINAL)

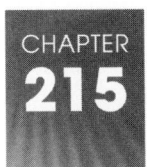

Balantidium coli Infection

PETER J. HOTEZ

Balantidium coli is the largest protozoan parasite and the only ciliate to infect humans.[6, 9, 15] The organism has a worldwide distribution, but it usually is found in the less developed nations of the tropics. Because pigs are a principal animal reservoir, most human infections have been reported in tropical regions where swine have close contact with humans, such as the islands of the South Pacific (including Papua New Guinea) and Central and South America.[10] Balantidiasis occurs in areas where other swine-associated parasitic zoonoses (e.g., taeniasis, trichinellosis, ascariasis) also are prevalent, although infection with *B. coli* still occurs rarely. Fewer than 1000 cases of human balantidiasis are reported in the literature.[9] The organism first was described in 1857 by P. H. Malmsten, who observed the ciliates from two patients in Sweden.[3]

Etiology and Pathogenesis

The organism has both trophozoite and cyst stages. The trophozoite is a large, pear-shaped organism covered with cilia. Estimates of size range from 50 to 100 μm in length and 40 to 70 μm in width.[6] This relatively enormous protozoan organism typically can be seen by light microscopy using only low-power magnification.[6] Subcellular organelles, such as a cytostome and many large vacuoles containing bacteria and debris, are visualized under higher magnification. Like many other ciliates, *B. coli* trophozoites have a macronucleus and a micronucleus. The trophozoites colonize the large intestine, where ultimately they round up and secrete a cyst wall as they pass down the lumen. The cysts measure 50 to 70 μm and also contain a macronucleus and a micronucleus. The cyst stages can survive in the outside environment and are infectious to a wide range of animals, including humans (discussed later).

Frequently, *B. coli* does not invade human tissues and, therefore, does not cause clinical disease. Under conditions that are not understood well, however, *B. coli* also has the potential for highly aggressive invasion and destruction of tissue. Whether the invasive potential of *B. coli* results from parasite virulence, compromised host defenses, or some combination of these two factors is not clear. The observation that invasive disease occurs more commonly in debilitated patients and in patients with polyparasitism suggests that host defenses have an important role in limiting tissue destruction by *B. coli*.[1, 9]

When parasite invasion occurs, it begins in the colonic mucosa, where ulcerations and secondary microabscesses can result. Extensive tissue damage in the cecum and appendix results in clinical presentations of typhlitis and appendicitis, respectively.[4, 5, 9] Histopathologic examination of these tissues reveals flask-shaped ulcerations and necrosis with an extensive inflammatory infiltrate composed predominantly of polymorphonuclear leukocytes.[4, 9] *B. coli* probably creates mucosal ulcerations through the release of histolytic enzymes similar to those described from *Entamoeba histolytica*.[12] Ulcerations can lead to hemorrhage or even colonic perforation. A second type of histopathology wherein patients harboring *B. coli* develop inflammatory polyposis of the rectum and sigmoid colon has been reported.[8]

When tissue invasion is extensive, the organism can metastasize to extraintestinal sites and cause hepatic and pulmonary involvement. Polymorphonuclear inflammatory cell infiltration results in abscesses at these sites.[3, 5, 8] Most patients with metastatic balantidiasis have recognizable defects in host defenses.[8]

Epidemiology

As noted earlier, human balantidiasis has a worldwide distribution, but epidemic foci have been reported in the swine-producing areas of Papua New Guinea, Micronesia, the Seychelles Islands, and Central and South America.[3, 10, 13] Incidence rates can be high among swine farmers and slaughterhouse workers. The potential for development of human *B. coli* infections is thought to be high in areas of poor hygiene where extensive contact occurs between humans and pigs. A notorious outbreak of human balantidiasis occurred after a devastating typhoon on the Pacific island of Truk caused widespread contamination of ground and surface water supplies with pig feces.[13] Many other animals, including nonhuman primates, guinea pigs, horses, cattle, and rats, also can serve potentially as reservoir hosts. *B. coli* also colonizes many great apes, including baboons, orangutans, chimpanzees, and gorillas, and clinical balantidiasis has been reported in these primates when they are maintained in captivity.[9] Human epidemics also have been described in institutional settings, especially where crowding mixes with low levels of personal hygiene.[13] In these instances, human-to-human spread has been postulated. Although not known as an opportunistic pathogen in patients infected with human immunodeficiency virus, at least one case of *B. coli* in this setting has been described.[3]

Clinical Manifestations

ASYMPTOMATIC INFECTION

Most infections are asymptomatic or cause occasional loose stools. This situation probably accounts for as many as 85 percent of patients harboring *B. coli*.[9] Asymptomatic infection may occur more commonly in children than in adults.[14]

DIARRHEA

The next most frequent presentation of *B. coli* infections is in patients who have intermittent diarrhea, abdominal pain, and weight loss.[14] Sometimes, discrete ulcerations can be observed during sigmoidoscopy.[9] A subset of these patients develop invasive disease subsequently.

INVASIVE COLONIC BALANTIDIASIS

The hallmark of *Balantidium* colitis is dysentery with bloody and mucous stools, colonic tenderness, leukocytosis, and fever. Sigmoidoscopy and colonoscopy of these patients reveal ulcerations and formation of mucosal granulomata.[1, 9, 11, 13] Involvement of the large intestine can be diffuse, although in some cases, right-sided colonic lesions predominate. Right-sided colonic lesions can progress to typhlitis or appendicitis.[4, 5, 9] Transmural involvement of the colon frequently results in intestinal obstruction, hemorrhage, and balantidial peritonitis. Colonic perforation is an ominous complication that is associated with extremely high mortality.[9]

METASTATIC BALANTIDIASIS

Highly invasive balantidiasis leading to metastatic disease of the mesenteric lymph nodes, liver, and lung is a rare complication that can occur in malnourished, debilitated, and immunocompromised patients.

Diagnosis

Stools from patients harboring *B. coli* have been described as having a pigpen odor.[14] The examination of wet preparations of fresh or concentrated stools usually demonstrates cyst and trophozoite forms of *B. coli*. Cilia motility and rapid rotary motion of the trophozoites occasionally can be appreciated under low-power magnification. Because the organism takes up heavy concentrations of dye, stained preparations typically do not reveal internal structures or even cilia.[6] These large organisms can be confused with helminth ova, especially on stained preparations.[6] As an adjunct to direct fecal examinations, sigmoidoscopy can demonstrate ulcerations from which abundant trophozoites may be obtained for diagnosis.[14]

Treatment

For the treatment of intestinal balantidiasis, numerous chemotherapeutic regimens have been tried, usually with some improvement. In many cases, however, the parasite is not eradicated.[9] For children older than 8 years of age, tetracycline (40 mg/kg/day in four doses for 10 days [maximum, 2 g/day]) is the treatment of choice. Tetracycline is considered to be investigational for this condition by the U.S. Food and Drug Administration. Also considered investigational for balantidiasis are the drugs iodoquinol (40 mg/kg/day in three doses for 20 days) and metronidazole (35 to 50 mg/kg/day in three doses for 5 days).[2, 7] Alternative chemotherapeutic agents that have been tried with varying degrees of success include paromomycin and chloroquine.[9] Surgical intervention often is required for gastrointestinal invasive complications of *B. coli,* such as typhlitis, appendicitis, and peritonitis.

REFERENCES

1. Arean, V. M., and Koppisch, E: Balantidiasis. A review and report of cases. Am. J. Pathol. *32*:1089–1116, 1956.
2. Beasley, J. W., and Walzer, P. D.: Ineffectiveness of metronidazole in treatment of *Balantidium coli* infections. Trans. R. Soc. Trop. Med. Hyg. *66*:519, 1972.
3. Clyti, E., Aznar, C., Couppie, P., et al.: A case of coinfection by *Balantidium coli* and HIV in French Guiana. Bull. Soc. Pathol. Exotique *91*:309–311, 1998.
4. Dodd, L. G.: *Balantidium coli* infestation as a cause of acute appendicitis. J. Infect. Dis. *163*:1392, 1991.
5. Dorfman, S., Rangel, O., and Bravo, L. G.: Balantidiasis: Report of a fatal case with appendicular and pulmonary involvement. Trans. R. Soc. Trop. Med. Hyg. *78*:833–834, 1984.
6. Garcia, L. S., and Bruckner, D. A.: Diagnostic Medical Parasitology. 2nd ed. Washington, D.C., American Society for Microbiology, 1993, pp. 44–46.
7. Garcia-Laverde, A., and DeBonilla, L.: Clinical trials with metronidazole in human balantidiasis. Am. J. Trop. Med. Hyg. *24*:781–783, 1975.
8. Ladas, S. D., Savva, S., Frydas, A., et al.: Invasive balantidiasis presented as chronic colitis and lung involvement. Dig. Dis. Sci. *34*:1621–1623, 1989.
9. Lee, R. V., Prowten, A. W., Anthone, S., et al.: Typhlitis due to *Balantidium coli* in captive lowland gorillas. Rev. Infect. Dis. *12*:1052–1059, 1990.
10. Radford, A. J.: Balantidiasis in Papua New Guinea. Med. J. Aust. *1*:238–241, 1971.
11. Swartzwelder, J. C.: Balantidiasis. Am. J. Dig. Dis. *17*:173–179, 1950.
12. Tempelis, C. H., and Lysenko, M. G.: The production of a hyaluronidase by *B. coli*. Exp. Parasitol. *6*:31–36, 1957.
13. Walzer, P. D., Judson, F. N., Murphy, K. B., et al.: Balantidiasis outbreak in Truk. Am. J. Trop. Med. Hyg. *22*:33–41, 1973.
14. Woody, N. C., and Woody, H. B.: Balantidiasis in infancy: Review of literature and report of a case. J. Pediatr. *56*:485–489, 1960.
15. Young, M. D.: Balantidiasis. J. A. M. A. *113*:580–584, 1939.

D. COCCIDIA, INICNOSPORIDIA (INTESTINAL)

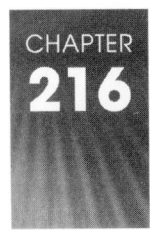

Cryptosporidiosis, *Cyclospora* Infection, Isosporiasis, and Microsporidiosis

JANE T. ATKINS ■ THOMAS G. CLEARY

The enteric coccidian parasites *(Cryptosporidium, Cyclospora,* and *Isospora)* and microsporidia are obligate intracellular protozoans that now are known to cause gastrointestinal disease in both immunocompetent and immunocompromised humans.[260, 289] *Sarcocystis,* another coccidian organism that may use humans as intermediate hosts, rarely causes disease. These pathogens were virtually unknown before the human immunodeficiency virus (HIV) epidemic. In an immunocompetent host, these enteric coccidian parasites typically cause an illness that is short lived, but in an immunodeficient host, they cause prolonged life-threatening diarrheal illness, as well as extraintestinal disease.

Cryptosporidiosis

Cryptosporidium is a coccidian protozoan that infects the gastric and respiratory epithelium of vertebrates.[67, 96] It first was identified in the gastric glands of laboratory mice by Tyzzer[325] in 1907 and for decades was considered to be nonpathogenic. However, not until 1976 were the first human cases of cryptosporidiosis reported.[218, 246] Before 1982, fewer than 10 cases of human cryptosporidiosis were reported in the literature.[96] With the advent of the acquired immunodeficiency syndrome (AIDS) epidemic, *Cryptosporidium* has emerged as a significant human pathogen and now is recognized as a common cause of diarrheal disease in immunocompetent as well as immunocompromised hosts.[67, 115]

MICROBIOLOGY

Cryptosporidium spp. are ubiquitous, small (2 to 6 μm), obligate intracellular parasites that infect the epithelium of the gastrointestinal and respiratory tracts of vertebrates.[64, 67] They are related to *Toxoplasma, Isospora, Plasmodium, Eimeria,* and *Sarcocystis.* The taxonomic classification of *Cryptosporidium, Isospora, Cyclospora,* and *Sarcocystis* is summarized in Figure 216–1.

Researchers initially assumed that *Cryptosporidium,* like other coccidia, was host-specific. Thus, cryptosporidia were speciated according to the animal that they infected.[67, 96] However, cross-transmission studies revealed that little host specificity for species of *Cryptosporidium* exists.[80, 96, 326] Molecular analysis has demonstrated substantial genetic heterogeneity among isolates of *Cryptosporidium* from different vertebrate hosts, thus suggesting a series of host-adopted genotype/strains/species.[238] Twenty-three species of *Cryptosporidium* have been described in the literature.[366] Presently, eight are recognized by taxonomists as valid species. Phylogenetic analysis of the 18S rDNA and heat shock protein-70 (HSP-70) sequences suggest that at least two unnamed avian species may exist.[234] The eight named species are *Cryptosporidium nasorum,* which infects fish, *Cryptosporidium serpentis,* which infects reptiles; *Cryptosporidium baileyi* and *Cryptosporidium meleagridis,* which infect birds; and *Cryptosporidium muris, Cryptosporidium felis, Cryptosporidium wrairi,* and *Cryptosporidium parvum,* which infect mammals. Several genotypes exist within these eight species. *C. parvum* genotypes 1 (human or anthroponotic genotype) and 2 (bovine or zoonotic genotype) are responsible for most human infections. The *C. parvum* dog genotype, *C. meleagridis,* and *C. felis* occasionally cause infection in immunocompetent children and HIV-infected patients.[237, 267, 366] *C. parvum* genotype 1 infects humans exclusively, with the exception of a single report of infection in a dugong *(Dugong dugon).*[239]

LIFE CYCLE

The life cycle of *Cryptosporidium* is monoxenous; that is, the entire life cycle is completed in a single host. Similar to other true coccidia, the life cycle of *Cryptosporidium* is characterized by six major developmental stages: (1) excystation, or release of infective sporozoites; (2) merogony, or asexual replication in the host; (3) gametogony, or the formation of microgametocytes and macrogametocytes; (4) fertilization, or the union of microgametocyte and macrogametocyte; (5) oocyst formation; and (6) sporogony, or the formation of infectious sporozoites within the oocyst wall.[58, 67, 68]

The life cycle of *Cryptosporidium* is summarized in Figure 216–2.

In humans, the life cycle begins with ingestion or possibly inhalation of the thick-walled oocyst from the environment. Excystation occurs in the small intestines and results in the release of four nonflagellated sporozoites that penetrate enterocytes by a flexing and twisting motion.[67] For most coccidia, excystation requires pancreatic enzymes, reducing conditions, and bile salt. Excystation of *Cryptosporidium* sporozoites can occur in an aqueous solution without these conditions, although it is optimal in the presence of trypsin and sodium taurocholate. The ability of *Cryptosporidium* to excyst without much stimulation may explain why it infects extraintestinal sites.[326] Once excystation has occurred, the sporozoite indents and invaginates the enterocyte surface in a glovelike manner to form a parasitiferous vacuole that is confined to the microvillous region. At the base of the parasitiferous vacuole is the "feeder organelle" (Fig. 216–3*A*). This organelle is formed at the attachment site by complex folding of the parasite membrane and serves as a source of sustenance.[203]

The sporozoite differentiates into a spherical, uninucleated trophozoite that undergoes merogony to form a

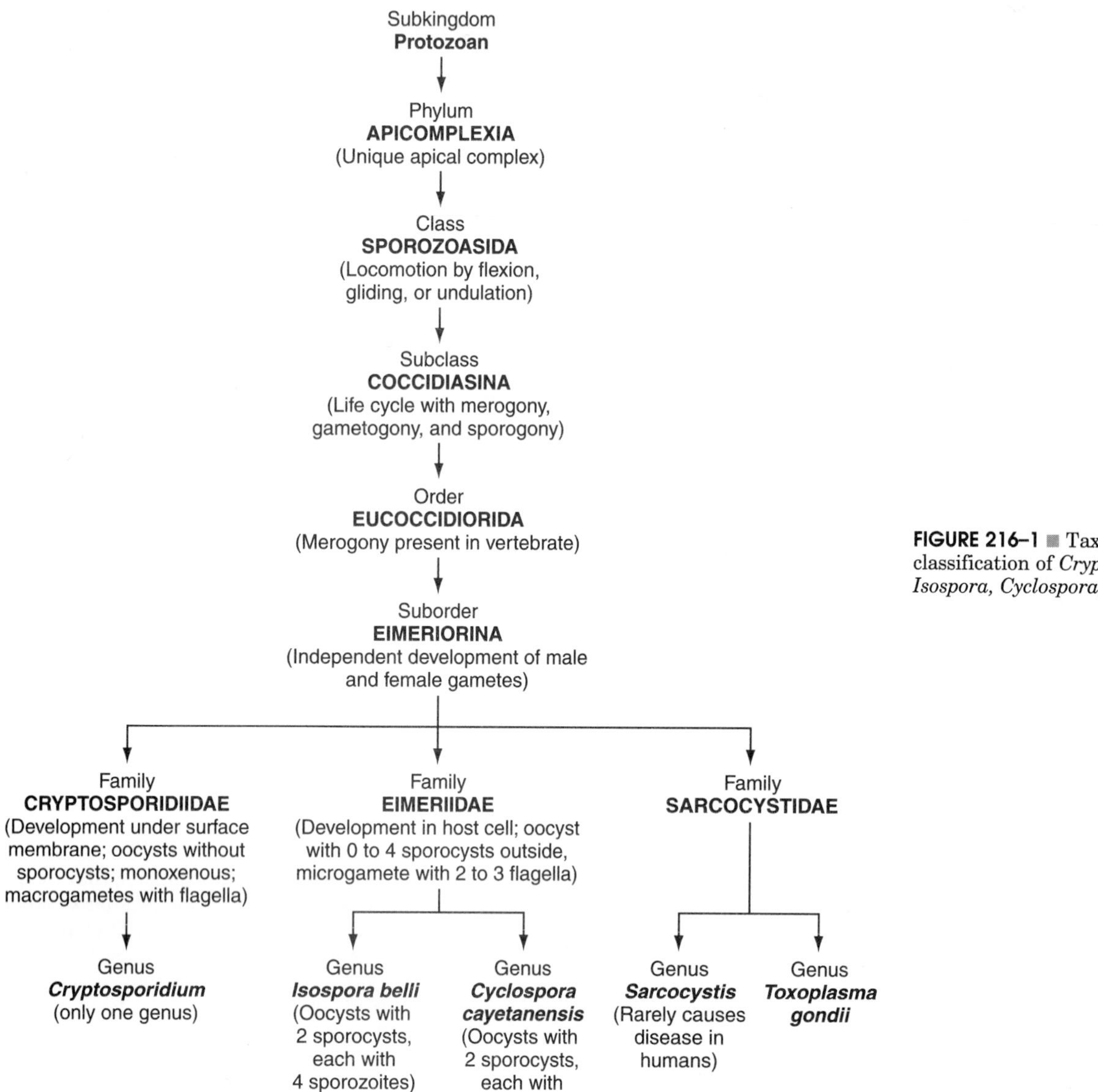

FIGURE 216–1 ■ Taxonomic classification of *Cryptosporidium, Isospora, Cyclospora,* and *Sarcocystis.*

type I meront. A mature type I meront contains six to eight merozoites (see Fig. 216–3*B*) that are released into the intestinal lumen and invade new uninfected enterocytes either to develop into more type I meronts (autoinfection) or to differentiate into type II meronts. A mature type II meront releases four merozoites that invade uninfected microvilli and undergo gametogony (sexual multiplication) to form either microgametocytes or macrogametocytes. The fourth developmental stage (fertilization) occurs when free microgametes make contact with the parasitiferous membrane covering the female macrogamete and penetrate into the macrogamete. The fertilized macrogametocyte matures into an oocyst that undergoes sporogony, thus completing the life cycle.[58, 67, 68] Approximately 80 percent of the oocysts are released into the environment in feces as dense, thick-walled cysts. The remaining 20 percent develop into thin-walled cysts that sporulate within the intestinal tract and autoinfect the host.[69] The presence of two autoinfective stages (type I meront and thin-walled oocyst) in the life cycle of *Cryptosporidium* may explain why severe infection can develop after the ingestion of small numbers of oocysts and why persistent, life-threatening illness can occur in immunocompromised hosts.[67]

EPIDEMIOLOGY

Cryptosporidium is distributed worldwide.[58, 67, 370] Prevalence rates in general are higher in developing countries than in industrialized countries. The prevalence of *Cryptosporidium* in stool has been reported to be 1 to 3 percent in the industrialized countries of North America and Europe; in undeveloped countries, it ranges from 5 percent in Asia to 10 percent in Africa.[67] The seroprevalence of antibodies to *Cryptosporidium* in industrialized regions of North America and Europe ranges from 25 to 35 percent and is as high as 64 percent in developing countries of South America.[39, 67, 137, 329] Travelers to endemic areas are at risk for acquiring cryptosporidiosis.[330]

Cryptosporidium has been reported more frequently in children than adults. Infection is particularly common in the first 2 years of life. In India, the prevalence rate for

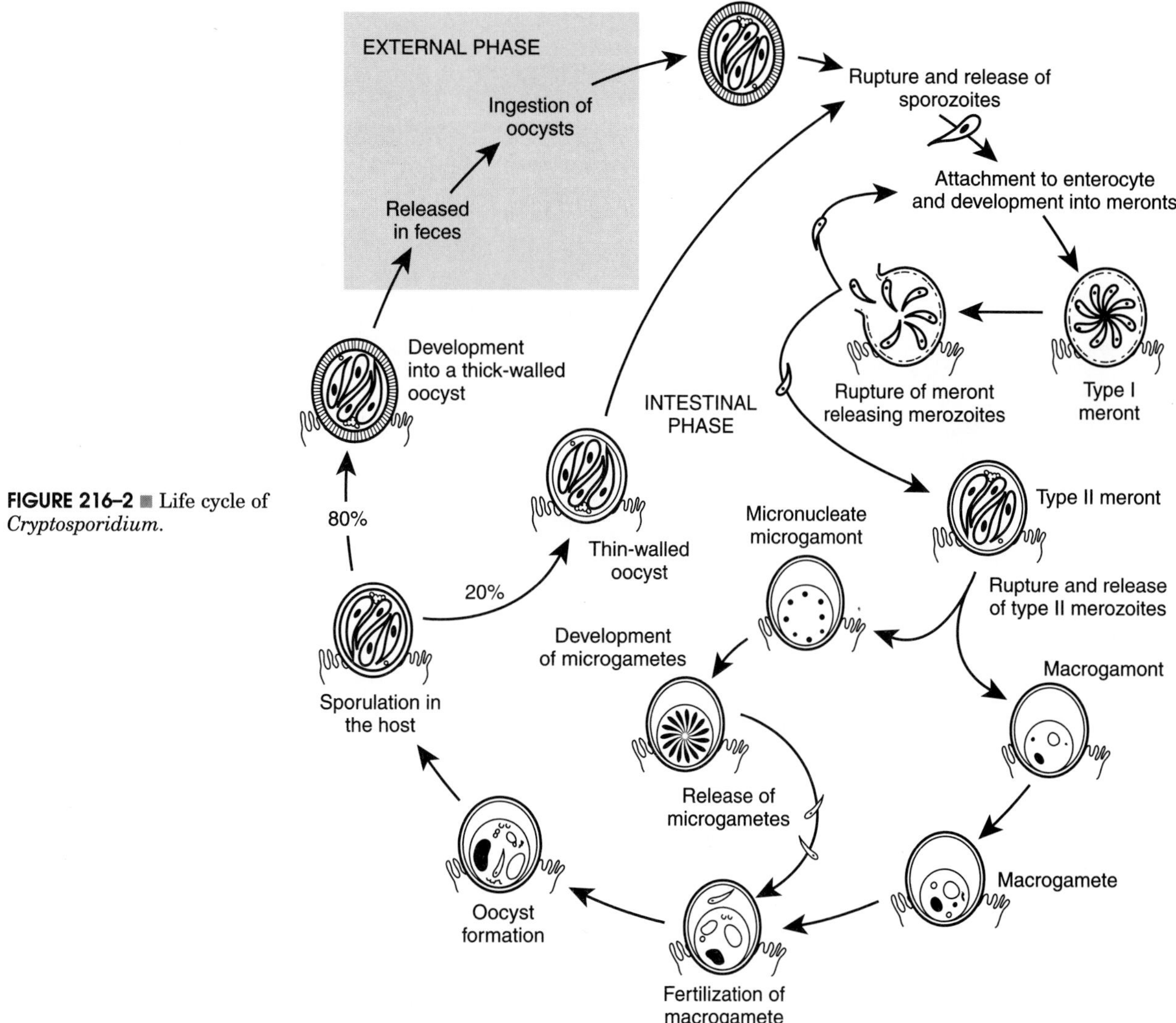

FIGURE 216–2 ■ Life cycle of *Cryptosporidium.*

children is 5.5 to 9.8 percent[74, 209]; in Liberia, it is 5.9 percent[150]; and in Guatemala it is 5.4 to 11.6 percent.[23, 60] The prevalence of asymptomatic infection with *Cryptosporidium* in children younger than 5 years varies with geographic location and is estimated to be less than 0.5 percent.[342] However, Pettoello-Mantovani and colleagues[266] reported a high prevalence of asymptomatic infection with *Cryptosporidium* in children from Naples, Italy (6.4% in immunocompetent children and 22% in immunodeficient children). Young children in the daycare setting are at high risk for acquiring infection.[54, 84] Outbreaks of cryptosporidiosis in childcare centers have been reported from the United States,[3, 51, 61, 138, 248, 303, 312, 317–319] Great Britain,[131] Australia,[59, 97] France,[31] Portugal,[219] Chile,[244, 358] and South Africa.[343]

Cryptosporidiosis is a common cause of diarrhea in patients infected with HIV.[49] Overall, in the United States, *Cryptosporidium* is reported as the AIDS-defining illness in 2.2 percent of HIV-infected patients reported to the Centers for Disease Control and Prevention (CDC). In children, 3.5 percent of cases reported to the CDC have cryptosporidiosis as the AIDS-defining illness.[166] Cryptosporidiosis occurs in an estimated 10 to 15 percent of patients with AIDS in United States and in 30 to 50 percent of patients with AIDS in developing countries.[201] In recent years, the widespread use of highly active antiretroviral therapy (HAART) has resulted in the restoration of immune function and, thus, a reduction in the incidence of cryptosporidiosis and other opportunistic infections.[200, 259]

Seasonal variation has been noted in some geographic locations. In tropical climates, the incidence of cryptosporidiosis is higher during the warm, humid months,[192, 208, 265, 298, 355] whereas in temperate climates, a late summer and early fall peak is observed.[199, 223, 231, 323, 362] In the United States, investigators have not observed a consistent seasonal variation.[16, 151, 163, 328, 362] However, daycare center outbreaks of cryptosporidiosis in the United States occur most often in the late summer and early autumn.[54]

TRANSMISSION

Person-to-person transmission through the fecal-oral route is the principal mechanism of transmission of *Cryptosporidium*. *Cryptosporidium* also is acquired by the ingestion of fecally contaminated water or food, by handling infected animals, or by contact with environmental surfaces contaminated with infected feces. Airborne transmission has been suggested but has not been proved.[22, 148] Secondary spread of *C. parvum* has been reported in the daycare setting,[54, 131] among household contacts,[65, 245] and in the hospital

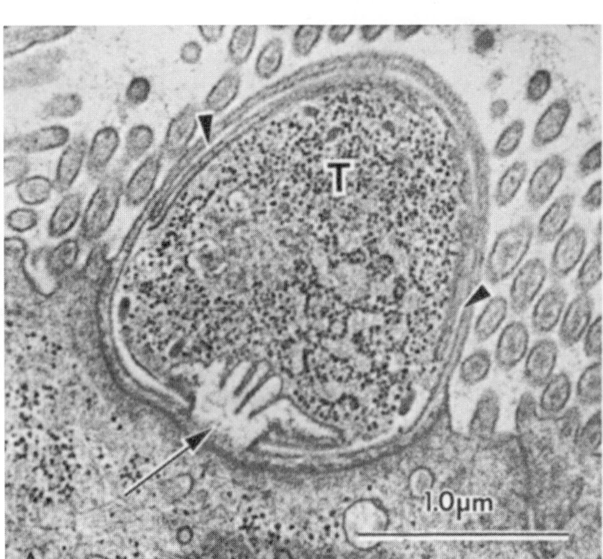

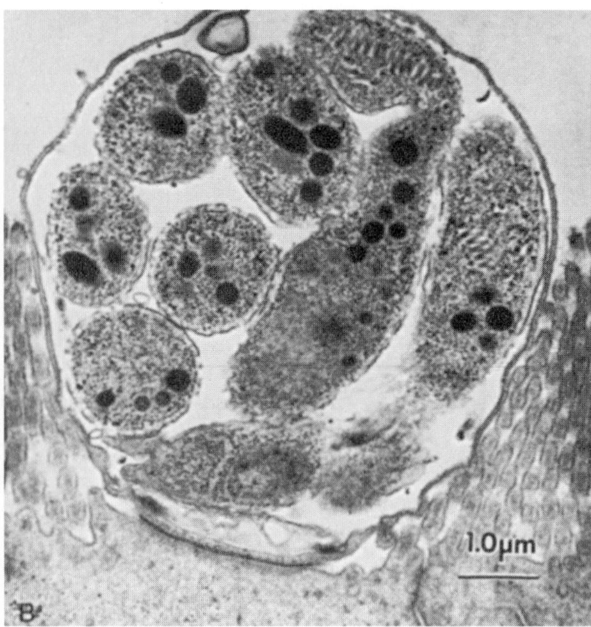

FIGURE 216–3 ■ Intestinal biopsy of a patient with AIDS infected with *Cryptosporidium. A,* Transmission electron micrograph of a trophozoite (T) within a parasitophorous vacuole. A space *(arrowheads)* separates the outer double membrane of the infected host intestinal cell from the inner double membrane surrounding the trophozoite. The "feeder organelle" *(arrow)* lies just above the dense attachment zone. *B,* Transmission electron micrograph of a type 1 meront containing portions of seven merozoites within the parasitophorous vacuole.

setting.[50, 87, 170, 207, 240, 242] The estimated median infective dose is 132 organisms, but as few as 30 organisms can cause infection in a susceptible host.[89] The incubation period of cryptosporidiosis in humans has been estimated to be 2 to 14 days.[58, 164]

During the acute diarrheal illness, large quantities of oocysts are excreted in stool and are highly infectious. Smaller quantities of oocysts are excreted with asymptomatic infections and during the convalescent phase.[3, 51] Asymptomatic shedding of oocysts may continue for up to 5 weeks after an acute episode of diarrhea.[312] Transmission to contacts can occur even when low quantities of oocysts are excreted.[3, 51] Fomites may play a role in the transmission of *Cryptosporidium,* especially in the daycare setting, where fecal contamination is a common occurrence.[3, 51, 335]

Cryptosporidium is a resilient organism. How long oocysts remain viable once they are excreted into the natural environment is not known. In the laboratory, oocysts suspended in calf feces are viable for at least 2 days on a dried wooden surface at room temperature.[5] Freezing at −20° C for 72 hours[279] and heating to 45° to 55° C for 20 minutes[4, 95] reduce the infectivity. An aqueous suspension of oocysts can be rendered noninfectious by exposure to 72.4° C for 1 minute, 64.2° C for longer than 2 minutes,[98] or ultraviolet light for 150 minutes.[190, 193] The parasite is resistant to disinfectants commonly used by hospitals and daycare centers, including 3 percent hypochlorite, sodium hydroxide, iodophors, cresylic acid, benzalkonium chloride, and 5 percent formaldehyde. It is sensitive to prolonged exposure to 70 to 100 percent bleach, 5 to 10 percent ammonia, and 10 percent formaldehyde.[7, 8, 35]

Infected water is a major source of transmission of *Cryptosporidium.*[107] Water-borne outbreaks of cryptosporidiosis have occurred in association with contaminated water from artesian wells,[73] surface water,[108, 110, 199] swimming pools,[45, 63, 162, 212, 311] and filtered public drinking water.[55, 137, 165, 276] *Cryptosporidium* has been found in treated water that meets the standard requirements for water purification, including filtration and chlorination.[73, 110, 121, 137] The largest water-borne outbreak of cryptosporidiosis caused by a contaminated public water supply occurred in Milwaukee, Wisconsin, in spring 1993; researchers estimated that more than 400,000 persons were infected.[196]

A wide variety of vertebrates, including fish, reptiles, birds, and mammals (e.g., horses, sheep, cows, primates, and domestic dogs and cats), are infected with *Cryptosporidium.*[7, 32, 81, 97, 153, 157, 202, 224, 326] Farmers and animal handlers are at increased risk for infection. However, zoonotic transmission is not as common as person-to-person and water-borne spread.[6, 70, 92, 274, 326] Transmission of *Cryptosporidium* from invertebrates rarely occurs. A case of *Cryptosporidium* detected in the gut of a common cockroach that was suspected to be the source of infection in a Peruvian child has been reported.[367, 368]

PATHOLOGY AND PATHOGENESIS

The proximal part of the small bowel is the primary site of infection.[41, 80, 326] In an immunocompromised patient, the entire intestinal tract from the oropharynx to the rectum may be infected. Histopathologic findings (Fig. 216–4) of cryptosporidiosis include patchy infection of the intestinal mucosa with mild to moderate villous atrophy, crypt hyperplasia, and mononuclear and polymorphonuclear cell infiltration of the lamina propria.[178, 180, 243] The stages in the life cycle of the parasite can be visualized with electron microscopy (see Fig. 216–3). In animals, an association exists between the extent of intestinal damage and clinical symptoms; however, this association has not been demonstrated in humans.[326]

The precise mechanism of diarrhea in human cryptosporidiosis has not been fully elucidated. Most enteric

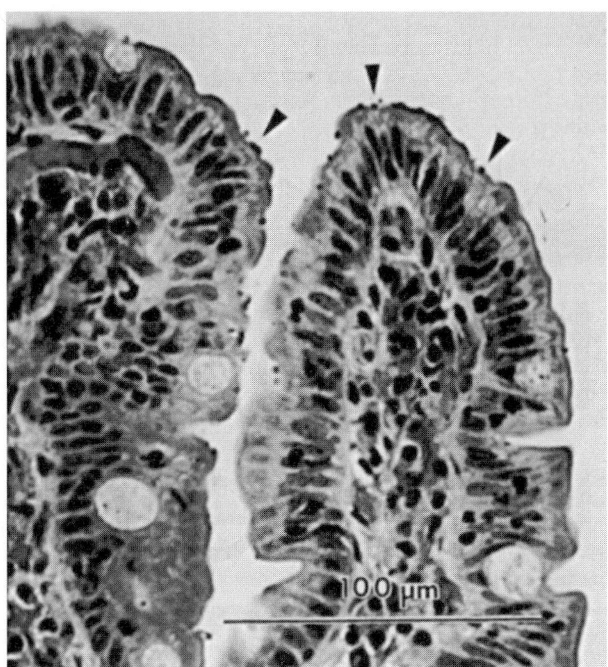

FIGURE 216–4 ■ Light micrograph of spherical, darkly stained cryptosporidia *(arrows)* embedded in the surfaces of jejunal villi from a boy with chronic diarrhea and congenital immunoglobulin deficiency. (From Heyworth, M. F., and Owen, R. L.: Gastrointestinal aspects of the acquired immunodeficiency syndrome. Surv. Dig. Dis. *3*:197, 1985.)

pathogens cause diarrhea by either impairing absorption or enhancing excretion. Clinically, impaired intestinal absorption and permeability have been observed in patients with AIDS infected with *Cryptosporidium.*[123] The profuse, watery diarrhea suggests a toxin-mediated process. Guarino and colleagues reported enterotoxin activity in fecal samples from patients with cryptosporidiosis.[129] However, these finding are controversial.[180] In the porcine model, *Cryptosporidium* impairs glucose-stimulated Na^+ and H_2O absorption or increases Cl^- excretion, or both.[10] Local production of prostaglandin contributes to the excretion of mucosal fluid and diarrheal illness in piglets with cryptosporidiosis.[9] In vitro, increased expression of prostaglandin H synthase-2 and production of prostaglandin E_2 and $F_{2\alpha}$ have been reported in human intestinal epithelium infected with *C. parvum.*[179] The cellular source of prostaglandin and the mechanism that leads to increased prostaglandin production are not known.[180] A protein with hemolytic activity (HemA) and its corresponding gene were identified in *C. parvum.* The peptide sequence of this hemolytic protein was similar to that of *Escherichia coli* O157 plasmid-encoded hemolysin. This hemolysin is speculated to play a role in formation of the parasitiferous vacuole and feeding organelle.[309]

IMMUNOLOGY

Innate immunity mediated by mucosal epithelium and acquired immunity mediated by B and T lymphocytes are both important in the defense and clearance of *C. parvum.* The importance of cell-mediated immunity (T_H1) is suggested by the chronic disease seen in AIDS; the relevance of humoral immunity (T_H2) is suggested by the observation that patients with hypogammaglobulinemia may have severe disease.[177, 192] Specific IgG, IgA, IgM, and IgE and secretory IgA antibodies can be measured by indirect fluorescent antibody (IFA) assay and enzyme-linked immunosorbent assay (ELISA), but the significance of these antibodies is not clear.[36, 39, 57, 66, 329, 330] High levels of specific serum and secretory antibodies have been observed in AIDS patients with protracted diarrhea, thus suggesting that a specific antibody response alone is not sufficient to control this infection.[57] $CD4^+$ lymphocytes and interferon-γ (INF-γ) are the two key components in the immune response necessary for clearance and prevention of cryptosporidiosis.[43, 47]

Although the experimental murine cryptosporidiosis models are not perfect models for human cryptosporidiosis, they have played a key role in our understanding of the immune response to *C. parvum* and the significance of $CD4^+$ lymphocytes and INF-γ.[43, 44, 175, 322] In the severe combined immunodeficiency (SCID) murine model of cryptosporidiosis, reconstitution of immune function with immunocompetent donor spleen cells resulted in resolution of infection with *C. parvum.* Reconstituted mice pretreated with anti-CD4 and anti–INF-γ could not clear infection with *C. parvum.*[43] Overwhelming infection developed in C57BL/6 mice with targeted disruption of the INF-γ gene (INF-γ knockout or GKO) and they died. INF-γ facilitates up-regulation of the expression of interleukin-12 (IL-12), inducible nitric oxide synthase (iNOS), and tumor necrosis factor–α (TNF-α). TNF-α appears to participate in the control of parasite development.[175]

In the neonatal murine cryptosporidiosis model, nitric oxide and other reactive nitrogen compounds appear to play a role in limiting the severity of infection. β-Defensins are small peptides that have broad-spectrum antimicrobial properties. A gene that expresses an enteric β-defensin has been demonstrated in the epithelial cells of the small bowel and colon of calves; expression of this gene was up-regulated 5- to 10-fold when calves were infected with *C. parvum.*[318]

Proinflammatory cytokines are produced by intestinal epithelium infected with *C. parvum* during the initial inflammatory response. In vitro, increased expression and secretion of the C-X-C chemokines IL-8 and GRO-α occur on the basolateral surface of human epithelial cell lines (HCT-8 and Caco-2) infected with *C. parvum.*[179] These chemokines are potent neutrophil chemoattractants, which explains the histologic finding of neutrophil infiltration of the subepithelium. In vitro studies using human intestinal xenograft in SCID mice infected with *C. parvum* also revealed increased production and excretion of IL-8 and GRO-α and subepithelial infiltration of neutrophils.[178, 180]

Gomez Morales and colleagues[122] noted antigen-specific in vitro proliferation of peripheral blood mononuclear cells from patients who were sensitized to *C. parvum.* They also found that the supernatant of peripheral blood mononuclear cells from immunocompetent persons contained IL-10 and INF-γ after exposure to *C. parvum* and that levels of INF-γ were significantly higher in persons who recovered from cryptosporidiosis. Children have much lower levels of INF-γ than adults do, and patients with AIDS also have impaired production of INF-γ, which may explain why some children and adults with AIDS have a more severe course with cryptosporidiosis.[122]

CLINICAL MANIFESTATIONS

The clinical spectrum of disease caused by *Cryptosporidium* is broad and depends on the immunologic status of the host.[135] In an immunocompetent host, *Cryptosporidium* infection usually is manifested by intestinal symptoms, whereas in immunodeficient patients, intestinal and extraintestinal involvement may occur. Regardless of the immunologic status of the patient, diarrhea is the most common clinical manifestation of cryptosporidiosis. In immunocompetent patients, the onset of diarrhea is abrupt and the illness is usually self-limited, with a duration of several days to 2 weeks.[168] In developing countries, severe diarrhea may develop in infants and toddlers[38, 205] and result in failure to thrive or contribute to malnutrition.[133, 156, 176, 195, 323] Malnourished children tend to have a protracted course and shed oocysts longer. They often require hospitalization for parenteral therapy, and their disease may have a fatal outcome.[26, 157, 176, 195, 323]

In AIDS patients, the onset of diarrhea is insidious, and the illness can last months and result in severe wasting that is life-threatening. Although intestinal cryptosporidiosis in patients with AIDS usually results in severe diarrhea, asymptomatic infection and spontaneous resolution of diarrhea have been reported in HIV-infected patients.[158] Four distinct gastrointestinal syndromes have been described in HIV-infected patients: (1) a cholera-like syndrome that requires rehydration, (2) a chronic diarrheal illness resulting in wasting, (3) transient diarrhea, and (4) relapsing diarrhea.[201] Intestinal cryptosporidiosis is characterized by a profuse, watery (cholera-like) diarrhea indistinguishable from that associated with other enteric coccidian parasites. Massive fluid loss is common. In patients with AIDS, the average fluid loss is 3 to 6 L/day, but it can be 17 to 20 L/day, and these patients may have 70 stools per day.[62] The stools rarely contain blood and fecal leukocytes; mucus is seen occasionally.[115] Charcot-Leyden crystals are not present. Other less common clinical findings include low-grade fever, crampy abdominal pain, flatulence, nausea, and vomiting.[133, 309] In addition, flulike symptoms such as myalgia, malaise, headache, and anorexia occasionally occur. Weight loss is a common finding in both immunocompetent and immunosuppressed hosts.[67, 115, 367] Chronic diarrhea usually is seen in markedly immunosuppressed HIV-infected individuals with CD4 counts less than 180 cells/mm^3.[101] The introduction of combination antiretroviral therapy has decreased the morbidity and mortality caused by *Cryptosporidium* and other opportunistic infections.[200, 259] Restoration of immune function with HAART has resulted in the resolution of chronic diarrhea associated with *Cryptosporidium*. The resolution of symptoms correlates with increasing CD4 counts rather than a reduction in viral load.[200] Relapse of cryptosporidiosis with discontinuation of antiretroviral therapy suggests that the organism may remain latent.

Other immunodeficient states associated with *Cryptosporidium* infection include cancer,[185, 217, 218, 225, 249, 315] hypogammaglobulinemia,[177, 304] SCID,[171] bone marrow[50, 169] and renal transplantation,[281, 357] and concurrent viral infections such as measles[78] and cytomegalovirus infection.[356] The severity and duration of illness generally depend on the degree of immune deficiency. In patients receiving immunosuppressive therapy, the diarrhea resolved with discontinuation of chemotherapy.[218, 225, 357] In immunodeficient patients, extraintestinal involvement may occur in the respiratory tract, biliary tract, or pancreas.

Respiratory *Cryptosporidium* infection causes cough, shortness of breath, wheezing, croup, and hoarseness.* *Cryptosporidium* has been reported as a cause of laryngobronchitis in children.[132] Not all patients have concurrent intestinal cryptosporidiosis. Oocysts can be identified in sputum, bronchoalveolar lavage fluid, tracheal aspirates, and lung and brush biopsy specimens.[68] *Cryptosporidium* has been identified as the only pathogen or as a co-infecting agent with cytomegalovirus, *Pneumocystis carinii,* and *Mycobacterium* spp.[268]

Cryptosporidiosis of the biliary tract usually is manifested as acalculous cholecystitis or cholangitis and less frequently as sclerosing cholangitis and hepatitis.[20, 25, 126, 128, 204, 269, 292, 334] Signs and symptoms associated with biliary cryptosporidiosis include fever, nonradiating right upper quadrant pain, jaundice, nausea, vomiting, and diarrhea.[20, 67, 323] Elevated levels of bilirubin, alkaline phosphatase, and transaminases may be noted.[20, 67, 323, 334] HIV-infected patients with CD4 counts less than 50/mm^3 are predisposed to biliary cryptosporidiosis.[334] Radiographic findings include dilation of extrahepatic and intrahepatic ducts, thickening of the wall of the gallbladder and extrahepatic ducts, pericholecystic fluid, and stenosis of the distal extrahepatic duct.[20, 323] Concomitant infection with cytomegalovirus can occur and frequently is associated with irregularities of the intrahepatic duct.[20, 144, 167, 323] A definitive diagnosis of biliary cryptosporidiosis is made by biopsy and demonstration of the various stages of *Cryptosporidium* in the biliary tree of a patient with compatible symptoms and abnormal radiographic results.[67, 334]

Pancreatitis is an uncommon manifestation of cryptosporidiosis but has been reported in both adults and children infected with HIV.[37, 126, 136, 144, 167, 171, 227, 320] Pancreatitis may occur concomitantly with cholecystitis.[144, 167, 323] *Cryptosporidium* oocysts have been identified in the pancreatic duct, usually near the head of the pancreas.[171, 323] The associated ductal epithelium generally is transformed to hyperplastic squamous metaplasia.[323]

DIAGNOSIS

Infection with *Cryptosporidium* is confirmed by detection of oocysts in stool or by identifying intracellular stages in tissue from intestinal or extraintestinal sites. Intestinal cryptosporidiosis usually is diagnosed by examination of stool for oocysts. The oocyst of *Cryptosporidium* is readily distinguished from the oocyst of other enteric coccidian parasites by its size and the presence of four mature sporozoites (Table 216–1 and Figs. 216–5 and 216–6). In acute cryptosporidiosis, oocysts are excreted in high concentration and can be seen in direct preparations. Several special staining methods have been explored, including auramine-rhodamine, auramine-carbolfuchsin, dimethyl sulfoxide stain, Giemsa stain, safranin–methylene blue stain, aniline–carbolmethyl violet, and acridine orange.[67, 100, 140, 197, 222, 232] The stains that are used routinely to detect other intestinal parasites (trichrome and iron hematoxylin) do not detect *Cryptosporidium*. Concentration techniques enhance recovery of the parasite from stool, especially when formed stools are examined.[67, 216, 343, 346] Several concentration techniques, including flotation methods (Sheather sugar solution, zinc sulfate, or saturated sodium chloride) and sedimentation methods (formalin–ethyl acetate and formalin-ether), have been used with varying degrees of success. Weber and colleagues[347] reported improved recovery of *Cryptosporidium* oocysts with a modified concentration technique that combines the sedimentation and flotation methods.[347]

Traditionally, the method of choice for clinical laboratories to detect *Cryptosporidium* oocysts in stool has been the modified acid-fast stain.[40, 100, 197] It is an inexpensive method; however, it lacks the sensitivity and specificity of

*See references 29, 67, 103, 132, 149, 169, 171, 194, 226, 233.

TABLE 216–1 ■ DIAGNOSTIC CHARACTERISTICS OF ENTERIC COCCIDIAN PROTOZOA AND MICROSPORIDIA

Organism	Oocyst Characteristics	Specimen	Recommended Diagnostic Procedure	Comments
Cryptosporidium	Spherical, 4–6 μm; oocyst is sporulated when passed in stool; sporulated oocyst contains 4 sporozoites	Stool Intestinal biopsy	Direct microscopy Modified acid-fast stain Monoclonal antibody stain Histopathology Electron microscopy	Concentration methods enhance recovery, especially when the stool is formed; fluorescence with auramine-rhodamine
Isospora belli	Oval, 20–30 × 10–19 μm; oocyst is unsporulated when passed in stool; sporulated oocyst contains 2 sporoblasts, each with 2 sporozoites	Stool Intestinal biopsy	Direct microscopy Modified acid-fast stain Histopathology Electron microscopy	Oocyst excreted intermittently; concentration methods enhance recovery; variable fluorescence with auramine–rhodamine
Cyclospora cayetanensis	Spherical, 8–10 μm; oocyst is unsporulated when passed in stool; sporulated oocyst contains 2 sporoblasts, each with 4 sporozoites	Stool Intestinal biopsy	Direct microscopy Modified acid-fast stain Histopathology Electron microscopy	Concentration methods enhance recovery; bright blue autofluorescence under ultraviolet light
Microsporidia	Spores with internal extrusion apparatus; variable size depends on species: 0.7–3.0 × 1.5–5 μm	Stool and body fluids Intestinal biopsy	Chromotrope stain Chemofluorescent Giemsa stain Histopathology Electron microscopy	Light microscopy of stool and tissue is sensitive when performed by someone with experience; electron microscopy is required to confirm the diagnosis

immunoassays.* Commercial immunoassay kits, including enzyme immunoassay (EIA) and IFA kits, are available for detection of *Cryptosporidium* in clinical and environmental samples.[47, 112, 124] These kits have excellent sensitivity and specificity when used on clinical specimens. False-positive EIA results on human feces are uncommon. Between November 1997 and March 1998, a pseudo-outbreak of cryptosporidiosis caused by nonspecific reaction with certain lot numbers of an EIA kit was reported in three states.[91] This pseudo-outbreak underscores the importance of quality assurance measures in the clinical laboratory. Serologic tests for *Cryptosporidium* (IFAs or ELISAs)[36, 39, 332] have been developed but are of limited value for the diagnosis of acute illness.[4, 39] These tests are useful to study the epidemiology or seroprevalence of *Cryptosporidium*.[329–332]

Several polymerase chain reaction (PCR)-based methods have been developed for the detection of *Cryptosporidium* oocysts in stool and environmental samples.[119, 181, 183, 235, 236] PCR-based detection methods are highly sensitive and specific and offer the added benefit of distinguishing non-*parvum Cryptosporidium* spp. from *C. parvum*. It is an excellent research tool and can be used for genotyping in epidemiologic investigations.[264] PCR-based technology has not been standardized for use in the clinical laboratory.

Biopsy of the intestine is not typically necessary for the diagnosis of intestinal infection, although the unique apical location within the intestinal epithelium is distinctive. However, identifying the various stages of the life cycle of *Cryptosporidium* in tissue is helpful in making the diagnosis of extraintestinal disease. The parasite can be visualized by light microscopy after staining with hematoxylin and eosin or by electron microscopy[68, 69, 120] (see Figs. 216–3 and 216–4). Indirect immunofluorescent antibody stains with *Cryptosporidium*-specific monoclonal antibodies also have been used.[189]

*See references 1, 11, 47, 109, 111, 112, 114, 124, 214, 250, 282, 287, 313.

TREATMENT AND PREVENTION

In an immunocompetent host, the illness is self-limited, and antimicrobial therapy is not necessary. In developing countries, it is commonly associated with malnutrition, although whether this association is causal is unclear. Optimal therapy in these settings is unknown. In immunocompromised hosts, especially patients with AIDS, management of intestinal cryptosporidiosis is problematic. Rehydration with oral or intravenous fluid is an essential part of management. Partial restoration of immune function with highly active antiretroviral therapy (HAART) is the best therapy for patients with AIDS.[47, 200]

More than 100 therapeutic agents have been investigated in humans or animals with variable success. Agents targeted at reducing diarrheal symptoms include peptidomimetics and antimotility drugs. Antimicrobials and passive immunotherapy have been used in an attempt to kill or eliminate the pathogen.[275]

The peptidomimetic agents octreotide and vapreotide are synthetic analogues of somatostatin. The mechanism of action of these compounds is inhibition of secretion of gastrointestinal hormones to enhance electrolyte and water absorption and decrease jejunal transit time.[89, 127] Octreotide also may act to inhibit HIV-induced activation of vasoactive intestinal peptide receptors in the gut.[286] Octreotide has been used to manage other causes of secretory diarrhea successfully.[241] Both octreotide[42, 48, 93, 174, 186, 280] and vapreotide[118, 125] have been used to treat HIV patients with chronic intestinal cryptosporidiosis. They have had limited success in reducing the symptoms, however. Adverse effects of octreotide include inhibition of gallbladder emptying and pancreatic secretion, which results in cholelithiasis and pancreatitis.[125, 221] These agents do not eradicate the pathogen. Antimotility agents such as loperamide and opiates control the diarrhea but, like the peptidomimetic agents, do not eradicate the parasite.[100, 278]

Combination therapy with azithromycin, an intracellular agent, and paromomycin, an intraluminal agent, has been considered first-line therapy for HIV-infected patients.[306] It is the best regimen for HIV-infected patients who have

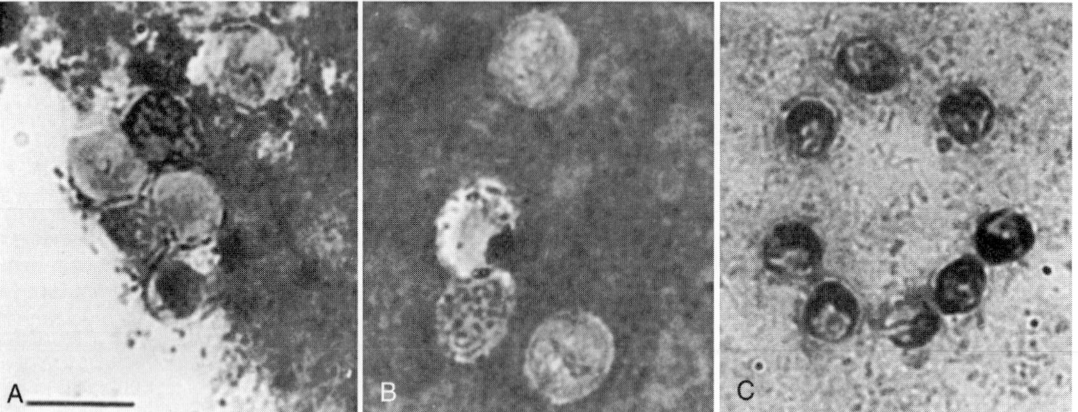

FIGURE 216–5 ■ Modified acid-fast stain of *Cyclospora* species *(A)*, *Cryptosporidium muris (B)*, and *Cryptosporidium parvum (C)*. Bar = 10 µm. (Reprinted, by permission, from Ortega, Y. R., Sterling, C. R., Gilman, R. H., et al.: Cyclospora species: A new protozoan pathogen of humans. N. Engl. J. Med. *328*:1308–1312, 1993.)

failed HAART or have drug-resistant HIV. This combination has not been studied in a randomized, controlled trial of malnourished children or other immunosuppressed patients (i.e., patients undergoing chemotherapy or organ transplantation). Some evidence has shown that in severely immunosuppressed HIV-infected patients, prophylaxis for *Mycobacterium avium* complex with clarithromycin, with or without rifabutin, may also protect against cryptosporidiosis.[152] Nitazoxanide has shown promise in several studies. In an uncontrolled trial involving AIDS patients from Africa, 95 percent of the patients had eradication or reduction of *C. parvum* oocyst shedding.[88] In a double-blind, placebo-controlled trial of AIDS patients from Mexico, parasitologic cure was observed in 86 percent of the treated patients.[284] In another double-blind, placebo-controlled study, nitazoxanide proved effective in the treatment of *C. parvum* infection in immunocompetent children and adults.[283, 284]

Successful use of hyperimmune bovine colostrum in immunodeficient patients has been documented in several anecdotal reports.[290, 299, 326, 327, 333] The only published double-blind, placebo-controlled study using hyperimmune bovine colostrum reported a significant reduction in shedding of oocysts in treated patients. However, this study was flawed because of a significant difference between the treated and control groups with respect to parasite load, clinical symptoms, and antiretroviral therapy.[247]

Bovine transfer factor is a purified bovine lymphocyte extract and was beneficial in five of eight patients with cryptosporidiosis.[191] A controlled trial using a bovine dialyzable leukocyte extract resulted in weight gain in six of seven patients and eradication of oocysts in five. When the five control patients subsequently were given the bovine dialyzable leukocyte extract, symptoms improved in two and oocysts were eradicated in two. Overall, the clinical response was favorable in 10 of 12 patients who received the bovine dialyzable leukocyte extract.[215] Human immunoglobulin administered orally appeared to be helpful in a child with leukemia and chronic cryptosporidiosis.[27, 28]

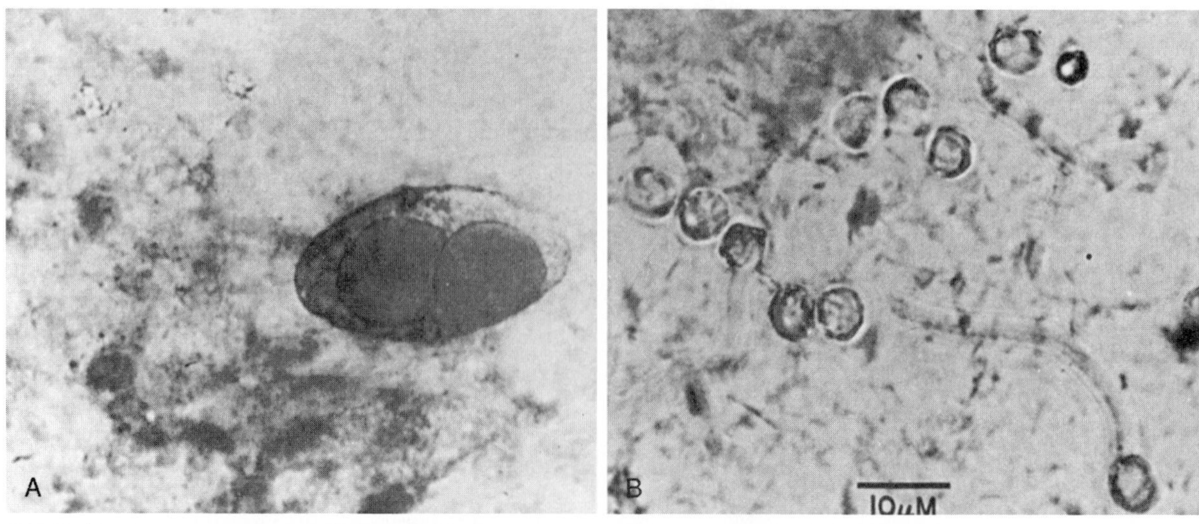

FIGURE 216–6 ■ Unconcentrated fresh stool sample from two patients with AIDS stained with modified Kinyoun stain. *Isospora belli (A)* and *Cryptosporidium (B)*. Note the difference in size and shape of the two coccidian parasites; *Isospora* averages 25 × 15 µm and contains two sporoblasts, whereas *Cryptosporidium* averages about 5 µm in diameter. (Reprinted, by permission, from DeHovitz, J. A., Pape, J. W., Boncy, M., et al.: Clinical manifestations and therapy of *Isospora belli* infection in patients with the acquired immunodeficiency syndrome. N. Engl. J. Med. *315*:87–90, 1986.)

In the hospital or child-care setting, handwashing is the single most important measure to prevent the spread of any enteric pathogen. In the hospital setting, enteric precautions (washing hands, wearing gloves, and wearing gowns if soiling is likely) are important measures to prevent nosocomial spread. Contaminated equipment such as endoscopes and bronchoscopes should be autoclaved.

Control of water-borne transmission of cryptosporidiosis is a major public health concern. This issue is complicated by the ability of *Cryptosporidium* to escape the filtration system used by most public water facilities and its resistance to chlorination. After the massive outbreak in Milwaukee, the CDC recommended that during outbreak situations, immunocompromised patients boil tap water for 1 minute, use a submicron personal-use filtration system to remove particles 1 μm or smaller in diameter, or use bottled water prepared by distillation or reverse osmotic filtration. In non-outbreak situations, no special measures are recommended. However, routinely using the outbreak measures outlined earlier for severely immunosuppressed patients may be prudent.[15] The CDC website contains an excellent patient fact sheet about *Cryptosporidium* and its prevention at www.cdc.gov/ncidod/dbd/parasites/cryptosporidios.

Cyclospora Infection

Cyclospora cayetanensis is a coccidian parasite that infects the gastrointestinal tract of both immunocompetent and immunocompromised patients.[263, 365] This organism was described in feces from humans without enteritis as early as 1979.[12] The first documented cases of diarrheal disease attributed to *Cyclospora* were reported in 1986 in four immunocompetent patients who had traveled from the United States to either Haiti or Mexico.[308] At that time, it was referred to as an unsporulated, coccidian body or a fungal spore. Before the mid-1980s, reports of diarrheal illness caused by *Cyclospora* were rare. With the advent of the AIDS epidemic, this organism has gained increasing recognition as an enteric pathogen.[263, 365]

MICROBIOLOGY AND LIFE CYCLE

Cyclospora is a round to ovoid, variable acid-fast organism that measures 8 to 10 μm in diameter[253] (see Fig. 216–5). It also has been referred to as a *Cyanobacterium*-like body, a blue-green alga, a coccidian-like body, *Cryptosporidium*-like, or big *Cryptosporidium*.[13, 19, 147, 253, 256, 258, 271, 300, 310] In 1993, Ortega and associates[253, 256] assigned this organism to the family Eimeriidae and the genus *Cyclospora* and proposed the name *C. cayetanensis* for the species that infects humans. This classification was based on its sporulation characteristics, and the name was derived from the institution where the original research was performed (Universidad Peruana Cayetano Heredia in Lima, Peru).[364]

Cyclospora, like *Isospora,* sporulates exogenously and has two sporocysts per oocyst. It differs from *Isospora* in that it has two sporozoites per sporocyst whereas *Isospora* has four per sporocyst. *Cyclospora* spp. are ubiquitous and infect a variety of animals, including vipers, moles, rodents, and myriapods. Humans are the only known host of *C. cayetanensis*. Organisms resembling *C. cayetanensis* have been found in the stool of chimpanzees living in Uganda.[364]

Both sexual and asexual stages of *Cyclospora* are found in jejunal biopsy specimens from infected individuals, thus demonstrating that this coccidian parasite can complete its entire life cycle in a single host.[254] Infected patients pass unsporulated oocysts into the environment. A period outside the host is required for maturation into an infectious, sporulated oocyst. A warm, moist environment appears to favor sporulation in nature. In vitro, sporulation occurs 1 to 2 weeks after incubation in distilled water or 2.5 percent potassium dichromate at 25° to 35° C.[307, 314] Sporulation has been delayed by storage of oocysts at 4° C for up to 6 months or by storage at 37° C for 14 days and can be completely aborted if oocyst are subjected to −20° C for longer than 24 hours or 60° C for longer than 1 hour.[305] In vivo, exocystation of mature sporulated oocysts most likely occurs in the small bowel. In vitro, a combination of bile salts, sodium taurocholate, and mechanical pressure is required for exocystation.[314]

EPIDEMIOLOGY

Cyclospora is distributed worldwide. Initial reports of cyclosporiasis involved residents of developing countries or travelers returning from such countries.[146, 253, 256, 271, 300] It has been identified in individuals residing in or traveling to numerous geographic areas, including North, Central, and South America, the Caribbean islands, England, eastern Europe, India, eastern Asia, South Africa, and Australia.[307, 314] In recent years, an increasing number of cases of food-borne outbreaks have been reported.[141–143] Seasonal variation has been described. In Nepal, most cases occur during the rainy season, between May and October.[146] In Peru, the peak is between April and June, during the fall.[256] The prevalence in endemic regions varies with the age and immunologic status of the host. Prevalence rates in children from Peru and Nepal are reported to range from 2 to 18 percent.[145, 256] In one series from Haiti, *Cyclospora* was reported in 11 percent of HIV-infected adults but was not detected in non–HIV-infected adults or infants younger than 6 months.[262]

Direct person-to-person transmission is unlikely because a period outside the host is required for maturation into a sporulated oocyst.[314] The infectious dose of *Cyclospora* is not known but is hypothesized to be low, as with other coccidian parasites. Contamination of the environment with oocysts plays a major role in the transmission of *Cyclospora.* Both food-borne and water-borne transmission of *Cyclospora* has been described.[314] Water-borne outbreaks have been reported in Chicago and in Nepal.[154, 258, 364]

Food-borne transmission of this organism via the consumption of uncooked meat and poultry was suspected as early as 1979.[12] Widespread recognition of this organism as a food-borne pathogen occurred in 1996 and 1997 when outbreaks of cyclosporiasis occurred in the United States and Canada and were associated with the consumption of raspberries imported from Guatemala.[141–143] Researchers postulated that the raspberries were contaminated with insecticide or fungicides that were mixed with contaminated water or that the irrigation water was contaminated with *Cyclospora* oocysts.[257, 307] During 1997, clusters of cases were identified in which fresh basil and mesclun lettuce were implicated.[272] *Cyclospora* oocysts contaminating vegetables are not easily removed by routine washing.[255]

CLINICAL MANIFESTATIONS

Cyclospora causes disease in both immunocompetent and immunocompromised patients.[256, 263, 271, 300, 364] The incubation period typically ranges from 2 to 11 days. In the Chicago outbreak, cases occurred 12 hours to 7 days after the suspected contamination of the water supply.[258] In an immunocompetent host, diarrheal symptoms may last up to 7 weeks and may be remitting.[364] A cyclic, relapsing pattern of diarrhea alternating with constipation may occur.[307] Resolution of symptoms usually correlates with disappearance of the organism from the stool.[146, 263] However, asymptomatic excretion of cysts has been reported.[19, 271] In immunocompromised hosts, the duration of diarrhea is highly variable and ranges from a few days to several months; in most cases it is protracted.

The illness is characterized by an abrupt onset of watery diarrhea. Flulike symptoms, including malaise, myalgia, and anorexia, also occur.[45, 364] Low-grade fever is reported in approximately 25 percent of patients.[258, 300, 364] Vomiting may occur but is less common than diarrhea. Other associated symptoms include abdominal cramping, heartburn, and indigestion.[307] Weight loss from malabsorption occurs in both immunocompetent and immunocompromised patients.[146, 308, 365] The median duration of disease in various U.S. outbreaks has been 10 to 20 days with a range of 1 to 60 days.[141] In HIV-infected patients, *Cyclospora* causes symptoms that are indistinguishable from those of *Cryptosporidium* and *Isospora* infection.[364] Biliary disease was reported in two AIDS patients infected with *Cyclospora*. These patients had clinical and radiographic confirmation of biliary disease and did not have evidence of infection with other pathogens. Both patients had acalculous cholecystitis that was responsive to therapy with trimethoprim-sulfamethoxazole.[301]

DIAGNOSIS

Cyclospora, unlike *Cryptosporidium,* can be visualized by light microscopy after formol-ether concentration of the stool. In fresh stool, the oocysts are unsporulated. They appear as refractile spherical bodies measuring 8 to 10 μm and have a central greenish morula that contains six to nine refractile globules.[253] Safranin staining enhances the outline of the membrane but does not stain internal structures. The sensitivity of wet mounts is 75 percent.[262] Oocysts exhibit bright blue autofluorescence when exposed to ultraviolet light. Staining is variable with modified Ziehl-Neelsen stain[256] (see Fig. 216–5). Fluorescence with auramine-rhodamine staining enhances the visualization of internal structures, but this stain is usually weak and irregular. *Cyclospora* is not visualized by Gram, Giemsa, Grocott-Gomori silver, Lugol-iodine, periodic acid–Schiff, or hematoxylin and eosin staining.[263, 364]

TREATMENT

The disease appears to be self-limited in immunocompetent hosts. When treatment is indicated because of the severity or persistence of symptoms, trimethoprim-sulfamethoxazole is the drug of choice. In a small, uncontrolled study, therapy with trimethoprim-sulfamethoxazole resulted in resolution of symptoms and reduction of the duration of shedding oocysts from 9 to 13 days.[198] In a placebo-controlled trial involving travelers to Nepal, trimethoprim-sulfamethoxazole for 7 days eradicated *Cyclospora* from the stool in 96 percent of patients.[146] In contrast, 88 percent of the placebo group still had detectable *Cyclospora* in the stool at the end of 7 days. Eradication of the organism correlated with resolution of symptoms. In one study, patients with *Cyclospora* did not improve when treated with empiric therapy (norfloxacin, tinidazole, quinacrine, nalidixic acid, and diloxanide furoate[300]) that was aimed at other enteric pathogens. Prophylaxis with trimethoprim-sulfamethoxazole 3 days a week appears to prevent recurrent episodes in HIV-infected patients.[262]

Isosporiasis

Isospora belli is an enteric coccidian parasite that is closely related to *Toxoplasma, Cryptosporidium, Sarcocystis,* and *Cyclospora* (see Fig. 216–1). Numerous species of *Isospora* infect reptiles, birds, and mammals. However, *I. belli* is the only species that infects humans.[90] *Isospora*, like the other enteric coccidian parasites, causes a self-limited diarrheal illness in immunocompetent hosts and a prolonged diarrheal illness in immunocompromised hosts. The first reported cases of human isosporiasis were in 1915.[359, 363] Like the other enteric coccidian diseases, isosporiasis was reported infrequently before the AIDS epidemic.

MICROBIOLOGY AND LIFE CYCLE

I. belli is a monoxenous coccidian parasite that is closely related to *Cyclospora.*[159] The mature oocyst of *I. belli* is oval-shaped, measures 10 to 20 × 20 to 33 μm, and has a translucent thin wall that contains two round sporoblasts, each with four crescent-shaped sporozoites[52] (see Fig. 216–6). Infection occurs after the ingestion of a mature sporulated oocyst. Excystation occurs in the proximal part of the small intestine and results in the release of sporozoites that invade enterocytes of the distal duodenum and proximal jejunum and develop into trophozoites. The trophozoites reproduce asexually to form merozoites. The merozoites undergo asexual replication (schizogony or merogony) or sexual replication (gametogony) that results in the production of an immature unsporulated oocyst. This latter form is excreted in stool and requires 12 to 48 hours to mature into the infectious form, a sporulated oocyst.[27]

EPIDEMIOLOGY AND TRANSMISSION

The true prevalence of *I. belli* is not known. It is more common in the tropical and subtropical regions[94, 188] of Africa, Southeast Asia, and Central and South America. In North America, it has been implicated as a cause of diarrhea in institutionalized patients[161] and as a cause of traveler's diarrhea.[117, 297] Before the AIDS pandemic, *Isospora* was an uncommon cause of diarrhea, even in endemic regions. Between 1976 and 1980, *Isospora* oocysts were detected in 0.17 percent of stool specimens from 1139 Southeast Asian refugees.[27] *Isospora* is found in 3 to 18 percent of AIDS patients from developing countries and in less than 0.2 percent of AIDS patients from the United States and Europe.[155, 261, 309] In Haiti, *Isospora* accounts for 15 percent of chronic diarrhea in patients with AIDS.[77]

The consensus is that humans are the only host of *I. belli* and that no animal reservoirs exist. However, organisms resembling *I. belli* have been identified in the stool of dogs.[116] Transmission is by the fecal-oral route. Sexual transmission of *Isospora* also has been suggested.[104] Infection occurs after the ingestion of oocysts in fecally contaminated food or water or from environmental sources.[104, 263, 309] The incubation period is thought to be 3 to 14 days.[27, 139] The infectious dose has not been established. In one investigation, symptoms developed in a single volunteer after ingesting 3000 organisms, but they failed to develop with a second challenge.[211] If untreated, the organism is shed in the stool for 11 to 120 days.[139] The oocysts of *I. belli* are highly resistant to commonly used disinfectants and may remain viable for months in a cool, moist environment.

PATHOGENESIS AND IMMUNOLOGY

The pathologic findings in patients with isosporiasis are nonspecific. Histopathologic changes include shortening of the villi, hypertrophy of the crypts, and infiltration of the lamina propria with plasma cells, lymphocytes, polymorphonuclear leukocytes, and eosinophils.[27, 30, 52, 261, 324] All stages of the life cycle have been identified within the villous epithelium (Fig. 216–7) and always are enclosed within a parasitiferous vessel.[30, 261, 324] Extracellular merozoites rarely are found in the intestinal lumen or the lamina propria.[52]

Isosporiasis is characterized by massive fluid loss suggestive of toxin-mediated hypersecretion, but no enterotoxin has been identified.[261] The pathophysiology of isosporiasis has not been defined; however, cell-mediated immunity appears to be important in the pathogenesis of villous changes. Activated T cells are mitogenic to enterocytes, and this mitogenic activity results in crypt hyperplasia, which in turn leads to villous atrophy. Local T-cell activation results in the release of lymphokines, increased intraepithelial lymphocytes, and enhanced expression of HLA-DR antigens on enterocytes of the villi and crypts. Intestinal mast cells also may play a role in the pathogenesis by releasing a collagen-IV protease.[33]

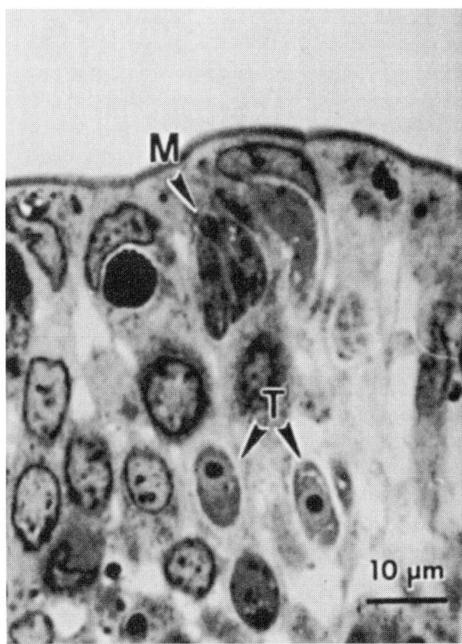

FIGURE 216–7 ■ *Isospora* infecting the jejunum of a patient with severe diarrhea. Trophozoites (T) divide within enterocytes by schizogony to form merozoites (M). (From Garcia, L. S., Owen, R. L., and Current, W. L.: Isosporiasis. *In* Balows, A., Hausler, W. J., Jr., Ohashi, M., and Turano, A. [eds.]: The Laboratory Diagnosis of Infectious Diseases: Principles and Practice. Vol. 1. New York, Springer-Verlag, 1988, pp. 899–903.)

CLINICAL MANIFESTATIONS

The clinical findings are indistinguishable from those of other enteric coccidian parasites. The spectrum of disease ranges from asymptomatic infection to severe, protracted, life-threatening diarrhea. Immunocompetent patients usually have a self-limited illness that spontaneously resolves over the course of several weeks.[261, 309, 361] Headache, malaise, vomiting, fever, and dehydration may be noted. Recurrent symptoms and chronic illness may occur.[188] The disease is more severe in infants and children than in adults,[187, 321] and intractable diarrhea has been reported in infants.[161] Patients with AIDS, alpha-chain disease, acute lymphoblastic leukemia, Hodgkin disease, and human T-cell lymphotropic virus type 1–related T-cell leukemia are predisposed to life-threatening illness.[285] In these patients, the onset of illness is insidious and associated with nonspecific symptoms such as low-grade fever, headache, malaise, myalgia, and anorexia.[77, 261] Nausea, vomiting, and diffuse crampy abdominal pain are also present. The stool is watery and may contain mucus but does not contain blood or leukocytes. Chronic intermittent diarrhea with a mean duration of 7.9 months (range, 2 to 26 months) is the major clinical manifestation.[263] Dehydration occurs in 70 percent of patients and requires intravenous fluids in 10 percent. The average daily fluid loss is 2 L, with some patients losing up to 20 L.[261] Malabsorption, steatorrhea, severe weight loss (>10% of body weight), and lactose intolerance have been reported.[30, 77, 324, 360] Charcot-Leyden crystals are a common finding in stool. Peripheral eosinophilia occurs in more than 50 percent of patients.[160, 263] Nonspecific radiographic findings include prominent mucosal folds, thickening of the intestinal wall, and disordered motility.[309]

Biliary disease and extraintestinal manifestations of *I. belli* are rare but have been reported in patients with AIDS.[33, 220, 275] The organism has been identified in tracheobronchial, mediastinal, and mesenteric lymph nodes, the spleen, and the liver.[220, 275] Acalculous cholecystitis has been reported.[18]

DIAGNOSIS

The diagnosis is made by identifying oocysts in stool or by visualizing the parasite in biopsy specimens of the small intestine.[27, 263, 309] Like *Cryptosporidium, Isospora* can be detected in stool by using modified acid-fast or auramine-rhodamine stain. Organisms are sparse, so concentration techniques such as zinc sulfate, hypertonic sodium chloride, formalin-ether sedimentation, and Sheather sucrose solution are used to enhance recovery.[261, 309] The thin translucent wall of the oocyst may be difficult to identify in stool preserved in polyvinyl alcohol.[206] *Isospora* oocysts are distinguished easily from *Cryptosporidium* oocysts. They are oval, contain one or two sporoblasts, and are 10 times larger than *Cryptosporidium* oocysts. In comparison, *Cryptosporidium* oocysts are round, contain four sporozoites, and measure 2 to 5 μm in diameter (see Fig. 216–6). The oocysts of *I. belli* exhibit autofluorescence with an ultraviolet epifluorescent illuminator (450 to 490 nm excitation filter).[206] The sensitivity and specificity of the different methods for detection of *Isospora* in stool are not known.[261] It is possible to detect the parasite by biopsy and not visualize oocysts in

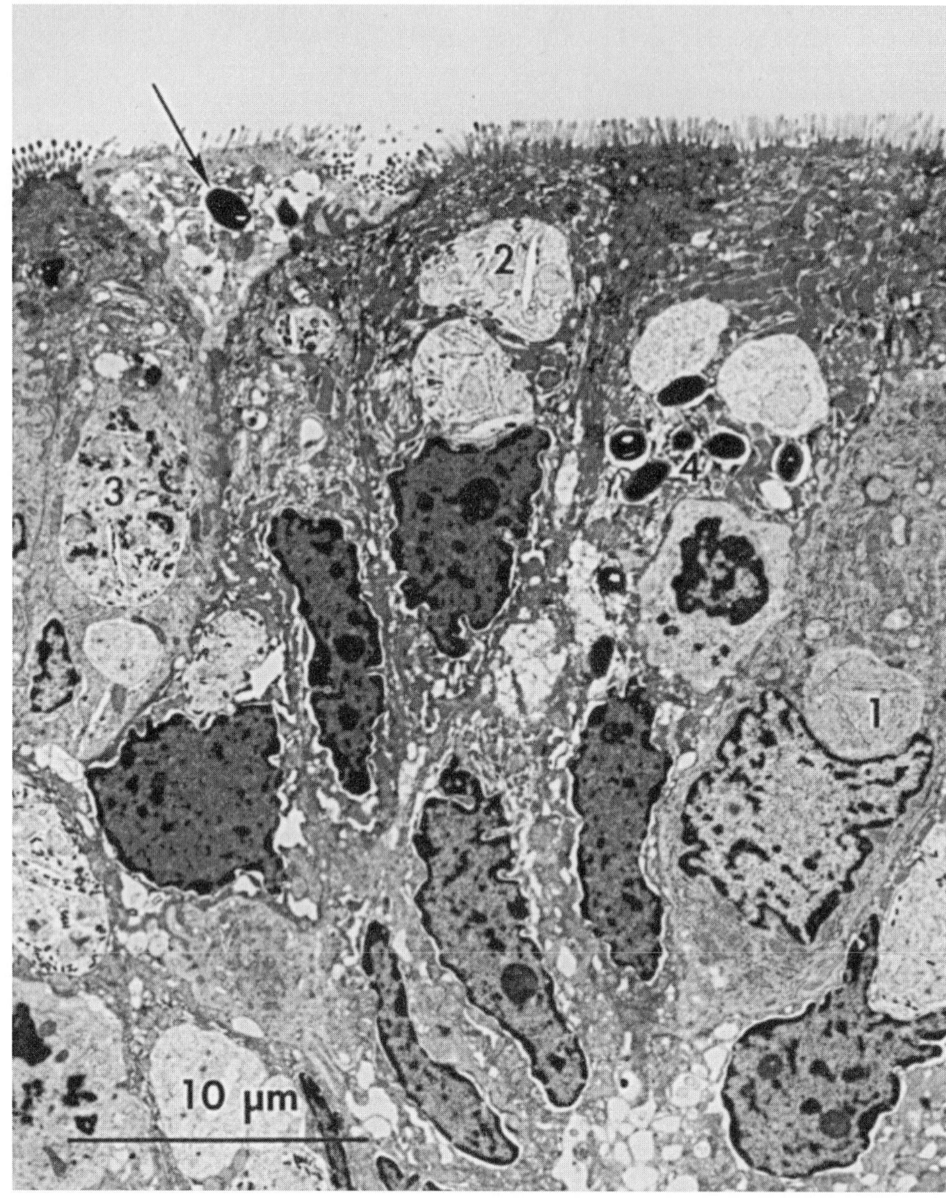

FIGURE 216–8 ■ Jejunal biopsy from a patient with AIDS and severe diarrhea. Various developmental stages of the intestinal microsporidian *Enterocytozoon* infect almost every enterocyte. Stages include proliferative plasmodia (1), early sporogonial plasmodia (2), late sporogonial plasmodia (3), and mature spores (4). A spore *(arrow)* can be seen within a necrotic enterocyte, which appears ready to slough into the lumen. (Reproduced from Cali, A., and Owen, R. L.: Intracellular development of *Enterocytozoon:* A unique microsporidian found in the intestine of AIDS patients. J. Protozool. *37*:145, 1990.)

stool.[30] The parasite usually is found in the proximal part of the small bowel (Fig. 216–8). However, in AIDS patients, it can be found in both the small and large intestines.

TREATMENT

The treatment of choice is trimethoprim-sulfamethoxazole given four times a day for 10 days.[77, 263, 309, 360] Patients who have been symptomatic for months usually have resolution in less than a week with this treatment. Pyrimethamine-sulfadiazine (Fansidar) is an alternative agent. For a sulfonamide-allergic patient, ciprofloxacin [340] or pyrimethamine[358] alone is an alternative agent. Ciprofloxacin [340] is not as effective as trimethoprim-sulfamethoxazole and is not approved by the U.S. Food and Drug Administration for children younger than 18 years. Data on the use of macrolides and metronidazole are limited to uncontrolled studies.[104, 188] Unfortunately, 50 percent of AIDS patients with isosporiasis have recurrences.[77, 263] Therefore, prophylaxis with trimethoprim-sulfamethoxazole 160 mg/800 mg three times a week or sulfadoxine-pyrimethamine (500 mg/25 mg) once a week is necessary to prevent relapse.[263] Ciprofloxacin can be used as an alternative prophylaxis agent for sulfonamide-allergic adolescent patients older than 17 years.[340] Pyrimethamine is an alternative prophylaxis agent, but data on its use are limited, especially in the pediatric age group.[358]

Microsporidiosis

Microsporidiosis is caused by an extensive group of obligate intracellular, phylogenetically ancient protozoan parasites that infect vertebrate and invertebrate animals.[17, 349] In humans, microsporidia first were detected in cerebrospinal fluid in 1959 in Japan in a child with seizures.[210] This infection has been reported infrequently in normal hosts. The number of cases described has increased since 1985, after recognition of the diarrhea and wasting syndrome in AIDS patients. The pathogenic role in other immunocompromised persons remains to be studied, as do the mode of transmission and sources of infection. The broad range of clinical manifestations includes keratoconjunctivitis, sinopulmonary infection, myositis, cholecystitis, hepatitis, and disseminated infection with tubulointerstitial nephritis.[349]

MICROBIOLOGY

Microsporidia are protozoan parasites belonging to the phylum Microspora that are characterized by the presence in the spore stage of an extrusion apparatus with a polar tubule that allows transfer of protoplasmic material into the host cell.[295, 349] One hundred forty-three microsporidial genera and more than 1200 species infect animals. Only 6 genera and 12 species have been described in humans: *Enterocytozoon, Encephalitozoon, Nosema, Trachipleistophora, Vittaforma,*[82] and *Pleistophora.* Unclassified microsporidia have been grouped under the term *Microsporidium.* Classification of the organisms traditionally has been based on morphologic characteristics of the stages of the parasite. However, recent advances in differentiation are based on phenotypic (protein antigenic patterns) and genotypic characteristics as determined by PCR techniques, small-subunit ribosomal RNA patterns, and restriction fragment length polymorphism.[76, 134, 293, 316, 341] These studies have allowed reclassification of the genus *Septata* into the previously known *Encephalitozoon.*[76] *Encephalitozoon hellem* is differentiated from *Encephalitozoon cuniculi* by antigenic and molecular analysis.[230, 288] A final taxonomic classification may develop after more precise molecular analysis is conducted.[349]

These spore-forming unicellular organisms are true eukaryotes, but their lack of mitochondria and the small rRNA and ribosomes resemble those of prokaryotes. The asexual life cycle in the host cell is divided into two phases: the merogonic or proliferative vegetative phase and the sporogonic phase, which results in the production of mature spores.[295] Intracellular stages proliferate by binary or multiple fission and appear as multinucleated elements that can be in direct contact with the cell cytoplasm (e.g., *Enterocytozoon bieneusi, Nosema* spp.) or engulfed in a parasitiferous vacuole (*Encephalitozoon* spp.). In the case of *Encephalitozoon intestinalis,* septa are formed by a fibrillar structure.[349] The spore consists of a surrounding protective three-layered wall and internal infective nucleated material that is injected into the host cell by extrusion of a coiled polar tubule attached to an anchoring disk. The average size of the vegetative stages ranges from 2 to 6 × 1 to 3 μm, and the average size of the spores ranges from 0.7 × 1.64 μm *(E. bieneusi)* to 3 × 5 μm *(Nosemaocularum).*

Cell culture systems are available for a few species, including *Nosema corneum, E. hellem,* and *E. intestinalis.*[76, 134, 229, 296, 337, 352] These isolated organisms are useful for the development of specific antisera that may allow differentiation of the microsporidial species.

EPIDEMIOLOGY

Precise data on the incidence, relevant reservoirs, source of infection, and mode of transmission are not defined. Symptomatic cases have been documented in non-AIDS patients, and half of them had evidence of altered immune status.[130, 345] Few cases of self-limited diarrhea have been reported in apparently normal hosts.[102, 345] In HIV-infected patients, approximately 25 to 50 percent of cases of chronic diarrhea of undetermined etiology or roughly 15 percent of the total cases of diarrhea may be caused by these organisms.[24, 173, 230, 338, 339] The percentages have varied, depending on the population studied and the diagnostic techniques used. Young homosexual or bisexual adults[14, 99, 273, 316] and severely immunosuppressed children with congenital HIV can be affected.[353] *E. bieneusi* has been the most prevalent microsporidium and is found mainly in persons with CD4 counts less than 100/mm^3.[83, 99] Asymptomatic infection and persistent carriage in immunosuppressed patients have been reported.[273] The other microsporidia infecting humans have been reported much less frequently.[82]

Microsporidia are ubiquitous in nature, and some of the species infecting humans are present in animals: *E. bieneusi* (pigs, nonhuman primates), *E. hellem* (parakeets), *E. cuniculi* (rabbits, dogs), and *Pleistophora* spp. (fish).[82] Cases of disease caused by contamination of water or food have been reported.[56] An aerosol route of bronchopulmonary infection with species that are not found in the gut, such as *Encephalitozoon,* is supported by histopathologic findings in the bronchial tract.[352] Direct contact with conjunctival mucosa is postulated to be the source of ocular infections.[252] Serologic surveys using *E. cuniculi* antigens have found antibodies in multiple population groups, but they probably represent cross-reactivity with either various microsporidia species or other organisms.[295] *Nosema* is the only member of this group not reported in AIDS patients; rather, it has been described as a disseminated infection in children with thymic aplasia and as local keratitis in normal hosts with or without previous trauma.[296, 349] *Pleistophora* infection may be manifested as myositis infiltrating muscle fibers and may cause atrophy and degeneration.[182]

Co-infection with other opportunistic agents, including cytomegalovirus, *Mycobacterium avium-intracellulare,* and *Cryptosporidium*[113] and other parasites, has been reported in 5 to 60 percent of cases.[14, 105, 173, 230, 251, 273] Unsuspected *Cryptosporidium* infection may be found in as many as 20 percent of patients with microsporidia.[114]

PATHOGENESIS AND PATHOLOGY

The mechanism of disease in humans is unknown.[349] Latent asymptomatic infection or acute disease has not been described fully in humans. With the exception of local ocular disease, the parasite proliferates when immunologic defenses are defective, especially cell-mediated immunity.

E. bieneusi almost always is limited to the intestinal and biliary tract; it has a preference for enterocytes in the small intestine. The organism produces a limited inflammatory reaction and abnormalities in villi,[99] but it rarely invades the lamina propria.[351] Exceptionally, respiratory epithelia may be infected. *E. intestinalis* can reach the submucosa; its presence in the kidneys and lower airways presumably results from systemic dissemination.[86, 229] Mucosal injury, characterized by partial villus atrophy and crypt hyperplasia, correlates with xylose malabsorption and decreased activity of mucosal disaccharidases.[172] Other types of encephalitozoonosis, including infection with *E. cuniculi* and *E. hellem,* have greater potential for dissemination.[293] *Encephalitozoon* infects macrophages and thus can disseminate to the liver, brain, kidneys, or sinuses and cause randomly distributed granulomatous lesions.[82] *E. cuniculi* has been reported in children with seizures,[21, 210] hepatitis, peritonitis, and disseminated infection. It has been found in conjunctival and sinopulmonary infections associated with colonization of the intestinal tract.[106] The portal of entry for the organism in these cases is uncertain. *E. hellem* may involve the urinary tract, bronchial epithelium, and conjunctiva.[293] In sections of corneal scrapings, the cytoplasm of superficial epithelial cells contains vacuoles with the granular organisms, but these vacuoles cause minimal nuclear distortion.[34]

CLINICAL MANIFESTATIONS

Intestinal and Biliary Tract Microsporidiosis

Chronic diarrhea and wasting syndrome are associated with microsporidial infection, particularly *E. bieneusi* and *E. intestinalis* infection, in severely immunodeficient HIV-infected patients (CD4 cell count <100/mm^3).[14, 230, 316] AIDS patients with more than 200 CD4$^+$ T cells/mL tend to have self-limited diarrhea. In some cases, microsporidiosis is the AIDS-defining opportunistic infection.[213, 251] Transplant patients are also at risk for acquiring these pathogens.[56] The usual symptom is afebrile, loose to watery, nonbloody, nonmucoid diarrhea consisting of 3 to 20 bowel movements per day that is worsened by food intake and associated with progressive weight loss, malabsorption, and anorexia.[14, 252] Absorption of fat, D-xylose, and zinc is abnormal.[14, 230] Persistent or intermittent symptoms may lead to severe cachexia by a combination of decreased intake and malabsorption.[316] Half of patients have abdominal pain; some complain of nausea and vomiting.[251] Affected children may suffer from failure to thrive, chronic diarrhea, and intermittent abdominal pain.[353] Sporadic cases of *E. bieneusi* and *E. intestinalis* causing self-limited diarrhea with diffuse abdominal pain and nausea in immunocompetent persons have been reported.[102, 344, 345]

Patients with cholangitis and acalculous cholecystitis have right upper quadrant abdominal pain. Imaging studies may reveal dilatation of the intrahepatic and common bile ducts or irregularities of the bile duct and gallbladder wall. The AIDS cholangiopathy is similar to that associated with cytomegalovirus and cryptosporidial infection.[270]

Ocular Infection

Immunocompetent patients with histologically confirmed ocular infection with *Microsporidium ceylonensis* and *Nosema* spp. (*N. corneum* and *N. ocularum*) have been reported.[71, 296, 349] The infection may be associated with previous trauma and lead to a progressive decrease in visual acuity secondary to severe corneal stroma disruption or corneal ulcer. *Encephalitozoon* spp., in particular, *E. hellem*, are a cause of keratoconjunctivitis and scleritis in HIV-infected patients; symptoms in these patients include conjunctival inflammation, photophobia, blurred vision, a foreign body sensation, decreased visual acuity, and punctate epithelial keratopathy.[252, 294] The lesion is usually bilateral and not associated with ocular trauma. Occasionally, the ocular involvement is accompanied by evidence of disseminated infection.[130]

Systemic Microsporidiosis

Disseminated systemic infection may develop in HIV-positive patients. Both *Encephalitozoon* spp. (*E. cuniculi* and *E. hellem*) have been associated with tubulointerstitial nephritis, ureteritis, cystitis, conjunctivitis, and colonization or infection of the respiratory tract; these findings may occur in the absence of gastrointestinal symptoms.[76, 130, 341, 345, 352] Flank pain, hematuria, and dysuria are symptoms of urinary tract involvement, and progressive nonproductive cough, wheezing, and pleuritic pain are seen with lower respiratory involvement. Disseminated *E. cuniculi* infection involving the intestinal tract has been reported.[106] *E. intestinalis* infection usually is limited to the intestinal tract, although systemic manifestations consisting of urinary tract involvement (interstitial nephritis) and sinopulmonary dissemination may occur after invasion of the intestinal lamina propria.[86, 130, 229]

Serologic evidence (EIA and counterimmunoelectrophoresis) shows that *E. intestinalis* causes central nervous system infection characterized by severe headache and seizures in HIV-infected patients.[339] Disseminated *Nosema conorii* infection has been described in an immunodeficient athymic child with chronic diarrhea, fever, and weight loss; the parasite was found in the myocardium, diaphragm, kidney tubules, liver, and lungs.[295]

Severely immunosuppressed hosts may be disposed to the development of myositis (caused by *Pleistophora* spp.) with nonspecific symptoms of generalized muscle weakness or myalgias and elevated creatinine phosphokinase. Muscle biopsy provides a definitive diagnosis.[184] Sinusitis with a mucopurulent nasal discharge or lower respiratory tract involvement with bronchiolitis, pneumonia, and respiratory failure has been described with *E. bieneusi* and *Encephalitozoon* spp.[351] The source of the organism is unknown and may represent primary respiratory acquisition or secondary dissemination from other mucosal surfaces.

DIAGNOSIS

A definitive diagnosis is made by direct morphologic demonstration of organisms in stool, body fluids (duodenal aspirates, bile, bronchoalveolar lavage fluid, nasal secretions, urine, conjunctival smears, cerebrospinal fluid), or tissue sections[46, 130, 229, 230, 349, 350]; microsporidia sometimes can be cultured.[229] Light microscopy is reliable, although the small size and the staining properties of microsporidia render recognition difficult. Electron microscopy is usually necessary to define the ultrastructural features of the different genera. Immunologic, molecular, antigenic, and biochemical analysis of isolated organisms can be performed if ultrastructure does not allow differentiation among similar species.[76, 134, 293, 352]

Weber chromotrope-based stain,[348] with modifications[288] that allow better resolution from background, has shown good sensitivity and specificity for the analysis of unconcentrated stool samples and other body fluids, including urine.[14, 75, 83, 86, 130, 352, 354] Under oil immersion, the pinkish-red spore wall of microsporidia must be differentiated morphologically from some yeast elements and bacteria.[316] Uvitex 2B[75, 336, 338] and calcofluor white[193] are useful, but fungi can give false-positive results.[83] Giemsa stain appears less satisfactory for stool analysis.[316] Whether intermittent shedding occurs is not clear, so multiple stool samples are needed for detection.[17, 230] Acid-fast staining has been attempted with some success in the cytologic examination of centrifuged fluids.[270]

Recognition of microsporidia by light microscopy[172, 230, 351] in paraffin-embedded tissue sections has been reported with routine techniques, including hematoxylin and eosin,[252, 293] tissue Gram,[252, 293, 316] periodic acid–Schiff, silver,[99] and Giemsa stains.[277, 316] The accuracy of each technique is related to the intensity of infection[338] and the level of training of the person performing the analysis. The spores are often on the surface of the villi; the multinucleated sporogonial stage appears as a collection of granules that is easily confused with cytoplasmic organelles.[251, 252] Some workers prefer touch preparations of small intestine stained with Giemsa.[17, 230, 302] Histologic examination of ultrathin plastic sections stained with toluidine blue or methylene blue azure II fuchsin stain may increase the sensitivity.[252, 316] Differentiation of the spores by IFA may allow identification of species.[11, 114, 294, 348, 352] Monoclonal antibodies produced against isolated microsporidia may permit speciation in cytologic and histologic analysis.[2, 341] Cross-reactivity of *Encephalitozoon* antisera has been used in the diagnosis of *E. bieneusi* infection in stool and intestinal biopsy tissue.[2, 369] In ocular microsporidiosis, conjunctival and corneal scrapings or biopsy samples prepared with Giemsa and other routine histologic stains can be used for diagnosis.[34, 252] Less invasive conjunctival swabs may be positive with the same stains as used for stool samples.[229, 352]

Electron microscopy of stool, body fluids, and tissue sections[130, 229, 252, 270, 273, 316, 352] is considered the gold standard for confirmation of infection; it allows evaluation of the multiple stages of the parasite in tissues. The sensitivity may be lower than that of other techniques for the detection of spores in stool and urine specimens.[72] Successful isolation of *Encephalitozoon* and *N. corneum* is possible with the use of several cell lines.[76, 134, 229, 296, 337, 352]

Serologic tests were available first for *E. cuniculi* infection.[21] The sensitivity and specificity are unknown, and cross-reactivity is likely. Presumed *E. intestinalis* infection has been diagnosed in AIDS patients by ELISA and counterimmunoelectrophoresis techniques.[339] PCR testing of intestinal biopsy specimens may be useful for the diagnosis[105, 228] and differentiation of species in disseminated disease.[76, 341, 352]

TREATMENT

Control of HIV infection is the most effective means of controlling infections caused by microsporidia. In patients who fail to respond to antiretroviral therapy, other measures may be necessary. Albendazole may be useful for infections caused by *E. intestinalis* and other *Encephalitozoon* spp.[14, 87, 99, 228, 229, 354] Intestinal *E. bieneusi* infection responds inconsistently to albendazole.[24, 344] Treatment with albendazole may lead to improvement in the diarrhea without eradication of spores in the stool specimens obtained; diarrhea eventually may recur.[229, 230, 354] Stool volume and frequency are reduced with a low-fat, low-residue diet.[14] Fumagillin, an antibiotic made by *Aspergillus fumigatus,* is effective topical therapy for microsporidial corneal disease but is too toxic for systemic administration.[85]

REFERENCES

1. Aarnaes, S. L., Blanding, J., Speier, S., et al.: Comparison of the ProSpecT and Color Vue enzyme-linked immunoassay for the detection of *Cryptosporidium* in stool specimens. Diagn. Microbiol. Infect. Dis. *19*: 221–225, 1994.
2. Aldras, A. M., Orenstein, J. M., Kotler, D. P., et al.: Detection of microsporidia by indirect immunofluorescence antibody test using polyclonal and monoclonal antibodies. J. Clin. Microbiol. *32*:608–612, 1994.
3. Alpert, G., Bell, L. M., Kirkpatrick, C. E., et al.: Outbreak of cryptosporidiosis in a day care center. Pediatrics *77*:152–157, 1986.
4. Anderson, B. C.: Moist heat inactivation of *Cryptosporidium* sp. Am. J. Public Health *75*:1433–1434, 1985.
5. Anderson, B. C.: Effects of drying on the infectivity of cryptosporidia-laden calf feces for 3- to 7-day-old mice. Am. J. Vet. Res. *47*:2272–2273, 1986.
6. Anderson, B. C., Donndelinger, T., Wilkins, R. M., et al.: Cryptosporidiosis in a veterinary student. J. Am. Vet. Med. Assoc. *180*:408–409, 1982.
7. Angus, K. W.: Cryptosporidiosis in man, domestic animals, and birds: A review. J. R. Soc. Med. *76*:62–70, 1983.
8. Angus, K. W., Sherwood, D., Hutchinson, G., et al.: Evaluation of the effect of two aldehyde-based disinfectants on the infectivity of fecal cryptosporidia for mice. Res. Vet. Sci. *33*:379–381, 1982.
9. Argenzio, R. A., Lecce, J., and Powell, D. W.: Prostanoids inhibit intestinal NaCl absorption in experimental porcine cryptosporidiosis. Gastroenterology *104*:440–447, 1993.
10. Argenzio, R. A., Liacos, J. A., Levy, M. L., et al.: Villous atrophy, crypt hyperplasia, cellular infiltration, and impaired glucose-Na absorption in enteric cryptosporidiosis of pigs. Gastroenterology *98*:1129–1140, 1990.
11. Arrowood, M. J., and Sterling, C. R.: Comparison of conventional staining methods and monoclonal antibody–based methods for *Cryptosporidium* oocyst detection. J. Clin. Microbiol. *27*:1490–1495, 1989.
12. Ashford, R. W.: Occurrence of an undescribed coccidian in man in Papua New Guinea. Ann. Trop. Med. Parasitol. *73*:497–500, 1979.
13. Ashford, R. W., Warhurst, D. C., and Reid, G. D. F.: Human infections with *Cyanobacterium*-like bodies. Lancet *341*:1034, 1993.
14. Asmuth, D. M., DeGirolami, P. C., Federman, M., et al.: Clinical features of microsporidiosis in patients with AIDS. Clin. Infect. Dis. *18*:819–825, 1994.
15. Assessing the public health threat associated with waterborne cryptosporidiosis: Report of a Workshop. M. M. W. R. Recomm. Rep. *44*(RR-6):1–19, 1995.
16. Baxby, D., and Hart, C. A.: The incidence of cryptosporidiosis: A two-year prospective survey in a children's hospital. J. Hyg. *96*:107–111, 1986.
17. Beauvais, B., Sarfati, C., Molina, J. M., et al.: Comparative evaluation of five diagnostic methods for demonstrating microsporidia in stool and intestinal biopsy specimens. Ann. Trop. Med. Parasitol. *87*:99–102, 1993.
18. Benator, D. A., French, A. L., Beaudet, L. M., et al.: *Isospora belli* infection associated with acalculous cholecystitis in a patient with AIDS. Ann. Intern. Med. *121*:663–664, 1994.
19. Bendell, R. P., Lucas S., Moody A., et al.: Diarrhoea associated with *Cyanobacterium*-like bodies: A new coccidian enteritis in man. Lancet *341*:590–592, 1993.
20. Benhamou, Y., Caumes E., Gerosa Y., et al.: AIDS-related cholangiopathy: Critical analysis of a prospective series of 26 patients. Dig. Dis. Sci. *38*:1113–1118, 1993.
21. Bergquist, N. R. G., Stintzing, L., Smedman, T., et al.: Diagnosis of encephalitozoonosis in man by serological tests. B. M. J. *288*:902, 1984.
22. Blagburn, B. L., and Current, W. L.: Accidental infection of a researcher with human *Cryptosporidium.* J. Infect. Dis. *148*:772–773, 1983.
23. Blanco, R. A., and Samayoa, J. C.: Diarrhea and *Cryptosporidium* in Guatemala. Bol. Med. Hosp. Infant. Mex. *45*:139–143, 1988.
24. Blanshard, C., Ellis, D. S., Tovey, D. G., et al.: Treatment of intestinal microsporidiosis with albendazole in patients with AIDS. AIDS *6*:311–313, 1992.
25. Blumberg, R. S., Kelsey, P., Perrone, T., et al.: Cytomegalovirus and *Cryptosporidium* associated with acalculous gangrenous cholecystitis. Am. J. Med. *76*:1118–1123, 1984.
26. Bogaerts, J., Lepage, P., Rouvroy, D., et al.: *Cryptosporidium* spp. a frequent cause of diarrhea in central Africa. J. Clin. Microbiol. *20*:874–876, 1984.
27. Bonnin, A., Dei-Cas, E., and Camerlynck, P.: *Cryptosporidium* and *Isospora. In* Myint, S., and Cann, A. (eds.): Molecular and Cell Biology of Opportunistic Infections in AIDS. London, Chapman & Hall, 1992, pp. 139–161.
28. Borowitz, S. M., and Saulsbury, F. T.: Treatment of chronic cryptosporidiosis with orally administered human serum immune globin. J. Pediatr. *119*:593–595, 1991.
29. Brady, E., Margolis M. L., and Korzeniowski, O. M.: Pulmonary cryptosporidiosis in acquired immune deficiency syndrome. J. A. M. A. *252*:89–90, 1984.
30. Brandborg, L. L., Goldberg, S. B., and Briedenbach, W. C.: Human coccidiosis, a possible cause of malabsorption: The life cycle in a small bowel mucosal biopsy as a diagnostic feature. N. Engl. J. Med. *283*:1306–1313, 1970.
31. Bretagne, S., Jacovella, J., Breuil, J., et al.: Cryptosporidiosis in children: Outbreaks and sporadic cases. Ann. Pediatr. *37*:381–386, 1990.
32. Brownstein, D. G., Strandberg, J. D., Montali, R. J., et al.: *Cryptosporidium* in snakes with hypertrophic gastritis. Vet. Pathol. *14*:606–617, 1977.
33. Buret, A., Gall, D. G., Nation, P. N., et al.: Intestinal protozoa and epithelia cell kinetics, structure and function. Parasitol. Today *6*: 375–380, 1990.
34. Cali, A., Meisler, D. M., Rutherford, I., et al.: Corneal microsporidiosis in a patient with AIDS. Am. J. Trop. Med. Hyg. *44*:463–468, 1991.
35. Campbell, I., Tzipori, S., Hutchinson, G., et al.: Effect of disinfectants on survival of *Cryptosporidium* oocyst. Vet. Rec. *111*:414–415, 1982.
36. Campbell, P. N., and Current, W. L.: Demonstration of serum antibodies to *Cryptosporidium* sp. in normal and immunodeficient humans with confirmed infections. J. Clin. Microbiol. *18*:165–169, 1983.
37. Cappell, M. S., and Hassan, T.: Pancreatic disease in AIDS: A review. J. Clin. Gastroenterol. *17*:254–263, 1993.

38. Carter, M. J., and Anziinlt, T.: *Cryptosporidium*: An important cause of gastrointestinal disease in immunocompetent patients. N. Z. Med. J. *99*:101–103, 1986.
39. Casemore, D. P.: The antibody response to *Cryptosporidium*: Development of a serological test and its use in a study of immunologically normal persons. J. Infect. Dis. *14*:125–134, 1987.
40. Casemore, D. P., and Roberts, C.: Guidelines for the screening for *Cryptosporidium* in stools: Report of a joint working group. J. Clin. Pathol. *46*:2–4, 1993.
41. Casemore, D. P., Sands, R. L., and Curry, A.: *Cryptosporidium* species a "new" human pathogen. J. Clin. Pathol. *38*:1321–1336, 1985.
42. Cello J. P., Grendell, J. H., Basuk, P., et al.: Effect of octreotide on refractory AIDS-associated diarrhea: A prospective, multicenter clinical trial. Ann. Intern. Med. *115*:705–710, 1991.
43. Chen, W., Harp, J. A., Harmsen, A. G.: Requirement for $CD4^+$ cells and gamma interferon in resolution of established *Cryptosporidium parvum* infection in mice. Infect. Immun. *61*:3928–3932, 1993.
44. Chen , W., Harp J. A., Harmsen, A. G., et al.: Gamma interferon functions in resistance to *Cryptosporidium parvum* infection in severe combined immunodeficient mice. Infect. Immun. *61*:3548–3551, 1993.
45. Chiodini, P. L.: A "new" parasite: Human infection with *Cyclospora cayetanensis.* Trans. R. Soc. Trop. Med. Hyg. *88*:369–371, 1994.
46. Chu, P., and West, A. B.: *Encephalitozoon (Septata) intestinalis:* Cytologic, histologic, and electron microscopic features of a systemic intestinal pathogen. Am. J. Clin. Pathol. *106*:606–614, 1996.
47. Clark, D. P.: New insights into human cryptosporidiosis. Clin. Microbiol. Rev. *12*:554–563, 1999.
48. Clotet, B., Sirera, G., Cofan, F., et al.: Efficacy of the somatostatin analogue (SMS-201-995), Sandostatin, for cryptosporidial diarrhoea in patients with AIDS. AIDS *3*:857–858, 1989.
49. Colford, J. M., Tager, I. B., Hirozawa, A. M., et al.: Cryptosporidiosis among patients infected with human immunodeficiency virus. Am. J. Epidemiol. *144*:807–816, 1996.
50. Collier, A. C., Miller, R. A., and Meyers, J. D.: Cryptosporidiosis after marrow transplantation, person to person transmission and treatment with spiramycin. Ann. Intern. Med. *101*:205–206, 1984.
51. Combee, C. L., Collinge, M. L., and Britt, E. M.: Cryptosporidiosis in a hospital-associated day care center. Pediatr. Infect. Dis. *5*:528–532, 1986.
52. Comin, C. E., and Santucci, M.: Submicroscopic profile of *Isospora belli* enteritis in a patient with acquired immune deficiency syndrome. Ultrastruct. Pathol. *18*:437–482, 1994.
53. Connor, B. A., and Shlim, D. R.: Foodborne transmission of *Cyclospora.* Lancet *346*:1634, 1995.
54. Cordell, R. L., and Addiss, D. G.: Cryptosporidiosis in child care setting: A review of the literature and recommendation for prevention and control. Pediatr. Infect. Dis. J. *13*:310–317, 1994.
55. Cordell, R. L., Thor, P. M., Addiss, D. G., et al.: Impact of a massive waterborne cryptosporidiosis outbreak on child care facilities in metropolitan Milwaukee, Wisconsin. Pediatr. Infect. Dis. J. *16*:639–644, 1997.
56. Cotte, L., Rabondonirina, M., Chapuis, F., et al.: Waterborne outbreak of intestinal microsporidiosis in persons with and without human immunodeficiency virus infection. J. Infect. Dis. *180*:2003–2008, 1999.
57. Cozon, G., Biron, F., Jeannin, M., et al.: Secretory IgA antibodies to *Cryptosporidium parvum* in AIDS patients with chronic cryptosporidiosis. J. Infect. Dis. *169*:696–699, 1994.
58. Crawford, F. G., and Vermund, S. H.: Human cryptosporidiosis. C. R. C. Crit. Rev. Microbiol. *16*:113–159, 1988.
59. Cruickshank, R., Ashdown, L., and Croese, J.: Human cryptosporidiosis in north Queensland. Aust. N. Z. J. Med. *18*:582–586, 1988.
60. Cruz, J. R., Cano, F., Caceres P., et al.: Infection and diarrhea caused by *Cryptosporidium spp.* among Guatemalan infants. J. Clin. Microbiol. *26*:88–91, 1988.
61. Cryptosporidiosis among children attending day-care centers—Georgia, Pennsylvania, Michigan, California, New Mexico. M. M. W. R. Morb. Mortal Wkly. Rep. *33*(42):599–601, 1984.
62. An assessment of chemotherapy of males with acquired immunodeficiency syndrome (AIDS). M. M. W. R. Morb. Mortal Wkly. Rep. *31*(44): 589–592, 1982.
63. *Cryptosporidium* infections associated with swimming pools—Dane County, Wisconsin, 1993. M. M. W. R. Morb. Mortal Wkly. Rep. *43*(31):561–563, 1994.
64. Current, W. L.: *Cryptosporidium*: Its biology and potential for environmental transmission. C. R. C. Crit. Rev. Environ. Control *17*:21–51, 1986.
65. Current, W. L.: *Cryptosporidium parvum*: Household transmission. Ann. Intern. Med. *120*:518–519, 1994.
66. Current, W. L., and Bick, P. H.: Immunobiology of *Cryptosporidium* spp. Pathol. Immunopathol. Res. *8*:141–160, 1989.
67. Current, W. L., and Garcia L. S.: Cryptosporidiosis. Clin. Microbiol. Rev. *4*:325–358, 1991.
68. Current, W. L., and Garcia L. S.: Cryptosporidiosis. Clin. Lab. Med. *11*:873–895, 1991.
69. Current, W. L., and Reese, N. C.: A comparison of endogenous development of three isolates of *Cryptosporidium* in suckling mice. J. Protozool. *33*:98–108, 1986.
70. Current, W. L., Reese, N. C., Ernst, J. V., et al.: Human cryptosporidiosis in immunocompetent and immunodeficient persons: Studies of an outbreak and experimental transmission. N. Engl. J. Med. *308*: 1252–1257, 1983.
71. Current, W. L., Upton, S. J., and Haynes, T. B.: The life cycle of *Cryptosporidium baileyi* n. sp. (Apicocomplexa: Cryptosporidiidae) infecting chickens. J. Protozool. *33*:289–296, 1986.
72. Curry, A., and Canning, E. U.: Human microsporidiosis. J. Infect. *27*:229–236, 1993.
73. D'Antonio, R. G., Win, R. E., Taylor, J. P., et al.: A waterborne outbreak of cryptosporidiosis in normal hosts. Ann. Intern. Med. *103*:886–888, 1985.
75. DeGirolami, P. C., Ezratty, C. R., Desai, G., et al.: Diagnosis of intestinal microsporidiosis by examination of stool and duodenal aspirate with Weber's modified trichrome and Uvitex 2B stains. J. Clin. Microbiol. *33*:805–810, 1995.
76. De Groote, M. A., Visvesvara, G., Wilson, M. L., et al.: Polymerase chain reaction and culture confirmation of disseminated *Encephalitozoon cuniculi* in patients with AIDS: Successful therapy with albendazole. J. Infect. Dis. *171*:1375–1378, 1995.
77. DeHovitz, J. A., Pape, J. W., Boncy, M., et al.: Clinical manifestations and therapy of *Isospora belli* infection in patients with the acquired immunodeficiency syndrome. N. Engl. J. Med. *315*:87–90, 1986.
78. DeMol, P., Mukashuma, S., Bogaerts, J., et al.: *Cryptosporidium* related to measles diarrhea in Rwanda. Lancet *2*:42–43, 1884.
79. De Oliveira, G. S., Barboso, W., and Dasilva, A. L.: Isosporose humana em Goias. Rev. Pat. Trop. 387–395, 1973.
80. De Rycke, J., Bernard, S., Laporte, J., et al.: Prevalence of various enteropathogens in the feces of diarrheic and healthy calves. Ann. Rech. Vet. *17*:159–168, 1986.
81. Dhillon, A. S., Thacker, H. L., Dietzel, A. V., et al.: Respiratory cryptosporidiosis in broiler chickens. Avian Dis. *25*:747–751, 1981.
82. Didier, E. S.: Microsporidiosis. Clin. Infect. Dis. *27*:1–7, 1998.
83. Didier, E. S., Orenstein, J. M., Aldras, A., et al.: Comparison of three staining methods for detecting microsporidia in fluids. J. Clin. Microbiol. *33*:3138–3145, 1995.
84. Diers, J., and McCallister, G. L.: Occurrence of *Cryptosporidium* in home day care centers in west central Colorado. J. Parasitol. *75*:637–638, 1989.
85. Diesenhouse, M. C., Wilson, L. A., Corrent, G. F., et al.: Treatment of microsporidial keratoconjunctivitis with topical fumagillin. Am. J. Ophthalmol. *115*:293–298, 1993.
86. Dore, G. J., Marriott, D. J., Hing, M. C., et al.: Disseminated microsporidiosis due to *Septata intestinalis* in nine patients infected with the human immunodeficiency virus: Response to therapy with albendazole. Clin. Infect. Dis. *21*:70–76, 1995.
87. Dryjanski, J., Gold, J. W., Ritchie, M. T., et al.: Cryptosporidiosis: Case report in a health team worker. Am. J. Med. *80*:751–752, 1986.
88. Doumbo O., Rossignol, J. F., Pichard, E., et al.: Nitazoxanide in the treatment of cryptosporidial diarrhea and other intestinal parasitic infections associated with acquired immunodeficiency syndrome in tropical Africa. Am. J. Trop. Med. Hyg. *56*:637–639, 1997.
89. DuPont, H. L., Chappell, C. L., Sterling, C. R., et al.: The infectivity of *Cryptosporidium parvum* in healthy volunteers. N. Engl. J. Med. *332*: 855–859, 1995.
90. Elsdon-Dew, R.: *Isospora natalensis* (sp. nov.) in man. J. Trop. Med. Hyg. *56*:149–150, 1953.
91. False-positive laboratory tests for *Cryptosporidium* involving an enzyme-linked immunosorbent assay—United States, November 1997–March 1998. M. M. W. R. Morb. Mortal Wkly. Rep. *48*(1):4–8, 1999.
92. Fang, G., Aruajo, V., and Guerrant, R. L.: Enteric infections associated with exposure to animals and animal products. Infect. Dis. Clin. North Am. *5*:681–701, 1991.
93. Fanning, M., Monte, M., Sutherland, L. R., et al.: Pilot study of Sandostatin (octreotide) therapy of refractory HIV-associated diarrhea. Dig. Dis. Sci. *36*:476–480, 1991.
94. Faust, E. C., Giraldo, L. E., Caicedo, G., et al.: Human isosporosis in the Western Hemisphere. Am. J. Med. *10*:343–349, 1983.
95. Fayer, R.: Effects of high temperature on infectivity of *Cryptosporidium parvum* oocyst in water. Appl. Environ. Microbiol. *60*:2732–2735, 1994.
96. Fayer, R., and Ungar, B. L. P.: *Cryptosporidium spp.* and cryptosporidiosis. Microbiol. Rev. *50*:458–483, 1986.
97. Ferson, M. J., and Young, L. C.: *Cryptosporidium* and coxsackievirus B5 causing epidemic diarrhoea in a child care center. Med. J. Aust. *156*:813, 1992.
98. Fichtenbaum, C. J., Ritchie, D. J., and Powderly, W. G.: Use of paromomycin for treatment of cryptosporidiosis in patients with AIDS. Clin. Infect. Dis. *16*:290–300, 1993.
99. Field, A. S., Hing, M. C., Miliken, S. T., et al.: Microsporidia in the small intestine of HIV-infected patients: A new diagnostic technique and a new species. Med. J. Aust. *158*:390–394, 1993.

100. Flanigan, T. P., and Soave, R.: Cryptosporidiosis. Prog. Clin. Parasitol. *3*:1–20, 1993.
101. Flanigan T., Whalen, C., Turner, J., et al.: *Cryptosporidium* infection and CD4 counts. Ann Intern. Med. *116*:840–842, 1992.
102. Flepp, M., Sauer, B., Luthy, R., et al.: Human microsporidiosis in HIV seronegative, immunocompetent patients. Abstract LM25. Paper presented at the 35th Interscience Conference on Chemotherapy and Antimicrobial Agents, San Francisco, 1995, p. 331.
103. Forgacs, P., Tarchis, A., Ma, P., et al.: Intestinal and bronchial cryptosporidiosis in an immunodeficient homosexual man. Ann. Intern. Med. *99*:793–794, 1983.
104. Forthal, D. N., and Guest, S. S.: *Isospora belli* enteritis in three homosexual men. Am. J. Trop. Med. Hyg. *33*:1060–1064, 1984.
105. Franzen, C., Muller, A., Hartmann, P., et al.: Polymerase chain reaction for diagnosis and species differentiation of microsporidia. Folia Parasitol. *45*:140–148, 1998.
106. Franzen, C., Schwartz, D. A., Visvesvara, G. S., et al.: Immunologically confirmed disseminated asymptomatic *Encephalitozoon cuniculi* infection of the gastrointestinal tract in a patient with AIDS. Clin. Infect. Dis. *21*:1480–1484, 1995.
107. Fricker, C. R. and Crabb, J. H.: Water-borne cryptosporidiosis detection methods and treatment options. Adv. Parasitol. *40*:241–278, 1998.
108. Gallaher, M. M., Herndon, J. L., Nims, L. J., et al.: Cryptosporidiosis and surface water. Am. J. Public Health *79*:39–42, 1989.
109. Garcia, L. S., Brewer, T. C., and Bruckner, D. A.: Fluorescent detection of *Cryptosporidium* oocyst in human fecal specimens by using monoclonal antibodies. J. Clin. Microbiol. *25*:119–121, 1987.
110. Garcia, L. S., Brewer, T. C., and Bruckner, D. A.: Incidence of *Cryptosporidium* in all patients submitting stool specimens for ova and parasites examination: Monoclonal antibody IFA method. Diagn. Microbiol. Infect. Dis. *11*:25–27, 1988.
111. Garcia, L. S., Owen, R. L., and Current W. L.: Isosporiasis. *In* Balows, A., Hausler, W. J., Jr., Ohashi, M., and Turano, A. (eds.): The Laboratory Diagnosis of Infectious Diseases: Principles and Practice. Vol. 1. New York, Springer-Verlag, 1988, pp. 897–903.
112. Garcia, L. S., and Shimizu, R. Y.: Evaluation of nine immunoassay kits (enzyme immunoassays and direct fluorescence) for detection of *Giardia lamblia* and *Cryptosporidium parvum* in human fecal specimens. J. Clin. Microbiol. *35*:1526–1529, 1997.
113. Garcia, L. S., Shimizu, R. Y., and Bruckner, D. A.: Detection of microsporidial spores in fecal specimens from patients diagnosed with cryptosporidiosis. J. Clin. Microbiol. *32*:1739–1741, 1994.
114. Garza, D., Hopfer, R. L., Eichelberger, C., et al.: Fecal staining for screening *Cryptosporidium* oocysts. J. Med. Technol. *1*:560–563, 1984.
115. Gellin, B. G., and Soave, R.: Coccidian infections in AIDS. Med. Clin. North Am. *76*:205–234, 1992.
116. Giraldo, L. E., Faust, E. C., Bonfante, R., et al.: Diagnostic findings from parasitological examination of excreta of dogs, human beings, and a hog collected in the streets of Ward Siloe, Cali, Colombia. J. Parasitol. *45*:46, 1959.
117. Girard, D. E., and Keefe, E. B.: *Isospora* and travelers diarrhea. Ann. Intern. Med. *106*:908, 1987.
118. Girard, P. M., Goldschmidt, E., Vittecoq, D., et al.: Vapreotide, a somatostatin analogue, in cryptosporidiosis and other AIDS-related diarrheal diseases. AIDS *6*:715–718, 1992.
119. Gobet, P., Buisson, J. C. Vagner, O., et al.: Detection of *Cryptosporidium parvum* DNA in formed human feces by a sensitive PCR-based assay including uracil-*N*-glycosylase inactivation. J. Clin. Microbiol. *35*: 254–256, 1997.
120. Goebel, E., and Brandler, U.: Ultrastructure of microgametogenesis, microgametes, and gametogomy of *Cryptosporidium sp.* in the intestine of mice. Prostistologica *18*:331–334, 1982.
121. Goldstein, S. T., Juranek D. D., Ravenholt O., et al.: Cryptosporidiosis: An outbreak associated with drinking water despite state-of-the art water treatment. Ann. Intern. Med. *124*:459–468, 1996.
122. Gomez Morales, M. A., Ausiello, C. M., Urbani, F., et al.: Crude extract and recombinant protein of *Cryptosporidium parvum* oocysts induce proliferation of human peripheral blood mononuclear cells in vitro. J. Infect. Dis. *172*:211–216, 1995.
123. Goodgame, R. W., Kimball, K., Ou, C. N., et al.: Intestinal function and injury in acquired immunodeficiency syndrome–related cryptosporidiosis. Gastroenterology *108*:1075–1082, 1995.
124. Graczyk, T. K., Cranfield, M. R., and Fayer, R.: Evaluation of commercial enzyme immunoassay (EIA) and immunofluorescent antibody (FA) test kits for detection of *Cryptosporidium* oocysts of species other than *Cryptosporidium parvum*. Am. J. Trop. Med. Hyg. *54*:274–279, 1996.
125. Gradon, J. D., Schulman, R. H., Chapnick, E. K., et al.: Octreotide-induced acute pancreatitis in a patient with acquired immunodeficiency syndrome. South. Med. J. *84*:1410–1411, 1991.
126. Gross, T. L., Wheat, J., Bartlett, M., et al.: AIDS and multiple system involvement with *Cryptosporidium*. Am. J. Gastroenterol. *81*:456–458, 1986.
127. Grossman, I., and Simon, D.: Potential gastrointestinal uses of somatostatin and its synthetic analogue octreotide. Am. J. Gastroenterol. *85*:1061–1072, 1990.
128. Guarda, L. A., Stein, S. A., Cleary, K. A., et al.: Human cryptosporidiosis in the acquired immune deficiency syndrome. Arch. Pathol. Lab. Med. *107*:562–566, 1983.
129. Guarino, A., Canani, R. B., Casola, A., et al.: Human intestinal cryptosporidiosis: Secretory diarrhea and enterotoxic activity in Caco-2 cells. *171*:976–983, 1995.
130. Gunnarson, G., Hurlbut, D., DeGirolami, P. C., et al.: Multiorgan microsporidiosis: Report of five cases and review. Clin. Infect. Dis. *21*: 37–44, 1995.
131. Hannah, J., and Riordan, T.: Case to case spread of cryptosporidiosis; evidence from a day nursery outbreak. Public Health *102*:539–544, 1988.
132. Harari, M. D., West, B., and Dwyer, B.: *Cryptosporidium* as a cause of laryngotracheitis in an infant. Lancet *1*:1207, 1986.
133. Hart, C. A., Baxby, D., and Blundell, N.: Gastroenteritis due to *Cryptosporidium:* A prospective survey in a children's hospital. J. Infect. *9*:264–270, 1984.
134. Hartskeerl, R. A., Van Gool, T., Schuitema, A. R., et al.: Genetic and immunological characterization of the microsporidian *Septata intestinalis* Cali, Kotler and Orenstein, 1993: Reclassification to *Encephalitozoon intestinalis*. Parasitology *110*:277–285, 1995.
135. Hashmey, R., Smith, N. H., and Cron, S.: Cryptosporidiosis in Houston, Texas. A report of 95 cases. Medicine (Baltimore) *76*:118–139, 1997.
136. Hawkins, S. P., Thomas, R. P., and Teasdale, C.: Acute pancreatitis: A new finding in *Cryptosporidium enteritis*. B. M. J. *294*:483–484, 1987.
137. Hayes, E. B., Matte, T. D., O'Brien, T. R., et al.: Large community outbreak of cryptosporidiosis due to contamination of a filtered public water supply. N. Engl. J. Med. *320*:1372–1376, 1989.
138. Heijbel, H., Slaine, K., Seigel, B., et al.: Outbreak of diarrhea in a day care center with spread to household members: The role of *Cryptosporidium*. Pediatr. Infect. Dis. J. *6*:532–535, 1987.
139. Henderson, A. E., Gillespie, G. W., Kaplan, P., et al.: The human *Isospora*. Am. J. Hyg. *78*:302–309, 1963.
140. Henricksen, S. A., and Pohlenz, J. F. L.: Staining of *Cryptosporidium* by a modified Ziehl-Neelsen technique. Acta Vet. Scand. *22*:594–596, 1981.
141. Herwaldt, B. L.: *Cyclospora cayetanensis*: A review, focusing on the outbreaks of *Cyclospora* in the 1990's. Clin. Infect. Dis. *31*:1040–1057, 2000.
142. Herwaldt, B. L., and Ackers, M. L.: An outbreak in 1996 of cyclosporiasis associated with imported raspberries. The *Cyclospora* Working Group. N. Engl. J. Med. *336*:1548–1556, 1997.
143. Herwaldt, B. L., and Beach, M. J.: The return of *Cyclospora* in 1997: Another outbreak of cyclosporiasis in North America associated with imported raspberries. *Cyclospora* Working Group. Ann. Intern. Med. *130*:210–220, 1999.
144. Hinnant, K., Swartz, A., Rotterdam, H., et al.: Cytomegaloviral and cryptosporidial cholecystitis in two patients with AIDS. Am. J. Surg. Pathol. *13*:57–60, 1989.
145. Hoge, C. W., Echeverria, P., Rajah, R., et al.: Prevalence of *Cyclospora* species and other enteric pathogens among children less than 5 years of age in Nepal. J. Clin. Microbiol. *33*:3058–3060, 1995.
146. Hoge, C. W., Shlim, D. R., Ghimire, M., et al.: Placebo-controlled trial of co-trimoxazole for *Cyclospora* infection among travellers and foreign residents in Nepal. Lancet *345*:691–693, 1995.
147. Hoge, C. W., Shlim, D. R., and Rajah, R.: Epidemiology of diarrhoeal illness associated with coccidian-like organism among travellers and foreign residents in Nepal. Lancet *341*:1175–1179, 1993.
148. Hojlyng, N., Holten-Anderson, W., and Jepsen, S.: Cryptosporidiosis: A case of airborne transmission. Lancet *2*:271–272, 1987.
149. Hojlyng, N., and Jensen, B. N.: Respiratory cryptosporidiosis in HIV-positive patients. Lancet *2*:590–591, 1988.
150. Hojlyng, N., Molbak, K., and Jepsen, S.: *Cryptosporidium* spp., a frequent cause of diarrhea in Liberian children. J. Clin. Microbiol. *23*:1109–1113, 1986.
151. Holley, H. P., Jr., and Dover, C.: *Cryptosporidium*: A common cause of parasitic diarrhea in otherwise healthy individuals. J. Infect. Dis. *153*:365–368, 1986.
152. Holmberg, S. D., Moorman, A. C., Von Bargen, J. C., et al.: Possible effectiveness of clarithromycin and rifabutin for cryptosporidiosis chemoprophylaxis in HIV disease. J. A. M. A. *279*:384–386, 1998.
153. Hoover, D. M., Hoerr, F. J., Carlton, W. W., et al.: Enteric cryptosporidiosis in a naso tang. *Naso lituratus* Block and Schneider. J. Fish Dis. *4*:425–428, 1981.
154. Huang, P., Weber, J. T., Sosin, D. M., et al. The first reported outbreak of diarrheal illness associated with *Cyclospora* in the United States. Ann. Intern. Med. *123*:409–414, 1995.
155. Hunter, G., Bagshawe, A. F., Baboo, K. S., et al.: Intestinal parasites in Zambian patients with AIDS. Trans. R. Soc. Trop. Med. Hyg. *86*:543–545, 1992.
156. Iseki, M.: *Cryptosporidium felis* sp. n. (Protozoa: Eimeriorina) from the domestic cat. Jpn. J. Parasitol. *28*:285–307, 1979.
157. Issacs, D., Hunt, G. H., Phillips, A. D., et al.: Cryptosporidiosis in immunocompetent children. J. Clin. Pathol. *38*:78–81, 1985.

158. Janoff, E. N., Limas C., and Gebhard, R. L.: Cryptosporidial carriage without symptoms in the acquired immunodeficiency syndrome (AIDS). Ann. Intern. Med. *112*:75–76, 1990.
159. Jarpa, A.: Isosporosis humana. Bol. Chileno Parasitol. *12*:31, 1957.
160. Jarpa Gana, A.: Coccidiosis humana. Biologica *39*:3–26, 1966.
161. Jeffrey, G. M.: Epidemiologic considerations of isosporiasis in a school for mental defective children. Ann. J. Hyg. *67*:251–255, 1958.
162. Joce, R. E., Bruce, J., Kiely, D., et al.: An outbreak of cryptosporidiosis associated with a swimming pool. Epidemiol. Infect. *107*:497–508, 1991.
163. Jokipii, A., Hemila, M., and Jokipii, L.: Prospective study of acquisition of *Cryptosporidium, Giardia lamblia,* and gastrointestinal illness. Lancet *2*:487–489, 1985.
164. Jokipii, L., and Jokipii, A. M.: Timing of symptoms and oocyst excretion in human cryptosporidiosis. N. Engl. J. Med. *315*:1643–1647, 1987.
165. Joseph, C., Hamilton, G., O'Connor M., et al.: Cryptosporidiosis in the Isle of Thanet: An outbreak associated with local drinking water. Epidemiol. Infect. *107*:509–519, 1991.
166. Juranek, D. D.: Cryptosporidiosis: Source of infection and guidelines for prevention. Clin. Infect. Dis. *21*:57–61, 1995.
167. Kahn, D. G., Garfinkle, J. M., Klonoff, D. C., et al.: Cryptosporidial and cytomegalovirus hepatitis and cholecystitis. Arch. Pathol. Lab. Med. *111*:879–881, 1987.
168. Keren, G., Barzilia A., Barzilay, Z., et al.: Life-threatening cryptosporidiosis in immunocompetent infants. Eur. J. Pediatr. *146*:187–189, 1987.
169. Kibbler, C. C., Smith, A., Hamilton-Dutoit, S. J., et al.: Pulmonary cryptosporidiosis occurring in a bone marrow transplant patient. Scand. J. Infect. *19*:581–584, 1987.
170. Koch, K. J., Phillips, D. J., Aber, R. C., et al.: Cryptosporidiosis in hospital personnel: Evidence for person-to-person transmission. Ann. Intern. Med. *102*:593–596, 1985.
171. Kocoshis, S. A., Cibull, M. L., Davis, T. E., et al.: Intestinal and pulmonary cryptosporidiosis in an infant with severe combined immune deficiency. J. Pediatr. Gastroenterol. Nutr. *3*:149–157, 1984.
172. Kotler, D. P., Giang, T. T., Garro, M. L., et al.: Light microscopic diagnosis of microsporidiosis in patients with AIDS. Am. J. Gastroenterol. *89*:540–544, 1994.
173. Kotler, D. P., and Orenstein, J. M.: Prevalence of intestinal microsporidiosis in HIV-infected individuals referred for gastroenterological evaluation. Am. J. Gastroenterol. *89*:1998–2002, 1994.
174. Kreinik, G., Burstein, O., and Landor, M., et al.: Successful management of intractable cryptosporidiosis diarrhea with intravenous octreotide, a somatostatin analogue. AIDS *5*:765–767, 1991.
175. Lacroix, S., Mancassola, R., Nacirl, M., et al.: *Cryptosporidium parvum*-specific mucosal immune response in C57BL/6 neonatal and gamma interferon–deficient mice: Role of tumor necrosis factor alpha in protection. Infect. Immun. *69*:1635–1642, 2001.
176. Lahdevirta, J., Jokipii, A. M. M., Sammalkorpi, K., et al.: Perinatal infection with *Cryptosporidium* and failure to thrive. Lancet *1*:48–49, 1987.
177. Lasser, K. H., Lewin, K. J., and Ryning, F. W.: Cryptosporidial enteritis in a patient with congenital hypogammaglobulinemia. Hum. Pathol. *10*:234–240, 1979.
178. Laurent, F., Eckmann, L., Savidge, T. C., et al.: *Cryptosporidium parvum* infection of human intestinal epithelial cells induces the polarized secretion of C-X-C chemokines. Infect. Immun. *65*:5067–5073, 1997.
179. Laurent, F., Kagnoff, M. F., Savidge, T. C., et al.: Human intestinal epithelial cells respond to *Cryptosporidium parvum* infection with increased prostaglandin H synthase 2 expression and prostaglandin E_2 and $F_{2\alpha}$ production. Infect. Immun. *66*:1787–1790, 1998.
180. Laurent, F., McCole, D., Eckmann, L., et al.: Pathogenesis of *Cryptosporidium parvum* infection. Microb. Infect. *2*:141–148, 1999.
181. Laxer, M. L., Timblin, B. K., Patel, R. J.: DNA sequence for the specific detection of *Cryptosporidium parvum* by polymerase chain reaction. Am. J. Trop. Med. Hyg. *45*:688–694, 1991.
182. Ledford, D. K., Overman, M. D., Gonzalvo, A., et al.: Microsporidiosis myositis in a patient with acquired immunodeficiency syndrome. Ann. Intern. Med. *102*:628–630, 1985.
183. Leng, X. D., Mosier, D. A., and Oberst, R. D.: Simplified method for recovery and PCR detection of *Cryptosporidium* DNA from bovine feces. Appl. Environ. Microbiol. *62*:643–647, 1996.
184. Levine, N. D.: Taxonomy and review of the coccidian genus *Cryptosporidium* (Protozoa, Apicocomplexa). J. Protozool. *31*:94–98, 1984.
185. Lewis, I. S., Hart, C. A., and Baxby, D.: Diarrhea due to *Cryptosporidium* in acute lymphoblastic leukemia. Arch. Dis. Child. *60*:60–62, 1985.
186. Liberti, A., Bisogno, A., and Izzo, E.: Octreotide treatment of secretory and cryptosporidial diarrhea with acquired immunodeficiency syndrome (AIDS): Clinical evaluation. J. Chemother. *4*:303–305, 1992.
187. Liebman, W. M., Thaler, M. M., DeLorimier, A., et al.: Intractable diarrhea of infancy due to intestinal coccidiosis. Gastroenterology *78*:579–584, 1980.
188. Lindsay, D. S., Dubey, J. P., and Blagburn, B. L.: Biology of *Isospora spp.* from humans, nonhuman primates, and domestic animals. Clin. Microbiol. Rev. *10*:19–34, 1997.
189. Loose, J. H., Sedergran, D. J., and Cooper, H. S.: Identification of *Cryptosporidium* in paraffin-embedded tissue sections with the use of a monoclonal antibody. Am. J. Clin. Pathol. *91*:206–209, 1989.
190. Lorenzo-Lorenzo, M. J., Ares-Mazas, M. E., Villacorta-Martinez de Maturana, I., et al.: Effect of ultraviolet disinfection of drinking water on the viability of *Cryptosporidium parvum* oocysts. J. Parasitol. *79*: 67–70, 1993.
191. Louie, E., Barkowsky, W., and Klesius, P. H.: Treatment of cryptosporidiosis with oral bovine transfer factor. Clin. Immunol. Immunopathol. *44*:329–334, 1987.
192. Loureiro, E. C., Linhares, A. da C., and Mata, L.: Acute diarrhoea associated with *Cryptosporidium sp.* in Belem, Brazil (preliminary report). Rev. Inst. Med. Trop. Sao Paulo *28*:138–140, 1986.
193. Luna, V. A., Stewart, B. K., Bergeron, D. L., et al.: Use of the fluorochrome calcofluor white in the screening of stool specimens for spores of microsporidia. Am. J. Clin. Pathol. *103*:656–659, 1995.
194. Ma, P., Villanueva, T. G., Kaufman, D., et al.: Respiratory cryptosporidiosis in the acquired immunodeficiency syndrome. J. A. M. A. *252*:1298–1301, 1984.
195. MacFarlane, D. E., and Horner-Bryce, J.: Cryptosporidiosis in well nourished and malnourished children. Acta Paediatr. Scand. *76*:474–477, 1987.
196. MacKenzie, W. R., Hoxie, N. J., Proctor, M. E., et al.: A massive outbreak in Milwaukee of *Cryptosporidium* infection transmitted through the public water supply. N. Engl. J. Med. *331*:161–167, 1994.
197. MacPherson, D. W., and McQueen, R.: Cryptosporidiosis: Multiattribute evaluation of six diagnostic methods. J. Clin. Microbiol. *31*:193–202, 1993.
198. Madico, G., Gilman, R., Miranda, E., et al.: Treatment of *Cyclospora* infections with co-trimoxazole. Lancet *342*:122–123, 1993.
199. Madore, M. S., Rose, J. B., Gerba, C. P., et al.: Occurrence of *Cryptosporidium* oocysts in sewage effluents and select surface waters. J. Parasitol. *73*:702–705, 1983.
200. Maggi, P., Larocca, A. M., Quarto, M., et al.: Effect of antiretroviral therapy on cryptosporidiosis and microsporidiosis in patients infected with human immunodeficiency virus type 1. Eur. J. Clin. Microbiol. Infect. Dis. *19*:213–217, 2000.
201. Manabe, Y. C., Clark, D. B., Moore, R. D., et al.: Cryptosporidiosis in patients with AIDS: Correlation of disease and survival. Clin. Infect. Dis. *27*:536–542, 1998.
202. Mann, E. D., Sekla, L. H., Nayer, G. P., et al.: Infection with *Cryptosporidium spp.* in humans and cattle in Manitoba. Can. J. Vet. Res. *50*:174–148, 1986.
203. Marcial, M. A., and Madara, J. L.: *Cryptosporidium*: Cellular localization, structural analysis of absorptive cell–parasite membrane–membrane interactions in guinea pigs, and suggestion of protozoan transport by M cells. Gastroenterology *90*:583–594, 1986.
204. Margulis, S. J., Honig, C. L., Soave, R., et al.: Biliary tract obstruction in the acquired immunodeficiency syndrome. Ann. Intern. Med. *105*: 207–210, 1986.
205. Marshall, A. R., Al-Jumaili, I. J., Fenwick, G. A., et al.: Cryptosporidiosis in patients in a large teaching hospital. J. Clin. Microbiol. *25*:172–173, 1987.
206. Marshall, M. M., Naumovitz, D., Ortega, Y., and Sterling, C. R.: Waterborne protozoan pathogens. Clin. Microbiol. Rev. *10*:67–85, 1997.
207. Martino, P., Gentile, G., Caprioli, A., et al.: Hospital acquired cryptosporidiosis in a bone marrow transplantation unit. J. Infect. Dis. *158*:647–648, 1988.
208. Mata, L., Bolanos, H., Pezarro, D., et al.: Cryptosporidiosis in children from some highland Costa Rican rural and urban areas. Am. J. Trop. Med. Hyg. *33*:24–29, 1984.
209. Mathan, M., Venkatesan, S., George, R., et al.: *Cryptosporidium* and diarrhoea in southern Indian children. Lancet *2*:1172–1175, 1985.
210. Matsubayashi, H., Koike, T., Mikata, T., et al.: A case of *Encephalitozoon*-like body infection in man. Arch. Pathol. *67*:181–187, 1959.
211. Matsubayashi, H., and Nozawa, T.: Experimental infection of *Isospora hominis* in man. Am. J. Trop. Hyg. *2*:633–637, 1948.
212. McAnulty, J. M., Flemming, D. W., and Gonzalez, A. H.: A community-wide outbreak of cryptosporidiosis associated with swimming in a wave pool. J. A. M. A. *272*:1597–1600, 1994.
213. McDougall, R. J., Tandy, M. W., Boreham, R. E., et al.: Incidental finding of microsporidian parasite from an AIDS patient. J. Clin. Microbiol. *31*:436–439, 1993.
214. McLaughlin, J., Casemore, D. P., Harrison, T. G., et al.: Identification of *Cryptosporidium* oocyst by monoclonal antibody. Lancet *1*:51, 1987.
215. McMeeking, A., Borkowsky, W., Klesius, P. H., et al.: A controlled trial of bovine dialyzable leukocyte extract for cryptosporidiosis in patients with AIDS. J. Infect. Dis. *161*:108–112, 1990.
216. McNabb, S. J. N., Hensel, D. M., Welch, D. F., et al.: Comparison of sedimentation and flotation techniques for identification of *Cryptosporidium sp.* oocysts in a large outbreak of human diarrhea. J. Clin. Microbiol. *22*:587–589, 1985.

217. Mead, G. M., Sweetenham, J. W., Ewins, D. L., et al.: Intestinal cryptosporidiosis: A complication of cancer treatment. Cancer Treat. Rep. *70*:769–770, 1986.
218. Meisel, J. L., Perera, D. R., Meligro, B. S., et al.: Overwhelming watery diarrhoea associated with a *Cryptosporidium* in an immunosuppressed patient. Gastroenterology *70*:1156–1160, 1976.
219. Melo Cristino, J. A. G., Carvalho, M. I. P., and Salgado, M. J.: An outbreak of cryptosporidiosis in a hospital day-care center. Epidemiol. Infect. *101*:355–359, 1988.
220. Michiels, J. F., Hofman P., Bernard, E., et al.: Intestinal and extraintestinal *Isospora belli* infection in an AIDS patient. Pathol. Res. Pract. *190*:1089–1093, 1994.
221. Michielsen, P. P., Fierens, H., and Van Maercke, Y. M.: Drug-induced gallbladder disease: Incidence, aetiology and management. Drug Saf. *7*:32–45, 1992.
222. Milacek, P., and Vitovec, J.: Differential staining of cryptosporidia beaniline-carbolmethyl violet and tartarzine in smears of feces and scrapping of intestinal mucosa. Folia Parasitol. *32*:50, 1985.
223. Miller, N. M., and VanDen, E. S.: Seasonal prevalence of *Cryptosporidium* associated diarrhea in young children. S. Afr. Med. J. *70*:636–637, 1986.
224. Miller, R. A., Bronsdon, M. A., and Morton, W. R.: Experimental cryptosporidiosis in a primate model. J. Infect. Dis. *161*:312–315, 1990.
225. Miller, R. A., Holmberg, R. E., and Clausen, C. R.: Life-threatening diarrhea caused by *Cryptosporidium* in a child undergoing therapy for acute lymphocytic leukemia. J. Pediatr. *103*:256–259, 1983.
226. Miller, R. A., Wasserheit, J. N., Kerihara, J., et al.: Detection of *Cryptosporidium* oocysts in sputum during screening for *Mycobacterium*. J. Clin. Microbiol. *20*:1191–1193, 1984.
227. Miller, T. L., Winter, H. S., Luginbuhl L. M., et al.: Pancreatitis in pediatric human immunodeficiency virus infection. J. Pediatr. *120*:223–227, 1992.
228. Molina, J. M., Chastang, C., Goguel, J., et al.: Albendazole for treatment and prophylaxis of microsporidiosis due to *Encephalitozoon intestinalis* in patients with AIDS: A randomized double-blind controlled trial. J. Infect. Dis. *177*:1371–1377, 1998.
229. Molina, J. M., Oksenhendler, E., Beauvais, B., et al.: Disseminated microsporidiosis due to *Septata intestinalis* in patients with AIDS: Clinical features and response to albendazole therapy. J. Infect. Dis. *171*:245–249, 1995.
230. Molina, J. M., Sarfati, C., Beauvais, B., et al.: Intestinal microsporidiosis in human immunodeficiency virus–infected patients with chronic unexplained diarrhea: Prevalence and clinical and biological features. J. Infect. Dis. *167*:217–221, 1993.
231. Montessori, G. A., and Bischoff, L.: Cryptosporidiosis cause of summer diarrhea in children. Can. Med. Assoc. J. *132*:1285, 1985.
232. Moodley, D., Jackson, T. F. H. G., Gathiram, B., et al.: A comparative assessment of commonly employed staining procedures for the diagnosis of cryptosporidiosis. S. Afr. Med. J. *79*:314–317, 1991.
233. Moore, J. A., and Frenkel, J. K.: Respiratory and enteric cryptosporidiosis in humans. Arch. Pathol. Lab. Med. *115*:1160–1162, 1991.
234. Morgan, U. M., Monis P. T., Xiao, L., et al.: Molecular and phylogentic characterization of *Cryptosporidium* from birds. Int. J. Parasitol. *31*: 289–296, 2001.
235. Morgan, U. M., O'Brien P. A., and Thompson, R. C. A.: The development of diagnostic PCR primers for *Cryptosporidium* using RAPD-PCR. Mol. Biochem. Parasitol. *77*:103–108, 1996.
236. Morgan, U. M., and Thompson, R. C. A.: PCR detection of *Cryptosporidium*: The way forward? Parasitol. Today *14*:241–246, 1998.
237. Morgan, U. M., Weber, R., Xioa, L., et al.: Molecular characterization of *Cryptosporidium* isolates obtained from human immunodeficiency virus–infected individuals living in Switzerland, Kenya, and the United States. J Clin. Microbiol. *38*:1180–1183, 2000.
238. Morgan, U. M., Xioa, L., Fayer, R., et al.: Variation in *Cryptosporidium*: Toward a taxonomic revision of the genus. Int. J. Parasitol. *29*: 1733–1751, 1999.
239. Morgan, U. M., Xiao, L., Hill, B. D., et al.: Detection of the *Cryptosporidium parvum* "human" genotype in a dugong (Dugong dugon). J Parasitol *86*:1352–1354, 2000.
240. Moskovitz, B. L., Stanton, T. L., and Kusmierek, J. J. E.: Spiramycin therapy for cryptosporidial diarrhea in immunocompromised patients. J. Antimicrob. Agents Chemother. *22*:189–191, 1988.
241. Mozzell, E. J., Woltering, E. A., and O'Dorisio, T. M.: Non-endocrine applications of somatostatin and octreotide acetate: Facts and flights of fancy. Dis. Mon. *12*:754–810, 1991.
242. Navarrett, S., Stetler, H. C., Avila, C., et al.: An outbreak of *Cryptosporidium* diarrhea in a pediatric hospital. Pediatr. Infect. Dis. J. *10*:248–250, 1991.
243. Navin, T. R., and Juranek, D. D.: Cryptosporidiosis: Clinical, epidemiological, and parasitological review. Rev. Infect. Dis. *6*:313–327, 1984.
244. Neira, P., Tardio, M. T., Carabelli, M., et al.: Cryptosporidiosis in the V region of Chile. III. Study of malnourished patients, 1985–1887. Bol. Chil. Parasitol. *44*:34–36, 1989.
245. Newman, R. D., Zu, S. X., Wuhib, T., et al.: Household epidemiology of *Cryptosporidium parvum* infection in an urban community in northeast Brazil. Ann. Intern. Med. *120*:500–505, 1994.
246. Nime, F. A., Burek, J. D., Page, D. L., et al.: Acute enterocolitis in a human being infected with the protozoan *Cryptosporidium*. Gastroenterology *70*:592–598, 1976.
247. Nord, J., Ma, P., and DiJohn, D.: Treatment with bovine hyperimmune colostrum of cryptosporidial diarrhea in AIDS patients. AIDS *4*:581–584, 1990.
248. Nwanyanwu, O. C., Baird, J. N., and Reeve, G. R.: Cryptosporidiosis in a day care center. Tex. Med. *85*:40–43, 1989.
249. Oh, S. H., Jaffe, N., Fainstein, V., et al.: Cryptosporidiosis and anticancer therapy. J. Pediatr. *104*:963–964, 1984.
250. Ongerth, J. E., and Stibbs, H. H.: Identification of *Cryptosporidium* oocysts in river water. Appl. Environ. Microbiol. *53*:672–676, 1987.
251. Orenstein, J. M.: Microsporidiosis in the acquired immunodeficiency syndrome. J. Parasitol. *77*:843–863, 1991.
252. Orenstein, J. M., Chiang, J., Steinberg, W., et al.: Intestinal microsporidiosis as a cause of diarrhea in human immunodeficiency virus–infected patients: A report of 20 cases. Hum. Pathol. *21*:475–481, 1990.
253. Ortega, Y. R., Gilman, R. H., and Sterling, C. R.: A new coccidian parasite (Apicomplexa: Eimeriidae) from humans. J. Parasitol. *80*:625–629, 1993.
254. Ortega, Y. R., Nagle R., Gilman R. H., et al.: Pathologic and clinical findings in patients with cyclosporiasis and a description of intracellular parasite life-cycle stages. J. Infect. Dis. *176*:1584–1589. 1997.
255. Ortega, Y. R., Roxas, C. R., Gilman, R. H., et al.: Isolation of *Cryptosporidium parvum* and *Cyclospora cayetanensis* from vegetables collected from markets of an endemic region in Peru. Am. J. Trop. Med Hyg. *57*:633–636, 1997.
256. Ortega, Y. R., Sterling C. R., Gilman, R. H., et al.: *Cyclospora* species: A new protozoan pathogen of humans. N. Engl. J. Med. *328*:1308–1312, 1993.
257. Osterholm, M. T.: Lessons learned again: Cyclosporiasis and raspberries. Ann. Intern. Med. *130*:233–234, 1999.
258. Outbreak of diarrheal illness associated with *Cyanobacteria* (blue-green algae)-like bodies—Chicago and Nepal, 1989 and 1990. M. M. W. R. Morb. Mortal Wkly. Rep. *40*(19):325–327, 1991.
259. Palella, F. J., Delaney, K. M., Moorman, A. C., et al.: Declining morbidity and mortality among patients with advanced human immunodeficiency virus infection. N. Engl. J. Med. *338*:853–860, 1998.
260. Panosian, C. B.: Parasitic diarrhea. Infect. Dis. Clin. North Am. *2*:685–703, 1988.
261. Pape, J. W., and Johnson, W. D., Jr.: *Isospora belli* infections. Prog. Clin. Parasitol. *2*:119–127, 1991.
262. Pape, J. W., Verdier, R., Boney, M., et al.: *Cyclospora* infection in adults infected with HIV: Clinical manifestations, treatment, and prophylaxis. Ann. Intern. Med. *121*:654–657, 1994.
263. Pape, J. W., Verdier, R., and Johnson, W. D.: Treatment and prophylaxis of *Isospora belli* infection in patients with the acquired immunodeficiency syndrome. N. Engl. J. Med. *320*:1044–1047, 1989.
264. Pedraza-Diaz, S., Amar, C., Nichols, G. L., et. al: Nested polymerase chain reaction for amplification of *Cryptosporidium* oocyst wall protein gene. Emerg. Infect. Dis. *7*:49–56, 2001.
265. Perez-Schael, I., Boher, Y., Mata, L., et al.: Cryptosporidiosis in Venezuelan children with acute diarrhea. Am. J. Trop. Med. Hyg. *34*:721–722, 1985.
266. Pettoello-Mantovani, M., Di Martino, L., Dettori, G., et al.: Asymptomatic carriage of intestinal *Cryptosporidium* in immunocompetent and immunodeficient children: A prospective study. Pediatr. Infect. Dis. J. *14*:1042–1047, 1995.
267. Pieniazek, N. J., Bornay-Llimares, F. J., Slemeda, S. B., et al.: New *Cryptosporidium* genotypes in HIV-infected persons. Emerg. Infect. Dis. *5*:444–449, 1999.
268. Pilla, A. M., Rybak, M. J., and Chandrasekar, P. H.: Spiramycin in the treatment of cryptosporidiosis. Pharmacotherapy *7*:188–190, 1987.
269. Pitlik, S., Fainstein V., Rios, A., et al.: Cryptosporidial cholecystitis. N. Engl. J. Med. *308*:967, 1983.
270. Pol, S., Romana, C. A., and Richard, S.: Microsporidia infection in patients with the human immunodeficiency virus and unexplained cholangitis. N. Engl. J. Med. *328*:95–99, 1993.
271. Pollok, R. C., Bendell, R. P., Moody, A., et al.: Traveller's diarrhoea associated with *Cyanobacterium*-like bodies. Lancet *340*:556–557, 1992.
272. Pritchett, R., Gossman, C., Radke, V., et al.: Outbreak of cyclosporiasis. Northern Virginia–Washington, D.C., Baltimore Maryland, Metropolitan Area, 1997. M. M. W. R. Morb. Mortal. Wkly. Rep. *46*:689–691, 1997.
273. Rabeneck, L., Gyorkey, F., Genta, R. M., et al.: The role of microsporidia in the pathogenesis of HIV-related chronic diarrhea. Ann. Intern. Med. *119*:895–899, 1993.
274. Rahaman, A. S. M. H., Sanyal, S. C., Al-Mahmud, K. A., et al.: Cryptosporidiosis in calves and their handlers in Bangladesh. Lancet *2*:221, 1984.

275. Restrepo, C., Macher, A. M., and Radany, E. H.: Disseminated extra-intestinal isosporiasis in a patient with acquired immunodeficiency syndrome. Am. J. Clin. Pathol. *87*:536–542, 1987.
276. Richardson, A. J., Frankenberg, R. A., Buck, A. C., et al.: An outbreak of waterborne cryptosporidiosis in Swindon and Oxfordshire. Epidemiol. Infect. *107*:485–495, 1991.
277. Rijpstra, A. C., Canning, E. U., van Ketel, R. J., et al.: Use of light microscopy to diagnose small intestinal microsporidiosis in patients with AIDS. J. Infect. Dis. *157*:827–831, 1988.
278. Ritchie, D. J., and Becker, E. S.: Update on the management of intestinal cryptosporidiosis in AIDS. Ann. Pharmacother. *28*:767–778, 1994.
279. Robertson, L. J., Campbell, A. T., and Smith, H. V.: Survival of *Cryptosporidium parvum* oocysts under various environmental pressures. Appl. Environ. Microbiol. *58*:3494–3500, 1992.
280. Romeu, J., Miro, J. M., Sirera, G., et al.: Efficacy of octreotide in the management of chronic diarrhoea in AIDS. AIDS *5*:1495–1499, 1991.
281. Roncoroni, A. J., Gomez, M. A., Mera, J., et al.: *Cryptosporidium* infection in renal transplant patients. J. Infect. Dis. *160*:559, 1989.
282. Rosenblatt, J. E., and Sloan, L. M.: Evaluation of an enzyme-linked immunosorbent assay for detection of *Cryptosporidium spp.* in stool specimens. J. Clin. Microbiol. *31*:1468–1471, 1993.
283. Rossignol, J. F., Ayoub, A., and Ayers, M. S.: Treatment of diarrhea caused by *Cryptosporidium parvum:* A prospective randomized, double-blind, placebo-controlled study of Nitazoxanide. J. Infect. Dis. *184*: 103–106, 2001.
284. Rossignol, J. F., Hidalgo, H., Feregrino, M., et al.: A double-'blind' placebo controlled study of nitazoxanide in treatment of cryptosporidial diarrhea in AIDS patients in Mexico. Trans. R. Soc. Trop. Med. Hyg. *92*:663–666, 1998.
285. Rotterdam, H., and Tsang, P.: Gastrointestinal disease in the immunocompromised patient. Hum. Pathol. *25*:1123–1140, 1994.
286. Ruff, M. R., Martin, B. M., Ginns, E. I., et al.: CD4 receptor binding peptides that block HIV infectivity cause human monocyte chemotaxis relationship to human monocyte chemotaxis. FEBS Lett. *211*:17–22, 1987.
287. Rusnak, J., Hadfield, T. L., Rhodes, M., et al.: Detection of *Cryptosporidium* oocysts in human fecal specimens by an indirect immunofluorescence assay with monoclonal antibodies. J. Clin. Microbiol. *27*:1135–1136, 1989.
288. Ryan, N. J., Sutherland, G., Coughlan, K., et al.: A new trichrome-blue stain for detection of microsporidial species in urine, stool and nasopharyngeal specimens. J. Clin. Microbiol. *31*:3264–3269, 1993.
289. Sallon, S., Deckelbaum, R. J., Schmid, I. I., et al.: *Cryptosporidium,* malnutrition, and chronic diarrhea in children. Am. J. Dis. Child. *142*: 312–315, 1988.
290. Saxon, A., and Weinstein, W.: Oral administration of bovine colostrum anti-cryptosporidia antibody failed to alter the course of human cryptosporidiosis. J. Parasitol. *73*:413–415, 1987.
291. Scaglia, M., Atzori, C., Marchetti, M., et al.: Effectiveness of aminosidine (Paromomycin) sulfate in chronic *Cryptosporidium* diarrhea in AIDS patients: An open, uncontrolled, prospective, clinical trial. J. Infect. Dis. *170*:1349–1350, 1994.
292. Schneiderman, D. J., Cello, J. P., and Laing, F. C.: Papillary stenosis and sclerosing cholangitis in the acquired immunodeficiency syndrome. Ann. Intern. Med. *106*:546–549, 1987.
293. Schwartz, D. A., Bryan, R. T., Hewan-Lowe, K. O., et al.: Disseminated microsporidiosis *(Encephalitozoon hellem)* and acquired immunodeficiency syndrome: Autopsy evidence for respiratory acquisition. Arch. Pathol. Lab. Med. *116*:660–668, 1992.
294. Schwartz, D. A., Visvesvara, G. S., Diesenhouse, M. C., et al.: Pathologic features and immunofluorescent antibody demonstration of ocular microsporidiosis *(Encephalitozoon hellem)* in seven patients with acquired immunodeficiency syndrome. Am. J. Ophthalmol. *115*: 285–292, 1993.
295. Shadduck, J. A., and Greeley, E.: Microsporidia and human infections. Clin. Microbiol. Rev. *2*:158–165, 1989.
296. Shadduck, J. A., Meccoli, R. A., Davis, R., et al.: Isolation of microsporidia from a human patient. J. Infect. Dis. *162*:773–776, 1990.
297. Shaffer, N., and Moore, L.: Chronic travelers' diarrhea in a normal host due to *Isospora belli.* J. Infect. Dis. *3*:596–597, 1989.
298. Shahid, N. S., Rahman, A. S., Anderson, B. C., et al.: Cryptosporidiosis in Bangladesh. B. M. J. *290*:114–115, 1985.
299. Sheild, J., Melville C., Novelli, V., et al.: Bovine colostrum immunoglobulin concentrate for cryptosporidiosis in AIDS. Arch. Dis. Child. *69*:451–453, 1993.
300. Shlim, D. R., Cohen, M. T., Easton, M., et al.: An alga-like organism associated with an outbreak of prolonged diarrhea among foreigners in Nepal. Am. J. Trop. Med. Hyg. *45*:383–389, 1991.
301. Sifuentes-Osornio, J., Porras-Cortes, G., and Bendall, R. P.: *Cyclospora cayetanensis* infection in patients with and without AIDS: Biliary disease as another clinical manifestation. Clin. Infect. Dis. *21*:1092–1097, 1995.
302. Simon, D., Weiss, L. M., Tanowitz, H. B., et al.: Light microscopic diagnosis of human microsporidiosis and variable response to octreotide. Gastroenterology *100*:271–273, 1991.
303. Skeel, M. R., Sokolow, R., Hubbard, C. V., et al.: *Cryptosporidium* infection in Oregon public health clinic patients 1985–88: The value of statewide laboratory surveillance. Am. J. Public Health *80*:305–308, 1990.
304. Sloper, K. S., Dourmashkin, R. R., Bird, R. B., et al.: Chronic malabsorption due to cryptosporidiosis in a child with immunoglobulin deficiency. Gut *23*:80–82, 1982.
305. Smith, H. V., Paton, C. A., Mtambo, M. M. A, et al.: Sporulation of *Cyclospora sp.* oocyst. Appl. Environ. Microbiol. *63*:1631–1632, 1997.
306. Smith N. H., Cron, S., Valdez, L. M., et al.: Combination drug therapy for cryptosporidiosis in AIDS. J Infect. Dis. *178*:900–903, 1998.
307. Soave, R.: *Cyclospora*: An overview. Clin Infect. Dis. *23*:429–437, 1996.
308. Soave, R., Dubey, J. P., Ramos, L. L., et al.: A new intestinal pathogen? Abstract. Clin. Res. *34*:533, 1986.
309. Soave, R., and Johnson, W. D.: *Cryptosporidium* and *Isospora belli* infections. J. Infect. Dis. *157*:225–229, 1988.
310. Soave, R., and Johnson, W. D.: *Cyclospora*: Conquest of an emerging pathogen. Lancet *345*:667–668, 1995.
311. Sorvillo, F. J., Fujioda, K., Nahlen, B., et al.: Swimming-associated cryptosporidiosis. Am. J. Public Health *82*:742–744, 1992.
312. Stehr-Green, J. K., McCaig, L., and Ramsen, H. M.: Shedding of oocysts in immunocompetent individuals infected with *Cryptosporidium.* Am. J. Trop. Med. Hyg. *36*:338–342, 1987.
313. Sterling, C. R., and Arrowood, M.: Detection of *Cryptosporidium* species infections using direct immunofluorescent assay. Pediatr. Infect. Dis. J. *5*(Suppl.):139–142, 1986.
314. Sterling, C. R., and Ortega, Y. R.: *Cyclospora:* An enigma worth unraveling. Emerg. Infect. Dis. *5*:48–53, 1999.
315. Stine, K. C., Harris, J. A., Lindsey, N. J., et al.: Spontaneous remission of cryptosporidiosis in a child with acute lymphoblastic leukemia. Clin. Pediatr. (Phila.) *24*:722–724, 1985.
316. Sun, T., Kaplan, M. H., Teichberg, S., et al.: Intestinal microsporidiosis: Report of five cases. Ann. Clin. Lab. Sci. *24*:521–532, 1994.
317. Tangermann, R. H., Gordon, S., Wiesner, P., et al.: An outbreak of cryptosporidiosis in a day-care center in Georgia. Am. J. Epidemiol. *133*:471–476, 1991.
318. Tarver, A. P., Clark, D. P., Diamond, G., et al.: Enteric β-defensin: Molecular cloning and characterization of a gene with inducible intestinal epithelial expression with *Cryptosporidium parvum* infection. Infect. Immun. *66*:1045–1056, 1998.
319. Taylor, J. P., Perdue, J. N., Dingley, D., et al.: Cryptosporidiosis outbreak in a day-care center. Am. J. Dis. Child. *139*:1023–1025, 1985.
320. Teixidor, H. S., Godwin, T. A., and Ramirez, E. A.: Cryptosporidiosis of the biliary tract. Radiology *180*:51–56, 1991.
321. Teschareon, S., Jariya, P., and Tipayadarapanich, C.: *Isospora belli* infection as a cause of diarrhoea. Southeast Asian J. Trop. Med. Public Health *14*:528–530, 1983.
322. Theodos, C. M., Sullivan, K. L., Griffiths, J. K., et al.: Profiles of healing and nonhealing *Cryptosporidium parvum* infection in C57BL/6 mice functional B and T lymphocytes: The extent of gamma interferon modulation determines outcome of infection. Infect. Immun. *65*:4761–4769, 1997.
323. Thomson, M. A., Benson, J. W., and Wright, P. A.: Two-year study of *Cryptosporidium* infection. Arch. Dis. Child. *62*:559–563, 1987.
324. Trier, J. S., Moxey, P. C., Schimmel, E. M., et al.: Chronic intestinal coccidiosis in man: Intestinal morphology and response to treatment. Gastroenterology *66*:923–925, 1974.
325. Tyzzer, E. E.: A sporozoan found in the peptic glands of the common mouse. Proc. Soc. Exp. Biol. Med. *5*:12–13, 1907.
326. Tzipori, S.: Cryptosporidiosis in animals and humans. Microbiol. Rev. *47*:84, 1983.
327. Tzipori, S., Roberton, D., and Chapman, C.: Remission of diarrhea due to cryptosporidiosis in an immunodeficient child with hyperimmune bovine colostrum. B. M. J. *293*:1276–1277, 1986.
328. Tzipori, S., Smith, M., Birch, C., et al.: Cryptosporidiosis in hospital patients with gastroenteritis. Am. J. Trop. Med. Hyg. *32*:931–934, 1983.
329. Ungar, B. L. P., Gilman, R. H., Lanata, C. F., et al.: Seroepidemiology of *Cryptosporidium* infection in two Latin American populations. J. Infect. Dis. *157*:551–556, 1988.
330. Ungar, B. L. P., Mulligan, M., and Nutman, T. B.: Serologic evidence of *Cryptosporidium* infection in US volunteers before and during Peace Corps service in Africa. Arch. Intern. Med. *149*:894–897, 1989.
331. Ungar, B. L. P., and Nash, T. E.: Quantification of specific antibody response to *Cryptosporidium* antigens by laser densitometry. Infect. Immun. *53*:124–128, 1986.
332. Ungar, B. L. P., Soave, R., Fayer, R., et al.: Enzyme immunoassay detection of immunoglobulin M and G antibodies to *Cryptosporidium* in immunocompetent and immunocompromised persons. J. Infect. Dis. *153*:570–578, 1986.
333. Ungar, B. L. P., Ward, D. S., Fayer, R., et al.: Cessation of *Cryptosporidium* associated diarrhea in an acquired immunodeficiency syndrome patient after treatment with hyperimmune bovine colostrum. Gastroenterology *98*:486–489, 1990.

334. Vakil, N. B., Schwartz, S. M., Buggy, B. P., et al.: Biliary cryptosporidiosis in HIV-infected people after the waterborne outbreak of cryptosporidiosis in Milwaukee. N. Engl. J. Med. *334*:19–23, 1996.
335. Van, R., Morrow, A. L., Reves, R. R., et al.: Environmental contamination in child day-care centers. Am. J. Epidemiol. *133*:460–470, 1991.
336. Van Gool, T., Canning, E. U., and Dankert, J.: An improved practical and sensitive technique for the detection of microsporidian spores in stool samples. Trans. R. Soc. Trop. Med. *88*:189–190, 1994.
337. Van Gool, T., Canning, E. U., Gilis, H., et al.: *Septata intestinalis* frequently isolated from stool of AIDS patients with a new cultivation method. Parasitology *109*:281–289, 1994.
338. Van Gool, T., Snijders, F., Reiss, P., et al.: Diagnosis of intestinal and disseminated microsporidial infections in patients with HIV by a new rapid fluorescence technique. J. Clin. Pathol. *46*:694–699, 1993.
339. Van Gool, T., Vetter, J. C., Van Dam, A. P., et al.: Serological diagnosis of *Septata intestinalis* infections. Abstract D79. Paper presented at the 35th Interscience Conference on Chemotherapy and Antimicrobial Agents. San Francisco, 1995, p. 80.
340. Verdier, R., Fitzgerald, D. W., Johnson, W. D., et al.: Trimethoprim-sulfamethoxazole compared with ciprofloxacin for treatment and prophylaxis of *Isospora belli* and *Cyclospora cayetanensis* infections in HIV-infected patients. Ann. Intern. Med. *132*:885–888, 2000.
341. Visvesvara, G. S., Leitch, G. J., Da Silva, A. J., et al.: Polyclonal and monoclonal antibody and PCR-amplified small-subunit rRNA identification of a microsporidian, *Encephalitozoon hellem,* isolated from an AIDS patient with disseminated infection. J. Clin. Microbiol. *32*:2760–2768, 1994.
342. Vuorio, A. F., Jokipii, A. M. M., and Jokipii, L.: *Cryptosporidium* in asymptomatic children. Rev. Infect. Dis. *13*:261–264, 1991.
343. Walters, I. N., Miller, N. M., Van den Ende, J., et al.: Outbreak of cryptosporidiosis among children attending a day-care center in Durban. S. Afr. Med. J. *74*:496–499, 1988.
344. Wanke, C. A., DeGirolami, P., and Federman, M.: *Enterocytozoon bieneusi* infection and diarrheal disease in patients who were infected with human immunodeficiency virus: Case report and review. Clin. Infect. Dis. *23*:816–818, 1996.
345. Weber, R., and Bryan, R. T.: Microsporidial infections in immunodeficient and immunocompetent patients. Clin. Infect. Dis. *19*:517–521, 1994.
346. Weber, R., Bryan, R. T., Bishop, H. S., et al.: Threshold of detection of *Cryptosporidium* oocyst in human stool specimens: Evidence for low sensitivity of current diagnostic methods. J. Clin. Microbiol. *29*:1323–1327, 1991.
347. Weber, R., Bryan, R. T., and Juranek, D. D.: Improved stool concentration procedures for the detection of *Cryptosporidium* oocyst in fecal specimens. J. Clin. Microbiol. *30*:2869–2873, 1992.
348. Weber, R., Bryan, R. T., Owen, R. L., et al.: Improved light microscopical detection of microsporidia spores in stool and duodenal aspirates. N. Engl. J. Med. *326*:161–166, 1992.
349. Weber, R., Bryan, R. T., Schwartz, D. A., et al.: Human microsporidial infections. Clin. Microbiol. Rev. *7*:426–461, 1994.
350. Weber, R., Deplazes, P., Flepp, M., et al.: Cerebral microsporidiosis due to *Encephalitozoon cuniculi* in a patient with immunodeficiency virus infection. N. Engl. J. Med. *336*:474–478, 1997.
351. Weber, R., Kuster, H., Keller, R., et al.: Pulmonary and intestinal microsporidiosis in a patient with the acquired immunodeficiency syndrome. Am. Rev. Respir. Dis. *146*:1603–1605, 1992.
352. Weber, R., Kuster, H., Visvesvara, G. S., et al.: Disseminated microsporidiosis due to *Encephalitozoon hellem:* Pulmonary colonization, microhematuria, and mild conjunctivitis in a patient with AIDS. Clin. Infect. Dis. *17*:415–419, 1993.
353. Weber, R., Sauer, B., Luthy, R., et al.: Intestinal coinfection with *Enterocytozoon bieneusi* and *Cryptosporidium* in a human immunodeficiency virus–infected child with chronic diarrhea. Clin. Infect. Dis. *17*:480–483, 1993.
354. Weber, R., Sauer, B., Spycher, M. A., et al.: Detection of *Septata intestinalis* in stool specimens and coprodiagnostic monitoring of successful treatment with albendazole. Clin. Infect. Dis. *19*:342–345, 1994.
355. Weikel, C. S., Johnson, L. I., DeSousa, M. A., et al.: Cryptosporidiosis in northeastern Brazil: Association with sporadic diarrhea. J. Infect. Dis. *151*:963–965, 1985.
356. Weinstein, L., Edelstein, S. M., Madura, J. L., et al.: Intestinal cryptosporidiosis complicated by disseminating cytomegalovirus infection. Gastroenterology *81*:584–591, 1981.
357. Weisburger, W. R., Hutcheon, D. F., Yardley, J. H., et al.: Cryptosporidiosis in an immunosuppressed renal-transplant recipient with IgA deficiency. Am. J. Clin. Pathol. *72*:473–478, 1979.
358. Weiss, L. M., Perlman, D. C., Sherman, J., et al.: *Isospora belli* infection: Treatment with pyrimethamine. Ann. Intern. Med. *109*:474–475, 1988.
359. Wenyon, C. M.: Observations on the common intestinal protozoa of men: Their diagnosis and pathogenicity. Lancet *2*:1173, 1915.
360. Whiteside, M. E., Barkin, J. S., and May, R. G.: Enteric coccidiosis among patients with the acquired immunodeficiency syndrome. Am. J. Trop. Med. Hyg. *33*:1065–1072, 1984.
361. Wittner, M., Tanowitz, H. B., and Weiss, L. M.: Parasitic infections in AIDS patients: Cryptosporidiosis, isosporiasis, microsporidiosis, cyclosporiasis. Infect. Dis. Clin. North Am. *7*:569–586, 1993.
362. Wolfson, J. S., Richter, J. M., Waldron, M. A., et al.: Cryptosporidiosis in immunocompetent patients. N. Engl. J. Med. *312*:1278–1282, 1985.
363. Woodcock, H. M.: Notes on the protozoan parasites in the excreta. Addendum to Ledingham, J. C. G., and Penfold, W. J.: Recent bacteriological experiences with typhoidal disease and dysentery. B. M. J. *2*:709, 1915.
364. Wurtz, R.: *Cyclospora*: A newly identified intestinal pathogen of humans. Clin. Infect. Dis. *18*:620–623, 1994.
365. Wurtz, R. M., Kocka, F. E., Peters, C. S., et al.: Clinical characteristics of seven cases of diarrhea associated with a novel acid-fast organism in stool. Clin. Infect. Dis. *16*:136–138, 1993.
366. Xiao, L., Bern, C., Limor, J., et al.: Identification of 5 types of *Cryptosporidium* parasites in children in Lima, Peru. J. Infect. Dis. *183*:492–497, 2001.
367. Zar, F., Geiseler, P. J., and Brown, V. A.: Asymptomatic carriage of *Cryptosporidium* in the stool of a patient with acquired immunodeficiency syndrome. J. Infect. Dis. *151*:195, 1985.
368. Zerpa, R., and Huicho, L.: Childhood cryptosporidial diarrhea associated with identification of *Cryptosporidium* sp. in the cockroach *Periplaneta americana.* Pediatr. Infect. Dis. *13*:546–548, 1994.
369. Zierdt, C. H., Gill, V. J., and Zierdt, W. S.: Detection of microsporidian spores in clinical samples by indirect fluorescent-antibody assay using whole-cell antisera to *Encephalitozoon cuniculi* and *Encephalitozoon hellem.* J. Clin. Microbiol. *31*:3071–3074, 1993.
370. Zu, S. X., and Guerrant, R. L.: Cryptosporidiosis. J. Trop. Med. *39*:132–135, 1993.

E. SPORAZIN, FLAGELLATES

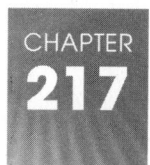

CHAPTER 217 Babesiosis

PETER J. KRAUSE

The first reference to babesiosis may have been in the Bible, where a widespread murrain or plague in cattle and other domestic animals is described in Exodus, Chapter 9, Verse 3: *"Behold, the hand of the Lord is upon thy cattle which is in the field, upon the horses, upon the asses, upon the camels, upon the oxen, and upon the sheep: there shall be a very grievous murrain."* The word "murrain" still is used to describe red-water fever, a form of babesiosis found in cattle in parts of Ireland.[20] Although babesiosis long has been recognized as an important disease in livestock, having a significant economic impact in many parts of the world, the first human case was not described until 1957.[29, 100]

Babesiosis is a disease caused by an intraerythrocytic protozoon that is transmitted by ticks and has many clinical features similar to those of malaria. The parasite first was described in animals in 1888 by Babes.[4] In 1893, it became the first microorganism shown to be transmitted by arthropods when Smith and Kilbourne[103] identified a tick as the vector for a species of babesiosis *(Babesia bigemina)* in Texas cattle. Since the initial report of babesiosis in humans, more than 300 clinical cases, including 5 in children, have been described.* Some evidence indicates that the disease occurs more commonly in both children and adults than these cases would suggest and that it is occurring more frequently than in the past.[21, 49, 51, 67] Since the 1970s, the epidemiology of the disease has changed from a few isolated cases to the establishment of endemic areas in southern New England, eastern Long Island, the north central Midwest, and a wide geographic range in North America and Europe.

Epidemiology

Worldwide, more than 90 species in the genus *Babesia* infect a wide variety of wild and domestic animals. For example, *B. bigemina, Babesia bovis, Babesia divergens,* and *Babesia major* are found in cattle; *Babesia equi* in horses; *Babesia canis* in dogs; *Babesia felis* in cats; and *Babesia microti* in rodents.[58] Previously, each species was thought to be host specific, but now the quite broad host range of some species is recognized.[36, 57, 58, 106, 113] Some confusion in taxonomy has occurred because the identification of different *Babesia* spp. has been based largely on morphology and the vertebrate host.[39] Most *Babesia* spp. are small (1 to 5 μm in length) and pear shaped, round, or oval.[57] Five *Babesia* spp. have been found to cause disease in humans: *B. microti,* WA1, and MO1 in North America, *B. divergens* in Europe, and TW1 in Taiwan.

Human babesiosis is a zoonotic disease transmitted by a tick vector from an infected animal reservoir (Fig. 217–1). Humans are a rare and terminal host for *Babesia* spp., which depend on other species for survival. The primary reservoir for *B. microti* in eastern North America is the white-footed mouse *(Peromyscus leucopus)*, but the parasite also has been found in shrews, chipmunks, voles, and rats.[36, 106, 112] As many as two thirds of *P. leucopus* have been found to be parasitemic in endemic areas.[107] *Babesia* spp. are transmitted by hard-bodied (ixodid) ticks. The primary vector in the northeastern United States is *Ixodes dammini* (also known as *Ixodes scapularis*), the same tick that transmits *Borrelia burgdorferi*, the etiologic agent of Lyme disease, and the agent of human granulocytic ehrlichiosis.[45, 47, 104, 105, 107–109, 114, 117] *I. dammini* ticks may be infected simultaneously with *B. burgdorferi, B. microti*, and the agent of human granulocytic ehrlichiosis.[63, 76, 117] Furthermore, both clinical and serologic evidence exists for simultaneous human infection with two or more of these pathogens.[5, 49–51, 60, 69, 115] Each of the three active stages in the life cycle of *I. dammini* (larva, nymph, and adult) takes a blood meal from a vertebrate host in order to mature to the next stage. Ingested babesial organisms infect intestinal tissue of the tick and subsequently travel to the salivary glands, from which they may be introduced into a new vertebrate host.[77] The *Babesia* spp. are transmitted to the subsequent tick stage (transstadial passage). In some species of babesia, such as *B. bovis*, the organisms may invade the ovaries and pass transovarially to the larvae.

In late summer, newly hatched larvae ingest the parasite with a blood meal from an infected rodent and maintain the parasite until it reaches the nymphal stage. Nymphs transmit the *Babesia* spp. to rodents in late spring and summer of the following year.[107, 108] Larvae, nymphs, and adults can feed on humans, but the nymph is the primary vector.[77] All active tick stages also feed on the white-tailed deer (*Odocoileus virginianus*), which is an important host for the tick but is not a reservoir for *B. microti*.[78, 107] An increase in the deer population during the past few decades is thought to be a major factor in the spread of *I. dammini* and the resulting increase in human cases.[34, 107, 108] Domestic animals such as the dog may carry the adult *I. dammini* but do not appear to be important hosts for the tick and are not infected with *B. microti*.[93, 105]

Most human cases of babesiosis occur in the summer. In areas where human *B. microti* infections have been reported, the tick, rodents, and deer are in close proximity to humans.[106, 110] *B. microti* has been identified in rodent populations in several regions of the United States,[2, 3, 87, 106] and human cases have been reported in Connecticut, Massachusetts, Rhode Island, New York, Minnesota, Wisconsin, and New Jersey.[15, 21, 24, 87, 110] Human babesiosis caused by organisms that are distinct morphologically from *B. microti* has been reported in California, Georgia, and Mexico, although the precise species in these cases have not been identified.[37, 73, 97] Moderately severe illness caused by a recently discovered babesia-like organism, designated WA1, has been reported in adults living in Washington state and California.[75, 80] WA1 is indistinguishable morphologically

*See references 15, 21, 23, 48, 51, 54, 62, 67, 98, 119.

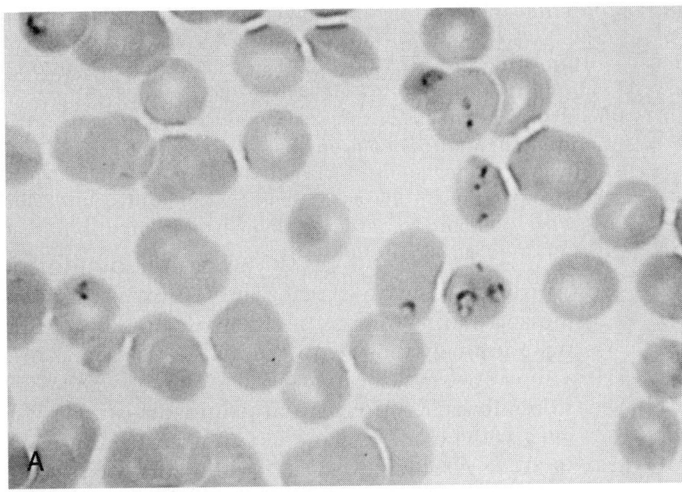

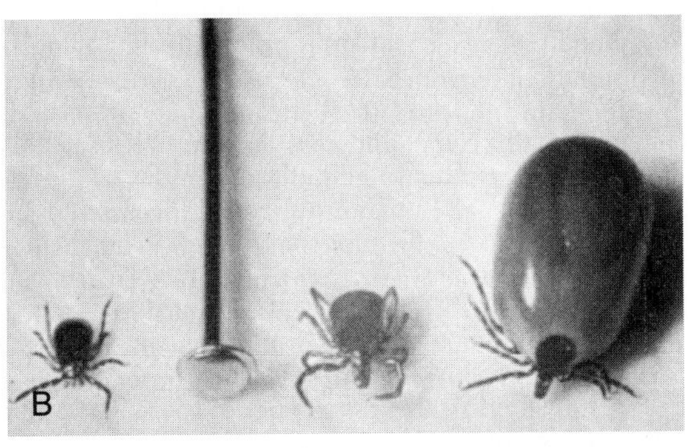

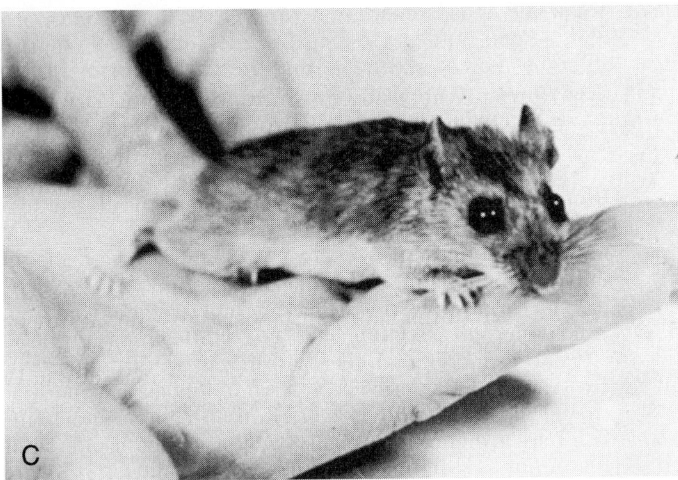

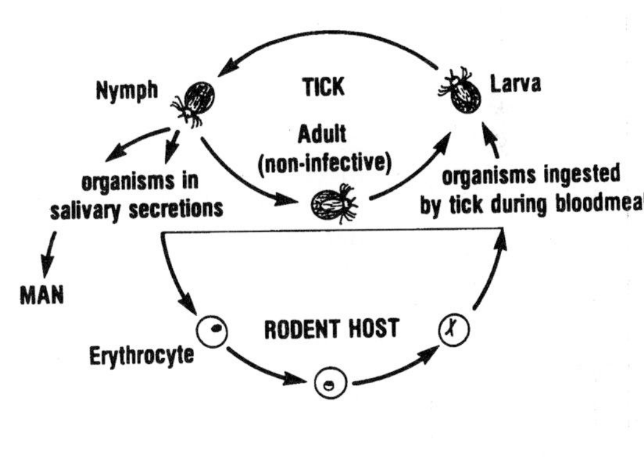

FIGURE 217–1 ■ Life cycle of *Babesia microti*. *A,* Ring forms of *Babesia microti* in human blood film (original magnfication × 1000). *B, Ixodes dammini* ticks and a common pin. The ticks are an adult male, an adult female, and an engorged female. (Courtesy of Mike Frigione, Pfizer, Inc., New York, NY.) *C,* White-footed mouse (*Peromyscus leucopus*). D, Life cycle of *B. microti*. (Modified from Ruebush, T. K., II: Babesiosis. In Strickland, G. T. [ed.]: Hunter's Tropical Medicine. Philadelphia, W. B. Saunders, 1984.)

from *B. microti* but is antigenically and genotypically distinct.[75, 80] A case of human babesiosis caused by MO1, a species that is similar to *B. divergens,* has been described in Missouri.[38] In Europe, *B. divergens* infections are believed to be transmitted by the cattle tick *Ixodes ricinus*.[39] Human cases have been reported in the former Yugoslavia, France, Ireland, Great Britain, and the former Soviet Union.[27, 28] Human cases in Asia and Africa also have been reported.[11, 40, 98a] An absence of clinical cases of babesiosis in the tropics may be due to cross-immunity from other endemic protozoal diseases.[46] Rarely, babesiosis is acquired through blood transfusions.[32, 43, 61, 102, 119] Whole blood, frozen erythrocytes, and platelets have been implicated. The incubation period in these cases appears to be 6 to 9 weeks. Transplacental and perinatal transmission of babesiosis also has been described.[23]

Pathogenesis and Pathology

Our understanding of the pathogenesis and pathology of babesiosis in humans is incomplete and is based in large part on information gathered from studies of babesiosis in other animals. *Babesia* spp. are intraerythrocytic protozoa, and extracellular forms are seen only in heavily parasitized cases.[1, 111] Jack and Ward[42] have presented data suggesting that *Babesia rodhani* gains entry into the erythrocyte by activation of the alternative complement pathway. They found that the C3b receptor plays a key role in modification of the parasite or red cell, allowing penetration of the parasite into the cell. Rudzinska and colleagues[47, 85, 86] have studied the life cycle of *B. microti* in erythrocytes using electron microscopy. After adhesion and entry into the erythrocyte, the organism multiplies by asexual budding into two to four daughter cells, or merozoites. Unlike *Plasmodium* spp. merozoites, which are released from the erythrocytes all at once (synchrony), *Babesia* spp. merozoites are released at varying intervals. New erythrocytes then are infected, and the cycle is repeated. Whether the initial merozoite release leads to destruction of the host erythrocyte is not known, but alteration of the erythrocyte membrane and eventually lysis occur.[85, 111] Erythrocyte lysis is responsible for many of the clinical manifestations and complications of the disease, including fever, hemolytic anemia, jaundice, hemoglobinemia, hemoglobinuria, and renal insufficiency. The absence of synchrony decreases the possibility of massive hemolysis and may explain why patients heavily parasitized with *Babesia* spp. may be less ill than are those with *Plasmodium* spp.[111] Ischemia and necrosis result from obstruction of blood vessels by parasitized erythrocytes, which may result in hepatomegaly and hepatic dysfunction, splenomegaly, and cerebral abnormalities.[20, 83, 89] Such clinical manifestations as hypotension, vascular congestion, and anoxia also may result from the activation of fibronectin, kallikreins, and complement.[22, 44, 122, 123]

Numerous immune mechanisms limit the severity of babesial infections, but immunity is incomplete because parasitemia may exist for months to years in animals and for as long as 27 months in humans after recovery from the initial illness.[54] Furthermore, reinfection may occur, although it is uncommon. Age is an important factor in host defense against babesial disease in both animals and humans. Most clinically apparent cases have occurred in adults, yet serologic surveys indicate that children are equally susceptible to infection and presumably are exposed to ticks to the same extent.[50, 87, 93] Four of the five pediatric cases reported have been in neonates.[23, 62, 98, 119] The increased severity of babesiosis observed in elderly people and in neonates has been postulated to have been the result of impaired splenic function because the spleen plays a critical role in protection against *Babesia* spp.[13, 23, 84, 98, 119, 122] The spleen is thought to protect against babesial infections by (1) removal of parasites from infected erythrocytes through a process known as "pitting," (2) ingestion of parasites by reticuloendothelial cells and mononuclear phagocytes, and (3) production of antibabesial antibody.[13, 19, 22, 122] That splenectomized animals have more severe babesiosis than do animals with intact spleens has been known for some time. Furthermore, animals that have recovered from babesiosis and have had negative blood smears have developed parasitemia again after undergoing splenectomy.[59, 94] Most fatal cases of babesiosis in humans have occurred in splenectomized individuals, although asplenia does not result always in death or even severe illness.[12, 84] Other host defense mechanisms that may help limit babesial infection include antibody[13, 44]; complement[8, 122]; a soluble nonantibody factor[18]; macrophages; and macrophage products such as tumor necrosis factor,[22, 122] B lymphocytes,[66] T lymphocytes,[13, 66, 91, 121] and polymorphonuclear leukocytes.[99]

Clinical Manifestations

The clinical manifestations of babesiosis range from subclinical illness to fulminating disease resulting in death. Overt signs and symptoms begin after an incubation period of 1 to 6 weeks from the beginning of tick feeding.[93] The unengorged *I. dammini* nymph is about 2 mm in length, and often the patient has no recollection of a tick bite. In most cases, the patient suffers a gradual onset of malaise, anorexia, and fatigue followed by intermittent temperature to as high as 40° C (104° F) and one or more of the following: chills, sweats, myalgia, arthralgia, nausea, and vomiting.[1, 28, 51, 55, 62, 87, 92, 110] Less commonly noted are emotional lability and depression, hyperesthesia, headache, sore throat, abdominal pain, conjunctival injection, photophobia, weight loss, and nonproductive cough.[48, 89, 110, 111] Unlike other tick-borne illnesses, such as Lyme disease, Rocky Mountain spotted fever, or tularemia, rash seldom is noted.[21] Ecchymoses and petechiae have been described.[48, 111] Erythema chronicum migrans has been noted in patients with babesiosis,[5] but these patients likely had Lyme disease as well.

The findings on physical examination generally are minimal, often consisting only of fever.[1, 37, 51, 92, 110] Mild splenomegaly, hepatomegaly, or both are noted occasionally.[89, 119] Slight pharyngeal erythema, jaundice, and retinopathy with splinter hemorrhages and retinal infarcts also have been reported.[48, 62, 72] Several abnormal laboratory findings in patients with babesiosis reflect the invasion and subsequent lysis of erythrocytes by the parasite.[48, 62, 87, 89] Mild to moderately severe hemolytic anemia, with an elevated reticulocyte count, is present. Elevated liver enzyme levels may be detected in serum.[87] The leukocyte count is normal to slightly decreased, with a "left shift." Thrombocytopenia may occur.[89] The erythrocyte sedimentation rate is elevated. Proteinuria and elevated blood urea nitrogen and creatinine levels also may be noted.[48, 62, 89] The illness usually lasts for a few weeks to several months, with prolonged recovery of up to 18 months.[1, 5, 54, 89, 92, 110] Parasitemia may continue even after the patient feels well. Persistent parasitemia and relapse of illness, as noted with malaria, has been described 27 months after the initial episode.[54]

Some patients, especially those with *B. divergens* infection or prior splenectomy, suffer a more severe form of the disease that consists of fulminant illness lasting about a week and ends in death or a prolonged convalescence.[28, 48, 60, 72, 111] Signs and symptoms include high fever, hemolytic anemia, hemoglobinemia and hemoglobinuria, jaundice, ecchymoses, petechiae, congestive heart failure, pulmonary edema, renal failure, adult respiratory distress syndrome, and coma.[30, 31, 48, 110, 111, 118] Patients with babesiosis who are co-infected with Lyme disease also have more severe acute illness than do those with babesiosis alone.[33, 51, 60, 115] Co-infected patients usually experience moderate to severe acute illness often followed by persistent fatigue. Between 10 and 66 percent of patients with antibody to *B. burgdorferi* also have been found to have antibody to *B. microti*.[7, 49, 50]

Inapparent infection also may occur. Data from seven serosurveys suggest that this form of the disease may be the most common. In a survey on Nantucket Island in Massachusetts, 2 percent of 577 random blood samples and 7.5 percent of 133 blood samples from patients with a history of tick bite or fever had *B. microti* indirect immunofluorescent antibody (IFA) titers of 1:64 or greater.[92] A survey of adults living on Shelter Island, New York, showed that 6 of 136 (4.4%) and 7 of 102 (6.9%) had *B. microti* IFA antibody at titers of 1:64 or greater.[25] In a survey of Massachusetts blood donors, 29 of 779 (37%) from Cape Cod had *B. microti* IFA antibody titers of 1:16, compared with 7 of 148 (4.7%) from metropolitan Boston.[79] In a serosurvey in Connecticut, 72 of 735 (9.5%) residents who were seropositive for *B. burgdorferi* had positive *B. microti* IFA antibody titers of 1:64, compared with 8 of 299 (2.7%) seronegative for *B. burgdorferi*.[49] Serosurveys in Mexico, Nigeria, and Taiwan also demonstrated high *B. microti* seroprevalence rates in comparison with the number of indigenous reported cases of babesiosis.[40, 56, 73]

Diagnosis

Specific diagnosis of babesiosis is made by microscopic identification of the organism by Giemsa or Wright stains of thick or thin blood smears and by detection of babesial antibodies by one of several serologic tests. *Babesia* spp. are round, oval, or pear shaped and have a blue cytoplasm with a red chromatin. The ring form is most common and is very similar to the rings of *Plasmodium falciparum*.[35] *Babesia* spp. can be distinguished from *Plasmodium* spp. by (1) the absence of pigment, which is present in older trophozoites of *Plasmodium* spp.; (2) the absence of schizonts and gametocytes; (3) the absence of synchronous stages within the erythrocytes; and (4) the presence of the infrequently noted tetrad or Maltese cross forms, in which four compact masses, each containing nuclear material, are joined by strands of cytoplasm.[35] Multiple thick and thin blood smears should be examined because only a few erythrocytes are infected in the early stage of the illness when most people seek medical attention.[35] Rapid automated differential blood analyzers may fail to distinguish erythrocytic inclusions.[10] In thick smears, the *Babesia* organism appears as a tiny red to purple nucleus with a thin tail of light blue cytoplasm. Maximum erythrocyte infection is about 10 percent in normal hosts but up to 85 percent in asplenic individuals.[110] Usually fewer than 1 percent of erythrocytes are parasitized early in the course of the illness, and the laboratory investigation of possible babesiosis should include more than an examination of blood smears.

Numerous serologic tests have been developed to detect babesial antibodies. Of the commonly used serologic tests, the IFA assay is the most reliable.[16, 52, 89] The IFA test is simpler, cheaper, and more rapid than is the complement-fixation test. Both immunoglobulin G and immunoglobulin M IFA antibodies can be detected.[16, 52] During the acute phase of the illness, titers usually exceed 1:1024 but decline to 1:64 or less within 8 to 12 months. Thus, a babesial IFA titer of 1:1024 or greater usually signifies active or recent infection.[16, 90] Although cross-reactions occur to different *Babesia* spp. and *Plasmodium* spp. with the IFA test, these titers almost always are low (1:16 or less).[16, 17] The problem of cross-reactivity with *Plasmodium* spp. is minimized in areas where no indigenous malaria exists. A reliable immunoblot assay for detection of *B. microti* antibody was developed recently.[96] Enzyme-linked immunosorbent assays for detection of *B. divergens* and *B. major* have been found to be superior to complement fixation and IFA procedures.[9, 82, 113, 116]

In cases in which the presence of *Babesia* spp. is suspected but not demonstrated by blood smears or antibody studies, babesial DNA can be amplified and detected using the polymerase chain reaction.[53, 74] Blood from the patient also can be injected by the intravenous or intraperitoneal route into small laboratory animals such as hamsters or gerbils. If present in the patient, *B. microti* usually appears in the blood of the inoculated animal within 2 to 4 weeks.[6] This diagnostic technique is less sensitive, more time consuming, and more costly than is polymerase chain reaction.[53]

Treatment and Prevention

The current therapy of choice for babesiosis is the combination of clindamycin (20 mg/kg/day in children; in adults, 300 to 600 mg every 6 hours given intravenously or orally) and quinine (25 mg/kg/day in children; in adults, 650 mg every 6 to 8 hours) taken for 7 to 10 days.[14, 30] This combination was used initially in the first reported case of babesiosis in a child, an 8-week-old infant who contracted babesiosis from a blood transfusion.[119] Initially, she was thought to have malaria. Clindamycin and quinine were given after failure with chloroquine. Her favorable outcome suggested the prospective use of this combination in adults. Numerous children and adults subsequently have been treated with clindamycin and quinine, with prompt clearing of parasitemia and resolution of clinical signs and symptoms.[14, 15, 23, 62, 98, 110]

The successful use of atovaquone and azithromycin for the treatment of malaria and for babesiosis in hamsters prompted a recent clinical trial to determine whether the combination would be effective in human babesiosis.[41, 120] Atovaquone and azithromycin were compared with clindamycin and quinine for treatment of babesiosis in adults.[55] Adverse effects were reported in 15 percent of subjects who received atovaquone and azithromycin compared with 72 percent of those who received clindamycin and quinine. In about one third of those taking clindamycin and quinine, the apparent drug reactions were so severe that the drugs were discontinued or the dosages decreased, compared with adverse reactions occurring in only 2 percent of those taking atovaquone and azithromycin. Both drug combinations were equally effective in clearing symptoms and parasitemia. Because the combination of atovaquone and azithromycin has not been tested in children, clindamycin and quinine remain the drugs of choice for treatment of babesiosis in this age group.

Other antimicrobial agents that have been used to treat babesiosis generally are ineffective. Chloroquine was used to treat babesiosis because of the occasional misdiagnosis of babesiosis as *P. falciparum* infection. Although chloroquine may give some symptomatic relief of fever and myalgia by its anti-inflammatory action, it often fails to clear parasitemia in guinea pigs and humans and is not recommended.[14, 68] Other antimalarial drugs, such as quinacrine, primaquine, pyrimethamine, pyrimethaminesulfadoxine, sulfadiazine, and tetracycline, have no effect on parasitemia in animals. Pentamidine isothionate has been found to decrease fever and parasitemia, but the organisms are not eradicated, and the drug has proved to be ineffective in animals and humans.[26] Diminazene aceturate was effective in clearing parasitemia and clinical symptoms in one patient, but he developed Guillain-Barré syndrome during recovery, possibly as a result of receiving the drug.[95] Pentamidine and trimethoprim-sulfamethoxazole were used successfully to treat a case of *B. divergens* infection in France.[81] Exchange blood transfusions have been used successfully in splenectomized patients with life-threatening *Babesia* spp. infections.[12, 43, 111] Transfusion can decrease the degree of parasitemia rapidly and remove toxic byproducts of babesial infections but should be used only in patients with the most severe infections.

Prevention of babesiosis can be accomplished by avoiding areas in May through September where ticks, deer, and mice are known to thrive. Asplenic individuals particularly should avoid contact with tall grass and brush in endemic areas where ticks may abound. Use of clothing that covers the lower part of the body and that is sprayed or impregnated with diethyltoluamide, dimethyl phthalate, or permethrin (Permanone) is recommended for those who travel in the foliage of endemic areas.[20, 101] A search for ticks on people and pets should be carried out and the ticks removed as soon as possible.[20] The latter is accomplished best by removal with tweezers by grasping the mouth parts without squeezing the body of the tick.[21, 71] Attempts to reduce the tick, mouse, or deer populations in endemic areas are less effective.[64, 101, 108]

Physicians have recommended that prospective blood donors who reside in endemic areas and who present with a history of fever within the preceding 1 to 2 months be excluded from giving blood in order to prevent transfusion-related cases.[88] The American Red Cross defers blood donors who have had a history of babesiosis.[65] Effective *B. bovis* and *B. bigemina* vaccines have been developed for use in cattle, but no *B. microti* vaccine exists.[70, 123]

REFERENCES

1. Anderson, A. E., Cassaday, P. B., and Healy, G. R.: Babesiosis in man: Sixth documented case. Am. J. Clin. Pathol. *62*:612–618, 1974.
2. Anderson, J. F., and Magnarelli, L. A.: Spirochetes in *Ixodes dammini* and *Babesia microti* on Prudence Island, Rhode Island. J. Infect. Dis. *148*:1124, 1983.

3. Anderson, J. F., Magnarelli, L. A., and Kurz, J.: Intraerythrocytic parasites in rodent populations of Connecticut: *Babesia* and *Grahamella* species. J. Parasitol. *65*:599–604, 1979.
4. Babes, V.: Sur l'hemoglubinurie bacterienne boeuf. Compt. Rend. Acad. Sci. *107*:692–694, 1888.
5. Benach, J. L., and Hibicht, G. S.: Clinical characteristics of human babesiosis. J. Infect. Dis. *144*:481, 1981.
6. Benach, J. L., White, D. J., and McGovern, J. P.: Babesiosis in Long Island: Host-parasite relationship of rodent- and human-derived *Babesia microti* isolates in hamsters. Am. J. Trop. Med. Hyg. *27*:1073–1078, 1978.
7. Benach, J. L., Coleman, J. L., Habicht, G. S., et al.: Serological evidence for simultaneous occurrences of Lyme disease and babesiosis. J. Infect. Dis. *152*:473–477, 1985.
8. Benach, J. L., Habicht, G. S., and Manburger, M. I.: Immunoresponsiveness in acute babesiosis in humans. J. Infect. Dis. *146*:369–380, 1982.
9. Bidwell, D. E., Turp, P., Joyner, L. P., et al.: Comparisons of serologic tests for *Babesia* in British cattle. Vet. Rec. *103*:446–449, 1978.
10. Bruckner, D. A., Garcia, L. S., Shimizu, R. Y., et al.: Babesiosis: Problems in diagnosis using autoanalyzers. Am. J. Clin. Pathol. *83*:320–321, 1985.
11. Bush, J. B., Isaacson M., Mohamed, A. S.: Human babesiosis: A preliminary report of two suspect cases in southern Africa. S. Afr. J. Med. *78*: 699, 1990.
12. Cahill, K. M., Benach, J. L., Reich, L. M., et al.: Red cell exchange: Treatment of babesiosis in a splenectomized patient. Transfusion *21*:193–198, 1981.
13. Carson, C. A., and Phillips, R. S.: Immunologic response of the vertebrate host to *Babesia. In* Ristic, M., and Kreier, J. P. (eds.): Babesiosis. New York, Academic Press, 1981, pp. 411–443.
14. Centers for Disease Control: Clindamycin and quinine treatment for *Babesia microti* infections. M. M. W. R. Morb. Mortal. Wkly. Rep. *32*:65–72, 1983.
15. Centers for Disease Control: Babesiosis in Connecticut. M. M. W. R. Morb. Mortal. Wkly. Rep. *38*:649–650, 1989.
16. Chisholm, E. S., Ruebush, T. K., II, Sulzer, A. J., et al.: *Babesia microti* infection in man: Evaluation of an indirect immunofluorescent antibody test. Am. J. Trop. Med. Hyg. *27*:14–19, 1978.
17. Chisholm, E. S., Sulzer, A. J., and Ruebush, T. K.: Indirect immunofluorescence test for human *Babesia microti* infection: Antigenic specificity. Am. J. Trop. Med. Hyg. *35*:921–925, 1986.
18. Clark, I. A., Wills, E. J., Richmond, J. E., et al.: Immunity to intraerythrocytic protozoa. Lancet *2*:1128–1129, 1973.
19. Cullen, J. M., and Levine, J. F.: Pathology of experimental *Babesia microti* infection in the Syrian hamster. Lab. Animal Sci. *37*:640–643, 1987.
20. Dammin, G. J.: Babesiosis. *In* Weinstein, L., and Fields, B. N. (eds.): Seminars in Infectious Disease. New York, Stratton, 1978, pp. 169–199.
21. Dammin, G. J., Spielman, A., Benach, J. L., et al.: The rising incidence of clinical *Babesia microti* infection. Hum. Pathol. *12*:398–400, 1981.
22. DeVos, A. J., Dalgliesh, R. J., and Callow, L. L.: Babesia. *In* Soulsby, E. J. L. (ed.): Immune Responses in Parasitic Infections: Immunology, Immunopathology, and Immunoprophylaxis. Vol. 3. Boca Raton, CRC Press, 1987, pp. 183–222.
23. Esernio-Jenssen, D., Scimeca, P. G., Benach, J. L., et al.: Transplacental/perinatal babesiosis. J. Pediatr. *110*:570–572, 1987.
24. Eskow E. S., Krause P. J., Spielman A., et al.: Southern extension of the range of human babesiosis in the eastern United States. J. Clin. Microbiol. *37*:2051–2052, 1999.
25. Filstein, M. R., Benach, J. L., White, D. J., et al.: Serosurvey for human babesiosis in New York. J. Infect. Dis. *141*:518–521, 1980.
26. Francioli, P. B., Keithly, J. S., Jones, T. C., et al.: Response of babesiosis to pentamidine therapy. Ann. Intern. Med. *94*:326–330, 1981.
27. Garnham, P. C. C.: Human babesiosis: European aspects. Trans. R. Soc. Trop. Med. Hyg. *74*:153–155, 1980.
28. Garnham, P. C. C., Donelly, J., Hoogstraal, H., et al.: Human babesiosis in Ireland: Further observations and the medical significance of this infection. Br. Med. J. *4*:768–770, 1969.
29. Gibbons, W. J.: Diseases of Cattle. 2nd ed. Wheaton, IL, Veterinary Publications, 1963, pp. 665–673.
30. Golightly, L. M., Hirschhorn, L. R., and Weller, P. F.: Fever and headache in a splenectomized woman. Rev. Infect. Dis. *11*:629–637, 1989.
31. Gordon, S., Cordon, R. A., Mazdzer, E. J., et al.: Adult respiratory distress syndrome in babesiosis. Chest *86*:633–634, 1984.
32. Grabowski, E. F., Giardina, P. J. V., Goldberg, D., et al.: Babesiosis transmitted by a transfusion of frozen-thawed blood. Ann. Intern. Med. *96*:466–467, 1982.
33. Grunwaldt, E., Barbour, A. G., and Benach, J. L.: Simultaneous occurrence of babesiosis and Lyme disease. N. Engl. J. Med. *308*:1166, 1983.
34. Healy, G.: The impact of cultural and environmental changes on the epidemiology and control of human babesiosis. Trans. R. Soc. Trop. Med. Hyg. *83*(Suppl.):35–38, 1989.
35. Healy, G. R., and Ruebush, T. K., II: Morphology of *Babesia microti* in human blood smears. Am. J. Clin. Pathol. *73*:107–109, 1980.
36. Healy, G. R., Spielman, A., and Gleason, N.: Human babesiosis: Reservoir of infection on Nantucket Island. Science *192*:479–480, 1976.
37. Healy, G. R., Walzer, P. D., and Sulzer, A. J.: A case of asymptomatic babesiosis in Georgia. Am. J. Trop. Med. Hyg. *25*:376–378, 1976.
38. Herwaldt, B. L., Persing, D. H., Precigont, E. A., et al.: A fatal case of babesiosis in Missouri: Identification of another piroplasm that infects humans. Ann. Intern. Med. *124*:643–650, 1996.
39. Hoare, C. A.: Comparative aspects of human babesiosis. Trans. R. Soc. Trop. Med. Hyg. *74*:143–148, 1980.
40. Hsu, N. H., and Cross, J. H.: Serologic survey for human babesiosis on Taiwan. J. Formosan Med. Assoc. *76*:950–954, 1977.
41. Hughes, W. T., and Oz, H. S.: Successful prevention and treatment of babesiosis with atovaquone. J. Infect. Dis. *172*:1042–1046, 1995.
42. Jack, R. M., and Ward, P. A.: *Babesia rodhaini* interactions with complement: Relationship to parasitic entry into red cells. J. Immunol. *124*:1566–1573, 1980.
43. Jacoby, G. A., Hunt, J. V., Kosinski, K. S., et al.: Treatment of transfusion-transmitted babesiosis by exchange transfusion. N. Engl. J. Med. *303*:1098–1100, 1980.
44. James, M. A.: Immunology of *Babesia* infections. *In* Ristic, M., Ambroise-Thomas, P., and Kreier, J. (eds.): Malaria and Babesiosis: Research Findings and Control Measures. Dordrecht, Martinus Nijhoff Publishers, 1984, pp. 53–63.
45. Johnson, R. C., Schmid, G. P., Hyde, F. W., et al.: *Borrelia burgdorferi*: Etiologic agent of Lyme disease. Int. J. Syst. Bacteriol. *34*:496–497, 1984.
46. Kakoma, I., and Ristic, M.: Pathogenesis of babesiosis. *In* Ristic, M., Ambroise-Thomas, P., and Kreier, J. (eds.): Malaria and Babesiosis: Research Findings and Control Measures. Dordrecht, Martinus Nijhoff Publishers, 1984, pp. 85–93.
47. Karakashian, S. J., Rudzinska, M. A., Spielman, A., et al.: Primary and secondary ookinetes of *Babesia microti* in the larval and nymphal stages of the tick *Ixodes dammini*. Can. J. Zool. *64*:328–339, 1986.
48. Kennedy, C. C.: Human babesiosis: Summary of a case in Ireland. Trans. R. Soc. Trop. Med. Hyg. *74*:156, 1980.
49. Krause, P. J., Telford, S. R., Ryan, R., et al.: Geographical and temporal distribution of babesial infection in Connecticut. J. Clin. Microbiol. *29*:1–4, 1991.
50. Krause, P. J., Telford, S. R., Pollack R. J., et al.: Babesiosis: An underdiagnosed disease of children. Pediatrics *89*:1045–1048, 1992.
51. Krause, P. J., Telford, S. R., Spielman, A., et al.: Concurrent Lyme disease and babesiosis: Evidence for increased severity and duration of illness. J. A. M. A. *275*:1657–1660, 1996.
52. Krause, P. J., Ryan, R., Telford, S. R., et al.: Efficacy of immunoglobulin M serodiagnostic test for rapid diagnosis of acute babesiosis. J. Clin. Microbiol. *34*:2014–2016, 1996.
53. Krause, P. J., Telford, S. R., Spielman, A., et al.: Comparison of PCR with blood smear and inoculation of small animals for diagnosis of *Babesia microti* parasitemia. J. Clin. Microbiol. *34*:2791–2794, 1996.
54. Krause, P. J., Spielman, A., Telford S., et al.: Persistent parasitemia after acute babesiosis. N. Engl. J. Med. *339*:160–165, 1998.
55. Krause, P. J., Lepore, T., Sikand, V. J., et al.: Atovaquone and azithromycin for the treatment of human babesiosis. N. Engl. J. Med. *343*:1454–1458, 2000.
56. Leeflang, P., Oomen, J. M. V., Zwart, D., et al.: The prevalence of *Babesia* antibody in Nigerians. Int. J. Parasitol. *6*:159–161, 1976.
57. Levine, N. D.: Protozoan Parasites of Domestic Animals and of Man. Minneapolis, Burgess Publishing, 1966, pp. 292–293.
58. Levine, N. D.: Taxonomy of the piroplasms. Trans. Am. Micros. Soc. *90*:2–33, 1971.
59. Lykins, J. D., Ristic, M., and Weisiger, R. M.: *Babesia microti*: Pathogenesis of parasite of human origin in the hamster. Exp. Parasitol. *37*:388–397, 1975.
60. Marcus, L. C., Steere, A. C., Duray, P. H., et al.: Fatal pancarditis in a patient with coexistent Lyme disease and babesiosis: Demonstration of spirochetes in the myocardium. Ann. Intern. Med. *103*:374–376, 1985.
61. Marcus, L. C., Valigorsky, J. M., Fanning, W. L., et al.: A case report of transfusion-induced babesiosis. J. A. M. A. *248*:465–467, 1982.
62. Mathewson, H. O., Anderson. A. E., and Hazard, G. W.: Self-limited babesiosis in a splenectomized child. Pediatr. Infect. Dis. *3*:148–149, 1984.
63. Mather, T. N., Telford, S. R., Moore, S. I., et al.: *Borrelia burgdorferi* and *Babesia microti:* Efficiency of transmission from reservoirs to vector ticks (*Ixodes dammini*). Exp. Parasitol. *70*:55–61, 1990.
64. Mather, T. N., Ribeiro, J. M. C., and Spielman, A.: Lyme disease and babesiosis: Acaricide focused on potentially infected ticks. Am. J. Trop. Med. Hyg. *36*:609–614, 1987.
65. McQuiston, J. H., Childs, J. E., Chamberland, M. E., et al. Transmission of tickborne agents by blood transfusions: A review of known and potential risks in the United States. Transfusion *40*:274–284, 2000.
66. Meeusen, E., Lloyd, S., and Soulsby, E. J. L.: *Babesia microti* in mice: Adoptive transfer of immunity with serum and cells. Aust. J. Exp. Biol. Med. Sci. *62*:551–566, 1984.
67. Meldrum, S. C., Birkhead, G. S., White, D. J., et al.: Human babesiosis in New York state: An epidemiological description of 136 cases. Clin. Infect. Dis. *15*:1019–1023, 1992.
68. Miller, L. H., Neva, F. A., and Gill, F.: Failure of chloroquine in human babesiosis *(Babesia microti)*: Case report and chemotherapeutic trials in hamsters. Ann. Intern. Med. *88*:200–202, 1978.
69. Mitchell, P. D., Reed, K. D., and Hofkes, J. M.: Immunoserologic evidence of coinfection with *Borrelia burgdorferi*, *Babesia microti*, and human

granulocytic ehrlichia species in residents of Wisconsin and Minnesota. J. Clin. Microbiol. *34*:724–727, 1996.

70. Montenegro-James, S.: Immunoprophylactic control of bovine babesiosis: Role of exoantigens of *Babesia*. Trans. R. Soc. Trop. Med. Hyg. *83*(Suppl.):85–94, 1989.
71. Needham, G. R.: Evaluation of five popular methods for tick removal. Pediatrics *75*:997–1002, 1985.
72. Ortiz, J. M., and Eagle, R. C., Jr.: Ocular findings in human babesiosis (Nantucket fever). Am. J. Ophthalmol. *93*:307–311, 1982.
73. Osorno, B. M., Vega, C., Ristic, M., et al.: Isolation of Babesia spp. from asymptomatic human beings. Vet. Parasitol. *2*:111–120, 1976.
74. Persing, D. H., Mathiesen, D., Marshall, W. F., et al.: Detection of *Babesia microti* by polymerase chain reaction. J. Clin. Microbiol. *30*:2097–2103, 1992.
75. Persing, D. H., Herwaldt, B. L., Glaser C., et al.: Infection with a *Babesia*-like organism in northern California. N. Engl. J. Med. *332*:298–303, 1995.
76. Piesman, J., Hicks, T. C., Sinsky, R. J., et al.: Simultaneous transmission of *Borrelia burgdorferi* and *Babesia microti* by individual nymphal *Ixodes dammini* ticks. J. Clin. Microbiol. *25*:2012–2013, 1987.
77. Piesman, J., and Spielman, A.: Human babesiosis on Nantucket Island: Prevalence of *Babesia microti* in ticks. Am. J. Trop. Med. Hyg. *29*:742–746, 1980.
78. Piesman, J., Spielman, A., Etkind, P., et al.: Role of deer in the epizootiology of *Babesia microti* in Massachusetts, U.S.A. J. Med. Entomol. *15*:537–540, 1979.
79. Popovsky, M. A., Lindbert, L. E., Syrek, A. L., et al.: Prevalence of *Babesia* antibody in a selected blood donor population. Transfusion *28*:59–61, 1987.
80. Quick, R. E., Herwaldt, B. L., Thomford, J. W., et al.: Babesiosis in Washington State: A new species of *Babesia*? Ann. Intern. Med. *119*:284–290, 1993.
81. Raoult, D., Soulayrol, L., Toga, B., et al.: Babesiosis, pentamidine, and cotrimoxazole. Ann. Intern. Med. *107*:944, 1987.
82. Reiter, I., and Weiland, G.: Recently developed methods for the detection of babesial infections. Trans. R. Soc. Trop. Med. Hyg. *83*(Suppl.):21–23, 1989.
83. Riek, R. F.: Babesiosis. *In* Weinman, D., and Ristic, M. (eds.): Infectious Blood Diseases of Man and Animals. Vol. 2. New York, Academic Press, 1968, pp. 219–268.
84. Rosner, F., Zarrabi, M. H., Benach, J. L., et al.: Babesiosis in splenectomized adults: Review of 22 reported cases. Am. J. Med. *76*:696–701, 1984.
85. Rudzinska, M. A.: Morphological aspects of host-cell-parasite relationships in babesiosis. *In* Ristic, M., and Kreier, J. P. (eds.): Babesiosis. New York, Academic Press, 1981, pp. 87–141.
86. Rudzinska, M. A., Spielman, A., Lewengrub, S., et al.: Sexuality in piroplasms as revealed by electron microscopy in *Babesia microti*. Proc. Natl. Acad. Sci. U. S. A. *80*:2966–2970, 1983.
87. Ruebush, T. K., II: Human babesiosis in North America. Trans. R. Soc. Trop. Med. Hyg. *74*:149–152, 1980.
88. Ruebush, T. K., II: Babesiosis. *In* Strickland, G. T. (ed.): Hunter's Tropical Medicine. Philadelphia, W. B. Saunders, 1984, pp. 608–611.
89. Ruebush, T. K., II, Cassaday, P. B., Marsh, H. J., et al.: Human babesiosis on Nantucket Island: Clinical features. Ann. Intern. Med. *86*:6–9, 1977.
90. Ruebush, T. K., II, Chisholm, E. S., Sulzer, A. J., et al.: Development and persistence of antibody in persons infected with *Babesia microti*. Am. J. Trop. Med. Hyg. *30*:291–292, 1981.
91. Ruebush, M. J., and Hanson, W. L.: Thymus dependence of resistance to infection with *Babesia microti* of human origin in mice. Am. J. Trop. Med. Hyg. *29*:507–515, 1980.
92. Ruebush, T. K., II, Juranek, D. D., Chisholm, E. S., et al.: Human babesiosis on Nantucket Island: Evidence for self-limited and subclinical infections. N. Engl. J. Med. *297*:825–827, 1977.
93. Ruebush, T. K., II, Juranek, D. D., Spielman. A., et al.: Epidemiology of human babesiosis on Nantucket Island. Am. J. Trop. Med. Hyg. *30*:937–41, 1981.
94. Ruebush, T. K., II, Piesman, J., Collins, W. E., et al.: Tick transmission of *Babesia microti* to rhesus monkeys *(Macaca mulatta)*. Am. J. Trop. Med. Hyg. *30*:555–559, 1981.
95. Ruebush, T. K., II, Rubin, R. H., Wolpow, E. R., et al.: Neurologic complications following the treatment of human *Babesia microti* infection with diminazene aceturate. Am. J. Trop. Med. Hyg. *28*: 184–189, 1979.
96. Ryan R., Krause P. J., Radolf J., et. al.: Diagnosis of babesiosis using an immunoblot serologic test. Clin. Diag. Lab. Immunol. *8*:1177–1180, 2001.
97. Scholtens, R. G., Braff, E. H., Healy, G. R., et al.: A case of babesiosis in man in the United States. Am. J. Trop. Med. Hyg. *17*:810–813, 1968.
98. Scimeca, P. G., Weinblatt, M. E., Schonfeld, G., et al.: Babesiosis in two infants from eastern Long Island, N. Y. Am. J. Dis. Child. *140*:971, 1986.

98a. Shih, C M., Liu, L. P., Chung, W. C., et al.: Human babeosis in Taiwan: Asymptomatic infection with a *Babesia microti*-like organism in a Taiwanese woman. J. Clin. Microbiol. *33*:450–454, 1997.
99. Simpson, C. F.: Phagocytosis of *Babesia canis* by neutrophils in the peripheral circulation. Am. J. Vet. Res. *35*:701–704, 1974.
100. Skrabalo, A., and Deanovic, A.: Piroplasmosis in man: Report on a case. Doc. Med. Geogr. Trop. *9*:11–16, 1957.
101. Smith, R. D., and Kakoma, I.: A reappraisal of vector control strategies for babesiosis. Trans. R. Soc. Trop. Med. Hyg. *83*(Suppl.):43–52, 1989.
102. Smith, R. P., Evans, A. T., Popovsky, M., et al.: Transfusion-acquired babesiosis and failure of antibiotic treatment. J. A. M. A. *256*:2726–2727, 1986.
103. Smith, T., and Kilbourne, F. L.: Investigation into the nature, causation, and prevention of southern cattle fever. U. S. Dept. Agr. Bur. Anim. Indust. Bull. *1*:1–301, 1893.
104. Spielman, A.: Human babesiosis on Nantucket Island: Transmission by nymphal *Ixodes* ticks. Am. J. Trop. Med. Hyg. *25*:784–787, 1976.
105. Spielman, A., Clifford, C. M., Piesman, J., et al.: Human babesiosis on Nantucket Island, U.S.A.: Description of the vector, *Ixodes (Ixodes) dammini*, n. sp. (Acarina: Ixodidae). J. Med. Entomol. *15*:218–234, 1979.
106. Spielman, A., Etkind, P., Piesman, J., et al.: Reservoir hosts of human babesiosis on Nantucket Island. Am. J. Trop. Med. Hyg. *30*:560–565, 1981.
107. Spielman, A., Wilson, M. L., Levine. J. F., et al.: Ecology of *Ixodes dammini*-borne human babesiosis and Lyme disease. Ann. Rev. Entomol. *30*:439–460, 1985.
108. Spielman, A.: Lyme disease and human babesiosis: Evidence incriminating vector and reservoir hosts. *In* Englund, P. T., and Sher, A. (eds.): The Biology of Parasitism. New York, Alan R. Liss, 1988, pp. 147–165.
109. Steere, A. C., and Malawista, S. E.: Cases of Lyme disease in the United States: Locations correlated with distribution of *Ixodes dammini*. Ann. Intern. Med. *91*:730–733, 1979.
110. Steketee, R. W., Eckman, M. R., Burgess, E. C., et al.: Babesiosis in Wisconsin: A new focus of disease transmission. J. A. M. A. *253*:2675–2678, 1985.
111. Sun, T., Tenenbaum, M. J., Greenspan, J., et al.: Morphologic and clinical observations in human infection with *Babesia microti*. J. Infect. Dis. *148*:239–248, 1983.
112. Telford, S. R., Mather, T. N., Adler, G. H., et al.: Short-tailed shrews as reservoirs of the agent of Lyme disease and human babesiosis. J. Parasitol. *76*:681–683, 1990.
113. Telford, S. R., Gorenflot, A., Brasseur P., et al.: Babesial infections in man and wildlife. *In* Kreirer, J. P., and Baker, J. R. (eds.): Parasitic Protozoa. 2nd ed. San Diego, Academic Press, 1991.
114. Telford, S. R., III, Dawson, J. E., Katavolos, P., et al.: Perpetuation of the agent of human granulocytic ehrlichiosis in a deer tick-rodent cycle. Proc. Nat. Acad. Sci. *93*:6209–6214, 1996.
115. Thompson, C., Krause, P., Telford, S., et al.: Increased severity of Lyme disease illness due to concurrent babesiosis and ehrlichiosis (abstract 1757). *In* Program and Abstracts of the 40th Interscience Conference on Antimicrobial Agents and Chemotherapy (Toronto). Washington, D.C.: American Society for Microbiology, 2000:500.
116. Todorovic, R. A., and Carson, C. A.: Methods for measuring the immunological response to *Babesia*. *In* Ristic, M., and Kreier, J. P. (eds.): Babesiosis. New York, Academic Press, 1981, pp. 381–410.
117. Varde, S., Beckley, J., and Schwartz, I.: Prevalence of tick-borne pathogens in *Ixodes scapularis* in a rural New Jersey County. Emerg. Infect. Dis. *4*:97–99, 1998.
118. William, H.: Human babesiosis. Trans. R. Soc. Trop. Med. Hyg. *74*:157, 1980.
119. Wittner, M., Rowin, K. S., Tanowitz, H. B., et al.: Successful chemotherapy of transfusion babesiosis. Ann. Intern. Med. *96*:601–604, 1982.
120. Wittner, M., Lederman, J., Tanowitz, H. B., et al.: Atovaquone in the treatment of *Babesia microti* infections in hamsters. Am. J. Trop. Med. Hyg. *55*:219–222, 1996.
121. Wolf, R. E.: Effects of antilymphocyte serum and splenectomy on resistance to *Babesia microti* infection in hamsters. Clin. Immunol. Immunopathol. *2*:381–394, 1974.
122. Wright, I. G., Goodger, B. V., Buffington, G. D., et al.: Immunopathophysiology of babesial infections. Trans. R. Soc. Trop. Med. Hyg. *83*(Suppl.):11–13, 1989.
123. Wright, I. G., and Mahoney, D. F.: The activation of kallikrein in acute *Babesia argentina* infections of splenectomized calves. Z. Parasitenkd. *43*:271–278, 1974.
124. Wright, I. G., Mirre, G. B., Rode-Bramanis, K., et al.: Protective vaccination against virulent *Babesia bovis* with a low-molecular-weight antigen. Infect. Immun. *48*:109–113, 1985.

CHAPTER 218 Malaria

ELIZABETH D. BARNETT

Malaria is a disease of global importance that results in 300 to 500 million cases and 1.5 to 2.7 million deaths yearly.[30] Half of the malaria deaths worldwide occur in children younger than 5 years.[55] Malaria is transmitted regularly in parts of Africa, Asia, the Middle East, Central and South America, Hispaniola, and Oceania. It has been imported by travel to nearly every part of the world. Because of the ubiquity of malaria, the ability to recognize its signs and symptoms and knowledge about methods of prevention and treatment are important for health care professionals wherever they practice.

Malaria usually is transmitted by bites of infected female anopheline mosquitoes. Disease results from infection with one or more of the four species of *Plasmodium (Plasmodium falciparum, Plasmodium vivax, Plasmodium ovale,* or *Plasmodium malariae)* that infect humans. These protozoa have complex life cycles involving both arthropod and vertebrate hosts. Untreated, *P. falciparum* malaria can progress to coma, renal failure, pulmonary edema, and death. Asymptomatic carriage may last decades in the case of *P. malariae.* Relapses are common with *P. vivax* and *P. ovale.* Resistance of the parasites to antimalarial agents and incomplete success in developing and maintaining programs to eradicate the mosquito vectors have contributed to making malaria a persistent worldwide challenge.

History

Malaria has been known since antiquity and probably affected prehistoric humans. Fossilized mosquitos have been found in geologic strata 30 million years old. Descriptions of the signs and symptoms of malaria have been found in early Hindu and Chinese writing, and Hippocrates described seasonal and geographic aspects of the disease.[91] Numerous references to malaria occur in literature, ranging from Shakespeare's *The Tempest* to Laura Ingalls Wilders' *Little House on The Prairie.* The name is derived from the Italian *mal aria* (bad air) based on recognition of the connection between malaria and swamps. The first methods of malaria control, draining of swamps, were based on this association.

The first malaria treatment known to Europeans, bark of the cinchona tree, was identified in the early 17th century almost 200 years before the active ingredient (quinine) was isolated. Not until the late 1800s was the vector-borne nature of malaria understood and described; for their roles in this discovery, the French military surgeon Laveran, working in Algeria, and the British military physician Ronald Ross, working in India, were awarded Nobel prizes. Further work by many investigators rounded out our current understanding of the life cycle of the malaria parasites and the complex interrelationships with vector mosquitoes.

During the 20th century, parallel efforts directed toward vector control and discovery and development of drugs to treat malaria were undertaken. The development of larvicides and insecticides permitted control of the mosquito vector.[102] Unquestionably, the spectacular success of house spraying with dichlorodiphenyltrichloroethane (DDT) was instrumental in eradication of malaria from most of North America and Europe and in significant decreases in prevalence in the Mediterranean area, the Middle East, the Far East, and parts of southern Africa.[76] The development of antimalarial drugs, stimulated largely by the need to protect soldiers during World Wars I and II during shortages of the standard antimalarial agent quinine, allowed for successful treatment of malaria cases.

The World Health Organization (WHO) launched a global campaign for eradication of malaria in 1957. Early successes, attributable to the efficacy of DDT and the development of new antimalarial agents, subsequently were hindered by resistance of mosquito vectors to DDT and resistance of the parasites to antimalarial drugs. In 1969, the WHO philosophy on malaria was altered to emphasize the development of health services and research. The goals of malaria control since have been refined and broadened to encompass an approach that incorporates the implementation of selective and sustainable preventive measures, early diagnosis and prompt treatment, early detection or prevention of epidemics, and strengthening of local infrastructures to allow better understanding of the determinants of local transmission and malaria control.[91]

During the last several decades, transmission of malaria has increased in many areas despite adoption of these measures. Factors contributing to increases in cases of malaria in many areas and re-emergence in areas thought free of disease include lapses in local control measures, resistance to antimalarial drugs, changes in climate, and population movement as a result of urbanization, mass displacement of populations, and international travel.[8, 46, 52, 55]

The Organism

The life cycle of malaria parasites is complex and requires a suitable population of anopheline mosquitos and infected humans for completion. Differences in the life cycle of the various species of *Plasmodium* do exist (Fig. 218–1; see Color Plate I).

To begin the cycle, the female anopheline mosquito injects sporozoites along with saliva in preparation for taking a blood meal from a vertebrate host. Sporozoites, the infective stage of *Plasmodium,* remain in the circulation for a relatively short period (less than an hour) and then migrate to the liver, where they invade hepatocytes and multiply asexually. Proliferation within hepatocytes takes approximately 1 week for *P. falciparum* and *P. vivax* and about 2 weeks for *P. malariae.* At the end of this period, mature tissue schizonts rupture and release thousands of merozoites, which then invade red blood cells (RBCs). *P. vivax* and *P. ovale* have a second type of exoerythrocytic form, the hypnozoite, which can remain dormant for weeks to years. Dormant hypnozoites may develop weeks, months, or years later into merozoites, which then can enter RBCs and cause relapse of malaria. Factors influencing which exoerythrocytic form develops are not understood.

Merozoites released from tissue schizonts invade RBCs, where the erythrocytic phase of the life cycle takes place. Two pathways exist in the erythrocytic, or blood, phase: asexual and sexual. In the asexual phase, development of the parasite begins with the youngest stage, the trophozoite, or ring form. The parasite then undergoes nuclear division to form schizonts and then merozoites in the asexual multiplication process called erythrocytic schizogony/merogony. Lysis of RBCs releases the merozoites, which invade other RBCs, thus perpetuating the asexual erythrocytic cycle. The cycle continues until interrupted by treatment or by the host's immune response.

In the sexual phase, subpopulations of merozoites in the erythrocytic phase differentiate into gametocytes, or sexual forms, which are then available for ingestion by mosquitoes to complete the life cycle within the mosquito. Female macrogametocytes and male microgametocytes appear in the circulation within 3 to 15 days of the onset of symptoms. Gametocytes of *P. vivax* may appear in 4 days, whereas those of *P. falciparum* may require as long as 10 days for development.

In the stomach (midgut) of the mosquito, male gametocyte nuclei divide into four to eight nuclei and form motile gametocytes that fertilize the female gametocytes. The zygotes become motile ookinetes that migrate through the wall of the midgut, attach to its outer surface, and form oocysts. The oocysts rupture 9 to 14 days later and release sporozoites that invade the mosquito salivary glands, where they are ready for inoculation into the next vertebrate host.

Epidemiology

Transmission of malaria occurs in large parts of Africa, the Indian subcontinent, Southeast Asia, the Middle East, Oceania, and Central and South America (Fig. 218–2; see Color Plate II). Although indigenous transmission of malaria has been eradicated almost completely from the United States and Canada, northern Europe, most of the Caribbean, parts of South America, Israel, Lebanon, Reunion, Singapore, Hong Kong, Japan, Korea, Taiwan, Brunei, and Australia, many cases of imported malaria occur in these countries each year.[91]

P. falciparum is the major malaria species in sub-Saharan Africa and the island of Hispaniola, with *P. malariae* assuming a more minor role. *P. vivax* occurs alongside *P. falciparum* in the Indian subcontinent, Central and South America, Mexico, Southeast Asia, and Oceania. *P. ovale* occurs mainly in Africa. *P. vivax* occurs rarely in sub-Saharan Africa because most Africans lack the Duffy blood group antigen necessary for parasite invasion.

Transmission

EPIDEMIOLOGIC TERMINOLOGY

Patterns of transmission of malaria include stable endemic malaria (natural transmission occurring over many years, with a predictable incidence of illness and prevalence of infection) and unstable malaria (transmission rates vary from year to year, and immunity is low, with a greater likelihood of epidemics). The degree of endemic malaria is based on the parasite rate in children between 2 and 9 years of age. Types of endemic malaria include hypoendemic (parasite rate of 0–10%), mesoendemic (parasite rate of 11–50%), hyperendemic (parasite rate consistently higher than 50%, with a high proportion of adults having enlarged spleens), and holoendemic (parasite rate consistently higher than 75%, with a low proportion of adults having enlarged spleens).[91]

Autochthonous malaria is acquired locally and may be indigenous or introduced. Introduced malaria may occur when migrant populations with asymptomatic infection provide blood meals for feeding anopheline mosquitoes under conditions that allow for the life cycle to be completed in the mosquito and thus enable the mosquito to infect others. Imported malaria cases may occur in nonendemic areas but result from infection in an endemic area. Induced malaria is acquired by exposure to infected blood, such as from blood transfusion, needle-stick injury, laboratory accident, or historically, medical treatments. Cryptic malaria cases are those for which no explanation can be found and no epidemiologic link to other cases can be identified.

MOSQUITO-BORNE TRANSMISSION

The most typical means of transmission of malaria is through the bite of an infected anopheline mosquito. Although more than 350 species of anopheline mosquito exist, only approximately 45 have been shown to be effective vectors of malaria. A population of infected humans is necessary to sustain transmission because of the short life span of mosquitoes (5 to 20 days) and the relatively long incubation period required in the mosquito (8 to 10 days or more).

BLOOD-BORNE TRANSMISSION

Transmission of malaria via blood transfusion is well documented.[59] Transmission also may occur through organ donation or needle-stick injury.[24, 101] Relapses of malaria cannot occur with blood-borne transmission, even if the infecting species is *P. vivax* or *P. ovale,* because the infection is produced by the transmission of infected RBCs rather than forms that invade the liver.

CONGENITAL MALARIA

Infants can acquire malaria from their mothers during pregnancy. Transplacental transmission of parasites has been proposed as the most likely route of transmission, although breakdown of placental barriers allowing transmission of maternal blood cells to the infant during labor or delivery also has been suggested as a mechanism of transmission.[31, 57] *P. vivax* most often is associated with this phenomenon, but it may occur with all species. Congenital malaria is less likely to occur in infants of semi-immune mothers because of passage of maternal antibody at the time of birth. As with transfusion-associated malaria, relapses do not occur.

CRYPTIC MALARIA

The category of cryptic malaria includes cases for which no source of infection can be identified. Typical cases might include confirmed malaria in U.S. residents who have never traveled to or resided in malarial areas, who have not received blood transfusions, and who are not linked epidemiologically with other cases.[44, 72, 101] Airport malaria, one kind of cryptic malaria, occurs in proximity to international airports and is thought to occur when mosquitoes arriving with airplanes from endemic areas infect individuals working in or living near airports.[38]

Host-Parasite Interaction

The intensity of transmission of malaria depends on factors that affect the density of vectors and the extent of vector-human contact. Transmission of malaria may be continuous or seasonal, or it may depend on local site-specific factors such as the presence of irrigation projects or intermittent flooding. Mosquito vectors differ in their efficiency to transmit malaria; the principal vector in sub-Saharan Africa, *Anopheles gambiense*, is known for being a highly effective vector. Variations in climate may affect the viability of mosquitoes.

The incidence and severity of malaria are affected by the intensity of exposure, the presence of immunity, and genetic factors. Distinction must be made between malaria infection (presence of parasitemia) and malaria illness. One of the major puzzles in malaria is why individuals with similar degrees of parasitemia may exhibit radically different clinical manifestations.

Individuals who reside in endemic areas and are continually exposed to infected mosquitoes acquire immunity to malaria illness. Adults in these areas continue to become infected, but they have lower levels of parasitemia. Infants born to mothers with acquired immunity may be protected transiently by placental passage of maternal antibody. The highest incidence of malaria infection occurs in infants and young children, those no longer protected by maternal antibody but too young for significant acquired immunity to have developed. Children also are more susceptible to certain manifestations of severe illness, such as cerebral malaria. Lack of acquired immunity in infants and young children accounts in part for their increased risk of acquiring disease and having severe manifestations. Acquired immunity diminishes during pregnancy, and pregnant women are the adults at greatest risk for severe complications of malaria. Individuals in the population who remain asymptomatic but harbor gametocytes in their blood are reservoirs of infection when bitten by mosquitoes.

The clinical manifestations of malaria may be severe in nonimmune patients. Malaria is the most common life-threatening infection acquired by travelers to malaria-endemic regions. Individuals with acquired immunity who then leave endemic areas for long periods may lose their immunity and be at risk for severe disease if re-exposed.

Genetic factors determine the risk of acquiring malaria and having severe infection. Individuals who have a Duffy-negative blood type lack specific receptors for invasion of the merozoites of *P. vivax* and are therefore resistant to infection with *P. vivax*. This resistance is the basis for the low incidence of vivax malaria in Africa. Specific human leukocyte antigens present in individuals from West Africa may protect against the development of severe complications of malaria, including cerebral malaria and severe anemia. The best-known example of the relationship between malaria and genetics is the association between sickle hemoglobinopathies and protection against severe falciparum malaria. This balanced polymorphism is thought to have helped ensure survival of the gene for hemoglobin S in the population because of the selective advantage provided on a population basis to those who are heterozygous for sickle-cell disease. An important note is that individuals with sickle hemoglobinopathies still may be infected and manifest signs and symptoms of malaria, although the risk of acquiring severe malaria or dying of malaria may be 60- to 70-fold less in children with hemoglobin AS than in those with hemoglobin AA.[40]

Pathophysiology

The pathogenesis of malaria is multifactorial because of the effects of blood-stage parasites, and it involves multiple organ systems. Pathophysiologic changes are caused by the destruction of RBCs, production of cytokines, stimulation of intravascular synthesis of nitric oxide (NO), and sequestration of infected erythrocytes.

Lysis of RBCs leads to anemia, which may be severe, and its attendant hemodynamic consequences. Anemia may develop as a result of hemolysis, impaired erythropoiesis, or bone marrow depression secondary to folic acid deficiency.[69] Intravascular hemolysis may be so severe that it results in pronounced hemoglobinuria ("blackwater fever"), which may be a precipitating event in the development of renal failure. This complication has been noted in association with quinine treatment. Hematopoiesis is suppressed during acute infection, and such suppression may not be reversed as readily in iron-deficient individuals, thereby contributing to chronic anemia.

Cytokines such as tumor necrosis factor (TNF) and interleukin-1 have important roles in the pathogenesis of malaria.[10] Severe disease has been associated with higher concentrations of TNF. Parasite factors responsible for release of cytokines have not been identified. One possible role of TNF in malaria is to stimulate NO, a short-lived neurotransmitter. NO may have a role in cerebral malaria, and its transient nature may provide a partial explanation for the complete recovery noted in some patients with severe cerebral malaria. Both TNF and NO have harmful and beneficial roles in the pathogenesis of malaria: both have been shown to be correlated with clearance of parasites and eventual recovery, as well as with the severity of illness.

Sequestration of infected RBCs has long been thought to contribute to the clinical manifestations of malaria, particularly that caused by *P. falciparum*. Late-stage parasites induce host cells to develop knobs on the surface of erythrocytes that facilitate adherence of these cells to vascular endothelium. The effects of these sequestered RBCs on the perfusion, nutrition, and oxygenation of surrounding tissues may be responsible for the complications of *P. falciparum* infection, including cerebral malaria, renal failure, and watery diarrhea.[60, 71] Consumption of glucose by metabolically active late-stage parasites contributes to hypoglycemia and lactic acidosis. Despite these changes, the histopathologic appearance of tissue is remarkably benign, consistent with the reversible nature of the changes. This phenomenon also lends support to the role of cytokines and secondary messengers in the pathogenesis of complications of cerebral malaria.[40, 91]

Clinical Features

The clinical manifestations of malaria depend on the species of malaria parasite causing the infection, the immune status of the individual, the mode of transmission of infection, whether the individual was taking prophylaxis, and host immune factors. Acute malaria generally is understood to refer to the signs and symptoms associated with disease caused by infection with malaria parasites. Recurrent infections are of three types: relapse, recrudescence, and reinfection. Relapses occur as a result of delayed maturation of the dormant liver stages (hypnozoites) of *P. vivax or P. ovale*. Recrudescence occurs when parasitemia caused by the same parasite responsible for the initial infection recurs after clearance or a significant reduction in the initial parasitemia. It occurs most commonly with *P. falciparum* because of drug

TABLE 218–1 ■ CHARACTERISTICS OF THE FOUR *PLASMODIUM* SPECIES RESPONSIBLE FOR HUMAN MALARIA

	P. falciparum	*P. vivax*	*P. ovale*	*P. malariae*
Incubation period in days (range)	12 (8–25)	14 (8–27)	17 (15–≥18?)	28 (15–≥40?)
Periodicity of febrile attacks (hr)	None	48	48	72
Earliest appearance of gametocytes (days)	10	3	?	?
Relapse	No	Yes	Yes	No
Duration of untreated infection (yr)	1–2	1.5–4	1.5–4	3–50
Red cell preference	Younger cells (but can invade cells of all ages)	Reticulocytes	Reticulocytes	Older cells
Characteristic morphology	Ring forms Multiply infected cells Banana-shape gametocytes	Schüffner dots Enlarged RBCs	Schüffner dots Somewhat enlarged RBCs	Normal sized cells Band or rectangular forms of trophozoites

resistance. Reinfection with different parasites, as well as infection with more than one type of *Plasmodium,* occurs especially in areas with a high intensity of transmission. Persistent infection is noted with *P. malariae.* Hypnozoites have not been identified with *P. malariae,* so the organism is thought to persist as a low-level parasitemia that can exist for years without causing symptoms.

The clinical manifestations of malaria depend on the infecting malaria species (Table 218–1). Most severe complications (cerebral malaria, renal failure) are associated with falciparum malaria. *P. vivax* infections rarely produce death because the inability of the parasite to enter RBCs other than reticulocytes limits the severity of the disease. Splenic rupture is a late complication, usually of vivax malaria, especially in those who have recently had their first infection.[105] The most characteristic syndrome produced by *P. malariae* is immune complex glomerulonephritis.

ACUTE MALARIA

A classic description of malaria would include features of the malaria paroxysm resulting from the lysis of parasitized RBCs and release of merozoites into the circulation at the completion of asexual reproduction. The paroxysm is characterized by fever and chills accompanied by constitutional symptoms consisting of headache, body ache, fatigue, dizziness, and malaise. Gastrointestinal symptoms may include nausea or vomiting, abdominal pain, or diarrhea. Cough and dyspnea may accompany an attack. Although periodicity of the paroxysms in primary attacks is thought to be pathognomonic for malaria species, this periodicity may take several days to become established, may not occur at all in asynchronous infections, or may be modified by previous immunity or treatment.

In children, fever and headache may be the sole symptoms, or gastrointestinal symptoms may predominate. Physical signs of malaria may include anemia, jaundice, and hepatosplenomegaly. Rash and lymphadenopathy typically are not associated with malaria, although malaria may precipitate recrudescence of latent herpes infections.

LABORATORY FINDINGS

Anemia is the most common abnormality in malaria. Thrombocytopenia is a common finding and may be the first manifestation in patients with uncomplicated malaria.[36, 40] Leukopenia also may occur, but high white blood cell counts are less usual and should provoke investigation for other conditions. Liver function test abnormalities may be present and can be mistaken for evidence of hepatitis, especially in patients with jaundice and tender hepatosplenomegaly. Hypoglycemia occurs frequently with falciparum malaria and may develop before or as a consequence of treatment with quinine. When present in children before treatment, hypoglycemia is associated with a poor prognosis.[90] Hyponatremia may occur as part of the syndrome of inappropriate secretion of antidiuretic hormone in some patients. Serum creatinine and blood urea nitrogen may be elevated transiently or may rise significantly with acute renal failure.

Malaria stimulates a polyclonal increase in immunoglobulins associated with rapid production of malaria-specific antibodies and reduced complement levels. False-positive tests for syphilis, rheumatoid factor, heterophil agglutinins, and cold agglutinins may occur.[91]

Malaria in Special Populations

MALARIA IN CHILDREN

The signs and symptoms of malaria in children range from asymptomatic infection to life-threatening illness. Severe anemia is most likely to develop in children younger than 2 years, whereas cerebral malaria is most likely to occur in older children (mean age of 3.5 years). In endemic areas, lack of diagnostic facilities, limited resources, and encroaching drug resistance complicate the ability to make a rapid, accurate diagnosis and provide expedient treatment to children with malaria. Malaria is often difficult to distinguish from other common illnesses such as pneumonia. Clinical algorithms that can distinguish children with malaria from those with pneumonia or other illnesses have been developed and studied but do not eliminate completely the overlap in conditions with similar clinical manifestations.[73, 74, 78] Risk factors for a fatal outcome in children with malaria were studied in Kenya; the presence of coma or respiratory distress, or both, at initial evaluation identified those at high risk of death.[54]

Imported malaria occurs in children in many nonendemic countries. The diagnosis often is delayed because of lack of consideration of malaria as a cause of illness and unfamiliarity with the disease. In children with acquired immunity, the signs and symptoms of disease may be subtle and nonspecific, but fever or a history of fever is universal.[17, 50] Other symptoms include anorexia, vomiting, diarrhea, headache, lethargy, and abdominal pain. Laboratory findings include anemia, thrombocytopenia, and leukopenia. The diagnosis of malaria should be considered in every child with fever or a history of recent fever who has visited an area where malaria occurs.

CONGENITAL MALARIA

All four types of human malaria can be transmitted congenitally, but the disease most often is associated with *P. vivax*. That congenital malaria is not seen more frequently is due in part to the effective barrier function of the placenta. Although congenital malaria develops in 0.1 percent of immune and 10 percent of nonimmune mothers in endemic areas, placental infection occurs in as many as one third of pregnant women.[34] In endemic areas, distinguishing malaria acquired congenitally from that acquired by transmission from mosquitoes is difficult.

The onset of symptoms is insidious and usually occurs at 2 to 8 weeks of age. The typical malaria paroxysm is absent, with the infant instead having poor feeding, fever, vomiting, diarrhea, irritability, and hepatosplenomegaly on physical examination.[31] The most common laboratory finding is anemia, but thrombocytopenia and hyperbilirubinemia are also common. Therapy for the infected species of malaria is curative, and the infant does not need treatment of the exoerythrocytic stages of the parasite (although the mother does).

MALARIA IN PREGNANCY

The effects of malaria on the mother depend on the degree of immunity that she has attained and her parity.[57] Relapses and recrudescence of malaria are common during pregnancy, probably because of the immunosuppression associated with the pregnant state. Malaria can exacerbate the anemia occurring during pregnancy, and hypoglycemia and renal insufficiency may complicate falciparum malaria during pregnancy.

Placental infection during pregnancy may be associated with low birth weight, particularly in primigravidas. Vivax malaria has been linked to maternal anemia and low birth weight in multigravidas as well as primigravidas.[62] Severe falciparum malaria is harmful to the fetus because of fetal tachycardia and distress secondary to maternal fever; disruption of maternal-fetal blood flow and exchange of metabolic substrates by malaria parasites trapped in the placenta; and the potential for reduction in fetal glucose supply, which may be exacerbated by treatment with quinine, a drug that is able to stimulate the release of insulin.[48] Heavy infection of the placenta interferes with transfer of tetanus antibodies from the mother to the fetus, but the effect on other antibodies is unknown.[9] Prompt treatment of pregnant women with severe malaria is critical to survival of both the mother and baby.

Complications of Malaria

SEVERE, COMPLICATED MALARIA

Nonimmune individuals are most susceptible to the severe complications of falciparum malaria, which include cerebral malaria, pulmonary failure or acute respiratory distress syndrome, renal failure, and severe anemia. Hypoglycemia and metabolic acidosis may occur. Falciparum malaria in nonimmune patients should be considered a medical emergency, and treatment of *P. falciparum* should be initiated in all ill patients with malaria until the species can be confirmed.

CEREBRAL MALARIA

Cerebral malaria is the most common complication of falciparum malaria in children and occurs most often in children 3 to 6 years of age.[70] Alteration of consciousness in a patient with falciparum malaria and no other explanation for the condition constitutes the general definition. Clinical manifestations are broad. Patients may be comatose without response to stimuli and may assume an opisthotonic posture. Generalized convulsions may occur, but focal findings are uncommon. Intracranial pressure often is increased in children with cerebral malaria, but a relationship between the presence of increased intracranial pressure and morbidity and mortality has not been established. Factors associated with neurologic sequelae include prolonged coma, severe anemia, and multiple seizures. Mortality rates range from 15 to 30 percent of affected children; most survivors recover completely, but approximately 10 percent may have neurologic sequelae. The most common neurologic sequelae in children noted in a study in the Gambia were hemiplegia, cortical blindness, aphasia, and ataxia.[10]

Many factors, including hypoglycemia, anemia, microvascular obstruction, acidosis, and elaboration of inflammatory mediators, contribute to the syndrome of cerebral malaria. Histopathologic features are minor, with occasional hemorrhages and perivascular infiltrates.

SEVERE ANEMIA

Children younger than 1 year, especially in sub-Saharan Africa, are those most likely to suffer from severe malarial anemia. This complication is thought to occur most often in areas with year-round transmission.

HYPOGLYCEMIA

Hypoglycemia (blood glucose <40 mg/dL) may be present on initial evaluation in as many as 20 percent of children with severe malaria and is associated with a poor prognosis. The etiology of pretreatment hypoglycemia is thought to be a combination of parasite consumption of glucose and inadequate gluconeogenesis in the liver. Hypoglycemia also can occur as a result of treatment, most typically with quinine. Rapid intravenous infusion may cause hypoglycemia by stimulating insulin secretion; pregnant women appear to be especially susceptible to this complication. In addition, hypoglycemia may occur several days into a course of oral quinine, presumably caused by resolution of the reduced tissue sensitivity to insulin that is a feature of acute malaria.

ACID-BASE CHANGES

Metabolic acidosis is a marker of severity and clinically may be manifested as hyperpnea. Acidosis often is associated with hypoglycemia. Fluid resuscitation and treatment with antimalarial drugs often result in rapid resolution of acidosis, although persistence of acidosis may occur in those who eventually die of malaria.

RENAL COMPLICATIONS

Acute renal failure is a potentially life-threatening consequence of acute malaria that occurs more commonly in adults than children. It is typically oliguric in nature and is often reversible if the patient can be supported by dialysis through the oliguric phase. It is rare in residents of endemic areas and long has been thought to occur more frequently in those treated with quinine or quinidine (blackwater fever). The histologic changes resemble those of acute tubular necrosis.

Nephrotic syndrome and chronic renal failure occur more frequently in areas where malaria is endemic and usually are associated with *P. malariae*. Symptoms occur before the age of 15 years in approximately half the cases, with gradual progression to renal failure over the course of 3 to 5 years. Most patients have asymptomatic proteinuria and the gradual development of hypertension and deterioration in renal function. Adults more commonly have hematuria and azotemia; both adults and children may have hematuria. The disease does not respond to antimalarial agents. Treatment with steroids, cyclophosphamide, and azathioprine has had variable results, with remission occurring in only those with mild changes on renal biopsy.[91]

PULMONARY EDEMA

Pulmonary edema typically develops late in the course of severe malaria when other complications are already present, and it occurs more commonly in adults than children. Its pathogenesis is more consistent with capillary leak syndrome.

HYPERREACTIVE MALARIAL SYNDROME (TROPICAL SPLENOMEGALY SYNDROME, HYPERREACTIVE MALARIAL SPLENOMEGALY)

Hyperreactive malarial syndrome (HMS) is characterized by massive splenomegaly, high concentrations of total serum IgM and malarial antibodies of multiple immunoglobulin classes, and clinical and immunologic response to antimalarial agents.[105] HMS is correlated with malaria endemicity, with an incidence varying from 0.5 to 80 percent of the adult population. Its pathogenesis is unknown but appears to involve chronic exposure to malaria resulting in chronic stimulation of the immune system, as well as genetic factors. Findings on physical examination include a huge spleen and an enlarged liver. Laboratory findings include anemia and an increased reticulocyte count; some patients may have thrombocytopenia or neutropenia. Patients may have an increased risk of acquiring bacterial infections, and some researchers have suggested that HMS is a premalignant condition.[5] Chronic, lifelong treatment with antimalarial agents is the treatment of choice for those who reside in endemic areas.[91]

Diagnosis

The most important first step in the diagnosis of malaria is to consider the diagnosis in all individuals with febrile illness, especially those with a history of travel to endemic areas. Manifestations of the disease are most classic in nonimmune individuals or in areas where malaria transmission is seasonal. The signs and symptoms of disease may be nonspecific in semi-immune individuals, those who have received malaria prophylaxis, or those who have been partially treated.

In nonendemic areas, a history of travel to an endemic area should suggest the diagnosis in all individuals with a febrile illness, regardless of the accompanying signs and symptoms. Common diagnoses mistakenly assigned to patients ultimately determined to have malaria include gastroenteritis and viral syndrome. The course of disease may be modified by exposure to antimalarial drugs, such as those that may have been used for prophylaxis, and the incubation period may be prolonged after the administration of antimalarial chemoprophylaxis.

Because malaria may be transmitted by blood transfusion or an organ transplant, may be congenitally acquired, and rarely, occurs cryptically, the diagnosis also should be entertained in patients with compatible signs and symptoms of malaria, anemia or thrombocytopenia (or both), and no other explanation for their illness.

Microscopy remains the technique most commonly used for the diagnosis of malaria. Alternatives to microscopic diagnostic techniques for malaria include tests using reagents based on parasite antigens or enzymes, fluorescent microscopy, DNA probes, polymerase chain reaction (PCR), antibody detection, and flow cytometry. Few of these methods meet the requirements of low cost, high reliability and reproducibility, and rapid turnaround time. Some of them, however, are suitable for use in field conditions and have been used in endemic areas under field conditions and for self-diagnosis.

MICROSCOPY

Microscopy is the gold standard for the diagnosis of malaria. Identification of typical parasite forms by an experienced microscopist is the mainstay of diagnosis worldwide (Figs. 218–3 to 218–5; see Color Plates III, IV, and V). The advantages of using light microscopy are many: it can be performed at low cost, it can be done rapidly, it allows both identification of the infecting species and estimation of parasite load, and it can be performed with a small amount of blood. The major disadvantage of microscopy is the need for an experienced microscopist. In settings where malaria is not endemic, the need for specialists to review microscope slides may lead to a delay in diagnosis.

Thin smears are the most useful in diagnosing malaria. They are easy to prepare, with only a single drop of blood required. The drop of blood is placed at one end of the slide, and the edge of a second slide is placed at the edge of the blood smear and drawn across the slide.[30] RBC morphology is preserved, so invasion of large RBCs by the parasites can be identified, and speciation of the organism is possible (see Table 218–1). Oil-immersion magnification (×1000) should be used for viewing the slide because many young asexual intraerythrocytic parasites are only 2 to 3 μm in diameter and may be missed when using high-dry (×440) magnification. Examining a thin smear is easiest, so the microscopist begins by looking at the thin edge of the blood film, farthest from where the drop of blood was placed. Giemsa stain is preferred to Wright stain when available because it preserves details such as Schüffner dots in *P. vivax* and *P. ovale* infections. When individual RBCs can be seen at low magnification (×100), switching to oil immersion allows examination for parasites within the cells. The major disadvantage of thin films is low sensitivity. With low parasite loads (less than 100 to 300/μL), the amount of blood on the smear may be too small to detect the parasites.

Thick smears have greater sensitivity than thin smears do as a result of the larger quantity of blood used. Because the RBCs are lysed during preparation of the slide, the types of cells containing parasites cannot be identified. To make a thick smear, a drop of blood is placed on the slide and spread in a circle. The slide then is stained without using methanol fixation, a procedure that lyses RBCs.

Estimating parasite density is often useful for assessing the likelihood of complications associated with high parasite density and for evaluating response to therapy. The density of parasites can be determined on thick or thin smears.[30, 40] When using thin smears, the proportion of RBCs infected is counted while viewing the smear under an oil-immersion lens.

FLUORESCENT MICROSCOPY

The quantitative buffy coat test relies on identification of parasitized RBCs stained with acridine orange in the RBC layer of centrifuged blood.[88] Experienced personnel can perform the test rapidly, but the reagents are costly when compared with those needed for microscopy, and the species of parasite cannot be identified. If a fluorescent microscope is available, identification of parasitized RBCs can be accomplished by staining a thick smear with acridine orange and examining under fluorescent light.

DETECTION OF PARASITE ANTIGEN

Antigen capture dipstick assays based on detection of either histidine-rich protein 2 (HRP-2; ParaSight F [Becton Dickinson] and ICT Malaria Pf [ICT Diagnostics]) or parasite lactate dehydrogenase (LDH; OptiMAL, Flow, Inc.) have been developed.[16, 51] Assays detecting HRP-2 are specific for *P. falciparum*, whereas the parasite LDH assay can identify both falciparum and vivax malaria.[12] The ParaSight F dipstick test, when studied in field trials in Kenya, showed a sensitivity of 96.5 to 100 percent in patients whose parasitemia was greater than 60 parasites per microliter, with lower sensitivity noted at lower levels of parasitemia. Antigen persisted to day 6 in 11.9 percent of children whose blood smears were clear at that time.[6] When studied in travelers, the sensitivity of the ParaSight F test ranged from 40 percent in those with fewer than 50 parasites per microliter to 93 percent or more in those with more than 100 parasites per microliter, and positive dipstick tests occurred in 68 percent of blood smear–negative patients on day 7 and in 20 percent on day 28.[32] The sensitivity of the dipstick test for detection of parasite LDH (OptiMAL) has noted to be in the range of 85 to 90 percent, and preliminary results suggest that positive tests do not persist after successful treatment.[67]

Dipstick tests may have a role in cost-effective malaria diagnosis in situations where laboratory services are inadequate, in mobile clinics, in locations where levels of malaria transmission are low and drug resistance is high, when the cost of treatment exceeds the cost of the dipstick test, and when blood films are negative and determining the diagnosis is critical. In developed countries, dipstick assays would benefit laboratories with less experienced microscopists by helping them make a rapid diagnosis, confirm a diagnosis made by microscopy, or speciate an infection.

Dipstick malaria tests have been proposed for use by travelers in the self-diagnosis of malaria and have been tested for this purpose. The use of these tests for self-diagnosis remains controversial, with some experts supporting this use and others believing that technical improvements in the tests are necessary before they can be used accurately to guide decisions about self-treatment of malaria.[33, 81]

DNA PROBE

Specific DNA probes for identification of *P. falciparum* have been developed and tested in field conditions in Thailand.[4] The technique compared favorably with microscopy and could be used to test large numbers of samples at a time, but it had the disadvantage of needing a radiolabeled probe. Non-isotope probes have been used in other field trials in Madagascar, where an enzyme-linked probe was compared with microscopy for the diagnosis of falciparum malaria. The results were comparable to examination of thick smears by microscopy for *P. falciparum* infection, but the assay could not identify infection with *P. vivax, P. ovale,* or *P. malariae* alone.[56]

POLYMERASE CHAIN REACTION

Field studies of PCR amplification of species-specific sequences of genes for sporozoite or merozoite proteins in Thailand and the Venezuelan Amazon demonstrated sensitivity greater than that of thick smears for the diagnosis of *P. falciparum* and *P. vivax* malaria.[3, 43] Major disadvantages of this technique include the need for expensive equipment and reagents. PCR may be better suited for use in large-scale epidemiologic surveys rather than the diagnosis of acute malaria in the clinical setting.

FLOW CYTOMETRY

Automated blood cell analyzers based on flow cytometry have been shown to display cells containing malaria pigment as a population of cells distinct from other blood components. To date, this discovery has been serendipitous in patients not suspected to have malaria, and the diagnosis must be confirmed by conventional methods.[23, 35] A future application of this technology could be to modify automated blood cell analyzers to flag specimens that need to be examined further by thin or thick smears (or both).[35]

ANTIBODY DETECTION

Malaria antibodies develop rapidly after infection and remain present for years; they are therefore of limited value in diagnosing malaria in individual patients. Occasionally, antibody tests might prove useful in the diagnosis of nonimmune individuals with cryptic febrile illnesses or on a population basis to assess the degree of community-wide immunity. Measurement of antibody may have a role in the diagnosis of HMS.[105]

Treatment

Treatment of malaria depends on identification of the species of *Plasmodium* causing infection, knowledge of the presence of resistance to chloroquine in the area in which malaria was contracted, and therapeutic goals (treatment of acute illness, eradication of the exoerythrocytic phase of malaria, or prevention of infection).[98] Drugs and classes of drugs currently in use for treating malaria include 4-aminoquinolines and related compounds (chloroquine, mefloquine, amodiaquine), primaquine, sulfadoxine-pyrimethamine, halofantrine, atovaquone-proguanil, artemisinin (qinghaosu) and other artemisinins (artemether, artesunate), cinchona alkaloids (quinine, quinidine), and doxycycline or tetracycline. Other combination drugs are available outside the United States, and multiple investigational compounds are in various stages of investigation. Drugs that may be used for the treatment of malaria are listed in Table 218–2. Drugs used for the prevention of malaria are discussed in a subsequent section.

The choice of agent for the treatment of symptomatic malaria depends on the presence of resistance to chloroquine and other antimalarial drugs, the availability of drugs in the local area, and the age of the patient. Local and national guidelines for the treatment of malaria differ, and practitioners treating patients with malaria should consult

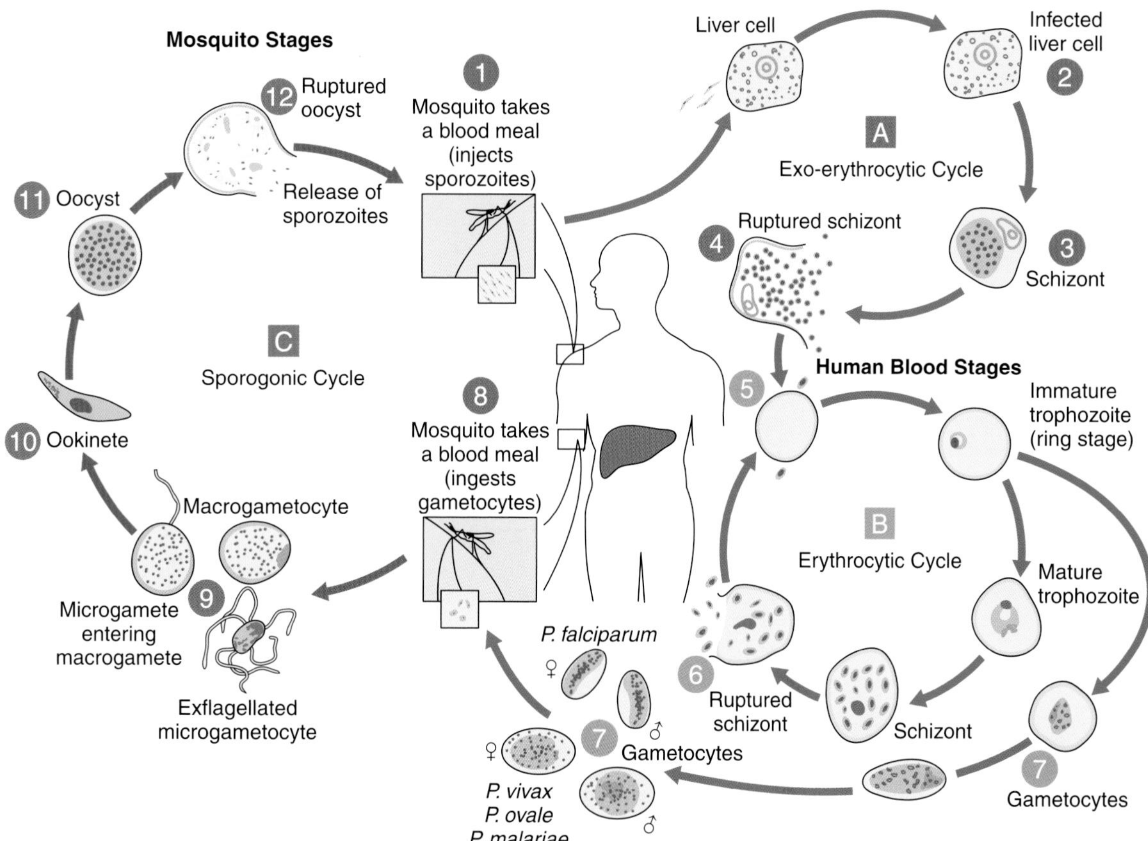

FIGURE 218–1 ■ Life cycle of the human malaria parasites.

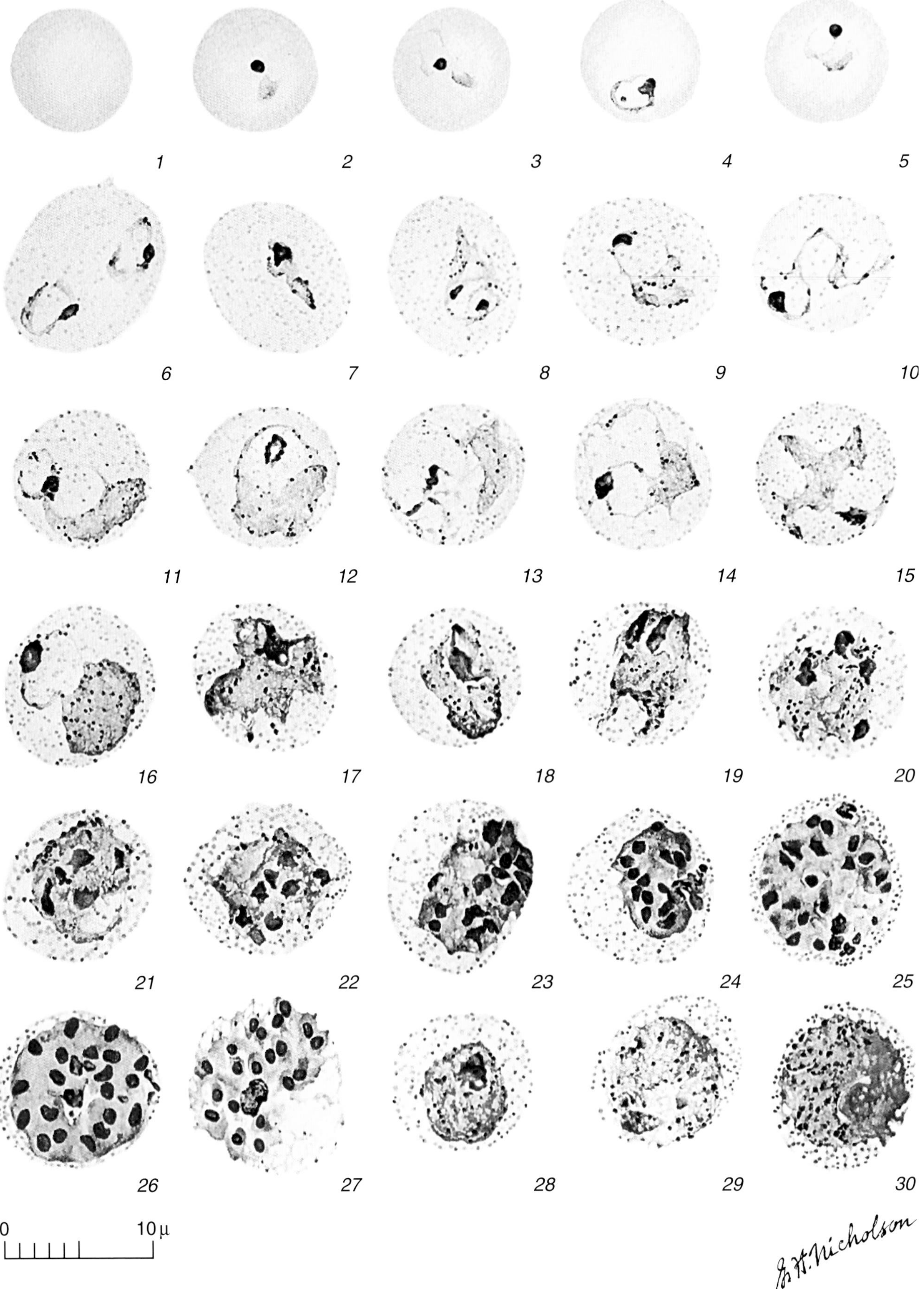

FIGURE 218–2 ■ *Plasmodium vivax.* 1, Normal erythrocyte; 2–5, young trophozoites; 6–16, growing trophozoites; 17, 18, mature trophozoites; 19–21, early schizonts; 22, 23, developing schizonts; 24–27, nearly mature and mature schizonts; 28, 29, nearly mature and mature macrogametocytes; 30, mature microgametocyte. (From Coatney, G. R., Collins, W. E., Warren, M., et al.: The Primate Malarias. Bethesda, MD, U.S. Department of Health and Human Services, National Institutes of Health, National Institute of Allergy and Infectious Diseases, 1971.)

TABLE 218–2 ■ DRUG REGIMENS FOR TREATMENT OF MALARIA

Infection	Drug	Adult Dosage	Pediatric Dosage	Comments
All *Plasmodium* except Chloroquine-Resistant *P. falciparum* and Chloroquine-Resistant *P. vivax*				
Patients able to take oral medications:				
	Chloroquine phosphate	1 g salt (600 mg base), then 500 mg salt (300 mg base) 6 hr later, then 500 mg salt (300 mg base) at 24 and 48 hr	10 mg base/kg (max, 600 mg base), then 5 mg base/kg 6 hr later, then 5 mg base/kg at 24 and 48 hr	Bitter taste; may be given by nasogastric tube
Patients not able to tolerate oral medications:				
	Quinidine gluconate (IV)	10 mg/kg loading dose (max, 600 mg) in normal saline slowly over 1 to 2 hr, followed by continuous infusion of 0.02 mg/kg/min until oral therapy can be started	Same as adult dose	
or				
	Quinine dihydrochloride (IV)	20 mg/kg loading dose IV in 5% dextrose over 4 hr, followed by 10 mg/kg over 2–4 hr q8h (max, 1800 mg/day) until oral therapy can be started	Same as adult dose	
Only if IV quinidine gluconate and IV quinidine dihydrochloride are unavailable and chloroquine phosphate cannot be given orally or by nasogastric tube:				
	Intramuscular chloroquine*	2.5 mg base/kg q4h or 3.5 mg base/kg q6h (total not to exceed 25 mg base/kg)	Same as adult dose, with care to avoid high IM or IV peak levels	See precautions in text
or				
	Intravenous chloroquine*	10 mg base/kg over 4 hr, followed by 5 mg base/kg q12h in a 2-hr infusion (total dose not to exceed 25 mg base/kg)	Same as adult dose, with care to avoid high IM or IV peak levels	See precautions in text
Chloroquine-Resistant *P. falciparum*				
Patients able to take oral medications:				
	Quinine sulfate	650 mg q8h × 3–7 days	25 mg/kg/day in 3 doses × 3–7 days	
plus				
	Doxycycline	100 mg bid × 7 days	2 mg/kg/day × 7 days	Not to be used in children <8 yr or pregnant women
or plus				
	Tetracycline	25 mg qid × 7 days	6.25 mg/kg qid × 7 days	Not to be used in children <8 yr or pregnant women
or plus				
	Clindamycin	900 mg tid × 5 days	20–40 mg/kg day in 3 doses × 5 days	May be used in pregnancy
or plus				
	Pyrimethamine-sulfadoxine	3 tablets at once on last day of quinine	<1 yr: 1/4 tablet 1–3 yr: 1/2 tablet 4–8 yr: 1 tablet 9–14 yr: 2 tablets	Tablets of Fanisdar contain 25 mg pyrimethamine and 500 mg sulfadoxine
	Alternative: Atovaquone	1000 mg daily × 3 days	11–20 kg: 250 mg 21–30 kg: 500 mg 31–40 kg: 750 mg	Malarone tablets: Adult: 250 mg atovaquone 100 mg proguanil Pediatric: 62.5 mg atovaquone, 25 mg proguanil

Continued

TABLE 218–2 ■ DRUG REGIMENS FOR TREATMENT OF MALARIA—cont'd

Infection	Drug	Adult Dosage	Pediatric Dosage	Comments
plus	Proguanil	400 mg daily × 3 days	11–20 kg: 100 mg 21–30 kg: 200 mg 31–40 kg: 300 mg	
or plus	Doxycycline	100 mg bid × 3 days	2 mg/kg/day × 3 days	Not to be used in children <8 yr pregnant women
	Alternative: Mefloquine	750 mg followed by 500 mg 12 hr later	15 mg/kg followed 8–12 hr later by 10 mg/kg (<45 kg)	See text for precautions and adverse events
	Alternative: Halofantrine*	500 mg q6h × 3 doses; repeat in 1 wk	8 mg/kg q6h x 3 doses (<40 kg); repeat in 1 wk	Do not use in patients with cardiac conduction defects or with drugs affecting the QT interval (quinine, quinidine, mefloquine). Should not be used in pregnancy
	Alternative: Artesunate*	4 mg/kg/day x 3 days		
plus	Mefloquine	750 mg followed by 500 mg 12 hr later		See text for precautions and adverse events
Patients not able to take oral medication:	Quinidine gluconate (IV)			
or	Quinine dihydrochloride (IV)			See above
	Alternative: Artemether*	3.2 mg/kg IM, then 1.6 mg/kg daily for ≥72 hr	Same as adult dose	
Multiply Resistant *P. falciparum*	Artesunate*	200 mg by rectum (pr) at 0, 4, 8, 12, 24, 36, 48 and 60 hr for a total pr dose of 1600 mg artesunate or 100 mg artesunate PO × 1, followed by 50 mg PO q12h × 5 days for total of 600 mg	4 mg/kg PO × 1, followed by 2 mg/kg/day × 3 days given in doses of 1 or 2 mg/kg q12h or q24h × 3 days for a total dose of 10 mg/kg	
plus	Mefloquine	750 mg PO at 72 hr and 500 mg PO at 84 hr	25 mg/kg PO on either day 1 or day 2	See text for precautions and adverse events
	Alternative: Mefloquine	750 mg followed by 500 mg PO 12 hr later	15 mg/kg followed 8–12 hr later by 10 mg/kg	See text for precautions and adverse events
	Alternative: Halofantrine*	500 mg PO q6h × 3 doses, repeat in 1 wk	8 mg/kg PO q6h × 3 doses; repeat in 1 wk	Do not use in patients with cardiac conduction defects or with drugs affecting the QT interval (quinine, quinidine, mefloquine). Should not be used in pregnancy

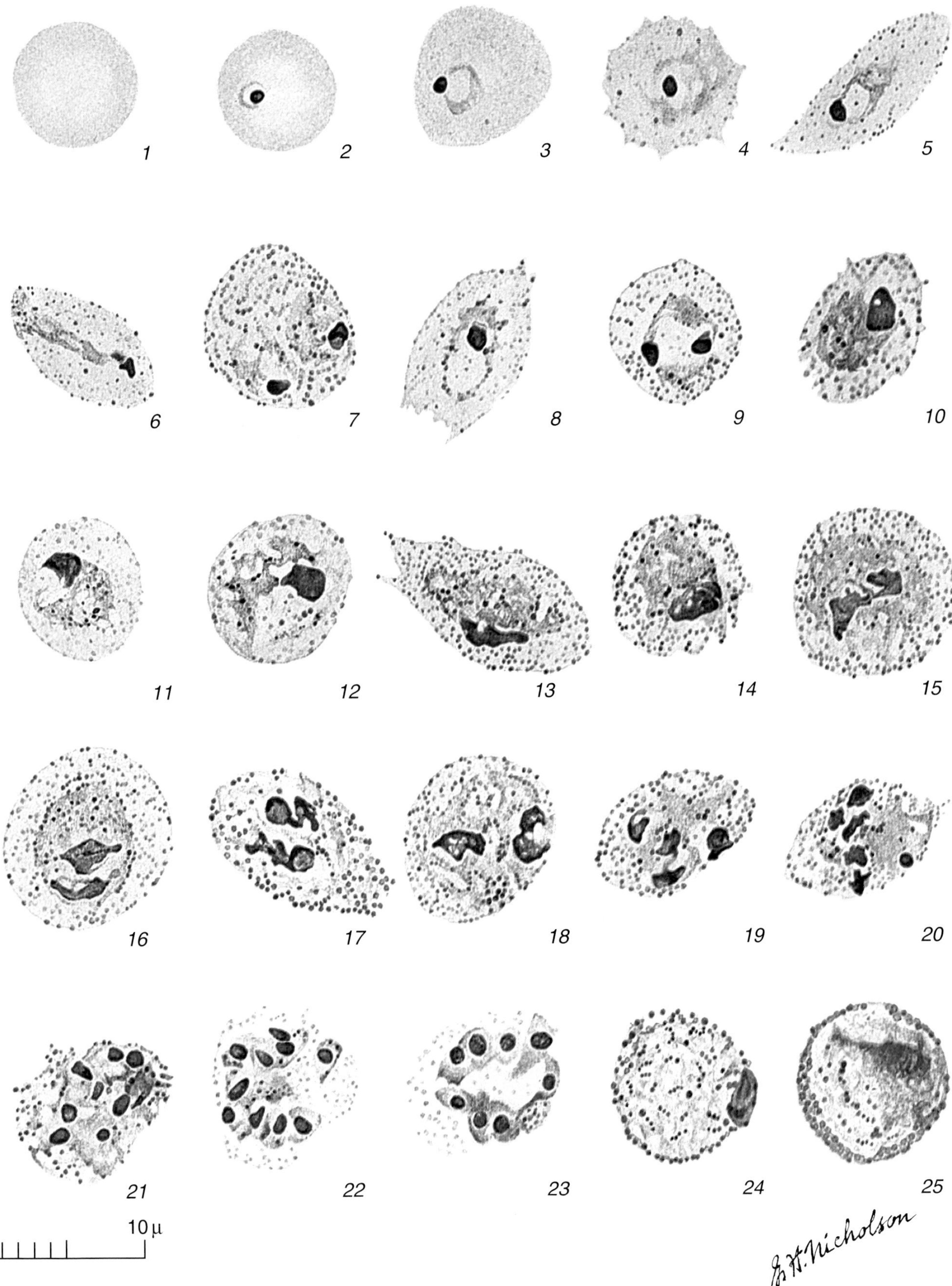

FIGURE 218–3 ■ *Plasmodium ovale.* 1, Normal erythrocyte; 2–5, young trophozoites; 6–16, growing trophozoites; 13–15, mature trophozoites; 16–22, developing schizonts; 23, mature schizont; 24, adult macrogametocyte; 25, adult microgametocyte. (From Coatney, G. R., Collins, W. E., Warren, M., et al.: The Primate Malarias. Bethesda, MD, U.S. Department of Health and Human Services, National Institutes of Health, National Institute of Allergy and Infectious Diseases, 1971.)

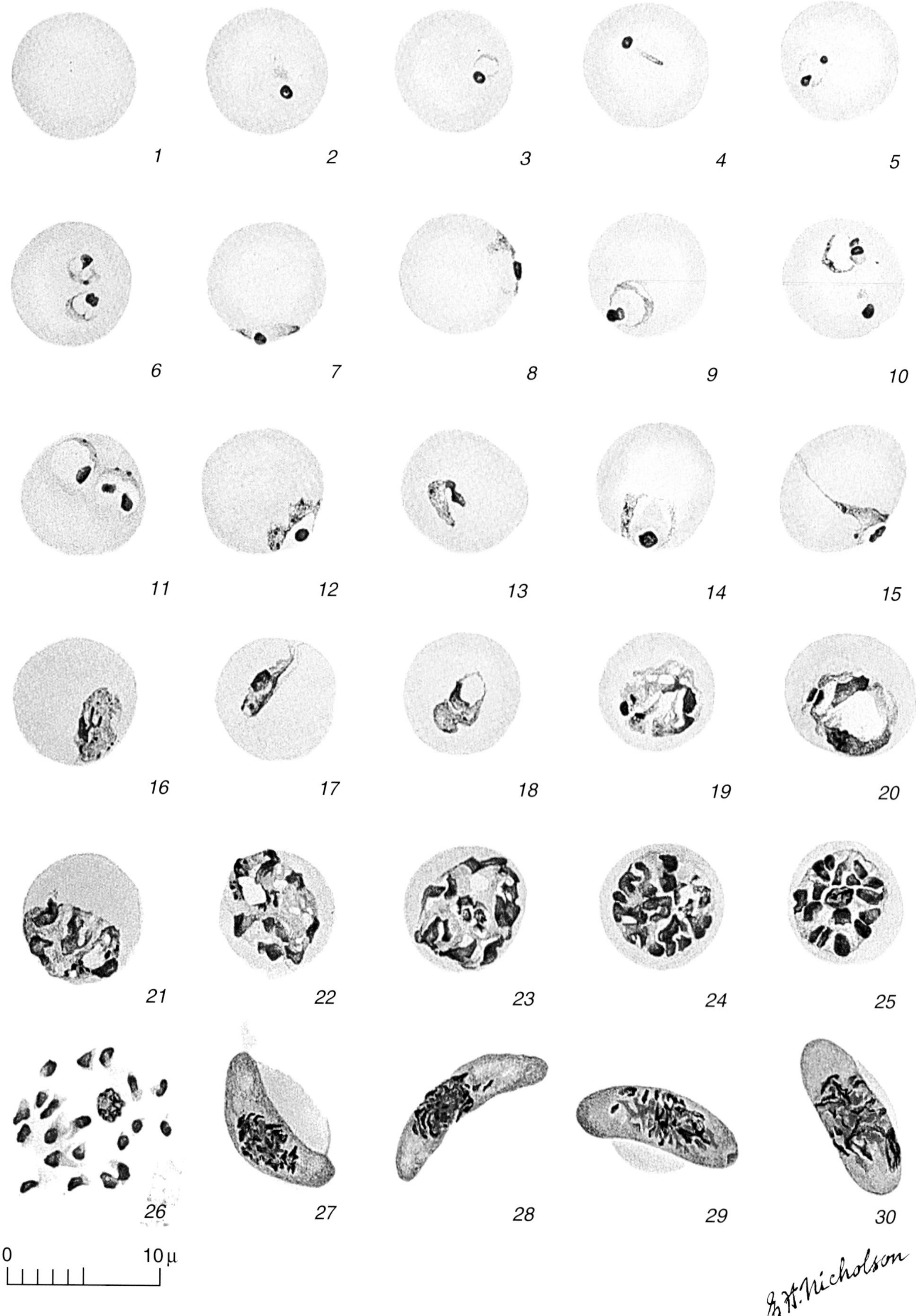

FIGURE 218–4 ■ *Plasmodium falciparum.* 1, Normal erythrocyte; 2–11, young trophozoites; 12–15, growing trophozoites; 16–18, mature trophozoites; 19–22, developing schizonts; 23–26, nearly mature and mature schizonts; 27, 28, mature macrogametocytes; 29, 30, mature microgametocytes. (From Coatney, G. R., Collins, W. E., Warren, M., et al.: The Primate Malarias. Bethesda, MD, U.S. Department of Health and Human Services, National Institutes of Health, National Institute of Allergy and Infectious Diseases, 1971.)

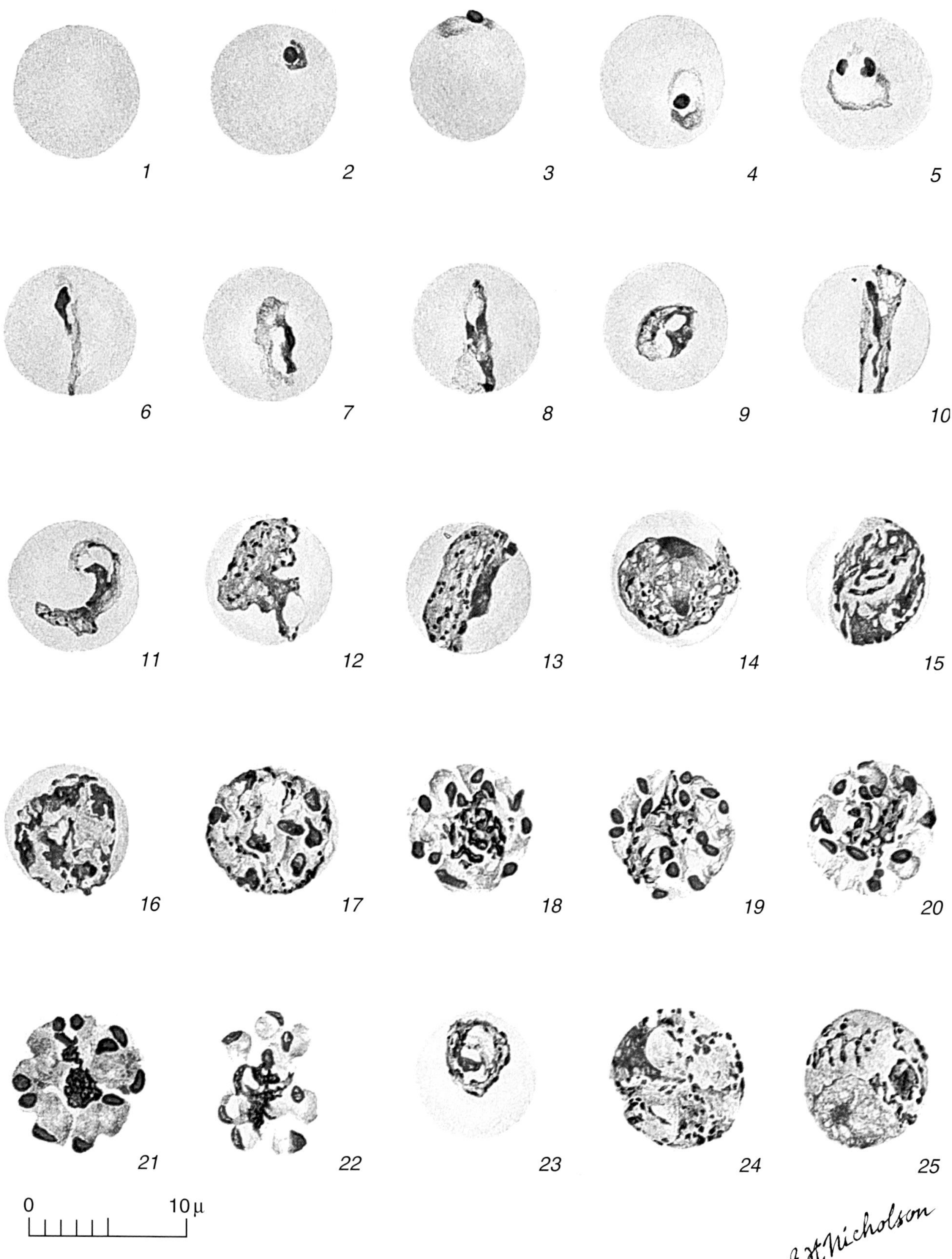

FIGURE 218–5 ■ *Plasmodium malariae.* 1, Normal erythrocyte; 2–5, young trophozoites; 6–11, growing trophozoites; 12, 13, nearly mature and mature trophozoites; 14–20, developing schizonts; 21, 22, mature schizonts; 23, developing gametocyte; 24, mature macrogametocyte; 25, mature microgametocyte. (From Coatney, G. R., Collins, W. E., Warren, M., et al.: The Primate Malarias. Bethesda, MD, U.S. Department of Health and Human Services, National Institutes of Health, National Institute of Allergy and Infectious Diseases, 1971.)

TABLE 218–2 ■ DRUG REGIMENS FOR TREATMENT OF MALARIA—cont'd

Infection	Drug	Adult Dosage	Pediatric Dosage	Comments
	Alternative: Atrovaquone	1000 mg/day × 3 days	11–20 kg: 250 mg 21–30 kg: 500 mg 31–40 kg: 750 mg	Malorone tablets: Adult: 250 atovaquone 100 mg proguanil Pediatric: 62.5 mg atovaquone, 25 mg proguanil
plus				
	Proguanil	400 mg/day × 3 days	11–20 kg: 100 mg 21–30 kg: 200 mg 31–40 kg: 300 mg	Same as above
	Alternative: Quinine sulfate	650 mg q8h × 3–7 days	25 mg/kg/day in 3 doses × 3–7 days	
plus				
	Doxycycline	100 mg bid × 7 days	2 mg/kg/day × 7 days	Not to be used in children <8 yr or pregnant women
or plus				
	Pyrimethamine-sulfadoxine	3 tablets at once on last day of quinine	<1 yr: ¼ tablet 1–3 yr: ½ tablet 4–8 yr: 1 tablet 9–14 yr: 2 tablets	
Prevention of Relapses: *P. vivax* and *P. ovale*				
	Primaquine phosphate	26.3 mg (15 mg base)/day × 14 days or 79 mg (45 mg base)/wk × 8 wk	0.3 mg base/kg/day × 14 days	Not to be used in glucose-6-phosphate dehydrogenase-deficient individuals or pregnant women; take with food

*Not available in the United States

local resources and experts. Information about countries and regions with chloroquine-resistant malaria is available in the United States from the Centers for Disease Control and Prevention (*www.cdc.gov*) and outside the United States from local and national health organizations.

CHLOROQUINE

Chloroquine is the drug of choice for chloroquine-susceptible malaria caused by *P. falciparum* and *P. vivax* and for all infections with *P. ovale* and *P. malariae*.[41] Chloroquine is a 4-aminoquinoline with rapid schizonticidal activity. It is not effective against exoerythrocytic forms of the parasite, and patients treated with chloroquine after acquiring *P. vivax* or *P. ovale* infection need to have additional treatment to eliminate these forms. Chloroquine is most active against late ring stages and mature trophozoites. Response to treatment is rapid, with disappearance of parasitemia within 48 to 72 hours after initiation of treatment when the parasite is susceptible.

Chloroquine is available as an oral preparation and, in many areas, as intramuscular and intravascular formulations. Oral absorption is excellent, and the drug is safe and effective when given by nasogastric or orogastric tube in comatose children.[99] Intramuscular and intravenous administration may be associated with an increased risk for cardiac arrhythmias.

Adverse reactions to chloroquine are rare at the doses used for suppression or treatment of malaria. Side effects include gastrointestinal symptoms such as nausea, vomiting and diarrhea, dizziness, headache, and fatigue. Pruritus may be a troubling adverse event, especially in black patients. Chloroquine has no known teratogenic effects, and it may be used in pregnant and lactating women. The drug is not contraindicated in glucose-6-phosphate dehydrogenase (G6PD)-deficient individuals. Serious adverse events, including hypotension, cardiac arrest, and circulatory failure, may occur after intravenous or intramuscular use of the drug, especially in children. Psychotic symptoms may occur rarely with chloroquine.[21] Chloroquine always should be given slowly when administered intravenously and in small doses when given by intramuscular injection; some experts discourage the use of parenteral chloroquine. Oral doses are absorbed rapidly. The risk of aspiration occurring while giving a dose by tube to a comatose patient must be weighed against the risk of complications developing when giving a dose by the intravenous or intramuscular route. The lethal dose of chloroquine in children is 1 g and in adults, 4 g. Cumulative doses exceeding 100 g are associated with an increased risk for retinopathy. Dose reduction may be required for patients with renal and hepatic disease.

MEFLOQUINE

The development of mefloquine was a major advance in the treatment of chloroquine-resistant malaria, although resistance has developed rapidly in some parts of the world where it is used widely. Mefloquine is a 4-quinolone-carbinolamine whose exact mechanism is unknown. Its main target is early trophozoites. Like chloroquine, it is not active against exoerythrocytic phases. Mefloquine has been associated with neurologic and psychiatric side effects when used for treatment or prophylaxis.[91] Vomiting occurs commonly when mefloquine is given to children younger than 5 years and may decrease its efficacy.[86] Mefloquine should not be administered concurrently with quinine, quinidine, or halofantrine because of concern about arrhythmias. The drug has been used in the second and third trimesters of pregnancy without adverse outcome.

AMODIAQUINE

Amodiaquine, like chloroquine, is a 4-aminoquinolone. It has similar efficacy but may have increased activity when compared with chloroquine for the treatment of strains of *P. falciparum* resistant to chloroquine.[66] It is available in an oral preparation and is more palatable. Significant adverse events such as agranulocytosis, hepatotoxicity, and deaths when used as a prophylactic agent have limited its use as a first-line agent. It is not licensed or marketed in the United States.

PRIMAQUINE

Primaquine, an 8-aminoquinoline derivative that is effective against exoerythrocytic hypnozoites, is used primarily to prevent relapses of *P. vivax* and *P. ovale,* although it may not be completely effective against some strains of *P. vivax.* It is not an effective blood schizonticide but is an active gametocidal and sporontocidal drug for all four species of human malaria. Primaquine can cause intravascular hemolysis in individuals with G6PD deficiency. Other adverse events include gastrointestinal symptoms such as nausea, epigastric pain, anorexia, and abdominal cramps. Other rare side effects include methemoglobinemia, hemoglobinuria, and bone marrow suppression. Safety in pregnancy has not been established, and the drug should not be used by pregnant women. Patients should be tested for G6PD deficiency before being treated with primaquine.

PYRIMETHAMINE-SULFADOXINE (FANSIDAR)

This combination drug (sulfonamide plus a dihydrofolate reductase inhibitor) exhibits synergy in its action against malaria parasites; the combination is active even against strains resistant to the individual drug components. Pyrimethamine-sulfadoxine often is used for presumptive treatment of malaria in travelers who are taking other drugs for prophylaxis in areas where chloroquine resistance occurs. An unacceptably high incidence of Stevens-Johnson reactions (fatalities in 1 in 11,000 to 25,0000 users) when the drug was used for prophylaxis resulted in withdrawal of the indication for this purpose. Although safety has not been established in pregnancy, the drug has been used effectively for intermittent presumptive treatment of pregnant women in endemic areas to decrease the risk for severe anemia.[85]

HALOFANTRINE

Halofantrine is a 9-phenanthrene-methanol that has been used for the treatment of malaria caused by chloroquine-resistant *P. falciparum.* Its major side effect is dose-related prolongation of the QT interval,[63] and it has been associated with cardiac arrhythmias and sudden death, especially in individuals taking mefloquine prophylaxis.[63, 89] Its major use was in uncomplicated malaria in areas of multidrug resistance, but cardiac toxicity at the doses required to be effective may limit its widespread use.[92] It is contraindicated in pregnant and lactating women because of embryotoxic effects. Resistance to halofantrine has limited its use in some areas.

ATOVAQUONE-PROGUANIL (MALARONE)

Malarone is a fixed-dose combination (available in both adult and pediatric formulations) of atovaquone and proguanil hydrochloride that is available for the treatment of malaria caused by *P. falciparum.* The combination is significantly more effective than either drug alone and is effective for the treatment of malaria strains resistant to other antimalarial drugs. The combination is also likely to be active against the blood stages of *P. vivax, P. ovale,* and *P. malariae,* but the regimen does not have activity against the hypnozoites of *P. vivax.* Atovaquone-proguanil is significantly more effective than mefloquine, chloroquine, amodiaquine, or pyrimethamine-sulfadoxine in locations where parasites are resistant to these drugs.[47]

ARTEMESININ DERIVATIVES

Artemesinin (qinghaosu) is a sesquiterpene lactone that along with its derivatives (artemether, artesunate, arteether, and others), has antimalarial activity thought to be due to the ability to cause free radical damage in parasite membrane systems.[27] These compounds are unique in their ability to cure malaria more rapidly than other agents do, with no apparent adverse events. Recrudescence rates are high, however, and the drug class seems to have limited potential for prophylaxis. Oral preparations, suppositories, and oil-based preparations for intramuscular injection are available, although standardization of preparations is lacking.[75] The major utility of these drugs at this time is for severe malaria in areas where quinine resistance is appearing or, in combination with other antimalarials, in areas of multidrug-resistant *P. falciparum.*[26] In clinical trials in the Gambia, artemether was as effective as quinine and chloroquine for treatment of cerebral malaria in children.[96, 100] When used in sequence with mefloquine, the combination was effective and tolerated well by patients with acute, uncomplicated falciparum malaria in Thailand, an area with multidrug resistance.[49] Later studies showed that the use of this combination may have helped halt the progressions of mefloquine resistance in the region.[65] At this time, no licensed preparations are available in the United States.

QUININE AND QUINIDINE

Quinine has been used for the treatment of malaria for centuries.[91] It is active against the mature asexual erythrocytic forms of all four species of human malaria and against the gametes of all species except *P. falciparum,* where it has activity against only immature gametes. It is not effective against exoerythrocytic forms. Quinine is the drug of choice for severe or complicated malaria. It may be given orally, but intravenous and intramuscular forms are available. Quinine crosses the placenta easily and may be used in the treatment of pregnant women, although close monitoring for hypoglycemia is warranted.[48]

Adverse reactions to quinine include tinnitus, headache, nausea, visual and hearing disturbances, and tremors, a constellation of symptoms called cinchonism. Symptoms may appear during the first 1 to 3 days of therapy and stop when treatment is terminated. Hypoglycemia may occur, particularly when the drug is used to treat pregnant women. Severe adverse events are rare, but may occur idiosyncratically. Blackwater fever (hemoglobinuria) seems to occur after treatment with quinine, but the causal mechanism is unknown.

Recrudescence rates may be high when quinine is used alone because of the presence of quinine-resistant strains of *P. falciparum*. A second drug usually is added to treat the remaining forms. Drugs used with quinine include doxycycline, tetracycline, clindamycin, and where resistance to this drug is not present, pryrimethamine-sufadoxine.[41]

Quinidine is a related drug that may be given intravenously; in some developed countries where intravenous quinine is unavailable, it is the drug of choice for severe malaria. The mechanisms of action and adverse events are similar, although cardiac arrhythmias occur more commonly with quinidine, and thus cardiac monitoring is advised.[98]

TETRACYCLINE AND DOXYCYCLINE

Tetracycline, doxycycline, and the related drug minocycline have very slow activity against malarial schizonts.[91] Doxycycline and minocycline may be given once daily. They are active against chloroquine- and pyrimethamine-sulfadoxine–resistant *P. falciparum*. Resistance to tetracycline has not been demonstrated. Because of their slow activity, they should be given in combination with a rapidly acting drug such as quinine. These drugs should not be used in children younger than 8 years or by pregnant or nursing women.

LUMEFANTRINE

Lumefantrine, available only in fixed combination with artemether, is available only in some tropical countries and some countries in Europe. It is well tolerated and very effective against multidrug-resistant falciparum malaria.[97a]

INVESTIGATIONAL DRUGS

Targets for new antimalarial drugs include malaria proteases, which play a critical role in malaria pathogenesis.[77] Adjuvant therapy that would modify or prevent the effects of inflammatory mediators also may have a role in the treatment of complications of malaria.

SUPPORTIVE AND ADJUNCTIVE THERAPY

The goals of supportive therapy are to maintain oxygenation and treat acidosis and hypoglycemia. Treatment with glucose infusion, oxygen, and blood transfusion may be necessary. In some cases, hemodialysis may be needed. Serial blood smears are necessary to assess the degree of parasitemia and response to therapy. Ruling out other conditions that may contribute concurrently to the clinical status of the patient is important. For example, bacterial meningitis should be ruled out in all patients with cerebral malaria.

Adjunctive therapies that have been demonstrated to have benefit include antipyretics and anticonvulsants. Exchange transfusion remains a controversial option.[40, 98] Some therapies, such as high-dose corticosteroids for cerebral malaria, have been shown to be harmful.[98, 103] The search for effective adjunctive therapy for severe and complicated malaria continues.

Prevention

Prevention of malaria can be accomplished by reduction of the mosquito population, use of personal protection methods to prevent mosquito bites, and chemoprophylaxis.[104] Reduction of mosquito vectors is most successful when locally controlled programs are developed and maintained.[39] Strategies that take into account local circumstances, such as applying insecticide to cattle in communities where families share their homes with domestic animals, are most likely to be successful.[79] Most programs will require a combination of preventive strategies and effective treatment modalities.

PERSONAL PROTECTIVE MEASURES

A significant reduction in the incidence of malaria in children in communities where bed nets, especially those impregnated with insecticide, are used consistently has been reported from many countries.[15, 22, 87] In northern Ghana, community-wide use of bed nets was associated with a reduction in all-cause child mortality in young children.[7] The use of bed nets, especially those impregnated with insecticide, is recommended for travelers to malarial areas. Other personal protective measures include using mosquito repellents and insecticide-impregnated clothing or gear, wearing clothing that covers areas likely to be bitten, and remaining, if possible, in air-conditioned or well-screened areas during times when mosquitoes are biting.

CHEMOPROPHYLAXIS

Country-specific information regarding recommendations for the use of antimalarial drugs may differ, and readers are urged to seek recommendations from national or local authorities. In the United States, these recommendations are available widely in publications from the Centers for Disease Control and Prevention[11] and worldwide from the WHO or national health information sources. Many excellent sources of health information for travelers include discussions of malaria prevention.[2, 18, 36, 80, 82, 88a] Some sources include lists of websites containing health information for travel.[19, 80] Drugs available for the prevention of malaria are listed in Table 218–3.

Chloroquine

A major determinant of appropriate chemoprophylaxis is whether a child will travel to an area of chloroquine resistance. In areas of the world that have no resistance to chloroquine, the drug of choice for prevention of malaria is chloroquine. This drug is tolerated well and may be given to children of all ages, including infants. Dosing of chloroquine in children is based on the child's weight and can be found in Table 218–3. In the United States, chloroquine is available only in tablets that have a very bitter taste. Pharmacies can prepare appropriate doses in capsules, and the contents of the capsule then can be mixed with a small amount of liquid or semisolid food for administration. Although liquid preparations are widely available overseas and are stable for long periods,[58] many U.S. pharmacies are reluctant to prepare liquid preparations. If patients are considering purchasing liquid preparations overseas, the family should be given information with the child's medication dose calculated as both the base and the salt because concentrations of liquid preparations may vary. Adverse events caused by chloroquine are uncommon when the medication is used at doses needed for malaria prophylaxis. Minor side effects can include gastrointestinal upset, headache, dizziness, blurred vision, and pruritus. Rarely do adverse events require discontinuation of medication. Chloroquine may be taken

TABLE 218–3 ■ DRUG REGIMENS USED FOR PREVENTION OF MALARIA

	Drug	Adult Dosage	Pediatric Dosage	Comments
Chloroquine-Sensitive Areas				
	Chloroquine phosphate (drug of choice)	500 mg salt (300 mg base) orally once/wk beginning the week before exposure and continuing for 4 wk after exposure	5 mg/kg base (8.3 mg/kg salt) once/wk, up to adult dose of 300 mg base beginning the week before exposure and continuing for 4 wk after exposure	May be used in pregnant women
Chloroquine-Resistant Areas				
	Mefloquine	250 mg salt (228 mg base) salt once/wk orally beginning the week before exposure and continuing for 4 wk after exposure	<15 kg: 5 mg/kg salt 15–19 kg: 1/4 tablet 20–30 kg: 1/2 tablet 31–45 kg: 3/4 tablet >45 kg: 1 tablet orally, once/wk before exposure beginning the week and continuing for 4 wk after exposure	See text for contraindications
or				
	Doxycycline	100 mg daily beginning 1–2 days before exposure and continuing for 4 wk after exposure	2 mg/kg/day up to 100 mg/day	Not to be used in children <8 yr or pregnant women
or				
	Atovaquone-proguanil	250 mg/100 mg (1 tablet) daily beginning 1-2 days before exposure and continuing for 7 days after exposure	11–20 kg: 62.5 mg/25 mg (1 pediatric tablet) 21–30 kg: 125 mg/50 mg (2 pediatric tablets) 31–40 kg: 187.5 mg/75 mg (3 pediatric tablets) >40 kg:1 adult tablet daily	
or				
	Alternatives: Primaquine	30 mg base daily	0.6 mg/kg base daily up to 30 mg daily	Contraindicated in pregnancy, lactation, and glucose-6-phosphate dehydrogenase deficiency Use in consultation with malaria experts
or				
	Chloroquine phosphate	Same as chloroquine-sensitive	Same as chloroquine-sensitive	
plus				
	Pyrimethamine-sulfadoxine for presumptive treatment	Carry a single dose (3 tablets) for self-treatment of febrile illness when medical care is not immediately available	<1 yr: 1/4 tablet 1–3 yr: 1/2 tablet 4–8 yr: 1 tablet 9–14 yr: 2 tablets	Seek medical attention after using this combination for presumptive treatment
or plus				
	Proguanil	200 mg daily	<2 yr: 50 mg daily 2–6 yr: 100 mg 7–10 yr: 150 mg >10 yr: 200 mg	Breakthroughs may occur frequently in areas of intense transmission with this combination

during pregnancy and is not contraindicated in children with G6PD deficiency.

The choice of antimalarial agents in locations where drug-resistant parasites have been identified is more challenging. Chloroquine-containing regimens are not recommended for travel to areas with known chloroquine-resistant *P. falciparum,* and deaths have occurred when these regimens have been used.[53] The choice of regimen depends on the type of drug resistance, length of stay, age of the traveler, and individual medical history. Drugs currently available in the United States include mefloquine (Lariam), doxycycline, and atovaquone-proguanil (Malarone); primaquine and tafenoquine may be available in the future.[29, 37, 84]

Mefloquine

Mefloquine generally is tolerated well in children and can be given to infants. Dosing is based on weight, and no liquid preparation is available. Doses for older children can be supplied by breaking tablets; when small fractions of tablets are needed, pharmacists can provide individual doses in capsules. The medication has a pasty consistency, but it is not bitter tasting. Infants tend to swallow doses better when given liquids or semisolid foods after the medication. Adverse events with mefloquine are self-limited in most cases and include gastrointestinal disturbance, insomnia, and dizziness.[45] Withdrawal rates in adults, presumably caused by the incidence of these adverse events, may impair the efficacy of mefloquine.[13] Rarely, serious adverse events such as psychosis or seizures have occurred after prophylactic doses of mefloquine. Consequently, mefloquine should not be used in those who have seizures or neuropsychiatric disorders or in patients who have had previous adverse events with mefloquine. Mefloquine also is contraindicated in patients with cardiac conduction abnormalities, although it may be used in those concurrently taking beta-blockers for indications other than arrhythmias. The drug must be taken weekly, beginning 1 to 2 weeks before travel and continuing weekly during travel and for 4 weeks after leaving the malarial area. Families may be counseled to choose a day of the week to take the medicine and to take their first dose or doses on that day of the week 1 to 2 weeks before departure. Mefloquine may be used by pregnant women, preferably after the first trimester.[64, 95]

Doxycycline

Doxycycline is an effective antimalarial drug in parts of the world where chloroquine resistance is present. It also has been shown to be effective in areas where mefloquine-resistant *P. falciparum* exists, such as portions of Cambodia, Burma (Myanmar), and Thailand. Limitations in the use of this drug include contraindications in children younger than 8 years, the need for daily dosing, and photosensitivity. In women, daily use of doxycycline may be associated with an increased risk of *Candida* vulvovaginitis. Gastrointestinal side effects, including nausea and vomiting, can be limited by taking the medication with meals and by avoiding bedtime dosing. Doxycycline must not be used by pregnant or lactating women. Prophylaxis with doxycycline needs to begin 1 to 2 days before travel and should be continued daily for 4 weeks after leaving the malarial area.

Atovaquone-Proguanil

Atovaquone-proguanil (Malarone) is the newest drug to be licensed in the United States for malaria prophylaxis. Currently, data about its use in children weighing less than 11 kg (25 lb) are limited. The drug is effective against most *P. falciparum,* including resistant strains. It is available in adult and pediatric dosing forms. The drug is started 1 to 2 days before travel and continued daily during travel and for 7 days after leaving the malarial area. The adverse events most commonly reported with atovaquone-proguanil are abdominal pain, nausea, vomiting, and headache.

Primaquine

Primaquine, used most often to eradicate the exoerythrocytic stages of *P. vivax* and *P. ovale,* shows promise as a prophylactic agent. The drug was put aside with the development of chloroquine but has received renewed attention as drug resistance has increased. It can be used to prevent vivax and falciparum malaria in non–G6PD-deficient individuals, and its efficacy compared favorably with that of mefloquine, doxycycline, and chloroquine plus proguanil in children in the holoendemic area of western Kenya.[20, 83, 97] At this time it is not licensed for this indication in the United States.

Tafenoquine

Tafenoquine is a long-acting primaquine analogue that kills parasites in the liver as well as in blood. It is thought to be more effective and less toxic than primaquine, but it cannot be used by individuals with G6PD deficiency or by pregnant women. No dosing regimen has been established, and it is not licensed for use.[84]

VACCINE

Vaccination against malaria has been a subject of active research for several decades, but a licensed vaccine still is not on the immediate horizon. The development of a vaccine is challenging because of the complexity of the parasite life cycle, heterogeneity of the host immune response, lack of animal models, and absence of surrogate markers of protection. Testing of vaccines is difficult because vaccine efficacy is dependent on conditions of transmission, as well as the degree of immunity present in the population being studied.[93] Targets for development of a vaccine include the sporozoite (prevention of infection), the merozoite (prevention of disease manifestations by preventing invasion of RBCs), or the gametocyte (prevention of transmission by interfering with development of the parasite within the mosquito).

The first malaria vaccines were directed against circumsporozoite antigen, an antigen present over most of the surface of the sporozoite. Development of these vaccines was based on the concept that sporozoites should be susceptible to antibody-mediated destruction in the extracellular space. Unfortunately, the results of studies involving the use of these vaccines have been disappointing, with inadequate protection provided against sporozoite challenge, inconsistent relationships between antibody response and clinical efficacy, and numerous local side effects.[25, 28] Investigators hypothesized that combination vaccines targeting antigens of more than one stage of the parasite might have greater efficacy.

Merozoite surface proteins are another group of antigens that have been studied in connection with the development of a blood-stage, or asexual, malaria vaccine.[68] The SPf66 vaccine, derived from three merozoite proteins linked to a 4-amino acid derived from a *P. falciparum* circumsporozoite protein, has been tested in clinical trials in Colombia, Tanzania, and the Gambia.[1, 14, 94] Although initial studies in countries in South America with low malaria endemicity showed promise, investigations in African countries with high endemicity have been disappointing, with protective efficacy ranging from 31 percent (95% confidence interval [CI], 0 to 52%) in Tanzania to 8 percent (95% CI, -18 to 29%) for first or only clinical episodes and 3% (95% CI, -24 to 24%) in overall incidence of clinical episodes in the Gambia. A study of this vaccine in northwest Thailand also failed to demonstrate efficacy.[61]

Vaccines that block transmission from humans to mosquitoes would reduce the reservoir of infected mosquitoes and thereby reduce transmission on a population level. The poor immunogenicity and diversity of gametocyte antigens have proved challenging to this approach to the development of a vaccine, and no vaccines of this type have been used yet in clinical trials. Future vaccines are likely to use a combination approach that incorporates target antigens from all three stages of the parasite.

Acknowledgments

With gratitude to Dr. Brant Viner for critical reading of the manuscript and helpful comments.

REFERENCES

1. Alonso, P. L., Smith, T., Armstrong Schellenberg, J. R. M., et al.: Randomised trial of efficacy of SPf66 vaccine against *Plasmodium falciparum* malaria in children in southern Tarzania. Lancet *344*: 1175–1181, 1994.
2. Baird, J. K., and Hoffman, S. L.: Prevention of malaria in travelers. Med. Clin. North Am. *83*:923–944, 1999.
3. Barker, R. H., Banchongaksorn, T., Courval, J. M., et al.: A simple method to detect *Plasmodium falciparum* directly from blood samples using the polymerase chain reaction. Am. J. Trop. Med. Hyg. *46*:416–426, 1992.
4. Barker, R. H., Suebsaeng, L., Rooney, W., and Wirth, D. F.: Detection of *Plasmodium falciparum* infection in human patients: A comparison of the DNA probe method to microscopic diagnosis. Am. J. Trop. Med. Hyg. *41*:266–272, 1989.
5. Bates, I., Bedu-Addo, G., Bevan, D. H., and Rutherford, T. R.: Use of immunoglobulin gene arrangements to show clonal lymphoproliferation in hyper-reactive malarial splenomegaly. Lancet *337*:505, 1991.
6. Beadle, C., Long, G. W., and Weiss, W. R.: Diagnosis of malaria by detection of *Plasmodium falciparum* HRP-2 antigen with a rapid dipstick antigen-capture assay. Lancet *343*:564–568, 1994.
7. Binka, F. N., Kubaje, A., Adjuik, M., et al.: Impact of permethrin impregnated bednets on child mortality in Kassena-Nankana district, Ghana: A randomized controlled trial. Trop. Med. Int. Health *1*:147–154, 1996.
8. Bouma, M. J., and Dye, C.: Cycles of malaria associated with El Niño in Venezuela. J. A. M. A. *278*:1772–1774, 1997.
9. Brair, M. E., Brabin, B. J., Milligan, P., et al.: Reduced transfer of tetanus antibodies with placental malaria. Lancet *343*:208–209, 1994.
10. Brewster, D. R., Kwiatkowski, D., and White, N. J.: Neurological sequelae of cerebral malaria in children. Lancet *336*:1039–1043, 1990.
11. Centers for Disease Control and Prevention: Health Information for International Travel, 2001–2002. Atlanta, U.S. Department of Health and Human Services, 2001.
12. Chiodini, P. L.: Non-microscopic methods for diagnosis of malaria. Lancet *351*:80–81, 1998.
13. Croft, A., and Garner, P.: Mefloquine to prevent malaria: A systematic review of trials. B. M. J. *315*:1412–1416, 1998.
14. D'Alessandro, U., Leach, A., Drakeley, C. J., et al.: Efficacy trial of malaria vaccine SPf66 in Gambian infants. Lancet *346*:462–467, 1995.
15. D'Alessandro, U., Olaleye, B. O., McGuire, W., et al.: Mortality and morbidity from malaria in Gambian children after introduction of an impregnated bednet programme. Lancet *345*:479–483, 1995.
16. Dietze, R., Perkins, M., Boulos, M., et al.: The diagnosis of *Plasmodium falciparum* infection using a new antigen detection system. Am. J. Trop. Med. Hyg. *52*:45–49, 1995.
17. Emanuel, B., Aronson, N., and Shulman, S.: Malaria in Children in Chicago. Pediatrics *92*:83–85, 1993.
18. Fischer, P. R.: Travel with infants and children. Infect. Dis. Clin. North Am. *12*:355–368, 1998.
19. Freedman, D. O.: Keeping current: Travel medicine resources available on the Internet. Infect. Dis. Clin. North Am. *12*:543–547, 1998.
20. Fryauff, D. J., Baird, J. K., Basri, H., et al.: Randomised placebo-controlled trial of primaquine for prophylaxis of falciparum and vivax malaria. Lancet *346*:1190–1193, 1995.
21. Garg, P., Mody, P., and Lall, K. B.: Toxic psychosis due to chloroquine—not uncommon in children. Clin. Pediatr. (Phila.) *29*:448–450, 1990.
22. Graves, P. M., Brabin, B. J., Charlwood, J. D., et al.: Reduction in incidence and prevalence of *Plasmodium falciparum* in under-5-year-old children by permethrin impregnation of mosquito nets. Bull. World Health Organ. *65*:869–877, 1987.
23. Hänscheid, T., Pinto, B. G., Pereira, I., et al.: Avoiding misdiagnosis of malaria: A novel automated method allows specific diagnosis, even in the absence of clinical suspicion. Emerg. Infect. Dis. *5*:836–837, 1999.
24. Haworth, F. L. M., and Cook, G. C.: Needlestick malaria. Lancet *346*:1361, 1995.
25. Heppner, D. G., Gordon, D. M., Gross, M., et al.: Safety, immunogenicity, and efficacy of *Plasmodium falciparum* repeatless circumsporozoite protein vaccine encapsulated in liposomes. J. Infect. Dis. *174*:361–366, 1996.
26. Hien, T. T., Day, N. P. J., Phu, N. H., et al.: A controlled trial of artemether or quinine in Vietnamese adults with severe falciparum malaria. N. Engl. J. Med. *335*:76–83, 1996.
27. Hien, T. T., and White, N. J.: Qinghaosu. Lancet *341*:603–608, 1993.
28. Hoffman, S. L., Edelman, R., Bryan, J. P., et al.: Safety, immunogenicity, and efficacy of a malaria sporozoite vaccine administered with monophosphoryl lipid A, cell wall skeleton of mycobacteria, and squalane as adjuvant. Am. J. Trop. Med. Hyg. *51*:603–612, 1994.
29. Høgh, B., Clarke, P. D., Camus, D., et al.: Atovaquone-proguanil versus chloroquine-proguanil for malaria prophylaxis in non-immune travellers: A randomised, double-blind study. Lancet *356*:1888–1894, 2000.
30. Holtz, T. M., Kachur, S. P., MacArthur, J. R., et al.: Malaria surveillance—United States 1998. M. M. W. R. CDC Surveill. Summ. *50*(SS-5):1–20, 2001.
31. Hulbert, T. V.: Congenital malaria in the United States: Report of a case and review. Clin. Infect. Dis. *14*:922–926, 1992.
32. Humar, A., Ohrt, C., Harrington, M. A., et al.: Parasight F test compared with the polymerase chain reaction and microscopy for the diagnosis of *Plasmodium falciparum* malaria in travelers. Am. J. Trop. Med. Hyg. *56*:44–48, 1997.
33. Jelinek, J., Amsler, L., Grobusch, M. P., and Nothdurft, H. D.: Self-use of rapid tests for malaria diagnosis by tourists. Lancet *354*:1609, 1999.
34. Joffe, A., and Jadavji, T.: Congenital malaria: A case report of a preventable disease. Pediatr. Infect. Dis. J. *9*:522–523, 1990.
35. Jones, K. N., Mascia, B., Waggoner-Fountain, L., and Pearson, R. D.: Diagnosis by automated blood analyzer (photo quiz). Clin. Infect. Dis. *33*:1886, 1944–1945, 2001.
36. Kain, K. C., and Keystone, J. S.: Malaria in travelers: Epidemiology, disease, and prevention. Infect. Dis. Clin. North Am. *12*:267–284, 1998.
37. Kain, K. C., Shanks, G. D., and Keystone, J. S.: Malaria chemoprophylaxis in the age of drug resistance. I. Currently recommended drug regimens. Clin. Infect. Dis. *33*:226–234, 2001.
38. Karch, S., Dellile, M.-F., Guillet, P., and Mouchet, J.: African malaria vectors in European aircraft. Lancet *357*:235, 2001.
39. Kitron, U., and Spielman, A.: Suppression of transmission of malaria through source reduction: antianopheline measures applied in Israel, the United States, and Italy. Rev. Infect. Dis. *11*:391–406, 1989.
40. Krogstad, D. J.: Malaria. *In* Guerrant, R. L., Walker, D. H., and Weller, P. F. (eds.): Tropical Infectious Diseases: Principles, Pathogens and Practice. 1st ed. New York, Churchill Livingstone, 1999, pp. 736–766.
41. Krogstad, D. J., Herwaldt, B. L., and Schlesinger, P. H.: Antimalarial agents: Specific treatment regimens. Antimicrob. Agents Chemother. *32*:957–961, 1988.
42. Kwiatkowski, D., Hill, A. V. S., Sambou, I., et al.: TNF concentration in fatal cerebral, non-fatal cerebral, and uncomplicated *Plasmodium falciparum* malaria. Lancet *336*:1201–1204, 1990.
43. Laserson, K. F., Petralanda, I., Hamlin, D. M., et al.: Use of the polymerase chain reaction to directly detect malaria parasites in blood samples from the Venezuelan Amazon. Am. J. Trop. Med. Hyg. *50*:169–180, 1994.
44. Layton, M., Parise, M. E., Campbell, C. C., et al.: Mosquito-transmitted malaria in New York City, 1993. Lancet *346*:729–731, 1995.
45. Lobel, H. O., Miani, M., Eng, T., et al.: Long-term malaria prophylaxis with weekly mefloquine. Lancet *341*:848–851, 1993.
46. Loevinsohn, M. E.: Climatic warming and increased malaria incidence in Rwanda. Lancet *343*:714–718, 1994.
47. Looareesuwan, S., Chulay, J. D., Canfield, C. J., and Hutchinson, D.: Malarone (atovaquone and proguanil hydrochloride): A review of its clinical development for treatment of malaria. Am. J. Trop. Med. Hyg. *60*:533–541, 1999.
48. Looareesuwan, S., Phillips, R. E., White, N. J., et al.: Quinine and severe falciparum malaria in late pregnancy. Lancet *2*:4–7, 1985.
49. Looareesuwan, S., Viravan, C., Vanijanonta, S., et al.: Randomised trial of artesunate and mefloquine alone and in sequence for acute uncomplicated falciparum malaria. Lancet *339*:821–824, 1992.
50. Lynk, A., and Gold, R.: Review of 40 children with imported malaria. Pediatr. Infect. Dis. J. *8*:745–750, 1989.
51. Makler, M. T., and Hinrichs, D. J.: Measurement of the lactate dehydrogenase activity of *Plasmodium falciparum* as an assessment of parasitemia. Am. J. Trop. Med. Hyg. *48*:205–210, 1993.
52. Malakooti, M. A., Biomndo, K., Shanks, G. D.: Reemergence of epidemic malaria in the highlands of western Kenya. Emerg. Infect. Dis. *4*:671–676, 1998.
53. Malaria deaths following inappropriate malaria chemoprophylaxis—United States, 2001. M. M. W. R. Morb. Mortal. Wkly. Rep. *50*(28): 597–599, 2001.
54. Marsh, K., Forster, D., Waruiru, C., et al.: Indicators of life-threatening malaria in African children. N. Engl. J. Med. *332*:1399–1404, 1995.
55. Martens, P., and Hall, L.: Malaria on the move: Human population movement and malaria transmission. Emerg. Infect. Dis. *6*:103–109, 2000.
56. McLaughlin, G. L., Subramanian, S., Lepers, J. P., et al.: Evaluation of a nonisotopic DNA assay kit for diagnosing *Plasmodium falciparum* malaria in Madagascar. Am. J. Trop. Med. Hyg. *48*:211–215, 1993.
57. Menendez, C.: Malaria during pregnancy: A priority area of malaria research and control. Parasitol. Today *11*:178–183, 1995.
58. Mirochnick, M., Barnett, E. D., Clarke, D. F., et al.: Stability of chloroquine in an extemporaneously prepared suspension stored at three temperatures. Pediatr. Infect. Dis. J. *13*:827–828, 1994.
59. Mungai, M., Tegtmeier, G., Chamberland, M., and Parise, M.: Transfusion-transmitted malaria in the United States from 1963 through 1999. N. Engl. J. Med. *344*:1973–1978, 2001.

60. Nagatake, T., Van Thuc, H., Tegoshi, T., et al.: Pathology of falciparum malaria in Vietnam. Am. J. Trop. Med. Hyg. *47*:259–264, 1992.
61. Nosten, F., Luxemburger, C., Kyle, D. E., et al.: Randomised double-blind placebo-controlled trial of SPf66 malaria vaccine in children in northwestern Thailand. Lancet *348*:701, 1996.
62. Nosten, F., McGready, R., Simpson, J. A., et al.: Effects of *Plasmodium vivax* malaria in pregnancy. Lancet *354*:546–549, 1999.
63. Nosten, F., ter Kuile, F. O., Luxemburger, C., et al.: Cardiac effects of antimalarial treatment with halofantrine. Lancet *341*:1054–1056, 1993.
64. Nosten, F., ter Kuile, F., Maelankiri, L., et al.: Mefloquine prophylaxis prevents malaria during pregnancy: A double-blind, placebo-controlled study. J. Infect. Dis. *169*:595–603, 1994.
65. Nosten, F., van Vugt, M., Price, R., et al.: Effects of artesunate-mefloquine combination on incidence of *Plasmodium falciparum* malaria and mefloquine resistance in western Thailand: A prospective study. Lancet *356*:297–302, 2000.
66. Olliaro, P., Nevill, C., LeBras, J., et al.: Systematic review of amodiaquine treatment in uncomplicated malaria. Lancet *348*:1196–1201, 1996.
67. Palmer, C. J., Lindo, J. F., Klaskala, W. I., et al.: Evaluation of the OptiMAL test for the rapid diagnosis of *Plasmodium vivax* and *Plasmodium falciparum* malaria. J. Clin. Microbiol. *36*:203–206, 1998.
68. Pasloske, B. L., and Howard, R. J.: The promise of asexual malaria vaccine development. Am. J. Trop. Med. Hyg. *50*(Suppl.):3–10, 1994.
69. Perrin, L. H., Mackey, L. J., and Miescher, P. A.: The hematology of malaria in man. Semin. Hematol. *19*:70–82, 1982.
70. Phillips, R. E., and Solomon, T.: Cerebral malaria in children. Lancet *336*:1355–1360, 1990.
71. Pongponratn, E., Riganti, M., Punpoowong, B., and Aikawa, M.: Microvascular sequestration of parasitized erythrocytes in human falciparum malaria: A pathological study. Am. J. Trop. Med. Hyg. *44*: 168–175, 1991.
72. Probable locally acquired mosquito-transmitted *Plasmodium vivax* infection—Suffolk County, New York, 1999. M. M. W. R. Morb. Mortal. Wkly. Rep. *49*(22):495–498, 2000.
73. Redd, S. C., Bloland, P. B., Kazembe, P. N., et al.: Usefulness of clinical case-definitions in guiding therapy for African children with malaria or pneumonia. Lancet *340*:1140–1143, 1992.
74. Redd, S. C., Kazembe, P. N., Luby, S. P., et al.: Clinical algorithm for treatment of *Plasmodium falciparum* malaria in children. Lancet *347*:223–227, 1996.
75. Rediscovering wormwood: Qinghaosu for malaria. Lancet *339*:649–651, 1992.
76. Roberts, D. R., Manguin, S., Mouchet, J.: DDT house spraying and re-emerging malaria. Lancet *356*:330–332, 2000.
77. Rosenthal, P. J.: Proteases of malaria parasites: New targets for chemotherapy. Emerg. Infect. Dis. *4*:49–57, 1998.
78. Rougemont, A., Breslow, N., Brenner, E., et al.: Epidemiological basis for clinical diagnosis of childhood malaria in endemic zone in West Africa. Lancet *338*:1292–1295, 1991.
79. Rowland, M., Durrani, N., Kenward, M., et al.: Control of malaria in Pakistan by applying deltamethrin insecticide to cattle: A community-randomised trial. Lancet *357*:1837–1841, 2001.
80. Ryan, E. T., and Kain, K. C.: Health advice and immunizations for travelers. N. Engl. J. Med. *342*:1716–1725, 2000.
81. Schlagenhauf, P., and Phillips-Howard, P. A.: Malaria: Emergency self-treatment by travelers. *In* Dupont, H. L., and Steffen, R. (eds.): Textbook of Travel Medicine and Health. 2nd ed. Hamilton, Ontario, B. C. Decker, 2001, pp. 205–213.
82. Schuman, A. J.: Preparing children and families to travel overseas. Contemp. Pediatr. *18*:45–59, 2001.
83. Schwartz, E., and Regev-Yochay, G.: Primaquine as prophylaxis for malaria for nonimmune travelers: A comparison with mefloquine and doxycycline. Clin. Infect. Dis. *29*:1502–1506, 1999.
84. Shanks, G. D., Kain, K. C., and Keystone, J. S.: Malaria chemoprophylaxis in the age of drug resistance. II. Drugs that may be available in the future. Clin. Infect. Dis. *33*:381–385, 2001.
85. Shulman, C. E., Dorman, E. K., Cutts, F., et al.: Intermittent sulphadoxine-pyrimethamine to prevent severe anaemia secondary to malaria in pregnancy: A randomised placebo-controlled trial. Lancet *353*:632–636, 1999.
86. Slutsker, L. M., Khoromana, C. O., Payne, D., et al.: Mefloquine therapy for *Plasmodium falciparum* malaria in children under 5 years of age in Malawi: In vivo/in vitro efficacy and correlation of drug concentration with parasitological outcome. Bull. World Health Organ. *68*:53–59, 1990.
87. Snow, R. W., Lindsay, S. W., Hayes, R. J., and Greenwood, B. M.: Permethrin-treated bed nets (mosquito nets) prevent malaria in Gambian children. Trans. R. Soc. Trop. Med. Hyg. *82*:838–842, 1988.
88. Spielman, A., Perrone, J. B., Teklehaimanot, A., et al.: Malaria diagnosis by direct observation of centrifuged samples of blood. Am. J. Trop. Med. Hyg. *39*:337–342, 1988.
88a. Spira, A. M.: Preparing the traveller. Lancet *361*:1368–1381, 2003.
89. Sudden death in a traveler following halofantrine administration—Togo, 2000. M. M. W. R. Morb. Mortal. Wkly. Rep. *50*(9):169–179, 2001.
90. Taylor, T. E., Molyneux, M. E., Wirima, J. J., et al.: Blood glucose levels in Malawian children before and during the administration of intravenous quinine for severe falciparum malaria. N. Engl. J. Med. *319*:1040–1047, 1988.
91. Taylor, T. E., and Strickland, G. T.: Malaria. *In* Strickland, G. T. (ed.): Hunter's Tropical Medicine and Emerging Infectious Diseases. 8th ed. Philadelphia, W. B. Saunders, 2000, pp. 614–643.
92. ter Kuile, F. O., Dolan, G., Nosten, F., et al.: Halofantrine versus mefloquine in treatment of multidrug-resistant falciparum malaria. Lancet *341*:1044–1049, 1993.
93. Towards a malarial vaccine. Lancet *339*:586–587, 1992.
94. Valero, M. V., Amador, L. R., Galindo, C., et al.: Vaccination with SPf66, a chemically synthesised vaccine, against *Plasmodium falciparum* malaria in Colombia. Lancet *341*:705–710, 1993.
95. Vanhauwere, B., Maradit, H., and Kerr, L.: Post-marketing surveillance of prophylactic mefloquine (Lariam) use in pregnancy. Am. J. Trop. Med. Hyg. *58*:17–21, 1998.
96. van Hensbroek, M. B., Onyiorah, E., Jaffar, S., et al.: A trial of artemether or quinine in children with cerebral malaria. N. Engl. J. Med. *335*:69–75, 1996.
97. Weiss, W. R., Oloo, A. J., Johnson, A., et al.: Daily primaquine is effective for prophylaxis against falciparum malaria in Kenya: Comparison with mefloquine, doxycycline, and chloroquine plus proguanil. J. Infect. Dis. *171*:1569–1575, 1995.
97a. White, N. J.: Malaria. *In* Cook, G. C., and Zumla, A. (eds.): Manson's Tropical Diseases. 21st ed. London, W. B. Saunders, 2003, pp. 1205–1295.
98. White, N. J.: The treatment of malaria. N. Engl. J. Med. *335*:800–806, 1996.
99. White, N. J., Miller, K. D., Churchill, F. C., et al.: Chloroquine treatment of severe malaria in children. N. Engl. J. Med. *319*:1493–1500, 1988.
100. White, N. J., Waller, D., Crawley, J., et al.: Comparison of artemether and chloroquine for severe malaria in Gambian children. Lancet *339*:317–321, 1992.
101. Williams, H. A., Roberts, J., Kachur, S. P., et al.: Malaria surveillance—United States, 1995. M. M. W. R. CDC Surveill. Summ. *48*(SS-1):1–23, 1998.
102. Wyler, D. J.: Malaria—resurgence, resistance, and research (first of two parts). N. Engl. J. Med. *308*:875–878, 1983.
103. Wyler, D. J.: Bark, weeds, and iron chelators—drugs for malaria. N. Engl. J. Med. *327*:1519–1521, 1992.
104. Wyler, D. J.: Malaria chemoprophylaxis for the traveler. N. Engl. J. Med. *329*:31–37, 1993.
105. Zingman, B. S., Viner, B. L.: Splenic complications in malaria: Case report and review. Clin. Infect. Dis. *16*:223–232, 1993.

CHAPTER 219 Leishmaniasis

MURRAY WITTNER ■ HERBERT B. TANOWITZ

Leishmaniasis consists of a diverse group of diseases that may affect the viscera, skin, or mucous membranes (or any combination of these sites) with a wide spectrum of clinical activity caused by obligate intracellular hemoflagellates of the genus *Leishmania.* Infection is transmitted by several genera and species of phlebotomine sandflies. Three major clinical syndromes usually are recognized: visceral (VL), cutaneous (CL), and mucocutaneous (MCL) leishmaniasis. In each type of disease, macrophages are parasitized.

The clinical manifestations of leishmaniasis appear to depend on a complex set of factors, including tropism and virulence of the parasite strain, as well as the susceptibility of the host, which may be determined genetically. Cell-mediated immune mechanisms appear to be the major factors in modulating these diseases (Table 219–1).

Each species of *Leishmania* has well-recognized clinical variants that seem to cause similar disease patterns in the same host species. Thus, in the case of VL (kala-azar), *Leishmania donovani, Leishmania chagasi,* and *Leishmania infantum* invade cells of the reticuloendothelium of viscera, usually causing splenomegaly and occasionally hepatomegaly and pancytopenia; untreated, the disease is progressive and generally fatal. In cutaneous disease, *Leishmania tropica* (with some notable exceptions), *Leishmania major, Leishmania aethiopica,* and *Leishmania mexicana* usually are restricted to reticuloendothelial cells of the skin, and infections generally are self-limited, with spontaneous healing. Similarly, *Leishmania braziliensis* invades the reticuloendothelial cells of the skin, although it may metastasize to the mucous membranes of the nose, mouth, and pharynx and result in serious disfigurement, if not death. Recent observations have shown that some strains of *L. tropica* may cause viscerotropic disease. Individuals with acquired immunodeficiency syndrome (AIDS) may have atypical manifestations.

It has been shown recently that the amount of a vasodilatory peptide, maxadilan, in sandfly saliva is a correlated with type of human infection. Thus, sandflies in Brazil that transmit *L. chagasi* VL have relatively large amounts of maxadilan, in their saliva, which causes marked vasodilation and may encourage visceralization of the parasites. The same complex of sandflies in Costa Rica, which have relatively small amounts of the vasodilatory peptide in their saliva, transmit a nonulcerating and nonvisceralizing *L. chagasi* infection that is constrained to the dermis. These studies appear to suggest that substances in sandfly saliva influence, at least in part, the tropism of the parasite and therefore the resulting disease.

The Organism

In vertebrate hosts, the various species of *Leishmania* are obligate intracellular parasites that exist only in the amastigote stage. The species that infect humans are usually morphologically indistinguishable from one another at both the light microscopic and ultrastructural levels. The organisms are round to oval bodies approximately 2 to 4 μm in diameter and possess a single nucleus and a specialized mitochondrial structure that has extranuclear DNA termed a *kinetoplast;* they lack a free flagellum. Amastigotes are engulfed by macrophages and reside within the parasitophorous vacuole of the macrophage host. In this environment, they multiply by binary fission and eventually destroy the host cell. Subsequently, they are phagocytized, and the process occurs repeatedly. No evidence indicates that *Leishmania* spp. actively penetrate host cells, as has been reported for *Trypanosoma cruzi.*

When the vector, a female sandfly, feeds on an infected person, it may ingest an infected cell from blood or tissue. Amastigotes are liberated in the fly's midgut, and within a few hours, transformation to the promastigote stage occurs. Promastigotes are elongated flagellates 15 to 25 μm long by 1.5 to 3.5 μm wide, each with an anterior, free flagellum that measures approximately 15 to 28 μm in length and may vary morphologically from a short and stumpy to an elongated form. Binary fission then begins, and large numbers of promastigotes are produced and gradually move forward to the pharynx, buccal cavity, and mouth parts. At 8 to 20 days, depending on temperature and the species of sandfly, the mouth parts of the fly may be blocked partially or completely by huge numbers of promastigotes. These organisms may be dislodged into the bite wound when the female sandfly *(Phlebotomus, Lutzomyia)* next takes a blood meal. Promastigotes have surface molecules that bind to several macrophage receptors. The phagocytized promastigote forms transform into amastigotes within the parasitophorous vacuole, and multiplication takes place.

Transmission is believed to also occur by contamination of the bite wound. Once they have been inoculated, many of the promastigotes do not survive because mammalian tissue fluids contain cytolytic substances. Organisms that are phagocytized transform to amastigotes and initiate replication. The organisms can be seen readily in tissues or smears by light microscopy, especially with Giemsa or Wright stain, with which the nucleus and kinetoplast stain bright red and the cytoplasm stains pale blue. In Novy-McNeal-Nicolle (NNN) culture medium at 24° C, the organisms grow readily and assume the promastigote or insect form.

At present, the taxonomic status of *Leishmania* remains unclear. Both specific and subspecific designations generally have been determined by the clinical syndrome caused by an isolate in a particular geographic area. However, these characteristics are imprecise and unreliable. Recently, various molecular biological techniques have been used to characterize the strains and species of clinical isolates: endonuclease restriction studies of kinetoplast DNA (K-DNA), buoyant density of K-DNA and mitochondrial DNA (M-DNA) on cesium chloride, leishmanial isozyme patterns, monoclonal antibody specificity, and exoantigen secretory factor 4 serotyping.

Epidemiology

The precise incidence of leishmaniasis is not known. However, the World Health Organization has estimated that 350

TABLE 219–1 ■ CLINICAL SYNDROMES CAUSED BY *LEISHMANIA* SPECIES AND THEIR GEOGRAPHIC DISTRIBUTION

Clinical Syndromes	*Leishmania* Species	Location
Visceral leishmaniasis		
Kala-azar: generalized involvement of the reticuloendothelial system (spleen, bone marrow, liver)	*L. (L.) donovani*	Indian subcontinent, northern and eastern China, Pakistan, Nepal
	L. (L.) infantum	Middle East, Mediterranean littoral, Balkans, central and southwestern Asia, northern and northwestern China, northern and sub-Saharan Africa
	L. (L.) donovani (archibaldi)	Sudan, Kenya, Ethiopia
	L. (L.) spp.	Kenya, Ethiopia, Somalia
	L. (L.) chagasi	Latin America
	L. (L.) amazonensis	Brazil (Bahia State)
	L. (L.) tropica	Israel, India, and viscerotropic disease in Saudi Arabia (U.S. troops)
Post-kala-azar dermal leishmaniasis	*L. (L.) donovani*	Indian subcontinent, East Africa
	L. (L.) spp.	Kenya, Ethiopia, Somalia
Old World cutaneous leishmaniasis		
Single or limited number of skin lesions	*L. (L.) major*	Middle East, northwestern China, northwestern India, Pakistan, Africa
	L. (L.) tropica	Mediterranean littoral, Middle East, western Asiatic area, Indian subcontinent
	L. (L.) aethiopica	Ethiopian highlands, Kenya, Yemen
	L. (L.) infantum	Mediterranean basin
	L. (L.) donovani (archibaldi)	Sudan and East Africa
	L. (L.) spp.	Kenya, Ethiopia, Somalia
Diffuse cutaneous leishmaniasis	*L. (L.) aethiopica*	Ethiopian highlands, Kenya, Yemen
New World cutaneous leishmaniasis		
Single or limited number of skin lesions	*L. (L.) mexicana* (chiclero ulcer)	Central America, Mexico, Texas
	L. (L.) amazonensis	Amazon basin and neighboring areas, Bahia and other states in Brazil
	L. (V.) braziliensis	Multiple areas of Central and South America
	L. (V.) guyanensis (forest yaws)	Guyana, Suriname, northern Amazon basin
	L. (V.) peruviana (uta)	Peru (western Andes) and Argentinean highlands
	L. (V.) panamensis	Panama, Costa Rica, Colombia
	L. (V.) pifanoi	Venezuela
	L. (V.) garnhami	Venezuela
	L. (V.) venezuelensis	Venezuela
	L. (V.) colombiensis	Colombia and Panama
	L. (L.) chagasi	Central and South America
Diffuse cutaneous leishmaniasis	*L. (L.) amazonensis*	Amazon basin and neighboring areas, Bahia and other states in Brazil
	L. (V.) pifanoi	Venezuela
	L. (L.) mexicana	Mexico and Central America
	L. (L.) spp.	Dominican Republic
Mucosal leishmaniasis	*L. (V.) braziliensis* (espundia)	Multiple areas in Latin America

(L.) subgenus *Leishmania*; (V.) subgenus *Viannia*.
Data from Laison, R., and Shaw, J.J.: Evolution, classification and geographic distribution. *In* Peters, W., Killick-Kendrick, R. (eds.): The Leishmaniases in Biology and Medicine. London, Academic Press, 1987, pp. 1–120; modified from Pearson, R. D., and Sousa, A. Q.: Clinical spectrum of leishmaniasis. Clin. Infect. Dis. *22*:1–13, 1996; from Pearson, R. D., Jeronimo, S. M. B., and de Queiroz, A.: Leishmaniasis. *In* Guerrant, R. L., Walker, D. H., and Weller, P. F. (eds.): Tropical Infectious Diseases: Principles, Pathogens and Practice. Philadelphia, Churchill Livingstone, 1999.

million individuals are at risk and that the disease is endemic in more than 80 countries. The estimated incidence of VL is 500,000 cases annually, and for CL and MCL, it is 1.5 million cases per year. Although the parasite usually is transmitted via the bite of the sandfly vector, it may be transmitted also as a result of a laboratory accident, direct person-to-person transmission, and blood transfusion. In addition, evidence indicates that it may be transmitted either in utero or during the peripartum period.

Visceral Leishmaniasis

VL is caused by various organisms in the *L. donovani* spp. complex, although recently, strains of *L. tropica* from the Middle East and *L. amazonensis* from Latin America have been found to cause this syndrome.

VL, or kala-azar, is found in a broad belt that extends from the Strait of Gibraltar across the Mediterranean through Asia to the east coast of China, at a latitude between 30 and 48 degrees north. It is transmitted by various species of sandfly, although occasionally, congenital and blood-borne infections also occur. VL has been reported from 47 countries, but the Sudan and India account for more than half the cases. In the Western Hemisphere, it is found in Brazil, northern Argentina, Paraguay, Venezuela, Colombia, Guatemala, and Mexico. Kala-azar appears to exist in at least three epidemiologic forms:

1. A Mediterranean type of VL, with a canine reservoir, in which young children (1 to 4 years of age) are infected and dogs, foxes, or feral animals are the reservoirs *(L. infantum)*. This type extends from the Mediterranean littoral through central Asia into China; it is also present in parts of South

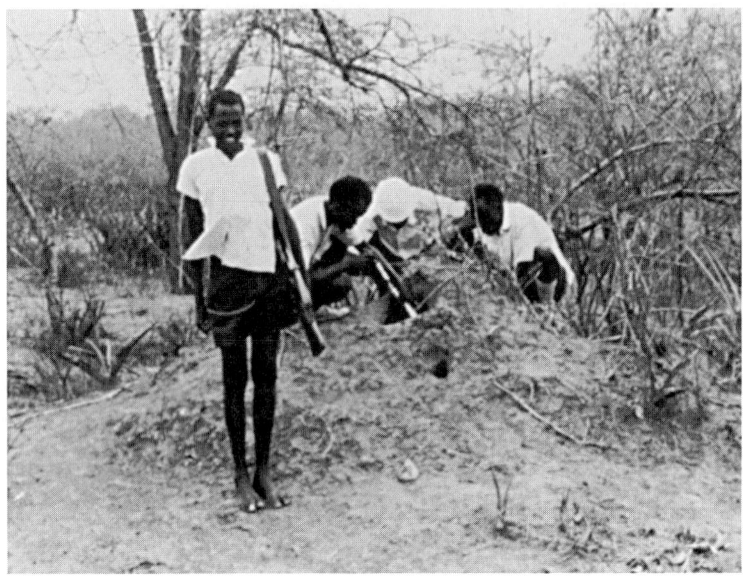

FIGURE 219–1 ■ Sandfly collecting by a medical team in East Africa. The flies are collected by sucking out the termite hill. (Courtesy of Dr. Leonard Marcus, Boston.)

America *(L. chagasi),* where foxes and dogs are reservoir hosts. In Brazil, young males most often are infected.

2. An Indian type *(L. donovani)* of VL, with a human reservoir, in which the disease predominates in Indian children between 5 and 15 years of age; humans are the only known reservoir. Though sought, evidence of natural infection in dogs has not been found. No evidence of rodent reservoirs exists.

3. An African type of VL in which rodents are the reservoir hosts. The Nile rat in the Sudan and probably the gerbil in Kenya are the reservoirs. In Kenya, researchers have noted that kala-azar often is related to old or eroded termite mounds where young males often congregate (Fig. 219–1).

PATHOLOGY

The principal pathologic lesions are the result of reticuloendothelial cell hyperplasia, especially in the spleen and liver. Later, the bone marrow and lymph nodes are filled with infected macrophages, and a concomitant leukopenia and anemia develop (i.e., pancytopenia). Similarly, the kidneys may be filled with infected macrophages, and invasion of the submucosa and mucosa of the digestive tract, especially in the duodenum and jejunum, results in hypertrophic congested and edematous villi. Small ulcerations and hemorrhages may occur. The spleen gradually enlarges, sometimes assuming enormous proportions, and eventually extends into the pelvis. Splenic infarcts are a frequent development. The capsule is thickened, and more deeply, the sinuses are dilated. Erythrophagocytosis by histiocytes is seen commonly, and the anemia so typical of kala-azar may in part be the result of such sequestration of red cells. Kupffer cells of the liver, filled with amastigotes, are swollen and hyperplastic, and centrilobular necrosis or fatty infiltration of the hepatic parenchyma often is observed. In late-stage or chronic disease, increased hepatic fibrosis may give a nodular cirrhotic appearance. Lymphadenopathy, especially of the mesenteric glands, is an early finding, and large numbers of parasite-filled macrophages are present. The bone marrow often is filled with parasitized histiocytes that replace the normal marrow elements; such replacement results in myelophthisic anemia.

The immunologic response to kala-azar infection is imperfectly understood. At the bite wound, a small, pea-sized, dermal lesion may form (i.e., a leishmanioma); the parasites, initially localized in dermal macrophages, disseminate within the macrophages to the spleen, liver, bone marrow, and lymph nodes.

The outcome of an infection seems to depend on the host's ability to raise a suitable cell-mediated immune response and the virulence of the invading organism. Experimentally, resistance in mice appears to be determined by a single autosomal gene. Researchers have shown in experimental infections that the disease is controlled by the T_H1 subset of $CD4^+$ and $CD8^+$ T cells; these cells are related to the production of cytokines such as interferon-γ (IFN-γ), interleukin-2, and tumor necrosis factor–α. Cytokines activate macrophages to kill intracellular amastigotes by oxidative and nonoxidative mechanisms. Studies in mice indicate that nitric oxide is an important factor in killing amastigotes. If the infection is not eliminated or controlled by the host's cellular immune response, it then becomes clinically evident. Lymphocytogenesis and histiocytogenesis occur in affected organs, with resultant hepatosplenomegaly and lymphadenopathy. Polyclonal B-cell activation ensues and causes hyperglobulinemia. This outpouring of humoral antibodies, chiefly IgG and largely nonspecific, is not protective and may represent more than half the total serum proteins of the patient. The specific antibodies produced during active disease have diagnostic significance. Fluorescent antibody, enzyme-linked immunosorbent assay (ELISA), indirect hemagglutination, and complement-fixation tests are reasonably reliable diagnostic procedures.

Resistance to kala-azar is essentially absent once the infection has become evident clinically. However, after chemotherapeutic cure, acquired immunity emerges; delayed hypersensitivity, as demonstrated by the Montenegro (leishmanin) skin test (see later), also becomes apparent. Moreover, the hypergammaglobulinemia abates concomitant with chemical cure and the appearance of delayed hypersensitivity. Usually, immunity to VL is complete and long lasting after chemotherapeutic cure. However, relapse, as seen in post–kala-azar dermal leishmaniasis (see later), is characterized by delayed hypersensitivity, dermal localization of parasites, and moderate hypergammaglobulinemia. Of interest is that although macrophage activation results in enhanced phagocytosis of parasites, macrophages remain unable to eliminate parasites. The appearance of dermal delayed hypersensitivity at the time that acquired immunity appears suggests that cell-mediated immunity plays an important role in protection. Further work on this aspect of VL is needed. The genetics of resistance in humans remains unclear.

CLINICAL MANIFESTATIONS

The incubation period varies widely from 6 weeks to 6 months but has been reported to be as short as 10 to 14 days and as long as 10 years. A primary skin nodule infrequently is seen, although in African leishmaniasis, it is a more regular feature. Infantile VL may begin either suddenly with high fever and vomiting or insidiously with irregular daily fever, anorexia, weight loss, lassitude, and pallor. When fever is present, double daily spikes are a characteristic sign, with temperatures reaching 40 to 40.6°C. The spleen gradually enlarges so that by the end of the first month, it usually can be palpated readily. If the symptoms continue unabated, the spleen may extend to the umbilicus or even into the pelvis. Diarrhea or frank dysentery is not unusual, and blood sometimes is observed. A general bleeding diathesis often becomes evident shortly before death. After several months, if the disease is untreated, patients usually die. Acute fulminant disease is seen more often in infants and young children.

In less fulminating cases, the clinical course is more protracted and generally ends fatally after a year or two. In older age groups, the disease tends to assume a more chronic course, with marked emaciation, brittle hair, massive splenomegaly, lymphadenopathy, and a dusky slate-gray complexion. Hyperglobulinemia, leukopenia, and anemia typically are found. As a result of general debility, death often results from intercurrent infections such as pneumonia, amebic or bacillary dysentery, malaria, or cancrum oris in more than 90 percent of cases. Infantile VL has been associated with alterations in lipoprotein metabolism. A handful of cases of presumed congenital VL have been reported. These infants were born of infected mothers, and in some, evidence of parasitism of the placenta was found. However, whether these cases represent congenital infection or peripartum infection is unclear because sophisticated serologic techniques were not available.

Cutaneous manifestations of kala-azar are encountered frequently. In India, the dark gray appearance of the skin is known as kala-azar (black sickness). In some cases of inadequately treated VL, a skin condition termed post–kala-azar dermal leishmaniasis may ensue if all parasites are not eradicated. In Indian VL, this complication is encountered in 15 to 20 percent of cases and appears several years after therapy. In African disease, it occurs much less commonly, often during therapy in approximately 2 to 3 percent of cases, and it heals spontaneously in a few months. The lesions are characterized by the appearance of hypopigmented, erythematous, or nodular lesions on the skin of the face, chest, neck, and buttocks. At times, the nodular lesions of the face may resemble lepromatous leprosy. The lesions are thought to represent a modified form of *L. (L.) donovani* infection in which the parasites no longer invade the viscera and are localized to the skin. These lesions seem to be related to the host's immune response. This change to dermal tropism is said to coincide with recovery from visceral disease and to disappear with relapse. Infection with *L.(L.). chagasi* causes VL in young children. Recently, atypical CL has been reported in older children with this infection.

Pancytopenia is not unusual. Characteristically, anemia is always evident, with hemoglobin levels below 8 g/dL. Survival of red cells is shortened as a result of several possible factors, including Coombs-positive hemolytic anemia and hypersplenism. Leukopenia of 2000 to 3000 cells/mm^3 typically is found with neutropenia, relative lymphocytosis, an almost total absence of eosinophils, and thrombocytopenia. Serum albumin is usually less than 3 g/dL, and globulin levels (mostly IgG) are often greater than 5 g/dL (5 to 10 g/dL).

Recently, kala-azar has been reported as an important opportunistic infection in patients infected with human immunodeficiency virus type 1 (HIV-1) and not known to have contracted *Leishmania* infection previously. These patients appear to have a more severe and fulminant form of kala-azar. In this regard, inapparent *Leishmania* infection may become evident after immunosuppression, such as chemotherapy for malignant disease. The diagnosis may be particularly difficult to make inasmuch as the findings are often atypical and consist of low-grade fever, fatigue, cough, and gastrointestinal complaints. Similarly, atypical visceral disease caused by *L. tropica* was seen in individuals who participated in Operation Desert Storm in the Persian Gulf.

DIAGNOSIS

VL is diagnosed by finding the organism in stained smears of spleen aspirate, peripheral blood, or bone marrow. In Indian kala-azar, the parasites may be found regularly in peripheral blood monocytes (i.e., buffy coat), but in the African and Mediterranean forms, they may be difficult to find by this technique. Blood and marrow cultures grown on NNN medium or in Schneider insect medium with 15 to 20 percent fetal calf serum are most useful. Some investigators regard splenic rather than bone marrow aspiration as the most sensitive procedure, although it can be especially hazardous in individuals with a bleeding diathesis. Contraindications include a soft or diffluent, acutely enlarging spleen. Patients with low platelet counts or a prolonged prothrombin time (or both) should not undergo the needle biopsy procedure. In children younger than 5 years, splenic aspiration should be performed only by a physician fully experienced in the procedure.

Spleen and bone marrow aspirates should be placed in culture medium and smeared on slides, and saline-diluted aspirates should be inoculated into the peritoneal cavity of hamsters (Fig. 219–2).

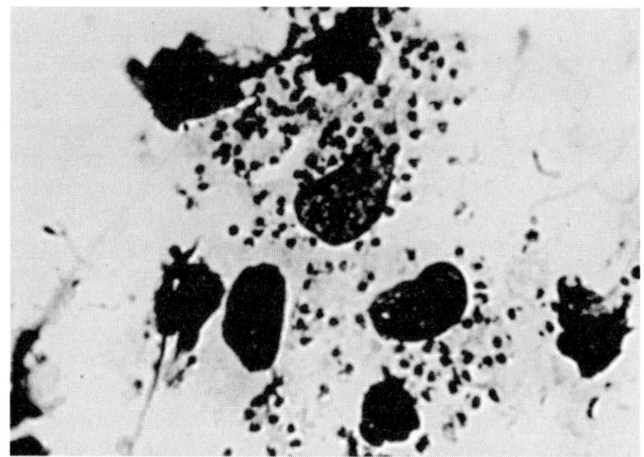

FIGURE 219–2 ■ *Leishmania donovani* in a liver touch preparation (original magnification × 288).

Nonspecific tests reflecting the markedly elevated serum globulins, such as the formol gel and Sia water tests, are helpful in acute disease and are performed readily in the field. Antileishmanial antibodies are usually present and can be used to aid in the diagnosis. The fluorescent antibody test is highly specific, as are the indirect hemagglutination and gel diffusion tests. The complement-fixation test, however, is positive in only 65 to 70 percent of cases. Sera from patients with VL are known to give false-positive results when antibodies to *T. cruzi* are present; consequently, in the Western Hemisphere, absorbing out these antibodies may be necessary. Of importance is to recognize that fluorescent antibody titers usually fall after complete cure, so a negative titer often is regarded as a sign of successful therapy. DNA-DNA hybridization tests are being evaluated and promise exquisite specificity and sensitivity for the diagnosis of leishmaniasis. Serologic tests may be positive as a result of past or subclinical inapparent infection. An ELISA that detects antibodies to a cloned recombinant antigen, K39, of *L. chagasi* has been shown to be specific in active VL and could detect antibodies in AIDS patients. A recent study has demonstrated that this test could be applied to field situations.

The usual diagnostic tests may be negative in patients with HIV or *L. tropica* infection or in otherwise profoundly immunocompromised patients. Recently, however, two genomic fragments encoding portions of a single 210-kd *L. tropica* protein have proved useful for the diagnosis of viscerotropic *L. tropica* infection in Desert Storm patients.

The leishmanin or Montenegro skin test, like the lepromin and tuberculin skin tests, is a measure of delayed hypersensitivity to leishmanial antigen. It consists of 10^6 phenol-killed, culture-grown promastigotes in 1 mL of 0.5 percent phenol in saline. The test is performed like the tuberculin test, that is, 0.1 mL is injected intradermally. A positive result is a palpable area of induration at least 5 mm in diameter in 48 to 72 hours. Because the leishmanin test can be positive in CL or VL, the results must be evaluated carefully. In VL, the test remains negative throughout the period of active disease. Once chemotherapeutic control starts to take effect and immunocompetent lymphocytes are able to respond, the test begins to turn positive. Thus, recovery from kala-azar is characterized by the development of cell-mediated immunity. The change from a negative to a positive leishmanin test in VL is regarded as an important prognostic sign that protective immunity is developing or has developed. Because numerous reports noting positive leishmanin tests in individuals who have had no history of VL have appeared recently, researchers have postulated that many individuals in an endemic area may become immune by previous inapparent infection.

PROGNOSIS

Untreated VL is fatal in 75 to 85 percent of infantile and 90 percent of adult cases. Properly treated at an early stage, it can be cured in 85 to 95 percent of cases. The prognosis for patients in whom pancytopenia or bleeding diatheses develop or in whom a delayed hypersensitivity skin reaction fails to develop usually is poor.

TREATMENT

VL generally responds to treatment with pentavalent antimonials such as stibogluconate sodium (Pentostam, Triostam), which is the usual drug of choice in the United States and is available through the Drug Service of the Centers for Disease Control and Prevention. Meglumine antimoniate (Glucantime) is available in French-speaking countries and Latin America. The pediatric and adult dose is 20 mg/kg daily administered intramuscularly or intravenously for 28 days. Treatment can be repeated. In areas where leishmanial parasites may have acquired relative resistance to pentavalent antimonials, such as India and East Africa, extending therapy for more than 4 weeks may be necessary. Side effects occur commonly and include nausea, vomiting, headache, anorexia, and abdominal pain. Elevated levels of serum amylase and lipase, indicative of pancreatitis, are encountered occasionally and can be severe. Electrocardiographic changes, including decreased T wave amplitude and T wave inversion, prolongation of the QTc, and nonspecific ST-T wave changes, are seen. They resolve shortly after therapy is concluded. (Treatment should be discontinued if the QTc interval exceeds 0.5 second.) Deaths, presumably caused by arrhythmias, have been reported in patients who were receiving more than 20 mg/kg/day. Primary antimony resistance, as well as relapses after receiving pentavalent antimony therapy, occurs with all types of VL but is most often encountered with the Indian form. In HIV-infected patients, almost 25 percent fail to respond to antimony therapy, and almost 40 percent of responders subsequently relapse.

Liposomal amphotericin B (AmBisome) has been approved by the Food and Drug Administration for the treatment of VL. This compound is taken up by cells of the reticuloendothelial system, where amastigotes reside, and is less nephrotoxic, thereby allowing for higher daily doses with shorter courses of therapy. The approved, recommended regimen for immunocompetent VL patients is 3 mg/kg/day on days 1 through 5 and days 14 and 21. In immunosuppressed and HIV patients, treatment of VL with AmBisome has resulted in an almost 100 percent response rate. However, most of these patients relapse. The recommended treatment is 4 mg/kg/day on days 1 through 5, 10, 17, 24, 31, and 38. Without maintenance therapy, almost all these patients relapse. Because resistance to pentavalent antimonials has developed in Bihar (India), amphotericin B is used and is highly efficacious. Several recent studies have used liposomal amphotericin B successfully for the treatment of VL presumably caused by *L. infantum* in immunocompetent children.

Parenteral pentamidine isethionate (Pentam 300) is administered intramuscularly (4 mg/kg is given three times weekly for up to 15 doses, depending on side effects such as hypotension, vomiting, and blood dyscrasias). Pentamidine occasionally may exacerbate diabetes mellitus or precipitate latent diabetes. Shock and liver and renal damage have been reported.

In several recent clinical trials, miltefosine, an oral alkyl phospholipid agent initially developed as an oral antineoplastic drug, has been used as an effective agent for the treatment of antimony-resistant Indian VL. The treatment dose was 2.5 mg/kg/day for 4 weeks.

Patients may require hospitalization for therapy; supportive and corrective measures should be instituted in the event that other infections are present. An occasional patient may be encountered who may require splenectomy to relieve the profound hypersplenism and the resulting anemia. Response to therapy often can be assessed by return of the patient's temperature to normal, a brisk reticulocytosis, a gradual reduction in spleen size, and the reappearance of eosinophils on the peripheral blood smear.

Recently, allopurinol has been used with pentavalent antimonials to treat cases of VL that did not respond to pentavalent antimonials alone. Several reports suggest that recombinant IFN-γ is helpful, along with pentavalent antimonial drugs, in successfully treating this disease. Because assessing whether a cure has been achieved is difficult, patients must be monitored at 6-month intervals for as long as 2 years. Fluorescent antibody titers should be absent by the end of 1 year and complement-fixation titers by 6 to 8 months. If post–kala-azar dermal leishmaniasis occurs, treatment should be reinstituted.

PREVENTION

Control of VL has many aspects. Sandflies *(Phlebotomus* and *Lutzomyia)* can be eliminated readily by residual spraying. Because sandflies ordinarily do not fly very high, sleeping quarters should be above ground level. Permethrin-impregnated bed nets can be highly effective in preventing sandfly bites. Animal reservoirs, such as infected dogs and rodents, should be destroyed. Early therapy will prevent family and neighborhood transmission.

Old World Cutaneous Leishmaniasis

DEFINITION AND EPIDEMIOLOGY

Old World CL is caused by *L. major* (rural), *L. tropica* (urban), and *L. aethiopica*. It is found throughout the Middle East, along the Mediterranean basin and islands, and in East and West Africa, India, and southwestern Asia. In humans, infection by *L. tropica* usually produces self-limited skin ulcers in which intracellular (amastigote) parasites can be found situated in macrophages in and about the lesions. These protozoan hemoflagellates almost never visceralize in humans. However, several recent reports have described *L. tropica* isolates from patients with VL (see the section on VL). In many areas, dogs or rodents are found to be naturally infected and are thought to be the natural reservoirs of infection. As with VL, various *Phlebotomus* spp. of sandfly transmit the infection, although person-to-person transmission is possible and is the basis of the long-time practice in middle and central Asia of immunizing inoculation, that is, "vaccination" to prevent possible disfigurement by a natural infection (Fig. 219–3).

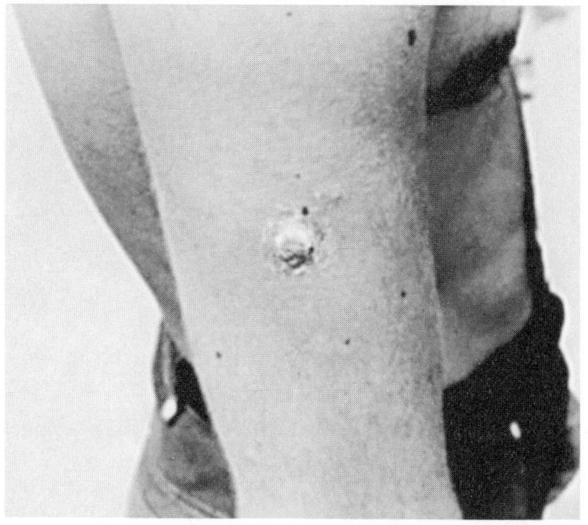

FIGURE 219–3 ■ *Leishmania tropica.* Immunization by an induced lesion. (From a nonprofit cooperative endeavor by numerous colleagues under the editorship of Dr. Herman Zaiman, New York.)

Old World leishmaniasis, or Oriental sore (Delhi boil, Aleppo button), often is classified into "wet" and "dry" types. The wet or rural form is caused by *L. major* and is found chiefly in various rodents on the edge of deserts. The dry or urban type is anthroponotic predominantly, caused by *L. tropica,* and transmitted by phlebotomine species that frequently feed on humans and dogs. The dry or urban form of Oriental sore is characterized by a long incubation period, long duration of active infection, and large numbers of parasites in the dermis. In contrast, the moist or rural type has a relatively short incubation period, with rapid healing and few parasites in the skin. *L. aethiopica* is restricted to the mountain valleys of the Rift Valley of Ethiopia and Kenya, where rock and tree hyraxes are infected regularly. Humans become infected when they intrude in these areas. This form of CL is usually self-limited, although in a small number of individuals (1/100,000), nonhealing diffuse cutaneous (DCL) disease has been reported.

PATHOLOGY

At the site of the bite wound, promastigotes are engulfed by histiocytes, in which they multiply repeatedly. The histiocytes are destroyed, and amastigotes are released into tissues, where the process is repeated. Lymphocytic and plasma cell infiltration along with histiocytic hyperplasia becomes evident. In some lesions, epithelioid and giant cells may be seen. Hypertrophy of the stratum corneum and hyperplasia of dermal papillae occur early in the course. Usually, they are followed by necrosis of the area caused by capillary obstruction and endothelial proliferation; eventually, the epithelium overlying the center of the lesion becomes necrotic and is sloughed, with the formation of a characteristic ulcer. Secondary neutrophil infiltration then is noted. At this point, a depressed ulcer with a raised purpuric indurated border and a base of friable granulation tissue is present. Amastigotes are usually located intracellularly, although during the period of necrosis, organisms may be seen outside cells but not dividing.

With *L. tropica,* development of the lesion may take weeks to months, and relatively few lymphocytes and plasma cells and large numbers of parasites in nests of macrophages are present. In *L. major* infection, the onset is rapid, with an outpouring of lymphocytes and plasma cells; parasites are sometimes difficult to find. In some cases, extensive satellite lesions form in the proximity of the primary lesion so that local spread often is seen. The pathologic reaction may be florid, with marked pseudoepitheliomatous hyperplasia that can be mistaken for carcinoma. Secondary bacterial infection may complicate the lesion and delay healing. Once the ulcer heals, however, usually by fibrosis, the patient has long-lasting immunity.

Several forms of CL have been described and seem to be associated with the ability of the patient to respond to the infection by cell-mediated immune mechanisms. Whether these mechanisms are directly responsible for protection in humans is still not certain. Thus, in a small number of patients, the inability to mount a suitable cell-mediated immune reaction is associated with specific anergy to leishmanin and an indolent nonhealing lesion. This condition is known as DCL, or leishmaniasis tegumentaria diffusa. Characteristically, lesions in DCL are filled with large, parasite-containing histiocytes, and lymphocytes are absent. Recent studies of DCL from the Dominican Republic suggest that immune suppression plays an important role in this form of the disease.

At the other extreme is a small group of patients whose cell-mediated immune response to infection with leishmanial organisms is exaggerated to such an extent that the lesions heal by scarring. At the edge of the scar, however, new lesions appear, so the disease seems to extend from the margins. Eventually, tissue damage may be rather extensive. On histologic examination, many lymphocytes, plasma cells, epithelioid cells, and large multinucleated giant cells are seen. Organisms are difficult to locate but sometimes can be cultured from these lesions. This form of CL is called leishmaniasis recidivans. Patients exhibit marked delayed hypersensitivity to leishmanin. Studies of Turk and Bryceson have provided the concept that CL may be a spectrum of diseases analogous to leprosy. They consider DCL to be at one end of the spectrum and representative of anergy and leishmaniasis recidivans to be at the other end and representative of marked delayed hypersensitivity, with an ordinary Oriental sore as the center in which balance exists.

CLINICAL MANIFESTATIONS

The disease usually begins with the appearance of a pruritic, red, vesicular papule that appears weeks to months after the bite of a sandfly. The papule gradually enlarges, often measuring 1 to 2 cm in diameter. When the surface of the papule dries, it encrusts and drops off to reveal a shallow ulcer. The ulcer may or may not enlarge progressively and characteristically has raised, sharp, indurated, deep purpuric margins. Healing usually takes place in 3 to 18 months, with an obvious hypopigmented or hyperpigmented depressed scar frequently remaining. However, single or multiple papules often heal directly without extensive ulceration. If the lesions do not become infected secondarily, usually no complications occur.

DIAGNOSIS

Microscopic examination of Giemsa- or Wright-stained smears of tissue obtained from non-necrotic areas of the ulcer or from the base should be performed. Aspiration and culture of tissue fluid taken from the ulcer margin can be rewarding. Biopsy material taken from the edge of the ulcer should be examined histologically, as should small fragments macerated in saline and inoculated into NNN medium or Schneider's insect medium, together with penicillin and streptomycin. Clinically, the lesions are often characteristic, so the diagnosis should be suspected in a patient who has visited an endemic area.

Although the leishmanin test is usually positive in patients with ulcerated lesions, the material is not readily available in the United States. However, a positive leishmanin skin test may help distinguish a variety of skin lesions such as syphilis, tropical phagedenic ulcer, yaws, tuberculosis, and various fungal diseases. The indirect fluorescent antibody test or direct agglutination test may be positive in this infection, although often at low titer and, therefore, of little value.

TREATMENT

Uncomplicated *L. tropica* lesions generally respond well to chemotherapy or to conservative management. Because Old World CL usually remains a local lesion, if the ulcer is not disfiguring and appears to be healing, allowing the lesion to heal spontaneously is not an unreasonable approach. Systemic therapy with stibogluconate sodium (see the section on VL) is very satisfactory in most cases. Several reports have indicated limited success in treating skin lesions with heat. Generally, raising intralesional temperature to 40° to 42° C for 12 hr/day was necessary to obtain a satisfactory result. Recently, recombinant IFN-γ has been reported to accelerate healing in this disease. Various parenteral, topical, and oral agents have been used, but the data are anecdotal or conflicting, or both. Thus, allopurinol and various imidazoles (e.g., ketoconazole, itraconazole) have been used and appear to have limited antileishmanial activity. Recently, an ointment containing paromomycin (aminosidine) and methylbenzethonium chloride (Leshcutan) has been reported to show some promise in treating cutaneous lesions, especially in Israel.

PREVENTION

Residual spraying for sandflies, eradication of reservoir hosts, and vaccination procedures have reduced and limited this disease in many areas of the Middle East and central Asia. Because of the indolent nature of the healing with vaccination and the possibility of visceralization, this practice has been discontinued in Israel.

American Cutaneous Leishmaniasis

The epidemiology and etiology of American CL have become extremely complex subjects. In South and Central America, many varieties of leishmaniasis exist, the mucocutaneous form, or espundia, being but one of them. In contrast to Old World CL, American cutaneous disease is tied closely to the forests of South and Central America, and each variety has its own distinct epidemiologic, pathologic, and clinical picture. Whether designating each of the clinical types of American CL by a separate species of *Leishmania* is justified remains unclear. With regard to the American cutaneous forms, two main groups of organisms are distinguished: the *L. mexicana* and *L. braziliensis* complexes (Figs. 219–4 to 219–6). The

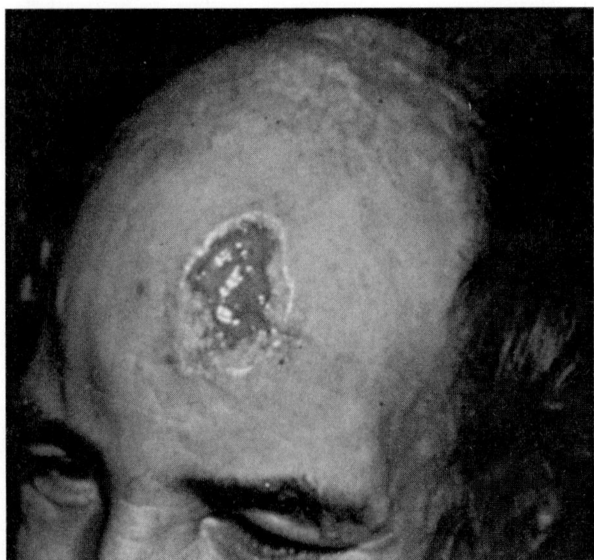

FIGURE 219–4 ■ Healing cutaneous leishmaniasis in a patient from Venezuela.

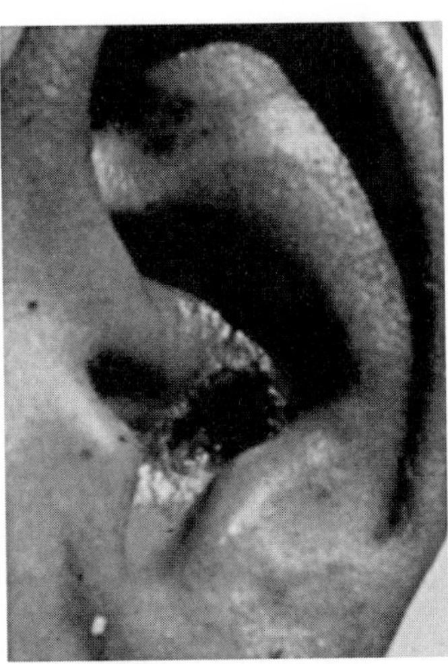

FIGURE 219–5 ■ Chiclero ulcer *Leishmania (mexicana) mexicana.* A typical chronic lesion of the external ear is evident. Such lesions never metastasize.

former are often characterized by rapid growth in culture medium and in hamsters, and the latter are organisms that grow slowly in culture and hamsters.

LEISHMANIA MEXICANA COMPLEX

1. *L. (mexicana) mexicana* is transmitted by species of sandflies of the genus *Lutzomyia.* Many rodent reservoir hosts exist. This species is found in Mexico, Guatemala, and Belize. It causes mild infection, often a single cutaneous lesion that is self-limited, or persistent chronic ear lesions, as well as chiclero ulcer. One case of disseminated disease has been reported. This species is probably responsible for the occasional cases of CL found in the southern portion of the United States.
2. *L. (mexicana) amazonensis* is found along the Amazon basin and in Trinidad. It rarely infects humans but is transmitted by various species of *Lutzomyia* in rodents. In humans, it causes a mild and self-limited skin lesion. Occasionally, disseminated disease reportedly develops.

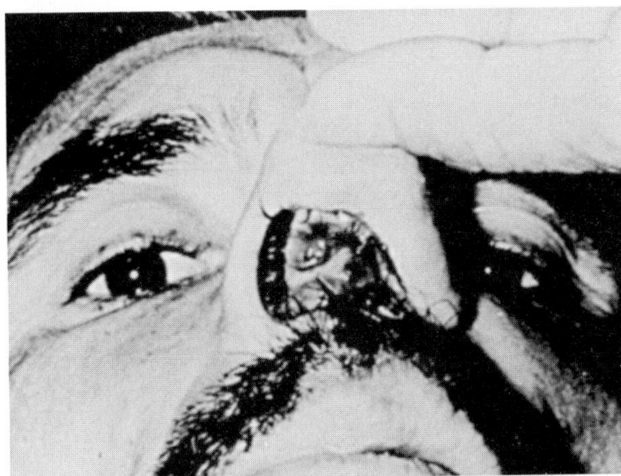

FIGURE 219–6 ■ Mucocutaneous leishmaniasis: *Leishmania (braziliensis) braziliensis.* The entire nasal septum has been eroded. Few organisms could be found by smear or biopsy; however, promastigote forms were cultured from the lesion.

LEISHMANIA BRAZILIENSIS COMPLEX

1. *L. (braziliensis) braziliensis* is transmitted by various species of *Lutzomyia* in Brazil and the forest areas east of the Andes. This organism is the "prototype" of American CL or MCL, or espundia. It may cause destructive ulcerative lesions of the naso-oropharynx as a result of early or late metastases from a more superficial site.
2. *L. (braziliensis) guyanensis* is transmitted by species of *Lutzomyia* in Guyana, Suriname, Brazil, and Venezuela. It causes single or multiple spreading cutaneous ulcers over many parts of the body and is believed to metastasize along the lymphatics but does not visceralize. The organism sometimes spreads to the naso-oropharynx and causes mucosal disease. It sometimes is referred to as pian bois, or forest yaws.
3. *L. (braziliensis) panamensis* is transmitted by species of *Lutzomyia* in Panama and possibly farther north and south. It may cause single to several superficial ulcers and may metastasize along the lymphatics to the naso-oropharynx.
4. *L. (braziliensis) peruviana* is seen in Peru on the western slopes of the Andes to an altitude of 3000 m. It causes a single or a few self-healing ulcers. No oronasopharyngeal spread occurs. Often, it is referred to as uta. Dogs are regarded as the reservoir hosts.

In MCL as represented by espundia, researchers estimate that nasal involvement may occur in as many as 80 percent of infections, up to 30 percent of which eventually may mutilate the mucous membranes of the mouth, nose, palate, larynx, and trachea. These cases are often fatal because of the intervening sepsis. Lesions of the mucous membranes often arise several years to decades after a cutaneous ulcer has healed. Once mucous membrane involvement occurs, the infection may be difficult to eradicate by chemotherapy.

DIAGNOSIS

The discussion of Old World CL includes the various methods for diagnosis. In mucocutaneous disease, the fluorescent antibody test using amastigote antigen is most useful in that it is positive in 75 to 85 percent of cases, with declining titers after therapeutic cure. A direct agglutination test using promastigotes also is used frequently, as is ELISA. Recently, a DNA-DNA hybridization or dot-blot test that is highly sensitive and species-specific in tissue or biopsy specimens has been used. Isozyme analysis of isolated organisms currently is being used to help identify the species causing the infection.

TREATMENT

As in Old World CL, treatment of most lesions will succeed if pentavalent antimonials are used. Because prompt and adequate therapy for primary cutaneous lesions is thought to reduce the risk of subsequent metastatic disease in potentially mucocutaneous infections, pentavalent antimony should be used. If lesions should prove unresponsive to antimony therapy, amphotericin B should be tried. There is no evidence that liposomal amphotericin is useful for this condition. Relapses with this form of leishmaniasis are not uncommon and must be treated again. Pentavalent antimonials are moderately effective in treating mild mucosal disease but are often unsatisfactory with severe mucosal involvement. Leishmaniasis tegumentaria diffusa, a disseminated form of the disease, should be treated with stibogluconate sodium; when relapses occur, amphotericin B should be used next because this disease is usually refractory to further antimony therapy. Pentamidine also has been used with limited success when lesions have proved resistant to antimony compounds. Pentavalent antimony-resistant cutaneous disease, such as leishmania recidivans, has been treated with limited success with ketoconazole, 400 to 600 mg daily for 4 weeks. Recently, miltefosine, an oral antileishmanial agent effective against VL, has shown promise for the treatment of American CL *(L. panamensis/ amazonensis).*

PREVENTION

This disease is extremely difficult to prevent because it is a forest disease. It can be avoided only by sleeping in tents under fine-mesh netting, wearing long-sleeved clothing, and using insect repellents.

BIBLIOGRAPHY

1. Arnot, D. E., and Barker, D. C.: Biochemical identification of cutaneous leishmaniasis by analysis of kinetoplast DNA. II. Sequence homologies in *Leishmania* kDNA. Mol. Biochem. Parasitol. *3*:47–56, 1981.
2. Ashford, R. W., Desjeux, P., and deRaadt, P.: Estimation of population at risk of infection and number of cases of leishmaniasis. Parasitol. Today *8*:104, 1992.
3. Badaro, R., Jones T. C., and Carvalho, E. M.: New perspectives on a subclinical form of VL. J. Infect. Dis. *154*:1003–1011, 1986.
4. Bekaert, E. D., Dole, E., Dubois, D. Y., et al.: Alterations in lipoprotein density classes in infantile leishmaniasis: Presence of apolipoprotein SAA. Eur. J. Clin. Invest. *22*:190–199, 1992.
5. Belli, A., Garcia, D., Palacios, X., et al.: Widespread atypical cutaneous leishmaniasis caused by *Leishmania (L.) chagasi* in Nicaragua. Am. J. Trop. Med. Hyg. *61*:380–385, 1999.
6. Berman, J. D.: Chemotherapy for leishmaniasis: Biochemical mechanisms, clinical efficacy, and future strategies. Rev. Infect. Dis. *10*:560–586, 1988.
7. Carvalho, E. M., Teixeira, R. S., and Johnson, W. D., Jr.: Cell-mediated immunity in American visceral leishmaniasis: Reversible immunosuppression during acute infection. Infect. Immun. *33*:498–500, 1981.
8. Chulay, J. D., and Bryceson, A. D. M.: Quantitation of amastigotes of *Leishmania donovani* in smears of splenic aspirates from patients with VL. Am. J. Trop. Med. Hyg. *32*:475–479, 1983.
9. Convit, J., Pinardi, M. E., and Rondon, A. J.: Diffuse cutaneous leishmaniasis: A disease due to an immunologic defect of the host. Trans. R. Soc. Trop. Med. Hyg. *66*:603–610, 1972.
10. Dillon, D. C., Day, C. H., Whittle, J. A., et al.: Characterization of a *Leishmania tropica* antigen that detects immune responses in Desert Storm viscerotropic leishmaniasis patients. Proc. Natl. Acad. Sci. U. S. A. *92*:7981–7985, 1995.
11. Eltoum, I. A., Zijlstra, E. E., Ali, M. S., et al.: Congenital kala-azar and leishmaniasis in the placenta. Am. J. Trop. Med. Hyg. *46*:57–62, 1992.
12. Grimaldi, G., Jr., and Tesh, R. B.: Leishmaniasis of the New World: Current concepts and implications for future research. Clin. Microbiol. Rev. *6*:230–250, 1993.
13 Handman, E.: Cell biology of *Leishmania*. Adv. Parasitol. *44*:1–39, 1999.
14. Herwaldt, B. L.: Leishmaniasis. Lancet *354*:1191–1199, 1999.
15. Herwaldt, B. L., and Berman, J. D.: Recommendations for treating leishmaniasis with sodium stibogluconate (Pentostam) and review of pertinent clinical studies. Am. J. Trop. Med. Hyg. *46*:296–306, 1992.
16. Jha, M. D., Sundar, S., Thakur, C. P., et al.: Miltefosine, an oral agent for the treatment of Indian VL. N. Engl. J. Med. *341*:1795–1800, 1999.
17. Locksley, R. M., Pingel, S., Lacy, D., et al.: Susceptibility to infectious diseases: *Leishmania* as a paradigm. J. Infect. Dis. *179*(Suppl. 2):305–308, 1999.
18. Mary, C., Auriault, V., Faugere, B., and Dessein, A. J.: Control of *Leishmania infantum* infection is associated with $CD8^+$ and gamma interferon– and interleukin-5–producing $CD4^+$ antigen-specific T cells. Infect. Immun. *67*:5559–5566, 1999.
19. Magill, A. J., Grogl, M., Gasser, R. A., et al.: Visceral infection caused by *Leishmania tropica* in veterans of Operation Desert Storm. N. Engl. J. Med. *328*:1383–1387, 1993.
20. Martino, L., Davidson, R. N., Giacchino, R. et al.: Treatment of VL in children with liposomal amphotericin B. J Pediatr. (on-line) *131*:1–8, 1997.
21. Medrano, F. J., Hernandez-Quero, J., Jimenez, E., et al.: VL in HIV-1–infected individuals: A common opportunistic infection in Spain? AIDS *6*:1499–1503, 1992.
22. Meyerhof, A.: U.S. Food and Drug Administration approval of AmBisome (liposomal amphotericin B) for treatment of VL. Clin. Infect. Dis. *28*:42, 1999.
23. Sacks, D., and Kamhawi, S.: Molecular aspects of parasite-vector and vector-host interactions in leishmaniasis. Annu. Rev. Microbiol. *55*:453–483, 2001.
24. Sampio, S., Castro, M. R., Dillon, N. L., et al.: Treatment of mucocutaneous leishmaniasis with amphotericin B: Report of 70 cases. Int. J. Dermatol. *10*:179–181, 1971.
25. Shaw, J. J., and Lainson, R.: Ecology and epidemiology: New World. *In* Peters, W., and Killick-Kendrick, R. (eds.): The Leishmaniases in Biology and Medicine. Vol. I. London, Academic Press, 1987, pp. 78–87.
26. Shaw, P. K., Quigg, L. T., Allain, D. S., et al.: Autochthonous dermal leishmaniasis in Texas. Am. J. Trop. Med. Hyg. *25*:788–796, 1976.
27. Soto, J., Toledo, J., Gutierrez, P., et al.: Treatment of American cutaneous leishmaniasis with miltefosine, an oral agent. Clin. Infect. Dis. *33*:e57–e61, 2001.
28. Sundar, S., Rosenkaimer, F., Makharia, M. K., et al.: Trial of oral miltefosine for VL. Lancet *352*:1821–1823, 1998.
29. Turk, J. L., and Bryceson, A. D.: Immunological phenomenon in leprosy and related diseases. Adv. Immunol. *13*:209–266, 1971.
30. Weigle, K. A., de Davalaos, M., Heredia, P., et al.: Diagnosis of cutaneous and mucocutaneous leishmaniasis in Columbia: A comparison of seven methods. Am. J. Trop. Med. Hyg. *36*:489–496, 1987.
31. Yadav, T. P., Gupta, H., Satteya, U., et al.: Congenital kala-azar. Ann. Trop. Med. Parasitol. *83*:535–537, 1989.

CHAPTER

220 Trypanosomiasis

MURRAY WITTNER ■ HERBERT B. TANOWITZ

American Trypanosomiasis

American trypanosomiasis, or Chagas disease, is caused by the protozoan hemoflagellate *Trypanosoma cruzi,* which first was discovered by Carlos Chagas in 1909 in the blood of a seriously ill, wasted Brazilian child suffering from fever, lymphadenopathy, and anemia. The disease, transmitted by reduviid bugs, is limited to the Western Hemisphere and is prevalent in South and Central America and Mexico. In areas where the disease is endemic, it occurs most commonly in the rural poor who live in an environment with many feral reservoir hosts. Several autochthonous and laboratory-acquired cases have been reported from the United States in recent years. Chagas disease in some endemic areas is the most important cause of heart disease and may result in serious chronic digestive tract pathology.

THE ORGANISM

T. cruzi is a pleomorphic, spindle-shaped organism whose size is quite variable, depending on the strain. The length of the blood forms (trypomastigote) in humans may vary widely, from 11 to 30 μm, including a free anterior flagellum. Most trypomastigotes assume a C or S shape, with the nucleus just anterior to the middle of the cell. The undulating membrane is small and originates from a very large posterior kinetoplast that often bulges the cell surface (Fig. 220–1). The kinetoplast contains thousands of minicircle and maxicircle DNA that serve in the synthesis of mitochondrial proteins.

The blood form trypomastigotes undergoes an obligatory developmental and reproductive cycle in the alimentary tract of the vector (reduviid or triatomine bugs) when ingested with a blood meal. The entire cycle takes place in the lumen of the gut during a 6- to 15-day period, depending on whether the bug is in its larval stage (6 or 7 days) or nymphal or adult stages (10 to 15 days). Within a few hours after taking an infective blood meal, short, spindle-shaped forms lacking a free flagellum can be found in the insect's foregut. These forms develop into small epimastigotes that continue to divide and give rise to large (35 to 40 μm) epimastigotes; by the third or fourth day after the blood meal, these organisms can be found attached to the rectal epithelium. By about the fifth day, the epimastigotes have begun to round up and gradually develop into short, stout trypomastigotes, which then proceed to elongate, and by the seventh and eighth days, they become the long, slender (17 to 22 μm), infective, metacyclic trypomastigotes. These forms do not divide again but are passed out with the feces some time after the blood meal. There may be 3000 to 4000 organisms per microliter of excreta. Transmission may occur by means of infected insect excreta, and metacyclic forms readily negotiate mucosa, conjunctiva, and abraded or otherwise broken skin (puncture site). Thus, extensive experimental evidence clearly has demonstrated that infection is by contamination rather than insect inoculation.

Once the infective metacyclic trypomastigotes traverse the skin, they invade and multiply locally in many cell types after having transformed into intracellular amastigote forms. Host-cell entry by the parasite is a complex process involving many host and parasite factors. Trypomastigotes released from infected host cells may infect adjacent uninfected cells or enter the bloodstream and lymphatics to infect distant tissues. No tissue is spared from infection, but *T. cruzi* strains may vary in tissue tropism. The cells of the reticuloendothelial system and nervous and muscular (striated and cardiac) systems appear to be particularly vulnerable. In the ensuing weeks, during which time repeated cycles of multiplication, cell destruction, and cell reinvasion have occurred, flagellates enter the bloodstream as trypomastigotes, and the infection becomes disseminated.

EPIDEMIOLOGY

Human Chagas disease is reported from Mexico to Chile and Argentina. Only the Caribbean Islands, Belize, Suriname, and Guyana are reported to be free of this infection. Just five autochthonous cases have been documented in the United States despite the presence of infected vectors. Estimating the number of persons infected with *T. cruzi* has been difficult, but various estimates are approximately 50,000 deaths and 10 to 20 million individuals at risk. Most workers believe that these figures are far too conservative. The vectors are found from the southern part of the United States to southern Argentina and Chile. Acute Chagas disease is reported in areas from Mexico to Rio Colorado in mid Argentina.

The vectors are distributed in rural wooded areas closely associated with feral animal species; humans intervene only occasionally. Thus, this infection is usually a zoonosis. However, many species have become adapted to houses, where they may live in cracks; on roofs, walls, and floors; and beneath little-moved objects. Other triatomine species have developed regular visiting habits to human dwellings but have not taken up residence as yet. Although Chagas disease always has been associated with rural areas and low socioeconomic groups, some vectors have adapted to areas undergoing urbanization. Various suitable hosts that often live close to humans, such as the opossum, may provide the transition between wild and domestic infection. Investigators frequently have observed that domestic animals such as pigs, cattle, goats, and sheep are kept in close contact with the domicile and that triatomines closely associated with these animals can be carried into the home.

Aside from natural transmission via the vector, other modes of transmission include congenital, blood transfusion, maternal milk, organ transplantation, and laboratory accident. The overall incidence of congenital Chagas disease is reported as 2 percent in 500 deliveries but is higher when the woman has acute infection.

Blood transfusion is an important mode of transmission. In many large urban areas of South America, 3 to 15 percent of blood donors were reported to have positive serology. The problem is compounded when one considers that in stored refrigerated blood, blood forms can live for weeks without losing their infectivity. In recent years, an influx of

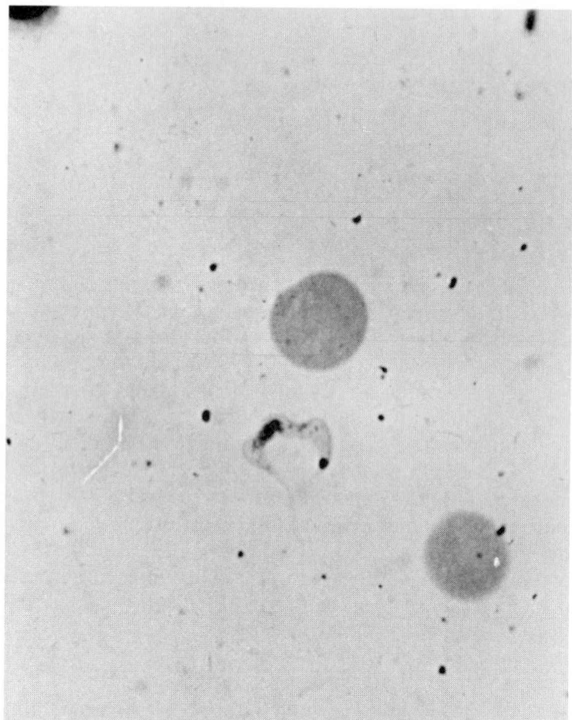

FIGURE 220–1 ■ *Trypanosoma cruzi* trypomastigote forms in a blood smear. Note the large posterior kinetoplast (original magnification ×288).

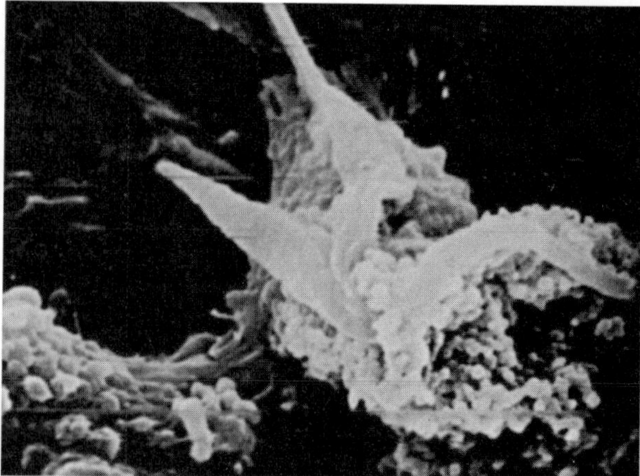

FIGURE 220–2 ■ *Trypanosoma cruzi* phagocytized by a mouse peritoneal macrophage (scanning electron micrograph ×6000).

immigrants has occurred from these areas into North America and Europe. Some of these individuals are seropositive for Chagas disease. With this immigration, an increase in the diagnosis of clinical Chagas disease has occurred in the United States, as has the recognition of blood transfusion–associated Chagas disease in nonendemic areas.

Ingestion of infected mice by cats or cannibalism among rodents has been shown to transmit the infection successfully. Furthermore, several reports have indicated the acquisition of infection by humans from infected meat. However, how important these routes of infection might be in maintaining the disease in nature or in humans remains unclear. In endemic areas, large numbers of feral and domestic reservoirs of *T. cruzi* exist. For example, dogs and cats, especially in Brazil and Chile, have been shown to have a high index of infection and are believed to represent important domestic reservoirs. In some areas, armadillos have been implicated. In the United States, naturally occurring Chagas disease has been reported from Louisiana, Oklahoma, and Texas. In addition, the wood rat, raccoon, armadillo, and opossum are important feral hosts.

PATHOGENESIS AND PATHOLOGY

Once metacyclic trypomastigotes traverse the skin or mucous membrane, they may be phagocytized by tissue macrophages or actively penetrate other cells (Figs. 220–2 and 220–3). Within the cell, trypomastigotes rapidly transform into rounded amastigotes, and division begins (Fig. 220–4). In vitro studies have demonstrated that parasites within macrophage vacuoles may be killed by the cytocidal mechanisms of the host cell, which include nitric oxide. The parasite may escape the parasitophorous vacuole by elaborating a hemolysin and reach the cytoplasm, where it reproduces. Within these cells, large numbers of amastigotes are formed, and within a few days, the greatly distended cell ruptures and frees trypomastigotes and amastigotes into tissues. They then actively invade previously uninfected cells, and the process is repeated. A nodular swelling, or chagoma, develops at the site of entry (Fig. 220–5). This area soon is infiltrated with macrophages surrounded by lymphocytes, eosinophils, and neutrophils. The process spreads to the regional lymph nodes, where focal lymphadenitis becomes evident. Shortly thereafter, blood forms appear and disseminate throughout the body. The acute pathologic process is related to the invasion and subsequent destruction of cells by the replicating intracellular parasites. Associated with these areas of cellular destruction is a marked host inflammatory reaction characterized by local accumulation of neutrophils, lymphocytes, and plasma cells. No tissue is spared, but cardiac and skeletal muscle and the cells of the reticuloendothelial and nervous systems most often are affected.

The myocardium reveals focal myonecrosis, contraction band necrosis, interstitial fibrosis, and lymphocytic infiltration. Interspersed among the degenerating fibers is a marked mixed inflammatory cell exudate, which with time becomes predominantly mononuclear. The course of the acute infection can be quite variable, with severe tissue destruction, or the infection can be silent, with little or no

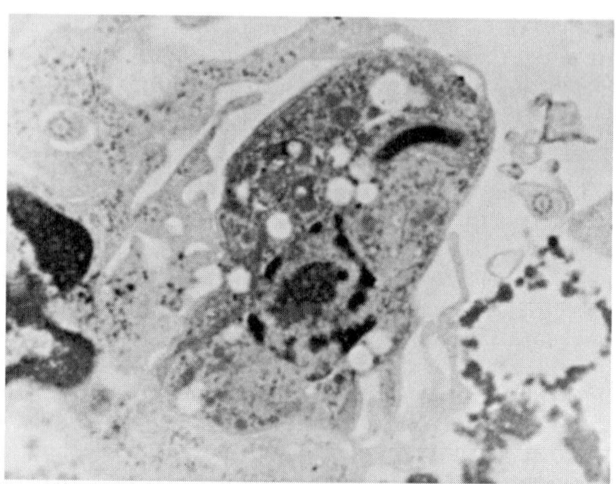

FIGURE 220–3 ■ *Trypanosoma cruzi* phagocytized by a mouse peritoneal macrophage (transmission electron micrograph ×7000).

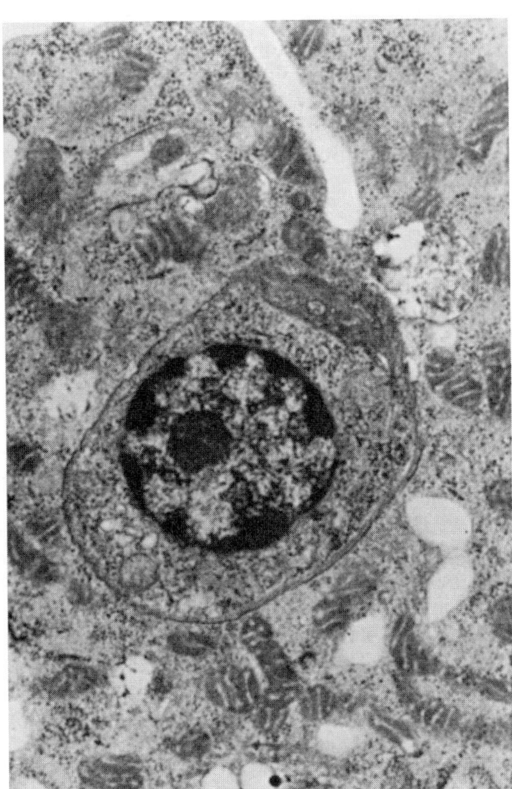

FIGURE 220–4 ■ *Trypanosoma cruzi* amastigote forms in the cytoplasm of a macrophage (transmission electron micrograph ×7000).

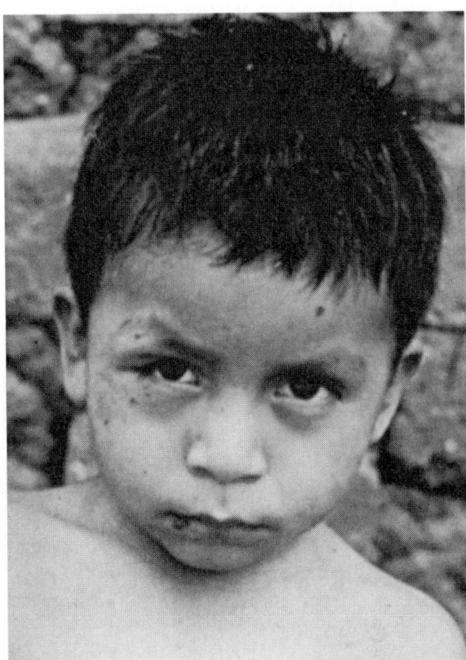

FIGURE 220–5 ■ Chagas disease. A chagoma on the mucocutaneous junction of the lip and moderate unilateral periorbital edema are present. (From a nonprofit cooperative endeavor by numerous colleagues under the editorship of Dr. Herman Zaiman, New York.)

obvious pathology. Nevertheless, the parasites have entered various cells of the body successfully and have formed pseudocysts, each containing hundreds to thousands of amastigotes (Fig. 220–6). Individuals who recover from the acute episode, including those who have had an inapparent infection, probably harbor these intracellular parasites for the rest of their lives.

The immunology of Chagas disease in experimental animals and humans has been investigated and is beyond the scope of this chapter. However, that both cell-mediated immunity and antibody play important roles in the immune response is clear. Cytokines such as interferon-γ and nitric oxide contribute to the intracellular killing of this parasite, as well as to myocardial and gastrointestinal tract dysfunction.

Chagasic heart disease represents the interplay of inflammation and ischemia. During acute infection, foci of myonecrosis, myocytolysis, and vasculitis are observed, along with an inflammatory exudate consisting primarily of leukocytes. Pseudocysts containing amastigotes can be found interspersed among the degenerating fibers. *T. cruzi* gains access to cardiac myocytes by first invading endothelial cells, the interstitial areas of the vascular wall, and the myocardium. Parasites can be seen in and around the endothelium of infected mice. The trypomastigotes pass two basal laminae and two layers of extracellular matrix (ECM). Parasite enzymes such as proteases, gelatinases, and collagenases degrade native type I collagen, heat-denatured type I collagen, and native type IV collagen. Proteolytic activities against laminin and fibronectin also have been detected. These enzymes may play an important role in the degradation of ECM and subsequent parasite invasion. Degradation of the collagen matrix, evident in acute murine Chagas disease, has been proposed to result in chronic pathology such as apical thinning of the ventricle. When damage such as that caused by ischemia and necrosis occurs, ECM degradation ensues and leads to slippage of the ventricular layers, with mural thinning and aneurysm formation. Damage to this area of the heart and remodeling of the wall frequently are encountered in chagasic heart disease. Remodeling refers to the structural changes associated with inflammation, necrosis, hypertrophy, and ventricular dilation. In the course of chronic chagasic heart disease, myonecrosis, myocytolysis, and contraction band necrosis are evident. The necrosis results from transient hypoperfusion followed by reperfusion, such as after local spasm of the coronary

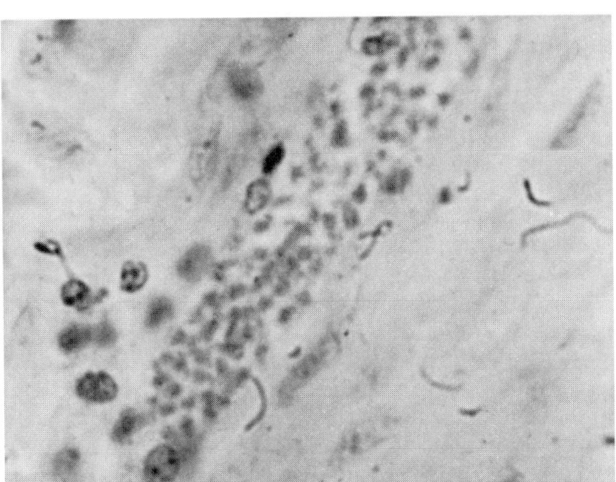

FIGURE 220–6 ■ *Trypanosoma cruzi* amastigote forms in cardiac muscle (original magnification ×288).

microvasculature. Focal and diffuse areas of myocellular hypertrophy may be observed with or without inflammatory infiltrates. In other areas, focal fibrosis replacing previously damaged myocardial tissue is evident. An important feature of chagasic heart disease is a dense accumulation of extracellular collagen that encloses fibers or groups of fibers. All areas of the heart may be involved, including the conduction pathways. Microvascular involvement, manifested by basement membrane thickening, has been demonstrated. These irreversible changes lead to functional disturbances. The remodeling process results in replacement of cardiac myocytes and cells of the vasculature by fibrous tissue, which leads to thinning of the myocardium and hypertrophy of the remaining cardiac myocytes. Chronic chagasic cardiomyopathy is characterized by focal lymphocytic infiltrates (predominately $CD8^+$), myocyte necrosis, and marked reactive and reparative fibrosis. The role of apoptosis in the pathogenesis of chronic chagasic cardiomyopathy is unclear.

In the chronic stage of Chagas disease, the heart is usually enlarged. The chambers may be dilated and associated with an apical left or right ventricular aneurysm, which rarely ruptures. Mural thrombi, especially of the right atrium and apex of the left ventricle, commonly are seen. They may cause widespread embolization, especially to the brain, lungs, spleen, and kidneys. The myocardium often reveals diffuse fibrosis with small numbers of mononuclear cells scattered throughout, and in many patients, finding parasites in the myocardium may be quite difficult. The apparent absence of parasites in the myocardium during routine histologic examination in chronic Chagas cardiomyopathy, even in the presence of marked morphologic and functional changes, has engendered much speculation regarding possible pathogenic etiologies. Parasite persistence, autoimmunity, disturbances in the autonomic nervous system, and vascular compromise have emerged as possible important factors. Recent experimental studies indicate that endothelin-1 and thromboxane A_2, potent vasoconstrictors, as well as nitric oxide may contribute to the pathogenesis of Chagas cardiomyopathy. In addition, genetic epidemiologic studies suggest that susceptibility to infection and progression to chronic disease may, in part, be genetically determined. Researchers have estimated that destruction of more than 95 percent of the ganglion cells of the myenteric plexus in the esophagus and colon is required for evidence of megaesophagus and megacolon. In experimental studies, destruction of ganglion cells mediated by inflammatory mediators is the result of parasitic destruction during the acute phase of the disease.

CLINICAL MANIFESTATIONS

Clinically, Chagas disease can be viewed as having three phases: acute, indeterminate, and chronic. Seroepidemiologic studies indicate that overt or clinically recognizable disease fails to develop in the vast majority of individuals infected with *T. cruzi,* and researchers estimate that as many as 99 percent of those infected have inapparent or subclinical infection. Most of those in whom clinical disease develops as a result of natural infection are infants unable to ward off the bite of triatomes, or "kissing bugs," as well as other young children up to 10 years of age. After an incubation period of approximately 7 to 14 days, acute clinical symptoms may begin with anorexia, lassitude, headache, and intermittent or remitting fever with temperatures of 38° to 40.5° C. In young infants, swelling and edema of the Bichet fat pad may make feeding painful. Locally, or near the site of initial infection, a characteristic unilateral, painless palpebral edema, often with conjunctivitis, may be recognized. This so-called Romaña sign, when present in an endemic area (25–30% of patients), is highly suggestive of early acute Chagas disease. However, the edema may be generalized and mistaken for nephrotic syndrome, or swelling of the preauricular region may be so severe that it suggests mumps. Generalized lymphadenopathy, hepatosplenomegaly, vomiting, and diarrhea, as well as signs of meningeal irritation, commonly are encountered. Skin lesions can vary from a generalized maculopapular or morbilliform eruption to urticaria. Neurologic symptoms, found more often in younger infants than in older patients, include focal to generalized seizures. Signs and symptoms of cardiac involvement are seen in almost every patient if sought for carefully. Such involvement includes tachycardia, cardiac enlargement, and congestive heart failure. In addition, the electrocardiogram may reveal prolongation of the PR interval, low-voltage QRS, and primary T wave changes. The early development of cardiac arrhythmias, such as premature ventricular contraction, atrial fibrillation, partial or complete atrioventricular (A-V) block, and congestive heart failure, does not bode well for the patient. During acute infection, echocardiography may reveal abnormal segmental left ventricular wall motion, most commonly in the anterior or apical (or both) regions. The overall size of the left ventricle and ejection fraction is typically normal. Fatal acute myocarditis may occur in a minority of patients. Examination of blood during the acute infection often reveals trypomastigote forms, leukocytosis with a relative lymphocytosis, and an elevated erythrocyte sedimentation rate. Trypomastigotes may be present in cerebrospinal fluid (CSF), even in the absence of neurologic abnormalities. Although the vast majority of patients recover, apparently without sequelae, 2 to 10 percent may die of severe myocarditis, meningoencephalitis, or an underlying bacterial or another intercurrent viral or bacterial infection. As the acute stage subsides in 8 to 12 weeks, fewer and fewer parasites can be found in the peripheral blood as antibody levels rise. The disease then enters the indeterminate period, and evidence of infection may be detected by special techniques described later. During acute infection, most of the antibody is IgM. Later, in the indeterminate and chronic stages, antibodies predominantly are IgG.

The indeterminate phase of Chagas disease represents the period between acute infection and the onset of chronic signs and symptoms. The duration of this period can span 10 to 40 years, and in the overwhelming majority of cases, overt clinical disease never develops despite the fact that in asymptomatic individuals, organisms often can be identified by culture or molecular methods and by xenodiagnosis. During the indeterminate phase, electrocardiographic or radiologic abnormalities may not be detectable. However, echocardiography often reveals significant changes. A substantial number of these individuals (10–30%) will eventually experience the serious and potentially fatal chronic phase of the disease. For example, a recent report from a hospital in Brazil identified Chagas heart disease in 11 percent of patients who died of a cardiovascular cause.

Chronic chagasic heart disease occurs insidiously or abruptly with an arrhythmia, dilated congestive cardiomyopathy, thromboembolic phenomena, and sudden death. An apical aneurysm, with or without thrombus formation, is one of the hallmarks of this disease and is found frequently, though not exclusively, in the left ventricle. Although significant major coronary artery lesions are usually absent, several instances of myocardial infarction in individuals with Chagas disease have been reported. Destruction of conduction tissue results in conduction abnormalities. In endemic areas, electrocardiographic abnormalities may be suggestive of chagasic cardiomyopathy. For example, a right bundle branch block (RBBB) and an RBBB together with an anterior fascicular block are highly suggestive of chagasic heart disease. These abnormalities have been reported in teenagers and young adults. In addition, premature ventricular contractions and RBBB occur in as many as 50 percent of cases, A-V block of varying degrees develops in about 30 percent of cases, complete A-V block is seen much less commonly, and left bundle branch block is not characteristic. Chest radiographs may reveal cardiomegaly. Heart sounds may be distant, and murmurs of functional mitral and tricuspid insufficiency sometimes are heard. In recent years, echocardiography and cardiac magnetic resonance imaging have been used in the diagnosis and prognosis of chronic chagasic cardiomyopathy. Once congestive heart failure ensues, it is usually intractable and difficult to treat.

Megaesophagus and megacolon are the result of destruction of the ganglion cells of the autonomic plexus. Although they are not usually fatal complications, except in congenital disease, the marked dilatation of the colon and esophagus is most distressing. Any hollow viscus, including the gallbladder and ureters, can be involved, but esophageal and colonic disease is encountered most frequently. Dysphagia, gastroesophageal reflux, and paroxysmal night coughs, presumably caused by aspiration while sleeping, are associated with megaesophagus; chronic constipation, long-term fecal retention, impaction, and volvulus are observed with megacolon. In some regions, patients with digestive disease have symptomatic chagasic heart disease as well. Wide geographic variation in the prevalence of cardiac and gastrointestinal disease has been noted. In Panama, Venezuela, and Colombia, "megas" almost never are encountered, whereas in parts of Brazil, both forms of Chagas disease may be seen in the same individual.

Congenital Chagas disease is caused by vertical transmission of the infection and has been appreciated since the initial descriptions. Pregnant women in endemic areas may experience abortion or placentitis and may give birth to infants with congenital infection associated with prematurity. In its acute stage, congenital Chagas disease often resembles the acquired disease. The onset may be at birth or a few months later, with the infant manifesting hepatosplenomegaly, anemia, jaundice, edema, thrombocytopenia, petechiae, tremors, and seizure disorders. The clinical and laboratory findings may resemble those of congenital toxoplasmosis, cytomegalovirus and herpes simplex virus, or erythroblastosis fetalis. Although frank meningoencephalitis has been observed, it is more likely to be silent. The prognosis of meningoencephalitis in congenital disease is better than in the acquired form of disease. Examination of CSF often reveals trypomastigotes. Necrotic and hemorrhagic lesions of the oral mucosa and skin are thought to represent hematogenously disseminated chagomas. Megacolon and megaesophagus can be present and cause constipation and aspiration pneumonitis.

Chagas disease now is appreciated as an opportunistic infection in patients with acquired immunodeficiency syndrome (AIDS) and in those infected with human immunodeficiency virus (HIV). Patients with these diseases and those receiving immunosuppressive therapy for malignancies and organ transplantation are susceptible to reactivation of *T. cruzi* infection. Similar to the experience with toxoplasmosis and HIV, patients with *T. cruzi* and HIV infection may present with necrotizing encephalitis. In addition, acute chagasic myocarditis is often the sole manifestation of reactivation, or it may accompany necrotizing encephalitis.

DIAGNOSIS

A presumptive diagnosis of Chagas disease rests on a history that the patient lives or once lived in an endemic area and that the cardiac or digestive tract lesions are compatible with Chagas disease. A definitive diagnosis depends on demonstration of the parasite in blood or tissues. It should be emphasized that examination of peripheral blood is of value only during the initial acute disease (6 to 12 weeks) or during chronic exacerbation. Inoculation of animals with the patient's blood often will aid in the diagnosis. In chronic stages, the investigator frequently must take 30 to 50 mL of the patient's blood and inoculate a large number of cultures to obtain a positive diagnosis. Liver biopsy, bone marrow aspiration, or splenic puncture often will provide the diagnosis. At times, xenodiagnosis may be the only means by which organisms can be found. In this technique, laboratory-reared reduviid bugs are permitted to feed on the patient or the patient's fresh blood; subsequently, the bugs are allowed to feed on uninfected guinea pigs. The latter are examined for trypomastigotes after approximately 45 days; though 100 percent specific, this test is less than 50 to 80 percent sensitive.

Serologic tests can be useful during various stages of the disease. The precipitin test may be positive during the acute episode, whereas complement fixation (Machado-Guerreiro test) is useful for the diagnosis of chronic disease. The indirect fluorescent antibody (IFA) and indirect hemagglutination tests are valuable tools for the diagnosis of Chagas disease. However, patients with leishmaniasis, malaria, collagen vascular disease, and syphilis may give false-positive reactions. In congenital disease, an IFA test using anti-IgM or an enzyme-linked immunosorbent assay (ELISA) for IgA antibodies may provide evidence of congenital disease. Tests also have been developed to detect antigen in serum and urine.

Tests using recombinant methods that have the potential for high specificity and high sensitivity have been developed during the past several years. During chronic infection, the number of circulating parasites is very low, but polymerase chain reaction (PCR)-based assays can detect low numbers of organisms because the parasite has highly repetitive nuclear and kinetoplast DNA sequences that can be amplified by PCR. During the chronic stage, serologic methods may be the only means to arrive at a diagnosis. The differential diagnosis of chronic chagasic cardiomyopathy includes rheumatic and arteriosclerotic heart disease and cardiomyopathies of other etiologies.

TREATMENT

No drug is uniformly effective for the treatment of Chagas disease. Nifurtimox (Lampit) is a nitrofuran derivative that has been used extensively with limited success. In some regions, the drug has had a high failure rate. It appears to reduce the period of acute disease and to decrease mortality associated with meningoencephalitis and myocarditis. The duration of parasitemia is shortened. Some researchers think that if treatment is instituted early in acute disease, therapy may cure patients with acute *T. cruzi* infection in as much as antibodies to *T. cruzi* fail to develop in such cases. Whether these individuals are then at risk for chronic Chagas disease at a later time is unknown. Nifurtimox is available in the United States from the Parasitic Drug Service of the Centers for Disease Control and Prevention. It is supplied in 30- and 120-mg tablets. The usual dose for adults is 8 to 10 mg/kg body weight per day. For adolescents

(11 to 16 years of age), it is 12.5 to 15 mg/kg/day, and for children (1 to 10 years of age), the dose is 15 to 20 mg/kg/day. It is given in four divided doses daily for 90 to 120 days. This drug has many untoward reactions, including abdominal pain, nausea, vomiting, anorexia, restlessness, disorientation, insomnia, twitching, paresthesia, polyneuritis, and seizures. Skin reactions also may be observed.

Benznidazole (Rochagan) is similar to nifurtimox and appears to have similar efficacy. Some researchers consider it to be tolerated well, with fewer adverse reactions. It is used extensively in Brazil at 5 mg/kg/day for 30 to 120 days in two divided doses (adult dose). For children up to 12 years of age, the dose is 10 mg/kg/day in two doses for 30 to 90 days. Bone marrow depression and peripheral neuritis have limited its use, however. No evidence has established that either drug is useful in the treatment of chronic Chagas disease, although some experts treat chronic chagasic cardiomyopathy with prolonged courses of nifurtimox or benznidazole.

Recently, interferon-γ has been used in conjunction with drug therapy because experimental data suggest that it is a useful adjunct in treatment by activating macrophage killing. Allopurinol and antifungal drugs have been suggested as alternatives in some patients. Patients with chronic chagasic cardiomyopathy may be helped for a varying period by implantation of a cardiac pacemaker, but the congestive heart failure is often refractory to cardiac glycosides and vasoactive drugs. More recently, inhibitors of angiotensin-converting enzymes have been advocated to reduce cardiac remodeling in these individuals. Heart transplantation also has been performed for the management of chronic cardiomyopathy. The use of high-fiber diets, occasional laxatives, and enemas may assist in the management of megacolon. When these measures fail, surgical resection may be required. Megaesophagus is usually amenable to therapy consisting of a combination of diet and dilatation of the esophagogastric region. In more severe disease, various surgical procedures have been used with variable success to relieve the symptoms of achalasia.

PREVENTION

Regular insecticide spraying programs with benzene hexachloride could reduce transmission of the infection, at least around domiciles. Proper screening and improved housing for those in endemic areas also would serve to reduce transmission. Careful screening of blood donors would help prevent transmission by transfusion in endemic areas. The development of a chemoprophylactic agent or vaccine holds the best hope for prevention and subsequent eradication of Chagas disease.

Transfusion-acquired disease is a major public health problem in endemic areas. Treatment of blood with gentian violet inactivates the parasite. Transfusion-acquired infection has been reported in North America. Because no effective rapid means of detecting the parasite exists, researchers have suggested that persons from endemic areas be rejected as blood donors.

African Trypanosomiasis

African sleeping sickness is caused by two morphologically identical subspecies of hemoflagellate protozoans: *Trypanosoma brucei gambiense,* the cause of West African or Gambian sleeping sickness, and *Trypanosoma brucei rhodesiense,* the cause of East African or Rhodesian disease. Although these parasites produce similar disease, the Gambian form is usually chronic and evolves slowly, often over the course of many years, and ends fatally if untreated, whereas the Rhodesian form is characterized by being acute, usually killing the host in a matter of weeks or months. These diseases exist wherever the various species of *Glossina,* the tsetse fly, are found.

THE ORGANISM

T. b. gambiense and *T. b. rhodesiense* are pleomorphic flagellates varying from 15 to 30 μm in length by 1.5 to 3.5 μm in breadth. In Giemsa-stained blood smears, they may appear long and slender with an undulating membrane and free anterior flagellum or appear short and broad without a free anterior flagellum. No intracellular forms exist. At various stages of disease, trypomastigote forms may be found in the peripheral blood, lymphatics, lymph nodes, CSF, and neural tissue. Thus, although the two species are morphologically indistinguishable and share major biochemical features, isozyme and molecular analysis has shown substantial variation among species. In addition, they maintain separate biologic characteristics, especially with regard to virulence in cross-inoculation experiments. Humans are the only important reservoir host for *T. b. gambiense,* whereas *T. b. rhodesiense* naturally infects wild game animals.

The haploid genome size of *T. brucei* spp. is approximately 40 mega-bases, with as much as 14 percent variation within the same subspp. and as much as 29 percent among different subspecies. Homologous chromosomes, when probed by Southern blot, can differ in size by up to 20 percent. In addition to the large chromosome pairs, *T. brucei* has approximately 100 linear minichromosomes ranging in size from 50 to 150 kb. These minichromosomes contain transcriptionally silent copies of variant surface glycoprotein *(VSG)* genes. *T. brucei* has approximately 1000 genes capable of coding for *VSG* genes; these genes are switched at a rate of 10^{-2} to 10^{-6} switches per generation, which serves as the main mechanism of immune evasion for *T. brucei.* Only one VSG expression site is active at any given time. Studies comparing homologous nuclear genes between *T. cruzi* and *T. brucei* have demonstrated large evolutionary divergence in codon usage. A comparison of the nuclear small- and large-subunit rRNA gene sequences yields genetic distances comparable to that between plants and animals.

Within the insect vector, the tsetse fly, trypomastigote forms that have ingested a blood meal settle in the posterior portion of the midgut and multiply by binary fission for approximately 7 to 10 days. The slender trypomastigotes then migrate anteriorly to the foregut, where they remain for the next 2 to 3 weeks. They next move further forward and finally enter the salivary glands, in which they transform into epimastigote forms, that is, forms in which the kinetoplast has migrated just anterior to the nucleus, and continue to replicate. After several cycles of division, they transform into infective metacyclic trypomastigote forms, which are the small, broad or "stumpy" forms that lack a free anterior flagellum. When next feeding, the infective tsetse fly may inoculate into the bite wound upward of several thousands of these infective trypomastigotes. The entire dipteran cycle spans a period of 15 to 35 days. Within the human host, trypomastigotes multiply by binary fission in blood, lymph, and extracellular spaces. The central nervous system (CNS) eventually is invaded, at which time multiplication continues unabated. Transmission by blood transfusion, hypodermic needle, other insects, and congenital transmission has been reported.

EPIDEMIOLOGY

African sleeping sickness *(T. b. gambiense* and *T. b. rhodesiense)* and veterinary trypanosomiasis caused by *T. brucei* subgroup parasites continue to be responsible for much human suffering and economic loss. These agents are restricted to an area spanning 10 million km^2 south of the Sahara, where the annual rainfall exceeds 500 mm (20 inches), because the larval stages of the tsetse fly are vulnerable to desiccation. The most recent estimates are that 25,000 new cases occur each year and a human population of 55 million is at risk, along with cattle and other species of agricultural importance. In the past, as many as 10,500 cases have been reported annually in Zaire. These figures are probably low in light of recent military activity in the Sudan, Democratic Republic of Congo (formerly Zaire), Angola, and Rwanda. Movement of populations in war areas has increased the risk of epidemics in these and neighboring regions.

The Gambian form occurs mainly in the western portion of tropical Africa, with focal incursions eastward north of Lake Victoria into the Sudan. *Glossina palpalis* is the main tsetse fly vector, although other related species, such as *Glossina tachinoides* and *Glossina fuscipes,* are implicated as well. The Rhodesian form is found in the southeastern portion of Africa.

Although *T. b. gambiense* can infect various mammals, humans appear to be more susceptible and maintain a high enough parasitemia to sustain the fly-human-fly cycle. The prolonged chronicity of Gambian disease with infectious individuals continually exposed to tsetse flies undoubtedly helps sustain the disease. Asymptomatic carriers of the infection also may be an important factor in maintaining the disease in a community. Furthermore, investigators have reported that among the important factors that may limit Gambian infection to humans is the transient and low parasitemia that results from an infective tsetse fly bite in mammals, usually ungulates. Thus, researchers have observed that Gambian disease usually is sustained only when a close and repeated relationship exists between humans and tsetse flies. The practical result of all this is that West African sleeping sickness is maintained by members of the *G. palpalis* group of tsetse flies that use or prefer human blood almost exclusively.

In contrast to Gambian disease, *T. b. rhodesiense* infection generally is maintained in wild mammals. Therefore, the fly-human-fly cycle tends to be unimportant inasmuch as the acute nature of the disease usually quickly removes acutely ill humans as an infective source. However, the intervention of wild game animals, in whom the disease tends to be less acute and whose blood appears to be more attractive, seems to have relegated humans to an occasional or facultative host for *T. b. rhodesiense.* The *Glossina morsitans* group of tsetse flies that inhabit the relatively dry East African savannah readily feed on wild ungulates, especially the bushbuck *Tragelaphus scriptus* and the hartebeest *Alcelaphus buselaphus.* On occasion, Rhodesian disease may reach epidemic proportions, and at these times, direct human-fly-human cycles may intervene. Although all age groups are susceptible to infection, the factors that influence human prevalence rest more on occupational exposure to suitable tsetse flies, as well as the flies' breeding and feeding habits. Young adult males are found most frequently to be infected. However, during epidemics, all groups are infected and mechanical transmission probably occurs. Tourists on safari are possibly at risk. In that regard, recently, reports of African trypanosomiasis in Europe, the United States, and Australia have been increasing.

PATHOGENESIS AND PATHOLOGY

The metacyclic infective trypomastigote forms are inoculated by the tsetse fly into the skin, where they multiply at the inoculation site. A characteristic, hard, sometimes painful chancre develops. By approximately the 10th day, long slender forms are found in the bloodstream and lymphatics, and for the next several days, their numbers increase logarithmically. Soon thereafter, the organisms nearly disappear from the bloodstream as a result of immune lysis, only to reappear again. The interval between waves of parasitemia may vary from 1 to 8 days, with clinical symptoms accompanying each bout of parasitemia. These parasitemic waves can be accounted for by the highly developed antigenic variation strategy of the parasite. Thus, the trypomastigote is covered with VSG, and with each peak of parasitemia, a predominant variable antigen type (VAT) is displayed by the organism. The specific antibody response to this coat protein (VSG) leads to the destruction of parasites that display the predominant VAT or homotype. Numerous heterotypes are found within each population of parasites, one of which, not recognized by the host's immune system, becomes the next homotype. The parasite in each successive wave of parasitemia bears a different VAT. A single trypomastigote may contain as many as 1000 genes, each encoding for a specific VSG. Each successive parasitemic wave represents a new antigenic variant that has emerged to elude the host's antibody response to the previous antigen. As a result of successive waves of immune lysis and parasitemia, a marked early humoral antibody response, predominantly involving IgM, is seen regularly. These macroglobulins contain not only antitrypanosomal antibodies, which are directed against the surface antigens, but also a variety of other antibodies such as heterophile and rheumatoid factor. Researchers have shown experimentally that because of polyclonal B-cell activation, many antibodies are produced to a wide variety of antigens, including brain-specific autoantibodies directed against myelin basic protein, gangliosides, and cerebrosides. Circulating immune complexes have been reported regularly and may be responsible for the glomerulonephritis, hypocomplementemia, and hemolytic anemia that often accompany acute and chronic disease. Cell-mediated immunity is also important in African trypanosomiasis, and increased production of nitric oxide may be important in depression of T-cell responsiveness and generalized immunodepression.

The main pathologic lesions involve the posterior cervical, submaxillary, supraclavicular, and mesenteric lymph nodes and the CNS. The lymphatic tissue usually reveals generalized hyperplasia with diffuse proliferation of lymphocytes. Later, the nodes may become small and fibrotic; however, they initially are markedly hemorrhagic and contain large numbers of trypomastigotes. The CNS remains normal until invaded by organisms, but then a progressive chronic leptomeningitis develops. The brain becomes edematous, and prominent perivascular cuffing by glial cells, lymphocytes, and plasma cells is present. When the latter become vacuolated with pyknotic nuclei, they often are referred to as the morula cells of Mott and Marshalko. Organisms often can be found in brain tissue in proximity to vessels and also may be detected in CSF. Glomerulonephritis, myocarditis, pericardial effusion, pulmonary edema, and hypoplastic bone marrow with associated anemia may be seen. The pathogenesis of the neuropsychiatric manifestations is not understood. Recent experimental studies suggest that changes in levels of brain neurotransmitters, deposition of immune complexes, and alteration in production of prostaglandin, cytokine, and nitric oxide may, in part, account for these behavioral changes.

CLINICAL MANIFESTATIONS

The clinical manifestations of *T. b. gambiense* and *T. b. rhodesiense* disease are similar, except that Rhodesian infection is a more fulminant, acute disease that may run its course in several weeks to 6 to 9 months whereas Gambian infection may last for years. Typically, the incubation period in Rhodesian infection is brief (3 to 21 days), whereas the onset of symptoms with Gambian infection may be delayed for several weeks or years. Approximately 1 week after infection and at the site of the tsetse fly bite, a hard and painful chancre sometimes appears and lasts several weeks. During the early stages when recurrent bouts of fever may be the only symptom, the blood and lymphatics primarily are involved and infection often is mistaken for malaria, especially if a chancre is not obvious or a history of exposure to tsetse flies is not obtained. The period of intermittent fever may last for months to years with Gambian infection. During this time, persistent headache and tachycardia often are encountered, and a circinate erythematous rash or erythema multiforme sometimes is noted. The fever abates gradually. In many patients, characteristic posterior cervical lymphadenopathy becomes evident (Winterbottom sign). The nodes are nontender and attain a diameter of approximately a centimeter. They tend to become small and fibrotic in approximately 6 months. Signs of CNS invasion often develop in untreated patients with Gambian disease. The initial signs and symptoms of neurologic involvement can be difficult to assess. They may consist of alterations in behavior or personality (or both) that eventually may be manifested as a severe psychosis. Severe headache, loss of nocturnal sleep, and a feeling of impending doom typically are described. Next, progressive mental deterioration may occur, and with unrelenting deterioration, patients become incapable of caring for themselves. Tremors, especially of the tongue, hands, or feet, and generalized or focal convulsive episodes may occur. Almost any neurologic or psychiatric manifestation can be seen, and with progressive mental deterioration, patients finally lapse into a coma and die. During the final period of the disease, patients often die of intercurrent infections such as bacterial pneumonia, amebiasis, and malaria. Wasting and malnutrition are a large component of the progressive deterioration in these patients. Sleeping sickness can be a difficult disease to diagnose early in young children. It usually is found only after a child is evaluated for obtundation, seizures, or psychomotor retardation.

DIAGNOSIS

A definitive diagnosis can be made only by finding trypanosomes in blood and bone marrow smears, in lymph node aspirates in early or acute disease, and in CSF in late or chronic disease. For examination of both thick and thin smears, as well as the buffy coat, 10 to 20 mL of citrated whole blood or the sediment from 5 mL of centrifuged CSF is essential. Numerous microscopic techniques, including capillary tube centrifugation, quantitative buffy coat examination, miniature anion-exchange centrifugation, density gradient centrifugation, and acridine orange staining, have been used to enhance parasite detection. Culture or animal inoculation, or both, is sometimes the only successful means of obtaining a diagnosis. In advanced CNS disease, lymphocytosis and elevated IgM are detected in the CSF.

A serologic diagnosis of African trypanosomiasis usually depends on detection of high levels of nonspecific serum IgM. Detection of specific antibody by IFA is helpful, especially when the serum is tested with trypanosomes of the homologous human species. Direct agglutination and a microscale version of ELISA are highly reliable methods for making a specific diagnosis of trypanosomiasis. Recently, antigen-detection and PCR tests have been developed to detect circulating parasites.

In advanced, untreated sleeping sickness, the IgM level in CSF often is elevated, but it has no relationship to the presence of trypanosomes in CSF. After successful treatment, the IgM level declines gradually and disappears after approximately 1 year. However, if 1 year after therapy a constant high level is present or an abrupt rise in IgM occurs, relapse should be suspected. Nonetheless, the IgM level should not be used as the sole method to arrive at a diagnosis or prognosis.

The differential diagnosis of African trypanosomiasis spans a wide spectrum of diseases, but chronic relapsing fever associated with enlarged cervical lymph nodes in an individual who has been to Africa is suggestive. As indicated earlier, considering such diseases as malaria, syphilis, lymphoma, visceral leishmaniasis, and leprosy is not unusual. Later, encephalitis of other etiologies must be excluded. An important diagnostic feature is the frequent finding of a strikingly elevated erythrocyte sedimentation rate, which is a reflection of the markedly increased serum macroglobulins.

PROGNOSIS

If therapy is initiated before significant CSF involvement, the outcome is usually favorable. Untreated infection often ends fatally.

TREATMENT

Chemotherapy for these diseases, both human and veterinary, has lagged remarkably behind that of other tropical diseases. The main chemotherapeutic agents for human trypanosomiasis remain pentamidine and suramin for early-stage disease and melarsoprol (Arsobal) for late-stage (CNS) disease. Eflornithine (difluoromethylornithine [DFMO]) is the only new practical addition to this list since the early 1950s. With the exception of suramin, resistance to the established agents is growing, and toxicity continues to be a disturbing factor in most cases.

Pentamidine is a water-soluble aromatic diamidine that has been in use for nearly 60 years. It is administered as either the isethionate form (Pentam 300) or methanesulfonate (Lomidine). The dose is 4 mg/kg/day for 10 days for both adults and children. Pentamidine is effective against early-stage *T. b. gambiense* infection but less effective against *T. b. rhodesiense* infection and ineffective against late-stage disease. African trypanosomes have a nucleoside (adenine/ adenosine: P_2) transporter that takes up pentamidine, which results in concentrations of the agent many times that in plasma. Although laboratory-induced resistant strains appear to have reduced transport properties, naturally derived clinical isolates seem to have retained transport, thus indicating that most resistance may be caused by alteration of a metabolic target rather than drug uptake.

Suramin is a sulfonated naphthylamine that has been used successfully against early-stage sleeping sickness caused chiefly by *T. b. rhodesiense*. It was first used in 1922 and was developed from the closely related azo dyes trypan red and trypan blue. Suramin is administered intravenously.

The adult dose is 100 to 200 mg (test dose), then 1 g on days 1, 3, 7, 14, and 21. The pediatric dose is 20 mg/kg on days 1, 3, 7, 14 and 21. Suramin has an extremely long half-life in humans, 44 to 54 days, the result of avid binding to serum proteins. Suramin binds to many plasma proteins, including low-density lipoprotein (LDL), which trypanosomes avidly bind and endocytose as a result of specific membrane receptors. LDL is a prime source of sterols for bloodstream trypanosomes. Suramin is taken up as a protein complex and has been shown to inhibit all the glycolytic enzymes in *T. b. brucei* in low concentrations, which in most cases are several-fold lower than for the corresponding mammalian enzyme. Suramin also has been found to affect thymidine kinase and dihydrofolate reductase.

Melarsoprol (Mel B; Arsobal) is an arsenical created by the efforts of Ernst Freidheim in the late 1940s. His initial compound, melarsen oxide, *p*-(4,6-diamino-*s*-triazinyl-2-yl) aminophenylarsenoxide, was complexed with dimercaptopropanol (British antilewisite) to form a less toxic complex, melarsoprol. Until 1990, it was the only agent available for curing the late-stage (CNS) disease of both East African and West African origin. Usually, each series is followed by a week interval before the next series. Melarsoprol is insoluble in water and must be dissolved in propylene glycol. It must be given intravenously; otherwise, it will induce a severe localized inflammatory reaction. This drug is administered intravenously. The adult dosing schedule is 2 to 3.6 mg/kg/day for 3 days. This is then followed in 1 week with 3.6 mg/kg/day for 3 days. This schedule is repeated after 10 to 21 days. The pediatric dose is 18 to 25 mg/kg total over 1 month; the initial dose is 0.36 mg/kg at intervals of 1 to 5 days for a total of 9 to 10 doses.

Reactive arsenical-induced encephalopathy (RAS) is an important toxicity of melarsoprol and is often followed by pulmonary edema and death within 48 hours in more than half the cases. The incidence of RAS has been estimated at 2 to 10 percent. In one clinical study, the co-administration of steroids significantly reduced the incidence of RAS-related deaths during therapy with melarsoprol. Although the mechanism of action of melarsoprol has been studied extensively, it still remains unclear.

DFMO is an enzyme-activated inhibitor of ornithine decarboxylase (ODC), the lead enzyme of polyamine biosynthesis. DFMO was developed as an antitumor agent. After initial testing in model infections, DFMO was studied extensively in human trials in Africa, with some trials in Europe and the United States. The standard treatment regimens resulting from trials indicate that DFMO is more than 95 percent active when given intravenously at 400 mg/kg/day in four doses every 6 hours for 14 days. In these studies, DFMO cured children as well as adults, patients with melarsoprol-refractory strains, and patients with late-stage disease. The short plasma half-life of DFMO necessitates constant dosing when given as an intravenous drip. The most frequent toxic reaction was reversible bone marrow suppression, which was reversed by reducing the dosage. The major drawback with respect to DFMO is its cost and the duration of treatment and availability. DFMO is not trypanocidal and depends on a functional immune system to rid the host of nondividing forms. It is curative for laboratory infections of *T. b. brucei* and *T. b. gambiense* but not all strains of *T. b. rhodesiense*. The reason for this selectivity is not completely evident, although it is not caused by uptake of DFMO because the drug enters by passive diffusion, not transport. DFMO treatment leads to intracellular concentrations of approximately 5 mmol/L, an increase of approximately 50-fold over untreated parasites. The basis for DFMO selectivity lies in the rapid turnover of the mammalian enzyme as opposed to trypanosome ODC. Because mammalian ODC is synthesized constantly at a high rate, DFMO must be continuously available, and this availability is made more difficult by rapid excretion.

PROPHYLAXIS AND PREVENTION

Chemoprophylaxis with suramin, 0.3 to 0.7 g intravenously every 2 to 3 months, is reported to be highly effective. With few exceptions, the vector has proved to be difficult to control. Preventing tsetse fly bites and chemoprophylaxis may be the best means of eliminating the disease from an area. Development of a vaccine has been hindered by antigenic variation.

BIBLIOGRAPHY

1. Adams, J. H., Haller, L., Boa, F. Y., et al.: Human African trypanosomiasis *(T. b. gambiense):* A study of 16 final cases of sleeping sickness with some observations on acute reactive encephalopathy. Neuropathol. Appl. Neurobiol. *12*:81–94, 1986.
2. Amole, B., Sharpless, N., Wittner, M., et al.: Neurochemical measurements in the brains of mice infected with *Trypanosoma brucei brucei* (TREU 667). Ann. Trop. Med. Parasitol. *83*:225–232, 1989.
3. Asonganyi, T., Doua, F., Kibona, S. N., et al.: A multicenter evaluation of the indirect agglutination test for trypanosomiasis (TrypTect CIATT). Ann. Trop. Med. Parasitol. *92*:837–844, 1998.
4. Azogue, E., LaFuente, C., and Darras, C.: Congenital Chagas' disease in Bolivia: Epidemiological aspects and pathological findings. Trans. R Soc. Trop. Med. Hyg. *79*:176–180, 1985.
5. Bittencourt, A. L.: Congenital Chagas' disease. Am. J. Dis. Child. *130*: 97–103, 1976.
6. Bittencourt, A. L., Vieira, G. O., Tavares, H. C., et al.: Esophageal involvement in congenital Chagas' disease: Report of a case with megaesophagus. Am. J. Trop. Med. Hyg. *33*:30–33, 1984.
7. Buyst, H.: Sleeping sickness in children. Ann. Soc. Belg. Med. Trop. *57*:201–212, 1977.
8. Corti, M.: AIDS and Chagas' Disease. A. I. D. S. Patient Care S. T. D. S. *14*:581–588, 2000.
9. Da-Costa-Pinto, E. A. L., Almeida, E. A., Figueiredo, D., et al.: Chagasic megaesophagus and megacolon diagnosed in childhood and probably caused by vertical transmission. Rev. Int. Med. Trop. Sao Paulo *43*:227–230, 2001.
10. de Oliviera, R. B., Troncon, L. E., Dantas, P. R., et al.: Gastrointestinal manifestations of Chagas disease. Am. J. Gastroenterol. *93*:884–889, 1998.
11. Di Pentima, M. C., and Edwards, M. S.: Enzyme-linked immunosorbent assay for IgA antibodies to *Trypanosoma cruzi* in congenital infection. Am. J. Trop. Hyg. *60*:211–214, 1999.
12. Donelson, I. E., Hill, K. L., and El Sayed, N. M. A.: Multiple mechanisms of immune evasion of African trypanosomes. Mol. Biochem. Parasitol. *91*:51–66, 1998.
13. Doua, F., Boa, F. Y., Schechter, P. F., et al.: Treatment of human late stage gambiense trypanosomiasis with alpha-difluoromethylornithine (eflornithine): Efficacy and tolerance in 14 cases in Cote d'Ivoire. Am. J. Trop. Med. Hyg. *37*:525–533, 1987.
14. Grant, I. H., Gold, J. W. M., Wittner, M., et al.: Transfusion associated acute Chagas' disease acquired in the United States. Ann. Intern. Med. *111*:849–851, 1989.
15. Greenwood, B. M., and Whittle, H. C.: The pathogenesis of sleeping sickness. Trans. R. Soc. Trop. Med. Hyg. *74*:716–725, 1980.
16. Kirchhoff, L. V.: American trypanosomiasis (Chagas' disease): A tropical disease now in the United States. N. Engl. J. Med. *329*:639–644, 1993.
17. Kirchhoff, L. V., Bacchi, C. J., Wittner, M., and Tanowitz, H. B.: American trypanosomiasis (Chagas' disease) Curr. Treat. Options Infect. Dis. *2*:59–65, 2000.
18. Kirchhoff, L. V., Bacchi, C. J., Wittner, M., and Tanowitz, H. B.: African trypanosomiasis (sleeping sickness) Curr. Treat. Options Infect. Dis. *2*:66–69, 2000.
19. Leiby, D. A., Wendel, S., Takaoka, D. T., et al.: Serologic testing *for Trypanosoma cruzi:* Comparison of radioimmune precipitation assay with commercially available immunofluorescence assay, indirect hemagglutination assay, and enzyme-linked immunosorbent assay kits. J. Clin. Microbiol. *38*:639–642, 2000.
20. Maguire, I. H., Hoff, R., Sherlock, I., et al.: Cardiac morbidity and mortality due to Chagas' disease: Prospective electrocardiographic study of a Brazilian community. Circulation *75*:1140–1145, 1987.
21. Mbala, L., Matendo, R, Kinkela, T., et al.: Congenital African trypanosomiasis in a newborn child with current neurologic symptomatology. Trop. Doctor *26*:186–187, 1996.

22. Parada, H., Carrasco, H., Anez, N., et al.: Cardiac involvement is a constant finding in acute Chagas' disease. A clinical, parasitological and histopathological study. Int. J. Cardiol. *60*:49–54, 1997.
23. Petkova, S. B., Huang, H., Factor, S. M., et al.: Role of endothelin in the pathogenesis of Chagas' disease. Int. J. Parasitol. *31*:499–511, 2000.
24. Reed, S. G.: Immunology of *Trypanosoma cruzi*. Chem. Immunol. *70*:124–143, 1998.
25. Sartori, A. M., Shikanai-Yasuda, M. A., Amato Neto, V., and Lopes, M. H.: Follow-up of 18 patients with human immunodeficiency virus infection and chronic Chagas' disease, with reactivation of Chagas' disease causing cardiac disease in three patients. Clin. Infect. Dis. *26*:177–179, 1998.
26. Sharafeldin, A., Eltayeb, R., Pashenkov, M., and Bakhiet, M.: Chemokines are produced in the brain early during the course of experimental African trypanosomiasis. J. Neuroimmunol. *103*:165–170, 2000.
27. Sinha, A., Grace, C., Alston, W. K., et al: African trypanosomiasis in two travelers from the United States. Clin. Infect. Dis. *29*:840–844, 1999.
28. Tanowitz, H. B., Kirchhoff, L. V., Simon, D., et al.: Chagas' disease. Clin. Microbiol. Rev. *5*:400–419, 1992.
29. Urbina, J. A.: Chemotherapy of Chagas' disease; the how and the why. J. Mol. Med. *77*:332–338, 1999.
30. Wery, M., Mulumba, P. M., Lambert, P. H., et al.: Hematologic manifestations, diagnosis and immunopathology of African trypanosomiasis. Semin. Hematol. *19*:83–92, 1982.

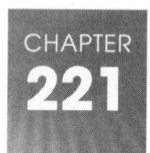

CHAPTER 221 *Naegleria, Acanthamoeba,* and *Balamuthia*

JAMES S. SEIDEL*

Potentially pathogenic free-living amebae of the genera *Acanthamoeba* and *Naegleria* and the newly recognized pathogenic leptomyxid ameba *Balamuthia mandrillaris* can produce disease in humans and animals. Two distinct entities exist. *Naegleria* is capable of producing a fatal fulminant primary meningoencephalitis, which usually results in death in 5 to 10 days, and *Acanthamoeba* and *Balamuthia* produce a more protracted granulomatous amebic encephalitis that leads to death in weeks to months. Contact lens wearers also may contract *Acanthamoeba* keratitis.

Although small free-living amebae occasionally were seen in stool specimens, they were considered harmless until 1957, when they were found to cause cytotoxic changes in green monkey tissue cultures.[33] Amebae were isolated from the brains of mice and monkeys who died of meningoencephalitis after intracerebral injection with tissue culture fluid. These isolates were instilled intranasally into mice, who also died of hemorrhagic meningoencephalitis.[16] Experimental infections with *Acanthamoeba* produced fulminant disease that killed animals in 4 to 7 days.[15, 17] The first human cases were reported in 1965 in Australia by Fowler and Carter[26] and in 1966 in Florida by Butt,[10] who named the disease primary amebic meningoencephalitis. The infection subsequently has been reported worldwide.[43, 62, 79, 83] Visvesvara and colleagues isolated a leptomyxid ameba from the brain of a baboon that died of meningoencephalitis and described a new agent of primary amebic meningoencephalitis, *B. mandrillaris*.[78]

Granulomatous amebic encephalitis caused by a leptomyxid ameba of the genus *Balamuthia* has been described in the literature.[2, 35, 38, 72] Most patients have been immunosuppressed, very young, or old[27]; however, amebic meningoencephalitis caused by *Balamuthia* also has been reported in normal children.[47, 60]

Epidemiology

Free-living amebae have a worldwide distribution and can be recovered from warm, natural bodies of water, including hot springs, quarries, lakes, rivers, improperly treated swimming pools and spas, moist soil, puddles, air conditioners, and other containers in which stagnant water may collect.[13, 36, 55] Free living amebae are predators controlling bacteria in the soil. They are an important component of the food chain that contributes to the organic material in soil. Factors affecting survival of amebae in soil include pH, temperature, salinity, and chemical composition. They are thus part of our natural environment and only in relatively rare circumstances cause disease.[59] Granulomatous encephalitis and disseminated disease have occurred in immunosuppressed patients with acquired immunodeficiency syndrome and cancer and after bone marrow transplantation.[3, 32, 51, 67] Patients who acquire *Naegleria* usually have a history of bathing in a warm body of water. Infections occur more commonly in the spring and summer. Pathogenic amebae were isolated year-round from aquatic water samples in the Tulsa, Oklahoma, area. Of 34 isolates, 38 percent were *Naegleria,* 38 percent were *Acanthamoeba,* and 9 percent were leptomyxid *(Balamuthia)*. Acquisition of *Acanthamoeba* and leptomyxid amebae probably occurs from contact with or inhalation of contaminated water or soil. Patients are usually debilitated or immunocompromised but may not have any history or indication of immunosuppression. Keratitis occurs from contaminated cleaning solutions for care of contact lenses and has been reported in wearers of both hard and soft lenses. The number of human infections caused by *Naegleria, Balamuthia,* and *Acanthamoeba* has increased dramatically. In 1996, 166 cases of granulomatous amebic encephalitis were reported, 103 caused by *Acanthamoeba* and 63 caused by *Balamuthia*. Seventy-two of these cases were reported in the United States.[49]

The Organisms

Amebae are not obligate parasites of humans, and the exact host factors that facilitate parasitic invasion are not well understood. Factors that contribute to virulence include the immune status of the host and the virulence properties of the organism, such as adherence, complement resistance,

*Deceased

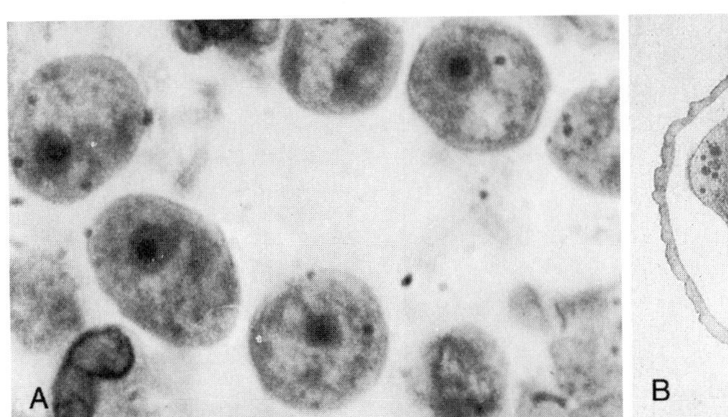

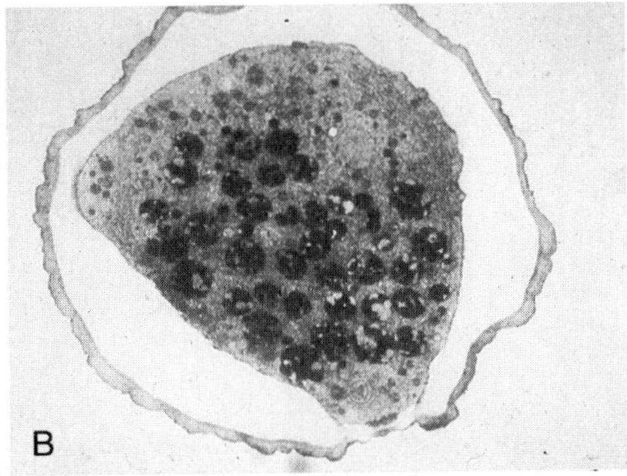

FIGURE 221–1 ■ *A,* Trophozoite of *Acanthamoeba. B,* Cyst of *Acanthamoeba* (scanning electron micrograph). (*A* from Jager, B. V., and Stamm, W. P.: Brain abscesses caused by free-living amoeba probably of the genus *Hartmannella* living in a patient with Hodgkin disease. Lancet *2*:1343–1345, 1972. © by The Lancet Ltd., 1972.)

cytopathic enzymes, and migration ability.[11, 39, 71] The genera *Naegleria* and *Acanthamoeba,* as well as *Balamuthia,* have been isolated from humans. Classification of these organisms has been described by Page[53] and Chang.[14]

Acanthamoeba is found as a trophozoite and cyst (Fig. 221–1). The trophozoite has multiple pseudopods with explosive movement of stellate extrusions of the cytoplasm and very little progressive motility. The cyst is smaller and has two distinct thick walls: an inner polyhedral or stellate cyst and an outer wall with an irregular shape. Both forms may be found in tissue[5, 64] (see Fig. 221–1). Species implicated in human disease include *Acanthamoeba culbertsoni, Acanthamoeba polyphaga, Acanthamoeba castellani,* and *Acanthamoeba astronyxis.*

Only the trophozoite of *Naegleria* is found in tissue or cerebrospinal fluid (CSF). The organism is 10 to 20 mm in size and has a large central nuclear karyosome. Progressive slow motility of the pseudopods may be noted on a warm saline preparation or in CSF (Fig. 221–2). The organism also may exist in a flagellate form when exposed to certain environmental conditions, such as instillation into fresh warm water (Fig. 221–3). Small cysts with a single outer wall rarely are seen.

The leptomyxid ameba *Balamuthia* is found in stagnant water and may be transmitted like *Acanthamoeba.* The portal of entry has been speculated to be the oral mucosa, skin, or respiratory tract, with subsequent hematogenous spread.[74] It may be seen in tissue as a trophozoite or cyst. The trophozoites are similar to those of *Acanthamoeba* (Fig. 221–4). The cyst may appear to have a double cyst wall similar to that of *Acanthamoeba;* however, electron microscopy reveals that the cyst has three walls (see Fig. 221–1). *Acanthamoeba* and *Naegleria* can be grown on nonnutrient agar with a lawn of bacteria, whereas *Balamuthia* can be cultured only in tissue culture cells.[36]

Some evidence indicates that *Acanthamoeba* may serve as a reservoir for *Legionella pneumophila.* Amebae isolated from sites of water collection in a hospital were found to have phagocytized the bacterial organisms. *Haemophilus influenzae* also may cohabitate with amebae, which supply necessary growth factors for the bacteria. Thus, these potentially pathogenic amebae may serve as a vector for both of these organisms within the respiratory tract.[1, 80]

Clinical Manifestations

NAEGLERIA FOWLERI

Infection with *N. fowleri* occurs in patients 5 to 15 days after bathing or swimming in warm, untreated water. Most people who have contracted the disease have been young, healthy individuals in their first, second, or third decades of life.[63] The exact factors responsible for development of disease in some individuals are unknown. Although many

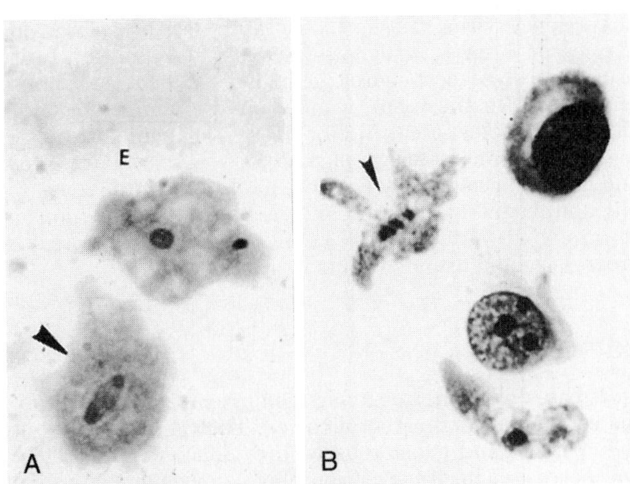

FIGURE 221–2 ■ *A* and *B,* Trophozoites of *Naegleria.*

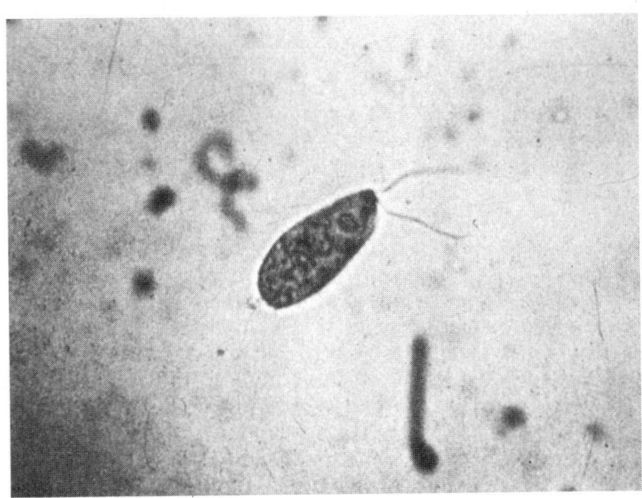

FIGURE 221–3 ■ Flagellate form of *Naegleria fowleri.*

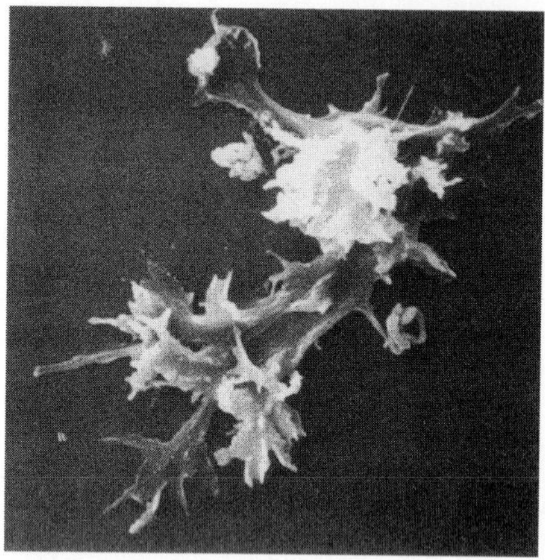
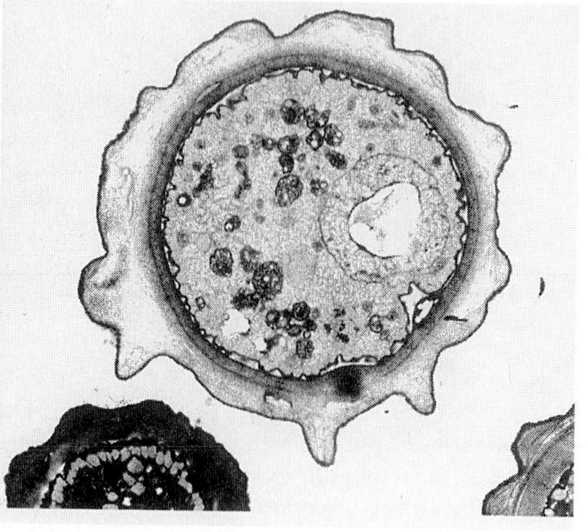

FIGURE 221–4 ■ Trophozoite and cyst of *Balamuthia mandrillaris*. (Courtesy of Dr. G. S. Visvesvara, Centers for Disease Control and Prevention.)

individuals may be exposed to contaminated water, illness develops in very few.[31] Invasive disease may be caused by predisposing factors such as the immune status of the host or by predisposing pathology such as inflammation or trauma to the respiratory tract. Strain differences in amebae also may play a role in the pathobiology of infection.

The prodrome is usually nonspecific and may consist of headache, fever, nausea, vomiting, and malaise. It may progress rapidly to meningitis with nuchal rigidity, abnormal reflexes, papilledema, seizures, and altered level of consciousness. Death may occur quickly unless the patient receives early diagnosis and treatment. This disease has no distinguishing characteristics to separate it from fulminant bacterial meningitis, except for a history of recent exposure to a warm body of water. Laboratory data are not helpful in distinguishing it from bacterial disease, except for the presence of amebae in CSF.

ACANTHAMOEBA

Acanthamoeba has been associated with primary amebic meningoencephalitis, granulomatous amebic encephalitis, and other infections. The organism has been isolated from chronic otitis media, skin, lungs, and patients with keratitis.[41, 50, 79] Those who contract granulomatous amebic encephalitis are usually very young, old, debilitated, immunosuppressed, or chronically ill.[52] The course of the disease is indolent, with acute, subacute, or chronic symptoms, including headache, nausea, vomiting, fever, somnolence, seizures, aphasia, hemiparesis, behavioral changes, and a clinical picture of encephalitis.[20] In some cases, the signs and symptoms resemble a tumor or space-occupying lesion of the brain.[32] Patients initially may have a chronic skin lesion that is culture-negative for bacteria and fungi. The lesion may be vesicular and pustular and increase in size until it becomes a large area of nodular indurated tissue with superficial ulcerations. Amebae are found in the skin and may serve as a nidus for later invasion of the central nervous system (CNS).[29] Organisms also have been recovered from cases of osteomyelitis and from the lungs and sinuses.[28, 41, 44]

Most patients who contract *Acanthamoeba* keratitis are healthy individuals who wear contact lenses. All types of lenses, including disposable soft and extended-wear lenses, have been implicated in infection. All contact lenses contain water, which serves as a medium for oxygen exchange. The water content of soft lenses is 50 to 75 percent. Thus, contact lenses can absorb pathogens, including bacteria and amebae, from cleaning solutions, carrying cases, hands, and water.[4, 11] When the lens comes in contact with contaminated water, amebae quickly adhere to the lens surface. If corneal trauma is present, the organisms invade the corneal tissue and produce infection[37] (Fig. 221–5). Persons who do not wear contact lenses also may be infected if they have corneal trauma and come in contact with contaminated water. The nidus for infection most likely is trauma to the cornea, but it also may be related to infection with herpesvirus or bacterial conjunctivitis. Symptoms may appear rapidly or after several weeks. Patients usually complain of a unilateral red eye, a foreign body sensation, tearing, photophobia, or severe pain. Often, the diagnosis is made in persons with keratitis who fail to respond to the usual antibacterial therapy. The disease may progress rapidly if not recognized and treated, and a deeply penetrating keratitis may lead to loss of the cornea. In addition, the infection has been associated with the complications of iritis, cataracts, hypopyon, glaucoma, scleritis, and penetrating keratitis.[6]

BALAMUTHIA

Chronic granulomatous encephalitis caused by leptomyxid amebae has no distinguishing clinical features. Patients may or may not be immunosuppressed or chronically ill and will have headache, meningismus, nausea, vomiting, seizures, and focal neurologic signs. Neuroimaging studies may show a hyperdense, space-occupying lesion that can be confused with a brain abscess or tumor. Cases have been reported in previously normal individuals.[40, 56–58] Multiple areas of the brain may be involved, and the condition may mimic fungal and bacterial abscesses in patients infected with human immunodeficiency virus. Tissue biopsy and electron microscopy may be necessary to diagnose infection. The clinical picture usually involves focal neurologic findings and may resemble a mass lesion in the brain. Cranial nerve findings, including sixth nerve palsy, occur in 50 percent of patients. CSF findings show a mononuclear pleocytosis with elevated protein and normal or low-normal glucose levels. Computed tomography and magnetic resonance imaging demonstrate lesions in the gray and white matter. The infection may be indolent or progressive and usually results in death.[60]

Pathology

Most cases of primary amebic meningoencephalitis involve the cerebellum and cerebral cortex. The tissue is generally soft, friable, and edematous with evidence of hemorrhage and necrosis. Uncal herniation may be evident. A purulent exudate may be seen on the brain surface and may be particularly prominent over the sulci and basal cisternae; the

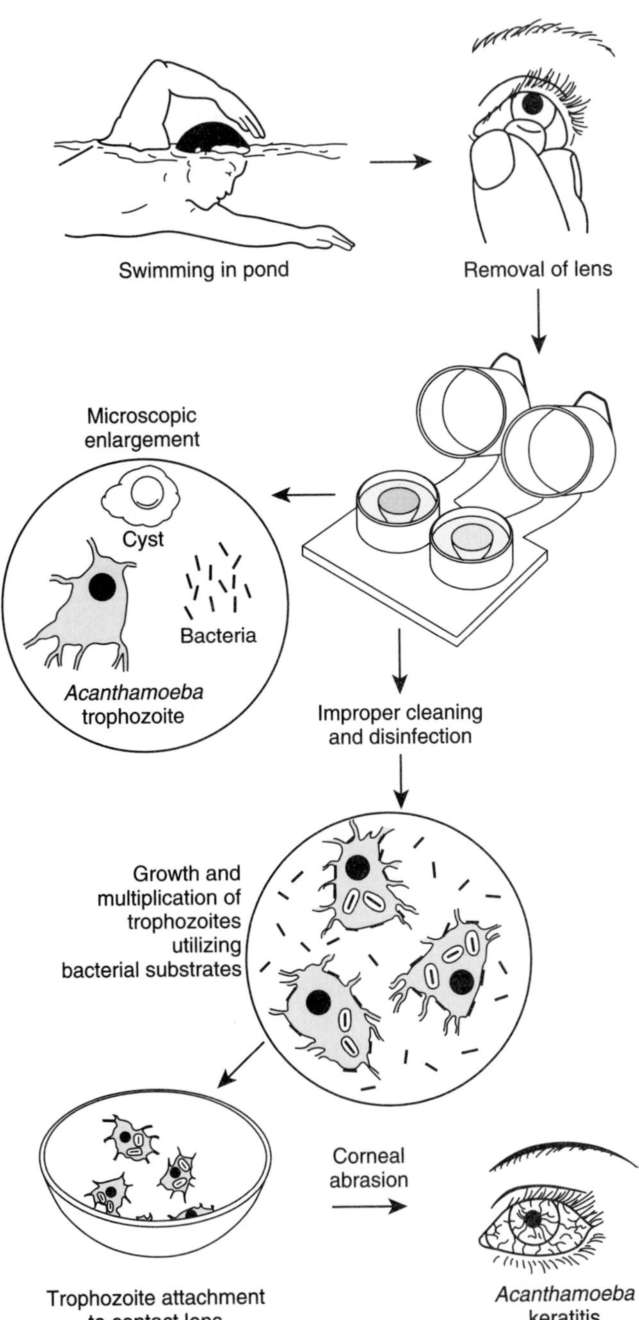

FIGURE 221–5 ■ Proposed mechanism for *Acanthamoeba* keratitis. Bacterial contaminants in the water on the lens support the growth of amebae, which leads to an increased number of invading organisms. The organisms adhere to the contact lens and enter tissue through the damaged cornea, with the subsequent development of keratitis.

olfactory bulbs may be necrotic (Fig. 221–6). The spinal cord often demonstrates necrotizing hemorrhagic myelitis. Microscopic examination of the tissue shows an acute meningeal and encephalitic inflammatory exudate of mononuclear and polymorphonuclear leukocytes that is prominent in the areas of the basal cistern, sulci, and sylvian fissures. The exudate may widen the Virchow-Robin spaces and extend into the cortex.[46]

Lesions of the brain, lungs, eyes, and skin can be associated with *Acanthamoeba* infection. The cerebral hemispheres have a mild focal edema with areas of necrosis and hemorrhage. Narrowing of the sulci and flattening of the gyri are

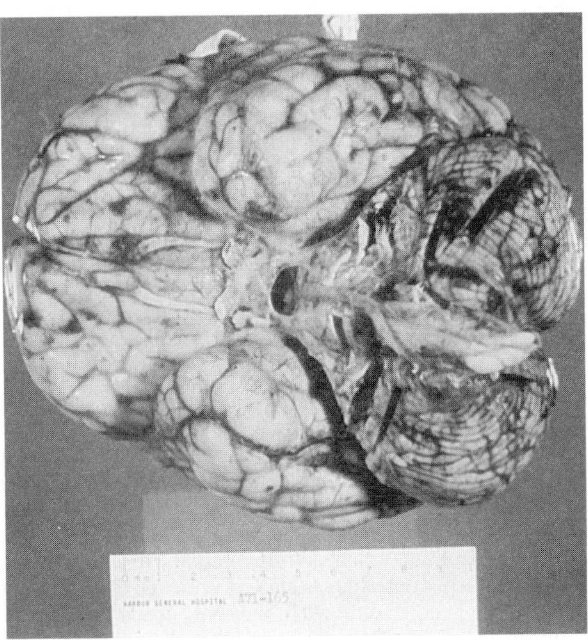

FIGURE 221–6 ■ Brain from a fatal case of *Naegleria* meningoencephalitis. Note the areas of necrosis on the basalar surface of the brain.

noted in areas of active infection. Other areas of the cerebral cortex may appear normal. The CNS lesions are associated with a chronic granulomatous reaction consisting of collections of macrophages and necrotic foci in the walls of arteries and arterioles, all of which suggest angiitis. The lesions may resemble brain abscesses. Both cysts and trophozoites are seen within brain tissue. Amebae may be observed in groups with little or no surrounding inflammatory reaction.[45] Trophozoites and cysts may be present in the alveoli, accompanied by a mononuclear cellular infiltrate. Skin lesions may be nodular and ulcerative, with subcutaneous inflammation and the formation of abscesses. Cysts and trophozoites are seen within the affected tissue.[45] A similar reaction may be detected in ulcerations of the cornea.[75]

Balamuthia is found in brain tissue in association with coagulation necrosis of gray and white matter, chronic perivascular inflammation, and microglial nodules in the white matter. Usually, diffuse cerebral edema with hemorrhagic necrotic lesions is present in the cortical lobar white matter, brain stem, and cerebellar deep white matter. Lesions may be seen in the hippocampus, temporal gyri, midbrain, and cerebellum.[19]

Laboratory Diagnosis

Routine laboratory tests do not distinguish amebic infection of the CNS from other causes of meningoencephalitis. The white blood cell count usually is elevated, with a preponderance of neutrophils and bands. Serum electrolyte analysis may be normal or show evidence of inappropriate secretion of antidiuretic hormone. Analysis of CSF reveals an elevated protein level with a normal or low glucose level and a pleocytosis with a high count of white and red blood cells. In granulomatous encephalitis, a mononuclear pleocytosis occurs, and organisms generally are not found on wet mount.[60]

The diagnosis of *B. mandrillaris* encephalitis should be considered when a previously healthy individual has focal or multifocal CNS lesions radiographically resembling infarcts. Definitive diagnosis is made by brain biopsy of the lesion. The periphery of the identified lesion may not contain amebae, and thus the site for biopsy must be chosen carefully.[21, 60]

DIRECT MICROSCOPIC IDENTIFICATION

Naegleria organisms may be identified on wet-mount examination of CSF by their morphology and motility. CSF should be kept warm before examination and should not be refrigerated. It should be placed directly on a slide with a coverslip or first gently centrifuged at 150 *g* for 5 minutes. The supernatant should be placed on a slide and covered with a No. 1 coverslip. Small (8- to 20-μm) trophozoites with progressive motility can be seen.[54] The cytoplasm may appear granular, and the nucleus is large and has a dense central karyosome (Fig. 221–7). One should note that activated macrophages often extrude pseudopods and may be mistaken for amebae. The supernatant also can be fixed for electron microscopy or dried on slides for staining. To ensure that the organism adheres to the slide, a drop of CSF should be placed in polyvinyl alcohol and smeared onto a slide. As an alternative method, a gelatin-coated glass slide may be used, or the dried specimen may be fixed with several drops of warmed Schaudinn solution. Wright, Giemsa, and trichrome stains may be used to stain the organism for identification. Tissue should be processed rapidly, fixed, and stained with hematoxylin and eosin. Gram stain is not useful in making the diagnosis because it often fails to stain the nuclear structure. The ultrastructure of the organism is well described, and material can be processed for electron microscopy by placing it in chilled 2.5 percent glutaraldehyde. The trophozoite shows an irregular cell border and a distinct polar orientation, with one end of the cell characterized by a uniformly appearing blunt or rounded pseudopod. The cell contains many vacuoles and a large nucleus with a prominent, dense central nucleolus. Numerous ribosomes and food vacuoles and occasional mitochondria that may or may not be dumbbell shaped are present.[31, 46]

B. *mandrillaris* trophozoites range in size from 12 to 60 μm (mean, 30 μm), are irregularly shaped, and sometimes have branched cytoplasm. They are uninucleated with a 5-μm nucleus and centrally located nucleolus. The cyst appears to have a double wall on light microscopy, but electron micrographs reveal that it has three layers.

Corneal scrapings may be stained with calcofluor white, which gives a fluorescence to the cysts of *Acanthamoeba*.[82] Indirect fluorescent antibody staining also may be performed for *Acanthamoeba* and *Naegleria*.

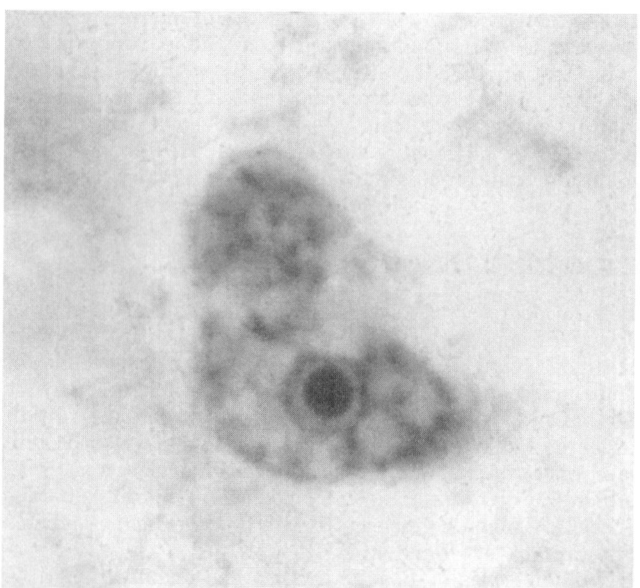

FIGURE 221–7 ■ Trichrome stain of a trophozoite of *Naegleria fowleri*.

CULTURE OF *NAEGLERIA* AND *ACANTHAMOEBA*

Naegleria may be cultured from CSF and tissue. CSF should be centrifuged at 2 *g* for 10 minutes. The supernatant should be removed and placed on a non-nutrient agar plate that has been covered with a suspension of *Escherichia coli* or *Enterobacter aerogenes*.[66] Tissue that has been ground up in sterile fashion may be planted on the same type of agar plate. Amebae will feed on the bacterial lawn and be isolated easily. *Acanthamoeba* can be cultured in a similar manner. A culture amplification technique for recovery of *Acanthamoeba* from corneal scrapings has been described.[11] Transformation of the cyst form in culture occurs after a few days, when the nutrient bacteria are not prevalent. Axenic culture techniques have been described by Nelson. Material also may be placed in monolayer cell cultures of monkey kidney, MRC human embryonic lung cells, and HeLa cells.[48, 64, 76] Transformation to the flagellate form may be accomplished by dropping the organisms into distilled water for several hours. Unlike *Naegleria* and *Acanthamoeba, Balamuthia* will not grow on non-nutrient agar and must be grown in tissue culture with E6 monkey kidney cells, MRC-5, or Hep-2 cells.

SEROLOGY

Routine commercial tests are not available. However, the Centers for Disease Control and Prevention will perform an indirect immunofluorescent antibody and immunoperoxidase test on the organism.

ANTIGENIC AND ISOENZYME ANALYSIS

Organisms can be classified by antigenic analysis with the use of gel diffusion, immunoelectrophoresis, immunofluorescence, and immunoblot assays (Figs. 221–8 and 221–9). Amebae also may be processed for isoenzyme analysis, which can distinguish the genera and species of amebae.[25, 48, 76, 77]

Treatment

NAEGLERIA MENINGOENCEPHALITIS

Meningoencephalitis caused by free-living amebae is a medical emergency. Only a few patients have survived, and treatment regimens have varied.[9, 54] Strain differences and host immunity probably play a role in the pathogenicity of the organism. Pathogenic strains of the organism are resistant to complement-mediated cell damage. In addition, early diagnosis and institution of therapy may have played a role in the handful of patients who have been treated successfully.

Several drugs have been shown to be active against *Naegleria* in vitro,[22] including amphotericin B, miconazole, and rifamycin.[12, 34, 70, 81] Synergism between drugs also has been demonstrated in vitro with tetracycline and amphotericin B and with amphotericin B and miconazole.[64, 70] Antagonism

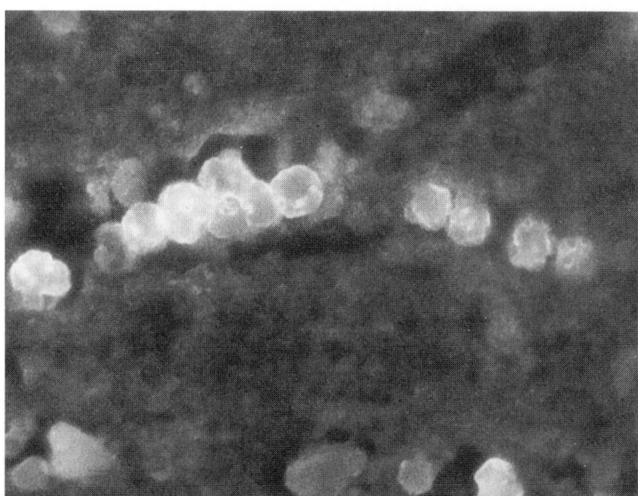

FIGURE 221–8 ■ Indirect fluorescent antibody examination of *Naegleria fowleri.* (Courtesy of Govinda S. Visvesvara, Centers for Disease Control and Prevention.)

between the two latter drugs has been demonstrated against *Candida albicans.*[61]

Therapy has included high-dose intravenous amphotericin B at 1 to 1.5 mg/kg/day alone or in combination with other drugs, including miconazole, rifampin, sulfa drugs, and tetracycline.[42] In addition, intrathecal amphotericin was used in one patient. Intrathecal drugs given via a cisternal reservoir have resulted in cerebral hypertension and death.

ACANTHAMOEBA INFECTION OF THE CENTRAL NERVOUS SYSTEM

Acanthamoeba infection of the CNS is difficult to treat because of the presence of cysts in tissue that are relatively resistant to chemotherapeutic agents. Immunosuppressed patients with disseminated disease have a poor prognosis. Both necrotizing acute meningoencephalitis and chronic granulomatous disease may respond to sulfadiazine and other sulfa drugs. However, the effects of therapy are inconsistent, and death often ensues in spite of therapy. Recovery from infection of the CNS has been reported after treatment with chloramphenicol and co-trimoxazole.[65] An immunosuppressed patient was treated successfully with intravenous pentamidine isethionate, topical chlorhexidine, and 2 percent ketoconazole cream, followed by oral itraconazole.[68]

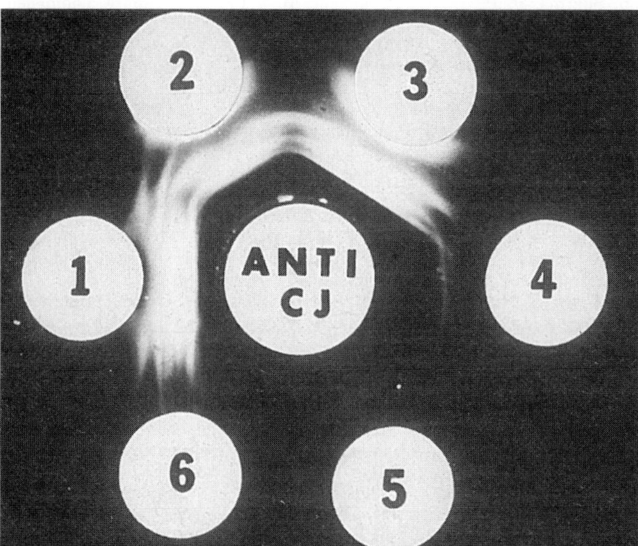

FIGURE 221–9 ■ Gel diffusion pattern showing the interaction between anti-CJ serum and the following amebae: (1) CJ strain of *Naegleria fowleri,* (2) HBSW pathogenic strain of *N. fowleri,* (3) HBC-1 California strain of *N. fowleri,* (4) and (5) EG strain of *Naegleria gruberi* (nonpathogenic), and (6) normal saline. (Courtesy of G. S. Visvesvara, Centers for Disease Control and Prevention.)

ACANTHAMOEBA KERATITIS

Medical treatment of keratitis has been inconsistent, and chemotherapy often is combined with surgical treatment. Cures have been reported with the use of 0.1 percent propamidine isethionate; a combination of chlorhexidine and propamidine; propamidine, neomycin, and polyhexamethylene biguanide; or propamidine isethionate, neomycin sulfate, and co-trimoxazole.[2, 8, 18, 30, 73, 84] Recently, a large number of patients were treated successfully with 0.02 percent topical polyhexamethylene biguanide.[23] Penetrating keratoplasty has been combined successfully with medical therapy to control infections that were severe or resistant to therapy.[7, 24] Topical or systemic corticosteroid therapy is contraindicated and results in severe complications.[69] Successful therapy for keratitis depends on early diagnosis and rapid intensive medical or surgical therapy (or both) directed at killing the cysts in tissue, removing infected tissue, and preventing secondary bacterial infections.

BALAMUTHIA

Treatment of *Balamuthia* infection remains empirical. Cases have been treated with miconazole, flucytosine, amphotericin, and ketoconazole with mixed results. Steroids are thought to be contraindicated.[21, 60]

REFERENCES

1. Allen, S. D., Place, D. A., and Culbertson C. G.: In vitro interaction of *Acanthamoeba* and *Haemophilus influenzae.* J. Protozool. *37*:48A–49A, 1990.
2. Alpuche-Arnada, C., and Santos Preciado, J. I.: Infeccion del sistema nervioso central de origen oscuro: Meningoencefalitis ambiana. Bol. Med. Hosp. Infect. Mex. *46*:581, 1989.
3. Andrelini, P., Przepiorka, D., Luna, M, et al.: *Acanthamoeba* meningoencephalitis after bone marrow transplantation. Bone Marrow Transplant. *14*:450–461, 1994.
4. Asbell, P. A.: *Acanthamoeba* keratitis: There and back again. Mount Sinai Med. J. *60*:279–282, 1993.
5. Ash, L. R., and Orihel, T. C.: Atlas of Human Parasitology. 3rd ed. Chicago, American Society of Clinical Pathologists, 1990.
6. Auran, J. D., Starr, M. B., and Jakobiec, F. A.: *Acanthamoeba* keratitis: A review of the literature. Cornea *6*:2–26, 1987.
7. Bacon, A. S., Frazer, D. G., Dart, J. K., et al.: A review of 72 consecutive cases of *Acanthamoeba* keratitis. Eye *7*:719–725, 1993.
8. Brasseur, G., Favennec, L., Perrine D., et al.: Successful treatment of *Acanthamoeba* keratitis by hexamindine. Cornea *13*:459–462, 1994.
9. Brown, R. L.: Successful treatment of primary amoebic meningoencephalitis. Arch. Intern. Med. *151*:1201–1202, 1991.
10. Butt, C. G.: Primary meningoencephalitis. N. Engl. J. Med. *274*: 1473–1476, 1966.
11. Buttone, E. J.: Free-living amoebas of the genera *Acanthamoeba* and *Naegleria*: An overview of basic microbiologic correlates. Mount Sinai Med. J. *60*:260–269, 1993.
12. Carter, R. F.: Sensitivity to amphotericin B of a *Naegleria* species isolated from a case of primary amoebic meningoencephalitis. J. Clin. Pathol. *22*:472–474, 1969.
13. Cerva, L., Novak, K., and Culbertson, C. G.: An outbreak of acute fatal amoebic meningoencephalitis. Am. J. Epidemiol. *88*:336–344, 1968.

14. Chang, S. L.: Small free-living amoebas: Cultivation, quantitation, identification, classification, pathogenesis, and resistance. Curr. Top. Comp. Pathobiol. *1*:201–254, 1971.
15. Culbertson, C. G., Ensminger, P. W. and Overton, W. M.: The isolation of additional strains of pathogenic *Hartmannella* sp.: Proposed culture method for application of biological material. Am. J. Pathol. *35*:383–387, 1965.
16. Culbertson, C. G., Smith, J. W., Cohen, H. K., et al.: Experimental infection of mice and monkeys by *Acanthamoeba*. Am. J. Pathol. *35*:185–197, 1959.
17. Culbertson, C. G, Smith, J. W., and Minner, J. D.: *Acanthamoeba* observation on animal pathogenicity. Science *127*:1506, 1958.
18. D'Aversa, G., Stern, G. A., and Driebe, W. T., Jr.: Diagnosis and successful medical treatment of *Acanthamoeba* keratitis. Arch. Opthalmol. *113*:1120–1123, 1995.
19. Denney C. F., Iragui, V. J., Uber-Zak, L. D., et al.: Amoebic meningocephalitis caused by *Balamuthia mandrillaris:* Case report and review Clin. Infect. Dis. *25*:1354–1358, 1997.
20. Di Gregorio, C., Rivasi, F., Mongiardo, N. et al.: *Acanthamoeba* meningoencephalitis in a patient with acquired immunodeficiency syndrome. Arch. Pathol. Lab. Med. *116*:1363–1365, 1992.
21. Duke, B. J., Tyson, R. W., DeBiasi, R., et al.: *Balamuthis mandrillaris* meningoencephalitis presenting with acute hyrodcephalis Pediatr. Neurosurg. *26*:107–111, 1997.
22. Duma, R. J., and Finley, R.: In vitro susceptibility of pathogenic *Naegleria* and *Acanthamoeba* species to a variety of chemotherapeutic agents. Antimicrob. Agents Chemother. *10*:370–376, 1976.
23. Elder, M. J., and Dart, K.: Chemotherapy for *Acanthamoeba* keratitis. Lancet *345*:791–792, 1995.
24. Ficker, L. A., Kirkness, C., and Wright, P.: Prognosis for keratoplasty in *Acanthamoeba* keratitis. Ophthalmology *100*:105–110, 1993.
25. Flores, B. M., Garcia, C. A., Stamm, W. E., et al.: Differentiation of *Naegleria fowleri* from *Acanthamoeba* species by using monoclonal antibodies and flow cytometry. J. Clin. Microbiol. *28*:1999–2002, 1990.
26. Fowler, M., and Carter, R. F.: Acute pyogenic meningitis probably due to *Acanthamoeba* sp.: A preliminary report. B. M. J. *2*:740–742, 1965.
27. Friedland, L. R., Rapheal, S. A., Deutsch, E. S., et al.: Disseminated *Acanthamoeba* infection in a child with symptomatic human immunodeficiency virus infection. Pediatr. Infect. Dis. J. *11*:404–407, 1993.
28. Gonzalez, M. D., Gould, E., Dickinson, G., et al.: Acquired immunodeficiency syndrome associated with *Acanthamoeba* and other opportunistic organisms. Arch. Pathol. Lab. Med. *110*:749–751, 1986.
29. Gutierrez, Y.: Diagnostic Pathology of Parasitic Infections with Clinical Correlations. Philadelphia, Lea & Febiger, 1990.
30. Hay, J., Kirkness, C. M., Seal, D. V., et al.: Drug resistance and *Acanthamoeba* keratitis: The quest for alternative antiprotozoal chemotherapy. Eye *8*:555–563, 1994.
31. Hecht, R. H., and Cohen, A. H.: Primary amoebic meningoencephalitis in California. West. J. Med. *117*:69–73, 1972.
32. Jager, B. V., and Stamm, W. P.: Brain abscesses caused by a free-living amoeba, probably of the genus *Hartmannella* in a patient with Hodgkin's disease. Lancet *2*:1343–1345, 1972.
33. Jahnes, W. G., Fullmer H. M., and Li, C. P.: Free-living amoebae as contaminants in monkey tissue culture. Proc. Soc. Exp. Biol. Med. *96*: 484–488, 1957.
34. Jamison, A.: The effects of clotrimazole on *Naegleria fowleri*. J. Clin. Pathol. *28*:446, 1975.
35. Jarmillo-Rodriguez, Y., Chavez-Macias, L. G., Olvera-Rabich, J. E., et al.: Encefalitis por una nueva amiba di vida libre, probablemente *Leptomyxid*. Patologia *27*:137–141, 1989.
36. John, D. T., and Howard, M. J.: Seasonal distribution of pathogenic free-living amoebae in Oklahoma waters. Parasitol. Res. *81*:193–201, 1995.
37. John, T., Desai, D., and Sahm, D.: Adherence of *Acanthamoeba castellani* cysts and trophozoites to unworn soft contact lenses. Am. J. Ophthalmol. *108*:658–664, 1989.
38. Katz, J. D., Ropper, A. H., Adelman, L., et al.: A case of *Balamuthia mandrillaris* meningoencephalitis. Arch. Neurol. *57*:1210–1212, 2000.
39. Kilvington, S., and Beeching, J.: Identification and epidemiological typing of *Naegleria fowleri* with DNA probes. Appl. Environ. Microbiol. *61*: 2071–2078, 1995.
40. Kodet, R., Nohynkova, E., Tichy, M., et al.: Amoebic encephalitis caused by *Balmuthia mandrillaris* in a Czech child: Description of the first case from Europe. Pathol. Res. Pract. *194*:423–429, 1998.
41. Lengy, J., Jakovljevich, R., and Talis, B.: Recovery of hartmannelloid amoeba from purulent ear discharge. Trop. Dis. Bull. *68*:818–819, 1971.
42. Loschiavo, F., Ventura-Spangolo, T., Sessa, E., et al.: Acute primary meningoencephalitis from entamoeba *Naegleria fowleri*: Report of a clinical case with a favorable outcome. Acta. Neurol. *15*:330–340, 1993.
43. Ma, P., Visvesvara, G. S., Martinez, A. J., et al.: *Naegleria* and *Acanthamoeba* infection. Rev. Infect. Dis. *12*:490–513, 1990.
44. Martinez, A. J.: Free Living Amoebas: Natural History, Prevention, Diagnosis, Pathology and Treatment of Disease. Boca Raton, FL, C. R. C. Press, 1985.
45. Martinez, A. J.: Free living amoebas: Infection of the central nervous system. Mount Sinai J. Med. *60*:271–278, 1993.
46. Martinez, A. J., dos Santos Neto, J. G., Nelson, E. C., et al.: Primary amoebic meningoencephalitis. Pathol. Ann. *2*:225–250, 1977.
47. Martinez, A. J., Guerra, A. E., Garcia-Tamayo, J., et al.: Granulomatous amoebic encephalitis: A review and report of a spontaneous case from Venezuela. Acta Neuropathol. *87*:430–434, 1994.
48. Martinez, A. J., and Visvesvara, G. S.: Laboratory diagnosis of pathogenic free-living amoebas: *Naegleria, Acanthamoeba* and Leptomyxida. Clin. Lab. Med. *11*:861–872, 1991.
49. Martinez, A. J., and Visvesvara, G. S.: Free-living amphizoic and opportunistic amoebas. Brain Pathol. *7*:583–598, 1997.
50. Moore, M. B., and McCulley, J. P.: *Acanthamoeba* keratitis associated with contact lenses: Six consecutive cases of successful management. Br. J. Ophthalmol. *73*:271–275, 1989.
51. Newsome, A. L., Curtis, F. T., and Culbertson C. G., et al.: Identification of *Acanthamoeba* in broncholalveolar lavage specimens. Diagn. Cytopathol. *8*:231–134, 1992.
52. Ofori-Kwakye, S. K., Sidebottom, D. G., Herbert, J., et al.: Granulomatous brain tumor caused by *Acanthamoeba*: Case report. J. Neurosurg. *64*:505–509, 1986.
53. Page, F. C.: Taxonomic criteria for limax amoebae with descriptions of three new species of *Hartmannella* and three of *Vahlkampfia*. J. Protozool. *14*:449–521, 1967.
54. Poungvarfian, N., and Jariya, P. L.: The fifth nonlethal case of primary amoebic meningoencephalitis. J. Med. Assoc. Thai. *74*:112–115, 1991.
55. Primary amebic meningoencephalitis—North Carolina, 1991. M. M. W. R. Morb. Mortal. Wkly. Rep. *41*(25):437–440, 1992.
56. Reed, R. P., Cooke-Yarborough, C. M., Jaquiery, A. L., et al.: Fatal granulomatous amoebic encephalitis caused by *Balamuthia mandrillaris*. Med. J. Aust. *167*:82–84, 1997.
57. Riestra-Castaneda, J. M., Riestra-Casteneda, R., Gonzalez-Garrido, A. A., et al.: Granulomatous amoebic encephalitis due to *Balmuthia mandrillaris* (Leptomyxidae): Report of four cases from Mexico. Am. J. Trop. Med. Hyg. *56*:603–607, 1997.
58. Rodriguez, R., Mendez, O., Molina, O., et al.: [Central nervous system infection by free-living amoebas: Report of 3 Venezuelan cases.] Rev. Neurol. *26*:1005–1008, 1998.
59. Rodriguez-Zaragosa, S.: Ecology of free-living amoebae. Crit. Rev. Microbiol. *20*:225–241, 1994.
60. Rowen, J. L., Doerr, C. A., Vogel, H., and Baker, C. J.: *Balmuthia mandrillaria:* A newly recognized agent for amoebic meningoencephalitis. Pediatr. Infect. Dis. J. *14*:705–710, 1995.
61. Schacter, L. P., Owellen R. J., Rathbun, H. K., et al.: Antagonism between miconazole and amphotericin B. Lancet *2*:318, 1976.
62. Schoeman, C. J., van der Vyver, A. E., and Visvesvara, G. S.: Primary amoebic meningo-encephalitis in southern Africa. J. Infect. *26*:211–214, 1993.
63. Seidel, J. S.: Primary amoebic meningoencephalitis. Pediatr. Clin. North Am. *32*:881–892, 1985.
64. Seidel, J. S., Harmatz, P., Visvesvara, G. S., et al.: Successful treatment of primary amoebic meningoencephalitis. N. Engl. J. Med. *30*:346–348, 1982.
65. Sharma, P. P., Gupta, P., Murali, M. V., et al.: Primary meningoencephalitis caused by *Acanthamoeba* successfully treated with cotrimoxazole. Indian Pediatr. *30*:1219–1222, 1993.
66. Singh, B. N.: Pathogenic and Non-Pathogenic Amoebae. New York, John Wiley & Sons, 1975.
67. Sison, J. P., Kemper, C. A., Loveless, M., et al.: Disseminated *Acanthamoeba* infection in patients with AIDS: Case reports and review. Clin. Infect. Dis. *20*:1207–1216, 1995.
68. Slater, C. A., Sickel, J. Z., Visvesvara, G. S., et al.: Brief report: Successful treatment of disseminated *Acanthamoeba* infection in an immunocompromised patient. N. Engl. J. Med. *331*:85–87, 1994.
69. Stern, G. A., and Buttross, M.: Use of corticosteroids in combination with antimicrobial drugs in the treatment of infectious corneal disease. Ophthalmology *98*:847–853, 1991.
70. Thong, Y. H., Rowan-Kelly, B., Shephard, C., et al.: Growth inhibition of *Naegleria fowleri* by tetracycline, rifamycin, and miconazole. Lancet *2*:876, 1977.
71. Toney, D. M., and Marciano-Cabral, F.: Modulation of complement resistance and virulence of *Naegleria fowleri* amoebae by alterations in growth media. J. Eukaryot. Microbiol. *41*:337–343, 1994.
72. Valenzuela, G., Lopez-Corella, E., and DeJonckheere, J. F.: Primary amoebic meningoencephalitis in a young male from northwestern Mexico. Trans. R. Soc. Trop. Med. Hyg. *78*:558–559, 1984.
73. Varga, J. H., Wolff, T. C., Jensen, H. G., et al.: Combined treatment of *Acanthamoeba* keratitis with propamidine, neomycin, and polyhexamethylene biguanide. Am. J. Ophthalmol. *115*:466–470, 1993.
74. Visvesvara, G. S.: Epidemiology of infections with free-living amoebas and laboratory diagnosis of microsporidiosis. Mt. Sinai J. Med. *60*:282–288, 1993.
75. Visvesvara, G. S., Jones, D. B., and Robinson, N. M.: Isolation, identification and biologic characterization of *Acanthamoeba polyphaga* from a human eye. Am. J. Trop. Med. Hyg. *24*:784–790, 1975.
76. Visvesvara, G. S., Mirra, S. S., Brandt, F. H., et al.: Isolation of two strains of *Acanthamoeba castellani* from human tissue and their pathogenicity and isoenzyme profiles. J. Clin. Microbiol. *18*:1405–1409, 1983.

77. Visvesvara, G. S., Peralta, M. J., Brandt, F. H., et al.: Production of monoclonal antibodies to *Naegleria fowleri,* agent of primary amoebic meningoencephalitis. J. Clin. Microbiol. *25*:1629–1631, 1987.
78. Visvesvara, G. C., Schuster, F. L., Martinez, A. J.: *Balamuthia mandrillaris.* N. G., N. Sp., agent of amoebic meningoencephalitis in humans and other animals. J. Eukaryot. Microbiol. *40*:504–514, 1993.
79. Visvesvara, G. S., and Stehr-Green, J. K.: Epidemiology of free-living amoeba infections. J. Protozool. *37*(Suppl.):25–33, 1990.
80. Wadowsky, R. M., Butler, L. J., Cook, M. K., et al.: Growth-supporting activity for *Legionella pneumophila* in tap water cultures and implication of Hartmannellid amoebae as growth factors. Appl. Environ. Microbiol. *54*:2677–2682, 1988.
81. Wang, A., Kay, R., Poon, W. S., et al.: Successful treatment of amoebic meningoencephalitis in a Chinese living in Hong Kong. Clin. Neurol. Neurosurg. *95*:249–252, 1993.
82. Wilhelmus, K. R., Osato, M. S., Font, R. L., et al.: Rapid diagnosis of *Acanthamoeba* keratitis using calcofluor white. Arch. Opthalmol. *104*: 1309–1321, 1986.
83. Willaert, E.: Primary amoebic meningoencephalitis: A selected bibliography and tabular survey of cases. Ann. Soc. Belg. Med. Trop. *54*: 429–440, 1974.
84. Wright, E., Warhurst, D., and Jones, B. R.: *Acanthamoeba* keratitis successfully treated medically. Br. J. Ophthalmol. *69*:778–782, 1985.

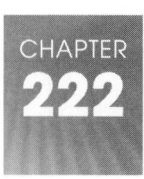

CHAPTER 222 Toxoplasmosis

KENNETH M. BOYER ■ JACK S. REMINGTON ■ RIMA L. McLEOD

Toxoplasma gondii is an obligate intracellular protozoan parasite (phylum Apicomplexa, class Sporozoasida, order Eucoccidiida). Infection may be clinically inapparent or result in disease. The disease produced by *T. gondii* is called toxoplasmosis. This parasite first was observed in 1908 by Nicolle and Manceaux[114, 115] in mononuclear cells in the spleen and liver of a North African rodent, the gundi *(Ctenodactylus gundi).* The organism soon was identified as a cause of disease in other animals,[150] and in 1923, Janku[68] first recognized a case in a human. He described a parasite found in the retina of an infant; it was recognized later by Levaditi[82] as *Toxoplasma.*

In 1937, Wolf and Cowen[159] reported a case of congenital granulomatous encephalitis that they considered to be caused by an "encephalitozoon." Sabin,[132] who previously had encountered *T. gondii* in guinea pigs, made the correct diagnosis. The discovery of *Toxoplasma* as a cause of disease acquired later in life has been credited to Pinkerton and Weinman,[119] who in 1940 described a generalized fatal illness caused by this organism in a young man. In retrospect, a case of acquired toxoplasmosis had been reported in 1908 by Darling.[35] In 1948, Sabin and Feldman[133] described a serologic test, the dye test, that allowed numerous investigators to study the epidemiologic and clinical aspects of toxoplasmosis and define the spectrum of disease in humans. Not until 1969, some 60 years after discovery of the parasite, did Frenkel and colleagues[46, 51, 53] establish that *Toxoplasma* was a coccidian protozoan and that its definitive host was the cat.

The Organism and Its Transmission

T. gondii exists in three forms, or stages: the proliferative stage, or *tachyzoite;* a tissue cyst that contains *bradyzoites;* and an oocyst, within which *sporozoites* develop. The cat family is the definitive host of the organism. The tachyzoite and tissue cyst are found in the extraintestinal tissues of cats, but they also are seen in other mammalian and avian hosts. The oocyst is formed during the intestinal epithelial stage of infection, exclusively in members of the cat family. Each stage of the organism has antigens in common with the other stages, as well as unique antigens. Many of these antigens have been cloned, sequenced, and localized to microanatomic structures.[100]

The tachyzoite form (Fig. 222–1*A* to *C*) is crescent shaped or oval, approximately 3 × 7 μm in size, and is seen during the acute stage of infection. It stains well with Wright or Giemsa stain. Ultrastructural features include the apical complex of microtubules and rings, secretory organelles called rhoptries, and a chloroplast-like structure with its own unique DNA.[23] Tachyzoites can invade all mammalian cells except perhaps non-nucleated red blood cells. They cannot withstand freezing and thawing, desiccation, or brief exposure to gastric or duodenal digestive juices. After penetration, the tachyzoite multiplies by endodyogeny, ultimately causing disruption of the cell.

The bradyzoite (see Fig. 222–1*D* to *F*) is able to persist in encysted form in all tissues and cause a chronic (latent) infection for the entire life span of the infected host. Cysts are demonstrable in tissues as early as the first week of infection and vary in size from approximately 10 to 100 μm. They have an argyrophilic wall but stand out most clearly from surrounding tissue when stained with periodic acid–Schiff stain. Usually, no inflammatory reaction occurs around cysts. Because this form may persist for many years in the tissues of clinically normal children and adults, its demonstration in histologic sections does not necessarily signify recent infection. Peptic or tryptic digestive fluids immediately disrupt the cyst wall, but the liberated bradyzoites (which resemble the tachyzoite form under light microscopy) can survive in these fluids for several hours, which allows time for invasion of local cells. The cyst is destroyed by heating to 66° C, by freezing (below –20° C) and thawing, and by desiccation. It can survive for some months at refrigeration temperatures (4° C) if it is in tissue. Therefore, infection in humans may be acquired by eating inadequately cooked meat that contains cysts (Fig. 222–2). In carnivorous animals, infection may be acquired by eating raw meat or prey species that contain encysted organisms.

The oocyst form (see Fig. 222–1*G* to *I*) is found only in feces of members of the cat family, the definitive host for *Toxoplasma,* and is the result of gametogony and schizogony, which occur in the intestinal epithelium.[66] The oocyst is ovoid and approximately 10 × 12 μm. Infected cats may shed as many as 10 million oocysts each day, which may be excreted for as long as 3 weeks after primary (acute) infection but rarely thereafter. Excreted oocysts become infectious only after they undergo sporulation (eight sporozoites form in each oocyst); sporulation occurs 1 to 21 days (most

TACHYZOITE (acute, active infection)

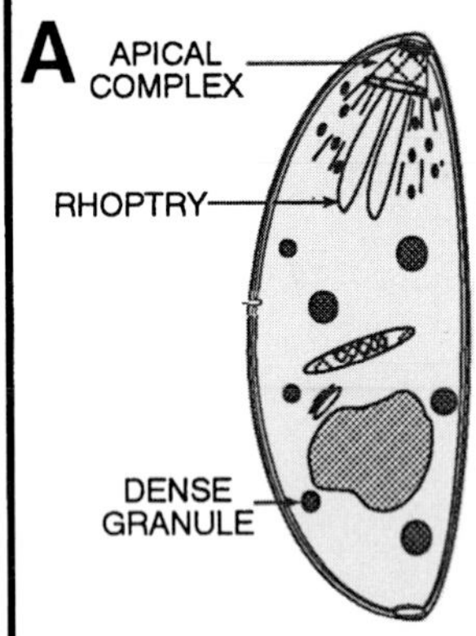

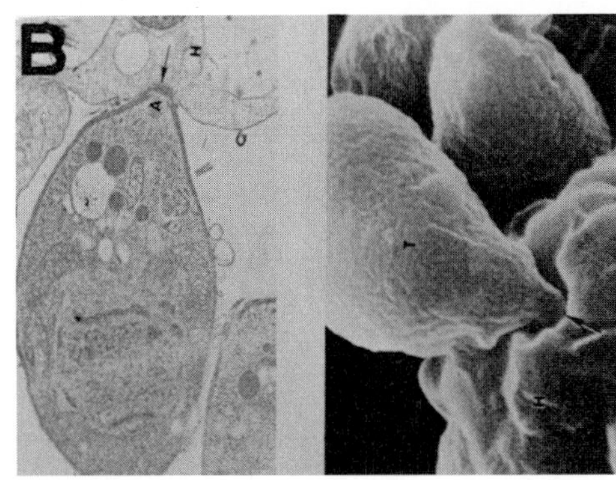

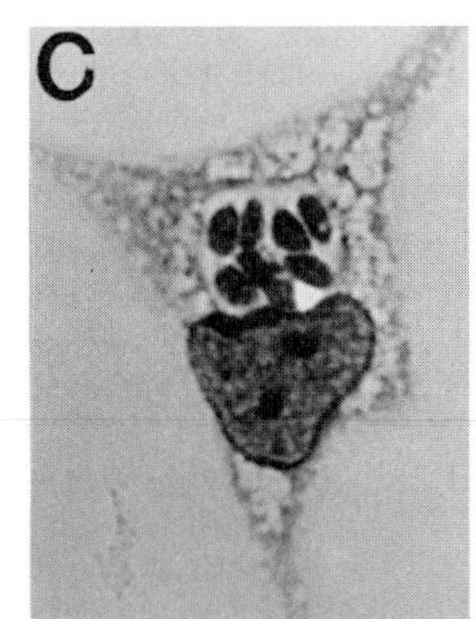

BRADYZOITE IN CYST (latent infection)

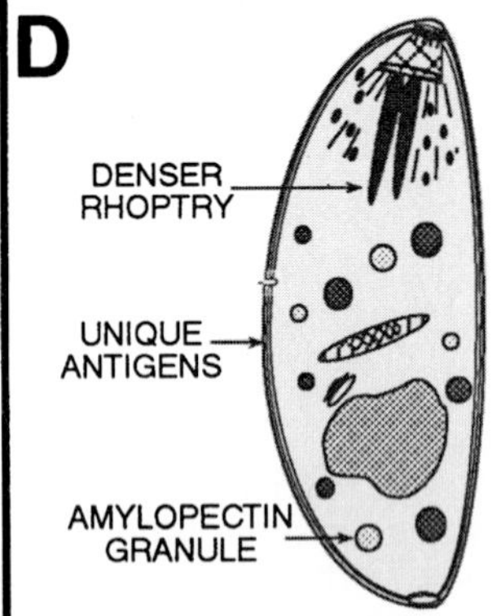

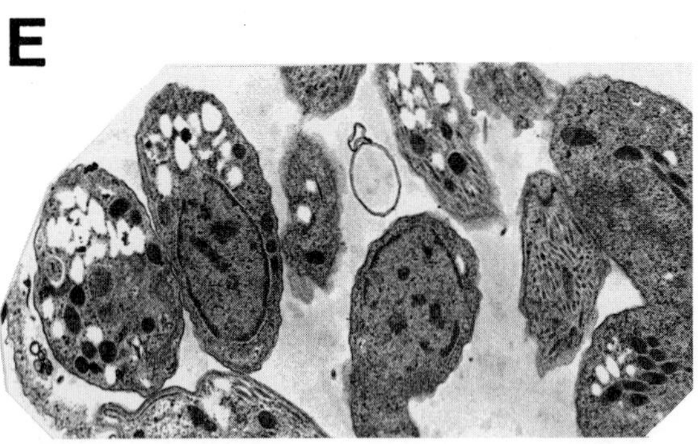

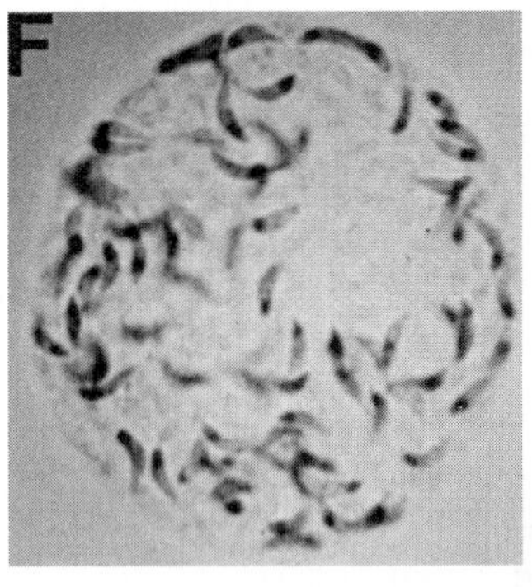

SPOROZOITE IN OOCYST (feline intestine and soil)

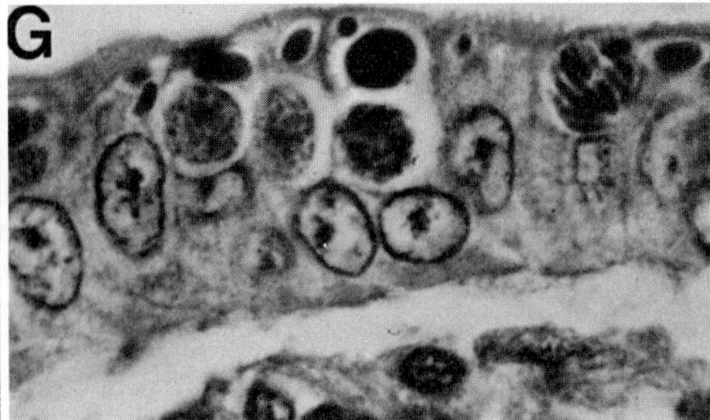

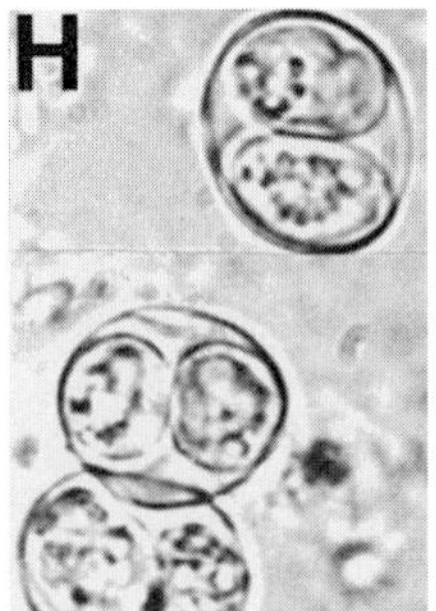

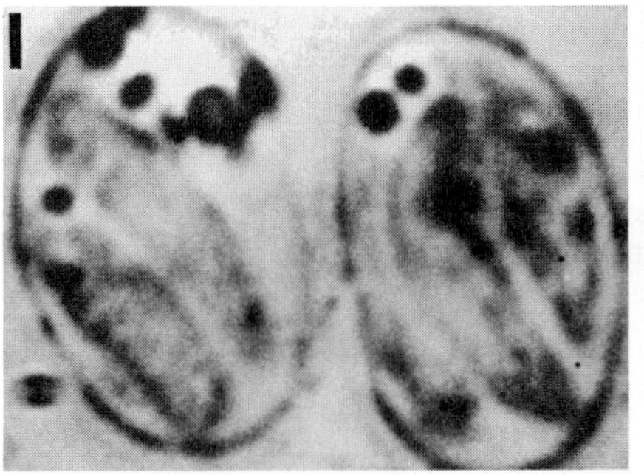

FIGURE 222–1 ■ Stages of *Toxoplasma gondii*. *A,* Schematic diagram of a tachyzoite. *B,* Transmission and scanning electron micrographs of a tachyzoite invading a host cell. *C,* Light micrograph of tachyzoites replicating within a parasitiferous vacuole in the host cell cytoplasm. *D,* Schematic diagram of a bradyzoite. *E,* Transmission electron micrograph of a cyst containing bradyzoites (the *arrow* indicates amylopectin granules). *F,* Light micrograph of a cyst containing bradyzoites. *G,* Development of oocysts in cat intestine. *H,* Oocysts in the lumen of cat intestine. *I,* Sporulating oocysts that contain sporozoites. (From Boyer, K. M., and McLeod, R. L.: *Toxoplasma gondii* [toxoplasmosis]. *In* Long, S. S., Pickering, L. K., and Prober, C. G. [eds.]: Principles and Practice of Pediatric Infectious Diseases. New York, Churchill Livingstone, 1997, p. 1423.)

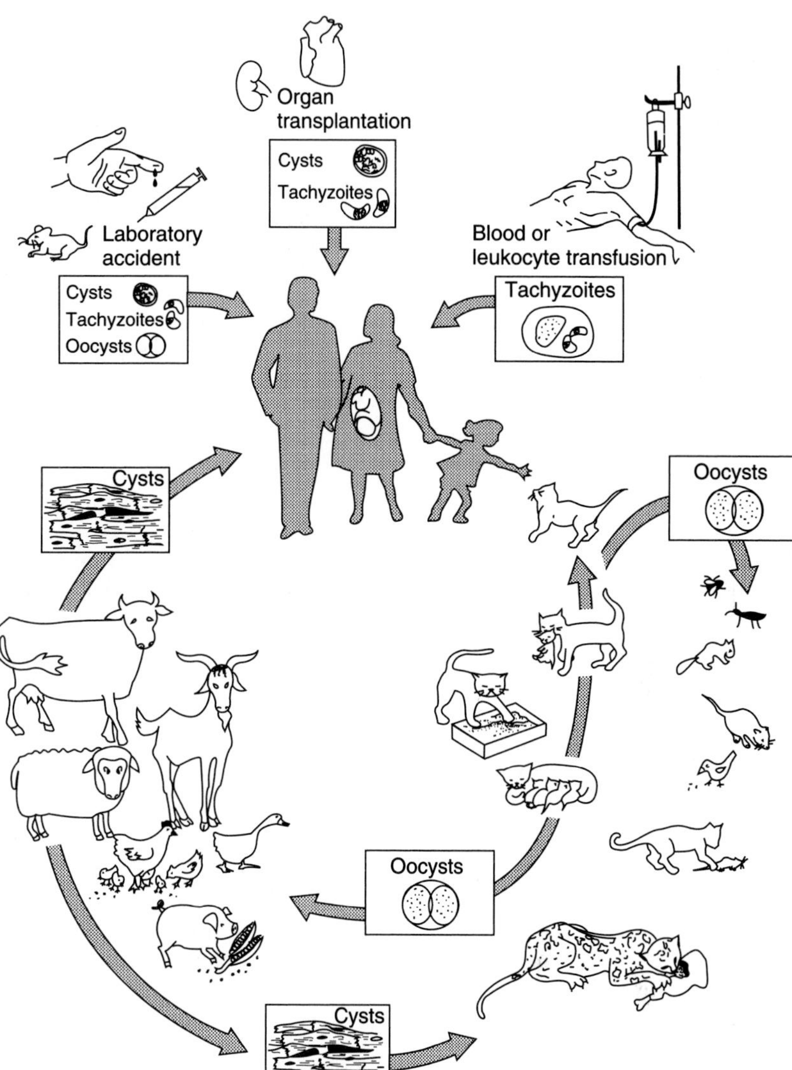

FIGURE 222–2 ■ Life cycle of *Toxoplasma gondii.* Cats are definitive hosts, with humans and other mammals being intermediate hosts. (From Remington, J. S., and McLeod, R.: Toxoplasmosis. *In* Braude, A. I. [ed.]: International Textbook of Medicine. Vol. II. Medical Microbiology and Infectious Disease. Philadelphia, W. B. Saunders, 1981, p. 1818.)

commonly 2 to 8 days) after excretion, depending on temperature and the availability of oxygen. The oocyst is far more resistant than the other life cycle forms and can survive for months in water and for a year or more in moist soil. Ingestion of sporulated oocysts transmits the infection. This fact suggests that the oocyst plays a major role in transmission by the fecal-oral route in animal reservoirs and, by inadvertent ingestion, in humans.

The genome of *T. gondii* consists of 8×10^7 base pairs distributed among 12 chromosomes. Much of the genome has been sequenced, and a genetic linkage map has been constructed.[70, 75, 139] The factors that regulate stage conversion from tachyzoite to bradyzoite are beginning to be defined.[100] The shikimate pathway, an enzyme system that is absent in animals, is important for the production of many essential aromatic compounds in plants, bacteria, and fungi. This biochemical pathway has been identified in *Toxoplasma,* as well as in other apicomplexan parasites such as *Plasmodium falciparum* and *Cryptosporidium parvum.*[127] Biochemical inhibition of this pathway suppresses the growth of these parasites.[124] Understanding of the regulation of life cycle stages and the unique pathways of intermediary metabolism in *T. gondii* may provide new approaches to therapy.

Epidemiology

ACQUIRED INFECTION

Infection with *Toxoplasma* occurs commonly in humans. The incidence of toxoplasmosis in the United States probably is decreasing at present, although data are relatively limited.[141] This decline may relate in part to widespread public awareness of the "dangers of kitty litter" for women who are pregnant, but people appear to be less informed about the potential for transmission of disease from raw or undercooked meat. However, the common practice of freezing commercial meat before releasing it for sale, combined with the use of home freezers, also may be having a beneficial effect.[141] Estimates are that approximately 8 percent of commercial beef, 20 percent of commercial pork, and 25 percent of commercial lamb contain encysted *Toxoplasma* bradyzoites.[122]

In the United States, the prevalence of seropositivity has been determined from studies of military recruits and surveys in major cities. In the early 1960s, the overall prevalence in military recruits was 14 percent, with the lowest rates in the Mountain (3%) and Pacific (8%) states and the highest rates in the Northeastern (20%) and East South

Central (19%) states.[141] A more recent study showed a similar geographic distribution but consistently lower prevalence.[141] Urban studies in U.S. women of child-bearing age have yielded variable rates: Denver, 3 percent; Palo Alto, 10 percent; Chicago, 12 percent; Boston, 14 percent; and Birmingham, 30 percent.[122] Internationally, rates are also variable: Thailand, 3 percent; Australia, 23 percent; Japan, 6 percent; United Kingdom, 35 percent; Poland, 36 percent; Belgium, 53 percent; Tahiti, 77 percent; and France, 87 percent.[122] In part, the prevalence of infection is determined by climate: colder regions and those that are hot and dry or at high altitude have lower rates of human infection than warmer, moister areas do.

The cat is central in the parasite's life cycle, and humans and other mammals are intermediate hosts. If infected tissue (e.g., a mouse) is consumed by a susceptible cat, the sexual cycle is induced in the cat intestine; oocysts are excreted and are infectious for mammals and birds, in whom the life cycle (tachyzoites and cysts) is perpetuated. Cats shed oocysts for only brief durations (days to weeks), but in extremely large numbers ($>10^7$/day). A cat is more likely to become infected if it is an outdoor cat or a predator or is fed fresh, uncooked table scraps. Humans come in contact with cat excrement either directly (e.g., emptying the litter pan) or by more insidious means (e.g., cleaning a horse stall, weeding the garden, playing in a sandbox). Meat for human consumption may serve as a source of infection if it is eaten raw or undercooked. Again, accidental ingestion may occur under circumstances that are unsuspected. Examples include an Amish farm wife preparing sausage, a couple consuming steak tartare in an expensive restaurant, and a rancher butchering a deer.[89]

Common-source outbreaks of acute acquired *Toxoplasma* infection have been authenticated. In some instances, unique and clear-cut sources have been documented to be highly likely, such as exposure to aerosolized cat excrement in a riding stable[148] or consumption of unpasteurized goat milk.[134] In other circumstances, extensive investigations have failed to yield convincing answers.[88, 138] Because of the possibility of common-source exposure, however, families of patients with acute acquired infection should be evaluated for subclinical infection.[85]

Accidental self-inoculation with a needle contaminated with *Toxoplasma* has resulted in many acquired infections in laboratory workers. Infections also have been ascribed to blood transfusions and organ transplantation.[50]

CONGENITAL INFECTION

Congenital infection is thought to occur, with rare exception, only after *primary* maternal infection with *Toxoplasma*.[40, 122] The only two well-documented exceptions to this rule occurred in immunodeficient pregnant women.[106, 122] In a large series that carefully studied more than 800 women who had given birth to congenitally infected children, however, not a single congenital infection occurred in subsequent pregnancies.[122] A general consensus is that only acute infection beginning *during* pregnancy can lead to congenital infection. Despite the existence of a few well-documented instances of biopsy-proven lymphadenopathic toxoplasmosis occurring 2 months *before* conception that resulted in congenitally infected babies,[150] this pattern of occurrence also appears to be extremely rare.[55]

The prevalence of congenital toxoplasmosis in a population, therefore, is determined by the risk of a woman's experiencing primary infection while she is pregnant. This risk depends in turn on three factors: the age-specific incidence of primary infection during the child-bearing years, the age distribution of pregnant women in the population, and the fetal transmission rate in primary infection. A theoretic analysis by Frenkel based on these three factors,[51] assuming a child-bearing age group of 20 to 29 years and an overall fetal transmission rate of 40 percent, showed that maximal risk occurs when the age-specific incidence rate in a population is 3 to 5 percent per year, which corresponds to a seropositivity rate of 50 to 80 percent in women of child-bearing age. In such a population, the predicted prevalence of congenital toxoplasmosis would be 4.4 to 4.6 per 1000 pregnancies. At higher age-specific incidences, rates of congenital toxoplasmosis would be lower because nearly all pregnant women already would be infected chronically. At lower incidences, rates also would be lower, but because of less frequent exposure.

Studies in the early 1970s revealed a prevalence of congenital toxoplasmosis in the United States of approximately 2 per 1000 births.[1, 10, 76, 122] The only prospective data currently available in the United States are derived from the screening of approximately 600,000 newborns in Massachusetts and New Hampshire with an IgM enzyme-linked immunosorbent assay (ELISA) as applied to filter paper blood samples.[60] The prevalence of infection identifiable at birth in this more recent study was approximately 1 in 12,000. The limitations of the testing method (small serum volumes, a test that yields positive results in only 75% of cases) undoubtedly render this estimate a conservative one, but it supports the notion that the prevalence has declined in recent years.

Pathology

After intracellular multiplication at the site of entry, tachyzoites are disseminated in blood and may invade all organs and tissues. The severity of infection is probably a function of strain virulence, host susceptibility, tissue tropism, and the immune privilege of the eyes and central nervous system (CNS).[58, 87, 123] Proliferation of tachyzoites results in death of the invaded cells and, eventually, small necrotic foci surrounded by intense cellular reaction. With recovery, cysts without an inflammatory response around them may persist in the brain, bone marrow, lymph nodes, liver, spleen, and lungs, as well as in skeletal, heart, and smooth muscle.[50–52]

In active infection of the CNS, *Toxoplasma*-filled cells are scattered throughout the gray matter, where they produce diffuse meningoencephalitis with miliary microglial nodules and foci of perivascular inflammation.[25] Large lesions may mimic cerebral tumors. Areas of basal ganglial and periventricular inflammation may calcify in the fetus.[44, 117] Obstruction of the aqueduct of Sylvius or the foramen of Monro may result in hydrocephalus in congenital infection.

The enlarged lymph nodes in acute acquired toxoplasmosis show characteristic pathologic changes that may warrant a presumptive diagnosis.[45, 150] Such changes include reactive follicular hyperplasia, epithelioid histiocytes encroaching on and blurring the margins of germinal centers, and distention of subcapsular and trabecular sinuses by monocytoid cells. Tachyzoites and cysts are seen rarely.[45]

In the eye, active chorioretinitis begins in the retina with severe inflammation and necrosis and exudation into the vitreous. Single or multiple foci occur, and secondary involvement of the choroid is always present. Both tachyzoites and cysts have been found in these lesions.[14, 15, 125, 126]

In immunocompromised hosts, widespread necrotizing lesions may be seen in the heart, muscle, brain, and other organs. These lesions, particularly those involving the CNS, have been found frequently with reactivation of toxoplasmosis in patients with acquired immunodeficiency syndrome (AIDS).[83]

Immunology

Cell-mediated immune responses are the major immunologic mechanisms that prevent reactivation of *T. gondii* in a chronically infected normal host.[24, 34] Numerous effector mechanisms contribute to protection in murine models and human infection: $CD8^+$ cytotoxic T lymphocytes, $CD4^+$ T lymphocytes, monocyte oxidative mechanisms, production of interferon-γ by natural killer cells, and activation of macrophages by interferon-γ and tumor necrosis factor–α.[57, 61, 71, 74, 139, 145] Killing of the parasite within activated macrophages is associated with the intracellular production of nitric oxide. Interleukin-2 and interleukin-12 enhance host resistance to *T. gondii*; interleukin-10 impairs the ability of macrophages to kill the parasite.[56]

In murine models, evidence exists for genetic determination of host resistance to infection.[16, 17, 87, 96] Presence of the DQ3 allele appears to be associated with toxoplasmic encephalitis in patients with AIDS and hydrocephalus in infants with congenital toxoplasmosis.[17] Successful immunization of mice[18] and sheep[19] with *T. gondii* components and live tachyzoites of an "incomplete" strain[20] raises the possibility of developing a human vaccine.[69, 97]

Clinical Syndromes

The disease in children may be considered in three categories: postnatally acquired, congenital, and ocular (which may be congenital or acquired). Clinically apparent infection in older children may have been acquired recently or caused by reactivation of latent congenital or postnatally acquired infection. Both congenital and acquired infections are usually subclinical, but congenital infection ultimately leads to serious sequelae in most cases.

ACUTE ACQUIRED TOXOPLASMOSIS

Acquired *Toxoplasma* infection is asymptomatic in most cases and frequently goes unrecognized because only 10 to 15 percent of infected persons have clinical symptoms and signs. However, in certain recent outbreaks related to infection by oocysts, more than half of infected patients have been symptomatic.[148] The most common findings are lymphadenopathy and fatigue without fever.[90] The nodes are discrete and may or may not be tender. They do not suppurate. The groups of nodes most commonly involved are the cervical, suboccipital, supraclavicular, axillary, and inguinal nodes. The adenopathy may be localized or involve multiple areas, including the retroperitoneal and mesenteric nodes. Uncommonly, the lymphadenopathy is accompanied by fever, malaise, fatigue, sore throat, and myalgia, a picture that closely simulates that of infectious mononucleosis but without serologic evidence of acute Epstein-Barr virus infection. The differential diagnosis of the lymphadenopathy often includes lymphoma. Chorioretinitis may develop, but it does not occur commonly.[88, 110] The liver may be involved, and liver function tests may reflect hepatocellular damage. In persons with normal immunologic function and no severe underlying disease, the infection is usually self-limited and rarely requires treatment.

In contrast, more severe and frequently fulminant infections are seen in patients receiving immunosuppressive therapy, in those who have disease of the bone marrow or reticuloendothelial system, in patients with agammaglobulinemia, in recipients of bone marrow transplants, and in those with AIDS.[37, 67, 80, 83, 131, 149] Encephalitis and rarely pneumonitis and myocarditis are the most important localized forms that may be encountered in immunocompromised patients. In toxoplasmic encephalitis, the predominant neurologic symptoms are headache, disorientation, and drowsiness. These symptoms may simulate aseptic meningitis or a mass lesion. In view of the variety of clinical manifestations of CNS involvement, of importance is to consider toxoplasmosis whenever evidence of acute CNS disease is present.

CONGENITAL TOXOPLASMOSIS

Congenital infection is most often the result of an asymptomatic acute infection in the mother.[48] In a small proportion of cases, spontaneous abortion, prematurity, or stillbirth may result. Congenital toxoplasmosis has a wide spectrum of clinical manifestations but is most often subclinical in newborn infants. When clinically apparent, it may mimic other diseases of the newborn. Fever, hydrocephalus or microcephaly, hepatosplenomegaly, jaundice, convulsions, chorioretinitis (usually bilateral), cerebral calcifications, and abnormal cerebrospinal fluid (markedly increased protein and mononuclear pleocytosis) are considered the classic features of congenital toxoplasmosis.[44, 104] These manifestations occurred commonly in an early series of patients reported by Eichenwald[47] (Table 222–1). The case-fatality rate was 12 percent. In survivors in this series, sequelae included mental retardation in 86 percent; convulsions, spasticity, and palsies in almost 75 percent; and severely impaired vision in 60 percent.[47] Other occasional findings included rash (maculopapular, petechial, or both), myocarditis, pneumonitis and respiratory distress, hearing defects, an erythroblastosis-like picture, thrombocytopenia, lymphocytosis, monocytosis, and nephrotic syndrome. These signs now are known to be most typical of the severe form of the infection in the absence of treatment.

The often subclinical nature of congenital toxoplasmosis in the newborn was demonstrated in a French prospective study of 154 mothers who had acquired *Toxoplasma* infection during pregnancy and did not receive treatment.[40] Nine pregnancies (6%) ended in stillbirth and 85 (55%) resulted in the birth of infected live-born infants. Of the live-born infants who were infected, 64 (75%) had subclinical infection, 14 (16%) had mild disease, and only 7 (8%) had clinically obvious severe disease.[40, 122]

The risk of transmission to the fetus varies significantly with the trimester of gestation in which the mother becomes infected. For untreated women, the rate is approximately 25 percent in the first trimester, 54 percent in the second trimester, and 65 percent in the third trimester; these figures are minimal estimates derived from placental isolation studies.[40] In contrast, the severity of clinical disease in congenitally infected infants is related inversely to the gestational age at the time of primary maternal infection. In two studies from France,[29, 40] severe disease or fetal/neonatal death occurred in approximately 40 to 79 percent of infants born to mothers with first-trimester infection, in 15 to 18 percent with second-trimester infection, and in 0 to 3 percent with third-trimester infection.

Another French prospective study of 210 congenitally infected infants born to mothers who were identified to have primary infection acquired during pregnancy revealed significant morbidity in 94 newborns.[29] Overall, 2 cases (0.9%)

TABLE 222–1 ■ SIGNS AND SYMPTOMS OCCURRING BEFORE DIAGNOSIS OR DURING THE COURSE OF UNTREATED ACUTE CONGENITAL TOXOPLASMOSIS IN 152 INFANTS AND 101 OF THESE SAME PATIENTS AFTER 4 YEARS OR MORE OF FOLLOW-UP*

	Frequency of Occurrence* in Patients with	
Signs and Symptoms	*Neurologic Disease*†	*Generalized Disease*‡
Infants	*N* = 108	*N* = 44
Chorioretinitis	102 (94)	29 (66)
Abnormal spinal fluid	59 (55)	37 (84)
Anemia	55 (51)	34 (77)
Jaundice	31 (29)	35 (80)
Splenomegaly	23 (21)	40 (90)
Convulsions	54 (50)	8 (18)
Fever	27 (25)	34 (77)
Intracranial calcification	54 (50)	2 (4)
Hepatomegaly	18 (17)	34 (77)
Lymphadenopathy	18 (17)	30 (68)
Vomiting	17 (16)	21 (48)
Hydrocephalus	30 (28)	0 (0)
Diarrhea	7 (6)	11 (25)
Pneumonitis	0 (0)	18 (41)
Microcephalus	14 (13)	0 (0)
Eosinophilia	6 (4)	8 (18)
Rash	1 (1)	11 (25)
Abnormal bleeding	3 (3)	8 (18)
Hypothermia	2 (2)	9 (20)
Cataracts	5 (5)	0 (0)
Glaucoma	2 (2)	0 (0)
Optic atrophy	2 (2)	0 (0)
Microphthalmos	2 (2)	0 (0)
Children 4 years or older	*N* = 70	*N* = 31
Mental retardation	62 (89)	25 (81)
Convulsions	58 (83)	24 (77)
Spasticity and palsies	53 (76)	18 (58)
Severely impaired vision	48 (69)	13 (42)
Hydrocephalus or microcephalus	31 (44)	2 (6)
Deafness	12 (17)	3 (10)
Normal	6 (9)	5 (16)

*Data indicate numbers of patients, with percentages in parentheses.
†Patients with central nervous system diseases in the first year of life.
‡Patients with non-neurologic diseases during the first 2 months of life.
Modified from Eichenwald, H.G.: A study of congenital toxoplasmosis, with particular emphasis on clinical manifestations, sequelae, and therapy. *In* Siim, J. C. (ed.): Human Toxoplasmosis. Copenhagen, Munksgaard, 1960, p. 44.

were fatal, 21 (10%) were severe, and 71 (33.8%) were mild; 116 cases were asymptomatic. Of note is that approximately 40 to 45 percent of the mothers in this study had been treated with spiramycin during pregnancy. These observations confirm that most congenital infections are subclinical at birth. Obvious manifestations occur relatively infrequently. In the same study by Couvreur and associates,[29] 116 infants initially were thought to not be infected on the basis of a routine newborn physical examination. On more intensive examination, however, 39 (34%) of them had one or more abnormalities. Twenty-two (19%) had abnormal cerebrospinal fluid on lumbar puncture, 17 (15%) had chorioretinitis on indirect ophthalmoscopic examination, and 10 (9%) had intracranial calcifications on head radiographs or computed tomographic scans. Guerina and colleagues[60] made remarkably similar observations in the congenitally infected newborns that they identified in New England by heelstick blood sampling.

Some infected children without overt disease as neonates may escape serious sequelae of the infection, whereas chorioretinitis, strabismus, blindness, hydrocephalus or microcephaly, cerebral calcifications, developmental delay, epilepsy, or deafness develop in most children months or even years later. Three studies provide data that define the incidence of these late sequelae.

In a study from Paris,[79] 26,402 apparently healthy infants were tested routinely for serologic evidence of *Toxoplasma* infection at 10 months of age. Fifty-one of these infants had positive serologic results for *Toxoplasma,* indicative of congenital infection. None had been treated for *Toxoplasma* infection in infancy. Of the 51, 5 were found to have chorioretinal scars by ophthalmologic examination, and chorioretinal lesions had developed in another 4 by 4 years of age, the longest period of follow-up. Some eventually lost functional vision in one eye. Three had intracranial calcifications.

Similarly, in a study from Holland in which a cohort of 1821 pregnant women were screened serologically, 12 congenitally infected infants were detected and 11 of them were monitored for 20 years.[76, 77] Of the 11, 5 were treated as neonates for 1 month only and 6 were not. Of the five treated infants, four had eye disease as neonates and one had parasites in cerebrospinal fluid, which prompted therapy. Nine of these 11 (82%) had chorioretinal scars by the time that they reached 20 years of age, and 4, including 2 who were initially normal, had severe visual impairment or blindness in one eye. The onset of disease leading to blindness occurred as late as 18 years of age. No neurologic or cognitive sequelae were observed.

The results of this prospective study are similar to those previously reported by Wilson and associates[158] from Alabama in a retrospective analysis of patients from the United States. Over a mean follow-up period of 8.3 years, sequelae developed in 11 of 13 congenitally infected children (85%) who had no signs of disease on detailed examination in the newborn period. Sequelae included chorioretinal lesions in 11 children (85%), severe neurologic disability in 1 child (8%), and mental retardation in 2 children (15%). Sequelae first were noted at ages ranging from 1 month to 9 years. These 13 children were detected either as a result of routine screening of cord serum for IgM antibodies to *Toxoplasma,*[9] performed because acute *Toxoplasma* infection was diagnosed in the mother,[2] or as a result of nonspecific findings in the neonatal period (two were small for gestational age, and one had transient borderline thrombocytopenia).

That treatment may decrease the frequency or severity of sequelae is suggested by the Alabama and Paris studies, in which chorioretinitis developed only in untreated infants between 10 months and 4 years of age. Taken together, these data indicate that most congenitally infected children who receive no or relatively brief treatment, including those with inapparent infection as neonates, suffer untoward sequelae during childhood. Current treatment regimens—prolonged for at least 1 year and often initiated before birth—appear to be associated with substantially less frequent and severe sequelae (see Treatment).

Congenital toxoplasmosis may mimic or coexist with infection by other organisms. It must be differentiated from other perinatal infections caused by cytomegalovirus (CMV), herpes simplex virus, rubella virus, *Treponema pallidum* (syphilis), human immunodeficiency virus type 1 (HIV-1), and certain bacteria (e.g., *Listeria).* Herpesvirus and CMV infection, syphilis, and rubella may cause chorioretinitis; CMV and HIV-1 may cause encephalopathies associated with cerebral calcifications. Degenerative encephalopathies and storage diseases in older children also may resemble congenital toxoplasmosis.

Many infants or preschool children with coexisting HIV infection and toxoplasmosis have been reported.[105, 106] In at least six of these patients, both HIV and *Toxoplasma* infection appear to have been acquired in utero. Of these six patients, all but one had clinical evidence of CNS disease, and in most of these children, the CNS disease was associated with other findings common in congenital infection. These findings included hepatosplenomegaly, fever, and chorioretinitis and were evident at birth (one infant) or developed by the time that the infant reached 4 months of age. Two of the other infants remained asymptomatic, one of whom was treated for *Toxoplasma* infection and the other was not. One additional infant who acquired HIV infection at 18 months of age from a blood transfusion died at 5 years of age of toxoplasmic encephalitis. The findings in this patient resembled those in adults with AIDS and toxoplasmic encephalitis.[83]

OCULAR TOXOPLASMOSIS

In active congenital toxoplasmosis, the retinal lesions are usually bilateral.[104] In older children, chorioretinitis may involve only one eye and may be the sole manifestation of congenital toxoplasmosis. Toxoplasmic chorioretinitis, even in older children and adults, usually is considered to be the result of congenital infection.[110] In some studies, *Toxoplasma* infection has accounted for as many as 5 percent of severe visual impairments in children.[72] Active lesions on the fundus appear as white or yellowish foci with elevated, edematous margins surrounded by a zone of hyperemia (Fig. 222–3). Cells and fibrinous exudate in the vitreous may obscure the fundus. Older lesions appear as glial scars, and in areas in which the retina has been destroyed, the choroid and sclera are visible. Around the depigmented areas, deposition of pigment from the destroyed retina is present. The position of the lesion may be macular, juxtapapillary, or peripheral.

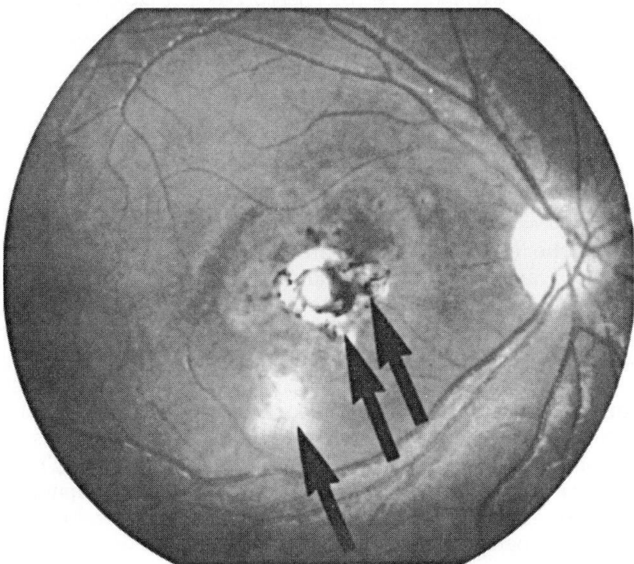

FIGURE 222–3 ■ An example of active and quiescent chorioretinitis caused by congenital toxoplasmosis in a 12-year-old patient. The active lesion *(single arrow)* is a satellite of an old chorioretinal scar *(two arrows)*. (From Mets, M., Holfels, E., Boyer, K. M., et al.: Eye manifestations of congenital toxoplasmosis. Am. J. Ophthalmol. *122*:309–324, 1996. Published with permission from the American Journal of Ophthalmology. Copyright by The Ophthalmic Publishing Company.)

Patients may experience loss of central vision (caused by a perimacular lesion), with hazy vision (caused by accumulated exudate) or "floaters" (caused by reactivation of peripheral foci). Neonates or infants with toxoplasmic eye disease may have microphthalmos, small corneas, posterior cortical cataract, anisometropia, strabismus, and nystagmus.[104] Strabismus and nystagmus in a child of any age should raise the possibility of congenital toxoplasmosis. The appearance of lesions in the fundus is not specific for toxoplasmosis. Similar lesions may occur with other less common granulomatous diseases in the eye, such as toxocariasis, cat-scratch disease, and tuberculosis. Chorioretinitis may be recurrent, most commonly with reactivation at the margins of preexisting lesions.

Laboratory Diagnosis

Acute infection can be diagnosed by isolation of *T. gondii* from blood or body fluids; demonstration of tachyzoites in histologic sections of tissue or cytologic preparations of body fluids; characteristic lymph node histology; demonstration of *Toxoplasma* cysts in the placenta, fetus, or neonate; detection of the *Toxoplasma* genome by polymerase chain reaction (PCR) in body fluids; and characteristic serologic test results.[13, 108] Each of these methods is discussed, but serologic tests are emphasized because they are the most common method of establishing the diagnosis (Table 222–2).

SEROLOGIC METHODS

Measurements of IgG Antibody

The most useful tests for detection of IgG antibodies to *Toxoplasma* include the Sabin-Feldman dye test,[133] the indirect immunofluorescent antibody (IFA) test, agglutination tests, and ELISA. Titers in ELISA are expressed in different terms for different commercial kits, thereby precluding a discussion of IgG ELISA titers per se in relation to the diagnosis of acute infection.[43, 152] In these tests, IgG antibodies appear within the first week of primary infection and reach peak titers (usually 1:500 or greater) within 1 to 2 months; detectable titers usually persist for life. Although the dye test is the most reliable method, it is available in only a few reference laboratories. The IFA test and ELISA are the most widely available and, when properly performed, yield results similar to those obtained with the dye test; however, many laboratories use commercially available kits that are not consistently reliable. Some sera that contain antinuclear antibodies yield false-positive IFA results. The direct agglutination tests that are currently available use formalin-fixed tachyzoites or antigen-coated latex particles, are simple to perform, and are accurate.[141]

Other tests vary in their reliability. Indirect hemagglutination is widely available, but the results are frequently negative in newborns with congenital infection.[154] This test should *not* be used for screening pregnant women because detectable rises in titer are delayed when compared with the rises detected by ELISA and by the dye, IFA, and agglutination tests.

Meaningful interpretation of changes in titer on sequential sera requires that assays on each sample be performed in the same run by a reliable laboratory.

TABLE 222–2 ■ GUIDELINES FOR INTERPRETATION OF SEROLOGIC TESTS FOR TOXOPLASMOSIS*

Test	Positive Titer	Titer in Congenital Infection (Infant) or Acute Infection (Older child, Adult)	Titer in Chronic Infection	Duration of Elevation of Titer
IgG				
Sabin-Feldman dye test	Undiluted	NC, S OCA, 1:4 to ≥1:1000 (usual)	1:4 to 1:2000	Years
Direct agglutination	≥1:20	NC, S OCA, rises slowly from negative to low to high titer (1:512)	Stable (≥1:1000) or slowly decreasing titer	≥1 yr
Indirect fluorescent IgG antibody	≥1:10	NC, S OCA, ≥1:1000	1:8 to 1:2000	Years
Indirect hemagglutination	≥1:16	NC, S OCA, ≥1:1000	1:16 to 1:256	Years
Complement fixation	≥1:4	NC, S OCA, varies among laboratories	Negative to 1:8	Years
IgM				
Indirect fluorescent IgM antibody	≥1:10 adults	OCA, ≥1:80 (use only for OCA, not NC)	Negative to 1:20	Weeks to months, occasionally years
Double-sandwich IgM EIA	≥ 0.2, newborn, fetus ≥1.7, older children, adults	NC, ≥0.2 OCA, ≥1.7	Negative to 1.7 (OCA)	Can be ≥1 yr
Immunosorbent test for IgM	≥3, infant 8, adult	NC, ≥3 OCA, >8	Negative to 1	Unknown, can be ≥1 yr
IgA				
IgA, EIA	≥1.0, infants ≥1.4, adults	NC, ≥1.0 OCA, >1.4	Negative to <1.0 Negative to ≤1.3	Weeks to months, occasionally longer
IgE				
IgE, EIA	≥1.9, infants and adults	NC and OCA, ≥1.9	Negative	Weeks to months, occasionally longer
Immunosorbent test for IgE	≥4, infants and adults	NC and OCA, ≥4	Negative	Weeks to months occasionally longer
AC/HS	See reference 33	See reference 33	See reference 33	Usually <9 mo
PCR (amniotic fluid; CSF)	Positive	Positive	Negative	Only when *Toxoplasma* DNA present during active infection

*Values are those of one reference laboratory; each laboratory must provide its own standards and interpretation of results in each clinical setting.
AC/HS, differential agglutinin test; CSF, cerebrospinal fluid; EIA enzyme immunoassay; NC, titer in newborn with congenital infection; OCA, titer in older child or adult with acute, acquired infection; PCR, polymerase chain reaction; S, usually the same as the mother.
Modified from McLeod, R., and Remington, J. S.: Toxoplasmosis. *In* Braunwald, E., Isselbacher, K. J., Petersdort, R. G., et al. (eds.): Harrison's Principles of Internal Medicine. New York, McGraw-Hill, 1987, p. 795. With permission from The McGraw-Hill Companies.

Measurements of IgM Antibody

IgM antibodies are detected most commonly by IgM IFA, IgM immunosorbent agglutination assay (ISAGA), or IgM ELISA. IgM antibodies appear in the first week of primary infection and peak within 1 month. Depending on the sensitivity of the method used, IgM antibodies may be demonstrable for 2 to 3 months to 1 year or longer. IgM ELISA and IgM ISAGA are much more sensitive than IgM IFA. Absence of IgM ELISA or IgM ISAGA antibodies in an immunologically normal older child (older than 1 year) or adult essentially rules out a recently acquired infection. A negative IgM IFA result is not as sensitive in ruling out recently acquired infection. Ninety-three percent of sera that were negative with IgM IFA and obtained from adults who had acquired toxoplasmosis recently were strongly positive in IgM ELISA.[113] IgM IFA detects specific IgM antibody in only 25 percent of infants with proven congenital infection, whereas IgM ELISA detects antibody in approximately 75 percent of such cases.[113] The presence of rheumatoid factor or antinuclear antibodies may cause false-positive results in IgM IFA.[2]

The "double-sandwich" IgM ELISA avoids both the false-positive results caused by the presence of rheumatoid factor, which the infant can produce in utero, and the false-negative results caused by competition from the high levels of maternal IgG antibody that occur in IgM IFA.[112] In addition, the false-positive results in IgM IFA caused by antinuclear antibodies are not found in IgM ELISA.[2, 111]

ISAGAs are used widely in Europe. Like IgM ELISA, they capture IgM on a solid surface, detect specific IgM, and involve the addition of whole formalin-fixed organisms or *Toxoplasma* antigen–coated latex particles.[42, 120] These assays are available commercially and give results comparable to those of IgM ELISA, are simpler to perform, and do not require expensive equipment.

Measurements of IgA and IgE Antibodies

Demonstration of IgA and IgE antibodies in the fetus or newborn infant by ELISA and ISAGA appears to be at least comparable in sensitivity for the diagnosis of congenital *Toxoplasma* infection to demonstration of IgM antibody.[36, 143, 160] The IgA test also seems to be more sensitive than the IgM test for detection of acquired infection. Specificity remains an issue, however, so neither ELISA nor ISAGA has superseded the IgM test for diagnosis of acquired infection. On the other hand, IgA and IgE antibodies have somewhat longer persistence than IgM does and thus may be useful in cases of subacute illness or when IgM titers are low.

Differential Agglutination

Acetone- and formalin-fixed *T. gondii* tachyzoites may yield differing agglutination titers depending on the acuity of the infection. The test based on this phenomenon is called the AC/HS differential agglutination test.[33] In general, a disproportionately high agglutination titer with acetone-fixed organisms suggests acute infection; a disproportionately high titer with formalin-fixed organisms suggests chronic infection. Interpretative norms for this test have been established.[33] This test, when combined with the dye test, IgM ELISA, IgA ELISA, IgE ELISA, and IgE ISAGA, yields a "toxoplasmic serologic profile" that permits the most accurate evaluation of infection acuity in pregnant women[109, 161] and often can resolve any inconclusive or discrepant results obtained in a hospital or commercial laboratory.

NONSEROLOGIC METHODS

Nonserologic methods are used less commonly for the diagnosis of *Toxoplasma* infection because they are not widely available and require tissue specimens.

Isolation of the Organism

Isolation of *Toxoplasma* from blood or body fluids (e.g., cerebrospinal fluid) establishes that the infection is acute. In the case of a neonate, isolation from the placenta or the infant's tissues is sufficient to diagnose congenital *Toxoplasma* infection. Isolation from the placenta usually (approximately 90% of the time), but not always is associated with congenital infection.[122] Isolation of *Toxoplasma* from the tissues of older children or adults, however, may reflect only the presence of latent infection (cyst form). The organism may be isolated by inoculation of body fluids, leukocytes, or tissue specimens into the peritoneal cavities of mice or into tissue cultures. Specimens should be processed and inoculated immediately; however, tissue and blood may be stored at 4° C overnight. Freezing and thawing or formalin treatment kills the organism. Definitive diagnosis by isolation of *Toxoplasma* from tissues usually takes 4 to 6 weeks by mouse inoculation; tissue culture is less sensitive for recovering *Toxoplasma,* but the results are available sooner.

Histology

Demonstration of tachyzoites, but not cysts, in tissue sections or smears of body fluids (e.g., cerebrospinal fluid) establishes a diagnosis of acute infection. The organism may be difficult to see with routine stains. The peroxidase-antiperoxidase technique is exquisitely sensitive and has been used with a high degree of sensitivity and specificity to demonstrate the organism in the CNS of patients with AIDS.[25] In older children and adults, the histopathologic changes in toxoplasmic lymphadenitis are sufficiently distinctive to enable pathologists to make a presumptive diagnosis of acute acquired toxoplasmosis (see "Pathology").[45, 150] Histologic demonstration of cysts establishes that a patient has *Toxoplasma* infection, but they are diagnostic of toxoplasmosis only in the placenta, fetus, or newborn infant.

Antigen-Specific Lymphocyte Transformation

Lymphocyte transformation in response to *Toxoplasma* antigens is a specific and sensitive indicator of previous *Toxoplasma* infection in adults and has been used successfully to diagnose congenital *Toxoplasma* infection in infants 2 months or older.[94, 144, 156] Lymphocyte transformation is often absent in the newborn period, particularly in more severely affected infants, because of specific immune tolerance.[94, 99]

Polymerase Chain Reaction

Amplification of the B1 genome of *T. gondii* DNA by PCR permits detection of the parasite in body fluids or tissues such as cerebrospinal fluid, amniotic fluid, and lymph nodes.[59, 62, 130, 150] Experience with the test in France, where PCR of amniotic fluid was compared with the results of percutaneous umbilical blood sampling in 339 pregnant women, has shown that agreement of the two methods is close to 100 percent for the diagnosis of intrauterine infection.[62] In view of the considerably lower risk of amniocentesis than percutaneous umbilical blood sampling and the fact that amniocentesis potentially can be performed earlier in gestation, this diagnostic procedure appears to be a major advance in prenatal diagnosis. A sobering recent prospective study in France, however, has shown that only 48 (64%) of 75 amniotic fluid specimens from congenitally infected infants were positive by PCR on a single sample obtained soon after maternal seroconversion. The test had a 100 percent positive predictive value, but a single negative assay did not rule out fetal infection.[130]

DIAGNOSIS IN SPECIFIC CLINICAL SITUATIONS

Acute Acquired Toxoplasmosis

If IgM or IgG antibody is not detectable, the diagnosis of acute *Toxoplasma* infection in an immunocompetent child virtually is excluded. The diagnosis of recently acquired infection is confirmed if seroconversion from a negative to a positive titer is noted or if a serial fourfold rise in titer to high levels is observed when sera drawn at 3-week intervals are run in parallel. A single high titer in any test is not diagnostic. A dye test or IFA titer of 1:500 or greater in the presence of a high IgM antibody titer is probably diagnostic of recent acute infection. The absence of IgM antibodies in IgM ELISA or IgM ISAGA essentially excludes the diagnosis of acute infection. In contrast, the absence of IgM antibodies in IgM IFA does not necessarily mean that the infection is not acute; in one series, 25 percent of results in adults with acute infection were negative by IgM IFA.[113]

Toxoplasma Infection in Immunodeficient Children

Serologic tests should be performed to identify persons at risk of acquiring toxoplasmosis, such as organ and bone marrow transplant recipients. The available serologic tests may be inadequate to detect acute active infection in some immunodeficient patients because their antibody response may be abnormal, which is especially the case in bone marrow transplant recipients.[38] Experience in the Palo Alto, California, reference laboratory has revealed that acute infection may be present in patients with AIDS and in bone marrow transplant recipients without any demonstrable IgM antibody and in some immunocompromised patients who have little or no IgG antibody. In patients with AIDS and active *Toxoplasma* infection, antibody titers in the modified direct agglutination test[43] clearly may be elevated in the presence of low or undetectable titers in the dye or IFA test.[91] These and other immunodeficient patients can have progressive, lethal toxoplasmosis. In almost all cases, encephalitis, brain abscesses, or both are the predominant findings; hepatic involvement, pneumonitis, and myocarditis may be present. A high index of suspicion is necessary in these patients, and immunoperoxidase staining of appropriate biopsy specimens often is required for diagnosis. For the special problem of interpretation of IgM and IgG antibody rises in organ transplant recipients, the reader is referred to an article by Luft and colleagues.[84]

Toxoplasma Infection in Pregnant Women

Toxoplasma infection acquired during pregnancy is associated with clinical signs (e.g., lymphadenopathy) in only 10 to 15 percent of patients. The fetus, however, is at risk for contracting the infection regardless of whether the mother is symptomatic. To detect acute infection in a pregnant woman in the absence of a routine screening program in which serologic tests are performed periodically throughout pregnancy, a suitable test for IgM antibody (IgM ELISA or IgM ISAGA) should be performed if other serologic tests are positive at any titer. If a suitable IgM antibody test is unavailable and the original serum contains IgG antibodies, the IgG antibody test should be repeated in 3 weeks, in parallel with the original serum, to determine whether the titer is stable or rising. If the IgM ELISA or IgM ISAGA result is negative and the IgG antibody titer is stable and less than 1:500, no further evaluation is necessary. Because IgG titers usually stabilize at high levels (e.g., the dye test or IFA titer ≥1:500) 6 to 8 weeks or longer after acquisition of the infection, if the dye test or IFA titer is 1:500 or less and stable (regardless of IgM antibody titer), infection was acquired at least 4 weeks and probably more than 8 weeks before the serum was obtained. However, in the United States, an asymptomatic woman commonly is evaluated for the first time more than 8 weeks after conception. If her dye test or IFA titer is 1:500 or higher, her IgM ELISA or IgM ISAGA result is negative, and no significant rise in titer in any test can be demonstrated, her infection almost certainly was acquired before conception. In women with elevated IgM titers or rising IgG test titers, infection possibly was acquired during pregnancy. A complete toxoplasmic serologic profile[109] in a reference serologic laboratory is recommended to settle the question.

Fetal Diagnosis

As noted earlier, severe disease almost always is associated with primary maternal infection in the first or second trimester of pregnancy, but only 25 and 54 percent, respectively, of such cases result in fetal infection. These rates may be reduced by half by maternal treatment with spiramycin. Identification of cases in which the fetus already is infected permits a parental decision to terminate the pregnancy or treat the fetal infection more aggressively with pyrimethamine-sulfadiazine.

Studies by workers in Paris have established an approach that allows definitive diagnosis and treatment of fetal infection in utero.[31, 41, 62] These researchers initially sought to establish the diagnosis of fetal infection at 20 to 29 weeks of gestation by isolation of *Toxoplasma* from amniotic fluid or from fetal blood obtained by percutaneous umbilical blood sampling and use of the sensitive mouse inoculation method. Prenatal diagnosis was attempted in 746 pregnancies in which seroconversion occurred near the time of conception or before the 26th week of gestation. In 39 of these pregnancies, fetal infection was diagnosed in utero. *Toxoplasma* was isolated from fetal blood alone in 12 cases, from amniotic fluid alone in 7 cases, and from both in 15 cases, for a total of 34. *Toxoplasma*-specific IgM antibodies were detected in fetal blood in only nine cases with the highly sensitive ISAGA, and none were positive before 24 weeks of gestation. By follow-up examination until 3 months post partum or by examination of aborted fetal tissue, a total of 42 cases were proved to have been infected. Thus, these researchers were able to successfully detect 39 (93%) of 42 cases of fetal infection occurring before the 26th week of gestation; no false-positive diagnoses occurred. These investigators subsequently extended their series and reported that a definitive diagnosis of infection was established in utero in 80 (90%) of 89 cases in which the fetus was infected.[63] These results may not be reproduced easily by others for various reasons: the ability to detect maternal infection soon after it occurs depends on monthly monitoring for new maternal infection, sampling of fetal blood and amniotic fluid on more than one occasion, the use of optimal laboratory methods and conditions, and experience in these procedures.

With the use of PCR to amplify the B1 gene of *Toxoplasma* in amniotic fluid obtained after 18 weeks of gestation, these same investigators were able to achieve a sensitivity and specificity for the diagnosis of fetal infection that approached 100 percent.[62] However, in the more recent multicenter collaborative French study, in which only single specimens were studied, the specificity and positive predictive value remained 100 percent, but the sensitivity was only 64 percent.[130] The sensitivity and specificity for this test as specimens currently are processed and handled in the United States remain to be determined.

Most of the mothers in these French studies had received treatment with spiramycin soon after primary maternal infection was diagnosed, with the intention of continuing therapy until delivery. In contrast to its beneficial effect on maternal-to-fetal transmission, spiramycin does not appear to decrease the severity of fetal infection once it has been established. Thus, the impetus for proving fetal infection in early to middle gestation is to allow for intervention either to terminate the pregnancy or to treat the fetus more aggressively. In an extended series of 89 infected fetuses reported by Hohlfeld and colleagues,[63] 34 pregnancies were terminated at the request of the parents. In each of these cases, which were selected either for detectable CNS disease on ultrasound examination or for onset of maternal infection before 12 weeks of gestation, brain necrosis was found on examination of tissue. These data indicate the value of specifically identifying fetuses that truly are infected and at high risk for acquiring severe disease because selective termination of these pregnancies allowed successful completion of most pregnancies in which fetal infection did not occur. In addition to the 34 terminated pregnancies with proved fetal infection, 52 pregnancies with 55 offspring were carried to term. In these 52, 43 had fetal infection proved prenatally, and 9 additional offspring were found to be infected by postnatal examination. In the 43 pregnancies in which prenatal diagnosis of fetal infection was established, more aggressive therapy with pyrimethamine and a sulfonamide compound alternating with spiramycin was given in the latter part of pregnancy. This treatment appeared to decrease the number of parasites, as indicated by an approximate

50 percent reduction in the fraction of placentas from which *Toxoplasma* was isolated at delivery in comparison to cases in which no treatment or spiramycin alone was given.

Regarding clinical outcome, the authors interpreted their data to indicate that such treatment decreased the incidence of severe disease.[63] However, this conclusion was based on a retrospective comparison to a group of historical controls in which information regarding fetal deaths and termination of pregnancy was not available. Because pregnancies with proven or probable severe fetal infection were terminated selectively at the parents' request, one cannot conclude with certainty that the outcome of the infants born to mothers with first-trimester infection was improved by the administration of more aggressive therapy; the outcome of those born to mothers with second-trimester infection appears to have been improved.[155] It would be desirable to have data from studies in which the effects of such therapy are compared directly in a randomized, concurrent study; such studies, however, are unlikely to be performed. Nonetheless, these studies have established the utility of an aggressive approach to prenatal diagnosis in allowing physicians to make an accurate, early diagnosis of fetal infection. If the fetus is infected and affected, as determined by ultrasonography, a decision for selective termination of pregnancy can be made rationally. Aggressive therapy with pyrimethamine-sulfadiazine may be offered in cases in which termination is not considered desirable, and it may improve the outcome.

Diagnosis of Congenital Toxoplasmosis after Birth

Performing a thorough clinical and laboratory evaluation is necessary to fully evaluate the existence and extent of congenital toxoplasmosis in a newborn (Table 222–3). Demonstration of IgM, IgA, or IgE antibody in an infant's blood or cerebrospinal fluid at any time is diagnostic of congenital infection if contamination by maternal blood reasonably can be excluded. Specimens obtained after the infant reaches 10 days of age are more reliable in this regard. If the much less sensitive IgM IFA is used, the presence of antinuclear antibody and rheumatoid factor also must be excluded. As mentioned earlier, the detection rate of congenitally infected infants is 25 percent for IgM IFA and 75 percent for IgM ELISA and IgM ISAGA. (Data are insufficient for prediction of how often IgA and IgE antibodies are detected.) IgM antibodies may be demonstrable in the first few days of life or may appear at varying times after birth.

If *Toxoplasma* is not isolated and IgM, IgA, or IgE antibodies are not detected, follow-up serologic testing is the only means of establishing the diagnosis. Maternally transmitted IgG antibodies may persist for 6 to 12 months or longer, depending on the original titer. The higher the original titer, the longer maternal antibody is detectable in the infant. Thus, the presence of IgG antibody at even 8 to 12 months of age does not necessarily prove that the infant is infected. Synthesis of IgG *Toxoplasma* antibody is usually demonstrable by the third month of life if the infant is not treated; it may be delayed until the sixth or ninth month if the infant is treated. At the time that the infant begins to synthesize IgG antibody, infection may be documented by computing the specific "antibody load," that is, the ratio of specific serum antibody titer to the level of serum IgG in the infant.[122] In the absence of infection, the antibody load decreases in the second or third month as the infant begins to produce IgG that does not contain specific *Toxoplasma* antibodies. In the presence of *Toxoplasma* infection, the infant produces specific antibodies, and thus the antibody load remains the same or increases. Most infected infants who are treated during the first year of life will have a

TABLE 222–3 ■ EVALUATION OF A NEONATE WHEN SEROLOGY OF THE MOTHER OR ILLNESS OF THE NEONATE INDICATES THAT A DIAGNOSIS OF CONGENITAL TOXOPLASMOSIS IS SUSPECTED OR PROBABLE

In addition to a careful general examination, the baby is examined by the following:

Clinical evaluation and nonspecific tests
- A pediatric ophthalmologist
- A pediatric neurologist
- Brain CT
- Blood tests
  - Complete blood cell count with differential and platelet counts
  - Serum total IgM, IgG, IgA, and albumin
  - Serum alanine aminotransferase, total and direct bilirubin
  - CSF cell count, glucose, protein, and total IgG

Toxoplasma gondii*–specific tests*
- Newborn serum analyzed for antibody detected by Sabin-Feldman dye test, IgM ISAGA, IgA EIA, IgE EIA/ISAGA (0.5 mL serum to *Toxoplasma* Serology Laboratory, Palo Alto Medical Foundation, 860 Bryant Street, Palo Alto, CA 94301, 415-326-8120)
- Newborn blood for inoculation into mice (1–2 mL clotted whole blood in red-topped tube to *Toxoplasma* Serology Laboratory)
- Lumbar puncture: CSF dye test and IgM EIA (0.5 mL CSF to *Toxoplasma* Serology Laboratory; consider PCR (1 mL frozen CSF to *Toxoplasma* Serology Laboratory)
- Sterile placental tissue (100 g in saline, from fetal side near insertion of cord, no formalin, to *Toxoplasma* Serology Laboratory for subinoculation)
- Maternal serum analyzed for antibody detected by dye test, IgM EIA, IgA EIA, IgE EIA/ISAGA, and AC/HS

AC/HS, differential agglutination test; CSF, cerebrospinal fluid; CT, computed tomography; EIA, enzyme immunoassay; ISAGA, immnosorbent test for IgM; PCR, polymerase chain reaction.
Modified from McLeod, R., Wisner, J., and Boyer, K.: Toxoplasmosis. *In* Krugman, S., Katz, S.L., and Gershon, A.A. (eds.): Infectious Diseases of Children. St. Louis, Mosby–Year Book, 1992, p. 539.

substantial increase in antibody after termination of therapy ("serologic rebound").[151] This phenomenon permits confirmation of the diagnosis in some uncertain cases.

Ocular Toxoplasmosis

Toxoplasma has been estimated to cause 35 percent of cases of chorioretinitis in the United States and central and western Europe.[135] Acquired toxoplasmosis usually is not accompanied by chorioretinitis. Most cases are thought to result from congenital infection that does not become clinically apparent until after reactivation. This event occurs most commonly in adolescence. Although the presence of chorioretinitis should prompt a search for *Toxoplasma* infection, proof that *Toxoplasma* caused the eye disease is often lacking. The titer of antibody in serum does not necessarily correlate with the presence of active lesions in the fundus. In fact, low titers of IgG antibody are the usual finding in patients with reactivation *Toxoplasma* chorioretinitis. IgM antibodies are generally absent.

Toxoplasma probably is excluded as a cause of chorioretinitis if the results of serologic tests are negative in undiluted serum. If the retinal lesions are characteristic and serologic test results are positive, the diagnosis is probable. If the retinal lesions are atypical and the serologic test results are positive, the diagnosis of *Toxoplasma* chorioretinitis is less certain because of the increasing prevalence of

Toxoplasma antibodies with age in the normal population. Finding *Toxoplasma* antibodies in the child's mother supports the possibility of congenital infection, as does detection of intracranial calcification on computed tomographic examination of the patient. Demonstration of local antibody production in aqueous humor obtained by paracentesis of the anterior chamber can be used to establish the diagnosis of *Toxoplasma* chorioretinitis in equivocal cases.[122] However, the risk of this procedure in a situation of threatened vision, when weighed against the relatively low risk of a short course of treatment, is such that it seldom is performed.

Treatment

The need for therapy and the duration of therapy are determined by the nature and severity of the clinical illness and by the immune status of the infected patient. Antibody titers are not useful indicators of therapeutic response, and an increasing antibody titer soon after discontinuation of therapy ("serologic rebound") is not an indication of therapeutic failure. Specific therapy acts primarily against the tachyzoite form; the drugs currently available do not eradicate the encysted form. Close, longitudinal follow-up and supportive interventions are extremely important contributors to therapeutic success.

THERAPEUTIC AGENTS

The therapeutic agents used, their dosages, and indications for their use in the management of toxoplasmosis are included in Table 222–4 and discussed next.

Spiramycin

This macrolide has been used extensively in Europe to reduce transmission of infection from an acutely infected mother to the fetus in utero.[26] It is concentrated in the placenta and is reported to reduce transmission by 50 to 60 percent. It reduces the ability to isolate the organism from the placentas of definitively infected newborns from 95 to 80 percent.[28] Spiramycin is less effective than pyrimethamine-sulfadiazine in the treatment of congenital infection and toxoplasmic encephalitis.[28, 39, 136, 137] Toxoplasmic encephalitis has developed in patients receiving spiramycin and then has been treated effectively with pyrimethamine-sulfadiazine. Toxicities include allergic manifestations, gastrointestinal intolerance, and paresthesias. Spiramycin does not appear to treat manifestations of *T. gondii* infection in the fetus in utero.[28, 39, 63, 136] It formerly was used in alternate-month regimens with pyrimethamine and sulfadiazine for treatment of congenital toxoplasmosis in France.[122] Spiramycin is not approved by the U.S. Food and Drug Administration (FDA) but may be obtained with compassionate clearance by calling 301-827-2127. The manufacturer (Aventis-Pasteur) provides the drug after documentation of the diagnosis and completion of FDA forms.

Pyrimethamine

Pyrimethamine has been demonstrated to be effective against *T. gondii* in vitro,[98, 101] in animal models,[54] and in human infections.[30, 32, 54, 86, 101, 161] When used in conjunction with sulfadiazine, synergy can be demonstrated. The pharmacokinetics of pyrimethamine has been studied in infants and adults.[99] Pyrimethamine is metabolized in the liver, and its pharmacokinetics is not altered by renal insufficiency but is affected by concomitantly administered drugs (e.g., phenobarbital). Pyrimethamine toxicities include reversible marrow suppression (most commonly) and allergy. Aplastic anemia, hepatotoxicity, and various allergic manifestations (including Stevens-Johnson syndrome) also have been listed as toxicities of this medication. Pyrimethamine always should be administered in conjunction with leukovorin (i.e., folinic acid) because human cells can use folinic acid for synthesis of nucleic acids, but *T. gondii* cannot.[99]

Leucovorin

Leucovorin always is administered during treatment with pyrimethamine. Increased doses of leukovorin are used in the event of marrow suppression. Because of the long half-life of pyrimethamine, continuation of leucovorin therapy for 1 week after discontinuing pyrimethamine is recommended.

Sulfadiazine, Sulfamerazine, and Sulfamethazine

These three sulfonamides (known as triple sulfa when used in combination) are the most active of the sulfonamides against *T. gondii* and are synergistic with pyrimethamine in their activity against *T. gondii*. Of the three, only sulfadiazine is currently available in the United States. All other sulfonamides are less active in vitro.[98] They are excreted by the kidney, and the dosage must be adjusted for patients with renal insufficiency. Toxicities include allergy, marrow suppression, and both hepatic and renal toxicity. Their pharmacokinetics has been studied in infants.[122]

Clindamycin

Although the effect of clindamycin is delayed, it does have an effect in vitro against *T. gondii* with prolonged time in culture.[118] It has been demonstrated to be effective in murine models as well. Clindamycin has been found to be comparable in efficacy to sulfadiazine for the treatment of toxoplasmic encephalitis in adult patients with AIDS when used in a combined high-dose regimen with pyrimethamine.[32, 86] Of note is that high-dosage pyrimethamine also is effective alone and that it was not compared directly with the other two regimens in the latter study.

Other Antimicrobial Agents

Numerous other antimicrobial agents have been demonstrated to be effective in vitro or in animal models against either tachyzoites or encysted bradyzoites,[3–6, 64, 65] but their role, if any, in the treatment of human disease remains to be defined. Atovaquone (5-hydroxynaphthoquinone), for example, was effective against bradyzoites within cysts in vitro.[65] Unfortunately, however, 40 percent of patients with AIDS had a relapse of their toxoplasmic encephalitis while being treated with this antimicrobial agent. Other antimicrobial agents with effect on *T. gondii* in vitro or in vivo include cycloguanil,[64] artemisinin,[64] pyrimethamine-sulfadoxine (Fansidar),[98] rifabutin,[7] trovafloxacin,[73] and the newer macrolides clarithromycin, azithromycin, and roxithromycin.[3, 5, 6]

Because the activity of sulfamethoxazole is less than that of sulfadiazine, trimethoprim-sulfamethoxazole has been considered less effective as treatment of toxoplasmosis. However, many investigators have used this combination successfully to treat toxoplasmic encephalitis in adults with AIDS. Doses of trimethoprim-sulfamethoxazole, as used to prevent *Pneumocystis carinii* pneumonia in the context of HIV infection, also may prevent episodes of reactivated

TABLE 222–4 ■ TREATMENT OF TOXOPLASMOSIS

Manifestation of Infection	Medication	Dosage	Duration of Therapy
Pregnant women with acute toxoplasmosis First 18 weeks of gestation or until term if fetus not infected	Spiramycin*	1 g q8h without food	Until fetal infection is documented or excluded at 18–20 wk; if documented, has been used in France in alternate months with pyrimethamine, sulfadiazine, and leucovorin until term†
Pregnant women with fetal infection confirmed after 17th wk of gestation or if maternal infection acquired in last few weeks of gestation (after amniocentesis and PCR to determine whether *Toxoplasma* infection is present in the fetus)	Pyrimethamine	Loading dose: 100 mg/day in 2 divided doses for 2 days, then 50 mg/day	Until term (leucovorin is continued 1 wk after pyrimethamine is discontinued)
	Sulfadiazine	Loading dose: 75 mg/kg day in 2 divided doses (maximum, 4 g/day) for 2 days, then 100 mg/kg/day in 2 divided doses (maximum, 4 g/day)	
	Leucovorin (folinic acid)	5–20 mg daily‡	
Congenital *Toxoplasma* infection in infants	Pyrimethamine§	Loading dose: 2 mg/kg/day for 2. days, then 1 mg/kg/day for 2 or 6 mo‖ then this dose every Monday, Wednesday, and Friday	1 yr¶ (leucovorin is continued 1 wk after pyrimethamine is discontinued)
	Sulfadiazine§	100 mg/kg/day in 2 divided doses	
	Leucovorin§	5–10 mg 3 times weekly‡	
CSF protein ≥1 g/dL or active chorioretinitis that threatens vision	Corticosteroids (prednisone)	1 mg/kg/day in 2 divided doses**	Until resolution of elevated CSF protein level or active chorioretinitis
Active chorioretinitis in older children	Pyrimethamine	Loading dose: 2mg/kg/day (maximum, 50 mg) for 2 days, then maintenance, 1 mg/kg/day (maximum, 25 mg)	Usually 1–2 wk beyond resolution of signs and symptoms (leucovorin is continued 1 wk after pyrimethamine is discontinued)
	Sulfadiazine	Loading dose: 75 mg/kg, then maintenace, 50 mg/kg q12 h	
	Leucovorin	5–20 mg 3 times weekly‡	
	Corticosteroids	1 mg/kg/day in 2 divided doses**	Until resolution**
Immunologically normal children			
Lymphadenopathy	No therapy		
Significant organ damage that is life-threatening	Pyrimethamine	Same as above for "active chorioretinitis in older children," no corticosteroids	Usually 4–6 wk, or 2 wk beyond resolution of signs and symptoms
	Sulfadiazine		
	Leucovorin		
Immunocompromised children			
Non-AIDS	Pyrimethamine	Same as above for "active chorioretinitis in older children," no corticosteroids	Usually 4–6 wk beyond complete resolution of signs and symptoms
	Sulfadiazine		
	Leucovorin		
AIDS	Pyrimethamine	Same as above for "active chorioretinitis in older children," no corticosteroids	Lifetime
	Sulfadiazine		
	Leucovorin		
	Clindamycin has been used in place of sulfadiazine	Reported trials for adults, but not infants and children	

*Available only by request from the Food and Drug Administration, telephone 301-443-5680.

†The only studies are those of Daffos and colleagues.[31] However, because Daffos and colleagues found pyrimethamine-sulfadiazine therapy to be superior to spiramycin for treatment of the fetus, continuous therapy with pyrimethamine, sulfadiazine, and leucovorin should be considered in the third trimester.

‡Adjusted for megaloblastic anemia, granulocytopenia, or thrombocytopenia; blood counts, including platelets, should be monitored as described in text.

§Optimal dosage, feasibility, and toxicity currently being evaluated or planned in ongoing Chicago-based National Collaborative Treatment Trial, telephone 312-791-4152.

¶In infants with AIDS. The duration of therapy is unknown. See discussion under the section on congenital toxoplasmosis and AIDS.

‖These two regimens currently are being compared in a randomized National Collaborative Treatment Trial. Data are not available to determine which, if either, is superior. Both regimens appear to be feasible and relatively safe.

**Corticosteroids should be continued until signs of inflammation (high CSF protein ≥1 g/dL) or active chorioretinitis that threatens vision have subsided; the dosage then can be tapered and discontinued. Use only with pyrimethamine, sulfadiazine, and leucovorin.

CSF, cerebrospinal fluid; PCR, polymerase chain reaction.

Modified from McLeod, R., Wisner, J., and Boyer, K.: Toxoplasmosis. *In* Krugman, S., Katz, S. L., and Gershon, A.A. (eds.): Infectious Diseases of Children. St. Louis, Mosby-Year Book, 1992, pp. 541–542.

toxoplasmosis.[21] Pyrimethamine combined with sulfadoxine, despite lower in vitro activity than that of pyrimethamine-sulfadiazine, also has been used in Europe to treat reactivated and congenital infection.[11]

THERAPY IN SPECIFIC CLINICAL SETTINGS

Acquired Toxoplasmosis

Most immunologically normal patients with the lymphadenopathic form of toxoplasmosis do not require specific treatment. Indications for treatment in these cases are the presence of severe and persistent symptoms or damage to vital organs. Because of the high incidence of severe morbidity and mortality in immunocompromised patients, toxoplasmosis should be treated in this population. Most immunocompromised patients in whom the diagnosis is established ante mortem improve when specific therapy is administered. The major problem lies in making the diagnosis early enough to institute treatment.

The optimal duration of specific therapy for toxoplasmosis is unknown. Patients who appear to be immunologically normal but who have severe and persistent symptoms or damage to vital organs should receive specific therapy for 2 to 6 weeks until symptoms resolve. In immunocompromised patients, therapy should continue at least 4 to 6 weeks beyond complete resolution of all signs and symptoms of active disease. Careful follow-up of these patients is imperative because relapse may occur and require prompt reinstitution of therapy. In patients with AIDS in whom toxoplasmosis develops, lifelong suppressive therapy with pyrimethamine-sulfadiazine or pyrimethamine-clindamycin should be used.

Pregnant Women

Treatment of an acutely infected woman during pregnancy may prevent transmission of the infection to her fetus. The rationale for such treatment is derived from the observation that the lag period between the onset of maternal infection and infection of the fetus may be significant. Data from France,[39, 40] where women were treated with spiramycin, and from Austria[8, 9] and Germany,[78] where women were treated with pyrimethamine and sulfonamides, indicate that the incidence of congenital infection in the offspring of mothers treated during gestation is at least 50 percent less than that in the offspring of untreated mothers. None of these studies were controlled rigidly. Nonetheless, the results of the large number of women studied by the group from France (154 untreated and 388 treated patients) strongly suggest that intrauterine treatment does reduce transmission of maternal infection to the fetus.[40, 122]

Of emphasis is that spiramycin treatment of pregnant women with recently acquired primary infection should be instituted empirically in the hope of preventing spread of infection to the fetus. Once fetal infection has occurred, however, maternal treatment with spiramycin does not appear to alter the evolution and severity of disease in the fetus, which is why evaluation of a potentially exposed fetus by PCR amplification of amniotic fluid permits informed decisions about termination of pregnancy or treatment of the fetus in utero with pyrimethamine-sulfadiazine.

Congenital Infection

POSTNATAL TREATMENT. Data regarding the efficacy of postnatal treatment of infants with congenital *Toxoplasma* infection are becoming available. Uncontrolled studies in humans and controlled studies in experimental animals[122] have been interpreted as indicating beneficial effects of postnatal treatment on the development of sequelae in both symptomatic and asymptomatic infants with congenital *Toxoplasma* infection. The controlled National Collaborative Treatment Trial is now in progress in Chicago. This study seeks to define optimal therapeutic regimens. Physicians treating patients with congenital *Toxoplasma* infection who are younger than 2.5 months may wish to contact this multidisciplinary group regarding potential enrollment of their patients in that study (312-791-4152).

Outcomes to date from the National Collaborative Treatment Trial are substantially better for most, but not all infants treated from the neonatal period for 12 months with pyrimethamine-sulfadiazine and leucovorin than for historical controls receiving no or short-course therapy.[92] Signs of active infection resolve within weeks of initiation of treatment. In substantial numbers of children, the appearance of brain computed tomographic scans has improved remarkably (Fig. 222–4). Cerebral calcifications have diminished in size or resolved in most such treated children.[117] In conjunction with this improvement in brain computed tomographic scans, cognitive function has been in the normal range for 69 percent of such treated children.[129, 146] This finding is in striking contrast to the 86 percent of children with "mental retardation" in the Eichenwald series noted earlier[47] (see Table 222–1). No significant diminution in cognitive function occurs over time, and most treated children are functioning well in regular school classrooms. Although the number of children compared is limited, for a small subset of these children, measures of cognitive function appear to be less than those for siblings. No sensorineural hearing loss has been ascribable to congenital toxoplasmosis in treated children.[93] Despite the much improved neurologic outlook for most of these children, a subset of children with significant irreversible neurologic damage already present in the perinatal period have manifested profound developmental delay, motor impairment, and seizures. For the most part, these were children with hydrocephalus, high cerebrospinal fluid protein (>1 g/dL), minimal improvement in brain computed tomographic scans after shunting, and often substantial delays in shunt placement or needed revision for shunt failure or other intercurrent medical problems.[146] This experience emphasizes the importance of recognizing hydrocephalus and managing it aggressively.

Although treatment during the first year of life arrests all signs of active disease, results in normal cognitive and motor outcome for most children, and may result in resolution of seizures without recurrence for some treated children, the drugs currently available do not eradicate all cysts containing bradyzoites. In most children, serologic titers of *T. gondii*–specific antibodies rebound in the 3 to 4 months after treatment.[89, 151] To date, new retinal lesions have occurred in 7 of 54 children in the National Collaborative Treatment Trial during 3 to 10 years' follow-up after the 1-year course of treatment.[104] These active lesions have responded to brief courses of treatment with pyrimethamine, sulfadiazine, and leucovorin without subsequent loss of visual acuity. Although follow-up durations are shorter, this result contrasts with the almost uniform eventual development of retinal lesions in studies of untreated or briefly treated children.[27, 47, 76, 77, 158] We recommend that infected children undergo retinal examination each month for 3 months after discontinuing treatment around their first birthday, then every 3 months until they are old enough to describe visual symptoms accurately, and then every 6 months. In addition, an ophthalmologic evaluation should be performed promptly for any acute visual signs or symptoms that may be related to recrudescence of congenital ocular toxoplasmosis.[104]

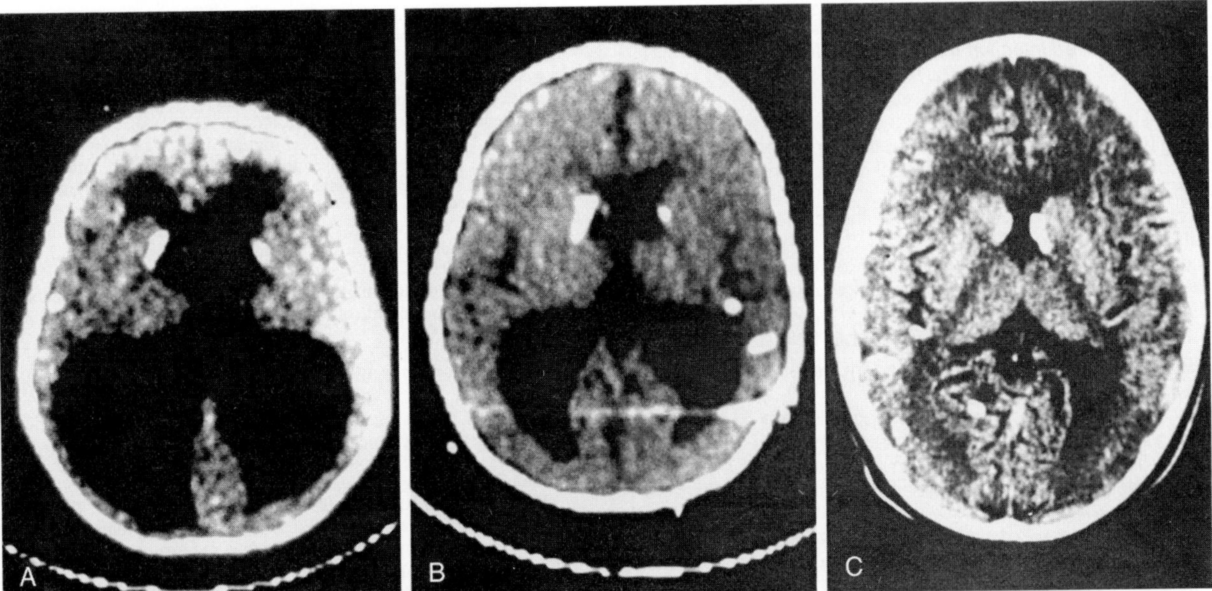

FIGURE 222–4 ■ An example of hydrocephalus and intracranial calcifications in a treated patient with congenital toxoplasmosis. *A,* Computed tomograph at 3 months of age showing hydrocephalus caused by aqueductal stenosis (before shunting), along with cortical and periventricular basal ganglion calcifications. *B,* Computed tomograph at 4 months of age after shunt placement. *C,* Computed tomograph at 8 years of age. The Stanford-Binet IQ was about 100 at 3 and 6 years of age. (From McAuley, J. B., Boyer, K. M., Patel, D., et al.: Early and longitudinal evaluations of treated infants and children and untreated historical patients with congenital toxoplasmosis: The Chicago Collaborative Treatment Trial. Clin. Infect. Dis. *18*:38–72, 1994.)

SEQUENTIAL FETAL AND POSTNATAL TREATMENT. Hohlfeld and colleagues[31, 63] described outcomes in patients treated in utero with continuing treatment during the first year of life. As noted earlier, however, pregnancies in which fetuses had obvious manifestations on ultrasound examination and most pregnancies with definite first-trimester infection were terminated.

Nonetheless, what is remarkable is that when this French method of initiating aggressive treatment of fetuses in utero was applied, retinal disease was reported in only 3 of 50 such infants monitored to 2 years of age. This finding contrasts with the presence of retinal or neurologic involvement in 50 percent of asymptomatic newborns detected by serologic screening in Massachusetts[60] and in 75 percent of children whose pediatricians referred them to our National Collaborative Treatment Trial for treatment in the perinatal period.[104] A prospective, carefully controlled study (as part of the National Collaborative Study) is under way to directly compare outcomes in infants identified and treated in utero, as detected by systematic neonatal screening and by pediatricians in the neonatal period and then referred. Of note is that the outcome of pregnancies with infection acquired in the first trimester after in utero treatment also has been reported to be favorable in another study[12] in which only pregnancies in which the fetus had hydrocephalus were terminated.

Though a rare occurrence when compared with adults with AIDS, the number of children with toxoplasmosis and coexistent HIV infection or AIDS appears to be increasing.[105] Most of these children have had congenital toxoplasmosis, and most have been symptomatic. For such children, therapy with pyrimethamine and sulfadiazine plus folinic acid is recommended in the doses described in Table 222–4. In adults, administration of maintenance therapy is necessary to prevent relapse after toxoplasmic encephalitis, and a recommendation of lifelong therapy for children with dual HIV and congenital *Toxoplasma* infection seems appropriate. Zidovudine antagonizes the toxoplasmacidal effect of pyrimethamine and its in vitro synergy with sulfonamide. Whether this effect occurs in vivo is unknown.[81] Consultation regarding dually infected children is available from Dr. Charles Mitchell in Miami (305-547-6676).

Ocular Toxoplasmosis

Prompt initiation of specific treatment in active ocular toxoplasmosis is mandatory to preserve vision. Inflammatory reactions in the vitreous are frequently a major pathogenetic phenomenon in patients with active disease, and in such cases, administration of corticosteroids in addition to specific anti-*Toxoplasma* therapy is recommended strongly.[116] Their use also is recommended for cases of retinochoroiditis involving the macula, maculopapillary bundle, or optic nerve. The initial daily dosage of prednisone is 1 mg/kg orally to a maximum of 75 mg in 24 hours. The equivalent dosage of another corticosteroid may be given. The dosage of corticosteroid may be reduced gradually when the lesion appears to be well demarcated and pigmentation has begun. Some physicians have used systemic or intraocular clindamycin to treat patients in whom the use of corticosteroids and pyrimethamine plus sulfadiazine has failed[147]; its efficacy has not been proved in humans.

Prevention

Congenital infection may be avoided by preventing primary *Toxoplasma* infection during pregnancy.[49, 92, 161] The responsibility of all physicians caring for pregnant women at risk is to inform them of specific hygienic measures (Table 222–5) for avoiding *Toxoplasma* infection. Similar measures are useful for prevention of acquired infection in other settings

TABLE 222–5 ■ PREVENTION OF *TOXOPLASMA* INFECTION

Prevention of Acquired Infection (Primary Prevention)

Cook meat to >150°F (>66°C), smoke it, or cure it in brine.
Wash fruits and vegetables before consumption.
Avoid touching mucous membranes of the mouth and eyes while handling uncooked meat or unwashed fruits or vegetables.
Wash hands and kitchen surfaces thoroughly after contact with raw meat or unwashed fruits or vegetables.
Prevent access of flies, cockroaches, and other coprophagic insects to fruits and vegetables.
Avoid contact with materials that potentially are contaminated with cat feces, such as cat litter boxes, or wear gloves when handling such materials and when gardening.
Disinfect cat litter boxes for 5 minutes with nearly boiling water.

Prevention of Congenital Infection (Secondary Prevention)

Identify women at risk by serologic testing.
Treatment during pregnancy results in an approximately 50 percent reduction in the incidence of infection in infants.
Therapeutic abortion prevents birth of an infected infant: consider only for women who acquire infection in the first or second trimester.

Adapted from Remington, J. S., and Wilson, C. B.: Toxoplasmosis. *In* Kass, E. H., and Platt, R. (eds.): Current Therapy in Infectious Disease: 1983–1984. Philadelphia, B. C. Decker, 1983, pp. 149–153.

as well. The ability of a 10-minute education program, offered as part of prenatal care, to reduce the risk of acquiring *Toxoplasma* infection by modifying the behavior of pregnant women with regard to cats, food, and personal hygiene has been demonstrated.[22] Pamphlets that describe methods to prevent toxoplasmosis in pregnant women are available from the March of Dimes (312-435-4007), from Abbott Diagnostics (800-323-9100), and on the Internet (http://www.iit.edu/~toxo/pamphlet).

Once primary maternal infection has occurred, several problems are inherent in the secondary prevention of congenital toxoplasmosis by therapeutic abortion or by treatment of the pregnant woman. Because 80 to 90 percent of women with primary *Toxoplasma* infection are asymptomatic, most primary infections are overlooked unless sequential serologic testing is performed routinely in pregnant women. The cost-effectiveness of routine screening in the prevention of congenital toxoplasmosis is clear in European countries where screening is mandated by law.[40] In countries with a lower incidence, cost-efficiency has not been proved.[128] In the absence of such data, physicians may choose to screen patients on an individual basis.[157] If screening is undertaken, a reliable serologic test for IgG antibodies (see Laboratory Diagnosis) should be performed before conception or as soon as possible thereafter and then repeated every 2 to 3 months until the time of delivery. Serologic test results that suggest the acquisition of primary infection during pregnancy should be confirmed by a reference laboratory. Decisions regarding treatment or therapeutic abortion should be based on a consideration of whether the fetus is infected or affected, as determined by amniocentesis and ultrasonography.

Acknowledgment

The authors acknowledge the contribution of Christopher B. Wilson, M.D., to this chapter in the previous edition of this text.

REFERENCES

1. Alford, C. A., Jr., Stagno, S., and Reynolds, D. W.: Congenital toxoplasmosis: Clinical, laboratory and therapeutic considerations, with special reference to subclinical disease. Bull. N. Y. Acad. Med. *50*:160, 1974.
2. Araujo, F. G., Barnett, E. V., Gentry, L. O., et al.: False positive anti-*Toxoplasma* fluorescent antibody tests in patients with antinuclear antibodies. Appl. Microbiol. *22*:270, 1971.
3. Araujo, F. G., Guptill D. R., and Remington, J. S.: Azithromycin, a macrolide antibiotic with potent activity against *Toxoplasma gondii*. Antimicrob. Agents Chemother. *32*:755–757, 1988.
4. Araujo, F. G., Lin, T., and Remington, J. S.: The activity of atovaquone (566C80) in murine toxoplasmosis is markedly augmented when used in combination with pyrimethamine or sulfadiazine. J. Infect. Dis. *167*: 494–497, 1993.
5. Araujo, F., Prokocimer, P., and Remington, J.: Clarithromycin-minocycline is synergistic in a murine model of toxoplasmosis. J. Infect. Dis. *165*:788, 1992.
6. Araujo, F., and Remington, J.: Recent advances in the search for new drugs for treatment of toxoplasmosis. Int. J. Antimicrob. Agents *1*:153–164, 1992.
7. Araujo, F. G., Slifer, T., and Remington, J. S.: Rifabutin is active in murine models of toxoplasmosis. Antimicrob. Agents Chemother. *38*:570–575, 1994.
8. Aspock, H.: Prevention of congenital toxoplasmosis by serological surveillance during pregnancy: Current strategies and future perspectives. *In* Marget, W., Lang, W., and Gabler-Sandberger, E. (eds.): Parasitic Infections, Immunology, Mycotic Infections, General Topics. Vol. 3. Munich, Medizin Verlag, 1986, pp. 69–72.
9. Aspock, H., Flamm, H., and Pilcher, O.: Die *Toxoplasmose*-Überwachung während der Schwangerschaft 10-jahre Erfahrungen in Österreich. Mitt. Oesterr. Ges. Trophenmed. Parasitol. *8*:105–113, 1986.
10. Beach, P. G.: Prevalence of antibodies to *Toxoplasma gondii* in pregnant women in Oregon. J. Infect. Dis. *140*:780, 1979.
11. Berger, R., Merkel, S., and Rudin, C.: Toxoplasmosis and pregnancy: Findings from umbilical cord blood screening in 30,000 newborn infants. Schweiz. Med. Wochenschr. *125*:1168–1173, 1995.
12. Berrebi, A., Kobuch, W. E., Bessieres, M. H., et al.: Termination of pregnancy for maternal toxoplasmosis. Lancet *344*:36–38, 1994.
13. Boyer, K. M.: Diagnostic testing for congenital toxoplasmosis. Pediatr. Infect. Dis. J. *20*:59–60, 2001.
14. Boyer, K. M., and McLeod, R.: *Toxoplasma gondii* (toxoplasmosis). *In* Long, S. S., Pickering, L. K., and Prober, C. G. (eds.): Principles and Practice of Pediatric Infectious Diseases. New York, Churchill Livingstone, 1997, pp. 1421–1448.
15. Brezin, A. P., Kasner, L., Thulliez, P., et al.: Ocular toxoplasmosis in the fetus: Immunohistochemistry analysis and DNA amplification. Retina *14*:19–26, 1994.
16. Brown, C. R., Estes, R. G., Bechmann, E., et al.: Definitive identification of a toxoplasmosis resistance gene. Res. Immunol. Ann. Inst. Pasteur. *144*:61–66, 1993.
17. Brown, C., and McLeod, R: Class I MHC genes and CDA+ T cells determine cyst number in *Toxoplasma gondii* infection. J. Immunol. *145*: 3438–3441, 1990.
18. Bnlow, R., and Boothroyd, J. C.: Protection of mice from fatal *Toxoplasma gondii* infection by immunization with p30 antigen in liposomes. J. Immunol. *147*:3496–3500, 1991.
19. Buxton, D.: Toxoplasmosis: The first commercial vaccine. Parasitol. Today *9*:335–337, 1993.
20. Buxton, D., and Innes, E. A.: A commercial vaccine for ovine toxoplasmosis. Parasitology *110*(Suppl.):11–16, 1995.
21. Carr, A., Tindall, B., Brew, B. J., et al.: Low-dose trimethoprim-sulfamethoxazole prophylaxis for toxoplasmic encephalitis in patients with AIDS. Ann. Intern. Med. *117*:106–111, 1992.
22. Carter, A. O., Gelmon, S. B., Wells, G. A., et al.: The effectiveness of a prenatal education programme for the prevention of congenital toxoplasmosis. Epidemiol. Infect. *103*:539–545, 1989.
23. Cesbron-Delau, M. F.: Dense-granule organelles of *Toxoplasma gondii*: Their role in the host-parasite relationship. Parasitol. Today *10*:293–296, 1994.
24. Cesbrons, M. F., Dubremetz, J. F., and Sher, A.: The immunobiology of toxoplasmosis. Res. Immunol. *144*:7–8, 1993.
25. Conley, F. K., Jenkins, H. T., and Remington, J. S.: *Toxoplasma gondii* infection of the central nervous system. Hum. Pathol. *12*:690, 1981.
26. Couvreur, J., and Desmonts, G.: Congenital and maternal toxoplasmosis: A review of 300 congenital cases. Dev. Med. Child. Neurol. *4*:519–530, 1962.
27. Couvreur, J., Desmonts, G., and Aron-Rosa, D.: Le pronostic oculaire de la toxoplasmosis congenital: Role du traitement. Ann. Pediatr. *31*: 855–858, 1994.
28. Couvreur, J., Desmonts, G., and Thulliez, P.: Prophylaxis of congenital toxoplasmosis: Effect of spiramycin on placental infection. J. Antimicrob. Chemother. *22*:193–200, 1988.
29. Couvreur, J., Desmonts, G., Tournier, G., et al.: Etude d'une serie homogene de 210 cas de toxoplasmose congenitale chez des nourrissons ages de 0 a 11 mois et depistes de facon prospective. Ann. Pediatr. *31*:815, 1984.
30. Couvreur, J., Thulliez, P., Daffos, F., et al.: Foetopathie toxoplasmique: Traitment in utero par l'association pyrimethamine-sulfamides. Arch. Fr. Pediatr. *48*:397–403, 1991.

31. Daffos, F., Forestier, F., Capella-Pavlovsky, et al.: Prenatal management of 746 pregnancies at risk for congenital toxoplasmosis. N. Engl. J. Med. *318*:271–275, 1988.
32. Dannemann, B., McCutchan, J. A., Israelski, D., et al.: Treatment of toxoplasmic encephalitis in patients with AIDS: A randomized trial comparing pyrimethamine plus clindamycin to pyrimethamine plus sulfonamides. Ann. Intern. Med. *116*:33–43, 1992.
33. Dannemann, B. R., Vaughan, W. C., Thulliez, P., et al.: The differential agglutination test for diagnosis of recently acquired infection with *Toxoplasma gondii.* J. Clin. Microbiol. *28*:1928–1933, 1990.
34. Darcy, F., and Santoro, F.: Toxoplasmosis. *In* Kierszenbaum, F. (ed.): Parasitic Infections and the Immune System. San Diego, CA, Academic Press, 1994, pp. 163–190.
35. Darling, S. T.: Sarcosporidiosis: With report of a case in man. Proc. Canal Zone Med. Assoc. *1*:141, 1908.
36. Decoster, A., Darcy, F., Caron, A., et al.: IgA antibodies against P30 as markers of congenital and acute toxoplasmosis. Lancet *2*:1104, 1988.
37. Derouin, F., Devergie, A., and Auber, P.: Toxoplasmosis in bone marrow-transplant recipients: Report of seven cases and review. Clin. Infect. Dis. *15*:267–270, 1992.
38. Derouin, F., Gluckman, E., Beauvais, B., et al.: *Toxoplasma* infection after human allogeneic bone marrow transplantation: Clinical and serological study of 80 patients. Bone Marrow Transplant. *1*:67, 1986.
39. Desmonts, G., and Couvreur, J.: Congenital toxoplasmosis: A prospective study of 378 pregnancies. N. Engl. J. Med. *290*:1110, 1974.
40. Desmonts, G., and Couvreur, J.: Congenital toxoplasmosis: A prospective study of the offspring of 54 women who acquired toxoplasmosis during pregnancy: Pathophysiology of congenital disease. *In* Thalhammer, O., Baumgarten, K., and Pollak, A. (eds.): Perinatal Medicine. Sixth European Congress, Vienna, 1978. Stuttgart, Georg Thieme, 1979.
41. Desmonts, G., Daffos, F., Forestier, F., et al.: Prenatal diagnosis of congenital toxoplasmosis. Lancet *1*:500, 1985.
42. Desmonts, G., Naot, Y., and Remington, J. S.: Immunoglobulin M–immunosorbent agglutination assay for diagnosis of infectious disease: Diagnosis of acute congenital and acquired *Toxoplasma* infections. J. Clin. Microbiol. *14*:486, 1981.
43. Desmonts, G., and Remington, J. S.: Direct agglutination test for diagnosis of *Toxoplasma* infection: Method for increasing sensitivity and specificity. J. Clin. Microbiol. *11*:562, 1980.
44. Diebler, C., Dussler, A., and Dulac, O.: Congenital toxoplasmosis: Clinical and neuroradiological evaluation of the cerebral lesions. Neuroradiology *27*:125–130, 1985.
45. Dorfman, R. F., and Remington, J. S.: Value of lymph node biopsy in the diagnosis of acute acquired toxoplasmosis. N. Engl. J. Med. *289*:878, 1973.
46. Dubey, J. P., Miller, N. L., and Frenkel, J. K.: The *Toxoplasma gondii* oocyst from cat feces. J. Exp. Med. *132*:636–662, 1970.
47. Eichenwald, H. G.: A study of congenital toxoplasmosis. *In* Siim, J. C. (ed.): Human Toxoplasmosis. Copenhagen, Munksgaard, 1960, pp. 41–49.
48. Featherstone, H.: A Difference in the Family. New York, Penguin, 1987.
49. Foulon, W., Naessens, A., and Ho-Yen, D.: Prevention of congenital toxoplasmosis. J. Perinat. Med. *28*:337–345, 2000.
50. Frenkel, J. K.: Toxoplasmosis. *In* Marcial-Rojas, R. A. (ed.): Pathology of Protozoal and Helminthic Diseases. Baltimore, Williams & Wilkins, 1971, pp. 254–290.
51. Frenkel, J. K.: Toxoplasmosis: A parasite life cycle, pathology, and immunology. *In* Hammond, D. M. (ed.): The Coccidian. Baltimore, University Park Press, 1973, pp. 343–410.
52. Frenkel, J. K.: Pathology and pathogenesis of congenital toxoplasmosis. Bull. N. Y. Acad. Med. 50:182–191, 1974.
53. Frenkel, J., Dubey, J. P., and Miller, N. L.: *Toxoplasma gondii* in cats: Fecal stage identified as coccidian oocysts. Science *167*:893–896, 1970.
54. Frenkel, J. K., Weber, R. W., and Lunde, M. N.: Acute toxoplasmosis: Effective treatment with pyrimethamine, sulfadiazine, leucovorin calcium and yeast. J. A. M. A. *173*:1471–1476, 1960.
55. Garcia, A. G. P.: Congenital toxoplasmosis in two successive sibs. Arch. Dis. Child. *43*:705–709, 1979.
56. Gazzinelli, R. T., Hayashi, S., Wysocka, M., et al.: Role of IL-12 in the initiation of cell-mediated immunity by *Toxoplasma gondii* and its regulation by IL-10 and nitric oxide. J. Eukaryot. Microbiol. *41*(Suppl.):9, 1994.
57. Gazzinelli, R. T., Oswald, I. P., James, S. L., et al.: IL-10 inhibits parasite killing and nitrogen oxide production by IFN-γ–activated macrophages: IL-10 prevents IFN-γ from inducing activity against *T. gondii* and increasing production of RNIs by murine macrophages. J. Immunol. *148*:1792–1796, 1992.
58. Grigg, M. E., Bonnefoy, S., Hehl, A. B., et al.: Success and virulence in *Toxoplasma* as the result of sexual recombination between two distinct ancestries. Science *294*:161–165, 2001.
59. Grover, C. M., Thulliez, P., Remington, J. S., et al.: Rapid prenatal diagnosis of congenital *Toxoplasma* infection using polymerase chain reaction and amniotic fluid. J. Clin. Microbiol. *28*:2297, 1990.
60. Guerina, N. G., Hsu, H.-W., Meissner, H. C., et al.: Neonatal serologic screening and early treatment for congenital *Toxoplasma gondii* infection. N. Engl. J. Med. *33*:1858–1863, 1994.
61. Hakim, F. T., Gazzinelli, R. T., Denkers, E., et al.: $CD8^+$ T cells from mice vaccinated against *Toxoplasma gondii* are cytotoxic for parasite-infected or antigen-pulsed host cells. J. Immunol. *147*:2310–2316, 1991.
62. Hohlfeld, P., Daffos, T., Costa, J. M., et al.: Prenatal diagnosis of congenital toxoplasmosis with a polymerase-chain reaction test on amniotic fluid. N. Engl. J. Med. *331*:695–699, 1994.
63. Hohlfeld, P., Daffos, F., Thulliez, P., et al.: Fetal toxoplasmosis: Outcome of pregnancy and infant follow-up after in utero treatment. J. Pediatr. *115*:765–769, 1989.
64. Holfels, E., McAuley, J., Mack, D., et al.: In vitro effects of artemisinin ether, cycloguanil hydrochloride (alone and in combination with sulfadiazine), quinine sulfate, mefloquine, primaquine phosphate, trifluoperazine hydrochloride, and verapamil on *Toxoplasma gondii.* Antimicrob. Agents Chemother. *38*:1392–1396, 1994.
65. Huskinson-Mark, J., Araujo, F. G., and Remington, J. S.: Evaluation of the effect of drugs on the cyst form of *Toxoplasma gondii.* J. Infect. Dis. *164*:170–177, 1991.
66. Hutchison, W. M., Dunachie, J. F., Siim, J. C., et al.: Coccidian-like nature of *Toxoplasma gondii.* B. M. J. *1*:142, 1970.
67. Ives, N. J., Gazzard, B. G., Easterbrook, P. J.: The changing pattern of AIDS-defining illnesses with the introduction of highly active antiretroviral therapy (HAART) in a London clinic. J. Infect. *42*:134–139, 2001.
68. Janku, J.: Pathogenesa a pathologicka anatomie tak nazveneho vrozeneho kolobomu slute skvrny v oku normalne velikem a mikrophthalmickem s nalezem parazitu v sitnici. Cas. Lek. Cesk. *60*:1021, 1923.
69. Johnson, A., McLeod, R., Cesbron-Delauw, M. F., et al.: Vaccine Development and Technology to Prevent Toxoplasmosis. Fontevraud, France, WHO Working Group, 1992, p. 1.
70. Joiner, K. A., and Dubremetz, J. F.: *Toxoplasma gondii:* A protozoan for the nineties. Infect. Immun. *61*:1169–1172, 1993.
71. Kasper, L. H., Khan, I. A., Ely, K. H., et al.: Antigen-specific (P30) mouse $CD8^+$ T cells are cytotoxic against *Toxoplasma gondii*–infected peritoneal macrophages. J. Immunol. *148*:1493, 1992.
72. Kazdan, J. J., McCulloch, J. C., and Crawford, J. S.: Uveitis in children. Can. Med. Assoc. J. *96*:385, 1967.
73. Khan, A. A., Slifer, T., Araujo, F. G., et al.: Trovafloxacin is active against *Toxoplasma gondii.* Antimicrob. Agents Chemother. *40*:1855–1859, 1996.
74. Khan, I. A., Ely, K. H., and Kasper, L. H.: A purified parasite antigen (p30) mediates $CD8^+$ T cell immunity against fatal *Toxoplasma gondii* infection in mice. J. Immunol. *147*:3501–3506, 1991.
75. Kim, K., Soldati, D., and Boothroyd, J. C.: Gene replacement in *Toxoplasma gondii* with chloramphenicol acetyltransferase as selectable marker. Science *262*:911–914, 1993.
76. Koppe, J. G., Kloosterman, G. J., deRoever-Bonnet, H., et al.: Toxoplasmosis and pregnancy, with a long-term follow-up of the children. Eur. J. Obstet. Gynecol. Reprod. Biol. *413*:101–110, 1974.
77. Koppe, J. G., Loewer-Sieger, D. H., and de Roever-Bonnet, H.: Results of 20-year follow-up of congenital toxoplasmosis. Lancet *1*:254–256, 1986.
78. Kräubig, H.: Preventive Behandlung der konatalen *Toxoplasmose. In* Kirchoff, H., and Kräubig, H. (eds.): *Toxoplasmose:* Praktische Fragen und Ergebnisse. Stuttgart, Georg Thieme Verlag, 1966.
79. Labadie, M. D., and Hazemann, J. J.: Apport des bilans de sante de l'-enfant pour le depistage et l'etude epidemiologique de la toxoplasmose congenitale. Ann. Pediatr. *31*:823, 1984.
80. Liesenfeld, O., Wong, S. Y., Remington, J. S.: Toxoplasmosis in the setting of AIDS. *In* Merigan, T. C., Bartlett, J. G., Bolognesi, D. (eds.): Textbook of AIDS Medicine. Baltimore, Williams & Williams, 1999, pp. 225–229.
81. Leport, C., Chakroun, M., Matheron, S., et al.: Zidovudine efficacy and tolerance in 32 patients with cerebral toxoplasmosis in the acquired immunodeficiency syndrome. Presse Med. *17*:1813–1814, 1988.
82. Levaditi, C.: Au sujet de certaines protozooses hereditaires humaines a localisations oculaires et nerveuses. C. R. Soc. Biol. *98*:297, 1928.
83. Luft, B. J., Conley, F., and Remington, J. S.: Outbreak of central-nervous-system toxoplasmosis in Western Europe and North America. Lancet *1*:781, 1983.
84. Luft, B. J., Naot, Y., Araujo, F. G., et al.: Primary and reactivated *Toxoplasma* infection in patients with cardiac transplants: Clinical spectrum and problems in diagnosis in a defined population. Ann. Intern. Med. *99*:27, 1983.
85. Luft, B. J., and Remington, J. S.: Acute *Toxoplasma* infection among family members of patients with acute lymphadenopathic toxoplasmosis. Arch. Intern. Med. *144*:53, 1984.
86. Luft, B. J., and Remington, J. S.: Toxoplasmic encephalitis in AIDS. Clin. Infect. Dis. *15*:211–222, 1992.
87. Mack, D. G., Johnson, J. J., Roberts, F., et al.: Murine and human MHC class II genes determine susceptibility to toxoplasmosis. Int. J. Parasitol. *29*:1351–1358, 1999.
88. Masur, H., Jones, T. C., Lempert, J. A., et al.: Outbreak of toxoplasmosis in a family and documentation of acquired retinochoroiditis. Am. J. Med. *64*:396, 1978.
89. McAuley, J. B., Boyer, K. M., Patel, D., et al.: Early and longitudinal evaluations of treated infants and children and untreated historical patients with congenital toxoplasmosis: The Chicago Collaborative Treatment Trial. Clin. Infect. Dis. *18*:38–72, 1994.

90. McCabe, R. E., Brooks, R. G., Dorfman, R. F., et al.: Clinical spectrum in 107 cases of toxoplasmic lymphadenopathy. Rev. Infect. Dis. *9*:754, 1987.
91. McCabe, R., Gibbons, D., Brooks, R. G., et al.: Agglutination test for diagnosis of toxoplasmosis in AIDS. Lancet *2*:680, 1983.
92. McCabe, R. E., and Remington, J. S.: Toxoplasmosis: The time has come. N. Engl. J. Med. *318*:313–315, 1988.
93. McGee, T., Wolters, C., Stein, L., et al.: Absence of sensorineural hearing abnormalities in treated infants with congenital toxoplasmosis. Otolaryngol. Head Neck Surg. *106*:75–80, 1992.
94. McLeod, R., Beem, M. O., and Estes, R. G.: Lymphocyte anergy specific to *Toxoplasma gondii* antigens in a baby with congenital toxoplasmosis. J. Clin. Lab. Immunol. *17*:149, 1985.
95. McLeod, R., Boyer, K. M., Roizen, N., et al.: The child with congenital toxoplasmosis. Curr. Clin. Top. Infect. Dis. *20*:189–208, 2000.
96. McLeod, R., Brown, C., and Mack, D.: Immunogenetics influence outcome of *Toxoplasma gondii* infection. J. Immunol. *142*:3247–3255, 1989.
97. McLeod, R., Frenkel, J. K., Estes, R. G., et al.: Subcutaneous and intestinal vaccination with tachyzoites of *Toxoplasma gondii* and acquisition of immunity to peroral and congenital *Toxoplasma* challenge. J. Immunol. *140*:1632–1637, 1988.
98. McLeod, R., and Mack, D.: A new micromethod to study the effects of antimicrobial agents of *Toxoplasma gondii:* Comparison of sulfadoxine and sulfadiazine individually and in combination with pyrimethamine and study of clindamycin, metronidazole, and cyclosporin A. Antimicrob. Agents Chemother. *26*:26–30, 1984.
99. McLeod, R., Mack, D. G., Boyer, K. M., et al.: Phenotypes and functions of lymphocytes in congenital toxoplasmosis. J. Lab. Clin. Med. *116*:623–635, 1990.
100. McLeod, R., Mack, D., and Brown, C.: New advances in cellular and molecular biology of *Toxoplasma gondii.* Exp. Parasitol. *72*:109–121, 1991.
101. McLeod, R., Mack, D., Foss, R., et al.: Levels of pyrimethamine in sera and cerebrospinal and ventricular fluids from infants treated for congenital toxoplasmosis. Antimicrob. Agents Chemother. *36*:1040–1048, 1992.
102. McLeod, R., and Remington, J. S.: Toxoplasmosis. *In* Braunwald, E., Isselbacher, K. J., Petersdorf, R. G., et al. (eds.): Harrison's Principles of Internal Medicine. New York, McGraw-Hill, 1987, p. 795.
103. McLeod, R., Wisner, J., and Boyer, K.: Toxoplasmosis. *In* Krugman, S., Katz, S. L., and Gershon, A. A. (eds.): Infectious Diseases of Children. St. Louis, Mosby–Year Book, 1992, pp. 539–542.
104. Mets, M. B., Holfels, E. M., Boyer, K. M., et al.: Eye manifestations of congenital toxoplasmosis. Am. J. Ophthalmol. *122*:309–324, 1996.
105. Miller, M. J., and Remington, J. S.: Toxoplasmosis in infants and children with HIV infection or AIDS. *In* Pizzo, P. A., and Wilfert, C. M. (eds.): Pediatric AIDS: The Challenge of HIV Infection in Infants, Children and Adolescents. Baltimore, Williams & Wilkins, 1990, pp. 299–307.
106. Mitchell, C. D., Erlich, S. S., Mastrucci, M. T., et al.: Congenital toxoplasmosis occurring in three infants perinatally infected with the human immunodeficiency virus (HIV-1). Pediatr. Infect. Dis. J. *9*:512, 1990.
107. Mitchell, W.: Neurological and developmental effects of HIV and AIDS in children and adolescents. Ment. Retard. Dev. Disabil. Res. Rev. *7*: 211–216, 2001.
108. Montoya, J. G.: Laboratory diagnosis of *Toxoplasma gondii* infection and toxoplasmosis. J. Infect. Dis. *185*(Suppl.):73–82, 2002.
109. Montoya, J. G., and Remington, J. S.: Studies on the serodiagnosis of toxoplasmic lymphadenitis. Clin. Infect. Dis. *20*:781–789, 1995.
110. Montoya, J. G., and Remington, J. S.: Toxoplasmic chorioretinitis in the setting of acute acquired toxoplasmosis. Clin. Infect. Dis. *23*:277–282, 1996.
111. Naot, Y., Barnett, E. V., and Remington, J. S.: Method for avoiding false positive results occurring in immunoglobulin M enzyme-linked immunosorbent assays due to presence of both rheumatoid factor and antinuclear antibodies. J. Clin. Microbiol. *14*:73, 1981.
112. Naot, Y., Desmonts, G., and Remington, J. S.: IgM enzyme-linked immunosorbent assay test for the diagnosis of congenital *Toxoplasma* infection. J. Pediatr. *98*:32, 1981.
113. Naot, Y., and Remington, J. S.: An enzyme-linked immunosorbent assay for detection of IgM antibodies to *Toxoplasma gondii:* Use for diagnosis of acute acquired toxoplasmosis. J. Infect. Dis. *142*:757, 1981.
114. Nicolle, C., and Manceaux, L.: Sur une infection à corps de Leishman (ou organisme voisins) du gondi. C. R. Acad. Sci. *147*:763, 1908.
115. Nicolle, C., and Manceaux, L.: Sur une protozoaire nouveau du gondi. C. R. Acad. Sci. *148*:369, 1909.
116. O'Connor, G. R.: Manifestations and management of ocular toxoplasmosis. Bull. N. Y. Acad. Med. *50*:192, 1974.
117. Patel, D. V., Hofels, E., Vogel, N., et al.: Resolution of intracerebral calcifications in children with treated congenital toxoplasmosis. Radiology *199*:433–440, 1996.
118. Pfefferkorn, E. R., Nothnagel, R. F., and Borotz, S. E.: Parasiticidal effect of clindamycin on *Toxoplasma gondii* grown in cultured cells and selection of a drug-resistant mutant. Antimicrob. Agents Chemother. *36*:1091–1096, 1992.
119. Pinkerton, H., and Weinman, D.: *Toxoplasma* infection in man. Arch. Pathol. *30*:374, 1940.
120. Remington, J., Eimstad, W., and Araujo, F.: Detection of immunoglobulin M antibodies with antigen-tagged latex particles in an immunosorbent assay. J. Clin. Microbiol. *17*:939, 1983.
121. Remington, J. S., and McLeod, R.: Toxoplasmosis. *In* Braude, A. I. (ed.): International Textbook of Medicine. Vol. II. Medical Microbiology and Infectious Disease. Philadelphia, W. B. Saunders, 1981, p. 1818.
122. Remington, J. S., McLeod, R., and Desmonts, G.: Toxoplasmosis. *In* Remington, J. S., and Klein, J. O. (eds.): Infectious Diseases of the Fetus and Newborn. 4th ed. Philadelphia, W. B. Saunders, 1995, pp. 140–263.
123. Remington, J. S., and Wilson, C. B.: Toxoplasmosis. *In* Kass, E. H., and Platt, R. (eds.): Current Therapy in Infectious Disease: 1983–1984. Philadelphia, B. C. Decker, 1983, pp. 149–153.
124. Roberts, C. W., Roberts, F., Lyons, R. E., et al.: The shikamate pathway and its branches in apicomplexan parasites. J. Infect. Dis. *185*(Suppl.):25–36, 2002.
125. Roberts, F., and McLeod, R.: Pathogenesis of toxoplasmic retinochoroiditis. Parasitol. Today *15*:51–57, 1999.
126. Roberts, F., Mets, M. B., Ferguson, D. J. P., et al.: Histopathological features of ocular toxoplasmosis in the fetus and infant. Arch. Ophthalmol. *19*:51–58, 2001.
127. Roberts, F., Roberts, C. W., Johnson, J. J., et al.: Evidence for the shikamate pathway in apicomplexan parasites. Nature *393*:801–805, 1998.
128. Roberts, T., and Frenkel, J. K.: Estimating income losses and other preventable costs caused by congenital toxoplasmosis in people in the United States. J. A. M. A. *2*:249–257, 1990.
129. Roizen, N., Swisher, C., Stein, M. A., et al.: Neurologic and developmental function in treated congenital toxoplasmosis. Pediatrics *95*:11–20, 1995.
130. Romand, D. S., Wallon, M., Franck, J., et al.: Prenatal diagnosis using polymerase chain reaction on amniotic fluid for congenital toxoplasmosis. Obstet. Gynecol. *97*:296–300, 2001.
131. Ruskin, J., and Remington, J. S.: Toxoplasmosis in the compromised host. Ann. Intern. Med. *84*:193, 1976.
132. Sabin, A. B.: Toxoplasmic encephalitis in children. J. A. M. A. *116*:801–807, 1941.
133. Sabin, A. B., and Feldman, H. A.: Dyes as microchemical indicators of a new immunity phenomenon affecting a protozoon parasite *(Toxoplasma).* Science *108*:660, 1948.
134. Sacks, J. J., Roberto, R. R., and Brooks, N. F.: Toxoplasmosis infection associated with raw goat's milk. J. A. M. A. *248*:1728, 1982.
135. Schlaegel, T. F.: Ocular Toxoplasmosis and Pars Planitis. New York, Grune & Stratton, 1978.
136. Schoondermark-Van de Ven, E., Galama, J., Camps, W., et al.: Pharmacokinetic of spiramycin in the rhesus monkey: Transplacental passage and distribution in tissue in the fetus. Antimicrob. Agents Chemother. *38*:1922–1929, 1994.
137. Schoondermark-Van de Ven, E., Melchers, W., Camps, W., et al.: Effectiveness of spiramycin for treatment of congenital *Toxoplasma gondii* infection in rhesus monkeys. Antimicrob. Agents Chemother. *38*:1930–1936, 1994.
138. Shenep, J. L., Barenkamp, S. J., Brammeier, S. A., et al.: An outbreak of toxoplasmosis on an Illinois farm. Pediatr. Infect. Dis. *3*:518, 1984.
139. Sher, A., Oswald, I. P., Hieny, S., et al.: *Toxoplasma gondii* induces a T-independent IFN-γ response in natural killer cells that requires both adherent accessory cells and tumor necrosis factor-α. J. Immunol. *150*: 3982–3989, 1993.
140. Sibley, L. D., Pfefferkorn, E. R., and Boothroyd, J. C.: Development of genetic systems for *Toxoplasma gondii.* Parasitol. Today *9*:392–395, 1993.
141. Smith, K. L., Wilson, M., Hightower, A. L., et al.: Prevalence of *Toxoplasma gondii* antibodies in U. S. military recruits in 1989: Comparison with data published in 1965. Clin. Infect. Dis. *23*:1182– 1183, 1996.
142. Splendore, A.: Un nuovo protozoa parassita dei conigli: Incontrato nelle lesioni anatomiche d'una malattia che ricorda in molti punti il Kalaazar dell'uomo. Rev. Soc. Sci. *3*:109, 1908.
143. Stepick-Biek, P., Thulliez, P., Araujo, F. G., et al.: IgA antibodies for diagnosis of acute congenital and acquired toxoplasmosis. J. Infect. Dis. *162*:270, 1990.
144. Stray-Pedersen, B.: Infants potentially at risk for congenital toxoplasmosis: A prospective study. Am. J. Dis. Child. *134*:638, 1980.
145. Suzuki, Y., Orellana, M. A., Schreiber, R. D., et al.: Interferon γ: The major mediator of resistance against *Toxoplasma gondii.* Science *240*:516, 1988.
146. Swisher, C. N., Boyer, K., and McLeod, R.: Congenital toxoplasmosis. The Toxoplasmosis Study Group. Semin. Pediatr. Neurol. *1*:4–25, 1994.
147. Tabbara, K., and O'Connor, R.: Treatment of ocular toxoplasmosis with clindamycin and sulfadiazine. Ophthalmology *87*:129, 1980.
148. Teutsch, S. M., Juranek, D. D., Sulzer, A., et al.: Epidemic toxoplasmosis associated with infected cats. N. Engl. J. Med. *300*:695, 1979.
149. Vietzke, W. M., Gelderman, A. H., Grimley, P. M., et al.: Toxoplasmosis complicating malignancy. Cancer *21*:816, 1968.

150. Vogel, N., Kirisits, M., Michael, E., et al.: Congenital toxoplasmosis transmitted from an immunologically competent mother infected before conception. Clin. Infect. Dis. *23*:1055–1060, 1996.
151. Wallon, M., Cogan, G., Ecochard, R., et al: Serological rebound in congenital toxoplasmosis. Long-term follow-up of 133 children. Eur. J. Pediatr. *160*:534–540, 2001.
152. Walls, K. W., and Remington, J. S.: Evaluation of a commercial latex agglutination method for toxoplasmosis. Diagn. Microbiol. Infect. Dis. *1*:265, 1983.
153. Weiss, L. M., Harris, C., Berger, M., et al.: Pyrimethamine concentrations in serum and cerebrospinal fluid during treatment of acute *Toxoplasma* encephalitis in patients with AIDS. J. Infect. Dis. *157*: 580–583, 1988.
154. Welch, P. C., Masur, H., Jones, T. C., et al.: Serologic diagnosis of acute lymphadenopathic toxoplasmosis. J. Infect. Dis. *142*:256, 1981.
155. Wilson, C. B.: Treatment of congenital toxoplasmosis during pregnancy. J. Pediatr. *116*:1003–1004, 1990.
156. Wilson, C. B., Desmonts, G., Couvreur, J., et al.: Lymphocyte transformation in the diagnosis of congenital *Toxoplasma* infection. N. Engl. J. Med. *302*:785, 1980.
157. Wilson, C. B., and Remington, J. S.: What can be done to prevent congenital toxoplasmosis? Am. J. Obstet. Gynecol. *138*:357, 1980.
158. Wilson, C. B., Remington, J. S., Stagno, S., et al.: Development of adverse sequelae in children born with subclinical congenital *Toxoplasma* infection. Pediatrics *66*:767, 1980.
159. Wolf, A., and Cowen, D.: Granulomatous encephalomyelitis due to an Encephalitozoon (encephalitozoic encephalomyelitis): A new protozoan disease of man. Bull. Neurol. Inst. N. Y. *6*:307, 1937.
160. Wong, S. Y., Hajdu, M. P., Ramirez, R., et al.: The role of specific immunoglobulin E in the diagnosis of acute *Toxoplasma* infection and toxoplasmosis. J. Clin. Microbiol. *31*:2952–2959, 1993.
161. Wong, S. Y., and Remington, J. S.: Toxoplasmosis in pregnancy. Clin. Infect. Dis. *18*:853–862, 1994.

Pneumocystis carinii Pneumonia

WALTER T. HUGHES ■ DONALD C. ANDERSON

Pneumocystis carinii (recently also referred to as *Pneumocystis jiroveci*)[150a] pneumonia (PCP) is an opportunistic infection of increasing importance to pediatricians. A marked increase in the prevalence of this disorder in the United States during the past 2 decades has paralleled therapeutic advances in the management of immunologic and neoplastic diseases, which has resulted in longer survival of children with these underlying disorders. Since 1980, the infection has occurred in epidemic proportions in association with acquired immunodeficiency syndrome (AIDS).

The Organism

As early as 1909, Chagas[16] identified what he interpreted as the spherical and sickle-shaped forms of the parasite *Trypanosoma cruzi* in the lungs of experimentally infected guinea pigs. The same organism was identified later by Carini[14] and others[168] in animals and human patients with trypanosome infections. In 1912, Delanoe and Delanoe[26] identified this parasite in the lungs of rats and guinea pigs not infected with trypanosomes and proposed an independent genus of *P. carinii*. These and other investigators, including Chagas, subsequently demonstrated that this agent was not related to the trypanosome.[44]

Attempts have been made to find a taxonomic place for *P. carinii*. Studies of DNA sequences coding for ribosomal RNA have shown that *P. carinii* has greater homology with certain fungi than with certain protozoa.[35] Unlike the dihydrofolate reductase of protozoa, the *P. carinii* enzyme is not a bifunctional polypeptide with thymidylate synthetase.[34] The cyst wall contains chitin and β-1,3-glucan, which are common components of fungal cell walls but also are found in certain protozoa and algae.[101, 167] However, unlike that of fungi, the cyst wall does not contain ergosterol or the characteristic protein elongation factor 3.[75] The antifungal drugs amphotericin B, ketoconazole, nystatin, 5-flucytosine, fluconazole, and miconazole have no effect against PCP, whereas the drugs with demonstrated anti–*P. carinii* activity are also antiprotozoan drugs: pentamidine *(Leishmania donovani* and *Trypanosoma gambiense),* trimethoprim-sulfamethoxazole *(Isospora belli, Toxoplasma gondii),* and pyrimethamine-sulfadiazine and atovaquone *(T. gondii* and *Plasmodium falciparum).* Although a fixed taxonomic position for *P. carinii* is desirable, elucidating the biologic characteristics of the organism to achieve effective and safe therapy is more important. Molecular probes for the detection and study of *P. carinii*[117, 165] and for identification of *P. carinii* chromosomes and mapping of genes[99] offer promise for further elucidation of this organism.

Three developmental forms of this organism have been identified by light microscopy: cysts, "sporozoites," and "trophozoites." Cysts occur in lung tissue or respiratory secretions as spherical or crescent-shaped structures approximately 5 μm in diameter (Figs. 223–1 and 223–2). They may contain as many as eight oval bodies or sporozoites 1 to 2 μm in diameter. A third extracystic pleomorphic structure, called a trophozoite, that varies in size from 2 to 5 μm in diameter is identified in association with cysts. The ultrastructural morphologic features identified by electron microscopy and scanning electron microscopy are well described in the literature.[12, 123, 126, 176] The major protein components of both trophozoites and cysts are referred to as major surface glycoproteins (MSGs) and have molecular weights ranging from 95 to 140 kd. Genes encoding the MSGs are repeated, highly polymorphic, and distributed among all of the 14 to 15 chromosomes.[87, 163] The MSGs are important factors in host-parasite interactions.

Pifer and associates[123] reported successful, though limited propagation of *P. carinii* in vitro in primary chick epithelial lung cells. Subsequently, propagation of *P. carinii* has been reported with Vero, Chang liver, and MRC-5 cells,[89] as well as WI-38[3] and A-549 cell lines.[23] Merali and colleagues[103] recently reported continuous axenic cultivation of *P. carinii* with a collagen-coated porous membrane and a modified minimal essential medium with Earle salt. To date, none of the culture systems have been established and standardized.

Transmission and Epidemiology

The mode of transmission in humans and the natural habitat of *P. carinii* remain largely unknown. This organism

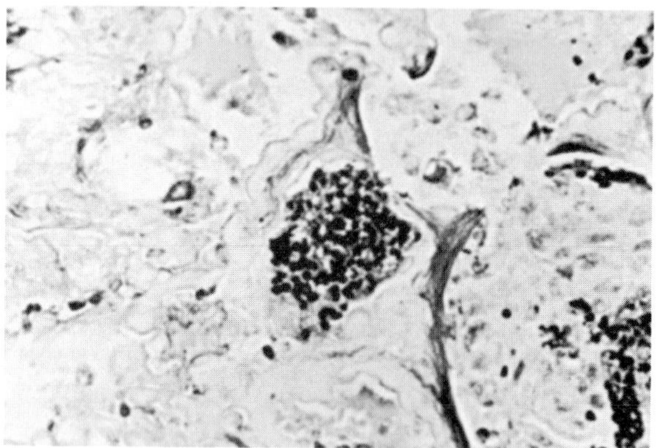

FIGURE 223–1 ■ Typical cyst forms demonstrated by Gomori silver methenamine stain of lung tissue obtained by open lung biopsy from a 20-month-old child with severe combined immunodeficiency disease (×100).

has been recognized in many wild and laboratory animal species over a wide geographic distribution. An association between animal reservoirs and human infection has not been established. Animal-to-animal transmission by the airborne route has been demonstrated in laboratory rats.[54, 58] Furthermore, DNA sequences identical to those of *P. carinii* have been detected in ambient air.[164] Evidence for transmission of *P. carinii* DNA from an infected infant to close hospital contacts has been reported.[159]

Before and during World War II, epidemics of interstitial plasma cell pneumonitis secondary to *P. carinii* were recognized in debilitated and premature infants throughout European institutions and nursing homes.[6, 138] In 1942, Van der Meer and Brug[156] identified *P. carinii* in the lungs of humans with interstitial plasma cell pneumonitis. Subsequent studies confirmed this organism as the cause of the pneumonitis. Interruption of outbreaks by the introduction of strict isolation of affected patients within these institutions suggests the probable importance of person-to-person spread of disease within that setting.[142]

In the United States, PCP was not reported until 1956.[25] In contrast to the early European patterns, American cases largely have been sporadic and have occurred almost exclusively in children with impaired host defenses.[118] A limited number of outbreaks of PCP within families[171] or among closely associated groups of hospitalized cancer patients have been reported, further suggesting the importance of contagion in the spread of this disease.[7, 136, 137, 147]

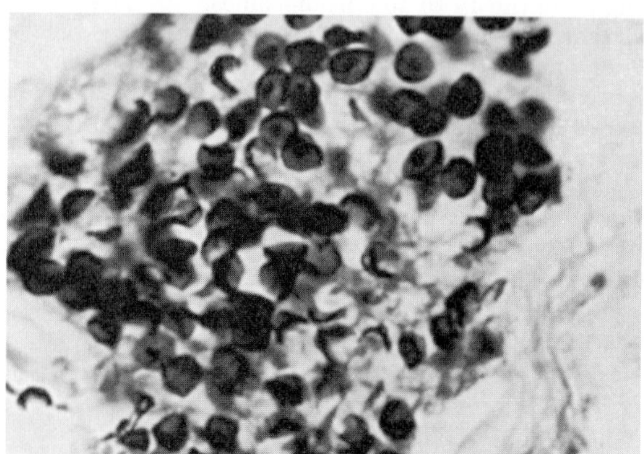

FIGURE 223–2 ■ Same as Figure 223–1 (× 1000).

Autopsy studies have demonstrated the occasional occurrence of *Pneumocystis* organisms in the lungs of patients without evidence of underlying host defense disorders or pulmonary disease.[93] Furthermore, autopsy studies have demonstrated that inapparent (asymptomatic) infection occurs frequently in cancer patients or other immunocompromised populations.[120, 175] An extensive review of autopsies at St. Jude Children's Research Center (1962 to 1969) demonstrated the occurrence of inapparent *Pneumocystis* infection in 4.7 percent of pediatric cancer patients as opposed to 0.1 percent of children who died without malignant disease.[121] The epidemiologic importance of these asymptomatic carriers in the transmission of *Pneumocystis* disease is unknown. Organisms are detected frequently in sputum, pharyngeal secretions, and tracheal aspirates of symptomatic patients.[51] Cysts have been shown to survive for several months in dried lung specimens maintained at room temperature.[68] These observations, in addition to the almost universal localization of disease within the lungs of affected patients, suggest that infection probably results from inhalation of the organism. In view of this possibility, respiratory isolation of symptomatic patients should be maintained to prevent exposure of other highly susceptible patients. No data support the isolation of such patients from otherwise healthy persons.

Asymptomatic *P. carinii* infection is highly prevalent in humans. Serologic studies have shown that more than 90 percent of adults have antibody to *P. carinii* and that approximately 75 percent had acquired *P. carinii* antibody before reaching 4 years of age.[85, 106, 119, 124] Recent molecular techniques show that during periods of immune suppression, PCP can occur either by reactivation or by the acquisition of new organisms.[57]

Persons infected with human immunodeficiency virus type 1 (HIV-1) have a remarkably high risk for the development of *P. carinii* pneumonitis. The pneumonitis was diagnosed in 1080 (39%) of the 2786 pediatric patients with AIDS reported to the Centers for Disease Control and Prevention (CDC) through 1990.[145] Pneumonitis develops in approximately 75 percent of adults with AIDS. Among children with AIDS, *P. carinii* pneumonitis may occur at any age, but most frequently it is found in those between the ages of 3 and 6 months.[84, 143, 145]

Although intrauterine transmission of *P. carinii* has been documented in one stillborn infant and has been implicated in three siblings with no demonstrable immunologic abnormalities who were infected in the neonatal period,[4] the paucity of such cases does not support the epidemiologic importance of this mode of transmission. Of the infants of eight women with AIDS and PCP during pregnancy, only one infant had evidence of *P. carinii* infection.[55, 112] Studies in severe combined immunodeficiency mice have failed to demonstrate transplacental passage of this organism.[72]

Recent studies in Santiago, Chile, and Oxford, United Kingdom, found *P. carinii* in 15 to 35 percent of infants with sudden infant death syndrome (SIDS) versus 2.9 percent of infants in the same age groups who died of other causes.[160] Because of the scarcity of organisms, the terminal event in SIDS cannot be explained by PCP; the association remains unexplained.

Pathogenesis

That *P. carinii* is an organism of low pathogenicity clearly is emphasized by the rare development of infection in intact hosts. Despite widespread occurrence in the lungs of healthy laboratory animals, it rarely causes pulmonary disease unless experimentally provoked.

Before the AIDS epidemic, PCP occurred almost exclusively in patients with primary immunologic disorders or in those receiving immunosuppressive therapy for oncologic disease or organ transplantation.[28, 46, 120, 161, 170] Of 194 cases reported to the CDC between 1967 and 1970, 29 occurred in infants younger than 1 year, 83 percent of whom had primary immunodeficiency disorders. In contrast, acute lymphocytic leukemia was the most common underlying disease in children older than 1 year.[170] Of 1251 children with malignancies at the St. Jude Research Hospital (1962 to 1971), PCP occurred in 51 (4.1%). In that series, the incidence of infection in 872 children with leukemia, Hodgkin disease, neuroblastoma, reticulum cell sarcoma, and Letterer-Siwe disease was 5.8 percent, whereas in 379 patients with other types of neoplasia and in 1669 children without malignant disease, *P. carinii* infection was not encountered.[68]

Within populations of cancer patients, *P. carinii* infection occurs more commonly in those with generalized lymphoproliferative malignancy than in patients with solid tumors.[9, 146] The extent of malignant disease and the intensity of the chemotherapy or radiotherapy provided are associated with an increased risk for the development of *Pneumocystis* infection.[59, 120, 146] In children with acute lymphocytic leukemia, mediastinal involvement or irradiation of the mediastinum, or both, also is associated with an increased incidence of PCP.[59]

The European outbreaks of PCP in debilitated infants, in addition to the well-known association of malnutrition and impaired resistance to a variety of infectious disorders, suggest the possible importance of malnutrition as an additional host determinant for the development of *P. carinii* infection.[69, 75, 76, 141]

Pneumocystis pneumonia has been reported in congenital and acquired hypogammaglobulinemia, severe combined immunodeficiency disease, partial immunodeficiency disease, and secondary immunodeficiency states. Only one patient with a pure T-cell deficiency (DiGeorge syndrome) has been reported with an associated *Pneumocystis* infection.[28]

No characteristic pattern of serum immunoglobulin abnormality has been demonstrated. Low levels of IgG were the most consistent finding in two reported series of children with immunodeficiency disease.[9, 170] In contrast, normal or elevated levels of IgG were documented in 70 percent of leukemic children with PCP. Administration of serum immunoglobulin to infected children with these disorders usually provided no therapeutic benefit.[170] The role of IgA antibody in host defense against *P. carinii* probably is not of major importance because secretory IgA levels are normal in most affected patients and those with immunodeficiency states characterized by IgA deficits are not unduly susceptible.[9, 170]

The development of specific antibodies to *P. carinii* in infected patients has been inconsistent. During the course of "epidemic" disease in malnourished infants, IgM values frequently increase markedly, with variable changes in IgG and IgA values. IgG antibody concentrations increase in serum 4 to 6 weeks after infection and are thought to provide permanent immunity in these infants.[83] In selected instances, specific antibody responses (IgG, IgA, and IgM) have been demonstrated in normal persons who have been associated closely with infected patients.[9, 105] The development of specific immunoglobulins (IgG and IgM) in two patients with lymphoreticular malignancies who recovered from PCP further emphasizes the probable importance of humoral immunity in determining the outcome of infection.[9]

Using immunofluorescent staining techniques, Brzosko and colleagues[8] demonstrated IgG and IgM antibody with smaller amounts of IgA antibody and beta$_{1c}$-globulin deposits on the surface of *Pneumocystis* organisms within the alveoli of infants with "epidemic" PCP. Late in the course of their disease, less immunoglobulin was present within alveoli, whereas increased numbers of plasma cells and alveolar macrophages containing fluorescent material were identified. Possibly, specific antibody fixes complement (beta$_{1c}$-globulin) on the surface of *Pneumocystis* organisms, thereby allowing subsequent phagocytosis by alveolar macrophages.[8]

The importance of impaired cellular immune responses in patients with PCP is evident. The ability of corticosteroids to induce *P. carinii* infection in laboratory animals, the occurrence of PCP in patients with AIDS and in at least one patient with a pure T-cell deficiency disease,[28] and the development of PCP in malnourished hosts with significantly impaired cellular immune responses[69, 75, 92, 141] provide indirect evidence of the potential importance of cellular immunity in protecting the host against this opportunist. Because corticosteroids, cytotoxic agents, and malnutrition variably depress both humoral and cellular immune mechanisms, as well as nonspecific immune responses (inflammation),[9, 19, 122] no absolute statement can be made regarding the relative importance of each defense mechanism. Strong evidence has implicated the importance of T-lymphocyte competence in the pathogenesis of PCP. Experimental studies in rats demonstrated provocation of the pneumonitis after the administration of cyclosporine.[71] This compound specifically affects T-cell–mediated immune responses related to impairment of interleukin-2 production and receptor site inhibition and has no direct effect on other components of the immune system. Especially convincing is the remarkable susceptibility of patients with AIDS to PCP. In this syndrome, host compromise is limited primarily to impaired T-cell function, and PCP develops in at least 50 percent of affected patients.[155]

In infants, children, and adults with AIDS, the quantity of peripheral blood CD4 (T4) helper T lymphocytes serves as a useful predictor of *P. carinii* pneumonitis. As the CD4 lymphocyte count decreases, the risk for acquiring *P. carinii* pneumonitis increases. In adults, a CD4 cell count less than 200/mm^3 is highly predictive of impending *P. carinii* pneumonitis. Because infants and children have relatively higher total lymphocyte counts, absolute CD4 cell counts are higher than those in adults. Therefore, the threshold for the risk of acquiring *P. carinii* infection is age related. Estimates indicate that risk of development of *P. carinii* pneumonitis in patients with AIDS warrants consideration of chemoprophylaxis if CD4 lymphocyte counts are less than 750/mm^3 in those 12 to 23 months of age, less than 500/mm^3 in children 24 months to 5 years of age, and less than 200/mm^3 in those 6 years or older.[84]

With any of the underlying causes of immunocompromise, patients recovering from *P. carinii* pneumonitis remain at high risk for the development of recurrent episodes.

For infants younger than 1 year, the CD4 lymphocyte count is less predictive of the risk for PCP and cannot be relied on for decisions about prophylaxis.[15, 144] However, most PCP episodes occur after the CD4 lymphocyte count decreases below 1500 cells/mm^3 during the first year of life.

Some evidence suggests that *P. carinii* pneumonitis may occur in immunocompetent infants in the United States.[150] In a prospective study of 67 infants 2 to 12 weeks of age with pneumonitis in Birmingham, Alabama, 10 were found to have serologic evidence of this infection. In 1 of the 10 babies, the diagnosis was proved by lung biopsy. In serial observations conducted every 2 months on a cohort of 107 normal healthy infants in Chile, *P. carinii* DNA was detected in nasopharyngeal aspirates obtained during episodes of mild respiratory infection in 24 (32%) of 74 infants from whom specimens were available. Three (12.5%) of those 24 infants versus 0 of 50 infants who tested negative for *P. carinii* had apnea episodes. Eighty-five percent of the infants seroconverted by 20 months of age.[158] Further delineation of the clinical features of *P. carinii* infection in normal hosts is needed.

Pathology

P. carinii infections are unique in that the pathologic findings, with rare exceptions, are limited to the lungs, even in fatal cases. In the infantile "epidemic" form of disease, essentially all alveoli contain large numbers of organisms. Extensive interstitial plasma cell infiltrates distend the alveolar walls 5 to 20 times over their normal thickness, and almost no intra-alveolar fibrinous exudate is noted.[32, 51] In the childhood and adult forms of PCP, the histogenesis has been described in three stages.[51, 68, 126] An initial stage is characterized by the presence of cysts and trophozoites attached by fibronectin to the alveolar walls.[125] No septal inflammatory or cellular response is evident, and no clinical disease is associated with this stage. A second stage, which may or may not be associated with clinical signs and symptoms, is characterized by desquamation of alveolar cells and an increase in the number of cysts within alveolar macrophages. Tumor necrosis factor may be a major mediator involved in the killing of *P. carinii* by activated alveolar macrophages and may be induced by oxidative stress in the alveoli.[121] The final stage is typified by extensive reactive and desquamative alveolitis manifested by marked cytoplasmic vacuolization of macrophages, mononuclear and plasma cell infiltrates within alveolar septa, and clusters of organisms located predominantly within macrophages in the lumen of alveoli. The histopathology of this final stage definitely is associated with clinical manifestations of pneumonitis.[126] In rare instances, *P. carinii* organisms have been detected in the lymph nodes, spleen, liver, retina, bone marrow, gastrointestinal tract, pancreas, heart, adrenals, and peripheral blood.[49, 127, 151] A fatal case of disseminated *P. carinii* infection in a 13-month-old infant with thymic alymphoplasia has been reported.[127]

Clinical Manifestations

The natural course of *P. carinii* infection in children varies highly and depends primarily on the status of host defenses in individual patients. The onset may be insidious, with a clinical course of 3 or more weeks, or be fulminant and rapidly progressive over a few days.

The clinical course of infantile epidemic pneumocystosis is typified in premature, debilitated, or marasmic infants between 2 and 6 months of age. These patients often have chronic diarrhea and weight loss before the development of respiratory symptoms. Characteristically, the onset is insidious, with progression of cough, tachypnea, and respiratory distress over the course of a 1- to 4-week interval. Fever is either absent or of low grade in most cases.[31]

Symptoms in immunosuppressed children or adults without AIDS may be more abrupt in onset and more rapidly progressive than those in infantile epidemic cases. Even with these patients, the course also varies highly.[9, 46, 51, 68, 129, 170] The mortality rate is approximately 100 percent in untreated cases because of the overall severity of the disease in immunocompromised patients.[51] In cases in children and adults, in contrast to infantile cases, fever is generally present and of high grade. It often precedes the onset of nonproductive cough, tachypnea, and severe dyspnea. Fever, tachypnea, and the radiographic appearance of pulmonary infiltrates, in that sequence from 1 to 21 days before diagnosis, occurred in a group of children with malignancy.[68] In half of these patients, signs and symptoms occurred within 5 days before initiation of treatment. In a select group of 10 untreated patients, the extent of fever, respiratory distress, and radiographic abnormalities varied from mild to severe. Pulmonary infiltrates were apparent 1 to 13 days before death, and the total course of infection ranged from 4 to 21 days.

The time of onset of clinical disease in non-AIDS, high-risk patients is unpredictable, but disease often occurs after discontinuance or a reduction in the dose of corticosteroid therapy. Rifkind and coworkers[131] noted the clinical onset of infection in transplant patients when the prednisone dosage was reduced below 1 mg/kg body weight per 24 hours. In another series, PCP developed in 9 of 46 patients while steroid therapy was being reduced.[9] However, the relationship may be to the duration of corticosteroid therapy rather than the withdrawal or reduction in dosage. A patient with severe combined immunodeficiency disease who received a bone marrow transplant subsequently contracted fulminant PCP when apparent immunologic reconstitution had taken place.[9] A similar case in Houston, Texas, occurred in a child with severe combined immunodeficiency disease who was the recipient of a thymic epithelial explant. This patient became clinically well, and evidence of engraftment and return of normal immunologic function was documented by in vitro studies approximately 6 weeks after the transplant. At that time, fulminant PCP developed, as determined by open lung biopsy (see Figs. 223–1 and 223–2). These observations imply that the development of clinical disease depends in part on normal inflammatory responses, which may be impaired somewhat as a result of the patient's underlying disease, the therapeutic regimen, or both.

Infants and children with AIDS usually are acutely ill with fever (79%), cough (86%), dyspnea (88%), tachypnea (88%), and an alveolar-arterial oxygen gradient greater than 30 mm Hg (95%) at the time of onset of *P. carinii* pneumonitis. The median length of survival after the diagnosis of *P. carinii* pneumonitis was only 2 months in a study by Connor and associates.[20]

In children and adults both with and without AIDS, physical examination at the time of initial evaluation may reveal tachypnea, nasal flaring, and intercostal, subcostal, or supracostal retractions. An ashen color or cyanosis may be present or may develop rapidly. Auscultation of the chest frequently is characterized by a conspicuous absence of adventitious sounds despite rapid (80 to 100/min), shallow respirations. Scattered rales, rhonchi, or wheezes most often are detected later in the clinical course as resolution occurs. Aside from variable elevation in temperature, few other physical abnormalities are noted, except those referable to pulmonary disease or secondary to the patient's underlying disease or treatment.[9, 51, 68, 170]

A variety of radiographic abnormalities have been observed in documented cases of isolated PCP.* These variations result partly from observations at different stages in the course of disease. Bilateral diffuse parenchymal infiltrates (Fig. 223–3) occur most commonly, but no pattern is

*See references 11, 13, 22, 29, 39, 42, 113, 128, 162, 174.

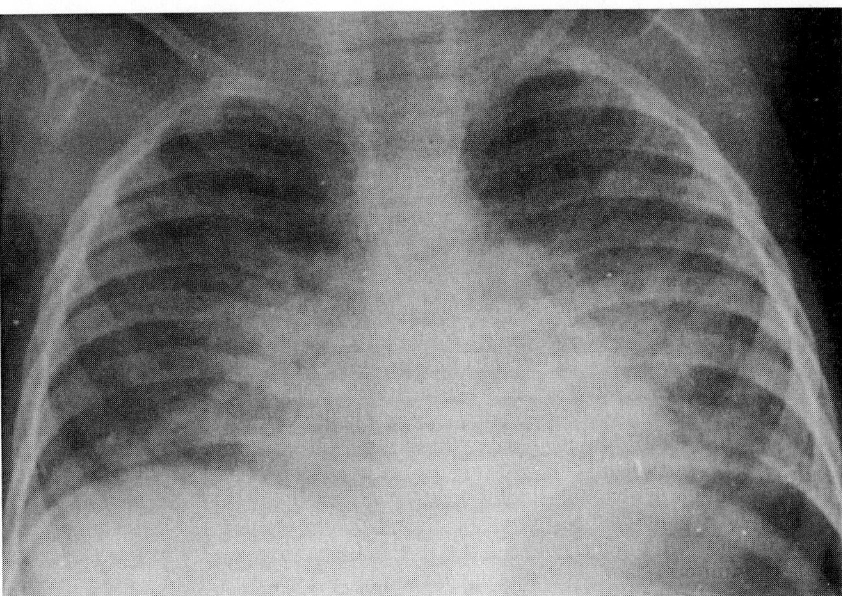

FIGURE 223–3 ■ Typical diffuse interstitial infiltrates seen in a 20-month-old child with severe combined immunodeficiency disease at the time of evaluation for clinical *Pneumocystis carinii* pneumonitis.

sufficiently specific to either exclude or confirm a consideration of *P. carinii* disease. Though initially a reticulogranular interstitial process, *Pneumocystis* pneumonitis progresses to a predominantly alveolar process with coalescence and air bronchogram formation. Late in the course of the disease, lung fields may opacify completely.[29, 39] Hilar adenopathy and pleural effusion are not characteristic unless they are a result of an underlying disorder. During treatment, radiographs show gradual clearing after a variable latent period, during which they may appear worse. Residual interstitial fibrosis occurs in a small percentage of patients.[174] Unusual radiographic findings, including an asymmetric distribution, consolidated lobar infiltrates,[11, 22, 39] pneumothorax and pneumomediastinum,[13] localized parenchymal nodular densities,[22, 29] and pleural effusion,[39] have been documented. One investigator noted the occurrence of at least one "atypical" radiographic finding in 56 percent of 30 cases of PCP.[29]

Diagnosis

Characteristic clinical features are not sufficiently specific to differentiate PCP from other opportunistic pulmonary infections in highly susceptible pediatric patients. Furthermore, mixed infections with viral, bacterial, fungal, or parasitic agents have been documented along with *P. carinii*.[9, 47, 88, 137, 152, 153] Implicit in these observations is the importance and urgency of establishing a definitive diagnosis before the institution of specific therapy. An etiologic diagnosis can be ascertained only by the demonstration of *P. carinii* organisms in lung tissue or respiratory secretions.

Numerous techniques have been used to obtain suitable material for diagnostic purposes. Although specimens obtained by noninvasive methods from sputum[40, 97] or pharyngeal,[37] tracheal,[91] or gastric[18] secretions occasionally reveal *P. carinii* in infected patients, these sources are not sufficiently reliable to exclude the diagnosis if organisms are not identified.[51] Bronchopulmonary lavage,[30, 51, 115] endobronchial brush biopsy,[38, 130] and transbronchial lung biopsy[50, 79] have been used successfully to establish a diagnosis of PCP in adult patients. Limited experience and the significant morbidity associated with these procedures in pediatric patients do not justify their routine use in children.

Invasive techniques, including open lung biopsy, closed needle biopsy, and percutaneous needle aspiration, are the most reliable methods for confirming a diagnosis.[51, 88, 108, 133, 169] Open lung biopsy provides the most dependable specimen from which identification of the organism, as well as the extent of the infection, can be ascertained. Its chief disadvantage is the need for general anesthesia. A closed needle biopsy procedure is less reliable in providing adequate tissue and is associated with significantly greater morbidity than open thoracotomy is.[80] Percutaneous needle aspiration has proved to be a relatively consistent and safe procedure in selected centers.[51, 81] Bronchoalveolar lavage has been safe and successful, especially in patients with AIDS, in whom organisms are in great abundance. Bye and colleagues[10] used bronchoalveolar lavage in infants as young as 2 months. Specimens thus obtained can be processed rapidly and stained by a method not adaptable to biopsy sections.[80] The optimal procedure used in obtaining a specimen depends on many factors, including the clinical status of the patient, the facilities available, and the preferential experience of the patient's physician. Regardless of the procedure selected, of critical importance is avoidance of undue delay in establishing a diagnosis before the patient's condition deteriorates sufficiently to preclude any definitive diagnostic procedure.

For diagnostic purposes, the methenamine silver nitrate method of Gomori[48] and the less widely used, but more rapid toluidine blue O stain[17] are most useful for demonstrating cyst forms in tissue sections, aspirates, or imprints. Because the Gomori stain as modified by Grocott requires approximately 4 hours for processing, a rapid methenamine silver nitrate procedure is used by some investigators and can be adapted to lung tissue aspirates but not to tissue sections.[149] For more detailed morphologic study of intracystic sporozoites and trophozoites, polychrome stains, including Giemsa, Wright, Gram, and methylene blue stains, are more suitable.[81] In tissue sections, the Gomori stain in combination with hematoxylin and eosin staining allows study of both the organism and host tissue.[60] An immunofluorescent monoclonal antibody technique has become commercially available (Meridian Diagnostics, Cincinnati, Ohio). This technique has no definite advantage over the more conventional methods, although one report describes slightly higher detection rates of *P. carinii* in sputum samples by the immunofluorescence method.[85, 86]

Serologic methods, including complement fixation, immunofluorescence,[114] enzyme-linked immunosorbent assay, and latex agglutination,[5] have been developed but are not generally useful for diagnostic purposes.[78] A lack of specificity or sensitivity inherent in the procedures themselves, in addition to the likelihood of impaired immune responses in affected patients, precludes interpretation of results in most cases. Antibody responses in infected patients with primary or secondary immune deficiency states, as well as those of healthy populations, have not been established clearly. Because *P. carinii* is possibly prevalent in a latent state in the general population, detection of specific antibody in selected patients may well be of no diagnostic value.[60]

A method for the detection of *P. carinii* antigenemia by counterimmunoelectrophoresis was described in 1978.[124] Although this study indicated promise for use as a diagnostic test, subsequent studies have yielded conflicting results.[100, 107] In one of these studies, more than 60 percent of bone marrow transplant recipients with viral or idiopathic pneumonia had demonstrable antigenemia.[107] Another controlled study of patients with AIDS found the test to be inadequate as a diagnostic test for *P. carinii* pneumonitis.[100]

Several investigators[98, 116, 139, 164, 166] have amplified *P. carinii* DNA by polymerase chain reaction (PCR) as a molecular diagnostic method. In a study of bronchoalveolar lavage or lung biopsy specimens (or both) from 47 HIV-infected patients, all of the 18 with documented PCP and 4 of 29 with other pulmonary conditions were positive by PCR analysis (sensitivity, 100%; specificity, 86%).[154] At this time, PCR remains a research tool and is not applicable to general clinical practice.

Hematologic studies are of no diagnostic value, primarily because of baseline abnormalities reflecting the underlying disease of afflicted patients. Eosinophilia has been reported in isolated cases but is not usually present.[78] Depressed serum total protein and albumin values frequently are noted because of the poor nutritional status of representative patients.[69] Lactic dehydrogenase activity is increased, but it is not a specific reaction for PCP and is of little diagnostic benefit.

Prognosis, Treatment, and Prevention

Before the availability of specific therapeutic agents, the overall prognosis of patients with PCP was poor. Despite supportive care, almost all infected patients with underlying neoplastic or immunodeficiency disorders died, whereas as many as 50 percent of affected infants in the European epidemics died as a result of this pulmonary infection.[55, 94, 109] To control the European epidemics, Ivády and Páldy[73] first suggested the use of pentamidine isethionate, a diamidine with previously demonstrated antifungal and antiprotozoal activity.[77, 160] Use of this therapeutic agent in infants during the next several years resulted in a dramatic reduction in the mortality rate from 50 to 3.5 percent.[74, 80]

Pentamidine became available to investigators in the United States through the CDC in 1967. During the next 3 years, of 163 children and adults with documented PCP who were treated with pentamidine, 43 percent recovered.[169, 172] However, of 404 patients to whom the drug was administered for suspected or documented *P. carinii* infection, 189 (47%) experienced significant toxic manifestations. Toxicity ranged from localized reaction at injection sites (18%) to systemic effects, including impaired renal function (24%), liver toxicity (10%), hypoglycemia (6%), hematologic abnormalities (4%), hypotension (10%), and hypocalcemia (1%).[168] Although pentamidine was effective in treating this disorder, the high incidence of toxicity emphasized the need for an alternative therapeutic agent. Before about 1982, essentially all administration of pentamidine was by the intramuscular route.[157] With the AIDS epidemic, that the drug could be given intravenously soon became apparent, which reduced the incidence of injection site reactions but produced little change in other adverse effects. Pentamidine (4 mg/kg/day) is now an alternative agent for children intolerant of trimethoprim-sulfamethoxazole or those who have not responded to trimethoprim-sulfamethoxazole after 5 to 7 days.

Early animal studies[41] and limited investigations in humans[137] suggested that a combination of pyrimethamine and sulfadiazine might be effective in the treatment of PCP. When a somewhat similar combination of trimethoprim and sulfamethoxazole (co-trimoxazole) became available, it also was investigated as an agent of potential therapeutic value in this disorder.[61] Initial studies in infected rats demonstrated therapeutic efficacy equal to that of pentamidine, as well as successful prevention of pneumocystic infection.[67] The efficacy of co-trimoxazole was demonstrated in the treatment of PCP complicating childhood leukemia. A controlled, randomized study involving 50 leukemic children with PCP was reported. Overall recovery rates of 75 percent for pentamidine and 77 percent for co-trimoxazole suggest that these drugs are equally effective in the treatment of PCP in this patient population. Of great importance was the fact that no significant toxicity secondary to co-trimoxazole therapy was observed in this investigation.[60] Subsequent studies have confirmed the efficacy of this drug combination in the treatment of pneumonitis.[52, 53, 90] At present, trimethoprim-sulfamethoxazole appears to be the drug of choice for the treatment and prevention of PCP. The therapeutic dosage is 20 mg of trimethoprim and 100 mg of sulfamethoxazole per kilogram per day orally in four equally divided doses. The intravenous dose is 15 mg of trimethoprim and 75 mg of sulfamethoxazole per kilogram per day in four doses. A minimum of 2 weeks of therapy is recommended; 3 weeks may be optimal for patients with AIDS.

Patients with AIDS have a remarkably high rate of adverse reactions to co-trimoxazole,[10] as well as pentamidine. Those who cannot take co-trimoxazole should be treated with intravenous pentamidine given as a single daily dose in an amount of 4.0 mg/kg.

Several other promising drugs are in various stages of clinical evaluation, although none has been investigated systematically in children. Those with evidence of efficacy include trimethoprim-dapsone,[62, 96] dapsone,[56] pyrimethamine and sulfadoxine,[82, 134] trimetrexate,[1] clindamycin and primaquine,[135] and atovaquone.[63, 66] Animal studies show that the combination of erythromycin-sulfisoxazole has strong anti–*P. carinii* activity through a synergistic mechanism.[64]

Some studies in adults with AIDS and *P. carinii* pneumonitis suggest that the administration of corticosteroids early in the course of moderately severe pneumonitis reduces the occurrence of respiratory failure and improves oxygenation.[21] Other studies show no benefit from corticosteroids.[27] More limited studies of this supportive therapy have been reported in children.[2, 148] If used, a reasonable approach seems to be to withdraw corticosteroids as soon as pulmonary function has become stabilized.

P. carinii pneumonitis can be prevented effectively by chemoprophylaxis with co-trimoxazole when given in a dosage of 150 mg of trimethoprim and 750 mg of sulfamethoxazole per square meter daily[65] or only 3 days a week.[70] *P. carinii* pneumonitis can be prevented in more than 95 percent of patients at high risk for acquiring the disease. Patients in high-risk groups, such as those with cancer or congenital immunodeficiency disorders and organ transplant recipients, should be placed on a chemoprophylaxis regimen

TABLE 223–1 ■ RECOMMENDATIONS FOR *PNEUMOCYSTIS CARINII* PNEUMONIA PROPHYLAXIS FOR HIV-EXPOSED INFANTS AND HIV-INFECTED CHILDREN

	Preventive Regimens	
Indications	**First Choice**	**Alternatives**
HIV-infected or HIV-indeterminant* infants aged 1–12 mo	Trimethoprim-sulfamethoxazole, 150/750 mg/m^2/day in 2 divided doses PO 3 times/wk on consecutive days	Dapsone (≥1 mo of age), 2 mg/kg (max, 100 mg) PO qd, or 4 mg/kg (max, 200 mg) PO per wk
HIV-infected children aged 1–5 yr with CD4 count <500/μL or CD4 percentage <15%	Acceptable alternative schedules:	Aerosolized pentamidine (≥5 yr of age), 300 mg every morning via Respirgard II neubulizer
HIV-infected children aged 6-12 yr with CD4 count <200/μL or CD4 percentage <15%	Single dose PO 3 times/wk on consecutive days	
Previous PCP	2 divided doses PO qd	Atovaquone (aged 1–3 mo and >24 mo), 30 mg/kg PO qd; (aged 4–24 mo), 45 mg/kg PO qd
	2 divided doses PO 3 times/wk on alternate days	

*No prophylaxis for infants younger than 1 month because of the rarity of *Pneumocystis carinii* pneumonia (PCP) at this age. HIV infection can be reasonably excluded in infants who have had two or more negative HIV diagnostic tests (i.e., HIV culture or polymerase chain reaction, both of which are performed at 1 month of age or older and one of which is performed at 4 months of age or older, or two or more negative HIV IgG antibody tests performed after 6 months of age in children who have no clinical evidence of HIV disease.

From 1999 USPHS/IDSA guidelines for the prevention of opportunistic infections in persons infected with human immunodeficiency virus: U.S. Public Health Service (USPHS) and Infectious Diseases Society of America (IDSA). M. M. W. R. Recomm. Rep. *48* (RR-10): 1–59, 61–66, 1999.

throughout the risk period. Generally, the patients within these categories who are the most severely immunosuppressed are the ones who require prophylaxis.

Revised guidelines for *P. carinii* prophylaxis in infants and children with AIDS have been proposed by an expert committee.[155] Because of the high risk for acquiring PCP during the first year of life, often before HIV infection is recognized,[143, 144] PCP prophylaxis should be initiated at 4 to 6 weeks of age in all infants born of HIV-infected women, regardless of CD4 lymphocyte cell counts. The use of chemoprophylaxis in this age group has been highly effective in HIV-infected infants.[132] Once infants are shown not to be infected with HIV, prophylaxis may be stopped. In addition, at 1 year of age and subsequently, the use of chemoprophylaxis is based on the CD4 lymphocyte count and other AIDS-defining features (Table 223–1). Co-trimoxazole given 3 days per week is the preferred drug. For those unable to take co-trimoxazole, dapsone (2.0 mg/kg/day or 4.0 mg/kg/wk) is suggested.[45, 110] An alternative to dapsone is aerosolized pentamidine (300 mg via Respirgard II inhaler monthly).[111] The dosage for aerosolized pentamidine is the same as that described for adults.[95, 110] Studies in adults show that daily doses of dapsone[104] or one dose of dapsone per week is effective prophylaxis.[58, 102] Atovaquone is effective and safe in both children[24] and adults.[36] Table 223–1 summarizes the approach to selection of patients at risk.

Several studies in adults[33, 43, 140, 173] show that PCP prophylaxis can be safely discontinued in those responding to highly active antiretroviral therapy (HAART) with a sustained increase in CD4 T lymphocytes from fewer than 200 cells/μL to more than 200 cells/μL. Similar consideration may be given to children in accordance with age-related CD4 T-lymphocyte counts (see Table 223–1).

Although the currently available anti–*P. carinii* drugs may prevent activation of latent infection, they do not eradicate the organism. Thus, patients are protected from pneumonitis only while receiving chemoprophylaxis and become susceptible again when use of the drugs is discontinued.

REFERENCES

1. Allegra, C. J., Chabner, B. A., Tuazon C. U., et al.: Trimetrexate for the treatment of *P. carinii* pneumonia in patients with the acquired immunodeficiency syndrome. N. Engl. J. Med. *317*:978–985, 1987.
2. Barone, S. R., Auito, L. T., and Krilov, L. R.: Increased survival of young infants with *Pneumocystis carinii* pneumonia and acute respiratory failure with early steroid administration. Clin. Infect. Dis. *19*:212–213, 1994.
3. Bartlett, M. S., Verbanac, P. A., and Smith, J. W.: Cultivation of *Pneumocystis carinii* with WI-38 cells. J. Clin. Microbiol. *10*:796–799, 1979.
4. Bazaz, G. R., Manfredi, O. L., Howard, P. G., et al.: *Pneumocystis carinii* pneumonia in three full-term siblings. J. Pediatr. *76*:767–773, 1970.
5. Benaz, P. J.: A propos du diagnostic immunologique des affections {grave a} *Pneumocystis carinii*. Le test d'agglutination au latex. Bull. Soc. Pathol. Exot. *66*:32–42, 1973.
6. Bommer, W.: Die interstitielle plasmacellul{umlaut a}re pneumoniae und *Pneumocystis carinii*. Ergeb. Mikrobiol. *38*:116–122, 1964.
7. Brazinsky, J. H., and Phillips, J. E.: *Pneumocystis* pneumonia transmission between patients with lymphoma. J. A. M. A. *209*:1527–1529, 1969.
8. Brzosko, W. J., Madalinski, K., Krawczynski, K., et al.: Immunohistochemistry in studies on the pathogenesis of *Pneumocystis* pneumonia in infants. Ann. N. Y. Acad. Sci. *177*:156–171, 1971.
9. Burke, B. A., and Good, R. A.: *Pneumocystis carinii* infection. Medicine (Baltimore) *52*:23–51, 1973.
10. Bye, M. R., Bernstein, L. J., Glaser, J., et al.: *P. carinii* pneumonia in young children with AIDS. Pediatr. Pulmonol. *9*:251–253, 1990.
11. Byrd, R. B., and Horn, B. R.: Infection due to *Pneumocystis carinii* simulating lobar bacterial pneumonia. Chest *70*:91–92, 1976.
12. Campbell, W. G., Jr.: Ultrastructure of pneumocystis in human lung: Life cycle in human pneumocystosis. Arch. Pathol. *93*:312–329, 1972.
13. Capitanio, M. A., and Kirkpatrick, J. A., Jr.: *Pneumocystis carinii* pneumonia. A. J. R. Am. J. Roentgenol. *97*:174–177, 1966.
14. Carini, A.: Formas de eschizogonia do trypanosoma Lewisii. Soc. Med. Cir. Sao Paulo, 16 Aout 1910, in Bulletin de l'Institut Pasteur *9*:937–939, 1911.
15. Centers for Disease Control and Prevention: 1999 USPHS/IDSA guidelines for the prevention of opportunistic infections in persons infected with human immunodeficiency virus: U.S. Public Health Service and Infectious Diseases Society of America. M. M. W. R. *48*(RR-10):1–66, 1999.
16. Chagas, C.: Nova trypanomiazaia humana. Mem. Inst. Oswaldo Cruz *1*:159, 1909.
17. Chalvardjian, A. M., and Growe, L. A.: A new procedure for the identification of *Pneumocystis carinii* in tissue sections and smears. J. Clin. Pathol. *16*:383–384, 1963.
18. Chan, H., Pifer, L., Hughes, W. T., et al.: Comparison of gastric contents to pulmonary aspirates for the cytologic diagnosis of *Pneumocystis carinii* pneumonia. J. Pediatr. *90*:243–244, 1977.
19. Chandra, R. K.: Immunocompetence in under-nutrition. J. Pediatr. *81*:1194–1200, 1972.
20. Connor, E., Bagarazzi, M., McSherry, G., et al.: Clinical and laboratory correlates of *P. carinii* pneumonia in children infected with HIV. J. A. M. A. *265*:1693–1697, 1991.
21. Consensus statement on the use of corticosteroids as adjunctive therapy for *Pneumocystis* pneumonia in the acquired immunodeficiency syndrome. National Institutes of Health–University of California Expert Panel for Corticosteroids as Adjunctive Therapy for *Pneumocystis* Pneumonia. N. Engl. J. Med. *323*:1500–1504, 1990.
22. Cross, A. S., and Steigbigel, R. T.: *Pneumocystis carinii* pneumonia presenting as localized nodular densities. N. Engl. J. Med. *291*:831–832, 1974.

23. Cushion, M. T., and Walzer, P. D.: Growth and serial passage of *Pneumocystis carinii* in the A549 cell line. Infect. Immun. *44*:245–251, 1984.
24. Dankner, W., Yogev, R., Hughes, W. T., et al.: Phase II/III, randomized, double-blind trial to compare atovaquone plus azithromycin to trimethoprim-sulfamethoxazole in the prevention of multiple opportunistic infections in HIV-infected children Abstract 1513. American Pediatric Society. Pediatr. Res. *47*:260, 2000.
25. Dauzier, G., Willis, T., and Barnet, R.: *Pneumocystis carinii* in an infant. Am. J. Clin. Pathol. *26*:787–793, 1956.
26. Delanoe, P., and Delanoe, M.: Sur les rapports des kystes de carinii du pneumon des rats avec le trypanosoma Lewisii. C. R. Acad. Sci. *155*:658, 1912.
27. Delclaux, C., Zahar, J.-R., Amraoui, G., et al.: Corticosteroids as adjunctive therapy for severe *Pneumocystis carinii* pneumonia in non-human immunodeficiency virus–infected patients: Retrospective study of 31 patients. Clin. Infect. Dis. *29*:670–672, 1999.
28. DiGeorge, A. M.: Congenital absence of the thymus and its immunologic consequences: Occurrence with congenital hypoparathyroidism. Birth Defects *4*:116–122, 1968.
29. Doppman, J. L., Geelhoed, G. W., and DeVita, V. T.: Atypical radiographic features in *Pneumocystis carinii* pneumonia. Radiology *114*:39–44, 1975.
30. Drew, W. L., Finley, T. N., Mintz, L., et al.: Diagnosis of *Pneumocystis carinii* pneumonia by bronchopulmonary lavage. J. A. M. A. *23*:713–715, 1974.
31. Dutz, W.: *Pneumocystis carinii* pneumonia. Pathol. Annu. *5*:309–341, 1970.
32. Dutz, W., Post, C., and Kohout, E.: Pneumocystosis: Cancer and therapy. Paper presented at the 13th International Congress of Pediatrics, 1971, Vienna.
33. Dworkin, M., Hanson, D., Jones, J., et al.: The risk of *Pneumocystis carinii* pneumonia and disseminated non-tuberculous mycobacteriosis after antiretroviral (ART) therapy associated with the CD4 T-lymphocyte count. Abstract 692. Paper presented at the 6th Conference on Retroviruses and Opportunistic Infections, 1999, Alexandria, VA.
34. Edman, J. C., Edman, U., Cao, M., et al.: Isolation and expression of the *P. carinii* dihydrofolate reductase gene. Proc. Natl. Acad. Sci. U. S. A. *86*:8625–8629, 1989.
35. Edman, J. C., Kovacs, J. A., Masur, H., et al.: Ribosomal RNA sequence shows *P. carinii* to be a member of the fungi. Nature *334*:519–522,1988.
36. El-Sadr, W. M., Murphy, R. L., McCabe, T., et al.: Atovaquone compared with dapsone for the prevention of *Pneumocystis carinii* pneumonia in patients with HIV infection who cannot tolerate trimethoprim, sulfonamides, or both. N. Engl. J. Med. *339*:1889–1895, 1998.
37. Erchol, J. E., Williams, L. P., and Murgham, P. P.: *Pneumocystis carinii* in hypopharyngeal material. N. Engl. J. Med. *267*:926–928, 1962.
38. Finley, R., Kieff, E., Thompson, S., et al.: Bronchial brushing in the diagnosis of pulmonary disease in patients at risk for opportunistic infection. Am. Rev. Respir. Dis. *109*:379–387, 1974.
39. Forest, J. V.: Radiographic findings in *Pneumocystis carinii* pneumonia. Radiology *103*:539–544, 1972.
40. Fortuny, I. E., Tempero, K. F., and Amsden, T. W.: *Pneumocystis carinii* pneumonia diagnosed from sputum and successfully treated with pentamidine isethionate. Cancer *26*:911–913, 1970.
41. Frenkel, J. K., Good, J. T., and Schulata, J. A.: Latent pneumocystis infection of rats: Relapse and chemotherapy. Lab. Invest. *15*:1559–1577, 1966.
42. Friedman, B. A., Wenglin, B. D., Hyland, R. N., et al.: Roentgenographically atypical *Pneumocystis carinii* pneumonia. Am. Rev. Respir. Dis. *111*: 89–93, 1975.
43. Furrer, H., Egger, M., Opravil, M., et al.: Discontinuation of primary prophylaxis against *Pneumocystis carinii* pneumonia in HIV-infected adults treated with combination antiretroviral therapy. N. Engl. J. Med. *340*:1301–1306, 1999.
44. Gajdusek, D. C.: *Pneumocystis carinii*: Etiologic agent of interstitial plasma cell pneumonia of premature and young infants. Pediatrics *19*:543–565, 1957.
45. Gatti, G., Loy, A., Casazza, R., et al.: Pharmacokinetics of dapsone in human immunodeficiency virus–infected children. Antimicrob. Agents Chemother. *39*:1101–1106, 1995.
46. Giebink, G. S., Sholler, L., Keenan, T. P., et al.: *Pneumocystis carinii* pneumonia in two Vietnamese refugee infants. Pediatrics *58*:115–118, 1976.
47. Gilbert, C. F., Fordham, C. C., and Benson, W. R.: Death resulting from pneumocystis pneumonia in an adult. Arch. Intern. Med. *112*:56–60, 1963.
48. Gomori, G. A.: New histochemical tests for glycogen and mucin. Am. J. Clin. Pathol. *10*:177–179, 1946.
49. Henderson, D. W., Humeniuk, V., Meadows, R., et al.: *Pneumocystis carinii* pneumonia with vascular and lymph nodal involvement. Pathology *6*:235–241, 1974.
50. Hodgkin, J. E., Anderson, H. A., and Rosenow, E. C.: Diagnosis of *Pneumocystis carinii* pneumonia by transbronchoscopic lung biopsy. Chest *64*:551–554, 1973.
51. Hughes, W. T.: Current status of laboratory diagnosis of *Pneumocystis carinii* pneumonitis. C. R. C. Crit. Rev. Clin. Lab. Sci. *6*:145–170, 1975.
52. Hughes, W. T.: Treatment of *Pneumocystis carinii* pneumonitis. N. Engl. J. Med. *295*:726–727, 1976.
53. Hughes, W. T.: Trimethoprim-sulfamethoxazole therapy for *Pneumocystis carinii* pneumonitis in children. Rev. Infect. Dis. *4*:602–607, 1982.
54. Hughes, W. T.: Natural mode of acquisition for de novo infection with *Pneumocystis carinii*. J. Infect. Dis. *145*:842–848, 1982.
55. Hughes, W. T.: *Pneumocystis carinii* infections in mothers, infants and non-AIDS elderly adults. *In* Sattler, F., and Walzer, P. (eds.): Baillieres Clin. Infect. Dis. *2*:1–10, 1995.
56. Hughes, W. T.: Use of dapsone in the prevention and treatment of *Pneumocystis carinii* pneumonia: A review. Clin. Infect. Dis. *27*:197–204, 1998.
57. Hughes, W. T.: Current issues in the epidemiology, transmission and reactivation of *Pneumocystis carinii*. Semin. Respir. Infect. *13*:283–288, 1998.
58. Hughes, W. T., Bartley, D. L., and Smith, B. M.: A natural source of infection due to *Pneumocystis carinii*. J. Infect. Dis. *147*:595, 1983.
59. Hughes, W. T., Feldman, S., Aur, R. J., et al.: Intensity of immunosuppressive therapy and the incidence of *Pneumocystis carinii* pneumonitis. Cancer *36*:2004–2009, 1975.
60. Hughes, W. T., Feldman, S., and Chaudhary, S., et al.: Comparison of pentamidine isethionate and trimethoprim-sulfamethoxazole in the treatment of *Pneumocystis carinii* pneumonitis. J. Pediatr. *92*:285–291, 1978.
61. Hughes, W. T., Feldman, S., and Sanyal, S. K.: Treatment of *Pneumocystis carinii* pneumonitis with trimethoprim-sulfamethoxazole. Can. Med. Assoc. J. *112*(Suppl.):47–50, 1975.
62. Hughes, W. T., Kennedy, W., Dugdale, M., et al.: Prevention of *P. carinii* pneumonitis in AIDS patients with weekly dapsone. Lancet *2*:1066, 1990.
63. Hughes, W. T., Kennedy, W., Shenep, J. L., et al.: Safety and pharmacokinetics of 566C80, a hydroxynaphthoquinone with anti–*P. carinii* activity: A phase I study in human immunodeficiency virus–infected men. J. Infect. Dis. *163*:843–848, 1991.
64. Hughes, W. T., and Killmar, J. T.: Synergistic anti–*P. carinii* effects of erythromycin and sulfisoxazole. J. Acquir. Immun. Defic. Syndr. *4*: 532–537, 1991.
65. Hughes, W. T., Kuhn, S., Chaudhary, S., et al.: Successful chemoprophylaxis for *Pneumocystis carinii* pneumonitis. N. Engl. J. Med. *297*: 1419–1426, 1977.
66. Hughes, W. T., Leoung, G., Kramer, F., et al.: Comparison of atovaquone (566C80) with trimethoprim-sulfamethoxazole to treat *Pneumocystis carinii* pneumonia in patients with AIDS. N. Engl. J. Med. *328*: 1521–1527, 1993.
67. Hughes, W. T., McNabb, P. C., and Makres, T. D.: Efficacy of trimethoprim and sulfamethoxazole in the prevention and treatment of *Pneumocystis carinii* pneumonitis. Antimicrob. Agents Chemother. *5*:289–293, 1974.
68. Hughes, W. T., Price, R. A., Kim, H., et al.: *Pneumocystis carinii* pneumonitis in children with malignancies. J. Pediatr. *82*:404–415, 1973.
69. Hughes, W. T., Price, R. A., Sisko, F., et al.: Protein-calorie malnutrition: A host determinant for *Pneumocystis carinii* infection. Am. J. Dis. Child. *128*:44–52, 1974.
70. Hughes, W. T., Rivera, G. K., Schell, M. J., et al.: Successful intermittent chemoprophylaxis for *Pneumocystis carinii* pneumonitis. N. Engl. J. Med. *316*:1627–1632, 1987.
71. Hughes, W. T., and Smith, B.: Provocation of *Pneumocystis carinii* by cyclosporin A. J. Infect. Dis. *145*:767, 1982.
72. Ito, M., Tsugane, T., Kobayashi, K., et al.: Study on placental transmission of *Pneumocystis carinii* in mice using immunodeficient SCID mice as a new animal model. J. Protozool. *38*(Suppl):218–219, 1991.
73. Ivády, G., and Páldy, L.: A new form of treatment for interstitial plasma-cell pneumonia in premature infants with pentavalent antimony and aromatic diamidines. Monatsschr. Kinderheilk. *106*:10–14, 1958.
74. Ivády, G., Páldy, L., Koltay, M., et al.: *Pneumocystis carinii* pneumonia. Lancet *1*:616–617, 1967.
75. Jackson, H. C., Colthurst, D., Hancock, V., et al.: No detection of characteristic fungal protein elongation factor EF-3 in *P. carinii*. J. Infect. Dis. *163*:675–677, 1991.
76. James, J. W.: Longitudinal study of the morbidity of diarrheal and respiratory infections in malnourished children. Am. J. Clin. Nutr. *25*:690–694, 1972.
77. Jonchere, H.: Treatment of the blood-lymph stage of human trypanosomiasis with diamidines in French West Africa. Bull. Soc. Pathol. Exot. *44*:603–612, 1951.
78. Jose, D. G., Gatti, R. A., and Good, R. A.: Eosinophilia with *Pneumocystis carinii* pneumonia and immune deficiency syndromes. J. Pediatr. *79*: 748–754, 1971.
79. Joyner, L. R., and Scheinhorn, D. J.: Transbronchial forceps lung biopsy through the fiberoptic bronchoscope. Chest *65*:532–535, 1975.
80. Kilman, J. W., Clatworthy, H. W., Hering, J., et al.: Open lung biopsy compared with needle biopsy in infants and children. J. Pediatr. Surg. *9*:347–353, 1974.
81. Kim, H. K., and Hughes, W. T.: Comparison of methods for identification of *Pneumocystis carinii* in pulmonary aspirates. Am. J. Clin. Pathol. *60*:462–466, 1973.

82. Kirby, H. B., Kenamore, B., and Guckian, J. G.: *Pneumocystis carinii* pneumonia treated with pyrimethamine and sulfadiazine. Ann. Intern. Med. *75*:505–509, 1971.
83. Koltay, M., and Illyes, M.: A study of immunoglobulins in the blood serum of infants with interstitial plasma cellular pneumonia. Acta Paediatr. *55*:489–496, 1966.
84. Kovacs, A., Frederick, T., Church, J., et al.: CD4 T-lymphocyte counts and *P. carinii* pneumonia in pediatric HIV infection. J. A. M. A. *265*:1698–1703, 1991.
85. Kovacs, J. A., Halpern, J. L., Swan, J. C., et al.: Identification of antigens and antibodies specific for *P. carinii*. J. Infect. Dis. *140*:2023–2025, 1988.
86. Kovacs, J. A., Ng, V., Masur, H., et al.: Diagnosis of *P. carinii*: Improved detection in sputum using monoclonal antibodies. N. Engl. J. Med. *318*:589–593, 1988.
87. Kovacs, J. A., Powell, F., Edman, J. C., et al.: Multiple genes encode the major surface glycoproteins of *Pneumocystis carinii*. J. Biol. Chem. *268*:6034–6040, 1993.
88. Kramer, R. I., Cirone, V. C., and Moore, H.: Interstitial pneumonia due to *Pneumocystis carinii* and cytomegalic inclusion disease and hypogammaglobulinemia occurring simultaneously in an infant. Pediatrics *29*:816–819, 1962.
89. Latorre, C. R., Sulzer, A. J., and Norman, L. G.: Serial propagation of *Pneumocystis carinii* in cell line cultures. Appl. Environ. Microbiol. *33*:1204–1206, 1977.
90. Lau, W. K., and Young, L. S.: Trimethoprim-sulfamethoxazole treatment of *Pneumocystis carinii* in adults. N. Engl. J. Med. *295*:716–718, 1976.
91. Lau, W. K., Young, L. S., and Remington, J. S.: *Pneumocystis carinii* pneumonia: Diagnosis by examination of pulmonary secretions. J. A. M. A. *236*:2399–2402, 1976.
92. Law, D. I., Dudrick, S. J., and Abdou, N. I.: Immunocompetence of patients with protein-calorie malnutrition. Ann. Intern. Med. *79*: 545–550, 1973.
93. LeClair, R. A.: *Pneumocystis carinii* and interstitial plasma cell pneumonia: A review. Am. Rev. Respir. Dis. *96*:1131–1136, 1967.
94. LeClair, R. A.: Descriptive epidemiology of interstitial pneumocystic pneumonia. Am. Rev. Respir. Dis. *99*:542–547, 1969.
95. Leoung, G. S., Feigal, D. W., Montgomery, A. B., et al.: Aerosolized pentamidine for prophylaxis against *P. carinii* pneumonia. N. Engl. J. Med. *323*:669–675, 1990.
96. Leoung, G. S., Mills, J., Hopewell, P. C., et al.: Dapsone-trimethoprim for *P. carinii* pneumonia in acquired immunodeficiency syndrome. Ann. Intern. Med. *105*:45–48, 1988.
97. Lim, S. K., Eveland, W. C., and Porter, R. J.: Direct fluorescent-antibody method for the diagnosis of *Pneumocystis carinii* pneumonitis from sputa or tracheal aspirates from humans. Appl. Microbiol. *27*:144–149, 1974.
98. Lipschik, G. Y., Gill, V. J., Lundgren, J. D., et al.: Improved diagnosis of *Pneumocystis carinii* infection by polymerase chain reaction on induced sputum and blood. Lancet *340*:203–206, 1992.
99. Lundgren, B., Cotton, R., Lundgren, J. D., et al.: Identification of *P. carinii* chromosomes and mapping of five genes. Infect. Immun. *58*:1705–1710, 1990.
100. Maddison, S. E., Wall, K. W., Haverkos, H. W., et al.: Evaluation of serologic tests for *Pneumocystis carinii* antibody and antigenemia in patients with acquired immunodeficiency syndrome. Diagn. Microbiol. Infect. Dis. *2*:69–73, 1984.
101. Matsumoto, Y., Matsuda, S., and Jegoshi, T.: Yeast glucan in cyst wall of *P. carinii*. J. Protozool. *36*(Suppl):21–22, 1989.
102. McIntosh, K., Cooper, E., Xu, J., et al.: Toxicity and efficacy of daily vs. weekly dapsone for prevention of *Pneumocystis carinii* pneumonia in children infected with HIV. Pediatr. Infect. Dis. J. *18*:432–439, 1999.
103. Merali, S., Frever, U., Williams, J. H., et al.: Continuous axenic cultivation of *Pneumocystis carinii*. Proc. Nat. Acad. Sci. U. S. A. *96*:2402–2407, 1999.
104. Metroka, C. E., Jacobus, D., and Lewis, N.: Successful chemoprophylaxis for *Pneumocystis* with dapsone or Bactrim. Paper presented at the 5th International Conference on AIDS, 1989, Montreal.
105. Meuwissen, J. H. E., Brzosko, W. J., Nowoslawski, A., et al.: Diagnosis of *Pneumocystis carinii* pneumonia in the presence of immunological deficiency. Lancet *1*:1124, 1970.
106. Meuwissen, J. H. E., Tauber, I., Leeuwenberg, A. D., et al.: Parasitologic and serologic observations of infection with *P. carinii* in humans. J. Infect. Dis. *136*:43–48, 1977.
107. Meyers, J. D., Pifer, L. L., Sale, G. E., et al.: The value of *Pneumocystis carinii* antibody and antigen detection for diagnosis of *Pneumocystis carinii* pneumonia after marrow transplantation. Am. Rev. Respir. Dis. *120*:1283–1287, 1979.
108. Michaelis, L. L., Leight, G. S., Powell, R. D., et al.: *Pneumocystis* pneumonia: The importance of early open lung biopsy. Ann. Surg. *183*:301–306, 1976.
109. Minielly, J. A., Mills, S. D., and Holley, K. E.: *Pneumocystis carinii* pneumonia. Can. Med. Assoc. J. *100*:846–854, 1969.
110. Mirochnick, M., Michaels, M., Clarke, D., et al.: Pharmacokinetics of dapsone in children. J. Pediatr. *122*:806–809, 1993.
111. Montaner, J. S. G., Lawson, L. M., Gervais, A., et al.: Aerosolized pentamidine for the prevention of AIDS-related *Pneumocystis carinii* pneumonia: Results of the Canadian Cooperative Trial. Abstract. Am. Rev. Respir. Dis. *141*:268, 1990.
112. Morlier, E., Pouchot, J., Boss, P., et al.: Maternal-fetal transmission of *Pneumocystis carinii* in human immunodeficiency virus infection. N. Engl. J. Med. *332*:825, 1995.
113. Munk, J.: The radiologic differentiation between acute diffuse interstitial pneumonia and pulmonary interstitial oedema in infancy and early childhood. Br. J. Radiol. *47*:752–757, 1974.
114. Norman, L., and Kagan, I. G.: A preliminary report of an indirect fluorescent-antibody test for detecting antibodies to cysts of *Pneumocystis carinii* in human sera. Am. J. Clin. Pathol. *58*:170–176, 1972.
115. Ognibene, F. P., Shelhamer, J., Gill, V., et al.: The diagnosis of *Pneumocystis carinii* pneumonia in patients with the acquired immunodeficiency syndrome using subsegmental bronchoalveolar lavage. Am. Rev. Respir. Dis. *129*:929–932, 1984.
116. Olsson, M., Elvin, K., Lofdahl, S., et al.: Detection of *Pneumocystis carinii* DNA in sputum and bronchoalveolar lavage samples by polymerase chain reaction. J. Clin. Microbiol. *32*:221–226, 1993.
117. Oz, H. S., and Hughes, W. T.: DNA amplification of nasopharyngeal aspirates in rats: A procedure to detect *Pneumocystis carinii*. Microb. Pathol. *27*:119–121, 1999.
118. Patterson, J. H., Lindsay, I. L., Edwards, E. S., et al.: *Pneumocystis carinii* pneumonia and altered host resistance: Treatment of one patient with pentamidine isethionate. Pediatrics *38*:388–392, 1966.
119. Peglow, S. L., Smulian, A. G., Linke, M. J., et al.: Serologic responses to *Pneumocystis carinii* antigens in health and disease. J. Infect. Dis. *161*:296–306, 1990.
120. Perera, D. R., Western, K. A., Johnson, H. D., et al.: *Pneumocystis carinii* pneumonia in a hospital for children: Epidemiologic aspects. J. A. M. A. *214*:1074–1078, 1970.
121. Pesanti, E. L.: Interaction of cytokines and alveolar cells with *Pneumocystis carinii* in vitro. J. Infect. Dis. *163*:611–616, 1991.
122. Pickering, L. K., Anderson, D. C., Choi, S., et al.: Leukocyte function in children with malignancies. Cancer *35*:1365–1371, 1974.
123. Pifer, L. L., Hughes, W. T., and Murphy, M. J.: Propagation of *Pneumocystis carinii* in vitro. Pediatr. Res. *11*:305–316, 1977.
124. Pifer, L. L., Hughes, W. T., Stagno, S., et al.: *Pneumocystis carinii* infection: Evidence for high prevalence in normal and immunosuppressed children. Pediatrics *61*:35–41, 1978.
125. Pottratz, S. T., and Martin, W. J., II: Role of fibronectin in *Pneumocystis carinii* attachment of cultured lung cells. J. Clin. Invest. *85*:351–356, 1990.
126. Price, R. A., and Hughes, W. T.: Histopathology of *Pneumocystis carinii* infestation and infection in malignant disease. Hum. Pathol. *5*:737–752, 1974.
127. Rahimi, S. A.: Disseminated *Pneumocystis carinii* in thymic alymphoplasia. Arch. Pathol. *97*:162–165, 1974.
128. Reed, J. C., and Maxwell, J. E.: The airbronchogram in interstitial disease of the lungs. Radiology *116*:1–8, 1975.
129. Remington, J. S., and Anderson, S. E.: Diagnosis and treatment of pneumocystosis and toxoplasmosis in the immunosuppressed host. Transplant. Proc. *5*:1263–1270, 1973.
130. Repsher, L. H., Schröter, G., and Hammond, W. S.: Diagnosis of *Pneumocystis carinii* pneumonitis by means of endobronchial brush biopsy. N. Engl. J. Med. *287*:340–341, 1972.
131. Rifkind, D., Starzl, T. E., Marchioro, T. Z., et al.: Transplantation pneumonia. J. A. M. A. *189*:808–821, 1964.
132. Rigaud, M., Pollack, H., Leibovitz, E., et al.: Efficacy of primary chemoprophylaxis against *Pneumocystis carinii* pneumonia during the first year of life in infants infected with human immunodeficiency virus type 1. J. Pediatr. *125*:476–480, 1994.
133. Rosen, P. R., Martini, R., and Armstrong, D.: *Pneumocystis carinii* pneumonia. Am. J. Med. *58*:794–802, 1975.
134. Ruf, B., and Phole, H. D.: Pyrimethamine-sulfadoxine (Fansidar) in primary and secondary chemoprophylaxis of *Pneumocystis carinii* pneumonia. Abstract. Am. Rev. Respir. Dis. *141*:154, 1990.
135. Ruf, B., Rohde, I., and Pohle, H. D.: Efficacy of clindamycin/primaquine vs treatment of *Pneumocystis carinii* pneumonia. Abstract. Am. Rev. Respir. Dis. *141*:154, 1990.
136. Ruskin, J., and Remington, J. S.: *Pneumocystis carinii* infection in the immunosuppressed host. Antimicrob. Agents Chemother. *7*:70–76, 1967.
137. Ruskin, J., and Remington, J. S.: The compromised host and infection. I. *Pneumocystis carinii* pneumonia. J. A. M. A. *202*:1070–1074, 1967.
138. Salfelder, K., and Schwarz, V.: Pneumocystosis. Am. J. Dis. Child. *114*:693–699, 1967.
139. Schluger, N., Godwin, T., Sepkowitz, K., et al.: Application of DNA amplification to pneumocystosis: Presence of serum *Pneumocystis carinii* DNA during human and experimentally induced pneumonia. J. Exp. Med. *176*:1327–1333, 1992.
140. Schneider, M. M. E., Borleffs, J. C. C., Stolk, R. P., et al.: Discontinuation of *Pneumocystis carinii* prophylaxis in HIV-1–infected patients treated with highly active antiretroviral therapy. Lancet *353*:201–203, 1999.

141. Scrimshaw, N. S.: Synergism of malnutrition and infection. J. A. M. A. *212*:1685–1691, 1970.
142. Sheldon, W.: Pulmonary *Pneumocystis carinii* infection. J. Pediatr. *61*:780–791, 1962.
143. Simonds, R. J., Hughes, W. T., Feinberg, J., et al.: Preventing *Pneumocystis carinii* pneumonia in persons infected with human immunodeficiency virus. Clin. Infect. Dis. *21*(Suppl. 1):544–548, 1995.
144. Simonds, R. J., Lindegren, M. L., Thomas, P., et al.: Prophylaxis against *Pneumocystis carinii* pneumonia among children with perinatally acquired HIV infection in the United States. N. Engl. J. Med. *332*: 786–790, 1995.
145. Simonds, R. J., Oxtoby, M. J., Caldwell, M. B., et al.: *Pneumocystis carinii* pneumonia among U.S. children with perinatally acquired HIV infection. J. A. M. A. *270*:470–473, 1993.
146. Simone, J. V., Aur, R. J., Hustu, H. O., et al.: Acute lymphocyte leukemia in children. Cancer *36*:770–774, 1975.
147. Singer, C., Armstrong, D., and Rosen, P. P.: *Pneumocystis carinii* pneumonia: A cluster of eleven cases. Ann. Intern. Med. *82*:772–777, 1975.
148. Sleasman, J. W., Hemenway, C., Klein, A. S., et al.: Corticosteroids improve survival of children with AIDS and *Pneumocystis carinii* pneumonia. Am. J. Dis. Child. *147*:30–34, 1993.
149. Smith, J. W., and Hughes, W. T.: A rapid staining technique for *Pneumocystis carinii*. J. Clin. Pathol. *25*:269–271, 1972.
150. Stagno, S., Pifer, L. L., Hughes, W. T., et al.: *Pneumocystis carinii* pneumonitis in young immunosuppressed infants. Pediatrics *66*:56–62, 1980.
151. Telzak, E. E., Cote, R. J., Gold, J. W. M., et al.: Extrapulmonary *Pneumocystis carinii* infections. Rev. Infect. Dis. *12*:380–386, 1990.
152. Theologides, A., Pflueger, O. H., and Kennedy, B. J.: Toxoplasmosis and *Pneumocystis carinii* pneumonitis. Minn. Med. *52*:737–742, 1969.
153. Tokumitsu, S., and Sajaki, T.: An autopsy case of generalized cytomegalic inclusion disease associated with *Pneumocystis carinii* pneumonia. Kumamoto Med. J. *28*:105–110, 1975.
154. Torres, J., Goldman, M., Wheat, L. F., et al.: Diagnosis of *Pneumocystis carinii* pneumonia in human immunodeficiency virus–infected patients with polymerase chain reaction: A blinded comparison to standard methods. Clin. Infect. Dis. *30*:141–145, 2000.
155. 1999 USPHS/IDSA guidelines for the prevention of opportunistic infections in persons infected with human immunodeficiency virus: U.S. Public Health Service (USPHS) and Infectious Diseases Society of America (IDSA). M. M. W. R. Recomm. Rep. *48*(RR-10):1–59, 61–66, 1999.
156. Van der Meer, G., and Brug, S. L.: Infection par pneumocystis chez l'homme et chez les animaux. Ann. Soc. Belge Med. Trop. *22*:301, 1942.
157. VanHoof, L., Herrard, C., and Peel, E.: Pentamidine in the prevention and treatment of trypanosomiasis. Trans. R. Soc. Trop. Med. Hyg. *37*:271–280, 1944.
158. Vargas, S. L., Hughes, W. T., Santolaya, M. E., et al.: Search for primary infection by *Pneumocystis carinii* in a cohort of normal, healthy infants. Clin. Infect. Dis. *32*:855–861, 2001.
159. Vargas, S. L., Ponce, C. A., Gigliotti, F., et al.: Transmission of *Pneumocystis carinii* DNA from a patient with *Pneumocystis carinii* pneumonia to immunocompetent contact health care workers. J. Clin. Microbiol. *38*:1536–1538, 2000.
160. Vargas, S. L., Ponce, C. A., Hughes, W. T., et al.: Association of primary *Pneumocystis carinii* infection and sudden infant death syndrome. Clin. Infect. Dis. *29*:1489–1493, 1999.
161. Vereerstraeten, P., Dekoster, J. P., Vereerstraeten, J., et al.: Pulmonary infections after kidney transplantation. Proc. Eur. Dial. Transplant. Assoc. *11*:300–307, 1975.
162. Vessal, K., Post, C., and Dutz, W.: Roentgenologic changes in infantile *Pneumocystis carinii* pneumonia. A. J. R. Am. J. Roentgenol. *120*: 254–260, 1974.
163. Wada, M., and Nakamura, Y.: Type II major-surface glycoprotein family of *Pneumocystis carinii* under the control of novel expression elements. DNA Res. *6*:211–217, 1999.
164. Wakefield, A. E.: Detection of DNA sequences identical to *Pneumocystis carinii* in samples of ambient air. J. Eukaryot. Microbiol. *41*(Suppl):116, 1994.
165. Wakefield, A. E., Banerji, S., Pixley, F. J., et al.: Molecular probes for the detection of *Pneumocystis carinii*. Trans. R. Soc. Trop. Med. Hyg. *84*(Suppl. 1):17–18, 1990.
166. Wakefield, A. E., Guiver, L., Miller, R. M., et al.: DNA amplification on induced sputum samples for diagnosis of *Pneumocystis carinii* pneumonia. Lancet *337*:1378–1379, 1993.
167. Walker, A. N., Garner, R. E., and Horst, M. N.: Immunocytochemical detection of chitin in *Pneumocystis carinii*. Infect. Immun. *58*:412–415, 1990.
168. Walker, C. L.: The schizogony of *Trypanosoma evansi* in the spleen of the vertebrate host. Philip. J. Sci. *7*:53–63, 1912.
169. Walzer, P., Perl, D. P., Krogstad, D. J., et al.: *Pneumocystis carinii* pneumonia in the United States. Ann. Intern. Med. *80*:83–93, 1974.
170. Walzer, P. D., Schultz, M. G., Western, K. A., et al.: *Pneumocystis carinii* pneumonia and primary immune deficiency diseases of infancy and childhood. J. Pediatr. *82*:416–422, 1973.
171. Watanabe, J. M., Chinchinian, J., Weitz, C., et al.: *Pneumocystis carinii* pneumonia in a family. J. A. M. A. *193*:685–686, 1965.
172. Western, K. A., Perera, D. R., and Schultz, M. G.: Pentamidine isethionate in the treatment of *Pneumocystis carinii* pneumonia. Ann. Intern. Med. *73*:695–699, 1970.
173. Weverling, G. J., Mocroft, A., Ledergerber, B., et al.: Discontinuation of *Pneumocystis carinii* pneumonia prophylaxis after start of highly active antiretroviral therapy in HIV-infection. Lancet *353*:1293–1298, 1999.
174. Whitcomb, M. E., Schwarz, M. I., and Charles, M. A.: Interstitial fibrosis after *Pneumocystis carinii* pneumonia. Ann. Intern. Med. *73*:761–764, 1970.
175. Winder, F. G., and Rooney, S. A.: *Pneumocystis carinii* in lungs of adults at autopsy. Am. Rev. Respir. Dis. *97*:935–937, 1968.
176. Yoshida, Y., Matsumoto, Y., Yamada, M., et al.: *Pneumocystis carinii* electron microscopic investigation on the interaction of trophozoite and alveolar lining cell. Zentralbl. Hyg. Umweltmed. *256*:390–399, 1984.

SUBSECTION **2**

NEMATODES

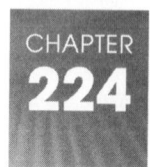

CHAPTER 224 Parasitic Nematode Infections

MICHAEL KATZ ■ PETER J. HOTEZ

Intestinal Nematodes

The three major intestinal nematodes of children, *Ascaris lumbricoides, Trichuris trichiura,* and the hookworms, together have a substantial impact on the health and well-being of children living in less developed nations of the world. This "unholy trinity" of soil-transmitted helminths (STHs), or "geohelminths," deprives hundreds of millions of young children of their full intellectual and growth potential. Current estimates suggest that 2 billion people are infected with STHs, 300 million of whom suffer from severe morbidity. An estimated 400 million schoolchildren are infected with STHs. Building on studies from the early part of this century,[9, 10] extensive new data from many different geographic regions confirm that chronic intestinal nematode infections during childhood suppress both cognitive and intellectual development[2, 5, 6] and impair physical growth and fitness.[3, 11–13] Because many of these detrimental effects are reversible with the use of anthelmintic drugs to eliminate nematodes from the intestinal tract,[12, 13] several investigators and international relief agencies have advocated the administration of benzimidazole anthelmintics as a cornerstone of public health programs directed at school-age children.[1, 7] However, because in highly endemic areas reinfection with *A. lumbricoides, T. trichiura,* and hookworms usually occurs within 6 months of receiving anthelmintic treatment,[14] this strategy is probably not a practical means of control unless the drugs are used frequently. Concern about the potential for emerging anthelmintic drug resistance also exists.[3] Some researchers have pointed to the use of genetically engineered antihelminth vaccines as one possible solution to the problem of worm reinfection and disease during childhood.[4]

In addition to the chronic effects seen when children harbor large numbers of intestinal nematodes are the increasingly recognized unique neonatal and infantile syndromes that new information indicates may result from vertical transmission of the infective stages of some intestinal nematodes, probably in colostrum and breast milk.[8] The best documented example of vertical transmission in infants results in the "swollen belly syndrome" caused by *Strongyloides fuelleborni,* although other perinatal nematode infections probably also occur (discussed later). Finally, children experience significant morbidity during zoonotic transmission of the infective stages of intestinal nematodes of companion animals such as dogs and cats. The resultant aberrant migration of these foreign nematode larvae (visceral larva migrans) has become a major pediatric public health problem in large urban areas of the United States and Europe.

ASCARIS LUMBRICOIDES

Ascariasis is among the most prevalent infections in the world, with an estimated 1.3 billion cases in the developing world.[21] Accurate determinations based on 1,477,742 fecal examinations indicate that more than 500 million cases of ascariasis occur in China alone![34] In parts of Africa, the average rate of infection is around 95 percent, and in Central and South America, the rate is about 45 percent. Surveys conducted in the rural southern communities of the United States during the 1970s indicated that the prevalence of ascariasis approached 20 to 67 percent.[16] However, that the rates still remain so high is doubtful.

Ascaris infection, when relatively light, is usually inapparent until the patient passes a worm through the rectum. In heavy infections, constitutional symptoms may occur during the early phase and intestinal malabsorption and even obstruction in the later phase. The infection is acquired by ingestion of the infective eggs, which hatch in the upper part of the small intestine and free the larvae. The larvae penetrate the intestinal wall, reach venules or lymphatics, and pass through the portal circulation to the liver, the right side of the heart, and the lungs.

In the lungs, the larvae break out of the capillaries and begin ascending through the respiratory radicles until they reach the glottis, and then, passing over the epiglottis, they enter the esophagus and are carried down to the small intestine, where they mature and become adult worms. The adult female *Ascaris* produces huge numbers of eggs, possibly as many as 200,000 a day. To ensure adequate quantities of egg-requiring cholesterol, the parasite sequesters oxygen through a specially modified hemoglobin.[22] The entire cycle, beginning with the infective eggs and resulting in ovipositing females, lasts approximately 2 months. Infection is maintained in the community by the deposition of human stool in soil, which permits embryonated eggs to develop into the infective stage. This process takes approximately 2 weeks. The high prevalence of infection results not only from deficient sanitary facilities for disposal of human excreta but also from the deliberate use of human feces as fertilizer.

Epidemiology

Ascaris is a ubiquitous parasite that is present in both temperate and tropical zones, but its highest prevalence is in warm countries where sanitation is deficient. All ages are affected by the parasite; young children, who are exposed more often to the contaminated soil, are affected most frequently. These children usually harbor greater numbers of adult worms in their intestine than do adults living under similar conditions.[11–13, 20] High worm burdens in children also occur with *Trichuris* infections (see later). This predisposition to "worminess" in childhood also may have a genetic or immunologic basis. Because *Ascaris* is extremely hardy and relatively resistant to extremes of temperature, a common finding is high rates of ascariasis in impoverished urban environments (e.g., Guatemala City, Mexico City), including those in some temperate zones, where the eggs can survive the ordinary freezing temperatures of winter months. The eggs are also resistant to chemical disinfectants and are not destroyed readily by sewage treatment. In some areas, pigs may serve as a reservoir for zoonotic *Ascaris* infection.[15]

Pathophysiology

During the migratory phase of the infection, the larvae evoke an inflammatory response associated with eosinophilic infiltration. *Ascaris* antigens—the so-called ABA-1 allergen—released during the molting of larvae evoke an immune response, and specific antibodies of the IgG class have been detected; IgE antibodies directed against ABA-1 may correlate with resistance.[30] An interesting but controversial role of IgE anti-Ascaris antibodies is in protecting children against atopic states, including asthma.[29] Little is known about the IgA response to this infection. The primary defense mechanism is most probably the cellular immune type in association with humoral immunity; in experimental animals infected with various nematodes, rejection of the worms by sensitized hosts has been reported.

During the intestinal stage of infection, symptoms derive primarily from the physical presence of the worms in the gut, from aberrant migration into other lumina, or from perforation into the peritoneum. Moreover, as a protective mechanism for its own survival, *Ascaris* secretes peptides that block the action of pancreatic digestive enzymes (trypsin, chymotrypsin, elastase),[23, 26] which may play a role in parasite-associated malabsorption. Whether malabsorption of nutrients, or even malnutrition at all, is the basis of *Ascaris*-associated physical growth retardation during childhood remains unknown, but chronic moderate and heavy *Ascaris* infections during childhood adversely affect physical growth and development.[3, 11–13, 20, 31]

Clinical Manifestations

The degree of disease induced by the migratory phase of *Ascaris* is related directly to the number of larvae migrating simultaneously. In light infections, this phase is unrecognized. Heavy infection, for example, that induced in himself by Koino,[28] who swallowed 2000 infected eggs, may cause severe pneumonitis.

In the lumen of the intestine, ascarid worms may become matted together and form a bolus large enough to cause intestinal obstruction. The incidence of this complication has been estimated at 2 per 1000 infected children per year.[16] When recognized early, the obstruction can be treated with medical management, but in many cases surgical intervention is mandatory.

Less common complications are perforation of the intestine and hepatobiliary and pancreatic ascariasis from blockage of the bile duct and pancreatic duct, respectively. Patients thus afflicted are subject to cholecystitis, acute cholangitis, "biliary colic," acute pancreatitis, or hepatic abscess.[27] Certain irritants such as halogenated hydrocarbons (e.g., carbon tetrachloride and tetrachloroethylene, used in the past to treat certain hookworm infections), elevation of body temperature, and general anesthesia have been known to precipitate aberrant migration. *Ascaris* screening by fecal examination should be considered before performing elective surgery on a child who might have immigrated recently from an impoverished area of the tropics.

Whatever the mechanism of interference by *Ascaris* with growth or nutrition, treatment with anthelmintics leads to substantial "catch-up" growth in previously parasitized children.[3, 11–13, 29, 31] Ascariasis in pregnant women results in intrauterine growth retardation.[33]

Most people with light infections are rarely symptomatic (such persons become aware of the parasites by passage of adult worms in stool or through regurgitating and vomiting the adult worms), although researchers have conjectured that even these persons may exhibit subtle deficits in cognitive and intellectual development.[2, 6]

Several cases of neonatal ascariasis have been described in the literature.[17, 18] The mode of acquisition of these infections is not known, but canine and feline ascarid infections commonly are acquired by a transplacental route, thus suggesting the possibility that this route also may occur in humans.

Differential and Specific Diagnoses

The differential diagnosis of pneumonia caused by *Ascaris* suggests a parasitic etiology because of the peripheral eosinophilia. However, any nematode with a migratory phase through the lungs can mimic this infection. *Ascaris* must be considered as a cause of intestinal obstruction in any geographic locale where its prevalence is high.

The diagnosis of intestinal ascariasis is established by identification of the characteristic ascarid eggs through microscopic examination of stool. Serologic tests are of limited value. The simpler tests are subject to cross-reactions; the more complicated ones are laborious and require sophisticated laboratory facilities. They stand in contrast to the simplicity of stool examination. Among these tests, radioimmunoprecipitation offers some opportunity for assessment of the intensity of the infection.[24] Detection of *Ascaris* metabolites in urine by gas-liquid chromatography also correlates with worm burden.[25]

Hepatobiliary and pancreatic ascariasis is suspected in heavily infected children who have signs of biliary obstruction, as noted earlier. Ultrasonography and endoscopic retrograde cholangiopancreatography are useful adjunctive diagnostic procedures for these patients.[27]

Treatment

For an ordinary *Ascaris* infection, either albendazole administered at a fixed dose of 400 mg once or mebendazole administered at a fixed dose of 100 mg twice daily for 3 days is effective. A single fixed dose of 500 mg of mebendazole also may be effective, but it may not be suitable for the treatment of other STH co-infections.[19] As an alternative, pyrantel pamoate administered in a single dose of 11 mg/kg, not to exceed 1 g, is effective. Neither the benzimidazoles nor pyrantel pamoate is approved yet for children younger than 2 years. Therefore, all the printed statements caution against the use of these drugs in the younger age group. Nevertheless, these drugs do not seem to act differently in this younger age group than they do in older children or adults, and widespread use overseas indicates that the benzimidazoles are probably safe.[19, 32] The risk of treatment in this younger age group currently is undergoing more rigorous investigation because of mounting evidence that the growth and cognitive delay caused by STHs may be corrected with albendazole or mebendazole.[19, 31] However, these drugs have a potential for embryotoxicity, so judicious use in young children is warranted. The World Health Organization (WHO) also is evaluating the use of benzimidazoles during pregnancy, particularly for use during the second and third trimesters.[19] In cases of intestinal obstruction, piperazine citrate may be effective because this drug paralyzes the myoneural junction of *Ascaris* and may result in relaxation of the matted bolus of worms. It is antagonistic to pyrantel pamoate, and therefore these two drugs should not be administered together.

Management of intestinal obstruction or hepatobiliary ascariasis is often surgical. For some patients, biliary decompression may be performed with endoscopic retrograde cholangiopancreatography.[27]

Prognosis

The prognosis is excellent in the great majority of cases of ascariasis. In patients with the complications of obstruction or perforation, the prognosis depends entirely on the speed of recognition and therapy.

Prevention

The infection could be eliminated entirely through proper disposal of human excreta. Unfortunately, as an isolated means of health improvement in the world, it has never been successful. Elimination of *Ascaris* from a community or a substantial reduction in the incidence of this infection usually occurs after general improvement in the standard of living. Periodic administration of community-wide therapy with anthelmintics has been effective in reducing worm burden as a short-term strategy. In the absence of aggressive sanitation and other control measures, however, reinfection often occurs within 6 months after treatment.[14]

TRICHURIS TRICHIURA

Trichuriasis has a prevalence approximating that of the other major intestinal nematode infections, or some 800 million cases worldwide,[35] but the infection is usually asymptomatic because in most cases it is light. However, children with so-called asymptomatic light infection may have deficits in cognition.[44]

The infection is acquired by the ingestion of embryonated eggs picked up from the soil on hands or through contaminated food. The eggs hatch in the upper part of the small intestine, and the liberated larvae penetrate the villi. Unlike the larvae of *Ascaris*, *Trichuris* larvae do not undergo extraintestinal migration but remain in situ for approximately

1 week, at which time they begin a progressive descent into the cecum and the colon. They mature there, and the attenuated anterior end of the adult worm embeds itself in the colonic mucosa. Creation of syncytial tunnels (derived from the columnar epithelium of the colon) is facilitated by the release of a parasite-derived, pore-forming protein.[38] The parasites derive their nourishment from these colonic mucosal tunnels. The entire cycle from the ingestion of embryonated ova to the development of sexually mature adults takes approximately 2 months. Persistence of the infection in a community depends on continual contamination of the soil with human feces.

Epidemiology

These parasites are found most commonly in the tropical regions, but they also are detected in subtropical areas such as the southern part of the United States. The distribution of this worm closely parallels that of *Ascaris*. In addition, as in the case of *Ascaris,* children with trichuriasis usually harbor greater numbers of worms than do adults living under similar conditions.[35, 36] Consequently, children suffer greater morbidity from trichuriasis than adults do. The mechanistic basis of added worminess in children is unknown, although researchers have observed that *Trichuris* infections are *aggregated,* with a minority of children suffering from particularly heavy infections. These heavily infected children appear to have a genetic or immunologic predisposition to *Trichuris* infection.[35, 36] Children also are the major source of *Trichuris* eggs in the environment, which when deposited in the soil become infective in approximately 1 month and remain viable for several months. They are killed by exposure to temperatures in excess of 40° C within 1 hour. Freezing temperatures below −8° C also destroy these eggs. Like ascarid eggs, they are relatively resistant to chemical disinfectants.

Pathophysiology

At the site of attachment, the adult worm elicits characteristic changes in the colonic mucosa as noted earlier. Inflammatory cells are also found at these sites, but they do not appear to account for the clinical resemblance of trichuriasis to some forms of inflammatory bowel disease.[35, 42] Like many other intestinal worms, *Trichuris* is expelled through the action of the host's immune system. This expulsion results from a combined effect of antibody and lymphoid cells.[45] Regulation of *Trichuris* populations in the gut has been ascribed to a carefully orchestrated balance of host-derived cytokines.[39] Although anemia has been attributed to trichuriasis,[40] the amount of blood loss caused by this parasite is much less than hookworm-associated blood loss and is not sufficient to account for anemia.[41] One possibility is that *Trichuris*-induced anemia results from chronic inflammation, similar to the anemia of inflammatory bowel disease.[35, 36]

Clinical Manifestations

Two major disease syndromes are caused by heavy *Trichuris* infection during childhood.[35, 36] The *Trichuris* dysentery syndrome (TDS) is associated with severe diarrhea with blood and mucus. Children with TDS are anemic and frequently manifest growth retardation and failure to thrive.[37] Infants and toddlers with TDS are at risk for protracted tenesmus, which leads to rectal prolapse. *Trichuris* colitis is a more chronic manifestation of moderate to heavy infection that is characterized by a form of inflammatory bowel disease similar to what happens in Crohn disease or ulcerative colitis. Children with this form of colitis also can have chronic malnutrition and short stature. Moderately and heavily infected (and possibly even lightly infected) children are at risk for deficits in cognition and intellectual development.[44]

Differential and Specific Diagnoses

The diagnosis is established by identification of the characteristic barrel-shaped eggs through microscopic examination of stool. Clinically, heavily infected children with TDS may resemble children with amebic or bacillary dysentery. Children with *Trichuris* colitis may have signs and symptoms that resemble other forms of inflammatory bowel disease. However, the erythrocyte sedimentation rate is not elevated in children with *Trichuris* colitis.

Treatment

In the past, when relatively noxious or toxic drugs had to be used, only patients with heavy infection were treated. Currently, any patient with this infection can be treated by the administration of either albendazole, administered as a single fixed dose of 400 mg (except for very heavy infections, in which consecutive doses for 3 days may be required), or mebendazole, 100 mg twice daily for 3 days.[43] The dose does not need to be adjusted to the weight of the patient because the drug is not well absorbed from the gastrointestinal tract. As noted earlier, the safety of the benzimidazoles in young children has not been established, but this may not preclude its use in the practice of pediatrics.[26] As an alternative, the drug oxantel is effective for the treatment of trichuriasis. In some countries, oxantel is formulated with pyrantel pamoate.[35]

Prevention

As in the case of other nematodes, sanitary disposal of excreta—but more important, improvement in the standard of living—tends to reduce the incidence of infection. Frequent mass treatments with mebendazole reduce the worm burden in a community.

HOOKWORMS

Hookworm infection is one of the most important infections of both adults and children in the developing world, with an estimated prevalence of 1 billion cases. Hookworms exert their pathogenic effect by causing intestinal blood loss, which leads to iron-deficiency anemia. By considering the average blood loss induced by each worm, the average number of worms per infected individual, and the prevalence, researchers have estimated that these parasites are responsible for a daily loss of more than 1 million L of blood in the world. Because loss of blood represents loss of erythrocytes *and* plasma, heavy infections, especially in malnourished populations, also contribute to malnutrition. Two major species of hookworms infect the human intestine: *Ancylostoma duodenale* and *Necator americanus.* Of the two, *A. duodenale* is more virulent and causes greater blood loss and morbidity leading to iron-deficiency anemia and hypoproteinemia.[50] Two other members of the genus *Ancylostoma, Ancylostoma ceylonicum* and the dog hookworm *Ancylostoma caninum,*[54] are much less frequent causes of intestinal pathology in humans.[50]

The infection is acquired either by exposure of skin to moist soil infested with the larvae of these worms *(A. duodenale* and *N. americanus)* or by ingestion of the infective larvae *(A. duodenale* only). The most propitious circumstances for infection are shady areas and sandy or loamy soil. Infection is particularly likely early in the morning, when the ground is moist with dew, or after a rainfall. After the larvae enter the host, they initiate a developmental program that continues until they enter the intestine.[4, 48, 52] Larvae that enter through the skin are carried by the venous circulation to the right side of the heart and there follow the route described for *Ascaris,* whereas larvae that are ingested may develop entirely within the gastrointestinal tract.

On reaching the small intestine, the larvae mature to adult worms, which become attached with their mouthparts to the intestinal mucosa. The worms sustain themselves by releasing hydrolytic enzymes that degrade the intestinal mucosa and then feeding on cellular and connective tissue debris.[50–52] During this process, capillaries and arterioles are eroded and lacerated, with subsequent extravasation of blood. The adult worms also ingest blood through the action of a parasite gut brush border metalloendopeptidase.[53] An anticoagulant that blocks the activity of host factor Xa facilitates blood flow and is responsible for continued bleeding from the original site after the worm has moved to a new one.[46] The entire cycle from penetration of the skin or ingestion of larvae to the development of mature worms usually takes approximately 6 to 8 weeks. At that time, hookworm eggs appear in the feces. However, *A. duodenale* larvae also may undergo a period of developmental arrest within the human host that lasts weeks or months. Thus, intestinal ancylostomiasis can occur up to a year (and possibly longer) after initial exposure to infective larvae.[56] Investigators have conjectured that the reservoir of arrested *A. duodenale* larvae enters the mammary glands and breast milk.[56] This sequence of events may account for cases of infantile ancylostomiasis noted in Africa, India, and China.[49] Humans are the major reservoir of these organisms, and this infection is maintained by continual contamination of soil by human feces.

Epidemiology

Although in ancient times these parasites had a worldwide distribution, they currently are most prevalent in tropical and subtropical zones and can be found in temperate climates only in isolated areas. *A. duodenale* predominates in many parts of the Indian subcontinent and focal areas of China north of the Yangtze River.[4] *A. duodenale* is also a major parasite in Egypt and other parts of the Mediterranean region, Africa, and a few focal areas in South America, including Paraguay and northern Argentina. A small Central American focus also exists in southern Honduras and El Salvador and among Aboriginal populations in western Australia. *N. americanus* is the predominant hookworm in the world, especially in the Western Hemisphere, most of Africa, China south of the Yangtze River, Southeast Asia and Indonesia, and certain islands of the Pacific. This differential distribution is not absolute, and small numbers of either parasite are present where the other predominates. Mixed infections with both species are extremely common. *A. ceylonicum* occurs in focally endemic areas of southern Asia,[50] whereas the dog hookworm *A. caninum* has been described as a cause of human eosinophilic enteritis in Australia and possibly elsewhere.[54]

Larvae survive in soil for 6 weeks. They are destroyed by drying, freezing temperatures, and heat in excess of 45° C. Hookworm infection occurs in areas with high agricultural intensity and is not found frequently in urban areas, where *Ascaris* and *Trichuris* might predominate. Because shade and moisture are essential for survival at the infective larval stage, a not surprising finding is high rates of hookworm infection in families that harvest tea in India and Bangladesh, mulberry leaves (for the silkworm industry) in eastern China, sweet potatoes and corn in western China, coffee and bananas in Central and South America, and rubber in Africa.

Like other STHs, hookworm infections usually are aggregated such that most persons harbor light worm burdens whereas a substantial minority harbor moderate or heavy infections.[57] Even after specific anthelmintic chemotherapy, moderately and heavily infected persons appear to be predisposed to the reacquisition of heavy infection.[57] A predisposition to hookworm infection may have a genetic or immunologic basis.

Unlike the other STHs, high rates of hookworm infection occur in both adults and children. In some regions, the age-associated prevalence and intensity increase linearly, with the heaviest infections occurring in elderly populations.[47]

Pathophysiology

During the migratory phase of the infection, the larvae evoke an inflammatory response associated with eosinophilic infiltration. Immune responses to the infection have been difficult to study in humans, but in an animal model, a dog infected with *A. caninum* can be rendered immune to challenge infection by repeated dosing with the infective larvae. This observation has provided a means of producing a live attenuated larval vaccine in the laboratory, but one that is not suitable for humans. Reproduction of this larval vaccine effect by using specifically genetically engineered polypeptides is in progress.[4, 52]

The major source of injury to the host is loss of blood. A single *A. duodenale* organism is responsible for the loss of approximately 0.2 mL of blood per day, and an *N. americanus* organism is responsible for 0.02 mL. Rarely, massive bleeding has been reported.[47] Iron-deficiency anemia results when iron loss exceeds the host's iron reserves. Hookworms may affect cognitive development because iron is important for the development of dopaminergic neurons and for the biosynthesis of some neurotransmitters. Heavy infections result in the characteristic features of severe iron deficiency. Loss of protein further contributes to malnutrition. The problem of malabsorption in hookworm infection is moot. Although malabsorption has been demonstrated in patients infected with these parasites, it appears to be a secondary effect, caused by hypoproteinemia, that can be corrected by a high-protein diet without deworming the patient.[55]

Clinical Manifestations

Penetration by larvae causes pruritus proportional in intensity to the number of infecting larvae. The "ground itch" or "dew itch," or pruritus of the soles after walking in the morning dew, is an example. The symptoms result from a hypersensitivity reaction.

The acute intestinal phase in heavy infections is characterized by abdominal pain, diarrhea, nausea, and anorexia.[53] After the acute phase abates, well-nourished persons with relatively light infections have no symptoms and no evidence of anemia or malnutrition. At the other extreme, heavily infected, malnourished children can have hemoglobin values as low as 2 g/dL and edema caused by hypoproteinemia. Infants with severe ancylostomiasis typically have failure to thrive, profound pallor, and melena.[49]

Deficits in physical and intellectual growth as a result of chronic hookworm infection in childhood have been reported since the early part of this century.[3, 4, 9, 10] Some recovery has been described after the administration of specific anthelmintic therapy or iron supplementation, although some deficits occurring in infancy may be irreversible.

Differential and Specific Diagnoses

As in the case of ascariasis, the differential diagnosis of pneumonia suggests a parasitic etiology because of peripheral eosinophilia. Anemia is caused by blood loss; therefore, it must be distinguished from all other causes of intestinal loss of blood. In the developing countries, where severe hookworm anemia is common, the probability of the occurrence of rarer causes of intestinal blood loss, such as Meckel diverticulum, polyps, and so on, is low. The opposite holds true for regions where hookworm infections are light or infrequent.

The diagnosis is established by identification of the characteristic eggs through microscopic examination of stool. The eggs of *A. duodenale* and *N. americanus* cannot be distinguished from each other easily, but the worms can be differentiated by direct examination of the infective larvae or adults. Therefore, one must assume that it is one or the other species on the basis of the geographic origin of the patient. Although this decision is not of paramount importance, it does have some therapeutic implications, including the possibility that arrested larvae of *A. duodenale* will become reactivated and either repopulate the intestine at some point after treatment or enter breast milk during or after parturition.

Treatment

For *N. americanus* infection, the drug of choice is either albendazole, administered at a fixed dose of 400 mg, or mebendazole (100 mg twice daily for 3 days). Pyrantel pamoate given as a single dose of 11 mg/kg, not to exceed 1 g, is a suitable alternative drug. In areas endemic for ancylostomiasis, the health provider should be aware of the potential of arrested tissue larvae to repopulate the intestine or enter breast milk and infect infants during the perinatal period. Iron supplementation and transfusion are occasional important adjunctive therapies for pediatric hookworm infection.

Prevention

As in all cases of nematode infection transmitted through soil, sanitary control of the disposal of excreta would eliminate the infection entirely. Unfortunately, accomplishing such elimination has not been feasible in most of the world. The popular recommendation to wear shoes is naive because the most virulent species of hookworm, *A. duodenale,* is orally infective and large segments of human populations go barefoot for economic and cultural reasons. Entry through the upper extremities is also a common mode of transmission. Moreover, contact with infested soil by any segment of the skin results in infection. Because infants often are placed on the soil and toddlers play in it, protection of the soles of the feet is inconsequential. Studies to investigate the possibility of vaccination against hookworm infection are in progress.[4, 52]

ENTEROBIUS VERMICULARIS

Pinworm infection (enterobiasis), or oxyuriasis (the older term), is the most frequent of all human helminth infections and one that is particularly common in North America and Europe.[63] However, some investigators think that the overall prevalence of enterobiasis is declining in the United States. Most infected persons are children, and the infection is found in all socioeconomic classes. It is acquired by the ingestion of infective eggs picked up on the perianal skin, in the air, or on bedclothes and underwear. Swallowed eggs, transmitted to the mouth by fingers or through inhalation, hatch in the duodenum, and the liberated larvae undergo additional maturational steps in the small intestine before reaching the cecum. There, the sexually mature worms copulate and then proceed to the rectum and eventually to the perianal skin, where the gravid females lay eggs. The eggs become infective within 2 to 4 hours after deposition. The entire cycle from ingestion of the egg to the egg-laying phase of the gravid female is 4 to 6 weeks. Rarely, a retrograde infection occurs in which eggs hatch on the anal mucosa and the larvae migrate up the bowel and mature to adult worms. Although enterobiasis is a human infection, anthropoid apes can be infected experimentally.

Epidemiology

The infection is worldwide in distribution, and children are infected most frequently. Communal living, especially assembling in school gymnasia and living in crowded households, promotes transmission of the infection. Adults tend to be infected through their contact with children; therefore, parents and teachers are the most vulnerable. Orphanages and daycare centers frequently are affected.[63]

Pathophysiology

No intestinal reactions occur during the migratory phase, and because no tissue migration takes place, no eosinophilia occurs to the degree seen with some of the other nematodes. Occasionally, hypersensitive persons may have a slight increase in eosinophils. The deposited ova induce pruritus on the perianal skin. No evidence indicates that some persons are more susceptible than others to this infection.

Enterobius occasionally has been found in vermiform appendixes removed at surgery. A causal relationship to appendicitis has not been established, but some evidence points to the possibility that this worm induces granuloma formation and, therefore, may cause obstruction of this vestigial structure.[58]

When the adult gravid female migrates along the perineal skin into the vagina, it may cause vulvitis as a reaction to the eggs deposited in that region. Some investigators speculate that migrating pinworms may introduce bacteria into the lower urinary tract and thereby result in urinary tract infection.[62] Other aberrant infections, such as those causing hepatic granuloma, occur more infrequently.[61]

Clinical Manifestations

Pruritus is the most common symptom; its intensity varies from mild itching to acute, intractable pain. Secondary cellulitis also may occur in severely pruritic cases.[60] Vaginal discharge and vulval itching are symptoms in the rare cases in which a worm has migrated into the vagina. Insomnia, restlessness, irritability, loss of appetite, loss of weight, and grinding of teeth all have been reported anecdotally in persons with pinworm infection, but no evidence has shown that any of these symptoms are related causally to *Enterobius* infection. Enuresis also has been blamed on the pinworm, but one epidemiologic study failed to determine the causality.[64] An unusual form of eosinophilic ileocolitis resulting from massive infestation with many *E. vermicularis* larvae has been described in an adult homosexual male patient.[59]

Specific Diagnosis

E. vermicularis eggs are identified readily by low-power microscopic examination of transparent adhesive tape previously applied to the perianal skin and then affixed to a microscope slide.

Treatment

Single-dose therapy with either mebendazole (100 mg), albendazole (400 mg), or pyrantel pamoate (11 mg/kg, not to exceed 1 g) is effective. With the current availability of these three highly effective drugs, the intensive laundering of underwear and bed clothing, recommended in the older literature, is no longer necessary. However, treating all members of the household is advisable because they all must be presumed to be infected. Re-treatment in 2 or 3 weeks to destroy any adult worms that have hatched from the eggs swallowed at the time of initial therapy may be necessary. None of these drugs destroy the eggs.

One of the most important aspects of management of this infection is reassurance that its ubiquity virtually precludes effective eradication. Therefore, reinfection can be anticipated in any family infected with pinworms because of the high prevalence of this worm in the community. Also important is to reassure families that the presence of pinworms does not suggest poor hygienic standards in the family.

STRONGYLOIDES STERCORALIS AND STRONGYLOIDES FUELLEBORNI

S. stercoralis and *S. fuelleborni* are among the most virulent helminthic pathogens of humans, although they are much less prevalent than *Ascaris* or hookworm. *S. stercoralis* has the unusual ability to cause autoinfection, which can lead to hyperinfection and disseminated infection in immunocompromised hosts.[68, 70, 72–77, 83, 84] *S. fuelleborni* causes an aggressive infantile protein-losing enteropathy that leads to ascites and high mortality.[65, 66]

S. stercoralis infection is acquired by the exposure of skin to infective larvae in the soil, much as in the case of hookworm infection. Similar circumstances that promote the survival of hookworm larvae in soil (i.e., moisture, sandy or loamy soil, and shade) promote the survival of *Strongyloides*. Larvae penetrate skin, facilitated by a potent histolytic protease that they secrete.[67, 80] From the moment of penetration of skin to arrival of the worms in the intestine, the cycle commonly is thought to be similar to that of hookworms, although experimental evidence suggests that *S. stercoralis* also may explore routes of migration that bypass the lungs.[86] Within the intestine, the small adult worms do not attach to the mucosa as hookworms do but, instead, lie embedded in its folds. The cycle from penetration of skin to development of mature worms in the intestine is approximately 28 days. No parasitic adult male worms exist to fertilize the eggs. Instead, the mature eggs develop by parthenogenesis. In addition, unlike those of other parasitic nematodes, these eggs usually are not found in feces but instead embryonate within the intestine and develop into larvae, which are deposited in soil with human stool. These so-called rhabditiform larvae must molt before they become infective.

This cycle has two variations. One permits the development of nonparasitic male and female adults in soil, which can maintain infestation of the soil for a certain period; this free-living phase sometimes is called the heterogonic life cycle. The second variation has much greater clinical relevance. Under certain conditions that are not well defined, the rhabditiform larvae molt to new infective larvae while still in the intestine. These new infective larvae can penetrate the intestine and set up a new cycle, commonly called autoinfection or the autoinfective cycle.[75] In this fashion, this nematode, unlike most other intestinal nematodes of humans, actually can increase in number without reinfection from the outside world. This phenomenon also is responsible for persistence of this infection for decades in an untreated host.[77] Some investigators think that low levels of autoinfection occur in most patients with strongyloidiasis.

When host defenses are impaired (discussed later), *S. stercoralis* can undergo multiple rounds of autoinfection leading to the production of thousands or even hundreds of thousands of adult parasites in the intestine. This phenomenon is known as hyperinfection.[68, 72, 76, 83] One possible consequence of hyperinfection is disseminated infection, in which larval and adult worms are identified at extraintestinal sites.

S. fuelleborni larvae are passed to infants by ingestion in breast milk.[65, 69] Transmammary infection by nematode larvae is an extremely common route of transmission in nonhuman nematode infections[8]; though not well studied, it probably also occurs commonly in humans.

Epidemiology

S. stercoralis infection has worldwide distribution, but it is most prevalent in tropical and subtropical regions. In North America, strongyloidiasis is focally endemic in some parts of Appalachia[70] and is common in Southeast Asian immigrants.[78] In one study, 76.6 percent of Kampuchean immigrants and 55.6 percent of Laotian immigrants were seropositive for *S. stercoralis* infection.[78] Strongyloidiasis is also endemic in Jamaica and presumably elsewhere in the Caribbean.[84] Because of the possibility of autoinfection and, by extension, infection through contamination of skin by infested feces, strongyloidiasis is highly prevalent in mental hospitals, prisons, and homes for retarded children. Dogs and anthropoid apes may serve as animal reservoir hosts for *S. stercoralis*. *S. fuelleborni* infection is endemic in Papua New Guinea and parts of sub-Saharan Africa.[65, 66]

Pathophysiology

During the migratory phase of the infection, the larvae of *S. stercoralis* evoke an inflammatory response associated with eosinophilic infiltration. The adult phase in the intestine, even in moderate infection, may be associated with an inflammatory reaction sufficient to be symptomatic. Some evidence suggests that *Strongyloides* induces a malabsorption syndrome, which has been treated effectively by deworming.[70, 82] Of interest is that this form of malabsorption involves steatorrhea, but D-xylose absorption is normal. An explanation for this dissociation is not available, but at least one speculation suggests that the malabsorption is caused by edema of the lamina propria as a result of the release of histamine from mast cells.[82] Young children with *S. stercoralis*–induced malabsorption experience growth stunting and failure to thrive.[70]

The deficits in host defense that promote hyperinfection and disseminated strongyloidiasis are not well understood. Although cell-mediated immune deficits, such as those occurring in immunosuppression, organ transplantation, severe malnutrition, and cytotoxic chemotherapy for neoplasms and collagen vascular disease, are associated with this phenomenon, certain established deficits in cell-mediated immunity, such as those in human immunodeficiency virus infection, do not necessarily trigger hyperinfection.[75]

Researchers have suggested that patients receiving large doses of corticosteroids are particularly susceptible to hyperinfection because the corticosteroids themselves function as direct signals or ligands for the parasite to undergo autoinfection.[75] Of interest is that patients in Japan and Jamaica with human T-cell lymphotropic virus type I appear to be at high risk for acquiring opportunistic strongyloidiasis,[73] possibly because of a specific deficit in their effector IgE immune response.[84]

The pathogenesis of the marked protein-losing enteropathy that leads to ascites in the swollen belly syndrome of *S. fuelleborni* infection has not been established.

Clinical Manifestations

During the migratory phase of larval strongyloidiasis, patients may be susceptible to the development of pneumonitis associated with eosinophilia. Larval migration through the skin can result in larva currens. Although most patients harboring *S. stercoralis* in their intestine are asymptomatic, those with moderate or heavy infection classically have intense diarrhea productive of watery, mucous stool. Periods of alternating diarrhea and constipation may occur. Anorexia and cachexia, which lead to failure to thrive and other deficits in physical growth, are common features of pediatric strongyloidiasis.[70]

In disseminated strongyloidiasis caused by the hyperinfective cycle, larvae may invade all tissues, including the central nervous system (CNS). Moreover, because larvae penetrate the intestine, they may carry with them enteric flora and cause sepsis or meningoencephalitis.[68] Although diarrhea is the most commonly recognized consequence of *Strongyloides* infection, it is the hyperinfective cycle that has the greatest portent for immunosuppressed patients.

Infants with *S. fuelleborni* infection may manifest the swollen belly syndrome with marked abdominal ascites and pleural effusions that can be fatal.

Differential and Specific Diagnoses

Strongyloides pneumonitis can resemble the clinical manifestations associated with the lung migration of other nematode parasites such as *Ascaris* and hookworm. The differential diagnosis of the diarrhea must include causes of chronic diarrheal disease. However, in view of its association with marked eosinophilia, diarrhea caused by *Strongyloides* ought not to be confused with diarrhea caused by enteric bacteria or pathogenic protozoa. Likewise, noninfectious causes of diarrhea, such as regional enteritis and ulcerative colitis, are not likely.

The diagnosis is established by identification of the characteristic larvae during microscopic examination of stool, which is not easy because rhabditiform larvae usually are not produced in abundance. Specific stool concentration techniques are available to increase the sensitivity of fecal examination, although they are not as effective as amplifying the heterogonic life cycle by the Baermann technique or by looking for characteristic larval tracks on nutrient agar plates.[87] The stool of all immunosuppressed persons, including those given corticosteroids for any reason, who have ever been in a region where *Strongyloides* is found must be examined to rule out this infection. If routine stool examination results are negative, the stool should be processed as outlined earlier. In addition, examination of duodenal contents can be attempted, either by aspiration or by the string test (Enterotest). This examination, however, only divulges the contents of the duodenum and can miss the larvae in the lower part of the small intestine. An enzyme-linked immunosorbent assay (ELISA) for detection of *Strongyloides*-specific antibodies is available on a research basis.[78, 84]

Children with the swollen belly syndrome from *S. fuelleborni* infection shed eggs rather than larvae in their feces. Large numbers of eggs are common findings in clinical cases.

Treatment

Previously, the drug of choice for both *S. stercoralis* and *S. fuelleborni* infection was thiabendazole, administered at a dose of 50 mg/kg/24 hr divided into two equal doses on each of 2 successive days. However, the drug has relatively high toxicity, which frequently includes nausea, vomiting, and vertigo and sometimes requires interruption of therapy. Rarely, it induces leukopenia, rash, and even Stevens-Johnson syndrome. Because the drug is detoxified in the liver, its dose may have to be reduced for patients with liver failure. In disseminated strongyloidiasis, thiabendazole should be continued for at least 5 days. Thiabendazole still is an effective drug with a cure rate in nondisseminated infection approaching 100 percent.[71] In the case of only partial removal of the worms, the therapy may be repeated.

Increasing experience with ivermectin suggests that this drug may be the new treatment of choice. It is administered at a dose of 200 μg/kg/day for 1 to 2 days. Treatment with ivermectin gives a cure rate of 80 percent.[79, 81] Because the mortality rate of patients with disseminated strongyloidiasis remains high despite thiabendazole therapy, a common practice is to treat first with ivermectin, often in a prolonged or repeated course. Secondary bacterial complications such as sepsis and meningitis are common with disseminated strongyloidiasis, so judicious use of broad-spectrum antimicrobial agents frequently is indicated for this condition. As an additional supportive measure, patients who have hyperinfective strongyloidiasis and are receiving high-dose corticosteroid therapy probably benefit from steroid taper. Curiously, patients with transplants and cyclosporine immunosuppression may benefit from some of the direct helminthotoxic properties of this compound.[85]

Prognosis

The prognosis is excellent in patients who do not have disseminated infection and are treated promptly. Unrecognized disseminated infection can be lethal.

Prevention

Proper disposal of human excreta substantially reduces the prevalence of strongyloidiasis in any community. In closed institutions, where control of direct spread is not likely to be achieved, identification plus treatment of infected persons is the only feasible control.[74]

Aberrant Infections with Intestinal Nematodes

TOXOCARA CANIS

As indicated in the previous sections, the life cycles of the intestinal nematodes are adjusted precisely through evolutionary selection. In many instances, only one host in which the cycle can be completed is parasitized by the nematode. Infection of an unnatural host, in most cases, leads to complete failure of development and causes no disease. In a few instances an infection may be established, but the cycle is not completed. Under such circumstances, the process of aberrant migration of larvae may be more pathogenic than steps in the natural cycle.

One of the most dramatic examples of an aberrant infection is visceral larva migrans, caused by infection with *T. canis*. This roundworm causes intestinal infection in the dog, in which its cycle resembles that of *A. lumbricoides* in humans. People become infected by *Toxocara* through the ingestion of an embryonated egg, much as in human infection with *Ascaris*. Larvae hatch in the small intestine, penetrate the villi, and begin a migration that takes them through every organ and tissue of the body. Because they cannot mature, the larvae tend to migrate for months until they are overcome by the inflammatory reaction of the host and die. Although larvae of other toxocarids such as *Toxocara cati* and *Toxascaris leonina* have been suggested as possible causes of visceral larva migrans, they are probably much less important as zoonotic pathogens in humans.

Epidemiology

The prevalence of toxocariasis is difficult to assess because of the failure of diagnosis in many cases. The disease has been reported from many parts of the world, and one can assume that it is found wherever humans and dogs coexist. Young children often come into contact with *T. canis* eggs while playing in sandboxes and on playgrounds that were contaminated by a family pet.[98–100] The level of contamination of public areas is also difficult to ascertain. In several studies, ova were present in 5 to 25 percent of soil samples obtained, and surveys of dogs in urban communities have shown the occurrence of frequent infections, particularly in puppies, which are infected almost universally with *T. canis* (canine infection occurs transplacentally).[94, 95] The seroprevalence of toxocariasis in the United States is high, and the parasite should be considered an emerging pathogen in some urban areas. In some groups of socioeconomically disadvantaged black children, the seroprevalence is as high as 30 percent,[98, 103] with even higher rates among U.S. inner-city Hispanic children.[105] Toxocariasis is endemic to Puerto Rico. Major risk factors for acquiring toxocariasis include having a litter of puppies in the home and the habit of geophagia.[101] The latter risk factor probably accounts for the observed association between toxocariasis and elevated lead levels.[101]

The presence of a positive skin test for toxocariasis is associated with poliomyelitis statistically.[108] No direct causal relationship exists; possibly, the circumstances leading to ingestion of *Toxocara* ova are also conducive to ingestion of poliomyelitis virus. Likewise, seizures are correlated with seropositivity for *Toxocara* antibodies, but a causal relationship has not been established.[88] Some investigators have postulated that toxocariasis may be an important cause of so-called idiopathic seizures in young children.[98]

Pathophysiology

The entire infection is restricted to the migratory phase and therefore represents an "exaggeration" of the symptoms found during the early phases of *A. lumbricoides* infection. Symptoms are protean and depend on which organ or tissue is infected. For unknown reasons, visceral migration through the liver, lungs, and brain occurs more commonly in toddlers and children younger than 5 years, whereas older children tend to have ocular involvement almost exclusively.[98–100] Thus, epidemiologic evidence suggests that this infection produces two distinct syndromes, visceral and ocular, because involvement of one tends to occur in the absence of the other.[97] Visceral migration elicits eosinophilic granuloma formation in the target organs and leads to hepatitis, pneumonitis, or cerebritis. Larval migration in the retina results in ocular larva migrans, which includes granuloma formation in the retina.[89, 93, 106] The lesion so resembles retinoblastoma that it is often confused with it. Endophthalmitis[93] or papillitis[92] also may develop. Invasion of other organs and tissues induces granuloma formation there.

Clinical Manifestations

Most patients infected with *T. canis* are thought to be asymptomatic. Some of these individuals have isolated findings, including eosinophilia, or wheezing and asthma. The term "covert toxocariasis" is used by some investigators to describe these patients, who often are identified by their circulating anti–*T. canis* antibody titers. An association between asthma and covert toxocariasis has been well described in Europe, but as yet this association is unproven in North America.[105]

Visceral larva migrans, the extreme form of toxocariasis, typically occurs in a toddler with the symptoms and signs of a multisystem disease. It is associated with fever, hepatosplenomegaly, lung infiltrates accompanied by wheezing, a high degree of eosinophilia (approaching 80%), and elevated immunoglobulin levels, particularly of the IgM class.[96, 99–101] Seizures and neuropsychiatric disturbances are also common. In one case report, the child's major neurologic manifestation was a static encephalopathy.[96]

In contrast, ocular larva migrans is characterized by a unilateral vision deficit and, sometimes, strabismus. Ophthalmologic examination frequently reveals one or more posterior poles or peripheral pole granulomas.[93, 100, 106] More global eye inflammation also can occur (discussed earlier). Children with ocular involvement usually have few, if any systemic manifestations. Often, no laboratory abnormalities are detected.

Differential and Specific Diagnoses

Visceral larva migrans must be distinguished from the migratory phase of the other nematode infections. Because of hepatosplenomegaly and hypereosinophilia, eosinophilic leukemia occasionally has been suspected, but it can be ruled out readily by examination of bone marrow.

T. canis larvae can be identified in tissues, for example, in liver biopsy specimens, but the diagnostic yield is low. Therefore, one must resort to indirect means and be aware that a multisystem disease with elevated IgM and hypereosinophilia fits the diagnostic criteria. An ELISA test available at the Centers for Disease Control and Prevention is highly specific and diagnostic.[100, 103, 104]

Ocular larva migrans usually is diagnosed by an experienced ophthalmologist who recognizes the characteristic granulomas and larval tracks on retinal examination. Presumably because of minimal antigen presentation by a few migrating larvae in the eye, often no measurable immune response occurs in this condition. For this reason, ELISA frequently is not reliable for making the diagnosis of ocular larva migrans.[98, 100, 101, 103, 104]

Treatment

Traditionally, treatment of visceral larva migrans was primarily symptomatic, especially because much of the morbidity is associated with immunopathologic responses against dying parasites. In the 1960s, thiabendazole and diethylcarbamazine were determined to be effective against migrating larvae.[102] Since then, new agents of the benzimidazole class have been claimed to be equally effective but associated with fewer drug toxicities.[99] In a comparative study with thiabendazole, the drug albendazole (10 mg/kg/day in two divided doses for 5 days) was shown to be well tolerated and less toxic.[107] Another benzimidazole, mebendazole, also may be effective when given in doses high enough to achieve significant extraintestinal levels.[90] Albendazole is the treatment of choice. Although anecdotal experience with albendazole and mebendazole overseas suggests that these drugs are safe in children,[91] the large doses required for the treatment of larva migrans may be associated with hepatic and other toxicities (including embryotoxicities), and therefore they have not been approved for this purpose.

Treatment of ocular larva migrans often requires surgical management, particularly in cases associated with tractional retinal detachment.[93, 106] Specific anthelmintic adjunctive chemotherapy appears to be of benefit in some cases.[94, 99, 106]

Prognosis

Except for patients in whom blindness develops as a consequence of retinal damage and a rare fatal case resulting from the intensity of the acute clinical reaction, the vast majority of patients recover. However, the recovery phase may be slow and take as long as 2 years.

Prevention

Theoretically, the disease can be prevented by elimination of dog feces from the human environment, but in practice, it is no less difficult to achieve than control of human excrement disposal.

OTHER ABERRANT INFECTIONS WITH INTESTINAL NEMATODES

Baylisascaris procyonis, a parasite of raccoons, also can cause visceral larva migrans. *Baylisascaris* infection occurs when humans accidentally ingest parasite eggs that are shed in barn lofts and attics accessible to raccoons.[101, 116, 118] In at least one reported human case, the infection was fatal in an infant.[116] Like *Toxocara* infection, *Baylisascaris* larvae within aberrant hosts cannot complete their cycle and continue their aimless migration through the tissues of these hosts. The lesions caused by the larvae are eosinophilic granulomas, which tend to be concentrated in the CNS and result in eosinophilic meningitis. Neither the frequency nor the range of severity of this infection in humans is known. Most human cases have been diagnosed at autopsy. Currently, no literature on specific anthelmintic chemotherapy exists.

Other less severe aberrant infections of importance to humans are those caused by the dog hookworm, primarily *Ancylostoma braziliense,* but also *A. caninum* and *Uncinaria stenocephala.*[50, 114, 115, 126] Infection with the larvae of *A. braziliense* and *U. stenocephala* cannot be completed, and they remain viable and migrate in the skin (usually between the epidermis and dermis); hence the terms *cutaneous larva migrans* and *creeping eruption* are used. Failure of these zoonotic hookworms to complete entry through the human skin may reflect differences in the hydrolytic enzymes released.[114, 115] Infection is acquired in the same fashion as that of the human hookworms. Children who expose their whole bodies to contaminated soil may be infected at any site. Adults are most likely to have infection in the lower extremities, but plumbers in the tropics, who often must crawl beneath houses, acquire infection on the elbows and knees. The interval from exposure to appearance of the first symptoms is approximately 2 weeks; papules 2 mm in diameter then begin to appear on the skin. Behind them usually are serpiginous, erythematous, intracutaneous tunnels. The entire area itches intensely. Left untreated, cutaneous larva migrans tends to last 2 months. Thiabendazole or albendazole is effective treatment when administered orally. Topical therapy with a 15 percent aqueous suspension of thiabendazole was successful in one reported series. Forty-seven of 50 patients achieved permanent cure in 2 weeks, and 2 more patients were cured after a third week.[129] Placebo-treated patients were used as controls in this study. In contrast with skin penetration of zoonotic hookworms, oral ingestion of the dog hookworm *A. caninum* results in an eosinophilic enteritis syndrome (discussed in the section on hookworm infection).

Rarer aberrant infections include those caused by various species of *Trichostrongylus, Oesophagostomum, Angiostrongylus, Capillaria,* and *Anisakis. Trichostrongylus* is a common parasite of many mammals, and it has been found in the small intestine of humans, mainly in Asia, Africa, and Australia. Ingestion of larvae leads to the development of adult worms in the small intestine. Whether this development results in any disease remains a moot point because infections tend to be mild and usually are associated with other helminth infections.[113] *Oesophagostomum bifurcum* is a common nematode of subhuman primates in Africa and has been reported to be a relatively common intestinal nematode that causes nodular disease of the intestines in humans living in West Africa.[120, 123] Human oesophagostomiasis has been treated successfully with pyrantel pamoate.[120]

Land snails and slugs serve as intermediate hosts for *Angiostrongylus* spp. *Angiostrongylus cantonensis* is a cause of eosinophilic meningitis throughout East Asia and Hawaii[111, 119, 124, 125]; *Angiostrongylus costaricensis* is a cause of mesenteric arteritis and abdominal pain in Central and South America and in Latin American immigrants to the United States.[117] The rat serves as the natural host of these parasites, which live either in the lung *(A. cantonensis)* or in mesenteric arteries *(A. costaricensis).* The rat eats the infected mollusks and thus ingests the larvae, which migrate to their final destination. An incomplete infection develops in people who ingest either the mollusks or food contaminated by the mollusks. *A. cantonensis* infection usually is limited to the CNS and is manifested as eosinophilic meningitis.[111, 119, 124, 125] Signs and symptoms include meningismus, severe headache, paresthesias, and less commonly, cranial nerve palsies. No specific treatment is available (although the anthelmintics thiabendazole and ivermectin are effective in some experimental animal models[111]), but the disease is self-limited and lasts no longer than 2 weeks. Symptomatic relief has been reported with the use of prednisone. In contrast, *A. costaricensis* infection typically is manifested as abdominal or right iliac fossa pain, fever, and eosinophilia. In children with this condition, appendicitis or Meckel diverticulum may be diagnosed.[117] High doses of mebendazole have been tried as therapy for this condition.

Capillaria philippinensis is a common parasite of water fowl in the Philippines.[110] The mode of transmission of this parasite to people is unknown, but human cases have been reported in which as many as 40,000 adult worms were found embedded in the crypts of the small intestine. *C. philippinensis,* like *S. stercoralis,* can undergo autoinfection and hyperinfection in humans.[110] No associated inflammatory reaction occurs, but flattening of villi, loss of epithelial surface area, and severe malabsorption have been reported.[110, 112, 128] In one series of 1000 cases of *C. philippinensis* infection, a mortality rate of 10 percent was reported.[112] Thiabendazole may be effective in shortening the course of the infection,[128] although albendazole has become the treatment of choice more recently.[110] Another member of the genus, *Capillaria hepatica,* a rare zoonosis of humans, has been known to disseminate to the lungs, liver, and other viscera.[122]

Anisakis spp. are nematode parasites of marine mammals, with fish being intermediate hosts. When the infective larvae of the parasite are ingested as a result of eating raw or poorly cooked fish, they may become embedded in the gastric mucosa and cause eosinophilic granuloma.[51, 109, 121, 127, 130, 131] In adults, it may resemble carcinoma of the stomach both clinically and radiographically. Human anisakiasis occurs with considerable frequency in Japan, where raw marine fish are eaten commonly, and in Holland, where lightly pickled herring is considered a delicacy.

Filarial Parasites

Except for rare instances of zoonotic *Brugia* infection,[132, 137] the filarial worms parasitizing humans affect people within the geographic area almost entirely limited by the two Tropics. Although accurate data are lacking, the latest estimates of the WHO suggest that 400 million people are infected with one or more filarial worms. The various human parasites in this category have certain characteristics in common. They all are spread by vectors, and the adults invade and occupy the lymphatics, skin, connective tissue, or blood. They produce live embryos called microfilariae that enter the bloodstream or skin, where they can survive for weeks or even years without further development. The range of disease caused by these worms is wide; some produce no symptoms, whereas others can be responsible for severe clinical disorders.

The life cycles of the filarial worms are similar in that infections are acquired through an insect bite, during which transmission of microfilariae is accomplished by transference of the infective larvae onto the skin of the host from the mouthparts of the insect. The larvae then enter the wound in the skin and make their way to the respective tissue, where they mature into adult worms. The adults mate and produce live larvae, which migrate to the blood through the walls of the lymphatics or through the thoracic duct. They are ingested by blood-sucking insects, in which they undergo metamorphosis through two larval stages until they reach the third, infective stage. The interval from the infective bite to the appearance of microfilariae in the blood of the host can be as long as 6 months.

Immunologic responses to the filarial infection develop in the host and can be used for immunodiagnosis. More significant, these immunologic host inflammatory responses themselves elicit pathology. Indeed, some of the most dramatic clinical manifestations of human filarial infection (e.g., elephantiasis, river blindness) usually result from immunopathologic-mediated damage occurring over a period of years. For that reason, these sequelae are not common in children.

LYMPHATIC FILARIASIS: *WUCHERERIA BANCROFTI* AND *BRUGIA* SPECIES

Epidemiology

Wuchereria bancrofti is prevalent primarily between the two Tropics but also is encountered north of the Tropic of Cancer in Africa. As many as 400 million people may suffer from lymphatic filariasis caused by this parasite. In each of its geographic locales, it has a specific anopheline or culicine mosquito vector. In the Caribbean area, South America, Asia, East and West Africa, and Papua New Guinea, the microfilariae of this worm exhibit nocturnal periodicity; in the South Pacific, their periodicity is diurnal. *W. bancrofti* has no animal hosts.

Brugia malayi occurs in India, Malaysia, and other parts of Southeast Asia. Some strains of *B. malayi* are associated with animal reservoirs, as are certain other members of the genus *Brugia* such as *Brugia timori.* In the United States, zoonotic *Brugia* infections caused by *Brugia beaveri* and *Brugia lepori* have been reported in humans.[132, 137]

Pathophysiology

The initial host response is that of inflammation around dead and dying adult worms in the lymphatics; such inflammation results in lymphangitis and in due course leads to enlargement of the affected lymph nodes and then hyperplasia, epithelioid granulomas, and eventually, fibrosis. It develops with a characteristic, painful, cordlike swelling associated with a reddish streak on the overlying skin. This manifestation usually is associated with a systemic reaction of fever, headache, and general malaise. Inflammatory reactions of other tissues, such as the testes and synovial membranes, likewise occur occasionally. The obstruction also may lead to chyluria and chylous diarrhea. In most infected persons, the response is not sufficiently severe to cause clinical disease, especially in children because the clinical manifestations are a result of years of repeated infection. The microfilariae themselves are apparently harmless.

Clinical Manifestations

Asymptomatic microfilaremia often develops in children living in endemic areas. With repeated exposure, these children may possibly later, as adolescents or young adults, begin to have occasional episodes of acute lymphangitis with some systemic manifestations. These "filarial fevers" frequently are accompanied by headache, malaise, and myalgia.[134] Benign lymphedema has been described in a few patients in the United States with zoonotic *Brugia* infection.[132, 137]

Clinical lymphatic filariasis results in lymphatic blockage through fibrosis, which causes lymphedema proximal to the obstruction and leads to the development of classic elephantiasis of the scrotum or labia majora and the lower extremities.

Chronic, recurrent pneumonitis associated with wheezing, cough, chest pain, pulmonary infiltrations, and hypereosinophilia is a hypersensitivity reaction caused by the migration of microfilariae through the lungs. This condition, known as tropical pulmonary eosinophilia, occurs commonly in young adult males living in parts of the Indian subcontinent.[135]

Differential and Specific Diagnoses

The differential diagnosis of lymphatic obstruction in children should rule out other more likely conditions before focusing on filariasis. In older children and adults, familial lymphedema (Milroy disease) can mimic filariasis.

The diagnosis becomes definitive only with identification of the characteristic microfilariae in blood. In view of the circadian periodicity of the appearance of large numbers of larvae in blood, a specimen should be collected at the appropriate time. It need not be examined immediately but may be placed in a large volume of formalin for subsequent concentration and staining. Migration of microfilariae into the peripheral circulation also can be provoked at other times by administering diethylcarbamazine. Immunodiagnostic tests that measure either specific antibody or even filarial antigen are undergoing development.[133, 134]

Treatment

New agents are needed that would be effective against the adult filarial worm and at the same time elicit minimal immunopathologic damage.[138] Currently, the major drugs used are effective mainly in eradicating microfilariae. Diethylcarbamazine is the treatment of choice. Side effects of specific antifilarial therapy include allergic and febrile reactions, which may be caused by the release of worm antigens rather than by the drug itself. This phenomenon occurs primarily in patients with high worm loads as evidenced by circulating microfilariae. These systemic manifestations can be treated symptomatically with antihistamines or corticosteroids. Some of the allergic manifestations also may be avoided by administering diethylcarbamazine in a graded, stepwise manner. This drug is also the treatment of choice for tropical pulmonary eosinophilia, a syndrome caused by circulating microfilariae, particularly in young adult males in India. Ivermectin also may have a role in the medical treatment of lymphatic filariasis and is effective in helping clear circulating microfilariae.[136]

The difficulty in management of filariasis by drugs is that late symptoms such as elephantiasis do not abate. The main usefulness of chemotherapy is in cases recognized early, before the anatomic abnormalities develop. The latter can be treated surgically if they are disfiguring or if they interfere with normal life.

As of this writing, the Clinical Center of the National Institutes of Health (Bethesda, MD) has extensive experience and expertise in the management and treatment of human filarial infections, including *W. bancrofti*, *Loa loa*, and *Onchocerca volvulus* infections.

Prevention

Prevention depends on vector control, which has been less than satisfactory, primarily because of the difficulty in developing effective insecticides that also would be nontoxic to the rest of the environment. Successful experience in China with supplementing dietary salt with diethylcarbamazine suggests that large-scale chemoprophylaxis approaches are possible in endemic countries. The WHO is directing a large-scale lymphatic filariasis control campaign on this principle.

LOA LOA

L. loa infection is limited to a small area of western and central Africa and is spread by *Chrysops* flies. Periodicity in *L. loa* microfilariae is diurnal. The parasite elicits numerous allergic inflammatory responses that are most evident in expatriates.[140–142] Infection leads to high eosinophilia and recurrent angioedema, which when localized develop into painful, pruritic, subcutaneous swellings on the extremities and the face known as Calabar swellings. Rarely, some cases of lymphatic obstruction of the lower extremities and hydroceles have been reported.

The most dramatic manifestation of this infection is the occasional appearance of a migrating *L. loa* adult under the conjunctiva of the eye. It does not damage the eye and can be removed surgically. Treatment with diethylcarbamazine, as indicated earlier, effectively destroys the adults, but reactions may be more intense than in the treatment of *Wuchereria* and *Brugia* infections.[139] Diethylcarbamazine should be administered in a gradual, stepwise manner as described earlier, particularly in patients with high levels of circulating microfilariae. Co-administration of corticosteroids often is required during treatment. Allergic encephalopathy has been described in patients receiving diethylcarbamazine.[139] Ivermectin appears to elicit fewer allergic symptoms during treatment and may be less toxic in general.

ONCHOCERCA VOLVULUS

O. volvulus infection is acquired through the bite of a *Simulium* fly, which tends to breed along rivers and streams (hence the name of the disease: river blindness).

Epidemiology

The disease is limited to Africa, Central America, and the northern parts of South America. In view of human dependence on water and the establishment of settlements along rivers, the frequency of infection tends to be high in areas where *Simulium* prevails. The development of hydroelectric power based on the construction of large dams has increased the breeding sites of *Simulium* and, hence, has increased the incidence of *Onchocerca* infection.

Pathophysiology

Larvae deposited by a *Simulium* bite remain in the subcutaneous tissue and develop into adult worms there. Adult worms tend to become coiled, and worms of both sexes become enveloped by fibrous tissue and form nodules within which they reproduce. The larvae produced by fertilized females invade the skin, where they remain until they are picked up by a *Simulium* bite or they die some 30 months later. In addition to the skin, microfilariae penetrate the eye and affect every layer from the conjunctiva to the optic nerve. In African onchocerciasis, chorioretinitis and optic atrophy occur commonly; in the Central American disease, iritis is the primary lesion.

The probability of the development of eye disease is related to the location of the adult worms. When the nodules are situated about the head, eye lesions are common; when they are in the lower parts of the body, eye lesions occur less frequently. In Africa, the nodules tend to be distributed primarily in the lower parts of the body, but because of the high prevalence of the infection, onchocercal blindness is a common occurrence. In Central America, the lesions tend to be on the upper part of the body.

Clinical Manifestations

The appearance of the skin nodules and the presence of live microfilariae within the eye (readily seen with an ophthalmoscope) are the manifestations of early and intermediate disease. Later, the eye involvement includes keratitis, iridocyclitis, chorioretinitis, and eventually, blindness. Microfilariae in the skin cause an inflammatory reaction that includes acute pruritus and chronic changes such as edema, hypertrophy, and reddish hyperpigmentation (peau d'orange).

Differential and Specific Diagnoses

Because the skin invasion is associated with itching, the pruritus of onchocercal infection must be differentiated from contact dermatitis, prickly heat, and insect bites.

Onchocerciasis is identified by examination of a skin snip. Examination of sectioned and stained tissue or a stained impression smear reveals microfilariae.

Treatment

Surgical removal of all visible nodules may radically extirpate the source of new microfilariae that invade the eye. Chemotherapy with ivermectin is the treatment of choice. Ivermectin also can be used in mass treatment to interrupt transmission by the vector and, thus, control the incidence of this infection.[143, 144]

Prevention

Vector control, periodic treatment of infected persons, and surgical removal of skin lesions by roving teams of physicians and other health care workers are currently the only means of prevention, but their success is limited.

MANSONELLA PERSTANS AND *MANSONELLA OZZARDI*

Neither *M. perstans* nor *M. ozzardi* is known to cause significant human pathology, but the microfilariae present in blood must be distinguished morphologically from those of the other more pathogenic filariae. *M. ozzardi* is found throughout the Caribbean (especially Haiti) and Central America. It has been suggested as a cause of chronic arthritis in these regions. *M. perstans* also is found in Africa, where it has been identified as a cause of painless nodules in the conjunctiva and secondary eyelid swelling. For that reason, it sometimes is called the Kampala or Ugandan eye worm.[145] Albendazole or mebendazole is the treatment of choice for *M. perstans* infection.

DIROFILARIA IMMITIS

D. immitis is a filarial worm commonly found in dogs, in which it occupies the right ventricle of the heart. The microfilariae produced circulate in blood and are transmitted to new animals through the bite of culicine mosquitoes. Fewer than 100 cases of human infection have been reported, none of them in children. Most human hosts infected with *Dirofilaria* were asymptomatic, but those who had symptoms complained of chest pain, wheezing, and cough. All infected persons had coin lesions detected on pulmonary radiographs.[146, 147] Lesions in the pediatric age group possibly have been missed because they might have been thought to represent a Ghon complex.

Human infection probably is transmitted through a mosquito bite, but this means has not been established. As with visceral larva migrans, the microfilariae of *D. immitis* cannot complete their cycle in humans. No microfilariae of this worm have ever been demonstrated in human peripheral blood. All patients evaluated for pulmonary dirofilariasis have had mild peripheral eosinophilia, usually not exceeding 10 percent. Because the radiographic picture is not diagnostic and in view of the potential seriousness of a coin lesion,[146] the lesion must be examined histologically. If a worm is found, the diagnosis of dirofilariasis can be made; if it is not found, the diagnosis is still tenable. In the presence of eosinophilia and pneumonitis, however, a whole range of other diagnostic possibilities must be considered, including eosinophilic pneumonia, polyarteritis nodosa, Wegener granulomatosis, and histiocytosis X. No treatment is necessary for this infection in humans.

DRACUNCULUS MEDINENSIS

Infection by *D. medinensis* also is limited largely to the tropics. The adult female worm lies in subcutaneous tissue and can extend over a length of 50 to 120 cm. No information about the fate of the male exists. The adult lives for as long as 18 months. At the end of the first year of infection, the adult female migrates to subcutaneous tissue, where it produces an indurated papule that tends to vesiculate and ulcerate. When the surface of the ulcer comes in contact with water, the worm discharges motile larvae. These larvae, in turn, are ingested by a crustacean, *Cyclops,* in which they undergo additional maturation and development. Humans become infected by swallowing *Cyclops* in drinking water. The larvae then penetrate through the gut into subcutaneous tissue by a route not fully understood. Multiple infections occur commonly. In Nigeria, this disease has been reported to be responsible for 25 percent of absenteeism in schoolchildren.[149] Secondary bacterial infections leading to cellulitis are common, as are secondary arthritis and contractures that can lead to permanent disability.[149]

Stagnant water is necessary for maintenance of the infection, which therefore tends to be infrequent when running water and properly constructed wells are available. The diagnosis is established readily by the observation of larvae emerging from a cutaneous ulcer. Moreover, the outline of the worm can be seen easily under the skin.

The classic treatment of this infection involves incision of the skin and tying the end of the worm to a small piece of wood. By turning the wood daily, the worm can be extracted over a period of several weeks. This therapy is unsatisfactory and often results in failure of complete extraction. If the worm tears, it releases larvae into subcutaneous tissue, which provokes an intense inflammatory reaction and skin sloughing. A far better approach is to continue to expose the protruding end of the worm to water so that the larvae can be extruded completely before forcible extraction is attempted.

Treatment with chemotherapeutic agents such as metronidazole is controversial. Some investigators report that treatment with these agents helps decrease inflammation and facilitate removal of the worm.

Because filtering of drinking water effectively would prevent this infection, authorities are optimistic that this parasite can be eradicated through appropriate control measures.[148–150] Through an initiative led by the Carter Center (Atlanta), success has been achieved in almost eradicating guinea worm infection in many parts of Africa and Asia. High rates of infection still exist in the Sudan because of the difficulty encountered in implementing public health control measures in this war-torn region.

REFERENCES

Intestinal Nematodes

1. Bundy, D. A. P.: New initiatives in the control of helminths. Trans. R. Soc. Trop. Med. Hyg. *84*:467–468, 1990.
2. Drake, L. J., Jukes, M. C. H., Sternberg, R. J., and Bundy, D. A. P.: Geohelminth infections (ascariasis, trichuriasis, and hookworm): Cognitive and developmental impacts. Semin. Pediatr. Infect. Dis. *11*:245–251, 2000.
3. Hotez, P. J.: Pediatric geohelminth infections: Trichuriasis, ascariasis, and hookworm infections. Semin. Pediatr. Infect. Dis. *11*:236–244, 2000.
4. Hotez, P. J., and Pritchard, D. I.: Hookworm infection. Sci. Am. *272*:68–75, 1995.
5. Kvalsvig, J. D., Cooppan, R. M., and Connolly, K. J.: The effects of parasite infections on cognitive processes in children. Ann. Trop. Med. Parasitol. *85*:551–568, 1991.
6. Nokes, C., Cooper, E. S., Robinson, B. A., et al.: Geohelminth infection and academic assessment in Jamaican children. Trans. R. Soc. Trop. Med. Hyg. *85*:272–273, 1991.
7. Savioli, L., Bundy, D., and Tomkins, A.: Intestinal parasitic infections: A soluble public health problem. Trans. R. Soc. Trop. Med. Hyg. *86*:353–354, 1992.
8. Shoop, W. L.: Vertical transmission of helminths: Hypobiosis and amphiparatenesis. Parasitol. Today 7:51–54, 1991.

9. Smillie, W. G., and Augustine, D. L.: Hookworm infestation: The effect of varying intensities on the physical condition of school children. Am. J. Dis. Child. *31*:151–168, 1926.
10. Smillie, W. G., and Spencer, C. R.: Mental retardation in school children infested with hookworms. J. Educ. Psychol. *17*:314–321, 1926.
11. Stephenson, L. S.: Helminth parasites, a major factor in malnutrition. World Health Forum *15*:169–172, 1994.
12. Stephenson, L. S., Latham, M. C., Kinoti, S. N., et al.: Improvements in physical fitness of Kenyan schoolboys infected with hookworm, *Trichuris trichiura,* and *Ascaris lumbricoides* following a single dose of albendazole. Trans. R. Soc. Trop. Med. Hyg. *84*:277–282, 1990.
13. Stephenson, L. S., Latham, M. C., Kurz, K. M., et al.: Treatment with a single dose of albendazole improves growth of Kenyan schoolchildren with hookworm, *Trichuris trichiura,* and *Ascaris lumbricoides* infections. Am. J. Trop. Med. Hyg. *41*:78–87, 1989.

ASCARIS LUMBRICOIDES

14. Albomico, M., Smith, P. G., Ercole, E., et al.: Rate of reinfection with intestinal nematodes after treatment of children with mebendazole or albendazole in a highly endemic area. Trans. R. Soc. Trop. Med. Hyg. *89*: 538–541, 1995.
15. Anderson, T. J. C.: *Ascaris* infections in humans from North America: Molecular evidence for cross-infection. Parasitology *110*:215–219, 1995.
16. Blumenthal, D. S., and Schultz, M. G.: Incidence of intestinal obstruction in children infected with *Ascaris lumbricoides.* Am. J. Trop. Med. Hyg. *24*:801–805, 1975.
17. Chu, W. G., Chen, P. M., Huang, C. C., et al.: Neonatal ascariasis. J. Pediatr. *81*:783–785, 1972.
18. Costa-Macedo, L. M., and Rey, L.: *Ascaris lumbricoides* in neonate: Evidence of congenital transmission of intestinal nematodes. Rev. Inst. Med. Trop. Sao Paulo *32*:351–354, 1990.
19. Cowden, J., and Hotez, P. J.: Mebendazole and albendazole treatment of geohelminth infections in children and pregnant women. Pediatr. Infect. Dis. J. *19*:657–680, 2000.
20. Crompton, D. W. T.: Ascariasis and childhood malnutrition. Trans. R. Soc. Trop. Med. Hyg. *86*:577–579, 1992.
21. DeSilva, N. R., Chan, M. S., and Bundy, D. A.: Morbidity and mortality due to ascariasis: Re-estimation and sensitivity analysis of global numbers at risk. Trop. Med. Int. Health *2*:519–528, 1997.
22. Goldberg, D. E.: Oxygen avid hemoglobin of ascariasis. Chem. Rev. *99*: 3371–3378, 1999.
23. Grasberger, B. L., Clore, G. M., and Gronenborn, A. M.: High resolution structure of *Ascaris* trypsin inhibitor in solution: Direct evidence for a pH-induced conformational transition in the reactive site. Structure *2*:669–678, 1994.
24. Hall, A., and Romanova, T.: *Ascaris lumbricoides*: Detecting its metabolites in the urine of the infected people using gas-liquid chromatography. Exp. Parasitol. *70*:35–42, 1990.
25. Haswell-Elkins, M. R., Kennedy, M. W., Maizels, R. M., et al.: Detection of *Ascaris* metabolites in the urine by gas-liquid chromatography also correlates with the worm burden. Parasite Immunol. *11*:615–627, 1989.
26. Huang, K., Strynadka, N. C., Bernard, V. D., et al.: The molecular structure of the complex of *Ascaris* chymotrypsin/elastase inhibitor with porcine elastase. Structure *2*:679–689, 1994.
27. Khuroo, M. S., Zargar S. A., and Mahajan, R.: Hepatobiliary and pancreatic ascariasis in India. Lancet *335*:1503–1506, 1990.
28. Koino, S.: Experimental infections on human body with ascarides. Jpn. Med. World *2*:317–320, 1922.
29. Lynch, N. R., Hagel, I. A., Palenque, M. E., et al. Relationship between helminthic infection and IgE response in atopic and nonatopic children in a tropical environment. J. Allergy Clin. Immunol. *101*:217–221, 1998.
30. McSharry, C., Xia, Y., Holland, C. V., and Kennedy, M. W.: Natural immunity to *Ascaris lumbricoides* associated with immunoglobulin E antibody to ABA-1 allergen and inflammation indicators in children. Infect. Immun. *67*:484–489, 1999.
31. Stephenson, L. S., Latham, M. C., Kurz, K. M., et al.: Treatment with a single dose of albendazole improves growth of Kenyan schoolchildren with hookworm, *Trichuris trichiura,* and *Ascaris lumbricoides* infections. Am. J. Trop. Med. Hyg. *41*:78–87, 1989.
32. Tankhiwalle, S. R., Kukade, A. L., Sarmah, H. C., et al.: Single dose therapy of ascariasis: A randomized comparison of mebendazole and pyrantel. J. Commun. Dis. *21*:71–74, 1989.
33. Villar, J., Klebanoff, M., and Kestler, E.: The effect on fetal growth of protozoan and helminthic infection during pregnancy. Obstet. Gynecol. *74*:915–929, 1989.
34. Xu, L., Jian, Z., Yu, S., et al.: Nationwide survey of the distribution of human parasites in China: Infection with parasite species in human population. Chin. J. Parasitol. Parasitic Dis. *13*:1–7, 1995.

TRICHURIS TRICHIURA

35. Bundy, D. A. P., and Cooper, E. S.: *Trichuris* and trichuriasis in humans. Adv. Parasitol. *28*:107–173, 1989.
36. Cooper E. S., and Bundy, D. A. P.: *Trichuris* is not trivial. Parasitol. Today *4*:301–305, 1988.
37. Cooper, E., Bundy, D., MacDonald, T., et al.: Growth suppression in the *Trichuris* dysentery syndrome. Eur. J. Clin. Nutr. *44*:285–291, 1990.
38. Drake, L., Korchev, Y., Bashford, L., et al.: The major secreted product of the whipworm *Trichuris* is a pore-forming protein. Proc. R. Soc. Lond. B *257*:255–261, 1994.
39. Else, K. J., Finkelman, F. D., Maliszewski, C. R., et al.: Cytokine-mediated regulation of chronic intestinal helminth infection. J. Exp. Med. *179*:347–351, 1994.
40. Layrisse, M., Aparcedo, L., Martinez Torres, C., et al.: Blood loss due to infection with *Trichuris trichiura.* Am. J. Trop. Med. Hyg. *16*:613–616, 1967.
41. Lotero, M., Tripathy, K., and Bolanos, O.: Gastrointestinal blood loss in *Trichuris* infection. Am. J. Trop. Med. Hyg. *23*:1203–1207, 1974.
42. MacDonald, T. T., Choy, M. Y., Spencer, J., et al.: Histopathology of the caecum in children with *Trichuris* dysentery syndrome. J. Clin. Pathol. *44*:194–199, 1991.
43. Maqbool, S., Lawrence, D., and Katz, M.: Treatment of trichuriasis with a new drug, mebendazole. J. Pediatr. *86*:463–465, 1975.
44. Simeon, D. T., Grantham-McGregor, S. M., and Wong, M. S.: *Trichuris trichiura* infection and cognition in children: Results of a randomized clinical trial. Parasitology *110*:457–464, 1995.
45. Wakelin, D., and Gelby, R. G.: Immune expulsion of *Trichuris muris* from resistant mice: Suppression by irradiation and restoration by transfer of lymphoid cells. Parasitology *72*:41–50, 1976.

HOOKWORMS

46. Cappello, M., Vlasuk, G. P., Bergum, P. W., et al.: *Ancylostoma caninum* anticoagulant peptide (AcAP): A novel hookworm-derived inhibitor of human coagulation factor Xa. Proc. Natl. Acad. Sci. U. S. A. *92*: 6152–6156, 1995.
47. Gandhi, N. S., Jizhang, C., Khoshnood, K., et al.: Epidemiology of *Necator americanus* hookworm infections in Xiulongkan Village, Hainan Province, China: High prevalence and intensity among middle-aged and elderly residents. J. Parasitol. *87*:739–743, 2001.
48. Hawdon, J. M., Jones, B., Perregaux, M., et al.: *Ancylostoma caninum*: Resumption of hookworm larval feeding coincides with metalloprotease release. Exp. Parasitol. *80*:205–211, 1995.
49. Hotez, P. J.: Hookworm disease in children. Pediatr. Infect. Dis. J. *8*:516–520, 1989.
50. Hotez, P. J.: Human hookworm infection. *In* Farthing, M. J. G., Keusch, G. T., and Wakelin, D. (eds.): Enteric Infection 2. Intestinal Helminths. London, Chapman & Hall, 1995, pp. 129–150.
51. Hotez, P. J., Cappello, M., Hawdon, J., et al.: Hyaluronidases from the gastrointestinal invasive nematodes *Ancylostoma caninum* and *Anisakis simplex:* Their function in the pathogenesis of human zoonoses. J. Infect. Dis. *170*:918–926, 1994.
52. Hotez, P. J., Ghosh, K., Hawdon, J. M., et al.: Experimental approaches to the development of a recombinant hookworm vaccine. Immunol. Rev. *171*:163–172, 1999.
53. Jones, B. F., and Hotez, P. J.: Molecular cloning and characterization of Ac-MEP-1, a developmentally regulated gut luminal metalloendopeptidase from adult *Ancylostoma caninum* hookworms. Mol. Biochem. Parasitol. *119*:107–116, 2002.
54. Prociv, P., and Croese, J.: Human eosinophilic enteritis caused by dog hookworm, *Ancylostoma caninum.* Lancet *335*:1299–1302, 1990.
55. Saraya, A. K., and Tandon, B. N.: Hookworm anemia and intestinal malabsorption associated with hookworm infestation. Prog. Drug Res. *19*:108–118, 1975.
56. Schad, G. A.: Hypobiosis and related phenomena in hookworm infection. *In* Warren, K. S., and Schad, G. A. (eds.): Hookworm Disease, Current Status and Future Directions. London, Taylor & Francis, 1990, pp. 71–88.
57. Schad, G. A., and Anderson, R. M.: Predisposition to hookworm infection. Science *228*:1537–1540, 1985.

ENTEROBIUS VERMICULARIS

58. Bhaskaran, C. S., Devi, E. S., and Rao, K. V.: *Enterobius vermicularis* and vermiform appendix. J. Indian Med. Assoc. *64*:334–336, 1975.
59. Liu, L. X., Chi, J., Upton, M. P., et al.: Eosinophilic colitis associated with larvae of the pinworm *Enterobius vermicularis.* Lancet *346*:410–412, 1995.
60. Mattia, A. R.: Perianal mass and recurrent and cellulitis due to *Enterobius vermicularis.* Am. J. Trop. Med. Hyg. *47*:811–815, 1992.
61. Mondou, E. N., and Gnepp, D. R.: Hepatic granuloma resulting from *Enterobius vermicularis.* Am. J. Clin. Pathol. *91*:97–100, 1989.
62. Simon, R. D.: Pinworm infestation and urinary tract infection in young girls. Am. J. Dis. Child. *128*:21–22, 1974.
63. Verumund, S. H.: Pinworm *(Enterobius vermicularis).* Semin. Pediatr. Infect. Dis. *11*:252–256, 2000.
64. Weller, T. H., and Gorenson, C. W.: Enterobiasis: Its incidence and symptomatology in a group of 505 children. N. Engl. J. Med. *224*:143–146, 1941.

STRONGYLOIDES STERCORALIS AND *STRONGYLOIDES FUELLEBORNI*

65. Ashford, R. W., Vince, J. D., Gratten, M. J., et al.: *Strongyloides* infection associated with acute infantile disease in Papua New Guinea. Trans. R. Soc. Trop. Med. Hyg. *72*:554, 1978.
66. Barnish, G., and Ashford, R. W.: *Strongyloides* cf. *fuelleborni* and hookworm in Papua New Guinea: Patterns of infection within the community. Trans. R. Soc. Trop. Med. Hyg. *83*:684–689, 1989.
67. Brindley, P. J., Gam, A. A., McKerrow, J. H., and Neva, F. A., et al.: Ss40: The zinc endopeptidase secreted by infective larvae of *Strongyloides stercoralis*. Exp. Parasitol. *80*:1–7, 1995.
68. Brown, H. W., and Perna, V. P.: An overwhelming *Strongyloides* infection. J. A. M. A. *168*:1648–1651, 1958.
69. Brown, R. C., and Girardeau, M. H. F.: Transmammary passage of *Strongyloides* sp. larvae in the human host. Am. J. Trop. Med. Hyg. *26*:215–219, 1977.
70. Burke, J. A.: Strongyloidiasis in childhood. Am. J. Dis. Child. *132*: 1130–1136, 1978.
71. Campbell, W. C., and Cuckler, A.: Thiabendazole in the treatment and control of parasitic infection in man. Tex. Rep. Biol. Med. *27*:665–692, 1964.
72. DeVault, G. A., King, J. W., Rohr, M. S., et al.: Opportunistic infections with *Strongyloides stercoralis* in renal transplantation. Rev. Infect. Dis. *12*:653–671, 1990.
73. Dixon, A. C., Yanaghihara, E. T., Kwock, D. W., et al.: Strongyloidiasis associated with human T-cell lymphotropic virus type 1 infection in a nonendemic area. West. J. Med. *151*:410–413, 1989.
74. Genta, R. M.: Global prevalence of strongyloidiasis: Critical review with epidemiologic insights into the prevention of disseminated disease. Rev. Infect. Dis. *11*:755–767, 1989.
75. Genta, R. M.: Dysregulation of strongyloidiasis: A new hypothesis. Clin. Microbiol. Rev. *5*:345–355, 1992.
76. Genta, R. M., Miles, P., and Fields, K.: Opportunistic *Strongyloides stercoralis* infection in lymphoma patients: Report of a case and review of the literature. Cancer *63*:1407–1411, 1989.
77. Gill, G. V., and Bell, D. R.: Longstanding tropical infections amongst former war prisoners of the Japanese. Lancet *1*:958–959, 1982.
78. Gyorkos, T. W., Genta, R. M., Viens, P., et al.: Seroepidemiology of *Strongyloides* infection in the southeast Asian refugee population in Canada. Am. J. Epidemiol. *132*:257–264, 1990.
79. Lyagoubi, M., Datry, A., Mayorga, R. et al.: Chronic persistent strongyloidiasis cured by ivermectin. Trans. R. Soc. Trop. Med. Hyg. *86*:541, 1992.
80. McKerrow, J. H., Brindley, P., Brown, M., et al.: *Strongyloides stercoralis*: Identification of a protease that facilitates penetration of skin by the infective larvae. Exp. Parasitol. *70*:134–143, 1990.
81. Naquira, C., Jimenez, G., Guerra, J. G., et al.: Ivermectin for human strongyloidiasis and other intestinal helminths. Am. J. Trop. Med. Hyg. *40*:304–309, 1989.
82. O'Brien, W.: Intestinal malabsorption in acute infection with *Strongyloides stercoralis*. Trans. R. Soc. Trop. Med. Hyg. *69*:69–77, 1975.
83. Purtillo, D. T., Meyers, W. M., and Connor, D. H.: Fatal strongyloidiasis in immunosuppressed patients. Am. J. Med. *56*:488–493, 1974.
84. Robinson, R. D., Lindo, J. F., Neva, F. A., et al.: Immunoepidemiologic studies of *Strongyloides stercoralis* and human T lymphotropic virus type I infections in Jamaica. J. Infect. Dis. *169*:692–696, 1994.
85. Schad, G. A.: Cyclosporine may eliminate the threat of overwhelming strongyloidiasis in immunosuppressed patients. J. Infect. Dis. *153*:178, 1986.
86. Schad, G. A., Aikens, L. M., and Smith, G.: *Strongyloides stercoralis*: Is there a canonical migratory route through the host? J. Parasitol. *75*: 740–749, 1989.
87. Sukhavat, K., Morakote, N., Chaiwong, P., et al.: Comparative efficacy of four methods for the detection of *Strongyloides stercoralis* in human stool specimens. Ann. Trop. Med. Parasitol. *88*:95–96, 1994.

Aberrant Infections with Intestinal Nematodes

TOXOCARA CANIS

88. Arpino, C., Gattinara, G. C., Piergili, D., et al.: *Toxocara* infection and epilepsy in children: A case-control study. Epilepsia *31*:33–36, 1990.
89. Ashton, N.: Larval granulomatosis of the retina due to *Toxocara*. Br. J. Ophthalmol. *44*:129–148, 1960.
90. Bekhti, A.: Mebendazole in toxocariasis. Ann. Intern. Med. *100*:463, 1984.
91. Biddulph, J.: Mebendazole and albendazole for infants. Pediatr. Infect. Dis. J. *9*:373, 1990.
92. Bird, A. C., Smith, J. L., and Curtin, V. T.: Nematode optic neuritis. Am. J. Ophthalmol. *69*:72–77, 1970.
93. Dinning, W. J., Gillespie, S. H., Cooling, R. J., et al.: Toxocariasis: A practical approach to management of ocular disease. Eye *2*:580–582, 1988.
94. Douglas, J. R., and Baker, N. F.: Some host-parasite relationships of canine helminths. *In* McCauley, J. E. (ed.): Host-Parasite Relationships. Proc. 26th Annual Biol. Colloq. Corvallis, Oregon State University Press, 1966, pp. 97–115.
95. Editorial: The public health significance of canine ascarid infections. Vet. Rec. *99*:37–38, 1976.
96. Fortenberry, J. D., Kenney, R. D., and Younger, J.: Visceral larva migrans producing static encephalopathy in an infant. Pediatr. Infect. Dis. J. *10*: 403–406, 1991.
97. Glickman, L. T., and Schantz, P. M.: Epidemiology and pathogenesis of zoonotic toxocariasis. Epidemiol. Rev. *10*:143–148, 1982.
98. Hotez, P. J.: Visceral and ocular larva migrans. Semin. Neurol. *13*:175–179, 1993.
99. Hotez, P. J.: *Toxocara canis*. *In* Burg, F. D., Ingelfinger, J. R., Wald, E. R., and Polin, R. A. (eds.): Gellis and Kagan's Current Pediatric Therapy. 15th ed. Philadelphia, W. B. Saunders, 1996.
100. Kazacos, K. R.: Visceral and ocular larva migrans. Semin. Vet. Med. Surg. (Small Animal) *6*:227–235, 1991.
101. Marmor, M., Glickman, L., Shofer, F., et al.: *Toxocara canis* infection of children: Epidemiologic and neuropsychologic findings. Am. J. Public Health *77*:554–559, 1987.
102. Nelson, J. D., McConnel, T. H., and Moore, D. V.: Thiabendazole therapy of visceral larva migrans: A case report. Am. J. Trop. Med. Hyg. *15*: 930–933, 1966.
103. Schantz, P. M.: *Toxocara* larva migrans now. Am. J. Trop. Med. Hyg. *41*(Suppl.):21–34, 1989.
104. Schantz, P. M., Meyer, D., and Glickman, L. T.: Clinical, serologic, and epidemiologic characteristics of ocular toxocariasis. Am. J. Trop. Med. Hyg. *28*:24–28, 1979.
105. Sharghi, N., Schantz, P. M., Caramico, L., et al.: Environmental exposure to *Toxocara* as a possible risk factor for asthma: A clinic-based case-control study. Clin. Infect. Dis. *32*:e111–e116, 2001.
106. Small, K. W., McCuen, B. W., De Juan, E., et al.: Surgical management of retinal retraction caused by toxocariasis. Am. J. Ophthalmol. *108*:10–14, 1989.
107. Sturchler, D., Schubarth, P., Fualzata, M., et al.: Thiabendazole vs. albendazole in treatment of toxocariasis. A clinical study. Ann. Trop. Med. Parasitol. *83*:473–478, 1989.
108. Woodruff, A. W., Bisseru, B., and Bowe, J. C.: Infection with animal helminths as a factor in causing poliomyelitis and epilepsy. B. M. J. *5503*:1576–1579, 1966.

OTHER ABERRANT INFECTIONS WITH INTESTINAL NEMATODES

109. Chitwood, M.: Nematodes of medical significance found in market fish. Am. J. Trop. Med. Hyg. *19*:599–602, 1970.
110. Cross, J.: Intestinal capillariasis. Clin. Microbiol. Rev. *5*:120–129, 1992.
111. Cuckler, A. C., Egerton, J. R., and Alicata, J. E.: Therapeutic effect of thiabendazole on *Angiostrongylus cantonensis* infections in rats. J. Parasitol. *51*:392–396, 1965.
112. Dauz, V., Cabrera, B. D., and Cancas, B.: Human intestinal capillariasis: I. Clinical features. Acta Med. Philipp. *4*:72–83, 1967.
113. Ghadirian, E., and Arfaa, F.: Present status of trichostrongyliasis in Iran. Am. J. Trop. Med. Hyg. *24*:935–941, 1975.
114. Hotez, P. J., Haggerty, J., Hawdon, J., et al.: Infective *Ancylostoma* hookworm larval metalloproteases and their possible functions in tissue invasion and ecdysis. Infect. Immun. *58*:3883–3892, 1990.
115. Hotez, P. J., Narasimhan, S., Haggerty, J., et al.: Hyaluronidase from *Ancylostoma* hookworm larvae and its function as a virulence factor in cutaneous larva migrans. Infect. Immun. *60*:1018–1023, 1992.
116. Huff, D. S., Neaffie, R. C., Binder, M. J., et al.: The first fatal *Baylisascaris* infection in humans: An infant with eosinophilic meningoencephalitis. Pediatr. Pathol. *2*:1–20, 1984.
117. Hurlbert, T. V., Larsen, R. A., and Chandrasoma, P. T.: Abdominal angiostrongyliasis mimicking acute appendicitis and Meckel's diverticulum: Report of a case in the United States and review. Clin. Infect. Dis. *14*:836–840, 1992.
118. Kazacos, K. R., and Boyce, W. M.: *Baylisascaris* larva migrans. J. Am. Vet. Med. Assoc. *195*:894–903, 1990.
119. Koo, J., Pien, F., and Kliks, M. M.: *Angiostrongylus (Parastrongylus)* eosinophilic meningitis. Rev. Infect. Dis. *10*:1155–1162, 1988.
120. Krepel, H. P., and Polderman, A. M.: Egg production of *Oesophagostomum bifurcum,* a locally common parasite of humans in Togo. Am. J. Trop. Med. Hyg. *46*:469–472, 1992.
121. McKerrow, J. H., Sakanari, J. A., and Deardorff, T. L.: Revenge of the "sushi parasite." N. Engl. J. Med. *319*:1228–1229, 1988.
122. Otto, G. I., Berthrong, M., Appleby, R. E., et al.: Eosinophilia and hepatomegaly due to *Capillaria hepatica* infection. Bull. Johns Hopkins Hosp. *94*:319–336, 1954.
123. Polderman, A. M., Kepel, H. P., Baeta, S., et al: Oesophagostomiasis, a common infection of man in northern Togo and Ghana. Am. J. Trop. Med. Hyg. *44*:336–344, 1991.
124. Rosen, L., Chappel, R., Laquer, G. L., et al.: Eosinophilic meningoencephalitis caused by a metastrongyloid lungworm of rats. J. A. M. A. *179*:620–624, 1962.
125. Rosen, L., Loisen, G., Laigret, J., et al.: Studies of eosinophilic meningitis. III. Epidemiologic and clinical observations on Pacific islands and the possible etiologic role of *Angiostrongylus cantonensis*. Am. J. Epidemiol. *85*:17–24, 1967.
126. Schad, G. A.: Hookworms: Pets to humans. Ann. Intern. Med. *120*: 434–435, 1994.

127. Schantz, P. M.: The dangers of eating raw fish. N. Engl. J. Med. *320*: 1143–1145, 1989.
128. Whalen, G. E., Rosenberg, E. B., Strickland, G. T., et al.: Intestinal capillariasis: A new disease in man. Lancet *1*:13–16, 1969.
129. Whitting, D. A.: The successful treatment of creeping eruption with topical thiabendazole. S. Afr. Med. J. *50*:253–255, 1976.
130. Wittner, M., Turner, J. W., and Jacquette, G.: Eustrongylidiasis: A parasitic infection acquired by eating sushi. N. Engl. J. Med. *320*: 1124–1126, 1989.
131. Yoshimura, H., Akao, N., Kondo, K., et al.: Clinicopathological studies on larval anisakiasis, with special reference to the report of extra-gastrointestinal anisakiasis. Jpn. J. Parasitol. *28*:347–354, 1979.

Filarial Parasites

LYMPHATIC FILARIASIS: *WUCHERERIA BANCROFTI* AND *BRUGIA* SPECIES

132. Baird, J. K., Alpert, L. I., and Friedman, R.: North American brugian filariasis: Report of nine infections of humans. Am. J. Trop. Med. Hyg. *35*:1205, 1986.
133. Grove, D. I., Cabrera, B. D., Valeza, F. S., et al.: Sensitivity and specificity of skin reactivity to *Brugia malayi* and *Dirofilaria immitis* antigens in bancroftian and Malayan filariasis in the Philippines. Am. J. Trop. Med. Hyg. *26*:220–229, 1977.
134. Nanduri, J., and Kazura, J. W.: Clinical and laboratory aspects of filariasis. Clin. Microbiol. Rev. *2*:39–60, 1986.
135. Ottesen, E. A., and Nutman, T. B.: Tropical pulmonary eosinophilia. Annu. Rev. Med. *43*:417–424, 1992.
136. Ottesen, E. A., Vijayasekaran, V., Kumaraswami, V., et al.: A controlled trial of ivermectin and diethylcarbamazine in lymphatic filariasis. N. Engl. J. Med. *322*:1113–1117, 1990.
137. Simmons, C. F., Jr., Winter, H. S., Berde, C., et al.: Zoonotic filariasis with lymphedema in an immunodeficient infant. N. Engl. J. Med. *310*: 1243–1245, 1984.
138. Vande, W. A. A.: Chemotherapy of filariases. Parasitol. Today *7*:194–199, 1991.

LOA LOA

139. Carme, B., Boulesteix, J., Boutes, H., et al.: Five cases of encephalitis during treatment of loiasis with diethylcarbamazine. Am. J. Trop. Med. Hyg. *44*:684–690, 1991.
140. Kilon, A. D., Massoughbodji, A., Sadeler, B. C., et al.: Loiasis in endemic and nonendemic populations: Immunologically mediated differences in clinical presentation. J. Infect. Dis. *163*:1318–1325, 1991.
141. Nutman, T. B., Reese, W., Poindexter, R. W., et al.: Immunologic correlates of the hyperresponsive syndrome of loiasis. J. Infect. Dis. *157*:544–550, 1988.
142. Olness, K., Franciosi, R. A., and Johnson, M. M.: Loiasis in an expatriate American child: Diagnostic and treatment difficulties. Pediatrics *80*:943, 1987.

ONCHOCERCA VOLVULUS

143. Taylor, H. R., and Greene, B. M.: The status of ivermectin in the treatment of human onchocerciasis. Am. J. Trop. Med. Hyg. *41*:460–466, 1989.
144. Taylor, H. R., Pacque, M., Munoz, B., et al.: Impact of mass treatment of onchocerciasis with ivermectin on the transmission of infection. Science *250*:116–118, 1990.

MANSONELLA PERSTANS AND *MANSONELLA OZZARDI*

145. Baird, J. K., Neafie, R. C., and Connor, D. H.: Nodules in the conjunctiva, bung-eye, and bulge-eye in Africa caused by *Mansonella perstans*. Am. J. Trop. Med. Hyg. *38*:553–557, 1988.

DIROFILARIA IMMITIS

146. Bloc, T., Glynn, T., and Hinshaw, M.: Human pulmonary dirofilariasis. Indiana Med. *83*:24–27, 1990.
147. Dayal, Y., and Neafie, R. C.: Human pulmonary dirofilariasis: A case report and review of the literature. Am. Rev. Respir. Dis. *112*:437–443, 1975.

DRACUNCULUS MEDINENSIS

148. Hopkins, D. R., and Ruiz-Tiben, E.: Strategies for dracunculiasis eradication. Bull. World Health Organ. *69*:533–540, 1991.
149. Ilegbodu, V. A., Oladele, K. O., Wise, R. A., et al.: Impact of guinea worm disease on children in Nigeria. Am. J. Trop. Med. Hyg. *35*:962–964, 1986.
150. Update: Dracunculiasis eradication—Ghana and Nigeria, 1990. M. M. W. R. Morb. Mortal. Wkly. Rep. *40*:245–247, 1991.

SUBSECTION 3

CESTODES

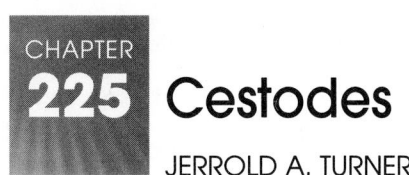

CHAPTER 225 Cestodes

JERROLD A. TURNER

The adult forms of tapeworms (cestodes) share common characteristics. They possess a specialized attachment organ called a scolex, which may have sucking grooves *(Diphyllobothrium, Spirometra)* or four circular suckers, as in the other medically important genera. In addition to having circular suckers, the scoleces of some species have hooks that assist in attaching to the mucosa of the definitive host. The body of the adult worm is ribbon-like and has no gastrointestinal tract or internal cavity. An undifferentiated neck region situated immediately behind the scolex is an area of great metabolic activity and growth. The remainder of the worm is differentiated into segments, or proglottids. Both male and female reproductive organs develop in each proglottid as it matures. The proglottids become increasingly mature the more distal they are to the neck region. Usually, the terminal proglottids are gravid and contain egg-filled uteri. The eggs of *Diphyllobothrium* and *Spirometra* require an aquatic environment, and larval development involves at least two intermediate hosts. The other species of tapeworm considered here parasitize their intermediate hosts when the eggs are ingested. In *Hymenolepis nana* infection, humans may serve as both definitive and intermediate hosts.

In certain circumstances, humans may be accidental intermediate hosts for tapeworms. Major examples of this phenomenon are cysticercosis, hydatid disease (echinococcosis), coenurosis, and sparganosis.

A review of cestode infections in children was published in 1997.[151]

Taeniasis Saginata *(Taenia Saginata* Infection, Beef Tapeworm Infection)

Goez in 1782 first recognized *T. saginata* as a separate species. In 1861, Leuckart defined the relationship between the adult worms and the larval forms found in cattle.

T. saginata is synonymous with *Taeniarhynchus saginatus*. Variations in morphology have led to the designation of species such as *Taenia confusa, Taenia hominis,* and *Taenia africana*. The validity of these species has been questioned, and *T. saginata* generally is used as an inclusive term.[147] If the recent description of *Taenia saginata asiatica* as a subspecies of *T. saginata* is accepted, the taxonomically correct designation for *T. saginata* will be *Taenia saginata saginata*.[88]

THE ORGANISM

The scolex of *T. saginata* measures 1 to 2 mm in diameter and has four cup-shaped muscular suckers but bears no hooks. The length of the parasite usually varies from 4 to 10 m but may reach 25 m. The size of the proglottids depends on their stage of development and their state of muscular relaxation. Gravid proglottids are 16 to 20 mm in length and 5 to 7 mm in width. The linear, central uterine stem has 12 to 30 main lateral branches on each side. The eggs measure 30 to 40 μm in diameter. The six-hooked embryo is surrounded by a brownish, radially striated embryophore.

When an intermediate host ingests the eggs of *T. saginata,* embryos hatch from the eggs and burrow through the intestinal mucosa, where they gain access to the circulation. After lodging in capillaries in various locations in the body of the intermediate host, each surviving embryo develops into a larval cysticercus or bladder worm. This cystic, ovoid structure measures 7 to 10 mm by 4 to 6 mm and contains an invaginated scolex.

Domestic bovine animals are the principal intermediate hosts, but infections have been found in reindeer and a variety of wild African herbivorous animals.[113] Humans are the only definitive host. Although rare reports of human cysticercosis caused by *T. saginata* cysticerci exist, the diagnosis is usually questionable.

TRANSMISSION

Completion of the life cycle of *T. saginata* requires transmission of the infection to the intermediate host and subsequently to humans. Contamination of pastures or feed lots with human feces or untreated sewage is the initial step. *Taenia* eggs ingested by cattle hatch in the intestine and develop into cysticerci in tissues. When humans eat raw or rare beef containing viable cysticerci, the scolex evaginates from the cysticercus and attaches to the intestinal wall, and development of the adult tapeworm begins. Gravid proglottids appear 84 to 120 days after infection is acquired.[113, 140] Infection may persist for the life of the human host. In most geographic areas, parasitization with more than a single worm is noted in less than 1 percent of infections, but in highly endemic areas, multiple infection may be found in more than 60 percent.[113]

Ova may be shed within the intestinal lumen by detached gravid proglottids, but dissemination of eggs more commonly occurs when single gravid proglottids actively migrate from the anus or out of the fecal mass. As these muscular proglottids crawl about, eggs are expressed from the anterior margin. Each proglottid contains approximately 80,000 eggs. Survival of eggs is optimal in a moist, cool environment. Although *T. saginata* eggs may survive for 1 to 3 months, they are rendered noninfectious rapidly under dry conditions.

Information on the longevity of cysticerci in cattle indicates wide variability, which may depend on the strain of parasite and the genetics and age of the host, as well as other factors. Viable cysticerci have been recovered from cattle several years after infection.

The ova of *Taenia solium* and *T. saginata* are not distinguishable on morphologic grounds. Although *T. saginata* eggs are not a hazard to humans, *T. solium* eggs can hatch within the intestine and cause cysticercosis. Therefore, until the diagnosis of *T. saginata* infection is confirmed, the patient should not be involved in food handling or preparation and should take extra care with personal hygiene and the disposition of underclothing.

EPIDEMIOLOGY

A review of taeniasis published in 1972[113] indicated the inadequacy of epidemiologic data from nearly all sources. In general, prevalence rates for human infection were below 1 percent in all but highly endemic areas. In the former Soviet Union, the areas of the Caucasus and the south-central Asian republics had prevalence rates ranging from 7 to 45 percent. Cattle-raising areas of Africa, excluding Egypt and South Africa, report rates above 10 percent. A review of the prevalence of taeniasis in 1982 showed no significant changes.[112] Although the incidence of taeniasis in the United States is low, transmission does occur. In 1988, less than 0.1 percent of fecal specimens examined in state health laboratories were positive for *Taenia* eggs.[76]

PATHOLOGY AND PATHOGENESIS

Little is known of the pathology or pathogenesis of intestinal taeniasis. Speculation regarding local mucosal trauma, irritation, production of toxic substances, or induction of clinically significant hypersensitivity has scant documentation. Rare, ectopic localization of worms or proglottids may stimulate local inflammatory reactions. Infections of the middle ear, nasopharynx, and gallbladder and an abdominal mass have been reported. Proglottids have been recovered from the uterine cavity, and acute appendicitis has been attributed to wandering proglottids on many occasions. Whether the appendiceal inflammation is a direct result of obstruction and irritation by proglottids or whether the presence of the parasite is merely a coincidental finding is not clear.

CLINICAL MANIFESTATIONS

The most common complaint is the discomfort and embarrassment caused by the migration of gravid proglottids from the anus. The patient's awareness of the infection frequently causes a preoccupation with gastrointestinal function. A summary of eight studies of *T. saginata* infection[113] revealed abdominal pain, nausea, weakness, and loss of weight as the most common symptoms recorded. Alterations in appetite and bowel habits were reported inconsistently.

Severe symptoms are especially likely to occur in infants, in whom vomiting, diarrhea, fever, weight loss, and irritability may develop.

Intestinal obstruction or symptoms related to ectopic localization of proglottids are extremely rare.

Although taeniasis usually is not associated with significant eosinophilia, one study of four patients showed transient eosinophilia that sometimes exceeded 30 percent between the sixth and ninth week after the initial infection. At the time that the patients first began passing proglottids, the eosinophilia had returned to normal or near normal.[61] Another series of observations showed a syndrome of marked eosinophilia and severe colicky abdominal pain that occurred approximately 1 month before the passage of *Taenia* proglottids.[9]

A single experimental infection produced symptoms of nausea, headache, and disturbed sleep at approximately the time that gravid proglottids appeared in the stool 84 days after infection. A 10.5 percent increase in eosinophils and a 13 percent increase in lymphocytes were noted.[140]

DIAGNOSIS

The scolex of *T. saginata* lacks hooks and may be differentiated easily from the scolex of *T. solium*, which bears a circle of hooks. However, the scolex usually is not recovered, even after successful treatment.

Eggs may be seen on routine fecal wet mounts, but the likelihood of detection is enhanced by concentration methods. Cellulose tape swabs applied to the anal and perianal skin, as used for the diagnosis of *Enterobius* infection, have been found to be even more efficient than fecal concentration.[95, 144]

The eggs of *T. saginata* and *T. solium* cannot be differentiated morphologically. Examination of gravid proglottids is the usual method for determining species. The patient is instructed to collect proglottids in a vial of saline and deliver the specimen to the laboratory as soon as possible. Fixatives such as alcohol or formalin tend to render the proglottids rigid and opaque. The proglottid should be compressed between two microscope slides. If the uterus contains enough ova, counting the main branches of the uterine stem is relatively easy. Visibility of the uterus may be enhanced by inserting a fine intradermal needle in the midportion of the proglottid and injecting a small amount of India ink. Counts of 13 or fewer branches on one side of the stem are considered diagnostic for *T. solium*. If the count is 14 or greater, the species is designated *T. saginata*. Because of morphologic variations, this method has been criticized, particularly when the decision is based on gravid proglottids with counts in the range of 12 to 15. Analysis of many specimens of *Taenia*, as identified by their scolex, showed that mature proglottids with fully developed sex organs could be differentiated by several characteristics.[117] The most prominent features are a vaginal sphincter seen only in *T. saginata* and a third ovarian lobe that is present only in *T. solium*. To define these and other features, the proglottids require painstaking staining and clearing, as well as examination by a skilled parasitologist. Many efforts to apply molecular techniques such as polymerase chain reaction (PCR) to the diagnosis of taeniasis and to the differentiation of species have been made. Recent approaches have developed PCR assays that may be able to distinguish *T. saginata* from *T. solium* effectively.[64] As yet, no practical application has been found for the molecular techniques in general clinical practice. Dot enzyme-linked immunosorbent assay (ELISA) dipsticks have been developed that can detect antigens from the genus *Taenia* in stool, but the results are not species-specific.[2]

Although many attempts have been made to develop diagnostic serologic tests and skin sensitivity tests for taeniasis, the antigens have not been sufficiently sensitive or specific to be helpful clinically. The use of excretory secretory antigens from tapeworms grown in immunosuppressed hamsters has allowed the development of a serologic test that can detect antibody in carriers of *T. solium* without cross-reacting with infections by other tapeworms or cysticercosis.[156] Preliminary data indicate that the test is 95 percent sensitive and 100 percent specific.

Occasionally, the diagnosis of tapeworm is made when larger portions of a worm appear as a ribbon-like defect in the barium column during contrast studies of the gastrointestinal tract. In plain films of the abdomen, a tapeworm may be seen as a linear density in a gas-filled loop of bowel.

TREATMENT

The drug of choice is praziquantel. This pyrazinoisoquinoline derivative is supplied as 600-mg, film-coated, scored tablets that are broken easily into 150-mg quarters. Praziquantel is administered in a single dose of 5 to 10 mg/kg. It is not recommended in pregnancy, and its safety in children younger than 4 years has not been established. Lactating mothers should avoid nursing for 72 hours after receiving treatment. Praziquantel must be administered with caution to patients at risk for neurocysticercosis (see later), and it has not been approved by the U.S. Food and Drug Administration for the treatment of infection with adult tapeworms. Therefore, use of this drug for this indication is considered investigational.

Quinacrine, used in the past for taeniasis, required multiple purges and frequently was associated with vomiting. It has been replaced by praziquantel. Niclosamide is a safe and effective taeniacidal drug that is approved for use in the United States, but it was withdrawn from the market by the manufacturer.

After treatment, the patient or parent is requested to watch for proglottids. Proglottids may be seen for up to 3 days after treatment. Proglottids or ova found 7 days after treatment indicate treatment failure, and the patient should be instructed to return for treatment. Four months after treatment, fecal examination should be performed for ova and proglottids.

PROGNOSIS

T. saginata infections are of little clinical significance except for the rare complications of ectopic location of the worm or intestinal obstruction. Symptoms, when present, may be annoying but do not alter health significantly. Treatment is highly effective.

PREVENTION

Meat inspection is effective in detecting all but light infections. Cooking beef to a temperature of 56° C kills cysticerci. Education of workers in the cattle-raising industry, coupled with detection and prompt treatment of human infection, may reduce transmission.

Mass examination and mass treatment have been helpful in decreasing the prevalence of infection in endemic areas of the former Soviet Union; however, this approach is not economically feasible in many developing countries that have high prevalence rates.

Asian Taeniasis

A tapeworm resembling *T. saginata* has been described from specimens recovered in Taiwan, China, Korea, Indonesia, the

Philippines, and Malaysia. This organism possesses a prominent protuberance in the center of the scolex called a rostellum. Gravid proglottids have 16 to 21 uterine branches on each side of the uterine stem, similar to the morphology of gravid proglottids of *T. saginata.* The cysticercus contains a scolex with a rostellum and rudimentary hooks. The outer surface of the cysticercus is covered with wart-like protuberances. Pigs are the most common and important intermediate hosts, but cattle, goats, monkeys, and wild boar also may be infected. The cysticerci are found in the livers of intermediate hosts. Most human infections have been reported from areas where raw or undercooked pork is eaten. An experimental infection demonstrated a period of 76 days between ingestion of the cysticercus and the appearance of gravid proglottids.[46] Although the parasite has been referred to as *Taenia asiatica,*[47] genetic studies suggest that this organism is a subspecies of *T. saginata,* and the name *Taenia saginata asiatica* has been proposed.[16, 88] The question of human cysticercosis occurring as a result of the ingestion of *T. saginata asiatica* eggs is yet to be resolved. However, no confirmed cases of cysticercosis attributable to this organism have been described.[58] A thorough review of Asian taeniasis was published in 1998.[51]

Taeniasis Solium (*Taenia solium* Infection, Pork Tapeworm Infection)

The life cycle of *T. solium* is similar to that of *T. saginata.* The pig is the intermediate host, and infection is acquired by the ingestion of inadequately cooked pork. The tapeworm is not as large as *T. saginata* and rarely exceeds 7 m in length. The gravid proglottids are less motile than those of *T. saginata* and usually are passed in feces. Humans are also susceptible to infection with the larval stage (cysticercus) of *T. solium.* This form of infection is called cysticercosis.

T. solium infection rarely occurs in the United States, but it is common in Mexico, Central and South America, parts of Africa, India, Korea, Thailand, and other Southeast Asian countries. In developed countries, cysticercosis usually is seen in immigrants from endemic areas, but transmission from tapeworm carriers occasionally occurs. A detailed review of the distribution and epidemiology of *T. solium* and cysticercosis was published in 1996.[28]

The diagnosis has been discussed in a previous section.

Clinical manifestations are similar to or perhaps even less prominent than those of *T. saginata* infection.

Treatment of infection with adult *T. solium* is identical to that recommended for *T. saginata;* however, the patient should be made aware of a theoretic risk for cysticercosis. This risk is based on the possibility that the gravid proglottids will liberate infective eggs within the intestine as a result of the treatment and that these eggs could be exposed to conditions that would induce hatching. This phenomenon never has been documented in humans, and the risk, if it exists, must be slight. Some authorities recommend administering a mild purgative after specific treatment, but whether doing so is necessary or advantageous is doubtful.[120]

Taenia solium Cysticercosis

T. solium assumes medical importance in that people can be intermediate as well as definitive hosts. Autopsy studies in heavily infected areas such as Mexico show that approximately 3.5 percent of the population has cysticercosis. Cysticercosis affects both sexes equally and may be manifested first in infancy. Human cysticercosis has been reviewed in detail.[19, 59, 159]

Cysticercosis usually is acquired by ingestion of the eggs of *T. solium* in food or drink contaminated with human feces. Persons harboring an adult worm are also a potential danger to themselves in that eggs can be introduced from the anus to the mouth (external autoinfection) or possibly by regurgitation of gravid proglottids into the stomach during vomiting. Only 20 percent of patients with cysticercosis have a history of having an intestinal tapeworm, but patients with such a history are more likely to have many cysticerci.[39]

PATHOLOGY AND PATHOGENESIS

Embryos are liberated from eggs in the intestine, enter the bloodstream, and are carried to distant sites. Any tissue may be affected. The most common locations are the brain, subcutaneous tissue, muscle, and eye. Full maturation of the cyst takes 3 to 4 months; the size of the mature cyst varies from 2 to 4 mm to 2 cm in diameter. The thin-walled cyst is fluid filled and contains a nodular area that extends from the cyst's inner wall. This nodule contains the invaginated scolex and a spiral canal that opens to the exterior of the cyst. In tissue other than brain, the cysticercus is enveloped in a fibrous capsule, where it may survive for 3 to 6 years or longer. A healthy cyst, "the vesicular stage," provokes little host reaction. The parasite has complex methods of evading host defense mechanisms.[155] Imaging studies of brain cysts at this stage show spherical lesions that are isointense with cerebrospinal fluid (CSF) and show no enhancement with contrast. However, as the cyst begins to die, an inflammatory reaction with infiltration of eosinophils, lymphocytes, granulocytes, and plasma cells occurs. Imaging studies show "ring enhancement" around the cyst, often with edema. The cyst contents become gelatinous and the organism's tissues begin hyaline degeneration as the process evolves into the "colloid stage." The cyst collapses, and its contents become semisolid as granulation tissue replaces the parasite. Neuroimaging shows an area of focal enhancement resembling a granuloma—the "granular nodular stage." Calcification begins in the area of the scolex and progresses to involve the cyst wall—the final "calcific stage." Approximately 20 percent of cerebral cysts eventually calcify. Calcified lesions once were assumed to be inactive. However, recent neuroimaging studies have shown that calcified lesions often have enhancement indicative of a reaction that may contribute to continuing seizure activity.[104, 132] A patient with multiple cysts may have individual cysts in different stages of evolution. Radiographically detectable calcifications rarely occur in muscle until at least 4 years after invasion of the muscle. Eye cysts, often subretinal, may lead to blindness as a consequence of retinal detachment or inflammatory changes.

Neurocysticercosis involving the brain or spinal cord has the potential for causing the most serious complications. The clinical manifestations depend on the numbers and locations of cysts and the degree of host response. Cysticerci can be found in the ventricles (Fig. 225–1) or subarachnoid space (Fig. 225–2) or can be embedded in brain parenchyma (Fig. 225–3). In the parenchyma, the cysts tend to localize in the cortex or at the junction between cortical gray matter and subcortical white matter. The organism often develops as a large irregular cyst or as grapelike clusters in the ventricles, basal cisterns, sylvian fissure, and subarachnoid space. This form of the cysticercus, which lacks a scolex, is known as a "racemose cyst." Young intact cysts induce little

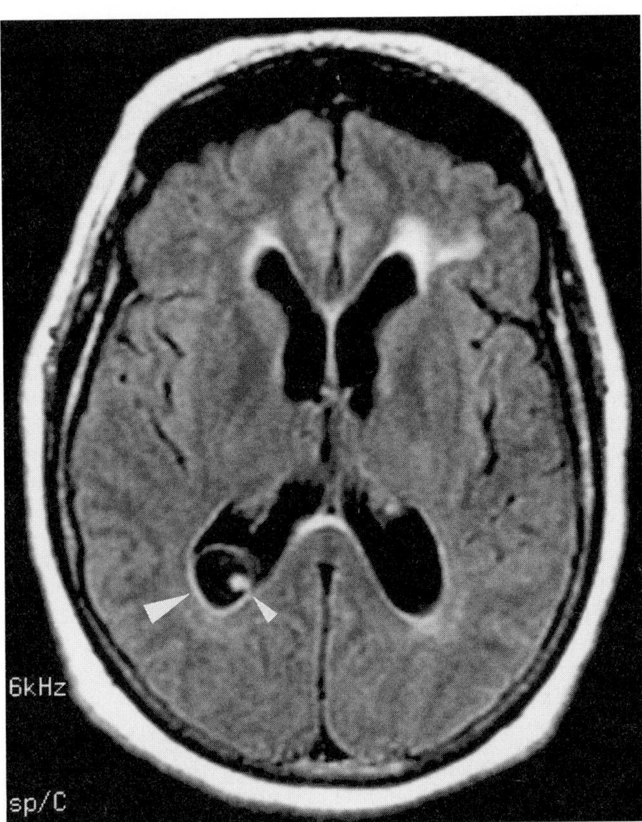

FIGURE 225–1 ■ Magnetic resonance image of an intraventricular cysticercus. The cyst wall is indicated by a *large arrow* and the scolex by a *small arrow*. (Courtesy of C. Mark Mehringer, M.D., Harbor-UCLA Medical Center.)

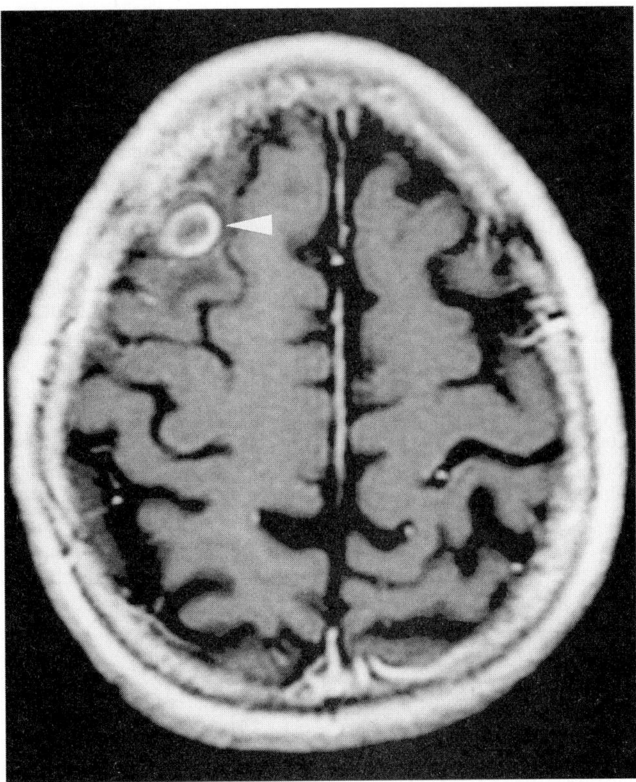

FIGURE 225–3 ■ Magnetic resonance image of an intraparenchymal cerebral ring-enhancing cysticercus. (Courtesy of C. Mark Mehringer, M.D., Harbor-UCLA Medical Center.)

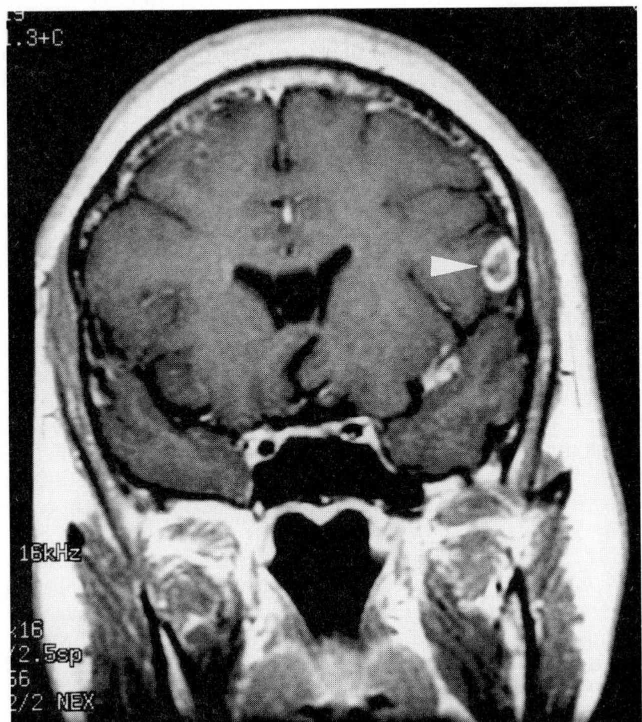

FIGURE 225–2 ■ Enhancing subarachnoid cysticercus. (Courtesy of C. Mark Mehringer, M.D., Harbor-UCLA Medical Center.)

reaction and rarely produce signs of nervous system disease unless present in large numbers or located in critical areas. The onset of symptoms usually coincides with development of the granulomatous reaction around dead or dying cysts. Parasitic membranes or inflammation induced by the parasite may interfere with the flow of spinal fluid and cause intracranial hypertension. Several reviews of neurocysticercosis are available.[19, 59, 98, 115, 134, 153, 154]

CLINICAL MANIFESTATIONS

Transient myalgia, fever, and eosinophilia may be present at the time of larval invasion, but this stage usually is unrecognized. Cysticerci that develop in subcutaneous tissue cause firm, mobile nodules that range in size from a few millimeters to several centimeters in diameter. The average size is 1 to 2 cm. These nodules are usually nontender and are found on the extremities and trunk more often than on the face. A review of the English language literature on subcutaneous cysticercosis has been published.[159]

Central nervous system (CNS) symptoms often appear 5 to 7 years after probable infection; latencies as short as 6 months and as long as 30 years have been documented.[39] In endemic areas such as Mexico, as many as one quarter of all suspected brain tumors prove to be cysticerci. Almost any combination of neurologic symptoms can be seen. Seizures are the most common symptom and occur separately or in combination with other manifestations. Generalized or focal motor seizures occur in most cases and may be the only symptom in as many as one third of cases. In a series of

238 patients with cysticercosis in California, 56 percent had seizures and 21 percent had increased intracranial pressure (ICP).[130] A condition referred to as cysticercotic encephalitis may develop when inflammation and edema around multiple intraparenchymal cysts cause cerebral swelling with papilledema, seizures, decreased visual acuity, and other signs of increased ICP. This condition also may simulate a psychotic illness with delirium or hallucinations. Although cysticercotic encephalitis occurs in less than 1 percent of patients with neurocysticercosis, it does so more commonly in children.[86] A recent study in Mexico has implicated this form of the disease in the genesis of behavioral disturbances that resemble attention-deficit disorder with hyperactivity and the subsequent development of learning disabilities.[122]

Psychiatric diagnoses of depression or psychosis have been described in a small series of patients with neurocysticercosis when given appropriate testing.[54] Cognitive impairment also was identified. Cysts at the base of the brain may cause signs and symptoms of intermittent or permanent hydrocephalus or acute or chronic meningitis. Subarachnoid cysts in this area have been implicated as a cause of vasculitis resulting in ischemic infarcts.[35] Subarachnoid cysts in the sylvian fissure or in a cerebral sulcus may develop into "giant" cysts 5 to 10 cm in diameter that compress the brain and produce symptoms of a space-occupying lesion. Intraventricular cysts may cause hydrocephalus through mechanical obstruction of CSF. If the cysts are floating free in the ventricles, the obstruction may be intermittent. As the cysts begin dying, the resulting inflammation often causes ependymitis and adherence of the degenerating cysts to the ventricular wall. Spinal cord involvement occurs in 1 to 5 percent of cases of neurocysticercosis. Symptoms usually are caused by extramedullary compression of the spinal cord or by arachnoiditis. Intramedullary cysts occur rarely. An uncommon form of cysticercosis that is limited largely to India is called disseminated cysticercosis. Massive involvement of muscle, subcutaneous tissue, and the brain occurs. The muscles enlarge (pseudohypertrophy), and multiple palpable subcutaneous nodules develop. Seizures and abnormal mental function are common findings.

Peripheral blood eosinophil and white blood cell counts are typically normal, as is the erythrocyte sedimentation rate. With meningeal involvement, the CSF is usually under increased pressure and shows pleocytosis. Typically, a moderate increase in protein is present. In approximately half the patients, spinal fluid glucose is low, and in some cases, it is very low (in the range of 5 mg/dL). The spinal fluid findings and clinical picture are readily confused with tuberculous or bacterial meningitis. Eosinophilia of the CSF may be helpful when present, but it is seen in less than half the cases of neurocysticercosis.

Skull radiographs showing spherical calcification of the 1- to 2-mm scolex, surrounded by a partially or totally calcified cyst 7 to 12 mm in diameter, are diagnostic. Computed tomography (CT) may be diagnostic when multiple cysts or typical calcifications are seen. Magnetic resonance imaging (MRI) is superior to CT for visualizing noncalcified cysts, especially in the diagnosis of ventricular and cisternal cysts and cysts near the base of the brain. Reviews of neuroimaging in cysticercosis should be consulted for detailed examples.[23, 110, 118, 126, 161]

DIAGNOSIS

Serologic tests are available, but results have been variable. An enzyme-linked immunoelectrotransfer blot assay using purified glycoprotein antigen was found to be 98 percent sensitive and 100 percent specific for human cysticercosis.[145] Unfortunately, this test often yields negative results in patients with a single intracerebral lesion, and 75 percent of children have single lesions.[137] The test is used on serum, and testing CSF offers no advantage.[137] Serum specimens for enzyme-linked immunoelectrotransfer blot assay are submitted to state public health department laboratories, which forward them to the Centers for Disease Control and Prevention (CDC), where the test is performed.

A defined set of criteria have been proposed to assist the clinician in the diagnosis of cysticercosis.[36] These criteria are based on information from imaging studies, clinical manifestations, serologic tests, and epidemiologic data. Various combinations of major criteria, minor criteria, and epidemiologic data are used to determine a definitive diagnosis, a probable diagnosis, or a possible diagnosis of cysticercosis. The authors consider this process to be valid for the diagnosis of all forms of human cysticercosis.

Subcutaneous cysticercosis usually is diagnosed by excisional biopsy. However, cytologic examination of fine-needle aspirates from a subcutaneous lesion is usually diagnostic.[8]

TREATMENT

No definitive agreement exists on the indications for drug treatment of neurocysticercosis. With the advent of the cysticidal drugs praziquantel and albendazole, great enthusiasm for treating neurocysticercosis, especially intraparenchymal cysts, has been generated. The reaction of the cysts and their reduction in size or number were measurable on imaging. Less well documented was improvement in clinical status. Because of the variability of the infection, performing controlled studies is not easy. Few of the many studies of drug therapy for neurocysticercosis meet the rigorous criteria for controlled trials. A carefully designed meta-analysis of the four available randomized, controlled trials of drug treatment of neurocysticercosis reported in November 1999 that there "is insufficient evidence to determine whether cysticidal therapy is of any clinical benefit to patients with neurocysticercosis."[127] The analysis was unable to exclude the possibility that more patients remain seizure-free when treated with cysticidal drugs, and the researchers recommended that additional placebo-controlled trials be performed. Reviews of neurocysticercosis specifically address the issue of treatment in children.[60, 97]

Praziquantel is an antiparasitic drug that is approved for use in the United States for schistosomiasis and certain liver fluke infections. It is active against cysticerci. Clinical trials have shown that treatment with praziquantel often causes lesions to disappear. It has been administered in a dose of 50 to 100 mg/kg of body weight daily divided into three equal doses for 30 days. Death of the parasites during administration of drug therapy causes an inflammatory response. Side effects occur in 80 percent or more of patients and may be more intense in those with greater numbers of cysts. Side effects include fever, headache, nausea, vomiting, seizures, and increased ICP. Cerebral infarction has been attributed to praziquantel treatment.[11, 158] The frequency and severity of side effects can be reduced with corticosteroids. However, the use of concomitant corticosteroids may lower the blood level of praziquantel by as much as 50 percent. Praziquantel levels also are reduced by concomitant use of phenytoin or carbamazepine. No firm evidence has established that the reduction in levels caused by these drugs interferes with the efficacy of treatment. Cimetidine has been found to increase praziquantel levels.

Albendazole, a benzimidazole compound, appears to be more effective than praziquantel in resolving intraparenchymal cysts. The standard course of albendazole has been 15 mg/kg of body weight per day (maximum, 800 mg) divided into two doses given for 8 to 30 days and repeated if necessary. Drug therapy is much less effective for ventricular and subarachnoid cysts. However, albendazole appears to be more active than praziquantel in these locations. Some authorities argue strongly that the use of drug therapy is contraindicated for ventricular or subarachnoid cysts.[50] They think that the arachnoiditis induced by death of the parasite has the potential to cause vasculitis with ischemia and infarcts, nerve entrapment, or hydrocephalus, even if corticosteroids are administered simultaneously. Ependymitis and obstruction of CSF flow often occur after the death of ventricular cysts. Side effects of albendazole treatment are similar in frequency and degree to those with praziquantel and probably result from the host reaction to death of the parasite. Administration of dexamethasone may increase plasma levels of albendazole. If drug treatment is to be used, corticosteroids usually are administered concomitantly to reduce the reaction to death of the parasites.[135]

Other investigators state that cysticidal drug treatment, if used at all, should be reserved for cystic parenchymal lesions that show no enhancement or surrounding edema on CT. Enhancement and edema signify that inflammation is occurring around a dying parasite and that spontaneous resolution or calcification can be expected. The rapid and spontaneous resolution of parenchymal cysts[99] and the improvement in symptoms[30] in the absence of cysticidal treatment in children indicate that a conservative approach seems appropriate for most of these infections. However, some physicians think that aggressive medical therapy is indicated to minimize residual calcification and, possibly, to reduce the persistence of seizures. One study of single enhancing lesions in children lends support to this approach.[12] If drug therapy is used, patients should be observed carefully for a prolonged period because of the occasional development or progression of hydrocephalus.

If cysts in the subarachnoid space of the brain or spinal cord or in ventricles have not undergone degeneration, they may be removed surgically. The use of fiberoptic endoscopes for neurosurgical procedures has enhanced the ability to extract the parasites before they cause inflammatory complications.[89] The general agreement is that administration of corticosteroids may be very beneficial in patients with active inflammatory processes. It is especially useful in cysticercotic encephalitis and subarachnoid cysticercosis with signs of meningitis. Long-term intermittent steroid therapy has been proposed for the management of chronic or relapsing arachnoiditis.[135] Surgical placement of ventricular shunts may be a lifesaving procedure in patients with progressive intracranial hypertension. If medical therapy is planned in those with increased ICP, placement of a shunt must precede initiation of drug treatment. Maintenance of shunts in patients with cysticercotic hydrocephalus is problematic because of inflammatory cells and debris compromising function of the shunt. The frequent need for revision of shunts causes an increase in morbidity and mortality. A recent study suggests that chronic steroid administration will reduce the likelihood of shunt obstruction.[121]

The surgical management of intraocular cysticercosis has been reviewed.[105]

Patients with cysticercosis always should be investigated for infection with the adult *T. solium*. In some circumstances, examination of family members or close contacts for *T. solium* infection is warranted. Fecal examination and perianal swabs suffer from poor patient compliance and low yield. The commercial availability of sensitive and specific coproantigen tests or serologic tests that identify tapeworm carriers would greatly enhance this screening process.

PROGNOSIS

The prognosis of neurocysticercosis varies greatly. Less than 10 percent of patients with cerebral lesions die, usually within the first 5 to 10 years of illness. Many more are incapacitated with seizures or deterioration in higher cerebral function. The clinical course often is characterized by spontaneous partial or complete remissions followed by one or more exacerbations. Usually, seizures occur less frequently over time, and the patient may improve gradually after several years. One series of 52 children with parenchymal cysts showed complete resolution of the lesions or residual punctate calcification within 2 to 9 months of observation. Sixty percent of the children were weaned successfully from anticonvulsants with no recurrence of seizures.[99]

PREVENTION

Successful attempts to decrease the prevalence of infection with *T. solium* in endemic areas by mass treatment[129] and by health education have been reported.[128] However, until the major problem of free-roaming pigs that have access to human feces is solved, the reduction in prevalence will be short lived. Until adequate sanitation and good pig husbandry practices can be introduced on a permanent basis, infection will be problematic. Adequate cooking of pork prevents infection with adult tapeworms, and protection of food and drink from contamination with human feces should prevent cysticercosis.

Taenia crassiceps Cysticercosis

T. crassiceps adult tapeworms are found in foxes, other canids, and cats in Europe, North America, and eastern and northern Asia. The larval stage, a cysticercus, has been detected in a variety of rodents, including field mice, where it develops in the peritoneal and pleural cavities and soft tissues. The cysticerci that develop in intermediate hosts after the ingestion of tapeworm eggs from the feces of the definitive hosts have the ability to continue to reproduce asexually by external budding and, less frequently, by internal budding. Cysticercosis with *T. crassiceps* rarely has been reported to occur in dogs or other non-rodent mammals. Three cases of human intraocular cysticercosis have been reported,[7, 25, 131] as have three cases of soft tissue cysticercosis in patients with acquired immunodeficiency syndrome (AIDS) in western Europe.[56, 82, 93] The ocular infections have been treated successfully by surgical techniques. The sites of involvement in patients with AIDS were (1) the paravertebral area, (2) the arm and pectoral area, and (3) the arm and forearm. The lesions appear as tumor-like masses. Incision or spontaneous rupture of the mass reveals a "tapioca-like" material containing granules and small vesicles representing the cysticerci. Treatment with praziquantel and albendazole appears to be suppressive but not curative.[93]

Diphyllobothriasis (Infection with *Diphyllobothrium latum* and Related Species, Fish Tapeworm Infection)

Diphyllobothriasis occurs in humans in areas where raw, pickled, or lightly smoked fresh-water fish are eaten frequently. The prevalence of infection increases with age in endemic areas. Nonspecific gastrointestinal complaints may occur. Megaloblastic anemia is a common finding in infected persons from certain geographic areas.

D. latum first was described in 1592 from specimens found in Switzerland. The life cycle was not known completely until the development of larval stages in copepods was demonstrated in 1917.

Several species of *Diphyllobothrium* have been reported in humans. A review of the taxonomy of the genus has led to the designation of *D. latum* of humans as a prototype for a complex of *latum*-like worms of the genus *Diphyllobothrium.*[149] Several of these species are primarily parasites of fish-eating birds, marine mammals, bears, dogs, and foxes. Humans who coexist in endemic areas may be infected incidentally.[31]

Dibothriocephalus latus is a synonym of *D. latum* that some authors prefer.

THE ORGANISM

The scolex of *D. latum* possesses two deep grooves rather than discrete suckers. The entire worm may be as long as 15 m. The gravid proglottids have a characteristic rosette-shaped central uterus. Eggs measure 55 to 61 μm by 37 to 56 μm and have light brown, operculated shells. The eggs are shed in an unembryonated state from a uterine pore into the fecal stream. The development of six-hooked embryos within the eggs takes place in fresh water. The ciliated embryos hatch from the eggs and must be ingested by copepods to develop further. The larval stages found in copepods then develop into more advanced stages in the muscles of fish that feed on the infected crustaceans. As the smaller fish are eaten by larger species, the larvae parasitize the muscles of the new host. Eventually, the larvae are found in fish that are sources of food for humans, such as species of pike, perch, turbot, lake trout, and whitefish. The forms found in fish are called plerocercoid larvae or spargana. They are whitish, ribbon-like worms approximately 5 cm in length.

TRANSMISSION

Plerocercoid larvae are infectious for humans when ingested in fish, fish liver, or roe that have not been treated adequately by heat, freezing, or chemical agents.

The cycle of infection is perpetuated by the discharge of untreated sewage into fresh-water lakes and streams.

Some fish-eating mammals also may serve as definitive hosts for *D. latum* and maintain the cycle of infection in the absence of humans. Because *D. latum* requires intermediate hosts, direct transmission is impossible, and no techniques of isolation or special precautions are required for infected patients.

EPIDEMIOLOGY

The prevalence of infection increases with age in endemic areas. However, infections have been reported in children younger than 1 year.[150] The disease is worldwide in distribution, but areas of endemicity are associated with cultures in which people traditionally eat roe or fresh-water fish raw, lightly salted, or pickled without cooking. Infection occurs frequently in the Baltic countries and the adjacent areas of the former Soviet Union; South America; Scandinavia; Switzerland and the adjacent lake regions of Italy, France, and Germany; the Danube River delta; the lake areas of the northern United States; Canada; and the river deltas of Alaska. A case of human infection in Cuba has been reported.[15] Prevalence rates in Finland have fallen from 70 percent to less than 2 percent. In one study in northern Canada, 83 percent of Eskimos older than 2 years were infected with *D. latum.*[6]

Salmonid fish (salmon, trout, whitefish) transmit *Diphyllobothrium nihonkaiense* to humans in Japan and *Diphyllobothrium dendriticum* to persons in South America, the circumpolar north, and other parts of the world. Pacific salmon are sources of infection with *Diphyllobothrium klebanovskii* in the far eastern part of the former Soviet Union and *Diphyllobothrium ursi* in northern Canada and Alaska. Infection of humans with a tapeworm parasite of seals, *Diphyllobothrium pacificum,* has been reported from Peru. Raw marine fish prepared with lemon juice (ceviche) is the usual source.[91]

In 1980, a small outbreak of diphyllobothriasis in southern California was associated with eating fresh Alaskan salmon. Several cases were linked to the raw fish dish sushi.[123] Megaloblastic anemia in *D. latum* infection rarely occurs outside Finland and the former Soviet Union, where it may develop in 2 percent of tapeworm carriers.[106]

PATHOLOGY AND PATHOGENESIS

Little is known about the direct effects of parasitization, with the exception of megaloblastic anemia.[4, 111] The following factors may be significant: (1) the strains of *D. latum* found in Finland, where anemia occurs, absorb seven times more vitamin B_{12} than do strains from North America, where anemia has not been reported; (2) interference with vitamin B_{12} absorption occurs in nonanemic carriers, as well as in those with anemia, and deficient stores of vitamin B_{12} plus B_{12} malabsorption may contribute to the anemic state; (3) dietary intake of vitamin B_{12} may be low in anemic patients, and oral B_{12} has been shown to cause reticulocytosis in the presence of the worm; (4) worms found in anemic patients take up more of an oral dose of vitamin B_{12} than do worms in asymptomatic carriers, and worms are attached more proximally in the small intestine in anemic patients; and (5) secretion of intrinsic factor is reduced in anemic patients.

CLINICAL MANIFESTATIONS

Most infections are asymptomatic, but patients may notice proglottids or chains of segments in their stool. In Finland, comparison of nonanemic infected patients with uninfected controls revealed an increase in the symptoms of fatigue, weakness, craving for salt, lack of well-being, dizziness, and numbness of the extremities in the infected group.[124]

Significant gastrointestinal symptoms occur infrequently. However, an experimental infection with seven larvae produced nausea, severe periumbilical pain, and marked weight loss.[139] Episodes of intestinal obstruction associated with the vomiting of masses of tapeworms have been reported.[150] Eosinophilia is uncommon.

Patients with *D. pacificum* complained of abdominal pain, vomiting, diarrhea, and flatulence.[91]

Megaloblastic anemia caused by *D. latum* infection is extremely rare outside Finland and neighboring endemic areas. Usually, it is seen in patients older than 50 years, but it has been reported in children as young as 9 years. The symptoms are identical to those seen in pernicious anemia, and neurologic involvement is not an uncommon finding.

DIAGNOSIS

Identification of the characteristic eggs or proglottids provides the diagnosis. The parasite produces nearly 1 million eggs per day, and ova usually are detected easily by fecal examination.

TREATMENT AND PREVENTION

Treatment with the regimen of praziquantel noted for *T. saginata* is highly effective. Tapeworm anemia is reversible by treating the infection, but it should be supplemented initially with vitamin B_{12}.

A significant reduction in the transmission of *D. latum* has been accomplished in many areas through the introduction of sewage treatment and targeted drug treatment of human infections. Preventing infection by other species of *Diphyllobothrium* that have sylvatic definitive hosts will be more difficult. Treating fish products by freezing or adequate cooking prevents infection.

Sparganosis (*Spirometra* Species Infection)

In 1854, the term *sparganum* was applied originally to the second-stage larvae of diphyllobothriid tapeworms whose adult forms were unknown. Human infection with these larvae is called sparganosis.

THE ORGANISM

Evidence indicates that the amorphous, thin, ribbon-like spargana recovered from human infections belong to the genus *Spirometra.* The adult tapeworms are found in dogs, cats, raccoons, and a variety of wild carnivores. Eggs passed in the feces of these definitive hosts hatch in fresh water. The embryo that emerges from the egg is ingested by a copepod, a common fresh-water crustacean, where it undergoes larval development. When a second intermediate host ingests the infected copepod, the larva develops into a sparganum (plerocercoid). The range of second intermediate hosts is extensive and includes amphibians, reptiles, birds, and mammals. Rodents, foxes, humans, and other primates also have been infected with spargana. When the second intermediate host is eaten by the definitive host, the sparganum attaches to the intestinal mucosa and develops into the adult tapeworm.

Little is known about the species of diphyllobothriid larvae found in humans. Because no distinguishing morphologic features of spargana exist, they must be fed to definitive hosts such as dogs and cats, and the adult worms must be recovered for study. This procedure is rarely possible, so the designation of species found in humans is based largely on epidemiologic relationships to species described in local animals. The species found in Africa, Asia, Europe, and South America usually is called *Spirometra mansoni* or *Spirometra erinacei,* and the species infecting humans in the United States is called *Spirometra mansonoides.*

A rare form of sparganosis that buds, branches, and multiplies asexually to massive numbers in humans is called sparganum proliferum. It may be an aberrant or mutant form, or it may be the result of viral infection of a sparganum.[17] Adult forms of sparganum proliferum are unknown.

TRANSMISSION

In parts of Asia, applying poultices of amphibian or reptile flesh to wounds or sores is a common practice and an apparent source for contact sparganosis when the spargana migrate from the poultice into human tissues. It probably is the most frequent cause of ocular sparganosis. Monkeys easily are infected experimentally by feeding them copepods containing the first larval stages. Human sparganosis in the United States often is associated with drinking well water or untreated surface water that could contain the minute copepods. Transmission by ingestion of the raw or inadequately cooked flesh of second intermediate hosts has been proved experimentally in humans.[160] Animal sources that have been incriminated in human infection are snakes, frogs, chickens, and pigs. Larval stages from crushed copepods can penetrate unbroken skin. Even though human infection has been induced in this manner, it seems an unlikely natural mode of transmission.

EPIDEMIOLOGY

Human infection is uncommon. In the United States, almost all reports have come from the southern or southeastern states and from Puerto Rico or were reported in persons who had been in these areas. The only report of infection in a child in the United States came from southern California.[27] Recent reports of sparganosis in feral hogs in Texas and in Florida indicate a significant reservoir in wild animals.[67] Reports of human infection have come from China, Korea, Southeast Asia, Japan, India, Indonesia, the Philippines, Australia, Africa, Italy, South America, and the former Soviet Union.

The extremely rare sparganum proliferum infections have been reported in Japan, the United States, and South America.

PATHOLOGY, PATHOGENESIS, AND CLINICAL MANIFESTATIONS

The larva penetrates tissue either on contact, as in poultice application, or through the intestinal mucosa. Ocular sparganosis, usually acquired by contact, may involve conjunctival, retro-orbital, or palpebral tissues and cause conjunctivitis, periorbital and palpebral edema, exophthalmos, chemosis, and corneal ulceration. Subcutaneous sparganosis is the most common form of the infection, with the trunk frequently involved. The lesion is usually nodular. Tenderness and inflammation may be absent, intermittent, or constant. Some lesions are migratory. The lesions have variable inflammatory responses.[146] Eosinophils may or may not be present. Some infections have had an associated peripheral eosinophilia, but it is not a constant finding. Other less common sites for spargana are the extremities, head, muscles, spermatic cord, jejunum, colon, urethra, bladder, and pulmonary artery. Sparganosis of the CNS usually causes seizures but may be associated with a variety of neurologic manifestations.[22, 75, 80, 83]

The disease caused by sparganum proliferum consists of progressive replacement of host tissues by the multiplying organisms. The patient may survive many years until the parasites impair the function of a vital organ. The initial evidence of proliferative sparganosis is often expression of a sparganum from a skin lesion. Eleven cases reported from the world literature were reviewed in 1990.[103]

DIAGNOSIS

The diagnosis may be suspected in persons with typical subcutaneous lesions and a suggestive epidemiologic background. Usually, however, the diagnosis is made during surgical removal of a painful or cosmetically disturbing lump without anticipating the parasitic etiology. Spargana vary considerably in width and length. They are usually several centimeters in length, whitish, and opaque, and they may have the grooved indentations on the anterior end that are precursors of the bothria or suckers of the scolex of the adult worm. A cross section of the parasite reveals the calcareous corpuscles seen in cestodes. Small portions of spargana are difficult to distinguish grossly or microscopically from cysticerci and other less common larval cestodes. Neuroimaging may yield characteristic findings in cerebral sparganosis.[22, 75] Obtaining an ELISA for serum and CSF antibody appears useful in endemic areas, but this test is not generally available. A sparganum-specific protein also has been used in an ELISA for the diagnosis of other forms of sparganosis.[107]

TREATMENT

Surgical removal is the only known form of therapy. Mebendazole and praziquantel have been tried in one case of proliferative sparganosis.[102] Although the patient improved while taking mebendazole, motile parasites were still present and new lesions were developing. Severe reactions to praziquantel caused cessation of treatment.

PREVENTION

Filtration of water prevents the ingestion of copepods from wells or ponds. Proper cooking of meat eliminates second intermediate hosts as sources of infection. Educational effort should be made to warn of the dangers of applying raw flesh poultices in areas where it is a cultural practice.

Dipylidiasis (*Dipylidium caninum* Infection, Dog Tapeworm Infection)

D. caninum, the common tapeworm of dogs and cats, also infects infants and young children. Transmission occurs through the accidental ingestion of infected fleas. Variable gastrointestinal symptoms may develop, or patients may be asymptomatic.

D. caninum was described first by Linnaeus in 1758, but it had been observed in an infected human by a student of Linnaeus in 1751. The life cycle was described fully in 1916.

THE ORGANISM

D. caninum adult worms have a scolex with four cup-shaped suckers and a central protrusible structure, the rostellum, that bears one to seven rows of small hooks. The worm ranges from 10 to 70 cm in length. The gravid proglottids resemble cucumber seeds in size and shape. The proglottids have two pairs of sex organs, and a genital pore opens on each lateral margin. The eggs measure 35 to 65 μm in diameter and appear in packets of 5 to 30 enclosed in a membrane. The gravid proglottids are excreted in feces or migrate actively from the anus. The eggs are liberated as the proglottid disintegrates. Several species of flea serve as intermediate hosts. The larval flea ingests the egg of *D. caninum*. Development of the tapeworm's larval stages takes place as the flea metamorphoses into an adult. When the flea is ingested by the definitive host, the adult worm develops in the small intestine.

TRANSMISSION

Humans acquire the infection by the accidental ingestion of infected fleas. Dogs may transfer infective larvae to humans by licking after nipping at fleas. Because of the motility of the proglottids, eggs may be disseminated widely in the environment of animal hosts. Fleas are so ubiquitous that transmission to the intermediate host is accomplished readily.

EPIDEMIOLOGY

Infection of dogs and cats occurs throughout the world. *D. caninum* also has been found in foxes, jackals, hyenas, dingoes, and a variety of wild felids. In view of the close relationship between children and their pets, the opportunity for infection appears to be great. Reports of dipylidiasis in humans in the United States, however, are uncommon.[70] It is generally agreed that human infections are far more frequent than reports indicate.

CLINICAL MANIFESTATIONS

Although the incubation period in humans is unknown, infection has been seen in infants 5 weeks of age.

Frequently, the only evidence of infection is the finding of proglottids in stool or in an infant's diapers. Varying degrees of abdominal pain, diarrhea, irritability, and pruritus have been recorded in symptomatic children.

DIAGNOSIS, PROGNOSIS, AND TREATMENT

The characteristic proglottids must be differentiated from other parasites. A frequent error is to assume, from the parents' description, that the small, motile proglottids that migrate from the anus are pinworms. Proglottids also may be mistaken for fly larvae.

Examination of stool specimens may be spuriously negative because proglottids tend to migrate from the fecal mass and disintegrate on the walls of the specimen container.

The infection has not been associated with serious symptoms, and response to treatment with praziquantel as used in *T. saginata* infection is excellent.

PREVENTION

Infected dogs and cats should be treated. Flea control requires the use of appropriate insecticides on pets. In addition, particular attention must be given to carpets and areas where pets sleep because these are the sites of development of the larval fleas. Aerosol insecticides specifically made for flea control are useful for large areas. In addition, oral medication may be used in pets to suppress flea development in the environment.

Hymenolepiasis (*Hymenolepis nana* Infection, Dwarf Tapeworm Infection)

Infection with *H. nana*, the dwarf tapeworm, occurs throughout the world and probably is maintained by direct fecal-oral transmission from person to person, although insects may serve as intermediate hosts. Infection may be asymptomatic, but gastrointestinal, neurologic, and allergic symptoms have been reported. Treatment with praziquantel is successful.

THE ORGANISM

H. nana first was reported from rodents in 1845. A human case was discovered at autopsy in 1851. In 1892, the development of adult worms from the ingestion of eggs was proved experimentally. Not until 1928 were insects shown to be effective intermediate hosts for the parasite.

Controversy exists about the identity of *H. nana* found in humans and morphologically identical organisms found in rodents. The rodent strains often are called *Hymenolepsis fraterna* or *H. nana* variety *fraterna.*

Adult worms of *H. nana* measure only 5 to 45 mm in length and are less than 1 mm in maximal width. The tiny scolex has four cup-shaped suckers and a protrusible rostellum with a circle of 20 to 30 small hooks. Gravid proglottids disintegrate within the intestine, and eggs are found in the feces. The eggs measure 30 to 50 μm in diameter and contain a six-hooked embryo within two envelopes. The space between the two envelopes contains filaments that extend from two small polar protrusions on the inner envelope. Larval stages develop in insect intermediate hosts after ingestion of the eggs. However, if the definitive host ingests eggs, larval stages develop in the intestinal villi in 4 to 5 days and then break into the lumen and develop into adult worms. Ova appear in feces 2 to 4 weeks after infection.

TRANSMISSION

Human infection is acquired most commonly by the ingestion of eggs from the feces of infected persons. Humans serve as both intermediate and definitive hosts in this direct cycle. Poor hygienic habits, overcrowding, lack of running water, and any other factor that fosters fecal-oral transmission enhance transmission via this route.

The rodent strains of *H. nana* are infectious for humans, and food contaminated by rodent feces is a possible source of infection. Pet rodents, such as rats, mice, and hamsters, often are infected, and close contact, as in playful fondling, could result in transmission by contaminated hands.

Ingestion of insect intermediate hosts accidentally or in infested food also may cause infection. This mode of infection may occur commonly in rodents but probably does so infrequently in people.

Adequate information on the duration of infection in humans is lacking. Eggs may be produced for periods longer than 1 year, but the possibility of recurrent autoinfection obscures determination of the duration of the initial infection.

Internal autoinfection may occur when ova from gravid proglottids are exposed to appropriate conditions within the intestinal lumen. Hatching occurs, and the embryos penetrate the mucosa, undergo larval development, and eventually emerge as adult worms.

Although little information exists concerning immunity to *H. nana* infection in humans, rodent experiments indicate that the larval stages occurring in the intestinal villi stimulate an immune response that is probably predominantly T cell–dependent.[90] Serum from infected animals also has been shown to protect uninfected mice from challenge infection.[38] Antibody has been demonstrated in infected humans.[63]

EPIDEMIOLOGY

H. nana is a common parasite of rats and mice throughout the world. The prevalence of infection in commercially supplied hamsters has been reported to be 44 percent.[138] Monkeys and chimpanzees rarely are infected. Flour beetles, mealworms, fleas, and cockroaches may serve as intermediate hosts.

The distribution of infection in humans is worldwide, with an increased prevalence in some urban areas.[53] Surveys have shown certain areas to have a high level of endemicity: rates of 46 percent have been reported in Sicily, 34 percent of schoolchildren in Algeria were infected, and the former southern Soviet Union had rates of 26 percent. Children between the ages of 4 and 10 years have the highest prevalence rates, and infections tend to affect several members of a family. The prevalence is also high in institutionalized children.

PATHOLOGY AND PATHOGENESIS

Little is known of the pathogenesis and pathology of *H. nana* infection in humans. Local reactions consisting of mucosal inflammation or atrophy may occur at the site of attachment of the adult worms in the small intestine.

The larval stage of *H. nana* is a cyst-like structure called a cysticercoid that is approximately 250 μm in diameter. In mice deprived of T cells, these larval stages may develop in an aberrant manner and produce multiple fluid-filled cysts several millimeters in diameter. These cysts spread from the intestinal villi to the lymphatics, liver, and lungs.[90] In a patient with Hodgkin disease who underwent radiation therapy and received immunosuppressive drugs, a disseminated larval cestode infection developed that was thought to be caused by sparganum proliferum. It now is thought that this case represented aberrant *H. nana* larvae.[90] A 13-year-old Egyptian girl with filariasis and a history of taking corticosteroids had dissemination of larval stages that were seen in a venous blood sample.[133]

CLINICAL MANIFESTATIONS

A wide variety of symptoms have been ascribed to *H. nana* infection, but well-controlled clinical studies are lacking. In a series of 43 patients with *H. nana* infection reported from South America, the following symptoms were noted in order of decreasing frequency: restlessness, irritability, diarrhea, abdominal pain, restless sleep, and anal and nasal pruritus.[41] Eosinophilia above 5 percent was noted in one third of these patients. In contrast, neither diarrhea nor eosinophilia was correlated with the presence of *H. nana* infection in an extensive epidemiologic study in western Pakistan.[18]

Symptoms reported from various series of infected cases include anorexia or an increase in appetite, nausea, vomiting, pains in the extremities, dizziness, and headache.

A study of 10 children in Thailand showed that worm burdens of 3000 or more were associated with abdominal pain, diarrhea or loose stools, malnutrition, growth retardation, and lethargy. Children with fewer than 100 worms appeared normal but occasionally had soft stools.[24]

One peculiar case of ectopic localization of *H. nana* was reported from Japan. An adult worm containing eggs was found in a mass on the chest wall of an elderly woman.[100]

Nervous system involvement with the production of seizures has received much attention in the former Soviet Union. It is thought to result from *H. nana* infection and occurs most frequently in children between the ages of 7 and 15 years.[65]

General experience suggests that patients either lack symptoms or have nonspecific gastrointestinal complaints.

DIAGNOSIS

Detecting the characteristic eggs in fecal material by examining direct saline wet mounts or by concentration techniques is not usually difficult. However, a single examination is not always adequate to rule out infection.

TREATMENT

Praziquantel is effective in treating *H. nana* infection in a single dose of 25 mg/kg. When praziquantel is used for *H. nana* infection in the United States, it is considered investigational.

A series of fecal examinations 3 to 4 weeks after the completion of treatment is necessary to assess the effectiveness of therapy. Family members should be examined and treated if infected.

PROGNOSIS

H. nana infection is not serious and responds well to appropriate treatment. Metastatic larval forms of *H. nana* are rare.[13, 90] The susceptibility of patients with impaired T-cell function, such as those with AIDS, has not been determined.

PREVENTION

Transmission of *H. nana* infection largely could be eliminated if proper methods of personal hygiene and disposal of human waste could be invoked throughout the world.

Infected food handlers always should be treated and monitored to ensure that treatment has been successful. Stored food should be protected from rodents and insects.

Echinococcosis (*Echinococcus* Species Infection, Hydatid Disease)

Humans may be infected with the larval stages of four species of *Echinococcus*. The larvae most frequently develop in the liver but may develop in many different tissues. Humans acquire the infection by the ingestion of ova from the feces of carnivorous definitive hosts. The disease in humans and intermediate hosts often is called hydatid disease. It also may be designated according to the morphology of the larval stages: cystic echinococcosis caused by *Echinococcus granulosus,* alveolar echinococcosis caused by *Echinococcus multilocularis,* and polycystic echinococcosis caused by *Echinococcus vogeli* or *Echinococcus oligarthrus.*

Excellent reviews of echinococcosis are available.[3, 14, 32, 87, 141]

THE ORGANISM

The life cycles of the species of *Echinococcus* are similar, but the geographic distribution, types of hosts, and morphology of the parasites differ significantly. *E. granulosus* is the most common species found in human infections. Considerable genetic variability exists within this species and has clinical and epidemiologic implications.[44] The taxonomic issues have been detailed.[142] Several strains of *E. granulosus* have been identified and categorized by the primary intermediate host. Significantly different strains are found in sheep, cattle, pigs, horses, camels, and cervids (deer, reindeer, moose, elk). Although much more information is needed, the pig, horse, and camel strains appear to have low infectivity for humans. Adult tapeworms of the sheep strain are found in dogs. The cervid strain primarily involves wolves, but dogs also may be infected. The adult tapeworm is only 3 to 8 mm long and has two to five segments. Dogs are often hosts to thousands of adult worms. When sheep or humans ingest eggs from the feces of infected dogs, the embryos hatch in the intestine and burrow through the intestinal wall to gain access to the portal circulation. Many embryos are destroyed, but those that survive are able to develop in many tissues, but most commonly the liver or lungs, where they become the cystic larval structures called hydatid cysts. A hydatid cyst is composed of an outer laminated, acellular membrane that is lined by a thin, cellular germinal membrane. Spherical structures called brood capsules grow from the germinal membrane. Protoscoleces develop within the brood capsules. Each protoscolex has suckers and hooks and the potential to become the scolex of an adult worm if eaten by a dog. Compression and reaction from growth of the cyst produce a "pericyst" of compact, collagen-rich host tissue around its exterior. In older cysts, so-called daughter cysts may develop within the primary cyst cavity.

E. multilocularis typically involves foxes as definitive hosts and rodents as intermediate hosts. The larval parasite does not form a large cystic structure but grows by progressive external budding. The laminated membrane and host pericyst are thin. The larval mass slowly enlarges and replaces liver tissue much as a malignancy does. The larvae may invade contiguous structures and rarely metastasize.

E. vogeli is a parasite of bush dogs and feral dogs in South America. The intermediate hosts are rodents (pacas, agoutis, spiny rats). When humans are infected, the germinal membrane grows externally to form additional cysts, and septa develop within the original cyst. This manifestation is the "polycystic" variety of hydatid disease. A rare cause of polycystic hydatid disease in humans has been attributed to *E. oligarthrus,* a fourth species that is found as adult tapeworms in wild felids such as pumas and jaguars. The intermediate hosts are the same as those for *E. vogeli.* Most infections occur in Central and South America.

TRANSMISSION

Humans acquire cystic hydatid disease by the ingestion of food or drink contaminated with feces from infected definitive hosts, usually dogs. Close contact with dogs can result in infection because tapeworm eggs can be found on the dog's perianal hair, muzzle, and paws. Flies and other insects may disseminate the eggs from dogs' feces. In Lebanon, the high prevalence rate of infection in shoemakers was linked to the practice of tanning leather with a mixture of water and dog feces.

Alveolar hydatid disease is acquired most often by exposure to foxes, although dogs, cats, and coyotes have been infected. Fur traders and hunters may be exposed by skinning foxes or by handling the fur. Sled dogs have been implicated as sources of infection in Arctic villages.

Polycystic hydatid disease caused by *E. vogeli* rarely occurs. Transmission is thought to occur from infected hunting dogs.[33]

EPIDEMIOLOGY

The sheep strain of *E. granulosus* is found worldwide in most areas where sheep are raised. The custom of feeding sheep viscera to sheep dogs maintains foci of infection. In the United States, Basques in central California, Mormon ranchers in Utah, and Native Americans in Arizona and New Mexico have been infected. The disease is endemic in the sheep-raising areas of South America, Australia, the Mediterranean basin, China, and the former Soviet Union. One of the highest morbidity rates is seen in rural Africans in Kenya and Uganda, where people live in close association with their dogs. The cervid strain of *E. granulosus* is found in northern parts of the Western Hemisphere. In Alaska and Canada, human infection usually is limited to Eskimos and Native Americans who have working dogs that are fed moose and reindeer viscera. The strain found in this region often is manifested as giant pulmonary cysts. The course of infection is usually benign.[52, 84] The cervid strain of *E. granulosus* also can be found in northern Scandinavia and the former Soviet Union, but human infection is uncommon. Recent reviews of the epidemiology of cystic echinococcosis in China,[21, 152] Latin America,[5] Europe,[42] and North Africa and the Middle East[34] are available.

Alveolar hydatid disease is found only in the Northern Hemisphere, where it is common in a cycle involving foxes and rodents. Infection in animals extends into the northern portion of many Midwestern states in the United States. The first human case of alveolar hydatid disease in the contiguous United States was diagnosed in Minnesota in 1977. The disease is endemic in large areas of the former Soviet Union, and human cases have been reported from China, northern Japan, Switzerland, and adjacent European countries. The geographic distribution of alveolar echinococcosis in foxes in Europe appears to be expanding and could become an increased risk to humans in this area.[42, 43]

The global epidemiology of cystic and alveolar echinococcosis has been reviewed in detail.[28]

Polycystic hydatid disease is limited to South and Central America, where fewer than 100 human infections have been reported.[32, 108]

PATHOLOGY AND PATHOGENESIS

In cystic hydatid disease, the pathology is related to compression or displacement of host tissue. Cyst growth is quite variable but probably averages about 1 cm in diameter per year. Rates of up to 4 to 5 cm/yr have been reported. The cyst may exceed 35 cm in diameter in the abdominal cavity. When rupture or leakage of a cyst occurs, an allergic reaction caused by the antigenic cyst contents may develop. Cysts may calcify after many years, which usually signifies death of the parasite. Hydatid cysts may form foci for secondary bacterial infection.

In alveolar hydatid disease, slow replacement of liver tissue by the parasite occurs and may continue for many years. The central area becomes a necrotic, pus-containing cavity. The margins of the lesion are indefinite. Microscopic examination shows multiple vesicles of different size advancing into normal hepatic tissue. The vesicles rarely contain protoscoleces. Metastatic lesions to the brain, lungs, and mediastinum occur in 2 percent of infections, and invasion of organs contiguous to the liver occurs in 15 percent.

Polycystic hydatid disease is characterized by multiple vesicles and cysts that measure from a few millimeters to several centimeters in diameter. Protoscoleces are usually abundant within blood capsules.

The complexity of the host-parasite interaction has been reviewed.[40]

CLINICAL MANIFESTATIONS

Most patients with *E. granulosus* infection have a single unilocular cyst, but multiple cysts are seen in 15 to 30 percent of patients, usually in a single organ system. Approximately one in five children with a pulmonary cyst also has a concurrent liver cyst. In adults and children, 10 percent of cysts are found in some site other than the liver or lung. The cervid strain of *E. granulosus* found in Canada and Alaska characteristically produces pulmonary cysts. Hydatid cysts have been reported in all organs, most notably the eye, brain, spleen, heart, endocrine glands, bone, and genitourinary tract. CNS hydatid disease occurs much more commonly in children than in adults.[20] Bone cysts, which may be seen in preschool children, occur most frequently in vertebral and long bones. Unlike cysts in other sites, bone cysts are characteristically multilocular and contain little fluid. Eye, bone, and brain cysts are typically small when discovered, whereas cysts in other sites may exceed 35 cm in diameter before being detected. Cysts grow approximately 1 to 3 cm in diameter each year. Serious morbidity is a consequence of enlargement, secondary infection, or cyst rupture. Some children with hydatid disease also have retarded growth patterns.[96] Infection of hydatid cysts and leakage or rupture with hypotension, urticaria, and eosinophilia are relatively uncommon complications of hydatid disease.

Symptoms are caused most often by the pressure produced by an expanding cyst; its location determines the clinical findings. Fever, cough, chest pain, and hemoptysis are common symptoms of patients with pulmonary cysts. As many as one third of pulmonary cysts rupture into the pleural space or into a bronchus. In the latter case, the patient may describe "coughing up grape skins." Symptomatic intrahepatic cysts cause constant or intermittent right upper quadrant pain or jaundice. In 5 to 15 percent of adults with hepatic hydatid cysts, the cyst ruptures into the biliary tract and simulates choledocholithiasis and ascending cholangitis with fever, pain, and jaundice; this complication occurs rarely during childhood.[77] Bone cysts are seen in patients with bone pain or pathologic fracture. Vertebral hydatid disease causes signs and symptoms of spinal cord and radicular compression; severe pain on palpation of the affected portion of the spine is characteristic. Fifty to 75 percent of intracranial cysts are seen in children.[48] Increased ICP with headache and vomiting is a common finding. Seizures also can occur. An extensive list of the symptoms and complications of cystic echinococcosis has been compiled.[3]

Symptoms of alveolar hydatid disease most often occur in older adults but have been reported in children as young as 5 years. The most common finding is hepatomegaly, often tender to palpation. Abdominal masses continuous with the liver are also common findings. Jaundice occurs in approximately 20 percent of infections. Metastases from the liver to the lung and brain may occur.

Polycystic hydatid disease usually occurs in adults, but it has been reported in children as young as 6 years. One third of the patients reported have been younger than 22 years. The clinical picture may resemble cirrhosis, hepatic tumor or abscess, or intra-abdominal tumor. Hepatomegaly, abdominal masses, fever, and jaundice are frequent initial signs.[32]

DIAGNOSIS

The diagnosis of cystic echinococcosis usually is suspected on the basis of clinical or radiologic findings plus a history of residence in an endemic area. Physical examination rarely is definitive. Only half of patients with hepatic cysts have abnormal liver function test results. Eosinophilia is more often absent than present, although serum IgE levels characteristically are elevated.[37] On occasion, scoleces of the parasite can be identified in vomitus, stool, urine, or sputum when the cyst has ruptured spontaneously, but usually the parasite is not seen until surgery.

The initial suspicion of cystic hydatid disease often is based on radiographic findings. An unruptured pulmonary hydatid cyst has a sharply demarcated, round or oval smooth border. It has a homogeneous "cannonball" appearance and sometimes is surrounded by a layer of atelectatic lung.[10, 68] After the cyst has ruptured into a bronchus, a crescent-shaped air layer may be seen that is virtually diagnostic. In addition to the arc of air between the parasite and the host cyst wall, air in the cyst lumen also may be present. The membrane of a collapsed cyst floating on the surface of the fluid in a ruptured pulmonary cyst has a characteristic "water lily" appearance.

Radiographically apparent cyst wall calcification occurs only in liver or spleen cysts and generally takes more than 5 to 10 years to develop; thus, it is rarely helpful for diagnosis in children. Cysts usually are seen easily and measured with CT. Ultrasound techniques are useful for defining most cysts within the abdomen and can differentiate fluid-filled cysts from solid tumors. Septa or daughter cysts, when present, produce echoes that are highly characteristic of hydatid cysts. Angiography is said to show a characteristic halo effect around the cyst in some cases. Bone cysts typically produce radiolucencies without periosteal reaction. MRI offers little advantage over CT for the imaging of cysts except in the CNS. Reviews of imaging modalities in a wide variety of manifestations of cystic echinococcosis are available.[66, 114]

Fine-needle aspiration of cysts for diagnosis was considered extremely dangerous because leakage of hydatid fluid can induce anaphylactic shock and possibly secondary cyst development. However, the percutaneous route has been used for both diagnosis and treatment, with few untoward events. The fluid obtained is examined for evidence of both protoscoleces and antigen. An algorithm for the use of diagnostic fine-needle aspiration has been proposed.[136] Diagnostic cytologic analysis of aspirated fluid was reported in one case of polycystic echinococcosis.[81]

The Casoni skin test is of historic interest only. Hydatid cyst fluid was injected into the skin. When positive, an erythematous papule developed at the injection site in less than 60 minutes. False-negative and false-positive results occurred in up to 30 percent. Serologic tests such as ELISA, indirect hemagglutination, and fluorescent antibody assays may be negative in 10 to 50 percent of patients with cystic hydatid disease. False-negative results seem to occur more commonly in patients with pulmonary cysts and in children. The tests available may cross-react with cysticercosis or other parasitic infections. The use of purified antigen B from *E. granulosus* shows promise. Immunoblotting techniques may be highly specific.[57] Currently, cystic hydatid disease cannot be ruled out on the basis of routine serologic testing. Attempts to develop tests to deal with cross-reactions appear promising.[116] Immunologic tests for alveolar hydatid disease that use the Em18 antigen are sensitive and specific. A recent report has indicated that cystic and alveolar disease can be differentiated by a combination of tests. One test uses fractions from *E. granulosus* (antigen B) that react with sera from cases of both types of hydatid disease. The second test uses the Em18 fraction from *E. multilocularis,* which is specific for alveolar disease.[74] Serologic tests may be useful in monitoring the effectiveness of treatment in alveolar echinococcosis.[92]

In approximately 70 percent of patients with alveolar echinococcosis, an abdominal radiograph will show scattered large areas of amorphous calcification containing 2- to 4-mm radiolucent areas surrounded by calcium.[143] The degree of liver invasion at surgery often is found to be much more extensive than the calcified area.

In the absence of a characteristic radiologic finding, the diagnosis of echinococcosis frequently is missed preoperatively. The diagnosis is confirmed at surgery by demonstration of the characteristic laminated membrane by periodic acid–Schiff staining or the presence of protoscoleces or hooklets.

A test has been developed that detects *E. multilocularis* antigen in the feces of foxes. It has been helpful in assessing control programs in Europe.

TREATMENT AND PROGNOSIS

Treatment of cystic echinococcosis is based on the location of the cyst or cysts, the nature and size of the cysts, and the condition of the patient. Surgery has been considered the treatment of choice for nearly all cases of cystic hydatid disease. The benzimidazoles mebendazole and albendazole provide a chemotherapeutic alternative to surgery or may be used as a supplement to surgery. The PAIR technique (*p*ercutaneous *a*spiration, *i*ntroduction of scolecide, and *r*easpiration), with or without medical therapy, offers a less invasive option than the traditional surgical approaches do.[94] It is now considered by many clinicians to be the treatment of choice for most cases of hepatic cystic echinococcosis.[1, 29, 79] Alcohol or hypertonic saline, or both, have been used as scolecides in this procedure.

Surgical success depends on the size and location of cysts and the skill of the surgeon. In cystic echinococcosis, rupture of the cyst contents at the time of surgery carries an immediate risk of anaphylaxis and a delayed risk of disseminated echinococcosis. The latter, relatively uncommon even after spillage, is a greatly feared complication. As a consequence, multiple surgical techniques are directed toward preventing spillage of viable cyst contents during surgery for hepatic cysts. These techniques include injection of hypertonic saline, alcohol, cetrimide, or other scolicide into the cyst. Scolicides must be used with caution because of the danger of causing sclerosing cholangitis. Evaluation of several scolecides in a mouse model showed that hydrogen peroxide and povidone-iodine were more effective than hypertonic saline and praziquantel.[85] Treatment of patients with albendazole before and after surgery has become a common practice.

It is administered with the expectation that pressure within the cyst will be reduced and removal of cyst membranes and contents will be facilitated. In addition, it is hoped that preoperative exposure to the drug will decrease the likelihood of secondary cyst development. The preoperative administration of praziquantel combined with a benzimidazole has been suggested because of the scolecidal properties of praziquantel.[69] One study reported that combined treatment with albendazole and praziquantel for a month before surgery resulted in decreased viability of cysts greater than that achieved with albendazole alone.[26]

Opinions differ regarding the optimal type of surgical procedure for hepatic cysts. Some surgeons prefer to sterilize and evacuate the cyst contents, refill the cyst with normal saline, and leave it in place. Other techniques are directed toward obliterating the large residual cavity after a cyst has been removed or emptied. Reviews of surgical management are available.[45, 62, 101, 109, 125]

In general, the surgical mortality rate is 3 to 5 percent, including surgery on multilocular cysts and reoperation. In some areas, one in five patients requires additional surgical procedures. Serologic and skin tests may remain positive for at least 10 years after successful surgery; a falling titer suggests cure, but a persistently elevated titer does not necessarily imply recurrence. Thoroughly calcified cysts in older persons rarely require treatment.

Pulmonary cysts have been treated successfully surgically,[119] medically,[78] and with PAIR.[94] The cervid strains of *E. granulosus* from Alaska and Canada do not produce anaphylaxis upon rupture, and pulmonary cysts spontaneously resolve after evacuating into bronchi.

Mebendazole was the first benzimidazole to be tried in hydatid disease. High doses had to be used because the drug is absorbed poorly from the gastrointestinal tract. The results were inconsistent. Albendazole now has replaced mebendazole. It is well absorbed and diffuses into cysts in effective concentrations. Levels of the active albendazole metabolite are increased with concomitant administration of cimetidine. The usual approach to the administration of albendazole is to give variable numbers of courses, depending on the individual response. Each course is 28 days in length and is followed by a 14-day rest period. In adults, albendazole is given at a total dose of 800 mg daily divided into two doses. If a response to albendazole is not evident after the administration of three courses of treatment, subsequent courses are unlikely to be beneficial. The results of clinical trials through 1996 have been summarized,[71] and a series of more than 400 cases monitored for 1 to 14 years have been reported.[55] Albendazole has shown beneficial effects in many, but not all, cases of hydatid disease. In children, the dose of albendazole is 15 mg/kg/day (maximum, 800 mg) divided into two doses for 28 days and repeated as necessary after a 14-day rest interval between cycles. Albendazole may cause reversible liver function abnormalities, transient leukopenia, and alopecia. Severe leukopenia or pancytopenia rarely has been reported. Severe hepatotoxicity associated with jaundice has been described in as many as 5 percent of patients treated. Liver function tests and blood counts should be monitored every 2 weeks during therapy. Albendazole is also helpful in inoperable cases of hydatid disease, and it may be used before or after surgery to reduce the risk of intraoperative dissemination and recurrence. A favorable response to albendazole has been reported in both alveolar and polycystic hydatid disease.[32, 157] Information on current drug therapy for hydatid disease may be obtained from the CDC in Atlanta.

The prognosis of hydatid disease varies widely. Hepatic cysts may undergo spontaneous death and calcification in as many as one quarter of cases. As many as two thirds of symptomatic patients die without intervention. Survivors usually experience spontaneous rupture and spontaneous evacuation of the cyst into a hollow viscus.

Untreated alveolar hydatid disease has a mortality rate exceeding 90 percent within 10 years of diagnosis. More than 70 percent of patients have lesions that are unresectable at the time of diagnosis. In some cases, partial hepatectomy or hepatic lobectomy can remove the entire multilocular cyst and still preserve sufficient organ function to sustain life. To eradicate the infection, all invaded tissue and a margin of normal tissue must be resected en bloc. Liver transplantation has been useful both as a curative approach in selected patients and as palliation in incurable disease. Chemotherapy with albendazole should be used as an adjunct to surgery. In inoperable patients, chemotherapy may arrest progression of the disease and possibly, in some patients, bring about a cure.[157] Albendazole treatment of alveolar echinococcosis is indicated for 2 years after radical surgery and longer (10 years or more) in inoperable patients or after incomplete surgical resection or liver transplantation.[69]

Albendazole is recommended as the initial treatment for all cases of polycystic echinococcosis.[32]

PREVENTION

Prevention of the disease requires elimination of the infection in dogs by using suitable veterinary taeniacides. Proper disposal of carcasses and entrails on ranges and from slaughterhouses prevents dogs from gaining access to them. The dog-sheep cycle is interrupted most easily; other cycles may be impossible to control. The effectiveness of dog control combined with educational efforts has been demonstrated best in Iceland. The disease initially was found in 22 percent of the population and now has been eradicated. Those who have contact with dogs that feed on carcasses of large deer should be warned against contamination of hands, food, or drink with dog feces. The hazards of exposure to wild foxes and dogs in the Arctic regions and foxes in Central and Western Europe also must be made known.

Coenurosis (Coenuriasis, *Taenia* (*Multiceps*) Species Infection)

Several species of *Taenia* have a larval stage called a coenurus that consists of a cystic membranous structure up to 6 cm in diameter from which multiple scoleces bud internally or externally. Because of this unique larval morphology, the parasite was given the species name *multiceps.* Currently, the preferred genus name is *Taenia* because of the morphology of the adult worms and the inability to justify genus designation based solely on the form of larvae.[49] Many publications still refer to the genus as *Multiceps.* The relationships of various species of coenurus-producing *Taenia (Multiceps)* are defined inadequately. The following species generally are accepted for purposes of discussion.

The adult tapeworm of *Taenia (Multiceps) multiceps* is found in dogs, and the larval stages occur in herbivores such as sheep, cattle, goats, and horses. These larvae often develop in the CNS and produce a condition known as gid or staggers in sheep. Because infection in sheep has not been seen in the United States for more than 60 years, this species is thought to be an unlikely candidate for the forms of human coenurosis found in this area. In sheep-raising areas of Europe and Asia, the infection is still endemic in animals.

TABLE 225–1 ■ LESS COMMON TAPEWORMS THAT CAN INFECT HUMANS

	Scolex	Approximate Length/Width	Proglottids	Eggs	Geographic Distribution	Intermediate Hosts	Transmission	Clinical Manifestations
Hymenolepis diminuta (rat tapeworm)	Four small suckers, no hooks	10–60 cm/ 4 mm max.	2.5 mm wide by 0.75 mm in length; usually not seen in feces	60–85 µm in diameter; embryo separated from egg shell by large space	Worldwide in rats and mice; human infections are uncommon but most frequent in children	Rat and mouse fleas; flour and grain beetles	Accidental ingestion of insect intermediate host, usually in uncooked or precooked cereal	Frequently asymptomatic; may have anorexia, nausea, vomiting, weight loss, abdominal pain, or diarrhea
Bertiella species	Four ovoid suckers, no hooks	26–45 cm/ 6 mm max.	6 mm wide by 0.75 mm in length; usually found in feces in chains of 10 or more	46–50 µm in diameter; irregularly ovoid; embryo envelope possesses a bicornuate protrusion	Found in primates worldwide; human infections are rare (fewer than 50 cases); usually in children in close contact with pet monkey or other primate	Oribatid mites	Accidental ingestion of mite; usually history of close contact with pet monkey	Usually asymptomatic; nonspecific gastrointestinal complaints have been reported
Raillietina species	Four suckers with tiny hooks; rostellum with double row of 80 or more hooks	Up to 12 m/3 mm	Resemble rice grains and appear motile in feces; contain egg capsules with several eggs in each capsule	Numbers of eggs included in capsule depend on species	Usually in infants and young children; found in South America (Ecuador is endemic), Philippines, Japan, Taiwan, Thailand, Indonesia, and Tahiti	Unknown, probably insects	Unknown	Reports from Ecuador[47] list nausea, vomiting, sialorrhea, flatulence, colic, diarrhea, nervous disorders, tachycardia, arrhythmia, syncope, anemia, and eosinophilia; asymptomatic infections also have been described

Inermicapsifer madagascariensis	Four suckers, no hooks	Up to 42 cm/ 2.6 mm	"Rice grains," similar to *Raillietina,* are passed in feces; eggs in capsules in gravid segments	Six or more eggs per capsule; 35–50 µm in diameter	Usually found in children younger than 6 yr; reported from Africa, also from Venezuela, Malaya, Thailand, and Philippines; more than 100 cases reported from Cuba	Unknown	Unknown	Not adequately described; probably asymptomatic
Mesocestoides species	Four suckers with slitlike openings	40 cm/2 mm (variable with species)	Passed in feces; beadlike; 1.5 mm wide by 2.5 mm in length; eggs located in a mass in the parauterine organ	Oval; approximately 20–26 µm in maximal diameter	Rare in humans; several infections in adults in Japan; few cases in children from United States and Africa; single case in Korea	Life cycle incompletely known; second intermediate hosts are birds, reptiles, frogs, and rodents	Probably ingestion of raw flesh of second intermediate hosts; Japanese cases associated with ingestion of raw reptile viscera and blood	Abdominal pain and severe diarrhea reported in Japanese adults; children have been asymptomatic

Taenia (Multiceps) serialis adult worms also are found in dogs and other canids, but common intermediate hosts are rabbits, hares, and rodents. The coenurus develops in subcutaneous and intramuscular tissue. In experimental infections in rodents, CNS involvement has been demonstrated. *T. serialis* has been reported from the United States, Canada, France, and Africa.

Taenia (Multiceps) brauni is the name given to the tapeworms of dogs, jackals, foxes, and genets found in tropical Africa. The larvae develop in gerbils and other rodents.

Humans are a rare accidental host for the larval stages of these worms. The disease is called coenurosis or coenuriasis. Fewer than 100 human infections have been recorded. Most infections are from Africa, with many in children. It is nearly impossible to give a species designation based solely on the morphology of organisms recovered from human tissue. The infection is presumed to be acquired by the ingestion of eggs excreted by the definitive hosts, usually dogs. Because of the subcutaneous and subconjunctival location of cysts in infections in tropical Africa, it has been suggested that direct contact of the eggs on skin or the conjunctiva is a mode of transmission. A review of the six human infections in North America has been published.[73]

The clinical manifestations of coenurosis are related to the location of the parasite. CNS involvement produces a spectrum of illness that resembles that of cysticercosis (discussed earlier), including meningeal reactions. Larvae have been seen in subconjunctival and subretinal tissue, extraocular muscles, the anterior chamber, and the vitreous. Subcutaneous and intramuscular lesions occur most commonly in the abdomen and chest wall.

A definitive diagnosis is made by demonstration of the characteristic morphology of the larva recovered at surgery. The multiple scoleces that bud from the delicate cyst membrane have double rows of hooklets of a typical shape, size, and number. In instances in which no scoleces are found, differentiating a coenurus from the racemose cysticercus of *T. solium* is impossible. The diagnosis of intramuscular coenurosis has been made by examination of fine-needle aspirates.[73] Radiographic studies such as CT are useful in cerebral coenurosis but do not differentiate the parasite from other cystic lesions.

Treatment is surgical. Mortality rates in cerebral disease are high. Organisms in other locations, with the exception of subretinal lesions, are removed easily. Praziquantel has been used successfully to treat sheep with cerebral coenurosis.[148] A combination of praziquantel and a corticosteroid administered to a patient with a subretinal coenurus caused death of the parasite, which resulted in a severe inflammatory reaction, retinal detachment, and permanent loss of vision.[72] Severe reactions were reported in the two additional cases described in this review. Praziquantel should be used with great caution, if at all, in cases of human coenurosis.

Although the exact mode of infection in humans has not been identified, avoiding close contact with dogs and dog excreta, which are the most likely sources of infection, is prudent.

Other, Less Common, Tapeworms

Table 225–1 summarizes data concerning the less common tapeworms that may infect humans. The recommended treatment for these infections is praziquantel, as used in *T. saginata* infection.

REFERENCES

1. Akhan, O., and Özmen, M. N.: Percutaneous treatment of liver hydatid cysts. Eur. J. Radiol. *32*:76–85, 1999.
2. Allan, J. C., Mencos, F., Garcia-Noval, J., et al.: Dipstick dot ELISA for the detection of *Taenia* coproantigens in humans. Parasitology *107*:79–85, 1993.
3. Ammann, R. W., and Eckert, J.: Cestodes. *Echinococcus.* Gastroenterol. Clin. North Am. *25*:655–689, 1996.
4. Anaemia and the fish-tapeworm. Lancet *1*:292, 1977.
5. Arambulo, P., III: Public health importance of cystic echinococcosis in Latin America. Acta Trop. *67*:113–124, 1997.
6. Arh, I.: Fish tapeworm in Eskimos in the Port Harrison area, Canada. Can. J. Public Health *51*:268–271, 1960.
7. Arocker-Mettinger, E., Huber-Spitzky, V., Auer, H., et al.: *Taenia crassiceps* in der Vorderkammer des menschlichen Auges. Klin. Monatsbl. Augenheilkd. *201*:34–37, 1992.
8. Arora, V. K., Gupta, K., Singh, N., and Bhatia, A.: Cytomorphologic panorama of cysticercosis on fine needle aspiration: A review of 298 cases. Acta Cytol. *38*:377–380, 1994.
9. Auche, Y., Bernard, J. P., and Faivre, J.: Grandes eosinophilies sanguines et taeniasis. Arch. Fr. Mal. Appl. Diagn. *60*:491–492, 1971.
10. Aytac, A., Yurdakul, Y., Ikizler, C., et al.: Pulmonary hydatid disease: Report of 100 patients. Ann. Thorac. Surg. *23*:145–151, 1977.
11. Bang, O. Y., Heo, J. H., Choi, S. A., and Kim, D. I.: Large cerebral infarction during praziquantel therapy in neurocysticercosis. Stroke *28*:211–213, 1997.
12. Baranwal, A. K., Singhi, P. D., Wal, N. K., and Singhi, S. C.: Albendazole therapy in children with focal seizures and single small enhancing computerized tomographic lesions: A randomized, placebo-controlled, double blind trial. Pediatr. Infect. Dis. J. *17*:696–700, 1998.
13. Beaver, P. C., and Rolon, F. A.: Proliferating larval cestode in man in Paraguay: A case report and review of the literature. Am. J. Trop. Med. Hyg. *30*:625–637, 1981.
14. Bhatia, G.: Echinococcus. Semin. Respir. Infect. *12*:171–187, 1997.
15. Bouza Suarez, M., Hormilla Manso, G., Dumenigo Ripoll, B., et al.: The first certain case of *Diphyllobothrium latum* in Cuba. Rev. Cubana Med. Trop. *42*:9–12, 1990.
16. Bowles, J., and McManus, D. P.: Genetic characterization of the Asian *taenia,* a newly described taeniid cestode of humans. Am. J. Trop. Med. Hyg. *50*:33–44, 1994.
17. Buergett, C. D., Greiner, E. C., and Senior, D. F.: Proliferative sparganosis in a cat. J. Parasitol. *70*:121–125, 1984.
18. Buscher, H. N., and Haley, A. J.: Epidemiology of *Hymenolepis nana* infections of Punjabi villagers in West Pakistan. Am. J. Trop. Med. Hyg. *21*:42–49, 1972.
19. Carpio, A., Escobar, A., and Hauser, W. A.: Cysticercosis and epilepsy: A critical review. Epilepsia *39*:1025–1040, 1998.
20. Carrea, R., Dowling, E., Jr., and Guevara, J. A.: Surgical treatment of hydatid cysts of the central nervous system in the pediatric age (Dowling's techniques). Childs Brain *1*:4–21, 1975.
21. Chai, J. J.: Epidemiological studies on cystic echinococcosis in China—a review. Biomed. Environ. Sci. *8*:122–136, 1995.
22. Chang, K. H., Chi, J. G., Cho, S. Y., et al.: Cerebral sparganosis: Analysis of 34 cases with emphasis on CT features. Neuroradiology *34*:1–8, 1992.
23. Chang, K. H., and Han, M. H.: MRI of CNS parasitic diseases. J. Magn. Reson. Imaging *8*:297–307, 1998.
24. Chitchang, S., Piamjinda, T., Yodmani, B., et al.: Relationship between severity of the symptom and the number of *Hymenolepis nana* after treatment. J. Med. Assoc. Thailand *68*:423–426, 1985.
25. Chuck, I. R. S., Olk, R. J., Weil, G. J., et al.: Surgical removal of a subretinal proliferating cysticercus of *Taeniaformis crassiceps.* Arch. Ophthalmol. *115*:562–563, 1997.
26. Cobo, F., Yarnoz, C., Sesma, B., et al.: Albendazole plus praziquantel versus albendazole alone as a pre-operative treatment in intra-abdominal hydatidosis caused by *Echinococcus granulosus.* Trop. Med. Int. Health *3*:462–466, 1998.
27. Corrall, C. J., II, and Appel, B. L.: Sparganosis: A clinical and pathologic observation of the first observed case in a child. Pediatr. Infect. Dis. J. *6*:481–485, 1987.
28. Craig, P. S., Rogan, M. T., and Allan, J. C.: Detection, screening and community epidemiology of Taeniid cestode zoonoses: Cystic echinococcosis, alveolar echinococcosis and neurocysticercosis. Adv. Parasitol. *38*:169–250, 1996.
29. Crippa, F. G., Bruno, R., Brunetti, E., and Filice, C.: Echinococcal liver cysts: Treatment with echo-guided percutaneous puncture PAIR for echinococcal liver cysts. Ital. J. Gastroenterol. Hepatol. *31*:884–892, 1999.
30. Cuéllar, R., Molinero, M., Ramírez, F., and Vallejo, V.: Manifestaciones clínicas de la neurocisticercosis cerebral activa en pediatría. Rev. Neurol. *29*:334–337, 1999.
31. Curtis, M. A., and Bylund, G.: Diphyllobothriasis: Fish tapeworm disease in the circumpolar north. Arct. Med. Res. *50*:18–24, 1991.
32. D'Alessandro, A.: Polycystic echinococcosis in tropical America: *Echinococcus vogeli* and *E. oligarthrus.* Acta Trop. *67*:43–65, 1997.
33. D'Alessandro, A., Rausch, R. L., Cuello, C., et al.: *Echinococcus vogeli* in man, with a review of polycystic hydatid disease in Colombia and neighboring countries. Am. J. Trop. Med. Hyg. *28*:303–317, 1979.
34. Dar, F. K., and Alkarmi, T.: Public health aspects of cystic echinococcosis in the Arab countries. Acta Trop. *67*:125–132, 1997.

35. Del Brutto, O. H.: Cysticercosis and cerebrovascular disease: A review. J. Neurol. Neurosurg. Psychiatry *55*:252–254, 1992.
36. Del Brutto, O. H., Wadia, N. H., Dumas, M., et al.: Proposal of diagnostic criteria for human cysticercosis and neurocysticercosis. J. Neurol. Sci. *142*:1–6, 1996.
37. Dessaint, J. P., Bout, D., Wattre, P., et al.: Quantitative determination of specific IgE antibodies to *Echinococcus granulosus* and IgE levels in sera from patients with hydatid disease. Immunology *29*:813–823, 1975.
38. Di Conza, J. J.: Protective action of passively transferred immune serum and immunoglobulin fractions against tissue invasive stages of the dwarf tapeworm *Hymenolepis nana*. Exp. Parasitol. *25*:368–375, 1969.
39. Dixon, H. B., and Lipscomb, F. M.: Cysticercosis: An analysis and follow-up of 450 cases. Med. Res. Spec. Rep. (Lond.) *299*:1–58, 1961.
40. Dixon, J. B.: Echinococcosis. Comp. Immunol. Microbiol. Infect. Dis. *20*:87–94, 1997.
41. Donckaster, R., and Habibe, O.: Contribución al estudio de la infección por *Hymenolepis nana:* Sintomalogía y eosinofilia relativa. Bol. Chil. Parasitol. *13*:9–11, 1958.
42. Eckert, J.: Epidemiology of *Echinococcus multilocularis* and *E. granulosus* in Central Europe. Parasitologia *39*:337–344, 1997.
43. Eckert, J., and Deplazes, P.: Alveolar echinococcosis in humans: The current situation in Central Europe and the need for countermeasures. Parasitol. Today *15*:315–319, 1999.
44. Eckert, J., and Thompson, R. C. A.: Intraspecific variation of *Echinococcus granulosus* and related species with emphasis on their infectivity to humans. Acta Trop. *64*:19–34, 1997.
45. Elburjo, M., and Gani, E. A.: Surgical management of pulmonary hydatid cysts in children. Thorax *50*:396–398, 1995.
46. Eom, K. S., and Rim, H. J.: Experimental human infection with Asian *Taenia saginata* metacestodes obtained from naturally infected Korean domestic pigs. Kisaengchunghak Chapchi *30*:21–24, 1992.
47. Eom, K. S., and Rim, H. J.: Morphologic descriptions of *Taenia asiatica* sp. N. Korean J. Parasitol. *31*:1–6, 1993.
48. Ersahin, Y., Mutluer, S., and Guzelbag, E.: Intracranial hydatid cysts in children. Neurosurgery *33*:219–224, 1993.
49. Esch, G. W., and Self, J. T.: A critical study of the taxonomy of *Taenia pisiformis* Bloch 1780; *Multiceps multiceps* (Leske, 1780); and *Hydatigera taeniaeformis* Batsch, 1786. J. Parasitol. *51*:932–937, 1965.
50. Estanol, B.: Medical treatment of cerebral cysticercosis. Eur. Neurol. *37*:124–131, 1997.
51. Fan, P. C., and Chung, W. C.: *Taenia saginata asiatica*: Epidemiology, infection, immunological and molecular studies. Chin. J. Microbiol. Immunol. *31*:84–89, 1998.
52. Finlay, J. C., and Speert, D. P.: Sylvatic hydatid disease in children: Case reports and review of endemic *Echinococcus granulosus* infection in Canada and Alaska. Pediatr. Infect. Dis. J. *11*:322–326, 1992.
53. Foresi, C.: Indagini sulla epidemiologia della imenolepiasi in Italia (Nota 1[a]). Arch. Ital. Sci. Med. Trop. *48*:251–262, 1967.
54. Forlenza, O. V., Filho, A. H., Nobrega, J. P., et al.: Psychiatric manifestations of neurocysticercosis: A study of 38 patients from a neurology clinic in Brazil. J. Neurol. Neurosurg. Psychiatry *62*:612–616, 1997.
55. Franchi, C., Di Vico, B., and Teggi, A.: Long-term evaluation of patients with hydatidosis treated with benzimidazole. Clin. Infect. Dis. *29*:304–309, 1999.
56. Francois, A., Favennec, L., Cambon-Michot, C., et al.: *Taenia crassiceps* invasive cysticercosis. A new human pathogen in acquired immunodeficiency syndrome? Am. J. Surg. Pathol. *22*:488–492, 1998.
57. Gadea, I., Ayala, G., Diago, M. T., et al.: Immunological diagnosis of human cystic echinococcosis: Utility of discriminant analysis applied to the enzyme-linked immunoelectrotransfer blot. Clin. Diagn. Lab. Immunol. *6*:504–508, 1999.
58. Galán-Puchades, M. T., and Fuentes, M. V.: The Asian *Taenia* and the possibility of cysticercosis. Korean J. Parasitol. *38*:1–7, 2000.
59. Garcia, H. H., and Del Brutto, O. H.: *Taenia solium* cysticercosis. Infect. Dis. Clin. North Am. *14*:97–119, 2000.
60. Garg, R. K.: Childhood neurocysticercosis: Issues in diagnosis and management. Indian Pediatr. *32*:1023–1029, 1995.
61. Garin, J. P., and Mojon, M.: L'eosinophilie sanguine au cours du taeniasis a *T. saginata*. Lyon Med. *228*:339–343, 1972.
62. Golematis, B. C., and Peveretos, P. J.: Hepatic hydatid disease: Current surgical treatment. Mt. Sinai J. Med. *62*:71–76, 1995.
63. Gomez-Priego, A., Godinez-Hana, A. L., and Gutierrez-Quiroz, M.: Detection of serum antibodies in human *Hymenolepis* infection by enzyme immunoassay. Trans. R. Soc. Trop. Med. Hyg. *85*:645–647, 1991.
64. González, L. M., Montero, E., Harrison, L. J., et al.: Differential diagnosis of *Taenia saginata* and *Taenia solium* infection by PCR. J. Clin. Microbiol. *38*:737–744, 2000.
65. Gordadze, G. N., and Gigitashvilli, M. S.: Epileptoid fits provoked by *Hymenolepis nana*. Med. Parazit. (Moskva) *28*:430–434, 1959.
66. Gossios, K. J., Kontoyiannis, D. S., Dascalogiannaki, M., and Gourtsoyiannis, N. C.: Uncommon locations of hydatid disease: CT appearances. Eur. Radiol. 7:1303–1308, 1997.
67. Gray, M. L., Rogers, F., Little, S., et al.: Sparganosis in feral hogs (*Sus scrofa*) from Florida. J. Am. Vet. Med. Assoc. *215*:204–208, 1999.
68. Grunebaum, M.: Radiological manifestations of lung echinococcosis in children. Pediatr. Radiol. *3*:65–69, 1975.
69. Guidelines for treatment of cystic and alveolar echinococcosis in humans. WHO Informal Working Group on Echinococcosis. Bull. World Health Organ. *74*:231–242, 1996.
70. Hamrick, H. J., Drake, W. R., Jr., Jones, H. M., et al.: Two cases of dipylidiasis (dog tapeworm infection) in children: Update on an old problem. Pediatrics *72*:114–117, 1983.
71. Horton, R. J.: Albendazole in treatment of human cystic echinococcosis: 12 years of experience. Acta Trop. *64*:79–93, 1997.
72. Ibechukwu, B. I., and Onwukeme, K. E.: Intraocular coenurosis: A case report. Br. J. Ophthalmol. *75*:430–431, 1991.
73. Ing, M. B., Schantz, P. M., and Turner, J. A.: Human coenurosis in North America: Case reports and review. Clin. Infect. Dis. *27*:519–523, 1998.
74. Ito, A., Ma, L., Schantz, P. M., et al.: Differential serodiagnosis for cystic and alveolar echinococcosis using fractions of *Echinococcus granulosus* cyst fluid (antigen B) and *E. multilocularis* protoscolex (EM18). Am. J. Trop. Med. Hyg. *60*:188–192, 1999.
75. Jeong, S. C., Bae, J. C., Hwang, S. H., et al.: Cerebral sparganosis with intracerebral hemorrhage: A case report. Neurology *50*:503–506, 1998.
76. Kappus, K. D., Lundgren, R. C., Juranek, D. D., et al.: Intestinal parasitism in the United States: Update on a continuing problem. Am. J. Trop. Med. Hyg. *50*:705–713, 1994.
77. Kattan, Y. B.: Intrabiliary rupture of hydatid cyst of the liver. Ann. R. Coll. Surg. Engl. *59*:108–114, 1977.
78. Keshmiri, M., Baharvahdat, H., Fattahi, S. H., et al.: A placebo controlled study of albendazole in the treatment of pulmonary echinococcosis. Eur. Respir. J. *14*:503–507, 1999.
79. Khuroo, M. S., Wani, N. A., Javid, G., et al.: Percutaneous drainage compared with surgery for hepatic hydatid cysts. N. Engl. J. Med. *337*:881–887, 1997.
80. Kim, C. Y., Cho, B. K., Kim, I. O., et al.: Cerebral sparganosis in a child. Pediatr. Neurosurg. *26*:103–106, 1997.
81. Kini, U., Shariff, S., Nirmala, V.: Aspiration cytology of *Echinococcus oligarthrus*: A case report. Acta Cytol. *41*:544–548, 1997.
82. Klinker, H., Tintelot, K., Joeres, R., et al.: *Taenia crassiceps* infektion bei AIDS. Dtsch. Med. Wochenschr. *117*:133–138, 1992.
83. Kudesia, S., Indira, D. B., Sarala, D., et al.: Sparganosis of brain and spinal cord: Unusual tapeworm infestation (report of two cases). Clin. Neurol. Neurosurg. *100*:148–152, 1998.
84. Lamy, A. L., Cameron, B. H., LeBlanc, J. G., et al.: Giant hydatid cysts in the Canadian northwest: Outcome of conservative treatment in three children. J. Pediatr. Surg. *28*:1140–1143, 1993.
85. Landa Garcia, J. I., Alonso, E., Gonzalez-Uriarte, J., and Rodriguez Romano, D.: Evaluation of scolicidal agents in an experimental hydatid disease model. Eur. Surg. Res. *29*:202–208, 1997.
86. Lang, E., and Vinas, F.: Cysticercosis of the brain. Surg. Clin. North Am. *38*:887–896, 1958.
87. Lewall, D. B.: Hydatid disease: Biology, pathology, imaging and classification. Clin. Radiol. *53*:863–874, 1998.
88. Loos-Frank, B.: An up-date of Verster's (1969) 'Taxonomic revision of the genus *Taenia* Linnaeus' (Cestoda) in table format. Syst. Parasitol. *45*:155–183, 2000.
89. Loyo-Varela, M.: Surgical treatment of cerebral cysticercosis. Eur. Neurol. *37*:129–130, 1997.
90. Lucas, S. B., Hassounah, O. A., Doeuhoff, M., et al.: Aberrant form of *Hymenolepis nana:* Possible opportunistic infection in immunosuppressed patients. Lancet *2*:1372–1373, 1979.
91. Lumbreras, H., Terashima, A., Alvarez, H., et al.: Single dose treatment with praziquantel (Cesol R, EmBay 8440) of human cestodiasis caused by *Diphyllobothrium pacificum*. Tropenmed. Parasitol. *33*:5–7, 1982.
92. Ma, L., Ito, A., Liu, Y., et al.: Alveolar echinococcosis: Em2^{plus}-ELISA^{TM} and Em18-Western blots for follow-up after treatment with albendazole. Trans. R. Soc. Trop. Med. Hyg. *91*:476–478, 1997.
93. Maillard, H., Marionneau, J., Prophette, B., et al.: *Taenia crassiceps* cysticercosis and AIDS. Letter. A. I. D. S. *12*:1551–1552, 1998.
94. Mawhorter, S., Temeck, B., Chang, R., et al.: Nonsurgical therapy for pulmonary hydatid cyst disease. Chest *112*:1432–1436, 1997.
95. Mazzoti, L.: Presencia de huevecillos de *Taenia* en la región perianal. Rev. Inst. Salubr. Enferm. Trop. Mex. *5*:153–155, 1944.
96. McIntyre, A.: Hydatid disease in children in South Australia. Med. J. Aust. *1*:1064–1065, 1971.
97. Mitchell, W. G.: Pediatric neurocysticercosis in North America. Eur. Neurol. *37*:126–129, 1997.
98. Mitchell, W. G.: Neurocysticercosis and acquired cerebral toxoplasmosis in children. Semin. Pediatr. Neurol. *6*:267–277, 1999.
99. Mitchell, W. G., and Crawford, T. O.: Intraparenchymal cerebral cysticercosis in children: Diagnosis and treatment. Pediatrics *82*:76–82, 1988.
100. Mori, Y., Shirayama, T., Agui, T., et al.: A case of chest wall tumor brought on by *Hymenolepis nana*. Bull. Osaka Med. Sch. *13*:52–54, 1967.
101. Morris, D. L., and Richards, K. S.: Hydatid Disease: Current Medical and Surgical Management. Oxford, Butterworth-Heinemann, 1992.

102. Moulinier, R., Martinez, E., Torres, J., et al.: Human proliferative sparganosis in Venezuela: Report of a case. Am. J. Trop. Med. Hyg. *31*:358–363, 1982.
103. Nakamura, T., Hara, M., Matsuoka, M., et al.: Human proliferative sparganosis. Am. J. Clin. Pathol. *94*:224–228, 1990.
104. Nash, T. E., and Patronas, N. J.: Edema associated with calcified lesions in neurocysticercosis. Neurology *53*:777–781, 1999.
105. Natarajan, S., Malpani, A., Nirmalan, P. K., and Dutta, B.: Management of intraocular cysticercosis. Graefes Arch. Clin. Exp. Ophthalmol. *237*:812–814, 1999.
106. Nyberg, W., Grasbeck, R., Saarni, M., et al.: Serum vitamin B_{12} levels and incidence of tapeworm anemia in a population heavily infected with *Diphyllobothrium latum*. J. Lab. Clin. Med. *57*:240–246, 1961.
107. Oh, S. J., Chi, J. G., and Lee, S. E.: Eosinophilic cystitis caused by vesical sparganosis: A case report. J. Urol. *149*:581–583, 1993.
108. Oostburg, B. F. J., Vrede, M. A., and Bergen, A. E.: The occurrence of polycystic echinococcosis in Suriname. Ann. Trop. Med. Parasitol. *94*:247–252, 2000.
109. Ozcelik, C., Inci, I., Toprak, M., et al.: Surgical treatment of pulmonary hydatidosis in children: Experience in 92 patients. J. Pediatr. Surg. *29*:392–395, 1994.
110. Palacios, E., Lujambio, P. S., and Jasso, R. R.: Computed tomography and magnetic resonance imaging of neurocysticercosis. Semin. Roentgenol. *32*:325–334, 1997.
111. Pathogenesis of tapeworm anaemia. B. M. J. *2*:1028, 1976.
112. Pawlowski, Z. S.: Taeniasis and cysticercosis. *In* Steele, J. H. (ed.): CRC Handbook Series in Zoonoses: Parasitic Zoonoses. Vol. 1. Boca Raton, FL, CRC Press, 1982, pp. 313–348.
113. Pawlowski, Z., and Schultz, M. G.: Taeniasis and cysticercosis *(Taenia saginata)*. Adv. Parasitol. *10*:269–343, 1972.
114. Pedrosa, I., Saíz, A., Arrazola, J., et al.: Radiologic and pathologic features and complications. Radiographics *20*:795–817, 2000.
115. Pittella, J. E.: Neurocysticercosis. Brain Pathol. *7*:681–693, 1997.
116. Poretti, D., Felleisen, E., Grimm, F., et al.: Differential immunodiagnosis between cystic hydatid disease and other cross-reactive pathologies. Am. J. Trop. Med. Hyg. *60*:193–198, 1999.
117. Proctor, E. M.: Identification of tapeworms. S. Afr. Med. J. *46*:234–238, 1972.
118. Rahalkar, M. D., Shetty, D. D., Kelkar, A. B., et al.: The many faces of cysticercosis. Clin. Radiol. *55*:668–674, 2000.
119. Rebhandl, W., Turnbull, J., Felberbauer, F. X., et al.: Pulmonary echinococcosis (hydatidosis) in children: Results of surgical treatment. Pediatr. Pulmonol. *27*:336–340, 1999.
120. Richards, F., Jr., and Schantz, P. M.: Treatment of *Taenia solium* infections. Lancet *1*:1264–1265, 1985.
121. Roman, R. A. S., Soto-Hernandez, J. L., and Sotelo, J.: Effects of prednisone on ventriculoperitoneal shunt function in hydrocephalus secondary to cysticercosis. J. Neurosurg. *84*:629–633, 1996.
122. Ruiz-García, M., González-Astiazarán, A., and Rueda-Franco, F.: Neurocysticercosis in children. Clinical experience in 122 patients. Childs Nerv. Syst. *13*:609–612, 1997.
123. Ruttenber, A. J., Weniger, B. G., Sorvillo, F., et al.: Diphyllobothriasis associated with salmon consumption in Pacific Coast states. Am. J. Trop. Med. Hyg. *33*:455–459, 1984.
124. Saarni, M., Nyberg, W., Grasbeck, R., et al.: Symptoms in carriers of *Diphyllobothrium latum*. Acta. Med. Scand. *173*:147–154, 1963.
125. Safioleas, M., Misiakos, E., Manti, C., et al.: Diagnostic evaluation and surgical management of hydatid disease of the liver. World J. Surg. *18*:859–865, 1994.
126. Salgado, P., Rojas, R., and Sotelo, J.: Cysticercosis. Clinical classification based on imaging studies. Arch. Int. Med. *157*:1991–1997, 1997.
127. Salinas, R., Counsell, C., Prasad, K., et al.: Treating neurocysticercosis medically: A systematic review of randomized, controlled trials. Trop. Med. Int. Health *4*:713–718, 1999.
128. Sarti, E., Flisser, A., Schantz, P. M., et al.: Development and evaluation of a health education intervention against *Taenia solium* in a rural community in Mexico. Am. J. Trop. Med. Hyg. *56*:127–132, 1997.
129. Sarti, E., Schantz, P. M., Avila, G., et al.: Mass treatment against human taeniasis for the control of cysticercosis: A population based intervention study. Trans. R. Soc. Trop. Med. Hyg. *94*:85–89, 2000.
130. Scharf, D.: Neurocysticercosis: Two hundred thirty-eight cases from a California hospital. Arch. Neurol. *45*:777–780, 1988.
131. Shea, M., Maberley, A. L., Walter, J., et al.: Intraocular *Taenia crassiceps* (Cestoda). Trans. Am. Acad. Ophthalmol. Otolaryngol. *77*:778–783, 1973.
132. Sheth, T. N., Pilon, L., Keystone, J., and Kucharczyk, W.: Persistent MR contrast enhancement of calcified neurocysticercosis lesions. A. J. N. R. Am. J. Neuroradiol. *19*:79–82, 1998.
133. Sidky, H. A., Hassan, Z. A., Hassan, R. R., et al.: Disseminated *Hymenolepis nana* in blood of a filarial patient. J. Egypt Soc. Parasitol. *17*:155–159, 1987.
134. Sotelo, J., and Del Brutto, O. H.: Brain cysticercosis. Arch. Med. Res. *31*:3–14, 2000.
135. Sotelo, J., and Jung, H.: Pharmacokinetic optimisation of the treatment of neurocysticercosis. Clin. Pharmacokinet. *34*:503–515, 1998.
136. Stefaniak, J.: Fine needle aspiration biopsy in the differential diagnosis of the liver cystic echinococcosis. Acta Trop. *67*:107–111, 1997.
137. St. Geme, J. W., III, Maldonado, Y. A., Enzmann, D., et al.: Consensus: Diagnosis and management of neurocysticercosis in children. Pediatr. Infect. Dis. J. *12*:455–461, 1993.
138. Stone, W. B., and Manwell, R. D.: Potential helminth infections in humans from pet or laboratory mice and hamsters. Public Health Rep. *81*:647–653, 1966.
139. Tarassov, V.: De l'immunite envers le bothriocephale *Diphyllobothrium latum* (L.). Ann. Parasitol. Hum. Comp. *15*:524–528, 1937.
140. Tesfa-Yohannes, T. M.: Observations on self-induced *Taenia saginata* infection. Ethiop. Med. J. *28*:91–93, 1990.
141. Thompson, R. C. A., and Lymbery, A. J. (eds.): *Echinococcus* and Hydatid Disease. Wallingford, Oxon, UK, CAB International, 1995.
142. Thompson, R. C. A., Lymbery, A. J., and Constantine, C. C.: Variation in *Echinococcus*: Towards a taxonomic revision of the genus. Adv. Parasitol. *35*:145–176, 1995.
143. Thompson, W. M., Chisholm, D. P., and Tank, R.: Plain film roentgenographic findings in alveolar hydatid disease: *Echinococcus multilocularis*. A. J. R. Radium Ther. Nucl. Med. *116*:345–358, 1972.
144. Thornton, H., and Goldsmid, J. M.: Cellophane tape as an aid to the detection of *Taenia saginata* eggs. Cent. Afr. J. Med. *19*:149–151, 1973.
145. Tsang, V. C., Brand, J. A., and Boyer, A. E.: An enzyme-linked immunoelectrotransfer blot assay and glycoprotein antigens for diagnosing human cysticercosis *(Taenia solium)*. J. Infect. Dis. *159*:50–59, 1989.
146. Tsou, M. H., and Huang, T. W.: Pathology of subcutaneous sparganosis: Report of two cases. J. Formos. Med. Assoc. *92*:649–653, 1993.
147. Verster, A.: A taxonomic revision of the genus *Taenia* Linnaeus, 1758. Onderstepoort J. Vet. Res. *36*:3–58, 1969.
148. Verster, A., and Tustin, R. C.: Treatment of the larval stage of *Taenia multiceps* with praziquantel. J. S. Afr. Vet. Assoc. *53*:107–108, 1982.
149. Vik, R.: The genus *Diphyllobothrium*: An example of the interdependence of systematics and experimental biology. Exp. Parasitol. *15*:361–380, 1964.
150. von Bonsdorff, B.: In which part of the intestinal canal is the fish tapeworm found? Acta Med. Scand. *129*:142–144, 1947.
151. Weisse, M. E., and Raszka, W. V., Jr.: Cestode infection in children. Adv. Pediatr. Infect. Dis. *12*:109–153, 1997.
152. Wen, H., and Yang, W. G.: Public health importance of cystic echinococcosis in China. Acta Trop. *67*:133–145, 1997.
153. White, A. C., Jr.: Neurocysticercosis: A major cause of neurological disease worldwide. Clin. Infect. Dis. *24*:101–115, 1997.
154. White, A. C., Jr.: Neurocysticercosis: Updates on epidemiology, pathogenesis, diagnosis, and management. Annu. Rev. Med. *51*:187–206, 2000.
155. White, A. C., Jr., Robinson, P., and Kuhn, R.: *Taenia solium* cysticercosis: Host-parasite interactions and the immune response. Chem. Immunol. *66*:209–230, 1997.
156. Wilkins, P. P., Allan, J. C., Verastegui, M., et al.: Development of a serologic assay to detect *Taenia solium* taeniasis. Am. J. Trop. Med. Hyg. *60*:199–204, 1999.
157. Wilson, J. F., Rausch, R. L., McMahon, B. J., et al.: Parasiticidal effect of chemotherapy in alveolar hydatid disease: Review of experience with mebendazole and albendazole in Alaskan Eskimos. Clin. Infect. Dis. *15*:234–249, 1992.
158. Woo, E., Yu, L., and Huang, C. Y.: Cerebral infarct precipitated by praziquantel in neurocysticercosis: A cautionary note. Trop. Geogr. Med. *40*:143–146, 1988.
159. Wortman, P. D.: Subcutaneous cysticercosis. J. Am. Acad. Dermatol. *25*:409–414, 1991.
160. Yokogawa, S., and Kobayashi, H.: On the species of *Diphyllobothrium mansoni* sensu lato and the infectious mode of human sparganosis. Far Eastern Association of Tropical Medicine. Transactions of the Eighth Congress. Bangkok, 1930, *2*:215–226, 1932.
161. Zee, C. S., Go, J. L., Kim, P. E., and DiGiorgio, C. M.: Imaging of neurocysticercosis. Neuroimaging Clin. N. Am. *10*:391–407, 2000.

TREMATODES

CHAPTER 226 Trematodes

JERROLD A. TURNER

The class of flatworms called trematodes or flukes contains several important species that cause infection in humans. Although schistosomes are trematodes, major differences in their morphology, biology, and clinical aspects require that they be considered separately. Trematodes other than schistosomes all have common characteristics. The adult worm usually is flat and leaf shaped, and it possesses an oral and ventral sucker and a bifurcated, blind-ended gastrointestinal tract. It is hermaphroditic and produces operculated eggs. The operculum, a lid-like structure at one end of the egg, covers the opening through which a ciliated larva will hatch. Snails are intermediate hosts for the trematodes. Depending on the species of fluke, the snail intermediate host is infected either by direct penetration by the ciliated larva or by ingestion of the unhatched egg. Complex larval development and multiplication occur within the snail host, with large numbers of larvae called cercariae ultimately produced. In most trematode life cycles, the cercariae emerge from aquatic snails and swim about until they attach to the appropriate second intermediate host, which may be fish, crustaceans, mollusks, or aquatic vegetation, depending on the species of fluke. After attachment, the larvae develop into metacercariae within protective cyst walls. At this stage, they are infectious for the definitive hosts. Researchers have estimated that more than 40 million people have food-borne trematode infections.[6] Many of the medically important flukes have a relatively wide range of definitive hosts. Fluke infections usually are diagnosed by demonstration of the characteristic ova. Advances in the identification of specific antigens and the use of enzyme-linked immunosorbent assays (ELISAs), immunoblotting techniques, DNA probes, and polymerase chain reaction may produce tests that are especially valuable in the diagnosis of lung and liver flukes. Intestinal and liver flukes have been reviewed.[25]

Fasciolopsiasis

THE ORGANISM

The adult form of *Fasciolopsis buski,* the giant intestinal fluke, measures up to 7.5 cm in length and attaches to the mucosa of the proximal end of the small intestine. It begins producing eggs approximately 3 months after infection, and the adult worm has a life span of approximately 6 months. The eggs are excreted in stool. The oval eggs of *Fasciolopsis* measure approximately 130 to 140 µm in length by 80 to 85 µm in breadth. A single parasite may excrete 25,000 eggs daily. After several weeks in fresh water, the ciliated larvae hatch from the eggs and penetrate snails, where they undergo further larval development. Cercariae emerge from the snail approximately 1 to 2 months later and encyst on a wide variety of aquatic vegetation.

TRANSMISSION

The infective larvae are encysted on aquatic plants, which if ingested raw, cause infection. Water chestnuts, caltrop, and water bamboo are common sources of infection. Water chestnuts often are peeled with the teeth, which fosters the ingestion of larvae attached to the outer coat of the nut.

EPIDEMIOLOGY

Fasciolopsiasis occurs most commonly in China, Southeast Asia, Bangladesh, and Assam State in India. Human infection has been reported in many other areas of India and the Far East, but the prevalence appears to be relatively low. A common reservoir host in many areas is the domestic pig. The level of infection in the human population correlates with the practice of cultivating edible aquatic vegetation in ponds that are fertilized with human feces. Infection rates are often highest in schoolchildren.

PATHOLOGY AND PATHOGENESIS

The parasites usually are found in the duodenum and jejunum but have been reported, in heavy infections, to involve the stomach, ileum, and colon. Inflammation, ulceration, and small abscesses may develop in the intestinal mucosa where the parasites are attached. Increased mucus secretion and minimal bleeding may occur. Intestinal obstruction may develop in massive infections. The edema and ascites accompanying severe infections have been attributed to toxic metabolites of the parasite or to a reaction to parasite allergens. More likely is that protein-losing enteropathy and malabsorption associated with hypoalbuminemia cause these findings. Children with heavy infections appear to be particularly vulnerable to the systemic manifestations.

CLINICAL MANIFESTATIONS

Usually, but not always, the severity of symptoms is correlated with the number of parasites. Epigastric pains resembling "hunger pains" or peptic ulcer disease and relieved by food intake have been reported as early as 30 days after exposure. Diarrhea and abdominal pain may be intermittent and may occur separately or simultaneously. In heavy infections, nausea and vomiting may develop. Facial edema, anasarca, and ascites are encountered in advanced, severe infections. Eosinophilia with counts greater than 30 percent is not uncommon. Leukocytosis and mild anemia may be noted.

In endemic areas, for a child to have multiple intestinal parasites and a borderline nutritional status is not unusual. Fasciolopsiasis adds an additional burden to the host defense mechanisms and may be responsible, in concert with the other stresses, for significant morbidity.

DIAGNOSIS

The eggs of *Fasciolopsis* are demonstrated easily by routine fecal examination, but they are virtually indistinguishable from those of the liver fluke *Fasciola hepatica* and the echinostomes. Epidemiologic information, such as travel history and exposure to sources of infection, may be helpful in determining the diagnosis. Because of the short life span of the adult worm, anyone who has been absent from an endemic area for longer than 9 months is not likely to have persisting infection with *Fasciolopsis*. Therefore, eggs present in stool would be attributable to the longer-lived *Fasciola*.

TREATMENT AND PROGNOSIS

Praziquantel, 75 mg/kg divided into three doses given in 1 day, is effective therapy and has few side effects. Although the U.S. Food and Drug Administration has approved praziquantel for use in clonorchiasis and opisthorchiasis, it is considered investigational for *Fasciolopsis* infection.

Infections treated early and most light infections, even when untreated, have an excellent prognosis. Heavy infections in children, especially when complicated by intestinal obstruction, edema, or concomitant secondary infections, have a much graver prognosis.

PREVENTION

Fasciolopsiasis is prevented easily by cooking aquatic vegetation or by immersing the plants or nuts briefly in boiling water. The use of human feces as fertilizer in aqua culture is a major cause of human infection, and this practice should be discouraged. Successful efforts in health education appear to have reduced the transmission of this parasite in some endemic areas.

Heterophyiasis

More than 10 different species of the family Heterophyidae have been reported to cause human infection. Except for two species, *Heterophyes heterophyes* and *Metagonimus yokogawai,* these infections are relatively uncommon and are incidental to the prevalence in other mammals and birds.

THE ORGANISMS

H. heterophyes and *M. yokogawai* adult worms attach to the mucosa of the small intestine. The parasites are only 1 to 2.5 mm long and less than 1 mm wide. They often burrow deeply into the mucosa. The eggs measure 26 to 30 μm in length and 15 to 17 μm in width. The eggs of the two species are essentially identical and also resemble the eggs of *Opisthorchis (Clonorchis)* spp. Careful study of egg size and shape has not provided a definitive method for differentiating these species.[7] Eggs excreted in stool are fully embryonated. The snail intermediate host becomes infected by ingesting the trematode egg. After multiplication in the snail, cercariae emerge and encyst under the scales or in the skin or flesh of a variety of fresh-water fish. After ingestion by the definitive host, the metacercariae are freed from their cysts and develop into adults in as little as 5 days.

TRANSMISSION AND EPIDEMIOLOGY

Humans acquire the infection by eating fresh-water fish that is raw, inadequately cooked, pickled, or salted.

Heterophyiasis occurs worldwide. Areas of endemic human infection are Southeast Asia, the Middle East, China, Japan, Taiwan, the Philippines, and parts of the former Soviet Union. Many reservoir hosts, such as dogs, cats, and fish-eating birds, may play an important role in maintenance of infection in some endemic areas. Detailed lists of the distribution and hosts of heterophyid species are available.[42]

PATHOLOGY AND PATHOGENESIS

The small heterophyid flukes may produce superficial inflammation and erosion at the sites of mucosal attachment. When the mucosa is penetrated, eggs may be deposited in tissues and produce granulomatous lesions that contain eosinophils. Eggs may gain access to the intestinal capillaries or lymphatics and embolize to distant sites. The myocardium, brain, spinal cord, liver, lungs, and spleen have been involved. The complications of embolic heterophyiasis appear to be particularly frequent in the Philippines, where heart disease often is attributed to heterophyiasis. The embolized eggs induce a granulomatous response, with the eventual production of fibrosis in the affected tissues.

CLINICAL MANIFESTATIONS

Light infections without the deposition of ectopic eggs are usually asymptomatic, although eosinophilia may be noted. In heavier infections, abdominal pain, often suggestive of peptic ulcer disease, is a common symptom. Intermittent diarrhea may occur. Seizures may result from eggs carried to the brain. Congestive heart failure or arrhythmias may occur after cardiac involvement.

DIAGNOSIS

Routine fecal examination demonstrates eggs, but differentiating *Opisthorchis* and *Clonorchis* eggs from heterophyid eggs is difficult. Eggs recovered from biliary drainage or from persons who have been out of endemic areas for more than 2 years can be assumed to be those of *Opisthorchis* or *Clonorchis.* The heterophyid worms have a relatively short life span when compared with that of the liver flukes.

TREATMENT AND PROGNOSIS

Praziquantel as used for fasciolopsiasis (discussed earlier) is effective.

With the exception of the complication of egg emboli to distant organs, the prognosis is excellent.

PREVENTION

If fresh-water fish were cooked adequately, heterophyiasis would disappear from the human population. Unfortunately, it is not an easy task to change human behavior or cultural traditions. Education concerning sources of infection and the need to prevent feeding raw fish to dogs and cats may reduce the prevalence of the disease.

Paragonimiasis

Paragonimus westermani is the species of lung fluke that causes most human infections. At least nine other species have been recovered from humans and in some instances have been found in distinct endemic foci. Reviews that include detailed discussion of the taxonomy and distribution of the genus are available.[4, 21]

THE ORGANISM

The adult forms of *Paragonimus* measure about 15 mm long by about 6 mm wide. They are nearly as thick as they are wide. The worms are located in the lungs. Eggs measuring 80 to 118 µm by 48 to 60 µm are discharged into the bronchi and are either expectorated or swallowed and excreted in feces. The larva hatches from the egg after at least 2 weeks of development in water. The free-swimming larva penetrates the snail intermediate host and undergoes development and multiplication for several weeks. Cercariae emerge and encyst in the tissues of fresh-water crabs and crayfish. When humans or reservoir hosts ingest the flesh of these second intermediate hosts, the larvae penetrate the wall of the intestine and migrate through or around the diaphragm to reach the lungs. In some instances, the worms may lodge in ectopic sites within the abdomen, in subcutaneous tissue, or in the central nervous system (CNS). The worms usually are found singly or in pairs within a capsule or cyst of reactive host tissue. Approximately 2 to 3 months are required from the time of ingestion until the worms are fully mature. In most infections, the worms die within 10 years; however, production of eggs for 20 years after the individual has left the endemic area has been reported.

TRANSMISSION AND EPIDEMIOLOGY

The infection is acquired by eating fresh-water crabs or crayfish that are raw, inadequately cooked, salted, pickled, or soaked in wine. Cooked foods may be contaminated with viable larvae from the hands, utensils, or cutting boards used in the preparation of crabs or crayfish.

Cats, civet cats, wild felids, foxes, wolves, dogs, pigs, and mongooses are significant reservoir hosts for *P. westermani*. Infection in humans is endemic in China, Taiwan, Korea, Japan, eastern India, Sri Lanka, Southeast Asia, Indonesia, and some areas of the former Soviet Union. Instances of paragonimiasis being acquired in North America are extremely rare.[29, 33]

More than nine different species of *Paragonimus* infect humans. In many areas, the distribution of these species often overlaps that of *P. westermani*. Significant foci of human infection with other species occur in West Africa and the Congo Valley, Mexico, South America, China, and Japan. The potential exists for transmission of paragonimiasis in the United States.[33]

The distribution and epidemiology of the various species of *Paragonimus* were reviewed in 1995.[6]

PATHOLOGY AND PATHOGENESIS

After penetration of the pleura, the worms locate near larger bronchioles or bronchi, where an exudate of neutrophils and eosinophils forms around them. In time, the area about the parasite organizes into a fibrotic wall, which may be thin or several millimeters thick. The cysts usually measure 1 to 2 cm in diameter and often are filled with a brownish material that probably contains hematin. The cyst often opens to a bronchiole or bronchus, which provides a route for discharge of the eggs into sputum. Secondary bacterial infection of the cysts or chronic bronchitis, bronchiectasis, and pneumonia are complications of the disease.

Cerebral paragonimiasis results when the parasites migrate into the brain. The theory that the parasites travel to the brain via the jugular foramina has not been confirmed. All areas of the brain and meninges are susceptible to invasion. The parasites and the eggs cause areas of central necrosis and granuloma formation with dense collagenous walls surrounded by lymphocytes, plasma cells, eosinophils, and Charcot-Leyden crystals. The lesions vary in size, may be several centimeters in diameter, and may appear cystic. Eventually, the wall may calcify. Spinal cord lesions are similar. Other sites at which worms may cause cysts or abscesses are the intestinal wall, mesentery, peritoneal cavity, liver, diaphragm, myocardium, and subcutaneous tissue.

CLINICAL MANIFESTATIONS

Migration of the worms from the intestinal tract to the lungs usually causes no symptoms, but diarrhea, abdominal pain, and urticaria may occur in the first 3 weeks after exposure. These symptoms may be followed closely by chest discomfort, cough, dyspnea, fever, and night sweats.

The established pulmonary infection is often asymptomatic, but frequently a chronic cough that is productive of mucoid, rust-colored, or blood-streaked sputum is present. Hemoptysis is usually intermittent and occasionally may be severe. Eosinophilia is a common finding in the early stages of infection but may return to normal over a period of months or years.

Complications of pneumothorax, pleural effusion, empyema, and pneumonia occur more often in association with heavy infections.

Cerebral paragonimiasis occurs in less than 1 percent of infections but results in serious morbidity and often death.[23] Cerebral involvement is more common in children, with more than half the infections occurring before the child reaches 10 years of age. This form of paragonimiasis may initially be manifested as a mass lesion, a seizure disorder, meningitis, or a cerebrovascular accident. Seizures often begin as the focal motor type but progress to generalized seizures as the disease worsens. Visual disturbances, headache, and elevated cerebrospinal fluid (CSF) pressure are common events. Pleocytosis with eosinophilia in the CSF may be noted.

The variety of neurologic manifestations depends on the number, location, and size of the lesions. Spinal cord lesions are often extradural and mimic mass lesions caused by tumors or infection.

Cutaneous paragonimiasis is identified by the appearance of subcutaneous nodules, which may be fixed or migratory. In China, species of *Paragonimus* found in the northern region often cause subcutaneous, migratory lesions associated with fever and eosinophilia. Worms recovered from these lesions are immature.

DIAGNOSIS

In light pulmonary infections, normal results on chest radiographs are not unusual. However, radiographic abnormalities may develop as the worms enter the lungs. Initially, the chest film shows basilar pneumonic infiltrates that are poorly defined. These areas become better demonstrated as cysts or nodules within a few weeks. Some initial pleural reaction, usually at the base of the lung, may occur and can be associated with effusion. Although the nodules and cysts of the chronic stage of infection may develop in any area of the lung, including the apices, they tend to localize in the periphery of the middle and lower lung fields. A common radiographic diagnostic feature is a "ring shadow." This finding represents the circular or oval thin-walled cyst with a crescent-shaped opacity along one side.

Cerebral paragonimiasis may be seen as an avascular mass on computed tomography. In long-standing cerebral infections, the cyst-like structures may calcify and be seen as a cluster of "soap bubbles." The individual oval or spherical bubbles may measure from 2 to 40 mm in diameter, and a cluster of these structures may extend 10 cm. Magnetic resonance imaging is not as effective in demonstrating calcification, but it is a useful supplement in defining the lesions of cerebral infection.[32]

Pulmonary paragonimiasis is diagnosed definitively by finding the characteristic eggs in sputum or stool. Several immunodiagnostic tests, complement fixation, ELISA, DNA probes, and immunoblotting have been developed.[29] Immunodiagnosis is especially useful in infections in which eggs are not demonstrated easily, such as in cerebral paragonimiasis. None of the immunologic tests appears to be consistently helpful in monitoring the success of treatment. Antigen-detection systems may be a more productive approach for this purpose.[44] Intradermal testing cannot distinguish between past and current infections, but it has been useful in performing epidemiologic studies.

Pulmonary paragonimiasis often is mistaken for tuberculosis. A careful history may provide information about travel and food habits that point to the correct diagnosis.

TREATMENT AND PROGNOSIS

Praziquantel, 75 mg/kg divided into three doses, is given daily for 2 days. In the United States, the drug is considered investigational when used for this purpose. Bithionol is an alternative drug that is available in the United States through the Centers for Disease Control and Prevention (CDC) in Atlanta. Bithionol is given in single doses of 30 to 50 mg/kg on alternate days for a total of 10 to 15 doses. Side effects occur much more commonly with bithionol than with praziquantel. Experimental administration of triclabendazole was at least as effective as praziquantel against *Paragonimus mexicana* infections in humans in Ecuador.[5]

The prognosis is good in most pulmonary infections, even if untreated, although symptoms may persist for many years. Treatment effectively resolves the pulmonary lesions and symptoms. The prognosis for CNS involvement depends on the location and extent of the lesions but is usually grave.

PREVENTION

The key in prevention is education of the population in endemic areas concerning the source of infection. Crabs and crayfish, prepared in a manner that transmits paragonimiasis, are delicacies in many parts of the world. Changing attitudes about food habits is no easy task, and that even mass treatment and improved sanitation could eliminate the occurrence of human infections is doubtful because of animal reservoirs.

Fascioliasis

The sheep liver fluke *Fasciola hepatica* causes fascioliasis. *Fasciola gigantica* is a closely related liver fluke that has a more limited geographic distribution and is reported as a cause of infection in humans much less frequently.

THE ORGANISM

The adult of *F. hepatica* measures up to 30 mm in length and 13 mm in width. The surface has scale-like spines, and the anterior portion of the worm is cone shaped. The worms reside in the bile ducts, and eggs appear in the bile and eventually are excreted in feces. Eggs measure approximately 130 μm in length and up to 90 μm in width. The eggs are indistinguishable from those of *F. buski*. After incubation in water for several days, the ciliated larva hatches from the egg and swims about in search of the snail intermediate host. The larva penetrates the snail and undergoes a complex cycle of asexual multiplication. Cercariae, which are the final stage of this asexual cycle, leave the snail and encyst on fresh-water vegetation, often watercress. These encysted metacercariae initiate infection when the mammalian host ingests the raw aquatic vegetation or drinks water contaminated with metacercariae. The metacercariae excyst in the intestine, penetrate the intestinal wall, and migrate in the peritoneal cavity to the liver. The developing worms penetrate the liver capsule and burrow through the parenchyma to the bile ducts. The adult worms feed on liver cells and duct epithelium.

TRANSMISSION AND EPIDEMIOLOGY

Ingestion of infected raw watercress is the most frequent cause of infection in humans. Water from ponds or marshes with infected vegetation may contain metacercariae. Infections occur in humans who have no history of eating watercress but have ingested water from sources that potentially are infected. The distribution of fascioliasis is worldwide, with the highest numbers of infected humans reported from Peru, Bolivia, Ecuador, Egypt, Iran, France, and Portugal. Autochthonous cases in the United States are rare. Sheep, goats, and cattle serve as the most common reservoir hosts, but many mammals are susceptible to infection. A detailed review of the epidemiology of fascioliasis has been published.[16] *F. gigantica* infections are predominantly infections in cattle. Human infection with *F. gigantica* occurs in Africa, the former Soviet Union, Vietnam, Hawaii, and Iraq.

PATHOLOGY AND PATHOGENESIS

Significant damage to liver tissues occurs as the juvenile worms migrate through the liver tissue to the bile ducts.

Linear necrotic lesions containing eosinophils form as worms progress through the liver parenchyma. Flukes that die before reaching the bile ducts may produce necrotic cavities that eventually evolve into fibrous scar tissue. Adult worms in the bile ducts cause inflammation and adenomatous changes in biliary epithelium. Ductal and periductal fibrosis occurs. The gallbladder and extrahepatic ducts may be invaded and undergo similar inflammatory and fibrotic reactions. Adult worms may migrate back into liver parenchyma through eroded biliary epithelium and cause abscess formation.

Heavy infections often are associated with anemia, which is attributed partially to blood loss from the biliary tract.

Juvenile flukes that fail to find their way into the liver may wander about and cause ectopic fascioliasis. They may appear in the intestine, pancreas, subcutaneous tissue, brain, eye, and other locations.

CLINICAL MANIFESTATIONS

The first symptoms of fascioliasis occur approximately 4 to 6 weeks after infection, but this period varies widely, depending on host response and the number of parasites. The acute stage of infection occurs during the migration of worms in the liver. Children often have severe symptoms of right upper quadrant or generalized abdominal pain, tender hepatomegaly, fever, anemia, and eosinophilia. Sweating, dizziness, wheezing, and urticaria may occur. This stage may last 1 to 3 months. The chronic form of the disease is less well defined and includes a variety of symptoms related to the biliary system. These symptoms are frequently identical to those of gallbladder disease, cholangitis, and pancreatitis caused by nonparasitic conditions. Elevation in alkaline phosphatase levels is common. Patients often endure years of biliary tract symptoms before the diagnosis of fascioliasis is considered. Heavy infections eventually may cause sufficient liver damage to produce cirrhosis with all of the classic complications of this condition. Chronic infection with *F. hepatica* also may be asymptomatic but often is associated with eosinophilia. If ectopic localization of immature *F. hepatica* flukes occurs, it is usually in the subcutaneous tissues of the thorax, back, and extremities. A detailed review of the clinical aspects of human fascioliasis has been published.[3] The manifestations of fascioliasis in a series of 16 Egyptian children also have been described.[11]

DIAGNOSIS

Routine stool examination using a formalin–ethyl acetate concentration technique should reveal ova of *Fasciola* in established infections. The problem of differentiating *Fasciolopsis* and *Fasciola* eggs was discussed in the section on fasciolopsiasis. False-positive stool examinations may occur if the patient ingests infected liver. Keeping the patient on a diet free of liver for 3 days before collecting the stool specimen eliminates this unusual possibility.

Because ova are not produced until approximately 4 months after infection (range, 3 to 18 months), diagnosis of fascioliasis during the acute stage of liver migration must rely on a combination of clinical findings, imaging studies, and immunologic tests. Obtaining a history of eating raw watercress or drinking surface water from an area that may be contaminated by domestic animals is helpful. The syndrome of fever, hepatomegaly, and eosinophilia is consistent with the diagnosis. Radiologic imaging of the liver may demonstrate findings of tract-like small abscesses, subcapsular lesions, and slow evolution of the lesions on follow-up examinations.[19] Computed tomography detects parenchymal lesions, and ultrasonography effectively evaluates the biliary tract and gallbladder. Magnetic resonance imaging findings have been reported.[20] A variety of immunologic tests have been developed. An ELISA using excretory-secretory products from adult worms has been useful in detecting serum antibodies without cross-reactivity with other trematode infections.[12, 13, 37] Serologic tests also should be useful in the diagnosis of ectopic fascioliasis.

Chronic fascioliasis may be detected during radiologic studies of the biliary tract or gallbladder. Adult worms may be seen on ultrasonography or appear as curvilinear lucent areas in the contrast medium at cholangiography.

TREATMENT AND PROGNOSIS

Unlike other trematode infections, fascioliasis is relatively resistant to praziquantel. Treatment with bithionol is effective. In the United States, this drug is available for investigational use only and must be obtained from the CDC. It usually is administered in a dose of 30 mg/kg given either daily for 5 days or on alternate days for a total of five doses.[14] More intense courses of 30 to 50 mg/kg on alternate days for 10 to 15 doses also have been recommended. Triclabendazole is a benzimidazole compound manufactured by Novartis Pharma AG of Switzerland as Fasinex. It is not available in the United States, but it has been registered in Egypt. The drug has been used successfully in a variety of open clinical trials in adults and children for both acute and chronic fascioliasis.[1, 2, 9, 10, 18, 26, 31, 43] It is given in a dosage of 10 mg/kg in a single dose with a meal to enhance absorption. Treatment failures usually respond to a second course of triclabendazole. Triclabendazole is effective against both migrating worms and established infections. After successful treatment, the eosinophilia resolves slowly and immunologic tests become negative.

In some instances, children with severe acute infections have been treated with 5 to 10 mg of prednisone before using specific fasciolicidal drugs.[15]

Heavy infections in children may be fatal during the acute stage of the disease. However, most become chronic or, possibly, asymptomatic. The variable reaction of the human host and the number of parasites determine the outcome. In heavy infections, hepatic damage may be significant, with fibrotic scarring or abscess formation. Chronic or recurrent biliary tract problems are common.

PREVENTION

Watercress grown for human consumption should be protected from human and animal fecal contamination. Animal fascioliasis can be targeted for chemotherapeutic control, and control of the snail intermediate hosts with molluscicides can be attempted. Effort should be made to educate the population at risk regarding the danger of eating raw watercress harvested from unprotected waters and the hazard of drinking untreated or filtered surface water.

Clonorchiasis and Opisthorchiasis

Three similar trematodes of the genus *Opisthorchis* infect the bile ducts of humans. Although the name *Opisthorchis sinensis* is proper parasitologically, this organism more commonly is called *Clonorchis sinensis,* and the name of the infection, clonorchiasis, is well entrenched in the clinical literature. This organism also is called the Chinese or Oriental liver fluke. *Opisthorchis viverrini* and *Opisthorchis felineus* have similar life cycles and produce similar lesions and illnesses in humans.

THE ORGANISMS

The adult flukes measure from 4 to 20 mm in length by 2 to 3 mm in breadth. They are found in the intrahepatic biliary ducts. The small operculate eggs, similar to those of the heterophyid flukes, appear in bile and are excreted in feces. The snail intermediate host ingests the embryonated egg, and free-swimming cercariae emerge from the snail approximately 6 to 8 weeks later. The cercariae encyst under the scales and in the flesh of a variety of fresh-water fish. When the raw, inadequately cooked, or pickled fish is eaten, the larvae excyst and migrate to the intrahepatic bile ducts, usually through the ampulla of Vater and the common duct. The worms probably survive for as long as 30 years.

TRANSMISSION AND EPIDEMIOLOGY

The ingestion of raw, inadequately cooked, or pickled fresh-water fish that have encysted larvae in their tissues initiates infection.

C. sinensis is endemic in China, Japan, Korea, Taiwan, and Vietnam. High prevalence rates in Hong Kong are attributed to the importation of fish from mainland China. Natural reservoir hosts are cats, dogs, pigs, and rats.

O. viverrini is fairly well localized to the northern areas of Thailand, where a dish prepared from chopped raw fish, called koi pla, is popular. Researchers have estimated that more than 7 million residents of that area are infected.[35] Cats, civet cats, dogs, and other fish-eating mammals serve as reservoirs. In China and other Asian countries, edible fish often are raised in ponds that are fertilized with human feces, thus providing perfect conditions for the entire life cycle of the parasite.

O. felineus is endemic in central Siberia and in eastern and southeastern Europe. Cats, dogs, and foxes serve as major reservoirs. Human infection is limited to groups that habitually consume raw, dried, or freshly salted fish or fish lightly pickled in garlic juice. Sporadic infections with *O. felineus* have been reported from several Asian countries.

The distribution of infection by all species in human infections depends on the eating habits of the population. In most areas, the prevalence is higher in older persons, but in Thailand, even infants are infected.

PATHOLOGY AND PATHOGENESIS

The epithelium of infected bile ducts reacts with desquamation, adenomatous hyperplasia, and metaplasia of goblet cells accompanied by an increase in mucus production. Mechanical damage from the flukes' suckers and metabolites from the worms are thought to be the cause. Ductal dilatation and bile stasis probably increase susceptibility to bacterial cholangitis. Inflammation of the bile duct wall usually indicates secondary infection.[8] Chronic infection may lead to considerable periductal fibrosis, but it does not progress to portal cirrhosis.[8] The presence of the parasites in addition to other factors appears to render the host susceptible to cholangiocarcinoma. Experiments in hamsters show that a nitrosamine carcinogen combined with *O. viverrini* infection induces cholangiocarcinoma, but infection alone or carcinogen alone does not.[40] An extensive analysis of the available data concerning cancer and liver flukes has concluded that infection with *O. viverrini* is carcinogenic to humans and that infection with *C. sinensis* is probably carcinogenic.[36] Data were not sufficient to determine the status of *O. felineus* infections. *O. viverrini* infections frequently involve the gallbladder. Complications may include cholecystitis and the formation of gallstones. The parasites often are found in the pancreatic ducts, where reactions of the epithelium are similar to those in the bile duct. Pancreatitis occurs infrequently in these liver fluke infections and is usually mild.

CLINICAL MANIFESTATIONS

The intensity of infection probably correlates with the occurrence of symptoms. Light and moderate infections in endemic areas appear asymptomatic. Patients with heavy infections may complain of right upper quadrant abdominal pain, weakness, or malaise and may have significant hepatic enlargement.[41] Studies of patients with chronic clonorchiasis who have left the endemic areas failed to find significant symptoms or any evidence of liver dysfunction associated with the infection.[30, 39] However, clonorchiasis has been detected in most cases of pancreatitis in Chinese immigrants.[6] An uncontrolled study of patients with *O. viverrini* infections in Thailand showed general improvement in well-being after treatment.[34] Symptoms of abdominal distress and epigastric pain declined significantly. A community study showed significant improvement in the infected population after receiving treatment based on symptoms, laboratory tests, and ultrasound abnormalities.[35]

Acute infections with fever, malaise, anorexia, diarrhea, tender hepatomegaly, and eosinophilia have been reported. These symptoms may develop in heavy infections 10 to 26 days after ingestion of the larvae. The eosinophilia of acute infection gradually decreases and, in chronic infection, disappears.[30]

Complications are probably more likely to occur in heavy infections. Relapsing cholangitis, cholecystitis, bilirubin gallstones, pancreatitis, and cholangiocarcinoma may occur in association with infection.[22]

DIAGNOSIS

Symptoms of acute infection may develop 3 to 4 weeks before eggs appear in the stool. Suspicion of the diagnosis may be based on epidemiologic information. Serologic tests would be helpful in this situation, but they are not readily available in the United States. In chronic infections, eggs should be evident in routine fecal examinations. Filtration of fluid obtained at duodenal intubation is claimed to be diagnostically more sensitive than examination of two fecal specimens.[17] A monoclonal antibody–based ELISA has been developed for the demonstration of *O. viverrini* antigen in fecal specimens. This test appears to be specific and highly sensitive.[38]

Cholangiography often shows multiple cystic dilatations of the ducts. A combination of large cystic dilatations and small cystic ectasias or mulberry-like dilatations is considered diagnostic. The flukes may be evident as linear radiolucencies on cholangiography.

The eggs of *O. viverrini* and *C. sinensis* are virtually identical. *O. felineus* is reported to have a narrower egg, as determined by the ratio of length to width. Differentiating between the eggs of these species of liver flukes and the eggs

TABLE 226–1 ■ LESS COMMON TREMATODES THAT CAN INFECT HUMANS

	Location in Human	Adult Length/ Width (mm)	Egg Length/ Width (μm)	Geographic Distribution	Second Intermediate Hosts	Reservoir Hosts	Transmission	Clinical Manifestations
Nanophyetus salmincola	Intestine	1.1/0.5	60–80/34–50	Pacific coast of Canada and north-west U.S. and Siberia	Salmonid fish	Dog, coyote, fox, skunk, mink, lynx, and others	Ingestion of raw, undercooked, or lightly smoked salmon or trout	Diarrhea, abdominal discomfort, nausea, vomiting, eosinophilia
Dicrocoelium dendriticum	Bile ducts	15/2.5	38–45/22–30	Widespread in animals. Sporadic human cases from Europe, the former Soviet Union, Middle East, South America, China, and elsewhere	Ant	Sheep, cattle, and many other ruminants	Accidental ingestion of ants contaminating food	Information is inadequate. Abdominal pain, nausea, diarrhea, constipation, and eosinophilia are reported. Spurious infection from eating infected liver
Echinostomes—several genera and many species	Small intestines	Wide range, up to 22/2.2. Collar of spines around oral sucker	Usually greater than 100 μm in length. Depends on species. Resembles *Fasciolopsis* and *Fasciola* eggs	Southeast Asia, Indonesia, Japan, Taiwan, Philippines, and sporadic cases elsewhere	Snails, clams, tadpoles, fish	Waterfowl and other birds, rats, dogs, muskrats, cats, and pigs	Ingestion of uncooked snails, clams, tadpoles, and fish	Scant information. Diarrhea, constipation, abdominal cramps, and eosinophilia. Light infections are asymptomatic
Gastrodiscoides hominis	Cecum and ascending colon	5–8/5–14. Pear shape, large disk-shaped posterior	150/60–70. Greenish brown, tapered at both ends	Common in Assam, India. Sporadic in Vietnam, Philippines, the former Soviet Union, and other areas	Unknown, possibly aquatic vegetation	Pigs	Unknown, possibly ingestion of raw vegetation	Mucous diarrhea

of small heterophyid flukes is difficult. Fortunately, treatment with praziquantel is identical for all these parasites.

TREATMENT AND PROGNOSIS

These liver fluke infections respond well to treatment with praziquantel, 75 mg/kg divided into three doses given in a single day. Side effects of headache and dizziness are common. Although untreated light and moderate infections appear asymptomatic and may have little, if any clinical significance, the availability of a safe, easily administered drug makes treatment seem appropriate, especially for those who have left endemic areas. Treatment also may decrease the risk of cholangiocarcinoma developing in those infected. Albendazole also has been found to be effective in clonorchiasis.[38] A dose of 10 mg/kg is given daily for 7 days. Effective treatment has reversed the biliary tract abnormalities in *O. viverrini* infections and would be expected to have a similar salutary effect in clonorchiasis and *O. felineus* infections.

The prognosis of heavy infections depends on the complications. Superimposed bacterial infections are the most common cause of morbidity and mortality.

PREVENTION

Education of the population at risk about the consumption of raw fish in its various forms (dried, pickled, salted, or smoked) is about the only hope for reducing prevalence in humans. A large reservoir exists in domestic and wild animals; therefore, attempts to eliminate infection in humans by mass treatment are unlikely to succeed. Prohibiting the fertilization of fishponds with raw human sewage surely would reduce transmission.

Metorchis Infection

Metorchis conjunctus, the North American liver fluke, is a member of the Opisthorchiidae family and has a life cycle similar to that of the other opisthorchids described earlier. A wide variety of fish-eating mammals may serve as definitive hosts. This infection is a significant cause of morbidity and mortality in sled dogs in Canada. It is an occasional incidental finding on fecal examination in native communities in northern Canada. An outbreak of 19 cases of *Metorchis* infection was related to fish prepared raw as sashimi.[27] The symptoms began 1 to 15 days after ingestion of the infected fish. The severity and duration of the symptoms correlated with the amount of fish eaten. Symptoms were fatigue, upper abdominal tenderness, fever, epigastric abdominal pain, headache, weight loss, anorexia, nausea, diarrhea, vomiting, muscle pain, backache, cough, and rash (in descending order of frequency). The degree of eosinophilia and elevation in liver enzyme levels were proportional to the amount of fish ingested. Eggs were noted in stools 10 days after infection. All symptoms resolved after treatment with the standard course of praziquantel. Serologic testing indicates that a similar liver fluke, *Metorchis bilis,* is a frequent parasite of residents of the Novosibirsk area of Russia.[24]

Less Common Trematode Infections

Table 226–1 summarizes information about some of the less common trematodes that may infect humans. All have snails as the first intermediate host, and the diagnosis is made by identification of eggs on fecal examination. Infections with trematodes listed in this table probably are treated effectively with praziquantel, 75 mg/kg divided into three doses given in a single day. *Nanophyetus salmincola* infection responds to a regimen of 60 mg/kg divided into three doses given in a single day.

REFERENCES

1. Abdul-Hadi, S., Contreras, R., Tombazzi, C., et al.: Hepatic fascioliasis: Case report and review. Rev. Inst. Med. Trop. Sao Paulo *38*:69–73, 1996.
2. Apt, W., Aguilera, X., Vega, F., et al.: Treatment of human chronic fascioliasis with triclabendazole: Drug efficacy and serologic response. Am. J. Trop. Med. Hyg. *52*:532–535, 1995.
3. Arjona, R., Riancho, J. A., Aguado, J. M., et al.: Fascioliasis in developed countries: A review of classic and aberrant forms of the disease. Medicine (Baltimore) *74*:13–23, 1995.
4. Blair, D., Xu, Z., and Agatsuma, T.: Paragonimiasis and the genus *Paragonimus*. Adv. Parasitol. *42*:113–222, 1999.
5. Calvopiña, M., Guderian, R. H., Paredes, W., et al.: Treatment of human pulmonary paragonimiasis with triclabendazole: Clinical tolerance and drug efficacy. Trans. R. Soc. Trop. Med. Hyg. *92*:566–569, 1998.
6. Control of foodborne trematode infections. Report of a WHO Study Group. World Health Organ. Tech. Rep. Ser. *849*:1–157, 1995.
7. Ditrich, O., Giboda, M., Scholz, T., et al.: Comparative morphology of eggs of the Haplorchiinae (Trematoda: Heterophyidae) and some other medically important heterophyid and opisthorchiid flukes. Folia Parasitol. (Praha) *39*:123–132, 1992.
8. Dooley, J. R., and Neafie, R. C.: *In* Binford, C. H., and Connor, D. H. (eds.): Pathology of Tropical and Extraordinary Diseases. Vol. 2. Washington, D. C., Armed Forces Institute of Pathology, 1976, pp. 509–516.
9. el-Karaksy, H., Hassanein, B., Okasha, S., et al.: Human fascioliasis in Egyptian children: Successful treatment with triclabendazole. J. Trop. Pediatr. *45*:135–138, 1999.
10. el-Morshedy, H., Farghaly, A., Sharaf, S., et al.: Triclabendazole in the treatment of human fascioliasis: A community-based study. Eastern Mediterranean Health J. *5*:888–894, 2000.
11. El-Shabrawi, M., El-Karaksy, H., et al.: Human fascioliasis: Clinical features and diagnostic difficulties in Egyptian children. J. Trop. Pediatr. *43*:162–166, 1997.
12. Espino, A. M., Dumenigo, B. E., Fernandez, R., et al.: Immunodiagnosis of human fascioliasis by enzyme-linked immunosorbent assay using excretory-secretory products. Am. J. Trop. Med. Hyg. *37*:605–608, 1987.
13. Espino, A. M., and Finlay, C. M.: Sandwich enzyme-linked immunosorbent assay for detection of excretory-secretory antigens in humans with fascioliasis. J. Clin. Microbiol. *32*:190–193, 1994.
14. Farag, H. F., Salem, A., el-Hifni, S. A., et al.: Bithionol (Bitin) treatment in established fascioliasis in Egyptians. J. Trop. Med. Hyg. *91*:240–244, 1988.
15. Farid, Z., Mansour, N., Kamal, M., et al.: The treatment of acute *Fasciola hepatica* infection in children. Trop. Geogr. Med. *42*:95–96, 1990.
16. [Fascioliasis.] Wkly. Epidemiol. Rec. *67*(44):326–329, 1992.
17. Feldmeier, H., and Horstmann, R. D.: Filtration of duodenal fluid for the diagnosis of opisthorchiasis. Ann. Trop. Med. Parasitol. *75*:462–465, 1981.
18. Hammouda, N. A., el-Mansoury, S. T., el-Azzouni, M. Z., and el-Gohari, Y.: Therapeutic effect of triclabendazole in patients with fascioliasis in Egypt. A preliminary study. J. Egyptian Soc. Parasitol. *25*:137–143, 1995.
19. Han, J. K., Choi, B. I., Cho, J. M., et al.: Radiological findings of human fascioliasis. Abdom. Imaging *18*:261–264, 1993.
20. Han, J. K., Han, D., Choi, B. I., and Han, M. C.: MR findings in human fascioliasis. Trop. Med. Int. Health *1*:367–372, 1996.
21. Kagawa, F. T.: Pulmonary paragonimiasis. Semin. Respir. Infect. *12*:149–158, 1997.
22. Kurathong, S., Lerdverasirikul, P., Wongpaitoon, V., et al.: *Opisthorchis viverrini* infection and cholangiocarcinoma: A prospective case-controlled study. Gastroenterology *89*:151–156, 1985.
23. Kusner, D. J., and King, C. H.: Cerebral paragonimiasis. Semin. Neurol. *13*:201–208, 1993.
24. Kuznetsova, V. G., Naumov, V. A., and Belov, G. F.: Metorchiasis in the residents of Novosibirsk area, Russia. Cytobios *102*:33–34, 2000.
25. Liu, L. X., and Harinasuta, K. T.: Liver and intestinal flukes. Gastroenterol. Clin. North Am. *25*:627–636, 1996.
26. López-Vélez, R., Domínguez-Castellano, A., and Garrón, C.: Successful treatment of human fascioliasis with triclabendazole. Eur. J. Clin. Microbiol. Infect. Dis. *18*:525–526, 1999.
27. MacLean, J. D., Arthur, J. R., Ward, B. J., et al.: Common-source outbreak of acute infection due to the North American liver fluke *Metorchis conjunctus*. Lancet *347*:154–158, 1996.
28. Maleewong, W.: Recent advances in diagnosis of paragonimiasis. Southeast Asian J. Trop. Med. Public Health *28*:134–138, 1997.

29. Mariano, E. G., Borja, S. R., and Vruno, M. J.: A human infection with *Paragonimus kellicotti* (lung fluke) in the United States. Am. J. Clin. Pathol. *86*:685–687, 1986.
30. Markell, E. K.: Laboratory findings in chronic clonorchiasis. Am. J. Trop. Med. Hyg. *15*:510–515, 1966.
31. Merino Alonso, J., Amérigo García, M. J., Alvarez Rubio, L., and Erdozaín Ruiz, I.: Fascioliasis humana con presentación atípica y grava. Tratamiento con triclabendazole. Enferm. Infecc. Microbiol. Clin. *16*:28–30, 1998.
32. Nomura, M., Nitta, H., Nakada, M., et al.: MRI findings of cerebral paragonimiasis in chronic stage. Clin. Radiol. *54*:622–624, 1999.
33. Procop, G. W., Marty, A. M., Scheck, D. N., et al.: North American paragonimiasis: A case report. Acta Cytol. *44*:75–80, 2000.
34. Pungpak, S., Chalermrut, K., Harinasuta, T., et al.: *Opisthorchis viverrini* infection in Thailand: Symptoms and signs of infection: A population-based study. Trans. R. Soc. Trop. Med. Hyg. *88*:561–564, 1994.
35. Pungpak, S., Viravan, C., Radomyos, B., et al.: *Opisthorchis viverrini* infection in Thailand: Studies on the morbidity of the infection and resolution following praziquantel treatment. Am. J. Trop. Med. Hyg. *56*:311–314, 1997.
36. Schistosomes, liver flukes and *Helicobacter pylori.* IARC Working Group on the Evaluation of Carcinogenic Risks to Humans. Lyon, 7–14 June 1994. I. A. R. C. Monogr. Eval. Carcinog. Risks Hum. *61*:1–241, 1994.
37. Shaheen, H., al Khafif, M., Farag, R. M., et al.: Serodifferentiation of human fascioliasis from schistosomiasis. Trop. Geogr. Med. *46*:326–327, 1994.
38. Sirisinha, S., Chawengkirttikul, R., Haswell-Elkins, M. R., et al.: Evaluation of the monoclonal antibody–based enzyme-linked immunosorbent assay for the diagnosis of *Opisthorchis viverrini* infection in an endemic area. Am. J. Trop. Med. Hyg. *52*:521–524, 1995.
39. Strauss, W. G.: Clinical manifestations of clonorchiasis: A controlled study of 105 cases. Am. J. Trop. Med. Hyg. *11*:625–630, 1962.
40. Thamavit, W., Bhamarapravati, N., Sahaphong, S., et al.: Effects of dimethylnitrosamine on induction of cholangiocarcinoma in *Opisthorchis viverrini*–infected Syrian golden hamsters. Cancer Res. *38*:4634–4639, 1978.
41. Upatham, E. S., Viyanant, V., Kurathong, S., et al.: Morbidity in relation to intensity of infection in *Opisthorchis viverrini:* Study of a community in Khon Kaen, Thailand. Am. J. Trop. Med. Hyg. *31*:1156–1163, 1982.
42. Velasquez, C. C.: Heterophydiasis. *In* Steele, J. H. (ed.): CRC Handbook Series in Zoonoses. Vol. 3. Boca Raton, FL, C. R. C. Press, 1982, pp. 99–107.
43. Yilmaz, H., Oner, A. F., Akdeniz, H., and Arslan, S.: The effect of triclabendazole (Fasinex) in children with fasciolosis. J. Eyptian Soc. Parasitol. *28*:497–502, 1998.
44. Zhang, Z., Zhang, Y., Zhiming, S., et al.: Diagnosis of active *Paragonimus westermani* infections with a monoclonal antibody–based antigen detection assay. Am. J. Trop. Med. Hyg. *49*:329–334, 1993.

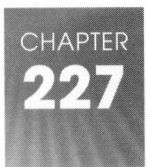

CHAPTER 227 Schistosomiasis

A. CLINTON WHITE, JR. ■ PHILIP R. FISCHER

Approximately 200,000,000 individuals are infected with parasites of the genus *Schistosoma.*[24, 54, 94, 124] Many are unaware of their infection, although approximately 20 million people have severe disease with portal hypertension, urinary tract involvement, renal failure, and bladder cancer, which may lead to death. Initial infection usually occurs during childhood. The prevalence typically peaks in the teen years, and although most of the morbidity occurs in adults, symptomatic disease develops in millions of children.

Historical evidence of schistosomiasis occurring as early as the second millennium before the Christian era exists.[110, 112] For example, *Schistosoma* eggs have been found in mummies from the 20th Dynasty in ancient Egypt and in ancient China. In 1851, Theodore Bilharz identified the parasitic etiology of endemic hematuria. At the same time, the association between *Schistosoma* and Katayama fever was recognized in Japan. The complete life cycle was identified during the first decades of the 20th century. Effective curative medication, however, became generally available only in the 1970s. Efforts to eradicate the disease are still in only the early stages.

Epidemiology

Schistosomiasis is caused by helminth parasites of the class Trematoda, which includes the flukes. Schistosomes differ from other human flukes in that they live within the vascular system and have separate male and female sexes. Humans are the definitive host for five species within the *Schistosoma* genus.[110, 112] *Schistosoma haematobium* is the cause of urinary schistosomiasis. *Schistosoma japonicum* and *Schistosoma mansoni* are common causes of disease resulting from infection of the intestinal vasculature. *Schistosoma mekongi* and *Schistosoma intercalatum* also cause infection along the intestinal tract but are restricted geographically. Other mammalian *Schistosoma* spp. occasionally infect humans. Avian species can cause symptoms when they enter through human skin but cause only local disease in the skin.

Each species of *Schistosoma* uses fresh-water snails as obligate intermediate hosts,[110, 112] and the geographic distribution of *Schistosoma* is limited by the habitat of these snails (Fig. 227–1). Updated World Health Organization figures on the prevalence and distribution of schistosomiasis are available at *http://www.who.int/ctd/schisto/epidemio.htm*. *Oncomelania* snails transmitting *S. japonicum* live in the moist soil along slow-flowing streams and irrigation canals. *S. japonicum* is limited primarily to parts of China, the Philippines, and Indonesia. The *Bulinus* snails associated with *S. haematobium* and the *Biomphalaria* snails associated with *S. mansoni* live in shaded, slow-flowing, shallow water. *S. haematobium* is seen primarily in tropical Africa, along the Nile River, and in the Middle East. *S. mansoni* causes disease across tropical Africa, along the Atlantic coast of South America, and on some Caribbean islands. *Tricula* is the snail host for *S. mekongi*, which is limited to the Mekong River in Laos and Cambodia. *S. intercalatum* and its snail host *Bulinus* are found in Cameroon and the Democratic Republic of Congo. In the United States, schistosomiasis occasionally is diagnosed in immigrants and travelers from endemic regions.

Most human infections occur when children come into contact with stool- or urine-contaminated fresh water in habitats where the snail hosts live[112] (Fig. 227–2). Sites of contact include streams, rivers, and lakes. Thus, for most of the world, transmission of disease occurs during routine activities such as obtaining water for household use,

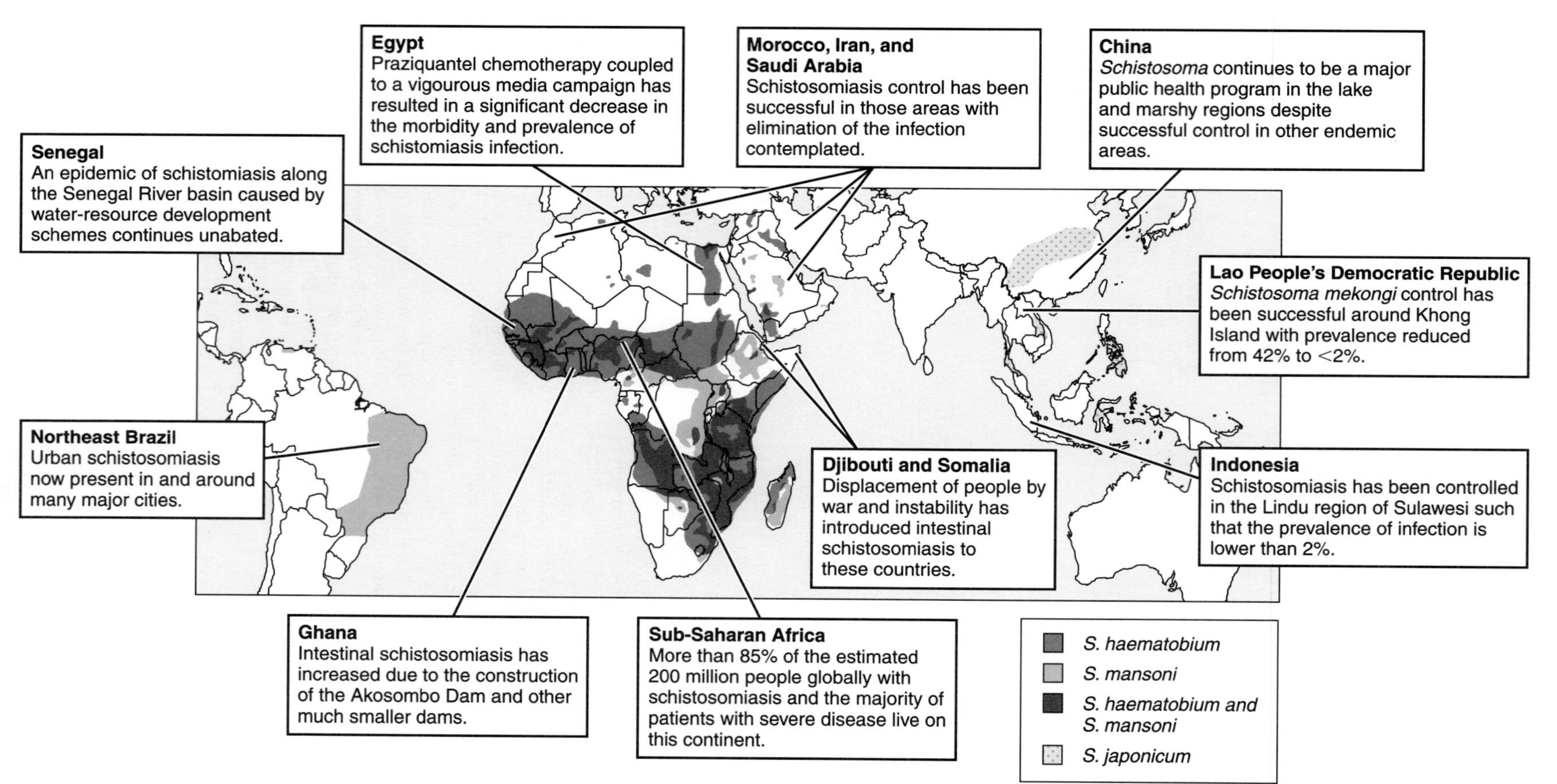

Senegal
An epidemic of schistomiasis along the Senegal River basin caused by water-resource development schemes continues unabated.
Egypt
Praziquantel chemotherapy coupled to a vigourous media campaign has resulted in a significant decrease in the morbidity and prevalence of schistomiasis infection.
Morocco, Iran, and Saudi Arabia
Schistosomiasis control has been successful in those areas with elimination of the infection contemplated.
China
Schistosoma continues to be a major public health program in the lake and marshy regions despite successful control in other endemic areas.
Lao People's Democratic Republic
Schistosoma mekongi control has been successful around Khong Island with prevalence reduced from 42% to <2%.
Northeast Brazil
Urban schistosomiasis now present in and around many major cities.
Djibouti and Somalia
Displacement of people by war and instability has introduced intestinal schistosomiasis to these countries.
Indonesia
Schistosomiasis has been controlled in the Lindu region of Sulawesi such that the prevalence of infection is lower than 2%.
Ghana
Intestinal schistosomiasis has increased due to the construction of the Akosombo Dam and other much smaller dams.
Sub-Saharan Africa
More than 85% of the estimated 200 million people globally with schistosomiasis and the majority of patients with severe disease live on this continent.
S. haematobium
S. mansoni
S. haematobium and S. mansoni
S. japonicum

FIGURE 227–1 ■ Geographic distribution of human schistosome species. (From *http://www.who.int/ctd/schisto/epidemio.htm.*)

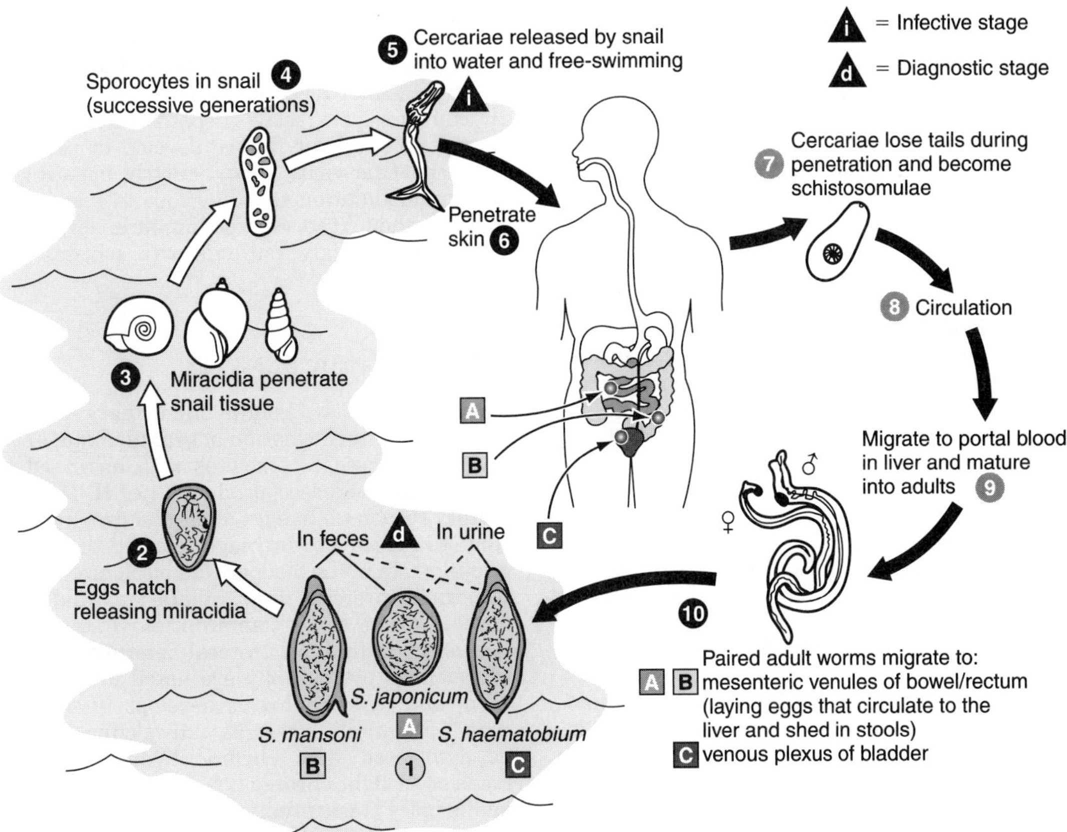

FIGURE 227–2 ■ Life cycle of the human schistosome species. (From Centers for Disease Control: *http://www.dpd.cdc.gov/dpdx/HTML/Schistosomiasis.htm.*)

bathing, fishing, and irrigating fields. Humans are infected in fresh water contaminated by the fork-tailed cercariae. Cercariae penetrate the skin with the aid of secretory proteases. During penetration, the parasites lose their tail and modify their tegument to form the schistosomula stage. Schistosomulae enter the bloodstream and then migrate to the lungs. They move from the pulmonary arterial to the venous circulation without exiting the vessels. The parasites then travel via the systemic circulation until they reach splanchnic vessels and gain access to the portal system.

Over the course of a few weeks, the schistosomulae develop into mature male and female adults, which mate continuously.[111, 112] Adult worms are 1 to 3 cm in length and usually live for 3 to 7 years. *S. haematobium* localizes to the venules of the urinary bladder, *S. japonicum* goes to the superior mesenteric vessels, and *S. mansoni* goes to the inferior mesenteric vessels. The gravid females migrate upstream to lay eggs near the bladder or intestines. Each adult female can produce hundreds to thousands of eggs per day. Most of the eggs become embedded in the walls of the peripheral vessel where they were laid. However, some of them flow with the blood and can stimulate reactions and cause disease at other sites. A localized granulomatous response allows the eggs to pass through the wall of the bladder (for *S. haematobium*) or the intestine (for other species) to be released in urine or stool. Released eggs mature in a week's time and then hatch to release miracidia. The miracidia penetrate the snail to continue their life cycle and eventually develop into hundreds of cercariae.

Whereas infection is seen in children as young as 6 months of age, exposure to cercariae is greatest in boys between the ages of 5 and 10 years.[54, 57, 110] The peak intensity of infection, as measured by egg excretion, occurs in children as young as 8 to 12 years in heavily infected areas and takes place during the teenage years in more lightly infected areas. The intensity and the incidence of excretion of eggs decline after the adolescent years.

Pathogenesis and Immunity

The cercariae use secretory serine proteases to enter the skin.[72, 98] Within hours of penetration, local erythema and inflammation may result, depending in part on the activity of parasite proteases.[114] In individuals previously sensitized, a delayed immune reaction may cause papular or vesicular lesions.[60, 110] The lesions result from infiltration of the epidermis and dermis with a mixture of mononuclear cells and eosinophils. This reaction (termed swimmer's itch) is more pronounced for avian schistosomes because the larvae are unable to enter the circulation and die in situ. During the initial migration of schistosomes through the lungs, fever, pneumonitis, pulmonary infiltrates, and eosinophilia develop in some patients. However, these reactions resolve spontaneously.

Acute schistosomiasis typically begins 4 to 8 weeks after exposure at the time that the female parasites begin to produce eggs.[33] This condition is recognized more commonly with *S. japonicum* than with *S. mansoni* and rarely is described with *S. haematobium*.[60, 110] Patients characteristically have marked eosinophilia along with IgE and IgG antibodies to the parasites, consistent with an active T_H2

response.[60, 110] However, recent studies suggest an important role for proinflammatory cytokines.[30] The antibodies react with egg antigens, which cross-react with antigens from the cercaria or schistosomula stages.[7, 50, 51] During early egg production, the quantity of antigen exceeds that of antibody, and soluble immune complexes are formed. Immune activation and immune complex deposition lead to the clinical manifestations, including fever, myalgia, urticarial rash, and bloody diarrhea. Pulmonary nodules and infiltrates also are noted commonly.[26, 99] In addition, acute infection can be complicated by ectopic egg production. Patients with acute *S. mansoni* or *S. haematobium* infection occasionally can have neurologic involvement.[19, 38, 88] Interestingly, acute disease occurs rarely in endemic populations, perhaps because of modulation of the immune response from exposure to parasite antigens in utero.

CHRONIC SCHISTOSOMIASIS

Despite the fact that the adult worms live within the bloodstream, they cause little host response. The parasite surface incorporates blood group glycoproteins and major histocompatibility antigens and down-regulates expression of its own surface proteins, which may help the adults evade immune system attack.[44, 86, 103]

Chronic infection is characterized by localized granulomata surrounding the parasite eggs.[60, 94, 110] Excretory products of the eggs (termed soluble egg antigen) are the major antigens. The egg antigens are cytotoxic to host cells, such that infection of mice lacking T cells results in increased localized necrosis surrounding the eggs; the granulomata help protect the host from the ravages of the eggs. The granulomata also seem to facilitate transit of the eggs into stool and urine inasmuch as immunodeficient hosts tend to have lower rates of shedding of eggs despite high concentrations of eggs in tissues.[32, 56]

The granulomata also contribute to the pathologic process. They are composed of a mixture of eosinophils, lymphocytes, macrophages, and granulocytes.[13] Late-stage granulomata also contain fibroblasts, collagen, and giant cells. Initially, antigen-presenting cells stimulate $CD4^+$ T cells to produce interleukin-2 (IL-2), tumor necrosis factor–α (TNF-α), and interferon-γ (IFN-γ).[81] Early expression of TNF-α plays a key role in the early formation of granulomata.[4] A subsequent shift occurs toward production of T_H2 cytokines (e.g., IL-4, IL-5, IL-10, and IL-13) along with antibody.[87] This event is accompanied by eosinophil recruitment. IL-4 and IL-13 also play a primary role in the development of hepatic granulomata, and IL-13 expression is linked closely to the development of fibrosis in murine models.[22, 23] Subsequent immunomodulation, largely mediated by IL-10 and transforming growth factor–β (TGF-β), results in down-sizing of the granuloma and suppression of the inflammation.[6, 36, 40, 52, 73, 80, 102, 121] When granulomata are limited to the intestines, the cytokine response is dominated by anti-inflammatory cytokines (e.g., IL-10 and TGF-β), and patients have few symptoms.[28] By contrast, patients with granulomata in the liver are more likely to be symptomatic. They express more inflammatory cytokines, including IL-13 and TNF-α. TGF-β also is associated with fibrosis in primate models,[36] whereas T_H1 cytokines (e.g., IFN-γ and IL-12) suppress fibrosis.[14, 125, 129]

IL-13 in particular stimulates the formation of fibrosis in the portal tracts.[22] This portal fibrosis leads to the development of portal hypertension, which can result in hepatosplenomegaly and the formation of ascites and esophageal varices.[60] Death from hepatic schistosomiasis typically results from gastrointestinal bleeding. In patients with isolated schistosomiasis, hepatocellular function is surprisingly normal.[13] Patients are thought to tolerate even gastrointestinal bleeding better than cirrhotic patients do. By contrast, progressive hepatocellular damage and rapid progression to liver failure develop in patients co-infected with hepatitis viruses, particularly hepatitis C.[5, 25, 55] The immunomodulation that develops in response to schistosomiasis is thought to suppress immune control of the hepatitis virus. Interestingly, patients with schistosomiasis are less prone to allergies.[118]

URINARY SCHISTOSOMIASIS

The pathogenesis of genital and urinary schistosomiasis also results from the formation of granulomata. For example, the severity of disease correlates with increased production of TNF-α and decreased production of IL-10.[61] Direct inflammatory responses to eggs along the ureters or from obstruction to ureteral drainage caused by space-occupying granulomata in the bladder wall block ureteral emptying.[58, 104] Abnormal ureteral flow, dilatation, and hydronephrosis develop.[104] In some communities where *S. haematobium* is a common finding, ureteral deformities demonstrable on intravenous pyelography are noted in half of affected children, and hydronephrosis develops in more than 10 percent.[59] Eventually, scarring and calcifications form and may be associated with chronic hydronephrosis, even with resolved or light chronic infection.[61, 104] The hydronephrosis and urinary stasis predispose patients to chronic bacteriuria and urinary tract infections.

In *S. mansoni* infection, immune complexes may mediate glomerulonephritis, as evidenced by the finding of schistosome-derived immune complex deposits in glomeruli.[9, 105] Nephrotic syndrome has been reported in association with chronic schistosomiasis.[74, 75] Amyloid deposits have been found in the kidneys of children with chronic schistosomiasis, and this condition probably is caused by immune responses that are altered by the chronic parasitic infection.[10, 119]

Squamous cell carcinoma of the bladder is a common occurrence in areas of heavy infection with *S. haematobium,* but otherwise, it is a rare form of bladder cancer.[61, 104, 110] The prolonged irritation of bladder epithelium by schistosome eggs and the resulting immune response are thought to trigger hyperplasia and subsequent malignancy.[64] This condition could be aggravated by urinary stasis in the bladder with secondary increases in pH that favor malignant transformation of epithelial cells. Carcinogenic tryptophan metabolites also have been postulated to link the nutritional activities of parasites near the bladder with subsequent carcinogenesis.

Clinical Manifestations

The main clinical manifestations of schistosomiasis vary with the stage of the parasite's life cycle and also differ among species. Many patients remain asymptomatic. Whereas heavy infections are most likely to cause initial symptoms and to carry the greatest risk for subsequent major health complications, any child with schistosomiasis is at risk for serious life-limiting disease. Patients with asymptomatic schistosomiasis may be identified during community screening programs in an endemic area, through immigrant or returned traveler evaluations in a nonendemic area, or when diagnostic tests such as urine or stool microscopy are performed when evaluating other, unrelated symptoms.

CERCARIAL PENETRATION

Within a few minutes of coming into contact with cercariae, pruritus develops in some children. This response to initial contact with the parasite occurs more commonly in nonimmune visitors to endemic areas than it does in indigenous residents of endemic areas, but it seems to be more pronounced after repeated exposure to cercariae than on the first exposure. It may occur after contact with any of the human *Schistosoma* spp., but it also is reported often after contact with the cercariae of avian schistosomes. An erythematous and, sometimes, papular rash may develop.[60, 110] The rash usually subsides over a period of 2 to 10 days without scarring, regardless of whether specific treatment is given.

ACUTE SCHISTOSOMIASIS

Acute schistosomiasis, referred to as Katayama fever, typically begins 4 to 8 weeks after exposure, at the time that the adult worms begin to produce eggs.[30, 33, 53] Acute symptoms initially were described for *S. japonicum*. They appear somewhat less commonly with *S. mansoni* and are seen much less often with *S. haematobium*.

Acute schistosomiasis usually is manifested as high fever, chills, myalgia, headache, and a general ill appearance.[30, 33] An urticarial rash, which may include giant urticariae, and diffuse lymphadenopathy may be seen.[92, 130] Cough, rales, and pulmonary infiltrates may be noted, even in the absence of fever.[26, 99] Gastrointestinal symptoms of anorexia, abdominal pain, and loose stools sometimes are observed. Bloody diarrhea may be seen acutely with heavy infections by *S. japonicum* and *S. mansoni*. Tender hepatomegaly and mild splenic enlargement develop in approximately 30 percent of children with Katayama fever. Recent reports suggest that myelopathies are a common accompaniment of acute schistosomiasis.[1, 38, 88] Genital symptoms (primarily hematospermia) are also frequent initial symptoms.[27, 90] Marked eosinophilia often is seen with acute schistosomiasis.

URINARY SCHISTOSOMIASIS

Hematuria is the classic finding of urinary schistosomiasis caused by *S. haematobium*.[16, 31, 58, 110, 123] In some highly endemic areas, for boys nearing puberty not to display this evidence of "male menstruation" is considered abnormal. Typically, hematuria results from the release of blood from irritated, inflamed areas around granulomata in the bladder wall as the bladder contracts during micturition.[104] Thus, the blood is most obvious at the end of the urine stream ("terminal hematuria"). The hematuria usually is not associated with pain or discomfort, but dysuria often is present.[1, 16] With chronic infection in children who either were not treated initially or were reinfected, obstructive uropathy can develop. In community surveys, as many as 40 percent of children were found to have significant renal or ureteral abnormalities (or both).[1, 49, 120] Hematuria and dysuria occur more commonly in children than adults, presumably because of heavier parasite loads. However, hydronephrosis, which develops more slowly, is seen more often in adults.[58, 59, 79, 104]

Bacterial urinary tract infection may coexist with urinary schistosomiasis, probably secondary to obstruction of urinary outflow.[104] However, bacteria such as *Salmonella* can "hide" within schistosomes and cause recurrent infections despite antimicrobial therapy. Thus, the bacteriuria usually clears only when the schistosomiasis is treated before treatment of the bacterial superinfection.

Chronic infection can lead to renal failure. Obstructive uropathy, with or without incident or recurrent urinary tract infections, can lead to loss of renal function. Children with schistosomal infection also can have glomerulonephritis and nephrotic syndrome. Bladder cancer usually develops in the setting of untreated, heavy chronic urinary schistosomiasis.

GENITAL SCHISTOSOMIASIS

Recent studies have emphasized the genital tract as an important site of schistosomiasis in both males and females.[18, 65, 66, 89, 90] In females, egg granulomata may be found in the cervix, vulva, or fallopian tubes.[37, 66, 89] Cervical irritation and ulceration, vaginal bleeding, or ectopic pregnancy may develop. Adolescent boys may have involvement of the prostate and seminal vesicles.[65, 90] Eggs were noted in semen from 43 percent of males in an area endemic for *S. haematobium*.[65] The main clinical finding is hematospermia,[65, 78] which may occur with acute infection or during chronic disease. In Africa in particular, genital schistosomiasis may be a cofactor in transmission of human immunodeficiency virus infection.

INTESTINAL DISEASE

Most children with intestinal schistosomiasis do not have intestinal symptoms.[108, 110] Thus, even finding eggs in stool does not mean that symptoms are related to schistosomiasis.[46] Nonetheless, both the small and large intestines may be involved with schistosomal disease. With irritation of the bowel wall as eggs stimulate inflammatory reactions, diarrhea may develop in children and can be bloody or contain mucus, or both.[20, 21, 108–110] Crampy abdominal pain and generalized malaise may occur. Endoscopy can reveal granular inflammation with hyperemic areas, ulceration, and hemorrhage. Polyps, which may develop around granulomata, may be identified by contrast radiography or endoscopy. Especially with small bowel disease, protein-losing enteropathy and blood loss can result in malnutrition and iron deficiency. The role of schistosomiasis in malnutrition was illustrated by studies of mass chemotherapy, which resulted in improved nutrition and a lower prevalence of anemia.[8, 82, 113]

HEPATOSPLENIC DISEASE (HEPATOMEGALY, SPLENOMEGALY, AND PORTAL HYPERTENSION)

The life-threatening complications caused by *S. japonicum* and *S. mansoni* are the result of eggs that remain in the venous vasculature and migrate back to the liver.[13] Egg burden seems to be the greatest predictor of hepatic involvement with schistosomiasis, but some link with HLA type has been suggested.[76, 78, 101, 122]

Children with compensated disease initially have few symptoms. These symptoms may include anorexia, malaise, and abdominal fullness.[13, 21, 62, 83, 90, 123] Children have hepatomegaly even without significant portal hypertension. The hepatomegaly is generally firm and either minimally tender or nontender. Splenic enlargement usually is noted as well. Liver function is affected only late in the course of hepatic schistosomiasis, so jaundice and liver enzyme elevations are unusual.

As fibrosis develops around eggs in the liver, portal hypertension ensues. Liver function usually remains intact, but esophageal varices can cause death during the late adolescent and early adult years.[13, 21, 83] Ascites gradually develops over a period of years, and the spleen may become very large. Bleeding esophageal varices are a common cause of demise in individuals who had heavy schistosomal infections in childhood. Such patients may come to medical attention for melena or hematemesis. Initial episodes are tolerated well. However, with progressive liver decompensation, variceal bleeding can be fatal.

Children with severe hepatosplenic schistosomiasis do not grow as well as other children. Debate has ensued regarding whether this deficiency is due to a direct effect of the parasitic infection or poor nutritional intake caused by poor general health. Some recent data suggest that a decrease in insulin-like growth factor type I activity is linked to hepatic schistosomiasis.[85] Extensive hepatic granuloma formation may hinder the liver's structure and function in such a way that growth-promoting factors are not produced normally.

PNEUMONITIS AND COR PULMONALE

Sometimes, children initially have low-grade fever and cough as schistosome larvae migrate through the lungs. This condition can occur with an initial heavy infection (when eggs will not be detectable) or with a heavy reinfection (when eggs will be detectable in urine or stool from the preceding underlying infection). This larval pneumonitis can be manifested on lung examination as basilar rales and wheezing.[26, 99] Radiographs may show basilar mottling in the lung fields. Eosinophilia is a common occurrence with such pneumonitis. Resolution, even without treatment, usually occurs in 2 to 4 weeks. Similar symptoms also may be seen as a reactive pneumonitis when patients with a heavy parasite burden are treated.

In children with advanced hepatosplenic schistosomiasis and portal hypertension, eggs may flow upstream from the abdominal and pelvic vessels where they are laid and end up lodging in small lung vessels. Over time, children may be subject to fatigue, cough, and right-sided heart failure. Medical therapy stops the progress of disease and might decrease the ongoing inflammatory responses, but it is not always fully curative of established right heart failure.

CENTRAL NERVOUS SYSTEM INVOLVEMENT

Neurologic manifestations of schistosomiasis are often dramatic even if not common.[38, 88, 100] Worms, and eggs for that matter, occasionally do not follow the typical routes described for urinary and intestinal schistosomiasis. Occasionally, worms migrate to cerebral blood vessels and cause seizures or headache, or both, in children.[88, 100] Sometimes, optic field defects and dysarthria are noted; these findings seem to result from localized space-occupying inflammatory reactions around worms or eggs. Spinal fluid pressure may be elevated, and both protein concentrations and lymphocyte counts in spinal fluid may be increased. This cerebral schistosomiasis occurs most commonly with *S. japonicum* infection and is thought to develop in as many as 2 percent of infected children.

Paraplegia and loss of bowel and bladder control can be initial problems in children with spinal schistosomiasis.[38, 100] This event usually occurs as a result of granuloma formation around an "ectopic" egg in a spinal vessel. Though unusual, this manifestation occurs more commonly with *S. mansoni* infection than with other *Schistosoma* spp.; *S. haematobium* also has caused this transverse myelitis.

CHRONIC OR RECURRENT SALMONELLOSIS

In endemic areas, some children have salmonellosis and schistosomiasis concurrently with chronic low-grade fever, fatigue, malaise, and poor growth.[43, 63, 91, 97, 128] Blood cultures frequently demonstrate *Salmonella* bacteremia, but stool may not contain these bacteria. Some children have chronic *Salmonella* bacteriuria. Sepsis and mortality are unusual findings despite these persistent bacterial infections. Relapse of the *Salmonella* infection occurs commonly unless the coexisting schistosomal infection is treated. Researchers have hypothesized that the bacteria hide within the parasitic worms, where antibiotic penetration is poor, and thereby elude the body's defenses and the effect of antibiotics.

Diagnosis

A clinical diagnosis of schistosomiasis is suggested by the presence of typical clinical features. These features might be as obvious as terminal hematuria in a child in a region endemic for *S. haematobium,* or portal hypertension may be noted late in the second decade of life in an otherwise well adolescent from an area known to be endemic for *S. mansoni* or *S. japonicum.*[90, 98] The other clinical findings described also should prompt the clinician to consider a diagnosis of schistosomiasis when the child has resided in or traveled through a *Schistosoma*-endemic area. In traveling children, the index of suspicion must be particularly high because patients may be asymptomatic or have atypical symptoms, they may not have any clear history of exposure to contaminated water, and parasitologic examinations are often negative.[12, 90]

Outside endemic areas, reinfection is not expected. Thus, a reasonable approach is to test all children, including asymptomatic children, who have had a significant exposure to fresh water in an area known to be endemic for schistosomes. Such testing would involve all travelers who swam in, waded in, or even touched suspicious water, and it could involve immigrants who have spent long periods in endemic areas. Certainly, any child outside an endemic area who has even a remote history of possible contact with cercariae and clinical findings suggestive of any form of schistosomiasis should be tested. Testing is appropriate because even late therapy can favorably alter the course and outcome of schistosomiasis. In some highly endemic areas, diagnostic testing is of limited feasibility or questionable reliability (or both), and curative medications are readily available. In such settings, a proven diagnosis might be less necessary, and mass treatment might be sensible. For example, in a highly endemic setting, a positive urine paper strip test for hematuria could provide sufficient suspicion of infection to warrant administration of specific antischistosomal therapy.

In established heavy infections, eggs are usually readily apparent on microscopic examination of urine or stool. For lighter infections, concentrating techniques are useful. Urine can be centrifuged and filtered to increase the yield of eggs. Urine is most likely to be positive when voided at midday and when collected at the end of the urine stream. In the event of high suspicion and negative urine findings, bladder wall biopsy can be performed. The procedure is not usually necessary, however, because urine microscopy, especially with filtered or concentrated samples, is generally positive. Examining multiple samples increases the yield.

The eggs of *S. haematobium* and *S. mansoni* are approximately 90 mm in diameter, whereas the eggs of *S. japonicum* are somewhat smaller. As demonstrated in Figure 227–3, identification of species is aided by observation of the spine—small for *S. japonicum,* at one end for *S. haematobium,* lateral for *S. mansoni,* and broad at each end for *S. intercalatum.* Eggs usually are detectable in voided urine. Plain radiographs might demonstrate some calcification in

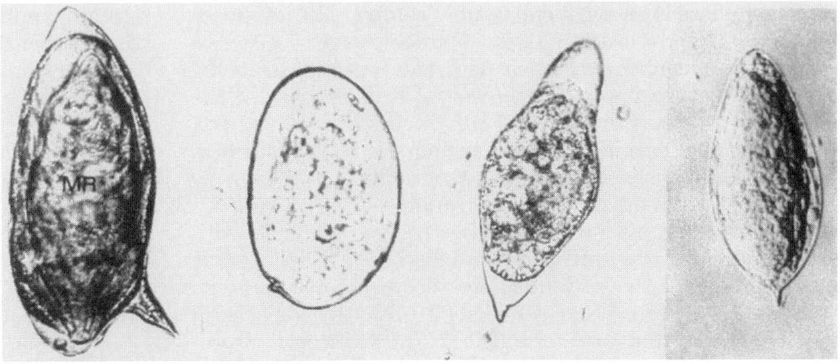

A B C D

FIGURE 227–3 ■ Human schistosome eggs: *A, S. mansoni; B, S. japonicum; C, S. intercalatum;* and *D, S. haematobium.* (From Mahmoud, A. A. F. [ed.]: Schistosomiasis. London, Imperial College Press, 2001. Reprinted with permission.)

the bladder wall around chronic granulomata. Cystoscopy, if performed, reveals hyperemia of the bladder wall and, subsequently, nodular lesions and fibrosis that give rise to "sandy patches" on the bladder wall. Granulomata may protrude from the bladder wall into the lumen. Both edema and granulomata may be seen obstructing ureteral orifices.

In light infections of the intestinal vessels, finding ova in stool samples is not always possible. Eggs may be shed intermittently or in low number. Thus, negative stool tests do not adequately rule out intestinal schistosomiasis.[12, 90] When repeated stools are negative for ova, rectal biopsy may be performed. Samples may be obtained by random pinch biopsy, but the yield is increased when samples are taken from inflamed sites under direct visualization. Eggs are detected in unstained smears made by pressing the tissue sample between a cover slip and a glass slide, but eggs also can be seen with standard histologic stains.

Nonviable eggs may be secreted for months or years after successful therapy. With good medical treatment, eggs are not usually viable when passed more than a week after the initiation of therapy. With partial treatment or reinfection, however, viable eggs may continue to be passed. On microscopic examination, living ova are transparent within the egg, and movement of the miracidia sometimes can be noted. For further documentation of their viability, the eggs may be hatched by placing them in fresh water exposed to light for 20 minutes; observation with a hand lens then can reveal swimming miracidia.

Serologic tests may be needed in acute infection, which may occur before the excretion of eggs or with eggs in ectopic locations.[48, 115] For travelers with limited exposure and the likelihood of, at most, a light infection, serology can be a useful diagnostic tool. Currently, the most common screening serologic test is the FAST-ELISA using *S. mansoni* adult worm microsomal antigen.[116] It also cross-reacts with *S. haematobium* but is less sensitive for *S. japonicum* or *S. mekongi* infection. Species can be confirmed by using an immunoblot assay (enzyme-linked immunotranfer blot).[116] An immunoblot assay is also available for *S. japonicum.* Antigen-detection assays may be helpful, but they are not available in the United States.[2]

Ultrasonography is the main imaging procedure used in schistosomiasis.[49] It can document involvement of the portal and urinary tracts and, in selected cases, can be diagnostic of schistosomiasis. Ultrasound can identify bladder polyps, ureteral dilatation, hydronephrosis, and calcifications within the urinary tract. An ultrasound evaluation of the urinary tract should be performed in any child found to be infected with *S. haematobium.* For children with persistent urinary symptoms (dysuria, suprapubic pain, hematuria) despite good medical treatment, cystoscopy should be performed to screen for bladder cancer. Other radiographs and tests of renal function and excretion generally are not indicated unless the ultrasound evaluation reveals significant urologic disease.

Treatment

Cercarial dermatitis resolves spontaneously and requires no curative treatment. Oral antihistaminic agents, however, may be given for severe itching.

Medical therapy for schistosomiasis caused by the human schistosomes is effective and well tolerated without significant complications. No good medical reason exists to allow schistosomiasis to go untreated. The cost of therapy, however, is a limiting factor in resource-poor areas of the world. Several different medications can be considered for curative treatment.

Praziquantel, a mixture of stereoisomers of pyrazinoisoquinoline ring structures, is a broad-spectrum oral anthelmintic agent that is effective against each of the five human schistosome species. The mechanism of action is not defined clearly, but the drug seems to stimulate tetanic muscle contractions in the parasites. Praziquantel is given in divided doses on a single day as full curative treatment. For infection with *S. haematobium, S. mansoni,* and *S. intercalatum,* the dose is 40 mg/kg in two divided doses given on the same day. For children infected by *S. japonicum* or *S. mekongi,* the dose is 60 mg/kg in either two or three divided doses given on the same day.[3, 34] Heavily infected children sometimes experience some nausea, vomiting, and abdominal cramping with treatment. Rare side effects, including headache, pruritus, bloody stools, and fever, are transient and resolve within 1 to 2 days after the initiation of treatment. Because praziquantel primarily kills mature adult worms, a second course is recommended for the treatment of acute infection. Praziquantel is effective in more than 90 percent of treated children. Some studies suggest that resistance may be emerging,[68, 69] in part as a consequence of reinfection (because juvenile forms are not as susceptible to praziquantel) or heavy infection. Studies from nonendemic areas continue to demonstrate excellent efficacy.[123]

An alternative treatment effective only against *S. mansoni* is oxamniquine, a tetrahydroquinoline compound.[107] The mechanism by which this agent acts is unknown. The effective dose has varied with the geographic origin of the schistosomal infection, but some resistance has been reported. Current recommendations are that children treated with oxamniquine be given 40 to 60 mg/kg divided into two doses administered on 1 day or four separate doses given over the course of 2 days. Mild side effects include nausea, headache, and fever. Seizures are a rare side effect, so administration of this medication should be avoided in children with seizure disorders. Cure rates of greater than 90 percent are reported with oxamniquine.

Metrifonate is an organophosphate compound that causes paralysis of the parasite. It is 70 to 80 percent effective against *S. haematobium* when used at a dose of 10 mg/kg orally once every 2 weeks for 6 weeks. It does decrease the child's own plasma and erythrocyte cholinesterase activity, but actual cholinergic symptoms seldom occur. This medication is less expensive than the other options, but it generally is not used when praziquantel is available.

Medical therapy is usually effective for children with schistosomiasis, even with advanced disease.[70, 95, 106, 128] Clear improvement in the patient's disease burden occurs when treatment is given. Even established uropathy and portal hypertension often are reversible.[72, 95, 106] Surgical procedures usually are reserved for children with complications related to long-term infection, such as persistent portal hypertension. Propranolol prophylaxis and sclerotherapy or banding can reduce rebleeding from esophageal varices.[35] Some cases require surgical decompression of portal hypertension. Splenorenal shunts are associated with high rates of hepatic encephalopathy. Comparative studies suggest that in experienced hands, esophagogastric devascularization with splenectomy is the procedure of choice.[39, 42]

Systemic steroids, however, may be useful for severely ill children with Katayama fever or severe larval pneumonitis. They also may be helpful in cases with granulomata in the central nervous system.[38, 41] However, corticosteroids have not been proved effective in other forms of the disease.

Prevention

The use of effective medical therapy coupled with improved urine and stool hygiene has the potential to eradicate schistosomiasis.[124] Elimination of the snails that serve as intermediate hosts also would be effective, but attempts at molluscicide have been unsuccessful to date. Recent control efforts have focused on mass chemotherapy, with particular emphasis on school-based therapy.[8, 47, 82, 84, 124] Treatment programs in which the entire school-age population is treated have resulted in overall improvement in levels of nutrition and in a reduction in the prevalence of anemia. However, the effects are of limited duration and must be repeated every 6 months to 1 year.

Several studies suggest that artemisinin derivatives can prevent infection and decrease the worm burden in those exposed to *S. mansoni* and *S. japonicum*.[67, 94, 117] However, they are less effective for chemotherapy than praziquantel is,[15, 29] probably because parasitologic activity is limited to the juvenile forms. Furthermore, the public health role of chemoprophylaxis in the prevention of infection has not been established.

Travelers and expatriates in endemic areas can prevent disease by limiting exposure to fresh water. The cercaria can be eliminated by chlorination or by allowing water to settle for 24 hours before bathing or washing.

Immunization of experimental animals with irradiated cercariae can prevent experimental schistosomiasis. Thus, development of a vaccine to prevent human schistosomiasis is theoretically possible. Several potentially protective antigens have been identified on schistosomes, and they are being used as targets for vaccine development. However, the correlates of protective immunity in humans are not well defined.[11] Currently, combinations of antigens are being studied for *S. mansoni*.[126] Early-stage clinical trials have been performed for *S. haematobium* glutathione-S-transferases.[17] Similar antigens also are being studied for *S. japonicum*.[77, 93] Whether development of a vaccine to prevent human infection is a possibility remains far from certain, and no vaccine is likely to be ready for clinical use in the near future.[45]

REFERENCES

1. Abdel-Wahab, M. F., Esmat, G., Ramzy, I., et al.: *Schistosoma haematobium* infection in Egyptian schoolchildren: Demonstration of both hepatic and urinary tract morbidity by ultrasonography. Trans. R. Soc. Trop. Med. Hyg. *86*:406–409, 1992.
2. Al-Sherbiny, M. M., Osman, A. M., Hancock, K., et al.: Application of immunodiagnostic assays: Detection of antibodies and circulating antigens in human schistosomiasis and correlation with clinical findings. Am. J. Trop. Med. Hyg. *60*:960–966, 1999.
3. American Academy of Pediatrics: Drugs for parasitic infections. *In* Pickering, L. K. (ed.): 2000 Red Book: Report of the Committee on Infectious Diseases. 25th ed. Elk Grove Village, IL, American Academy of Pediatrics, 2000, pp. 693–725.
4. Amiri, P., Locksley, R. M., Parslow, T. G., et al.: Tumour necrosis factor alpha restores granulomas and induces parasite egg-laying in schistosome-infected SCID mice. Nature *356*:604–607, 1992.
5. Aquino, R. T., Chieffi, P. P., Catunda, S. M., et al.: Hepatitis B and C virus markers among patients with hepatosplenic mansonic schistosomiasis. Rev. Inst. Med. Trop. Sao Paulo *42*:313–320, 2000.
6. Araujo, M. I., de Jesus, A. R., Bacellar, O., et al.: Evidence of a T helper type 2 activation in human schistosomiasis. Eur. J. Immunol. *26*:1399–1403, 1996.
7. Aronstein, W. S., and Strand, M.: Gender-specific and pair-dependent glycoprotein antigens of *Schistosoma mansoni*. J. Parasitol. *70*:545–757, 1984.
8. Assis, A. M., Barreto, M. L., Prado, M. S., et al.: *Schistosoma mansoni* infection and nutritional status in schoolchildren: A randomized, double-blind trial in northeastern Brazil. Am. J. Clin. Nutr. *68*:1247–1253, 1998.
9. Barsoum, R. S.: Schistosomal glomerulopathies. Kidney Int. *44*:1–12, 1993.
10. Barsoum, R. S., Bassily, S., Soliman, M. M., et al.: Renal amyloidosis and schistosomiasis. Trans. R. Soc. Trop. Med. Hyg. *73*:367–374, 1979.
11. Bergquist, R., Al-Sherbiny, M., Barakat, R., and Olds, R.: Blueprint for schistosomiasis vaccine development. Acta Trop. *82*:183–192, 2002.
12. Bialek, R., and Knobloch, J.: Schistosomiasis in German children. Eur. J. Pediatr. *159*:530–534, 2000.
13. Bica, I., Hamer, D. H., and Stadecker, M. J.: Hepatic schistosomiasis. Infect. Dis. Clin. North Am. *14*:583–604, viii, 2000.
14. Boros, D. L., and Whitfield, J. R.: Enhanced Th1 and dampened Th2 responses synergize to inhibit acute granulomatous and fibrotic responses in murine schistosomiasis mansoni. Infect. Immun. *67*:1187–1193, 1999.
15. Borrmann, S., Szlezak, N., Faucher, J. F., et al.: Artesunate and praziquantel for the treatment of *Schistosoma haematobium* infections: A double-blind, randomized, placebo-controlled study. J. Infect. Dis. *184*:1363–1366, 2001.
16. Browning, M. D., Narooz, S. I., Strickland, G. T., et al.: Clinical characteristics and response to therapy in Egyptian children infected with *Schistosoma haematobium*. J. Infect. Dis. *149*:998–1004, 1984.
17. Capron, A., Capron, M., Dombrowicz, D., and Riveau, G.: Vaccine strategies against schistosomiasis: From concepts to clinical trials. Int. Arch. Allergy Immunol. *124*:9–15, 2001.
18. Carey, F. M., Quah, S. P., Hedderwick, S., et al.: Genital schistosomiasis. Int. J. S.T.D. A.I.D.S. *12*:609–611, 2001.
19. Cetron, M. S., Chitsulo, L., Sullivan, J. J., et al.: Schistosomiasis in Lake Malawi. Lancet *348*:1274–1278, 1996.
20. Chen, M. C., Wang, S. C., Chang, P. Y., et al.: Granulomatous disease of the large intestine secondary to schistosome infestation. A study of 229 cases. Chin. Med. J. (Engl.) *4*:371–378, 1978.
21. Chen, M. G.: *Schistosoma japonicum* and *S. japonicum*-like infections: Clinical and pathological aspects. *In* Jordan, P., Webbe, G., and Sturrock, R. F. (eds.): Human Schistosomiasis. Wallingford, UK, CAB International, 1993, pp. 237–270.
22. Chiaramonte, M. G., Cheever, A. W., and Malley, J. D.: Studies of murine schistosomiasis reveal interleukin-13 blockade as a treatment for established and progressive liver fibrosis. Hepatology *34*:273–282, 2001.
23. Chiaramonte, M. G., Schopf, L. R., Neben, T. Y., et al.: IL-13 is a key regulatory cytokine for Th2 cell-mediated pulmonary granuloma formation and IgE responses induced by *Schistosoma mansoni* eggs. J. Immunol. *162*:920–930, 1999.
24. Chitsulo, L., Engels, D., Montresor, A., and Savioli, L.: The global status of schistosomiasis and its control. Acta Trop. *77*:41–51, 2000.
25. Conceicao, M. J., Argento, C. A., Chagas, V. L., et al.: Prognosis of schistosomiasis mansoni patients infected with hepatitis B virus. Mem. Inst. Oswaldo Cruz *93*:255–258, 1998.
26. Cooke, G. S., Lalvani, A., Gleeson, F. V., and Conlon, C. P.: Acute pulmonary schistosomiasis in travelers returning from Lake Malawi, sub-Saharan Africa. Clin. Infect. Dis. *29*:836–839, 1999.
27. Corachan, M., Valls, M. E., Gascon, J., et al.: Hematospermia: A new etiology of clinical interest. Am. J. Trop. Med. Hyg. *50*:580–584, 1994.

28. Correa-Oliveira, R., Malaquias, L. C., Falcao, P. L., et al.: Cytokines as determinants of resistance and pathology in human *Schistosoma mansoni* infection. Braz. J. Med. Biol. Res. *31*:171–177, 1998.
29. De Clercq, D., Vercruysse, J., Kongs, A., et al.: Efficacy of artesunate and praziquantel in *Schistosoma haematobium* infected schoolchildren. Acta Trop. *82*:61–66, 2002.
30. de Jesus, A. R., Silva, A., Santana, L. B., et al.: Clinical and immunologic evaluation of 31 patients with acute schistosomiasis mansoni. J. Infect. Dis. *185*:98–105, 2002.
31. Delegue, P., Picquet, M., Shaw, D. J., et al.: Morbidity induced by *Schistosoma haematobium* infections, as assessed by ultrasound before and after treatment with praziquantel, in a recently expanded focus (Senegal River basin). Ann. Trop. Med. Parasitol. *92*:775–783, 1998.
32. Doenhoff, M. J., Hassounah, O., Murare, H., et al.: The schistosome egg granuloma: Immunopathology in the cause of host protection or parasite survival? Trans. R. Soc. Trop. Med. Hyg. *80*:503–514, 1986.
33. Doherty, J. F., Moody, A. H., Wright, S. G.: Katayama fever: An acute manifestation of schistosomiasis. B. M. J. *313*:1071–1072, 1996.
34. Drugs for parasitic infections. Med. Lett. Drugs. Ther. *March*:1–12, 2002.
35. el Tourabi, H., el Amin, A. A., Shaheen, M., et al.: Propranolol reduces mortality in patients with portal hypertension secondary to schistosomiasis. Ann. Trop. Med. Parasitol. *88*:493–500, 1994.
36. Farah, I. O., Mola, P. W., Kariuki, T. M., et al.: Repeated exposure induces periportal fibrosis in *Schistosoma mansoni*-infected baboons: Role of TGF-beta and IL-4. J. Immunol. *164*:5337–5343, 2000.
37. Feldmeier, H., Daccal, R. C., Martins, M. J., et al.: Genital manifestations of schistosomiasis mansoni in women: Important but neglected. Mem. Inst. Oswaldo Cruz *93*:127–133, 1998.
38. Ferrari, T. C.: Spinal cord schistosomiasis. A report of 2 cases and review emphasizing clinical aspects. Medicine (Baltimore) *78*:176–190, 1999.
39. Ferraz, A. A., Bacelar, T. S., Silveira, M. J., et al.: Surgical treatment of schistosomal portal hypertension. Int. Surg. *86*:1–8, 2001.
40. Flores-Villanueva, P. O., Zheng, X. X., Strom, T. B., et al.: Recombinant IL-10 and IL-10/Fc treatment down-regulate egg antigen–specific delayed hypersensitivity reactions and egg granuloma formation in schistosomiasis. J. Immunol. *156*:3315–3320, 1996.
41. Fowler, R., Lee, C., and Keystone, J. S.: The role of corticosteroids in the treatment of cerebral schistosomiasis caused by *Schistosoma mansoni:* Case report and discussion. Am. J. Trop. Med. Hyg. *61*:47–50, 1999.
42. Gawish, Y., El-Hammadi, H. A., Kotb, M., et al.: Devascularization procedure and DSRS: A controlled randomized trial on selected haemodynamic portal flow patterns in schistosomal portal hypertension with variceal bleeding. Int. Surg. *85*:325–330, 2000.
43. Gendrel, D., Kombila, M., Beaudoin-Leblevec, G., et al.: Nontyphoidal salmonellal septicemia in Gabonese children infected with *Schistosoma intercalatum.* Clin. Infect. Dis. *18*:103–105, 1994.
44. Goldring, O. L., Clegg, J. A., Smithers, S. R., and Terry, R. J.: Acquisition of human blood group antigens by *Schistosoma mansoni.* Clin. Exp. Immunol. *26*:181–187, 1976.
45. Gryseels, B.: Schistosomiasis vaccines: A devil's advocate view. Parasitol. Today *16*:46–48, 2000.
46. Guyatt, H., Gryseels, B., Smith, T., and Tanner, M.: Assessing the public health importance of *Schistosoma mansoni* in different endemic areas: Attributable fraction estimates as an approach. Am. J. Trop. Med. Hyg. *53*:660–667, 1995.
47. Guyatt, H. L., Brooker, S., Kihamia, C. M., et al.: Evaluation of efficacy of school-based anthelmintic treatments against anaemia in children in the United Republic of Tanzania. Bull. World Health Organ. *79*:695–703, 2001.
48. Hamilton, J. V., Klinkert, M., and Doenhoff, M. J.: Diagnosis of schistosomiasis: Antibody detection, with notes on parasitological and antigen detection methods. Parasitology *117*(Suppl.):41–57, 1998.
49. Hatz, C. F.: The use of ultrasound in schistosomiasis. Adv. Parasitol. *48*:225–284, 2001.
50. Hiatt, R. A., Ottesen, E. A., Sotomayor, Z. R., and Lawley, T. J.: Serial observations of circulating immune complexes in patients with acute schistosomiasis. J. Infect. Dis. *142*:665–670, 1980.
51. Hiatt, R. A., Sotomayor, Z. R., Sanchez, G., et al.: Factors in the pathogenesis of acute schistosomiasis mansoni. J. Infect. Dis. *139*:659–666, 1979.
52. Hoffmann, K. F., Cheever, A. W., and Wynn, T. A.: IL-10 and the dangers of immune polarization: Excessive type 1 and type 2 cytokine responses induce distinct forms of lethal immunopathology in murine schistosomiasis. J. Immunol. *164*:6406–6416, 2000.
53. Istre, G. R., Fontaine, R. E., Tarr, J., and Hopkins, R. S.: Acute schistosomiasis among Americans rafting the Omo River, Ethiopia. J. A. M. A. *251*:508–510, 1984.
54. Jordan, P., and Webbe, G.: Epidemiology. *In* Jordan, P., Webbe, G., and Sturrock, R. F. (eds.): Human Schistosomiasis. Wallingford, UK, CAB International, 1993, pp. 87–158.
55. Kamal, S. M., Rasenack, J. W., Bianchi, L., et al.: Acute hepatitis C without and with schistosomiasis: Correlation with hepatitis C–specific CD4(+) T-cell and cytokine response. Gastroenterology *121*:646–656, 2001.
56. Karanja, D. M., Colley, D. G., Nahlen, B. L., et al.: Studies on schistosomiasis in western Kenya: I. Evidence for immune-facilitated excretion of schistosome eggs from patients with *Schistosoma mansoni* and human immunodeficiency virus coinfections. Am. J. Trop. Med. Hyg. *56*:515–521, 1997.
57. King, C. H.: Epidemiology of schistosomiasis: Determinants of transmission of infection. *In* Mahmoud, A. A. F. (ed.): Schistosomiasis. London, Imperial College Press, 2001, pp. 115–132.
58. King, C. H.: Disease due to schistosomiasis haematobia. *In* Mahmoud, A. A. F. (ed.): Schistosomiasis. London, Imperial College Press, 2001, pp. 265–295.
59. King, C. H., Keating, C. E., Muruka, J. F., et al.: Urinary tract morbidity in schistosomiasis haematobia: Associations with age and intensity of infection in an endemic area of Coast Province, Kenya. Am. J. Trop. Med. Hyg. *39*:361–368, 1988.
60. King, C. L.: Initiation and regulation of disease in schistosomiasis. *In* Mahmoud, A. A. F. (ed.) Schistosomiasis. London, Imperial College Press, 2001, pp. 213–264.
61. King, C. L., Malhotra, I., Mungai, P., et al.: *Schistosoma haematobium*-induced urinary tract morbidity correlates with increased tumor necrosis factor-alpha and diminished interleukin-10 production. J. Infect. Dis. *184*:1176–1182, 2001.
62. Lambertucci, J. R.: *Schistosoma mansoni:* Pathological and clinical aspects. *In* Jordan, P., Webbe, G., and Sturrock, R. F. (eds.): Human Schistosomiasis. Wallingford, UK, CAB International, 1993, pp. 195–235.
63. Lambertucci, J. R., Rayes, A. A., and Gerspacher-Lara, R.: *Salmonella–S. mansoni* association in patients with acquired immunodeficiency syndrome. Rev. Inst. Med. Trop. Sao Paulo *40*:233–235, 1998.
64. Lemmer, L. B., and Fripp, P. J.: Schistosomiasis and malignancy. S. Afr. Med. J. *84*:211–215, 1994.
65. Leutscher, P., Ramarokoto, C. E., Reimert, C., et al.: Community-based study of genital schistosomiasis in men from Madagascar. Lancet *355*:117–118, 2000.
66. Leutscher, P., Ravaoalimalala, V. E., Raharisolo, C., et al.: Clinical findings in female genital schistosomiasis in Madagascar. Trop. Med. Int. Health *3*:327–332, 1998.
67. Li, S., Wu, L., Liu, Z., et al.: Studies on prophylactic effect of artesunate on schistosomiasis japonica. Chin. Med. J. (Engl.) *109*:848–853, 1996.
68. Liang, Y. S., Coles, G. C., Dai, J. R., et al.: Biological characteristics of praziquantel-resistant and -susceptible isolates of *Schistosoma mansoni.* Ann. Trop. Med. Parasitol. *95*:715–723, 2001.
69. Liang, Y. S., Coles, G. C., and Doenhoff, M. J.: Detection of praziquantel resistance in schistosomes. Trop. Med. Int. Health *5*:72, 2000.
70. Liang, Y. S., Dai, J. R., Ning, A., et al.: Susceptibility of *Schistosoma japonicum* to praziquantel in China. Trop. Med. Int. Health *6*:707–714, 2001.
71. Lim, K. C., Sun, E., Bahgat, M., et al.: Blockage of skin invasion by schistosome cercariae by serine protease inhibitors. Am. J. Trop. Med. Hyg. *60*:487–492, 1999.
72. Lischer, G. H., and Sweat, S. D.: 16-year-old boy with gross hematuria. Mayo Clin. Proc. *77*:475–478, 2002.
73. Malaquias, L. C., Falcao, P. L., Silveira, A. M., et al.: Cytokine regulation of human immune response to *Schistosoma mansoni:* Analysis of the role of IL-4, IL-5 and IL-10 on peripheral blood mononuclear cell responses. Scand. J. Immunol. *46*:393–398, 1997.
74. Martinelli, R., Noblat, A. C., Brito, E., and Rocha, H.: *Schistosoma mansoni*-induced mesangiocapillary glomerulonephritis: Influence of therapy. Kidney Int. *35*:1227–1233, 1989.
75. Martinelli, R., Pereira, L. J., Brito, E., and Rocha, H.: Clinical course of focal segmental glomerulosclerosis associated with hepatosplenic schistosomiasis mansoni. Nephron *69*:131–134, 1995.
76. May, J., Kremsner, P. G., Milovanovic, D., et al.: HLA-DP control of human *Schistosoma haematobium* infection. Am. J. Trop. Med. Hyg. *59*:302–306, 1998.
77. McManus, D. P.: The search for a vaccine against schistosomiasis—a difficult path but an achievable goal. Immunol. Rev. *171*:149–161, 1999.
78. McManus, D. P., Ross, A. G., Williams, G. M., et al.: HLA class II antigens positively and negatively associated with hepatosplenic schistosomiasis in a Chinese population. Int. J. Parasitol. *31*:674–680, 2001.
79. Medhat, A., Zarzour, A., Nafeh, M., et al.: Evaluation of an ultrasonographic score for urinary bladder morbidity in *Schistosoma haematobium* infection. Am. J. Trop. Med. Hyg. *57*:16–19, 1997.
80. Mola, P. W., Farah, I. O., Kariuki, T. M., et al.: Cytokine control of the granulomatous response in *Schistosoma mansoni*-infected baboons: Role of exposure and treatment. Infect. Immun. *67*:6565–6571, 1999.
81. Montenegro, S. M., Miranda, P., Mahanty, S., et al.: Cytokine production in acute versus chronic human schistosomiasis mansoni: The cross-regulatory role of interferon-gamma and interleukin-10 in the responses of peripheral blood mononuclear cells and splenocytes to parasite antigens. J. Infect. Dis. *179*:1502–1514, 1999.
82. Olds, G. R., King, C., Hewlett, J., et al.: Double-blind placebo-controlled study of concurrent administration of albendazole and praziquantel in schoolchildren with schistosomiasis and geohelminths. J. Infect. Dis. *179*:996–1003, 1999.
83. Olveda, R. M.: Disease due to schistosomiasis japonicum. *In* Mahmoud, A. A. F. (ed.): Schistosomiasis. London, Imperial College Press, 2001, pp. 361–389.

84. Olveda, R. M., Daniel, B. L., Ramirez, B. D., et al.: Schistosomiasis japonica in the Philippines: The long-term impact of population-based chemotherapy on infection, transmission, and morbidity. J. Infect. Dis. *174*:163–172, 1996.
85. Orsini, M., Rocha, R. S., Disch, J., et al.: The role of nutritional status and insulin-like growth factor in reduced physical growth in hepatosplenic *Schistosoma mansoni* infection. Trans. R. Soc. Trop. Med. Hyg. *95*:453–456, 2001.
86. Pearce, E. J., Basch, P. F., and Sher, A.: Evidence that the reduced surface antigenicity of developing *Schistosoma mansoni* schistosomula is due to antigen shedding rather than host molecule acquisition. Parasite Immunol. *8*:79–94, 1986.
87. Pearce, E. J., Caspar, P., Grzych, J. M., et al.: Downregulation of Th1 cytokine production accompanies induction of Th2 responses by a parasitic helminth, *Schistosoma mansoni.* J. Exp. Med. *173*:159–166, 1991.
88. Pittella, J. E.: Neuroschistosomiasis. Brain Pathol. *7*:649–662, 1997.
89. Poggensee, G., Kiwelu, I., Weger, V., et al.: Female genital schistosomiasis of the lower genital tract: Prevalence and disease-associated morbidity in northern Tanzania. J. Infect. Dis. *181*:1210–1213, 2000.
90. Roca, C., Balanzo, X., Gascon, J., et al.: Comparative, clinico-epidemiologic study of *Schistosoma mansoni* infections in travellers and immigrants in Spain. Eur. J. Clin. Microbiol. Infect. Dis. *21*:219–223, 2002.
91. Rocha, H., Kirk, J. W., and Hearey, C. D., Jr.: Prolonged *Salmonella* bacteremia in patients with *Schistosoma mansoni* infection. Arch. Intern. Med. *128*:254–257, 1971.
92. Rocha, M. O., Greco, D. B., Pedroso, E. R., et al.: Secondary cutaneous manifestations of acute schistosomiasis mansoni. Ann. Trop. Med. Parasitol. *89*:425–430, 1995.
93. Ross, A. G., Sleigh, A. C., Li, Y., et al.: Schistosomiasis in the People's Republic of China: Prospects and challenges for the 21st century. Clin. Microbiol. Rev. *14*:270–295, 2001.
94. Ross, A. G. P., Bartley, P. B., Sleigh, A. C., et al.: Schistosomiasis. N. Engl. J. Med. *346*:1212–1220, 2002.
95. Saconato, H., and Atallah, A.: Interventions for treating schistosomiasis mansoni. Cochrane Database Syst. Rev. 2, 2000.
96. Salih, S. Y., Subaa, H. A., Asha, H. A., and Satir, A. A.: Salmonellosis complicating schistosomiasis in the Sudan. J. Trop. Med. Hyg. *80*:14–18, 1977.
97. Salter, J. P., Lim, K. C., Hansell, E., et al.: Schistosome invasion of human skin and degradation of dermal elastin are mediated by a single serine protease. J. Biol. Chem. *275*:38667–38673, 2000.
98. Samuel, M., Misra, D., Larcher, V., and Price, E.: *Schistosoma haematobium* infection in children in Britain. B. J. U. Int. *85*:316–318, 2000.
99. Schwartz, E., Rozenman, J., and Perelman, M.: Pulmonary manifestations of early schistosome infection among nonimmune travelers. Am. J. Med. *109*:718–722, 2000.
100. Scrimgeour, E. M., and Gajdusek, D. C.: Involvement of the central nervous system in *Schistosoma mansoni* and *S. haematobium* infection. A review. Brain *108*:1023–1038, 1985.
101. Secor, W. E., del Corral, H., dos Reis, M. G., et al.: Association of hepatosplenic schistosomiasis with HLA-DQB1*0201. J. Infect. Dis. *174*:1131–1135, 1996.
102. Sher, A., Fiorentino, D., Caspar, P., et al.: Production of IL-10 by CD4+ T lymphocytes correlates with down-regulation of Th1 cytokine synthesis in helminth infection. J. Immunol. *147*:2713–2716, 1991.
103. Simpson, A. J., Singer, D., McCutchan, T. F., et al.: Evidence that schistosome MHC antigens are not synthesized by the parasite but are acquired from the host as intact glycoproteins. J. Immunol. *131*: 962–965, 1983.
104. Smith, J. H., and Christie, J. D.: The pathobiology of *Schistosoma haematobium* infection in humans. Hum. Pathol. *17*:333–345, 1986.
105. Sobh, M. A., Moustafa, F. E., el-Housseini, F., et al.: Schistosomal specific nephropathy leading to end-stage renal failure. Kidney Int. *31*: 1006–1011, 1987.
106. Squires, N.: Interventions for treating schistosomiasis haematobium. Cochrane Database Syst. Rev. 2, 2000.
107. Stelma, F. F., Sall, S., Daff, B., et al.: Oxamniquine cures *Schistosoma mansoni* infection in a focus in which cure rates with praziquantel are unusually low. J. Infect. Dis. *176*:304–307, 1997.
108. Strickland, G. T.: Gastrointestinal manifestations of schistosomiasis. Gut *35*:1334–1337, 1994.
109. Strickland, G. T., Merritt, W., El-Sahly, A., and Abdel-Wahab, F.: Clinical characteristics and response to therapy in Egyptian children heavily infected with *Schistosoma mansoni.* J. Infect. Dis. *146*:20–29, 1982.
110. Strickland, G. T., and Ramirez, B. L.: Schistosomiasis. *In* Strickland, G. T. (ed.): Hunter's Tropical Medicine. 8th ed. Philadelphia, W. B. Saunders, 1999, pp. 804–832.
111. Sturrock, R. F.: The parasites and their life cycles. *In* Jordan, P., Webbe, G., and Sturrock, R. F., (eds.): Human Schistosomiasis. Wallingford, UK, CAB International, 1993.
112. Sturrock, R. F.: The schistosomes and their intermediate hosts. *In* Mahmoud, A. A. F. (ed.): Schistosomiasis. London, Imperial College Press, 2001, pp. 7–83.
113. Taylor, M., Jinabhai, C. C., Couper, I., et al.: The effect of different anthelmintic treatment regimens combined with iron supplementation on the nutritional status of schoolchildren in KwaZulu-Natal, South Africa: A randomized controlled trial. Trans. R. Soc. Trop. Med. Hyg. *95*:211–216, 2001.
114. Teixeira, M. M., Doenhoff, M. J., McNeice, C., et al.: Mechanisms of the inflammatory response induced by extracts of *Schistosoma mansoni* larvae in guinea pig skin. J. Immunol. *151*:5525–5534, 1993.
115. Tsang, V. C., and Wilkens, P. P.: Immunodiagnosis of schistosomiasis. Immunol. Invest. *26*:175–188, 1997.
116. Tsang, V. C. W., and Wilkens, P. P.: Immunodiagnosis of schistosomiasis. Screen with FAST-ELISA and confirm with immunoblot. Clin. Lab. Med. *11*:1029–1039, 1991.
117. Utzinger, J., N'Goran, E. K., N'Dri, A., et al.: Oral artemether for prevention of *Schistosoma mansoni* infection: Randomised controlled trial. Lancet *355*:1320–1325, 2000.
118. van den Biggelaar, A. H., van Ree, R., Rodrigues, L. C., et al.: Decreased atopy in children infected with *Schistosoma haematobium:* A role for parasite-induced interleukin-10. Lancet *356*:1723–1727, 2000.
119. Veress, B., Musa, A. R., Osman, H., et al.: The nephrotic syndrome in the Sudan with special reference to schistosomal nephropathy. A preliminary morphological study. Ann. Trop. Med. Parasitol. *72*:357–361, 1978.
120. Vester, U., Kardorff, R., Traore, M., et al.: Urinary tract morbidity due to *Schistosoma haematobium* infection in Mali. Kidney Int. *52*:478–481, 1997.
121. Wahl, S. M., Frazier-Jessen, M., Jin, W. W., et al.: Cytokine regulation of schistosome-induced granuloma and fibrosis. Kidney Int. *51*:1370–1375, 1997.
122. Waine, G. J., Ross, A. G., Williams, G. M., et al.: HLA class II antigens are associated with resistance or susceptibility to hepatosplenic disease in a Chinese population infected with *Schistosoma japonicum.* Int. J. Parasitol. *28*:537–542, 1998.
123. Whitty, C. J., Mabey, D. C., Armstrong, M., et al.: Presentation and outcome of 1107 cases of schistosomiasis from Africa diagnosed in a non-endemic country. Trans. R. Soc. Trop. Med. Hyg. *94*:531–534, 2000.
124. World Health Organization: Report of the WHO informal consultation on schistosomiasis control. Geneva, WHO, 1998.
125. Wynn, T. A., Cheever, A. W., Jankovic, D., et al.: An IL-12–based vaccination method for preventing fibrosis induced by schistosome infection. Nature *376*:594–596, 1995.
126. Yang, W., Jackson, D. C., Zeng, Q., and McManus, D. P.: Multi-epitope schistosome vaccine candidates tested for protective immunogenicity in mice. Vaccine *19*:103–113, 2000.
127. Young, S. W., Higashi, G., Kamel, R., et al.: Interaction of salmonellae and schistosomes in host-parasite relations. Trans. R. Soc. Trop. Med. Hyg. *67*:797–802, 1973.
128. Yu, D. B., Li, Y., Sleigh, A. C., et al.: Efficacy of praziquantel against *Schistosoma japonicum:* Field evaluation in an area with repeated chemotherapy compared with a newly identified endemic focus in Hunan, China. Trans. R. Soc. Trop. Med. Hyg. *95*:537–541, 2001.
129. Zhang, L., Mi, J., Yu, Y., et al.: IFN-gamma gene therapy by intrasplenic hepatocyte transplantation: A novel strategy for reversing hepatic fibrosis in *Schistosoma japonicum*–infected mice. Parasite Immunol. *23*:11–17, 2001.
130. Zuidema, P. J.: The Katayama syndrome; an outbreak in Dutch tourists to the Omo National Park, Ethiopia. Trop. Geogr. Med. *33*:30–35, 1981.

ARTHROPODS

CHAPTER 228 Arthropods

JAN E. DRUTZ

Arthropods constitute nearly three fourths of the world's animal species. Although some arthropods are capable of damaging agriculture and homes and others serve as reservoirs, hosts, and vectors of human and animal pathogens, most have no significant impact in causing human disease.[48] However, among the more significant diseases transmitted to humans by arthropods are Chagas disease, malaria, dengue, and bubonic plague. In the United States, ticks transmit more vector-borne diseases caused by bacteria, rickettsia, viruses, and protozoa than do any other species. Tularemia, tick paralysis, tick-borne relapsing fever, Rocky Mountain spotted fever, Colorado tick fever, babesiosis, Lyme disease, human monocytic ehrlichiosis, and human granulocytic ehrlichiosis are the diseases most commonly transmitted by ticks in the United States.[44]

Ticks

Ticks, mites, spiders, and scorpions all belong to a class of arthropods known as Arachnida. Two of three families of ticks belonging to this class contain species capable of transmitting pathogens to humans. Ixodidae, the hard tick family, and Argasidae, the soft tick family, serve as both vectors and reservoirs for many rickettsiae (Table 228–1). Using a fluorescent technique, these rickettsiae can be identified in the tick hemolymph.

Hard ticks are so named because of their scotum, a dorsal sclerotized shield. Owing to the limited scotum coverage of the female, she is more capable of becoming engorged with blood than is the male, a factor significant in the reproductive process. During feedings, these ticks remain attached to the host for hours or days at a time.[13, 43] Three genera of Ixodidae are known to transmit disease to humans in the United States: *Amblyomma*, *Dermacentor*, and *Ixodes*.[42]

Soft ticks have no scotum and tend to live for long periods of time, often surviving for years without eating. Both the nymph form and the adult tick have a tendency to eat often, but for brief periods often lasting less than 30 minutes.[13, 43] Of the family Argasidae, only ticks of the genus *Ornithodoros* are known to transmit pathogens to humans in the United States.[42] Specifically, they are the vectors of tick-borne relapsing fever.

Local reaction from tick bites appears to be mediated by complement. The reaction from these bites may persist and subsequently develop into a so-called tick bite granuloma. Systemic reactions such as fever, chills, nausea, vomiting, abdominal pain, and headache can be associated with tick bites.

TICK PARALYSIS

Tick paralysis is a neurologic syndrome characterized chiefly by an ascending flaccid paralysis in association with the attachment of certain species of ticks. A well-known disease of animals, it was first reported to occur in humans in North America in 1912.[46] Most cases have occurred in the Pacific Northwest and Rocky Mountain states during spring and summer.[44] It has been reported to occur more frequently in children, especially girls between 2 and 5 years of age, than in adults. Numerous genera of ticks are known to be associated with tick paralysis. In North America, *Dermacentor andersoni* (wood tick) and *Dermacentor variabilis* (dog tick) are the primary species responsible for tick paralysis.[28] In Australia, ticks implicated most commonly are *Ixodes holocyclus* and *Ixodes cornatus*. Both adult female and male, as well as immature, ticks have been implicated in this nervous system disorder.

Pathogenesis

Tick paralysis is thought to be caused by a neurotoxin (holocyclotoxin) produced in the tick's salivary glands.[26] It usually is released by gravid female ticks at the site of attachment, usually the scalp. The neurotoxin is a protein with temperature-dependent activity.[11] The exact mechanism and location of the toxin's action are not known but may include decreased entry of calcium into motor-nerve terminals or interference with presynaptic excitation-secretion coupling, which leads to a reduction of acetylcholine release at the motor end-plate.

Investigations in children with tick paralysis have implicated primarily peripheral nerve dysfunction because nerve conduction velocities were noted to be diminished somewhat.[21, 45] Compound muscle action potentials that are abnormally low or low-normal in amplitude when the patient has maximal neurologic deficits generally are reversed rapidly once the tick is removed.[28] Swift and Ignacio[45] postulate that the major effect of the toxin is to prevent depolarization in the terminal portions of the motor neurons.

Clinical Manifestations

The symptoms of tick paralysis usually occur within 2 to 7 days after the tick begins feeding. Symmetric weakness of the lower extremities progresses to an ascending flaccid paralysis over several hours or days. Sensory function usually is spared, and the sensorium is clear.[44] Alternatively, the disease can present as acute ataxia without muscle weakness.[29] If the paralysis involves the cranial nerves, the

TABLE 228–1 ■ HUMAN INFECTIOUS DISEASES FOR WHICH TICKS ARE A VECTOR

Disease	Agent
Relapsing fever	*Borrelia duttonii*
Q fever	*Coxiella burnetii*
Tularemia	*Francisella tularensis*
Queensland tick typhus	*Rickettsia australis*
Fiévre boutonneuse	*R. conorii*
Rocky Mountain spotted fever	*R. rickettsii*
Asian tick typhus	*R. sibirica*
Colorado tick fever	Arbovirus
Encephalitis	Arbovirus
Lyme disease	*Borrelia burgdorferi*
Human monocytic ehrlichiosis	*Ehrlichia chaffeensis*
Human granulocytic ehrlichiosis	*Ehrlichia* species
Babesiosis	*Babesia microti*

patient may have changes in voice and difficulty swallowing and handling secretions. Nystagmus, strabismus, and convulsions may occur as well.[21] Temperature elevation generally is not present. After removal of the tick, symptoms tend to resolve within several hours or days. Left untreated, tick paralysis can be fatal, with reported mortality rates of 10 to 12 percent.[39]

Routine laboratory tests are not helpful in establishing diagnosis. The white blood cell count, urine analysis, cerebrospinal fluid, and erythrocyte sedimentation rate usually are normal.

Diagnosis

The diagnosis of tick paralysis can be established when the patient shows the typical clinical picture and improves when a tick is removed. The differential diagnosis of tick paralysis includes Guillain-Barré syndrome, poliomyelitis, myelitis, spinal cord neoplasm, syringomyelia, porphyria, and botulism.

Treatment

The earlier the tick is removed in the course of the syndrome, the more promptly the syndrome will clear. Forceps, not fingers, should be used to remove the tick. The tick's head should be gently but firmly grasped and slow, reverse traction should be applied to remove all body parts. Recovery generally is complete within 1 to 5 days. In one reported case, weakness did not resolve for several months.[14] Intensive supportive care is required if the patient has cranial nerve dysfunction. Ineffective ventilation and ensuing respiratory failure require assisted ventilation.

Myiasis

Myiasis is the invasion of a host's tissues by the larval stage (maggot) of nonbiting flies. Because of the immaturity of maggots, differentiating the various species is difficult. Myiasis can be classified according to the anatomic site of infestation (i.e., aural myiasis, ophthalmomyiasis, or cutaneous myiasis) or on the basis of clinical syndrome (i.e., furuncular cutaneous myiasis, migratory cutaneous myiasis, or wound myiasis).[41] In the past, parasitic diseases were limited to their endemic areas. With the relative ease of worldwide travel, however, they are appearing with increasing frequency in the United States and other developed countries.[20]

ETIOLOGY

The true flies of the order Diptera undergo metamorphosis in four stages: the egg, larva, pupa, and adult. Some larvae of the suborder Cyclorrhapha have adapted to a parasitic relationship with humans to different degrees. Some are classified as obligate, facultative, or accidental parasites in humans. In each case, the larval stage of the fly is able to invade the tissues of the host and progress in the stages of metamorphosis.

EPIDEMIOLOGY

The occurrence of human myiasis has been linked to humid and warm climates that favor the breeding of flies. Epizootics in livestock, marginal housing, poor disposal of refuse, and undernutrition also are important factors in the development of human myiasis.[32] In the United States, myiasis has been reported from both flies native to North America and the larvae of flies acquired during foreign travel. More than 50 species of flies have been reported to cause human myiasis.

PATHOGENESIS

The pathogenesis of human myiasis differs with the degree of parasitic adaptation of each fly. *Dermatobia hominis* (the human botfly) uses a bloodsucking insect as a vector to deposit its eggs on a warm-blooded host. The larvae emerge from the eggs and then penetrate the host's skin, frequently using the puncture site of the carrier insect. The larvae develop within the dermal layer of skin, which leads to a boil-like swelling. During this period, the human host develops clinical symptoms. *D. hominis* and *Cochliomyia hominivorax*, the primary screwworm, are examples causing obligate myiasis.[32] *C. hominivorax* can be responsible for aural or nasal myiasis.

The genus *Sarcophaga* (flesh flies) is capable of causing facultative myiasis. The adult fly is attracted to wounds or ulcers containing purulent and necrotic material. The adult fly deposits eggs in the open wound where the larvae hatch.

Maggots seldom are found in the human intestinal or urinary tract.[41] Accidental myiasis can occur when humans ingest eggs or larvae and the larvae remain in the intestinal tract. Genitourinary myiasis is thought to occur by the deposition of eggs around the external urethral orifice. The larvae then may migrate into and up the urethra. Such situations should be called *pseudomyiasis*[51] because the maggots are not living parasitically.

CLINICAL MANIFESTATIONS

The lesions of cutaneous myiasis generally are located over the exposed area of the body. Early in the course of cutaneous myiasis, pruritus is the predominant symptom. As the larvae grow after the first week of infestation, a serous exudate may drain from the penetrating site. At this point, pain and pruritus are prominent symptoms, and the lesion appears as a small furuncle (furuncular myiasis). Destruction of tissue by the larvae may continue, and secondary bacterial infection can occur. *Staphylococcus aureus* and group A streptococci, as well as gram-negative organisms, have been isolated from infected cutaneous myiasis wounds.

Abdominal pain, diarrhea, and anal bleeding are the symptoms of intestinal myiasis, which is self-limited and may last 2 to 6 weeks. Larvae within the genitourinary tract may lead to proteinuria, dysuria, hematuria, and pyuria. Nasal myiasis can extend into bone, sinus cavities, and even the meninges.[3] Aural myiasis has been described in a child without underlying pathology.[12] Ophthalmomyiasis is characterized by an acute catarrhal conjunctivitis.[15] Penetration into the brain has been associated with intracerebral hematomas.[27]

DIAGNOSIS

A careful history of travel, occupation, and exposure is necessary for diagnosis when the physician is confronted with unusual skin lesions that are pruritic and have not resolved with usual local care.[19, 25] Myiasis is confirmed if larvae are demonstrated within the wound. A parasitologist or entomologist may be able to identify the species of larvae responsible.

TREATMENT

The removal of the larvae is necessary in any of the forms of myiasis. Endoscopic removal of nasal infestation is recommended. Surgical intervention may be required to expose the larvae in the wound. Forceps are used to pick out the larvae; the application of 5 percent chloroform in olive oil may facilitate removal. Occlusive coverings of the wound opening are helpful in extruding *Dermatobia* larvae because this maneuver diminishes the oxygen supply to the larvae. A thick layer of petroleum jelly (Vaseline) effectively interrupts air flow to larvae. Local or systemic antibiotics may be required if secondary bacterial infection is present.

The prevention of human myiasis requires good wound care, adequate personal hygiene, screening to protect against flies, and the prevention of myiasis in domestic animals.

Mites

As mentioned earlier, mites belong to the same class of arthropods (Arachnida) as do ticks, spiders, and scorpions. They too can be vectors for infectious agents. The house mite, *Liponyssoides sanguineus*, is the vector for the rickettsial pox agent. Chiggers, which are larvae of mites (family Trombiculidae), transmit to humans the agent responsible for scrub typhus, *Rickettsia tsutsugamushi*.

Scabies, an extremely pruritic skin infestation, has been known for more than 2500 years. The etiologic agent for this condition, *Sarcoptes scabiei*, is an obligate human parasite that burrows into the epidermis, no deeper than the stratum granulosum.[10] Scabies appears to have an increased incidence in 15-year cycles,[40] transmitted person-to-person through direct and usually prolonged contact.

PATHOGENESIS

Mites of all developmental stages tunnel into the stratum corneum and deposit feces (scybala) behind them. Characteristically, the gravid female lays eggs in the tunnels. Clothing and bed items are thought to be less important in the transmission of the *Sarcoptes* mite. Because scabies is transmitted by skin-to-skin contact, sexual transmission is a common occurrence, as is nonsexual spread in family settings.[10] Epidemic outbreaks of scabies have been reported in hospitals and other institutions where people were living closely together and especially where poor sanitation predominated.[5]

Hypersensitivity of both immediate and delayed types has been implicated in the development of lesions other than burrows.[10] Papulovesicular scabies is characterized by perivascular lymphohistiocytic infiltrates with eosinophils. The papillary dermis is edematous. The histologic appearance of nodular scabies is one of a dense, superficial, and deep perivascular lymphohistiocytic infiltrate with many plasma cells and eosinophils. Various vascular changes also may be apparent. Norwegian scabies (crusted scabies) is distinguished by numerous mites that are found in histologic sections of the stratum corneum, and hyperkeratosis is noted.[17] This form of scabies occurs most commonly in debilitated individuals, such as institutionalized retarded children or immunosuppressed children, including children with human immunodeficiency virus infection.

CLINICAL MANIFESTATIONS

Scabies is characterized by moderate to severe pruritus that starts several weeks to months after infestation, at which time the host has become hypersensitive to the mite or its products. Itching, most evident at night, is the primary symptom of infection. A papular or vesicular eruption with pustules and linear burrows occurs and classically involves the webs between the fingers, flexures of the arms, axillae, and genital regions. In infants and children, scabitic lesions more typically occur on the palms, soles, head, and neck in the form of vesicles, pustules, or nodules. In this age group, scabies often is not suspected because of the atypical skin lesions that result from vigorous scratching and secondary infections.[24]

Acute glomerulonephritis may be associated with pyoderma in scabies. A careful history may reveal that other family members or child caretakers have pruritus and skin lesions consistent with scabies. Examination of the skin of family members for signs of scabies frequently is helpful. Norwegian scabies may present not with the typical pruritic papules but rather with a nonspecific hyperkeratosis that may be generalized or localized to the hands or feet.[16]

DIAGNOSIS

Definitive diagnosis can be made by microscopic identification of the mites, eggs, or mite feces.[25] To obtain this material, skin scrapings should be taken from papules or the end of a burrow and from the underneath surface of fingernails. In some cases, a variety of biopsy techniques can be useful.[8]

The diagnosis should be considered when the physician is faced with an unusual papular or bullous rash. The differential diagnosis of scabies in children includes impetigo, atopic eczema, seborrheic or contact dermatitis, psoriasis, histiocytosis, and chickenpox.[23, 24]

TREATMENT

The management of scabies involves the application of a topical scabicide to all areas of skin (except the face) and subsequent removal in 8 to 24 hours, depending on the product applied. Effective scabicides are gamma benzene hexachloride (lindane), permethrin 5 percent, and 10 percent crotamiton.

The agent of choice for infants and young children is permethrin topical cream, which can be applied to the entire head, neck, and body of the infant.[24] All family members should be treated simultaneously.[35] Antibiotics may be necessary if secondary bacterial infection is present.

Ivermectin has proved to be highly efficacious as an oral therapy for scabies in a single dose for otherwise healthy or human immunodeficiency virus–infected adults.[33] It works against several different parasites by interrupting γ-aminobutyric acid–induced neurotransmission.[10] Approval has not been granted for use of ivermectin in children, especially those weighing less than 15 kg.

Articles of clothing and bed sheets should be washed in hot water by machine washing at 60° C. Insecticidal powder or aerosol should be reserved for materials that cannot be washed.[10] Some evidence indicates that gamma benzene hexachloride may not be safe for use in infants and young children because of transcutaneous absorption and subsequent adverse central nervous system effects.[24, 30] These adverse effects possibly may be prevented by a careful explanation of the application and removal of lindane after 8 to 12 hours.[16, 22] Pruritus often persists for some time after successful treatment with a scabicide and may be relieved by an oral antihistamine or mild to moderate topical steroids.[8, 35] In hospitalized patients, contact isolation is recommended to lessen the potential for nosocomial transmission.

Pediculosis

Arthropods of the order Anoplura (sucking lice) are important as vectors of rickettsial or spirochetal illnesses. The body louse *Pediculus humanus humanus* is the vector for epidemic typhus *(Rickettsia prowazekii)*, trench fever *(Bartonella quintana)*, and louse-borne relapsing fever *(Borrelia recurrentis)*. The body louse, head louse *(Pediculus humanus capitis)*, and crab louse *(Phthirus pubis)* all are capable of human infestation. Pediculosis has been a problem for humans for more than 10,000 years.[10]

PATHOGENESIS

Head lice are the most common type of louse. Tiny, they measure no more than 1 to 4 mm in length. They have six legs, each with powerful claws allowing for firm attachment. Mouth parts consist of stylets (retracted when not in use) modified for piercing and sucking. When not feeding, lice are translucent with grayish white bodies, but when engorged with blood, they become red. Each female is capable of laying up to 300 eggs (nits) in a brief lifetime of 1 to 3 months. These eggs are less than 1 mm in diameter and hatch in 6 to 10 days, giving rise to nymphs. Over a period of 10 days, the nymphs become adults. Schoolchildren of all socioeconomic groups are affected, with head-to-head contact being the most common means of transmission.

CLINICAL MANIFESTATIONS

Children or adults with head lice usually present with white or opalescent nits attached to individual strands of hair. The lice themselves firmly adhere to the base of the hair shaft, millimeters from the scalp. Once a louse pierces the skin, a poisonous salivary secretion is exuded, resulting in pruritic dermatitis. Itching is the primary symptom in acute cases.

Body lice occur when poor socioeconomic conditions exist. Infestation occurs when people fail or are unable to wash their clothes regularly, such as those in living in refugee camps. Intense itching is a major problem, with noticeable excoriations and occasional secondary infections.

Pubic lice primarily are transmitted through sexual contact, although not exclusively so. In children, pubic lice generally occur as a result of non–sexually transmitted contact with an infected parent. Again, itching is a major presenting symptom. Pubic lice may become attached to other hairy areas of the body such as the axillae of adolescents, the eyelashes of children, and the scalp hair of any age group.[10]

As mentioned, body lice can function as vectors for the transmission of several diseases. One of these diseases is trench fever caused by *Bartonella quintana*. Whereas some patients may have no symptoms, others may present with fever, myalgias, headache, meningoencephalitis, transient maculopapular rashes, or chronic adenopathies. Another of these diseases is epidemic typhus caused by *Rickettsia prowazekii*. Symptoms of this infection may include fever, headache, rash, or confusion. Relapsing fever caused by *Borrelia recurrentis* is the third of the group of louse vector-transmitted diseases.[10]

DIAGNOSIS

Head, body, and pubic lice are visibly recognizable. Nits are firmly attached to hair shafts and are distinguished readily from dandruff flakes, lint, and other debris easily removed from the hair. Viable nits, located close to the scalp, are oval shaped and grayish to yellow-white in color. Empty nonviable nits, attached at some distance from the scalp, are almost completely clear. Although they are difficult to see with the naked eye, nits visibly fluoresce yellow-green under a Wood's lamp. Polymerase chain reaction allows for the identification of host DNA from lice through their blood meal, providing valuable information for rape, homicide, and child-abuse cases.[31]

The body louse has been demonstrated only lately as the true vector of trench fever by polymerase chain reaction detection of *B. quintana* DNA in lice from infected patients.[7] Detection of rickettsial DNA in lice indicates current human typhus.

TREATMENT

Head Lice

Numerous forms of treatment for the eradication of head lice have been used. Gamma benzene hexachloride (lindane) shampoo was used almost exclusively until the early 1970s. Because of concern regarding potential neurotoxic effects for the patient, it no longer is recommended as a first-line medication for children. Subsequently, a 1 percent permethrin crème rinse used as a single treatment became the preferred form of therapy. This biodegradable and generally very safe product is recommended to be applied to wet hair and left in place for about 10 minutes before rinsing. To remove the firmly adherent nits, a fine-toothed stainless-steel comb (LiceMeister) has been recommended.

Over time, resistance to several forms of therapy has developed. Additional therapeutic intervention has included pyrethrin plus piperonyl butoxide, ivermectin, malathion, trimethoprim-sulfamethoxazole, and the use of smothering agents including olive oil, margarine, and petroleum jelly. Some success has been reported using a 5 percent permethrin preparation and wearing a shower cap overnight.[37]

Malathion, an organophosphate, when applied to hair and left in place for 8 to 12 hours, provides residual protection.

A combination of 0.5 percent malathion and 78 percent isopropanol has been approved for use by the U.S. Food and Drug Administration. Because it is hydrolyzed and detoxified by plasma carboxylesterases much more rapidly in mammals than in insects, it is considered safe.[1] However, it is flammable and is not recommended for use in children younger than 6 months of age.[10]

Ivermectin in the form of a lotion, shampoo, and oral preparation has been tried. The single oral dose has been about 0.2 mg/kg. A second dose has been given to children when lice have remained active 24 hours after the first dose.[4]

The use of the antibiotic combination trimethoprim-sulfamethoxazole works by destroying essential gut bacteria in the louse. These bacteria, responsible for the production of vitamin B, are essential for life.

Body Lice

A general recommendation has been thorough washing of the body with soap and water followed by the application of a pyrethrin, pyrethroid, or malathion for 8 to 24 hours. Again, caution should be taken in the use of these latter preparations in children. Decontamination of clothing and bed linens is essential either by washing them in hot soapy water at a temperature of 130° F for 10 minutes or placing them in a hot clothes drier for 20 minutes.

Pubic Lice

Treatment should be similar to that used for managing head lice. Clothes and bed linen should be decontaminated. In the case of children, parents also should be treated, and in the case of adolescents, sexual partners require treatment.

Spiders

Of the thousands of species in the United States, only a few pose a threat to humans. Species of the genus *Loxosceles* are the spiders predominantly responsible for necrotic arachnidism in the United States. The two most common ones are the black widow spider and the brown recluse spider. Both spiders prefer dark, undisturbed habitats, such as outdoor lavatories, woodpiles, ground under stones, or dark corners of garages and attics. The black widow has a characteristic red hourglass shape on its ventral surface. The brown recluse has a violin-shaped marking over its dorsal surface. In the Pacific Northwest area of the United States, the hobo spider (*Tegeenaria agrestis*) produces an envenomation similar to that of the brown recluse spider.[9]

PATHOGENESIS

Venom from the black widow contains a neurotoxin (α-lactrotoxin), not a tissue toxin. The main effect is at the presynaptic membrane of the neuromuscular junction. Venom from the brown recluse spider contains sphingomyelinase D, a phospholipase that induces dermal necrosis and also causes systemic effects through its interaction with red blood cells, platelets, and endothelium.[38] The necrosis caused by the venom is dependent on neutrophils, but the neutrophils are not activated by the venom itself. Rather, the venom is a potent stimulus for the inflammatory response of endothelial cells, which in turn activates the polymorphonuclear neutrophils to cause tissue destruction.[34]

CLINICAL MANIFESTATIONS

The bite of the black widow spider generally is painless, but a target lesion may develop. Within 30 to 120 minutes, some patients complain of regional lymph node tenderness.[50] The primary symptom that develops after the bite is muscle cramping, generally involving the abdomen, chest, or back, depending on the location of the bite. Autonomic symptoms, including profuse sweating, nausea and vomiting, and tachycardia, may occur.[38] Hypertension can be a significant problem. The degree of systemic symptoms depends on the amount of venom injected and the number of bites. Severe cases may progress to internal hemorrhage, paralysis, and, rarely, even death.

The brown recluse spider bite may produce a mild or sharp stinging sensation. After several hours, the pain intensifies and itching occurs.[2] Eventually, a blister forms at the site with surrounding erythema. Over time, the lesion becomes larger, and central necrosis develops. Systemic signs developing in the first 24 to 48 hours may include headache, fever, nausea, vomiting, or joint pain. Disseminated intravascular coagulation, multiorgan failure, and death have been reported in children.[18, 49]

Like that of the brown recluse spider, the hobo spider bite also may result in a central necrotic area. The most common systemic symptom is a severe headache. Protracted systemic effects, including aplastic anemia, intractable vomiting, or profuse secretory diarrhea, are rare occurrences but may be associated with death.[47]

TREATMENT

For patients with black widow spider bites, analgesia is the mainstay of care.[38]

An antivenin is available, but only for the most severe cases of envenomation that are unresponsive to other measures.[6]

For brown recluse spider bites, numerous treatments have been used, including hyperbaric oxygen therapy, early excision, antibiotics, dapsone, and corticosteroids. Careful supportive care, including monitoring of electrolytes and renal function, is required if symptoms are severe.[38] Systemic corticosteroid therapy may be of some benefit if the patient has systemic symptoms. Dapsone, an inhibitor of neutrophil function, appears to decrease the development of wound complications and subsequent need for surgical excision.[36]

REFERENCES

1. Abramowicz, M.: Malthion for treatment of head lice. Med. Lett. Drugs Ther. *41*:73–74, 1999.
2. Allen, C.: Arachnid envenomations. Emerg. Med. Clin. North Am. *10*:269–298, 1992.
3. Badia, L., and Lund, V.: Vile bodies: An endoscopic approach to nasal myiasis. J Laryngol. Otol. *108*:1083–1085, 1994.
4. Bell, T. A.: Treatment of *Pediculus humanus* var. capitis infestation in Cowlitz County, Washington, with ivermectin and the LiceMeister comb. Pediatr. Infect. Dis. J. *17*:923–924, 1998.
5. Bernstein, B., and Mihan, R.: Hospital epidemic of scabies. J. Pediatr. *83*:1086–1087, 1973.
6. Bond, G. R.: Snake, spider and scorpion envenomation in North America. Pediatr. Rev. *20*:147–150, 1999.
7. Brouqui, D., Lascola, B., Roux. V., et al.: Chronic *Bartonella quintana* bacteremia in homeless patients. N. Engl. J. Med. *340*:184–189, 1999.
8. Burgess, I.: *Sarcoptes scabiei* and scabies. Adv. Parasitol. *35*:235–292, 1994.
9. Centers for Disease Control and Prevention: Necrotic arachnidism—Pacific Northwest, 1988–1996. M. M. W. R. *45*:433–436, 1996.
10. Chosidow, O.: Scabies and pediculosis. Lancet *355*:819–826, 2000.
11. Cooper, B. J., and Spence, I.: Temperature-dependent inhibition of evoked acetylcholine release in tick paralysis. Nature *263*:693–695, 1976.

12. Cunningham, D. G., and Zonga, J. R.: Myiasis of the external auditory canal. J. Pediatr. *84*:856–858, 1974.
13. Cupp, E. W.: Biology of ticks. Vet. Clin. North Am. Small Animal Pract. *21*:1–26, 1991.
14. Donat, J. R., and Donat, J. F.: Tick paralysis with persistent weakness and electromyographic abnormalities. Arch. Neurol. *38*:59–61, 1981.
15. Elgart, M. L.: Flies and myiasis. Dermatol. Clin. *8*:237–244, 1990.
16. Elgart, M. L.: Scabies. Dermatol. Clin. *8*:253–263, 1990.
17. Fernandez, N., Torres, A., and Ackerman, A. B.: Pathologic findings in human scabies. Arch. Dermatol. *113*:320–324, 1977.
18. Ginsburg, C. M., and Weinberg, A. G.: Hemolytic anemia and multiorgan failure associated with localized cutaneous lesion. J. Pediatr. *112*:496–499, 1988.
19. Guillozet, N.: Diagnosing myiasis. J. A. M. A. *244*:698–699, 1980.
20. Hall, M., and Wall, R.: Myiasis of humans and domestic animals. Adv. Parasitol. *35*:257–334, 1995.
21. Haller, J. S., and Fabara, J. A.: Tick paralysis: Case report with emphasis on neurological toxicity. Am. J. Dis. Child *124*:915–917, 1972.
22. Honig, P. J.: Bites and parasites. Pediatr. Clin. North Am. *30*:563–581, 1983.
23. Hurwitz, S.: Scabies in babies. Am. J. Dis. Child *126*:226–228, 1973.
24. Hurwitz, S. (ed.): Clinical Pediatric Dermatology. 2nd ed. Philadelphia, W. B. Saunders, 1993, pp. 405–412.
25. Iannini, P. B., Brandt, D., and La Force, F. M.: Furuncular myiasis. J. A. M. A. *233*:1375–1376, 1975.
26. Kaire, G. H.: Isolation of tick paralysis toxin from *Ixodes holocyclus*. Toxicon *4*:91–97, 1996.
27. Kalelioglu, M., Akturkm G., Akturk, F., et al.: Intracerebral myiasis from *Hypoderma bovis* larva in a child. J. Neurosurg. *71*:929–931, 1989.
28. Kincaid, J. C.: Tick bite paralysis. Semin. Neurol. *10*:32–34, 1990.
29. Lagos, J. C., and Thies, R. E.: Tick paralysis without muscle weakness. Arch. Neurol. *21*:471–474, 1969.
30. Lee, B., and Croth, P.: Scabies: Transcutaneous poisoning during treatment. Pediatrics *59*:643, 1977.
31. Lord, W. D., DiZonno, J. A., Wilson, M. R., et al.: Isolation, amplification and sequencing of human mitochondrial DNA obtained from human crab louse, *Pthirus pubis* (L), blood meals. J. Forensic Sci. *43*:1097–1100, 1998.
32. Macias, E. G., Graham, A. J., Green, M., et al.: Cutaneous myiasis in South Texas. N. Engl. J. Med. *289*:1239–1241, 1973.
33. Meinking, T. L., Taplin, D., Hermida, J. L., et al.: The treatment of scabies with ivermectin. N. Engl. J. Med. *333*:26–30, 1995.
34. Patel, K. D., Modur, V., Zimmerman, G. A., et al.: The necrotic venom of the brown recluse spider induces dysregulated endothelial cell-dependent neutrophil activation: Differential induction of GM-CSF, IL-8, and E-selectin expression. J. Clin. Invest. *94*:631–642, 1994.
35. Rasmussen, J. E.: Scabies. Pediatr. Rev. *15*:110–114, 1994.
36. Rees, R. S., Altenbern, D. P., Lynch, J. B., et al.: Brown recluse spider bites: A comparison of early surgical excision versus dapsone and delayed surgical excision. Ann. Surg. *202*:659–663, 1985.
37. Schachner, L. A.: Treatment resistant head lice: Alternative therapeutic approaches. Pediatr. Dermatol. *14*:409–410, 1997.
38. Schexnayder, S. M., and Schexnayder, R. E.: Bites, stings, and other painful things. Pediatr. Ann. *29*:354–358, 2000.
39. Schmitt, N., Bowmer, E. J., and Gregson, J. D.: Tick paralysis in British Columbia. Can. Med. Assoc. J. *100*:417–421, 1969.
40. Shaw, P. K., and Juranek, D. D.: Recent trends in scabies in the United States. J. Infect. Dis. *134*:414–416, 1976.
41. Sherman, R. A.: Wound myiasis in urban and suburban United States. Arch. Intern. Med. *160*:2004–2014, 2000.
42. Sonenshine, D. E., and Azad, A. F.: Ticks and mites in disease transmission. *In* Strickland, G. T. (ed.): Hunter's Tropical Medicine. 7th ed. Philadelphia, W. B. Saunders, 1991, pp. 971–981.
43. Sonenshine, D. E.: Biology of ticks. Vol. 1. New York, Oxford University Press, 1992.
44. Spach, D. H., Liles, W. C., Campbell, G. L., et al.: Medical progress: Tick-borne diseases in the United States. N. Engl. J. Med. *329*:936–947, 1993.
45. Swift, T. R., and Ignacio, O. J.: Tick paralysis: Electrophysiologic studies. Neurology *25*:1130–1133, 1975.
46. Todd, J. L.: Does a human tick-borne disease exist in British Columbia? Can. Med. Assoc. J. *2*:686, 1912.
47. Vest, D. K.: Protracted reactions following probable hobo spider (*Tegenaria agrestis*) envenomation [Abstract]. Am. Arachnol. *48*:10, 1993.
48. Vetter, R. S., and Visscher, P. K.: Bites and stings of medically important venomous arthropods. Int. J. Dermatol. *37*:481–496, 1998.
49. Vorse, H., Seccareccio, P., Woodruff, K., et al.: Disseminated intravascular coagulopathy following fatal brown spider bite. J. Pediatr. *80*:1035–1037, 1972.
50. Walter, F. G., Bilden, E. F., and Gibly, R. L.: Envenomations. Crit Care Clin *15*:353–386, 1999.
51. Zumpt, F.: Myiasis in man and animals in the old world. London, Butterworths, 1965.

Health Information for International Travel

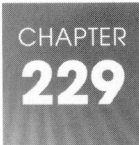

CHAPTER 229

International Travel Issues for Children

MICHELLE WEINBERG ■ SUSAN A. MALONEY

International Travel and Travel-Related Illness

During the past half century, the number of persons traveling internationally has increased tremendously. Between 1950 and 1999, the number of international arrivals worldwide grew from 25 million to 664 million, an annual growth rate of 7 percent. Close to 26.9 million residents of the United States traveled overseas in 2000. Approximately 50 percent of U.S. residents traveled to destinations other than Europe; these destinations included almost 5 million trips to Asia, more than 2.2 million trips to South and Central America, 1.3 million trips to the Middle East, and 500,000 trips to the African continent.[96] These data represent "overseas" trips taken by U.S. residents and do not include travel to Canada or Mexico.

International travelers may be exposed to a variety of health risks, depending on the travel destination, trip itinerary, duration of stay, planned travel activities (i.e., business versus adventure), individual risk factors, and preventive measures taken. For persons from industrialized countries visiting developing countries, travel may expose them to a variety of infectious pathogens and environmental hazards, some of which they may rarely encounter at home. An estimated 15 to 70 percent of adult travelers report health problems during international travel; 1 to 5 percent of travelers seek medical care during travel, 0.1 to 1 percent are hospitalized abroad, 0.01 to 0.1 percent require emergency evacuation, and 1 in 100,000 dies.[89, 91] Infectious diseases are a major cause of morbidity among international travelers. Numerous authors have studied and estimated the incidence of infectious diseases in international travelers, [15, 16, 20, 76, 91] and the most common illness reported on is diarrhea, which develops in an estimated 40 percent of persons traveling annually from industrialized to developing countries.[15, 16, 18, 22, 76, 86, 91] Malaria occurs less frequently but is a potentially life-threatening problem for travelers, with an estimated 30,000 North American and European travelers contracting malaria annually.[50] Other infectious diseases reported in travelers include hepatitis A and B, sexually transmitted diseases, animal bites with a risk of rabies, typhoid, cholera, legionellosis, human immunodeficiency virus (HIV) infection, and meningococcal disease.* Fewer data have been collected on the incidence of noninfectious health problems among adult travelers, but those available suggest that injuries (especially from motor vehicle and sporting accidents and drowning) and complications from preexisting medical conditions are substantial causes of serious morbidity and mortality.[88] Noninfectious health problems are also more common causes of mortality among adult travelers than infectious diseases are. In separate studies of deaths in adult international travelers (from the United States, Australia, and Scotland), the most common cause of death was cardiovascular disease; among U.S. travelers, cardiovascular disease in men older than 60 years accounted for 50 percent of all deaths.[28, 29, 68, 74, 85]

*See references 2, 5, 21, 26, 34, 45, 47, 52, 59, 60, 62, 70, 80, 83, 87, 90, 91, 99.

Pediatric Travelers and Health Risks Abroad

Less specific information is available on the number of children traveling internationally or living abroad. Extrapolating from overseas travel data for U.S. residents, a conservative estimate is that at least 1.9 million children travel overseas annually (i.e., 7% of the 26.9 million U.S. residents traveling internationally in 2000 reported traveling with children). Information is also more limited on the causes of serious morbidity and mortality among pediatric travelers, and efforts to collect these data should be undertaken to direct prevention measures so that morbidity and mortality in pediatric travelers can be decreased.[3, 33, 73] The data available include a 1-year prospective hospital-based study in the United Kingdom of children admitted with fever who had recently traveled to the tropics.[44] In this study, 31 children with a median age of 4 years (range, 5 months to 15 years) met the study entry criteria. Fourteen of these children had nonspecific, self-limited illnesses of presumed viral origin, and 17 children had conditions requiring hospital management and antimicrobial therapy. Conditions requiring hospital management included four cases of malaria (three of *Plasmodium falciparum* malaria and one of *Plasmodium vivax* malaria), three cases of bacillary dysentery, two cases each of dengue and typhoid fever, and one case each of acute hepatitis A infection, pneumonia (unspecified), *Pneumocystis carinii* pneumonia (in a child with newly diagnosed HIV infection), bacterial lymphadenitis, streptococcal throat infection, and acute myeloid leukemia; no deaths occurred. In another retrospective study of traveler's diarrhea in Swiss children who had visited the tropics or subtropics, Pitzinger and colleagues found incidence rates of 40, 8.5, 21.7, and 36 percent in children aged 0 to 2, 3 to 6, 7 to 14, and 15 years and older, respectively.[73] Other authors have reported substantial health risks for pediatric travelers from noninfectious causes such as injuries, including automobile accidents and drowning.[33]

Although data from adult travelers can be extrapolated to use in the management of pediatric travelers, infants and children have special vulnerabilities and needs when preparing for travel abroad. These needs include (1) up-to-date and appropriate vaccinations (at times through accelerated or altered routine childhood vaccine schedules and also including special travel-related vaccines); (2) appropriate malaria and other chemoprophylaxis regimens tailored for use in pediatric travelers; (3) prevention counseling, particularly in the areas of insect barriers, food and water safety, and injury prevention; and (4) anticipatory guidance for the management of potential illness and successful location of medical resources overseas. This chapter will provide recommendations for conducting a pediatric pretravel assessment to ensure that the child has received the appropriate vaccination and chemoprophylaxis regimens, pretravel prevention counseling, and means of accessing additional sources of travel information about health risks and the availability of medical resources at specific travel destinations.

General Approach to Pretravel Assessment for Children

Before international travel, children should have a pretravel health assessment performed by a health care provider. The number of physicians who specialize in travel medicine for children is relatively limited, and most pretravel assessments are performed by general pediatricians or pediatricians who specialize in infectious diseases. The visit should be conducted with the goal of preventing travel-related illnesses. Depending on the destination and the vaccinations recommended or required, the assessment should optimally be conducted up to 6 months before travel. Because families may not be aware of the need for multiple vaccinations, health care providers should be proactive and routinely ask patients and their families if they are anticipating any international travel in the next 6 months, especially before holiday periods.

During the pretravel assessment, the provider should

1. Review the child's current and past medical history, including the status of routine childhood vaccinations
2. Obtain specific details about the travel itinerary and planned activities

Then, after reviewing endemic diseases and recent outbreaks in travel destinations,

3. Administer indicated routine and travel-related vaccinations
4. Prescribe antimalarial and other prophylactic medication (based on risk assessment from the medical history, travel itinerary, and planned activities)
5. Counsel about prevention of travel-related illnesses
6. Provide guidance about seeking medical assistance for travel-related illness

The age, immunization status, and medical history of the child are important information to have when conducting the pretravel assessment. The provider should consider three categories of vaccinations: routine childhood vaccinations, required travel-related vaccinations, and recommended travel-related vaccinations. Some routine vaccinations should be administered at an earlier age or after an accelerated schedule in preparation for international travel. In addition, the provider should review and administer travel-related vaccinations that are required for entry by various countries to prevent the importation of disease and development of outbreaks, as well as vaccinations recommended for the prevention of illness in the individual traveler. Currently, only two vaccines, yellow fever and meningococcal vaccine, are required for entry by selected countries; however, these requirements may change in the future. In addition, some countries require documentation of HIV testing before allowing entry of long-term travelers (see International Travel Information Resources). Guidelines for standard and accelerated schedules for routine childhood immunizations and for required and recommended travel-related vaccinations by specific travel destinations are summarized in this chapter under Vaccination for International Travel. A review of medical conditions and contraindications is critical before administering vaccinations or prescribing medications such as antimalarial chemoprophylaxis.

The pretravel assessment should include a detailed review of the trip itinerary. The health care provider should ask about sources of water and food (local eating establishments versus hotel restaurants), type of accommodations (e.g., camping, hotel chains, or residing with local families), extent of contact with the local population, and planned activities during travel (adventure travel with exposure to animals, water, high altitude, or any combination of these factors). A template of a pretravel assessment questionnaire for children that can be completed by the family at the visit is shown in Figure 229–1. Recommendations to prevent vector-borne diseases, including malaria, should be determined by a comprehensive review of the travel itinerary and planned activities. Guidance for determining appropriate regimens for antimalarial chemoprophylaxis in pediatric travelers is provided in this chapter under Malaria Prevention. In addition, the risk of acquiring an infectious disease differs and is probably greater for an adolescent who is participating in a rural home stay program for 3 months than for a 5-year-old child traveling with parents to a beach resort. Furthermore, expatriates who live abroad and foreign-born persons, especially immigrants, refugees, and their children visiting friends and relatives in their home country, have different health risks than do short-term travelers who are visiting tourist destinations. These differential risk profiles should be taken into account during the pretravel assessment because such knowledge is essential for devising a specific pretravel management plan.

Based on risk assessment, preventive health counseling should include information about prevention of vector-borne illnesses, food and water safety, and prevention of other infectious and noninfectious illnesses such as automobile accidents. General and specific prevention counseling recommendations are addressed later in the chapter. In addition, families should clarify with their health insurance company whether they are covered for health care provided abroad. If not, insurance can be purchased from several companies; such insurance may include coverage for health care providers in a specific country and airlift/medical evacuation (see International Travel Information Resources). If assistance for illness acquired abroad is needed, the U.S. embassy or consulate can provide names and addresses of English-speaking health care providers at the travel destination. This information can be obtained before departure by accessing embassy Internet sites or by calling the embassy. In addition, names of physicians abroad also can be obtained from some worldwide directories (see International Travel Information Resources). Parents should be told to carry all health-related documents with them for easy retrieval, including written prescriptions for medications, health insurance information, and medical contacts abroad. Counseling on ensuring the use of sterile needles and the safety of the local blood supply

Name: ____

Age: ____________________ Date of birth:__________________

Medical history and recent changes in medical history:

____

____

____

Routine vaccinations	Total number of doses	Date of last dose
Hepatitis B		
DaPT/DPT/DT/dT		
Hib		
Polio		
MMR		
Varicella		
Pneumococcal		
Hepatitis A (in selected areas)		

Current medications: ____

Date of departure _________ Date of return ________

Destination Information

Location	Country	Urban	Rural	Purpose/Activities	Duration

Food preparation (check all that apply):
_____ self _____ fast food _____ small restaurants _____ hotel restaurants ____ local homes

Anticipated water source (check all that apply):
_____ bottled _____ boiled _____ tap _____ filtered _____ treated

Accommodations (check all that apply):
_____ large hotel chains _____ small local hotels _____ living with local families _____ camping
_____ other (specify) ____

Adventure activities (check all that apply):
_____ freshwater activities (lakes, streams) _____ ocean activities
_____ high-altitude/mountain climbing _____ backpacking/trekking _____ jungle

Anticipated animal exposures: ___ yes ___no
If yes, type(s) of animal(s) : ____

Exposures in health care setting (working in health care environment): ___ yes _____no

FIGURE 229–1 ■ Pretravel assessment questionnaire for children.

also should be included in pretravel prevention counseling topics; blood screening and infection control practices may not be as stringent in some countries as in the United States.

Special consideration must be given to children who have chronic diseases. Children with medical conditions should take a summary of their medical history and treatment record. If the child has cardiac disease, the family should consider taking a copy of the child's recent electrocardiogram and echocardiography report. Children with diabetes who are traveling through more than one time zone should consult their pediatrician or endocrinologist for guidance on the need for altering insulin dosing. Prescription medications should be carried in original bottles, and a sufficient supply for the length of the planned trip should be taken. Required medications should be carried on the plane rather than packed in luggage because bags may be lost or exposed to unfavorable environmental conditions. Families should be counseled about the potential hazards of obtaining medications in pharmacies in developing countries, where many medications can be purchased over the counter without a prescription and where the names, content, and concentration of medications may be different from those of U.S. products. Parents carrying medical equipment (such as nebulizers) should remember to take adaptors for foreign electric current and bring a letter from a physician that documents the need for the equipment.[17] Similar documentation is encouraged for anaphylaxis kits that include syringes. Additional information on travel considerations for immunocompromised children is provided later in the chapter.

Vaccination for International Travel

Vaccination before international travel is among the most critical and complex components of the pretravel assessment for children. The pretravel assessment should include a review of both recommended routine childhood vaccinations and required and recommended travel-related vaccines.

ROUTINE CHILDHOOD VACCINATIONS FOR PEDIATRIC TRAVELERS

For children who will be traveling internationally, having their routine immunizations brought up to date is essential because many vaccine-preventable diseases are more prevalent in developing countries than in the United States. The pretravel visit also may give the health care provider a unique opportunity to update the routine vaccination status of a patient who has fallen behind schedule. In certain cases, routine vaccinations may need to be accelerated to maximize protection, particularly against polio, diphtheria/tetanus/pertussis, and measles (for example, measles vaccination may be recommended for children younger than 12 months).[72] The management plan for routine vaccinations will be determined by the travel destination and itinerary. For example, diphtheria and pertussis are prevalent in eastern Europe and many developing countries, and measles is still endemic in the developing world; therefore, if travel to developing countries is planned, ensuring immunity is imperative and accelerated schedules should be considered. In addition, parents should check their own immune status because traveling with children can increase their risk of exposure to measles and other vaccine-preventable diseases. Trip activities also may increase the risk of acquiring infectious diseases such as measles; recently, an epidemiologic investigation identified numerous cases of serologically confirmed measles in internationally adopted children and their new parents and siblings who had traveled to China to accompany them home (Centers for Disease Control and Prevention [CDC], unpublished data). Data suggest that the exposure to measles occurred in China, probably at the orphanage, where an outbreak of measles was occurring. In addition, travel in large groups on conveyances such as cruise ships can facilitate the transmission of infectious and vaccine-preventable diseases.[54] The CDC recently has provided consultation on managing outbreaks of varicella and meningococcal disease in pediatric travelers on international cruise ships (CDC, unpublished data).

Worldwide polio eradication efforts have decreased the number of countries where travelers are at risk for acquiring polio from more than 120 in 1988 to approximately 50 in 1998 (with most poliovirus transmissions now occurring in two large endemic areas in south Asia and sub-Saharan Africa).[7] However, outbreaks of polio still occur; in July 2000, an outbreak of vaccine-derived poliovirus type 1 was reported in the Dominican Republic and Haiti.[102] To ensure protection, pediatric travelers visiting countries where polio is epidemic or still endemic should be fully immunized. Hepatitis B, *Haemophilus influenzae* type b, *Streptococcus pneumoniae,* and varicella are endemic in many developing countries, and vaccination should be ensured, particularly for young pediatric travelers to these regions. For detailed information about accelerating routine childhood vaccinations and indications for use in pediatric travelers, see Table 229–1.

COMMON TRAVEL-RELATED VACCINES FOR CHILDREN

An important consideration when determining travel vaccination needs is "required" versus "recommended" vaccinations. The most recent travel requirements and recommendations for vaccinations can be obtained from the CDC Travelers' Health Internet site (see International Travel Information Resources). Few vaccinations are required. The United States does not require arriving travelers to have any vaccinations for entry or return to the United States. However, immigrants, refugees, asylum seekers, and internationally adopted children migrating to the United States for permanent residence have different requirements. Some other countries may require proof of vaccination against yellow fever for entry, especially if the traveler is arriving from a country where yellow fever is present. Yellow fever vaccine is available only from certified yellow fever vaccination centers; providers can contact their state public health department to locate certified centers in their areas. Saudi Arabia requires meningococcal vaccine for travelers to the Hajj in Mecca. Some countries previously have required cholera vaccination, but currently no countries do so. However, non-U.S. customs officials who "unofficially" request proof of vaccination have been reported. Cholera vaccine is not available in the United States.

Table 229–2 provides general guidelines and indications for the use of selected travel-related vaccines based on U.S. recommendations[1, 35, 36, 72]; World Health Organization (WHO) recommendations may differ.[7, 111] Depending on the complexity of the travel itinerary and the patient's medical history, the vaccination plan may need to be developed in consultation with a travel medicine or infectious disease specialist. Travel-related vaccine recommendations should be carefully tailored to the trip itinerary and based on the travel destination, season when the travel will occur, duration of the trip, and activities to be undertaken.[95] For example, hepatitis A is endemic in most of the world, and travelers are at risk in any area where sanitation is poor. Vaccination is recommended for pediatric travelers 2 years or older who

TABLE 229–1 ■ ROUTINE CHILDHOOD VACCINATIONS AND ACCELERATED SCHEDULES AND MODIFICATIONS FOR PEDIATRIC TRAVELERS

Vaccine*	Minimal Age	Routine Schedule: Number of Doses and Recommended Ages[†]	Accelerated Schedule and Modifications: Number of Doses and Minimum Intervals between Doses (Note: Interval Represents Time from Dose)	Indications for Use and Other Information[‡]
DTaP/DTP/DT	6 wk	5 doses at ages 2, 4, 6, and 15–18 mo and 4–6 yr	5 doses Minimal interval (MI) from dose 1 to 2: 4 wk MI from dose 2 to 3: 4 wk MI from dose 3 to 4: 6 mo Minimal age for dose 4: 12 mo MI from doses 4 and 5: 6 mo Minimal recommended age for dose 5: 4–6 yr	Use for children 6 wk to 7 yr of age Use DT for children <7 yr of age for primary series (instead of DTaP/DTP) when pertussis vaccination is contraindicated
Td	7 yr	1 dose at age 11–12 yr followed by 1 booster dose every 10 yr Children 11–16 yr + 5 yr since primary series: 1 booster dose Children >17 yr + 10 yr since last tetanus vaccine: 1 booster dose	Booster for adventure travel: 1 dose every 5 yr	Use for children and adults ≥7 yr of age
Hepatitis B[§]	Birth	3 doses at ages 0–2, 1–4, and 6–18 mo For children aged 11–12 yr: 3 doses at 0 -, 1 -, 4 -mo intervals For unvaccinated adolescents aged 11–15 yr: 2-dose vaccine series (only Recombivax HB, adult dose) at 0, 4–6 mo or 3 doses of other vaccine brands as for children 11–12 yr old	3 doses (except 2 doses of Recombivax HB, adult dose for adolescents) MI from dose 1 to 2: 4 wk MI from dose 2 to 3: 8 wk MI from dose 1 to 3: 16 wk Minimal age for dose 3: 6 mo	Use for travelers to endemic areas, including Africa, Asia, Latin America, who plan to 1. Travel abroad for ≥6 mo 2. Have intimate or sexual contact with local population 3. Work in health care setting or may have contact with blood, blood products, or body fluids Count all doses; do not restart series even if time lapse between doses is greater than recommended interval Accelerated schedules that may be associated with decreased immunogenicity: 4 doses at 0, 1, 3 wk and 6–12 mo *or* 4 doses at 0, 7, 21 days and booster at 1 yr
Hib	6 wk	4 doses at ages 2, 4, 6, and 12–15 mo *or* 3 doses at ages 2, 4, and 12–15 mo (PRP-OMP vaccines only) Unvaccinated child >15 mo: 1 dose	Accelerated schedule available but varies by vaccine brand; see package insert for vaccine used MI between doses: 4–8 wk	Vaccinate all children <5 yr of age and children >5 yr of age with special indications (e.g., asplenia, immunodeficiency)
MMR	6 mo	2 doses at ages 12–15 mo and 4–6 yr	Children aged 6–11 mo: 1 dose then revaccinate at 12–15 mo and 4–6 yr of age Children >12 mo vaccinated with 1 previous dose: 1 additional dose at least 4 wk after dose 1 Unvaccinated children >12 mo: 2 doses separated by 4 wk MI between doses: 4 wk	Do not administer MMR for 3 mo after immunoglobulin for hepatitis A prophylaxis; see *Red Book* for deferral times for blood products and immunoglobulin administered for other indications Defer immunoglobulin administration for 2 wk after MMR vaccination Monovalent vaccines available for measles, mumps, and rubella

Continued

TABLE 229–1 ■ ROUTINE CHILDHOOD VACCINATIONS AND ACCELERATED SCHEDULES AND MODIFICATIONS FOR PEDIATRIC TRAVELERS—cont'd

Vaccine*	Minimal Age	Routine Schedule: Number of Doses and Recommended Ages†	Accelerated Schedule and Modifications: Number of Doses and Minimum Intervals between Doses (Note: Interval Represents Time from Dose)	Indications for Use and Other Information‡
Pneumococcal conjugate —7 valent	6 wk	4 doses at ages 2, 4, 6, and 12–15 mo	Children <7 mo of age: 4 doses MI from dose 1 to 2: 4 wk MI from dose 2 to 3: 4 wk MI from dose 3 to 4: 8 wk Minimal age for dose 4: 12 mo Children aged 7–11 mo: 3 doses MI from dose 1 to 2: 4 wk MI from dose 2 to 3: 8 wk Minimal age for dose 3: 12 mo Children aged 12–23 mo: 2 doses MI from dose 1 to 2: 6 wk Children aged >24 mo to 9 yr: 1 dose	Consider vaccinating children <9 yr old who are traveling to areas with limited access to medical care Pneumococcal polysaccharide vaccine (PPV23) is routinely recommended for high-risk persons. See Pediatrics *106*:362–366, 2000
Polio—IPV	6 wk	4 doses at ages 2, 4, and 6–18 mo and 4–6 yr	Previously unvaccinated children: 3 doses separated by minimum of 4 wk Previously unvaccinated children <4 yr of age at completion of dose 3: 4 doses Previously unvaccinated children ≥4 years of age at completion of dose 3: 3 doses Previously vaccinated adult (≥18 years of age): 1 booster recommended for travel to risk area MI between doses: 4 wk	Primary series recommended for all travelers; booster dose for adults recommended for international travelers to Africa or Asia; not routinely recommended for travel to Latin America except to Haiti or Dominican Republic, where an outbreak occurred in 2001 Single booster for previously vaccinated adults confers lifetime immunity
Polio—OPV	U.S.: 6 wk WHO: birth	Not routinely recommended for use in U.S.	Previously unvaccinated children and adults: 3 doses MI between doses: 4 wk	Not routinely recommended except for unvaccinated children who will be traveling in less than 4 wk to risk areas Consider for children <6 wk of age traveling to high-risk areas
Varicella	12 mo	1 dose at age 12–18 mo Unvaccinated children <13 yr: 1 dose Unvaccinated children ≥13 yr: 2 doses separated by 4 wk	MI from dose 1 to 2: 4 wk	All international travelers >1 yr of age should have previous vaccination or history of disease Give simultaneously with MMR/ yellow fever or wait for 4 wk Defer varicella vaccination for 3 mo after immunoglobulin administration for hepatitis A prevention. See *Red Book* for deferral times for immunoglobulin administered for other indications Defer immunoglobulin administration for hepatitis A prevention for 2 wk after varicella vaccination unless the benefits outweigh those of the vaccine. In this case, revaccinate 5 mo later or check antibody titer at 6 mo and revaccinate if seronegative

*Hepatitis A vaccine is recommended for children older than 2 years who live in selected areas. See M. M. W. R. Recomm. Rep. *48* (RR-12):1–37, 1999. Influenza vaccine is recommended annually for children age ≥6 months with certain risk factors. See M. M. W. R. Recomm. Rep. *52* (RR-8):1–36, 2003.

†The minimal age is the U.S. recommendation unless otherwise noted. Recommendations in the U.S. schedule may be different from those of the World Health Organization and other countries.

‡Contraindications: anaphylactic reaction to a previous dose or any vaccine component or moderate to severe acute illness (or both) is a contraindication for all vaccines.

§Combination hepatitis A–hepatitis B (Twinrix) is now available for use in persons 18 years or older. The vaccine, which is composed of inactivated viral components, is administered intramuscularly. The schedule involves three doses at 0, 1, and 6 months. It can be administered at an accelerated schedule of four doses at 0, 7, and 21 days and 1 year.

DT, diphtheria and tetanus toxoids (pediatric type); DTaP, diphtheria and tetanus toxoids and acellular pertussis; DTP, diphtheria and tetanus toxoids and pertussis; Hib, *Haemophilus influenzae* type b; IPV, inactivated poliovirus vaccine; MMR, measles-mumps-rubella; Td, tetanus and diphtheria toxoids (adult type); WHO, World Health Organization.

TABLE 229–2 ■ COMMON TRAVEL-RELATED VACCINES AND IMMUNOGLOBULIN FOR CHILDREN

Vaccine*	Vaccine Type	Route	Minimal Age	Primary Series: Number of Doses and Recommended Ages and Intervals (Note: Interval Represents Time from Dose)	Booster or Revaccination: Number of Doses and Recommended Ages and Intervals	Accelerated Schedule	Protection After	General Indications for Use[†]
Bacille Calmette Guérin (BCG)	Live attenuated bacteria	ID, SC	Birth	1 dose	None	None	2 mo after dose (WHO)	Consider for children <1 yr who will be long-term travelers residing in high-risk areas to protect against meningeal and military tuberculosis
Hepatitis A[‡]	Inactivated virus	IM	2 yr	2 doses at 0 and 6- to 12-mo intervals	Unknown	None	4 wk after dose 1 Protective antibody titers 2 wk after dose 1: 69–98% of vaccinees studied Protective antibody titers 4 wk after dose 1: 95–100% of vaccinees studied Dose 2 required for long-term protection	Use for travel to Latin America, Africa, Asia (except Japan), Oceania (except Australia, New Zealand), Middle East, and selected areas of Europe Give immunoglobulin in addition to or instead of vaccine to travelers who are departing within 4 wk Count all doses and do not restart series even if time lapse between doses is greater than recommended interval Hepatitis A vaccine is recommended routinely for children >2 yr who live in selected areas of the U.S. See M. M. W. R. Recomm. Rep. *48* (RR-12):1–37, 1999
Immuno-globulin (IG)	Antibody from pooled human plasma	IM	Birth	1 dose See *Red Book* for IG dosing	3–6 mo	None	Immediate	Use to prevent hepatitis A infection in children <2 yr of age who are traveling to risk areas or for persons departing within 4 wk Defer MMR vaccination for 3 mo after IG administered for hepatitis A prevention; defer administration of IG for hepatitis A prevention for 2 wk after MMR vaccination Defer varicella vaccination for 3 mo after IG administered for hepatitis A prevention; defer administration of IG for hepatitis A prevention for 2 wk after varicella vaccination

Continued

TABLE 229–2 ■ COMMON TRAVEL-RELATED VACCINES AND IMMUNOGLOBULIN FOR CHILDREN—cont'd

Vaccine*	Vaccine Type	Route	Minimal Age	Primary Series: Number of Doses and Recommended Ages and Intervals (Note: Interval Represents Time from Dose)	Booster or Revaccination: Number of Doses and Recommended Ages and Intervals	Accelerated Schedule	Protection After	General Indications for Use†
Influenza	Inactivated virus	IM	6 mo	Previously unvaccinated children <9 yr of age: 2 doses separated by 1 mo Previously vaccinated children <9 yr of age: 1 dose Children ≥9 yr of age: 1 dose	1 yr	None	14 days after completed age-dependent series	Consider for travelers who are at high risk for complications from influenza for travel to 1. Tropics any time of year 2. Southern Hemisphere from April through September 3. Any destination with large groups of tourists at any time of year 4. Any destination where influenza outbreaks are occurring Vaccine may not be available in U.S. during summer months Do not administer to children with severe anaphylactic reaction to eggs
Japanese encephalitis	Inactivated virus	SC	1 yr	3 doses at 0, 7, and 14 or 30 days	2–3 yr Booster: 1 dose	None	10–14 days after dose 3	Use for travelers to selected areas of Asia, Oceania (Australia and Papua New Guinea), Russia, especially long-term travelers to rural, agricultural endemic areas or epidemic regions during seasonal transmission (usually May to September) Allergic reaction (urticaria, angioedema, respiratory distress,anaphylaxis) occur in approximately 0.6% of persons. Anaphylaxis can occur up to 10 days after vaccination, so all doses of vaccine should be administered at least 10 days before departure. Persons vaccinated should remain in areas with access to health care. Observe for 30 minutes after vaccine administration and counsel about possible delayed hypersensitivity reactions. Persons with history of urticaria are at greater risk for allergic reactions

								Mild adverse reactions (headache, fever, local reactions) occur in approximately 20% of vaccines
Meningococcal (quadrivalent A, C, Y, W-135; bivalent A, C)§	Polysaccharide inactivated bacterial components	SC	2 yr	1 dose	3–5 yr except that children who were vaccinated at <4 yr of age should receive booster after 2–3 yr	None	7–10 days after dose	Required for travelers to annual Hajj in Mecca, Saudi Arabia Recommended for travel to sub-Saharan Africa during dry season (December through June) or for travel to any country where an epidemic is occurring Bivalent A, C vaccine available outside U.S.
Rabies Human diploid-cell vaccine (HDCV) Rabies vaccine adsorbed (RVA) Purified chick embryo cell culture vaccine (PCEC)	Inactivated virus; cell culture derived	IM, ID (HDCV only)	U.S.: None WHO: 1 yr	3 doses at 0, 7, and 21 or 28 days	6 mo to 3 yr, depending on risk or serologic tests Continuous risk: check antibody titer every 6 mo Frequent exposure: check antibody titer after 2 yr WHO: 1 yr after primary series then every 2–3 yr Booster: 1 dose	None	14 days after dose 3	Use for travelers to rabies-endemic countries. Recommended for long-term travel in rural areas or regions with limited access to health care. Travelers with extensive exposure in rural areas, such as backpacking, should consider vaccination even for trips of short duration Widespread worldwide rabies distribution. See Health Information for International Travel[7] for list of countries that have not reported cases of rabies recently Complete intradermal rabies vaccine series atleast 7 days before starting chloroquine or mefloquine Postexposure vaccination is required even for persons who receive vaccination before exposure After exposure in vaccinated person: 2 doses at 0 and 3 days (no rabies IG required) After exposure in unvaccinated person: rabies IG (20, IU/kg) plus vaccination with 5 doses at 0, 3, 7, 14, and 28 days

Continued

TABLE 229–2 ■ COMMON TRAVEL-RELATED VACCINES AND IMMUNOGLOBULIN FOR CHILDREN—cont'd

Vaccine*	Vaccine type	Route	Minimal Age	Primary Series: Number of Doses and Recommended Ages and Intervals (Note: Interval Represents Time from Dose)	Booster or Revaccination: Number of Doses and Recommended Ages and Intervals	Accelerated Schedule	Protection After	General Indications for Use[†]
Typhoid (ViCPS)	Capsular poly-saccharide	SC	2 yr	1 dose	2 yr	None	14 days after dose	Use recommended for travelers to Africa, Asia, and Latin America for long-term stay; travel outside usual tourist destinations; or travelers who desire maximal protection Patients should be counseled regarding protective efficacy of vaccine (approximately 50–74% when studied in endemic areas) and importance of other preventive measures
Typhoid oral (Ty21a)	Live attenuated bacteria	Oral	6 yr	4 doses at 0, 2, 4, and 6 days	5 yr	None	7–10 days after last dose	See indications for Typhoid ViCPS Patients should be counseled regarding protective efficacy of vaccine (approximately 60–85% when studied in endemic areas) and importance of other preventive measures Must be swallowed (cannot be chewed) 1 hr before meal, and vaccine must be refrigerated until administration Do not administer within 24 hr of mefloquine, atovaquone-proguanil, doxycycline, or any other antibiotic Contraindicated for immunocompromised patients

Yellow fever	Live attenuated virus	SC	6 mo	1 dose	10 yr	None	10 days after dose	Use for travelers to selected areas of Africa and South America Yellow fever has not been reported in Asia; however, some countries require vaccination if the traveler is arriving from a yellow fever–endemic country Yellow fever vaccination for children aged 6–9 mo should be discussed with an expert to weigh risk of adverse events versus risk of yellow fever Recent reports of rare serious adverse events of multiorgan system failure after vaccination Contraindicated for patients who are immunocompromised or have allergy to eggs

*Cholera vaccine is no longer available in the United States. It is administered as a two-dose series at 1- to 4-week intervals. It has limited efficacy and was associated with frequent adverse effects. Tick-borne encephalitis vaccine is not available in the United States. It is administered as a four-dose series at 0, 28, and 42 days and 1-year intervals with booster doses required every 3 to 5 years. The vaccine is available in Europe.

†Contraindications: anaphylactic reaction to a previous dose or any vaccine component or moderate to severe acute illness (or both) is a contraindication for all vaccines.

‡Combination hepatitis A–hepatitis B (Twinrix) is now available for use in persons 18 years or older. The vaccine, which is composed of inactivated viral components, is administered intramuscularly. The schedule involves three doses at 0, 1, and 6 months. It can be administered at an accelerated schedule of four doses at 0,7 and 21 days and 1 year.

§Meningococcal vaccine: serogroup A is immunogenic in children 3 months or older. Responses to other serogroup components are poor or unknown in children 2 years or younger. Group A meningococcal vaccine can be administered to children younger than 18 months; it is administered as two doses separated by a 3-month interval. Quadrivalent vaccine can also be administered to children younger than 18 months but may induce a limited immunologic response.

IO, intradermal; MMR, measles mumps rubella; WHO, World Health Organization.

will be visiting countries with intermediate to high endemicity (areas other than the United States, Canada, Australia, New Zealand, Western Europe, and Scandinavia). Intramuscular immunoglobulin is recommended for immunoprophylaxis against hepatitis A in children younger than 2 years. In addition, for children 2 years or older who will be departing sooner than 4 weeks after the pretravel visit (and therefore may not have sufficient time for immunity to develop after hepatitis A vaccination), both immunoglobulin and vaccine can be given concurrently at different sites to ensure more immediate protection. Shortages of immunoglobulin have occurred recently, so obtaining it for hepatitis A prophylaxis may be difficult. Studies have demonstrated that 2 weeks after the first dose of hepatitis A vaccine, protective antibody titers are present in 69 to 98 percent of vaccinees, whereas after 4 weeks, protective antibody titers are present in 95 to 100 percent.

Meningococcal disease occurs sporadically worldwide. Epidemic disease has been reported in India, Saudi Arabia, and sub-Saharan Africa; indeed, recurrent epidemics of meningococcal disease occur in sub-Saharan Africa, mainly from December to June (the dry season). Serogroup A is the most common cause of epidemics outside the United States, but serogroup C and other serogroups also have been associated with epidemics. Serogroup W-135 meningococcal infection has been reported recently in travelers returning from Saudi Arabia after visiting the Hajj.[99] The meningococcal vaccine available in the United States is the quadrivalent polysaccharide A/C/Y/W-135. It is recommended for pediatric travelers 2 years or older who are visiting sub-Saharan Africa during the dry season or any country where an epidemic caused by a vaccine serogroup is occurring. The vaccine can be administered to children younger than 2 years, but they may have a limited immunologic response (other than to serogroup A).[72]

Yellow fever occurs year-round in the predominately rural areas of sub-Saharan Africa and South America, but of late, outbreaks have been increasing. The recent resurgence of yellow fever in Brazil has raised concern about increased risk in other areas of Latin America and the possibility of urban yellow fever transmission.[104, 105] Though a rare disease, yellow fever continues to be reported in travelers, particularly unvaccinated travelers, and it is usually fatal. Preventive measures taken against yellow fever should include the use of personal protection against mosquitoes and vaccination. As discussed previously, some countries require yellow fever vaccination for travelers arriving from endemic regions; current requirements and recommendations for vaccination based on travel destination can be obtained from the CDC Travelers' Health Internet site. Yellow fever vaccine is largely considered to be a safe and effective vaccine. However, the vaccine has been found to be associated with an increased risk of encephalitis and other severe reactions in young infants.[72] The vaccine should not be used in children younger than 6 months. It should be used with caution in children 6 to 9 months of age after discussion with a travel medicine expert to weigh the risks and benefits.[7] Medical waivers can be given to children who are too young for vaccination and to those who have other contraindications to vaccination, such as immunodeficiency. More recently, life-threatening severe illness with major organ system failure has been reported in association with yellow fever vaccination. The syndrome usually consists of fever, jaundice, and multiple organ system failure, and more than half of the people who have developed these adverse effects have died. The risk is thought to be approximately 1 per 200,000 to 300,000 doses in persons younger than 60 years of age, and 1 per 40,000 to 50,000 doses in persons 60 years of age and older. Further studies are being conducted.[11, 55, 104] In the interim, the CDC has stated that given the risk of serious illness and death from yellow fever,[57] evidence of increasing transmission of the disease,[79] and the known effectiveness of the vaccine, clinicians should continue to use yellow fever vaccine to protect travelers. However, the CDC recommends that health care providers carefully review travel itineraries to ensure that only people traveling to yellow fever–endemic areas or areas where yellow fever activity is reported receive yellow fever vaccine.[23, 24]

Japanese encephalitis (JE) is a viral infection transmitted by *Culex* mosquitoes that bite from dusk to dawn. JE occurs year-round in tropical regions and primarily from May through October in temperate zones. The risk is greatest for travelers to rural Asia, where the mosquito breeds in rice fields and other agricultural areas. JE is associated with a high case-fatality rate and severe neurologic sequelae, especially in young children and the elderly. Vaccination should be considered for pediatric travelers 1 year or older who will visit and reside in areas where JE is endemic or epidemic, especially during the transmission season, or for pediatric travelers whose activities include trips to rural farming areas. Short-term travelers (less than 30 days) who visit only major urban areas are at lower risk for acquiring JE and generally do not need to be vaccinated.[7]

Rabies occurs worldwide except in Antarctica. In certain areas of the world, including (but not limited to) parts of Brazil, Bolivia, Colombia, Ecuador, El Salvador, Guatemala, India, Mexico, Nepal, Peru, the Philippines, Sri Lanka, Thailand, and Vietnam, canine rabies remains highly endemic. Rabies also occurs in other wild animals, including bats. Rabies vaccine should be considered for children visiting rabies-endemic countries for longer than 1 month, those undertaking extensive outdoor activities such as backpacking or camping in endemic countries, or children traveling to areas where access to health care is limited. To reduce the risk of acquiring rabies, children and their families should be counseled to stay away from stray dogs and other animals, especially if traveling to Latin America, Asia, or Africa.[7]

Typhoid vaccine is recommended for pediatric travelers visiting developing countries, especially for prolonged periods, or traveling outside the usual tourist destinations. Parents should be cautioned, however, that vaccination is not 100 percent effective, and precautions regarding safe food and water should be followed.

Finally, bacille Calmette-Guérin (BCG) vaccine is a live vaccine prepared from attenuated strains of *Mycobacterium bovis;* BCG is used primarily in young infants to prevent disseminated and other forms of life-threatening disease caused by tuberculosis (TB), such as tuberculous meningitis. BCG is recommended by the WHO for administration at birth; in the United States, BCG is recommended in only limited circumstances, such as unavoidable risk of exposure to *Mycobacterium tuberculosis*. Vaccination of a young pediatric traveler (non–HIV infected and with a negative TB skin test) might be considered, therefore, if long-term stay is planned in a country with a high prevalence of TB and prolonged contact with active TB cases is thought to be a potential problem.[72, 94] BCG vaccine can be obtained from the Canadian subdivisions of Aventis Pasteur or Organon. More generally, children traveling to countries with a high prevalence of TB should be skin-tested before and after travel to document possible exposure to TB. According to reports, U.S. children who had traveled to countries with a high prevalence of TB within the previous 12 months were 3.9 times more likely to have positive TB skin tests than were children who lived in the same U.S. areas but had not traveled.[49] Additional information about preventing other infectious diseases is provided in this chapter under Preventing Other Infectious Diseases in Pediatric Travelers.

One limitation to performing adequate travel-related vaccination is that patients may not seek medical assessment in sufficient time to complete vaccination and acquire protective immunity. Providers should routinely ask patients whether they are planning any travel in the future, particularly in the months before holidays and summer vacations. Multiple doses are required for some travel-related vaccines. In addition, other time-related vaccination issues also should be considered; for example, a patient who receives JE vaccine should complete the series of three doses at least 10 days before travel so that the patient can be observed for delayed allergic reactions.

Malaria Prevention

EPIDEMIOLOGY OF MALARIA

Malaria is a parasitic infection caused by one of four species of *Plasmodium: Plasmodium falciparum, Plasmodium vivax, Plasmodium ovale, or Plasmodium malariae.* It is transmitted by the bite of an infective female *Anopheles* mosquito. Malaria is endemic in more than 100 countries on five continents; transmission occurs primarily in the tropic and subtropical regions of sub-Saharan Africa, Asia, Latin America, the Caribbean, the Middle East, and Oceania. Globally, malaria is responsible for 300 to 500 million clinical infections and 1.5 to 2.7 million deaths annually, with most caused by *P. falciparum,* principally in young children and pregnant women.[112]

Recently, an estimated 10,000 to 30,000 travelers from industrialized countries were thought to contract malaria each year, but these numbers probably are underestimated because they do not include travelers in whom malaria was diagnosed and treated abroad.[39, 40, 50] In the United States, 5794 cases of malaria in U.S. civilians were reported to the CDC from 1992 through 2000. Of 5662 U.S. civilian cases with information about the country of acquisition, 3289 (58%) were acquired in Africa, 1054 (19%) in Asia, 1059 (19%) in Latin America or the Caribbean, and 260 (4%) in Oceania. During this period, 976 (17%) of the cases occurred in children younger than 18 years. Among children with malaria, 343 (35%) were 1 month to 5 years old, 215 (22%) were 6 to 9 years old, 226 (23%) were 10 to 14 years old, and 192 (20%) were 15 to 17 years old (CDC, unpublished data). A recent review of malaria cases in U.S. civilians (adults and children) reported that the largest percentage of cases (38.5%) occurred in persons who were visiting friends or relatives in malaria-endemic areas.[32] Retrospective reviews of malaria in children also have found that a substantial proportion of cases occurred in recent immigrants and the children of former immigrants who had traveled to visit their family's country of origin.[3, 78] These data highlight the importance of pretravel assessment and counseling, particularly for foreign-born persons, who may assume that they are protected by natural immunity or do not perceive the risk of malaria developing in their children who accompany them when returning to visit their home country.

PREVENTING MALARIA IN PEDIATRIC TRAVELERS

The substantial proportion of U.S. civilian malaria cases reported in children younger than 18 years underscores the importance of pretravel counseling and strategies for malaria prevention. Young children and nonimmune persons of any age are at greater risk for severe complications from malaria. Prevention of malaria in pediatric travelers depends first on obtaining current and accurate information about the risk of acquiring malaria in proposed travel destinations and determining whether planned activities, such as rural versus urban travel and the season of travel, place the traveler at increased risk of exposure. Information on the geographic- and country-specific risk of acquiring malaria is available from multiple sources. Selected websites with information about the country-specific risk of acquiring malaria are listed in this chapter under International Travel Information Resources.

After a thorough assessment of the risk of acquiring malaria has been made, prevention strategies for pediatric travelers are twofold: personal protection measures against contact with mosquitoes and antimalarial chemoprophylaxis. The first mainstay of prevention of malaria is appropriate and effective use of personal protection measures. All travelers to malaria-endemic areas should be counseled on recommended measures to avoid bites from *Anopheles* mosquitoes, which typically are evening and nighttime feeders. Such measures include wearing clothing that reduces the amount of exposed skin (such as long-sleeved shirts, long pants tucked into socks, hats) and, whenever possible, remaining in well-screened or enclosed air-conditioned areas. Travelers staying overnight in facilities without air conditioning or screens should use insecticide-treated mosquito nets over the beds. Bed nets that have been treated with insecticide such as permethrin or deltamethrin are more effective in preventing malaria than are untreated bed nets and are safe for children.[64] Travelers can purchase permethrin to spray on the bed nets or purchase pretreated (or impregnated) bed nets. Permethrin also can be sprayed on clothing, but it should not be applied directly to skin. During the evening, insecticide also can be sprayed inside rooms. Another important focus of counseling for personal protection measures should be appropriate use of insect repellent such as *N,N*-diethylmetatoluamide (DEET) on exposed skin. Because of reports of seizures in children, physicians previously thought that products formulated with lower concentrations of DEET would be safer for children; therefore, the American Academy of Pediatrics (AAP) had recommended using repellents with less than 10 percent DEET. However, recent studies reviewed by the Environmental Protection Agency (EPA) suggest that products with lower concentrations of DEET are not necessarily safer than products with higher concentrations. In 1998, the EPA reassessed the safety and labeling of DEET and stated that as long as consumers follow label directions and take proper precautions, insect repellents containing DEET do not present a health concern. The EPA concluded that the scientific data on DEET do not support product label claims of child safety based on the percentage of DEET and, therefore, no longer allows labeling of insect repellents with indications specifically for children. The AAP currently is considering a recommendation for the use of products with concentrations of approximately 30 percent for children.[107] DEET should not be used on children younger than 2 months or applied to the hands or mouth or near the eyes of young children. Clinicians are encouraged to stress the importance of the use of personal protection measures to parents and children alike. Despite the demonstrated efficacy of these measures, studies have found that only 17 percent of adult travelers with malaria reported using insect protection methods and only 11 percent took the recommended chemoprophylaxis.[39]

The second mainstay of malaria prevention is chemoprophylaxis. Selection of the appropriate drug for antimalarial chemoprophylaxis must be based on numerous factors, including the most recent information available about malaria in the proposed travel destinations; the trip itinerary; the age, weight, and medical history of the traveler; personal preference regarding the frequency of dosing and the duration of chemoprophylaxis on return from the trip; and the cost of medication. These decisions can be challenging for primary care providers and clinicians with limited experience in infectious disease and travel medicine, so when in doubt, clinicians should seek the advice of a travel medicine or infectious disease expert. In addition, the CDC provides resources with guidance on appropriate use and recommended regimens for antimalarial chemoprophylaxis (listed in "International Travel Information Resources").

Figure 229–2 outlines an algorithm for determining appropriate antimalarial chemoprophylaxis regimens for pediatric travelers. Maps of malaria-endemic areas and zones of drug resistance, which can be used as visual aids, are presented in Figures 229–3 and 229–4. Because data on the distribution of drug-resistant malaria are evolving constantly, in addition to using the information in this chapter, clinicians should always obtain the most recent information about the risk of malaria and zones of drug resistance before prescribing malaria chemoprophylaxis.[84] The first decision point in selecting appropriate antimalarial chemoprophylaxis is whether travel is occurring in a region of chloroquine-sensitive or chloroquine-resistant malaria. For travel to areas with chloroquine-sensitive malaria, chloroquine is the drug of choice for antimalarial chemoprophylaxis. *P. ovale, P. malariae,* and most *P. vivax* are widely sensitive to chloroquine; however, chloroquine-resistant *P. vivax* is an emerging problem and has been reported from Guyana, Papua New Guinea, India, Myanmar (Burma), and areas of Indonesia.[41] In addition to chloroquine-resistant *P. vivax,* chloroquine-resistant *P. falciparum* has been reported from these areas, and consequently, chloroquine would not be recommended as chemoprophylaxis for travelers to these regions.

If the traveler is visiting a region with chloroquine-resistant malaria, the next decision point is whether travel will include regions with chloroquine-resistant malaria only or both chloroquine- and mefloquine-resistant malaria. Chloroquine-resistant *P. falciparum* is widespread and exists in all malaria-endemic areas except Mexico, the Caribbean, Central America west of the former Panama Canal Zone, Argentina, and parts of the Middle East and China.[41] In some regions, *P. falciparum* may be resistant to both chloroquine and mefloquine; these areas currently are limited to the borders of Thailand with Myanmar (Burma) and Cambodia, the western provinces of Cambodia, and the eastern states of Myanmar.[7, 41] For travel to areas with chloroquine-resistant malaria, three current antimalarial chemoprophylaxis options are mefloquine (Lariam), atovaquone-proguanil

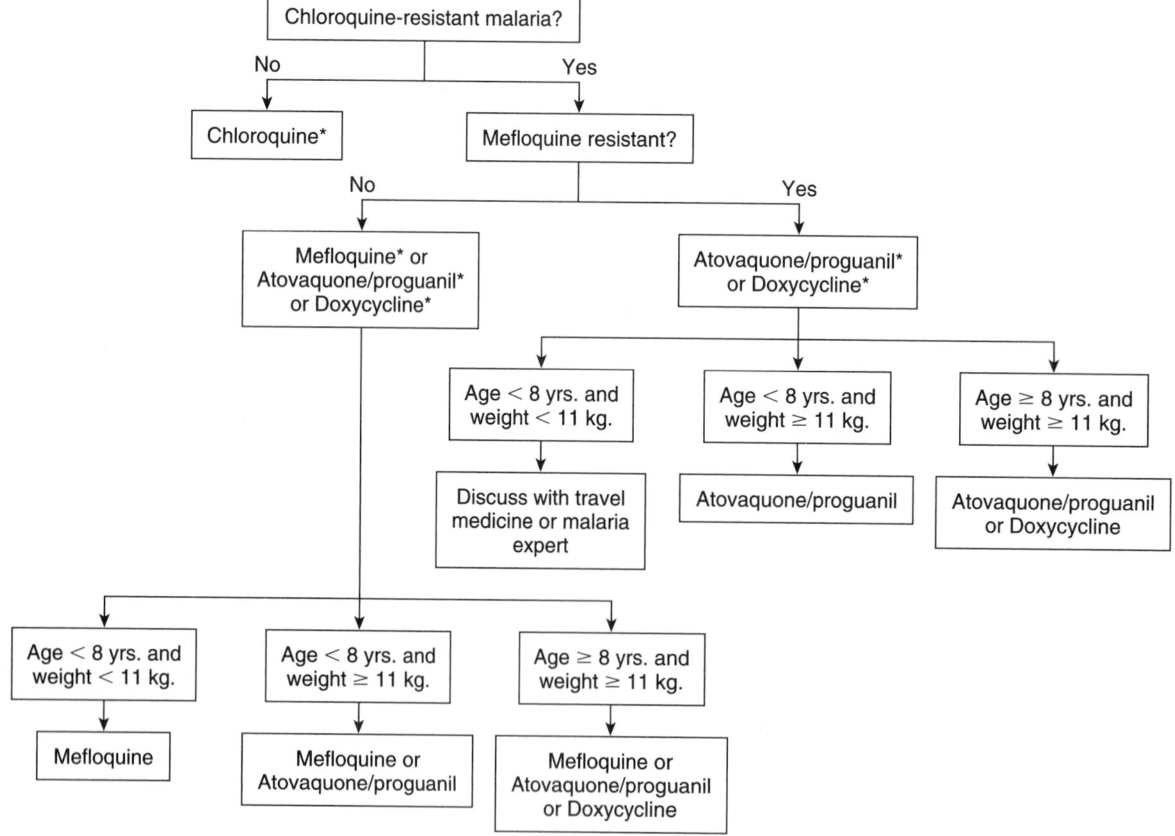

FIGURE 229–2 ■ Algorithm for determining appropriate antimalarial chemoprophylaxis regimens for pediatric travelers.

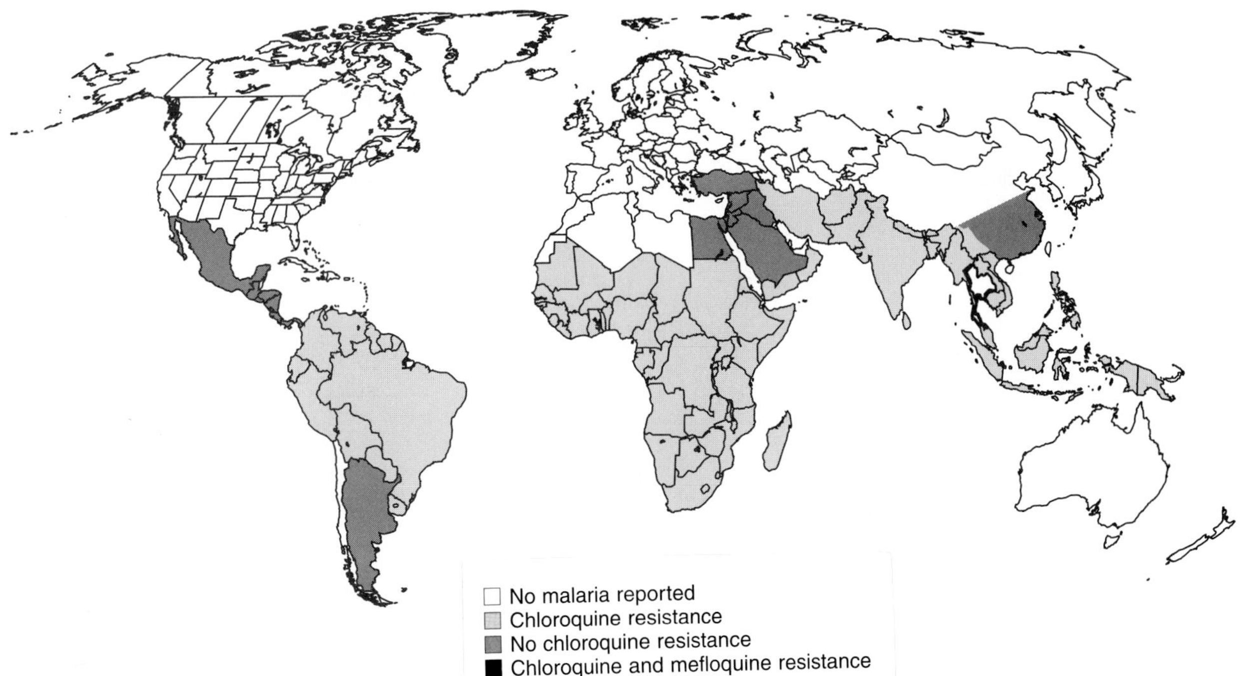

FIGURE 229–3 ■ Map of areas in which malaria is endemic and zones of drug resistance. This map is for use as a visual aid only; more detailed information about country-specific malaria risk is available through on-line resources (see International Travel Information Resources). (From Kain, K., Shanks, G., and Keystone, J.: Malaria chemoprophylaxis in the age of drug resistance. I. Currently recommended drug regimens. Curr. Infect. Dis. Rep. *33*:228, 2001.)

(Malarone), and doxycycline. The CDC no longer recommends the use of chloroquine-proguanil for chemoprophylaxis in chloroquine-resistant areas. For travel to areas with chloroquine- and mefloquine-resistant malaria, either atovaquone-proguanil or doxycycline can be used. Primaquine can be used as an option for primary prophylaxis in special circumstances. Clinicians should contact the CDC Malaria Hotline (770-488-7788) for additional information. Primaquine can also be used for terminal prophylaxis to prevent relapses of *P. vivax* or *P. ovale*. In general, terminal prophylaxis is indicated only for persons who have had prolonged exposure to malaria-endemic areas (missionaries, expatriates).[7] Tafenoquine, a long-acting primaquine analog is being investigated and may be approved for malaria chemoprophylaxis in the future.[41, 46]

In evaluating options for antimalarial chemoprophylaxis, each medication should be reviewed for contraindications and weight and age restrictions (see Table 229–3). Chloroquine is relatively well tolerated in children. In the United States, chloroquine is available in tablet form; in Europe and other countries, it is also available as a syrup. Mefloquine can be used safely in children weighing less than 15 kg and may be useful for longer trips because it is administered once weekly.[51] However, it must be continued for 4 weeks after leaving the malarious area, and no liquid preparation is available. Doses for children are 1/4, 1/2, and 3/4 of a tablet, depending on weight. No data are available on the use of atovaquone-proguanil in children weighing less than 11 kg; however, studies are in progress. For children who weigh more than 11 kg and are at risk of acquiring chloroquine-resistant *P. falciparum* infection, atovaquone-proguanil can be advantageous for short trips because it is started 1 to 2 days before the trip commences and can be stopped 7 days after the trip. However, the patient or parent must remember to take or administer the medication daily. It is available in pediatric tablet form. Doxycycline is contraindicated in children younger than 8 years because of concern about the

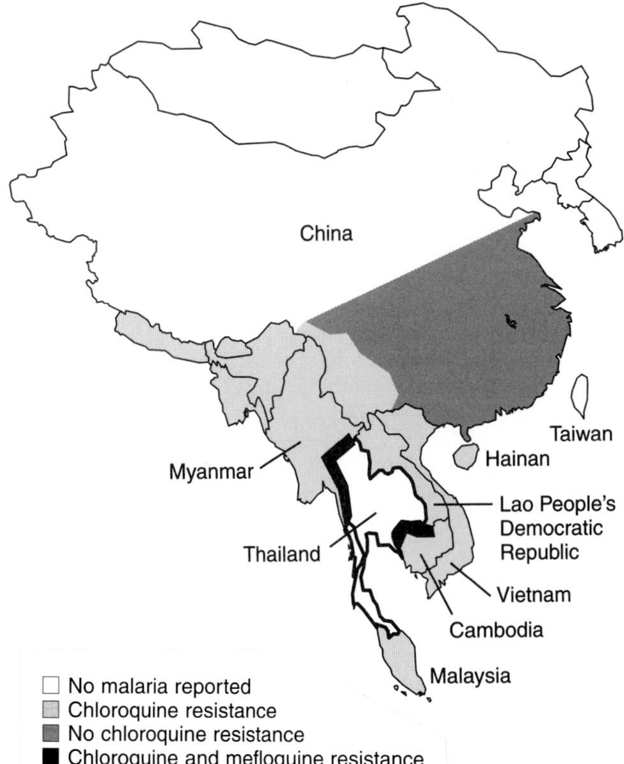

FIGURE 229–4 ■ Zones of antimalarial drug resistance in Southeast Asia. This map is for use as a visual aid only; more detailed information about country-specific malaria risk is available through on-line resources (see International Travel Information Resources). (From Kain, K., Shanks, G., and Keystone, J.: Malaria chemoprophylaxis in the age of drug resistance. I. Currently recommended drug regimens. Curr. Infect. Dis. Rep. *33*:229, 2001.)

TABLE 229–3 ■ ANTIMALARIAL CHEMOPROPHYLAXIS REGIMENS FOR PEDIATRIC TRAVELERS

Medication	Regimen	Dose	Contraindications and Precautions	Side Effects	General Indications and Information for Use
Chloroquine (Aralen)	Weekly starting 1–2 wk before trip; continue weekly during trip and for 4 wk after trip	5 mg base/kg (8.3 mg salt/kg) up to 300 mg base (500 mg salt) *Tablets: 300 mg base (500 mg salt)*	Previous retinal or visual field changes Psoriasis (may be exacerbated by chloroquine) Do not administer with intradermal human diploid-cell rabies vaccine (intradermal rabies vaccine series must be completed at least 7 days before starting chloroquine)	Gastrointestinal symptoms, seizures, rash, headache, dizziness, pruritus (especially in dark-skinned persons), blurred vision, decreased hearing, tinnitus, retinal damage at high cumulative doses* High toxicity in overdoses; keep out of reach of children	Use only in areas of chloroquine-sensitive malaria Limited usefulness because of widespread chloroquine resistance Bitter taste
Mefloquine (Lariam)	Weekly starting 1 wk before trip; continue weekly during trip and for 4 wk after trip	≤15 kg: 4.6 mg/kg base (5 mg/kg salt) 15–19 kg: ¼ tablet 20–30 kg: ½ tablet 31–45 kg: ¾ tablet ≥46 kg: 1 tablet *Tablets: 228 mg base (250 mg salt)*	Psychiatric conditions, cardiac conduction disorders, seizure disorders, persons with known hypersensitivity to mefloquine Should not take with quinine-like drugs Do not administer with intradermal human diploid-cell rabies vaccine (intradermal rabies vaccine series must be completed at least 7 days before starting mefloquine) Do not administer oral typhoid vaccine within 24 hr of mefloquine	Gastrointestinal symptoms, dizziness, insomnia Occasional serious adverse effects: seizures, nightmares, depression, anxiety, psychosis, especially in persons with these preexisting medical conditions	Use in areas with chloroquine-resistant malaria Advantageous for long-term travelers because of weekly dosing and lower cost than atovaquone-proguanil Bitter taste
Atovaquone-proguanil (Malarone)	Daily starting 1–2 days before trip; continue daily during trip and for 7 days after trip	11–20 kg: 1 pediatric tablet (62.5 kg/25 mg) 21–30 kg: 2 pediatric tablets (125 mg/50 mg) 31–40 kg: 3 pediatric tablets (187.5 mg/75 mg) ≥40 kg: 1adult tablet (250 mg atovaquone and 100 mg proguanil hydrochloride) *Pediatric tablets:* 62.5 mg atovaquone and 25 mg proguanil hydrochloride *Adult tablets:* 250 mg atovaguone and 100 mg proguanil hydrochloride	Contraindicated in severe renal failure. Not recommended or use with caution in children <11 kg, pregnant or lactating women Do not take with tetracycline, metoclopramide, rifampin, rifabutin (all reduce concentrations of atovaquone) Do not administer oral typhoid vaccine within 24 hr of atovaquone-proguanil	Gastrointestinal symptoms, headache, loss of appetite, dizziness, pruritus	Use in areas with chloroquine-resistant or mefloquine-resistant malaria Advantageous for short-term travelers because can stop prophylaxis 1 wk after leaving malaria area Available in pediatric tablets Take with food or milk

Continued

TABLE 229–3 ■ ANTIMALARIAL CHEMOPROPHYLAXIS REGIMENS FOR PEDIATRIC TRAVELERS—cont'd

Medication	Regimen	Dose	Contraindications and Precautions	Side Effects	General Indications and Information for Use
Doxycycline	Daily starting 1–2 days before trip; continue daily during trip and for 4 wk after trip	2 mg/kg up to 100 mg daily *Tablets: 50, 100 mg*	Do not use for children <8 yr of age, pregnant or lactating women Do not give simultaneously with antacids or Pepto-Bismol Do not administer oral typhoid vaccine within 24 hr of doxycycline	Gastrointestinal symptoms, photosensitivity, increased blood urea nitrogen, hypersensitivity reactions, blood dyscrasias, vaginal candidiasis May decrease the effectiveness of oral contraceptives	Use in areas with chloroquine-resistant and mefloquine-resistant malaria (borders of Thailand Myanmar and with Cambodia, western Cambodia, and eastern Myanmar) Take with food; taking with food or milk can decrease gastric irritation (absorption of doxycycline is not significantly decreased by simultaneous administration of milk or food)
Primaquine	Daily Primary chemoprophylaxis: contact CDC Malaria Hotline Terminal chemoprophylaxis: daily for 14 days leaving malaria-endemic area	0.6 mg/kg base (1.0 mg/kg salt) up to 30 mg	G6PD deficiency, pregnancy, and lactation unless infant being breast-fed has a documented normal G6PD level	Fatal hemolysis in persons with G6PD deficiency	Must document normal G6PD level before use Primary chemoprophylaxis: contact CDC Malaria Hotline (770-488-7788) for information about use in special circumstances Terminal chemoprophylaxis: to prevent relapses of *P. vivax* or *P. ovale* infection. Generally indicated only for persons who have had prolonged exposure to malaria endemic areas (missionaries, expatriates)

*Despite the use of chloroquine as an antimalarial chemoprophylaxis agent for decades and the use of high-dose chloroquine for certain chronic diseases, the literature is inconclusive regarding the potential risk of retinopathy associated with the long-term use of chloroquine for antimalarial prophylaxis. Retinopathy rarely has been reported in patients receiving weekly prophylaxis. Retinopathy appears to be related to the dosage and accumulated dosage.

propensity of tetracyclines to stain growing teeth or to potentially affect developing bones. For older children, doxycycline must be administered daily and continued for 4 weeks after departing the malarious area.[41, 46]

The importance of determining appropriate antimalarial chemoprophylaxis regimens for travelers and counseling to improve compliance cannot be overemphasized. A review of malaria cases among U.S. civilians in 1998 found that close to 60 percent had not taken any chemoprophylaxis and another 13 percent had not taken the CDC-recommended drug for the area visited.[32] In retrospective reviews of pediatric malaria cases, between 75 and 100 percent of infected children had received no or inadequate chemoprophylaxis.[78, 106] Indeed, the inappropriate use of antimalarial chemoprophylaxis has been shown to be an important cause of mortality and serious morbidity in travelers. From 1992 through early 2001, the CDC received reports of seven U.S. travelers who died of malaria after using inappropriate chemoprophylaxis. All these travelers had received prescriptions for chloroquine for travel to areas with widespread chloroquine resistance. Among 4685 cases of imported malaria with information about chemoprophylaxis during 1992 through early 2001, 2616 (56%) took no chemoprophylaxis and 893 (19%) took an inappropriate chemoprophylaxis regimen.[53] Finally, effective pretravel malaria prevention counseling includes anticipatory guidance for parents about recognition and response to symptoms of malaria infection in young pediatric travelers. Parents should be counseled that although compliance with personal protection measures and chemoprophylaxis will decrease the risk, it cannot guarantee prevention of malaria infection. They should be instructed about the symptoms of malaria infection, such as fever, headache, vomiting, diarrhea, and myalgia, and be counseled to seek immediate medical attention if symptoms occur. Delay in recognition and treatment of malaria is associated directly with an increase in morbidity and mortality; therefore, prompt and appropriate initiation of effective therapy is paramount.[27, 39, 40, 92, 110] Parents also should be advised that some types of malaria can become symptomatic several weeks to months after exposure, and, therefore, prompt medical attention should be sought even if illness develops in a child months after international travel to malarious areas.

Preventing Other Infectious Diseases in Pediatric Travelers

Because the epidemiology of many diseases is evolving over time, prevention hinges on clinicians being knowledgeable about information regarding current outbreaks and risk in planned travel destinations, evaluating risk based on planned activities and the season of travel, and providing appropriate counseling and vaccination, if available. Information about specific infectious disease risks can be obtained from numerous sources listed in "International Travel Information Resources." More detailed information about specific vaccinations is included under "Vaccination for International Travel."

A variety of pathogens increasingly are being recognized as emerging infectious diseases in travelers. In addition to malaria, other vector-borne infectious diseases are among the important diseases for consideration in travelers. Dengue is one of the most significant vector-borne viral infections worldwide and is endemic in Asia, the South Pacific, Africa, Latin America, and the Caribbean. Epidemics of dengue hemorrhagic fever, the more severe clinical form of dengue fever, occur every 3 to 5 years in Southeast Asia and are an emerging problem in Latin America.[69] Recently, outbreaks of dengue fever occurred in Hawaii and along the U.S.-Mexican border.[9, 75, 98] Worldwide, an estimated 50 to 100 million cases of dengue fever occur annually; of these cases, 200,000 to 500,000 are dengue hemorrhagic fever. Every year, cases of dengue fever in U.S. travelers are reported to the CDC. Dengue is transmitted primarily by day-biting *Aedes aegypti* mosquitoes, which breed in flower vases, barrels, and discarded tires that collect water. Transmission occurs in rural and urban areas, but the risk is greatest in urban areas. Prevention should focus on protection against mosquito bites. Travelers to areas of risk should be counseled to apply repellent during the day, even while visiting cities. No vaccine is available, and previous infection with one of the four serotypes does not protect against infection with another serotype. The risk of contracting dengue hemorrhagic fever may actually increase after subsequent infection with a different serotype.[93]

African trypanosomiasis (sleeping sickness), a parasitic infection transmitted by the bite of a tsetse fly, occasionally has been reported in travelers. Infection can result in severe neurologic sequelae and is 100 percent fatal if untreated. In 2001, significant increases in cases were reported among U.S. and European travelers to game parks in Tanzania and Kenya. Between 1967 and 2000, an imported case occurred on average every 1 to 2 years; however, in 2001, seven cases were reported in U.S. travelers.[61, 97]

Schistosomiasis, another parasitic infection caused by flukes that live part of their life cycle in fresh-water snail hosts, affects more than 200 million people worldwide. Schistosomiasis has been reported in travelers to endemic areas of Africa, Asia, South America, and the Caribbean who participated in high-risk activities such as swimming or wading in fresh water.[7, 10, 14, 37] Because most acute infections are asymptomatic, preventive counseling is critical. Children and their families should be counseled against swimming or wading in fresh water in risk areas. Tick-borne encephalitis is transmitted primarily by the bite of *Ixodes* ticks. It also can be transmitted by the ingestion of unpasteurized dairy products from infected livestock. Transmission occurs during the summer months in western and central Europe, Scandinavia, and parts of the former Soviet Union. Persons who will be traveling for longer than 3 weeks in endemic rural areas or travelers who will be engaging in high-risk activities, such as camping, should be considered for vaccination. The vaccine is not available in the United States but can be obtained in Europe.[7]

Adventure travel can increase the risk of acquiring a variety of infectious diseases. Examples of recent outbreaks or cases of unusual pathogens affecting adventure travelers include fungal organisms (such as histoplasmosis and coccidioidomycosis), leptospirosis, and leishmaniasis. Histoplasmosis is a fungal infection acquired by the inhalation of spores, usually through exposure to bat, bird, or chicken droppings in barnyards and caves. The organism is endemic in the United States, Latin America, eastern Asia, parts of Europe, Africa, and Australia. Coccidioidomycosis, a fungal infection associated with the inhalation of organisms in soil from high-risk areas, is endemic in the southwestern part of the United States and Latin America. Both infections can cause a spectrum of illness from asymptomatic infection to acute pulmonary infection to severe, disseminated disease, especially in immunocompromised persons. Several outbreaks of histoplasmosis have been reported in groups of U.S. visitors who entered a cave with bats in Costa Rica (CDC, unpublished data),[6] Ecuador,[103] Peru,[63] and Nicaragua.[108] Recently, more than 200 college students became infected with histoplasmosis during a spring break trip to Acapulco, Mexico.[66, 101] Two outbreaks of coccidioidomycosis have been reported in youth missionary groups involved in construction work in Mexico.[4, 12] Most of these fungal outbreaks have two common features: high-risk, group activities and high attack rates, even in young, non-immunocompromised individuals. Because no vaccine is available, prevention involves counseling travelers regarding the avoidance of exposure or the use of special masks for high-risk individuals who cannot avoid exposure.[8] Leptospirosis is a zoonotic infection that is transmitted by exposure to water or soil contaminated with organisms excreted by domestic and wild animals. Outbreaks have been reported in white-water rafters in Costa Rica[67] and in athletes from 26 countries who participated in the Eco-Challenge multisport expedition race in Borneo, Malaysia, in 2000.[65, 100] Because no vaccine against leptospirosis exists, persons engaging in high-risk activities should be counseled to avoid exposure to water that may be contaminated or to wear protective clothing. The CDC recommends that persons engaging in high-risk activities consider the use of doxycycline for prophylaxis. Leishmaniasis, a parasitic infection transmitted by the bite of a sandfly, can lead to cutaneous or visceral infection. It has been reported in students who traveled to the rain forest in Costa Rica and other travelers.[30, 31, 58, 108, 109] The appropriate use of insect repellent and other personal protection measures against sandfly bites is the only prevention tool available.

Finally, studies of sexual practices among travelers have shown that 5 to 50 percent of short-term travelers engage in casual sex while abroad; 40 to 60 percent of long-term travelers have reported engaging in casual sex while abroad.[56] A recent study of British travelers reported that 18.6 percent had had new sexual partners, two thirds of those who were sexually active did not use condoms on every occasion, and 5.7 percent contracted sexually transmitted diseases.[76] Adolescents should be counseled about the risks and prevention of sexually transmitted diseases, hepatitis B, and HIV infection associated with sexual contact, sharing needles, or receiving acupuncture or tattoos.

Prevention of Travelers' Diarrhea in Children

EPIDEMIOLOGY OF TRAVELERS' DIARRHEA

One of the most difficult tasks faced by international travelers of any age is ensuring the safety of food and water. Travelers' diarrhea, caused by the ingestion of contaminated food and water, typically is defined as the occurrence of four or more unformed stools in a 24-hour period or three or more unformed stools in an 8-hour period with at least one of the following signs or symptoms: temperature greater than 38° C, abdominal cramping, nausea, vomiting, fecal urgency, tenesmus, or blood or mucus in stools.[19, 22, 71] Travelers' diarrhea affects between approximately 20 and 50 percent of adult travelers and is the health problem most frequently reported by travelers to developing countries.[18, 19] It can occur any time during travel but typically occurs within the first week or two of the trip. The illness is usually self-limited, and for adults the average duration of illness has been reported to be 3 to 5 days.[22] Less information about travelers' diarrhea in children is known. A retrospective study of Swiss children who had visited the tropics or subtropics conducted by Pitzinger and associates reported finding similar incidence rates of traveler's diarrhea in children: 40, 8.5, 21.7, and 36 percent in children aged 0 to 2, 3 to 6, 7 to 14, and 15 years and older, respectively.[73] In this study the authors also found that small children (0 to 2 years old) most frequently were affected with travelers' diarrhea and that the clinical course tended to be more severe and prolonged than in older pediatric age groups. Overall, children were found to have longer-lasting illness than noted in adults, with an average duration of 11 days for all children combined and 29 days for small children.

Enteric pathogens typically are isolated from approximately 50 to 75 percent of stool specimens from adult travelers with diarrhea; in the remainder, usually no pathogen is isolated. *Escherichia coli*, especially *enterotoxigenic E. coli*, is the most common overall cause of travelers' diarrhea (although the incidence can vary by destination), followed by *Campylobacter*, *Salmonella*, and *Shigella*. Other etiologic agents include pathogenic bacteria such as *Aeromonas* and *Plesiomonas*, protozoa (e.g., *Giardia lamblia*, *Entamoeba histolytica*, *Cryptosporidium* spp., and *Cyclospora cayetanensis)*, viruses such as rotavirus or Norwalk-like viruses, and rarely, helminths.[71] Numerous risk factors for traveler's diarrhea, including the consumption of certain high-risk foods (raw foods such as meats, seafood, and vegetables, unpasteurized dairy products, and ice and tap water) and travel to certain destinations, also have been identified.[86] Other authors previously categorized destinations by high, intermediate, and low levels of risk for acquiring travelers' diarrhea. Destinations generally considered to have the highest associated risk for contracting travelers' diarrhea include Latin America, Africa, Asia, and the Middle East; destinations with intermediate risk include southern Europe and the Caribbean; and low-risk travel destinations include North America, northern Europe, Australia, and New Zealand.[7] The location of food preparation is also a recognized risk factor for acquiring traveler's diarrhea, with a higher risk shown for travelers eating from street vendors and in local restaurants and a lower risk in luxury hotels and private homes. Although fewer data on travelers' diarrhea in children are available, children (especially toddlers) are probably more vulnerable to food- and water-borne pathogens for many reasons, including their propensity to touch multiple surfaces and to mouth objects. Of note, one study found that only 40 percent of parents said that they had practiced dietary prevention measures consistently, and only 5 percent reported using oral rehydration solutions (the mainstay of treatment of diarrhea in children).[73]

PREVENTIVE COUNSELING FOR TRAVELERS' DIARRHEA

Counseling parents of pediatric travelers about appropriate preventive behavior to avoid traveler's diarrhea and anticipatory guidance to ensure successful management of diarrhea are important aspects of the pretravel assessment.

Food and Beverage Precautions

The most important aspect of preventive counseling for parents of pediatric travelers is appropriate food and beverage precautions (Table 229–4). In addition to preventing the diarrheal diseases already listed, compliance with food and water precautions also will decrease the risk of contracting other food-borne diseases such as hepatitis A. Parents should be counseled that in areas where chlorinated tap water is not available or where hygiene and sanitation are poor, tap water (including ice cubes) should be considered contaminated and avoided. In addition, travelers also should

TABLE 229–4 ■ FOOD AND BEVERAGE PRECAUTIONS FOR INTERNATIONAL TRAVEL

Generally Safe Food and Beverages	Generally Unsafe Food and Beverages
Boiled or chemically disinfected water	Tap water and ice
Powdered drink mixes made with boiled water (e.g., formula, tea, Kool-Aid)	Unpasteurized milk and dairy products (including cheese and ice cream)
Canned or bottled water or beverages	Cooled, standing, or reheated foods
Peeled fruits and vegetables	Raw fruit and vegetables,
Breads and cereals	Raw fruit and vegetables,
Hot, fully cooked pasta, vegetables, meat, fish	Undercooked or raw meats
	Undercooked or raw fish and shellfish; fish with suspected biotoxins

Modified from Jenista, J. A.: The international child traveler. *In* Jensen, H. B., and Baltimore, R. S. (eds.): Pediatric Infectious Diseases: Principles and Practice. Norwalk, CT, Appleton & Lange, 1995, p.1518.

be advised to avoid brushing their teeth with tap water. Breast-feeding, boiled or bottled water, and bottled carbonated beverages are recommended as typically safe beverages for children; powdered drink mixes made with boiled water (e.g., formula, tea, Kool-Aid) also generally can be considered safe. Parents should dry wet cans and bottles before opening and wipe drinking surfaces clean before serving.[38]

In areas where access to bottled water is poor, water may be boiled for 1 minute (or for 3 minutes at altitudes greater than 2000 m [6562 ft]). These procedures will kill bacterial, parasitic, and viral pathogens. Chemical disinfection with iodine is an alternative method for water treatment when the water cannot be boiled; however, this method cannot be trusted to kill *Cryptosporidium* unless the water stands for 15 minutes after boiling before drinking. Two well-tested methods are the use of tincture of iodine and tetraglycine hydroperiodide tablets (e.g., Globaline, Potable Aqua, or Coughlan's); these tablets are available at pharmacies, sporting goods stores, and camping outfitters. Chlorine also can be used for chemical disinfection, but its germicidal activity varies with pH, temperature, and the organic content of the water; it can therefore provide less consistent levels of disinfection in many types of water. Portable filters are available and provide various degrees of protection against microbes. Reverse-osmosis filters afford protection against viruses, bacteria, and protozoa, but they are large and expensive, and the small pores can be plugged by cloudy or muddy water. Microstrainer filters with pore sizes in the 0.1- to 0.3-μm range can remove bacteria and protozoa from drinking water, but they do not remove viruses. To kill viruses, parents using microstrainer filters should be advised to chemically disinfect water with iodine after filtration. Data are inadequate at the present time to evaluate the efficacy of specific brands or models of filters, and therefore the CDC cannot identify or recommend specific brands or models of filters most likely to remove bacteria and viruses.[7]

Parents of pediatric travelers also should be counseled on the importance of advance planning for food and beverage items, especially for infants and young children. Breast-feeding infants are considered relatively safe from contracting travelers' diarrhea because they are not exposed to local food and water; therefore, traveling mothers should be encouraged to continue breast-feeding for as long as practical. For infants receiving formula, formula concentrate and powdered forms are the most convenient for travel, but a clean water supply must be available or water must be boiled or chemically disinfected before preparation. For feeding toddlers and older children, the travel adage of "boil it, cook it, peel it, or forget it" applies. In general, unless beverages and food come from a can or can be completed cooked or peeled, they should be considered unsafe (including raw fruits and vegetables). Travelers should avoid unpasteurized dairy products, including cheese and ice cream. In addition, travelers should be advised to not consume raw seafood, shellfish, and meats. Freshly prepared steaming hot food, breads and cereals, hot pasta (including rice and noodles), and well-cooked meat or fish generally can be considered safe for consumption. Bringing crackers and peanut butter is a good suggestion for parents of hungry children when the availability of safe foods is uncertain. The incidence of travelers' diarrhea in children also can be reduced potentially by advising parents to encourage or supervise frequent handwashing and trying to prevent them from placing objects in their mouth.

Some species of fish and shellfish can contain poisonous biotoxins such as ciguatoxin and scombrotoxin, even when well cooked. Ciguatera poisoning is a potential risk in all subtropical and tropical regions of the West Indies and the Pacific and Indian oceans where the implicated fish are consumed; such fish include barracuda, red snapper, grouper, amberjack, and sea bass. Symptoms of ciguatera poisoning include gastroenteritis and neurologic manifestations such as dysesthesias and weakness. Scombroid poisoning occurs in tropical as well as temperate regions and is caused by high levels of histidine in the flesh of fish such as bluefin, yellowfin tuna, mackerel, bonito, mahi-mahi, herring, amberjack, and bluefish; if improperly refrigerated, histidine is converted to histamine, which can cause flushing, headache, nausea, vomiting, diarrhea, and urticaria.[7]

MANAGING TRAVELERS' DIARRHEA IN CHILDREN

When diarrhea develops in a pediatric traveler, oral rehydration solution (ORS) to maintain hydration is the treatment of choice. Parents also should be educated about the signs of mild, moderate, and severe dehydration and instructed in the management of diarrhea, especially oral rehydration therapy (Table 229–5). Parents traveling with children, especially those younger than 5 years, should include oral rehydration packets in their travel kit because young children are at particular risk of dehydration, even from mild diarrheal disease. In the United States, premixed liquid ORS formulations are available but are generally too heavy to pack; powdered WHO ORS packets (glucose-based citrate formula) are manufactured and distributed by Jianas Brothers, Kansas City, Missouri (816-421-2880), and powdered rice-based Ceralyte ORS packets are available from Cera Products in Columbia, Maryland (410-997-2334, 888-237-2598, or www.ceralyte.com). In addition, in most destinations overseas, inexpensive formulations of ORS may be available in pharmacies and grocery stores. If travelers are in a remote area where ORS is not available, a recipe for preparing a similar solution also is presented in Table 229–5. In addition, parents should be told that ORS can protect the child from serious complications of dehydration but typically will not decrease the number of stools or the duration of illness. Antimotility agents such as Lomotil (active

TABLE 229–5 ■ ANTICIPATORY GUIDANCE FOR MANAGEMENT OF TRAVELERS' DIARRHEA IN CHILDREN

1. Include oral rehydration solution (ORS) packets in travel kit
   Jianas Brothers, Kansas City, MO: 816-421-2880 (WHO ORS packets (glucose-based formula))
   Cera Products, Columbia, MD: 888-237-2598 or www.ceralyte.com (rice-based formula)
2. Recognize the signs and symptoms of mild, moderate, and severe dehydration[7]

	Mild Dehydration	Moderate Dehydration	Severe Dehydration
General condition	Thirsty, restless	Thirsty (variable); restless, agitated	Withdrawn, lethargic, or comatose
Pulse	Normal	Rapid, weak	Rapid, weak
Anterior fontanelle	Normal	Sunken	Sunken
Eyes	Normal	Sunken	Sunken
Tears	Present	Absent	Absent
Urine output	Normal	Reduced, concentrated	None
Weight loss	4–5%	6–9%	≥10%

3. Begin ORS with first episode of watery stools or >1 vomiting episode
4. Mix 1 ORS packet with 1 L of bottled of boiled water in a clean container; discard after 12 hr at room temperature
5. If ORS not available, a similar solution can be prepared[48, 82]
   ½ tsp salt
   ½ tsp baking soda
   4 tbsp sugar
   1 L clean water (boiled or bottled)
6. Administer ORS appropriately:
   In a nondehydrated child: give 0.5–1 cup of ORS for each diarrheal stool
   In a mildly dehydrated child: give ORS replacement of 50–100 mL/kg (1 oz/lb) over 4-hr period.
   For vomiting children: give smaller, more frequent amounts (i.e., 1 tsp (5 mL)) every 15–20 min)
7. Continue normal feeding throughout illness if possible
   In infants: formula and/or breast-feeding
   In older children: encourage bananas, cooked rice, potatoes, toasted bread, or crackers
8. Antimotility agents (i.e., Lomotil (active ingredient, diphenoxylate) and Imodium (active ingredient, loperamide) generally are not recommended
9. Empiric treatment with antimicrobials is not recommended generally
10. Seek urgent medical attention for diarrhea with high fever, bloody stools, moderate to severe dehydration, lethargy, severe vomiting, or diarrhea lasting more than 3 days

Modified from Jenista, J. A.: The international child traveler. *In* Jensen H. B., and Baltimore, R. (eds.): Pediatric Infectious Diseases: Principles and Practice. Norwalk, CT, Appleton & Lange, 1995, p. 1520.

ingredient, diphenoxylate) and Imodium (active ingredient, loperamide) are not recommended for use in children because of potential toxic megacolon, toxicity (extrapyramidal symptoms with diphenoxylate), and prolongation of the illness. Empiric treatment of traveler's diarrhea with antimicrobial agents, typically ciprofloxacin because of resistance to other agents such as trimethoprim-sulfamethoxazole, is used for adults. Few studies of empiric antimicrobial treatment in children exist, and it is not a routinely recommended intervention for children. Parents should be advised that severe diarrheal disease consisting of fever or bloody stools (or both), moderate to severe dehydration, lethargy, severe vomiting, or diarrhea lasting longer than 3 days requires urgent medical attention, especially in younger pediatric travelers. Prophylaxis for travelers' diarrhea with medications such as bismuth subsalicylate (the active ingredient in Pepto-Bismol) is not recommended because of the accumulation of salicylate. Prophylactic regimens with antimicrobial agents also are not recommended in children; the benefits usually are outweighed by the potential risks, including allergic drug reactions, antimicrobial-associated colitis, widespread resistance caused by the pervasive use of certain agents, and limited information about destinationspecific antimicrobial resistance patterns.[72]

Special Considerations for Immunocompromised Pediatric Travelers

Travel preparations for a child with an immunocompromising condition, including congenital immunodeficiencies and acquired immunodeficiencies (such as HIV), need to be tailored to the specific underlying condition. Limited data are available on health risks in immunocompromised pediatric travelers, but data from adult travelers can be used to guide the management of children. A key component of the pretravel assessment should be a careful review of routine and travel-related vaccinations. In addition, the child and family should receive individualized preventive counseling about how to reduce disease risk while traveling. The health care provider should ensure that parents of immunocompromised children are knowledgeable about the type of immune defect or condition, the types of infections to which their children will be more susceptible, and how these risks may be affected by planned travel and activities. As previously discussed, parents should be advised to carry the following items with them for easy retrieval: (1) a summary of their child's medical history and treatment record, (2) copies of all important health-related documents (i.e., written prescriptions for medications, health insurance information, and medical contacts abroad, including specialists in planned travel destinations), and (3) all required prescription medications (in original bottles and sufficient supply for the length of the trip). Physicians should stress the importance of bringing an adequate supply of prescription medications, especially for HIV-infected travelers, because many medications are unavailable outside the United States. At the present time, no countries require proof of a negative HIV test for entry for tourism purposes; however, some countries require HIV testing for students and workers and for persons wishing to stay in the country longer than 3 months.[13]

VACCINATION OF IMMUNOCOMPROMISED PEDIATRIC TRAVELERS

The AAP, Committee on Infectious Diseases, reports that experience with vaccine administration in immunocompromised children is limited. In most situations, theoretic considerations are used to guide decisions about vaccine administration because data about specific vaccines in children with specific disorders are lacking.[72] Vaccination recommendations may change, so clinicians should obtain the most recent recommendations before vaccinating immunocompromised patients (see "International Travel Information Resources"). In general, children with immunocompromising conditions, including primary and secondary immune deficiencies, should receive all inactivated vaccines that are recommended for non-immunocompromised pediatric travelers. The risk of complications from the administration of inactivated vaccines and immunoglobulin preparations has not been shown to be increased in immunocompromised persons; however, immune responses may vary and may be suboptimal (thereby substantially reducing vaccine immunogenicity). Children with a deficiency in antibody-synthesizing capacity are usually incapable of mounting an antibody response to vaccines and should receive regular doses of immunoglobulin to provide passive protection against many infectious diseases. Children with milder B-lymphocyte and antibody deficiencies have an intermediate degree of vaccine responsiveness and may require monitoring of postimmunization antibody titers to confirm vaccine immunogenicity.[72] Consideration should be given to timing the dosing of intravenous immunoglobulin to coincide with the immediate pretravel period.[13, 72]

In general, immunocompromised children should not receive live vaccines, either viral or bacterial, because of the risk of disease developing from vaccine strains. The AAP, Committee on Infectious Diseases, notes, however, that some immunocompromised children may benefit from special-use as well as routinely administered immunizations.[72] In patients with primary immunodeficiencies, live vaccines are contraindicated for most individuals with B-lymphocyte defects except IgA deficiency and for all patients with T-lymphocyte–mediated disorders. Fatal poliomyelitis and measles vaccine virus infections have occurred in children with disorders in T-cell function after the administration of live viral vaccines. Children with phagocytic function disorders, including chronic granulomatous disease and leukocyte adhesion defect, can receive all immunizations except live bacterial vaccines (BCG and Ty21a *Salmonella typhi*). Live vaccines are generally contraindicated in patients with secondary immunodeficiencies (including children with HIV infection or acquired immunodeficiency syndrome [AIDS]), cancer, and organ transplants and in children receiving immunosuppressive or radiation therapy. Exceptions to this proviso are children with HIV infection who are not severely immunocompromised; measles-mumps-rubella vaccines are recommended in these children, and varicella vaccine should be considered if age-specific $CD4^+$ T-lymphocyte values are 25 percent or more. In the United States, BCG is contraindicated for HIV-infected children, although the WHO recommends giving BCG to asymptomatic HIV-infected children in regions with high TB prevalence. All HIV-infected children should, however, have tuberculin skin testing performed before and after travel. Yellow fever vaccination is contraindicated in HIV-infected persons by the Advisory Committee on Immunization Practices, but it is recommended by the WHO for those with asymptomatic HIV infection who reside in endemic areas.[72, 111]

MALARIA PREVENTION IN IMMUNOCOMPROMISED CHILDREN

No data have been published to indicate that immunocompromised travelers are at increased risk for acquiring malaria; however, if acquired, the disease is suspected to be more severe in these populations. Therefore, counseling should emphasize the importance of personal protection measures against malaria and the use of recommended chemoprophylaxis. In addition, some groups, such as those infected with HIV, may have an increased risk for adverse effects associated with some antimalarial chemoprophylaxis regimens and should be counseled specifically on recognizing these effects. Immunocompromised patients, particularly HIV-infected individuals, may be at risk for acquiring a variety of infections that are manifested as febrile illnesses; parents should be advised to seek expert medical advice early in the course of a febrile illness to ensure that the child receives the appropriate diagnosis and effective treatment.[13]

PREVENTING TRAVELERS' DIARRHEA AND OTHER INFECTIOUS DISEASES IN IMMUNOCOMPROMISED CHILDREN

During travel to developing countries, immunocompromised children may be at higher risk for acquiring food- and waterborne diseases than when they are in the United States. At present, data are too limited to determine whether the risk and incidence of travelers' diarrhea are increased in this population; however, good evidence indicates that the disease is more severe or prolonged in immunocompromised travelers.[13] Intensive counseling on the effective use of food and beverage precautions for this population is essential to minimize and prevent morbidity and mortality. Water-borne infections also can result from swallowing water during recreational water activities. To reduce the risk of acquiring diseases such as cryptosporidiosis and giardiasis, parents should be advised that children should avoid swimming in water that might be contaminated and that their children should be encouraged to not swallow water during swimming. In addition, many tropical and developing countries have high rates of TB; some immunocompromised persons, such as HIV-infected travelers, may be at greater risk for acquiring TB, especially during long-term travel.[77] BCG vaccination is contraindicated in HIV-infected persons, but some evidence suggests that isoniazid chemoprophylaxis may be effective.

TABLE 229–6 ■ INTERNATIONAL TRAVELERS HEALTH INFORMATION, RECOMMENDATIONS, AND OUTBREAK NOTICES

Resource	Contact Information	Information/Services Provided
Centers for Disease Control and Prevention (CDC) Travelers' Health Information	877-394-8747 (phone) 888-232-3299 (fax)	Recorded health information Documents on U.S. recommendations for specific travel destinations and regions, including malaria prophylaxis
	www.cdc.gov/travel/	U.S. recommendations, malaria prophylaxis; links to other sites, travel advisories, and outbreak notices
CDC Health Information for International Travel (Yellow Book)	*www.cdc.gov/travel/yellowbook.pdf* or order from Public Health Foundation at *http://bookstore.phf.org* 877-252-1200 or 301-645-7773 (international orders)	General travelers' health information, region- and destination-specific recommendations, including malaria prophylaxis
CDC Malaria Branch	770-488-7788 (8:00 AM to 4:30 PM EST, Monday through Friday) 404-639-2888 (4:30 PM to 8:00 AM EST, weekends and holidays; ask operator for staff on call for Malaria Epidemiology Branch)	Information about malaria prophylaxis and treatment, intended for use by health care professionals
CDC MMWR weekly and summaries	*www.cdc.gov/mmwr*	Reports on outbreak investigations and surveillance summaries (domestic and international)
CDC National Immunization Program	*www.cdc.gov/nip*	Immunization information
National Network for Immunization Information (NNII)	*www.immunizationinfo.org* 877-341-6644	Immunization information for health care practitioners and parents
U.S. State Department	*www.travel.state.gov*	General information about travel, including safety, visa requirements, links to individual embassies and consulates
U.S. Department of Defense	*www.geis.ha.osd.mil*	Worldwide network providing information on emerging infections to U.S. military
World Health Organization (WHO) Infectious Disease Health Topics	*www.who.int/health-topics/*	Information and maps of travel-related diseases
WHO Yellow Book, "International Travel and Health"	*www.who.int/ith/*	General travelers' health recommendations; country-specific malaria risks and recommendations
WHO, Outbreak News	*www.who.int/disease-outbreak-news/*	Monthly newsletter with notifications of recent infectious disease outbreaks
WHO, *Weekly Epidemiological Record*	*www.who.int/wer*	Global disease surveillance and WHO program updates
Health Canada, Travel Medicine Program	*www.travelhealth.gc.ca*	Canadian recommendations for travelers health; outbreak information
EuroSurveillance	*www.eurosurveillance.org*	Surveillance and outbreak information for European nations; weekly and monthly surveillance reports and outbreak notices
PROMED (Program for Monitoring Emerging Diseases)	*www.promedmail.org*	E-mail postings; verified and unverified reports on emerging diseases and outbreaks

Chemoprophylaxis may be appropriate for some individuals visiting or living in high-risk areas for a prolonged period. When immunocompromised children travel abroad, they may encounter new organisms not endemic in their own countries; these organisms will pose variable risks based on their degree of immunocompromise. Health care providers should identify travel-specific risks and instruct parents in ways to reduce the risk of contracting infection. Other pathogens that can lead to more severe infection in immunocompromised travelers include visceral leishmaniasis and fungal infections (including *Penicillium marneffei*, coccidioidomycosis, and histoplasmosis).[7] Leishmaniasis is endemic in the Mediterranean coastal regions of southern Europe and northern Africa. *P. marneffei* poses a risk for travelers to the Far East, and histoplasmosis affects those traveling to Latin America. Few data exist on the efficacy of primary prophylaxis for opportunistic infections such as leishmaniasis and penicilliosis; therefore, avoiding areas of high prevalence may be prudent if the child has severe immunodeficiency or advanced HIV disease.[42]

General Travel Health Counseling for Children

During the pretravel assessment, the clinician should provide the parents with general advice and preventive counseling to avoid health risks and injuries in children. Simple personal protection measures can prevent children from incurring many types of travel-associated injuries and conditions. The most common skin condition reported by travelers is sunburn. To prevent sunburn and the subsequent risk of skin malignancies later in life, children should avoid sun exposure during peak hours and use sunscreen appropriate for the child's age. When sunscreen and insect repellent are used concomitantly, the former should be applied first. Injuries and motor vehicle accidents pose a great risk for morbidity and mortality among international travelers.[29, 76] The risk of motor vehicle–related death is generally many times higher in developing countries than in the United States. Parents traveling with infants or young children should be advised to bring their own child safety restraint seats for use during travel. The use of car seats and seat belts for children, preferably sitting in the rear seat, should be emphasized. Unfortunately, in some developing countries, cars with seat belts may not be readily available. Night driving can be more hazardous, especially outside urban areas in developing countries, and should be avoided.[7] Use of a helmet is imperative for bicycle travel. Fire injuries can be prevented by advising parents to inquire whether hotels have smoke detectors and sprinkler systems (they also may consider bringing their own smoke detector). Other major causes of injury and trauma include drowning and boating accidents. Parents and children should be counseled to be aware of weather conditions and forecasts, and parents should be advised that an adult should accompany children at all times when swimming. Personal floatation devices should be used when boating or skiing regardless of the distance to be traveled or swimming ability.[81]

Swimming in contaminated water can result in skin, eye, ear, and some intestinal infections; for prevention of infectious diseases, generally only pools that contain chlorinated water can be considered safe. Parents should also be advised that swimming in fresh-water lakes and streams in developing countries carries a risk of contracting schistosomiasis,

TABLE 229–7 ■ TRAVEL-RELATED MEDICAL SERVICES, INSURANCE, AND INTERNET RESOURCES FOR TRAVELERS

Resource	Contact Information	Information/Services Provided
International Society of Travel Medicine (ISTM)	*www.istm.org* 800-433-5256	Directory of travel medicine clinics and practitioners with ISTM affiliation
American Society of Tropical Medicine and Hygiene (ASTMH)	*www.astmh.org* 847-480-9592	Directory of travel medicine clinics and practitioners certified by ASTMH
International Association for Medical Assistance to Travelers (IAMAT)	716-754-4883 736 Center Street Lewiston, NY 14092	Health information packets for travelers, including worldwide directories of English-speaking physicians with travel medicine experience
International S.O.S. Assistance	*www.intsos.com* 800-523-8930	Overseas assistance and coverage for emergency evacuation; requires fee
Travel Assistance International	800-821-2828	Individual health insurance for travel and coverage for emergency evacuation
Highway to Health (Radnor, PA)	*www.hthworldwide.com* 610-293-2062	Information on physicians overseas; requires fee
Medex	*www.medexassist.com* 800-527-0218	Overseas assistance, insurance, and evacuation; requires fee
TEN (St. Petersburg, FL)	*www.tenweb.com* 800-ASK-4TEN	Overseas assistance and insurance; requires fee
Travelhealth On-line (Shoreland)	*www.tripprep.com*	Travelers' health information; country-specific recommendations
Mdtravel Health	*www.Mdtravelhealth.com*	Travelers' health information; country-specific recommendations
Fit for Travel, Travax On-line	*www.fitfortravel.scot.nhs.us*	Travelers' health information from the Travel Medicine Division of the Scottish Centre for Infection and Environmental Health; outbreak information
Medicine Planet	*www.travelhealth.com*	Travelers' health information and fee-for-service health care access for travelers
University of Texas at Austin: world maps on-line	*www.lib.utexas.edu/maps*	World maps on-line

leptospirosis, and primary amebic meningoencephalitis.[7] In salt-water bodies, biting and stinging fish, corals, and jellyfish also can be a risk. Parents of pediatric travelers, especially to areas endemic for rabies, should be reminded to warn children that they should not attempt to pet, handle, or feed domestic or wild animals (including monkeys). Travelers also should avoid snakes because most bites are the direct result of handling, harassing, or trying to kill snakes. In general, children should wear covered footwear rather than sandals, including when wading on reefs and swimming.[7, 81] Children should avoid walking barefoot, particularly in rural areas, to prevent cutaneous larva migrans, hookworm, and *Strongyloides* infections.

International Travel Information Resources

One of the most important functions that a clinician can fulfill in preparing a pediatric patient and parents for international travel is to provide up-to-date and accurate travel health information and recommendations for preventing illness. Many varied sources of information are available, including software packages and databases designed specifically for use in travel medicine and pretravel care, such as TRAVAX.[25, 43] Increasingly, the Internet and computer-based travel resources are being used by both practitioners and consumers alike because they provide current information to appropriately and effectively counsel and treat international travelers. Two recent reviews have provided comprehensive summaries of travel medicine resources.[25, 43] Included in this section is a summary of some selected travel health resources that can be useful for providing health care professionals and parents with essential information on (1) health risks in specific travel destinations (including endemic or epidemic diseases) and current travel health recommendations (including immunizations and chemoprophylaxis) (Table 229–6) and (2) health insurance and emergency evacuation coverage during travel and medical assistance in the event of a travel-related illness (Table 229–7). This summary is not meant to be comprehensive; because resources are constantly changing, clinicians are advised to review and compare sites for availability and updated information and recommendations.

REFERENCES

1. American Academy of Pediatrics. Committee on Infectious Diseases. Policy statement: Recommendations for the prevention of pneumococcal infections, including the use of pneumococcal conjugate vaccine (Prevnar), pneumococcal polysaccharide vaccine, and antibiotic prophylaxis. Pediatrics *106*:362–366, 2000.
2. Bernard, K., and Fishbein, D.: Pre-exposure rabies prophylaxis for travellers: Are the benefits worth the cost? Vaccine *9*:833–836, 1991.
3. Brabin, B., and Ganley, Y.: Imported malaria in children in the UK. Arch. Dis. Child. *77*:76–81, 1997.
4. Cairns, L., Blythe, D., Kao, A., et al.: Outbreak of coccidioidomycosis in Washington state residents returning from Mexico. Clin. Infect. Dis. *30*: 61–64, 2000.
5. Castellani-Pastoris, M., Monaco, R., Goldoni, P., et al.: Legionnaires' disease on a cruise ship linked to the water supply system: Clinical and public health implications. Clin. Infect. Dis. *28*:33–38, 1999.
6. Cave-associated histoplasmosis—Costa Rica. M. M. W. R. Morb. Mortal. Wkly. Rep. *37*(20):312–313, 1988.
7. Centers for Disease Control and Prevention: Health Information for International Travel 2003–2004. Atlanta, U.S. Department of Health and Human Services, Public Health Service, 2003.
8. Centers for Disease Control and Prevention: National Institute for Occupational Safety and Health. Histoplasmosis: Protecting workers at risk, revised guidelines for preventing histoplasmosis. 1997. Available at *http://www.cdc.gov/niosh/97–146.html*.
9. Centers for Disease Control and Prevention: Travelers' Health Notice: Dengue Fever, Hawaii. *http://www.cdc.gov/travel/other/dengue-hawaii-oct2001.htm*.
10. Cetron, M., Chitsulo, L., Sullivan, J., et al.: Schistosomiasis in Lake Malawi. Lancet *348*:1274–1278, 1996.
11. Chen, R., Penney, D., Little, D., et al.: Hepatitis and death following vaccination with 17D-204 yellow fever vaccine. Lancet *358*:121–122, 2001.
12. Coccidioidomycosis in travelers returning from Mexico—Pennsylvania, 2000. M. M. W. R. Morb. Mortal. Wkly. Rep. *49*(44):1004–1006, 2000.
13. Conlon, C.: The immunocompromised traveler. *In* Dupont, H. L., and Steffen, R. (eds.): Textbook of Travel Medicine and Health. 2nd ed. Hamilton, Ontario, Canada, B. C. Decker, 2001, pp. 464–469.
14. Cooke, G., Lalvani, A., Gleeson, F., et al.: Acute pulmonary schistosomiasis in travelers returning from Lake Malawi, sub-Saharan Africa. Clin. Infect. Dis. *29*:836–839, 1999.
15. Cossar, J., Reid, D., Fallon, R., et al.: A cumulative review of studies on travelers, their experience of illness and the implications of these findings. J. Infect. *21*:27–42, 1990.
16. Cossar, J., Reid, D., Grist, N., et al.: Illness associated with travel. Travel Med. Int. *3*:13–18, 1985.
17. Dawson, A.: Medical aspects of air travel. *In* Dupont, H. L., and Steffen, R. (eds.): Textbook of Travel Medicine and Health. 2nd ed. Hamilton, Ontario, Canada, B. C. Decker, 2001, pp. 390–403.
18. Dupont, H., and Capsuto, E.: Persistent diarrhea in travelers. Clin. Infect. Dis. *22*:124–128, 1996.
19. Dupont, H., and Ericsson, C.: Prevention and treatment of traveler's diarrhea. N. Engl. J. Med. *328*:1821–1827, 1993.
20. Dupont, H., and Khan, F.: Travelers' diarrhea: Epidemiology, microbiology, prevention, and therapy. J. Travel Med. *1*:84–93, 1994.
21. Eng, T., O'Brien, R., Bernard, K., et al.: HIV-1 and HIV-2 infections among U.S. Peace Corps volunteers returning from West Africa. J. Travel Med. *2*:174–177, 1995.
22. Ericsson, C., and Dupont, H.: Travelers diarrhea: Approaches to prevention and treatment. Clin. Infect. Dis. *16*:616–624, 1993.
23. Fatal yellow fever in a traveler returning from Venezuela, 1999. M. M. W. R. Morb. Mortal. Wkly. Rep. *49*(14):303–305, 2000.
24. Fever, jaundice, and multiple organ system failure associated with 17D-derived yellow fever vaccination, 1996–2001. M. M. W. R. Morb. Mortal. Wkly. Rep. *50*(30):643–645, 2001.
25. Freedman, D., and Leuthold, C.: Information sources in travel medicine. *In* Dupont, H. L., and Steffen, R. (eds.): Textbook of Travel Medicine and Health. 2nd ed. Hamilton, Ontario, Canada, B. C. Decker, 2001, pp. 37–45.
26. Foster, J., Watson, B., and Bell, L.: Travel with infants and children. Emerg. Med. Clin. North Am. *15*:71–92, 1997.
27. Greenberg, A., and Lobel, H.: Mortality from *Plasmodium falciparum* malaria in travelers from the United States. Ann. Intern. Med. *113*: 326–327, 1990.
28. Guptill, K., Hargarten, S., and Baker, T.: American travel deaths in Mexico: Causes and prevention strategies. West. J. Med. *154*:169–171, 1991.
29. Hargarten, S., Baker, T., and Guptill, K.: Overseas fatalities of United States citizen travelers: An analysis of deaths related to international travel. Ann. Emerg. Med. *20*:622–626, 1991.
30. Hatchette, T., Green, P., Schlech, W., et al.: Lesion on the arm of a returning traveler. Clin. Infect. Dis. *33*:815, 897–898, 2001.
31. Herwaldt, B., Stokes, S., and Juranek, D.: American cutaneous leishmaniasis in US travelers. Ann. Intern. Med. *118*:779–784, 1993.
32. Holtz, T., Kachur, S., Macarthur, J., et al.: Malaria surveillance—United States, 1998. M. M. W. R. Surveill. Summ. *50*(SS-5):1–18, 2001.
33. Hostetter, M.: Epidemiology of travel-related morbidity and mortality in children. Pediatr. Rev. *20*:228–233, 1999.
34. Houweling, H., and Coutinho, R.: HIV infections, needlesticks and sexual behavior among Dutch expatriates in sub-Saharan Africa. *In* Lobel, H., Steffen, R., and Kozarsky, P. E. (eds.): Travel Medicine 2. Proceedings of the Second Conference on International Travel Medicine. Atlanta, International Society of Travel Medicine, 1991, pp. 204–206.
35. Immunization Action Coalition: Summary of rules for childhood immunization. St. Paul, MN, March 2001.
36. Immunization Action Coalition: Summary of recommendations for adult immunization. St. Paul, MN, April 2001.
37. Jelinek, T., Nothdurft, H., and Loscher, T.: Schistosomiasis in travelers and expatriates. J. Travel Med. *3*:160–164, 1996.
38. Jenista, J.: The international child traveler. *In* Jensen, H. B., and Baltimore, R. S. (eds.): Pediatric Infectious Diseases: Principles and Practice. Norwalk, CT, Appleton & Lange, 1995, pp. 1509–1523.
39. Kain, K., Harrington, M., Tennyson, S., and Keystone, J.: Imported malaria: Prospective analysis of problems in diagnosis and management. Clin. Infect. Dis. *27*:142–149, 1998.
40. Kain, K., and Keystone, J.: Malaria in travelers: Epidemiology, disease, and prevention. Infect. Dis. Clin. North Am. *12*:267–284, 1998.
41. Kain, K., Shanks, G., and Keystone, J.: Malaria chemoprophylaxis in the age of drug resistance. I. Currently recommended drug regimens. Clin. Infect. Dis. *33*:226–234, 2001.
42. Karp, C. L.: Preparation of the HIV-infected traveler to the tropics. Curr. Infect. Dis. Rep. *3*:50–58, 2001.

43. Keystone, J., Kozarsky, P., and Freedman, D.: Internet and computer-based resources for travel medicine practitioners. Clin. Infect. Dis. *32*: 757–765, 2001.
44. Klein, J., and Millman, G.: Prospective, hospital based study of fever in children in the United Kingdom who had recently spent time in the tropics. B. M. J. *316*:1425–1426, 1998.
45. Koch, S., and Steffen, R.: Meningococcal disease in travelers: Vaccination recommendations. J. Travel Med. *1*:4–7, 1994.
46. Labbe, A., Lautfy, M., and Kain, K.: Recent advances in the prophylaxis and treatment of malaria. Curr. Infect. Dis. Rep. *3*:68–76, 2001.
47. Laga, M.: Risk of infection and other sexually transmitted diseases in travellers. *In* Lobel, H. O., Steffe, R., and Kozarsky, P. E. (eds.): Travel Medicine 2. Proceedings of the Second Conference on International Travel Medicine. Atlanta, International Society of Travel Medicine, 1992, pp. 201–203.
48. Larson, S.: Traveler's diarrhea. Emerg. Med. Clin. North Am. *15*: 179–189, 1997.
49. Lobato, M., and Hopewell, P.: *Mycobacterium tuberculosis* infection after travel to or contact with visitors from countries with a high prevalence of tuberculosis. Am. J. Respir. Crit. Care Med. *158*:1871–1875, 1998.
50. Lobel, H., and Kozarsky, P.: Update on prevention of malaria in travelers. J. A. M. A. *278*:1767–1771, 1997.
51. Luxemberger, C., Price, R., Nosten, F., et al.: Mefloquine in infants and young children. Ann. Trop. Paediatr. *16*:281–286, 1996.
52. Mahon, B., Mintz, E., Green, K., et al.: Reported cholera in the United States, 1990–1994. J. A. M. A. *276*:307–312, 1996.
53. Malaria deaths following inappropriate malaria chemoprophylaxis—United States, 2001. M. M. W. R. Morb. Mortal. Wkly. Rep. *50*(28): 597–599, 2001.
54. Maloney, S., and Cetron, M.: Investigation and management of infectious diseases on international conveyances (airplanes and cruiseships). *In* Dupont, H. L., and Steffen, R. (eds.): Textbook of Travel Medicine and Health. 2nd ed. Hamilton, Ontario, Canada, B. C. Decker, 2001, pp. 519–530.
55. Martin, M., Tsai, T., Cropp, B., et al.: Fever and multisystem organ failure associated with 17D-204 yellow fever vaccination: A report of four cases. Lancet *358*:98–104, 2001.
56. Matteelli, A., and Carosi, G.: Sexually transmitted diseases in travelers. Clin. Infect. Dis. *32*:1063–1067, 2001.
57. McFarland, J., Baddour, L., Nelson, J., et al.: Imported yellow fever in a United States citizen. Clin. Infect. Dis. *25*:1143–1147, 1997.
58. Melby, P., Kreutzer, R., McMahon-Pratt, D., et al.: Cutaneous leishmaniasis: Review of 58 cases seen at the National Institutes of Health. Clin. Infect. Dis. *15*:924–937, 1992.
59. Memish, Z.: Meningococcal disease and travel. Clin. Infect. Dis. *34*:84–90, 2002.
60. Mermin, J., Townes, J., Gerber, M., et al.: Typhoid fever in the United States, 1985–1994. Arch. Intern. Med. *158*:633–638, 1998.
61. Moore, A.: African trypanosomiasis in U.S. travelers. Presented at the 50th Annual Meeting of the American Society of Tropical Medicine and Hygiene, November 2001, Atlanta.
62. Moore, P., Harrison, L., Telzak, E., et al.: Group A meningococcal carriage in travelers returning from Saudi Arabia. J. A. M. A. *260*: 2686–2689, 1988.
63. Nasta, P., Donisi, A., Cattane, A., et al.: Acute histoplasmosis in spelunkers returning from Mato Grosso, Peru. J. Travel Med. *4*:176–178, 1997.
64. Nevill, C., Some, E., Mug'ala, V. et al.: Insecticide-treated bednets reduce mortality and severe morbidity from malaria among children. Trop. Med. Int. Health *1*:139–146, 1996.
65. Outbreak of acute febrile illness among participants in Eco-Challenge-Sabah 2000—Malaysia, 2000. M. M. W. R. Morb. Mortal. Wkly. Rep. *49*:816–817, 2000.
66. Outbreak of acute respiratory febrile illness among college students—Acapulco, Mexico, March 2001. M. M. W. R. Morb. Mortal. Wkly. Rep. *50*(14):261–262, 2001.
67. Outbreak of leptospirosis among white-water rafters—Costa Rica, 1996. M. M. W. R. Morb. Mortal. Wkly. Rep. *46*(25):577–579, 1997.
68. Paixao, M., Dewar, R., Cossar, J., et al.: What do Scots die of when abroad? Scott. Med. J. *36*:114–116, 1991.
69. Pan American Health Organization: Reemergence of dengue in the Americans. Epidemiol. Bull. Pan Am. Health Organ. *18*:1–10, 1997.
70. Phanuphak, P., Ubolyam, S., and Sirivichayakul, S.: Should travellers in rabies endemic areas receive pre-exposure rabies immunization? Ann. Med. Interne (Paris) *145*:409–411, 1994.
71. Peltola, H., and Gorbach, S.: Travelers' diarrhea: Epidemiology and clinical aspects. *In* Dupont, H. L., and Steffen, R. (eds.): Textbook of Travel Medicine and Health. 2nd ed. Hamilton, Ontario, Canada, B. C. Decker, 2001, pp. 151–159.
72. Pickering, L. K. (ed.): 2000 Red Book: Report of the Committee on Infectious Diseases. 25th ed. Elk Grove Village, IL, American Academy of Pediatrics, 2000.
73. Pitzinger, B., Steffen, R., and Tschopp, A.: Incidence and clinical features of traveler's diarrhea in infants and children. Pediatr. Infect. Dis. J. *10*: 719–723, 1991.
74. Prociv, P.: Deaths of Australian travelers overseas. Med. J. Aust. *163*: 27–30, 1995.
75. Rawlings, J., Hendricks, K., Burgess, C., et al.: Dengue surveillance in Texas, 1995. Am. J. Trop. Med. Hyg. *59*:95–99, 1998.
76. Reid, D., Keystone, J., and Cossar, J.: Health risks abroad: General considerations. *In* Dupont, H. L., and Steffen, R. (eds.): Textbook of Travel Medicine and Health. 2nd ed. Hamilton, Canada, B. C. Decker, 2001, pp. 3–10.
77. Rieder, H.: Risk of travel-associated tuberculosis. Clin. Infect. Dis. *33*: 1393–1396, 2001.
78. Rivera-Matos, I., Atkins, J., Doerr, C., and White, A., Jr.: Pediatric malaria in Houston, Texas. Am. J. Trop. Med. Hyg. *57*:560–563, 1997.
79. Robertson, S., Hull, B., Tomori, O., et al.: Yellow fever: A decade of reemergence. J. A. M. A. *276*:1157–1162, 1996.
80. Rosmini, F., Castellani-Patoris, M., Mazzoti, M., et al.: Febrile illness in successive cohorts of tourists to a hotel on the Italian Adriatic Coast: Evidence of a persistent foci of *Legionella* infection. Am. J. Epidemiol. *119*:124–134, 1984.
81. Ryan, E., and Kain, K.: Health advice and immunizations for travelers. N. Engl. J. Med. *342*:1716–1725, 2000.
82. Sears, S., and Sack, D.: Medical advice for the international traveler. *In* Barker, L., Burton, J., and Zieve, P. (eds.): Ambulatory Medicine, 4th ed. Baltimore, Williams & Wilkins, 1995, p. 402.
83. Serogroup W-135 meningococcal disease among travelers returning from Saudi Arabia—United States, 2000. M. M. W. R. Morb. Mortal. Wkly. Rep. *49*(16):345–346, 2000.
84. Shanks, G., Kain, K., and Keystone, J.: Malaria chemoprophylaxis in the age of drug resistance. II. Drugs that may be available in the future. Clin. Infect. Dis. *33*:381–385, 2001.
85. Sniezek, J., and Smith, S.: Injury mortality among non-US residents in the United States 1979–1984. Int. J. Epidemiol. *19*:225–229, 1991.
86. Steffen, R.: Epidemiologic studies of travelers diarrhea, severe gastrointestinal infections, and cholera. Rev. Infect. Dis. *8*(Suppl. 2):122–130, 1986.
87. Steffen, R.: Risk of hepatitis B for travelers. Vaccine *8*:31–32, 1990.
88. Steffen, R.: Travel medicine: Prevention based on epidemiological data. Trans. R. Soc. Trop. Med. Hyg. *85*:156–162, 1991.
89. Steffen, R., and Jong, E.: Travelers' and immigrants' health. *In* Guerrant, R. L., Walker, D. H., and Wyler, P. F. (eds.): Tropical Infectious Diseases: Principles, Pathogens and Practice. Philadelphia, Churchill Livingstone, 1999, pp. 106–114.
90. Steffen, R., Kane, M., Shapiro, C., et al.: Epidemiology and prevention of hepatitis A in travelers. J. A. M. A. *272*:885–889, 1994.
91. Steffen, R., Rickenbach, M., Wilhelm, U., et al.: Health problems after travel to developing countries. J. Infect. Dis. *156*:84–91, 1987.
92. Svenson, J., MacLean, J., Gyorkos, T., et al.: Imported malaria: Clinical presentation and examination of symptomatic travelers. Arch. Intern. Med. *155*:861–868, 1995.
93. Thein, S., Aung, M., Shwe, T., et al.: Risk factors in dengue shock syndrome. Am. J. Trop. Med. Hyg. *56*:566–572, 1997.
94. The role of BCG vaccine in the prevention and control of tuberculosis in the United States. A joint statement by the Advisory Council for the Elimination of Tuberculosis and the Advisory Committee on Immunization Practices. M. M. W. R. Recomm. Rep. *45*(RR-4):1–18, 1996.
95. Thompson, R.: Travel and Routine Immunizations: A Practical Guide for the Medical Office, 2001. Milwaukee, WI, Shoreland, Inc., 2001.
96. Tourism Industries Office, Trade Department, International Trade Administration, U.S. Department of Commerce. http://www.tinet.ita.doc.gov.
97. Tropneteurop: Outbreak of African trypanosomiasis among travelers to the Serengeti National Park in Tanzania. Abstract FC05.06. Paper presented at the 7th Conference of the International Society of Travel Medicine, May 29, 2001, Innsbruck, Austria, p. 89.
98. Underdiagnosis of dengue—Laredo, Texas, 1999. M. M. W. R. Morb. Mortal. Wkly. Rep. *50*(4):57–59, 2001.
99. Update: Assessment of risk for meningococcal disease associated with the Hajj 2001. M. M. W. R. Morb. Mortal. Wkly. Rep. *50*(12):221–222, 2001.
100. Update: Outbreak of acute febrile illness among athletes participating in Eco-Challenge-Sabah 2000—Borneo, Malaysia, 2000. M. M. W. R. Morb. Mortal. Wkly. Rep. *50*(2):21–24, 2001.
101. Update: Outbreak of acute febrile respiratory illness among college students —Acapulco, Mexico, March 2001. M. M. W. R. Morb. Mortal. Wkly. Rep. *50*(18):359–360, 2001.
102. Update: Outbreak of poliomyelitis—Dominican Republic and Haiti, 2000–2001. M. M. W. R. Morb. Mortal. Wkly. Rep. *50*(39):855–856, 2001.
103. Valdez, H., and Salata, R.: Bat-associated histoplasmosis in returning travelers: Case presentation and description of a cluster. J. Travel Med. *6*:258–260, 1999.
104. Vasconcelos, P., Luna, E., Galler, R., et al.: Serious adverse events associated with yellow fever 17DD vaccine in Brazil: A report of two cases. Lancet *358*:9107, 2001.
105. Vasconcelos, P., Travassos da Rosa, A., Pinheiro, F., et al.: *Aedes aegypti*, dengue and re-urbanization of yellow fever in Brazil and other South American countries: Past and present situation and future perspectives. W. H. O. Dengue Bull. *23*:55–56, 1999.
106. Viani, R., and Bromberg, K.: Pediatric imported malaria in New York: Delayed diagnosis. Clin. Pediatr. (Phila.) *38*:333–337, 1999.

107. Weil, W.: New information leads to changes in DEET recommendations. Am. Acad. Pediatr. News *19*:52, 2001.
108. Weinberg, M.: An outbreak of acute febrile illness among travelers to Nicaragua. Paper presented at the 50th Annual Meeting of the American Society of Tropical Medicine and Hygiene, November 2001, Atlanta.
109. Wilson, M., and Lucchina, L.: Healthy student with a papule. Clin. Infect. Dis. *33*:816, 899–900, 2001.
110. Winters, R., and Murray, H.: Malaria—the mime revisited: Fifteen more years of experience at a New York City teaching hospital. Am. J. Med. *93*:243–246, 1992.
111. World Health Organization: International Travel and Health: Vaccination Requirements and Health Advice. Geneva, World Health Organization, 2001.
112. World Health Organization: [World malaria situation in 1994. Part I. Population at risk.] Wkly. Epidemiol. Rec. *72*:269–276, 1997.

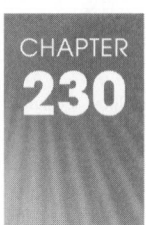

Infectious Disease Problems of International Adoptees and Refugees

MARGARET K. HOSTETTER

Infectious Diseases in Internationally Adopted Children

More than 15,000 internationally adopted children enter the United States each year to begin life with their new families. The demographics of this process have changed considerably since the mid-1980s, when approximately 70 percent of internationally adopted children spent their infancy in two-parent foster homes in Korea. Since 1991, China, Russia, and eastern Europe are the countries of origin for more than 70 percent of internationally adopted children; the vast majority of these children spend weeks to years in orphanages and other state-run institutions variably called nurseries, baby homes, or hospitals. Although all internationally adopted children have special health needs, institutionalized children are particularly at risk for acquiring any of numerous infectious diseases, as well as for developmental and emotional handicaps ascribable to institutional care.

PRE-ADOPTION ENVIRONMENTS IN THE COUNTRIES OF ORIGIN

Children coming from the state-subsidized foster homes of Korea receive optimal nutrition, nurturing, and preventive health care. The Korean foster home system chooses only two-parent families who have successfully raised their own children. Foster parents must meet defined dates for medical follow-up, continuity of care, and immunizations. Both boys and girls may be adopted, although numerous Korean stipulations exist regarding age, physical condition, and household income of the prospective adoptive parents. Korean infants typically are adopted when they are between 6 and 13 months of age.

Because Chinese culture stipulates that the son care for the aging parents, most infants surrendered for adoption under China's "one-child" policy are girls. These children typically are adopted in the United States when they are between 8 and 15 months of age. The standard of care in Chinese orphanages certainly is acceptable in terms of nutrition, but hygiene and immunization practices can be variable. At times, the child's stated age may be younger than the actual age because growth parameters and developmental attainments then appear more favorable.

Children coming from Russian or eastern European orphanages have highly variable lengths of stay and pre-adoption care. A substantial proportion of Russian adoptees have remained in institutions for more than 2 years. Children can be removed from their biologic families at any time, and finding sibling groups that have been separated because of parental abuse or alcoholism is not uncommon. Immunizations may be erratic and, though recorded, may not have been administered. Anecdotal reports of caseworkers filling out immunization sheets as the child is leaving with the parents are not unusual. The varying backgrounds of Russian or eastern European adoptees, the variable ages at adoption, and the unpredictable nature of the pre-adoption environment carries implications for not only medical but also developmental health.

Other countries also serving as resources for international adoption include Central and South America, India, Vietnam, and Cambodia. In Guatemala, adoptions typically are arranged by lawyers, who place the children in foster homes for which subsidies are paid by the potential adopting parents. Often, little or no information about the child's birth circumstances or the foster home is available. Orphanages run by religious groups in Central America and Colombia often provide prenatal care for single mothers and excellent postnatal care for their infants. Most children from India come from orphanages where limited resources may impair the ability of the orphanage workers to meet all the needs of the children in their care. Children from Vietnam and Cambodia often are adopted at an early age, which mitigates the effects of less than optimal nutrition and truncates the potential time of exposure to cases of tuberculosis among caregivers.

To our knowledge, screening for tuberculosis is not required in any of the countries in which children are adopted from orphanage settings, nor have the routine standards of sanitation that have been mandated or accepted worldwide been established in orphanages. As a result, the highly varying environments from which these children come carry substantial implications for their health. This chapter addresses many of the issues with which infectious disease specialists must be familiar.

TABLE 230–1 ■ SCREENING TESTS FOR INTERNATIONALLY ADOPTED CHILDREN

Hepatitis B profile—to include HbsAg and antibodies to hepatitis B surface and core antigens
HIV antibodies by ELISA*
Stool sample for ova and parasites
VDRL (or RPR) and FTA-ABS
Mantoux skin test with control for adequacy of the delayed hypersensitivity response
Complete blood count with erythrocyte indices
Urinalysis

*Some experts recommend polymerase chain reaction for HIV RNA because as long as 3 months can be required for antibodies to develop.
ELISA, enzyme-linked immunosorbent assay; FTA-ABS, fluorescent treponemal antibody absorption test; HbsAg, hepatitis B surface antigen; HIV, human immunodeficiency virus; RPR, rapid plasma reagin; VDRL, Venereal Disease Research Laboratory.

SPECIFIC DISEASES

Screening tests currently recommended by the American Academy of Pediatrics (AAP) should be applied to internationally adopted children without regard to age, sex, or country of origin (Table 230–1). Many pre-adoption referrals will report the results of medical testing performed in the country of origin, but any test done in the country of origin should be repeated when the child arrives in the United States. In my experience, testing performed in the country of origin is wrong approximately 10 percent of the time, especially with regard to hepatitis B.

Secondary screening tests are recommended by the AAP for children from China, Russia, or eastern European orphanages, but some experts apply them to all adoptees, especially because hepatitis C is not confined to these countries (Table 230–2). As shown in Table 230–3, the reported prevalence of hepatitis B and hepatitis C may vary widely depending on the country of origin. The remainder of this section will discuss specific infectious diseases of particular importance to children, parents, and physicians.

Hepatitis B

The prevalence of hepatitis B in internationally adopted children varies with the carriage rate for this virus among women of child-bearing age (see Table 230–3). As a result, parents planning to adopt from most countries in Asia (Cambodia, China, India, or Vietnam) should be informed that the chance of a hepatitis B infection may be as high as 10 percent in unvaccinated children; parents planning to adopt from Russia or eastern Europe should know that the prevalence of hepatitis B ranges from 2 to 20 percent, the latter rate occurring in some regions of Romania.[6]

Table 230–4 delineates common patterns of serologic responses to the three components of the hepatitis B profile: hepatitis B surface antigen (HBsAg) and antibodies to hepatitis B surface and core antigens (antisurface and anticore antibodies). The use of all three tests is essential to enable the practitioner to determine which category best fits the child's serologic pattern. A substantial proportion of hepatitis B infections in internationally adopted children are misdiagnosed as the "carrier state" when HBsAg is positive but testing for IgG core antibodies is omitted.[4] A child who is positive for HBsAg and IgG anticore antibodies for more than 6 months meets the definition for having chronic hepatitis B; chronic infection will develop in approximately 90 percent of children exposed to hepatitis B during the first 12 months of life, and in approximately 10 percent of these children, cirrhosis or hepatocellular carcinoma will eventually develop. Therefore, the finding of a positive HBsAg never should be dismissed as a "carrier state."

Additional testing in children positive for HBsAg should include hepatitis B antigen, aspartate/alanine transaminase (AST/ALT), and testing for hepatitis D antibodies. Hepatitis D (delta virus) occurs only in conjunction with hepatitis B and typically is acquired in regions such as in southern Italy, parts of eastern Europe, South America, Africa, and the Middle East. Practitioners should be aware that administration of hepatitis B vaccine can lead to a brief period of antigenemia if testing for HBsAg is performed within 2 to 3 days of vaccination.

Hepatitis B immunization is given appropriately in Korea, and this national policy has eliminated hepatitis B infection completely in Korean adoptees.[4] However, although the Korean government has practiced universal immunization for hepatitis B since 1989, premature infants or the rare abandoned child may not have been vaccinated within the first week of life. Hepatitis B immunizations are given erratically if at all in every other country from which internationally adopted children come. Health care providers should review the timing of hepatitis B immunizations: the first is given optimally within the first week of life; the second, 1 month later; and the third, 6 months after the first. In many countries, the initial hepatitis B immunization is delayed for

TABLE 230–2 ■ SECONDARY SCREENING TESTS*

Hepatitis C EIA
Lead level
TSH

*Some experts recommend these tests only for children from China, Russia, and eastern Europe.
EIA, enzyme immunoassay; TSH, thyroid-stimulating hormone.

TABLE 230–3 ■ PREVALENCE OF HEPATITIS B AND C BY COUNTRY OF ORIGIN

Country	Hepatitis B[10]	Hepatitis C[1,5,7,9,13,15]
Central/South America	2–7%	0–2.3%
China	8–10%	3–8%
Eastern Europe	2–7%	2–8%
Russia/USSR	2–10%	1–10%
South Korea	8–10%	1.7%

TABLE 230–4 ■ INTERPRETATION OF HEPATITIS B PROFILE

Status	HbsAg	Anti-HBc	Anti-HBs	AST/ALT
Carrier	+	–	–	Normal
Acute infection	+	IgM	–	Elevated
Chronic infection	+	IgG	–	Normal/elevated
Past infection	–	IgG	IgG	Normal
Passive transfer	–	IgG	IgG	Normal
Vaccination	–	–	IgG	Normal

ALT, alanine transaminase; AST, aspartate transaminase; HBc, hepatitis B core; HbsAg, hepatitis B surface antigen.

several weeks or months. This delay, of course, means that the child is not protected from the acquisition of hepatitis B either by vertical transmission from the mother or by horizontal transmission in the orphanage during this time.

Most children who have received at least two hepatitis B vaccines should have positive antisurface antibodies. Anticore antibodies are negative after vaccination. Children who do not have antisurface antibodies after two or more recorded vaccines probably have not received the immunizations on their certificates, and the entire hepatitis B series should be initiated again.

Hepatitis B vaccination also is essential for household contacts, including family members, home daycare contacts, and providers of home daycare. Although most infants in the United States will have received hepatitis B vaccine and are thereby protected from horizontal transmission in a daycare center, daycare mothers or other daycare workers themselves often are not immunized. The primary caregiver is the one to whom hepatitis B most frequently is transmitted; therefore, the physician should provide counseling to the adoptive parents regarding the necessity of immunizing household contacts and home daycare providers who will be caring for any child who is HBsAg-positive. The coexistence of hepatitis B e antigen increases the risk of infectivity.

Hepatitis C

The epidemiology of hepatitis C is somewhat more obscure. Although numerous publications place the incidence as high as 8 percent (see Table 230–3), no study on the prevalence of this infection in internationally adopted children has been published. Approximately 6 percent of infants born to infected mothers will acquire the virus; data on transmissibility from breast milk are somewhat more controversial. A number of studies have documented the presence of hepatitis C RNA in breast milk, but studies looking for infection after breast-feeding typically have found little if any evidence that breast-feeding is a major source of infection.[12, 14]

The hepatitis C enzyme immunoassay (EIA) is the test of choice. If it is positive, the physician may choose either the recombinant immunoblot assay (RIBA) or a direct measure of viral RNA by polymerase chain reaction (PCR) for confirmation. The latter test is preferred by many adoption medicine specialists because it is quite specific for infection and very helpful for identifying infection in infants in whom passive transfer of maternal antibody may confound the clinical picture. Documenting AST and ALT levels for children who are positive by the antibody test also is of importance.

The prognosis of children with hepatitis C infection is unclear. Although in many children the disease is thought to be benign, anecdotal reports of internationally adopted children with more aggressive manifestations do exist. Children with bridging necrosis or active cirrhosis on liver biopsy or with persistently elevated serum transaminase concentrations exceeding twice the upper limit of normal should be referred to a gastroenterologist for further management, which typically includes tests for alpha-fetoprotein and abdominal ultrasonography. INF-α therapy unfortunately is not approved for patients younger than 18 years; thus, despite anecdotal reports of its efficacy in children, no prospective treatment trials in this age group have been undertaken.

Syphilis

Maternal syphilis is a major problem in Russia, eastern Europe, and Guatemala. Treatment in these countries often is erratic or inadequate; foreshortened courses, the use of oral agents, and poor documentation of treatment are common findings in pregnant women. Referral paperwork on many adoptees states that "preventive treatment for syphilis was given," but these regimens can vary dramatically from a few days of oral antibiotic therapy to the more appropriate 21-day course of intramuscular penicillin.

As a result, testing for syphilis with both a nontreponemal (Venereal Disease Research Laboratory [VDRL] or rapid plasma reagin [RPR]) and a treponemal (fluorescent treponemal antibody absorption test [FTA-ABS]) test is essential in internationally adopted children, despite purportedly negative test reports from abroad. The combination of the VDRL and FTA-ABS is extremely useful, especially in infants young enough to have passive transfer of maternal antibodies. In the case of mothers who are truly infected with syphilis, the FTA-ABS will be positive and antibody will be passed to the young infant, even if the child's VDRL has been obliterated by partial therapy in the nursery or orphanage. When the FTA-ABS or VDRL test is positive, consideration should be given to obtaining spinal fluid, long bone films, and hepatic transaminase concentrations before the initiation of parenteral penicillin therapy. Because syphilis is an entirely curable disease and the complications of untreated or partially treated syphilis involve not only intellectual impairment but also disfiguring physical complications such as Hutchinson incisors, saber shins, and gummas, accurate determination of the adoptee's syphilis status is essential.

Tuberculosis

The AAP has mandated that the purified protein derivative (PPD) (Mantoux) test be used for evaluating skin test reactivity in children coming from areas in which tuberculosis is endemic. Despite this recommendation, many pediatricians still use the Tine test or do not test at all if the adoptee has received bacille Calmette-Guérin (BCG) vaccine. Both these practices are incorrect. All internationally adopted children should be tested with a PPD (and a *Candida* skin test or other control for delayed-type hypersensitivity) as soon after adoption as feasible. Children who have received the BCG vaccine by report and whose left or right deltoid shows the typical scar may be tested with the PPD approximately 12 months after administration of the BCG vaccine without inducing a false-positive reaction. Prospective studies in Native American children given BCG at birth have demonstrated that cross-reactivity between BCG and PPD is maximal 6 months after vaccination and thereafter wanes.[8] Concern regarding a sloughing reaction if a PPD test is performed after administration of BCG vaccine is exaggerated and should not stand in the way of performing a Mantoux skin test.

The Mantoux test should be read by trained medical personnel, not by parents. If the PPD shows more than 10 mm of induration in transverse diameter, chest radiography should be performed. If the chest radiograph is negative, the child should receive 10 mg/kg of isoniazid once a day for 9 months. The 6-month course of isoniazid for prophylactic therapy no longer is recommended. Parents should be instructed that isoniazid as prepared by many commercial pharmacies may be tolerated poorly from the standpoint of taste and gastrointestinal complaints. Under these circumstances, physicians should contact Compounded Solutions (877-796-3337; *Compounds1@aol.com*) for a low-sucrose preparation in various appealing flavors. A little extra work by the physician to ensure the palatability of isoniazid goes a long way toward maintaining parental compliance.

A child with a positive PPD and a positive chest radiograph should be managed by an infectious disease specialist. Resistance to multiple antituberculous agents can be a problem in the countries of Southeast Asia and in some areas of Russia and eastern Europe; as a result, unusual regimens may need to be implemented for individual patients based on the drug susceptibility of their isolates.

In children older than 5 years with a positive PPD and a negative chest radiograph, consideration should be given to extrapulmonary disease of the spine or genitourinary tract. Standard evaluation in these cases should include a sedimentation rate, imaging of the lumbosacral spine with appropriate shielding, and three first-morning voided urine specimens as well as urinalysis to look for hematuria and sterile pyuria.

Transmission of tuberculosis to school or family contacts is a rare event in children younger than 6 years because they cannot generate sufficient tussive force to spread respiratory droplets. However, cavitary disease, though a rare occurrence in children, virtually always is infectious for others, and failure to perform a Mantoux skin test or to interpret it correctly can lead to widespread dissemination among multiple contacts.[3]

Intestinal Pathogens

The presence of intestinal parasites is a common concomitant of orphanage confinement. We have yet to find intestinal parasites in any child coming from Korea in the more than 750 children whom we have examined; however, intestinal parasitosis is found in children coming from virtually any other country. The use of albendazole abroad may limit the number of parasites found in internationally adopted children, but certain parasites such as *Giardia lamblia* are not killed by this regimen. Because of the potential to transmit parasites in the daycare setting, most children should be treated, even when asymptomatic.

A single stool sample for ova and parasite is informative approximately 85 percent of the time.[2] Eggs of *Ascaris lumbricoides* will not be found in the stool sample if the harbored worm is either a male or an unfertilized female, but subsequent passage of the worm may cause great consternation for the parent. Apprising the parents of this possibility obviates recriminations later.

Treatment of *Blastocystis hominis, Chilomastix mesnili, Trichomonas hominis* or *tenax, Entamoeba coli,* and *Iodamoeba buetschlii* is not necessary because these organisms are not pathogenic, although some experts recommend treatment of immunocompromised children with *Blastocystis*. Repeat stool samples for ova and parasites should be performed at the close of a treatment course if the child remains persistently symptomatic or if more than one organism was isolated at the original screening.

Some practitioners also test for *Salmonella*; although this organism can be present in asymptomatic children, treatment prolongs excretion and, therefore, is not recommended for otherwise normal children older than 3 months. Children with explosive diarrhea obviously should undergo evaluation for a number of other pathogens, including rotavirus and *Shigella*.

Human Immunodeficiency Virus Infection

Only a small number of cases of human immunodeficiency virus (HIV) infection in internationally adopted children have been detected after their arrival in the United States. However, because of the confusion that can be introduced by the presence of passively transferred maternal antibodies in young children, some experts recommend the use of PCR testing on arrival. A secondary advantage of this test is that horizontal transmission within the previous 1 to 2 months theoretically will be detected, even though time has not been sufficient for an antibody response to develop. Other experts recommend repeat testing for HIV by enzyme-linked immunosorbent assay 6 months after the child's arrival.

Other Tests for Infectious Diseases in International Adoptees

A microcephalic child represents a perplexing dilemma. Studies have shown that head circumference can be affected by length of time in an orphanage,[6] and a downward trend of head circumference from the percentile recorded at birth is quite common in adoptees reared in orphanages. Microcephaly is a common feature of fetal alcohol syndrome (FAS), but testing for treatable etiologies such as toxoplasmosis or syphilis should be undertaken before a diagnosis of FAS is made. Entities such as rubella, cytomegalovirus (CMV), or herpes simplex virus are highly important prognostically and should be evaluated.

Internationally adopted children from Mediterranean regions, Middle Eastern countries, and China should be tested for glucose-6-phosphate dehydrogenase deficiency if administration of nalidixic acid, nitrofurantoin, or sulfonamide is contemplated. Routine screening tests for malaria and CMV are not warranted in internationally adopted children. Some physicians have advocated prospective screening for *Helicobacter pylori* in all adoptees because of the increased incidence of carriage in developing nations; however, no data support treatment of asymptomatic children at this time.

MANAGEMENT ISSUES

Validity of Medical Records and Medical Testing in the Country of Origin

Parents often are encouraged to believe what they read in medical records from abroad, especially with regard to screening that is performed in the country of origin. Parents should be cautioned that many countries have no standard accreditation of laboratory personnel and that testing results may be haphazard, inaccurate, or falsified. For these reasons, medical testing should be repeated once the child arrives in the United States.

Immunization for Diphtheria, Pertussis, and Tetanus

A major area of debate at present is the validity of immunizations obtained abroad. A careful analysis of both the number of immunizations and the interval between them more often than not detects aberrancies. Immunizations that antedate a child's recorded birth date, that are given on the same day of the month (e.g., 8/7/00, 9/7/00, 2/7/01), or that are administered in orphanages without refrigeration are suspect. One prospective study of more than 155 internationally adopted children predominantly from Chinese, Russian, or eastern European orphanages whose immunization certificates recorded three or more diphtheria-pertussis-tetanus (DPT) vaccines found protective antibodies to diphtheria and tetanus present in only 38 percent by hemagglutination assay. A second study of approximately 50 international adoptees found the presence of protective antibodies in 70 percent by EIA. A third prospective study evaluated the presence of antisurface antibodies in children who supposedly had received three vaccinations for hepatitis B; only 50 percent of these children had detectable surface antibodies, thereby confirming the discrepancy between written immunization certificates and the presence of protective antibodies in children immunized in orphanages.

Based on these reports, the Advisory Committee on Immunization Practices has recommended re-administration of the entire DPT series (and inactivated poliovirus vaccine) if the child's record has any departure from the U.S. vaccination schedule in terms of the number of vaccinations, the interval between them, or the child's age at immunization. In my experience of more than 16 years with reimmunization of children with questionable vaccination certificates, I have encountered not a single incident of toxicity with this approach. At issue here is not so much an infant who may have received one immunization abroad and will certainly receive a protective complement here in the United States; rather, the focus of concern should be older children aged 4 to 6 whose immunization certificate may be inaccurate. Such children, if not reimmunized, are at risk for acquiring tetanus in the United States or for other diseases such as polio or diphtheria that may be acquired during international travel.

Immunization for Measles, Mumps, and Rubella

Countries other than Korea either omit measles-mumpsrubella (MMR) vaccine entirely or give only the measles component, typically at 6 to 12 months of age. MMR vaccine should be given to all international adoptees at 12 to 16 months of age, at 4 to 6 years of age, and again in middle school.

TRAVEL MEDICAL KIT

Many parents are encouraged by adoption agencies or by information on the Internet to take antibiotics to the country of origin. Although this tactic may seem prudent, no antibiotic known to the author is a panacea for all infectious diseases. A child with a fever whose parents are carrying a first-generation cephalosporin may not respond to the drug and may have needed treatment delayed if the real cause of the illness is *Salmonella* bacteremia. For these reasons, in our clinic we instruct parents that fever should prompt medical attention, not random dosing with an antibiotic. Teaching parents how to take a rectal temperature accurately is more important than supplying them with an antibiotic that may be outdated, inefficacious, or contaminated with nonsterile water on dilution.

INTERNET RESOURCES

Informative websites for prospective adoptive parents can be found at *eeadopt.org* and *www.adopting.com*. A plethora of websites also provide first-hand information from parents, but subjective reports should not be confused with objective information. Physicians may find the website *adoptmed.edu* of value if questions arise with regard to individual patients.

Infectious Diseases in Refugee Children

The widely varying conditions from which internationally adopted children come are no more predictable for refugee children. Some children will have experienced only recent disruption, whereas in other cases, children may have been displaced from parents for months to years. An accompanying parent often is helpful in providing information regarding immunizations and illnesses in the past, but refugees from war or persecution may arrive without a knowledgeable adult.

TABLE 230–5 ■ COMPARISON OF REFUGEES AND ADOPTEES

Refugees	Adoptees
Organized screening in camps	No organized screening
Most diseases already identified	Many medical illnesses unidentified
Medical testing accurate in camps	Medical testing inaccurate
Preventive health care under way	Preventive health care delayed

Adapted from Hostetter, M. K.: *In* Long, S., Pickering, L., and Prober, C. (eds.): *Principles and Practice of Pediatric Infectious Diseases*. New York, Churchill Livingstone, 1997, p. 39.

Except in the most chaotic circumstances, refugee children who have spent some time in a camp supervised by responsible international health organizations have many advantages over internationally adopted children, for whom no globally accepted screening protocols exist (Table 230–5).

SCREENING TESTS

No universally accepted recommendations exist for medical evaluation of refugee children. In general, in the absence of documentation of immunizations or screening undertaken in refugee camps, the most prudent course is to screen for transmissible infectious diseases that are more common in the child's country of origin or that may have been transmitted during the period of displacement. Such entities include, but are not limited to hepatitis B, hepatitis C, tuberculosis, HIV, and diarrheal pathogens such as *Salmonella, Shigella, Campylobacter,* and *Yersinia.* Illnesses such as melioidosis, typhoid fever, malaria, filariasis, and flukes may be more common in refugees than in adoptees because of regional prevalence. In refugees or immigrants from regions such as Asia, the Middle East, sub-Saharan Africa, eastern Europe, and Latin America and the Caribbean, the frequency of intestinal parasitosis may be high; therefore, some experts recommend providing presumptive treatment of adults with albendazole as a more cost-effective strategy than screening.[11] Practitioners should be aware that such treatment is not effective against *G. lamblia*. The pediatric dosage is 400 mg given once.

A careful history and physical examination may suggest diseases caused by geographically circumscribed entities such as leprosy, schistosomiasis, and other rarely encountered parasitic diseases. Many travel medicine clinics find it particularly helpful to have a parasitologist on staff or at least have ready access to informed consultation. Finally, consideration of sickle hemoglobinopathies in Africa, India, and Central/South America; hemoglobin E in Southeast Asia; glucose-6-phosphate dehydrogenase deficiency in Africa, the Mediterranean, the Middle East, and China; and delta hepatitis (hepatitis D) in hepatitis B–infected individuals from southern Italy, eastern Europe, South America, Africa, and the Middle East is indicated for both refugees and adoptees.

REFERENCES

1. Barham, W. B., Figueroa, R., Phillips, I. A., and Hyams, K. C.: Chronic liver disease in Peru: Role of viral hepatitis. J. Med. Virol. *42*:129–132, 1994.
2. Bass, J. L., Mehta, K. A., and Eppes, B.: Parasitology screening of Latin American children in a primary care clinic. Pediatrics *89*:279–283, 1992.

3. Curtis, A. B., Ridzon, R., Vogel, R., et al.: Extensive transmission of *Mycobacterium tuberculosis* from a child. N. Engl. J. Med. *341*: 1491–1495, 1999.
4. Hostetter, M. K., Iverson, S., Thomas, W. E., et al.: Prospective medical evaluation of internationally adopted children. N. Engl. J. Med. *325*: 479–485, 1991.
5. Ivan, A., Azoicai, D., Filimon, R., et al.: The epidemiological aspects and prevalence of markers in those with viral hepatitis C in some population categories in 1994–1997 in Iasi County. Bacteriol. Virusol. Parazitol. Epidemiol. *43*:275–279, 1998.
6. Johnson, D. E., Miller, L. C., Iverson, S., et al.: The health of children adopted from Romania. J. A. M. A. *268*:3446–3451, 1992.
7. Kim, Y. S., Pai, C. H., Chi, H. S., et al.: Prevalence of hepatitis C virus antibody among Korean adults. J. Korean Med. Sci. 7:333–336, 1992.
8. Lifschitz, M.: The value of the tuberculin skin test as a screening test for tuberculosis among BCG-vaccinated children. Pediatrics *36*:624–627, 1965.
9. Lvov, D. K., Samokhvalov, E. I., Tsuda, F., et al.: Prevalence of hepatitis C virus and distribution of its genotypes in Northern Eurasia. Arch. Virol. *141*:1613–1622, 1996.
10. Mahoney, F. J.: Hepatitis B virus. *In* Long, S., Pickering, L., and Prober, C. (eds.): Principles and Practice of Pediatric Infectious Diseases. New York, Churchill Livingstone, 1997, p. 1195.
11. Muennig, P., Pallin, D., Sell, R. L., and Chan, M. S.: The cost effectiveness of strategies for the treatment of intestinal parasites in immigrants. N. Engl. J. Med. *340*:773–779, 1999.
12. Polywka, S., Schroter, M., Feucht, H. H., et al.: Low risk of vertical transmission of hepatitis C virus by breast milk. Clin. Infect. Dis. *29*:1327–1329, 1999.
13. Robinson, J. W., Rosas, M., Guzman, F., et al.: Comparison of prevalence of anti–hepatitis C virus antibodies in differing South American populations. J. Med. Virol. *50*:188–192, 1996.
14. Ruiz-Extremera, A., Salmeron, J., Torres, C., et al.: Follow-up of transmission of hepatitis C to babies of human immunodeficiency virus–negative women: The role of breast feeding in transmission. Pediatr. Infect. Dis. J. *19*:511–516, 2000.
15. Shimbo, S., Zhang, Z. W., Gao, W. P., et al.: Prevalence of hepatitis B and C infection markers among adult women in urban and rural areas in Shaanxi Province, China. Southeast Asian J. Trop. Med. Public Health *29*:263–268, 1998.

PART IV

Infection Control

SECTION XXIV

Hospital Control of Infections

CHAPTER 231

Nosocomial Infections

W. CHARLES HUSKINS ■ DONALD A. GOLDMANN

Nosocomial infections generally have been defined as infections that develop in hospitalized patients and were neither present nor incubating at the time of their admission to the hospital.[229] The term *nosocomial* originates from the Greek words *nosos* (disease) and *komeion* (to take care of).[583] In light of this entomology, a more inclusive definition is infections that occur as a consequence of health care, regardless of whether they arise during hospitalization. This definition includes surgical-site infections after outpatient surgical procedures and cases of varicella acquired during an emergency room visit. Infections in hospital personnel caused by microorganisms acquired in the hospital are also nosocomial infections. This expanded view of nosocomial infections fits well with recent trends in medicine that have placed increased emphasis on outpatient care, more comprehensive assessment of outcomes of medical care, and the risk of acquiring occupational diseases facing medical personnel.

In some cases, determining whether an infection is a consequence of receiving health care may be difficult. Infections with long or variable incubation periods, such as hepatitis B or late-onset prosthetic-valve endocarditis, may become manifested long after medical procedures are performed, thus raising doubt regarding their causation. Infections such as cytomegalovirus (CMV) pneumonia occurring in immunocompromised patients during hospitalization often are perceived as being attributable to the patients' underlying risk of acquiring infection and previous colonization rather than being a result of health care.

Despite these ambiguities, defining nosocomial infections as infections that occur in persons who are exposed to the health care environment is logical because it identifies the population at risk. This definition affords us the opportunity to better understand the mechanisms leading to the acquisition of these infections and to design and evaluate interventions to prevent their occurrence. This chapter discusses the general epidemiology of nosocomial infections (including those that are introduced into the hospital from the community); infections related to invasive devices, procedures, and treatments; and infections in special populations. Programmatic approaches to the prevention and control of nosocomial infections are discussed in Chapter 232.

Historical Aspects

The history of nosocomial infections and their control is linked tightly to developments in institutional medical care. Two publications have described this history in considerable detail.[363, 583] Unfortunately, historical data regarding nosocomial infections in children are relatively limited. Nonetheless, ample evidence suggests that efforts to study and prevent infections in hospitalized children have contributed significantly to the development of nosocomial infection control and prevention efforts in general.

Hospitals in Europe during the Middle Ages and the Renaissance were notorious for their overcrowding and unsanitary conditions, and one can imagine that children suffered greatly from the epidemics of contagious diseases that spread through hospitals during this period. By the 18th and 19th centuries, sketchy information regarding the impact of nosocomial infections in pediatric patients began to emerge. These data, summarized in a report presented in a landmark seminar regarding nosocomial infections in pediatric patients at the Sixth Northern Pediatric Congress in Stockholm in 1934,[219] provide dramatic evidence that nosocomial infections were the cause of considerable morbidity and mortality in hospitalized children.

Semmelweis' classic studies of puerperal fever in the Vienna Lying-In Hospital in the mid-1800s provide insight into the etiology of perinatal infections in newborn infants, not just their afflicted mothers.[584] Semmelweis noted that rates of mortality in infants born to women in the First Division of the hospital (the division where medical students who had come from the autopsy table cared for women in labor) were several-fold higher than rates in infants born to women in the Second Division of the hospital (the division where midwives cared for women in labor). In support of his theories regarding the infectious etiology of puerperal fever, he noted that rates of infant mortality closely paralleled rates of maternal mortality from puerperal fever and that autopsy findings were remarkably similar in infants and mothers.

The opening of wards and entire hospitals designated for the treatment of patients with infectious diseases in the early 20th century stimulated interest in the study of "cross-infection" with measles, chickenpox, scarlet fever, whooping cough, diphtheria, and invasive meningococcal disease.[583] The potential for the occurrence of cross-infection with these classic contagious diseases on pediatric wards, especially wards caring for infants, was well recognized in the leading hospitals of the day and stimulated the implementation of numerous interventions to minimize this problem. Quarantine areas for new admissions, confinement of each child in an individual cubicle, cohorting of patients admitted during community epidemics, use of masks by persons caring for patients, exclusion of visitors, and strict control of the health of nurses and physicians caring for the patients were implemented to minimize the spread of contagious diseases.[63, 75, 283, 381, 394] Some hospitals even used closed cubicles with outside exhaust of air for patients with measles or varicella.[283] Analysis of the effectiveness of these interventions contributed to a better understanding of how contagious diseases are spread in hospitals.

Undoubtedly because of this vigilance, the first systematic surveys of nosocomial infections in pediatric patients in hospitals in Europe and the United States published in the 1930s and 1940s demonstrated that nosocomial spread of the classic contagious diseases did occur, but relatively uncommonly.[283, 381, 436, 512, 667] However, nosocomial respiratory infections of various types were encountered frequently; gastrointestinal and skin infections also were relatively common events.[283, 381, 436, 667]

Although nosocomial infections caused by beta-hemolytic streptococci had been a scourge of obstetric and surgical wards for centuries, advances in diagnostic microbiology and serotyping of streptococci in the mid-1900s led to greater appreciation of the etiologic role of this organism in nosocomial scarlet fever, postpartum infection, postoperative infection, and secondary infection in patients with burns, measles, and influenza.[571, 583] The decline of this organism as a major nosocomial pathogen coincided with the introduction of antibiotic therapy in the 1940s and 1950s, although a causal link between these events has not been established.[571]

Outbreaks of *Staphylococcus aureus* infection in hospitalized newborn infants had been documented in the late 1800s and early 1900s,[84, 338] but the pandemic of *S. aureus* infections that plagued hospitals in the 1950s and 1960s drew special attention to the impact of nosocomial infections with this organism. Outbreaks of staphylococcal disease were particularly devastating in newborn nurseries, where epidemics caused by specific phage types were responsible for substantial morbidity and mortality.[571, 575]

This serious problem of nosocomial staphylococcal infection spawned more comprehensive efforts to document the impact and consequences of nosocomial infections and served as the impetus to develop organized infection control programs, particularly in Great Britain (with its tradition of infection control sisters) and North America. A 1-year study of nosocomial infections in pediatric patients at The Hospital for Sick Children in Toronto was conducted in 1959.[555–557] The cumulative incidence of nosocomial infection was 6.5 percent; respiratory and gastrointestinal infections occurred most commonly. *S. aureus* caused infection in only 2.6 percent of patients overall but accounted for the vast majority of surgical-site infections. Even this early study recognized the important consequences of nosocomial infection when it reported that 16 deaths and 2070 extra hospital days were the result of these infections.

In 1970, a nosocomial infection surveillance and control program was established at Children's Hospital in Boston, and data were reported to the nascent National Nosocomial Infections Study (NNIS) at the Centers for Disease Control and Prevention (CDC).[223] The cumulative incidence of infection was 4.6 percent. *S. aureus* was the most common pathogen, but more than 60 percent of the pathogens were gram-negative bacilli, including *Pseudomonas aeruginosa, Escherichia coli,* and *Klebsiella*, *Enterobacter*, *Proteus*, and *Serratia* spp. Of note is that study of the epidemiology of specific nosocomial pathogens in this period was hampered because few clinical laboratories performed extensive speciation at the time. Moreover, detection of nosocomial viral infections was hindered by the limited availability of suitable diagnostic techniques. The Children's Hospital study emphasized the association of nosocomial infections with exposure to invasive devices and procedures (e.g., surgical-site infections in patients undergoing surgery, urinary tract infections in patients with indwelling urinary catheters, bloodstream infections and septic phlebitis associated with intravascular catheters, and ventriculitis associated with cerebrospinal fluid [CSF] shunts). Additional epidemiologic studies of nosocomial infections in newborn infants and children who received care in intensive care units (ICUs) during the 1970s and early 1980s strengthened awareness of the association between the use of invasive devices and procedures and nosocomial infection.[249, 288, 296, 405]

Advances in viral diagnostics in the 1970s led to greater appreciation of the importance of viruses as a significant cause of nosocomial infection, particularly in pediatric patients.[653, 676] Nosocomial spread of respiratory and gastrointestinal viruses, especially respiratory syncytial virus (RSV) and rotavirus, was documented to be a severe problem on pediatric wards.[173, 263, 444, 560, 679]

The past 25 years have witnessed several major new developments. Gram-positive bacteria, including coagulase-negative staphylococci, *S. aureus,* enterococci, and streptococci, have reemerged as significant nosocomial pathogens.[205, 319, 463] Antimicrobial-resistant bacteria such as methicillin-resistant *S. aureus* (MRSA), vancomycin-resistant enterococci (VRE), and gram-negative bacilli resistant to third-generation cephalosporins, aminoglycosides, carbapenems, and quinolones have become especially troublesome.[309, 463, 649, 650] With the increasing numbers of severely ill and immunosuppressed children who receive care in hospitals, the incidence of nosocomial fungal infection has increased dramatically, especially *Candida* and *Aspergillus* infection.[1, 205, 213, 319, 320] Finally, the potential for nosocomial infection by blood-borne pathogens such as human immunodeficiency virus (HIV), hepatitis B, and hepatitis C in patients as well as health care workers is now well recognized.[62, 86, 238, 503, 684]

In summary, the history of nosocomial infections in children is closely tied to the progress of medicine itself. New therapies and invasive procedures have had the unwanted side effect of increasing the risk for nosocomial infection. Longer survival from conditions formerly causing early death and increasing numbers of immunocompromised children have resulted in a growing population of children with impaired host defenses who have an increased risk for infection. The selective pressure of the widespread use of new, broad-spectrum antimicrobial agents has resulted in the development of previously unknown forms of antimicrobial resistance and the emergence of fungi as serious nosocomial pathogens.

General Epidemiology of Nosocomial Infections

Perhaps more than any other area of infectious disease epidemiology, the methodology used to study the epidemiology of nosocomial infections has itself been subjected to intense investigation and validation. This section describes the epidemiology of nosocomial infections in pediatric patients in general terms while highlighting important methodologic issues. The epidemiology of specific nosocomial infections and pathogens is discussed in later sections.

RATES OF NOSOCOMIAL INFECTION

During the 1960s to 1980s, a number of hospital surveys examined rates of nosocomial infection in pediatric patients.[138, 205, 223, 319, 438, 555–557, 676] These surveys were useful in documenting the nature and frequency of nosocomial infections and illustrating trends in infections caused by various pathogens (see "Historical Aspects"). However, methodologic differences rendered evaluation and comparison of infection rates among these studies difficult. Considerable variability occurred in the types of nosocomial infections studied and the definitions used to identify infections. The sensitivity of the case-finding techniques used and the vigor with which viral infections were sought and confirmed also varied greatly. In most cases, insufficient adjustment was made for length of hospitalization, exposure to invasive devices and procedures, case mix, and severity of illness, all of which increase the risk for nosocomial infection.

Many, but not all of these methodologic concerns have been alleviated by examining rates of nosocomial infection in pediatric patients provided by the NNIS System under the coordination of the Division of Healthcare Quality Promotion at the CDC. Similar methods have been used in other countries for surveillance of nosocomial infections in pediatric patients.[529] As of 2000, more than 320 U.S. acute care hospitals, including 70 pediatric ICUs and more than 120 high-risk nurseries (the term used by the NNIS System for newborn ICUs), were reporting data regarding the incidence of nosocomial infections to the NNIS.[618] Participating hospitals follow NNIS surveillance methods, which include the use of published definitions of nosocomial infections,[229] standardized coding of data, structured data collection sheets, and a microcomputer surveillance software program designed to report data to the NNIS System.[188, 299] Case-finding methods are not specified in the NNIS methodology, although the vast majority of hospitals identify nosocomial infections by reviewing microbiology reports and patient charts.[188] Post-discharge surveillance for infections such as surgical-site infection is highly variable among participating hospitals.

The accuracy of data reported to the NNIS has been evaluated in a small subset of ICUs that did not include any pediatric ICUs or high-risk nurseries.[189] The accuracy of the reported data varied by site of infection. The sensitivity of surveillance for bloodstream infection, pneumonia, surgical-site infection, urinary tract infection, and other sites of infection was 85, 68, 67, 59, and 30 percent, respectively; the specificity was 98, 98, 98, 99, and 99 percent, respectively. Consequently, whereas current surveillance procedures in these hospitals fail to identify some infections, the infections that are reported are very likely to be true infections.

Table 231–1 contains overall infection rates by service for NNIS hospitals from 1986 to 1990. Though dated, these data illustrate that the cumulative incidence of nosocomial infections (number of nosocomial infections per 100 discharges) for pediatric services and normal newborn nurseries is generally lower than that for most other services. Newborn ICUs, on the other hand, have a comparatively high cumulative incidence of infection that rivals the incidence in burn services.

Length of hospitalization is an important factor in assessing rates of nosocomial infection because the cumulative probability that an individual will experience at least one nosocomial infection increases with longer duration of exposure to the hospital. To minimize the impact of differences in length of hospitalization, rates of nosocomial infection are expressed as an incidence density (the number of nosocomial infections per 1000 patient days). Table 231–1 also contains the incidence density of nosocomial infections by service for NNIS hospitals from 1986 to 1990. When expressed as incidence density, the frequency of nosocomial infections in newborn ICUs is not as striking in comparison to other services, probably because of adjustment for length of hospitalization, which can be very long for premature infants and severely ill full-term infants.

The invasive devices that are a routine part of modern hospital care are especially important risk factors for nosocomial infection, and additional adjustment of infection rates is necessary to accurately reflect these risks. Central venous catheters increase the risk for bloodstream infection, mechanical ventilation increases the risk for pneumonia, and indwelling urinary catheters increase the risk of contracting a urinary tract infection. To adjust for exposure (as well as the duration of exposure) to these devices, infection rates can be expressed as the number of infections in individuals exposed to the device per 1000 device exposure days. Table 231–2 contains data regarding the device-associated incidence density of bloodstream infection, pneumonia, and urinary tract infection for adult and pediatric ICUs in hospitals participating in the NNIS System.[463] Table 231–3 contains data regarding the device-associated incidence density of bloodstream infections and pneumonia stratified by birth weight for high-risk nurseries in hospitals participating in the NNIS System.[463] These data illustrate that the pooled mean rate of bloodstream infection is higher in pediatric ICUs and high-risk nurseries, particularly for lower birth weight categories, than in adult ICUs (except for adult trauma and burn ICUs). Conversely, the pooled mean rate of pneumonia is substantially lower in pediatric ICUs and high-risk nurseries than in adult ICUs. The pooled mean rate of urinary tract infections in pediatric ICUs is comparable to that in adult ICUs.

Based on seminal studies by Freeman and others, birth weight long has been recognized as an important risk factor for nosocomial infection in newborn infants.[210, 288] For this

TABLE 231–1 ■ OVERALL MEDIAN NOSOCOMIAL INFECTION RATES BY SERVICE IN HOSPITALS PARTICIPATING IN THE NATIONAL NOSOCOMIAL INFECTION SURVEILLANCE SYSTEM

Service	Infections/100 Discharges	Infections/1000 Patient-Days
Medicine	3.5	5.7
Oncology	5.1	8.1
Burn	14.9	11.9
Cardiac surgery	9.8	13.8
Orthopedics	3.9	5.8
Ophthalmology	0.0	0.0
Obstetrics	0.9	5.0
Pediatrics	0.4	0.9
Newborn ICU	14.0	9.9
Normal newborn nursery	0.4	1.1

Data are from 1986 to 1990.

TABLE 231–2 ■ POOLED MEANS OF DEVICE-ASSOCIATED INFECTION RATES BY TYPE OF INTENSIVE CARE UNIT IN HOSPITALS PARTICIPATING IN THE NATIONAL NOSOCOMIAL INFECTION SURVEILLANCE SYSTEM

	Pooled Mean		
Type of ICU	Central Line-Associated Bloodstream Infection/1000 Central Line Days	Ventilator-Associated Pneumonia/1000 Ventilator Days	Catheter-Associated Urinary Tract Infection/1000 Urinary Catheter Days
Adult ICUs			
Coronary	4.5	8.4	5.8
Cardiothoracic	2.9	10.5	3.1
Medical	5.9	7.3	6.6
Medical/surgical			
Major teaching	5.3	10.5	5.8
All others	3.8	8.7	3.9
Neurosurgical	4.7	14.9	7.8
Respiratory	3.4	4.3	5.5
Surgical	5.3	13.2	5.2
Trauma	7.9	16.2	6.7
Burn	9.7	15.9	9.7
Pediatric ICUs	7.6	4.9	4.9

Data are from January 1995 to June 2001.
Modified from National Nosocomial Infection Surveillance System: National Nosocomial Infection Surveillance (NNIS) System report, data summary from January 1992–June 2001, issued August 2001. Am. J. Infect. Control. *29*:404–421, 2001.

reason, rates of device-associated bloodstream infection and pneumonia from high-risk nurseries participating in the NNIS System are stratified into four birth weight groups (see Table 231–3): 1000 g or less, 1001 to 1500 g, 1501 to 2500 g, and more than 2500 g.[463] A progressive and marked increase is found in rates of bloodstream infection in sequentially lower birth weight categories such that the rate of infection in infants weighing 1000 g or less is nearly threefold higher than the rate in infants weighing more than 2500 g. Higher rates of pneumonia also occur in lower birth weight categories, but this trend is much less marked than that for bloodstream infections.

TABLE 231–3 ■ POOLED MEANS OF DEVICE-ASSOCIATED INFECTION RATES BY BIRTH WEIGHT CATEGORY IN HIGH-RISK NURSERIES IN HOSPITALS PARTICIPATING IN THE NATIONAL NOSOCOMIAL INFECTION SURVEILLANCE SYSTEM

	Pooled Means	
Birth Weight Category (g)	Central or Umbilical Intravascular Catheter-Associated Bloodstream Infection/1000 Central or Umbilical Line Days	Ventilator-Associated Pneumonia/1000 Ventilator Days
≤1000	11.3	4.8
1001–1500	6.9	3.6
1501–2500	4.0	2.9
>2500	3.8	2.6

Data are from January 1995 to June 2001.
Modified from National Nosocomial Infection Surveillance System: National Nosocomial Infection Surveillance (NNIS) System report, data summary from January 1992–June 2001, issued August 2001. Am. J. Infect. Control. *29*:404–421, 2001.

Despite adjustment for length of hospitalization, exposure to invasive devices, and birth weight (for neonates), nosocomial infection rates still vary considerably among ICUs. Box plots of the distribution of device-associated infection rates reported by pediatric ICUs and high-risk nurseries in hospitals participating in the NNIS System are displayed in Figures 231–1 and 231–2, respectively.[463] These figures illustrate that device-associated infection rates vary as much as 10-fold among units.

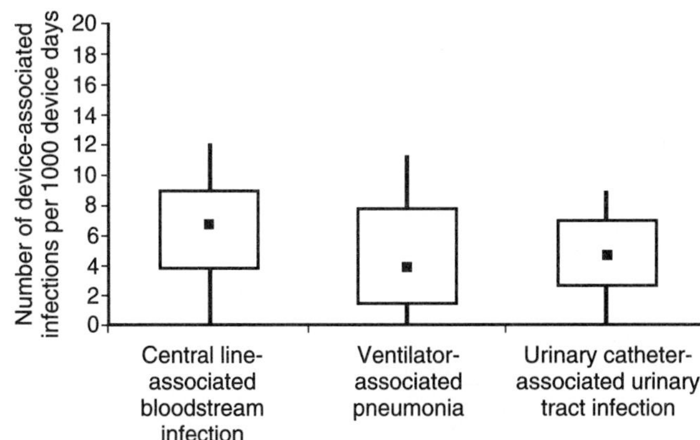

FIGURE 231–1 ■ Distribution of device-associated infection rates in pediatric intensive care units in hospitals participating in the National Nosocomial Infection Surveillance System. Box plots of the distribution of device-associated infection rates in pediatric intensive care units indicate the following: the *solid square* represents the 50th percentile (median). The lower and upper bounds of the *open vertical rectangle* represent the 25th and 75th percentiles, respectively. The lower and upper bounds of the *lines* extending above and below the open vertical rectangle represent the 10th and 90th percentiles, respectively. (Modified from National Nosocomial Infection Surveillance System: National Nosocomial Infection Surveillance [NNIS] System report, data summary from January 1992–June 2001, issued August 2001. Am. J. Infect. Control *29*:404–421, 2001.)

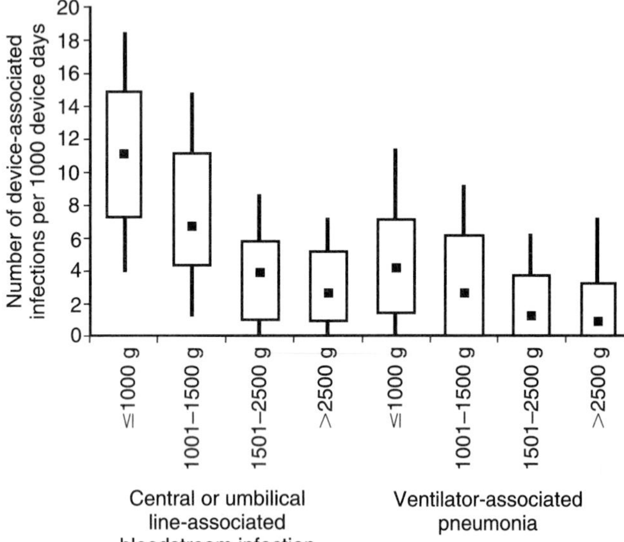

FIGURE 231–2 ■ Distribution of device-associated infection rates in high-risk nurseries in hospitals participating in the National Nosocomial Infection Surveillance System. Box plots of the distribution of device-associated infection rates in pediatric intensive care units indicate the following: the *solid square* represents the 50th percentile (median). The lower and upper bounds of the *open vertical rectangle* represent the 25th and 75th percentiles, respectively. The lower and upper bounds of the *lines* extending above and below the open vertical rectangle represent the 10th and 90th percentiles, respectively. (Modified from National Nosocomial Infection Surveillance System: National Nosocomial Infection Surveillance [NNIS] System report, data summary from January 1992–June 2001, issued August 2001. Am. J. Infect. Control *29*:404–421, 2001.)

A portion of this variability probably is due to differences in the nature and severity of patients' underlying illnesses. Simple systems for classifying severity of illness, such as the system proposed by McCabe and Jackson[427] and the American Society of Anesthesiologists Physical Status Classification (ASA score), have been in existence for decades.[334] In the 1980s and 1990s, investigators developed and refined scoring systems of severity of illness for adult, pediatric, and newborn ICUs. Use of these measures to adjust rates of nosocomial infection in pediatric and newborn ICUs is discussed in the following paragraphs.

The Physiologic Stability Index (PSI) was developed and validated as a measure of severity of illness for pediatric ICU patients.[695] The Pediatric Risk of Mortality (PRISM) score subsequently provided a streamlined scoring system by reducing the number of variables in the PSI through regression analysis and weighting of physiologic variables to better reflect their contribution to the risk of mortality.[507] Although the utility of this score and its subsequent modifications in predicting mortality in pediatric ICU patients has been studied extensively,[505–507] only three studies have examined use of the PRISM score as a predictor of nosocomial infection.[508, 607, 608] The most recent study developed a multivariable model, including the PRISM III-24 score, for assessing the risk of acquiring a nosocomial infection.[608] The model consisted of three factors assessed on the day of admission: use of invasive devices (i.e., central venous catheter, mechanical ventilation, indwelling urinary catheter), administration of parenteral nutrition, and an interaction of the PRISM III-24 score and postoperative care. As a whole, the model predicted the risk of acquiring nosocomial infection well. However, the data sets used to develop and validate the model were limited in size and derived from only one pediatric ICU. In addition, the most common nosocomial infection was tracheitis, which accounted for over a third of all nosocomial infections analyzed; bloodstream infections and pneumonia represented only 25 and 7 percent, respectively, of the infections analyzed. The implication of these observations on the generalizability of the model is not clear.

Several severity-of-illness measures have been developed for newborn ICU patients.[253, 302, 539–541, 646] The most extensively tested and applied score, the Score for Neonatal Acute Physiology (SNAP), was shown by Gray and colleagues to be a strong predictor of nosocomial coagulase-negative staphylococcal bacteremia in very low birth weight (<1500 g) infants in an early study.[254] However, rates of infection in this study were not adjusted for exposure to central or umbilical lines, and information regarding other significant risk factors, such as the administration of lipid emulsions, was not available. Two subsequent studies have examined SNAP in more detail as a predictor of the risk for development of bacteremia. In a follow-up case-control study conducted in the same units used by Gray, Avila-Figueroa and colleagues found that after adjustment for birth weight, length of hospital stay, and nearest date of discharge, SNAP on day 7 of hospitalization did not show any association with the development of nosocomial coagulase-negative bacteremia.[34] In addition, Brodie and colleagues conducted a cohort study in six newborn ICUs and found that after adjustment for birth weight and the presence of small size for gestational age, SNAP was not a significant predictor of nosocomial bloodstream infection.[77] Therefore, in these two studies, SNAP did not add to the adjustments by other intrinsic (i.e., host) risk factors. Consistent with a previous work,[209] both studies identified administration of parenteral nutrition with lipid emulsion as a highly significant risk factor for acquiring infection.[34, 77] Interestingly, the study by Brodie and associates found substantial variability in infection rates among newborn ICUs, even after applying rigorous methods of risk adjustment, thus suggesting that other patient care practices also may play a role in the observed variability in infection rates among newborn ICUs.[77] Though not explored in Brodie and colleagues' study, higher patient-to-nurse staffing ratios have been linked to higher rates of nosocomial infection in various inpatient settings, including ICUs.[27, 214, 263, 265, 281, 466, 546]

Another approach to risk adjustment—use of a composite risk index calculated by using several individual risk factors—has been applied to analysis of surgical-site infections by the NNIS System. Developed by analysis of 4 years of data on surgical-site infections reported to the NNIS, the NNIS Basic Surgical-Site Infection Risk Index is an example of a composite risk index that has been incorporated into routine surveillance in many hospitals.[149, 233] This risk index is calculated by counting 1 point for each of the following three risk factors: a preoperative ASA score of 3, 4, or 5; an operation classified as either contaminated or dirty-infected; and an operation with a duration of more than T hours, where T depends on the operative procedure performed.[149] The duration of a particular procedure is thought to reflect the complexity of the procedure. As seen in Table 231–4, this risk index provides a much better assessment of risk than does traditional wound classification alone. This index has not been applied to pediatric patients undergoing surgery. Moreover, although the NNIS Basic Surgical-Site Infection Risk Index works well across a broad range of different surgical procedures, it does not work as well for some specific procedures such as cardiac surgery, neurosurgery, and cesarean section.[190, 231, 298, 536, 554] Procedure-specific

TABLE 231–4 ■ SURGICAL SITE INFECTION RATES* BY TRADITIONAL WOUND CLASSIFICATION AND THE NATIONAL NOSOCOMIAL INFECTION SURVEILLANCE SYSTEM BASIC SURGICAL SITE INFECTION RISK INDEX†

	Basic Surgical Site Infection Risk Index				
Wound Classification	**0**	**1**	**2**	**3**	**Cumulative**
Clean	1.0	2.3	5.4	—	2.1
Clean-contaminated	2.1	4.0	9.5	—	3.3
Contaminated	—	3.4	6.8	13.2	6.4
Dirty-infected	—	3.1	8.1	12.8	7.1
Cumulative	1.5	2.9	6.8	13.0	

*Surgical site infections per 100 operative procedures.

†Calculated by counting 1 point for each of the following three risk factors: a preoperative American Society of Anesthesiologists score of 3, 4, or 5; an operation classified as either contaminated or dirty-infected; an operation with a duration of more than *T* hours (*T* is the 75th percentile for the duration of surgery rounded to the nearest hour for procedures included in the NNIS database; see reference below).

Modified from Culver, D. H., Horan,T. C., Gaynes, R. P. et al.: Surgical wound infection rates by wound class, operative procedure, and patient risk index. Am. J. Med. *91*(Suppl.):152–157, 1991.

composite risk indices are being developed with the use of NNIS data and multivariate modeling techniques.[232, 297] The standardized infection ratio (a ratio that compares the observed rate of infection with the expected rate of infection generated by using the regression equation developed by multivariate modeling) has been proposed as means of using procedure-specific composite risk indices for benchmarking surgical-site infection rates.[232, 297] A similar approach could be applied to other infections.[608]

In summary, the methodology for obtaining meaningful comparison of rates of nosocomial infection among ICUs or hospitals has advanced remarkably in the past 2 decades. Hospitals have used risk-adjusted infection rates, such as those provided by the NNIS System, to benchmark their institution-specific rates and to target areas for improvement. They probably have achieved some measure of success in this effort because rates of device-associated bloodstream infection, pneumonia, and urinary tract infection all have declined in adult and pediatric ICUs participating in the NNIS System during the 1990s.[103, 618] In high-risk nurseries during the same period, rates of catheter-associated bloodstream infection decreased in infants in all birth weight categories, and rates of ventilator-associated pneumonia decreased in all but the smallest infants.[618] The reasons for these declines have not been established and could be due, in part, to artifacts of reporting or the limitations of current surveillance methods. Nonetheless, they are encouraging indications that rates of nosocomial infection may be reduced despite the substantial risks inherent in modern medical care. Future efforts to identify additional risk factors for acquiring infection and to refine risk adjustment methods to facilitate additional improvement are challenges for the future.

SITES OF NOSOCOMIAL INFECTION

Figures 231–3 and 231–4 illustrate the site distribution of nosocomial infections in patients in pediatric ICUs and high-risk nurseries in hospitals participating in the NNIS System.[234, 538] Bloodstream infection, pneumonia, urinary tract infection, other types of lower respiratory tract infection (e.g., tracheitis), and surgical-site infection constitute the vast majority of nosocomial infections among patients in pediatric ICUs (see Fig. 231–3). The distribution of infections does not vary substantially by age group, although bacteremia occurs more commonly and urinary tract infection less commonly in the youngest children (≤2 months). Bloodstream infection; pneumonia; eye, ear, nose, and throat infection; gastrointestinal infection; and skin and soft tissue infection account for the vast majority of nosocomial infections among patients in high-risk nurseries (Fig. 231–4).

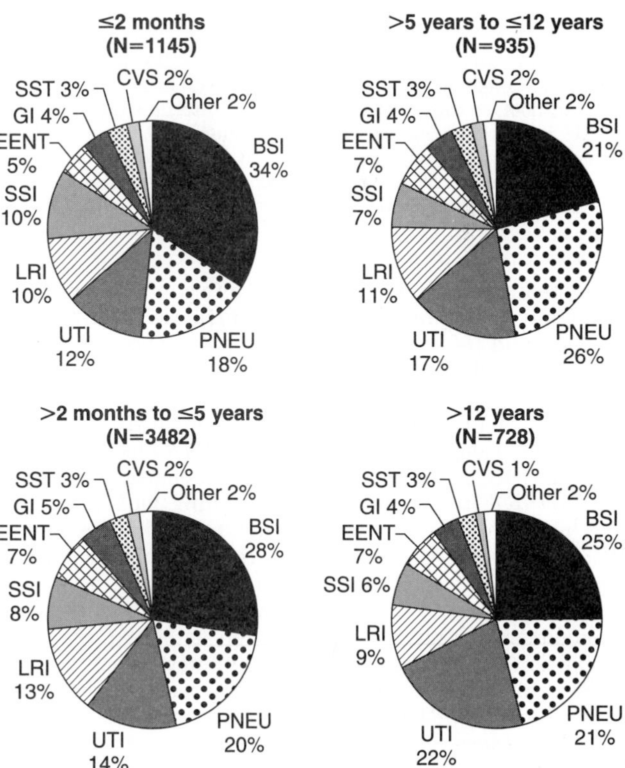

FIGURE 231–3 ■ Site distribution of nosocomial infections in pediatric intensive care units in hospitals participating in the National Nosocomial Infection Surveillance System. BSI, bloodstream infection; CVS, cardiovascular infection; EENT, eye, ear, nose, or throat infection; GI, gastrointestinal infection; LRI, lower respiratory tract infection other than pneumonia; PNEU, pneumonia; SSI, surgical site infection; SST, skin or soft tissue infection; UTI, urinary tract infection. (Modified from Richards, M. J., Edwards, J. R., Culver, D. H., et al.: Nosocomial infections in pediatric intensive care units in the United States. Pediatrics *103*:e39, 1999.)

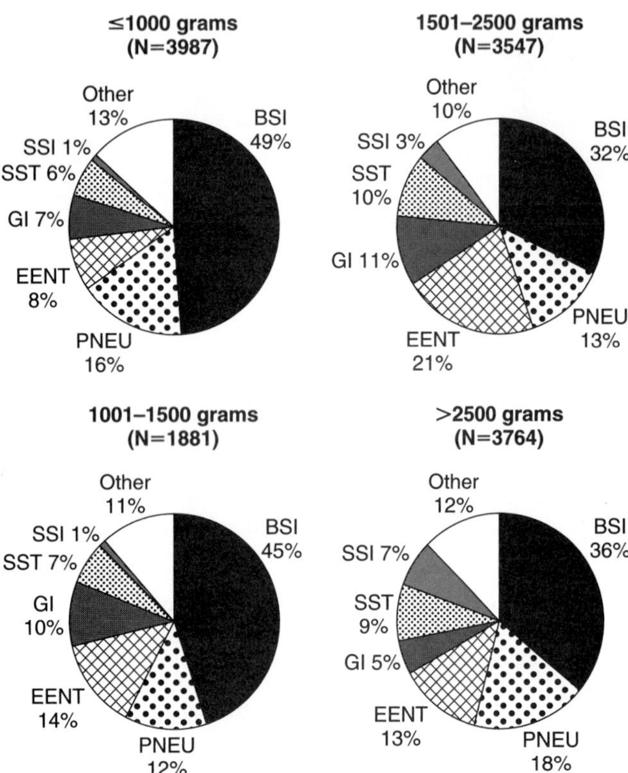

FIGURE 231–4 ■ Site distribution of nosocomial infections in high-risk nurseries in hospitals participating in the National Nosocomial Infection Surveillance System. BSI, bloodstream infection; EENT, eye, ear, nose, or throat infection; GI, gastrointestinal infection; PNEU, pneumonia; SSI, surgical site infection; SST, skin or soft tissue infection. (Modified from Gaynes, R. P., Edwards, J. R., Jarvis, W. R., et al.: Nosocomial infections among neonates in high-risk nurseries in the United States. Pediatrics *98*:357–361, 1996.)

As noted previously, bloodstream infection occurs most commonly in infants in the lower birth weight categories (≤1000 g and 1001 to 1500 g). A point prevalence survey conducted in pediatric and newborn ICUs in 29 U.S. hospitals participating in the Pediatric Prevention Network (PPN), a research collaboration between the National Association of Children's Hospitals and Related Institutions (NACHRI) and the CDC, confirmed these general conclusions.[259, 617]

The site distribution of nosocomial infections in children and newborns differs substantially from that in adults. Bloodstream infection represents a considerably greater proportion of nosocomial infections in children and newborns; conversely, urinary tract infection and, to a lesser extent, pneumonia and surgical-site infection account for a lower proportion of infections in children and newborns.

Some of these differences are due to variations in exposure to invasive devices, but others are not. For example, because urinary catheters are used much less frequently in pediatric and newborn ICUs than in adult ICUs,[463] the overall frequency of urinary tract infection is decreased, although the per-day risk of acquiring infection is probably similar. In contrast, the greater frequency of bloodstream infections in children and newborns is not attributable to catheter exposure because central lines (including central venous and umbilical catheters) are used less frequently in pediatric and newborn ICUs.[463] Indeed, as discussed previously (see "Rates of Nosocomial Infection"), rates of bloodstream infection are higher in children and newborns than in adults, even after adjustment for catheter exposure.[463] Children in pediatric ICUs and very low birth weight infants (≤1000 g) in newborn ICUs are mechanically ventilated roughly as frequently as adults in ICUs, thus indicating that other factors must play a role in the lower proportion and rates of pneumonia in children and newborns. Other factors playing a role in these differences are discussed in greater detail in other portions of this chapter (see "Nosocomial Infections Related to Invasive Devices, Procedures, and Treatments" and "Nosocomial Infections in Special Populations").

Nosocomial respiratory and gastrointestinal infections caused by seasonal pathogens circulating in the community, especially viruses such as RSV, influenza virus, and rotavirus, are important because of their impact on children and newborn infants. These infections are discussed in detail in other portions of this chapter (see "Nosocomial Infections Caused by Spread of Infections Common in the Community").

NOSOCOMIAL PATHOGENS

Tables 231–5 and 231–6 list the distribution of pathogens for major sites of nosocomial infection among patients in pediatric ICUs and high-risk nurseries participating in the NNIS System.[234, 538] *S. aureus*, coagulase-negative staphylococci, enterococci, a variety of gram-negative bacilli, and *Candida* spp. are responsible for the vast majority of nosocomial infections. Pathogens responsible for specific nosocomial infections are discussed in more detail in other portions of this chapter (see "Nosocomial Infections Caused by Spread of Infections Common in the Community"; "Nosocomial Infections Related to Invasive Devices, Procedures, and Treatments"; and "Nosocomial Infections in Special Populations").

Several general trends in the microbial etiology of nosocomial infections that are relevant for children should be emphasized. Coagulase-negative staphylococcal infections have increased dramatically in the past 2 decades, almost entirely as a result of an increase in the frequency of bloodstream infections caused by these microorganisms.[234, 538, 574] This trend is particularly impressive in newborns,[234] which is explained, at least in part, by the increased survival rates of very low birth weight infants who have long hospital stays and are highly dependent on intravascular catheters and parenteral nutrition.[209–211, 599] Several studies using molecular epidemiologic techniques indicate that specific strains of coagulase-negative staphylococci may become endemic in newborn ICUs and may be transmitted via the hands of caregivers.[81, 308, 398, 484, 611, 661] The frequency of *Candida* spp., especially *Candida albicans,* has increased for all major sites of infection.[213, 320, 574] Infections caused by these fungi have had a major impact on critically ill and immunocompromised children and premature infants.[213, 320, 524, 567] The frequency of infections caused by *S. aureus,* enterococci, *Pseudomonas aeruginosa,* and *Enterobacter* spp. has increased slightly.[574]

More alarming is the dramatic increase in antimicrobial resistance in common nosocomial pathogens. Project ICARE (Intensive Care Antimicrobial Resistance Epidemiology) studied the prevalence of antimicrobial resistance in adult and pediatric ICUs in more than 40 U.S. hospitals during 1996 to 1997.[215] This surveillance project subsequently has become a part of the NNIS System.[462, 463] In its 2001 report, the NNIS reported that the overall prevalence of methicillin resistance in *S. aureus* strains causing nosocomial infection was 55 percent (an increase of 29% in 2000 in comparison to 1995 to 1999) and that the prevalence of vancomycin resistance in enterococci was 26 percent (an increase of 31% in 2000 in comparison to 1995 to 1999).[463] Resistance to methicillin now is virtually ubiquitous in coagulase-negative staphylococci.

TABLE 231–5 ■ COMMONLY REPORTED PATHOGENS BY SITE OF NOSOCOMIAL INFECTION IN PEDIATRIC INTENSIVE CARE UNITS PARTICIPATING IN THE NATIONAL NOSOCOMIAL INFECTION SURVEILLANCE SYSTEM

Pathogen	Bloodstream Infection, % (*N* = 1887)	Pneumonia, % (*N* = 1459)	Urinary Tract Infection, % (*N* = 1045)	Lower Respiratory Tract Infection, % (*N* = 935)	Surgical Site Infection, % (*N* = 544)
Coagulase-negative staphylococci	37.8	0.9	4.3	1.5	14.0
Enterococcus	11.2	1.0	10.0	1.2	8.1
Staphylococcus aureus	9.3	16.9*	1.5	18.8	20.2†
Enterobacter spp.	6.2	9.3†	10.3	12.2	8.1
Candida albicans	5.5*‡	1.6	14.3‡§	3.6	5.0
Pseudomonas aeruginosa	4.9	21.8	13.1‡	15.1	14.5‖
Klebsiella pneumoniae	4.1	5.3	7.3	3.5	3.7
Other *Candida* spp.	3.4*	0.4	6.2	1.1	2.0
Escherichia coli	2.9	3.6	19.0‖	3.2	5.1
Acinetobacter spp.	2.0	3.1	0.4	3.1	0.7
Serratia marcescens	2.0	3.6	1.2	3.6	2.8
Streptococcus pneumoniae	0.6	3.4	0	2.6	0.6
Citrobacter	0.5	0.5	4.3	1.1	1.8
Candida glabrata	0.4*	0	0.6	0	0
Other fungi	0.2*	0.7	1.6	0.1	0.2
Group B streptococcus	0.1	0.2	0.1	0	0.4
Haemophilus influenzae	0.1	10.2	0	5.8	0.9
Aspergillus	0.1	0.5	0	0.1	0.7
Viruses	0.1	2.5†	0.2	10.1	0

Data are from 1992 to 1997.
*Reports of fungi from bloodstream infections and *S. aureus* from pneumonia were more common in children older than 5 years than they were in younger children ($p < .001$).
†Reports of *Enterobacter* spp. and viruses from patients with pneumonia and *S. aureus* from wound infections were more common in children 2 months and younger than in older children ($p < .001$).
‡Pathogens associated with use of an invasive device.
‖Reports of *E coli* from urinary tract infections and *P. aeruginosa* from surgical site infections were more common in children older than 2 months ($p < .02$) than in neonates.
§Reports of *C. albicans* from urinary tract infections were more common in children older than 12 years than in younger children ($p < .002$).
Modified from Richards, M. J., Edwards, J. R., Culver, D. H., et al.: Nosocomial infections in pediatric intensive care units in the United States. Pediatrics *103*:E39, 1999.

TABLE 231–6 ■ COMMONLY REPORTED PATHOGENS BY SITE OF NOSOCOMIAL INFECTION IN HIGH-RISK NURSERIES PARTICIPATING IN THE NATIONAL NOSOCOMIAL INFECTION SURVEILLANCE SYSTEM

Pathogen	Bloodstream Infections, % (*N* = 7521)	Eye, Ear, Nose, and Throat Infections, % (*N* = 2685)	Gastrointestinal Infection, % (*N* = 1058)	Pneumonia, % (*N* = 2665)	Surgical Site Infection, % (*N* = 619)
Coagulase-negative staphylococci	51.0	29.3	9.6	16.5	19.2
Staphylococcus aureus	7.5	15.4	0	16.7	22.3
Group B streptococci	7.9*	0	0	5.7*	
Enterococci	6.2	3.4	0	4.6	8.9
Candida spp.	6.9	0	0	0	0
Escherichia coli	4.3	6.1	13.9	5.8	12.0
Other *Streptococcus* spp.	2.7	7.4	0	3.3	0
Enterobacter spp.	2.9	4.5	5.5	8.2	7.6
Klebsiella pneumoniae	2.5	2.8	9.8	5.8	6.3
Pseudomonas aeruginosa	0	6.6	0	11.7	0
Haemophilus influenzae	0	2.7	0	1.4	0
Viruses	0	5.1	30.0†	0	0
Gram-positive anaerobes	0	0	9.4	0	0
Other enteric bacilli	0	0	0.8	0	0
Others	8.1	16.7	21.0	21.7	23.7

Data are from 1986 to 1993.
*Group B streptococcal bloodstream infections and pneumonia were more common in infants weighing more than 2500 g.
†Rotavirus constitutes 96.4% of viruses isolated from gastrointestinal infections.
Modified from Gaynes, R. P., Edwards, J. R., Jarvis, W. R., et al.: Nosocomial infections among neonates in high-risk nurseries in the United States. National Nosocomial Infections Surveillance System. Pediatrics *98*:357–361, 1999.

Resistance to third-generation cephalosporins is common in gram-negative rods such as *E. coli, Klebsiella pneumoniae, Enterobacter* spp., and *P. aeruginosa,* and resistance to imipenem and quinolones is a rapidly growing problem with *P. aeruginosa.*[463]

Hospitals caring for children have not escaped these trends, although the frequency of problems of specific resistance differs somewhat between pediatric and adult ICUs.

Infections caused by MRSA in pediatric patients have been recognized in children's hospitals since the 1980s, and numerous outbreaks of infection with these bacteria have been reported.[322, 471, 530, 534, 535, 542] However, data from Project ICARE indicate that the prevalence of MRSA in pediatric and neonatal ICUs is far less than that in adult ICUs.[462] Similarly, a study of the prevalence of colonization with antimicrobial-resistant bacteria in patients in eight U.S. pediatric and newborn ICUs participating in the PPN found that colonization with this microorganism was an uncommon occurrence.[600] Reasons for this difference are not known but may relate to the greater proportion of adult patients who are transferred to the ICU from long-term care facilities, where colonization occurs more commonly, and the greater success of various control measures in containing or eradicating MRSA from an individual unit when the overall prevalence rate in the unit is relatively low.[42, 140, 180, 265, 294, 324, 530, 595, 632] Unfortunately, community acquisition of MRSA is occurring more commonly,[199, 290, 311] and this fact may complicate control efforts in hospitalized children in the future.

The first reported infection by *S. aureus* with reduced susceptibility to vancomycin occurred in a child with a wound infection after cardiac surgery in Japan,[293] although the experience thus far in the United States has involved infections in only a handful of adults.[104, 602, 615]

As previously noted, methicillin resistance among coagulase-negative staphylococci encountered in the hospital setting is now nearly universal in all inpatient care settings. Infections caused by *Staphylococcus epidermidis* with reduced susceptibility to vancomycin also have been reported in adults.[230, 603]

Viridans streptococci have emerged as a major cause of bloodstream infection in neutropenic patients, and the prevalence of resistance to penicillins and cephalosporins is increasing in these bacteria.[185, 591]

Resistance in enterococci has become a particularly alarming problem, especially given the increasing frequency of nosocomial infections caused by these organisms. Enterococci are intrinsically resistant to many antimicrobial agents, including all cephalosporins, clindamycin, and trimethoprim-sulfamethoxazole.[114] In addition, enterococci, especially *Enterococcus faecium,* always have been relatively resistant to penicillin, but high-level resistance caused by mutations in penicillin-binding proteins is now relatively common.[114] High-level resistance to aminoglycosides emerged in the 1970s and became widespread in the 1980s; enterococci resistant to both streptomycin and gentamicin are resistant to the synergistic activity of all known antimicrobial combinations.[114] Penicillin resistance as a result of β-lactamase production in conjunction with high-level gentamicin resistance also has been reported.[533, 677] As alarming as these trends were, the rapid increase in the rate of colonization and infection with VRE observed across the United States during the 1990s was truly astounding.[92, 463] Recent work has demonstrated that treatment of VRE-colonized adults with anti-anaerobic antibiotics promotes high-density colonization with VRE, which may facilitate dissemination of these bacteria.[177] Although colonization and infection with VRE have been demonstrated in pediatric patients,[60, 61, 255, 390, 417, 558, 606, 651] data from Project ICARE and the PPN colonization study indicate that the problem is much less widespread in hospitalized children than adults.[462, 600]

In contrast, antimicrobial-resistant gram-negative bacilli are both a common and a serious threat to hospitalized children. The introduction plus widespread use of third-generation cephalosporins in the 1980s was followed quickly by the emergence and dissemination of gram-negative bacilli, with mutations resulting in constitutive expression of chromosomally encoded AmpC β-lactamases.[389] In the late 1980s and throughout the 1990s, plasmid-borne extended-spectrum β-lactamases (ESBLs) capable of inactivating third-generation cephalosporins were identified in gram-negative rods from around the world, including *Klebsiella, Enterobacter, E. coli, Citrobacter, Morganella morganii,* and *P. aeruginosa.*[71, 389] These pathogens often carry genes for resistance to aminoglycosides and other front-line antibiotics on their plasmids.[71, 389] More recently, some gram-negative rods have been demonstrated to produce both an AmpC β-lactamase and an ESBL, with both enzymes encoded on a plasmid.[497] Gram-negative rods producing AmpC β-lactamases or ESBLs have caused numerous outbreaks involving pediatric patients,[29, 212, 464, 587] and data from Project ICARE and the PPN colonization study indicate that these bacteria, especially *Enterobacter* spp. and *P. aeruginosa,* are a significant and widespread problem in pediatric and newborn ICUs.[462, 600] Aminoglycoside resistance caused by the production of aminoglycoside-inactivating enzymes by gram-negative rods has been a persistent but less pervasive problem. Resistance to imipenem and fluoroquinolones is a newer and growing concern, particularly among *P. aeruginosa* strains,[462] although the impact of these problems in pediatric patients has been limited thus far. Other gram-negative bacilli, including *Stenotrophomonas maltophilia, Acinetobacter, Citrobacter, Alcaligenes,* and *Burkholderia cepacia,* infrequently cause nosocomial infection, but they are notable because they usually exhibit multiple drug resistance.[54, 169, 222, 295, 429, 430, 492, 662, 663]

Multicenter studies of bloodstream infections caused by *Candida* spp. have revealed considerable variability among institutions in the frequency of resistance to the azole group of antifungal agents.[493, 494, 496] Non-*albicans* species of *Candida,* which more frequently demonstrated resistance to fluconazole than *C. albicans* did, have become more prominent in some locales.[493] Limited data on trends in antifungal susceptibility among *Candida* spp. from a single institution suggest that the frequency of azole resistance has not changed substantially[495]; however, data from additional multicenter studies are needed.

ANTIMICROBIAL USE

The emergence, selection, amplification, and dissemination of antimicrobial-resistant microorganisms are related closely to the use of antimicrobial agents, although this connection may be easier to demonstrate at a population level than in an individual patient. Data regarding the use of antimicrobial agents in hospitals providing care to pediatric patients are very limited, but two multicenter studies provide general descriptive information.

Project ICARE tracked the use of antimicrobial agents in adult and pediatric ICUs. The initial Project ICARE report provided data from only a small number of pediatric ICUs,[215] but the 2001 NNIS System report included data from 16 pediatric ICUs.[463] Antimicrobial use in this report is quantified as the number of "defined daily doses" (DDD) per 1000 patient days. The DDD is a metric designed to quantify medication use in adult patients and does not make any adjustment for weight (e.g., the DDD for cefotaxime is 3 g/day, whereas the usual dose prescribed for a child is 150 mg/kg/day). Consequently, the data in the NNIS System report probably underestimate the use of antimicrobial agents in children versus adults. Despite this caveat, these data provide a qualitative assessment of the frequency of use of specific agents in pediatric ICUs. In the participating units, third-generation cephalosporins are by far the most commonly used agents, followed by parenteral vancomycin, first-generation cephalosporins, ampicillin- or amoxicillin-containing agents, second-generation cephalosporins, antistaphylococcal penicillins, trimethoprim-sulfamethoxazole, antipseudomonal penicillins, fluoroquinolones, carbapenems, penicillins, oral vancomycin, and aztreonam.

The PPN point prevalence survey cited earlier found somewhat different results.[256] In this study, the antimicrobial agent most commonly used in pediatric ICUs was a first-generation cephalosporin, followed by third-generation cephalosporins and vancomycin. Most patients receiving cefazolin had undergone surgery recently. The agent most commonly used in neonatal ICUs was gentamicin, followed by ampicillin and vancomycin.

The reason for the discrepant results between the NNIS System report and the PPN study are not clear and may relate to differences in the ICUs and their patient populations or methodologic differences in measuring antimicrobial use. Although these two studies provide data on the relative frequency of use of specific antimicrobial agents, the determinants or the appropriateness of antimicrobial use in hospitals providing care to children in the United States has not been described in any detail. Moreover, a standardized approach to the measurement of antimicrobial use in children has not been defined and validated.

INTERACTIONS BETWEEN HOSTS AND PATHOGENS

Generally, newborns begin life devoid of microbial flora but quickly become colonized with a broad array of microorganisms. The vast majority of these microorganisms will not produce disease unless their human host's natural defenses against infection are compromised. In contrast, exposure to microbial pathogens may lead to infection unless the host has effective innate or specific immunity to these microorganisms. In hospitalized children, weakened host defenses, coupled with the aggressive medical care required to sustain critically ill children, tend to be more important factors than the pathogenic potential of the specific microorganisms that happen to be circulating in the institution at any given moment.

Neonates are at particular risk for acquiring infection because of the relative immaturity of their immune systems, especially if they are born prematurely. A full review of the deficits in newborn immune function is available in other texts,[379] but a few of the most important problems deserve emphasis. Infants born before approximately 28 weeks of gestation do not have the benefit of transplacentally acquired maternal antibody, and even more mature newborns lack specific antibodies to many of the pathogens that they can expect to encounter early in life. The alternative pathway of complement activation is designed to protect the host in the absence of specific antibody, but it may not function adequately against newborn pathogens. Neonates have limited neutrophil reserves, which may be exhausted quickly in the face of aggressive pathogens. In addition, neutrophil migration is decreased, phagocytosis is less effective, and production of antibiotic proteins and peptides, such as bactericidal/permeability-increasing protein, is decreased.[378] Not surprisingly, opsonophagocytosis is compromised by the combination of inadequate specific antibody, suboptimal complement activation, and qualitative defects in neutrophil recruitment, migration, and function. Immature cellular immunity also compromises the response of neonates to viral and other intracellular pathogens. Moreover, the neonate's lack of an established normal bacterial flora provides no natural "colonization resistance" against pathogens entering the upper respiratory or alimentary tracts, and the fragile skin of premature infants is less resistant to trauma and the resulting microbial invasion.

Even after their immune system has matured and they are capable of mounting their own vigorous immune response to infection, infants and young children remain susceptible to communicable diseases that may be spread in hospitals, such as varicella, measles, and parvovirus, if they lack specific immunity. Some pathogens, such as RSV, provoke such a limited immune response that infants become susceptible again a short time after infection. Others, such as influenza virus, change their antigenic properties so rapidly that immunity acquired in 1 year is of limited value in the next.

Underlying diseases, especially those that compromise the immune system, predispose the host to infection by a wide array of microorganisms that ordinarily do not cause disease in normal hosts. For instance, neutropenic children are particularly susceptible to filamentous fungal infections that rarely affect other children, such as invasive pulmonary aspergillosis.[1, 664] Immunocompromised children also may suffer more severe consequences from infections that would be relatively trivial in normal hosts. For example, RSV and adenovirus may cause prolonged lower respiratory tract infection or even fatal pneumonia in transplant recipients; rotavirus and *Cryptosporidium* may cause chronic diarrhea in children with acquired immunodeficiency syndrome (AIDS). Pathogens that remain well localized in normal hosts may disseminate widely in compromised children (e.g., disseminated candidiasis in neutropenic children).

Medical treatment also has an important impact on the risk of acquiring infection. Common features of modern medical care include the use of intravascular catheters and infusions, indwelling urinary catheters, and mechanical ventilation. Many pediatric patients require much more sophisticated care, including invasive hemodynamic monitoring, extracorporeal membrane oxygenation, intensive chemotherapy, bone marrow and solid organ transplantation, hemodialysis, plasmapheresis, and intracranial pressure monitoring. Aggressive surgical procedures, such as reconstructive surgery and sophisticated cardiovascular surgery, not only are performed more frequently but also are performed on children at a very young age. Overuse of antibiotics in critically ill children predisposes them to colonization and infection with antimicrobial-resistant bacteria or fungi.

Although considerable knowledge about host factors that influence the risk of acquiring nosocomial infection exists, substantially less is known about the properties of specific microorganisms that render them more or less pathogenic in hospitalized patients. For the most part, why some microorganisms do not disseminate widely in a hospital whereas others do and why some microorganisms colonize many patients but produce few infections whereas others cause devastating epidemics of disease remain mysteries. Why, for example, did the *S. aureus* phage type 80/81 cause a worldwide pandemic of staphylococcal disease, especially in nurseries, whereas other phage types have a much more limited range, appeared to disseminate less readily on hospital wards, and produced serious infections less frequently?[571]

Contemporary laboratory techniques gradually are unraveling the pathogenic properties of specific microorganisms. For example, the genome of nosocomially acquired and community-acquired MRSA has been sequenced and analyzed by using a new strategy, called genomic island allotyping, that can help predict the pathogenic potential and antimicrobial susceptibility of specific strains.[39, 358] Studies of coagulase-negative staphylococci have determined that these bacteria produce a capsular polysaccharide that facilitates their adherence to prosthetic materials and a "slime" that protects them from clearance by host defense mechanisms[307, 347, 435];

Citrobacter diversus elaborates a surface protein that contributes to its propensity to produce destructive meningitis and cerebral abscesses[345, 346]; *E. coli* with the K1 capsular serotype is more likely to invade the meninges[318]; group A streptococci that produce an exuberant hyaluronic acid capsule are more likely to evade opsonophagocytosis[681]; and *E. coli* strains that produce P pili, are hemolytic, and have specific capsular serotypes and colicin types are more likely to produce urinary tract infections.[326] Nonetheless, we are a long way from understanding the factors that govern the ecology and pathogenic potential of most nosocomial microorganisms and using this knowledge to prevent infections caused by these microorganisms.

MODES OF TRANSMISSION OF NOSOCOMIAL INFECTIONS

Modes of transmission are the general mechanisms involved in the transfer of microorganisms from the reservoirs where they live and replicate to susceptible hosts. Table 231–7 lists the important modes of transmission. Examples of specific nosocomial infections, including the relevant reservoirs, sources, and modes of transmission of microorganisms causing these infections, are listed. Because reservoirs often cannot be eliminated, strategies must be designed to interrupt modes of transmission. Such strategies are discussed in detail in Chapter 232.

The three basic types of airborne transmission are dissemination of droplet nuclei, "shedding" of skin squames (or "rafts") by colonized or infected individuals, and aerosolization of fungal spores. Droplet nuclei are small particles (<5 μm) generated by the desiccation of larger droplets expelled by coughing, sneezing, or speaking letters such as "T" or "P" forcefully. Because they are extremely light, droplet nuclei can travel over very long distances on air currents. If ventilation is poor and the microorganisms in the droplet nuclei are hardy, these infectious particles may remain suspended in the air of enclosed spaces for relatively long periods in concentrations sufficient to cause infection, even if the index patient is no longer present. Because they are so small, droplet nuclei can remain suspended in inhaled air, evade the mechanical host defenses of the upper respiratory tract, and reach the lungs.[455] Classic diseases spread by respiratory droplet nuclei include measles, tuberculosis, smallpox, and in certain circumstances, influenza and varicella.[151, 374, 456, 531, 670] Legionnaires' disease may be spread by small aerosolized droplets generated by devices such as cooling towers, showerheads, and even bedpan cleaners.[639]

TABLE 231–7 ■ MODES OF TRANSMISSION WITH EXAMPLES OF SPECIFIC NOSOCOMIAL INFECTIONS AND THE RESERVOIRS AND SOURCES INVOLVED IN THE TRANSMISSION OF THESE INFECTIONS

Mode of Transmission	Nosocomial Infection	Reservoir	Source
Airborne	Measles, varicella,* pulmonary tuberculosis	Infected persons	Airborne droplet nuclei
Contact			
Direct	Neonatal staphylococcal skin infection	Infected/colonized caregiver	Drainage from infected wound on hand of a caregiver
Indirect	Respiratory syncytial virus infection	Infected persons	Hands of caregivers, fomites
	Infection with antimicrobial-resistant bacteria	Infected/colonized persons	Hands of caregivers, fomites
Droplet	Pertussis, invasive meningococcal disease, group A streptococcal infection	Infected/colonized persons	Large respiratory droplets
Endogenous (autoinfection)†	Coagulase-negative staphylococcal bacteremia associated with central venous line	Skin at site of catheter insertion	Intravascular catheter
	Escherichia coli urinary tract infection associated with an indwelling urinary catheter	Periurethral skin and mucous membranes	Indwelling urinary catheter
Common vehicle	Gram-negative bacteremia associated with intravenous infusion	Liquid substances in environment	Intrinsically or extrinsically contaminated intravenous fluids
	Post-transfusion infection with blood-borne pathogen (human immunodeficiency virus, hepatitis B virus, hepatitis C virus, cytomegalovirus)	Infected persons	Blood products from infected donors
	Salmonellosis	Infected/colonized persons	Contaminated food
Vector	Enteric infection	Infected person or infectious material	Files, pharaoh ants

*Varicella-zoster virus may be transmitted by airborne, direct contact, and droplet contact transmission.
†See text.

Certain individuals are heavy "shedders" of skin squames contaminated by staphylococci or, more rarely, by group A streptococci and other skin microorganisms (e.g., *Rhodococcus*).[571] Shedders may have obvious dermatitis or a clinical infection but often are asymptomatic. Shedders have been implicated in outbreaks of infection, especially in operating rooms, but the vast majority of personnel who are colonized with potential pathogens do not dispense large numbers of bacteria and do not pose a threat to patients.[571]

Spores of filamentous fungi, such as *Aspergillus* and *Zygomycetes,* are ubiquitous in the environment, especially where decaying organic matter and moisture are present. Their small size (<3 μm) and aerodynamic shape permit dispersion over long distances and facilitate penetration of hospital air handling systems and the respiratory tract of susceptible individuals.

Aerosolization of other organisms, such as *Coxiella burnetii,* can occur in hospitals in special circumstances. For example, an outbreak of Q fever among personnel occurred when sheep were transported through the corridor of a university hospital for a research study.[439]

Contact transmission is the principal mode of transmission for most nosocomial infections. Direct contact transmission involves physical contact between a person harboring the microorganism and the host, such as a staphylococcal infection on the hands of a caregiver. Indirect contact transmission involves the transfer of microorganisms via an intermediary person or object. The hands of caregivers are the most common source of indirect contact transmission, but fomites are also important for certain pathogens (e.g., RSV, *Clostridium difficile).* Droplet contact transmission involves the transfer of microorganisms by large respiratory droplets, such as those generated by coughing or sneezing; these organisms typically travel no farther than 3 ft in the air before settling. Important nosocomial pathogens spread by this route include *Bordetella pertussis, Neisseria meningitidis,* and group A streptococci.

Endogenous infection (or autoinfection) is caused by a patient's own flora. These generally harmless commensals cause disease when the patient's host defenses are compromised by severe underlying disease, immunosuppressive therapy, or invasive devices and procedures. Microorganisms that produce endogenous infections are not always part of the normal flora that the patient brought into the hospital from the community. Commonly, these microorganisms are transferred from other patients via the hands of caregivers and become part of a patient's colonizing endogenous flora. Consequently, these infections can be considered a special case of contact transmission.

Common-vehicle (common-source) transmission involves the widespread dissemination of a microorganism to many persons via a contaminated item or substance. Many outbreaks of infection in hospitals have been caused by nonenteric gram-negative bacilli such as *P. aeruginosa,* which thrives in medications, solutions, or wet equipment and is relatively resistant to antimicrobial preservatives, antiseptics, and disinfectants.

Vector transmission of microorganisms either on (extrinsic) or within (intrinsic) insects is a rare event in hospitals. Extrinsic vector transmission of enteric pathogens may occur when these microorganisms are transported on the legs of flies, roaches, or ants.[49, 115, 206] Intrinsic vector transmission, such as transmission of malaria or dengue, involves more than physical transfer of the microorganism because a portion of the life cycle of the microorganism is completed in the vector. Although intrinsic vector transmission in the hospital is theoretically possible, to our knowledge, no cases have been reported.

Some infections may be spread by more than one mode of transmission. For example, varicella-zoster virus (VZV) may be spread by airborne and direct contact transmission.

CONSEQUENCES AND COSTS OF NOSOCOMIAL INFECTIONS

Valid, well-controlled studies of the consequences and costs of nosocomial infections in pediatric patients are limited, partly because of the difficulty of determining whether the consequences or costs are directly attributable to the patient's nosocomial infection as opposed to the patient's underlying disease. To attribute a consequence to nosocomial infection, investigators must match infected and noninfected patients carefully by using criteria such as age, sex, presence of underlying conditions, severity of illness, operative procedures, and length of stay, or they must adjust for these potential confounding factors by using multivariate statistical analyses. In addition, studies must quantify hospital costs, as opposed to hospital charges, which may be difficult to do precisely.[562]

Pediatric studies that have made an effort to rigorously measure attributable risk indicate that nosocomial infections have a substantial adverse impact on hospitalized children. For example, Valenti and colleagues matched infected and uninfected patients by age, sex, underlying illness, and time of year of admission and found that nosocomial infections increased the length of stay by an average of 9 days.[653] Patients infected with RSV and influenza had average increases in length of stay of 6 and 5 days, respectively.[653] Appropriately designed cohort studies of coagulase-negative staphylococcal bacteremia in newborn ICUs (including adjustment for birth weight and severity of illness) have found increased length of stay (approximately 14 days), increased use of antibiotics, and increased hospital charges (about $25,000), but no increased rate of mortality from this infection.[208, 254] A study by Leroyer and associates in France found that infants in a neonatal ICU who suffered a nosocomial infection were hospitalized 5 days longer than matched, uninfected controls were and that hospital costs were $10,000 higher for infected infants.[375]

Controlled studies performed in hospitalized adult patient populations also indicate that the consequences and cost of nosocomial infections are substantial. For instance, a matched case-control study of nosocomial bloodstream infections in adult surgical ICU patients estimated that this infection had an attributable mortality rate of 35 percent, increased the length of stay in the ICU by 8 days, prolonged the overall hospital stay by 24 days, and cost $40,000 per survivor.[500] Studies of bloodstream infections caused by specific pathogens, such as *Candida* and *Enterococcus,* have documented comparable outcomes.[367, 682] However, a small matched case-control study found that the attributable mortality associated with bloodstream infection decreased substantially after additional adjustments were made for the severity of illness after 1 week of ICU stay.[619] A case-control study of pneumonia in patients who were mechanically ventilated estimated that the attributable mortality rate of this infection was 27 percent and that it prolonged the ICU stay by 13 days.[194] A subsequent cohort study performed by the same investigators found that nosocomial pneumonia and nosocomial bloodstream infection were independent predictors of mortality.[195] Surgical-site infection has been estimated to increase the length of hospital stay by an average of 8 days and resulted in average extra hospital costs of more than 1000 British pounds.[133] A study of nosocomial infection after cardiac surgery found that infection was an independent predictor of multiorgan dysfunction but did not contribute to mortality directly.[351] Finally, through a series of observational studies, Kollef and colleagues associated increased mortality rates in adult ICU patients with inadequate treatment of nosocomial infection.[350–353]

Nosocomial Infections Caused by Spread of Infections Common in the Community

Nosocomial infections that occur as a result of in-hospital transmission of infections common in the community are a major concern for all facilities providing health care to children. Several principles regarding the general epidemiology of these infections, modified from those initially published by Hall in relation to the epidemiology of nosocomial respiratory viruses,[266] are summarized in this section. First, their appearance and spread on the wards closely parallel the disease activity in the community. Second, significant exposure to these pathogens generally results in infection in any host who lacks specific immunity; consequently, a susceptible child is at risk regardless of the nature or severity of the underlying disease or specific medical treatment. Third, these infections are often more severe in hospitalized patients who have underlying diseases (e.g., pulmonary or cardiac disease) or who are immunocompromised. Fourth, children hospitalized as a result of community-acquired infections are the most important reservoir for microorganisms causing these infections, but mildly symptomatic or asymptomatically colonized adult caregivers may be important reservoirs for some agents (e.g., RSV, pertussis). Fifth, prevention is dependent primarily on timely implementation of and compliance with isolation precautions specifically designed to interrupt transmission of the microorganisms involved. In some infections, other interventions, such as antimicrobial therapy to reduce the risk of transmission from children with pertussis and passive immunization with varicella-zoster immune globulin (VZIG) to protect high-risk individuals exposed to varicella, also are indicated. Finally, unless post-discharge surveillance is performed, reports of the frequency of these infections are likely to be gross underestimations, especially given recent trends toward a shorter length of hospital stay, because many of these infections may be in the incubation period at the time of discharge and become manifested only after the child returns home.

RESPIRATORY INFECTIONS

Respiratory Viruses

RSV is the most common nosocomial respiratory virus infection, especially in the first 2 years of life.[205, 268, 653, 676] Community outbreaks occur every year in the late fall or winter, although the precise timing, intensity, and duration of these outbreaks may vary.[275] Population-based studies indicate that RSV infection may account for a substantial number of hospital admissions in young children during epidemic periods, especially those with underlying medical conditions.[70, 589]

Children admitted to the hospital with community-acquired RSV infection represent a substantial reservoir for nosocomial transmission of RSV to other hospitalized children and health care workers. In a study conducted during a community outbreak in the 1970s, 45 percent of children who were hospitalized for 1 week or longer on an infant ward and 40 percent of the caregivers on this ward acquired nosocomial RSV infection.[273] A more recent study actively surveyed the frequency of nosocomial RSV infection in all children admitted to eight leading Canadian children's hospitals during the mid-1990s.[368] The percentage of nosocomial RSV cases among all RSV cases (community and nosocomial) in the hospital varied from 2.8 to 13.0 percent in the participating hospitals. As demonstrated in several studies, risk factors for acquisition of nosocomial infection are prematurity, heart and lung disease, and immunocompromising conditions.[274, 275, 368, 400, 502] Outbreaks in newborn ICUs have been reported, some in association with other viruses.[274, 440, 616, 652, 688]

In the absence of effective control programs, attack rates tend to be high because immunity after infection is short lived and inoculation of virus into the nose or eyes reliably leads to infection.[267, 268, 270] Moreover, RSV survives for relatively long periods in the environment, and infected children excrete high titers of virus in their copious secretions.[267, 268, 2725] Not surprisingly, the duration of hospitalization (and thus the duration of potential exposure) correlates strongly with the risk of acquiring infection because a greater opportunity exists for direct or indirect contact transmission.[273] One study used polymerase chain reaction (PCR) to detect RSV nucleic acid in the air samples of patient rooms, including samples taken as far as 7 m from the bedside.[8] However, the implication of this finding on infectivity is unclear.

Scrupulous attention to hand hygiene and the use of barriers (gloves and gowns) when touching patients or their immediate inanimate environment can markedly reduce transmission of RSV.[372] Goggles or masks, or both, may be effective in reducing the RSV attack rate in personnel,[6, 221] which in turn can reduce transmission of virus to patients. However, whether masks and eye protection are effective because they prevent direct deposition of respiratory droplets on the eyes or nose or merely because they reduce the likelihood that staff will rub their eyes or noses with contaminated hands is unclear. Covering only the nose and mouth with a mask is probably not very effective.[271] Masks and eye protection are not recommended in the CDC's isolation precautions guidelines,[228] and use of these barriers has not achieved wide popularity, perhaps because of cost and inconvenience. Some investigators have demonstrated that cohorting infected patients, combined with the use of barriers, can reduce the spread of RSV.[175, 356, 403] However, whether cohorting by clinical symptoms alone is effective or whether all admitted patients must be screened for RSV infection to identify children with minimal symptoms who may be excreting the virus is not clear. Moreover, the added value of strict cohorting, which may be expensive or difficult to implement, as opposed to the rigorous use of barrier techniques has not been demonstrated. A variety of multidisciplinary programs to promote awareness of the potential for nosocomial transmission of RSV and to optimize the use of prevention measures have been described.[330, 372, 399] Two studies estimated that the cost savings associated with their programs were substantial.[330, 399]

One group of investigators used a screening approach to reduce the frequency of RSV infection in children undergoing cardiac surgery.[11] They screened all children 16 days to 4 years of age admitted for cardiac surgery between September and March with an RSV enzyme-linked immunoassay. Surgery was delayed in patients with symptomatic disease, as well as asymptomatic patients with positive RSV tests (most of whom had symptoms in the subsequent days after the positive test). Although it was not a controlled trial, postoperative infections with RSV and the attendant complications were reduced substantially during the screening period.

Treatment of RSV infection with ribavirin reduces shedding of RSV,[172] which may decrease the potential for nosocomial transmission. However, use of this agent has been limited because of a lack of clear evidence of clinical benefit.[18] RSV immune globulin and palivizumab, a humanized murine monoclonal antibody, have demonstrated efficacy in preventing or reducing the severity of RSV infection in high-risk patients,[19] but they are unlikely to have a profound effect on nosocomial transmission. Palivizumab has been used to help control an outbreak of RSV in a neonatal unit.[143] The development of vaccines against RSV is under way, and they may lead to more effective prevention strategies in the future.[268]

Nosocomial infections caused by parainfluenza virus are similar to RSV in their epidemiology and prevention.[268, 452]

Population-based studies indicate that rates of hospitalization in young children are substantially lower for influenza than RSV infection.[70, 315, 467, 589] However, the potential for nosocomial transmission of influenza virus is still significant. Nosocomial influenza is a common cause of intercurrent fever in hospitalized children during epidemic periods,[269] and outbreaks in neonatal ICUs have been described.[150, 457]

Although the modes of transmission of influenza have not been defined precisely, direct, indirect, and droplet contact are likely to be most important in health care settings. Nonetheless, data from animal models and the rapid spread of influenza in confined human populations suggest that airborne transmission may occur in some situations.[247, 456] In addition to the precautions described for RSV, masks should be worn during close contact because of the potential for droplet transmission. The need for isolation rooms with negative air pressure relative to hallways has not been established; however, use of these rooms is encouraged, if possible.[228, 639] If the use of such rooms is not feasible, placement of a patient in a private room without special air handling and cohorting of patients with proven influenza are alternative control strategies.[228, 639]

Annual influenza vaccination of high-risk individuals and hospital staff can limit the potential for large outbreaks of influenza if the vaccination is both offered at the appropriate time and well accepted by patients and staff.[76] A live attenuated intranasal vaccine is under development and may help boost vaccination rates.[141] Amantadine is approved for prophylaxis and treatment of high-risk children 1 year and older during outbreaks of influenza A.[141] Rimantadine is approved only for prophylaxis of influenza A in this age group, but experience with its use for treatment exists as well.[141] Resistance to these agents has been documented to emerge during treatment.[141] The neuraminidase inhibitors oseltamivir and zanamivir are active against both influenza A and B. Oseltamivir is approved for treatment and prophylaxis in children 1 year and older; zanamivir is approved for treatment only in children 7 years and older.[141] These agents may reduce the risk of nosocomial transmission, although such reduction has not been demonstrated.

Nosocomial adenovirus infections occur sporadically throughout the year, and outbreaks of respiratory infection and pharyngoconjunctival fever in hospitalized children are well described.[202, 237, 459, 498, 511, 605, 634, 680] Outbreaks in ICUs have been associated with severe disease and substantial mortality.[605, 680] Children undergoing liver transplantation are also at high risk for severe disease in the immediate post-transplant period.[443] In addition to direct and indirect contact, adenovirus may be spread by droplet contact, thus necessitating the use of masks with eye protection during close contact.

Nosocomial rhinovirus infections are generally mild, although serious lower respiratory tract disease has been documented in children with underlying disorders.[126, 310] The mode of transmission of rhinovirus infection remains controversial. Some studies suggest direct and indirect contact transmission as the primary mode of transmission; others suggest that droplet contact may be more important.[247] Hand hygiene is sufficient as a control measure in most situations.

Pertussis

Outbreaks of pertussis in hospitals and chronic care institutions are well documented.[203, 359, 386, 590, 627, 643, 654] In many situations, health care workers were responsible for spreading pertussis to hospitalized children.[125, 359, 386, 652] Indeed, two studies have demonstrated that infection among health care workers occurs relatively commonly, even in the absence of a defined nosocomial outbreak.[171, 692]

Prevention of nosocomial pertussis is dependent on the appropriate isolation of children in whom the infection is suspected, the use of masks to prevent droplet contact transmission, antimicrobial treatment of confirmed cases to minimize the potential for transmission, and prophylactic treatment of exposed individuals. In addition, hospital staff who have symptoms suggesting pertussis (upper respiratory tract infection with severe, prolonged coughing) must be evaluated and treated promptly. The availability of clarithromycin and azithromycin has enhanced treatment of exposed individuals because most adults tolerate these agents much better than erythromycin.

The beneficial impact, but relatively high cost of aggressive steps to control the nosocomial spread of pertussis was illustrated during a large community-wide epidemic of pertussis in Cincinnati in 1993.[127] During this epidemic, 102 patients were hospitalized with pertussis, and 87 hospital staff had pertussis diagnosed on clinical or microbiologic grounds. Fifteen strict control measures, including prompt investigation of all suspected cases among patients and staff, appropriate isolation of proven and suspected cases among patients, furloughs for all staff with suspected pertussis until they had completed 5 days of antimicrobial therapy, and antimicrobial therapy for all close contacts of confirmed cases, were implemented to prevent transmission within the hospital. Only one case of nosocomial pertussis occurred—an infant who was infected by a symptomatic nurse later confirmed to be culture-positive. Among 274 culture-confirmed cases in the community, only 2 were epidemiologically linked to hospital staff with pertussis. The cost of these measures was more than $85,000.

Acellular pertussis vaccine is effective in boosting antibody titers in adults[186] and may provide an opportunity to boost immunity in hospital staff. Acellular pertussis vaccine was used as an adjunctive control measure in a hospital outbreak of pertussis.[590] The vaccine was reasonably well tolerated, but no data regarding its efficacy were reported.

Diphtheria

The potential for nosocomial transmission of diphtheria was emphasized by a large outbreak in Russia and the Ukraine in the 1990s. Diphtheria acquired during travel to these regions has been reported in U.S. citizens, and imported cases have been documented in other European countries.[97] An imported case of diphtheria in a child from Haiti resulted in exposure of a large number of hospital contacts in Florida. Secondary cases were reported in household, but not hospital contacts.[198] Health care workers should wear masks during the care of patients with pharyngeal diphtheria. Investigation and prophylaxis of contacts should be pursued aggressively.[198]

GASTROINTESTINAL INFECTIONS

Gastrointestinal Viruses

Rotavirus is the most common cause of endemic and epidemic nosocomial gastrointestinal virus infection.* The risk of infection developing is closely associated with the length of hospitalization.[136, 167] Infection is usually self-limited, although prolonged diarrhea may occur in immunocompromised patients. One study associated an outbreak of necrotizing enterocolitis in a newborn nursery with concurrent rotavirus infection.[551]

Patients infected with rotavirus in the hospital or community may shed the virus in their stool for many days after symptomatic infection.[686] Asymptomatically infected patients also may shed virus.[136, 686] Together, these patients represent a substantial reservoir of virus that may be transmitted easily to other patients. In addition, rotavirus can be transferred via hands and can survive for extended periods on environmental surfaces.[26, 572] The primary mode of transmission is indirect contact via the contaminated hands of caregivers, and the scrupulous use of barriers (gowns and gloves), hand hygiene, and appropriate disinfection of environmental surfaces is critically important. An experimental study suggests that rotavirus infection also can be spread by the respiratory route,[514] although this finding has not been demonstrated clinically.

A randomized, double-blind, placebo-controlled trial demonstrated that *Lactobacillus* GG decreased the incidence of nosocomial diarrhea in hospitalized children 1 to 36 months of age.[638] The frequency of symptomatic diarrhea (defined as a new onset of three or more loose or watery stools per day during hospitalization) was 7 percent in the treated group and 33 percent in the placebo group. Although the frequency of identification of rotavirus in the stools of children in the two groups was equivalent, the frequency of rotavirus-associated diarrhea was 2 percent in the treated group and 17 percent in the placebo group.

A variety of other gastrointestinal viruses, including enteric adenoviruses,[354] Norwalk-like viruses,[623] calicivirus,[624] astrovirus,[166, 360] and torovirus, also have been documented to cause endemic and epidemic nosocomial gastrointestinal infection.[317]

*See references 101, 119, 205, 240, 252, 365, 520, 526, 547, 548, 653, 665, 676.

Clostridium difficile

Although toxin-producing *C. difficile* is a well-recognized cause of antimicrobial-associated diarrhea in adults, investigation of the role of this organism as a cause of nosocomial diarrhea in hospitalized children and infants has been quite limited.

Studies conducted in the 1980s illustrated that toxin-producing *C. difficile* often can be found in the stool of neonates and young infants.[132] Because *C. difficile* seldom is found in the stool of healthy women and because clusters of colonized infants often can be detected in nurseries,[132] one may presume that nosocomial, as opposed to vertical, transmission plays a role in the acquisition of this microorganism by neonates. Nonetheless, *C. difficile* rarely produces significant disease in newborns or young infants,[132] although one study has reported that infants whose stools are positive for *C. difficile* toxin A have more stools per day than do infants whose stools are negative.[191]

On the other hand, numerous reports indicate that symptomatic *C. difficile*–associated diarrhea can develop in older children and even infants and that severe disease, including pseudomembranous colitis, may develop in some children.[79, 88, 200, 282, 431, 476, 479, 515, 699] Disease usually occurs in association with antimicrobial therapy, and several reports have described the occurrence of disease in children with cancer.[79, 88, 515, 699]

Two recent studies have explored the relationship of humoral immunity and *C. difficile*–associated diarrhea in elderly hospitalized adults.[361, 362] In one study, hospitalized adults who became asymptomatically colonized with *C. difficile* but in whom disease did not develop had significantly higher serum levels of IgG antibody against toxin A than did those in whom disease developed.[361] A second study of patients with an initial case of *C. difficile*–associated diarrhea found that recurrent disease was less likely to develop in patients with higher serum concentrations of IgM and IgG antibodies against toxin A than in patients with lower concentrations of antibody.[362] The implications of these findings on the epidemiology of this disease in children have not been investigated.

C. difficile can be found on the hands of personnel and in the patient's immediate environment,[432] where *C. difficile* spores can survive for prolonged periods and are relatively resistant to disinfectants. Therefore, direct or indirect contact is responsible for the spread of this microorganism from patient to patient. Barriers (gowns and gloves) and hand hygiene may reduce transmission. Vigorous environmental cleaning is probably important and certainly is prudent, although the use of specific disinfecting agents in preventing transmission has not been defined well. However, because asymptomatic carriage of this microorganism occurs more commonly than symptomatic disease and because excretion often continues for long periods,[432] the impact of these interventions may be somewhat limited unless all patients are screened and precautions are implemented for colonized patients—an expensive and usually impractical approach.

If possible, antibiotic therapy should be discontinued. Diarrhea resolves spontaneously in 15 to 25 percent of patients without further intervention, although predicting which patients will respond to conservative management is difficult. Oral metronidazole and vancomycin are equivalent in terms of response and relapse rates,[644] but metronidazole is considerably less expensive. Vancomycin may be preferable treatment in severely ill patients. Oral metronidazole is not effective in eliminating carriage in asymptomatic patients; oral vancomycin may reduce carriage temporarily, but recrudescence of carriage occurs commonly.[327] *Saccharomyces boulardii* and *Lactobacillus* GG have shown promise in the primary treatment and prevention of recurrence of *C. difficile*–associated diarrhea in adults, but these agents have not been tested systematically in children.[159]

Other Bacteria

Bacterial pathogens are rare causes of endemic nosocomial diarrhea in U.S. hospitals.[181] Consequently, in the absence of an outbreak, the yield of routine stool cultures in the evaluation of nosocomial diarrhea is extremely low.[73, 144, 698] One study developed and evaluated simple screening criteria for rejecting stool bacterial cultures for patients who were hospitalized for more than 3 days.[698] The reduction in volume of tests processed by the laboratory led to cost savings of $25,082 in the 6-month trial period. Outbreaks of nosocomial salmonellosis have been documented throughout the world, although they are reported more commonly from developing countries.* Neonates are

*See references 261, 277, 337, 406, 454, 483, 564, 609, 631, 693.

particularly susceptible to infection by *Salmonella,* and invasive disease such as bacteremia, meningitis, and osteomyelitis is a common occurrence.[261, 277, 337, 406, 609, 631, 693] Transmission occurs through a variety of means, including contaminated food, direct contact between patients, and indirect contact transmission via contaminated hands or instruments.

Outbreaks of nosocomial shigellosis are much less common. Only one hospital outbreak has been reported in the United States,[52] although shigellosis can be a major problem in institutions caring for disabled children.[41, 182] A study in a hospital in Kenya cultured *Shigella* organisms from the stools of 2.5 percent of patients with nosocomial diarrhea.[483] *Shigella* is transmitted easily by direct or indirect contact, and only a small inoculum is required to establish infection.[181]

Nosocomial cholera has been documented in developing countries.[442, 561] One of these reports is notable because it provides evidence that nosocomial acquisition of *Vibrio cholerae* by children who were discharged home before becoming symptomatic was instrumental in initiating and sustaining an outbreak of cholera in the surrounding community.[442] The mechanism involved in nosocomial transmission of cholera in these studies is not clear, but direct or indirect contact transmission, as opposed to transmission via contaminated water, was suspected.

Other bacterial pathogens have caused outbreaks of diarrhea, including *Campylobacter,*[82, 291, 332, 656] *Yersinia,*[85, 525] and various strains of *E. coli*.[236, 585]

Protozoa

Nosocomial infections caused by protozoa rarely occur. An outbreak of cryptosporidiosis was reported from a pediatric hospital in Mexico.[465] The index case was a patient with AIDS who had chronic diarrhea caused by infection with *Cryptosporidium.* Although giardiasis is a common cause of diarrhea in institutionalized children,[645] infections in hospitalized children or neonates have not been reported. Given the large number of severely immunocompromised children in U.S. hospitals and the relative ease of transmitting protozoa by direct or indirect transmission in families and daycare centers, it is somewhat surprising that nosocomial gastroenteritis caused by *Giardia, Cryptosporidium, Microsporidium,* and other intestinal protozoa has not been reported more frequently.

VARICELLA-ZOSTER VIRUS

Outbreaks of nosocomial varicella in hospitals have been documented in numerous reports.[218, 262, 374, 576] These reports demonstrate conclusively that varicella can be transmitted by the airborne route, although spread via direct and droplet contact may well be more efficient. In these outbreaks, secondary infections occurred in patients who had no face-to-face contact with the index patient and were separated from the index patient by considerable physical distances (in some cases more than 30 m).[262, 374] Air flow studies indicated that air in the rooms of index patients flowed into the hallway and into other patient rooms.[262, 374] In one report, air flowed through an open window in the index patient's room, traveled along the exterior of the building, and entered other patient rooms via through-the-wall ventilation units.[374] Most secondary infections in each of these outbreaks occurred in patients who had been discharged and were detected only by telephone contact or home visit.[262, 374] Several susceptible hospital staff members also were infected.

These clinical observations of airborne spread of VZV are supported by a study that used PCR to detect airborne virus in the hospital rooms of patients with active infection.[573] VZV was detected in air samples collected 1.2 to 5.5 m from patients' beds for 1 to 6 days after the onset of rash. VZV DNA also could be detected in some air samples obtained in the hallway just outside the patient's negative-pressure isolation rooms.

Nosocomial transmission of varicella can be minimized if infected patients receive care in single rooms with separate exhaust systems and negative air pressure relative to the hallway.[21] Because infected persons are infectious for 24 to 48 hours before distinctive symptoms and signs appear, prompt recognition and isolation of patients and visitors who may be in the contagious phase of varicella are also critical. A simple series of screening questions can help identify these individuals (see Chapter 232). Barriers to prevent direct and indirect contact transmission (gloves and gowns) can dramatically reduce the nosocomial spread of this infection. In addition, caregivers who are not immune to varicella should not care for such patients. VZIG can prevent infection or mitigate the consequences of infection in high-risk, exposed, susceptible individuals if administered within 96 hours, but preferably within 48 hours of exposure.[16] Intravenous acyclovir should be administered to these individuals to limit the replication of virus if infection develops.[16] Hospitalized exposed children should remain in isolation from day 8 to day 21 after exposure. If VZIG is administered, isolation should be continued until day 28 after exposure.[16] Management of exposed health care workers is discussed in Chapter 232.

The use of VZV vaccine should diminish the risk of nosocomial varicella by decreasing the number of children hospitalized with varicella, reducing the size of the pool of susceptible children in hospital wards, and providing protective immunity to health care workers who do not have a history of having a previous infection. However, data demonstrating these effects have not been published. The use of this vaccine in health care workers is discussed in Chapter 232.

CYTOMEGALOVIRUS

Perhaps no issue is the subject of as much concern and misinformation among health care workers as the risk of acquiring nosocomial CMV. Concern among caregivers undoubtedly has been heightened by reports of CMV infection in daycare center staff. Daycare centers provide optimal conditions for transmission of CMV because many children are excreting CMV in their saliva or urine and abundant opportunities exist for sustained contact with contaminated secretions. However, even in the daycare setting, transmission of CMV to susceptible care providers occurs slowly.[5] This delay reflects the relative inefficiency of direct or indirect contact transmission of CMV, a virus that is easily inactivated by soaps, detergents, and disinfectants and is not stable on environmental surfaces for long periods.[5]

In hospitals, the risk to staff appears to be negligible. A meta-analysis of numerous studies that have examined the risk of CMV developing in pediatric nurses has indicated that CMV infection in this population occurs at a rate that is comparable to that in control populations (persons of comparable age and sex who are not nurses).[5] A subanalysis of these data suggests that nursery nurses may have a slightly higher rate of infection than control populations do.[5] However, studies of CMV infection in nursery nurses involving restriction enzyme analysis of CMV isolates have shown that the nurses did not acquire CMV from the infants in their care[5]; presumably, they contracted their infections from children in their own households, through sexual contact, or from other community sources.

In conclusion, little, if any data suggest that nosocomial transmission of CMV is a significant risk to health care workers. Given the frequency of asymptomatic CMV excretion in children (for example, approximately 1% of newborns excrete the virus), health care workers should assume that any child may be excreting virus and should practice handwashing and the use of standard precautions (see Chapter 232) as a part of routine patient care. Additional interventions are not indicated, and pregnant staff need not be given special assignments.

Two restriction enzyme studies have documented probable patient-to-patient spread of CMV in a newborn ICU and a chronic care unit.[165, 621] In both situations, the infected children had been in close proximity and received care from common caregivers for extended periods.

HERPES SIMPLEX VIRUS

Nosocomial transmission of herpes simplex virus (HSV) type 1 to newborn infants has been confirmed through restriction enzyme analysis.[278, 385, 569, 657] The mode of transmission is not clear in all these cases, however. Direct contact with a hospital worker with herpes labialis was implicated in one case.[657] In the other cases, indirect contact transmission from one infected infant to another is most likely, although direct contact transmission from an asymptomatic parent or caregiver cannot be eliminated.[278, 385, 569] Nosocomial HSV infection in health care workers, patients, and family members also has been described in ICUs.[4, 490] Herpetic whitlow is a common manifestation in nurses, presumably as a result of direct transmission during suctioning of oral and respiratory secretions from infected patients.[4] The risk associated with this procedure is substantial given recent data indicating that HSV is found commonly in mucosal and orofacial cultures obtained from intubated patients, including those without obvious lesions.[280] When present, lesions are often atypical in appearance and are found commonly in the distribution of tape used to secure endotracheal tubes.[280] Substantial risk of transmission from immunocompromised patients, in whom reactivation of latent HSV infection is common, also exists.[666, 690] The implementation of standard precautions (see Chapter 232), particularly the use of gloves during contact with oral and respiratory sections and hand hygiene, will prevent transmission of HSV.

Surveys of nosocomial infections in pediatric wards indicate that nosocomial HSV infections are uncommon.[205, 653, 676] When documented, these infections usually are attributed to reactivation of preexisting endogenous infection rather than primary infection.[653] However, as with ICU patients, subclinical infection in other hospitalized children may occur more commonly than presently recognized.

MEASLES, MUMPS, AND RUBELLA VIRUSES

Transmission of measles in health care facilities is an uncommon event, but it has the potential to serve as a nidus for community-wide infection.[434, 519, 545] Nosocomial infection may be initiated by the unrecognized introduction of measles by patients from the immediate community or visitors or by immigrants from foreign countries. Conversely, patients who acquire measles in the hospital can serve as a nidus for spread of infection in the community when they return to their homes.

Nosocomial measles represented a small, but important proportion of all measles cases in the 1980s (3.5% in 1985 to 1989).[31] Although the incidences of measles in the United States has been reduced significantly,[108] the risk of nosocomial transmission remains a threat.[626]

Measles may be transmitted on hospital wards and also in ambulatory care facilities such as emergency rooms and medical clinics.[161, 170, 197, 314, 519, 545, 626] During a community outbreak in Los Angeles in 1988, 6 children with unrecognized measles were hospitalized, which resulted in the exposure of 107 other hospitalized children and 24 hospital staff members.[545] Nosocomial measles developed in four patients, one of whom died of measles-related pneumonia, and four hospital staff members, two of whom required hospitalization for pneumonia. One of the patients who had been exposed to measles in this hospital subsequently was admitted to another hospital and exposed eight additional patients before isolation precautions were instituted. In an outbreak of measles in two counties in Florida, transmission of measles in the hospital was linked directly to the initiation and propagation of the outbreak in the community.[519] In one of the involved hospitals, inadequate isolation of patients with measles and failure to vaccinate or passively immunize exposed, susceptible individuals contributed to transmission.[519] Investigation of every reported case of measles in Oklahoma from 1981 to 1985 found that 27 percent of cases were associated with nosocomial transmission in medical offices and clinics and an additional 18 percent were secondary cases resulting from exposure to nosocomially infected individuals.[314] Another survey of measles cases during outbreaks in Los Angeles and Houston found that exposure to emergency rooms was a substantial risk factor for acquiring infection.[197]

Measles is transmitted by airborne droplet nuclei, as demonstrated by a report of an outbreak in a pediatrician's office.[531] Measles subsequently developed in four susceptible children visiting the office on the same day as the index child, even though none of these children had face-to-face contact with the index child or were even in the same room at the same time. Three children visited the office 60 to 75 minutes after the index child had left.

Prevention of nosocomial measles hinges on prompt recognition of infected or potentially infected patients and placement of these patients in isolation rooms with negative air pressure relative to the hallway.[228] Prophylactic vaccination of exposed susceptible individuals within 3 days of the exposure reliably prevents measles, whereas administration of immune globulin within 3 days attenuates the disease but does not guarantee that contagious infection will not develop in the exposed individual.[15] To avoid outbreaks of nosocomial measles in health care workers, health care facilities are advised to require that new employees involved in patient care provide evidence of immunity or appropriate vaccination or receive vaccination with either measles vaccine or MMR (measles, mumps, rubella) as a condition of employment (see Chapter 232).[357] Individuals born before 1957 generally are thought to be immune to measles because childhood measles was widespread at the time, but occasional cases have developed in this age group during hospital outbreaks.[581]

Outbreaks of nosocomial mumps and rubella have been reported less commonly than nosocomial measles.[292, 504, 633, 683] The primary concern with regard to nosocomial spread of both these infections relates to potential complications in health care workers. Mumps orchitis in adult males can cause sterility; rubella in pregnant staff can result in fetal infection and congenital rubella syndrome. Information regarding the transmission of both these viruses is limited, but it probably occurs primarily via droplet contact. Masks should be worn during close contact with infected patients.[228] Patients with congenital rubella syndrome may excrete large amounts of virus in their urine and respiratory secretions, and excretion of virus in urine may persist for months or even years. Consequently, gowns and gloves should be worn for contact with these patients during their first year of life unless nasopharyngeal and urine cultures are negative by the time that they are 3 months of age.[228] No effective postexposure prophylaxis for exposed individuals is known. As with prevention of nosocomial measles, health care facilities are advised to require that new employees involved in patient care provide evidence of immunity or appropriate vaccination or receive vaccination with MMR as a condition of employment (see Chapter 232).[357]

PARVOVIRUS B19

Parvovirus B19 causes the relatively benign syndrome of erythema infectiosum (occasionally accompanied by arthritis, particularly in older children and adults), acute aplastic crisis in children with hemoglobinopathies, and chronic infection and anemia in immunocompromised children. Some reports have suggested an association with vasculitis and other immunologically mediated diseases.[201, 691] An experimental study of acute parvovirus B19 infection in normal adults detected virus in the respiratory secretions of three of four patients during a period of viremia and systemic symptoms 6 to 13 days after inoculation.[25] Detectable virus in respiratory secretions disappeared as the viremia and systemic symptoms diminished, and virus was not demonstrable in respiratory secretions when rash, arthralgias, and arthritis occurred several days later.[25] Recognition of the wide spectrum of disease caused by parvovirus, coupled with well-documented nosocomial outbreaks of infection, has fueled efforts to understand the transmission and control of this virus in hospitals.[53, 193, 396, 499, 528]

Two outbreaks of nosocomial parvovirus B19 infection occurred among hospital staff members after exposure to adolescents with sickle-cell disease and aplastic crisis.[53] Both outbreaks were recognized when symptoms and signs consistent with erythema infectiosum developed in nurses. Of the 40 health care workers who were exposed to the two index cases, 8 (20%) had evidence of past infection and were not susceptible; 12 (38%) of the remaining 32 susceptible health care workers showed evidence of infection by serologic testing, and all but 1 had symptomatic disease. None of the infected individuals were pregnant, and no other complications were reported. All but one of the infected individuals were nurses, and all but two had contact with an index case in the first several days of hospitalization, when titers of virus in the bloodstream and respiratory secretions of patients with aplastic crisis would have been highest. A play therapist was infected after infection control measures had been instituted during the second outbreak, apparently as a consequence of spending less than 5 minutes in the isolation room of one of the patients. She did not wear a mask or have any physical contact with the patient. No community outbreak of erythema infectiosum was noted at the time of these outbreaks.

In another outbreak of parvovirus B19 infection on a children's ward, infection developed in two nurses on the same day.[499] Whether they acquired their infection from an undetected case in the hospital or in the community is not clear, but they apparently transmitted parvovirus to numerous hospital workers and patients. In all, infection occurred in 10 of 30 (33%) exposed, susceptible staff members and in 2 of 9 (22%) exposed, susceptible immunocompromised patients. All but one of the infected staff were symptomatic, but symptoms did not develop in either of the two infected immunocompromised patients, perhaps because they were given prophylactic immune globulin when the outbreak first was recognized.

A third study that used serologic studies to document recent infection with parvovirus B19 found that the risk of parvovirus B19 infection developing in nonimmune health care workers exposed to patients with transient aplastic crisis was equivalent to the risk in nonimmune, nonexposed health care workers on other wards.[528] The risk of infection in the exposed health care workers was low despite failure to place the patients in isolation at the onset of hospitalization.

The risk of infection being acquired from chronically infected immunocompromised patients is less clear. In one study, 10 susceptible health care workers had substantial exposure to an immunocompromised patient with pure red blood cell aplasia and chronic parvovirus B19 infection. Infection did not develop in any of them even though no isolation precautions were instituted for the first 3½ weeks of hospitalization.[355] In another study of an outbreak in a renal transplant unit, an index immunocompromised patient transmitted parvovirus infection to two other immunocompromised patients.[396] Notably, the index case transmitted infection many weeks after the onset of her clinical symptoms. The virus strains from all three patients were confirmed to be identical by molecular techniques.

From these studies, it is apparent that parvovirus B19 infection can be transmitted by acutely infected patients, probably as a result of the high levels of virus in their blood, as well as their respiratory sections. The likelihood of transmission from chronically infected, immunocompromised patients is less clear; however, from the report just described, these patients clearly can transmit infection. The mode of transmission is not apparent, but it probably involves direct or indirect contact with respiratory secretions or droplet contact transmission. Therefore, gloves and gowns should be worn during contact with infected patients or fomites contaminated with respiratory secretions, and a mask should be worn during close contact.[228] The transmission of parvovirus to the play therapist described earlier despite her lack of close contact with an infected patient has led to concern about possible airborne transmission, but the need for the use of isolation rooms with negative air pressure has not been established, and they are not recommended.[228]

Limited data in one of the outbreaks described earlier suggest that standard immune globulin preparations may be useful in mitigating the consequences of infection in high-risk, exposed susceptible contacts.[499] However, data are insufficient at present to recommend the routine use of immune globulin for postexposure prophylaxis.

HEPATITIS A VIRUS

Although nosocomial outbreaks of hepatitis A are uncommon, this pathogen can cause major epidemics before infection is detected and contained. The largest outbreak of hepatitis A occurred as a result of blood transfusion from a single donor who was viremic but symptomatic disease had not yet developed; 11 newborns received contaminated transfusions, and 55 secondary cases occurred in two hospitals.[470] Other transfusion outbreaks have been described,[37, 343] as have outbreaks traced to asymptomatic excretion by an infected child[178] and vertical transmission from mother to infant.[668]

Because children, particularly newborns and young infants, usually have subclinical infection, outbreaks generally are detected only when secondary symptomatic infections develop in adult caregivers.[37, 178, 343, 470, 668] Given the long incubation period of this infection, ample opportunity exists for transmission of virus to caregivers and other hospitalized children before secondary symptomatic cases are recognized. Secondary cases in hospitalized children and their young siblings are usually asymptomatic, thus facilitating amplification of the outbreak in both the hospital and the community through successive cycles of infection and transmission. Direct contact is responsible for transmission of the virus from infected children to caregivers; indirect contact is generally responsible for transmission of the virus from one child to another in the hospital setting.

Given this epidemiology, controlling a nosocomial hepatitis A outbreak is difficult and usually requires assistance of the local health department, especially if nonhospitalized contacts or more than one institution is involved. To limit the potential for indirect contact transmission, hospitalized infected children should be cohorted. Hand hygiene and the use of barrier precautions should be emphasized to prevent direct contact transmission to caregivers and indirect contact transmission to other children.[228] These precautions should be maintained for the duration of hospitalization in children younger than 3 years and for 2 weeks in children 3 to 14 years of age.[228] Older children hospitalized with symptomatic disease have rapidly decreasing titers of virus in their stool by the time that they become symptomatic, and they are not very contagious. Nevertheless, barrier precautions should be used for 7 days.[228]

Immune globulin should be administered to all exposed, susceptible individuals.[14] Symptomatic health care providers should be furloughed until 1 week after the onset of symptomatic infection or until all susceptible persons have received immune globulin.[14] Tracing contacts is necessary to prevent additional secondary cases. Hepatitis A vaccine can be administered concurrently with immune globulin to previously unimmunized patients if vaccination is indicated for these individuals.[15]

ENTEROVIRUSES

Numerous outbreaks of nosocomial enterovirus have been reported, and the majority have occurred in newborn nurseries.[43, 117, 287, 325, 341, 522, 640] In most cases, adult caregivers infected in the community transmitted the virus to one or more hospitalized children through direct contact, with subsequent indirect contact transmission from one child to another. In one nursery outbreak, the virus was introduced by a perinatally infected child.[522] Newborns with severe underlying illness were more likely to be infected, presumably because the prolonged and intensive care that these infants required provided more opportunities for transmission.[341, 522] Nosocomial enterovirus infections in newborn infants can be severe—even fatal—but mild and subclinical illness also may occur.[450, 522] The presence of maternally derived antibody may play a role in limiting the severity of disease in some infants.[450, 522]

Surveys of nosocomial infections in pediatric wards indicate that nosocomial enterovirus infections are uncommon,[205, 653, 676] but the potential for nosocomial transmission of these viruses is substantial. Large community outbreaks of echovirus and coxsackievirus infection occur predictably every summer and fall. Because virus is excreted in stool for long periods, a large number of hospitalized children and caregivers certainly are excreting virus during these periods. Detection of nosocomial infection may be compromised because viral cultures may not be readily available, some enteroviruses are difficult to cultivate in tissue culture, and infection may not become evident until after discharge.

Like hepatitis A, enteroviruses are picornaviruses; the use of hand hygiene and barrier precautions is of paramount importance to prevent transmission, and cohorting of infected infants is prudent.[228] A recent report has demonstrated the value of early diagnosis with PCR and aggressive control measures.[33] The upper respiratory tract may be involved in acute enteroviral infection, but most authorities do not recommend the use of masks during the care of infected patients.[228] These same principles should be applied to confirmed or suspected enteroviral infections in children, especially young diapered children, although the need for cohorting is debatable and it may not be feasible during summer and fall epidemics. The efficacy of immune globulin as treatment prophylaxis for individuals exposed during the course of an outbreak is unclear, but it may be helpful if the preparation used has significant titers of antibody to the outbreak strain, especially in newborn infants, who are at risk for severe disease.[2] A new antiviral agent, pleconaril, may be useful in treating serious infection.[552]

RABIES

Rabies has been transmitted by corneal transplants,[24] but spread via contact with infected patients has not been reported.

TUBERCULOSIS

The number of new cases of tuberculosis in the United States has reached an all-time low.[107] In addition, the number and proportion of cases of multidrug-resistant *Mycobacterium tuberculosis* (MDRTB) have decreased in comparison to the early 1990s. However, the threat of nosocomial transmission of tuberculosis is still important because of the increasing proportion of tuberculosis cases in the United States that occur in foreign-born persons and continuing problems with MDRTB in many regions of the world.[107, 192]

This risk was demonstrated dramatically by outbreaks of MDRTB in adult patients and health care workers in several hospitals in New York and Florida in the 1990s.[50, 139, 184, 216, 323, 487] One of these outbreaks involved transmission of MDRTB in the hospital nursery and resulted in infection in infants, mothers, and health care workers.[469] This outbreak and others illustrate that nosocomial tuberculosis in hospitals caring for pediatric patients occurs almost exclusively as a result of transmission of *M. tuberculosis* from infected adults—parents, visitors, and health care workers—to other children and adults.[38, 235, 469, 629, 671] Probable transmission from infected children in health care settings has been described.[423, 521] However, the risk of transmission from a child is very small because children infrequently have cavitary disease and, consequently, have fewer tubercle bacilli in their endobronchial secretions and young children do not tend to generate aerosols of airborne droplet nuclei.[625] Nonetheless, transmission from children can occur, as evidenced by extensive transmission from a 9-year-old child with bilateral cavitary disease.[151]

The risk of nosocomial tuberculosis occurring in adult hospitals has been minimized by prompt recognition and treatment of pulmonary tuberculosis, adequate isolation of infectious patients in rooms with negative air pressure relative to the hallway, and proper use of personal protective equipment.[65, 96, 418, 635, 678] If rooms with appropriate ventilation are unavailable, alternative engineering solutions may be useful, such as well-placed and maintained ultraviolet lights.[95, 460] Personnel entering the rooms of infected patients should wear respiratory protection devices. Particulate respirators with a National Institute for Occupational Safety and Health certification of N95 or better satisfy the CDC specifications for these devices.[96, 461] These devices must be fit-tested on the individuals using them according to the standards of the Occupational Health and Safety Administration.[96] Prompt identification of tuberculosis in parents, visitors, and health care workers in hospitals caring for pediatric patients is an integral part of reducing the risk of transmission of nosocomial tuberculosis.

INVASIVE BACTERIAL INFECTIONS

Nosocomial transmission of *N. meningitidis* is a rare occurrence and has been demonstrated in hospitalized patients only when the index patient has meningococcal pneumonia,[134, 550] an uncommon clinical manifestation of disease in children. Other situations in which nosocomial transmission has occurred have involved special circumstances. For instance, a mother became infected after nursing her infant who was hospitalized with meningococcemia,[416] and fatal disease developed in several microbiology laboratory workers after working with cultures of this microorganism.[91] Hospital personnel caring for patients, on the other hand, appear to be at minimal risk unless they have extensive face-to-face contact and fail to wear a mask.

Nosocomial transmission of *Haemophilus influenzae* and *Streptococcus pneumoniae* also has been regarded as a rare phenomenon, but it may be more common than previously recognized. A few reports from the 1980s documented transmission of *H. influenzae* type b (Hib) among pediatric patients,[40, 47] and cases in elderly adults and even hospital workers were reported in the late 1980s and early 1990s.[305, 433, 485, 613] Widespread immunization of infants with Hib conjugate vaccine has greatly reduced the risk of nosocomial transmission of this microorganism in pediatric patients. Numerous outbreaks of nosocomial infection caused by nonencapsulated *H. influenzae* in elderly patients and hospital staff also have been reported.[22, 305]

In recent years, many outbreaks of nosocomial infection in hospitalized adults and residents of nursing homes by penicillin-resistant *S. pneumoniae* have been documented in North America and Europe.[164, 419, 446, 473, 674] Fewer reports of nosocomial multidrug-resistant pneumococcocal infections in pediatric patients exist,[128, 157] although this problem has been well documented in hospitalized children in South Africa for many years.[217]

N. meningitidis, H. influenzae, and *S. pneumoniae* are spread by droplet contact transmission. Masks should be worn by health care workers during the care of patients with suspected invasive meningococcal disease until the patient has completed 24 hours of parenteral antimicrobial therapy.[228] In the past, the use of masks during care of patients with Hib infection was variable in many hospitals. However, a CDC guideline recommends the use of masks to prevent droplet contact transmission from patients infected with *H. influenzae* until they have completed 24 hours of parenteral antimicrobial therapy.[228] The guideline does not recommend the use of a mask when caring for patients with *S. pneumoniae* or even penicillin-resistant *S. pneumoniae,*[228] perhaps because nosocomial transmission of this microorganism has not been a problem in United States in the past. However, given the reports of nosocomial transmission of *S. pneumoniae* discussed earlier, we recommend the use of masks when caring for patients with infections caused by penicillin-resistant *S. pneumoniae.* Antimicrobial prophylaxis should be administered to persons who have close, unprotected contact with patients infected with *N. meningitidis,* but it is not recommended for exposure to patients infected with *H. influenzae* or *S. pneumoniae* unless an outbreak is clearly in progress.

Invasive bacterial infections in neonates, including infections caused by *S. aureus,* group B streptococci, *Citrobacter* spp., and *Enterobacter sakazakii,* are discussed in another section of this chapter ("Nosocomial Infections in Special Populations," "Newborn Infants").

ECTOPARASITES

Scabies and pediculosis are common infections in children, and incidental diagnosis of these infections in hospitalized children is not an uncommon occurrence. A large number of outbreaks of scabies have been reported from a variety of health care institutions.[377] The presence of crusted scabies, which is associated with defects in cellular immunity, including HIV infection, increases the risk of transmission occurring because of the large number of mites in these lesions.[377] Although nosocomial transmission of pediculosis is possible, the direct or indirect contact necessary to spread this infection (i.e., head-to-head contact or sharing of combs) is less likely to occur in medical settings than at home.

INTESTINAL HELMINTHS

Person-to-person transmission of four intestinal helminths, *Enterobius vermicularis* (pinworm), *Strongyloides stercoralis, Hymenolepis nana,* and *Taenia solium,* is possible because these microorganisms do not require an intermediate host and the eggs or larvae excreted in stool are infectious.[376] However, evidence for nosocomial transmission of these microorganisms is limited.[376]

UNUSUAL INFECTIONS, INCLUDING INFECTIONS CAUSED BY AGENTS OF BIOLOGIC WARFARE

A variety of unusual, potentially fatal infections may be nosocomially transmitted. Because international air travel has increased the mobility of the world's population, persons may travel long distances during the incubation period of infections acquired in remote settings. In addition, some of the potential agents of bioterrorism (e.g., smallpox virus, *Yersinia pestis,* hemorrhagic fever viruses) are highly transmissible and could result in secondary nosocomial cases after a primary bioterrorism attack.[28, 68, 168, 289, 312] A high index of suspicion for these infections and prompt institution of appropriate isolation precautions as indicated are necessary to reduce the risk of nosocomial transmission.

Smallpox is the most feared of the potential agents of biologic warfare because it can be transmitted via droplet nuclei over large distances, the case-fatality ratio is approximately 30 percent, no effective treatment exists, and much of the world's population is either nonimmune or was immunized in the distant past.[289] Even a very limited number of cases of smallpox would be a global public health emergency, and detailed plans for containment would be needed. Airborne and contact isolation precautions must be instituted for hospitalized patients, and health care workers caring for these patients must be vaccinated.[112, 113, 289]

Plague is endemic in portions of the western United States and other countries. No person-to-person transmission of plague has been identified in the United States for more than a half century,[312] but an outbreak in India illustrated the potential for importation of plague to other countries.[94, 95] Droplet transmission of *Y. pestis* is well documented from persons with pulmonary involvement. Health care workers should wear masks during the care of patients with signs or symptoms of pulmonary involvement.[312] Tetracycline, doxycycline, sulfonamides, chloramphenicol, and perhaps fluoroquinolones can be used for prophylaxis of contacts.[312]

Ebola, Marburg, Lassa, and Crimean-Congo viruses and the New World arenaviruses have been spread in hospitals by close contact with infectious body fluids or reuse of contaminated needles.[45, 68, 333, 335, 453, 491, 537, 612, 636] Nosocomial transmission of hantavirus in the United States has not been reported but has occurred with Andes virus, another cause of hantavirus pulmonary syndrome.[481] Ebola, Marburg, Lassa, New World arenaviruses, Rift Valley fever, yellow fever, Omsk hemorrhagic fever, and Kyasanur Forest disease viruses have been proposed as potential biologic weapons.[68] Of these viruses, only Ebola, Marburg, and Lassa viruses and the New World arenaviruses are spread from person to person (see earlier).[68] The bulk of evidence suggests that airborne transmission of these viruses does not occur in clinical settings, although epidemiologic data are insufficient to exclude this possibility.[98] When caring for these patients, airborne isolation precautions should be instituted, as well as additional viral hemorrhagic fever–specific precautions. Emphasis should be placed on enhanced barrier precautions to avoid contact with the copious amounts of infected material typically encountered in the care of such patients.[68]

Nosocomial Infections Related to Invasive Devices, Procedures, and Treatments

INFECTIONS RELATED TO INTRAVASCULAR CATHETERS AND INFUSIONS

Local infections associated with the use of intravascular catheters include infection at the site where the catheter exits the skin (exit-site infection), infection along the subcutaneous tract of a tunneled catheter (tunnel infection), and infection in the subcutaneous pocket containing an implanted catheter (pocket infection).[441, 475] Phlebitis is a common local complication related to the use of intravascular catheters, but it usually is caused by chemical or mechanical irritation and occurs less commonly in children than adults.[226] Suppurative thrombophlebitis is a rare event in children.[336]

Systemic infections related to the use of intravascular catheters include bloodstream infections occurring as a result of microbial colonization of the catheter (catheter-related bloodstream infection) and contamination of fluids or medications infused through the catheter (infusate-related bloodstream infection).[441, 475] Endocarditis, septic thrombophlebitis, and infection at other body sites as a result of hematogenous seeding (e.g., meningitis, pyelonephritis, hepatic or splenic abscesses, osteomyelitis, septic arthritis, and endophthalmitis) are serious complications of bloodstream infection.

The risk of endemic local and systemic infection associated with intravascular catheters varies with the type of catheter in use. Percutaneously inserted peripheral intravenous catheters, especially catheters made with modern pliant, nonthrombogenic material, are associated with a very low rate of local infection in children, and bloodstream infections are rare occurrences.[226, 227, 596]

Rates of local and bloodstream infection are also low in newborn infants,[225] but infusion of parenteral nutrition with lipid emulsion through these catheters significantly increases the risk for bloodstream infection with coagulase-negative staphylococci and *Candida*.[34, 77, 209, 567] Peripheral arterial catheters generally also have a low rate of endemic local and systemic infectious complications; two reports studying a total of more than 400 arterial catheters did not identify any catheter-related bloodstream infections.[179, 220]

The vast majority of endemic catheter-related bloodstream infections in pediatric patients are associated with central venous catheters.[321] As shown in Tables 231–2 and 231–3, rates of bloodstream infection associated with central venous catheters in pediatric ICUs and central venous and umbilical catheters in newborn ICUs are higher than in adult ICUs in hospitals participating in the NNIS System.[463] Rates of infection in low-birth-weight infants (<1000 g) in newborn ICUs are higher than those of any other ICU population.[463] These data do not distinguish rates of infection associated with specific catheter types, nor do they distinguish whether a specific catheter is the source of the infection in patients with multiple catheters in place at the same time.

Comparisons of bloodstream infection rates associated with different types of central venous catheters in pediatric patients are confounded by numerous factors.[685] The patient populations in which these catheters are used have diverse underlying diseases (e.g., cancer, cystic fibrosis, prematurity, short-bowel syndrome, AIDS) with a widely varying intrinsic risk for the development of bloodstream infection. Even in pediatric oncology patients, the risk varies considerably with the type of cancer and the intensity of chemotherapy,[313] and younger children have a higher risk of acquiring infection, even when the underlying disease and the type of catheter used are similar.[313, 694] Use of the catheter for multiple purposes and infusion of parenteral nutrition with lipid emulsion also increase the risk for infection.[34, 77, 339]

With these caveats, a review suggests that rates of bloodstream infection are lower in totally implanted (0.1 to 0.7 infections/1000 catheter days) than tunneled (0.4 to 7.8 infections/1000 catheter days) catheters.[685] This conclusion is supported by several studies that directly compared rates of infection between these two types of catheters.[371, 447, 586, 694] These studies demonstrated lower rates of infection with implanted catheters, although statistically significant differences were not seen in every report.

In adults, rates of bloodstream infection associated with percutaneously inserted central venous catheters are at least several-fold higher than rates associated with either tunneled or implanted catheters,[146] and this observation appears to be true in infants and children as well.[306, 628] Rates of infection associated with hemodialysis catheters or intracardiac catheters in pediatric patients after cardiac surgery have not been reported. The use of midline and peripherally inserted central venous catheters is increasing in newborn ICUs, pediatric ICUs, and pediatric wards. A randomized trial of peripherally inserted central venous catheters versus peripheral intravenous catheters in very low birth weight infants found no difference in rates of bloodstream infection associated with these two types of catheters. A study of umbilical catheters in neonates found that bloodstream infection occurred in 5 percent of neonates with umbilical artery catheters and in 3 percent of neonates with umbilical venous catheters (rates of infections per 1000 catheter days were not reported).[366]

In contrast to endemic infections, which are associated closely with the type of catheter used, epidemics of bloodstream infection generally are related to other factors.[51] Improperly disinfected pressure transducers are the most common cause of epidemics of bloodstream infection.[51] The use of disposable domes with reusable transducers may reduce, but does not obviate, this risk. Microorganisms contaminating the transducer head may be transferred to the dome and the infusion system by the hands of workers who manipulate these components of the apparatus during setup, calibration, and blood drawing.[51] Detailed investigation of practices is often necessary to identify and eliminate causes of bloodstream infection outbreaks, as illustrated by an outbreak of candidemia in a newborn ICU related to retrograde administration of medications through intravenous tubing.[592]

The principal risk factors for catheter-related nosocomial bloodstream infection in adults have been identified.[146, 147, 475, 486] Heavy colonization of the skin at the catheter exit site is an important risk factor for colonization of the external surface of catheters of all types and is correlated with an increased risk for bloodstream infection.[146, 147, 475] Colonization of the catheter hub is also an important risk factor for bloodstream infection, especially disease occurring late in the course of central venous catheterization.[163, 383] Other risk factors related to central venous catheters include longer duration of insertion (>3 days), insertion in the internal jugular vein as opposed to the subclavian vein, use of catheters with multiple lumina as opposed to a single lumen, and the presence of a mural or atrial thrombus.[146, 147, 475] Both the level and the composition of nurse staffing have been associated with bloodstream infections in adult surgical ICUs—a low nurse-to-patient ratio and a low regular nurse (as opposed to pool nurse)-to-patient ratio were associated with a higher risk for bloodstream infection.[214, 546]

Information regarding risk factors in children and newborn infants is far more limited than that in adults. Two studies of peripheral intravenous catheters in pediatric patients found that the likelihood of colonization of the external surface of the catheter was slightly greater with increasing duration of insertion, but bloodstream infections were extremely uncommon events even in patients with colonized catheters.[226, 227] A study of catheter colonization in newborn ICU patients found that duration of insertion longer than 3 days was a significant risk factor for colonization of peripheral intravenous and umbilical catheters.[148] A similar trend was seen with central venous catheters in this patient population, although the number of catheters studied was limited and no conclusions could be drawn with regard to the risk for development of bloodstream infection.[148] Current information is not sufficient to state whether the site of insertion of central venous catheters has an impact on the risk for infection, although one study in pediatric ICU patients found similar rates of infection between catheters inserted in the femoral vein and catheters inserted into veins at other sites.[628] As in adult patients, the risk for infection is higher with the use of larger catheters (i.e., multiple-lumen versus single-lumen catheters).[130] Finally, a series of studies of coagulase-negative staphylococcal bloodstream infections in patients in newborn ICUs found that length of stay, birth weight, and administration of lipid emulsions were significant risk factors.[34, 209, 210] No studies in children or newborn infants have examined colonization of the catheter hub.

Microorganisms associated with catheter-related bloodstream infections in pediatric and newborn ICUs participating in the NNIS System are displayed in Tables 231–5 and 231–6.[234, 538] In both populations, the most common cause of bloodstream infection is coagulase-negative staphylococci. Other gram-positive bacteria, including *S. aureus*, enterococci, and various streptococci, also are relatively common causes. Ten to 20 percent of infections are caused by gram-negative bacteria, including *E. coli, P. aeruginosa, K. pneumoniae, Enterobacter, Acinetobacter, Serratia marcescens, Citrobacter,* and other aerobic gram-negative bacilli. *C. albicans,* other *Candida* spp., and other fungi together cause 5 to 10 percent of infections. Atypical mycobacteria occasionally cause bloodstream infections.[424]

The mechanisms involved in the pathogenesis of infections associated with intravascular catheters and infusions are depicted in Figure 231–5. A large number of studies,

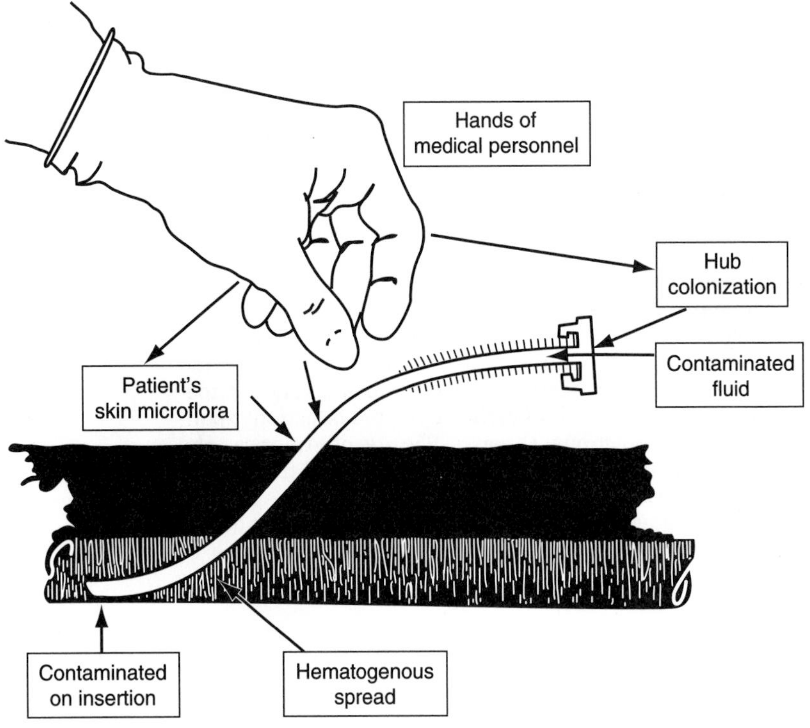

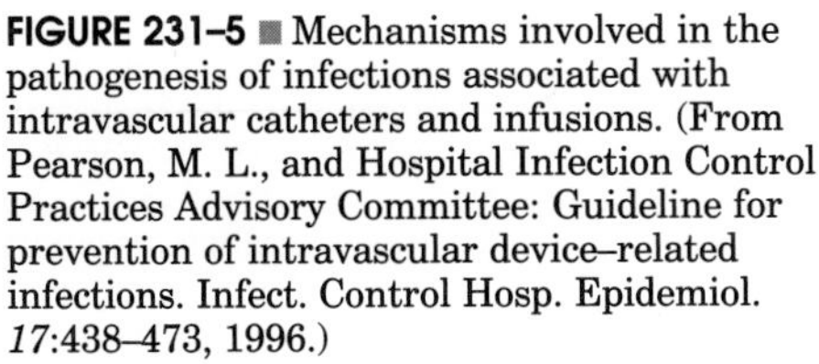
FIGURE 231–5 ■ Mechanisms involved in the pathogenesis of infections associated with intravascular catheters and infusions. (From Pearson, M. L., and Hospital Infection Control Practices Advisory Committee: Guideline for prevention of intravascular device–related infections. Infect. Control Hosp. Epidemiol. *17*:438–473, 1996.)

including studies involving molecular typing of isolates, have demonstrated that most infections arise from microorganisms colonizing the skin at the insertion site that migrate along the external surface of the catheter through its subcutaneous tract and into the blood vessel.[146, 147, 475] Colonization of the interior surface of the catheter occurs via contamination of the catheter hub.[146, 147, 475] The relative contributions of these two mechanisms may depend on the duration of catheterization.[516] Detailed microbiologic studies and scanning electron microscopy have demonstrated that colonization of the external surface predominates in the first 10 days after insertion whereas colonization of the internal surface increases with the length of catheterization and is significantly more common in catheters that have been in place for more than 30 days.[516] Microorganisms on the hands of health care workers can contaminate the catheter, the insertion site, or the hub during insertion and maintenance of the infusion system.

A variety of microbial and host factors play a role in the pathogenesis of bloodstream infection. For example, capsular polysaccharide adhesin, which is a component of the capsule of coagulase-negative staphylococci, facilitates adherence of these bacteria to prosthetic material, as well as the formation of biofilm ("slime") and intercellular adhesion.[307, 435] *Candida* spp. also may produce slime, particularly in the presence of glucose-containing fluids.[74] Interactions among organisms in mixed biofilms likewise may contribute to colonization of catheter surfaces.[3]

Catheter materials are important in catheter colonization and infection. Catheters made of polyvinyl chloride or polyethylene are less resistant to colonization in vitro than are catheters made of Teflon, silicon elastomer, or polyurethane. Trauma to blood vessels is more likely to occur with the use of stiff plastics (e.g., polyvinyl chloride) than the newer plastic materials (Teflon, silicon elastomer, or polyurethane); such trauma predisposes to the development of phlebitis and infection. Other factors such as surface irregularities and the thrombogenicity of catheter material also may play a role. Catheters that are coated or impregnated with anti-infective agents (e.g., benzalkonium chloride, chlorhexidine–silver sulfadiazine, minocycline-rifampin) to resist bacterial colonization have been developed (see additional discussion later).[146]

Other mechanisms involved in the pathogenesis of these infections are depicted in Figure 231–5. Contaminated intravenous infusions,[412, 592] medications,[55, 258] and narcotics (as a result of criminal tampering)[408, 480]; blood products[100]; and hemodynamic monitoring systems[51] have resulted in serious outbreaks of infection. Purposeful contamination of infusates as a form of child abuse also has been reported.[388] The frequency of hematogenous seeding of the catheter from a distant site of infection is unknown but is likely to be uncommon.

Table 231–8 lists clinical and culture criteria for the diagnosis of infections related to intravascular catheters and infusions.[441] These criteria are drawn from a detailed guideline for the management of catheter-related infections sponsored by the Infectious Diseases Society of America, the American College of Critical Care Medicine, and the Society for Healthcare Epidemiology of America. Definitions used by the NNIS System are similar but do not specifically define separate local infections and include two subcategories of bloodstream infection (laboratory-confirmed bloodstream infection and clinical sepsis).[229]

Potential bloodstream infections should be evaluated with two blood cultures at a minimum before the institution of antimicrobial therapy, including at least one blood sample drawn by venipuncture.[441] If indications for removal of the

TABLE 231–8 ■ DIAGNOSTIC CRITERIA FOR INFECTIONS RELATED TO INTRAVASCULAR CATHETERS AND INFUSIONS

Infection	Diagnostic Criteria
Catheter colonization	Significant growth of a microorganism in a quantitative or semiquantitative culture of the catheter tip, subcutaneous catheter segment, or catheter hub
Phlebitis	Induration or erythema, warmth, and pain or tenderness around the catheter exit site
Exit-site infection	
Microbiologic	Exudate at the catheter exit site yields a microorganism with or without concomitant bloodstream infection
Clinical	Erythema, tenderness, and/or induration within 2 cm of the catheter exit sites; may be associated with other signs and symptoms of infection such as fever or pus emerging from the exit site, with or without concomitant bloodstream infection
Tunnel infection	Tenderness, erythema, and/or induration >2 cm from the exit site, along the subcutaneous tract of a tunneled catheter, with or without concomitant bloodstream infection
Pocket infection	Infected fluid in the subcutaneous pocket of a totally implanted intravascular device. Often associated with tenderness, erythema, and/or induration over the pocket; spontaneous rupture and drainage; or necrosis of the overlying skin, with or without concomitant bloodstream infection
Bloodstream infection	
Infusate related	Concordant growth of the same organism from infusate and cultures of percutaneously obtained blood samples with no other identifiable source of infection
Catheter related	Bacteremia or fungemia in a patient who has an intravascular device and ≥1 positve result of a culture of blood samples obtained from the peripheral vein, clinical manifestations of infection (e.g., fever, chills, and/or hypotension), and no apparent source for bloodstream infection (with the exception of the catheter). One of the following should be present: a positive result of semiquantitative (≥15 CFU per catheter segment) or quantitative (≥10^2 CFU per catheter segment) catheter culture and the same organism (species and antibiogram) isolated from a catheter segment and a peripheral blood sample, simultaneous quantitative cultures of blood samples with a ratio of ≥5:1 (CVC vs. peripheral), and differential time to positivity (i.e., a positive result of culture from a CVC is obtained at least 2 hours earlier than a positive result of a culture from peripheral blood)

CFU, colony forming units; CVC, central venous catheter.
Modified from Mermel, I., A., Farr, B. M., Sherertz, R. J., et al.: Guidelines for the management of intravascular catheter-related infections. Clin. Infect. Dis. *32*:1249–1272, 2001.

catheter exist (see additional discussion later), it should be removed by aseptic technique and culture performed to determine whether it is colonized. Nontunneled central venous catheters may be changed over a wire or removed and cultured. The semiquantitative roll-plate culture technique is the traditional and most widely available method for culturing of the catheter.[415] The presence of more than 15 colony-forming units (CFU) is regarded as evidence of colonization of the external surface of the catheter but does not reliably predict the risk of bloodstream infection; the presence of more than 100 CFU has greater positive predictive value for bloodstream infection.[415] However, the roll-plate technique does not detect colonization of the catheter hub or the intraluminal surface of the catheter. Quantitative culturing of catheter segments (i.e., the catheter tip, subcutaneous segment, or hub), which involves flushing the segment with broth culture media or sonicating the segment in broth followed by serial dilution of the broth and plating on blood agar, is more sensitive than the roll-plate technique because it detects colonization of both the external and internal surfaces of the catheter.[518, 593, 594, 601] One study suggests that sonication is the most important procedure for increasing the recovery of bacteria from removed catheters.[593] Unfortunately, quantitative catheter cultures are time-consuming and expensive, and they are not universally available.

Because these techniques require removal of the catheter, some investigators have attempted to diagnose catheter-related bloodstream infection by comparing quantitative culture on blood drawn through the catheter with culture of blood obtained by venipuncture (paired cultures) or by culturing multiple samples drawn through the catheter only (unpaired cultures). A small study of paired cultures from children with tunneled catheters found that either a 10-fold higher concentration in the catheter specimen in comparison to the venipuncture specimen or a concentration of more than 2000 CFU/mL in the catheter specimen was predictive of catheter-related bloodstream infection.[527] However, a meta-analysis of studies performed in adults and children found that paired and unpaired blood cultures were equivalent in their performance characteristics.[601] A subsequent study examined the time to positivity of paired specimens analyzed by an automated blood culture incubator/detector.[64] In cases of confirmed catheter-related infection, this study found that the sample drawn through the catheter was positive at least 2 hours earlier than the venipuncture sample, presumably because of the larger number of organisms in the specimen drawn through the catheter. This technique is attractive because it uses information (time to positivity) already provided by existing automated systems and avoids the necessity of performing labor-intensive quantitative culture procedures. However, this study was relatively small, and the technique requires that consistent volumes of blood be inoculated into each of the paired culture bottles.

Other investigators have examined rapid techniques. In a study of infants, Gram stain and an acridine-orange leukocyte Cytospin test of blood drawn through a central venous catheter had 87 percent sensitivity and 94 percent specificity for the diagnosis of catheter-related bloodstream infections when compared with quantitative culture of blood samples drawn from the catheter and by venipuncture.[559] A follow-up study of this technique in an adult population demonstrated that the test had a sensitivity of 96 percent and a specificity of 92 percent.[342] An advantage of this test is that it can be completed in less than 1 hour. Buffy coat Gram stain of a blood sample drawn from the catheter may reveal yeast forms in some patients with candidemia. If the catheter is removed, Gram staining of adherent material also may facilitate rapid diagnosis.

In practice, several difficulties arise in the diagnosis of nosocomial bloodstream infections. Physicians' designation of microorganisms isolated from blood cultures as pathogens or contaminants may be confounded by the patient's age and underlying condition and the presence of an intravascular catheter, particularly a central venous catheter. For example, in one study, physicians were more likely to interpret the coagulase-negative staphylococci in blood cultures from very low birth weight infants as clinically significant.[211]

The terminology used to describe the clinical manifestations of bloodstream infections in pediatric patients requires standardization. Consensus definitions of the systemic inflammatory response syndrome (a condition arising from a variety of processes, including bloodstream infection), sepsis, severe sepsis, and septic shock in adult patients have been published.[67] An epidemiologic study of these conditions found that bloodstream infections occurred in 17 percent of patients with sepsis, 25 percent of patients with severe sepsis, and 69 percent of patients with septic shock.[523] Although the pathophysiology and management of sepsis in pediatric patients also have been reviewed,[563] precise definitions of sepsis in children and newborn infants have not been promulgated and validated. The definition of bloodstream infection used by the NNIS System lists clinical criteria for the diagnosis of sepsis, including criteria for use in children younger than 12 months, but the sensitivity and specificity of these criteria have not been examined.

In many instances, sufficient culture information is not available to satisfy the diagnostic criteria in Table 231–8. Obtaining samples for culture by venipuncture is difficult in young children, and clinicians may be reluctant to obtain blood for more than one culture from low-birth-weight infants. Central venous catheters often are not removed for culture because of potential complications associated with reinsertion of a new catheter and the fact that many catheter-related bloodstream infections can be treated with the catheter in place. Finally, unless infusate-related bloodstream infection is suspected, obtaining cultures of intravenous fluids or medications often is overlooked.

Empiric antimicrobial therapy given for suspected bloodstream infection while awaiting culture results should be based on the severity of the patient's clinical disease, the nature and severity of the patient's underlying condition, and knowledge of the relative frequency and local susceptibility patterns of nosocomial pathogens. The guideline cited previously contains detailed recommendations for the management of these infections.[441] In most situations, empiric therapy should include an agent effective against gram-positive bacteria, such as nafcillin, oxacillin, or vancomycin, and an agent effective against most gram-negative bacteria, including *Pseudomonas,* such as ceftazidime or cefepime, with or without an aminoglycoside. In institutions where infection with MRSA is common, the use of vancomycin is appropriate; otherwise, nafcillin or oxacillin is reasonable. Gentamicin is generally equivalent to ceftazidime or cefepime in activity against gram-negative rods, is synergistic with vancomycin against susceptible *Enterococcus* spp., and is much less costly. Unless renal toxicity or ototoxicity is a major concern, gentamicin may be appropriate empiric coverage against gram-negative rods. Empiric use of two agents with activity against gram-negative rods (e.g., ceftazidime or cefepime plus gentamicin) is appropriate in a severely ill patient or when infection with a resistant gram-negative rod is suspected. Empiric antifungal therapy can be initiated in situations in which suspicion of fungemia is very high (i.e., a severely ill patient who is colonized with *Candida* or a neutropenic patient who is already receiving broad-spectrum antibacterial therapy). Once culture information is available, the treatment regimen can be tailored accordingly or discontinued if no infection is identified.

The aforementioned management guideline also reviews the efficacy of the "antibiotic lock" technique for treatment of tunneled catheter–related bacteremia.[441] The concept behind this approach is that organisms embedded in biofilms on the luminal surfaces of long-term, tunneled catheters may be killed more effectively by antibiotic concentrations 100 to 1000 higher than standard concentrations of therapeutic parenteral antibiotics.[441] An antibiotic solution (usually vancomycin or gentamicin) in a concentration of 1 to 5 mg/mL with an appropriate concentration of heparin (usually 50 to 100 U) is infused into the catheter in sufficient volume (2 to 5 mL) to fill the lumen and is left in place while the catheter is not being used.[441] The volume of instilled antibiotic is removed before infusion of the next dose of antibiotic or intravenous medication or solution. This treatment approach may be used with or without concomitant systemic therapy in carefully selected patients with tunneled catheter–related bacteremia caused by intraluminal colonization of the catheter.[441]

No evidence indicates that the use of thrombolytic agents as adjunctive treatment of catheter-related bloodstream infection provides any benefit. Two noncontrolled studies reported good responses to treatment of catheter-related bloodstream infection with a combination of antimicrobial therapy and low-dose urokinase.[329, 580] However, two subsequent randomized, controlled trials found no benefit from the combination of urokinase and antimicrobial therapy.[30, 370] Recombinant tissue plasminogen activator has proved effective in restoring flow to occluded central venous catheters,[316, 510] but this agent has not been studied as adjunctive therapy for catheter-related bloodstream infection.

Substantial evidence indicates that most uncomplicated bloodstream infections associated with central venous catheters can be treated effectively without removing the catheter.[441, 685] However, treatment of catheter-associated fungemia without removal of the catheter has a relatively low success rate and may be associated with higher mortality rates, as well as other complications.[156, 441] Strong consideration also should be given to removing catheters associated with difficult-to-treat bacteria, such as antimicrobial-resistant enterococci or gram-negative rods. In our experience, in situ treatment is not as likely to be successful with implanted catheters, but little published data specifically address this issue. Percutaneously inserted central venous catheters may be changed over a wire and the catheter tip sent for culture. If culture of the tip is negative, the replacement catheter can be left in place. If culture of the tip is positive, the replacement catheter should be removed and a new catheter inserted at a different site. Catheters should be removed immediately if evidence of embolic phenomena, septic thrombophlebitis, or endocarditis is present or if the patient is hemodynamically unstable.

Few data exist regarding the optimal duration of therapy for bloodstream infection if the catheter remains in place, but experience suggests that 10 to 14 days is usually adequate. If the catheter is removed, shorter courses of therapy (5 to 7 days) are appropriate for uncomplicated infections caused by less virulent pathogens such as coagulase-negative staphylococci.

Persistently positive blood cultures despite the administration of antimicrobial therapy or recrudescence of infection shortly after therapy is completed should prompt removal of the catheter. The need to remove catheters from patients with persistent fever but no positive culture results and no evidence of infection at another site is controversial and should be approached on a case-by-case basis.

Some success has been reported in treating uncomplicated exit-site infections with the catheter in place.[441, 685] A trial of a combination of local and systemic antimicrobial treatment is warranted before a decision to remove the catheter is made. In contrast, treatment outcomes of tunnel or pocket infections are generally poor if the catheter is left in place.[424, 441, 685]

A guideline for the prevention of infections related to intravascular catheters and infusions has been published recently.[475] In addition, a recent review has focused on the role of novel technologies in the prevention of these infections.[146, 147] Key aspects of the prevention of these infections are emphasized in the following paragraphs.

Intravascular catheters and infusions should be used only when necessary and only for as long as necessary. Caregivers should monitor catheterized patients closely for signs of local and systemic infection. Interventions directed at minimizing contamination of the catheter during insertion include the use of an effective skin antiseptic (chlorhexidine-based agents are more effective than povidone-iodine– or alcohol-based agents).[116, 146, 225, 413] Full sterile barrier precautions (e.g., sterile gowns, gloves, and large drapes) should be used during the insertion of central venous catheters.[517]

Several studies, including a study involving neonates, have examined the efficacy of a chlorhexidine-impregnated sponge placed at the catheter insertion site.[224, 279, 411] This sponge reduced cutaneous colonization at the insertion site and colonization of the catheter tip; however, only one study demonstrated that use of the sponge resulted in lower bloodstream infection rates.[411] In the neonatal study, localized contact dermatitis from the sponge occurred in 15 percent of neonates weighing less than 1000 g.[224] Routine application of topical antimicrobials to the catheter exit site is not recommended.[146, 475] Transparent semipermeable dressings facilitate inspection of the catheter site. However, some studies suggest that they may increase microbial proliferation at the site of insertion and predispose to bloodstream infection, whereas others have shown no difference in colonization of the site or infection rates in comparison to gauze and tape dressings.[486] Despite the controversy, transparent dressings are in widespread use, often in combination with a small piece of gauze at the site of insertion to absorb moisture.

A recent publication has reviewed data on the effect of central venous catheters impregnated with antimicrobials and silver-impregnated subcutaneous catheter cuffs on the incidence of catheter-related bloodstream infection.[146] These studies have not involved any pediatric patients. Catheters impregnated with chlorhexidine–silver sulfadiazine (coating the external surface only) and minocycline-rifampin (coating both the internal and external surfaces) both significantly reduced rates of bloodstream infection when compared with unmedicated catheters.[146] The minocycline-rifampin–coated catheter was associated with lower rates of bloodstream infection than the chlorhexidine–silver sulfadiazine–coated catheter was in a head-to-head trial.[154] However, a new chlorhexidine–silver sulfadiazine catheter has been designed with a higher level of antiseptic in the catheter material and with coating of the internal and external surfaces.[146] New silver-impregnated catheters and catheters using active iontophoresis also are being developed.[146] The long-term impact of these catheters on antimicrobial resistance has not been evaluated.[146]

Catheter hubs containing antiseptic agents also have been tested. A randomized controlled trial of a central venous catheter hub with a chamber containing 3 percent iodinated alcohol demonstrated a fourfold reduction in the rate of catheter-related bloodstream infection,[582] although these results were not confirmed in a subsequent study performed by a different group.[397] A small randomized controlled trial of a povidone-iodine–saturated sponge to encase the hub demonstrated a significant reduction in bloodstream infections.[276] These devices have not gained widespread acceptance, and the amount of iodine that may enter the bloodstream if these devices are used routinely is unclear.

Needleless connectors for intravenous tubing are important to reduce the risk of needle-stick injury in health care workers. However, increased rates of bloodstream infection have been observed when these devices have been used incorrectly.[137, 153, 428]

Studies of the use of "prophylactic" vancomycin or other antibiotics added to intravenous fluids and flush solutions to prevent catheter-related infections have shown some promise.[475] However, this practice is controversial, and further studies are needed to assess the efficacy of this practice and its impact on the emergence of resistant pathogens.[257] Manipulation of the catheter and infusion sets should be minimized, and these sets should be maintained as closed systems whenever possible. When manipulation is necessary, hand hygiene and the use of aseptic technique should be practiced, and hubs should be disinfected with an alcohol swab. Infusion sets used for standard intravenous fluid administration need not be changed more frequently than every 72 hours.[475] If parenteral nutrition or blood products are administered, infusion sets should be changed at least every 24 hours.[475]

The apparatus for hemodynamic monitoring should be maintained as a closed system, and manipulation of this system should be minimized.[475] When manipulation is necessary, hand hygiene and the use of aseptic technique should be practiced. Disposable domes and transducers used for hemodynamic monitoring should be changed every 96 hours.[475] Reused transducers should be reprocessed appropriately between use.[475]

Stopcocks are common components of intravenous infusion and hemodynamic monitoring systems and are used as portals for the injection of medications, infusion of fluids (e.g., parenteral nutrition), and collection of blood samples. These devices can become contaminated during use, although their role in bloodstream infections is not studied well. Manipulation of these devices should be minimized, and the access port should be disinfected before it is entered.

INFECTIONS RELATED TO RESPIRATORY THERAPY

The vast majority of cases of nosocomial pneumonia are caused by bacteria and are associated with mechanical ventilation. Pneumonia also can be caused by respiratory viruses, but such infections are the result of intrahospital transmission of common community infections rather than exposure to medical devices or ICUs (see Nosocomial Infections Caused by Spread of Infections Common in the Community, Respiratory Infections, Respiratory Viruses). *Legionella* and filamentous fungi also cause pneumonia, but these infections occur almost exclusively in immunocompromised patients and are related to inhalation of contaminated aerosols or fungal spores, not respiratory therapy (see Nosocomial Infections in Special Populations, Immunocompromised Children).

Tables 231–2 and 231–3 display rates of pneumonia associated with mechanical ventilation in pediatric ICUs and newborn ICUs in U.S. hospitals participating in the NNIS System.[463] Rates of pneumonia are considerably lower in pediatric and newborn ICUs than in adult ICUs.[463] In general, discrepancies in rates of pneumonia among studies using differing definitions must be interpreted cautiously. No pediatric studies have been performed with rigorous bronchoscopic techniques for diagnosing criteria for pneumonia (see additional discussion later).

Nosocomial pneumonia related to the use of equipment generating contaminated mists has not been reported recently in pediatric patients, although numerous outbreaks caused by "water bacteria" (e.g., *Flavobacterium meningosepticum, P. aeruginosa, Achromobacter)* in pediatric patients in the 1950s and 1960s were linked to the use of centrifugal, Venturi, and ultrasonic mechanical nebulizers.[451] Such devices can aerosolize droplets that are small enough to reach the distal airways, so contamination of their fluid reservoirs is extremely hazardous. Large-volume mechanical nebulizers have been replaced for the most part by heated humidifiers. These devices are considerably less dangerous because they do not generate small-particle aerosols and are less prone to heavy contamination because heating the reservoir retards the growth of most potential pathogens. The mist tents used today for patients with bronchiolitis and croup do have mechanical nebulizers, but they generate larger particles that are deposited in the environment, mouth, and pharynx and generally do not reach the lower respiratory tract. Nonetheless, an effective cleaning and disinfection program is required to minimize the likelihood of infection.

On the other hand, the small-volume, hand-held nebulizers used commonly for inhalation therapy in pediatric patients are designed intentionally to generate particles small enough to reach the distal airways, and the potential for development of nosocomial pneumonia related to the use of these devices is underappreciated by most caregivers. An outbreak of *Legionella* pneumonia caused by contaminated medication administered through small-volume nebulizers has been reported.[422] In addition, the small-volume nebulizers used in conjunction with mechanical ventilators can become contaminated by bacteria colonizing the ventilator circuit and thereby generate bacteria-laden aerosols.[145]

Mechanical ventilation is a major risk factor not only for nosocomial pneumonia but also for sinusitis and otitis media because the nasotracheal tube interferes with normal drainage of the ostia of the sinuses and the eustachian tube.[56, 260] Detection of these infections requires a high index of suspicion because they are often "silent," with little in the way of symptoms other than fever.

Risk factors for the development of pneumonia in adults have been summarized in a review.[639] This review groups risk factors into several categories: (1) host factors, such as chronic pulmonary disease and immunosuppression, which increase general susceptibility to pneumonia; (2) factors that enhance bacterial colonization of the oropharynx and stomach with pathogenic bacteria, such as severe underlying disease, administration of antimicrobials, and possibly, agents that raise gastric pH (e.g., antacids, H_2 blockers); (3) factors that increase the likelihood of reflux of gastric contents and aspiration into the lower airway, such as depressed mental status, supine positioning, nasogastric tubes, and enteral feeding; (4) conditions that require prolonged ventilation and, hence, increase potential exposure to contaminated respiratory equipment and contact with contaminated hands of caregivers; and (5) factors that hinder adequate pulmonary toilet, such as thoracic or abdominal surgery and immobilization.[639] No comparable studies have been performed in patients in pediatric and newborn ICUs, but at least some of these risk factors are probably important in children as well.

Microorganisms associated with nosocomial pneumonia in pediatric and newborn ICUs participating in the NNIS System are displayed in Tables 231–5 and 231–6.[234, 538]

Not reflected in these tables is the fact that most cases of pneumonia are polymicrobial and often include both gram-positive and gram-negative bacteria.[639] Gram-negative bacilli, including *P. aeruginosa* and *Enterobacter* and *Klebsiella* spp., are major pathogens, as is *S. aureus*. *S. pneumoniae* and *H. influenzae* have been recognized increasingly as causes of early-onset nosocomial pneumonia in adults.[639] *Moraxella catarrhalis* is an occasional pathogen. Anaerobic bacteria are implicated uncommonly as a cause of pneumonia,[639] but they may play a role in some polymicrobial infections, especially when pneumonia is caused by aspiration. Although *C. albicans* and other *Candida* spp. are isolated in some cases, they rarely, if ever are the primary cause of nosocomial pneumonia. The distribution of microorganisms causing sinusitis and otitis media in nasotracheally intubated patients is similar to that of pneumonia, although anaerobic bacteria may play a greater role.[78]

The pathogenesis of ventilator-associated pneumonia is complex but can be reduced to two general mechanisms: aspiration of microorganisms colonizing the stomach and oropharynx and inhalation of contaminated aerosols.[639] Aspiration is responsible for most cases of endemic pneumonia, whereas inhalation of contaminated aerosols tends to occur in the context of common-source outbreaks of infection.

A variety of factors facilitate colonization of the oropharynx and upper respiratory tract with pathogenic bacteria. Adherence of gram-negative bacteria to mucosal cells is enhanced in severely ill or debilitated patients by exposure of epithelial bacterial receptors and by changes in the amount and character of respiratory secretions.[639] Bacterial factors, such as the presence of pili in *P. aeruginosa,* also play a role.[639] Antimicrobial therapy reduces the concentration of normal flora, thereby reducing "colonization resistance" and allowing antimicrobial-resistant nosocomial microorganisms to gain a foothold. Bacteria may reach the pharynx via the hands of caregivers or from contaminated equipment or aerosols, or they may be regurgitated into the pharynx from the stomach. Normal gastric pH prevents heavy contamination of stomach contents, but bacteria proliferate to high levels when stomach acid is neutralized by antacids or H_2 blockers.[639] Although the role of these agents in fostering gastric colonization is supported by most studies, the degree to which they are associated with an increased risk for nosocomial pneumonia is less clear.[639] Factors that increase reflux of gastric contents into the upper airway, such as bolus enteral feeding, nasogastric tubes, and supine position, probably increase the risk substantially, but they have not been studied intensively.

Regardless of how nosocomial microorganisms reach the upper respiratory tract, contaminated secretions can be aspirated into the lower respiratory tract of mechanically ventilated patients during changes in position or deflation of the endotracheal tube cuff. Uncuffed endotracheal tubes are used in most pediatric patients, so a constant potential for aspiration exists.

Pneumonia associated with the inhalation of contaminated aerosols occurs much less commonly than does colonization of the oropharynx and aspiration.[639] As noted previously, such infections are likely to be caused by *P. aeruginosa, Legionella,* and a variety of other nonenteric gram-negative bacilli that are capable of surviving and proliferating in the medications and solutions used in respiratory therapy.[639]

Once microorganisms have entered the lower airway, the status of normal defense mechanisms is extremely important in determining whether infection results. Diseases that compromise the mucociliary clearance system (i.e., cystic fibrosis, chronic lung disease) and the ability of the immune system to contain and inactivate these microorganisms (i.e., chemotherapy, HIV infection) dramatically increase the risk for development of infection.

Methods used to diagnose community-acquired pneumonia, such as auscultation of the chest, examination of sputum, and chest radiography, are helpful but much less precise tools for the diagnosis of nosocomial pneumonia in mechanically ventilated patients. Auscultation often is hindered by sounds of the ventilation system itself. Furthermore, a variety of underlying pulmonary diseases (e.g., bronchopulmonary dysplasia, adult respiratory distress syndrome, cystic fibrosis) and conditions (e.g., fluid overload) may produce sounds indistinguishable from those present in pneumonia. Cultures of tracheal aspirates may be misleading because the endotracheal tube often is colonized with potential pathogens, especially in patients ventilated for more than a few days.[243] A Gram stain of the tracheal aspirate can semiquantitatively assess both the number of neutrophils and the number and type of microbial flora, but localized irritation or superficial infection of the trachea related to the endotracheal tube may produce purulent secretions that are laden with bacteria on Gram stain. Finally, the presence of new radiographic findings consistent with pneumonia may be extraordinarily difficult to assess in patients with underlying lung disease or those recovering from thoracic or complicated cardiac surgery.

A variety of techniques to improve the diagnosis of nosocomial pneumonia in mechanically ventilated patients have been tested. These techniques have been reviewed in detail in a recent publication.[426] Originally studied by Chastre and colleagues in Europe,[121–123] bronchoscopic techniques (e.g., quantitative culture of protected brush specimens, bronchoalveolar lavage, and protected bronchoalveolar lavage) offer greater sensitivity and specificity in diagnosing ventilator-associated pneumonia in adult patients than do traditional clinical and laboratory diagnostic criteria.[426] However, these techniques have not been used as widely in the United States because they are invasive, they may be difficult to perform safely in severely ill patients, and their results can be difficult to interpret in patients who have recently (<72 hours before bronchoscopy) begun antibiotic treatment or had their existing antibiotic therapy modified to empirically treat nosocomial pneumonia. In addition, proper procedures for obtaining and processing cultures must be followed to obtain interpretable results.[426] Bronchoscopic techniques have not been studied rigorously in ventilated children or infants.

Blind catheterization of the distal airway to obtain specimens for Gram stain and quantitative culture of the endotracheal aspirate is more practical than bronchoscopy is, although data validating this technique are limited.[426] In a study of blind catheterization of the distal airway in a pediatric ICU, positive cultures correlated strongly with the independent diagnosis of bacterial nosocomial pneumonia by specific clinical, laboratory, and radiographic criteria.[48] However, nearly a third of patients with pulmonary infiltrates of a noninfectious nature also had positive cultures.

Future study may lead to better diagnostic methods, but at present, the diagnosis of ventilator-associated nosocomial pneumonia in pediatric patients usually is made by a constellation of clinical, laboratory, and radiographic criteria. Our institution uses the following definition: a new or worsening infiltrate on chest radiograph compatible with pneumonia (by the pediatric radiologist's report) after more than 48 hours of mechanical ventilation, purulent tracheobronchial secretions (described as tan, beige, yellow, or green in the hospital record or showing moderate or abundant numbers of neutrophils per high-power field on Gram stain), and growth of a pathogen in moderate or abundant amounts from an endotracheal aspirate culture. Other definitions for use in pediatric patients also have been published.[48, 229] Viral pneumonia requires demonstration of the pathogen by direct detection, culture, or serology.

Evaluation of fever in a mechanically ventilated patient should include examination for otitis media. If an etiology of the fever is not established, consideration should be given to radiographic studies of the sinuses (e.g., sinus films or a computed tomographic scan), especially if the child has a nasotracheal tube. If otitis media or sinusitis is diagnosed, tympanocentesis or a tap of the sinuses for culture should be considered in an attempt to guide antimicrobial therapy.

Empiric antimicrobial therapy for nosocomial pneumonia in a mechanically ventilated patient should be guided by Gram stain of the endotracheal aspirate. Once culture information is available, the treatment regimen can be tailored accordingly or discontinued if no infection is identified. Prolonged treatment of patients in whom the diagnosis is questionable should be avoided because it often leads to endotracheal colonization with antimicrobial-resistant bacteria. The duration of treatment has not been studied. We usually treat uncomplicated cases with approximately 10 days of therapy. If a necrotizing gram-negative pneumonia is diagnosed (rare in pediatric patients), at least 14 days of therapy should be administered.

Nasotracheally intubated patients with otitis media or sinusitis should have the nasotracheal tube changed to an orotracheal tube. Short-term treatment with a decongestant and lavage of the sinuses (often performed at the time of sinus tap) may be beneficial in the treatment of sinusitis. Treatment of these infections also has not been studied extensively, but we generally use approximately 10 days of therapy for otitis media; extensive sinusitis warrants at least 14 days of therapy.

A comprehensive guideline for the prevention of nosocomial pneumonia has been developed by the CDC and the Hospital Infection Control Practices Advisory Committee (HICPAC).[639] Key features of this guideline are emphasized in the following text.

Mechanical ventilation should be used only when necessary and only as long as necessary. New approaches to weaning patients from mechanical ventilation can reduce the period of mechanical ventilation significantly.[648] Caregivers should monitor ventilated patients carefully for signs of pneumonia, otitis media, and sinusitis. Prevention of cross-colonization with "hospital flora," especially antimicrobial-resistant bacteria, should be stressed. Hand hygiene and the use of gloves during contact with respiratory secretions or objects or surfaces contaminated with respiratory secretions are important, especially in busy ICUs caring for many sick patients. Suctioning should be performed gently with a sterile, single-use catheter, and sterile fluids should be used to loosen secretions and clear the suction catheter. Data are insufficient to recommend sterile versus clean, nonsterile gloves or multiuse, closed-system suction catheters versus single-use, open-system catheters.

Endotracheal tubes and ventilator circuits become contaminated with the patient's own oropharyngeal flora very quickly, and repeatedly changing this equipment does not reduce the risk of infection. Ventilator circuits and humidifiers should be changed no more frequently than every 48 hours. The maximal "permissible" period of use has not been established.[639] Care should be taken to prevent the condensate that collects in the ventilator tubing from draining into the endotracheal tube because this fluid can be contaminated with a very large number of microorganisms. Tubing should be maintained in a dependent position relative to the endotracheal tube, and condensate should be discarded routinely. The impact of various innovations, such as traps to collect condensate, bacterial filters, hygroscopic condenser-humidifiers, or heat exchange humidifiers, on the risk of development of pneumonia has not been determined.

Large-volume mechanical nebulizers should not be used unless they are scrupulously cleaned and reprocessed on a daily basis. Only sterile water should be used in these devices. Small, hand-held medication nebulizers should be rinsed with sterile water and allowed to air-dry between use. These devices should be reprocessed before use in another patient. Only sterile, aseptically dispensed medications should be used in these devices. Other respiratory therapy equipment should be reprocessed between patients.

The development and application of effective procedures for reprocessing all reused respiratory therapy and ventilator equipment have played a major role in reducing the risk of serious gram-negative pneumonia. Items that have direct or indirect contact with the mucous membranes or respiratory secretions should be cleaned thoroughly and either sterilized or disinfected in a manner consistent with high-level disinfection.

Many issues related to prevention of oropharyngeal or gastric colonization, reflux of gastric contents, and aspiration are unresolved. Several procedures to prevent reflux of gastric contents during enteral feeding, such as elevating the head of the bed, avoiding rapid infusion of large fluid volumes, and avoiding external pressure on the stomach, are simple to implement and probably helpful. The use of continuous versus intermittent bolus feeding and duodenal versus gastric placement of the feeding tube has not been studied in sufficient detail. If a regimen to prevent gastric stress ulcers is needed, the use of agents that do not elevate gastric pH (e.g., sucralfate) is prudent, but whether it actually reduces the incidence of nosocomial pneumonia is not clear. Finally, the effectiveness of selective decontamination of the digestive tract has been debated extensively. A systematic review found that a combination of topical and systemic antibiotics reduced the incidence of ventilator-associated pneumonia and mortality rates in adult patients.[380] The review could not recommend a specific regimen, but topical polymyxin, tobramycin, and amphotericin combined with systemic cefotaxime is the regimen used most commonly. The review emphasizes that the issue of whether this approach leads to the emergence of resistant bacteria has not been addressed adequately.[380]

INFECTIONS RELATED TO INSTRUMENTATION OF THE URINARY TRACT

Urinary tract infections are the most common nosocomial infection in hospitalized adults, and they account for approximately 40 percent of all infections in this group.[264] In contrast, urinary tract infections are a much smaller proportion (10% or less) of nosocomial infections in hospitalized children.[205, 319, 369, 676] This difference can be explained in part by differences in urinary tract catheterization in these two populations. Data from the NNIS System indicate that indwelling urinary catheters are used approximately half as frequently in pediatric ICUs as they are in adult ICUs.[463] Indwelling urinary catheters are used infrequently in newborn ICU patients. On the other hand, the infectious risk associated with the use of indwelling urinary catheters is similar in adults and children. As shown in Table 231–2, rates of urinary tract infection associated with indwelling urinary catheters are only slightly lower in pediatric ICUs than in adult ICUs in U.S. hospitals participating in the NNIS System.[463]

The descriptive epidemiology of urinary tract infections in pediatric patients has been examined in several studies.[160, 369, 391, 392, 478] In a prospective cohort study, catheterized patients were identified and prospectively monitored for symptoms and signs of urinary tract infection (in which case, urinalysis and culture were performed) and by weekly urinalysis and urine culture regardless of symptoms.[392] Nosocomial urinary tract infections in noncatheterized patients also were studied. Urinary tract infections were detected in 11 percent of all catheterized patients, including 11 percent of those in whom only indwelling catheterization was used, 9 percent with both indwelling and intermittent catheterization, and 12 percent with intermittent catheterization alone. The incidence density of infection was not reported. The median duration of catheterization preceding infection was 7 days (range, 2 to 77 days). Three quarters of the infections identified were symptomatic. No definite cases of secondary bacteremia were detected.

Additional information regarding the spectrum of nosocomial urinary tract infections in this study was provided by combining data from catheterized and noncatheterized patients.[392] Catheterization and female sex were identified as risk factors for the development of urinary tract infection: 77 percent of all infections occurred in catheterized patients and 75 percent of all infections occurred in females. The vast majority of infections in noncatheterized patients occurred in the newborn ICU and the preschool-age ward. A wide range of underlying diagnoses were reported, but neurologic, renal, oncologic, orthopedic, and trauma-related diagnoses accounted for 50 percent of cases.

No data have been published on rates of urinary tract infection associated with different types of indwelling catheters (e.g., urethral, suprapubic, ureteral, nephrostomy) in pediatric patients. In our experience, infection (or at least bacteriuria or candiduria) is a common occurrence in patients with catheters that remain in place for long periods (i.e., more than 1 to 2 weeks), regardless of the type of catheter used. Data regarding the incidence of infection after cystoscopy, renal transplantation, and other types of urinary tract instrumentation in pediatric patients are not available. In our experience, infections seldom occur after cystoscopy alone or urologic surgery in which preexisting infection or bacteriuria is not present and long-term use of indwelling catheters is not necessary. Bacteriuria and urinary tract infection appear to occur more commonly in patients undergoing renal transplantation, although determining whether this increased incidence is due to the use of urinary catheters in this population or inherent risks of the transplantation procedure itself is difficult.

Outbreaks in adult patients in the 1970s and 1980s were attributed to contamination of the urinary collecting system by nosocomial pathogens on the hands of hospital personnel, contaminated drainage pans and measuring containers, and the use of inadequate or contaminated antiseptics, or both.[80] Several outbreaks demonstrated that the use of urinary catheters contributed to the emergence of antimicrobial resistance among gram-negative bacilli.[80] Antibiotics excreted in urine provide selective pressure for the emergence of resistant populations of bacteria colonizing urine collection systems, and the large numbers of different types of bacteria present in these systems facilitate transfer of resistance plasmids between species.[80]

Microorganisms causing urinary tract infections in pediatric ICUs participating in the NNIS System are displayed in Table 231–5.[538] Roughly a fifth of infections are caused by *E. coli* alone, and another quarter are caused by a number of other gram-negative bacteria. *Enterococcus* and various *Candida* spp. account for 10 and 14 percent of infections, respectively. These data are similar to those reported from individual studies.[160, 391, 392] The percentage of urinary tract infections attributed to coagulase-negative infections in newborn ICU patients has been reported to be in excess of 30 percent.[160, 391]

Microbial colonization of the urine is the first step in the pathogenesis of urinary tract infection. A detailed culturing study of catheterized patients suggests that roughly two thirds of infections are caused by microorganisms that migrate up the extraluminal surface of the catheter and that the other third of infections arise from microorganisms that gain access to the bladder via the internal lumen of the catheter.[641] In addition, numerous studies in catheterized adults have correlated microorganisms colonizing the urethral meatus with those most frequently causing infection.[80] These microorganisms can be carried into the bladder during catheter insertion, or more commonly, once the catheter is in place, they can migrate along the external surface of the catheter into the bladder. The shorter length of the urethra in females has been suggested as an explanation for the increased risk of infection in females. However, meatal colonization with pathogenic microorganisms, which also occurs more commonly in females, likewise may be important.[80] Distention of the urethra by the catheter, obstruction of the periurethral glands, adherence of pathogenic microbes to the uroepithelium and the external surface of the catheter, and the formation of a biofilm composed of host proteins and microbial exopolysaccharide on the external surface of the catheter all play roles in initiating infection, but the relative contribution of each of these factors is poorly understood.[80]

Microorganisms also may be introduced into the bladder from exogenous reservoirs. Although modern catheters and urine collecting systems are "closed" systems, microorganisms may be introduced into the interior of the catheter collecting system at three points: the junction between the urinary catheter and the collecting system, the port used to aspirate urine specimens and irrigate the catheter, and the drainage spigot attached to the collection container. Some urinary catheters are fused to the collection system during manufacture, thereby eliminating the possibility of junction disconnection, but such catheters are not in widespread use. Improper technique in use of the aspiration/irrigation port or the spigot also may result in contamination of the interior surfaces of the system. Once microorganisms gain access to the interior of the catheter or collecting system, they can multiply quickly and reach concentrations in the collection container exceeding 10^5 CFU/mL of urine in a matter of a few days. Encrustations on the interior surface of the system may serve as sites for microbial attachment and proliferation. Movement of microorganisms into the bladder is facilitated by obstruction of urine flow and reflux of urine into the bladder (i.e., raising the collection system above the level of the bladder), but many gram-negative bacteria are motile and can "swim" upstream even if the system is maintained properly.

Microorganisms that reach the bladder multiply in the small, but persistent reservoir of urine that is not drained completely by the catheter.[80] Infection (i.e., symptoms and signs of tissue invasion) is not an inevitable result of colonization of the bladder, and many chronically catheterized patients go for long periods with gross urine colonization but no clinical evidence of infection. Because many young children have vesicoureteral reflux, ascending infection involving the kidneys is a significant concern, but the epidemiologic studies discussed earlier have not demonstrated pyelonephritis and secondary bacteremia to be common problems.

The diagnosis of nosocomial urinary tract infection depends heavily on the results of quantitative urine culture.

Urine specimens from noncatheterized patients should be obtained aseptically by one of three techniques: midstream clean-catch collection, "straight" catheterization of the bladder, or suprapubic aspiration. Cultures of urine specimens obtained from external bag collectors are of dubious value because they frequently are contaminated. Specimens from patients with indwelling urinary catheters should be obtained from the aspiration port because urine collected from the collection container may reflect colonization of this reservoir rather than infection.

Although diagnostic criteria for catheter-associated urinary tract infection vary, several definitions established for surveillance purposes are generally well accepted.[229] Symptomatic urinary tract infection is defined as the presence of symptoms or signs of infection (e.g., fever, urgency, frequency, dysuria, or suprapubic tenderness), a quantitative urine culture with more than 10^5 CFU/mL of urine, and no more than two different species. Asymptomatic bacteriuria or candiduria (also termed asymptomatic urinary tract infection in some studies, including the cohort study discussed earlier[392]) is defined as the absence of symptoms or signs of infection, a quantitative urine culture with more than 10^5 CFU/mL of urine, and no more than two different species.[229] The diagnosis of asymptomatic bacteriuria is complicated by the fact that approximately 5 percent of healthy school-age and adolescent girls in the community have asymptomatic bacteriuria that may be detected only after hospitalization. A urinalysis showing evidence of pyuria (e.g., dipstick positive for leukocyte esterase or ≥10 white blood cells/mL^3 of urine) or nitrate provides corroborating evidence of infection. Pyuria is a reasonably good predictor of the presence of significant concentrations of gram-negative rods in the urine of catheterized patients, but it is a poor predictor for the presence of significant concentrations of enterococci or *Candida*.[642] A Gram stain of an unspun urine specimen is useful in guiding initial treatment decisions. However, one should note that patients with indwelling catheters and low-level bacteriuria ($<10^5$ CFU/mL) tend to progress to frank bacteriuria with 10^5 CFU/mL or more within a few days if antibiotics are not administered.

The diagnosis of symptomatic urinary tract infection in patients with urinary catheters is often complicated by the fact that these patients do not have symptoms such as urgency, frequency, or dysuria, and assessing abdominal pain and tenderness may be difficult in newborns and severely ill children in ICUs. Consequently, fever is the most commonly identified sign of infection in these patients, thus emphasizing the importance of quantitative urine culture in the evaluation of a new fever in a hospitalized child.

Therapy for nosocomial urinary tract infection is similar to that for community-acquired infection, although parenteral therapy usually is administered initially until secondary bacteremia is excluded. Empiric therapy should be based on knowledge of the relative frequency and susceptibility patterns of nosocomial pathogens in a given hospital. In our institution, ampicillin plus gentamicin is the parenteral regimen most commonly used for empiric therapy. If renal toxicity from the use of an aminoglycoside is a serious concern, the use of trimethoprim-sulfamethoxazole, a third-generation cephalosporin, aztreonam, or a quinolone in older children is appropriate. If Gram stain reveals only gram-negative bacilli, gentamicin alone is used because enterococcal infection is unlikely. If the Gram stain reveals only yeast, antifungal therapy (e.g., bladder irrigation with amphotericin, oral or parenteral fluconazole, or parenteral amphotericin) is initiated instead. Once culture information is available, the treatment regimen can be tailored accordingly or discontinued if no infection is identified. Whenever possible, indwelling urinary catheters should be removed. Cases of asymptomatic bacteriuria (or asymptomatic candiduria) often resolve with removal of the catheter alone.

Data are limited regarding the appropriate duration of therapy for nosocomial urinary tract infection. Although simple community-acquired cystitis in older children and adolescents often can be treated successfully with 1 to 3 days of oral therapy, treating uncomplicated hospital-acquired urinary tract infections for at least 7 days is prudent. If the infection is uncomplicated and the child has responded to therapy, oral therapy can be used to complete the course. Even pyelonephritis may be treated with oral agents if the pathogen is susceptible, but therapy should be extended to at least 14 days. Secondary bacteremia generally is treated parenterally. Treatment of asymptomatic candiduria with a short course (i.e., 5 days) of therapy is sufficient, but infection is likely to recur unless the catheter is removed. Likewise, infections involving nephrostomy or suprapubic catheters often recur if these catheters must remain in place. For cases in which nephrostomy tubes must be used for extended periods, we often use suppressive antimicrobial therapy after treatment is completed. Although this approach poses a risk of secondary infection with resistant bacteria or yeast, it has not proved to be a significant problem.

The prospective cohort study discussed previously examined the consequences of nosocomial urinary tract infection during the 6 months after infection.[392] Four (7.8%) patients had relapses, and one (2.0%) patient suffered a reinfection. No deaths occurred, and no additional complications were identified. The need for evaluation of vesicoureteral reflux or anatomic abnormalities of the kidney or urinary collecting system after nosocomial urinary tract infections has not been evaluated in infants or young children. We do not perform these studies routinely if the infection appears to be related to a urinary catheter.

A guideline for the prevention of nosocomial urinary tract infections was published in the mid-1980s.[689] Key features of the prevention of these infections are emphasized in the next paragraph.

Reducing unnecessary use of urinary catheters is the most effective preventive measure. Davies and colleagues reduced the rate of nosocomial urinary tract infection in a pediatric ICU by 90 percent over an 8-month period simply by instituting a policy whereby nurses automatically removed urinary catheters from patients after 48 to 72 hours unless a physician indicated that continued catheterization was necessary.[160] Urinary catheters should be inserted by trained personnel using careful aseptic technique after the meatus has been cleansed and an effective antiseptic (e.g., povidone-iodine) has been applied to the meatus and surrounding skin.[689] Contamination of the interior surfaces of the catheter and collection system can be minimized by maintaining a closed system (i.e., avoiding disruption of the connection between the catheter and the collection system), disinfecting the aspiration/irrigation port before accessing this port, and minimizing contamination of the spigot on the collection container.[689] The collecting system should be examined regularly to ensure that urine flow is not impeded, and care should be taken to always maintain the collection system in a dependent position relative to the bladder to prevent reflux of urine.[689] Treating preexisting urinary tract infections is important, especially in patients with underlying renal, urologic, or neurologic disease, in whom these infections occur commonly.[689] Systemic antibiotics are effective in preventing urinary tract infections for short periods (5 days or less)[80]; however, routine use of antibiotics for this purpose is likely to facilitate the emergence of resistant pathogens. Numerous other interventions have been studied, most with limited or variable benefit.[80, 414] Manufacturers continue to attempt to design a catheter that will resist the adherence of microorganisms or minimize urethral trauma, or both. A new silver-hydrogel catheter that inhibits adherence of microorganisms to the catheter surface and two antibiotic-impregnated catheters (one using nitrofurazone and the other using minocycline and rifampin) have shown promise in several clinical trials.[155, 331, 409, 410, 414] No studies of novel urinary catheters have been performed in pediatric patients.

INFECTIONS RELATED TO SURGICAL PROCEDURES

Patients undergoing surgical procedures are at risk for a variety of nosocomial infections. A 1-year study of more than 600 pediatric patients undergoing surgical procedures found that surgical-site infection was the most common nosocomial infection after surgery (3.5% of patients).[58] Bloodstream infection developed in 2.3 percent of patients, with half of these infections occurring in patients whose surgical procedure was insertion of a tunneled central venous catheter. Other reported infections included pneumonia (1.6%), urinary tract infection (0.8%), gastrointestinal infection caused by rotavirus (0.3%), and necrotizing enterocolitis (0.2%). A report of nosocomial infections in pediatric patients undergoing cardiovascular surgery found that surgical-site infection and bacteremia accounted for 28 and 27 percent of all infections, respectively.[509]

Data from the handful of reports that have described the epidemiology of surgical-site infections in general pediatric surgery patients are displayed in Table 231–9.[57, 158, 162, 176, 402, 588] These studies were performed in pediatric referral hospitals and used prospective case-finding methods and definitions of surgical-site infection that are identical or similar to published criteria.[9] Outpatient surgery was excluded in studies performed in the United States[57, 162]; studies in other countries did not specifically state whether these patients were included in their reports.[158, 176, 588] Postdischarge follow-up is an important aspect of surveillance because 20 to 70 percent of surgical-site infections may not be detected until after the patient has been discharged.[647] Follow-up methods have included direct observation by the investigators,[57, 588] a questionnaire mailed to surgeons 1 month after the surgery,[162] and automated systems using pharmacy and administrative information.[501] The latter approach is more accurate and much less time-consuming than other methods.

As can be seen in Table 231–9, wound class was a powerful predictor of the likelihood of surgical-site infection in these studies. This finding is expected because wound classification was devised to predict the degree of microbial contamination of the wound and, consequently, the risk of development of infection.[9] Rates of infection by wound class in adult patients from U.S. hospitals participating in the NNIS System also are displayed in Table 231–9 and show similar, though less dramatic step-ups in the risk of development of infection with increasing contamination of the wound. Considerable variability in infection rates within wound class categories is noted in the pediatric studies, thus suggesting that other factors must have a strong impact on the risk for infection. In fact, this factor has been demonstrated in adult patients. Through analysis of data from the NNIS System, a composite risk index was developed that includes measures of severity of illness (the ASA score) and duration of surgery, in addition to wound class; this index is a much better predictor of the risk of surgical-site infection than wound class alone is (see Table 231–4).[149]

The studies listed in Table 231–9 identified other specific risk factors for surgical-site infection in pediatric patients. Longer duration of surgery has been recognized consistently as an important risk factor.[58, 158, 162, 176] This variable was identified as the strongest independent predictor of infection in the only study to use logistic regression analysis.[162]

Several studies have found higher rates of infection in young children, especially neonates,[176, 402, 588] but others have not.[57, 162] Other identified risk factors have included prolonged preoperative hospital stay,[158, 162, 176] emergency surgery,[57, 176] longer incision length,[158, 176] and the presence of underlying disease.[57] The experience of the surgeon (i.e., resident versus attending surgeon) performing the surgery was not found to be a risk factor for the development of infection in any of these studies.

Two types of surgical procedures—cardiovascular procedures and neurosurgical procedures—are discussed in the following paragraphs because of the particularly serious nature of surgical-site infections associated with these procedures.

A study of more than 300 children undergoing cardiovascular surgery found an infection rate of 7.1 percent.[509] Surprisingly, infection rates in this study were lower in patients undergoing open heart surgery with cardiopulmonary bypass (6.7%) than in those undergoing closed heart surgery without bypass (8.1%), but this difference was not statistically significant. Infection rates were higher in patients in whom the sternum was left open after surgery (27.6% in patients with open sternums versus 5.0% in patients with closed sternums, $p < .001$) and in patients with higher PRISM scores (10.7% in patients with PRISM scores ≥10 versus 2.3% in patients with PRISM scores <10, $p < .01$). Whether an open sternum after surgery was an independent risk factor for infection or whether the increased risk of infection in patients with open sternums was attributable all or in part to an increased severity of illness (i.e., higher PRISM score) is not clear from the data presented in this study.

Rates of infection after the performance of CSF shunting procedures vary widely, but many studies are dated, report rates of infection related to ventriculoatrial and ventriculoperitoneal shunts, involve small numbers of patients, or did not routinely incorporate perioperative antimicrobial prophylaxis into the regimen of care.[697] A large pediatric series from the 1980s involving more than 500 patients undergoing ventriculoperitoneal shunting procedures, the vast majority of whom received perioperative antimicrobial prophylaxis, reported an infection rate of 11 percent.[474] Rates of infection were higher in patients with myelomeningocele and those who had undergone previous shunting procedures. Half the infections occurred in the 2 weeks after surgery and were not associated commonly with simultaneous incisional infection.

Microorganisms causing surgical-site infections in pediatric ICUs participating in the NNIS System are displayed in Table 231–5.[538] Gram-positive cocci account for nearly half the isolates. *S. aureus* is the most frequent isolate, but coagulase-negative staphylococci and *Enterococcus* spp. are also common. Gram-negative bacilli of various types account for approximately 40 percent of the isolates. *Bacteroides fragilis* and other anaerobic bacteria seldom are isolated, but how frequently anaerobic cultures were performed is unclear. *C. albicans* and other *Candida* spp. are isolated from a minority (4%) of surgical-site infections. This distribution of microorganisms is similar in the several studies of surgical-site infection in the general pediatric surgery patients cited previously.[58, 158, 588] Studies of pediatric cardiovascular surgery patients have described a similar distribution of microorganisms.[187, 509] Gram-positive bacteria more commonly are the cause of CSF shunt infections. In the large study cited previously, gram-positive bacteria accounted for

TABLE 231–9 ■ CUMULATIVE INCIDENCE OF SURGICAL SITE INFECTION RATES BY WOUND CLASS* IN PEDIATRIC AND ADULT PATIENTS

					Cumulative Incidence of Surgical Site Infection by Wound Class (%)				
Ref	**Location**	**Year(s) of Study**	**Age Group**	**No. of Patients**	Clean	Clean-Contaminated	Contaminated	Dirty-Infected	Overall
176	England	1973	Overall	329	3.5	16.0	37.5†	—	13.7
			Neonates	65	18.5	45.0	55.6†	—	38.4
			1 mo–1 yr	54	16.0	20.0	33.3f†	—	24.1
			1–5 yr	73	2.5	33.3	44.4†	—	19.2
			>5 yr	137	5.6	15.8	72.7†	—	12.4
162	USA	1980–81	Overall	1045	3.1	7.8	16.7	9.7	4.2
588	India	NS	Overall	1325	1.8	5.8	27.0†	—	5.4
			Neonates	160	5.3	21.2	42.9†	—	13.8
			1 mo–1 yr	326	2.4	3.9	33.3†	—	6.7
			1–5 yr	396	1.0	5.0	25.5†	—	3.8
			>5yr	443	0.5	3.2	17.1†	—	2.9
158	England	1974–87	Neonates	1094	11.1	20.9	20.5†	—	18.0
57	USA	1986–88	Overall	676	1.0	2.9	7.9	6.3	2.5
			Neonates	137	—	—	—	—	0.7
			1 mo–1yr	197	—	—	—	—	4.1
			>1 yr	342	—	—	—	—	2.3
402	England	NS	Neonates	143	3.9	11.3		16.7†	9.1
149	USA‡	1987–90	Adults	84,691	2.1	3.3	6.4	7.1	

*Wound class as defined in Altemeier, W. A., Burke, J. F., and Sandusky, W. R. (eds.): Manual on Control of Infection in Surgical Patients. 2nd ed. Philadelphia, J. B. Lippincott, 1984.

†Combined contaminated and dirty-infected categories.

‡Data from U. S. hospitals participating in the National Nosocomial Infection Surveillance System; modified from Culver, D. H., Horan, T. C., Gaynes, R. P., et al.: Surgical wound infection rates by wound class, operative procedure, and patient risk index. Am. J. Med. *91* (Suppl.):152–157, 1991.

NS, not stated in the report.

three fourths of the infections; coagulase-negative staphylococci were the cause of 40 percent of the infections.[474]

The pathogenesis of surgical-site infection is related to the degree of microbial contamination of the wound, the condition of the host (both resistance to infection and the ability to heal the wound), and performance of the procedure itself. Microbial contamination of the surgical site occurs almost exclusively during the time that the incision is open, which probably is the reason that a longer duration of surgery is associated with an increased risk for infection, although longer procedures also may be reflective of other factors that influence risk (i.e., complexity of the surgery, skill of the surgeon, care in dissection). If the incision is closed primarily, subsequent contamination of the site from external sources (i.e., use of contaminated antiseptics or dressings) seldom occurs. The vast majority of the microorganisms contaminating open wounds are endogenous in origin (i.e., microorganisms colonizing the skin and respiratory, gastrointestinal, and genitourinary tracts). Indeed, carriage of *S. aureus* in the anterior nares is associated with postoperative infection caused by this organism.[348, 420] Infrequent outbreaks of surgical-site infections caused by *S. aureus*, group A streptococci, and group C streptococci have been traced to personnel in the operating room (but not necessarily participating in the surgery itself) who are heavy shedders of these microorganisms, usually as a result of rectal, vaginal, or nasal carriage.[248, 544, 571] The inanimate environment of the operating room (e.g., walls, floors, other surfaces, and surgical instruments) is a very uncommon source of microorganisms causing surgical-site infection.[35] Postoperative hematogenous seeding of the surgical site can occur but is uncommon.

Host factors, such as underlying diseases (e.g., malignancy, uremia), the competence of the immune system, and nutritional status, are likely to be important, but the nature and degree to which these factors affect the risk for infection are not described well.

Even with careful skin preparation in clean surgery, small numbers of microorganisms are present at the surgical site in virtually every procedure, and careful surgical technique is necessary to avoid conditions that favor the growth of these microorganisms in the postoperative period. Damaged and devascularized tissue created by rough tissue handling and the overuse of electrocautery is less resistant to infection.[9] Hematomas and seromas, which provide optimal growth conditions for bacteria, may develop if dead spaces are not obliterated or if hemostasis is inadequate.[9] Low-pressure suction drains are indicated to facilitate drainage of blood and secretions, facilitate adherence of tissues and surfaces, and promote wound healing.[9] To the extent that they accomplish this goal, surgical drains are useful. However, unnecessary use of drains should be avoided because they provide a portal for entry of microorganisms and may inhibit healing.

Consensus criteria for surgical-site infections developed through the collaborative efforts of the CDC, surgeons, and infection control professionals have been published.[300] Surgical-site infections are subcategorized into superficial incisional infections (involving the skin or subcutaneous tissue), deep incisional infections (involving the muscle or fascia), and organ/space infections (involving visceral organs or deep body spaces or cavities). For the most part, these criteria rely on observations made by direct inspection of the surgical site. Cultures of wound drainage are useful to determine the microbial etiology of the infection, but these criteria rely on the results of wound cultures only when wound drainage is not clearly purulent (i.e., serosanguineous drainage must be culture-positive for it to be considered evidence of an infection). Stitch abscesses are not considered surgical-site infections.

Principles of the treatment of surgical-site infections are described in other sources.[9] Significant fluid collections should be drained, especially collections of purulent material. In some cases, fluid collections may be inaccessible, or an attempt at drainage may seriously compromise the patient. In such cases, antimicrobial therapy alone may be successful in resolving the infection, although therapy needs to be chosen carefully to ensure adequate penetration into the area and minimize the potential for emergence of antimicrobial resistance. Clinical response must be monitored closely. Devitalized tissue should be débrided, and any tension, pressure, or obstruction in the area should be relieved to allow adequate blood flow and drainage. Foreign bodies should be removed. For instance, CSF shunt infections are unlikely to resolve without removal of the shunt.[697] In some special cases, antimicrobial therapy can dramatically suppress infection with foreign bodies in place while postoperative healing takes place (i.e., plates and screws to stabilize bones during healing after orthopedic procedures). However, these devices generally require eventual removal to achieve complete cure. Systemic antimicrobial therapy should be prescribed for serious infections, but many superficial infections resolve with local care and application of topical antimicrobial agents.

A guideline for the prevention of surgical-site infections is available.[420] Key prevention measures that have the common goal of minimizing microbial contamination of the surgical site are summarized in the following paragraphs.

Preoperative interventions have a major impact on the nature and degree of microbial contamination of the surgical site. To minimize preoperative hospitalization is prudent because hospitalized patients are more likely to become colonized with "hospital flora" (e.g., methicillin-resistant staphylococci). Treatment of preexisting infections is very important because the microorganisms causing these infections may contaminate the surgical site, but unnecessary therapy should be avoided because it increases the likelihood of colonization with antimicrobial-resistant microorganisms.

Preoperative bathing with an agent that has antimicrobial activity is a logical prevention measure. This practice does reduce colony counts of bacteria on the skin but has not been shown to definitively reduce the rate of surgical-site infections.[420] A comparative study of the use of chlorhexidine versus iodophor shampoos before performing neurosurgical procedures in children demonstrated that chlorhexidine shampoos reduced the number of microorganisms on the scalp before surgery and the frequency of wound contamination; however, the number of patients studied was not sufficient to demonstrate any effect on infection rates.[373]

A randomized trial examined the effect of topical mupirocin applied to the nares preoperatively to prevent surgical-site infections after general, gynecologic, neurologic, or cardiothoracic surgical procedures.[489] Children were not included in this trial. The overall surgical-site infection rate was not different in patients receiving topical mupirocin versus those receiving placebo. However, the risk of development of nosocomial infection with *S. aureus* at any site (surgical site, bloodstream, catheter, lower respiratory tract) in patients with nasal carriage of *S. aureus* was significantly lower in those who received mupirocin than in those who received placebo.

Although removing hair appears to provide a "cleaner" operative site, shaving the skin, especially when performed the day before surgery, has the paradoxical effect of increasing skin colonization by liberating resident skin flora from deeper skin structures and causing microscopic skin trauma that facilitates the growth of bacteria. If hair removal is necessary, hair should be clipped instead of shaved. If shaving is necessary, it should be done immediately before surgery.

Appropriately administered perioperative antimicrobial prophylaxis eradicates or at least retards the growth of bacteria that gain access to the surgical site. Numerous studies have examined the effectiveness of perioperative antimicrobial prophylaxis for various surgical procedures performed on adults, but few such studies have included pediatric patients. Consequently, recommendations regarding perioperative antimicrobial prophylaxis for pediatric surgery largely follow the regimens recommended for use in adults.[17] Prophylaxis should be administered within 2 hours before making the surgical incision.[131] If prophylaxis is administered outside this 2-hour window, effectiveness is diminished greatly; administration more than 6 hours after the incision has essentially no effect.[131] If the surgical procedure is prolonged, another dose should be administered after two half-lives of the administered agent has elapsed (i.e., 4 to 6 hours for cefazolin). Administration of additional doses in the postoperative period is unnecessary. Ensuring appropriate use and timing of perioperative antimicrobial prophylaxis is an important quality-of-care issue (see Chapter 232); likewise, ensuring that prophylaxis is not used unnecessarily is important for cost containment.

A variety of intraoperative practices and procedures are intended to prevent microbial contamination of the surgical site.[420] However, the effectiveness of many of these measures is either minimal or has not been studied rigorously. Cleaning the skin plus application of an antiseptic (e.g., alcohols, iodophors, chlorhexidine) reduces the number of viable bacteria at the surgical site. Surgical hand scrubbing with an effective antiseptic (e.g., alcohols, iodophors, chlorhexidine) by members of the operative team reduces the number of bacteria on the hands and the potential for contamination of the surgical site through visible or microscopic breaks in surgical gloves. The practice of wearing barriers (i.e., masks, caps, gowns) by the surgical team is a logical operating room practice and provides protection for the operative team against exposure to blood and body fluids, but little evidence suggests that this practice has a substantial impact on the risk of development of surgical-site infections. Traffic and activity in the operating room increase the bacterial count in the air, and keeping the number of persons and movement to a minimum is reasonable, but the effect on the risk for development of infection is likely to be minimal. Bacterial counts in the air also can be minimized by regularly servicing the operating room ventilation system and by maintaining adequate ventilation parameters (15 air changes with 3 changes of outside air per hour).[20] Laminar air flow and ultraviolet lights can decrease bacterial counts in the air to very low levels, but their effectiveness in reducing the incidence of infections remains controversial.

Proper surgical technique also is important in prevention of surgical-site infections, as discussed previously. Many studies have demonstrated that confidential feedback of surgeon-specific rates of infection to individual surgeons reduces rates of infection.[647] This approach has been endorsed by the CDC, surgeons, and infection control professionals as a means by which individual surgeons may examine their own rates of infection and adjust their operative techniques accordingly.[647]

INFECTIONS RELATED TO ADMINISTRATION OF BLOOD PRODUCTS

The infectious risks associated with the administration of blood products have been summarized in several comprehensive reviews.[250, 251, 610] Blood-borne infections in health care personnel as a consequence of exposure that occurs in the workplace are discussed in Chapter 232.

The blood supply in the United States is now safer than ever because of implementation of procedures to minimize infectious risks during blood donation and preparation of blood products. Prospective donors are provided written information on possible risk factors for blood-borne infections to encourage self-deferral of donation.[242, 250] In addition, screening procedures include a self-administered questionnaire about risk factors, health, and international travel history and direct questions by trained staff about specific high-risk behavior.[242, 250] Donors are given additional opportunities to self-defer use of their blood for any reason after it is obtained. These screening processes alone substantially reduce the risk of transmission of blood-borne infections.[242, 250]

Donated blood is tested routinely for the following laboratory markers of infection: HIV-1 and HIV-2 antibody, HIV p24 antigen, hepatitis B surface antigen (HBsAg), hepatitis B core antibody, hepatitis C antibody, hepatitis C nucleic acid amplification tests, human T-lymphotropic virus type I/II (HTLV-I/II) antibody, and nontreponemal antibody. If these tests are negative, a small threat of acquiring a transfusion-related infection remains because of the "window" period between the time of infection in the donor and the time that these markers of infection are detectable in the donor's blood. The likelihood of transmission after transfusion of infected blood is high (80 to 90%) for HIV-1, hepatitis B virus, and hepatitis C virus, but lower (20 to 30%) for HTLV-I/II.[610] The risk of acquiring an infection from a single unit of screened blood is estimated at 1:200,000 to 2,000,000 for HIV-1, 1:30,000 to 250,000 for hepatitis B virus, 1:30,000 to 150,000 for hepatitis C virus, and 1:250,000 to 2,000,000 for HTLV-I/II.[250]

The incidence of bloodstream infection as a result of bacterial contamination of blood products is not as well defined, but it is estimated to be substantially more likely than transfusion-associated infection with HIV or hepatitis B virus.[250] The risk of acquiring a bloodstream infection associated with platelet transfusion is estimated to be 1 in 12,000 and may be greater with transfusion of pooled platelet concentrates from multiple donors,[344] in part because of the fact that platelets are stored at room temperature (20 to 24° C). A variety of skin flora, including coagulase-negative staphylococci, *S. aureus*, and diphtheroids, as well as gram-negative bacteria, have been found to contaminate blood products.[174, 344] *Yersinia enterocolitica* bloodstream infections have occurred after transfusion of contaminated red blood cells, presumably as a result of unrecognized bacteremia in donors.[100] Transfusion-associated syphilis occurs extremely rarely because of screening of donated blood and the fact that spirochetes do not survive in refrigerated, citrate-anticoagulated blood for longer than 72 hours.[610] Transmission of *Rickettsiae, Ehrlichia,* and *Brucella* has been reported, but transmission of *Borrelia burgdorferi* has not been documented.[174]

Transfusion-associated CMV infection occurs uncommonly despite the fact that most blood donors are positive for antibody to CMV.[610] Transfusion-acquired infection with CMV is mild or asymptomatic in most immunocompetent hosts but may be severe in CMV antibody–negative immunocompromised recipients and newborns.[610] Superinfection with a new strain of CMV in a CMV antibody–positive immunocompromised individual has been described.[610] The risk of acquiring infection is confined to the transfusion of cellular components and can be nearly eliminated by procedures that ensure depletion of white blood cells, either by filtration or by additional centrifugation.[610] Transfusion of blood products from CMV antibody–negative donors is another strategy to prevent transmission to high-risk recipients, but this approach limits the potential donor pool substantially.

Hepatitis A virus may be transmitted by transfusion from donors who are viremic but have not yet manifested clinical features of infection. Transfusion-associated infection has been reported primarily in relation to hepatitis A virus outbreaks in newborn nurseries and neonatal ICUs (see "Nosocomial Infections Caused by Spread of Infections Common in the Community," "Hepatitis A Virus").

Other viruses, including hepatitis G, TT virus, and parvovirus B19, are transmissible by transfusion, but the significance of post-transfusion infection with these agents is unclear.[10, 120, 395, 468]

Approximately two cases of transfusion-related malaria occur each year.[174] Persons who have lived in areas of the world where malaria is prevalent are excluded from donation for a period of 3 years; those who have visited these areas are excluded for 1 year.[174]

Immigration of persons from rural areas of Central and South America where infection with the protozoan *Trypanosoma cruzi* (the etiologic agent of Chagas disease) occurs commonly has raised concern regarding the potential for transfusion-associated infection with this agent in the United States.[174] Transfusion-associated infections are well described in other countries, and several cases have been reported in the United States and Canada.[174] This organism survives well in blood and in components frozen or stored for 21 days at 4° C.[610] The risk of acquiring this infection is highest in areas with substantial immigrant populations, particularly southern California and Texas. Tests to screen donated blood for antibody against *T. cruzi* are used in Latin America but are not performed routinely in the United States.[174]

As demonstrated by an outbreak of hepatitis C infection in recipients of a contaminated intravenous immunoglobulin preparation,[93] plasma and immunoglobulin preparations, which include pooled specimens from many donors, are particularly vulnerable to viral contamination. Manufacturing processes for these blood products subsequently have been modified to include solvent-detergent treatment, which is designed to inactivate contaminating viruses.[32] However, the process does not inactivate nonenveloped viruses such as hepatitis A, parvovirus B19, and TT virus, although antibodies against these viruses contained in pooled preparations may be sufficient to inactivate the viruses.[251]

No cases of transmission of Creutzfeldt-Jakob disease (CJD) or new variant Creutzfeldt-Jakob disease (vCJD) by blood or blood products have been documented in humans, but concern exists about the potential for such an event.[549] In addition, transmission of bovine spongiform encephalopathy to a sheep by transfusion of whole blood from another sheep during the symptom-free phase of experimental infection has been documented.[304] Because of these concerns, the U.S. Food and Drug Administration has recommended exclusion criteria to eliminate donors who might transmit vCJD or CJD.[89]

Nosocomial infection with blood-borne pathogens also may occur through means other than transfusion of blood products. Indirect transmission of hepatitis B has been demonstrated to occur as a result of inadequately disinfected instruments, such as a device used for fingerstick glucose measurements,[503] and it is a well-documented problem for both patients and health care workers in hemodialysis units.[106] For this reason, most dialysis units physically separate HBsAg-positive patients from uninfected patients.[106] Administration of hepatitis B vaccine is strongly encouraged for all dialysis patients and health care workers in dialysis units.[106] The risk of hepatitis C transmission occurring through indirect transmission is not clear, although studies in hemodialysis units suggest that hepatitis C transmission may occur in this setting.[106] An outbreak of hepatitis C virus infection in a pediatric oncology ward has been reported.[349] HIV transmission has been documented in a dialysis center in South America as a result of inadequate disinfection procedures[659] and in other countries as a result of reuse of needles.[66, 696] A possible case of HIV transmission in a pediatric ward in the United States has been reported, although extensive investigation failed to reveal a source of the infection.[62]

INFECTIONS RELATED TO ENDOSCOPY

Few systematic, prospective studies of infection after endoscopy have been conducted, and essentially no data exist regarding rates of infection specifically in children. In general, however, infectious complications after endoscopy are uncommon,[36, 421, 577, 620] especially given the large number of procedures performed.

Endoscopy-related infections may be exogenous (i.e., contamination of the endoscope) or endogenous (i.e., transfer of microorganisms from one body site to another during the procedure).[36, 421] Exogenous infections have been reported more frequently.[36, 421, 620] Improper cleaning and disinfection procedures may result in transmission of microorganisms from one patient to another,[102, 620] and even conscientious reprocessing may be foiled by the complicated design or intrinsic design defects of many endoscopes.[109, 620] Exogenous infections also can be caused by contamination of endoscopes during the reprocessing procedure itself. Even apparently sophisticated, automated reprocessing machines are not immune to this problem, as evidenced by recent reports.[12, 90, 102, 620] An outbreak of pseudoinfection (i.e., exogenous contamination of culture specimens) from contaminated endoscopes also has been described.[90]

The most common endogenous infection is transient bacteremia, which can occur after instrumentation of the gastrointestinal, respiratory, or genitourinary tract.[36, 421] Clinical symptoms do not develop in most patients, but endocarditis has been reported.[36, 421] Cholangitis is a significant complication of endoscopic retrograde cholangiopancreatography (ERCP), especially when biliary tract obstruction occurs.[36, 421] Pneumonia developing after bronchoscopy, wound infection and perforation of the intestine associated with operative endoscopy (e.g., cholecystectomy), and joint infection occurring after arthroscopy also have been reported.[36, 102, 109]

A summary of published reports found that *Salmonella* spp. and *P. aeruginosa* were the most common etiologic agents of infections related to gastrointestinal endoscopy.[620] Infection by other gram-negative enteric bacilli (e.g., *Klebsiella, Enterobacter,* and *S. marcescens*), enterococci, and *Helicobacter pylori* also occurs.[620] *M. tuberculosis,* atypical mycobacteria, and *P. aeruginosa* were the causes of pneumonia most commonly reported after bronchoscopy.[620] One case of hepatitis B virus transmission via gastrointestinal endoscopy has been described.[620]

Proper reprocessing procedures are critical for the prevention of exogenous infection after endoscopic procedures. Reprocessing requirements vary according to the intended use of the endoscope (i.e., entry into sterile tissue or cavities versus contact only with mucous membranes), tolerance of the equipment to various reprocessing methods (i.e., steam sterilization or immersion in liquid disinfectants/sterilants), and the specified turnaround time. Detailed reviews of reprocessing procedures have been published recently.[36, 421, 620]

Antimicrobial prophylaxis for endoscopy is controversial. At a minimum, it is prudent to administer appropriate antimicrobial prophylaxis to patients at risk for endocarditis during procedures with a potential for transient bacteremia (e.g., procedures involving instrumentation of the gastrointestinal, respiratory, and genitourinary tracts), during ERCP, and during cystoscopy performed in the presence of probable or confirmed bacteriuria.[36]

Nosocomial Infections in Special Populations

NEWBORN INFANTS

Healthy newborns are thrust into the world quickly and become colonized with microorganisms derived from their mothers and the immediate environment within several days. Predominant colonizers are coagulase-negative staphylococci on the skin and umbilicus and in the nose and alpha-hemolytic streptococci in the mouth. Colonization of the gastrointestinal tract is more complex. Lactobacilli predominate in breast-fed babies, whereas more "adult" flora composed of *Bacteroides* spp., other anaerobes, and *E. coli* colonize formula-fed babies.[244] These commensals help resist colonization with pathogenic microorganisms. Because pathogens can spread quickly in crowded nurseries, rooming-in and early discharge reduce the potential for transmission to normal newborns. However, early discharge also renders detection of significant problems when they occur more difficult. For instance, the incubation period for *S. aureus* infection is generally longer than a newborn's stay in the hospital, and significant outbreaks can escape detection unless an aggressive reporting system is established.[286, 401]

Premature and full-term infants requiring care in newborn ICUs face a far different fate. Colonization of these infants is delayed substantially, perhaps because of limited contact with their mothers, delayed enteral feeding, and administration of parenteral antimicrobial agents.[239, 244] When colonization does occur, it is with markedly different microorganisms. Coagulase-negative staphylococci colonize the skin, umbilicus, and nose of these infants as well.[244] However, recent molecular typing studies have demonstrated that particular strains of coagulase-negative staphylococci can persist in newborn ICUs over extended periods; they are transmitted on the hands of caregivers and cause bloodstream infection in some infants.[308, 398, 484] *S. aureus* may colonize a variety of sites, particularly the umbilicus and nose.[244] Although lactobacilli and anaerobes still colonize the gut, aerobic gram-negative bacilli, including *E. coli, Klebsiella, Enterobacter, P. aeruginosa, S. marcescens,* and *Citrobacter,* represent a much larger proportion of the intestinal flora than is the case in normal newborns.[239, 244] Antimicrobial-resistant strains of these bacteria are a particular problem in many newborn ICUs. Because these bacteria can reach concentrations in the stool of 10^6 to 10^8 CFU/g, the hands of caregivers are contaminated easily and provide an important route of nosocomial transmission. *Enterococcus* and *Candida* can become established on the skin and umbilicus and in the gut,[244] again as a result of contamination of the hands of caregivers and selection pressure imposed by treatment with antimicrobial agents. Unfortunately, the medical devices that help sustain these infants, such as intravascular catheters and mechanical ventilation, provide portals of entry for these microorganisms to invade sterile sites and cause infection.

The preceding sections have described a variety of microorganisms generally regarded as community pathogens that often cause outbreaks of nosocomial infection in nurseries and newborn ICUs, including RSV and other respiratory viruses, rotavirus, *Salmonella* and other enteric bacterial pathogens, HSV, CMV, hepatitis A virus, and enteroviruses, as well as infections related to the use of invasive devices in neonates (see "Nosocomial Infections Caused by Spread of Infections Common in the Community," "Nosocomial Infections Related to Invasive Devices, Procedures, and Treatments").

Other important pathogens in normal newborn nurseries and newborn ICUs are highlighted in the following text.

S. aureus remains a significant pathogen in newborn infants, though not nearly to the degree that it was in the 1950s and 1960s. Staphylococcal skin and soft tissue infections, including superficial skin infections, mastitis, and omphalitis, are the most common infections; severe staphylococcal pneumonia is now a rarity.[571] Because newborns are not colonized with this organism at birth, it must be transmitted to them postnatally. Direct contact with colonized caregivers is the predominant mode of transmission.[571] Indirect contact transmission from infected or colonized infants and droplet contact transmission from infants with coexisting viral respiratory tract infection (so-called "cloud babies") seldom occur.[571] Colonization of the skin, nose, umbilicus, or rectum precedes infection, but correlation between rates of colonization and infection is poor. Typically, the number of colonized infants far exceeds the number of infected infants; conversely, outbreaks of staphylococcal infection can occur in nurseries with low colonization rates.[571] For this reason and because of cost considerations, surveillance cultures to detect colonized infants are not recommended except in outbreak conditions.

Hand hygiene and the use of barrier precautions (e.g., gloves and gowns) are effective means of preventing transmission of *S. aureus* from heavily colonized or infected infants. The use of hexachlorophene (3%) for bathing is effective in reducing colonization,[246, 284] but this agent was found to cause cystic degenerative changes in the white matter of premature infants,[513, 597, 598] although no evidence was found that this agent poses a hazard to full-term infants. A warning against the use of hexachlorophene was issued by the Food and Drug Administration in 1972. Use of this agent for infant bathing remains an option during outbreaks of *S. aureus* infection, but it should be diluted 1:4 or 1:5 in water and should not be used for bathing very low birth weight infants.[246] Chlorhexidine is a reasonable alternative because it has good antistaphylococcal activity and studies in neonates have demonstrated negligible absorption after bathing or cord care and no recognized toxicity.[7, 142, 328] The use of iodophors may cause adsorption of iodine, and alcohols may cause chemical burns, so these agents should not be used for bathing. A variety of agents, including triple dye (an aqueous mixture of brilliant green, proflavine hemisulfate, and crystal violet), alcohol, bacitracin, chlorhexidine, and mupirocin, have been used for cord care, although extensive efficacy and safety data are not available for any of these compounds.[246, 284]

Fifty to seventy-five percent of women with group B streptococcal vaginal colonization will transmit this microorganism to their newborn infants, but only 1 to 2 percent of colonized infants will become infected. The CDC defines these and other infections transmitted via the birth canal as nosocomial infections.[229, 234] The logic behind this designation has not been explicitly stated, but because these infections occur after an event (i.e., delivery) usually associated with medical care, to consider them nosocomial infections is reasonable. However, the impact of conventional infection control interventions on early-onset (i.e., within the first

7 days of life) invasive group B streptococcal infection is likely to be limited. Intrapartum prophylaxis of women is a far more effective intervention to reduce infection rates in newborns.[99, 579] An important note is that group B streptococci can be associated with nosocomial infection, not just perinatal infection. Outbreaks of group B streptococcal infection caused by indirect contact transmission in nurseries have been documented well.[183, 245, 472]

Preterm infants are particularly susceptible to infection with a variety of yeasts and, to a lesser extent, filamentous fungi. *Candida* spp. are the most common pathogens. Infants probably become colonized in their gastrointestinal tracts from the carriage of *Candida,* especially *Candida parapsilosis,* on the hands of health care workers.[566] Cutaneous colonization also may lead to invasive infection.[553] Risk factors for colonization with *Candida* are treatment with H_2 blockers or third-generation cephalosporins and delayed enteral feeding.[566] Risk factors for infection include a low 5-minute Apgar score, shock, disseminated intravascular coagulopathy, central venous catheterization, administration of parenteral nutrition (including Intralipid), use of H_2 blockers, and prolonged mechanical ventilation and length of stay.[567] Risk factors for *Malassezia furfur* infection are similar to those for *Candida,* but the association with lipid emulsion is particularly strong because this organism is obligatively lipophilic.[152, 393, 543] Outbreaks of *Malassezia pachydermatis* infection have been reported, in one case in association with colonization of health care workers' dogs.[118, 675] Infections caused by filamentous fungi rarely occur but usually are associated with contaminated devices or practices that facilitate cutaneous invasion.[448, 553]

C. diversus has been responsible for numerous outbreaks of nosocomial infection in newborn infants.[382, 482, 687] Although clinical disease does not develop in most infants colonized with this microorganism, infection almost always results in meningitis because of the particular neurotropism of this organism (see General Epidemiology of Nosocomial Infections, Interactions Between Hosts and Pathogens) and usually is accompanied by the formation of one or more brain abscesses. Outbreaks of infection caused by this organism may occur sporadically over an extended period.[382, 482, 687] Transmission of this bacterium on the hands of caregivers has been implicated in several of these outbreaks.[482, 687] On the other hand, molecular techniques have demonstrated that *C. diversus* also can be acquired perinatally by vertical transmission.[285]

E. sakazakii is a rare cause of nosocomial infection in neonates. Like infection by *C. diversus*, infection with this bacterium is usually severe, often involving meningitis and brain abscess.[59, 110, 129, 364, 604, 655] Outbreaks of infection by *E. sakazakii* have been linked conclusively to the consumption of intrinsically contaminated powdered milk formulas.[59, 110, 458, 604, 655] A variety of products have been implicated in these outbreaks.[110, 364] Because powdered formulas are not marketed as sterile products, feeding practices in neonatal ICUs need to balance the relative nutritional benefits of particular products against the small, but real risk of acquiring infection with *E. sakazakii* and other potential pathogens.

New obstetric practices, such as water birth, may pose infectious threats to infants, as demonstrated by the report of a case of *Legionella* pneumonia in an infant after prolonged delivery in a pool with contaminated water.[207]

Hand hygiene is the most effective intervention to prevent the spread of pathogenic microorganisms.[69] However, the hands of some staff may remain colonized with these microorganisms for prolonged periods despite scrupulous handwashing.[244] In addition, the use of artificial nails or nail wraps has been associated with carriage of *P. aeruginosa* on the hands of health care workers in a neonatal ICU.[204] The use of these devices should be banned in such units.[565] Alcohol-based hand rubs are the most effective agents in reducing hand colonization with pathogenic bacteria and are the preferred method for hand hygiene when hands are not visibly soiled.[69]

The preceding sections contain specific recommendations for the prevention of nosocomial infections caused by community pathogens and infections related to the use of invasive devices (see Nosocomial Infections Caused by Spread of Infections Common in the Community and Nosocomial Infections Related to Invasive Devices, Procedures, and Treatments). Other general recommendations for the prevention of nosocomial infections in normal nurseries and newborn ICUs, including recommendations regarding the design of facilities, appropriate staffing, and general infection prevention procedures, have been published.[13, 284]

Several interventions designed specifically to prevent nosocomial infections in high-risk infants deserve additional comment.

The NIC/Q Collaborative is a large multicenter network of neonatal units organized for the purpose of implementing evidenced-based interventions to improve the quality of care of newborn infants (*www.nicq.org*).[301] A subgroup of six units used quality improvement methods to implement 17 practices designed to reduce the incidence of nosocomial infections. The range of the number of these practices implemented per unit was 10 to 16. When compared with 65 units that did not participate in this initiative, overall rates of nosocomial infection and rates of coagulase-negative staphylococcal bacteremia declined more rapidly in the 6 units implementing these interventions.[303]

Many investigators have colonized infants in newborn ICUs purposefully with nonpathogenic microorganisms, including viridans streptococci and *Lactobacillus*, to "interfere" with colonization by potential pathogens.[246, 445, 532] Some of the studies using viridans streptococci demonstrated favorable results, but this approach has not been pursued, in part because of concern about the potential for development of adverse events.[246] Studies using *Lactobacillus* have demonstrated little or no beneficial effect.[445, 532]

Because premature infants lack sufficient levels of opsonizing antibodies, several well-designed trials have examined the efficacy of intravenous immunoglobulin in preventing nosocomial infection in premature infants.[44, 196, 340, 404, 673] Only one of these trials demonstrated any benefit in reducing overall nosocomial infection rates.[44] A systematic review of studies addressing the efficacy of intravenous immunoglobulin in preterm (<37 weeks) or low-birth-weight (<2500 g) infants found an overall 3 percent reduction in sepsis and a 4 percent reduction in serious infections associated with the administration of immunoglobulin. However, no evidence was found of an impact on other outcomes, such as necrotizing enterocolitis, intraventricular hemorrhage, length of stay, or mortality.[477] An evaluation of commercially available intravenous immunoglobulin preparations found a large degree of variability in opsonic activity against common neonatal pathogens among lots produced by various manufacturers.[672] Individual lots also demonstrated variable levels of opsonic activity against different pathogens. This variability appeared to be a function of the donor pool rather than the manufacturing method. Whether intravenous preparations with known pathogen-specific antibody content may be effective in reducing nosocomial infections by specific agents remains to be seen.

Because preterm infants have limited neutrophil pools, as well as limited neutrophil function, several randomized, controlled studies have examined the prophylactic and therapeutic effect of granulocyte-macrophage colony-stimulating factor (GM-CSF) and granulocyte colony-stimulating factor (G-CSF) on nosocomial infections in preterm infants. In all these studies, infants receiving these agents had higher peripheral blood neutrophil counts than did infants receiving placebo. However, the benefit of treatment with these agents has been limited. A study of prophylactic treatment with GM-CSF for 5 days beginning shortly after birth found a trend toward decreased infection rates in treated infants, although the study was powered to address whether treatment reduced neutropenia, not whether it reduced infection.[87] A second study of prophylactic treatment with GM-CSF during the first 28 days of life failed to demonstrate any benefit in terms of decreased nosocomial infection rates.[83] A study of the therapeutic effect of 3 days of treatment with G-CSF administered to infants with the clinical diagnosis of early-onset sepsis did not demonstrate any reduction in mortality rates but did find that nosocomial infection rates were lower in treated infants in the 2 weeks after treatment.[449]

The use of postnatal corticosteroids to prevent or treat chronic lung disease in preterm infants has been associated with higher rates of nosocomial infection,[630] as well as other short- and long-term adverse outcomes.[135]

IMMUNOCOMPROMISED CHILDREN

The principal nosocomial infectious threats to immunocompromised children are those discussed previously (see Nosocomial Infections Caused by Spread of Infections Common in the Community and Nosocomial Infections Related to Invasive Devices, Procedures, and Treatments). However, several issues regarding the epidemiology and prevention of nosocomial infections in these high-risk patients deserve additional comment.

Candida and other yeasts (e.g., *Trichosporon beigelii)* are significant nosocomial pathogens in immunocompromised children, both because these hosts have impaired defenses and because they often require invasive devices (such as central venous catheters), parenteral nutrition, and broad-spectrum antimicrobial therapy. The spectrum of disease includes superficial infection (e.g., mucocutaneous candidiasis), bloodstream infection associated with central venous catheters, and disseminated infection (e.g., meningitis, hepatosplenic infection, renal infection, ophthalmitis). Neutropenia greatly increases the risk of development of disseminated disease.[320] Although specific *Candida* strains generally are regarded as endogenous flora, molecular epidemiologic studies demonstrate that they can be acquired within the hospital by indirect contact transmission.[570, 658] Handwashing and the use of standard precautions (see Chapter 232) when caring for high-risk patients are likely to be helpful in reducing nosocomial transmission of *Candida* spp.

HSV, CMV, and VZV are also common causes of infection in hospitalized immunocompromised patients. However, reactivation of a preexisting latent infection occurs more frequently than primary infection does. Development of a lymphoproliferative disorder secondary to reactivation of Epstein-Barr virus is a significant complication of solid organ transplantation (particularly liver, bowel, heart, and heart/lung transplants) and T-cell–depleted allogeneic bone marrow transplantation. Primary nosocomial CMV infection is a particular problem in allogeneic bone marrow or solid organ transplant recipients because the scarcity of suitable donors does not allow selection of CMV-negative donors for CMV-negative recipients. Prophylaxis to prevent herpesvirus disease in immunocompromised patients is discussed in detail in other chapters.

Nosocomial respiratory viral infections can be severe and prolonged in patients with profoundly compromised immune systems (see Nosocomial Infections Caused by Spread of Infections Common in the Community). Nosocomial multidrug-resistant tuberculosis is a problem in adult patients with HIV infection, although it has not been demonstrated to be a significant problem in HIV-infected children.

Though far less common, *Legionella* and filamentous fungi cause serious, potentially lethal disease in immunocompromised children.[1, 23, 72, 664]

The principal reservoir for *Legionella* is the hospital water supply, particularly aging systems with large dead spaces.[639] Contaminated aerosols generated by showerheads, faucet aerators, and even bedpan cleaners may lead to the development of nosocomial disease.[639] Decontamination of the water supply is a difficult and expensive endeavor. The most cost-effective approach among those described in the CDC/HICPAC guideline for prevention of nosocomial pneumonia has not been determined.[639]

Spores of *Aspergillus* and other filamentous fungi are virtually ubiquitous wherever decaying organic matter or moisture is found. Airborne spores may enter the hospital through inadequate air filtration systems and open windows or doors. Spores also may originate from within the hospital (e.g., air ducts, wet wood or plaster, fireproofing materials, soil of plants, and even pepper). Hospital construction may release clouds of fungal spores, and once in the hospital, spores can survive indefinitely in dust. Ventilation systems designed to reduce the frequency of infections caused by airborne fungi are described in a guideline for the prevention of nosocomial pneumonia.[639]

Comprehensive, multidisciplinary guidelines for the prevention of opportunistic infections in hematopoietic stem cell transplant recipients and HIV-infected patients have been published.[105, 111] Similar multidisciplinary guidelines for the prevention of infection in solid organ transplant recipients do not exist.

CHILDREN WITH BURNS

Information regarding the epidemiology of nosocomial infections in pediatric burn patients is limited.[578, 669] The experience of a single pediatric burn facility that performed prospective surveillance with the use of modified CDC definitions has been reported.[669] The definitions used in this study were modified to describe nosocomial burn infection and secondary bloodstream infection more accurately in the burn population. Based on this and other studies, new definitions for burn infection have been proposed.[488] The overall frequency of nosocomial infection in this unit was 14 percent, or 16 infections per 1000 patient-days.[669] The frequency of burn infection was 10 percent, or 5.6 burn infections per 1000 patient-days. Gram-positive cocci, including *S. aureus* and MRSA, were the most frequent cause of burn infections in patients with relatively small burns (<30% of body surface area). Gram-positive cocci and gram-negative bacteria (especially *P. aeruginosa)* were common causes in patients with extensive burns (>30% of body surface area). Rates of device associated infections were 4.9 bloodstream infections per 1000 central venous catheter-days, 11.4 cases of ventilator pneumonia per 1000 ventilator-days, and 13.2 urinary tract infections per 1000 urinary catheter-days. These rates are somewhat lower than the pooled means for adult burn units (see Table 231–2) and are roughly comparable to rates of infection in pediatric ICUs (see Table 231–2 and Fig. 231–1), although the incidence of urinary tract infection is somewhat higher. When infection rates in this study were stratified by the extent of the burn, the incidence of bloodstream infection secondary to burn infection and catheter-associated urinary tract infection increased with increasing burn size, although rates based on the number of patient-days or device-days reflected the risk of infection more accurately over time. In an older study of viral infections in pediatric burn patients, CMV infection was a relatively common occurrence, perhaps in part because of transfusion-related infection.[384] Isolation of HSV from pharyngeal and perioral cultures also was common, but clinical symptoms were infrequent findings.

Interventions to reduce the incidence of nosocomial infections in burn patients include the use of barrier techniques to decrease cross-colonization of patients, prevention of cross-colonization during hydrotherapy treatment, use of topical antibiotics to retard the growth of microorganisms in the burn wound, appropriate use of systemic antibiotics, and early excision and closure of the burn wound.[425] A randomized, controlled trial of selective decontamination of the digestive tract with polymyxin E, tobramycin, and amphotericin B in severely burned children found no evidence of benefit.[46] Care of high-risk patients in single-bed isolation rooms (as opposed to beds on open wards) appears to reduce the risk of acquiring infection,[437] although this intervention has not been subjected to a controlled trial. A study outlining an effective program for the control of MRSA in a pediatric burn unit may be applicable to the control of other antimicrobial-resistant microorganisms.[595]

CHILDREN WITH CYSTIC FIBROSIS

Saiman and colleagues reviewed the epidemiology of important pathogens in persons with cystic fibrosis in a document summarizing the conclusions of an international consensus conference convened to develop evidence-based guidelines for standardized microbiologic and infection control practices for persons with cystic fibrosis.[568] They found substantial evidence for transmission of *B. cepacia* complex, *P. aeruginosa,* and MRSA to persons with cystic fibrosis in health care settings. They concluded that the evidence was insufficient to determine whether *S. maltophilia, Achromobacter xylosoxidans,* nontuberculous mycobacteria, or filamentous fungi could be transmitted from person to person. One report of a large hospital outbreak of *B. cepacia* complex found evidence for transmission to patients with cystic fibrosis and patients who did not have cystic fibrosis.[295] Another report documented transmission of MRSA from hospitalized patients to patients with cystic fibrosis.[241] Given these data, transmission of *P. aeruginosa* from a patient with cystic fibrosis to a patient who did not have cystic fibrosis has never been reported, even though patients with cystic fibrosis are heavily colonized with *P. aeruginosa* and frequently have a productive cough during inpatient admission for treatment of pulmonary exacerbation.

At least nine distinct species of *B. cepacia* complex exist. Most patients colonized with *B. cepacia* complex are colonized with genomovar III.[386, 622] Investigators have been studying genomovar III strains intensively to identify bacterial factors associated with transmissibility and virulence. Transmission has been associated with the presence of cable pili and the *B. cepacia* epidemic strain marker (BCESM).[295, 407, 622, 637] However, considerable geographic variability in the prevalence of these markers has been observed, and transmission of strains with neither marker has occurred.[124, 387]

The aforementioned guideline emphasizes standard infection control practices in the care of patients with cystic fibrosis, including appropriate hand hygiene and the use of barriers by health care workers, proper use of isolation precautions, and effective procedures for cleaning and disinfecting/sterilizing reused equipment contaminated with respiratory secretions.[568]

In inpatient settings, the guideline recommends contact isolation and a private room for patients who are colonized or infected with MRSA, *B. cepacia* complex, and multidrug-resistant *P. aeruginosa.* Patients who are not colonized with these bacteria may share a room with a patient who does not have cystic fibrosis and who is at low risk for acquiring infection with these bacteria. All patients, regardless of whether they are colonized with these bacteria, should avoid contact with other patients who have cystic fibrosis.

The guideline makes no recommendation regarding the use of masks by patients with cystic fibrosis in either inpatient or outpatient settings because of the lack of sufficient evidence for or against the efficacy of this practice.

In ambulatory settings, the guideline recommends that patients with cystic fibrosis who are colonized or infected with *B. cepacia* complex be segregated from other cystic fibrosis patients and other patients colonized or infected with *B. cepacia* (to avoid replacement of one strain with another), that their visits be scheduled at the end of the clinic session or on another day, and that they be placed in an examination room immediately instead of sitting with other patients in the waiting room. Patients colonized or infected with multidrug-resistant *P. aeruginosa* also should be placed in an examination room immediately. For other patients, the guideline recommends a variety of clinic logistics to minimize the time that patients spend in waiting areas and emphasizes education of patients regarding appropriate waiting area behavior to minimize contact among patients (e.g., discouraging hand shakes and physical contact among patients, maintaining at least 3 ft between patients, avoiding contact with common-use items). All patients should receive annual influenza vaccination and age-appropriate pneumococcal vaccination.

CHILDREN IN LONG-TERM CARE FACILITIES

The preceding sections have described a variety of microorganisms that have caused disease in long-term care facilities for children, including various viral infections and enteric pathogens. Specific interventions to prevent these infections have been discussed previously (see Nosocomial Infections Caused by Spread of Infections Common in the Community).

A prospective, longitudinal study in a pediatric long-term care facility illustrates the spectrum of endemic nosocomial infections in this population.[660] The cumulative incidence of infection was 40 percent in the more than 400 patients who received care in this facility over a 2-year period. Upper respiratory tract infections and urinary tract infections accounted for 37 and 31 percent of the infections, respectively. Nearly 80 percent of the urinary tract infections occurred in a small group of patients with neural tube defects or neuromuscular disorders, but the study did not differentiate between symptomatic infection and asymptomatic bacteriuria. The rate of infection in children exposed to indwelling or intermittent catheterization (or both) also was not reported. Upper and lower respiratory tract infections were common in young children with tracheostomies. Skin infections accounted for 16 percent of the infections, but the specific percentage of decubitus ulcers was not reported. Gastrointestinal infections were remarkably uncommon events (4% of all nosocomial infections).

A guideline for the prevention of nosocomial infections in long-term care residents has been published, although this document does not deal with issues specific to the care of children.[614] Key prevention measures are effective hand hygiene, appropriate use of barriers and isolation precautions, proper care of patients who have indwelling devices (e.g., tracheostomies) or require invasive procedures (e.g., bladder catheterization), prevention of decubitus ulcers, age-appropriate immunization (including yearly influenza vaccine, conjugate or polysaccharide pneumococcal vaccine, hepatitis B vaccine, and hepatitis A vaccine, depending on local epidemiologic conditions), and early detection and control of outbreaks of infection.

REFERENCES

1. Abbasi, S., Shenep, J. L., Hughes, W. T., and Flynn, P. M.: Aspergillosis in children with cancer: A 34-year experience. Clin. Infect. Dis. *29*: 1210–1219, 1999.
2. Abzug, M. J., Keyserling, H. L., Lee, M. L., et al.: Neonatal enterovirus infection: Virology, serology, and effects of intravenous immune globulin. Clin. Infect. Dis. *20*:1201–1206, 1995.
3. Adam, B., Baillie, G. S., and Douglas, L. J.: Mixed species biofilms of *Candida albicans* and *Staphylococcus epidermidis*. J. Med. Microbiol. *51*:344–349, 2002.
4. Adams, G., Stover, B. H., Keenlyside, R. A., et al.: Nosocomial herpetic infections in a pediatric intensive care unit. Am. J. Epidemiol. *113*: 126–132, 1981.
5. Adler, S. P.: Hospital transmission of cytomegalovirus. Infect. Agents Dis. *1*:43–49, 1992.
6. Agah, R., Cherry, J. D., Garakian, A. J., and Chapin, M.: Respiratory syncytial virus infection rate in personnel caring for children with RSV infections: Routine isolation procedure vs routine procedure supplemented by use of masks and goggles. Am. J. Dis. Child. *141*:695–697, 1987.
7. Aggett, P. J., Cooper, L. V., Ellis, S. H., and McAinsh, J.: Percutaneous absorption of chlorhexidine in neonatal cord care. Arch. Dis. Child. *56*: 878–880, 1981.
8. Aintablian, N., Walpita, P., and Sawyer, M. H.: Detection of *Bordetella pertussis* and respiratory syncytial virus in air samples from hospital rooms. Infect. Control Hosp. Epidemiol. *19*:918–923, 1998.
9. Altemeier, W. A., Burke, J. F., and Sandusky, W. R.: Manual on Control of Infection in Surgical Patients. 2nd. ed. Philadelphia, J. B. Lippincott, 1984.
10. Alter, H. J., Nakatsuji, Y., Melpolder, J., et al.: The incidence of transfusion-associated hepatitis G virus infection and its relation to liver disease. N. Engl. J. Med. *336*:747–754, 1997.
11. Altman, C. A., Englund, J. A., Demmler, G., et al.: Respiratory syncytial virus in patients with congenital heart disease: A contemporary look at epidemiology and success of preoperative screening. Pediatr. Cardiol. *21*:433–438, 2000.
12. Alvarado, C. J., Stolz, S. M., and Maki, D. G.: Nosocomial infections from contaminated endoscopes: A flawed automated endoscope washer. An investigation using molecular epidemiology. Am. J. Med. *91*(Suppl.): 272–280, 1991.
13. American Academy of Pediatrics, American College of Obstetricians and Gynecologists: Guidelines for Perinatal Care. 4th ed. Elk Grove Village, IL, American Academy of Pediatrics, 1997.
14. American Academy of Pediatrics: Hepatitis A. *In* Pickering, L. K. (ed.): 2000 Red Book: Report of the Committee on Infectious Diseases. 25th ed. Elk Grove Village, IL, American Academy of Pediatrics, 2000, pp. 280–289.
15. American Academy of Pediatrics: Measles. *In* Pickering, L. K. (ed.): 2000 Red Book: Report of the Committee on Infectious Diseases. 25th ed. Elk Grove Village, IL, American Academy of Pediatrics, 2000, pp. 385–396.
16. American Academy of Pediatrics: Varicella-zoster infections. *In* Pickering, L. K. (ed.): 2000 Red Book: Report of the Committee on Infectious Diseases. Elk Grove Village, IL, American Academy of Pediatrics, 2000, pp 624–636.
17. American Academy of Pediatrics: Antimicrobial prophylaxis in pediatric surgical patients. *In* Pickering, L. K. (ed.): 2000 Red Book: Report of the Committee on Infectious Diseases. 25th ed. Elk Grove Village, IL, American Academy of Pediatrics, 2000, pp. 730–735.
18. American Academy of Pediatrics Committee on Infectious Diseases: Reassessment of the indications for ribavirin therapy in respiratory syncytial virus infections. Pediatrics *97*:137–140, 1996.
19. American Academy of Pediatrics Committee on Infectious Diseases and Committee of Fetus and Newborn: Prevention of respiratory syncytial virus infections: Indications for the use of palivizumab and update on the use of RSV-IGIV. Pediatrics *102*:1211–1216, 1998.
20. American Institute of Architects, Academy of Architecture for Health: Guidelines for Design and Construction of Hospital and Health Care Facilities. 1996–1997 ed. The American Institute of Architects Press, Washington, D. C., 1996.
21. Anderson, J. D., Bonner, M., Scheifele, D. W., and Schneider, B. C.: Lack of nosocomial spread of varicella in a pediatric hospital with negative pressure ventilated patient rooms. Infect. Control *6*:120–121, 1985.
22. Anderson, J. R., Smith, M. D., Kibbler, C. C., et al.: A nosocomial outbreak due to non-encapsulated *Haemophilus influenzae:* Analysis of plasmids coding for antibiotic resistance. J. Hosp. Infect. *27*:17–27, 1994.
23. Anderson, K., Morris, G., Kennedy, H., et al.: Aspergillosis in immunocompromised paediatric patients: Associations with building hygiene, design, and indoor air. Thorax *51*:256–261, 1996.
24. Anderson, L. J., Williams, L., Jr., Layde, J. B., et al.: Nosocomial rabies: Investigation of contacts of human rabies cases associated with a corneal transplant. Am. J. Public Health *74*:370–372, 1984.
25. Anderson, M. J., Higgins, P. G., Davis, L. R., et al.: Experimental parvoviral infection in humans. J. Infect. Dis. *152*:257–265, 1985.
26. Ansari, S. A., Sattar, S. A., Springthorpe, V. S., et al.: Rotavirus survival on human hands and transfer of infectious virus to animate and nonporous inanimate surfaces. J. Clin. Microbiol. *26*:1513–1518, 1988.
27. Archibald, L. K., Manning, M. L., Bell, L. M., et al.: Patient density, nurse-to-patient ratio and nosocomial infection risk in a pediatric cardiac intensive care unit. Pediatr. Infect. Dis. J. *16*:1045–1048, 1997.
28. Arnon, S. S., Schechter, R., Inglesby, T. V., et al.: Botulinum toxin as a biological weapon: Medical and public health management. J. A. M. A. *285*:1059–1070, 2001.
29. Asensio, A., Oliver, A., Gonzalez-Diego, P., et al.: Outbreak of a multiresistant *Klebsiella pneumoniae* strain in an intensive care unit: Antibiotic use as risk factor for colonization and infection. Clin. Infect. Dis. *30*:55–60, 2000.
30. Atkinson, J. B., Chamberlin, K., and Boody, B. A.: A prospective randomized trial of urokinase as an adjuvant in the treatment of proven Hickman catheter sepsis. J. Pediatr. Surg. *33*:714–716, 1998.
31. Atkinson, W. L., Markowitz, L. E., Adams, N. C., and Seastrom, G. R.: Transmission of measles in medical settings—United States, 1985–1989. Am. J. Med. *91*(Suppl.):320–324, 1991.
32. AuBuchon, J. P., and Birkmeyer, J. D.: Safety and cost-effectiveness of solvent-detergent–treated plasma. In search of a zero-risk blood supply. J. A. M. A. *272*:1210–1214, 1994.
33. Austin, B. J., Croxson, M. C., Powell, K. F., and Gunn, T. R.: The successful containment of Coxsackie B4 infection in a neonatal unit. J. Paediatr. Child Health *35*:102–104, 1999.
34. Avila-Figueroa, C., Goldmann, D. A., Richardson, D. K., et al.: Intravenous lipid emulsions are the major determinant of coagulase-negative staphylococcal bacteremia in very low birth weight newborns. Pediatr. Infect. Dis. J. *17*:10–17, 1998.
35. Ayliffe, G. A.: Role of the environment of the operating suite in surgical wound infection. Rev. Infect. Dis. *13*(Suppl.):800–804, 1991.
36. Ayliffe, G. A.: Nosocomial infections associated with hemodialysis. *In* Mayhall, C. G. (ed): Hospital Epidemiology and Infection Control. Philadelphia, Lippincott Williams & Wilkins, 1999, pp. 881–895.
37. Azimi, P. H., Roberto, R. R., Guralnik, J., et al.: Transfusion-acquired hepatitis A in a premature infant with secondary nosocomial spread in an intensive care nursery. Am. J. Dis. Child. *140*:23–27, 1986.
38. Aznar, J., Safi, H., Romero, J., et al.: Nosocomial transmission of tuberculosis infection in pediatrics wards. Pediatr. Infect. Dis. J. *14*:44–48, 1995.
39. Baba, T., Takeuchi, F., Kuroda, M., et al.: Genome and virulence determinants of high virulence community-acquired MRSA. Lancet *359*: 1819–1827, 2002.
40. Bachrach, S.: An outbreak of *Haemophilus influenzae* type b bacteraemia in an intermediate care hospital for children. J. Hosp. Infect. *11*:121–126, 1988.
41. Bachrach, S. J.: Successful treatment of an institutional outbreak of shigellosis. Clin. Pediatr. (Phila.) *20*:127–131, 1981.
42. Back, N. A., Linnemann, C. C., Jr., Staneck, J. L., and Kotagal, U. R.: Control of methicillin-resistant *Staphylococcus aureus* in a neonatal intensive-care unit: Use of intensive microbiologic surveillance and mupirocin. Infect. Control Hosp. Epidemiol. *17*:227–231, 1996.
43. Bailly, J. L., Beguet, A., Chambon, M., et al.: Nosocomial transmission of echovirus 30: Molecular evidence by phylogenetic analysis of the VP1 encoding sequence. J. Clin. Microbiol. *38*:2889–2892, 2000.
44. Baker, C. J., Melish, M. E., Hall, R. T., et al.: Intravenous immune globulin for the prevention of nosocomial infection in low-birth-weight neonates. The Multicenter Group for the Study of Immune Globulin in Neonates. N. Engl. J. Med. *327*:213–219, 1992.
45. Baron, R. C., McCormick, J. B., and Zubeir, O. A.: Ebola virus disease in southern Sudan: Hospital dissemination and intrafamilial spread. Bull. World Health Organ. *61*:997–1003, 1983.
46. Barret, J. P., Jeschke, M. G., and Herndon, D. N.: Selective decontamination of the digestive tract in severely burned pediatric patients. Burns *27*:439–445, 2001.
47. Barton, L. L., Granoff, D. M., and Barenkamp, S. J.: Nosocomial spread of *Haemophilus influenzae* type b infection documented by outer membrane protein subtype analysis. J. Pediatr. *102*:820–824, 1983.
48. Barzilay, Z., Mandel, M., Keren, G., and Davidson, S.: Nosocomial bacterial pneumonia in ventilated children: Clinical significance of culture-positive peripheral bronchial aspirates. J. Pediatr. *112*:421–424, 1988.
49. Beatson, S. H.: Pharaoh's ants as pathogen vectors in hospitals. Lancet *1*:425–427, 1972.

50. Beck-Sague, C., Dooley, S. W., Hutton, M. D., et al.: Hospital outbreak of multidrug-resistant *Mycobacterium tuberculosis* infections. Factors in transmission to staff and HIV-infected patients. J. A. M. A. *268*: 1280–1286, 1992.
51. Beck-Sague, C. M., and Jarvis, W. R.: Epidemic bloodstream infections associated with pressure transducers: A persistent problem. Infect. Control Hosp. Epidemiol. *10*:54–59, 1989.
52. Beers, L. M., Burke, T. L., and Martin, D. B.: Shigellosis occurring in newborn nursery staff. Infect. Control Hosp. Epidemiol. *10*:147–149, 1989.
53. Bell, L. M., Naides, S. J., Stoffman, P., et al.: Human parvovirus B19 infection among hospital staff members after contact with infected patients. N. Engl. J. Med. *321*:485–491, 1989.
54. Benaoudia, F., and Bingen, E.: Evidence for the genetic unrelatedness of nosocomial *Alcaligenes xylosoxidans* strains in a pediatric hospital. Infect. Control Hosp. Epidemiol. *18*:132–134, 1997.
55. Bennett, S. N., McNeil, M. M., Bland, L. A., et al.: Postoperative infections traced to contamination of an intravenous anesthetic, propofol. N. Engl. J. Med. *333*:147–154, 1995.
56. Berman, S. A., Balkany, T. J., and Simmons, M. A.: Otitis media in the neonatal intensive care unit. Pediatrics *62*:198–201, 1978.
57. Bhattacharyya, N., and Kosloske, A. M.: Postoperative wound infection in pediatric surgical patients: A study of 676 infants and children. J. Pediatr. Surg. *25*:125–129, 1990.
58. Bhattacharyya, N., Kosloske, A. M., and Macarthur, C.: Nosocomial infection in pediatric surgical patients: A study of 608 infants and children. J. Pediatr. Surg. *28*:338–343, 1993.
59. Biering, G., Karlsson, S., Clark, N. C., et al.: Three cases of neonatal meningitis caused by *Enterobacter sakazakii* in powdered milk. J. Clin. Microbiol. *27*:2054–2056, 1989.
60. Bingen, E. H., Denamur, E., Lambert-Zechovsky, N. Y., and Elion, J.: Evidence for the genetic unrelatedness of nosocomial vancomycin-resistant *Enterococcus faecium* strains in a pediatric hospital. J. Clin. Microbiol. *29*:1888–1892, 1991.
61. Bingen, E., Lambert-Zechovsky, N., Mariani-Kurkdjian, P., et al.: Bacteremia caused by a vancomycin-resistant *Enterococcus*. Pediatr. Infect. Dis. J. *8*:475–476, 1989.
62. Blank, S., Simonds, R. J., Weisfuse, I., et al.: Possible nosocomial transmission of HIV. Lancet *344*:512–514, 1994.
63. Blatt, M. L.: Cross-infection: Its prevention in a children's hospital. Illinois Med. J. *70*:483–487, 1936.
64. Blot, F., Nitenberg, G., Chachaty, E., et al.: Diagnosis of catheter-related bacteraemia: A prospective comparison of the time to positivity of hub-blood versus peripheral-blood cultures. Lancet *354*:1071–1077, 1999.
65. Blumberg, H. M., Watkins, D. L., Berschling, J. D., et al.: Preventing the nosocomial transmission of tuberculosis. Ann. Intern. Med. *122*:658–663, 1995.
66. Bobkov, A., Garaev, M. M., Rzhaninova, A., et al.: Molecular epidemiology of HIV-1 in the former Soviet Union: Analysis of env V3 sequences and their correlation with epidemiologic data. A. I. D. S. *8*:619–624, 1994.
67. Bone, R. C., Balk, R. A., Cerra, F. B., et al.: Definitions for sepsis and organ failure and guidelines for the use of innovative therapies in sepsis. Chest *101*:1644–1655, 1992.
68. Borio, L., Inglesby, T., Peters, C. J., et al.: Hemorrhagic fever viruses as biological weapons: Medical and public health management. J. A. M. A. *287*:2391–2405, 2002.
69. Centers for Disease Control and Prevention: Guidelines for hand hygiene in the health-care settings: Recommendations of the Healthcare Infection Control Practices Advisory Committee and the HICPAC/SHEA/APIC/IDSA Hand Hygiene Task Force. M. M. W. R. Recomm. Rep. *51*(RR-16):1–48, 2002.
70. Boyce, T. G., Mellen, B. G., Mitchel, E. F., Jr., et al.: Rates of hospitalization for respiratory syncytial virus infection among children in Medicaid. J. Pediatr. *137*:865–870, 2000.
71. Bradford, P. A.: Extended-spectrum beta-lactamases in the 21st century: Characterization, epidemiology, and detection of this important resistance threat. Clin. Microbiol. Rev. *14*:933–951, 2001.
72. Brady, M. T.: Nosocomial legionnaires disease in a children's hospital. J. Pediatr. *115*:46–50, 1989.
73. Brady, M. T., Pacini, D. L., Budde, C. T., and Connell, M. J.: Diagnostic studies of nosocomial diarrhea in children: Assessing their use and value. Am. J. Infect. Control *17*:77–82, 1989.
74. Branchini, M. L., Pfaller, M. A., Rhine-Chalberg, J., et al.: Genotypic variation and slime production among blood and catheter isolates of *Candida parapsilosis*. J. Clin. Microbiol. *32*:452–456, 1994.
75. Brennemann, J.: The infant ward. Am. J. Dis. Child. *43*:577–584, 1932.
76. Bridges, C. B, Fukuda, K., Cox, N. J., and Singleton, J. A.: Prevention and control of influenza. Recommendations of the Advisory Committee on Immunization Practices (ACIP). M. M. W. R. Recomm. Rep. *50*(RR-4):1–44, 2001.
77. Brodie, S. B., Sands, K. E., Gray, J. E., et al.: Occurrence of nosocomial bloodstream infections in six neonatal intensive care units. Pediatr. Infect. Dis. J. *19*:56–65, 2000.
78. Brook, I.: Microbiology of nosocomial sinusitis in mechanically ventilated children. Arch. Otolaryngol. Head Neck Surg. *124*:35–38, 1998.
79. Brunetto, A. L., Pearson, A. D., Craft, A. W., and Pedler, S. J.: *Clostridium difficile* in an oncology unit. Arch. Dis. Child. *63*:979–981, 1988.
80. Burke, J. P., and Zavasky, D. M.: Nosocomial urinary tract infections. *In* Mayhall, C. G. (ed): Hospital Epidemiology and Infection Control. Philadelphia, Lippincott Williams & Wilkins, 1999, pp. 173–187.
81. Burnie, J. P., Naderi-Nasab, M., Loudon, K. W., and Matthews, R. C.: An epidemiological study of blood culture isolates of coagulase-negative staphylococci demonstrating hospital-acquired infection. J. Clin. Microbiol. *35*:1746–1750, 1997.
82. Butzler, J. P., Goossens, H.: *Campylobacter jejuni* infection as a hospital problem: An overview. J. Hosp. Infect. *11*:374–377, 1988.
83. Cairo, M. S., Agosti, J., Ellis, R., et al.: A randomized, double-blind, placebo-controlled trial of prophylactic recombinant human granulocyte-macrophage colony-stimulating factor to reduce nosocomial infections in very low birth weight neonates. J. Pediatr. *134*:64–70, 1999.
84. Call, E. L.: An epidemic of pemphigus neonatorum. Am. J. Obstet. *50*: 473, 1904.
85. Cannon, C. G., and Linnemann, C., Jr.: *Yersinia enterocolitica* infections in hospitalized patients: The problem of hospital-acquired infections. Infect. Control Hosp. Epidemiol. *13*:139–143, 1992.
86. Cardo, D. M., and Bell, D. M.: Bloodborne pathogen transmission in health care workers. Risks and prevention strategies. Infect. Dis. Clin. North Am. *11*:331–346, 1997.
87. Carr, R., Modi, N., Dore, C. J., et al. A randomized, controlled trial of prophylactic granulocyte-macrophage colony-stimulating factor in human newborns less than 32 weeks gestation. Pediatrics *103*:796–802, 1999.
88. Cartwright, C. P., Stock, F., Beekmann, S. E., et al.: PCR amplification of rRNA intergenic spacer regions as a method for epidemiologic typing of *Clostridium difficile*. J. Clin. Microbiol. *33*:184–187, 1995.
89. Center for Biologics Evaluation and Research, Food and Drug Administration, U.S. Department of Health and Human Services: Guidance for industry: Revised preventative measures to reduce the possible risk of transmission of Creutzfeldt Jakob disease and variant Creutzfeldt Jakob disease by blood and blood products. Available at http://www.fda.gov/cber/gdlns/cjdvcjd.pdf; accessed on 1 June 2002. 2002.
90. Centers for Disease Control and Prevention: Laboratory-acquired meningococcemia—California and Massachusetts. M. M. W. R. Morb. Mortal. Wkly. Rep. *40*(3):46–47, 55, 1991.
91. Centers for Disease Control and Prevention: Nosocomial infection and pseudoinfection from contaminated endoscopes and bronchoscopes—Wisconsin and Missouri. M. M. W. R. Morb. Mortal. Wkly. Rep. *40*(39): 675–678, 1991.
92. Centers for Disease Control and Prevention: Nosocomial enterococci resistant to vancomycin—United States, 1989–1993. M. M. W. R. Morb. Mortal. Wkly. Rep. *42*(30):597–599, 1993.
93. Centers for Disease Control and Prevention: Outbreak of hepatitis C associated with intravenous immunoglobulin administration—United States, October 1993–June 1994. M. M. W. R. Morb. Mortal. Wkly. Rep. *43*(28):505–509, 1994.
94. Centers for Disease Control and Prevention: Update: Human plague—India, 1994. M. M. W. R. Morb. Mortal. Wkly. Rep. *43*(41):722–723, 1994.
95. Centers for Disease Control and Prevention: Detection of notifiable diseases through surveillance for imported plague—New York, September–October 1994. M. M. W. R. Morb. Mortal. Wkly. Rep. *43*(44): 805–807, 1994.
96. Centers for Disease Control and Prevention: Guidelines for preventing the transmission of *Mycobacterium tuberculosis* in health-care facilities, 1994. M. M. W. R. Recomm. Rep. *43*(RR-13):1–132, 1994.
97. Centers for Disease Control and Prevention: Diphtheria acquired by U.S. citizens in the Russian Federation and Ukraine—1994. M. M. W. R. Morb. Mortal. Wkly. Rep. *44*(12):237, 243–234, 1995.
98. Centers for Disease Control and Prevention: Update: Management of patients with suspected viral hemorrhagic fever—United States. M. M. W. R. Morb. Mortal. Wkly. Rep. *44*(25):475–479, 1995.
99. Centers for Disease Control and Prevention: Prevention of perinatal group B streptococcal disease: a public health perspective. M. M. W. R. Recomm. Rep. *45*(RR-7):1–24, 1996.
100. Centers for Disease Control and Prevention: Red blood cell transfusions contaminated with *Yersinia enterocolitica*—United States, 1991–1996, and initiation of a national study to detect bacteria-associated transfusion reactions. M. M. W. R. Morb. Mortal. Wkly. Rep. *46*(24):553–555, 1997.
101. Centers for Disease Control and Prevention: Laboratory-based surveillance for rotavirus—United States, July 1996–June 1997. M. M. W. R. Morb. Mortal. Wkly. Rep. *46*(46):1092–1094, 1997.
102. Centers for Disease Control and Prevention: Bronchoscopy-related infections and pseudoinfections—New York, 1996 and 1998. M. M. W. R. Morb. Mortal. Wkly. Rep. *48*(26):557–560, 1999.
103. Centers for Disease Control and Prevention: Monitoring hospital-acquired infections to promote patient safety—United States, 1990–1999. M. M. W. R. Morb. Mortal. Wkly. Rep. *49*(8):149–153, 2000.
104. Centers for Disease Control and Prevention: *Staphylococcus aureus* with reduced susceptibility to vancomycin—Illinois, 1999. M. M. W. R. Morb. Mortal. Wkly. Rep. *48*(51–52):1165–1167, 2000.
105. Centers for Disease Control and Prevention: Guidelines for preventing opportunistic infections among hematopoietic stem cell transplant recipients. M. M. W. R. Recomm. Rep. *49*(RR-10):1–125, CE1–CE7, 2000.

106. Centers for Disease Control and Prevention: Recommendations for preventing transmission of infections among chronic hemodialysis patients. M. M. W. R. Recomm. Rep. *50*(RR-5):1–43, 2001.
107. Centers for Disease Control and Prevention: Tuberculosis morbidity among U.S.-born and foreign-born populations—United States, 2000. M. M. W. R. Morb. Mortal. Wkly. Rep. *51*(5):101–104, 2002.
108. Centers for Disease Control and Prevention: Measles—United States 2000. M. M. W. R. Morb. Mortal. Wkly. Rep. *51*(6):120–123, 2002.
109. Centers for Disease Control and Prevention: *Pseudomonas aeruginosa* infections associated with defective bronchoscopes. M. M. W. R. Morb. Mortal. Wkly. Rep. *51*:190, 2002.
110. Centers for Disease Control and Prevention: *Enterobacter sakazakii* infections associated with the use of powdered infant formula—Tennessee, 2001. M. M. W. R. Morb. Mortal. Wkly. Rep. *51*(14):297–300, 2002.
111. Centers for Disease Control and Prevention: Guidelines for preventing opportunistic infections among HIV-infected persons—2002 recommendations of the U.S. Public Health Service and the Infectious Diseases Society of America. M. M. W. R. Recomm. Rep. *51*(RR-8):1–52, 2002.
112. Centers for Disease Control and Prevention: Interim smallpox response plan and guidelines. Available at http://www.bt.cdc.gov/DocumentsApp/Smallpox/RPG/index.asp; accessed on 1 June 2002.
113. Centers for Disease Control and Prevention: Draft supplemental recommendation of the ACIP on the use of smallpox (vaccinia) vaccine. Available at http://www.cdc.gov/nip/smallpox/supp_recs.htm; accessed on 21 June 2002.
114. Cetinkaya, Y., Falk, P., and Mayhall, C. G.: Vancomycin-resistant enterococci. Clin. Microbiol. Rev. *13*:686–707, 2000.
115. Chadee, D. D., and Le Maitre, A.: Ants: Potential mechanical vectors of hospital infections in Trinidad. Trans. R. Soc. Trop. Med. Hyg. *84*:297, 1990.
116. Chaiyakunapruk, N., Veenstra, D. L., Lipsky, B. A., and Saint, S.: Chlorhexidine compared with povidone-iodine solution for vascular catheter-site care: A meta-analysis. Ann. Intern. Med. *136*:792–801, 2002.
117. Chambon, M., Bailly, J. L., Beguet, A., et al.: An outbreak due to echovirus type 30 in a neonatal unit in France in 1997: Usefulness of PCR diagnosis. J. Hosp. Infect. *43*:63–68, 1999.
118. Chang, H. J., Miller, H. L., Watkins, N., et al.: An epidemic of *Malassezia pachydermatis* in an intensive care nursery associated with colonization of health care workers' pet dogs. N. Engl. J. Med. *338*:706–711, 1998.
119. Chapin, M., Yatabe, J., and Cherry, J. D.: An outbreak of rotavirus gastroenteritis on a pediatric unit. Am. J. Infect. Control *11*:88–91, 1983.
120. Charlton, M., Adjei, P., Poterucha, J., et al.: TT-virus infection in North American blood donors, patients with fulminant hepatic failure, and cryptogenic cirrhosis. Hepatology *28*:839–842, 1998.
121. Chastre, J., Fagon, J. Y., Bornet-Lecso, M., et al.: Evaluation of bronchoscopic techniques for the diagnosis of nosocomial pneumonia. Am. J. Respir. Crit. Care Med. *152*:231–240, 1995.
122. Chastre, J., Fagon, J. Y., Soler, P., et al.: Diagnosis of nosocomial bacterial pneumonia in intubated patients undergoing ventilation: Comparison of the usefulness of bronchoalveolar lavage and the protected specimen brush. Am. J. Med. *85*:499–506, 1988.
123. Chastre, J., Viau, F., Brun, P., et al.: Prospective evaluation of the protected specimen brush for the diagnosis of pulmonary infections in ventilated patients. Am. Rev. Respir. Dis. *130*:924–929, 1984.
124. Chen, J. S., Witzmann, K. A., Spilker, T., et al.: Endemicity and intercity spread of *Burkholderia cepacia* genomovar III in cystic fibrosis. J. Pediatr. *139*:643–649, 2001.
125. Cherry, J. D.: Nosocomial pertussis in the nineties. Infect. Control Hosp. Epidemiol. *16*:553–555, 1995.
126. Chidekel, A. S., Rosen, C. L., and Bazzy, A. R.: Rhinovirus infection associated with serious lower respiratory illness in patients with bronchopulmonary dysplasia. Pediatr. Infect. Dis. J. *16*:43–47, 1997.
127. Christie, C. D. C., Glover, A. M., Willke, M. J., et al.: Containment of pertussis in the regional pediatric hospital during the Greater Cincinnati epidemic of 1993. Infect. Control Hosp. Epidemiol. *16*:556–563, 1995.
128. Cimolai, N., Cogswell, A., and Hunter, R.: Nosocomial transmission of penicillin-resistant *Streptococcus pneumoniae*. Pediatr. Pulmonol. *27*: 432–434, 1999.
129. Clark, N. C., Hill, B. C., O'Hara, C. M., et al.: Epidemiologic typing of *Enterobacter sakazakii* in two neonatal nosocomial outbreaks. Diagn. Microbiol. Infect. Dis. *13*:467–472, 1990.
130. Clark-Christoff, N., Watters, V. A., Sparks, W., et al.: Use of triple-lumen subclavian catheters for administration of total parenteral nutrition. J. P. E. N. J. Parenter. Enteral Nutr. *16*:403–407, 1992.
131. Classen, D. C., Evans, R. S., Pestotnik, S. L., et al.: The timing of prophylactic administration of antibiotics and the risk of surgical-wound infection. N. Engl. J. Med. *326*:281–286, 1992.
132. Cleary, T. G., Guerrant, R. L., and Pickering, L. K.: Microorganisms responsible for neonatal diarrhea. *In* Remington, J. S., and Klein, J. O. (ed.): Infectious Diseases of the Fetus & Newborn Infant. Philadelphia, W. B. Saunders, 2001, pp. 1249–1326.
133. Coello, R., Glenister, H., Fereres, J., et al.: The cost of infection in surgical patients: A case-control study. J. Hosp. Infect. *25*:239–250, 1993.
134. Cohen, M. S., Steere, A. C., Baltimore, R., et al.: Possible nosocomial transmission of group Y *Neisseria meningitidis* among oncology patients. Ann. Intern. Med. *91*:7–12, 1979.
135. Committee on the Fetus and Newborn, American Academy of Pediatrics, Canadian Paediatric Society: Postnatal corticosteroids to treat or prevent chronic lung disease in preterm infants. Pediatrics *109*:330–338, 2002.
136. Cone, R., Mohan, K., Thouless, M., and Corey, L.: Nosocomial transmission of rotavirus infection. Pediatr. Infect. Dis. J. *7*:103–109, 1988.
137. Cookson, S. T., Ihrig, M., O'Mara, E. M., et al.: Increased bloodstream infection rates in surgical patients associated with variation from recommended use and care following implementation of a needleless device. Infect. Control Hosp. Epidemiol. *19*:23–27, 1998.
138. Cooper, R. G., and Sumner, C.: Hospital infection data from a children's hospital. Med. J. Aust. *2*:1110–1113, 1970.
139. Coronado, V. G., Beck-Sague, C. M., Hutton, M. D., et al.: Transmission of multidrug-resistant *Mycobacterium tuberculosis* among persons with human immunodeficiency virus infection in an urban hospital: Epidemiologic and restriction fragment length polymorphism analysis. J. Infect. Dis. *168*:1052–1055, 1993.
140. Cosseron-Zerbib, M., Roque Afonso, A. M., Naas, T., et al.: A control programme for methicillin-resistant *Staphylococcus aureus* containment in a paediatric intensive care unit: Evaluation and impact on infections caused by other micro-organisms. J. Hosp. Infect. *40*:225–235, 1998.
141. Couch, R. B.: Prevention and treatment of influenza. N. Engl. J. Med. *343*:1778–1787, 2000.
142. Cowen, J., Ellis, S. H., and McAinsh, J.: Absorption of chlorhexidine from the intact skin of newborn infants. Arch. Dis. Child. *54*:379–383, 1979.
143. Cox, R. A., Rao, P., and Brandon-Cox, C.: The use of palivizumab monoclonal antibody to control an outbreak of respiratory syncytial virus infection in a special care baby unit. J. Hosp. Infect. *48*:186–192, 2001.
144. Craven, D., Brick, D., Morrisey, A., et al.: Low yield of bacterial stool culture in children with nosocomial diarrhea. Pediatr. Infect. Dis. J. *17*: 1040–1044, 1998.
145. Craven, D. E., Lichtenberg, D. A., Goularte, T. A., et al.: Contaminated medication nebulizers in mechanical ventilator circuits: Source of bacterial aerosols. Am. J. Med. *77*:834–838, 1984.
146. Crnich, C. J., and Maki, D. G.: The promise of novel technology for the prevention of intravascular device–related bloodstream infection. I. Pathogenesis and short-term devices. Clin. Infect. Dis. *34*:1232–1242, 2002.
147. Crnich, C. J., and Maki, D. G.: The promise of novel technology for the prevention of intravascular device–related bloodstream infection. II. Long-term devices. Clin. Infect. Dis. *34*:1362–1368, 2002.
148. Cronin, W. A., Germanson, T. P., and Donowitz, L. G.: Intravascular catheter colonization and related bloodstream infection in critically ill neonates. Infect. Control Hosp. Epidemiol. *11*:301–308, 1990.
149. Culver, D. H., Horan, T. C., Gaynes, R. P., et al.: Surgical wound infection rates by wound class, operative procedure, and patient risk index. National Nosocomial Infections Surveillance System. Am. J. Med. *91*(Suppl. 3B):152–157, 1991.
150. Cunney, R. J., Bialachowski, A., Thornley, D., et al.: An outbreak of influenza A in a neonatal intensive care unit. Infect. Control Hosp. Epidemiol. *21*:449–454, 2000.
151. Curtis, A. B., Ridzon, R., Vogel, R., et al.: Extensive transmission of *Mycobacterium tuberculosis* from a child. N. Engl. J. Med. *341*: 1491–1495, 1999.
152. Dankner, W. M., Spector, S. A., Fierer, J., and Davis, C. E.: *Malassezia* fungemia in neonates and adults: Complication of hyperalimentation. Rev. Infect. Dis. *9*:743–753, 1987.
153. Danzig, L. E., Short, L. J., Collins, K., et al.: Bloodstream infections associated with a needleless intravenous infusion system in patients receiving home infusion therapy. J. A. M. A. *273*:1862–1864, 1995.
154. Darouiche, R. O., Raad, I. I., Heard, S. O., et al.: A comparison of two antimicrobial-impregnated central venous catheters. N. Engl. J. Med. *340*:1–8, 1999.
155. Darouiche, R. O., Smith, J. A., Jr., Hanna, H., et al.: Efficacy of antimicrobial- impregnated bladder catheters in reducing catheter-associated bacteriuria: A prospective, randomized, multicenter clinical trial. Urology *54*:976–981, 1999.
156. Dato, V. M., and Dajani, A. S.: Candidemia in children with central venous catheters: Role of catheter removal and amphotericin B therapy. Pediatr. Infect. Dis. J. *9*:309–314, 1990.
157. Daum, R. S., Nachman, J. P., Leitch, C. D., and Tenover, F. C.: Nosocomial epiglottitis associated with penicillin- and cephalosporin-resistant *Streptococcus pneumoniae* bacteremia. J. Clin. Microbiol. *32*: 246–248, 1994.
158. Davenport, M., and Doig, C. M.: Wound infection in pediatric surgery: A study in 1,094 neonates. J. Pediatr. Surg. *28*:26–30, 1993.
159. Davidson, G. P., and Butler, R. N.: Probiotics in pediatric gastrointestinal disorders. Curr. Opin. Pediatr. *12*:477–481, 2000.
160. Davies, H. D., Jones, E. L., Sheng, R. Y., et al.: Nosocomial urinary tract infections at a pediatric hospital. Pediatr. Infect. Dis. J. *11*:349–354, 1992.
161. Davis, R. M., Orenstein, W. A., Frank, J., Jr., et al.: Transmission of measles in medical settings, 1980 through 1984. J. A. M. A. *255*: 1295–1298, 1986.

162. Davis, S. D., Sobocinski, K., Hoffman, R. G., et al.: Postoperative wound infections in a children's hospital. Pediatr. Infect. Dis. J. *3*:114–116, 1984.
163. de Cicco, M., Panarello, G., Chiaradia, V., et al.: Source and route of microbial colonisation of parenteral nutrition catheters. Lancet *2*: 1258–1261, 1989.
164. de Galan, B. E., van Tilburg, P. M., Sluijter, M., et al.: Hospital-related outbreak of infection with multidrug-resistant *Streptococcus pneumoniae* in the Netherlands. J. Hosp. Infect. *42*:185–192, 1999.
165. Demmler, G. J., Yow, M. D., Spector, S. A., et al.: Nosocomial cytomegalovirus infections within two hospitals caring for infants and children. J. Infect. Dis. *156*:9–16, 1987.
166. Dennehy, P. H., Nelson, S. M., Spangenberger, S., et al.: A prospective case-control study of the role of astrovirus in acute diarrhea among hospitalized young children. J. Infect. Dis. *184*:10–15, 2001.
167. Dennehy, P. H., and Peter, G.: Risk factors associated with nosocomial rotavirus infection. Am. J. Dis. Child. *139*:935–939, 1985.
168. Dennis, D. T., Inglesby, T. V., Henderson, D. A., et al.: Tularemia as a biological weapon: Medical and public health management. J. A. M. A. *285*:2763–2773, 2001.
169. Denton, M., and Kerr, K. G.: Microbiological and clinical aspects of infection associated with *Stenotrophomonas maltophilia.* Clin. Microbiol. Rev. *11*:57–80, 1998.
170. de Swart, R. L., Wertheim-van Dillen, P. M., van Binnendijk, R. S., et al.: Measles in a Dutch hospital introduced by an immuno-compromised infant from Indonesia infected with a new virus genotype. Lancet *355*:201–202, 2000.
171. Deville, J. G., Cherry, J. D., Christenson, P. D., et al.: Frequency of unrecognized *Bordetella pertussis* infections in adults. Clin. Infect. Dis. *21*:639–642, 1995.
172. DeVincenzo, J. P.: Therapy of respiratory syncytial virus infection. Pediatr. Infect. Dis. J. *19*:786–790, 2000.
173. Ditchburn, R. K., McQuillin, J., Gardner, P. S., and Court, S. D.: Respiratory syncytial virus in hospital cross-infection. B. M. J. *3*: 671–673, 1971.
174. Dodd, R. Y.: Transmission of parasites and bacteria by blood components. Vox Sang. *78*:239–242, 2000.
175. Doherty, J. A., Brookfield, D. S., Gray, J., and McEwan, R. A.: Cohorting of infants with respiratory syncytial virus. J. Hosp. Infect. *38*:203–206, 1998.
176. Doig, C. M., and Wilkinson, A. W.: Wound infection in a children's hospital. Br. J. Surg. *63*:647–650, 1976.
177. Donskey, C. J., Chowdhry, T. K., Hecker, M. T., et al.: Effect of antibiotic therapy on the density of vancomycin-resistant enterococci in the stool of colonized patients. N. Engl. J. Med. *343*:1925–1932, 2000.
178. Drusin, L. M., Sohmer, M., Groshen, S. L., et al.: Nosocomial hepatitis A infection in a paediatric intensive care unit. Arch. Dis. Child. *62*: 690–695, 1987.
179. Ducharme, F. M., Gauthier, M., Lacroix, J., and Lafleur, L.: Incidence of infection related to arterial catheterization in children: A prospective study. Crit. Care Med. *16*:272–276, 1988.
180. Dunkle, L. M., Naqvi, S. H., McCallum, R., and Lofgren, J. P.: Eradication of epidemic methicillin-gentamicin-resistant *Staphylococcus aureus* in an intensive care nursery. Am. J. Med. *70*:455–458, 1981.
181. DuPont, H. L.: Nosocomial salmonellosis and shigellosis. Infect. Control Hosp. Epidemiol. *12*:707–709, 1991.
182. DuPont, H. L., Gangarosa, E. J., Reller, L. B., et al.: Shigellosis in custodial institutions. Am. J. Epidemiol. *92*:172–179, 1970.
183. Easmon, C. S., Hastings, M. J., Clare, A. J., et al.: Nosocomial transmission of group B streptococci. B. M. J. *283*:459–461, 1981.
184. Edlin, B. R., Tokars, J. I., Grieco, M. H., et al.: An outbreak of multidrug-resistant tuberculosis among hospitalized patients with the acquired immunodeficiency syndrome. N. Engl. J. Med. *326*:1514–1521, 1992.
185. Edmond, M. B., Wallace, S. E., McClish, D. K., et al.: Nosocomial bloodstream infections in United States hospitals: A three-year analysis. Clin. Infect. Dis. *29*:239–244, 1999.
186. Edwards, K. M., Decker, M. D., Graham, B. S., et al.: Adult immunization with acellular pertussis vaccine. J. A. M. A. *269*:53–56, 1993.
187. Edwards, M. S., and Baker, C. J.: Median sternotomy wound infections in children. Pediatr. Infect. Dis. J. *2*:105–109, 1983.
188. Emori, T. G., Culver, D. H., Horan, T. C., et al.: National nosocomial infections surveillance system (NNIS): Description of surveillance methods. Am. J. Infect. Control *19*:19–35, 1991.
189. Emori, T. G., Edwards, J. R., Culver, D. H., et al.: Accuracy of reporting nosocomial infections in intensive-care-unit patients to the National Nosocomial Infections Surveillance System: A pilot study. Infect. Control Hosp. Epidemiol. *19*:308–316, 1998.
190. Emori, T. G., Edwards, J. R., Horan, T. C., et al.: Risk factors for surgical site infection following craniotomy operation reported to the National Nosocomial Infection Surveillance System. Abstract. Infect. Control Hosp. Epidemiol. *21*:144, 2000.
191. Enad, D., Meislich, D., Brodsky, N. L., and Hurt, H.: Is *Clostridium difficile* a pathogen in the newborn intensive care unit? A prospective evaluation. J Perinatol. *17*:355–359, 1997.
192. Espinal, M. A., Laszlo, A., Simonsen, L., et al.: Global trends in resistance to antituberculosis drugs. World Health Organization–International Union against Tuberculosis and Lung Disease Working Group on Anti-Tuberculosis Drug Resistance Surveillance. N. Engl. J. Med. *344*:1294–1303, 2001.
193. Evans, J. P. M., Rossiter, M. A., Kumaran, T. O., and Marsh, G. W.: Human parvovirus aplasia: Case due to cross infection in a ward. B. M. J. *288*:681, 1984.
194. Fagon, J. Y., Chastre, J., Hance, A. J., et al.: Nosocomial pneumonia in ventilated patients: A cohort study evaluating attributable mortality and hospital stay. Am. J. Med. *94*:281–288, 1993.
195. Fagon, J. Y., Chastre, J., Vuagnat, A., et al.: Nosocomial pneumonia and mortality among patients in intensive care units. J. A. M. A. *275*: 866–869, 1996.
196. Fanaroff, A. A., Korones, S. B., Wright, L. L., et al.: A controlled trial of intravenous immune globulin to reduce nosocomial infections in very-low- birth-weight infants. National Institute of Child Health and Human Development Neonatal Research Network. N. Engl. J. Med. *330*: 1107–1113, 1994.
197. Farizo, K. M., Stehr-Green, P. A., Simpson, D. M., and Markowitz, L. E.: Pediatric emergency room visits: A risk factor for acquiring measles. Pediatrics *87*:74–79, 1991.
198. Farizo, K. M., Strebel, P. M., Chen, R. T., et al.: Fatal respiratory disease due to *Corynebacterium diphtheriae:* Case report and review of guidelines for management, investigation, and control. Clin. Infect. Dis. *16*:59–68, 1993.
199. Fergie, J. E., and Purcell, K.: Community-acquired methicillin-resistant *Staphylococcus aureus* infections in south Texas children. Pediatr. Infect. Dis. J. *20*:860–863, 2001.
200. Ferroni, A., Merckx, J., Ancelle, T., et al.: Nosocomial outbreak of *Clostridium difficile* diarrhea in a pediatric service. Eur. J. Clin. Microbiol. Infect. Dis. *16*:928–933, 1997.
201. Finkel, T. H., Torok, T. J., Ferguson, P. J., et al.: Chronic parvovirus B19 infection and systemic necrotising vasculitis: Opportunistic infection or aetiological agent? Lancet *343*:1255–1258, 1994.
202. Finn, A., Anday, E., and Talbot, G. H.: An epidemic of adenovirus 7a infection in a neonatal nursery: Course, morbidity, and management. Infect. Control Hosp. Epidemiol. *9*:398–404, 1988.
203. Fisher, M. C., Long, S. S., McGowan, K. L., et al.: Outbreak of pertussis in a residential facility for handicapped people. J. Pediatr. *114*:934–939, 1989.
204. Foca, M., Jakob, K., Whittier, S., et al.: Endemic *Pseudomonas aeruginosa* infection in a neonatal intensive care unit. N. Engl. J. Med. *343*: 695–700, 2000.
205. Ford-Jones, E. L., Mindorff, C. M., Langley, J. M., et al.: Epidemiologic study of 4684 hospital-acquired infections in pediatric patients. Pediatr. Infect. Dis. J. *8*:668–675, 1989.
206. Fotedar, R., Banerjee, U., Singh, S., et al.: The housefly *(Musca domestica)* as a carrier of pathogenic microorganisms in a hospital environment. J. Hosp. Infect. *20*:209–215, 1992.
207. Franzin, L., Scolfaro, C., Cabodi, D., et al.: *Legionella pneumophila* pneumonia in a newborn after water birth: A new mode of transmission. Clin. Infect. Dis. *33*:e103–e104, 2001.
208. Freeman, J., Epstein, M. F., Smith, N. E., et al.: Extra hospital stay and antibiotic usage with nosocomial coagulase-negative staphylococcal bacteremia in two neonatal intensive care unit populations. Am. J. Dis. Child. *144*:324–329, 1990.
209. Freeman, J., Goldmann, D. A., Smith, N. E., et al.: Association of intravenous lipid emulsion and coagulase-negative staphylococcal bacteremia in neonatal intensive care units. N. Engl. J. Med. *323*:301–308, 1990.
210. Freeman, J., Platt, R., Epstein, M. F., et al.: Birth weight and length of stay as determinants of nosocomial coagulase-negative staphylococcal bacteremia in neonatal intensive care unit populations: Potential for confounding. Am. J. Epidemiol. *132*:1130–1140, 1990.
211. Freeman, J., Platt, R., Sidebottom, D. G., et al.: Coagulase-negative staphylococcal bacteremia in the changing neonatal intensive care unit population. Is there an epidemic? J. A. M. A. *258*:2548–2552, 1987.
212. French, G. L., Shannon, K. P., and Simmons, N.: Hospital outbreak of *Klebsiella pneumoniae* resistant to broad-spectrum cephalosporins and beta-lactam-beta-lactamase inhibitor combinations by hyperproduction of SHV-5 beta-lactamase. J. Clin. Microbiol. *34*:358–363, 1996.
213. Fridkin, S. K., and Jarvis, W. R.: Epidemiology of nosocomial fungal infections. Clin. Microbiol. Rev. *9*:499–511, 1996.
214. Fridkin, S. K., Pear, S. M., Williamson, T. H., et al.: The role of understaffing in central venous catheter–associated bloodstream infections. Infect. Control Hosp. Epidemiol. *17*:150–158, 1996.
215. Fridkin, S. K., Steward, C. D., Edwards, J. R., et al.: Surveillance of antimicrobial use and antimicrobial resistance in United States hospitals: Project ICARE phase 2. Project Intensive Care Antimicrobial Resistance Epidemiology (ICARE) hospitals. Clin. Infect. Dis. *29*:245–252, 1999.
216. Frieden, T. R., Sherman, L. F., Maw, K. L., et al.: A multi-institutional outbreak of highly drug-resistant tuberculosis: Epidemiology and clinical outcomes. J. A. M. A. *276*:1229–1235, 1996.
217. Friedland, I. R., and Klugman, K. P.: Antibiotic-resistant pneumococcal disease in South African children. Am. J. Dis. Child. *146*:920–923, 1992.

218. Friedman, C. A., Temple, D. M., Robbins, K. K., et al.: Outbreak and control of varicella in a neonatal intensive care unit. Pediatr. Infect. Dis. J. *13*:152–154, 1994.
219. Frölich, T.: Infections nosocomiales dans les crèches et hôpitaux pour enfants. Acta Pediatr. *17*:18–23, 1935.
220. Furfaro, S., Gauthier, M., Lacroix, J., et al.: Arterial catheter–related infections in children. A 1-year cohort analysis. Am. J. Dis. Child. *145*:1037–1043, 1991.
221. Gala, C. L., Hall, C. B., Schnabel, K C., et al.: The use of eye-nose goggles to control nosocomial respiratory syncytial virus infection. J. A. M. A. *256*:2706–2708, 1986.
222. Garcia de Viedma, D., Marin, M., Cercenado, E., et al.: Evidence of nosocomial *Stenotrophomonas maltophilia* cross-infection in a neonatology unit analyzed by three molecular typing methods. Infect. Control Hosp. Epidemiol. *20*:816–820, 1999.
223. Gardner, P., and Carles, D. G.: Infections acquired in a pediatric hospital. J. Pediatr. *81*:1205–1210, 1972.
224. Garland, J. S., Alex, C. P., Mueller, C. D., et al.: A randomized trial comparing povidone-iodine to a chlorhexidine gluconate–impregnated dressing for prevention of central venous catheter infections in neonates. Pediatrics *107*:1431–1436, 2001.
225. Garland, J. S., Buck, R. K., Maloney, P., et al.: Comparison of 10% povidone-iodine and 0.5% chlorhexidine gluconate for the prevention of peripheral intravenous catheter colonization in neonates: A prospective trial. Pediatr. Infect. Dis. J. *14*:510–516, 1995.
226. Garland, J. S., Dunne, W. M., Jr., Havens, P., et al.: Peripheral intravenous catheter complications in critically ill children: A prospective study. Pediatrics *89*:1145–1150, 1992.
227. Garland, J. S., Nelson, D. B., Cheah, T., et al.: Infectious complications during peripheral intravenous therapy with Teflon catheters: A prospective study. Pediatr. Infect. Dis. J. *6*:918–921, 1987.
228. Garner, J. S.: Guideline for isolation precautions in hospitals. The Hospital Infection Control Practices Advisory Committee. Infect. Control Hosp. Epidemiol. *17*:53–80, 1996.
229. Garner, J. S., Jarvis, W. R., Emori, T. G., et al.: CDC definitions for nosocomial infections, 1988. Am. J. Infect. Control *16*:128–140, 1988.
230. Garrett, D. O., Jochimsen, E., Murfitt, K., et al.: The emergence of decreased susceptibility to vancomycin in *Staphylococcus epidermidis*. Infect. Control Hosp. Epidemiol. *20*:167–170, 1999.
231. Gaynes, R. P.: Surgical-site infections and the NNIS SSI Risk Index: Room for improvement. Infect. Control Hosp. Epidemiol. *21*:184–185, 2000.
232. Gaynes, R. P.: Surgical-site infections (SSI) and the NNIS Basic SSI Risk Index, part II: Room for improvement. Infect. Control Hosp. Epidemiol. *22*:266–267, 2001.
233. Gaynes, R. P., Culver, D. H., Horan, T. C., et al.: Surgical site infection (SSI) rates in the United States, 1992–1998: The National Nosocomial Infections Surveillance System basic SSI risk index. Clin. Infect. Dis. *33*(Suppl. 2):69–77, 2001.
234. Gaynes, R. P., Edwards, J. R., Jarvis, W. R., et al.: Nosocomial infections among neonates in high-risk nurseries in the United States. National nosocomial Infections Surveillance System. Pediatrics *98*: 357–361, 1996.
235. George, R. H., Gully, P. R., Gill, O. N., et al.: An outbreak of tuberculosis in a children's hospital. J. Hosp. Infect. *8*:129–142, 1986.
236. Gerards, L. J., Hennekam, R. C., von Dijk, W. C., et al.: An outbreak of gastroenteritis due to *Escherichia coli* O142:H6 in a neonatal department. J. Hosp. Infect. *5*:283–288, 1984.
237. Gerber, S. I., Erdman, D. D., Pur, S L., et al.: Outbreak of adenovirus genome type 7d2 infection in a pediatric chronic-care facility and tertiary-care hospital. Clin. Infect. Dis. *32*:694–700, 2001.
238. Gerberding, J. L.: Management of occupational exposures to blood-borne viruses. N. Engl. J. Med. *332*:444–451, 1995.
239. Gewolb, I. H., Schwalbe, R. S., Taciak, V. L., et al.: Stool microflora in extremely low birthweight infants. Arch. Dis. Child Fetal Neonatal Ed. *80*:F167–F173, 1999.
240. Gianino, P., Mastretta, E., Longo, P., et al.: Incidence of nosocomial rotavirus infections, symptomatic and asymptomatic, in breast-fed and non–breast-fed infants. J. Hosp. Infect. *50*:13–17, 2002.
241. Givney, R., Vickery, A., Holliday, A., et al.: Methicillin-resistant *Staphylococcus aureus* in a cystic fibrosis unit. J. Hosp. Infect. *35*:27–36, 1997.
242. Glynn, S. A., Kleinman, S. H., Schreiber, G. B., et al.: Trends in incidence and prevalence of major transfusion-transmissible viral infections in US blood donors, 1991 to 1996. J. A. M. A. *284*:229–235, 2000.
243. Golden, S. E., Shehab, Z. M., Bjelland, J. C., et al.: Microbiology of endotracheal aspirates in intubated pediatric intensive care unit patients: Correlations with radiographic findings. Pediatr. Infect. Dis. J. *6*: 665–669, 1987.
244. Goldmann, D. A.: Bacterial colonization and infection in the neonate. Am. J. Med. *70*:417–422, 1981.
245. Goldmann, D. A.: Strategies for preventing neonatal group B streptococcal disease. Infect. Control *7*:137–139, 143, 1986.
246. Goldmann, D. A.: Prevention and management of neonatal infections. Infect. Dis. Clin. North Am. *3*:779–813, 1989.
247. Goldmann, D. A.: Epidemiology and prevention of pediatric viral respiratory infections in health-care institutions. Emerg. Infect. Dis. *7*:249–253, 2001.
248. Goldmann, D. A., and Breton, S. J.: Group C streptococcal surgical wound infections transmitted by an anorectal and nasal carrier. Pediatrics *61*:235–237, 1978.
249. Goldmann, D. A., Durbin, W., Jr., and Freeman, J.: Nosocomial infections in a neonatal intensive care unit. J. Infect. Dis. *144*:449–459, 1981.
250. Goodnough, L. T., Brecher, M. E., Kanter, M. H., and AuBuchon, J. P.: Transfusion medicine. First of two parts—blood transfusion. N. Engl. J. Med. *340*:438–447, 1999.
251. Goodnough, L. T., Brecher, M. E., Kanter, M. H., and AuBuchon, J. P.: Transfusion medicine. Second of two parts—blood conservation. N. Engl. J. Med. *340*:525–533, 1999.
252. Graman, P. S., and Hall, C. B.: Epidemiology and control of nosocomial viral infections. Infect. Dis. Clin. North Am. *3*:815–841, 1989.
253. Gray, J. E., Richardson, D. K., McCormick, M C., et al.: Neonatal therapeutic intervention scoring system: A therapy-based severity-of-illness index. Pediatrics *90*:561–567, 1992.
254. Gray, J. E., Richardson, D. K., McCormick, M. C., and Goldmann, D. A.: Coagulase-negative staphylococcal bacteremia among very low birth weight infants: Relation to admission illness severity, resource use, and outcome. Pediatrics *95*:225–230, 1995.
255. Gray, J. W., and George, R. H.: Experience of vancomycin-resistant enterococci in a children's hospital. J. Hosp. Infect. *45*:11–18, 2000.
256. Grohskopf, L. A., Huskins, W. C., Sinkowitz-Cochran, R., et al.: Use of antimicrobial agents in U.S. neonatal and pediatric intensive care unit patients. Abstract. Presented at the 11th Annual Scientific Meeting of the Society for Healthcare Epidemiology of America, October 25–28, 2001, Toronto, p. 92.
257. Grohskopf, L. A., Maki, D. G., Sohn, A. H., et al.: Reality check: Should we use vancomycin for the prophylaxis of intravascular catheter–associated infections? Infect. Control Hosp. Epidemiol. *22*:176–179, 2001.
258. Grohskopf, L. A., Roth, V. R., Feikin, D. R., et al.: *Serratia liquefaciens* bloodstream infections from contamination of epoetin alfa at a hemodialysis center. N. Engl. J. Med. *344*:1491–1497, 2001.
259. Grohskopf, L. A., Sinkowitz-Cochran, R. L., Garrett, D. O., et al.: A national point-prevalence survey of pediatric intensive care unit–acquired infections in the United States. J. Pediatr. *140*:432–438., 2002.
260. Guerin, J. M., Lustman, C., Meyer, P., and Barbotin-Larrieau, F.: Nosocomial sinusitis in pediatric intensive care patients. Crit. Care Med. *18*:902, 1990.
261. Gupta, P., Ramachandran, V. G., Sharma, P. P., et al.: *Salmonella senftenberg* septicemia: A nursery outbreak. Indian Pediatr. *30*:514–516, 1993.
262. Gustafson, T. L., Lavely, G. B., Brawner, E., Jr., et al.: An outbreak of airborne nosocomial varicella. Pediatrics *70*:550–556, 1982.
263. Haley, R. W., and Bregman, D. A.: The role of understaffing and overcrowding in recurrent outbreaks of staphylococcal infection in a neonatal special-care unit. J. Infect. Dis. *145*:875–885, 1982.
264. Haley, R. W., Culver, D. H., White, J. W., et al.: The nationwide nosocomial infection rate: A new need for vital statistics. Am. J. Epidemiol. *121*:159–167, 1985.
265. Haley, R. W., Cushion, N. B., Tenover, F. C., et al.: Eradication of endemic methicillin-resistant *Staphylococcus aureus* infections from a neonatal intensive care unit. J. Infect. Dis. *171*:614–624, 1995.
266. Hall, C. B.: Nosocomial viral respiratory infections: Perennial weeds on pediatric wards. Am. J. Med. *70*:670–676, 1981.
267. Hall, C. B.: Nosocomial respiratory syncytial virus infections: The "Cold War" has not ended. Clin. Infect. Dis. *31*:590–596, 2000.
268. Hall, C. B.: Respiratory syncytial virus and parainfluenza virus. N. Engl. J. Med. *344*:1917–1928, 2001.
269. Hall, C. B., and Douglas, R., Jr.: Nosocomial influenza infection as a cause of intercurrent fevers in infants. Pediatrics *55*:673–677, 1975.
270. Hall, C. B., and Douglas, R., Jr.: Modes of transmission of respiratory syncytial virus. J. Pediatr. *99*:100–103, 1981.
271. Hall, C. B., and Douglas, R., Jr.: Nosocomial respiratory syncytial viral infections: Should gowns and masks be used? Am. J. Dis. Child. *135*:512–515, 1981.
272. Hall, C. B., Douglas, R., Jr., and Geiman, J. M.: Possible transmission by fomites of respiratory syncytial virus. J. Infect. Dis. *141*:98–102, 1980.
273. Hall, C. B., Douglas, R., Jr., Geiman, J. M., and Messner, M. K.: Nosocomial respiratory syncytial virus infections. N Engl J Med. *293*:1343–1346, 1975.
274. Hall, C. B., Kopelman, A. E., Douglas, R., Jr., et al.: Neonatal respiratory syncytial virus infection. N. Engl. J. Med. *300*:393–396, 1979.
275. Hall, C. B., Powell, K. R., MacDonald, N. E., et al.: Respiratory syncytial viral infection in children with compromised immune function. N. Engl. J. Med. *315*:77–81, 1986.
276. Halpin, D. P., O'Byrne, P., McEntee, G., et al.: Effect of a Betadine connection shield on central venous catheter sepsis. Nutrition *7*:33–34, 1991.
277. Hammami, A., Arlet, G., Ben Redjeb, S., et al.: Nosocomial outbreak of acute gastroenteritis in a neonatal intensive care unit in Tunisia caused by multiple drug resistant *Salmonella wien* producing SHV-2 betalactamase. Eur. J. Clin. Microbiol. Infect. Dis. *10*:641–646, 1991.

278. Hammerberg, O., Watts, J., Chernesky, M., et al.: An outbreak of herpes simplex virus type 1 in an intensive care nursery. Pediatr. Infect. Dis. J. *2*:290–294, 1983.
279. Hanazaki, K., Shingu, K., Adachi, W., et al.: Chlorhexidine dressing for reduction in microbial colonization of the skin with central venous catheters: A prospective randomized controlled trial. J. Hosp. Infect. *42*:165–168, 1999.
280. Hanley, P. J., Conaway, M. M., Halstead, D. C., et al.: Nosocomial herpes simplex virus infection associated with oral endotracheal intubation. Am. J. Infect. Control *21*:310–316, 1993.
281. Harbarth, S., Sudre, P., Dharan, S., et al.: Outbreak of *Enterobacter cloacae* related to understaffing, overcrowding, and poor hygiene practices. Infect. Control Hosp. Epidemiol. *20*:598–603, 1999.
282. Harmon, T., Burkhart, G., and Applebaum, H.: Perforated pseudomembranous colitis in the breast-fed infant. J. Pediatr. Surg. *27*:744–746, 1992.
283. Harries, E. H. R.: Infection and its control in children's wards. Lancet *2*:173–178, 1935.
284. Harris, J. S., and Goldmann, D. A.: Infections acquired in the nursery: Epidemiology and control. *In* Remington, J. S., and Klein, J. O. (eds.): Infectious Diseases of the Fetus & Newborn Infant. Philadelphia, W. B. Saunders, 2001, pp. 1371–1418.
285. Harvey, B. S., Koeuth, T., Versalovic, J., et al.: Vertical transmission of *Citrobacter diversus* documented by DNA fingerprinting. Infect. Control Hosp. Epidemiol. *16*:564–569, 1995.
286. Hedberg, K., Ristinen, T. L., Soler, J. T et al.: Outbreak of erythromycin-resistant staphylococcal conjunctivitis in a newborn nursery. Pediatr. Infect. Dis. J. *9*:268–273, 1990.
287. Helin, I., Widell, A., Borulf, S., et al.: Outbreak of coxsackievirus A-14 meningitis among newborns in a maternity hospital ward. Acta Paediatr. *76*:234–238, 1987.
288. Hemming, V. G., Overall, J., Jr., and Britt, M. R.: Nosocomial infections in a newborn intensive-care unit: Results of forty-one months of surveillance. N. Engl. J. Med. *294*:1310–1316, 1976.
289. Henderson, D. A., Inglesby, T. V., Bartlett, J. G., et al.: Smallpox as a biological weapon: Medical and public health management. Working Group on Civilian Biodefense. J. A. M. A. *281*:2127–2137, 1999.
290. Herold, B. C., Immergluck, L. C., Maranan, M. C., et al.: Community-acquired methicillin-resistant *Staphylococcus aureus* in children with no identified predisposing risk. J. A. M. A. *279*:593–598, 1998.
291. Hershkowici, S., Barak, M., Cohen, A., and Montag, J.: An outbreak of *Campylobacter jejuni* infection in a neonatal intensive care unit. J. Hosp. Infect. *9*:54–59, 1987.
292. Heseltine, P. N., Ripper, M., and Wohlford, P.: Nosocomial rubella—consequences of an outbreak and efficacy of a mandatory immunization program. Infect. Control *6*:371–374, 1985.
293. Hiramatsu, K., Hanaki, H., Ino, T., et al.: Methicillin-resistant *Staphylococcus aureus* clinical strain with reduced vancomycin susceptibility. J. Antimicrob. Chemother. *40*:135–136, 1997.
294. Hitomi, S., Kubota, M., Mori, N., et al.: Control of a methicillin-resistant *Staphylococcus aureus* outbreak in a neonatal intensive care unit by unselective use of nasal mupirocin ointment. J. Hosp. Infect. *46*: 123–129, 2000.
295. Holmes, A., Nolan, R., Taylor, R., et al.: An epidemic of *Burkholderia cepacia* transmitted between patients with and without cystic fibrosis. J. Infect. Dis. *179*:1197–1205, 1999.
296. Hoogkamp-Korstanje, J. A., Cats, B., Senders, R. C., and van Ertbruggen, I.: Analysis of bacterial infections in a neonatal intensive care unit. J. Hosp. Infect. *3*:275–284, 1982.
297. Horan, T., and Culver, D.: Comparing surgical site infection rates. *In* Pfeiffer, J. (ed.): APIC Text of Infection Control and Epidemiology. Association for Professionals in Infection Control and Epidemiology, 2000, Washington, D.C., pp. 14-1–14-7.
298. Horan, T. C., Culver, D. H., Gaynes, R. P., National Nosocomial Infections Surveillance System: Results of a multicenter study on risk factors for surgical site infections following C-section. Abstract. Am. J. Infect. Control *24*:84, 1996.
299. Horan, T. C., and Emori, T. G.: Definitions of key terms used in the NNIS System. Am. J. Infect. Control *25*:112–116, 1997.
300. Horan, T. C., Gaynes, R. P., Martone, W. J., et al.: CDC definitions of nosocomial surgical site infections, 1992: A modification of CDC definitions of surgical wound infections. Am. J. Infect. Control *20*:271–274, 1992.
301. Horbar, J. D.: The Vermont Oxford Network: Evidence-based quality improvement for neonatology. Pediatrics *103*:350–359, 1999.
302. Horbar, J. D., Onstad, L., and Wright, E.: Predicting mortality risk for infants weighing 501 to 1500 grams at birth: A National Institutes of Health Neonatal Research Network report. Crit. Care Med. *21*:12–18, 1993.
303. Horbar, J. D., Rogowski, J., Plsek, P. E., et al.: Collaborative quality improvement for neonatal intensive care. NIC/Q Project Investigators of the Vermont Oxford Network. Pediatrics *107*:14–22, 2001.
304. Houston, F., Foster, J. D., Chong, A., et al.: Transmission of BSE by blood transfusion in sheep. Lancet *356*:999–1000, 2000.
305. Howard, A. J.: Nosocomial spread of *Haemophilus influenzae*. J. Hosp. Infect. *19*:1–3, 1991.
306. Hruszkewycz, V., Holtrop, P. C., Batton, D. G., et al.: Complications associated with central venous catheters inserted in critically ill neonates. Infect. Control Hosp. Epidemiol. *12*:544–548, 1991.
307. Huebner, J., and Goldmann, D. A.: Coagulase-negative staphylococci: Role as pathogens. Annu. Rev. Med. *50*:223–236, 1999.
308. Huebner, J., Pier, G. B., Maslow, J. N., et al.: Endemic nosocomial transmission of *Staphylococcus epidermidis* bacteremia isolates in a neonatal intensive care unit over 10 years. J. Infect. Dis. *169*:526–531, 1994.
309. Huskins, W. C.: Antimicrobial resistance and its control in pediatrics. Semin. Pediatr. Infect. Dis. *12*:138–146, 2001.
310. Huskins, W. C., Potter-Bynoe, G., Spencer, S., et al.: An outbreak of rhinovirus respiratory tract infection associated with serious complications among residents of a pediatric skilled nursing facility. Abstract. Presented at the Fourth Decennial International Conference on Nosocomial and Healthcare-Associated Infections, March 5–9, 2000, Atlanta, p. 150.
311. Hussain, F. M., Boyle-Vavra, S., and Daum, R. S.: Community-acquired methicillin-resistant *Staphylococcus aureus* colonization in healthy children attending an outpatient pediatric clinic. Pediatr. Infect. Dis. J. *20*: 763–767, 2001.
312. Inglesby, T. V., Dennis, D. T., Henderson, D. A., et al.: Plague as a biological weapon: Medical and public health management. Working Group on Civilian Biodefense. J. A. M. A. *283*:2281–2290, 2000.
313. Ingram, J., Weitzman, S., Greenberg, M. L., et al.: Complications of indwelling venous access lines in the pediatric hematology patient: A prospective comparison of external venous catheters and subcutaneous ports. Am. J. Pediatr. Hematol. Oncol. *13*:130–136, 1991.
314. Istre, G. R., McKee, P. A., West, G. R., et al.: Measles spread in medical settings: An important focus of disease transmission? Pediatrics *79*: 356–358, 1987.
315. Izurieta, H. S., Thompson, W. W., Kramarz, P., et al.: Influenza and the rates of hospitalization for respiratory disease among infants and young children. N. Engl. J. Med. *342*:232–239, 2000.
316. Jacobs, B. R., Haygood, M., and Hingl, J.: Recombinant tissue plasminogen activator in the treatment of central venous catheter occlusion in children. J. Pediatr. *139*:593–596, 2001.
317. Jamieson, F. B., Wang, E. E., Bain, C., et al.: Human torovirus: A new nosocomial gastrointestinal pathogen. J. Infect. Dis. *178*:1263–1269, 1998.
318. Jann, K., and Jann, B.: Capsules of *Escherichia coli,* expression and biological significance. Can. J. Microbiol. *38*:705–710, 1992.
319. Jarvis, W. R.: Epidemiology of nosocomial infections in pediatric patients. Pediatr. Infect. Dis. J. *6*:344–351, 1987.
320. Jarvis, W. R.: Epidemiology of nosocomial fungal infections, with emphasis on *Candida* species. Clin. Infect. Dis. *20*:1526–1530, 1995.
321. Jarvis, W. R., Edwards, J. R., Culver, D. H., et al.: Nosocomial infection rates in adult and pediatric intensive care units in the United States. Am. J. Med. *91*(Suppl.):185–191, 1991.
322. Jarvis, W. R., Thornsberry, C., Boyce, J., and Hughes, J. M.: Methicillin-resistant *Staphylococcus aureus* at children's hospitals in the United States. Pediatr. Infect. Dis. J. *4*:651–655, 1985.
323. Jereb, J. A., Klevens, R. M., Privett, T D., et al.: Tuberculosis in health care workers at a hospital with an outbreak of multidrug-resistant *Mycobacterium tuberculosis*. Arch. Intern. Med. *155*:854–859, 1995.
324. Jernigan, J. A., Titus, M. G., Groschel, D. H., et al.: Effectiveness of contact isolation during a hospital outbreak of methicillin-resistant *Staphylococcus aureus*. Am. J. Epidemiol. *143*:496–504, 1996.
325. Johnson, I., Hammond, G. W., and Verma, M. R.: Nosocomial coxsackie B4 virus infections in two chronic-care pediatric neurological wards. J. Infect. Dis. *151*:1153–1156, 1985.
326. Johnson, J. R.: Virulence factors in *Escherichia coli* urinary tract infection. Clin. Microbiol. Rev. *4*:80–128, 1991.
327. Johnson, S., Homann, S. R., Bettin, K. M., et al.: Treatment of asymptomatic *Clostridium difficile* carriers (fecal excretors) with vancomycin or metronidazole: A randomized, placebo-controlled trial. Ann. Intern. Med. *117*:297–302, 1992.
328. Johnsson, J., Seeberg, S., and Kjellmer, I.: Blood concentrations of chlorhexidine in neonates undergoing routine cord care with 4% chlorhexidine gluconate solution. Acta Paediatr. *76*:675–676, 1987.
329. Jones, G. R., Konsler, G. K., Dunaway, R. P., et al.: Prospective analysis of urokinase in the treatment of catheter sepsis in pediatric hematology-oncology patients. J. Pediatr. Surg. *28*:350–355, 1993.
330. Karanfil, L. V., Conlon, M., Lykens, K., et al.: Reducing the rate of nosocomially transmitted respiratory syncytial virus. Am. J. Infect. Control *27*:91–96, 1999.
331. Karchmer, T. B., Giannetta, E. T., Muto, C. A., et al.: A randomized crossover study of silver-coated urinary catheters in hospitalized patients. Arch. Intern. Med. *160*:3294–3298, 2000.
332. Karmali, M. A., Norrish, B., Lior, H., et al.: *Campylobacter* enterocolitis in a neonatal nursery. J. Infect. Dis. *149*:874–877, 1984.
333. Keane, E., and Gilles, H. M.: Lassa fever in Panguma Hospital, Sierra Leone, 1973–6. B. M. J. *1*:1399–1402, 1977.
334. Keats, A. S.: The ASA classification of physical status—a recapitulation. Anesthesiology *49*:233–236, 1978.
335. Kerstiens, B., and Matthys, F.: Interventions to control virus transmission during an outbreak of Ebola hemorrhagic fever: experience from

Kikwit, Democratic Republic of the Congo, 1995. J. Infect. Dis. *179* (Suppl. 1):263–267, 1999.

336. Khan, E. A., Correa, A. G., and Baker, C. J.: Suppurative thrombophlebitis in children: A ten-year experience. Pediatr. Infect. Dis. J. *16*: 63–67, 1997.
337. Khan, M. A., Abdur-Rab, M., Israr, N., et al.: Transmission of *Salmonella worthington* by oropharyngeal suction in hospital neonatal unit. Pediatr. Infect. Dis. J. *10*:668–672, 1991.
338. Kilham, E. B.: An epidemic of pemphigus neonatorum. Am. J. Obstet. *22*:1039, 1889.
339. King, D. R., Komer, M., Hoffman, J., et al.: Broviac catheter sepsis: The natural history of an iatrogenic infection. J. Pediatr. Surg. *20*:728–733, 1985.
340. Kinney, J., Mundorf, L., Gleason, C., et al.: Efficacy and pharmacokinetics of intravenous immune globulin administration to high-risk neonates. Am. J. Dis. Child. *145*:1233–1238, 1991.
341. Kinney, J. S., McCray, E., Kaplan, J. E., et al.: Risk factors associated with echovirus 11 infection in a hospital nursery. Pediatr. Infect. Dis. J. *5*:192–197, 1986.
342. Kite, P., Dobbins, B. M., Wilcox, M. H., and McMahon, M. J.: Rapid diagnosis of central-venous-catheter–related bloodstream infection without catheter removal. Lancet *354*:1504–1507, 1999.
343. Klein, B. S., Michaels, J. A., Rytel, M. W., et al.: Nosocomial hepatitis A. A multinursery outbreak in Wisconsin. J. A. M. A. *252*:2716–2721, 1984.
344. Klein, H. G., Dodd, R. Y., Ness, P. M., et al.: Current status of microbial contamination of blood components: Summary of a conference. Transfusion *37*:95–101, 1997.
345. Kline, M. W., Kaplan, S. L., Hawkins, E. P., and Mason, E. O., Jr.: Pathogenesis of brain abscess formation in an infant rat model of *Citrobacter diversus* bacteremia and meningitis. J. Infect. Dis. *157*: 106–112, 1988.
346. Kline, M. W., Mason, E. O., Jr., and Kaplan, S. L.: Characterization of *Citrobacter diversus* strains causing neonatal meningitis. J. Infect. Dis. *157*:101–105, 1988.
347. Kloos, W. E., and Bannerman, T. L.: Update on clinical significance of coagulase-negative staphylococci. Clin. Microbiol. Rev. 7:117–140, 1994.
348. Kluytmans, J. A., Mouton, J. W., Ijzerman, E. P., et al.: Nasal carriage of *Staphylococcus aureus* as a major risk factor for wound infections after cardiac surgery. J. Infect. Dis. *171*:216–219, 1995.
349. Knoll, A., Helmig, M., Peters, O., and Jilg, W.: Hepatitis C virus transmission in a pediatric oncology ward: analysis of an outbreak and review of the literature. Lab. Invest. *81*:251–262, 2001.
350. Kollef, M. H.: Inadequate antimicrobial treatment: An important determinant of outcome for hospitalized patients. Clin. Infect. Dis. *31*(Suppl. 4):131–138, 2000.
351. Kollef, M. H., Sharpless, L., Vlasnik, J., et al.: The impact of nosocomial infections on patient outcomes following cardiac surgery. Chest *112*:666–675, 1997.
352. Kollef, M. H., Sherman, G., Ward, S., and Fraser, V. J.: Inadequate antimicrobial treatment of infections: A risk factor for hospital mortality among critically ill patients. Chest *115*:462–474, 1999.
353. Kollef, M. H., Ward, S., Sherman, G., et al.: Inadequate treatment of nosocomial infections is associated with certain empiric antibiotic choices. Crit. Care Med. *28*:3456–3464, 2000.
354. Kotloff, K. L., Losonsky, G. A., Morris, J., Jr., et al.: Enteric adenovirus infection and childhood diarrhea: An epidemiologic study in three clinical settings. Pediatrics *84*:219–225, 1989.
355. Koziol, D. E., Kurtzman, G., Ayub, J., et al.: Nosocomial human parvovirus B19 infection: Lack of transmission from a chronically infected patient to hospital staff. Infect. Control Hosp. Epidemiol. *13*:343–348, 1992.
356. Krasinski, K., LaCouture, R., Holzman, R. S., et al.: Screening for respiratory syncytial virus and assignment to a cohort at admission to reduce nosocomial transmission. J. Pediatr. *116*:894–898, 1990.
357. Krause, P. J., Gross, P. A., Barrett, T. L., et al.: Quality standard for assurance of measles immunity among health care workers. Infect. Control Hosp. Epidemiol. *15*:193–199, 1994.
358. Kuroda, M., Ohta, T., Uchiyama, I., et al.: Whole genome sequencing of methicillin-resistant *Staphylococcus aureus*. Lancet *357*:1225–1240, 2001.
359. Kurt, T. L., Yeager, A. S., Guenette, S., and Dunlop, S.: Spread of pertussis by hospital staff. J. A. M. A. *221*:264–267, 1972.
360. Kurtz, J. B., Lee, T. W., and Pickering, D.: Astrovirus associated gastroenteritis in a children's ward. J. Clin. Pathol. *30*:948–952, 1977.
361. Kyne, L., Warny, M., Qamar, A., and Kelly, C. P.: Asymptomatic carriage of *Clostridium difficile* and serum levels of IgG antibody against toxin A. N. Engl. J. Med. *342*:390–397, 2000.
362. Kyne, L., Warny, M., Qamar, A., and Kelly, C. P.: Association between antibody response to toxin A and protection against recurrent *Clostridium difficile* diarrhoea. Lancet *357*:189–193, 2001.
363. LaForce, F. M.: The control of infections in hospitals: 1750 to 1950. *In* Wenzel, R. P. (ed.): Prevention and Control of Nosocomial Infections. Baltimore, Williams & Wilkins, 1997, pp. 3–17.
364. Lai, K. K.: *Enterobacter sakazakii* infections among neonates, infants, children, and adults. Case reports and a review of the literature. Medicine (Baltimore) *80*:113–122, 2001.
365. Lam, B. C., Tam, J., Ng, M. H., and Yeung, C. Y.: Nosocomial gastroenteritis in paediatric patients. J. Hosp. Infect. *14*:351–355, 1989.
366. Landers, S., Moise, A. A., Fraley, J. K., et al.: Factors associated with umbilical catheter–related sepsis in neonates. Am. J. Dis. Child. *145*:675–680, 1991.
367. Landry, S. L., Kaiser, D. L., and Wenzel, R. P.: Hospital stay and mortality attributed to nosocomial enterococcal bacteremia: A controlled study. Am. J. Infect. Control *17*:323–329, 1989.
368. Langley, J. M., LeBlanc, J. C., Wang, E. E., Law B. J. et al.: Nosocomial respiratory syncytial virus infection in Canadian pediatric hospitals: A Pediatric Investigators Collaborative Network on Infections in Canada Study. Pediatrics. *100*:943–946, 1997.
369. Langley, J. M., Hanakowski, M., and Leblanc, J. C.: Unique epidemiology of nosocomial urinary tract infection in children. Am. J. Infect. Control *29*:94–98, 2001.
370. La Quaglia, M. P., Caldwell, C., Lucas, A., et al.: A prospective randomized double-blind trial of bolus urokinase in the treatment of established Hickman catheter sepsis in children. J. Pediatr. Surg. *29*:742–745, 1994.
371. La Quaglia, M. P., Lucas, A., Thaler, H. T., et al.: A prospective analysis of vascular access device–related infections in children. J. Pediatr. Surg. *27*:840–842, 1992.
372. Leclair, J. M., Freeman, J., Sullivan, B. F., et al.: Prevention of nosocomial respiratory syncytial virus infections through compliance with glove and gown isolation precautions. N. Engl. J. Med. *317*:329–334, 1987.
373. Leclair, J. M., Winston, K. R., Sullivan, B. F., et al.: Effect of preoperative shampoos with chlorhexidine or iodophor on emergence of resident scalp flora in neurosurgery. Infect. Control *9*:8–12, 1988.
374. Leclair, J. M., Zaia, J. A., Levin, M. J., et al.: Airborne transmission of chickenpox in a hospital. N. Engl. J. Med. *302*:450–453, 1980.
375. Leroyer, A., Bedu, A., Lombrail, P., et al.: Prolongation of hospital stay and extra costs due to hospital-acquired infection in a neonatal unit. J. Hosp. Infect. *35*:37–45, 1997.
376. Lettau, L. A.: Nosocomial transmission and infection control aspects of parasitic and ectoparasitic diseases: Part I. Introduction/enteric parasites. Infect. Control Hosp. Epidemiol. *12*:59–65, 1991.
377. Lettau, L. A.: Nosocomial transmission and infection control aspects of parasitic and ectoparasitic diseases. Part III. Ectoparasites/summary and conclusions. Infect. Control Hosp. Epidemiol. *12*:179–185, 1991.
378. Levy, O., Martin, S., Eichenwald, E., et al.: Impaired innate immunity in the newborn: Newborn neutrophils are deficient in bactericidal/permeability- increasing protein. Pediatrics *104*:1327–1333, 1999.
379. Lewis, D. B., and Wilson, C. B.: Developmental immunology and role of host defenses in fetal and neonatal susceptibility to infection. *In* Remington, J. S., and Klein, J. O. (eds.): Infectious Diseases of the Fetus & Newborn Infant. Philadelphia, W. B. Saunders, 2001, pp. 25–138.
380. Liberati, A., D'Amico, R., Pifferi, S., et al.: Antibiotics for preventing respiratory tract infections in adults receiving intensive care. Cochrane Database Syst. Rev. *2002*(2):2002.
381. Lichtenstein, A.: Nosocomial infections in children's hospitals and institutions. Our means for combating these infections. Acta Paediat. *17*:36–49, 1935.
382. Lin, F. C., Devoe, W. F., Morrison, C., et al.: Outbreak of neonatal *Citrobacter diversus* meningitis in a suburban hospital. Pediatr. Infect. Dis. J. *6*:50–55, 1987.
383. Linares, J., Sitges-Serra, A., Garau, J., et al.: Pathogenesis of catheter sepsis: A prospective study with quantitative and semiquantitative cultures of catheter hub and segments. J. Clin. Microbiol. *21*:357–360, 1985.
384. Linnemann, C. C., and MacMillan, B. G.: Viral infections in pediatric burn patients. Am. J. Dis. Child. *135*:750–753, 1981.
385. Linnemann, C. C., Jr., Buchman, T. G., Light, I. J., and Ballard, J. L.: Transmission of herpes-simplex virus type 1 in a nursery for the newborn. Identification of viral isolates by DNA "fingerprinting." Lancet. *1*:964–966, 1978.
386. Linnemann, C. C., Jr., Ramundo, N., Perlstein, P. H., et al.: Use of pertussis vaccine in an epidemic involving hospital staff. Lancet *2*:540–543, 1975.
387. LiPuma, J. J., Spilker, T., Gill, L. H., et al.: Disproportionate distribution of *Burkholderia cepacia* complex species and transmissibility markers in cystic fibrosis. Am. J. Respir. Crit. Care Med. *164*:92–96, 2001.
388. Liston, T. E., Levine, P. L., and Anderson, C.: Polymicrobial bacteremia due to Polle syndrome: The child abuse variant of Munchausen by proxy. Pediatrics *72*:211–213, 1983.
389. Livermore, D. M.: Beta-lactamases in laboratory and clinical resistance. Clin. Microbiol. Rev. *8*:557–584, 1995.
390. Livingston, R. A., Froggatt, J. W., McLaughlin, J. M., et al.: Vancomycin resistant enterococci: Infection and colonization within a children's center. Abstract. Pediatr. Res. *29*:178, 1991.
391. Lohr, J. A., Donowitz, L. G., and Sadler, J. E.: Hospital-acquired urinary tract infection. Pediatrics *83*:193–199, 1989.
392. Lohr, J. A., Downs, S. M., Dudley, S., and Donowitz, L. G.: Hospital-acquired urinary tract infections in the pediatric patient: A prospective study. Pediatr. Infect. Dis. J. *13*:8–12, 1994.
393. Long, J. G., and Keyserling, H. L.: Catheter-related infection in infants due to an unusual lipophilic yeast—*Malassezia furfur*. Pediatrics *76*: 896–900, 1985.

394. Lövegren, E.: Infection risks in nursing institutions for infants and young children and measures for their prevention. Acta Paediatr. *17*:50–55, 1935.
395. Luban, N. L.: Human parvoviruses: Implications for transfusion medicine. Transfusion *34*:821–827, 1994.
396. Lui, S. L., Luk, W. K., Cheung, C Y., et al.: Nosocomial outbreak of parvovirus B19 infection in a renal transplant unit. Transplantation *71*: 59–64, 2001.
397. Luna, J., Masdeu, G., Perez, M., et al.: Clinical trial evaluating a new hub device designed to prevent catheter-related sepsis. Eur. J. Clin. Microbiol. Infect. Dis. *19*:655–662, 2000.
398. Lyytikainen, O., Saxen, H., Ryhanen, R et al.: Persistence of a multiresistant clone of *Staphylococcus epidermidis* in a neonatal intensive-care unit for a four-year period. Clin. Infect. Dis. *20*:24–29, 1995.
399. Macartney, K. K., Gorelick, M. H., Manning, M. L., et al.: Nosocomial respiratory syncytial virus infections: The cost-effectiveness and cost-benefit of infection control. Pediatrics *106*:520–526, 2000.
400. MacDonald, N. E., Hall, C. B., Suffin, S. C., et al.: Respiratory syncytial viral infection in infants with congenital heart disease. N. Engl. J. Med. *307*:397–400, 1982.
401. Mackenzie, A., Johnson, W., Heyes, B., et al.: A prolonged outbreak of exfoliative toxin A–producing *Staphylococcus aureus* in a newborn nursery. Diagn. Microbiol. Infect. Dis. *21*:69–75, 1995.
402. Madden, N. P., Levinsky, R. J., Bayston, R., et al.: Surgery, sepsis, and nonspecific immune function in neonates. J. Pediatr. Surg. *24*:562–566, 1989.
403. Madge, P., Paton, J. Y., McColl, J. H., and Mackie, P. L.: Prospective controlled study of four infection-control procedures to prevent nosocomial infection with respiratory syncytial virus. Lancet *340*:1079–1083, 1992.
404. Magny, J. F., Bremard-Oury, C., Brault, D., et al.: Intravenous immunoglobulin therapy for prevention of infection in high-risk premature infants: Report of a multicenter, double-blind study. Pediatrics *88*: 437–443, 1991.
405. Maguire, G. C., Nordin, J., Myers, M. G., et al.: Infections acquired by young infants. Am. J. Dis. Child. *135*:693–698, 1981.
406. Mahajan, R., Mathur, M., Kumar, A., et al.: Nosocomial outbreak of *Salmonella typhimurium* infection in a nursery intensive care unit (NICU) and paediatric ward. J. Commun. Dis. *27*:10–14, 1995.
407. Mahenthiralingam, E., Vandamme, P., Campbell, M. E., et al.: Infection with *Burkholderia cepacia* complex genomovars in patients with cystic fibrosis: Virulent transmissible strains of genomovar III can replace *Burkholderia multivorans*. Clin. Infect. Dis. *33*:1469–1475, 2001.
408. Maki, D. G., Klein, B. S., McCormick, R. D., et al.: Nosocomial *Pseudomonas pickettii* bacteremias traced to narcotic tampering. A case for selective drug screening of health care personnel. J. A. M. A. *265*: 981–986, 1991.
409. Maki, D. G., Knasinski, V., Halvorson, K. T., et al.: A prospective, randomized, investigator-blinded trial of a novel nitrofurazone-impregnated urinary catheter. Abstract. Infect. Control Hosp. Epidemiol. *18*(Suppl.):50, 1997.
410. Maki, D. G., Knasinski, V., Halvorson, K., and Tambyah, P. A.: A novel silver-hydrogel–impregnated indwelling catheter reduces catheter associated urinary tract infections: A prospective, double-blind trial. Abstract. Infect. Control Hosp. Epidemiol. *19*:682, 1998.
411. Maki, D. G., Mermel, L. A., Kluger, D. M., et al.: The efficacy of a chlorhexidine-impregnated sponge for the prevention of intravascular catheter–related infection—a prospective, randomized, controlled, multicenter trial. Abstract 1430.Presented at the 40th Interscience Conference on Antimicrobial Agents and Chemotherapy, Toronto, 2000, p. 422.
412. Maki, D. G., Rhame, F. S., Mackel, D. C., and Bennett, J. V.: Nationwide epidemic of septicemia caused by contaminated intravenous products. I. Epidemiologic and clinical features. Am. J. Med. *60*:471–485, 1976.
413. Maki, D. G., Ringer, M., and Alvarado, C. J.: Prospective randomised trial of povidone-iodine, alcohol, and chlorhexidine for prevention of infection associated with central venous and arterial catheters. Lancet *338*:339–343, 1991.
414. Maki, D. G., and Tambyah, P. A.: Engineering out the risk for infection with urinary catheters. Emerg. Infect. Dis. *7*:342–347, 2001.
415. Maki, D. G., Weise, C. E., and Sarafin, H. W.: A semiquantitative culture method for identifying intravenous-catheter–related infection. N. Engl. J. Med. *296*:1305–1309, 1977.
416. Malhotra, V. L., Prakash, K., and Lakshmy, A.: Hospital-acquired meningococcaemia. J. Hosp. Infect. *18*:332, 1991.
417. Malik, R. K., Montecalvo, M. A., Reale, M. R., et al.: Epidemiology and control of vancomycin-resistant enterococci in a regional neonatal intensive care unit. Pediatr. Infect. Dis. J. *18*:352–356, 1999.
418. Maloney, S. A., Pearson, M. L., Gordon, M. T., et al.: Efficacy of control measures in preventing nosocomial transmission of multidrug-resistant tuberculosis to patients and health care workers. Ann. Intern. Med. *122*:90–95, 1995.
419. Mandigers, C. M., Diepersloot, R. J., Dessens, M., et al.: A hospital outbreak of penicillin-resistant pneumococci in The Netherlands. Eur. Respir. J. 7:1635–1639, 1994.
420. Mangram, A. J., Horan, T. C., Pearson, M. L., et al.: Guideline for prevention of surgical site infection, 1999. Centers for Disease Prevention and Control (CDC) Hospital Infection Control Practices Advisory Committee. Am. J. Infect. Control *27*:97–132, 1999.
421. Martin, M. A., and Reichelderfer, M.: APIC guidelines for infection prevention and control in flexible endoscopy. Association for Professionals in Infection Control and Epidemiology, Inc. 1991, 1992, and 1993, APIC Guidelines Committee. Am. J. Infect. Control *22*:19–38, 1994.
422. Mastro, T. D., Fields, B. S., Breiman, R. F., et al.: Nosocomial legionnaires' disease and use of medication nebulizers. J. Infect. Dis. *163*: 667–671, 1991.
423. Matlow, A. G., Harrison, A., Monteath, A., et al.: Nosocomial transmission of tuberculosis (TB) associated with care of an infant with peritoneal TB. Infect. Control Hosp. Epidemiol. *21*:222–223, 2000.
424. Mayhall, C. G.: Diagnosis and management of infections of implantable devices used for prolonged venous access. Curr. Clin. Top. Infect. Dis. *12*:83–110, 1992.
425. Mayhall, C. G.: Nosocomial burn wound infections. *In* Mayhall, C. G. (ed): Hospital Epidemiology and Infection Control. Philadelphia, Lippincott Williams & Wilkins, 1999, pp. 275–286.
426. Mayhall, C. G.: Ventilator-associated pneumonia or not? Contemporary diagnosis. Emerg. Infect. Dis. *7*:200–204, 2001.
427. McCabe, W. R., Jackson, G. G.: Gram-negative bacteremia. I. etiology and ecology. Arch. Intern. Med. *110*:847–853, 1962.
428. McDonald, L. C., Banerjee, S. N., and Jarvis, W. R.: Line-associated bloodstream infections in pediatric intensive-care-unit patients associated with a needleless device and intermittent intravenous therapy. Infect. Control Hosp. Epidemiol. *19*:772–777, 1998.
429. McDonald, L. C., Banerjee, S. N., and Jarvis, W. R.: Seasonal variation of *Acinetobacter* infections: 1987–1996. Nosocomial Infections Surveillance System. Clin. Infect. Dis. *29*:1133–1137, 1999.
430. McDonald, L. C., Walker, M., Carson, L., et al.: Outbreak of *Acinetobacter* spp. bloodstream infections in a nursery associated with contaminated aerosols and air conditioners. Pediatr. Infect. Dis. J. *17*: 716–722, 1998.
431. McFarland, L. V., Brandmarker, S. A., and Guandalini, S.: Pediatric *Clostridium difficile:* A phantom menace or clinical reality? J. Pediatr. Gastroenterol. Nutr. *31*:220–231, 2000.
432. McFarland, L. V., Mulligan, M. E., Kwok, R. Y., and Stamm, W. E.: Nosocomial acquisition of *Clostridium difficile* infection. N. Engl. J. Med. *320*:204–210, 1989.
433. McGechie, P. B.: Nosocomial bacteraemia in hospital staff caused by *Haemophilus influenzae* type b. J. Hosp. Infect. *21*:159–160, 1992.
434. McGrath, D., Swanson, R., Weems, S., et al.: Analysis of a measles outbreak in Kent County, Michigan in 1990. Pediatr. Infect. Dis. J. *11*: 385–389, 1992.
435. McKenney, D., Hubner, J., Muller, E., et al.: The ica locus of *Staphylococcus epidermidis* encodes production of the capsular polysaccharide/adhesin. Infect. Immun. *66*:4711–4720, 1998.
436. McKhann, C. F., Steeger, A., and Long, A. P.: Hospital infections: A survey of the problem. Am. J. Dis. Child. *55*:579–599, 1938.
437. McManus, A. T., Mason, A., Jr., McManus, W. F., and Pruitt, B., Jr.: A decade of reduced gram-negative infections and mortality associated with improved isolation of burned patients. Arch. Surg. *129*:1306–1309, 1994.
438. McNamara, M. J., Hill, M. C., Balows, A., and Tucker, E. B.: A study of the bacteriologic patterns of hospital infections. Ann. Intern. Med. *66*:480–488, 1967.
439. Meiklejohn, G., Reimer, L. G., Graves, P. S., and Helmick, C.: Cryptic epidemic of Q fever in a medical school. J. Infect. Dis. *144*:107–113, 1981.
440. Meissner, H. C., Murray, S. A., Kiernan, M. A., et al.: A simultaneous outbreak of respiratory syncytial virus and parainfluenza virus type 3 in a newborn nursery. J. Pediatr. *104*:680–684, 1984.
441. Mermel, L. A., Farr, B. M., Sherertz, R. J., et al.: Guidelines for the management of intravascular catheter–related infections. Clin. Infect. Dis. *32*:1249–1272, 2001.
442. Mhalu, F. S., Mtango, F. D., and Msengi, A. E.: Hospital outbreaks of cholera transmitted through close person-to-person contact. Lancet *2*:82–84, 1984.
443. Michaels, M. G., Green, M., Wald, E. R., and Starzl, T. E.: Adenovirus infection in pediatric liver transplant recipients. J. Infect. Dis. *165*:170–174, 1992.
444. Middleton, P. J., Szymanski, M. T., and Petric, M.: Viruses associated with acute gastroenteritis in young children. Am. J. Dis. Child. *131*:733–737, 1977.
445. Millar, M. R., Bacon, C., Smith, S. L., et al.: Enteral feeding of premature infants with *Lactobacillus* GG. Arch. Dis. Child. *69*:483–487, 1993.
446. Millar, M. R., Brown, N. M., Tobin, G. W., et al.: Outbreak of infection with penicillin-resistant *Streptococcus pneumoniae* in a hospital for the elderly. J. Hosp. Infect. *27*:99–104, 1994.
447. Mirro, J., Jr., Rao, B. N., Kumar, M., et al.: A comparison of placement techniques and complications of externalized catheters and implantable port use in children with cancer. J. Pediatr. Surg. *25*:120–124, 1990.
448. Mitchell, S. J., Gray, J., Morgan, M. E., et al.: Nosocomial infection with *Rhizopus microsporus* in preterm infants: Association with wooden tongue depressors. Lancet *348*:441–443, 1996.

449. Miura, E., Procianoy, R. S., Bittar, C., et al.: A randomized, double-masked, placebo-controlled trial of recombinant granulocyte colony-stimulating factor administration to preterm infants with the clinical diagnosis of early-onset sepsis. Pediatrics *107*:30–35, 2001.
450. Modlin, J. F.: Perinatal echovirus and group B coxsackievirus infections. Clin. Perinatol. *15*:233–246, 1988.
451. Moffet, H. L., and Allan, D.: Colonization of infants exposed to bacterially contaminated mists. Am. J. Dis. Child. *114*:21–25, 1967.
452. Moisiuk, S. E., Robson, D., Klass, L., et al.: Outbreak of parainfluenza virus type 3 in an intermediate care neonatal nursery. Pediatr. Infect. Dis. J. *17*:49–53, 1998.
453. Monath, T. P., Mertens, P. E., Patton, R., et al.: A hospital epidemic of Lassa fever in Zorzor, Liberia, March–April 1972. Am. J. Trop. Med. Hyg. *22*:773–779, 1973.
454. Morosini, M. I., Canton, R., Martinez-Beltran, J., et al.: New extended-spectrum TEM-type beta-lactamase from *Salmonella enterica subsp. enterica* isolated in a nosocomial outbreak. Antimicrob. Agent Chemother. *39*:458–461, 1995.
455. Morrow, P. E.: Physics of airborne particles and their deposition in the lung. Ann. N. Y. Acad. Sci. *353*:71–80, 1980.
456. Moser, M. R., Bender, T. R., Margolis, H. S., et al.: An outbreak of influenza aboard a commercial airliner. Am. J. Epidemiol. *110*:1–6, 1979.
457. Munoz, F. M., Campbell, J. R., Atmar, R. L., et al.: Influenza A virus outbreak in a neonatal intensive care unit. Pediatr. Infect. Dis. J. *18*: 811–815, 1999.
458. Muytjens, H. L., Roelofs-Willemse, H., and Jaspar, G. H.: Quality of powdered substitutes for breast milk with regard to members of the family Enterobacteriaceae. J. Clin. Microbiol. *26*:743–746, 1988.
459. Nakayama, M., Miyazaki, C., Ueda, K., et al.: Pharyngoconjunctival fever caused by adenovirus type 11. Pediatr. Infect. Dis. J. *11*:6–9, 1992.
460. Nardell, E. A.: Interrupting transmission from patients with unsuspected tuberculosis: A unique role for upper-room ultraviolet air disinfection. Am. J. Infect. Control *23*:156–164, 1995.
461. National Institute for Occupational Safety and Health, Centers for Disease Control and Prevention, Public Health Service, Department of Health and Human Services: Respiratory protective devices: Final rules and notice. Fed. Reg. *60*:30336–30404, 1995.
462. National Nosocomial Infections Surveillance System: Intensive Care Antimicrobial Resistance Epidemiology (ICARE) Surveillance Report, data summary from January 1996 through December 1997. Am. J. Infect. Control *27*:279–284, 1999.
463. National Nosocomial Infections Surveillance System: National Nosocomial Infections Surveillance (NNIS) System Report, data summary from January 1992–June 2001, issued August 2001. Am. J. Infect. Control *29*:404–421, 2001.
464. Naumovski, L., Quinn, J. P., Miyashiro, D., et al.: Outbreak of ceftazidime resistance due to a novel extended-spectrum beta-lactamase in isolates from cancer patients. Antimicrob. Agents Chemother. *36*: 1991–1996, 1992.
465. Navarrete, S., Stetler, H. C., Avila, C., et al.: An outbreak of *Cryptosporidium* diarrhea in a pediatric hospital. Pediatr. Infect. Dis. J. *10*:248–250, 1991.
466. Needleman, J., Buerhaus, P., Mattke, S., et al.: Nurse-staffing levels and the quality of care in hospitals. N. Engl. J. Med. *346*:1715–1722, 2002.
467. Neuzil, K. M., Mellen, B. G., Wright, P. F., et al.: The effect of influenza on hospitalizations, outpatient visits, and courses of antibiotics in children. N. Engl. J. Med. *342*:225–231, 2000.
468. Nishizawa, T., Okamoto, H., Konishi, K., et al.: A novel DNA virus (TTV) associated with elevated transaminase levels in posttransfusion hepatitis of unknown etiology. Biochem. Biophys. Res. Commun. *241*:92–97, 1997.
469. Nivin, B., Nicholas, P., Gayer, M., et al.: A continuing outbreak of multidrug- resistant tuberculosis, with transmission in a hospital nursery. Clin. Infect. Dis. *26*:303–307, 1998.
470. Noble, R. C., Kane, M. A., Reeves, S. A., and Roeckel, I.: Posttransfusion hepatitis A in a neonatal intensive care unit. J. A. M. A. *252*:2711–2715, 1984.
471. Noel, G. J., Kreiswirth, B. N., Edelson, P. J., et al.: Multiple methicillin-resistant *Staphylococcus aureus* strains as a cause for a single outbreak of severe disease in hospitalized neonates. Pediatr. Infect. Dis. J. *11*: 184–188, 1992.
472. Noya, F. J., Rench, M. A., Metzger, T. G., et al.: Unusual occurrence of an epidemic of type Ib/c group B streptococcal sepsis in a neonatal intensive care unit. J. Infect. Dis. *155*:1135–1144, 1987.
473. Nuorti, J. P., Butler, J. C., Crutcher, J. M., et al.: An outbreak of multidrug-resistant pneumococcal pneumonia and bacteremia among unvaccinated nursing home residents. N. Engl. J. Med. *338*:1861–1868, 1998.
474. Odio, C., McCracken, G. H., Jr., and Nelson, J. D.: CSF shunt infections in pediatrics. A seven-year experience. Am. J. Dis. Child. *138*:1103–1108, 1984.
475. Centers for Disease Control and Prevention: Guideline for the prevention of intravascular catheter-related infections. M. M. W. R. Recomm. Rep. *51*(RR-10):1–29, 2002.
476. Oguz, F., Uysal, G., Dasdemir, S., et al.: The role of *Clostridium difficile* in childhood nosocomial diarrhea. Scand. J. Infect. Dis. *33*:731–733, 2001.
477. Ohlsson, A., and Lacy, J. B.: Intravenous immunoglobulin for preventing infection in preterm and/or low-birth-weight infants. Cochrane Database Syst. Rev. *2002*(2):2002.
478. Orrett, F. A., Brooks, P. J., Richardson, E. G., and Mohammed, S.: Paediatric nosocomial urinary tract infection at a regional hospital. Int. Urol. Nephrol. *31*:173–179, 1999.
479. Oskarsdottir, S., Mellander, L., Marky, I., and Seeberg, S.: *Clostridium difficile* in children with malignant disease. Pediatr. Hematol. Oncol. *8*:269–272, 1991.
480. Ostrowsky, B. E., Whitener, C., Bredenberg, H. K., et al.: *Serratia marcescens* bacteremia traced to an infused narcotic. N. Engl. J. Med. *346*:1529–1537, 2002.
481. Padula, P. J., Edelstein, A., Miguel, S. D., et al.: Hantavirus pulmonary syndrome outbreak in Argentina: Molecular evidence for person-to-person transmission of Andes virus. Virology *241*:323–330, 1998.
482. Parry, M. F., Hutchinson, J. H., Brown, N. A., et al.: Gram-negative sepsis in neonates: A nursery outbreak due to hand carriage of *Citrobacter diversus.* Pediatrics *65*:1105–1109, 1980.
483. Paton, S., Nicolle, L., Mwongera, M., et al.: *Salmonella* and *Shigella* gastroenteritis at a public teaching hospital in Nairobi, Kenya. Infect. Control Hosp. Epidemiol. *12*:710–717, 1991.
484. Patrick, C. H., John, J. F., Levkoff, A. H., and Atkins, L. M.: Relatedness of strains of methicillin-resistant coagulase-negative *Staphylococcus* colonizing hospital personnel and producing bacteremias in a neonatal intensive care unit. Pediatr. Infect. Dis. J. *11*:935–940, 1992.
485. Patterson, J. E., Madden, G. M., Krisiunas, E. P., et al.: A nosocomial outbreak of ampicillin-resistant *Haemophilus influenzae* type b in a geriatric unit. J. Infect. Dis. *157*:1002–1007, 1988.
486. Pearson, M. L.: Guideline for prevention of intravascular device–related infections. Hospital Infection Control Practices Advisory Committee. Infect. Control Hosp. Epidemiol. *17*:438–473, 1996.
487. Pearson, M. L., Jereb, J. A., Frieden, T. R., et al.: Nosocomial transmission of multidrug-resistant *Mycobacterium tuberculosis.* A risk to patients and health care workers. Ann. Intern. Med. *117*:191–196, 1992.
488. Peck, M. D., Weber, J., McManus, A., et al.: Surveillance of burn wound infections: A proposal for definitions. J. Burn Care Rehabil. *19*:386–389, 1998.
489. Perl, T. M., Cullen, J. J., Wenzel, R. P., et al.: Intranasal mupirocin to prevent postoperative *Staphylococcus aureus* infections. N. Engl. J. Med. *346*:1871–1877, 2002.
490. Perl, T. M., Haugen, T. H., Pfaller, M. A., et al.: Transmission of herpes simplex virus type 1 infection in an intensive care unit. Ann. Intern. Med. *117*:584–586, 1992.
491. Peters, C. J., Kuehne, R. W., Mercado, R. R., et al.: Hemorrhagic fever in Cochabamba, Bolivia, 1971. Am. J. Epidemiol. *99*:425–433., 1974.
492. Pfaller, M. A., Jones, R. N., Marshall, S. A., et al.: Inducible amp C beta-lactamase producing gram-negative bacilli from blood stream infections: Frequency, antimicrobial susceptibility, and molecular epidemiology in a national surveillance program (SCOPE). Diagn. Microbiol. Infect. Dis. *28*:211–219, 1997.
493. Pfaller, M. A., Jones, R. N., Messer, S. A., et al.: National surveillance of nosocomial blood stream infection due to species of *Candida* other than *Candida albicans:* Frequency of occurrence and antifungal susceptibility in the SCOPE Program. Diagn. Microbiol. Infect. Dis. *30*:121–129, 1998.
494. Pfaller, M. A., Jones, R. N., Messer, S. A., et al.: National surveillance of nosocomial blood stream infection due to *Candida albicans:* Frequency of occurrence and antifungal susceptibility in the SCOPE Program. Diagn. Microbiol. Infect. Dis. *31*:327–332, 1998.
495. Pfaller, M. A., Messer, S. A., Hollis, R. J., et al.: Trends in species distribution and susceptibility to fluconazole among blood stream isolates of *Candida* species in the United States. Diagn. Microbiol. Infect. Dis. *33*:217–222, 1999.
496. Pfaller, M. A., Messer, S. A., Houston, A., et al.: National epidemiology of mycoses survey: A multicenter study of strain variation and antifungal susceptibility among isolates of *Candida* species. Diagn. Microbiol. Infect. Dis. *31*:289–296, 1998.
497. Philippon, A., Arlet, G., and Jacoby, G. A.: Plasmid-determined AmpC-type beta-lactamases. Antimicrob. Agents Chemother. *46*:1–11, 2002.
498. Piedra, P. A., Kasel, J. A., Norton, H. J., et al.: Description of an adenovirus type 8 outbreak in hospitalized neonates born prematurely. Pediatr. Infect. Dis. J. *11*:460–465, 1992.
499. Pillay, D., Patou, G., Hurt, S., et al.: Parvovirus B19 outbreak in a children's ward. Lancet *339*:107–109, 1992.
500. Pittet, D., Tarara, D., and Wenzel, R. P.: Nosocomial bloodstream infection in critically ill patients. Excess length of stay, extra costs, and attributable mortality. J. A. M. A. *271*:1598–1601, 1994.
501. Platt, R., Yokoe, D. S., and Sands, K. E.: Automated methods for surveillance of surgical site infections. Emerg. Infect. Dis. *7*:212–216, 2001.
502. Pohl, C., Green, M., Wald, E. R., and Ledesma-Medina, J.: Respiratory syncytial virus infections in pediatric liver transplant recipients. J. Infect. Dis. *165*:166–169, 1992.

503. Polish, L. B., Shapiro, C. N., Bauer, F., et al.: Nosocomial transmission of hepatitis B virus associated with the use of a spring-loaded finger-stick device. N. Engl. J. Med. *326*:721–725, 1992.
504. Polk, B. F., White, J. A., DeGirolami, P. C., and Modlin, J. F.: An outbreak of rubella among hospital personnel. N. Engl. J. Med. *303*: 541–545, 1980.
505. Pollack, M. M., Patel, K. M., and Ruttimann, U. E.: PRISM III: An updated Pediatric Risk of Mortality score. Crit. Care Med. *24*:743–752, 1996.
506. Pollack, M. M., Patel, K. M., and Ruttimann, U. E.: The Pediatric Risk of Mortality III—Acute Physiology Score (PRISM III-APS): A method of assessing physiologic instability for pediatric intensive care unit patients. J. Pediatr. *131*:575–581, 1997.
507. Pollack, M. M., Ruttimann, U. E., and Getson, P. R.: Pediatric risk of mortality (PRISM) score. Crit. Care Med. *16*:1110–1116, 1988.
508. Pollock, E., Ford-Jones, E. L., Corey, M., et al.: Use of the Pediatric Risk of Mortality score to predict nosocomial infection in a pediatric intensive care unit. Crit. Care Med. *19*:160–165, 1991.
509. Pollock, E. M., Ford-Jones, E. L., Rebeyka, I., et al.: Early nosocomial infections in pediatric cardiovascular surgery patients. Crit. Care Med. *18*:378–384, 1990.
510. Ponec, D., Irwin, D., Haire, W. D., et al.: Recombinant tissue plasminogen activator (alteplase) for restoration of flow in occluded central venous access devices: A double-blind placebo-controlled trial—the Cardiovascular Thrombolytic to Open Occluded Lines (COOL) efficacy trial. J. Vasc. Interv. Radiol. *12*:951–955, 2001.
511. Porter, J. D., Teter, M., Traister, V., et al.: Outbreak of adenoviral infections in a long-term paediatric facility, New Jersey, 1986/87. J. Hosp. Infect. *18*:201–210, 1991.
512. Poulsen, V.: Über das heutige Auftreten der nosocomialen Infektionen au Kinderkrankenhäusern, insbesondere in Bezug auf dei Häufigkeit und die Infektionswege. Acta Pediatr. *17*:25–35, 1935.
513. Powell, H., Swarner, O., Gluck, L., and Lampert, P.: Hexachlorophene myelinopathy in premature infants. J. Pediatr. *82*:976–981, 1973.
514. Prince, D. S., Astry, C., Vonderfecht, S., et al.: Aerosol transmission of experimental rotavirus infection. Pediatr. Infect. Dis. J. *5*:218–222, 1986.
515. Qualman, S. J., Petric, M., Karmali, M. A., et al.: *Clostridium difficile* invasion and toxin circulation in fatal pediatric pseudomembranous colitis. Am. J. Clin. Pathol. *94*:410–416, 1990.
516. Raad, I., Costerton, W., Sabharwal, U., et al.: Ultrastructural analysis of indwelling vascular catheters: A quantitative relationship between luminal colonization and duration of placement. J. Infect. Dis. *168*:400–407, 1993.
517. Raad, I. I., Hohn, D. C., Gilbreath, B. J., et al.: Prevention of central venous catheter–related infections by using maximal sterile barrier precautions during insertion. Infect. Control Hosp. Epidemiol. *15*:231–238, 1994.
518. Raad, I. I., Sabbagh, M. F., Rand, K. H., and Sherertz, R. J.: Quantitative tip culture methods and the diagnosis of central venous catheter–related infections. Diagn. Microbiol. Infect. Dis. *15*:13–20, 1992.
519. Raad, I. I., Sherertz, R. J., Rains, C. S., et al.: The importance of nosocomial transmission of measles in the propagation of a community outbreak. Infect. Control Hosp. Epidemiol. *10*:161–166, 1989.
520. Raad, I. I., Sherertz, R. J., Russell, B. A., and Reuman, P. D.: Uncontrolled nosocomial rotavirus transmission during a community outbreak. Am. J. Infect. Control *18*:24–28, 1990.
521. Rabalais, G., Adams, G., and Stover, B.: PPD skin test conversion in health-care workers after exposure to *Mycobacterium tuberculosis* infection in infants. Lancet *338*:826, 1991.
522. Rabkin, C. S., Telzak, E. E., Ho, M. S., et al.: Outbreak of echovirus 11 infection in hospitalized neonates. Pediatr. Infect. Dis. J. *7*:186–190, 1988.
523. Rangel-Frausto, M. S., Pittet, D., Costigan, M., et al.: The natural history of the systemic inflammatory response syndrome (SIRS). A prospective study. J. A. M. A. *273*:117–123, 1995.
524. Rangel-Frausto, M. S., Wiblin, T., Blumberg, H. M., et al.: National epidemiology of mycoses survey (NEMIS): Variations in rates of bloodstream infections due to *Candida* species in seven surgical intensive care units and six neonatal intensive care units. Clin. Infect. Dis. *29*:253–258, 1999.
525. Ratnam, S., Mercer, E., Picco, B., et al.: A nosocomial outbreak of diarrheal disease due to *Yersinia enterocolitica* serotype 0:5, biotype 1. J. Infect. Dis. *145*:242–247, 1982.
526. Ratner, A. J., Neu, N., Jakob, K., et al.: Nosocomial rotavirus in a pediatric hospital. Infect. Control Hosp. Epidemiol. *22*:299–301, 2001.
527. Raucher, H. S., Hyatt, A. C., Barzilai, A., et al.: Quantitative blood cultures in the evaluation of septicemia in children with Broviac catheters. J. Pediatr. *104*:29–33, 1984.
528. Ray, S. M., Erdman, D. D., Berschling, J. D., et al.: Nosocomial exposure to parvovirus B19: Low risk of transmission to healthcare workers. Infect. Control Hosp. Epidemiol. *18*:109–114, 1997.
529. Raymond, J., and Aujard, Y.: Nosocomial infections in pediatric patients: A European, multicenter prospective study. European Study Group. Infect. Control Hosp. Epidemiol. *21*:260–263, 2000.
530. Reboli, A. C., John, J., Jr., and Levkoff, A. H.: Epidemic methicillin-gentamicin-resistant *Staphylococcus aureus* in a neonatal intensive care unit. Am. J. Dis. Child. *143*:34–39, 1989.
531. Remington, P. L., Hall, W. N., Davis, I. H., et al.: Airborne transmission of measles in a physician's office. J. A. M. A. *253*:1574–1577, 1985.
532. Reuman, P. D., Duckworth, D. H., Smith, K. L., et al.: Lack of effect of *Lactobacillus* on gastrointestinal bacterial colonization in premature infants. Pediatr. Infect. Dis. *5*:663–668, 1986.
533. Rhinehart, E., Smith, N. E., Wennersten, C., et al.: Rapid dissemination of beta-lactamase–producing, aminoglycoside-resistant *Enterococcus faecalis* among patients and staff on an infant-toddler surgical ward. N. Engl. J. Med. *323*:1814–1818, 1990.
534. Ribner, B. S.: Endemic, multiply resistant *Staphylococcus aureus* in a pediatric population. Clinical description and risk factors. Am. J. Dis. Child. *141*:1183–1187, 1987.
535. Ribner, B. S., Landry, M. N., Kidd, K., et al.: Outbreak of multiply resistant *Staphylococcus aureus* in a pediatric intensive care unit after consolidation with a surgical intensive care unit. Am. J. Infect. Control *17*:244–249, 1989.
536. Richards, C., Gaynes, R. P., Horan, T., et al.: Risk factors for surgical site infection following spinal fusion surgery in the United States. National Nosocomial Infections Surveillance System. Abstract. Infect. Control Hosp. Epidemiol. *21*:147, 2000.
537. Richards, G. A., Murphy, S., Jobson, R., et al.: Unexpected Ebola virus in a tertiary setting: Clinical and epidemiologic aspects. Crit. Care Med. *28*:240–244, 2000.
538. Richards, M. J., Edwards, J. R., Culver, D. H, and Gaynes, R. P.: Nosocomial infections in pediatric intensive care units in the United States. National Nosocomial Infections Surveillance System. Pediatrics *103*(4):e39, 1999.
539. Richardson, D. K., Corcoran, J. D., Escobar, G. J., and Lee, S. K.: SNAP-II and SNAPPE-II: Simplified newborn illness severity and mortality risk scores. J. Pediatr. *138*:92–100, 2001.
540. Richardson, D. K., Gray, J. E., McCormick, M. C., et al.: Score for Neonatal Acute Physiology: A physiologic severity index for neonatal intensive care. Pediatrics *91*:617–623, 1993.
541. Richardson, D. K., Phibbs, C. S., Gray, J. E., et al.: Birth weight and illness severity: Independent predictors of neonatal mortality. Pediatrics *91*:969–975, 1993.
542. Richardson, J. F., Quoraishi, A. H., Francis, B. J., and Marples, R. R.: Beta-lactamase–negative, methicillin-resistant *Staphylococcus aureus* in a newborn nursery: Report of an outbreak and laboratory investigations. J. Hosp. Infect. *16*:109–121, 1990.
543. Richet, H. M., McNeil, M. M., Edwards, M. C., and Jarvis, W. R.: Cluster of *Malassezia furfur* pulmonary infections in infants in a neonatal intensive-care unit. J Clin Microbiol. *27*:1197–1200, 1989.
544. Richman, D. D., Breton, S. J., and Goldman, D. A.: Scarlet fever and group A streptococcal surgical wound infection traced to an anal carrier. J. Pediatr. *90*:387–390, 1977.
545. Rivera, M. E., Mason, W. H., Ross, L. A., and Wright, H., Jr.: Nosocomial measles infection in a pediatric hospital during a community-wide epidemic. J. Pediatr. *119*:183–186, 1991.
546. Robert, J., Fridkin, S. K., Blumberg, H. M., et al.: The influence of the composition of the nursing staff on primary bloodstream infection rates in a surgical intensive care unit. Infect. Control Hosp. Epidemiol. *21*:12–17, 2000.
547. Rodriguez, W. J., Kim, H. W., Brandt, C. D., et al.: Rotavirus: A cause of nosocomial infection in the nursery. J. Pediatr. *101*:274–277, 1982.
548. Rogers, M., Weinstock, D. M., Eagan, J., et al.: Rotavirus outbreak on a pediatric oncology floor: Possible association with toys. Am. J. Infect. Control *28*:378–380, 2000.
549. Roos, R. P.: Controlling new prion diseases. N. Engl. J. Med. *344*: 1548–1551, 2001.
550. Rose, H. D., Lenz, I. E., and Sheth, N. K.: Meningococcal pneumonia. A source of nosocomial infection. Arch. Intern. Med. *141*:575–577, 1981.
551. Rotbart, H. A., Levin, M. J., Yolken, R. H., et al.: An outbreak of rotavirus-associated neonatal necrotizing enterocolitis. J. Pediatr. *103*:454–459, 1983.
552. Rotbart, H. A., and Webster, A. D.: Treatment of potentially life-threatening enterovirus infections with pleconaril. Clin. Infect. Dis. *32*: 228–235, 2001.
553. Rowen, J. L., Atkins, J. T., Levy, M. L., et al.: Invasive fungal dermatitis in the < or = 1000-gram neonate. Pediatrics *95*:682–687, 1995.
554. Roy, M. C., Herwaldt, L. A., Embrey, R., et al.: Does the Centers for Disease Control's NNIS system risk index stratify patients undergoing cardiothoracic operations by their risk of surgical-site infection? Infect. Control Hosp. Epidemiol. *21*:186–190, 2000.
555. Roy, T. E., McDonald, S., Patrick, M. L., et al.: A survey of hospital infection in a pediatric hospital. Part I. Description of hospital, organization of survey, population studied and some general findings. Can. Med. Assoc. J. *87*:531–538, 1962.
556. Roy, T. E., McDonald, S., Patrick, M. L., et al.: A survey of hospital infection in a pediatric hospital. Part II. The distribution of hospital infections in different areas of the hospital, postoperative wound infections and the consequences of infection. Can. Med. Assoc. J. *87*:592–599, 1962.

557. Roy, T. E., McDonald, S., Patrick, M. L., et al.: A survey of hospital infection in a pediatric hospital. Part III. Staphylococcal infections, notes on antibiotic sensitivity of the staphylococci from postoperative wound and other infections, discussion and summary. Can. Med. Assoc. J. *87*: 656–660, 1962.
558. Rubin, L. G., Tucci, V., Cercenado, E., et al.: Vancomycin-resistant *Enterococcus faecium* in hospitalized children. Infect. Control Hosp. Epidemiol. *13*:700–705, 1992.
559. Rushforth, J. A., Hoy, C. M., Kite, P., and Puntis, J. W.: Rapid diagnosis of central venous catheter sepsis. Lancet *342*:402–403, 1993.
560. Ryder, R. W., McGowan, J. E., Hatch, M. H., and Palmer, E. L.: Reovirus-like agent as a cause of nosocomial diarrhea in infants. J. Pediatr. *90*:698–702, 1977.
561. Ryder, R. W., Rahman, A. S., Alim, A. R., et al.: An outbreak of nosocomial cholera in a rural Bangladesh hospital. J. Hosp. Infect. *8*:275–282, 1986.
562. Sachdeva, R. C.: Cost of nosocomial infections in the pediatric intensive care unit. Semin. Pediatr. Infect. Dis. *10*:239–242, 1999.
563. Saez-Llorens, X., and McCracken, G. H., Jr.: Sepsis syndrome and septic shock in pediatrics: Current concepts of terminology, pathophysiology, and management. J. Pediatr. *123*:497–508, 1993.
564. Saha, M. R., Sircar, B. K., Dutta, P., and Pal, S. C.: Occurrence of multiresistant *Salmonella typhimurium* infection in a pediatric hospital at Calcutta. Indian Pediatr. *29*:307–311, 1992.
565. Saiman, L., Lerner, A., Saal, L., et al.: Banning artificial nails from health care settings. Am. J. Infect. Control *30*:252–254, 2002.
566. Saiman, L., Ludington, E., Dawson, J. D., et al.: Risk factors for *Candida* species colonization of neonatal intensive care unit patients. Pediatr. Infect. Dis. J. *20*:1119–1124, 2001.
567. Saiman, L., Ludington, E., Pfaller, M., et al.: Risk factors for candidemia in neonatal intensive care unit patients. The National Epidemiology of Mycosis Survey Study Group. Pediatr. Infect. Dis. J. *19*:319–324, 2000.
568. Saiman, L., and Siegel, J. D.: Infection control recommendations for patients with cystic fibrosis: Microbiology, important pathogens, and infection control practices to prevent patient-to-patient transmission. Cystic Fibrosis Foundation Consensus Conference on Infection Control. Am. J. Infect. Control. *31*:56–562, 2003.
569. Sakaoka, H., Saheki, Y., Uzuki, K., et al.: Two outbreaks of herpes simplex virus type 1 nosocomial infection among newborns. J. Clin. Microbiol. *24*:36–40, 1986.
570. Sanchez, V., Vazquez, J. A., Barth-Jones, D., et al.: Epidemiology of nosocomial acquisition of *Candida lusitaniae*. J. Clin. Microbiol. *30*: 3005–3008, 1992.
571. Sands, K. E. F., and Goldmann, D. A.: Epidemiology of *Staphylococcus aureus* and group A streptococci. *In* Bennett, J. V., and Brachman, P. S. (ed.): Hospital Infections. 4th ed. Philadelphia, Lippincott-Raven, 1998, pp. 621–636.
572. Sattar, S. A., Lloyd-Evans, N., Springthorpe, V. S., and Nair, R. C.: Institutional outbreaks of rotavirus diarrhoea: Potential role of fomites and environmental surfaces as vehicles for virus transmission. J. Hyg. *96*:277–289, 1986.
573. Sawyer, M. H., Chamberlin, C. J., Wu, Y. N., et al.: Detection of varicella-zoster virus DNA in air samples from hospital rooms. J. Infect. Dis. *169*:91–94, 1994.
574. Schaberg, D. R., Culver, D. H., and Gaynes, R P.: Major trends in the microbial etiology of nosocomial infection. Am. J. Med. *91*(Suppl.):72–75, 1991.
575. Schaffer, T. E., Sylvester, R. F., Jr., and Baldwin, J. N.: Staphylococcal infections in newborn infants. II. Report of 19 epidemics caused by an identical strain of *Staphylococcus pyogenes*. Am. J. Public Health. *47*:990–1008, 1957.
576. Scheifele, D., and Bonner, M.: Airborne transmission of chickenpox. N. Engl. J. Med. *303*:281–282, 1980.
577. Schembre, D. B.: Infectious complications associated with gastrointestinal endoscopy. Gastrointest. Endosc. Clin. North Am. *10*:215–232, 2000.
578. Schlager, T., Sadler, J., Weber, D., et al.: Hospital-acquired infections in pediatric burn patients. South Med. J. *87*:481–484, 1994.
579. Schrag, S. J., Zywicki, S., Farley, M. M., et al.: Group B streptococcal disease in the era of intrapartum antibiotic prophylaxis. N. Engl. J. Med. *342*:15–20, 2000.
580. Schuman, E. S., Winters, V., Gross, G. F., and Hayes, J. F.: Management of Hickman catheter sepsis. Am. J. Surg. *149*:627–628, 1985.
581. Schwarcz, S., McCaw, B., and Fukushima, P.: Prevalence of measles susceptibility in hospital staff. Evidence to support expanding the recommendations of the Immunization Practices Advisory Committee. Arch. Intern. Med. *152*:1481–1483, 1992.
582. Segura, M., Alvarez-Lerma, F., Tellado, J. M., et al.: A clinical trial on the prevention of catheter-related sepsis using a new hub model. Ann. Surg. *223*:363–369, 1996.
583. Selwyn, S.: Hospital infection: The first 2500 years. J. Hosp. Infect. *18*:5–64, 1991.
584. Semmelweis, I. F.: The Etiology, the Concept and the Prophylaxis of Childbed Fever. The Classics of Medicine Library, 1981.
585. Senerwa, D., Olsvik, O., Mutanda, L. N., et al.: Enteropathogenic *Escherichia coli* serotype O111:HNT isolated from preterm neonates in Nairobi, Kenya. J. Clin. Microbiol. *27*:1307–1311, 1989.
586. Severien, C., and Nelson, J. D.: Frequency of infections associated with implanted systems vs cuffed, tunneled Silastic venous catheters in patients with acute leukemia. Am. J. Dis. Child. *145*:1433–1438, 1991.
587. Shannon, K., Fung, K., Stapleton, P., et al.: A hospital outbreak of extended-spectrum beta-lactamase–producing *Klebsiella pneumoniae* investigated by RAPD typing and analysis of the genetics and mechanisms of resistance. J. Hosp. Infect. *39*:291–300, 1998.
588. Sharma, L. K., and Sharma, P. K.: Postoperative wound infection in a pediatric surgical service. J. Pediatr. Surg. *21*:889–891, 1986.
589. Shay, D. K., Holman, R. C., Newman, R. D., et al.: Bronchiolitis-associated hospitalizations among US children, 1980–1996. J. A. M. A. *282*:1440–1446, 1999.
590. Shefer, A., Dales, L., Nelson, M., et al.: Use and safety of acellular pertussis vaccine among adult hospital staff during an outbreak of pertussis. J. Infect. Dis. *171*:1053–1056, 1995.
591. Shenep, J. L.: Viridans-group streptococcal infections in immunocompromised hosts. Int. J. Antimicrob. Agents *14*:129–135, 2000.
592. Sherertz, R. J., Gledhill, K. S., Hampton, K. D., et al.: Outbreak of *Candida* bloodstream infections associated with retrograde medication administration in a neonatal intensive care unit. J. Pediatr. *120*: 455–461, 1992.
593. Sherertz, R. J., Heard, S. O., and Raad, I. I.: Diagnosis of triple-lumen catheter infection: Comparison of roll plate, sonication, and flushing methodologies. J. Clin. Microbiol. *35*:641–646, 1997.
594. Sherertz, R. J., Raad, I., Belani, A., et al.: Three-year experience with sonicated vascular catheter cultures in a clinical microbiology laboratory. J. Clin. Microbiol. *28*:76–82, 1990.
595. Sheridan, R. L., Weber, J., Benjamin, J., et al.: Control of methicillin-resistant *Staphylococcus aureus* in a pediatric burn unit. Am. J. Infect. Control *22*:340–345, 1994.
596. Shimandle, R. B., Johnson, D., Baker, M., et al.: Safety of peripheral intravenous catheters in children. Infect. Control Hosp. Epidemiol. *20*:736–740, 1999.
597. Shuman, R. M., Leech, R. W., and Alvord, E. C., Jr.: Neurotoxicity of hexachlorophene in the human: I. A clinicopathologic study of 248 children. Pediatrics *54*:689–695, 1974.
598. Shuman, R. M., Leech, R. W., and Alvord, E. C., Jr.: Neurotoxicity of hexachlorophene in humans. II. A clinicopathological study of 46 premature infants. Arch. Neurol. *32*:320–325, 1975.
599. Sidebottom, D. G., Freeman, J., Platt, R., et al.: Fifteen-year experience with bloodstream isolates of coagulase-negative staphylococci in neonatal intensive care. J. Clin. Microbiol. *26*:713–718, 1988.
600. Siegel, J. D., Krishner, K. K., Levine, G. L., et al.: Prevalence of antimicrobial resistant bacteria in Pediatric Prevention Network intensive care units. Presented at the 39th Annual Meeting of the Infectious Diseases Society of America, October 25–28, 2001, San Francisco, pp. 92.
601. Siegman-Igra, Y., Anglim, A. M., Shapiro, D. E., et al.: Diagnosis of vascular catheter-related bloodstream infection: A meta-analysis. J. Clin. Microbiol. *35*:928–936, 1997.
602. Sieradzki, K., Roberts, R. B., Haber, S. W., and Tomasz, A.: The development of vancomycin resistance in a patient with methicillin-resistant *Staphylococcus aureus* infection. N. Engl. J. Med. *340*:517–523, 1999.
603. Sieradzki, K., Roberts, R. B., Serur, D., et al.: Heterogeneously vancomycin-resistant *Staphylococcus epidermidis* strain causing recurrent peritonitis in a dialysis patient during vancomycin therapy. J. Clin. Microbiol. *37*:39–44, 1999.
604. Simmons, B. P., Gelfand, M. S., Haas, M., et al.: *Enterobacter sakazakii* infections in neonates associated with intrinsic contamination of a powdered infant formula. Infect. Control Hosp. Epidemiol. *10*:398–401, 1989.
605. Singh-Naz, N., Brown, M., and Ganeshananthan, M.: Nosocomial adenovirus infection: Molecular epidemiology of an outbreak. Pediatr. Infect. Dis. J. *12*:922–925, 1993.
606. Singh-Naz, N., Sleemi, A., Pikis, A., et al.: Vancomycin-resistant *Enterococcus faecium* colonization in children. J. Clin. Microbiol. *37*: 413–416, 1999.
607. Singh-Naz, N., Sprague, B. M., Patel, K. M., and Pollack, M. M.: Risk factors for nosocomial infection in critically ill children: A prospective cohort study. Crit. Care Med. *24*:875–878, 1996.
608. Singh-Naz, N., Sprague, B. M., Patel, K. M., and Pollack, M. M.: Risk assessment and standardized nosocomial infection rate in critically ill children. Crit. Care Med. *28*:2069–2075, 2000.
609. Sirinavin, S., Hotrakitya, S., Suprasongsin, C., et al.: An outbreak of *Salmonella urbana* infection in neonatal nurseries. J. Hosp. Infect. *18*:231–238, 1991.
610. Sloand, E. M., Pitt, E., and Klein, H. G.: Safety of the blood supply. J. A. M. A. *274*:1374–1379, 1995.
611. Sloos, J. H., Horrevorts, A. M., Van Boven, C. P., and Dijkshoorn, L.: Identification of multiresistant *Staphylococcus epidermidis* in neonates of a secondary care hospital using pulsed field gel electrophoresis and quantitative antibiogram typing. J. Clin. Pathol. *51*:62–67, 1998.
612. Smith, D. H., Johnson, B. K., Isaacson, M., et al.: Marburg-virus disease in Kenya. Lancet *1*:816–820, 1982.
613. Smith, P. F., Stricof, R. L., Shayegani, M., and Morse, D. L.: Cluster of *Haemophilus influenzae* type b infections in adults. J. A. M. A. *260*:1446–1449, 1988.

614. Smith, P. W., and Rusnak, P. G.: Infection prevention and control in the long-term-care facility. Infect. Control Hosp. Epidemiol. *18*:831–849, 1997.
615. Smith, T. L., Pearson, M. L., Wilcox, K. R., et al.: Emergence of vancomycin resistance in *Staphylococcus aureus*. Glycopeptide-Intermediate *Staphylococcus aureus* Working Group. N. Engl. J. Med. *340*:493–501, 1999.
616. Snydman, D. R., Greer, C., Meissner, H. C., and McIntosh, K.: Prevention of nosocomial transmission of respiratory syncytial virus in a newborn nursery. Infect. Control Hosp. Epidemiol. *9*:105–108, 1988.
617. Sohn, A. H., Garrett, D. O., Sinkowitz-Cochran, R. L., et al.: Prevalence of nosocomial infections in neonatal intensive care unit patients: Results from the first national point-prevalence survey. J. Pediatr. *139*:821–827, 2001.
618. Sohn, A. H., and Jarvis, W. R.: Benchmarking in pediatric infection control: Results from the National Nosocomial Infections Surveillance (NNIS) System and the Pediatric Prevention Network. Semin. Pediatr. Infect. Dis. *12*:254–265, 2001.
619. Soufir, L., Timsit, J. F., Mahe, C., et al.: Attributable morbidity and mortality of catheter-related septicemia in critically ill patients: A matched, risk-adjusted, cohort study. Infect. Control Hosp. Epidemiol. *20*:396–401, 1999.
620. Spach, D. H., Silverstein, F. E., and Stamm, W. E.: Transmission of infection by gastrointestinal endoscopy and bronchoscopy. Ann. Intern. Med. *118*:117–128, 1993.
621. Spector, S. A.: Transmission of cytomegalovirus among infants in hospital documented by restriction-endonuclease-digestion analyses. Lancet *1*:378–381, 1983.
622. Speert, D. P., Henry, D., Vandamme, P., et al.: Epidemiology of *Burkholderia cepacia* complex in patients with cystic fibrosis, Canada. Emerg. Infect. Dis. *8*:181–187, 2002.
623. Spender, Q. W., Lewis, D., and Price, E. H.: Norwalk like viruses: Study of an outbreak. Arch. Dis. Child. *61*:142–147, 1986.
624. Spratt, H. C., Marks, M. I., Gomersall, M., et al.: Nosocomial infantile gastroenteritis associated with minirotavirus and calicivirus. J. Pediatr. *93*:922–926, 1978.
625. Starke, J. R.: Tuberculosis in children. Curr. Opin. Pediatr. *7*:268–277, 1995.
626. Steingart, K. R., Thomas, A. R., Dykewicz, C. A., and Redd, S. C.: Transmission of measles virus in healthcare settings during a communitywide outbreak. Infect. Control Hosp. Epidemiol. *20*:115–119, 1999.
627. Steketee, R. W., Burstyn, D. G., Wassilak, S. G., et al.: A comparison of laboratory and clinical methods for diagnosing pertussis in an outbreak in a facility for the developmentally disabled. J. Infect. Dis. *157*:441–449, 1988.
628. Stenzel, J. P., Green, T. P., Fuhrman, B. P., et al.: Percutaneous femoral venous catheterizations: A prospective study of complications. J. Pediatr. *114*:411–415, 1989.
629. Stewart, C. J.: Tuberculosis infection in a paediatric department. B. M. J. *1*:30–32, 1976.
630. Stoll, B. J., Temprosa, M., Tyson, J. E., et al.: Dexamethasone therapy increases infection in very low birth weight infants. Pediatrics *104*:e63, 1999.
631. Stone, A., Shaffer, M., and Sautter, R. L.: *Salmonella poona* infection and surveillance in a neonatal nursery. Am. J. Infect. Control *21*:270–273, 1993.
632. Stover, B. H., Duff, A., Adams, G., et al.: Emergence and control of methicillin-resistant *Staphylococcus aureus* in a children's hospital and pediatric long-term care facility. Am. J. Infect. Control *20*:248–255, 1992.
633. Strassburg, M. A., Imagawa, D. T., Fannin, S. L., et al.: Rubella outbreak among hospital employees. Obstet. Gynecol. *57*:283–288, 1981.
634. Straube, R. C., Thompson, M. A., Van Dyke, R. B., et al.: Adenovirus type 7b in a children's hospital. J. Infect. Dis. *147*:814–819, 1983.
635. Stroud, L. A., Tokars, J. I., Grieco, M. H., et al.: Evaluation of infection control measures in preventing the nosocomial transmission of multidrug-resistant *Mycobacterium tuberculosis* in a New York City hospital. Infect. Control Hosp. Epidemiol. *16*:141–147, 1995.
636. Suleiman, M. N., Muscat-Baron, J. M., Harries, J. R., et al.: Congo/Crimean haemorrhagic fever in Dubai. An outbreak at the Rashid Hospital. Lancet *2*:939–941, 1980.
637. Sun, L., Jiang, R. Z., Steinbach, S., et al.: The emergence of a highly transmissible lineage of cbl+ *Pseudomonas (Burkholderia) cepacia* causing CF centre epidemics in North America and Britain. Nat. Med. *1*:661–666, 1995.
638. Szajewska, H., Kotowska, M., Mrukowicz, J. Z., et al.: Efficacy of *Lactobacillus* GG in prevention of nosocomial diarrhea in infants. J. Pediatr. *138*:361–365, 2001.
639. Tablan, O. C., Anderson, L. J., Arden, N. H., et al.: Guideline for prevention of nosocomial pneumonia. The Hospital Infection Control Practices Advisory Committee. Infect. Control Hosp. Epidemiol. *15*:587–627, 1994.
640. Takami, T., Sonodat, S., Houjyo, H., et al.: Diagnosis of horizontal enterovirus infections in neonates by nested PCR and direct sequence analysis. J. Hosp. Infect. *45*:283–287, 2000.
641. Tambyah, P. A., Halvorson, K. T., and Maki, D. G.: A prospective study of pathogenesis of catheter-associated urinary tract infections. Mayo Clin. Proc. *74*:131–136, 1999.
642. Tambyah, P. A., and Maki, D. G.: The relationship between pyuria and infection in patients with indwelling urinary catheters: A prospective study of 761 patients. Arch. Intern. Med. *160*:673–677, 2000.
643. Tanaka, Y., Fujinaga, K., Goto, A., et al.: Outbreak of pertussis in a residential facility for handicapped people. Dev. Biol. Stand. *73*:329–332, 1991.
644. Teasley, D. G., Gerding, D. N., Olson, M. M., et al.: Prospective randomised trial of metronidazole versus vancomycin for *Clostridium-difficile* -associated diarrhoea and colitis. Lancet *2*:1043–1046, 1983.
645. Thacker, S. B., Kimball, A. M., Wolfe, M., et al.: Parasitic disease control in a residential facility for the mentally retarded: Failure of selected isolation procedures. Am. J. Public Health. *71*:303–305, 1981.
646. The International Neonatal Network: The CRIB (clinical risk index for babies) score: A tool for assessing initial neonatal risk and comparing performance of neonatal intensive care units. Lancet *342*:193–198, 1993.
647. The Society for Hospital Epidemiology of America, Association for Practitioners in Infection Control, Centers for Disease Control, Surgical Infection Society: Consensus paper on the surveillance of surgical wound infections. Infect. Control Hosp. Epidemiol. *13*:599–605, 1992.
648. Tobin, M. J.: Advances in mechanical ventilation. N. Engl. J. Med. *344*: 1986–1996, 2001.
649. Toltzis, P., and Blumer, J. L.: Problems with resistance in pediatric intensive care. New Horiz. *4*:353–360, 1996.
650. Toltzis, P., and Blumer, J. L.: Nosocomial acquisition and transmission of antibiotic-resistant gram-negative organisms in the pediatric intensive care unit. Pediatr. Infect. Dis J. *20*:612–618, 2001.
651. Tucci, V., Haran, M. A., and Isenberg, H. D.: Epidemiology and control of vancomycin-resistant enterococci in an adult and children's hospital. Am. J. Infect. Control *25*:371–376, 1997.
652. Valenti, W. M., Clarke, T. A., Hall, C. B et al.: Concurrent outbreaks of rhinovirus and respiratory syncytial virus in an intensive care nursery: Epidemiology and associated risk factors. J. Pediatr. *100*:722–726, 1982.
653. Valenti, W. M., Menegus, M. A., Hall, C. B., et al.: Nosocomial viral infections: I. Epidemiology and significance. Infect. Control *1*:33–37, 1980.
654. Valenti, W. M., Pincus, P. H., and Messner, M. K.: Nosocomial pertussis: Possible spread by a hospital visitor. Am. J. Dis. Child. *134*:520–521, 1980.
655. van Acker, J., de Smet, F., Muyldermans, G., et al.: Outbreak of necrotizing enterocolitis associated with *Enterobacter sakazakii* in powdered milk formula. J. Clin. Microbiol. *39*:293–297, 2001.
656. van Dijk, W. C., and van der Straaten, P. J.: An outbreak of *Campylobacter jejuni* infection in a neonatal intensive care unit. J. Hosp. Infect. *11*:91–92, 1988.
657. Van Dyke, R. B., and Spector, S. A.: Transmission of herpes simplex virus type 1 to a newborn infant during endotracheal suctioning for meconium aspiration. Pediatr. Infect. Dis. J. *3*:153–156, 1984.
658. Vazquez, J. A., Sanchez, V., Dmuchowski, C., et al.: Nosocomial acquisition of *Candida albicans*: An epidemiologic study. J. Infect. Dis. *168*: 195–201, 1993.
659. Velandia, M., Fridkin, S. K., Cardenas, V., et al.: Transmission of HIV in dialysis centre. Lancet *345*:1417–1422, 1995.
660. Vermaat, J. H., Rosebrugh, E., Ford-Jones, E. L., et al.: An epidemiologic study of nosocomial infections in a pediatric long-term care facility. Am. J. Infect. Control *21*:183–188, 1993.
661. Villari, P., Sarnataro, C., and Iacuzio, L.: Molecular epidemiology of *Staphylococcus epidermidis* in a neonatal intensive care unit over a three-year period. J. Clin. Microbiol. *38*:1740–1746, 2000.
662. Villarino, M. E., Stevens, L. E., Schable, B., et al.: Risk factors for epidemic *Xanthomonas maltophilia* infection/colonization in intensive care unit patients. Infect. Control Hosp. Epidemiol. *13*:201–206, 1992.
663. Villers, D., Espaze, E., Coste-Burel, M., et al.: Nosocomial *Acinetobacter baumannii* infections: Microbiological and clinical epidemiology. Ann. Intern. Med. *129*:182–189, 1998.
664. Walmsley, S., Devi, S., King, S., et al.: Invasive *Aspergillus* infections in a pediatric hospital: A ten-year review. Pediatr. Infect. Dis. J. *12*: 673–682, 1993.
665. Walther, F. J., Bruggeman, C., and Daniels-Bosman, M. S.: Rotavirus infections in high-risk neonates. J. Hosp. Infect. *5*:438–443, 1984.
666. Wasserman, R., August, C. S., and Plotkin, S. A.: Viral infections in pediatric bone marrow transplant patients. Pediatr. Infect. Dis. J. *7*: 109–115, 1988.
667. Watkins, A. G., and Lewis-Fanning, E.: Incidence of cross-infection in children's wards. B. M. J. *2*:616–619, 1949.
668. Watson, J. C., Fleming, D. W., Borella, A. J., et al.: Vertical transmission of hepatitis A resulting in an outbreak in a neonatal intensive care unit. J. Infect. Dis. *167*:567–571, 1993.
669. Weber, J. M., Sheridan, R. L., Pasternack, M. S., and Tompkins, R. G.: Nosocomial infections in pediatric patients with burns. Am. J. Infect. Control *25*:195–201, 1997.
670. Wehrle, P. F., Posch, J., Richter, K. H., and Henderson, D. A.: An airborne outbreak of smallpox in a German hospital and its significance with respect to other recent outbreaks in Europe. Bull. World Health Organ. *43*:669–679, 1970.
671. Weinstein, J. W., Barrett, C. R., Baltimore, R. S., and Hierholzer, W. J., Jr.: Nosocomial transmission of tuberculosis from a hospital visitor on a pediatrics ward. Pediatr. Infect. Dis. J. *14*:232–234, 1995.

672. Weisman, L. E., Cruess, D. F., and Fischer, G. W.: Opsonic activity of commercially available standard intravenous immunoglobulin preparations. Pediatr. Infect. Dis. J. *13*:1122–1125, 1994.
673. Weisman, L. E., Stoll, B. J., Kueser, T. J., et al.: Intravenous immune globulin prophylaxis of late-onset sepsis in premature neonates. J. Pediatr. *125*:922–930, 1994.
674. Weiss, K., Restieri, C., Gauthier, R., et al.: A nosocomial outbreak of fluoroquinolone-resistant *Streptococcus pneumoniae.* Clin. Infect. Dis. *33*:517–522, 2001.
675. Welbel, S. F., McNeil, M. M., Pramanik, A., et al.: Nosocomial *Malassezia pachydermatis* bloodstream infections in a neonatal intensive care unit. Pediatr. Infect. Dis. J. *13*:104–108, 1994.
676. Welliver, R. C., and McLaughlin, S.: Unique epidemiology of nosocomial infection in a children's hospital. Am. J. Dis. Child. *138*:131–135, 1984.
677. Wells, V. D., Wong, E. S., Murray, B. E., et al.: Infections due to beta-lactamase–producing, high-level gentamicin-resistant *Enterococcus faecalis.* Ann. Intern. Med. *116*:285–292, 1992.
678. Wenger, P. N., Otten, J., Breeden, A., et al.: Control of nosocomial transmission of multidrug-resistant *Mycobacterium tuberculosis* among health-care workers and HIV-infected patients. Lancet *345*:235–240, 1995.
679. Wenzel RP, Deal EC, Hendley JO: Hospital-acquired viral respiratory illness on a pediatric ward. Pediatr. *60*:367–371, 1977.
680. Wesley, A. G., Pather, M., and Tait, D.: Nosocomial adenovirus infection in a paediatric respiratory unit. J. Hosp. Infect. *25*:183–190, 1993.
681. Wessels, M. R., Moses, A. E., Goldberg, J. B., and DiCesare, T. J.: Hyaluronic acid capsule is a virulence factor for mucoid group A streptococci. Proc. Natl. Acad. Sci. U. S. A. *88*:8317–8321, 1991.
682. Wey, S. B., Mori, M., Pfaller, M. A., et al.: Hospital-acquired candidemia. The attributable mortality and excess length of stay. Arch. Intern. Med. *148*:2642–2645, 1988.
683. Wharton, M., Cochi, S. L., Hutcheson, R. H., and Schaffner, W.: Mumps transmission in hospitals. Arch. Intern. Med. *150*:47–49, 1990.
684. Widell, A., Christensson, B., Wiebe, T., et al.: Epidemiologic and molecular investigation of outbreaks of hepatitis C virus infection on a pediatric oncology service. Ann. Intern. Med. *130*:130–134, 1999.
685. Wiener, E. S.: Catheter sepsis: The central venous line Achilles' heel. Semin. Pediatr. Surg. *4*:207–214, 1995.
686. Wilde, J., Yolken, R., Willoughby, R., and Eiden, J.: Improved detection of rotavirus shedding by polymerase chain reaction. Lancet *337*: 323–326, 1991.
687. Williams, W. W., Mariano, J., Spurrier, M., et al.: Nosocomial meningitis due to *Citrobacter diversus* in neonates: New aspects of the epidemiology. J. Infect. Dis. *150*:229–235, 1984.
688. Wilson, C. W., Stevenson, D. K., and Arvin, A. M.: A concurrent epidemic of respiratory syncytial virus and echovirus 7 infections in an intensive care nursery. Pediatr. Infect. Dis. J. *8*:24–29, 1989.
689. Wong, E. S.: Guideline for prevention of catheter-associated urinary tract infections. Am. J. Infect. Control *11*:28–36, 1983.
690. Wood, D. J., and Corbitt, G.: Viral infections in childhood leukemia. J. Infect. Dis. *152*:266–273, 1985.
691. Woolf, A. D., and Cohen, B. J.: Parvovirus B19 and chronic arthritis—causal or casual association? Ann. Rheum. Dis. *54*:535–536, 1995.
692. Wright, S. W., Decker, M. D., and Edwards, K. M.: Incidence of pertussis infection in healthcare workers. Infect. Control Hosp. Epidemiol. *20*:120–123, 1999.
693. Wu, S. X., and Tang, Y.: Molecular epidemiologic study of an outbreak of *Salmonella typhimurium* infection at a newborn nursery. Chin. Med. J. *106*:423–427, 1993.
694. Wurzel, C. L., Halom, K., Feldman, J. G., and Rubin, L. G.: Infection rates of Broviac-Hickman catheters and implantable venous devices. Am. J. Dis. Child. *142*:536–540, 1988.
695. Yeh, T. S., Pollack, M. M., Ruttimann, U. E., et al.: Validation of a physiologic stability index for use in critically ill infants and children. Pediatr. Res. *18*:445–451, 1984.
696. Yerly, S., Quadri, R., Negro, F., et al.: Nosocomial outbreak of multiple bloodborne viral infections. J. Infect. Dis. *184*:369–372, 2001.
697. Yogev, R.: Cerebrospinal fluid shunt infections: A personal view. Pediatr. Infect. Dis. J. *4*:113–118, 1985.
698. Zaidi, A. K., Macone, A., and Goldmann, A. D.: Impact of simple screening criteria on utilization of low-yield bacterial stool cultures in a Children's Hospital. Pediatrics *103*:1189–1192, 1999.
699. Zwiener, R. J., Belknap, W. M., and Quan, R.: Severe pseudomembranous enterocolitis in a child: Case report and literature review. Pediatr. Infect. Dis. J. *8*:876–882, 1989.

CHAPTER 232 Prevention and Control of Nosocomial Infections in Health Care Facilities That Serve Children

W. CHARLES HUSKINS ■ DONALD A. GOLDMANN

The history of formal hospital programs designed to prevent and control nosocomial infections generally is traced to the organized efforts of hospitals in Great Britain and North America to control the pandemic of *Staphylococcus aureus* infection in the 1950s and early 1960s. However, programs to study and control the nosocomial spread of contagious diseases were well established in the leading pediatric hospitals in several European countries and North America even in the mid-1930s.[12, 17, 52, 71, 72, 78]

In the past half century, the scope and complexity of hospital programs for prevention and control of infection have expanded dramatically. Today, hospital inpatient populations include more severely ill children and children with compromised immune systems. Advances in medical care and technology have improved the survival of these vulnerable patients; however, this progress has gone hand in hand with an increased risk of acquiring nosocomial infection caused by a wide spectrum of microbial pathogens. The shift in the site of patient care from the inpatient to the outpatient setting has expanded the focus of infection control programs from the hospital to the entire health care system. The risk of occupationally acquired infection among medical professionals has required that infection control programs work with employee health services to develop policies and procedures to prevent these infections. Finally, many infection control professionals have taken on additional responsibilities to address more general issues of health care quality and patient safety.

This chapter highlights key elements of a comprehensive program to prevent and control nosocomial infections in pediatric patients and health care workers. A detailed description of how to develop, implement, and maintain an effective program is beyond the scope of this chapter, and the reader is referred to several excellent and authoritative sources.[1, 7, 33, 76, 114] Specific nosocomial infections are discussed in Chapter 231.

External Organizations Influencing Health Care Infection Prevention and Control Programs

The nature and activity of the large number of external organizations that have significant influence on health care infection prevention and control programs in the United States are described elsewhere.[77] A few of the most influential of these organizations are discussed in this section.

The Division of Healthcare Quality Promotion (DHQP), formerly the Hospital Infections Program, is a part of the National Center for Infectious Diseases of the Centers for Disease Control and Prevention (CDC) (*http://www.cdc.gov/ncidod/hip*). The DHQP has a major role in providing information and guidance to health care infection control programs, as well as in conducting its own investigations. It has the single largest experience in investigation of nosocomial infection outbreaks and can provide assistance to individual health care institutions.[57]

Coordinated by the DHQP, the National Nosocomial Infection Surveillance (NNIS) System collects data on the incidence of nosocomial infections in more than 300 U.S. hospitals.[103] Participation in the NNIS System is voluntary; consequently, data reported by the NNIS System are not necessarily representative of the universe of U.S. hospitals. Nonetheless, these data are very useful in detecting and describing broad-based trends in the incidence and microbial etiology of nosocomial infections in the United States. In addition, the NNIS System regularly reports several key device-associated, exposure-adjusted infection rates (e.g., number of central venous catheter infections per 1000 central venous catheter–days), device utilization rates in intensive care units (ICUs) (i.e., number of central venous catheters used per 100 patients), and risk-adjusted surgical-site infection rates for specific operative procedures.[82] Although comparisons of infection rates among hospitals still is hampered by incomplete adjustment for severity of illness and case mix, hospitals analyzing their performance relative to these benchmarks may identify areas for improvement.[44] Moreover, hospitals as a whole probably have achieved some measure of success in this effort because rates of device-associated bloodstream infection, pneumonia, and urinary tract infection all have declined in adult and pediatric ICUs participating in the NNIS System during the 1990s.[24, 103] In high-risk nurseries during the same period, rates of catheter-associated bloodstream infection declined among infants in all birth weight categories, and rates of ventilator pneumonia declined among all but the smallest infants.[103]

The Healthcare Infection Control Practices Advisory Committee (HICPAC) was established in 1991 to provide advice and guidance to the DHQP and the CDC regarding the practice of infection control and strategies for surveillance, prevention, and control of nosocomial infections in U.S. health care systems (*http://www.cdc.gov/ncidod/hip/HICPAC/Hicpac.htm*). HICPAC issues evidence-based guidelines for infection control.[13, 15, 42, 55, 75, 86, 104]

A large number of professional and trade associations also develop recommendations and guidelines related to infection control. The most prominent among these associations in the United States are the Society of Healthcare Epidemiology of America (SHEA) and the Association for Professionals in Infection Control and Epidemiology (APIC). In Europe, a variety of organizations also are developing evidence-based guidelines, the most prominent of which has been the *epic* program in England.[92]

During the past several decades, the Joint Commission on Accreditation of Healthcare Organizations (JCAHO), a private, not-for-profit organization, has had a major influence on the structure and activity of health care infection prevention and control programs (*http://www.jcaho.org*).[87] JCAHO's standards regarding these programs have evolved consistent with the commission's Agenda for Change, an initiative to place greater emphasis on organizational performance regarding processes that have a significant impact on patient care.[87] One of the major goals of this effort has been to develop the ORYX Initiative—a series of performance indicators that are being incorporated into JCAHO's core measures and will be necessary for accreditation. These indicators can be used not only to track organizational performance but also to facilitate comparisons of quality of care (benchmarking) among hospitals. In addition, the JCAHO survey process has moved away from assessment of the structural elements of an infection control program, such as the existence of an infection control committee, toward integration of nosocomial infection prevention and control into the everyday activities of the health care system as a whole. In the future, JCAHO plans to develop surveys that are more "data-driven, less predictable, and more customized to individual organizations."[59]

Responding to the hazards of occupational exposure to blood-borne pathogens and tuberculosis, the U.S. Department of Labor's Occupational Safety and Health Administration (OSHA) has issued regulations that have had a major impact on the structure and activity of infection prevention and control activities. In 1991, OSHA issued regulations regarding blood-borne pathogens, "Occupational Exposure to Bloodborne Pathogens: Final Rule," that mandated specific exposure prevention strategies, health care worker education, evaluation and management of exposure situations, voluntary hepatitis B vaccination at no cost to employees, and detailed record keeping.[85] OSHA also is considering regulations regarding occupational exposure to *Mycobacterium tuberculosis*.

Integration of Health Care Infection Prevention and Control and Quality Improvement and Patient Safety Efforts

Many hospitals have implemented continuous quality improvement (CQI) initiatives (also called total quality management [TQM]) as a means for improving the quality of health care.[10, 29, 30, 66] Some individuals involved in health care infection prevention and control programs have been leaders in this effort because they know how to apply epidemiologic principles to the collection, analysis, and interpretation of data, and they have extensive experience in improving systems of care—both central components of the CQI approach. Systems of care that have an impact on the risk of acquiring nosocomial infection are typically complex and involve personnel from many departments. Infection control personnel do not "own" any of these systems. Therefore, they must assist others in using epidemiologically valid methods to study and improve systems of care critical for prevention of nosocomial infection. This section provides an illustration of how epidemiologic studies and systems improvement can be integrated into an overall CQI effort.

A system of care can be analyzed in terms of its structure (i.e., essential facilities, equipment, supplies, personnel, and organizational networks), processes (i.e., the relationships and interactions among structural elements), and outcomes (i.e., nosocomial infection rates or mortality, the cost of nosocomial infections, patient satisfaction).[32] The systems of care critical for the prevention of surgical-site infections provide an excellent illustration of this conceptual model.

Structural elements important for the prevention of surgical-site infections (e.g., presence of skilled surgeons, a program for surveillance and feedback of surgical-site infection rates to surgeons, guidelines for perioperative antimicrobial prophylaxis, effective sterilization methods for surgical instruments, adequately designed and equipped operating rooms) are well described,[75] although not all of the individual contributions of each of these elements have been confirmed by rigorous experimental trials. Processes important in the prevention of surgical-wound infection (e.g., methods of preoperative hair removal, procedures for preparation of the skin at the site of the incision, the timing of perioperative antimicrobial prophylaxis) have been studied extensively.[75] Methods for collecting data regarding surgical-site infections and calculating risk-adjusted rates of surgical-site infection for specific surgical procedures are well described as a result of decades of methodologic investigation.[75, 105]

Epidemiologic studies (e.g., experimental clinical trials, cohort studies, and case-control studies) have defined the impact of various structures and processes on surgical-site infection rates. For example, many clinical trials have examined the effectiveness of various regimens for perioperative antimicrobial prophylaxis in the prevention of surgical-site infections. Based on these studies, guidelines for perioperative antimicrobial prophylaxis have been developed.[2, 4] Nonetheless, studies have shown that utilization of perioperative prophylaxis often is less than optimal.[28, 35, 101] Currier and colleagues found that only 60 percent of patients with indications for prophylaxis actually received it; conversely, prophylaxis was administered to 41 percent of patients with no indication.[28] Prophylaxis is continued for excessively long periods (>2 days) in many instances.[28, 35, 101] The critical importance of the timing of perioperative antimicrobial prophylaxis in the prevention of surgical-site infections was demonstrated in a cohort study. Classen and colleagues showed that the effectiveness of prophylaxis was maximized only if it was administered during a 2-hour window period before the start of the procedure; prophylaxis administered before or after this period was much less effective, and prophylaxis administered 6 or more hours after the start of the procedure essentially had no effect.[26] Nearly 40 percent of patients in this study did not receive prophylaxis within this critical window period.[26]

CQI is ideally suited to address multidisciplinary, interdepartmental systems problems, such as timely administration of perioperative antimicrobial prophylaxis. With the help of personnel intimately involved in this system (e.g., surgeons, nurses, pharmacists, anesthesiologists), the reasons why patients do not receive prophylaxis at the appropriate time can be examined and the system for ordering, dispensing, delivering, and administrating prophylactic agents can be streamlined. A recent study described how CQI was used to improve the use and timing of perioperative antimicrobial prophylaxis for cesarean section.[110] A comprehensive guide to assist hospitals in using CQI to improve utilization of antimicrobial agents and prevent and control the emergence and dissemination of antimicrobial-resistant microorganisms also has been published.[45]

More recently, some infection control professionals have applied their skills in epidemiology and systems improvement to the general area of patient safety, especially the detection and prevention of adverse drug events. The genesis of this trend came from two major studies of adverse events and an influential report in 2000 by the Institute of Medicine that emphasized the substantial deficiencies in patient safety that exist in U.S. hospitals.[16, 106] Adverse drug events are among the most common nonsurgical adverse events, comparable in incidence between hospitalized adults and children and similar to nosocomial infections in terms of their cost and associated morbidity.[5, 6, 62] The same systems analysis and multidisciplinary approach to the prevention of nosocomial infection can be applied to the prevention of adverse drug events.

Organization and Activities of Health Care Infection Control Programs

The Study on the Efficacy of Nosocomial Infection Control (SENIC) conducted in U.S. hospitals in the mid-1970s found that hospitals with a trained, effective infection control physician, one infection control nurse per 250 acute care hospital beds, and a system for reporting surgical-site infection rates to surgeons could reduce their nosocomial infection rates by 32 percent in comparison to hospitals with no infection control program.[49] However, because relatively few hospitals implemented these maximally effective programs, only 6 percent of the theoretically preventable infections nationwide were, in fact, prevented. In 1983, a repeat survey of a sample of the participating hospitals found that the percentage of hospitals with one infection control nurse per 250 acute care hospital beds had increased from 22 to 57 percent[50]; however, the percentage with a physician trained in infection control remained low (15%), and the percentage of hospitals performing surgical-site infection surveillance and reporting these rates to surgeons actually decreased. The percentage of preventable infections that were avoided had risen to 9 percent. Apart from the landmark SENIC project, objective evaluation of the efficacy of various components of infection control programs has been minimal.

Nonetheless, a large amount of practical experience has guided the development of health care infection control programs. In 1998, the report of a consensus panel of national experts on the requirements for infrastructure and the essential activities of these programs was published with the endorsement of SHEA, APIC, and other key organizations (including DHQP and JCAHO).[100] The report stated that the principal goals of these programs are to protect the patient, the health care worker, visitors, and others in the health care environment and to accomplish these goals in a cost-effective manner whenever possible.[100] The specific recommendations of the panel were accompanied by an indication of the strength of the recommendation. The recommendations are described in more detail in the published report and are listed in Table 232–1.[100] A guideline for the prevention of nosocomial infection in long-term care residents also has been published.[102] Neither of these publications deals with specific pediatric issues, although the recommendations are generally applicable to facilities providing care to children.

Surveillance Strategies

Surveillance of nosocomial infections is necessary to understand the specific nosocomial infection problems of individual hospitals. Surveillance data can focus prevention and control efforts on the patients at highest risk and provide a means of evaluating the effectiveness of these interventions. By establishing endemic rates of nosocomial infection, surveillance also facilitates detection of outbreaks. For these reasons, surveillance traditionally has been regarded as an essential component of a hospital infection prevention and control program—a view that was validated by the SENIC project.[49] Recommended practices for surveillance have been defined and published.[70]

TABLE 232–1 ■ CONSENSUS PANEL RECOMMENDATIONS REGARDING THE REQUIREMENTS FOR INFRASTRUCTURE AND ESSENTIAL ACTIVITIES OF INFECTION CONTROL AND EPIDEMIOLOGY IN HOSPITALS

Recommendation	Category*
Critical Data and Information	
Surveillance of nosocomial infections must be performed.	I
Surveillance data must be analyzed appropriately and used to monitor and improve infection control and health care outcomes.	I
Clinical performance and assessment indicators used to support external comparative measurement should meet the criteria delineated by SHEA and APIC.	II
Polices and Procedures	
Written infection prevention and control policies and procedures must be established, implemented, and updated periodically.	II and III
Policies and procedures should be monitored periodically for performance.	II and III
Regulations, Guidelines, and Accreditation Requirements	
Health care facilities should use infection control personnel to assist in maintaining compliance with relevant regulatory and accreditation requirements.	II
Infection control personnel should have appropriate access to medical or other relevant records and to staff members who can provide information on the adequacy of the institution's compliance with regard to regulations, standards, and guidelines.	II
The infection control program should collaborate with and provide liaison to appropriate local and state health departments for reporting of communicable diseases and related conditions and to assist with the control of infectious diseases.	II and III
Employee Health	
The infection control program personnel should work collaboratively with the facility's employee health program personnel.	II
At the time of employment, all facility personnel should be evaluated by the employee health program for conditions related to communicable diseases.	II and III
Appropriate employees or other health care workers should have periodic medical evaluations to assess for new conditions related to infectious diseases that may have an impact on patient care, the employee, or other health care workers; the evaluation should include review of immunization and tuberculosis skin test status, if appropriate.	II and III
Employees must be offered appropriate immunizations for communicable diseases.	I and III
The employee health program should develop policies and procedures for the evaluations of ill employees, including assessment of disease communicability, indications for work restrictions, and management of employees who have been exposed to infectious diseases, including postexposure prophylaxis and work restrictions.	I
Prevention of Transmission of Infectious Diseases	
All health care facilities must have the capacity to identify the occurrence of outbreaks or clusters of infectious diseases.	I
All health care facilities must have access to the services of personnel trained and experienced in conducting outbreak investigations.	II
When an outbreak occurs, the infection control team must have adequate resources and the authority to ensure a comprehensive and timely investigation and the implementation of appropriate control measures.	II
Education and Training of Health Care Workers	
Health care facilities must provide ongoing education programs in infection prevention and control to health care workers.	II and III
Education programs should be evaluated periodically for effectiveness, and attendance should be monitored.	II and III
Personnel	
The personnel and supporting resources, including secretarial services, available to the hospital epidemiology and infection control program should be proportional to the size, complexity, and estimated risk of the population served by the institution.	II
All hospitals should have the continuing services of a trained hospital epidemiologist(s) and infection control professional(s).	I
Infection control professional should be encouraged to obtain certification in infection control.	II
Health care facilities should provide or make available, in a timely fashion, sufficient office space, equipment, statistical and computer support, and clinical microbiology and pathology laboratory services to support the surveillance, prevention, and control program of the institution.	II

*I, strongly recommended for implementation based on evidence from at least one properly randomized, controlled trial, evidence from at least one well-designed clinical trial without randomization, evidence from cohort or case-control analytic studies (preferably from more than one center), or evidence from multiple time-series studies; II, recommended for implementation based on published clinical experience or descriptive studies, reports of expert committees, or opinions of respected authorities; III, recommended when required by government rules or regulations.

APIC, Association of Professionals in Infection Control and Epidemiology; SHEA, Society for Healthcare Epidemiology of America.

From Scheckler, W. E., Brimhall, D., Buck, A. S., et al.: Requirements for infrastructure and essential activities of infection control and epidemiology in hospitals: A consensus panel report. Infect. Control Hosp. Edpidemiol. *19*:114–124, 1998.

Prevalence surveys can be used to quickly gain a perspective of the nature and scope of nosocomial infection problems. These surveys also can be used to validate the sensitivity and specificity of ongoing surveillance. For hospitals that focus surveillance efforts on high-risk patients, periodic prevalence surveys can provide reassurance that previously low-risk populations or low-priority problems have not become more problematic. In general, however, surveillance systems that measure the incidence of nosocomial infections provide a more detailed assessment of infection risk and are much more likely to detect outbreaks.

Hospital-wide surveillance, frequently performed by programs in the 1970s and 1980s, largely has been abandoned because of the substantial time commitment required for data collection, although some hospitals have developed computerized systems for case finding that have improved the efficiency of this approach considerably.[19, 36] Most hospitals currently favor focused (or targeted) surveillance that concentrates on specific high-risk groups (e.g., patients in ICUs, surgical patients), specific sites of infection (e.g., bloodstream infections, surgical-site infections), or specific pathogens (e.g., respiratory virus infections, toxin-producing *Clostridium difficile,* multidrug-resistant microorganisms). This approach is designed to maximize the efficiency of surveillance and focus on particularly problematic infections or pathogens. Haley has advocated a refinement of focused surveillance that he calls "surveillance by objective."[48] This approach ensures that surveillance will support specific program goals and provides concrete measures of success. It is suited only for mature surveillance programs that have a clear understanding of their priorities and are confident of their capacity to detect outbreaks through means other than ongoing analysis of endemic infection rates. Hospitals with advanced CQI programs will find this data-driven approach to advancing institutional priorities quite familiar.

A surveillance plan for an individual health care facility may incorporate various types of surveillance. A written plan for surveillance activity should be reviewed yearly and modified as necessary. For each surveillance component, the plan should include a description of (1) the rationale for surveillance, (2) the target population, (3) infection definitions, (4) case-finding methods, (5) source of denominators used for rate calculations, (6) collection of additional data regarding risk factors, (7) calculation of infection rates (including stratification by risk factors, if planned), (8) frequency of reporting to specific target groups (e.g., clinicians, infection control committee, leadership), and (9) estimated time commitment of staff for data collection, analysis, and reporting.

When choosing a particular surveillance strategy, consideration of its sensitivity and specificity is important. For example, self-reporting by clinicians is notoriously insensitive, and surveillance that relies on microbiology culture results alone is likely to be both insensitive and nonspecific. Considerable research regarding case-finding methods has been performed.[43, 88] In general, active, concurrent case finding —that is, active searching for cases by trained persons— should be used. The "gold standard" for case finding includes bedside examination, interviews with ward staff, review of patient charts and all kardexes, and verification of all related microbiologic information by a trained surveyor.[40] However, few programs have the staff for this labor-intensive effort. Many programs rely on positive microbiology culture reports as a starting point for the investigation of infections for which cultures are obtained routinely, such as bloodstream infections, with subsequent review of patient charts to confirm or refute the presence of a nosocomial infection. Nosocomial infections that are not evaluated by microbiologic cultures will, of course, be missed by this approach. Strategies for surveillance that use electronic information also have been developed.[19, 36, 37, 91] Sands and colleagues have conducted detailed studies of the usefulness of this approach in performing surveillance of surgical-site infections.[99]

Calculations of infection rates should include appropriate adjustments whenever possible (see Chapter 231). The simplest technique is merely to adjust for exposure to a particular device or procedure (e.g., number of bloodstream infections per 100 patients with central venous catheters). Adjustment for the duration of exposure to the hospital (e.g., number of infections per 1000 patient-days) or device exposure (e.g., number of bloodstream infections per 1000 central venous catheter–days) is more useful if the necessary denominator data can be obtained. Surgical-site infections should be stratified by wound class, preferably by the surgical-site infection risk index.[27] Some investigators have used severity of illness to adjust infection rates, but this type of adjustment has yet to be incorporated widely into routine surveillance data analysis (see Chapter 231).

Feedback of infection rates to clinicians should be done regularly in an easy-to-understand format. Graphic displays of data, such as statistical process control charts, are particularly effective.[8, 9] Surveillance data also should be used to target areas for further investigation, additional staff education, and specific interventions. High-priority problems should be addressed by a systematic approach to problem solving as discussed earlier (see Integration of Hospital Infection Prevention and Control and Quality Improvement and Patient Safety Efforts).

Surveillance plus reporting of communicable infections to state departments of health is a duty retained by some hospital infection prevention and control programs, although others delegate this responsibility primarily to the microbiology laboratory.

Outbreak Investigation

Researchers have estimated that a community hospital can expect to experience at least one nosocomial infection outbreak per year[51]; teaching hospitals can expect to have several outbreaks every year.[114] Because outbreaks of nosocomial infection often are associated with significant patient morbidity and mortality, clusters of infection should be investigated promptly. A single, highly unusual infection, such as a postoperative group A streptococcal infection, is sufficient cause for an investigation. Clusters of nosocomial infection caused by an uncommon microorganism, a common microorganism with an unusual antimicrobial susceptibility pattern, or a series of infections at the same anatomic site (i.e., an outbreak of diarrhea) also are obvious indications for an investigation. However, some outbreaks are more difficult to recognize because they occur intermittently, involve multiple microorganisms, or involve infection at various anatomic sites.

A guide to the investigation of a cluster of nosocomial infections is provided in Table 232–2. Detailed discussions of the methodology for outbreak investigation also are found in other sources.[58, 112] The large number of published outbreak investigations are an invaluable resource because they often provide insight into potential causes of the outbreak. For example, an outbreak caused by *Stenotrophomonas (Xanthomonas) maltophilia, Burkholderia (Pseudomonas) cepacia,* or *Pseudomonas* spp. should suggest the possibility of a common-source outbreak caused by a contaminated solution or medication or an inadequately disinfected piece of equipment. On the other hand, to jump to conclusions regarding the cause of a particular cluster of infections based on the results of a previous investigation is hazardous. Careful investigation is necessary to establish or refute epidemiologic links between cases and potential causes.

Molecular genotyping techniques are an essential adjunct to investigations of outbreaks. Despite rapid advances in recent years, "gold standard" techniques do not exist for all microorganisms, and testing is not generally available outside academic medical centers. Genotyping is most helpful when it is applied to test a hypothesis about the relatedness of various isolates recovered during the course of a thorough outbreak investigation in which traditional epidemiologic methods (cohort or case-control studies) are used.

Policies and Procedures

Policies and procedures are necessary to optimize and standardize hospital routines and patient care practices.

TABLE 232–2 ■ APPROACH TO THE INVESTIGATION OF CLUSTERS OF NOSOCOMIAL INFECTIONS

1. Confirm the diagnosis.
2. Make a case definition.
3. Search for additional cases.
4. Plot the epidemic curve.
5. Compare pre-epidemic rates with current rates by using statistical tests to prove that an epidemic exists.
6. Perform a literature review.
7. Open lines of communication with leaders of relevant departments, the microbiology laboratory, and the hospital administration.
8. Keep detailed records of events and conversations.
9. Review the charts of all cases and compile a line listing of relevant information.
10. Formulate a hypothesis about a likely reservoir and mode of transmission.
11. Institute temporary control measures.
12. Perform a case-control study to develop epidemiologic evidence to support or refute the hypotheses.
13. Update control measures.
14. Document the reservoir and mode of transmission microbiologically. Confirm the relatedness of isolates with molecular genotyping techniques if necessary.
15. Document the efficacy of control measures.
16. Write a report and distribute it to appropriate individuals.
17. Change policies and procedures if necessary.

Certain generic policies and procedures apply to all departments, such as those for handwashing, isolation precautions, prevention of transmission of infectious diseases from and to visitors and health care workers, reprocessing of reusable patient care items, and disposal of medical waste. Other policies and procedures should be tailored to the potential infection risks relevant to specific departmental activities. Numerous guidelines have been published that can help hospitals develop policies and procedures.*

A number of studies have documented poor compliance with policies for handwashing and isolation precautions.[67, 68] Unfortunately, relatively few studies have attempted to elucidate the reasons for noncompliance or to investigate methods for modifying the behavior of staff.[68, 84, 115] To have any chance of improving performance in such critical aspects of infection prevention, hospital and departmental leaders must make compliance an organizational priority.[45, 68, 69] Staff members responsible for implementation should be included in the process of developing policies and procedures to ensure that the resulting documents are workable, as well as to develop their sense of ownership and responsibility for successful implementation and sustained compliance. Staff education is important, but not sufficient in and of itself. Prompt feedback of data concerning key outcome and process measures is also critical in motivating staff, and barriers to improvement must be identified and removed.[45, 68, 69] For example, clinicians cannot be expected to comply with an isolation precaution policy if gloves are not available or are located inconveniently. Additional investigation into engineering solutions, cognitive approaches, behavioral modification, and training strategies also is needed.

HAND HYGIENE

Proper hand hygiene, which encompasses both handwashing with soap and water and hand antisepsis with a waterless (alcohol-based) agent, reduces carriage of potential nosocomial pathogens on the hands of health care workers.[67] Hand hygiene is regarded widely as the quintessential infection prevention measure.

Indications and procedures for hand hygiene are reviewed in detail in a recent HICPAC guideline.[15] In general, hand hygiene should be practiced before and after patient contact; after contact with body fluids and substances, mucous membranes, nonintact skin, and objects that probably are contaminated; before performing invasive procedures; and after removing gloves (see Isolation Precautions). Handwashing must be performed when hands are visibly soiled to remove organic material and associated microorganisms. When hands are not visibly soiled, hand antisepsis is preferred because is it likely to reduce the number of pathogenic bacteria that transiently colonize the hands more effectively than handwashing does.[15, 89] Hand hygiene also is necessary after removing gloves—an indication that many health care professionals fail to fully appreciate—because gloves may have macroscopic and microscopic holes that lead to hand contamination[64] and because hands may be contaminated in the process of removing soiled gloves.

Before the widespread availability of alcohol-based agents, compliance with hand hygiene (accomplished solely by handwashing) was notoriously poor among health care workers.[15, 67] However, the hope is that wider use of alcohol-based agents will boost hand hygiene compliance because these agents are faster and more convenient to use (i.e., they can be placed near the patient's bedside and require less than 30 seconds to use), are less drying and irritating to the skin than handwashing is,[14] and are more effective in reducing numbers of transient flora.[89] Programs that combine ready access to these products at the point of care (i.e., close to the patient's bedside) with active effort to promote their use have demonstrated improved compliance with hand hygiene.[11, 90] One before-after study reported a concomitant reduction in infections caused by methicillin-resistant *S. aureus*. For these reasons, a HICPAC guideline on hand hygiene in health care facilities strongly recommends that these agents be used preferentially for hand hygiene (when hands are not visibly soiled) and that facilities develop active programs to promote the use of these agents.[15]

Persons wearing artificial nails are more likely to harbor pathogenic gram-negative bacilli and yeast on their fingertips, and these organisms are less effectively cleared on artificial nails with use of an alcohol-based agent than on natural nails.[53, 79] The use of artificial nails or nail wraps was associated with carriage of *Pseudomonas aeruginosa* on the hands of health care workers and infection of high-risk infants in a neonatal ICU.[39] For these reasons, the HICPAC guideline on hand hygiene recommends that health care workers not wear artificial fingernails or extenders when providing patient care and that natural nails be kept less than 1/4 inch long.[15]

ISOLATION PRECAUTIONS

Proper use of isolation precautions is important for all health care facilities, but it is especially critical in facilities caring for pediatric patients. Children hospitalized as a result of infections acquired in the community represent a substantial proportion of pediatric admissions, and nosocomial transmission of these infections to other susceptible patients is a significant problem (see Chapter 231). Effective use of appropriate isolation precautions markedly reduces nosocomial transmission of these agents.[3, 69]

A HICPAC guideline recommends the use of two tiers of precautions, standard precautions and transmission-based

*See references 13, 15, 23, 42, 55, 75, 85, 86, 93, 94, 104.

precautions, which are described in greater detail in the following sections.[42]

Standard Precautions

Standard precautions synthesizes the elements of two previous precautions systems: universal precautions (UP) and body substance isolation (BSI). UP was a strategy developed in 1985, largely in response to the human immunodeficiency virus (HIV) epidemic, to protect health care workers from exposure to blood-borne pathogens, including HIV and hepatitis B virus.[21, 22] Because many persons requiring health care may have unrecognized infection with a blood-borne pathogen, UP were to be used during the care of all patients to prevent health care workers from being exposed to blood and other specific body fluids potentially contaminated with a blood-borne pathogen. BSI was developed in 1987 with the intention of providing a simpler, easy-to-use alternative to the isolation precautions systems in use at that time.[73] BSI was similar to UP in that it was to be used during the care of all patients; however, it differed from UP in that it advocated the use of barriers to prevent contact by health care workers with all moist body substances and mucous membranes, not just blood and body fluids potentially contaminated with blood-borne pathogens. BSI was designed not only to protect health care workers from blood-borne pathogens but also to prevent cross-infection caused by hand contamination while caring for patients who may have undetected colonization with a nosocomial pathogen. The advantages and disadvantages of these two systems and the confusion regarding the interpretation and implementation of these systems by health care workers are described in detail in the HICPAC guideline.[42]

Standard precautions synthesizes the goals of protecting health care workers from blood-borne pathogens and protecting health care workers and patients from transmission of microorganisms from moist body substances.[42] Standard precautions apply to any planned or potential contact with blood; all body fluids, secretions, and excretions except sweat, regardless of whether they contain visible blood; nonintact skin; and mucous membranes. Standard precautions should be used in the care of all patients at all times, regardless of their diagnosis or presumed infection status.[42] Table 232–3 lists the components of standard precautions.

One should note that OSHA's blood-borne pathogens standard includes the prevention measures embodied in UP (see "Occupational Health").[85] The prevention measures included in Standard Precautions comply with the provisions of the OSHA standard.

Transmission-Based Precautions

Other precautions are needed to prevent the transmission of contagious diseases (e.g., varicella, measles, tuberculosis, and pertussis) and other epidemiologically important microorganisms (e.g., multidrug-resistant microorganisms, toxin-producing *C. difficile)* from infected or colonized patients. Transmission-based precautions are designed to provide the necessary measures, in addition to those already specified by standard precautions, to interrupt known modes of transmission of these microorganisms (see Chapter 231).[42] The three types of transmission-based precautions are airborne, droplet, and contact precautions.

Airborne precautions (Table 232–4) are designed to prevent the transmission of microorganisms spread by droplet nuclei (e.g., measles, varicella, tuberculosis), which can be carried on air currents over substantial distances.[42] Special air handling and ventilation are required.[42] Droplet precautions (see Table 232–4) are designed to prevent the transmission of microorganisms spread by large respiratory droplets, which travel only short distances (<3 feet) before settling.[42] Special air handling and ventilation are not required. Contact precautions (see Table 232–4) are designed to prevent the transmission of microorganisms spread by direct and indirect contact.[42] Some infections are spread by more than one mode of transmission, so precaution systems may need to be combined for these infections (i.e., varicella requires airborne precautions and contact precautions). Patients infected or colonized with more than one microorganism also may require a combination of precaution systems (i.e., a patient with active pulmonary tuberculosis and *C. difficile* enterocolitis requires airborne precautions and contact precautions).

Table 232–5 lists clinical syndromes and conditions warranting the empiric use of transmission-based precautions, in addition to standard precautions, to prevent the transmission of epidemiologically important pathogens until infection with these microorganisms is excluded.[42] To ensure that appropriate empiric precautions are implemented promptly, hospitals must have systems in place to evaluate patients for these infections as part of their routine pre-admission and admission care. Table 232–6 lists the type and duration of transmission-based precautions, to be used in addition to standard precautions, for specific clinical syndromes and infectious agents. Only agents requiring one or more of the three transmission-based precautions are listed.

The HICPAC guideline recommends only standard precautions for infections caused by penicillin-resistant *Streptococcus pneumoniae.* Based on reports of nosocomial transmission of penicillin-resistant *S. pneumoniae* in a variety of settings and the possibility that these infections were spread by droplet transmission,[31, 41, 74, 80, 83, 111] the authors recommend the use of droplet precautions until 24 hours of effective antimicrobial therapy has been completed.

VISITORS

Visitors with communicable diseases can expose hospitalized patients and health care workers inadvertently unless procedures to identify and exclude them are in place. Varicella, measles, and tuberculosis are the most problematic infections because they are spread by airborne transmission, which enables infected visitors to expose a large number of individuals in a short period. In addition, visitors with pertussis, viral respiratory and gastrointestinal infections, parvovirus B19 infection, rubella, and mumps can pose a significant hazard to patients and health care workers with whom they have close contact.

Procedures to identify potentially infected visitors should be targeted toward visiting children because they are the persons most likely to be infected with these agents. The parents or guardians of all visiting children younger than 12 years should be asked a set of screening questions regarding the presence of fever, rash, and respiratory and gastrointestinal symptoms in the visiting child, as well as any recent exposure to other children with chickenpox, measles, or whooping cough. Children without any significant symptoms or exposure should be allowed to visit with no restrictions. Children with a history of fever or vomiting in the past 24 hours or an upper respiratory tract infection in the past week can be allowed to visit, but with restrictions, including avoidance of close contact (<3 feet) with any patient, no visits to the activity room, and no sharing of food, drinks, or toys. Children with upper respiratory tract infections should not be allowed to visit children with congenital heart disease, bronchopulmonary dysplasia,

TABLE 232–3 ■ STANDARD PRECAUTIONS*

Handwashing

Wash hands after touching blood, body fluids, secretions, excretions, and contaminated items, regardless of whether gloves are worn.

Wash hands immediately after gloves are removed, between patient contact, and when otherwise indicated to avoid transfer of microorganisms to other patients or environments.

When necessary, wash hands between performance of tasks and procedures on the same patient to prevent cross-contamination of different body sites.

Use a plain (non-antimicrobial) soap for handwashing.

Use an antimicrobial agent or a waterless antiseptic agent for specific circumstances (e.g., control of outbreaks or hyperendemic infections), as defined by the infection control program. (See Table 232–4, Contact Precautions, for additional recommendations on using antimicrobial agents.)

Gloves

Wear gloves (clean nonsterile gloves are adequate) when touching blood, body fluids, secretions, excretions, and contaminated items.

Put on clean gloves just before touching mucous membranes and nonintact skin.

Change gloves between tasks and procedures on the same patient after contact with material that may contain a high concentration of microorganisms.

Remove gloves promptly after use, before touching noncontaminated items and environmental surfaces, and before going to another patient, and wash hands immediately to avoid transfer of microorganisms to other patients or environments.

Mask, Eye Protection, and Face Shield

Wear a mask and eye protection or a face shield to protect mucous membranes of the eyes, nose, and mouth during procedures and patient care activities that are likely to generate splashes or sprays of blood, body fluids, secretions, and excretions.

Gown

Wear a gown (a clean nonsterile gown is adequate) to protect skin and prevent soiling of clothing during procedures and patient care activities that are likely to generate splashes or sprays of blood, body fluids, secretions, or excretions.

Select a gown that is appropriate for the activity and amount of fluid likely to be encountered.

Remove a soiled gown as promptly as possible, and wash hands to avoid transfer of microorganisms to other patients or environments.

Patient Care Equipment

Handle used patient care equipment soiled with blood, body fluids, secretions, or excretions in a manner that prevents skin and mucous membrane exposure, contamination of clothing, and transfer of microorganisms to other patients and environments.

Ensure that reusable equipment is not used for the care of another patient until it has been appropriately cleaned and reprocessed.

Ensure that single-use items are discarded properly.

Environmental Control

Ensure that the hospital has adequate procedures for the routine care, cleaning, and disinfection of environmental surfaces, beds, bed rails, bedside equipment, and other frequently touched surfaces, and ensure that these procedures are followed.

Linen

Handle, transport, and process used linen soiled with blood, body fluids, secretions, or excretions in a manner that prevents skin and mucous membrane exposure and contamination of clothing and that avoids transfer of microorganisms to other patients and environments.

Occupational Health and Blood-Borne Pathogens

Take care to prevent injuries when using needles, scalpels, and other sharp instruments or devices, when handling sharp instruments after procedures, when cleaning used instruments, and when disposing of used needles.

Never recap used needles or otherwise manipulate them with both hands or use any other technique that involves directing the point of a needle toward any part of the body; instead, use either a one-handed "scoop" technique or a mechanical device designed for holding the needle sheath.

Do not remove used needles from disposable syringes by hand, and do not bend, break, or otherwise manipulate used needles by hand.

Place used disposable needles and syringes, scalpel blades, and other sharp items in appropriate puncture-resistant containers that are located as close as practical to the area in which the items were used, and place reusable syringes and needles in a puncture-resistant container for transport to the reprocessing area.

Use mouth pieces, resuscitation bags, or other ventilation devices as an alternative to mouth-to-mouth resuscitation methods in areas where the need for resuscitation is predictable.

Patient Placement

Place a patient who contaminates the environment or who does not (or cannot be expected to) assist in maintaining appropriate hygiene or environmental control in a private room.

If a private room is not available, consult with infection control professionals regarding patient placement or other alternatives.

*Standard precautions apply to all patients regardless of their diagnosis or presumed infection status. Standard precautions apply to any planned or potential contact with (1) blood; (2) all body fluids, secretions, and excretions except sweat, regardless of whether they contain visible blood: (3) nonintact skin; and (4) mucous membranes.

From Garner, J. S.: Guideline for isolation precautions in hospitals. The Hospital Infection Control Practices Advisory Committee. Infect. Control Hosp. Epidemiol. *17*:53–80, 1996.

cellular immunodeficiency, or other conditions that predispose to severe infection with respiratory viruses. Children with significant exposure to chickenpox, measles, or whooping cough who may be in the incubation period of the disease should not be allowed to visit the hospital. This screening process should be repeated each day that the child visits the hospital. This procedure does not guarantee that a child may not be in the incubation phase of a contagious disease at the time of the visit—varicella is an obvious example—but it can be useful in limiting potential exposure.

OCCUPATIONAL HEALTH

Health care workers require protection from the significant infectious risks inherent in patient care; conversely, patients and health care workers need to be protected from exposure to health care workers with communicable diseases. Integrating management and prevention strategies to accomplish these two goals requires close collaboration between hospital infection prevention and control programs and employee health departments. A HICPAC guideline for infection control in health care workers contains comprehensive recommendations for evaluation of illnesses, postexposure evaluation and management, and prevention of occupationally acquired infections in health care workers.[13]

Evaluation of Ill Health Care Workers

Hospital staff and volunteers with symptoms such as persistent fever, conjunctivitis, skin lesions or rash, diarrhea, and

TABLE 232–4 ■ TRANSMISSION-BASED PRECAUTIONS*

Airborne Precautions

Patient Placement

Place the patient in a private room that has (1) monitored negative air pressure in relation to the surrounding areas, (2) 6 to 12 air changes per hour, and (3) appropriate discharge or air outdoors or monitored high-efficiency filtration of room air before the air is circulated to other areas in the hospital.

Keep the room door closed and the patient in the room.

When a private room is not available, place the patient in a room with a patient who has active infection with the same microorganism, unless otherwise recommended, but with no other infection.

When a private room is not available and cohorting is not desirable, consultation with infection control professionals is advised before patient placement.

Respiratory Protection

Wear respiratory protection when entering the room of a patient with known or suspected infectious pulmonary tuberculosis.

Susceptible persons should not enter the room of patients known or suspected to have measles (rubeola) or varicella (chickenpox) if other immune caregivers are available.

If susceptible persons must enter the room of a patient known or suspected to have measles or varicella, they should wear respiratory protection.

Persons immune to measles or varicella need not wear respiratory protection.

Patient Transport

Limit movement and transport of the patient from the room to essential purposes only.

If transport or movement is necessary, minimize dispersal of droplet nuclei by placing a surgical mask on the patient, if possible.

Additional Precautions for Preventing Transmission of Tuberculosis

Consult the CDC "Guidelines for Preventing the Transmission of *Mycobacterium tuberculosis* in Health Care Facilities 1994,[11] for additional prevention strategies.[23]

Droplet Precautions

Patient Placement

Place the patient in a private room.

When a private room is not available, place the patient in a room with a patient(s) who has active infection with the same microorganism, but with no other infection.

When a private room is not available and cohorting is not achievable, maintain spatial separation of at least 3 feet between the infected patient and other patients and visitors.

Special air handling and ventilation are not necessary, and the door may remain open.

Mask

Wear a mask when working within 3 feet of the patient. (Logistically, some hospitals may want to implement the wearing of a mask to enter the room.)

Patient Transport

Limit movement and transport of the patient from the room to essential purposes only.

If transport or movement is necessary, minimize dispersal of droplets by placing a surgical mask on the patient, if possible.

Contact Precautions

Patient Placement

Place the patient in a privation room.

When a private room is not available, place the patient in a room with a patient(s) who has active infection with the same microorganism, but with no other infection.

When a private room is not available and cohorting is not achievable, consider the epidemiology of the microorganism and the patient population when determining patient placement; consultation with infection control professionals is advised before patient placement.

Gloves

Wear gloves (clean nonsterile gloves are adequate) when entering the room.

During the course of providing care for a patient, change gloves after having contact with infective material that may contain high concentrations of microorganisms (fecal material and wound drainage).

Remove gloves before leaving the patient's environment and wash hands immediately with an antimicrobial agent or a waterless antiseptic agent.

After glove removal and handwashing, ensure that hands do not touch potentially contaminated environmental surfaces or items in the patient's room to avoid transfer of microorganisms to other patients or environments.

Gown

Wear a gown (a clean, nonsterile gown is adequate) when entering the room if you anticipate that your clothing will have substantial contact with the patient, environmental surfaces, or items in the patient's room or if the patient is incontinent or has diarrhea, an ileostomy, a colostomy, or wound drainage not contained by a dressing.

Remove the gown before leaving the patient's environment.

After gown removal, ensure that clothing does not contact potentially contaminated environmental surfaces to avoid transfer of microorganisms to other patients or environments.

Patient Transport

Limit movement and transport of the patient from the room to essential purposes only.

If the patient is transported out of the room, ensure that precautions are maintained to minimize the risk of transmission of microorganisms to other patients and contamination of environmental surfaces or equipment.

Patient Care Equipment

When possible, dedicate the use of noncritical patient care equipment to a single patient (or a cohort of patients infected or colonized with the pathogen requiring precautions) to avoid sharing between patients.

If use of common equipment or items is unavoidable, adequately clean and disinfect them before use for another patient.

Additional Precautions for Preventing the Spread of Vancomycin Resistance

Consult the HICPAC report on preventing the spread of vancomycin resistance for additional prevention strategies.[55]

*Transmission-based precautions are followed, when indicated, in addition to standard precautions.

From Garner, J. S.: Guideline for isolation precautions in hospitals. The Hospital Infection Control Practices Advisory Committee. Infect. Control Hosp. Epidemiol. *17*:53–80, 1996.

persistent cough should be evaluated for the presence of a contagious disease. Possible cases of varicella, herpes zoster on an exposed area of the body, herpetic whitlow, adenoviral conjunctivitis, measles, mumps, rubella, pertussis, staphylococcal skin infection, enteric infection in a food service worker, and active pulmonary tuberculosis should be investigated promptly and confirmed with laboratory tests if necessary. Although many health care workers will choose to have these problems evaluated by their primary care providers, employee health departments have an interest in completing these assessments, especially if a question arises regarding whether the condition was acquired in the workplace, requires a furlough from work, or may have exposed patients or other health care workers. Infection control staff can provide assistance in these evaluations as needed and should be kept abreast of the results.

TABLE 232–5 ■ CLINICAL SYNDROMES OR CONDITIONS WARRANTING EMPIRIC USE OF TRANSMISSION-BASED PRECAUTIONS TO PREVENT TRANSMISSION OF EPIDEMIOLOGICALLY IMPORTANT PATHOGENS UNTIL INFECTION WITH THESE MICROORGANISMS IS EXCLUDED*

Clinical Syndrome or Condition†	Potential Pathogens‡	Empiric Precautions
Diarrhea		
Acute diarrhea with a probable infectious cause in an incontinent or diapered patient	Enteric pathogens§	Contact
Diarrhea with a history of recent antibiotic use	*Clostridium difficile*	Contact
Meningitis	*Neisseria meningitidis*	Droplet
Rash or exanthems, generalized, etiology unknown		
Petechial/ecchymotic with fever	*Neisseria meningitidis*	Droplet
Vesicular	Varicella	Airborne and contact
Maculopapular with coryza and fever	Rubeola (measles)	Airborne
Respiratory infections		
Cough/fever/upper lobe pulmonary infiltrate in an HIV-negative patient or a patient at low risk for HIV infection	*Mycobacterium tuberculosis*	Airborne
Cough/fever/pulmonary infiltrate in any lung location in an HIV-infected patient or a patient at high risk for HIV infection	*Mycobacterium tuberculosis*	Airborne
Paroxysmal or severe persistent cough during periods of pertussis activity	*Bordetella pertussis*	Droplet
Respiratory infections, particularly bronchiolitis and croup, in infants and young children	Respiratory syncytial or parainfluenza virus	Contact
Risk of multidrug-resistant microorganisms		
History of infection or colonization with multidrug-resistant organisms‖	Resistant bacteria	Contact
Skin, wound, or urinary tract infection in a patient with recent hospital or long-term care in a facility where multidrug-resistant organisms are prevalent	Resistant bacteria	Contact
Skin or wound infection		
Abscess or draining wound that cannot be covered	*Staphylococcus aureus*, group A streptococci	Contact

*Infection control professionals are encouraged to modify or adapt this table according to local conditions. To ensure that appropriate empiric precautions are implemented in every case, hospitals must have systems in place to evaluate patients routinely according to these criteria as a part of their pre-admission and admission care.

†Patients with the syndromes or conditions listed may have atypical signs or symptoms (e.g., pertussis in neonates and adults may not be associated with paroxysmal or severe cough). The clinician's index of suspicion should be guided by the prevalence of specific conditions in the community, as well as clinical judgment.

‡The microoganisms listed are not intended to represent the complete or even the most likely diagnosis, but rather possible etiologic agents that require additional precautions in addition to standard precautions until they can be ruled out.

§These pathogens include enterohemorrhagic *Escherichia coli* O157:H7, *Shigella*, hepatitis A, and rotavirus.

‖Resistant bacteria judged by the infection control program, based on current state, regional, or national recommendations, to be of special clinical or epidemiologic significance.

From Garner, J. S.: Guideline for isolation precautions in hospitals. The Hospital Infection Control Practices Advisory Committee. Infect. Control Hosp. Epidemiol. *17*:53–80, 1996.

Postexposure Evaluation and Management of Health Care Workers

A structured approach to the assessment and management of exposure of health care workers to patients with infectious diseases is critical to promptly provide postexposure prophylaxis, if indicated, and allay anxiety while avoiding unnecessary interventions and loss of workdays. The first step is to develop criteria for assessing the nature of the exposure because many reported encounters are not significant. Some exposures (e.g., varicella, hepatitis B) may require an assessment of the susceptibility of the health care worker to infection, and procedures should describe the indications for laboratory tests, as well as the interpretation of results. Postexposure prophylaxis regimens are discussed in Chapter 231 and in the following paragraphs. Finally, counseling regarding the risks and consequences of the exposure is an important component of this service.

Postexposure evaluation and management of varicella, blood-borne pathogens, and tuberculosis are highlighted because they are common focal points for interactions between the hospital infection prevention and control program and the occupational health department.

Exposure to varicella is a common occurrence in hospitals caring for pediatric patients. Fortunately, the vast majority of hospital staff have protective immunity.[34] A previous history of varicella is a reliable indicator of immunity, and even most adult health care workers without a past history of varicella have serologic evidence of immunity.[34] Nonetheless, some health care workers are susceptible to varicella, particularly workers born and reared in tropical and subtropical countries. Varicella vaccine is recommended for susceptible staff, especially those who will have contact with patients who are at significant risk of acquiring severe disease.[13] Immunization with this vaccine has been demonstrated to reduce the incidence of varicella among susceptible staff who subsequently are exposed to wild-type varicella, as well as lessen the severity of the disease.[98] Prevaccination testing for antibody to varicella-zoster virus among workers without a history of varicella at the time of hiring is not necessary, and postvaccination testing for an antibody response is not recommended.[13] Proper, cost-efficient procedures for managing staff who have been vaccinated and then subsequently exposed to varicella are not well established. A reasonable procedure is to test these individuals for immunity to

TABLE 232–6 ■ TYPE AND DURATION OF TRANSMISSION-BASED PRECAUTIONS NEEDED FOR SELECTED INFECTIONS AND CONDITIONS

Infection/Condition	Precautions: Type*	Precautions: Duration†
Abscess, draining (no dressing or dressing does not contain drainage adequately)	C	DI
Adenovirus infection, in infants and young children	D, C	DI
Bordetella pertussis (see Pertussis)		
Campylobacter species (see Gastroenteritis, *Campylobacter* species)		
Cellulitis, uncontrolled drainage	C	DI
Chickenpox (varicella)	A, C	F[1]
Chickenpox (varicella) exposure	A[2]	F[2]
Cholera (see Gastroenteritis, *Vibrio cholerae*)		
Clostridium difficile	C	DI
Congenital rubella	C	F[3]
Conjunctivitis, acute viral (acute hemorrhagic)	C	DI
Decubitus ulcer, infected (no dressing or dressing does not contain drainage adequately)	C	DI
Diphtheria		
Cutaneous	C	CN[4]
Pharyngeal	D	CN[4]
Ebola viral hemorrhagic fever	C[5]	DI
Enterococcus species (see Multidrug-resistant organisms if epidemiologically significant or vancomycin-resistant)		
Enterocolitis, *Clostridium difficile*	C	DI
Enteroviral infections, infants and young children	C	DI
Epiglottitis caused by *Haemophilus influenzae*	D	$U^{24\,hr}$
Furunculosis—staphylococcal, infants and young children	C	DI
Gastroenteritis		
Campylobacter species	C[6]	DI
Vibrio cholerae (cholera)	C[6]	DI
Clostridium difficile	C	DI
Crytposporidium species	C[6]	DI
Escherichia coli		
Enterohemorrhagic O157:H7	C[6]	DI
Other species	C[6]	DI
Giardia lamblia	C[6]	DI
Rotavirus	C[6]	DI
Salmonella species (including *S. typhi*)	C[6]	DI
Shigella Species	C[6]	DI
Vibrio parahaemolyticus	C[6]	DI
Viral, other than rotavirus	C[6]	DI
Yersinia enterocolitica	C[6]	DI
German measles (rubella; also see Congenital rubella)	D	F[7]
Giardiasis (see Gastroenteritis, *Giardia lamblia*)		
Haemophilus influenzae	D	$U^{24\,hr}$
Hand, foot, and mouth disease (see Enteroviral infections)		
Hemorrhagic fevers (e.g., Lassa, Ebola, Marburg)	C[5]	DI
Hepatitis A, diapered or incontinent patients	C	F[8]
Herpes simplex		
Neonatal infection	C	DI
Neonatal exposure	C[9]	DI
Mucocutaneous, disseminated or primary, severe	C	DI
Herpes zoster (varicella-zoster), disseminated or localized in immunocompromised patient	A, C[10]	DI
Impetigo	C	$U^{24\,hr}$
Influenza	D[11]	DI
Lassa fever	C[5]	DI
Lice (pediculosis)	C	$U^{24\,hr}$
Marburg virus disease	C[5]	DI
Measles (rubeola), all manifestations	A	DI
Meningitis		
Enterovirus, known or suspected in infants and young children	C	DI
Haemophilus influenzae, known or suspected	D	$U^{24\,hr}$
Neisseria meningitidis, known or suspected	D	$U^{24\,hr}$
Streptococcus pneumoniae, penicillin-resistant, known or suspected	D[12]	$U^{24\,hr}$
Meningococcemia (meningococcal sepsis)	D	$U^{24\,hr}$
Multidrug-resistant organisms, infection or colonization[13]		
Gastrointestinal	C	CN
Respiratory	C	CN
Skin, wound, or burn	C	CN
Mumps (infectious parotitis)	D	F[14]
Mycobacterium tuberculosis (see Tuberculosis)		
Mycoplasma pneumoniae (see Pneumonia, *Mycoplasma*)		
Neisseria meningitidis	D	$U^{24\,hr}$
Parainfluenza virus infection, respiratory in infants and young children	C	DI
Parvovirus B19	D	F[15]
Pediculosis (lice)	C	$U^{24\,hr}$
Pertussis (whooping cough)	D	F[16]
Plague, pneumonic	D	$U^{72\,hr}$
Pneumococcemia (pneumococcal sepsis), penicillin-resistant	D[12]	$U^{24\,hr}$
Pneumonia		
Adenovirus	D, C	DI
Haemophilus influenzae, in infants and children (any age)	D	$U^{24\,hr}$
Mycoplasma pneumoniae (primary atypical pneumonia)	D	DI
Neisseria meningitidis	D	$U^{24\,hr}$
Streptococcus, group A, in infants and young children	D	$U^{24\,hr}$
Streptococcus pneumoniae, penicillin-resistant	D[12]	$U^{24\,hr}$
Viral, in infants and young children (see Respiratory infectious disease, acute)		
Respiratory infectious disease, acute (if not covered elsewhere), in infants and young children	C	DI
Respiratory syncytial virus infection, in infants, young children, and immunocompromised adults	C	DI
Rotavirus (see Gastroenteritis, Rotavirus)		
Rubella (German measles; also see Congenital rubella)	D	F[7]
Rubeola (measles)	A	DI
Salmonellosis (see Gastroenteritis, *Salmonella* species)		
Scabies	C	$U^{24\,hr}$
Shigellosis (see Gastroenteritis, *Shigella* species)		
Staphylococcal disease (*Staphylococcus aureus*)		
Skin, wound, or burn, major (no dressing or dressing does not contain drainage adequately)	C	DI
Streptococcal disease (group A streptococci)		
Skin, wound, or burn, major (no dressing or dressing does not contain drainage adequately)	C	$U^{24\,hr}$
Pharyngitis in infants and young children	D	$U^{24\,hr}$
Pneumonia in infants and young children	D	$U^{24\,hr}$

Continued

TABLE 232–6 ■ TYPE AND DURATION OF TRANSMISSION-BASED PRECAUTIONS NEEDED FOR SELECTED INFECTIONS AND CONDITIONS—cont'd

Infection/Condition	Precautions Type*	Precautions Duration†	Infection/Condition	Precautions Type*	Precautions Duration†
Scarlet fever in infants and younger children	D	U[24 hr]	*Vibrio parahaemolyticus* (see Gastroenteritis, *Vibrio parahaemolyticus)*		
Streptococcus pneumoniae, penicillin-resistant	D[12]	U[24 hr]			
Tuberculosis, pulmonary or laryngeal, confirmed or suspected	A	F[17]	Whooping cough	D	F[16]
Varicella (chickenpox)	A,C	F[1]	Wound infections, major, (no dressing or dressing does not contain drainage adequately)	C	DI
Varicella (chickenpox) exposure	A[2]	F[2]	*Yersinia enterocolitica* (see Gastroenteritis, *Yersinia enterocolitica)*		
Vibrio cholerae (see Gastroenteritis, Cholera)					

*A, airborne; C, contact; D, droplet. Standard precautions apply to all patients at all times in addition to the specified transmission-based precautions.
†CN, until antimicrobial agents are discontinued and culture-negative; DI, duration of illness (with wound lesions, DI means until they stop draining); F, see footnote number; U, until time specified in hours (hr) after initiation of effective therapy.
[1]Maintain precautions until all lesions are crusted.
[2]Place exposed, susceptible patients on airborne precautions beginning 8 days after exposure and continuing until 21 days after the last exposure (up to 28 days if varicella-zoster immune globulin has been given).
[3]Place infant on contact precautions during any admission until 1 year of age, unless nasopharyngeal and urine cultures are negative for virus after the age of 3 months.
[4]Until two cultures taken at least 24 hours apart are negative.
[5]Call the state health department and CDC for specific advice about management of a suspected case.
[6]Use contact precautions for diapered or incontinent children and any child younger than 6 years for the duration of the illness.
[7]Until 7 days after onset of the rash.
[8]Maintain precautions in infants and children younger than 3 years for the duration of the hospitalization; in children 3 to 14 years of age, until 2 weeks after the onset of symptoms; and in others until 1 week after the onset of symptoms.
[9]For infants delivered vaginally or by cesarean section and if the mother has active infection and membranes have been ruptured for more than 4 to 6 hours.
[10]Persons susceptible to varicella are also at risk for varicella when exposed to patients with herpes zoster lesions; therefore, susceptibles should not enter the room if other immune caregivers are available.
[11]The "Guideline for Prevention of Nosocomial Pneumonia"[104] recommends surveillance, vaccination, antiviral agents, and the use of private rooms with negative air pressure as much as feasible for patients in whom influenza is suspected or diagnosed. Many hospitals ecounter logistic difficulties and physical plant limitations when admitting multiple patients with suspected influenza during community outbreaks. If sufficient private rooms are unavailable, consider cohorting patients or, at the very least, avoid sharing with high-risk patients. See "Guideline for Prevention of Nosocomial Pneumonia"[104] for additional prevention and control strategies.
[12]The CDC/HICPAC guideline recommends only standard precautions for infections caused by penicillin-resistant *Streptococcus pneumoniae*. Based on reports of nosocomial transmission of penicillin-resistant *S. pneumoniae* in hospitals outside the United States and the possibility that these infections were spread by droplet transmission,[31, 41, 74, 80, 83, 111] the authors recommend the use of droplet precautions until 24 hours of effective antimicrobial therapy has been completed.
[13]Resistant bacteria judged by the infection control program, based on current state, regional, or national recommendations, to be of special clinical or epidemiologic significance.
[14]For 9 days after the onset of parotid swelling.
[15]Maintain precautions for the duration of hospitalization when chronic disease occurs in an immunodeficient patient. For patients with transient aplastic or red cell crisis, maintain precautions for 7 days.
[16]Maintain precautions until 5 days after the initiation of effective therapy.
[17]Discontinue precautions only when the patient is receiving effective tuberculosis (TB) therapy, is improving clinically, and has three consecutive negative sputum smears collected on different days or TB is ruled out. Also see CDC "Guidelines for Preventing the Transmission of *Mycobacterium tuberculosis* in Health Care Facilities, 1994."[23]
Modified from Garner, J. S.: Guideline for isolation precautions in hospitals. The Hospital Infection Control Practices Advisory Committee. Infect. Control Hosp. Epidemiol. 17: 53–80, 1996.

varicella and, if the initial test is negative, repeat the test 5 to 6 days later to determine whether an anamnestic response has developed.[13] Persons who remain antibody-negative, as well as susceptible, unvaccinated staff, should be furloughed beginning 10 and 8 days, respectively, after their initial exposure until 21 days after their last exposure (28 days if they received varicella-zoster immune globulin [VZIG]), unless they become infected and recover sooner. Alternative strategies to allow these individuals to continue to work with specific safeguards may substantially reduce the number of lost workdays, but they may result in preventable secondary exposure of patients and other hospital workers.[47, 60] Administration of VZIG should be considered for high-risk individuals (pregnant and immunocompromised persons); some physicians advocate VZIG for all exposed, susceptible adults because of the potential severity of varicella in this population. Acyclovir may decrease the severity of the disease if started as soon as infection is noted.

The OSHA blood-borne pathogens standard requires hospitals to test the source patient for evidence of a blood-borne infection, when consent can be obtained, and to provide postexposure prophylaxis in accordance with CDC recommendations.[25, 85] Significant exposure is defined as percutaneous, mucous membrane, or nonintact skin exposure to blood, other potentially infectious body fluids (cerebrospinal fluid, pericardial fluid, pleural fluid, peritoneal fluid, synovial fluid, amniotic fluid, semen, cervical/vaginal secretions), tissue, or visibly bloody fluids, excretions, or secretions.[25]

Summary risk estimates are helpful in counseling persons who have suffered an exposure, although many factors may affect the risk of acquiring infection in an individual case (e.g., level of viremia in the source patient, amount of blood involved in the exposure, the nature of the exposure). Hepatitis B is by far the most infectious of the blood-borne viruses, probably because titers of virus in the blood are higher for hepatitis B than for other agents.[25] The risk of hepatitis B infection developing after percutaneous exposure to blood is estimated to be 23 to 37 percent for hepatitis B e antigen–negative blood and 37 to 62 percent for hepatitis B e antigen–positive blood; the risk of clinical hepatitis is

1 to 6 percent and 22 to 31 percent in each of these scenarios, respectively. The risk of hepatitis B infection after mucous membrane or nonintact skin exposure is not well quantified, but infection can occur.[25] The risk of hepatitis C infection after percutaneous exposure is estimated to be 1.8 percent. Transmission of hepatitis C virus after mucous membrane exposure to blood is rare, and no transmission has been documented after intact or nonintact skin exposure to blood.[25] The risk of HIV infection is estimated to be 0.3 percent after percutaneous exposure to blood and 0.09 percent after mucous membrane exposure.[25]

Recommendations for postexposure prophylaxis after percutaneous or mucous membrane exposure to hepatitis B virus are listed in Table 232–7.[25] No known effective prophylaxis is available for hepatitis C infection.

The efficacy of postexposure prophylaxis for HIV has not been established definitively. Nonetheless, the use of antiretroviral agents as postexposure prophylaxis is supported by several lines of evidence, including a case-control study conducted among exposed health care workers,[20] and this practice has become widespread in the United States.[25] The use of postexposure prophylaxis for HIV is complex and requires careful consideration of the source patient, the nature of the exposure, any preexisting conditions in the exposed persons, and the risk of adverse reactions from antiretroviral agents or interactions with other medications.[25] A 2001 CDC guideline contains recommendations for the use of multiple drug regimens and the advantages and disadvantages of specific agents.[25] Exposed health care workers should be encouraged strongly to report exposure as soon as possible to persons who are expert in the evaluation of such exposure and in the prescription of postexposure prophylaxis and who have access to the most recent prophylaxis recommendations, such as those available at the DHQP website (*http://www.cdc.gov/ncidod/hip*).

Persons exposed to active pulmonary tuberculosis should be evaluated by purified protein derivative (PPD) skin testing if they do not have a history of PPD reactivity. A skin test should be administered after the exposure and, if negative, 12 weeks later.[23] Skin test converters and persons with signs of active tuberculosis should be treated according to published recommendations.[23] All skin tests should be performed and interpreted by trained personnel according to the CDC guideline.[23]

Because exposure to tuberculosis may be unrecognized, hospitals should require health care workers to undergo periodic PPD skin testing.[23] Persons who do not have a history of previous PPD reactivity and who do not have a documented negative PPD reaction within the preceding 12 months should have a baseline PPD skin test performed with the two-step method to detect the booster phenomenon that could be misinterpreted as a skin test conversion. Thereafter, persons can be screened with a single PPD skin test, with the frequency of testing dictated by the risk of exposure. Persons with a history of previous PPD reactivity should be assessed periodically for evidence of active disease. To ensure compliance, many hospitals currently require periodic skin tests as a prerequisite for reappointment of physicians or continuing employment of other hospital staff.

Prevention of Occupationally Acquired Infections in Health Care Workers

Because vaccination against infectious diseases is a highly cost-effective prevention strategy, hospitals should offer vaccinations free of charge. Vaccination against measles is so effective that ensuring immunity to measles (as a result of either previous infection or vaccination) among hospital staff is regarded widely as an appropriate quality-of-care indicator for occupational health programs.[65] Because the combined measles, mumps, rubella (MMR) vaccine is readily available,[109] immunity against mumps and rubella can be ensured in an analogous fashion. Influenza vaccination of health care workers is recommended by the Immunization Practices Advisory Committee.[18] However, acceptance of this vaccine by health care workers is often suboptimal.[108] Consequently, employee health departments need to consider aggressive and innovative strategies to encourage annual influenza vaccination. Given the significant occupational risk of acquiring hepatitis B infection in hospitals, hepatitis B vaccination should be offered routinely to health care workers. The OSHA blood-borne pathogens standard requires hospitals to offer hepatitis B vaccination free of charge; workers who do not wish to be vaccinated must sign

TABLE 232–7 ■ RECOMMENDATIONS FOR POSTEXPOSURE PROPHYLAXIS TO HEPATITIS B VIRUS

Vaccination and Antibody Response Status of Exposed Person	Treatment		
	Source is HBs-Ag Positive	Source is HBsAg-Negative	Source is Unknown or Not Available for Testing
Unvaccinated	HBIG* × 1, initiate HBV series†	Initiate HBV series†	Initiate HBV series†
Previously vaccinated			
Known responder‡	No treatment	No treatment	No treatment
Known nonresponder‡	HBIG* × 1 and reinitiate HBV series† or HBIG* × 2	No treatment	If known high-risk source, treat as though source were HBsAg-positive
Antibody response unknown	Test exposed person for anti-HBs: If adequate‡ no treatment is necessary If inadequate,‡ administer HBIG* × 1 and HBV† booster	No treatment	Test exposed person for anti-HBs: If adequate,‡ no treatment is necessary If inadequate,‡ administer HBV† booster and recheck titer in 1–2 mo

*The HBIG dose is 0.06 mL/kg intramuscularly.
†HBV dosing requirements vary according to the manufacturer, the age of the recipient, and other factors (persons undergoing dialysis and immunocompromised persons require higher doses); follow the manufacturer's dosing recommendations.
‡An adequate anti-HBs level is 10 mIU/mL or higher.
anti-HBs, antibody to hepatitis B surface antigen; HBIG, hepatitis B immune globulin; HBsAg, hepatitis B surface antigen; HBV, hepatitis B vaccine.
Modified from Centers for Disease Control: Updated U.S. Public Health Service guidelines for the management of occupational exposures to HBV, HCV, and HIV and recommendations for postexposure prophylaxis. M. M. W. R. Recomm. Rep. *50* (RR-11):1–52, 2001.

a specific "informed refusal." Other vaccine advances, such as the development of acellular pertussis vaccine and licensure of a varicella vaccine, offer the hope that hospitals may soon be able to eliminate or at least drastically reduce occupational acquisition of these diseases as well.

In addition to providing standards for hepatitis B vaccination, the OSHA blood-borne pathogens standard mandates other specific prevention measures, including (1) the development of an exposure control plan that identifies employees with an occupational risk of exposure to blood-borne pathogens; (2) annual training for these individuals regarding the risk of blood-borne infection and prevention measures; (3) provision of personal protective clothing and equipment; (4) work practice controls, including equipment and procedures for the safe handling and disposal of sharp implements; and (5) procedures for identification, transportation, storage, and disposal of contaminated items and waste.[85]

The CDC's "Guidelines for Preventing the Transmission of *Mycobacterium tuberculosis* in Health Care Facilities, 1994" emphasizes a hierarchy of prevention and control measures.[23] The first level consists of administrative controls, including (1) developing and implementing effective written policies and protocols to ensure rapid identification, isolation, diagnostic evaluation, and treatment of persons likely to have tuberculosis; (2) implementing effective work practices among health care workers (e.g., using and correctly wearing respiratory protection, keeping doors to isolation rooms closed); (3) educating, training, and counseling health care workers about tuberculosis; and (4) screening health care workers for *M. tuberculosis* infection and disease. The second level is the use of engineering controls to eliminate or reduce the concentration of droplet nuclei (i.e., controlling the amount, direction, and exhaust of ventilation systems and using high-efficiency particulate air [HEPA] filtration or ultraviolet irradiation). Because eliminating infectious droplet nuclei is not possible in some areas of the hospital (e.g., patient isolation rooms, treatment rooms where cough-inducing procedures are performed), the third level involves the use of personal respiratory protection devices by health care workers to prevent the inhalation of droplet nuclei. Particulate respirators with a National Institute for Occupational Safety and Health certification of N95 or better and personal respirators with HEPA filtration satisfy the CDC specifications for these devices.[23, 81] These devices must be fit-tested on the individuals using them according to OHSA standards.[23] Additional regulations from OSHA may be forthcoming.

REPROCESSING OF REUSABLE PATIENT CARE ITEMS

A large number of nosocomial infection outbreaks have been related to the use of contaminated equipment. Consequently, hospital infection prevention and control programs must work closely with all hospital departments reprocessing reusable patient care items to ensure proper selection, implementation, and quality monitoring of reprocessing methods. An APIC guideline discusses the characteristics and efficacy of various classes of disinfectants and provides recommendations for methods used to reprocess specific patient care items.[94] New methods for sterilization and disinfection have been reviewed recently.[96, 97]

REGULATED MEDICAL WASTE

Regulated medical waste refers to waste that has at least the potential to transmit infectious agents to humans. However, of importance is to recognize that infections resulting from exposure to regulated medical waste (other than those related to percutaneous exposure within hospitals) have not been documented.[95] Moreover, waste from hospitals represents 1 percent or less of the total municipal waste generated annually and has been demonstrated to have a lower microbial burden than common household waste does.[95]

Nonetheless, a variety of national, state, and local regulations pertain to the identification, packaging, transport, storage, and disposal of regulated medical waste.[46] A full discussion of this topic is beyond the scope of this chapter, but hospital infection prevention and control programs can provide valuable input into the design of rational approaches for complying with these regulations. Because the management of regulated medical waste is considerably more expensive than the management of traditional waste, ensuring proper sorting of regulated medical waste from nonregulated hospital waste can result in considerable cost savings.

Education and Training of Health Care Workers

Providing education and training in both general principles and specific aspects of hospital infection prevention and control is one of the primary responsibilities of program staff. Program staff in many hospitals are responsible for providing training regarding the risks of acquiring blood-borne pathogens and for implementing the prevention measures mandated by OSHA. Program staff need to be familiar with the principles of adult learning, assessing the educational needs of the audience, defining learning objectives, determining optimal instructional formats, using effective teaching and communication skills, and weighing the merits of various educational tools.[54]

Antibiotic Utilization and Antimicrobial-Resistant Microorganisms

Data from the NNIS System indicate that the prevalence of antimicrobial resistance among important nosocomial bacterial pathogens (e.g., methicillin-resistant *S. aureus*, vancomycin-resistant enterococci, gram-negative bacteria resistant to third-generation cephalosporins) in ICUs continues to increase.[82] The mechanisms involved in the emergence and spread of antimicrobial resistance are complex but no doubt are facilitated by the intense selection pressure caused by the overuse and misuse of antimicrobial agents in hospitals, particularly newer, broad-spectrum agents. Dissemination of resistant strains is facilitated by suboptimal compliance with hand hygiene and isolation precautions.

Solutions to this problem are complex and require a multidisciplinary, systems-oriented approach, catalyzed and supported by hospital leadership.[45] In 1994, a workshop sponsored by the National Foundation for Infectious Diseases and the CDC developed strategic goals related to improving the use of antimicrobial agents and reducing the transmission of antimicrobial-resistant microorganisms in hospitals[45] (Table 229–8). Outcome and process measurements useful in gauging progress toward these strategic goals, as well as potential barriers to success and effective countermeasures, are described in the workshop report.[45]

The literature for specific interventions to improve antimicrobial use and reduce the spread of resistant bacteria, including studies relevant to pediatrics, has been reviewed in several publications.[38, 56, 63, 107] Evidence has been presented

TABLE 232–8 ■ STRATEGIC GOALS RELATED TO THE USE OF ANTIMICROBIAL AGENTS AND TRANSMISSION OF ANTIMICROBIAL-RESISTANT MICROORGANISMS IN HOSPITALS

Strategies to Optimize the Prophylactic, Empiric, and Therapeutic Use of Antimicrobial Agents

- Optimize antimicrobial prophylaxis for operative prophylaxis.
- Optimize the choice and duration of empiric antimicrobial therapy.
- Improve antimirobial prescribing practices by educational and administrative means.
- Establish a system to monitor and provide feedback on the occurrence and impact of antimicrobial resistance.
- Define and implement institutional or health care system delivery guidelines for important types of antimicrobial use.

Strategies for Detecting, Reporting, and Preventing Transmission of Antimicrobial-Resistant Microorganisms

- Develop a system to recognize and promptly report significant changes and trends in antimicrobial resistance to hospital and physician leaders; medical, nursing, infection control, and pharmacy staff; and others who need to know.
- Develop a system for rapid detection and reporting of resistant microorganisms in individual patients to appropriate personnel (caregivers and infection control staff) and for rapid response by caregivers.
- Increase adherence to policies and procedures, especially hand hygiene, barrier precautions, and environmental control measures.
- Incorporate the detection, prevention, and control of antimicrobial resistance into institutional strategic goals and provide the required resources (e. g., by providing adequate facilities and resources for handwashing, isolation, and environmental hygiene; funding ongoing monitoring and data collection, including infection control/hospital epidemiology and quality improvement in the planning process; and setting managerial goals and accountability for reductions in colonization and infection with resistant microorganisms).
- Develop a plan for identifying, transferring, discharging, and re-admitting patients colonized with specified antimicrobial-resistant microorganisms.*

*Each hospital should specify a list of problematic pathogens, such as methicillin-resistant *Staphylococcus aureus*, vancomycin-resistant and high-level gentamicin-resistant enterococci, and gram-negative bacilli resistant to third-generation cephalosporins and aminoglycosides.

From Goldmann, D. A., Weinstein, R. A., Wenzel, R. P., et al.: Strategies to prevent and control the emergence and spread of antimicrobial-resistant microorganisms in hospitals. A challenge to hospital leadership. J. A. M. A. *275*: 234-240, 1996.

for the efficacy of interventions such as reducing the number of prescriptions for third-generation cephalosporins for the control of resistant gram-negative rods, using alcohol-based agents for hand hygiene, and using barrier precautions in the care of colonized patients for the control of resistant gram-positive bacteria.[38, 56, 63, 107] However, these conclusions are supported largely by reports of the successful control of outbreaks caused by resistant bacteria and a handful of observational, quasi-experimental, and small-scale, single-center clinical trials. Well-designed trials are needed to test new prevention strategies.

Product Evaluation

A large number of new medical products are introduced to the health care market every year. Although some of these products have the potential to reduce infectious risks, data to substantiate the safety and efficacy claims of manufacturers often are limited. Many devices marketed to hospitals caring for children actually have never been tested in children. Because these products are often substantially more expensive than existing products, a compelling rationale for their use must exist. Hospital infection prevention and control staff can provide valuable assistance to hospital committees evaluating new products and, in some cases, can design and conduct appropriate clinical trials.[61]

REFERENCES

1. Abrutyn, E., Goldmann, D. A., and Scheckler, W. E. (ed.): Saunders Infection Control Reference Service. 2nd ed. Philadelphia, W. B. Saunders, 2001.
2. American Academy of Pediatrics: Antimicrobial prophylaxis in pediatric surgical patients. *In* Pickering, L. K. (ed.): 2000 Red Book: Report of the Committee on Infectious Diseases. Elk Grove Village, IL, American Academy of Pediatrics, 2000, pp. 730–735.
3. Anderson, J. D., Bonner, M., Scheifele, D. W., and Schneider, B. C.: Lack of nosocomial spread of varicella in a pediatric hospital with negative pressure ventilated patient rooms. Infect. Control *6*:120–121, 1985.
4. Antimicrobial prophylaxis in surgery. Med. Lett. Drugs Ther. *43*:92–97, 2001.
5. Bates, D. W., Cullen, D. J., Laird, N., et al.: Incidence of adverse drug events and potential adverse drug events: Implications for prevention. ADE Prevention Study Group. J. A. M. A. *274*:29–34, 1995.
6. Bates, D. W., Spell, N., Cullen, D. J., et al.: The costs of adverse drug events in hospitalized patients. Adverse Drug Events Prevention Study Group. J. A. M. A. *277*:307–311, 1997.
7. Bennett, J. V., and Brachman, P. S. (eds.): Hospital Infections. 3rd ed. Boston, Little, Brown, 1992.
8. Benneyan, J. C.: Statistical quality control methods in infection control and hospital epidemiology, part I: Introduction and basic theory. Infect. Control Hosp. Epidemiol. *19*:194–214, 1998.
9. Benneyan, J. C.: Statistical quality control methods in infection control and hospital epidemiology, part II: Chart use, statistical properties, and research issues. Infect. Control Hosp. Epidemiol. *19*:265–283, 1998.
10. Berwick, D. M.: Continuous improvement as an ideal in health care. N. Engl. J. Med. *320*:53–56, 1989.
11. Bischoff, W. E., Reynolds, T. M., Sessler, C. N., et al.: Handwashing compliance by health care workers: The impact of introducing an accessible, alcohol-based hand antiseptic. Arch. Intern. Med. *160*:1017–1021, 2000.
12. Blatt, M. L.: Cross-infection: Its prevention in a children's hospital. Illinois Med. J. *70*:483–487, 1936.
13. Bolyard, E. A., Tablan, O. C., Williams, W. W., et al.: Guideline for infection control in healthcare personnel, 1998. Hospital Infection Control Practices Advisory Committee. Control Hosp. Epidemiol. *19*:407–463, 1998.
14. Boyce, J. M., Kelliher, S., and Vallande, N.: Skin irritation and dryness associated with two hand-hygiene regimens: Soap-and-water hand washing versus hand antisepsis with an alcoholic hand gel. Infect. Control Hosp. Epidemiol. *21*:442–448, 2000.
15. Centers for Disease Control and Prevention: Guideline for hand hygiene in health-care settings: Recommendations of the Healthcare Infection Control Practices Advisory Committee and the HIPAC/SHEA/APIC/IDSA Hand Hygiene Task Force. M. M. W. R. Recomm. Rep. *51*(RR-16):1–48, 2002.
16. Brennan, T. A., Leape, L. L., Laird, N. M., et al.: Incidence of adverse events and negligence in hospitalized patients. Results of the Harvard Medical Practice Study I. N. Engl. J. Med. *324*:370–376, 1991.
17. Brennemann, J.: The infant ward. Am. J. Dis. Child. *43*:577–584, 1932.
18. Bridges, C. B., Fukuda, K., Uyeki, T. M., et al.: Prevention and control of influenza. Recommendations of the Advisory Committee on Immunization Practices (ACIP). M. M. W. R. Recomm. Rep. *51*(RR-3): 1–31, 2002.
19. Broderick, A., Mori, M., Nettleman, M. D., et al.: Nosocomial infections: Validation of surveillance and computer modeling to identify patients at risk. Am. J. Epidemiol. *131*:734–742, 1990.
20. Cardo, D. M., Culver, D. H., Ciesielski, C. A., et al.: A case-control study of HIV seroconversion in health care workers after percutaneous exposure. Centers for Disease Control and Prevention Needlestick Surveillance Group. N. Engl. J. Med. *337*:1485–1490, 1997.
21. Centers for Disease Control and Prevention: Recommendations for preventing transmission of infection with human T-lymphotropic virus type III/lymphadenopathy-associated virus in the workplace. M. M. W. R. Morb. Mortal. Wkly. Rep. *34*:681–686, 691–695, 1985.
22. Centers for Disease Control and Prevention: Recommendations for prevention of HIV transmission in health-care settings. M. M. W. R. Morb. Mortal. Wkly. Rep. *36*(Suppl.):1–18, 1987.
23. Centers for Disease Control and Prevention: Guidelines for preventing the transmission of *Mycobacterium tuberculosis* in health care facilities, 1994. M. M. W. R. Morb. Mortal. Wkly. Rep. *43*(RR-13):1–132, 1994.
24. Centers for Disease Control and Prevention: Monitoring hospital-acquired infections to promote patient safety—United States, 1990–1999. M. M. W. R. Morb. Mortal. Wkly. Rep. *49*(8):149–153, 2000.

25. Centers for Disease Control and Prevention: Updated U.S. Public Health Service guidelines for the management of occupational exposures to HBV, HCV, and HIV and recommendations for postexposure prophylaxis. M. M. W. R. Recomm. Rep. *50*(RR-11):1–52, 2001.
26. Classen, D. C., Evans, R. S., Pestotnik, S. L., et al.: The timing of prophylactic administration of antibiotics and the risk of surgical-wound infection. N. Engl. J. Med. *326*:281–286, 1992.
27. Culver, D. H., Horan, T. C., Gaynes, R. P., et al.: Surgical wound infection rates by wound class, operative procedure, and patient risk index. National Nosocomial Infections Surveillance System. Am. J. Med. *91*(Suppl.):152–157, 1991.
28. Currier, J. S., Campbell, H., Platt, R., and Kaiser, A. B.: Perioperative antimicrobial prophylaxis in middle Tennessee, 1989–1990. Rev. Infect. Dis. *13*(Suppl.):874–878, 1991.
29. Decker, M. D.: Continuous quality improvement. Infect. Control Hosp. Epidemiol. *13*:165–169, 1992.
30. Decker, M. D.: The application of continuous quality improvement to healthcare. Infect. Control Hosp. Epidemiol. *13*:226–229, 1992.
31. de Galan, B. E., van Tilburg, P. M., Sluijter, M., et al.: Hospital-related outbreak of infection with multidrug-resistant *Streptococcus pneumoniae* in the Netherlands. J. Hosp. Infect. *42*:185–192, 1999.
32. Donabedian, A.: Contributions of epidemiology to quality assessment and monitoring. Infect. Control Hosp. Epidemiol. *11*:117–121, 1990.
33. Donowitz, L. G. (ed.): Hospital-Acquired Infection in the Pediatric Patient. Baltimore, Williams & Wilkins, 1988.
34. Donowitz, L. G., Hunt, E. H., Pugh, V. G., et al.: Comparison of historical and serologic immunity to varicella-zoster virus in 373 hospital employees. Am. J. Infect. Control. *15*:212–214, 1987.
35. Durbin, W., Jr., Lapidas, B., and Goldmann, D. A.: Improved antibiotic usage following introduction of a novel prescription system. J. A. M. A. *246*:1796–1800, 1981.
36. Evans, R. S., Burke, J. P., Classen, D. C., et al.: Computerized identification of patients at high risk for hospital-acquired infection. Am. J. Infect. Control *20*:4–10, 1992.
37. Evans, R. S., Larsen, R. A., Burke, J. P., et al.: Computer surveillance of hospital-acquired infections and antibiotic use. J. A. M. A. *256*:1007–1011, 1986.
38. Farr, B. M., Salgado, C. D., Karchmer, T. B., and Sherertz, R. J.: Can antibiotic-resistant nosocomial infections be controlled? Lancet Infect. Dis. *1*:38–45, 2001.
39. Foca, M., Jakob, K., Whittier, S., et al.: Endemic *Pseudomonas aeruginosa* infection in a neonatal intensive care unit. N. Engl. J. Med. *343*: 695–700, 2000.
40. Freeman, J., and McGowan, J. E., Jr.: Methodologic issues in hospital epidemiology. I. Rates, case-finding, and interpretation. Rev. Infect. Dis. *3*:658–667, 1981.
41. Friedland, I. R., and Klugman, K. P.: Antibiotic-resistant pneumococcal disease in South African children. Am. J. Dis. Child. *146*:920–923, 1992.
42. Garner, J. S.: Guideline for isolation precautions in hospitals. The Hospital Infection Control Practices Advisory Committee. Infect. Control Hosp. Epidemiol. *17*:53–80, 1996.
43. Gaynes, R. P., and Horan, T. C.: Surveillance of nosocomial infections. *In* Mayhall, C. G. (ed.): Hospital Epidemiology and Infection Control. Baltimore, Williams & Wilkins, 1995, pp. 1017–1031.
44. Gaynes, R. P., and Solomon, S.: Improving hospital-acquired infection rates: The CDC experience. Jt. Comm. J. Qual. Improv. *22*:457–467, 1996.
45. Goldmann, D. A., Weinstein, R. A., Wenzel, R. P., et al.: Strategies to prevent and control the emergence and spread of antimicrobial-resistant microorganisms in hospitals. A challenge to hospital leadership. J. A. M. A. *275*:234–240, 1996.
46. Gordon, J. G., Reinhardt, P. A., Denys, G. A., and Alvarado, C. J.: Medical waste management. *In* Mayhall, C. G. (ed.): Hospital Epidemiology and Infection Control. Baltimore, Williams & Wilkins, 1999, pp. 1387–1397.
47. Haiduven, D. J., Hench, C. P., and Stevens, D. A.: Postexposure varicella management of nonimmune personnel: An alternative approach. Infect. Control Hosp. Epidemiol. *15*:329–334, 1994.
48. Haley, R. W.: Surveillance by objective: A new priority-directed approach to the control of nosocomial infections. Am. J. Infect. Control *13*:78–89, 1985.
49. Haley, R. W., Culver, D. H., White, J. W., et al.: The efficacy of infection surveillance and control programs in preventing nosocomial infections in US hospitals. Am. J. Epidemiol. *121*:182–205, 1985.
50. Haley, R. W., Morgan, W. M., Culver, D. H., et al.: Update from the SENIC project. Hospital infection control: Recent progress and opportunities under prospective payment. Am. J. Infect. Control *13*:97–108, 1985.
51. Haley, R. W., Tenney, J. H., Lindsey, J. D., et al.: How frequent are outbreaks of nosocomial infection in community hospitals? Infect. Control *6*:233–236, 1985.
52. Harries, E. H. R.: Infection and its control in children's wards. Lancet *2*:173–178, 1935.
53. Hedderwick, S. A., McNeil, S. A., Lyons, M. J., and Kauffman, C. A.: Pathogenic organisms associated with artificial fingernails worn by healthcare workers. Infect. Control Hosp. Epidemiol. *21*:505–509, 2000.
54. Hoffmann, K. K., and Clontz, E. P.: Education of health care workers in the prevention of nosocomial infections. *In* Mayhall, C. G. (ed.): Hospital Epidemiology and Infection Control. Baltimore, Williams & Wilkins, 1999, pp. 1373–1380.
55. Hospital Infection Control Practices Advisory Committee: Recommendations for preventing the spread of vancomycin resistance. Infect. Control Hosp. Epidemiol. *16*:105–113, 1995.
56. Huskins, W. C.: Antimicrobial resistance and its control in pediatrics. Semin. Pediatr. Infect. Dis. *12*:138–146, 2001.
57. Jarvis, W. R.: Nosocomial outbreaks: The Centers for Disease Control's Hospital Infections Program experience, 1980–1990. Am. J. Med. *91*(Suppl.):101–106, 1991.
58. Jarvis, W. R., and Zaza, S.: Investigation of outbreaks. *In* Mayhall, C. G. (ed.): Hospital Epidemiology and Infection Control. Baltimore, Williams & Wilkins, 1999, pp. 111–120.
59. Joint Commission on Accreditation of Healthcare Organizations: The accreditation process circa 2004. *2002*:2002. http://www.jcaho.org/accredited+organizations/api/accredited+process+04.htm. Accessed on August 19, 2002.
60. Josephson, A., Karanfil, L., and Gombert, M. E.: Strategies for the management of varicella-susceptible healthcare workers after a known exposure. Infect. Control Hosp. Epidemiol. *11*:309–313, 1990.
61. Karanfil, L. V., and Gershon, R. R. M.: Evaluating and selecting products that have infection control implications. *In* Mayhall, C. G. (ed.): Hospital Epidemiology and Infection Control. Baltimore, Williams & Wilkins, 1999, pp. 1367–1371.
62. Kaushal, R., Bates, D. W., Landrigan, C., et al.: Medication errors and adverse drug events in pediatric inpatients. J. A. M. A. *285*:2114–2120, 2001.
63. Kollef, M. H., and Fraser, V. J.: Antibiotic resistance in the intensive care unit. Ann. Intern. Med. *134*:298–314, 2001.
64. Korniewicz, D. M., Kirwin, M., Cresci, K., and Larson, E.: Leakage of latex and vinyl exam gloves in high and low risk clinical settings. Am. Ind. Hyg. Assoc. J. *54*:22–26, 1993.
65. Krause, P. J., Gross, P. A., Barrett, T. L., et al.: Quality standard for assurance of measles immunity among health care workers. Infect. Control Hosp. Epidemiol. *15*:193–199, 1994.
66. Kritchevsky, S. B., and Simmons, B. P.: Continuous quality improvement: Concepts and applications for physician care. J. A. M. A. *266*:1817–1823 1991.
67. Larson, E.: Skin hygiene and infection prevention: More of the same or different approaches? Clin. Infect. Dis. *29*:1287–1294, 1999.
68. Larson, E., and Kretzer, E. K.: Compliance with handwashing and barrier precautions. J. Hosp. Infect. *30*:88–106, 1995.
69. Leclair, J. M., Freeman, J., Sullivan, B. F., et al.: Prevention of nosocomial respiratory syncytial virus infections through compliance with glove and gown isolation precautions. N. Engl. J. Med. *317*:329–334, 1987.
70. Lee, T. B., Baker, O. G., Lee, J. T., et al.: Recommended practices for surveillance. Association for Professionals in Infection Control and Epidemiology, Inc. Surveillance Initiative Working Group. Am. J. Infect. Control *26*:277–288, 1998.
71. Lichtenstein, A.: Nosocomial infections in children's hospitals and institutions. Our means for combating these infections. Acta Paediatr. *17*:36–49, 1935.
72. Lövegren, E.: Infection risks in nursing institutions for infants and young children and measures for their prevention. Acta Paediatr. *17*:50–55, 1935.
73. Lynch, P., Jackson, M. M., Cummings, M. J., and Stamm, W. E.: Rethinking the role of isolation practices in the prevention of nosocomial infections. Ann. Intern. Med. *107*:243–246, 1987.
74. Mandigers, C. M., Dieperloot, R. J., Dessens, M., et al.: A hospital outbreak of penicillin-resistant pneumococci in The Netherlands. Eur. Respir. J. *7*:1635–1639, 1994.
75. Mangram, A. J., Horan, T. C., Pearson, M. L., et al.: Guideline for prevention of surgical site infection, 1999. Centers for Disease Control and Prevention (CDC) Hospital Infection Control Practices Advisory Committee. Am. J. Infect. Control *27*:97–132, 1999.
76. Mayhall, C. G. (ed.): Hospital Epidemiology and Infection Control. Philadelphia, Lippincott Williams & Wilkins, 1999.
77. McDonald, L. L., and Pugliese, G.: Regulatory, accreditation, and professional agencies influencing infection control programs. *In* Wenzel, R. P. (ed.): Prevention and Control of Nosocomial Infections. Baltimore, Williams & Wilkins, 1997, pp. 57–70.
78. McKhann, C. F., Steeger, A., and Long, A. P.: Hospital infections. A survey of the problem. Am. J. Dis. Child. *55*:579–599, 1938.
79. McNeil, S. A., Foster, C. L., Hedderwick, S. A., and Kauffman, C. A.: Effect of hand cleansing with antimicrobial soap or alcohol-based gel on microbial colonization of artificial fingernails worn by health care workers. Clin. Infect. Dis. *32*:367–372, 2001.
80. Millar, M. R., Brown, N. M., Tobin, G. W., et al.: Outbreak of infection with penicillin-resistant *Streptococcus pneumoniae* in a hospital for the elderly. J. Hosp. Infect. *27*:99–104, 1994.
81. National Institute for Occupational Safety and Health, Centers for Disease Control and Prevention, Public Health Service, Department of Health and Human Services: Respiratory protective devices: Final rules and notice. Fed. Reg. *60*:30336–30404, 1995.
82. National Nosocomial Infections Surveillance System: National Nosocomial Infections Surveillance (NNIS) System Report, data summary

from January 1992–June 2001, issued August 2001. Am. J. Infect. Control *29*:404–421, 2001.

83. Nuorti, J. P., Butler, J. C., Crutcher, J. M., et al.: An outbreak of multidrug-resistant pneumococcal pneumonia and bacteremia among unvaccinated nursing home residents. N. Engl. J. Med. *338*:1861–1868, 1998.
84. O'Boyle, C. A., Henly, S. J., and Larson, E.: Understanding adherence to hand hygiene recommendations: The theory of planned behavior. Am. J. Infect. Control *29*:352–360, 2001.
85. Occupational Safety and Health Administration, Department of Labor: Occupational exposure to bloodborne pathogens: Final rule. Fed. Reg. *56*:64175–64182, 1991.
86. Centers for Disease Control and Prevention: Guideline for the prevention of intravascular catheter-related infections. M. M. W. R. Recomm. Rep. *51*(RR-10):1–29, 2002.
87. Patterson, C. H.: Joint Commission on Accreditation of Healthcare Organizations. Infect. Control. Hosp. Epidemiol. *16*:36–42, 1995.
88. Perl, T. M.: Surveillance, reporting, and the use of computers. *In* Wenzel, R. P. (ed.): Prevention and Control of Nosocomial Infections. Baltimore, Williams & Wilkins, 1993, pp. 139–176.
89. Pittet, D., Dharan, S., Touveneau, S., et al.: Bacterial contamination of the hands of hospital staff during routine patient care. Arch. Intern. Med. *159*:821–826, 1999.
90. Pittet, D., Hugonnet, S., Harbarth, S., et al.: Effectiveness of a hospital-wide programme to improve compliance with hand hygiene. Lancet *356*:1307–1312, 2000.
91. Platt, R., Yokoe, D. S., and Sands, K. E.: Automated methods for surveillance of surgical site infections. Emerg. Infect. Dis. *7*:212–216, 2001.
92. Pratt, R. J., Pellowe, C., Loveday, H. P., et al.: The *epic* project: Developing national evidence-based guidelines for preventing healthcare associated infections. Phase I: Guidelines for preventing hospital-acquired infections. Department of Health (England). J. Hosp. Infect. *47*(Suppl.):3–82, 2001.
93. Pugliese, G., Lamberto, B., and Kroc, K. A.: Development and implementation of infection control policies and procedures. *In* Mayhall, C. G. (ed.): Hospital Epidemiology and Infection Control. Baltimore, Williams & Wilkins, 1999, pp. 1357–1366.
94. Rutala, W. A.: APIC guideline for selection and use of disinfectants. 1994, 1995, and 1996 APIC Guidelines Committee. Association for Professionals in Infection Control and Epidemiology, Inc. Am. J. Infect. Control *24*:313–342, 1996.
95. Rutala, W. A., and Weber, D. J.: Infectious waste—mismatch between science and policy. N. Engl. J. Med. *325*:578–582, 1991.
96. Rutala, W. A., and Weber, D. J.: Disinfection of endoscopes: Review of new chemical sterilants used for high-level disinfection. Infect. Control Hosp. Epidemiol. *20*:69–76, 1999.
97. Rutala, W. A., and Weber, D. J.: New disinfection and sterilization methods. Emerg. Infect. Dis. 7:348–353, 2001.
98. Saiman, L., LaRussa, P., Steinberg, S. P., et al.: Persistence of immunity to varicella-zoster virus after vaccination of healthcare workers. Infect. Control Hosp. Epidemiol. *22*:279–283, 2001.
99. Sands, K., Vineyard, G., Livingston, J., et al.: Efficient identification of postdischarge surgical site infections: Use of automated pharmacy dispensing information, administrative data, and medical record information. J. Infect. Dis. *179*:434–441, 1999.
100. Scheckler, W. E., Brimhall, D., Buck, A. S., et al.: Requirements for infrastructure and essential activities of infection control and epidemiology in hospitals: A consensus panel report. Infect. Control Hosp. Epidemiol. *19*:114–124, 1998.
101. Shapiro, M., Townsend, T. R., Rosner, B., and Kass, E. H.: Use of antimicrobial drugs in general hospitals: Patterns of prophylaxis. N. Engl. J. Med. *301*:351–355, 1979.
102. Smith, P. W., and Rusnak, P. G.: Infection prevention and control in the long-term-care facility. Infect. Control Hosp. Epidemiol. *18*:831–849, 1997.
103. Sohn, A. H., and Jarvis, W. R.: Benchmarking in pediatric infection control: Results from the National Nosocomial Infections Surveillance (NNIS) System and the Pediatric Prevention Network. Semin. Pediatr. Infect. Dis. *12*:254–265, 2001.
104. Tablan, O. C., Anderson, L. J., Arden, N. H., et al.: Guideline for prevention of nosocomial pneumonia. The Hospital Infection Control Practices Advisory Committee, Centers for Disease Control and Prevention. Infect. Control Hosp. Epidemiol. *15*:587–627, 1994.
105. The Society for Hospital Epidemiology of America, the Association for Practitioners in Infection Control, the Centers for Disease Control, the Surgical Infection Society: Consensus paper on the surveillance of surgical wound infections. Infect. Control Hosp. Epidemiol. *13*:599–605, 1992.
106. Thomas, E. J., Studdert, D. M., Burstin, H. R., et al.: Incidence and types of adverse events and negligent care in Utah and Colorado. Med. Care *38*:261–271, 2000.
107. Toltzis, P., and Blumer, J. L.: Nosocomial acquisition and transmission of antibiotic-resistant gram-negative organisms in the pediatric intensive care unit. Pediatr. Infect. Dis. J. *20*:612–618, 2001.
108. Watanakunakorn, C., Ellis, G., and Gemmel, D.: Attitude of healthcare personnel regarding influenza immunization. Infect. Control Hosp. Epidemiol. *14*:17–20, 1993.
109. Watson, J. C., Hadler, S. C., Dykewicz, C. A., et al.: Measles, mumps, and rubella—vaccine use and strategies for elimination of measles, rubella, and congenital rubella syndrome and control of mumps: Recommendations of the Advisory Committee on Immunization Practices (ACIP). M. M. W. R. Recomm. Rep. *47*(RR-8):1–57, 1998.
110. Weinberg, M., Fuentes, J. M., Ruiz, A. I., et al.: Reducing infections among women undergoing cesarean section in Colombia by means of continuous quality improvement methods. Arch. Intern. Med. *161*: 2357–2365, 2001.
111. Weiss, K., Restieri, C., Gauthier, R., et al.: A nosocomial outbreak of fluoroquinolone-resistant *Streptococcus pneumoniae*. Clin. Infect. Dis. *33*:517–522, 2001.
112. Wendt, C., and Herwaldt, L. A.: Epidemics: Identification and management. *In* Wenzel, R. P. (ed.): Prevention and Control of Nosocomial Infections. Baltimore, Williams & Wilkins, 1997, pp. 175–213.
113. Wenzel, R. P. (ed.): Prevention and Control of Nosocomial Infections. 3rd ed. Baltimore, Williams & Wilkins, 1997.
114. Wenzel, R. P., Thompson, R. L., Landry, S. M., et al.: Hospital-acquired infections in intensive care unit patients: An overview with emphasis on epidemics. Infect. Control *4*:371–375, 1983.
115. Williams, C. O., Campbell, S., Henry, K., and Collier, P.: Variables influencing worker compliance with universal precautions in the emergency department. Am. J. Infect. Control *22*:138–148, 1994.

PART V

Therapeutics

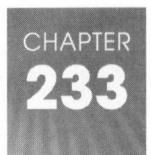

CHAPTER 233 Antibiotic Resistance

PHILIP TOLTZIS ■ JEFFREY L. BLUMER

Soil bacteria developed mechanisms of resistance to antibiotics millions of years ago as a means of protecting themselves against other antibiotic-producing microorganisms or their own antimicrobial products. The current crisis of antibiotic resistance, however, was prompted by the intense selective pressure posed by the worldwide use of antibiotics during the past half-century. The problem of antimicrobial resistance in humans has been exacerbated by the widespread administration of antibiotics to farm animals[198, 284, 321]; resistant zoonotic bacteria selected by this practice contaminate the food supply and thereby spread to human consumers.

To fully understand antibiotic resistance, one must make a distinction between the in vitro phenomenon of resistance and the less frequently observed clinical consequences of this in vitro phenomenon. Much of the discussion of bacterial resistance to antibiotics derives from the apparent changes in susceptibility of pathogenic bacteria to the concentrations of antibiotic achieved in blood after standard antibiotic dosing.[138] These concentrations have been established as "breakpoints" based on integration of data derived from both clinical and animal studies, as well as measurement of plasma/serum drug concentrations associated with successful outcomes. Unfortunately, such breakpoints are not absolute. Rather, they depend on an intricate interrelationship between the pharmacokinetics and pharmacodynamics of the drug in question.[249] Hence, if one component of this complex interrelationship is changed, the apparent breakpoint distinguishing susceptibility from resistance possibly and probably also will change. Consequently, in presenting information concerning the mechanisms of antibiotic resistance and their clinical contexts, one must remember that the discussion derives, in part, from certain artificial pretexts. Any changes in a drug-dosing paradigm (e.g., dose, infusion duration, formulation) might have a dramatic impact on the clinical relevance of the in vitro observations.

Bacteria acquire resistance to antimicrobial agents through three principal cellular mechanisms (Table 233–1). In some microorganisms, more than one mechanism of resistance to a given agent exists simultaneously. Antibiotic resistance genes may be encoded either on the bacterial chromosome or on extrachromosomal DNA. The spread of antibiotic resistance among bacteria has been facilitated by the inclusion of many resistance genes on transmissible extrachromosomal genetic elements. To date, three interrelated genetic elements have been implicated in the expression and spread of antibiotic resistance, namely, *plasmids, transposons,* and *integrons.*

TABLE 233–1 ■ CELLULAR MECHANISMS OF ANTIBIOTIC RESISTANCE AND THEIR TRANSFER

Mechanisms
Genes that encode enzymes that modify or degrade antibiotics
Genes that modify the molecular targets of antibiotics
Genes that code for changes in cell wall channels or active pumping mechanisms
Transfer
Plasmids—extrachromosomal genetic elements made of circular double-stranded DNA<10 to >400 kilobase pairs; autonomous, self-reproducing; may be conjugative or nonconjugative
Transposon—a mobile genetic element in the bacterial chromosome or plasmid that confers a recognizable phenotype characteristic; incapable of self-replication
Integron—DNA sequences on a bacterial chromosome or plasmid often linked to a resistance gene that facilitates recombination between nonhomologous DNA sequences

Plasmids are composed of circular double-stranded extrachromosomal DNA. Although plasmids characteristically use bacterial DNA polymerase to replicate, their replication occurs autonomously.[300] Many different plasmids exist in nature and vary in size, in the complexity of their genetic machinery, in their host range and ability to conjugate, and in their stability within the bacterium. Minimal plasmids (replicons) contain genetic sequences encoding the site at which their replication begins and sequences that determine the copy number produced per cell. However, many more genetic elements can be inserted into the replicon. Indeed, plasmids range in size from 1 kb to more than 400 kb; because additional genetic machinery is required for conjugation, conjugative plasmids are at least 30 kb in size.[273] Groups of plasmids containing homologous replicative sequences are generally unable to be maintained in the same bacterial cell. This property has been exploited to categorize plasmids into different "incompatibility groups."

The importance of plasmids to human disease increased substantially when researchers discovered that these elements could incorporate one or more antibiotic resistance genes. These so-called resistance plasmids are found in a wide variety of gram-positive and gram-negative bacteria and encode determinants conferring resistance to a large number of antibiotics. Resistance-conferring sequences that produce resistance to several drugs may be included on the same plasmid, and multiple, different plasmids expressing different determinants can be included in the same microorganism.[28, 300] Several additional classes of plasmid-borne determinants besides antibiotic resistance genes can confer selective advantage to the bacterium. Such determinants include genes rendering resistance to environmental heavy metals (e.g., mercury, antimony, arsenic, and silver) and a variety of toxic organic compounds (e.g., camphor and toluene); genes leading to the synthesis of virulence factors, such as adhesion ligands promoting bacterial attachment to epithelial surfaces and those encoding exotoxins; and genes encoding compounds enabling the acquisition of chemicals necessary for bacterial survival (e.g., siderophores).[300] The coexistence of these genes on plasmids carrying antibiotic resistance determinants serves to maintain the plasmid even in the absence of antibiotic exposure.

Plasmids are transmitted from microorganism to microorganism both vertically and horizontally.[300] Vertical transmission occurs during bacterial division as the plasmids segregate to each daughter cell. Horizontal transmission is effected through conjugation, or transmission of the plasmid from one bacterium to another. At a minimum, all conjugal plasmids encode a genetic sequence that serves as the origin of transmission, and most encode additional mobilization genes.[297] However, plasmids that are unable to conjugate on their own frequently are able to do so when a conjugal plasmid co-resides in the same cell.[300] Especially in gram-negative bacteria, the donor-recipient contact required for conjugation is effected through sex pili. Conjugation frequently is restricted to intragenus transfer, but conjugation across bacterial genera may occur, particularly in gram-negative organisms, and conjugation occurs across Gram stain barriers.[193, 297]

A second group of bacterial nucleic acid elements that carry antibiotic resistance genes are termed *transposons*. Transposons move segments of nucleic acid from one location to another, such as from different sites on the bacterial chromosome or from chromosome to plasmid.[268, 274] Unlike chromosomal and plasmid DNA, transposons do not replicate independently, and therefore, to propagate they must be integrated into a molecule capable of replication. Antibiotic resistance genes may be encoded on conjugative transposons, which unlike nonconjugative transposons, are able to transfer from one bacterium to another.[274] Most antibiotic resistance conjugative transposons characterized to date have been identified in gram-positive organisms, although transposons in *Bacteroides* have been well characterized and transposons in some facultative gram-negative bacteria also have been discovered.[263] Conjugative transposons are very promiscuous in two senses. First, they move easily from one species of bacterium to another.[263, 274] Second, integration of transposons into other nucleic acid elements is relatively sequence-nonspecific. Although the preference is for integrating into host DNA sequences with long stretches rich in adenine and thymidine, integration of conjugative transposons targets no detectable consensus sequences.[263]

Intracellular shuttling of a transposon from DNA to DNA begins with the production of a staggered cut on either side of the transposon sequence to produce single-stranded overhangs. These overhang sequences (termed "coupling sequences") join covalently to produce a circularized double-stranded intermediate that contains the non–base-paired coupling sequences derived from opposite ends of the transposon.[263, 274] Integration of the circle into the target double-stranded DNA also results in flanking non–base-paired regions, which become complementary only after a round of replication.[274] Conjugation of the transposon from cell to cell likewise begins with the circularized intermediate, which after nicking at a presumed origin site is transferred as a single strand from donor bacterium to recipient bacterium, whereupon it recircularizes. Complementary strands then are added to both single strands in the donor and the recipient, and integration into target DNA in both cells ensues.[263]

Excision and integration of transposons are catalyzed by a transposon-encoded integrase.[263, 274] The efficiency of excision varies widely and accounts for differences in rates of transposon transfer. Conjugation of many transposons appears to be regulated.[263] Unlike some plasmids, conjugative transposons do not exclude the entry of other transposons.[263] Indeed, some transposons promote the conjugation of other transposons, as well as co-resident plasmids, thereby resulting in the dissemination of resistance determinants that are not encoded on the transposon itself.[274]

Integrons, a third type of bacterial DNA important in antibiotic resistance, are composed of segments of DNA that are able to capture and excise gene cassettes coding for antibiotic-resistance genes. They are unable to transfer from bacterium to bacterium by themselves. To disseminate, the integron first must insert into a plasmid or transposon.[86, 242, 246] To date, integrons have been identified primarily in gram-negative organisms.[242, 246] Integrons contain an integrase that catalyzes the incorporation and excision of the cassette into the integron, as well as a promoter that mediates expression of the resistance determinant, both situated 5′ to the cassette. The cassettes themselves are small segments usually encoding a single antibiotic resistance determinant. Cassettes have been identified that confer resistance to a broad range of antibiotics, including the β-lactam agents, the aminoglycosides, trimethoprim, and choramphenicol.[86, 242, 246] At the 3′ end of each cassette is a variable region commonly termed the "59–base pair element," although these sites vary in length from cassette to cassette; this element contains the sequences recognized by the integrase for incorporation of the gene cassette into the integron.[86, 246] A single integron may contain multiple cassettes in tandem, all of which are controlled by the single integron promoter. Transcription of tandem cassettes may terminate prematurely, however, such that the cassettes closest to the integron promoter are transcribed at the highest level.[242, 246] Cassettes also have been identified on transposons and less commonly on the bacterial genome.[246]

Resistance to Specific Antibiotics

β-LACTAM ANTIBIOTICS

The β-lactam antibiotics are a diverse, highly effective family of drugs with broad activity against a wide variety of hospital- and community-acquired pathogens. The β-lactams are composed of four subgroups: the penicillins, the cephalosporins, the monobactams, and the carbapenems. Resistance to the β-lactams is mediated by one of two principal mechanisms: production of enzymes capable of hydrolyzing the β-lactam ring and alteration of the target bacterial molecules, the penicillin-binding proteins (PBPs).

β-Lactamase Production

CLINICAL RELEVANCE. The explosive development in antimicrobial therapeutics during the past 40 or 50 years has been driven, to a great extent, by the impact of β-lactamase activity on the response to antibiotic therapy in the clinical setting.[249] Shortly after penicillin became incorporated into the clinical armamentarium for the treatment of systemic infections, clinical failures were reported in patients being treated for infections caused by *Staphylococcus aureus*. On further analysis, these failures were attributed to the presence of an enzyme, penicillinase, elaborated and excreted by the bacteria that inactivated the antibiotic before it could manifest its clinical effect. This finding led to the development of numerous new antistaphylococcal penicillins (i.e., the isoxazolyl penicillins) that were not substrates for this enzyme.

At the same time, a new class of β-lactam agents, the cephalosporins, was developed. One of the criteria used in moving candidate drugs from this class to the clinic was their resistance to inactivation by the penicillinase elaborated by staphylococci. Further development of all four of the subgroups in the β-lactam family (i.e., penicillins, cephalosporins, monobactams, and carbapenems) was influenced significantly by the recognition that the penicillinase elaborated by staphylococci was representative of a larger class of enzymes that were also present in gram-negative organisms. In this regard, history repeated itself. As gram-negative organisms such as *Escherichia coli* emerged as important clinical pathogens, their increasing resistance to aminopenicillins on the basis of β-lactamase elaboration spawned the development of a group of enzyme inhibitors that included clavulanic acid, sulbactam, and tazobactam.[179, 252] Moreover, even as expansion of the spectrum of both the penicillins and cephalosporins to include some of the more itinerant gram-negative organisms such as *Serratia, Enterobacter,* and even *Pseudomonas* became necessary, β-lactamase stability emerged as a necessary attribute for clinical success.[179, 252] This stability was accomplished either through the addition of one of the β-lactamase inhibitors to members of the carboxy and acylureido class of penicillins or through structural engineering such as that seen with development of the second- and third-generation cephalosporins and carbapenems.

In pediatric practice, the importance of β-lactamase became apparent soon after the widespread use of antibiotics in hospitalized patients began. Outbreaks of serious staphylococcal infections in neonatal nurseries prompted the early adoption of antistaphylococcal penicillins into pediatric practice; however, two sentinel clinical events probably were most responsible for establishing β-lactamase as a prominent pediatric clinical problem. In 1974, the first case of bacterial meningitis caused by an ampicillin-resistant *Haemophilus influenzae* type b strain was reported.[217, 296] This report resulted in marked changes in clinical practice. First, all infants and children with suspected bacterial meningitis were treated empirically with both ampicillin and chloramphenicol (a drug not susceptible to degradation by bacterial β-lactamase) instead of ampicillin alone.[249] In addition, numerous newer antibiotics, particularly the second- and third-generation cephalosporins, were evaluated for their efficacy in this clinical setting. From these studies, ceftriaxone and cefotaxime emerged as the drugs of choice for the empiric treatment of suspected or proven bacterial meningitis in children. This selection was based on both their greater potency against *H. influenzae* type b and their stability to β-lactamase.

The other mitigating circumstances resulting in the affirmation of β-lactamase as an important clinical problem in pediatrics were the recognition of *Moraxella catarrhalis,* a β-lactamase–producing organism, as the third leading cause of acute otitis media in infants and children and the emergence of amoxicillin resistance among the nontypeable strains of *H. influenzae.*[23] β-Lactamase production in the latter organism was thought to be associated particularly with therapeutic failure, thereby spawning the development of oral second- and third-generation cephalosporins and newer macrolides as therapeutic alternatives for childhood otitis media.

MECHANISM OF RESISTANCE. The β-lactamases constitute a broad array of enzymes that hydrolyze the β-lactam ring of selected antibiotics (Fig. 233–1). Most β-lactamases are structurally similar to the PBPs, and at least some of the β-lactamases are thought to be evolutionarily derived from them.[201] β-Lactamases can be identified in both gram-positive and gram-negative bacteria. In the former, the enzyme is secreted into the cell-free environment, whereas in the latter, most enzymes are confined to and concentrated in the periplasmic space between the cell wall and the outer membrane.

By the late 1990s, nearly 200 β-lactamases had been characterized,[34] and doubtless, many more exist in nature. They have been categorized variously according to substrate preference, isoelectric focus, whether they are encoded on the bacterial chromosome or an episome, their ability to be inhibited by clavulanate, and their molecular structure. The molecular classification of Ambler[2] proposed in the early 1980s still is used widely. This classification divides the β-lactamases into four categories, A through D, although all but B, the metallo-enzymes, have proved to have similar three-dimensional conformations.

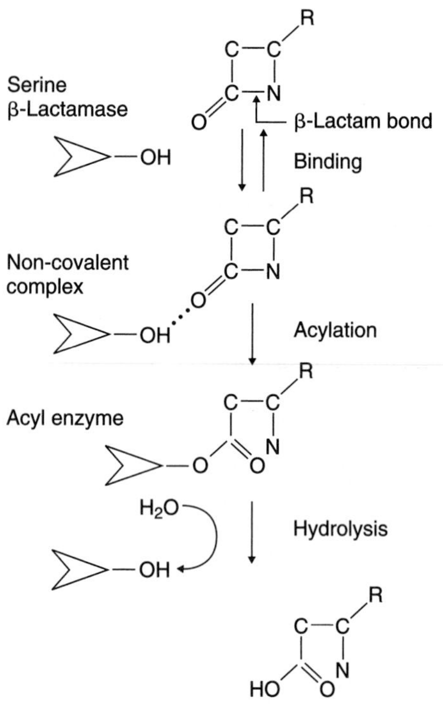

FIGURE 233–1 ■ Mode of action of β-lactamases. (classes A, C, and D).

The updated classification system of Bush, Jacoby, and Medeiros, proposed in 1995,[34] divides these enzymes into four groups (with subcategories) by using virtually all the aforementioned properties to discriminate one class of enzyme from the others. The properties of the three most important groups according to this system are summarized in Table 233–2. The group 1 enzymes (also referred to as "AmpC" β-lactamases) hydrolyze virtually all β-lactam antibiotics except the carbapenems and are resistant to inhibition by clavulanate. These enzymes are chromosomally encoded on a sequence labeled *ampC* in a wide range of gram-negative bacteria; however, the AmpC β-lactamases are expressed in quantities sufficient to produce clinically important resistance only in selected species, including *Enterobacter cloacae, Serratia marcescens, Citrobacter*

TABLE 233–2 ■ PROPERTIES OF THE MAJOR GROUPS OF β-LACTAMASES

BJM* Group	1	2	3
Ambler Class	C	A, D	B
Substrate preference	All but carbapenems	Variable†	Variable (carbapenems)
Chromosomal/plasmid	C	P	C/P
Distribution	Gram-neg	Gram-neg/gram-pos	Gram-neg
Clavulanate inhibition	No	Yes	No
Inducible‡	Yes	No	No

*Bush, Jacoby, and Medeiros.
†May be divided into subgroups including penicillinases, cephalosporinases, cloxacillinases, and carbapenemases. Enzymes frequently can hydrolyze more than one group of β-lactam.
‡Indicates that normally repressed β-lactamase production can be induced by β-lactam exposure.

freundii, *Pseudomonas aeruginosa*, and *Morganella morganii*. In the absence of drug exposure, expression of the group 1 AmpC β-lactamases in these species is repressed by an upstream sequence labeled *amp*R[19, 201, 236] (Fig. 233–2). However, exposure of the bacteria to a β-lactam leads to the production and cytoplasmic processing of a bacterial cell wall metabolite by the enzyme AmpD.[141, 178] The AmpD product interacts with *amp*R to reverse the repression, and relevant quantities of the AmpC β-lactamase are subsequently synthesized.

β-Lactam antibiotics differ in their ability to induce AmpC β-lactamases by this mechanism. Ampicillin, cefoxitin, and imipenem are potent inducers, whereas most of the third-generation cephalosporins are weak. However, spontaneous mutations leading to a dysfunctional AmpD enzyme, which occur at high frequency in nature, lead to the accumulation of peptidoglycan degradation products that in turn results in permanent de-repression of the *amp*C gene and constitutive, large-quantity production of the AmpC β-lactamase (see Fig. 233–2). De-repressed organisms are rendered highly resistant after this single mutational step. The third-generation cephalosporins are particularly prone to selecting such AmpD mutants, and the clinical emergence of resistant de-repressed isolates during the course of treatment with a third-generation cephalosporin has been documented.[50]

The Bush, Jacoby, and Medeiros group 2 β-lactamases include a wide variety of enzymes that are encoded primarily on plasmids.[34, 123, 157, 209, 219, 236] These plasmids commonly contain resistance determinants to other antibiotic classes as well. The plasmids are stable in nature and frequently are maintained within the bacteria even in the absence of antibiotic pressure. Moreover, they can be transmitted by conjugation from organism to organism and across species,

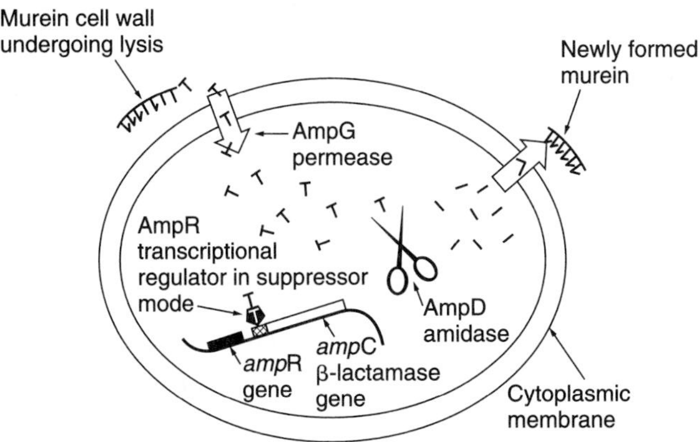

FIGURE 233–2 ■ A model for peptidoglycan recycling and β-lactamase induction in enterobacteria. The lytic transglycosylases in the periplasm cleave the bond between *N*-acetylglucosamine (GlcNac) and *N*-acetyluramic acid (MurNac) and form the peptidoglycan degradation product *N*-acetylglucosaminyl-1,6-anhydro-*N*-acetylmuramyl-L-alanyl-D-glutamyl-meso-diaminopimelic acid (T). The AmpG permease transports T into the cytoplasm. The AmpD amidase specifically recognizes substrate containing anhydro muramic acid and cleaves the bond between it and L-alanine, with subsequent release of the stem tripeptide L-Ala-D-Glu-m-A_2pm (I). Unprocessed T activates the AmpR transcriptional regulator, thereby inducing β-lactamase production. The tripeptide I, on the other hand, recycles to form new peptidoglycan. By regulating the relative amounts of T versus I, AmpD may control peptidoglycan composition.

sometimes leading to a "plasmid outbreak" in a confined environment (e.g., a nursing home or intensive care unit) caused by different species containing the same plasmid.[323] The group 2 enzymes have a range of substrate preferences that have become more and more extensive with the introduction of each new class of β-lactam antibiotic; this enhanced range of substrates has resulted in the evolution of "extended-spectrum β-lactamases" (ESBLs). Characteristically, the group 2 enzymes are inhibited by clavulanate and are found in both gram-positive and gram-negative bacteria[34, 157, 201] (see Table 233–2).

The prototypic group 2 β-lactamases are included in the TEM and SHV families of enzymes, although a large number of group 2 enzymes not belonging to either of these families also have been characterized. TEM-1, first identified in Europe in 1963, hydrolyzed ampicillin. During the ensuing decades, the TEM sequence mutated in a stepwise fashion (with each new iteration labeled sequentially: TEM-2, TEM-3, and so on), which has resulted in the ability of each new enzyme to degrade an ever-increasing number of β-lactam antibiotics.[75, 201] Many of these mutations widen a critical cavity formed by the three-dimensional configuration of the molecule; this cavity contains a serine active site at its bottom, which is key to hydrolysis of the β-lactam.[103] Although these mutations render the enzymes kinetically less efficient than their parents, they allow entry of the newer β-lactams with their bulky side chains into the cavity and thereby enable the serine active site at the bottom to reach the β-lactam ring.[75, 201]

The Bush, Jacoby, and Medeiros group 3 β-lactamases are composed of the metallo-enzymes.[33, 34] These β-lactamases are genetically heterogeneous and structurally dissimilar to those of groups 1 and 2. To date, they remain relatively infrequent and geographically confined.[33] Initially, they were identified on the bacterial chromosome, but more recent varieties have been plasmid-borne. Their substrate preference varies, but organisms identified in Japan in the latter 1990s hydrolyze the carbapenems. These enzymes are not inhibited by clavulanate. Frequently, organisms encoding a metallo-enzyme express other chromosomal and plasmid-encoded β-lactamases as well.

Although the properties summarized in Table 233–2 apply to most of the enzymes in each group, many exceptions have been noted. For example, enzymes that are genetically homologous to the group 2 family, typically plasmid-borne, have been identified on the bacterial chromosome in some isolates of *S. marcescens* and *E. cloacae*.[201] Conversely, group 1 AmpC enzymes, typically located on the bacterial chromosome, recently have been identified on plasmids.[219, 236] Some rare group 2–type enzymes are inducible.[201] TEM-type enzymes that are resistant to clavulanate have been identified (the so-called inhibitor-resistant TEMs [IRTs]).[33, 43, 157]

The degree of resistance exhibited by an organism encoding a β-lactamase frequently depends not only on the enzyme's in vitro substrate specificity and kinetics but also on the amount of enzyme produced. Hyperproduction of β-lactamase is usually the result of some alteration in a controlling sequence or an increase in copy number of the β-lactamase gene within the bacterium.[89, 102, 227, 327, 330] High-level resistance results, and the susceptibility of the organism diminishes with increasing numbers of such altered bacteria. Consequently, the organism may appear clinically unresponsive to a β-lactam antibiotic if hyperproduction occurs in the context of a high-inoculum disease. In some circumstances, hyperproduction operates in concert with other mechanisms to derive a resistant phenotype. Thus, some isolates of *E. cloacae* and *P. aeruginosa* have been rendered carbapenem-resistant through a combination of hyperproduction of an AmpC β-lactamase, which is normally ineffective in hydrolyzing the carbapenems, and simultaneous loss of the outer-membrane porin through which imipenem traverses to reach the PBP.[47, 51]

Alteration of Penicillin-Binding Proteins

CLINICAL RELEVANCE. Not until recognition of penicillin-resistant *Streptococcus pneumoniae* did pediatricians began to realize that alterations in PBPs in the bacterial cell wall might pose a major clinical problem.[40, 153, 195] These organisms seemed to emerge as pediatric pathogens in the late 1980s at just about the time that the challenges associated with β-lactamase–producing organisms appeared to be reasonably addressed. Before this occurrence, the experience with altered penicillin binding as a mechanism of antibiotic resistance had been limited to a few patients with infections caused by methicillin-resistant *S. aureus* (MRSA). The identification of patients with pneumococcal infections caused by organisms resistant to penicillin created tremendous consternation within the pediatric infectious disease community. However, to date, the precise clinical importance of these organisms remains unclear.

Part of the problem in assessing the clinical importance of altered penicillin binding among pneumococci is that rather than simply conferring penicillin resistance, the gene or genes coding for this altered enzyme activity often cosegregate with genes coding for resistance to other antibiotics such as trimethoprim-sulfamethoxazole (TMP-SMX) and the macrolides.[68, 285, 286] Thus, unlike resistance associated with the elaboration of β-lactamase, for which simply selecting a different class of antibiotic often will provide a reasonable solution, resistance associated with alteration in PBPs is multifarious and, if clinically important, may require significant alterations in clinical practice to provide an effective antimicrobial regimen. The more limited menu of antibiotic choices for the treatment of infections caused by these organisms has led to some interesting therapeutic conventions. For example, because the basis for this type of resistance is akin to altered enzyme affinity, researchers recognized in the mid-1990s that they might be able to overcome the apparent decrease in efficacy by simply increasing the dose of β-lactam.[153, 196, 197] Of the available agents, only amoxicillin had the requisite therapeutic index to support the increased dosing strategy. On this basis (almost exclusively), the high-dose amoxicillin regimen (80 to 100 mg/kg/day), which currently is recommended, was adopted. Additionally, the perceived need for a drug effective against antibiotic-resistant *S. pneumoniae* has led to widespread use of the parenteral third-generation cephalosporin ceftriaxone in the setting of common upper and lower respiratory tract infections because of its in vitro activity against these organisms.

As the clinical impact of the emergence of antibiotic-resistant *S. pneumoniae* has been examined more carefully in recent years, several trends have surfaced.[153, 195, 329] In immunocompetent patients with pneumonia and most other non–central nervous system (CNS) pneumococcal infections, no difference in outcome appears to exist between patients infected with organisms that are susceptible to penicillin and those infected with organisms showing decreased susceptibility to penicillin.[226] Moreover, no association between the intrinsic virulence of the organism and its antibiotic susceptibility has been found. In contrast, in patients with pneumococcal meningitis caused by organisms with decreased penicillin susceptibility, a delay in cerebrospinal fluid (CSF) sterilization appears to occur with standard treatment.[182, 328] For this reason, the current recommendation for empiric treatment of bacterial meningitis in infants and children consists of a combination of ceftriaxone or cefotaxime and vancomycin until the identity of the organism and its antibiotic susceptibility are known.

S. pneumoniae remains the most prevalent bacterial cause of acute otitis media in infants and children.[23] The clinical importance of the antibiotic susceptibility of these organisms in this clinical setting remains difficult to ascertain. The infection has a high rate of spontaneous resolution, and virtually all treatment is provided on an empiric basis. Consequently, any improved cure rate related to altered prescribing practices aimed at greater activity against organisms with decreased antibiotic susceptibility would be difficult to substantiate. Finally, the importance and virulence of these organisms in children who are either immunocompromised or immunosuppressed remains to be determined unequivocally.

MECHANISM OF RESISTANCE. β-Lactam antibiotics must bind to PBPs to confer their activity, and alteration of PBP structure results in diminished affinity for drug and, consequently, antibiotic resistance. The PBPs are a heterogeneous group of compounds normally responsible for maintaining the peptidoglycan matrix supporting the bacterial cell wall. PBPs vary from species to species in number, size, copy number per cell, and affinity for β-lactam agents.[100, 117, 265] Typically, four to eight PBPs are present in any given bacterial isolate; they range in molecular weight from 35 to 120 kd.[100] By convention, the PBPs are numbered in order of decreasing molecular weight. PBPs possess two principal enzymatic activities. In general, the larger PBPs are responsible for peptidoglycan transpeptidase activity, whereas the smaller PBPs usually carry D,D-carboxypeptidase activity.[100] They constitute the final reactions in formation of the peptidoglycan matrix and are responsible for the cross-linkage that significantly adds to the tensile strength of the bacterial cell surface.

Examination of PBP-mediated β-lactam resistance in *S. pneumoniae* and *S. aureus* serves to exemplify some of the features of this mechanism of resistance. Detailed investigations indicate that penicillin resistance in pneumococcus is associated with alternations in PBP types 1A, 1B, 2A, 2X, and 2B; cephalosporin resistance has been correlated with structural abnormalities in PBP types 1A, 2A, and 2X.[17, 55, 110, 116, 118, 137, 214] Confirmation that the resistant phenotype is related directly to structural abnormalities in various pneumococcal PBPs has been achieved through transformation experiments.[17, 55, 110, 214] In these studies, penicillin-susceptible strains are converted to resistant ones by the addition of amplified DNA encoding the putative resistant PBPs. Patterns of PBPs from resistant pneumococci vary considerably from geographic location to location, thus indicating that PBP-related pneumococcal resistance probably arose independently in various parts of the world.[116]

PBPs from penicillin-resistant *S. pneumoniae* contain blocks of amino acid sequences that are remarkably divergent from those seen in susceptible pneumococci. These sequences are homologous to those coding for PBPs from other streptococcal species (e.g., *Streptococcus oralis* and *Streptococcus mitis*), which suggests that resistant pneumococci contain mosaic PBPs that arose after transformation and recombination of homologous genes from closely related bacteria.[72, 73, 115, 165] These sequences then developed point mutations conferring resistance. A similar pattern of "resistance blocks" of amino acids has been identified in the PBPs of penicillin-resistant *Neisseria gonorrhoeae*; these blocks likewise appear to have originated from other *Neisseria* spp.[117] The degree of resistance conferred by a single mutated PBP is relatively small.[100, 110] Acquisition of multiple abnormal PBPs results in incremental resistance and, ultimately, an organism that can survive routine β-lactam therapy.

The complexity of the genetics underlying PBP-associated β-lactam resistance is apparent in MRSA. All isolates of MRSA contain the *mecA* gene, a 2130-bp chromosomal sequence encoding PBP-2A, which unlike other staphylococcal PBPs, has low affinity for β-lactam antibiotics.[61, 62, 117] In the presence of methicillin concentrations inhibitory to susceptible staphylococci, MRSA PBP-2A assumes virtually all responsibility for peptidoglycan synthesis, with the resultant production of a matrix of unusual muropeptide composition. Some MRSA strains encode regulatory sequences for *mecA* termed *mecRI*, whose product is a transmembrane sensor needed for induction of *mecA* expression in the presence of β-lactam, and an inhibitory controlling sequence (*mecI*).[117] However, the degree of methicillin resistance is not well correlated with the amount of expressed PBP-2A,[61, 62] thus indicating that other cellular factors are important for production of the resistant phenotype. Transposon inactivation experiments have identified multiple additional sites on the staphylococcal chromosome critical for methicillin resistance. These sequences, termed *fem* (*f*actors *e*ssential for *m*ethicillin resistance) genes, express abundant substrate for PBP-2A, which in turn is available to successfully compete with methicillin and other β-lactam antibiotics for the PBP-2A active site.[117] Dysfunction of the *fem* genes and absence of these peptidoglycan precursors result in reversion to the methicillin-susceptible phenotype, even in the presence of *mecA*-encoded PBP-2A. Similar mechanisms appear to operate in methicillin-resistant, coagulase-negative staphylococci.

MACROLIDES, LINCOSAMIDES, AND STREPTOGRAMINS

CLINICAL RELEVANCE. The macrolides are compounds that contain 14-member (e.g., erythromycin and clarithromycin), 15-member (e.g., azithromycin), or 16-member (e.g., spiramycin) lactone rings. Their activity is directed primarily against gram-positive organisms and some gram-negative respiratory tract pathogens. In many bacteria, resistance to macrolides occurs concomitantly with that of the structurally unrelated lincosamide (including clindamycin) and streptogramin B families of antibiotics, two classes with activity also primarily against gram-positive bacteria. Because these three families of antibiotics interact competitively for ribosomal binding, they probably are associated with the same ribosomal site.

Resistance to the macrolides was noted in staphylococcal species soon after the introduction of erythromycin. More recently, however, macrolide resistance in streptococcal species has emerged and assumed major clinical importance. The late 20th century witnessed dramatic increases in the incidence of macrolide resistance in *S. pneumoniae* in many areas of the world.[124] In Southeast Asia, surveys have indicated that nearly 40 percent of pneumococcal isolates are resistant to all macrolide antibiotics, whereas sampling of organisms from Europe and the Western Hemisphere showed similar, but less dramatic trends.[124, 156, 262] In Atlanta, pneumococcal isolates causing invasive disease became increasingly resistant to erythromycin throughout the 1990s (31% by 1999), and the mean minimal inhibitory concentration (MIC) of these resistant isolates against the macrolides increased as well.[98] Macrolide resistance among *S. pneumoniae* is a result of both international dissemination of resistant clones and horizontal transmission of resistance determinants.[99, 262] Perhaps most troubling, resistance to macrolides among pneumococci is found particularly frequently in isolates co-expressing resistance to penicillin and other oral antibiotics.[136]

Increasing macrolide resistance also has been noted in other streptococcal species, specifically two organisms for which macrolides are the preferred agent in a penicillin-allergic host: *Streptococcus pyogenes* (group A streptococci) and *Streptococcus agalactiae* (group B streptococci). Macrolide resistance in group A streptococci has been distributed unevenly geographically.[154] By the early 21st century, most surveys in the Western Hemisphere, including the United States, indicated an incidence of resistance of approximately 10 percent or less,[152, 225, 318] although the city-wide clonal outbreak of macrolide-resistant group A streptococcus experienced in Pittsburgh in 2001 highlights the potential for this phenotype to spread rapidly within a community.[187] In Finland, by contrast, resistance in group A streptococci approached 20 percent in the 1990s, and in Turin, Italy, the incidence of resistance was greater than 40 percent.[266] Similarly, surveys of group B streptococci have demonstrated erythromycin resistance in 20 to 40 percent of isolates in the United States,[210] France,[63] and Taiwan.[133]

The increase in macrolide resistance occurred concomitantly with increased worldwide use of these compounds for respiratory tract infections in the 1980s and 1990s,[53, 108, 136, 275, 292] thus suggesting a biologic association between these two phenomena. A nationwide survey of macrolide susceptibility among pneumococcal isolates in the United States, for example, documented an increase in erythromycin resistance from 10.6 percent in 1995 to 20.4 percent in 1999, a time when the number of prescriptions for macrolides increased by 13 percent across the board and by 320 percent in pediatric patients.[136] Seppälä and colleagues reported an increase in resistance among *S. pyogenes* isolates in Finland from 5 percent in 1988 to 13 percent in 1990 after national macrolide use doubled through the 1980s. In response, a national campaign to reduce macrolide-prescribing practices in Finland was launched in the early 1990s, after which macrolide resistance fell by half.[275]

The relationship between macrolide exposure and the emergence of macrolide resistance at the individual patient level is more complicated. The incidence of nasopharyngeal colonization with macrolide-resistant organisms usually decreases after dosing with a macrolide antibiotic, but less so than when colonized with susceptible organisms. Consequently, the proportion of resistant organisms versus susceptible ones increases, even as the absolute incidence of colonization with resistant organisms is lowered.[156, 167, 211, 310] Moreover, in most persons, the ecology of nasopharyngeal colonization gradually returns to baseline after the course of antibiotics is completed.

Although the epidemiologic trends in macrolide resistance are alarming, the clinical consequences of the increase in macrolide resistance among streptococci are unknown. Current convention uses an MIC of 2 μg/mL or greater to define resistance. The newer macrolide compounds, however, achieve tissue and intracellular concentrations that are many-fold higher.[81, 204] The relationship between infection with a macrolide-resistant pathogen and clinical failure after prescription of a macrolide antibiotic is not well established. Case reports of clinical failure of macrolides in the face of bacteremia caused by resistant organisms have been published.[88] Italian investigators, on the other hand, noted a very high incidence of erythromycin resistance among group A streptococcal throat isolates, but neither clinical nor microbiologic failures were associated clearly with macrolide treatment.[309]

A new group of related antibiotics, the ketolides, which contain chemical modifications of the lactone ring, are in development. To date, they have proven in vitro activity against organisms that express high-level macrolide resistance.[204, 212]

Although the MICs of ketolides for macrolide-resistant organisms are higher than those for macrolide-susceptible bacteria, they remain well within the range of concentrations achieved with standard dosing. The ketolides also have shown excellent cure rates in animal models infected with organisms expressing different macrolide resistance phenotypes.[204]

MECHANISM OF RESISTANCE. Two principal resistance phenotypes to macrolides and related antibiotics have been detected. The first, denoted the MLS_B phenotype, is characterized by resistance to all macrolides regardless of ring size, as well as to the lincosamides and type B streptogramins. Most organisms expressing the MLS_B phenotype remain susceptible to the combination streptogramins (e.g., quinupristin-dalfopristin).[94, 270] The second phenotype, denoted the M phenotype, is associated with resistance to the 14- and 15-member macrolides (including erythromycin, azithromycin, and clarithromycin), but not to those with 16-member rings. The degree of resistance to the affected macrolides is lower on average than that seen with MLS_B resistance. In addition, in organisms with the M phenotype, susceptibility to clindamycin is preserved.[98, 191, 290]

Most MLS_B resistance results from methylation of the 23S ribosomal RNA (rRNA) in the 50S subunit of the bacterial ribosome within the peptidyltransferase circle in domain V.[64, 143, 295, 320] The methylases are encoded on transposons, with sequences found both on plasmids and in the bacterial chromosome. Methylation of the 23S rRNA is encoded by a family of related genes labeled *erm* (*e*rythromycin *r*esistance *m*ethylases).[64, 143, 295, 320] Historically, these methylases have been described and named in a haphazard fashion. Recently, investigators have suggested a classification scheme based on genetic homology in which 21 different groups of *erm* genes are enumerated.[255]

Methylation is both inducible and constitutively expressed. Unlike many other inducible antibiotic resistance factors, the mechanism of MLS_B resistance induction is at the level of translation rather than transcription.[317] In the uninduced state, the leader sequence of the mRNA encoding ErmC, one of the methylases found in *S. aureus*, forms two stem loop structures that stall the ribosome's movement along the message, thereby preventing synthesis of the methylase enzyme. Attachment of erythromycin to the ribosome leads to a conformational alteration in this leader sequence that uncovers the appropriate ribosomal binding sites and allows the stalled ribosomes to proceed to translation.[317] Through the 1990s, greater numbers of *erm*-containing bacteria produced the rRNA methylase constitutively, a consequence of mutation of the leader sequence.

In the mid-1990s, macrolide resistance mediated through a genetically transferable efflux pump was identified.[290] The majority of organisms expressing the M phenotype are resistant through this mechanism. Most macrolide-resistant pneumococci in North America express the macrolide efflux pump, and much of the expansion of macrolide resistance through the 1990s was a result of the appearance of organisms exhibiting this mechanism.[136, 149, 177] A family of related genes, termed *mef,* encode the macrolide efflux pumps. The *mef* genes are included on transposons encoding associated functions, in particular, an adenosine triphosphate (ATP)-binding protein.[98, 99, 191] As expected, ribosomes isolated from organisms resistant through *mef* genes bind to macrolide antibiotics as readily as do ribosomes from susceptible organisms. Radiolabeled erythromycin is excluded from the intracellular space in *mef*-positive bacteria, a phenomenon that is reversed by compounds that poison ATP-dependent pumps.[290]

Mechanisms of macrolide resistance besides rRNA methylation and efflux pumps have been identified but to date occur rarely. Some organisms modify the antibiotic by hydrolysis, acetylation, phosphorylation, or esterification.[255] Evidence indicates that some erythromycin resistance is caused by altered ribosomal proteins, which results in the production of ribosomes with diminished affinity for drug.[48]

TRIMETHOPRIM AND SULFAMETHOXAZOLE

CLINICAL RELEVANCE. The combination antibiotic TMP-SMX inhibits bacterial folate synthesis at two successive steps. This mechanism accounted for its broad activity against a wide variety of gram-positive and gram-negative bacteria when it was introduced in 1968. Despite its dual activity, resistance to TMP-SMX has risen steadily over the decades of its use and now is commonplace. Acquisition of resistance is potentiated by recent exposure to TMP-SMX.[82, 287, 326] When resistance occurs, the MIC expressed is usually very high,[134, 135] and the affected organisms are frequently co-resistant to multiple other classes of antibiotics. Indeed, TMP-SMX resistance is sufficiently widespread that it largely precludes use of the drug as a first-line antibiotic in clinical circumstances in which it formerly was the agent of choice, namely, respiratory tract infections, urinary tract infections (UTIs), and *Shigella*-associated dysentery.

Respiratory Tract Infections (Otitis Media and Pneumonia). The frequency of TMP-SMX resistance in organisms causing respiratory tract infection has increased dramatically. Among *S. pneumoniae,* resistance to TMP-SMX was identified during the 1990s in many geographic locations, with resistance detected in 12 percent to over 50 percent of isolates.[67, 124, 132, 186, 230, 258, 288] A worldwide survey conducted in the late 1990s noted the highest incidence of TMP-SMX pneumococcal resistance in the Asian Pacific region and Latin America.[124] In surveys of American isolates, TMP-SMX resistance is the most common resistance phenotype found in *S. pneumoniae,*[322] although the incidence of resistance varies widely from region to region.[67] TMP-SMX resistance is associated strongly with resistance to other classes of antibiotics commonly used in respiratory tract infections, particularly penicillin and the macrolides. Among other organisms implicated in respiratory tract infections, TMP-SMX resistance also has been documented with increasing frequency in *H. influenzae,* with resistance ranging from 7 percent in Finland[186] to more than 50 percent in Taiwan.[132] TMP-SMX resistance among *M. catarrhalis* isolates remains uncommon.[124, 186, 336]

The clinical consequences of TMP-SMX resistance are not well defined. Direct evidence of an association between isolation of a TMP-SMX–resistant organism from the middle ear and failure of TMP-SMX therapy in acute otitis media, for example, is lacking, but such an association is assumed to exist. The issue of the clinical relevance of TMP-SMX resistance in respiratory tract infections is particularly pressing in underdeveloped countries, where World Health Organization guidelines recommend TMP-SMX as a first-line agent for pneumonia. A comparison of amoxicillin and TMP-SMX for pneumonia in Pakistan demonstrated superiority of amoxicillin in producing clinical cure, but failure was not associated with resistance in the infecting organism.[289] These data and others[155, 257] support continued use of TMP-SMX therapy for pneumonia in the developing world, as least at present.

Urinary Tract Infections. Through the 1990s, TMP-SMX resistance in urinary tract isolates of *E. coli,* the most prominent pathogen implicated in UTIs, rose to 15 to 25 percent in the developed world and to as high as 60 percent in nonindustrialized countries.[113, 114, 185, 326, 336] Studies in the

1990s indicated that TMP-SMX–resistant *E. coli* can be transmitted to household contacts.[259] Indeed, one analysis suggested that TMP-SMX–resistant urinary tract isolates from geographically disparate areas of the United States may have emanated from a single clone.[185] Although urinary concentrations of both trimethoprim and sulfamethoxazole are several-fold higher than concomitant concentrations in serum, resistance to TMP-SMX nonetheless is associated with treatment failure in UTIs. Bacterial and clinical response rates to TMP-SMX are approximately 80 to 95 percent for cystitis and pyelonephritis caused by susceptible organisms, but response falls to approximately 50 percent when the infecting agent is TMP-SMX–resistant.[190, 194, 293] Consequently, because of the additional expense of clinical failure, analyses have indicated that the total cost of treatment of UTIs with TMP-SMX begins to exceed that incurred by therapy with more expensive antibiotics, such as the fluoroquinolones, when community resistance rates of urinary pathogens exceeds about 20 percent.[166, 293]

Shigellosis. Resistance of *Shigella* spp. to TMP-SMX rose dramatically during the 1980s in many parts of the world, including Bangladesh,[20] Thailand,[125] Somalia,[39] Israel,[8] and Canada.[119] In these surveys, the incidence of disease caused by TMP-SMX–resistant *Shigella* increased twofold to threefold, to well over half the isolates; by 1998, more than 90 percent of *Shigella* in Thailand,[125] as well as *Shigella* cultured from patients with acquired immunodeficiency syndrome in Kenya,[163] were resistant to TMP-SMX. A large proportion of these *Shigella* strains express extraordinarily high levels of resistance, with MICs to trimethoprim exceeding 1000 μg/mL. In the United States, TMP-SMX resistance among *Shigella* organisms initially was confined to closed populations.[111] A more recent survey in Oregon, however, indicated that by the late 1990s, the incidence of TMP-SMX resistance among *Shigella* isolates in that state approached 60 percent. Resistant isolates were found disproportionately frequently in migrant workers traveling from Mexico and other areas of Latin America,[250] thus emphasizing the importance of geographic spread of resistance in modern society. The incidence of TMP-SMX resistance in *Shigella* mirrors the increased TMP-SMX resistance among other enteric species as well,[111, 306] notably *Salmonella*.[1]

TMP-SMX resistance in *Shigella* virtually always is borne on conjugative plasmids, and frequently these plasmids contain resistance determinants to several other antibiotic classes.[39, 111, 163, 176, 306] Co-resistance to four or more unrelated antibiotics, including β-lactams, chloramphenicol, tetracycline, and the aminoglycosides, is a common finding. Molecular analysis in a given geographic environment usually indicates a fluid epidemiology, with multiple dominant chromosomal genotypes containing a variety of resistance plasmids.[26, 176] Exchange of these determinants among enteric species in the gut is suspected strongly.

MECHANISMS OF RESISTANCE. In susceptible bacteria, TMP-SMX inhibits sequential steps in the de novo synthesis of folate (Fig. 233–3). Sulfamethoxazole inhibits the enzyme dihydropteroate synthetase (DHPS), which catalyzes the conversion of para-aminobenzoic acid to dihydrofolate. Trimethoprim inhibits the next enzyme in the pathway, namely, dihydrofolate reductase (DHFR), which catalyzes the conversion of dihydrofolate to tetrahydrofolate. The resulting depletion of folate within the bacterium interrupts the synthesis of critical cellular substrates, including purine nucleotides.[256] Eukaryotic DHFR is resistant to the activity of sulfonamides, and eukaryotic cells do not express DHPS activity at all, which accounts for the selective activity of these drugs against bacteria.[134, 135]

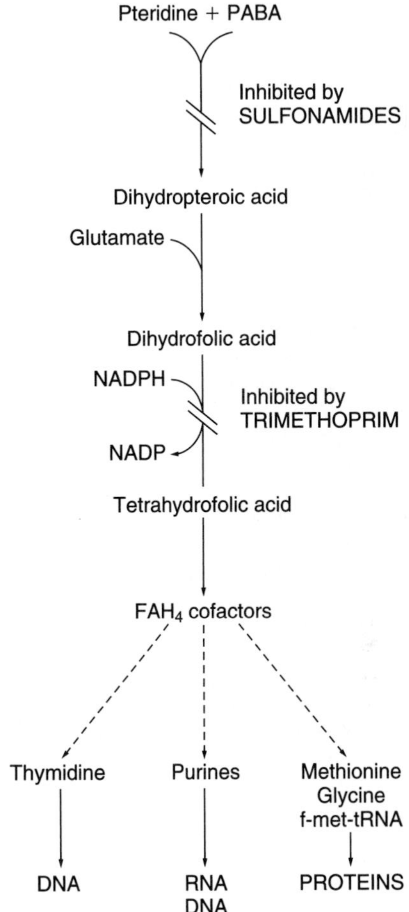

FIGURE 233–3 ■ Trimethoprim-sulfamethoxazole inhibition of de novo folate synthesis.

The principal mechanism of resistance to TMP-SMX is alteration of the target enzymes. Altered genes for DHFR with reduced susceptibility to trimethoprim have been identified on the chromosomes of intrinsically resistant organisms from a variety of species,[241] as well as on transferable elements. Many of the transferable resistance genes are encoded on transposons that can shuttle between plasmids and chromosomal DNA. Approximately 20 different transferable *dhfr* resistance genes have been identified.[135] Resistance usually is conferred by a single point mutation that results in disruption of the three-dimensional conformation of DHFR; a hydrogen bond normally available for binding the antibiotic is interrupted, but the affinity for its natural substrate is left intact.[58, 135, 241] These structural changes may occur in concert with mutations in controlling sequences that lead to overproduction of the altered DHFR.[241] Similarly, sulfonamide resistance is usually the result of mutated *dhps* genes. In TMP-SMX–resistant *Neisseria meningitidis,* the abnormal chromosomal *dhps* sequence is different from that found in susceptible isolates over a large portion of the gene, thus implying that resistance resulted from a recombination event after horizontal transfer from an unrelated *Neisseria* spp.[244] Similar recombination events may account for sulfonamide resistance in pneumococci. In other species, the abnormal *dhps* gene is the result of a single amino acid mutation, and the resistance gene is encoded on a transmissible transposon,[224] frequently linked to a *dhfr* resistance gene.[135]

Some organisms, particularly *P. aeruginosa,* are intrinsically resistant to TMP-SMX on the basis of the expression of multidrug efflux pumps.[158] The same pumps are responsible for resistance to a wide variety of other antibiotics, including fluoroquinolones, chloramphenicol, and β-lactams. Homologous pumps occasionally have been identified in other gram-negative species as well. Finally, in some isolates, the mechanism of resistance to TMP-SMX is not attributable to any of the aforementioned mechanisms and remains undefined.[135, 224]

AMINOGLYCOSIDES

CLINICAL RELEVANCE. The aminoglycosides are parenteral antibiotics that are used primarily for serious infections in hospitalized patients. Resistance to aminoglycosides is encoded on transmissible elements that have disseminated throughout the world, both among gram-negative and among gram-positive pathogens. In gram-negative species, resistance to the aminoglycosides varies widely from one geographic location to another.[269, 271] Surveys of hospital isolates conducted throughout Europe in the late 1990s indicated resistance rates of 1 to 15 percent among enteric bacilli and 10 to 40 percent among non–lactose fermenters.[85, 162, 269, 271, 308] In all cases, the incidence of resistance was lowest to amikacin.[269, 271] Aminoglycoside resistance occurs with much higher frequency in gram-negative organisms with coexisting resistance to other antibiotics.[14, 96] Not surprisingly, fecal colonization with aminoglycoside-resistant bacilli seldom occurs in healthy persons.[139, 172, 174, 221] Although resistance to some of the older aminoglycosides, such as streptomycin and kanamycin, has disseminated into the community, carriage of organisms resistant to gentamicin is a rare occurrence in ambulatory populations.[139, 172, 174, 221]

Few data exist on the endemic incidence of aminoglycoside resistance in gram-negative organisms specifically in hospitalized children. In a survey of pediatric patients in an intensive care unit (ICU) in Cleveland in the mid-1990s, approximately 10 percent of patients were colonized before discharge with a tobramycin-resistant, gram-negative bacillus.[303] A survey in the neonatal ICU in the same institution, where gentamicin was used frequently, recorded an approximate 5 percent endemic incidence of colonization with gentamicin-resistant bacilli.[302] However, outbreaks caused by gram-negative rods resistant to aminoglycoside have been reported from numerous neonatal ICUs during the past 20 years.[57, 146, 199]

Although the aminoglycosides have no utility in the treatment of infections with gram-positive organisms when used alone, they improve killing when administered in combination with cell wall–active agents. For this reason, they frequently are added to β-lactam agents or vancomycin when treating difficult or persistent infections caused by *S. aureus*, coagulase-negative staphylococci, or enterococci. However, resistance to aminoglycosides has been documented in all these gram-positive microorganisms. Recent surveys in Europe have indicated 20 to 30 percent resistance to aminoglycosides among hospital isolates of *S. aureus*.[269] The incidence of aminoglycoside resistance is 15-fold higher in MRSA than in bacteria that are methicillin-susceptible.[85] As with gram-negative bacilli, aminoglycoside resistance among *S. aureus* strains varies greatly from region to region[162, 271] but correlates largely with the incidence of MRSA. Several surveys from France in the late 1990s actually reported a decrease in aminoglycoside resistance among MRSA, largely attributed to the introduction of dominant strains expressing a more heterogeneous resistance to methicillin as well.[10, 21, 171] Aminoglycoside resistance in coagulase-negative staphylococci also occurs commonly. As with *S. aureus*, resistance occurs much more frequently in organisms that are methicillin-resistant (seen in over half the isolates tested from centers around the world), as opposed to the unusual hospital-acquired, methicillin-susceptible, coagulase-negative staphylococci, which have a recorded resistance to aminoglycosides of less than 10 percent.[65, 269]

Since the 1970s, a proliferation of enterococci that express MICs to the aminoglycosides exceeding 2000 μg/mL has occurred, thus rendering the organisms resistant to all synergistic effects when used with a cell wall–active agent.[78, 232] Such high-level aminoglycoside resistance has been recorded in approximately 30 percent of enterococcal samples from hospitals throughout the world.[180, 280, 307] Organisms expressing high-level aminoglycoside resistance frequently test highly resistant to ampicillin as well.[232] High-level aminoglycoside resistance also is a common finding in vancomycin-resistant enterococci, especially those identified in the United States.[180]

MECHANISM OF RESISTANCE. The aminoglycosides are hydrophilic sugars composed of one to four rings, with amino groups substituting for some of the hydroxyl groups at sites that vary from drug to drug. The amino groups render the drugs polycationic, and this property allows them to bind with high affinity to selected sequences of nucleic acid.[248] The antibacterial activity of these drugs is due to their binding to specific sites on the 16S rRNA, which in turn interferes with the recognition of transfer RNA during translation and the translocation of tRNA to the peptidyl-tRNA site. Three-dimensional studies of the aminoglycoside-rRNA interaction suggest that this interference is the result of conformational changes in the shape of the rRNA.[161] The affinity of the aminoglycosides to rRNA is 10-fold higher in prokaryotes than in eukaryotes.[247]

The principal mechanism of resistance to the aminoglycosides is through the expression of aminoglycoside-modifying enzymes (Table 233–3). Many of these enzymes are encoded on transposons that reside in plasmids along with other resistance determinates. Three groups of modifying enzymes have been identified: acetyltransferases (AAC), nucleotidyltransferases (ANT), and phosphotransferases (APH), each of which adds its respective moieties to selected side groups of the aminoglycoside sugar rings.[161, 276] Researchers have hypothesized that these genes originated from bacterial housekeeping enzymes and then expanded to include aminoglycosides among their substrates through mutational evolution.[276] Transcription of these resistance genes is constitutive. Most members of each group of modifying enzymes share structural homologies, with minor amino acid variations resulting in specific substrate profiles.[276] The enzymes are subdesignated by the site that they modify and by the resistance profile that they confer (Fig. 233–4). Thus, for example, AAC(6′)-II denotes an aminoglycoside acetyltransferase that substitutes an acetyl group for the amino group at the 6′ site of the aminoglycoside, thereby resulting in resistance pattern II (including in this case, resistance to gentamicin, tobramycin, and sisomicin, but not amikacin). At least one enzyme has been discovered that possesses both acetyltransferase and phosphotransferase activity (designated AAC(6′)-Ie-APH(2″)-Ia).[49, 276] The modifications conferred by these enzymes result in altered electrostatic qualities of the antibiotic and a consequently reduced ability to interact with rRNA.

The pharmaceutical industry has altered the structure of the aminoglycoside compounds to render them poorer substrates for the modifying enzymes. Such alteration has been most successful in the development of amikacin, a kanamycin derivative with a relatively long aminohydroxybutyrate added at the 1 position.[203] This substitution does

TABLE 233–3 ■ AMINOGLYCOSIDE-MODIFYING ENZYMES

Drug	Aminoglycoside* Acetyltransferase (Acetylation)	Aminoglycoside* Nucleotidyltransferase (Adenylation)	Aminoglycoside* Phosphotransferase (Phosphorylation)
Amikacin	X	X	
Gentamicin	X	X	X
Kanamycin	X	X	X
Netilmicin	X		
Neomycin	X	X	X
Streptomycin		X	X
Tobramycin	X	X	X

*The number of susceptible sites on each molecule varies.
Data from Welton, A., and Neu, H. C. (eds.): The Aminoglycosides. New York, Marcel Dekker, 1982.

not interfere with rRNA binding but protects the compound from alteration by many of the modifying enzymes. Consequently, organisms resistant to gentamicin, for example, may remain susceptible to amikacin. Not all positions are protected, however, and amikacin-resistant phenotypes are conferred by numerous modifying enzymes, most notably AAC(6′)-I.[203]

Moderate-level resistance to the aminoglycosides has been achieved by some bacteria through decreased uptake of drug.[203] This mechanism has been noted most frequently in *Pseudomonas.* To date, modification of the ribosomal binding sequences has been identified only rarely as a mechanism of resistance to the aminoglycosides.[203] The sequences involved in aminoglycoside binding are probably sufficiently critical to survival of the organism that mutations within this site are usually fatal.[161]

GLYCOPEPTIDES

CLINICAL RELEVANCE. Vancomycin is one of two glycopeptides available for clinical use. The second, teicoplanin, is licensed in Europe but not the United States. Since the late 1980s, the prevalence of vancomycin resistance in organisms belonging to the genus *Enterococcus* (vancomycin-resistant enterococci [VRE]) has risen alarmingly. VRE are frequently highly resistant to many other antibiotics as well, and

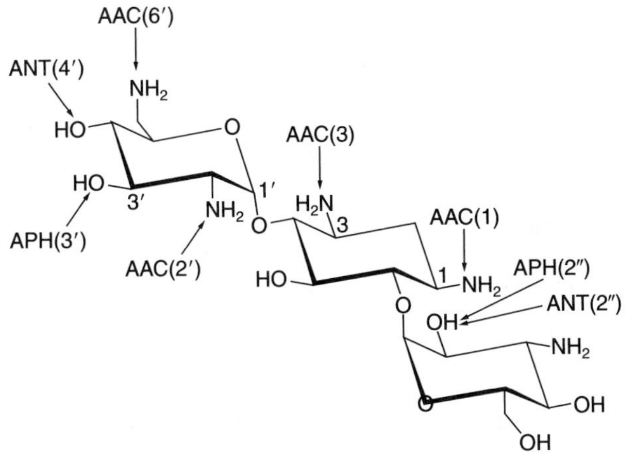

Kanamycin B

FIGURE 233–4 ■ Sites of modification on kanamycin B by various aminoglycoside-modifying enzymes. The *arrows* point to the sites of modification by the specific enzymes—acetyltransferases, phosphotransferases, and nucleotidyltransferases.

reported mortality rates from infection with these resistant organisms exceed 30 percent.[213, 279]

The appearance of VRE in the late 1980s occurred coincident with an increased use of vancomycin in the United States and addition of the glycopeptide avoparcin as a growth promoter in animal feed in Europe, a practice that was banned by the European Union in 1997.[215] The incidence of VRE colonization and disease is much more prevalent in the United States than in other areas of the world.[180] Approximately 17 percent of American enterococcal isolates investigated in a survey in 1999 were resistant to vancomycin.[180] A disproportionate number of VRE in the United States are found in patients in ICUs, especially those with prolonged hospitalization and severe disease.[121, 180, 181, 279, 281] Additionally, a high incidence of VRE is seen among oncology recipients,[77, 206, 279] transplant patients,[15, 223] and those with chronic renal failure treated by dialysis.[9, 313] Some surveys have documented VRE in adults in chronic care facilities, who then export the organism into the community after acquisition in an acute care setting.[304]

Surveys of European centers also indicate a concentration of VRE in ICUs, but in substantially smaller numbers than in the United States.[59, 180, 220, 307, 319] A continent-wide survey of enterococcal isolates in Europe in 1997 indicated that VRE were found in only 10 of 27 countries surveyed, and then only infrequently.[272]

The genetic machinery conferring vancomycin resistance to enterococci is complex, and resistance does not develop de novo by spontaneous mutation under antibiotic pressure.[215] The initial event in the appearance of VRE in a given unit is importation of the resistant organism into the environment. The association between antecedent treatment with vancomycin and acquisition of VRE has been documented by many,[9, 59, 92, 279, 319] but not all investigators.[37, 70, 181] Some have established a stronger connection between the appearance of VRE and the use of extended-spectrum cephalosporins[25, 59, 223] and antibiotics with potent anti-anaerobic activity.[77, 181] A study conducted in a Veteran's Affairs Hospital reported that the stool density of VRE in patients who were treated with anti-anaerobic antibiotics increased exponentially whereas the density decreased in those whose antibiotics had limited anaerobic activity.[69] The principal role of antecedent antibiotic exposure in VRE is possibly to open ecologic niches in the gastrointestinal tract that allow a stable presence of VRE once the patient is exposed to the resistant organism.

Horizontal transmission of VRE is prominent in any closed environment and may outweigh antecedent antibiotic exposure as the principal determinant for acquisition.[121] Patient-to-patient spread in an ICU, presumably through the hands of caregivers, has been documented repeatedly,[206, 223, 281] as has contamination of the immediate environment of a VRE-positive patient.[281] Indeed, perhaps the most significant risk factor for acquisition of VRE is the number of neighboring patients colonized with the organism at the same time.[12, 25]

In many American ICUs, multiple clones of VRE are present at any given moment, some imported into the unit and others spread after admission has occurred,[223] thus rendering control and containment very difficult to achieve. Extreme barrier isolation precautions, including surveillance for VRE on admission to a given unit, single-room isolation with dedicated medical instruments, and strict use of gowns and gloves, are frequently necessary to contain VRE once it has established an endemic presence, and even then these precautions may not be entirely effective.[145, 164, 281] Some units have had improved success with the implementation of cohorting of staff and patients.[207]

With some exceptions,[109, 200, 301] to date VRE have posed less of a threat to pediatric patients than to adults despite the wide use of vancomycin among hospitalized pediatric patients and their geographic proximity in many hospitals to sick adults colonized with the organism. Several outbreaks of VRE in the newborn nursery have been reported,[170, 183, 200] but they have been due primarily to dissemination of a single clone within the unit and have been eradicated with relatively simple barrier isolation and cohorting measures. The presence of VRE among adult patients, however, started with poorly controlled single-clone outbreaks that subsequently disseminated to other hospitals and into the community,[121] and the outlook for VRE in pediatrics is uncertain.

In the latter half of the 1990s, a second phenomenon involving reduced susceptibility to vancomycin was identified, namely, vancomycin-intermediate *S. aureus* (VISA).[91, 283] These organisms express MICs to vancomycin in the intermediate range of 8 μg/mL. Virtually all such isolates are co-resistant to methicillin, but several of them have retained susceptibility to many other antimicrobial agents. To date, VISA strains have been identified primarily in patients who have been treated with prolonged courses of vancomycin for MRSA infection. A disproportionate number of patients have been maintained by dialysis.[283] Eradication of VISA has been difficult but is achievable with high doses of vancomycin in combination with other antibiotics.[91, 283] At present, infection with VISA is a very rare occurrence, both in adults and in children.[11, 90]

In 2002, the first two cases of true vancomycin-resistant *S. aureus* (VRSA) in the United States were reported, one from Michigan and the other from Pennsylvania (vancomycin MICs >128 μg/mL and equal to 32 μg/mL, respectively).[41, 42] Both patients were suffering from chronic foot ulcers from which the organisms were isolated. In both instances, the bacteria were susceptible to alternative agents and the patients remained clinically stable. The potential for VRSA to emerge as a major public health hazard is substantial, however, but as of 2002, this potential had not been realized.

MECHANISMS OF RESISTANCE. By the year 2001, five genotypes for vancomycin resistance in enterococci were defined and labeled VanA through VanE, each associated with phenotypic nuances[5, 84, 215, 235] (Table 233–4). These genotypes differ in the species of enterococci affected, the relative resistance conferred to vancomycin and teicoplanin, and whether they are inducible or constitutively expressed (Table 233–4). The VanC phenotype is distinct from the others in that it is an intrinsically expressed, species-specific product of *Enterococcus gallinarum, Enterococcus casseliflavus,* and *Enterococcus flavescens.*[216] The other vancomycin phenotypes are acquired, although VanD and VanE resistance is not readily transferable.

In susceptible bacteria, the glycopeptides are large molecules that interfere with cell wall peptidoglycan synthesis at a point proximal to that targeted by the β-lactam antibiotics. Specifically, the synthesis of peptidoglycan in vancomycin-susceptible bacteria includes the incorporation of a D-alanyl-D-alanine dipeptide onto the carboxyl end of the growing glycopeptide chain to form a pentapeptide precursor. The D-Ala-D-Ala carboxy-terminal end of this pentapeptide is critical for continued synthesis of the peptidoglycan chain and, ultimately, for formation of a stable cell wall. Vancomycin binds to the D-Ala-D-Ala moiety of the pentapeptide through several hydrogen bonds,[18] thereby blocking synthesis of the remaining macromolecule.

The molecular basis for vancomycin resistance results from the complex, coordinated interactions of multiple genes usually encoded on a single genetic element. They have been defined best for the VanA phenotype, although genetic homologues are found in organisms expressing the other vancomycin resistance phenotypes. The genetic machinery for VanA resides on the 10,851–base pair transposon Tn*1546*.[5, 314] The molecules central to conferring the resistant phenotype are encoded by the contiguous genes labeled *vanH, vanA,* and *vanX,* all of which are essential for expression of vancomycin resistance and all of which appear to be controlled by a single promoter. The *vanA* gene encodes a ligase that unlike the native enterococcal ligase, produces an abnormal D-alanyl-D-lactate dimer instead of the normal D-alanyl-D-alanine.[29, 76, 80] This process results in formation of the peptidoglycan precursor UDP-MurNAc-L-Ala-D-Glu-L-Lys-D-Ala-D-Lac, whose C-terminus has profoundly reduced affinity for vancomycin.[30] The homologous ligase in VanC- and VanE-expressing organisms synthesizes D-Ala-D-serine (see Table 233–4) with similar consequences.[215] VanH catalyzes the reaction taking pyruvate to D-Lac, thereby increasing the availability of this substrate to VanA for production of the D-Ala-D-Lac dimer.[30] *vanX* encodes a cleaving enzyme for the D-Ala-D-Ala dipeptide that reduces the natural cellular substrate for the D-Ala-D-Ala adding enzyme and results in greater relative incorporation of D-Ala-D-Lac into the peptidoglycan precursor.[251]

The *vanS* and *vanR* genes included on the same vancomycin resistance transposon regulate expression of resistance. The products of these genes are homologous to other compounds of so-called two-component regulatory systems.[120, 126, 305] The functions of the last two gene products, VanY and VanZ, are not essential for expression of the resistant phenotype.[6, 7]

None of the VISA organisms studied to date contain the genetic machinery present in VRE. The mechanism of resistance is uncertain, but several isolates have acquired unusual extracellular material around the cell wall, as detected by electron microscopy,[31, 283] that may interfere with the association of the drug and its cell wall targets. Other vancomycin resistance phenomena in *S. aureus* have been described and include those in which subpopulations express MICs twofold to eightfold higher than those of the parent population (termed "hetero-resistance")[91, 151] and those in which *S. aureus* can be inhibited but not readily killed by vancomycin (termed "tolerance").[192] The clinical consequences of these phenomenon and whether the organisms involved are precursors of VISA are unknown. By contrast, the recently identified strains of VRSA contained both the *mecA* and *vanA* genes.[41, 42] This finding indicates that true VRSA results from conjugal transfer of the vancomycin resistance transposon from VRE to MRSA, a phenomenon that can be replicated in vitro.[218]

QUINOLONES

CLINICAL RELEVANCE. The quinolone family of antibiotics possesses activity against a broad variety of microorganisms. As of the early 21st century, the quinolones have

TABLE 233–4 ■ CHARACTERISTICS OF THE TYPES OF RESISTANCE TO GLYCOPEPTIDE ANTIBIOTICS FOUND IN ENTEROCOCCI

	Type				
Characteristics	VanA	VanB	VanC	VanD	VanE*
Genetic characteristics	Acquired (e.g., *Tn1546*)	Acquired (e.g., *Tn1547*)	Intrinsic (chromosomally encoded characteristic of the species)	Acquired	Acquired
Terminus of peptidoglycan precursor	D-Ala-D-Lac	D-Ala-D-Lac	D-Ala-D-Ser	D-Ala-D-Lac	D-Ala-D-Ser
Minimal inhibitory concentration (μg/mL)					
Vancomycin	64 to >1000	4 to >1000	2 to 32	16 to 64	16
Teicoplanin	16 to 512	0.5 to >32†	0.5 to 1	2 to 4	0.5
Ligase gene	*vanA*	*vanB*	*vanC-1* and *vanC-2/VanC-3*‡	*VanD*	*VanE*
Bacteria found to have these genes for resistance in nature	*Enterococcus faecium, E. faecalis, E. durans, E. mundtii, E. avium, E. gallinarum, E. casseliflavus, Bacillus circulans, Streptococcus gallolyticus,* §corynebacteria, arcanobacteria, lactococci, Oerskovia	*E. faecalis, E. faecium, S. bovis, S. gallolyticus*§	*E. gallinarum* and *E. casseliflavus, E. flavescens*‖	*E. faecium*	*E. faecalis*
Bacteria to which vancomycin resistance has been transferred from enterococci in the laboratory setting	*Streptococcus sanguis, S. pyogenes, Listeria, Staphylococcus aureus*	*E. faecalis, E. faecium*			

*The designation VanE also has been used for a different resistance type in *Bacillus popiliae.*
†Most *vanB*-containing isolates are susceptible to teicoplanin on testing, but the development of resistance in vivo and in vitro has been documented.
‡The *vanC-3* gene is 98 percent identical to *VanC-2.*
§This organism was formerly considered part of the *Streptococcus bovis* group.
‖*Enterococcus flavescens* is probably the same species as *E. casseliflavus.*
Reprinted, by permission, from Murray, B. E.: Vancomycin-resistant enterococcal infections. N. Engl. J. Med. *342*:710–721, 2000.

not been labeled for pediatric use. However, the safety profile of the more recently developed quinolones (i.e., the fluoroquinolones) in children is similar to that recorded in adults,[144] and selected antibiotics from this family probably will be approved soon for treating pediatric infections. The following discusses clinical circumstances in which quinolone resistance most likely will be relevant to pediatric practice.

Cystic Fibrosis. The lungs of patients with cystic fibrosis (CF) are infected chronically early in life, primarily with *S. aureus* and later with *P. aeruginosa*. Exacerbations of pulmonary symptoms are treated effectively with antibiotics directed toward these microorganisms. Ciprofloxacin is the first oral agent with significant anti-*Pseudomonas* activity and has potency generally superior to that of the other fluoroquinolones.[239] As a result, experts in many centers have begun to use ciprofloxacin to treat patients with CF, even when the recipients are younger than 18 years. In most circumstances, pediatric patients with CF who are treated with ciprofloxacin have experienced improvement in their respiratory status.[52, 267]

Surveys of *Pseudomonas* isolated from patients with and without CF that were conducted during the mid to late 1990s indicated susceptibility to ciprofloxacin in approximately 60 to 90 percent of strains, with CF isolates tending to express resistance more frequently than others did.[38, 87, 122, 261, 278] Several investigators have documented that decreased susceptibility of *Pseudomonas* lung isolates to ciprofloxacin occurs frequently during the course of ciprofloxacin treatment in CF patients.[66, 71] However, as a general rule, patients who improve clinically during therapy for an acute pulmonary exacerbation do not eradicate the infecting organisms, and the importance of the emergence of bacteria during therapy that are resistant to any of the commonly used antibiotics is uncertain, as long as the infecting organisms were susceptible initially. Moreover, *Pseudomonas* frequently reverts back to a quinolone-susceptible phenotype several weeks after ciprofloxacin treatment has been completed.[66, 71] As a result, ciprofloxacin appears to be a useful option at present for patients with CF and worsening pulmonary disease if at least one of the organisms in the initial sputum culture is susceptible.

The usefulness of ciprofloxacin in a patient with CF who is infected with *S. aureus* also probably depends on the susceptibility of the pretreatment isolates. A worldwide survey conducted in the late 1990s indicated that most methicillin-susceptible strains of *S. aureus* also were susceptible to ciprofloxacin and other fluoroquinolones. However, fluoroquinolone susceptibility among methicillin-resistant strains was less than 20 percent, and susceptibility to ciprofloxacin was extraordinarily low in particular.[85, 112]

Enteric Gram-Negative Bacilli: Uropathogens, Nosocomial Bacteria, and Agents of Bacterial Enteritis. Quinolone resistance among enteric gram-negative rods, particularly among uropathogens, has been an uncommon finding in North America. Studies of enteric urinary tract isolates in the United States and Canada have documented excellent susceptibility rates to ciprofloxacin during the 1990s in nonelderly patients and supported the use of quinolones for routine, community-acquired cystitis and uncomplicated pyelonephritis.[74, 113, 114, 166, 194, 293, 336] In contrast, in some regions of Europe, the incidence of quinolone resistance among uropathogens has increased to more than 5 percent as administration of this class of antibiotics has become more widespread.[106, 131] A survey of urinary tract isolates from Latin America conducted in 1998 indicated an even more dramatic incidence of quinolone resistance: 22 percent of *E. coli,* 30 percent of *Proteus mirabilis,* and over 35 percent of *Enterobacter* spp. were ciprofloxacin-resistant.[96] Quinolone resistance also has increased gradually among lactose-fermenting, gram-negative isolates from bloodstream infections in some locations.[46, 85] Resistance has been noted among nosocomially acquired *Klebsiella* spp., the majority of which co-express ESBLs and other resistance determinants.[4, 27, 231]

Antibiotic therapy for bacterial enteritis, including treatment with a quinolone, usually is not indicated.[324] That said, with the exception of *Campylobacter* spp., most agents that cause bacterial enteritis have remained susceptible to the quinolones by in vitro testing.[8, 44, 105, 324] *Salmonella typhimurium* DT104, which spread rapidly throughout Europe and the United States in the late 1990s, was resistant to nalidixic acid, but most isolates (except for some identified in the United Kingdom) were susceptible to the newer fluoroquinolones.[94, 105, 205]

In contrast to that of other enteritis-associated bacteria, quinolone resistance among *Campylobacter* isolates from many parts of the world has become prominent and high level.[125, 237, 282, 299, 325] *Campylobacter* spp. can acquire quinolone resistance shortly after exposure to the antibiotic. Indeed, clinical relapse with quinolone-resistant organisms in patients who have received therapy for *Campylobacter* enteritis occurs relatively commonly.[237, 325] The introduction of quinolones into the poultry feed of animals bred for food has exacerbated the spread of *Campylobacter* resistance in humans.[282] In chicken obtained from several different supermarkets in Minnesota in the mid-1990s, nearly 90 percent of samples were culture-positive for *Campylobacter,* and approximately 20 percent of these strains were resistant to ciprofloxacin.[282] Unlike most other bacteria, *Campylobacter* spp. become highly resistant to the quinolones after a single mutation,[104, 315] so most quinolone-resistant clinical isolates demonstrate MICs of 32 μg/mL or higher, well above the conventional cutoff for defining quinolone resistance.

Community-Acquired Respiratory Tract Infections. The applicability of quinolones to respiratory tract infections has been shadowed by the marginal activity of the first modern quinolones (ciprofloxacin, ofloxacin, and norfloxacin) against *S. pneumoniae.* MICs of these antibiotics against most clinical isolates of *S. pneumoniae* average 1 to 2 μg/mL, concentrations that are close to that achievable in bronchial secretions.[239] Several reports of clinical failure surfaced when ciprofloxacin was applied to pneumococcal disease in the respiratory tract.[159, 168, 234] Moreover, even when *S. pneumoniae* has not been the intended target of therapy, wide use of the early quinolone agents in treating community-acquired infections during the 1990s resulted in the inadvertent exposure of respiratory tract colonizers to these drugs, including *S. pneumoniae.* This exposure has led to an even greater, albeit gradual increase in the MICs of community-acquired *S. pneumoniae* isolates to ciprofloxacin.[22, 45, 83, 148, 260, 294]

Most of the more recently introduced fluoroquinolones are substantially more potent against *S. pneumoniae* than ciprofloxacin is, with MICs that are easily achieved in the respiratory tract. Susceptibility is maintained even in isolates resistant to the older quinolone agents.[95, 150, 239, 253, 254] However, MICs against the newer quinolones roughly correlate with those expressed against ciprofloxacin.[45, 148, 150, 254] This observation suggests that if the average MICs of *S. pneumoniae* to ciprofloxacin continue to increase over time, MICs against the newer agents may increase concomitantly to the point that they become clinically irrelevant as well. Noteworthy is that to date, the susceptibility of other respiratory tract pathogens, including *H. influenzae, M. catarrhalis,*[22, 83, 142, 239, 253] and the bacterial agents causing atypical pneumonia, remains excellent to all the fluoroquinolones.

MECHANISMS OF RESISTANCE. The two principal molecular targets of the quinolone antibiotics are topoisomerase II, also called DNA gyrase, and topoisomerase IV. These enzymes mediate the three-dimensional topologic configuration of the bacterial duplex DNA ring during cell division and transcription.[127] Several reactions have been identified as being mediated by these two bacterial DNA topoisomerases and include negative supercoiling and catenation.[128, 291] Both DNA gyrase and topoisomerase IV are composed of two nonidentical subunits. In DNA gyrase, they are labeled GyrA and GyrB, which are constructed into an A_2B_2 tetramer.[128, 291] Quinolones bind to the GyrA subunit of the DNA gyrase-DNA-ATP complex, thereby preventing a key conformational change and further progress of the enzyme along the nucleic acid.[128] Two equivalent subunits of topoisomerase IV labeled ParC and ParE share sequence homologies with GyrA and GyrB, respectively.[129]

Quinolone resistance is conferred through several molecular mechanisms. To date, virtually all quinolone resistance determinants are encoded on the bacterial chromosome. Most organisms resistant to the fluoroquinolones demonstrate one or more mutations in DNA gyrase, topoisomerase IV, or both. Resistance to quinolones by gram-negative bacilli usually is mediated through mutations in DNA gyrase, whereas resistance in gram-positive organisms is caused by alterations in topoisomerase IV.[228, 340] However, this pattern varies from organism to organism (the primary target in *S. pneumoniae,* for example, appears to be DNA gyrase) and from quinolone to quinolone.[129] In gram-negative bacilli, most first-step, resistance-conferring mutations occur in *gyrA,* the gene encoding the GyrA subunit. These mutations are clustered in a segment termed the quinolone resistance determining region (QRDR).[238, 264, 332, 334] Hybrid DNA gyrase molecules composed of the A subunit from a resistant bacterial strain and the B subunit from a susceptible isolate confer quinolone resistance.[36] Within the QRDR, most mutations have involved the substitution of a serine for a bulkier, nonpolar amino acid at a single, specific site. This mutation, first identified in *E. coli,*[311, 332] has been documented since then in a variety of organisms.[60, 140, 160, 208, 245] Other amino acid substitutions near this site also have been described, with multiple-site mutations resulting in increased quinolone resistance in comparison to mutation in a single site alone.[311] Mutations of the GyrB subunit that lead to a quinolone-resistant phenotype also have been identified. In general, mutations affecting the GyrB subunit result in lower levels of resistance than do those noted with GyrA.[334] As with GyrA mutations, those affecting GyrB preferentially localize to specific amino acids.[36, 334]

In most quinolone-resistant, gram-positive organisms, mutations of topoisomerase IV occur at locations that are equivalent to those observed in DNA gyrase. First-step mutations are noted most frequently in *parC,* which like *gyrA,* contains a hot-spot segment around which most resistance-conferring mutations occur.[128, 129, 238] *GyrA* mutations in these organisms are frequently clinically silent unless they occur concomitantly with a mutation in *parC.*[128]

Two additional mechanisms of quinolone resistance, which may appear together and in conjunction with a topoisomerase mutation in the same cell, have been identified. Both these additional mechanisms result in diminished intracellular accumulation of drug. The first mechanism involves decreased entry of antibiotic into the cell caused by alterations in porin composition, a mutation that generally results in only moderate drug resistance and that affects individual quinolones differentially depending on their hydrophilicity.[264] Particular attention has centered on alterations in the outer-member protein F (OmpF).[56, 130, 338] This mutation, identified principally in *E. coli,* frequently is associated with resistance to other classes of antibiotics as well, including chloramphenicol, tetracycline, and some of the β-lactams. The diminished expression of OmpF in these resistant isolates does not appear to be caused by mutations in the corresponding structural gene or its regulatory sequences. Rather, decreased expression of this outer-membrane protein is mediated through enhanced expression of the gene *micF,* which transcribes an antisense RNA complementary to the 5′ end of the *ompF* message[3] that destabilizes its binding to the ribosome. Occasional mutants involving additional strains of Enterobacteriaceae have demonstrated other alterations in outer-membrane porin composition.[36]

Several quinolone-resistant species mediate their resistance through increased drug efflux.[173, 175, 188] Both bacterial and eukaryotic cells normally encode several efflux pumps that provide protection from a range of potential exogenous toxins.[233] Growing evidence indicates that quinolone resistance mediated through overexpression of an efflux pump may account, at least in part, for the resistant phenotype in many clinical isolates.[188] Individual efflux pumps probably select substrates based on their physicochemical properties (e.g., hydrophobicity and net charge) rather than gross structural similarities; therefore, the various quinolone compounds, which differ from one another regarding these properties, may be differentially susceptible to organisms expressing these pumps.[233]

The gene encoding the quinolone efflux pump in *S. aureus,* labeled *norA,*[333] has been cloned and sequenced. Transformation of susceptible bacteria with the putative gene results in a resistant phenotype, but the resistance can be abolished by the addition of inhibitors of energy-dependent cellular pumps.[56, 333] This pump, however, appears to be able to transport only hydrophilic quinolones; intracellular accumulation of the hydrophobic drug sparfloxacin, for example, is unaffected.

A range of additional genes encoding efflux pumps capable of producing quinolone resistance have been identified in other species, such as *prmA* in *S. pneumoniae,*[238] *marA* in *E. coli,*[184] and the *mexAmexB-oprM* complex in *P. aeruginosa.*[189] This last complex gene encodes components that transport the drug through both the cell wall and across the periplasmic space, as well as an outer-membrane protein.[233] Most of these pumps are able to extrude a wide variety of exogenous substances from the bacterial cytoplasm, such as detergents, dyes, and other antibiotics.[188]

Quinolone resistance occurs incrementally as the organism experiences a series of topoisomerase mutations, altered outer-membrane proteins, and overexpression of efflux pumps.[79] Thus, in gram-negative species, mutations of *gyrA* usually occur in first-step mutants and result in relatively small increases in the MIC to the antibiotic. Additional mutations to *gyrA,* or added mutations to *parC* or the overexpression of an efflux pump, which may in themselves confer undetectable or only minor resistance to the quinolones, result in substantial quinolone resistance when they operate in concert.[129, 264] Therefore, choosing a fluoroquinolone that can achieve a concentration at the site of infection 5- to 10-fold above the MIC may suppress the emergence of resistance because this concentration is sufficient to suppress growth of both the parent organism and first-step mutants.[264] Moreover, because the different fluoroquinolones are affected to differing degrees by *gyrA* and *parC* mutations and are variably efficient substrates for the many efflux pumps, resistance to one quinolone does not necessarily predict resistance to another.[264, 298] This phenomenon, termed "dissociative resistance," justifies the in vitro susceptibility testing of multiple fluoroquinolones, even after resistance to one of them has been demonstrated.

CHLORAMPHENICOL

CLINICAL RELEVANCE. In industrialized nations, chloramphenicol has been supplanted by other agents with similar or improved antibacterial potency and less toxicity. However, the antibiotic remains a staple for pediatric bacteremia and meningitis in the developing world because of its broad antibacterial activity, low cost, favorable achievable serum concentrations after oral or intramuscular administration, and excellent penetration across the blood-brain barrier. The incidence of resistance to chloramphenicol among the principal organisms causing bacteremia and meningitis in children, namely, *H. influenzae, S. pneumoniae, N. meningitidis,* and *Salmonella,* varies greatly by geographic location. During the late 1980s and 1990s, surveys of *H. influenzae,* both type b and non–type b, were completed in several areas of the world. In vitro resistance to chloramphenicol was noted in 0 percent of isolates from the Central African Republic[257] and various locations in South America,[316] in approximately 10 percent in Indonesia[101] and Egypt,[222] and in more than 50 percent in India,[147] where co-resistance with ampicillin was a common occurrence. Recent studies of *H. influenzae* isolates in Canada and the United States, where infection by these organisms almost always is treated with an alternative agent, indicated chloramphenicol resistance in less than 0.5 percent of tested bacteria.[67, 124, 337]

Recent surveys measuring the in vitro susceptibility of *S. pneumoniae* to chloramphenicol indicate resistance rates exceeding 10 to 20 percent in many areas of the world.[169, 222, 257] International surveys completed in the late 1990s detected chloramphenicol resistance in approximately 10 percent of European isolates of *S. pneumoniae* and 5 percent of those identified in the United States and Canada.[124] Resistance to chloramphenicol occurs more commonly and is of a higher grade in penicillin-resistant pneumococci than in isolates that are penicillin-susceptible.[124, 169] Even in penicillin-intermediate or penicillin-resistant strains that retain in vitro susceptibility to chloramphenicol, the clinical response to the latter antibiotic in meningitis is poor. Some investigators have suggested that such bacteria express high minimal bactericidal concentrations to chloramphenicol; as a result, concentrations of drug achieved in CSF with routine dosing are below those required for a good outcome in CNS infection.[93]

Chloramphenicol retains excellent activity against most strains of *N. meningitidis.* However, investigators recently described meningococcal strains from Vietnam and Paris that possessed high-level resistance to chloramphenicol while maintaining susceptibility to penicillin and the cephalosporins.[97] Finally, chloramphenicol resistance in *Salmonella* spp., a fourth group of organisms that cause disseminated disease and meningitis in pediatrics, varies geographically. High rates of susceptibility continue in Bangladesh[335] and Malawi.[107] By contrast, significant rates of chloramphenicol resistance among typhoidal and nontyphoidal strains recently have been recorded in India (12%),[35] Spain (26%),[243] Turkey (38%),[13] and Taiwan (67%).[331] Resistance to chloramphenicol in *Salmonella* frequently is co-expressed with resistance to multiple other agents; in an outbreak of typhoid fever caused by contaminated drinking water in Tajikistan during the latter 1990s, for example, 93 percent of the organisms tested demonstrated resistance to ampicillin, nalidixic acid, streptomycin, sulfisoxazole, and tetracycline, as well as chloramphenicol.[202] In the United States, the strain *S. typhimurium* DT104, which typically co-expresses resistance to several classes of antibiotics, including chloramphenicol, has become a widespread health hazard.[1, 54, 312]

MECHANISMS OF RESISTANCE. The antibacterial activity of chloramphenicol is conferred by its interference with the peptidyltransferase region of the 50S prokaryotic ribosome. The principal mechanism of resistance is through expression of the modifying enzyme chloramphenicol acetyltransferase (CAT), which catalyzes acetylation of the C3-hydroxy group of the drug, thereby preventing its binding to the bacterial ribosome.[277] CAT actually represents a family of enzymes. Many CATs share chemical properties and structural homologies, especially around the active site.[16, 277] CATs frequently reside on plasmids or transposons that carry other antibiotic resistance determinants, although occasional gram-negative organisms encode CAT on genomic sequences. Expression in gram-negative bacteria is constitutive, whereas the expression of CAT in many gram-positive species is inducible.[229, 277]

Alternative mechanisms of resistance to chloramphenicol also has been identified in numerous gram-negative species. In most of these organisms, resistance is linked to decreased intracellular accumulation of drug. In chloramphenicol-resistant *Pseudomonas* spp., this phenomenon has been associated with the overproduction of an approximately 50-kd outer-membrane protein,[175] which in the past has led to speculation that entry of drug into the bacterium is diminished by an abnormal porin. More recently, however, cell membrane proteins of this size have been identified as components of complex efflux apparatuses that include both the pump itself and proteins that channel the extruded substance across the periplasmic space through the outer membrane.[233] More direct evidence of such multidrug resistance efflux pumps has been identified in chloramphenicol-resistant *Pseudomonas,*[175] *Burkholderia,*[32] *Stenotrophomonas,*[339] and *Salmonella* spp.[24, 240] Usually, these pumps result in co-resistance to multiple other antimicrobial agents, including tetracycline, sulfonamides, aminoglycosides, quinolones, and selected detergents.

REFERENCES

1. Ackers, M. L., Puhr, N. D., Tauxe, R. V., and Mintz, E. D.: Laboratory-based surveillance of *Salmonella* serotype *typhi* infections in the United States: Antimicrobial resistance on the rise. J. A. M. A. *283*:2668–2673, 2000.
2. Ambler, R. P.: The structure of beta-lactamases. Philos. Trans. R. Soc. Lond. B Biol. Sci. *289*:321–331, 1900.
3. Andersen, J., and Delihas, N.: micF RNA binds to the 5′ end of ompF mRNA and to a protein from *Escherichia coli.* Biochemistry *29*:9249–9256, 1990.
4. Araque, M., and Velazco, E.: In vitro activity of fleroxacin against multiresistant gram-negative bacilli isolated from patients with nosocomial infections. Intensive Care Med. *24*:839–844, 1998.
5. Arthur, M., and Courvalin, P.: Genetics and mechanisms of glycopeptide resistance in enterococci. Antimicrob. Agents Chemother. *37*:1563–1571, 1993.
6. Arthur, M., Depardieu, F., Molinas, C., et al.: The vanZ gene of Tn1546 from *Enterococcus faecium* BM4147 confers resistance to teicoplanin. Gene *154*:87–92, 1995.
7. Arthur, M., Depardieu, F., Snaith, H. A., et al.: Contribution of VanY D,D-carboxypeptidase to glycopeptide resistance in *Enterococcus faecalis* by hydrolysis of peptidoglycan precursors. Antimicrob. Agents Chemother. *38*:1899–1903, 1994.
8. Ashkenazi, S., May-Zahav, M., Sulkes, J., et al.: Increasing antimicrobial resistance of *Shigella* isolates in Israel during the period 1984 to 1992. Antimicrob. Agents Chemother. *39*:819–823, 1995.
9. Atta, M. G., Eustace, J. A., Song, X., et al.: Outpatient vancomycin use and vancomycin-resistant enterococcal colonization in maintenance dialysis patients. Kidney Int. *59*:718–724, 2001.
10. Aubry-Damon, H., Legrand, P., Brun-Buisson, C., et al.: Reemergence of gentamicin-susceptible strains of methicillin-resistant *Staphylococcus aureus:* Roles of an infection control program and changes in aminoglycoside use. Clin. Infect. Dis. *25*:647–653, 1997.
11. Aucken, H. M., Warner, M., Ganner, M., et al.: Twenty months of screening for glycopeptide-intermediate *Staphylococcus aureus.* J. Antimicrob. Chemother. *46*:639–640, 2000.
12. Austin, D. J., Bonten, M. J., Weinstein, R. A., et al.: Vancomycin-resistant enterococci in intensive-care hospital settings: Transmission dynamics, persistence, and the impact of infection control programs. Proc. Natl. Acad. Sci. U. S. A. *96*:6908–6913, 1999.
13. Aysev, A. D., Guriz, H., and Erdem, B.: Drug resistance of *Salmonella* strains isolated from community infections in Ankara, Turkey, 1993–99. Scand. J. Infect. Dis. *33*:420–422, 2001.
14. Babini, G. S., and Livermore, D. M.: Antimicrobial resistance amongst *Klebsiella* spp. collected from intensive care units in Southern and Western Europe in 1997–1998. J. Antimicrob. Chemother. *45*:183–189, 2000.
15. Bakir, M., Bova, J. L., Newell, K. A., et al.: Epidemiology and clinical consequences of vancomycin-resistant enterococci in liver transplant patients. Transplantation *72*:1032–1037, 2001.
16. Bannam, T. L., and Rood, J. I.: Relationship between the *Clostridium perfringens* catQ gene product and chloramphenicol acetyltransferases from other bacteria. Antimicrob. Agents Chemother. *35*:471–476, 1991.
17. Barcus, V. A., Ghanekar, K., Yeo, M., et al.: Genetics of high level penicillin resistance in clinical isolates of *Streptococcus pneumoniae.* F. E. M. S. Microbiol. Lett. *126*:299–303, 1995.
18. Barna, J. C., and Williams, D. H.: The structure and mode of action of glycopeptide antibiotics of the vancomycin group. Annu. Rev. Microbiol. *38*:339–357, 1984.
19. Bartowsky, E., and Normark, S.: Interactions of wild-type and mutant AmpR of *Citrobacter freundii* with target DNA. Mol. Microbiol. *10*:555–565, 1993.
20. Bennish, M. L., Salam, M. A., Hossain, M. A., et al.: Antimicrobial resistance of *Shigella* isolates in Bangladesh, 1983–1990: Increasing frequency of strains multiply resistant to ampicillin, trimethoprim-sulfamethoxazole, and nalidixic acid. Clin. Infect. Dis. *14*:1055–1060, 1992.
21. Bertrand, X., Thouverez, M., and Talon, D.: Antibiotic susceptibility and genotypic characterization of methicillin-resistant *Staphylococcus aureus* strains in eastern France. J. Hosp. Infect. *46*:280–287, 2000.
22. Blondeau, J. M., Vaughan, D., Laskowski, R., and Borsos, S.: Susceptibility of Canadian isolates of *Haemophilus influenzae, Moraxella catarrhalis* and *Streptococcus pneumoniae* to oral antimicrobial agents. Int. J. Antimicrob. Agents *17*:457–464, 2001.
23. Bluestone, C. D., and Klein, J. D.: Otitis Media in Infants and Children. 2nd ed. Philadelphia, W. B. Saunders, 1995.
24. Bolton, L. F., Kelley, L. C., Lee, M. D., et al.: Detection of multidrug-resistant *Salmonella enterica* serotype *typhimurium* DT104 based on a gene which confers cross-resistance to florfenicol and chloramphenicol. J. Clin. Microbiol. *37*:1348–1351, 1999.
25. Bonten, M. J., Slaughter, S., Ambergen, A. W., et al.: The role of "colonization pressure" in the spread of vancomycin-resistant enterococci: An important infection control variable. Arch. Intern. Med. *158*:1127–1132, 1998.
26. Bratoeva, M. P., John, J. F., and Barg, N. L.: Molecular epidemiology of trimethoprim-resistant *Shigella boydii* serotype 2 strains from Bulgaria. J. Clin. Microbiol. *30*:1428–1431, 1992.
27. Brisse, S., Milatovic, D., Fluit, A. C., et al.: Epidemiology of quinolone resistance of *Klebsiella pneumoniae* and *Klebsiella oxytoca* in Europe. Eur. J. Clin. Microbiol. Infect. Dis. *19*:64–68, 2000.
28. Brubaker, R. R.: Mechanisms of bacterial virulence. Annu. Rev. Microbiol. *39*:21–50, 1985.
29. Bugg, T. D., Dutka-Malen, S., Arthur, M., et al.: Identification of vancomycin resistance protein VanA as a D-alanine:D-alanine ligase of altered substrate specificity. Biochemistry *30*:2017–2021, 1991.

30. Bugg, T. D., Wright, G. D., Dutka-Malen, S., et al.: Molecular basis for vancomycin resistance in *Enterococcus faecium* BM4147: Biosynthesis of a depsipeptide peptidoglycan precursor by vancomycin resistance proteins VanH and VanA. Biochemistry *30*:10408–10415, 1991.
31. Burnie, J., Matthews, R., Jiman-Fatami, A., et al.: Analysis of 42 cases of septicemia caused by an epidemic strain of methicillin-resistant *Staphylococcus aureus:* Evidence of resistance to vancomycin. Clin. Infect. Dis. *31*:684–689, 2000.
32. Burns, J. L., Wadsworth, C. D., Barry, J. J., and Goodall, C. P.: Nucleotide sequence analysis of a gene from *Burkholderia (Pseudomonas) cepacia* encoding an outer membrane lipoprotein involved in multiple antibiotic resistance. Antimicrob. Agents Chemother. *40*:307–313, 1996.
33. Bush, K.: Metallo-beta-lactamases: A class apart. Clin. Infect. Dis. *27*(Suppl. 1):48–53, 1998.
34. Bush, K., Jacoby, G. A., and Medeiros, A. A.: A functional classification scheme for beta-lactamases and its correlation with molecular structure. Antimicrob. Agents Chemother. *39*:1211–1233, 1995.
35. Butler, T., Sridhar, C. B., Daga, M. K., et al.: Treatment of typhoid fever with azithromycin versus chloramphenicol in a randomized multicentre trial in India. J. Antimicrob. Chemother. *44*:243–250, 1999.
36. Cambau, E., and Gutmann, L.: Mechanisms of resistance to quinolones. Drugs *45*:15–23, 1993.
37. Carmeli, Y., Samore, M. H., and Huskins, C.: The association between antecedent vancomycin treatment and hospital-acquired vancomycin-resistant enterococci: A meta-analysis. Arch. Intern. Med. *159*:2461–2468, 1999.
38. Carmeli, Y., Troillet, N., Eliopoulos, G. M., and Samore, M. H.: Emergence of antibiotic-resistant *Pseudomonas aeruginosa:* comparison of risks associated with different antipseudomonal agents. Antimicrob. Agents Chemother. *43*:1379–1382, 1999.
39. Casalino, M., Nicoletti, M., Salvia, A., et al.: Characterization of endemic *Shigella flexneri* strains in Somalia: Antimicrobial resistance, plasmid profiles, and serotype correlation. J. Clin. Microbiol. *32*:1179–1183, 1994.
40. Centers for Disease Control and Prevention: Geographic variation in penicillin resistance in *Streptococcus pneumoniae*—selected sites, United States, 1997. M. M. W. R. Morb. Mortal. Wkly. Rep. *48*:(30):656–661, 1999.
41. Centers for Disease Control and Prevention: *Staphylococcus aureus* resistant to vancomycin—United States, 2002. M. M. W. R. Morb. Mortal. Wkly. Rep. *51*(26):565–567, 2000.
42. Centers for Disease Control and Prevention: Vancomycin-resistant *Staphylococcus aureus*—Pennsylvania, 2002. M. M. W. R. Morb. Mortal. Wkly. Rep. *51*(40):902, 2000.
43. Chaibi, E. B., Sirot, D., Paul, G., and Labia, R.: Inhibitor-resistant TEM beta-lactamases: Phenotypic, genetic and biochemical characteristics. J. Antimicrob. Chemother. *43*:447–458, 1999.
44. Cheasty, T., Skinner, J. A., Rowe, B., and Threlfall, E. J.: Increasing incidence of antibiotic resistance in shigellas from humans in England and Wales: Recommendations for therapy. Microb. Drug Resist. *4*:57–60, 1998.
45. Chen, D. K., McGeer, A., de Azavedo, J. C., and Low, D. E.: Decreased susceptibility of *Streptococcus pneumoniae* to fluoroquinolones in Canada. Canadian Bacterial Surveillance Network. N. Engl. J. Med. *341*:233–239, 1999.
46. Cheong, H. J., Yoo, C. W., Sohn, J. W., et al.: Bacteremia due to quinolone-resistant *Escherichia coli* in a teaching hospital in South Korea. Clin. Infect. Dis. *33*:48–53, 2001.
47. Chevalier, J., Pages, J. M., Eyraud, A., and Mallea, M.: Membrane permeability modifications are involved in antibiotic resistance in *Klebsiella pneumoniae.* Biochem. Biophys. Res. Commun. *274*:496–499, 2000.
48. Chittum, H. S., and Champney, W. S.: Ribosomal protein gene sequence changes in erythromycin-resistant mutants of *Escherichia coli.* J. Bacteriol. *176*:6192–6198, 1994.
49. Chow, J. W.: Aminoglycoside resistance in enterococci. Clin. Infect. Dis. *31*:586–589, 2000.
50. Chow, J. W., Fine, M. J., Shlaes, D. M., et al.: *Enterobacter* bacteremia: Clinical features and emergence of antibiotic resistance during therapy. Ann. Intern. Med. *115*:585–590, 1991.
51. Chow, J. W., and Shlaes, D. M.: Imipenem resistance associated with the loss of a 40 kDa outer membrane protein in *Enterobacter aerogenes.* J. Antimicrob. Chemother. *28*:499–504, 1991.
52. Church, D. A., Kanga, J. F., Kuhn, R. J., et al.: Sequential ciprofloxacin therapy in pediatric cystic fibrosis: Comparative study vs. ceftazidime/tobramycin in the treatment of acute pulmonary exacerbations. The Cystic Fibrosis Study Group. Pediatr. Infect. Dis. J. *16*:97–105, 123–126, 1997.
53. Cizman, M., Pokorn, M., Seme, K., et al.: The relationship between trends in macrolide use and resistance to macrolides of common respiratory pathogens. J. Antimicrob. Chemother. *47*:475–477, 2001.
54. Cody, S. H., Abbott, S. L., Marfin, A. A., et al.: Two outbreaks of multidrug-resistant *Salmonella* serotype *typhimurium* DT104 infections linked to raw-milk cheese in Northern California. J. A. M. A. *281*:1805–1810, 1999.
55. Coffey, T. J., Daniels, M., McDougal, L. K., et al.: Genetic analysis of clinical isolates of *Streptococcus pneumoniae* with high-level resistance to expanded-spectrum cephalosporins. Antimicrob. Agents Chemother. *39*:1306–1313, 1995.
56. Cohen, S. P., McMurry, L. M., and Levy, S. B.: marA locus causes decreased expression of OmpF porin in multiple-antibiotic-resistant (Mar) mutants of *Escherichia coli.* J. Bacteriol. *170*:5416–5422, 1988.
57. Cook, L. N., Davis, R. S., and Stover, B. H.: Outbreak of amikacin-resistant Enterobacteriaceae in an intensive care nursery. Pediatrics *65*:264–268, 1980.
58. Dale, G. E., Broger, C., D'Arcy, A., et al.: A single amino acid substitution in *Staphylococcus aureus* dihydrofolate reductase determines trimethoprim resistance. J. Mol. Biol. *266*:23–30, 1997.
59. Dan, M., Poch, F., Leibson, L., et al.: Rectal colonization with vancomycin-resistant enterococci among high-risk patients in an Israeli hospital. J. Hosp. Infect. *43*:231–238, 1999.
60. Deguchi, T., Yasuda, M., Asano, M., et al.: DNA gyrase mutations in quinolone-resistant clinical isolates of *Neisseria gonorrhoeae.* Antimicrob. Agents Chemother. *39*:561–563, 1995.
61. de Jonge, B. L., and Tomasz, A.: Abnormal peptidoglycan produced in a methicillin-resistant strain of *Staphylococcus aureus* grown in the presence of methicillin: Functional role for penicillin-binding protein 2A in cell wall synthesis. Antimicrob. Agents Chemother. *37*:342–346, 1993.
62. de Lencastre, H., de Jonge, B. L., Matthews, P. R., and Tomasz, A.: Molecular aspects of methicillin resistance in *Staphylococcus aureus.* J. Antimicrob. Chemother. *33*:7–24, 1994.
63. De Mouy, D., Cavallo, J. D., Leclercq, R., and Fabre, R.: Antibiotic susceptibility and mechanisms of erythromycin resistance in clinical isolates of *Streptococcus agalactiae:* French multicenter study. Antimicrob. Agents Chemother. *45*:2400–2402, 2001.
64. Depardieu, F., and Courvalin, P.: Mutation in 23S rRNA responsible for resistance to 16-membered macrolides and streptogramins in *Streptococcus pneumoniae.* Antimicrob. Agents Chemother. *45*:319–323, 2001.
65. Diekema, D. J., Pfaller, M. A., Schmitz, F. J., et al.: Survey of infections due to *Staphylococcus* species: Frequency of occurrence and antimicrobial susceptibility of isolates collected in the United States, Canada, Latin America, Europe, and the Western Pacific region for the SENTRY Antimicrobial Surveillance Program, 1997–1999. Clin. Infect. Dis. *32*(Suppl. 2):114–132, 2001.
66. Diver, J. M., Schollaardt, T., Rabin, H. R., et al.: Persistence mechanisms in *Pseudomonas aeruginosa* from cystic fibrosis patients undergoing ciprofloxacin therapy. Antimicrob. Agents Chemother. *35*:1538–1546, 1991.
67. Doern, G. V., Heilmann, K. P., Huynh, H. K., et al.: Antimicrobial resistance among clinical isolates of *Streptococcus pneumoniae* in the United States during 1999–2000, including a comparison of resistance rates since 1994–1995. Antimicrob. Agents Chemother. *45*:1721–1729, 2001.
68. Doern, G. V., Pfaller, M. A., Kugler, K., et al.: Prevalence of antimicrobial resistance among respiratory tract isolates of *Streptococcus pneumoniae* in North America: 1997 results from the SENTRY antimicrobial surveillance program. Clin. Infect. Dis. *27*:764–770, 1998.
69. Donskey, C. J., Chowdhry, T. K., Hecker, M. T., et al.: Effect of antibiotic therapy on the density of vancomycin-resistant enterococci in the stool of colonized patients. N. Engl. J. Med. *343*:1925–1932, 2000.
70. Donskey, C. J., Schreiber, J. R., Jacobs, M. R., et al.: A polyclonal outbreak of predominantly VanB vancomycin-resistant enterococci in northeast Ohio. Northeast Ohio Vancomycin-Resistant Enterococcus Surveillance Program. Clin. Infect. Dis. *29*:573–579, 1999.
71. Dostal, R. E., Seale, J. P., and Yan, B. J.: Resistance to ciprofloxacin of respiratory pathogens in patients with cystic fibrosis. Med. J. Aust. *156*:20–24, 1992.
72. Dowson, C. G., Hutchison, A., Brannigan, J. A., et al.: Horizontal transfer of penicillin-binding protein genes in penicillin-resistant clinical isolates of *Streptococcus pneumoniae.* Proc. Natl. Acad. Sci. U. S. A. *86*:8842–8846, 1989.
73. Dowson, C. G., Hutchison, A., and Spratt, B. G.: Extensive re-modelling of the transpeptidase domain of penicillin-binding protein 2B of a penicillin-resistant South African isolate of *Streptococcus pneumoniae.* Mol. Microbiol. *3*:95–102, 1989.
74. Drago, L., De Vecchi, E., Mombelli, B., et al.: Activity of levofloxacin and ciprofloxacin against urinary pathogens. J. Antimicrob. Chemother. *48*:37–45, 2001.
75. Du Bois, S. K., Marriott, M. S., and Amyes, S. G.: TEM- and SHV-derived extended-spectrum beta-lactamases: Relationship between selection, structure and function. J. Antimicrob. Chemother. *35*:7–22, 1995.
76. Dutka-Malen, S., Molinas, C., Arthur, M., and Courvalin, P.: Sequence of the vanC gene of *Enterococcus gallinarum* BM4174 encoding a D-alanine:D-alanine ligase-related protein necessary for vancomycin resistance. Gene *112*:53–58, 1992.
77. Edmond, M. B., Ober, J. F., Weinbaum, D. L., et al.: Vancomycin-resistant *Enterococcus faecium* bacteremia: Risk factors for infection. Clin. Infect. Dis. *20*:1126–1133, 1995.
78. Eliopoulos, G. M., Wennersten, C., Zighelboim-Daum, S., et al.: High-level resistance to gentamicin in clinical isolates of *Streptococcus (Enterococcus) faecium.* Antimicrob. Agents Chemother. *32*:1528–1532, 1988.

79. Everett, M. J., Jin, Y. F., Ricci, V., and Piddock, L. J.: Contributions of individual mechanisms to fluoroquinolone resistance in 36 *Escherichia coli* strains isolated from humans and animals. Antimicrob. Agents Chemother. *40*:2380–2386, 1996.
80. Evers, S., Sahm, D. F., and Courvalin, P.: The vanB gene of vancomycin-resistant *Enterococcus faecalis* V583 is structurally related to genes encoding D-Ala:D-Ala ligases and glycopeptide-resistance proteins VanA and VanC. Gene *124*:143–144, 1993.
81. Facinelli, B., Spinaci, C., Magi, G., et al.: Association between erythromycin resistance and ability to enter human respiratory cells in group A streptococci. Lancet *358*:30–33, 2001.
82. Feikin, D. R., Dowell, S. F., Nwanyanwu, O. C., et al.: Increased carriage of trimethoprim/sulfamethoxazole-resistant *Streptococcus pneumoniae* in Malawian children after treatment for malaria with sulfadoxine/pyrimethamine. J. Infect. Dis. *181*:1501–1505, 2000.
83. Felmingham, D., Robbins, M. J., Tesfaslasie, Y., et al.: Antimicrobial susceptibility of community-acquired lower respiratory tract bacterial pathogens isolated in the UK during the 1995–1996 cold season. J. Antimicrob. Chemother. *41*:411–415, 1998.
84. Fines, M., Perichon, B., Reynolds, P., et al.: VanE, a new type of acquired glycopeptide resistance in *Enterococcus faecalis* BM4405. Antimicrob. Agents Chemother. *43*:2161–2164, 1999.
85. Fluit, A. C., Jones, M. E., Schmitz, F. J., et al.: Antimicrobial susceptibility and frequency of occurrence of clinical blood isolates in Europe from the SENTRY antimicrobial surveillance program, 1997 and 1998. Clin. Infect. Dis. *30*:454–460, 2000.
86. Fluit, A. C., and Schmitz, F. J.: Class 1 integrons, gene cassettes, mobility, and epidemiology. Eur. J. Clin. Microbiol. Infect. Dis. *18*:761–770, 1999.
87. Fluit, A. C., Verhoef, J., and Schmitz, F. J.: Antimicrobial resistance in European isolates of *Pseudomonas aeruginosa*. European SENTRY Participants. Eur. J. Clin. Microbiol. Infect. Dis. *19*:370–374, 2000.
88. Fogarty, C., Goldschmidt, R., and Bush, K.: Bacteremic pneumonia due to multidrug-resistant pneumococci in 3 patients treated unsuccessfully with azithromycin and successfully with levofloxacin. Clin. Infect. Dis. *31*:613–615, 2000.
89. Fournier, B., Lagrange, P. H., and Philippon, A.: Beta-lactamase gene promoters of 71 clinical strains of *Klebsiella oxytoca*. Antimicrob. Agents Chemother. *40*:460–463, 1996.
90. Franchi, D., Climo, M. W., Wong, A. H., et al.: Seeking vancomycin resistant *Staphylococcus aureus* among patients with vancomycin-resistant enterococci. Clin. Infect. Dis. *29*:1566–1568, 1999.
91. Fridkin, S. K.: Vancomycin-intermediate and -resistant *Staphylococcus aureus:* What the infectious disease specialist needs to know. Clin. Infect. Dis. *32*:108–115, 2001.
92. Fridkin, S. K., Edwards, J. R., Courval, J. M., et al.: The effect of vancomycin and third-generation cephalosporins on prevalence of vancomycin-resistant enterococci in 126 U.S. adult intensive care units. Ann. Intern. Med. *135*:175–183, 2001.
93. Friedland, I. R., and Klugman, K. P.: Failure of chloramphenicol therapy in penicillin-resistant pneumococcal meningitis. Lancet *339*:405–408, 1992.
94. Frost, J. A., Kelleher, A., and Rowe, B.: Increasing ciprofloxacin resistance in salmonellas in England and Wales 1991–1994. J. Antimicrob. Chemother. *37*:85–91, 1996.
95. Fuentes, F., Gimenez, M. J., Marco, F., et al.: In vitro susceptibility to gemifloxacin and trovafloxacin of *Streptococcus pneumoniae* strains exhibiting decreased susceptibility to ciprofloxacin. Eur. J. Clin. Microbiol. Infect. Dis. *19*:137–139, 2000.
96. Gales, A. C., Jones, R. N., Gordon, K. A., et al.: Activity and spectrum of 22 antimicrobial agents tested against urinary tract infection pathogens in hospitalized patients in Latin America: Report from the second year of the SENTRY antimicrobial surveillance program (1998). J. Antimicrob. Chemother. *45*:295–303, 2000.
97. Galimand, M., Gerbaud, G., Guibourdenche, M., et al.: High-level chloramphenicol resistance in *Neisseria meningitidis.* N. Engl. J. Med. *339*:868–874, 1998.
98. Gay, K., Baughman, W., Miller, Y., et al.: The emergence of *Streptococcus pneumoniae* resistant to macrolide antimicrobial agents: A 6-year population-based assessment. J. Infect. Dis. *182*:1417–1424, 2000.
99. Gay, K., and Stephens, D. S.: Structure and dissemination of a chromosomal insertion element encoding macrolide efflux in *Streptococcus pneumoniae*. J. Infect. Dis. *184*:56–65, 2001.
100. Georgopapadakou, N. H.: Penicillin-binding proteins and bacterial resistance to beta-lactams. Antimicrob. Agents Chemother. *37*:2045–2053, 1993.
101. Gessner, B. D., Sutanto, A., Steinhoff, M., et al.: A population-based survey of *Haemophilus influenzae* type b nasopharyngeal carriage prevalence in Lombok Island, Indonesia. Pediatr. Infect. Dis. J. *17*(Suppl.):179–182, 1998.
102. Gheorghiu, R., Yuan, M., Hall, L. M., and Livermore, D. M.: Bases of variation in resistance to beta-lactams in *Klebsiella oxytoca* isolates hyperproducing K1 beta-lactamase. J. Antimicrob. Chemother. *40*:533–541, 1997.
103. Ghuysen, J. M.: Serine beta-lactamases and penicillin-binding proteins. Annu. Rev. Microbiol. *45*:37–67, 1991.
104. Gibreel, A., Sjogren, E., Kaijser, B., et al.: Rapid emergence of high-level resistance to quinolones in *Campylobacter jejuni* associated with mutational changes in gyrA and parC. Antimicrob. Agents Chemother. *42*:3276–3278, 1998.
105. Glynn, M. K., Bopp, C., Dewitt, W., et al.: Emergence of multidrug-resistant *Salmonella enterica* serotype *typhimurium* DT104 infections in the United States. N. Engl. J. Med. *338*:1333–1338, 1998.
106. Goettsch, W., van Pelt, W., Nagelkerke, N., et al.: Increasing resistance to fluoroquinolones in *Escherichia coli* from urinary tract infections in the Netherlands. J. Antimicrob. Chemother. *46*:223–228, 2000.
107. Gordon, M. A., Walsh, A. L., Chaponda, M., et al.: Bacteraemia and mortality among adult medical admissions in Malawi—predominance of non-*typhi* salmonellae and *Streptococcus pneumoniae.* J. Infect. *42*:44–49, 2001.
108. Granizo, J. J., Aguilar, L., Casal, J., et al.: *Streptococcus pyogenes* resistance to erythromycin in relation to macrolide consumption in Spain (1986–1997). J. Antimicrob. Chemother. *46*:959–964, 2000.
109. Gray, J. W., and George, R. H.: Experience of vancomycin-resistant enterococci in a children's hospital. J. Hosp. Infect. *45*:11–18, 2000.
110. Grebe, T., and Hakenbeck, R.: Penicillin-binding proteins 2b and 2x of *Streptococcus pneumoniae* are primary resistance determinants for different classes of beta-lactam antibiotics. Antimicrob. Agents Chemother. *40*:829–834, 1996.
111. Griffin, P. M., Tauxe, R. V., Redd, S. C., et al.: Emergence of highly trimethoprim-sulfamethoxazole–resistant *Shigella* in a Native American population: An epidemiologic study. Am. J. Epidemiol. *129*:1042–1051, 1989.
112. Guirao, G. Y., Martinez Toldos, M. C., Mora Peris, B., et al.: Molecular diversity of quinolone resistance in genetically related clinical isolates of *Staphylococcus aureus* and susceptibility to newer quinolones. J. Antimicrob. Chemother. 47:157–161, 2001.
113. Gupta, K., Hooton, T. M., and Stamm, W. E.: Increasing antimicrobial resistance and the management of uncomplicated community-acquired urinary tract infections. Ann. Intern. Med. *135*:41–50, 2001.
114. Gupta, K., Sahm, D. F., Mayfield, D., and Stamm, W. E.: Antimicrobial resistance among uropathogens that cause community-acquired urinary tract infections in women: A nationwide analysis. Clin. Infect. Dis. *33*:89–94, 2001.
115. Hakenbeck, R., Balmelle, N., Weber, B., et al.: Mosaic genes and mosaic chromosomes: Intra- and interspecies genomic variation of *Streptococcus pneumoniae.* Infect. Immun. *69*:2477–2486, 2001.
116. Hakenbeck, R., Briese, T., Chalkley, L., et al.: Antigenic variation of penicillin-binding proteins from penicillin-resistant clinical strains of *Streptococcus pneumoniae.* J. Infect. Dis. *164*:313–319, 1991.
117. Hakenbeck, R., and Coyette, J.: Resistant penicillin-binding proteins. Cell. Mol. Life Sci. *54*:332–340, 1998.
118. Hakenbeck, R., Tarpay, M., and Tomasz, A.: Multiple changes of penicillin-binding proteins in penicillin-resistant clinical isolates of *Streptococcus pneumoniae.* Antimicrob. Agents Chemother. *17*:364–371, 1980.
119. Harnett, N.: High level resistance to trimethoprim, cotrimoxazole and other antimicrobial agents among clinical isolates of *Shigella* species in Ontario, Canada—an update. Epidemiol. Infect. *109*:463–472, 1992.
120. Hashimoto, Y., Tanimoto, K., Ozawa, Y., et al.: Amino acid substitutions in the VanS sensor of the VanA-type vancomycin- resistant *Enterococcus* strains result in high-level vancomycin resistance and low-level teicoplanin resistance. F. E. M. S. Microbiol. Lett. *185*:247–254, 2000.
121. Hayden, M. K.: Insights into the epidemiology and control of infection with vancomycin-resistant enterococci. Clin. Infect. Dis. *31*:1058–1065, 2000.
122. Henwood, C. J., Livermore, D. M., James, D., and Warner, M.: Antimicrobial susceptibility of *Pseudomonas aeruginosa:* Results of a UK survey and evaluation of the British Society for Antimicrobial Chemotherapy disc susceptibility test. J. Antimicrob. Chemother. *47*:789–799, 2001.
123. Heritage, J., M'Zali, F. H., Gascoyne-Binzi, D., and Hawkey, P. M.: Evolution and spread of SHV extended-spectrum beta-lactamases in gram-negative bacteria. J. Antimicrob. Chemother. *44*:309–318, 1999.
124. Hoban, D. J., Doern, G. V., Fluit, A. C., et al.: Worldwide prevalence of antimicrobial resistance in *Streptococcus pneumoniae, Haemophilus influenzae,* and *Moraxella catarrhalis* in the SENTRY Antimicrobial Surveillance Program, 1997–1999. Clin. Infect. Dis. *32*(Suppl. 2):81–93, 2001.
125. Hoge, C. W., Gambel, J. M., Srijan, A., et al.: Trends in antibiotic resistance among diarrheal pathogens isolated in Thailand over 15 years. Clin. Infect. Dis. *26*:341–345, 1998.
126. Holman, T. R., Wu, Z., Wanner, B. L., and Walsh, C. T.: Identification of the DNA-binding site for the phosphorylated VanR protein required for vancomycin resistance in *Enterococcus faecium.* Biochemistry *33*:4625–4631, 1994.
127. Hooper, D. C.: Quinolone mode of action—new aspects. Drugs *45*:8–14, 1993.
128. Hooper, D. C.: Bacterial topoisomerases, anti-topoisomerases, and anti-topoisomerase resistance. Clin. Infect. Dis. *27*(Suppl. 1):54–63, 1998.

129. Hooper, D. C.: Mechanisms of action of antimicrobials: Focus on fluoroquinolones. Clin. Infect. Dis. *32*(Suppl. 1):9–15, 2001.
130. Hooper, D. C., Wolfson, J. S., Bozza, M. A., and Ng, E. Y.: Genetics and regulation of outer membrane protein expression by quinolone resistance loci nfxB, nfxC, and cfxB. Antimicrob. Agents Chemother. *36*:1151–1154, 1992.
131. Howard, A. J., Magee, J. T., Fitzgerald, K. A., and Dunstan, F. D.: Factors associated with antibiotic resistance in coliform organisms from community urinary tract infection in Wales. J. Antimicrob. Chemother. *47*:305–313, 2001.
132. Hsueh, P. R., Liu, Y. C., Shyr, J. M., et al.: Multicenter surveillance of antimicrobial resistance of *Streptococcus pneumoniae, Haemophilus influenzae,* and *Moraxella catarrhalis* in Taiwan during the 1998–1999 respiratory season. Antimicrob. Agents Chemother. *44*:1342–1345, 2000.
133. Hsueh, P. R., Teng, L. J., Lee, L. N., et al.: High Incidence of erythromycin resistance among clinical isolates of *Streptococcus agalactiae* in Taiwan. Antimicrob. Agents Chemother. *45*:3205–3208, 2001.
134. Huovinen, P.: Resistance to trimethoprim-sulfamethoxazole. Clin. Infect. Dis. *32*:1608–1614, 2001.
135. Huovinen, P., Sundstrom, L., Swedberg, G., and Skold, O.: Trimethoprim and sulfonamide resistance. Antimicrob. Agents Chemother. *39*:279–289, 1995.
136. Hyde, T. B., Gay, K., Stephens, D. S., et al.: Macrolide resistance among invasive *Streptococcus pneumoniae* isolates. J. A. M. A. *286*:1857–1862, 2001.
137. Ikeda, F., Yokota, Y., Ikemoto, A., et al.: Interaction of beta-lactam antibiotics with the penicillin-binding proteins of penicillin-resistant *Streptococcus pneumoniae.* Chemotherapy *41*:159–164, 1995.
138. Inderlied, C. B., and Nash, K. A.: Antimicrobial agents: In vitro susceptibility testing, spectra of activity, mechanisms of action and resistance and assays for activity in biological fluids. *In* Lorian, V. (ed.): Antibiotics in Laboratory Medicine. 4th ed., Baltimore, Williams & Wilkins, 1996, pp. 127–175.
139. Ismaeel, N. A.: Resistance of bacteria from human faecal flora to antimicrobial agents. J. Trop. Med. Hyg. *96*:51–55, 1993.
140. Ito, H., Yoshida, H., Bogaki-Shonai, M., et al.: Quinolone resistance mutations in the DNA gyrase gyrA and gyrB genes of *Staphylococcus aureus.* Antimicrob. Agents Chemother. *38*:2014–2023, 1994.
141. Jacobs, C., Joris, B., Jamin, M., et al.: AmpD, essential for both beta-lactamase regulation and cell wall recycling, is a novel cytosolic N-acetylmuramyl-L-alanine amidase. Mol. Microbiol. *15*:553–559, 1995.
142. Jacobs, M. R., Bajaksouzian, S., Zilles, A., et al.: Susceptibilities of *Streptococcus pneumoniae* and *Haemophilus influenzae* to 10 oral antimicrobial agents based on pharmacodynamic parameters: 1997 U.S. surveillance study. Antimicrob. Agents Chemother. *43*:1901–1908, 1999.
143. Jenssen, W. D., Thakker-Varia, S., Dubin, D. T., and Weinstein, M. P.: Prevalence of macrolides-lincosamides-streptogramin B resistance and erm gene classes among clinical strains of staphylococci and streptococci. Antimicrob. Agents Chemother. *31*:883–888, 1987.
144. Jick, S.: Ciprofloxacin safety in a pediatric population. Pediatr. Infect. Dis. J. *16*:130–134, 160–162, 1997.
145. Jochimsen, E. M., Fish, L., Manning, K., et al.: Control of vancomycin-resistant enterococci at a community hospital: Efficacy of patient and staff cohorting. Infect. Control Hosp. Epidemiol. *20*:106–109, 1999.
146. John, J. F., Jr., McKee, K. T., Jr., Twitty, J. A., and Schaffner, W.: Molecular epidemiology of sequential nursery epidemics caused by multiresistant *Klebsiella pneumoniae.* J. Pediatr. *102*:825–830, 1983.
147. John, T. J., Cherian, T., and Raghupathy, P.: *Haemophilus influenzae* disease in children in India: A hospital perspective. Pediatr. Infect. Dis. J. *17*(Suppl.):169–171, 1998.
148. Johnson, A. P., Warner, M., George, R. C., and Livermore, D. M.: Activity of moxifloxacin against clinical isolates of *Streptococcus pneumoniae* from England and Wales. J. Antimicrob. Chemother. *47*:411–415, 2001.
149. Johnston, N. J., De Azavedo, J. C., Kellner, J. D., and Low, D. E.: Prevalence and characterization of the mechanisms of macrolide, lincosamide, and streptogramin resistance in isolates of *Streptococcus pneumoniae.* Antimicrob. Agents Chemother. *42*:2425–2426, 1998.
150. Jorgensen, J. H., Weigel, L. M., Swenson, J. M., et al.: Activities of clinafloxacin, gatifloxacin, gemifloxacin, and trovafloxacin against recent clinical isolates of levofloxacin-resistant *Streptococcus pneumoniae.* Antimicrob. Agents Chemother. *44*:2962–2968, 2000.
151. Kantzanou, M., Tassios, P. T., Tseleni-Kotsovili, A., et al.: Reduced susceptibility to vancomycin of nosocomial isolates of methicillin-resistant *Staphylococcus aureus.* J. Antimicrob. Chemother. 43:729–731, 1999.
152. Kaplan, E. L., Johnson, D. R., Del Rosario, M. C., and Horn, D. L.: Susceptibility of group A beta-hemolytic streptococci to thirteen antibiotics: Examination of 301 strains isolated in the United States between 1994 and 1997. Pediatr. Infect. Dis. J. *18*:1069–1072, 1999.
153. Kaplan, S. L., and Mason, E. O., Jr.: Management of infections due to antibiotic-resistant *Streptococcus pneumoniae.* Clin. Microbiol. Rev. *11*:628–644, 1998.
154. Kataja, J., Huovinen, P., and Seppälä, H.: Erythromycin resistance genes in group A streptococci of different geographical origins. The Macrolide Resistance Study Group. J. Antimicrob. Chemother. *46*:789–792, 2000.
155. Keeley, D. J., Nkrumah, F. K., and Kapuyanyika, C.: Randomized trial of sulfamethoxazole + trimethoprim versus procaine penicillin for the outpatient treatment of childhood pneumonia in Zimbabwe. Bull. World Health Organ. *68*:185–192, 1990.
156. Kellner, J. D., and Ford-Jones, E. L.: *Streptococcus pneumoniae* carriage in children attending 59 Canadian child care centers. Toronto Child Care Centre Study Group. Arch. Pediatr. Adolesc. Med. *153*:495–502, 1999.
157. Knox, J. R.: Extended-spectrum and inhibitor-resistant TEM-type beta-lactamases: Mutations, specificity, and three-dimensional structure. Antimicrob. Agents Chemother. *39*:2593–2601, 1995.
158. Kohler, T., Kok, M., Michea-Hamzehpour, M., et al.: Multidrug efflux in intrinsic resistance to trimethoprim and sulfamethoxazole in *Pseudomonas aeruginosa.* Antimicrob. Agents Chemother. *40*:2288–2290, 1996.
159. Korner, J. R., Reeves, S. D., and MacGowan, P. A.: Dangers of oral fluoroquinolone treatment in community acquired upper respiratory tract infections. B. M. J. *308*:191–192, 1994.
160. Korten, V., Huang, W. M., and Murray, B. E.: Analysis by PCR and direct DNA sequencing of gyrA mutations associated with fluoroquinolone resistance in *Enterococcus faecalis.* Antimicrob. Agents Chemother. *38*:2091–2094, 1994.
161. Kotra, L. P., Haddad, J., and Mobashery, S.: Aminoglycosides: Perspectives on mechanisms of action and resistance and strategies to counter resistance. Antimicrob. Agents Chemother. *44*:3249–3256, 2000.
162. Kristensen, B., Smedegaard, H. H., Pedersen, H. M., et al.: Antibiotic resistance patterns among blood culture isolates in a Danish county 1981–1995. J. Med. Microbiol. *48*:67–71, 1999.
163. Kruse, H., Kariuki, S., Soli, N., and Olsvik, O.: Multiresistant *Shigella* species from African AIDS patients: Antibacterial resistance patterns and application of the E-test for determination of minimum inhibitory concentration. Scand. J. Infect. Dis. *24*:733–739, 1992.
164. Lai, K. K., Kelley, A. L., Melvin, Z. S., et al.: Failure to eradicate vancomycin-resistant enterococci in a university hospital and the cost of barrier precautions. Infect. Control Hosp. Epidemiol. *19*:647–652, 1998.
165. Laible, G., Spratt, B. G., and Hakenbeck, R.: Interspecies recombinational events during the evolution of altered PBP 2x genes in penicillin-resistant clinical isolates of *Streptococcus pneumoniae.* Mol. Microbiol. *5*:1993–2002, 1991.
166. Le, T. P., and Miller, L. G.: Empirical therapy for uncomplicated urinary tract infections in an era of increasing antimicrobial resistance: A decision and cost analysis. Clin. Infect. Dis. *33*:615–621, 2001.
167. Leach, A. J., Shelby-James, T. M., Mayo, M., et al.: A prospective study of the impact of community-based azithromycin treatment of trachoma on carriage and resistance of *Streptococcus pneumoniae.* Clin. Infect. Dis. *24*:356–362, 1997.
168. Lee, B. L., Padula, A. M., Kimbrough, R. C., et al.: Infectious complications with respiratory pathogens despite ciprofloxacin therapy. N. Engl. J. Med. *325*:520–521, 1991.
169. Lee, H. J., Park, J. Y., Jang, S. H., et al.: High incidence of resistance to multiple antimicrobials in clinical isolates of *Streptococcus pneumoniae* from a university hospital in Korea. Clin. Infect. Dis. *20*:826–835, 1995.
170. Lee, H. K., Lee, W. G., and Cho, S. R.: Clinical and molecular biological analysis of a nosocomial outbreak of vancomycin-resistant enterococci in a neonatal intensive care unit. Acta Paediatr. *88*:651–654, 1999.
171. Lelievre, H., Lina, G., Jones, M. E., et al.: Emergence and spread in French hospitals of methicillin-resistant *Staphylococcus aureus* with increasing susceptibility to gentamicin and other antibiotics. J. Clin. Microbiol. *37*:3452–3457, 1999.
172. Lester, S. C., del Pilar Pla, M., Wang, F., et al.: The carriage of *Escherichia coli* resistant to antimicrobial agents by healthy children in Boston, in Caracas, Venezuela, and in Qin Pu, China. N. Engl. J. Med. *323*:285–289, 1990.
173. Levy, S. B.: Active efflux mechanisms for antimicrobial resistance. Antimicrob. Agents Chemother. *36*:695–703, 1992.
174. Levy, S. B., Marshall, B., Schluederberg, S., et al.: High frequency of antimicrobial resistance in human fecal flora. Antimicrob. Agents Chemother. *32*:1801–1806, 1988.
175. Li, X. Z., Livermore, D. M., and Nikaido, H.: Role of efflux pump(s) in intrinsic resistance of *Pseudomonas aeruginosa:* Resistance to tetracycline, chloramphenicol, and norfloxacin. Antimicrob. Agents Chemother. *38*:1732–1741, 1994.
176. Lima, A. A., Sidrim, J. J., Lima, N. L., et al.: Molecular epidemiology of multiply antibiotic-resistant *Shigella flexneri* in Fortaleza, Brazil. J. Clin. Microbiol. *35*:1061–1065, 1997.
177. Lina, G., Quaglia, A., Reverdy, M. E., et al.: Distribution of genes encoding resistance to macrolides, lincosamides, and streptogramins among staphylococci. Antimicrob. Agents Chemother. *43*:1062–1066, 1999.
178. Lindberg, F., Lindquist, S., and Normark, S.: Inactivation of the ampD gene causes semiconstitutive overproduction of the inducible *Citrobacter freundii* beta-lactamase. J. Bacteriol. *169*:1923–1928, 1987.

179. Livermore D. M., and Williams, J. D.: Beta-lactams: Mode of action and mechanisms of bacterial resistance. *In* Lorian, V. (ed.): Antibiotics in Laboratory Medicine. 4th ed. Baltimore, Williams & Wilkins, 1996, pp. 502–578.
180. Low, D. E., Keller, N., Barth, A., and Jones, R. N.: Clinical prevalence, antimicrobial susceptibility, and geographic resistance patterns of enterococci: Results from the SENTRY Antimicrobial Surveillance Program, 1997–1999. Clin. Infect. Dis. *32*(Suppl. 2):133–145, 2001.
181. Lucas, G. M., Lechtzin, N., Puryear, D. W., et al.: Vancomycin-resistant and vancomycin-susceptible enterococcal bacteremia: Comparison of clinical features and outcomes. Clin. Infect. Dis. *26*:1127–1133, 1998.
182. Lutsar, I., McCracken, G. H., Jr., and Friedland, I. R.: Antibiotic pharmacodynamics in cerebrospinal fluid. Clin. Infect. Dis. *27*:1117–1127, 1998.
183. Malik, R. K., Montecalvo, M. A., Reale, M. R., et al.: Epidemiology and control of vancomycin-resistant enterococci in a regional neonatal intensive care unit. Pediatr. Infect. Dis. J. *18*:352–356, 1999.
184. Maneewannakul, K., and Levy, S. B.: Identification for mar mutants among quinolone-resistant clinical isolates of *Escherichia coli*. Antimicrob. Agents Chemother. *40*:1695–1698, 1996.
185. Manges, A. R., Johnson, J. R., Foxman, B., et al.: Widespread distribution of urinary tract infections caused by a multidrug-resistant *Escherichia coli* clonal group. N. Engl. J. Med. *345*:1007–1013, 2001.
186. Manninen, R., Huovinen, P., and Nissinen, A.: Increasing antimicrobial resistance in *Streptococcus pneumoniae, Haemophilus influenzae* and *Moraxella catarrhalis* in Finland. J. Antimicrob. Chemother. *40*:387–392, 1997.
187. Martin, J. M., Green, M., Barbadora, K. A., and Wald, E. R.: Erythromycin-resistant group A streptococci in schoolchildren in Pittsburgh. N. Engl. J. Med. *346*:1200–1206, 2002.
188. Martinez, J. L., Alonso, A., Gomez-Gomez, J. M., and Baquero, F.: Quinolone resistance by mutations in chromosomal gyrase genes. Just the tip of the iceberg? J. Antimicrob. Chemother. *42*:683–688, 1998.
189. Maseda, H., Yoneyama, H., and Nakae, T.: Assignment of the substrate-selective subunits of the MexEF-OprN multidrug efflux pump of *Pseudomonas aeruginosa*. Antimicrob. Agents Chemother. *44*:658–664, 2000.
190. Masterton, R. G., and Bochsler, J. A.: High-dosage co-amoxiclav in a single dose versus 7 days of co-trimoxazole as treatment of uncomplicated lower urinary tract infection in women. J. Antimicrob. Chemother. *35*:129–137, 1995.
191. Matsuoka, M., Janosi, L., Endou, K., and Nakajima, Y.: Cloning and sequences of inducible and constitutive macrolide resistance genes in *Staphylococcus aureus* that correspond to an ABC transporter. F. E. M. S. Microbiol Lett *181*:91–100, 1999.
192. May, J., Shannon, K., King, A., and French, G.: Glycopeptide tolerance in *Staphylococcus aureus*. J. Antimicrob. Chemother. *42*:189–197, 1998.
193. Mazodier, P., and Davies, J.: Gene transfer between distantly related bacteria. Annu. Rev. Genet. *25*:147–171, 1991.
194. McCarty, J. M., Richard, G., Huck, W., et al.: A randomized trial of short-course ciprofloxacin, ofloxacin, or trimethoprim/sulfamethoxazole for the treatment of acute urinary tract infection in women. Ciprofloxacin Urinary Tract Infection Group. Am. J. Med. *106*:292–299, 1999.
195. McCracken, G. H., Jr.: Emergence of resistant *Streptococcus pneumoniae:* A problem in pediatrics. Pediatr. Infect. Dis. J. *14*:424–428, 1995.
196. McCracken, G. H., Jr.: Treatment of acute otitis media in an era of increasing microbial resistance. Pediatr. Infect. Dis. J. *17*:576–580, 1998.
197. McCracken, G. H., Jr.: Prescribing antimicrobial agents for treatment of acute otitis media. Pediatr. Infect. Dis. J. *18*:1141–1416, 1999.
198. McDonald, L. C., Rossiter, S., Mackinson, C., et al.: Quinupristin-dalfopristin–resistant *Enterococcus faecium* on chicken and in human stool specimens. N. Engl. J. Med. *345*:1155–1160, 2001.
199. McKee, K. T., Jr., Cotton, R. B., Stratton, C. W., et al.: Nursery epidemic due to multiply-resistant *Klebsiella pneumoniae:* Epidemiologic setting and impact on perinatal health care delivery. Infect. Control *3*:150–156, 1982.
200. McNeeley, D. F., Brown, A. E., Noel, G. J., et al.: An investigation of vancomycin-resistant *Enterococcus faecium* within the pediatric service of a large urban medical center. Pediatr. Infect. Dis. J. *17*:184–188, 1998.
201. Medeiros, A. A.: Evolution and dissemination of beta-lactamases accelerated by generations of beta-lactam antibiotics. Clin. Infect. Dis. *24*(Suppl. 1):19–45, 1997.
202. Mermin, J. H., Villar, R., Carpenter, J., et al.: A massive epidemic of multidrug-resistant typhoid fever in Tajikistan associated with consumption of municipal water. J. Infect. Dis. *179*:1416–1422, 1999.
203. Mingeot-Leclercq, M. P., Glupczynski, Y., and Tulkens, P. M.: Aminoglycosides: Activity and resistance. Antimicrob. Agents Chemother. *43*:727–737, 1999.
204. Mitten, M. J., Meulbroek, J., Nukkala, M., et al.: Efficacies of ABT-773, a new ketolide, against experimental bacterial infections. Antimicrob. Agents Chemother. *45*:2585–2593, 2001.
205. Molbak, K., Baggesen, D. L., Aarestrup, F. M., et al.: An outbreak of multidrug-resistant, quinolone-resistant *Salmonella enterica* serotype *typhimurium* DT104. N. Engl. J. Med. 341:1420–1425, 1999.
206. Montecalvo, M. A., Horowitz, H., Gedris, C., et al.: Outbreak of vancomycin-, ampicillin-, and aminoglycoside-resistant *Enterococcus faecium* bacteremia in an adult oncology unit. Antimicrob. Agents. Chemother. *38*:1363–1367, 1994.
207. Montecalvo, M. A., Jarvis, W. R., Uman, J., et al.: Infection-control measures reduce transmission of vancomycin-resistant enterococci in an endemic setting. Ann. Intern. Med. *131*:269–272, 1999.
208. Moore, R. A., Beckthold, B., Wong, S., et al.: Nucleotide sequence of the gyrA gene and characterization of ciprofloxacin-resistant mutants of *Helicobacter pylori*. Antimicrob. Agents Chemother. *39*:107–111, 1995.
209. Moosdeen, F.: The evolution of resistance to cephalosporins. Clin. Infect. Dis. *24*:487–493, 1997.
210. Morales, W. J., Dickey, S. S., Bornick, P., and Lim, D. V.: Change in antibiotic resistance of group B streptococcus: Impact on intrapartum management. Am. J. Obstet. Gynecol. *181*:310–314, 1999.
211. Morita, J. Y., Kahn, E., Thompson, T., et al.: Impact of azithromycin on oropharyngeal carriage of group A *Streptococcus* and nasopharyngeal carriage of macrolide-resistant *Streptococcus pneumoniae*. Pediatr. Infect. Dis. J. *19*:41–46, 2000.
212. Morosini, M. I., Canton, R., Loza, E., et al.: In vitro activity of telithromycin against Spanish *Streptococcus pneumoniae* isolates with characterized macrolide resistance mechanisms. Antimicrob. Agents Chemother. *45*:2427–2431, 2001.
213. Morris, J. G., Jr., Shay, D. K., Hebden, J. N., et al.: Enterococci resistant to multiple antimicrobial agents, including vancomycin. Establishment of endemicity in a university medical center. Ann. Intern. Med. *123*:250–259, 1995.
214. Munoz, R., Dowson, C. G., Daniels, M., et al.: Genetics of resistance to third-generation cephalosporins in clinical isolates of *Streptococcus pneumoniae*. Mol. Microbiol. *6*:2461–2465, 1992.
215. Murray, B. E.: Vancomycin-resistant enterococcal infections. N. Engl. J. Med. *342*:710–721, 2000.
216. Navarro, F., and Courvalin, P.: Analysis of genes encoding D-alanine-D-alanine ligase-related enzymes in *Enterococcus casseliflavus* and *Enterococcus flavescens*. Antimicrob. Agents Chemother. *38*:1788–1793, 1994.
217. Nelson, J. D.: Should ampicillin be abandoned for treatment of *Haemophilus influenzae* disease? Editorial. J. A. M. A. *229*:322–324, 1974.
218. Noble, W. C., Virani, Z., and Cree, R. G.: Co-transfer of vancomycin and other resistance genes from *Enterococcus faecalis* NCTC 12201 to *Staphylococcus aureus*. F. E. M. S. Microbiol. Lett. *72*:195–198, 1992.
219. Nordmann, P.: Trends in beta-lactam resistance among Enterobacteriaceae. Clin. Infect. Dis. *27*(Suppl. 1):100–106, 1998.
220. Nourse, C., Byrne, C., Kaufmann, M., et al.: VRE in the Republic of Ireland: Clinical significance, characteristics and molecular similarity of isolates. J. Hosp. Infect. *44*:288–293, 2000.
221. Osterblad, M., Hakanen, A., Manninen, R., et al.: A between-species comparison of antimicrobial resistance in enterobacteria in fecal flora. Antimicrob. Agents Chemother. *44*:1479–1484, 2000.
222. Ostroff, S. M., Harrison, L. H., Khallaf, N., et al.: Resistance patterns of *Streptococcus pneumoniae* and *Haemophilus influenzae* isolates recovered in Egypt from children with pneumonia. The Antimicrobial Resistance Surveillance Study Group. Clin. Infect. Dis. *23*:1069–1074, 1996.
223. Ostrowsky, B. E., Venkataraman, L., D'Agata, E. M., et al.: Vancomycin-resistant enterococci in intensive care units: High frequency of stool carriage during a non-outbreak period. Arch. Intern. Med. *159*:1467–1472, 1999.
224. Padayachee, T., and Klugman, K. P.: Novel expansions of the gene encoding dihydropteroate synthase in trimethoprim-sulfamethoxazole–resistant *Streptococcus pneumoniae*. Antimicrob. Agents Chemother. *43*:2225–2230, 1999.
225. Palavecino, E. L., Riedel, I., Berrios, X., et al.: Prevalence and mechanisms of macrolide resistance in *Streptococcus pyogenes* in Santiago, Chile. Antimicrob. Agents Chemother. *45*:339–341, 2001.
226. Pallares, R., Linares, J., Vadillo, M., et al.: Resistance to penicillin and cephalosporin and mortality from severe pneumococcal pneumonia in Barcelona, Spain. N. Engl. J. Med. *333*:474–480, 1995.
227. Palucha, A., Mikiewicz, B., and Gniadkowski, M.: Diversification of *Escherichia coli* expressing an SHV-type extended-spectrum beta-lactamase (ESBL) during a hospital outbreak: Emergence of an ESBL-hyperproducing strain resistant to expanded-spectrum cephalosporins. Antimicrob. Agents Chemother. *43*:393–396, 1999.
228. Pan, X. S., and Fisher, L. M.: DNA gyrase and topoisomerase IV are dual targets of clinafloxacin action in Streptococcus pneumoniae. Antimicrob. Agents Chemother. *42*:2810–2816, 1998.
229. Parent, R., and Roy, P. H.: The chloramphenicol acetyltransferase gene of Tn2424: A new breed of cat. J. Bacteriol. *174*:2891–2897, 1992.
230. Parry, C. M., Diep, T. S., Wain, J., et al.: Nasal carriage in Vietnamese children of *Streptococcus pneumoniae* resistant to multiple antimicrobial agents. Antimicrob. Agents Chemother. *44*:484–488, 2000.
231. Paterson, D. L., Mulazimoglu, L., Casellas, J. M., et al.: Epidemiology of ciprofloxacin resistance and its relationship to extended-spectrum beta-lactamase production in *Klebsiella pneumoniae* isolates causing bacteremia. Clin. Infect. Dis. *30*:473–478, 2000.
232. Patterson, J. E., and Zervos, M. J.: High-level gentamicin resistance in *Enterococcus:* Microbiology, genetic basis, and epidemiology. Rev. Infect. Dis. *12*:644–652, 1990.

233. Paulsen, I. T., Brown, M. H., and Skurray, R. A.: Proton-dependent multidrug efflux systems. Microbiol. Rev. *60*:575–608, 1996.
234. Perez-Trallero, E., Garcia-Arenzana, J. M., Jimenez, J. A., and Peris, A.: Therapeutic failure and selection of resistance to quinolones in a case of pneumococcal pneumonia treated with ciprofloxacin. Eur. J. Clin. Microbiol. Infect. Dis. *9*:905–906, 1990.
235. Perichon, B., Reynolds, P., and Courvalin, P.: VanD-type glycopeptide-resistant *Enterococcus faecium* BM4339. Antimicrob. Agents Chemother. *41*:2016–2018, 1997.
236. Philippon, A., Dusart, J., Joris, B., and Frere, J. M.: The diversity, structure and regulation of beta-lactamases. Cell. Mol. Life Sci. *54*:341–346, 1998.
237. Piddock, L. J.: Quinolone resistance and *Campylobacter* spp. J. Antimicrob. Chemother. *36*:891–898, 1995.
238. Piddock, L. J.: Mechanisms of fluoroquinolone resistance: An update 1994–1998. Drugs *58*:11–18, 1999.
239. Piddock, L. J., Johnson, M., Ricci, V., and Hill, S. L.: Activities of new fluoroquinolones against fluoroquinolone-resistant pathogens of the lower respiratory tract. Antimicrob. Agents Chemother. *42*:2956–2960, 1998.
240. Piddock, L. J., White, D. G., Gensberg, K., et al.: Evidence for an efflux pump mediating multiple antibiotic resistance in *Salmonella enterica* serovar *typhimurium*. Antimicrob. Agents Chemother. *44*:3118–3121, 2000.
241. Pikis, A., Donkersloot, J. A., Rodriguez, W. J., and Keith, J. M.: A conservative amino acid mutation in the chromosome-encoded dihydrofolate reductase confers trimethoprim resistance in *Streptococcus pneumoniae*. J. Infect. Dis. *178*:700–706, 1998.
242. Ploy, M. C., Lambert, T., Couty, J. P., and Denis, F.: Integrons: An antibiotic resistance gene capture and expression system. Clin. Chem. Lab. Med. *38*:483–488, 2000.
243. Prats, G., Mirelis, B., Llovet, T., et al.: Antibiotic resistance trends in enteropathogenic bacteria isolated in 1985–1987 and 1995–1998 in Barcelona. Antimicrob. Agents Chemother. *44*:1140–1145, 2000.
244. Radstrom, P., Fermer, C., Kristiansen, B. E., et al.: Transformational exchanges in the dihydropteroate synthase gene of *Neisseria meningitidis:* A novel mechanism for acquisition of sulfonamide resistance. J. Bacteriol. *174*:6386–6393, 1992.
245. Rahman, M., Mauff, G., Levy, J., et al.: Detection of 4-quinolone resistance mutation in gyrA gene of *Shigella dysenteriae* type 1 by PCR. Antimicrob. Agents Chemother. *38*:2488–2491, 1994.
246. Recchia, G. D., and Hall, R. M.: Gene cassettes: A new class of mobile element. Microbiology *141*:3015–3027, 1995.
247. Recht, M. I., Douthwaite, S., and Puglisi, J. D.: Basis for prokaryotic specificity of action of aminoglycoside antibiotics. EMBO J. *18*:3133–3138, 1999.
248. Recht, M. I., Fourmy, D., Blanchard, S. C., et al.: RNA sequence determinants for aminoglycoside binding to an A-site rRNA model oligonucleotide. J. Mol. Biol. *262*:421–436, 1996.
249. Reed, M. D., and Blumer, J. A.: Anti-infective therapy. *In* Jenson, H. B., and Baltimore, R. S. (eds.): Pediatric Infectious Diseases. Principles and Practice. 2nd ed. Philadelphia, W. B. Saunders, 2002, pp. 147–231.
250. Replogle, M. L., Fleming, D. W., and Cieslak, P. R.: Emergence of antimicrobial-resistant shigellosis in Oregon. Clin. Infect. Dis. 30:515–519, 2000.
251. Reynolds, P. E., Depardieu, F., Dutka-Malen, S., et al.: Glycopeptide resistance mediated by enterococcal transposon Tn1546 requires production of VanX for hydrolysis of D-alanyl-D-alanine. Mol. Microbiol. *13*:1065–1070, 1994.
252. Rice, L. B., and Bonomo, R. A.: Genetic and Biochemical Mechanisms of Bacterial Resistance to Antimicrobial Agents. *In* Lorian, V. (ed.): Antibiotics in Laboratory Medicine. 4th ed. Baltimore, Williams & Wilkins, 1996, pp. 453–501.
253. Richard, M. P., Aguado, A. G., Mattina, R., and Marre, R.: Sensitivity to sparfloxacin and other antibiotics, of *Streptococcus pneumoniae, Haemophilus influenzae* and *Moraxella catarrhalis* strains isolated from adult patients with community-acquired lower respiratory tract infections: A European multicentre study. SPAR Study Group. Surveillance Programme of Antibiotic Resistance. J. Antimicrob. Chemother. *41*:207–214, 1998.
254. Rittenhouse, S., McCloskey, L., Broskey, J., et al.: In vitro antibacterial activity of gemifloxacin and comparator compounds against common respiratory pathogens. J. Antimicrob. Chemother. *45*(Suppl. 1):23–27, 2000.
255. Roberts, M. C., Sutcliffe, J., Courvalin, P., et al.: Nomenclature for macrolide and macrolide-lincosamide-streptogramin B resistance determinants. Antimicrob. Agents Chemother. *43*:2823–2830, 1999.
256. Roland, S., Ferone, R., Harvey, R. J., et al.: The characteristics and significance of sulfonamides as substrates for *Escherichia coli* dihydropteroate synthase. J. Biol. Chem. *254*:10337–10345, 1979.
257. Rowe, A. K., Deming, M. S., Schwartz, B., et al.: Antimicrobial resistance of nasopharyngeal isolates of *Streptococcus pneumoniae* and *Haemophilus influenzae* from children in the Central African Republic. Pediatr. Infect. Dis. J. *19*:438–444, 2000.
258. Rudolph, K. M., Parkinson, A. J., Reasonover, A. L., et al.: Serotype distribution and antimicrobial resistance patterns of invasive isolates of *Streptococcus pneumoniae:* Alaska, 1991–1998. J. Infect. Dis. *182*:490–496, 2000.
259. Rydberg, J., and Cederberg, A.: Intrafamilial spreading of *Escherichia coli* resistant to trimethoprim. Scand. J. Infect. Dis. *18*:457–460, 1986.
260. Sahm, D. F., Peterson, D. E., Critchley, I. A., and Thornsberry, C.: Analysis of ciprofloxacin activity against *Streptococcus pneumoniae* after 10 years of use in the United States. Antimicrob. Agents Chemother. *44*:2521–2524, 2000.
261. Saiman, L., Mehar, F., Niu, W. W., et al.: Antibiotic susceptibility of multiply resistant *Pseudomonas aeruginosa* isolated from patients with cystic fibrosis, including candidates for transplantation. Clin. Infect. Dis. *23*:532–537, 1996.
262. Sa-Leao, R., Tomasz, A., Sanches, I. S., et al.: Carriage of internationally spread clones of *Streptococcus pneumoniae* with unusual drug resistance patterns in children attending day care centers in Lisbon, Portugal. J. Infect. Dis. *182*:1153–1160, 2000.
263. Salyers, A. A., Shoemaker, N. B., Stevens, A. M., and Li, L. Y.: Conjugative transposons: An unusual and diverse set of integrated gene transfer elements. Microbiol. Rev. *59*:579–590, 1995.
264. Sanders, C. C.: Mechanisms responsible for cross-resistance and dichotomous resistance among the quinolones. Clin. Infect. Dis. *32*(Suppl. 1):1–8, 2001.
265. Satta, G., Cornaglia, G., Mazzariol, A., et al.: Target for bacteriostatic and bactericidal activities of beta-lactam antibiotics against *Escherichia coli* resides in different penicillin-binding proteins. Antimicrob. Agents Chemother. *39*:812–818, 1995.
266. Savoia, D., Avanzini, C., Bosio, K., et al.: Macrolide resistance in group A streptococci. J. Antimicrob. Chemother. *45*:41–47, 2000.
267. Schaad, U. B., Wedgwood, J., Ruedeberg, A., et al.: Ciprofloxacin as antipseudomonal treatment in patients with cystic fibrosis. Pediatr. Infect. Dis. J. *16*:106–111, 123–126, 1997.
268. Schmitt, R.: Molecular biology of transposable elements. J. Antimicrob. Chemother. *18*(Suppl. C):25–34, 1986.
269. Schmitz, F. J., Fluit, A. C., Gondolf, M., et al.: The prevalence of aminoglycoside resistance and corresponding resistance genes in clinical isolates of staphylococci from 19 European hospitals. J. Antimicrob. Chemother. *43*:253–259, 1999.
270. Schmitz, F. J., Sadurski, R., Kray, A., et al.: Prevalence of macrolide-resistance genes in *Staphylococcus aureus* and *Enterococcus faecium* isolates from 24 European university hospitals. J. Antimicrob. Chemother. *45*:891–894, 2000.
271. Schmitz, F. J., Verhoef, J., and Fluit, A. C.: Prevalence of aminoglycoside resistance in 20 European university hospitals participating in the European SENTRY Antimicrobial Surveillance Programme. Eur. J. Clin. Microbiol. Infect. Dis. *18*:414–421, 1999.
272. Schouten, M. A., Hoogkamp-Korstanje, J. A., Meis, J. F., and Voss, A.: Prevalence of vancomycin-resistant enterococci in Europe. Eur. J. Clin. Microbiol. Infect. Dis. *19*:816–822, 2000.
273. Scott, J. R.: Regulation of plasmid replication. Microbiol. Rev. *48*:1–23, 1984.
274. Scott, J. R., and Churchward, G. G.: Conjugative transposition. Annu. Rev. Microbiol. *49*:367–397, 1995.
275. Seppälä, H., Klaukka, T., Vuopio-Varkila, J., et al.: The effect of changes in the consumption of macrolide antibiotics on erythromycin resistance in group A streptococci in Finland. Finnish Study Group for Antimicrobial Resistance. N. Engl. J. Med. *337*:441–446, 1997.
276. Shaw, K. J., Rather, P. N., Hare, R. S., and Miller, G. H.: Molecular genetics of aminoglycoside resistance genes and familial relationships of the aminoglycoside-modifying enzymes. Microbiol. Rev. *57*:138–163, 1993.
277. Shaw, W. V.: Bacterial resistance to chloramphenicol. Br. Med. Bull. *40*:36–41, 1984.
278. Shawar, R. M., MacLeod, D. L., Garber, R. L., et al.: Activities of tobramycin and six other antibiotics against *Pseudomonas aeruginosa* isolates from patients with cystic fibrosis. Antimicrob. Agents Chemother. *43*:2877–2880, 1999.
279. Shay, D. K., Maloney, S. A., Montecalvo, M., et al.: Epidemiology and mortality risk of vancomycin-resistant enterococcal bloodstream infections. J. Infect. Dis. *172*:993–1000, 1995.
280. Silverman, J., Thal, L. A., Perri, M. B., et al.: Epidemiologic evaluation of antimicrobial resistance in community-acquired enterococci. J. Clin. Microbiol. *36*:830–832, 1998.
281. Slaughter, S., Hayden, M. K., Nathan, C., et al.: A comparison of the effect of universal use of gloves and gowns with that of glove use alone on acquisition of vancomycin-resistant enterococci in a medical intensive care unit. Ann. Intern. Med. *125*:448–456, 1996.
282. Smith, K. E., Besser, J. M., Hedberg, C. W., et al.: Quinolone-resistant *Campylobacter jejuni* infections in Minnesota, 1992–1998. Investigation Team. N. Engl. J. Med. *340*:1525–1532, 1999.
283. Smith, T. L., Pearson, M. L., Wilcox, K. R., et al.: Emergence of vancomycin resistance in *Staphylococcus aureus.* Glycopeptide-Intermediate *Staphylococcus aureus* Working Group. N. Engl. J. Med. *340*:493–501, 1999.
284. Sorensen, T. L., Blom, M., Monnet, D. L., et al.: Transient intestinal carriage after ingestion of antibiotic-resistant Enterococcus faecium from chicken and pork. N. Engl. J. Med. *345*:1161–1166, 2001.
285. Spangler, S. K., Jacobs, M. R., and Appelbaum, P. C.: Susceptibilities of penicillin-susceptible and -resistant strains of *Streptococcus pneumoniae*

to RP 59500, vancomycin, erythromycin, PD 131628, sparfloxacin, temafloxacin, win 57273, ofloxacin, and ciprofloxacin. Antimicrob. Agents Chemother. *36*:856–859, 1992.

286. Spangler, S. K., Jacobs, M. R., and Appelbaum, P. C.: In vitro susceptibilities of 185 penicillin-susceptible and -resistant pneumococci to WY-49605 (SUN/SY 5555), a new oral penem, compared with those to penicillin G, amoxicillin, amoxicillin-clavulanate, cefixime, cefaclor, cefpodoxime, cefuroxime, and cefdinir. Antimicrob. Agents Chemother. *38*:2902–2904, 1994.
287. Steinke, D. T., Seaton, R. A., Phillips, G., et al.: Factors associated with trimethoprim-resistant bacteria isolated from urine samples. J. Antimicrob. Chemother. *43*:841–843, 1999.
288. Stratchounski, L. S., Kretchikova, O. I., Kozlov, R. S., et al.: Antimicrobial resistance of *Streptococcus pneumoniae* isolated from healthy children in day-care centers: Results of a multicenter study in Russia. Pediatr. Infect. Dis. J. *19*:196–200, 2000.
289. Straus, W. L., Qazi, S. A., Kundi, Z., et al.: Antimicrobial resistance and clinical effectiveness of co-trimoxazole versus amoxycillin for pneumonia among children in Pakistan: Randomised controlled trial. Pakistan Co-trimoxazole Study Group. Lancet *352*:270–274, 1998.
290. Sutcliffe, J., Tait-Kamradt, A., and Wondrack, L.: *Streptococcus pneumoniae* and *Streptococcus pyogenes* resistant to macrolides but sensitive to clindamycin: A common resistance pattern mediated by an efflux system. Antimicrob. Agents Chemother. *40*:1817–1824, 1996.
291. Sutcliffe, J. A., Gootz, T. D., and Barrett, J. F.: Biochemical characteristics and physiological significance of major DNA topoisomerases. Antimicrob. Agents Chemother. *33*:2027–2033, 1989.
292. Syrogiannopoulos, G. A., Grivea, I. N., Davies, T. A., et al.: Antimicrobial use and colonization with erythromycin-resistant *Streptococcus pneumoniae* in Greece during the first 2 years of life. Clin. Infect. Dis. *31*:887–893, 2000.
293. Talan, D. A., Stamm, W. E., Hooton, T. M., et al.: Comparison of ciprofloxacin (7 days) and trimethoprim-sulfamethoxazole (14 days) for acute uncomplicated pyelonephritis in women: A randomized trial. J. A. M. A. *283*:1583–1590, 2000.
294. Tarasi, A., Capone, A., Tarasi, D., et al.: Comparative in-vitro activity of moxifloxacin, penicillin, ceftriaxone and ciprofloxacin against pneumococci isolated from meningitis. J. Antimicrob. Chemother. *43*:833–835, 1999.
295. Thakker-Varia, S., Jenssen, W. D., Moon-McDermott, L., et al.: Molecular epidemiology of macrolides-lincosamides-streptogramin B resistance in *Staphylococcus aureus* and coagulase-negative staphylococci. Antimicrob. Agents Chemother. *31*:735–743, 1987.
296. Thomas, W. J., McReynolds, J. W., Mock, C. R., and Bailey, D. W.: Ampicillin-resistant *Haemophilus influenzae* meningitis. Letter. Lancet *1*:313, 1974.
297. Thompson, R.: R plasmid transfer. J. Antimicrob. Chemother. *18*(Suppl. C):13–23, 1986.
298. Thomson, K. S., and Sanders, C. C.: Dissociated resistance among fluoroquinolones. Antimicrob. Agents Chemother. *38*:2095–2100, 1994.
299. Thwaites, R. T., and Frost, J. A.: Drug resistance in *Campylobacter jejuni, C coli,* and *C lari* isolated from humans in north west England and Wales, 1997. J. Clin. Pathol. *52*:812–814, 1999.
300. Timmis, K. N., Gonzalez-Carrero, M. I., Sekizaki, T., and Rojo, F.: Biological activities specified by antibiotic resistance plasmids. J. Antimicrob. Chemother. *18*(Suppl. C):1–12, 1986.
301. Toledano, H., Schlesinger, Y., Raveh, D., et al.: Prospective surveillance of vancomycin-resistant enterococci in a neonatal intensive care unit. Eur. J. Clin. Microbiol. Infect. Dis. *19*:282–287, 2000.
302. Toltzis, P., Dul, M. J., Hoyen, C., et al.: Molecular epidemiology of antibiotic-resistant gram-negative bacilli in a neonatal intensive care unit during a nonoutbreak period. Pediatrics *108*:1143–1148, 2001.
303. Toltzis, P., Yamashita, T., Vilt, L., and Blumer, J. L.: Colonization with antibiotic-resistant gram-negative organisms in a pediatric intensive care unit. Crit. Care Med. *25*:538–544, 1997.
304. Trick, W. E., Kuehnert, M. J., Quirk, S. B., et al.: Regional dissemination of vancomycin-resistant enterococci resulting from interfacility transfer of colonized patients. J. Infect. Dis. *180*:391–396, 1999.
305. Ulijasz, A. T., and Weisblum, B.: Dissecting the VanRS signal transduction pathway with specific inhibitors. J. Bacteriol. *181*:627–631, 1999.
306. Urbina, R., Prado, V., and Canelo, E.: Trimethoprim resistance in enterobacteria isolated in Chile. J. Antimicrob. Chemother. *23*:143–149, 1989.
307. van den Braak, N., Ott, A., van Belkum, A., et al.: Prevalence and determinants of fecal colonization with vancomycin-resistant *Enterococcus* in hospitalized patients in The Netherlands. Infect. Control Hosp. Epidemiol. *21*:520–524, 2000.
308. Vanhoof, R., Nyssen, H. J., Van Bossuyt, E., and Hannecart-Pokorni, E.: Aminoglycoside resistance in gram-negative blood isolates from various hospitals in Belgium and the Grand Duchy of Luxembourg. Aminoglycoside Resistance Study Group. J. Antimicrob. Chemother. *44*:483–488, 1999.
309. Varaldo, P. E., Debbia, E. A., Nicoletti, G., et al.: Nationwide survey in Italy of treatment of *Streptococcus pyogenes* pharyngitis in children: Influence of macrolide resistance on clinical and microbiological outcomes. Artemis-Italy Study Group. Clin. Infect. Dis. *29*:869–873, 1999.
310. Varon, E., Levy, C., De La Rocque, F., Boucherat, M., et al.: Impact of antimicrobial therapy on nasopharyngeal carriage of *Streptococcus pneumoniae, Haemophilus influenzae,* and *Branhamella catarrhalis* in children with respiratory tract infections. Clin. Infect. Dis. *31*:477–481, 2000.
311. Vila, J., Ruiz, J., Marco, F., et al.: Association between double mutation in gyrA gene of ciprofloxacin-resistant clinical isolates of *Escherichia coli* and MICs. Antimicrob. Agents Chemother. *38*:2477–2479, 1994.
312. Villar, R. G., Macek, M. D., Simons, S., et al.: Investigation of multidrug-resistant *Salmonella* serotype *typhimurium* DT104 infections linked to raw-milk cheese in Washington State. J. A. M. A. *281*:1811–1816, 1999.
313. von Baum, H., Schehl, J., Geiss, H. K., and Schaefer, F.: Prevalence of vancomycin-resistant enterococci among children with end-stage renal failure. Mid-European Pediatric Peritoneal Dialysis Study Group. Clin. Infect. Dis. *29*:912–916, 1999.
314. Walsh, C. T.: Vancomycin resistance: Decoding the molecular logic. Science *261*:308–309, 1993.
315. Wang, Y., Huang, W. M., and Taylor, D. E.: Cloning and nucleotide sequence of the *Campylobacter jejuni* gyrA gene and characterization of quinolone resistance mutations. Antimicrob. Agents Chemother. *37*:457–463, 1993.
316. Weinberg, G. A., Spitzer, E. D., Murray, P. R., et al.: Antimicrobial susceptibility patterns of *Haemophilus* isolates from children in eleven developing nations. BOSTID *Haemophilus* Susceptibility Study Group. Bull. World Health Organ. *68*:179–184, 1990.
317. Weisblum, B.: Insights into erythromycin action from studies of its activity as inducer of resistance. Antimicrob. Agents Chemother. *39*:797–805, 1995.
318. Weiss, K., De Azavedo, J., Restieri, C., et al.: Phenotypic and genotypic characterization of macrolide-resistant group A *Streptococcus* strains in the province of Quebec, Canada. J. Antimicrob. Chemother. *47*:345–348, 2001.
319. Wendt, C., Krause, C., Xander, L. U., et al.: Prevalence of colonization with vancomycin-resistant enterococci in various population groups in Berlin, Germany. J. Hosp. Infect. *42*:193–200, 1999.
320. Westh, H., Hougaard, D. M., Vuust, J., and Rosdahl, V. T.: Prevalence of erm gene classes in erythromycin-resistant *Staphylococcus aureus* strains isolated between 1959 and 1988. Antimicrob. Agents Chemother. *39*:369–373, 1995.
321. White, D. G., Zhao, S., Sudler, R., et al.: The isolation of antibiotic-resistant salmonella from retail ground meats. N. Engl. J. Med. *345*:1147–1154, 2001.
322. Whitney, C. G., Farley, M. M., Hadler, J., et al.: Increasing prevalence of multidrug-resistant *Streptococcus pneumoniae* in the United States. N. Engl. J. Med. *343*:1917–1924, 2000.
323. Wiener, J., Quinn, J. P., Bradford, P. A., et al.: Multiple antibiotic-resistant *Klebsiella* and *Escherichia coli* in nursing homes. J. A. M. A. *281*:517–523, 1999.
324. Wistrom, J., and Norrby, S. R.: Fluoroquinolones and bacterial enteritis, when and for whom? J. Antimicrob. Chemother. *36*:23–39, 1995.
325. Wretlind, B., Stromberg, A., Ostlund, L., et al.: Rapid emergence of quinolone resistance in *Campylobacter jejuni* in patients treated with norfloxacin. Scand. J. Infect. Dis. *24*:685–686, 1992.
326. Wright, S. W., Wrenn, K. D., and Haynes, M. L.: Trimethoprim-sulfamethoxazole resistance among urinary coliform isolates. J. Gen. Intern. Med. *14*:606–609, 1999.
327. Wu, P. J., Shannon, K., and Phillips, I.: Mechanisms of hyperproduction of TEM-1 beta-lactamase by clinical isolates of *Escherichia coli.* J. Antimicrob. Chemother. *36*:927–939, 1995.
328. Wubbel, L., and McCracken, G. H., Jr.: Management of bacterial meningitis: 1998. Pediatr. Rev. *19*:78–84, 1998.
329. Wubbel, L., Muniz, L., Ahmed, A., et al.: Etiology and treatment of community-acquired pneumonia in ambulatory children. Pediatr. Infect. Dis. J. *18*:98–104, 1999.
330. Xiang, X., Shannon, K., and French, G.: Mechanism and stability of hyperproduction of the extended-spectrum beta-lactamase SHV-5 in *Klebsiella pneumoniae.* J. Antimicrob. Chemother. *40*:525–532, 1997.
331. Yang, Y. J., Liu, C. C., Wang, S. M., et al.: High rates of antimicrobial resistance among clinical isolates of nontyphoidal *Salmonella* in Taiwan. Eur. J. Clin. Microbiol. Infect. Dis. *17*:880–883, 1998.
332. Yoshida, H., Bogaki, M., Nakamura, M., and Nakamura, S.: Quinolone resistance-determining region in the DNA gyrase gyrA gene of *Escherichia coli.* Antimicrob. Agents Chemother. *34*:1271–1272, 1990.
333. Yoshida, H., Bogaki, M., Nakamura, S., et al.: Nucleotide sequence and characterization of the *Staphylococcus aureus* norA gene, which confers resistance to quinolones. J. Bacteriol. *172*:6942–6949, 1990.
334. Yoshida, H., Bogaki, M., Nakamura, M., et al.: Quinolone resistance-determining region in the DNA gyrase gyrB gene of *Escherichia coli.* Antimicrob. Agents Chemother. 35:1647–1650, 1991.
335. Zahurul Haque Asna, S. M., and Ashraful Haq, J.: Decrease of antibiotic resistance in *Salmonella typhi* isolated from patients attending hospitals of Dhaka City over a 3 year period. Int. J. Antimicrob. Agents *16*:249–251, 2000.

336. Zhanel, G. G., Karlowsky, J. A., Harding, G. K., et al.: A Canadian national surveillance study of urinary tract isolates from outpatients: Comparison of the activities of trimethoprim-sulfamethoxazole, ampicillin, mecillinam, nitrofurantoin, and ciprofloxacin. The Canadian Urinary Isolate Study Group. Antimicrob. Agents Chemother. *44*:1089–1092, 2000.
337. Zhanel, G. G., Karlowsky, J. A., Low, D. E., and Hoban, D. J.: Antibiotic resistance in respiratory tract isolates of *Haemophilus influenzae* and *Moraxella catarrhalis* collected from across Canada in 1997–1998. J. Antimicrob. Chemother. *45*:655–662, 2000.
338. Zhanel, G. G., Karlowsky, J. A., Saunders, M. H., et al.: Development of multiple-antibiotic-resistant (Mar) mutants of *Pseudomonas aeruginosa* after serial exposure to fluoroquinolones. Antimicrob. Agents Chemother. *39*:489–495, 1995.
339. Zhang, L., Li, X. Z., and Poole, K.: Multiple antibiotic resistance in *Stenotrophomonas maltophilia:* Involvement of a multidrug efflux system. Antimicrob. Agents Chemother. *44*:287–293, 2000.
340. Zhao, X., Xu, C., Domagala, J., and Drlica, K.: DNA topoisomerase targets of the fluoroquinolones: A strategy for avoiding bacterial resistance. Proc. Natl. Acad. Sci. U. S. A. *94*:13991–13996, 1997.

The Pharmacokinetic-Pharmacodynamic Interface: Determinants of Anti-infective Drug Action and Efficacy in Pediatrics

SUSAN M. ABDEL-RAHMAN ■ GREGORY L. KEARNS

The success of anti-infective treatment of any infection wholly depends on proper drug selection and use. Without question, consideration of in vitro data that define the offending pathogen and provide information with regard to drug susceptibility is both valuable and vital. However, consideration of in vitro data in the absence of information that determines and governs drug exposure often can result in a therapeutic act of omission sufficient to bring about treatment failure. Thus, the conjoint consideration of drug action (i.e., pharmacodynamics) and drug disposition (i.e., pharmacokinetics) is of critical importance in the selection and evaluation of any anti-infective drug regimen.

The "pharmacokinetic-pharmacodynamic interface" reflects an association between two determinants of drug effect, delivery of drug to the site of action and the intrinsic activity of a drug to alter cellular function once it reaches that site. In much of the contemporary literature in clinical pharmacology and therapeutics, "kinetics" generally is associated with a description of the rate processes associated with drug absorption, distribution, metabolism, and excretion (ADME). Though accurate in its definition concerning the movement of drugs into and out of the body, "kinetics" as a determinant of drug effect must be viewed in a much broader context, specifically, the sojourn and fate of a drug molecule in both the extracellular and intracellular milieu. Although understanding this facet of drug behavior admittedly is difficult because of a relative inability in the clinical context to track the intracellular fate of a drug in humans, achieving a high degree of control over anti-infective therapy by the application of well-characterized and understood "kinetic" principles is quite possible.

The focus of this chapter is to profile the pharmacologic considerations necessary for the prudent use of anti-infective agents in pediatric patients, specifically, the pharmacokinetic and pharmacodynamic principles that if embraced, can be the key to optimizing drug treatment and maximizing therapeutic efficacy and safety. The context of the pediatric patient presents a particular challenge to the clinician. Although pediatric practitioners generally recognize that "children are not just miniature adults," one may not appreciate that the dramatic changes associated with normal human growth and development can, and many times do, exert a profound influence on drug disposition, drug action, and ultimately, therapeutic outcome.[100] Failure to compensate for developmental differences in pharmacokinetics in the context of therapeutic drug use in pediatrics can increase the risk of occurrence of adverse drug effects associated with either overdose (i.e., drug toxicity) or underdose (i.e., lack of efficacy).[68, 100]

The following sections of this chapter present the basic principles required to understand the pharmacokinetic-pharmacodynamic interface in pediatrics, namely, general principles in pharmacokinetics, the impact of development on drug disposition, the pharmacokinetic determinants of drug action, and methods to facilitate clinical integration of the pharmacokinetic and pharmacodynamic properties necessary to optimize anti-infective therapy.

Pharmacokinetic Determinants of Exposure

Implicit in the production of any pharmacologic effect is the association of a drug molecule with one or more receptors and the subsequent propagation of intracellular events that ultimately translate into drug action. In general terms, successful drug-receptor interactions are characterized by three principles: (1) *avidity,* the ability of a drug to combine with a receptor; (2) *affinity,* the physical combination of a drug with a receptor, and (3) *intrinsic activity,* the ability of the drug-receptor combination to generate one or more "impulses" or "signals" capable of activating biologic effector systems. The primary determinants of both avidity and affinity reside with the maintenance of structural specificity of both the drug and receptor to ensure that an association with one or more physicochemically distinct active sites can occur. Simply stated, a drug molecule must fit into a receptor like a "key fits into a lock" before intrinsic activity becomes a possibility. The receptor or receptors thus function in the role of cellular targets for drug molecules when an effective combination is required for drug effect and, ultimately, therapeutic efficacy. The pharmacodynamic implications of these "targets" are discussed in the second half of this chapter and in other chapters in this textbook for specific anti-infective agents.

The onset and offset of drug action are determined not only by receptor-modulated intrinsic activity but also by receptor occupancy. In almost all instances, these events are both concentration- and time-dependent. Hence, the disposition of a drug in the body (e.g., ADME) becomes the "driver" for its pharmacodynamics. This action is particularly true for anti-infective drugs when the therapeutic "target," the infecting organism, must be exposed to a sufficient concentration of pharmacologically active (i.e., free) drug for a period sufficient for drug binding to critical cellular elements (e.g., penicillin-binding proteins [PBPs], intracellular enzymes) to occur and subsequent disruption of normal cellular function (e.g., inhibition of protein biosynthesis, inhibition of cell wall synthesis) to result in cellular demise. Thus, the clinical determinants of drug efficacy (and safety), such as proper selection of both dose and dosing interval relative to the intrinsic sensitivity of the infecting pathogen or pathogens, and factors that determine delivery of the drug to the site or sites of infection embody the importance of pharmacokinetics in the selection and clinical use of anti-infective drugs.

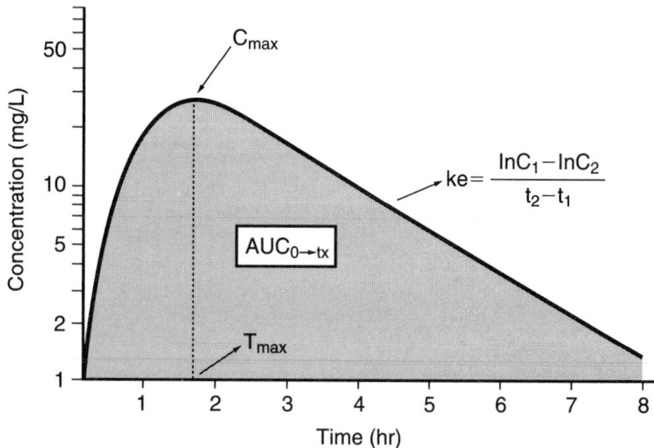

FIGURE 234–1 ■ Representative plasma concentration versus time curve illustrating commonly referenced pharmacokinetic parameters, including AUC, area under the curve; C_{max}, maximal plasma concentration; ke, elimination rate constant; T_{max}, time to achieve maximal plasma concentration.

BASIC TERMS

A complete discussion of pharmacokinetics is beyond the scope of this chapter because it would require a description of theory and a presentation of relatively sophisticated mathematic concepts. This information can be found in many excellent textbooks that provide both theoretic[67] and conceptual[100, 166, 208] presentations of pharmacokinetics and through Internet-based programmed instruction courses.[20] However, well within the scope of this chapter is a "definition and glossary" of pharmacokinetic terms sufficient to equip the reader with a conceptual, working knowledge of this pharmacotherapeutic "tool." These definitions and concepts are presented as follows:

Absolute bioavailability (F) is the extent or fraction of drug absorbed after extravascular administration. It is determined by comparing the area under the plasma concentration versus time curve (AUC) after administration of an oral dose of a drug with the AUC after administration of an intravenous dose (e.g., $F = AUC_{po} * dose_{iv}/AUC_{iv} * dose_{po}$).

Absorption of drugs describes the process of drug uptake from a site of extravascular administration (e.g., oral, intramuscular, subcutaneous, intraperitoneal, intraosseous, intratracheal, intravaginal, intraurethral, sublingual, buccal, rectal, and dermal) into the systemic circulation. Drug absorption is conceptualized most accurately by considering both rate (e.g., absorption half-life, time to peak concentration) and extent (e.g., bioavailability), either of which can be influenced by biopharmaceutical (e.g., drug formulation), physicochemical (e.g., pH, solubility, hydrophilicity and lipophilicity, protein binding, complexation characteristics with food or drugs, etc.), and physiologic factors (e.g., barrier integrity, motility, volume and pH of body fluids at the absorptive site, protein binding capacity, degradation/biotransformation potential, etc.).

Area under the curve (AUC) is, conceptually, a measure of both the extent of drug absorbed and its persistence in the body. It is the integral of drug blood levels over time from zero to either a predetermined post-dose time point (i.e., $AUC_{0\rightarrow tx}$) or extrapolated to infinity (i.e., $AUC_{0\rightarrow\infty}$) by using the apparent terminal elimination rate constant (similarly calculated from the observed plasma concentration versus time plot) (Fig. 234–1). AUC is therefore a pharmacokinetic parameter that is both time- and concentration-dependent.

Bioequivalence of a drug product is achieved if its extent and rate of absorption are not significantly different (i.e., within 80–125%) from those of a reference standard drug product when administered at the same molar dose. A note to be stressed is that bioequivalence is a pharmacokinetically determined parameter and does not entail a relative comparison of drug action/efficacy. Therefore, if a drug product (e.g., a generic drug) produces a rate and extent of absorption sufficiently similar to those of the reference formulation, the effect and toxicity profiles of the two drugs are assumed to be virtually identical.

Biopharmaceutics deals with the physical and chemical properties of the drug substance, the dosage form, and the body, as well as the biologic actions of a drug or drug product after administration. Biopharmaceutical considerations (e.g., rate and extent of the disintegration or dissolution of a dosage form, liberation of the active drug from a dosage form, solubility or binding of the drug at the site of absorption, etc.) can be "rate limiting" for drug absorption or bioavailability, or for both, and thus may limit the efficacy of drug therapy.

Clearance of a drug is represented conceptually by the volume of blood from which a certain amount of unmetabolized drug is removed (i.e., cleared) per unit time by any and all pathways capable of drug removal (e.g., renal, hepatic, biliary, pulmonary, breast milk, sweat). In pharmacokinetics, clearance (Cl) generally is represented as total-body (or plasma) clearance, renal clearance (Cl_{ren}), or nonrenal clearance (Cl_{nr}). Cl is determined easily from knowledge of the drug dose and AUC and can be calculated as follows: Cl = Dose (mg/kg)/AUC (mg/L * hr), where AUC can represent either the $AUC_{0\rightarrow tx}$ for single-dose administration or the AUC from time zero to the end of the dosing interval at steady state (i.e., $AUCss_{0\rightarrow\tau}$). Calculation of Cl_{ren} requires a complete, quantitative collection of urine (usually over 24 hours) to determine the amount of drug excreted (Ae) unchanged. Cl_{nr} generally is determined as the difference between Cl and Cl_{ren}. For drug administration *by any extravascular route,* calculation of Cl yields an "apparent" value (e.g., Cl/F) in that it must be corrected for the extent of the drug dose absorbed (i.e., the bioavailability) from the site of administration.

A *compartment* in pharmacokinetics represents a *hypothetic space* into and out of which drug partitions as a function of time. *Compartment models* are used in pharmacokinetics to characterize the relationship between drug dose and concentration as a function of time. The most simple of all pharmacokinetic models is a one-compartment open model in which the only applicable rate processes represent drug ingress and egress from a single theoretic or "central" space. A two-compartment model has been used to characterize the disposition of many anti-infective agents in both pediatric and adult subjects. This particular model is composed of a "central compartment" and a "peripheral compartment," both of which represent the various fluids and tissues where a drug might reside. Although a compartment often may not correspond to a true physiologic space that can be characterized by a specific volume of biologic fluid, compartment models can be used to conceptualize both drug distribution between physiologic spaces and elimination from the body. In the two-compartment model, for example, the central compartment often is used to represent drug resident within the intravascular space and the highly exchangeable extracellular fluid of tissues and organs that are well perfused, whereas the peripheral compartment represents drug distribution to intracellular fluid and tissues and organs that are less well perfused and, in some instances, association of drug (e.g., binding) to specific tissues or tissue components. In all instances, compartmental models oversimplify the true processes of ADME. However, they have been demonstrated repeatedly to be useful as a means to reliably model and, therefore, predict the relationship between drug dose and concentration in both plasma and tissue.

Disposition refers collectively to the processes of ADME, all of which occur simultaneously after administration of drug as opposed to being discrete pharmacologic events.

Dose-response curve is a graphic representation of the pharmacologic effect as a function of either the drug dose or the concentration of drug. A log dose-response curve is sigmoidal in shape, whereas a Cartesian concentration-effect curve is hyperbolic (Fig. 234–2). Theoretically, a drug concentration of zero indicates no drug effect (i.e., E_0). As a drug travels to and interacts with a receptor, the effect (E) increases in a concentration-dependent manner (i.e., $E=[(E_{max} * C)/(E_{50}+C)]$) to a point where a maximal effect (E_{max}) is attained and above which higher drug concentrations fail to enhance the effect. A pharmacologically important term that can be derived easily from a concentration-effect curve is the EC_{50}, or the drug concentration for which the observed effect is 50 percent of the E_{max}.

Elimination half-life of a drug is the time necessary to reduce the drug concentration (in blood serum or plasma) by

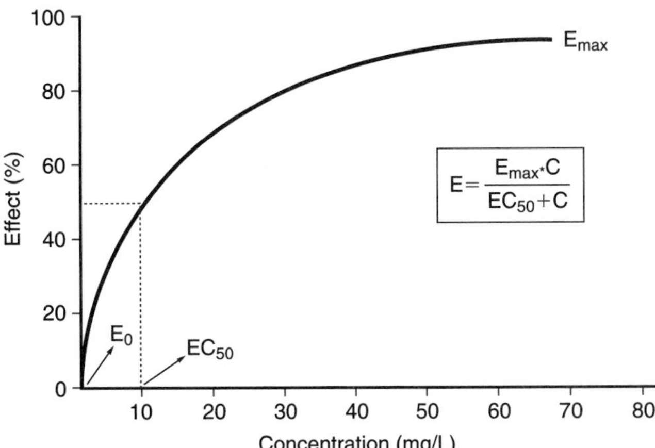

FIGURE 234–2 ■ Representative nonlinear concentration versus effect profile.

50 percent after absorption is complete and distribution between body compartments has attained equilibrium. Loss of drug from the body, as represented by the elimination half-life, reflects elimination of the administered parent drug molecule (i.e., not its metabolites) by metabolism, urinary excretion, or other pathways capable of resulting in elimination of drug. Accordingly, many individuals use elimination half-life as a "surrogate" indicator of drug clearance. Such a determination should be made cautiously because this particular pharmacokinetic parameter is dependent on both clearance and the apparent volume of distribution as illustrated by the following equation: $t_{1/2}$ elimination $=[(0.693 * VD)/Cl]$. Practically speaking, the elimination half-life is an important pharmacokinetic parameter because it can be used to determine the period of time required for a drug dosing regimen to produce steady-state plasma concentrations (e.g., $5 * t_{1/2}$ elimination) and the dosing interval required to produce a desired excursion (i.e., peak and trough) in plasma drug concentrations.

First-pass effect describes a phenomenon whereby drugs may be metabolized or chemically degraded (or both) after extravascular administration before they reach the systemic circulation. Specific examples include biotransformation of selected drugs (e.g., cytochrome CYP3A4 substrates) in the enterocyte and nonenzymatic hydrolysis of an active drug (e.g., aspirin) in the lumen of the gastrointestinal tract (e.g., stomach, intestine, rectum). Drugs subject to a first-pass effect generally have a reduced rate or extent of relative bioavailability, or both, when compared with that achieved by parenteral administration.

Protein binding is the phenomenon that occurs when a drug (or metabolite) combines with plasma or extracellular or tissue proteins to form a reversible drug-protein complex. In general, drug-protein binding is usually nonspecific and depends on the drug's affinity for the protein molecule (i.e., binding site), the number of protein-binding sites, and the drug and protein concentrations. With few exceptions, drugs that are bound to proteins are pharmacologically inactive and cannot be metabolized or excreted readily. The pharmacokinetic consequences of drug-protein binding can influence the drug dose versus plasma concentration versus effect relationship. For example, drugs with extensive tissue binding have apparent volumes of distribution that are far in excess of the total-body water space and, in general, have relatively long elimination half-lives. Conditions in which intravascular proteins escape to extravascular sites (e.g., nephrotic syndrome, severe burns, ascites) can increase the apparent volume (and elimination half-life) of drugs that are extensively (i.e., >70%) bound to albumin.

Relative bioavailability reflects the extent of drug absorbed from one dosage form given by an extravascular route of administration in comparison to a dose of a "standard" drug formulation administered by the same route. Generally, it reflects the relative extent of systemic availability (F) and is calculated by comparing the AUC of the test regimen relative to the standard formulation (e.g., $F = AUC_{test} * dose_{standard}/AUC_{standard} * dose_{test}$).

Steady state reflects the level of drug accumulation in blood and tissue after multiple dosing when input (i.e., the amount of drug placed into the systemic circulation) and output (i.e., drug clearance) are at equilibrium. When drugs are given at fixed doses and dosing intervals, the steady-state concentrations fluctuate between a maximum (C_{max}) and minimum (C_{min}) within a given dose interval that is identical between doses, provided that the size of the dose, method of administration, dosing interval, or drug pharmacokinetics (or any combination of these parameters) does not change. For drugs that follow first-order pharmacokinetics, steady-state plasma concentrations for a given dosing regimen are attained over a period that corresponds to four to five times the elimination half-life. In general, the pharmacokinetics of a drug at steady state provides the most accurate correlate for examining drug effect.

Volume of distribution (apparent volume of distribution) (VD) represents a hypothetic volume of body fluid that would be required to dissolve the total amount of drug at the same concentration as that found in the blood and is illustrated by the following equation: $VD = Dose/Cp^0$, where Cp^0 represents the highest attainable plasma concentration after the administration of a single dose. As a proportionality constant, VD is a determinant of plasma drug concentrations attained after administration of a given drug dose. For drugs that are not distributed extensively or that bind with great affinity to proteins and tissues, the apparent VD may correspond dimensionally to physiologic/anatomic body spaces (e.g., VD < 0.1 L/kg approximates the intravascular space, 0.1 to 0.3 L/kg for the extracellular space, 0.6 to 0.7 L/kg approximates the total-body water space), which when altered by disease or development, or by both, will influence the apparent VD and thus the achievable concentration for a given drug.

A working knowledge of these pharmacokinetic definitions makes possible an understanding of the relationships among drug dose, concentration, and effect. The use of knowledge related to the physicochemical and pharmacologic properties of a drug, the impact of isolated or concurrent variables that can have an effect on drug disposition, and predictors of pharmacodynamics/drug response enables the clinician to optimize the selection of agents and dosing regimens and, thus, individualize drug therapy. To accomplish this goal, it is imperative that the relationship between drug pharmacokinetics and pharmacodynamics not be compartmentalized but rather, as illustrated in Figure 234–3, be conceptualized as multifactorial, where the determinants of drug concentration and effect are dynamic and change as a function of disease state and drug therapy.

IMPACT OF ONTOGENY ON PHARMACOKINETICS

Development represents a continuum of biologic events that enable adaptation, somatic growth, neurobehavioral maturation, and eventually, reproduction. The impact of development on the pharmacokinetics of a given drug is determined, to a great degree, by age-related changes in body composition and the acquisition of function in organs and organ systems that are important in determining drug metabolism and excretion. Although classifying pediatric patients on the basis of postnatal age (e.g., neonates, ≤1 month of age; infants, 1 to 24 months of age; children, 2 to 12 years of age; and adolescents, 12 to 18 years of age) is often convenient for provision of drug therapy, recognizing that the changes in physiology are not linearly related to age and may not correspond to these age-defined breakpoints is important.

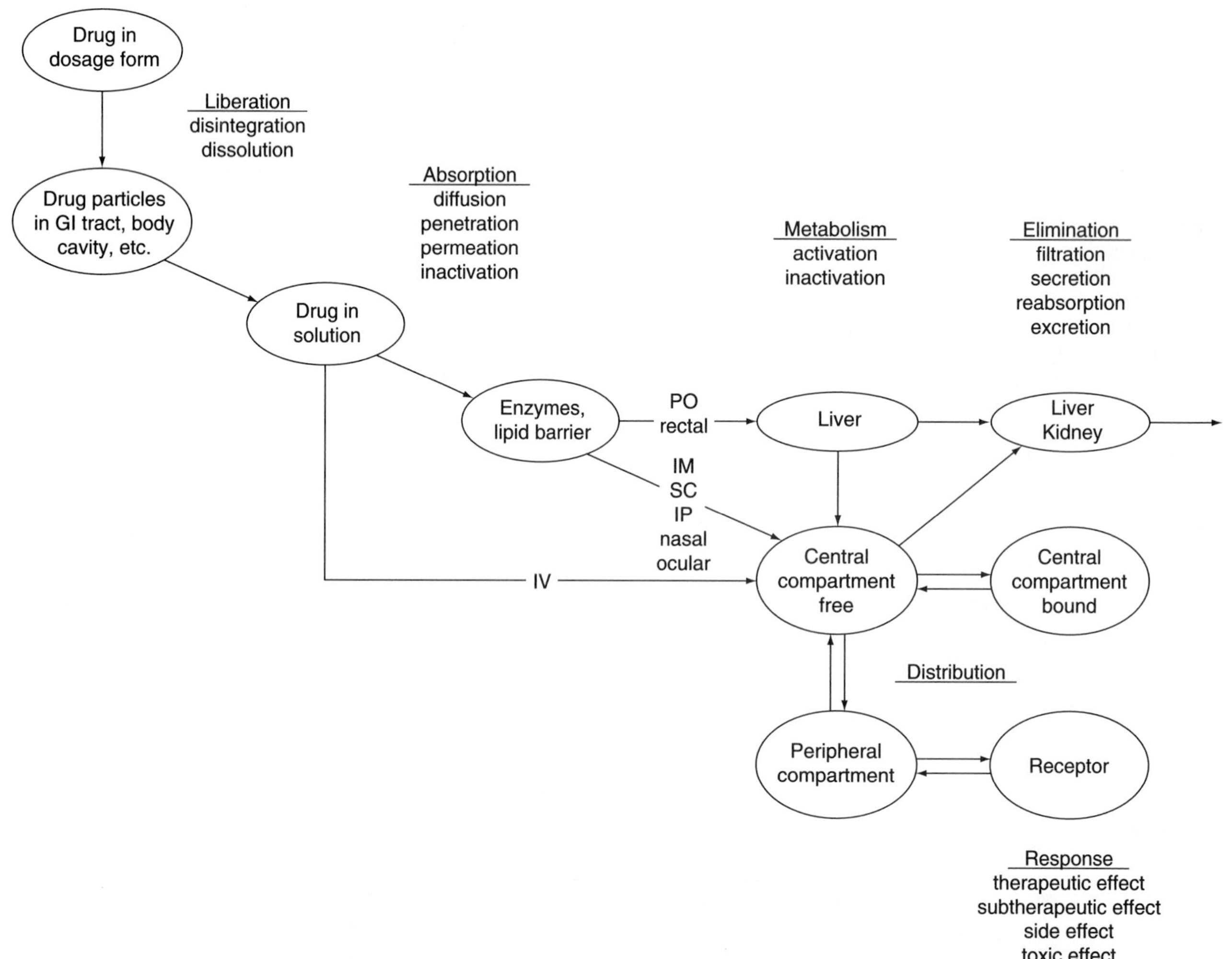

FIGURE 234–3 ■ Graphic representation of the pharmacokinetic-pharmacodynamic interface.

In fact, the most dramatic changes in drug disposition occur during the first 18 months of life, when the acquisition of organ function is most dynamic. Additionally, an important note is that the pharmacokinetics of a given drug may be altered in pediatric patients as a result of intrinsic (e.g., gender, genotype, ethnicity, inherited diseases) or extrinsic (e.g., acquired disease states, xenobiotic exposure, diet) factors that may occur during the first 2 decades of life.

Selection of an appropriate drug dose for a neonate, infant, child, or adolescent requires an understanding of the basic pharmacokinetic properties of a given compound and how the process of development affects each facet of drug disposition. Accordingly, conceptualizing pediatric pharmacokinetics by examining the impact of development on the physiologic variables that govern ADME is most useful.

DRUG ABSORPTION. The rate and extent of gastrointestinal (GI) absorption primarily depend on pH-dependent passive diffusion and motility of the stomach and small intestine, both of which control transit time. In full-term neonates, gastric pH ranges from 6 to 8 at birth and drops to 2 to 3 within the first few hours. After the first 24 hours of extrauterine life, gastric pH increases to approximately 6 to 7 as a result of immaturity of the parietal cells. A relative state of achlorhydria remains until adult values and diurnal patterns of gastric pH are reached at 20 to 30 months of age. Although basal gastric acid output can be quite similar in neonates, young infants, and adults, stimulated acid output can be threefold to fourfold higher than that seen in adults.[46, 47]

In neonates, GI transit time is prolonged as a result of reduced motility and peristalsis. Gastric emptying is both irregular and erratic and only partially dependent on feeding. Gastric emptying rates approximate adult values by the time that the infant reaches 6 to 8 months of age. During infancy, intestinal transit time generally is reduced relative to adult values because of increased intestinal motility.[100] In contrast to developmental changes in motility, histologic examination of the luminal absorptive surface suggests that the adult pattern of architecture (and, hence, absorptive surface area relative to body size) is present at birth.[71, 205] In neonates and young infants, additional factors may play a role in intestinal drug absorption, including diminished splanchnic blood flow, immature biliary function, variable microbial colonization, and an apparent reduction in the activity of intestinal drug-metabolizing enzymes.[36, 160]

These developmental changes in GI function/structure in the newborn period and early infancy produce alterations in drug absorption that are quite predictable. In general, the oral bioavailability of acid-labile compounds (e.g., β-lactam antibiotics) is increased, whereas that of weak organic acids (e.g., phenobarbital, phenytoin) is decreased. For orally administered drugs with limited water solubility (e.g., phenytoin, carbamazepine), the rate of absorption (i.e., T_{max}) can be altered dramatically as a result of changes in GI motility.[160] The pharmacokinetics of the antiviral agent pleconaril similarly provides an example of developmental differences in drug absorption. After administration of a 5-mg/kg dose, the AUC was much lower in neonates than either children or adults, thus demonstrating that the extent of pleconaril bioavailability in neonates was reduced. The reason for this difference may be attributed to the lipid-based pleconaril formulation and developmental differences in the ability to absorb lipids as a consequence of biliary immaturity and reduced lipase secretion in neonates.[102]

In newborns and young infants, both rectal and percutaneous absorption is highly efficient for properly formulated drug products. The bioavailability of many drugs administered by the rectal route is increased as a result of not only efficient translocation across the rectal mucosa but also a reduced first-pass effect caused by the immaturity of a number of drug-metabolizing enzymes in the liver. Both the rate and extent of percutaneous drug absorption are increased because of the thinner and more well hydrated stratum corneum in young infants. As a consequence, systemic toxicity can occur with the percutaneous application of some drugs (e.g., hexachlorophene) to seemingly small areas of skin during the first 8 to 12 months of life. In contrast to older infants and children, the rate of bioavailability for drugs administered by the intramuscular route may be altered (i.e., delayed T_{max}) more than the extent of absorption in a neonate. This developmental pharmacokinetic alteration is the consequence of relatively low muscular blood flow in the first few days of life, the relative inefficiency of muscular contractions (useful in dispersing an intramuscular drug dose), and an increased percentage of water per unit of muscle mass.[160]

Developmental differences in drug absorption among neonates, infants, and older children are summarized in Table 234–1. One must recognize that the data contained therein reflect developmental differences that might be

TABLE 234–1 ■ SUMMARY OF DRUG ABSORPTION IN NEONATES, INFANTS, AND CHILDREN*

	Neonates	Infants	Children
Physiologic Alteration			
Gastric emptying time	Irregular	Increased	Slightly increased
Gastric pH	>5	4 to 2	Normal (2–3)
Intestinal motility	Reduced	Increased	Slightly increased
Intestinal surface area	Reduced	Near adult	Adult pattern
Microbial colonization	Reduced	Near adult	Adult pattern
Biliary function	Immature	Near adult	Adult pattern
Muscular blood flow	Reduced	Increased	Adult pattern
Skin permeability	Increased	Increased	Near adult pattern
Possible Pharmacokinetic Consequences			
Oral absorption	Erratic—reduced	Increased rate	Near adult pattern
Intramuscular absorption	Variable	Increased	Adult pattern
Percutaneous absorption	Increased	Increased	Near adult pattern
Rectal absorption	Very efficient	Efficient	Near adult pattern
Presystemic clearance	Less than adult	Greater than adult	Greater than adult (increased rate)

*The direction of alteration is given relative to the expected normal adult pattern.
Adapted from Ritschel, W. A., and Kearns, G. L.: Pediatric pharmacokinetics. *In* Ritschel, W. A., and Kearns, G. L. (eds.): Handbook of Basic Pharmacokinetics. 5th ed. Washington, D.C., American Pharmaceutical Association, 1999, pp. 304–321.

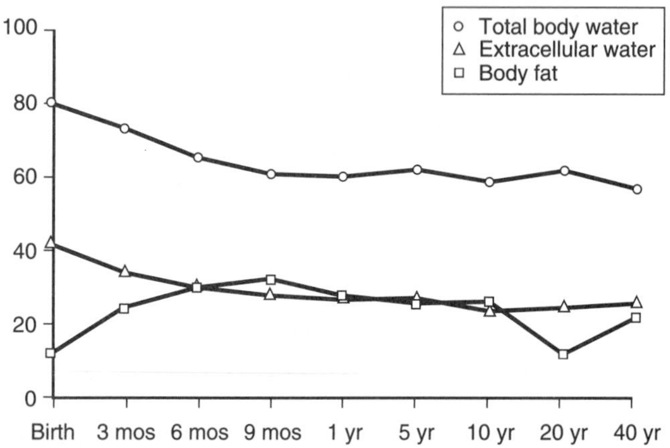

FIGURE 234–4 ■ Body composition reflected as a percentage (y-axis) of total-body mass for total-body water (TBW), extracellular water (ECW), and body fat as a function of age (x-axis). (From Ritschel, W. A., Kearns, G. L.: Pediatric pharmacokinetics. *In* Ritschel, W. A., and Kearns, G. L. [eds.]: Handbook of Basic Pharmacokinetics. 5th ed. Washington, D.C., American Pharmaceutical Association, 1999, pp. 304–321.)

expected to occur in healthy pediatric patients. Certain conditions/disease states that might modify the function or structure, or both, of the absorptive surface area, GI motility, or systemic blood flow can further affect either the rate or the extent of absorption for extravascularly administered drugs in pediatric patients.

DISTRIBUTION. Development is associated with marked changes in body composition as reflected by examination of total-body water, extracellular water, and stores of body fat (Fig. 234–4). The most dynamic changes occur in the first year of life, with the exception of total-body fat, which has a distinctly different pattern in males and females. Furthermore, another important note is that the adipose tissue of neonates may contain as much as 57 percent water and 35 percent lipids, whereas values in adults approach 26.3 percent and 71.7 percent, respectively.[160]

In addition to age-related alterations in body composition, several physiologic changes that occur during the neonatal period are capable of altering the plasma protein binding of drugs (Table 234–2). In neonates, the free fraction of drugs that are bound extensively to circulating plasma proteins is increased markedly, largely because of lower concentrations of drug-binding proteins, reduced binding affinity of these proteins, the presence of a relatively acidic plasma pH, and endogenous competing ligands (e.g., bilirubin, free fatty acids). This consideration is exemplified by ceftriaxone, a weak acid that is approximately 95 percent bound to albumin in adults but only 70 percent bound in neonates and, thus, is capable of producing significant displacement of bilirubin.[80, 129] The reduced plasma protein binding in combination with absolute and relative differences in the size of various body compartments (e.g., total-body water, extracellular fluid, composition of body tissues) frequently influences (i.e., increases) the apparent volume of distribution for many drugs and also their localization (i.e., both uptake and residence) in tissue, which in turn can alter their plasma elimination half-life.

RENAL EXCRETION. The renal excretion of many drugs is directly proportional to age-dependent patterns in the acquisition of renal function, primarily glomerular filtration and active tubular secretion. Accordingly, developmental differences in renal function may serve as a major determinant of drug clearance in neonates and young infants for compounds that are not metabolized extensively.[160]

In preterm infants, renal function is reduced dramatically because of the continued development of functioning nephron units (i.e., nephrogenesis). In contrast, the acquisition of renal function in a term neonate represents, to a great degree, the recruitment of fully developed nephron units. In both term neonates and preterm infants who have birth weights greater than 1500 g, glomerular filtration rates increase dramatically during the first 2 weeks of postnatal life (Fig. 234–5). This particular dynamic change in function is a direct consequence of postnatal adaptations in the distribution of renal blood flow (i.e., medullary distribution to the corticomedullary border) and results in dramatic recruitment of functioning nephron units.[100] In addition, a glomerular/tubular imbalance exists in which maturation of glomerular function is more advanced than proximal tubular secretion. This imbalance may persist for up to 6 to 10 months of age, when both tubular function and glomerular function approach values approximately equal to those observed in healthy, young adults.[160]

The impact of development on each of the components of renal function can be characterized by a definable pattern during the first year of life[146] (see Fig. 234–5). Accordingly, the renal handling and, hence, excretion/elimination characteristics of virtually any drug in neonates, infants, and children can be predicted largely by considering the ontogeny of

TABLE 234–2 ■ PLASMA PROTEIN BINDING AND DRUG DISTRIBUTION*

	Neonates	Infants	Children
Physiologic Alteration			
Plasma albumin	Reduced	Near normal	Near adult pattern
Fetal albumin	Present	Absent	Absent
Total protein	Reduced	Decreased	Near adult pattern
Serum bilirubin	Increased	Normal	Normal adult pattern
Serum free fatty acids	Increased	Normal	Normal adult pattern
Blood pH	7.1–7.3	7.4 (normal)	7.4 (normal)
Possible Pharmacokinetic Consequences			
Free fraction	Increased	Increased	Slightly increased
Apparent volume of distribution			
Hydrophilic drugs	Increased	Increased	Slightly increased
Hydrophobic drugs	Reduced	Reduced	Slightly decreased
Tissue/plasma ratio	Increased	Increased	Slightly increased

*The direction of alteration is given relative to the expected normal adult pattern.
Adapted from Ritschel, W. A., and Kearns, G. L.: Pediatric pharmacokinetics. *In* Ritschel, W. A., and Kearns, G. L. (eds.): Handbook of Basic Pharmacokinetics. 5th ed. Washington, D. C., American Pharmaceutical Association, 1999, pp. 304–321.

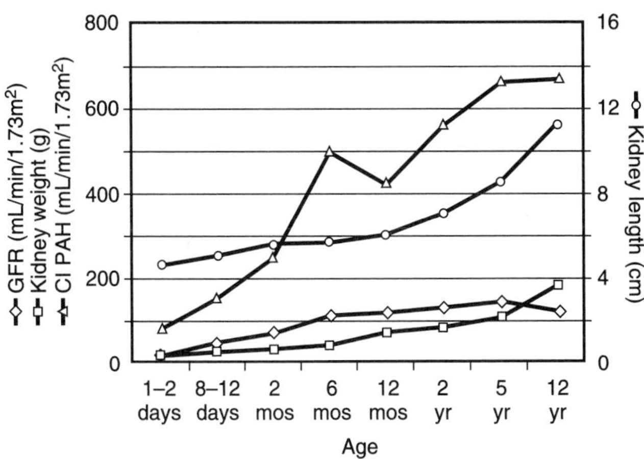

FIGURE 234–5 ■ Ontogeny of renal function. Cl, clearance; GFR, glomerular filtration rate; PAH, para-aminohippuric acid. (Adapted from Papadopoulou, Z. L., Tina, L. U., Sandler, P., et al.: Size and function of the kidneys. *In* Johnson, T. R., Moore, W. M., and Jeffries, J. E. [eds.]: Children Are Different: Developmental Physiology. 2nd ed. Ross Laboratories, Columbus, OH, 1978, pp. 97–104.)

renal function and the specific pharmacologic characteristics of a given drug with regard to its renal excretion (e.g., routes of renal excretion, the percentage of a given dose excreted unchanged in urine) in adults. For antimicrobial agents, the impact of the ontogeny of renal function on pharmacokinetics is reflected largely by alterations in plasma drug clearance. As summarized by van den Anker and Kearns,[197] the elimination half-life of antimicrobial agents from different classes that share predominantly renal pathways of excretion is increased substantially in neonates and young infants (Table 234–3). This increase is not the case for antimicrobial and other agents that are not excreted primarily by the kidneys (e.g., ceftriaxone) (Table 234–3).

METABOLISM. Simply stated, drug metabolism (or biotransformation) involves the modification of a drug molecule by one or more enzymes such that the hydrophilicity of the product is increased relative to the parent drug, thus enhancing elimination/excretion. In most instances, drug metabolism produces products that are either less pharmacologically active than the parent drug (e.g., desacetylcefotaxime) or devoid of pharmacologic activity altogether (e.g., cefotaxime lactone metabolites).[99] In other instances,

TABLE 234–3 ■ IMPACT OF ONTOGENY ON THE ELIMINATION HALF-LIFE OF DRUGS WITH PREDOMINANT RENAL ROUTES OF EXCRETION*

			Elimination $t_{1/2}$ (hr)	
Drug	Cl (mL/hr/kg)	VD (mL/kg)	Neonate	Adult
Gentamicin	35–72	350–500	4.4–11.4	2.5
Tobramycin	41–74	590–840	8.2–11.3	2.0
Amikacin	50	570	8.4	2.5
Cefotaxime	50–100	310–790	3.4–6.4	1.2
Ceftriaxone	44–60	530–610	7.7–8.4	6.5
Ceftazidine	31–42	292–363	5.0–8.7	1.8
Vancomycin	36–78	480–680	8.0–17	6.0

*Data represent average or a range of average values reported from individual studies and summarized by van den Anker and Kearns[197] (for preterm infants) and Ritschel and Kearns[160] for adults.

Cl, total plasma clearance; $t_{1/2}$, half-life; VD, apparent volume of distribution.

metabolism can result in drug bioactivation and produce metabolites with pharmacologic activity from an inactive parent drug (i.e., prodrug) or generate metabolites that can result in cellular toxicity in the host (e.g., sulfamethoxazole's nitroso and hydroxylamine reactive metabolites, acetaminophen's NAPQI reactive metabolite).

Virtually every tissue has some ability to carry out drug biotransformation reactions. Although the liver is quantitatively the most important organ capable of drug metabolism, the small intestine, lungs, skin, and kidneys also display substantial drug biotransformation activity. In infants, children, and adolescents, developmental variations in drug metabolism have been associated with age, gender, maturation, and genetic constitution. For compounds that are extensively metabolized, developmental differences in drug metabolism can serve as the primary determinant for age-appropriate dose selection.[115] Much of the existing information regarding the impact of ontogeny on drug metabolism has been derived as a byproduct of pharmacokinetic investigations designed, in part, to determine whether age-dependent differences in drug disposition were evident.[100] The following paragraphs highlight important general issues regarding drug metabolism and its relationship to development.

Phase I Pathways. Phase I biotransformation reactions include oxidation, reduction, and hydrolysis reactions that in general, introduce or unmask a functional group (e.g., hydroxyl, amine, sulfhydryl, etc.) that makes a drug more polar. Quantitatively, the P-450 cytochromes are the most important of the phase I enzymes and represent a superfamily of heme-containing proteins that catalyze the metabolism of many lipophilic endogenous substances (e.g., steroids, fatty acids and fat-soluble vitamins, prostaglandins, leukotrienes, and thromboxanes) and exogenous compounds. In humans, the P-450 cytochromes can be divided functionally into two distinct classes: steroidogenic enzymes expressed in specialized tissues such as the adrenal glands, gonads, and placenta and enzymes involved in the metabolism of drugs, pesticides, and environmental contaminants. P-450 cytochromes that have been identified as being important in human drug metabolism are found predominantly in the CYP1, CYP2, and CYP3 gene families.[115]

As reviewed by Leeder and Kearns,[115] considerable interindividual variability exists in the hepatic expression of P-450 enzymes, and for a given individual, the pathway and rate of a compound's metabolic clearance constitute that individual's unique phenotype with respect to the forms and amounts of P-450 species expressed. Of the P-450 cytochromes involved in drug biotransformation, CYP2C19, CYP2C9, and CYP2D6 are polymorphically expressed in humans. Polymorphic expression of CYP1A2 and CYP3A4 has been reported in the literature but not definitively established with regard to functional consequences. Within a P-450 subfamily, several isoforms can exist (e.g., CYP3A4, CYP3A5, and CYP3A7), each of which can demonstrate substrate specificity and a distinct developmental pattern with regard to enzyme activity. In addition, certain P-450 cytochromes (e.g., CYP3A4) can work cooperatively with transporters (e.g., MDR-1 or P-glycoprotein) located in distinct cells or tissues to alter the availability of specific drugs to the systemic circulation (e.g., first-pass metabolism of CYP3A4 substrates in the enterocyte). Moreover, for certain polymorphically expressed P-450 cytochromes (e.g., CYP2C19, CYP2D6), enzyme activity has been shown to vary as a consequence of racial or ethnic origin[156] and, within a given phenotypic distribution (e.g., extensive metabolizers for CYP2D6), as a function of single nucleotide polymorphisms that exist in either the gene or its regulatory regions.[154] Finally, of importance is that throughout development, the activities of the

P-450 cytochromes can vary widely (e.g., 5- to 25-fold) among individuals of the same phenotype,[115] an important factor with respect to their ability for induction or inhibition and, thus, the prediction of drug-drug or drug-xenobiotic interactions in vivo.

Phase II Pathways. In general, phase II reactions involve the coupling of a drug or drug metabolite with an endogenous substance to further enhance its hydrophilicity and facilitate drug excretion in either urine or bile. These reactions require the participation of specific transferase enzymes (e.g., epoxide hydrolase, glucuronosyltransferases, glutathione *S*-transferases, sulfotransferases, N-acetyltransferases, methyltransferases, transacylases) and high-energy, activated endogenous substances. Although most conjugation reactions result in drug detoxification, examples of bioactivation by phase II enzymes do exist.[159] Similar to what has been found for certain of the P-450 cytochromes, different isoforms of phase II enzymes also exist in humans. This finding is exemplified by the recent review of de Wildt and colleagues,[35] who described substrate specificity for 10 different glucuronosyltransferase isoforms in humans and known polymorphisms in five different isoforms of this enzyme. The impact of age on the disposition of several glucuronosyltransferase substrates (e.g., morphine, acetaminophen, zidovudine, chloramphenicol) suggests that isoform-specific, age-related differences in activity occur to a degree sufficient to produce profound effects on drug clearance that translate directly into age-specific differences in drug dose.[35]

Normal growth and development can have a profound effect on the activity of drug-metabolizing enzymes. Traditionally, the impact of ontogeny for all enzymes was viewed as being extremely limited in newborn infants, rapidly increasing in the first year of life to levels in toddlers and older children that may exceed adult capacity, and declining to adult levels by the conclusion of puberty. Experimental and clinical data previously reviewed demonstrate that this theory is indeed not the case.[100, 115] As illustrated by the summary data contained in Table 234–4, the impact of ontogeny on the activity of both phase I and phase II drug-metabolizing enzymes is very much a substrate- and isoform-specific event, development being one dynamic factor in a multitude of conditions (e.g., nutritional status, gender, diurnal variation, menstrual cycle, disease states/organ dysfunction, pregnancy, concomitant drug therapy) capable of altering the activity of drug-metabolizing enzymes and, thus, the clearance of drugs (and their metabolites) from plasma. Although discussion of the impact of ontogeny on the disposition (pharmacokinetics) of specific drugs is beyond the scope of this chapter, the clinician can use much of the information concerning specific enzymes provided in Table 234–4 as a tool to facilitate inquiry or clinical decision making, or both. It can be done simply by using readily available, updated information describing which enzymes are responsible for drug metabolism and then searching the published or unpublished (e.g., information available from pharmaceutical companies for drugs under development) literature for information describing the pharmacokinetics of the drug being considered.[51]

Clinicians must recognize that age-dependent differences in the activity of enzymes that catalyze drug biotransformation are not limited solely to P-450 cytochromes or the host of transferase enzymes responsible for phase II drug metabolism and that in many cases, these differences represent a critical determinant for successful anti-infective drug therapy. This factor is exemplified by considering the example of two antimicrobial agents that have unique places in pediatric therapy: cefotaxime and linezolid. In the case of cefotaxime, non–P-450 enzymes (probably an esterase) capable of generating the active desacetylcefotaxime metabolite appear to be present and fully active by the third trimester of gestation.[104] Nonetheless, the elimination half-life of cefotaxime in neonates is approximately threefold greater (i.e., approximately 3 to 4 hours) than that observed in older infants and children (i.e., approximately 1 to 1.5 hours), a difference that permits extension of the dosing interval for the use of cefotaxime in neonates. The reasons for this developmental difference reside not with the enzymes responsible for generation of an active metabolite but, instead, appear to be age-associated reductions in the activity of enzymes responsible for the generation of inactive metabolites of cefotaxime (e.g., cefotaxime lactone) and pathways involved in the renal clearance of desacetylcefotaxime.[103] Linezolid, a new oxazolidinone antimicrobial approved in the United States for use in pediatric patients, undergoes extensive biotransformation in humans, not via a cytochrome P-450 enzyme, but rather by nonselective chemical oxidation.[105] As recently demonstrated by Kearns and associates,[101] the mean plasma clearance of linezolid in children was approximately threefold higher than that observed previously for adults, with the greatest increase noted in infants younger than 1 year.

TABLE 234–4 ■ DEVELOPMENTAL PATTERNS FOR THE ONTOGENY OF IMPORTANT DRUG-METABOLIZING ENZYMES IN HUMANS

Enzyme(s)	Known Developmental Pattern
Phase I Enzymes	
CYP2D6	Low to absent in fetal liver but present at 1 wk of age. Poor activity (i.e., 20% of adult) by 1 mo. Adult competence by 3 to 5 yr of age
CYP2C9	Apparently absent in fetal liver. Low activity in first 2 to 4 wk of life, with adult activity reached by approximately 6 mo. Activity may exceed adult levels during childhood and declines to adult levels after conclusion of puberty
CYP1A2	Not present in appreciable levels in human fetal liver. Adult levels reached by approximately 4 mo and exceeded in children at 1 to 2 yr of age. Adult activity reached after puberty
CYP3A7	Fetal form of CYP3A that is functionally active (and inducible) during gestation. Virtually disappears by 1 to 4 wk of postnatal life when CYP3A4 activity predominates, but remains present in approximately 5% of individuals
CYP3A4	Extremely low activity at birth, reaching approximately 30 to 40% of adult activity by 1 mo, and full adult activity by 6 mo. May exceed adult activity between 1 to 4 yr of age, decreasing to adult levels after puberty
Phase II Enzymes	
NAT2	Some fetal activity by 16 wk gestation. Poor activity between birth and 2 mo of age. Adult phenotype distribution reached by 4 to 6 mo, with adult activity reached by 1 to 3 yr
TPMT	Fetal levels approximately 30% of adult values. In newborns, activity is approximately 50% higher than in adults, with phenotype distribution approximating that of adults. Exception is Korean children, in whom adult activity is seen by 7 to 9 yr of age
UGT	Ontogeny is isoform-specific. In general, adult activity is reached by 6 to 24 mo of age
ST	Ontogeny is isoform-specific and appears more rapid than that for UGT. Activity for some isoforms may exceed adult levels during infancy and early childhood

CYP, cytochrome P-450; NAT2, *N*-acetyltransferase-2; ST, sulfotransferase; TPMT, thiopurine methyltransferase; UGT, glucuronosyltransferase.
Adapted from Leeder, J. S., and Kearns, G. L.: Pharmacogenetics in Pediatrics: Implications for Practice. Pediatr. Clin. North Am. *44*:55–57, 1997.

Given the mechanism of action for linezolid and properties that reflect time-dependent killing,[105] the clinical implications of the age-dependent pattern of increased plasma clearance for this drug in young infants and children suggest that for infections with selected pathogens that have relatively high (90 percent) minimal inhibitory concentration (MIC_{90}) values for the drug, shorter dosing intervals (e.g., every 8 hours) may be necessary to ensure sufficient exposure of the organism in blood and tissue through most of a dosing interval.[101]

Pharmacokinetic Determinants of Effect

Collectively, the most important determinants of efficacy for anti-infective agents are the pharmacokinetic profile of the drug, the physicochemical and biochemical characteristics of the local environment (i.e., site of infection), and the susceptibility of the infecting organisms under local growth conditions. As previously reviewed by Barza,[9] the mechanisms and pharmacokinetics of drug transport to and accumulation at the site or sites of infection, as well as the subcellular localization of drugs, are critical to success and poorly understood. In many circumstances, plasma drug concentrations may not be reflective of those in tissue. Pathophysiologic processes related to the host, the infection, and the physicochemical properties of the drug work in concert to regulate distribution into and retention of active drug at the site of infection. Because these considerations should be embraced by the clinician when a particular anti-infective drug is selected for treatment and its therapy is monitored for clinical evidence of success, some general examples are presented as follows.

In addition to age (as discussed earlier), many disease processes (e.g., trauma, malignancy, renal/hepatic disease) have an impact on both the quantity of circulating plasma proteins (e.g., albumin, α_1-acid glycoprotein) and their affinity to bind anti-infective agents. Given that only free drug is available to enter tissue, the degree of binding to protein components in the blood will affect tissue concentrations. Thus, despite the presence of total (i.e., free and bound) plasma drug concentrations well in excess of the MIC, they may not be predictive of concentrations of highly bound (i.e., >70%) drug at the site of infection. Properties of the capillary bed feeding the site of infection also dictate drug penetration. Highly vascularized tissue with a large capillary surface area–to-volume ratio can be expected to accumulate higher drug concentrations than can tissue that is poorly vascularized, principally because of the rate and extent to which drug can be delivered to the site. As with protein binding, variability in capillary density may be a function of disease (e.g., severe atherosclerosis, diabetes), infection (e.g., abscess, cardiac vegetation), and age, and it should be expected to have an impact on drug delivery. Similarly, tissues with tight junctions and few fenestrations (e.g., eye, central nervous system [CNS]) will afford lower tissue concentrations, given that drug entry is restricted to transport across the lipid bilayer of the endothelial cell (i.e., transcellular versus paracellular transport). Here, adequate drug penetration is restricted to agents with a favorable lipid-water partition coefficient and ionization constant. As such, many infectious processes warrant direct instillation of antibiotic at the site of infection (e.g., intracisternal, intrathecal, intra-articular). Additionally, cellular transporters (e.g., P-glycoprotein at the blood-brain barrier, organic anion/cation transporters at the choroid plexus) capable of "pumping" drug from the cell can limit distribution and retention of drug at the tissue level. Finally, the pH at the site of infection (e.g., in tissue fluids, exudates, transudates) relative to the pH in plasma also can govern distribution of a drug. For example, in cases of bacterial meningitis, the pH that occurs in the CNS is lower relative to plasma. Weak acids (e.g., penicillin) are more highly ionized in plasma than in cerebrospinal fluid (CSF) and pass more readily from the CSF into plasma than in the reverse direction. Similarly, when the pH of the local environment drops in the face of infection, as occurs in lung abscesses, aminoglycoside efficacy is reduced because of chemical inactivation of the drug by ionization and the formation of stable adducts with high DNA concentrations found in purulent secretions. Finally, the physicochemical association of an intact (i.e., unmetabolized) drug with a particular physiologic fluid as part of its normal excretion profile can serve to localize drug at the site of infection (e.g., accumulation of drugs excreted by the biliary route in patients with cholangitis and in the urine in patients with nephritis).

Pharmacodynamic Determinants of Effect

The desired effect of any drug is realized when sufficient concentrations are achieved and maintained at the active site for an adequate period. In many models of disease for which the treatment targets of modern chemotherapy remain fixed, the concentration-effect (i.e., pharmacodynamic) relationships can be described with relatively modest effort. In contrast, evaluating the concentration-effect relationship for antimicrobials can be anything but straightforward given the dynamic nature of infection. The intended target of the anti-infective agent is in constant flux as the number of organisms changes, the quantity and affinity of target receptors evolve, and the contribution of the host response adapts accordingly during the course of infection. Moreover, antimicrobials demonstrate variable effects at different concentrations and under different physicochemical environments. In fact, evaluating whether an organism survives in the presence of antibiotic is only one criterion by which to predict or define drug effect. Rather, a variety of effects related to antimicrobial concentration—from the extremes of complete eradication to complete survival—can be observed in the invading organism. The previous sections of this chapter reviewed the principles of pharmacokinetics, specifically, factors that link dose to concentration. The sections that follow explore the pharmacodynamics of anti-infective therapy and detail the multitude of factors that link concentration with effect.

EFFECTS DESCRIBED BY PHARMACOKINETIC PARAMETERS AND CONVENTIONAL SUSCEPTIBILITY END-POINTS

Clinicians have many decision-making tools at their disposal, including qualitative (e.g., breakpoints) and quantitative (e.g., MIC, minimal bactericidal concentration [MBC]) estimates of susceptibility, to guide in the selection of antimicrobial therapy. Although numerous studies and years of clinical evidence support the correlation between qualitative end-points and clinical outcome, their predictive power drops in the face of immunocompromise, severe underlying disease, mixed infections, and infection with organisms demonstrating heterogeneic resistance patterns.[25, 31, 50, 123, 131] Quantitative end-points provide a better assessment of dose-effect relationships, with antibiotic concentration serving as a surrogate for dose. However, these data alone do not reveal the complete picture relative to the anticipated bacterial response because laboratory-based quantitative tests contain a notable number of artificial aspects. Factors appreciated to influence the activity of antimicrobial agents in vivo (e.g., protein binding, fluctuating drug concentrations, serial drug

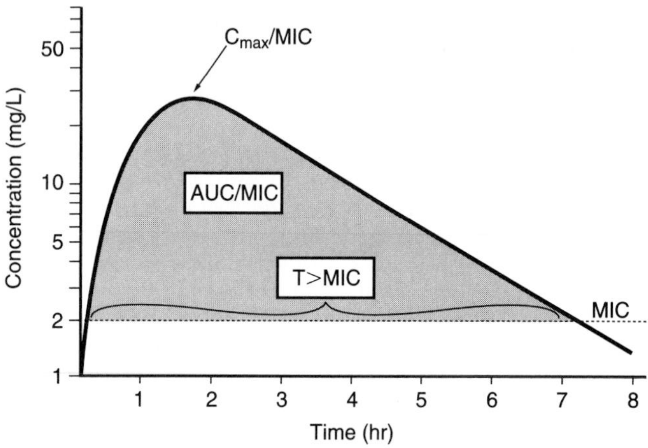

FIGURE 234–6 ■ Representative plasma concentration versus time curve illustrating commonly referenced pharmacodynamic parameters.

exposure, inoculum size, immune defense status, physicochemical environment, compound stability) essentially are neglected when determining MIC values. As such, agents with comparable MIC values in vitro may, in fact, demonstrate markedly different effect profiles in a patient.[1, 24, 57, 95, 109]

In an attempt to move beyond reliance on quantitative tests as the sole marker for predicting antimicrobial activity in vivo, the integration of susceptibility information with population- and patient-specific pharmacokinetic data continues to be explored. Surrogate end-points, defined by a combination of pharmacokinetic parameters and quantitative susceptibility data, have been suggested to more reliably predict the efficacy of different antimicrobials. By far, pharmacodynamic determinants of antimicrobial effect most frequently link attainable drug concentrations or estimates of total-body exposure (or both) with in vitro estimates of pathogen sensitivity. For antimicrobials for which the mechanism of action is determined to be time-dependent (concentration-independent), the percentage of time that plasma or tissue concentrations remain above the MIC has been closely linked to therapeutic response (Fig. 234–6). By comparison, the C_{max}-to-MIC ratio has demonstrated a similar relationship for drugs with concentration-dependent killing (see Fig. 234–6). Furthermore, the AUC-to-MIC ratio, which reflects the concentration profile over time, has been used with both classes of agents (see Fig. 234–6).

Evidence to support the application of specific pharmacodynamic surrogates is reviewed in the following paragraphs. One should note, however, that a large degree of interdependence exists among these pharmacokinetic parameters. With few exceptions, when the dose of a drug is increased, C_{max} and the total AUC increase, and with no change in clearance, so too does the percentage of time that plasma drug concentrations remain above the MIC. Accordingly, making distinctions among the various pharmacokinetic parameters in an attempt to determine the optimal pharmacodynamic end-point can be misleading. Given that many studies evaluate a limited number of doses or dosing intervals, restrict the number of pharmacokinetic parameters that are calculated, or neglect to perform multivariate analysis on the data such that clear distinctions cannot be made between parameters, an appropriate degree of caution should be exercised when evaluating such data.[200]

TIME ABOVE THE MIC (T > MIC). Among the first class of antimicrobial agents to be discussed in the context of their concentration-effect relationships were the β-lactams, specifically penicillin. Although limited supporting evidence existed at the time, investigators were concerned with maintaining adequate blood levels of the drug in the host for a fixed period. This concern was reflected in their attempts to inhibit clearance pathways and formulate sustained-release preparations designed specifically for the purpose of extending the time spent above some minimal concentration.[12, 162] As it turns out, in vitro studies support the relative concentration independence of penicillin and demonstrate that a maximal rate of killing can be observed that is quickly saturated at reasonably low multiples of the MIC (Fig. 234–7*A*). As concentrations increase above this maximal level, no faster rates of kill can be demonstrated.[28] Rather, penicillin displays time-dependent killing in which the duration of time spent above some minimal concentration (typically ±1 to 2 dilutions of the MIC or MBC) appears to be the most important determinant of activity.[43] As newer antimicrobial

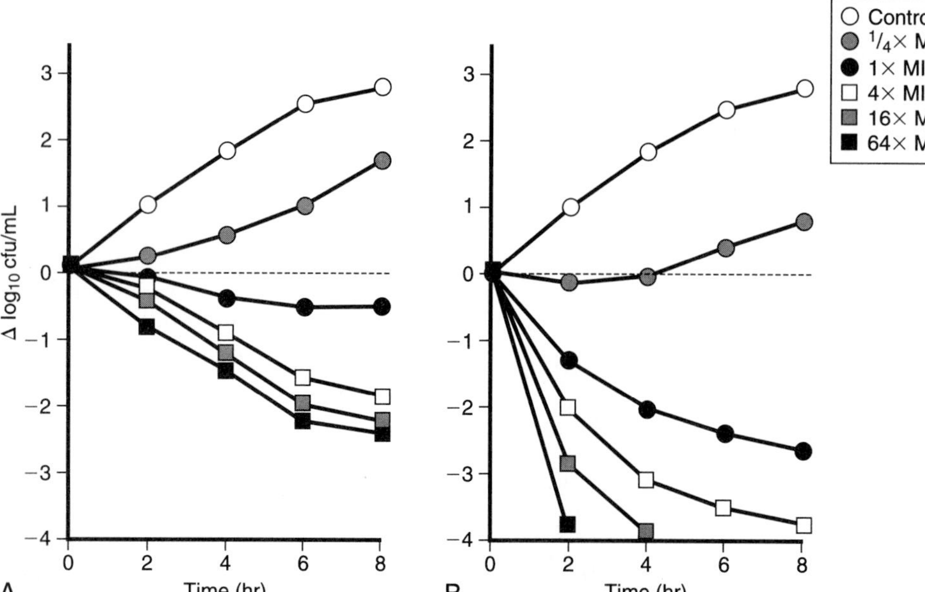

FIGURE 234–7 ■ Representative log-kill curves illustrating the response to concentration-independent *(A)* (time-dependent) and concentration-dependent *(B)* antimicrobial agents. (Adapted from Craig, W. A., and Ebert, S. C.: Killing and regrowth of bacteria in vitro: A review. Scand. J. Infect. Dis. *74*[Suppl.]:63–70, 1991.)

agents with putative time-dependent activity became available for evaluation, those with longer plasma and tissue terminal elimination half-lives demonstrated enhanced bactericidal activity when compared with similar drugs. Those that simply resulted in higher maximal peak concentrations, with no extension of the time above the MIC, produced minimal if any differences in effect.[5, 72, 168, 206] This time-dependent activity has been observed in vitro with virtually all β-lactams (e.g., cephalosporins, carbapenems, monobactams) against both gram-positive and gram-negative organisms.[52, 72, 181, 212] Similarly, other drug classes, namely, the macrolides, azalides, glycylcyclines, glycopeptides, and ketolides, appear to possess this same characteristic.[77, 126, 198, 199]

When evaluating whether the time-dependent activity observed in vitro can be reproduced in vivo by distilling antibiotic activity in the host to its purest sense through restriction of observations to animals in which the element of both humoral and cell-mediated immunity has been removed, the strongest relationship between antimicrobial concentration and effect for the aforementioned agents remains the time spent above the MIC.[163] Although most investigations represent models of tissue infection, elegant studies evaluating extensive numbers of dosing regimens and drug-microbe combinations demonstrate that β-lactam and macrolide efficacy correlates best with the percentage of time spent above the MIC, irrespective of whether gram-positive or gram-negative pathogens are involved.[200] Given the same total daily dose, therapy administered at more frequent intervals is required for a successful outcome.[7, 116] Even when the drug-microbe interaction is such that only bacteriostatic activity results, a regimen consisting of more frequent doses is able to maintain an environment of no net growth, whereas positive net growth is observed with larger doses administered less frequently.[65] From such data, the efficacy of time-dependent agents appears to be maximized by maintaining antibiotic concentrations above the MIC for as much of the dosing interval as possible.

When evaluating whether these agents obey the same relationship in the presence of a competent immune system, animal models similarly demonstrate a significant correlation between antimicrobial efficacy and the percentage of time spent above the MIC.[3, 58] In contrast to immunocompromised animals, however, it is not necessary that virtually 100 percent of the dosing interval be spent above the MIC for adequate antimicrobial activity in animals with a functional immune system. Although the bactericidal activity of penicillin ceases when concentrations fall below the MIC, the remaining organisms do not resume multiplication for many hours, well in excess of the time observed for the same organisms in vitro.[44, 97] This difference may reflect the time required for the organism to recover from the initial antibiotic insult, coupled with the complementary activity of subinhibitory antibiotic concentrations and the immune system (these pharmacodynamic principles will be explored later in further detail).[63] Irrespective of the mechanism by which the protracted antimicrobial effect occurs, the pharmacodynamic goals for time-dependent agents are not as stringent in vivo as they are in vitro. As would be expected, the persistent suppression of bacterial growth is not indefinite, and a maximal amount of time can be spent below the MIC before a reduction in efficacy becomes apparent. Thus, a maximal dosing interval for these agents appears to exist in immunocompetent hosts, beyond which a decrease in efficacy can be expected.[42, 173]

Clinical studies further confirm that for the agents discussed earlier, time above the MIC is a suitable pharmacodynamic end-point in patients. In clinical studies of upper respiratory tract infection, the highest bacterial eradication rates for the β-lactams are observed when the time above the MIC exceeds 40 to 50 percent of the dosing interval.[32] For cefuroxime, cure rates drop from greater than 90 percent to approximately 75 percent when the time above the MIC falls below 40 percent.[61, 69] Patients with a susceptible organism show 92 percent efficacy with a continuous-infusion regimen of cefamandole versus 63 percent efficacy when receiving intermittent administration of the agent. Finally, in neutropenic patients, an overall efficacy rate of 65 percent was observed after continuous infusion of cefamandole as opposed to 21 percent efficacy in patients receiving intermittent administration.[19] For macrolide-susceptible pathogens, cure rates approaching 100 percent were observed when concentrations remained above the MIC for greater than 80 percent of the dosing interval.[32] As the MIC increases such that the percentage of time spent above the MIC falls, so too do cure rates. Macrolide concentrations rarely exceed the MIC for *Haemophilus influenzae,* and cure rates are comparable to those seen in placebo-treated individuals.[32] A handful of studies appear to contradict the aforementioned data, thus indicating that little difference in clinical response is observed when the same total daily dose of selected agents is administered as a continuous infusion or with increased frequency versus less frequent intermittent administration; however, a prolonged post-antibiotic effect (PAE) or protracted half-life, such that both of the regimens evaluated spend nearly 100 percent of the dosing interval above the MIC, may explain these discrepancies.[23, 112, 201]

CONCENTRATION ABOVE THE MIC (C_{MAX}/MIC). In contrast to the aforementioned agents, a smaller group of agents demonstrate concentration dependence, with the magnitude of antimicrobial effect increasing in direct proportion to increasing drug concentrations[11, 128] (see Fig. 234–7*B*). The aminoglycoside and fluoroquinolone antibiotics are the prototypic drugs of this pharmacodynamic class; however, concentration-dependent activity also has been observed with the lipopeptides and metronidazole.[34, 180, 196] Unlike the time-dependent agents, for which shortening the dosing interval results in increased efficacy, extending the dosing interval for concentration-dependent drugs affords an ability to increase the dose, which results in a greater reduction in bacterial inoculum and, for some agents, a diminution in adaptive resistance.[33] Though highly variable, optimal peak plasma concentration to MIC ratios that result in complete killing have been defined for many drug-microbe combinations. Similarly, C_{max}/MIC ratios can be defined below which the organism is afforded the opportunity to regrow with increased selection of resistant subpopulations.[17, 39, 40]

Concentration-dependent killing for many of these agents has been demonstrated in both animal models and human clinical trials. In neutropenic mice with pseudomonal soft tissue infection, dosing schemes that deliver larger aminoglycoside doses less frequently result in greater killing than do schemes with the same total daily dose administered more frequently, despite the fact that all regimens achieved serum concentrations in excess of the MIC.[65] In patients receiving quinolone therapy for the treatment of respiratory tract, urinary tract, and skin and soft tissue infections, several pharmacodynamic parameters proved to correlate with clinical response; however, the best correlation was observed with the C_{max}-to-MIC ratio.[151] In clinical trials in which patients received aminoglycoside therapy for gram-negative infections, the strongest association between pharmacokinetic indices and clinical response was observed with the C_{max}-to-MIC ratio. In fact, the relationship between C_{max}/MIC and clinical response appeared to be linear over the range of clinically relevant plasma concentrations. An important note is that no significant difference occurred in the time to achieve C_{max} between responders and nonresponders; therefore, the improved response rates in patients achieving higher peak plasma concentrations were not simply an artifact of drug accumulation as a result of longer duration of therapy.[134, 136]

In addition to the absolute peak plasma concentration, the time that optimal peak levels are achieved appears to play a critical role in the response to concentration-dependent antimicrobial agents. A significant correlation with clinical improvement and reduction in mortality is observed if therapeutic peak plasma concentrations are reached early during the course of treatment.[135, 139] This effect is probably due to the fact that the response of the bacterial population to the same antibiotic concentration can change with subsequent doses. As alluded to earlier, subtherapeutic peak plasma concentrations serve to select out fewer susceptible variants within the population.[17, 18, 64] Based on these data, a key goal of therapy (i.e., in addition to proper drug selection) for concentration-dependent agents appears to be the attainment of high peak plasma concentrations early in therapy to afford rapid initial killing and minimize adaptive resistance.

Although prolonging the dosing interval affords the luxury of increasing the dose to optimize killing, the law of diminishing returns applies even for concentration-dependent agents, and it is possible to increase the dosing interval to excess and decrease efficacy. Despite the clear concentration dependence with escalating doses of fluoroquinolones, a simulated every-12-hour regimen was less effective than a regimen using the same total daily dose administered every 8 hours.[10] Similarly, animal models of gram-negative lung and soft tissue infection suggest that delayed clearance of the infecting organism is observed in response to aminoglycoside and fluoroquinolone therapy when administered in protracted dosing regimens (e.g., dosing interval much greater than the half-life) as opposed to shorter dosing intervals.[116, 138, 163] Again, scattered studies appear to contradict these findings; however, they use agents with a longer half-life, and therefore, the dosing interval may in fact not exceed the time spent above the MIC plus the residual PAE.[37] Thus, despite their concentration dependence, an element of time appears to be involved in the response to these agents. Unless peak concentrations are achieved in excess of those necessary to obtain maximal kill rates and the dosing interval does not markedly exceed time above the MIC plus the PAE, the efficacy of such agents is not only dose- but also dose interval–dependent.

TOTAL-BODY EXPOSURE ABOVE THE MIC (AUC/MIC). The AUC, a reflection of total-body exposure, is a pharmacokinetic parameter that integrates both time and drug concentration. Estimates of AUC reflect the magnitude of the dose received and the drug half-life relative to the dosing interval. Accordingly, researchers have proposed that the AUC/MIC ratio may serve as a better surrogate of pharmacodynamic activity for both time- and concentration-dependent agents. In several studies, the AUC/MIC ratio serves as the best correlate of the reduction in number of organisms for aminoglycosides, quinolones, streptogramins, and evernimicin.[38, 48, 111, 119, 163] Because of the interdependence between AUC and the pharmacokinetic parameters previously noted, studies also can be identified that demonstrate a relationship between clinical or microbiologic outcome and the AUC/MIC ratio for agents with time-dependent activity (e.g., the β-lactams and glycopeptides). Often, however, these studies fail to evaluate multiple pharmacokinetic parameters.[133, 172]

In an elegant study evaluating a number of aminoglycoside dosing regimens against *Pseudomonas aeruginosa* and *Escherichia coli* infection, the log-normalized AUC provided the best correlation with efficacy. However, as was observed with concentration-dependent agents, when the dosing interval exceeded the time above the MIC plus the residual PAE, the best correlation with efficacy was the percentage of time spent above the MIC, thus reaffirming that the dosing interval can be too long with the aminoglycosides.[200] A meta-analysis of 19 studies evaluating eight quinolones and six different organisms in experimental endocarditis similarly demonstrated a correlation between the AUC/MIC and reduction in $\log_{10}$ colony-forming units (CFU) per vegetation. However, given the relationship between the pharmacokinetic parameters, C_{max}/MIC and T > MIC also proved to correlate with a decrease in the size of the inoculum.[2] In human investigations, AUC/MIC appears to serve as the best predictor of clinical response, microbiologic response, and bacterial eradication for the fluoroquinolones. Nonetheless, C_{max}/MIC and T > MIC can be linked similarly to bacterial eradication for this class of agents.[55, 56, 148]

Clearly, the optimal AUC/MIC ratio will be different for different organisms despite sharing a similar quantitative susceptibility end-point. Likewise, optimal AUC/MIC ratios are highly variable and depend on the antimicrobial agent being evaluated. For example, effective eradication of organisms implicated in nosocomial pneumonia is observed with an AUC/MIC ratio of 540 for cefmenoxime, 34 for tobramycin, and 23 for ciprofloxacin.[171] Consequently, attempts have been made to standardize this pharmacodynamic end-point, with investigators proposing a value of 125 as the cutoff below which a reduction in efficacy and increase in resistance may be expected.[88, 170] However, optimal AUC/MIC ratios may differ depending not only on a given organism and agent but also on the desired outcome and the disease state involved. A ratio greater than 125 resulted in bacterial eradication roughly 7 days after the initiation of β-lactam and quinolone therapy; however, an AUC/MIC ratio of 250 resulted in eradication of the pathogen within 1 to 2 days after initiating quinolone therapy.[170] For patients with acute exacerbations of chronic bronchitis who are receiving fluoroquinolones, an AUC/MIC ratio less than 276 was associated with longer time to clinical success, whereas a ratio greater than 576 was associated with a reduction in coughs per day and a ratio greater than 212 with decreasing days to a reduction in the volume of sputum.[132] In an animal model of bacterial endocarditis, significantly lower numbers of organism were found in the vegetation after 3 to 6 days of therapy when the AUC/MIC ratio exceeded 100.[2] Moreover, a value of 100 appeared to be the cutoff below which an increased risk of resistance was observed in a retrospective review of 107 acutely ill patients with lower respiratory tract infection.[191] Furthermore, in vitro models evaluating fluoroquinolone activity against *Streptococcus pneumoniae* demonstrate effective eradication with an AUC/MIC ratio between 30 and 65, well less than the value of 125 reported as optimal for other pathogens.[111, 119]

Although this hybrid parameter bridges concentration and time (i.e., extent of systemic drug exposure from a given dose) and has been demonstrated to correlate with efficacy for numerous drug classes, optimal criteria appear to vary with the organism, agent, disease state, and desired outcome. In addition, established relationships may no longer hold for some agents when a protracted dosing interval is used in therapy. As such, a general classification and standard outcome are not straightforward, and agents need to be evaluated with respect to known mechanisms of activity and the specific clinical and microbiologic scenarios in which they are used.

OPTIMAL SURROGATES FOR DRUGS IN COMBINATION. Combination antimicrobial therapy is initiated in numerous circumstances to ensure broad-spectrum coverage early in therapy, to treat polymicrobial infections, and to combat organisms that require multiple agents for effective eradication. Often, combination therapy entails the use of agents from different classes or agents that have different mechanisms of action (or both). This particular scenario raises the question of how one applies the aforementioned pharmacodynamic principles to selecting or evaluating the efficacy of drug therapy when confronted with the combined use of agents that do not share similar pharmacodynamic targets. Although optimization of combination therapy may be possible by choosing the interval for one agent,[66] efficacy appears to be best explained when a combination of both pharmacodynamic properties is considered.[65, 137]

Reasonable models of a concentration-effect relationship have been proposed for numerous agents alone and in combination; however, optimal ratios remain to be defined for many drug-microbe combinations. Moreover, it is probably more complex than simply defining the optimal ratio for specific combinations. Even though one can define the best correlate, killing rates in fact may vary with the site of infection because penetration of drug into or clearance from tissue varies from site to site. For example, logAUC proves to be the best predictor for clearance of organisms from the lung regardless of the dosing interval used. In contrast, given faster drug clearance from the thigh, the time above the MIC was a more important predictor of eradication when a longer dosing interval was used, whereas the logAUC was the best predictor of clearance of organisms with the use of shorter dosing intervals.[117] Similarly, in animal models of bacterial meningitis, greater kill rates were observed as T > MBC increased. However, when concentrations remained above the MBC for the entire dosing interval, which may not be unexpected in situations in which the antibiotic half-life is longer in CSF than plasma, kill rates were directly proportional to both peak/MBC and AUC/MBC ratios.[127] These data suggest that we may need to expand the characterization of pharmacodynamic surrogates to look at the pharmacokinetic-pharmacodynamic interface at the site of infection rather than simply defining dosing strategies based on in vitro susceptibility data and the disposition characteristics of drugs in plasma. Without question, a great deal of data need to be collected and verified in the human host. The maximal dose and dosing regimen ideally are selected so that the resultant pharmacokinetic profile affords optimal pharmacodynamic activity without causing the unnecessary adverse events and therapeutic failure (e.g., underdosing, acquisition of resistance with suboptimal dosing) that might be observed with inappropriate dosing. Development of a successful therapeutic strategy requires incorporation of knowledge regarding the infecting pathogen; the physicochemical, pharmacologic, and pharmacokinetic properties of the anti-infective agent; and specific factors of the host or disease that are capable of altering either drug disposition or action. Such an approach enables the clinician to make clearer distinctions among agents with similar susceptibility profiles, yet different mechanistic or pharmacokinetic profiles and to select an optimal drug regimen that will be most likely to result in successful therapy.

EFFECT OF SUPRAINHIBITORY ANTIMICROBIAL CONCENTRATIONS (EAGLE EFFECT, PARADOXICAL ZONE PHENOMENON, CONCENTRATION QUENCHING)

In simplest terms, one typically thinks of anti-infective activity increasing with increasing antimicrobial concentration. More sophisticated models describe increasing activity with increasing drug concentration to a maximal effect until activity reaches a plateau and remains relatively constant despite further increases in drug concentration (e.g., the sigmoid E_{max} model; see Fig. 234–4). However, for many antibiotics, an increase in drug concentration can, in fact, result in a reduction in antimicrobial activity[84] (Fig. 234–8). This paradoxical effect was observed as early as 1945 and described 3 years later by Eagle and Musselman, who reported the existence of antibiotic concentrations above the maximally effective concentration at which the killing rate of bacteria is paradoxically reduced.[45, 107] This phenomenon has been described with a host of organisms and, though originally observed with penicillin, has been confirmed with other β-lactams, glycopeptides, aminoglycosides, and fluoroquinolones.[125, 141, 149, 186, 209] Given the diversity of agents that demonstrate a paradoxical reduction in activity with increasing drug concentration, this phenomenon probably cannot be explained by a single mechanism, and though not definitively elucidated, numerous mechanisms have been proposed to explain these observations.

For certain β-lactam antimicrobials, induction of β-lactamase may be responsible for the paradoxical effects observed in selected organisms. In vitro experiments performed with *Proteus vulgaris* suggested that the greatest paradoxical response seen with β-lactams was observed with agents that demonstrated the highest β-lactamase–inducing capacity and the poorest stability to degradation by this enzyme. When a mutant strain of this organism that was unable to induce β-lactamase production was evaluated, no paradoxical effect was noted.[92] In animal models of peritoneal infection, antibiotics with strong dose-dependent induction of β-lactamase similarly demonstrated a paradoxical effect against β-lactamase–positive strains of *P. vulgaris.* However, no paradoxical effect was observed against β-lactamase–negative strains. Agents that were only weak inducers of β-lactamase demonstrated no evidence of a paradoxical effect, regardless of whether the *P. vulgaris* strains produced β-lactamase.[91]

Because this paradoxical effect can be demonstrated with the β-lactams against organisms that do not produce β-lactamase, other mechanisms also must be responsible. One such mechanism may involve dysregulation of the bacterial autolytic system, which often confers tolerance to an organism but also may uncover an Eagle-type effect.[79] A paradoxical

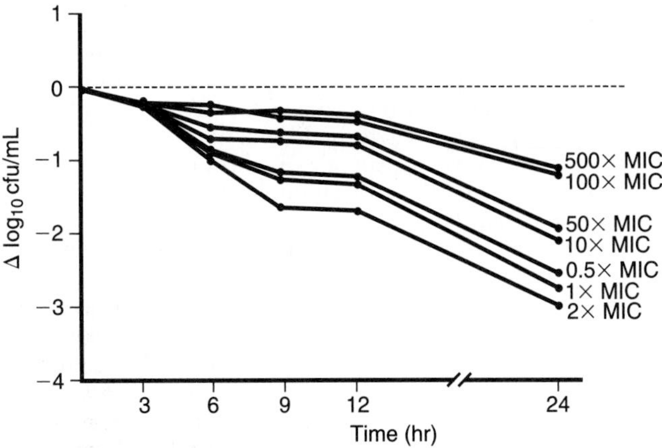

FIGURE 234–8 ■ Representative log-kill curve demonstrating the paradoxical effects that can be observed with suprainhibitory antimicrobial concentrations. (Adapted from Holm, S. E., Odenholdt-Tornqvist, I., and Cars, O.: Paradoxical effects of antibiotics. Scand. J. Infect. Dis. Suppl. *74*:113–117, 1991.)

reduction in antimicrobial activity at high doses may be related to differences in regulation or expression of these autolytic enzymes. In *Enterococcus* strains that fully express only one of two recognized autolytic enzymes, diminished or deficient production of the second enzyme resulted in a paradoxical response to penicillin. Strains in which both enzymes were produced remained susceptible to the antibiotic irrespective of concentration, thus suggesting that a proportional dose-response relationship may require the synergistic activity of both enzymes.[53, 54] Further investigation into the paradoxical effect observed in tolerant organisms suggests that organisms in the exponential growth phase demonstrate this response more consistently than do those in the stationary phase.[150, 152] Animal models of *Staphylococcus aureus* endocarditis provide in vivo confirmation of the paradoxical response observed with tolerant organisms in vitro. Administration of continuous-infusion cloxacillin to animals infected with a nontolerant strain produced a dose-proportional reduction in bacterial density ($\log_{10}$CFU/g) within the vegetation, whereas animals infected with a tolerant strain demonstrated a reduction and subsequent paradoxical increase in bacterial density with increasing dose. Of note is that no statistical difference was observed in bacterial density within other organs or in overall survival, which raises questions regarding the in vivo significance of these observations.[202]

For antibiotics that demonstrate polyfunctional activity at supratherapeutic concentrations, a paradoxical response may occur as a result of secondary alterations in cellular functions that are requisite for antimicrobial activity. Despite a principal mechanism of action for the fluoroquinolones at the site of DNA gyrase, these agents appear to be bactericidal only in cells able to synthesize protein. As quinolone concentrations increase above those that are bactericidal, RNA synthesis, and therefore protein synthesis, is progressively inhibited, thus explaining the reduced rate of bactericidal activity observed at high quinolone concentrations.[161] Incompletely characterized genetic modifications also may confer a paradoxical response to antibiotics. β-Lactam resistance in methicillin-resistant *S. aureus* (MRSA) is mediated by de-repressing the production of a low-affinity PBP. However, because the modified PBP serves as an inefficient transpeptidase, it is regarded as an internal selective pressure in the bacterium and a countermutation has arisen. Though not completely understood, the phenotypic expression of this countermutation is manifested as an Eagle-type resistance to methicillin.[108, 167] Finally, an observed paradoxical response may not be a result of the drug-microbe combination alone but a result of the chemical environment as well. A paradoxical effect with penicillin, in which both cell count and the rate of killing were affected, was demonstrated in *Streptococcus agalactiae* when the pH was reduced under in vitro conditions.[90]

Most studies investigating the Eagle effect have been conducted in vitro, and the clinical implications of the paradoxical phenomenon have yet to be fully elucidated. However, anecdotal evidence appears to suggest that the clinical efficacy of antimicrobials can be compromised by high-dose antibiotic therapy. Case reports of β-lactam–susceptible streptococcal endocarditis and staphylococcal pneumonia describe patients who failed to respond to high-dose β-lactam therapy (plasma concentrations $>100\times$ MIC in one case), with subsequent improvement in each case when the dose was lowered.[63a, 73, 189] For many agents, it is clearly advantageous to establish high peak drug concentrations early, the benefits of which include increasing log kill, preventing the selection of resistant mutants, overcoming refractoriness, and enhancing penetration of tissue. However, the relative safety of many drug classes (e.g., the β-lactams) often results in the use of doses that may be higher than necessary. When clear evidence is lacking for enhanced bactericidal activity at higher concentrations coincident with the potential for diminished efficacy, escalation of antibiotic doses should be considered judiciously.

EFFECTS OF SUBINHIBITORY ANTIMICROBIAL CONCENTRATION

Individuals may be exposed to subtherapeutic antimicrobial concentrations for many reasons, including underdosing, poor compliance, and perhaps most commonly, the inability of the pharmacokinetic profile of the agent in question to afford adequate penetration to the site of infection. Exposure of bacteria to antibiotic concentrations below the MIC can have variable effects, depending on the organism and the antimicrobial agent involved. In fact, the effects observed with subinhibitory levels are not simply a milder extension of those observed at inhibitory concentrations but, instead, are qualitatively different from the effects observed at concentrations that equal or exceed the MIC.[121] Subinhibitory concentrations can enhance or impair opsonization and phagocytosis; have an impact on the virulence of the bacteria by modifying the bacterial cell surface; alter adherence properties, antigen expression, or the excretion of enzymes and toxins (or any combination of these effects); and inhibit bacterial growth.[143, 144, 194] The result can be an increase or decrease in responsiveness to therapy, both of which are discussed later in this section. Before reviewing the current data, however, one should note that this discussion does not refer to subinhibitory concentrations occurring after initial suprainhibitory drug levels. These particular effects are distinguished as PAE and will be addressed separately.

Despite the fact that antibiotic concentrations may fail to equal or exceed the MIC, these agents still can affect the growth of an invading organism adversely.[121, 122, 124] In fact, the term minimal antibacterial concentration (MAC), usually a fraction of the MIC, was coined to describe the lowest concentration of antibiotic required to produce either structural changes in the bacterium, a one $\log_{10}$ decrease in the number of organisms present, or a 10 percent delay in turbidimetric growth in vitro.[62, 185] Rather than resulting in treatment failure, subinhibitory antimicrobial concentrations in concert with defenses in an immunocompetent host may be sufficient to clear the infection.[194] A multitude of effects have been observed to occur as a result of exposure to subinhibitory antimicrobial concentrations and are mediated by a variable number of mechanisms.

Increased susceptibility to phagocytosis may be seen with subinhibitory antibiotic concentrations and can occur in many ways. Subinhibitory concentrations may induce morphologic changes in the bacterium such that its size and shape are altered markedly and, as a result, the immune system is signaled to clear the bacterium.[6, 185, 203] However, subinhibitory concentrations of drugs that share a common intracellular target cannot be expected to have the same effects on bacterial morphology. Despite the fact that both penicillins and cephalosporins act via PBPs, subinhibitory concentrations of penicillins induce filaments in *Proteus mirabilis*, whereas cephalosporins induce the formation of globules.[122, 124, 189] A likely explanation lies in their different affinity for the various PBPs, whereby they can be expected to bind selectively at low concentrations and rather nonspecifically at therapeutic or supratherapeutic concentrations. The preferential binding of ceftibuten to PBP-3 of

E. coli at subinhibitory concentrations results in filamentation because this PBP allows crosswall but not sidewall synthesis.[21] Similarly, subinhibitory concentrations of the same drug applied to different organisms can produce different morphologic changes. In *S. aureus,* subinhibitory concentrations of loracarbef induce no morphologic changes, whereas similar concentrations lead to elongated forms and short-chain forms in *E. coli* and elongated and filamentous forms in *H. influenzae.*[195]

Although size may be one factor stimulating enhanced clearance of the organism, increased uptake by the immune system can be demonstrated even for cells with little gross morphologic alteration. Subinhibitory antibiotic concentrations can impair the synthesis of antiphagocytic surface factors or liberate their release, thereby enhancing complement binding, opsonization, phagocytosis, and ultimately, bacterial killing.[81, 86, 113] Production of the antiphagocytic A protein of *S. aureus* can be inhibited by subinhibitory concentrations of selected protein synthesis inhibitors and fluoroquinolones.[130, 179] Subinhibitory concentrations of β-lactam agents, but not vancomycin or protein synthesis inhibitors, increase the susceptibility of *S. agalactiae* to uptake by polymorphonuclear leukocytes (PMNs) because of the loss of antiphagocytic capsular material.[85] Carbapenems and cephalosporins at subinhibitory concentrations increase the serum sensitivity of K1-positive *E. coli* by reducing expression of the K1 capsular polysaccharide.[187]

Even drugs with no inherent bacteriostatic or bactericidal activity against a specific organism can induce sufficient changes in the cell surface to affect serum sensitivity. Preincubation of *P. aeruginosa* with subinhibitory concentrations of certain macrolides decreases cell surface hydrophobicity and enhances the sensitivity of the organism to human serum bactericidal activity.[190] Subinhibitory β-lactam concentrations are capable of sufficiently altering the peptidoglycan structure in MRSA to enhance susceptibility of the organism to the lysozyme present in sputum despite the fact that the organism, because of altered PBP production, is no longer susceptible to the bactericidal activity of these agents.[89] Although most effects stimulating bacterial clearance by the host occur as a direct result of cellular changes in the organism, immune cells also can be altered by subinhibitory antibiotic concentrations. Erythromycin does not affect the generation of serum-derived leuko-attractants, nor does it increase PMN cell numbers, yet it appears to be capable of stimulating the migration of PMNs. Researchers have suggested that this effect probably results from the ability of erythromycin to sustain cellular migration by reducing the level of leuko-attractant–induced auto-oxidation mediated by the myeloperoxidase–hydrogen peroxide–halide system.[49]

In addition to enhancing bacterial clearance, subinhibitory antibiotic concentrations also can impair bacterial virulence mechanisms. For many organisms, pili, fimbriae, and fimbriae-associated adhesins are responsible for the initial events surrounding adherence and colonization at the site of entry or infection.[169] Subinhibitory quinolone and clindamycin concentrations are capable of decreasing the adherence of nosocomial pathogens (e.g., *Staphylococcus epidermidis*) to the synthetic materials of implantable catheters.[26, 177] Subinhibitory concentrations of penicillins, cephalosporins, azalides, and quinolones all have demonstrated the ability to decrease the formation of fimbriae or alter structures that mediate adherence. Specific examples include decreased adherence to oral and urinary tract epithelial cells for organisms such as *Porphyromonas gingivalis, E. coli, Salmonella typhimurium,* and *P. aeruginosa.*[21, 120, 179, 188, 203] Moreover, these effects do not appear to be growth phase–specific for select drug-microbe combinations.[22]

Subtherapeutic antibiotic concentrations also can have an impact on virulence by down-regulating bacterial toxin production. Subinhibitory concentrations of clindamycin can inhibit toxin production in *S. epidermidis* markedly without appreciably altering bacterial growth.[177] *Pseudomonas* exoenzymes that facilitate disease pathogenesis (e.g., exotoxin A, exoenzyme S, phospholipase C, total protease, elastase) are suppressed after exposure to subinhibitory concentrations of ciprofloxacin, tobramycin, and ceftazidime.[74] Finally, given the ability of subinhibitory fluoroquinolone concentrations to disrupt DNA structure sufficiently to interfere with effective mRNA production, continuous exposure of *S. aureus* to fluoroquinolones at subinhibitory concentrations decreases the production of nuclease and hemolytic alpha-toxin production.[179]

Although discerning which of these effects alone or in combination are responsible for the subinhibitory effects is difficult, one might see in vivo that the impact of the sum total of these effects can be observed at the level of the host. In a non-neutropenic rat model of *Klebsiella pneumoniae* pneumonia, a continuous infusion of ceftazidime resulting in steady-state concentrations of 0.06 mg/L protected all the animals from death, despite a MIC for the pathogen of 0.2 mg/L. The same could not be said, however, for immunocompromised animals, which required steady-state concentrations of 0.38 mg/L for adequate protection.[164, 165] In a similar model of intraperitoneal *K. pneumoniae* infection, subinhibitory clindamycin concentrations resulted in an increase in bacterial clearance and a decrease in the $\log_{10}$CFU in blood at 72 hours.[4] In humans, low-dose ampicillin (such that concentrations in urine were no greater than a fourth to a half times the MIC) combined with large water intake was demonstrated to clear documented *E. coli* urinary tract infection in 16 of 20 patients within 2 days of initiating therapy, whereas none of the 18 control subjects receiving the fluid intervention alone demonstrated resolution.[158] Despite the resistance of *Pseudomonas* in patients with cystic fibrosis, the fluoroquinolones remain capable of eliciting a significant reduction in sputum colony counts and improvement in clinical signs and symptoms.[175, 178]

One must recognize that subinhibitory antimicrobial concentrations can be as potentially disadvantageous to the host as they can be of benefit. They can impair the ability of the host to respond to the bacterial inoculum, can augment bacterial defenses, and can serve to inactivate the antibiotic. For organisms that are susceptible to β-lactamase induction, strong inducers can up-regulate β-lactamase synthesis at concentrations below the MIC. Although β-lactamase induction is typically a reversible phenomenon, many antibiotics demonstrate the ability to select out genetically de-repressed mutants at subinhibitory concentrations.[176, 182] Irrespective of whether this induction is phenotypic or genotypic in nature, many antibiotics to which the organism originally may have been susceptible no longer retain their efficacy in light of β-lactamase production. This type of adaptive resistance, observed in response to sublethal antibiotic concentrations, also can be nonenzymatic in nature. A single one-time exposure of *P. aeruginosa* to subinhibitory concentrations of chlorhexidine results in unstable resistance, and repeated exposure leads to stable expression of altered cell surface macromolecules or efflux systems responsible for resistance.[192] In a clinical strain of this same organism exposed to subinhibitory concentrations of fluoroquinolones and carbapenems for 5 days, a 16- to 32-fold increase in MIC has been observed to occur in concert with an alteration in overall protein expression.[27]

Sublethal antibiotic concentrations also can stimulate the production of toxins that may be detrimental to the host.

Exposure of enterohemorrhagic *E. coli* to subinhibitory concentrations of fluoroquinolones, cephalosporins, tetracyclines, and inhibitors of folic acid synthesis induces enhanced expression of a Shiga-like toxin (SLT-1), which is proposed to mediate events surrounding the development of hemolytic-uremic syndrome. Subinhibitory fluoroquinolone concentrations also can stimulate the production of verotoxins in this same organism.[204, 210] Lincomycin and tetracycline at subinhibitory concentrations stimulate the production of heat-labile enterotoxin in enterotoxigenic *E. coli,* as well as *Vibrio cholerae* enterotoxin, despite the fact that these agents are principally protein synthesis inhibitors. Researchers have shown that the copy number of plasmids does not increase and have proposed that the rate of enterotoxin liberation is enhanced as a result of antibiotic inhibition of the synthesis of proteins responsible for degrading the toxin.[118, 211] The alpha-toxin of *S. aureus* is demonstrated to be hemolytic, dermonecrotic, and antichemotactic and appears to be up-regulated in the presence of subinhibitory nafcillin concentrations irrespective of whether the isolate is susceptible to the agent. Greater hemolytic activity and increased lethality of the broth filtrate in a murine intraperitoneal model are observed, and this activity is ablated when incubated with anti–alpha-toxin antibody.[106] Other β-lactams (with the exception of aztreonam), ofloxacin, and trimethoprim are similarly capable of inducing alpha-toxin expression at subinhibitory concentrations.[145]

The up-regulation of protein expression by subinhibitory antibiotic concentrations not only is responsible for contributing to antibiotic and cellular destruction but also can enhance the binding of pathogens to host proteins and implantable devices. Subinhibitory concentrations of ciprofloxacin increase the transcription of fibronectin-binding proteins in *S. aureus* isolates and thereby result in greater adhesion to immobilized fibronectin and fibronectin-coated polymers, a particular concern with subcutaneously implanted devices that have polymer surfaces.[14, 15] Subinhibitory concentrations of antibiotic also can alter the immunogenicity of the pathogen such that the host can no longer mount the same degree of immune response. *S. aureus* isolates co-incubated with subinhibitory concentrations of oxacillin demonstrated a diminished capacity to stimulate proinflammatory cytokine production (e.g., tumor necrosis factor–α, interleukin-1β [IL-1β], and IL-6) in human monocytes. Given that activation of the complement system and cytokine release are stimulated by peptidoglycan molecules of a certain size or tertiary structure, subinhibitory β-lactam concentrations probably distort the peptidoglycan structure sufficiently that the immune system no longer effectively responds to these immunostimulatory components.[174]

Unless unusual circumstances prevail, the goal of therapy probably will not be to target plasma concentrations below the MIC. However, given the reality of encountering this situation in the clinical setting, practitioners certainly need to be aware of the potential implications for therapeutic response associated with subinhibitory concentrations of antimicrobial agents.

EFFECTS THAT PERSIST AFTER ANTIMICROBIAL EXPOSURE (PAE, PALE, AND PLIE)

Early investigations into antibiotic activity described a delay in the recovery and regrowth of penicillin-exposed staphylococci and streptococci when the drug was removed by enzymatic inactivation or the organism was removed to drug-free media.[13, 41, 147] In addition, in vivo evaluations of penicillin activity suggested that the effects of penicillin in an immunocompetent animal lasted well beyond the time when blood levels remained above quantifiable concentrations. Despite a half-life of minutes, many hours could elapse after the administration of a dose of penicillin before bacterial growth resumes.[44, 97, 173] The term *post-antibiotic effect* was coined to describe the suppression of bacterial growth that persists after brief exposure of the organism to an antimicrobial agent.[30] Unlike the subinhibitory effects discussed earlier in the chapter, the PAE occurs as a result of residual antimicrobial activity after initial exposure at inhibitory concentrations as opposed to the subinhibitory concentrations themselves. The PAEs described to date typically are reversible and, although the mechanisms have not been elucidated fully, are probably caused by either nonlethal damage or persistence of antibiotic at the site of action. In the same vein as the PAEs, the term post–β-lactamase inhibitor effect (PLIE) was coined to describe the residual effects of β-lactamase inhibitors after exposure to inhibitory concentrations.[193] Similarly, one will encounter the term post-antibiotic leukocyte enhancement (PALE), which is used to account for a PAE in vivo that lasts longer than that observed in vitro and is defined as exposure to subinhibitory concentrations of an antibiotic that render the organism more susceptible to the phagocytic and bactericidal action of neutrophils.

The PAE is dependent on many factors, the most discernible being the drug-microbe combination.[94] Since the initial descriptions with penicillin were reported, similar observations have been noted for a broad range of organisms, and essentially all antibiotic classes demonstrate a PAE against select organisms.[30] Virtually all agents evaluated demonstrate a PAE against susceptible gram-positive cocci. Inhibitors of protein and nucleic acid synthesis produce longer-lasting PAEs in vitro than cell wall–acting agents do, with an average of approximately 1 to 2 hours for β-lactams, 1 to 3 hours for fluoroquinolones, and 3 to 5 hours for protein synthesis inhibitors. For resistant gram-positive cocci, descriptions of a PAE are mixed. Against gram-negative bacilli, no appreciable PAE is observed for trimethoprim or the β-lactams in vitro, with the exception of the carbapenems, which demonstrate a PAE of approximately 1 to 2 hours. The fluoroquinolones and protein synthesis inhibitors have PAEs of roughly 1 to 3 hours and 3 to 8 hours, respectively. Within this group of organisms, *P. aeruginosa* serves as an exception, and the fluoroquinolones and protein synthesis inhibitors display slightly shorter PAEs, 1 to 2 hours and 2 to 3 hours on average for the respective drug classes. Similar observations have been described for the gram-negative anaerobes, with little or no PAE seen with the β-lactams but a measurable PAE observed for protein synthesis inhibitors.[30]

Given that most drug classes demonstrate a PAE, multiple mechanisms must exist by which this effect arises. For the β-lactams, researchers have proposed that the PAE corresponds to the time required for the organism to synthesize new PBPs. The initial high β-lactam concentrations are thought to bind irreversibly to and thus inactivate the PBPs. As such, cell multiplication subsequently is prolonged until a critical number of PBPs are resynthesized and cell division can resume.[194] Within the large class of β-lactam agents, however, further distinctions can be made based on the specific PBP bound and the subsequent morphologic alteration that is induced. Against *E. coli,* the longest lasting PAEs are observed for agents that induce the formation of spheroplasts and the shortest for agents that induce the formation of filaments. On drug removal, filaments (which may contain a biomass corresponding to more than 20 bacteria) readily separate into individual bacteria, whereas spheroplasts require a longer period to resynthesize a normal cell wall and resume replication.[78] Analogous to the β-lactams, the time required for the resynthesis or recovery of ribosomal proteins is probably responsible for the PAEs observed after the administration of an aminoglycoside. Evaluation of the intracellular events taking place in *E. coli* during aminoglycoside-induced PAEs suggests that both DNA and RNA synthesis resumes immediately after drug removal; however, synthesis of structural and functional protein does not resume for nearly 5 hours.[8, 94] For the fluoroquinolones, the proposed mechanism behind the PAE is not as consistent with the antimicrobial activity of these agents. A progressive increase in ^{3}H-thymidine incorporation in *S. aureus* during the PAE suggests that DNA synthesis continues to occur, and thus, the PAE might represent the time needed to repair the damage to DNA gyrase, the time required to re-establish the function of DNA gyrase after dissociation of the antibiotic from the enzyme, or the time required to synthesize new DNA gyrase.[70]

In addition to the specific drug-microbe combination, the magnitude and duration of drug exposure also will have an impact on the PAE. Cell wall–acting agents (e.g., β-lactams and glycopeptides) demonstrate a concentration-dependent PAE. An increase in the concentration and duration of exposure, (i.e., increasing AUC) will prolong the PAE in both gram-positive and gram-negative organisms to a point of maximal effect, typically 2 to 6 hours, although the time may be shorter for some members of this class. In fact, the PAE appears to be related to the log-normalized AUC in a sigmoidal manner.[29, 78, 110] Similarly, an increasing concentration of protein synthesis inhibitors is associated with progressive prolongation in PAE to a point of maximal effect. However, it can be difficult to establish with the aminoglycosides and fluoroquinolones because complete killing at supratherapeutic concentrations can obscure accurate determination of the PAE.[30, 94] Bacteriostatic agents generally demonstrate concentration-independent PAEs such that increasing the duration of antibiotic exposure, but not the concentration, results in an increase in PAE to some maximal effect.[30]

As expected, the magnitude of the PAE also depends on whether antimicrobial agents are administered alone or in combination. Indifferent, additive, and synergistic PAEs all have been described with the use of combination therapy.[59, 76, 94] However, for some drug-microbe combinations, the magnitude of the PAE may differ with the phenotypic expression of resistance. For *Enterococcus faecalis* isolates that demonstrate only low-level resistance to streptomycin or gentamicin, the effect of a penicillin-aminoglycoside combination on the PAE is markedly synergistic. In contrast, for isolates with high-level resistance to the aminoglycosides, no synergistic PAE is observed.[207] Additionally, physicochemical factors can affect in vitro determination of PAEs, and although the in vivo relevance is questionable, some are worthy of consideration. In *S. aureus,* the PAEs of penicillin and gentamicin are markedly protracted at the slightly acidic pH 6 as compared with a physiologic pH of 7.4. Given that a relatively acidic pH can occur at the site of active infection, a disease-PAE interaction is possible. A similar pH-dependent effect on PAE is not observed with the fluoroquinolones or macrolides against *S. aureus,* nor is it noted for *E. coli* and *P. aeruginosa* with the β-lactams, fluoroquinolones, and macrolides.[60, 75] An increase in PAE in vitro also is observed as temperature drops, which raises the question of whether the PAE is truly altered or the generation time is lengthened. Regardless, the temperatures evaluated were well below physiologic and probably have no clinical impact in the face of infection. Finally, anaerobic conditions are observed to increase the PAE for ciprofloxacin–*E. coli* and gentamicin–*S. aureus* combinations, but not with other combinations.[60]

The attention paid to PAE of late highlights its significance, which lies in the flexibility that it affords to extend the dosing interval before re-exposure to drug, essentially redosing, is necessary. Researchers have suggested that agents with a small PAE require that a dosing interval be selected that will maintain concentrations above the MIC throughout most of the interval. Agents with a more protracted PAE can be given less often and thus at higher doses, thereby supporting the argument for once-daily dosing with drugs such as the aminoglycosides. However, many nuances can be identified between the in vitro conditions under which PAEs are determined and the in vivo conditions of infection such that the ultimate clinical (i.e., therapeutic) implications of these data have yet to be determined. In vitro, attempts are made to remove drug completely (i.e., abruptly terminate drug exposure to the microbe) after initial exposure when determining the PAE. In contrast, drug concentrations fall in a more controlled, typically first-order fashion in vivo. The impact of this distinction on PAEs in patients remains unknown. Variable growth rates or metabolic states of the organism when growing in vivo may similarly have an impact on the PAE. In vitro, a prolonged PAE is observed when *Enterococcus faecium* is exposed to the combination of gentamicin and penicillin; yet when the same drug concentrations and the same inoculum size are achieved in the vegetation of a murine aortic valve endocarditis model, no prolongation of PAE can be observed.[83] Similarly, a rat model of *P. aeruginosa* endocarditis failed to demonstrate a PAE in vivo for the combination of imipenem and gentamicin despite a PAE of nearly 5 hours determined in vitro; however, an observable PAE in vitro and in vivo is noted in the same model when ciprofloxacin is evaluated.[82, 93]

IMPACT OF INOCULUM SIZE ON THE CONCENTRATION-EFFECT RELATIONSHIP

The antimicrobial effect observed at any given drug concentration may vary with the number of organisms at the site of infection. Accordingly, the size of the inoculum can be a primary determinant of drug efficacy. Early investigations clearly demonstrate that the duration of the infection before treatment is a significant predictor of clinical response.[96] When therapy is delayed, presumably leading to a larger inoculum, the efficacy of that therapy often is affected adversely. In non-neutropenic rats, larger doses of antibiotic were needed to treat *K. pneumoniae* pneumonia, whether administered by continuous or intermittent infusion, when the infection was allowed to progress 34 hours before therapy was initiated versus 5 hours.[164] Many potential mechanisms have been proposed to account for this event. Large inocula perhaps generate a higher local density of enzymes that effectively reduce active (i.e., functional) antibiotic concentrations at the site of infection. Large bacterial populations also are statistically more likely to contain resistant organisms that arise by spontaneous mutation and predominate within the population as a result of the selective pressure posed by the antibiotic. One such example has been observed in a murine model of group A streptococcal myositis, in which the activity of penicillin is most severely compromised in the presence of a large inoculum (10^8 to 10^9 CFU/mL), with relatively little impact on the activity of clindamycin. Given that the isolate did not produce β-lactamase and any residual PAE was irrelevant because both regimens maintained drug concentrations above the MIC for the duration of the dosing interval, this effect of the inoculum was attributed in part to the selection of a cell wall–deficient mutant.[183] Clindamycin, however, is not devoid of susceptibility to the inoculum effect for all organisms; an increase in the size of the inoculum or an increase in the time until therapy resulted in a lower reduction in $\log_{10}$CFU in a murine *Bacillus fragilis* abscess model.[98] Another proposed mechanism for the effect of the inoculum lies in the fact that dense populations of organisms may grow at a slower rate or be metabolically inactive when compared with their less dense counterparts. An effect arising by this mechanism probably will not affect antimicrobial agents that are bactericidal against both rapidly growing and stationary-phase organisms (e.g., fluoroquinolones). However, for agents that exert their bactericidal effects primarily on rapidly dividing organisms (e.g., β-lactams), activity may be compromised in the presence of an established infection in which the bacterial population is large and as many as 90 percent of the organisms may be slowly dividing and, thus, metabolically inactive. For clinical isolates of group G streptococci, time-kill studies demonstrated rapid complete bacterial killing when the organism was primarily in log-phase growth, regardless of whether 10^4 or 10^7 organisms were involved. In contrast, when the organism was principally in the stationary phase, rapid and complete killing was observed only for the smaller inoculum (10^4 organisms), with no appreciable killing at 10^8 organisms. Furthermore, patients with a protracted clinical course of infection or recalcitrant infection failed therapy despite receiving high doses and having a susceptible isolate.[114]

Attempting to link multiple pharmacodynamic effects in evaluating the outcome of anti-infective therapy poses an arduous task from both a theoretic and practical perspective, and hence, a complete discussion will not be undertaken in this chapter. Nonetheless, the combination of such effects has received some attention in the literature and thus merits mention. Specifically, large inocula appear to be capable of modulating the PAE and subinhibitory effects observed with numerous agents. Exposure of *E. coli* to subinhibitory sparfloxacin concentrations produces a pronounced inoculum-dependent subinhibitory effect. At a dose that was 0.3 times the MIC, growth of the organism was delayed by 0.3, 0.9, and 3.3 hours with inocula of 10^8, 10^6, and 10^4 CFU, respectively, with similar observations noted for other drug-microbe combinations.[29, 142]

CONCENTRATION-DEPENDENT COMBINATION EFFECTS (SYNERGY/ANTAGONISM)

As discussed earlier and elsewhere in this text, antimicrobial combinations are used for many purposes: to prevent or delay the emergence of resistance, to enable dosage reduction and thereby minimize dose-related toxicities, and to treat polymicrobial infections. Combination therapy can be designed with the goal of synergistic/additive activity in mind, or alternatively, these effects can occur without conscious consideration or forethought. Moreover, the undesirable outcomes of indifference or antagonism similarly can result through the combination of agents. Although a complete review of antagonism and synergy is beyond the scope of this section, we would be remiss to not mention concentration-dependent combination effects. We provide this brief discussion specifically to point out that a simple classification of drug combinations as synergistic, antagonist, and so forth is not always feasible. As discussed elsewhere, disagreement in the classification certainly can arise when different methods are used for evaluation.[16, 140]

However, even when restricted to evaluations using the same experimental methods, certain combinations can be classified differently, depending on antibiotic concentration. Synergy is observed with cefoperazone and low imipenem concentrations against MRSA; however, higher concentrations of imipenem antagonize the activity of cefoperazone. Although antagonism with imipenem often is explained away as being β-lactamase mediated, the concentration-dependent antagonism observed remains unexplained via this mechanism because antagonism was shown for strains that lacked β-lactamase production.[155] The combination of penicillin and clindamycin at subinhibitory concentrations demonstrates synergy against group A beta-hemolytic streptococci. At concentrations ranging from two to four times the MIC, the combination demonstrates antagonism, and at clinically relevant concentrations (approximately 100 times the MIC), indifference is observed, with the combination exhibiting no advantage over either agent alone.[184] Against isolates of vancomycin-intermediate *S. aureus,* antagonism is observed when methicillin and vancomycin are combined at subinhibitory concentrations. However, when the methicillin concentration exceeds the MIC, synergy is observed with the same combination. Although the mechanism behind this differential activity remains unclear, researchers have proposed that the antagonism observed at lower methicillin concentrations results from an increase in the density of non–cross-linked D-alanyl-D-alanine side chains, the target site for vancomycin and a substrate for the PBPs. This increase would decrease the efficacy of methicillin as a PBP inhibitor by substrate competition.[87] For certain strains of methicillin-sensitive *S. aureus,* a combination of rifampin and methicillin below the MIC is synergistic, but above the MBC it is antagonistic. Similarly, a rifampin-vancomycin combination is synergistic at concentrations close to the MBC but indifferent as concentrations rise.[213] Furthermore, for some drug-microbe combinations, it is not the classification per se that is affected by the concentration, but rather the magnitude of the effect observed. Against *E. faecium,* fixed piperacillin and variable teicoplanin concentrations are synergistic. However, the degree of synergy is dependent on the teicoplanin concentration, with comparable synergistic activity occurring at teicoplanin concentrations of 2, 4, or 8 mg/L; reduced synergistic activity at teicoplanin concentrations of 16 and 32 mg/L; and the greatest degree of synergy observed at a concentration of 64 mg/L.[157]

Thus, the available data support the fact that in many cases, the clinical assignment or "expectation" of synergy, additivity, or antagonism by specific combinations of anti-infective agents cannot be assumed simply by virtue of the drug class or drug-specific mechanisms of action (or both). With drug combinations for which the activity against an infecting pathogen is potentially concentration-dependent, prediction of therapeutic outcome must entail some assessment, be it actual or theoretic (e.g., the use of pharmacokinetic modeling), of the time-dependent drug concentration profile at the site or sites of infection.

Conclusions

Since the mid-1950s, the development of pharmacokinetics has produced a powerful and valuable tool, with applications for both science and clinical medicine. For the clinical scientist, pharmacokinetics can be used to characterize a given drug by providing a "profile" of its absorption, distribution, metabolism, and excretion in individuals with and without disease, during "normal" alterations of human physiology (e.g., pregnancy), and under conditions of normal altered organ function or body composition (e.g., growth and development, senescence). For the clinical practitioner, the tool of pharmacokinetics can provide a means to individualize drug therapy by characterizing the relationship between drug dose and resultant drug concentrations in plasma or other relevant biologic fluids (e.g., urine, CSF, synovial fluid, pleural fluid, peritoneal fluid). When linked with information regarding the pharmacodynamic behavior of the antibiotic, the susceptibility of the organism, and the status of the host, the application of pharmacokinetics affords the practitioner the ability to exercise some degree of adaptive control over drug therapy by selecting a drug and dosing regimen that have the greatest likelihood of producing both efficacy and safety.

REFERENCES

1. Anderson, E. T., Young, L. S., and Hewitt, W. L.: Simultaneous antibiotic levels in "breakthrough" gram-negative rod bacteremia. Am J Med *61*:493–497, 1976.
2. Andes, D. R., and Craig, W. A.: Pharmacodynamics of fluoroquinolones in experimental models of endocarditis. Clin. Infect. Dis. *27*:47–50, 1998.
3. Andes, D., and Craig, W. A.: In vivo activities of amoxicillin and amoxicillin-clavulanate against *Streptococcus pneumoniae:* Application to breakpoint determinations. Antimicrob. Agents Chemother. *42*:2375–2379, 1998.
4. Arbo, A., Mancilla, J., Alpuche, C., and Santos, J. I.: In vitro and in vivo effects of subinhibitory concentrations of clindamycin on experimental *Klebsiella pneumoniae* sepsis. Chemotherapy *36*:337–344, 1990.
5. Azoulay-Dupuis, E., Vallee, E., Bedos, J. P., et al.: Prophylactic and therapeutic activities of azithromycin in a mouse model of pneumococcal pneumonia. Antimicrob. Agents Chemother. *35*:1024–1028, 1991.
6. Baker, P. J., Busby, W. F., and Wilson, M. E.: Subinhibitory concentrations of cefpodoxime alter membrane protein expression of *Actinobacillus actinomycetemcomitans* and enhance its susceptibility to killing by neutrophils. Antimicrob. Agents Chemother. *39*:406–412, 1995.
7. Bakker-Woudenberg, I. A. J. M., van Gerwen, A. L. E. M., and Michel, M. F.: Efficacy of antimicrobial therapy in experimental rat pneumonia: Antibiotic treatment schedules in rats with impaired phagocytosis. Infect. Immun. *25*:376–387, 1979.
8. Barmada, S., Kohlhepp, S., Leggett, J., et al.: Correlation of tobramycin-induced inhibition of protein synthesis with postantibiotic effect in *Escherichia coli.* Antimicrob. Agents Chemother. *37*:2678–2683, 1993.
9. Barza, M.: Challenges to antibiotic activity in tissue. Clin. Infect. Dis. *19*:910–915, 1994.
10. Baurenfiend, A.: Questioning dosing regimens of ciprofloxacin. J. Antimicrob. Chemother. *31*:789–798, 1993.
11. Begg, E. J., Peddie, B. A., Chambers, S. T., and Boswell, D. R.: Comparison of gentamicin dosing regimens using an in vitro model. J. Antimicrob. Chemother. *29*:427–433, 1992.
12. Beyer, K. H., Woodward, R., Peters, L., et al.: The prolongation of penicillin retention in the body by means of para-aminohippuric acid. Science *100*:107–108, 1944.
13. Bigger, J. W.: The bactericidal action of penicillin on *Staphylococcus pyogenes.* Ir. J. Med. Sci. *227*:533–568, 1944.
14. Bisognano, C., Vaudaux, P. E., Lew, D. P., et al.: Increased expression of fibronectin-binding proteins by fluoroquinolone-resistant *Staphylococcus aureus* exposed to subinhibitory levels of ciprofloxacin. Antimicrob. Agents Chemother. *41*:906–913, 1997.
15. Bisognano, C., Vaudaux, P., Rohner, P., et al.: Induction of fibronectin-binding proteins and increased adhesion of quinolone-resistant *Staphylococcus aureus* by subinhibitory levels of ciprofloxacin. Antimicrob. Agents Chemother. *44*:1428–1437, 2000.
16. Blaser, J.: Interactions of antimicrobial combinations in vitro: The relativity of synergism. Scand. J. Infect. Dis. Suppl. *74*:71–79, 1991.
17. Blaser, J., Stone, B. B., Groner, M. C., and Zinner, S. H.: Comparative study with enoxacin and netilmicin in a pharmacodynamic model to determine importance of ratio of antibiotic peak concentration to MIC for bactericidal activity and emergence of resistance. Antimicrob. Agents Chemother. *31*:1054–1060, 1987.
18. Blaser, J., Stone, B. B., and Zinner, S. H.: Efficacy of intermittent versus continuous administration of netilmicin in a two-compartment in vitro model. Antimicrob. Agents Chemother. *27*:343–349, 1985.
19. Bodey, G. P., Ketchel, S. J., and Rodriguez, V.: A randomized trial of carbenicillin plus cefamandole or tobramycin in the treatment of febrile episodes in cancer patients. Am. J. Med. *67*:608–616, 1979.
20. Bourne, D. (ed.): A First Course in Pharmacokinetics and Biopharmaceutics. *http://gaps.cpb.ouhsc.edu*, 2001.
21. Braga, P. C., and Piatti, G.: Kinetics of filamentation of *Escherichia coli* induced by different sub-MICs of ceftibuten at different times. Chemotherapy *39*:272–277, 1993.
22. Breines, D. M., and Burnham, J. C.: Modulation of *Escherichia coli* type 1 fimbrial expression and adherence to uroepithelial cells following exposure of logarithmic phase cells to quinolones at subinhibitory concentrations. J. Antimicrob. Chemother. *34*:205–221, 1994.
23. Brewin, A., Arango, L., Hadley, W. K., and Murray, J. F.: High-dose penicillin therapy and pneumococcal pneumonia. J. A. M. A. *230*:409–413, 1974.
24. Bryan, C. S., Reynolds, K. L., and Brenner, E. R.: Analysis of 1,186 episodes of gram-negative bacteremia in non-university hospitals: The effects of antimicrobial therapy. Rev. Infect. Dis. *5*:629–638, 1983.
25. Chalmers, J. P., and Tiller, D. J.: Effects of treatment on the mortality rate in septicemia. B. M. J. *2*:338–341, 1969.
26. Chaudhry, A. Z., Knapp, C. C., Sierra-Madero, J., and Washington, J. A.: Antistaphylococcal activities of sparfloxacin (CI-978 AT-4140), ofloxacin, and ciprofloxacin. Antimicrob. Agents Chemother. *34*:1843–1845, 1990.
27. Cipriani, P., Giordano, A., Magni, A., et al.: Outer membrane alterations in *Pseudomonas aeruginosa* after five-day exposure to quinolones and carbapenems. Drugs Exp. Clin. Res. *2*:139–144, 1995.
28. Craig, W. A.: Choosing an antibiotic on the basis of pharmacodynamics. Ear Nose Throat J. *77*(Suppl.):7–11, 1998.
29. Craig, W. A., and Ebert, S. C.: Killing and regrowth of bacteria in vitro: A review. Scand. J. Infect. Dis. *74*(Suppl.):63–70, 1991.
30. Craig, W. A., and Gudmundsson, S.: Postantibiotic effect. *In* Lorian, V. (ed.): Antibiotics in Laboratory Medicine. 4th ed. Baltimore, Williams & Wilkins, 1996, pp. 296–329.
31. Craven, D. E., Kollisch, N. R., Hsieh, C. R., et al.: Vancomycin treatment of bacteremia caused by oxacillin-resistant *Staphylococcus aureus:* Comparison with beta-lactam antibiotic treatment of bacteremia caused by oxacillin-sensitive *Staphylococcus aureus.* J. Infect. Dis. *147*:137–143, 1983.
32. Dagan, R., Klugman, K. P., Craig, W. A., and Baquero, F.: Evidence to support the rationale that bacterial eradication in respiratory tract infection is an important aim of antimicrobial therapy. J. Antimicrob. Chemother. *47*:129–140, 2001.
33. Daikos, G. L., Jackson, G. G., Lolans, V. T., and Livermore, D. M.: Adaptive resistance to aminoglycoside antibiotics from first-exposure down-regulation. J. Infect. Dis. *162*:414–420, 1990.
34. Daikos, G. L., Lolans, V. T., and Jackson, G. G.: First-exposure adaptive resistance to aminoglycoside antibiotics in vivo with meaning for optimal clinical use. Antimicrob. Agents Chemother. *35*:117–123, 1991.
35. de Wildt, S. N., Kearns, G. L., Leeder, J. S., and van den Anker, J. N.: Glucuronidation in humans: Pharmacogenetic and developmental aspects. Clin. Pharmacokinet. *36*:439–452, 1999.
36. deWildt, S. N., Kearns, G. L., Hop, W. C., et al.: Pharmacokinetics and metabolism of oral midazolam in preterm infants. Br. J. Clin. Pharmacol. *53*:390–392, 2002.
37. Drusano, G. L., Johnson, D., Rosen, M., and Standiford, M. C.: Pharmacodynamics of a fluoroquinolone antimicrobial agent in a neutropenic rat model of *Pseudomonas* sepsis. Antimicrob. Agents Chemother. *37*:483–490, 1993.
38. Drusano, G. L., Preston, S. L., Hardalo, C., et al.: Use of preclinical data for selection of a phase II/III dose for evernimicin and identification of a preclinical MIC breakpoint. Antimicrob. Agents Chemother. *45*:13–22, 2001.
39. Dudley, M. N., Blaser, J., Gilbert, D., et al.: Combination therapy with ciprofloxacin plus azlocillin against *Pseudomonas aeruginosa:* Effect of simultaneous versus staggered administration in an in vitro model. J. Infect. Dis. *164*:499–506, 1991.
40. Dudley, M. N., Mandler, H. D., Gilbert, D., et al.: Pharmacokinetics and pharmacodynamics of intravenous ciprofloxacin. Studies in vivo and in an in vitro dynamic model. Am. J. Med. *82*(4A):363–368, 1987.
41. Eagle, H.: The recovery of bacteria from the toxic effects of penicillin. J. Clin. Invest. *28*:832–836, 1949.
42. Eagle, H., Fleishman, R., and Levy, M.: On the duration of penicillin action in relation to its concentration in the serum. J. Lab. Clin. Med. *41*:122–132, 1953.
43. Eagle, H., Fleishman, R., and Levy, M.: "Continuous" vs. "discontinuous" therapy with penicillin: The effect of the interval between injections on therapeutic efficacy. N. Engl. J. Med. *248*:481–488, 1953.
44. Eagle, H., Fleischman, R., and Musselman, A. D.: The bactericidal action of penicillin in vivo: The participation of the host, and slow recovery of the surviving organisms. Ann. Intern. Med. *33*:544–571, 1950.
45. Eagle, H., and Musselman, A. D.: The rate of bactericidal action of penicillin in vitro as a function of its concentration, and its paradoxically reduced activity at high concentration against certain organisms. J. Exp. Med. *88*:99–131, 1948.
46. Euler, A., Byrne, W., and Campbell, M.: Basal and pentagastrin-stimulated gastric acid secretory rates in normal children and those with peptic ulcer disease. J. Pediatr. *103*:766–768, 1983.
47. Euler, A., Byrne, W., Meis, P., et al.: Basal and pentagastrin stimulated acid secretion in newborn human infants. Pediatr. Res. *13*:36–37, 1979.
48. Fantin, B., Leclercq, R., Merle, Y., et al.: Critical influence of resistance to streptogramin B–type antibiotics on activity of RP 59500 (quinupristin-dalfopristin) in experimental endocarditis due to *Staphylococcus aureus.* Antimicrob. Agents Chemother. *39*:400–405, 1995.

49. Fernandes, A. C., Anderson, R., Theron, A. J., et al.: Enhancement of human polymorphonuclear leucocyte motility by erythromycin in vitro and in vivo. S. Afr. Med. J. *66*:173–177, 1984.
50. Flick, M. R., and Cluff, L. E.: *Pseudomonas* bacteremia. Review of 108 cases. Am. J. Med. *60*:501–508, 1976.
51. Flockhart, D. A.: Clinically used drugs metabolized by cytochrome P450. *http://medicine.iupui.edu/flockhart/clinlist.html.*
52. Fluckiger, U., Segessenmann, C., and Gerber, A. U.: Integration of pharmacokinetics and pharmacodynamics of imipenem in a human-adapted mouse. Antimicrob. Agents Chemother. *35*:1905–1910, 1991.
53. Fontana, R., Amalfitano, G., Rossi, L., and Staat, G.: Mechanisms of resistance to growth inhibition and killing by beta-lactam antibiotics in enterococci. Clin. Infect. Dis. *15*:486–489, 1992.
54. Fontana, R., Boaretti, M., Grossato, A., et al.: Paradoxical response of *Enterococcus faecalis* to the bactericidal activity of penicillin is associated with reduced activity of one autolysin. Antimicrob. Agents Chemother. *34*:314–320, 1990.
55. Forrest, A., Ballow, C. H., Nix, D. E., et al.: Development of a population pharmacokinetic model and optimal sampling strategy for intravenous ciprofloxacin. Antimicrob. Agents Chemother. *37*:1065–1072, 1993.
56. Forrest, A., Nix, D. E., Ballow, C. H., et al.: Pharmacodynamics of intravenous ciprofloxacin in seriously ill patients. Antimicrob. Agents Chemother. *37*:1073–1081, 1993.
57. Freid, M. A., and Vosti, K. L.: The importance of underlying disease in patients with gram-negative bacteremia. Arch. Intern. Med. *121*:418–423, 1968.
58. Frimodt-Moller, N., Bentzon, M. W., and Thomsen, V. F.: Experimental infection with *Streptococcus pneumoniae* in mice: Correlation of in vitro activity and pharmacokinetic parameters with in vivo effect for 14 cephalosporins. J. Infect. Dis. *154*:511–517, 1986.
59. Fuursted, K.: Comparative killing activity and postantibiotic effect of streptomycin combined with ampicillin, ciprofloxacin, imipenem, piperacillin or vancomycin against strains of *Streptococcus faecalis* and *Streptococcus faecium.* Chemotherapy *34*:229–234, 1988.
60. Fuursted, K.: Postexposure factors influencing the duration of postantibiotic effect: Significance of temperature, pH, cations, and oxygen tension. Antimicrob. Agents Chemother. *41*:1693–1696, 1997.
61. Gehanno, P., Lenoir, G., and Berche, P.: In vivo correlates for *Streptococcus pneumoniae* penicillin resistance in acute otitis media. Antimicrob. Agents Chemother. *39*:271–272, 1995.
62. Gemmell, C. G., and Lorian, V.: Effects of low concentrations of antibiotics on bacterial ultrastructure, virulence and susceptibility to immunodefenses: Clinical significance. *In* Lorian, V. (ed.): Antibiotics in Laboratory Medicine. Baltimore, Williams & Wilkins, 1996, pp. 397–452.
63. Gengo, F. M., Mannion, T. W., Nightingale, C. H., and Schentag, J. J.: Integration of pharmacokinetics and pharmacodynamics of methicillin in curative treatment of experimental endocarditis. J. Antimicrob. Chemother. *14*:619–631, 1984.
63a. George, R. H., and Dyas, A.: Paradoxical effect of penicillin in vivo. J Antimicrob. Chemother. *17*:684–685, 1986.
64. Gerber, A. U., and Craig, W. A.: Aminoglycoside-selected subpopulations of *Pseudomonas aeruginosa.* J. Lab. Clin. Med. *100*:671–681, 1982.
65. Gerber, A. U., Craig, W. A., Brugger, H. P., et al.: Impact of dosing intervals on activity of gentamicin and ticarcillin against *Pseudomonas aeruginosa* in granulocytopenic mice. J. Infect. Dis. *147*:910–917, 1983.
66. Gerber, A. U., Kozac, S., Segessenmann, C., et al.: Once daily versus thrice-daily administration of netilmicin in combination therapy of *Pseudomonas aeruginosa* infection in a man-adapted neutropenic animal model. Eur. J. Clin. Microbiol. Infect. Dis. *8*:233–237, 1989.
67. Gibaldi, M., and Perrier, D. (eds.): Pharmacokinetics. 2nd ed., revised and expanded. New York, Marcel Dekker, 1982.
68. Gilman, J. T., and Gal, P.: Pharmacokinetic and pharmacodynamic data collection in children and neonates. A quiet frontier. Clin. Pharmacokinet. *23*:1–9, 1992.
69. Ginsburg, C. M., McCraken, G. H., Jr., Petruska, M., and Olson, K.: Pharmacokinetics and bactericidal activity of cefuroxime axetil. Antimicrob. Agents Chemother. *28*:504–507, 1985.
70. Gottfredsson, M., Erlendsdottir, H., Kolka, R., and Gudmundsson, S.: Metabolic and ultrastructural effects induced by ciprofloxacin in *Staphylococcus aureus* during the postantibiotic effect (PAE) phase. Scand. J. Infect. Dis. Suppl. *74*:124–128, 1991.
71. Grand, R. J., Watkins, J. G., and Torti, F. M.: Development of the human gastrointestinal tract. Gastroenterology *70*:790–810, 1976.
72. Grasso, S., Meinardi, G., de Carneri, I., and Taassia, V.: New in vitro models to study the effect of antibiotic concentration and rate of elimination on antibacterial activity. Antimicrob. Agents Chemother. *13*:570–576, 1978.
73. Griffiths, L. R., and Green, H. T.: Paradoxical effect of penicillin in-vivo. J. Antimicrob. Chemother. *15*:507–508, 1985.
74. Grimwood, K., To, M., Rabin, H. R., and Woods, D. E.: Inhibition of *Pseudomonas aeruginosa* exoenzyme expression by subinhibitory antibiotic concentrations. Antimicrob. Agents Chemother. *33*:41–47, 1989.
75. Gudmundsson, A., Erlendsdottir, H., Gottfredsson, M., and Gudmundsson, S.: Impact of pH and cationic supplementation on in vitro postantibiotic effect. Antimicrob. Agents Chemother. *35*:2617–2624, 1991.
76. Gudmundsson, S., Erlensdottir, H., Gottfredsson, M., and Gudmundsson, A.: The postantibiotic effect induced by antimicrobial combinations. Scand. J. Infect. Dis. Suppl. *74*:80–93, 1991.
77. Gustafsson, I., Hjelm, E., and Cars, O.: In vitro pharmacodynamics of the new ketolides HMR 3004 and HMR 3647 (telithromycin) against *Chlamydia pneumoniae.* Antimicrob. Agents Chemother. *44*:1846–1849, 2000.
78. Hanberger, H., Nilsson, L. E., Maller, R., and Nilsson, M.: Pharmacodynamics of beta-lactam antibiotics on gram-negative bacteria: Initial killing, morphology and post-antibiotic effect. Scand. J. Infect. Dis. Suppl. *74*:118–123, 1991.
79. Handwerger, S., and Tomasz, A.: Antibiotic tolerance among clinical isolates of bacteria. Rev. Infect. Dis. *7*:368–386, 1985.
80. Hayton, W. L., and Stoeckel, K.: Age-associated changes in ceftriaxone pharmacokinetics. Clin. Pharmacokinet. *11*:76–86, 1986.
81. Herrera-Insua, I., Perez, P., Ramos, C., et al.: Synergistic effect of azithromycin on the phagocytic killing of *Staphylococcus aureus* by human polymorphonuclear leukocytes. Eur. J. Clin. Microbiol. Infect. Dis. *16*:13–16, 1997.
82. Hessen, M. T., Pitsakis, P. G., and Levison, M. E.: Absence of a postantibiotic effect in experimental *Pseudomonas* endocarditis treated with imipenem with or without gentamicin. J. Infect. Dis. *158*:542–548, 1988.
83. Hessen, M. T., Pitsakis, P. G., and Levison, M. E.: Postantibiotic effect of penicillin plus gentamicin versus *Enterococcus faecalis* in vitro and in vivo. Antimicrob. Agents Chemother. *33*:608–611, 1989.
84. Holm, S. E., Odenholdt-Tornqvist, I., and Cars, O.: Paradoxical effects of antibiotics. Scand. J. Infect. Dis. Suppl. *74*:113–117, 1991.
85. Horne, D., and Tomasz, A.: Hypersusceptibility of penicillin treated group B streptococci to bactericidal activity of human polymorphonuclear leukocytes. Antimicrob. Agents Chemother. *19*:745–753, 1981.
86. Hostacka, A.: Changes in serum sensitivity and hydrophobicity in a clinical isolate of *Klebsiella pneumoniae* treated with subinhibitory concentrations of aminoglycosides. Zentralbl. Bakteriol. *288*:519–526, 1998.
87. Howe, R. A., Wootton, M., Bennett, P. M., et al.: Interactions between methicillin and vancomycin in methicillin-resistant *Staphylococcus aureus* strains displaying different phenotypes of vancomycin susceptibility. J. Clin. Microbiol. *37*:3068–3071, 1999.
88. Hyatt, J. M., Nix, D. E., and Schentag, J. J.: Pharmacokinetic and pharmacodynamic activities of ciprofloxacin against strains of *Streptococcus pneumoniae, Staphylococcus aureus* and *Pseudomonas aeruginosa* for which MIC's are similar. Antimicrob. Agents Chemother. *38*:2730–2737, 1994.
89. Igarashi, K., and Matsuyama, T.: Alternative activity of beta-lactam antibiotics against methicillin- and cephem-resistant *Staphylococcus aureus* in the presence of respiratory tract mucus. J. Infect. Dis. *161*:250–254, 1990.
90. Ikeda, N., Hanaki, H., Hiramatsu, K., and Kuwabara, Y.: In vitro susceptibility of *Streptococcus agalactiae* clinical isolates to beta-lactam antibiotics. Kansenshogaku Zasshi *73*:163–171, 1999.
91. Ikeda, Y., Fukuoka, Y., Motomura, K., et al.: Paradoxical activity of beta-lactam antibiotics against *Proteus vulgaris* in experimental infection in mice. Antimicrob. Agents Chemother. *34*:94–97, 1990.
92. Ikeda, Y., and Nishino, T.: Paradoxical antibacterial activities of beta-lactams against *Proteus vulgaris:* Mechanism of the paradoxical effect. Antimicrob. Agents Chemother. *32*:1073–1077, 1988.
93. Ingerman, M. J., Pitsakis, P. G., Rosenberg, A. F., and Levison, M. E.: The importance of pharmacodynamics in determining the dosing interval in therapy for experimental *Pseudomonas* endocarditis in the rat. J. Infect. Dis. *153*:707–714, 1986.
94. Isaksson, B., Hanberger, H., Maller, R., et al.: The postantibiotic effect of amikacin alone and in combination with piperacillin on gram-negative bacteria. Scand. J. Infect. Dis. Suppl. *74*:129–132, 1991.
95. Isenberg, H. D.: Clinical evaluation of laboratory guidance to antibiotic therapy. Health Lab. Sci. *4*:164–180, 1967.
96. Eagle, H: The effect of the size of inoculum and the age of the infection and the curative dose of penicillin in experimental infections with streptococci, pneumococci and *Treponema pallidum.* J. Exp. Med. *90*:595–607, 1949.
97. Jawetz, E.: Dynamics of the action of penicillin in experimental animals. Arch. Intern. Med. *77*:1–15, 1946.
98. Joiner, K., Lowe, B., Dzink, J., and Bartlett, J. G.: Comparative efficacy of 10 antimicrobial agents in experimental infection with *Bacteroides fragilis.* J. Infect. Dis. *145*:561–568, 1982.
99. Kearns, G. L.: Desacetylcefotaxime: Clinical implications of an active metabolite in infants and children. Drug Invest. *4*(Suppl. 2):9–17, 1992.
100. Kearns, G. L.: Impact of developmental pharmacology on pediatric study design: Overcoming the challenges. J. Allergy Clin. Immunol. *106*(Suppl.):128–138, 2000.
101. Kearns, G. L., Abdel-Rahman, S. M., Blumer, J. L., et al.: Single dose pharmacokinetics of linezolid in infants and children. Pediatr. Infect. Dis. J. *19*:1178–1184, 2000.
102. Kearns, G. L., Bradley, J. S., Jacobs, R. F., et al.: Single dose pharmacokinetics of pleconaril in neonates. Pediatric Pharmacology Research Unit Network. Pediatr. Infect. Dis. J. *19*:833–839, 2002.
103. Kearns, G. L., and Young, R. A.: Pharmacokinetics of cefotaxime and desacetylcefotaxime in the young. Diagn. Microbiol. Infect. Dis. *22*:97–104, 1995.

104. Kearns, G. L., Young, R. A., and Jacobs, R. F.: Cefotaxime dosing in infants and children: Pharmacokinetic and clinical rationale for an extended dosing interval. Clin. Pharmacokinet. *4*:284–297, 1992.

105. Kennedy, M. J., Abdel-Rahman, S. M., and Kearns, G. L.: Oxazolidinones: Clinical pharmacology and use in the treatment of infections caused by resistant gram-positive pathogens. Semin. Pediatr. Infect. Dis. *12*:186–199, 2001.

106. Kernodle, D. S., McGraw, P. A., Barg, N. L., et al.: Growth of *Staphylococcus aureus* with nafcillin in vitro induces alpha-toxin production and increases the lethal activity of sterile broth filtrates in a murine model. J. Infect. Dis. *172*:410–419, 1995.

107. Kirby, W. M. M.: Bacteriostatic and lytic actions of penicillin on sensitive and resistant staphylococci. J. Clin. Invest. *24*:165–169, 1945.

108. Kondo, N., Kuwahara-Arai, K., Kuroda-Murakami, H., et al.: Eagle-type methicillin resistance: New phenotype of high methicillin resistance under mec regulator gene control. Antimicrob. Agents Chemother. *45*:815–824, 2001.

109. Kreger, B. E., Craven, D. E., and McCabe, W. R.: Gram-negative bacteremia. IV. Re-evaluation of clinical features and treatment in 612 patients. Am. J. Med. *68*:344–355, 1980.

110. Kuenzi, B., Segessenmann, C., and Gerber, A. U.: Postantibiotic effect of roxithromycin, erythromycin, and clindamycin against selected gram-positive bacteria and *Haemophilus influenzae*. J. Antimicrob. Chemother. *20*(Suppl. B):39–46, 1987.

111. Lacy, M. K., Lu, W., Xu, X., et al.: Pharmacodynamic comparisons of levofloxacin, ciprofloxacin and ampicillin against *Streptococcus pneumoniae* in an in vitro model of infection. Antimicrob. Agents Chemother. *43*:672–677, 1999.

112. Lagast, H., Meunier-Carpienter, F., and Klastersky, J.: Treatment of gram-negative bacillary septicaemia with cefoperazine. Eur. J. Clin. Microbiol. *2*:554–558, 1983.

113. Lam, C., Georgopoulos, A., Laber, G., and Schultze, E.: Therapeutic relevance of penicillin-induced hypersensitivity of *Staphylococcus aureus* to killing by polymorphonuclear leukocytes. Antimicrob. Agents Chemother. *26*:149–154, 1984.

114. Lam, K., and Bayer, A. S.: Serious infections due to group G streptococci: Report of 15 cases with in vitro–in vivo correlations. Am. J. Med. *75*:561–570, 1983.

115. Leeder, J. S., Kearns, G. L.: Pharmacogenetics in pediatrics: Implications for practice. Pediatr. Clin. North Am. *44*:55–57, 1997.

116. Leggett, J. E., Ebert, S., Fantin, B., and Craig, W. A.: Comparative dose-effect relations at several dosing intervals for beta-lactam, aminoglycoside and quinolone antibiotics against gram-negative bacilli in murine thigh-infection and pneumonitis models. Scand. J. Infect. Dis. Suppl. *74*:179–184, 1991.

117. Leggett, J. E., Fantin, B., Ebert, S., et al.: Comparative antibiotic dose-effect relations at several dosing intervals in murine pneumonitis and thigh infection models. J. Infect. Dis. *159*:281–292, 1989.

118. Levner, M., Weiner, F. P., and Rubin, B. A.: Induction of *Escherichia coli* and *Vibrio cholerae* enterotoxins by an inhibitor of protein synthesis. Infect. Immun. *15*:132–137, 1977.

119. Lister, P. D., and Sanders, C. C.: Pharmacodynamics of levofloxacin and ciprofloxacin against *Streptococcus pneumoniae*. J. Antimicrob. Chemother. *43*:79–86, 1999.

120. Lo Bue, A. M., Rossetti, B., Cali, G., et al.: Antimicrobial interference of a subinhibitory concentration of azithromycin on fimbrial production of *Porphyromonas gingivalis*. J. Antimicrob. Chemother. *40*:653–657, 1997.

121. Lorian, V.: Some effects of subinhibitory concentrations of antibiotics on bacteria. Bull. N. Y. Acad. Med. *51*:1046–1055, 1975.

122. Lorian, V., and Atkinson, B.: Abnormal forms of bacteria produced by antibiotics. Am. J. Clin. Pathol. *64*:678–688, 1975.

123. Lorian, V., and Burns, L.: Predictive value of susceptibility tests for the outcome of antibacterial therapy. J. Antimicrob. Chemother. *25*:175–181, 1990.

124. Lorian, V., and Sabath, L. D.: Penicillin and cephalosporin: Differences in morphologic effects on *Proteus mirabilis*. J. Infect. Dis. *125*:560–564, 1972.

125. Lorian, V., Silletti, R. P., Biondo, F. X., and De Freitas, C. C.: Paradoxical effect of aminoglycoside antibiotics on the growth of gram-negative bacilli. J. Antimicrob. Chemother. *5*:613–616, 1979.

126. Lowdin, E., Odenholt, I., and Cars, O.: In vitro studies of pharmacodynamic properties of vancomycin against *Staphylococcus aureus* and *Staphylococcus epidermidis*. Antimicrob. Agents Chemother. *42*:2739–2744, 1998.

127. Lutsar, I., Friedland, I. R., Wubbel, L., et al.: Pharmacodynamics of gatifloxacin in cerebrospinal fluid in experimental cephalosporin-resistant pneumococcal meningitis. Antimicrob. Agents Chemother. *42*:2650–2655, 1998.

128. MacArthur, R. D., Lolans, V., Zar, F., and Jackson, G. G.: Biphasic, concentration-dependent and rate-limited, concentration independent bacterial killing by an aminoglycoside antibiotic. J. Infect. Dis. *150*:778–779, 1984.

129. Martin, E., Fanconi, S., Kalin, P., et al.: Ceftriaxone-bilirubin-albumin interactions in the neonate, an in vivo study. Eur. J. Pediatr. *152*:530–540, 1993.

130. Mascellino, M. T., De Vito, M. L., Maclean Feeney, E., et al.: Phagocytosis and killing of A-protein positive *Staphylococcus aureus* in the presence of low doses of antibiotics. Drugs Exp. Clin. Res. *15*:63–69, 1989.

131. McCabe, W. R., and Jackson, G. G.: Gram-negative bacteremia. II. Clinical and therapeutic observations. Arch. Intern. Med. *110*:856–864, 1962.

132. Meinl, B., Hyatt, J. M., Forrest, A., et al.: Pharmacokinetic/pharmacodynamic predictors of time to clinical resolution in patients with acute bacterial exacerbations of chronic bronchitis treated with a fluoroquinolone. Int. J. Antimicrob. Agents *16*:273–280, 2000.

133. Moise, P. A., Forrest, A., Bhavnani, S. M., et al.: Area under the inhibitory curve and a pneumonia scoring system for predicting outcomes of vancomycin therapy for respiratory infections by *Staphylococcus aureus*. Am. J. Health Syst. Pharm. *57*(Suppl. 2):4–9, 2000.

134. Moore, R. D., Lietman, P. S., and Smith, C. R.: Clinical response to aminoglycoside therapy: Importance of the ratio of peak concentration to minimum inhibitory concentration. J. Infect. Dis. *155*:93–99, 1987.

135. Moore, R. D., Smith, C. R., and Lietman, P. S.: The association of aminoglycoside plasma levels with mortality in patients with gram negative bacteremia. J. Infect. Dis. *149*:443–448, 1984.

136. Moore, R. D., Smith, C. R., and Lietman, P. S.: Association of aminoglycoside plasma levels with therapeutic outcome in gram-negative pneumonia. Am. J. Med. *77*:657–662, 1984.

137. Mouton, J. W., van Ogtrop, M. L., Andes, D., and Craig, W. A.: Use of pharmacodynamic indices to predict efficacy of combination therapy in vivo. Antimicrob. Agents Chemother. *43*:2473–2478, 1999.

138. Nishi, T., and Tsuchiya, K.: Experimental respiratory tract infection with *Klebsiella pneumoniae* DT-S in mice: Chemotherapy with kanamycin. Antimicrob. Agents Chemother. *17*:494–505, 1980.

139. Noone, P., Parsons, T. M. S., Pattison, J. R., et al.: Experience in monitoring gentamicin therapy during treatment of serious gram negative sepsis. B. M. J. *1*:477–481, 1974.

140. Norden, C. W., Wentzel, H., and Keleti, E.: Comparison of techniques for measurement of in vitro antibiotic synergism. J. Infect. Dis. *140*:629–633, 1979.

141. Odenholt-Tornqvist, I.: Pharmacodynamics of beta-lactam antibiotics. Scand. J. Infect. Dis. Suppl. *58*:1–55, 1989.

142. Odenholt-Tornqvist, I., and Bengtsson, S.: Postantibiotic effect, and postantibiotic effect of subinhibitory concentrations, of sparfloxacin on gram-negative bacteria. Chemotherapy *40*:30–36, 1994.

143. Odenholt-Tornqvist, I., Lowdin, E., and Cars, O.: Pharmacodynamic effects of subinhibitory concentrations of β-lactam antibiotics in vitro. Antimicrob. Agents Chemother. *35*:1834–1839, 1991.

144. Odenholt-Tornqvist, I., Lowdin, E., and Cars, O.: Postantibiotic sub-MIC effect of vancomycin, roxithromycin, sparfloxacin and amikacin. Antimicrob. Agents Chemother. *36*:1852–1858, 1992.

145. Ohlsen, K., Ziebuhr, W., Koller, K. P., et al.: Effects of subinhibitory concentrations of antibiotics on alpha-toxin (hla) gene expression of methicillin-sensitive and methicillin-resistant *Staphylococcus aureus* isolates. Antimicrob. Agents Chemother. *42*:2817–2823, 1998.

146. Papadopoulou, Z. L., Tina, L. U., Sandler, P., et al.: Size and function of the kidneys. *In* Johnson, T. R., Moore, W. M., and Jeffries, J. E. (eds.): Children Are Different: Developmental Physiology. 2nd ed. Ross Laboratories, Columbus, OH, 1978, pp. 97–104.

147. Parker, R. F., and Luse, S.: The action of penicillin on staphylococcus: Further observations on the effect of a short exposure. J. Bacteriol. *56*:75–84, 1948.

148. Peloquin, C. A., Cumbo, T. J., Nix, D. E., et al.: Evaluation of intravenous ciprofloxacin in patients with nosocomial lower respiratory tract infections. Arch. Intern. Med. *149*:2269–2273, 1989.

149. Piddock, L. J., Walters, R. N., and Diver, J. M.: Correlation of quinolone MIC and inhibition of DNA, RNA, and protein synthesis and induction of the SOS response in *Escherichia coli*. Antimicrob. Agents Chemother. *34*:2331–2336, 1990.

150. Powley, L., Meeson, J., and Greenwood, D.: Tolerance to penicillin in streptococci of viridans group. J. Clin. Pathol. *42*:77–80, 1989.

151. Preston, S. L., Drusano, G. L., Berman, A. L., et al.: Pharmacodynamics of levofloxacin: A new paradigm for early clinical trials. J. A. M. A. *279*:125–129, 1998.

152. Puntorieri, M., Primavera, A., Privitera, O., et al.: Observations on the tolerance and the paradoxical effect in enterococci. J. Chemother. *6*:377–382, 1994.

153. Queiroz, M. L. S., Bathirunathan, N., and Mawer, G. E.: Influence of dosage interval on the therapeutic response to gentamicin in mice infected with *Klebsiella pneumoniae*. Chemotherapy *33*:68–76, 1987.

154. Raimundo, S., Fischer, J., Eichelbaum, M., et al.: Elucidation of the genetic basis of the common "intermediate" metabolizer phenotype for drug oxidation by CYP2D6. Pharmacogenomics *10*:577–581, 2000.

155. Rand, K. H., and Brown, P.: Concentration-dependent synergy and antagonism between cefoperazone and imipenem against methicillin-resistant *Staphylococcus aureus*. Antimicrob. Agents Chemother. *39*:1173–1177, 1995.

156. Raucy, J. L., and Allen, S. W.: Recent advances in P450 research. Pharmacogenomics J. *1*:178–186, 2001.

157. Ravizzola, G., Cabibbo, E., Peroni, L., et al.: In vitro study of the synergy between β-lactam antibiotics and glycopeptides against enterococci. J. Antimicrob. Chemother. *39*:461–470, 1997.
158. Redjeb, S. B., Slim, A., Horchani, A., et al.: Effects of ten milligrams of ampicillin per day on urinary tract infections. Antimicrob. Agents Chemother. *22*:1084–1086, 1982.
159. Riddick, D. S.: Drug biotransformation. *In* Kalant, H., and Roschlau, W. H. E. (eds.): Principles of Medical Pharmacology. 6th ed. New York, Oxford University Press, 1998, pp. 38–66.
160. Ritschel, W. A., and Kearns, G. L.: Pediatric pharmacokinetics. *In* Ritschel, W. A., and Kearns, G. L. (eds.): Handbook of Basic Pharmacokinetics. 5th ed. Washington, D.C., American Pharmaceutical Association, 1999, pp. 304–321.
161. River, J. M., and Wise, R.: Morphological and biochemical changes in *E. coli* after exposure to ciprofloxacin. J. Antimicrob. Chemother. *18*(Suppl. D):31–41, 1986.
162. Romansky, M. J., and Rittman, G. E.: A method of prolonging the action of penicillin. Science *100*:196–198, 1944.
163. Roosendaal, R., and Bakker-Woudenberg, I. A. J. M.: Impact of the antibiotic dosage schedule on efficacy in experimental lung infections. Scand. J. Infect. Dis. Suppl. *74*:155–162, 1991.
164. Roosendaal, R., Bakker-Woudenberg, I. A. J. M., van den Berg, J. C., and Michel, M. F.: Therapeutic efficacy of continuous versus intermittent administration of ceftazidime in an experimental *Klebsiella pneumoniae* pneumonia in rats. J. Infect. Dis. *152*:373–378, 1985.
165. Roosendaal, R., Bakker-Woudenberg, I. A. J. M., van den Berghe-van Raffe, M., and Michel, M. F.: Continuous vs. intermittent administration of ceftazidime in experimental *Klebsiella pneumoniae* pneumonia in normal and leukopenic rats. Antimicrob. Agents Chemother. *30*:403–408, 1986.
166. Rowland, M., and Tozer, T. N. (eds.): Clinical Pharmacokinetics: Concepts and Applications. 2nd ed. Philadelphia, Lea & Febiger, 1989.
167. Ryffel, C., Strassle, A., Kayser, F. H., and Berger-Bachi, B.: Mechanisms of heteroresistance in methicillin-resistant *Staphylococcus aureus*. Antimicrob. Agents Chemother. *38*:724–728, 1994.
168. Scaglione, F., Demartini, G., Dugnani, S., and Fraschini, F.. In vitro comparative dynamics of modified-release clarithromycin and of azithromycin. Chemotherapy *46*:342–352, 2000.
169. Schaeffer, A. J., Amundsen, S. K., and Schmidt, L. N.: Adherence of *Escherichia coli* to human urinary tract epithelial cells. Infect. Immun. *24*:753–759, 1979.
170. Schentag, J. J.: Antimicrobial action and pharmacokinetics/pharmacodynamics: The use of AUIC to improve efficacy and avoid resistance. J. Chemother. *11*:426–439, 1999.
171. Schentag, J. J., Nix, D. E., and Adelman, M. H.: Mathematical examination of dual individualization principles (I): Relationships between AUC above MIC and area under the inhibitory curve for cefmenoxime, ciprofloxacin and tobramycin. Ann. Pharmacother. *25*:1050–1057, 1991.
172. Schentag, J. J., Smith, I. L., Swanson, D. J., et al.: Role for individualization with cefmenoxime. Am. J. Med. *77*(Suppl. 6A):43–50, 1984.
173. Schmidt, L. H., Walley, A., and Larson, R. D.: The influence of the dosage regimen on the therapeutic activity of penicillin G. J. Pharmacol. Exp. Ther. *96*:258–268, 1949.
174. Schmitz, F. J., Verhoef, J., Hadding, U., et al.: Reduction in cytokine release from human monocytes by modifications in cell wall structure of *Staphylococcus aureus* induced by subinhibitory concentrations of oxacillin. J. Med. Microbiol. *47*:533–541, 1998.
175. Shalit, I., Stutman, H. R., Marks, M. I., et al.: Randomized study of two dosage regimens of ciprofloxacin for treating chronic bronchopulmonary infection in patients with cystic fibrosis. Am. J. Med. *82*(Suppl. 4A):189–195, 1987.
176. Shannon, K., and Phillips, I.: The effects on β-lactam susceptibility of phenotypic induction and genotypic derepression of β-lactamase synthesis. J. Antimicrob. Chemother. *18*(Suppl. E):15–22, 1968.
177. Shibl, A. M., Ramadan, M. A., and Tawfik, A. F.: Differential inhibition by clindamycin on slime formation, adherence to Teflon catheters and hemolysin production by *Staphylococcus epidermidis*. J. Chemother. *6*:107–110, 1994.
178. Smith, A. L.: Antibiotic resistance is not relevant in infections in cystic fibrosis. Pediatr. Pulmonol. *8*(Suppl. 5):93, 1990.
179. Sonstein, S. A., and Burnham, J. C.: Effect of low concentrations of quinolone antibiotics on bacterial virulence mechanisms. Diagn. Microbiol. Infect. Dis. *16*:277–289, 1993.
180. Sorberg, M., Hanberger, H., Nilsson, M., and Nilsson, L. E.: Pharmacodynamic effects of antibiotics and acid pump inhibitors on *Helicobacter pylori*. Antimicrob. Agents Chemother. *41*:2218–2223, 1997.
181. Soriano, F., Garcia-Corbeira, P., Ponte, C., et al.: Correlation of pharmacodynamic parameters of five beta-lactam antibiotics with therapeutic efficacies in an animal model. Antimicrob. Agents Chemother. *40*:2686–2690, 1996.
182. Stapleton, P., Shannon, K., and Phillips, I.: The ability of beta-lactam antibiotics to select mutants with derepressed beta-lactamase synthesis from *Citrobacter freundii*. J. Antimicrob. Chemother. *36*:483–496, 1995.
183. Stevens, D. L., Gibbons, A. E., Bergstrom, R., and Winn, V.: The Eagle effect revisited: Efficacy of clindamycin, erythromycin, and penicillin in the treatment of streptococcal myositis. J. Infect. Dis. *158*:23–28, 1988.
184. Stevens, D. L., Madaras-Kelly, K. J., and Richards, D. M.: In vitro antimicrobial effects of various combinations of penicillin and clindamycin against four strains of *Streptococcus pyogenes*. Antimicrob. Agents Chemother. *42*:1266–1268, 1998.
185. Stille, W.: Dose-activity relationships in chemotherapy. Infection Suppl. 1:14–20, 1980.
186. Stratton, C. W., Liu, C., Ratner, H. B., and Weeks, L. S.: Bactericidal activity of daptomycin (LY146032) compared with those of ciprofloxacin, vancomycin, and ampicillin against enterococci as determined by kill-kinetic studies. Antimicrob. Agents Chemother. *31*:1014–1016, 1987.
187. Suerbaum, S., Leying, H., Meyer, B., and Opferkuch, W.: Influence of beta-lactam antibiotics on serum resistance of K1-positive blood culture isolates of *Escherichia coli*. Antimicrob. Agents Chemother. *34*:628–631, 1990.
188. Svanborg-Eden, C., Sandberg, T., Stenqvist, K., and Ahlstedt, S.: Decrease in adhesion of *Escherichia coli* to human urinary tract epithelial cells in vitro by subinhibitory concentrations of ampicillin. Infection *6*(Suppl. 1):121–123, 1978.
189. Svenungsson, B., Kalin, M., and Lindgren, L. G.: Therapeutic failure in pneumonia caused by a tolerant strain of *Staphylococcus aureus*. Scand. J. Infect. Dis. *14*:309–311, 1982.
190. Tateda, K., Hirakata, Y., Furuya, N., et al.: Effects of sub-MICs of erythromycin and other macrolide antibiotics on serum sensitivity of *Pseudomonas aeruginosa*. Antimicrob. Agents Chemother. *37*:675–680, 1993.
191. Thomas, J. K., Forrest, A., Bhavnani, S. M., et al.: Pharmacodynamic evaluation of factors associated with the development of bacterial resistance in acutely ill patients during therapy. Antimicrob. Agents Chemother. *42*:521–527, 1998.
192. Thomas, L., Maillard, J. Y., Lambert, R. J., and Russell, A. D.: Development of resistance to chlorhexidine diacetate in *Pseudomonas aeruginosa* and the effect of a "residual" concentration. J. Hosp. Infect. *46*:297–303, 2000.
193. Thorburn, C. E., Molesworth, S. J., Sutherland, R., and Rittenhouse, S.: Postantibiotic and post–β-lactamase inhibitor effects of amoxicillin plus clavulanate. Antimicrob. Agents Chemother. *40*:2796–2801, 1996.
194. Tornqvist, I. O., Holm, S. E., and Cars, O.: Pharmacodynamic effects of subinhibitory antibiotic concentrations. Scand. J. Infect. Dis. Suppl. *74*:94–101, 1991.
195. Tripodi, M. F., Adinolfi, L. E., Utili, R., et al.: Influence of subinhibitory concentrations of loracarbef (LY 163892) and daptomycin (LY 146032) on bacterial phagocytosis, killing and serum sensitivity. J. Antimicrob. Chemother. *26*:491–501, 1990.
196. Vance-Bryan, K., Larson, T. A., Rotschafer, J. C., and Toscano, J. P.: Investigation of the early killing of *Staphylococcus aureus* by daptomycin by using an in vitro pharmacodynamic model. Antimicrob. Agents Chemother. *36*:2334–2337, 1992.
197. van den Anker, J. N., and Kearns, G. L.: Pharmacology of antimicrobial agents in preterm infants. *In* Tibboel, D., and van der Voort, E. (eds.): Intensive Care in Childhood: A Challenge to the Future. Springer, New York, 1996, pp. 400–410.
198. van Ogtrop, M. L., Andes, D., Stamstad, T. J., et al.: In vivo pharmacodynamic activities of two glycylcyclines (GAR-936 and WAY 152,288) against various gram-positive and gram-negative bacteria. Antimicrob. Agents Chemother. *44*:943–949, 2000.
199. Veber, B., Vallee, E., Desmonts, J. M., et al.: Correlation between macrolide lung pharmacokinetics and therapeutic efficacy in a mouse model of pneumococcal pneumonia. J. Antimicrob. Chemother. *32*:473–482, 1993.
200. Vogelman, B., Gudmundsson, S., Leggett, J., et al.: Correlation of antimicrobial pharmacokinetic parameters with therapeutic efficacy in an animal model. J. Infect. Dis. *158*:831–847, 1988.
201. Vogelman, B., Gudmundsson, S., Turnridge, J., et al.: In vivo post-antibiotic effect in a thigh infection in neutropenic mice. J. Infect. Dis. *157*:287–298, 1988.
202. Voorn, G. P., Thompson, J., Goessens, W. H., et al.: Paradoxical dose effect of continuously administered cloxacillin in treatment of tolerant *Staphylococcus aureus* endocarditis in rats. J. Antimicrob. Chemother. *33*:585–593, 1994.
203. Vranes, J., Zagar, Z., and Kurbel, S.: Influence of subinhibitory concentrations of ceftazidime, ciprofloxacin and azithromycin on the morphology and adherence of P-fimbriated *Escherichia coli*. J. Chemother. *8*:254–260, 1996.
204. Walterspiel, J. N., Ashkenazi, S., Morrow, A. L., and Cleary, T. G.: Effect of subinhibitory concentrations of antibiotics on extracellular Shiga-like toxin I. Infection *20*:25–29, 1992.
205. Weaver, L. T., Austin, S., and Cole, T. J.: Small intestinal length: A factor essential for gut adaptation. Gut *32*:1321–1323, 1991.
206. White, C. A., and Toothaker, R. D.: Influence of ampicillin elimination half-life on in-vitro bactericidal effect. J. Antimicrob. Chemother. *15*(Suppl. A):257–260, 1985.

207. Winstanley, T. G., and Hastings, J. G. M.: Penicillin-aminoglycoside synergy and post-antibiotic effect for enterococci. J. Antimicrob. Chemother. *23*:189–199, 1989.
208. Winter, M. E., Koda-Kimble, M. A., and Young, L. Y. (eds.): Basic Clinical Pharmacokinetics. 2nd ed. Vancouver, WA, Applied Therapeutics, 1988.
209. Woolfrey, B. F., and Enright, M. A.: Ampicillin killing curve patterns for ampicillin-susceptible nontypeable *Haemophilus influenzae* strains by the agar dilution plate count method. Antimicrob. Agents Chemother. *34*:1079–1087, 1990.
210. Yoh, M., Frimpong, E. K., Voravuthikunchai, S. P., and Honda, T.: Effect of subinhibitory concentrations of antimicrobial agents (quinolones and macrolide) on the production of verotoxin by enterohemorrhagic *Escherichia coli* O157:H7. Can. J. Microbiol. *45*:732–739, 1999.
211. Yoh, M., Yamamoto, K., Honda, T., et al.: Effects of lincomycin and tetracycline on production and properties of enterotoxins of entertoxigenic *Escherichia coli*. Infect. Immun. *42*:778–782, 1983.
212. Zinner, S. H., Dudley, M. N., Gilbert, D., and Bassignani, M.: Effect of dose and schedule on cefoperazone pharmacodynamics in an in vitro model of infection in a neutropenic host. Am. J. Med. *85*(Suppl. 1A):56–58, 1988.
213. Zinner, S. H., Lagast, H., and Klastersky, J.: Antistaphylococcal activity of rifampin with other antibiotics. J. Infect. Dis. *144*:365–375, 1981.

Antibacterial Therapeutic Agents

IAN C. MICHELOW ■ GEORGE H. McCRACKEN, Jr.

This review of the use of antimicrobial agents is divided into two sections: (1) the clinical pharmacology of currently available antibacterial drugs and (2) the various aspects of administration of antimicrobial agents to infants and children. The second section includes dosage schedules and routes, prophylactic use of antimicrobial agents, considerations in writing orders and prescriptions, and other aspects of administration. Drugs of value in the treatment of disease caused by viruses, fungi, mycobacteria, and parasites are discussed in other chapters dealing with these pathogens. For the most part, only antimicrobial agents approved for use in infants and children by the Food and Drug Administration (FDA) are discussed.

Clinical Pharmacology

The antimicrobial agents of value in treating infectious diseases in infants and children may be classified into five groups:

1. The β-lactams, including penicillins, cephalosporins, carbacephems, monobactams, and carbapenems
2. The glycopeptides (i.e., vancomycin)
3. The aminoglycosides
4. The macrolides, including erythromycin, clarithromycin, and azithromycin
5. Miscellaneous antibacterial agents, including chloramphenicol, clindamycin, fluoroquinolones, rifamycins, the sulfonamides, and the tetracyclines

The following properties that govern the use of each group of drugs in infants and children are considered: mechanism of action, mechanisms of resistance, in vitro efficacy, pharmacokinetics, therapeutic uses, available preparations, and side effects and toxicity.

β-LACTAMS

BIOCHEMICAL STRUCTURE

The β-lactams are a large group of compounds that have in common a four-membered β-lactam ring. The subclasses of β-lactams differ from one another with regard to their side chains and the presence of other ring structures: the penicillins contain a 5-membered thiazolidine α-ring fused to the β-lactam ring,[127] the cephalosporins have a six-membered dihydrothiazine instead of the five-membered thiazolidine ring, and the carbacephems have a methylene group replacing the sulfur atom in the dihydrothiazine ring of the cephalosporin nucleus. The β-lactam ring is essential for antibacterial activity, whereas the side chains influence the pharmacologic properties of the β-lactam and the spectrum of antibacterial activity.

MECHANISM OF ACTION

The exact mechanism of action of the β-lactams remains elusive. Previously, researchers thought that binding of β-lactam to a bacterial cell membrane–associated enzyme (transpeptidase) blocked the terminal step in synthesis of the peptidoglycan layer of the bacterial cell wall. Cell death would ensue because the weakened cell wall could not withstand the osmotic and mechanical pressure resulting from a growing bacterium.[242, 243] Recent evidence suggests that it is a more complex process involving inhibition of cell wall synthesis and activation of endogenous autolytic systems.[173, 244] The known targets of β-lactams are penicillin-binding proteins (PBPs), which are vital for cell division, cell shape, and structural integrity. Because the specific PBPs within each bacterial species and the affinity of each β-lactam antibiotic for a particular PBP differ, some β-lactams have better activity than do others against particular bacteria. The various β-lactam antibiotics can have different morphologic effects on the same bacterial species, which is thought to be related to specific functions of the PBP to which the β-lactam binds.[230] Some bacteria have a deficiency in the system of autolytic enzymes that results in inhibition, but not killing of the bacteria by a β-lactam that otherwise would be bactericidal. This phenomenon is called *tolerance* and is demonstrated in vitro by a minimal inhibitory concentration (MIC) in the susceptible range and a minimal bacterial concentration (MBC)/MIC ratio of 32 or greater.[101]

β-Lactam antibiotics are bactericidal against most susceptible bacteria. The nature of the bactericidal activity has been described as concentration-independent and time-dependent, as opposed to the concentration-dependent bactericidal activity of aminoglycosides.[74, 139, 254] Bactericidal activity is believed to be optimal when the concentration of β-lactam antibiotic at the site of infection is 4 to 10 times greater than that of the MIC (MBC) of the infecting organism. The rapidity and extent of killing are not increased when concentrations exceed that ratio. A more important determinant of bactericidal activity for β-lactams is the length of time during the dosing interval that the concentration of antibiotic exceeds the MIC or MBC for the infecting organism.

MECHANISMS OF RESISTANCE

Bacteria can acquire resistance to an antibiotic by at least three mechanisms: alteration in the antimicrobial target, decreased uptake of the antibiotic, and production of an enzyme that inactivates the antibiotic.[184] With respect to β-lactam antibiotics, resistance involves alterations in PBPs leading to decreased affinity for the β-lactam, decreased permeability of the bacterial cell wall resulting in diminished amounts of β-lactam reaching the PBPs, or production of β-lactamases that hydrolyze the β-lactam ring. Hydrolysis of β-lactam is the mechanism that is most significant clinically. Gram-positive bacteria excrete their β-lactamases outside the cell wall, whereas the β-lactamases of gram-negative bacteria remain in the periplasmic space. The spectrum of β-lactamase activity involves narrow-spectrum penicillinases that preferentially hydrolyze penicillins; broad-spectrum β-lactamases that hydrolyze penicillins and cephalosporins equally well; cephalosporinases that preferentially hydrolyze cephalosporins and are resistant to inhibition by clavulanic acid; extended-spectrum β-lactamases that hydrolyze first-, second-, and third-generation cephalosporins but are susceptible to inhibition by clavulanic acid; and carbapenemases that inactivate all β-lactams, including imipenem-cilastatin.[40]

TABLE 235–1 ■ CLASSIFICATION SCHEME FOR PENICILLINS

Generic Name	Trade Name	Route
Natural Penicillins		
Penicillin G	Many	PO,* IM, IV
Penicillin V	Many	PO
Aminopenicillins		
Ampicillin	Many	PO, IM, IV
Amoxicillin	Many	PO
Amoxicillin/clavulanate	Augmentin	PO
Ampicillin/sulbactam†	Unasyn	IM, IV
Bacampicillin	Spectrobid	PO
Penicillinase-Resistant Penicillins		
Cloxacillin	Cloxapen, Tegopen*	PO
Dicloxacillin	Dycill, Dynapen, Pathocil	PO
Methicillin	Celbenin,* Staphcillin	IM, IV
Nafcillin	Nafcil, Nallpen, Unipen,	IM, IV, PO
Oxacillin	Bactocill, Prostaphlin	IM, IV, PO
Extended-Spectrum Penicillins		
Carbenicillin (Indanyl)	Geocillin	PO
Ticarcillin	Ticar	IM, IV
Ticarcillin/clavulate†	Timentin	IV
Mezlocillin	Mezlin	IM, IV
Piperacillin†	Pipracil	IM, IV
Piperacillin/tazobactam†	Zosyn	IV

*No longer available.
†Safety and efficacy have not been established for children younger than 12 years.
IM, Intramuscularly; IV, intravenously; PO, orally.
Modified from USP DI: Information for the Health Care Professional. Vol. 1, Thomson MICROMEDEX, 2003.

Penicillins

Though first discovered by Fleming in the late 1920s, penicillin G was not available for general use in the United States for another 20 years. Since that time, numerous semisynthetic penicillins have been developed. The penicillins can be classified into four groups based on their antimicrobial activity, with some overlap (Table 235–1). The spectrum of activity among the compounds within each group is usually similar to the major differences related to pharmacologic properties (Table 235–2).

PENICILLIN G AND PENICILLIN V

Despite the more than 50 years that penicillin G has been in use, some bacteria continue to be exquisitely susceptible. Resistant strains of *Streptococcus pyogenes* (group A *Streptococcus)* and *Streptococcus agalactiae* (group B *Streptococcus)* have not emerged. Penicillin G remains the drug of choice for the treatment of disease caused by a wide variety of microorganisms (Table 235–3).

TABLE 235–2 ■ PHARMACOKINETICS OF PENICILLINS

Antibiotic	Oral Absorption (%)	Protein Binding (%)	Metabolized (%)	Urinary Recovery* (%)	Approximate Half-Life† (hr)
Natural Penicillins					
Penicillin G	15-30	60	20	20/60–90	0.5–0.7
Penicillin V	60–73	80	55	20–40	0.5–1
Aminopenicillins					
Ampicillin	35–50	20	10	40–45/75–90	1-1.5
Amoxicillin	75-90	20	10	60–75	1
Penicillinase-Resistant Penicillins					
Cloxacillin	50	95	20	30–60	0.5–1
Dicloxacillin	37–50	95–98	10	50–70	0.5–1
Methicillin		40	10	60–80	0.3–1
Nafcillin	Erratic	90	60–70	11–30	0.5–1.5
Oxacillin	30–35	90–94	45	55–60	0.4–0.7
Extended-Specturm Penicillins					
Carbenicillin indanyl	30	50	0–2	36	1.0–1.5
Ticarcillin		45–60	15	60–80	1.0–1.2
Mezlocillin		16–42	20–30	55–60	0.8–1.1
Piperacillin		16	20–30	60–80	0.6–1.2

*Urinary recovery after oral/parenteral administration.
†With normal renal function.
Modified from USP DI: Information for the Health Care Professional. Vol. 1, Thomson MICROMEDEX, 2003.

TABLE 235–3 ■ MICROORGANISMS FOR WHICH PENICILLIN G OR V IS THE DRUG OF CHOICE

Actinomyces israelii
Bacillus anthracis
Clostridium species
Corynebacterium diphtheriae
Erysipelothrix rhusiopathiae
Leptospira species
*Neisseria gonorrhoeae**
Neisseria meningitidis
Pasteurella multocida
Spirillum minus
*Staphylococcus aureus**
Streptobacillus moniliformis
Streptococcus groups A, B, C, D, G; viridans group† anaerobic strains
Streptococcus pneumoniae†
Treponema pallidum

*Strains that do not produce β-lactamase.
†Only those without altered penicillin-binding proteins.

The mechanism by which most bacteria have acquired resistance to penicillin G is that of β-lactamase production; resistance caused by altered PBPs occurs less commonly. The great majority of strains of *Staphylococcus aureus* and *Staphylococcus epidermidis* produce penicillinase. *Neisseria gonorrhoeae* was thought to be uniformly susceptible to penicillin G, but some strains that produce a β-lactamase and are highly resistant to penicillin G have been identified, first in the Far East and later in military personnel and their contacts in the United States. Although geographic variation in the prevalence of penicillinase-producing strains of *Haemophilus influenzae* occurs, recent surveillance studies estimate that approximately 30 percent of type b and 15 percent of nontypeable strains are penicillin-resistant.[120] Most *Moraxella catarrhalis* isolates produce β-lactamase. Penicillinase or cephalosporinase production is the most common cause of β-lactam resistance in gram-negative anaerobes, including *Bacteroides* spp.[189] Though uncommon, strains of *Neisseria meningitidis* resistant to penicillin because of altered PBPs and β-lactamase production have been reported from Spain and from South Africa and Britain, respectively.

Of most recent concern are reports of disease caused by strains of *Streptococcus pneumoniae* resistant to penicillin G as a result of altered PBPs.[36] The first documented clinical case of infection caused by penicillin-resistant pneumococcus was reported in 1967 from Australia. Recently, resistant pneumococcal infections have been seen worldwide, with most cases occurring in Spain, South Africa, Hungary, and the Far East. In the United States, the percentage of pneumococci resistant to penicillin varies geographically and ranges from 4 to 48 percent.[155] Many strains of penicillin-resistant pneumococci, especially those with an MIC of 2 μg/mL or greater, are also resistant to other commonly used antibiotics such as trimethoprim-sulfamethoxazole (TMP-SMX), erythromycin, chloramphenicol, clindamycin, and third-generation cephalosporins. Although penicillin-resistant pneumococcal meningitis has developed in patients while receiving vancomycin for pneumococcal sepsis,[46] no treatment failures have been documented when the appropriate dosage of vancomycin has been administered.

Several oral and parenteral forms of penicillin G are available. Selection of a preparation is based on the pattern of antimicrobial activity, including the peak and duration of activity in serum and tissues, and factors that reflect absorption, distribution, and excretion of the drug. These characteristics of penicillins are as follows:

1. Aqueous (water-soluble) penicillin G produces high peak concentrations of antibacterial activity in serum within 30 minutes after intramuscular administration but is excreted rapidly; thus, the concentration in serum is low within 2 to 4 hours. If aqueous penicillin G is given by the intravenous route, the peak is higher and occurs earlier and the duration of antibacterial activity in serum is shorter (approximately 2 hours). Aqueous penicillin G given intramuscularly or intravenously is used for severe disease such as meningitis, pneumonia, and endocarditis. In such cases, the drug should be administered at frequent intervals, usually every 4 hours, until the infection has been controlled.

2. Procaine penicillin G given intramuscularly produces lower concentrations of serum antibacterial activity (approximately 10–30% of the peak concentration achieved by the same dosage of the aqueous form), but activity persists in serum for as long as 12 hours. Intramuscular administration of procaine penicillin G should be reserved for patients with mild to moderate disease who cannot tolerate oral preparations.

3. Benzathine penicillin G given intramuscularly is a repository preparation that provides low concentrations of serum activity (approximately 1–2% of the peak concentration achieved by the same dosage of the aqueous form). After administration of this drug, concentrations of penicillin are measurable in serum for 3 weeks or more and in urine for several months. Pain at the site of injection is the major deterrent to widespread use of this unique antibiotic. A combination of the benzathine and procaine salts (900,000 and 300,000 U, respectively) is a less painful treatment and is comparable in efficacy to benzathine alone (1,200,000 U) for the treatment of streptococcal pharyngitis.[15] Benzathine penicillin G is appropriate for only highly sensitive organisms present in tissues that are well vascularized so that the drug can diffuse readily to the site of infection. Thus, benzathine penicillin G is suitable for treatment of children with group A streptococcal pharyngitis or impetigo and for prophylaxis of streptococcal infection in children who have had rheumatic carditis. Current recommendations by the Centers for Disease Control and Prevention (CDC)[99] for management of syphilis include the use of benzathine penicillin G for primary, secondary, and early latent syphilis (<1 year's duration). Benzathine penicillin G also is recommended for infants with suspected congenital syphilis who do not meet the criteria for therapy with a 10-day course of aqueous or procaine penicillin G and whose follow-up can be ensured for repeat serologic testing.

4. Oral preparations of buffered penicillin G and phenoxymethylpenicillin (penicillin V) are absorbed well from the gastrointestinal tract. The peak concentration of serum activity of penicillin V is approximately 40 percent and that of buffered penicillin G is approximately 20 percent of the concentration achieved by the same dosage of aqueous penicillin G administered intramuscularly. Therefore, oral penicillins may be satisfactory for treating mild to moderately severe infections by susceptible organisms. Penicillin V and penicillin G have equivalent activity in vitro against gram-positive cocci, but penicillin V is less active than penicillin G against *N. meningitidis, N. gonorrhoeae,* and *H. influenzae.*[127] The benefit of treating streptococcal tonsillopharyngitis with a 10-day regimen of penicillin V for the prevention of acute rheumatic fever is based on indirect evidence derived from rates of pharyngeal eradication of *S. pyogenes* equivalent to those of injectable penicillin, the treatment with proven efficacy.[67, 224] From a practical standpoint, oral formulations of penicillin G no longer are available in the United States.

All penicillins are excreted by both glomerular filtration and tubular secretion. The concomitant use of probenecid, a drug that blocks tubular secretion of organic acids, with a penicillin can produce higher peak and more sustained concentrations of antimicrobial activity. Dosages and dosing intervals may need adjustment when penicillins are administered to persons with altered renal function.

PENICILLINASE-RESISTANT PENICILLINS

The semisynthetic penicillinase-resistant penicillins were developed in response to the emergence of penicillinase-producing staphylococci. The acyl side chain, by means of steric hindrance, prevents hydrolysis of the β-lactam ring by penicillinases.

Most strains of *S. aureus* produce penicillinase, regardless of whether the infection is nosocomial or community acquired. Thus, penicillinase-resistant penicillins are the drugs of choice for the initial management of patients with suspected staphylococcal disease. With the exception of methicillin, these agents are active against streptococci and can be used for empiric treatment of infections commonly caused by both staphylococci and streptococci. Because these agents are less active than penicillin G against streptococci, penicillin G should be used instead of these agents if streptococci alone are isolated from culture. Penicillinase-resistant penicillins have no activity against gram-negative bacteria or enterococci.[152]

Methicillin was the first penicillinase-resistant penicillin to be introduced and was available in parenteral form only. Oxacillin and nafcillin are available in both parenteral and oral preparations and have greater in vitro activity against gram-positive cocci than methicillin does. Cloxacillin and dicloxacillin are available in oral forms only and are absorbed more efficiently from the gastrointestinal tract than the other oral drugs are. Differences among these five penicillins include routes of elimination, degree of binding to proteins and degradation by β-lactamases, and in vitro susceptibility[183]; however, all are effective in the treatment of staphylococcal disease, and clinical studies have shown them to be equivalent when used at appropriate dosage schedules.

Disease caused by methicillin-resistant staphylococci was reported shortly after introduction of the drug. Resistance is caused by alterations in PBPs rather than production of β-lactamase.[45] The *mecA* gene, a transposon integrated into the chromosome, encodes a new PBP (2a) that has low affinity for β-lactams, thereby resulting in resistance to all β-lactam antibiotics currently available, including penicillinase-resistant penicillins, cephalosporins, and carbapenems. Many of these methicillin-resistant strains are also resistant to other antimicrobial agents for which the mechanism of action is unrelated to PBPs, including the macrolides and clindamycin, fusidic acid, some aminoglycosides, and sulfonamides. This resistance can be plasmid mediated or chromosomal.[150]

Coagulase-negative staphylococci, including *S. epidermidis,* are residents of the normal microbial flora of the skin and are occasional contaminants of body fluid cultures. These organisms can be pathogens in certain settings, such as in neonates, or in infections of prosthetic devices, such as heart valves or cerebrospinal fluid (CSF) shunts. Most strains of coagulase-negative staphylococci produce a penicillinase that inactivates penicillin G, penicillin V, and ampicillin, and many strains have an altered PBP (2a) leading to methicillin resistance. In addition, these methicillin-resistant, coagulase-negative staphylococci are frequently resistant to cephalosporins, erythromycin, and clindamycin. Vancomycin is the drug of choice for disease known or suspected to be caused by methicillin-resistant *S. aureus* or *S. epidermidis.*

AMINOPENICILLINS

The aminopenicillins are semisynthetic β-lactam antibiotics formed by the addition of an amino group to benzylpenicillin. Amoxicillin differs from ampicillin by the presence of a hydroxyl group on the phenyl side chain. The aminopenicillins were the first penicillins that had activity against some gram-negative organisms, including *H. influenzae, Escherichia coli, Proteus mirabilis, Salmonella* spp., and *Shigella* spp., while retaining activity against penicillin-susceptible, gram-positive bacteria.[182]

When compared with penicillin G, aminopenicillins are significantly more active against *Listeria monocytogenes;* slightly more active against enterococci; equally active against *Actinomyces, N. meningitidis,* and clostridial and corynebacteria species; and slightly less active against group A streptococci, group B streptococci, and pneumococci. Aminopenicillins are the drugs of choice for the treatment of infections caused by *L. monocytogenes* and enterococci. Other organisms susceptible in vitro to ampicillin and amoxicillin include non–penicillinase-producing strains of *H. influenzae, M. catarrhalis, N. gonorrhoeae, S. aureus, E. coli, Salmonella,* and *Shigella.* The in vitro spectrum of activity for amoxicillin and ampicillin is identical, except that amoxicillin is two times less active against *Shigella* and two to four times more active against enterococci and *Salmonella* than ampicillin is.[182]

As seen with penicillin G, the primary means of acquired resistance to aminopenicillins is the production of β-lactamase. However, organisms that are resistant to penicillin G or to methicillin because of altered PBPs—*S. pneumoniae* and *S. aureus,* respectively—are also resistant to aminopenicillins.

The broad-spectrum activity of ampicillin and amoxicillin provides the basis for their use against susceptible pathogens causing (1) lower respiratory infections; (2) acute otitis media, for which amoxicillin remains the drug of choice[71]; (3) acute bacterial meningitis (ampicillin only in the United States); (4) acute and chronic infections of the urinary tract; and (5) acute diarrheal disease when therapy is indicated for shigellosis or salmonellosis. By bacteriologic and clinical measures, amoxicillin is significantly less effective than ampicillin for the treatment of shigellosis.[180]

Both drugs are available for oral administration; ampicillin alone is available in a parenteral form. Amoxicillin provides higher and more prolonged serum concentrations than those achieved with equivalent dosages of ampicillin; thus, amoxicillin can be given in lower dosage, two or three times a day rather than four times as required for ampicillin. An additional advantage of amoxicillin is that absorption is not altered when the antibiotic is administered with food whereas absorption of ampicillin is decreased significantly when it is given with food. Ampicillin is associated more frequently with diarrhea than amoxicillin is.

EXTENDED-SPECTRUM PENICILLINS

Extended-spectrum penicillins are semisynthetic derivatives of ampicillin that have better activity against gram-negative organisms because of a higher affinity for PBPs and greater penetration through the gram-negative outer membrane. Carbenicillin and ticarcillin, the carboxypenicillins, have a carboxyl group replacing the amino group side chain of ampicillin, whereas the acylureidopenicillins have a ureido (urea) side chain (mezlocillin) or ureido and piperazine side chains (piperacillin). Their pharmacologic properties are similar and include susceptibility to hydrolysis by staphylococcal penicillinases and, to a lesser extent, the β-lactamases of gram-negative bacteria. They differ somewhat in their toxicities and spectrum of activity.

The activity of carbenicillin is equivalent to or slightly less than that of ampicillin against non–β-lactamase–producing *N. gonorrhoeae, N. meningitidis, H. influenzae, E. coli, P. mirabilis, Salmonella* spp., and *Shigella* spp. It is less active than ampicillin against group A streptococci, pneumococci, and enterococci. Its activity is variable against many *Bacteroides fragilis, Enterobacter,* and *Serratia* organisms, and it is not active against *Klebsiella.* The intravenous preparation of carbenicillin is not marketed any longer in the United States; however, an oral preparation, carbenicillin indanyl, is available but seldom used.

The activity of ticarcillin is similar to that of carbenicillin, but it is two to four times more active against some strains of *Pseudomonas aeruginosa* and less active against gram-positive cocci. In addition, ticarcillin can be used for infections caused by susceptible strains of *Acinetobacter.* Because of its increased activity, ticarcillin may be used in smaller doses than needed with carbenicillin for the treatment of disease caused by gram-negative organisms.

Piperacillin and mezlocillin are parenteral penicillins with a spectrum of activity similar to that of ticarcillin but greater activity in vitro against some gram-negative bacilli and anaerobic bacteria.[73] Piperacillin is more active than carbenicillin, ticarcillin, or mezlocillin against *P. aeruginosa.* Piperacillin and mezlocillin are more active in vitro than carbenicillin or ticarcillin against susceptible strains of *E. coli, Klebsiella, Enterobacter, Serratia,* and *B. fragilis.*[252] Furthermore, piperacillin, mezlocillin, and ticarcillin are effective in the treatment of infections caused by susceptible strains of *Citrobacter,* indole-positive *Proteus,* and *Providencia.* Combination therapy with an aminoglycoside results in synergy against some gram-negative enteric bacilli.[87]

Ticarcillin, a disodium salt, contains 5.2 mEq (120 mg) of sodium per gram. The acylureidopenicillins are monosodium salts that have a lower sodium content than the carboxypenicillins do. The amount of sodium administered may be of concern when treating certain patients with renal or cardiac disease. Hypokalemia with metabolic alkalosis occasionally occurs with the administration of extended-spectrum penicillins, especially the carboxypenicillins. The penicillin acts as a nonreabsorbable anion in the distal renal tubules, where it affects normal hydrogen exchange and secondarily results in loss of potassium.[42] These extended-spectrum penicillins can bind to platelet adenosine diphosphate receptors and thereby result in abnormal platelet aggregation and prolonged bleeding times.[37] This dose-related phenomenon occurs more frequently with the administration of ticarcillin than with the acylureidopenicillins. The effects on platelet function may be a consideration when choosing empiric therapy for a thrombocytopenic patient with suspected gram-negative infection.

These penicillins (usually combined with an aminoglycoside) have been used in adults for the treatment of intra-abdominal, gynecologic, and urinary tract infections and sepsis in patients with altered host defenses. Patients with susceptible organisms causing urinary tract infections or sepsis had a better clinical response to ticarcillin than did those with lower respiratory tract infections caused by ticarcillin-susceptible bacteria.[193] All the extended-spectrum penicillins, except for carbenicillin, are available in parenteral formulations only. Because of limited clinical experience in infants and children, piperacillin has not been approved for use in patients younger than 12 years.

β-LACTAM/β-LACTAMASE INHIBITOR COMBINATIONS

β-Lactamase inhibitors are compounds that have weak antibacterial activity but can bind irreversibly to many β-lactamases and render them inactive. The inhibitors currently in use are clavulanic acid, sulbactam, and tazobactam, the latter of which are halogenated penicillanic acid derivatives. All three inhibitors are identical in their mode of activity but differ to some degree in their potency and spectrum of enzyme inhibition. These β-lactamase inhibitors are not effective against Bush group 1–inducible chromosomal β-lactamases produced by strains of *Pseudomonas, Serratia, Citrobacter,* and *Enterobacter* and against some plasmid-mediated enzymes. Furthermore, clavulanate actually can induce Bush group 1 enzymes. Disks containing β-lactamase inhibitors can be used in the clinical microbiology laboratory to detect pathogens that produce extended-spectrum β-lactamases of the TEM and SHV types that may be overlooked otherwise.[41] β-Lactamase inhibitors have been formulated in a fixed ratio with a β-lactam antibiotic. The spectrum of activity of each combination is determined primarily by the spectrum of activity of the β-lactam. However, many determinants of the inhibitor influence its activity, including its affinity for the β-lactamase and its ability to traverse the gram-negative cell wall to bind to periplasmic β-lactamases.[141] The main indication for the use of these combination antimicrobial agents is for the treatment of nosocomial infections or polymicrobial infections caused by susceptible β-lactamase–producing pathogens.

AMOXICILLIN–CLAVULANIC ACID. Amoxicillin combined with potassium clavulanate was introduced in 1984 for oral administration. The pharmacokinetics of the two drugs are similar; both are absorbed rapidly and are not affected when taken with meals. Gastrointestinal side effects, including nausea, vomiting, and diarrhea, occur more commonly with amoxicillin-clavulanate than with amoxicillin alone.[231]

The combination drug is equivalent to amoxicillin alone in activity against amoxicillin-susceptible organisms. The addition of clavulanic acid extends the in vitro activity of amoxicillin to include β-lactamase–producing strains of *S. aureus* (but not methicillin-resistant strains), *H. influenzae, M. catarrhalis, N. gonorrhoeae, E. coli, Proteus, Klebsiella,* and some anaerobic bacteria, including *B. fragilis.* Some β-lactamase–producing strains of *E. coli* are resistant to amoxicillin–clavulanic acid because of either hyperproduction of the β-lactamase or production of a β-lactamase that is not susceptible to clavulanate.

Ampicillin or amoxicillin alone is considered the preferred therapy for children with mild to moderately severe disease of the respiratory tract, including initial empiric therapy for otitis media. Alternative therapy, including amoxicillin–clavulanic acid, should be considered if a β-lactamase–producing organism is known or suspected to be the cause of the disease.[71] Recently, a new formulation of amoxicillin–clavulanic acid was approved that provides a larger dosage (90 mg/kg/day in two divided doses) for the treatment of high-risk patients with acute otitis media. The combination drug is useful in areas where the proportion of β-lactamase–producing strains of *H. influenzae* is large (>30%) and where *M. catarrhalis* organisms (most of which are β-lactamase producers) are identified more frequently as pathogens in otitis media, sinusitis, and other respiratory tract infections. Amoxicillin-clavulanate also has been used successfully for the oral treatment of urinary tract, skin, and soft tissue infections, as well as for the treatment of human and animal bite wounds.[41]

AMPICILLIN-SULBACTAM. Ampicillin was combined with sulbactam to have a parenteral β-lactam/β-lactamase inhibitor combination. The spectrum of activity of ampicillin-sulbactam is similar to that of amoxicillin-clavulanate. It is most useful as monotherapy for potential polymicrobial infections, such as intra-abdominal, gynecologic, and soft tissue infections. Ampicillin-sulbactam has been shown to be safe and efficacious for the treatment of skin and skin structure infections caused by susceptible organisms in children aged 3 months to 12 years.[9] The combination of ampicillin-sulbactam and an aminoglycoside has efficacy equivalent to that of a combination of ampicillin, clindamycin, and an aminoglycoside for empiric treatment of intra-abdominal infections in children.[50]

TICARCILLIN–POTASSIUM CLAVULANATE. Ticarcillin combined with potassium clavulanate extends the spectrum of activity of ticarcillin to include β-lactamase–producing strains of staphylococci, *H. influenzae, M. catarrhalis, E. coli, Klebsiella, Proteus, Providencia, N. gonorrhea,* and *B. fragilis.*[48] Ticarcillin-clavulanate is also often active against multidrug-resistant *Stenotrophomonas maltophilia.* Enterococci are moderately resistant to this agent. Because clavulanic acid does not inhibit Bush group 1–inducible chromosomal β-lactamases, derepressed mutant strains of *Pseudomonas aeruginosa* that are resistant to ticarcillin because of inducible cephalosporinases are also resistant to ticarcillin–potassium clavulanate. Ticarcillin–potassium clavulanate is approved for use in children older than 3 months for lower respiratory, skin and skin structure, urinary tract, bone and joint, and intra-abdominal infections caused by susceptible pathogens.[27]

PIPERACILLIN-TAZOBACTAM. Piperacillin combined with tazobactam was approved for use in adults in 1993. It extends the spectrum of activity of piperacillin to include β-lactamase–producing strains of methicillin-susceptible *S. aureus*, many members of the Enterobacteriaceae, and virtually all gram-positive and gram-negative anaerobes; its spectrum of activity is superior to that of ceftazidime and other β-lactam/β-lactamase inhibitor combinations. Penicillin-resistant pneumococci, methicillin-resistant staphylococci, *Corynebacterium jeikeium*, and most *Enterococcus faecium* strains are resistant to piperacillin-tazobactam.[41] Although studies have shown piperacillin-tazobactam to be safe and effective for the treatment of lower respiratory tract, intra-abdominal, and skin and skin structure infections in adults, as well as for empiric treatment of febrile episodes in neutropenic adults,[41] the experience in children is limited. The safety and efficacy of piperacillin-tazobactam have not been established for children.

ADVERSE EFFECTS AND SENSITIZATION

The penicillins are unique among antimicrobial agents in having little dose-related toxicity (Table 235–4). Seizures may occur under circumstances that result in high concentrations of penicillin in nervous tissue: rapid intravenous infusion of single large dosages, substantial dosages for prolonged periods in patients with impaired renal function, high concentrations given by the intrathecal route, or direct application of penicillin to brain tissue, as might occur inadvertently during a neurosurgical procedure. Confusion, dizziness, seizures, and psychosis caused by toxic concentrations of procaine have been associated with the administration of procaine penicillin G.[227] Nephritis has been associated with the administration of some penicillins, most frequently after the use of methicillin. Bleeding because of drug-induced platelet aggregation has been noted after the administration of carbenicillin and penicillin G.

Although toxicity may not be a significant concern with the penicillins, sensitization is an important factor.[140] Penicillins are haptens, that is, they are low-molecular-weight compounds too small to elicit an immune response alone, but when bound to a carrier molecule (such as host tissues or proteins), they are highly immunogenic in humans. The native penicillin molecule can bind to a protein, as can its penicilloyl and penicillanic metabolites, the major and minor determinants, respectively. Four types of

TABLE 235–4 ■ ADVERSE REACTIONS TO PENICILLINS

Type of Reaction	Frequency (%)	Most Frequent*
Electrolyte disturbance		
Sodium overload	Variable	Ticar
Hypokalemia	Variable	Ticar
Hyperkalemia, acute	Rare	PCN G
Gastrointestinal		
Diarrhea	2–5	Amp
Enterocolitis	<1	Amp
Hematologic		
Hemolytic anemia	Rare	PCN G
Neutropenia	1–4	PCN G, Naf, Ox, Pip
Platelet dysfunction	3	Carben, Ticar
Hepatic		
Elevated AST	1–4	Ox, Naf, Carben
Neurologic		
Seizures	Rare	PCN G
Bizarre sensations		Procaine PCN
Renal		
Interstitial nephritis	1–2	Meth
Hemorrhagic cystitis	Rare	Meth
Allergic		
IgE mediated	0.004–0.4	PCN G
Cytotoxic antibody	Rare	PCN G
Immune complexes	Rare	PCN G
Delayed hypersensitivity	4–8	Amp
Idiopathic	4–8	Amp

*All reactions can occur with any penicillin.
Amp, ampicillin; AST, aspartate transaminase; Carben, carbenicillin; Meth, methicillin; Naf, nafcillin; Ox, oxacillin; PCN G, penicillin G; Pip, piperacillin; Ticar, ticarcillin.
Modified from Chambers, H. F., and Neu, H.C.: Penicillins. *In* Mandell, G.L., Bennett, J.E., and Dollin, R. (eds.): Mandell, Douglas and Bennett's Principles and Practice of Infectious Diseases. 4th ed. New York, Churchill-Livingstone, 1995.

immune-mediated reactions can occur after the administration of a penicillin (or any drug or antigen): immediate hypersensitivity (IgE-mediated) reactions, cytotoxic antibody reactions, immune complex reactions (Arthus reaction), and delayed (cell-mediated) hypersensitivity.[258] Researchers have estimated that an immediate serious reaction occurs in 2 of every 10,000 courses and fatal reactions occur in 1 of 100,000 treatment courses.[17]

1. *Type 1 immediate hypersensitivity reactions* usually occur within 30 minutes after administration and are life-threatening events. The interaction of preformed mast cell–bound IgE antibody to the antigenic determinants of penicillin results in the release of mast cell mediators.[30] Clinical signs include hypotension or shock, urticaria, laryngeal edema, and bronchospasm. Acute anaphylaxis is rare after the administration of penicillin, but a significant number of fatalities occur each year because of the extensive use of these drugs. Children are thought to have fewer systemic reactions than adults do, presumably because of fewer previous exposures to penicillin antigens. Oral preparations are less likely to result in an immediate reaction than parenteral forms are, perhaps because antigens are altered in the gastrointestinal tract, absorption is slower, dosages are smaller, or a combination of these factors.

2. *Type 2 cytotoxic antibody reactions* can occur after passive absorption of the penicilloyl hapten by the membrane of circulating blood cells or by renal interstitial cells, especially when high dosages of penicillins are used for prolonged periods. IgM antibody, IgG antibody, or both antibodies to the penicilloyl antigen bind to the altered cell surface; complement can be activated, and damage to the

cell ensues. Cytotoxic antibody reactions usually are manifested more than 72 hours after initiation of antibiotic therapy and include hemolytic anemia, leukopenia, thrombocytopenia, and drug-induced nephritis.

3. *Type 3 immune complex (Arthus) reactions* occur after the formation of immune complexes between soluble penicillin antigens and IgG and IgM antibodies. The complexes lodge in the skin, joints, kidneys, or other tissue sites. Complement activation occurs, and the clinical manifestations of serum sickness ensue: cutaneous symptoms (urticaria, maculopapular rash, erythema multiforme), polyarthralgia, and fever. The onset is typically 7 to 21 days after initiation of penicillin therapy but can occur after use of the antibiotic has been discontinued. Although serum sickness has been associated with the administration of penicillins, it occurs more frequently after cefaclor.

4. *Type 4 delayed hypersensitivity reactions* involve cellular rather than humoral immunity. Thymus-derived lymphocytes react to penicillin haptens bound to host tissue after the topical administration of penicillins. Contact dermatitis is rare now that topical penicillins are not used any longer.

Idiopathic reactions are those for which an immune-mediated mechanism has not been proved. Included in this category are the morbilliform exanthems, erythema multiforme, photosensitivity reactions, exfoliative dermatitis, and pruritus. Approximately 4 percent of courses of penicillin and up to 9 percent of courses of ampicillin or amoxicillin therapy are associated with a maculopapular rash. In some of these patients, the rash is a manifestation of a primary viral infection for which the penicillin was prescribed inappropriately.

Identifying patients who will have a significant reaction if penicillin is administered remains difficult. Serologic assays (radioallergosorbent tests) for the detection of IgE antibodies to major and minor penicillin determinants are available but are time consuming, expensive, and less sensitive than skin testing. Because the immediate reaction is mediated largely by IgE reagin or skin-sensitizing antibody, patients who are likely to respond subsequently with a life-threatening reaction can be identified by the use of intradermal tests with appropriate antigens. Selecting the most appropriate antigens to be used for skin testing, however, has been problematic because many different antigens may play roles in the allergic reaction. At least 10 metabolic breakdown products of the penicillin nucleus have been identified. Other potential antigens include macromolecular impurities present in solutions of the drug, high-molecular-weight penicillin polymers found in poorly buffered penicillin solutions standing for prolonged periods, side chains of the various penicillins, and the bacterial enzymes (amidases) used to prepare semisynthetic penicillins. Thus, investigators have had difficulty choosing sensitive and specific antigens to use for skin-testing purposes.

The most promising studies of skin test antigens have been those of Levine,[137] who identified two antigens, penicilloyl polylysine (Pre-Pen, Taylor Pharmacal, Decatur, IL) and a "minor determinant mixture," a preparation of a dilute solution of aqueous crystalline penicillin G that includes metabolic breakdown products. Only the Pre-Pen reagent is available commercially in the United States; a solution of benzylpenicillin has been used as a less effective minor determinant skin test reagent. The CDC recommends the use of major and minor determinants, a positive control (histamine), and a negative control (diluent, phenol saline) after a protocol prepared by Beall.[17, 99] A prick test is performed first. If the patient's penicillin allergy is that of a mild reaction, the skin test reagent can be used at full strength; however, if the previous history is suggestive of anaphylaxis, a 1:100 dilution of the reagent should be used for the first prick test, followed by a full-strength test if no reaction with the diluted reagent occurs. If the prick test result is negative, an intradermal test is performed and the skin observed for 20 minutes. A positive result is indicated by a wheal-and-flare reaction in 10 to 15 minutes and suggests a significant chance of a reaction occurring on subsequent administration of a penicillin. A negative result suggests that a significant allergic reaction will not take place. Although much effort has gone into clinical tests of these antigens, the predictive value of positive and negative results in children remains uncertain. Because of the risk of severe life-threatening reactions when a skin test is performed, having a physician present and resuscitation equipment and medications readily available is prudent.

At present, the physician must rely on the patient's history of an adverse reaction after administration of a penicillin to identify who is likely to be allergic. If the reaction appears to be related to the administration of a penicillin, the drug should be avoided for minor infections. Because no proven alternative therapies to penicillin are recommended for treating patients with neurosyphilis or syphilis in pregnancy, the CDC recommends skin testing and desensitization of patients considered to have reacted positively to the skin test antigens.[99] If a life-threatening infection should occur and penicillin is clearly the drug of choice, the physician may choose to administer the drug under carefully controlled conditions after desensitization. All penicillins are cross-reactive with regard to sensitization; allergy to any one implies sensitization to all, although cross-sensitivity is considerably less than 100 percent.

Cephalosporins

The cephalosporins have a broad range of activity that includes gram-positive cocci, gram-negative enteric bacilli, and anaerobic bacteria. Most cephalosporins are relatively resistant to hydrolysis by β-lactamases produced by *S. aureus*, but many are susceptible to gram-negative β-lactamases. Unlike other antimicrobial agents, this group has a high therapeutic-to-toxic index. For simplicity, the cephalosporins have been categorized as first, second, third, and fourth generation (Table 235–5) based on the pattern of in vitro activity.

PHARMACOKINETICS

The cephalosporins are available as parenteral and oral products (Table 235–6). Most of the parenteral drugs can be administered by the intravenous or intramuscular routes. Most of the oral products are absorbed well from the gastrointestinal tract. Esterification of the base compounds of cefuroxime and cefpodoxime is required to enhance gastrointestinal absorption. The presence of food does not alter absorption and, for some antibiotics, even can enhance absorption. Cephalosporins penetrate well into most tissues and body fluids except for CSF. The first- and second-generation cephalosporins, other than cefuroxime, do not achieve adequate CSF concentrations. CSF penetration of third-generation drugs varies. Cefepime, a fourth-generation cephalosporin, reaches adequate CSF concentrations for the treatment of most common invasive pathogens. Because glomerular filtration and tubular secretion are the major modes of excretion, the urinary concentrations achieved are sufficient for the treatment of urinary tract infections. Ceftriaxone has dual excretion via the kidneys and the biliary tract and achieves high concentrations in urine and bile. The presence of moderate to severe renal insufficiency may require adjustment of the dosage or dosing interval for all cephalosporins except those with biliary excretion. Hepatic

TABLE 235–5 ■ CLASSIFICATION SCHEME FOR CEPHALOSPORINS

Generic Name	Trade Name	Route
First Generation		
Cephalexin	Keflex, Keftab*	PO
Cefadroxil	Duricef	PO
Cepharadine	Velosef	PO,
Cephalothin†		IM, IV
Cefazolin	Ancef, Kefzol	IM, IV
Cephapirin	Cefadyl	IM, IV
Second Generation		
Cefaclor‡	Ceclor	PO
Cefuroxime axetil§	Ceftin	PO
Cefprozil*	Cefzil	PO
Ceftibuten*	Cedax	PO
Cefamandole‡	Mandol	IM, IV
Cefonicid‖	Monocid	IM, IV
Cefuroxime	Zinacef, Kefurox	IM, IV
Cephamycins		
Cefoxitin	Mefoxin	IM, IV
Cefotetan‖	Cefotan	IM, IV
Third Generation		
Cefixime*	Suprax	PO
Cefpodoxime proxetil¶	Vantin	PO
Cefdinir*	Omnicef	PO
Cefditoren pivoxil**	Spectracef	PO
Ceftizoxime*	Cefizox	IM, IV
Cefotaxime	Claforan	IM, IV
Ceftriaxone	Rocephin	IM, IV
Ceftazidime	Fortax, Tazicef, Tazidime, Ceptaz	IM, IV
Cefoperazone‖	Cefobid	IM, IV
Fourth Generation		
Cefepime††	Maxipime	IM, IV

*Safety and efficacy have not been determined for infants younger than 6 months.
†No longer available in the United States.
‡Safety and efficacy have not been determined for infants younger than 1 month.
§Safety and efficacy have not been established for infants younger than 3 months.
‖Not approved for use in children.
¶Safety and efficacy have not been established for infants younger than 5 months.
**Safety and efficacy have not been established for children younger than 12 years.
††Safety and efficacy have not been established for infants younger than 2 months.
IM, intramuscularly; IV, intravenously; PO, orally.
Modified from USP DI: Information for the Healthcare Professional, Vol. 1. Thomson MICROMEDEX, 2003.

insufficiency can affect the metabolism of cephalosporins that undergo biliary excretion; however, adjustments in ceftriaxone dosage or dosing interval are required only in the presence of both hepatic and renal insufficiency.

Therapeutic advantages of cephalosporins include concentration-independent bactericidal activity, broad-spectrum antibacterial activity, lack of significant dose-related toxicity, and relative stability against staphylococcal β-lactamases. Certain cautions must be kept in mind when prescribing cephalosporins: none is effective against enterococci, methicillin-resistant staphylococci, *L. monocytogenes,* chlamydial species, and *Clostridium difficile,* and resistance may develop rapidly in closed communities, such as neonatal or pediatric intensive care units, because of inducible chromosomal β-lactamases produced by gram-negative bacteria. Some products may cause unexpected reactions, such as the serum sickness–like disease described with cefaclor and the bile sludge attributed to ceftriaxone. All new products are expensive, especially when compared with generic preparations. Recommended daily dosage schedules are shown in Table 235–10.

FIRST-GENERATION CEPHALOSPORINS

First-generation cephalosporins are effective against gram-positive cocci, including β-lactamase–producing *S. aureus,* and they have variable activity against gram-negative enteric bacilli. Five first-generation cephalosporins are currently available for infants and children: the parenteral drugs cephapirin and cefazolin; the oral products cephalexin and cefadroxil; and cephradine. Because cephapirin is painful in intramuscular injections, the intravenous route is preferred. Cefazolin produces higher concentrations in blood than do the other parenteral first-generation drugs. Cefadroxil can be administered in twice-daily dosing because of its longer serum half-life. None of these agents attain appreciable concentrations in the central nervous system (CNS).

These drugs are of value as alternatives to penicillin for disease caused by *S. aureus, S. pyogenes,* and susceptible *S. pneumoniae,* and they are active against some strains of community-acquired gram-negative enteric bacilli such as *E. coli, P. mirabilis,* and *Klebsiella pneumoniae.* The three oral preparations have comparable activity in vitro and in vivo. Both cefazolin and cephalexin are active against methicillin-susceptible *S. aureus;* however, cefazolin is less stable with staphylococcal β-lactamases than cephalothin is,[82] the clinical significance of which has not been established. Antibacterial activity against gram-negative bacteria is similar for all first-generation cephalosporins, except for cefazolin, which has slightly increased gram-negative activity.[215] First-generation cephalosporins are not the initial drug of choice for any pediatric infection but are of value in children who have a history of minor allergy to penicillin. They have been used to treat staphylococcal and streptococcal skin and skin structure infections, bone and joint infections, pharyngitis, and uncomplicated community-acquired urinary tract infections caused by susceptible bacteria. Cefadroxil is effective for the treatment of streptococcal pharyngitis in a once-a-day dosage schedule. Cephalexin has been used for sequential parenteral-oral treatment of staphylococcal osteomyelitis and arthritis occurring after surgical intervention and an initial period of parenteral antibiotic therapy. Cefazolin has been used for perioperative prophylaxis in selected surgical procedures. Because first-generation cephalosporins have minimal if any activity against *H. influenzae* and *M. catarrhalis* and inadequate activity against penicillin-resistant *S. pneumoniae,* they should not be used for empiric treatment of respiratory tract infections. Empiric therapy for suspected gram-negative nosocomial infections would be covered better with a third-generation cephalosporin, an aminoglycoside, or both. The safety and efficacy of cephalexin and cephapirin have not been established for infants younger than 1 month and 3 months, respectively.

SECOND-GENERATION CEPHALOSPORINS

The second-generation cephalosporins that are approved for use in children consist of two parenteral drugs (cefamandole and cefuroxime) and three oral preparations (cefaclor, cefuroxime axetil, and cefprozil). Also classified with the second-generation cephalosporins are the cephamycins, of which only one, cefoxitin, is approved for use in children. When compared with the first-generation cephalosporins, the true second-generation agents have similar or somewhat less activity against gram-positive cocci but better activity against *H. influenzae, M. catarrhalis, N. meningitidis, N. gonorrhoeae,* and some members of the Enterobacteriaceae. The cephamycins are more active than the first- or true

TABLE 235–6 ■ PHARMACOKINETICS OF CEPHALOSPORINS

Antibiotic	Bioavailability* (%)	Protein Binding (%)	Metabolized (%)	Urinary Recovery (%/hr)	Approximate Half-Life[†] (hr)
First Generation					
Cephalexin	95	10–15	0	90/8	0.9–1.2
Cefadroxil	95	15–20	0	93/24	1.2–1.5
Cephradine	95	8–17	0	60–80/6	0.8–1.3
Cephalothin		70	20–30	60–70/6	0.5–1.0[‡]
Cefazolin		85	0	80–100/24	1.4–1.8[‡]
Cephapirin		44–50	40	70/6	0.5–0.8
Second Generation					
Cefaclor	95	25	0	60–85/8	0.6–0.9
Cefuroxime axetil	37/52	50	0[§]	32–48/12	1.3[‡]
Cefprozil	95	36	0	60/8	1.3
Ceftibuten	75–90/<75[‖]	65–77	10[¶]	95/24	1.4–2.6
Cefamandole		70–80	0	60–85/8	0.5–1.2
Cefonicid		>90	0	99/24	4.5
Cefuroxime		50	0	89/8	1.3–1.7
Cefoxitin		70–80	<5	85/6	0.7–1.1
Third Generation					
Cefixime	40–50	65–70	0	50/24	3–4
Cefpodoxime proxetil	50/>50	40	0[§]	29–33/12	2.1–2.8
Cefdinir	16–25**	60–70	0	3–13/12	1.5–1.7
Cefditoren pivoxil	13–19	88	0		1.6
Ceftizoxime		30	0	85–95/24	1.7
Cefotaxime		38	30–50	60/6	1.0
Ceftriaxone		85–95	0	33–67[††]/24	4.3–8.7
Ceftazidime		<10	0	80–90/24	1.9
Fourth Generation					
Cefepime	100	20	15	80–85/12	2.0

*Fasting/nonfasting.
†Normal renal function.
‡Elimination half-life prolonged in neonates.
§Prodrug rapidly metabolized to active drug; otherwise, no significant metabolism.
‖Because the bioavailability of suspensions is decreased by food, ceftibuten should be administered at least 2 hours before or 1 hour after a meal.
¶*Cis*-isomer converted to *trans*-isomer.
**Suspension formulation has greater bioavailability than the capsule formulation.
††Forty to 75 percent eliminated unchanged in bile.
Modified from USP DI: Information for the Health Care Professional. Vol. 1. Thomson MICROMEDEX, 2003.

second-generation cephalosporins against gram-negative enteric bacteria and *B. fragilis,* but they have poor activity against gram-positive cocci.

CEFACLOR. Cefaclor is more active than cephalexin against *H. influenzae, M. catarrhalis, E. coli,* and *P. mirabilis* and has activity against staphylococci similar to that of cephalexin. Cefaclor is an unstable compound and is destroyed within 2 hours in human plasma. It is susceptible to hydrolysis by the β-lactamases produced by some strains of *Haemophilus* and *M. catarrhalis.* It is relatively effective therapy for otitis media, sinusitis, and mild to moderate cases of pneumonia. Cefaclor is a suitable alternative to amoxicillin for treating children with infections caused by susceptible organisms and suspected allergy to penicillin or when a β-lactamase–producing strain of *H. influenzae* is known or suspected to be a cause of the disease. The rare but potential risk of serum sickness, as well as its variable stability to some β-lactamases, has limited its use. Cefaclor is ineffective against penicillin-intermediate and penicillin-resistant strains of *S. pneumoniae*. The safety and efficacy of cefaclor have not been established for infants younger than 1 month, although it has been used successfully to treat neonatal otitis media. Cefaclor is ineffective against penicillin-intermediate and penicillin-resistant *S. pneumoniae*.

CEFAMANDOLE. Cefamandole is active against gram-positive cocci, including β-lactamase–producing *S. aureus,* and some gram-negative enteric bacteria, and it was the first cephalosporin to be effective for infections caused by *H. influenzae,* including β-lactamase–producing strains.[86, 165] Before the development of cefuroxime, cefamandole was used for respiratory tract, skin, and soft tissue infections in infants and children.[8, 212] Once cefuroxime was approved for use, cefamandole seldom was used because although its spectrum of activity was comparable with that of cefuroxime, some of its pharmacologic features made it less favorable. Cefamandole does not penetrate well into the CSF, and because it contains a methylthiotetrazole side chain, altered hemostasis may occur. Clinical and microbiologic failure in cases of meningitis caused by *H. influenzae* (despite in vitro susceptibility and evidence of CSF penetration) has limited the use of cefamandole to disease in which the development of sepsis is not a concern. The safety and efficacy of this agent have not been established for infants younger than 1 month. Alternative drugs are preferred in pediatric patients.

CEFOXITIN. Cefoxitin has excellent activity against anaerobic organisms and is the most active cephalosporin against *B. fragilis.*[21] It has selective activity against gram-negative enteric bacilli but is never active against *Enterobacter* or *Pseudomonas.* Cefoxitin is resistant to hydrolysis by the β-lactamases produced by gram-positive bacteria and some of the gram-negative β-lactamases. Because it is a potent inducer of Bush group 1 chromosomal β-lactamases,[209] its indiscriminate use should be avoided.

Cefoxitin has been shown to be effective for infections involving facultative gram-negative bacilli and anaerobes, such as intra-abdominal, pelvic, and gynecologic infections. When combined with doxycycline, cefoxitin is effective for the treatment of pelvic inflammatory disease.[44, 99] The use of β-lactam/β-lactamase inhibitor combinations or metronidazole rather than cefoxitin should be considered for empiric treatment of patients with life-threatening anaerobic infections because as many as 15 percent of *B. fragilis* organisms can be resistant to cephamycins.

CEFPROZIL. Cefprozil has a structure similar to that of the first-generation cephalosporin cefadroxil. It is more active than the oral first-generation agents against *S. pyogenes, S. pneumoniae, Neisseria* spp., *H. influenzae, M. catarrhalis, E. coli, P. mirabilis, Klebsiella,* and to a lesser extent staphylococci. It has relatively poor activity against *H. influenzae.* When compared with cefaclor, cefprozil is more stable against many β-lactamases. Because of its relatively long serum half-life, cefprozil can be administered twice daily. Cefprozil is comparable to penicillin, cefaclor, and erythromycin in the treatment of pharyngitis[159] and is equal or superior to cefaclor and erythromycin in the treatment of mild to moderate skin and skin structure infections.[188] Cefprozil is approved for the treatment of acute otitis media, mild lower respiratory tract infections, acute sinusitis, and skin and skin structure infections. It is unlikely to be effective in children with penicillin-nonsusceptible *S. pneumoniae* or *H. influenzae* on the basis of unfavorable pharmacodynamic parameters.[245] Cefprozil is safe and effective as part of a parenteral-oral antibiotic regimen for the treatment of suppurative skeletal infections in children.[246] The safety and efficacy of cefprozil have not been established for infants younger than 6 months.

CEFUROXIME. When compared with first-generation cephalosporins, cefuroxime is slightly less active against staphylococci but is more active against group A streptococci and pneumococci. Cefuroxime has excellent activity against many members of the Enterobacteriaceae.[185] Its stability to β-lactamases is greater than that of first-generation agents or cefamandole, and it is the only first- or second-generation antibiotic that achieves adequate CSF concentrations, except against *H. influenzae* in some patients. Cefuroxime has been approved for the treatment of skin and skin structure infections, lower respiratory tract infections, bone and joint infections, uncomplicated gonorrhea, and uncomplicated urinary tract infections caused by susceptible bacteria. Cefuroxime is most useful for the treatment of infections in which both *S. aureus* and *H. influenzae* type b are probable pathogens, that is, septic arthritis, orbital cellulitis, and severe pneumonia. Cefuroxime offers the advantage of single-drug therapy for these diseases, whereas the combination of a penicillinase-resistant penicillin and chloramphenicol was required previously. Because of persistently positive 24-hour CSF cultures in some infants and children with *H. influenzae* meningitis treated with cefuroxime, third-generation cephalosporins (cefotaxime and ceftriaxone) are preferred for the treatment of known or suspected meningitis or invasive bacterial disease that may progress to meningitis.[223] With the dramatic reduction in the incidence of invasive *H. influenzae* type b infection in the United States after the introduction of *H. influenzae* type b conjugate vaccines, using an antibiotic that provides coverage against both *S. aureus* and *H. influenzae* type b no longer is imperative.

CEFUROXIME AXETIL. Cefuroxime axetil is an oral form of cefuroxime with a similar spectrum of activity. It is an ester prodrug of cefuroxime that is metabolized to the active drug by intestinal esterases. Oral absorption is increased by the presence of food. When crushed, the tablet has a bitter taste that renders it unpalatable. The suspension has an unpleasant flavor that makes it difficult for some children to tolerate and therefore may limit compliance. The drug may be considered a suitable alternative to amoxicillin for the treatment of otitis media[71] and sinusitis when coverage must include β-lactamase–producing bacteria. Cefuroxime axetil has limited activity against penicillin-nonsusceptible pneumococci. It has been approved for the treatment of uncomplicated urinary tract infection, skin and soft tissue infection, acute bacterial maxillary sinusitis, and lower respiratory tract infection caused by susceptible bacteria. Cefuroxime axetil can be used as an alternative to penicillin for the treatment of group A streptococcal pharyngitis. The safety and efficacy of cefuroxime axetil have not been established for infants younger than 3 months.

THIRD-GENERATION CEPHALOSPORINS

Third-generation cephalosporins approved for use in children include the parenteral agents cefotaxime, ceftizoxime, ceftriaxone, and ceftazidime and the oral agents cefixime, cefpodoxime proxetil, ceftibuten, cefdinir, and cefditoren pivoxil. They are the most potent cephalosporins against gram-negative enteric bacteria.[241] Most of them have excellent activity against *H. influenzae, M. catarrhalis, N. gonorrhoeae, N. meningitidis,* group A streptococci, and penicillin-susceptible pneumococci, but relatively poor activity against staphylococci. Ceftazidime is the only agent with activity against *P. aeruginosa.* Increasing resistance to third-generation cephalosporins by members of the Enterobacteriaceae on the basis of plasmid-mediated production of extended-spectrum β-lactamases is of concern.[118] The parenteral cephalosporins provide high concentrations of drug in serum and adequate concentrations in CSF.

CEFOTAXIME. Cefotaxime has excellent activity against group A streptococci, penicillin-susceptible pneumococci, *H. influenzae, N. meningitidis,* and *N. gonorrhoeae.* Because cefotaxime can be hydrolyzed by Bush group 1–inducible chromosomal β-lactamases and by extended-spectrum β-lactamases, it is not active against strains of Enterobacteriaceae that produce these β-lactamases. Cefotaxime is metabolized in the liver to desacetyl cefotaxime, a less active metabolite that may act synergistically with cefotaxime. Though metabolized in the liver, cefotaxime is excreted by the kidneys. High serum and tissue concentrations of cefotaxime can be achieved at the recommended dosages. The rapid development of resistance of gram-negative enteric bacilli when cefotaxime was used extensively for initial treatment of neonatal sepsis raised concern that extensive use of newer cephalosporins in the nursery or intensive care units might lead to more rapid emergence of drug-resistant bacteria than had been identified with the traditional regimens of a penicillin and an aminoglycoside. Because of its broad spectrum of activity against many of the common pathogens causing pediatric infections, cefotaxime is used widely for inpatient treatment of lower respiratory tract infections, urinary tract infections, sepsis, intra-abdominal infections, bone and joint infections, and meningitis or ventriculitis caused by susceptible organisms.

CEFTIZOXIME. Ceftizoxime is a parenteral agent with a spectrum of activity similar to that of cefotaxime, except that it has better activity against *B. fragilis.* Its safety and efficacy have not been established for infants younger than 6 months, and it rarely is used in pediatrics.

CEFTRIAXONE. The antibacterial spectrum of ceftriaxone is similar to that of cefotaxime, with activity against group A streptococci, penicillin-susceptible pneumococci, *H. influenzae, Neisseria* spp., and many members of the Enterobacteriaceae. The activity of ceftriaxone and cefotaxime against methicillin-susceptible *S. aureus* is inconsistent; neither should be used as empiric monotherapy for infections presumed to be caused by staphylococci. Ceftriaxone is not active against most strains of *Pseudomonas.* It differs from cefotaxime in its pharmacokinetic properties. Ceftriaxone undergoes extensive protein binding and has a long serum half-life. Because of its broad spectrum of activity against many of the pathogens that commonly cause sepsis, meningitis, and respiratory tract infections in older infants and children, along with its unique pharmacokinetic features, ceftriaxone has been used excessively for outpatient management of febrile infants and young children being evaluated for possible systemic bacterial infection. Single-dose therapy was approved for the treatment of acute otitis media in 1997; a 3-day regimen is recommended as alternative therapy for refractory cases.[71, 136]

Ceftriaxone is effective for various sexually transmitted diseases, including chancroid, proctitis, epididymitis (in combination with doxycycline), and different forms of gonococcal disease (neonatal ophthalmia); for uncomplicated urethral, endocervical, rectal, or pharyngeal gonorrhea (in combination with doxycycline for treatment of possible coexisting chlamydial infection); and for disseminated gonococcal infection, meningitis, or endocarditis.[99] Ceftriaxone therapy for 5 days is comparable in effectiveness to conventional chloramphenicol therapy for typhoid fever in children.[172] However, short-course treatment may result in confirmed bacteriologic relapse in children with multidrug-resistant strains of *Salmonella typhi.*[20] A 14-day regimen of ceftriaxone is equally effective as a 21-day course of oral doxycycline for clinical cure of acute disseminated Lyme disease without meningitis in children older than 8 years and adults.[62] Although third-generation cephalosporins have been used for empiric treatment of nosocomial pneumonia, wound infections, and urinary tract infections caused by gram-negative bacteria, administering an aminoglycoside instead of or in addition to a third-generation cephalosporin is often prudent because of the risk of encountering plasmid-mediated extended-spectrum β-lactamase resistance or inducing the expression of chromosomal-mediated β-lactamases.

For infections requiring prolonged therapy (e.g., septic arthritis, osteomyelitis, brain abscess) and caused by susceptible organisms, ceftriaxone therapy is cost-effective for use outside the hospital. Once the acute signs of disease have diminished and the child remains in the hospital for only parenteral therapy, discharge and once-daily administration of ceftriaxone in the home or clinic can be considered.

Because of its extensive protein binding, ceftriaxone can displace bilirubin from albumin-binding sites, although to date no evidence of adverse clinical effects has been reported. Cefotaxime is administered to neonates more often than ceftriaxone is because of considerably more information about its safety and the potential but unproven risk of kernicterus. Ceftriaxone is excreted and concentrated in bile. Gallbladder "sludge" diagnosed by abdominal sonography (and not identifiable by other radiographic techniques) has been demonstrated in some patients who received ceftriaxone. The material appears to be a calcium-ceftriaxone complex and resolves with cessation of the drug. Most patients with ceftriaxone-associated "sludge" are asymptomatic, but occasionally, patients have symptoms of gallbladder disease, and incidents of acute cholecystitis occurring in a few children have been reported.

CEFTAZIDIME. When compared with cefotaxime and ceftriaxone, ceftazidime has poor antibacterial activity against *S. aureus,* is less active against penicillin-susceptible *S. pneumoniae,* is slightly less active against group A streptococci, but is more active against *P. aeruginosa.* On a weight basis, ceftazidime is the most effective of all β-lactam antimicrobial agents in vitro against *P. aeruginosa.* It is frequently active in vitro against *P. aeruginosa* strains that are resistant to antipseudomonal penicillins. Resistance to ceftazidime can develop in gram-negative bacteria by the production of extended-spectrum β-lactamases or because of decreased bacterial cell permeability, as seen with *P. aeruginosa, Acinetobacter,* and some *Serratia* strains. Ceftazidime is indicated for use in infections that are suspected to be caused by *Pseudomonas,* including acute exacerbations of chronic pulmonary infections in cystic fibrosis patients, chronic suppurative otitis media or malignant otitis externa, and febrile illnesses in neutropenic cancer patients.

CEFIXIME. Cefixime has a vinyl group instead of a chlorine atom at position 3 of the cephem nucleus and an aminothiazole oxime group rather than a phenyl glycine side chain. These biochemical changes result in potent gram-negative activity. Cefixime was introduced in 1989 as an oral third-generation cephalosporin with a broad spectrum of activity, including activity against group A streptococci, *H. influenzae, M. catarrhalis,* penicillin-susceptible *S. pneumoniae,* and many members of the Enterobacteriaceae, including *Shigella, Salmonella, E. coli, Klebsiella,* and *P. mirabilis.*[13] Cefixime, like ceftibuten, is distinguished from other extended-spectrum oral cephalosporins by its lack of activity against *S. aureus.* It is also inactive against *P. aeruginosa, Serratia, Enterobacter,* and *Citrobacter freundii.* Although cefixime has in vitro activity against penicillin-susceptible pneumococci, lower bacteriologic cure rates occurred with cefixime than with amoxicillin when used to treat children with pneumococcal acute otitis media.[111] Cefixime is highly resistant to degradation by β-lactamases. Administration of cefixime is facilitated by once-daily dosing,[76] pleasant taste, and stability of the suspension at room temperature. Cefixime is effective therapy for uncomplicated gonorrhea, uncomplicated urinary tract infections caused by *E. coli* or *P. mirabilis,* shigellosis, and acute otitis media or sinusitis caused by *H. influenzae* or *M. catarrhalis.*[25] Clinical studies indicate that the rate of laboratory-confirmed eradication of *Shigella sonnei* in an epidemic setting is higher with a 5-day than with a 2-day cefixime regimen,[154] cefixime alone is equally effective as sequential therapy with intravenous and oral antibiotics in selected febrile infants with urinary tract infections,[108] and a 14-day cefixime regimen for treatment of multidrug-resistant *S. typhi* septicemia in children has efficacy comparable to that of a 5-day course of ceftriaxone therapy.[92] Cefixime is not recommended for the treatment of infections frequently caused by staphylococci, such as skin or soft tissue infections, and it is not the most effective agent for the treatment of pneumococcal infections. The safety and efficacy of cefixime have not been established for infants younger than 6 months.

CEFPODOXIME PROXETIL. The antibacterial activity of cefpodoxime proxetil is similar to that of cefixime, with the exception of improved activity against staphylococci. Cefpodoxime is active against group A streptococci; penicillin-susceptible pneumococci; β-lactamase–producing strains of *N. gonorrhoeae, H. influenzae,* and *M. catarrhalis;* methicillin- susceptible *S. aureus;* and many members of the Enterobacteriaceae. It is not active against *Enterobacter, Pseudomonas, Serratia,* or *Morganella.* Cefpodoxime proxetil, the ester prodrug of cefpodoxime, is cleaved by intestinal esterases to the active drug. Oral absorption is increased by the presence of food. Because of its longer serum half-life, cefpodoxime proxetil can be administered in twice-daily dosing intervals. Cefpodoxime is hydrolyzed by some extended-spectrum β-lactamases. The unfavorable palatability of cefpodoxime proxetil may adversely affect compliance.[232]

Treatment of group A streptococcal pharyngitis with a 5-day cefpodoxime proxetil regimen is equivalent to therapy with penicillin V and has been approved for this indication by the FDA.[60] A 5-day regimen is approved for the treatment of acute otitis media based on clinical outcomes that are comparable or superior to therapy with amoxicillin-clavulanate, cefaclor, or cefixime.[49] Cefpodoxime is not likely to be effective for the treatment of acute otitis media caused by penicillin-nonsusceptible pneumococci because of its unfavorable pharmacodynamic parameters.[251] It also has been approved for outpatient treatment of community-acquired respiratory tract infections, uncomplicated urinary tract infections, and mild skin and skin structure infections. The safety and efficacy of cefpodoxime proxetil have not been established for infants younger than 2 months.

CEFTIBUTEN. Ceftibuten was approved by the FDA for pediatric use in 1995. The primary active component is formulated as a *cis*-isomer that is converted in serum to the less active *trans*-isomer. The chemical structure and spectrum of antimicrobial activity are similar to those of cefixime. Ceftibuten, like cefixime, is distinguished from other extended-spectrum oral cephalosporins by its lack of activity against *S. aureus.* Its antimicrobial activity against groups A, C, F, and G beta-hemolytic streptococci is good, whereas its activity against groups B and D, as well as viridans streptococci, is poor. Ceftibuten exhibits MICs for penicillin-susceptible pneumococci in the susceptible range, whereas penicillin-nonsusceptible strains are ceftibuten-resistant. When compared with other oral cephalosporins, ceftibuten is the most stable to hydrolysis by β-lactamases produced by Neisseriaceae, *Moraxella, Haemophilus,* and Enterobacteriaceae, including most strains of *E. coli* and *K. pneumoniae* that produce plasmid-mediated extended-spectrum β-lactamases of the TEM, SHV, and OXA types. Ceftibuten is variably active against strains of *Citrobacter, Serratia,* and *Morganella* but it is inactive against *Acinetobacter, Pseudomonas, Enterobacter, Bordetella,* and anaerobic species. It is also a weak inducer of AmpC Bush group 1 β-lactamases produced by *Serratia marcescens, Enterobacter cloacae,* and *Enterobacter aerogenes.*[97]

Ceftibuten has excellent bioavailability and a favorable pharmacokinetic profile that facilitates a once-daily dosing schedule.[12] Ten-day treatment regimens have been approved for streptococcal tonsillopharyngitis and acute otitis media caused by *H. influenzae, M. catarrhalis,* or *S. pyogenes* because of superior clinical and microbiologic efficacy data for ceftibuten in comparison to penicillin V in children with streptococcal tonsillopharyngitis[197] and comparable clinical efficacy data for ceftibuten versus amoxicillin, amoxicillin-clavulanate, cefaclor, and cefprozil for the treatment of children with clinically defined acute otitis media with or without effusion. However, cumulative data from clinical trials indicate that microbiologic cure rates of pneumococcal otitis media are lower for ceftibuten than for comparable antimicrobial agents.[97] Because of the increased prevalence of nonsusceptible *S. pneumoniae* isolates, ceftibuten has almost no place in the treatment of acute otitis media, especially in young or otherwise at-risk infants and children. Ceftibuten also should be considered as alternative therapy for sinusitis caused by susceptible organisms. Furthermore, ceftibuten achieved equivalent clinical success and superior bacterial eradication than TMP-SMX did in the treatment of complicated or recurrent urinary tract infections in children.[11] Adverse reactions to ceftibuten, which are limited mainly to the gastrointestinal tract, occur in approximately 10 percent of children, a rate similar to comparable oral β-lactam antibiotics. The safety and efficacy of ceftibuten have not been established for infants younger than 6 months.

CEFDINIR. Cefdinir was approved in 1999 for the treatment of acute otitis media in children. It has a broad spectrum of in vitro antimicrobial activity, favorable pharmacokinetics, a convenient once- or twice-daily dosage schedule, superior palatability, a low rate of adverse events, and proven clinical efficacy against common childhood pathogens.[128] When compared with cephalexin, cefaclor, cefuroxime, cefixime, and cefpodoxime, cefdinir has equivalent or superior MICs for groups A, B, C, F, and G streptococci, viridans streptococci, and methicillin-susceptible staphylococci. Its in vitro activity against penicillin-susceptible and penicillin-nonsusceptible strains of *S. pneumoniae* is equivalent to that of cefuroxime and cefpodoxime but superior to that of other oral cephalosporins. Cefixime and cefpodoxime have superior activity against *H. influenzae* (including β-lactamase–producing strains), whereas cefdinir and cefuroxime have comparable activity against this pathogen. The activity of cefdinir against *M. catarrhalis* is similar to that of cefixime, cefpodoxime, and cefuroxime but superior to that of earlier-generation cephalosporins. Cefdinir is stable to hydrolysis by some Enterobacteriaceae produced β-lactamases. However, activity against these pathogens is variable. Cefdinir is inactive against strains of enterococci, methicillin-resistant staphylococci, *P. aeruginosa, Acinetobacter, Enterobacter, Citrobacter, Serratia, Stenotrophomonas, Listeria, Legionella,* and most anaerobes.[98]

Based on comparative clinical and microbiologic efficacy trials, administration of cefdinir should be considered for (1) children with acute bacterial otitis media caused by β-lactamase–positive or β-lactamase–negative strains of *H. influenzae* and *M. catarrhalis* or penicillin-susceptible or penicillin-intermediate resistant strains of *S. pneumoniae* as either a 5- or 10-day regimen; cefdinir has efficacy equivalent to that of cefuroxime and cefpodoxime but superior palatability and therefore should be considered as an alternative to other second-line regimens that include amoxicillin-clavulanate or three single daily doses of parenteral ceftriaxone if treatment with amoxicillin has failed[71, 128]; (2) group A streptococcal tonsillopharyngitis in 5- or 10-day dosage schedules[196]; (3) acute maxillary sinusitis caused by susceptible organisms; and (4) uncomplicated skin and skin structure infections caused by *S. aureus* or group A streptococci. The safety and efficacy of cefdinir have not been established for infants younger than 6 months.

CEFDITOREN PIVOXIL. Cefditoren pivoxil was approved by the FDA in 2002 for oral treatment of acute exacerbations of chronic bronchitis, pharyngitis, tonsillitis, and uncomplicated skin and soft tissue infections in adults and children aged 12 years or older. Cefditoren is similar to cefdinir and cefpodoxime in its antibacterial activity. However, cefditoren has the greatest in vitro antimicrobial activity of all oral cephalosporins against *S. pneumoniae.* The inactive metabolite pivalate is eliminated by the kidneys in combination with carnitine as pivaloylcarnitine. Although cefditoren transiently decreases serum concentrations of carnitine, the clinical significance of this is not clear, but no adverse effects have been reported.

FOURTH-GENERATION CEPHALOSPORINS

CEFEPIME. Cefepime, the prototypic agent of this class of antibiotics, was approved by the FDA in 1996. It is distinguished from other cephalosporins by the following characteristics: rapid penetration of outer-membrane porins into the periplasmic space of gram-negative bacteria, facilitated by its net neutral charge; enhanced stability against hydrolysis by inducible or constitutively expressed chromosomal-mediated AmpC Bush group 1 β-lactamases and plasmid-mediated SHV- and TEM-type extended-spectrum β-lactamases; and increased binding affinity to multiple PBPs. These factors contribute to cefepime's expanded spectrum of activity and improved efficacy against gram-negative pathogens when compared with third-generation cephalosporins.

The in vitro activity of cefepime encompasses a broad range of gram-positive and gram-negative organisms, including methicillin-susceptible staphylococci; more than 80 percent of penicillin-resistant strains of *S. pneumoniae*; viridans streptococci; most strains of Enterobacteriaceae, including most notably, extended-spectrum β-lactamase–producing strains of *E. coli* and *K. pneumoniae;* and AmpC-mediated resistant *Enterobacter* spp. and *Citrobacter* spp., as well as *P. aeruginosa.* Furthermore, bacteria in which resistance to third-generation cephalosporins develops by means of single-step mutations usually remain susceptible to cefepime. Clinical and laboratory data also indicate that selection of cefepime resistance, specifically among *Enterobacter* spp. and *P. aeruginosa,* is rare. As with other cephalosporins, cefepime is inactive against enterococci, methicillin-resistant staphylococci, *S. maltophilia,* and many anaerobic organisms.[124]

Cefepime is indicated for the parenteral treatment of lower respiratory tract, urinary tract, skin and skin structure, and intra-abdominal (in combination with anaerobic antibacterial agents) infections, as well as for empiric monotherapy in pediatric cancer patients with fever and neutropenia. In comparative clinical and microbiologic efficacy trials, cefepime as a single antibacterial agent was equivalent to third-generation cephalosporins for the most common childhood pathogens. In addition, cefepime is as safe and well tolerated, as are other cephalosporin antibiotics.[33, 177, 222]

Cefepime should be reserved for complicated community-acquired, nosocomial, or polymicrobial infections, penicillin-resistant and third-generation cephalosporin–resistant pathogens, and patients with cystic fibrosis and *P. aeruginosa* lung infections. Cefepime concentrations in CSF reach approximately 3 to 6 μg/mL (9% of the peak plasma concentration) in children with bacterial meningitis. Therefore, achievable CSF concentrations exceed the MICs of common CNS pathogens by at least 10-fold, except for penicillin- and cephalosporin-resistant *S. pneumoniae.*[29] Currently, data are insufficient to recommend cefepime as single-agent therapy for meningitis caused by penicillin- and cephalosporin-resistant *S. pneumoniae.* The safety and efficacy of cefepime have not been established for neonates.

ADVERSE EFFECTS

The cephalosporins, like the penicillins, are safe for children and have almost no dose-related toxicity. The most common reactions are local ones, including pain at the injection site or thrombophlebitis with parenteral administration, and mild gastrointestinal complaints with oral dosing. Hypersensitivity reactions occur in approximately 1 to 3 percent of treatment courses and include morbilliform rash, urticaria, and pruritus. Anaphylaxis is rare in children. Drug fever has been associated with the administration of cephalosporin. Nonspecific antibiotic-associated diarrhea and, less commonly, *C. difficile* toxin–mediated colitis can occur after cephalosporin use.

Other adverse effects are rare, and some are unique to one or a few cephalosporins. Physicians should be alert for uncommon reactions, including reversible neutropenia, which can occur after prolonged use of high-dosage cephalosporins, Coombs-positive hemolytic anemia, and bleeding. Altered hemostasis because of hypoprothrombinemia can result when using any cephalosporin that contains a methylthiotetrazole side chain (cefamandole, cefotetan, and moxalactam). These agents act as competitive inhibitors of vitamin K–dependent carboxylase, which converts clotting factors II, VII, IX, and X to their active forms. These methylthiotetrazole antibiotics also have been associated with a disulfiram-like (Antabuse) response in patients drinking alcoholic beverages. Nephrotoxicity has been reported in adults who received cephalothin combined with gentamicin[14]; however, whether cephalosporins can potentiate aminoglycoside nephrotoxicity remains uncertain.[153] Nephrotoxicity is a rare complication of the currently available cephalosporins. Gallbladder sludging, biliary pseudolithiasis, and symptomatic obstructive biliary disease rarely have been associated with the administration of ceftriaxone.[265]

The cephalosporins may produce allergic reactions similar to those caused by the penicillins. Cross-sensitization exists among the cephalosporins, and allergy to one cephalosporin implies allergy to all. Various degrees of immunologic cross-reaction of penicillins and cephalosporins have been demonstrated in vitro and in animal models.[194] Previously quoted studies have suggested that the frequency of allergic reactions to cephalosporins ranges from 5.4 to 16.5 percent in adult patients with a history of penicillin allergy and from 1 to 2.5 percent in those without such a history. The incidence of hypersensitivity to unrelated drugs is increased in some patients who are allergic to penicillin, thus suggesting that excipients in antibiotic preparations may be responsible for these reactions. Consequently, whether a penicillin-allergic patient reacts to a cephalosporin because of cross-allergenicity is uncertain.[219] Most patients who are thought to be allergic to penicillin receive cephalosporins without adverse reaction. Although a cephalosporin may be used with caution as an alternative to penicillin in children who have an ambiguous history of rash, cephalosporins should be avoided in patients with a known immediate or accelerated reaction to a penicillin. Currently, skin testing to evaluate for cephalosporin hypersensitivity is not possible because the potential cephalosporin haptens are unknown and no standardized antigen exists.

An unusual serum sickness–like reaction has been reported in children who received cefaclor. A generalized pruritic rash, similar to erythema multiforme, developed in some cases along with fever, purpura, and arthritis with pain and swelling in the knees and ankles. The signs appeared 5 to 19 days after the start of therapy and generally disappeared within 4 to 5 days after discontinuing use of the drug. The children had no previous history of allergy to a penicillin or cephalosporin.[176] Three hundred eleven cases, including 289 children, were reported to the manufacturer by 1982. At that time, approximately 3 million courses of cefaclor had been administered, which suggested a minimal (considering the likelihood of underreporting) incidence of 1 reaction per 10,000 courses.* Levine[138] compared adverse reactions in children who received cefaclor (1017 patients, 2513 courses) or amoxicillin (1009 patients, 2358 courses). Serum sickness (defined as arthritis/arthralgia plus a rash or urticaria) or erythema multiforme occurred in 11 children (1.1%) who received cefaclor but in none of those who received amoxicillin. Recent studies suggest that serum sickness–like reactions to cefaclor are associated with lymphocyte sensitization.[122]

*Data provided by J. Getty, Marketing Plans Manager, Eli Lilly Co., and published in *Pediatric Infectious Disease Newsletter,* edited by J. D. Nelson and G. H. McCracken, Jr., May/June 1982, Vol. 8, No. 3.

Carbacephems

Carbacephems have a carbon atom at position 1 of the dihydrothiazine ring (cephem nucleus) rather than a sulfur atom. The only carbacephem currently available is loracarbef. Loracarbef is structurally similar to cefaclor but has greater chemical stability in solution. The antibacterial spectrum of loracarbef is similar to that of second-generation cephalosporins. When compared with cefaclor, loracarbef has similar activity against penicillin-susceptible pneumococci, group A streptococci, and methicillin-susceptible *S. aureus* and greater activity against *H. influenzae* and *M. catarrhalis,* including β-lactamase–producing strains.[70] Loracarbef is not active against *P. aeruginosa, Enterobacter, Citrobacter,* indole-positive *Proteus,* or *B. fragilis.*

Loracarbef is more stable than cefaclor to hydrolysis by β-lactamases but can be hydrolyzed by extended-spectrum β-lactamases. Loracarbef is available for oral administration only. It is absorbed rapidly and well; however, absorption is decreased when taken with food. Loracarbef has a longer serum half-life than some of the penicillins do and can be given twice daily. It is excreted by the kidneys. Loracarbef is relatively well tolerated. Gastrointestinal complaints, including diarrhea, nausea, and vomiting, are the adverse effects most frequently reported, but they occur in less than 5 percent of treatment courses. The safety and efficacy of loracarbef have not been established for infants younger than 6 months.

Loracarbef can be used as an alternative to penicillin or erythromycin for the treatment of group A streptococcal pharyngitis.[69] The effectiveness of loracarbef is similar to that of amoxicillin and amoxicillin-clavulanate for the treatment of acute otitis media caused by susceptible bacteria.[83] It is not effective against penicillin-nonsusceptible pneumococci. For the treatment of mild to moderate skin and skin structure infections, the efficacy of loracarbef is comparable to that of cefaclor.[103] It has been approved for use in the treatment of acute bacterial sinusitis and uncomplicated urinary tract infections caused by susceptible bacteria.

Monobactams

Aztreonam is the prototype monobactam, a name that refers to the unique monocyclic nucleus. It has aerobic, gram-negative antibacterial activity similar to that of ceftazidime, but it has no significant gram-positive activity. Unlike most β-lactam antibiotics, aztreonam has the advantage of not inducing β-lactamase activity, and its molecular structure confers a high degree of stability to hydrolysis by β-lactamases. Although it is a β-lactam, aztreonam is weakly immunogenic and can be used in patients with minor forms of β-lactam allergy. Its use in pediatrics is indicated as a secondary agent for the intravenous treatment of lower respiratory tract, skin and soft tissue, urinary tract, and intra-abdominal infections caused by susceptible pathogens. Higher doses of aztreonam may be warranted for pediatric patients with cystic fibrosis. The safety and efficacy of aztreonam have not been established for infants younger than 9 months or for children with impaired renal function.

Carbapenems

Carbapenems differ from penicillin by virtue of the substitution of a sulfur atom by a carbon atom at position 1 of the β-lactam ring and possession of an unsaturated bond between carbon atoms at positions 2 and 3 in the structure. The carbapenem class of antimicrobial agents exhibits the broadest spectrum of activity of all β-lactam antibiotics; they are active against most clinically significant gram-positive and gram-negative pathogens, including anaerobic organisms. Because they are acid-labile in the stomach, they must be administered parenterally.[55]

IMIPENEM-CILASTATIN. Imipenem-cilastatin was the first carbapenem evaluated for the treatment of severe bacterial infections in children. Extensive hydrolysis of imipenem by dehydropeptidase I in the proximal renal tubule results in the production of a potentially nephrotoxic inactive metabolite. Consequently, imipenem must be administered with cilastatin, an inhibitor of dehydropeptidase I. Despite favorable in vitro efficacy against a broad spectrum of bacterial pathogens, the clinical suitability of this antibiotic is limited because of the drug's epileptogenic potential, especially in children with bacterial meningitis. Imipenem causes seizures presumably by acting as a competitive inhibitor of γ-aminobutyric acid, an inhibitory neurotransmitter.[55] Imipenem-cilastatin is indicated for children with severe non-CNS infections caused by susceptible organisms. The dose must be reduced for children with impaired renal function. With the advent of meropenem, imipenem-cilastatin is used less frequently in pediatrics.

MEROPENEM. Meropenem was approved for use in children in 1996. It is structurally related to imipenem. However, it is more stable against degradation by renal dehydropeptidase I and, therefore, does not require coadministration with cilastatin. On the basis of its superior safety and efficacy, meropenem generally is considered the preferred carbapenem for treatment of childhood infections.

MECHANISMS OF ACTION

As with other β-lactam antibiotics, meropenem is bactericidal against susceptible bacteria because it inhibits bacterial cell wall synthesis. The *trans* configuration of the hydroxyethyl side chain and hydrogen atoms protect the parent β-lactam structure from inactivation by the most common β-lactamases, including AmpC Bush group 1–inducible cephalosporinases produced by strains of *Enterobacter, Serratia, Citrobacter,* and *Pseudomonas* and the extended-spectrum β-lactamases commonly found in *E. coli* and *Klebsiella* spp. In addition, the pyrrolidine side chain enhances the compound's antipseudomonal activity.[28]

MECHANISMS OF RESISTANCE

Resistance may be intrinsic or acquired and is mediated by numerous mechanisms: (1) some strains of *P. aeruginosa* are deficient in the cell wall porin proteins that usually facilitate intracellular penetration; (2) efflux pumps in some gram-negative bacteria are capable of excreting carbapenems; (3) *S. multophilia* and some other gram-negative pathogens possess uncommon metallo-β-lactamases (Bush groups 3a and 3b) and clavulanic acid–inhibited carbapenemases (group 2f) that are mediated by transferable R-plasmids; and (4) methicillin-resistant *S. aureus* strains and *E. faecium* have altered PBPs, which accounts for their inherent resistance.[32, 115] At present, the risk of a single-step spontaneous mutation causing resistance among *Pseudomonas* spp. appears to be low.

IN VITRO ACTIVITY

Meropenem has equivalent or slightly less in vitro potency than imipenem does against gram-positive pathogens, but it is significantly more active against gram-negative organisms. Its spectrum of activity encompasses streptococci (excluding some strains of penicillin-resistant *S. pneumoniae),* methicillin-susceptible staphylococci, ampicillin-susceptible enterococci, *L. monocytogenes, H. influenzae, N. meningitidis,* Enterobacteriaceae, most strains of *P. aeruginosa,* and anaerobes (including β-lactamase–positive strains of *B. fragilis).* Pathogens resistant to meropenem are *Stenotrophomonas,* methicillin-resistant *S. aureus, E. faecium,* and some strains of *Pseudomonas* and *S. pneumoniae.*[32] In vitro tests indicate that meropenem acts synergistically with aminoglycoside antibiotics against some isolates of *P. aeruginosa.*[115]

PHARMACOKINETICS. Meropenem exhibits nearly linear pharmacokinetics, which indicates that increases in dosage result in approximately proportional increases in the peak plasma concentration and area under the plasma concentration-time curve (AUC).[26] Only 2 percent of the drug is bound to plasma proteins, and the drug is distributed widely into tissues and fluids.[55] The elimination half-life declines with increasing age (premature neonates, 2.9 hours; term neonates, 2 hours; children, 1.1 hours; adults, 1 hour) and is longer than that for imipenem. Because meropenem is cleared primarily by glomerular filtration, the dosage should be reduced in children with renal dysfunction.[32] Furthermore, meropenem is cleared efficiently by hemodialysis; therefore, it should be administered after the patient undergoes this procedure. Pharmacodynamic studies indicate that a favorable bacteriologic outcome is best predicted by the duration of the dosing interval for which the meropenem plasma concentration exceeds the MIC_{90} of the target pathogen.[55] Accordingly, a dose of 20 mg/kg every 8 hours achieves optimal plasma concentrations (50 to 60 μg/mL) for systemic infections that do not involve the CNS,[28] whereas 40 mg/kg every 8 hours is recommended for patients with cystic fibrosis because of accelerated drug excretion.[109] Penetration of meropenem through inflamed meninges is approximately 8 percent of the mean plasma concentration. Consequently, a dose of 40 mg/kg every 8 hours is required to achieve mean peak CSF concentrations of 0.9 to 6.5 μg/mL and to ensure effective treatment of bacterial meningitis.[55, 59, 191] An every-12-hour administration schedule is probably appropriate for neonates because of their immature renal function.[26]

INDICATIONS FOR USE

The FDA has approved meropenem as monotherapy for susceptible organisms causing intra-abdominal infections and bacterial meningitis in children older than 2 months. Meropenem should be reserved for the treatment of cephalosporin-resistant nosocomial pathogens, severe polymicrobial infections with favorable susceptibility profiles, and infections that fail to respond to other antimicrobial agents. Meropenem monotherapy has clinical and microbiologic efficacy equivalent to that of third-generation cephalosporin-based regimens for septicemia and infections of the CNS, abdominal cavity, lower respiratory tract, urinary tract, and skin.[34, 129, 191] In addition, meropenem monotherapy has been shown to be equivalent to ceftazidime and amikacin for empiric treatment of febrile children with neutropenia.[51] Clinical efficacy against cephalosporin-resistant pathogens also has been demonstrated in patients with cystic fibrosis.[109] In view of increasing resistance of pneumococci to β-lactam antibiotics, some experts recommend co-administration of vancomycin with meropenem for empiric treatment of meningitis caused by gram-positive cocci until susceptibility to meropenem can be confirmed and CSF can be re-evaluated. Combination therapy with aminoglycosides should be considered for suspected or proven *P. aeruginosa* infections in view of emerging resistant strains and potential antibiotic synergy. The effectiveness of meropenem for neonatal infections has been assessed in small noncomparative studies that demonstrated a favorable clinical response in neonates who previously had failed conventional therapy.[115]

ADVERSE EFFECTS

Data from well-designed clinical trials indicate that meropenem has clinical and laboratory adverse event profiles that are equivalent to those of comparable antibiotic regimens. In contrast to treatment with imipenem-cilastatin, no increased risk of seizures exists in children with or without meningitis who are treated with meropenem,[129] presumably because meropenem has less affinity than imipenem does for the γ-aminobutyric acid receptor. Meropenem can be given intravenously as small-volume bolus injections (over a course of 3 to 5 minutes) without inducing nausea or vomiting. The most common adverse reactions include diarrhea (4%), rash (2%), and vomiting (1%).[32]

β-Lactam Antibiotics Not Approved for Use in Children

Several β-lactam antibiotics are available in the United States, but they are not approved for use in children. These agents include cefonicid, a second-generation cephalosporin; cefotetan, a cephamycin; and cefoperazone, a third-generation cephalosporin. New cephalosporins such as cefpirome are undergoing clinical investigation.

VANCOMYCIN

Vancomycin, first isolated from *Amycolatopsis orientalis* (formerly called *Streptomyces,* then *Nocardia)* in soil samples from Borneo, is a high-molecular-weight, complex, soluble glycopeptide.[195] Because of a lack of adequate therapy for penicillinase-producing staphylococci, it was approved expeditiously by the FDA in 1956 before exhaustive pharmacologic and toxicologic studies had been performed. Once the penicillinase-resistant penicillins were developed, vancomycin no longer was indispensable until the emergence of methicillin-resistant staphylococci in the late 1970s.

MECHANISMS OF ACTION

Vancomycin is bactericidal against most susceptible gram-positive bacteria except for enterococci, for which it is bacteriostatic. Its major mechanism of action involves prevention of polymerization of the phosphodisaccharide-pentapeptide-lipid complex during the second stage of peptidoglycan cell wall synthesis. Because its site of action is distinct from that of β-lactam antibiotics, no cross-resistance between the drugs and no competitive inhibition exist. Additionally, vancomycin alters cytoplasmic membrane permeability and impairs RNA synthesis. In vitro studies suggest that it exhibits concentration-independent/time-dependent bactericidal activity against susceptible organisms, similar to that of β-lactams.[72, 139] A lag phase before the onset of rapid killing has been demonstrated in serum-killing studies.[3]

MECHANISMS OF RESISTANCE

Resistance can be categorized into three types: tolerance, acquired resistance, and inherent resistance. Some susceptible gram-positive bacteria, especially enterococci, are tolerant to the bactericidal activity of vancomycin; that is, vancomycin inhibits but does not kill the bacteria (MBC/MIC ratio >32). Staphylococci tolerant to vancomycin can have autolysin deficiencies. Although most resistance to vancomycin by gram-positive bacteria is acquired, three genera of gram-positive organisms are inherently resistant to vancomycin: *Erysipelothrix, Leuconostoc,* and *Pediococcus.* Five genes code for acquired vancomycin resistance in enterococci: *VanA, VanB, VanC, VanD,* and *VanE.*[175] The mechanism of resistance has been characterized best for the *VanA* cluster of genes. The presence of an inducer such as vancomycin or teicoplanin, another glycopeptide that has not been approved for use in the United States, activates the transcription of genes that encode ligases necessary for resistance to vancomycin. Some enzymes make cell wall precursors ending in D-alanyl-D-lactate located at the end of the pentapeptide side chain, to which vancomycin binds with very low affinity. Other enzymes inhibit or alter the synthesis of endogenous cell wall precursors ending in D-alanyl-D-alanine, to which vancomycin is unable to bind. Vancomycin resistance genes can be transferred experimentally among enterococci and other gram-positive pathogens. This finding highlights the potential risk of spread of resistance by means of naturally occurring plasmid- or transposon-mediated conjugative systems.[175] Although vancomycin resistance can affect susceptibility to other investigational glycopeptides, no cross-resistance exists between other unrelated antibiotics. Resistance to vancomycin rarely develops during appropriate therapy, perhaps because of its multiple mechanisms of action, but prolonged or indiscriminate use can contribute to selective pressure resulting in the development of vancomycin-resistant enterococci colonizing the gut. Of greatest concern is the emergence of enterococci resistant to all currently available antibiotics (vancomycin, ampicillin, and high-level aminoglycosides) and spread of vancomycin resistance to pneumococci and staphylococci. Clinical evidence corroborating these concerns was provided when the first cases of glycopeptide-intermediate *S. aureus* (GISA) strains, defined as having MICs of 8 or 16 μg/mL, were detected in the United States in 1997. GISA isolates were found to have thicker extracellular matrices on electron microscopy. However, no evidence was found of gene transfer from enterococci, and the precise mechanism of resistance remains to be elucidated.[149] Pneumococci tolerant to vancomycin were described first in 1999.[190] These strains escape lysis and killing by vancomycin because of an alteration in the regulation of autolysin. Their prevalence is 3 to 8 percent based on several studies, and when etiologic in meningitis, they can be difficult to treat.

IN VITRO ACTIVITY

The in vitro spectrum of activity for vancomycin is limited to gram-positive bacteria, with little if any activity against aerobic or anaerobic gram-negative bacilli except for *Flavobacterium meningosepticum.*[256] Group A streptococci, pneumococci, *Corynebacteria* spp., and *C. difficile* are highly susceptible to vancomycin, whereas *L. monocytogenes,* microaerophilic and anaerobic streptococci, enterococci, staphylococci, *Bacillus anthracis, Lactobacillus, Actinomyces,* and other *Clostridium* spp. have higher MIC values that are still in the susceptible range. The bactericidal activity of vancomycin combined with gentamicin has been shown to be synergistic in vitro against strains of enterococci, nonenterococcal group D streptococci, viridans streptococci, and *S. aureus.* Although vancomycin has activity against many gram-positive bacteria, it is not the most active agent for these organisms, except for multidrug-resistant bacteria such as methicillin-resistant staphylococci and highly penicillin- and cephalosporin-resistant pneumococci. Clinical studies indicate that vancomycin is safe and effective therapy for staphylococcal infections in children.

PHARMACOKINETICS

Intravenous administration of vancomycin is preferred because intramuscular injection causes pain and tissue necrosis. Intravenous preparations must be diluted further in normal saline or dextrose solutions before beginning slow infusion. Vancomycin is approximately 55 percent bound to serum proteins and diffuses well into most body tissues, with adequate concentrations achieved in pericardial, pleural, ascitic, and synovial fluids. Vancomycin does not diffuse well into CSF in the absence of inflamed meninges, but adequate CSF concentrations can be achieved during therapy for meningitis when higher dosages (15 mg/kg every 6 hours) are administered. Intrathecal or intraventricular administration has been used infrequently for CNS infections that are difficult to eradicate.[148] Vancomycin is not metabolized significantly and is excreted by glomerular filtration. The mean serum elimination half-life in adults with normal renal function is 6 hours. For children, it ranges from 5 to 10 hours in newborns, 4 hours in older infants, and 2 to 3 hours in children. In anephric patients, the elimination half-life extends to 7 or more days. Vancomycin is not removed effectively by either peritoneal dialysis or hemodialysis, although cases of increased clearance with recently developed hemodialysis filters have been reported. Nomograms[170] and patient-individualized bayesian dosing regimens[132] have been used for vancomycin dosing in renal failure.

INDICATIONS FOR USE

Because of the possibility of toxicity and the potential for development of resistance, vancomycin should be reserved for patients with moderate to severe infections caused by vancomycin-susceptible bacteria that are resistant to other antibiotics. Vancomycin can be used for the treatment of infections caused by β-lactam– and vancomycin-susceptible bacteria in patients with hypersensitivity reactions to β-lactam antimicrobial agents. Empiric therapy for patients with ventricular shunt– and catheter-associated infections frequently includes vancomycin to provide activity against coagulase-negative staphylococci. Vancomycin can be used in combination with gentamicin or streptomycin for bactericidal synergistic activity to treat methicillin-resistant staphylococcal endocarditis or endocarditis caused by high-level penicillin-resistant, aminoglycoside-susceptible strains of enterococci. In addition, vancomycin is the drug of choice in patients with immediate-type hypersensitivity to penicillins and other β-lactam antibiotics for the treatment of endocarditis caused by streptococci, enterococci, and staphylococci.[260] Empiric treatment of bacterial meningitis suspected or proved to be caused by *S. pneumoniae* in children 1 month or older should consist of vancomycin in addition to a third-generation cephalosporin until susceptibility data are available. However, vancomycin need not be used if compelling evidence implicates pathogens other than *S. pneumoniae,* such as the observation of gram-negative diplococci on a CSF smear. Vancomycin also is indicated for the treatment of penicillin-resistant streptococci, *C. jeikeium,* and *Bacillus* spp., as well as for bacteremia, pneumonia, cellulitis, and osteomyelitis caused by methicillin-resistant staphylococci. Although nonabsorbable oral vancomycin is effective therapy for *C. difficile* colitis, oral metronidazole represents first-line therapy; vancomycin should be given only for metronidazole treatment failures to limit the development of vancomycin-resistant enterococci. Vancomycin is among the agents of choice for the treatment of meningitis caused by *F. meningosepticum.*

ADVERSE EFFECTS

The purification of vancomycin allegedly decreased the frequency of adverse reactions noted several decades ago. The most common adverse effect is "red man" or "red neck" syndrome, or glycopeptide-induced anaphylactoid reaction,[198] manifested as flushing of the face and upper part of the trunk and pruritus during vancomycin infusion. Vancomycin directly causes release of histamine from mast cells by non–immune-mediated mechanisms. Because it is a dose- and rate-dependent reaction, administering doses less than 500 mg, prolonging the infusion period to at least 1 hour, or doing both decreases the risk of occurrence. Pretreatment with H_1-receptor antagonists (diphenhydramine, hydroxyzine) prevents its development, and symptoms usually resolve promptly after discontinuation of the infusion. The spectrum of severity ranges from pruritus with a macular rash to hypotension.

Controversy surrounds the issue of vancomycin-induced ototoxicity and nephrotoxicity.[38] Such toxicity has not been demonstrated in experimental animal models. Although numerous cases of toxicity in humans have been reported, the literature is difficult to interpret because of confounding variables, including recent or concurrent use of aminoglycosides or other ototoxic or nephrotoxic agents, lack of identification of antecedent otologic or renal disease, and inconsistencies in sampling methods when measuring serum vancomycin concentrations. Tinnitus and high-tone hearing loss have been associated with the administration of vancomycin, but they are generally reversible after discontinuation. If vancomycin is ototoxic, whether toxic peak or toxic trough serum concentrations are responsible certainly is not clear. Several studies suggest an increased risk of nephrotoxicity when aminoglycosides are used concurrently with vancomycin, especially when administered for longer than 21 days.[93] Other adverse effects seen occasionally with the use of vancomycin include reversible neutropenia, thrombocytopenia, macular rash, and rarely, cardiovascular collapse.

The usefulness of serum vancomycin concentration determinations has been argued because a definitive relationship between vancomycin concentration and either adverse effects or clinical outcome has not been proved.[43, 169] Until the significance of vancomycin serum concentration determinations has been clarified, monitoring has been suggested for the following clinical situations only: (1) patients with altered renal function, including premature infants; (2) patients receiving larger than normal dosages, especially those with meningitis in whom adequate CSF values are necessary; (3) anephric patients undergoing hemodialysis (to avoid sub-therapeutic vancomycin concentrations during prolonged dosing intervals); and (4) patients receiving concomitant therapy with nephrotoxic agents.[169] Further studies evaluating the relationship between serum vancomycin concentrations and clinical outcome and adverse effects are warranted.

AMINOGLYCOSIDES

Aminoglycosides are natural and semisynthetic compounds that consist of at least two amino sugars bound by a glycosidic linkage to a hexose nucleus, the aminocyclitol ring. A more appropriate name would be aminoglycosidic aminocyclitols. Streptomycin, isolated from *Streptomyces griseus,* was the first aminoglycoside and was available for use in 1944. Many aminoglycosides have been isolated or developed since that time. The suffix denotes the origin of the aminoglycoside: those ending with the suffix *-mycin* were derived from *Streptomyces* spp., whereas those ending with *-micin* were derived from *Micromonospora* spp. Currently, eight aminoglycosides are approved for use in the United States (Table 235–7), and several more are available in other countries. Despite the development of less toxic antibiotics with broad-spectrum activity, aminoglycosides continue to fulfill an essential role in the treatment of severe infections caused by aerobic gram-negative bacilli and enterococci.

TABLE 235–7 CLASSIFICATION SCHEME FOR AMINOGLYCOSIDES

Aminocyclitol Ring	Family	Member
Streptidine	Streptomycin	Streptomycin
2-Deoxystreptamine	Kanamycin	Kanamycin Amikacin Tobramycin
2-Deoxystreptamine	Gentamicin	Gentamicin Netilmicin
2-Deoxystreptamine	Neomycin	Neomycin Paromomycin

MECHANISMS OF ACTION

Against susceptible bacteria, aminoglycosides demonstrate rapid, concentration-dependent bactericidal activity.[72, 139] They exert their effect by binding irreversibly to the 30S subunit of the bacterial ribosome, which results in inhibition of protein synthesis and induction of translational errors. Bacterial uptake of aminoglycosides can be facilitated by concomitant therapy with cell wall–active antibiotics such as vancomycin or β-lactams. Extensive research has expanded our understanding of the mechanisms of uptake and action. Penetration of the outer membrane of gram-negative bacteria is mediated by a self-promoted uptake process involving aminoglycoside-induced disruption of magnesium bridges between adjacent lipopolysaccharide molecules. Passage through porin channels is unlikely because of the large size of aminoglycosides. Subsequent transport into cytoplasm plus attachment to the 30S ribosomal subunit requires two energy- and oxygen-dependent steps, energy-dependent phases I and II (EDP-I and EDP-II), that use an electrochemical proton gradient. EDP-I is inhibited by hyperosmolarity, low pH, and anaerobic conditions.[166] Unlike other protein synthesis inhibitors, which are usually bacteriostatic, aminoglycosides are bactericidal. Binding of aminoglycosides to the 30S subunit does not prevent formation of the initiation complex of peptide synthesis. However, it disrupts elongation of the peptide chain by impairing the proofreading process, which results in translational inaccuracy. Aberrant protein products may be inserted in the cell membrane and cause altered permeability. The primed amino sugar and 2-deoxystreptamine groups are essential for the ribosome-specific activity of aminoglycosides.[166]

MECHANISMS OF RESISTANCE

The prevalence of acquired aminoglycoside resistance is relatively low, and its development during therapy is an unusual event. Bacteria can acquire resistance to aminoglycosides because of alterations in the bacterial target, reduced bacterial cell permeability or uptake, or modification of the antibiotic by bacterial enzymes, the last being most significant clinically.[63] Mutations in the aminoglycoside-binding site of the 30S ribosome have been associated with high-level resistance to streptomycin but not to other aminoglycosides, possibly because, unlike streptomycin, they bind to multiple sites on the ribosome. Facultative aerobic bacteria causing infection in sites with reduced oxygen tension, anaerobic bacteria, and such fermentative bacteria as streptococci are inherently resistant to aminoglycosides because they are unable to generate an electrochemical proton gradient sufficient for aminoglycoside transport into the cytoplasm. Other bacteria can acquire resistance because of reduced permeability or lack of transport, as demonstrated in staphylococci, in which resistance to aminoglycosides quickly develops when monotherapy is administered. *P. aeruginosa*, other nonfermenting gram-negative bacilli, and less frequently, members of the Enterobacteriaceae can acquire a moderate level of resistance to all aminoglycosides as a result of various mechanisms that interfere with uptake, cytoplasmic transport, or regulation of the anaerobic respiratory pathway. Plasmid-mediated production of aminoglycoside-modifying enzymes is the most common mechanism of acquired resistance. Many enzymes have different substrate specificities, several of which can be elaborated simultaneously in the same bacterium. These acetyltransferases, nucleotidyltransferases, and phosphotransferases interact with amino or hydroxyl groups on the aminoglycoside and modify the aminoglycoside so that it binds poorly to the 30S ribosome, thereby usually resulting in high-level resistance.[166] Gentamicin and tobramycin each are susceptible to at least five modifying enzymes, whereas amikacin possesses an aminohydroxybutyryl group that prevents enzymatic modification at multiple sites. Consequently, more than 80 percent of gentamicin-resistant strains of Enterobacteriaceae and 25 to 85 percent of gentamicin-resistant *P. aeruginosa* strains are susceptible to amikacin.[130]

IN VITRO ACTIVITY

The in vitro antibacterial spectrum of aminoglycosides includes a wide range of aerobic gram-negative bacilli, many methicillin-susceptible staphylococci, many enterococci, and some mycobacteria.[168] Some gram-negative bacilli, including *Burkholderia cepacia* and *S. maltophilia,* are consistently resistant to all aminoglycosides. The spectrum of activity of gentamicin, tobramycin, and netilmicin is similar, and strains resistant to one are usually resistant to the others. The major advantage of tobramycin is its activity against some strains of *P. aeruginosa* that are resistant to gentamicin and netilmicin. Because many aminoglycoside-modifying enzymes are active against gentamicin, tobramycin, and netilmicin but inactive against amikacin, amikacin frequently is prescribed for empiric treatment of nosocomial gram-negative bacillary infections. Amikacin also has activity against the *Mycobacterium avium* complex (MAC), some rapidly growing mycobacteria, and *Nocardia asteroides.* Netilmicin is less active than other aminoglycosides against *P. aeruginosa,* but it can have activity against some gentamicin-resistant aerobic gram-negative bacilli. Although gentamicin, tobramycin, amikacin, and netilmicin have similar spectra of activity, susceptibility testing is recommended because of geographic and interhospital variation in resistance patterns. Lack of activity against *P. aeruginosa, Klebsiella,* and *Serratia* has limited the use of kanamycin. Streptomycin is inactive against many gram-negative enteric bacilli but does have activity against *Francisella tularensis, Yersinia pestis,* and *Mycobacterium tuberculosis.*

PHARMACOKINETICS

Aminoglycosides have in common many pharmacokinetic characteristics. They are highly polar, water-soluble compounds that are positively charged cations at neutral pH. Their antibacterial activity is pH-dependent, with increased activity at higher pH. They are relatively resistant to degradation at various temperatures and pH values, but in vitro inactivation after exposure to extended-spectrum penicillins, particularly ticarcillin and carbenicillin, has been described.[255] After parenteral administration, aminoglycosides are distributed rapidly in extracellular body water, with slow accumulation in tissues. The volume of distribution is decreased (with respect to total body weight) in obese patients and increased in patients with illnesses associated with edema, such as severe infections, burns, and ascites. With the exception of proximal renal tubular cells and possibly inner ear hair cells, penetration into other body compartments is impaired because of lipid insolubility, polycationic charge, and size of the aminoglycoside. Proximal renal tubular cells absorb aminoglycosides via carrier-mediated pinocytosis, and as a result, renal cortical concentrations exceed those in plasma. Aminoglycosides do not penetrate the blood-brain barrier in the absence of meningeal inflammation, but with inflammation, approximately 20 to 25 percent of the serum concentration penetrates into CSF. Because of the narrow therapeutic/toxic index, monotherapy for gram-negative bacillary meningitis with aminoglycosides is not recommended. Aminoglycosides are not metabolized and, after parenteral administration, are excreted unchanged in the kidney by glomerular filtration, with approximately 5 percent of excreted drug reabsorbed in the proximal tubular cells. Minimal amounts are excreted in saliva and feces. Urine concentrations exceed those in plasma by 25 to 100 times.

After intramuscular injection, aminoglycosides are absorbed completely and peak serum concentrations are achieved within 90 minutes, except in some disease states that interfere with tissue perfusion, such as hypotension. When administered intravenously, the infusion should be given slowly over the course of 30 to 60 minutes to avoid the development of potential adverse effects. Peak serum concentrations are achieved within 30 to 60 minutes after infusion. Because of their polar nature, absorption after oral administration is insignificant and inadequate to treat systemic infections, but aminoglycosides can accumulate in the presence of renal failure and result in concentrations sufficient to cause toxicity. Although aminoglycosides are nonirritating when instilled into pleural or peritoneal spaces, their absorption is rapid and can result in significant toxicity. In contrast, instillation into the lateral ventricles or irrigation of the bladder has not been associated with significant systemic absorption. When compared with parenteral administration, aerosol administration of aminoglycoside results in higher concentrations in bronchial secretions and less toxicity.[205] Aminoglycosides should not be used topically as ointments or creams because of the rapid development of resistant strains after extensive topical use.

Antimicrobial dosing in newborns and young infants differs from that in older children and adults because of developmental changes in renal function and increased total-body water composition. Neonates and young infants have a larger volume of distribution and a reduced glomerular filtration rate; these differences are more pronounced in very-low-birth-weight premature neonates.[200] Aminoglycoside dosing protocols that incorporate these pharmacokinetic variabilities have been developed, with dosage and dosing intervals based on postconceptual age (gestational age plus postnatal age) rather than postnatal age.[145]

The aminoglycoside dosing schedule currently approved for use in older children and adults incorporates a twice- (streptomycin) or three-times-daily regimen. Several pharmacodynamic features of aminoglycosides may work in concert to allow once-daily dosing. Because aminoglycosides demonstrate concentration-dependent bactericidal activity, higher peak serum concentrations result in more extensive and more rapid killing.[254] Aminoglycosides also demonstrate a post-antibiotic effect against susceptible aerobic gram-negative bacilli in vitro and in vivo,[56, 263] as well as enhanced phagocytosis of aminoglycoside-exposed bacteria in vitro by host leukocytes, referred to as post-antibiotic leukocyte enhancement.[81] The higher the peak serum concentration, the longer the duration of the post-antibiotic effect.[116] When the entire daily dosage of aminoglycoside is administered at one time, a peak serum concentration in the range of 15 to 20 μg/mL can be achieved. In the presence of normal renal function, the serum concentration is low or undetectable before the administration of the next dose, but antibacterial activity continues because of the post-antibiotic effect. In vitro studies,[23] experimental animal models, and clinical studies in adults suggest that once-daily aminoglycoside dosing may be at least as efficacious as traditional dosing for the treatment of some aerobic gram-negative infections.[89] Ototoxicity and nephrotoxicity occurred less frequently in experimental animal models after once-daily administration.[89] Few clinical studies of once-daily aminoglycoside dosing in children exist, but data from the small studies available suggest that efficacy and toxicity are comparable to those seen with traditional dosing schedules.[65, 81] Further clinical studies must be performed, however, before this dosing regimen can be recommended.

INDICATIONS FOR USE

The major use of aminoglycosides in children is for serious infections caused by gram-negative enteric bacilli, including neonatal sepsis, sepsis in a child with malignancy or an immunologic defect, abdominal and systemic infections associated with spillage of fecal contents into the peritoneum, and complicated urinary tract infections. Because gentamicin is the least expensive aminoglycoside and the one with which physicians have the most experience, it often is considered the first-line agent for empiric treatment of suspected aerobic gram-negative bacillary infections in institutions with minimal background resistance. Combinations of an aminoglycoside and a cell wall–active antibiotic have been used for synergistic bactericidal activity. Gentamicin or streptomycin, in combination with penicillin G, ampicillin, or vancomycin, is recommended for the treatment of endocarditis caused by enterococci, viridans streptococci, or *Streptococcus bovis*. Administration of gentamicin for 3 to 5 days, in combination with an antistaphylococcal agent, should be considered for the treatment of staphylococcal endocarditis.[260] Gentamicin or tobramycin combined with ceftazidime or an acylureidopenicillin has been used to treat serious infections caused by *P. aeruginosa*. Amikacin often is used for empiric treatment of nosocomial aerobic gram-negative bacillary infections in institutions with significant resistance to gentamicin and tobramycin. Streptomycin is indicated for use alone or in combination with other antibiotics for the treatment of tularemia and plague and in combination with other agents for the treatment of tuberculosis, brucellosis, and enterococcal endocarditis. Paromomycin is too toxic for parenteral use but, when administered orally, has been useful in the treatment of asymptomatic intestinal amebiasis,[1] *Dientamoeba fragilis, Giardia lamblia* during pregnancy, or cryptosporidiosis in patients with acquired immunodeficiency syndrome (AIDS).[79]

ADVERSE EFFECTS

Although aminoglycosides have intrinsic toxicity, allergic reactions are uncommon. All aminoglycosides can injure the proximal renal tubules, the cochlea, the vestibular apparatus, or a combination thereof and can cause neuromuscular blockade, but the risk varies with each agent. Because aminoglycosides do not induce a significant inflammatory response, pain at intramuscular injection sites and phlebitis at intravenous infusion sites are unusual. Hypersensitivity reactions and drug fever are rare events.

Many theories have been postulated regarding the mechanism of nephrotoxicity,[167] including inhibition of lysosomal phospholipases within the proximal renal tubules.[248] Clinical findings include a mild, nonoliguric decrease in the glomerular filtration rate that is typically reversible. When compared with traditional dosing, once-daily dosing was less nephrotoxic in experimental animal models.[18] Some studies suggest that neomycin is the most nephrotoxic and streptomycin the least nephrotoxic aminoglycoside. In humans, nephrotoxicity has been associated with prolonged duration of therapy at high dosages, previous aminoglycoside therapy, administration of drugs to critically ill patients with intravascular volume depletion or hyponatremia and to those with impaired kidney function, and concomitant administration of other potentially nephrotoxic agents such as amphotericin B and loop diuretics.[66] Debate continues regarding the causal association of these factors to nephrotoxicity and the risk of toxicity with each aminoglycoside.[164] Clearly, factors that increase renal cortical uptake of aminoglycoside, such as the duration of therapy and the dosage regimen, influence the risk of nephrotoxicity.[81, 157]

The mechanism by which aminoglycosides cause vestibular and cochlear ototoxicity has not been elucidated fully. Cochlear damage is manifested as tinnitus or high-frequency hearing loss, whereas vestibular toxicity is associated with vertigo, nystagmus, and ataxia.[7] Damage can be unilateral or bilateral. Occasionally, the ototoxicity is reversible, but permanent damage occurs commonly. Mild cochlear damage may not be recognized because the high-frequency hearing range is affected first. Conventional audiograms that do not test high-frequency ranges may not detect cochlear injury. Delayed onset of high-frequency hearing loss has been observed in humans. Factors that increase the risk for aminoglycoside ototoxicity in humans include impaired renal function and prolonged duration of treatment. Though not proved, some studies suggest that streptomycin, gentamicin, and tobramycin are more likely to affect vestibular function and amikacin and kanamycin are more likely to damage the cochlear apparatus, but both functions may be affected by each drug. Although elevated serum peak and trough concentrations are thought to contribute to ototoxicity, a specific threshold for peak or trough concentrations has not been established. Some studies suggest that children are less susceptible to aminoglycoside-induced ototoxicity, but this suggestion has not been proved.[7]

Neuromuscular blockade can occur after rapid intravenous infusion, after extensive peritoneal irrigation, or during routine parenteral aminoglycoside administration in patients with underlying conditions that affect the neuromuscular junction, such as myasthenia gravis and botulism, or during concomitant administration of agents that act on the neuromuscular junction, such as succinylcholine.

To avoid toxicity and ensure therapeutic values, concentrations of aminoglycosides in serum should be monitored in all patients with impaired renal function. Additionally, serum concentrations should be measured in patients who receive other nephrotoxic medications or treatment for longer than 2 or 3 days (empiric therapy for suspected sepsis); such monitoring is particularly relevant to preterm, low-birth-weight infants. Monitoring also should be considered in obese and undernourished children, children with severe burns, and those with chronic disease, for which the volume of distribution of the drug can be altered (e.g., cystic fibrosis).

MACROLIDES

Erythromycin, isolated from *Streptomyces erythreus* found in a soil sample in the Philippines, was the first macrolide and was available for use in 1952. Many natural and semi-synthetic erythromycin derivatives have been developed since then, three of which are approved for use in pediatrics: erythromycin, clarithromycin, and azithromycin. Macrolide antibiotics consist of a large lactone ring attached by a glycosidic bond to one or more amino or neutral sugar moieties. Erythromycin and clarithromycin have 14-membered lactone rings, whereas azithromycin, an azalide antibiotic that is grouped with the macrolides, has a tertiary amino group inserted in its 15-membered ring. In addition to similarities in chemical structure, these macrolides have similar antibacterial spectra, mechanisms of action, and mechanisms of resistance, but they differ in their pharmacokinetic characteristics.

MECHANISMS OF ACTION

Macrolide antibiotics reversibly bind to the 50S ribosomal subunit and inhibit protein synthesis. Initial studies suggested that the antibacterial activity of erythromycin was usually bacteriostatic, but against some actively growing, susceptible bacteria, large concentrations of erythromycin were bactericidal.[100] Clarithromycin and azithromycin are usually bacteriostatic, but they are bactericidal against *S. pyogenes, S. pneumoniae,* and *H. influenzae.*[266] As Mazzei and colleagues[158] noted, the specific interaction resulting in inhibition of protein synthesis is uncertain but thought to involve dissociation of peptidyl-tRNA from ribosomes during the elongation step. Although the exact target or targets are controversial, several studies suggest that macrolides bind to 23S ribosomal RNA and several ribosomal proteins. Erythromycin interferes with binding to the 50S ribosome by chloramphenicol and clindamycin, thus suggesting common or overlapping binding sites for these agents.

MECHANISMS OF RESISTANCE

Many gram-negative bacteria are inherently resistant to macrolides because of the relative impermeability of their outer membrane. Other bacteria can acquire resistance by production of enzymes that modify the macrolide, active efflux of the antibiotic, and altered ribosomal targets, the latter occurring most frequently.[134, 135, 257] Two mechanisms by which bacteria can alter their ribosomes and acquire macrolide resistance have been identified. High-level resistance because of an altered protein component of the 50S ribosomal subunit has occurred after a one-step chromosomal mutation. Such resistance has been demonstrated in *Bacillus subtilis, E. coli,* and group A streptococci. Plasmid-mediated macrolide, lincosamide, streptogramin B (MLS_B) resistance occurs when adenine residues on the 23S RNA component of the 50S ribosomal subunit are methylated; such methylation results in an altered target that confers cross-resistance to macrolides, including clarithromycin, azalides, lincosamides, and streptogramin B. The production of methylases is encoded by a class of genes referred to as *erm* (erythromycin ribosome methylation), approximately 30 of which have been characterized.[211] *Erm*-mediated resistance can be constitutive or inducible. When bacteria with inducible MLS_B resistance are exposed to subinhibitory concentrations of erythromycin, production of adenine methylase is turned on and resistance is induced, but when they are exposed to higher concentrations, protein synthesis is inhibited and induced resistance is blocked. This variable response is called dissociated resistance and can be seen in staphylococci, streptococci, and *Bacteroides* spp. Less commonly, bacteria produce enzymes that inactivate the macrolide, including acetyltransferases, esterases, phosphorylases, or glycosylases found in some strains of Enterobacteriaceae.[211] A macrolide and streptogramin B (MS) pattern of resistance that is plasmid-mediated results in macrolide resistance because of active efflux encoded by the *mef*(A) (macrolide efflux) and *msr*(A) (macrolide and streptogramin B resistant) genes. Isolates with these resistance genotypes are resistant to macrolides and streptogramin B but not to clindamycin, a lincosamide.[211] A causal association between erythromycin resistance and antibiotic use, probably mediated by selection pressure, was suggested by a nationwide epidemiologic study in Finland in which reduction of the use of erythromycin over time was associated with a steady decline in erythromycin resistance among *S. pyogenes* isolates from throat swabs and pus specimens.[225]

IN VITRO ACTIVITY

Erythromycin is effective in vitro against a diverse group of microorganisms, including *Bordetella pertussis,* the bacterium of legionnaires' disease *(Legionella pneumophila), Corynebacterium diphtheriae,* spirochetes *(Treponema pallidum),* mycoplasmas *(Mycoplasma pneumoniae* and *Ureaplasma urealyticum),* chlamydiae, anaerobic and aerobic gram-positive cocci *(S. pneumoniae, S. pyogenes,* and penicillinase-producing and non–penicillinase-producing strains of methicillin-susceptible *S. aureus),* and *Bacteroides* spp. Although methicillin-susceptible staphylococci and many streptococci are frequently susceptible, erythromycin-resistant group A streptococci have been reported in Scandinavian countries, France, and Japan.[226] Resistance in these countries occurred in association with increased use of erythromycin by the general population. Penicillin-resistant pneumococci are frequently resistant to macrolides. Erythromycin is highly active against *Campylobacter jejuni* and has adequate activity against *N. meningitidis* and *N. gonorrhoeae* and less activity against *H. influenzae.*

The newer macrolides have spectra of activity similar to that of erythromycin. When compared with erythromycin, clarithromycin has equivalent or greater activity against *M. catarrhalis, H. influenzae, M. pneumoniae, Chlamydia pneumoniae, Chlamydia trachomatis, L. pneumophila, U. urealyticum,* and *N. gonorrhoeae.* Clarithromycin is two to four times more active against most erythromycin-susceptible streptococci and staphylococci. However, pneumococci that are resistant to erythromycin (approximately 5 to 20%) are also resistant to clarithromycin and azithromycin; rates of macrolide resistance tend to correlate with rates of penicillin resistance.[266] The active metabolite of clarithromycin, 14-hydroxyclarithromycin, is more active than clarithromycin against *H. influenzae* and *M. catarrhalis,* and when combined with clarithromycin, their activities are additive or synergistic.[103, 144] Clarithromycin also has activity against organisms that are resistant to erythromycin, including *Toxoplasma gondii, Mycobacterium leprae,* MAC, and *Mycobacterium chelonae.*

When compared with erythromycin, azithromycin has less activity against gram-positive bacteria, including *S. pneumoniae,* but has better activity against gram-negative bacteria, including some Enterobacteriaceae such as *Shigella* spp., although the clinical importance of these findings is uncertain. The in vitro activity of azithromycin against *M. pneumoniae, C. pneumoniae,* and *L. pneumophila* is similar to that of erythromycin and clarithromycin. Azithromycin is more active than erythromycin against *C. trachomatis* and *U. urealyticum* and twofold to eightfold more active than erythromycin or clarithromycin against *M. catarrhalis* and *H. influenzae.*[10, 161] Azithromycin has activity against *T. gondii* and, though less than that of clarithromycin, against MAC organisms. Azithromycin and clarithromycin are highly effective in vitro against *Borrelia burgdorferi,*[199] *Bartonella henselae,* and *Bartonella quintana.*

PHARMACOKINETICS

The macrolides differ in pharmacokinetic properties (Table 235–8). Clarithromycin[96] and azithromycin[179] are gastric acid–stable and relatively well absorbed from the gastrointestinal tract, whereas erythromycin is acid-labile and absorption varies with the oral preparation. Macrolides undergo metabolism by the hepatic microsomal cytochrome P-450 system. Most of the metabolites are inactive with the exception of 14-(*R*)-hydroxyclarithromycin, an active metabolite that can act additively or synergistically with clarithromycin. The lipophilic macrolides are distributed well in tissues and fluids with the exception of CSF. High intracellular concentrations are achieved, but with the exception of azithromycin, the macrolides rapidly diffuse out of cells when extracellular concentrations are low. Clarithromycin and azithromycin are transported actively into leukocytes and macrophages. High concentrations of clarithromycin are present in the nasal mucosa, tonsils, and pulmonary epithelial lining fluid and alveolar cells.[52] Tissue concentrations of clarithromycin and azithromycin exceed those found in plasma by 2 to 20 times and 10 to 100 times, respectively. The favorable cellular penetration probably contributes to the efficacy of clarithromycin and azithromycin in the treatment of intracellular pathogens. Furthermore, sustained intracellular concentrations of azithromycin facilitate short-course therapy for pharyngitis and acute otitis media and single-dose therapy for chlamydial sexually transmitted diseases. Isolated cases of intravascular bacterial infections developing during macrolide therapy for focal infections have been reported[208] and evoke concern that despite elevated tissue concentrations, low serum concentrations may not treat systemic infections consistently. Erythromycin and azithromycin are eliminated primarily by biliary excretion, whereas clarithromycin is excreted predominantly by the kidneys. A reduction in clarithromycin dosage may be required in patients with moderate to severe renal insufficiency. Because of their longer serum half-life, azithromycin and clarithromycin can be administered in a once- and twice-daily regimen, respectively, as compared with the three- or four-times-daily dosing necessary for erythromycin.

Because erythromycin base is unstable at the low pH of the stomach, better-absorbed products were prepared by the addition of protective enteric coating or by alteration of the chemical structure through the formation of salts and esters. Salt and ester derivatives include ethylsuccinate or propionate (esters), stearate (a salt), and estolate (salt of an ester). Estolate provides the highest concentration of antimicrobial activity in serum, but controversy continues about which preparation provides the most biologically active drug at the site of infection. Because the base is the active component, all erythromycin preparations must be hydrolyzed to the base after absorption. Formulations of erythromycin base include tablets, delayed-release tablets, and capsules. Erythromycin estolate is marketed in capsule form, suspension, tablets, and chewable tablets. Erythromycin ethylsuccinate is available in suspension and tablet form. Parenteral preparations of erythromycin include the lactobionate and gluceptate derivatives. Intramuscular administration of these forms is painful and should be avoided. Clarithromycin can be taken without regard to food, whereas azithromycin should be taken at least 1 hour before or 2 hours after a meal. Clarithromycin is available in suspension (125 and 250 mg/5 mL) and in tablet (250 and 500 mg) form. Azithromycin is manufactured in 250-mg capsules and as a suspension (100 and 200 mg/5 mL). Azithromycin for intravenous injection has not been approved for use in children.

TABLE 235–8 ■ PHARMACOKINETICS OF MACROLIDE ANTIBIOTICS

	Erythromycin	Clarithromycin*	Azithromycin†
Bioavailability (%)	30–65‡	55	37
Protein binding (%)	70–90	65–75	7–50§
Half-life (hr)	1.4–2	Nonlinear‖	11–14 (48–96)
C_{max} (μg/mL)¶	0.8–3‡	3–7 (1–2)** 2–3 (≤1)††	0.4 (0.25)
Elimination route			
Biliary excretion	Majority	Minimal	>50%
Renal excretion (%)	2–15	20–40 (10–15)	4.5

*Values in parentheses are for the active metabolite 14-OH-clarithromycin.
†After one 500-mg dose; values in parentheses are at steady state after 500 mg × 1 day, then 250 mg/day (oral dosage forms).
‡Varies with the oral preparation and the presence of food.
§Protein binding varies with serum concentration.
‖Varies with dosing; 250 mg twice a day: clarithromycin = 3 to 4 hours, 14-OH-C = 5 to 6 hours; 500 mg twice a day: clarithromycin = 5 to 7 hours, 14-OH-C = 7 hours.
¶C_{max} = peak serum concentration.
**In adults given clarithromycin suspension, 7.5 mg/kg twice a day.
††In adults given clarithromycin tablets, 500 mg twice a day.
Modified from USP DI: Information for the Health Care Professional. Vol. 1. Thomson MICROMEDEX, 2003.

INDICATIONS FOR USE

Erythromycin is the drug of choice for the treatment of chlamydial conjunctivitis, pneumonia, and urethritis; mycoplasmal and *Legionella* pneumonia; and pertussis. It also is approved for use as a preoperative bowel preparation and for treatment of group A streptococcal sinusitis and pharyngitis, mild pneumococcal pneumonia, uncomplicated skin and soft tissue infections caused by susceptible organisms, diphtheria, and erythrasma. It is approved for use in penicillin-allergic persons as prophylaxis for bacterial endocarditis and rheumatic fever and for the treatment of syphilis in nonpregnant individuals.

Clarithromycin is approved for the treatment of bacterial exacerbations of bronchitis; streptococcal pharyngitis; mycoplasmal, chlamydial, and pneumococcal community-acquired pneumonia; acute maxillary sinusitis; and uncomplicated skin and soft tissue infections caused by susceptible bacteria. Clinical studies suggest that clarithromycin is as safe and effective as amoxicillin for the treatment of acute otitis media in children[201] and is as safe and effective as cefadroxil for the treatment of skin infections.[105] Clarithromycin, in combination with amoxicillin and bismuth compounds or H_2-receptor antagonists, is indicated for the treatment of *Helicobacter pylori*–associated peptic ulcer disease. Clarithromycin also is approved for prophylaxis of disseminated MAC infections in children and adults with advanced human immunodeficiency virus (HIV) infection. Furthermore, clarithromycin, in combination with other antimycobacterials, is an effective therapeutic agent for disseminated MAC infections. The safety and efficacy of clarithromycin have not been established for infants younger than 6 months.

In adults, azithromycin is approved for the treatment of bacterial exacerbations of bronchitis, chlamydial cervicitis and urethritis, chancroid, streptococcal tonsillitis and pharyngitis, uncomplicated skin and soft tissue infections caused by susceptible bacteria, and pneumonia caused by *H. influenzae* and *S. pneumoniae*. Pediatric indications include group A streptococcal pharyngitis[236]; acute otitis media caused by *H. influenzae, M. catarrhalis,* and *S. pneumoniae*[163]; and mild community-acquired pneumonia caused by *S. pneumoniae, H. influenzae, M. pneumoniae,* or *C. pneumoniae*. Five-day regimens have been approved for the treatment of pharyngitis (12 mg/kg/day) and otitis media (single dose of 10 mg/kg followed by 5 mg/kg/day). A randomized clinical trial comparing azithromycin and amoxicillin-clavulanate for the treatment of acute otitis media indicated that the β-lactam–containing regimen achieved superior bacteriologic and clinical outcomes for all bacterial pathogens and for *H. influenzae* specifically.[58] Consequently, consensus guidelines do not recommend azithromycin or clarithromycin for empiric treatment of acute otitis media.[71] Clinical studies have suggested benefit with a 5-day regimen of azithromycin for localized lymphadenopathy caused by *B. henselae* (cat-scratch disease)[16] and with one to six doses of azithromycin for trachoma, regimens that were equivalent to prolonged topical treatment with oxytetracycline/polymyxin ointment.[64] The U. S. Public Health Service recommends azithromycin for the treatment of chlamydial genital infections, nongonococcal urethritis, and chancroid[99] (a single 10-mg/kg dose; maximal dose, 1 g) and for prophylaxis of disseminated MAC infection in HIV-infected children.[250] Although no well-controlled studies comparing the use of erythromycin versus azithromycin or clarithromycin for the prophylaxis of pertussis have been performed, limited data suggest that 3- or 5-day azithromycin regimens may eradicate *B. pertussis* effectively from the nasopharynx of hospitalized children.[126] The safety and efficacy of azithromycin have not been determined for infants younger than 6 months.

ADVERSE EFFECTS

The macrolides are usually well tolerated and relatively safe. The most common adverse effect is gastrointestinal disturbance, which can occur with the administration of any macrolide but is associated most commonly with the use of erythromycin.[44] It is a dose-related phenomenon. Because it acts as a motilin receptor agonist, gastrointestinal symptoms (nausea, vomiting, diarrhea, flatulence, and abdominal cramps) can occur with orally or parenterally administered erythromycin. Enteric coating of erythromycin does not decrease the incidence. Rapid intravenous infusions of erythromycin can result in thrombophlebitis. Cholestatic hepatitis is an unusual, but serious macrolide toxicity. It occurs more commonly in adults and possibly in pregnant women and is associated most frequently with the estolate preparation.[35] The onset typically begins approximately 16 days after beginning therapy and is manifested as fever, pruritus, jaundice, elevated liver function tests, and occasionally, rash, leukocytosis, and eosinophilia. Signs and symptoms resolve after discontinuation of the macrolide but recur with subsequent therapy. Other adverse reactions seldom occur. Manifestations of hypersensitivity, including rash, fever, and eosinophilia, rarely occur. Transient hearing loss has been described after the administration of large dosages of erythromycin lactobionate. *Torsades de pointes* is an uncommon reaction to intravenous infusions of erythromycin and occasionally occurs during concomitant therapy with cisapride. Gastrointestinal overgrowth of *Candida* is an infrequent occurrence. A sevenfold increase in the rate of infantile hypertrophic pyloric stenosis was associated temporally with and was probably causally related to the prophylactic use of erythromycin in neonates during a pertussis outbreak in a community hospital.[110] Gastrointestinal disturbances occur less frequently with clarithromycin[54] and azithromycin, principally because lower dosages are required for effective therapy.

A common and potentially serious toxicity is that of drug interactions.[91] Macrolides are metabolized by hepatic microsomal cytochrome P-450 enzymes. Drug interactions can occur during concomitant therapy with two or more drugs that undergo hepatic microsomal P-450 metabolism. One proposal for this drug interaction suggests that the macrolide is *N*-demethylated to a nitrosoalkane that interacts with and inactivates the microsomal enzyme. Toxicity can occur because of interference with metabolism and consequent accumulation of the second drug. The ability to inactivate the enzyme varies with each macrolide; erythromycin is a more potent inhibitor than clarithromycin is. Azithromycin has not been associated yet with nitrosoalkane formation and resulting drug interactions, but caution should be exercised with concomitant administration of other drugs known to interact with macrolides. Drugs with which macrolides can interact include astemizole, carbamazepine, cisapride, cyclosporine, digoxin, methylprednisolone, rifampin, tacrolimus, terfenadine, theophylline, triazolam, valproate, warfarin, and zidovudine.

MISCELLANEOUS ANTIBIOTICS

Lincosamides

Lincosamide antibiotics consist of an amino acid linked to an amino sugar. Lincomycin, elaborated by *Streptomyces lincolnensis* variety *lincolnensis,* originally isolated from a soil sample near Lincoln, Nebraska, was the first lincosamide available for use. Clindamycin, a semisynthetic derivative of lincomycin produced by the substitution of a chlorine atom for a hydroxyl group at position 7,[151] was available for use in the early 1970s. Because clindamycin has increased antibacterial activity and better oral absorption than lincomycin does, lincomycin rarely is used.

MECHANISMS OF ACTION

Lincosamides bind to the 50S subunit of susceptible bacterial ribosomes and thereby inhibit protein synthesis. The exact mechanism of action is not known but probably involves interference with transpeptidation.[75] Because the ribosomal binding sites for lincosamides overlap with those of chloramphenicol and erythromycin, concurrent use of these agents can result in antagonism and should be avoided. Lincosamides are usually bacteriostatic but can be bactericidal against highly susceptible microorganisms in the presence of high lincosamide concentrations. Even subinhibitory concentrations can potentiate opsonization and phagocytosis of bacteria.

MECHANISMS OF RESISTANCE

Some bacteria, including members of the Enterobacteriaceae and *Pseudomonas* and *Acinetobacter* spp., are inherently resistant to lincosamides, most likely because of relative impermeability of the outer membrane of the cell wall. Acquired resistance can develop as a result of altered ribosomal targets and, less commonly, lincosamide inactivation, whereas resistance as a result of reduced lincosamide uptake has not been described.[134, 135] Two mechanisms by which bacteria can alter their ribosomes and acquire lincosamide resistance have been identified. High-level resistance because of an altered protein component of the 50S ribosomal subunit after a one-step chromosomal mutation confers resistance to erythromycin and often to the lincosamides. Plasmid-mediated MLS_B resistance occurs when adenine residues on the 23S RNA component of the 50S ribosomal subunit are methylated and an altered target is created that confers cross-resistance to macrolides, lincosamides, and streptogramin B. The production of methylases is encoded by a class of genes referred to as *erm*.[211] This resistance can be constitutive or inducible and can be seen in staphylococci, streptococci, and *Bacteroides* spp. Erythromycin is the most potent inducer of MLS_B resistance in staphylococci, whereas any macrolide, lincosamide, or streptogramin B can be an inducer in streptococci. Some strains of *B. fragilis* can have inducible MLS_B resistance that is not detected easily by disk agar diffusion susceptibility testing[233] but recognizable because of frequently concurrent high-level erythromycin resistance. An MS pattern of resistance that is plasmid mediated results in macrolide resistance as a result of active efflux encoded by the *mef*(A) and *msr*(A) genes. Isolates with these resistance genotypes are resistant to macrolides and streptogramin B but not to clindamycin.[211] Rarely, staphylococci produce a plasmid-mediated, nonconjugative nucleotidyltransferase that inactivates lincosamides and results in high-level resistance to lincomycin and tolerance to clindamycin (MBC/MIC ratio >32).

IN VITRO ACTIVITY

Both lincosamides are effective in vitro against gram-positive cocci, whereas clindamycin is also active against a wide range of anaerobic bacteria. Clindamycin is many times more active than lincomycin[162] and as active as or slightly more active than erythromycin against staphylococci, pneumococci, group A streptococci, and viridans streptococci. Unlike erythromycin, the lincosamides do not have clinically significant activity against *H. influenzae, M. pneumoniae,* or *Neisseria* spp. Clindamycin is active against many gram-positive cocci, including penicillinase- and non–penicillinase-producing staphylococci and groups A, B, C, and G beta-hemolytic streptococci and pneumococci, but it is not active against enterococci or most nosocomial methicillin-resistant staphylococci.[68] Many erythromycin-resistant *S. aureus* organisms are resistant to clindamycin, and in those that are not, resistance often rapidly develops during clindamycin therapy. Most community-acquired isolates of methicillin-resistant *S. aureus* have been susceptible to clindamycin. Erythromycin and lincosamide resistance in pneumococci and group A streptococci has been increasing. Clindamycin has been shown to be active against most penicillin-resistant pneumococci. Most facultative aerobic gram-negative bacilli, with the exception of *Campylobacter* spp. (including *C. jejuni* and *C. fetus*) and *H. pylori,* are inherently resistant to clindamycin. Anaerobes frequently susceptible to clindamycin include the anaerobic gram-negative bacilli *Bacteroides, Fusobacterium, Prevotella,* and *Porphyromonas* spp.; the non–spore-forming gram-positive bacilli *Propionibacterium, Eubacterium,* and actinomyces; the anaerobic gram-positive cocci *Peptococcus, Peptostreptococcus,* and microaerophilic streptococci; and many *Clostridium* organisms, excluding *C. difficile, Clostridium sporogenes,* and *Clostridium tertium.* Clindamycin resistance does occur, especially in *Fusobacterium varium,* the non-*fragilis Bacteroides* group, as many as 7 percent of *B. fragilis* isolates, and as many as 20 percent of anaerobic gram-positive cocci. When combined with other agents, clindamycin is active against certain other pathogens such as *Babesia, Plasmodium, Pneumocystis carinii,* and *T. gondii.*

PHARMACOKINETICS

Oral absorption of lincosamides occurs rapidly. The presence of food delays, but does not decrease the absorption of clindamycin, but it does reduce the absorption of lincomycin. Concomitant administration of kaolin- or attapulgite-containing antidiarrheal agents can decrease absorption; therefore, these agents should not be administered within 2 hours before or 3 to 4 hours after oral lincosamides are given. Lincosamides are distributed rapidly and widely to most tissues and fluids, including saliva, sputum, respiratory tissue, pleural fluid, soft tissues, bones and joints, prostate, semen,[192] appendix, and peritoneal fluid.[178] Lincosamides are transported actively into macrophages and polymorphonuclear leukocytes, and high concentrations are achieved in bile, urine, and bone. Penetration into CSF is limited, unless inflammation is present. In experimental pneumococcal meningitis, concentrations of clindamycin in CSF were approximately 10 percent of the corresponding serum values. Lincosamides are highly protein-bound, with values ranging from 70 to 75 percent for lincomycin and 92 to 94 percent for clindamycin. The inactive palmitate and phosphate esters are hydrolyzed in the liver to clindamycin, the active agent. Clindamycin undergoes hepatic biotransformation to active and inactive metabolites. Ten percent of absorbed lincomycin is excreted unchanged in urine, 3 percent is excreted unchanged in feces, and the remainder is excreted as inactive metabolites, primarily in the biliary system. Elimination is delayed in the presence of severe hepatic insufficiency alone or severe concurrent renal and hepatic impairment, and therefore adjustments in dosages may be necessary. Formulations of lincosamides available for use include lincomycin hydrochloride in 250- and 500-mg capsules and in solution for parenteral use. Clindamycin phosphate, a water-soluble ester of clindamycin and phosphoric acid, is available for parenteral use. Oral formulations include clindamycin palmitate hydrochloride granules reconstituted to 75 mg base per 5 mL and clindamycin hydrochloride capsules in 75, 150, and 300 mg of the base compound. Clindamycin is also available as a topical solution, gel, lotion, and vaginal cream.

INDICATIONS FOR USE

Lincomycin can be used for the treatment of serious infections caused by susceptible strains of staphylococci, pneumococci, other streptococci, or anaerobic organisms, but it rarely is used in pediatric patients. Clindamycin is effective against and has been approved for the treatment of staphylococcal bone and joint infections[77]; anaerobic pelvic infections, including pelvic inflammatory disease, nongonococcal tubo-ovarian abscess, and postsurgical vaginal cuff infections; anaerobic intra-abdominal infections, including peritonitis and abscesses; pneumonitis, empyema, and lung abscesses caused by anaerobes and as a second-line agent for infections caused by pneumococci and staphylococci; anaerobic septicemia; and skin and soft tissue infections caused by anaerobes, staphylococci, and streptococci. It is also effective and has been approved as a topical agent for acne vulgaris. Unconfirmed retrospective data suggest that clindamycin in combination with a β-lactam antibiotic, with surgery if indicated, might be the most effective treatment of invasive *S. pyogenes* infections.[264] Other infections for which clindamycin may be effective but has not been approved for therapy include chronic suppurative otitis media or chronic sinusitis in which anaerobes may play a role, chronic pharyngeal carriers of group A streptococci,[235] odontogenic infections, toxoplasmosis of the CNS (in combination with pyrimethamine), uncomplicated falciparum malaria[131] or babesiosis (in combination with quinine), and mild to moderate *P. carinii* pneumonia in patients with AIDS (in combination with primaquine).[22] Because of poor penetration into CSF, it is not approved for the treatment of meningitis. Clindamycin is a third-line agent for endocarditis prophylaxis for upper respiratory tract, dental, or oral procedures in persons allergic to or intolerant of amoxicillin and erythromycin. Oral and intravenous formulations of clindamycin are approved for use in infants and children of all ages. The bitter taste of the oral suspension may limit compliance.

ADVERSE EFFECTS

The most frequent side effects include generalized morbilliform-like rash and mild, self-limited diarrhea occurring in as many as 10 percent and in 2 to 20 percent of patients, respectively. Other gastrointestinal disturbances include anorexia, nausea, vomiting, flatulence, abdominal pain, and a metallic taste. Pseudomembranous colitis, a serious and sometimes fatal illness, is the adverse event posing the most concern. Most antibiotics have been associated with pseudomembranous colitis, but those most frequently implicated include ampicillin, lincosamides, and cephalosporins. The incidence of lincosamide-associated pseudomembranous colitis varies from 0.1 to 10 percent. Antibiotic-associated pseudomembranous colitis is caused by overgrowth of toxin-producing strains of *C. difficile*[238]; at least two extracellular toxins are elaborated: toxin A or D-1, a potent enterotoxin, and toxin B or D-2, a cytotoxin.[228] The risk of disease developing is increased in elderly patients and those with chronic debilitating conditions. It is unrelated to the total dosage, duration of therapy, route of administration, or underlying disease. The onset most frequently occurs between days 4 and 9 of therapy, but signs and symptoms develop in one third of patients 2 to 10 weeks after discontinuation of the antibiotic. More than 80 percent of patients have fever, leukocytosis, crampy abdominal pain, and watery diarrhea, and 5 to 10 percent have bloody diarrhea. Sigmoidoscopic findings include plaque-like lesions on colonic or rectal mucosa consisting of polymorphonuclear leukocytes, chronic inflammatory cells, fibrin, and epithelial debris. Treatment includes prompt discontinuation of the antibiotic, avoidance of antiperistaltic agents, and oral administration of metronidazole. Use of a nonabsorbable oral vancomycin formulation is potentially effective. However, it may induce resistance to this agent in enterococci, and therefore it should be reserved for children who fail to respond to metronidazole therapy.

Other less common adverse events include hypersensitivity reactions such as urticarial rash, drug fever, and eosinophilia; transient neutropenia, agranulocytosis, or thrombocytopenia; and a mild, reversible elevation in hepatic transaminases. Hypotension and cardiac arrest have been reported after rapid intravenous infusion of lincomycin. Caution must be exercised when administering lincosamides to newborns; fatal gasping syndromes have been described, possibly related to the preservative benzyl alcohol.

Drug interactions include incompatibility with many agents in solution, including aminophylline, ampicillin, barbiturates, calcium gluconate, diphenylhydantoin, and magnesium sulfate, and interaction with hydrocarbon-containing inhalational anesthetics. Lincosamides are weak neuromuscular blockers[229] but can enhance neuromuscular blockade when administered concurrently with neuromuscular blockers. Chloramphenicol and macrolides can have an antagonistic effect when administered concurrently with lincosamides because of competition for ribosomal binding sites.

Chloramphenicol

Chloramphenicol, originally derived from *Streptomyces venezuela* obtained from soil near Caracas, Venezuela, in 1947, now is prepared synthetically. It is a chemically unique agent that contains an aromatic nitro group, an *N*-dichloroacetyl substituent, and two chiral centers. The availability of less toxic and equally or more effective agents has limited the usefulness of chloramphenicol in the United States.

MECHANISMS OF ACTION

Chloramphenicol reversibly binds to the 50S subunit of 70S bacterial ribosomes and thereby inhibits protein synthesis. The exact mechanism remains uncertain but most likely involves suppression of peptidyltransferase activity with a resultant inability to form peptide bonds.[261] Because the ribosomal binding sites of chloramphenicol overlap with those of macrolides and clindamycin, concomitant use with a macrolide or clindamycin can result in antagonism and should be avoided. Chloramphenicol is usually bacteriostatic but can be bactericidal when high concentrations are achieved against highly susceptible organisms.

MECHANISMS OF RESISTANCE

The most common mechanism of acquired resistance is plasmid-mediated production of chloramphenicol acetyltransferase, which acetylates chloramphenicol and renders it unable to bind to the ribosomal target.[261] This resistance has been documented in many different genera of bacteria, including *H. influenzae,* members of the Enterobacteriaceae, *Neisseria,* streptococci, and *S. aureus.* Less commonly, chromosomal or plasmid-mediated alterations in permeability have been a cause of chloramphenicol resistance in *E. coli, H. influenzae, P. aeruginosa,* and *B. cepacia.* Isolated cases of resistance in *B. subtilis* because of altered ribosomes and in anaerobes because of inactivation of chloramphenicol by nitroreduction have been reported.

IN VITRO ACTIVITY

Chloramphenicol has broad-spectrum activity against aerobic and anaerobic gram-positive and gram-negative bacteria, chlamydiae, mycoplasmas, spirochetes, and rickettsiae.[210] It is bactericidal against susceptible strains of *H. influenzae, N. meningitidis,* and penicillin-susceptible *S. pneumoniae,* whereas it is bacteriostatic against most other susceptible microorganisms.[203] Frequently susceptible aerobic gram-positive cocci include groups A and B beta-hemolytic streptococci, viridans streptococci, and penicillin-susceptible pneumococci. Because penicillin-resistant pneumococci may be tolerant to chloramphenicol in vitro,[85] verifying chloramphenicol susceptibility by MBC testing is prudent, especially when treating meningitis. Usually, chloramphenicol is active against methicillin-susceptible *S. aureus,* but susceptibility patterns vary with the use of chloramphenicol, and more suitable alternatives for therapy exist. Susceptible gram-positive bacilli include *Bacillus* spp., *L. monocytogenes, C. diphtheriae, Clostridium* spp., and *Eubacterium.* Most *N. meningitidis* and *N. gonorrhoeae* organisms are susceptible. However, several high-level chloramphenicol-resistant strains of meningococcus belonging to serogroup B recently were isolated from the CSF of children in Vietnam.[88] The susceptibility of Enterobacteriaceae, including that for *Salmonella* and *Shigella* spp., is variable. Other gram-negative bacilli frequently susceptible to chloramphenicol include *H. influenzae, Brucella, B. pertussis, Pasteurella multocida, Y. pestis, F. tularensis, Pseudomonas pseudomallei, B. cepacia, Vibrio cholerae,* and *C. jejuni.* Virtually all obligate anaerobes are susceptible.

PHARMACOKINETICS

After oral administration, absorption of chloramphenicol is rapid and complete. Bioavailability is approximately 80 percent after oral administration but only 70 percent after an intravenous dose because approximately 30 percent of the parenterally administered dose is excreted in urine before hydrolysis of the succinate ester to the active form. Intramuscular injection results in peak serum concentrations comparable to those achieved after intravenous infusion. Because of its lipid solubility, chloramphenicol diffuses rapidly and widely into tissues and fluids.[210] The highest concentrations are achieved in the liver and kidneys, with high concentrations present in urine, and therapeutic concentrations are achieved in aqueous and vitreous humor. CSF concentrations range from 21 to 50 percent and from 45 to 89 percent of serum values in the presence of uninflamed and inflamed meninges, respectively. Brain tissue concentrations exceed those in plasma. Chloramphenicol also is distributed into pleural, ascitic, and synovial fluids; saliva; and breast milk. Protein binding ranges from 32 percent in premature newborns to 50 to 60 percent in adults. Chloramphenicol palmitate and chloramphenicol sodium succinate are esterified prodrugs of chloramphenicol. Orally administered chloramphenicol palmitate is hydrolyzed to active drug by pancreatic esterases in the small intestine before absorption. After intravenous infusion, chloramphenicol sodium succinate is hydrolyzed rapidly to active drug in the kidneys, liver, and lungs. Ninety percent of active chloramphenicol is conjugated to the inactive glucuronide primarily by the liver. Immature metabolic function of the liver in the fetus and newborn results in inadequate conjugation of chloramphenicol, with subsequent accumulation of toxic concentrations of active drug. Peak serum concentrations in children after a dose of 25 mg/kg range from 19 to 28 μg/mL, whereas in adults receiving doses of 12.5 mg/kg, peak serum values of 11 to 18 μg/mL can be achieved. Though metabolized to inactive metabolites by the liver, chloramphenicol is excreted by the kidneys: 5 to 10 percent as active drug and 80 percent as inactive metabolites. The elimination half-life is significantly longer but variable, and serum concentrations are unpredictable in neonates.[210] Dosage adjustments should be considered in persons with severe hepatic insufficiency or combined hepatic and renal insufficiency and in patients receiving drugs that compete for hepatic P-450 cytochrome oxidases, such as phenytoin, phenobarbital, and rifampin. Chloramphenicol is not removed by peritoneal dialysis or hemodialysis, but charcoal hemoperfusion may lower serum concentrations.

Formulations of chloramphenicol available include chloramphenicol palmitate in an oral suspension of 150 mg base/5 mL, 250-mg capsules of chloramphenicol base, and chloramphenicol sodium succinate for parenteral use. Other formulations include 1 percent cream for topical use, 0.5 percent otic solution, 0.5 percent ophthalmic solution, and 1 percent ophthalmic ointment.

INDICATIONS FOR USE

Because of its low therapeutic/toxic index, use of chloramphenicol should be reserved for serious infections for which less toxic agents are ineffective or contraindicated. In some developed countries, chloramphenicol has been replaced by third-generation cephalosporins for the treatment of bacterial meningitis and by clindamycin or metronidazole for the treatment of anaerobic infections. Ceftriaxone is a safe and effective alternative to chloramphenicol for the treatment of acute typhoid fever.[172] Infections for which chloramphenicol may be indicated include pneumococcal, meningococcal, and *H. influenzae* meningitis in β-lactam–allergic persons; brain abscesses caused by susceptible anaerobic bacteria resistant to other agents; acute typhoid fever; rickettsial infections (typhus, Q fever, Rocky Mountain spotted fever); and ehrlichiosis in young patients with a relative contraindication to the use of tetracyclines. Chloramphenicol is not indicated for the treatment of trivial infections, prophylaxis of infections, or treatment of typhoid carrier states.

ADVERSE EFFECTS

Hematologic adverse events associated with the use of chloramphenicol include hemolytic anemia in patients with the Mediterranean type of glucose-6-phosphate dehydrogenase deficiency, reversible bone marrow suppression, and aplastic anemia. Reversible bone marrow suppression is a dose-related phenomenon. It usually occurs when serum concentrations exceed 25 μg/mL, as can be seen when administering large dosages, during prolonged therapy, or in patients with impaired liver function. Although mammalian cells contain 80S ribosomes rather than the 70S ribosomes found in prokaryotes, mitochondria possess 70S ribosomes. A proposed mechanism of myelosuppression involves inhibition of host mitochondrial protein synthesis.[261] Dose-related bone marrow suppression is manifested by peripheral anemia with or without reticulocytopenia, leukopenia, and thrombocytopenia and bone marrow findings of increased cellularity, cytoplasmic vacuolization, and maturation arrest of erythroid and myeloid precursors. In contrast, aplastic anemia is a rare, often fatal idiosyncratic reaction that is unrelated to the dosage, duration, or route of therapy.[259] The pathogenesis is understood less well but possibly is related to DNA damage from toxic metabolites of chloramphenicol produced by nitroreduction.[261] The incidence ranges from 1 in 25,000 to 40,000 courses. Onset can begin during therapy but typically occurs weeks to months or rarely years after therapy has been discontinued. Manifestations include peripheral pancytopenia and hypoplastic or aplastic marrow.

Gray syndrome or gray baby syndrome is a rare, but serious and potentially fatal adverse event that usually occurs in newborns but has been described in older children and adults with hepatic insufficiency. Most often it occurs when serum chloramphenicol concentrations exceed 40 μg/mL, and it is thought to be a result of inhibition of mitochondrial electron transport in liver, skeletal muscle, and myocardium. The onset typically begins 2 to 9 days after initiating therapy. Manifestations include hypothermia, tachypnea, blue-gray skin color (cyanosis), abdominal distention, emesis, unresponsiveness, and refractory metabolic acidosis that can progress to vasomotor collapse and death within 2 days.

Uncommon side effects include hypersensitivity reactions such as drug fever, rash, urticaria, anaphylaxis, and a Herxheimer-like reaction during therapy for syphilis, typhoid fever, and brucellosis; gastrointestinal symptoms, including nausea, emesis, diarrhea, and an unpleasant taste; and neurologic symptoms such as peripheral neuritis, headache, mental confusion, and optic neuritis,[204] the last of which may not be entirely reversible.

Chloramphenicol can inhibit the metabolism of other drugs metabolized by the hepatic microsomal cytochrome P-450 system and thus result in the accumulation of alfentanil, barbiturates, cyclophosphamide, phenytoin, antidiabetic sulfonylureas (more common with chlorpropamide and tolbutamide than with glyburide and glipizide), and warfarin during concomitant therapy.[4] Because some agents such as rifampin,[123] phenobarbital, and phenytoin are potent inducers of hepatic microsomal enzymes, when they are given concomitantly with chloramphenicol, metabolism is enhanced and serum concentrations of active chloramphenicol are reduced. Other drug interactions include a reduction in the effectiveness of estrogen-containing oral contraceptives when used concurrently with chloramphenicol and a delay in the response to vitamin B_{12}, folic acid, and iron. A mild disulfiram-like reaction can occur when alcohol is ingested during chloramphenicol therapy. Both cimetidine and chloramphenicol have rare associations with aplastic anemia; a few reports of concomitant use resulting in aplastic anemia have been documented, thus suggesting a potential for additive or synergistic risk.[259] Concomitant acetaminophen therapy has been the subject of controversy; some studies suggest that co-administration can prolong the elimination half-life of chloramphenicol, but other reports suggest no effect or enhanced metabolism of chloramphenicol. Lincosamides and macrolides can have an antagonistic effect when administered concurrently with chloramphenicol because of competition for ribosomal binding sites. Chloramphenicol can inhibit the in vitro bactericidal activity of cefotaxime and ceftriaxone against susceptible strains of gram-negative bacilli, group B streptococci, and *S. aureus*.[6] Chloramphenicol is physically incompatible in solution with many drugs, including tetracyclines and vancomycin.

Because of considerable variability in serum chloramphenicol concentrations, the narrow therapeutic/toxic index, and the potential for drug interactions, monitoring serum concentrations of chloramphenicol and peripheral blood counts during therapy is prudent.

Sulfonamides

Sulfachrysoidine (Prontosil), discovered in the 1930s, was the first sulfonamide developed. Sulfonamides are broad-spectrum antimicrobial agents derived from sulfanilamide (para-aminobenzene sulfonamide) and are structural analogues of para-amino benzoic acid (PABA); they compete with PABA and result in interference with nucleotide synthesis. Sulfanilamide was manipulated to form other compounds with expanded antimicrobial activity and reduced toxicity. Sulfonamides are distributed widely in fluids and tissues. The preparations currently available have greater solubility and are less likely to cause crystalluria than earlier compounds were. Sulfonamides available for single-agent use include sulfacytine (Renoquid), sulfadiazine, sulfamethizole (Thiosulfil Forte), sulfamethoxazole (Gantanol), and sulfisoxazole (Gantrisin). Sulfonamide combinations, including TMP-SMX and erythromycin ethylsuccinate–sulfisoxazole, are used frequently in pediatrics.

TRIMETHOPRIM-SULFAMETHOXAZOLE. TMP is a diaminopyrimidine antibiotic available for single-agent use. Combinations of TMP and sulfonamides were used in the late 1960s because of presumed synergistic antibacterial activity, although clinical evidence of synergy is equivocal.[114] Because SMX has rates of absorption and elimination similar to those of TMP, it was the sulfonamide selected for combination.

MECHANISMS OF ACTION

SMX competitively inhibits dihydropteroate synthetase, the bacterial enzyme that assimilates PABA into dihydrofolic acid; such inhibition results in a reduction in dihydrofolic acid synthesis and, therefore, a reduction in the amount of tetrahydrofolic acid, a cofactor for nucleotide synthesis.[107] Only bacteria that must synthesize folic acid are potentially susceptible. SMX is bacteriostatic when used alone and can be inhibited by PABA and its derivatives (procaine and tetracaine). TMP reversibly binds and inhibits dihydrofolate reductase, an enzyme that reduces dihydrofolic acid to tetrahydrofolic acid; this activity results in diminished amounts of folic acid, an essential cofactor in nucleic acid production.[39] TMP is bacteriostatic when used alone, but in combination with SMX against susceptible bacteria, bactericidal activity can be achieved by blockade of sequential steps in folic acid metabolism. The effect of sulfonamide on bacteria is circumvented in mammals, which obtain folate from food sources. The reaction inhibited by TMP is similar in bacteria and mammals but differs quantitatively in the extent of binding of the drug to the enzyme; mammalian dihydrofolate reductase is 60,000 times less sensitive to TMP than is the enzyme in susceptible bacteria.

MECHANISMS OF RESISTANCE

Bacteria can be inherently resistant to either agent or can acquire resistance to TMP, SMX, or both agents. Resistance to SMX and other sulfonamides is associated with hyperproduction of PABA, as demonstrated in strains of *Neisseria* and staphylococci, or is caused by an altered dihydropteroate synthetase enzyme with lower affinity for sulfonamides, as found in *E. coli*, *N. meningitidis,* and *S. pneumoniae.*[240] Chromosomal-mediated resistance to TMP has been observed in strains of *S. pneumoniae, H. influenzae, E. coli, Pediococcus, B. fragilis,* and *Nocardia* and *Clostridium* spp.[114] Furthermore, *P. aeruginosa* is inherently resistant to TMP because of cell wall impermeability. Acquired resistance to TMP can be plasmid mediated or chromosomal and occurs in members of the Enterobacteriaceae, staphylococci, and streptococci. Mechanisms of acquired TMP resistance include cell wall impermeability, thymine auxotrophy, resistant dihydrofolate reductase, and overproduction of dihydrofolate reductase,[113] the most common being plasmid-mediated production of dihydrofolate reductases, which are encoded by at least 17 genes. Resistance to sulfonamides is encoded by the *sul*I and *sul*II genes. Despite the reduced use of sulfonamides, the genetic determinants for sulfonamide resistance probably persist because of the efficient integron transfer mechanisms.[114] Bacterial resistance to both TMP and SMX can develop as a result of altered cell wall permeability or alternative metabolic pathways (e.g., thymine auxotrophy), whereby they obtain thymine or thymidine from the environment.[240]

IN VITRO ACTIVITY

TMP-SMX has significant activity against a broad spectrum of gram-positive cocci and gram-negative enteric pathogens. TMP is more active than the sulfonamide, but the mixture is significantly more effective than either drug alone. Synergism is more likely if the bacteria are susceptible to both drugs, but it can occur even when the bacteria are resistant to only one agent. Bacteria with potential susceptibility to the combination include *Brucella, B. cepacia, E. coli, H. influenzae, M. catarrhalis, N. gonorrhoeae, Nocardia, Proteus, Salmonella, Shigella, Serratia marcescens,* methicillin-susceptible *S. aureus, S. maltophilia,* penicillin-susceptible *S. pneumoniae,* some environmental mycobacteria, *Yersinia enterocolitica, Aeromonas hydrophila,* and *P. carinii.* However, increasing rates of resistance to TMP-SMX among strains of penicillin-nonsusceptible *S. pneumoniae,* methicillin-resistant staphylococci, *M. catarrhalis, H. influenzae, E. coli, Klebsiella, Shigella,* and *Salmonella* limit the usefulness of this antibacterial agent.[114]

PHARMACOKINETICS

Optimal synergistic activity occurs when a 1:20 ratio of TMP and SMX serum concentrations is attained, which can be achieved after the administration of a fixed 1:5 ratio of TMP to SMX. Both agents are absorbed rapidly and fairly well when administered alone and in combination. Both penetrate most body fluids and tissues, although TMP frequently penetrates extravascular tissues to a greater degree than SMX does. Both agents cross the placenta, are excreted in breast milk, and diffuse into pleural, peritoneal, and synovial fluid and CSF. Protein binding varies from 40 to 60 percent for TMP and from 60 to 70 percent for SMX. Both are metabolized in the liver to inactive metabolites. The primary route of elimination is by the kidneys, with small amounts excreted in bile and feces. Dosage adjustments are required for renal impairment.

Available preparations include an oral suspension containing 40 mg of TMP and 200 mg of SMX per 5 mL, tablets containing 80 mg of TMP and 400 mg of SMX, double-strength tablets consisting of 160 mg of TMP and 800 mg of SMX, and a parenteral solution.

INDICATIONS FOR USE

TMP-SMX is approved for the treatment of acute exacerbations of chronic bronchitis in adults, enterocolitis caused by susceptible *Shigella* organisms, acute otitis media caused by *H. influenzae* or susceptible pneumococcus, *P. carinii* pneumonia, traveler's diarrhea caused by *Shigella* and enterotoxigenic *E. coli,* and acute or chronic urinary tract infections. Though not approved for use and not usually prescribed as a first-line antibiotic, TMP-SMX has been effective therapy for typhoid fever, brucellosis, nocardiosis, sinusitis, biliary tract infections, and bone and joint infections caused by susceptible organisms. It also has been used for *P. carinii* pneumonia prophylaxis in immunosuppressed children with cancer and patients infected with HIV and for prophylaxis of recurrent bacterial urinary tract infections. Because early studies did not evaluate the effect of prolonged or recurrent therapy on somatic growth or bone marrow function in children, TMP-SMX was not approved for prophylaxis or prolonged treatment of otitis media. It is not recommended for treatment of group A streptococcal tonsillopharyngitis because it does not eradicate the organism or reliably prevent the nonsuppurative sequelae.

ADVERSE EFFECTS

Most of the side effects occurring during administration of TMP-SMX are caused by the sulfonamide. Gastrointestinal disturbances and hypersensitivity reactions are the adverse events most commonly observed. Anorexia, nausea, vomiting, diarrhea, drug eruption, and photosensitivity reactions can occur in 1 to 4 percent of patients. Hypersensitivity reactions that develop less frequently include erythema nodosum, erythema multiforme (including Stevens-Johnson syndrome), urticaria, anaphylaxis, and thyroid damage. Drug-induced hepatitis has been described but is an unusual event. CNS side effects include vertigo, ataxia, headache, and aseptic meningitis. TMP-SMX can affect renal function when administered to persons with underlying renal disease, but it is usually reversible after discontinuation of therapy. Crystalluria occurred more commonly with earlier preparations because of low solubility. SMX has a greater tendency to cause crystalluria than do other sulfonamides that are currently available because of slower absorption and excretion, but with adequate fluid intake, alkalinization of the urine is usually unnecessary. Interstitial nephritis and tubular necrosis seldom are associated with the use of TMP-SMX. Blood dyscrasias can be a limiting factor to the administration of TMP-SMX. Acute hemolytic anemia has been described after the use of TMP-SMX in patients with glucose-6-phosphate dehydrogenase deficiency. Though uncommon in patients with normal hematopoietic systems, aplastic anemia, agranulocytosis, leukopenia, and thrombocytopenia can occur. Prolonged use can result in megaloblastic anemia because of impaired folate utilization. Administration of sulfonamide can trigger an acute attack of porphyria. Sulfonamides can displace bilirubin from albumin-binding sites. In neonates, especially premature infants, the activity of sulfonamides can be increased as a result of reduced conjugation by the immature liver. Because of the increased risk of kernicterus from sulfonamide displacement of bilirubin, the use of sulfonamides during the last month of pregnancy and in neonates is discouraged.

Drug-drug interactions with TMP-SMX are numerous. Sulfonamides can displace other drugs from albumin-binding sites and thereby result in increased effective activity of the second drug, as can be seen with the concurrent administration of methotrexate,[78] phenytoin, sulfonylurea hypoglycemic agents, thiazide diuretics, and warfarin. Drugs that when co-administered can displace sulfonamides from binding sites and lead to increased effective sulfonamide activity include indomethacin, phenylbutazone, probenecid, salicylates, and sulfinpyrazone. Agents that reduce the effect of sulfonamides include methenamine, which results in insoluble urinary precipitates of the sulfonamide, and derivatives of PABA. Sulfonamides are physically incompatible with many drugs, among them aminoglycosides, chloramphenicol, insulin, lincomycin, methicillin, tetracycline, and vancomycin.

ERYTHROMYCIN ETHYLSUCCINATE–SULFISOXAZOLE ACETYL. The combination of erythromycin ethylsuccinate and sulfisoxazole acetyl (EES-SSX) in a fixed ratio expands the spectrum of antibacterial activity. The mechanism of action, mechanisms of resistance, pharmacokinetics, and adverse events for EES-SSX are the same as those for each individual drug. Because EES-SSX is effective in vitro against common pathogens causing otitis media in children,[31] it was approved for the treatment of acute otitis media. Though not approved for use, it can be effective therapy for sinusitis caused by *H. influenzae,* susceptible pneumococci, and *M. catarrhalis.* Its principal use today in pediatrics is for the treatment of acute otitis media in patients with β-lactam hypersensitivity.

Tetracyclines

Chlortetracycline, also known as Aureomycin, was the first natural tetracycline discovered when isolated from *Streptomyces aureofaciens* in 1948.[80] Many tetracyclines have been developed since then. Those currently marketed include the natural agents tetracycline, oxytetracycline, and demeclocycline and the semisynthetic agents doxycycline and minocycline. Their basic structure consists of a hydronaphthacene nucleus with four fused rings. They differ from each other biochemically by substituent variations at carbons 5, 6, or 7. Their mechanisms of action and mechanisms of resistance, as well as their spectra of activity, are similar, but the analogues differ in the degree of activity and in pharmacokinetic properties. Glycylcyclines, a new generation of tetracyclines with improved activity against drug-resistant bacteria, are in clinical trials.[234]

MECHANISMS OF ACTION

Tetracyclines are bacteriostatic agents that reversibly bind to the 30S subunit of 70S bacterial ribosomes and inhibit protein synthesis. Because attachment of aminoacyl-tRNA to the ribosome acceptor site is prevented, the bacteria are unable to add amino acids to the growing peptide chain. According to studies of tetracycline in *E. coli,* tetracyclines passively diffuse through outer-membrane porins and then traverse the cytoplasmic membrane by energy-independent and energy-dependent mechanisms; the precise molecular nature of the latter is inconclusive.[47]

MECHANISMS OF RESISTANCE

In many bacteria, including members of the Enterobacteriaceae, *P. aeruginosa,* staphylococci, streptococci, and *Bacteroides,* resistance to tetracyclines has developed. Resistance most often is carried on plasmids but can be chromosomal. The genes encoding for resistance are called *tet,* or tetracycline resistance determinants. Resistance to one tetracycline usually implies resistance to all; however, many tetracycline-resistant bacteria are susceptible to doxycycline, minocycline, or both. The most common mechanism of resistance results from active efflux. *Tet* genes encode for membrane proteins that mediate energy-dependent efflux. These proteins are different in gram-positive and gram-negative bacteria. Efflux has been found in the Enterobacteriaceae, enterococci, streptococci, staphylococci, *V. cholerae, Bacteroides, Peptostreptococcus, Eubacterium,* and others. Less commonly, ribosomal protection by a soluble protein (ribosomal protection protein) encoded by different *tet* genes and an *otr* gene has been found in a wide variety of aerobic and anaerobic gram-positive and gram-negative bacteria, as well as in mycoplasmas and ureaplasmas. The precise mechanism by which ribosomal protection protein mediates resistance to tetracyclines is being investigated. Researchers have suggested, though not verified, that these protection determinants are transferred from antibiotic-producing bacteria to pathogenic strains.[237] Enzymatic inactivation of tetracycline, encoded for by another *tet* gene, has been demonstrated in in vitro studies of aerobically grown *E. coli,* but the clinical significance has not been established.

IN VITRO ACTIVITY

Tetracyclines are broad-spectrum antibiotics with activity against aerobic and anaerobic gram-positive and gram-negative bacteria, chlamydiae, mycoplasmas, rickettsiae, and spirochetes. Activity against gram-negative bacteria has been limited by the emergence of tetracycline-resistant strains. Most *P. aeruginosa* and many *Shigella* and *Salmonella* organisms are resistant. Penicillin-susceptible strains of *N. gonorrhoeae* and *N. meningitidis* are usually susceptible to tetracyclines, but penicillin-resistant strains of *N. gonorrhoeae* are not. Gram-negative organisms with continued susceptibility to tetracyclines include *A. hydrophila, Brucella, Campylobacter,* some *Haemophilus* organisms, *Helicobacter, P. multocida, Plesiomonas shigelloides,* and *Vibrio.* Tetracyclines are active against some gram-positive bacilli, including *Actinomyces israelii, B. anthracis,* many clostridia, *Listeria,* and *Nocardia.* Tetracyclines have excellent activity against *Chlamydia, M. pneumoniae,* and rickettsiae. Other organisms for which tetracyclines have activity include *Mycobacterium marinum* and *B. burgdorferi.* The more lipophilic agents doxycycline and minocycline are generally more active than the others. Minocycline has excellent activity against staphylococci, and both doxycycline and minocycline are more active than tetracycline against *S. aureus* and some streptococci, but they have no activity against enterococci and group B streptococci. Because of extensive plasmid-mediated resistance in pneumococci, therapy with tetracycline should be avoided.

TABLE 235–9 ■ PHARMACOKINETICS OF TETRACYCLINES

Drug	Oral Absorption (%)	Protein Binding (%)	Primary Route of Excretion	Approximate Half-Life* (hr)
Short Acting				
Oxytetracycline	58	35	Renal	6–10
Tetracycline	75–77	65	Renal	6–11
Intermediate Acting				
Demeclocycline	66	91	Renal	10–17
Long Acting				
Doxycycline	90–100	93	Biliary	12–22
Minocycline	90–100	76	Biliary	11–23

*Normal renal function.
Modified from USP DI: Information for the Health Care Professional. Vol. 1. Thomson MICROMEDEX, 2003.

Doxycycline and minocycline are more active than the other agents against anaerobic bacteria.

PHARMACOKINETICS

The five tetracycline compounds available for systemic use can be classified by duration of activity: tetracycline and oxytetracycline are short-acting agents, demeclocycline is intermediate-acting, and doxycycline and minocycline are long-acting agents (Table 235–9). Oral administration is the preferred route because thrombophlebitis is associated with intravenous infusion and pain is associated with intramuscular injections. Oral absorption ranges from 58 percent for the short-acting agents to 100 percent for the long-acting ones. The presence of food decreases the absorption of demeclocycline, oxytetracycline, and tetracycline. Because tetracyclines form insoluble complexes in the gut with aluminum, calcium, iron, magnesium, zinc, and other bivalent and trivalent cations, co-administration with milk and other dairy products, antacids, calcium or iron supplements, cathartics, and other agents can reduce absorption and should be avoided. Differences in lipid solubility affect penetration of tissues by the various tetracyclines. All agents readily penetrate many tissues and fluids, among which are pleural, ascitic, and synovial fluids, sinus secretions, sputum, bone, teeth, and breast milk. Tetracyclines can cross the placenta. The highest concentrations are achieved in bile and can exceed serum concentrations by 5 to 20 times. Therapeutic concentrations of doxycycline can be achieved in tonsillar and pulmonary tissues, the eye, and the prostate,[57] and high concentrations are achieved in myometrial and endometrial tissue[217] and the kidney. Minocycline penetrates into sputum, saliva, and tears and into cells of the vestibular apparatus.[119] Minocycline is biotransformed to inactive metabolites by the liver; the other tetracyclines are not metabolized, although whether doxycycline is metabolized is not clear. Oxytetracycline, demeclocycline, and tetracycline are eliminated unchanged in urine. Approximately 10 percent of minocycline is excreted unchanged in urine, 20 to 35 percent is excreted unchanged in feces, and the remainder is excreted as inactive metabolites in urine and feces. Thirty to forty percent of doxycycline is excreted in urine; the remainder is excreted by the biliary tract and by diffusion through the intestinal wall, where some of it is chelated and prevented from reabsorption and enterohepatic cycling. Dosing of short- and intermediate-acting tetracyclines must be adjusted for renal failure.

Systemic formulations available in the United States include tablets, capsules, delayed-release capsules, and suspensions for many of the tetracyclines, as well as parenteral preparations of doxycycline, minocycline, and oxytetracycline. Ophthalmic and topical preparations are also available.

INDICATIONS FOR USE

With few exceptions, tetracyclines are no longer the drug of choice for many infections because of the availability of cephalosporins and semisynthetic penicillins with equivalent or greater activity and less frequent side effects. As a result of the potential for dental toxicity, tetracyclines are not recommended for use in children younger than 9 years, except for specific infections for which alternative therapy is potentially more toxic, such as chloramphenicol for Rocky Mountain spotted fever[2] and ehrlichiosis. Approved indications in the United States include treatment of actinomycosis, anthrax, brucellosis, inclusion conjunctivitis,[218] psittacosis, Q fever, rickettsialpox, Rocky Mountain spotted fever, typhus, relapsing fever, syphilis, trachoma,[218] yaws, and Vincent necrotizing gingivostomatitis caused by *Fusobacterium,* as well as infections caused by *Bacteroides* spp., *Bartonella bacilliformis, C. fetus, F. tularensis, M. pneumoniae, V. cholerae, Y. pestis,* and others. Because of its excellent tissue penetration and spectrum of activity, doxycycline is the preferred tetracycline for treatment of atypical pneumonia caused by *M. pneumoniae* and *C. pneumoniae,* intra-abdominal or pelvic infections, and several sexually transmitted diseases, including granuloma inguinale, chlamydial infections, *U. urealyticum* infection, nongonococcal urethritis, pelvic inflammatory disease (plus cefoxitin), proctitis (plus ceftriaxone), and prostatitis. Doxycycline is an alternative drug for (nonpregnant) penicillin-allergic patients with primary, secondary, or late latent syphilis. Although minocycline is effective in eradicating nasopharyngeal carriage of meningococcus, its potential for vestibular toxicity precludes its use for this purpose. Topical tetracyclines have been used extensively for the treatment of acne vulgaris and other dermatologic illnesses.[112]

ADVERSE EFFECTS

Gastrointestinal disturbances are the most common side effects associated with tetracycline and include anorexia, nausea, emesis, flatulence, and diarrhea. These symptoms occur less frequently with minocycline. Esophageal ulceration has been associated with the oral administration of tetracyclines.[84] All tetracyclines except doxycycline can cause a negative nitrogen balance, with an elevation in blood urea nitrogen that is not usually significant except in the presence of underlying renal insufficiency. Demeclocycline can cause nephrogenic diabetes insipidus and, for this reason, has been used for treatment of the syndrome of inappropriate antidiuretic hormone secretion. Rarely, tetracyclines have been associated with hepatic injury as manifested by elevated transaminases and diffuse vacuolar fatty metamorphosis on biopsy, with or without pancreatitis. It is dose related, and the risk is increased with pregnancy, malnutrition, and preexisting renal or hepatic disease and in patients receiving other hepatotoxic agents. The use of tetracyclines in children younger than 9 years is relatively contraindicated because tetracyclines chelate with calcium and can be deposited in developing bones and teeth and lead to a transient decrease in bone growth, permanent tooth discoloration, and enamel hypoplasia. The risk of these side effects occurring with one course at an appropriate dosage is low; the degree of tooth discoloration is associated with the total dosage administered.[95] Minocycline has been associated with reversible vestibular toxicity. All tetracyclines have been noted to cause pseudotumor cerebri, a benign elevation in intracranial pressure that is reversible after discontinuation of the drug. Some data suggest that an increased risk may exist with the concurrent use of tetracycline and isotretinoin. Tetracyclines have been associated with an exaggerated sunburn reaction after sun exposure. This risk occurs most frequently with demeclocycline and rarely with minocycline. Hypersensitivity reactions occur infrequently and include morbilliform rash, urticaria, exfoliative dermatitis, and rarely, anaphylaxis. Hyperpigmentation of the mucosal membranes, skin, and nails has been reported with the use of tetracycline, particularly minocycline.

Drug-drug interactions are numerous. A decrease in absorption of tetracyclines can occur with the co-administration of oral antacids, bismuth subsalicylate, iron, kaolin or pectin, zinc sulfate, and other divalent or trivalent cations that chelate the antibiotic. A reduced effect of tetracyclines because of increased metabolism is associated with the concomitant use of doxycycline with barbiturates, carbamazepine, phenytoin, rifampin, and alcohol in heavy drinkers. Co-administration with tetracyclines can increase the effect of oral anticoagulants, digoxin, lithium, and theophylline and can decrease the effect of oral contraceptive agents and oral iron. Tetracyclines can inhibit the in vitro bactericidal activity of penicillins and aminoglycosides. Other drug-drug interactions include benign intracranial hypertension with the concomitant administration of vitamin A, severe nephrotoxicity with the co-administration of methoxyflurane and tetracycline, and localized hemosiderosis with amitriptyline and minocycline.

Rifamycins

The rifamycins are a group of complex macrocyclic antibiotics that were isolated from *Streptomyces mediterranei* in the early 1960s. Rifampin (rifampicin) and rifabutin are structurally related, semisynthetic broad-spectrum antibiotics derived from rifamycin B and S, respectively. These bactericidal agents avidly bind to DNA-dependent RNA polymerase and thereby prevent attachment of the enzyme to DNA and thus block initiation of RNA transcription and protein synthesis. Rifabutin was approved in 1992 for prevention of disseminated MAC disease in adults with advanced HIV infection. Single point mutations rapidly develop when rifamycins are used alone. Therefore, administering these antibiotics in combination with other antimicrobial agents when indicated is preferable.[207]

IN VITRO ACTIVITY

Rifamycins have excellent in vitro activity against many gram-positive cocci, including many methicillin-resistant staphylococci and penicillin-nonsusceptible *S. pneumoniae,* some gram-negative organisms, *Legionella, C. trachomatis, T. gondii, M. tuberculosis,* and *M. leprae.* Rifampin is active against *Mycobacterium kansasii,* but not most other species of atypical mycobacteria. In contrast, rifabutin is active against most atypical mycobacteria except *M. chelonae.* Rifabutin is also more active than rifampin against rifampin-susceptible strains of *M. tuberculosis* and is active against approximately one third of rifampin-resistant strains.[143, 171]

PHARMACOKINETICS

Rifampin and rifabutin are highly lipid-soluble and highly protein-bound (72–89%) molecules. Consequently, they are well absorbed from the gastrointestinal tract and have excellent intracellular and CNS penetration, particularly in the presence of inflammation of the meninges, where they reach therapeutic concentrations. They are metabolized primarily by the liver via deacetylation, and 30 to 40 percent of the drug is excreted via the biliary system. In the presence of hepatic dysfunction, dosage adjustments are necessary, whereas no alteration in dosage is required for children with renal dysfunction. In adults, rifabutin has a significantly longer mean terminal half-life than rifampin does (45 verus 2 to 5 hours).[207]

INDICATIONS FOR USE

Prophylaxis with rifampin monotherapy is used to eradicate nasopharyngeal colonization in close contacts of individuals with infections caused by *H. influenzae* type b[94, 174] and *N. meningitidis,*[53] as well as index cases with these infections unless they were treated with third-generation cephalosporins. Rifampin also has been used alone or in combination with other antimicrobial agents to eradicate carriage of group B streptococci, penicillin-nonsusceptible *S. pneumoniae,* and *S. aureus* in high-risk children. It rarely is used for this purpose now. The use of rifampin combined with two or three other bactericidal antituberculosis agents for the treatment of active tuberculosis, as well as its combined use with clofazimine and dapsone for the treatment of leprosy, is considered an essential component of effective regimens. In some patients, rifampin can be considered as part of a combination regimen for the treatment of (1) meningitis caused by penicillin- and cephalosporin-resistant *S. pneumoniae* in combination with a third-generation cephalosporin and vancomycin; (2) complicated or severe *B. henselae* infection (cat-scratch disease); (3) shunt- or catheter-associated staphylococcal infections, often with removal of the foreign material; (4) *S. aureus* implant-related orthopedic infections in combination with a fluoroquinolone; (5) prosthetic valve endocarditis caused by staphylococci; (6) brucellosis in combination regimens with TMP-SMX, a tetracycline, or an aminoglycoside[125, 147]; and (8) MAC-associated disseminated disease or lymphadenitis, if not completely resectable, in combination with ethambutol and azithromycin or clarithromycin.[143] Furthermore, rifampin- and minocycline-impregnated central venous catheters have been used successfully in adults to prevent catheter colonization and bloodstream infection with gram-positive and gram-negative pathogens, as well as *Candida* spp.[61] In the last circumstance, surveillance for resistance is important.

Rifabutin is effective for the treatment of most mycobacterial species, *H. pylori,* and *T. gondii* in adults. Limited data are available for the treatment of MAC infections in children with HIV infection. Clinical studies in adults with advanced HIV infection indicate that administration of daily clarithromycin or weekly azithromycin is superior to rifabutin alone for prophylaxis of MAC infection.[171] The safety and efficacy of rifabutin for prophylaxis of MAC infection in children have not been established.

Rifampin is available in capsule (150 and 300 mg) and intravenous formulations. Rifabutin is available only in capsule (150 mg) form. A suspension can be compounded by the pharmacy, or the capsule contents can be mixed with thick, sweet food for infants and young children. Absorption of rifampin is optimal if administered 1 hour before or 2 hours after a meal, whereas a high-fat meal decreases the rate, but not the total amount of absorption of rifabutin. The use of fixed-dose combinations of rifampin, isoniazid, and pyrazinamide is not recommended for children. The safety and efficacy of rifapentine, a rifamycin antibiotic similar in structure and activity to rifampin and rifabutin, have not been established for children younger than 12 years.

ADVERSE EFFECTS

Adverse events associated with rifampin include gastrointestinal disorders, rash, hepatotoxicity, hypersensitivity, and a flulike syndrome. Adverse reactions to rifabutin include gastrointestinal disorders, rash, leukopenia, neutropenia, and rarely, uveitis, although safety data in children are limited. The parenteral form of rifampin is associated with thrombophlebitis. Routine determination of serum aminotransferase concentrations is not recommended for children receiving brief or prolonged courses of therapy, except for those with clinical evidence of hepatitis or severe or disseminated tuberculosis. In these situations, at least monthly measurements should be performed. In addition, patients should be warned that rifamycins discolor urine, tears, sweat, and feces and permanently stain soft contact lenses. Because rifamycins induce hepatic cytochrome P-450 enzyme activity, they may interact with other medications administered concurrently and cause decreased concentrations of some antiretroviral agents, particularly protease inhibitors, azole antifungal agents, barbiturates, oral contraceptives, warfarin (Coumadin), clarithromycin, and cyclosporine. Conversely, rifamycin serum drug concentrations may increase if administered with other drugs that inhibit hepatic enzymes, and the dose of rifamycin antibiotic may need to be reduced by as much as 50 percent. Rifabutin induces hepatic enzymes to a lesser extent than rifampin does and, therefore, has less potential for drug interactions.[143, 171]

Fluoroquinolones

Fluoroquinolone antibiotics are derivatives of nalidixic acid. When compared with nalidixic acid, fluoroquinolones have a broader spectrum of activity that includes gram-negative enteric organisms, *P. aeruginosa,* staphylococci, some streptococci, *Mycoplasma,* and *Chlamydia;* better penetration into tissues; good intracellular penetration; and rapid bactericidal activity. In vitro studies of investigational fluoroquinolones against penicillin- and cephalosporin-resistant pneumococci look promising. In addition, the limited available data indicate that fluoroquinolones have favorable pharmacokinetic properties in children and their efficacy correlates best with the 24-hour AUC/MIC ratio, as would be expected for an antibiotic with concentration-dependent killing and a post-antibiotic effect. These properties suggest that large doses given at relatively infrequent intervals would be most effective.[220] However, based on pharmacokinetic studies, dosages for patients with cystic fibrosis should be higher and more frequent than for patients without cystic fibrosis, and the dosage should be decreased in proportion to increasing body weight.

Fluoroquinolones have been used extensively in adults for the treatment of skin and soft tissue infections, skeletal infections, and infections of the urinary and respiratory tracts. Use in pediatric patients has been limited because of the potential for induction of arthropathy, as demonstrated in juvenile animal studies. However, no unequivocal evidence suggests that quinolone-induced arthropathy occurs in humans. Reversible arthralgia and tendinopathy have a temporal association with fluoroquinolone use. Fluoroquinolones are not approved for use in children and adolescents younger than 18 years, but they have been used in certain settings, primarily because, apart from carbenicillin, they are the only oral antibiotics with activity against *P. aeruginosa.* These agents, particularly ciprofloxacin, have been used to treat exacerbations of chronic pseudomonal pulmonary infections in patients with cystic fibrosis, complicated urinary tract infections caused by multidrug-resistant bacteria, chronic suppurative otitis media, enteric infections in developing countries, including multidrug-resistant typhoid fever, infections in neutropenic cancer patients, and multidrug-resistant bacterial meningitis in more than 10,000 children worldwide.[221, 253] Fluoroquinolones also effectively eradicate nasopharyngeal carriage of meningococci. Clinical adverse events associated with fluoroquinolone therapy occur in 5 to 15 percent of adult and pediatric patients and cause discontinuation of treatment in 1 to 2 percent. The most common reactions are gastrointestinal, minor CNS disorders, and allergic rashes.[220] The current recommendation is that fluoroquinolones not be used if effective and nonrestricted alternative antimicrobial agents are available.

Selected Aspects of the Administration of Antimicrobial Agents

DOSAGE SCHEDULES FOR INFANTS AND CHILDREN

Dosage schedules of antimicrobial agents commercially available in the United States for infants (beyond the newborn period) and children are listed in Table 235–10. The list is subdivided into dosage schedules for mild to moderate and for severe disease. Oral regimens are used for mild to moderate infections caused by susceptible organisms in areas that are well vascularized and in which adequate concentrations of drug are achieved at the site of infection. Parenteral administration should be considered for severe infections, especially those caused by less susceptible organisms producing disease in areas in which diffusion of drug is limited.

DOSAGE SCHEDULES FOR NEWBORN INFANTS

The clinical pharmacology of antimicrobial agents administered to newborn infants is unique and cannot be extrapolated from data derived from older children or adults.[216] The physiologic and metabolic processes that affect the distribution, metabolism, and excretion of drugs undergo rapid changes during the child's first few weeks of life. The increased efficiency of kidney function after the infant's first 7 days requires an increase in dosage and a decrease in the interval between doses of penicillins and aminoglycosides for maintaining therapeutic concentrations of drug in blood and tissues. Thus, different dosage schedules are provided for the first week of life and for the subsequent weeks of the neonatal period (Tables 235–11 and 235–12). With survival of very-low-birth-weight, premature infants, more data are needed on the use of antimicrobial agents in these infants with immature metabolic and physiologic mechanisms.[200, 216]

SHOULD DOSAGES BE DETERMINED BY WEIGHT OR BY SURFACE AREA?

In most standard pediatric texts and in the package inserts prepared by manufacturers, dosages of antibiotics for children are based on body weight. Body surface area correlates more closely with extracellular fluid volume. Some investigators suggest that more predictable serum concentrations can be achieved by using calculations of dosages based on surface area[104] than by using those based on weight. This method may be more reliable for drugs that are distributed in extracellular fluid, such as aminoglycosides, especially when prescribed for obese or malnourished children. Currently, however, the convenience of calculating dosage on the basis of weight appears to be the more important consideration.

USE OF ORAL PREPARATIONS FOR SERIOUS INFECTIONS

Oral preparations of antimicrobial agents vary in their degree of absorption from individual to individual and within an individual, depending on the illness being treated and the formulation used. Because higher and more consistent serum

TABLE 235–10 ■ DAILY DOSAGE SCHEDULES FOR ANTIMICROBIAL AGENTS IN PEDIATRIC PATIENTS BEYOND THE NEWBORN PERIOD

Agent, Generic (Trade name)	Route	Mild to Moderate Infections*	Severe Infections*
Penicillin G, crystalline (numerous)	IV, IM	25,000-50,000 U ÷ into 4 doses	250,000-400,000 U ÷ into 6 doses
Penicillin G, procaine (numerous)	IM	25,000-50,000 U ÷ into 1-2 doses	Inappropriate
Penicillin G, benzathine (Bicillin)	IM	<30 lb = 600,000 U; 30-60 lb = 1,200,000 U; >60 lb = 2,400,000 U†	Inappropriate
Penicillin G, potassium (numerous)	PO	25-50 mg ÷ into 3-4 doses	Inappropriate
Penicillin V, phenoxymethyl penicillin (numerous)	PO	25-50 mg ÷ into 3-4 doses	Inappropriate
Penicillinase-resistant penicillins			
Methicillin (Staphcillin)	IV, IM	100-200 mg ÷ into 4 doses	200-300 mg ÷ into 4-6 doses
Oxacillin (Prostaphlin, Bactocill)	IV, IM	100-150 mg ÷ into 4 doses	150-200 mg ÷ into 4-6 doses
Nafcillin (Nafcil, Unipen, Nallpen)	IV, IM	50-100 mg ÷ into 4 doses	100-200 mg ÷ into 4-6 doses
Cloxacillin (Cloxapen)	PO	50-100 mg ÷ into 4 doses	Inappropriate
Dicloxacillin (Dynapen, Pathocil)	PO	25-50 mg ÷ into 4 doses	Inappropriate
Aminopenicillins			
Ampicillin (numerous)	IV, IM	100-200 mg ÷ into 4 doses	200-400 mg ÷ into 4 doses
	PO	50-100 mg ÷ into 4 doses	Inappropriate
Ampicillin + sulbactam (Unasyn)	IV	Inappropriate	150-400 mg of ampicillin ÷ into 4 doses
Amoxicillin (Amoxil, Polymox, Trimox, Wymox)	PO	25-90 mg ÷ into 2-3 doses	Inappropriate
Amoxicillin + clavulanate (Augmentin)	PO	45-90 mg ÷ into 2-3 doses	Inappropriate
Extended-spectrum penicillins			
Carbenicillin indanyl (Geocillin)	PO	30-50 mg ÷ into 4 doses	Inappropriate
Ticarcillin (Ticar)	IV, IM	100-200 mg ÷ into 4 doses	200-300 mg ÷ into 4-6 doses
Ticarcillin + clavulanate (Timentin)	IV	Inappropriate	200-300 mg ÷ into 4-6 doses
Mezlocillin (Mezlin)	IV, IM	Inappropriate	200-300 mg ÷ into 4-6 doses
Piperacillin (Pipracil)	IV, IM	Inappropriate	200-300 mg ÷ into 4-6 doses
Piperacillin + tazobactam (Zosyn)	IV	Inappropriate	240 mg of piperacillin ÷ into 3 doses
Monobactams			
Aztreonam (Azactam)	IV, IM	irappropriate	120 mg ÷ into 4 doses
Cephalosporins			
Cephalothin (Keflin)‡	IV, IM	80-100 mg ÷ into 4 doses	100-150 mg ÷ into 4-6 doses
Cefazolin (Ancef, Kefzol)	IV, IM	50 mg ÷ into 3 doses	50-100 mg ÷ into 3-4 doses
Cephalexin (Keflex, Keftab)	PO	25-50 mg ÷ into 4 doses	Inappropriate
Cefadroxil (Duricef)	PO	30 mg ÷ into 2 doses	Inappropriate
Cefaclor (Ceclor)	PO	40 mg ÷ into 3 doses	Inappropriate
Cefprozil (Cefzil)	PO	30 mg ÷ into 2 doses	Inappropriate
Loracarbef (Lorabid)	PO	15-30 mg ÷ into 2 doses	Inappropriate
Cefuroxime axetil (Ceftin)	PO	30-40 mg ÷ into 2 doses	Inappropriate
Cefuroxime (Kefurox, Zinacef)	IV, IM	Inappropriate	100-200 mg ÷ into 3 doses
Cefoxitin (Mefoxin)	IV	Inappropriate	80-160 mg ÷ into 4-6 doses
Cefixime (Suprax)	PO	8 mg ÷ into 1-2 doses	Inappropriate
Cefpodoxime proxetil (Vantin)	PO	10 mg ÷ into 2 doses	Inappropriate
Ceftibuten (Cedax)	PO	9 mg once daily	Inappropriate
Cefdinir (Omnicef)	PO	14 mg ÷ into 1-2 doses	Inappropriate
Cefditoren (Spectracef)	PO	200-400 mg twice daily†§	Inappropriate
Cefotaxime (Claforan)	IV, IM	Inappropriate	100-200 mg ÷ into 3-4 doses
Ceftriaxone (Rocephin)	IV, IM	Inappropriate	50-100 mg ÷ into 1-2 doses
Ceftazidime (Fortaz, Tazicef, Tazidime)	IV, IM	Inappropriate	100-150 mg ÷ into 3 doses
Cefepime (Maxipime)	IV, IM	Inappropriate	100-150 mg ÷ into 2-3 doses
Carbapenems			
Imipenem-cilastatin (Primaxin)	IV, IM	Inappropriate	60-100 mg ÷ into 4 doses
Meropenem (Merrem)	IV	Inappropriate	60-120 mg ÷ into 3 doses
Macrolides			
Erythromycin gluceptate (Ilotycin)	IV	Inappropriate	20-50 mg ÷ into 4 doses
Erythromycin lactobionate (Erythrocin)	IV	Inappropriate	20-50 mg ÷ into 4 doses
Erythromycin base (numerous)	PO	30-50 mg ÷ into 4 doses	Inappropriate
Erythromycin ethylsuccinate (E.E.S., EryPed, Erythro)	PO	30-50 mg ÷ into 4 doses	Inappropriate
Erythromycin Stearate (Erythrocin Stearate, Erythrocot, My-E)	PO	30-50 mg ÷ into 4 doses	Inappropriate
Erythromycin estolate (Ilosone)	PO	30-50 mg ÷ into 4 doses	Inappropriate
Clarithromycin (Biaxin)	PO	15 mg ÷ into 2 doses	Inappropriate

TABLE 235–10 ■ DAILY DOSAGE SCHEDULES FOR ANTIMICROBIAL AGENTS IN PEDIATRIC PATIENTS BEYOND THE NEWBORN PERIOD—cont'd

Agent, Generic (Trade name)	Route	Mild to Moderate Infections*	Severe Infections*
Azithromycin (Zithromax)	PO	10 mg on day 1, then 5 mg thereafter; 12 mg for pharyngitis	Inappropriate
Lincosamides			
Clindamycin (Cleocin)	IV, IM	Inappropriate	25–40 mg ÷ into 4 doses
	PO	20–30 mg ÷ into 4 doses	Inappropriate
Vancomycin (Vancocin)	IV	Inappropriate	40–60 mg ÷ into 4 doses
Aminoglycosides			
Amikacin (Amikin)	IV, IM	Inappropriate	15–22.5 mg ÷ into 3 doses
Gentamicin (Garamycin)	IV, IM	Inappropriate	5–7.5 mg ÷ into 3 doses‖
Kanamycin (Kantrex)	IV, IM	Inappropriate	15–30 mg ÷ into 3 doses
Netilmicin (Netromycin)	IV, IM	Inappropriate	3–7.5 mg ÷ into 3 doses
Paramomycin (numerous)	PO	30 mg ÷ into 3 doses	Inappropriate
Streptomycin (numerous)	IM	Inappropriate	20–40 mg ÷ into 2 doses
Tobramycin (Nebcin)	IV, IM	Inappropriate	5–7.5 mg ÷ into 3 doses
Tetracyclines			
Tetracycline (numerous)	PO	25–50 mg ÷ into 4 doses	Inappropriate
Doxycycline (Doryx, Vibramycin, Vibratabs, Monodox)	PO	2–4 mg ÷ into 1–2 doses	Inappropriate
Chloramphenicol (Chloromycetin)	IV	Inappropriate	50–100 mg ÷ into 3–4 doses
	PO	Inappropriate	50–100 mg ÷ into 3–4 doses
Sulfonamides			
Sulfadiazine (numerous)	PO	100–150 mg ÷ into 4 doses	Inappropriate
Sulfisoxazole (Gantrisin)	PO	120–150 mg ÷ into 4 doses	Inappropriate
Trimethoprim-sulfamethoxazole (Bactrim, Septra, Sulfatrim, Cotrim)	PO	8–12 mg trimeth/40–60 mg sulfa ÷ into 2 doses	Inappropriate
	IV	Inappropriate	10–20 mg trimeth/50–100 mg sulfa ÷ into 4 doses
Erythromycin ethylsuccinate-sulfisoxazole (Pediazole, Eryzole)	PO	50 mg erythro/150 mg sulfa ÷ into 4 doses	Inappropriate
Fluoroquinolones			
Ciprofloxacin (Cipro)	PO	20–30 mg ÷ into 2 doses	Inappropriate
	IV	Inappropriate	20–30 mg ÷ into 2 doses
Rifampin (Rifadin, Rimactane)	PO	10–20 mg ÷ into 1–2 doses	20 mg ÷ into 2 doses
	IV	Inappropriate	20 mg ÷ into 2 doses
Metronidazole (Flagyl)	PO	15–35 mg ÷ into 3–4 doses	Inappropriate
	IV	Inappropriate	30 mg ÷ into 4 doses
Linezolid (Zyvox)	PO	Inappropriate	20–30 mg ÷ into 2 or 3 doses
	IV	Inappropriate	20–30 mg ÷ into 2 or 3 doses
Quinupristin-Dalfopristine (Synercid)	IV	Inappropriate	22.5 mg ÷ 3 doses

*Total daily dosage (per kg). For larger children, maximal dosages may apply.
†Total dose.
‡No longer available in the United States.
§Not approved for children younger than 12 years of age.
‖A dose of 5–6 mg/kg once daily is investigational.
IM, intramuscularly; IV, intravenously; PO, orally; SC, subcutaneously.

concentrations of drug are achieved after parenteral administration, parenteral routes are preferable for serious infections. Sequential parenteral-oral antimicrobial therapy may be an option in patients with uncomplicated pneumonia, pyelonephritis, and suppurative skeletal infections.[160] Results of studies[181, 239] of orally administered antibiotics in children with skeletal infections indicate that this mode of administration can be used successfully for a portion of the therapeutic course.

Specific guidelines for oral treatment of serious infections are recommended: (1) the patient should be able to swallow and retain the medication, (2) the dosage should be sufficiently large to provide adequate bactericidal concentrations of drug at the site of infection, and (3) the hospital laboratory should be able to determine serum antimicrobial concentrations and serum minimal inhibitory titers to ensure therapeutic values.

Oral therapy can be considered for osteomyelitis and suppurative arthritis only after an initial period of parenteral therapy (5 to 7 days), after results are available from cultures and susceptibility tests, and after the patient shows definite signs of resolution of inflammation. Oral therapy should be initiated before discharge from the hospital to ascertain compliance, determine serum antimicrobial concentrations, and observe for significant side effects that would preclude use of the oral antibiotic.

FOOD INTERFERES WITH THE ABSORPTION OF SOME ORAL ANTIBIOTICS

The absorption of some oral antimicrobial agents is decreased significantly when the drug is taken with food or near mealtime. These drugs include unbuffered penicillin G,

TABLE 235–11 ■ DOSAGE SCHEDULES FOR ANTIMICROBIAL AGENTS FREQUENTLY USED IN NEONATES

		Dosage (mg/kg) and Interval of Administration				
		Weight < 1200 g	*Weight 1200–2000 g*		*Weight > 2000 g*	
Antibiotic	**Route**	**Age 0–4 wk**	**Age 0–7 Days**	**Age >7 Days**	**Age 0–7 Days**	**Age >7 Days**
Penicillin G, crystalline (U)	IV	25,000–50,000 q12h	25,000–50,000 q12h	25,000–50,000 q8h	25,000–50,000 q8h	25,000–50,000 q6h
Penicillin G, procaine (U)	IM		50,000 q 24h	50,000 q 24h	50,000 q 24h	50,000 q 24h
Penicillin G, benzathine (U)	IM		50,000 once	50,000 once	50,000 once	50,000 once
Penicillinase-resistant penicillins						
Methicillin	IV, IM	25 q12h	25–50 q12h	25–50 q8h	25–50 q8h	25–50 q6h
Oxacillin	IV, IM	25 q12h	25–50 q12h	25–50 q8h	25–50 q8h	37.5–50 q6h
Nafcillin	IV, IM	25 q12h	25–50 q12h	25–50 q8h	25–50 q8h	37.5–50 q6h
Broad-spectrum penicillins						
Ampicillin	IV, IM					
Meningitis		50 q12h	50 q12h	50 q8h	50 q8h	50 q6h
Other infections		25 q12h	25 q12h	25 q8h	25 q8h	25 q6h
Ticarcillin	IV, IM	75 q12h	75 q12h	75 q8h	75 q8h	75 q6h
Cephalosporins						
Cefazolin	IV, IM	20 q12h	20 q12h	20 q12h	20 q12h	20 q8h
Cefotaxime	IV, IM	50 q12h	50 q12h	50 q8h	50 q12h	50 q6h or q8h
Ceftriaxone	IV, IM	50 q24h	50 q24h	50 q24h	50 q24h	75 q24h
Ceftazidime	IV, IM	50 q12h	50 q12h	50 q8h	50 q8h	50 q8h
Chloramphenicol*	IV	25 q24h	25 q24h	25 q24h	25 q24h	25 q12h
Clindamycin	IV, IM	5 q 12h	5 q12h	5 q8h	5 q8h	5–7.5 q6h
Erythromycin	PO	10 q12h	10 q12h	10 q8h	10 q12h	10 q6h or q8h

*Use with caution in neonates. The appropriate dosage schedule should be based on serum concentration measurements.
IM, intramuscularly; IV, intravenously; PO, orally.
Modified from Sáez-Llorens, X., and McCracken, G.H., Jr.: Clinical pharmacology of antibacterial agents. *In* Remington, J.S., and Klein, J.O. (eds.): Infectious Diseases of the Fetus and Newborn Infant. 4th ed. Philadelphia, W.B. Saunders, 1995, p. 1325.

TABLE 235–12 ■ DOSAGE SCHEDULE FOR ANTIBIOTICS BASED ON POSTCONCEPTUAL AGE

		Dosage (mg/kg) and Interval of Administration: Gestational Age plus Weeks of Life			
Antibiotic	Route	*≤26*	*27-34*	*35-42*	*≥43*
Amikacin	IV, IM	7.5 q24h	7.5 q18h	10 q12h	10 q8h
Gentamicin	IV, IM	2.5 q24h	2.5 q18h	2.5 q12h	2.5 q8h
Tobramycin	IV, IM	2.5 q24h	2.5 q18h	2.5 q12h	2.5 q8h
Vancomycin	IV	10–15 q24h	10–15 q18h*	10–15 q12h*	10–15 q8h*

*At 28 days of life, vancomycin is administered at 20 mg/kg per dose; the interval remains the same.
IM, intramuscularly; IV, intravenously.

penicillinase-resistant penicillins (nafcillin, oxacillin, cloxacillin, and dicloxacillin), ampicillin, and lincomycin. Dairy products and other foods or medications containing calcium or magnesium salts interfere with the absorption of tetracyclines. Absorption of penicillin V, buffered penicillin G, amoxicillin, cephalexin, cefaclor, chloramphenicol, erythromycin, and clindamycin is affected only slightly by food. When absorption is affected by the concurrent ingestion of food, antibiotics should be taken 1 or more hours before or 2 or more hours after meals. A four-times-daily dosage schedule, rarely used for common infections, can be arranged for the drug to be given on arising, 1 hour before lunch and supper, and at bedtime. Most orally administered antibiotics can be administered twice or three times daily, a schedule that is accommodated easily by most parents.

INTRAVENOUS VERSUS INTRAMUSCULAR ADMINISTRATION

Although a brief period occurs when the serum antimicrobial concentration is higher after intravenous administration of an antimicrobial agent than after intramuscular administration, no therapeutic advantage of intravenous as opposed to intramuscular administration has been demonstrated. Intravenous administration should be used if the patient is in shock or is suffering from a bleeding diathesis. If prolonged parenteral therapy is anticipated, the pain of injection and the small muscle mass of infants and young children preclude the intramuscular route and make intravenous therapy preferable. The physician must be alert for thrombophlebitis, which can result from prolonged intravenous administration, and for sterile abscesses, which can develop after intramuscular administration.

Chloramphenicol, tetracyclines, erythromycin, and vancomycin should be administered intravenously rather than intramuscularly. Chloramphenicol was thought to be absorbed poorly from intramuscular sites, although recent data suggest that such is not the case. Intramuscular injection of parenteral tetracyclines and erythromycin causes local irritation and pain, and intramuscular injection of vancomycin causes tissue necrosis. Care should be given to the administration of intramuscular injections.[19, 146] Sites that minimize the risk of local neural, vascular, or tissue injury should be selected. The preferred site varies with the age of the child: the upper anterolateral aspect of the thigh in infants, the ventrogluteal area in children older than 2 years, and the deltoid area for older children. Inadvertent intra-arterial injection of benzathine penicillin G can cause tissue damage.

"PUSH" VERSUS "STEADY" OR "CONTINUOUS DRIP" INTRAVENOUS ADMINISTRATION

Antimicrobial agents can be administered intravenously by the "push" method, in which case the drug is infused in 5 to 15 minutes; by "steady drip" in 1 to 2 hours; or by "continuous drip," whereby the drug is given throughout the period of administration. The push method results in high antibacterial activity in serum for short periods, whereas the steady and continuous drip methods produce lower, but more sustained activity. The risk of adverse effects influences whether an antimicrobial agent should be administered by push or by steady drip. Recent pharmacodynamic studies suggest optimization of bactericidal activity when aminoglycosides are given by push or steady drip once daily and when β-lactams are given in many small, frequent doses or by a continuous drip to maintain concentrations of drug at the infection site that exceed the MIC of the pathogen for much of the dosing interval. Rapid administration (<5 minutes) of large intravenous doses of penicillin should be avoided because of possible adverse CNS effects. Aminoglycosides given by the intravenous route should be infused in 20 to 60 minutes rather than as a bolus because high concentrations of drug can cause eighth nerve toxicity. Antimicrobial activity, especially for penicillins, can deteriorate if drugs are kept in solution at room temperature for prolonged periods, as might occur with use of the continuous drip method. Fresh solutions of penicillins should be administered every 6 to 8 hours when the continuous drip method is used.

DIFFUSION OF ANTIMICROBIAL AGENTS ACROSS BIOLOGIC MEMBRANES

Diffusion of any drug across a biologic membrane depends on the molecular size of the drug, the degree of protein binding (only the unbound portion of the drug crosses), the degree of ionization at physiologic pH (only the un-ionized portion is available for equilibration), and solubility in lipids. Thus, the lipid solubility of the un-ionized and unbound fraction of an antimicrobial agent determines the capability of the drug to diffuse to the site of infection. Antibiotics usually are not distributed evenly throughout the body.[186, 187]

Diffusion of antimicrobial agents from blood into a joint space, pleural and pericardial fluid, and middle ear fluid is relatively unimpeded, and high concentrations of many drugs are achieved in these sites after systemic administration. More than 60 percent of the peak serum concentration of various penicillins and cephalosporins is present in the inflamed joint space.[181] Loculations of fluid in the presence of fibrous adhesions may limit the passage of antimicrobial agents into infected areas.

Diffusion of antibiotics from blood into CSF or into the aqueous humor of the eye is more limited. Drugs that are highly soluble in lipids, un-ionized, and minimally bound to proteins (e.g., isoniazid, chloramphenicol, sulfonamides) pass into CSF in high concentrations, even in the absence of inflammation, whereas drugs such as the macrolides diffuse into CSF little, if at all. Penicillins, cephalosporins, and aminoglycosides pass into CSF only when the membrane is inflamed; variable, but often low concentrations of drug in CSF can be present even in the early stages of meningitis. The β-lactams are pumped actively out of the CSF space by the choroid plexus, a process that is inhibited partially by inflammation.

DURATION OF THERAPY

Physicians must rely on empirically derived schedules of therapy for rapid and complete resolution of disease and minimal risk in terms of clinical or microbiologic failure or drug toxicity. Numerous studies evaluating the duration of therapy have been performed for streptococcal pharyngitis. The results are consistent in suggesting that 10 days of oral therapy with penicillin V, erythromycin, or cefadroxil, 5 days of azithromycin, or a single intramuscular dose of benzathine penicillin G is appropriate. Opinions vary and data are conflicting regarding the duration of treatment for diseases such as osteomyelitis, suppurative arthritis, and infections of the urinary tract. Radetsky[202] has written an enlightening history of the recommendations for the duration of treatment in bacterial meningitis and has pointed out that "Even in the absence of specific data certain numbers have an unaccountable power to satisfy and reassure ... 7, 10, 14 and 21 days have consistently appeared. Even in the trials performed at the dawn of the antimicrobial era, these numbers were chosen."

DOSAGE SCHEDULES IN CHILDREN WITH RENAL OR HEPATIC INSUFFICIENCY

The kidneys are the major organs of excretion for most antimicrobial agents, including penicillins, cephalosporins, aminoglycosides, and tetracyclines (with the exception of doxycycline). Because impaired excretion can result in high and possibly toxic serum and tissue antimicrobial concentrations, alterations in dosage schedules should be considered in children with diminished renal function. Antibiotics that require careful dosage adjustment for renal impairment include imipenem-cilastatin, meropenem, ticarcillin, aminoglycosides, tetracyclines, and vancomycin. Agents requiring dosage adjustments only when renal failure is severe include most penicillins, cephalosporins, and clindamycin. Drugs that are eliminated by nonrenal mechanisms and therefore do not require adjustment of the dosage schedule for renal impairment include chloramphenicol, cloxacillin, dicloxacillin, doxycycline, erythromycin (including the newer macrolides), metronidazole, nafcillin, oxacillin, and rifampin.

Dosage schedules for patients with renal insufficiency can be altered by administering the usual dosage for the initial dose and increasing the interval between doses or decreasing individual doses (or both in the case of renal shutdown). Although numerous guidelines have been developed to assist the physician,[142] these formulas have been generated from studies of adults with renal impairment, and pediatricians must be cautious in adapting the formulas for use in infants and young children. Serum antimicrobial concentrations should be monitored when aminoglycosides, vancomycin, and other drugs of potential toxicity are administered to children with renal insufficiency. Serum specimens are obtained at the time of the anticipated peak and trough concentrations on the first day and repeated on subsequent days to ensure a safe and effective dosage schedule.[106]

Hepatic disorders can alter plasma protein binding, tissue binding, hepatic metabolism, and the distribution of antimicrobials that are metabolized or excreted by the liver.[247] Few data exist regarding adjustment of dosage schedules for antibiotics that are metabolized by the liver in patients with hepatic insufficiency.[133] It would be prudent to avoid the use of tetracyclines and to exercise caution when prescribing macrolides, chloramphenicol, clindamycin, rifampin, and metronidazole to patients with underlying hepatic disease.

TOPICAL USE OF ANTIMICROBIAL AGENTS

Topical antimicrobial agents[249] are used for a variety of indications: bacitracin or polymyxin ointments are available (in many cases without prescription) for first aid of minor cuts, abrasions, and burns; tetracycline, erythromycin, and clindamycin have been used for the treatment of pustular acne; and metronidazole is approved for the topical treatment of inflammatory lesions and erythema associated with rosacea. Erythromycin, chloramphenicol, sulfonamide, gentamicin, tobramycin, tetracycline, and a combination of TMP and polymyxin B ointment or drops are used for the treatment of conjunctivitis, sties, and other minor infections of the eye. Silver nitrate drops or either erythromycin or tetracycline ointment is used for the prevention of gonococcal ophthalmia in newborn infants. A controlled trial involving newborn infants in Africa demonstrated equivalent or superior efficacy of a 2.5 percent ophthalmic solution of povidone-iodine in comparison to topical silver nitrate or erythromycin for prophylaxis against ophthalmia neonatorum caused by *C. trachomatis, N. gonorrhoeae,* staphylococci, or gram-negative bacteria.[117] Ofloxacin drops (Floxin Otic) are approved for the treatment of otitis externa, chronic suppurative otitis media, and acute otitis media in children with tympanostomy tubes.[24, 213] Mupirocin is effective in vitro against *S. aureus* (including methicillin-resistant strains) and group A streptococci and is approved for the treatment of impetigo. Mupirocin applied to the anterior nares may be of value in eradicating nasal carriage of methicillin-resistant staphylococci. However, a large randomized, placebo-controlled study demonstrated marginal efficacy of topical mupirocin in eradicating methicillin-resistant *S. aureus* carriage from multiple body sites in adolescents and adults.[102] Most antibiotics used topically, such as bacitracin, neomycin, and polymyxin B, are of limited use as systemic agents.

Absorption after application to the conjunctivae or large areas of denuded skin can be significant, but application to normal skin does not result in detectable concentrations of antimicrobial activity in blood or urine. Sensitization does not appear to be an important problem with most topical antibiotics, although some patients with chronic dermatoses may react to certain agents such as neomycin. Antimicrobial agents of value for systemic use should not be applied extensively to the surface of the body or used routinely in closed units (e.g., burn units) because of the risk of inducing resistance.

The Committee on Drugs of the American Academy of Pediatrics (AAP) concluded that topical antimicrobial agents may prevent infection after minor cuts, abrasions, and burns but that in most instances, gentle cleansing of minor wounds and burns is sufficient antisepsis.[5] Systemic antibiotics rather than topical drugs are recommended for chronic pyoderma, including impetigo, especially when more than several lesions are present.

Intermittent administration of inhaled tobramycin (twice daily for 4 weeks followed by 4 drug-free weeks) is indicated for the management of children and adults with cystic fibrosis and *P. aeruginosa* infection. Clinical data from a large randomized, placebo-controlled trial indicate that tobramycin treatment improves pulmonary function, decreases the density of *P. aeruginosa* in sputum, reduces the risk of hospitalization, and is well tolerated. The diminished microbial reduction during the third cycle of treatment was not explained by the development of resistance to tobramycin.[206]

The use of antimicrobial-coated central venous catheters is not accepted practice in pediatrics, but limited evidence supports its potential usefulness. Rates of bacterial colonization and bloodstream infections associated with the use of central venous catheters in high-risk adult patients were found to be lower in patients whose catheters were impregnated with minocycline and rifampin versus those impregnated with chlorhexidine and silver sulfadiazine.[61]

CURRENT USE OF ANTIMICROBIAL AGENTS FOR PROPHYLAXIS

Chemoprophylaxis refers to the use of drugs to prevent infection. Antimicrobial treatment refers to the use of drugs after infection has taken place or when early signs of infectious disease are present or infection is suspected. The use of antimicrobial agents for prophylaxis has proved to be of value in many circumstances (Table 235–13) and currently is considered to be of probable value or is investigational for the prevention of infections in many other situations. Prophylaxis is of greatest value when the following criteria are met: use of a single drug with a narrow spectrum of activity, use of a drug with limited side effects or toxicity, and prevention of colonization by an organism of known susceptibility and one that is unlikely to become resistant during the period of drug use.

USE OF ANTIMICROBIAL AGENTS FOR CHILDREN IN SCHOOL OR GROUP DAYCARE

Infants and children usually return to their school or daycare during a course of antimicrobial therapy. Because of problems with the administration of drugs outside the home, physicians should prescribe medications that are given infrequently, are relatively stable at ambient temperatures, and need only simple directions. Drugs that are administered in once- or twice-daily schedules are preferred. Chewable tablets, when available, may be of value in reducing the need for the school or daycare provider to measure specific amounts of liquid suspension and to refrigerate suspensions. Single-dosage regimens, such as intramuscular benzathine penicillin G for group A streptococcal infections, may be advantageous. Guidelines for administration of medications in school have been published by the Committee of School Health of the AAP and should be useful to the physician for prescribing drugs to young children in daycare.[262]

RESTRICTION ON USE OF ANTIMICROBIAL AGENTS FOR INFANTS AND CHILDREN

Many antimicrobial agents are approved for use in adults but have not been approved by the FDA for use in infants and children. The reasons for lack of approval include recently released drugs with insufficient experience in children, such as piperacillin-tazobactam (Zosyn); agents with real or suspected toxicity in children (e.g., damage to articular cartilage in juvenile animals associated with administration of the fluoroquinolones) that preclude use; and antibiotics for which the manufacturers have chosen not to submit data on use in children to the FDA, such as

TABLE 235–13 ■ ANTIMICROBIAL PROPHYLAXIS IN CHILDREN

Prevention of Infection in Certain Patients	Antimicrobial Agent
Group A streptococcal infection in patients with a history of rheumatic fever	Benzathine penicillin G IM, penicillin G or V PO
Bacterial endocarditis in patients at risk during surgical procedures:	
Dental procedures, surgery on the upper respiratory tract	Amoxicillin PO; erythromycin or clindamycin in penicillin-allergic patients
Gastrointestinal or genitourinary tract surgery or instrumentation	Penicillin G or ampicillin IM + gentamicin
Neonatal sepsis caused by group B *Streptococcus*	Ampicillin IM or IV (intrapartum)
Staphylococcal disease in newborn infants	Hexachlorophene
Gonococcal ophthalmia in newborn infants	Silver nitrate or erythromycin ophthalmic ointment
Malaria in travelers to endemic areas	Chloroquine, mefloquine (if chloroquine resistance is endemic)
Meningococcal disease in contacts	Rifampin, ceftriaxone
Haemophilus influenzae type b disease in contacts	Rifampin
Recurrent episodes of acute otitis media	Amoxicillin, sulfisoxazole
Postoperative infections	Penicillinase-resistant penicillins or first- or second-generation cephalosporins
Tuberculosis infections in household contacts	Isoniazid
Recurrent urinary tract infections	Trimethoprim-sulfamethoxazole, nitrofurantoin
Pneumocystis carinii pneumonia in immunosuppressed transplant recipients or patients with AIDS	Trimethoprim-sulfamethoxazole
Influenza A	Amantadine, rimantidine
Influenza A or B	Oseltamivir (children older than 12 yr)
Sepsis in patients with functional asplenia	Penicillin, amoxicillin, trimethoprim-sulfamethoxazole

IM, Intramuscularly; IV, intravenously; PO, orally.

metronidazole (Flagyl), piperacillin (Pipracil), and cefotetan (Cefotan). Although a drug that has been approved for adults may be used in children at the discretion of the physician, the prudent physician chooses to use such a drug only when it is uniquely appropriate for the infectious illness and records the basis for choice of the unapproved drug.

Two restricted antibiotics were approved recently for use in adults and have potential usefulness in the management of some pediatric patients with infections caused by multidrug-resistant gram-positive cocci. Linezolid (Zyvox), an oxazolidinone, has unique activity against methicillin-resistant *S. aureus* and *S. epidermidis* strains and vancomycin-resistant enterococci. The recommended dosage is 10 mg/kg given intravenously or orally two or three times daily (the half-life is shorter in the first year of life). The second agent is quinupristin-dalfopristin (Synercid), a semisynthetic streptogramin. This combination drug has synergistic activity against the same organisms as linezolid does and has been used extensively in adults in Europe. The dosage for children is 7.5 mg/kg given intravenously three times daily. Both drugs have been well tolerated by children, with diarrhea being the most common adverse effect. Neutropenia was noted in 6 percent of children treated for pneumonia in one study.[121]

HOME INTRAVENOUS ANTIBIOTIC THERAPY

Home intravenous antibiotic therapy is now available in most communities and enables discharge from the hospital earlier than in the past. The safety, effectiveness, and cost-efficiency of such a program have been proved, and it is of particular value for children who require 4 to 6 weeks of therapy for osteomyelitis or septic arthritis or who have chronic disease that can be managed in the home, such as cystic fibrosis or malignancy. In many cases, home care enables the patient to resume normal activities, including return to school. The following are factors that are necessary before consideration of home care:

1. Availability of a team that includes the physician, the pharmacist, a vendor who will supply the drug and supplies, and an intravenous specialty nurse
2. A disease that is stable and requires only continued antimicrobial therapy
3. Unavailability of a suitable oral antibacterial agent and availability of a parenteral antibiotic with low toxicity that the patient can tolerate (as demonstrated in the hospital) and preferably with a long half-life to allow infrequent dosing
4. A member of the household who is able to administer the antibiotic and provide aseptic care of the venous access device
5. Appropriate follow-up that can be maintained for monitoring safety and effectiveness

If problems with venous access arise and ceftriaxone is appropriate therapy, the drug can be administered in the home once a day by a nurse via the intramuscular route with success.[90, 214]

DRUG-DRUG INTERACTIONS

Drug-drug interactions can lead to therapeutic failure because of lack of effective activity of one or both drugs or serious adverse events because of toxic serum concentrations of one or both drugs.[91] Most children do not require daily medications for chronic diseases; thus, drug-drug interactions occur less commonly in pediatric than in geriatric patients, but the potential for interactions exists and must be considered when prescribing antibiotics. Because drug-drug interactions are not limited to prescription medications, inquiry into the use of over-the-counter medications should be made. Mechanisms for drug-drug interactions are physiochemical, whereby one drug is physically incompatible in solution with another; pharmacokinetic, whereby one drug interferes with the absorption, distribution, metabolism, or excretion of the other; and pharmacodynamic, whereby one drug affects the activity of a second drug. Examples of each mechanism include inactivation of aminoglycosides by extended-spectrum penicillins, decreased absorption of tetracyclines with co-administration of antacids, and antagonism of sulfonamide activity by procaine as a result of competition for PABA-binding sites.

Summary and Conclusions

A summary of the information contained in this chapter is presented in a format of questions that the physician must consider for appropriate use of antimicrobial agents in children.

1. Before the drug is administered:
   a. Have appropriate cultures been obtained for a specific microbiologic diagnosis?
   b. Has the patient received the drug previously? If so, did the patient tolerate the drug? Were there any signs of toxicity or sensitization?
   c. Does the patient have a condition that requires exclusion of some drugs? For example, children with glucose-6-phosphate dehydrogenase deficiency may have induced hemolysis when a sulfonamide, nitrofurantoin, or primaquine is administered.
2. Factors to be considered when writing orders for the administration of antimicrobial agents in a hospital:
   a. If the drug is given by mouth, will co-administration with food interfere with absorption, or is diarrhea a risk?
   b. If a parenteral route is used, should the drug be administered by the intravenous or the intramuscular route?
   c. If the drug is administered by the intravenous route, is push, steady drip, or continuous drip preferred?
   d. Should the drug be instilled directly at the site of infection?
   e. Will the drug diffuse to the site of infection?
   f. Should incision and drainage of the infected area be performed before or after beginning therapy? Incision and drainage should be considered whenever a significant collection of pus is present. If the drainage procedure is performed before administration of the antibiotic, material should be obtained for culture and susceptibility testing.
   g. Does the patient have renal or hepatic insufficiency that requires alteration of the dosage schedule?
   h. Are any special precautions required for household contacts? Prophylaxis may be warranted in special circumstances of infection occurring in the household, daycare center, or nursery school.
3. Use of antimicrobial agents in children who are treated as outpatients[156]:
   a. Have the names and functions of the drugs been communicated to the patient and the parent? Do any of the drugs prescribed interact with each other?
   b. Is the dosage schedule simple and satisfactory for the family circumstances (e.g., the child's school schedule, the schedule of the working parents)?
   c. Does the child have an adequate supply of the drug until it can be purchased? If not, the use of starter packages is of value. Administration of the first dose in the clinic is advantageous because it provides knowledge of acceptance and tolerability of the drug by the child.
   d. Are parents given instructions for reporting the clinical course by telephone? Is an appointment made for the next visit?
   e. Does the patient or parent know how to assess adequacy of response to the drug? Does the parent know how to take the child's temperature?
   f. Is the total amount of drug prescribed adequate for the course? Will refills of the prescription be needed?
   g. Is the drug provided in a convenient dosage form? Will the package be provided with an adequate means of measuring the drug? Does the agent require refrigeration?
   h. Has the patient or parent been informed of signs of side effects or toxicity?
   i. Are generic equivalents of the drug adequate?
   j. Will the patient be able to pay for the drug if it is purchased elsewhere (away from the clinic)? If applicable, will a third party pay for this prescription? (In some states, prescriptions by brand name may not be filled because reimbursement by the third-party payer, such as Medicaid, is insufficient.)
4. After the patient's course:
   a. How long should the patient take the drug?
   b. When should the initial choice of antimicrobial agents be reconsidered? When the results of cultures and appropriate susceptibility tests are available, the initial choice should be re-evaluated and altered, if necessary.
   c. What studies should be performed to monitor the safety and adequacy of the regimen? Hematologic indices must be measured during the administration of certain antibiotics to detect any adverse reaction.
   d. Are repeat cultures necessary? In certain cases, the most appropriate criterion of efficacy is evaluation of the results of cultures.
   e. What clinical and laboratory signs of efficacy should be monitored? Signs may differ for different diseases and various drugs but should be considered by the physician when the course of therapy is designed.
5. What factors should be considered if the patient fails to respond to the antimicrobial agent? If the patient does not respond appropriately to the course of therapy, various factors must be considered, including those related to the disease, host, drug, or organism (Table 235–14).

TABLE 235–14 ■ FACTORS CONTRIBUTING TO ANTIMICROBIAL FAILURE

Host Related
Foreign body present
Anatomic defect
Defect in immune response to infection
Disease Related
Antibiotic inappropriate for the disease
Ancillary therapy not instituted
Sequestered focus of infection (undetected or inaccessible)
Organism Related
Acquired resistance to an antimicrobial agent
Superinfection with resistant bacteria
Drug Related
Inadequate compliance
Improper dosage schedule—route, dose, or duration
Inadequate diffusion to the site of infection
Drug-drug interactions—antibiotic inactivation or antagonism
Deterioration of drug during storage

Acknowledgments

We would like to acknowledge the contributions of Dr. Jerome Klein and Dr. Sheila Hickey, who were instrumental in preparation of this chapter in previous editions. Many of the sections have been modified to reflect recently published information or the availability of new antimicrobial agents.

REFERENCES

1. Abramowicz, M.: Drugs for parasitic infections. Med. Lett. Drugs Ther. *37*:99–108, 1995.
2. Abramson, J. S., and Givner, L. B.: Should tetracycline be contraindicated for therapy of presumed Rocky Mountain spotted fever in children less than 9 years of age? Editorial. Pediatrics *86*:123–124, 1990.
3. Ackerman, B. H., Vannier, A. M., and Eudy, E. B.: Analysis of vancomycin time-kill studies with *Staphylococcus* species by using a curve stripping program to describe the relationship between concentration and pharmacodynamic response. Antimicrob. Agents Chemother. *36*:1766–1769, 1992.
4. Ambrose, P. J.: Clinical pharmacokinetics of chloramphenicol and chloramphenicol succinate. Clin. Pharmacokinet. *9*:222–238, 1984.
5. American Academy of Pediatrics, Committee on Drugs: Topical antibiotics. Pediatrics *59*(Suppl.):1041–1042, 1977.
6. Asmar, B. I., Prainito, M., and Dajani, A. S.: Antagonistic effect of chloramphenicol in combination with cefotaxime or ceftriaxone. Antimicrob. Agents Chemother. *32*:1375–1378, 1988.
7. Assael, B. M., Parini, R., and Rusconi, F.: Ototoxicity of aminoglycoside antibiotics in infants and children. Pediatr. Infect. Dis. J. *1*:357–365, 1982.
8. Azimi, P. H.: Clinical and laboratory investigation of cefamandole therapy of infections in infants and children. J. Infect. Dis. *137*(Suppl.):155–160, 1978.
9. Azimi, P. H., Barson, W. J., Janner, D., et al.: Efficacy and safety of ampicillin/sulbactam and cefuroxime in the treatment of serious skin and skin structure infections in pediatric patients. UNASYN Pediatric Study Group. Pediatr. Infect. Dis. J. *18*:609–613, 1999.
10. Bahal, N., and Nahata, M. C.: The new macrolide antibiotics: Azithromycin, clarithromycin, dirithromycin, and roxithromycin. Ann. Pharmacother. *26*:46–55, 1992.
11. Banfi, A., Gabriele, G., Hill-Juarez, J. M., et al.: Multinational comparative trial of ceftibuten and trimethoprim-sulfamethoxazole in the treatment of children with complicated or recurrent urinary tract infections. Ceftibuten Urinary Tract Infection International Study Group. Pediatr. Infect. Dis. J. *12*(Suppl.):84–91, 1993.
12. Barr, W. H., Affrime, M., Lin, C. C., et al.: Pharmacokinetics of ceftibuten in children. Pediatr. Infect. Dis. J. *14*(Suppl.):93–101, 1995.
13. Barry, A. L., and Jones, R. N.: Cefixime: Spectrum of antibacterial activity against 16,016 clinical isolates. Pediatr. Infect. Dis. J. *6*:954–957, 1987.
14. Barza, M.: The nephrotoxicity of cephalosporins: An overview. J. Infect. Dis. *137*(Suppl.):60–73, 1978.
15. Bass, J. W., Crast, F. W., Knowles, C. R., et al.: Streptococcal pharyngitis in children. A comparison of four treatment schedules with intramuscular penicillin G benzathine. J. A. M. A. *235*:1112–1116, 1976.
16. Bass, J. W., Freitas, B. C., Freitas, A. D., et al.: Prospective randomized double blind placebo-controlled evaluation of azithromycin for treatment of cat-scratch disease. Pediatr. Infect. Dis. J. *17*:447–452, 1998.
17. Beall, G. N.: Penicillins. *In* Saxon, A. (moderator): Immediate hypersensitivity reactions to beta-lactam antibiotics [clinical conference]. Ann. Intern. Med. *107*:204–215, 1987.
18. Bennett, W. M., Plamp, C. E., Gilbert, D. N., et al.: The influence of dosage regimen on experimental gentamicin nephrotoxicity: Dissociation of peak serum levels from renal failure. J. Infect. Dis. *140*:576–580, 1979.
19. Bergeson, P. S., Singer, S. A., and Kaplan, A. M.: Intramuscular injections in children. Pediatrics *70*:944–948, 1982.
20. Bhutta, Z. A., Khan, I. A., and Shadmani, M.: Failure of short-course ceftriaxone chemotherapy for multidrug- resistant typhoid fever in children: A randomized controlled trial in Pakistan. Antimicrob. Agents Chemother. *44*:450–452, 2000.
21. Birnbaum, J., Stapley, E. O., Miller, A. K., et al.: Cefoxitin, a semi-synthetic cephamycin: A microbiological overview. J. Antimicrob. Chemother. *4*:15–32, 1978.
22. Black, J. R., Feinberg, J., Murphy, R. L., et al.: Clindamycin and primaquine therapy for mild-to-moderate episodes of *Pneumocystis carinii* pneumonia in patients with AIDS: AIDS Clinical Trials Group 044. Clin. Infect. Dis. *18*:905–913, 1994.
23. Blaser, J.: Efficacy of once- and thrice-daily dosing of aminoglycosides in in-vitro models of infection. J. Antimicrob. Chemother. *27*(Suppl. C):21–28, 1991.
24. Bluestone, C. D.: Efficacy of ofloxacin and other ototopical preparations for chronic suppurative otitis media in children. Pediatr. Infect. Dis. J. *20*:111–115, 2001.
25. Blumer, J. L.: Cefixime. Drug Ther. *19*:60–84, 1989.
26. Blumer, J. L.: Pharmacokinetic determinants of carbapenem therapy in neonates and children. Pediatr. Infect. Dis. J. *15*:733–737, 1996.
27. Blumer, J. L.: Ticarcillin/clavulanate for the treatment of serious infections in hospitalized pediatric patients. Pediatr. Infect. Dis. J. *17*:1211–1215, 1998.
28. Blumer, J. L., Reed, M. D., Kearns, G. L., et al.: Sequential, single-dose pharmacokinetic evaluation of meropenem in hospitalized infants and children. Antimicrob. Agents Chemother. *39*:1721–1725, 1995.
29. Blumer, J. L., Reed, M. D., and Knupp, C.: Review of the pharmacokinetics of cefepime in children. Pediatr. Infect. Dis. J. *20*:341–346, 2001.
30. Boguniewicz, M., and Leung, D. Y.: Hypersensitivity reactions to antibiotics commonly used in children. Pediatr. Infect. Dis. J. *14*:221–231, 1995.
31. Bonacorsi, S., and Bingen, E.: Bactericidal activity of erythromycin associated with sulphisoxazole against the infectious agents most frequently responsible for acute infantile otitis media. Letter. J. Antimicrob. Chemother. *33*:885–886, 1994.
32. Bradley, J. S.: Meropenem: A new, extremely broad spectrum beta-lactam antibiotic for serious infections in pediatrics. Pediatr. Infect. Dis. J. *16*:263–268, 1997.
33. Bradley, J. S., and Arrieta, A.: Empiric use of cefepime in the treatment of lower respiratory tract infections in children. Pediatr. Infect. Dis. J. *20*:347–353, 2001.
34. Bradley, J. S., Faulkner, K. L., and Klaugman, K. P.: Efficacy, safety and tolerability of meropenem as empiric antibiotic therapy in hospitalized pediatric patients. Pediatr. Infect. Dis. J. *15*:749–757, 1996.
35. Braun, P.: Hepatotoxicity of erythromycin. J. Infect. Dis. *119*:300–306, 1969.
36. Breiman, R. F., Butler, J. C., Tenover, F. C., et al.: Emergence of drug-resistant pneumococcal infections in the U.S. J. A. M. A. *271*:1831–1835, 1994.
37. Brown, C. H., III, Natelson, E. A., Bradshaw, M. W., et al.: Study of the effects of ticarcillin on blood coagulation and platelet function. Antimicrob. Agents Chemother. *7*:652–657, 1975.
38. Brummett, R. E.: Ototoxicity of vancomycin and analogues. Otolaryngol. Clin. North Am. *26*:821–828, 1993.
39. Burchall, J. J.: Mechanism of action of trimethoprim-sulfamethoxazole. II. J. Infect. Dis. *128*(Suppl.):437–441, 1973.
40. Bush, K., Jacoby, G. A., and Medeiros, A. A.: A functional classification scheme for beta-lactamases and its correlation with molecular structure. Antimicrob. Agents Chemother. *39*:1211–1233, 1995.
41. Bush, L. M., and Johnson, C. C.: Ureidopenicillins and beta-lactam/beta-lactamase inhibitor combinations. Infect. Dis. Clin. North Am. *14*:409–433, 2000.
42. Cabizuca, S. V., and Desser, K. B.: Carbenicillin-associated hypokalemic alkalosis. J. A. M. A. *236*:956–957, 1976.
43. Cantu, T. G., Yamanaka-Yuen, N. A., and Lietman, P. S.: Serum vancomycin concentrations: Reappraisal of their clinical value. Clin. Infect. Dis. *18*:533–543, 1994.
44. Carter, B. L., Woodhead, J. C., Cole, K. J., et al.: Gastrointestinal side effects with erythromycin preparations. Drug Intell. Clin. Pharmacol. *21*:734–738, 1987.
45. Chambers, H. F., and Sachdeva, M.: Binding of beta-lactam antibiotics to penicillin-binding proteins in methicillin-resistant *Staphylococcus aureus*. J. Infect. Dis. *161*:1170–1176, 1990.
46. Chesney, P. J., Davis, Y., English, B. K., et al.: Occurrence of *Streptococcus pneumoniae* meningitis during vancomycin and cefotaxime therapy of septicemia in a patient with sickle cell disease. Pediatr. Infect. Dis. J. *14*:1013–1015, 1995.
47. Chopra, I., Hawkey, P. M., and Hinton, M.: Tetracyclines, molecular and clinical aspects. J. Antimicrob. Chemother. *29*:245–277, 1992.
48. Clarke, A. M., and Zemcov, S. J.: Clavulanic acid in combination with ticarcillin: An in-vitro comparison with other beta-lactams. J. Antimicrob. Chemother. *13*:121–128, 1984.
49. Cohen, R.: Clinical experience with cefpodoxime proxetil in acute otitis media. Pediatr. Infect. Dis. J. *14*(Suppl.):12–18, 1995.
50. Collins, M. D., Dajani, A. S., Kim, K. S., et al.: Comparison of ampicillin/sulbactam plus aminoglycoside vs. ampicillin plus clindamycin plus aminoglycoside in the treatment of intraabdominal infections in children. The Multicenter Group. Pediatr. Infect. Dis. J. *17*(Suppl.):15–18, 1998.
51. Cometta, A., Calandra, T., Gaya, H., et al.: Monotherapy with meropenem versus combination therapy with ceftazidime plus amikacin as empiric therapy for fever in granulocytopenic patients with cancer. Antimicrob. Agents Chemother. *40*:1108–1115, 1996.
52. Conte, J. E., Jr., Golden, J. A., Duncan, S., et al.: Intrapulmonary pharmacokinetics of clarithromycin and of erythromycin. Antimicrob. Agents Chemother. *39*:334–338, 1995.
53. Control and prevention of meningococcal disease: Recommendations of the Advisory Committee on Immunization Practices. M. M. W. R. Recomm. Rep. *46*(RR-5):1–10, 1997.
54. Craft, J. C., Siepman, N.: Overview of the safety profile of clarithromycin suspension in pediatric patients. Pediatr. Infect. Dis. J. *12*(Suppl.):142–147, 1993.
55. Craig, W. A.: The pharmacology of meropenem, a new carbapenem antibiotic. Clin. Infect. Dis. *24*(Suppl. 2):266–275, 1997.
56. Craig, W. A., and Ebert, S. C.: Killing and regrowth of bacteria in vitro: A review. Scand. J. Infect. Dis. *74*:63–70, 1990.
57. Cunha, B. A., Sibley, C. M., and Ristuccia, A. M.: Doxycycline. Ther. Drug Monit. *4*:115–135, 1982.
58. Dagan, R., Johnson, C. E., McLinn, S., et al.: Bacteriologic and clinical efficacy of amoxicillin/clavulanate vs. azithromycin in acute otitis media. Pediatr. Infect. Dis. J. *19*:95–104, 2000.

59. Dagan, R., Velghe, L., Rodda, J. L., et al.: Penetration of meropenem into the CSF of patients with inflamed meninges. J. Antimicrob. Chemother. *34*:175–179, 1994.
60. Dajani, A. S.: Pharyngitis/tonsillitis: European and U.S. experience with cefpodoxime proxetil. Pediatr. Infect. Dis. J. *14*(Suppl.):7–11, 1995.
61. Darouiche, R. O., Raad, I. I., Heard, S. O., et al.: A comparison of two antimicrobial-impregnated central venous catheters. N. Engl. J. Med. *340*:1–8, 1999.
62. Dattwyler, R. J., Luft, B. J., Kunkel, M. J., et al.: Ceftriaxone compared with doxycycline for the treatment of acute disseminated Lyme disease. N. Engl. J. Med. *337*:289–294, 1997.
63. Davies, J. E.: Resistance to aminoglycosides: Mechanisms and frequency. Rev. Infect. Dis. *5*(Suppl. 2):261–266, 1983.
64. Dawson, C. R., Schachter, J., Sallam, S., et al.: A comparison of oral azithromycin with topical oxytetracycline/polymyxin for the treatment of trachoma in children. Clin. Infect. Dis. *24*:363–368, 1997.
65. de Alba Romero, C., Gomez Castillo, E., Manzanares Secades, C., et al.: Once daily gentamicin dosing in neonates. Pediatr. Infect. Dis. J. *17*:1169–1171, 1998.
66. De Broe, M. E., Giuliano, R. A., and Verpooten, G. A.: Choice of drug and dosage regimen. Two important risk factors for aminoglycoside nephrotoxicity. Am. J. Med. *80*:115–118, 1986.
67. Denny, F. W., Wannamaker, L. W., Brink, W. R., et al.: Prevention of rheumatic fever: Treatment of the preceding streptococcal infection. J. A. M. A. *143*:151–153, 1950.
68. Dhawan, V. K., and Thadepalli, H.: Clindamycin: A review of fifteen years of experience. Rev. Infect. Dis. *4*:1133–1153, 1982.
69. Disney, F. A., Hanfling, M. J., and Hausinger, S. A.: Loracarbef (LY163892) vs. penicillin VK in the treatment of streptococcal pharyngitis and tonsillitis. Pediatr. Infect. Dis. J. *11*(Suppl.):20–26, 1992.
70. Doern, G.: In vitro activity of loracarbef and effects of susceptibility test methods. Am. J. Med. *92*(Suppl.):7–15, 1992.
71. Dowell, S. F., Butler, J. C., Giebink, G. S., et al.: Acute otitis media: Management and surveillance in an era of pneumococcal resistance. A report from the Drug-Resistant *Streptococcus pneumoniae* Therapeutic Working Group. Pediatr. Infect. Dis. J. *18*:1–9, 1999.
72. Drusano, G. L.: Role of pharmacokinetics in the outcome of infections. Antimicrob. Agents Chemother. *32*:289–297, 1988.
73. Drusano, G. L., Schimpff, S. C., and Hewitt, W. L.: The acylampicillins: Mezlocillin, piperacillin, and azlocillin. Rev. Infect. Dis. *6*:13–32, 1984.
74. Ebert, S. C., and Craig, W. A.: Pharmacodynamic properties of antibiotics: Application to drug monitoring and dosage regimen design. Infect. Control Hosp. Epidemiol. *11*:319–326, 1990.
75. Falagas, M. E., and Gorbach, S. L.: Clindamycin and metronidazole. Med. Clin. North Am. *79*:845–867, 1995.
76. Faulkner, R. D., Yacobi, A., Barone, J. S., et al.: Pharmacokinetic profile of cefixime in man. Pediatr. Infect. Dis. J. *6*:963–970, 1987.
77. Feigin, R. D., Pickering, L. K., Anderson, D., et al.: Clindamycin treatment of osteomyelitis and septic arthritis in children. Pediatrics *55*:213–223, 1975.
78. Ferrazzini, G., Klein, J., Sulh, H., et al.: Interaction between trimethoprim-sulfamethoxazole and methotrexate in children with leukemia. J. Pediatr. *117*:823–826, 1990.
79. Fichtenbaum, C. J., Ritchie, D. J., and Powderly, W. G.: Use of paromomycin for treatment of cryptosporidiosis in patients with AIDS. Clin. Infect. Dis. *16*:298–300, 1993.
80. Finland, M.: Twenty-fifth anniversary of the discovery of Aureomycin: The place of the tetracyclines in antimicrobial therapy. Clin. Pharmacol. Ther. *15*:3–8, 1974.
81. Fisman, D. N., and Kaye, K. M.: Once-daily dosing of aminoglycoside antibiotics. Infect. Dis. Clin. North Am. *14*:475–487, 2000.
82. Fong, I. W., Engelking, E. R., and Kirby, W. M.: Relative inactivation by *Staphylococcus aureus* of eight cephalosporin antibiotics. Antimicrob. Agents Chemother. *9*:939–944, 1976.
83. Foshee, W. S., and Qvarnberg, Y.: Comparative U.S. and European trials of loracarbef in the treatment of acute otitis media. Pediatr. Infect. Dis. J. *11*(Suppl.):12–19, 1992.
84. Foster, J. A., and Sylvia, L. M.: Doxycycline-induced esophageal ulceration. Ann. Pharmacother. *28*:1185–1187, 1994.
85. Friedland, I. R., Shelton, S., and McCracken, G. H., Jr.: Chloramphenicol in penicillin-resistant pneumococcal meningitis. Letter. Lancet *342*:240–241, 1993.
86. Fu, K. P., and Neu, H. C.: A comparative study of the activity of cefamandole and other cephalosporins and analysis of the beta-lactamase stability and synergy of cefamandole with aminoglycosides. J. Infect. Dis. *137*(Suppl.):38–50, 1978.
87. Fu, K. P., and Neu, H. C.: Piperacillin, a new penicillin active against many bacteria resistant to other penicillins. Antimicrob. Agents Chemother. *13*:358–367, 1978.
88. Galimand, M., Gerbaud, G., Guibourdenche, M., et al.: High-level chloramphenicol resistance in *Neisseria meningitidis*. N. Engl. J. Med. *339*:868–874, 1998.
89. Gilbert, D. N.: Aminoglycosides. *In* Mandell, G. L., Bennett, J. E., and Dolin, R. (eds.): Mandell, Douglas, and Bennett's Principles and Practice of Infectious Disease, 4th ed. New York, Churchill-Livingstone, 1995, pp. 279–306.
90. Gilbert, D. N., Dworkin, R. J., Raber, S. R., et al.: Drug therapy: Outpatient parenteral antimicrobial-drug therapy. N. Engl. J. Med. *18*:829–838, 1997.
91. Gillum, J. G., Israel, D. S., and Polk, R. E.: Pharmacokinetic drug interactions with antimicrobial agents. Clin. Pharmacokinet. *25*:450–482, 1993.
92. Girgis, N. I., Sultan, Y., Hammad, O., et al.: Comparison of the efficacy, safety and cost of cefixime, ceftriaxone and aztreonam in the treatment of multidrug-resistant *Salmonella typhi* septicemia in children. Pediatr. Infect. Dis. J. *14*:603–605, 1995.
93. Goetz, M. B., and Sayers, J.: Nephrotoxicity of vancomycin and aminoglycoside therapy separately and in combination. [Published erratum appears in J Antimicrob Chemother 1993 Dec;32(6):925.] J. Antimicrob. Chemother. *32*:325–334, 1993.
94. Green, M., Li, K. I., Wald, E. R., et al.: Duration of rifampin chemoprophylaxis for contacts of patients infected with *Haemophilus influenzae* type b. Antimicrob. Agents Chemother. *36*:545–547, 1992.
95. Grossman, E. R., Walchek, A., and Freedman, H.: Tetracyclines and permanent teeth: The relation between dose and tooth color. Pediatrics *47*:567–570, 1971.
96. Guay, D. R., and Craft, J. C.: Overview of the pharmacology of clarithromycin suspension in children and a comparison with that in adults. Pediatr. Infect. Dis. J. *12*(Suppl.):106–611, 1993.
97. Guay, D. R. P.: Ceftibuten: A new expanded-spectrum oral cephalosporin. Ann. Pharmacother. *31*:1022–1033, 1997.
98. Guay, D. R. P.: Pharmacodynamics and pharmacokinetics of cefdinir, an oral extended spectrum cephalosporin. Pediatr. Infect. Dis. J. *19*(Suppl.):141–146, 2000.
99. 1998 Guidelines for the treatment of sexually transmitted diseases. M. M. W. R. Recomm. Rep. *47*(RR-1):1–118, 1998.
100. Haight, T. H., and Finland, M.: Observations on mode of action of erythromycin. Proc. Soc. Exp. Biol. Med. *81*:188–193, 1952.
101. Handwerger, S., and Tomasz, A.: Antibiotic tolerance among clinical isolates of bacteria. Rev. Infect. Dis. *7*:368–386, 1985.
102. Harbarth, S., Dharan, S., Liassine, N., et al.: Randomized, placebo-controlled, double-blind trial to evaluate the efficacy of mupirocin for eradicating carriage of methicillin-resistant *Staphylococcus aureus*. Antimicrob. Agents Chemother. *43*:1412–1416, 1999.
103. Hardy, D. J., Swanson, R. N., Rode, R. A., et al.: Enhancement of the in vitro and in vivo activities of clarithromycin against *Haemophilus influenzae* by 14-hydroxy-clarithromycin, its major metabolite in humans. Antimicrob. Agents Chemother. *34*:1407–1413, 1990.
104. Haycock, G. B., Schwartz, G. J., and Wisotsky, D. H.: Geometric method for measuring body surface area: A height-weight formula validated in infants, children, and adults. J. Pediatr. *93*:62–66, 1978.
105. Hebert, A. A., Still, J. G., and Reuman, P. D.: Comparative safety and efficacy of clarithromycin and cefadroxil suspensions in the treatment of mild to moderate skin and skin structure infections in children. Pediatr. Infect. Dis. J. *12*(Suppl.):112–117, 1993.
106. Hewitt, W. L., and McHenry, M. C.: Blood level determinations of antimicrobial drugs. Some clinical considerations. Med. Clin. North Am. *62*:1119–1140, 1978.
107. Hitchings, G. H.: Mechanism of action of trimethoprim-sulfamethoxazole. I. J. Infect. Dis. *128*(Suppl.):433–436, 1973.
108. Hoberman, A., Wald, E. R., Hickey, R. W., et al.: Oral versus initial intravenous therapy for urinary tract infections in young febrile children. Pediatrics *104*:79–86, 1999.
109. Hoiby, N., Ciofu, O., Jensen, T., et al.: Use of carbapenems and other antibiotics for pulmonary infections in patients with cystic fibrosis. Pediatr. Infect. Dis. J. *15*:738–743, 1996.
110. Honein, M. A., Paulozzi, L. J., Himelright, I. M., et al.: Infantile hypertrophic pyloric stenosis after pertussis prophylaxis with erythromycin: A case review and cohort study. Lancet *354*:2101–2105, 1999.
111. Howie, V. M., and Owen, M. J.: Bacteriologic and clinical efficacy of cefixime compared with amoxicillin in acute otitis media. Pediatr. Infect. Dis. J. *6*:989–991, 1987.
112. Humbert, P., Treffel, P., Chapuis, J. F., et al.: The tetracyclines in dermatology. J. Am. Acad. Dermatol. *25*:691–697, 1991.
113. Huovinen, P.: Trimethoprim resistance. Antimicrob. Agents Chemother. *31*:1451–1456, 1987.
114. Huovinen, P.: Increases in rates of resistance to trimethoprim. Clin. Infect. Dis. *24*(Suppl. 1):63–66, 1997.
115. Hurst, M., and Lamb, H. M.: Meropenem: A review of its use in patients in intensive care. Drugs *59*:653–680, 2000.
116. Isaksson, B., Nilsson, L., Maller, R., et al.: Postantibiotic effect of aminoglycosides on gram-negative bacteria evaluated by a new method. J. Antimicrob. Chemother. *22*:23–33, 1988.
117. Isenberg, S. J., Apt, L., and Wood, M.: A controlled trial of povidone-iodine as prophylaxis against ophthalmia neonatorum. N. Engl. J. Med. *332*:562–566, 1995.
118. Jacoby, G. A., and Medeiros, A. A.: More extended-spectrum beta-lactamases. Antimicrob. Agents Chemother. *35*:1697–1704, 1991.
119. Jonas, M., and Cunha, B. A.: Minocycline. Ther. Drug Monit. *4*:137–145, 1982.
120. Jorgensen, J. H., Doern, G. V., Maher, L. A., et al.: Antimicrobial resistance among respiratory isolates of *Haemophilus influenzae*, *Moraxella*

catarrhalis, and *Streptococcus pneumoniae* in the U.S. Antimicrob. Agents Chemother. *34*:2075–2080, 1990.
121. Kaplan, S. L., Patterson, L., Edwards, K. M., et al.: Linezolid for the treatment of community-acquired pneumonia in hospitalized children. Pediatr. Infect. Dis. J. *20*:488–494, 2001.
122. Kearns, G. L., Wheeler, J. G., Childress, S. H., et al.: Serum sickness–like reactions to cefaclor: Role of hepatic metabolism and individual susceptibility. J. Pediatr. *125*:805–811, 1994.
123. Kelly, H. W., Couch, R. C., Davis, R. L., et al.: Interaction of chloramphenicol and rifampin. J. Pediatr. *112*:817–820, 1988.
124. Kessler, R. E.: Cefepime microbiologic profile and update. Pediatr. Infect. Dis. J. *20*:335–340, 2001.
125. Khuri-Bulos, N. A., Daoud, A. H., and Azab, S. M.: Treatment of childhood brucellosis: Results of a prospective trial on 113 children. Pediatr. Infect. Dis. J. *12*:377–381, 1993.
126. Klein, J. O.: Clarithromycin and azithromycin. Pediatr. Infect. Dis. J. *17*:516–517, 1998.
127. Klein, J. O., and Finland, M.: The new penicillins. N. Engl. J. Med. *269*:1019–1025, 1963.
128. Klein, J. O., and McCracken, G. H., Jr.: Summary: Role of a new oral cephalosporin, cefdinir, for therapy of infections of infants and children. Pediatr. Infect. Dis. J. *19*(Suppl.):181–183, 2000.
129. Klugman, K. P., Dagan, R.: Randomized comparison of meropenem with cefotaxime for treatment of bacterial meningitis. Meropenem Meningitis Study Group. Antimicrob. Agents Chemother. *39*:1140–1146, 1995.
130. Kotra, L. P., Haddad, J., and Mobashery, S.: Aminoglycosides: Perspectives on mechanisms of action and resistance and strategies to counter resistance. Antimicrob. Agents Chemother. *44*:3249–3256, 2000.
131. Kremsner, P. G., Winkler, S., Brandts, C., et al.: Clindamycin in combination with chloroquine or quinine is an effective therapy for uncomplicated *Plasmodium falciparum* malaria in children from Gabon. J. Infect. Dis. *169*:467–470, 1994.
132. Leader, W. G., Chandler, M. H., and Castiglia, M.: Pharmacokinetic optimisation of vancomycin therapy. Clin. Pharmacokinet. *28*:327–342, 1995.
133. Lebel, M. H.: Pharmacology of antimicrobial agents in children with hepatic dysfunction. Pediatr. Infect. Dis. J. *5*:686–690, 1986.
134. Leclercq, R., and Courvalin, P.: Bacterial resistance to macrolide, lincosamide, and streptogramin antibiotics by target modification. [Published erratum appears in Antimicrob Agents Chemother 1991 Oct;35(10):2165.] Antimicrob. Agents Chemother. *35*:1267–1272, 1991.
135. Leclercq, R., and Courvalin, P.: Intrinsic and unusual resistance to macrolide, lincosamide, and streptogramin antibiotics in bacteria. Antimicrob. Agents Chemother. *35*:1273–1276, 1991.
136. Leibovitz, E., Piglansky, L., Raiz, S., et al.: Bacteriologic efficacy of a three-day intramuscular ceftriaxone regimen in nonresponsive acute otitis media. Pediatr. Infect. Dis. J. *17*:1126–1131, 1998.
137. Levine, B. B.: Immunologic mechanisms of penicillin allergy. A haptenic model system for the study of allergic diseases of man. N. Engl. J. Med. *275*:1115–1125, 1966.
138. Levine, L. R.: Quantitative comparison of adverse reactions to cefaclor vs. amoxicillin in a surveillance study. Pediatr. Infect. Dis. J. *4*:358–361, 1985.
139. Levison, M. E.: Pharmacodynamics of antimicrobial agents. Bactericidal and postantibiotic effects. Infect. Dis. Clin. North Am. *9*:483–495, 1995.
140. Lin, R. Y.: A perspective on penicillin allergy. Arch. Intern. Med. *152*:930–937, 1992.
141. Livermore, D. M.: Determinants of the activity of beta-lactamase inhibitor combinations. J. Antimicrob. Chemother. *31*(Suppl. A):9–21, 1993.
142. Livornese, L. L., Jr., Slavin, D., Benz, R. L., et al.: Use of antibacterial agents in renal failure. Infect. Dis. Clin. North Am. *14*:371–390, 2000.
143. Loeffler, A. M.: Uses of rifampin for infections other than tuberculosis. Pediatr. Infect. Dis. J. *18*:631–632, 1999.
144. Logan, M. N., Ashby, J. P., Andrews, J. M., et al.: The in-vitro and disc susceptibility testing of clarithromycin and its 14-hydroxy metabolite. J. Antimicrob. Chemother. *27*:161–170, 1991.
145. Lopez-Samblas, A. M., Torres, C. L., Wang, H., et al.: Effectiveness of a gentamicin dosing protocol based on postconceptional age: Comparison to published neonatal guidelines. Ann. Pharmacother. *26*:534–538, 1992.
146. Losek, J. D., and Gyuro, J.: Pediatric intramuscular injections: Do you know the procedure and complications? Pediatr. Emerg. Care *8*:79–81, 1992.
147. Lubani, M. M., Dudin, K. I., Sharda, D. C., et al.: A multicenter therapeutic study of 1100 children with brucellosis. Pediatr. Infect. Dis. J. *8*:75–78, 1989.
148. Luer, M. S., and Hatton, J.: Vancomycin administration into the CSF: A review. Ann. Pharmacother. *27*:912–921, 1993.
149. Lundstrom, T. S., and Sobel, J. D.: Antibiotics for gram-positive bacterial infections. Vancomycin, teicoplanin, quinupristin/dalfopristin, and linezolid. Infect. Dis. Clin. North Am. *14*:463–474, 2000.
150. Lyon, B. R., and Skurray, R.: Antimicrobial resistance of *Staphylococcus aureus:* Genetic basis. Microbiol. Rev. *51*:88–134, 1987.
151. Magerlein, B. J.: Modification of lincomycin. Adv. Appl. Microbiol. *14*:185–229, 1971.
152. Marcy, S. M., and Klein, J. O.: The isoxazolyl penicillins: Oxacillin, cloxacillin, and dicloxacillin. Med. Clin. North Am. *54*:1127–1143, 1970.
153. Marsh, F. P.: Do cephalosporins potentiate or antagonize aminoglycoside nephrotoxicity? J. Antimicrob. Chemother. *4*:103–106, 1978.
154. Martin, J. M., Pitetti, R., Maffei, F., et al.: Treatment of shigellosis with cefixime: Two days vs. five days. Pediatr. Infect. Dis. J. *19*:522–526, 2000.
155. Mason, E. O., Jr., Kaplan, S. L.: Penicillin-resistant pneumococci in the U.S. Letter. Pediatr. Infect. Dis. J. *14*:1017–1018, 1995.
156. Mattar, M. E., Markello, J., and Yaffe, S. J.: Inadequacies in the pharmacologic management of ambulatory children. J. Pediatr. *87*:137–141, 1975.
157. Mattie, H., Craig, W. A., and Pechere, J. C.: Determinants of efficacy and toxicity of aminoglycosides. J. Antimicrob. Chemother. *24*:281–293, 1989.
158. Mazzei, T., Mini, E., Novelli, A., et al.: Chemistry and mode of action of macrolides. J. Antimicrob. Chemother. *31*(Suppl. C):1–9, 1993.
159. McCarty, J. M., and Renteria, A.: Treatment of pharyngitis and tonsillitis with cefprozil: Review of three multicenter trials. Clin. Infect. Dis. *14*(Suppl. 2):224–230, 1992.
160. McCracken, G. H., Jr.: New era for orally administered antibiotics: Use of sequential parenteral-oral antibiotic therapy for serious infectious diseases of infants and children. Pediatr. Infect. Dis. J. *6*:951–953, 1987.
161. McCracken, G. H., Jr.: Microbiologic activity of the newer macrolide antibiotics. Pediatr. Infect. Dis. J. *16*:432–437, 1997.
162. McGehee, R. F., Jr., Smith, C. B., Wilcox, C., Finland, M.: Comparative studies of antibacterial activity in vitro and absorption and excretion of lincomycin and clinimycin. Am. J. Med. Sci. *256*:279–292, 1968.
163. McLinn, S.: Double blind and open label studies of azithromycin in the management of acute otitis media in children: A review. Pediatr. Infect. Dis. J. *14*(Suppl.):62–66, 1995.
164. Meyer, R. D.: Risk factors and comparisons of clinical nephrotoxicity of aminoglycosides. Am. J. Med. *80*:119–125, 1986.
165. Meyers, B. R., and Hirschman, S. Z.: Antibacterial activity of cefamandole in vitro. J. Infect. Dis. *137*(Suppl.):25–31, 1978.
166. Mingeot-Leclercq, M. P., Glupczynski, Y., and Tulkens, P. M.: Aminoglycosides: Activity and resistance. Antimicrob. Agents Chemother. *43*:727–737, 1999.
167. Mingeot-Leclercq, M. P., and Tulkens, P. M.: Aminoglycosides: Nephrotoxicity. Antimicrob. Agents Chemother. *43*:1003–1012, 1999.
168. Moellering, R. C., Jr.: In vitro antibacterial activity of the aminoglycoside antibiotics. Rev. Infect. Dis. *5*(Suppl. 2):212–231, 1983.
169. Moellering, R. C., Jr.: Monitoring serum vancomycin levels: Climbing the mountain because it is there? Editorial. [Published erratum appears in Clin Infect Dis 1994 Aug;19(2):379.] Clin. Infect. Dis. *18*:544–546, 1994.
170. Moellering, R. C., Jr., Krogstad, D. J., and Greenblatt, D. J.: Vancomycin therapy in patients with impaired renal function: A nomogram for dosage. Ann. Intern. Med. *94*:343–346, 1981.
171. Mofenson, L. M.: Rifabutin. Pediatr. Infect. Dis. J. *17*:71–72, 1998.
172. Moosa, A., and Rubidge, C. J.: Once daily ceftriaxone vs. chloramphenicol for treatment of typhoid fever in children. Pediatr. Infect. Dis. J. *8*:696–699, 1989.
173. Moreillon, P., Markiewicz, Z., Nachman, S., et al.: Two bactericidal targets for penicillin in pneumococci: Autolysis-dependent and autolysis-independent killing mechanisms. Antimicrob. Agents Chemother. *34*:33–39, 1990.
174. Murphy, T. V., Chrane, D. F., McCracken, G. H., Jr., et al.: Rifampin prophylaxis v placebo for household contacts of children with *Hemophilus influenzae* type b disease. Am. J. Dis. Child. *137*:627–632, 1983.
175. Murray, B. E.: Vancomycin-resistant enterococcal infections. N. Engl. J. Med. *342*:710–721, 2000.
176. Murray, D. L., Singer, D. A., Singer, A. B., et al.: Cefaclor: A cluster of adverse reactions. Letter. N. Engl. J. Med. *303*:1003, 1980.
177. Mustafa, M. M., Carlson, L., Tkaczewski, I., et al.: Comparative study of cefepime *versus* ceftazidime in the empiric treatment of pediatric cancer patients with fever and neutropenia. Pediatr. Infect. Dis. J. *20*:366–373, 2001.
178. Nagar, H., Berger, S. A., Hammar, B., et al.: Penetration of clindamycin and metronidazole into the appendix and peritoneal fluid in children. Eur. J. Clin. Pharmacol. *37*:209–210, 1989.
179. Nahata, M. C.: Pharmacokinetics of azithromycin in pediatric patients: Comparison with other agents used for treating otitis media and streptococcal pharyngitis. Pediatr. Infect. Dis. J. *14*(Suppl.):39–44, 1995.
180. Nelson, J. D., and Haltalin, K. C.: Amoxicillin is less effective than ampicillin against *Shigella* in vitro and in vivo: Relationship of efficacy to activity in serum. J. Infect. Dis. *129*(Suppl.):222–227, 1974.
181. Nelson, J. D., Howard, J. B., and Shelton, S.: Oral antibiotic therapy for skeletal infections of children. I. Antibiotic concentrations in suppurative synovial fluid. J. Pediatr. *92*:131–134, 1978.
182. Neu, H. C.: Antimicrobial activity and human pharmacology of amoxicillin. J. Infect. Dis. *129*(Suppl.):123–131, 1974.
183. Neu, H. C.: Antistaphylococcal penicillins. Med. Clin. North Am. *66*:51–60, 1982.
184. Neu, H. C.: The crisis in antibiotic resistance. Science *257*:1064–1073, 1992.
185. Neu, H. C., and Fu, K. P.: Cefuroxime, a beta-lactamase–resistant cephalosporin with a broad spectrum of gram-positive and -negative activity. Antimicrob. Agents Chemother. *13*:657–664, 1978.

186. Nix, D. E., Goodwin, S. D., Peloquin, C. A., et al.: Antibiotic tissue penetration and its relevance: Models of tissue penetration and their meaning. Antimicrob. Agents Chemother. *35*:1947–1952, 1991.
187. Nix, D. E., Goodwin, S. D., Peloquin, C. A., et al.: Antibiotic tissue penetration and its relevance: Impact of tissue penetration on infection response. Antimicrob. Agents Chemother. *35*:1953–1959, 1991.
188. Nolen, T. M.: Clinical trials of cefprozil for treatment of skin and skin-structure infections: Review. Clin. Infect. Dis. *14*(Suppl. 2):255–263, 1992.
189. Nord, C. E.: Mechanisms of beta-lactam resistance in anaerobic bacteria. Rev. Infect. Dis. *8*(Suppl. 5):543–548, 1986.
190. Novak, R., Henriques, B., Charpentier, E., et al.: Emergence of vancomycin tolerance in *Streptococcus pneumoniae.* Nature *399*:590–593, 1999.
191. Odio, C. M., Puig, J. R., Feris, J. M., et al.: Prospective, randomized, investigator-blinded study of the efficacy and safety of meropenem vs. cefotaxime therapy in bacterial meningitis in children. Pediatr. Infect. Dis. J. *18*:581–590, 1999.
192. Panzer, J. D., Brown, D. C., Epstein, W. L., et al.: Clindamycin levels in various body tissues and fluids. J. Clin. Pharmacol. New Drugs *12*:259–262, 1972.
193. Parry, M. G., and Neu, H. C.: Ticarcillin for treatment of serious infections with gram-negative bacteria. J. Infect. Dis. *134*:476–485, 1976.
194. Petz, L. D.: Immunologic cross-reactivity between penicillins and cephalosporins: A review. J. Infect. Dis. *137*(Suppl.):74–79, 1978.
195. Pfeiffer, R. R.: Structural features of vancomycin. Rev. Infect. Dis. *3*(Suppl.):205–209, 1981.
196. Pichichero, M. E., and Gooch, W. M.: Comparison of cefdinir and penicillin V in the treatment of pediatric streptococcal tonsillopharyngitis. Pediatr. Infect. Dis. J. *19*(Suppl.):171–173, 2000.
197. Pichichero, M. E., McLinn, S. E., Gooch, W. M., et al.: Ceftibuten vs. penicillin V in group A beta-hemolytic streptococcal pharyngitis. Members of the Ceftibuten Pharyngitis International Study Group. Pediatr. Infect. Dis. J. *14*(Suppl.):102–107, 1995.
198. Polk, R. E.: Anaphylactoid reactions to glycopeptide antibiotics. J. Antimicrob. Chemother. *27*(Suppl. B):17–29, 1991.
199. Preac-Mursic, V., Wilske, B., Schierz, G., et al.: Comparative antimicrobial activity of the new macrolides against *Borrelia burgdorferi.* Eur. J. Clin. Microbiol. Infect. Dis. *8*:651–653, 1989.
200. Prober, C. G., Stevenson, D. K., and Benitz, W. E.: The use of antibiotics in neonates weighing less than 1200 grams. Pediatr. Infect. Dis. J. *9*:111–121, 1990.
201. Pukander, J. S., Jero, J. P., Kaprio, E. A., et al.: Clarithromycin vs. amoxicillin suspensions in the treatment of pediatric patients with acute otitis media. Pediatr. Infect. Dis. J. *12*(Suppl.):118–121, 1993.
202. Radetsky, M.: Duration of treatment in bacterial meningitis: A historical inquiry. Pediatr. Infect. Dis. J. *9*:2–9, 1990.
203. Rahal, J. J., Jr., and Simberkoff, M. S.: Bactericidal and bacteriostatic action of chloramphenicol against meningeal pathogens. Antimicrob. Agents Chemother. *16*:13–18, 1979.
204. Ramilo, O., Kinane, B. T., and McCracken, G. H., Jr.: Chloramphenicol neurotoxicity. Pediatr. Infect. Dis. J. *7*:358–359, 1988.
205. Ramsey, B. W., Dorkin, H. L., Eisenberg, J. D., et al.: Efficacy of aerosolized tobramycin in patients with cystic fibrosis. N. Engl. J. Med. *328*:1740–1746, 1993.
206. Ramsey, B. W., Pepe, M. S., Quan, J. M., et al.: Intermittent administration of inhaled tobramycin in patients with cystic fibrosis. Cystic Fibrosis Inhaled Tobramycin Study Group. N. Engl. J. Med. *340*:23–30, 1999.
207. Reed, M. D., and Blumer, J. L.: Clinical pharmacology of antitubercular drugs. Pediatr. Clin. North Am. *30*:177–193, 1983.
208. Reid, R., Jr., Bradley, J. S., and Hindler, J.: Pneumococcal meningitis during therapy of otitis media with clarithromycin. Pediatr. Infect. Dis. J. *14*:1104–1105, 1995.
209. Richards, G. A., and Klugman, K. P.: Implications of bacterial resistance for the use of beta-lactam agents in clinical practice. Editorial. S. Afr. Med. J. *83*:163–164, 1993.
210. Ristuccia, A. M.: Chloramphenicol: Clinical pharmacology in pediatrics. Ther. Drug Monit. *7*:159–167, 1985.
211. Roberts, M. C., Sutcliffe, J., Courvalin, P., et al.: Nomenclature for macrolide and macrolide-lincosamide-streptogramin B resistance determinants. Antimicrob. Agents Chemother. *43*:2823–2830, 1999.
212. Rodriguez, W. J., Ross, S., Khan, W. N., et al.: Clinical and laboratory evaluation of cefamandole in infants and children. J. Infect. Dis. *137*(Suppl.):150–154, 1978.
213. Ruben, R. J.: Efficacy of ofloxacin and other otic preparations for otitis externa. Pediatr. Infect. Dis. J. *20*:108–110, 2001.
214. Russo, T. A., Cook, S., and Gorbach, S. L.: Intramuscular ceftriaxone in home parenteral therapy. Antimicrob. Agents Chemother. *32*:1439–1440, 1988.
215. Sabath, L. D., Wilcox, C., Garner, C., et al.: In vitro activity of cefazolin against recent clinical bacterial isolates. J. Infect. Dis. *128*(Suppl.): 320–326, 1973.
216. Sáez-Llorens, X., and McCracken, G. H., Jr.: Clinical pharmacology of antibacterial agents. *In* Remington, J. S., and Klein, J. O. (eds.): Infectious Diseases of the Fetus and Newborn Infant. 4th ed. Philadelphia, W. B. Saunders, 1995, pp. 1287–1336.
217. Saivin, S., and Houin, G.: Clinical pharmacokinetics of doxycycline and minocycline. Clin. Pharmacokinet. *15*:355–366, 1988.
218. Salamon, S. M.: Tetracyclines in ophthalmology. Surv. Ophthalmol. *29*:265–275, 1985.
219. Saxon, A.: Immediate hypersensitivity reactions to β-lactam antibiotics. Rev. Infect. Dis. 5(*Suppl.)*:368–378, 1983.
220. Schaad, U. B.: Pediatric use of quinolones. Pediatr. Infect. Dis. J. *18*:469–470, 1999.
221. Schaad, U. B., Abdus Salam, M., Aujard, Y., et al.: Use of fluoroquinolones in pediatrics: Consensus report of an International Society of Chemotherapy Commission. Pediatr. Infect. Dis. J. *14*:1–9, 1995.
222. Schaad, U. B., Eskola, J., Kafetzis, D., et al.: Cefepime vs. ceftazidime treatment of pyelonephritis: A European, randomized, controlled study of 300 pediatric cases. European Society for Pediatric Infectious Diseases (ESPID) Pyelonephritis Study Group. Pediatr. Infect. Dis. J. *17*:639–644, 1998.
223. Schaad, U. B., Suter, S., Gianella-Borradori, A., et al.: A comparison of ceftriaxone and cefuroxime for the treatment of bacterial meningitis in children. N. Engl. J. Med. *322*:141–147, 1990.
224. Schwartz, R. H., Wientzen, R. L., Pedreira, F., et al.: Penicillin V for group A streptococcal pharyngotonsillitis. A randomized trial of seven vs ten days' therapy. J. A. M. A. *246*:1790–1795, 1981.
225. Seppala, H., Klaukka, T., Vuopio-Varkila, J., et al.: The effect of changes in the consumption of macrolide antibiotics on erythromycin resistance in group A streptococci in Finland. Finnish Study Group for Antimicrobial Resistance. N. Engl. J. Med. *337*:441–446, 1997.
226. Seppala, H., Nissinen, A., Jarvinen, H., et al.: Resistance to erythromycin in group A streptococci. N. Engl. J. Med. *326*:292–297, 1992.
227. Silber, T. J., and D'Angelo, L.: Psychosis and seizures following the injection of penicillin G procaine. Hoigne's syndrome. Am. J. Dis. Child. *139*:335–337, 1985.
228. Silva, J., Jr.: Update on pseudomembranous colitis. West. J. Med. *151*:644–648, 1989.
229. Snavely, S. R., and Hodges, G. R.: The neurotoxicity of antibacterial agents. Ann. Intern. Med. *101*:92–104, 1984.
230. Spratt, B. G.: Distinct penicillin binding proteins involved in the division, elongation, and shape of *Escherichia coli* K12. Proc. Natl. Acad. Sci. U. S. A. *72*:2999–3003, 1975.
231. Stapleton, P., Wu, P. J., King, A., et al.: Incidence and mechanisms of resistance to the combination of amoxicillin and clavulanic acid in *Escherichia coli.* Antimicrob. Agents Chemother. *39*:2478–2483, 1995.
232. Steele, R. W., Thomas, M. P., and Begue, R. E.: Compliance issues related to the selection of antibiotic suspensions for children. Pediatr. Infect. Dis. J. *20*:1–5, 2001.
233. Tally, F. P., Cuchural, G. J., Jr., and Malamy, M. H.: Mechanisms of resistance and resistance transfer in anaerobic bacteria: Factors influencing antimicrobial therapy. Rev. Infect. Dis. *6*(Suppl. 1):260–269, 1984.
234. Tally, F. T., Ellestad, G. A., and Testa, R. T.: Glycylcyclines: A new generation of tetracyclines. J. Antimicrob. Chemother. *35*:449–452, 1995.
235. Tanz, R. R., Poncher, J. R., Corydon, K. E., et al.: Clindamycin treatment of chronic pharyngeal carriage of group A streptococci. J. Pediatr. *119*:123–128, 1991.
236. Tarlow, M. J.: Macrolides in the management of streptococcal pharyngitis/tonsillitis. Pediatr. Infect. Dis. J. *16*:444–448, 1997.
237. Taylor, D. E., and Chau, A.: Tetracycline resistance mediated by ribosomal protection. Antimicrob. Agents Chemother. *40*:1–5, 1996.
238. Tedesco, F. J.: Pseudomembranous colitis: Pathogenesis and therapy. Med. Clin. North Am. *66*:655–664, 1982.
239. Tetzlaff, T. R., McCracken, G. H., Jr., and Nelson, J. D.: Oral antibiotic therapy for skeletal infections of children. II. Therapy of osteomyelitis and suppurative arthritis. J. Pediatr. *92*:485–490, 1978.
240. Then, R. L.: Mechanisms of resistance to trimethoprim, the sulfonamides, and trimethoprim-sulfamethoxazole. Rev. Infect. Dis. *4*:261–269, 1982.
241. Thornsberry, C.: Review of in vitro activity of third-generation cephalosporins and other newer beta-lactam antibiotics against clinically important bacteria. Am. J. Med. *79*:14–20, 1985.
242. Tipper, D. J.: Mode of action of beta-lactam antibiotics. Pharmacol. Ther. *27*:1–35, 1985.
243. Tipper, D. J., and Strominger, J. L.: Mechanism of action of penicillins: A proposal based on their structural similarity to acyl-D-alanyl-D-alanine. Proc. Natl. Acad. Sci. U. S. A. *54*:1133–1141, 1965.
244. Tomasz, A.: From penicillin-binding proteins to the lysis and death of bacteria: A 1979 view. Rev. Infect. Dis. *1*:434–467, 1979.
245. Trujillo, M., Correa, N., Olsen, K., et al.: Cefprozil concentrations in middle ear fluid of children with acute otitis media. Pediatr. Infect. Dis. J. *19*:268–269, 2000.
246. Trujillo, M., Ehrett, S., Hoyt-Sehnert, M. J., et al.: Safety and efficacy of cefprozil as part of a parenteral-oral antibiotic regimen for the treatment of suppurative skeletal infections in children. Clin. Infect. Dis. *23*:843, 1996.
247. Tschida, S. J., Vance-Bryan, K., and Zaske, D. E.: Anti-infective agents and hepatic disease. Med. Clin. North Am. *79*:895–917, 1995.

248. Tulkens, P. M.: Experimental studies on nephrotoxicity of aminoglycosides at low doses. Mechanisms and perspectives. Am. J. Med. *80*:105–114, 1986.
249. Tunkel, A. R.: Topical antibacterials. *In* Mandell, G. L., Bennett, J. E., and Dolin, R. (eds.): Mandell, Douglas, and Bennett's Principles and Practice of Infectious Disease. 4th ed. New York, Churchill-Livingstone, 1995, pp. 381–389.
250. 1999 USPHS/IDSA guidelines for the prevention of opportunistic infections in persons infected with human immunodeficiency virus. M. M. W. R. Recomm. Rep. *48*(RR-10):15–16, 1999.
251. van Dyk, J. C., Terespolsky, S. A., Meyer, C. S., et al.: Penetration of cefpodoxime into middle ear fluid in pediatric patients with acute otitis media. Pediatr. Infect. Dis. J. *16*:79–81, 1997.
252. Verbist, L.: Comparison of the activities of the new ureidopenicillins piperacillin, mezlocillin, azlocillin, and Bay k 4999 against gram-negative organisms. Antimicrob. Agents Chemother. *16*:115–119, 1979.
253. Vinh, H., Wain, J., Vo, T. N. H., et al.: Two or three days of ofloxacin treatment for uncomplicated multidrug-resistant typhoid fever in children. Antimicrob. Agents Chemother. *40*:958–961, 1996.
254. Vogelman, B., and Craig, W. A.: Kinetics of antimicrobial activity. J. Pediatr. *108*:835–840, 1986.
255. Wallace, S. M., and Chan, L. Y.: In vitro interaction of aminoglycosides with beta-lactam penicillins. Antimicrob. Agents Chemother. *28*:274–281, 1985.
256. Watanakunakorn, C.: The antibacterial action of vancomycin. Rev. Infect. Dis. *3*(Suppl.):210–215, 1981.
257. Weisblum, B.: Erythromycin resistance by ribosome modification. Antimicrob. Agents Chemother. *39*:577–585, 1995.
258. Weiss, M. E., and Adkinson, N. F., Jr.: Beta-lactam allergy. *In* Mandell, G. L., Bennett, J. E., and Dolin, R. (eds.): Mandell, Douglas, and Bennett's Principles and Practice of Infectious Disease. 4th ed. New York, Churchill-Livingstone, 1995, pp. 272–278.
259. West, B. C., DeVault, G. A., Jr., Clement, J. C., et al.: Aplastic anemia associated with parenteral chloramphenicol: Review of 10 cases, including the second case of possible increased risk with cimetidine. Rev. Infect. Dis. *10*:1048–1051, 1988.
260. Wilson, W. R., Karchmer, A. W., Dajani, A. S., et al.: Antibiotic treatment of adults with infective endocarditis due to streptococci, enterococci, staphylococci, and HACEK microorganisms. American Heart Association. J. A. M. A. *274*:1706–1713, 1995.
261. Yunis, A. A.: Chloramphenicol: Relation of structure to activity and toxicity. Annu. Rev. Pharmacol. Toxicol. *28*:83–100, 1988.
262. Zanga, J., Donlan, M. A., Newton, J., et al.: Administration of medication in school. American Academy of Pediatrics. Committee on School Health. Pediatrics *74*:433–436, 1984.
263. Zhanel, G. G., and Craig, W. A.: Pharmacokinetic contributions to postantibiotic effects. Focus on aminoglycosides. Clin. Pharmacokinet. *27*:377–392, 1994.
264. Zimbelman, J., Palmer, A., and Todd, J.: Improved outcome of clindamycin compared with beta-lactam antibiotic treatment for invasive *Streptococcus pyogenes* infection. Pediatr. Infect. Dis. J. *18*:1096–1100, 1999.
265. Zinberg, J., Chernaik, R., Coman, E., et al.: Reversible symptomatic biliary obstruction associated with ceftriaxone pseudolithiasis. Am. J. Gastroenterol. *86*:1251–1254, 1991.
266. Zuckerman, J. M.: The newer macrolides: Azithromycin and clarithromycin. Infect. Dis. Clin. North Am. *14*:449–462, 2000.

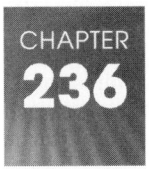

CHAPTER 236 Antimicrobial Prophylaxis

ADNAN S. DAJANI ■ WALID ABUHAMMOUR

Antimicrobial prophylaxis is the practice of administering an antimicrobial agent or agents with the intent of preventing an infection. Prevention, rather than treatment, always is preferred, provided that the means are available and the risk-benefit and cost-benefit ratios are acceptable. This chapter focuses on the prevention of morbidity and mortality from bacterial infections through the prophylactic and often empiric use of antimicrobial agents.

General Principles of Prophylaxis

Several factors that influence the efficacy of prophylaxis are related to the potential pathogen, the prophylactic agent, the host, and the disease to be prevented (Table 236–1). Failure to consider all these factors will lead to ineffective prophylaxis, overuse of antimicrobial agents, promotion of resistant microorganisms, economic waste, and risk of toxicity or side effects. These factors are discussed here in general and more specifically in later sections.

TABLE 236–1 ■ FACTORS INFLUENCING EFFECTIVE PROPHYLAXIS

Single versus multiple potential pathogens
Time of exposure to the pathogen
Source of pathogens
Severity of the disease to be prevented
Targeted organ(s) that could become infected
Spectrum of activity of the antimicrobial agent
Pharmacokinetics and the pharmacodynamics of the selected agent
Duration of chemoprophylaxis
Cost, toxicity, side effects, and acceptability of the agent
Likelihood and consequences of emerging resistance

THE BACTERIAL PATHOGEN

Prophylaxis is more effective when a single pathogen is targeted as opposed to multiple pathogens. In general, the greater the number of targeted pathogens, the less effective, the more toxic, and the more expensive the regimen becomes. Ideally, prophylaxis should be administered at the time of exposure to the potential pathogen or shortly thereafter. If exposure is prolonged or continuous, prophylaxis becomes less effective and less desirable. Bacteria that are not endogenous to the host (i.e., not part of the host's normal flora) generally are targeted more effectively if the exposure is known and identified.

THE DISEASE

The severity of the disease to be prevented is a major consideration. Potentially fatal infections (e.g., meningococcemia) or infections that result in high morbidity (e.g., endocarditis) are justifiably targeted diseases. On the other hand, prophylaxis usually is not required for minor illnesses (e.g., cuts, abrasions). The site of infection to be prevented is also important. Adequate concentrations of antimicrobials are achieved readily in organs that are highly vascular and have no barriers, whereas infections in compartments (e.g., middle ear) or involving prosthetic materials may require special considerations.

THE ANTIMICROBIAL AGENT

The most desirable prophylactic agent is narrow spectrum, inexpensive, easily administered, and well tolerated and has minimal side effects. The less frequently an agent is given, the more reliable the adherence (compliance) of the patient.[65] Situations in which prophylaxis can be achieved effectively with a single administration of the antimicrobial agent are ideal.

Prophylaxis in Newborn Infants

OPHTHALMIA NEONATORUM

Prophylaxis is targeted against *Neisseria gonorrhoeae* and *Chlamydia trachomatis*. Ideally, prophylaxis should be directed at infants who are exposed to these two pathogens; however, identifying this group with certainty is impossible. Routine prophylaxis has been discontinued in some countries (United Kingdom, Sweden)[25]; however, it is required in the United States.

Topical 1 percent silver nitrate solutions are available in single-dose ampules or single-dose tubes of an ophthalmic ointment containing 0.5 percent erythromycin or 1 percent tetracycline. All agents are effective and recommended for prophylaxis of gonococcal ophthalmia neonatorum.[59] Silver nitrate has been in use for such prophylaxis for more than 100 years. Because silver nitrate frequently causes chemical conjunctivitis, its use has been challenged, and alternative regimens have been sought. Erythromycin and tetracycline ophthalmic ointments appear to be as effective as silver nitrate solution for routine prophylaxis of gonococcal ophthalmia[77, 123]; however, silver nitrate probably is the most effective agent against penicillinase-producing *N. gonorrhoeae*. The effectiveness of erythromycin or tetracycline in the prevention of ophthalmia caused by penicillinase-producing *N. gonorrhoeae* has not been established. No topical regimen has proven efficacy against *Chlamydia* conjunctivitis.[13, 26, 60] Furthermore, topical regimens do not eliminate *C. trachomatis* from the nasopharynx and do not prevent pneumonia.

Prophylaxis should be administered as soon as possible after birth. Each eyelid should be wiped gently with sterile cotton before local prophylaxis is administered. Care must be exercised to ensure that the solution or ointment is in the conjunctival sac and that it is not flushed from the eye after instillation.

GROUP B *STREPTOCOCCUS* INFECTIONS

Prophylaxis is aimed at prevention of early-onset neonatal group B *Streptococcus* (GBS) infections.[3, 4, 15, 93, 102, 104] No recommendations for prophylaxis against late-onset infections exist.

Several regimens have been used in attempts to reduce vertical transmission of GBS. Multiple studies involving the use of oral antimicrobial agents to eradicate GBS colonization prepartum (antepartum chemoprophylaxis) have not been successful, even when sexual partners were treated concurrently.[93] Prophylaxis of newborn infants with penicillin G or ampicillin soon after birth (postnatal chemoprophylaxis) is ineffective in preventing early-onset GBS disease, primarily because in most patients, infection occurs in utero and the infants are asymptomatic at or within a few hours after birth.

Current recommendations focus on targeting colonized women who fall into special-risk categories (selective intrapartum maternal chemoprophylaxis).[1, 3, 4] The American Academy of Pediatrics recommends that lower vaginal and anorectal (single swab) specimens for culture be obtained at 35 to 37 weeks' gestation, placed into selective broth medium, transported, and subcultured onto solid media.[3] Women who have no prenatal GBS culture results available and who begin labor with an identified risk factor (Table 236–2) may be tested for GBS by the rapid antigen test or by culture. Maternal GBS carriers identified prepartum or those without culture but with one or more risk factors should be given intrapartum intravenous ampicillin (2 g initially, then 1 to 2 g every 4 to 6 hours) or penicillin G (5 million U every 6 hours) until delivery.[24] Penicillin-allergic women may be given clindamycin or erythromycin intravenously. Previous delivery of an infant with invasive GBS disease warrants intrapartum maternal chemoprophylaxis for each subsequent pregnancy, regardless of maternal colonization.

Intrapartum antibiotic prophylaxis will prevent substantial numbers but not all cases of early-onset GBS neonatal infection and will decrease the incidence of maternal GBS postpartum endometritis.[80, 88] Since the institution of intrapartum antimicrobial prophylaxis, the rate of invasive GBS disease has declined approximately 65 percent. Administration of intravenous ampicillin reduces the risk of development of early-onset GBS infection by 36 percent in infants born to women with premature rupture of membranes.[11] Treatment of women with chorioamnionitis with ampicillin and gentamicin during labor reduces the likelihood of GBS infection developing by 86 percent. In some reports, the decrease in the rate of GBS disease was associated with an increased rate of disease caused by gram-negative pathogens. Although many obstetric care providers take some measures to prevent the development of GBS disease, reported practices are often inconsistent with the existing recommendations.[66] The major contended issue is timing of the antepartum screening cultures.[80]

Management of infants whose mothers received intrapartum chemoprophylaxis remains empiric and should be based on clinical manifestations and gestational age.

TABLE 236–2 ■ RISK FACTORS FOR EARLY-ONSET GROUP B *STREPTOCOCCUS* (GBS) INFECTION

Risk Factors
Maternal Risk Factors
Premature onset of labor of <37 weeks' gestation
Premature rupture of membranes at <37 weeks' gestation
Rupture of membranes (>18 hr) at any gestation
Maternal fever during labor
Multiple births
High GBS genital inoculum
GBS bacteriuria
Low type-specific GBS capsular polysaccharide antibody
Maternal age <20 yr
Black race
Diabetes mellitus
Infant Risk Factors
Low birth weight
Prematurity

If indicated, appropriate cultures should be performed and antimicrobial therapy initiated, pending culture results.[3]

NECROTIZING ENTEROCOLITIS

Bacterial proliferation and invasion of the intestinal wall are part of the pathogenesis of necrotizing enterocolitis (NEC). Therefore, suppression of gastrointestinal flora with nonabsorbable oral antimicrobials was attempted in an effort to prevent the development of NEC in premature infants. Administration of oral kanamycin or gentamicin prophylactically in the first few hours of life generated contradictory data. Furthermore, selective overgrowth of resistant organisms in the bowel and significant systemic absorption of aminoglycosides from the injured mucosa are potential risk factors. Currently, oral aminoglycosides are not recommended for the prophylaxis of NEC.

One report[92] suggests that oral vancomycin given for 48 hours before the introduction of oral feeding may be beneficial in preventing NEC. These observations have not been confirmed, and such prophylaxis is not practiced routinely or recommended.

INTRAVASCULAR CATHETER INSERTION

Infection with coagulase-negative staphylococci, primarily *Staphylococcus epidermidis,* is likely to occur in premature infants or infants who have indwelling vascular catheters. Low-grade sepsis is the most common clinical manifestation; however, meningitis, endocarditis, omphalitis, cellulitis, and other focal infections may occur. Two randomized trials of low-dose vancomycin added to total parenteral nutrition fluids (25 μg of vancomycin per milliliter of fluid) suggested that such a prophylactic regimen significantly reduces coagulase-negative staphylococcal infections in small premature infants in neonatal intensive care units.[68, 115] Widespread use of this regimen will not be recommended until more data are collected and the issue of emergence of vancomycin-resistant organisms is addressed adequately.[8]

Disease-Targeted Prophylaxis

RHEUMATIC FEVER

Group A *Streptococcus* (GAS) infections of the pharynx are the precipitating cause of rheumatic fever. Appropriate antibiotic treatment of streptococcal pharyngitis prevents the development of acute rheumatic fever in most cases.[38] Because at least one third of episodes of acute rheumatic fever result from inapparent streptococcal infections[30] and some symptomatic patients do not seek medical care, not all instances of rheumatic fever are preventable. Prevention of first attacks (primary prevention) is accomplished by proper identification, adequate antibiotic treatment, and eradication of this streptococcal infection. An individual who has suffered an attack of rheumatic fever is at very high risk for recurrence after subsequent GAS pharyngitis and needs continuous chemoprophylaxis to prevent such recurrence (secondary prevention).[34]

Primary Prevention

In selecting a regimen for the treatment of GAS pharyngitis, physicians should consider various factors, including bacteriologic and clinical efficacy, ease of adherence to the recommended regimen (frequency of daily administration, duration of therapy, palatability), cost, spectrum of activity of the selected agent, and potential side effects. No single regimen eradicates GAS from the pharynx in 100 percent of treated patients.

Penicillin is the antimicrobial agent of choice for the treatment of GAS,[2, 9, 34] except in penicillin-allergic individuals (Table 236–3). Penicillin has a narrow spectrum of activity, has long-standing proven efficacy, and is the least expensive regimen. GAS organisms that are resistant to penicillin have not been documented. Even when started as long as 9 days after the onset of acute illness, penicillin effectively prevents primary attacks of rheumatic fever.[24] Therefore, a brief delay (24 to 48 hours) for processing the throat culture before initiation of antibiotic therapy does not increase the risk of development of rheumatic fever. Patients are considered noncontagious 24 hours after initiation of therapy.[114]

TABLE 236–3 ■ PREVENTION OF RHEUMATIC FEVER

Agent	Dose	Mode	Duration
	Primary Prevention		
Benzathine penicillin G	600,000 U for patients ≤27 kg 1,200,000 U for patients >27 kg	Intramuscularly	Once
Penicillin V	Children: 250 mg 2–3 times daily Adolescents and adults: 500 mg 2–3 times daily	Orally	10 days
	For Individuals Allergic to Penicillin		
Erythromycin	40 mg/kg/day 2–4 times daily (maximum, 1 g/day)	Orally	10 days
	Secondary Prevention		
Benzathine penicillin G	1,200,000 U every 3–4 wk *or*	Intramuscularly	See text
Penicillin V	250 mg twice daily *or*	Orally	See text
Sulfadiazine	0.5 g once daily for patients ≤27 kg (60 lb) 1.0 g once daily for patients >27 kg (60 lb)	Orally	See text
	For Individuals Allergic to Penicillin and Sulfadiazine		
Erythromycin	250 mg twice daily	Orally	See text

From Dajani, A., Taubert, K., Ferrieri, P., et al.: Treatment of acute streptococcal pharyngitis and prevention of rheumatic fever: A statement for health professionals. Pediatrics *96*:758–764, 1995. Copyright American Academy of Pediatrics 1995.

Intramuscular benzathine penicillin G is preferred to oral penicillin, particularly for patients who are unlikely to complete a 10-day course of oral therapy and patients with a personal or family history of rheumatic fever, rheumatic heart disease, or other environmental factors that place them at substantial risk for rheumatic fever.[34] Benzathine penicillin injections should be given as a single dose in a large muscle mass. This formulation is painful; injections that contain procaine penicillin in addition to benzathine penicillin G are less painful. The combination of 900,000 U of benzathine penicillin G and 300,000 U of procaine penicillin G is satisfactory therapy for most children.[10] The efficacy of this combination for heavier patients, such as teenagers and adults, requires further study. Less discomfort is associated with intramuscular benzathine penicillin G if the medication is warmed to room temperature before administration.

The oral antibiotic of choice is penicillin V (phenoxymethyl penicillin) (see Table 236–3). All patients should continue to take oral penicillin regularly for an entire 10-day period, even though they probably will be asymptomatic after the first few days. Penicillin V is preferred to penicillin G because it is more resistant to gastric acid. Although the broader-spectrum penicillins, ampicillin and amoxicillin, often are used for treatment of GAS pharyngitis, they offer no microbiologic advantage over penicillin.

Oral erythromycin is acceptable for patients allergic to penicillin.[34] Treatment also should be prescribed for 10 days. Erythromycin estolate (20 to 40 mg/kg/day in two to four divided doses) or erythromycin ethyl succinate (40 mg/kg/day in two to four divided doses) is effective in treating streptococcal pharyngitis; however, the efficacy of a twice-daily regimen in adults requires further study. The maximal dose of erythromycin is 1 g/day. Although strains of GAS resistant to erythromycin are prevalent in some areas of the world and have resulted in treatment failure,[107] they are uncommon findings in most parts of the United States.[28]

The new macrolide azithromycin has a similar susceptibility pattern to that of erythromycin against GAS but may cause less frequent gastrointestinal side effects. Azithromycin can be administered once daily and produces high tonsillar tissue concentrations.[117] A 5-day course of azithromycin is approved by the Food and Drug Administration (FDA) as second-line therapy for individuals 16 years or older with GAS pharyngitis. The recommended dosage is 500 mg as a single dose on the first day, followed by 250 mg once daily for 4 days.[64]

A 10-day course of an oral cephalosporin is an acceptable alternative, particularly for penicillin-allergic individuals. Narrower-spectrum cephalosporins such as cefadroxil and cephalexin are probably preferable to the broader-spectrum cephalosporins such as cefaclor, cefuroxime, cefixime, and cefpodoxime.[34] Some penicillin-allergic persons (<15%) are also allergic to cephalosporins, and these agents should not be used in patients with immediate (anaphylactic-type) hypersensitivity to penicillin. Several reports indicate that a 10-day course with an oral cephalosporin is superior to 10 days of oral penicillin in eradicating GAS from the pharynx.[14, 33, 54, 98] Recent reports suggest that a 5-day course with selected oral cephalosporins is comparable to a 10-day course of oral penicillin in eradicating GAS from the pharynx.[5, 31, 97, 117] Such regimens currently are not approved by the FDA, and further studies are warranted to expand and confirm these observations.

Secondary Prevention

An individual in whom streptococcal pharyngitis develops after a previous attack of rheumatic fever is at high risk for a recurrent attack of rheumatic fever. A GAS infection need not be symptomatic to trigger a recurrence. Furthermore, recurrence of rheumatic fever can take place even when a symptomatic infection is treated optimally. For these reasons, prevention of recurrent rheumatic fever requires continuous antimicrobial prophylaxis rather than recognition and treatment of acute episodes of streptococcal pharyngitis.[34] Continuous prophylaxis is recommended for patients with a well-documented history of rheumatic fever (including cases manifested solely by Sydenham chorea) and those with definite evidence of rheumatic heart disease. Such prophylaxis should be initiated as soon as acute rheumatic fever or rheumatic heart disease is diagnosed. A full therapeutic course of penicillin should be given first to patients with acute rheumatic fever to eradicate residual GAS, even if a throat culture is negative at that time. Streptococcal infections occurring in family members of rheumatic patients should be treated promptly.

An injection of 1,200,000 U of benzathine penicillin G every 4 weeks is the recommended regimen for secondary prevention in most circumstances in the United States (see Table 236–3). In countries where the incidence of rheumatic fever is particularly high, in special circumstances, or in certain high-risk individuals, such as patients with residual rheumatic carditis, administration of benzathine penicillin G every 3 weeks is justified and recommended.[82, 83] Long-acting penicillin is of particular value in patients with a high risk of rheumatic fever recurrence, especially those with rheumatic heart disease, in whom recurrence is very serious. The advantages of giving benzathine penicillin G must be weighed against the inconvenience to the patient and the pain of injection, which causes some individuals to discontinue prophylaxis.

Successful oral prophylaxis (penicillin V or sulfadiazine, see Table 236–3) depends primarily on the patient's adherence to prescribed regimens.[32] Patients need detailed, careful, and repeated instructions about the importance of continuing prophylaxis. Most failures of prophylaxis occur in nonadherent patients. Even with optimal patient adherence, the risk of having a recurrence is higher in individuals receiving oral prophylaxis than in those receiving intramuscular benzathine penicillin G.[47] Oral agents are more appropriate for patients at lower risk for rheumatic recurrence. Accordingly, some physicians elect to switch therapy to oral prophylaxis when patients have reached late adolescence or young adulthood and have remained free of rheumatic attacks for at least 5 years.

Although sulfonamides are not effective in the eradication of GAS, they do prevent infection. Sulfonamide prophylaxis is contraindicated in late pregnancy because of transplacental passage of such drugs and potential competition with bilirubin for albumin-binding sites.

For patients who are allergic to penicillin and sulfisoxazole, erythromycin is recommended. No data have been published about the use of other penicillins, macrolides, or cephalosporins for the secondary prevention of rheumatic fever.

The appropriate duration of prophylaxis must be determined for each individual situation.[34] Patients who have had rheumatic carditis are at relatively high risk for recurrence of carditis and are likely to sustain increasingly severe cardiac involvement with each recurrence. Therefore, patients who have had rheumatic carditis should receive long-term antibiotic prophylaxis, perhaps for life. Prophylaxis should continue, even after valve surgery, including prosthetic valve replacement. Patients who have had rheumatic fever without rheumatic carditis are at considerably less risk of having cardiac involvement with a recurrence. Therefore, a physician may consider discontinuing prophylaxis in these individuals after several years.[12] In general, prophylaxis should continue until 5 years has elapsed since the last rheumatic fever attack or the age of 21 years, whichever is longer.[34]

The decision to discontinue prophylaxis or reinstate it should be made after discussion with the patient regarding the potential risks and benefits and careful consideration of various epidemiologic risk factors.[34] The risk of having a recurrence increases with multiple previous attacks, whereas the risk decreases as the interval since the most recent attack lengthens. In addition, the likelihood of acquiring a streptococcal upper respiratory tract infection is an important consideration. Individuals with increased exposure to streptococcal infections include children and adolescents, parents of young children, teachers, physicians, nurses and allied health personnel in contact with children, military recruits, and others living in crowded situations. A higher risk for recurrence has been demonstrated in economically disadvantaged populations.

BACTERIAL ENDOCARDITIS

Prophylactic antibiotics are recommended for children who are at risk for endocarditis when they undergo procedures that may induce bacteremia with organisms likely to cause endocarditis. Recommended prophylaxis regimens are based primarily on in vitro studies, data collected from experimental animal models, epidemiologic observations, and clinical experience. No adequately controlled clinical trials to validate the efficacy of such prophylaxis have been performed. Prevention of all episodes of bacteremia is impossible, and endocarditis may occur despite appropriate antimicrobial prophylaxis.[35]

The relative risk for endocarditis varies with the underlying condition (Table 236–4). Although intravenous drug abuse and indwelling central venous catheters are high-risk situations, prophylaxis in these situations is not practical. In general, dental or surgical procedures that induce bleeding from the gingiva or from the mucosal surfaces of the oral, respiratory, gastrointestinal, and genitourinary tracts may cause bacteremia and require prophylaxis (Table 236–5).

Poor dental hygiene and periodontal or periapical infections may produce bacteremia even in the absence of dental or oral procedures. Maintenance of optimal dental care and oral hygiene is important for the prevention of endocarditis in children with underlying cardiac disease. Patients in whom prosthetic valves or other devices are to be placed should undergo needed dental procedures to establish optimal oral hygiene before cardiac surgery is performed. Prophylaxis is most effective when given perioperatively, starting shortly before a procedure and maintained for approximately 10 hours. Doses should ensure that adequate serum concentrations are achieved during and after a particular procedure.

Alpha-hemolytic streptococci are the most common cause of endocarditis after dental, oral, upper respiratory tract, or esophageal procedures.[35] Prophylaxis after such procedures should be directed specifically against these organisms, which generally are very susceptible to penicillin, ampicillin, or amoxicillin (Table 236–6). The standard general prophylaxis regimen is recommended, even in patients who are at high risk for endocarditis. For penicillin-allergic patients, clindamycin is recommended. Azithromycin and clarithromycin are also acceptable alternatives.

Bacterial endocarditis that occurs after genitourinary or gastrointestinal tract surgery or instrumentation is caused primarily by enterococci.[35] Bacteremia developing after

TABLE 236–4 ■ RELATIVE RISK OF ENDOCARDITIS FOR VARIOUS CONDITIONS

High Risk
Prosthetic valves
Previous episode of endocarditis
Surgically constructed systemic artery-to-pulmonary artery shunts
Intravenous drug abuse
Indwelling central venous catheters
Complex cyanotic congenital heart disease

Moderate Risk
Uncorrected patent ductus arteriosus
Ventricular septal defect
Uncorrected atrial septal defect (other than secundum)
Bicuspid aortic valve
Mitral valve prolapse with regurgitation and/or dysplastic leaflets
Rheumatic mitral or aortic valve disease
Other acquired valvar diseases
Hypertrophic cardiomyopathy

TABLE 236–5 ■ DENTAL AND SURGICAL PROCEDURES FOR WHICH PROPHYLAXIS IS RECOMMENDED

Dental procedures known to induce gingival or mucosal bleeding
- Gingival surgery
- Subgingival scaling or polishing
- Subgingival orthodontic banding
- Extractions
- Matrix retainers and wedges
- Periodontal surgery
- Prophylactic teeth cleaning

Tonsillectomy and/or adenoidectomy
Bronchoscopy with a rigid bronchoscope
Esophageal stricture dilatation
Cystoscopy
Urethral dilatation
Urethral catheterization if urinary tract infection is present*
Urinary tract surgery if urinary tract infection is present*
Incision and drainage of infected tissue*

*Antibiotic therapy should be directed against the most likely bacterial pathogen.

TABLE 236–6 ■ RECOMMENDED PROPHYLAXIS FOR DENTAL, ORAL, RESPIRATORY TRACT, AND ESOPHAGEAL PROCEDURES

Standard General Prophylaxis	
Amoxicillin	50 mg/kg (maximum, 2 g) orally 1 hr before procedure
Unable to Take Oral Medications	
Ampicillin	50 mg/kg (maximum, 2 g) intravenously or intramuscularly within ½ hr before procedure
Penicillin-Allergic	
Clindamycin	20 mg/kg (maximum, 300 mg) orally 1 hr before procedure
or	
Azithromycin	15 mg/kg (maximum, 500 mg) orally 1 hr before procedure
or	
Clarithromycin	
Penicillin-Allergic and Unable to Take Oral Medications	
Clindamycin	20 mg/kg (maximum, 600 mg) intravenously within ½ hr before procedure

For patients in the high-risk category for endocarditis, half the dose may be repeated 6 hours after the initial dose (except for azithromycin; a second dose is not necessary).

gastrointestinal endoscopy is very rare in children[22, 43] and occurs more commonly after genitourinary tract procedures. Gram-negative bacilli may induce bacteremia after such procedures; however, endocarditis rarely is caused by these organisms. Therefore, prophylaxis is directed primarily against enterococci (Table 236–7).

In special situations, the aforementioned recommendations may not apply. Surgical procedures through infected tissue require antimicrobial therapy directed against the most likely pathogen. Children who are receiving penicillin prophylaxis for prevention of rheumatic fever recurrence may have alpha-hemolytic streptococci in their oral cavities that are relatively resistant to penicillins. In such cases, an agent other than amoxicillin (e.g., clindamycin) should be selected for endocarditis prophylaxis. Finally, prophylaxis is recommended for patients who undergo open heart surgery, but such prophylaxis should be aimed primarily against *Staphylococcus aureus* and coagulase-negative staphylococci (see the section on cardiovascular surgery later). A first-generation cephalosporin or vancomycin is a reasonable choice and should be used only perioperatively and for no longer than 48 hours.

RECURRENT OTITIS MEDIA

Acute otitis media is one of the most common infections in infants and children and has a tendency to recur, particularly during the first few years of life. In addition to tympanostomy tube placement and adenoidectomy, antimicrobial prophylaxis is one of the options recommended for the management of recurrent otitis media.[23, 42, 101]

Antimicrobial prophylaxis currently is recommended for a child who has had three or more episodes of acute otitis media in 6 months or four episodes within a year, with the last episode occurring during the previous 6 months.[53, 95] Patients who are most likely to benefit from prophylaxis include those younger than 2 years, those in out-of-home childcare, and Native American children.[73, 95] Prophylaxis is directed against the most common potential pathogens that cause otitis media: *Streptococcus pneumoniae, Moraxella catarrhalis,* and nontypable *Haemophilus influenzae.* Amoxicillin, at a dose of 20 mg/kg, or sulfisoxazole, at a dose of 50 mg/kg, may be given orally each evening for a period of 3 to 6 months or during the winter months. Although many other antimicrobial agents are used for the treatment of otitis media, only amoxicillin and sulfisoxazole currently are recommended as prophylactic agents. Antimicrobial prophylaxis must be used with great caution and balanced against the potential for increasing the emergence of resistant organisms, particularly *S. pneumoniae.* Other measures that may decrease the incidence of recurrent acute otitis media include eliminating smoking in the home, reducing daycare attendance, eliminating pacifiers, and administering influenza vaccine. Conjugated pneumococcal vaccines also may be beneficial. If these measures do not prevent recurrent infections, referral to an otolaryngologist is recommended for evaluation and possible tympanostomy tube placement or adenoidectomy, or both procedures.

TABLE 236–7 ■ RECOMMENDED PROPHYLAXIS FOR GENITOURINARY OR GASTROINTESTINAL TRACT PROCEDURE IN CHILDREN

High Risk	
Ampicillin	50 mg/kg (maximum, 2 g) intravenously or intramuscularly within ½ hr before procedure
plus	
Gentamicin	1.5 mg/kg (maximum, 120 mg) intravenously or intramuscularly within ½ hr before procedure (6 hr) later, may use ampicillin, 25 mg/kg intravenously or intramuscularly, or amoxicillin, 25 mg/kg orally)
High Risk, Penicillin-Allergic	
Vancomycin	20 mg/kg (maximum, 1 g) intravenously over a period of 1 hr. Complete the infusion within ½ hr before procedure
plus	
Gentamicin	1.5 mg/kg (maximum, 120 mg) intravenously or intramuscularly. Complete the infusion/injection within ½ hr before procedure
Moderate Risk	
Amoxicillin	50 mg/kg (maximum, 2 g) orally 1 hr before procedure
or	
Ampicillin	50 mg/kg (maximum, 2 g) intravenously or intramuscularly within ½ hr before procedure
Moderate Risk, Penicillin-Allergic	
Vancomycin	20 mg/kg (maximum, 1 g) intravenously over a period of 1 hr. Complete the infusion within ½ hr before procedure

RECURRENT URINARY TRACT INFECTION

Urinary tract infection (UTI) occurs in approximately 5 percent of females and 1 to 2 percent of males.[126] Recurrent UTIs are noted in roughly 30 to 50 percent of children with UTIs, with most recurrences taking place within 3 months after the initial episode. Eighty percent of recurrences are new infections caused by different colonic bacterial species that have become resistant to recently administered antibiotics. The recurrence rate is not altered by extending the duration of treatment.

Renal parenchymal infections and renal scarring are well-recognized complications of UTIs in children.[63, 87, 110] Parenchymal scarring is found in 10 to 15 percent of children with UTIs,[113, 126] hypertension will develop in an estimated 10 percent of children with this complication, and renal insufficiency may develop in a smaller number.[67] Vesicoureteral reflux is noted in 30 to 50 percent of children with UTIs,[87] the frequency being directly related to the number of UTI episodes and inversely related to age. Children with reflux have a much higher incidence (30 to 60%) of pyelonephritic scarring than do children without reflux. More than 90 percent of children with renal parenchymal scarring have had vesicoureteral reflux and a history of UTI.[113, 126]

Children who have three or more UTIs in a 12-month period may benefit from suppressive antibiotic therapy for as long as 6 months to allow repair of intrinsic bladder defense mechanisms.[126] In children with anatomic defects or reflux, suppressive therapy may be needed for as long as the underlying defect exists.

Appropriate prophylactic agents should result in low serum but high urinary levels of the medication, have minimal effect on fecal flora, be well tolerated, and be inexpensive.[86] Methenamine mandelate (75 mg/kg divided every 12 hours) is a suitable agent for prophylaxis because it releases formaldehyde in an acid medium. A pH of 5.5 or lower must be maintained in the urine to obtain optimal results. Ascorbic acid or other acidifying agents should be used to achieve the desired urine acidity. Other useful agents for prophylaxis in children with normal renal function are trimethoprim-sulfamethoxazole (TMP-SMX), nitrofurantoin, and nalidixic acid.[17, 61, 67, 87, 108] TMP-SMX can be given at 2 mg of TMP and 10 mg of SMX per kilogram in a single daily dose or at 5 mg of TMP and 25 mg of SMX per kilogram twice a week.

TMP has the additional unique characteristic of diffusing into vaginal and urethral fluids, thereby decreasing bacterial colonization with members of the Enterobacteriaceae and diminishing ascending reinfection.[61, 116] Nitrofurantoin is recommended at 1 to 2 mg/kg taken each night. It has been used effectively as prophylaxis for recurrent UTIs in infants and children. Pulmonary, neurologic, and hepatic adverse effects have been reported but are rare.[87] Nalidixic acid (not recommended for children) is administered at 30 mg/kg divided every 12 hours. It is a bactericidal agent for most of the common gram-negative uropathogens. More recently, various cephalosporins and amoxicillin–clavulanic acid have been used as prophylactic agents with good results.[86] Prophylactic agents are best administered as a single dose at bedtime.

Postexposure Prophylaxis

Prophylaxis targeted against specific organisms after an individual is exposed is discussed in this section.

PERTUSSIS

When a case of pertussis is identified, prompt use of erythromycin prophylaxis in close contacts is effective in limiting secondary transmission. Close contacts are household members, attendees of childcare facilities, and other individuals who are in contact with the index case for 4 or more hours a day. Chemoprophylaxis is recommended irrespective of age or vaccination status because immunity after receiving pertussis immunization is not absolute and may not prevent infection.[2] The recommended dose of erythromycin is 40 to 50 mg/kg/day (maximum, 2 g/day) to be given orally in four divided doses for 14 days. Individuals who are allergic to erythromycin or cannot tolerate it may be given TMP-SMX, although the efficacy of this regimen has not been documented. The dose is 8 mg/kg/day (TMP) and 40 mg/kg/day (SMX) orally in two divided doses for 14 days.

Persons who have been in contact with an infected individual should be monitored closely for respiratory symptoms for 2 weeks after the last contact with the index case. The risk of contracting pertussis in adults providing medical care to children should be recognized. Symptoms may be mild and not readily recognized as pertussis; however, such individuals can transmit the infection.

MENINGOCOCCAL INFECTIONS

Close contacts of patients with invasive disease caused by *Neisseria meningitidis* (meningococcemia, meningitis, or both) are at higher risk for infection than the general population is. Secondary cases and outbreaks may occur in households, childcare centers, nursery schools, colleges, and military camps.[2] The attack rate for household contacts is 0.3 to 1.0 percent (300 to 1000 times the rate in the general population). Spread from patients to medical care providers occurs infrequently unless intimate contact (e.g., mouth-to mouth resuscitation, intubation, suctioning) occurs. Respiratory tract cultures are not recommended and are not of value in deciding who should receive prophylaxis.[2]

Chemoprophylaxis should be administered as soon as possible, preferably within 24 hours of identifying the index case.[2] Systemic antimicrobial therapy for meningococcal disease does not eradicate nasopharyngeal carriage of *N. meningitidis* reliably; therefore, antimicrobial chemoprophylaxis should be administered to the index patient before discharge from the hospital. The antibiotic of choice in most instances is rifampin. The recommended regimen is 10 mg/kg (maximum, 600 mg) every 12 hours for a total of four doses in 2 days. A liquid preparation can be formulated, or the powder can be mixed with applesauce or a similar vehicle. The rifampin prophylaxis regimen recommended for *H. influenzae* type b disease (see later) is also effective for meningococcal prophylaxis.

Rifampin prophylaxis has several shortcomings.[105] It fails to eradicate *N. meningitidis* in 10 to 20 percent of pharyngeal carriers.[90] It is not recommended for pregnant women. Side effects occur frequently and include headache, dizziness, gastrointestinal symptoms, discoloration of body secretions (saliva, tears, urine), staining of contact lenses, and hepatotoxicity. Finally, several studies have documented the emergence of resistant meningococcal strains after the administration of rifampin prophylaxis.[105]

If the meningococcal isolate is known to be susceptible to sulfonamides, sulfisoxazole is recommended. The dose is 500 mg/day for infants, 500 mg every 12 hours for children 1 to 12 years of age, and 1 g every 12 hours for children older than 12 years and adults. The duration of prophylaxis is 2 days.

In one study,[105] a single intramuscular injection of ceftriaxone was compared with oral rifampin in eradicating pharyngeal carriage of group A *N. meningitidis* during an outbreak. Ceftriaxone was significantly more effective than rifampin in eradicating meningococci at 1 week (97 versus 75%) and at 2 weeks (97 versus 81%) after prophylaxis. Ceftriaxone was administered as a single intramuscular dose (125 mg for children younger than 15 years and 250 mg for adults). Although at this stage ceftriaxone is not recommended for routine prophylaxis, it has the advantages of ease of administration, possibly greater efficacy, and safety in pregnancy. For high-risk contacts 18 years or older, a single 500-mg oral dose of ciprofloxacin is a third option for meningococcal prophylaxis.

HAEMOPHILUS INFLUENZAE TYPE b INFECTIONS

The risk for secondary invasive disease with *H. influenzae* type b (Hib) is age-dependent.[7] Household contacts younger than 1 year have the highest risk (6%) for secondary illness; the risk in children 4 years or younger remains high (2.1%). Children older than 6 years and adults are at little or no risk. The risk for children attending childcare centers may be increased but appears to be less than that for household contacts.[19, 48, 85, 91, 94] Exposed hospital personnel do not require antimicrobial prophylaxis.

Postexposure Hib prophylaxis may prove unnecessary eventually, given the widespread childhood immunization with conjugate vaccines. In addition to protecting vaccinated children against invasive disease, conjugate vaccines appear to decrease pharyngeal colonization, which would reduce Hib transmission to unvaccinated children. Prophylaxis currently is recommended for all household contacts, regardless of age, if at least one of the contacts is younger than 4 years and not immunized completely.[2] Complete immunization is defined as having received a conjugate vaccine: (1) at least one dose at 15 months or older, (2) two doses between 12 and 14 months of age, or (3) two or more doses when younger than 12 months with a booster at 12 months or older.

Prophylaxis for nursery and daycare center contacts is less well defined, and definitive recommendations are lacking. In general, prophylaxis is recommended for childcare centers with the same regimen as recommended for households if (1) the center is attended by unvaccinated or incompletely vaccinated children younger than 2 years where contact is 25 hr/wk or more or (2) two or more cases of invasive Hib disease occur among attendees within 60 days and unvaccinated or incompletely vaccinated children attend the facility.[2] In facilities where all contacts are older than 2 years, prophylaxis need not be given, regardless of vaccination status.

Rifampin in a single dose of 20 mg/kg/day (maximum, 600 mg) for 4 days effectively eliminates oropharyngeal carriage of Hib in 95 percent of treated individuals.[2] This regimen has been shown to be effective in preventing secondary cases of invasive Hib disease in household members, daycare settings, and classroom contacts.[2, 7, 19] Prophylaxis should be initiated as soon as possible because most secondary cases occur during the first week after identification of the index case.[7] The index case also should receive rifampin prophylaxis, usually initiated during hospitalization and just before discharge.

If prophylaxis is given to limit secondary spread to a cohort (household or daycare), children vaccinated with any Hib vaccine and unvaccinated susceptible children should receive prophylaxis.[2] Prophylaxis is not recommended for pregnant women.

TUBERCULOSIS

The three goals of preventive therapy for tuberculosis are to (1) prevent asymptomatic (latent) infection from progressing to clinical (active) disease, (2) prevent recurrence of past disease, and (3) prevent initial infection in individuals who have negative tuberculin skin tests. The first two goals are covered in detail elsewhere; prevention of initial infection is addressed herein. Chemoprophylaxis is given in an attempt to prevent the establishment of infection, and the recipient is protected only as long as antituberculous therapy is continued.

In the United States, isoniazid is the only drug approved by the FDA for chemoprophylaxis against *Mycobacterium tuberculosis.* The recommended dose is 10 to 15 mg/kg/day (maximum, 300 mg/day) to be given as a single dose.

Persons exposed to an infectious case of tuberculosis should undergo tuberculin skin testing, have a chest radiograph, and receive isoniazid prophylaxis.[2] If the tuberculin test and chest radiograph are negative and the individual is not anergic, isoniazid should be administered for 12 weeks and contact with the index case should be broken. Isoniazid may be discontinued if a repeat skin test after 12 weeks of prophylaxis remains negative. If the skin test becomes positive, isoniazid is continued for a total of 9 months. Candidates for prophylaxis include persons with impaired immunity; household contacts, particularly children younger than 4 years; recent contacts, especially human immunodeficiency virus–positive contacts; and persons known to be anergic from populations with a high prevalence of tuberculosis.

Management of a newborn infant whose mother or other household contact has tuberculosis should be based on individual considerations.

Host-Targeted Prophylaxis

HUMAN AND ANIMAL BITES

Human and animal bites are relatively common. According to the Centers for Disease Control and Prevention, more than 1 million animal bites that occur each year require medical attention.[119] Human bites accounted for 1 in 600 pediatric emergency visits and dog bites for 1 percent of all such visits.[106] Dog bites account for 80 to 90 percent of animal bites that require medical care.[18] The organisms most frequently isolated in human bites are *S. aureus*, gamma-hemolytic streptococci, *Bacteroides* spp., *Eikenella corrodens,* and *Fusobacterium* spp. In animal bites, *Pasteurella multocida, S. aureus,* and anaerobic cocci are the main pathogens.

Data on the use of prophylactic antimicrobial agents after bites are sparse, and the role of prophylaxis in patients who seek medical care early for bite wounds is uncertain.[6, 40, 106, 112] However, because these wounds are usually contaminated with potential pathogens, administering prophylaxis is advisable for patients who have the following risk factors: delay of 18 hours or more between the time of injury and the time of initial physician assessment, facial and hand bites, deep puncture wounds, bites that are difficult to irrigate and cleanse adequately before repair, delay in primary closure of wounds, and wounds in immunocompromised individuals.[6, 18, 39, 84, 106, 127]

Because most human and animal bites result in polymicrobial aerobic and anaerobic infections, prophylaxis should target these organisms. For initial prophylaxis, amoxicillin–clavulanic acid (30 to 50 mg/kg/day) is probably optimal therapy.[16, 18, 46, 1128] Prophylaxis is recommended for 3 to 5 days. Combination therapy with penicillin and cephalexin or dicloxacillin has been suggested by some authorities. Though only moderately active against *P. multocida,* erythromycin (30 to 50 mg/kg/day) is an accepted alternative in penicillin-allergic children.

ASPLENIA

The spleen constitutes approximately 25 percent of the lymphoid mass. It filters blood at a rate of 150 mL/min and plays an important role in the primary defense against bacteria that gain access to the circulation.[118] The spleen has an active role in phagocytosis, is a major source of T lymphocytes, and produces IgM antibodies, complement, opsonins, and "tuftsin" (a phagocytosis-promoting tetrapeptide).

Asplenia may be congenital or acquired. Splenectomy is not uncommonly performed and is done for a variety of indications. Overwhelming and often fatal septicemia and meningitis occur with increased frequency in asplenic individuals.[125] The frequency of sepsis is 60 times greater in children who undergo splenectomy than in normal children. Fatality from sepsis in splenectomized individuals is 200 times more common than that in the normal population.[118] The risk of sepsis developing is greatest in patients who have undergone splenectomies for underlying immunologic or reticuloendothelial disorders, and the risk is lowest in children after splenectomy for trauma.[74] In all categories, the risk is highest in young infants and children, but it extends to teenagers and adults as well. The period of heightened susceptibility to infection is the initial 1 to 2 years after splenectomy; however, fulminant infection has been reported as long as 25 years after splenectomy.

S. pneumoniae is the most common cause of septicemia in splenectomized individuals. Despite prompt diagnosis and treatment, pneumococcal septicemia is associated with a fatality rate as high as 50 percent. Overall, 80 percent of post-splenectomy infections are caused by bacteria with capsular polysaccharides: *S. pneumoniae, H. influenzae,* and *N. meningitidis.*[111, 118]

To reduce the likelihood of serious infections occurring after splenectomy, several measures are advisable. Splenectomy should be performed only when absolutely indicated. If possible, the best approach is to delay the surgical intervention until the child is 5 or 6 years of age.

Although multivalent pneumococcal polysaccharide vaccine provides incomplete protection for patients undergoing splenectomy, especially infants and young children, it should be administered to all these patients, ideally 2 weeks before performing the splenectomy.[111] Vaccination against Hib and *N. meningitidis* types A and C also should be provided. For antibiotic prophylaxis, penicillin is the agent of choice. Penicillin V given twice daily significantly decreases the frequency of invasive pneumococcal infection. Erythromycin or TMP-SMX is an alternative option in patients with documented hypersensitivity to penicillin. The duration of prophylactic coverage remains controversial; current practice is to provide penicillin prophylaxis indefinitely in immunocompromised patients.[111]

HEMOGLOBINOPATHIES

Functional asplenia is the primary reason for susceptibility to pneumococcal infection in children with sickle-cell anemia. Serum immunoglobulins are normal or increased in these children; however, they have a dysfunctional alternative complement pathway and decreased opsonic activity (which is mediated by both the alternative and the classic components) against *S. pneumoniae.* Leukocyte function is also defective in patients with sickle-cell anemia; intracellular production of hydrogen peroxide, respiratory stimulation, and hexose monophosphate shunt activity are inadequate during phagocytosis. In contrast, leukocytes from splenectomized patients without sickle-cell anemia exhibit normal phagocytic function accompanied by adequate metabolic stimulation. Immunologic dysfunction occurs less rapidly and less commonly in children with hemoglobin C–sickle-cell anemia and hemoglobin C–beta-thalassemia.[78]

Patients with sickle-cell disease are at risk for overwhelming infection (septicemia and meningitis) by encapsulated bacteria, including *S. pneumoniae,* Hib, and *N. meningitidis. S. pneumoniae* is the most important and frequent cause of septicemia and meningitis in these patients.[121] The risk is particularly high in children younger than 3 years.[51] A trend toward increased frequency of invasive disease occurring in the first 2 to 5 years after undergoing splenectomy also has been noted. Unlike very young children, preschool children appear to be less vulnerable to pneumococcal invasive infection, even though they remain functionally asplenic.[52, 121, 124]

The efficacy of penicillin prophylaxis in preventing pneumococcal infection in infants and young children with sickle-cell disease has been well documented in several reports.[44, 51, 52, 96, 124] The recommended dose of penicillin V is 125 mg twice daily in children younger than 3 years and 250 mg twice daily in children 3 years or older. Some physicians recommend using amoxicillin (20 mg/kg/day) or TMP-SMX (4 mg TMP plus 20 mg SMX/kg/day) in children younger than 5 years to include coverage against Hib, which is less likely to be a concern in patients who are immunized adequately.

Because overwhelming infection can occur in infants as young as 3 months, detection of sickle-cell anemia should be accomplished in the neonatal period. Babies in whom sickle-cell anemia is diagnosed should start a prophylactic antibiotic regimen no later than 3 to 4 months of age.[52] The optimal duration of prophylaxis is not defined clearly, and the age at which prophylactic penicillin can be discontinued safely is determined arbitrarily. A concern is that penicillin prophylaxis may decrease the development of natural immunity against pneumococcal infection in children receiving prophylaxis, thereby rendering them more prone to infection after discontinuing prophylaxis.[20] Another concern is the accelerated development of penicillin-resistant strains of *S. pneumoniae.*[45, 121] A multicenter study by the Prophylactic Penicillin Study II group suggests that in children with sickle-cell anemia who have not had a previous severe pneumococcal infection or surgical splenectomy and are receiving comprehensive care, prophylaxis may be stopped safely at 5 years of age.[45] Continuous prophylaxis has limitations, and serious overwhelming infection can occur while patients are receiving prophylaxis. Patients or parents (or both) should be aware that any febrile illness is potentially serious and immediate medical attention should be sought.[29, 96]

CEREBROSPINAL FLUID LEAKAGE

The value of antibiotic prophylaxis in patients with cerebrospinal fluid (CSF) leakage is debatable.[49, 89] In the absence of meningeal inflammation, many antibiotics do not penetrate the blood-brain barrier and do not attain adequate levels in CSF. Antibiotic prophylaxis often fails and frequently alters the normal flora of the respiratory tract, thereby resulting in colonization with resistant bacteria. Prophylaxis may be considered for a short duration while surgical repair is being planned.[89]

Surgical Prophylaxis

GENERAL SURGICAL PROCEDURES

Postoperative infection always has been a feared complication of surgical procedures. Skin incision, organ manipulation, and surgical trauma increase the likelihood of local infection. Surgical procedures traditionally are classified as clean, clean-contaminated, and contaminated (Table 236–8). Prophylactic antibiotics are effective in reducing postoperative infections after contaminated and clean-contaminated surgical procedures, whereas their efficacy is more controversial for clean surgical procedures. Clean surgical procedures generally carry a risk of postoperative wound infection that is less than 5 percent and, in many hospitals, less than 1 percent.

The critical period for development of infection is short, and optimal prophylaxis should be restricted to the perioperative period. Antibiotic prophylaxis of less than 24 hours' duration is effective both clinically and experimentally. Administration of antibiotics should be started at the time of anesthesia induction or immediately before the surgical incision is made and discontinued within 24 hours.

TABLE 236–8 ■ SURGICAL PROCEDURES AND PROBABLE PATHOGENS

Surgical Category	Most Likely Pathogens
Clean	
Neurosurgical	CNS, *Staphylococcus aureus*
Cardiovascular	CNS, *S. aureus*
Orthopedics	CNS, *S. aureus*
Clean-Contaminated	
Burn	Group A streptococci, *S. aureus* GNB
Gastrointestinal	GNB, anaerobes, enterococci
Urogenital	GNB, enterococci
Respiratory	Alpha-hemolytic streptococci, anaerobes
Contaminated	
Ruptured viscera	GNB, anaerobes, enterococci
Traumatic wounds	*S. aureus,* group A streptococci, clostridia

CNS, coagulase-negative staphylococci; GNB, gram-negative bacilli.

Addressing all situations of surgical prophylaxis is beyond the scope of this chapter, and the reader is referred to several recent publications and reviews on the subject.[36, 62, 68, 70, 99, 120]

NEUROSURGICAL PROCEDURES

The use of prophylactic antibiotics for clean neurosurgical procedures remains controversial.[50, 57, 89, 100] However, because of the suggested benefit of prophylactic antibiotics in uncontrolled trials involving a large number of patients, of whom adults were the majority, and in view of the scarcity of definitive studies, the literature supports the use of a short-course prophylactic regimen.[21, 41, 55, 122] Prophylaxis for clean neurosurgical procedures is particularly valuable for high-risk groups (e.g., patients undergoing operative procedures in excess of 4 hours, operations in which craniotomies are performed, or patients with major underlying pathology).[37, 109]

Placement of CSF shunts is one of the most common neurosurgical procedures in pediatric patients. An estimated 10,000 new shunt insertions and 6000 revisions are performed annually in the United States. The frequency of shunt infection varies from 1.5 to 39 percent (average, 10 to 15%).[75, 103] The major route of infection is colonization of the device or the operative wounds during placement.[55] Retrograde spread from the distal end of the catheter or hematogenous seeding accounts for some instances of infection.

Most infections are noted within 15 days to 2 months of shunt placement.[79, 103] Commensal skin flora are the predominant pathogens. Coagulase-negative staphylococci are the most common pathogens and account for approximately 70 percent of shunt infections. *S. aureus* is less common. Gram-negative bacilli are the least common and are often the result of retrograde infection from the peritoneum.[75, 103]

The role of prophylactic antibiotics for placement of CSF shunts has been controversial. A meta-analysis of 1359 patients in 12 randomized, controlled trials indicated that short-term perioperative antimicrobial prophylaxis at the time of placement of a CSF shunt significantly decreases the risk for subsequent device-related infection.[79] Various antimicrobial regimens, including antistaphylococcal penicillins, cephalosporins, TMP-SMX, vancomycin, gentamicin, and combinations, were used in these trials. The choice of an appropriate prophylactic regimen in a particular setting should be based on the local epidemiology of suspected pathogens, local patterns of antimicrobial susceptibility, cost, and expected toxicity. The duration of perioperative prophylaxis should not exceed 48 hours.[72, 79] A longer duration of prophylaxis increases cost and the risk for adverse reactions and promotes alteration of the normal flora and the emergence of resistant bacteria.

CARDIOVASCULAR SURGERY

Infectious complications of cardiovascular surgery can be very serious and life-threatening, and antimicrobial prophylaxis is used commonly in most medical centers.[71, 76] Most available data are based on reports from adult patients,[27, 58] with little specific information on prophylactic antibiotic use in pediatric patients. The goal of prophylactic therapy is prevention of wound infection, mediastinitis, and endocarditis. A survey of 43 North American academic centers with pediatric cardiovascular surgery programs indicated that all centers use prophylactic antibiotics for all operative procedures.[81] Monotherapy prophylaxis was used by 91 percent of respondents and consisted almost exclusively of a first- or second-generation cephalosporin. In 95 percent of centers, prophylaxis was started just before surgery or intraoperatively. Prophylaxis was continued for 48 hours or less in most (68%) instances. Prophylactic antibiotics often were continued while thoracostomy tubes, mediastinal tubes, or transthoracic vascular catheters were in place but usually not for endotracheal tubes, arterial or percutaneous central venous catheters, or temporary pacing wires.

REFERENCES

1. Allen, U. D., Navas, L., and King, S. M.: Effectiveness of intrapartum penicillin prophylaxis in preventing early-onset group B streptococcal infection: Results of a meta-analysis. Can. Med. Assoc. J. *149*:1659–1665, 1993.
2. American Academy of Pediatrics: 1994 Red Book: Report of the Committee on Infectious Diseases. Elk Grove Village, IL, American Academy of Pediatrics, 1994.
3. American Academy of Pediatrics: Group B streptococcal infections. *In* Pickering, L. D. (ed.): 2000 Red Book: Report of the Committee on Infectious Diseases. 25th ed. Elk Grove Village, IL, American Academy of Pediatrics, 2000, p. 537.
4. American College of Obstetricians and Gynecologists: Group B Streptococcal Infections in Pregnancy. ACOG Technical Bulletin No. 170. Washington, D.C., American College of Obstetricians and Gynecologists, 1992.
5. Aujard, Y., Boucot, I., Brahimi, N., et al.: Comparative efficacy and safety of four-day cefuroxime axetil and ten-day penicillin treatment of group A beta-hemolytic streptococcal pharyngitis in children. Pediatr. Infect. Dis. J. *14*:295–300, 1995.
6. Baker, D. M., and Moore, S. E.: Human bites in children: A six-year experience. Am. J. Dis. Child. *141*:1285–1290, 1987.
7. Band, J. D., Fraser, D. W., Ajello, G., et al.: Prevention of *Haemophilus influenzae* type B disease. J. A. M. A. *251*:2381–2386, 1984.
8. Barefield, E. S., and Philips, J. B., III: Vancomycin prophylaxis for coagulase-negative staphylococcal bacteremia. J. Pediatr. *125*:230–232, 1994.
9. Bass, J. W.: Antibiotic management of group A streptococcal pharyngotonsillitis. Pediatr. Infect. Dis. J. *10*(Suppl.):43–49, 1991.
10. Bass, J. W., Crast, F. W., Knowles, C. R., et al.: Streptococcal pharyngitis in children: A comparison of four treatment schedules with intramuscular penicillin G benzathine. J. A. M. A. *235*:1112–1116, 1976.
11. Benitz, W. E., Gould, J. B., and Druzin, M. L.: Antimicrobial prevention of early-onset group B streptococcal sepsis: Estimates of risk reduction based on a critical literature review. Pediatrics *103*:1278, 1999.
12. Berrios, X., del Campo, E., Guzman, B., et al.: Discontinuing rheumatic fever prophylaxis in selected adolescents and young adults. Ann. Intern. Med. *118*:401–406, 1993.
13. Black-Payne, C., Bocchini, J. A., Jr., and Cedotal, C.: Failure of erythromycin ointment for postnatal ocular prophylaxis of chlamydial conjunctivitis. Pediatr. Infect. Dis. J. *8*:491–498, 1989.
14. Block, S. L., Hedrick, J. A., and Tyler, R. D.: Comparative study of the effectiveness of cefixime and penicillin V for the treatment of streptococcal pharyngitis in children and adolescents. Pediatr. Infect. Dis. J. *11*:919–925, 1992.
15. Boyer, K. M., and Gotoff, S. P.: Prevention of early-onset neonatal group B streptococcal disease with selective intrapartum chemoprophylaxis. N. Engl. J. Med. *314*:1665–1669, 1986.
16. Brakenbury, P. H., and Muwanga, C.: A comparative double blind study of amoxicillin/clavulanate vs. placebo in the prevention of infection after animal bites. Arch. Emerg. Med. *6*:251–256, 1989.
17. Brendstrup, L., Hjelt, K., Petersen, K. E., et al.: Nitrofurantoin versus trimethoprim prophylaxis in recurrent urinary tract infection in children: A randomized, double blind study. Acta Paediatr. Scand. *79*:1225–1234, 1990.
18. Brook, I.: Microbiology of human and animal bite wounds in children. Pediatr. Infect. Dis. J. *6*:29–32, 1987.
19. Broome, C. V., Mortimer, E. A., Katz, S. L., et al.: Use of chemoprophylaxis to prevent the spread of *Hemophilus influenzae* B in day-care facilities. N. Engl. J. Med. *316*:1226–1228, 1987.
20. Buchanan, G. R., and Smith, S. J.: Pneumococcal septicemia despite pneumococcal vaccine and prescription of penicillin prophylaxis in children with sickle cell anemia. Am. J. Dis. Child. *140*:428–432, 1986.
21. Bullock, R., Van Dellen, J. R., Ketelbey, W., et al.: A double-blind placebo-controlled trial of perioperative prophylactic antibiotics for elective neurosurgery. J. Neurosurg. *69*:687–691, 1988.
22. Byrne, W., Euler, A., Campbell, M., et al.: Bacteremia in children following upper gastrointestinal endoscopy or colonoscopy. J. Pediatr. Gastroenterol. Nutr. *1*:551–553, 1982.

23. Casselbrant, M. L., Kaleida, P. H., Rockette, H. E., et al.: Efficacy of antimicrobial prophylaxis and of tympanostomy tube insertion for prevention of recurrent acute otitis media: Results of a randomized clinical trial. Pediatr. Infect. Dis. J. *11*:278–286, 1992.
24. Catanzaro, F. J., Stetson, C. A., Morris, A. J., et al.: Symposium on rheumatic fever and rheumatic heart disease. Am. J. Med. *17*:749–756, 1954.
25. Chandler, J. W.: Controversies in ocular prophylaxis of newborns. Arch. Ophthalmol. *107*:814–815, 1989.
26. Chen, J. Y.: Prophylaxis of ophthalmia neonatorum: Comparison of silver nitrate, tetracycline, erythromycin and no prophylaxis. Pediatr. Infect. Dis. J. *11*:1026–1030, 1992.
27. Conte, J. E., Jr., Cohen, S. N., Roe, B. B., et al.: Antibiotic prophylaxis and cardiac surgery: A prospective double-blind comparison of single-dose versus multiple-dose regimens. Ann. Intern. Med. *76*:943–949, 1972.
28. Coonan, K. M., and Kaplan, E. L.: In vitro susceptibility of recent North American group A streptococcal isolates to eleven oral antibiotics. Pediatr. Infect. Dis. J. *13*:630–635, 1994.
29. Cummins, D., Heuschkel, R., and Davies, S. C.: Penicillin prophylaxis in children with sickle cell disease in Brent. B. M. J. *302*:989–990, 1991.
30. Dajani, A. S.: Current status of nonsuppurative complications of group A streptococci. Pediatr. Infect. Dis. J. *10*(Suppl.):25–27, 1991.
31. Dajani, A. S.: Pharyngitis/tonsillitis: European and United States experience with cefpodoxime proxetil. Pediatr. Infect. Dis. J. *14*(Suppl.):7–11, 1995.
32. Dajani, A. S.: Adherence to physicians' instructions as a factor in managing streptococcal pharyngitis. Pediatrics *97*:976–980, 1996.
33. Dajani, A. S., Kessler, S. L., Mendelson, R., et al.: Cefpodoxime proxetil vs. penicillin V in pediatric streptococcal pharyngitis/tonsillitis. Pediatr. Infect. Dis. J. *12*:275–279, 1993.
34. Dajani, A., Taubert, K., Ferrieri, P., et al.: Treatment of acute streptococcal pharyngitis and prevention of rheumatic fever: A statement for health professionals. Pediatrics *96*:758–764, 1995.
35. Dajani, A. S., Taubert, K. A., Wilson, W., et al.: Prevention of bacterial endocarditis: Recommendations by the American Heart Association. J. A. M. A. *277*:1794–1801, 1997.
36. Dellinger, E. P., Gross, P. A., Barrett, T. L., et al.: Quality standard for antimicrobial prophylaxis in surgical procedures. Clin. Infect. Dis. *18*:422–427, 1994.
37. Dempsey, R., Rapp, R. P., Young, B., et al.: Prophylactic parenteral antibiotics in clean neurosurgical procedures: A review. J. Neurosurg. *69*:52–57, 1988.
38. Denny, F. W., Wannamaker, L. W., Brink, W. R., et al.: Prevention of rheumatic fever: Treatment of the preceding streptococcal infection. J. A. M. A. *143*:151–153, 1950.
39. Dire, D. J.: Cat bite wounds: Risk factors for infection. Ann. Emerg. Med. *20*:973–979, 1991.
40. Dire, D. J., Hogan, D. E., and Walker, J. S.: Prophylactic oral antibiotics for low-risk dog bite wounds. Pediatr. Emerg. Care *8*:194–199, 1992.
41. Djindjian, M., Lepresel, E., and Homs, J. B.: Antibiotic prophylaxis during prolonged clean neurosurgery. J. Neurosurg. *73*:383–386, 1990.
42. Dowell, S. F., Marcy, S. M., Phillips, W. R., et al.: Otitis media—principles of judicious use of antimicrobial agents. Pediatrics *101*:165–171, 1998.
43. El-Baba, M., Tolia, V., Lin, C., et al.: Absence of bacteremia after gastrointestinal procedures in children. Gastrointest. Endosc. *44*:378–381, 1996.
44. El-Hazmi, M. A. F., Bahakim, H. M., Babikar, M. A., et al.: Symptom-free intervals in sicklers: Does pneumococcal vaccination and penicillin prophylaxis have a role? J. Trop. Pediatr. *36*:56–62, 1990.
45. Falletta, J. M., Woods, G. M., Verter, J. I., et al.: Discontinuing penicillin prophylaxis in children with sickle cell anemia. J. Pediatr. *127*:685–690, 1995.
46. Feder, H., Jr., Shanley, J. D., and Barbera, J. A.: Review of 59 patients hospitalized with animal bites. Pediatr. Infect. Dis. J. *6*:24–28, 1987.
47. Feinstein, A. R., Harrison, F. W., Epstein, J. A., et al.: A controlled study of three methods of prophylaxis against streptococcal infection in a population of rheumatic children. N. Engl. J. Med. *260*:697–702, 1959.
48. Fleming, D. W., Leibenhaut, M. H., Albanes, D., et al.: Secondary *Haemophilus influenzae* type B in day-care facilities. J. A. M. A. *254*:509–514, 1985.
49. Frazee, R. C., Mucha, P., Jr., Farnell, M. B., et al.: Meningitis after basilar skull fracture: Does antibiotic prophylaxis help? Postgrad. Med. *83*:267–274, 1988.
50. Gardner, B. P., and Gordon, D. S.: Postoperative infection in shunts for hydrocephalus: Are prophylactic antibiotics necessary? B. M. J. *284*:1914–1915, 1982.
51. Gaston, M. H., and Verter, J.: Sickle cell anaemia trial. Stat. Med. *9*:45–51, 1990.
52. Gaston, M. H., Verter, J. I., Woods, G., et al.: Prophylaxis with oral penicillin in children with sickle cell anemia. N. Engl. J. Med. *314*:1593–1599, 1986.
53. Giebink, G. S.: Preventing otitis media. Ann. Otol. Rhinol. Laryngol. *103*:20–23, 1994.
54. Gooch, W. M., McLinn, S. E., Aronovitz, G. H., et al.: Efficacy of cefuroxime axetil suspension compared with that of penicillin V suspension in children with group A streptococcal pharyngitis. Antimicrob. Agents Chemother. *37*:159–163, 1993.
55. Guevara, J. A., Zuccaro, G., Trevisan, A., et al.: Bacterial adhesion to cerebrospinal fluid shunts. J. Neurosurg. *67*:438–445, 1987.
56. Haines, S. J.: Efficacy of antibiotic prophylaxis in clean neurosurgical operations. Neurosurgery *24*:401–405, 1989.
57. Haines, S. J., and Goodman, M. L.: Antibiotic prophylaxis of postoperative neurosurgical wound infection. J. Neurosurg. *56*:103–105, 1982.
58. Hall, J. C., Christiansen, K., Carter, M. J., et al.: Antibiotic prophylaxis in cardiac operations. Ann. Thorac. Surg. *56*:916–922, 1993.
59. Hammerschlag, M. R.: Neonatal ocular prophylaxis. Pediatr. Infect. Dis. J. *7*:81–82, 1988.
60. Hammerschlag, M. R., Cummings, C., Roblin, P., et al.: Efficacy of neonatal ocular prophylaxis for the prevention of chlamydial and gonococcal conjunctivitis. N. Engl. J. Med. *320*:769–772, 1989.
61. Hanson, E., Hansson, S., and Jodol, U.: Trimethoprim-sulfadiazine prophylaxis in children with vesicoureteral reflux. Scand. J. Infect. Dis. *21*:201–204, 1989.
62. Hirschmann, J. V., and Inui, T. S.: Antimicrobial prophylaxis: A critique of recent trials. Rev. Infect. Dis. *2*:1–23, 1980.
63. Holland, N. H., Jackson, E. C., Kazee, M., et al.: Relation of urinary tract infection and vesicoureteral reflux to scars: Follow-up of thirty-eight patients. J. Pediatr. *116*(Suppl.):65–71, 1990.
64. Hooton, T. M.: A comparison of azithromycin and penicillin V for the treatment of streptococcal pharyngitis. Am. J. Med. *91*(Suppl.):23–30, 1991.
65. Hussar, D. A.: Importance of patient compliance in effective antimicrobial therapy. Pediatr. Infect. Dis. J. *6*:971–975, 1987.
66. Jafari, H. S., Schuchat, A., Hilsdon, R., et al.: Barriers to prevention of perinatal group B streptococcal disease. Pediatr. Infect. Dis. J. *14*:662–667, 1995.
67. Jodal, U., Koskimies, O., Hanson, E., et al.: Infection pattern in children with vesicoureteral reflux randomly allocated to operation or long-term antibacterial prophylaxis. J. Urol. *148*:1650–1652, 1992.
68. Jones, R. N., Wojeski, W., Bakke, J., et al.: Antibiotic prophylaxis of 1,036 patients undergoing elective surgical procedures: A prospective, randomized comparative trial of cefazolin, cefoxitin, and cefotaxime in a prepaid medical practice. Am. J. Surg. *153*:341–346, 1987.
69. Kacica, M. A., Horgan, M. J., Ochoa, L., et al.: Prevention of gram-positive sepsis in neonates weighing less than 1500 grams. J. Pediatr. *125*:253–258, 1994.
70. Kaiser, A. B.: Antimicrobial prophylaxis in surgery. N. Engl. J. Med. *315*:1129–1138, 1986.
71. Kaiser, A. B., Petracek, M. R., Lea, J. W., Jr., et al.: Efficacy of cefazolin, cefamandole, and gentamicin as prophylactic agents in cardiac surgery. Ann. Surg. *206*:791–797, 1987.
72. Kestle, J. R. W., Hoffman, H. J., Soloniuk, D., et al.: A concerted effort to prevent shunt infection. Childs Nerv. Syst. *9*:163–165, 1993.
73. Klein, J. O.: Preventing recurrent otitis: What role for antibiotics? Contemp. Pediatr. *11*:44–60, 1994.
74. Konradsen, H. B., and Henrichsen, J.: Pneumococcal infections in splenectomized children are preventable. Acta Paediatr. Scand. *80*:423–427, 1991.
75. Kontny, U., Hofling, B., Gutjahr, P., et al.: CSF shunt infections in children. Infection *21*:89–92, 1993.
76. Kreter, B., and Woods, M.: Antibiotic prophylaxis for cardiothoracic operations: Metaanalysis of thirty years of clinical trials. J. Thorac. Cardiovasc. Surg. *104*:590–599, 1992.
77. Laga, M., Plummer, F. A., Piot, P., et al.: Prophylaxis of gonococcal and chlamydial ophthalmia neonatorum: A comparison of silver nitrate and tetracycline. N. Engl. J. Med. *318*:653–657, 1988.
78. Lane, P. A., Rogers, Z. R., Woods, G. M., et al.: Fatal pneumococcal septicemia in hemoglobin SC disease. J. Pediatr. *124*:859–862, 1994.
79. Langley, J. M., LeBlanc, J. C., Drake, J., et al: Efficacy of antimicrobial prophylaxis in placement of cerebrospinal fluid shunts: Meta-analysis. Clin. Infect. Dis. *17*:98–103, 1993.
80. Larsen, J. W., and Dooley, S. L.: Group B streptococcal infections: An obstetrical viewpoint. Pediatrics *91*:148–149, 1993.
81. Lee, K. R., Ring, J. C., and Leggiadro, R. J.: Prophylactic antibiotic use in pediatric cardiovascular surgery: A survey of current practice. Pediatr. Infect. Dis. J. *14*:267–269, 1995.
82. Lue, H. C., Wu, M. H., Hsieh, K. H., et al.: Rheumatic fever recurrences: Controlled study of a 3-week versus 4-week benzathine penicillin prevention program. J. Pediatr. *108*:299–304, 1986.
83. Lue, H. C., Wu, M. H., Wang, J. K., et al.: Long-term outcome of patients with rheumatic fever receiving benzathine penicillin G prophylaxis every three weeks versus every four weeks. J. Pediatr. *125*:812–816, 1994.
84. Maimaris, C., and Quinton, D. N.: Dog-bite lacerations: A controlled trial of primary wound closure. Arch. Emerg. Med. *5*:156–161, 1988.
85. Makintubee, S., Istre, G. R., and Ward, J. I.: Transmission of invasive *Haemophilus influenzae* type B disease in day care settings. J. Pediatr. *111*:180–186, 1987.
86. Mangiarotti, P., Pizzini, C., and Fanos, V.: Antibiotic prophylaxis in children with relapsing urinary tract infections: Review. J. Chemother. *12*:115–123, 2000.
87. McCracken, G. H., Jr.: Options in antimicrobial management of urinary tract infections in infants and children. Pediatr. Infect. Dis. J. *8*:552–555, 1989.

88. Mohle-Boetani, J. C., Schuchat, A., Plikaytis, B., et al.: Comparison of prevention strategies for neonatal group B streptococcal infection: A population-based economic analysis. J. A. M. A. *270*:1442–1448, 1993.
89. Mollman, D. H., and Haines, S. J.: Risk factors for postoperative neurosurgical wound infection: A case-control study. J. Neurosurg. *64*:902–906, 1986.
90. Munford, R. S., Vasconcelos, Z. J. S., Phillips, C. J., et al.: Eradication of carriage of *Neisseria meningitidis* in families: A study in Brazil. J. Infect. Dis. *129*:644–649, 1974.
91. Murphy, T. V., Clements, J. F., Breedlove, J. E., et al.: Risk of subsequent disease among day-care contacts of patients with systemic *Hemophilus influenzae* type B disease. N. Engl. J. Med. *316*:5–10, 1987.
92. Ng, P. C., Dear, P. R. F., and Thomas, D. F. M.: Oral vancomycin in prevention of necrotising enterocolitis. Arch. Dis. Child. *63*:1390–1393, 1988.
93. Noya, F. J. D., and Baker, C. J.: Prevention of group B streptococcal infection. Infect. Dis. Clin. North Am. *6*:41–54, 1992.
94. Osterholm, M. T., Pierson, L. M., White, K. E., et al.: The risk of subsequent transmission of *Hemophilus influenzae* type B disease among children in day care. N. Engl. J. Med. *316*:1–5, 1987.
95. Paradise, J. L.: Antimicrobial prophylaxis for recurrent acute otitis media. Ann. Otol. Rhinol. Laryngol. *155*:33–36, 1992.
96. Pegelow, C. H., Armstrong, F. D., Light, S., et al.: Experience with the use of prophylactic penicillin in children with sickle cell anemia. J. Pediatr. *118*:736–738, 1991.
97. Pichichero, M. E., Gooch, W. M., Rodriguez, W., et al.: Effective short-course treatment of acute group A beta-hemolytic streptococcal tonsillopharyngitis: Ten days of penicillin V vs. 5 days or 10 days of cefpodoxime therapy in children. Arch. Pediatr. Adolesc. Med. *148*:1053–1060, 1994.
98. Pichichero, M. E., and Margolis, P. A.: A comparison of cephalosporins and penicillin in the treatment of group A streptococcal pharyngitis: A meta-analysis supporting the concept of microbial copathogenicity. Pediatr. Infect. Dis. J. *10*:275–281, 1991.
99. Platt, R.: Methodologic aspects of clinical studies of perioperative antibiotic prophylaxis. Rev. Infect. Dis. *13*(Suppl.):810–814, 1991.
100. Pons, V. G., Denlinger, S. L., Guglielmo, B. J., et al.: Ceftizoxime versus vancomycin and gentamicin in neurosurgical prophylaxis: A randomized, prospective, blinded clinical study. Neurosurgery *33*:416–423, 1993.
101. Principi, N., Marchisio, P., Massironi, E., et al.: Prophylaxis of recurrent acute otitis media and middle-ear effusion. Am. J. Dis. Child. *143*:1414–1418, 1989.
102. Pylipow, M., Gaddis, M., and Kinney, J. S.: Selective intrapartum prophylaxis for group B *Streptococcus* colonization: Management and outcome of newborns. Pediatrics *93*:631–635, 1994.
103. Schoenbaum, S. C., Gardner, P., and Shillito, J.: Infections of cerebrospinal fluid shunts: Epidemiology, clinical manifestations, and therapy. J. Infect. Dis. *131*:543–551, 1975.
104. Schuchat, A., Oxtoby, M., Cochi, S., et al.: Population-based risk factors for neonatal group B streptococcal disease: Results of a cohort study in metropolitan Atlanta. J. Infect. Dis. *162*:672–677, 1990.
105. Schwartz, B., Al-Ttobaiqi, A., and Al-Ruwais, A.: Comparative efficacy of ceftriaxone and rifampicin in eradicating pharyngeal carriage of group A *Neisseria meningitidis*. Lancet *1*:1239–1242, 1988.
106. Schweich, P., and Fleisher, G.: Human bites in children. Pediatr. Emerg. Care *1*:51–53, 1985.
107. Seppala, H., Nissinen, A., Jarvinen, H., et al.: Resistance to erythromycin in group A streptococci. N. Engl. J. Med. *326*:292–297, 1992.
108. Shapiro, E. D.: Infections of the urinary tract. Pediatr. Infect. Dis. J. *11*:165–168, 1992.
109. Shapiro, M.: Prophylaxis in otolaryngologic surgery and neurosurgery: A critical review. Rev. Infect. Dis. *13*(Suppl. 10):858–868, 1991.
110. Shortliffe, L. M. D.: The management of urinary tract infections in children without urinary tract abnormalities. Urol. Clin. North Am. *22*:67–73, 1995.
111. Siddins, M., Downie, J., and Wise, K.: Prophylaxis against postsplenectomy pneumococcal infection. Aust. N. Z. J. Surg. *60*:183–187, 1990.
112. Skurka, J., Willert, C., and Yogev, R.: Wound infection following dog bite despite prophylactic penicillin. Infection *14*:134–135, 1986.
113. Smellie, J. M., and Normand, I. C. S.: Urinary infections in children, 1985. Postgrad. Med. J. *61*:895–905, 1985.
114. Snellman, L. W., Stang, H. J., Stang, J. M., et al.: Duration of positive throat cultures for group A streptococci after initiation of antibiotic therapy. Pediatrics *91*:1166–1170, 1993.
115. Spafford, P. S., Sinkin, R. A., Cox, C., et al.: Prevention of central venous catheter–related coagulase-negative staphylococcal sepsis in neonates. J. Pediatr. *125*:259–263, 1994.
116. Stamay, T. A., Condy, M., and Mibara, G.: Prophylactic efficacy of nitrofurantoin macrocrystals and trimethoprim-sulfamethoxazole in urinary infections: Biologic effect on the vaginal and rectal flora. N. Engl. J. Med. *296*:780–783, 1977.
117. Still, J. G.: Management of pediatric patients with group A beta-hemolytic *Streptococcus pharyngitis*: Treatment options. Pediatr. Infect. Dis. J. *14*(Suppl.):57–61, 1995.
118. Terezhalmy, G. T., and Hall, E. H.: The asplenic patient: A consideration for antimicrobial prophylaxis. Oral Surg. *57*:114–117, 1984.
119. U.S. Public Health Service: Annual Summary 1976. Publication No. CDC 77-8241. M. M. W. R. Morb. Mortal. Wkly. Rep. 25:43, 1977.
120. Waldvogel, F. A., Vaudaux, P. E., Pittet, D., et al.: Session I. Theoretical and preclinical experimental bases of prophylaxis: Perioperative antibiotic prophylaxis of wound and foreign body infections: Microbial factors affecting efficacy. Rev. Infect. Dis. *13*(Suppl.):782–789, 1991.
121. Wong, W. Y., Overturf, G. D., and Powars, D. R.: Infection caused by *Streptococcus pneumoniae* in children with sickle cell disease: Epidemiology, immunologic mechanisms, prophylaxis, and vaccination. Clin. Infect. Dis. *14*:1124–1136, 1992.
122. Young, R. F., and Lawner, P. M.: Perioperative antibiotic prophylaxis for prevention of postoperative neurosurgical infections: A randomized clinical trial. J. Neurosurg. *66*:701–705, 1987.
123. Zanoni, D., Isenberg, S., and Apt, L.: A comparison of silver nitrate with erythromycin for prophylaxis against ophthalmia neonatorum. Clin. Pediatr. (Phila.) *31*:295–298, 1992.
124. Zarkowsky, H. S., Gallagher, D., Gill, F. M., et al.: Bacteremia in sickle hemoglobinopathies. J. Pediatr. *109*:579–585, 1986.
125. Zarrabi, M. H., and Rosner, F.: Serious infections in adults following splenectomy for trauma. Arch. Intern. Med. *144*:1421–1424, 1984.
126. Zelikovic, I., Adelman, R. D., and Nancarrow, P. A.: Urinary tract infections in children: An update. West. J. Med. *157*:554–561, 1992.
127. Zubowicz, V. N., and Gravier, M.: Management of early human bites of the hand: A prospective randomized study. Plast. Reconstr. Surg. *88*:111–114, 1991.

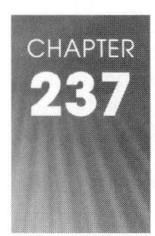

CHAPTER 237

Outpatient Intravenous Antibiotic Therapy for Serious Infections

JOHN S. BRADLEY

Community outpatient parenteral anti-infective therapy (CoPAT) is the means by which children can receive the benefits of parenteral (intravenous or intramuscular) therapy in an outpatient setting, usually the home, without requiring hospitalization. The widespread acceptance of CoPAT by physicians, families, and insurers has led to a tremendous increase in the outpatient treatment of serious infectious diseases.[18, 20, 32] The standard of care provided to children through CoPAT should equal or surpass that provided to hospitalized children. National guidelines for CoPAT in adults and children, published by the Infectious Diseases Society of America in 1997 and 2003, define the potential benefits and risks.[42, 49] This chapter explains the basic concepts behind CoPAT for children. The CoPAT team, which includes the physician, CoPAT coordinator, nurse, pharmacist, parent or caregiver, and third-party payer, needs to work together to ensure a successful outcome for the child.

Evaluating a Child and Parents for CoPAT

Broad criteria are used to determine the medical feasibility of CoPAT (Table 237–1). The most important aspect in the assessment of a newborn, infant, or child for CoPAT is a determination that ongoing parenteral therapy is required to appropriately treat the infection and that skilled nursing observation and care are not necessary for the infection being treated. Complications of the infection in the child should be considered to be highly unlikely so that unskilled observations by the parents or caregivers will be adequate for care. No additional significant risk should be placed on the child's recovery by enrollment in a CoPAT program. If feasible, oral antibiotic therapy should be used instead of parenteral therapy.

A child usually is placed on a CoPAT regimen from either a hospital setting with previous intravenous therapy or an outpatient setting such as a clinic or emergency department. For a child being discharged from the hospital, an unequivocal response to parenteral anti-infective therapy should be demonstrated. Most often, appropriate cultures will have directed anti-infective therapy. For children with no positive cultures, the signs and symptoms of the infection should be resolving with empiric therapy, as demonstrated by decreasing fever and improving function. No need should be anticipated for any further surgical or medical interventions, further laboratory tests, or imaging procedures that are important for bringing the infection under control. The child should have no need for 24-hour skilled pediatric nursing observation or care.

From the outpatient setting, the child's condition should not be so severe that inpatient care is required. The child's infection should be judged by the clinician to be unlikely to progress and result in complications. Because the child's clinical course during therapy will need to be monitored to be certain that the anticipated response occurs, an outpatient visit the following day usually is made.

Before enrolling a child in CoPAT, an assessment of the parents or caregivers also is required (see Table 237–1). Because the parents are responsible for the nursing care of their child in the home, they must be willing and capable participants. Although most parents are very interested and highly motivated to return home with their child, not all are willing or capable of performing the necessary and required nursing functions. Most parents are capable of limited medical assessment of their children, but some are not. In addition, the home environment should have the resources for the proposed medical care. For example, intravenous therapy administered to a child through a tunneled, central catheter requires a sterile environment to be present for anti-infective infusions and dressing changes. Less stringent criteria for the home would apply for a child receiving daily intramuscular injections in an outpatient clinic. Communication between the parents and medical personnel is essential. For parents or caregivers, telephone access to nurses and clinicians is critical. In addition, the parents should be able to bring their child back to the hospital or clinic for re-evaluation if complications arise from either the infection or therapy, which requires having adequate transportation to a medical facility. Families with no car or access to transportation, families who live in rural areas far from a medical facility, and hostile environmental/weather conditions that prevent transportation all should be considered before

TABLE 237–1 ■ MEDICAL AND SOCIAL CRITERIA FOR CoPAT

Medical Criteria for CoPAT
Medical diagnosis of infection with a suspected or documented pathogen
Clinical response to anti-infective therapy (if therapy is started in the hospital)
No assessed need for urgent medical, surgical, or laboratory interventions to achieve a clinical response to anti-infective therapy
No significant risk of complications of the infection
No assessed need for skilled nursing care
Social Criteria for CoPAT
Parents interested and motivated
Parents capable of assessing the child for complications of infection and therapy
24-hr telephone access to the CoPAT team
Transportation for urgent return to the clinic or hospital, if needed
Home environment acceptable and resources available
Parents documented to be capable, before CoPAT begins, of administering anti-infective agents if required

CoPAT, community outpatient parenteral anti-infective therapy.

starting CoPAT. In addition to teaching the parents to observe their child and communicate information to medical providers, some parents may be asked to infuse anti-infective agents into their children. Doing so requires an additional level of skill in the parent or caregiver and further assessment of parental competence by the CoPAT nursing and medical personnel.

The CoPAT Program

The roles of physicians, CoPAT coordinators, nurses, pharmacists, and parents/patients have been defined previously[42, 49] (Table 237–2). Once the clinician believes that the child's condition is sufficiently stable (either to be discharged from a hospital ward or to pursue outpatient therapy from a clinic or emergency department setting), the coordinator of the outpatient treatment program is notified. This person is capable of assessing the feasibility of CoPAT for that particular child. The CoPAT coordinator interviews parents and medical staff to determine the parents' willingness and their abilities and to assess the home environment. After the clinician prescribes the anti-infective agents, required nursing visits, ongoing laboratory and imaging tests, and follow-up clinic visits, the CoPAT coordinator puts together the resources required for successful therapy. With knowledge of the parents' abilities and resources, the medication and equipment requirements, and the home nursing visits required, the coordinator makes the final determination regarding the feasibility of the program. The coordinator also determines whether the costs of CoPAT are to be borne by the parents or a third-party payer and obtains authorization from the third-party payer if required before CoPAT can begin. An example of a CoPAT physician's order form that includes catheter management and medication orders, laboratory and imaging test orders, and clinic visits is reproduced in Figure 237–1. The coordinator of the CoPAT program, whether clinic or hospital based, should ensure that open lines of communication exist among the clinician, the home visiting nurse, the pharmacist, and the parents. A defined, written plan for medical and nursing care should be established. All members of the CoPAT team should be aware of their responsibilities before initiating outpatient therapy.

The frequency of the home pediatric nursing visits required needs to be individualized for each child and depends on many factors: the clinical course while receiving therapy, the seriousness of the infection, the ability of parents to effectively examine the child, and anticipated complications with therapy that can be related to either anti-infective agents or the infection. For most children, the frequency of home nursing visits will be greatest at the beginning of CoPAT, often once daily. After treatment at home has been delivered as anticipated and recovery from infection is proceeding as expected, visits may be decreased to two or three times each week, particularly if the parents have demonstrated competency in providing nursing care, managing the catheter, and providing clinical assessment. The home visiting nurse also will have the opportunity to evaluate the parents' ability to administer anti-infective agents in the home. Physical assessment of neonates may be particularly difficult, and daily visits through the entire course of therapy by pediatric home visiting nurses are usually important. Daily visits are also important for children with less stable infections, such as central nervous system infections, because subtleties in the neurologic examination not appreciated by parents or caregivers may provide clues to impending problems. Nursing aspects of pediatric CoPAT have been outlined by successful programs.[21, 27, 39]

Pediatric competency in nursing is not standardized. Each state government licenses nurses based on criteria specific for that state. However, just as for inpatient pediatric care, pediatric experience is an important qualification for the home visiting nurse. Because no licensing requirements include the stipulation that home nursing agencies providing care to children have expertise in pediatric nursing, considerable discrepancies exist in pediatric competency among nursing agencies. Given the importance of pediatric expertise in evaluation and management, the home nursing agency contracted to provide care is expected to have personnel with the experience and training necessary and equivalent to those of nurses providing care in a pediatric inpatient setting. The home nursing agency providing care should be able to provide to the clinician and CoPAT coordinator reasonable assurance of proficiency in dealing with newborns, infants, and children.

In many states, only licensed nurses (RN, LVN) may infuse anti-infective agents. However, most states have no legislation prohibiting parents from administering drugs.

TABLE 237–2 ■ ROLES OF PHYSICIAN, CoPAT COORDINATOR, NURSE, PHARMACIST, AND PARENT

Role	Physician*	CoPAT Coordinator*	Pediatric Nurse*	Pediatric Pharmacist*	Parent or Patient
Assess medical stability for home therapy	+	+	–	–	–
Assess family for capability for CoPAT	+	+	+	–	–
Create and implement CoPAT treatment plan	+	+	+	+	–
Order nursing visits	+	–	–	–	–
Order clinic visits, laboratory tests, imaging examinations	+	–	–	–	–
Educate parents regarding infection and complications	+	+	+	–	–
Educate parents regarding therapy and complications	+	+	+	+	–
Manage treatment	+	+	+	–	+
Monitor IV catheter status	+	–	+	–	+
Monitor clinical status	+	–	+	–	+
Monitor anti-infective therapy	+	–	+	+	+
Prepare anti-infective therapy	–	–	+	+	+
Availability for complications	+	–	+	+	+
Outcome assessment	+	+	+	+	+

*Certification or experience in pediatrics.
CoPAT, community outpatient parenteral anti-infective therapy.

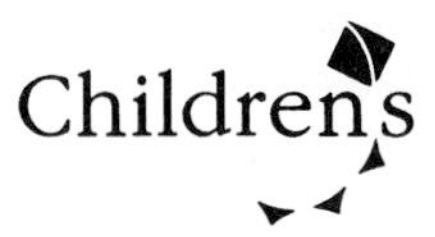

Children's Hospital - San Diego
3020 Children's Way
San Diego, California 92123-4282

Home Care Order Sheet for Infectious Diseases

Patient: ______________________

MR# ______________________

Account # ______________________

1. DISCHARGE DIAGNOSIS

2. NURSING REQUIREMENTS

a. Frequency of visits:

b. Complications to watch for (include with assessment at each visit):

c. Other nursing requirements

3. MEDICATIONS/ANTIBIOTICS (type, dose, dosing interval, duration):

a.

b.

c.

d. NS FLUSH ______ cc q ______ hrs e. Heparin flush ______ u/cc ______ cc ______ q hrs

4. LABORATORY TESTING:

☐ Via Venipuncture or ☐ Venous Access Device ☐ Other

a. Antibiotic levels

b. CBC

c. ESR, CRP

d. Chem 20

e. Cultures

5. OUTPATIENT VISITS (frequency while on therapy):

a. Infectious Disease Clinic (specify attending physician)

b. Other specialists

c. Primary care physician

6. OTHER TESTS TO BE SCHEDULED (imaging, etc.):

7. DC IV AND DC FROM HOMECARE WHEN THERAPY COMPLETE:

☐ YES ☐ RE-EVAL

8. ATTENDING PHYSICIAN

Dr. NOTIFIED OF PLAN BY

Signature ______________________ Date ______________

NON STOCK / RBF 1898 (06/96) ORIGINAL - Chart CANARY - Home Care Agency PINK - Infectious Diseases GOLD - Primary Care Physician

FIGURE 237–1 ■ An example of a physician's order sheet for outpatient intravenous antibiotic therapy for serious infections (CoPAT) (Children's Hospital and Health Center, San Diego, California).

Accordingly, parents are expected to infuse medications to their children if licensed nurses are not deemed by the home care agency to be necessary or are not available to provide these services. The physician should be aware of the qualifications of the personnel responsible for the intravenous infusion of anti-infective agents.

The home visiting nurse should communicate with the physician regarding the status of the child as determined by the physician before starting CoPAT. Analogous to inpatient care, the nurses and physicians are expected to be on call 24 hours each day.

Similarly, the pharmacist providing anti-infective therapy for CoPAT should be familiar with the dosages and side effects of therapy provided to all pediatric age groups, from newborns to adolescents. Dosing errors in infants and children are not uncommon given the broad range of doses prescribed and administered.[24]

The parents should have written instructions for the tasks that they are required to perform in the home, including information on sterile technique, administration of antibiotics, flushing of catheters, and dressing changes. Their proficiency in management of the catheter and infusion of anti-infective agents should be demonstrated before discharging the child from the hospital, emergency department, or clinic. Telephone numbers should be provided for the 24-hour on-call nursing and physician personnel. A list of complications of the medications and procedures and information on clinical assessment of the child's infection should be provided, along with a set of parameters requiring immediate notification of medical personnel. Plans for disposal of needles, dressings, and other medical waste also should be made before sending the child home.

Visits to clinicians (primary care providers, surgeons, subspecialists) are scheduled as necessary according to the clinical status of the child and the degree of expertise required by the examiner. If the child is stable in an outpatient setting, once-weekly visits to a physician are usually sufficient unless the home visiting nurse or parent observes problems requiring more immediate attention. For any high-risk, unstable child, daily physician visits are important, particularly if skilled pediatric home nursing is not available.

Although abuse of intravenous access seldom occurs, for an adolescent who may have a history of alcohol or drug dependence, the clinician should be particularly cautious in approving CoPAT. For younger children with indwelling catheters, Munchausen syndrome by proxy may be a concern for those who do not recover as anticipated.

TABLE 237–3 ■ INFECTIONS TREATED WITH CoPAT

Infection Treated	Reference	Design*
Collections of various infections	4, 6, 7, 14, 39	III
Appendicitis	3, 12, 37, 45	II
Catheter infection	25	III
Chronic suppurative otitis media	10	II
Cystic fibrosis	50	I
	8	II
	13, 19, 23, 27, 35, 38	III
Fever in immunocompromised children	28, 33, 47	I
	9, 36	II
	21, 46	III
Meningitis	1, 2, 11	III
Mastoiditis	31	II
Neonatal infections	43	II
	5, 11	III
UTI	30	III
Peritonitis, peritoneal catheter related	26	III

*I, randomized, prospective, comparative trial; II, prospective evaluation; III, retrospectively reviewed clinical experience.
CoPAT, community outpatient parenteral anti-infective therapy; UTI, urinary tract infection.

Infections Suitable for CoPAT

Virtually any infection can be treated by CoPAT at some point in the course of therapy by following the aforementioned guidelines (Table 237–1). For each child, a thorough assessment of the risks of complications for the infection must be made before outpatient therapy is considered. A partial list of infections treated with CoPAT is given in Table 237–3; most of the studies are not prospective, randomized investigations comparing children receiving all of their therapy in the hospital with those who receive at least a portion out of the hospital. The variety of infections that may be treated with CoPAT at some point include bloodstream infections such as bacteremia, catheter sepsis, and endocarditis; central nervous system infections, including meningitis and brain abscess; osteomyelitis and septic arthritis; urinary tract infections; upper respiratory tract infections, including severe acute otitis media, chronic suppurative otitis, and mastoiditis; lower respiratory tract infections; fever with or without neutropenia in low-risk immunocompromised children; neonatal bacterial sepsis; intra-abdominal infections; and postoperative wound infections.

Delivery of Anti-infective Therapy

SELECTION OF AN ANTI-INFECTIVE AGENT. Selection of anti-infective therapy for CoPAT is similar to selection of therapy for any child in that the primary goal is to achieve clinical and microbiologic cure with the most efficacious, least toxic, and most cost-effective agents. Selecting an agent that may not be effective simply because it is more convenient and less expensive to administer is not appropriate. However, of the agents that demonstrate equivalent activity against the child's pathogen, the preferred agent is the one that is given least frequently, is nontoxic, and requires the least frequent monitoring. Preferred agents for the most common community-acquired pathogens are given in Table 237–4. Almost any pathogen, community acquired or nosocomial, bacterial, fungal, or viral, can be treated in the home if the medical and social criteria for CoPAT can be met.

In general, β-lactam agents (penicillins, cephalosporins, carbapenems) require less frequent monitoring than do aminoglycosides (gentamicin, tobramycin, amikacin) or glycopeptides (vancomycin or teicoplanin). Agents that can be given intravenously over a short period (less than 15 minutes), such as β-lactam agents, are preferred to those that require up to an hour with each infusion (aminoglycosides and glycopeptides). Agents that can be given intramuscularly if intravenous access is temporarily lost are preferred to those that may be given only intravenously. Not only are these parameters designed to provide the optimal clinical outcome with minimal toxicity, they also are designed to facilitate therapy in the home. Dosing more frequently than every 8 hours poses a formidable challenge to many families, particularly those without extensive support. These parameters maximize the potential for parents to provide care at home with minimal risk. Although more frequent nursing visits may provide relief to parents, the charges for home nursing visits to administer therapy and provide nursing

TABLE 237–4 ■ SELECTION OF ANTI-INFECTIVE AGENTS FOR COMMON PATHOGENS IN COMMUNITY-ACQUIRED INFECTIONS

Pathogen	Anti-infective Agent	Dosing Frequency (hr)	Toxicity
Gram-Positive Bacteria			
Streptococcus pneumoniae	Penicillin G*	6	
	Ampicillin*	6–8	
	Cefuroxime*	8	
	Cefotaxime*	6–8	
	Ceftriaxone*†	24	
	Vancomycin (for penicillin and cephalosporin nonsusceptible strains)‡	8–12	Renal toxicity, ototoxicity
Staphylococcus aureus	Oxacillin*	6–8	
	Cefazolin†	8–12	
	Clindamycin*	8	Colitis
	Vancomycin‡	8–12	Renal toxicity, ototoxicity
Streptoccocus pyogenes	See *S. pneumoniae*		
Enterococcus	Ampicillin plus gentamicin*†	Ampicillin: 6–8 Gentamicin: 8	Renal toxicity, ototoxicity (gentamicin)
	Vancomycin plus gentamicin*‡	Vancomycin: 8–12 Gentamicin: 8	Renal toxicity ototoxicity (both gentamicin and vancomycin
Gram-Negative Bacteria			
Haemophilus influenzae	Ampicillin*	6–8	
	Cefuroxime	8	
	Cefotaxime	8	
	Ceftriaxone†	24	
Escherichia coli	Ceftriaxone†	24	
	Ampicillin*	6–8	
	Cefotaxime‡	6–8	
	Gentamicin‡ or tobramycin	8–24	Renal: toxicity, ototoxicity
	Amikacin‡	12–24	Renal: toxicity, ototoxicity
Enterobacter, Serratia, Citrobacter (pathogens with inducible AmpC beta-lactamases)	Cefepime†	8–12	
	Meropenem†	8	
	Imipenem/cilastatin	6–8	
	Cefotaxime* or ceftriaxone plus an aminoglycoside‡ (gentamicin, tobramycin, amikacin)	Cefotaxime: 6–8 Ceftriaxone: 24 Gentamicin and tobramycin: 8–24 Amikacin: 24	Renal toxicity, ototoxicity (aminoglycoside)
Pseudomonas aeruginosa	Meropenem†	8	
	Cefepime	8	
	Ceftazidime* plus an aminoglycoside‡	Ceftazidime: 8 Aminoglycoside: see above	Renal toxicity, ototoxicity (aminoglycoside)
	Imipenem-cilastatin	6–8	CNS irritability in children with underlying CNS inflammation
	Ticarcillin-clavulanate* plus an aminoglycoside‡	T-C:6 Aminoglycoside: see above	Renal toxicity, ototoxicity (aminoglycoside)
	Piperacillin-tazobactam* plus an aminoglycoside‡	P-T: 6 Aminoglycoside: see above	Renal: toxicity, (aminoglycoside)
	Ciprofloxacin§	8–12	Possible arthropathy
Neisseria meningitidis	Ceftriaxone†	24	
	Penicillin G	6	
Fungal Pathogens			
Candida	Fluconazole IV†	24	
	Amphotericin B (lipid preparations are better tolerated)	24, or every other day; may return to infusion center for each injection to manage side effects	Fever, chills, anemia, hyponatremia, decreased glomerular function
Viral Pathogens			
Herpes simplex virus	Acyclovir	8	Neutropenia, renal toxicity
Cytomegalovirus	Ganciclovir	12–24	Neutropenia

*If organisms are documented to be susceptible.
†Preferred agents based on dosing frequency and side effects.
‡Requires monitoring of renal function and serum concentrations.
§Not indicated for therapy unless no other therapy options exist.

care (e.g., wound dressing changes) are substantial; the charges for three nursing visits each day approaches the cost of a day in the hospital for a stable child.

Depending on the agent used, monitoring in the outpatient setting should occur with the same frequency as that for the inpatient setting. Monitoring of renal function and serum antibiotic concentrations is important for children being treated with aminoglycosides or vancomycin. For children receiving long-term β-lactam therapy, periodic monitoring of the peripheral white blood count and renal and hepatic function every 2 to 4 weeks may detect the uncommon antibiotic-mediated toxicities of this class of antibiotics before the occurrence of clinical manifestations. The vast majority of abnormalities induced by β-lactam drugs are completely reversible.

DELIVERY OF ANTI-INFECTIVE AGENTS. CoPAT can be delivered by intramuscular or intravenous injection. In general, the need for more than two or three injections necessitates intravenous therapy, although intramuscular therapy lasting 1 week or longer has not been associated with short-term complications in anecdotal reports.[5, 6] The short polyethylene catheters normally used for inpatient intravenous therapy may be used for short-term therapy lasting less than 5 to 7 days. Occasionally, intravenous access will be lost and the child will need to be re-evaluated for replacement of the catheter; if clinical improvement exceeds expectations, an early switch to oral therapy may be possible. If not, intravenous access may need to be re-established. It may be performed in the home but more often will require the child and parent to return to the clinic or hospital. An intramuscular injection or injections may be given temporarily in the home until the intravenous catheter can be replaced.

For therapy lasting longer than 5 to 7 days, central catheters are preferred. Peripherally inserted Silastic central catheters are practical and cost-effective and have become the intravenous access of choice for extended therapy.[40] These catheters may be inserted through many different peripheral sites (usually the antecubital vein) by physicians or nurses with training in the placement of central catheters. Sedation usually is required for younger infants and children. Alternatively, more traditional subcutaneously tunneled central catheters with multiple ports (e.g., Hickman, Groshong) may be placed by a surgeon in the operating room with the child under general anesthesia. These catheters are preferred for children requiring several weeks of therapy with agents that call for periodic monitoring of organ function and serum antibiotic concentrations. Tunneled central catheters are more suited for frequent blood sampling because of the larger catheter lumen size. Each type of central catheter requires sterile technique for accessing the catheter and close monitoring of the catheter exit site during therapy. The home visiting nurse agency should have written protocols for the care and use of central catheters that are consistent with standards set by the Joint Commission on Accreditation of Healthcare Organizations (JCAHO) for inpatients and for use by home visiting nurses and parents.

Anti-infective agents may be infused directly into the catheter by the caregiver by way of a syringe attached to the catheter hub ("IV push"), followed by flushing the catheter with saline or a heparin-containing solution. Alternatively, particularly for agents that cannot be infused quickly, an intravenous drip system must be used, or the agent must be infused by a pump. Pumps come in three basic designs: those with no electronic or moving parts; syringe pumps in which the syringe containing the anti-infective agent is placed in a motorized pump designed to administer the dose over a certain period; and electronic programmable pumps, which may have a variety of pump mechanisms and are computer chip driven to control infusions of one or more agents administered over different periods.

The least expensive pumps are those with no moving parts in which the agent is placed either into a thick elastomeric "balloon" that propels the agent through an infusion rate–limiting valve into the child, or into a bag that is then placed into a device in which spring-loaded plates press on the anti-infective agent contained in the bag, again pushing the agent into the child through an infusion rate–limiting valve. These pumps are generally disposable and are adequate for treatment with a single agent administered a few times each day.

New tools for CoPAT are becoming available each year. Resource guides to the equipment used for CoPAT are available in handbooks[41] and on the Internet.[52] Most of the equipment and resources available are designed for adults.

Outcome Analysis

The anticipated outcome in the treatment of an infection is clinical and microbiologic cure with no complications of therapy. Although the psychosocial benefits of CoPAT for children from a secure home environment were the original impetus for pediatric programs, the economic benefits of outpatient therapy have been easier to document for both adults and children.[3, 16, 17, 23, 29, 44, 48, 50, 51] The cost of treatment is substantially less for outpatient therapy when neither hospital facilities nor 24-hour skilled nursing care is necessary. With shorter hospitalizations, the risk of acquiring a nosocomial viral or bacterial infection should diminish and further decrease the overall cost of care to the health care system.

However, complications may occur in children receiving CoPAT, just as they occur in inpatients.[15] The infection being treated may not be under control or may relapse while being monitored by parents or home nursing personnel. Errors in antibiotic dosing and administration may occur,[24] particularly if parents are given the responsibility for preparing and administering antibiotics in the home. Complications of anti-infective therapy may increase when the number of doses administered to a child increases as multiple anti-infective agents and frequent dosing of certain agents are required. Catheter- and pump-related complications may arise during therapy.[34] Parents may not be compliant with clinic visits and may not be in the home when the home nursing agency has scheduled a visit. Family members other than those trained to care for the child may provide care without the knowledge of the home nursing agency or physician. The clinician may rehospitalize the child if doing so is required to complete parenteral therapy safely.

JCAHO now reviews home care outcomes by evaluating specified parameters,[22] including unscheduled inpatient admissions, early discontinuation of parenteral therapy, interruptions in parenteral therapy, catheter-related infections, and adverse drug reactions. Until recently, data on outcomes from various home nursing agencies were not made available to contracting physicians, hospitals, or payers. Outcome data now are required to be collected by home health organizations, which eventually will help standardize the assessment of CoPAT programs. The physician or CoPAT coordinator should request outcomes data from any home nursing agency proposing to care for a child who requires CoPAT.

Summary

Successful CoPAT requires integrated delivery of care for children who are assessed to be at low risk for complications from their infections and therapy. Parents fulfill the role of the skilled pediatric nurse in the hospital and should be capable of providing a focused, limited assessment of their child and communicating any changes in the child's medical condition to the appropriate medical personnel. The anti-infective agents, infusion equipment, and medical follow-up all should be designed for the outpatient setting compatible with the training and resources available to parents or caregivers in the home. Outcomes of pediatric CoPAT should be equivalent to or better than those achieved in an inpatient setting.

REFERENCES

1. Al-Howasi, M.: The use of a modified out-patient infusion therapy for lowering the cost in Suleimania Children's Hospital. J. Kuwait Med. Assoc. *28*:455–457, 1996.
2. Arditi, M., and Yogev, R.: Convalescent outpatient therapy for selected children with acute bacterial meningitis. Semin. Pediatr. Infect. Dis. *1*:404–410, 1990.
3. Bradley, J. S., Behrendt, C. E., Arrieta, A. C., et al.: Convalescent phase outpatient parenteral antiinfective therapy for children with complicated appendicitis. Pediatr. Infect. Dis. J. *20*:19–24, 2001.
4. Bradley, J. S., Ching, D. K., and Phillips, S. E.: Outpatient therapy of serious pediatric infections with ceftriaxone. Pediatr. Infect. Dis. *7*:160–164, 1988.
5. Bradley, J. S., Ching, D. L., Wilson, T. A., and Compogiannis, L. S.: Once-daily ceftriaxone to complete therapy of uncomplicated group B streptococcal infection in neonates. A preliminary report. Clin. Pediatr. (Phila.) *31*:274–278, 1992.
6. Bradley, J. S., Farhat, C., Stamboulian, D., et al.: Ceftriaxone therapy of bacterial meningitis: Cerebrospinal fluid concentrations and bactericidal activity after intramuscular injection in children treated with dexamethasone. Pediatr. Infect. Dis. J. *13*:724–728, 1994.
7. Dagan, R., Philip, M., Watemberg, N. M., et al.: Outpatient treatment of serious outpatient community-acquired pediatric infections using once-daily intramuscular ceftriaxone. Pediatr. Infect. Dis. J. *12*:1080–1084, 1987.
8. Donati, M. A., Guenette, G., and Auerbach, H.: Prospective controlled study of home and hospital therapy of cystic fibrosis. J. Pediatr. *111*:28–33, 1987.
9. Egerer, G., Goldschmidt, H., Muller, I., et al.: Ceftriaxone for the treatment of febrile episodes in nonneutropenic patients with hematooncological disease or HIV infection: Comparison of outpatient and inpatient care. Chemotherapy *47*:219–225, 2001.
10. Esposito, S., Noviello, S., Ianniello, F., et al: Ceftazidime for outpatient parenteral antibiotic therapy (OPAT) of chronic suppurative otitis media due to *Pseudomonas aeruginosa*. J. Chemother. *12*:88–93, 2000.
11. Ferris, E. W.: A neonatal home intravenous antibiotic therapy program. J. Intraven. Nurs. *13*:383–387, 1991.
12. Fishman, S. J., Pelosi, L., Klavon, S. L., et al: Perforated appendicitis: Prospective outcome analysis for 150 children. J. Pediatr. Surg. *35*:923–926, 2000.
13. Gilbert, J., Robinson, T., and Littlewood, J. M.: Home intravenous antibiotic treatment in cystic fibrosis. Arch. Dis. Child. *63*:512–517, 1988.
14. Goldenberg, R. I., Poretz, D. M., Eron, L. J., et al.: Intravenous antibiotic therapy in ambulatory pediatric patients. Pediatr. Infect. Dis. *3*:514–517, 1984.
15. Gomez, M., Maraqa, N., Alvarez, A., and Rathore, M.: Complications of outpatient parenteral antibiotic therapy in childhood. Pediatr. Infect. Dis. J. *20*:541–543, 2001.
16. Grainger-Rousseau, T. J., and Segal, R.: Economic, clinical and psychosocial outcomes of home infusion therapy: A review of published studies. Pharm. Pract. Manage. Q. *15*:57–77, 1995.
17. Grizzard, M. B., Harris, G., and Karns, H.: Use of outpatient parenteral antibiotic therapy in a health maintenance organization. Rev. Infect. Dis. *13*(Suppl.):174–179, 1991.
18. Gutierrez, K.: Continuation of antibiotic therapy for serious bacterial infections outside of the hospital. Pediatr. Ann. *25*:639–645, 1996.
19. Hammond, L. J., Caldwell, S., and Campbell, P. W.: Cystic fibrosis, intravenous antibiotics, and home therapy. J. Pediatr. Health Care *5*:24–30, 1991.
20. Harris, J. A.: Antimicrobial therapy of pneumonia in infants and children. Semin. Respir. Infect. *11*:139–147, 1996.
21. Hooker, L., and Kohler, J.: Safety, efficacy, and acceptability of home intravenous therapy administered by parents of pediatric oncology patients. Med. Pediatr. Oncol. *32*:421–426, 1999.
22. Joint Commission on Accreditation of Healthcare Organizations: Accreditation Manual for Home Care. Oak Brook Terrace, IL, JCAHO, 1995.
23. Kane, R. E., Jennison, K., Wood, C., et al.: Cost savings and economic considerations using home intravenous antibiotic therapy for cystic fibrosis patients. Pediatr. Pulmonol. *4*:84–89, 1988.
24. Kaushal, R., Bates, D. W., Landrigan, C., et al.: Medication errors and adverse drug events in pediatric inpatients. J. A. M. A. *285*:2114–2120, 2001.
25. Kinsey, S. E.: Experience with teicoplanin in non-inpatient therapy in children with central line infections. Eur. J. Haematol. Suppl. *62*:11–14, 1998.
26. Kuizon, B., Melocoton, T. L., Holloway, M., et al.: Infectious and catheter-related complications in pediatric patients treated with peritoneal dialysis at a single institution. Pediatr. Nephrol. *9*(Suppl.):12–17, 1995.
27. Leaver, J., Radivan, F., Patel, L., et al.: Home intravenous antibiotic therapy: Practical aspects in children. J. R. Soc. Med. *90*:26–33, 1997.
28. Mullen, C. A., Petropoulos, D., Roberts, W. M., et al.: Outpatient treatment of fever and neutropenia for low risk pediatric cancer patients. Cancer *86*:126–134, 1999.
29. Mullen, C. A., Petropoulos, D., Roberts, W. M., et al.: Economic and resource utilization analysis of outpatient management of fever and neutropenia in low-risk pediatric patients with cancer. J. Pediatr. Hematol. Oncol. *21*:212–218, 1999.
30. Nelson, D. S., Gurr, M. B., Schunk, J. E.: Management of febrile children with urinary tract infections. Am. J. Emerg. Med. *16*:643–647, 1998.
31. Niv, A., Nash, M., Peiser, J., et al.: Outpatient management of acute mastoiditis with periosteitis in children. Int. J. Pediatr. Otorhinolaryngol. *46*:9–13, 1998.
32. Patrick, C. C., and Shenep, J. L.: Outpatient management of the febrile neutropenic child with cancer. Adv. Pediatr. Infect. Dis. *14*:29–47, 1999.
33. Petrilli, A. S., Dantas, L. S., Campos, M. C., et al.: Oral ciprofloxacin vs. intravenous ceftriaxone administered in a outpatient setting for fever and neutropenia in low-risk pediatric oncology patients: Randomized prospective trial. Med. Pediatr. Oncol. *34*:87–91, 2000.
34. Porea, T. J., Margolin, J. F., and Chintagumpala, M. M.: Radiological case of the month: Pulmonary air embolus with home antibiotic infusion. Arch. Pediatr. Adolesc. Med. *155*:963–964, 2001.
35. Rucker, R. W., and Harrison, G. M.: Outpatient intravenous medications in the management of cystic fibrosis. Pediatrics *54*:358–360, 1974.
36. Shemesh, E., Yaniv, I., Drucker, M., et al.: Home intravenous antibiotic treatment for febrile episodes in immune-compromised pediatric patients. Med. Pediatr. Oncol. *30*:95–100, 1998.
37. Stovroff, M. C., Totten, M., and Glick, P. L.: PIC lines save money and hasten discharge in the care of children with ruptured appendicitis. J. Pediatr. Surg. *29*:245–247, 1994.
38. Strandvik, B., Hjelte, L., Malmborg, A.-S., and Widén, B.: Home intravenous antibiotic treatment of patients with cystic fibrosis. Acta Paediatr. *81*:340–344, 1992.
39. Sudela, K. D.: Nursing aspects of pediatric home infusion therapy for the treatment of serious infections. Semin. Pediatr. Infect. Dis. *1*:306–317, 1990.
40. Thiagarajan, R. R., Ramamoorthy, C., Gettmann, T., et al.: Survey of the use of peripherally inserted central venous catheters in children. Pediatrics *99*:E4, 1997.
41. Tice, A. D.: Handbook of Outpatient Parenteral Therapy for Infectious Diseases. New York, Scientific American, 1997.
42. Tice, A. D., Williams, D. N., Rehm, S. J., et al.: Practice guidelines for community-based parenteral anti-infective therapy. Clin. Infect. Dis. In press.
43. Wagner, C. L., Wagstaff, P., Cox, T. H., and Annibale, D. J.: Early discharge with home antibiotic therapy in the treatment of neonatal infection. J. Perinatol. *20*:346–350, 2000.
44. Wai, A. O., Frighetto, L., Marra, C. A., et al.: Cost analysis of an adult outpatient parenteral antibiotic therapy (OPAT) programme. A Canadian teaching hospital and Ministry of Health perspective. Pharmacoeconomics *18*:451–457, 2000.
45. Warner, B. W., Kulick, R. M., Stoops, M. M., et al.: An evidenced-based clinical pathway for acute appendicitis decreases hospital duration and cost. J. Pediatr. Surg. *33*:1371–1375, 1998.
46. Wiernikowski, T. J., Rothney, M., Dawson, S., et al.: Evaluation of a home intravenous antibiotic program in pediatric oncology. Am. J. Pediatr. Hematol. Oncol. *13*:144–147, 1991.
47. Wilimas, J. A., Flynn, P. M., Harris, S., et al.: A randomized study of outpatient treatment with ceftriaxone for selected febrile children with sickle cell disease. N. Engl. J. Med. *329*:472–476, 1993.
48. Williams, D. N., Bosch, D., Boots, J., et al.: Safety, efficacy and cost savings in an outpatient intravenous antibiotic program. Clin. Ther. *15*:169–179, 1993.
49. Williams, D. N., Rehm, S. J., Tice, A. D., et al.: Practice guidelines for community-based parenteral anti-infective therapy. Clin. Infect. Dis. *25*:787–801, 1997.
50. Wolter, J. M., Bowler, S. D., Nolan, P. J., et al.: Home intravenous therapy in cystic fibrosis: A prospective randomized trial examining clinical, quality of life and cost aspects. Eur. Respir. J. *10*:896–900, 1997.
51. Woodin, K. A., and Davis, C. J.: The economic and psychosocial impact of outpatient parenteral antibiotic therapy in pediatrics. Semin. Pediatr. Infect. Dis. *1*:419–428, 1990.
52. www.idlinks.com (information on CoPAT, 2002).

CHAPTER

238 Antiviral Agents

GAIL J. DEMMLER

History and Background

The age of modern antiviral therapy began in the early 1950s, when methisazone, a derivative of the thiosemicarbazones (early antituberculosis compounds), was found to also have activity against vaccinia and variola viruses.[26, 27, 184, 371, 453, 479] In 1959, the first antiherpes compound, idoxuridine, was synthesized, and in 1962 it was approved for the topical treatment of herpetic keratitis.[244, 358] Shortly thereafter, in 1964, trifluridine also was used to treat herpetic keratitis.[245, 246] Also in 1964, the first description of vidarabine as an antiviral agent active against herpes simplex virus (HSV) was published, and amantadine was shown to have activity against influenza virus.[104, 396] Two years later, amantadine was approved first for the prophylaxis and subsequently for the treatment of influenza A virus infection.[481] Shortly thereafter, in 1972, vidarabine was approved for the treatment of herpes encephalitis.[471] The year 1972 also marked the first description of ribavirin as a broad-spectrum antiviral agent, with activity against both DNA and RNA viruses, and in 1985 the aerosolized form of the drug was approved for the treatment of respiratory syncytial virus (RSV) bronchiolitis.[107, 405] In 1977, acyclovir was reported to be a potent and selective inhibitor of the replication of both HSV and varicella-zoster virus (VZV) and boasted the added advantage of a favorable safety profile.[106, 127, 392] Subsequently, several structural analogues of acyclovir led to the development of antiviral agents with expanded antiviral spectra, such as ganciclovir, and agents with more favorable bioavailability, such as with the prodrugs valacyclovir and valganciclovir.[97, 297] Most recently, the introduction of cidofovir, a broad-spectrum, long-lasting antiviral agent, and the neuraminidase inhibitors zanamivir and oseltamivir, which treat both influenza A and influenza B viruses, has added new dimensions to antiviral therapy.[94, 274, 418] The research now being conducted no doubt will expand our antiviral armamentarium to combat viruses that may be used as biologic weapons, as well as prevent the emergence of resistant viruses and spawn creative strategies such as multidrug therapy and targeted delivery systems.[162, 194]

Even though diseases caused by viruses (Table 238–1) now may be treated with a variety of antiviral agents, the close relationship between the viral replicative cycle and its host-cell metabolism unfortunately has caused the development of safe and effective antiviral agents during the past 50 years to lag behind the development of other antimicrobials such as antibiotics. Clinically successful antiviral agents target and inhibit virus-specific functions while keeping cellular toxicity to a minimum. In addition, as a further testament to the co-dependency between viruses and host cells, some antiviral agents actually require cellular metabolism for antiviral activity, such as the terminal phosphorylation of acyclovir monophosphate to the active triphosphate form.

Antiviral agents can be categorized as virucidals, antiviral chemotherapeutic agents or drugs, and immunomodulators. Virucidal agents inactivate the virus on contact and include detergents, solvents, and ultraviolet light. These agents are not useful for treating human viral disease because healthy tissue also is destroyed. They may, however, be used to inactivate viruses on the surface of the skin or inanimate objects. Antiviral treatments that physically destroy both virus and the tissues infected or transformed by them include cryotherapy, laser therapy, or podophyllin and are used primarily to treat recalcitrant or life-threatening warts on mucocutaneous or laryngeotracheal tissue. These agents are discussed in Chapter 159. The host immune response also is important and, in many cases, essential for recovery from viral disease or even maintenance of a latent or inactivated state of the virus. Therefore, successful antiviral treatment may necessitate relief from immunosuppression when feasible, such as for patients with Epstein-Barr virus (EBV)– induced lymphoproliferative disease who are undergoing cancer chemotherapy or organ transplantation. It also may include the use of biologic response modifiers, or immunomodulators, that manipulate the immune system to enhance its ability to contain viral infection. Examples of immune modulators include immune globulin and monoclonal antibody preparations, cytokines such as interferons, and even novel approaches such as virus-specific cytotoxic T-cell lines designed to reconstitute host immunity.[15, 24] Finally, the explosion of new knowledge about specific antiretroviral therapy is reviewed in Chapter 193.

Antiviral chemotherapeutic agents usually inhibit virus-specific events, such as adsorption or attachment to the host cell (pleconaril), penetration and uncoating of the viral genome (amantadine), viral gene expression and nucleic acid synthesis (acyclovir, ganciclovir), or even viral assembly of intact, infectious viral particles (interferons) (Fig. 238–1). Therefore, antiviral agents exhibit their "antiviral effect" primarily while viral replication is active at the host-cell level. If the antiviral compound is withdrawn or discontinued, viral replication resumes. Furthermore, the currently available antiviral agents do not appear to eliminate viruses that are latent or in other dormant or nonreplicative states. The goal of antiviral therapy, for the most part, is to inhibit active viral replication to such a degree that the host immune response is able to contain or, in some instances, even eliminate the infection.

Antiviral agents usually have a narrow range of activity that can be predicted by their molecular mechanism of action. For example, rimantadine and amantadine have high activity against the RNA-containing influenza A virus, very limited activity against influenza B virus, and virtually no activity against the DNA herpesviruses,[94, 104] whereas acyclovir, a deoxyguanosine analogue that requires monophosphorylation by the viral enzyme thymidine kinase (TK) for activation, has significant activity against DNA viruses (HSV), which carry TK, but no activity against RNA viruses such as influenza virus. Viruses infecting a host also may become resistant to a specific agent to which they originally were susceptible, usually by induced or selected mutations. Resistance is therefore most likely to occur in viruses that infect the host with a high viral load and that have a high intrinsic viral mutation rate, as well as in hosts who are exposed to selective drug pressure during chronic, low-dose,

TABLE 238–1 ■ VIRUS-ASSOCIATED DISEASES THAT MAY BE TREATED WITH ANTIVIRAL AGENTS THAT ARE CURRENTLY AVAILABLE OR UNDER CLINICAL DEVELOPMENT

DNA Viruses
Herpes simplex virus
  Gingivostomatitis
  Keratoconjunctivitis
  Eczema herpeticum
  Whitlow
  Genital ulcers
  Esophagitis
  Hepatitis
  Encephalitis
  Aseptic meningitis
  Neonatal disease
Varicella-zoster virus
  Chickenpox
  Zoster
  Acute retinal necrosis
  Pneumonitis
  Hepatitis
  Cerebral vasculitis/stroke
Cytomegalovirus
  Retinitis
  Pneumonitis
  Esophagitis and colitis
  Fever and leukopenia syndrome
  Congenital disease
Epstein-Barr virus
  Mononucleosis syndrome
  Post-transplant lymphoproliferative disease
Herpes B virus
  Encephalitis
Adenoviruses
  Disseminated disease
  Hemorrhagic cystitis
  Pneumonitis
  Colitis
  Conjunctivitis
Hepatitis B virus
  Acute and chronic hepatitis
Varioloa virus
  Smallpox
Vaccinia virus
  Vaccine-associated complications
Papillomaviruses
  Cutaneous and genital warts
  Laryngeal papillomatosis
Polyomaviruses (BK, JC, SV40)
  Hemorrhagic cystitis
  Progressive multifocal encephalopathy

RNA Viruses
Influenza viruses
  Influenza syndrome and complications
Parainfluenza viruses
  Laryngotracheobronchitis
  Pneumonitis
Respiratory syncytial virus
  Bronchiolitis
  Pneumonitis
Measles virus
  Measles syndrome
  Encephalitis
Pneumonitis
Enteroviruses
  Aseptic meningitis and meningoencephalitis
  Myocarditis
  Neonatal disease
Arenavirus
  Lassa fever
Hepatitis C virus
  Acute and chronic hepatitis

or repeated treatment with an antiviral agent.[213] Both resistant and sensitive viruses are capable of causing serious disease, especially in an immunocompromised host. Currently, most antiviral agents are administered alone. However, in the future, combination antiviral therapy, now a routine therapy in modern antiretroviral regimens, may someday be evaluated in clinical trials.[189, 194] Such a strategy may increase antiviral effectiveness, prevent the emergence of drug resistance, and allow the administration of lower, less toxic dosages.

Antiviral Agents Active against RNA Viruses (Table 238–2)

AMANTADINE AND RIMANTADINE

Spectrum of Activity

Amantadine (1-adamantanamine hydrochloride) and rimantadine (α-methyl-1-adamantane methylamine hydrochloride) are tricyclic amines with specific activity against influenza A viruses (Fig. 238–2). Mean inhibitory concentrations of 0.1 to 0.4 μg/mL for amantadine have been reported, and rimantadine is 4 to 10 times more active than amantadine against influenza A virus.[56, 192] Amantadine also has in vitro activity against rubella virus, but efficacy was not confirmed in animal models.[341, 342, 432] Much higher concentrations (10 to 50 μg/mL) appear to inhibit influenza B virus and parainfluenza viruses, but these high concentrations cannot be achieved safely in humans.[432] These agents also have activity against hepatitis C virus (HCV).[415]

Mechanism of Action and Resistance

The mechanism of action of both amantadine and rimantadine against influenza A virus appears to be primarily inhibition of the ion channel function of the M2 protein in the membrane of the virus, possibly affecting two stages of viral replication, uncoating and, to a lesser extent, assembly.[94, 188] Amantadine and rimantadine resistance occurs when mutations cause an amino acid change in one of four critical sites (amino acids 26, 27, 30, or 31) in the transmembrane channel or domain of the M2 viral protein.[262] Such mutations occur frequently and rapidly during therapy because approximately 30 percent of adults and children who receive amantadine or rimantadine therapy for at least 5 days shed resistant influenza virus.[190, 193] These resistant strains are genetically stable, may be transmitted to close contacts, and can produce disease.[31, 190, 489] Immunocompromised patients may shed drug-resistant influenza viruses for prolonged periods, and resistant strains can persist even after drug administration has been discontinued.[262] Evidence supporting the notion that these resistant strains will produce community outbreaks, epidemics, or pandemics is scant at this time.[31, 190, 489] However, debate has begun among experts concerning whether patients in whom a resistant strain is identified should be isolated somehow until viral shedding has ceased.[180] Strains of influenza A virus resistant to amantadine also are resistant to rimantadine, and vice versa, but they are usually susceptible to ribavirin and neuraminidase inhibitors.

Pharmacokinetics

Amantadine is absorbed rapidly and nearly completely after oral administration, with peak plasma concentrations of 0.5 to 0.8 μg/mL attained within 2 hours of administration.[39, 198]

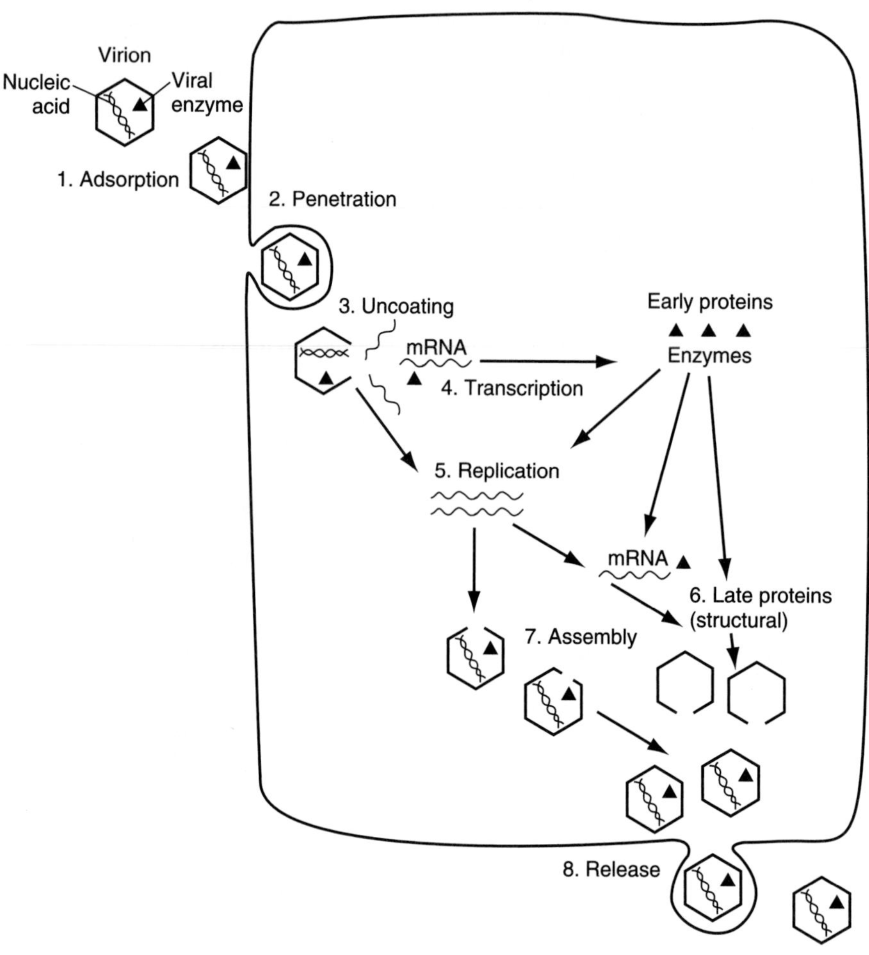

FIGURE 238–1 ■ Basic steps in intracellular (DNA) replication. *1,* Adsorption of virion to the cell membrane. *2,* Penetration. *3,* Uncoating, removal of the protein coat. *4,* Early gene expression, transcription of viral proteins. *5,* Replication, synthesis of DNA strands. *6,* Late gene expression, transcription of messenger RNA, and translation of late protein synthesis. *7,* Maturation and assembly of virions. *8,* Release.

It is excreted almost unchanged in urine. Nasal and salivary secretions also contain high levels of amantadine, and the drug is present in cerebrospinal fluid (CSF) as well, at approximately half the plasma level. Dose reductions, adjusted according to creatinine clearance, are required in patients with renal insufficiency and renal failure.[222, 423, 481] Rimantadine, on the other hand, is more slowly absorbed than amantadine, with peak plasma levels of 0.4 to 0.6 μg/mL achieved within 2 to 4 hours of administration.[9, 198, 330]

TABLE 238–2 ■ CLINICAL INDICATIONS AND USUAL TREATMENT DOSAGES FOR ANTIVIRAL AGENTS ACTIVE AGAINST RNA VIRUSES

Agent	Indication	Dosage
Amantadine	Influenza A	2.2–4.4 mg/kg/dose PO bid (max, 100–200 mg daily)
Rimantadine	Influenza A	2.5 mg/kg/dose PO bid (max, 150 mg daily)
Oseltamivir	Influenza A and B	2 mg/kg/dose PO bid (max, 150 mg daily)
Zanamivir	Influenza A and B	5 mg/dose inhaled bid
Ribavirin	RSV	6 g/300 mL inhaled daily over 18-hr period *or* 2–6 g/100 mL inhaled over 2-hr period tid
	Hepatitis C	600 mg PO bid (with interferon-α)

Rimantadine is also present in high concentration in nasal secretions. It is excreted in urine, but only after extensive metabolism by the liver. Dose reduction, therefore, is recommended in patients with renal or hepatic disease.[63, 474] Hemodialysis does not appear to clear either drug, so supplemental doses usually are not recommended after dialysis.[423] When administered to chronically ill, institutionalized elderly patients, dosages also may need to be adjusted.[322, 347] In addition, aerosolized forms of amantadine and rimantadine have been evaluated in human volunteers.[196, 202]

Clinical Indications, Dosage, and Adverse Effects

CLINICAL INDICATIONS

Amantadine and rimantadine are equally effective for the treatment of disease caused by influenza A virus.[94, 262, 475] If administered within the first 48 hours of symptoms, both agents significantly reduce the signs and symptoms of

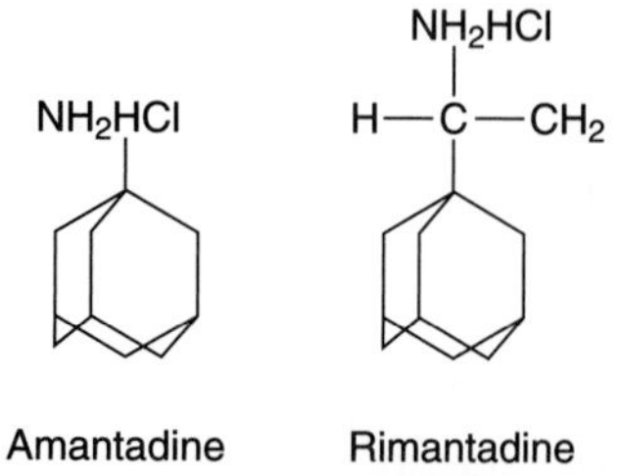

NH_2HCl Amantadine

NH_2HCl, H—C—CH_2 Rimantadine

FIGURE 238–2 ■ Structure of amantadine and rimantadine.

influenza in both adults and children by significantly shortening the duration of fever and respiratory and systemic symptoms by 1 day.[94, 109, 287, 454, 475, 484] The duration and amount of viral shedding from the nasopharyngeal tract also are decreased, and otologic complications may be reduced.[118] Both agents are effective for prophylaxis against influenza A virus infection and disease, with approximately 50 percent overall effectiveness in preventing infection with the virus and approximately 60 to 70 percent overall effectiveness (up to 90% in some studies) in preventing clinical disease and, in individuals with breakthrough clinical disease, in reducing the severity of the disease.* The emergence of resistant strains during rimantadine or amantadine therapy and subsequent transmission of these resistant strains may lessen the effectiveness of prophylaxis in some families and nursing homes.[190, 303] Amantadine and rimantadine are both available as tablets (100 mg) and syrup (50 mg/5 mL) for oral administration.

DOSAGE

The usual dose of amantadine for children is 4.4 to 8.8 mg/kg/day divided twice daily (many experts recommend 5 mg/kg/day), with a maximal recommended daily dose of 200 mg. The usual dose of rimantadine for children is 5 mg/kg/day divided twice daily, with a maximal recommended daily dose of 150 mg.[9, 180, 330, 474] Older children and adolescents may take the usual adult dose for each drug, which is 200 mg/day given once daily or, for better tolerance, divided into two 100-mg doses daily.[9] Elderly patients should receive 100 mg daily, or less if renal insufficiency is present. To be effective, these agents should be given as soon as possible after the onset of symptoms.[94, 95] The duration of treatment of established influenza should be 3 to 7 days, or at least 2 days after the cessation of systemic signs and symptoms.[94] Prevention of influenza is accomplished best through annual vaccination; however, rimantadine and amantadine may be used to prevent or lessen influenza symptoms in both adults and children.[83, 94, 96] Prophylaxis should be administered during the period of risk, whether exposure is in the family, community, or nosocomial setting. In general, prophylaxis should continue for at least 10 days after a known exposure occurs in an unprotected individual. For patients who receive the combination of inactivated vaccine and oral prophylaxis, rimantadine or amantadine should be continued for at least 2 to 4 weeks after vaccination, when maximal antibody response from the vaccine is expected to occur. For patients who are at high risk but did not receive the vaccine, oral prophylaxis should be continued for as long as the period of risk is anticipated and may be extended to the end of the community's influenza season. Doses of both drugs should be adjusted for patients with renal disease, as well as doses of rimantadine for patients with hepatic disease.[63, 222, 423, 474] Prolonged treatment may be associated with side effects, especially in the elderly.[347] If side effects occur, the daily dose may be reduced to 100 mg and still be effective in most cases. The emergence of resistant strains during the period of drug administration may lessen the effectiveness of prophylaxis in some patients.[190, 303] Combination with aerosolized ribavirin may enhance the antiviral effect of amantadine or rimantadine against influenza A virus.[189, 194]

ADVERSE EFFECTS

The adverse effects of both amantadine and rimantadine include central nervous system (CNS) effects such as anxiety, depression, insomnia, dizziness, and impaired concentration; in children, these side effects appear to be rare, but they may be manifested as behavioral changes.[83, 94, 116, 421] Rimantadine reportedly has fewer CNS side effects than amantadine does.[94, 116, 197, 318] Hallucinations, tremors, and seizures also may occur, especially in patients with renal failure who have high plasma levels of amantadine. In addition, rare cases of coma and fatal cardiac dysrhythmia have been reported.[352, 388] A prudent procedure is to administer amantadine and rimantadine with caution to individuals being treated for seizures or neuropsychiatric disorders or to patients also receiving other medications that affect the nervous system, such as antihistamines.[318] Furthermore, the institutionalized elderly may have increased plasma levels and experience side effects more often than younger patients do.[347] Occasionally, gastrointestinal symptoms such as nausea and vomiting may accompany the oral administration of these agents in all age groups. Most reported adverse effects of these two agents have been reversible, with significant long-term complications being exceedingly rare. Of note, amantadine also is used to treat parkinsonism and drug-induced extrapyramidal reactions.[398]

NEURAMINIDASE INHIBITORS (ZANAMIVIR AND OSELTAMIVIR)

Spectrum of Activity

Zanamivir (5-[acetylamino]-4-[(aminoiminomethyl)-amino]-2,6-anhydro-3,4,5-trideoxy-D-glycero-D-galacto-non-2-eonic acid) and oseltamivir ([3R, 4R, 5S]-4-acetylamino-5-amino-3[1-ethylpropoxy]-1-cyclohexene-1-carboxylic acid, ethyl ester, phosphate [1:1]) are both analogues of *N*-acetylneuraminic acid, the cell surface receptor for influenza viruses, and were designed to inhibit the viral neuraminidase of influenza viruses (Fig. 238–3). Both agents are potent and specific

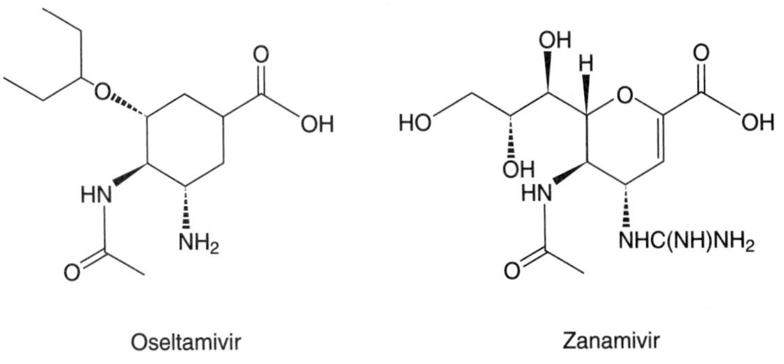

Oseltamivir

Zanamivir

FIGURE 238–3 ■ Structure of the neuraminidase inhibitors oseltamivir and zanamivir.

*See references 94, 110, 116, 156, 231, 232, 323, 338, 380, 467, 490.

inhibitors of the neuraminidases of influenza A and B viruses, with 90 percent of the strains inhibited at concentrations of 0.05 to 100 μmol/L.[254, 456] The compounds also are capable of inhibiting neuraminidases from other pathogens and mammalian cells, but only at extremely high concentrations.

Mechanism of Action and Resistance

Neuraminidase permits influenza virus to penetrate through the mucoproteins present in respiratory secretions to the surfaces of cells, and inhibition of this enzyme prevents viral access and infection of cells. Neuraminidase also destroys receptors recognized by viral hemagglutinin and is therefore necessary for optimal release of influenza virus particles from infected cells. Inhibition prevents cell-to-cell spread of virus within the respiratory tract and lessens the intensity of the initial infection.[87, 94, 254, 332, 456] Mutations that induce amino acid changes in viral neuraminidase alter enzyme stability or activity, mutations in hemagglutinin produce a reduced affinity for cell receptors, and mutations in both produce resistant influenza viruses.[94, 172–175] Cross-resistance to both zanamivir and oseltamivir also can occur, especially if the mutation is in the hemagglutinin portion.[313] Resistance has been documented not only by in vitro passage of the virus in increasing concentrations of the agents, but also in patients receiving these agents. Clinical trials of oral oseltamivir for the treatment of naturally occurring influenza detected resistance in 1 to 2 percent of post-treatment isolates from adults and adolescents and in 5 to 8 percent of isolates from younger children.[94, 174, 222, 486] Zanamivir resistance has been documented in one immunocompromised child receiving the drug for 2 weeks, but not in large, randomized trials of healthy individuals.[172, 195, 199, 203, 320] Preliminary evidence suggests that mutant resistant strains may have reduced infectivity or virulence in comparison to susceptible strains.[442]

Pharmacokinetics

Zanamivir is administered topically as an inhaled dry powder and is deposited in the oropharynx and, to a lesser extent, in the tracheobronchial tree and lungs.[94] Approximately 4 to 17 percent of inhaled drug is absorbed systemically, and levels of 17 to 142 ng/mL can be detected in serum 1 to 2 hours after administration of a typical inhaled dose of 10 mg to adults.[64] Serum levels in pediatric patients who received an inhaled dose were extremely low (less than 10 ng/mL) or undetectable, which may be related to the ability of the patient to cooperate with the inhaled drug delivery system. The oral bioavailability of zanamivir is extremely low, with less than 5 percent of the administered dose absorbed, and therefore it is not administered in this form. Intravenous preparations of zanamivir also have been tested in clinical trials, but this form is not available clinically at this time.[62, 64, 153] The drug is excreted unchanged in urine.

Oseltamivir, in contrast, has good oral bioavailability. The prodrug compound oseltamivir phosphate is metabolized by hepatic esterases to the parent active compound oseltamivir carboxylate.[94] Approximately 75 to 80 percent of the administered dose is absorbed, and peak plasma concentrations are reached within 3 to 4 hours but may be delayed, but not reduced, if the drug is given with food. A typical 75-mg dose will provide plasma concentrations of 0.3 to 0.5 μg/mL. Both the prodrug and the active form are eliminated unchanged through the kidneys, and dosages should be adjusted for patients with renal insufficiency or renal failure. Whether the drug dosage should be adjusted for patients with hepatic disease or liver failure is unclear from the available evidence. Information from a small number of pediatric patients suggests that the drug may be eliminated faster in younger children. Elderly, geriatric patients, however, appear to metabolize the drug similar to young adults.

Clinical Indications, Dosage, and Adverse Effects

CLINICAL INDICATIONS

Zanamivir and oseltamivir have been shown to be effective in treating both influenza A and influenza B infection. When administered within the first 2 days of illness, they provide relief from symptoms up to 1.5 days earlier than placebo does and reduce the quantity and duration of viral shedding.* In some studies, the frequency of secondary complications such as sinusitis, bronchitis, and otitis media with effusion (but not pneumonia) also was reduced.[94, 461] Both antiviral agents are effective for the prophylaxis of influenza A and influenza B infection in both adults and children in family, community, and nursing home situations. They appear to be 30 to 50 percent effective in preventing viral infection and 64 to 84 percent effective in preventing disease.[94, 195, 201, 305, 324, 461] However, up to 89 percent efficacy in preventing disease in families has been reported, and in elderly patients in nursing homes, 92 percent of cases of influenza may be prevented if the agents are administered to those who also have received influenza vaccine.[94, 195, 305]

DOSAGE

Zanamivir is administered by oral inhalation with an inhalation device provided with the product. Each inhalation dose is 5 mg, and two inhalations twice daily for 5 days is the usual recommended dosage for all age groups. Use of this drug and device is dependent on the understanding and cooperation of the patient, and therefore, it is not indicated for use in children younger than 7 years and may be of limited use in older children and adults who are unable to cooperate with the delivery system. No reduction in dosage is needed for patients with impaired renal function because very little of the inhaled drug is absorbed systemically. Oseltamivir is administered orally and is available in 75-mg capsules and a 12-mg/mL suspension. The usual adult dosage is 75 mg twice daily for treatment and once or twice daily for as long as 6 weeks for prophylaxis. The pediatric dose is 2 mg/kg per dose given twice daily (4 mg/kg/day divided twice daily).[94]

ADVERSE EFFECTS

Both neuraminidase inhibitors are generally well tolerated, with very few, if any serious adverse effects observed in clinical trials. Zanamivir inhalation, however, may produce local irritation or bronchospasm in some patients, and oseltamivir has been associated with nausea and vomiting, which may be lessened by administering the drug with food.[94]

RIBAVIRIN

Spectrum of Activity

Ribavirin (1-β-D-ribofuranosyl-1,2,4-triazole-3-carboxamide) is a synthetic guanosine analogue with broad-spectrum antiviral activity[412] (Fig. 238–4). It inhibits the in vitro replication of a wide variety of RNA viruses, including orthomyxoviruses such as influenza A and B viruses; paramyxoviruses such as RSV, parainfluenza viruses, and

*See references 61, 94, 199, 262, 305, 320, 325, 355, 450, 473.

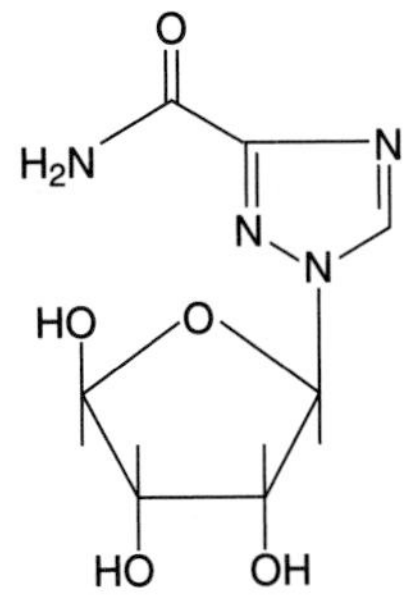

Ribavirin

FIGURE 238–4 ■ Structure of ribavirin.

measles virus; arenaviruses such as Lassa fever virus; bunyaviruses that cause viral encephalitis; togaviruses such as HCV; enteroviruses such as polioviruses and coxsackie B virus; and retroviruses, including human immunodeficiency virus (HIV) type 1.[136, 225, 252, 275, 277, 340, 405] Also inhibited by ribavirin are many DNA viruses, such as adenoviruses; herpesviruses, including HAV and cytomegalovirus (CMV); and poxviruses, such as vaccinia virus.[117] It inhibits most orthomyxoviruses and paramyxoviruses at concentrations of 3 to 10 μg/mL and Lassa fever virus at 4 to 40 μmol/L.[224] Because most of its clinical use has been for the treatment of RNA viruses, especially RSV, ribavirin is included in this section of the chapter.

Mechanism of Action and Resistance

Ribavirin most likely exerts it antiviral effects by altering the cellular nucleotide pools and by interfering with viral mRNA formation.[55, 136, 434] The compound is phosphorylated by host-cell enzymes to monophosphate, diphosphate, and triphosphate active forms, each with specific antiviral actions.[410] For example, ribavirin monophosphate competitively interferes with the synthesis of guanosine triphosphate and, subsequently, with viral nucleic acid synthesis. Ribavirin triphosphate inhibits the RNA polymerase of influenza virus and also interferes with the capping of its viral mRNA.[136, 252, 340, 480] In addition, the diphosphate and triphosphate forms of ribavirin appear to inhibit the reverse transcriptase activity of HIV-1.[140] The mechanism of action of ribavirin against HCV and other viruses, however, is not well understood. Ribavirin also exerts an effect on the host immune system by inhibiting mast cell secretory responses and diminishing IgE responses.[298] Antiviral resistance is not well characterized and appears to be a rare occurrence. No ribavirin-resistant RSV isolates have been identified during clinical trials, and information is scant regarding the resistance of other viruses to ribavirin.[182, 293, 393]

Pharmacokinetics

Ribavirin can be administered topically by aerosol, orally, and intravenously. Aerosol administration of ribavirin with a small-particle aerosol generator delivers very high concentrations (over 1000 μg/mL) of the drug to the respiratory tract.[264] The aerosolized drug also is absorbed systemically, and peak plasma levels after 8 hours of continuous aerosol administration range from 0.5 to 2.2 μg/mL; after 20 hours, they reach 0.8 to 3.3 μg/mL. After oral administration, bioavailability is 33 to 45 percent, and peak plasma levels of 1.3 to 3.2 μg/mL have been observed 1 to 2 hours after administration. Intravenous administration of ribavirin produces 10-fold higher plasma levels in less than 1 hour than after the administration of equivalent doses by different routes.[345] The higher doses used to treat Lassa fever produce plasma levels of up to 24 μg/mL. Ribavirin also crosses the blood-brain barrier and is present in CSF at approximately 70 percent of the plasma level.[91, 223] The drug is metabolized by the liver, and approximately 40 percent of the dose is excreted by the kidneys.[345] The triphosphate form also concentrates in erythrocytes at an erythrocyte-to-plasma ratio of 40:1 and is slowly eliminated with a half-life ($t_{1/2}$) of 40 days or longer. Hemodialysis and hemofiltration do not remove significant amounts of ribavirin from the body.[267]

Clinical Indications, Dosage, and Adverse Effects

CLINICAL INDICATIONS

Ribavirin aerosol is licensed for the treatment of RSV bronchiolitis and pneumonia in children.[179] Treatment shortens the duration of viral shedding and improves the fever, respiratory rate, arterial oxygen saturation, and lower respiratory tract signs on physical examination in severely ill patients who receive the antiviral agent early in the course of their illness.*

No clear benefit has been observed in patients with mild disease or in those who receive treatment late in the course of the disease. Studies of infants receiving mechanical ventilation have reported conflicting results regarding clinical benefit.[310, 321, 413] However, despite numerous clinical studies, indications for treatment remain controversial because efficacy has not been documented convincingly in all studies and the benefits observed generally have been mild and difficult to quantitate objectively.[179] Nonetheless, because antiviral treatment clearly appeared to provide benefit to some children, in 1996, the American Academy of Pediatrics recommended that ribavirin be considered for the treatment of hospitalized infants and children with severe lower respiratory tract infection caused by RSV, and these recommendations remain in effect.

Patients thought to potentially benefit the most from treatment were those younger than 6 weeks, those with chronic illnesses such as congenital heart disease and chronic lung disease, premature infants, immunosuppressed children, and those with neurologic or neuromuscular disorders. Treatment with ribavirin also appears to decrease nasopharyngeal secretion of RSV-specific IgE and IgA responses.[378] Long-term follow-up of treated patients suggests no adverse effects but possible improvement in pulmonary function.[206, 238, 290] Treatment may benefit immunocompromised children who have serious or prolonged RSV infection, such as those with congenital severe combined immunodeficiency.[308] Aerosolized or intravenous ribavirin, especially when combined with intravenous immune globulin or hyperimmune globulin, also may be of benefit to bone marrow transplant recipients with RSV lower tract disease.[290, 292, 470] Anecdotal reports suggest that early administration of ribavirin to immunocompromised patients during upper respiratory tract disease may be more efficacious than supportive care alone in preventing progression to lower tract disease or pneumonia.[132, 308] Laboratory confirmation of RSV infection by viral culture or rapid diagnostic tests that detect viral antigen in respiratory secretions is recommended for all patients before treatment with ribavirin is initiated or continued beyond 12 to 24 hours. Ribavirin also is licensed in capsule form for the treatment of chronic hepatitis caused by HCV, and when

*See references 171, 181, 206, 238, 310, 321, 359, 413, 441, 469.

combined with interferon-α, it produces a sustained decrease in HCV RNA levels, improvement in systemic symptoms such as fatigue, reduction in transaminases, and improvement in liver histology. These clinical benefits have been observed during initial treatment in previously untreated patients, in individuals initially unresponsive to interferon alone, and in patients treated for relapse.[38, 41, 105, 114, 152, 221, 307, 365] Treatment with high doses of orally or intravenously administered ribavirin significantly reduces mortality rates in patients with Lassa fever.[237, 306] Ribavirin also appears to benefit patients suffering from other hemorrhagic fever syndromes, including Argentine, Sabia, Bolivian, and Crimean-Congo hemorrhagic fever, as well as those who have hemorrhagic fever with renal failure syndrome.[134, 143, 226, 227, 253] In addition, ribavirin may benefit patients with viral encephalitis, but clinical trials have not been performed.[65] Oral ribavirin also may be of benefit prophylactically in individuals who are exposed to hemorrhagic fever syndromes, including Lassa fever.[220] Treatment of hantavirus pulmonary syndrome with intravenously administered ribavirin is being evaluated in clinical trials. Ribavirin also may benefit individuals with influenza A or B virus infection. In one randomized study of young adults suffering from influenza, aerosol treatment significantly reduced fever, systemic signs and symptoms, and virus titer in respiratory secretions.[412] Another study showed clinical benefit with high-dose oral ribavirin, but other studies have not confirmed a measurable clinical benefit or virologic response consistently with aerosolized or oral ribavirin.[34, 263, 412, 431] Intravenous ribavirin also has been used anecdotally to treat serious, life-threatening influenza.[200, 361] Early treatment with aerosolized or intravenous ribavirin in bone marrow and stem cell transplant recipients infected with parainfluenza virus may help prevent progression to lower tract disease and pneumonia, but controlled trials documenting efficacy and effect on overall mortality rates have not been published.[128, 200, 468] Ribavirin also has been used to treat measles pneumonia in immunocompetent and immunocompromised patients, with clinical benefit reported in some.[146, 176, 242]

Clinical benefit, but not cure, also has been documented in case reports of children with subacute sclerosing panencephalitis (SSPE) caused by measles virus.[223, 224, 329, 443] In these reports, repeated courses of large doses of ribavirin administered intravenously, when combined with interferon-α, provided serum and CSF levels that exceeded the minimal inhibitory concentrations (MICs) needed to inhibit the virus in vitro and improved or stabilized seizures and neurologic status in treated patients.[223] Case reports and small series using ribavirin to treat serious adenoviral disease, including pneumonia and disseminated adenoviral disease, have been published, but no controlled trials documenting clinical benefit have been published.[22, 46, 69, 160, 302, 327] Despite documented antiretroviral activity, treatment of HIV-infected patients with oral ribavirin has not shown clinical, virologic, or immunologic benefits consistently.[91, 140, 239]

DOSAGE

A number of different dosages and routes of administration have been used to administer ribavirin to a variety of patients experiencing various infections. In normal and immunocompromised patients of all ages, the usual dosage of ribavirin, when administered topically by aerosol to the respiratory tract for treatment of influenza and lower respiratory tract disease caused by RSV, parainfluenza virus, and measles virus, is 6 g of drug reconstituted in a final volume of 300 mL of sterile water (final concentration, 20 mg/mL); a small-particle aerosol generator (SPAG-2 unit) is used to administer the drug continuously over a period of 12 to 18 hours for 3 to 7 days.* The drug may be delivered to an infant oxygen hood or tent, by facemask, or through pressure- or volume-cycled ventilators, provided that ventilatory pressure is monitored and the device is checked for precipitation, which may cause ventilator dysfunction.[151, 339]

Intermittent high-dose therapy, with drug administered at 60 mg/mL for 2 hours three times daily for 5 days, also appears to be effective and may be better tolerated in some older patients.[131] Longer courses of aerosolized therapy for up to 14 days have been used in severely immunocompromised patients with prolonged viral shedding and severe disease.[285] Oral doses of up to 600 mg twice daily for 24 to 48 weeks, usually combined with interferon-α, are used to treat HCV in adults.[38, 41, 105, 114, 221, 307, 365] High doses of oral ribavirin also appear to be effective in treating influenza in normal hosts.[432] Even higher doses of oral ribavirin (2-g loading dose, followed by 2 g/day divided every 8 hours for 10 days) have been used for the treatment of Lassa fever and other hemorrhagic fever syndromes in adults.[134, 143, 220, 227, 237, 253, 306] The intravenous dose of ribavirin used to treat Lassa fever is a 2-g loading dose (25 to 33 mg/kg estimated pediatric dose), followed by 1-g doses (16 mg/kg estimated pediatric dose) every 6 hours for 4 days and then 500-mg doses (8 mg/kg estimated pediatric dose) every 8 hours for 3 days to complete a 7- to 10-day course of treatment.[237, 306] This intravenous dosage regimen also has been used to treat measles pneumonia, severe influenza with complications, pneumonia caused by parainfluenza virus in immunocompromised patients, and disseminated adenovirus disease.[146, 176, 292, 361] Continuous intravenous infusions of ribavirin have been used in patients with severe disease caused by influenza and parainfluenza viruses.[200] Doses used to treat SSPE in children have been considerably higher and administered for longer periods.[223, 329] In one report, pediatric patients received interferon-α combined with 10 mg/kg of ribavirin administered intravenously every 8 hours daily for 7 days. Escalating doses of 20 and then 30 mg/kg given every 8 hours daily for 7 days at 7-day intervals then were administered.[223] The highest dose tolerated was given for 7 days, repeated in 7-day intervals, and administered for a period of 6 months.

ADVERSE EFFECTS

Adverse effects of aerosolized ribavirin are unusual but include local irritation causing facial rash and conjunctivitis. Abnormalities in pulmonary function, including worsening of respiratory distress and bronchospasm, also have been reported.[165, 182, 441] In addition, one case of water intoxication associated with aerosolized ribavirin administration has been reported.[447] Older children, adolescents, and adults may be noncompliant with treatment or may even have anxiety attacks or experience other forms of psychologic stress as they are being confined for continuous treatment for a 12- to 18-hour period. In these cases, intermittent, high-dose regimens may be better tolerated and might enhance patient compliance.[131] Precipitation of the drug in ventilator tubing systems and on filtering devices may cause ventilator dysfunction and respiratory distress or failure in mechanically ventilated patients, especially those receiving high-dose intermittent administration, but such events may be minimized by frequently monitoring ventilator pressure and changing the filters.[151, 310, 321, 339] Adverse hematologic effects such as anemia have not been documented consistently in

*See references 34, 128, 171, 181, 182, 242, 263, 285, 302, 310, 321, 327, 412, 413, 441, 470.

patients who received aerosolized ribavirin. The environmental exposure to aerosolized ribavirin by health care workers providing direct care to a virus-infected patient may, in some instances, cause headache, conjunctivitis, contact lens damage, watery eyes, and bronchospasm in those with underlying reactive airway disease.[49, 165, 372, 404] These potential adverse effects are probably more likely to be seen in instances in which ribavirin is administered by hood, tent, or facemask than when administered to mechanically ventilated patients.[50] Environmental exposure of health care workers and family members may be reduced by providing routine patient care during periods when the aerosol generator has been turned off, by turning off the aerosol generator during periods of more urgent care, and by using protective equipment such as masks and goggles. Dose-related, reversible, usually mild anemia occurs frequently during and after long-term oral therapy and intravenous administration of ribavirin.[221, 239] Rarely, severe anemia may occur and necessitate dose reduction or cessation of therapy. Reversible increases in serum bilirubin, serum iron, and uric acid concentrations also have been documented during oral therapy. On rare occasion, intravenous administration of ribavirin has produced chills and rigors.[142, 165] Ribavirin has shown teratogenic, mutagenic, and embryotoxic effects in preclinical animal models.[211] Therefore, investigators recommend that exposure of pregnant women to ribavirin, either therapeutically or through environmental exposure, be minimized or prevented whenever possible or practical.

PLECONARIL

Spectrum of Activity

Pleconaril (3-[3,5-dimethyl-4-[[3-(3-methyl-5-isoxazolyl) propyl]]-olyl]phenyl]-5-(trifluoromethyl)-1,2,4-oxadiazole) is an antiviral agent with significant and specific activity against picornaviruses, both enteroviruses and rhinoviruses (Fig. 238–5). In vitro, pleconaril inhibits the replication of most serotypes of enteroviruses at concentrations between 0.01 and 0.1 μg/mL.[351] Echovirus 11, a commonly isolated enterovirus in the United States, appears to be the most sensitive enterovirus tested to date (inhibited at a mean concentration of 0.006 μg/mL). Most rhinovirus serotypes are inhibited at slightly higher concentrations of 0.21 to 0.78 mg/mL, but still within ranges safely achievable in patients.

Mechanism of Action and Resistance

Pleconaril binds efficiently to a specific hydrophobic pocket within the viral capsid of picornaviruses and exhibits an antiviral effect by interfering with uncoating, attachment, and cell-to-cell transmission of infectious viral particles.[379] The drug induces a more rigid structure within the viral capsid, which then interferes with viral uncoating and release of viral RNA.[148, 309, 350, 351, 373, 379] Pleconaril also appears to change the conformation of the canyon floor of the virus capsid when it integrates with the underlying pocket, thereby interfering with attachment of the virus to host-cell receptors.[350, 379] Resistance of picornaviruses to pleconaril has not been reported.

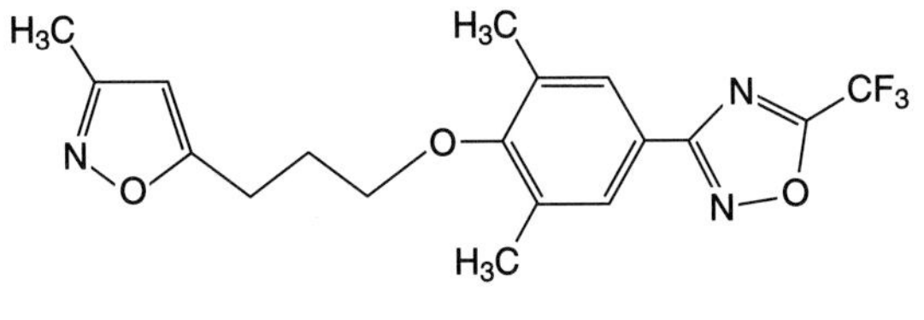

Pleconaril

FIGURE 238–5 ■ Structure of pleconaril.

Pharmacokinetics

The pharmacokinetics of pleconaril varies with the age of the group tested. After oral administration of single doses of 200 to 400 mg to adults, peak plasma concentrations of 1.1 to 2.4 μg/mL are achieved in 1.5 to 5 hours, with an average elimination $t_{1/2}$ of 25 hours.[2] Repeated dosing for a 7-day period increases plasma concentrations to 1.33 to 3.4 μg/mL. When taken with food, especially a meal high in fat, absorption of pleconaril is enhanced significantly.[1, 248] Single oral doses of 5 mg/kg in children provide plasma concentrations of approximately 1.3 μg/mL with a more rapid elimination $t_{1/2}$ of approximately 6 hours.[247] Neonates also absorb pleconaril well, but they do not exhibit dose-proportionate pharmacokinetics like adults do.[248] The drug also has a large volume of distribution and concentrates in tissues such as the liver, brain, and nasal epithelium, where viral replication and viral-induced disease are likely to occur.[248] Pleconaril appears to be excreted in feces and urine.

Clinical Indications, Dosage, and Adverse Effects

CLINICAL INDICATIONS

Pleconaril currently is not licensed for therapeutic use, but because it is in advanced clinical development, information is included in this chapter. Efficacy is being evaluated in clinical trials, and for some patients, the agent can be obtained for compassionate use from the manufacturer. Pleconaril has shown efficacy in early clinical trials against picornavirus infections in adults, children, and neonates. In pretreated adults experimentally infected with coxsackie A21 virus, pleconaril significantly reduced viral titers, as well as the clinical parameters of fever, nasal mucus production, and systemic symptoms, when compared with placebo.[191, 379, 394] In another trial, pleconaril resolved the symptoms of illness 2 days earlier than placebo did, and patients who received pleconaril did not require as much concomitant medication for symptomatic relief as did those who received placebo.[379] In two placebo-controlled trials in adults with aseptic meningitis caused by enterovirus, pleconaril treatment reduced the duration of headache and other symptoms of meningitis by 2 to 3 days and allowed treated patients to return to work and routine daily activities 2 days earlier than patients who received placebo.[379, 394] In a placebo-controlled trial in pediatric patients with aseptic meningitis caused by enterovirus, pleconaril significantly improved illness scores and reduced the duration of headache in older children, but clinical efficacy was difficult to assess in infants and younger children. Viral shedding from the throat also was reduced in the treatment group.[379] In addition to treatment for the "common cold" and for "viral meningitis," another potential use for pleconaril is for the treatment of serious, persistent, or life-threatening illness caused by enteroviruses. More than 90 patients with unusual or life-threatening infections with enterovirus have received pleconaril on a compassionate-use basis.[148] These patients included immunocompromised patients with chronic meningitis, neonates with disseminated disease, patients with myocarditis,[374] and individuals with poliomyelitis associated with vaccine or wild-type poliovirus. In all groups, most of the patients showed clinical and virologic responses.

DOSAGE

Pleconaril is manufactured as a hard gelatin capsule and an oral solution. The capsule contains 200 mg of drug, and doses used in adults and older children have been 200 to 400 mg every 8 hours for 7 days (21 doses). An oral solution also has been prepared for pediatric use. It contains 40 mg/mL of pleconaril, medium-chain triglycerides, two surfactants (Tween 80 and Arlacel), 1.5% saccharin, and cherry-peppermint flavoring. Doses of 5 to 7.5 mg/kg of the oral solution administered every 8 to 12 hours for 7 days (14 to 21 doses) have been used in clinical trials of young children, infants, and neonates.[379] Oral pleconaril is generally well tolerated by all age groups.

ADVERSE EFFECTS

Adverse effects associated with pleconaril treatment include nausea, diarrhea, stomach upset or discomfort, and headache. Serious toxicities have not been documented to date, and preclinical studies did not show teratogenicity or fetal toxicity.

Antiviral Agents Active against DNA Viruses (Table 238–3)

ACYCLOVIR

Spectrum of Activity

Acyclovir (9-[(2-hydroxyethoxy)methyl]-9H-guanine; a.k.a. acycloguanosine) is an analogue of the nucleoside deoxyguanosine that has selective activity against the herpes family of viruses[101, 127] (Fig. 238–6). It has the most potent antiviral activity against HSV type 1 and inhibits the virus at concentrations of 0.02 to 0.9 μg/mL.[459, 472] Inhibitory concentrations of HSV type 2 and VZV are also high, at 0.3 to 2.2 μg/mL and 0.8 to 4.0 μg/mL, respectively.[37, 392, 459, 472] In addition, EBV replication is inhibited by acyclovir at a mean concentration of 1.6 μg/mL, but the drug has no effect on cells latently infected with EBV.[85, 286] CMV also is inhibited by very high concentrations of acyclovir (2 to 57 μg/mL).[37] Acyclovir has in vitro activity against simian herpesvirus B and hepatitis B virus (HBV).[33, 219, 459]

Mechanism of Action and Resistance

Acyclovir is phosphorylated to acyclovir monophosphate by viral TK. Cellular enzymes then convert the monophosphate form to acyclovir triphosphate, the active form of the drug.[472] Acyclovir triphosphate is present in HSV-infected cells at 40 to 100 times the concentration found in uninfected cells, and it competitively inhibits viral DNA polymerase in infected cells. Acyclovir triphosphate also is incorporated into viral DNA and, because it lacks the 3′-hydroxyl group, acts as a chain terminator during viral DNA synthesis. The DNA polymerase enzymes of the various herpesviruses differ in their degree of inhibition by acyclovir triphosphate, and for EBV and CMV, which do not contain viral TK, this inhibition accounts for most of the antiviral effect of the drug.[111, 154] Host cellular growth also can be inhibited by acyclovir, but only at levels thousands of times higher than those that inhibit viral replication. This relatively selective mechanism of antiviral action provides a uniquely high therapeutic index.

Three basic mechanisms of resistance have been identified for herpesviruses to become resistant to acyclovir: deficient TK activity caused by absent or low production of viral TK, altered TK activity caused by abnormal substrate specificity so that the enzyme is present and able to phosphorylate but just does not phosphorylate acyclovir, and altered

TABLE 238–3 ■ CLINICAL INDICATIONS AND USUAL TREATMENT DOSAGES FOR ANTIVIRAL AGENTS ACTIVE AGAINST DNA VIRUSES

Agent	Indication	Dosage
Acyclovir	HSV—mucocutaneous	5% ointment 6x daily; 15 mg/kg/dose PO 5x daily (max, 200 mg/dose); 5–10 mg/kg/dose IV q8h
	HSV—encephalitis	10–20 mg/kg/dose IV q8h
	HSV—neonatal	20 mg/kg/dose IV q8h
	VZV—chickenpox and zoster	20 mg/kg/dose (max, 800 mg) PO q6h; 10 mg/kg/dose (500 mg/m^2/dose) IV q8h
Valacyclovir	HSV	500–1000 mg/dose PO bid*
	VZV—zoster	1000 mg/dose PO bid*
Penciclovir	HSV—mucocutaneous	1% cream q2h
Famciclovir	HSV—mucocutaneous	125–500 mg PO bid*
	VZV—zoster	500 mg PO tid*
Ganciclovir	CMV	5–6 mg/kg/dose IV q12h—induction; 5 mg/kg/dose qd 5 days/wk *or* 1000 mg PO tid* *or* 500 mg PO 6x daily*—maintenance
Valganciclovir	CMV	900 mg PO bid*—induction; 900 mg PO qd*—maintenance
Foscarnet	CMV	60 mg/kg/dose IV q8h—induction; 90–120 mg/kg/dose daily—maintenance
Cidofovir	CMV	5 mg/kg/dose IV weekly *or* 1 mg/kg/dose IV 3x/wk—induction; 5 mg/kg q2wk—maintenance

*Only adult dosages are available at this time.
CMV, cytomegalovirus; HSV, herpes simplex virus; VZV, varicella-zoster virus.

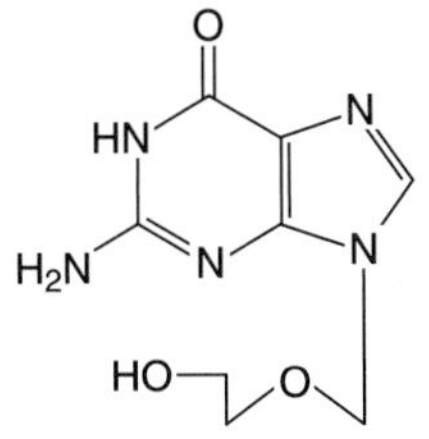

Acyclovir

FIGURE 238–6 ■ Structure of acyclovir.

DNA polymerase.[70] Most clinical isolates of HSV that are resistant to acyclovir have deficient TK activity, and most resistant VZV isolates have altered TK activity or altered DNA polymerase.[346] The prevalence of acyclovir-resistant HSV isolates in normal hosts is less than 1 percent, but it can be as high as 10 to 20 percent in immunocompromised hosts receiving acyclovir therapy for 2 weeks or longer.[79, 100, 133, 159, 208] Resistant strains of VZV, on the other hand, are unusual.[86] Resistant HSV and VZV isolates retain virulence and can cause disease, especially extensive mucocutaneous lesions in immunocompromised hosts, but invasive diseases such as keratitis, uveitis, meningoencephalitis, and pneumonia also have occurred with resistant strains of HSV.[79, 133, 159, 208, 233, 417] Immunocompromised hosts may shed resistant strains of HSV for prolonged periods and may experience recurrent disease with either sensitive or resistant strains. Such mutants are also cross-resistant to other antiviral agents that require viral TK for phosphorylation and activation (e.g., penciclovir and ganciclovir), but they are inhibited by antiviral agents that have different mechanisms of action (e.g., foscarnet, cidofovir, and trifluridine).

Pharmacokinetics

Acyclovir is available for topical, oral, and intravenous administration. Systemic absorption of acyclovir after topical application to intact skin is minimal (<0.01 μg/mL), and in one study in which acyclovir ointment was applied to zoster lesions in immunocompromised patients, plasma concentrations of less than 0.1 to 0.78 μg/mL were observed, thus suggesting some degree of percutaneous absorption.[93, 459] The bioavailability of oral acyclovir is low (15 to 21%), with peak plasma concentrations of 0.4 to 0.8 μg/mL observed after the intake of one 200-mg capsule and concentrations of up to 1.6 μg/mL observed after an 800-mg dose.[40] When an equivalent dose in liquid suspension is administered to children, slightly lower peak plasma levels of 1.0 μg/mL were observed.[438] Intravenous infusion of 5 mg/kg for 1 hour provides peak plasma levels of 9.8 μg/mL, whereas plasma levels of 20.7 μg/mL are produced after a 10-mg/kg infusion. Most of the administered dose of acyclovir is excreted unchanged in urine.[459] The elimination $t_{1/2}$ of acyclovir is 2.5 to 3 hours in adult patients with normal renal function, slightly longer (3.8 hours) in neonates, and up to 20 hours in anuric patients.[40, 150, 212] Therefore, dose adjustment, according to creatinine clearance, is needed in patients with renal insufficiency or renal failure.[278] Probenecid administration decreases renal clearance and prolongs the $t_{1/2}$ of acyclovir. Acyclovir is distributed widely into a variety of body fluids, including saliva (13% of plasma levels), vaginal secretions (15 to 170% of plasma levels), zoster vesicular fluid (90 to 100% of plasma levels), aqueous humor (37% of plasma levels), breast milk (>300% of plasma levels), amniotic fluid and placenta (>200% of plasma levels), and CSF (50% of plasma levels.[150, 229, 259, 279, 316] More than half the drug is removed by hemodialysis, but very little after peritoneal dialysis.[268, 278]

Clinical Indications, Dosage, and Adverse Effects

CLINICAL INDICATIONS

Topical acyclovir may decrease healing time and viral shedding slightly in mucocutaneous lesions of patients experiencing primary infection with HSV.[93] Little, if any clinical benefit has been documented in patients with recurrent herpes simplex lesions; however, some patients report a soothing sensation after application of ointment to the lesions. Topical therapy also may produce a mild clinical benefit in immunocompromised patients with zoster lesions.[459] Oral acyclovir significantly reduces viral shedding, clinical symptoms, and time until lesion healing in normal and immunocompromised patients with a variety of mucocutaneous lesions (e.g., orolabial, pharyngeal, genital, rectal, gingivostomatitis, whitlow, skin) associated with primary HSV infection.[8, 375, 472] It also has been used to treat eye disease, including dendritic corneal ulcers.[90, 205]

Oral acyclovir provides benefit to normal and immunocompromised children, adolescents, and adults with primary infection with VZV (varicella or chickenpox). Treatment reduces the duration of fever by 24 hours, the mean number of skin lesions, and the time to total crusting of lesions by 2 days. Postexposure prophylaxis with oral acyclovir also may reduce the risk of acquiring varicella by close and household contacts of patients with varicella. Administration of oral acyclovir during pregnancy is likely to clinically benefit a mother with varicella, but whether it reduces the risk of congenital or neonatal disease is not clear at this time. Recurrent HSV disease also is improved with oral acyclovir therapy. When administered during the prodrome or at the very first sign of lesions, treatment reduces viral shedding and time to lesion healing by 1.5 to 2 days.[366, 460] Long-term, continuous suppressive therapy with oral acyclovir may be of benefit in some patients with frequent episodes of recurrent mucocutaneous disease, but asymptomatic shedding and person-to-person transmission still may occur.[166, 376] Patients with recurrent skin disease, whitlow, or erythema multiforme may benefit from long-term suppressive therapy with oral acyclovir. Oral acyclovir suppression also reduces recurrences of genital herpes simplex during the last trimester of pregnancy and decreases the need for cesarean section delivery.[53, 397, 399, 400, 401] Short-term prophylaxis administered during a period of risk for recurrence (sunlight exposure, for example) may reduce the clinical recurrence of mucocutaneous disease. Oral acyclovir reduces virus shedding, time to skin lesion healing, and the duration of zoster-associated pain.[29, 84] Treatment combined with steroids also appears to decrease the frequency and severity of postherpetic neuralgia in older patients and the elderly, but specific trials conducted in children have not been performed because children seldom experience postherpetic neuralgia. Oral acyclovir also may reduce recurrences of HSV and VZV in bone marrow and solid organ transplant recipients. Its effect on CMV and EBV disease in these patients, however, is minimal, if any. Continuous suppressive therapy with oral acyclovir reduces cutaneous recurrences after neonatal infection when administered after a 14- to 21-day course of intravenous therapy has been completed.[258] Whether long-term oral suppressive therapy in neonates also prevents CNS recurrence is unclear at this time. Bell palsy associated with HSV infection may be treated with a combination of acyclovir and prednisone.[4] EBV-associated diseases have been treated with acyclovir, with variable clinical benefit.[397, 439] Oral hairy leukoplakia, however, appears to respond to oral acyclovir treatment.[368] Treatment of patients with infectious mononucleosis reduces viral shedding but does not alter the disease course.[451] No clinical benefit has been documented when acyclovir was used to treat chronic hepatitis B.[33]

Intravenous acyclovir is used to treat all severe or life-threatening diseases caused by HSV and VZV, including encephalitis, hepatitis, neonatal disease, acute retinal necrosis syndrome, mucocutaneous disease, and zoster, with or without visceral dissemination, in both normal and immunocompromised patients.[177, 256, 261, 270, 344, 458, 483] Pediatric patients suffering from severe herpetic gingivostomatitis may benefit as well.[8] Early clinical trials also showed efficacy in the treatment of primary genital HSV infection.[92] In addition, normal patients with complications of varicella, including pneumonitis, encephalitis, and hepatitis, should receive intravenous acyclovir.[177] Other diseases associated with VZV in which acyclovir treatment is beneficial include zoster ophthalmicus with complications such as keratitis, anterior uveitis, or contralateral hemiplegia, as well as acute retinal necrosis syndrome.[344, 417] Intravenous acyclovir is also highly effective in reducing the incidence of disease associated with HSV and VZV in marrow and solid organ transplant recipients. Moreover, it may help reduce serious CMV disease in selected marrow and solid organ transplant recipients, although it clearly is not as effective as ganciclovir or other antiviral agents with specific activity against CMV.[18, 19, 43, 317, 455] Treatment of human herpes infection with simian virus B requires high doses of intravenous acyclovir administered over a prolonged period, followed by suppressive therapy.[219] Despite in vitro activity, clinical benefit has not been documented in patients with hepatitis B.[33]

DOSAGE

Topical acyclovir as a 5 percent ointment can be applied to local lesions every 3 to 4 hours five to six times daily for 7 days.[93] If the disease is unresponsive or severe, systemic therapy with oral or intravenous acyclovir should be initiated.

Oral acyclovir is formulated as 200-mg capsules, 800-mg tablets, or a 200-mg/5mL banana-flavored suspension. The usual dose used to treat mucocutaneous lesions caused by primary infection with HSV in adults and adolescents is 200 mg administered five times daily for 10 days. The usual pediatric oral dose is 15 mg/kg per dose (maximum, 200 mg per dose) administered five times daily for 10 days. Recurrent HSV disease in adults and adolescents may be treated with a variety of different regimens: 800 mg three times daily for 2 days, 400 mg three times daily for 5 days, or 200 mg five times daily for 5 days.[244, 245, 460] Suppressive doses of 400 mg administered twice daily, often for many years, seem to be safe and effective.[166] This dose, administered to pregnant women with recent primary or recurrent genital herpes, also appears to decrease recurrences at or near delivery and diminish the need for cesarean section delivery.[53, 259, 401] After intravenous therapy has been completed, the usual dose for neonatal suppressive therapy is 300 mg/m^2 per dose administered three times daily for 6 months.[258] Because neonatal prophylaxis decreases, but does not eliminate the risk for CNS recurrence and because the emergence of resistant strains has been documented, all early cutaneous recurrences that occur despite compliance with oral prophylaxis, as well as other signs and symptoms suggestive of recurrent visceral or CNS disease, should be evaluated carefully in young infants, and the need for systemic therapy should be considered.[258] Oral acyclovir must be administered in higher doses to treat varicella and other VZV-associated diseases.[472] Adults and adolescents require 800-mg doses administered five times daily for 7 to 10 days or until lesions have crusted over.[23, 462] The pediatric dose of acyclovir to treat varicella or chickenpox is 20 mg/kg (up to 800 mg maximum) per dose (80 mg/kg/day) administered four times daily for 5 days or until lesions have crusted.[7, 124]

The usual dose for intravenous administration of acyclovir to treat serious disease associated with HSV is 5 to 10 mg/kg per dose administered as a 1-hour infusion every 8 hours.[357, 459, 472] Treatment for a duration of 7 days is usually sufficient for mucocutaneous disease, but it should be continued until all lesions are healed. Herpes encephalitis should be treated for at least 10 to 14 days or longer, depending on clinical response and clearance of HSV DNA from the CSF.[255, 256, 271, 471] The usual recommend dose to treat neonatal HSV disease with disseminated visceral involvement or encephalitis is a high-dose regimen of 20 mg/kg per dose administered every 8 hours (60 mg/kg/day) for at least 21 days or until HSV DNA has cleared from the CSF, whichever is longer.[255, 256] Some experts use a slightly lower dose (15 mg/kg per dose or 45 mg/kg/day) and a slightly shorter duration of therapy (14 days) for neonates with proven skin/eye/mouth disease without clinical and laboratory evidence of visceral or CNS involvement. Clinical studies have documented that these higher doses are safe in neonates, but it has not been established clearly that they have superior efficacy over lower doses. Treatment of VZV-associated disease requires higher doses of acyclovir: 500 mg/m^2 per dose (10 to 20 mg/kg per dose) administered every 8 hours (total, 1500 mg/m^2/day) for at least 5 to 7 days or until all lesions have been crusted over for 24 to 48 hours.[459, 472] In all clinical indications, the dosage of intravenously administered acyclovir should be adjusted according to creatinine clearance in patients with renal insufficiency and renal failure.

ADVERSE EFFECTS

Adverse effects of acyclovir are unusual.[250] Topical application of the ointment may cause pain or local irritation, usually caused by the polyethylene glycol base.[93, 459] Handwashing must be performed after each local application to lesions to avoid autoinoculation or person-to-person transmission. Oral acyclovir may cause nausea and diarrhea, rash, or headache.[459] Long-term oral acyclovir appears to be safe in adults but may be associated with neutropenia in 46 percent of infants who receive suppression after treatment of neonatal HSV infection.[258, 319] Intravenous acyclovir is generally well tolerated. However, extravasation of the drug (pH 9 to 11) can cause inflammation, ulceration, and necrosis of surrounding tissue.[250, 440] Phlebitis also can develop. Neurotoxicity occurs rarely, usually in patients with renal insufficiency who have high serum concentrations.[28, 139, 178, 457] Neurotoxicity associated with acyclovir is characterized by lethargy, confusion, tremor, and rarely, seizures and coma. Renal tubular damage, crystalline nephropathy, or interstitial nephritis may occur in approximately 5 percent of patients.[360, 390] These renal complications are more likely to develop in patients who are not adequately hydrated or in whom the drug has been infused at a rate faster than the recommended infusion time of 1 hour. No excess frequency of adverse events has been reported to date in pregnant women who receive acyclovir or in their fetuses or newborns.[53, 67, 259, 397, 401, 483] Therefore, based on available information, acyclovir seems to be safe when administered during pregnancy, especially during the last trimester, and does not appear to have any significant adverse effects.

VALACYCLOVIR

Spectrum of Activity

Valacyclovir (L-valine, 2-[(2-amino-1,6-dihydro-6-oxo-9H-purin-9-yl)methoxy]ethylester monohydrochloride, a.k.a. valacyclovir hydrochloride) is the hydrochloride salt of the L-valine ester of acyclovir.[30] It has essentially the same selective spectrum of antiviral activity against the herpesviruses as acyclovir does.[35]

Mechanism of Action and Resistance

Valacyclovir is converted rapidly to acyclovir and therefore has the same mechanisms of action and resistance as acyclovir does.[35] Viral isolates that are resistant to acyclovir will be resistant to valacyclovir.

Pharmacokinetics

The pharmacokinetics of valacyclovir has not been studied in the pediatric population, but information gained from adults can be applied, in many ways, to pediatric patients. After oral administration, valacyclovir is absorbed rapidly from the gastrointestinal tract. It is metabolized by first pass through the intestinal tract and also by the liver into acyclovir and L-valine.[35] It has the advantage over acyclovir of having 54 percent bioavailability (versus 20% for acyclovir), which is not altered by food.[422] A single dose of 1 g of valacyclovir administered to an adult produces plasma levels of 0.4 to 0.8 μg/mL. The $t_{1/2}$ is 2.5 to 3 hours, similar to acyclovir, and is prolonged in patients with renal insufficiency or renal failure.[464, 466] The drug is removed by hemodialysis. The rate, but not the extent of conversion of valacyclovir to acyclovir is prolonged in patients with liver disease.

Clinical Indications, Dosage, and Adverse Effects

CLINICAL INDICATIONS

Valacyclovir has been reported to be effective in treating primary and recurrent mucocutaneous disease caused by HSV-1, HSV-2, and VZV.[35, 36, 42, 284, 367, 429] Randomized clinical trials conducted in adult patients showed valacyclovir to be superior to placebo and comparable to acyclovir in reducing the number and duration of lesions, pain, and time to healing in patients with primary and recurrent genital herpes and zoster.[42, 367, 429] It is also comparable to acyclovir for suppression of genital herpes recurrences. Furthermore, in a study of 27 CMV-seropositive heart transplant recipients, valacyclovir appeared to be equal or superior to oral acyclovir in preventing both laboratory and clinical parameters of CMV reactivation.[126] Because valacyclovir is converted to acyclovir, it is likely to be effective for all the clinical indications for which acyclovir has been shown to be effective.

DOSAGE

Valacyclovir is available only in 500-mg caplets; therefore, a pediatric liquid formulation is not available at this time. The usual dose is 1 g twice daily for 10 days for primary genital herpes and 500 mg twice daily for 3 to 5 days for recurrent disease.[35, 42, 284, 429] A daily dose of 500 mg has been used safely for longer than a year to suppress recurrences of HSV disease.[298] The dose to treat VZV-associated disease is higher than that for HSV-associated disease. A dose of 1 g three times a day for at least 7 days is usually necessary to treat zoster, and therapy should be continued until the lesions have dried.[36] The dose of valacyclovir should be adjusted according to creatinine clearance in patients with renal insufficiency or renal failure.

ADVERSE EFFECTS

The adverse effects of oral valacyclovir are similar to the those of oral acyclovir and include gastrointestinal disturbances such as nausea, vomiting, and diarrhea.[35] Headache and behavioral changes also have been observed. Overdosage may produce precipitation of acyclovir in the renal tubules, as well as CNS toxicity.

PENCICLOVIR

Spectrum of Activity

Penciclovir (9-[4-hydroxy-3-hydroxymethylbut-1-yl]guanine) is an acyclic guanosine analogue with a selective spectrum of activity against the herpesviruses similar to that of acyclovir[48] (Fig. 238–7). This compound inhibits HSV-1 at very low concentrations (0.2 to 0.6 μg/mL) and HSV-2 at slightly higher concentrations (0.3 to 2.4 μg/mL).[16, 48, 167, 465] At even higher concentrations (0.9 to 4.0 μg/mL), it inhibits VZV.[16, 17] The compound has very little activity against CMV, with concentrations greater than 50 μg/mL required to inhibit CMV. However, penciclovir does have activity against hepatitis B virus.[89, 266, 403]

Mechanism of Action and Resistance

Like acyclovir, penciclovir is preferentially phosphorylated by viral TK in virus-infected cells to penciclovir monophosphate and by cellular enzymes to penciclovir triphosphate, which is the active form of the drug.[125] Penciclovir triphosphate competitively inhibits viral DNA polymerase. It is approximately 100 times less potent than acyclovir triphosphate in inhibiting viral DNA polymerase, but an antiviral effect is achieved because it is present in high concentrations for a prolonged period (7 to 20 hours) in virus-infected cells. However, unlike acyclovir, penciclovir is not a chain terminator during DNA synthesis. Penciclovir triphosphate also inhibits the DNA polymerase of HBV. Emergence of HSV strains resistant to penciclovir has been minimal.[282] Similar to HSV isolates resistant to acyclovir, isolates resistant to penciclovir may have viral TK gene mutations that produce mutants with deficient or altered TK activity, or they may have mutations in DNA polymerase genes.[74] Strains of acyclovir-resistant HSV that are TK-deficient mutants also will be resistant to penciclovir, but strains of acyclovir-resistant HSV that are TK altered may be susceptible to penciclovir.[49, 348]

Pharmacokinetics

Penciclovir is poorly absorbed after oral administration.[147] Adults who received a 10-mg/kg intravenous infusion of

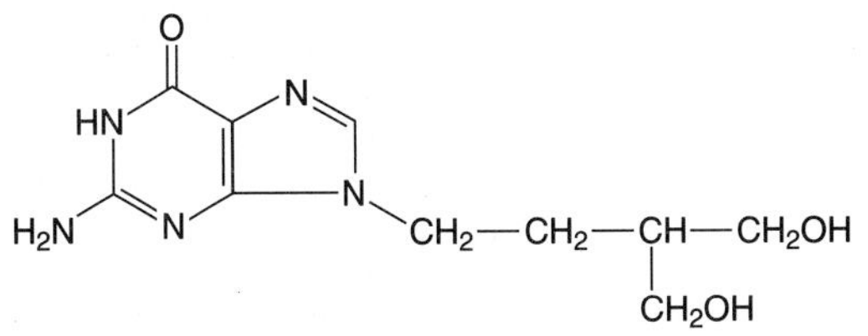

Penciclovir

FIGURE 238–7 ■ Structure of penciclovir.

penciclovir had plasma levels of 12 μg/mL, but no pediatric information is available. Penciclovir 1 percent cream is not absorbed systemically. The systemic pharmacokinetics of penciclovir is discussed under "Famciclovir."

Clinical Indications, Dosage, and Adverse Effects

Penciclovir is available in the United States as a 1 percent cream in a propylene glycol base and is licensed for the treatment of herpes labialis lesions on the lips and face. Maximal clinical benefit occurs when the cream is applied to the lesions early, at the first clinical sign of disease, every 2 hours while awake for 3 to 5 days.[428] Application of penciclovir cream may be associated with local skin reactions, most likely caused by the propylene glycol base. An intravenous form of penciclovir has been tested in Europe, but it is not available in the United States. Penciclovir is not absorbed orally, but it is available as the oral prodrug famciclovir, which is converted rapidly to penciclovir. Dosages and systemic adverse effects of penciclovir are discussed under "Famciclovir."

FAMCICLOVIR

Spectrum of Activity

Famciclovir (2-[(2-amino-9H-purin-9-yl)]-1, 3-propanedial diacetate) is the prodrug of the antiviral agent penciclovir, which has selective activity against HSV-1, HSV-2, VZV, and HBV.

Mechanism of Action and Resistance

Famciclovir undergoes rapid transformation to penciclovir, which is monophosphorylated by viral TK to penciclovir monophosphate; the monophosphate, in turn, is converted by cellular enzymes to penciclovir triphosphate, the active form of the antiviral compound. Penciclovir then competitively inhibits viral DNA polymerase and, thereby, viral replication. The prolonged intracellular $t_{1/2}$ observed with penciclovir also is observed with famciclovir. Penciclovir-resistant strains of HSV and VZV occur when mutations produce deficient or altered TK or altered DNA polymerase. Most TK-deficient acyclovir-resistant strains of HSV are also resistant to penciclovir.

Pharmacokinetics

Famciclovir is the diacetyl-6-deoxy analogue of the antiviral compound penciclovir. After oral administration, famciclovir is absorbed rapidly from the gastrointestinal tract with excellent (77%) bioavailability, and then it is metabolized in the liver by deacetylation and oxidation to form penciclovir. Single oral doses of 250 and 500 mg of famciclovir administered to adults produce peak plasma penciclovir levels of 1.6 to 1.9 μg/mL and 2.7 to 4.0 μg/mL, respectively. Administration of famciclovir with food reduces peak plasma concentrations by slowing the absorption time but does not alter the overall bioavailability of the drug. The $t_{1/2}$ for penciclovir is 2 to 3 hours, after which it is excreted by filtration and active tubular secretion by the kidneys. Nonrenal clearance by fecal excretion also occurs for as much as one third of the oral dose. Excretion of penciclovir is decreased in patients with renal insufficiency and renal failure, and in patients with liver disease, peak plasma levels may be reduced.[44] Penciclovir is removed from the body by hemodialysis. After oral administration of famciclovir to rats, penciclovir is concentrated in breast milk; however, no studies have been performed in lactating mothers to confirm such concentration in humans.

Clinical Indications, Dosage, and Adverse Effects

CLINICAL INDICATIONS

In adult clinical trials, oral famciclovir was as effective as oral acyclovir and superior to placebo in treating recurrent mucocutaneous infections with HSV and VZV in both normal and immunocompromised patients.[82, 299, 381, 452] When given early in the course of illness, time to lesion crusting and healing, duration of viral shedding, and length of acute pain all were shortened by treatment with famciclovir. In some studies, the duration of postherpetic neuralgia in elderly patients with zoster also was shortened.[452] Although to date it has not been studied specifically in clinical trials of patients with primary HSV and VZV infection, famciclovir probably also will provide clinical benefit in these conditions.[291] In addition, famciclovir is effective as suppressive therapy to reduce HSV recurrences and viral shedding.[113, 315] Famciclovir also has been used to treat chronic HBV infection and for prophylaxis against recurrent HBV infection in liver transplant recipients.[183, 299, 406] No clinical trials in pediatric patients have been conducted.

DOSAGE

Famciclovir is available in 125-, 250-, and 500-mg tablets. An oral suspension for pediatric use is not available. The usual recommended oral dose of famciclovir to treat primary and recurrent mucocutaneous HSV disease is 125 mg twice daily for 5 days.[381] Dosages of suppressive therapy are slightly higher, 250 mg twice daily for as long as 1 year. Of note is that clinical trials showed that single daily doses of 250 mg were not as effective as the twice-daily regimen in suppressing recurrences. For immunocompromised patients, especially those infected with HIV, even higher doses (500 mg twice daily for 7 days) may be necessary.[391] Treatment of VZV-associated disease such as zoster also requires higher doses, 500 mg twice or three times daily for 10 days.[452] All dosage regimens should be reduced, according to creatinine clearance, in patients with renal insufficiency or renal failure.

ADVERSE EFFECTS

Adverse effects of treatment with oral famciclovir are unusual and include gastrointestinal disturbances such as nausea and diarrhea; rash; CNS complaints such as confusion, hallucinations, and disorientation; neutropenia; and elevated liver transaminases.[82, 103, 386]

GANCICLOVIR

Spectrum of Activity

Ganciclovir (9-[1,3-dihydroxy-2-propoxymethyl] guanine, a.k.a. DHPG) is an analogue of deoxyguanosine, similar to acyclovir, yet different in that it has an additional hydroxymethyl group on the acyclic side chain[138, 141, 354, 409] (Fig. 238–8). This antiviral compound has selective activity against the herpesviruses, with uniquely potent antiviral activity against CMV. Ganciclovir inhibits HSV-1 and HSV-2 at 0.05 to 0.6 μg/mL, VZV at 0.4 to 10 μg/mL, CMV at 0.02 to 3.4 μg/mL, and EBV at 1.5 μg/mL. Human herpesvirus-6 (HHV-6), HHV-7, and HHV-8 also may be inhibited by ganciclovir.[249] It has in vitro activity against adenoviruses

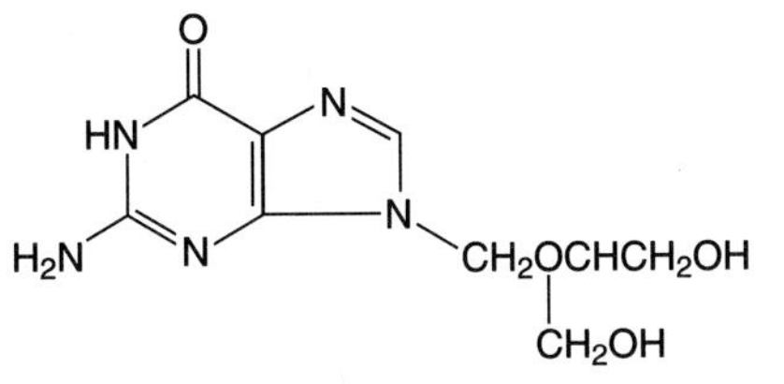

Ganciclovir

FIGURE 238–8 ■ Structure of ganciclovir.

and HBV as well.[138, 164, 327, 446] High concentrations (30 to >700 µg/mL) of ganciclovir will inhibit the growth of most uninfected mammalian cells; bone marrow–derived cells, however, appear to be uniquely sensitive and can be inhibited at much lower concentrations (<0.7 µg/mL).

Mechanism of Action and Resistance

Ganciclovir is monophosphorylated in infected cells by virus-induced enzymes: TK in HSV-infected cells and protein kinases that are encoded by the *UL97* phosphotransferase gene in CMV-infected cells.[37, 138, 288, 409] Cellular enzymes complete the phosphorylation to ganciclovir triphosphate, the active form of the compound, which is concentrated in infected cells. Ganciclovir triphosphate competitively inhibits the incorporation of deoxyguanosine triphosphate into viral DNA, where it slows and stops viral DNA chain elongation and produces short, noninfectious viral DNA fragments.[185] Ganciclovir also preferentially inhibits viral DNA polymerase.[294] Ganciclovir resistance has been detected in 8 to 38 percent of immunocompromised adult and pediatric patients who have received prolonged administration of ganciclovir, and such resistance is an important clinical problem.[76, 121, 163, 430]

Patients may be infected with single or multiple strains of CMV, with both drug-sensitive and drug-resistant strains mixed in the population.[135] Resistant strains may be induced or infect a patient primarily, emerge quickly after only weeks of therapy, or evolve more slowly and emerge sequentially after several months of antiviral prophylaxis or therapy.[77, 135, 230, 377, 478] These resistant mutants also retain virulence and are capable of producing serious and progressive disease.[45, 135, 230, 420, 448] Ganciclovir resistance in CMV strains occurs by at least two mechanisms: (1) point mutations or deletions in the *UL97* gene that reduce intracellular phosphorylation of ganciclovir and (2) point mutations in the viral DNA polymerase *UL54 (pol)* gene that alter the function of the polymerase.[76, 294, 414, 430] Most strains of CMV that are resistant to ganciclovir have *UL97* mutations (most commonly at codons 460, 520, 594, and 595) and reduced phosphorylation, but they remain susceptible to foscarnet and cidofovir.[75, 76, 430] However, CMV strains that are resistant to ganciclovir because of a mutation in the *UL54* DNA polymerase gene also may be resistant to foscarnet or cidofovir, or to both.[294, 387] Moreover, multiple highly resistant strains of CMV may occur if both *UL97* phosphotransferase and *UL54* DNA polymerase gene mutations are present.[77, 414] Resistance conferred by *UL54* mutations usually emerges after *UL97* mutations have occurred.[163, 414] Ganciclovir resistance in HSV occurs in TK-deficient, acyclovir-resistant strains of the virus.

Pharmacokinetics

Intravenous administration of a 5-mg/kg dose of ganciclovir in adults produces peak plasma levels of 8 to 11 µg/mL.[138, 144] Similar pharmacokinetics in 10 pediatric patients aged 9 months to 12 years has been observed.[155] A study of the pharmacokinetics of ganciclovir in 27 neonates aged 2 to 49 days who were administered intravenous ganciclovir to treat congenital CMV disease showed a dose of 6 mg/kg to be the most appropriate dose for that age group.[449, 488] After intravenous administration, ganciclovir is distributed in CSF at 24 to 70 percent of plasma levels, and 38 percent of plasma levels enter brain tissue.[82] Drug levels in aqueous, vitreous, and subretinal fluid in the eye are comparable to serum levels, and even higher levels can be achieved with intravitreal implants.[13, 144, 269, 301, 328] Ganciclovir also accumulates in breast milk in animal models.[5] The plasma $t_{1/2}$ is 2 to 4 hours in adults with normal renal function and longer than 24 hours in patients with renal insufficiency and renal failure.[419] The drug is eliminated by renal excretion, and dose reduction is required for patients with impaired creatinine clearance. Hydration will enhance elimination of the drug, and hemodialysis removes 60 percent of ganciclovir in plasma.[419] Ganciclovir also can be administered orally. Its oral bioavailability is rather poor: 5 percent under fasting conditions and 6 to 9 percent if administered with food.[10, 280] Oral doses of 1000 mg administered to adults every 8 hours produce plasma levels of 0.9 to 1.2 µg/mL.[10, 424] A recently licensed valine ester prodrug of ganciclovir, valganciclovir, has high oral bioavailability.[300]

Clinical Indications, Dosage, and Adverse Effects

CLINICAL INDICATIONS

Ganciclovir is used for the treatment of established CMV disease, for early or preemptive therapy in immunocompromised patients with virologic markers of active infection that are predictive of CMV disease, and for prophylaxis of high-risk patients such as those who are CMV-seropositive or who have received transplants from CMV-seropositive donors. Ganciclovir is licensed for treatment and chronic suppression of sight-threatening CMV retinitis in immunocompromised patients and for prevention of CMV disease in transplant recipients. Clinical trials have demonstrated efficacy in these conditions.* Treatment with ganciclovir also is beneficial in immunocompromised individuals with other forms of invasive CMV disease, including pneumonia, colitis, esophagitis, myocarditis, encephalitis, persistent fever and leukopenia syndrome, and viral sepsis syndrome.† Treating established CMV pneumonia in bone marrow and stem cell transplant recipients is difficult, and the disease may not respond to ganciclovir treatment, with or without immune modulators or globulins. Most clinical trials have been performed in adults, but children and infants with CMV disease benefit from treatment as well. Ganciclovir treatment also has been evaluated in newborns congenitally infected with CMV with CNS involvement.[257, 449, 488] In addition, ganciclovir is used for preemptive therapy for patients (primarily recipients of solid organ, marrow, and stem cell transplants) with virologic markers that are predictive of serious CMV disease.[52, 169, 207, 426] Prophylaxis with ganciclovir to prevent CMV infection and disease in immunocompromised patients, including solid organ and bone marrow transplant recipients and patients with acquired immunodeficiency syndrome (AIDS), also has been beneficial in most groups studied.[52, 123, 168, 426, 476, 477] Prophylaxis reduces the risk for the acquisition of serious CMV disease or, in some groups, prolongs the incubation period, but it does not eliminate the risk.[123, 168, 395, 476] Ganciclovir prophylaxis is also effective

*See references 52, 99, 123, 168, 169, 207, 218, 314, 395, 476.
†See references 60, 80, 88, 115, 119, 129, 363, 364, 424, 426, 427.

in preventing HSV infection in immunocompromised patients.[168] Ganciclovir appears to decrease HBV DNA levels and to improve hepatic enzymes in patients with post-transplantation infection or reactivation with HBV.[164] In addition, ganciclovir has been used to treat patients with serious disease associated with adenovirus infection, but clinical trials proving efficacy have not been performed.[446]

DOSAGE

Ganciclovir is supplied as a solution for intravenous infusion and as 250- and 500-mg capsules for oral administration. The intravenous infusions are delivered best in a concentration of 10 mg/mL or less and administered over a 1-hour period. Intravitreal implants are also available and are designed to slowly release relatively large doses of ganciclovir locally into the eye over a period of many months. Ganciclovir therapy for serious CMV disease usually is administered in two phases, induction and maintenance. The recommended dose for induction therapy for serious CMV disease in adults and children with normal renal function is 5 mg/kg per dose administered intravenously every 12 hours for 2 to 3 weeks. Successful induction therapy is accompanied by clinical and virologic response. Maintenance therapy at doses of 5 mg/kg/day administered intravenously should be continued in severely immunocompromised patients who are at risk for relapse. Selected patients may receive oral ganciclovir for maintenance therapy. The usual recommended dose for adults is 1000 mg three times daily or, alternatively, 500 mg administered six times daily. The pediatric dose for maintenance oral therapy has not been established. The duration of maintenance therapy should be individualized for each patient, but such therapy usually lasts through the period of greatest risk, such as rejection or immune suppression, or may be lifelong, as in patients with AIDS. Some patients who experience CMV disease, such as solid organ transplant recipients with minimal immune suppression and minimal or no rejection, will respond dramatically to induction therapy and will not require long-term maintenance therapy. A dose of 6 mg/kg administered every 12 hours for 6 weeks has been used to treat newborns with congenital CMV disease.[257, 276, 488] This dose appears to be adequate for term newborns and premature newborns as young as 32 weeks' gestation, provided that renal function seems to be normal for age. The dose for extremely premature newborns is not known and should be individualized according to the clinical judgment of the infectious diseases specialist. Preemptive therapy, 5 mg/kg per dose administered every 12 hours, is initiated when virologic markers for active, invasive infection, such as positive cultures for CMV from bronchoalveolar lavage samples or the presence of CMV DNA-emia or antigenemia, are identified by routine virologic surveillance.[395, 425] After an induction period of 7 to 14 days, maintenance therapy usually is continued for 100 to 120 days after transplantation or longer if the patient remains at high risk for relapse of CMV disease. Prophylaxis with ganciclovir is administered immediately pretransplant and for a defined period post-transplant in patients who are high risk, such as those who are CMV-seropositive pretransplant and those who receive marrow or solid organ transplants from a CMV-seropositive donor.[51, 123, 157, 168, 395, 426, 476, 477] Patients who do not respond to induction therapy or who relapse or progress during maintenance therapy with ganciclovir may have a resistant strain of CMV. The addition of another antiviral with different mechanisms of action, such as foscarnet or cidofovir, may be beneficial. If clinical or virologic responses still are not maintained, the possibility of a multiply resistant CMV strain should be considered. Patients with disseminated adenovirus disease have received doses of 5 mg/kg every 12 hours for 14 or more days, but clinical benefit has not been proved.[327]

ADVERSE EFFECTS

Adverse effects of ganciclovir can be both local and systemic. Local reactions such as phlebitis, irritation, blistering, or ulceration at or around the infusion site can occur and usually are attributed to the alkaline pH (pH 11) of the intravenous solution. Local reactions can be minimized by paying careful attention to the infusion site or by administering the antiviral agent through a central venous catheter. The most common systemic toxicity associated with ganciclovir administration is dose-dependent, reversible neutropenia, which occurs in a third to a half of patients (adults, children, and newborns) who receive this antiviral for longer than 2 weeks.[99, 138] Thrombocytopenia also can occur, most often in patients with AIDS who are receiving other antiviral agents, including antiretrovirals.[216] If the neutropenia is severe (absolute neutrophil count below 500/mm^3), ganciclovir administration should be halted temporarily until the neutrophil count recovers. Ganciclovir then may be readministered, if still clinically indicated, at the same or half the original dose while carefully monitoring the patient for recurrence of the neutropenia. Some experts have used recombinant granulocyte-macrophage colony-stimulating factor successfully to treat ganciclovir-induced neutropenia.[187] Anemia associated with ganciclovir administration is an unusual occurrence. Other adverse effects associated with ganciclovir include CNS disturbances such as headache, behavioral changes, psychosis, seizures, and coma; mild nephrotoxicity with azotemia; liver dysfunction with elevated transaminases; and rash. Ganciclovir also is mutagenic, carcinogenic, and immunosuppressive. In addition, preclinical animal studies showed reproductive toxicity, with teratogenicity, embryotoxicity, and testicular atrophy.[138] Long-term studies in children who received ganciclovir as newborns are being conducted to determine the long-term effects of ganciclovir administration, if any. Also, caretakers who prepare and administer ganciclovir to patients should take precautions to minimize direct exposure to the antiviral agent.

VALGANCICLOVIR

Spectrum of Activity

Valganciclovir (L-valine 2[(2-amino-1,6-dihydro-6-oxy-9H-purin-9-yl)methoxy]-3-hydroxypropyl ester) is a prodrug of ganciclovir and therefore has the same selective spectrum of activity as ganciclovir against herpesviruses, especially CMV, as well as limited activity against adenoviruses and HBV.

Mechanism of Action and Resistance

Valganciclovir is the L-valyl ester (prodrug) of ganciclovir.[300] It is metabolized rapidly in the body to ganciclovir. Ganciclovir then is monophosphorylated by viral protein kinase (coded for by *UL97* genes) in CMV-infected cells and further phosphorylated to the active form ganciclovir triphosphate by cellular kinases. Viral DNA synthesis is inhibited by ganciclovir triphosphate (see "Ganciclovir" for details). Isolates of CMV become resistant to valganciclovir by mutations in *UL97,* the viral kinase gene, or in *UL54,* the viral DNA polymerase gene. Mutations in *UL97* confer resistance to ganciclovir and, therefore, to valganciclovir, whereas mutations in *UL54* confer double or triple resistance to ganciclovir, foscarnet, and cidofovir. Mutations in both genes can produce highly resistant strains of CMV.

Pharmacokinetics

Valganciclovir is well absorbed after oral administration and is rapidly hydrolyzed in the intestine and liver to ganciclovir.[349] The bioavailability of valganciclovir is high, approximately 60 percent (versus 6 to 9% for ganciclovir), and an oral dose of 900 mg administered to adults produces ganciclovir blood levels equivalent to a 5-mg/kg dose administered intravenously.[54, 241, 300] Absorption is enhanced significantly with the ingestion of food, so physicians recommend that valganciclovir be taken with food or meals. The drug is excreted by the kidneys, and renal insufficiency produces prolonged excretion and a longer $t_{1/2}$ (see "Ganciclovir"). The pharmacokinetics of valganciclovir in pediatric patients has not been published; however, a clinical trial studying the pharmacokinetics in newborns congenitally infected with CMV is in progress.

Clinical Indications, Dosage, and Adverse Effects

Valganciclovir is available in 450-mg tablets, and the usual adult dose is 900 mg (two 450-mg tablets) twice daily for 14 days (induction therapy), followed by a maintenance dose of 900 mg administered once daily.[300] Valganciclovir is licensed for induction and maintenance treatment of CMV retinitis in immunocompromised patients, but clinical trials are likely to show that valganciclovir is beneficial to a variety of patients with a number of different CMV infections.[300] A liquid, pediatric formulation is not available at this time. Similar to ganciclovir, if a patient treated with valganciclovir experiences progression of disease or recurrence during maintenance therapy, a resistant strain of CMV should be considered a possibility. Adverse effects associated with the oral administration of valganciclovir are similar to those with oral ganciclovir and include diarrhea and dose-dependent, reversible neutropenia.[300]

FOSCARNET

Spectrum of Activity

Foscarnet (phosphonoformic acid or trisodium phosphonoformate hexahydrate) is a pyrophosphate analogue that selectively inhibits herpesviruses[337] (Fig. 238–9). It also has activity against HIV and HBV.[20, 137] At concentrations of 100 to 300 μmol/L CMV is inhibited, whereas slightly lower concentrations (80 to 200 μmol/L) inhibit HSV types 1 and 2, VZV, EBV, and HHV-8.[337] Concentrations between 20 and 200 μmol/L appear to inhibit HBV. Foscarnet also inhibits most, but not all acyclovir-resistant HSV and VZV strains and most, but not all ganciclovir-resistant CMV strains.[149, 296, 382] Combinations of ganciclovir and foscarnet are synergistic against CMV, and combinations of zidovudine and foscarnet appear to be synergistic against HIV.[137, 296] At high concentrations (500 to 1000 μmol/L), foscarnet inhibits cellular DNA synthesis in uninfected cells.[78]

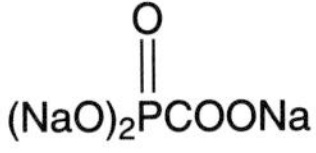

FIGURE 238–9 ■ Structure of foscarnet.

Mechanism of Action and Resistance

Foscarnet is not a nucleoside analogue, and it does not require phosphorylation or any other form of intracellular metabolism to be activated. Rather, it is a pyrophosphate analogue that directly inhibits viral and cellular DNA polymerase.[98, 112] Selective viral inhibition is accomplished by noncompetitively and reversibly blocking the pyrophosphate binding site of the viral polymerase, in much lower concentrations than it inhibits cellular DNA polymerases. Because foscarnet does not require phosphorylation by viral TK or other kinases, it inhibits TK-deficient and altered strains of HSV and VZV that are resistant to acyclovir, as well as *UL97* phosphotransferase mutants of CMV that are resistant to ganciclovir. However, strains of herpesviruses of all types that are resistant to acyclovir or ganciclovir by mutation of the viral DNA polymerase gene are also resistant to foscarnet.[21, 384]

Pharmacokinetics

Intravenous administration of 60 mg of foscarnet every 8 hours to adults produces plasma levels of 450 to 575 μmol/L; 90 mg administered every 12 hours produces plasma levels of 420 to 746 μmol/L.[112, 382] CSF levels are usually approximately 60 percent of plasma levels, and vitreous concentrations in the eye are the same or slightly higher than plasma levels.[204] Most (80%) of the dose of foscarnet is eliminated unmetabolized from the body through the kidneys, and plasma clearance decreases if renal function is impaired. The remaining 20 percent appears to be deposited in teeth and bone, where it accumulates and remains for months. The drug is removed by hemodialysis, but not appreciably by peritoneal dialysis.[6, 295] Oral foscarnet has poor bioavailability (less than 10%) and causes diarrhea, and it is unlikely to be available for patient use.[336] Pharmacokinetic data in infants and children have not been published. However, preclinical studies showed that deposition of foscarnet in teeth and bones is greater in younger than older animals.

Clinical Indications, Dosage, and Adverse Effects

CLINICAL INDICATIONS

Foscarnet is licensed for both induction and maintenance treatment of CMV retinitis in immunocompromised patients and for treatment of mucocutaneous disease caused by acyclovir-resistant HSV.* Foscarnet also may be of benefit in patients with zoster caused by acyclovir-resistant VZV.[382] Because the combination of foscarnet and ganciclovir appears to be synergistic in vitro, immunocompromised patients who experience progression or relapse of CMV disease while receiving therapy with one or the other antiviral agent may benefit from combination therapy in some instances.[122, 149, 234] Foscarnet also may be used for the treatment or prophylaxis of serious or life-threatening CMV disease when ganciclovir is contraindicated or otherwise deemed clinically undesirable because of its myelosuppressive effects.[369, 482] The antiretroviral properties of foscarnet, when combined with other antiviral agents, also may be beneficial in patients with HIV infection or AIDS.[32, 236, 343]

DOSAGE

Treatment with foscarnet usually is divided into two phases, induction and maintenance. The usual dosage of foscarnet for induction therapy is 60 mg/kg per dose administered intravenously every 8 hours for 3 weeks; maintenance

*See references 112, 122, 234, 281, 295, 343, 384, 435, 436,463.

therapy is 90 to 120 mg/kg day administered indefinitely or through the period of risk.[243] The dose of foscarnet should be given slowly, over the course of 2 hours (or no faster than 1 mg/kg/min), to reduce renal toxicity. Creatinine clearance should be used to adjust dosage regimens in patients with renal insufficiency or renal failure. Published experience on the use of foscarnet in pediatric patients is limited, but undoubtedly, certain pediatric patients benefit from receiving foscarnet therapy.[463] In these cases, the same per-kilogram dosage regimens can be used for most patients.

ADVERSE EFFECTS

Foscarnet is associated with serious adverse effects and should be used only after thorough consideration of the risks and benefits involved.[78, 112] Renal toxicity with azotemia, proteinuria, crystalluria, renal tubular acidosis or necrosis, and interstitial nephritis can occur in as many as a third of patients who receive foscarnet.[110, 240] Renal toxicity generally occurs after the first week of therapy and usually is reversible. The risk for the development of renal toxicity is increased if the drug is given by rapid infusion or administered in high doses, if the patient is dehydrated, or if other nephrotoxic drugs are administered concomitantly with foscarnet.[333] Hydration, including saline loading, and administering each dose over the course of at least 2 hours appear to reduce the risk of renal toxicity developing. Foscarnet binds divalent metal ions such as calcium in the body, and metabolic abnormalities, including hypocalcemia and hypercalcemia (total or ionized), hypophosphatemia and hyperphosphatemia, hypomagnesemia, and hypokalemia may occur in approximately a third of patients who receive foscarnet.[235] Symptoms of these acute metabolic abnormalities include perioral tingling, numbness or paresthesias of the limbs, and if severe, seizures, tetany, and cardiac dysrhythmias. Administration of the dose over the course of at least 2 hours also reduces the risk for development of metabolic abnormalities. Foscarnet also can be deposited and concentrate in bone, with as yet unclear long-term consequences.[112] CNS side effects also occur in approximately a fourth of patients and include headache, tremor, seizures, and behavioral changes. Abnormal liver function tests have been noted, and high urinary concentrations of foscarnet may produce painful genital ulcerations and rash in some patients.[417] Preclinical studies showed foscarnet to be mutagenic and associated with anomalies of skeletal development in young animals.[109]

CIDOFOVIR

Spectrum of Activity

Cidofovir (1-[S]-3-hydroxy-2-[phosphonomethoxypropyl]) cytosine dihydrate, a.k.a. HPMPC) is an acyclic phosphonate nucleotide analogue of deoxycytidine monophosphate with broad-spectrum in vitro antiviral activity against all DNA viruses, including herpesviruses (HSV types 1 and 2, CMV, EBV, VZV, and HHV types 6, 7, and 8), adenoviruses, polyomaviruses (JC and BK viruses), papillomaviruses, and poxviruses (vaccinia, variola or smallpox, cowpox, monkeypox, camelpox, and molluscum contagiosum and orf viruses) (Fig. 238–10).* Cidofovir exhibits its most specific and potent antiviral activity against CMV (MIC, 0.25 μmol/L).[71, 72, 120, 130] The compound also is very active against VZV (0.79 μmol/L),

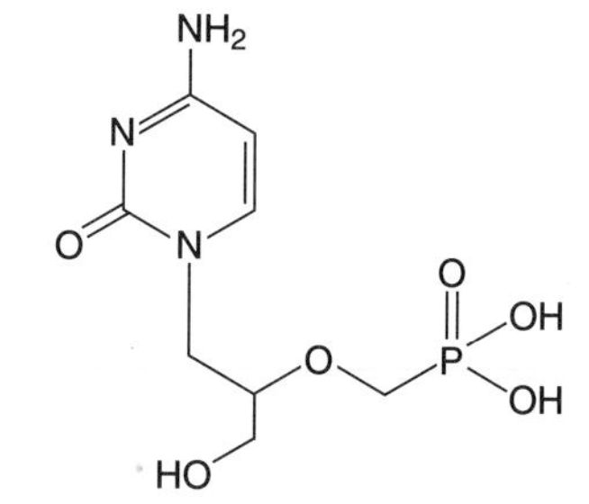

Cidofovir

FIGURE 238–10 ■ Structure of cidofovir.

HSV-1 (12.7 μmol/L), and acyclovir-resistant, TK-deficient HSV-1 strains (6.24 μmol/L).[214, 312, 418] Cidofovir inhibits HSV-2 at concentrations of 31.7 μmol/L, adenoviruses at 10.8 μmol/L, and vaccinia virus at 12.7 μmol/L.[108, 170, 411] Strains of CMV *UL97* mutants that are resistant to ganciclovir are inhibited by cidofovir, and cidofovir in combination with ganciclovir or foscarnet shows synergistic inhibition of CMV in vitro.[383]

Mechanisms of Action and Resistance

Cidofovir inhibits the replication of CMV and other viruses by selective inhibition of viral DNA polymerase.[72, 214, 312] The compound is phosphorylated by cellular enzymes to the active form cidofovir diphosphate. Cidofovir diphosphate inhibits both viral and cellular DNA polymerase; however, because the concentration necessary to inhibit cellular DNA synthesis is hundreds of times higher than that needed to inhibit viral DNA synthesis, cidofovir appears to selectively inhibit viral DNA synthesis at concentrations safely administered to humans. Cidofovir diphosphate has a long intracellular $t_{1/2}$ that provides prolonged and persistent antiviral activity and allows for infrequent dosing regimens in humans.[145, 215, 418] Because the compound does not require TK for initial phosphorylation, it is active against TK-deficient and TK-altered acyclovir-resistant HSV strains.[312] Resistance to cidofovir is unusual but can occur by mutations in viral DNA polymerase genes (codons 375 to 540 and possibly 978 to 988), most likely in patients who have received prolonged or repeated periods of treatment with ganciclovir or foscarnet. Strains of CMV that are resistant to cidofovir are also usually resistant to ganciclovir, and occasionally, triple mutants resistant to ganciclovir, foscarnet, and cidofovir occur.[120, 445]

Pharmacokinetics

After an intravenous infusion of 5 mg/kg of cidofovir, peak plasma levels range from 11.6 to 26.1 μg/mL, with the latter occurring after administration of probenicid.[102, 383, 445] The plasma $t_{1/2}$ is 2 to 3 hours, but the intracellular $t_{1/2}$ is very prolonged (between 17 and 65 hours).[418] CSF penetration by cidofovir is not well studied, but in at least one patient, the drug did not appear to cross the blood-brain barrier in detectable amounts. After topical administration to the eye or intact skin, systemic absorption is low, with peak plasma levels usually less than 0.5 μg/mL.[273, 274] However, patients with abraded or denuded skin may have significant absorption.[36] The systemic absorption that occurs after intralesional or subcutaneous administration is not well characterized at this time. Intravitreal administration produces sustained antiviral effects in animal models.[145] Cidofovir is not well absorbed orally, with less than 5 percent bioavailability. However, bioavailable alkoxyalkyl esters of cidofovir are in development and may lead to an oral compound in the near future.[251]

*See references 11, 71, 72, 108, 120, 130, 161, 170, 214, 312, 334, 335, 383, 407, 408, 411, 418, 453.

Aerosolized cidofovir also is being studied in animal models and appears to deliver high concentrations of antiviral to the lungs.[51] Cidofovir is eliminated through the kidney by glomerular filtration and active tubular secretion, and more than 90 percent of the original dose can be recovered unchanged in urine.

Clinical Indications, Dosage, and Adverse Effects

CLINICAL INDICATIONS

Cidofovir is licensed for induction and maintenance treatment of CMV retinitis in immunocompromised adults with AIDS.[383] Clinical trials have shown that cidofovir significantly delays progression of CMV retinitis in previously untreated patients, as well as those who previously failed or were intolerant of foscarnet or ganciclovir therapy.[273, 274, 356, 437] Cidofovir also has been shown to be effective for the treatment of CMV infection and disease in marrow and stem cell transplant recipients. In addition, it has been used, in selected patients, for preemptive treatment of CMV infection after marrow and stem cell transplantation.[68, 289, 353] One study also showed that cidofovir helped prevent post-transplantation CMV-associated atherosclerosis in rats.[57] Patients infected with CMV strains resistant to ganciclovir or foscarnet, or both, may benefit from receiving cidofovir treatment.[120] Cidofovir is used by clinicians to treat immunocompromised children with serious CMV disease despite the lack of published experience in children.[59, 66] Cidofovir has broad-spectrum antiviral activity, and published case reports show that it has been used to treat patients with serious infections caused by a wide variety of DNA viruses. For example, patients with acyclovir- and foscarnet-resistant HSV infection have been treated successfully with topical and systemic cidofovir.[58, 265, 272, 274] It also may be effective in treating selected patients with acyclovir-resistant VZV infections.[444] Moreover, one report showed that treatment with cidofovir and anti-CD20 monoclonal antibody was associated with remission and regression of post-transplant EBV-associated lymphoproliferative disease.[186] The use of cidofovir to treat patients with AIDS and HHV-8 viremia and disease also has been reported.[47, 304] Human papillomavirus-induced epithelial cell proliferation may be responsive to treatment with topical and intralesional administration of cidofovir. Several small, uncontrolled case series have described the successful use of cidofovir to treat juvenile laryngeal papillomatosis, hypopharyngeal and esophageal papillomatous lesions, anogenital condylomas, and cervical intraepithelial neoplasia.[14, 73, 416, 433, 485] Furthermore, intravenous therapy with cidofovir has been used to treat individual patients, including at least one child, with refractory disseminated respiratory papillomatosis of the lung.[14] Human BK polyomavirus–associated acute hemorrhagic cystitis in immunocompromised patients has been treated with cidofovir, with varying results.[25] Case reports and small clinical trials evaluating cidofovir treatment in patients with progressive multifocal leukoencephalopathy who have AIDS or other immunocompromising conditions have not shown consistent benefit in survival or sustained improvement in neurologic status.[12, 81, 158, 228, 326, 362, 385, 402] Successful cidofovir treatment of adenovirus disease in marrow and stem cell transplant recipients has been published in reports of case series, with the best results noted in patients in whom the disease was localized and treatment was initiated early.[46, 160, 217, 283, 370] Controlled clinical trials evaluating eye drops containing an investigational topical solution of cidofovir to treat patients with acute keratoconjunctivitis caused by adenovirus have not shown consistent benefit in the doses used.[209, 210] Poxviruses are inhibited by cidofovir in concentrations safely achievable in humans, and at least one case report of successful treatment of orf (ecthyma contagiosum) has been published.[161] In addition, in vitro and animal model data suggest that cidofovir may be effective in the treatment and short-term, postexposure prophylaxis of smallpox and other related poxvirus infections in humans, as well as in the treatment of complications that may occur after inoculation with smallpox (vaccinia-like) vaccine.[11, 71, 72, 108, 120, 383, 411] However, no clinical trials in humans to evaluate the efficacy of cidofovir for the treatment of poxvirus infections have been published.

DOSAGE

The usually recommended dose for induction therapy with cidofovir is 5 mg/kg given as an intravenous infusion over the course of 1 hour administered once weekly for 2 consecutive weeks. Some clinicians suggest a reduced dosage regimen of 1 mg/kg administered three times weekly to reduce the risk of renal toxicity.[217] Maintenance therapy usually is administered as 1-hour infusions of 5 mg/kg once very 2 weeks to complete a total of at least five doses. These doses should be decreased to 1 to 3 mg/kg if renal insufficiency is present and discontinued if significant elevation of serum creatinine or proteinuria occurs. Probenecid must be administered orally with each dose of cidofovir, 3 hours before and then 2 and 8 hours after completion of the intravenous infusion. Prehydration with normal saline before each infusion also is recommended. Investigational topical preparations of eye drops containing 0.2 to 1 percent cidofovir and creams containing 1 percent cidofovir are being investigated.[209, 210] The usual concentration used for intralesional injection is 2.5 mg/mL.[433]

ADVERSE EFFECTS

Cidofovir is nephrotoxic and produces clinically apparent proximal tubular dysfunction, including Fanconi syndrome and acute renal failure, in as many as half the patients who receive the drug.[311, 383] Early laboratory signs of renal toxicity include proteinuria, glycosuria, azotemia, and metabolic acidosis. Therefore, patients receiving cidofovir should have a urinalysis and serum tests for renal function performed before taking each dose. The risk of development of renal toxicity can be reduced, but not eliminated by probenecid and saline prehydration. Moreover, renal toxicity is more likely to occur if other nephrotoxic agents, such as aminoglycosides, amphotericin B, or foscarnet, are administered concurrently with cidofovir.[487] In clinical trials of patients with AIDS, administration of cidofovir also was associated with neutropenia. Ocular toxicity, including ocular hypotony (decreased intraocular pressure) and anterior uveitis and iritis, also has been reported in patients receiving cidofovir therapy.[3] Therefore, frequent monitoring by an ophthalmologist, including measurement of intraocular pressure, is recommended for patients receiving cidofovir therapy. Intravitreal administration of cidofovir has produced uveitis, vitreitis, reduced intraocular pressure, and loss of vision.[260, 331] Local or topical treatment with cidofovir may produce local reactions in the skin.

REFERENCES

1. Abdel-Rahman, S. M., and Kearn, G. L.: Single dose pharmacokinetics of pleconaril (VP63843) oral solution: Effect of food. Antimicrob. Agents Chemother. *43*:2706–2709, 1998.
2. Abdel-Rahman, S. M., and Kearn, G. L.: Single oral dose escalation pharmacokinetics of pleconaril (VP63843) capsules in adults. J. Clin. Pharmacol. *39*:613–618, 1999.

3. Accorinti, M., Ciapparoni, V., Pirraglia, M., and Pivetti-Pezzi, P.: Treatment of severe ocular hypotony in AIDS patients with cytomegalovirus retinitis and cidofovir-associated uveitis. Ocul. Immunol. Inflamm. *9*:211–217, 2001.
4. Adour, K. K., Ruboyianes, J., Von Doersten, P. G., et al.: Bell's palsy treatment with acyclovir and prednisone compared with prednisone alone: A double-blind, randomized, controlled trial. Ann. Otol. Rhinol. Laryngol. *105*:371-378, 1996.
5. Alcorn, J., McNamara, P.: Acyclovir, ganciclovir, and zidovudine transfer into rat milk. Antimicrob. Agents Chemother. *46*:1831–1836, 2002.
6. Alexander, A., Akers, A., Matzke, G., et al.: Disposition of foscarnet during peritoneal dialysis. Ann. Pharmacol. Ther. *30*:1106–1109, 1996.
7. American Academy of Pediatrics Committee on Infectious Diseases. The use of oral acyclovir on otherwise healthy children with varicella. Pediatrics *91*:674–676, 1993.
8. Amir, J., Harel, L., Smetana, Z., et al.: Treatment of herpes simplex gingivostomatitis with acyclovir in children: A randomized, double blind, placebo-controlled study. B. M. J. *314*:1800–1803, 1997.
9. Anderson, E. L., Van Voris, L. P., Bartram, J., et al.: Pharmacokinetics of a single dose of rimantadine in young adults and children. Antimcirob. Agents Chemother. *31*:1140–1142, 1987.
10. Anderson, R. D., Griffy, K. G., Jung, D., et al.: Ganciclovir absolute bioavailability steady-state pharmacokinetics after oral administration of two 300 mg/d dosing regimens in human immunodeficiency virus- and cytomegalovirus-positive patients. Clin. Ther. *17*:435–432, 1995.
11. Andrei, G., Snoeck, R., Vandeputte, M., and De Clercq, E.: Activities of various compounds against murine and primate polyomaviruses. Antimicrob. Agents Chemother. *41*:587–593, 1997.
12. Angelini, L., Pietrogrande, M., Delle Piano, M., et al.: Progressive multifocal leukoencephalopathy in a child with hyperimmunoglobulin E recurrent infection syndrome and review of the literature. Neuropediatrics *32*:250–255, 2001.
13. Arevalo, J. F., Gonzalez, C., Capparelli, E. V., et al.: Intravitreous and plasma concentrations of ganciclovir and foscarnet after intravenous therapy in patients with AIDS and cytomegalovirus retinitis. J. Infect. Dis. *172*:951-956, 1995.
14. Armbruster, C., Kreuzer, A., Vorbach, H., et al.: Successful treatment of severe respiratory papillomatosis with intravenous cidofovir and interferon alpha-2b. Eur. Respir. J. *17*:830–831, 2001.
15. Arvin, A. M., Feldman, S., and Merigan, T. C.: Human leukocyte interferon in the treatment of varicella in children with cancer: A preliminary controlled trial. Antimicrob. Agents Chemother. *13*:605–607, 1978.
16. Bacon, T. H., Howard, B. A., Spender, L. C., Boyd, M. R.: Activity of penciclovir in antiviral assays against herpes simplex virus. J. Antimicrob. Chemother. *37*:303–313, 1996.
17. Bacon, T. H., and Schimazi, R. F.: An overview of the further evaluation of penciclovir against herpes simplex virus and varicella-zoster virus in cell culture highlighting contrasts with acyclovir. Antiviral Chem. Chemother. *4*:25–26, 1993.
18. Bailey, A. D., Seaberg, E. C., Porayko, M. D., et al.: Prophylaxis of cytomegalovirus infection in liver transplantation: A randomized trial comparing a combination of ganciclovir and acyclovir to acyclovir. Liver Transplantation Database. Transplantation *64*:66–73, 1997.
19. Bailey, T. C., Ettinger, N. A., Storch, G. A., et al.: Failure of high-dose oral acyclovir with or without immune globulin to prevent primary cytomegalovirus disease in recipients of solid organ transplants. Am. J. Med. *95*:273–278, 1993.
20. Bain, V., Daniels, H., Chanas, A., et al.: Foscarnet therapy in chronic hepatitis B virus E antigen carriers. J. Med. Virol. *29*:152–155, 1989.
21. Baldanti, F., Underwood, M. Stanat, S., et al.: Single amino acid changes in the DNA polymerase confer foscarnet resistance and slow growth phenotype, while mutations in the UL97-encoded phosphotransferase confer ganciclovir resistance in three double-resistant human cytomegalovirus strains recovered form patients with AIDS. J. Virol. *70*:1390–1395, 1996.
22. Baldwin, A., Kingman, H., Darville, M., et al.: Outcome and clinical course of 100 patients with adenovirus infection following bone marrow transplantation. Bone Marrow Transplant. *26*:1333–1338, 2000.
23. Balfour, H., Rotbart, H. A., Feldman, S., et al.: Acyclovir treatment of varicella in otherwise healthy adolescents. The Collaborative Acyclovir Varicella Study Group. J. Pediatr. *120*:627–633, 1992.
24. Baron, S., Brunell, P. A., and Grossbert, S. E.: Mechanisms of action and pharmacology: The immune and interferon systems. *In* Galasso, G. J., et al.: (eds.): Antiviral Agents and Viral Diseases in Man. New York, Raven Press, 1979, pp. 151–208.
25. Barouch, D. H., Faquin, W. C., Chen, Y., et al.: BK virus-associated hemorrhagic cystitis in a human immunodeficiency virus-infected patient. Clin. Infect. Dis. *35*:326-329, 2002.
26. Bauer, D. J.: The antiviral and synergistic actions of isatin thiosemicarbazone and certain phenoxypyrimidines in vaccinia infection in mice. Br. J. Exp. Pathol. *36*:105–114, 1955.
27. Bauer, D. J., St. Vincent, L., Kempe, C. H., and Downie, A. W.: Prophylactic treatment of smallpox contacts with N-methylisatin beta-thiosemicarbazone. Lancet *2*:494–496, 1963.
28. Bean, B., and Aeppli, D.: Adverse effects of high-dose intravenous acyclovir in ambulatory patients with acute herpes zoster. J. Infect. Dis. *151*:262–265, 1985.
29. Bean, B., Braun, C., and Balfour, H.: Acyclovir therapy for acute herpes zoster. Lancet *2*:118–121, 1982.
30. Beauchamp, L. M., Orr, G. F., deMiranda, P., et al.: Amino ester prodrugs of acyclovir. Antiviral Chem. Chemother. *3*:157–164, 1992.
31. Belshe, R. B., Burk, B., Newman, F., et al.: Resistance of influenza A virus to amantadine and rimantadine: Results of one decade of surveillance. J. Infect. Dis. *159*:430–435, 1989.
32. Berghdal, S., Jacobsen, B., Moberg, L., et al.: Pronounced anti-HIV activity of foscarnet in patients without cytomegalovirus infection. J. Acquir. Immune Defic. Syndr. Hum. Retrovirol. *18*:51–53, 1998.
33. Berk, L., and Schalm, S. W.: Failure of acyclovir to enhance the antiviral effect of alpha lymphoblastoid interferon on HBe-seroconversion in chronic hepatitis B: A multi-center randomized controlled trial. J. Hepatol. *14*:305–309, 1992.
34. Bernstein, D. I., Reuman, P. D., Sherwood, J. R., et al.: Ribavirin small particle aerosol treatment of influenza B virus infection. Antimicrob. Agents Chemother. *32*:761–764, 1988.
35. Beutner, K. R.: Valacyclovir: A review of antiviral activity, pharmacokinetic properties, and clinical efficacy. Antiviral Res. *28*:281–290, 1995.
36. Beutner, K. R., Friedman, D. J., Forszpaniak, C., et al.: Valacyclovir compared with acyclovir for improved therapy for herpes zoster in immunocompetent adults. Antimicrob. Agents Chemother. *39*:1546–1553, 1995.
37. Biron, K. K., Stanat, S. C., Sorell, J. R., et al.: Metabolic activation of the nucleoside analog 9-[(2-hydroxy-1-(hydroxymethyl)ethoxy]methyl)guanine] in human diploid fibroblasts infected with human cytomegalovirus. Proc. Natl. Acad. Sci. U. S. A. *82*:2473–2477, 1985.
38. Bizollon, T., Palazzo, U., Ducerf, C., et al.: Pilot study of the combination of interferon alpha and ribavirin as therapy of recurrent hepatitis C after liver transplantation. Hepatology *26*:500–504, 1997.
39. Bleidner, W. E., Harmon, J. B., Hewes, U. E., et al.: Absorption, distribution, and excretion of amantadine hydrochloride. J. Pharmacol. Exp. Ther. *150*:484–490, 1965.
40. Blum, M. R., and Liao, S. H.: Overview of acyclovir pharmacokinetic disposition in adults and children. Am. J. Med. *73*:186–192, 1982.
41. Bodenheimer, H. J., Lindsey, K. L., Davis, G. L., et al.: Tolerance and efficacy of oral ribavirin treatment of chronic hepatitis C: A multicenter trial. Hepatology 26:473–477, 1997.
42. Bodsworth, N. J., Crooks, R. J., Borelli, S., et al.: Valacyclovir versus acyclovir in patient initiated treatment of recurrent genital herpes: A randomized, double blind clinical trial. International Valacyclovir HSV Study Group. Genitourin. Med. *73*:110–116, 1997.
43. Boekth, M., Gooley, T. A., Reusser, P., et al.: Failure of high-dose acyclovir to prevent cytomegalovirus disease after autologous marrow transplantation. J. Infect. Dis. *172*:939–943, 1995.
44. Boike, S. C., Pue, M., Audet, P. R., et al.: Pharmacokinetics of famciclovir in subjects with chronic hepatitis disease. J. Clin. Pharmacol. *34*:1199–1207, 1994.
45. Boivin, G., Chou, S., Quirk, M., et al.: Detection of ganciclovir resistance mutations and quantitation of cytomegalovirus (CMV) DNA in leukocytes of patients with fatal disseminated CMV disease. J. Infect. Dis. *173*:523–528, 1996.
46. Bordigoni, P., Carnet, A., Vernard, V., et al.: Treatment of adenovirus infections in patients undergoing allogeneic hematopoietic stem cell transplantation. Clin. Infect. Dis. *32*:1290–1297, 2001.
47. Boulanger, E., Agbalika, F., Maarek, O., et al.: A clinical, molecular, and cytogenetic study of 12 cases of human herpesvirus 8 associated primary effusion lymphoma in HIV-infected patients. Hematol. J. *2*:172–179, 2001.
48. Boyd, M. R., Bacon, T. H., Sutton, D., and Cole, M.: Antiherpes activity of 9-(4-hydroxy-3-hydroxy-methylbut-1-yl) guanine (BRL 39123) in cell culture. Antimicrob. Agents Chemother. *31*:1238–1242, 1987.
49. Boyd, M. R., Kern, E. R., and Safrin, S.: Penciclovir: A review of its spectrum of activity, selectivity and cross-resistance pattern. Antiviral Chem.y Chemother. *4*:3–11, 1993.
50. Bradley, J. S., Connor, J. D., Compogiannis, L. S., et al.: Exposure of health care workers to ribavirin during therapy for respiratory syncytial virus infections. Antimicrob. Agents Chemother. *34*:668–670, 1990.
51. Bray, M., Martinez, M., Kefauver, D., et al.: Treatment of aerosolized cowpox virus infection in mice with aerosolized cidofovir. Antiviral Res. *54*:129–142, 2002.
52. Brennan, D., Garlock, K., Singer, G., et al.: Prophylactic oral ganciclovir compared with deferred therapy for control of cytomegalovirus in renal transplant recipients. Transplantation *64*:1843–1846, 1997.
53. Brocklehurst, P., Kinghorn, G., Carney, O., et al.: A randomized placebo controlled trial of suppressive acyclovir in late pregnancy in women with recurrent genital herpes infection. Br. J. Obstet. Gynaecol *105*:275–280, 1998.
54. Brown, F., Banken, L., Saywell, K., and Arum, I.: Pharmacokinetics of valganciclovir and ganciclovir following multiple oral dosages of valganciclovir in HIV- and CMV-seropositive volunteers. Clin. Pharmacokinet. *37*:167–196, 1999.

55. Browne, M. J.: Mechanism and specificity of action of ribavirin. Antimicrob. Agents Chemother. *15*:740–753, 1979.
56. Browne, M. J., Moss, M. Y., and Boyd, M. R.: Comparative activity of amantadine and ribavirin against influenza virus in vitro: Possible clinical relevance. Antimicrob. Agents Chemother. *23*:503–505, 1983.
57. Bruning, J., Persoons, M., Lemstrom, K., et al.: Enhancement of transplantation-associated atherosclerosis by CMV, which can be prevented by antiviral therapy in the form of HPMPC. Transpl. Int. *7*(Suppl. 1): 365–370, 1994.
58. Bryant, P., Sasadeusz, J., Carapetis, J., et al.: Successful treatment of foscarnet-resistant herpes simplex stomatitis with intravenous cidofovir in a child. Pediatr. Infect. Dis. J. *20*:1083–1086, 2001.
59. Bueno, J., Ramil, C., and Green, M.: Current management strategies for the prevention and treatment of cytomegalovirus infection in pediatric transplant recipients. Paediatr. Drugs *4*:279–290, 2002.
60. Buhles, W. C., Jr., Mastre, B. J., Tinker, A. J., et al.: Ganciclovir treatment of life- or sight-threatening cytomegalovirus infection: Experience in 314 immunocompromised patients. Rev. Infect. Dis *10*(Suppl. 3): 495–506, 1988.
61. Calfree, D. P., and Hayden, F. G.: New approaches to influenza chemotherapy: Neuraminidase inhibitors. Drugs *56*:537–553, 1998.
62. Calfree, D. P., Peng, A. W., Cass, L. M., et al.: Safety and efficacy of intravenous zanamivir in preventing experimental human influenza A virus infection. Antimicrob. Agents Chemother. *43*:1616–1620, 1999.
63. Capparelli E. V., Stevens, R. C., Chow, M. S., et al.: Rimantadine pharmacokinetics in healthy subjects and patients with end stage renal disease. Clin. Pharmacol. Ther. *43*:536–541, 1988.
64. Cass, L. M. R., Efthymiopoulos, C., and Bye, A.: Pharmacokinetics of zanamivir after intravenous, oral, inhaled or intranasal administration to healthy volunteers. Clin. Pharmacokinet. *36*(Suppl. 1):1–11, 1999.
65. Cassidy, L. F., and Patterson, J. L.: Mechanism of La Crosse virus inhibition by ribavirin. Antimicrob. Agents Chemother. *33*:2009–2011, 1989.
66. Castagnola, E., Cristina, E., Dallorso, S., et al.: Failure of cidofovir to reduce CMV-antigenemia in a child transplanted from a matched unrelated donor. J. Chemother. *13*:100–101, 2001.
67. Centers for Disease Control and Prevention: Pregnancy outcomes following systemic prenatal acyclovir exposure: June 1, 1984–June 30, 1993. M. M. W. R. Morb. Mortal. Wkly. Rep. *42*(41):806–809, 1993.
68. Chakrabarti, S., Collingham, K. E., Osman, H., et al.: Cidofovir primary preemptive therapy for post-transplant cytomegalovirus infections. Transplantation *28*:879–881, 2001.
69. Chakrabarti, S., Mauther, V., Osman, H., et al.: Adenovirus infections following allogeneic stem cell transplantation: Incidence and outcome in relation to graft manipulation, immunosuppression, and immune recovery. Blood *100*:1619–1627, 2002.
70. Chatis, P. A., and Crumpacker, C. S.: Resistance of herpes viruses to antiviral drugs. Antimicrob. Agents Chemother. *36*:1589–1595, 1992.
71. Cherrington, J. M., Fuller, M. D., Larry, P. D., et al.: In vitro antiviral susceptibilities of isolates from CMV retinitis patients receiving first or second line cidofovir therapy: Relationship to clinical outcome. J. Infect. Dis. *178*:1821–1825, 1998.
72. Cherrington, J., M., Miner, R., Hitchcock, M., et al.: Susceptibility of human cytomegalovirus to cidofovir is unchanged after limited in vivo exposure to various regimens of drug. J. Infect. Dis. *173*:987–992, 1996.
73. Chhetri, D., Blumin, J., Shapiro, N., and Berke, G.: Office-based treatment of laryngeal papillomatosis with percutaneous injection of cidofovir. Otolaryngol. Head Neck Surg. *126*:642–648, 2002.
74. Chiou, H. C., Kumara, K., Hu, A., et al.: Penciclovir-resistance mutations in the herpes simplex virus DNA polymerase gene. Antiviral Chem. Chemother. *6*:281–288, 1995.
75. Chou, S., Erice, A., Jordan, M. C., et al.: Analysis of the UL97 phosphotransferase coding sequence in clinical cytomegalovirus isolates and identification of mutations conferring ganciclovir resistance. J. Infect. Dis. *171*:576–583, 1995.
76. Chou, S., Guentzel, S., Michels, K. R., et al.: Frequency of UL97 phosphotransferase mutations related to ganciclovir resistance in clinical cytomegalovirus isolates. J. Infect. Dis. *172*:239–242, 1995.
77. Chou, S., Marousek, G., Guentzel, S., et al.: Evolution of mutations conferring multidrug resistance during prophylaxis and therapy for cytomegalovirus disease. J. Infect. Dis. *176*:786–789, 1997.
78. Chrisp, P., and Clissold, S.: Foscarnet: A review of its antiviral activity, pharmacokinetic properties, and therapeutic use in immunocompromised patients with cytomegalovirus retinitis. Drugs *41*:104–129, 1991.
79. Christophers, J., Clayton, J., Craske, J., et al.: Survey of resistance of herpes simplex virus to acyclovir in Northwest England. Antimicrob. Agents Chemother. *42*:868–872, 1998.
80. Cinque, P., Baldanti, F., Vago, L., et al.: Ganciclovir therapy for cytomegalovirus (CMV) infection of the central nervous system in AIDS patients: Monitoring by CMV DNA detection in cerebrospinal fluid. J. Infect. Dis. *171*:1603–1606, 1995.
81. Cinque, P., Pierotti, C., Vigano, M., et al.: The good and evil of HAART in HIV-related progressive multifocal leukoencephalopathy. J. Neurovirol. *7*:358–363, 2001.
82. Cirelli, R., Herne, K., McCrary, M., et al.: Famciclovir: Review of clinical efficacy and safety. Antiviral Res. *29*:141–145, 1996.
83. Clover, R. D., Crawford, S. A., Abell, T. D., et al.: Effectiveness of rimantadine prophylaxis of children within families. Am. J. Dis. Child. *140*:706–709, 1986.
84. Cobo, L. M., Foulks, G. N., Liesegang, T., et al.: Oral acyclovir in the treatment of acute herpes zoster ophthalmicus. Opthalmology *93*:763–770, 1986.
85. Colby, B. M., Shaw, J. E., Elion, G. B., et al.: Effect of acyclovir [9-(2-hydroxyethoxymethyl)guanine] on Epstein-Barr virus DNA replication. J. Virol. *34*:560–568, 1980.
86. Cole, N. L., and Balfour, H.: Varicella-zoster virus does not become more resistant to acyclovir during therapy. J. Infect Dis. *153*:605–608, 1986.
87. Coleman, P. M.: Influenza virus neuraminidase: Structure, antibodies and inhibitors. Protein Sci. *3*:1687–1696, 1994.
88. Collaborative DHPG Treatment Study Group: Treatment of serious cytomegalovirus infections with 9-(1,3-dihydroxy-2-propoxymethyl) guanine in patients with AIDS and other immunodeficiencies. N. Engl. J. Med. *314*:801–805, 1986.
89. Colledge, D., Locarnini, S., and Shaw, T.: Synergistic inhibition of hepadnaviral replication by lamivudine in combination with penciclovir in vitro. Hepatology *26*:216–225, 1997.
90. Collum, L. M., Benedict-Smith, A., and Hillary, I. B.: Randomized double blind trial of acyclovir and idoxuridine in dendritic corneal ulceration. Br. J. Ophthalmol. *64*:766–769, 1980.
91. Connor, E. S., Morrison, J., Lane, J., et al.: Safety, tolerance, and pharmacokinetics of systemic ribavirin in children with human immunodeficiency virus infection. Antimicrob. Agents Chemother. *37*:532–539, 1993.
92. Corey, L., Fite, K. H., Benedetti, J. K., et al.: Intravenous acyclovir for the treatment of primary genital herpes. Ann. Intern. Med. *98*:914–921, 1983.
93. Corey, L., Nahmias, A. J., Guinan, M. D., et al.: A trial of topical acyclovir in genital herpes simplex virus infections. N. Engl. J. Med. *306*:914–921, 1983.
94. Couch, R. B.: Prevention and treatment of influenza. N. Engl. J. Med. *343*:1778–1787, 2000.
95. Couch, R. B., Jackson, G.: Antiviral agents in influenza: Summary of Influenza Workshop VIII. J. Infect. Dis. *134*:516–527, 1976.
96. Crawford, S. A., Clover, R. D., Abell, T. D., et al.: Rimantadine prophylaxis in children: A followup study. Pediatr. Infect. Dis. J. *7*:379–383, 1988.
97. Crooks, R. J., and Murray, A.: Valacyclovir: A review of a promising new antiherpes agent. Antiviral Chem. Chemother. *5*(Suppl. 1):31–37, 1994.
98. Crumpacker, C.: Mechanism of action of foscarnet against viral polymerases. Am. J. Med. *92*:35–75, 1992.
99. Crumpacker, C.: Ganciclovir. N. Engl. J. Med. *335*:721–729, 1996.
100. Crumpacker, C., Schnipper, L. E., Marlowe, S. I., et al.: Resistance to antiviral drugs of herpes simplex virus isolated from a patient treated with acyclovir. N. Engl. J. Med. *306*:343–345, 1979.
101. Crumpacker, C., Schnipper, L. E., Zaia, J. A., et al.: Growth inhibition by acycloguanosine of herpesviruses isolated from human infections. Antimicrob. Agents. Chemother. *15*:642–645, 1979.
102. Cundy, K. C., Petty, B. G., Flaberty, F., et al.: Clinical pharmacokinetics of cidofovir in human immunodeficiency virus–infected patients. Antimicrob. Agents Chemother. *39*:1247–1252, 1995.
103. Daniels, S., and Schentage, J. J.: Drug interaction studies and safety of famciclovir in healthy volunteers: A review. Antiviral Chem. Chemother. *4*:57–64, 1993.
104. Davies, W. L., Grunert, R. R., Haff, J. W., et al.: Antiviral activity of L-adamantanamine (amantadine). Science *144*:862–863, 1964.
105. Davis, G. I., Esteban-Mur, R., Rustigi, V., et al.: Interferon alfa–2b alone or in combination with ribavirin for the treatment of relapse of chronic hepatitis C. International Hepatitis Interventional Therapy Group. N. Engl. J. Med. *339*:1493–1499, 1998.
106. DeClercq, E.: Antivirals for the treatment of herpesvirus infections. J. Antimicrob. Chemother. *32*(Suppl. A):121–132, 1993.
107. DeClercq, E.: Perspectives for the chemotherapy of respiratory syncytial virus (RSV) infections. Int. J. Antimicrob. Agents *7*:193–202, 1996.
108. de Oliveira, C. B., Stevenson, D., LaBree, L., et al.: Evaluation of cidofovir (HPMPC, GS-504) against adenovirus type 5 infection in vitro and in a New Zealand rabbit ocular model. Antiviral Res. *31*:165–172, 1996.
109. Demicheli, V., Jefferson, T., Rivetti, D., and Deeks, J.: Prevention and early treatment of influenza in healthy adults. Vaccine *18*:957–1030, 2000.
110. Deray, G., Martinez, F., Katlama, C., et al.: Foscarnet nephrotoxicity: Mechanism, incidence and prevention. Am. J. Nephrol. *9*:316–321, 1989.
111. Derse, D., Cheng, Y. C., Furman, P. A., et al.: Inhibition of purified human and herpes simplex virus–induced DNA polymerase by 9-(2-hydroxyethoxymethyl) guanine triphosphate: Effects on primer template function. J. Biol. Chem. *256*:11447–11451, 1981.
112. DeTorres, O.: Focus on foscarnet: A pyrophosphate analog for use in CMV retinitis and other viral infections. Hosp. Formul. *26*:929–946, 1991.
113. Diaz-Mitoma, F., Sibbald, R. G., and Shafram, S. D.: Oral famciclovir for the suppression of recurrent genital herpes: A randomized controlled trial. J. A. M. A. *200*:887–892, 1998.

114. DiBisceglie, A. M., Conjeevram, H. S., Friet, M. S., et al.: Ribavirin as therapy for chronic hepatitis C: A randomized, double blind, placebo controlled trial. Ann. Intern. Med. *123*:897–903, 1995.
115. Dietrick, D., Kotler, D., Busch, D., et al.: Ganciclovir treatment of cytomegalovirus colitis in AIDS: A randomized, double blind, placebo controlled multicenter study. J. Infect. Dis. *167*:278–282, 1993.
116. Dolin, R., Reichman, R. C., Madore, H. Q., et al.: A controlled trial of amantadine and rimantadine in the prophylaxis of influenza A infection. N. Engl. J. Med. *307*:580–584, 1982.
117. Dowling, J. N., Postic, B., and Buevarra, L. O.: Effect of ribavirin on murine cytomegalovirus infection. Antimicrob. Agents. Chemother. *10*:809–813, 1976.
118. Doyle, W. J., Skoner, D. P., Alper, C. M., et al.: Effect of rimantadine treatment on clinical manifestation and otologic complications in adults experimentally infected with influenza A (H1N1) virus. J. Infect. Dis. *177*:1260–1265, 1998.
119. Drew, W. L.: Cytomegalovirus infection in patients with AIDS. Clin. Infect. Dis. *14*:608–615, 1992.
120. Drew, W. L.: Treatment of drug-resistant CMV disease in HIV-infected patients. Infect. Med. *17*:737–744, 2000.
121. Drew, W. L., Miner, R. C., Busch, D. F., et al.: Prevalence of resistance in patients receiving ganciclovir for serious cytomegalovirus infection. J. Infect. Dis. *163*:716–719, 1991.
122. Drobyski, W., Knox, K., Carrigan, D., et al.: Foscarnet therapy of ganciclovir-resistant cytomegalovirus in marrow transplantation. Transplantation *52*:155–157, 1991.
123. Duncan, S., Paradis, I., Dauber, J., et al.: Ganciclovir prophylaxis for cytomegalovirus infections in pulmonary allograft recipients. Am. Rev. Respir. Dis. *146*:1213–1215, 1992.
124. Dunkle, L., Arvin, A, Whitley, R. J., et al.: A controlled trial of acyclovir for chickenpox in normal children. N. Engl. J. Med. *325*:1539–1544, 1991.
125. Earnshaw, D. L., Bacon, T. H., Darlison, S. J., et al.: Mode of antiviral action of penciclovir in MRC-5 cells infected with herpes simplex virus type 1 (HSV-1), HSV-2, and varicella-zoster virus. Antimicrob. Agents Chemother. *36*:2747–2757, 1992.
126. Egan, J. J., Carroll, K. B., Yonan, N., et al.: Valacyclovir prevention of cytomegalovirus reactivation after heart transplantation: A randomized trial. J. Heart Lung Transplant. *21*:460–466, 2002.
127. Elion, G. B., Furman, P. A., Fyfe, J. A., et al.: Selectivity of action of an anti-herpetic agent, 9-(2-hydroxyethoxymethyl) guanine. Proc. Natl. Acad. Sci. U. S. A. *74*:5716–5720, 1077.
128. Elizaga, J., Olavarria, E., Apperley, J. F., et al.: Parainfluenza virus 3 infection after stem cell transplant: Relevance to outcome of rapid diagnosis and ribavirin treatment. Clin. Infect. Dis. *32*:413–418, 2001.
129. Emanuel, D., Cuningham, I., Jules-Eluseek, et al.: Cytomegalovirus pneumonia after bone marrow transplantation successfully treated with the combination of ganciclovir and high-dose intravenous globulin. Ann. Intern. Med. *109*:777–782, 1988.
130. Emery, V. C.: Progress in understanding cytomegalovirus drug resistance. J. Clin. Virol. *21*:223–228, 2001.
131. Englund, J. A., Piedra, P. A., Jefferson, L. S., et al.: High dose, short duration ribavirin aerosol therapy in children with suspected respiratory syncytial virus infection. J. Pediatr. *117*:313–320, 1990.
132. Englund, J. A., Piedra, P. A., and Whimbey, E.: Prevention and treatment of respiratory syncytial virus and parainfluenza viruses in immunocompromised patients. Am. J. Med. *102*:61–70, 1997.
133. Englund, J. A., Zimmerman, M. D., Swierkosz, E. M., et al.: Herpes simplex virus resistant to acyclovir: A study in a tertiary care center. Ann. Intern. Med. *112*:416–422, 1990.
134. Enria, D. A., and Maiziegui, J. I.: Antiviral treatment of Argentine hemorrhagic fever. Antiviral Res. *23*:23–31, 1994.
135. Erice, A., Chou, S., Biron, K., et al.: Progressive disease due to ganciclovir-resistant cytomegalovirus in immunocompromised patients. N. Engl. J. Med. *320*:289–293, 1989.
136. Eriksson, B. E., Helgstrand, N. G., Johansson, A., et al.: Inhibition of influenza virus ribonucleic acid polymerase by ribavirin triphosphate. Antimicrob. Agents Chemother. *11*:946–951, 1977.
137. Eriksson, B., and Schinazi, R.: Combination of 3'-azido-3'-deoxythymidine (zidovudine) and phosphonoformate (foscarnet) against human immunodeficiency virus type 1 and cytomegalovirus replication in vitro. Antimicrob. Agents Chemother. *33*:663–669, 1989.
138. Faulds, D., and Heel, R.: Ganciclovir: A review of its antiviral activity, pharmacokinetic properties, and therapeutic efficacy in cytomegalovirus infections. Drugs *39*:597–638, 1990.
139. Feldman, S., Rodman, J., and Gregory, B.: Excessive serum concentration of acyclovir and neurotoxicity. J. Infect. Dis. *157*:385–388, 1986.
140. Fernandez-Larson, R., and Patterson, J. L.: Ribavirin is an inhibitor of human immunodeficiency virus reverse transcriptase. Mol. Pharmacol. *38*:766–770, 1990.
141. Field, A. K., Davies, M. E., DeWitt, C., et al.: 9-([2-hydroxy-1-(hydroxymethyl)ethoxy]methyl) guanine: A selective inhibitor of herpes group virus replication. Proc. Natl. Acad. Sci. U. S. A. *80*:4139–4143, 1983.
142. Fischer-Hoch, S. P., Gborie, S., and Parker, L.: Unexpected adverse reactions during a clinical trial in rural West Africa. Antiviral Res. *19*:139–147, 1992.
143. Fischer-Hoch, S. P., Khan, J. A., Rehman, S., et al.: Crimean-Congo hemorrhagic fever treated with oral ribavirin. Lancet *346*:472–475, 1995.
144. Fletcher, C., Sawchuk, R., Chinnock, B., et al.: Human pharmacokinetics of the antiviral drug DHPG. Clin. Pharmacol. Ther. *40*:281–286, 1986.
145. Flores-Aguilar, M., Huang, J. S., Wiley, C. A., et al.: Long-acting therapy of retinitis with (S)-1-(3-hydroxy-2-phosphonylmethoxypropyl) cytosine. J. Infect. Dis. *169*:642–647, 1994.
146. Forni, A. L., Schluger, N. W., and Roberts, R. B.: Severe measles pneumonitis in adults: Evaluation of clinical characteristics and therapy with intravenous ribavirin. Clin. Infect. Dis. *19*:454–462, 1994.
147. Fowler, S. E., Pierce, D. M., Prince, W. T., et al.: The tolerance to and pharmacokinetics of penciclovir (BRL39, 123A), a novel antiherpes agent, administered by intravenous infusion to healthy subjects. Eur. J. Clin. Pharmacol. *43*:513–516, 1992.
148. Fox, M. P., McKinlay, M. A., Diana, G. D., and Dutko, F. J.: Binding affinities of structurally related human rhinovirus capsid-binding compounds are related to their activities against human rhinovirus type 14. Antimicrob. Agents Chemother. *35*:1040–1047, 1991.
149. Freitas, V., Fraser-Smith, E., and Matthews, T.: Increased efficacy of ganciclovir in combination with foscarnet against cytomegalovirus and herpes simplex virus type 2 in vitro and in vivo. Antiviral Res. *12*:205–212, 1989.
150. Frenkel, L., Brown, Z. A., Bryson, Y. J., et al.: Pharmacokinetics of acyclovir in the term human pregnancy and neonate. Am. J. Obstet. Gynecol. *164*:569–576, 1991.
151. Frenkel, L. R., Wilson, C. W., Demers, R. R., et al.: A technique for the administration of ribavirin to mechanically ventilated infants with severe respiratory syncytial virus infection. Crit. Care Med. *15*:1051–1054, 1987.
152. Fried, M. W., Shiffman, M. L., Reddy, R., et al.: Peginterferon alfa-2a plus ribavirin for chronic hepatitis C virus infection. N. Engl. J. Med. *347*:975–982, 2002.
153. Fritz, R. S., Hayden, F. G., Calfee, D. P., et al.: Nasal cytokine and chemokine responses in experimental influenza A virus infection: Results of a placebo-controlled trial of intravenous zanamivir treatment. J. Infect. Dis. *180*:586–593, 1999.
154. Furman, P. A., St. Clair, M. A., and Spector, T.: Acyclovir triphosphate is a suicide inactivator of the herpes simplex virus DNA polymerase. J. Biol. Chem. *359*:9575–9579, 1984.
155. Gaines, K., Jung, D., and Tan, S.-J.: Final report of study GANS51788. An open label evaluation of the safety and pharmacokinetics of ganciclovir in children. Clinical Research Report CL6791. August 1994.
156. Galbraith, A. W., Oxford, J. S., Schild, G. C., et al.: Study of L-amantanamine hydrochloride used prophylactically during the Hong Kong influenza epidemic in the family environment. Bull. World Health Organ. *41*:677–682, 1969.
157. Game, E., Saliba, F., Valdecassas, G., et al.: Randomized trial of efficacy and safety of oral ganciclovir in the prevention of cytomegalovirus disease in liver transplant recipients. Lancet *350*:1729–1733, 1997.
158. Gasnault, J., Kousignian, P., Kahraman, M., et al.: Cidofovir in AIDS-associated progressive multifocal leukoencephalopathy: A monocenter observational study with clinical and JC viral load monitoring. J. Neurovirol. *7*:375–381, 2001.
159. Gaudreau, A., Hill, E., Balfour, H., et al.: Phenotypic and genotypic characterization of acyclovir-resistant herpes simplex viruses from immunocompromised patients. J. Infect. Dis. *178*:297–303, 1998.
160. Gavin, P. J., and Katz, B. Z.: Intravenous ribavirin treatment for severe adenovirus disease in immunocompromised children. Pediatrics *110*:e9–e12, 2002.
161. Geerinck, K., Lukito, G., Snoeck, R., et al.: A case of human orf in an immunocompromised patient treated successfully with cidofovir cream. J. Med. Virol. *64*:543–549, 2001.
162. Gilbert, B. E., and Knight, V.: Pulmonary delivery of antiviral drugs in liposome aerosols. Semin. Pediatr. Infect. Dis. *7*:148–154, 1996.
163. Gilbert, C., Roy, J., Belanger, R., et al.: Lack of emergence of cytomegalovirus UL97 mutations conferring ganciclovir (GCV) resistance following pre-emptive GCV therapy in allogeneic stem cell transplant recipients. Antimicrob. Agents Chemother. *215*:3669–3671, 2001.
164. Gish, R. G., Lau, J. Y., and Brooks, L.: Ganciclovir treatment of hepatitis B virus infection in liver transplant recipients. Hepatology *23*:1–7, 1996.
165. Glada, J. M., and Ecobichon, D. J.: Evaluation of exposure of healthcare personnel to ribavirin. J. Toxicol. Environ. Health *28*:1–12, 1989.
166. Goldberg, L. H., Kaufman, R., Kurtz, T. O., et al.: Long term suppression of recurrent genital herpes with acyclovir: A 5 year benchmark. Acyclovir Study Group. Arch. Dermatol. *129*:582–587, 1993.
167. Goldthorpe, S. E., Boud, M. R., and Field, H. J.: Effects of penciclovir and famciclovir in a murine model of encephalitis induced by intranasal inoculation of herpes simplex virus type 1. Antimicrob. Agents Chemother. *3*:37–47, 1992.
168. Goodrich, J., Bowden, R., Fisher, L., et al.: Ganciclovir prophylaxis to prevent cytomegalovirus disease after allogeneic marrow transplant. Ann. Intern. Med. *118*:173–178, 1993.

169. Goodrich, J., Morci, M., and Gleaves, C.: Early treatment with ganciclovir to prevent cytomegalovirus disease after allogeneic bone marrow transplantation: N. Engl. J. Med. *325*:1601–1607, 1991.
170. Gordon, Y. J., Ramanowski, E., Araullo-Cruz, T., et al.: Inhibitory effect of (S)-HPMPC, (S)-HPMPA, and 2′-nor-cyclic GMP on clinical ocular adenoviral isolates is serotype-dependent in vitro. Antiviral Res. *16*:11–16, 1991.
171. Groothius, J. R., Woodin, K. A., Katz, R., et al.: Early ribavirin treatment of respiratory syncytial viral infections in high risk children. J. Pediatr. *117*:792–798, 1990.
172. Gubareva, L. V., Matrosovich, M. N., Brenner, M. K., et al.: Evidence for zanamivir resistance in an immunocompromised child infected with influenza B virus J. Infect. Dis. *178*:1257–1262, 1998.
173. Gubareva, L. V., Robinson, M. J., Bethall, R. C., and Webster, R. G.: Catalytic and framework mutations in the neuraminidase active site of influenza viruses that are resistant to 4-guanidino-Neu5AcZen. J. Virol. *71*:3385–3390, 1997.
174. Gubareva, L. V., Webster, R. G., and Hayden, F. G.: Comparison of the activities of zanamivir, oseltamivir, and RWJ-270201 against clinical isolates of influenza virus and neuraminidase inhibitor–resistant variants. Antimicrob. Agents Chemother. *45*:3403–3408, 2001.
175. Gubareva, L. V., Webster, R. G., and Hayden, F. G.: Detection of influenza virus resistance to neuraminidase inhibitors by an enzyme inhibition assay. Antiviral Res. *53*:47–61, 2002.
176. Gururangan, S., Stevens, N., and Morrisa, D.: Ribavirin response in measles pneumonia. J. Infect. Dis. *20*:219–221, 1990.
177. Haake, D. A., Zakowski, P. C., Haake, D. L., Bryson, Y. J.: Early treatment with acyclovir for varicella pneumonia in otherwise healthy adults: Retrospective controlled study and review. Rev. Infect. Dis. *12*:788–798, 1990.
178. Haefleri, W. E., Schonenberger, R. A., Weiss, P. P., et al.: Acyclovir-induced neurotoxicity: Concentration side effect relationship in acyclovir overdose. Am. J. Med. *94*:212–215, 1993.
179. Hall, C. B.: Respiratory syncytial virus and parainfluenza virus. N. Engl. J. Med. *344*:1917–1928, 2001.
180. Hall, C. B., Dolin, R., Gala, C. L., et al.: Children with influenza A infection: Treatment with rimantadine. Pediatrics *80*:275–282, 1987.
181. Hall, C. B., McBride, J. T., Gala, C. L., et al.: Ribavirin treatment of respiratory syncytial viral infection in infants with underlying cardiopulmonary disease. J. A. M. A. *254*:3047–3051, 1985.
182. Hall, C. B., McBride, J. T., Walsh, E. E., et al.: Aerosolized ribavirin treatment of infants with respiratory syncytial viral infection: A randomized, double blind study. N. Engl. J. Med. *308*:1443–1447, 1983.
183. Haller, G. W., Bechstein, W. O., Neuhaus, R., et al.: Famciclovir therapy for recurrent hepatitis B virus infection after liver transplantation. Transpl. Int. *9*(Suppl. 1):210–212, 1996.
184. Hamre, D., Brownlea, K. A., and Donovick, R.: Studies on the chemotherapy of vaccinia virus. II. The activity of some thiosemicarbazones. J. Immunol. *67*:305–312, 1951.
185. Hamzeh, F. M., and Lietman, P. J.: Intranuclear accumulation of subgenomic noninfectious human cytomegalovirus DNA in infected cells in the presence of ganciclovir. Antimicrob. Agents Chemother. *35*:1818–1823, 1991.
186. Hanel, M., Fiedler, F., and Thornis, C.: Anti-CD20 monoclonal antibody (rituximab) and cidofovir as successful treatment of an EBV-associated lymphoma with CNS involvement. Onkolgie *24*:491–494, 2001.
187. Hardy, W.: Combined ganciclovir and recombinant human granulocyte-macrophage colony stimulating factor in the treatment of cytomegalovirus retinitis in AIDS patients. J. Acquir. Immune Defic. Syndr. *4*:(Suppl):22–28, 1991.
188. Hay, A. J.: The action of adamananamines against influenza A viruses: Inhibition of the M2 ion channel protein. Semin. Virol. *3*:21–30, 1992.
189. Hayden, F. G.: Combined antiviral therapy for respiratory virus infections. Antiviral Res. *29*:45–48, 1996.
190. Hayden, F. G., Belshe, R. B., Clover, R. D., et al.: Emergence and apparent transmission of rimantadine-resistant influenza A virus in families. N. Engl. J. Med. *321*:1696–1702, 1989.
191. Hayden, F. G., Coats, T., Kim, K., et al.: Oral pleconaril treatment of picornavirus-associated viral respiratory illness in adults: Efficacy and tolerability in phase II clinical trials. Antiviral Ther. *7*:53–56, 2002.
192. Hayden, F. G., Cote, K. M., and Douglas, R. G.: Plaque inhibition assay for drug susceptibility testing of influenza viruses. Antimicrob. Agents Chemother. *17*:865–870, 1980.
193. Hayden, F. G., and Couch, R. B.: Clinical and epidemiological importance of influenza A virus resistant to amantadine and rimantadine. Rev. Med. Virol. *2*:89–96, 1992.
194. Hayden, F. G., Douglas, R. G., Jr., and Simons, R.: Enhancement of activity against influenza viruses by combinations of antibacterial agents. Antimicrob. Agents Chemother. *18*:536–541, 1980.
195. Hayden, F. G., Gubareva, L. V., Monto, A. S., et al.: Inhaled zanamivir for the prevention of influenza in families. Zanamivir Family Study Group. N. Engl. J. Med. *18*:1282–1289, 2000.
196. Hayden, F. G., Hall, W. J., Douglas, R. G., Jr., et al.: Amantadine aerosols in normal volunteers: Pharmacology and safety testing. Antimcirob. Agents Chemother. *16*:644–650, 1979.
197. Hayden, F. G., Hoffman, H. E., and Spyker, D. A.: Differences in side effects of amantadine hydrochloride and rimantadine hydrochloride relate to differences in pharmacokinetics. Antimicrob. Agents. Chemother. *23*:458–464, 1983.
198. Hayden, F. G., Minoha, A., Spyker, D. A., et al.: Comparative single dose pharmacokinetics of amantadine hydrochloride and rimantadine hydrochloride in young and elderly adults. Antimicrob. Agents Chemother. *28*:216–221, 1985.
199. Hayden, F. G., Osterhaus, A. D., Treanor, J. J., et al.: Efficacy and safety of the neuraminidase inhibitor zanamivir in the treatment of influenza virus infections. N. Engl. J. Med. *337*:874–878, 1997.
200. Hayden, F. G., Sable, C. A., Connor, J. D., and Lane, J.: Intravenous ribavirin by constant infusion for serious influenza and parainfluenza virus infection. Antiviral Ther. *1*:51–56, 1996.
201. Hayden, F. G., Treanor, J. J., Belts, R. F., et al.: Safety and efficacy of the neuraminidase inhibitor GG167 in experimental human influenza. J. A. M. A. *275*:295–299, 1996.
202. Hayden, F. G., Zlydnikov, D. M., Ijenko, V. I., et al.: Comparative therapeutic effect of aerosolized and oral rimantadine HCl in experimental human influenza A virus infection. Antiviral Res. *2*:142–153, 1982.
203. Hedrick, J. A., Barzilai, A., Behre, U., et al.: Zanamivir for treatment of symptomatic influenza A and B infection in children five to twelve years of age: A randomized controlled trial. Pediatr. Infect. Dis. J. *19*:410–417, 2000.
204. Hengge, U., Brockmeyer, N., Malessa, R., et al.: Foscarnet penetrates the blood brain barrier: Rationale for therapy of cytomegalovirus encephalitis. Antimicrob. Agents Chemother. *37*:1010–1014, 1998.
205. Herpetic Eye Disease Study Group: Acyclovir for the prevention of recurrent herpes simplex virus eye disease. N. Engl. J. Med. *339*:300–306, 1998.
206. Hiatt, P. W., Treece, D., Morris, L., et al.: Longitudinal pulmonary function (PF) following treatment with ribavirin in infants hospitalized with RSV bronchiolitis. Am. J. Respir. Crit. Care Med. *179*:209–213, 1993.
207. Hibberd, P., Tolkoff-Rubin, N., Conti, D., et al.: Pre-emptive ganciclovir therapy to prevent cytomegalovirus disease in cytomegalovirus antibody positive renal transplant recipients: A randomized controlled trial. Ann. Intern. Med. *123*:18–26, 1995.
208. Hill, E. L., Hunter, G. A., Ellis, M. N., et al.: In vitro and in vivo characterization of herpes simplex virus clinical isolates recovered from patients infected with human immunodeficiency virus. Antimicrob. Agents Chemother. *35*:2322–2328, 1991.
209. Hillenkamp, J., Reinhard, T., Bohringer, D., et al.: Topical treatment of acute adenoviral keratoconjunctivitis with 0.2% cidofovir and 1% cyclosporin: A controlled clinical pilot study. Arch. Ophthalmology *119*:1487–1491, 2001.
210. Hillenkamp, J. Reinhard, T., Bohringer, D., et al.: The effects of cidofovir 1% with and without cyclosporin A 1% as a topical treatment of acute adenoviral keratoconjunctivitis: A controlled clinical pilot study. Ophthalmology *109*:845–850, 2002.
211. Hillyard, I. W.: The preclinical toxicology and safety of ribavirin. *In* Smith, R. A., Kirkpatrick, W. (eds.): Ribavirin: A Broad Spectrum Antiviral Agent. New York, Academic Press, 1980, pp. 59–60.
212. Hintz, M., Connor, J. D., Spector, S. A., et al.: Neonatal acyclovir pharmacokinetics in patients with herpes virus infections. Am. J. Med. *73*:210–214, 1982.
213. Hirsch, M. S., and Shooley, R. T.: Resistance to antiviral drugs: The end of innocence. N. Engl. J. Med. *320*:313–314, 1989.
214. Hitchcock, M. J., Jaffee, A. S., Martin, J. C., et al.: Cidofovir: A new agent with potent anti-herpes activity. Antiviral. Chem. Chemother. 7:115–127, 1996.
215. Ho, H. T., Woods, K. L., Bronzon, J. J., et al.: Intracellular metabolism of the anti-herpes agent (S)-1-[3-hydroxy-2-(phosphonylmethoxy) propyl] cytosine. Mol. Pharmacol. *41*:197–202, 1992.
216. Hochster, H., Dietrich, D., Bozzette, S., et al.: Toxicity of combined ganciclovir and zidovudine for cytomegalovirus disease associated with AIDS: An AIDS Clinical Trial Group Study. Ann. Intern. Med. *113*:111–117, 1990.
217. Hoffman, J., Shah, A., Ross, L., and Kapoor, N.: Adenoviral infections and a prospective trial of cidofovir in pediatric hematopoietic stem cell transplantation. Biol. Blood Marrow Transplant. 7:388–394, 2001.
218. Holland, G., Sidikraro, Y., Kreiger, A., et al.: Treatment of cytomegalovirus retinopathy with ganciclovir. Ophthalmology *94*:815–823, 1987.
219. Holmes, G. P., Chapman, L. E., Stewart, J. A., et al.: Guidelines for the prevention and treatment of B-virus infections in exposed persons: The B Virus Working Group. Clin. Infect. Dis. *20*:421–439, 1995.
220. Holmes, G. P., Mccormick, J. B., Trock, S. C., et al.: Lassa fever in the United States: Investigation of a case and new guidelines for management. N. Engl. J. Med. *323*:1120–1123, 1990.
221. Hoofnagle, J. H., and Di Bisceglie, A. M.: Drug therapy: The treatment of chronic viral hepatitis. N. Engl. J. Med. *336*:347–356, 1997.
222. Horadam, V. W., Sharp, J. G., Smilack, J. D., et al.: Pharmacokinetics of amantadine hydrochloride in subjects with normal and impaired renal function. Ann. Intern. Med. *94*:454–458, 1981.

223. Hosoya, M., Shigeta, S., Mori, S., et al.: High dose intravenous ribavirin therapy for subacute sclerosing panencephalitis. Antimicrob. Agents Chemother. *45*:943–945, 2001.
224. Hosoya, M., Shigeta, A., Nakamura, K., and DeClercq, E.: Inhibitory effect of selected antiviral compounds on measles (SSPE) virus replication in vitro. Antiviral Res. *12*:87–98, 1989.
225. Hruska, J. F., Morrow, P. E., Suffin, S. C., et al.: In vivo inhibition of respiratory syncytial virus by ribavirin. Antimicrob. Agents Chemother. *21*:125–130, 1982.
226. Huggins, J. W.: Prospects for treatment of viral hemorrhagic fevers with ribavirin, a broad spectrum antiviral drug. Rev. Iinfect. Dis. *11*(Suppl. 4):750–761, 1989.
227. Huggins, J. W., Hsiang, C. M., Cosgriff, T. M., et al.: Prospective, double blind, concurrent, placebo controlled clinical trial of intravenous ribavirin therapy of hemorrhagic fever with renal syndrome. J. Infect. Dis. *164*:1119–1127, 1991.
228. Hugonenq, C., Lethal, V., Chambost, H., et al.: Progressive multifocal leukoencephalopathy revealing AIDS in a 13 year old girl. Arch. Pediatr. *9*:32–35, 2002.
229. Hung, S. O., Patterson, A., and Rees, P. J.: Pharmacokinetics of oral acyclovir (Zovirax) in the eye. Br. J. Ophthalmol. *68*:192–195, 1984.
230. Jabs, D. A., Enger, C., Dunn, J. P., et al.: Cytomegalovirus retinitis and viral resistance: Ganciclovir resistance. J. Infect. Dis. *177*:770–773, 1998.
231. Jackson, G. G., Muldoon, R. C., and Akers, L. W.: Serologic evidence for prevention of influenzal infection in volunteers by an anti-influenzal drug, amantadine hydrochloride. Antimicrob. Agents Chemother. *3*:703–707, 1963.
232. Jackson, G. G., and Stanley, E. D.: Prevention and control of influenza by chemoprophylaxis and chemotherapy: Prospects from examination of recent experience. J. A. M. A. *235*:2739–2742, 1976.
233. Jacobsen, M. A., Berger, T. G., Fikrig, S., et al.: Acyclovir-resistant varicella-zoster virus infection after chronic oral acyclovir therapy in patients with the acquired immunodeficiency syndrome (AIDS). Ann. Intern. Med. *112*:187–191, 1990.
234. Jacobsen, M. A., Drew, W., Feinberg, J., et al.: Foscarnet therapy for ganciclovir-resistant cytomegalovirus retinitis in patients with AIDS. J. Infect. Dis. *163*:1318–1351, 1991.
235. Jacobsen, M., Gambertoglio, J., Aweeka, T., et al.: Foscarnet-induced hypocalcemia and effects of foscarnet on calcium metabolism. J. Clin. Endocrinol. Metab. *72*:1130–1135, 1991.
236. Jacobsen, M., van der Hurst, C., Causey, D., et al.: In vivo additive antiretroviral effect of combined zidovudine and foscarnet therapy for human immunodeficiency virus infection (ACTG Protocol 053). J. Infect. Dis. *163*:1219–1222, 1991.
237. Jahrling, P. B., Hesse, R. A., Eddy, G. A., et al.: Lassa fever infection of rhesus monkeys: Pathogenesis and treatment with ribavirin. J. Infect. Dis. *141*: 580–589, 1980.
238. Janai, H. K., Stutman, H. R., Zaleska, M., et al.: Ribavirin effect on pulmonary function in young infants with respiratory syncytial virus bronchiolitis. Pediatr. Infect. Dis. J. *12*:214–218, 1993.
239. Japour, A. J., Lertora, J. J., Meehan, P. M., et al.: A phase-1 study of the safety, pharmacokinetics, and antiviral activity of combination didanosine and ribavirin in patients with HIV-1 disease. AIDS Clinical Trials Group 231 Protocol Team. J. Acquir. Immune Defic. Syndr. Hum. Retrovirol. *13*:235–246, 1996.
240. Jayaweera, D.: Minimizing the dosage-limiting toxicities of foscarnet induction therapy. Drug Saf. *16*:258–266, 1997.
241. Jung, D., and Dorr, A.: Single-dose pharmacokinetics of valganciclovir in HIV- and CMV-seropositive subjects. J. Clin. Pharmacol. *39*:800–804, 1999.
242. Kaplan, I. J., Daum, R. S., Smaron, M., et al.: Severe measles in immunocompromised patients. J. A. M. A. *267*:1237–1241, 1992.
243. Katlama, C., Dobin, E., Caumes, E., et al.: Foscarnet induction therapy for cytomegalovirus retinitis in AIDS: Comparison of twice-daily and three-times-daily regimens. J. Acquir. Immune Defic. Syndr. *5*(Suppl. 1): 18–24, 1992.
244. Kaufman, H. E.: Clinical cure of herpes simplex keratitis by 5-iodo-2'-deoxyuridine. Proc. Soc. Exp. Biol. Med. *109*:251–252, 1962.
245. Kaufman, H. E., and Heidelberger, C.: Therapeutic antiviral action of 5-trifluoromethyl-s'-deoxyuridine in herpes simplex keratitis. Science. *145*:585–586, 1964.
246. Kaufman, H. E., Martola, E., and Dohlman, C.: Use of 5-iodo-2'-deoxyuridine (IDU) in treatment of herpes simplex keratitis. Arch. Ophthalmol. *68*:235–239, 1962.
247. Kearns, G. L., Abdel-Rahman, S. M., James, L. P., et al.: Single-dose pharmacokinetics of a pleconaril (VP63843) oral solution in children and adolescents. Antimicrob. Agents Chemother. *43*:634–638, 1999.
248. Kearns, G. L., Bradley, J. S., Jacobs, R. F., et al.: Single dose pharmacokinetics of pleconaril in neonates. Pediatr. Infect. Dis. J. *19*:833–839, 2000.
249. Kedes, D., and Ganem, D.: Sensitivity of sarcoma-associated herpesvirus replication to antiviral drugs: Implications for potential therapy. J. Clin. Invest. *99*:2082–2086, 1997.
250. Keeney, R. E., Kirk, L. E., and Bridgen, D.: Acyclovir tolerance in humans. Am. J. Med. *73*:176–181, 1982.
251. Kern, E. R., Hartline, C., Harden, E., et al.: Enhanced inhibition of orthopoxvirus replication in vitro by alkoxyalkylesters of cidofovir and cyclic cidofovir. Antimicrob. Agents Chemother. *46*:991–995, 2002.
252. Khare, G. P., Sidwell, R. W., Witkowski, J. T., et al.: Suppression by 1-beta-D-ribofuranosyl-1,2,4-triazole-3-carboxamide (Virazol, ICN1229) of influenza virus–induced infections in mice. Antimicrob. Agents Chemother. *3*:517–522, 1973.
253. Kilgore, P. E., Ksiazek, T. G., Rollin, P. E., et al.: Treatment of Bolivian hemorrhagic fever with intravenous ribavirin. Clin. Infect. Dis. *24*:718–722, 1997.
254. Kim, C. U., Lew, W., Williams, M. A., et al.: Influenza neuraminidase inhibitors possessing a novel hydrophobic interaction in the enzyme active site: Design, synthesis, and structural analysis of carbyclic sialic acid analogues with potent anti-influenza activity. J. Am. Chem. Soc. *119*:681–690, 1997.
255. Kimberlin, D., Lakeman, F., Arvin, A., et al.: Application of the polymerase chain reaction to the diagnosis and management of neonatal herpes simplex virus disease. J. Infect. Dis. *174*:1162–1167, 1996.
256. Kimberlin, D. W., Chin, Y. Y., Jacobs, R. F., et al.: Safety and efficacy of high-dose intravenous acyclovir in the management of neonatal herpes simplex virus infections. Pediatrics *108*:230–238, 2000.
257. Kimberlin, D. W., Lin, C.-Y., Sanchez, P., et al.: Antiviral treatment of symptomatic congenital cytomegalovirus (CMV) infections: Results of a phase III randomized trial. Abstract 1942. Presented at the 40th Annual Meeting of the Interscience Conference on Antimicrobial Agents and Chemotherapy, September 17–20, 2000, Toronto.
258. Kimberlin, D. W., Powell, D., Gruber, W., et al.: Administration of oral acyclovir, suppressive therapy after neonatal herpes simplex virus disease limited to the skin, eye and mouth: Results of a phase I/II trial. Pediatr. Infect. Dis. J. *15*:247–254, 1996.
259. Kimberlin, D. W., Weller, S., Whitley, R. J., et al.: Pharmacokinetics of oral valacyclovir and acyclovir in late pregnancy. Am. J. Obstet. Gynecol. *179*:846–851, 1998.
260. Kirsch, L. S., Arevalo, J., Chavez, D., et al.: Intravitreal cidofovir (HPMPC) treatment of cytomegalovirus retinitis in patients with acquired immune deficiency syndrome. Ophthalmology *102*:702–709, 1995.
261. Klein, N. A., Mabie, W. C., Shaver, D. C., et al.: Herpes simplex virus hepatitis in pregnancy: Two patients successfully treated with acyclovir. Gastroenterology *100*:239–244, 1991.
262. Klimov, A. I., Rocha, E., Hayden, F. G., et al.: Prolonged shedding of amantadine-resistant influenza A viruses by immunodeficient patients: Detection by polymerase chain reaction-restriction analysis. J. Infect. Dis. *172*:1352–1355, 1995.
263. Knight, V., and Gilbert, B. E.: Ribavirin aerosol treatment of influenza. Infect. Dis. Clin. North Am. *1*:441–457, 1987.
264. Knight, V., Yu, C. P., Gilbert, B. E., et al.: Estimating the dosage of ribavirin aerosol according to age and other variables. J. Infect. Dis. *158*:443–448, 1988.
265. Kopp, T., Geusau, A., Rieger, A., and Stinge, G.: Successful treatment of an acyclovir-resistant herpes simplex type 2 infection with cidofovir in an AIDS patient. Br. J. Dermatol. *147*:134–138, 2002.
266. Korba, B. E., and Boyd, M. R.: Penciclovir is a selective inhibitor of hepatitis B virus replication in cultured human hepatoblastoma cells. Antimicrob. Agents Chemother. *40*:1282–1284, 1996.
267. Kramer, T. H., Gaar, G. G., Ray, C. G., et al.: Hemodialysis clearance of intravenously administered ribavirin. Antimicrob. Agents Chemother. *34*:489–490, 1990.
268. Krasny, H. C., Liao, S. H., deMiranda, P., et al.: Influence of hemodialysis on acyclovir pharmacokinetics in patients with chronic renal failure. Am. J. Med. *73*:202–204, 1982.
269. Kupperman, B., Quicenco, J., Flores-Aguilar, M., et al.: Intravitreal ganciclovir concentration after intravenous administration in AIDS patients with cytomegalovirus retinitis: Implications for therapy. J. Infect. Dis. *168*:1506–1509, 1993.
270. Kusne, S., Schwartz, M., Breinig, M. K., et al.: Herpes simplex virus hepatitis after solid organ transplantation in adults. J. Infect. Dis. *163*:1001–1007, 1991.
271. Lakeman, F., and Whitley, R.: Diagnosis of herpes simplex encephalitis: Application of polymerase chain reaction to cerebrospinal fluid from brain-biopsied patients and correlation with disease. NIAID Collaborative Antiviral Study Group. J. Infect. Dis. *171*:857–863, 1995.
272. Lalezari, J. P., Drew, W. L., Glutzer, E., et al.: Treatment with intravenous (S)-1-[3-hydroxy-2-(phosphonylmethoxy)propyl]-cytosine of acyclovir-resistant mucocutaneous infection with herpes simplex virus in patient with AIDS. J. Infect. Dis. *170*:570–572, 1994.
273. Lalezari, J. P., Holland, G. N., Kramer, F., et al.: Randomized, controlled study of the safety and efficacy of intravenous cidofovir for the treatment of relapsing cytomegalovirus retinitis in patients with AIDS. J. Acquir. Immune Defic. Syndr. Hum. Retrovirol. *17*:339–344, 1998.
274. Lalezari, J. P., Stagg, R., Kuppermann, B., et al.: Intravenous cidofovir for peripheral cytomegalovirus retinitis in patients with AIDS. A randomized, controlled trial. Ann. Intern. Med. *126*:257–263, 1997.
275. Larson, E. W., Stephen, E. C., and Walker, J. S.: Therapeutic effects of small-particle aerosols of ribavirin in parainfluenza (Sendai) virus infections in mice. Antimicrob. Agents Chemother. *10*:770–772, 1976.

276. Laskin, O. L., Cederberg, D., Mills, J., et al.: Ganciclovir for the treatment and suppression of serious infections caused by cytomegalovirus. Am. J. Med. *83*:201–207, 1987.
277. Laskin, O. L., Longstreth, J. A., Hart, C. C., et al.: Ribavirin disposition in high-risk patients for acquired immunodeficiency syndrome. Clin. Pharmacol. Ther. *41*:546–555, 1987.
278. Laskin, O. L., Longstreth, J. A., Shelton, A., et al.: Effect of renal failure on the pharmacokinetics of acyclovir. Am. J. Med. *73*:197–201, 1982.
279. Lau, R. J., Emery, M. J., Galinsky, B. E., et al.: Unexpected accumulation of acyclovir in breast milk with estimate of infant exposure. Obstet. Gynecol. *69*:468–471, 1987.
280. Lavelle, J., Fallansbee, S., Trapnell, C. B., et al.: Effect of food on the relative bioavailability of oral ganciclovir. J. Clin. Pharmacol. *36*:238–241, 1996.
281. Lawell, D., Rosenthal, D., Aoki, F., et al.: Efficacy and safety of foscarnet for recurrent orolabial herpes: A multicentre randomized double-blind study. C. M. A. J. *138*:329–333, 1988.
282. Leary, J. J., Wittrock, R., Sarisky, R., et al.: Susceptibilities of herpes simplex viruses to penciclovir and acyclovir in eight cell lines. Antimicrob. Agents Chemother. *46*:762–768, 2002.
283. Legrand, F., Berrebi, D., Houhou, N., et al.: Early diagnosis of adenovirus infection and treatment with cidofovir after bone marrow transplantation in children. Bone Marrow Transplant. *27*:621–626, 2001.
284. Leone, P. A., Trottier, S., Miller, J. M.: Valacyclovir for episodic treatment of genital herpes: A shorter 3-day treatment course compared with 5-day treatment. Clin. Infect. Dis *34*:958–962, 2002.
285. Lewis, V. A., Champlin, R., Englund, J., et al.: Respiratory disease due to parainfluenza virus in adult bone marrow transplant recipients. Clin. Infect. Dis. *23*:1033–1037, 1996.
286. Lin, J. C., Smith, M. C., Cheng, Y. C., et al.: Epstein-Barr virus: Inhibition of replication by three new drugs. Science *221*:578–579, 1983.
287. Little, J. W., Hall, H. J., and Douglas, R. G., Jr.: Amantadine effect on peripheral airways abnormalities in influenza. Ann. Intern. Med. *85*:177–180, 1976.
288. Littler, E., Stuart, A. D., and Chee, M. S.: Human cytomegalovirus UL97 open reading frame encodes a protein that phosphorylates the antiviral nucleoside analogue ganciclovir. Nature *358*:160–162, 1992.
289. Ljungman, P., Deliliers, G., Platzbecker, V., et al.: Cidofovir for cytomegalovirus infection and disease in allogeneic stem cell transplant recipients. The Infectious Diseases Working Party of the European Group for Blood and Marrow Transplantation. Blood *97*:388–392, 2001.
290. Long, C. E., Voter, K. Z., Barker, W. H., et al.: Long term followup of children hospitalized with respiratory syncytial virus lower respiratory tract infection and randomly treated with ribavirin or placebo. Pediatr. Infect. Dis. *16*:1023–1028, 1997.
291. Loveless, M., Sacks, S. L., and Harris, R. J: Famciclovir in the management of first episode genital herpes. Infect. Dis. Clin. Pract. *6*:512–516, 1997.
292. Lowensohn, D. M., Bowden, R. A., Mattson, A., et al.: Phase I study of intravenous ribavirin treatment of respiratory syncytial virus pneumonia after marrow transplantation. Antimicrob. Agents. Chemother. *40*:2555–2557, 1996.
293. Lugo, R. A., and Nahata, M. C.: Pathogenesis and treatment of bronchiolitis. Clin. Pharm. *12*:95–116, 1993.
294. Lurain, N. S., Thompson, K. D., Holes, E. W., et al.: Point mutations in the DNA polymerase gene of human cytomegalovirus that result in resistance to antiviral agents. J. Virol. *66*:7146–7152, 1992.
295. MacGregor, R., Graziani, A., Weiss, R., et al.: Successful foscarnet therapy for cytomegalovirus retinitis in an AIDS patient undergoing hemodialysis: Rationale for empiric dosing and plasma level monitoring. J. Infect. Dis. *164*:785–787, 1991.
296. Manischewitz, J., Quinnan, G., Lane, H., et al.: Synergistic effect of ganciclovir and foscarnet on cytomegalovirus replication in vitro. Antimicrob. Agents Chemother. *34*:373–375, 1990.
297. Markham, A., and Faulds, D.: Ganciclovir: An update of its therapeutic use in cytomegalovirus infection. Drugs *48*:455–484, 1994.
298. Marquaidt, D. L., Gruber, H. E., and Walker, L. L.: Ribavirin inhibits mast cell mediator release. J. Pharmacol. Exp. Ther. *240*:145–149, 1990.
299. Marques, A. R., Lau, D. T., McKenzie, R., et al.: Combination therapy with famciclovir and interferon-alpha for the treatment of chronic hepatitis B. J. Infect. Dis. *178*:1483–1487, 1998.
300. Martin, D. F., Sierra-Madero, J., Walmsley, S., et al.: Controlled trial of valganciclovir as induction therapy for cytomegalovirus retinitis. N. Engl. J. Med. *346*:1119–1126, 2002.
301. Marx, J. L., Kapusta, M., Patel, S., et al.: Use of the ganciclovir implant in the treatment of recurrent cytomegalovirus retinitis. Arch. Ophthalmol. *114*:815–820, 1996.
302. Maslo, C., Girard, P. M., Urban, T., et al.: Ribavirin therapy for adenovirus pneumonia in an AIDS patient. Am. J. Respir. Crit. Care Med. *156*:911–914, 1997.
303. Mast, E. E., Harmon, M. W., Gravenstein, S., et al.: Emergence and possible transmission of amantadine-resistant viruses during nursing home outbreaks of influenza A (H3N2) Am. J. Epidemiol. *13*:988–997, 1991.
304. Mazzi, R., Parisi, S., Sarmati, L., et al.: Efficacy of cidofovir on human herpesvirus 8 viraemia and Kaposi's sarcoma progression in two patients with AIDS. *15*:2061–2062, 2001.
305. McClellan, K., and Perry, C. M.: Oseltamivir: A review of its use in influenza. Drugs *61*:263–283, 2001.
306. McCormick, J. B., King, I. J., Webb, P. A., et al.: Lassa fever: Effective therapy with ribavirin. N. Engl. J. Med. *314*:20–26, 1986.
307. McHutchison, J. G., Gordon, S. C., Schiff, E. R., et al.: Interferon alfa-2b alone or in combination with ribavirin as initial treatment for chronic hepatitis C. Hepatitis Interventional Therapy Group. N. Engl. J. Med. *339*:1485–1492, 1998.
308. McIntosh, K., Kurachek, S. C., Cairns, et al.: Treatment of respiratory syncytial viral infection in an immunodeficient infant with ribavirin aerosol. Am. J. Dis. Child. *138*:305–308, 1984.
309. McKinlay, M. A., Pevear, D. C., and Rossman, M. G.: Treatment of the picornavirus common cold by inhibitors of viral uncoating and attachment. Annu. Rev. Microbiol. *46*:635–654, 1992.
310. Meert, K. L., Sarnaik, A. P., Gelmini, M. I., et al.: Aerosolized ribavirin in mechanically ventilated children with respiratory syncytial virus lower respiratory tract disease: A prospective, double-blind, randomized trial. Crit. Care Med. *22*:566–572, 1994.
311. Meier, P., Dautheville-Gaibal, S., Ronco, P., and Rossert, J.: Cidofovir-induced end-stage renal failure. Nephrol. Dial. Transplant. *17*:148–149, 2002.
312. Mendel, D. B., Barkhimer, D. B., and Chen, M. S.: Biochemical basis for increased susceptibility to cidofovir of herpes simplex viruses with altered or deficient thymidine kinase activity. Antimicrob. Agents Chemother. *39*:2120–2122, 1995.
313. Mendel, D. B., and Sidwell, R. W.: Influenza virus resistance to neuraminidase inhibitors. Drug Resistance Updates *1*:184–189, 1998.
314. Merigan, T. C., Renlund, D., Keay, S., et al.: A controlled trial of ganciclovir to prevent cytomegalovirus disease after heart transplantation. N. Engl. J. Med. *326*:1182–1186, 1992.
315. Mertz, G. J., Loveless, M. O., Levin, M. J., et al.: Oral famciclovir for suppression of recurrent genital herpes simplex virus infection in women: A multicenter, double-blind placebo-controlled trial. Collaborative Famciclovir Genital Herpes Research Group. Arch. Intern. Med. *157*:343–349, 1997.
316. Meyer, L. J., Smith, M. P., Sheth, N., et al.: Acyclovir in human breast milk. Am. J. Obstet. Gynecol. *158*:586–588, 1988.
317. Meyers, J. D., Reed, E. C., Shepp, D. H., et al.: Acyclovir for prevention of cytomegalovirus infection and disease after allogeneic marrow transplantation. N. Engl. J. Med. *318*:70–75, 1988.
318. Millet, V. M., Dreisbach, M., and Bryson, Y. J.: Double blind controlled study of central nervous system side effects of amantadine, rimantadine, and chlorpheniramine. Antimicrob. Agents Chemother. *21*:1–4, 1982.
319. Mindel, A., Faherty, A., Carney, O., et al.: Dosage and safety of long term suppressive acyclovir therapy for recurrent genital herpes. Lancet *1*:926–928, 1988.
320. MIST Study Group: Randomized trial of efficacy and safety of inhaled zanamivir in treatment of influenza A and B virus infections. Lancet *352*:1877–1881, 1998.
321. Moler, F. W., Steinhart, C. M., Ohmit, S. E., and Stidham, G. I.: Effectiveness of ribavirin in otherwise well infants with respiratory syncytial virus associated respiratory failure. Pediatric Critical Care Study Group. J. Pediatr. *128*:422–428, 1996.
322. Montanaki, C., Farrari, P., and Bavazzand, A.: Urinary excretion of amantadine by the elderly. Eur. J. Clin. Pharmacol. *8*:349–356, 1975.
323. Monto, A. S., Gunn, R. A., and Bardyk, M. G.: Prevention of Russian influenza by amantadine. J. A. M. A. *241*:1003–1007, 1979.
324. Monto, A. S., Robinson, D. P., Herlocher, M. L., et al.: Zanamivir in the prevention of influenza among healthy adults: A randomized controlled trial. J. A. M. A. *282*:31–35, 1999.
325. Monto, A. S., Webster, A., and Keene, O.: Randomized, placebo controlled studies of inhaled zanamivir in the treatment of influenza A and B: Pooled efficacy analysis. J. Antimicrob. Chemother. *44*(Suppl. B): 23–29, 1999.
326. Morra, C., Rajicic, N., Barker, D., et al.: A pilot study of cidofovir for progressive multifocal leukoencephalopathy in AIDS. A. I. D. S. *16*:1791–1797, 2002.
327. Munoz, F., and Demmler, G. J.: Disseminated adenovirus disease in immunocompromised and immunocompetent children. Clin. Infect. Dis. *27*:1194–1200, 1998.
328. Musch, D. C., Martin, D. F., Gordon, J., et al.: Treatment of cytomegalovirus retinitis with a sustained-release ganciclovir implant. The Ganciclovir Implant Study Group. N. Engl. J. Med. *337*:83–90, 1997.
329. Mustafa, M. M., Witman, S. D., Wirick, N. J., et al.: Subacute measles encephalitis in the young immunocompromised host: Report of two cases diagnosed by polymerase chain reaction and treated with ribavirin and review of the literature. Clin. Infect. Dis. *16*:654–660, 1993.
330. Nahata, M. C., and Brady, M. T.: Serum concentrations and safety of rimantadine in pediatric patients. Eur. J. Clin. Pharmacol. *30*:719–722, 1986.
331. Neau, D., Renaud-Rougier, M. B., Viallard, J., et al.: Intravenous cidofovir induced iritis. Clin. Infect. Dis. *28*:1257–158, 1999.
332. Nedyalkova, M. S., Hayden, F. G., Webster, R. G., and Gubareva, L. V.: Accumulation of defective neuraminidase (NA) genes by influenza A

viruses in the presence of NA inhibitors as a marker of reduced dependence on NA. J. Infect. Dis. *185*:591–598, 2002.
333. Nevarro, J., Quereda, C., Gallego, N., et al.: Nephrogenic diabetes insipidus and renal tubular acidosis secondary to foscarnet therapy. Am. J. Kidney Dis. *27*:431–434, 1996.
334. Neyts, J., and DeClercq, E.: Efficacy of (S)-1-(3-hydroxy-2-phosphonylmethoxypropyl)-purine for the treatment of lethal vaccinia virus infections in severe combined immune deficiency (SCID) mice. J. Med. Virol. *41*:242–246, 1993.
335. Neyts, J., and DeClercq, E.: Effect of 5-iodo-2′-deoxyuridine on vaccinia virus (orthopoxvirus) infections in mice. Antimicrob. Agents Chemother. *46*:2842–2847, 2002.
336. Noormohamed, F., Youle, M., Higgs, C., et al.: Pharmacokinetics and absolute bioavailability of oral foscarnet in human immunodeficiency virus positive patients. Antimicrob. Agents Chemother. *42*:293–297, 1998.
337. Oberg, B.: Antiviral effects of phosphonoformate (PFA, foscarnet sodium). Pharmacol. Ther. *19*:387–415, 1983.
338. O'Donoghue, J. M., Ray, C. G., Terry, D. W., et al.: Prevention of nosocomial influenza infection with amantadine. Am. J. Epidemiol. *97*:276–282, 1973.
339. Outwater, K. M., Meissner, H. C., and Peterson, M. B.: Ribavirin administration to infants receiving mechanical ventilation. Am. J. Dis. Child. *142*:512–515, 1988.
340. Oxford, J. S.: Effects of 1-beta-D-ribofuranosyl-1,2,4-triazole-3-carboxamide on influenza virus replication and polypeptide synthesis. J. Antimicrob. Agents Chemother. *1*(Suppl.):71–76, 1973.
341. Oxford, J. S., and Schild, G. C.: In vitro inhibition of rubella virus by 1-amantanamine hydrochloride. Arch. Gesamte Virusforsch. *17*:313–329, 1965.
342. Oxford, J. S., and Schild, G. C.: The evaluation of antiviral compounds for rubella virus using organ cultures. Arch. Gesamte Virusforsch. *22*:349–356, 1967.
343. Palestine, A. G., Polis, M. A., DeSmet, M. D., et al.: A randomized controlled trial of foscarnet in the treatment of cytomegalovirus retinitis in patients with AIDS. Ann. Intern. Med. *115*:665–673, 1991.
344. Palsey, D. A., Sternberg, P. J., Davis, J., et al.: Decrease in the risk of bilateral acute retinal necrosis by acyclovir therapy. Am. J. Ophthalmol. *112*:250–255, 1991.
345. Paroni, R., Borghi, C., Sirtori, C. R., et al.: Pharmacokinetics of ribavirin and urinary excretion of the major metabolite 1,2,4-triazole-3-carboxamide in normal volunteers. Int. J. Clin. Pharmacol. Ther. Toxicol. *27*:302–307, 1989.
346. Parris, D. S., and Harrington, J. E.: Herpes simplex virus variants resistant to high concentrations of acyclovir exist in clinical isolates. Antimicrob. Agents Chemother. *22*:71–77, 1982.
347. Patriarca, P. A., Kater, N. A., Kendeal, A. P., et al.: Safety of prolonged administration of rimantadine hydrochloride in the prophylaxis of influenza A virus infection in nursing homes. Antimicrob. Agents Chemother. *26*:101–103, 1984.
348. Pelosi, E., Mulamba, G. B., and Coen, D. M.: Penciclovir and pathogenic phenotypes of drug resistant herpes simplex virus mutants. Antiviral Res. *37*:17–28, 1998.
349. Pescovitz, M. D., Rabkin, J., Merion, R., et al.: Valganciclovir results in improved oral absorption of ganciclovir in liver transplant recipients. Antimicrob. Agents Chemother. *44*:2811–2815, 2000.
350. Pevear, D. C., Fancher, M. J., Felock, P. J., et al.: Conformational changes in the floor of the human rhinovirus blocks adsorption to HeLa cell receptors. J. Virol. *63*:2002–2007, 1989.
351. Pevear, D. C., Tull, T. M., Seipel, M. E., and Broarke, J. M.: Activity of pleconaril against enteroviruses. Antimicrob. Agents Chemother. *43*:2109–2115, 1999.
352. Pimentel, L., and Hughes, B.: Amantadine toxicity presenting with complex ventricular ectopy and hallucinations. Pediatr. Emerg. Care *7*:89–92, 1991.
353. Platzbecker, U., Bandt, U., Thiede, C., et al.: Successful preemptive cidofovir treatment for CMV antigenemia after dose reduced conditioning and allogeneic blood stem cell transplantation. Transplantation *15*:880–885, 2001.
354. Plotkin, S. A., Drew, W. L., Felsenstein, D., et al.: Sensitivity of clinical isolates of human cytomegalovirus to 9-(1,3-dihydroxy-2-propoxymethyl)guanine. J. Infect. Dis. *152*:833–834, 1985.
355. Poehling, K. A., and Edwards, K. M.: Prevention, diagnosis, and treatment of influenza: Current and future options. Curr. Opin. Pediatr. *13*:60–64, 2001.
356. Polis, M., Spooner, K., Baird, B., et al.: Anticytomegaloviral activity and safety of cidofovir in patients with human immunodeficiency virus infection and cytomegalovirus viruria. Antimicrob. Agents Chemother. *39*:882–886, 1995.
357. Prober, C. G., Kirk, L. E., and Keeney, R. E.: Acyclovir therapy for chickenpox in immunosuppressed children: A collaborative study. J. Pediatr. *101*:622–625, 1982.
358. Prusoff, W. H.: Synthesis and biological activities of iododeoxyuridine, an analogue of thymidine. Biochem. Biophys. Acta *32*:295–296, 1959.
359. Randolph, A. G., and Wang, E.: Ribavirin therapy for respiratory syncytial virus lower respiratory tract infection: A systematic overview. Arch. Pediatr. Adolesc. Med. *150*:942–947, 1996.
360. Rashed, A., Azadek, B., and Abu, R. H.: Acyclovir induced acute tubulo-interstitial nephritis. Nephron *56*:436–438, 1990.
361. Ray, C. G., Isenogle, T. B., Minnich, L. L., et al.: The use of intravenous ribavirin to treat influenza-associated acute myocarditis. J. Infect. Dis. *159*:829–836, 1989.
362. Razonable, R. R., Aksamit, A., Wright, A., and Wilson, J.: Cidofovir treatment of progressive multifocal leukoencephalopathy in a patient receiving highly active antiretroviral therapy. Mayo Clin. Proc. *76*:1171–1175, 2001.
363. Reed, E. C., Bowden, R., and Dandliker, P. S.: Treatment of cytomegalovirus pneumonia with ganciclovir and intravenous cytomegalovirus immunoglobulin in patients with bone marrow transplants. Ann. Intern. Med. *109*:783–788, 1988.
364. Reed, E., Wolford, S., Koppecky, K., et al.: Ganciclovir for the treatment of cytomegalovirus gastroenteritis in bone marrow transplant patients: A randomized, placebo-controlled trial. Ann. Intern. Med. *112*:505–510, 1990.
365. Reichard, O., Norkrans, G., Fryden, A., et al.: Randomized, double-blind placebo controlled trial of interferon alpha-2b with and without ribavirin for chronic hepatitis C. Lancet *351*:83–87, 1998.
366. Reichman, R. C., Badger, G. J., Mertz, G. J., et al.: Treatment of recurrent genital herpes simplex infections with oral acyclovir: A controlled trial. J. A. M. A. *251*:2103–2107, 1984.
367. Reitano, M., Tyring, S., Lang, W., et al.: Valacyclovir for the suppression of recurrent genital herpes simplex virus infection: A large scale dose range finding study. J. Infect. Dis. *178*:603–610, 1998.
368. Resnick, L., Herbst, J. S., Abashi, D. V., et al.: Regression of oral hairy leukoplakia after orally administered acyclovir therapy. J. A. M. A. *259*:384–388, 1988.
369. Reusser, P., Gambertoglio, J., Lilleby, K., et al.: Phase I/II trial of foscarnet for prevention of cytomegalovirus infection in autologous and allogeneic marrow transplant recipients. J. Infect. Dis. *166*:473–479, 1992.
370. Ribaud, P., Scieux, D., Freymouth, F., et al.: Successful treatment of adenovirus disease with intravenous cidofovir in an unrelated stem cell transplant recipient. Clin. Infect. Dis. *28*:690–691, 1999.
371. Ribeiro de Valle, L. A., Resposo de Melo, P., de Salles Gomez, L. F., et al.: Methisazone in prevention of variola minor among contacts. Lancet *2*:976–978, 1965.
372. Rodriguez, W. J., Bui, R. H., Connor, J. D., et al.: Environmental exposure of primary care personnel to ribavirin aerosol when supervising treatment of infants with respiratory syncytial virus infections. Antimicrob. Agents Chemother. *31*:1143–1146, 1987.
373. Rombart, B., Vrjsen, R., and Boeye, A.: Comparison of arildone and 3-methylquercatin as stabilizers of poliovirus. Antivir. Res. *1*(Suppl.): 67–73, 1985.
374. Romero, J. R., Gross, T., Abromowitch, M., and Jung, L.: Pleconaril treatment of vaccine-acquired poliovirus. Abstract. Pediatr. Res. *45*:173, 1999.
375. Rompalo, A. M., Mertz, G. J., Davis, L. G., et al.: Oral acyclovir for treatment of first episode herpes simplex virus proctitis. J. A. M. A. *259*:2879–2881, 1988.
376. Rooney, J. F., Felser, J. M., Ostrove, J. M., et al.: Acquisition of genital herpes from an asymptomatic sexual partner. N. Engl. J. Med. *314*:1561–1564, 1986.
377. Rosh, H. R., Benner, K. G., Flora, K. D., et al.: Development of ganciclovir resistance during treatment of primary cytomegalovirus infection after liver transplantation. Transplantation *63*:476–478, 1996.
378. Rosner, I. K., Welliver, R. C., Edelson, P. J., et al.: Effect of ribavirin therapy on respiratory syncytial virus specific IgE and IgA responses after infection. J. Infect. Dis. *155*:1043–1047, 1987.
379. Rotbart, H. A.: Pleconaril treatment of enterovirus and rhinovirus infections. Infect. Med. *17*:488–494, 2000.
380. Sabin, A. B.: Amantadine hydrochloride: Analysis of data related to its proposed use for prevention of A2 influenza virus disease in human beings. J. A. M. A. *200*:943–950, 1967.
381. Sacks, S. L., Aoki, F. Y., Diaz-Mitoma, F., et al.: Patient-initiated, twice-daily oral famciclovir for early recurrent genital herpes: A randomized double blind multicenter trial. Canadian Famciclovir Study Group. J. A. M. A. *276*:44–49, 1996.
382. Safrin, S., Berger, T., Gilson, I, et al.: Foscarnet therapy in five patients with AIDS and acyclovir-resistant varicella-zoster virus infection. Ann. Intern. Med. *115*:19–21, 1991.
383. Safrin, S., Cherrington, J., and Jaffe, H. S.: Clinical uses of cidofovir. Rev. Med. Virol. *7*:145–156, 1997.
384. Safrin, S., Kemmerly, S., Plotkin, B., et al.: Foscarnet resistant herpes simplex virus infection in patients with AIDS. J. Infect. Dis. *169*:193–196, 1994.
385. Salmaggi, A., Maccagnano, E., Castagna, A., et al.: Reversal of CSF positivity for JC virus genome by cidofovir in a patient with systemic lupus erythematosus and progressive multifocal leukoencephalopathy. Neurol. Sci. *22*:17–20, 2001.

386. Salzman, R., Jurewicz, R., and Boon, R.: Safety of famciclovir in patients with herpes zoster and genital herpes. Antimicrob. Agents Chemother. *38*:2454–2457, 1994.
387. Sarasini, A., Baldanti, F., Furione, M., et al.: Double resistance to ganciclovir and foscarnet of four human cytomegalovirus strains recovered from AIDS patients. J. Med. Virol. *47*:237–244, 1995.
388. Sartori, M., Pratt, C. M., and Young, J. B.: Malignant cardiac arrhythmia induced by amantadine poisoning. Am. J. Med. *77*:388–391, 1984.
389. Sawyer, M. H., Saez-Llorenz, Y., Luiz-Aviles, C., et al.: Oral pleconaril reduces the duration and severity of enteroviral meningitis in children. Abstract. Pediatr. Res. *45*:173, 1999.
390. Sawyer, M. H., Webb, D. E., Balow, J. E., et al.: Acyclovir induced renal failure: Clinical course and histology. Am. J. Med. *84*:1067–1071, 1988.
391. Schacker, T., Hui-lin, H., Koelle, D. M., et al.: Famciclovir for the suppression of symptomatic and asymptomatic herpes simplex virus reactivation in HIV infected persons. Ann. Intern. Med. *128*:21–28, 1998.
392. Schaeffer, H. J., Beauchamp, L., DeMiranda, P., et al.: 9-(2-hydroxyethoxymethyl)guanine activity against viruses of the herpes group. Nature *272*:583–585, 1978.
393. Scheibel, L. M., Durbin, R. K., and Stollar, V.: Sindbis virus mutants resistant to mycophenolic acid and ribavirin. Virology *158*:1–7, 1987.
394. Schiff, G. M., and Sherwood, J. R.: Clinical activity of pleconaril in an experimentally induced coxsackievirus A21 respiratory infection. J. Infect. Dis. *181*:20–26, 2000.
395. Schmidt, G., Horak, D., Niland, J., et al.: A randomized controlled trial of prophylactic ganciclovir for cytomegalovirus pulmonary infection in recipients of allogeneic bone marrow transplants. The city of Hope Stanford Syntex CMV Study Group. N. Engl. J. Med. *324*:1005–1011, 1991.
396. Schnabel, F. M., Jr.: The antiviral activity of 9-beta-D-arabinofuranosyladenine (ara-A). Chemotherapy *13*:321–338, 1968.
397. Schooley, R. T., Carey, R. W., Miller, G., et al.: Chronic Epstein-Barr virus infection associated with fever and interstitial pneumonitis: Clinical and serologic features and response to antiviral chemotherapy. Ann. Intern. Med. *104*:636–643, 1986.
398. Schwab, R. S., England, A. C., Jr., Poskanzer, D. C., et al.: Amantadine in the treatment of Parkinson's disease. J. A. M. A. *209*:1168–1170, 1969.
399. Scott, L. L.: Perinatal herpes: Current status and obstetric management strategies. Pediatr. Infect. Dis. J. *14*:827–832, 1995.
400. Scott, L. L.: Prevention of perinatal herpes: Prophylactic antiviral therapy. Clin. Obstet. Gynecol. *42*:134–148, 1999.
401. Scott, L. L., Sanchez, P. J., Jackson, G. L., et al.: Acyclovir suppression to prevent cesarean delivery after first episode genital herpes. Obstet. Gynecol. *87*:69–73, 1996.
402. Segarra-Newnham, M., and Vodolo, K.: Use of cidofovir in progressive multifocal leukoencephalopathy. Ann. Pharmacol. *35*:741–744, 2001.
403. Shaw, T., Mok, S. S., and Locarnini, S. A.: Inhibition of hepatitis B virus DNA polymerase by enantiomers of penciclovir triphosphate and metabolic basis for selective inhibition of HBV replication by penciclovir. Hepatology *24*:996–1002, 1996.
404. Shults, R. A., Baron, S., Decker, J., et al.: Health care worker exposure to aerosolized ribavirin: Biological and air monitoring. J. Occup. Environ. Med. *38*:257–263, 1996.
405. Sidwell, R. W., Huffmann, J. H., Khare, G. P., et al.: Broad spectrum antiviral activity of virazole: 1-beta-D-ribofuranosyl-1,2,4-triazole-3-carboxamide. Science *17*:705–706, 1972.
406. Singh, N., Gayowski, T., Wannstedt, C. F., et al.: Pretransplant famciclovir as prophylaxis for hepatitis B virus recurrence after liver transplantation. Transplantation *63*:1415–1419, 1997.
407. Smee, D. F., Bailey, K. W., and Sidwell, R. W.: Treatment of lethal vaccinia virus respiratory infections in mice with cidofovir. Antiviral Chem. Chemother. *12*:71–76, 2001.
408. Smee, D. F., Bailey, K. W., Wong, M. H., and Sidwell, R. W.: Effects of cidofovir on the pathogenesis of a lethal vaccinia virus respiratory infection in mice. Antiviral Res. *52*:55–62, 2001.
409. Smee, D. F., Martin, J. C., Verheyden, T. P., et al.: Antiherpesvirus activity of the acyclic nucleoside 9-(1,3-dihydroxy-2-propoxymethyl) guanine. Antimicrob. Agents Chemother. *23*:676–682, 1983.
410. Smee, D. F., and Matthews, T. R.: Metabolism of ribavirin in respiratory syncytial virus infected and uninfected cells. Antimicrob. Agents Chemother. *30*:117–121, 1986.
411. Smee, D. F., Sidwell, R. W., Kefauver, D., et al.: Characterization of wild type and cidofovir resistant strains of camelpox, cowpox, monkeypox and vaccinia viruses. Antimicrob. Agents Chemother. *46*:1329–1335, 2002.
412. Smith, C. B., Charette, R. P., Fox, J. P., et al.: Double blind evaluation of ribavirin in naturally occurring influenza. *In* Smith, R. A., and Kilpatrick, W. (eds.): Ribavirin: A Broad-Spectrum Antiviral Agent. New York, Academic Press, 1980, pp. 147–164.
413. Smith, D. W., Frankel, L. R., Mathers, L. H., et al.: A controlled trial of aerosolized ribavirin in infants receiving mechanical ventilation for severe respiratory syncytial virus infection. N. Engl. J. Med. *325*:24–29, 1991.
414. Smith, I. L., Cherrington, J. M., Jules, R. E., et al.: High level resistance of cytomegalovirus to ganciclovir is associated with alterations in both the UL 97 and DNA polymerase genes. J. Infect. Dis. *176*:69–77, 1997.
415. Smith, J. P.: Treatment of chronic hepatitis C with amantadine. Dig. Dis. Sci. *42*:1681–1687, 1997.
416. Snoeck, R., Andrei, G., and Declercq, E.: Cidofovir in the treatment of HPV-associated lesions. Verh. Acad. Geneeskd. Belg. *63*:93–120, 2001.
417. Snoeck, R., Gerand, M., Sadzot-Delvaux, S., et al.: Meningoradiculoneuritis due to acyclovir-resistant varicella-zoster virus in a patient with AIDS. J. Infect. Dis. *168*:1330–1331, 1993.
418. Soike, K. F., Huang, J. L., Zahang, J.-Y., et al.: Evaluation of infrequent dosing regimens with (5)-1-[3-hydroxy-2-(phosphonylmethoxy) propyl] cytosine (5-HPMPC) in simian varicella infection in monkeys. Antiviral Res. *16*:17–28, 1991.
419. Sommadassi, J. P., Bevan, R., Ling, T., et al.: Clinical pharmacokinetics of ganciclovir in patients with normal and impaired renal function. Rev. Infect. Dis *10*(Suppl. 3):507–514, 1988.
420. Soo, S. K., Regan, A., Cihlar, T., et al.: Cytomegalovirus ventriculoencephalitis in a bone marrow transplant recipient receiving antiviral maintenance: Clinical and molecular evidence of drug resistance. Clin. Infect. Dis. *33*:e105–e108, 2001.
421. Soo, W.: Adverse effects of rimantadine: Summary from clinical trials. J. Respir. Dis *10* (Suppl):526–531, 1989.
422. Soul-Lawton, J., Seaber, E., Oh, N., et al.: Absolute bioavailability and metabolic disposition of valacyclovir, the L-valyl ester of acyclovir, following oral administration to humans. Antimicrob. Agents Chemother. *39*:2759–2764, 1995.
423. Soung, L. S., Ing, T. S., Daugirdas, J. T., et al.: Amantadine hydrochloride pharmacokinetics in hemodialysis patients. Ann. Intern. Med. *93*:46–49, 1980.
424. Spector, S. A., Busch, D., Follanskee, S., et al.: Pharmacokinetic, safety, and antiviral profiles of oral ganciclovir in persons infected with human immunodeficiency virus: A phase I/II study. J. Infect. Dis. *171*:1431–1437, 1995.
425. Spector, S., Hsia, K., Wolf, D., et al.: Molecular detection of human cytomegalovirus and determination of genotypic ganciclovir resistance in clinical specimens. Clin. Infect. Dis. *21*(Suppl. 2):170–173, 1995.
426. Spector, S. A., McKinley, G., Lalezari, J., et al.: Oral ganciclovir for the prevention of cytomegalovirus disease in persons with AIDS. Roche Cooperative Oral Ganciclovir Study Group. N. Engl. J. Med. *334*:1491–1497, 1996.
427. Spector, S. A., Weingeist, T., Pollard, R. B., et al.: A randomized, controlled study of intravenous ganciclovir therapy for cytomegalovirus peripheral retinitis in patients with AIDS. J. Infect. Dis. *168*:557–563, 1993.
428. Spruance, S. L., Rea, T. L., Thorning, C., et al.: Penciclovir cream for the treatment of herpes simplex labialis: A randomized multicenter double blind placebo controlled trial. Topical Penciclovir Collaborative Study Group. J. A. M. A. *277*:1374–1379, 1997.
429. Spruance, S. L., Tyring, S. K., Degregorio, B., et al.: A large scale, placebo controlled, dose ranging trial of peroral valacyclovir for episodic treatment of recurrent herpes genitalis. Valacyclovir Study Group. Arch. Intern. Med. *156*:1729–1735, 1996.
430. Stanat, S. C., Reardon, J. E., Erice, A., et al.: Ganciclovir-resistant cytomegalovirus clinical isolates: Mode of resistance to ganciclovir. Antimicrob. Agents Chemother. *35*:2191–2197, 1991.
431. Stein, D. S., Creticos, C. M., Jackson, G. G., et al.: Oral ribavirin treatment of influenza A and B. Antimicrob. Agents Chemother. *31*:1285–1287, 1987.
432. Stephenson, J. A., Artenstein, M. S., Parkman, P. D., et al.: Effect of amantadine hydrochloride on rubella virus infection in the rhesus monkey. Antimicrob. Agents Chemother. *5*:548–552, 1965.
433. Stragier, I., Snoeck, R., DeClercq, E., et al.: Local treatment of HPV-induced skin lesions by cidofovir. J. Med. Virol. *67*:241–245, 2002.
434. Streeter, D. G., Witkowski, J. T., Khare, T, et al.: Mechanism of action of 1-D-ribofuranosyl-1,2,3-triazole-3-carboxamide (Virazole), a new broad spectrum antiviral agent. Proc. Natl. Acad. Sci. U. S. A. *70*:1174–1178, 1973.
435. Studies of Ocular Complications of AIDS Research Group in collaboration with the AIDS Clinical Trial Group: Mortality in patients with the acquired immunodeficiency syndrome treated with either foscarnet or ganciclovir for cytomegalovirus retinitis. N. Engl. J. Med. *326*:213–220, 1992.
436. Studies of the Ocular Complications of AIDS Research Group in collaboration with the AIDS Clinical Trials Group: Combination foscarnet and ganciclovir therapy versus monotherapy for the treatment of relapsed cytomegalovirus retinitis in patients with AIDS: The Cytomegalovirus Retreatment Trial. Arch. Ophthalmol. *114*:23–33, 1996.
437. Studies of Ocular Complications of AIDS Research Group: Parenteral cidofovir for cytomegalovirus retinitis in patients with AIDS: The HPMPC Peripheral Cytomegalovirus Retinitis Trial. A randomized controlled trial. Ann. Intern. Med. *126*:264–274, 1997.
438. Sullender, W. M., Arvin, A. M., and Diaz, P. S.: Pharmacokinetics of acyclovir suspension in infants and children. Antimicrob. Agents Chemother. *31*:1722–1726, 1987.

439. Sullivan, J. L., Byron, K. S., Brewster, F. E., et al.: Treatment of life threatening Epstein-Barr virus infection with acyclovir. Am. J. Med. *73*:262–266, 1982.
440. Sylvester, R. K., Ogden, W. B., Draxler, C. A., et al.: Vesicular eruption: A local complication of concentrated acyclovir infusions. J. A. M. A. *255*:365–386, 1986.
441. Taber, L. H., Knight, V., Gilbert, B. E., et al.: Virazole aerosol treatment of bronchiolitis associated with respiratory tract infection in infants. Pediatrics *72*:613–618, 1983.
442. Tai, C. Y., Escarpe, P. A., Sidwell, R. W., et al.: Characterization of human influenza virus variants selected in vitro in the presence of the neuraminidase inhibitor 654071. Antimicrob. Agents Chemother. *42*:3224–3241, 1998.
443. Takahasi, T. M., Hosoya, K., Kimura, K., et al.: The cooperative effective of interferon and ribavirin on subacute sclerosing panencephalitis (SSPE) virus infections, in vitro and in vivo. Antiviral Res. *37*:29–35, 1998.
444. Talarico, C. L., Phelps, W., and Biron, K.: Analysis of the thymidine kinase genes from acyclovir-resistant mutants of varicella-zoster virus isolated from patients with AIDS. J. Virol. *67*:1024–1033, 1993.
445. Tatarowicz, W. A., Lurain, N. S., and Thompson, K. D.: A ganciclovir-resistant clinical isolate of human cytomegalovirus exhibiting cross-resistance to other DNA polymerase inhibitors. J. Infect. Dis. *166*:904–907, 1992.
446. Taylor, D. L., Jeffries, D. J., and Taylor-Robinson, D.: The susceptibility of adenovirus infection to the anti-cytomegalovirus drug, ganciclovir (DHPG). F. E. M. S. Microbiol. Lett. *49*:337–341, 1988.
447. Titus, B. J., Perez, A. F., and Arcata, B. I.: Water intoxication after nebulized ribavirin. Lancet *345*:1116, 1995.
448. Tokumoto, J. I., and Hollander, H: Cytomegalovirus polyradiculopathy caused by a ganciclovir-resistant strain. Clin. Infect. Dis. *17*:854–856, 1993.
449. Trang, J. M., Kidd, L., Gruber, W., et al.: And the NIAID collaborative Antiviral Study Group. Linear single dose pharmacokinetics of ganciclovir in newborns with congenital cytomegalovirus infection. Clin. Pharmacol. Ther. *53*:15–21, 1993.
450. Treanor, J. J., Hayden, F. G., Vrooman, P. S., et al.: Efficacy and safety of the oral neuraminidase inhibitor oseltamivir in treating acute influenza: A randomized controlled trial. J. A. M. A. *283*:1016–1024, 2000.
451. Tynell, E., Aurelius, E., Brandell, A., et al.: Acyclovir and prednisolone treatment of acute infectious mononucleosis: A multicenter, double-blind placebo-controlled study. J. Infect. Dis. *174*:324–331, 1996.
452. Tyring, S., Barbarash, R. A., Nahlik, J. E., et al.: Famciclovir for the treatment of acute herpes zoster: Effects on acute disease and post-herpetic neuralgia. Ann. Intern. Med. *123*:89–96, 1995.
453. van Rooyen, C. E., Casey, J., Lee, S. H., et al.: Vaccinia gangrenosa and 1-methylisatin-3-thiosemicarbozone (methisazone). Can. Med. Assoc. J. *97*:160–165, 1967.
454. van Voris, L. P., Betts, R. F., Hayden, F. G., et al.: Successful treatment of naturally occurring influenza A/USSR/77H1N1. J. A. M. A. *245*:1128–1131, 1981.
455. Vasquez, E. M., Sanchez, T., Pollak, J., et al.: High dose oral acyclovir prophylaxis for primary cytomegalovirus infection in seronegative renal allograft recipients. Transplantation *55*:448–450, 1993.
456. von Itzstein, M., Wu, W. Y., Kok, G. B., et al.: Rational design of potent sialidase-based inhibitors of influenza virus replication. Nature *36*:418–423, 1993.
457. Wade, J. C., and Meyers, J. D.: Neurologic symptoms associated with parenteral acyclovir treatment after marrow transplantation. Ann. Intern. Med. *98*:921–925, 1983.
458. Wade, J. C., Newton, B., McLaren, C., et al.: Intravenous acyclovir to treat mucocutaneous herpes simplex virus infection after marrow transplantation: A double blind trial. Ann. Intern. Med. *96*:265–269, 1982.
459. Wagstaff, A. J., Faulds, D., and Goa, K. C.: Acyclovir: A reappraisal of its antiviral activity, pharmacokinetic properties, and therapeutic efficacy. Drugs *47*:153–205, 1994.
460. Wald, A., Carrell, D., Remington, M., et al.: Two day regimen of acyclovir for treatment of recurrent genital herpes simplex virus type 2 infection. Clin. Infect. Dis. *34*:944–948, 2002.
461. Walker, J. B., Hussey, E. K., and Treanor, J. J.: Effects of the neuraminidase inhibitor zanamivir on otologic manifestations of experimental human influenza. J. Infect. Dis. *176*:1417–1422, 1997.
462. Wallace, M. R., Bowler, W. A., Murray, N. B., et al.: Treatment of adult varicella with oral acyclovir: A randomized, placebo controlled trial. Ann. Intern. Med. *117*:358–363, 1992.
463. Walsh, J. E., Abinun, M., Peiris, J. S., et al.: Cytomegalovirus infection in severe combined immune deficiency: Eradication with foscarnet. Pediatr. Infect. Dis. J. *14*:911–912, 1995.
464. Wang, L. H., Schultz, M., Weller, S., et al.: Pharmacokinetics and safety of multiple dose valacyclovir in geriatric volunteers with and without concomitant diuretic therapy. Antimicrob. Agents Chemother. *40*:80–85, 1996.
465. Weinberg, A., Bate, B. J., Masters, H., et al.: In vitro activities of penciclovir and acyclovir against herpes simplex virus types 1 and 2. Antimicrob. Agents Chemother. *36*:2037–2038, 1992.
466. Weller, S., Blum, M. R., Doucette, M., et al.: Pharmacokinetics of the acyclovir pro-drug valacyclovir after escalating single and multiple dose administration to normal volunteers. Clin. Pharmacol. Ther. *54*:595–605, 1993.
467. Wendel, H. A., Snyder, M. T., and Pell, S.: Trial of amantadine in epidemic influenza. Clin. Pharmacol. Ther. *7*:38–43, 1966.
468. Wendt, C. H., Weisdorf, D. J., Jordan, M. C., et al.: Parainfluenza virus respiratory infection after bone marrow transplantation. N. Engl. J. Med. *326*:921–926, 1992.
469. Wheeler, J. G., Wofford, J., and Turner, R. B.: Historical cohort evaluation of ribavirin efficacy in respiratory syncytial virus infection. Pediatr. Infect. Dis. J. *12*:209–213, 1993.
470. Whimbey, E., Champlin, R. E., Englund, J. A., et al.: Combination therapy with aerosolized ribavirin and intravenous immunoglobulin for respiratory syncytial virus disease in adult bone marrow transplant recipients. Bone Marrow Transplant. *16*:393–399, 1995.
471. Whitley, R., Alford, C., Hirsch, M., et al.: Vidarabine versus acyclovir therapy in herpes simplex encephalitis. N. Engl. J. Med. *314*:144–149, 1986.
472. Whitley, R. J., and Gnann, J. J.: Acyclovir: A decade later. N. Engl. J. Med. *327*:782–789, 1992.
473. Whitley, R. J., Hayden, F. G., Relsenger, K. S., et al.: Oral oseltamivir treatment of influenza in children. Pediatr. Infect. Dis. J. *20*:127–133, 2001.
474. Wills, R. J., Belshe, R., Tomlinsin, D., et al.: Pharmacokinetics of rimantadine hydrochloride in patients with chronic liver disease. Clin. Pharmacol. Ther. *42*:449–454, 1987.
475. Wingfield, W. L., Pollack, D., and Grunert, R. R.: Therapeutic efficacy of amantadine HCl and rimantadine in naturally occurring influenza A2 respiratory illness in man. N. Engl. J. Med. *281*:579–584, 1969.
476. Winston, D., Ho, W., and Baroni, K.: Ganciclovir prophylaxis of cytomegalovirus infection and disease in allogeneic bone marrow transplant recipients: Results of a placebo controlled, double blind trial. Ann. Intern. Med. *118*:179–184, 1993.
477. Winston, D., Wirin, D., Shaked, A., et al.: Randomized comparison of ganciclovir and high-dose acyclovir for long term cytomegalovirus prophylaxis in liver transplant recipients. Lancet *346*:69–74, 1995.
478. Wolf, D. G., Yaniv, I., Honigman, A., et al.: Early emergence of ganciclovir-resistant human cytomegalovirus strains in children with primary combined immunodeficiency. J. Infect. Dis. *178*:535–538, 1998.
479. Woodson, B., and Joklik, W. K.: The inhibition of vaccinia virus multiplication by isatin–3-thiosemicarbazone. Proc. Natl. Acad. Sci. U. S. A. *54*:946–953, 1965.
480. Wray, S. K., Gilbert, P. E., and Knight, V.: Effect of ribavirin triphosphate on primer generation and elongation during influenza virus transcription in vitro. Antiviral Res. *5*:39–48, 1985.
481. Wu, M. J., Ing, T. S., Soung, L. S., et al.: Amantadine hydrochloride pharmacokinetics in patients with impaired renal function. Clin. Nephrol. *17*:19–23, 1982.
482. Youle, M., Chanas, A., and Gazzard, B.: Treatment of acquired immune deficiency syndrome (AIDS)-related pneumonia with foscarnet: A double blind placebo controlled study. J. Infect. Dis. *20*:41–50, 1990.
483. Young, E., Chafizadeh, E., Oliveira, V., and Genta, R.: Disseminated herpesvirus infection during pregnancy. Clin. Infect. Dis. *22*:51–58, 1996.
484. Younsin, S. W., Betts, R. F., Roth, F. K., et al.: Reduction in fever and symptoms in young adults with influenza A/Brazil/78H1N1 infection after treatment with aspirin or amantadine. Antimicrob. Agents Chemother. *23*:577–582, 1983.
485. Zabawski, E. J.: A review of topical and intralesional cidofovir. Dermatol. Online J. *6*:3–10, 2000.
486. Zambon, M., and Hayden, F. G.: Position statement: Global neuraminidase inhibitor susceptibility network. Antiviral Res. *49*:147–156, 2001.
487. Zedtwitz-Liebenstein, K., Prester, E., and Graninger, W.: Acute renal failure in a lung transplant patient after therapy with cidofovir. Transplant. Int. *14*:445–446, 2001.
488. Zhou, X. J., Gruber, W., Demmler, G., et al.: Population pharmacokinetics of ganciclovir in newborns with congenital cytomegalovirus infections. NIAID Collaborative Antiviral Study Group. Antimicrob. Agents Chemother. *40*:2202–2205, 1996.
489. Ziegler, T., Hamphill, M. I., Ziegler, M.-L., et al.: Low incidence of rimantadine resistance in field isolates of influenza A virus. J. Infect. Dis. *180*:935–939, 1999.
490. Zlydnikov, D. M., Kubar O., I., and Kovaleva, R. P.: Study of rimantadine in the USSR: A review of the literature. Rev. Infect. Dis. *3*:408–421, 1981.

CHAPTER
239 Antifungal Agents

ANDREAS H. GROLL ■ THOMAS J. WALSH

Invasive fungal infections are important causes of morbidity and mortality in children with severe underlying illnesses. These infections remain difficult to diagnose and can be rapidly fatal. As a consequence, early and aggressive antifungal chemotherapy is pivotal for successful management and survival. For some time, options for antifungal chemotherapy have been limited to amphotericin B deoxycholate (D-AmB), with or without the addition of flucytosine (5-FC). The past decade, however, has witnessed major progress through the introduction of fluconazole and itraconazole and the development of less toxic formulations of amphotericin B. More recent advances include the design of a series of novel, potent, and broad-spectrum antifungal triazoles and the clinical development of echinocandins, a new class of antifungal lipopeptides that target the fungal cell wall (Fig. 239–1). This chapter is devoted to the clinical pharmacology of approved and currently investigational antifungal agents for the treatment of invasive as well as superficial fungal infections; emphasis is placed on pharmacokinetics, dosing, and safety in pediatric age groups.

Agents for Treatment of Invasive Mycoses

POLYENE ANTIBIOTICS

Amphotericin B Deoxycholate

Despite an expanded antifungal armamentarium, amphotericin B remains the cornerstone of chemotherapy in critically ill patients with invasive fungal infections. First isolated in the 1950s as a natural product of a soil actinomycete,[123] amphotericin B belongs to a family of approximately 200 polyene macrolide antibiotics and consists of seven conjugated double bounds, an internal ester, a free carboxyl group, and a glycoside side chain with a primary amino group (Fig. 239–2). The compound is amphoteric, not orally or intramuscularly absorbed, and virtually insoluble in water. For parenteral use, amphotericin B has been solubilized with deoxycholate as a micellar suspension, and this formulation has been available for more than 40 years.[32]

MECHANISM OF ACTION. Amphotericin B, similar to other polyenes, primarily acts by binding to ergosterol, the principal sterol in the cell membrane of most fungi. This interaction with ergosterol results in the formation of ion channels, loss of protons and monovalent cations, depolarization, and concentration-dependent cell death. Though with less avidity, the compound also binds to cholesterol, the main sterol of mammalian cell membranes, which accounts for most of its toxicity. A second mechanism of action of amphotericin B may involve oxidative damage to the cell through a cascade of oxidative reactions linked to its own oxidation with the formation of free radicals or an increase in membrane permeability. In addition to its antifungal activity, amphotericin B has stimulatory effects on phagocytic cells that also are related to oxidation-dependent events.[50, 141]

ANTIFUNGAL ACTIVITY. Amphotericin B has a broad spectrum of antifungal activity that includes most fungi pathogenic in humans. This characteristic is sustaining amphotericin B as the gold standard for other antifungal agents. True microbiologic resistance to antifungal polyenes has been associated with qualitative or quantitative differences in the sterol composition of the cell membrane, but it also may be related to increased catalase activity along with decreased susceptibility to oxidative damage.[141] Resistance to amphotericin B remains rare in *Candida* spp. other than *Candida lusitaniae*, although the compound appears to be somewhat less active against *Candida guilliermondii*, *Candida parapsilosis*, and *Candida tropicalis*.[365, 376, 398] *Aspergillus* spp. and other opportunistic molds,[65] but not the dimorphic molds, tend to have more variable susceptibility to amphotericin B; *Aspergillus terreus*[181, 347] and some of the emerging pathogens such as *Trichosporon beigelii*,[12, 379, 380] *Fusarium* spp.,[48, 296] *Pseudallescheria boydii*,[354, 382] *Scedosporium prolificans*,[37, 226] and other dematiaceous fungi[146] may be completely resistant to amphotericin B at concentrations achievable in patients by

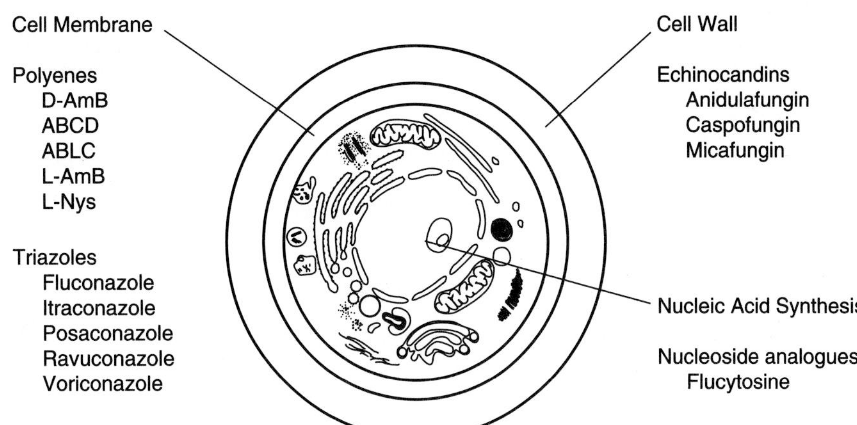

FIGURE 239–1 ■ Cellular targets of approved and investigational antifungal agents for treatment of invasive mycoses at the beginning of the 21st century. (Modified from Groll, A. H., Piscitelli, S. C., and Walsh, T. J.: Clinical pharmacology of systemic antifungal agents: A comprehensive review of agents in clinical use, current investigational compounds, and putative targets for antifungal drug development. Adv. Pharmacol. *44*:343–500, 1998.)

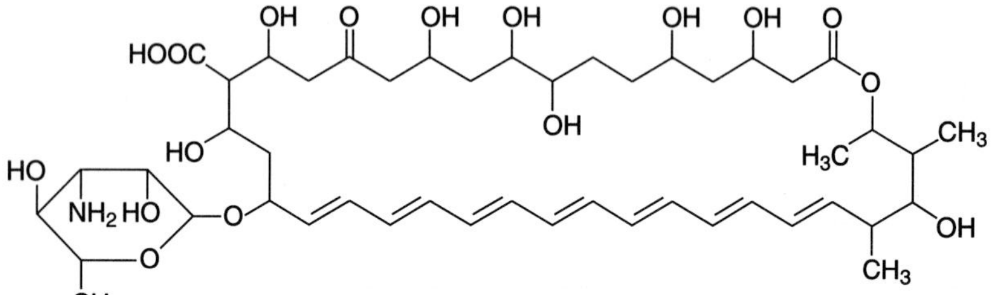

Amphotericin B

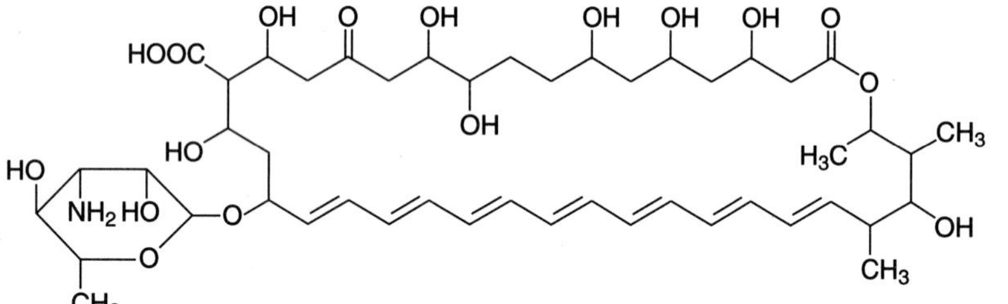

Nystatin A1

FIGURE 239–2 ■ Structural formulas of antifungal polyenes: amphotericin B and nystatin A1.

maximally tolerated dosages. Acquisition of secondary resistance seldom occurs and has not been a clinical problem.[141]

PHARMACODYNAMICS. In time-kill studies, amphotericin B displays concentration-dependent fungicidal activity against susceptible *Candida albicans*, *Cryptococcus neoformans*, and *Aspergillus fumigatus*.[197, 198, 290] In addition to its concentration-dependent fungicidal dynamics, a prolonged post-antifungal effect of amphotericin B of up to 12 hours' duration has been demonstrated in *C. albicans* and *C. neoformans*.[101, 360] Studies in laboratory animals support the concentration-dependent kill kinetics of amphotericin B in vitro. In a neutropenic pharmacokinetic/pharmacodynamic mouse model of disseminated candidiasis, C_{max}/MIC (peak plasma concentration/minimal inhibitory concentration) was the parameter that provided the best correlation with outcome as measured by the residual organism burden in kidney tissue.[18] These laboratory findings indicate that large doses will be most effective and that achievement of optimal peak concentrations is important. Therefore, the dosage of amphotericin B should not be reduced without careful consideration, and infusion for longer durations than recommended by the manufacturer should be avoided. Furthermore, dose escalation may be a valid approach for the treatment of clinically refractory infections by amphotericin-susceptible organisms.

PHARMACOKINETICS. After intravenous administration, amphotericin B rapidly dissociates from its vehicle and becomes highly protein-bound before distributing into tissues.[68] The disposition of the compound follows a three-compartment model, with rapid initial clearance from plasma followed by a biphasic pattern of elimination with a β-half life of 24 to 48 hours and a terminal (γ) half-life of 15 days or longer.[24] Tissue levels of amphotericin B in laboratory animals are highest in the liver, spleen, bone marrow, kidney, and lung; concentrations in body fluids other than plasma are generally low.[182, 212] However, despite mostly undetectable concentrations in cerebrospinal fluid (CSF) and comparatively low concentrations in brain tissue across all species, amphotericin B is effective in the treatment of fungal infections of the central nervous system. Although no metabolites of amphotericin B have been identified, only small quantities of parent compound are excreted into urine and bile, thus suggesting that tissue accumulation accounts for most drug disposition.[75, 302] Accordingly, dose adjustment is not necessary in patients with unrelated renal or hepatic dysfunction. Because of its high protein binding, hemodialysis usually does not affect plasma concentrations of amphotericin B.[76]

Reported pharmacokinetic data in pediatric age groups are characterized by high interindividual variability, which probably is related to differences in underlying disease and modes of administration[27, 35, 200, 255, 343] (Table 239–1). However, infants and children appear to clear the drug from plasma more rapidly than adults do, as indicated by a significant negative correlation between age and clearance in two

TABLE 239–1 ■ PHARMACOKINETIC PARAMETERS OF AMPHOTERICIN B DEOXYCHOLATE IN PEDIATRIC PATIENTS

Population	Dosage (mg/kg)	C_{max} (µg/mL)	$AUC_{0\to\infty}$ (µg/mL·hr)	Vd_{ss} (L/kg)	Cl (L/hr/kg)	$t_{1/2}$ (hr)
Preterm neonates[343] (*n* = 5, 0.5–7.5 mo)	1.0/md	0.96	n/a	4.1	0.122	39
Preterm neonates[27] (*n* = 13, 0.06–1.8 mo)	0.5/md	0.96	n/a	1.5	0.036	14.8
Infants/children[200] (*n* = 13, 0.08–18 yr)	0.5/sd	1.5	n/a	0.37	0.026	9.9
Infants/children[35] (*n* = 12, 0.3–14 yr)	0.68/md	2.9	n/a	0.76	0.027	18.1
Infants/children[255] (*n* = 20, 2.2–14.3 yr)	0.98/sd	2.43	22.0	0.92	0.039	15.1
Children/adults[8] (*n* = 20, 4–66 yr)	1.0/md	2.9	36	1.1	0.028	39

All values are given as means.

$AUC_{0\to\infty}$, area under the concentration versus time curve from time zero to infinity; Cl, plasma clearance; C_{max}, peak plasma concentration; md, multiple-dose data; n/a, not assessed; sd, single-dose data; $t_{1/2}$, elimination half-life; Vd_{ss}, apparent volume of distribution of steady state.

separate studies.[35, 200] Because distribution into tissues seems to be the main route of clearance from plasma, the faster clearance in individuals of younger age may be explained by their larger relative volume of parenchymatous organs in comparison to adults.[194, 249] Whether the enhanced clearance from the bloodstream has implications for dosing remains unknown. Currently, dosage recommendations for all pediatric age groups do not differ from those in adult patients.

ADVERSE EFFECTS. Infusion-related reactions and nephrotoxicity are major problems associated with the use of conventional amphotericin B, and they often limit successful therapy. Infusion-related reactions (fever, rigors, chills, myalgia, arthralgia, nausea, vomiting, and headaches) are thought to be mediated by the release of cytokines from monocytes in response to the drug.[21] They can be noted in as many as 73 percent of patients prospectively monitored at the bedside.[374] In a recent prospective interventional study in pediatric cancer patients, fever or rigors (or both) associated with the infusion of conventional amphotericin B were observed in 19 of 78 treatment courses (24%).[255] Interestingly, however, these characteristic adverse effects of amphotericin B are observed only rarely in the neonatal setting.[195] In clinical practice, infusion-related reactions associated with amphotericin B therapy may be blunted by slowing the infusion rate, but premedication with acetaminophen (10 to 15 mg/kg), hydrocortisone (0.5 to 1.0 mg/kg), or meperidine (0.2 to 0.5 mg/kg) often is required.[376] Less common acute adverse effects include hypotension, hypertension, flushing, and vestibular disturbances; bronchospasm and true anaphylaxis are rare occurrences.[141] Cardiac arrhythmias and cardiac arrest caused by acute potassium release may occur with rapid infusion (<60 minutes), especially if preexisting hyperkalemia or renal impairment, or both, are present.[59, 126]

The hallmarks of nephrotoxicity associated with amphotericin B are azotemia and wasting of potassium and magnesium; tubular acidosis and impaired urinary concentrating ability are rarely of clinical significance.[323] Relevant electrolyte wasting occurs in approximately 12 percent of prospectively monitored patients[374]; of note, hypokalemia can be quite refractory to replacement until hypomagnesemia is corrected.[323] Azotemia occurs commonly. In a large prospective clinical trial, the baseline serum creatinine level rose by more than 100 percent in 34 percent of 344 unstratified pediatric and adult patients receiving conventional amphotericin B for empirical treatment of fever and neutropenia.[374] Azotemia can be exacerbated by concomitant nephrotoxic agents, in particular, cyclosporine and tacrolimus. In a recent clinical trial involving persistently febrile neutropenic patients, renal toxicity occurred in 67 percent of patients receiving these drugs versus 31 percent of patients not receiving them concurrently with amphotericin B.[395] Data from another recent clinical trial have suggested a somewhat lower rate of azotemia in children than adults,[289] but this difference does not appear to be a consistent observation.[395] Interestingly, a frequency of amphotericin B–associated azotemia of only 2 percent has been reported for pediatric cancer patients receiving the drug at 1 mg/kg/day for empirical antifungal therapy.[255] In a recent series reporting the safety data of conventional amphotericin B (0.5 to 1.0 mg/kg) in premature neonates, the incidence of azotemia ranged from zero to 15 percent,[58, 121, 195, 216] thus indicating that the compound is much better tolerated in this setting than earlier reported.[26]

Renal toxicity associated with the use of conventional amphotericin B has the potential to lead to renal failure and the need for dialysis,[399] but azotemia often stabilizes with therapy and usually is reversible after discontinuation of the drug.[376] Avoidance of concomitant nephrotoxic agents, appropriate hydration, and normal saline loading (10 to 15 mL NaCl/kg/day)[22, 163] may greatly lessen the likelihood and severity of azotemia associated with amphotericin B therapy.

Other potentially relevant adverse effects of amphotericin B include a demyelinizing encephalopathy in bone marrow transplant recipients conditioned with total-body irradiation or receiving cyclosporine and concomitant high-dose amphotericin B therapy (or both)[250] and a normocytic, normochromic anemia associated with low erythropoietin levels after chronic administration.[76] D-AmB is topically irritating; therefore, a central line should be used for infusion, and local instillation of amphotericin B should be considered only in conjunction with expert consultation.

THERAPEUTIC MONITORING. Historically, 1-hour postinfusion plasma concentrations of twice the MIC of the fungal isolate have been proposed as the target for treatment of yeast infections.[93] However, monitoring of amphotericin B concentrations in plasma or CSF appears to be of little value because relationships between plasma and tissue concentrations and clinical efficacy or toxicity have not been characterized adequately.[142]

The toxicity of amphotericin B and the practice of normal saline loading necessitate close monitoring of related laboratory parameters. The drug must not be infused in less than 60 minutes and only with particularly careful cardiac monitoring in newborns and patients with hyperkalemia and renal impairment, circumstances in which arrhythmias caused by acute potassium release have been observed.[59, 126]

DRUG INTERACTIONS. Drug-drug interactions caused by shared metabolic pathways are unknown for amphotericin B. Hypokalemia may be aggravated by corticosteroids and, in turn, can potentiate digoxin toxicity, cause rhabdomyolysis, and enhance the effects of nonpolarizing muscle relaxants. Similarly, hypomagnesemia may become especially profound in cancer patients with platinum-associated nephropathy. Impairment of glomerular filtration by amphotericin B may enhance plasma levels and, consequently, the toxicity of many renally cleared drugs, including aminoglycosides, vancomycin, fluorocytosine, and cyclosporine.[141] Finally, the simultaneous infusion of granulocytes has been associated with acute pulmonary reactions[404] and therefore should be avoided.

INDICATIONS. Despite its toxicity profile, D-AmB still is considered the drug of choice for the initial treatment of most life-threatening fungal diseases (Tables 239–2 to 239–4). Infections by *C. lusitaniae*, *T. beigelii*, *A. terreus*, *Paecilomyces lilacinus*, *Fusarium* spp., *P. boydii*, and *S. prolificans* may not be amenable to amphotericin B and may require therapy with alternative agents,[147] again underscoring the importance of microbiologic identification and development of in vitro testing methods that predict microbiologic resistance and potential therapeutic failure. Depending on both the type of infection and the host, the recommended daily dosage ranges from 0.5 to 1.5 mg/kg/day administered over a period of 2 to 4 hours as tolerated.[141]

For empiric antifungal therapy in a persistently febrile neutropenic host, the historical standard dosage is 0.5 to 0.6 mg/kg/day.[98, 284] The efficacy of prophylactic intravenous amphotericin B in the setting of anticancer therapy has not been documented,[143] and recently, a large randomized multicenter study failed to show any preventive benefit of aerosolized amphotericin B in treating neutropenic patients at high risk for invasive mold infections.[333]

As a principle, treatment should be started at the full target dosage with careful bedside monitoring during the first hour of infusion to allow for prompt intervention for infusion-related reactions.[376] The duration of treatment is ill

TABLE 239–2 ■ MEDICAL MANAGEMENT OF INVASIVE INFECTIONS BY OPPORTUNISTIC YEASTS

Fungal Disease	Management
Invasive candidiasis	
Esophageal	Fluconazole,* 3–12 mg/kg qd Itraconazole, 2.5 mg/kg bid Amphotericin B deoxycholate, 0.5–1.0 mg/kg qd
Uncomplicated fungemia	Amphotericin B deoxycholate, 0.5–1.0 mg/kg qd Fluconazole,*† 6–12 mg/kg qd Echinocandin lipopeptides (*investigational*)‡
Acute single-site or disseminated candidiasis ± fungemia	Amphotericin B deoxycholate 0.5–1.0 (1.5) mg/kg qd, ± 5-FC,§ 100 mg/kg/day divided into 3 to 4 doses Fluconazole,*† (6)–12 mg/kg qd Amphotericin B lipid formulations,‖ 5 mg/kg qd
***Trichosporon* infection**	
Single site, disseminated, or fungemia	Fluconazole,* (6)–12 mg/kg qd, plus amphotericin B in neutropenic patients at risk for breakthrough infections 2nd-generation triazoles¶ (*investigational*)
Cryptococcosis	
Cerebral, extracerebral, or fungemia	Amphotericin B deoxycholate, 0.7 mg/kg qd 5-FC,§ 100 mg/kg/day divided into 3 to 4 doses for a minimum of 2 wk (induction), followed in stable patients by fluconazole,* 8 mg/kg qd, for consolidation and maintenance Liposomal amphotericin,‖ 5 mg/kg qd

*Loading dose: twice the target dose up to 12 mg/kg on the first day of treatment. Dose adjustment is required in patients with reduced creatinine clearance and high dosages. The maximal daily dose is 800 mg.
†Only for typed and in vitro susceptible isolate of *Candida*.
‡Includes anidulafungin, caspofungin, and micafungin.
§Monitoring of serum levels is required (<100 µg/mL; target, 40–60 µg/mL). Dose adjustment is required in patients with reduced creatinine clearance.
‖In patients refractory to or intolerant of amphotericin B deoxycholate.
¶Includes posaconazole, ravuconazole, and voriconazole.
5-FC, 5-fluorocytosine.

TABLE 239–3 ■ MEDICAL MANAGEMENT OF INVASIVE INFECTIONS BY OPPORTUNISTIC MOLDS

Fungal Disease	Management
Aspergillus infections	Amphotericin B deoxycholate, 1.0–1.5 mg/kg qd Amphotericin B lipid formulations,* 5 mg/kg qd Itraconazole,†‡ 2.5 (max. of 5) mg/kg bid PO Caspofungin,§ (*investigational*) 2nd-generation triazoles‖ (*investigational*)
Fusarium infections	Amphotericin B deoxycholate, 1.0–1.5 mg/kg qd Amphotericin B lipid formulations,* 5 mg/kg qd 2nd-generation triazoles‖ (*investigational*)
Zygomycetes infections	Amphotericin B deoxycholate, 1.0–1.5 mg/kg qd Amphotericin B lipid formulations,* 5 mg/kg qd
Infections by dematiaceous molds	Amphotericin B deoxycholate, 1.0–1.5 mg/kg qd, ±5-FC¶ 100 mg/kg/day divided into 3 or 4 doses Itraconazole,†‡ 2.5 (max. of 5) mg/kg bid PO Amphotericin B lipid formulations,* 5 mg/kg qd 2nd-generation triazoles,‖ (*investigational*)

*In patients intolerant of or refractory to amphotericin B deoxycholate.
†In patients intolerant of or refractory to amphotericin B or for consolidation/maintenance in stable patients.
‡Monitoring of itraconazole serum levels is required (≥0.50 µg/mL (high-performance liquid chromatography) or >2.0 µg/mL (bioassay) before the next dose). Suggested loading dose: 2.5 mg tid over period of 3 days. Intravenous therapy (≥18 yr): 200 mg bid for 2 days, followed by 200 mg qd for maximum of 14 days. Not indicated for creatinine clearance of 30 mL/min or less.
§In patients intolerant of or refractory to standard therapy. Dosage in patients 18 years or older: 70 mg on day 1, followed by 50 mg qd. Investigational in pediatric patients.
‖Includes posaconazole, ravuconazole, and voriconazole.
¶Monitoring of serum levels required (<100 µg/mL: target, 40 to 60 µg/mL). Dose adjustment is needed with reduced creatinine clearance.
5-FC, 5-fluorocytosine.

TABLE 239–4 ■ MEDICAL MANAGEMENT OF INVASIVE INFECTIONS BY DIMORPHIC MOLDS

Fungal Disease	Management
Histoplasmosis	Amphotericin B deoxycholate, 0.5–1.0 mg/kg qd Itraconazole,*† 2.5 (max. 5) mg/kg bid PO Liposomal amphotericin,‡ 5 mg/kg qd Fluconazole,§ (6)–12 mg/kg qd
Coccidioidomycosis	Amphotericin B deoxycholate, 0.5–1.0 mg/kg qd Fluconazole,‖ (6)–12 mg/kg qd Itraconazole,†¶ 2.5 (max. 5) mg/kg bid PO
Blastomycosis	Amphotericin B deoxycholate, 0.5–1.0 mg/kg qd Itraconazole,*† 2.5 (max. 5) mg/kg bid PO Fluconazole,** (6)–12 mg/kg qd
Paracoccidioidomycosis	Amphotericin B deoxycholate, 0.5–1.0 mg/kg qd Itraconazole,*† 2.5 (max. 5) mg/kg bid PO
Sporotrichosis	Amphotericin B deoxycholate, 0.5–1.0 mg/kg qd Itraconazole,*† 2.5 (max. 5) mg/kg bid PO Fluconazole,** (6)–12 mg/kg qd Terbinafine: <20 kg, 62.5 mg qd; 20–40 kg, 125 mg qd; >40 kg, 250 mg qd (*investigational*)††
Penicilliosis	Amphotericin B deoxycholate, 0.5–1.0 mg/kg qd Itraconazole,*† 2.5 (max. 5) mg/kg bid PO

*In stable patients with mild to moderate non-CNS disease or for maintenance.

†Monitoring of itraconazole serum levels is required (≥0.50 µg/mL (high-performance liquid chromatography) or >2.0 µg/mL (bioassay) before the next dose). Suggested loading dose: 2.5 mg tid over period of 3 days. Intravenous therapy (≥18 yr): 200 mg bid for 2 days, followed by 200 mg qd for maximum of 14 days. Not indicated for creatinine clearance of 30 mL/min or less.

Note that ketoconazole is effective in the treatment of endemic mycoses but has generally been replaced by itraconazole due to this compound's better absorption and greater specificity.

‡In patients intolerant of or refractory to amphotericin B deoxycholate.

§For consolidation therapy for meningeal histoplasmosis.

‖Preferred agent for coccidioidal meningitis; loading dose: twice the target dose on the first day of treatment.

Dose adjustment may be required with reduced creatinine clearance and high dosages.

¶Non-CNS disease only.

**Secondary alternative; loading dose: twice the target dose on the first day of treatment.

Dose adjustment may be required with reduced creatinine clearance and high dosages.

††Cutaneous forms only.

Data from references 66, 113, 192, 393.

defined for most infections. Prolonged and individualized therapy, including the use of lipid formulations of amphotericin B, triazoles and echinocandins for salvage, or consolidation therapy, often is required until complete resolution of the individual disease process.

Amphotericin B Lipid Formulations

During the late 1990s, three novel formulations of amphotericin B were approved in the United States and most of Europe: amphotericin B colloidal dispersion (ABCD [Amphocil, Amphotec]), amphotericin B lipid complex (ABLC [Abelcet]), and a small unilamellar vesicle (SUV) liposomal formulation (L-AmB [AmBisome]). Because of their reduced nephrotoxicity in comparison to D-AmB, these compounds allow for the safe delivery of higher dosages of amphotericin B. However, data from animal models suggest that higher dosages are required for equivalent antifungal efficacy.[168, 403]

PHYSICOCHEMICAL PROPERTIES AND PHARMACOKINETICS. The carriers of the lipid formulations are made up of biodegradable, amphiphilic bilayered membranes in which the hydrophilic heads of the lipid molecules face outward to shield the hydrophobic tails. The membranes may form either spherical vesicles called liposomes or bilayered complexes or dispersions with no specific vesicular structure. When incorporated into these water-soluble carriers, amphotericin B becomes soluble in plasma and available for distribution. Each of the lipid formulations of amphotericin B possesses distinct physicochemical and pharmacokinetic properties. All three, however, are preferentially distributed to organs of the mononuclear phagocytic system (MPS) and functionally spare the kidney. Whereas the micellar dispersion of ABCD behaves very similar kinetically to that of D-AmB, the unilamellar liposomal preparation has a prolonged circulation time in plasma, achieves strikingly high peak plasma concentrations and area under the concentration (AUC) values, and is only slowly taken up by the MPS. In contrast, the large ribbon-like aggregates of ABLC are efficiently opsonized by plasma proteins and rapidly taken up by the MPS, thereby resulting in lower peak plasma and AUC values[139, 168] (Table 239–5). Whether and how the distinct physicochemical and pharmacokinetic features of each formulation translate into different pharmacodynamic properties in vivo are largely unknown. However, recent experimental head-to-head comparisons of all four formulations of amphotericin B against defined invasive mycoses suggest important differences in antifungal efficacy, depending on the agent, dose, and type and site of infection.[70, 132, 268]

TABLE 239–5 ■ PHYSICOCHEMICAL PROPERTIES AND MULTIPLE-DOSE PHARMACOKINETIC PARAMETERS OF THE FOUR CURRENTLY MARKETED AMPHOTERICIN B FORMULATIONS

	D-AmB	ABCD	ABLC	L-AmB
Lipids (molar ratio)	Deoxycholate	Cholesterylsulfate	DMPC/DMPG (7:3)	HPC/CHOL/DSPG (2:1:0.8)
Mol% AmB	34%	50%	50%	10%
Lipid configuration	Micelles	Micelles	Membrane-like	SUVs
Diameter (μm)	0.05	0.12–0.14	1.6–11	0.08
Dosage (mg AmB/kg)	1	5	5	5
C_{max} (μg/mL)	2.9	3.1	1.7	58
$AUC_{0\rightarrow\infty}$ (μg/mL-hr)	36	43	14	713
Vd_{ss} (L/kg)	1.1	4.3	131	0.22
Cl (L/hr/kg)	0.028	0.117	0.476	0.017

Data represent mean values, stem from adult patients, and were obtained after different rates of infusion.
$AUC_{0\rightarrow\infty}$, area under the concentration versus time curve from time zero to infinity; CHOL, cholesterol; Cl, plasma clearance; C_{max}, peak plasma concentration; DMPC, dimiristoyl phosphatidylcholine; DMPG, dimiristoyl phosphatidylglycerol; DSPG, disteaoryl phosphatidylglycerol; HPC, hydrogenated phosphatidylcholine; SUV, small unilamellar vesicle; Vd_{ss}, apparent volume of distribution at steady state.
Modified from Groll, A. H., Muller, F. M., Piscitelli, S. C., and Walsh, T. J.: Lipid formulations of amphotericin B: Clinical perspectives for the management of invasive fungal infections in children with cancer. Klin. Padiatr. *210*: 264–273, 1998.

SAFETY AND ANTIFUNGAL EFFICACY. The safety and antifungal efficacy of ABCD, ABLC, and L-AmB have been demonstrated in open phase I/II studies in immunocompromised, mostly adult patients with a wide spectrum of underlying disorders.[164, 304, 378, 394] The overall response rates in these trials ranged from 53 to 84 percent in patients with invasive candidiasis and from 34 to 59 percent, respectively, in patients with presumed or documented invasive aspergillosis.[139] A few randomized, controlled trials have been completed in which one of the new formulations has been compared with D-AmB. These studies consistently have shown at least equivalent therapeutic efficacy and reduced nephrotoxicity in comparison to D-AmB. Infusion-related side effects of fever, chills, and rigor appear to occur less frequently with L-AmB only.[16, 374, 395] Several individual cases of substernal chest discomfort, respiratory distress, and sharp flank pain have been noted during infusion of L-AmB,[186] and in a comparative study, hypoxic episodes associated with fever and chills occurred more frequently in ABCD recipients than D-AmB recipients.[395] Mild increases in serum bilirubin and alkaline phosphatase have been observed with all three formulations and mild increases in serum transaminases with L-AmB. However, no case of fatal liver disease has occurred.[139, 168, 403]

EXPERIENCE IN PEDIATRIC PATIENTS. A considerable number of pediatric patients have been treated with ABCD, ABLC, or L-AmB on protocol in the aforementioned clinical trials; separately published pediatric data are discussed in the following paragraphs.

ABCD. ABCD is a complex of amphotericin B and sodium cholesteryl sulfate in an approximate 1:1 molar ratio, and it forms disk-like colloidal structures on dissolution.[139] Population-based multiple-dose pharmacokinetic studies with ABCD in bone marrow transplant patients with systemic fungal infections included the compartmental analysis of five children younger than 13 years who received the compound at 7.0 and 7.5 mg/kg/day. Estimated pharmacokinetic parameters in these children were not significantly different from those obtained in a dose-matched cohort of adult patients: under conditions of steady state, the mean AUC_{0-24} was 7.10 μg/mL·hr (normalized to a 1-mg/kg/day dose), the mean volume distribution (Vd) was 4.57 L/kg, and the mean total clearance was 0.144 L/hr/kg.[8]

A double-blind, randomized trial comparing ABCD (4 mg/kg/day) with D-AmB (0.8 mg/kg/day) for empirical antifungal treatment of febrile neutropenic patients separately reported safety data from 46 children (≥2 to <16 years of age) randomized to receive either ABCD (n = 25) or D-AmB (n = 21). Overall, ABCD was significantly less nephrotoxic than D-AmB, and no differences in adverse events and efficacy in comparison to the (much larger) adult study population were reported.[395] An additional 70 children (0 to 15 years; mean, 8.8 years) with presumed or proven invasive fungal infections refractory to or intolerant of amphotericin B were treated in five different open-label studies of ABCD. Dosages ranged from 0.8 to 7.5 mg/kg (mean, 4.5 mg/kg), administered for a mean of 30 days (range, 1 to 192). Although 67 percent of patients reported infusion-related reactions, nephrotoxicity, defined as an increase in serum creatinine to two times the baseline value or greater, was reported in only 12 percent. Other unexpected toxicities were not observed.[322]

The published experience in the neonatal setting is limited to 16 very low-birth-weight infants (779 ± 170 g; 25 ± 2 weeks) with invasive candidiasis and a serum creatinine value of 1.2 mg/dL or greater.[221] The infants received 3 mg/kg ABCD on day 1, followed by 5 mg/kg/day thereafter; a second agent was permitted for candidemia that persisted for 7 days or longer. Thirteen of 14 evaluable patients cleared the organism after therapy with ABCD alone (n = 8) or in combination with another agent (n = 5), and the overall survival rate was 75 percent. ABCD was well tolerated, without infusion-related reactions, increases in serum creatinine, or hepatotoxicity.

These data indicate no overall fundamental differences in the disposition, safety, and antifungal efficacy of ABCD in comparison to adult populations. The Food and Drug Administration (FDA)-approved indication is treatment of probable or proven invasive aspergillosis, and the approved dosage is 3 to 6 mg/kg/day administered over a 2-hour period.

ABLC. ABLC is composed of dimyristoyl phosphatidylcholine (DMPC) and dimiristoyl phosphatidylglycerol (DMPG) in a 1:1 molar ratio of lipid to amphotericin B and forms large ribbon-like structures. The pharmacokinetics of ABLC has been studied in whole blood from three pediatric cancer patients who received the compound at 2.5 mg/kg over the course of 6 weeks for hepatosplenic candidiasis.[384] Steady state was achieved by day 7 of therapy; after the final dose, the mean AUC_{0-24} was 11.9 ± 2.6 μg/mL·hr, the mean C_{max} was 1.69 ± 0.75, and clearance was 0.218 L/kg/hr.

In the six patients evaluable for assessment of safety, mean serum creatinine levels were stable at the end of therapy and at 1-month follow-up, and no increase in hepatic transaminases occurred. Five of the patients had infusion-related reactions to the first dose, which was monitored prospectively without premedication; however, infusion-related adverse reactions were well controlled thereafter by conventional premedication. All evaluable patients responded to therapy.

The safety and antifungal efficacy of ABLC were studied in 111 treatment episodes in pediatric patients (21 days to 16 years of age) refractory of or intolerant to conventional antifungal agents through an open-label, emergency-use protocol in the United States.[383] ABLC was administered at a mean daily dosage of 4.85 mg/kg (range, 1.1 to 9.5 mg/kg/day) for a mean duration of 38.9 days (range, 1 to 198 days). The mean serum creatinine concentration for the entire study population did not change significantly in the 6 weeks between baseline (1.23 ± 0.11 mg/dL) and cessation of ABLC therapy (1.32 ± 0.12 mg/dL). No significant differences were observed between baseline and end-of-therapy levels of serum potassium, magnesium, hepatic transaminases, alkaline phosphatase, and hemoglobin. However, an increase in mean total bilirubin (3.66 ± 0.73 to 5.13 ± 1.09 mg/dL) was noted at the end of therapy (p = .054). In seven patients (6%), ABLC therapy was discontinued because of one or more adverse effects, and in six patients (5%), ABLC was discontinued because of progression of disease. Of 54 patients fulfilling the criteria for evaluation of antifungal efficacy, a complete or partial therapeutic response was obtained in 38 (70%).

A retrospective study from Europe investigated the safety and efficacy of ABLC in 46 immunocompromised pediatric patients (9.7 ± 4.8 years of age) with invasive fungal infections, including a large proportion who were refractory to or intolerant of conventional therapy. ABLC was administered at a mean daily dose of 4.11 mg/kg/day, and the mean duration of therapy was 38.7 days. Overall, ABLC was well tolerated without any increase in mean serum creatinine from baseline to the end of therapy. Thirty-eight patients (83%) responded to treatment with ABLC, including 18 of 23 with aspergillosis and 17 of 19 with candidiasis.[165]

Eleven infants 6 months of age and younger with candidemia were enrolled in the U.S. open-label emergency-use protocol[383] and received 5 to 41 daily doses of ABLC; they were between 3 and 13 weeks of age and weighed between 0.8 and 5 kg. Seven of the 11 patients maintained a stable mean serum creatinine concentration; in 4 patients, a rise in serum creatinine was observed, but in each case, the increase was less than 40 percent of the baseline value. No differences were observed between baseline and end-of-therapy mean bilirubin levels. Among the eight evaluable infants, a complete response was observed in 6 (75%).[383] ABLC was effective and well-tolerated in 11 neonates (0.7 to 5 kg; median, 1.4 kg) with systemic *Candida* infections who received the drug at a median dose of 4.9 mg/kg (range, 3.2 to 6.5 mg/kg) for a median duration of 23 days (range, 4 to 41 days). In no infant was ABLC discontinued because of adverse effects.[4]

Current data suggest no fundamental difference in the disposition, safety, or antifungal efficacy of ABLC in children versus adults. The FDA-approved dosage for the treatment of probable or proven invasive infections is 5 mg/kg/day administered over the course of 2 hours.

L-AMB. L-AmB consists of small, unilamellar spherical vesicles (true liposomes) composed of hydrogenated soy phosphatidylcholine and disteaoryl phosphatidylglycerol stabilized by cholesterol and combined with amphotericin B in a 2:0.8:1:0.4 molar ratio.[139] The pharmacokinetics and safety of L-AmB at dosages of 2.5, 5.0, and 7.5 mg/kg were investigated in a phase I/II clinical trial involving immunocompromised children and adolescents. L-AmB was tolerated well without dose-limiting toxicity, and no substantial differences in the compound's plasma pharmacokinetics were noted in comparison to adults.

Many pediatric patients have been enrolled in clinical trials with L-AmB but have not been reported separately.[7, 243, 374] Two hundred four children (mean age, 7 years) with neutropenia and fever of unknown origin were randomized in an open-label, multicenter trial to receive D-AmB, 1 mg/kg/day (n = 63), L-AmB, 1 mg/kg/day (n = 70), or L-AmB, 3 mg/kg/day (n = 71) for empirical antifungal therapy.[289] Twenty-nine percent of the patients treated with 1 mg L-AmB, 39 percent of the patients treated with 3 mg L-AmB, and 54 percent of patients treated with D-AmB experienced adverse effects (p = .01); nephrotoxicity, defined as a 100 percent or greater increase in serum creatinine from baseline, was noted in 8, 11, and 21 percent, respectively (not significant [NS]). Hypokalemia (<2.5 mmol/L) occurred in 10, 11, and 26 percent of patients (p = .02); increases in serum transaminase levels (≥110 U/L) in 17, 23, and 17 percent (NS); and increases in serum bilirubin (≥35 μmol/L) in 11, 12, and 10 percent of patients, respectively. Efficacy assessment by intent-to-treat analysis indicated successful therapy in 51 percent of children treated with D-AmB and in 64 and 63 percent of children treated with L-AmB at either 1 or 3 mg/kg/day (p = .22). L-AmB at either 1 or 3 mg/kg/day was significantly safer and at least equivalent to D-AmB with regard to resolution of fever of unknown origin. Moreover, L-AmB was well tolerated and effective in small cohorts of immunocompromised children requiring antifungal therapy for proven or suspected infection, including patients with bone marrow transplants as primary immunodeficiencies[276] and cancer patients.[303]

The safety and efficacy of L-AmB in the neonatal population have been comparatively well studied. L-AmB (2.5 to 7 mg/kg/day administered over a 1-hour period) was evaluated prospectively in 25 episodes of invasive candidiasis occurring in 24 very low-birth-weight infants (mean birth weight, 847 ± 244 g; mean gestational age 26 weeks).[188] Thirteen of the infants had failed previous antifungal therapy consisting of conventional amphotericin B with or without 5-FC. The mean duration of L-AmB therapy was 21 days, and the mean cumulative dose was 94 mg/kg. Fungal eradication was achieved in 92 percent; 20 (83%) infants were considered clinically cured at end of therapy. Four infants (17%) died; in 2 of them, the cause of death was attributed directly to the infection. No major adverse effects were observed. Increased bilirubin and hepatic transaminase levels developed in one infant during therapy.

A retrospective case series from Italy reported on the safety and efficacy of L-AmB in 40 preterm (mean birth weight, 1090 g [range, 80 to 1840 g]; mean gestational age, 28.35 [range, 5 to 3 weeks]) and 4 full-term (mean birth weight, 3080 ± 118 g; mean gestational age, 39 ± 0.7 weeks) newborn infants with invasive yeast infections.[327] The initial daily dosage of 1 mg/kg/day was increased stepwise by 1 mg/kg to a maximal dose of 5 mg/kg, depending on the patient's response. Six infants received the initial dosage of 1 mg/kg throughout treatment; in 22 cases, the daily dosage was increased to a maximum of 3 mg/kg/day, in 14 to a maximum of 4 mg/kg/day, and in 2 to a maximum of 5 mg/kg/day. The mean duration of therapy was 22 days (range, 7 to 49 days). Administration of L-AmB was tolerated without apparent infusion-associated reactions. Though not listed in detail, blood pressure and hepatic, renal, or hematologic indices were reported as within the normal range, except for transient hypokalemia in 16 infants. Treatment was successful in

72 percent of the patients altogether; however, 12 of the 40 preterm infants (30%) succumbed to the fungal infection. All these infants had a birth weight of 1500 g or less. The mean duration of therapy in the fatal cases was 14 ± 6 days.

A second retrospective case series analyzed changes in serum creatinine and serum potassium in 21 very-low-birth weight infants (median gestational age, 25 weeks [range, 23 to 31]; median birth weight, 730 g [range, 450 to 1370 g]) who received the compound for presumed or documented yeast infections.[389] Antifungal therapy was started after a median age of 13 days (range, 1 to 49). The median dose was 2.6 mg/kg/day (range, 1 to 5 mg/kg/day), and the median duration of therapy was 2 days (range, 11 to 79). Hypokalemia (<3 mmol/L) was observed in 30 percent before and in 15 percent during treatment. The median maximal creatinine level before treatment was 121 μmol/L (range, 71 to 221) and fell to 68 μmol/L (range, 31 to 171) during treatment and 46 μmol/L (range, 26 to 62) 21 days after termination of therapy. All patients responded to therapy with liposomal amphotericin B, although the number of proven invasive fungal infections was small (7/21, 33%).

Current data indicate no substantial differences in the pharmacokinetics and pharmacodynamics of L-AmB between pediatric and adult patients. FDA-approved dosages are 3 mg/kg/day (empirical antifungal therapy in febrile neutropenic patients) and 3 to 5 mg/kg/day (therapy for probable and proven invasive infections) administered over a 2-hour period.

INDICATIONS. The lipid formulations of amphotericin B are an important therapeutic advance in the management of invasive opportunistic fungal infections in immunocompromised patients. All three compounds have less renal toxicity than conventional amphotericin B does, as defined by the development of azotemia; distal tubular toxicity also may be somewhat reduced. The infusion-related reactions of fever, chills, and rigor appear to occur substantially less frequently only with L-AmB, and no new toxicities have been noted. Preliminary pharmacokinetic and safety data from children thus far indicate no fundamental differences from those obtained in the adult population.

Therapeutically, the lipid formulations are at least as effective as conventional amphotericin B for the treatment of most opportunistic human mycoses, and they can be effective if conventional amphotericin B has failed. They may be indicated when toxicity prohibits the administration of effective dosages of D-AmB and when standard therapies fail to induce a therapeutic response against an amphotericin B–susceptible organism. The experience with life-threatening endemic mycoses, however, is limited. The lipid formulations are approved for the treatment of patients with invasive mycoses refractory to or intolerant of D-AmB and limited to L-AmB for empirical treatment of persistently neutropenic patients (see Tables 239–2 to 239–4).

The optimal dosages of each formulation for the various types and sites of invasive fungal infection remain to be defined. Considerable uncertainty exists in most physicians regarding dosage, which is mainly driven by the high costs of these compounds. Based on animal data[168] and the few randomized studies that have used D-AmB as a comparator,[16, 215] we and most other experts in the field consider a dosage of 5 mg/kg/day of ABCD, ABLC, and L-AmB to be equivalent to a dosage of 1 mg/kg/day of D-AmB. Accordingly, an initial dosage of 5 mg/kg/day of ABCD, ABLC, or L-AmB is recommended for the treatment of suspected or documented invasive fungal infection, and a dosage of 3 mg/kg/day when L-AmB is chosen for empirical antifungal therapy in persistently febrile neutropenic patients (see Table 239–5).

Liposomal Nystatin

Nystatin, the first antifungal polyene, was discovered as a natural fermentation product of *Streptomyces noursei* in the early 1950s.[160] It is a tetraene-diene macrolide, and its carbon skeleton differs from that of amphotericin B only by the lack of one double bound (see Fig. 239–2). Though generally less potent on a molar basis, the compound has broad-spectrum activity similar to that of amphotericin B; resistance in clinical isolates occurs rarely.[62] In vitro time-kill studies of *Candida* spp. demonstrate concentration-dependent, rapid fungicidal activity at concentrations exceeding the MIC, and prolonged, concentration-dependent post-antifungal effects of as long as 15 hours have been noted.[97, 150] Although nystatin has been available for many years for topical use, problems with solubilization and toxicity precluded its development for systemic treatment.[141]

However, laboratory research performed by Mehta and coworkers in the mid-1980s demonstrated that incorporation of nystatin into multilamellar liposomes consisting of DMPC and DMPG protects human erythrocytes from toxicity while preserving the compound's antifungal activity in vitro.[239] The liposomal formulation of nystatin was well tolerated and effective in murine screening models of disseminated candidiasis[240] and disseminated aspergillosis[84, 373] and showed promising activity in persistently neutropenic rabbit models of invasive pulmonary aspergillosis[133] and subacute disseminated candidiasis.[140] Pharmacokinetic studies in healthy rabbits established nonlinear pharmacokinetics with decreasing clearance at higher dosage levels; the compound reached relatively high peak plasma levels and then was rapidly distributed and eliminated from plasma with a half-life of 1 to 2 hours.[138]

CLINICAL TRIALS. The plasma pharmacokinetics of liposomal nystatin were investigated in HIV-infected patients who received the drug every other day for as long as 15 days at dosages ranging from 2 to 7 mg/kg. After achieving comparatively high peak plasma concentrations in the range of 4.8 to 24.1 μg/mL, the drug was distributed rapidly and eliminated from plasma with a half-life of 5 to 7 hours, a pharmacokinetic profile different from that of all four amphotericin B formulations.[74] In a phase I study in 32 patients with hematologic malignancies and refractory febrile neutropenia, liposomal nystatin was relatively well tolerated at multiple dosages of up to 8 mg/kg without reaching a maximal tolerated dose. Nephrotoxicity occurred at the higher end of the dosage range, but it did not exceed grade II.[49] The antifungal efficacy of liposomal nystatin in the treatment of candidemia was investigated in a phase II multicenter study involving 109 non-neutropenic patients who received the compound at 2 (n = 91) or 4 mg/kg (n = 18) once daily for a mean duration of 10.6 days. Successful treatment was noted in 60 of 72 evaluable patients (83%) with no trend for superior efficacy at the higher dosage.[397] Nine of 15 patients who entered the study with candidemia refractory to standard therapies responded to treatment with liposomal nystatin.[307] Liposomal nystatin also was investigated as salvage therapy in 24 patients with probable or definite invasive aspergillosis who were either intolerant of or refractory to conventional amphotericin B. Patients received liposomal nystatin at 4 mg/kg once daily for a median of 27 days (range, 1 to 48 days). Complete or partial responses were noted in 6 of 19 evaluable patients (31%); 7 of 16 evaluable patients were alive on day 30 after end of treatment (44%).[266] Finally, in two large multinational randomized trials involving 538 patients, liposomal nystatin (2 mg/kg) was compared with conventional amphotericin B (0.6 to 0.8 mg/kg) for empirical antifungal therapy in persistently

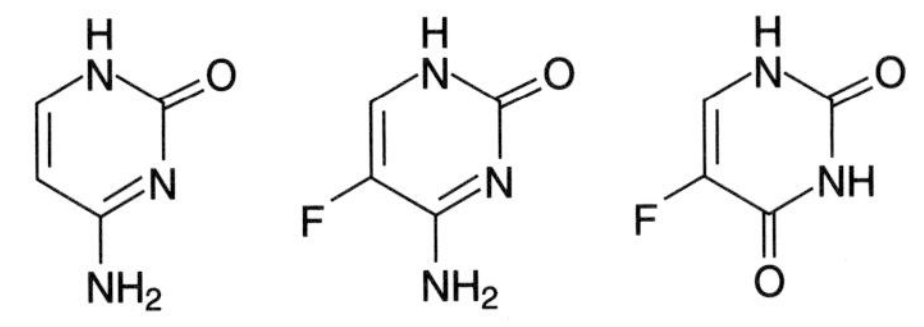

Cytosine Flucytosine Fluorouracil

FIGURE 239–3 ■ Structural formulas of cytosine, flucytosine, and fluorouracil.

febrile neutropenic cancer patients. Both compounds had similar efficacy, but nephrotoxicity was significantly less in the nystatin arm.[287]

No pediatric studies have been completed thus far; filing for a new drug application is expected.

FLUCYTOSINE

5-FC is low-molecular-weight, water-soluble, synthetic fluorinated pyrimidine analogue (Fig. 239–3). It is taken up into the fungal cell by the fungus-specific enzyme cytosine permease and converted in the cytoplasm by cytosine deaminase to 5-fluorouracil, a potent antimetabolite that causes RNA miscoding and inhibits DNA synthesis[90] (Fig. 239–4). 5-FC is relatively nontoxic to mammalian cells because of the absence or very low level of activity of cytosine deaminase. In the United States, 5-FC is available only as an oral formulation; an intravenous formulation is available outside the United States in certain countries.

ANTIFUNGAL ACTIVITY. The antifungal activity of 5-FC in vitro is limited essentially to *Candida* spp., *C. neoformans*, *Saccharomyces cerevisiae*, and selected dematiaceous molds.[108, 169, 281] 5-FC has no or only weak activity against *Aspergillus* and other hyaline molds.[116, 232] Notably, whereas *Candida krusei* appears less susceptible to 5-FC, the compound is highly active against *Candida glabrata*.[90, 108] Synergistic or additive effects in combination with amphotericin B have been observed against *Candida* spp.[237, 248] and in combination with amphotericin B or fluconazole against *C. neoformans*.[156, 237, 260]

Two mechanisms of resistance have been reported: mutations in enzymes necessary for cellular uptake and transport of 5-FC or its metabolism and increased synthesis of pyrimidine, which competes with fluorinated antimetabolites of the compound.[369] The exact frequency of primary resistance among yeast-like organisms is not clear but is highly dependent on the testing method; in pretreatment isolates, intrinsic resistance to 5-FC has been found in 7 to 8 percent of *C. albicans* strains, in as many as 22 percent of non-*albicans* *Candida* spp., and in 2 percent or less of *C. neoformans* isolates.[238] Development of resistance to 5-FC can be observed during treatment[108] and is thought to be caused predominantly by selection of resistant clones.[369] As a consequence, 5-FC rarely is given alone; instead, it is given in combination with amphotericin B or, more recently, fluconazole.

PHARMACODYNAMICS. Time-kill assays of *Candida* spp. and *C. neoformans* have demonstrated a predominantly concentration-independent fungistatic (99% reduction in colony-forming units [CFU]) activity of 5-FC at concentrations exceeding the MIC of the investigated isolates.[218, 362] A prolonged post-antifungal effect against these organisms

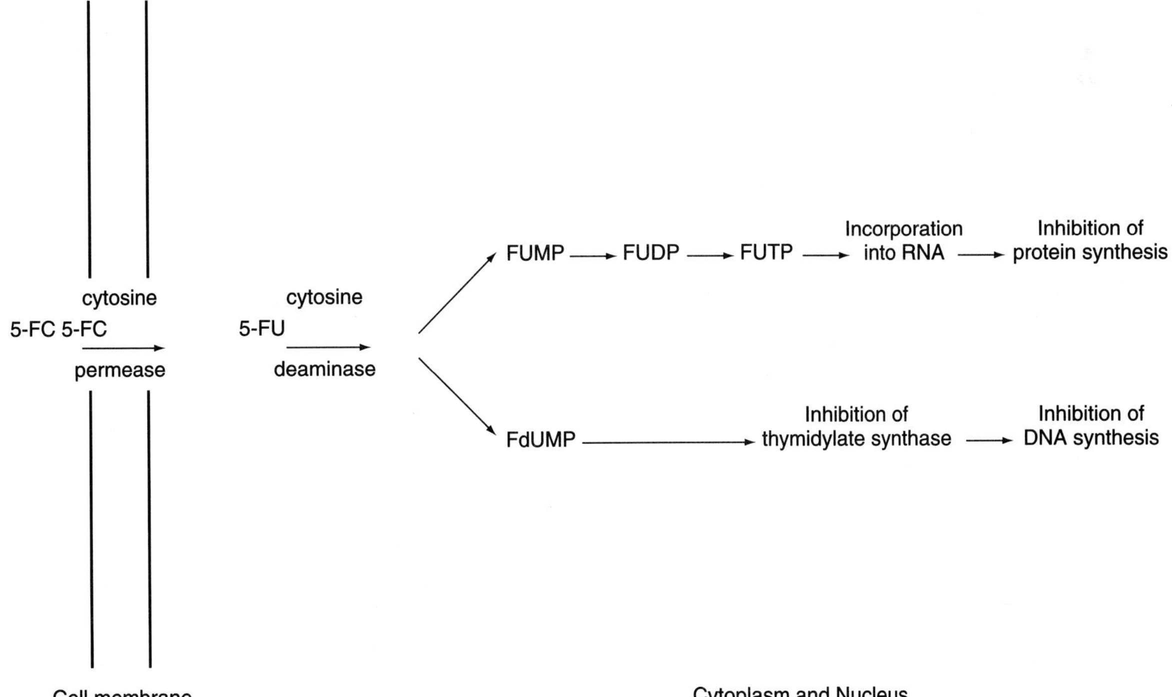

FIGURE 239–4 ■ Schematic of the intracellular pathways and mechanism of action of flucytosine. 5-FC, flucytosine; FdUMP, 5-fluorodeoxyuridine monophosphate; 5-FU, 5-fluorouracil; FUDP, 5-fluoridine diphosphate; FUMP, 5-fluoridine monophosphate; FUTP, 5-fluoridine triphosphate. (Modified from Groll, A. H., Piscitelli, S. C., and Walsh, T. J.: Clinical pharmacology of systemic antifungal agents: A comprehensive review of agents in clinical use, current investigational compounds, and putative targets for antifungal drug development. Adv. Pharmacol. *44*:343–500, 1998; and Vermes, A., Guchelaar, H. J., and Dankert, J.: Flucytosine: A review of its pharmacology, clinical indications, pharmacokinetics, toxicity and drug interactions. J. Antimicrob. Chemother. *46*:171–179, 2000.)

has been noted consistently that was dependent on the concentration of 5-FC and the duration of exposure and ranged from 0.8 to as long as 10 hours.[325, 407] In addition, synergistic post-antifungal effects were demonstrated with 5-FC plus fluconazole and amphotericin B, respectively, against *C. albicans*.[245, 325, 326] Investigation of the pharmacokinetic and pharmacodynamic relationships in a neutropenic mouse model of disseminated candidiasis, with the residual fungal burden in kidney tissue used as the end-point of antifungal efficacy, revealed that both the time above the MIC and AUC/MIC were important in predicting efficacy, whereas peak level/MIC was the least important parameter. Maximal efficacy was observed when levels exceeded the MIC for only 20 to 25 percent of the 24-hour dosing interval.[20] These data collectively suggest that lower dosages or less frequent dosing may yield identical antifungal efficacy while further reducing potential toxicities of 5-FC that are thought to be concentration-dependent.[108]

PHARMACOKINETICS. Flucytosine is absorbed readily from the gastrointestinal tract, and oral bioavailability exceeds 80 percent (Table 239–6). Peak concentrations in plasma occur 1 to 2 hours after administration. As a water-soluble compound, 5-FC has negligible protein binding (4%) and is widely distributed in the body, with a Vd that approximates that of total-body water. Mean CSF concentrations are usually 65 to 90 percent of simultaneous plasma concentrations. The drug penetrates well into peritoneal fluid, inflamed joints, and other fluid compartments, including the eye.[76, 141]

In humans, less than 1 percent of a given dose of 5-FC is thought to undergo hepatic metabolism. In addition to 5-fluorouracil, several other metabolites of yet unclear toxic potential have been identified.[228] Some evidence indicates that bacteria of the gastrointestinal flora deaminate 5-FC to resorbable 5-fluorouracil,[158, 228] which may account for some of the toxicity observed after oral administration of the drug. Approximately 95 percent of a given dose of 5-FC is excreted into urine in unchanged, active form by simple glomerular filtration, and the plasma elimination half-life is 3 to 6 hours in adult patients with normal renal function.[141] Because the compound's elimination parallels the glomerular filtration rate, adjustment in dosage is necessary for patients with impaired renal function.[76] In patients undergoing hemodialysis, a dose of 37.5 mg/kg is recommended after dialysis,[40] and in those undergoing hemofiltration, the dosage needs to be adjusted according to the individual filtration rate.[180, 210] In patients treated by peritoneal dialysis, the compound can be administered systemically or intraperitoneally.[244]

TABLE 239–6 ■ PHARMACOKINETICS OF FLUCYTOSINE IN ADULTS

Parameter or Characteristic	Value
Oral bioavailability	≥80%
C_{max}	50–120 µg/mL*
T_{max}	1–2 hr
Protein binding	4%
Vd_{ss}	0.6–0.7 L/kg
$t_{1/2}\beta$	3–6 hr
Clearance	≥95% renal
Unchanged drug in urine	≥95%
Relative cerebrospinal fluid levels	65–90%

*At steady state in patients with cryptococcal meningitis receiving 4 × 2 g/day orally.

Modified from Groll, A. H., Piscitelli, S. C., and Walsh, T. J.: Clinical pharmacology of systemic antifungal agents: A comprehensive review of agents in clinical use, current investigational compounds, and putative targets for antifungal drug development. Adv. Pharmacol. *44*:343–500, 1998.

Although data are limited, studies indicate that impaired liver function does not appear to alter the disposition of 5-FC.[76]

In infants and children, the pharmacokinetics of 5-FC has not been characterized systematically. However, because of very similar physicochemical and pharmacokinetic properties, developmental changes in disposition similar to those found with fluconazole can be anticipated. Indeed, a similarly marked interindividual variability in clearance and Vd has been reported in neonates,[27] thus rendering uniform dosing recommendations in this population impossible.

A starting dosage of 100 mg/kg daily divided into three or four doses is recommended for both adults and children. Monitoring of plasma concentrations is essential for adjusting the dosage to changing renal function and to avoid toxicity. After oral administration, the near-peak levels achieved 2 hours after dosing overlap with trough levels as patients reach steady state and are thus sufficient for therapeutic monitoring.[108] Peak plasma levels between 40 and 60 µg/mL correlate with antifungal efficacy and seldom are associated with hematologic adverse effects.[108, 370]

ADVERSE EFFECTS. Common adverse effects associated with 5-FC include gastrointestinal intolerance and reversible elevation of hepatic transaminases and alkaline phosphatase in 5 to 6 percent of patients. More infrequent side effects are rashes, blood eosinophilia, and crystalluria.[141]

Hematologic adverse effects have been reported in an overall 6 percent of patients receiving oral 5-FC and may include neutropenia, thrombocytopenia, or pancytopenia. Although they are usually reversible after discontinuation of the drug or a reduction in dosage, fatal outcomes have been reported.[108, 141] Some of the adverse effects of 5-FC may be caused by the compound's conversion to 5-fluorouracil by gastrointestinal bacterial flora[158, 228] or the toxic effects of endogenously produced metabolites. Notably, hematologic adverse effects occur less frequently if plasma levels of 5-FC do not exceed 100 µg/mL.[108, 370] However, this relationship is not absolute, and hematologic toxicity may occur at levels well below this threshold.

DRUG INTERACTIONS. Oral administration of nonresorbable antibiotics and aluminum/magnesium hydroxide–based antacids may delay but does not impair absorption of the compound from the gastrointestinal tract.[141] 5-FC undergoes only minor hepatic metabolism, and it is not known to interfere with the cytochrome P-450 (CYP450) enzyme system. However, any drug that can cause a reduction in the glomerular filtration rate may lead to increased 5-FC serum levels and thereby has the potential to enhance 5-FC–associated toxicity. This phenomenon is encountered almost invariably with concomitant administration of amphotericin B, but it can occur similarly with many antimicrobial agents, anticancer drugs, and cyclosporine, to name only the most common examples.[76] The anticancer drug cytosine arabinoside competitively inhibits the action of 5-FC, and both drugs should not be given concomitantly.[63]

CLINICAL INDICATIONS. Because of the propensity of susceptible organisms to acquire resistance in vitro,[285] 5-FC traditionally is not administered as a single agent.

Ample laboratory and clinical experience exists regarding the combination of conventional amphotericin B and 5-FC[90, 141, 369] (see Table 239–2). Randomized clinical trials have established the use of amphotericin B in combination with 5-FC as the current standard for induction therapy for cryptococcal meningitis in patients who were and were not infected with human immunodeficiency virus (HIV).[34, 363] Although no comparative trials have been performed, the cumulative clinical experience supports the combination of amphotericin B with 5-FC for the treatment of *Candida* infections involving deep tissues, particularly in critically ill patients and when non-*albicans Candida* spp. are involved.[108, 173, 233, 349] These infections include *Candida* meningitis, endophthalmitis, endocarditis, vasculitis, and peritonitis, as well as osteoarticular, renal, and chronic disseminated candidiasis.[141, 376] Susceptibility of *Aspergillus* spp. to 5-FC in vitro occurs infrequently,[116, 232] and high-dose amphotericin B plus 5-FC versus high-dose amphotericin B alone in the treatment of invasive aspergillosis never has been investigated. Although the combination has been used successfully for invasive aspergillosis,[55, 82, 190] its role remains unclear.

More recently, investigators also have begun to explore combinations of 5-FC with fluconazole.[141] This combination was studied in a prospective study of 32 patients with acquired immunodeficiency syndrome (AIDS) and cryptococcal meningitis. Clinical and microbiologic responses were superior to those reported with either amphotericin B or fluconazole alone but not as good as those documented for the combination of amphotericin B and 5-FC.[209] Thus, 5-FC in combination with fluconazole may be used for cryptococcal meningitis when treatment with conventional or liposomal amphotericin B is not feasible. In addition, this combination also may be useful as second-line therapy for individual patients with invasive *Candida* infections involving aqueous body compartments.

5-FC has demonstrated impressive therapeutic efficacy against chromoblastomycosis[223] and significant activity in murine models of phaeohyphomycosis.[41, 88] Given the high case-fatality rate of invasive phaeohyphomycosis in humans, further experimental investigation of 5-FC in combination with other antifungal compounds against these infections appears warranted.

ANTIFUNGAL TRIAZOLES

The antifungal azoles are a class of synthetic compounds that have one or more azole rings and, attached to one of the nitrogen atoms, a more or less complex side chain. Whereas the imidazoles have two, the triazoles have three nitrogen atoms in the five-member ring. The triazole ring confers improved resistance to metabolic degradation, greater target specificity, and an expanded spectrum of activity.[127, 128]

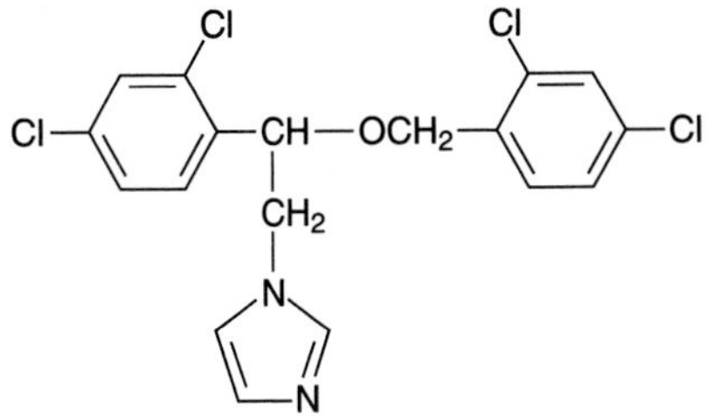

Miconazole

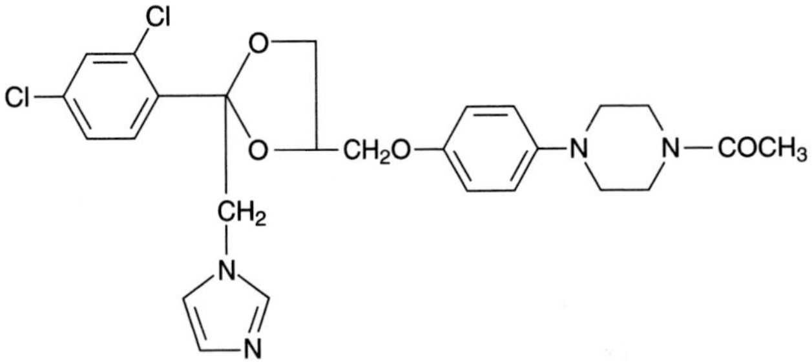

Ketoconazole

FIGURE 239–5 ■ Structural formulas of systemic antifungal imidazoles: miconazole and ketoconazole.

The imidazoles miconazole and ketoconazole (Fig. 239–5) were the first azole compounds developed for systemic treatment of human mycoses. Severe toxicities associated with the drug carrier (miconazole) and erratic absorption and significant interference with the human CYP450 system (ketoconazole), however, have limited their clinical usefulness.[141] The triazoles fluconazole and itraconazole (Fig. 239–6), in contrast, have become extremely useful components of the antifungal armamentarium. Overall, they are well tolerated and have a broad spectrum of activity. Whereas fluconazole and itraconazole have been available for more than a decade, several new triazoles are in advanced stages of clinical development. These second-generation triazoles include voriconazole, posaconazole, and ravuconazole.

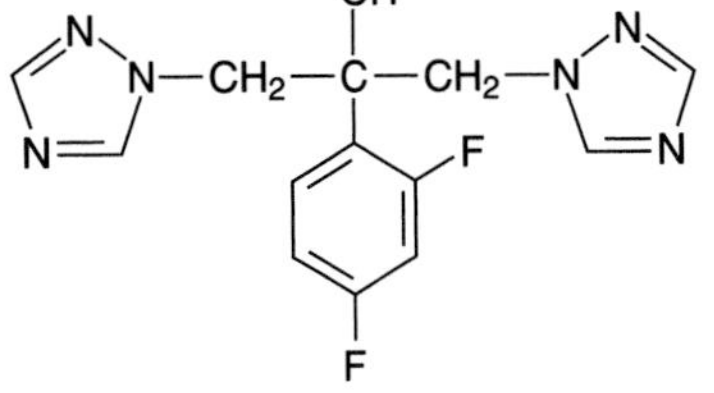

Fluconazole

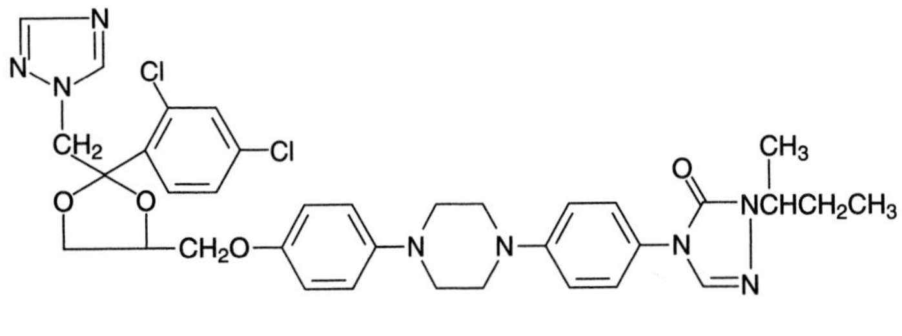

Itraconazole

FIGURE 239–6 ■ Structural formulas of first-generation systemic antifungal triazoles: fluconazole and itraconazole.

MECHANISM OF ACTION. The antifungal azoles, as a class, target ergosterol biosynthesis by inhibiting the fungal CYP450-dependent enzyme lanosterol 14α-demethylase. This inhibition interrupts the conversion of lanosterol to ergosterol, which leads to the accumulation of aberrant 14α-methylsterols and depletion of ergosterol in the fungal cell membrane (Fig. 239–7). This process alters cell membrane properties and function and, depending on the organism and compound, may lead to cell death or inhibition of cell growth and replication. In addition, the azoles also inhibit CYP450-dependent enzymes of the fungal respiration chain. Of note, interaction with mammalian CYP450-dependent enzyme systems is responsible for most of the toxicities and drug interactions of this class of compounds.[141, 366]

ANTIFUNGAL ACTIVITY. Fluconazole and itraconazole are principally active against dermatophytes, *Candida* spp., *C. neoformans*, *T. beigelii*, and other uncommon yeast-like organisms and against dimorphic fungi such as *Histoplasma capsulatum*, *Coccidioides immitis*, *Blastomyces dermatitidis*, *Paracoccidioides brasiliensis*, and *Sporothrix schenkii*.[127, 128] They have less activity against *C. glabrata* and none against *C. krusei*.[298, 299] Clinically useful activity against *Aspergillus* spp. and dematiaceous molds is restricted to itraconazole, and both itraconazole and fluconazole are quite inactive against *Fusarium* spp. and the zygomycetes.[141] The second-generation triazoles voriconazole, posaconazole, and ravuconazole have an enhanced target activity and are active against a wide spectrum of clinically important fungi, including *Candida*, *T. beigelii*, *C. neoformans*, *Aspergillus*, *Fusarium*, other hyaline molds, and dematiaceous as well as dimorphic molds.[67, 141] At present, no fundamental differences in potency and spectrum have been noted among these agents.

RESISTANCE. Selection and nosocomial spread of azole-resistant *Candida* spp. has become a matter of increasing concern. During the past few years, several mechanisms of resistance have been identified and include, but are not limited to alterations at the target binding site, increased target expression, and induction of cellular efflux pumps.[396] In contrast to pathogenic bacteria, genetic exchange mechanisms are largely unknown in fungi. Exposure-induced cumulative molecular events that lead to stable azole resistance have been reported; however, in the clinical setting, resistance is encountered most commonly in the form of a primarily resistant species or through selection of resistant subclones during exposure to azoles.[223, 396]

Acquisition of microbiologic and clinical azole resistance first was reported in patients with chronic mucocutaneous candidiasis receiving long-term therapy with ketoconazole.[174] In the 1990s, before the advent of highly active antiretroviral therapy (HAART), azole-resistant oropharyngeal and esophageal candidiasis became a major clinical conundrum in patients with advanced HIV infection.[291, 310] The emergence of *C. glabrata* and *C. krusei* infection in association with fluconazole prophylaxis has been observed in several bone marrow transplant centers.[183, 235, 400, 401] However, a large prospective series from Seattle showed an altogether low incidence of breakthrough candidemia (4.6%; in two thirds caused by *C. glabrata* or *C. krusei*) and a low attributable mortality rate (20%) in patients receiving fluconazole prophylaxis despite frequent colonization with fluconazole-resistant *Candida* spp.[235] Although cross-resistance of *Candida* spp. to antifungal azoles is a common occurrence,[124, 251, 277] it is not obligate; for example, patients with microbiologic and clinical fluconazole-resistant mucosal candidiasis may respond to itraconazole or second-generation triazoles.[162, 316]

Acquired azole resistance has been documented in a few patients with *C. neoformans* meningitis receiving maintenance therapy, but little is known about the frequency and mechanisms of secondary azole resistance in filamentous fungi.[141]

Fluconazole

Fluconazole is a synthetic low-molecular-weight, water-soluble bis-triazole (see Fig. 239–6). When compared with ketoconazole, the compound has similar potency at the target enzyme

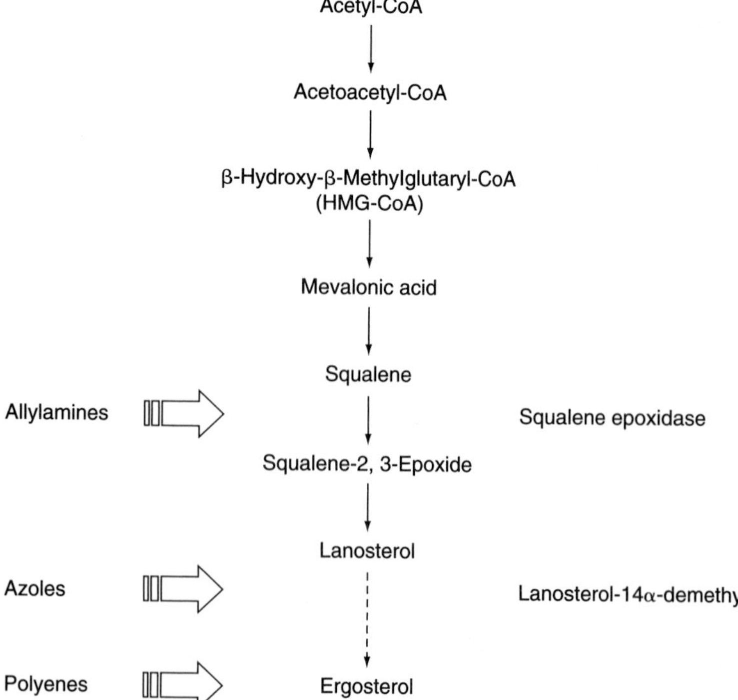

FIGURE 239–7 ■ Ergosterol biosynthesis and targets of current antifungal agents. (Modified from Groll, A. H., and Walsh, T. J.: Antifungal triazoles. *In* Yu, V. L., Merigan, T. C., and Barriere, S. [eds.]: Antimicrobial Chemotherapy and Vaccines. Baltimore, Williams & Wilkins, 1998, pp. 1158–1170.)

but is much more specific and, therefore, better tolerated. Fluconazole is active against *Candida*, *C. neoformans*, *T. beigelii*, and endemic dimorphic fungi, but not against *Aspergillus* and other hyaline or dematiaceous molds. Fluconazole has intermediate activity against *C. glabrata* and is inactive against *C. krusei*.[122, 128]

PHARMACODYNAMICS. Fluconazole generally is considered to be a fungistatic agent.[142] Time-kill assays of susceptible *Candida* spp. and *C. neoformans* performed over the course of 24- to 48-hour incubation periods show fungistatic activity of fluconazole with variable concentration-related growth effects.[56, 57, 197, 198] However, time-kill studies that used extended periods of incubation of up to 14 days and nonproliferating growth conditions have demonstrated direct fungicidal activity of fluconazole against *C. albicans*.[341] These observations indicate that ultimately, fluconazole may be able to eliminate *Candida* without help from host defenses. In serum-free growth media, fluconazole displays no measurable post-antifungal effect against *C. albicans* and *C. neoformans*, but concentration-dependent, post-antifungal effects of 1 to 3.6 hours were observed in the presence of fresh serum. Finally, pretreatment of *C. albicans* with fluconazole increased its vulnerability to killing by polymorphonuclear leukocytes.[101, 246]

In vivo pharmacodynamic studies of fluconazole in murine models of disseminated *C. albicans* candidiasis, with the fungal burden in kidney tissue used as the end-point for antifungal efficacy, collectively suggest that the AUC/MIC ratio is the pharmacodynamic parameter that best predicts the antifungal efficacy of fluconazole.[19, 225, 342] Pharmacodynamic studies of fluconazole in patients with fungal infections have not been presented to date. The dose-independent pharmacokinetics and the available experimental and clinical data are in support of once-daily dosing regimens. The current susceptibility breakpoints and dosing recommendations for fluconazole against *Candida* spp. have been derived from MIC and outcome information of patients with mostly superficial *Candida* infections.[298] The principal feasibility of this approach is supported by the pharmacodynamic models discussed earlier and several animal studies that have demonstrated a correlation between MIC and antifungal efficacy.[13, 29, 306, 377] However, in view of the evolving state of antifungal susceptibility testing and the limited clinical correlation, treatment of serious invasive mycoses caused by organisms in the susceptible–dose-dependent MIC range by dose escalation remains controversial and warrants further investigation.

PHARMACOKINETICS. Fluconazole has very favorable pharmacokinetic properties. It is available for oral and parenteral use, and its disposition is independent of route and formulation. Fluconazole exhibits linear plasma pharmacokinetics that best fit a two-compartment open model.[52]

Independent of food or intragastric pH, the oral bioavailability of fluconazole is greater than 90 percent. Peak plasma concentrations occur 1 to 2 hours after ingestion. Multiple dosing increases peak plasma concentration approximately 2.5-fold. Steady state generally is reached within 4 to 7 days after initiation of once-daily dosing, but it can be achieved rapidly by doubling the dose on the first day.[122, 128] Because of fluconazole's free solubility in water, protein binding is low. Fluconazole is distributed well in virtually all tissue sites and body fluids. The ratio of CSF and serum concentrations ranges from 0.5 to 0.9 during the dosing interval, and penetration into brain tissue and the different compartments of the eye is excellent. Fluconazole is relatively stable to metabolic conversion; more than 90 percent of a dose is excreted via the kidney, with approximately 80 percent recovered as unchanged, active drug and 11 percent recovered as inactive metabolites. Most of the drug is excreted in unchanged form into the urine.[52, 122, 128] Because excretion of fluconazole parallels the glomerular filtration rate, the dosage must be adjusted in patients with renal failure. A 50 percent reduction is required in patients with a creatinine clearance of 50 mL/min or less and a 75 percent reduction in patients with a creatinine clearance below 21 mL/min; the initial loading dose need not be adjusted.[38, 128] Fluconazole is dialyzable; in patients undergoing hemodialysis, 100 percent of the target dose is given after each dialysis session. In continuous hemofiltration, standard dosing has been suggested. A dose of 150 mg in a single 2-L dialysate bag has been used for continuous ambulatory peritoneal dialysis.[122, 261, 331, 352] Hepatic insufficiency per se does not require dose adjustment, but careful monitoring for additional hepatic toxicity is essential.[311]

The plasma pharmacokinetics of fluconazole in pediatric age groups reflects developmental changes in Vd and clearance that are characteristic for a highly water-soluble drug with minor metabolism and predominantly renal elimination (Table 239–7). Except for premature neonates, in whom clearance is decreased initially, pediatric patients tend to have an increased weight-normalized clearance rate from plasma that leads to a shorter half-life than in adults.[51, 205, 214, 324, 334, 352] As a consequence, dosages at the high end of the recommended dosage range are necessary for the treatment of invasive mycoses in children. Because exposure over time appears to be the most predictive pharmacodynamic parameter,[19, 225] fractionating of the dose may not be required in infants and children despite the shorter half-life in these age groups.

ADVERSE EFFECTS. In adults, fluconazole has been administered safely for prolonged periods at dosages of up to 1200 mg/day; dose escalation to 1600 mg/day resulted mainly in increased hepatotoxicity, and dose-limiting neurotoxicity was observed at 2000 mg/day.[14] Data compiled from adult patients who received the drug at dosages of 100 to 400 mg/day for at least 7 days indicate an overall incidence of possibly related adverse effects of 16 percent; significant adverse effects or laboratory abnormalities leading to the discontinuation of the drug were noted in 2.8 percent overall.[128] Nausea, vomiting, and other gastrointestinal symptoms are seen in less than 5 percent, rash and headaches in less than 2 percent, and usually reversible, asymptomatic hepatic transaminase elevations in as many as 7 percent of adult patients.[71, 128]

In pediatric patients of all age groups, fluconazole generally is well tolerated at dosages of up to 12 mg/kg/day. The most common reported side effects in pediatric patients include gastrointestinal disturbances (8%), increases in hepatic transaminases (5%), and skin reactions (1%); discontinuation of therapy with fluconazole for toxicity-related reasons

TABLE 239–7 ■ PHARMACOKINETIC PARAMETERS OF FLUCONAZOLE IN PEDIATRIC PATIENTS

Age Group	Vd_{ss} (L/kg)	Cl (L/hr/kg)	$t_{1/2}\beta$ (hr)
Preterm (<1500 g)			
Day 1	1.18	0.010	88
Day 6	1.84	0.019	67
Day 12	2.25	0.031	55
Term neonates	1.43	0.036	28
Infants >1 to 6 mo	1.02	0.037	19
Children, 5 to 15 yr	0.84	0.031	18
Adult volunteers	0.65	0.015	30

Data represent mean values and are compiled from six studies.[51,205,214,252,324,334] Cl, total plasma clearance; $t_{1/2}\beta$, elimination half-life; Vd_{ss}, apparent volume of distribution at steady state.

occurs in approximately 3 percent of patients.[264] Severe side effects, including severe hepatotoxicity and exfoliative skin reactions, have been reported anecdotally in association with fluconazole therapy. Fluconazole does not appear to affect the synthesis of human steroid hormones at the currently used dosages.[71, 141]

DRUG INTERACTIONS. Fluconazole undergoes minimal CYP-mediated metabolism, inhibits CYP3A4 and several other CYP isoforms in vitro, and interacts with enzymes involved in glucuronidation, thereby leading to numerous significant drug-drug interactions[71, 131, 148, 283] (Table 239–8). Most importantly, concurrent therapy with cisapride and newer antihistamines results in inhibition of the metabolic pathways of these drugs and potentially serious cardiac arrhythmias and is therefore strictly contraindicated.[141] By similar mechanisms, fluconazole can precipitate phenytoin toxicity[247]; may lead to increased plasma concentrations of cyclosporine, tacrolimus, and all-*trans*-retinoic acid[213, 270, 332]; and may potentiate the effects of warfarin, sulfonylurea drugs, rifabutin, benzodiazepines, carbamazepine, and nifedipine.[213, 253, 267] At small dosages, fluconazole can decrease the plasma clearance of theophylline and zidovudine.[199, 320] Fluconazole also may interfere with the plasma clearance of cyclophosphamide, a widely used anticancer agent that must be metabolized by CYP450 enzymes to produce the alkylating species. This interaction may result in a potentially relevant reduction in the therapeutic efficacy of cyclophosphamide.[406]

On the other hand, drugs notorious for hepatic enzyme induction may lead to decreased fluconazole levels and therapeutic failure as the ultimate consequence.[71, 128] In addition, the potential for added hepatotoxicity must be monitored when fluconazole is given in combination with these compounds.[128, 253]

CLINICAL INDICATIONS. Clinical indications for fluconazole are summarized in Tables 239–2, 239–4, 239–10, and 239–12. Fluconazole is highly effective against superficial infections caused by dermatophytes and *Pityrosporum* spp.[109, 153] and has excellent activity in the treatment of mucosal candidiasis, including vaginal, oropharyngeal, esophageal, and chronic mucocutaneous candidiasis.[105, 128, 130, 153, 166, 231]

Several controlled studies including both neutropenic and non-neutropenic adult patients indicate that intravenous fluconazole (400 to 800 mg/day or 3 to 6 mg/kg/day) is as effective as D-AmB (0.5 to 1.0 mg/kg/day) against candidemia and other forms of documented or suspected invasive candidiasis and is better tolerated.[11, 15, 282, 297] Fluconazole thus can be used for invasive *Candida* infections caused by susceptible organisms in patients who are in stable condition.[300] In patients who have received antifungal azoles for prophylaxis, the role of fluconazole as a therapeutic agent is very limited; breakthrough infections are highly likely to be caused by fluconazole-resistant *Candida* spp.,[235] and amphotericin B remains the current agent of choice in this setting.

Fluconazole is a useful agent for the treatment of invasive *Candida* infections in the neonatal setting. In six published series including 10 or more patients, each with proven invasive *Candida* infection, treatment with fluconazole at a daily dosage of mostly 5 to 6 mg/kg was successful in 83 to 97 percent of patients, and crude mortality rates ranged from 10 to 33 percent. In none of the 125 total patients was fluconazole discontinued because of toxicity.[39, 47, 91, 92, 104, 179, 372] The recommended dosage range for pediatric patients of all age groups is 6 to 12 mg/kg/day. However, in view of the faster clearance rate, the larger Vd, and the safety profile of fluconazole, 12 mg/kg/day may be the more appropriate dosage for treatment of serious infections in term neonates, infants, and children. In preterm neonates less than 1500 g, a dosing

TABLE 239–8 ■ DRUG-DRUG INTERACTIONS WITH FLUCONAZOLE AND ITRACONAZOLE

Mechanism and Drug Involved	Triazole Involved	Comment
Decreased Plasma Concentration of Triazole		
Decreased absorption of triazole	Itra*	Take antacids and antifungal agent at least 2 hr apart
Antacids, H_2 antagonists, omeprazole, sucralfate, didanosine, grapefruit juice		
Increased metabolism of triazole	Itra,* Flu	Potential for therapy failure; increased potential for hepatotoxiciy
Isoniazid, rifampin, rifabutin, phenytoin, phenobarbital, carbamazepine		
Increased Plasma Concentration of Co-administered Drug through Inhibition of Its Metabolism by Triazole		
Terfenadine, astemizole, cisapride	Flu,‡ Itra‡	Concomitant use prohibited
Lovastatin, simvastatin, atorvastatin	Itra,‡ Flu‡	Concomitant use prohibited
Phenytoin	Flu*, Itra*	Monitor levels
Benzodiazepines	Flu†, Itra†	Monitor closely
Carbamazepine	Flu†	Monitor closely
Haloperidol	Itra†	Monitor closely
Rifampin, rifabutin	Flu,† Itra†	Monitor closely
Clarithromycin	Itra†	Monitor closely
Indinavir, ritonavir	Itra†	Monitor closely
Vincristine, busulfan	Itra†	Avoid concomitant use
All *trans*-retinoic acid	Flu†	Monitor closely
Nifedipine, felodipine	Itra,† Flu†	Monitor closely
Cyclosporine A, tacrolimus	Flu,† Itra†	Monitor serum level
Sulfonylurea drugs, warfarin, prednisolone	Flu,† Itra†	Monitor closely
Digoxin, quinidine	Itra†	Monitor levels (digoxin)
Zidovudine, theophylline	Flu†	Monitor closely

*Major significance.
†Moderate significance.
‡Contraindicated.
Modified from Groll, A. H., Piscitelli, S. C., and Walsh, T. J.: Clinical pharmacology of systemic antifungal agents: A comprehensive review of agents in clinical use, current investigational compounds, and putative targets for antifungal drug development. Adv. Pharmacol. *44*:343–500, 1998.

regimen of 6 to 12 mg/kg once every 72 hours has been advocated during the first week of life based on an initially decreased clearance of fluconazole.[324] However, this dosage regimen has not been validated in the therapeutic setting; given the extreme variability in extravascular water content and renal function in many of these children, predictably effective and safe treatment with fluconazole may not be possible in the early postnatal period.

Fluconazole has been useful in the treatment of focal *Candida* urinary tract infection and uncomplicated funguria and has been used successfully in treating *Candida* peritonitis, endocarditis, osteomyelitis, meningitis, and endophthalmitis.[141, 217] Additional potential indications for fluconazole beyond the treatment of acute invasive *Candida* infection include consolidation therapy for chronic disseminated candidiasis[10, 191] and cryptococcal meningitis.[315, 363] High-dose fluconazole is the agent of choice for treating systemic infections caused by the yeast *T. beigelii* in nonneutropenic hosts; because of potential for the development of breakthrough infections by other opportunistic fungi, the addition of D-AmB is recommended in persistently neutropenic patients.[146] Fluconazole has become the drug of choice for the treatment of coccidioidal meningitis[114, 321] and has been proved to have effectiveness in nonmeningeal coccidioidal infections.[95] It appears to be comparatively less active than itraconazole for the treatment of paracoccidioidomycosis, blastomycosis, histoplasmosis, and sporotrichosis.[86, 155, 193, 274, 275, 392]

Fluconazole can prevent mucosal candidiasis in patients with HIV infection or cancer[134, 263, 286] and has proven efficacy in preventing the development of invasive *Candida* infections in high-risk patients with acute leukemia or bone marrow or liver transplants.[125, 308, 402] A randomized, double-blind, placebo-controlled trial in adult patients with allogeneic bone marrow transplants has shown that fluconazole, given at 400 mg/day from the start of the conditioning regimen until day 75, can reduce the frequency of invasive *Candida* infection and lower mortality rates at day 110.[339] Moreover, 8 years after completion of the study, patients treated with fluconazole had persistent protection against invasive candidiasis and *Candida*-related death, a decreased frequency of severe, gut-related graft-versus-host disease, and an independent overall survival benefit of 17 percent.[234] A recent study including 278 pediatric patients has shown that treatment with fluconazole, simultaneously initiated with empirical antibacterial chemotherapy at the onset of fever, might reduce the frequency of candidemia, persistent fever, and the use of empirical amphotericin B in neutropenic patients.[385]

Itraconazole

Itraconazole is a high-molecular-weight, highly lipophilic bistriazole (see Fig. 239–6). Closely related structurally to ketoconazole, it has a broader spectrum of antifungal activity that includes dermatophytes, *Candida* spp. (*C. krusei* excluded), *C. neoformans*, *Aspergillus* spp., various dematiaceous molds, *Paecilomyces* spp., and the dimorphic fungi.[5] Itraconazole binds more avidly to its fungal target than ketoconazole does, but only weakly to human CYP450, thus leading to comparatively fewer mechanism-associated adverse effects.[127]

PHARMACODYNAMICS. In vitro, itraconazole exerts species- and strain-dependent fungistatic or fungicidal pharmacodynamics. Time-kill experiments in serum-free and serum-containing media have demonstrated concentration-independent, fungistatic activity of itraconazole against *Candida* and *C. neoformans*.[56, 57, 112, 407] Against *Aspergillus* spp., however, itraconazole displayed time- and concentration-dependent fungicidal activity with greater than 87 to greater than 97 percent killing, respectively, within 24 hours of drug exposure.[229] Persistent effects have not been reported thus far.

The principal feasibility of a correlation between in vitro susceptibility and outcome has been demonstrated in mice with experimental disseminated aspergillosis.[81] Relationships between drug concentrations and the antifungal efficacy of itraconazole have been assessed in a model of invasive pulmonary aspergillosis in methylprednisolone/cyclosporine-immunosuppressed rabbits. In this model, an inhibitory sigmoid maximal-effect model predicted a significant pharmacodynamic relationship ($r = .87$, $p < .001$) between itraconazole concentrations in plasma and antifungal efficacy as a function of the burden of *A. fumigatus* in lung tissue.[36]

In patients, however, the main rationale for monitoring plasma levels has been the erratic oral bioavailability of itraconazole, particularly in neutropenic patients. Historically, the target plasma level for itraconazole has been estimated at 0.25 µg/mL (high-performance liquid chromatography [HPLC]) at trough based on the 90 percent inhibitory concentration (IC_{90}) of a large set of clinical isolates.[46, 77] More recently, the predictive value of threshold concentrations of prophylactic itraconazole has been analyzed in a large cohort of patients undergoing intensive chemotherapy for acute leukemia. The median itraconazole trough concentration after the first week of prophylaxis was significantly lower in patients in whom invasive fungal infections developed (0.46 versus 0.82 µg/mL, $p = .008$). Multivariate logistic regression analysis demonstrated a significant ($p = .028$) statistical association of trough concentrations less than 0.5 µg/mL with the development of invasive fungal infections. A threshold of 0.25 µg/mL did not influence the occurrence of invasive mycoses in univariate and multivariate analyses.[120]

In a phase I/II clinical trial of oral cyclodextrin itraconazole in HIV-infected children with oropharyngeal candidiasis, the relationships between pharmacodynamic parameters and therapeutic response as assessed by standardized scoring of mucosal disease after 14 days of therapy corresponded to pharmacodynamic models of the inhibitory maximal effect. Best fits were observed for AUC, AUC/MIC, C_{max}, and C_{max}/MIC ($r = .483$ to $.595$, $p < .01$). Of note, no significant correlations were found in this study between the MIC values of itraconazole for the fungal isolates at baseline and therapeutic response.[135]

PHARMACOKINETICS. Itraconazole is available as capsules, as an oral solution in hydroxypropyl-β-cyclodextrin (HP-β-CD), and as a parenteral solution that also uses HP-β-CD as a solubilizer. Absorption of itraconazole in the capsule form is dependent on a low intragastric pH and is compromised by the fasting state, and it becomes erratic in granulocytopenic cancer patients and in patients with hypochlorhydria.[71, 141, 144] Absorption can be somewhat improved when the capsules are taken with food or an acidic cola beverage.[78, 144] The novel oral solution of itraconazole in HP-β-CD, however, leads to improved oral bioavailability of the parent compound that is further enhanced in the fasting state.[30, 301]

After oral administration of the drug, peak plasma concentrations are measured within 1 to 4 hours; after once-daily dosing, steady state is achieved after 7 to 14 days, and peak plasma levels are two to five times higher than those achieved after a single dose.[127, 141] Steady state can be reached more rapidly by doubling the dose during the first 2 to 3 days. In adult patients with cancer who are receiving the standard regimen of 2.5 mg/kg of itraconazole in HP-β-CD twice a day, mean peak plasma levels were 1.2 µg/mL and trough levels were 0.8 µg/mL under conditions of steady state[288]; systemic absorption of the carrier is negligible.[85] After administration of intravenous itraconazole in HP-β-CD, the drug and carrier rapidly dissociate and follow their own disposition. After administration of 200 mg twice a day for 2 days followed by 200 mg daily for 5 days to patients with hematologic malignancies, mean peak levels immediately after completion of the 1-hour infusion were 2.25 μg/mL, and mean trough levels 24 hours after the last dose were 0.53 μg/mL.[45] The carrier HP-β-CD is not metabolized significantly, and virtually 100 percent is eliminated from plasma within 24 hours in unchanged form via glomerular filtration.[408]

Itraconazole exhibits dose-dependent pharmacokinetics with hyperproportional increases in the area under the concentration versus time curve with increasing and split dosages.[127, 135, 288] Itraconazole is highly (95%) protein-bound; only 0.2 percent circulates as free drug, whereas the remainder is bound to blood cells.[167] The compound is extensively distributed throughout the body. Whereas concentrations in nonproteinaceous body fluids are negligible, tissue concentrations in many organs, including the brain, exceed corresponding plasma levels by 2 to 10 times.[78, 167]

Itraconazole is metabolized extensively in the liver by numerous pathways to more than 30 metabolites and excreted in metabolized form into bile and urine. The major metabolite, hydroxy-itraconazole, possesses antifungal activity similar to that of itraconazole. It is eliminated more rapidly, but its plasma concentrations at steady state are 1.5 to 2 times higher than those of the parent compound.[78, 141] As a consequence, plasma concentrations of itraconazole measured by bioassay are approximately 3.5 times higher than those determined by HPLC.[386] Elimination of itraconazole from plasma follows a biphasic pattern. In healthy adult volunteers, the elimination half-life of the compound is 20 to 24 hours after single dosing and 35 to 40 hours under terms of steady state because of saturable excretion mechanisms.[157] The dosage of oral itraconazole does not need to be adjusted in patients with renal insufficiency or dialysis. Because the elimination of HP-β-CD parallels the glomerular filtration rate, intravenous itraconazole is contraindicated in patients with a creatinine clearance of less than 30 mL/min; no data are available for its use in patients undergoing dialysis. In patients with severe hepatic insufficiency, the elimination half-life of itraconazole can be prolonged, so additional hepatic toxicity or possible drug interactions should be carefully monitored.

Data on the plasma pharmacokinetics of itraconazole in pediatric patients are limited to the oral HP-β-CD solution[85, 135, 328] (Table 239–9). In 26 infants and children aged 6 months to 12 years with cancer (n = 20) or liver transplants who received the compound at 5 mg/kg once daily for documented mucosal candidiasis or as antifungal prophylaxis for 2 weeks,[85] cyclodextrin itraconazole was well tolerated. However, plasma concentrations were substantially lower than those reported in adult cancer patients, particularly in children younger than 2 years.[288] In contrast, in a pharmacokinetic study in 16 neutropenic children (1.7 to 14.3 years of age) who received cyclodextrin itraconazole for antifungal prophylaxis in a split dosing regimen of 2.5 mg/kg twice a day, peak and trough levels of itraconazole were substantially higher; nevertheless, a similar trend toward lower plasma concentrations in the group of children 5 years or younger was noted.[328] Finally, in a cohort of 26 HIV-infected children and adolescents (1.25 to 18 years old), cyclodextrin itraconazole was safe and effective for the treatment of oropharyngeal candidiasis at dosages of 2.5 mg/day or 2.5 mg twice a day given for at least 14 days.[135] A high percentage (77%) of the patients were receiving concomitant therapy with protease-inhibitors or clarithromycin (or both), drugs that are strong inhibitors of the CYP3A4-dependent metabolism of itraconazole.[283] Peak and trough levels measured after administration of the split-dosage regimen were similar to those observed in cancer patients receiving the same dosage regimen.[328]

Despite the tremendous interpatient variability that results from both variable absorption and hepatic metabolism, the pharmacokinetics of itraconazole apparently are not fundamentally different from those in adults. Although oral cyclodextrin itraconazole is not approved for the treatment of pediatric age groups, a starting dosage of 2.5 mg/kg twice

TABLE 239–9 ■ PHARMACOKINETICS OF ITRACONAZOLE AND HYDROXY-ITRACONAZOLE AFTER ADMINISTRATION OF HYDROXYPROPYL-β-CYCLODEXTRIN ORAL SOLUTION TO IMMUNOCOMPROMISED INFANTS AND CHILDREN

	Children with Cancer/Liver Transplant* (n = 8, 0.5–2 yr)	Children with Cancer* (n = 7, 2–5 yr)	Children with Cancer* (n = 11, 6–12 yr)	Children with Cancer† (n = 9, 2–5 yr)	Children with Cancer† (n = 6, 6–12 yr)
Itraconazole					
C_{max} (μg/mL)	0.571 ± 0.416	0.534 ± 0.431	0.631 ± 0.358	1.024 ± 0.351	1.524 ± 0.770
T_{max} (hr)	1.9 ± 0.1	2.9 ± 2.5	3.1 ± 2.1	n/a	n/a
C_{min}	0.159 ± 0.218	0.179 ± 0.100	0.233 ± 0.14	0.711 ± 0.251	1.072 ± 0.408
$AUC_{0\to\infty}$ (μg/mL·hr)	6.930 ± 5.83	7.33 ± 5.42	8.77 ± 5.05	n/a	n/a
$t_{1/2}\beta$ (hr)	47.4 ± 55.0	30.6 ± 25.3	28.3 ± 9.6	n/a	n/a
Acc. factor	6.2 ± 5.0	3.3 ± 3.0	8.6 ± 7.4	n/a	n/a
OH-Itraconazole					
C_{max} (μg/mL)	0.690 ± 0.445	0.687 ± 0.419	0.699 ± 0.234	1.358 ± 0.373	2.180 ± 0.753
T_{max} (hr)	4.4 ± 2.3	4.8 ± 2.7	10.8 ± 14.3	n/a	n/a
C_{min}	0.308 ± 0.430	0.487 ± 0.310	0.437 ± 0.240	1.275 ± 0.322	1.964 ± 0.562
$AUC_{0\to\infty}$ (μg/mL·hr)	13.20 ± 11.40	13.4 ± 9.1	13.45 ± 7.19	n/a	n/a
$t_{1/2}\beta$ (hr)	18.0 ± 18.1	17.1 ± 14.5	17.9 ± 8.7	n/a	n/a
Acc· factor	11.4 ± 16.0	2.3 ± 1.9	6.4 ± 5.6	n/a	n/a

Pharmacokinetic parameters were obtained over a period of 14 days after daily dosing. All values represent mean values ± SD.
*Cyclodextrin dosage: 5.0 mg/kg/day for 14 days. Data from de Repentigny, L., Ratelle, J., Leclerc, J. M., et al.: Repeated-dose pharmacokinetics of an oral solution of itraconazole in infants and children. Antimicrob. Agents Chemother. 42:404–408, 1998.
†Cyclodextrin dosage: 2.5 mg/kg twice daily for 14 days. Data from Schmitt, C., Perel, Y., Harousseau, J. I., et al.: Pharmacokinetics of itraconazole oral solution in neutropenic children during long-term prophylaxis. Antimicrob. Agents Chemother. 45:1561–1564, 2001.
Acc. factor, accumulation factor (AUC_{0-24} day 14/$AUC_{0\to\infty}$ day 1); $AUC_{0\to\infty}$ area under the concentration versus time curve from zero to infinity; C_{max}, peak plasma levels; n/a, not assessed; $t_{1/2}\beta$, elimination half-life; T_{max}, time until occurrence of C_{max}.

a day can be advocated based on the available pharmacokinetic data.[85, 135, 328] The recommended dosage range for the capsule formulation is 5 to 8 (12) mg/kg/day (corresponding to dosages of 200 to 400 [600] mg/day recommended for adults), with a loading dose of 4 mg/kg three times a day for the first 3 days. Data on the use of intravenous itraconazole in pediatric patients are lacking; the dosage regimen used in the published adult studies is 200 mg twice a day for 2 days, followed by 200 mg four times a day for a maximum of 12 days.[45, 61] Because some evidence supports the existence of a relationship between trough concentrations and antifungal efficacy,[120] trough levels should be monitored and dosing adjusted to maintain plasma concentrations of the parent itraconazole above 0.5 μg/mL. Only anecdotal reports have been published on the use of itraconazole in the neonatal setting.

ADVERSE EFFECTS. Itraconazole is usually well tolerated, with a similar pattern and an approximately identical frequency of adverse effects as noted with fluconazole.[71] In 189 adult patients treated for systemic fungal infections at dosages of 50 to 400 mg/day for a median of 5 months, the rate of possibly or definitely related adverse effects was 39 percent.[359] Most of the observed reactions were transient and included nausea and vomiting (<10%), hypertriglyceridemia (9%), hypokalemia (6%), elevated hepatic transaminases (5%), rash or pruritus (or both) (2%), headaches or dizziness (<2%), and pedal edema (1%). Four percent of patients discontinued itraconazole treatment because of adverse effects. Gastrointestinal intolerance appears to be the dose-limiting toxicity of the oral cyclodextrin formulation; in a comparative study in adult patients with acute leukemia, 46 percent of patients receiving a daily dose of 800 mg stopped treatment early because of severe nausea and vomiting. Crossover to the identical dose of the capsule formulation was well tolerated by all patients; patients receiving 400 mg/day of the solution had no gastrointestinal adverse effects.[119] Only a few cases of more severe hepatic injury or hepatitis have been described.[211] Itraconazole can have negative inotropic effects; because of a low, but possible risk of cardiac toxicity, itraconazole should not be administered to patients with ventricular dysfunction.

Cyclodextrin itraconazole solution was safe and well tolerated for at least 14 days in the reported phase I/II pharmacokinetic studies in immunocompromised pediatric patients.[85, 135, 328] Vomiting (12%), abnormal liver function test results (5%), and abdominal pain (3%) were the most common adverse effects considered definitely or possibly related to cyclodextrin itraconazole solution in an open study of 103 neutropenic pediatric cancer patients who received the drug at 5 mg/kg/day or 2.5 mg/kg twice a day for antifungal prophylaxis for a median duration of 37 days; 18 percent of patients withdrew from the study because of adverse events.[106]

DRUG INTERACTIONS. When compared with fluconazole, itraconazole has a greater propensity for and extent of drug-drug interactions[141] (see Table 239–8). Itraconazole is a substrate of CYP3A4, but it also interacts with the heme moiety of CYP3A and thereby results in noncompetitive inhibition of the oxidative metabolism of many CYP3A substrates. An interaction also can result from inhibition of P-glycoprotein–mediated efflux; P-glycoprotein is extensively co-localized and exhibits overlapping substrate specificity with CYP3A. Finally, the systemic availability of itraconazole depends in part on gastric acidity and the activity of intestinal CYP3A4 and P-glycoprotein.[131, 148] Inhibition of hepatic CYP450 enzyme systems may lead to increased and potentially toxic concentrations of co-administered drugs. Most important, co-administration of cisapride, terfenadine, and astemizole with itraconazole can lead to serious cardiac arrhythmias and is thus strictly contraindicated.[171, 283] Similarly contraindicated is the co-administration of cholesterol-lowering agents such as lovastatin, simvastatin, and atorvastatin, which has been associated with rhabdomyolysis.[259] Potentially toxic levels of the co-administered drug also can be reached when itraconazole is given along with phenytoin, benzodiazepines, cyclosporine, tacrolimus, methylprednisolone, digoxin, quinidine, warfarin, sulfonylurea compounds, rifampin, rifabutin, ritonavir, indinavir, haloperidol, clarithromycin, felodipine, and vincristine.[43, 152, 204, 267, 283, 319, 367] Increased metabolism of itraconazole resulting in decreased plasma levels can be induced by rifampin, rifabutin, isoniazid, carbamazepine, phenobarbital, and phenytoin.[283, 358] As a consequence, patients who receive itraconazole along with one of the listed drugs should be followed closely, and the plasma concentrations of ideally both compounds as well as hepatic function should be monitored carefully.

CLINICAL INDICATIONS. Clinical indications for itraconazole are summarized in Tables 239–2, 239–3, 239–4, 239–10, and 239–12. Itraconazole is a useful agent for treating dermatophytic infections, pityriasis versicolor,[3, 109, 127, 151] and vaginal candidiasis.[344] It is effective in the treatment of oropharyngeal and esophageal candidiasis, including cases in adult and pediatric patients in which resistance to fluconazole has developed.[1, 85, 135, 316] The clinical efficacy of itraconazole in candidemia and other deeply invasive *Candida* infections has not been evaluated systematically. Although the experience with itraconazole in the primary treatment of cryptococcal meningitis is scant, itraconazole has been used with success for long-term treatment of cryptococcal meningitis in patients with HIV infection.[315, 363]

Itraconazole is approved as a second-line agent for treatment of invasive *Aspergillus* infections. Two separate uncontrolled studies have investigated oral itraconazole for the treatment of proven or probable invasive aspergillosis; the results suggest a response rate comparable to that of conventional amphotericin B.[83, 345] The published experience with the intravenous formulation for this indication is promising but limited.[61] Because few data exist on the use of itraconazole for first-line treatment of invasive aspergillosis in neutropenic patients, we reserve its use in this population for consolidation therapy in patients who no longer are neutropenic. Beyond being used to treat invasive aspergillosis, itraconazole may be useful in the management of infections caused by certain dematiaceous molds.[146, 338] However, the compound has no documented activity against zygomycosis and fusariosis.

Itraconazole is the current treatment of choice for lymphocutaneous sporotrichosis[193, 295] and non–life-threatening, nonmeningeal paracoccidioidomycosis, blastomycosis, and histoplasmosis in non-immunocompromised patients.[66, 87, 254, 257, 351, 393] It also has established efficacy in both induction and maintenance therapy for mild to moderate, nonmeningeal histoplasmosis in HIV-infected patients.[390, 391, 393] Whereas earlier uncontrolled clinical trials suggested a somewhat inferior efficacy against nonmeningeal and meningeal coccidioidomycosis in comparison to fluconazole,[129, 356, 357] a recent randomized, double-blind comparative study in patients with progressive, nonmeningeal coccidioidomycosis showed a trend toward slightly greater efficacy when both drugs were given at a daily dosage of 400 mg.[115] Of emphasis, however, is that amphotericin B remains the treatment of choice for most immunocompromised patients and for those with life-threatening forms of endemic mycoses.[141]

No clinical trials have been published on the use of itraconazole as antifungal prophylaxis after undergoing allogeneic stem cell transplantation. A randomized, placebo-controlled, double-blind multicenter study that evaluated the use of itraconazole, 2.5 mg/kg twice a day, as antifungal prophylaxis in a total of 405 neutropenic patients with hematologic malignancies found a significant reduction in the incidence of proven or suspected invasive fungal infections in the itraconazole arm[242] that mainly was due to a reduction in the occurrence of candidemia. However, the number of documented cases of invasive aspergillosis was too low (1%, or five cases in total) to allow for any assessment of prophylactic efficacy against this important disease. In the same patient population, itraconazole (200 mg four times a day intravenously for ≤12 days, followed by 200 mg twice a day of the oral solution for ≤14 day) also was compared in a prospective, open, randomized study with amphotericin B (0.7 to 1.0 mg/kg four times a day) for empirical antifungal therapy in a total of 384 persistently febrile neutropenic patients.[44] Itraconazole was at least as effective as conventional amphotericin B and was superior with respect to its safety profile, which has led to approval of this indication by the FDA.

Second-Generation Antifungal Triazoles: Posaconazole, Ravuconazole, and Voriconazole

Further improvement of the structure-activity relationship has led to a new generation of synthetic antifungal triazoles that are in advanced stages of clinical development. These new triazoles include posaconazole (SCH 56592; Schering-Plough Inc., Kenilworth, NJ), ravuconazole (Bristol-Myers Squibb Inc., Wallingford, CT), and voriconazole (Pfizer Ltd., Sandwich, UK) (Fig. 239–8). Whereas ravuconazole and voriconazole are structurally related to fluconazole, the structure of posaconazole is similar to that of itraconazole.

The second-generation triazoles possess enhanced target activity and specificity. They are active against a wide spectrum of clinically important fungi, including *Candida*, *T. beigelii*, *C. neoformans*, *Aspergillus*, *Fusarium*, and other hyaline molds, as well as dematiaceous and dimorphic molds.[67] Similar to itraconazole, these novel triazoles appear to exert fungistatic activity against susceptible yeast-like organisms and strain-dependent fungicidal activity against susceptible filamentous fungi,[69, 103, 112, 185, 196, 229, 230] and they appear to display exposure-dependent antifungal efficacy in vivo.[17, 137]

Thus far, fundamental differences in potency, spectrum, and antifungal efficacy among posaconazole, ravuconazole, and voriconazole have not surfaced. Although all three agents display some nonlinearity in their disposition, undergo hepatic metabolism, and have the potential for drug-drug interactions through their affinity to CYP450 isoenzymes, key pharmacokinetic parameters (oral bioavailability, protein binding, plasma clearance, and Vd) vary. Whether these differences are of clinical significance, however, remains to be elucidated.[170]

CLINICAL TRIALS. Whereas clinical trials of only ravuconazole have been initiated, posaconazole and voriconazole have been studied in several phase II and III studies.

The antifungal efficacy of posaconazole was studied in two large randomized comparative studies in HIV-infected individuals with oropharyngeal candidiasis. Treatment with posaconazole (50 to 400 mg orally) was well tolerated and was as effective as fluconazole (100 mg) at the end of 14 days of treatment.[262, 368] Moreover, in an open, noncomparative multicenter salvage study including 97 patients with a variety of invasive fungal infections refractory to or intolerant of standard therapies, response rates (defined as complete or partial response) in subjects with aspergillosis, fusariosis, cryptococcosis, candidiasis, and phaeohyphomycosis after 4 to 8 weeks of therapy with 800 mg/day orally ranged from 44 to 80 percent.[154] Additional clinical trials and development of an intravenous formulation are under way.

Voriconazole has demonstrated excellent clinical efficacy in a noncomparative phase I/II study in HIV-infected patients with oropharyngeal candidiasis[162] and was as effective as fluconazole for the treatment of esophageal candidiasis in a double-blind, randomized multicenter trial.[94] In a phase II study of 102 patients with acute invasive aspergillosis refractory to or intolerant of standard therapy, a complete or partial response was observed in 53 percent of patients,[80] and in a different study, 11 of 19 non-neutropenic patients with chronic invasive aspergillosis responded to treatment with voriconazole.[95] A large, randomized, multicenter trial has been completed that compared voriconazole with liposomal amphotericin B for empirical antifungal therapy.[381] The preliminary results of this study showed comparable composite

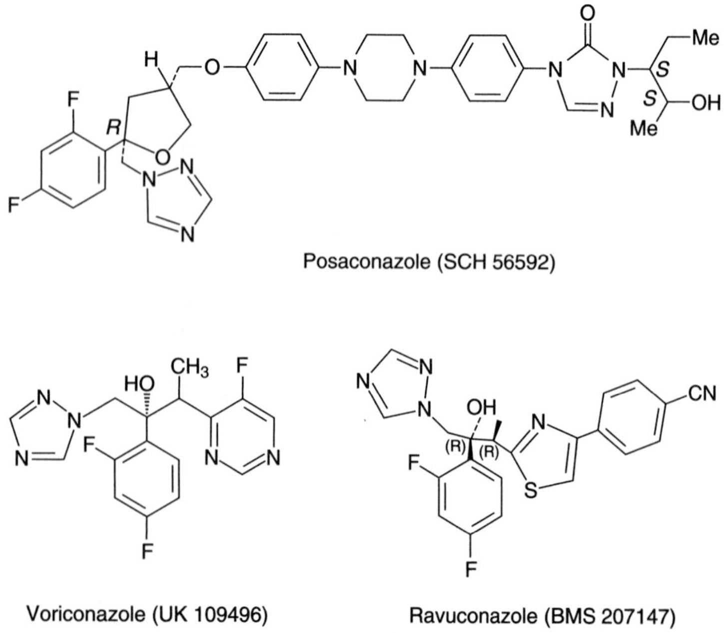

Posaconazole (SCH 56592)

Voriconazole (UK 109496)

Ravuconazole (BMS 207147)

FIGURE 239–8 ■ Structural formulas of second-generation systemic antifungal triazoles: posaconazole, ravuconazole, and voriconazole.

success rates but fewer proven and probable breakthrough infections, less infusion-related toxicity, and less nephrotoxicity in the voriconazole-treated cohort. However, patients receiving voriconazole had significantly more frequent episodes of transient visual disturbances and hallucination.

PEDIATRIC EXPERIENCE. Data on pediatric patients are limited to voriconazole. The safety and efficacy of voriconazole in immunocompromised pediatric patients treated within the voriconazole compassionate-use program have been reported.[375] Sixty-one patients 15 years or younger received voriconazole at a dosage of 4 mg/kg twice a day (6 mg/kg twice a day on the first day) for a median of 84 days (range, 1 to 800) for definite or probable invasive fungal infections refractory to or intolerant of previous antifungal therapy. *Aspergillus* and *Scedosporium* were the most common infecting species. Altogether, a complete or partial response to therapy with voriconazole was demonstrated in 40 percent of patients. Long-term therapy with voriconazole was well tolerated: the treatment-related adverse events most commonly reported included increased liver function test parameters (21%), rash (19.6%), transient visual disturbances (8.1%), and nausea or vomiting (6.5%). A formal phase II pharmacokinetic study in pediatric patients has been completed but not yet published.

ECHINOCANDIN LIPOPEPTIDES: ANIDULAFUNGIN, CASPOFUNGIN, AND MICAFUNGIN

The echinocandins are a novel class of semisynthetic amphiphilic lipopeptides that are composed of a cyclic hexapeptide core linked to a variably configured lipid side chain. Three compounds are in advanced stages of clinical development: anidulafungin (VER-002, formerly LY303366; Versicor Inc, Freemont, CA), caspofungin (MK-0991; Merck & Co., Inc., Rahway, NJ), and micafungin (FK463; Fujisawa Inc., Deerfield, IL) (Fig. 239–9). The current data indicate that these agents have very similar pharmacological properties. Of note, caspofungin recently received limited approval by the FDA for third-line treatment of invasive aspergillosis.

MECHANISM OF ACTION. The echinocandins act by noncompetitive inhibition of the synthesis of 1,3-β-glucan, a polysaccharide in the cell wall of many pathogenic fungi (Fig. 239–10). Together with chitin, the rope-like glucan fibrils are responsible for the cell wall's strength and shape. They are important in maintaining osmotic integrity of the fungal cell and play a key role in cell division and cell growth.[79, 118, 147, 161] The proposed molecular target of the echinocandins, glucan synthase, is a heteromeric enzyme complex composed of at least one large integral membrane protein encoded by the *FKS* genes that bind the substrate (uridine diphosphate [UDP]-glucose) and one small regulatory subunit, Rho1p, a guanosine triphosphate (GTP)-binding protein; additional, yet unidentified components also may be involved.[206, 350]

ANTIFUNGAL ACTIVITY. All three compounds have potent broad-spectrum fungicidal activity in vitro against *Candida* spp. and potent inhibitory activity against *Aspergillus;* their antifungal efficacy against these organisms in vivo has been demonstrated in various animal models. The current echinocandins have variable activity against dematiaceous and endemic molds but are inactive against most hyalohyphomycetes, zygomycetes, and *C. neoformans* and *T. beigelii*. Of note, all echinocandins have demonstrated preventive and therapeutic activity in animal models of *Pneumocystis carinii* pneumonitis.[145, 147, 159]

As expected from their mechanism of action, the echinocandins show no cross-resistance to amphotericin B– and fluconazole-resistant *Candida* isolates. Inherited resistance to echinocandins in otherwise susceptible fungal yeast species is a rare finding; most mutations conferring resistance have been mapped to the *FKS* gene.[206] The results of resistance-induction studies with caspofungin demonstrate a low potential for induced resistance in *Candida* spp.[31] The frequency of primary echinocandin resistance among clinical isolates of *Aspergillus* and induction of secondary resistance in vitro have not been studied.

PHARMACODYNAMICS. The echinocandins demonstrate a species-dependent mode of antifungal activity. Although similarly potent activity at the target enzyme has been demonstrated in membrane preparations of *Candida* and *Aspergillus* spp., whole-cell in vitro assays reveal fungicidal activity against most *Candida* but not against *Aspergillus* spp.[31, 348] Microscopic examination of exposed organisms shows a dose-dependent formation of microcolonies with progressively truncated, swollen hyphal elements that appear to be cell wall deficient but are able to regain their cell walls after subculture in the absence of drug.[89, 207, 265, 294] These observations indicate differences in functional target sensitivity in both species that are not fully understood.

Time-kill studies in *Candida* spp. have demonstrated predominantly concentration-dependent fungicidal activity (99.9% reduction in CFU) and rate of kill above the MIC for all three compounds.[100, 102, 278] In addition, a concentration-dependent prolonged post-antifungal effect exceeding 12 hours at concentrations above the MIC has been demonstrated for anidulafungin and caspofungin.[101] Pharmacodynamic studies in neutropenic animals with disseminated candidiasis and a murine thigh infection model have demonstrated similar concentration-dependent activity of anidulafungin and micafungin, respectively.[36, 136, 236]

PHARMACOKINETICS. At present, all current echinocandins are available only for intravenous administration. They exhibit dose-proportional plasma pharmacokinetics with a triexponential elimination pattern. The β-half-life is between 10 and 15 hours, thus allowing for once-daily dosing without major accumulation after multiple dosing. All echinocandins are highly (>95%) protein-bound and are distributed into all major organ sites, including the brain; however, concentrations in uninfected CSF are low. The echinocandins are metabolized by the liver and slowly excreted into urine and feces, with only small fractions (<2%) of a dose being excreted into urine in unchanged form.[145, 147, 159] Whether differences in individual pharmacokinetic parameters such as AUC, peak plasma levels, Vd, and clearance of the echinocandins are of clinical significance remains to be elucidated.

ADVERSE EFFECTS. At their currently investigated dosages, all echinocandins are generally well tolerated, and only a small fraction of patients enrolled in the various clinical trials (<5%) discontinued echinocandin therapy because of drug-related adverse events.[53, 227, 280, 318] Detailed safety data have been published for caspofungin only: the adverse effects most frequently reported as being possibly, probably, or definitely associated with caspofungin treatment included fever (3.6 to 26%), increased liver transaminases (10.6 to 13%), phlebitis (1.5 to 15.7%), nausea (2.5 to 6%), and headache (6.0 to 11.3%).[273] Like other basic polypeptides, the echinocandins have the theoretic potential to cause histamine release. Symptoms such as rash, facial swelling, pruritus, or a sensation of warmth, which could potentially have been mediated through endogenous histamine release, have been reported in isolated cases; a reversible anaphylactic reaction occurred in one patient during initial administration of caspofungin.[317]

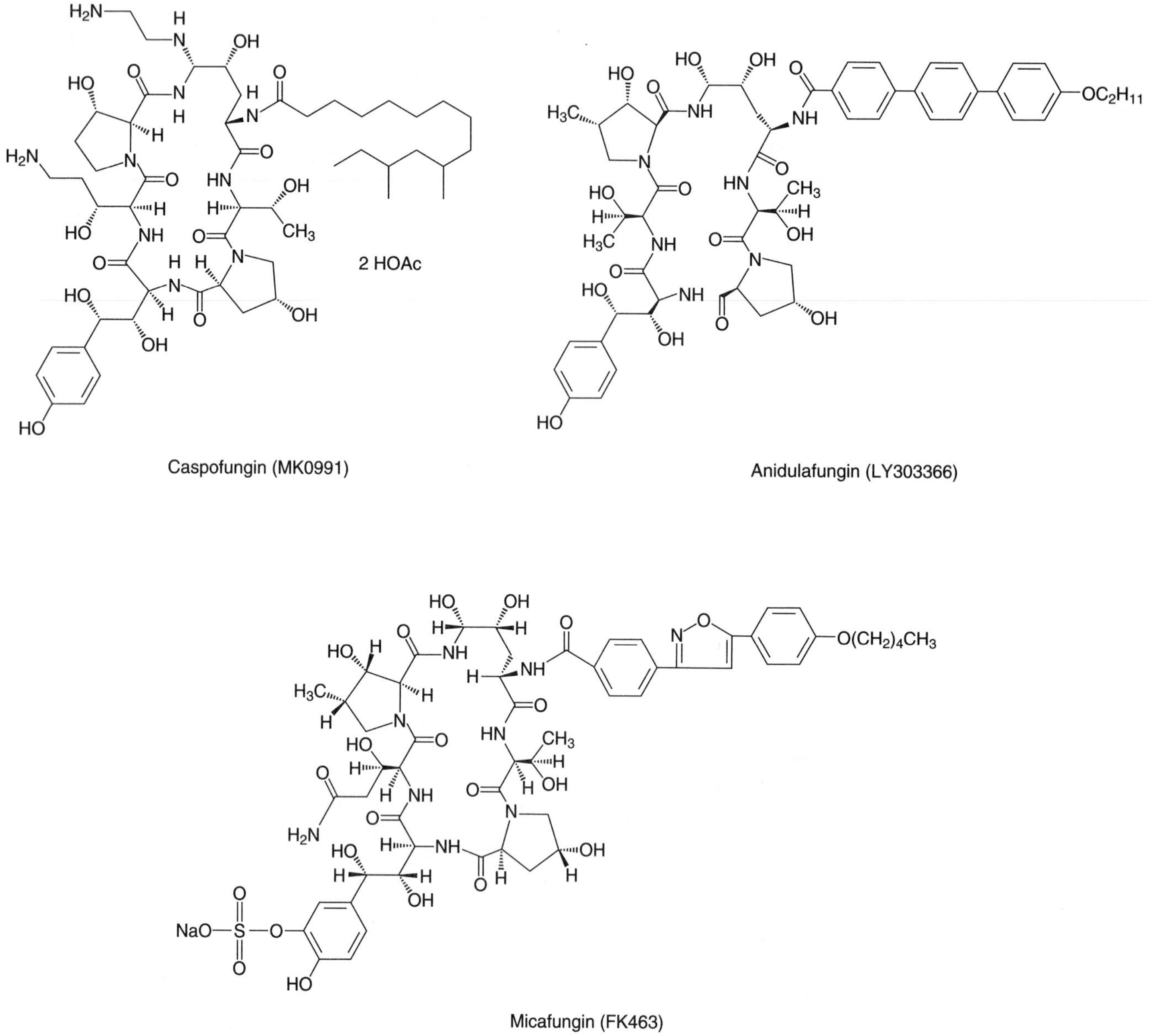

Caspofungin (MK0991)

Anidulafungin (LY303366)

Micafungin (FK463)

FIGURE 239–9 ■ Structural formulas of echinocandin lipopeptides: anidulafungin, caspofungin, and micafungin.

DRUG INTERACTIONS. The current echinocandins appear to have no significant potential for drug interactions mediated by the CYP450 enzyme system. In vitro biotransformation studies of caspofungin revealed that the compound is not a substrate of P-glycoprotein and is a poor substrate and a weak inhibitor of CYP450 enzymes.[25, 405] Thus far, no pharmacokinetic interactions were noted between caspofungin and itraconazole, D-AmB, and the immunosuppressant mycophenolate.[273, 346] Caspofungin can reduce the AUC of tacrolimus by approximately 20 percent but has no effect on cyclosporine levels. However, cyclosporine increased the AUC of caspofungin by approximately 35 percent; because of transient elevations of hepatic transaminases in single-dose interaction studies, the concomitant use of both drugs is not recommended.[273] Finally, regression analysis of patient pharmacokinetic data suggests that inducers of drug clearance or mixed inducer/inhibitors, namely, efavirenz, nelfinavir, nevirapine, phenytoin, rifampin, dexamethasone, and carbamazepine, may reduce caspofungin concentrations.[273]

CLINICAL STUDIES. The antifungal efficacy of anidulafungin has been studied in 36 immunocompromised adult patients who were randomized to receive either a 50-mg loading dose with 25-mg maintenance or a 70-mg loading dose with 35-mg maintenance for a total of 14 to 21 days for treatment of esophageal candidiasis. Based on endoscopy scoring at the completion of therapy, treatment was effective in 81 and 85 percent of patients, respectively. Anidulafungin was well tolerated, and no drug-related serious adverse events were noted.[53]

In a randomized, double-blind, multicenter trial performed in South America, caspofungin at 50 mg/day and 70 mg/day for a total of 14 days was compared with conventional amphotericin B (0.5 mg/kg/day for the same duration) for the treatment of esophageal candidiasis in 128 immunocompromised patients. Clinical response (symptoms plus endoscopy) was noted in 85.1 percent of patients in the combined caspofungin group versus 66.7 percent in the amphotericin B group. Caspofungin appeared to be well tolerated; no serious adverse events were associated with caspofungin.[318] The clinical

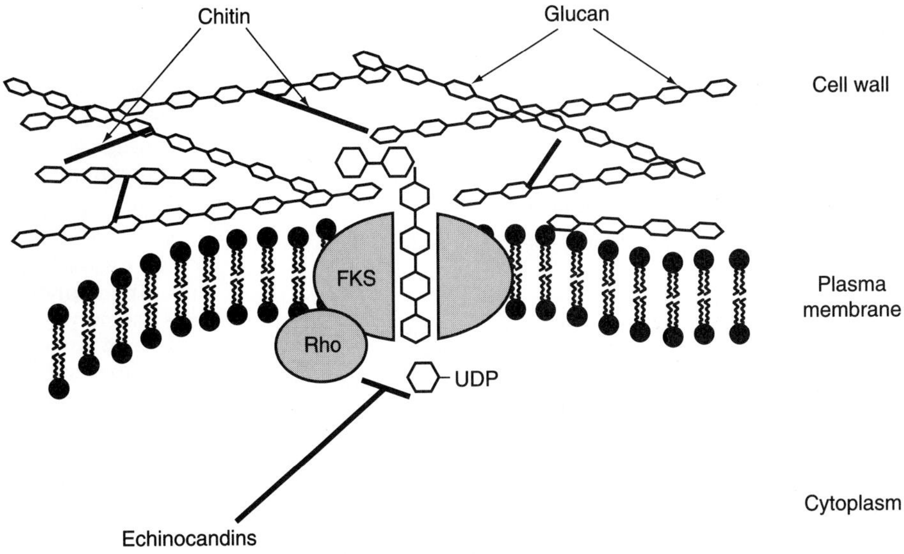

FIGURE 239–10 ■ Schematic of the proposed mechanism of action of echinocandin lipopeptides. Echinocandins inhibit the synthesis of cell wall 1,3-β-glucan at the level of the cell membrane. FKS is the proposed catalytic subunit, and Rho is the proposed regulatory subunit of the glucan synthase complex. (Modified from Kurtz, M. B., and Douglas, C. M.: Lipopeptide inhibitors of fungal glucan synthase. J. Med. Vet. Mycol. *35*:79–86, 1997.)

efficacy of caspofungin (70 mg on day 1, followed by 50 mg once daily) against invasive aspergillosis has been studied in a multicenter phase II trial in patients with definite or probable invasive aspergillosis refractory to or intolerant of standard therapies. A total of 63 patients received caspofungin for a mean duration of 33.7 days (range, 1 to 162 days). Most patients (66%) had hematologic malignancies or had undergone bone marrow transplantation, and most patients had infections that were refractory to standard therapies (53/63, 84%). Twenty-two percent (14/63) of patients were neutropenic, and 37 percent (23/63) received 20 mg or more of prednisolone equivalent at study entry. As determined by an independent expert panel, a favorable response (defined as either complete or partial response) was observed in 41 percent of patients receiving at least one dose of caspofungin; in patients receiving the drug for a period longer than 7 days, a favorable response was seen in 50 percent.[277]

A multicenter, dose de-escalation study has been completed that evaluated the safety and minimally effective dose of micafungin in 74 HIV-infected patients with endoscopically documented *Candida* esophagitis.[279] In patients who received the drug for at least 8 days, resolution or improvement in clinical signs and symptoms was observed in 21 of 21 (100%) patients receiving 50 mg, in 18 of 20 (90%) receiving 25 mg, and in 17 of 21 (81%) of patients receiving 12.5 mg. One serious adverse event (diarrhea and dehydration) was reported that was assessed as possibly related to FK463. Infusion-related toxicity or reactions attributable to the release of histamine were not reported, and no nephrotoxicity or hepatotoxicity was noted.[279] Further dose escalation to a daily dosage of 75 and 100 mg/kg and end-point evaluation by endoscopy demonstrated consistent results in clearing or improvement of endoscopic lesions in 35 of 36 (97%) patients who received at least 10 days of therapy, without any safety issues.[280]

Phase III efficacy studies of echinocandins for the treatment of invasive candidiasis and for empiric antifungal therapy in persistently febrile neutropenic patients are ongoing or have been initiated.

PEDIATRIC EXPERIENCE. Pediatric data are limited to micafungin. The safety and plasma pharmacokinetics of micafungin have been investigated in a phase I dose escalation study in febrile neutropenic pediatric patients (2 to 12 years old) who received the compound for a mean of 8 days (range, 1 to 14 days) at dosages ranging from 0.5 to 4 mg/kg administered once daily over the course of 1 hour. Noncompartmental analysis revealed linear pharmacokinetics with dose-proportional increases in the $AUC_{0–8}$ and minor increases equal to or less than 130 percent at steady state. The mean elimination half-life was 11 to 17 hours and did not vary with time. On day 1, mean clearance ranged from 0.257 to 0.419 mL/kg/ min, and the mean terminal-phase volume of distribution was 0.266 to 0.466 L/kg. The compound was well tolerated without evidence of differences in pharmacokinetics, safety, and efficacy in comparison to adults.[335, 353] A phase I/II clinical pharmacology study of caspofungin in pediatric patients has been initiated.

CLINICAL INDICATIONS. At the time of the writing of this chapter, only caspofungin has been approved for the treatment of invasive fungal infections. Caspofungin may be indicated in patients with probable or proven invasive aspergillosis refractory to or intolerant of other approved therapies[227] (see Table 239–3). The currently recommended dose regimen of caspofungin in adults consists of a single 70-mg loading dose on day 1, followed by 50 mg daily thereafter administered by slow intravenous infusion for approximately 1 hour.

Current data indicate a major role for the echinocandins in the treatment of proven or suspected, superficial and invasive *Candida* infections in immunocompetent and immunocompromised patients in the future. They also may be useful for the prevention of infection in neutropenic patients with cancer or after hematopoietic stem cell transplantation. Because most in vitro studies showed synergistic or additive effects, great potential exists for investigation of combination therapies including amphotericin B and the antifungal triazoles. Finally, the echinocandins also may prove useful for the treatment and prevention of *P. carinii* pneumonitis.

Agents for Systemic Treatment of Mycoses of the Skin and Its Appendages

GRISEOFULVIN

Griseofulvin (Fig. 239–11) was originally isolated in 1939 as a natural product of *Penicillium griseofulvum*.[272] However, not until the late 1950s was it reported to be effective as an antifungal agent.[117] It since has been used extensively for the systemic treatment of superficial dermatophyte infections in both adults and children.

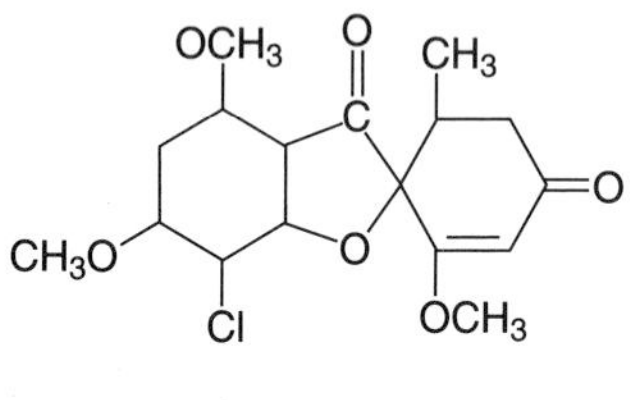

Griseofulvin

FIGURE 239–11 ■ Structural formula of griseofulvin.

MECHANISM OF ACTION. Griseofulvin interferes with fungal microtubule formation. It disrupts formation of the cell's mitotic spindle and thus arrests the metaphase of cell division.[149] Several additional mechanisms of action have been proposed, including inhibition of nucleic acid synthesis, interference with the synthesis of cell wall chitin, and anti-inflammatory properties.[153] Griseofulvin is deposited in keratin precursor cells and produces an unfavorable environment for fungal invasion; infected skin, hair, or nails are replaced with tissue not infected by the dermatophyte.

ANTIFUNGAL ACTIVITY. As evident from its mechanism of action, griseofulvin is a fungistatic compound. It is active against *Trichophyton*, *Microsporon*, and *Epidermophyton* spp. The drug has no activity against yeast-like organisms such as *Candida*, *Pityrosporum*, and *C. neoformans*. It also is inactive against opportunistic hyaline and dematiaceous molds and the dimorphic (endemic) molds.[110]

PHARMACOKINETICS. Griseofulvin is available commercially for oral administration only as griseofulvin microsize and griseofulvin ultramicrosize. Microsize griseofulvin contains predominantly particles on the order of 4 μm in diameter, and ultramicrosize griseofulvin contains predominantly particles less than 1 μm in diameter. Griseofulvin is weakly water-soluble and poorly absorbed from the gastrointestinal tract. When compared with nonmicronized drug preparations, micronized and ultramicronized formulations display enhanced absorption, particularly when polyethylene glycol is used as a dispersion carrier in the ultramicronized formulations. Oral bioavailability of the micronized formulation is variable and ranges from 25 to 70 percent; ultramicronized griseofulvin, in contrast, is almost completely absorbed.[42, 153]

After oral administration, peak plasma concentrations occur approximately 4 hours after dosing. Griseofulvin is distributed to keratin precursor cells and is concentrated in skin, hair, nails, liver, adipose tissue, and skeletal muscles. In skin, a concentration gradient is established over time, with the highest concentrations in the outermost stratum corneum.[99, 337] Non–protein-bound drug is carried in extracellular fluid and sweat and eliminated through transepidermal fluid loss; in addition, reversible protein binding and high lipid solubility cause griseofulvin to partition into the stratum corneum, where its concentration exceeds that in serum. Within 48 to 72 hours after discontinuation, plasma concentrations of griseofulvin are markedly reduced, and the compound no longer is detectable in the stratum corneum.[42, 153]

Griseofulvin is oxidatively demethylated and conjugated with glucuronic acid primarily in the liver; its major metabolite, 6-desmethylgriseofulvin, is microbiologically inactive.[219] Elimination of the compound from plasma is bi-exponential with a terminal elimination half-life of 9 to 21 hours.[309] Approximately one third of a single dose of micronized griseofulvin is excreted in feces and 50 percent in urine within 5 days. In urine, the drug is excreted mainly as free and glucuronized 6-desmethylgriseofulvin. Unchanged drug in urine accounts for less than 1 percent of the dose.[219, 220]

Separate pharmacokinetic data for pediatric patients have not been published; however, the compound is approved for children older than 2 years. The recommended pediatric dosage of microsize griseofulvin is 10 to 20 mg/kg/day (maximum, 1 g) administered in two divided doses; the recommended pediatric dosage of ultramicronized griseofulvin is 5 to 10 mg/kg/day (maximum, 750 mg), also into two divided doses.[9]

ADVERSE EFFECTS. Griseofulvin is generally well tolerated. More common adverse effects of griseofulvin include headaches and a variety of gastrointestinal symptoms. Griseofulvin can cause photosensitivity and exacerbate lupus and porphyria. Cases of erythema multiforme–like reactions, toxic epidermal necrolysis, and a reaction resembling serum sickness have been described. Proteinuria, nephrosis, hepatotoxicity, leukopenia, and menstrual irregularities have been reported rarely in association with griseofulvin therapy. Griseofulvin has been found to produce estrogen-like effects in children and reversible diminution of hearing.[42, 110, 153] Griseofulvin is contraindicated in patients with porphyria or hepatocellular failure. The compound has been shown to be teratogenic in animals and should not be administered to pregnant women. Griseofulvin also has mutagenic and carcinogenic potential; the significance of these observations for humans, however, is unclear.[110]

DRUG INTERACTIONS. Griseofulvin has been noted to enhance the clearance of oral contraceptives, cyclosporine, theophylline, aspirin, and warfarin. Concurrent use of phenobarbital may lead to decreased griseofulvin levels. Finally, concurrent alcohol ingestion may lead to a disulfiram-like reaction.[110]

INDICATIONS. Griseofulvin remains an important agent for the treatment of tinea capitis and refractory tinea corporis (Table 239–10). For tinea capitis, 6 to 8 weeks of treatment generally is required[96, 175]; the usual duration of therapy for refractory tinea corporis is 4 weeks.[9] Nail infections, which rarely occur in the pediatric population, usually fail to respond to therapy with griseofulvin and are better treated with itraconazole or terbinafine. Because griseofulvin is not effective against other fungal infections, the infecting organism always should be identified as a dermatophyte before the initiation of therapy. Of note, in vitro resistance of dermatophytes to griseofulvin has been reported and may be the cause of therapeutic failure.[23]

TERBINAFINE

The synthetic allylamine terbinafine (Fig. 239–12) is a relatively novel antifungal agent that is useful for topical and systemic (oral) treatment of superficial infections of the skin and its appendages by dermatophytes and yeasts and possibly for cutaneous sporotrichosis. It acts by inhibiting the biosynthesis of fungal ergosterol at the level of squalene epoxidase (see Fig. 239–7), thereby leading to depletion of ergosterol and accumulation of toxic squalenes in the fungal cell membrane.[28]

ANTIFUNGAL ACTIVITY. Terbinafine has exceptionally potent and fungicidal in vitro activity against dermatophytes. It is also highly active against *Aspergillus*, *Fusarium*, dematiaceous and dimorphic fungi, and *P. carinii*. Its in vitro activity against yeasts appears to be more variable.[141, 184, 312] Comparative studies have indicated that terbinafine may be more active against *Aspergillus* than itraconazole[336] or amphotericin B[330] is and that it is less or comparably active than the azoles against yeasts.[336] Of note, synergy with triazoles against *C. albicans*,[107, 388] *C. neoformans*,[107] *A. fumigatus*,[313]

TABLE 239–10 ■ MEDICAL MANAGEMENT OF SUPERFICIAL INFECTIONS BY DERMATOPHYTES

Fungal Disease	Management
Tinea capitis	Griseofulvin: micronized, 5 to 10 mg/kg bid; ultramicronized, 2.5–5 mg/kg bid, for a total of 6–8 wk Fluconazole, 6 mg/kg qd for 4 wk Itraconazole, 2.5 mg/kg bid for 4 wk* Terbinafine: <20 kg, 62.5 mg qd; 20–40 kg, 125 mg qd; >40 mg, 250 mg qd for 4 wk*
Tinea unguinum	Itraconazole, 2.5 mg/kg bid 1 wk per mo for 3-4 mo* Terbinafine: <20 kg, 62.5 mg qd; 20–40 kg, 125 mg qd; >40 kg, 250 mg qd for 6 wk (fingernail) or 12 wk (toenail)*
Tinea corporis Tinea facialis Tinea pedis	Topical antifungal azoles: Miconazole, clotrimazole, econazole, ketoconazole, sulconazole, oxiconazole, bid for 2–4 wk Topical allyl/benzylamines: thiocarbamates: Terbinafine, naftifine, butenafine, tolnaftate, qd/bid for 2–4 wk Other topical agents: Ciclopirox olamine, bid for 2–4 wk Refractory infections/immunocompromised patients: Griseofulvin: micronized 5–10 mg/kg bid, ultramicronized 2.5–5 mg/kg bid for 2–4 wk Fluconazole, 3–6 mg/kg qd for 2–4 wk Itraconazole, 2.5 mg/kg bid for 2–4 wk* Terbinafine, <20 kg, 62.5 mg qd; 20–40 kg, 125 mg qd; >40 kg, 250 mg qd for 2–4 wk*

*Not approved by the U.S. Food and Drug Administration in individuals of younger than 18 years.
Data from Friedlander, S. F., and Suarez, S.: Pediatric antifungal therapy. Dermatol. Clin. *16*:527–537, 1998; and Howard, R. M., and Frieden, I. J.: Dermatophyte infections in children. Adv. Pediatr. Infect. Dis. *14*:73–107, 1999.

and other hyalohyphomycetes[241, 312] has been reported. Though more variable, synergy with amphotericin B also has been demonstrated for filamentous and yeast-like fungi.[312]

PHARMACOKINETICS. The pharmacokinetics of terbinafine in adults is well characterized.[28] Independent of food, oral bioavailability is 70 to 80 percent. The adult dosage range of 125 to 750 mg once daily displays linear plasma pharmacokinetics. Peak plasma concentrations of 0.5 to 2.7 μg/mL are measured within 2 hours,[201] and steady state is reached in 10 to 14 days after only twofold accumulation.[28] As a lipophilic drug, terbinafine is strongly bound to plasma proteins. The compound is distributed extensively to tissues and accumulates throughout adipose tissue, dermis, epidermis, and nails. It exhibits a triphasic distribution pattern in plasma with a terminal half-life of up to 3 weeks; microbiologically active concentrations can be measured in plasma for weeks to months after the last dose, which is consistent with slow redistribution from peripheral tissue and adipose tissue sites.[28, 201, 256]

Terbinafine undergoes extensive and complex hepatic biotransformation that involves at least seven CYP450 enzymes.[371] Fifteen metabolites have been identified, mainly in urine; none of them has been shown to be mycologically active.[202] Studies using radiolabeled drug have demonstrated that urinary excretion accounts for more than 70 percent and fecal elimination for 10 percent of the radioactivity; the extent of enterohepatic recycling is yet unknown.[177, 178] As a consequence of the compound's extensive hepatic metabolism and urinary excretion, caution is warranted in patients with severe hepatic and renal impairment.[28]

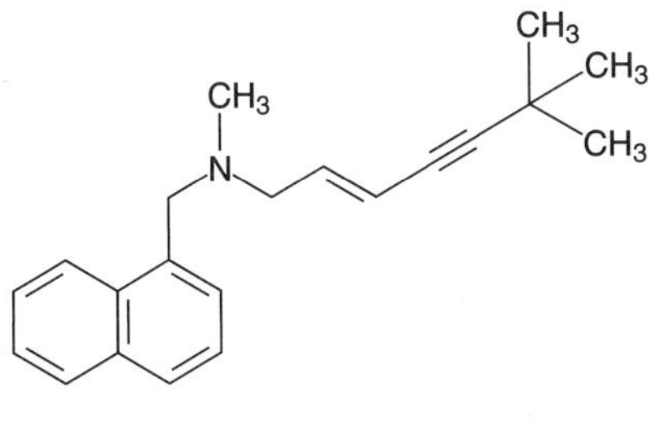

Terbinafine

FIGURE 239–12 ■ Structural formula of terbinafine.

Several studies have been conducted to evaluate the safety, pharmacokinetics, and antifungal efficacy in the pediatric population.[54, 178, 187, 203, 258]

The pharmacokinetics of terbinafine and five known major metabolites in plasma and urine have been investigated carefully after single and repeated oral administration of 125 mg/day to 12 pediatric patients for as long as 56 days (mean age, 8 years; age range, 5 to 11 years; weight range, 17 to 34 kg) (Table 239–11). No differences were found regarding the metabolism of terbinafine in comparison to healthy adults. Steady state was reached at least on day 21, and no further accumulation occurred between days 21 and 56.[177, 258] Comparison of the kinetic parameters of terbinafine after single administration of 125 mg showed comparable C_{max} and T_{max} values and a 40 percent higher AUC; when the dose was calculated as milligrams per kilogram or square meter, children had a lower AUC (range, –29 to –45%) than adults did as a result of a higher, weight-normalized Vd into lipophilic tissue. Children had shorter β-phase elimination half-lives, but the γ-phase terminal half-life determined after multiple dosing during washout was similar to that in adults. Thus, in children weighing 17 to 34 kg, a dose of 125 mg terbinafine yields pharmacokinetics similar to that in adults without drug accumulation, and the use of milligrams per kilogram or square meter would lead to lower drug levels than those recorded in adults.[178, 187, 258] Evaluation of lower doses (62.5 mg/day) in eight children weighing 19 to 35 kg revealed an approximate 50 percent reduction in drug levels, thus

TABLE 239–11 ■ PHARMACOKINETIC PARAMETERS OF TERBINAFINE IN CHILDREN AFTER A SINGLE DOSE OF 125 mg COMPARED WITH SIMILAR PARAMETERS IN HEALTHY ADULTS

	Children with Tinea Capitis (n = 12)	Healthy Adults (n = 16)	Statistical Comparison
Age (yr)	8 ± 2* (5–11)	26 ± 4 (21–34)	—
Weight (kg)	26 ± 5 (17–34)	64 ± 6 (54–80)	—
C_{max} (μg/mL)	0.706 ± 0.277 (0.333–1.212)	0.565 ± 0.329 (0.196–1.172)	NS
T_{max} (hr)	2.1 ±1.1 (1.0–4.0)	5 ± 0.7 (0.7–2.5)	NS
$AUC_{0\rightarrow\infty}$ (μg/mL·hr)	2.967 ± 0.965 (1.474–4.841)	2.135 ± 1.131 (0.758–4.435)	$p < .05$
$t_{1/2}\beta$ (hr)	14.7 ± 4.3 (10–26)	27 ± 12 (12–58)	$p < .001$

*Mean values ± SD (range).
$AUC_{0\rightarrow\infty}$, area under the concentration versus time curve from zero to infinity; C_{max}, peak plasma levels; $t_{1/2}\beta$, elimination half-life; T_{max}, time until occurrence of C_{max}.
Modified from Jones T. C.: Overview of the use of terbinafine (Lamisil) in children. Br. J. Dermatol. *132*:683–689, 1995.

demonstrating the linearity of plasma pharmacokinetics in children.[187]

Based on the experience with dosages of 10 mg/kg and less in adults and the described pharmacokinetic profile of the compound in children, a dose of 250 mg/day has been proposed for children weighing more than 40 kg, a dose of 125 mg/day for children weighing 20 to 40 kg, and 62.5 mg/day for children weighing less than 20 kg.[187]

ADVERSE EFFECTS. In adults, terbinafine is usually well tolerated at dosages of up to 500 mg/day and has a relatively low incidence of adverse effects. The primary adverse effects associated with terbinafine include gastrointestinal upset and skin reactions in 2 to 7 percent of patients. Terbinafine can cause hepatitis and liver failure. Potentially severe hepatotoxicity is estimated to occur in 1 in 120,000 patients, and asymptomatic rises in liver enzyme activity are likely to occur at a frequency of 1 in 200. Although hepatotoxicity may develop in patients with or without chronic or active liver disease, the drug should not be administered to patients with an underlying liver problem, and liver function tests should be obtained before prescribing terbinafine. Less common significant adverse effects have included reversible loss of taste, severe skin eruptions, Stevens-Johnson syndrome, and blood dyscrasias.[2] No evidence exists that these idiosyncratic effects are increasing in incidence with the increasing use of terbinafine.[271]

Several clinical studies have documented the safety of terbinafine in pediatric patients.[54, 60, 111, 187, 203, 258] Terbinafine administered for a median duration of 4 weeks (range, 1 to 28 weeks) was safe in children between 2 and 17 years of age who received the drug for various dermatophyte and yeast infections of the skin. Of a total of 196 patients enrolled in six studies, 22 adverse events were observed in 15 patients. Adverse events probably associated with the use of terbinafine occurred in six of these patients (3%), but terbinafine therapy was not discontinued in any of them.[187]

DRUG INTERACTIONS. Multiple CYP450 enzymes are involved in the metabolism of terbinafine. However, with the possible exception of CYP2D6 substrates, in vitro studies revealed little or no effect on the metabolism of many characteristic CYP substrates.[371] Inhibition of CYP2D6-mediated metabolism may be relevant with the concomitant use of tricyclic antidepressants, beta-blockers, selective serotonin reuptake inhibitors, and type B monoamine oxidase inhibitors.

In clinical interaction studies, no pharmacokinetic or pharmacodynamic interactions have been observed with the concomitant administration of terfenadine[305] and midazolam.[6] Terbinafine can reduce the clearance of theophylline,[355] increase levels of nortryptiline,[364] increase or reduce warfarin exposure,[152, 387] and reduce the trough cyclosporine concentration in transplant recipients.[222] The metabolism of terbinafine may be decreased by cimetidine and increased by rifampin.[141]

CLINICAL INDICATIONS. Terbinafine is indicated for the treatment of superficial infections of the skin and its appendages by dermatophytes[2, 28, 109] and possibly for cutaneous sporotrichosis[176] (see Tables 239–4 and 239–10). The recommended duration of treatment for tinea capitis, tinea corporis and pedis, fingernail onychomycosis, and toenail onychomycosis in adults is 4, 2, 6, and 12 weeks, respectively.[187] Several studies have demonstrated the safety and clinical efficacy of terbinafine in the pediatric population.[54, 60, 111, 187, 203, 258] The overall mycologic and clinical efficacy for 152 children between 2 and 17 years of age with various dermatophyte and yeast infections of the skin exceeded 95 percent.[187] In a prospective, randomized clinical trial in 210 children that compared treatment with 4 weeks of terbinafine versus 8 weeks of griseofulvin for tinea capitis, both regimens showed overall similar efficacy.[111]

Its broad-spectrum fungicidal in vitro activity, systemic availability, and lack of significant side effects have suggested potential usefulness of terbinafine against deep-seated fungal infections. However, terbinafine was ineffective against rodent models of pulmonary aspergillosis,[329] systemic sporotrichosis,[189] cerebral phaeohyphomycosis,[88] disseminated candidiasis, and pulmonary cryptococcosis,[314] which has been explained by nonsaturable protein-binding kinetics.[329] Nevertheless, terbinafine was as effective as trimethoprim-sulfamethoxazole in a rat model of pulmonary pneumocystosis,[72, 73] thus indicating that the compound may have therapeutic potential beyond fungal infections of the skin and its appendages.

Topical Antifungal Agents

Apart from fungal keratitis, the use of topical antifungal agents is confined to superficial infections of the skin and mucosal surfaces. The decision to treat superficial infections of the skin and mucosal surfaces with a topical or systemic agent depends mainly on the site and extent of the infection. Immunocompromised children, however, usually require systemic therapy, as do patients with tinea capitis and onychomycosis[96] (Table 239–12; see also Table 239–10).

TABLE 239–12 ■ MEDICAL MANAGEMENT OF SUPERFICIAL INFECTIONS BY YEAST-LIKE FUNGI

Fungal Disease	Management
Candida dermatitis Tinea versicolor	Topical antifungal azoles: Miconazole, sulconazole, econazole, oxiconazole, clotrimazole, bid for 2–4 wk Topical polyenes: Amphotericin B or nystatin, bid/qid for 2–4 wk Other topical agents: Ciclopirox olamine, bid for 2–4 wk Refractory infections/immunocompromised patients: Fluconazole, 3–6 mg/kg qd for 2–4 wk Itraconazole, 2.5 mg/kg bid for 2–4 wk*
Oropharyngeal candidiasis	Topical polyenes: Nystatin, 200–600,000 U, or amphotericin B, 100 mg four times daily for ≥2 wk Topical antifungal azoles: Clotrimazole lozenges, 10 mg five times daily for ≥2 wk Refractory infections/immunocompromised patients: Fluconazole, 3–6 mg/kg qd for ≥2 wk Itraconazole, 2.5 mg/kg bid for ≥2 wk Amphotericin B deoxycholate 0.5–1 mg/kg qd
Vulvovaginal candidiasis	Topical antifungal azoles: Miconazole, clotrimazole, butoconazole, terconazole, tioconazole, qhs for ≤7 days Topical polyenes: Nystatin, qhs for 14 days Systemic antifungal azoles: Fluconazole, 150 mg PO × 1 day/50 mg PO × 3 days, Refractory infections/immunocompromised patients: Fluconazole, 3–6 mg/kg qd for ≥2 wk Itraconazole, 2.5 mg/kg bid for ≥2 wk Amphotericin B deoxycholate, 0.5–1 mg/kg qd

*Not approved by the U.S. Food and Drug Administration for individuals younger than 18 years.
Data from Bennett, J. E.: Antifungal agents. *In* Mandell, G. L. Bennett, J. E. and Dolin, R. (eds).: Principles and Practice of Infections Diseases. 4th ed. New York, Churchill Livingstone, 1995, pp. 401–410; and Walsh, T. J., Gonzalez, C., Lyman, C. A., et al.: Invasive fungal infections in children: Recent advances in diagnosis and treatment. Adv. Pediatr. Infect. Dis. *11*:187–290, 1996.

TOPICAL THERAPEUTICS FOR SUPERFICIAL SKIN INFECTIONS

Dermatophytosis is caused by the filamentous fungi *Microsporon*, *Trichophyton*, and *Epidermophyton floccosum*. A large variety of agents and formulations, including allylamines and azoles, are available for topical treatment of dermatophytic skin infections (tinea corporis, facialis, or pedis). Agents for the treatment of *Candida* dermatitis and tinea (pityriasis) versicolor (caused by *Malassezia furfur* or *Malassezia pachydermatis*) include various topical azoles and topical polyenes. Most topical agents usually are applied twice daily well beyond clinical resolution of the infection. A detailed review of the pharmacologic properties of these topical drugs and the treatment of cutaneous mycoses is beyond the scope of this chapter and can be found elsewhere.[96, 110, 175]

TOPICAL THERAPEUTICS FOR MUCOSAL CANDIDIASIS

Agents for the topical treatment of vulvovaginal candidiasis include a large variety of antifungal azoles and the polyene nystatin.[33, 340] Of note, azole agents may be absorbed to a minor extent and potentially can interfere with the metabolism of concomitant drugs. For example, potentiation of the anticoagulatory effects of acenocoumarol was noted after vaginal administration of miconazole capsules to two postmenopausal patients[208] and after oral administration of miconazole gel to three elderly patients with oral candidiasis.[269]

Antifungal azoles such as clotrimazole and miconazole and antifungal polyenes such as amphotericin B and nystatin are effective in the treatment of oropharyngeal candidiasis. Many clinical trials have evaluated the usefulness of these agents for prevention of fungal infections in immunocompromised cancer or hematopoietic stem cell transplant patients. Although most agents have documented efficacy in the prevention of oropharyngeal candidiasis, they are not effective in preventing invasive mycoses and improving infection-related and overall mortality rates in this setting.[143, 172, 224, 361]

Future Directions

The past decade has seen considerable expansion in antifungal drug research and the clinical development of several new compounds targeted against invasive fungal infections. Knowledge of the pharmacokinetics of these compounds in pediatric patients is pivotal for their safe and effective use in this population. Developmental differences in a drug's distribution, metabolism, or excretion potentially can result in serious untoward effects or suboptimal therapeutic efficacy. For these reasons, simple extrapolation of adult dosages to pediatric patients is not generally feasible, and separate pharmacokinetic studies are required to establish the appropriate dosage regimens for further assessment of safety and efficacy.[194, 292] Although progress has been made during the past few years in retrospectively establishing pharmacokinetics and dosage regimens, not all of the currently available antifungal agents are yet approved for pediatric age groups. However, new regulatory requirements that request the early incorporation of pediatric studies in the clinical development of important new therapeutics before their approval in adult patients[293] offer hope to achieve access to safe and effective drug therapy and participation of children in therapeutic progress more rapidly than in the past.

REFERENCES

1. Aanpreung, P., and Veerakul, G.: Itraconazole for treatment of oral candidosis in pediatric cancer patients. J. Med. Assoc. Thai. *80*:358–362, 1997.
2. Abdel-Rahman, S. M., and Nahata, M. C.: Oral terbinafine: A new antifungal agent. Ann. Pharmacother. *31*:445–456, 1977.
3. Abdel-Rahman, S. M., Powell, D. A., and Nahata, M. C.: Efficacy of itraconazole in children with *Trichophyton tonsurans* tinea capitis. J. Am. Acad. Dermatol. *38*:443–446, 1998.
4. Adler-Shohet, F., Waskin, H., and Lieberman, J. M.: Amphotericin B lipid complex for neonatal invasive candidiasis. Arch. Dis. Child. Fetal Neonatal Ed. *84*:F131–F133, 2001.
5. Aguilar, C., Pujol, I., Sala, J., and Guarro, J.: Antifungal susceptibilities of *Paecilomyces* species. Antimicrob. Agents Chemother. *42*:1601–1604, 1998.
6. Ahonen, J., Olkkola, K. T., and Neuvonen, P. J.: Effect of itraconazole and terbinafine on the pharmacokinetics and pharmacodynamics of midazolam in healthy volunteers. Br. J. Clin. Pharmacol. *40*:270–272, 1995.
7. al Arishi, H., Frayha, H. H., Kalloghlian, A., and al Alaiyan, S.: Liposomal amphotericin B in neonates with invasive candidiasis. Am. J. Perinatol. *41*:573–576, 1998.
8. Amantea, M. A., Bowden, R. A., Forrest, A., et al.: Population pharmacokinetics and renal function-sparing effects of amphotericin B colloidal dispersion in patients receiving bone marrow transplants. Antimicrob. Agents Chemother. *39*:2042–2047, 1995.
9. American Academy of Pediatrics: Tinea capitis. *In* Peter, G. (ed.): 1997 Red Book: Report of the Committee on Infectious Diseases. 24th ed. Elk Grove Village, IL, American Academy of Pediatrics, 1997, pp. 523–525.
10. Anaissie, E., Bodey, G. P., Kantarjian, H., et al.: Fluconazole therapy for chronic disseminated candidiasis in patients with leukemia and prior amphotericin B therapy. Am. J. Med. *91*:142–150, 1991.
11. Anaissie, E. J., Darouiche, R. O., Abi-Said, D., et al.: Management of invasive candidal infections: Results of a prospective, randomized, multicenter study of fluconazole versus amphotericin B and review of the literature. Clin. Infect. Dis. *23*:964–972, 1996.
12. Anaissie, E., Gokoslan, A., Hachem, R., and Rubin, R.: Azole therapy for trichosporonosis: Clinical evaluation of eight patients, experimental therapy for murine infection, and review. Clin. Infect. Dis. *15*:781–787, 1992.
13. Anaissie, E. J., Karyotakis, N. C., Hachem, R., et al.: Correlation between in vitro and in vivo activity of antifungal agents against *Candida* species. J. Infect. Dis. *170*:384–389, 1994.
14. Anaissie, E. J., Kontoyiannis, D. P., Huls, C., et al.: Safety, plasma concentrations, and efficacy of high-dose fluconazole in invasive mold infections. J. Infect. Dis. *172*:599–602, 1995.
15. Anaissie, E. J., Vartivarian, S. E., Abi-Said, D., et al.: Fluconazole versus amphotericin B in the treatment of hematogenous candidiasis: A matched cohort study. Am. J. Med. *101*:170–176, 1996.
16. Anaissie, E., White, M., Uzun, O., et al.: Amphotericin B lipid complex (ABLC) versus amphotericin B (AMB) for treatment of hematogenous and invasive candidiasis: A prospective, randomized, multicenter trial. Abstract LM 21. *In* Abstracts of the 35th Interscience Conference on Antimicrobial Agents and Chemotherapy. Washington, D.C., American Society for Microbiology, 1995, p. 330.
17. Andes, D. R., Stamstad, T., and Conklin, R.: In vivo characterization of the pharmacodynamics of ravuconazole in a neutropenic murine disseminated candidiasis model. Abstract 840. *In* Abstracts of the 40th Interscience Conference on Antimicrobial Agents and Chemotherapy. Washington, D.C., American Society for Microbiology, 2000, p. 22.
18. Andes, D., Stamsted, T., and Conklin, R.: Pharmacodynamics of amphotericin B in a neutropenic-mouse disseminated-candidiasis model. Antimicrob. Agents Chemother. *45*:922–926, 2001.
19. Andes, D., and van Ogtrop, M.: Characterization and quantitation of the pharmacodynamics of fluconazole in a neutropenic murine disseminated candidiasis infection model. Antimicrob. Agents Chemother. *43*:2116–2120, 1999.
20. Andes, D., and van Ogtrop, M.: In vivo characterization of the pharmacodynamics of flucytosine in a neutropenic murine disseminated candidiasis model. Antimicrob. Agents Chemother. *44*:938–942, 2000.
21. Arning, M., Kliche, K. O., Heer-Sonderhoff, A. H., et al.: Infusion-related toxicity of three different amphotericin B formulations and its relation to cytokine plasma levels. Mycoses *38*:459–465, 1995.
22. Arning, M., and Scharf, R. E.: Prevention of amphotericin B induced nephrotoxicity by loading with sodium-chloride: A report of 1291 days of treatment with amphotericin B without renal failure. Klin. Wochenschr. *67*:1020–1028, 1989.
23. Artis, W. M., Odle, B. M., and Jones, H. E.: Griseofulvin-resistant dermatophytosis correlates with in vitro resistance. Arch. Dermatol. *117*:16–19, 1981.
24. Atkinson, A. J., Jr., and Bennett, J. E.: Amphotericin B pharmacokinetics in humans. Antimicrob. Agents Chemother. *13*:271–276, 1978.
25. Balani, S. K., Xu, X., Arison, B. H., et al.: Metabolites of caspofungin acetate, a potent antifungal agent, in human plasma and urine. Drug Metab. Dispos. *28*:1274–1278, 2000.
26. Baley, J. E., Kliegman, R. M., and Fanaroff, A. A.: Disseminated fungal infections in very low-weight infants: Therapeutic toxicity. Pediatrics *73*:153–157, 1984.
27. Baley, J. E., Meyers, C., Kliegman, R. M., et al.: Pharmacokinetics, outcome of treatment, and toxic effects of amphotericin B and 5-fluorocytosine in neonates. J. Pediatr. *116*:791–797, 1990.
28. Balfour, J. A., and Faulds, D.: Terbinafine. A review of its pharmacodynamic and pharmacokinetic properties, and therapeutic potential in superficial mycoses. Drugs *43*:259–284, 1992.
29. Barchiesi, F., Najvar, L. K., Luther, M. F., et al.: Variation in fluconazole efficacy for *Candida albicans* strains sequentially isolated from oral cavities of patients with AIDS in an experimental murine candidiasis model. Antimicrob. Agents Chemother. *40*:1317–1320, 1996.
30. Barone, J. A., Moskovitz, B. L., Guarnieri, J., et al.: Enhanced bioavailability of itraconazole in hydroxypropyl-beta-cyclodextrin solution versus capsules in healthy volunteers. Antimicrob. Agents Chemother. *42*:1862–1865, 1998.
31. Bartizal, K., Gill, C. J., Abruzzo, G. K., et al.: In vitro preclinical evaluation studies with the echinocandin antifungal MK-0991 (L-743,872). Antimicrob. Agents Chemother. 41:2326–2332, 1997.
32. Barton, E., Zinnes, H., Moe, R. A., and Kulesza, J. S.: Studies on a new solubilized preparation of amphotericin B. *In* Antibiotics Annual, 1957–1958. New York, Medical Encyclopedia, 1958, pp. 53–57.
33. Bennett, J. E.: Antifungal agents. *In* Mandell, G. L., Bennett, J. E., Dolin, R. (eds.): Principles and Practice of Infectious Diseases. 4th ed. New York, Churchill Livingstone, 1995, pp. 401–410.
34. Bennett, J. E., Dismukes, W. E., Haywood, M., et al.: A comparison of amphotericin B alone and in combination with flucytosine in the treatment of cryptococcal meningitis. N. Engl. J. Med. *301*:126–131, 1979.
35. Benson, J. M., and Nahata, M. C.: Pharmacokinetics of amphotericin B in children. Antimicrob. Agents Chemother. *33*:1989–1993, 1989.
36. Berenguer, J., Ali, N. M., Allende, M. C., et al.: Itraconazole for experimental pulmonary aspergillosis: Comparison with amphotericin B, interaction with cyclosporin A, and correlation between therapeutic response and itraconazole concentrations in plasma. Antimicrob. Agents Chemother. *38*:1303–1308, 1994.
37. Berenguer, J., Rodriguez-Tudela, J. L., Richard, C., et al.: Deep infections caused by *Scedosporium prolificans*. A report on 16 cases in Spain and a review of the literature. *Scedosporium Prolificans* Spanish Study Group. Medicine (Baltimore) *76*:256–265, 1997.
38. Berl, T., Wilner, K. D., Gardner, M., et al.: Pharmacokinetics of fluconazole in renal failure. J. Am. Soc. Nephrol. *6*:242–247, 1995.
39. Bilgen, H., Ozek, E., Korten, V., et al.: Treatment of systemic neonatal candidiasis with fluconazole. Infection *23*:394, 1995.
40. Block, E. R., and Bennett, J. E.: Pharmacological studies with 5-fluorocytosine. Antimicrob. Agents Chemother. *1*:476–482, 1992.
41. Block, E. R., Jennings, A. E., and Bennet, J. E.: Experimental therapy of cladosporiosis and sporotrichosis with 5-fluorocytosine. Antimicrob. Agents Chemother. *3*:95–98, 1973.
42. Blumer, J. L.: Pharmacologic basis for the treatment of tinea capitis. Pediatr. Infect. Dis. J. *18*:191–199, 1999.
43. Bohme, A., Ganser, A., and Hoelzer, D.: Aggravation of vincristine-induced neurotoxicity by itraconazole in the treatment of adult ALL. Ann. Hematol. *71*:311–312, 1995.
44. Boogaerts, M., Garber, G., Winston, D., et al.: Itraconazole compared with amphotericin B as empirical therapy for persistent fever of unknown origin in neutropenic patients. Bone Marrow Transplant. *23*(Suppl. 1): 111, 1999.
45. Boogaerts, M., Michaux, J. L., Bosly, A., et al.: Pharmacokinetics and safety of seven days intravenous itraconazole followed by two weeks oral itraconazole solution in patients with hematological malignancies. Abstract A87. *In* Program and Abstracts of the 36th Interscience Conference on Antimicrobial Agents and Chemotherapy. Washington, D.C., American Society for Microbiology, 1996, p. 17.
46. Boogaerts, M. A., Verhoef, G. E., Zachee, P., et al: Antifungal prophylaxis with itraconazole in prolonged neutropenia: Correlation with plasma levels. Mycoses *32*(Suppl. 1):103–108, 1989.
47. Botas, C. M., Kurlat, I., Young, S. M., and Sola, A.: Disseminated candidal infections and intravenous hydrocortisone in preterm infants. Pediatrics *95*:883–887, 1995.
48. Boutati, E. I., and Anaissie, E. J.: *Fusarium*, a significant emerging pathogen in patients with hematologic malignancy: Ten years' experience at a cancer center and implications for management. Blood *90*:999–1008, 1997.
49. Boutati, E., Maltezou, H. C., Lopez-Berestein, G., et al.: Phase I study of maximum tolerated dose of intravenous liposomal nystatin for the treatment of refractory febrile neutropenia in patients with hematological malignancies. Abstract LM22. *In* Program and Abstracts of the 35th Interscience Conference on Antimicrobial Agents and Chemotherapy. Washington, D.C., American Society for Microbiology, 1995, p. 330.
50. Brajtburg, J., Powderly, W. G., Kobayashi, G. S., and Medoff, G.: Amphotericin B: Current understanding of mechanisms of action. Antimicrob. Agents Chemother. *34*:183–188, 1990.
51. Brammer, K. W., and Coates, P. E.: Pharmacokinetics of fluconazole in pediatric patients. Eur. J. Clin. Microbiol. Infect. Dis. *13*:325–329, 1994.
52. Brammer, K. W., Farrow, P. R., and Faulkner, J. K.: Pharmacokinetics and tissue penetration of fluconazole in humans. Rev. Infect. Dis. *12*(Suppl. 3):318–326, 1990.

53. Brown, G. L., White, R. J., and Turik, M.: Phase II, randomized, open label study of two intravenous dosing regimens of V-echinocandin in the treatment of esophageal candidiasis. Abstract 1106. *In* Abstracts of the 40th Interscience Conference on Antimicrobial Agents and Chemotherapy. Washington, D.C., American Society for Microbiology, 2000, p. 371.
54. Bruckbauer, H. R., and Hofmann, H.: Systemic antifungal treatment of children with terbinafine. Dermatology *195*:134–136, 1997.
55. Burch, P. A., Karp, J. E., Merz, W. G., et al.: Favorable outcome of invasive aspergillosis in patients with acute leukemia. J. Clin. Oncol. *5*:1985–1993, 1987.
56. Burgess, D. S., and Hastings, R. W.: A comparison of dynamic characteristics of fluconazole, itraconazole, and amphotericin B against *Cryptococcus neoformans* using time-kill methodology. Diagn. Microbiol. Infect. Dis. *38*:87–93, 2000.
57. Burgess, D. S., Hastings, R. W., Summers, K. K., et al.: Pharmacodynamics of fluconazole, itraconazole, and amphotericin B against *Candida albicans*. Diagn. Microbiol. Infect. Dis. *36*:13–18, 2000.
58. Butler, K. M., Rench, M. A., and Baker, C. J.: Amphotericin B as a single agent in the treatment of systemic candidiasis in neonates. Pediatr. Infect. Dis. J. *9*:51–56, 1990.
59. Butler, W. T., Bennett, J. E., Alling, D. W., et al.: Nephrotoxicity of amphotericin B: Early and late effects in 81 patients. Ann. Intern. Med. *62*:175–187, 1964.
60. Caceres-Rios, H., Rueda, M., Ballona, R., and Bustamante, B.: Comparison of terbinafine and griseofulvin in the treatment of tinea capitis. J. Am. Acad. Dermatol. *42*:80–84, 2000.
61. Caillot, D., Bassaris, H., Seifert, W. F., et al.: Efficacy, safety, and pharmacokinetics of intravenous followed by oral itraconazole in patients with invasive pulmonary aspergillosis. Abstract 1646. *In* Abstracts of the 39th International Conference on Antimicrobial Agents and Chemotherapy. Washington, D.C., American Society for Microbiology, 1999, p. 575.
62. Carrillo-Munoz, A. J., Quindos, G., Tur, C., et al.: In vitro antifungal activity of liposomal nystatin in comparison with nystatin, amphotericin B cholesteryl sulphate, liposomal amphotericin B, amphotericin B lipid complex, amphotericin B deoxycholate, fluconazole and itraconazole. J. Antimicrob. Chemother. *44*:397–401, 1999.
63. Cartwright, R. Y.: Use of antibiotics: Antifungals. B. M. J. *2*:101–111, 1978.
64. Catanzaro, A., Galgiani, J. N., Levine, B. E., et al.: Fluconazole in the treatment of chronic pulmonary and non-meningeal disseminated coccidioidomycosis. Am. J. Med. *98*:249–256, 1995.
65. Chan-Tack, K. M., Thio, C. L., Miller, N. S., et al.: *Paecilomyces lilacinus* fungemia in an adult bone marrow transplant recipient. Med. Mycol. *37*:57–60, 1999.
66. Chapman, S. W., Bradsher, R. W., Jr., Campbell, G. D., Jr., et al.: Practice guidelines for the management of patients with blastomycosis. Infectious Diseases Society of America. Clin. Infect. Dis. *30*:679–683, 2000.
67. Chiou, C. C., Groll, A. H., and Walsh, T. J.: New drugs and novel targets for treatment of invasive fungal infections in patients with cancer. Oncologist *5*:120–135, 2000.
68. Christiansen, K. J., Bernard, E. M., Gold, J. W. M., and Armstrong, D.: Distribution and activity of amphotericin B in humans. J. Infect. Dis. *152*:1037–1043, 1985.
69. Clancy, C. J., and Nguyen, M. H.: In vitro efficacy and fungicidal activity of voriconazole against *Aspergillus* and *Fusarium* species. Eur. J. Clin. Microbiol. Infect. Dis. *17*:573–575, 1998.
70. Clemons, K. V., and Stevens, D. A.: Comparison of Fungizone, Amphotec, AmBisome, and Abelcet for treatment of systemic murine cryptococcosis. Antimicrob. Agents Chemother. *42*:899–902, 1998.
71. Como, J. A., and Dismukes, W. E.: Oral azole drugs as systemic antifungal therapy. N. Engl. J. Med. *330*:263–272, 1994.
72. Contini, C., Colombo, D., Cultrera, R., et al.: Employment of terbinafine against *Pneumocystis carinii* infection in rat models. Br. J. Dermatol. *134*(Suppl. 46):30–32, 1996.
73. Contini, C., Manganaro, M., Romani, R., et al.: Activity of terbinafine against *Pneumocystis carinii* in vitro and its efficacy in the treatment of experimental pneumonia. J. Antimicrob. Chemother. *34*:727–735, 1994.
74. Cossum, P. A., Wyse, J., Simmons, Y., et al.: Pharmacokinetics of Nyotran (liposomal nystatin) in human patients. Abstract A88. *In* Program and Abstracts of the 36th Interscience Conference on Antimicrobial Agents and Chemotherapy. Washington, D.C., American Society for Microbiology, 1996, p. 17.
75. Craven, P. C., Ludden, T. M., Drutz, D. J., et al.: Excretion pathways of amphotericin B. J. Infect. Dis. *140*:329–341, 1979.
76. Daneshmend, T. K., and Warnock, D. W.: Clinical pharmacokinetics of systemic antifungal drugs. Clin. Pharmacokinet. *8*:17–42, 1983.
77. De Beule, K.: Itraconazole: Pharmacology, clinical experience and future development. Int. J. Antimicrob. Agents *6*:175–181, 1996.
78. De Beule, K., and Van Gestel, J.: Pharmacology of itraconazole. Drugs *61*(Suppl. 1):27–37, 2001.
79. Debono, M., and Gordee, R. S.: Antibiotics that inhibit fungal cell wall development. Annu. Rev. Microbiol. *48*:471–497, 1994.
80. Denning, D. W., del Favero, A., Gluckman, E., et al.: UK 109946, a novel wide spectrum triazole derivative for the treatment of fungal infections: Clinical efficacy in acute invasive aspergillosis. Abstract F80. *In* Abstracts of the 35th International Conference on Antimicrobial Agents and Chemotherapy. Washington, D.C., American Society for Microbiology, 1995, p. 126.
81. Denning, D. W., Radford, S. A., Oakley, K. L., et al.: Correlation between in vitro susceptibility testing to itraconazole and in vivo outcome of *Aspergillus fumigatus* infection. J. Antimicrob. Chemother. *40*:401–414, 1997.
82. Denning, D. W., and Stevens, D. A.: Antifungal and surgical treatment of invasive aspergillosis: Review of 2,121 published cases. Rev. Infect. Dis. *12*:1147–1201, 1992.
83. Denning, D. W., Tucker, R. M., Hanson, L. H., and Stevens, D. A.: Treatment of invasive aspergillosis with itraconazole. Am. J. Med. *86*:791–800, 1989.
84. Denning, D. W., and Warn, P.: Dose range evaluation of liposomal nystatin and comparisons with amphotericin B and amphotericin B lipid complex in temporarily neutropenic mice infected with an isolate of *Aspergillus fumigatus* with reduced susceptibility to amphotericin B. Antimicrob. Agents Chemother. *43*:2592–2599, 1999.
85. de Repentigny, L., Ratelle, J., Leclerc, J. M., et al.: Repeated-dose pharmacokinetics of an oral solution of itraconazole in infants and children. Antimicrob. Agents Chemother. *42*:404–408, 1998.
86. Diaz, M., Negroni, R., Montero-Gei, F., et al.: A Pan-American 5-year study of fluconazole therapy for deep mycoses in the immunocompetent host. Pan-American Study Group. Clin. Infect. Dis. *14*(Suppl. 1):68–76, 1992.
87. Dismukes, W. E., Bradsher, R. W., Cloud, G. C., et al.: Itraconazole therapy for blastomycosis and histoplasmosis. Am. J. Med. *93*:489–497, 1992.
88. Dixon, D. M., and Polak, A.: In vitro and in vivo drug studies with three agents of central nervous system phaeohyphomycosis. Chemotherapy *33*:129–140, 1987.
89. Douglas, C. M., Bowman, J. C., Abruzzo, G. K., et al.: The glucan synthesis inhibitor caspofungin acetate (Cancidas, MK-0991, L-743872) kills *Aspergillus fumigatus* hyphal tips in vitro and is efficacious against disseminated aspergillosis in cyclophosphamide induced chronically leukopenic mice. Abstract 1683. *In* Program and Abstracts of the 40th Interscience Conference on Antimicrobial Agents and Chemotherapy. Washington, D.C., American Society for Microbiology, 2000, p. 387.
90. Drew, R. H., and Perfect, J. R.: Flucytosine. *In* Yu, V. L., Merigan, T. C., and Barriere S. (eds.): Antimicrobial Chemotherapy and Vaccines. Baltimore, Williams & Wilkins, 1998, pp. 1170–1184.
91. Driessen, M., Ellis, J. B., Cooper, P. A., et al.: Fluconazole vs. amphotericin B for the treatment of neonatal fungal septicemia: A prospective randomized trial. Pediatr. Infect. Dis. J. *15*:1107–1112, 1996.
92. Driessen, M., Ellis, J. B., Muwazi, F., and De Villiers, F. P.: The treatment of systemic candidiasis in neonates with oral fluconazole. Ann. Trop. Paediatr. *7*:263–271, 1997.
93. Drutz, D. J., Spickard, A., Rogers, D. E., and Koenig, M. G.: Treatment of disseminated mycotic infections. A new approach to amphotericin B therapy. Am. J. Med. *45*:405–418, 1968.
94. Dupont, B., Ally, R., Burke, J., et al.: A double-blind, randomized, multicenter trial of voriconazole vs. fluconazole in the treatment of esophageal candidiasis in immunocompromised adults. Abstract 706. *In* Abstracts of the 40th Interscience Conference on Antimicrobial Agents and Chemotherapy. Washington, D.C., American Society for Microbiology, 2000, p. 365.
95. Dupont, B., Denning, D., Lode, H., et al.: UK-109,496, a novel, wide-spectrum triazole derivative for the treatment of fungal infections: Clinical efficacy in chronic invasive aspergillosis. Abstract F81. *In* Program and Abstracts of the 35th Interscience Conference on Antimicrobial Agents and Chemotherapy. Washington, D.C., American Society for Microbiology, 1995, p. 126.
96. Elewski, B. E.: Cutaneous mycoses in children. Br. J. Dermatol. *134*(Suppl. 46):7–11, 1996.
97. Ellepola, A. N., and Samaranayake, L. P.: The in vitro post-antifungal effect of nystatin on *Candida* species of oral origin. J. Oral. Pathol. Med. *28*:112–116, 1999.
98. EORTC International Antimicrobial Therapy Cooperative Group: Empiric antifungal therapy in febrile granulocytopenic patients. Am. J. Med. *86*:668–672, 1986.
99. Epstein, W. L., Shah, V. P., and Riegelman, S.: Griseofulvin levels in stratum corneum. Study after oral administration in man. Arch. Dermatol. *106*:344–348, 1992.
100. Ernst, E. J., Klepser, M. E., Ernst, M. E., et al.: In vitro pharmacodynamic properties of MK-0991 determined by time-kill methods. Diagn. Microbiol. Infect. Dis. *33*:75–80, 1999.
101. Ernst, E. J., Klepser, M. E., and Pfaller, M. A.: Postantifungal effects of echinocandin, azole, and polyene antifungal agents *Candida albicans* and *Cryptococcus neoformans*. Antimicrob. Agents. Chemother. *44*:1108–1111, 2000.
102. Ernst, M. E., Klepser, M. E., Wolfe, E. J., and Pfaller, M. A.: Antifungal dynamics of LY 303366, an investigational echinocandin B analog, against *Candida* ssp. Diagn. Microbiol. Infect. Dis. *26*:125–131, 1996.
103. Espinel-Ingroff, A.: Comparison of in vitro activities of the new triazole SCH56592 and the echinocandins MK-0991 (L-743,872) and LY303366 against opportunistic filamentous and dimorphic fungi and yeasts. J. Clin. Microbiol. *36*:2950–2956, 1998.

104. Fasano, C., O'Keeffe, J., and Gibbs, D.: Fluconazole treatment of neonates and infants with severe fungal infections not treatable with conventional agents. Eur. J. Clin. Microbiol. Infect. Dis. *13*:351–354, 1994.
105. Flynn, P. M., Cunningham, C. K., Kerkering, T., et al.: Oropharyngeal candidiasis in immunocompromised children: A randomized, multicenter study of orally administered fluconazole suspension versus nystatin. J. Pediatr. *127*:322–328, 1995.
106. Foot, A., Veys, P., and Gibson, B.: Itraconazole oral solution as antifungal prophylaxis in children undergoing stem cell transplantation or intensive chemotherapy for haematological disorders. Bone Marrow Transplant. *24*:1089–1093, 1999.
107. Fothergill, A. W., Leitner, I., Meingassner, J. G., et al.: Combination antifungal susceptibility testing of terbinafine and the triazoles fluconazole and itraconazole. Abstract E53. *In* Abstracts of the 36th Interscience Conference on Antimicrobial Agents and Chemotherapy. Washington, D.C., American Society for Microbiology, 1996, p. 91.
108. Francis, P., and Walsh, T. J.: Evolving role of flucytosine in immunocompromised patients: New insights into safety, pharmacokinetics, and antifungal therapy. Clin. Infect. Dis. *15*:1003–1018, 1992.
109. Friedlander, S. F.: The evolving role of itraconazole, fluconazole and terbinafine in the treatment of tinea capitis. Pediatr. Infect. Dis. J. *18*:205–210, 1999.
110. Friedlander, S. F., and Suarez, S.: Pediatric antifungal therapy. Dermatol. Clin. *16*:527–537, 1998.
111. Fuller, L. C., Smith, C. H., Cerio, R., et al.: A randomized comparison of 4 weeks of terbinafine vs. 8 weeks of griseofulvin for the treatment of tinea capitis. Br. J. Dermatol. *144*:321–327, 2001.
112. Fung-Tomc, J. C., Huczko, E., Minassian, B., and Bonner, D. P.: In vitro activity of a new oral triazole, BMS-207147 (ER-30346). Antimicrob. Agents Chemother. *42*:313–318, 1998.
113. Galgiani, J. N., Ampel, N. M., Catanzaro, A., et al.: Practice guideline for the treatment of coccidioidomycosis. Infectious Diseases Society of America. Clin. Infect. Dis. *30*:658–661, 2000.
114. Galgiani, J. N., Catanzaro, A., Cloud, G. A., et al.: Fluconazole therapy for coccidioidal meningitis. Ann. Intern. Med. *119*:28–35, 1993.
115. Galgiani, J. N., Catanzaro, A., Cloud, G. A., et al.: Comparison of oral fluconazole and itraconazole for progressive, nonmeningeal coccidioidomycosis. A randomized, double-blind trial. Mycoses Study Group. Ann. Intern. Med. *133*:676–686, 2000.
116. Gehrt, A., Peter, J., Pizzo, P. A., and Walsh, T. J.: Effect of increasing inoculum sizes of pathogenic filamentous fungi on MICs of antifungal agents by broth microdilution method. J. Clin. Microbiol. *33*:1302–1307, 1995.
117. Gentles, J. C.: Experimental ringworm in guinea pigs: Oral treatment with griseofulvin. Nature *182*:476–477, 1958.
118. Georgopapadakou, N. H.: Update on antifungals targeted to the cell wall: Focus on beta-1,3-glucan synthase inhibitors. Expert Opin. Investig. Drugs *10*:269–280, 2001.
119. Glasmacher, A., Hahn, C., Molitor, E., et al.: Itraconazole through concentrations in antifungal prophylaxis with six different dosing regimens using hydroxypropyl-beta-cyclodextrin oral solution or coated-pellet capsules. Mycoses *42*:591–600, 1999.
120. Glasmacher, A., Hahn, C., Molitor, E., et al.: Definition of itraconazole target concentration for antifungal prophylaxis. Abstract 700. *In* Abstracts of the 40th Interscience Conference on Antimicrobial Agents and Chemotherapy. Washington, D.C., American Society for Microbiology, 2000, p. 363.
121. Glick, C., Graves, G. R., and Feldman, S.: Neonatal fungemia and amphotericin B. South. Med. J. *86*:1368–1371, 1993.
122. Goa, K. L., and Barradell, L. B.: Fluconazole. An update of its pharmacodynamic and pharmacokinetic properties and therapeutic use in major superficial and systemic mycoses in immunocompromised patients. Drugs *50*:658–690, 1995.
123. Gold, W., Stout, H. A., Pagona, I. F., and Donovick, R.: Amphotericins A and B, antifungal antibiotics produced by a streptomycete. I. In vitro studies. *In* Antibiotics Annual, 1955–1956. New York, Medical Encyclopedia, 1955, pp. 579–586.
124. Goldman, M., Cloud, G. A., Smedema, M., et al.: Does long-term itraconazole prophylaxis result in in vitro azole resistance in mucosal *Candida albicans* isolates from persons with advanced human immunodeficiency virus infection? Antimicrob. Agents Chemother. *44*:1585–1587, 2000.
125. Goodman, J. L., Winston, D. J., Greenfield, R. A., et al.: A controlled trial of fluconazole to prevent fungal infections in patients undergoing bone marrow transplantation. N. Engl. J. Med. *326*:845–851, 1992.
126. Googe, J. H., and Walterspiel, J. N.: Arrhythmia caused by amphotericin B in a neonate. Pediatr. Infect. Dis. J. 7:73, 1988.
127. Grant, S. M., and Clissold, S. P.: Itraconazole: A review of its pharmacodynamic and pharmacokinetic properties, and therapeutic use in superficial and systemic mycoses. Drugs *37*:310–344, 1989.
128. Grant, S. M., and Clissold, S. P.: Fluconazole: A review of its pharmacodynamic and pharmacokinetic properties, and therapeutic potential in superficial and systemic mycoses. Drugs *39*:877–916, 1990.
129. Graybill, J. R., Stevens, D. A., Galgiani, J. N., et al.: Itraconazole treatment of coccidioidomycosis. Am. J. Med. *89*:282–290, 1990.
130. Groll, A., Nowak-Goettl, U., Wildfeuer, A., et al.: Fluconazole treatment of oropharyngeal candidosis in pediatric cancer patients with severe mucositis following antineoplastic chemotherapy. Mycoses *35*(Suppl.): 35–40, 1992.
131. Groll, A. H., Chiou, C. C., and Walsh, T. J.: Antifungal drugs: Drug interactions with antifungal azole derivatives. *In* Aronson, J. K., and van Boxtel, C. J. (eds.): Side Effects of Drugs. Annual 24. Amsterdam, Elsevier Science. In press.
132. Groll, A. H., Giri, N., Petraitis, V., et al.: Comparative central nervous system distribution and antifungal activity of lipid formulations of amphotericin B in rabbits. J. Infect. Dis. *182*:274–282, 2000.
133. Groll, A. H., Gonzalez, C. E., Giri, N., et al.: Liposomal nystatin against experimental pulmonary aspergillosis in persistently neutropenic rabbits: Efficacy, safety and non-compartmental pharmacokinetics. J. Antimicrob. Chemother. *43*:95–103, 1999.
134. Groll, A. H., Just-Nuebling, G., Kurz, M., et al.: Fluconazole versus nystatin in the prevention of *Candida* infections in children and adolescents undergoing remission induction or consolidation chemotherapy for cancer. J. Antimicrob. Chemother. *40*:855–862, 1997.
135. Groll, A. H., Mickiene, D., McEvoy, M., et al.: Pharmacokinetics and pharmacodynamics of cyclodextrin itraconazole in pediatric patients with HIV infection and oropharyngeal candidiasis. Abstract 1647. *In* Abstracts of the 39th Interscience Conference on Antimicrobial Agents and Chemotherapy. Washington, D.C., American Society for Microbiology, 1999, p. 575.
136. Groll, A. H., Mickiene, D., Petraitiene, R., et al.: Disposition and pharmacokinetic/pharmacodynamic relationships of the echinocandin LY303366 in a neutropenic animal model of disseminated candidiasis. Abstract 2001. *In* Abstracts of the 39th Interscience Conference on Antimicrobial Agents and Chemotherapy. Washington, D.C., American Society for Microbiology, 1999.
137. Groll, A. H., Mickiene, D., Petraitiene, R., et al.: Pharmacokinetics and pharmacodynamics of posaconazole (SCH 56592) in a neutropenic animal model of invasive pulmonary aspergillosis. Abstract 1675. *In* Abstracts of the 40th Interscience Conference on Antimicrobial Agents and Chemotherapy. Washington, D.C., American Society for Microbiology, 2000, p. 385.
138. Groll, A. H., Mickiene, D., Werner, K., et al.: Compartmental pharmacokinetics and tissue distribution of multilamellar liposomal nystatin in rabbits. Antimicrob. Agents Chemother. *44*:950–957, 2000.
139. Groll, A. H., Muller, F. M., Piscitelli, S. C., and Walsh, T. J.: Lipid formulations of amphotericin B: Clinical perspectives for the management of invasive fungal infections in children with cancer. Klin. Padiatr. *210*:264–273, 1998.
140. Groll, A. H., Petraitis, V., Petraitiene, R., et al.: Safety and efficacy of multilamellar liposomal nystatin against disseminated candidiasis in persistently neutropenic rabbits. Antimicrob. Agents Chemother. *43*:2463–2467, 1999.
141. Groll, A. H., Piscitelli, S. C., and Walsh, T. J.: Clinical pharmacology of systemic antifungal agents: A comprehensive review of agents in clinical use, current investigational compounds, and putative targets for antifungal drug development. Adv. Pharmacol. *44*:343–500, 1998.
142. Groll, A. H., Piscitelli, S. C., and Walsh, T. J.: Antifungal pharmacodynamics. Concentration-effect relationships in vitro and in vivo. Pharmacotherapy *21*(Suppl. 8):133–148, 2001.
143. Groll, A. H., Ritter, J., and Mueller, F. M. C.: [Prevention of fungal infections in children and adolescents with cancer.] Klin. Paediatr. *213*(Suppl. 1):A50–A68, 2001.
144. Groll, A. H., and Walsh, T. J.: Antifungal triazoles. *In* Yu, V. L., Merigan, T. C., and Barriere, S. (eds.): Antimicrobial Chemotherapy and Vaccines. Baltimore, Williams & Wilkins, 1998, pp. 1158–1170.
145. Groll, A. H., and Walsh, T. J.: FK-463. Curr. Opin. Antiinfect. Investig. Drugs *2*:405–412, 2000.
146. Groll, A. H., and Walsh, T. J.: Uncommon opportunistic fungi: New nosocomial threats. Clin. Microbiol. Infect. 7(Suppl. 2):8–24, 2001.
147. Groll, A. H., and Walsh, T. J.: Caspofungin: Pharmacology, safety, and therapeutic potential in superficial and invasive fungal infections. Expert Opin. Investig. Drugs *10*:1545–1558, 2001.
148. Gubbins, P. O., McConnell, S. A., and Penzak, S. R.: Antifungal agents. *In* Piscitelli, S. C., Rodvold, K. A. (eds.): Drug Interactions in Infectious Diseases. Totowa, NJ, Humana Press, 2001, pp. 185–217.
149. Gull, K., and Trinci, A. P.: Griseofulvin inhibits fungal mitosis. Nature *244*:292–294, 1973.
150. Gunderson, S. M., Hoffman, H., Ernst, E. J., et al.: In vitro pharmacodynamic characteristics of nystatin including time-kill and postantifungal effect. Antimicrob. Agents Chemother. *44*:2887–2890, 2000.
151. Gupta, A. K., Nolting, S., de Prost, Y., et al.: The use of itraconazole to treat cutaneous fungal infections in children. Dermatology *199*:248–252, 1999.
152. Gupta, A. K., and Ross, G. S.: Interaction between terbinafine and warfarin. Dermatology *196*:266–267, 1998.
153. Gupta, A. K., Sauder, D. N., and Shear, N. H.: Antifungal agents: An overview. J. Am. Acad. Dermatol. *30*:677–698, 911–933, 1994.
154. Hachem, R. Y., Raad, I. I., Afif, C. M., et al.: An open, non-comparative multicenter study to evaluate efficacy and safety of posaconazole

(SCH 56592) in the treatment of invasive fungal infections refractory to or intolerant to standard therapy. Abstract 1109. *In* Abstracts of the 40th International Conference on Antimicrobial Agents and Chemotherapy. American Society for Microbiology, Washington, D.C., 2000, p. 372.

155. Hamill, R. J., Thomas, C. J., and Dismukes, W. E.: Fluconazole therapy for histoplasmosis. The National Institute of Allergy and Infectious Diseases Mycoses Study Group. Clin. Infect. Dis. *23*:996–1001, 1996.
156. Hamilton, J. D., and Elliott, D. M.: Combined activity of amphotericin B and 5-fluorocytosine against *Cryptococcus neoformans* in vitro and in vivo in mice. J. Infect. Dis. *131*:129–137, 1975.
157. Hardin, T. C., Graybill, J. R., Fetchick, R., et al.: Pharmacokinetics of itraconazole following oral administration to normal volunteers. Antimicrob. Agents Chemother. *32*:1310–1313, 1988.
158. Harris, B. E., Manning, B. W., and Federle, T. W.: Conversion of 5-fluorocytosine to 5-fluorouracil by human intestinal microflora. Antimicrob. Agents Chemother. *29*:44–48, 1986.
159. Hawser, S.: LY-303366. Curr. Opin. Antiinfect. Investig. Drugs *1*:353–360, 1999.
160. Hazen, E. L., and Brown, R.: Two antifungal agents produced by a soil actinomycete. Science *112*:423, 1950.
161. Hector, R. F.: Compounds active against cell walls of medically important fungi. Clin. Microbiol. Rev. *6*:1–21, 1993.
162. Hegener, P., Troke, P. F., Fakenheuer, G., et al.: Treatment of fluconazole-resistant candidiasis with voriconazole in patients with AIDS. A. I. D. S. *12*:2227–2228, 1998.
163. Heidemann, H. T., Gerkens, J. F., Spickard, W. A., et al.: Amphotericin B nephrotoxicity in humans decreased by salt repletion. Am. J. Med. *75*:476–481, 1983.
164. Herbrecht, R.: Safety of amphotericin B colloidal dispersion. Eur. J. Clin. Microbiol. Infect. Dis. *16*:74–80, 1997.
165. Herbrecht, R., Auvrignon, A., Andres, E., et al.: Efficacy of amphotericin B lipid complex in the treatment of invasive fungal infections in immunosuppressed paediatric patients. Eur. J. Clin. Microbiol. Infect. Dis. *20*:77–82, 2001.
166. Hernandez-Sempelayo, T.: Fluconazole vs. ketoconazole in the treatment of oropharyngeal candidiasis in HIV-infected children. Eur. J. Clin. Microbiol. Infect. Dis. *13*:340–344, 1994.
167. Heykants, J., Michiels, M., Meuldermans, W., et al.: The pharmacokinetics of itraconazole in animals and man: An overview. *In* Fromtling, R. A. (ed.): Recent Trends in the Discovery, Development and Evaluation of Antifungal Agents. Barcelona, Spain, J. R. Prous, 1987, pp. 223–249.
168. Hiemenz, J. W., and Walsh, T. J.: Lipid formulations of amphotericin B: Recent progress and future directions. Clin. Infect. Dis. *22*(Suppl. 2):133–144, 1996.
169. Hoban, D. J., Zhanel, G. G., and Karlowsky, J. A.: In vitro susceptibilities of *Candida* and *Cryptococcus neoformans* isolates from blood cultures of neutropenic patients. Antimicrob. Agents Chemother. *43*:1463–1464, 1999.
170. Hoffman, H. L., Ernst, E. J., and Klepser, M. E.: Novel triazole antifungal agents. Expert Opin. Investig. Drugs *9*:593–605, 2000.
171. Honig, P. K., Wortham, D. C., Hull, R., et al.: Itraconazole affects single-dose terfenadine pharmacokinetics and cardiac repolarization pharmacodynamics. J. Clin. Pharmacol. *33*:1201–1206, 1993.
172. Hoppe, J. E.: Treatment of oropharyngeal candidiasis and candidal diaper dermatitis in neonates and infants: Review and reappraisal. Pediatr. Infect. Dis. J. *16*:885–894, 1997.
173. Horn, R., Wong, B., Kiehn, T. E., and Armstrong, D.: Fungemia in a cancer hospital: Changing frequency, earlier onset, and results of therapy. Rev. Infect. Dis. *7*:646–655, 1985.
174. Horsburgh, C. R., Jr., and Kirkpatrick, C. H.: Long-term therapy of chronic mucocutaneous candidiasis with ketoconazole: Experience with twenty-one patients. Am. J. Med. *74*:23–29, 1983.
175. Howard, R. M., and Frieden, I. J.: Dermatophyte infections in children. Adv. Pediatr. Infect. Dis. *14*:73–107, 1999.
176. Hull, P. R., and Vismer, H. F.: Treatment of cutaneous sporotrichosis with terbinafine. J. Dermatol. *126*(Suppl. 39):51–55, 1992.
177. Humbert, H., Cabiac, M. D., Denouel, J., and Kirkesseli, S.: Pharmacokinetics of terbinafine and of its five main metabolites in plasma and urine, following a single oral dose in healthy subjects. Biopharm. Drug Dispos. *16*:685–694, 1995.
178. Humbert, H., Denouel, J., Cabiac, M. D., et al.: Pharmacokinetics of terbinafine and five known metabolites in children, after oral administration. Biopharm. Drug Dispos. *19*:417–423, 1998.
179. Huttova, M., Hartmanova, I., Kralinsky, K., et al.: *Candida* fungemia in neonates treated with fluconazole: Report of forty cases, including eight with meningitis. Pediatr. Infect. Dis. J. *17*:1012–1015, 1998.
180. Ittel, T. H., Legler, U. F., Polak, A., et al.: 5-Fluorocytosine kinetics in patients with acute renal failure undergoing continuous hemofiltration. Chemotherapy *33*:77–84, 1987.
181. Iwen, P. C., Rupp, M. E., Langnas, A. N., et al.: Invasive pulmonary aspergillosis due to *Aspergillus terreus:* 12-year experience and review of the literature. Clin. Infect. Dis. *26*:1092–1097, 1998.
182. Jagdis, F. A., Hoeprich, P. D., Lawrence, R. M., and Schaffner, C. P.: Comparative pharmacology of amphotericin B and amphotericin B methyl ester in the non-human primate, *Macacca mulatta.* Antimicrob. Agents Chemother. *12*:582–590, 1977.
183. Jarque, I., Saavedra, S., Martin, G., et al.: Delay of onset of candidemia and emergence of *Candida krusei* fungemia in hematologic patients receiving prophylactic fluconazole. Haematologica *85*:441–443, 2000.
184. Jessup, C. J., Ryder, N. S., and Ghannoum, M. A.: An evaluation of the in vitro activity of terbinafine. Med. Mycol. *38*:155–159, 2000.
185. Johnson, E. M., Szekely, A., and Warnock, D. W.: In vitro activity of voriconazole, itraconazole and amphotericin B against filamentous fungi. J. Antimicrob. Chemother. *42*:741–745, 1998.
186. Johnson, M. D., Drew, R. H., and Perfect, J. R.: Chest discomfort associated with liposomal amphotericin B: Report of three cases and review of the literature. Pharmacotherapy *18*:1053–1061, 1998.
187. Jones, T. C.: Overview of the use of terbinafine (Lamisil) in children. Br. J. Dermatol. *132*:683–689, 1995.
188. Juster-Reicher, A., Leibovitz, E., Linder, N., et al.: Liposomal amphotericin B (AmBisome) in the treatment of neonatal candidiasis in very low birth weight infants. Infection *28*:223–226, 2001.
189. Kan, V. L., and Bennett, J. E.: Efficacies of four antifungal agents in experimental murine sporotrichosis. Antimicrob. Agents Chemother. *32*:1619–1623, 1988.
190. Karp, J. E., Burch, P. A., and Merz, W. G.: An approach to intensive antileukemia therapy in patients with previous invasive aspergillosis. Am. J. Med. *85*:203–206, 1988.
191. Kauffman, C. A., Bradley, S. F., Ross, S. C., and Weber, D. R.: Hepatosplenic candidiasis: Successful treatment with fluconazole. Am. J. Med. *91*:137–141, 1991.
192. Kauffman, C. A., Hajjeh, R., and Chapman, S. W.: Practice guidelines for the management of patients with sporotrichosis. For the Mycoses Study Group. Infectious Diseases Society of America. Clin. Infect. Dis. *30*:684–687, 2000.
193. Kauffman, C. A., Pappas, P. G., McKinsey, D. S., et al.: Treatment of lymphocutaneous and visceral sporotrichosis with fluconazole. Clin. Infect. Dis. *22*:46–50, 1996.
194. Kearns, G. L., and Reed, M. D.: Clinical pharmacokinetics in infants and children, a reappraisal. Clin. Pharmacokinet. *17*(Suppl. 1):29–67, 1989.
195. Kingo, A. R., Smyth, J. A., and Waisman, D.: Lack of evidence of amphotericin B toxicity in very low birth weight infants treated for systemic candidiasis. Pediatr. Infect. Dis. J. *16*:1002–1003, 1997.
196. Klepser, M. E., Malone, D., Lewis, R. E., et al.: Evaluation of voriconazole pharmacodynamics using time-kill methodology. Antimicrob. Agents Chemother. *44*:1917–1920, 2000.
197. Klepser, M. E., Wolfe, E. J., Jones, R. N., et al: Antifungal pharmacodynamic characteristics of fluconazole and amphotericin B tested against *Candida albicans.* Antimicrob. Agents Chemother. *41*:1392–1395, 1997.
198. Klepser, M. E., Wolfe, E. J., and Pfaller, M. A.: Antifungal pharmacodynamic characteristics of fluconazole and amphotericin B against *Cryptococcus neoformans.* J. Antimicrob. Chemother. *41*:397–401, 1998.
199. Konishi, H., Morita, K., and Yamaji, A.: Effect of fluconazole on theophylline disposition in humans. Eur. J. Clin. Pharmacol. *46*:309–312, 1994.
200. Koren, G., Lau, A., Klein, J., et al.: Pharmacokinetics and adverse effects of amphotericin B in infants and children. J. Pediatr. *113*:559–563, 1988.
201. Kovarik, J. M., Kirkesseli, S., Humbert, H., et al.: Dose-proportional pharmacokinetics of terbinafine and its N-demethylated metabolite in healthy volunteers. Br. J. Dermatol. *126*(Suppl. 39):8–13, 1992.
202. Kovarik, J. M., Mueller, E. A., Zehender, H., et al.: Multiple-dose pharmacokinetics and distribution in tissue of terbinafine and metabolites. Antimicrob. Agents Chemother. *39*:2738–2741, 1995.
203. Krafchik, B., and Pelletier, J.: An open study of tinea capitis in 50 children treated with a 2-week course of oral terbinafine. J. Am. Acad. Dermatol. *41*:60–63, 1998.
204. Kramer, M. R., Marshall, S. E., Denning, D. W., et al.: Cyclosporine and itraconazole interaction in heart and lung transplant recipients. Ann. Intern. Med. *113*:327–329, 1990.
205. Krzeska, I., Yeates, R. A., and Pfaff, G.: Single dose intravenous pharmacokinetics of fluconazole in infants. Drugs Exp. Clin. Res. *19*:267–271, 1993.
206. Kurtz, M. B., and Douglas, C. M.: Lipopeptide inhibitors of fungal glucan synthase. J. Med. Vet. Mycol. *35*:79–86, 1997.
207. Kurtz, M. B., Heath, I. B., Marrinan, J., et al.: Morphological effects of lipopeptides against *Aspergillus fumigatus* correlate with activities against (1,3)-beta-D-glucan synthase. Antimicrob. Agents Chemother. *38*:1480–1489, 1994.
208. Lansdorp, D., Bressers, H. P., Dekens-Konter, J. A., and Meyboom, R. H.: Potentiation of acenocoumarol during vaginal administration of miconazole. Br. J. Clin. Pharmacol. *47*:225–226, 1999.
209. Larsen, R. A., Bozette, S. A., Jones, B. E., et al.: Fluconazole combined with flucytosine for treatment of cryptococcal meningitis in patients with AIDS. Clin. Infect. Dis. *19*:741–745, 1994.
210. Lau, A. H., and Kronfol, N. O.: Elimination of flucytosine by continuous hemofiltration. Am. J. Nephrol. *15*:327–331, 1995.
211. Lavrijsen, A. P. M., Balmus, K. J., Nugteren-Huyning, W. M., et al.: Hepatic injury associated with itraconazole. Lancet *340*:251–252, 1992.

212. Lawrence, R. M., Hoeprich, P. D., Jagdis, F. A., et al.: Distribution of doubly radiolabelled amphotericin B methyl ester and amphotericin B in the non-human primate, *Macaca mulatta.* J. Antimicrob. Chemother. *6*:241–249, 1980.
213. Lazar, J. D., and Wilner, K. D.: Drug interactions with fluconazole. Rev. Infect. Dis. *12*(Suppl. 3):327–333, 1990.
214. Lee, J. W., Seibel, N. L., Amantea, M., et al.: Safety, tolerance, and pharmacokinetics of fluconazole in children with neoplastic diseases. J. Pediatr. *120*:987–993, 1992.
215. Leenders, A. C., Daenen, S., Jansen, R. L., et al.: Liposomal amphotericin B compared with amphotericin B deoxycholate in the treatment of documented and suspected neutropenia-associated invasive fungal infections. Br. J. Haematol. *103*:205–212, 1998.
216. Leibovitz, E., Iuster-Reicher, A., Amitai, M., and Mogilner, B.: Systemic candidal infections associated with use of peripheral venous catheters in neonates: A 9-year experience. Clin. Infect. Dis. *14*:485–491, 1992.
217. Leibovitz, E., Rigaud, M., Chandwani, S., et al.: Disseminated fungal infection in children with human immunodeficiency virus. Pediatr. Infect. Dis. J. *10*:888–894, 1991.
218. Lewis, R. E., Klepser, M. E., and Pfaller, M. A.: In vitro pharmacodynamic characteristics of flucytosine determined by time-kill methods. Diagn. Microbiol. Infect. Dis. *36*:101–105, 2000.
219. Lin, C. C., Magat, J., Chang, R., et al.: Absorption, metabolism and excretion of ^{14}C-griseofulvin in man. J. Pharmacol. Exp. Ther. *187*:415–422, 1973.
220. Lin, C., and Symchowicz, S.: Absorption, distribution, metabolism, and excretion of griseofulvin in man and animals. Drug Metab. Rev. *4*:75–95, 1975.
221. Linder, N., Shalit, I., Tallen-Gozani, E., et al.: Amphotericin B colloidal dispersion use in very low birth weight infants. Abstract 2438. *In* Abstracts of the 2000 Pediatric Academic Societies and American Academy of Pediatrics Joint Meeting, Chicago, 2000.
222. Lo, A. C. Y., Lui, S. L., Lo, W. K., et al.: The interaction of terbinafine and cyclosporine A in renal transplant patients. Br. J. Clin. Pharmacol. *43*:340–341, 1997.
223. Lopez, C. F.: Recent developments in the therapy for chromoblastomycosis. Bull. Pan Am. Health. Org. *15*:58–64, 1981.
224. Lortholary, O., Dupont, B.: Antifungal prophylaxis during neutropenia and immunodeficiency. Clin. Microbiol. Rev. *10*:477–504, 1997.
225. Louie, A., Drusano, G. L., Banerjee, P., et al.: Pharmacodynamics of fluconazole in a murine model of systemic candidiasis. Antimicrob. Agents Chemother. *42*:1105–1109, 1998.
226. Maertens, J., Lagrou, K., Deweerdt, H., et al.: Disseminated infection by *Scedosporium prolificans:* An emerging fatality among haematology patients. Case report and review. Ann. Hematol. *79*:340–344, 2000.
227. Maertens, J., Raad, I., Sable, C. A., et al.: Multicenter, noncomparative study to evaluate safety and efficacy of caspofungin in adults with invasive aspergillosis refractory or intolerant to amphotericin B, amphotericin B lipid formulations, or azoles. Abstract 1103. *In* Abstracts of the 40th International Conference on Antimicrobial Agents and Chemotherapy. Washington, D.C., American Society for Microbiology, 2000, p. 371.
228. Malet-Martino, M. C., Martino, R., deForni, M., et al.: Flucytosine conversion to fluorouracil in humans: Does a correlation with gut flora status exist? A report of two cases using fluorine-19 magnetic resonance spectroscopy. Infection *19*:178–180, 1991.
229. Manavathu, E. K., Cutright, J. L., and Chandrasekar, P. H.: Organism-dependent fungicidal activities of azoles. Antimicrob. Agents Chemother. *42*:3018–3021, 1998.
230. Manavathu, E. K., Cutright, J. L., Loebenberg, D., and Chandrasekar, P. H.: A comparative study of the in vitro susceptibilities of clinical and laboratory-selected resistant isolates of *Aspergillus* spp. to amphotericin B, itraconazole, voriconazole and posaconazole (SCH 56592). J. Antimicrob. Chemother *46*:229–234, 2000.
231. Marchisio, P., and Principi, N.: Treatment of oropharyngeal candidiasis in HIV-infected children with oral fluconazole. Eur. J. Clin. Microbiol. Infect. Dis. *13*:338–340, 1994.
232. Marco, F., Pfaller, M. A., Messer, S. A., and Jones, R. N.: Antifungal activity of a new triazole, voriconazole (UK-109,496), compared with three other antifungal agents tested against clinical isolates of filamentous fungi. Med. Mycol. *36*:433–436, 1998.
233. Marina, N. M., Flynn, P. M., Rivera, G. K., and Hughes, W. T.: *Candida tropicalis* and *Candida albicans* fungemia in children with leukemia. Cancer *68*:594–599, 1991.
234. Marr, K. A., Seidel, K., Slavin, M. A., et al.: Prolonged fluconazole prophylaxis is associated with persistent protection against candidiasis-related death in allogeneic marrow transplant recipients: Long-term follow-up of a randomized, placebo-controlled trial. Blood *96*:2055–2061, 2000.
235. Marr, K. A., Seidel, K., White, T. C., and Bowden, R. A.: Candidemia in allogeneic blood and marrow transplant recipients: Evolution of risk factors after the adoption of prophylactic fluconazole. J. Infect. Dis. *181*:309–316, 2000.
236. Matsumoto, S., Warabe, E., Wakai, Y., et al.: Pharmacodynamics of FK463 in a thigh infection model with *Candida albicans*. Abstract 1687. *In* Abstracts of the 40th Interscience Conference on Antimicrobial Agents and Chemotherapy. Washington, D.C., American Society for Microbiology, 2000, p. 388.
237. Medoff, G., Comfort, M., and Kobayashi, G. S.: Synergistic action of amphotericin B and 5-fluorocytosine against yeast-like organisms. Proc. Soc. Exp. Biol. Med. *138*:571–574, 1971.
238. Medoff, G., and Kobayashi, G. S.: Strategies in the treatment of systemic fungal infections. N. Engl. J. Med. *302*:1451–1455, 1980.
239. Mehta, R. T., Hopfer, R. L., Gunner, L. A., et al.: Formulation, toxicity, and antifungal activity in vitro of liposome-encapsulated nystatin as therapeutic agent for systemic candidiasis. Antimicrob. Agents Chemother. *31*:1897–1900, 1987.
240. Mehta, R. T., Hopfer, R. L., McQueen, T., et al.: Toxicity and therapeutic effects in mice of liposome-encapsulated nystatin for systemic fungal infections. Antimicrob. Agents Chemother. *31*:1901–1903, 1987.
241. Meletiadis, J., Mouton, J. W., Rodriguez-Tudela, J. L., et al.: In vitro interaction of terbinafine with itraconazole against clinical isolates of *Scedosporium prolificans*. Antimicrob. Agents Chemother. *44*:470–472, 2000.
242. Menichetti, F., Del Favero, A., Martino, P., et al.: Itraconazole oral solution as prophylaxis for fungal infections in neutropenic patients with hematologic malignancies: A randomized, placebo-controlled, double-blind, multicenter trial. GIMEMA Infection Program. Gruppo Italiano Malattie Ematologiche dell' Adulto. Clin. Infect. Dis. *28*:250–255, 1999.
243. Meunier, F., Prentice, H. G., and Ringden, O.: Liposomal amphotericin B (AmBisome): Safety data from a phase II/III clinical trial. J. Antimicrob. Chemother. *28*(Suppl. B):83–91, 1991.
244. Michel, C., Courdavault, L., al Khayat, R., et al.: Fungal peritonitis in patients on peritoneal dialysis. Am. J. Nephrol. *14*:113–120, 1994.
245. Mikami, Y., Scalarone, G. M., Kurita, N., et al.: Synergistic postantifungal effect of flucytosine and fluconazole on *Candida albicans*. J. Med. Vet. Mycol. *30*:197–206, 1992.
246. Minguez, F., Chiu, M. L., Lima, J. E., et al.: Activity of fluconazole: Postantifungal effect, effects of low concentrations and of pretreatment on the susceptibility of *Candida albicans* to leucocytes. J. Antimicrob. Chemother. *34*:93–100, 1994.
247. Mitchell, A. S., and Holland, J. T.: Fluconazole and phenytoin: A predictable inter-action. B. M. J. *298*:1315, 1989.
248. Montgomerie, J. Z., Edwards, J. E., Jr., and Guze, L. B.: Synergism of amphotericin B and 5-fluorocytosine for *Candida* species. J. Infect. Dis. *132*:82–86, 1975.
249. Morselli, P. L.: Clinical pharmacology of the perinatal period and early infancy. Clin. Pharmacokinet. *17*(Suppl. 1):13–28, 1989.
250. Mott, S. H., Packer, R. J., Vezina, L. G., et al.: Encephalopathy with parkinsonian features in children following bone marrow transplantation and high dose amphotericin B. Ann. Neurol. *37*:810–814, 1995.
251. Mueller, F. M., Weig, M., Peter, J., and Walsh, T. J.: Azole cross-resistance to ketoconazole, fluconazole, itraconazole and voriconazole in clinical *Candida albicans* isolates from HIV-infected children with oropharyngeal candidosis. J. Antimicrob. Chemother. *46*:338–340, 2000.
252. Nahata, M. C., Tallian, K. B., Force, R. W.: Pharmacokinetics of fluconazole in young infants. Eur. J. Drug Metab. Pharmacokinet. *24*:155–157, 1999.
253. Narang, P. K., Trapnell, C. B., Schoenfelder, J. R., et al.: Fluconazole and enhanced effect of rifabutin prophylaxis. N. Engl. J. Med. *330*:1316–1317, 1994.
254. Naranjo, M. S., Trujillo, M., Munera, M. I., et al.: Treatment of paracoccidioidomycosis with itraconazole. J. Med. Vet. Mycol. *28*:67–76, 1990.
255. Nath, C. E., Shaw, P. J., Gunning, R., et al.: Amphotericin B in children with malignant disease: A comparison of the toxicities and pharmacokinetics of amphotericin B administered in dextrose versus lipid emulsion. Antimicrob. Agents Chemother. *43*:1417–1423, 1999.
256. Nedelman, J. R., Gibiansky, E., Robbins, B. A., et al.: Pharmacokinetics and pharmacodynamics of multiple-dose terbinafine. J. Clin. Pharmacol. *36*:452–461, 1996.
257. Negroni, R., Palmieri, O., Koren, F., et al.: Oral treatment of paracoccidioidomycosis and histoplasmosis with itraconazole in humans. Rev. Infect. Dis. *9*(Suppl. 1):47–50, 1987
258. Nejjam, F., Zagula, M., Cabiac, M. D., et al.: Pilot study of terbinafine in children suffering from tinea capitis: Evaluation of efficacy, safety and pharmacokinetics. Br. J. Dermatol. *132*:98–105, 1995.
259. Neuvonen, P. J., and Jalava, K. M.: Itraconazole drastically increases plasma concentrations of lovastatin and lovastatin acid. Clin. Pharmacol. Ther. *60*:54–61, 1996.
260. Nguyen, M. H., Barchiesi, F., McGough, D. A., et al.: In vitro evaluation of combination of fluconazole and flucytosine against *Cryptococcus neoformans* var. *neoformans*. Antimicrob. Agents Chemother. *39*:1691–1695, 1995.
261. Nicolau, D. P., Crowe, H., Nightingale, C. H., and Quintiliani, R.: Effect of continuous arteriovenous hemofiltration on the pharmacokinetics of fluconazole. Pharmacotherapy *14*:502–505, 1994.
262. Nieto, L., Northland, R., Pittisuttithum, P., et al.: Posaconazole equivalent to fluconazole in the treatment of oropharyngeal candidiasis. Abstract 1108. *In* Abstracts of the 40th Interscience Conference on Antimicrobial Agents and Chemotherapy. Washington, D.C., American Society for Microbiology, 2000, p. 372.

263. Ninane, J., Gluckman, E., Hann, I., et al.: A multicentre study of fluconazole versus oral polyenes in the prevention of fungal infection in children with hematological or oncological malignancies. Eur. J. Clin. Microbiol. Infect. Dis. *13*:330–337, 1994.
264. Novelli, V., and Holzel, H.: Safety and tolerability of fluconazole in children. Antimicrob. Agents Chemother. *43*:1955–1960, 1999.
265. Oakley, K. L., Moore, C. B., and Denning, D. W.: In vitro activity of the echinocandin antifungal agent LY303,366 in comparison with itraconazole and amphotericin B against *Aspergillus* spp. Antimicrob. Agents Chemother. *42*:2726–2730, 1998.
266. Offner, F. C. J., Herbrecht, R., Engelhard, D., et al.: EORTC-IFCG phase II study on liposomal nystatin in patients with invasive aspergillosis refractory or intolerant to conventional/lipid amphotericin B. Abstract 1102. *In* Abstracts of the 40th Interscience Conference on Antimicrobial Agents and Chemotherapy. Washington, D.C., American Society for Microbiology, 2000, p. 372.
267. Olkkola, K. T., Ahonen, J., and Neuvonen, P. J.: The effects of the systemic antimycotics, itraconazole and fluconazole, on the pharmacokinetics and pharmacodynamics of intravenous and oral midazolam. Anesth. Analg. *82*:511–516, 1996.
268. Olson, J., Satorius, A., McAndrews, B., and Adler-Moore, J.: Treatment of systemic murine candidiasis with amphotericin B or different amphotericin B lipid formulations. Abstract B-11. *In* Abstracts of the 37th Interscience Conference on Antimicrobial Agents and Chemotherapy. Washington, D.C., American Society for Microbiology, 1997, p. 28.
269. Ortin, M., Olalla, J. I., Muruzabal, M. J., et al.: Miconazole oral gel enhances acenocoumarol anticoagulant activity: A report of three cases. Ann. Pharmacother. *33*:175–177, 1999.
270. Osowski, C. L., Dix, S. P., Lin, L. S., et al.: Evaluation of the drug interaction between intravenous high-dose fluconazole and cyclosporine or tacrolimus in bone marrow transplant patients. Transplantation *61*:1268–1272, 1996.
271. O'Sullivan, D. P., Needham, C. A., Bangs, A., et al.: Postmarketing surveillance of oral terbinafine in the UK: Report of a large cohort study. Br. J. Clin. Pharmacol. *42*:559–565, 1996.
272. Oxford, A. E., Raistrick, H., and Simonart, P.: Studies in the biochemistry of microorganisms: Griseofulvin, C17H17O6Cl, a metabolic product of *Penicillium griseofulvum*. Biochem. J. *33*:240–248, 1939.
273. Package Circular: Cancidas (caspofungin acetate for injection). January 2001.
274. Pappas, P. G., Bradsher, R. W., Chapman, S. W., et al.: Treatment of blastomycosis with fluconazole: A pilot study. Clin. Infect. Dis. *20*:267–271, 1995.
275. Pappas, P. G., Bradsher, R. W., Kauffman, C. A., et al.: Treatment of blastomycosis with higher doses of fluconazole. The National Institute of Allergy and Infectious Diseases Mycoses Study Group. Clin. Infect. Dis. *25*:200–205, 1997.
276. Pasic, S., Flannagan, L., and Cant, A. J.: Liposomal amphotericin B (AmBisome) is safe in bone marrow transplantation for primary immunodeficiency. Bone Marrow Transplant. *19*:1229–1232, 1997.
277. Pelletier, R., Peter, J., Antin, C., et al.: Emergence of resistance of *Candida albicans* to clotrimazole in human immunodeficiency virus–infected children: In vitro and clinical correlations. J. Clin. Microbiol. *38*:1563–1568, 2000.
278. Petraitis, V., Petraitiene, R., Groll, A., et al.: Comparative antifungal efficacy of the echinocandin FK463 against disseminated candidiasis and invasive pulmonary aspergillosis in persistently neutropenic rabbits. Abstract 1684. *In* Abstracts of the 40th Interscience Conference on Antimicrobial Agents and Chemotherapy. Washington, D.C., American Society for Microbiology, 2000, p. 387.
279. Pettengell, K., Mynhardt, J., Kluyts, T., and Soni, P.: A multicenter study to determine the minimal effective dose of FK463 for the treatment of esophageal candidiasis in HIV-positive patients. Abstract 1421. *In* Abstracts of the 39th Interscience Conference on Antimicrobial Agents and Chemotherapy. Washington, D.C., American Society for Microbiology, 1999, p. 567.
280. Pettengell, K., Mynhardt, J., Kluyts, T., et al.: A multicenter study of the echinocandin antifungal FK463 for the treatment of esophageal candidiasis in HIV positive patients. Abstract 1104. *In* Abstracts of the 40th Interscience Conference on Antimicrobial Agents and Chemotherapy. Washington, D.C., American Society for Microbiology, 2000, p. 371.
281. Pfaller, M. A., Messer, S. A., and Coffman, S.: In vitro susceptibilities of clinical yeast isolates to a new echinocandin derivative, LY303366, and other antifungal agents. Antimicrob. Agents Chemother. *41*:763–766, 1997.
282. Phillips, P., Shafran, S., Garber, G., et al.: Multicenter randomized trial of fluconazole versus amphotericin B for treatment of candidemia in non-neutropenic patients. Canadian Candidemia Study Group. Eur. J. Clin. Microbiol. Infect. Dis. *16*:337–345, 1997.
283. Piscitelli, S. C., and Gallicano, K. D.: Interactions among drugs for HIV and opportunistic infections. N. Engl. J. Med. *344*:984–996, 2001.
284. Pizzo, P. A., Robichaud, K. J., Gill, F. A., et al.: Empiric antibiotic and antifungal therapy for cancer patients with prolonged fever and granulocytopenia. Am. J. Med. *72*:101–111, 1982.
285. Polak, A.: Mode of action studies. *In* Ryley, J. F. (ed.): Handbook of Experimental Pharmacology. Vol. 96. Berlin, Springer-Verlag, 1990, pp. 153–182.
286. Powderly, W. G., Finkelstein, D., Feinberg, J., et al.: A randomized trial comparing fluconazole with clotrimazole troches for the prevention of fungal infections in patients with AIDS. N. Engl. J. Med. *332*:700–705, 1995.
287. Powles, R., Mawhorter, S., and Williams, A. H.: Liposomal nystatin (Nyotran) vs. amphotericin B (Fungizone) in empiric treatment of presumed fungal infections in neutropenic patients. Abstract LB-4. *In* Program and Abstracts of the 39th Interscience Conference on Antimicrobial Agents and Chemotherapy. Washington, D.C., American Society for Microbiology, 1999, p. 14.
288. Prentice, A. G., Warnock, D. W., Johnson, S. A., et al.: Multiple dose pharmacokinetics of an oral solution of itraconazole in patients receiving chemotherapy for acute myeloid leukaemia. J. Antimicrob. Chemother. *36*:657–663, 1995.
289. Prentice, H. G., Hann, I. M., Herbrecht, R., et al.: A randomized comparison of liposomal versus conventional amphotericin B for the treatment of pyrexia of unknown origin in neutropenic patients. Br. J. Haematol. *98*:711–718, 1997.
290. Ralph, E. D., Khazindar, A. M., Barber, K. R., and Grant, C. W. M.: Comparative in vitro effects of liposomal amphotericin B, amphotericin B-deoxycholate, and free amphotericin B against fungal strains determined by using MIC and minimal lethal concentration susceptibility studies and time-kill curves. Antimicrob. Agents Chemother. *35*:188–191, 1991.
291. Redding, S., Smith, J., Farinacci, G., et al.: Resistance of *Candida albicans* to fluconazole during treatment of oropharyngeal candidiasis in a patient with AIDS: Documentation by in vitro susceptibility testing and DNA subtype analysis. Clin. Infect. Dis. *18*:240–242, 1994.
292. Reed, M. D., and Besunder, J. B.: Developmental ontogenic basis of drug disposition. Pediatr. Clin. North. Am. *36*:1053–1074, 1989.
293. Regulations requiring manufacturers to assess the safety and effectiveness of new drugs and biological products in pediatric patients. Fed. Reg. *63*:66632–66672, 1998.
294. Rennie, R., Sand, C., and Sherburne, R.: Electron microscopic evidence of the effect of LY303366 on *Aspergillus fumigatus*. Abstract p451. *In* Abstracts of the 13th Meeting of the International Society for Human and Animal Mycology. Parma, Italy, 1997, p. 191.
295. Restrepo, A., Robledo, J., Gomez, I., et al.: Itraconazole therapy in lymphangitic and cutaneous sporotrichosis. Arch. Dermatol. *122*:413–417, 1986.
296. Reuben, A., Anaissie, E., Nelson, P. E., et al.: Antifungal susceptibility of 44 clinical isolates of *Fusarium* species determined by using a broth microdilution method. Antimicrob. Agents Chemother. *33*:1647–1649, 1989.
297. Rex, J. H., Bennett, J E., Sugar, A M., et al.: A randomized trial comparing fluconazole with amphotericin B for the treatment of candidemia in patients without neutropenia. N. Engl. J. Med. *331*:1325–1330, 1994.
298. Rex, J. H., Pfaller, M. A., Galgiani, J. N., et al.: Development of interpretive breakpoints for antifungal susceptibility testing: Conceptual framework and analysis of in vitro–in vivo correlation data for fluconazole, itraconazole, and *Candida* infections. Subcommittee on Antifungal Susceptibility Testing of the National Committee for Clinical Laboratory Standards. Clin. Infect. Dis. *24*:235–247, 1997.
299. Rex, J. H., Rinaldi, M. G., and Pfaller, M. A.: Resistance of *Candida* species to fluconazole. Antimicrob. Agents Chemother. *39*:1–8, 1995.
300. Rex, J. H., Walsh, T. J., Sobel, J. D., et al.: . Practice guidelines for the treatment of candidiasis. Infectious Diseases Society of America. Clin. Infect. Dis. *30*:662–678, 2000.
301. Reynes, J., Bazin, C., Ajana, F., et al.: Pharmacokinetics of itraconazole (oral solution) in two groups of human immunodeficiency virus–infected adults with oral candidiasis. Antimicrob. Agents Chemother. *41*:2554–2558, 1997.
302. Reynolds, E. S., Tomkiewicz, Z. M., and Dammin, G. J.: The renal lesion related to amphotericin B treatment for coccidioidomycosis. Med. Clin. North Am. *47*:1149–1154, 1993.
303. Ringden, O.: Clinical use of AmBisome with special emphasis on experience in children. Bone Marrow Transplant. *12*(Suppl. 4):149–150, 1993.
304. Ringden, O., Meunier, F., Tollemar, J., et al.: Efficacy of amphotericin B encapsulated in liposome (AmBisome) in the treatment of invasive fungal infections in immunocompromised patients. J. Antimicrob Chemother. *28*(Suppl. B):73–82, 1991.
305. Robbins, B., Chang, C. T., Cramer, J. A., et al.: Safe coadministration of terbinafine and terfenadine: A placebo-controlled crossover study of pharmacokinetic and pharmacodynamic interactions in healthy volunteers. Clin. Pharmacol. Ther. *59*:275–283, 1996.
306. Rogers, T. E., and Galgiani, J. N.: Activity of fluconazole (UK 49,858) and ketoconazole against *Candida albicans* in vitro and in vivo. Antimicrob. Agents Chemother. *30*:418–422, 1986.
307. Rolston, K., Baird, I., Graham, D. R., and Jauregui, L.: Treatment of refractory candidemia in non-neutropenic patients with liposomal

nystatin (Nyotran). Abstract LB-1. *In* Program and Abstracts of the 38th Interscience Conference on Antimicrobial Agents and Chemotherapy. Washington, D.C., American Society for Microbiology, 1998, p. 24.

308. Rotstein, C., Bow, E. J., Laverdiere, M., et al.: Randomized placebo-controlled trial of fluconazole prophylaxis for neutropenic cancer patients: Benefit based on purpose and intensity of cytotoxic therapy. The Canadian Fluconazole Prophylaxis Study Group. Clin. Infect. Dis. *28*:331–340, 1999.
309. Rowland, M., Riegelman, S., and Epstein, W. L.: Absorption kinetics of griseofulvin in man. J. Pharm. Sci. *57*:984–989, 1968.
310. Ruhnke, M., Eigler, A., Tennagen, I., et al.: Emergence of fluconazole-resistant strains of *Candida albicans* in patients with recurrent oropharyngeal candidosis and human immunodeficiency virus infection. J. Clin. Microbiol. *32*:2092–2098, 1994.
311. Ruhnke, M., Yeates, R. A., Pfaff, G., et al.: Single-dose pharmacokinetics of fluconazole in patients with liver cirrhosis. J. Antimicrob. Chemother. *35*:641–647, 1995.
312. Ryder, N. S.: Activity of terbinafine against serious fungal pathogens. Mycoses *42*(Suppl. 2):115–119, 1999.
313. Ryder, N. S., and Leitner, I.: Synergistic interaction of terbinafine with triazoles or amphotericin B against *Aspergillus* species. Med. Mycol. *39*:91–95, 2001.
314. Ryley, J. F., and McGregor, S.: A multiinfection model for antifungal screening in vivo. J. Antimicrob. Chemother. *22*:353–358, 1988.
315. Saag, M. S., Cloud, G. A., Graybill, J. R., et al.: A comparison of itraconazole versus fluconazole as maintenance therapy for AIDS-associated cryptococcal meningitis. National Institute of Allergy and Infectious Diseases Mycoses Study Group. Clin. Infect. Dis. *28*:291–296, 1999.
316. Saag, M. S., Fessel, W. J., Kaufman, C. A., et al.: Treatment of fluconazole-refractory oropharyngeal candidiasis with itraconazole oral solution in HIV-positive patients. A. I. D. S. Res. Hum. Retroviruses *15*:1413–1417, 1999.
317. Sable, C. A, Nguyen, B. Y., Chodakewitz, J. A., et al.: Safety of caspofungin acetate in the treatment of fungal infections. Abstract 021. *In* Program and Abstracts of Focus on Fungal Infections 11. Alpharetta, GA, Immedex Inc., 2000.
318. Sable, C. A., Villanueva, A., Arathon, E., et al.: A randomized, double-blind, multicenter trial of MK-0991 (L-743,872) vs amphotericin B (AmB) in the treatment of *Candida* esophagitis in adults. Abstract LB-33. *In* Abstracts of the 37th Interscience Conference on Antimicrobial Agents and Chemotherapy. Washington, D.C., American Society for Microbiology, 1997, p. 15.
319. Sachs, M. K., Blanchard, L. M., and Green, P. J.: Interaction of itraconazole and digoxin. Clin. Infect. Dis. *16*:400–403, 1993.
320. Sahai, J., Gallicano, K., Pakuts, A., and Cameron, D. W.: Effect of fluconazole on zidovudine pharmacokinetics in patients infected with human immunodeficiency virus. J. Infect. Dis. *169*:1103–1107, 1994.
321. Saitoh, A., Homans, J., and Kovacs, A.: Fluconazole treatment of coccidioidal meningitis in children: Two case reports and a review of the literature. Pediatr. Infect. Dis. J. *19*:1204–1208, 2000.
322. Sandler, E. S., Mustafa, M. M., Tkaczewski, I., et al.: Use of amphotericin B colloidal dispersion in children. J. Pediatr. Hematol. Oncol. *22*:242–246, 2000.
323. Sawaya, B. P., Briggs, J. P., and Schnermann, J.: Amphotericin B nephrotoxicity: The adverse consequences of altered membrane properties. J. Am. Soc. Nephrol. *6*:154–164, 1995.
324. Saxen, H., Hoppu, K., and Pohjavuori, M.: Pharmacokinetics of fluconazole in very low birth weight infants during the first two weeks of life. Clin. Pharmacol. Ther. *54*:269–277, 1993.
325. Scalarone, G. M., Mikami, Y., Kurita, N., et al.: The postantifungal effect of 5-fluorocytosine on *Candida albicans*. J. Antimicrob. Chemother. *29*:129–136, 1992.
326. Scalarone, G. M., Mikami, Y., Kurita, N., et al.: Comparative studies on the postantifungal effect produced by the synergistic interaction of flucytosine and amphotericin B on *Candida albicans*. Mycopathologia *120*:133–138, 1992.
327. Scarcella, A., Pasquariello, M. B., Giugliano, B., et al.: Liposomal amphotericin B treatment for neonatal fungal infections. Pediatr. Infect. Dis. J. *17*:146–148, 1998.
328. Schmitt, C., Perel, Y., Harousseau, J., et al.: Pharmacokinetics of itraconazole oral solution in neutropenic children during long-term prophylaxis. Antimicrob. Agents Chemother. *45*:1561–1564, 2001.
329. Schmitt, H. J., Andrade, J., Edwards, F., et al.: Inactivity of terbinafine in a rat model of pulmonary aspergillosis. Eur. J. Clin. Microbiol. Infect. Dis. *9*:832–835, 1990.
330. Schmitt, H. J., Bernard, E. M., Andrade, J., et al.: MIC and fungicidal activity of terbinafine against clinical isolates of *Aspergillus* spp. Antimicrob. Agents Chemother. *32*:780–781, 1988.
331. Scholz, J., Schulz, M., Steinfath, M., et al.: Fluconazole is removed by continuous venovenous hemofiltration in a liver transplant patient. J. Mol. Med. *73*:145–147, 1995.
332. Schwartz, E. L., Hallam, S., Gallagher, R. E., and Wiernik, P. H.: Inhibition of all-*trans*-retinoic acid metabolism by fluconazole in vitro and in patients with acute promyelocytic leukemia. Biochem. Pharmacol. *50*:923–928, 1995.
333. Schwartz, S., Behre, G., Heinemann, V., et al.: Amphotericin B inhalations as prophylaxis of invasive *Aspergillus* infections during prolonged neutropenia: Results of a prospective randomized multicenter trial. Blood *93*:3654–3661, 1999.
334. Seay, R. E., Larson, T. A., Toscano, J. P., et al.: Pharmacokinetics of fluconazole in immunocompromised children with leukemia or other hematologic diseases. Pharmacotherapy *15*:52–58, 1995.
335. Seibel, N., Schwartz, C., Arrieta, A., et al.: A phase I study to determine the safety and pharmacokinetics of FK463 in febrile neutropenic pediatric patients. Abstract 18. *In* Abstracts of the 40th Interscience Conference on Antimicrobial Agents and Chemotherapy. Washington, D.C., American Society for Microbiology, 2000, p. 1.
336. Shadomy, S., Espinel-Ingroff, A., and Gebhart, R. J.: In-vitro studies with SF 86-327, a new orally active allylamine derivative. Sabouraudia *23*:125–132, 1985.
337. Shah, V. P., Riegelman, S., and Epstein, W. L.: Determination of griseofulvin in skin, plasma, and sweat. J. Pharm. Sci. *61*:634–636, 1972.
338. Sharkey, P. A., Graybill, J. R., Rinaldi, M. G., et al.: Itraconazole treatment of phaeohyphomycosis. J. Am. Acad. Dermatol. *23*:577–586, 1990.
339. Slavin, M. A., Osborne, B., Adams, R., et al.: Efficacy and safety of fluconazole prophylaxis for fungal infections after marrow transplantation—a prospective, randomized, double-blind study. J. Infect. Dis. *171*:1545–1552, 1995.
340. Sobel, J. D., Faro, S., Force, R. W., et al.: Vulvovaginal candidiasis: Epidemiologic, diagnostic, and therapeutic considerations. Am. J. Obstet. Gynecol. *178*:203–211, 1998.
341. Sohnle, P. G., Hahn, B. L., and Erdmann, M. D.: Effect of fluconazole on viability of *Candida albicans* over extended periods of time. Antimicrob. Agents Chemother. *40*:2622–2625, 1996.
342. Sorensen, K., Corcoran, E., Chen, S., et al.: Pharmacodynamic assessment of efflux- and target based resistance to fluconazole on efficacy against C. *albicans* in a mouse kidney infection model. Abstract 1271. *In* Abstracts of the 39th Interscience Conference on Antimicrobial Agents and Chemotherapy. Washington, D.C., American Society for Microbiology, 1999, p. 328.
343. Starke, J. R., Mason, O., Kramer, W. G., et al.: Pharmacokinetics of amphotericin B in infants and children. J. Infect. Dis. *155*:766–774, 1987.
344. Stein, G. E., and Mummaw, N.: Placebo-controlled trial of itraconazole for treatment of acute vaginal candidiasis. Antimicrob. Agents Chemother. *37*:89–92, 1993.
345. Stevens, D. A., and Lee, J. Y.: Analysis of compassionate use itraconazole therapy for invasive aspergillosis by the NIAID Mycoses Study Group criteria. Arch. Intern. Med. *157*:1857–1862, 1997.
346. Stone, J. A., McCrea, J., Wickersham, P., et al.: A phase I study of caspofungin evaluating the potential for drug interactions with itraconazole, the effect of gender and the use of a loading dose regimen. Abstract 854. *In* Program and Abstracts of the 40th Interscience Conference on Antimicrobial Agents and Chemotherapy. Washington, D.C., American Society for Microbiology, 2000, p. 26.
347. Sutton, D. A., Sanche, S. E., Revankar, S. G., et al.: In vitro amphotericin B resistance in clinical isolates of *Aspergillus terreus*, with a head-to-head comparison to voriconazole. J. Clin. Microbiol. *37*:2343–2345, 1999.
348. Tang, T. R., Parr, R., Turner, W., et al.: LY-303366: A non-competitive inhibitor of (1,3)-b-D glucan synthases from *Candida albicans* and *Aspergillus fumigatus*. Abstract 367. *In* Abstracts of the 33rd Interscience Conference on Antimicrobial Agents and Chemotherapy. Washington, D.C., American Society for Microbiology, 1993.
349. Thaler, M., Pastakia, B., Shawker, T. H., et al.: Hepatic candidiasis in cancer patients: The evolving picture of the syndrome. Ann. Intern. Med. *108*:88–100, 1988.
350. Thompson, J. R., Douglas, C. M., Li, W., et al.: A glucan synthase FKS1 homolog in *Cryptococcus neoformans* is single copy and encodes an essential function. J. Bacteriol. *181*:444–453, 1999.
351. Tobon, A. M., Franco, L., Espinal, D., et al.: Disseminated histoplasmosis in children: The role of itraconazole therapy. Pediatr. Infect. Dis. J. *15*:1002–1008, 1996.
352. Toon, S., Ross, C. E., Gokal, R., and Rowland, M.: An assessment of the effects of impaired renal function and haemodialysis on the pharmacokinetics of fluconazole. Br. J. Clin. Pharmacol. *29*:221–226, 1990.
353. Townsend, R., Bekersky, I., Buell, D. N., and Seibel. N.: Pharmacokinetic evaluation of the echinocandin FK463 in pediatric and adult patients. Abstract 024. *In* Program and Abstracts of Focus on Fungal Infections 11. Alpharetta, GA, Immedex Inc., 2001.
354. Travis, L. B., Roberts, G. D., Wilson, W. R.: Clinical significance of *Pseudallescheria boydii:* A review of 10 years' experience. Mayo Clin. Proc. *60*:531–537, 1985.
355. Trepanier, E. F., Nafziger, A. N., and Amsden, G. W.: Effect of terbinafine on theophylline pharmacokinetics in healthy volunteers. Antimicrob. Agents Chemother. *42*:695–697, 1998.
356. Tucker, R. M., Denning, D. W., Arathoon, E. G., et al.: Itraconazole therapy for nonmeningeal coccidioidomycosis: Clinical and laboratory observations. J. Am. Acad. Dermatol. *23*:593–601, 1990.

357. Tucker, R. M., Denning, D. W., Dupont, B., and Stevens, D. A.: Itraconazole therapy for chronic coccidioidal meningitis. Ann. Intern. Med. *112*:108–112, 1990.
358. Tucker, R. M., Denning, D. W., Hanson, L. H., et al.: Interaction of azoles with rifampin, phenytoin, and carbamazepine: In vitro and clinical observations. Clin. Infect. Dis. *14*:165–174, 1992.
359. Tucker, R. M., Haq, Y., Denning, D. W., and Stevens, D. A.: Adverse events associated with itraconazole in 189 patients on chronic therapy. J. Antimicrob. Chemother. *26*:561–566, 1990.
360. Turnidge, J. D., Gudmundsson, S., Vogelman, B., and Craig W. A.: The postantibiotic effect of antifungal agents against common pathogenic yeasts. J. Antimicrob. Chemother. *34*:83–92, 1994.
361. Uzun, O., and Anaissie, E. J.: Antifungal prophylaxis in patients with hematologic malignancies: A reappraisal. Blood *86*:2063–2072, 1995.
362. Van der Auwera, P., Ceuppens, A. M., Heymans, C., and Meunier, F.: In vitro evaluation of various antifungal agents alone and in combination by using an automatic turbidimetric system combined with viable count determinations. Antimicrob. Agents Chemother. *29*:997–1004, 1986.
363. van der Horst, C. M., Saag, M. S., Cloud, G. A., et al.: Treatment of cryptococcal meningitis associated with the acquired immunodeficiency syndrome. N. Engl. J. Med. *337*:15–21, 1997.
364. van der Kuy, P. H., and Hooymans, P. M.: Nortriptyline intoxication induced by terbinafine. B. M. J. *316*:441, 1998.
365. Vanden Bossche, H., Dromer, F., Improvisi, I., et al.: Antifungal drug resistance in pathogenic fungi. Med. Mycol. *36*(Suppl. 1):119–128, 1998.
366. Vanden Bossche, H., and Koymans, L.: Cytochromes P450 in fungi. Mycoses *41*(Suppl. 1):32–38, 1998.
367. Varhe, A., Olkkola, K. T., and Neuvonen, P. J.: Oral triazolam is potentially hazardous to patients receiving systemic antimycotics ketoconazole or itraconazole. Clin. Pharmacol. Ther. *56*:601–607, 1994.
368. Vazquez, J. A., Northland, R., Miller, S., et al.: Posaconazole compared to fluconazole for oral candidiasis in HIV-positive patients. Abstract 1107. *In* Abstracts of the 40th Interscience Conference on Antimicrobial Agents and Chemotherapy. Washington, D.C., American Society for Microbiology, 2000, p. 370.
369. Vermes, A., Guchelaar, H. J., and Dankert, J.: Flucytosine: A review of its pharmacology, clinical indications, pharmacokinetics, toxicity and drug interactions. J. Antimicrob. Chemother. *46*:171–179, 2000.
370. Vermes, A., van Der Sijs, H., and Guchelaar, H. J.: Flucytosine: Correlation between toxicity and pharmacokinetic parameters. Chemotherapy *46*:86–94, 2000.
371. Vickers, A. E., Sinclair, J. R., Zollinger, M., et al.: . Multiple cytochrome P-450s involved in the metabolism of terbinafine suggest a limited potential for drug-drug interactions. Drug Metab. Dispos. *27*:1029–1038, 1999.
372. Wainer, S., Cooper, P. A., Gouws, H., and Akierman, A.: Prospective study of fluconazole therapy in systemic neonatal fungal infection. Pediatr. Infect. Dis. J. *16*:763–767, 1997.
373. Wallace, T. L., Paetznick, V., Cossum, P. A., et al.: Activity of liposomal nystatin against disseminated *Aspergillus fumigatus* infection in neutropenic mice. Antimicrob. Agents Chemother. *41*:2238–2243, 1997.
374. Walsh, T. J., Finberg, R. W., Arndt, C., et al.: Liposomal amphotericin B for empirical therapy in patients with persistent fever and neutropenia. National Institute of Allergy and Infectious Diseases Mycoses Study Group. N. Engl. J. Med. *340*:764–771, 1999.
375. Walsh, T. J., Gharamani, P., Hodges, M. R., and Lutsar, I.: Efficacy and safety of voriconazole in the treatment of invasive fungal infections in children. Abstract 1100. *In* Abstracts of the 40th Interscience Conference on Antimicrobial Agents and Chemotherapy. Washington, D.C., American Society for Microbiology, 2000, p. 372.
376. Walsh, T. J., Gonzalez, C., Lyman, C. A., et al.: Invasive fungal infections in children: Recent advances in diagnosis and treatment. Adv. Pediatr. Infect. Dis. *11*:187–290, 1996.
377. Walsh, T. J., Gonzalez, C. E., Piscitelli, S., et al.: Correlation between in vitro and in vivo antifungal activities in experimental fluconazole-resistant oropharyngeal and esophageal candidiasis. J. Clin. Microbiol. *38*:2369–2373, 2000.
378. Walsh, T. J., Hiemenz, J. W., Seibel, N., et al.: Amphotericin B lipid complex for invasive fungal infections: Analysis of safety and efficacy in 556 cases. Clin. Infect. Dis. *26*:1383–1396, 1998.
379. Walsh, T. J., Melcher, G., Rinaldi, M., et al.: *Trichosporon beigelii:* An emerging pathogen resistant to amphotericin B. J. Clin. Microbiol. *28*:1616–1622, 1990.
380. Walsh, T. J., Newman, K. R., Moody, M., et al.: Trichosporonosis in patients with neoplastic disease. Medicine (Baltimore) *65*:268–279, 1986.
381. Walsh, T. J., Pappas, P., Winston, D., et al.: Voriconazole versus liposomal amphotericin B for empirical antifungal therapy of persistently febrile neutropenic patients: A randomized, international multicenter trial. Abstract L-1. *In* Abstract Addendum of the 40th International Conference on Antimicrobial Agents and Chemotherapy. Washington, D.C., American Society for Microbiology, 2000, p. 20.
382. Walsh, T. J., Peter, J., McGough, D. A., et al.: Activities of amphotericin B and antifungal azoles alone and in combination against *Pseudallescheria boydii.* Antimicrob. Agents Chemother. *39*:1361–1364, 1995.
383. Walsh, T. J., Seibel, N. L., Arndt, C., et al.: Amphotericin B lipid complex in pediatric patients with invasive fungal infections. Pediatr. Infect. Dis. J. *18*:702–708, 1999.
384. Walsh, T. J., Whitcomb, P., Piscitelli, S., et al.: Safety, tolerance, and pharmacokinetics of amphotericin B lipid complex in children with hepatosplenic candidiasis. Antimicrob. Agents Chemother. *41*:1944–1948, 1997.
385. Walsh, T. J., White, M., Seibel, N., et al.: Efficacy of early empirical fluconazole therapy in febrile neutropenic patients: Results of a randomized, double-blind, placebo-controlled, multicenter trial. Abstract LB-22. *In* Program addendum and late-breaker abstracts of the 36th Interscience Conference on Antimicrobial Agents and Chemotherapy. Washington, D.C., American Society for Microbiology, 1996.
386. Warnock, D. W., Turner, A., and Burke, J.: Comparison of high performance liquid chromatography and microbiological methods for determination of itraconazole. J. Antimicrob. Chemother. *21*:93–100, 1986.
387. Warwick, J. A., and Corrall, R. J.: Serious interaction between warfarin and oral terbinafine. B. M. J. *316*:440, 1998.
388. Weig, M., and Muller, F. M.: Synergism of voriconazole and terbinafine against *Candida albicans* isolates from human immunodeficiency virus–infected patients with oropharyngeal candidiasis. Antimicrob. Agents Chemother. *45*:966–968, 2001.
389. Weitkamp, J. H., Poets, C. F., Sievers, R., et al.: *Candida* infection in very low birth-weight infants: Outcome and nephrotoxicity of treatment with liposomal amphotericin B (AmBisome). Infection *26*:11–15, 1998.
390. Wheat, J., Hafner, R., Korzun, A. H., et al.: Itraconazole treatment of disseminated histoplasmosis in patients with the acquired immunodeficiency syndrome. Am. J. Med. *98*:336–342, 1995.
391. Wheat, J., Hafner, R., Wulfsohn, M., et al.: Prevention of relapse of histoplasmosis with itraconazole in patients with the acquired immunodeficiency syndrome. Ann. Intern. Med. *118*:610–616, 1993.
392. Wheat, J., McWhinney, S., Hafner, R., et al.: Treatment of histoplasmosis with fluconazole in patients with acquired immunodeficiency syndrome. National Institute of Allergy and Infectious Diseases Acquired Immunodeficiency Syndrome Clinical Trials Group and Mycoses Study Group. Am. J. Med. *103*:223–232, 1997.
393. Wheat, J., Sarosi, G., McKinsey, D., et al.: Practice guidelines for the management of patients with histoplasmosis. Infectious Diseases Society of America. Clin. Infect. Dis. *30*:688–695, 2000.
394. White, M. H., Anaissie, E. J., Kusne, S., et al.: Amphotericin B colloidal dispersion vs. amphotericin B as therapy for invasive aspergillosis. Clin. Infect. Dis. *24*:635–642, 1997.
395. White, M. H., Bowden, R. A., Sandler, E. S., et al.: Randomized, double-blind clinical trial of amphotericin B colloidal dispersion vs. amphotericin B in the empirical treatment of fever and neutropenia. Clin. Infect. Dis. *27*:296–302, 1998.
396. White, T. C.: Increased mRNA levels of ERG16, CDR, and MDR1 correlate with increases in azole resistance in *Candida albicans* isolates from a patient infected with human immunodeficiency virus. Antimicrob. Agents Chemother. *41*:1482–1487, 1997.
397. Williams, A. H., and Moore, J. E.: Multicenter study to evaluate the safety and efficacy of various doses of liposomal encapsulated nystatin in nonneutropenic patients with candidemia. Abstract 1420. *In* Program and Abstracts of the 39th Interscience Conference on Antimicrobial Agents and Chemotherapy. Washington, D.C., American Society for Microbiology, 1999, p. 567.
398. Wingard, J. R.: Infections due to resistant *Candida* species in patients with cancer who are receiving chemotherapy. Clin. Infect. Dis. *19*(Suppl. 1): 49–53, 1994.
399. Wingard, J. R., Kubilis, P., Lee, L., et al.: Clinical significance of nephrotoxicity in patients treated with amphotericin B for suspected or proven aspergillosis. Clin. Infect. Dis. *29*:1402–1407, 1999.
400. Wingard, J. R., Merz, W. G., Rinaldi, M. G., et al.: Increase in *Candida krusei* infection among patients with bone marrow transplantation and neutropenia treated prophylactically with fluconazole. N. Engl. J. Med. *325*:1274–1277, 1991.
401. Wingard, J. R., Merz, W. G., Rinaldi, M. G., et al.: Association of *Torulopsis glabrata* infections with fluconazole prophylaxis in neutropenic bone marrow transplant patients. Antimicrob. Agents Chemother. *37*:1847–1849, 1993.
402. Winston, D. J., Pakrasi, A., and Busuttil, R. W.: Prophylactic fluconazole in liver transplant recipients. A randomized, double-blind, placebo-controlled trial. Ann. Intern. Med.*131*:729–737, 1999.
403. Wong-Beringer, A., Jacobs, R. A., and Guglielmo, B. J.: Lipid formulations of amphotericin B: Clinical efficacy and toxicities. Clin. Infect. Dis. *27*:603–618, 1997.
404. Wright, D. G., Robichaud, K. J., Pizzo, P. A., and Deisseroth, A. B.: Lethal pulmonary reactions associated with the combined use of amphotericin B and leukocyte transfusions. N. Engl. J. Med. *304*:1185–1189, 1981.
405. Xu, X., Deluna, F., Nishime, J., et al.: Lack of metabolism-based drug interactions of MK-0991, a potent antifungal agent, in rats. Pharm. Res. *14*(Suppl. 11):558, 1997.
406. Yule, S. M., Walker, D., Cole, M., et al.: The effect of fluconazole on cyclophosphamide metabolism in children. Drug Metab. Dispos. *27*:417–421, 1999.

407. Zhanel, G. G., Saunders, D. G., Hoban, D. J., and Karlowsky, J. A.: Amphotericin B, azole, and 5-flucytosine pharmacodynamic parameters in the presence of human serum. Abstract 542. *In* Abstracts of the 39th Interscience Conference on Antimicrobial Agents and Chemotherapy. Washington, D.C., American Society for Microbiology, 1999, p. 23.

408. Zhou, H., Goldman, M., Wu, J., et al.: A pharmacokinetic study of intravenous itraconazole followed by oral administration of itraconazole capsules in patients with advanced human immunodeficiency virus infection. J. Clin. Pharmacol. *38*:593–602, 1998.

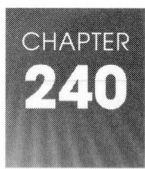

Drugs for Parasitic Infections

THE MEDICAL LETTER (PETER J. HOTEZ)

Parasitic infections are found throughout the world. With increasing travel, immigration, use of immunosuppressive drugs, and the spread of acquired immunodeficiency syndrome (AIDS), physicians anywhere may see infections caused by previously unfamiliar parasites. The table below lists first-choice and alternative drugs for most parasitic infections. The manufacturers of the drugs are listed at the end of the chapter. The table was modified from *The Medical Letter*—Drugs for Parasitic Infections.

Infection		Drug	Adult Dosage	Pediatric Dosage
Acanthamoeba keratitis				
Drug of choice:		See footnote 1		
AMEBIASIS *(Entamoeba histolytica)*				
asymptomatic				
Drug of choice:		Iodoquinol	650 mg tid × 20 d	30–40 mg/kg/d (max. 2 g) in 3 doses × 20 d
	OR	Paromomycin	25–35 mg/kg/d in 3 doses × 7 d	25–35 mg/kg/d in 3 doses × 7 d
Alternative:		Diloxanide furoate*	500 mg tid × 10 d	20 mg/kg/d in 3 doses × 10 d
mild to moderate intestinal disease[2]				
Drug of choice:		Metronidazole	500–750 mg tid × 7–10 d	35–50 mg/kg/d in 3 doses × 7–10 d
	OR	Tinidazole[3]*	2 g/d divided tid × 3 d	50 mg/kg (max. 2 g) qd × 3 d
severe intestinal and extraintestinal disease				
Drug of choice:[2]		Metronidazole	750 mg tid × 7–10 d	35–50 mg/kg/d in 3 doses × 7–10 d
	OR	Tinidazole[3]*	600 mg bid to 800 mg tid × 5 d	50–60 mg/kg/d (max. 2 d) × 5 d
AMEBIC MENINGOENCEPHALITIS, PRIMARY				
Naegleria				
Drug of choice:		Amphotericin B[4, 5]	1 mg/kg/d IV, uncertain duration	1 mg/kg/d IV, uncertain duration
Acanthamoeba				
Drug of choice:		See footnote 6		
Balamuthuia mandrillaris				
Drug of choice:		See footnote 7		

*Availability problems. See table on page 3119.

1. For treatment of keratitis caused by *Acanthamoeba*, concurrent topical use of 0.1% propamidine isethionate *(Brolene)* plus neomycin-polymyxin B-gramicidin ophthalmic solution has been successful (SL Hargrave et al, Ophthalmology, 106:952, 1999). In addition, 0.02% topical polyhexamethylene biguanide (PHMB) and/or chlorhexadine has been used successfully in a large number of patients (CF Radford et al, Br J Ophthalmol, 82:1387, 1998). PHMB is available as *Baquacil* (ICI America), a swimming pool disinfectant (E Yee and TK Winarko, Am J Hosp Pharm, 50:2523, 1993).
2. Treatment should be followed by a course of iodoquinol or paromomycin in the dosage used to treat asymptomatic amebiasis.
3. A nitro-imidazole similar to metronidazole, but not marketed in the United States, tinidazole appears to be at least as effective as metronidazole and better tolerated. Ornidazole, a similar drug, is also used outside the United States. Higher dosage is for hepatic abscess.
4. A *Naegleria* infection was treated successfully with intravenous and intrathecal use of both amphotericin B and miconazole, plus rifampin (J Seidel et al, N Engl J Med, 306:346, 1982). Other reports of successful therapy are questionable.
5. An approved drug, but considered investigational for this condition by the U.S. Food and Drug Administration.
6. Strains of *Acanthamoeba* isolated from fatal granulomatous amebic encephalitis are usually susceptible in vitro to pentamidine, ketoconazole (Nizoral), flucytosine (Ancobon) and (less so) to amphotericin B. One patient with disseminated cutaneous infection was treated successfully with intravenous pentamidine isethionate, topical chlorhexidine and 2% ketoconazole cream, followed by oral itraconazole (CA Slater et al, N Engl J Med, 331:85,1994).
7. A recently described free-living leptomyxid ameba that causes subacute to chronic granulomatous disease of the CNS. In vitro pentamidine isethionate 10 µg/ml is amebastatic (CF Denney et al, Clin Infect Dis, 25:1354, 1997). One patient, according to Medical Letter consultants, was successfully treated with clarithromycin (Biaxin) 500 mg tid, fluconazole (Diflucan) 400 mg once daily, sulfadiazine 1.5 g q6h and flucytosine (Ancobon) 1.5 g q6h.

Infection	Drug	Adult Dosage	Pediatric Dosage
ANCYLOSTOMA caninum (Eosinophilic enterocolitis)			
Drug of choice:	Albendazole[5]	400 mg once	400 mg once
	OR Mebendazole	100 mg bid × 3 d	100 mg bid × 3 d
	OR Pyrantel pamoate[5]	11 mg/kg (max. 1 g) × 3 d	11 mg/kg (max. 1 g) × 3 d
Ancylostoma duodenale, see HOOKWORM			
ANGIOSTRONGYLIASIS			
Angiostrongylus cantonensis			
Drug of choice:[8]	Mebendazole[5]	100 mg bid × 5 d	100 mg bid × 5 d
Angiostrongylus costaricensis			
Drug of choice:	Mebendazole[5]	200–400 mg tid × 10 d	200–400 mg tid × 10 d
Alternative:	Thiabendazole[5]	75 mg/kg/d in 3 doses × 3 d (max. 3 g/d)[9]	75 mg/kg/d in 3 doses × 3 d (max. 3 g/d)[9]
ANISAKIASIS (*Anisakis*)			
Treatment of choice:	Surgical or endoscopic removal		
ASCARIASIS (*Ascaris lumbricoides*, roundworm)			
Drug of choice:	Albendazole[5]	400 mg once	400 mg once
	OR Mebendazole	100 mg bid × 3 d or 500 mg once	100 mg bid × 3 d or 500 mg once
	OR Pyrantel pamoate[5]	11 mg/kg once (max. 1 g)	11 mg/kg once (max. 1 g)
BABESIOSIS (*Babesia microti*)			
Drugs of choice:[10]	Clindamycin[5]	1.2 g bid IV or 600 mg tid PO × 7 d	20–40 mg/kg/d PO in 3 doses × 7 d
	plus quinine	650 mg tid PO × 7 d	25 mg/kg/d PO in 3 doses × 7 d
	OR Atovaquone[5]	750 mg bid PO × 7–10 d	20 mg/kg bid PO × 7–10 d
	plus azithromycin[5]	1000 mg daily PO × 3d, then 500 mg daily × 7 d	12 mg/kg daily PO × 7–10 d
Balamuthuia mandrillaris, see AMEBIC MENINGOENCEPHALITIS, PRIMARY			
BALANTIDIASIS (*Balantidium coli*)			
Drug of choice:	Tetracycline[5, 11]	500 mg qid × 10 d	40 mg/kg/d (max. 2 g) in 4 doses × 10 d
Alternatives:	Iodoquinol[5]	650 mg tid × 20 d	40 mg/kg/d in 3 doses × 20 d
	Metronidazole[5]	750 mg tid × 5 d	35–50 mg/kg/d in 3 doses × 5 d
BAYLISASCARIASIS (*Baylisascaris procyonis*)			
Drug of choice:	See footnote 12		
BLASTOCYSTIS hominis infection			
Drug of choice:	See footnote 13		
CAPILLARIASIS (*Capillaria philippinensis*)			
Drug of choice:	Mebendazole[5]	200 mg bid × 20 d	200 mg bid × 20 d
Alternatives:	Albendazole[5]	400 mg daily × 10 d	400 mg daily × 10 d
Chagas disease, see TRYPANOSOMIASIS			
Clonorchis sinensis, see FLUKE infection			
CRYPTOSPORIDIOSIS (*Cryptosporidium*)			
Drug of choice:[14]	Nitazoxanide	500 mg bid	100–200 mg bid

*Availability problems. See table on page 3119.

8. Antiparasitic drugs can provoke neurologic symptoms, and most patients recover spontaneously without them. Analgesics, corticosteroids, and careful removal of CSF at frequent intervals can relieve symptoms (FD Pien and BC Pien, Int J Infect Dis, 3:161, 1999). Albendazole, levamisole (Ergamisol), or ivermectin have been used successfully in animals.
9. This dose is likely to be toxic and may have to be decreased.
10. Exchange transfusion has been used in severely ill patients with high (>10%) parasitemia (MR Boustani and JA Gelfard, Clin Infect Dis, 22:611, 1996). Combination therapy with atovaquone and azithromycin may be better tolerated (PJ Krause et al, American Society of Tropical Medicine and Hygiene Annual Meeting, 46:247, 1997, abstract 430). Concurrent use of pentamidine and trimethoprim-sulfamethoxazole has been reported to cure an infection with *B. divergens* (D Raoult et al, Ann Intern Med, 107:944, 1987).
11. Use of tetracyclines is contraindicated in pregnancy and in children less than 8 years old.
12. No drugs have been demonstrated to be effective. However, albendazole, mebendazole, thiabendazole, levamisole (Ergamisol) and ivermectin could be tried. Steroid therapy may be helpful, especially in eye and CNS infections. Ocular baylisascariasis has been treated successfully using laser photocoagulation therapy to destroy the intraretinal larvae.
13. Clinical significance of these organisms is controversial, but metronidazole 750 mg tid × 10 d or iodoquinol 650 mg tid × 20 d has been reported to be effective (DJ Stenzel and PFL Borenam, Clin Microbiol Rev, 9:563, 1996). Metronidazole resistance may be common (K Haresh et al, Trop Med Int Health, 4:274, 1999). Trimethoprim-sulfamethoxazole is an alternative regimen (UZ Ok et al, Am J Gastroenterol, 94:3245, 1999).
14. Treatment is not curative in immunocompromised patients and infection is self-limited in immunocompetent patients. Combination therapy with azithromycin 600 mg daily has been effective in some patients (NH Smith et al, J Infect Dis, 178:900, 1998). Nitazoxanide (an investigational drug in the USA manufactured by Romark Laboratories, Tampa, Florida, 813-282-8544, *www.romarklaboratories.com)* 500–1000 mg PO bid may be used as an alternative (J-F Rossignol et al, Trans R Soc Trop Med Hyg, 92:663, 1998). Duration of therapy is uncertain.

Infection	Drug	Adult Dosage	Pediatric Dosage
CUTANEOUS LARVA MIGRANS (creeping eruption, dog and cat hookworm)			
Drug of choice:	Albendazole[5]	400 mg daily × 3 d	400 mg daily × 3 d
	OR Ivermectin[5]	200 µg/kg daily × 1–2 d	200 µg/kg daily × 1–2 d
	OR Thiabendazole[15]	Topically	Topically
CYCLOSPORA **infection**			
Drug of choice:	Trimethoprim-sulfamethoxazole[5, 16]	TMP 160 mg, SMX 800 mg bid × 7 d	TMP 5 mg/kg, SMX 25 mg/kg bid × 7 d
CYSTICERCOSIS, see TAPEWORM infection			
DIENTAMOEBA fragilis infection			
Drug of choice:	Iodoquinol	650 mg tid × 20 d	30–40 mg/kg/d (max. 2 g) in 3 doses × 20 d
	OR Paromomycin[5]	25–35 mg/kg/d in 3 doses × 7 d	25–30 mg/kg/d in 3 doses × 7 d
	OR Tetracycline[5, 11]	500 mg qid × 10 d	40 mg/kg/d (max. 2 g) in 4 doses × 10 d
Diphyllobothrium latum, see TAPEWORM infection			
DRACUNCULUS medinensis (guinea worm) infection			
Drug of choice:	Metronidazole[5,17]	250 mg tid × 10 d	25 mg/kd/d (max. 750 mg) in 3 doses × 10 d
Echinococcus, see TAPEWORM infection			
Entamoeba histolytica, see AMEBIASIS			
ENTAMOEBA polecki infection			
Drug of choice:	Metronidazole[5]	750 mg tid × 10 d	35–50 mg/kg/d in 3 doses × 10 d
ENTEROBIUS vermicularis (pinworm) infection			
Drug of choice:	Pyrantel pamoate	11 mg/kg base once (max. 1 g); repeat in 2 wk	11 mg/kg once (max. 1 g) repeat in 2 wk
	OR Mebendazole	100 mg once; repeat in 2 wk	100 mg once; repeat in 2 wk
	OR Albendazole[5]	400 mg once; repeat in 2 wk	400 mg once; repeat in 2 wk
Fasciola hepatica, see FLUKE infection			
FILARIASIS			
Wuchereria bancrofti, Brugia malayi			
Drug of choice: [18, 19]	Diethylcarbamazine[20]*	Day 1: 50 mg, p.c. Day 2: 50 mg tid Day 3: 100 mg tid Days 4 through 14: 6 mg/kg/d in 3 doses	Day 1: 1 mg/kg p.c. Day 2: 1 mg/kg tid Day 3: 1–2 mg/kg tid Days 4 through 14: 6 mg/kg/d in 3 doses
Loa loa			
Drug of choice:[19, 21]	Diethylcarbamazine[20]*	Day 1: 50 mg p.c. Day 2: 50 mg tid Day 3: 100 mg tid Days 4 through 21: 9 mg/kg/d in 3 doses	Day 1: 1 mg/kg p.c. Day 2: 1 mg/kg tid Day 3: 1–2 mg/kg tid Days 4 through 21: 9 mg/kg/d in 3 doses
Mansonella ozzardi			
Drug of choice:	See footnote 22		
Mansonella perstans			
Drug of choice:	Mebendazole[5]	100 mg bid × 30 d	100 mg bid × 30 d
	OR Albendazole[5]	400 mg bid × 10 d	400 mg bid × 10 d

*Availability problems. See table on page 3119.

15. HD Davis et al, Arch Dermatol, 129: 588, 1993.
16. HIV infected patients may need higher dosage and long-term maintenance.
17. Not curative, but decreases inflammation and facilitates removing the worm. Mebendazole 400–800 mg/d for 6 d has been reported to kill the worm directly.
18. A single dose of ivermectin, 200 µg/kg, is effective for treatment of microfilaremia but does not kill the adult worm. In a limited study, single-dose diethylcarbamazine (6 mg/kg) was as macrofilaricidal as a multidose regimen against *W. bancrofti* (J Norões et al, Trans R Soc Trop Med Hyg, 91:78, 1997).
19. Antihistamines or corticosteroids may be required to decrease allergic reactions due to disintegration of microfilariae in treatment of filarial infections, especially those caused by *Loa loa*.
20. For patients with no microfilariae in the blood, full doses can be given from day one.
21. In heavy infections with *Loa loa*, rapid killing of microfilariae can provoke an encephalopathy. Apheresis has been reported to be effective in lowering microfilarial counts in patients heavily infected with *Loa loa* (EA Ottesen, Infect Dis Clin North Am, 7:619, 1993). Albendazole or ivermectin has also been used to reduce microfilaremia but because of slower onset of action, albendazole is preferred (AD Klion et al, J Infect Dis, 168: 202; 1993; M Kombila et al, Am J Trop Med Hyg, 58:458, 1998). Albendazole may be useful for treatment of loiasis when diethylcarbamazine is ineffective or cannot be used but repeated courses may be necessary (AD Klion et al, Clin Infect Dis, 29:680, 1999). Diethylcarbamazine, 300 mg once weekly, has been recommended for prevention of loiasis (TB Nutman et al, N Engl J Med, 319:752, 1988).
22. Diethylcarbamazine has no effect. Ivermectin, 200 µg/kg once, has been effective.

Infection	Drug	Adult Dosage	Pediatric Dosage
FILARIASIS—*(continued)*			
Mansonella streptocerca			
Drug of choice:[23]	Diethylcarbamazine*	6 mg/kg/d × 14 d	6 mg/kg/d × 14 d
	Ivermectin[5]	150 μg/kg once	150 μg/kg once
Tropical Pulmonary Eosinophilia (TPE)			
Drug of choice:	Diethylcarbamazine*	6 mg/kg/d in 3 doses × 21 d	6 mg/kd/d in 3 doses × 21 d
Onchocerca volvulus (River blindness)			
Drug of choice:	Ivermectin[24]	150 μg/kg once, repeated every 6–12 mo until asymptomatic	150 μg/kg once, repeated every 6–12 mo until asymptomatic
FLUKE, hermaphroditic, infection			
***Clonorchis sinensis* (Chinese liver fluke)**			
Drug of choice:	Praziquantel	75 mg/kg/d in 3 doses × 1 d	75 mg/kd/d in 3 doses × 1 d
	OR Albendazole[5]	10 mg/kg × 7 d	10 mg/kg × 7 d
***Fasciola hepatica* (sheep liver fluke)**			
Drug of choice:[25]	Triclabendazole*	10 mg/kg once	10 mg/kg once
Alternative:	Bithionol*	30–50 mg/kg on alternate days × 10–15 doses	30–50 mg/kg on alternate days × 10–15 doses
***Fasciolopsis buski, Heterophyes heterophyes, Metagonimus yokogawai* (intestinal flukes)**			
Drug of choice:	Praziquantel[5]	75 mg/kg/d in 3 doses × 1 d	75 mg/kg/d in 3 doses × 1 d
***Metorchis conjunctus* (North American liver fluke)[26]**			
Drug of choice:	Praziquantel[5]	75 mg/kg/d in 3 doses × 1 d	75 mg/kg/d in 3 doses × 1 d
Nanophyetus salmincola			
Drug of choice:	Praziquantel[5]	60 mg/kg/d in 3 doses × 1 d	60 mg/kg/d in 3 doses × 1 d
***Opisthorchis viverrini* (Southeast Asian liver fluke)**			
Drug of choice:	Praziquantel	75 mg/kg/d in 3 doses × 1 d	75 mg/kg/d in 3 doses × 1 d
***Paragonimus westermani* (lung fluke)**			
Drug of choice:	Praziquantel[5]	75 mg/kg/d in 3 doses × 2 d	75 mg/kg/d in 3 doses × 2 d
Alternative:[27]	Bithionol*	30–50 mg/kg on alternate days × 10–15 doses	30–50 mg/kg on alternate days × 10–15 doses
GIARDIASIS *(Giardia lamblia)*			
Drug of choice:	Metronidazole[5]	250 mg tid × 5 d	15 mg/kg/d in 3 doses × 5 d
Alternatives:[28]	Quinacrine[29]	100 mg PO tid × 5 d (max. 300 mg/d)	2 mg/kg PO tid × 5 d (max. 300 mg/d)
	Tinidazole*	2 g once	50 mg/kg once (max. 2 g)
	Furazolidone	100 mg qid × 7–10 d	6 mg/kg/d in 4 doses × 7–10 d
	Paromomycin[5, 30]	25–35 mg/kg/d in 3 doses × 7 d	25–35 mg/kg/d in 3 doses × 7 d
GNATHOSTOMIASIS *(Gnathostoma spinigerum)*			
Treatment of choice:[31]	Surgical removal		
	OR Albendazole[5]	400 mg bid × 21 d	400 mg bid × 21 d
GONGYLONEMIASIS *(Gongylonema* sp.*)*			
Treatment of choice:[32]	Surgical removal		
	OR Albendazole[5]	10 mg/kg/d × 3 d	10 mg/kg/d × 3 d
HOOKWORM infection *(Ancylostoma duodenale, Necator americanus)*			
Drug of choice:	Albendazole[5]	400 mg once	400 mg once
	OR Mebendazole	100 mg bid × 3 d or 500 mg once	100 mg bid × 3 d or 500 mg once
	OR Pyrantel pamoate[5]	11 mg/kg (max. 1 g) × 3 d	11 mg/kg (max. 1 g) × 3 d

*Availability problems. See table on page 3119.

23. Diethylcarbamazine is potentially curative due to activity against both adult worms and microfilariae, but is not available in the United States for this indication from the CDC. Ivermectin is only active against microfilariae.
24. Annual treatment with ivermectin 150 μg/kg can prevent blindness due to ocular onchocerciasis (D Mabey et al, Ophthalmology, 103:1001, 1996).
25. Unlike infections with other flukes, *Fasciola hepatica* infections may not respond to praziquantel. Triclabendazole (Fasinex–Novartis), a veterinary fasciolide, may be safe and effective but data are limited (R López-Vélez et al, Eur J Clin Microbiol, 18:525, 1999). It should be given with food for better absorption.
26. JD MacLean et al, Lancet, 347:154, 1996.
27. Triclabendazole may be effective in a dosage of 5 mg/kg once daily for 3 days or 10 mg/kg twice in one day (M Calvopiña et al, Trans R Soc Trop Med Hyg, 92:566, 1998).
28. Albendazole 400 mg daily × 5 d may be effective (A Hall and Q Nahar, Trans R Soc Trop Med Hyg, 87:84, 1993). Bacitracin zinc or bacitracin 120,000 U bid for 10 days may also be effective (BJ Andrews et al, Am J Trop Med Hyg, 52:318, 1995).
29. Quinacrine is not available commercially, but as a service can be compounded by Medical Center Pharmacy, New Haven, CT (203-688-6816) or Panorama Compounding Pharmacy 6744 Balboa Blvd, Van Nuys, CA 91406 (800-247-9767).
30. Not absorbed; may be useful for treatment of giardiasis in pregnancy.
31. Ivermectin has been reported to be effective in animals but there are few data in humans (MT Anantaphruti et al, Trop Med Parasitol, 43:65, 1992; R Ruiz-Maldonado and MA Mosqueda-Cabrera, Int J Dermatol, 38:52, 1999).
32. M Eberhard et al, Am J Trop Med Hyg, 61:51, 1999.

Infection	Drug	Adult Dosage	Pediatric Dosage
Hydatid cyst, see TAPEWORM infection			
Hymenolepis nana, see TAPEWORM infection			
ISOSPORIASIS *(Isospora belli)*			
Drug of choice:	Trimethoprim-sulfamethoxazole[5, 33]	160 mg TMP, 800 mg SMX qid × 10 d, then bid × 3 wk	TMP 5 mg/kg, SMX 25 mg/kg bid × 10 d
LEISHMANIASIS (Cutaneous due to *L. mexicana, L. tropica, L. major, L. braziliensis;* mucocutaneous mostly due to *L. braziliensis;* visceral due to *L. donovani* (Kala-azar), *L. infantum, L. chagasi)*			
Drug of choice:[34]	Sodium stibogluconate*	20 mg Sb/kg/d IV or IM × 20–28 d[35]	20 mg Sb/kg/d IV or IM × 20–28 d[35]
	OR Meglumine antimonate*	20 mg Sb/kg/d IV or IM × 20–28 d[35]	20 mg Sb/kg/d IV or IM × 20–28 d[35]
	OR Amphotericin B[5]	0.5 to 1 mg/kg IV daily or every 2 d for up to 8 wk	0.5 to 1 mg/kg IV daily or every 2 d for up to 8 wk
	OR Liposomal Amphotericin B[36]	3 mg/kg/d (days 1-5) and 3 mg/kg/d days 14, 21[37]	3 mg/kg/d (days 1-5) and 3 mg/kg/d days 14, 21[37]
Alternatives:	Pentamidine	2–4 mg/kg daily or every 2 d IV or IM for up to 15 doses[38]	2–4 mg/kg daily or every 2 d IV or IM for up to 15 doses[38]
	OR Paromomycin[39]*	Topically twice daily × 10–20 d	
LICE infestation *(Pediculus humanus, P. capitis, Phthirus pubis)*[40]			
Drug of choice:	1% Permethrin[41]	Topically	Topically
	OR 0.5% Malathion[42]	Topically	Topically
Alternative:	Pyrethrins with piperonyl butoxide[41]	Topically	Topically
	OR Ivermectin[5, 43]	200 µg/kg once	200 µg/kg once
Loa loa, see FILARIASIS			
MALARIA, Treatment of *(Plasmodium falciparum, P. ovale, P. vivax,* and *P. malariae)*			
Chloroquine-resistant *P. falciparum*[44]			
ORAL			
Drugs of choice:	Quinine sulfate	650 mg q8h × 3–7 d[45]	25 mg/kg/d in 3 doses × 3–7 d[45]
	plus doxycycline[5, 11]	100 mg bid × 7 d	2 mg/kg/d × 7 d
	or plus tetracycline[5, 11]	250 mg qid × 7 d	6.25 mg/kg qid × 7 d
	or plus pyrimethamine-sulfadoxine[46]	3 tablets at once on last day of quinine	<1 yr: ¼ tablet 1–3 yr: ½ tablet 4–8 yr: 1 tablet 9–14 yr: 2 tablets
	or plus clindamycin[5, 47]	900 mg tid × 5 d	20–40 mg/kg/d in 3 doses × 5 d

*Availability problems. See table on page 3119.

33. In sulfonamide-sensitive patients, pyrimethamine 50–75 mg daily in divided doses has been effective (JP Ackers, Semin Gastrointest Dis, 8:33, 1997).
34. For treatment of kala-azar, oral miltefosine 100–150 mg daily for 4 weeks was 97% effective after 6 months. Gastrointestinal adverse effects are common and the drug is contraindicated in pregnancy (TK Jha et al, N Engl J Med, 341: 1795, 1999).
35. May be repeated or continued. A longer duration may be needed for some forms of visceral leishmaniasis (BL Herwaldt, Lancet, 354:1191, 1999).
36. Three preparations of lipid-encapsulated amphotericin B have been used for treatment of visceral leishmaniasis. Largely based on clinical trials in patients infected with *L. infantum*, the FDA approved liposomal amphotericin B (AmBisome) for treatment of visceral leishmaniasis (A Meyerhoff, Clin Infect Dis, 28:42, 1999; JD Berman, Clin Infect Dis, 28:49, 1999). Amphotericin B lipid complex (Abelcet) and amphotericin B cholesteryl sulfate (Amphotec) have also been used with good results. Some studies indicate that *L. donovani* resistant to pentavalent antimonial agents may respond to lipid-encapsulated amphotericin B (S Sundar et al, Ann Trop Med Parasitol, 92:755, 1998).
37. The dose of immunocompromised patients with HIV is 4 mg/kg/d (days 1–5) and 4 mg/kg/d on days 10, 17, 24, 31, 38. The relapse rate is high, suggesting that maintenance therapy may be indicated.
38. 4 mg/kg qod × 15 doses for *L. donovani*; 2 mg/kg qod × 7 or 3 mg/kg qod × 4 doses for cutaneous disease.
39. Two preparations of paromomycin have been studied. The first, a formulation of 15% paromomycin and 12% methylbenzethonium chloride in soft white paraffin for topical use, has been reported to be effective in some patients against cutaneous leishmaniasis due to *L. major* (O Ozgoztasi and I Baydar, Int J Dermatol, 36:61, 1997). The second, injectable paromomycin (aminosidine, not available in the United States), has been used successfully for the treatment of kala-azar in India where antimony resistance is common (TK Jha et al, BMJ, 316:1200, 1998).
40. For infestation of eyelashes with crab lice, use petrolatum. For pubic lice, treat with 5% permethrin or ivermectin as for scabies (see page 3116).
41. A second application is recommended one week later to kill hatching progeny. Some lice are resistant to pyrethrins and permethrin (RJ Pollack, Arch Pediatr Adolesc Med, 153:969, 1999).
42. Medical Letter, 41:73, 1999.
43. Ivermectin is effective against adult lice but has no effect on nits (TA Bell, Pediatr Infect Dis J, 17:923, 1998).
44. Chloroquine-resistant *P. falciparum* occur in all malarious areas except Central America west of the Panama Canal Zone, Mexico, Haiti, the Dominican Republic, and most of the Middle East (chloroquine resistance has been reported in Yemen, Oman, Saudi Arabia, and Iran).
45. In Southeast Asia, relative resistance to quinine has increased and the treatment should be continued for seven days.
46. Fansidar tablets contain 25 mg of pyrimethamine and 500 mg of sulfadoxine. Resistance to pyrimethamine-sulfadoxine has been reported from Southeast Asia, the Amazon basin, sub-Saharan Africa, Bangladesh, and Oceania.
47. For use in pregnancy.

Infection	Drug	Adult dosage	Pediatric Dosage
MALARIA, Treatment of *(continued)*			
Chloroquine-resistant *P. falciparum* *(continued)*			
Alternatives[48]:	Mefloquine[49, 50]	750 mg followed by 500 mg 12 hr later	15 mg/kg PO followed by 10 mg/kg PO 8-12 hr later (<45 kg)
	Halofantrine[51]*	500 mg q6h × 3 doses; repeat in 1 wk[52]	8 mg/kg q6h × 3 doses (<40 kg); repeat in 1 wk[52]
	OR Atovaquone/ proguanil[53]	2 adult tablets bid × 3d	11-20 kg: 1 adult tablet/day × 3d 21-30 kg: 2 adult tablets/day × 3d 31-40 kg: 3 adults tablets/day × 3d >40 kg: 2 adult tablets bid × 3d
Alternatives[54]:	Mefloquine[55, 56]	750 mg followed by 500 mg 12 hr later	<45 kg: 15 mg/kg PO followed by 10 mg/kg PO 8-12 hr later
	Halofantrine[57]*	500 mg q6h × doses; repeat in 1 wk[58]	<40 kg: 8 mg/kg q6h × 3 doses; repeat in 1 wk[58]
	OR Artesunate[59]*	4 mg/kg/d × 3d	
	plus mefloquine[55, 56]	750 mg followed by 500 mg 12 hr later	15 mg/kg followed 8–12 hr later by 10 mg/kg
Chloroquine-resistant *P. vivax*[54]			
Drug of choice:	Quinine sulfate	650 mg q8h × 3–7 d[45]	25 mg/kg/d in 3 doses × 3–7 d[45]
	plus doxycycline[5, 11]	100 mg bid × 7 d	2 mg/kg/d × 7 d
	OR Mefloquine	750 mg followed by 500 mg 12 hr later	15 mg/kg followed 8–12 hr later by 10 mg/kg
Alternatives:	Halofantrine[51, 55]*	500 mg q6h × 3 doses	8 mg/kg q6h × 3 doses
	Chloroquine	25 mg base/kg in 3 doses over 48 hr	
	plus primaquine[56]	2.5 mg base/kg in 3 doses over 48 hr	

*Availability problems. See table on page 3119.

48. For treatment of multiple-drug-resistant *P. falciparum* in Southeast Asia, especially Thailand, where resistance to mefloquine and halofantrine is frequent, a 7-day course of quinine and tetracycline is recommended (G Watt et al, Am J Trop Med Hyg, 47:108, 1992). Artesunate plus mefloquine (C Luxemburger et al, Trans R Soc Trop Med Hyg, 88:213, 1994), artemether plus mefloquine (J Karbwang et al, Trans R Soc Trop Med Hyg, 89:296, 1995) or mefloquine plus doxycycline are also used to treat multiple-drug-resistant *P. falciparum*.
49. At this dosage, adverse effects including nausea, vomiting, diarrhea, dizziness, disturbed sense of balance, toxic psychosis, and seizures can occur. Mefloquine is teratogenic in animals and should not be used for treatment of malaria in pregnancy. It should not be given together with quinine, quinidine, or halofantrine, and caution is required in using quinine, quinidine, or halofantrine to treat patients with malaria who have taken mefloquine for prophylaxis. The pediatric dosage has not been approved by the FDA. Resistance to mefloquine has been reported in some areas, such as the Thailand-Myanmar and -Cambodia borders and in the Amazon basin, where 25 mg/kg should be used.
50. In the United States, a 250-mg tablet of mefloquine contains 228 mg mefloquine base. Outside the United States, each 275-mg tablet contains 250 mg base.
51. May be effective in multiple-drug-resistant *P. falciparum* malaria, but treatment failures and resistance have been reported, and the drug has caused lengthening of the PR and QTc intervals and fatal cardiac arrhythmias. It should not be used for patients with cardiac conduction defects or with other drugs that may affect the QT interval, such as quinine, quinidine, and mefloquine. Cardiac monitoring is recommended. Variability in absorption is a problem; halofantrine should not be taken one hour before to two hours after meals because food increases its absorption. It should not be used in pregnancy.
52. A single 250-mg dose can be used for repeat treatment in mild to moderate infections (JE Touze et al, Lancet, 349:255, 1997).
53. Atovaquone plus proguanil is available as a fixed-dose combination tablet: adult tablets (250 mg atovaquone/100 mg proguanil, Malarone) and pediatric tablets (62.5 mg atovaquone/25 mg proguanil, Malarone pediatric). To enhance absorption, it should be taken within 45 minutes after eating (S Looareesuwan et al, Am J Trop Med Hyg 1999;60:533). Although approved for once daily dosing, to decrease nausea and vomiting the dose for treatment is usually divided in two.
54. For treatment of multiple-drug-resistant *P. falciparum* in Southeast Asia, especially Thailand where resistance to mefloquine and halofantrine is frequent, a 7-day course of quinine and tetracycline is recommended (G Watt et al, Am J Trop Med Hyg 1992; 47:108). Artesunate plus mefloquine (C Luxemburger et al, Trans R Soc Trop Med Hyg 1994; 88:213), artemether plus mefloquine plus mefloquine (J Karbwang et al, Trans R Soc Trop Med Hyg 1995; 89:296), mefloquine plus doxycycline, or atovaquone/Proguanil may also be used to treat multiple-drug-resistant *P. falciparum*.
55. At this dosage, adverse effects including nausea, vomiting, diarrhea, dizziness, disturbed sense of balance, toxic psychosis, and seizures can occur. Mefloquine is teratogenic in animals and should not be used for treatment of malaria in pregnancy. It should not be given together with quinine, quinidine, or halofantrine, and caution is required in using quinine, quinidine, or halofantrine to treat patients with malaria who have taken mefloquine for prophylaxis. The pediatric dosage has not been approved by the FDA. Resistance to mefloquine has been reported in some areas, such as the Thailand-Myanmar and -Cambodia borders and in the Amazon basin, where 25 mg/kg should be used.
56. In the United States, a 250-mg tablet of mefloquine contains 228 mg mefloquine base. Outside the United States, each 275-mg tablet contains 250 mg base.

Infection	Drug	Adult Dosage	Pediatric Dosage
MALARIA, Treatment of *(continued)*			
All *Plasmodium* except Chloroquine-resistant *P. falciparum*[44] and Chloroquine-resistant *P. vivax*[54]			
ORAL			
Drug of choice:	Chloroquine phosphate[57]	1 gram (600 mg base), then 500 mg (300 mg base) 6 hr later, then 500 mg (300 mg base) at 24 and 48 hr	10 mg base/kg (max. 600 mg base), then 5 mg base/kg 6 hr later, then 5 mg base/kg at 24 and 48 hr
All *Plasmodium*			
PARENTERAL			
Drug of choice:[58]	Quinidine gluconate[59, 60]	10 mg/kg loading dose (max. 600 mg) in normal saline slowly over 1–2 hr, followed by continuous infusion of 0.02 mg/kg/min until oral therapy can be started	Same as adult dose
	OR Quinine dihydrochloride[59, 60]	20 mg/kg loading dose IV in 5% dextrose over 4 hr, followed by 10 mg/kg over 2–4 hr q8h (max. 1800 mg/d) until oral therapy can be started	Same as adult dose
Alternative:	Artemether[61]*	3.2 mg/kg IM, then 1.6 mg/kg daily × 5–7 d	Same as adult dose
Prevention of relapses: *P. vivax* and *P. ovale* only			
Drug of choice:	Primaquine phosphate[56, 62]	26.3 mg (15 mg base)/d × 14 d or 79 mg (45 mg base)/wk × 8 wk	0.3 mg base/kg/d × 14 d
MALARIA, Prevention of[63]			
Chloroquine-sensitive areas[44]			
Drug of choice:	Chloroquine phosphate[64, 65]	500 mg (300 mg base), once/wk[66]	5 mg/kg base once/wk, up to adult dose of 300 mg base[66]
Chloroquine- resistant areas[44]			
Drug of choice:	Mefloquine [50, 65, 67]	250 mg once/wk[66]	<15 kg: 5 mg/kg[66] 15–19 kg: ¼ tablet[66] 20–30 kg: ½ tablet[66] 31–45 kg: ¾ tablet[66] >45 kg: 1 tablet[66]
	OR Doxycycline[5, 65]	100 mg daily[68]	2 mg/kg/d, up to 100 mg/day[68]
	OR Atovaquone/ Proguanil[53]	250 mg/100 mg (1 tablet) daily[69]	11–20 kg: 62.5 mg/25 mg[69] 21–30 kg: 125 mg/50 mg[69] 31–40 kg: 187.5 mg/75 mg[69]
Alternative:	Primaquine[5, 56, 70]	30 mg base daily	0.5 mg/kg base daily

*Availability problems. See table on page 3119.

57. If chloroquine phosphate is not available, hydroxychloroquine sulfate is as effective; 400 mg of hydroxychloroquine sulfate is equivalent to 500 mg of chloroquine phosphate.
58. Exchange transfusion has been helpful for some patients with high-density (>10%) parasitemia, altered mental status, pulmonary edema, or renal complications (KD Miller et al, N Engl J Med, 321:65, 1989).
59. Continuous EKG, blood pressure, and glucose monitoring are recommended, especially in pregnant women and young children. For problems with availability, call the manufacturer (Eli Lilly, 800-821-0538) or the CDC Malaria Hotline (770-488-7788).
60. Quinidine may have greater antimalarial activity than quinine. The loading dose should be decreased or omitted in those patients who have received quinine or mefloquine. If more than 48 hours of parenteral treatment is required, the quinine or quinidine dose should be reduced by ⅓ to ½.
61. NJ White, N Engl J Med, 335:800,1996. Not available in the United States.
62. Relapses have been reported with this regimen, and should be treated with a second 14-day course of 30 mg base/day.
63. No drug regimen guarantees protection against malaria. If fever develops within a year (particularly within the first two months) after travel to malarious areas, travelers should be advised to seek medical attention. Insect repellents, insecticide-impregnated bed nets, and proper clothing are important adjuncts for malaria prophylaxis.
64. In pregnancy, chloroquine prophylaxis has been used extensively and safely.
65. For prevention of attack after departure from areas where *P. vivax* and *P. ovale* are endemic, which includes almost all areas where malaria is found (except Haiti), some experts prescribe in addition primaquine phosphate 15 mg base (26.3 mg)/d or, for children, 0.3 mg base/kg/d during the last 2 weeks of prophylaxis. Others prefer to avoid the toxicity of primaquine and rely on surveillance to detect cases when they occur, particularly when exposure was limited or doubtful. See also footnotes 56 and 62.
66. Beginning 1 to 2 weeks before travel and continuing weekly for the duration of stay and for 4 weeks after leaving.

Infection	Drug	Adult Dosage	Pediatric Dosage
MALARIA, Prevention of *(continued)*			
Chloroquine-resistant areas[49]			
Alternatives:	Chloroquine phosphate	500 mg (300 mg base) once/wk[71]	5 mg/kg base once/week, up to adult dose of 300 mg base[71]
	plus proguanil[74]	200 mg once/day	<2yr: 50 mg once/day 2–6 yr: 100 mg once/day 7–10 yr: 150 mg once/day >10 yr: 200 mg once/day
Presumptive treatment	Atovaquone/ proguanil[53]	2 adult tablets bid × 3 d[73]	11–20 kg: one adult tablet/day × 3 d[73] 21–30 kg: 2 adult tablets/day × 3 d[73] 31–40 kg: 3 adult tablets/day × 3 d[73] >40 kg: 2 adult tablets bid × 3 d[73]
	OR Pyrimethamine-sulfadoxine[51]	Carry a single dose (3 tablets) for self treatment of febrile illness when medical care is not immediately available	<1 yr: 1/4 tablet 1–3 yrs: 1/2 tablet 4–8 yrs: 1 tablet 9–14 yrs: 2 tablets
MICROSPORIDIOSIS			
Ocular *(Encephalitozoon hellem, Encephalitozoon cuniculi, Vittaforma corneae (Nosema corneum))*			
Drug of choice:	Albendazole[7] plus fumagillin[72]*	400 mg bid	
Intestinal *(Enterocytozoon bieneusi, Encephalitozoon (Septata) intestinalis)*			
E. bieneusi[75]			
Drug of choice:	Fumagillin*	60 mg/d PO × 14d	
E. intestinalis			
Drug of choice:	Albendazole[7]	400 mg bid × 21d	
Disseminated *(E. hellem, E. cuniculi, E. intestinalis, pleistophora* sp., *Trachipleistophora* sp. and *Brachiola vesicularum)*			
Drug of choice[76]	Albendazole[7]	400 mg bid	
Mites, see SCABIES			
MONILIFORMIS moniliformis infection			
Drug of choice:	Pyrantel pamoate[5]	11 mg/kg once, repeat twice, 2 wk apart	11 mg/kg once, repeat twice, 2 wk apart
Naegleria species, see AMEBIC MENINGOENCEPHALITIS, PRIMARY			
Necator americanus, see HOOKWORM infection			
OESOPHAGOSTOMUM bifurcum			
Drug of choice:	See footnote 74		
Onchocerca volvulus, see FILARIASIS			
Opisthorchis viverrini, see FLUKE infection			
Paragonimus westermani, see FLUKE infection			
Pediculus capitis, humanus, Phthirus pubis, see LICE			
Pinworm, see ENTEROBIUS			

*Availability problems. See table on page 3119.

67. The pediatric dosage has not been approved by the FDA, and the drug has not been approved for use during pregnancy. However, it has been reported to be safe for prophylactic use during the second or third trimester of pregnancy and possibly during early pregnancy as well (CDC Health Information for International Travel, 1999–2000, p. 120; BL Smoak et al, J Infect Dis, 176:831, 1997). Mefloquine is not recommended for patients with cardiac conduction abnormalities. Patients with a history of seizures or psychiatric disorders should avoid mefloquine (Medical Letter, 32:13, 1990). Resistance to mefloquine has been reported in some areas, such as Thailand; in these areas, doxycycline should be used for prophylaxis. In children less than 8 years old, proguanil plus sulfisoxazole has been used (KN Suh and JS Keystone, Infect Dis Clin Pract, 5:541, 1996).
68. Beginning 1–2 days before travel and continuing for the duration of stay and for 4 weeks after leaving. Use of tetracyclines is contraindicated in pregnancy and in children less than 8 years old. Doxycycline can cause gastrointestinal disturbances, vaginal moniliasis, and photosensitivity reactions.
69. GE Shanks et al, Clin Infect Dis, 27:494, 1998; B Lell et al, Lancet, 351:709, 1998. Beginning 1 to 2 days before travel and continuing for the duration of stay and for 1 week after leaving.
70. Several studies have shown that daily primaquine beginning one day before departure and continued until two days after leaving the malaria area provides effective prophylaxis against chloroquine-resistant *P. falciparum* (E Schwartz and G Regev-Yochay, Clin Infect Dis, 29:1502, 1999). Some studies have shown less efficacy against *P. vivax*.
71. In areas with strains resistant to pyrimethamine-sulfadoxine, atovaquone/proguanil or atovaquone plus doxycycline can also be used for presumptive treatment. See page 3113 for dosage.
72. Ocular lesions due to *E. hellem* in HIV-infected patients have responded to fumagillin eyedrops prepared from Fumidil-B, a commercial product (Mid-Continent Agrimarketing, Inc., Olathe, Kansas, 1-800-547-1392) used to control a microsporidial disease of honey bees (MC Diesenhouse, Am J Ophthalmol, 115:293, 1993). For lesions due to *V. corneae*, topical therapy is generally not effective and keratoplasty may be required (RM Davis et al, Ophthalmology, 97:953, 1990).
73. Octreotide (Sandostatin) has provided symptomatic relief in some patients with large-volume diarrhea. Oral fumagillin (see footnote 73) has been effective in treating *E. bieneusi* (J-M Molina et al, AIDS, 11:1603, 1997), but has been associated with thrombocytopenia. Highly active antiretroviral therapy may lead to microbiologic and clinical response in HIV-infected patients with microsporidial diarrhea (NA Foudraine et al, AIDS, 12:35, 1998; A Carr et al, Lancet, 351:256, 1998).
74. Albendazole or pyrantel pamoate may be effective (HP Krepel et al, Trans R Soc Trop Med Hyg, 87:87, 1993)
75. Oral fumagillin (see footnote 72, Sanofi Recherche, Gentilly France) has been effective in treating *E. bieneusi* (J-M Molina et al, AIDS 2000; 14:1341), but has been associated with thrombocytopenia. Highly active antiretroviral therapy (HAART) may lead to microbiologic and clinical response in HIV-infected patients with microsporidial diarrhea (NA Foudraine et al, AIDS 1998; 12:35; A Carr et al, Lancet 1998; 351:256). Octreotide (Sandostatin) has provided symptomatic relief in some patients with large volume diarrhea.
76. J-M Molina et al, J Infect Dis 1995; 171:245. There is no established treatment for *Pleistophora*.

Infection	Drug	Adult Dosage	Pediatric Dosage
***PNEUMOCYSTIS** carinii* pneumonia (PCP)[77]			
Drug of choice:	Trimethoprim-sulfamethoxazole	TMP 15 mg/kg/d, SMX 75 mg/kg/d,oral or IV in 3 or 4 doses × 14–21 d	Same as adult dose
Alternatives:	Pentamidine	3–4 mg/kg IV daily × 14–21 d	Same as adult dose
	OR Trimethoprim[5]	5 mg/kg PO tid × 21 d	
	plus dapsone[5]	100 mg PO daily × 21 d	
	OR Atovaquone	750 mg bid PO × 21 d	
	OR Primaquine[5,56]	30 mg base PO daily × 21 d	
	plus clindamycin[5]	600 mg IV q6h × 21 d, or 300–450 mg PO q6h × 21 d	
Primary and secondary prophylaxis			
Drug of Choice:	Trimethoprim-sulfamethoxazole	1 tab (single or double strength) PO daily or 1 DS tab 3 × /week	TMP 150 mg/m^2, SMX 750 mg/m^2 in 2 doses PO on 3 consecutive d/wk
Alternatives:[78]	Dapsone[5]	50 mg PO bid, or 100 mg PO daily	2 mg/kg (max. 100 mg) PO daily OR 4 mg/kg (max. 200 mg each week)
	OR Dapsone[5]	50 mg PO daily or 200 mg each wk	
	plus pyrimethamine[79]	50 mg or 75 mg PO/each wk	
	OR Pentamidine aerosol	300 mg inhaled monthly via Respirgard II nebulizer	>5 yr: same as adult dose
	OR Atovaquone[5]	1500 mg daily PO	
Roundworm, see ASCARIASIS			
SCABIES *(Sarcoptes scabiei)*			
Drug of choice:	5% Permethrin	Topically	Topically
Alternatives:	Ivermectin[5, 80]	200 μg/kg PO once	200 μg/kg PO once
	10% Crotamiton	Topically	Topically
SCHISTOSOMIASIS *(Bilharziasis)*			
S. haematobium			
Drug of choice:	Praziquantel	40 mg/kg/d in 2 doses × 1 d	40 mg/kg/d in 2 doses × 1 d
S. japonicum			
Drug of choice:	Praziquantel	60 mg/kg/d in 3 doses × 1 d	60 mg/kg/d in 3 doses × 1 d
S. mansoni			
Drug of choice:	Praziquantel	40 mg/kg/d in 2 doses × 1 d	40 mg/kg/d in 2 doses × 1 d
Alternative:	Oxamniquine[81]	15 mg/kg once[82]	20 mg/kg/d in 2 doses × 1 d[82]
S. mekongi			
Drug of choice:	Praziquantel	60 mg/kg/d in 3 doses × 1 d	60 mg/kg/d in 3 doses × 1 d
Sleeping sickness, see TRYPANOSOMIASIS			
STRONGYLOIDIASIS *(Strongyloides stercoralis)*			
Drug of choice:[83]	Ivermectin	200 μg/kg/d × 1–2 d	200 μg/kg/d × 1–2 d
Alternative:	Thiabendazole	50 mg/kg/d in 2 doses (max. 3 g /d) × 2 d[9]	50 mg/kg/d in 2 doses (max. 3 g /d) × 2 d[9]

*Availability problems. See table on page 3119.

77. In severe disease with room air Po_2 ≤70 mm Hg or Aa gradient ≥35 mm Hg, prednisone should also be used (S Gagnon et al, N Engl J Med, 323:1444, 1990; E Caumes et al, Clin Infect Dis, 18:319, 1994).
78. Weekly therapy with sulfadoxine 500 mg/pyrimethamine 25 mg/leucovorin 25 mg was effective PCP prophylaxis in liver transplant patients (J Torre-Cisneros et al, Clin Infect Dis, 29:771, 1999).
79. Plus leucovorin 25 mg with each dose of pyrimethamine.
80. Effective for crusted scabies in immunocompromised patients (M Larralde et al, Pediatr Dermatol, 16:69, 1999; A Patel et al, Australas J Dermatol, 40:37, 1999).
81. Oxamniquine has been effective in some areas in which praziquantel is less effective (FF Stelma et al, J Infect Dis, 176:304, 1997). Oxamniquine is contraindicated in pregnancy.
82. In East Africa, the dose should be increased to 30 mg/kg, and in Egypt and South Africa, 30 mg/kg/d × 2d. Some experts recommend 40–60 mg/kg over 2–3 days in all of Africa (KC Shekhar, Drugs, 42:379, 1991).
83. In immunocompromised patients or disseminated disease, it may be necessary to prolong or repeat therapy or use other agents. A veterinary parenteral formulation of invermectin was used in one patient (PL Chiodini et al, Lancet, 355:43, 2000).

Infection	Drug	Adult Dosage	Pediatric Dosage
TAPEWORM infection — **Adult (intestinal stage)**			
Diphyllobothrium latum **(fish),** ***Taenia saginata*** **(beef),** ***Taenia solium*** **(pork),** ***Dipylidium caninum*** **(dog)**			
Drug of choice:	Praziquantel[5]	5–10 mg/kg once	5–10 mg/kg once
Alternative:	Niclosamide	2 g once	50 mg/kg once
Hymenolepis nana **(dwarf tapeworm)**			
Drug of choice:	Praziquantel[5]	25 mg/kg once	25 mg/kg once
-Larval (tissue stage)			
Echinococcus granulosus **(hydatid cyst)**			
Drug of choice:[84]	Albendazole	400 mg bid × 1–6 mo	15 mg/kg/d (max. 800 mg) × 1–6 mo
Echinococcus multilocularis			
Treatment of choice:	See footnote 85		
Cysticercus cellulosae **(cysticercosis)**			
Treatment of choice:	See footnote 86		
Alternative:	Albendazole	400 mg bid × 8–30 d; can be repeated as necessary	15 mg/kg/d (max. 800 mg) in 2 doses × 8–30 d: can be repeated as necessary
	OR Praziquantel[5]	50–100 mg/kg/d in 3 doses × 30 d	50–100 mg/kg/d in 3 doses × 30 d
Toxocariasis, see VISCERAL LARVA MIGRANS			
TOXOPLASMOSIS *(Toxoplasma gondii)*[87]			
Drugs of choice:[88]	Pyrimethamine[89]	25–100 mg/d × 3–4 wk	2 mg/kg/d × 3 d, (max. 25 mg/d) × 4 wk[90]
	plus sulfadiazine	1–1.5 g qid × 3–4 wk	100–200 mg/kg/d × 3–4 wk
Alternative:[91]	Spiramycin*	3–4 g/d × 3–4 wk	50–100 mg/kg/d × 3–4 wk
TRICHINOSIS *(Trichinella spiralis)*			
Drugs of choice:	Steroids for severe symptoms		
	plus mebendazole[5]	200–400 mg tid × 3 d, then 400–500 mg tid × 10 d	200–400 mg tid × 3 d, then 400–500 mg tid × 10 d
Alternative:	Albendazole[5]	400 mg PO bid × 8–14 d	400 mg PO bid × 8–14 d
TRICHOMONIASIS *(Trichomonas vaginalis)*			
Drug of choice:[92]	Metronidazole	2 g once; or 250 mg tid or 375 mg bid PO × 7 d	15 mg/kg/d orally in 3 doses × 7 d
	OR Tinidazole[3]*	2 g once	50 mg/kg once (max. 2 g)

*Availability problems. See table on page 3119.

84. Patients may benefit from or require surgical resection cysts. Praziquantel is useful preoperatively or in case of spill during surgery. Percutaneous drainage with ultrasound guidance plus albendazole therapy has been effective for management of hepatic hydatid cyst disease (MS Khuroo et al, N Engl J Med. 337:881, 1997).
85. Surgical excision is the only reliable means of treatment. Some reports have suggested use of albendazole or mebendazole (W Hao et al, Trans R Soc Trop Med Hyg, 88:340, 1994; WHO Group, Bull WHO, 74:231, 1996).
86. Initial therapy of parenchymal disease with seizures should focus on symptomatic treatment with anticonvulsant drugs. Treatment of parenchymal disease with albendazole and praziquantel is controversial and randomized trials have not shown a benefit. Obstructive hydrocephalus is treated with surgical removal of the obstructing cyst or CSF diversion. Prednisone 40 mg PO may be given in conjunction with surgery. Arachnoiditis, vasculitis, or cerebral edema is treated with prednisone 60 mg daily or dexamethasone 4–16 mg/d combined with albendazole or praziquantel (AC White, Jr. Annu Rev Med, 51:187, 2000). Any cysticercocidal drug may cause irreparable damage when used to treat ocular or spinal cysts, even when corticosteroids are used. An ophthalmic exam should always be done before treatment to rule out intraocular cysts.
87. In ocular toxoplasmosis with macular involvement, corticosteroids are recommended for an anti-inflammatory effect on the eyes.
88. To treat CNS toxoplasmosis in HIV-infected patients, some clinicians have used pyrimethamine 50 to 100 mg daily (after a loading dose of 200 mg) with a sulfonamide and, when sulfonamide sensitivity developed, have given clindamycin 1.8 to 2.4 g/d in divided doses instead of the sulfonamide (JS Remington et al, Lancet, 338:1142, 1991; BJ Luft et al, N Engl J Med, 329:995, 1993). Atovaquone plus pyrimethamine appears to be an effective alternative in sulfa-intolerant patients (JA Kovacs et al, Lancet, 340:637, 1992). Treatment is followed by chronic suppression with lower dosage regimens of the same drugs. For primary prophylaxis in HIV patients with <100 CD4 cells, either trimethoprim-sulfamethoxazole, pyrimethamine with dapsone of atovaquone with or without pyrimethamine can be used (USPHS/IDSA, MMWR, Morb Mortal Wkly Rep, 48, RR-10:41, 1999). See also footnote 89.
89. Plus leucovorin 10 to 25 mg with each dose of pyrimethamine.
90. Congenitally infected newborns should be treated with pyrimethamine every two or three days and a sulfonamide daily for about one year (JS Remington and G Desmonts in JS Remington and JO Klein, eds, *Infectious Disease of the Fetus and Newborn Infant,* 4th ed, Philadelphia:W.B.Saunders, 1995. p. 140).
91. For prophylactic use during pregnancy. If it is determined that transmission has occurred in utero, therapy with pyrimethamine and sulfadiazine should be started.
92. Sexual partners should be treated simultaneously. Metronidazole-resistant strains have been reported and should be treated with metronidazole 2–4 g/d × 7–14 d. Desensitization has been recommended for patients allergic to metronidazole (MD Pearlman et al, Am J Obstet Gynecol, 174:934, 1996).

Infection	Drug	Adult Dosage	Pediatric Dosage
TRICHOSTRONGYLUS infection			
Drug of choice:	Pyrantel pamoate[5]	11 mg/kg base once (max. 1 g)	11 mg/kg once (max.1 g)
Alternative:	Mebendazole [5]	100 mg bid × 3 d	100 mg bid × 3 d
	OR Albendazole[5]	400 mg once	400 mg once
TRICHURIASIS (*Trichuris trichiura*, whipworm)			
Drug of choice:	Mebendazole	100 mg bid × 3 d or 500 mg once	100 mg bid × 3 d or 500 mg once
Alternative:	Albendazole[5]	400 mg once[93]	400 mg once[93]
TRYPANOSOMIASIS			
T. cruzi (American trypanosomiasis, Chagas disease)			
Drug of choice:	Benznidazole*	5–7 mg/kg/d in 2 divided doses × 30–90 d	Up to 12 yr: 10 mg/kg/d in 2 doses × 30–90 d
	OR Nifurtimox[94]*	8–10 mg/kg/d in 3–4 doses × 90–120 d	1–10 yr: 15–20 mg/kg/d in 4 doses × 90 d; 11–16 yr: 12.5–15 mg/kg/d in 4 doses × 90 d
T. brucei gambiense (West African trypanosomiasis, sleeping sickness) hemolymphatic stage			
Drug of choice:[95]	Pentamidine isethionate[5]	4 mg/kg/d IM × 10 d	4 mg/kg/d IM × 10 d
Alternative:	Suramin*	100–200 mg (test dose) IV, then 1 g IV on days 1, 3, 7, 14, and 21	20 mg/kg on days 1, 3, 7, 14, and 21
	OR Eflornithine*	See footnote 96	
T.b. rhodesiense (East African trypanosomiasis, sleeping sickness) hemolymphatic stage			
Drug of choice:	Suramin*	100–200 mg (test dose) IV, then 1 g IV on days 1, 3, 7, 14, and 21	20 mg/kg on days 1, 3, 7, 14, and 21
	OR Eflornithine*	See footnote 96	
late disease with CNS involvement (*T.b. gambiense* or *T.b. rhodesiense*)			
Drug of choice:	Melarsoprol[97]*	2–3.6 mg/kg/d IV × 3 d; after 1 wk 3.6 mg/kg/ d IV × 3 d; repeat again after 10–21 d	18–25 mg/kg total over 1 mo; initial dose of 0.36 mg/kg IV, increasing gradually to max. 3.6 mg/kg at intervals of 1–5 d for total of 9–10 doses
	OR Eflornithine	See footnote 96	
VISCERAL LARVA MIGRANS[98] (Toxocariasis)			
Drug of choice:	Albendazole[5]	400 mg bid × 5 d	400 mg bid × 5 d
	Mebendazole[5]	100–200 mg bid × 5 d	100–200 mg bid × 5 d
Whipworm, see TRICHURIASIS			
Wuchereria bancrofti, see FILARIASIS			

*Availability problems. See table on page 3119.

93. In heavy infection, it may be necessary to extend therapy to 3 days.

94. No longer manufactured, but available from CDC in selected cases. The addition of gamma interferon to nifurtimox for 20 days in a limited number of patients and in experimental animals appears to have shortened the acute phase of Chagas disease (RE McCabe et al, J Infect Dis, 163:912, 1991).

95. Suramin is the drug of choice for treatment of *T.b. rhodesiense*. For treatment of *T.b. gambiense*, pentamidine, and suramin have equal efficacy but pentamidine is better tolerated.

96. Eflornithine is highly effective in *T.b. gambiense* and variably effective in *T.b. rhodesiense* infections. It is available in limited supply only from the WHO, and is given 400 mg/kg/d IV in 4 divided doses for 14 days.

97. In frail patients, begin with as little as 18 mg and increase the dose progressively. Pretreatment with suramin has been advocated for debilitated patients. Corticosteroids have been used to prevent arsenical encephalopathy (J Pepin et al, Trans R Soc Trop Med Hyg 89:92, 1995). Up to 20% of patients fail to respond to melarsoprol (MP Barrett, Lancet, 353:1113, 1999).

98. For severe symptoms of eye involvement, corticosteroids can be used in addition.

MANUFACTURERS OF SOME ANTIPARASITIC DRUGS

albendazole—*Albenza* (SmithKline Beecham)
§ aminosidine, see paromomycin
§ artemether—*Artenam* (Arenco, Belgium)
§ artesunate—(Guilin No. 1 Factory, People's Republic of China)
atovaquone—*Mepron* (Glaxo-Wellcome)
atovaquone/proguanil—*Malarone* (Glaxo-Wellcome)
bacitracin—many manufacturers
§ bacitracin-zinc—(Apothekernes Laboratorium A.S.,Oslo, Norway)
§ benznidazole—*Rochagan* (Roche, Brazil)
† bithionol—*Bitin* (Tanabe, Japan)
chloroquine HCl and chloroquine phosphate—*Aralen* (Sanofi), others
crotamiton—*Eurax* (Westwood-Squibb)
dapsone—(Jacobus)
† diethylcarbamazine citrate USP—(University of Iowa School of Pharmacy)
§ diloxanide furoate—*Furamide* (Boots, United Kingdom)
§ eflornithine (Difluoromethylornithine, DFMO)—*Ornidyl* (Ilex-Oncology, Inc)
furazolidone—*Furoxone* (Roberts)
§ halofantrine—*Halfan* (SmithKline Beecham)
iodoquinol—*Yodoxin* (Glenwood), others
ivermectin—*Stromectol* (Merck)
malathion—*Ovide* (Medicis)
mebendazole—*Vermox* (McNeil)
mefloquine—*Lariam* (Roche)
§ meglumine antimonate—*Glucantime* (Aventis, France)
§ melarsoprol—*Arsobal* (Aventis)
metronidazole—*Flagyl* (Searle), others
§ miltefosine—(Asta Medica, Germany)
§ niclosamide—*Yomesan* (Bayer, Germany)
† nifurtimox—*Lampit* (Bayer, Germany)
§ nitazoxanide—*Cryptaz* (Romark)
§ ornidazole—*Tiberal* (Hoffman-LaRoche, Switzerland)
oxamniquine—*Vansil* (Pfizer)
paromomycin—*Humatin* (Parke-Davis); aminosidine (topical and parenteral formulations not available in United States)
pentamidine isethionate—*Pentam 300, NebuPent* (Fujisawa)
permethrin—*Nix* (Glaxo-Wellcome), *Elimite* (Allergan)
praziquantel—*Biltricide* (Bayer)
primaquine phosphate USP
§ proguanil—*Paludrine* (Wyeth Ayerst, Canada; Zeneca, United Kingdom)
§ propamidine isethionate—*Brolene* (Aventis, Canada)
pyrantel pamoate—*Antiminth* (Pfizer)
pyrethrins and piperonyl butoxide—*RID* (Pfizer), others
pyrimethamine USP—*Daraprim* (Glaxo-Wellcome)
quinine sulfate—many manufacturers
§ quinine dihydrochloride
† sodium stibogluconate—*Pentostam* (Glaxo-Wellcome, United Kingdom)
* spiramycin—*Rovamycine* (Aventis)
† suramin sodium—(Bayer, Germany)
thiabendazole—*Mintezol* (Merck)
§ tinidazole—*Fasigyn* (Pfizer)
§ triclabendazole—*Fasinex* (Novartis Agribusiness)
trimetrexate—*Neutrexin* (US Bioscience)

*Available in the United States only from the manufacturer.
§Not available in the United States.
†Available under an Investigational New Drug (IND) protocol from the CDC Drug Service, Centers for Disease Control and Prevention, Atlanta, GA 30333; 404-639-3670 (evenings, weekends, or holidays: 404-639-2888).

CHAPTER 241 Immunomodulating Agents

TIMOTHY R. LA PINE ■ HARRY R. HILL

During the past 2 decades, considerable basic science research and clinical interest has been generated in determining the functional mechanisms of the immune response and identifying the specific biologic factors that modulate this response. This research has established that a critical and delicate balance in regulation of both humoral and cellular function is essential for complete immunologic responsiveness to invasive pathogens and that alteration of this regulation may have potential clinical significance. Recent attempts to augment immune function in challenged hosts or during specific immunodeficiency states have focused on numerous specific immune biologic response modifiers. These efforts, in combination with advances in hybridoma and recombinant DNA technology, have resulted in numerous clinical trials that have explored the therapeutic utility of immunomodulating agents for treating specific human disease states.

We review the biologic agents used to manipulate immune regulation for the prevention and management of infectious diseases in infants and children. In addition, we identify the actions of potentially useful immunomodulators derived from in vitro or animal model experiments, or both, that may be used in future human clinical trials. We discuss the historical and current use of monoclonal antibodies that either are directed at bacterial pathogens and their components or are used to regulate mediators of the proinflammatory cascade leading to septic shock. We specifically focus on modulation of the clinically important activities of the cytokine family, the members of which play many key roles in orchestration of the immune response. These cytokines include the lymphokines and monokines (interleukins [ILs] and tumor necrosis factor–α [TNF-α], as well as the hematopoietic growth factors); colony-stimulating factors (CSFs); and interferon-α, (INF-α), INF-β, and INF-γ. In addition, we explore the potential clinical utility of modulating neutrophil functions, which include the integrins and selectins, bactericidal/permeability-increasing protein (BPI), and the defensins, as well as complement component activation. We also discuss platelet-activating factor (PAF) and nitric oxide, which are emerging as important immunoregulators of the acute inflammatory response.

Monoclonal Antibodies

The use of serum antibody therapy in the late 1800s was among the first clinical attempts to modulate the immune response in the treatment of human sepsis. By the mid-1930s, serum-based therapy was the standard of care for many infectious illnesses, particularly pneumonia. Controlled trials during that time demonstrated that the administration of type-specific pneumococcal serum reduced the mortality rate of patients with pneumococcal pneumonia by 50 percent.[39, 40, 69] With the introduction of antimicrobial pharmacologic agents in the 1940s, the use of serum antibody therapy as treatment of sepsis became less popular. The development of hybridoma technology by Kohler and Milstein in 1975, however, provided the means to generate virtually unlimited amounts of monoclonal antibodies for potential clinical use.[131] This development, in combination with the advances achieved during the past 2 decades in recombinant DNA technology, has allowed researchers to generate highly specific human monoclonal antibodies and to humanize murine monoclonal antibodies.[27, 252] Monoclonal antibodies are considered attractive molecules for potential clinical use as antimicrobial agents and immunomodulators for delivering pharmacologic substances to sites of inflammation or even for targeting certain cancerous tissues. This potential has led to recent resurgence in the development of monoclonal antibody–based therapies to treat sepsis, septic shock, and numerous inflammatory diseases in infants, children, and adults.

A monoclonal antibody that would alter the clinical course of any infectious or inflammatory disease state could, in theory, be generated. This hypothesis has fostered numerous studies evaluating the use of monoclonal antibodies in a variety of clinical diseases, particularly those related to alloimmune and autoimmune phenomena.[48, 60, 94, 156, 197] The use of monoclonal antibodies to alter the pathogenesis of sepsis and septic shock also has received considerable recent experimental and clinical attention. These efforts have focused on two phases in development of the septic shock syndrome: blocking bacteria and their components that induce shock and modifying the release and action of proinflammatory mediators that lead to septic shock.

The initial use of monoclonal antibody preparations in early studies to block bacteria or their components in the development of septic shock involved type-specific antisera against *Streptococcus pneumoniae, Neisseria meningitidis,* and *Haemophilus influenzae* type b.[40] More recent attempts to use monoclonal antibody therapy to alter the pathogenesis of bacterial sepsis leading to septic shock have focused on group B streptococcus (GBS) and *Escherichia coli.* These two bacteria are significant causes of neonatal morbidity and mortality. Infants usually acquire these bacterial infections from exposure in the birth canal, but bacterial sepsis actually develops in only a small fraction of exposed infants. Factors predisposing infants to infection with these organisms include prematurity, prolonged rupture of membranes, and maternal sepsis. Neonatal infections occur more commonly with bacteria that possess specific capsular polysaccharides, such as the type III polysaccharide of GBS or the K-1 capsule of *E. coli.* Bacteria bearing these capsular components are able to avoid opsonization and subsequent phagocytic killing by polymorphonuclear leukocytes (PMNs). Newborns with a deficiency of type-specific antibody to these bacterial capsular antigens, whether because of prematurity, which contributes to decreased maternal transplacental antibody transport, or inadequate maternal stores, are predisposed to GBS and *E. coli* infections.[106] These observations led investigators to hypothesize that passive antibody administration may be beneficial in preventing or reducing the neonatal morbidity and mortality observed with these bacterial infections.

Rebecca Lancefield in 1933 originally demonstrated protective efficacy of GBS antibody therapy with rabbit antisera.

She established that this protective efficacy is type specific and classified three types of GBS bacterial strains. Antisera raised against type II or type III GBS did not protect against infection with type I bacteria. These experiments also suggested that antibodies to group B non–type-specific determinants (i.e., expressed on all GBS bacteria) are not protective.[77, 140, 141] Further experiments by Lancefield and coworkers with type I GBS demonstrated that antibodies to both carbohydrate and protein capsular components can be protective.[139, 141] The first human studies to suggest that the administration of antibody to the infecting strain of bacteria could improve survival after early-onset GBS in infants occurred in the mid-1970s. In these studies, fresh whole blood either containing or lacking opsonic antibody was administered to infants with early-onset GBS disease. All nine infants who demonstrated a rise in opsonic antibody post-transfusion survived. In contrast, three of the six infants who received blood lacking antibody to their infection strain died.[218] Subsequently, studies have suggested that intravenous immunoglobulins (IVIGs) could offer some protection against GBS infection in experimental animal models.[72, 111] Because of their lack of specificity and decreased opsonic activity, however, polyclonal-type IVIG antibody preparations have had only variable and limited ability to alter the course and outcome of GBS or other bacterial infections in clinical trials.[102]

The development of monoclonal antibodies to GBS type III occurred in the early 1980s. GBS type III–specific antibodies, which were of the IgM class, protected rats against intraperitoneal infection with homologous-type group B streptococci. Survival rates were 95 to 100 percent for rats protected by monoclonal antibody versus 17 percent for unprotected rats. Protection was afforded even when therapy was delayed as long as 24 hours after inoculation. Antibody administration resulted in the rapid accumulation of PMNs at the site of infection and prevented the depletion of bone marrow granulocyte stores commonly seen in animal models and human neonates with GBS infection.[220] Monoclonal IgG and IgA antibody preparations to type III GBS also have been generated.[17, 108, 219] A protective effect in animal models of GBS infection for all three immunoglobulin isotypes has been established.[221] In GBS infections, the ability of an antibody isotype preparation to activate the complement system is related directly to its protective and opsonic activity. IgM is much more active in triggering complement than monoclonal IgG and IgA preparations are,[145] which may explain why monoclonal IgM is quantitatively more effective against GBS infection.[105, 204] Although human monoclonal IgM antibodies to GBS are available and have demonstrated effectiveness in reducing mortality rates in animal models of GBS sepsis, they have yet to be used clinically in an attempt to prevent or attenuate GBS sepsis and septic shock in human neonates.[200, 222]

Concomitant with the studies of monoclonal antibody preparations for use in experimental models of GBS infection were similar studies using monoclonal preparations in *E. coli* sepsis. *E. coli* is an antigenically complex gram-negative bacterium with more than 150 somatic (O) and 100 capsular (K) antigens. Several factors associated with *E. coli* have been implicated as contributing to the virulence of these organisms. Among these factors, K-1 capsular polysaccharide and lipopolysaccharide (LPS) have received the most attention.[22] Robbins and colleagues in 1974 first suggested that the K-1 capsular polysaccharide on *E. coli* was a contributing factor to the virulence of this organism.[204] Researchers subsequently established that *E. coli* strains that possess the K-1 capsular polysaccharide are resistant to opsonization via the alternate complement pathway.[24, 227] Several investigators have shown that antibody preparations to the K-1 capsular polysaccharide are opsonic and protective against lethal *E. coli* bacteremia in animals.[23] Although protection has been demonstrated primarily with IgM antibody, polyclonal hyperimmune IgG has shown some protection in animal models of lethal *E. coli* sepsis.[199] Because the serum from newborn infants is deficient in opsonic activity for *E. coli,* researchers suggested that administration of antibody against *E. coli* K-1 would enhance neonatal resistance to infections with this organism.[25, 47] Investigators since have developed murine and human monoclonal IgM antibodies to *E. coli* K-1 and have demonstrated that these antibodies are opsonic and protective against lethal *E. coli* infection in animal models.[199] Human clinical trials using monoclonal antibodies to *E. coli* K-1 have not been initiated to our knowledge.

Staphylococci are a major cause of acquired infections in infants born prematurely. Antibiotic resistance among staphylococcal species in these immunocompromised patients is of significant concern. Most recently, a human chimeric monoclonal antibody has been generated that is opsonic for *Staphylococcus epidermidis* and *Staphylococcus aureus.* In an animal model of *S. epidermidis* and *S. aureus* sepsis, this monoclonal antibody enhanced bacterial clearance and significantly improved survival. Clinical trials with this monoclonal antibody are under way to determine the clinical usefulness of monoclonal antibody preparations in preventing nosocomial staphylococcal infections in high-risk preterm neonates.[73, 242]

During the past 2 decades, the importance of pneumococcal vaccination for individuals at risk of acquiring infection has been underscored by the emergence of antibiotic resistance among pneumococcal strains and the increased prevalence of invasive pneumococcal disease in immunocompromised patients. Unfortunately, pure pneumococcal capsular polysaccharide vaccines are poorly immunogenetic in many immunodeficient patients who are at risk for infection. This factor has led to the development of monoclonal antibodies against type-specific pneumococcal infections. Recently, a human monoclonal IgM antibody has been generated and shown to provide type-specific protection against lethal pneumococcal infection in mice, even in the presence of complement deficiency.[255] Thus, type-specific monoclonal antibody preparations probably could provide protection against pneumococcal infection in high-risk immunocompromised humans.

The use of monoclonal antibodies as single-agent therapy to treat or prevent bacterial sepsis has been limited to experimental animal models, primarily because of the narrow spectrum of monoclonal antibody therapy and the exceedingly large number of patients required to demonstrate the efficacy of human monoclonal antibody therapy in clinical trials. The future clinical use of monoclonal antibodies directed at bacteria or their components in the treatment of sepsis requires many clinical considerations: (1) because antibodies are more effective in preventing an infection than in treating an established infection, monoclonal antibody therapy is most useful when administered early in the course of a disease; (2) successful implementation of monoclonal antibody therapy directed at a specific pathogen requires refinements in diagnostic laboratory methodology to hasten pathogen identification and thereby lead to early treatment; (3) monoclonal antibody therapy is pathogen specific, which is problematic when dealing with unknown infections early during their course and with mixed infections with multiple organisms or serotypes; for pathogens that are antigenically variable, the use of monoclonal antibody cocktail preparations that combine monoclonal antibodies to common antigenic serotypes may be useful, and antibody cocktails also may be designed to include monoclonal antibodies of different isotypes (IgM, IgG, IgA) to further enhance their effectiveness; (4) combination therapy with monoclonal antibodies and antimicrobial chemotherapeutic agents may be an alternative means of treating bacteria and their components and preventing the development of septic shock, could potentially reduce the amount or length of antibiotic treatment and decrease the effect of antibiotic-resistant pathogens, and may be clinically beneficial in cases in which the antimicrobial agents are themselves toxic; and (5) monoclonal antibodies may elicit self-neutralizing antibodies. Thus, administration of a monoclonal antibody could promote the production of antibody against the monoclonal antibody itself, which would diminish the clinical response and potentially cause severe anaphylaxis in cases of antibody re-treatment. Likewise, widespread use of monoclonal antibody therapy could select for antibody-resistant pathogens or other serotypes or even entirely different infecting organisms.[144]

During the past 2 decades, researchers have examined the possibility of blocking the proinflammatory cascade that accompanies severe infections.[1, 9, 81, 143] Experimental attempts to use monoclonal antibodies to modify the release and action of the proinflammatory mediators that lead to septic shock have focused on the proinflammatory effects of the cytokine family, endotoxin, and the functions of neutrophils and complement.

The Cytokines

LYMPHOKINES AND MONOKINES

The cytokines are a family of small soluble protein molecules that are responsible for cell-to-cell communication. They are produced by several cell types and play crucial roles in many biologic processes, including growth, inflammation, immunity, and hematopoiesis. During infection, genes for nearly all the cytokines are expressed. The biologic activity of the prototype cytokines, the lymphokines and monokines, include ILs and TNF-α; these molecules, along with granulocyte CSFs, have received considerable attention as potential immunomodulatory agents. In response to pathogen invasion, these cytokines perform a complex series of interactions to initiate a cascade of biologic events that result in propagation and subsequent regulation of the inflammatory response leading to pathogen alienation while maintaining host preservation. Thus, the cytokine family, through a complex web of interactions, functions to initiate and then both up-regulate and down-regulate the inflammatory response. Based on their roles of either up-regulating or down-regulating immune responsiveness, the cytokines generally and historically have been classified as either proinflammatory or anti-inflammatory molecules. Although numerous cytokines, either directly or indirectly, have the potential to perform dual functions, their proinflammatory or anti-inflammatory properties are of considerable basic science and clinical therapeutic interest.[21, 41, 57, 76, 143, 146, 155, 192]

The proinflammatory cytokines and their cellular sources are listed in Table 241–1. TNF-α and IL-1 generally are considered to be prominent early proinflammatory mediators. They induce gene expression of other proinflammatory cytokines, including IL-6, IL-8, and IL-9, and in this manner lead to neutrophil activation, recruitment, and degranulation. TNF-α and IL-1 also activate a secondary cascade of inflammatory mediators, including arachidonic acid–derived prostaglandin I_2, thromboxane A_2, prostaglandin E_2, PAF, and the complement system. The CSFs and IL-3 are additional proinflammatory cytokines that induce stem cell production of granulocytes and monocytes in bone marrow, in addition to activating neutrophils and inducing the production of IL-1 and TNF-α.[21, 41, 57, 76, 143, 146, 155]

Prominent among the anti-inflammatory cytokines (Table 241–2) are IL-4, IL-10, IL-13, and transforming growth factor–β (TGF-β). These cytokines block endotoxin induction of IL-1 and TNF-α and suppress lymphocyte and monocyte function. In addition, IL-1 receptor antagonist (IL-1ra) blocks the proinflammatory action of IL-1 by binding its receptor.[21, 41, 57, 76, 143, 146, 155]

Considerable experimental and clinical interest has focused on the proinflammatory cytokines TNF-α and IL-1 as important early mediators in the pathogenesis of sepsis and septic shock syndrome. The basis for the potential therapeutic utility of these two cytokines in human disease states involves two clinically distinct hypotheses: excessive production of cytokine results in host immune injury leading to severe shock, and deficient production of cytokine renders a host susceptible to infection by invasive pathogens.[143]

The hypothesis that overproduction of cytokine can lead to severe lethal shock has been demonstrated in several animal models and has been suggested in patients with overwhelming sepsis. The outer membranes of gram-negative bacteria contain LPS or endotoxin that induces early production of the proinflammatory cytokines TNF-α and IL-1. Although these cytokines may protect the host from infection, if expressed in excessive amounts, their effects can result in multiple organ failure and death. During severe sepsis, levels of both TNF-α and IL-1 increase proportionately with the degree of hypotension and organ failure. The combination of two cytokines can result in synergistic effects by several-fold and lead to lethal septic shock syndrome.[31, 32] In animal models of shock and gram-negative sepsis, TNF-α levels rise rapidly after bacterial or endotoxin injection and reach peak concentrations at 60 to 90 minutes, whereas IL-1 levels rise more slowly and peak at 180 minutes. A similar time-course response has been observed in human subjects injected with endotoxin.[32, 174] In children with septicemia and purpura fulminans and children with meningococcal disease, an association was demonstrated between morbidity and mortality and high serum levels of TNF-α and IL-1.[82, 182] These studies and others implicate TNF-α and IL-1 as prominent modulators in the development of septic shock syndrome and suggest that a potential therapeutic benefit may be obtained by inhibiting the production of these cytokines and reducing their proinflammatory effects.

Experimental attempts to attenuate the excessive proinflammatory cytokine activity of TNF-α and IL-1 have focused on (1) inhibiting endotoxin release, (2) blocking endotoxin–target cell binding and preventing the transmembrane signaling mechanisms leading to TNF-α and IL-1 production, (3) controlling the synthesis of TNF-α and IL-1 by inhibiting or suppressing specific cytokine gene transcription and translation, (4) inhibiting TNF-α and IL-1 release, (5) administering TNF-α and IL-1 neutralizing antibodies and soluble receptors, (6) producing and administering TNF-α and IL-1 receptor antagonists that block specific cytokine binding to target cell receptors, and (7) blocking TNF-α or IL-1 intracellular transmembrane signaling mechanisms and preventing their action on target cells.[146]

The use of monoclonal anti-endotoxin antibodies to inhibit the binding of endotoxin to its target cells has received considerable attention. Numerous in vitro and in vivo animal experiments have suggested that blocking endotoxin leads to improved survival by inhibiting proinflammatory cytokine production and expression.[183] The initial clinical studies in patients with gram-negative bacteremia treated with immunoglobulin preparations directed against endotoxin

TABLE 241–1 ■ PROINFLAMMATORY CYTOKINES

Cytokine	Function	Predominant Cell Source
Tumor necrosis factor–α	Stimulates interleukin-6 and colony-stimulating factors. Depresses erythropoiesis. Stimulates interleukin-8 and interleukin-9. Promotes tumor necrosis and endotoxic shock	Monocytes and macrophages
Interleukin-1	Stimulates proliferation and differentiation of T and B lymphocytes. Stimulates T lymphocytes to produce interleukin-2. Promotes colony-stimulating factor, interleukin-8, and interleukin-9 production and endotoxic shock	Macrophages, astrocytes, monocytes, fibroblasts, keratinocytes, B cells, corneal epithelium, and other cell types
Interleukin-2	Stimulates grow of T lymphocytes. Stimulates B-lymphocyte and monocyte differentiation. Increases cytotoxicity of T lymphocytes and natural killer cells	Activated T lymphocytes
Interleukin-3	Multipotential hematopoietic cell growth factor, stimulates early B and T lymphocytes. Mast cell growth factor	Activated T lymphocytes, natural killer cells
Interleukin-5	Stimulates eosinophil formation and differentiation. Augments T-lymphocyte cytotoxicity and proliferation of B lymphocytes	T lymphocytes, mast cells
Interleukin-7	Supports growth of pre-B lymphocytes. Stimulates T lymphocytes	B lymphocytes, bone marrow fibroblasts, monocytes
Interleukin-8	Stimulates neutrophil, monocyte, and lymphocyte activation and chemotaxis	Monocytes
Interleukin-9	Stimulates neutrophil, monocyte, and lymphocyte activation and chemotaxis. Stimulates erythroid progenitors, helper T-lymphocyte growth factor	T lymphocytes
Interleukin-11	T-lymphocyte–dependent stimulator of B lymphocytes	Bone marrow fibroblasts
Interleukin-12	Stimulates helper T-lymphocyte differentiation and interleukin-2 production. Stimulates IFN-γ production. Increases cytotoxicity of natural killer cells	T and B lymphocytes, lymphoblastoid cells
Interleukin-14	Stimulates proliferation of activated B lymphocytes. Inhibits immunoglobulin secretion from B lymphocytes	T lymphocytes
Interleukin-15	Stimulates T lymphocyte function and proliferation. Enhances natural killer cell function	Monocytes and macrophages
Interleukin-16	Promotes migration of T lymphocytes	T lymphocytes
Interleukin-17	Stimulates interleukin-6 and interleukin-8 production	T lymphocytes
Interleukin-18	Stimulates IFN-γ and TNF-α production	Macrophages, mononuclear cells, and dendritic cells
Granulocyte colony-stimulating factor	Stimulates neutrophil colony formation	Monocytes and fibroblasts
Granulocyte-macrophage colony-stimulating factor	Stimulates granulocyte and monocyte formation. Induces TNF	T lymphocytes, natural killer cells, endothelial cells, fibroblasts, and keratinocytes
Macrophage colony-stimulating factor	Activates monocytes and granulocytes. Stimulates macrophage colony formation. Induces interleukin-1 and TNF	Fibroblasts, monocytes, and endothelial cells

INF, interferon; TNF, tumor necrosis factor.

demonstrated a significant reduction in mortality rates.[10, 211] Further studies suggested a reduction in septic shock in similarly treated high-risk surgical patients.[10] These observations led to the development of several clinical trials using human monoclonal anti-endotoxin antibodies. HA-1A is a human monoclonal antibody directed against the lipid A moiety of bacterial endotoxin. The mechanism of HA-1A action is to block endotoxin from triggering the intracellular events leading to the synthesis of proinflammatory cytokines. In placebo-controlled clinical trials of HA-1A, either HA-1A or placebo was infused over the course of 20 minutes to patients with severe sepsis. These patients received cardiopulmonary support and antibacterial therapy. The etiologic agents of sepsis included *E. coli*, *Pseudomonas*, and *Klebsiella* and *Enterobacter* spp. The authors reported that HA-1A significantly reduced mortality in adults with septic shock and gram-negative bacteremia. Patients who were in severe shock before the administration of HA-1A had a 42 percent reduction in mortality rates.[256] Although these early clinical studies using HA-1A were encouraging, a protective role for anti-endotoxin antibodies has not been established in subsequent clinical trials.[159] Anti-endotoxin therapy may be more effective if given earlier during the sepsis syndrome before the development of shock. Because bacterial lysis by antibiotics is an ongoing process and results in further release of endotoxin, multiple dosing of anti-endotoxin antibodies also may prove beneficial in treating sepsis. The future clinical use of anti-endotoxin antibodies may be in combination with other immunomodulation therapies directed at simultaneously blocking several steps in both the propagation and action of proinflammatory cytokines.

Studies on cytokine inhibition have focused on controlling TNF-α and IL-1 with anti–TNF-α antibodies directed at these specific cytokines and their receptors. Control of proinflammatory cytokine synthesis is specific for each individual cytokine and requires an understanding of the unique temporal relationships that these molecules have during the propagation of inflammatory responses. A critical aspect of

TABLE 241–2 ■ ANTI-INFLAMMATORY CYTOKINES

Cytokines	Function	Predominant Cell Source
Interleukin-4	Stimulates proliferation of T and B lymphocytes and megakaryocytes and is a growth factor for mast cells and erythroid precursors	T lymphocytes
Interleukin-6	Blocks endotoxin induction of interleukin-1 and tumor necrosis factor. B- and T-lymphocyte–stimulating activity	Monocytes, T and B lymphocytes, fibroblasts, epithelial and endothelial cells
Interleukin-10	Blocks production of interleukin-1 and tumor necrosis factor. Inhibits primary allogeneic T-lymphocyte responses. Inhibits interleukin-2, interleukin-8, and GM-CSF	T and B lymphocytes, macrophages and monocytes
Interleukin-13	Blocks production of interleukin-1, tumor necrosis factor, and interleukin-8. Suppresses nitric oxide formation	T lymphocytes
Interleukin-1 receptor antagonist	Binds interleukin-1 receptors, thereby blocking interleukin-1 effects	Monocytes and macrophages
Transforming growth factor-β	Reduces endotoxin-induced interleukin-1 and tumor necrosis factor production	Monocytes and macrophages

GM-CSF, granulocyte-macrophage colony-stimulating factor.

TNF-α and IL-1 gene expression in a variety of cell types has been the reported exquisite sensitivity of these cytokines to bacterial endotoxin.[41, 57, 143, 146] Human blood monocytes synthesize TNF-α and IL-1 in the presence of endotoxin. In the absence of endotoxin, however, gene expression occurs, but protein translation does not take place.[212] Thus, these cells may be viewed as being primed for exposure to bacterial endotoxin. TNF-α and IL-1 transcription is suppressed by the anti-inflammatory cytokines IL-4, IL-10, IL-13, and TGF-β, but the clinical therapeutic benefit that these cytokines have in treating septic shock remain to be defined.[43, 98, 176, 213] Agents blocking the lipoxygenase pathway of arachidonate metabolism also have been implicated in the reduction of TNF-α and IL-1 synthesis, and corticosteroids have been shown to suppress both TNF-α and IL-1 transcription and synthesis, but only when administered before transcription has been initiated.[74, 210] The use of corticosteroids in infants and children with bacterial meningitis has demonstrated that treatment with a combination of dexamethasone and antibiotics results in lower cerebrospinal fluid levels of TNF-α than does treatment with placebo and antibiotics.[182] In addition, patients treated with corticosteroids had fewer neurologic symptoms.[126] Multicenter trials conducted subsequently, however, have failed to establish a protective effect of corticosteroid use in the treatment of children with meningitis.[237] One possible explanation for this discrepancy may be that corticosteroids almost exclusively suppress endotoxin-induced proinflammatory cytokine gene transcription but have little or no effect on proinflammatory cytokine translation.[57, 223] Thus, researchers have suggested that the early administration of corticosteroids, before transcription has been initiated, would block cytokine synthesis. The timing of corticosteroid administration, therefore, may account for some of the clinical variability seen with its use in children with meningitis. Current clinical trials are focusing on blocking TNF-α and IL-1 synthesis with the administration of corticosteroids either before or during antibiotic administration. Similarly, the concurrent use of antibiotics, corticosteroids, and anti-endotoxin therapy may result in an additive therapeutic benefit.

Neutralizing monoclonal antibodies against murine or human TNF-α have been shown to decrease mortality rates in several experimental animal models of sepsis.[14, 166, 232] Studies involving soluble TNF-α receptors or their immunoadhesion constructs also have demonstrated an immunoprotective effect of TNF-α blockade in animal models of endotoxemia or bacteremia.[13] Although anti–TNF-α antibodies are being used with caution in humans, in a limited number of patients with established septic shock, anti–TNF-α treatment has resulted in increased vascular hemodynamics and left ventricular stroke volume.[92] The in vitro use of free soluble TNF-α receptors to bind TNF-α results in a 10- to 50-fold increase in binding affinity over that observed with anti–TNF-α monoclonal antibodies.[93] Results from phase II clinical trials using soluble TNF-α receptors, however, have not shown improvement in survival rates; moreover, high doses actually increased mortality rates.[93, 208]

Certain naturally occurring substances inhibit IL-1 synthesis and action, but they also have effects on many of the other cytokines. Specific inhibitors of IL-1, however, have been identified. Most prominent of these inhibitors is the IL-1 receptor inhibitor that competes with binding of IL-1 to its cell surface receptor. The administration of recombinant IL-1ra to block the effects of IL-1 has been studied in various animal models.[2, 190] For instance, IL-1ra prevents death from endotoxic shock in rabbits.[190] The therapeutic use of IL-1ra in treating septic shock in early phase II human clinical trials showed improved survival at 28 days.[75] Subsequent randomized phase III trials, however, failed to show improvement in patients with severe shock.[74] Further clinical studies are ongoing. IL-1ra also has been used in treatment trials of acute myelogenous leukemia (AML). Uncontrolled production of IL-1 by leukemic blasts is proposed to result in continued proliferation of these cells and the development of AML. Recent studies have shown that IL-1ra blocks the spontaneous proliferation and production of granulocyte-macrophage colony-stimulating factor (GM-CSF), IL-1, and IL-6 in the peripheral blood and bone marrow cells of these patients.[201] The potential clinical use of IL-1ra is being investigated in patients with psoriasis, rheumatoid arthritis, and myelogenous leukemia.[95] Similarly, combination therapy with simultaneous blockade of both TNF-α and IL-1 is being investigated in endotoxin models of shock and numerous clinical disease states.[207]

Another promising approach to attenuate excessive proinflammatory cytokine responses is the use of pharmacologic agents. Salyer and associates[209] demonstrated that pentoxifylline, a methylxanthine derivative that blocks TNF-α transcription and production, could override some of the effects of TNF-α on PMNs. In her study, the profound decrease in human PMN chemotactic ability caused by excessive TNF-α was restored to normal by treatment with pentoxifylline. The specific mechanisms of pentoxifylline's effect are not known, but it has been shown to restore the PMN membrane fluidity inhibited by TNF-α that is critical for cell movement.[187] Furthermore, pentoxifylline can block PMN adhesion to endothelium and thereby result in decreased PMN respiratory burst activity, an effect thought to be responsible for the improved survival rates seen in animal models of endotoxin-induced septic shock treated with pentoxifylline.[191] Some of the clinical trials using pentoxifylline in surgical patients with early evidence of systemic inflammation have suggested a cardioprotective effect, but other studies have been less convincing.[67, 226] Pentoxifylline also has been evaluated in preterm infants with sepsis.[148] A total of 78 infants with documented sepsis were randomly assigned to receive pentoxifylline (5 mg/kg/hr for 6 hours on 6 successive days) or placebo. Infants treated with pentoxifylline had significantly lower levels of TNF-α but not IL-1. Only 1 of 40 infants in the pentoxifylline-treated group died as compared with 6 of 38 in the control group ($p < .05$). Amrinone, a phosphodiesterase inhibitor, also has been shown to reduce TNF-α levels in LPS-challenged mice.[83] Thus, these and other pharmacologic agents may be useful in preventing or reducing some of the adverse and even fatal effects mediated by proinflammatory cytokines.

IVIG therapy may have a potential inhibitory effect on proinflammatory cytokine activity. Patients in the active phase of Kawasaki disease have increased levels of TNF-α and IL-1. These cytokines are postulated to stimulate local inflammatory responses by regulating leukocyte adherence and activation, thereby leading to the vascular damage that is a critical clinical aspect of this disease. Researchers also have suggested that the effects of IVIG therapy in Kawasaki disease, and perhaps in other diseases as well, may be achieved by attenuating production of the proinflammatory cytokines TNF-α and IL-1.[3, 6, 105, 149] Animal models of LPS-induced TNF-α and IL-1 synthesis demonstrate a suppression of mononuclear cell synthesis of these proinflammatory cytokines when treated with IVIG.[8] The peripheral blood mononuclear cells of Kawasaki disease patients receiving IVIG therapy, however, showed decreased synthesis of IL-1 but not TNF-α.[150] The role of IVIG as an immunomodulator has been suggested in an ever-growing number of clinical disease states because of its broad immunoregulatory potential.[6, 101] Its specific role in arresting proinflammatory cytokine activity, either directly or indirectly, warrants further clinical investigation.

The hypothesis that diminished levels of cytokines may render a host susceptible to infection was introduced by Weatherstone and Rich.[240] They suggested that the increased susceptibility to infection observed in premature neonates may be secondary to deficient proinflammatory cytokine production. In their study, they measured cord blood monocyte secretion of TNF-α and IL-1 with and without LPS stimulation. IL-1 activity by stimulated preterm monocytes did not differ from that observed by LPS-stimulated adult monocytes. TNF-α activity, however, in the LPS-stimulated monocytes from preterm neonates was significantly lower than that of both stimulated and unstimulated adult monocytes. Thus, they concluded that diminished production of TNF-α may predispose preterm infants to infection. This suggestion has not been supported by studies of infected animals that show markedly elevated TNF-α levels, and subsequent studies in preterm infants have not established a deficiency in TNF-α.[247] Williams and colleagues and Peat and coworkers, in contrast, have shown that mononuclear cells from term newborns produce enhanced levels of TNF-α in response to GBS or endotoxin.[193, 247] Ongoing studies are defining the role of cytokine production in neonatal and other infections.

The proinflammatory cytokine IL-2 acts on activated T cells and to some extent on B cells and natural killer cells and causes them to proliferate or differentiate. IL-2 is synthesized by both T cells and natural killer cells.[175, 238] Decreased production of IL-2 or IL-2 receptor expression has been noted in numerous clinical disease states, most notably in cases of severe combined immunodeficiency disease. Lesser degrees of abnormality may occur in acquired immunodeficiency syndrome (AIDS), type 1 diabetes mellitus, systemic lupus erythematosus, and hypogammaglobulinemia.[143, 146, 155] The most intriguing potential for IL-2 in the treatment of disease involves its use in tumor therapy.[206] IL-2 is approved for the treatment of metastatic renal carcinoma. The use of IL-2–activated natural killer cells results in a decrease in tumor burden in approximately 20 percent of patients, although serious side effects do occur. In addition to its potential role as an antitumor agent, IL-2 shares many of the same effects as IFN-γ and someday may function as a therapeutic agent in infection, autoimmunity, and immunodeficiency.[146, 206]

Both IL-8 and IL-9 are being investigated in various human disease states, primarily because of their powerful role in stimulating neutrophil function, including activation, adhesion, and chemotaxis. Patients with cystic fibrosis, bronchiectasis, and chronic bronchitis have been shown to have elevated levels of IL-8 in their sputum.[202] Sputum from these patients is highly chemotactic to neutrophils, but when treated with monoclonal antibodies to IL-8, this chemotactic effect was inhibited. Aerosolized IL-8 inhibitors have been used in patients with cystic fibrosis and have resulted in decreased inflammation in these patients.[168, 202] IL-8 inhibitors are being evaluated in infants with bronchopulmonary dysplasia. Researchers speculate that the persistently elevated levels of IL-8 seen in the tracheal fluid of ventilated preterm infants leads to an accumulation of neutrophils and the development of pulmonary fibrosis, which may be reduced by IL-8 inhibitors.[123, 133] Similar studies are being conducted with IL-9 inhibitors. Thus, these cytokines may play an important role in the acute inflammatory response leading to chronic disease states, and blocking this response may be of therapeutic benefit. The proinflammatory IL-5 has not been associated with a specific human disease state, but its strong B-cell proliferative effects suggest a possible role in the pathogenesis of immunodeficiency, and its potent effects on eosinophil production, activation, and migration implicate its action in allergic responses.[29]

The proinflammatory activities of IL-12 and IL-18 are of current immunologic interest as well. IL-12 is an integral immune regulator that is produced primarily by macrophages and dendritic cells.[188] IL-12 has been shown to induce the production of INF-γ by T cells and natural killer cells.[161, 163, 188] IL-18, another recently described cytokine with many proinflammatory functions,[170] was defined initially as INF-γ–inducing factor.[33, 58, 147] IL-12 and IL-18 both alone and in synergy regulate INF-γ production in response to infection with intracellular parasites and bacteria and in certain autoimmune diseases.* Regulation of these cytokines may be therapeutically beneficial in certain disease states.[62, 88] The other proinflammatory cytokines are also in various developmental stages of experimental investigation. As we learn more about their specific actions, we will be better able to determine their use as potential immunomodulating agents.

*See references 58, 115, 125, 165, 189, 224, 228, 236, 241, 253.

Clinical use of the anti-inflammatory cytokines is limited. IL-4 can block both IL-1 and TNF-α transcription[98, 213] and has been shown to inhibit human neutrophil adhesion to human endothelial cells while enhancing the adhesion of eosinophils.[179] These effects have not been implicated in specific human diseases, but IL-4 action is suggested in allergic responses. Although IL-6 has both anti-inflammatory and proinflammatory effects, levels of this cytokine were found to correlate with mortality rates in children with gram-negative and gram-positive sepsis, thus suggesting that monitoring IL-6 levels may be of prognostic value.[235] Similarly, IL-10 has been shown to block the production of IL-1, IL-6, IL-8, IL-12, and TNF-α, as well as GM-CSF, in animal models.[51, 54] It also has effects on mast cells, T cells, and natural killer cells and inhibits primary allogeneic T-cell responses. Thus, IL-10 may have a potential role in treating acute and chronic inflammation and may be effective in suppressing transplant rejection.[11, 51] Recent studies examining the safety and immunomodulatory effects of the intravenous injection of IL-10 in humans demonstrate that it is well tolerated and results in decreased production of both TNF-α and IL-1.[21] Additional clinical studies are being conducted on the potential immunoregulatory effects of the anti-inflammatory cytokines and may indicate their therapeutic use in human disease states.

COLONY-STIMULATING FACTORS

CSFs are involved principally in the production of neutrophils and monocytes. They were discovered because of their ability to stimulate the formation of colonies of granulocytes and monocytes/macrophages in cultured bone marrow cells and were named according to the primary cell colony type that they elicited. GM-CSF induces the production of peripheral blood macrophages and granulocytes. It also has other pleiotropic effects, including stimulation of precursors of megakaryocytes, mast cells, and eosinophils. In addition, GM-CSF has effects on neutrophil migration and phagocytosis. Granulocyte CSF (G-CSF) induces the production of peripheral blood granulocytes. Its actions involve both the production and function of neutrophils, including migration, phagocytosis, and superoxide generation. Macrophage CSF (M-CSF) induces the production of peripheral mononuclear phagocytes. IL-3 increases mast cell populations as well as the induction of granulocytes, macrophages, eosinophils, and megakaryocytes.[59, 91, 146, 147, 154, 173]

Clinical studies with GM-CSF and G-CSF as adjuvant therapy have been performed in individuals with distinct lymphopoietic disorders (i.e., congenital agranulocytosis, cyclic neutropenia, Schwachman-Diamond syndrome) or disorders resulting from the consequences of cytotoxic chemotherapy, AIDS, and aplastic anemia. The CSFs can stimulate granulocyte and monocyte populations in these individuals, but the response is restricted to the number of available stem cells. CSF treatment can partially or completely reverse congenital neutropenia and has shown great promise in the regeneration of lymphopoietic cells after cytotoxic chemotherapy and high-dose chemotherapy followed by autologous bone marrow transplantation. Recombinant human GM-CSF (rhGM-CSF) also has been shown to be beneficial in patients with aplastic anemia.[5, 233]

Hammond and colleagues[96] demonstrated a dramatic increase in neutrophil counts in children with cyclic neutropenia treated with recombinant human G-CSF (rhG-CSF). Cyclic neutropenia is a rare disorder characterized by regular 21-day cyclic fluctuations in the number of blood neutrophils, monocytes, eosinophils, lymphocytes, platelets, and reticulocytes. Although the exact mechanism of this disorder is not known, it is attributed to a regulatory abnormality affecting stem cell proliferation. These infants have recurrent aphthous stomatitis, pharyngitis, lymphadenopathy, fever, and numerous infections during the periods of neutropenia. The length of cycling in treated infants decreased from 21 to 1 day, and the neutrophil turnover rate increased nearly fourfold, thereby significantly reducing the frequency of infection. Recombinant G-CSF also has shown promise in infants and children with neutrophil production disorders. Infants with congenital agranulocytosis, Kostmann syndrome, and Schwachman-Diamond syndrome have disorders characterized by a severe, persistent absolute neutropenia that shows a dramatic increase in neutrophil count after treatment with rhG-CSF.[20] In addition, rhG-CSF and rhGM-CSF have been used in neutropenic patients with AIDS. Although a concern is that the effects of GM-CSF in activating macrophages may in turn promote the replication of human immunodeficiency virus (HIV), current studies are defining the role of rhGM-CSF and rhG-CSF in patients with AIDS.[90, 154]

Thus, CSFs are emerging as significant modulators of human immune function and lymphopoiesis. Recombinant G-CSF and GM-CSF have demonstrated promising effects in clinical trials, and the utility of M-CSF and IL-3 is being investigated. Because the CSFs also can functionally activate mature granulocytes and monocytes, considerable attention has focused on their future role in treating individuals at risk for acquiring infection. English and coauthors[61] reported decreased GM-CSF production by neonatal T cells. Because a major factor contributing to the increased susceptibility of human neonates to the development of severe infections is their inability to produce adequate numbers of neutrophils in response to bacterial infections, these neonates may benefit from CSF treatment for severe infection.[16] Similar treatment in immunologically stressed burn and trauma patients also may prove beneficial.[50, 186]

Interferons

INTERFERON-α AND INTERFERON-β

The interferons are glycoproteins that were discovered because of their antiviral properties. They are known to possess antitumor and immunomodulatory activity in addition to their antiviral effect. The interferons have been classified into three major groups: INF-α, INF-β, and INF-γ. INF-α and INF-β were known previously as type I interferon and have similar protein structures and bind the same receptor. INF-γ, formerly type II interferon, has a much different structure and its own receptor.[7] IFN-α is produced by leukocytes. The earliest demonstration of its clinical usefulness was in the treatment of AIDS-related Kaposi sarcoma (KS). In these initial studies, a KS response occurred in 30 to 50 percent of the patients treated with recombinant IFN-α.[89, 136, 177, 181] IFN-α is speculated to exert its antitumor effect by activating cytotoxic T cells. Since then, placebo-controlled clinical trials have shown that IFN-α also may have a significant antiretroviral effect in HIV-infected patients.[135, 142] Clinical trials are under way to determine the effect of early treatment with IFN-α in reducing the progression of HIV disease and to determine the therapeutic effect of IFN-α in combination with other drugs in the treatment of HIV and HIV-related diseases.[134]

IFN-α also has been used in various parts of the world for the treatment of chronic myeloid leukemia, hairy-cell leukemia, basal cell carcinoma, multiple myeloma, hepatitis B and C, and condylomata acuminata. In chronic myeloid leukemia, early treatment with IFN-α has been reported to elicit complete hematologic remission in more than 70 percent of the patients treated. Many of these patients had total elimination of the Philadelphia chromosome, which is a hallmark of the disease.[229-231] Complete to 80 percent remissions also have been reported in the treatment of hairy-cell leukemia.[198] Intralesional injection of IFN-α into basal cell carcinoma of the skin resulted in 81 percent tumor remission as determined by biopsy.[46, 120] Despite the variability in reported outcomes with the use of IFN-α in the treatment of multiple myeloma, it has been approved as therapy for these patients in numerous European countries.[164] IFN-α also is used for the treatment of hepatitis B and C.[147] Clinical responses have been reported to be of long duration, often with complete loss of both hepatitis B surface antigen and evidence of viral replication. In chronic hepatitis C, complete response to therapy as determined by a decline in serum aspartate aminotransferase to normal levels has been reported in 50 to 70 percent of the patients treated. Although serum aspartate aminotransferase levels returned to pretreatment levels within 6 to 12 months after discontinuation of therapy in half the patients who had improved, nearly 20 percent achieved sustained remission.[53, 56, 114, 132, 194] Studies also have shown that IFN-α is useful in treating genital warts, or condylomata acuminata caused by papillomaviruses.[28] Intralesional injections of IFN-α completely eliminated warts in more than 50 percent of the patients treated. In addition, IFN-α therapy is suggested to reduce the number of lesions in juvenile laryngeal papillomatosis after systemic use.[160] Thus, IFN-α has therapeutic potential as both an antitumor and an antiviral agent.

IFN-β also has received attention as an antiviral and antitumor agent. Its clinical usefulness as single-agent therapy is suggested in relapsing multiple sclerosis. The mechanism of therapeutic action of IFN-β in multiple sclerosis is unknown, however.[121] Current studies are investigating IFN-β therapy in combination with IFN-α for the treatment of various malignancies.

INTERFERON-γ

IFN-γ is produced by CD4 and CD8 cells, as well as by natural killer cells.[103] Investigators have reported that circulating mononuclear cells and T lymphocytes from neonates are markedly deficient in their ability to produce IFN-γ in response to a variety of stimuli in comparison to adult cells.[153, 215, 248] Studies using recombinant IFN-γ have shown that pre-incubation of neonatal neutrophils, which are deficient in chemotactic ability, with recombinant IFN-γ enhances their chemotactic response to a level equal to that of adult neutrophils.[103] Other studies have shown that neonatal mixed mononuclear cells are deficient in production of the IFN-γ–stimulating cytokines IL-12 and IL-18 in response to GBS.[107, 109, 124] In vitro treatment with recombinant IL-12 and IL-18 can correct this defect in IFN-γ production in response to GBS. These findings suggest a potential role for the regulation of IFN-γ in neonatal host defense.

Job syndrome was described first by Davis, Schaller, and Wedgwood in 1965 in two patients with recurrent staphylococcal abscesses.[52] Chronic sinopulmonary infections and mucocutaneous *Candida* infections often develop in patients with this syndrome. Hill and coworkers[110] observed that patients with Job syndrome also have a profound defect in neutrophil chemotactic responsiveness, along with extreme hyperimmunoglobulinemia E. This defect in neutrophil chemotaxis is intermittent and occurs predominantly when the patient is symptomatic.[49, 104, 110] Because IFN-γ production by mononuclear leukocytes in patients with hyperimmunoglobulinemia E is markedly deficient or absent, in vitro studies were conducted to determine the effect of recombinant IFN-γ on the chemotactic responsiveness of neutrophils from patients with this syndrome. After pretreatment with IFN-γ, the chemotactic response of neutrophils from patients with Job syndrome increased significantly, with an average enhancement of 300 percent above baseline to levels not significantly different from those of matched healthy controls.[122] Preliminary trials of IFN-γ therapy in four patients with Job syndrome and hyperimmunoglobulinemia E suggested clinical benefit in three, with a significant decrease in eczema and in pulmonary symptoms and secretions.

Patients with chronic granulomatous disease (CGD) have an inherited deficiency in the proteins required for nicotinamide-adenine dinucleotide phosphate oxidase activity. Phagocytes with this enzymatic defect are able to engulf bacteria but cannot generate the respiratory burst necessary to kill the organisms. Consequently, patients with CGD suffer severe chronic, recurrent life-threatening infections. The value of using IFN-γ to treat patients with CGD was suggested by studies showing that this lymphokine can stimulate the respiratory burst of normal phagocytes. The results of studies by Ezekowitz and colleagues[65] and Sechler and associates[214] showed that when macrophages from patients with CGD were treated with IFN-γ in vitro, a respiratory burst occurred and superoxide anion was generated. Sechler and coworkers[214] further demonstrated a partial correction in neutrophils and monocytes from patients with CGD after subcutaneous treatment with recombinant IFN-γ. These initial results suggested that recombinant IFN-γ could partially correct the defective ability of phagocytes to kill bacteria when administered in vivo to patients with CGD. Ezekowitz and colleagues[66] extended these findings in a double-blind, placebo-controlled trial. They showed that recombinant IFN-γ significantly decreased the relative risk of serious infection developing in patients with CGD. Patients who received IFN-γ had a 70 percent reduction in the risk for serious infection when compared with controls. Overall, IFN-γ decreases the risk of acquiring infection and the length of hospitalization in patients with CGD. When administered with prophylactic antibiotics, an additive effect occurs, with a nearly 20 percent increase, in comparison to IFN-γ alone, in the infection-free rate of CGD patients.[66] IFN-γ was license by the Food and Drug Administration in December 1990 for the treatment of patients with CGD. The authors of the collaborative studies recommended its use with the addition of prophylactic antibiotics for the treatment of children with CGD.[79]

Neutrophils and Complement

Recruitment of neutrophils from the bloodstream to extravascular sites of inflammation is a critical event in host defense against bacterial infection and in the repair of tissue damage. In certain circumstances, accumulation of neutrophils may contribute to vascular and tissue injury. Thus, the regulatory mechanisms involved in neutrophil activation, recruitment, and subsequent degranulation are of potential clinical significance. Neutrophil adherence to and migration through capillary endothelium is a critical early event in the acute inflammatory response. The adhesive interactions between leukocytes and endothelial cell surfaces are regulated by two novel families of glycoproteins: the integrins and the selectins. The β_2 integrins are membrane-bound glycoprotein receptors found on the surface of PMNs.

β_2 Integrins, CD11/CD18, are required for PMN adherence to endothelial cell surfaces. The selectins are also membrane-bound glycoproteins that mediate neutrophil adhesion to endothelial cells. They include L-selectin, which is found on the surface of PMNs, and P-selectin and E-selectin, which are expressed on the surface of activated endothelial cells.[15, 38, 225, 243, 258]

The interaction between β_2 integrins and the selectins serves to regulate PMN responses during inflammation. In general, P- and E-selectins on activated endothelial cell surface and L-selection on the PMN cell surface function to facilitate PMN rolling and tethering to activated capillary endothelium. Once this tethering has occurred and the PMN itself is activated, the β_2 integrin CD11/CD18 receptors on the PMN form a tight adhesion to the endothelial cell surface that facilitates PMN polarization and subsequent migration.[15, 38, 225, 258] Congenital β_2 integrin CD11/CD18 deficiency states have been described (leukocyte adhesion deficiency type I [LAD-I]). These patients have profound defects in PMN adhesion and motility and recurrent life-threatening infections, along with delayed separation of the umbilical cord and juvenile periodontitis.[64, 78] A second type of leukocyte adhesion deficiency, LAD-II, has been described and is caused by a deficiency in sialyl Lewis X, the PMN ligand for E-selectin on endothelial cells.[195] Tethering of PMNs to P-selectin on activated endothelial cells also has been shown to be critical for PMN priming by PAF, and monoclonal antibodies to P-selectin can block this response.[157] Monoclonal antibodies to P-selectin have been used in animal models of ischemia and reperfusion injury and have been shown to significantly reduce the severe edema and endothelial cell injury observed after reperfusion.[249] Similarly, monoclonal antibodies to P-selectin have resulted in significant endothelial cell preservation in animal models of lung injury and cardiac ischemia.[180, 244] Monoclonal antibodies to E-selectin and L-selectin also are being tested in animal models.[169] With the rapid advancements in identifying new molecules that influence endothelial cell–leukocyte interactions, we will gain greater understanding of the complexity of cellular communication during inflammation.

BACTERICIDAL/PERMEABILITY-INCREASING FACTOR AND DEFENSINS

In addition to their respiratory burst activity in antimicrobial defense, human neutrophils recently have been shown to contain a variety of granule-associated antibacterial proteins and peptides,[203] including BPI and the defensin family of peptides. BPI is a 55-kd receptor present in neutrophil granules that contains two domains. One of the domains binds with LPS to increase membrane permeability and lysis of gram-negative bacteria, whereas the other promotes opsonization of gram-negative bacteria.[112] Neutrophil BPI functions best in inflamed tissues, where it acts in concert with defensins and the membrane attack complex of complement to cause cell lysis.

Meningococcemia is a severe gram-negative infection that occurs predominantly in infants and young adults. Mortality rates in meningococcemia range from 10 to 20 percent.[26, 100, 217, 245, 251] Endotoxin levels may be profoundly elevated and correlate with the severity of the illness.[26] Recombinant BPI (rBPI) has been used as an adjunct to antimicrobial therapy in children with severe meningococcal sepsis[151]; 14 of 193 patient with severe meningococcal disease who received rBPI (2 mg/kg over a 30-minute period) died versus 20 of 203 control infants, an insignificant difference. Among the surviving treated patients, however, a modest improvement in long-term functional outcome was noted, thus suggesting a possible beneficial effect in decreasing the complications associated with septic shock.[84, 151] Neonates recently have been shown to have reduced release and activity of BPI, which may contribute to their enhanced susceptibility to gram-negative bacterial infection.[152] Future studies are exploring the clinical effects of rBPI in sepsis syndromes.

The defensins are strongly cationic, single-chain peptides contained in neutrophil primary, or azurophilic, granules with molecular weights between 3 and 4.5 kd. Defensins account for 50 percent of the protein content of the neutrophil primary granules.[80, 254] These peptides possess broad antimicrobial activity against gram-positive and gram-negative bacteria, fungi, mycobacteria, and some viruses. The defensins create voltage-sensitive pores in microbial membranes that result in cell lysis. They are divided into α- and β-defensins. Humans have six human α-defensins (HAD-1 to HAD-6) and two human β-defensins (HBD-1 and HBD-2).

The α-defensins, HAD-1 to HAD-6, are made by neutrophils and represent 30 to 50 percent of the primary granule content.[99] Defensins appear at the site of inflammation. They are present after neutrophil degranulation induced by LPS, IL-8, C5a, and other stimuli. In addition, they are found on the epithelial surfaces of bronchi and in bronchial lavage fluid from patients with various types of inflammatory lung disease. The antimicrobial activity of defensins is inhibited by high salt content, which may be clinically important in the immune response of cystic fibrosis patients.[86]

β-Defensins are produced by epithelial cells of the respiratory and gastrointestinal tracts.[18, 216] HBD-1 is expressed constitutively by epithelial cells in the bronchi and the intestine, whereas HBD-2 synthesis is up-regulated by inflammatory stimuli, including LPS, TNF-α, bacterial infection, and injury. Thus, HBD-1 acts to kill organisms in the absence of inflammation, whereas HBD-2 acts primarily as part of the inflammatory process.

In inflammatory lung disease such as chronic bronchitis and chronic obstructive pulmonary disease, both α-defensins (HAD-1 to HAD-6) and the β-defensin HBD-2 may be increased significantly, perhaps contributing to airway inflammation.[254] No clinical disorders of defensin production have been reported. A potential role for the defensins as immunoregulatory-antimicrobial agents is being investigated.

Endotoxin and other proinflammatory mediators activate the complement system and the chemotactic properties of C5a, which recruits neutrophils to sites of infection. Interrupting this process at various levels may be possible by using monoclonal antibody strategies that counteract the effects of complement in leading to septic shock. Although the use of monoclonal antibodies directed at the specific components of the complement cascade has not been tested in human clinical trials, the use of monoclonal antibodies to inhibit C5a in primates challenged with *E. coli* improved the survival rate and reduced the development of adult respiratory distress syndrome.[4, 19]

PLATELET-ACTIVATING FACTOR

PAF is a potent phospholipid inflammatory mediator with many biologic effects. Its synthesis is regulated by phospholipase A_2, an enzyme associated with the arachidonic acid pathway. PAF has a very short half-life in vivo because of its rapid degradation by PAF acetylhydrolase. PAF is synthesized by many cell types, including macrophages, neutrophils, platelets, eosinophils, endothelial cells, and hepatocytes.[246] Intravenous infusion of PAF in animals results in pulmonary hypertension, bronchoconstriction, neutropenia, thrombocytopenia, and ischemic bowel necrosis.[12, 42, 97] Production of PAF is stimulated in numerous clinical disease states, including hypoxia and ischemia, and after the administration of biologic agents such as LPS, GM-CSF, TNF-α, IL-1, bradykinin, and thrombin.[68, 137, 172, 196, 205, 250] Corticosteroids decrease PAF levels by induction of its natural inhibitor PAF acetylhydrolase.[87] PAF has been shown to stimulate the production of many other mediators of inflammation, including TNF-α, complement breakdown products, oxygen radicals, catecholamines, prostaglandins, thromboxane, and the leukotrienes.[70, 118, 137, 205, 234, 257] It also activates endothelial cells and neutrophils and monocytes, thereby leading to their adherence and migration.[171] Thus, PAF is a ubiquitous phospholipid mediator with many biologic effects and interactions within the inflammatory cascade.

Regulation of PAF has been studied in numerous potential clinical disease states, including sepsis and septic shock.[116] The clinical phase III trials in septic patients and patients in septic shock who received a PAF antagonist did show a significant reduction in mortality.[55] The role of PAF, however, in the pathogenesis of necrotizing enterocolitis (NEC) has received considerable recent attention.[35, 36] NEC is a gastrointestinal disease that is often fatal and affects predominantly premature infants. Exogenous administration of PAF into the rat mesenteric circulation causes ischemic bowel necrosis and pathology similar to that of neonatal NEC.[117] Endotoxin-induced intestinal injury is associated with increased levels of PAF, and infusion of high doses of endotoxin into animals produces a similar pathologic model of NEC that can be prevented by the administration of dexamethasone, PAF acetylhydrolase, or PAF receptor antagonists.[34, 119] These animal studies suggest a link between PAF and its regulation and the development of NEC and implicate PAF as a potential endogenous inflammatory mediator in the pathogenesis of neonatal NEC.

Evidence in humans supports an association between PAF and human neonatal NEC. PAF levels are higher in infants with NEC than in controls, and PAF acetylhydrolase activity is lower in infants with NEC.[37] PAF acetylhydrolase is suppressed with prematurity.[33] Because enteral feeding is necessary for the development of NEC, PAF levels were measured in feeding premature infants. In these studies, feedings alone increased circulating PAF levels but not PAF acetylhydrolase, and infants fed human breast milk had lower PAF levels and a lower incidence of NEC, thus suggesting a protective effect of human milk through PAF regulation.[162] Human milk is known to have many factors that are protective against infectious disease, including PAF acetylhydrolase.[30, 85] Because PAF acetylhydrolase activity is present in human milk and absent in formulas, researchers have suggested that the protective activity observed in human milk against the development of NEC may result from blocking of PAF-related inflammatory responses.[30] Modulation of the many interactions of PAF within the inflammatory cascade may have future clinical potential in regulating neonatal NEC and other inflammatory disease states.

NITRIC OXIDE

Nitric oxide is a membrane-permeable gas that functions in the regulation of vascular tone and inhibition of platelet aggregation and leukocyte adhesion. In addition, nitric oxide has been shown to have antitumor as well as antimicrobial activity. Under normal conditions, nitric oxide synthase induces endothelial cell production of nitric oxide. The signal transduction pathway for nitric oxide is linked to pathways involving vasodilation. Evidence exists for activation of the L-arginine–nitric oxide pathway in sepsis, in which the effects of nitric oxide on the vasculature are associated with the severe vascular failure observed during septic shock.[44, 130, 178, 184, 185] Thus, inhibition of nitric oxide production has been proposed as a novel approach for treatment of the severe hypotension associated with septic shock.[239]

The increased production of nitric oxide observed during septic shock may have several harmful effects. Nitric oxide may be largely responsible for sepsis-induced hypotension. In vitro studies implicate nitric oxide in sepsis-induced myocardial depression, although nitric oxide synthase inhibitors have not been shown to prevent endotoxin-induced myocardial depression in vivo. Nitric oxide also has direct cytotoxic effects, and its overproduction in septic shock can lead to tissue injury and organ failure.[45, 71, 128] In addition, in vitro experiments suggest that nitric oxide may enhance the release of proinflammatory cytokines during septic shock.[63, 184] Production of nitric oxide may have some beneficial effects during septic shock, however. It is implicated in maintaining visceral and other microvasculature blood flow, both as a counter-regulatory mechanism to the vasoconstrictive mediators released during sepsis and by its ability to block platelet adhesion and thereby reduce potential microvasculature stasis and thrombosis.[129, 167] In addition, high levels of nitric oxide have antimicrobial activity and enhance LPS-induced cytokine production,[138] although whether these levels of nitric oxide reflect actual physiologic states has not been determined.

Because hypotension during sepsis is an important predictor of organ injury and death, the use of nitric oxide synthase inhibitors may improve survival rates in severe septic shock by increasing mean arterial pressure. Nitric oxide synthase inhibitors have been shown to restore vascular responsiveness to catecholamines in animal models of endotoxin-induced septic shock.[113] In addition, nitric oxide synthase inhibition has been shown to normalize mean arterial pressure in anesthetized animals challenged with endotoxin or TNF-α without causing hypertension.[128] These considerations have led to the use of nitric oxide synthase inhibitors to treat hypotension in patients with sepsis and in those receiving cytokine therapy for cancer.[127, 158] Although these agents can alter mean arterial pressure, beneficial effects on clinical outcomes, including survival, are only suggested in human clinical trials.[184] Studies of endotoxin-challenged rats showed that partial nitric oxide synthase inhibition improves survival, whereas complete inhibition of nitric oxide production is clearly harmful, thus suggesting a beneficial effect with selective partial nitric oxide inhibition. Currently, studies of nitric oxide inhibition that are more selective are being explored, and in the future such therapy may have clinical utility in the treatment of infectious disease states.

Conclusion

Initial attempts to augment immune function in the treatment of sepsis consisted of serum antibody therapy. The development and refinements in hybridoma and recombinant technologies have provided the means to generate highly specific monoclonal antibodies. Although monoclonal antibodies directed toward bacteria and their components are not used during sepsis, their future may be in combination with antimicrobial pharmacologic agents to treat certain pathogens. Recent advances in basic science and clinical research also have demonstrated that the cytokines play many crucial roles in the pathogenesis of septic shock. Interaction among the proinflammatory cytokines initiates the development of a cascade of biologic events leading to the propagation and regulation of inflammation. Although the proinflammatory cytokines are effective in augmenting immune responses, their overexpression can often result in severe septic shock. The use of neutralizing monoclonal antibodies to endotoxin, anti–TNF-α antibodies, and soluble TNF-α and IL-1 receptors, as well as IL-1ra, in human clinical trials of septic shock, however, have shown limited therapeutic potential. The future clinical use of cytokine inhibition probably may include a combination of numerous recombinant and pharmacologic agents concurrently administered to regulate multiple proinflammatory cytokine–mediated steps in the development of septic shock. The hematopoietic growth factors have demonstrated considerable clinical effect, especially in individuals with distinct lymphopoietic disorders and in patients receiving immunosuppressive chemotherapy. IFN-α, IFN-β, and IFN-γ have received considerable attention during the past decade as potential immunomodulators. IFN-α has shown broad clinical application as an antitumor as well as an antiviral agent, and IFN-β is being used with some success in patients with relapsing multiple sclerosis. The stimulatory effect of IFN-γ on human neutrophils has been demonstrated in infants and children with specific neutrophil disorders and in neonatal sepsis. Investigations defining the actions of the integrins and the selectins, BPI, and the defensins, as well as PAF and nitric oxide, may provide novel future clinical therapeutic approaches to attenuate acute inflammatory responses. As we learn more about the complexity of intracellular and extracellular interactions and the delicate balance that these molecules have in regulating immune responses, we will be better able to implement their clinical use in regulating infectious disease states in infants and children.

REFERENCES

1. Abraham, E.: Why immunomodulatory therapies have not worked in sepsis. Intensive Care Med. *25*:556–566, 1999.
2. Alexander, H. R., Doherty, G. M., Buresh, C. M., et al.: A recombinant human receptor antagonist to interleukin-1 improves survival after lethal endotoxemia in mice. J. Exp. Med. *173*:1029, 1991.
3. Andersson, J. P., and Andersson, U. G.: Human intravenous immunoglobulin modulates monokine production in vitro. Immunology *71*:372, 1990.
4. Andrews, E., Feldhoff, P. A., and Lassiter, H. A.: Modulation of the complement system in the prevention and treatment of sepsis. Semin. Pediatr. Infect. Dis. *12*:54–63, 2001.
5. Antman, K. S., Griffin, J. D., Elias, A., et al.: Effect of recombinant human granulocyte-macrophage colony-stimulating factor on chemotherapy-induced myelosuppression. N. Engl. J. Med. *319*:593, 1988.
6. Ballow, M.: Mechanisms of action of intravenous immune serum globulin therapy. Pediatr. Infect. Dis. J. *13*:806, 1994.
7. Baron, S., Tyring, S. K., Fleischmann, W. R., et al.: The interferons: Mechanism of action and clinical applications. J. A. M. A. *266*:1375, 1991.
8. Basta, M., Kirshborn, P., Frank, M. M., et al.: Mechanisms of therapeutic effects of high-dose intravenous immunoglobulin: Attenuation of acute complement-dependent immune damage in a guinea pig model. J. Clin. Invest. *84*:1974, 1989.
9. Baumgartner, J. D., and Calandra, T.: Treatment of sepsis: Past and future avenues. Drugs *57*:127–132, 1999.
10. Baumgartner, J. D., Glauser, M. P., McCutchan, J. A., et al.: Prevention of gram-negative shock and death in surgical patients by antibody to endotoxin core glycolipid. Lancet *2*:59, 1985.
11. Berg, D. J., Kühn, R., and Rajewsky, K.: Interleukin-10 is a central regulator of the response to LPS in murine models of endotoxic shock and the Shwartzman reaction but not endotoxin tolerance. J. Clin. Invest. *96*:2339, 1995.
12. Bernat, A., Herbert, J. M., Salel, V., et al.: Protective effect of SR 27417, a novel PAF antagonist, on PAF- or endotoxin-induced hypotension in the rat and the guinea-pig. J. Lipid Mediat. *5*:41–48, 1992.
13. Bertini, R., Delgado, R., Faggioni, R., et al.: Urinary TNF-binding protein (TNF soluble receptor) protects mice against the lethal effect of TNF and endotoxin shock. Eur. Cytokine Netw. *4*:39, 1993.
14. Beutler, B., Milsark, I. W., and Cerami, A. C.: Passive immunization against cachectin/tumor necrosis factor protects mice from lethal effect of endotoxin. Science *229*:869–871, 1985.
15. Bevilacqua, M. P., and Nelson, R. M.: Selectins. J. Clin. Invest. *91*:379, 1993.
16. Bilgin, K., Yaramis, A., Haspolat, K., et al.: A randomized trial of granulocyte-macrophage colony-stimulating factor in neonates with sepsis and neutropenia. Pediatrics *107*:36–41, 2001.
17. Bohnsack, J. F., Hawley, M. M., Pritchard, D. G., et al.: An IgA monoclonal antibody directed against type III antigen on group B streptococci acts as an opsonin. J. Immunol. *143*:3338–3342, 1989.
18. Boman, H. G.: Innate immunity and the normal microflora. Immunol. Rev. *173*:5–16, 2000.
19. Bone, R. C.: Inhibitors of complement and neutrophils: A critical evaluation of their role in the treatment of sepsis. Crit. Care Med. *20*:891–898, 1992.
20. Bonilla, M. A., Gillio, A. P., Ruggeno, M., et al.: Effect of recombinant human granulocyte colony-stimulating factor on neutropenia in patients with congenital agranulocytosis. N. Engl. J. Med. *320*:1574, 1989.
21. Borish, L., and Rosenwasser, L. J.: Update on cytokines. J. Allergy Clin. Immunol. *97*:719, 1996.
22. Bortolussi, R.: Potential for intravenous gamma-globulin use in neonatal gram-negative infection: An overview. Pediatr. Infect. Dis. *5*(Suppl.): 198–200, 1986.
23. Bortolussi, R., and Ferrieri, P.: Protection against *Escherichia coli* K1 infection in newborn rats by antibody to K1 capsular polysaccharide antigen. Infect. Immun. *28*:111–117, 1980.
24. Bortolussi, R., Ferrieri, P., and Quie, P. G.: Influence of growth temperature of *Escherichia coli* on K1 capsular antigen production and resistance to opsonization. Infect. Immun. *39*:1136–1141, 1983.
25. Bortolussi, R., and Fischer, G. W.: Opsonic and protective activity of immunoglobulin, modified immunoglobulin, and serum against neonatal *Escherichia coli* K1 infection. Pediatr. Res. *20*:175–178, 1986.
26. Brandtzaeg, P., Kierulf, P., Gaustad, P., et al.: Plasma endotoxin as a predictor of multiple organ failure and death in systemic meningococcal disease. J. Infect. Dis. *159*:195–204, 1989.
27. Breedveld, F. C.: Therapeutic monoclonal antibodies. Lancet *355*:735–740, 2000.
28. Brodell, R. T.: The use of natural alpha interferon in the treatment of condyloma acuminata. Infect. Med. *13*:56, 1996.
29. Broide, D. H., Paine, M. M., and Firestein, G. S.: Eosinophils express interleukin-5 and granulocyte macrophage-colony stimulating factor mRNA at sites of allergic inflammation in asthmatics. J. Clin. Invest. *90*:1414, 1992.
30. Buescher, E. S.: Host defense mechanisms of human milk and their relations to enteric infections and necrotizing enterocolitis. *In* Stoll, B. J., and Kliegman, R. M. (eds.): Clinics in Perinatology. Philadelphia, W. B. Saunders, 1994, pp. 247–262.
31. Calandra, T., Baumgartner, J. D., Grau, G. E., et al.: Prognostic values of tumor necrosis factor/cachectin, interleukin-1, interferon-alpha, interferon-gamma in the serum of patients with septic shock. J. Infect. Dis. *161*:982, 1990.
32. Cannon, J. G., Tompkins, R. G., Gelfand, J. A., et al.: Circulating interleukin-1 and tumor necrosis factor in septic shock and experimental endotoxin fever. J. Infect. Dis. *161*:79, 1990.
33. Caplan, M., Hsueh, W., Kelly, A., Donovan, M.: Serum PAF acetylhydrolase increases during neonatal maturation. Prostaglandins *39*:705–714, 1990.
34. Caplan, M. S., Kelly, A., and Hsueh, W.: Endotoxin and hypoxia induced intestinal necrosis in rats: The role of platelet activating factor. Pediatr. Res. *31*:428, 1992.
35. Caplan, M. S., and MacKendrick, W.: Inflammatory mediators and intestinal injury. Clin. Perinatol. *21*:235–246, 1994.
36. Caplan, M. S., Sun, X. M., and Hsueh, W.: Hypoxia, PAF and necrotizing enterocolitis. Lipids *26*:1340, 1991.
37. Caplan, M. S., Sun, X. M., Hsueh, W., et al.: Role of platelet activating factor and tumor necrosis factor-alpha in neonatal necrotizing enterocolitis. J. Pediatr. *116*:960, 1990.
38. Carlos, T. M., and Harlan, J. M.: Leukocyte-endothelial adhesion molecules. Blood *84*:2068, 1994.
39. Casadevall, A., and Scharff, M. D.: Serum therapy revisited: Animal models of infection and development of passive antibody therapy. Antimicrob. Agents Chemother. *38*:1695–1702, 1994.
40. Casadevall, A., and Scharff, M. D.: Return to the past: The case for antibody-based therapies in infectious disease. Clin. Infect. Dis. *21*:150–161, 1995.
41. Cerami, A.: Inflammatory cytokines. Clin. Immunol. Pathol. *62*:53, 1992.
42. Chang, S. W., Feddersen, C. O., Henson, P. M., et al.: Platelet activating factor mediates hemodynamic changes and lung injury in endotoxin-treated rats. J. Clin. Invest. *79*:1498, 1987.
43. Chantry, D., Turner, M., Abney, E., et al.: Modulation of cytokine production by transforming growth factor-beta. J. Immunol. *142*:4295, 1989.
44. Cobb, J. P., Cunnion, R. E., and Danner, R. L.: Nitric oxide as a target for therapy in septic shock. Crit. Care Med. *21*:1261, 1993.
45. Cobb, J. P., Natanson, C., Hoffman, W. D., et al.: N-omega-amino-L-arginine, an inhibitor of nitric oxide synthase, raises vascular resistance but increases mortality rates in awake canines challenged with endotoxin. J. Exp. Med. *176*:1175–1182, 1992.

46. Cornell, R. C., Greenway, H. T., Tucker, S. B., et al.: Intralesional interferon therapy for basal cell carcinoma. J. Am. Acad. Dermatol. *23*:694, 1990.
47. Cross, A. S., Wooldridge, W. H., and Zollinger, W. D.: Monoclonal antibody 2-2-B kills K1-positive *Escherichia coli* in conjunction with cord blood neutrophils and sera, but not with spinal fluid. Pediatr. Res. *18*:770–772, 1984.
48. Czuczman, M. S., Grillo-Lopez, A. J., White, C. A., et al.: Treatment of patients with low-grade B-cell lymphoma with the combination of chimeric anti-CD20 monoclonal antibody and CHOP chemotherapy. J. Clin. Oncol. *17*:268–276, 1999.
49. Dahl, M. V., Greene, W. H., Jr., and Quie, P. G.: Infection, dermatitis, increased IgE, and impaired neutrophil chemotaxis. A possible relationship. Arch. Dermatol. *112*:1387, 1976.
50. Dale, D. C.: Potential role of colony-stimulating factors in the prevention and treatment of infectious diseases. Clin. Infect. Dis. *18*(Suppl.):180, 1994.
51. D'Andrea, A., Aste-Amezaga, M., Vaiante, N. M., et al.: Interleukin-10 (IL-10) inhibits human lymphocyte interferon-g production by suppressing natural killer cell stimulatory factor IL-12 synthesis in accessory cells. J. Exp. Med. *178*:1041, 1993.
52. Davis, D. S., Schaller, J., and Wedgwood, R. J.: Job's syndrome. Recurrent "cold" staphylococcal abscesses. Lancet *1*:1013–1015, 1965.
53. Davis, G. L., Balart, L. A., Shiff, E. R., et al.: Treatment of chronic hepatitis C with recombinant interferon alpha: A multicenter randomized controlled trial. N. Engl. J. Med. *321*:1501, 1989.
54. de Malefyt, R., Yssel, H., Roncarolo, M. G., et al.: Interleukin-10. Curr. Opin. Immunol. *4*:314, 1992.
55. Dhainaut, J. F., Tenaillon, A., Le Tulzo, Y., et al.: Platelet-activating factor receptor antagonist BN52021 in the treatment of severe sepsis: A randomized, double-blind, placebo-controlled, multicenter clinical trial. Crit. Care Med. *22*:1720, 1994.
56. DiBisceglie, A. M., Martin, P., Kassianides, C., et al.: Recombinant interferon alpha therapy for chronic hepatitis C: A randomized, double-blind, placebo-controlled trial. N. Engl. J. Med. *321*:1506, 1989.
57. Dinarello, C. A.: The proinflammatory cytokines, interleukin-1 and tumor necrosis factor and the treatment of the septic shock syndrome. J. Infect. Dis. *163*:1177, 1991.
58. Dinarello, C. A.: IL-18: A Th-1–inducing, proinflammatory cytokine and new member of the IL-1 family. J. Allergy Clin. Immunol. *103*:11, 1999.
59. Donahue, R. E.: Colony-stimulating factors: Their biological activities and clinical promise. Adv. Vet. Sci. Comp. Med. *36*:291, 1991.
60. Elliott, M. J., Maini, R. N., Feldmann, M., et al.: Randomised double-blind comparison of chimeric monoclonal antibody to tumor necrosis factor alpha (cA2) versus placebo in rheumatoid arthritis. Lancet *344*:1105–1110, 1994.
61. English, K. B., Hammond, W. P., Lewis, D. B., et al.: Decreased granulocyte-macrophage colony stimulating factor production by human neonatal blood mononuclear cells and T cells. Pediatr. Res. *31*:211, 1992.
62. Esfandiari, E., McInnes, I. B., Lindop, G., et al.: A proinflammatory role of IL-18 in the development of spontaneous autoimmune disease. J. Immunol. *167*:5338, 2001.
63. Estrada, C., Gomez, C., Martin, C., et al.: Nitric oxide mediates tumor necrosis factor alpha cytotoxicity in endothelial cells. Biochem. Biophys. Res. Commun. *186*:475, 1992.
64. Etzloni, A., Frydman, M., Pollack, S., et al.: Brief report: Recurrent severe infections caused by a novel leukocyte adhesion deficiency. N. Engl. J. Med. *327*:1789, 1992.
65. Ezekowitz, R. A., Dinauer, M. C., Jaffe, H. S., et al.: Partial correction of the phagocytic defect in patients with X-linked chronic granulomatous disease by subcutaneous interferon gamma. N. Engl. J. Med. *319*:146–151, 1988.
66. Ezekowitz, R. A. B., and International Collaborative Study Group to Assess the Efficiency of rIFN-gamma in CGD: Clinical efficacy of recombinant human interferon-gamma (rIFN-gamma) in chronic granulomatous disease (CGD). Abstract. Clin. Res. *38*:465, 1990.
67. Faist, E., Schinkel, C., and Zimmer, S.: Update on the mechanisms of immune suppression of injury and immune modulation. World J. Surg. *20*:454, 1996.
68. Feuerstein, G., and Hallenbeck, J. M.: Prostaglandins, leukotrienes and platelet activating factor in shock. Annu. Rev. Pharmacol. Toxicol. *27*:301, 1987.
69. Finberg, S. M.: The therapy of (horse) serum reactions, general rules in the administration of therapeutic serums. J. A. M. A. *107*:1717–1719, 1936.
70. Fink, M. P.: Platelet-activating factor, eicosanoids, and bradykinin as targets for adjuvant therapies for sepsis. Semin. Pediatr. Infect. Dis. *12*:30–41, 2001.
71. Finkel, M. S., Oddis, C. V., Jacob, T. D., et al.: Negative inotropic effects of cytokines on the heart mediated by nitric oxide. Science *257*:387, 1992.
72. Fischer, G. W., Hemming, V. G., Hunter, K. W., Jr., et al.: Intravenous immunoglobulin in the treatment of neonatal sepsis: Therapeutic strategies and laboratory studies. Pediatr. Infect. Dis. *5*(Suppl.):171–175, 1986.
73. Fischer, G., Schuman, R., Wilson, S., et al.: Monoclonal antibody enhances survival in neonatal models of lethal staphylococcal sepsis. Abstract. E. S. P. I. D. *17*:27, 1999.
74. Fisher, C. J., Dhainaut, J.-F. A., Opal, S. M., et al.: Recombinant human interleukin 1 receptor antagonist in the treatment of patients with sepsis syndrome. J. A. M. A. *271*:1836, 1994.
75. Fisher, C. J., Slotman, G. J., Opal, S. M., et al.: Initial evaluation of human recombinant interleukin-1 receptor antagonist in the treatment of sepsis syndrome: A randomized, open label, placebo controlled multicentric trial. Crit. Care Med. *22*:12, 1994.
76. Fisher, C. J., Jr., and Zheng, Y.: Potential strategies for inflammatory mediator manipulation: Retrospect and prospect. World J. Surg. *20*:447, 1996.
77. Freimer, E. H., and Lancefield, R. C.: Type-specific polysaccharide antigens of group B streptococci. J. Hyg. (Lond.) *64*:191–203, 1966.
78. Frydman, M., Etzioni, A., Eidlitz-Markus, T., et al.: Rambam-Hasharon syndrome of psychomotor retardation, short stature, defective neutrophil motility and Bombay phenotype. Am. J. Med. Genet. *44*:297, 1992.
79. Gallin, J. I.: Interferon-gamma in the management of chronic granulomatous disease: The evolving use of biologicals in the treatment and prevention of infectious diseases. Rev. Infect. Dis. *13*:973, 1991.
80. Ganz, T., and Weiss, J.: Antimicrobial peptides of phagocytes and epithelia. Semin. Hematol. *34*:343–354, 1997.
81. Gaur, S., Kesarwala, H., Gavai, M., et al.: Clinical immunology and infectious diseases. Pediatr. Clin. North Am. *41*:745–782, 1994.
82. Girardin, E., Grau, G. E., Dayer, J. M., et al.: Tumor necrosis factor and interleukin-1 in the serum of children with severe infectious purpura. N. Engl. J. Med. *319*:397, 1988.
83. Giroir, B. P., and Beutler, B.: Effect of amrinone on tumor necrosis factor production in endotoxic shock. Circ. Shock *36*:200–207, 1992.
84. Giroir, B. P., Quint, P. A., Barton, P., et al.: Preliminary evaluation of recombinant amnio-terminal fragment of human bactericidal/permeability-increasing protein in children with severe meningococcal sepsis. Lancet *350*:1539–1443, 1997.
85. Goldman, A. S.: The immune system of human milk: Antimicrobial anti-inflammatory and immunomodulating properties. Pediatr. Infect. Dis. J. *12*:664, 1993.
86. Goldman, M. J., Anderson, G. M., Stolzenberg, E. D., et al.: Human β-defensin-1 is a salt-sensitive antibiotic in lung that is inactivated in cystic fibrosis. Cell *88*:553–560, 1997.
87. Goppelt-Struebe, M., and Rehfeldt, W.: Glucocorticoids inhibit TNF alpha induced cytosolic phospholipase A_2 activity. Biochim. Biophys. Acta *1127*:163, 1992.
88. Gracie, J. A., Forsey, R. J., Chan, W. L., et al.: A proinflammatory role for IL-18 in rheumatoid arthritis. J. Clin. Invest. *104*:1393, 1999.
89. Groopman, J. E., Gottlieb, M. S., Goodman, J., et al.: Recombinant alpha-2 interferon therapy for Kaposi's sarcoma associated with acquired immune deficiency syndrome. Ann. Intern. Med. *100*:671, 1984.
90. Groopman, J. E., Mitsuyasu, R. T., DeLeo, M. J., et al.: Effect of recombinant human granulocyte-macrophage colony-stimulating factor on myelopoiesis in the acquired immunodeficiency syndrome. N. Engl. J. Med. *317*:593, 1987.
91. Grosh, W. W., Quesenberry, P. J.: Recombinant human hematopoietic growth factors in the treatment of cytopenias. Clin. Immunol. Immunopathol. *62*(Suppl.):25, 1992.
92. Guirao, X., and Lowry, S. F.: Biological control of injury and inflammation: Much more than too little or too late. World J. Surg. *20*:437, 1996.
93. Haak-Frendscho, M., Marseters, S. A., Mordenti, J., et al.: Inhibition of TNF by a TNF receptor immunoadhesin. Comparison to an anti-TNF monoclonal antibody. J. Immunol. *152*:1347, 1994.
94. Hamm, C. W., Heeschen, C., Goldmann, B., et al.: Benefit of abciximab in patients with refractory unstable angina in relation to serum troponin T levels. c7E3 Fab Antiplatelet Therapy in Unstable Refractory Angina (CAPTURE) study investigators. N. Engl. J. Med. *340*:1623–1629, 1999.
95. Hammerberg, C., Arend, W. P., Fisher, G. J., et al.: Interleukin-1 receptor agonist in normal and psoriatic epidermis. J. Clin. Invest. *90*:571, 1992.
96. Hammond, W. P., 4th, Price, T. H., Souza, L. M., et al.: Treatment of cyclic neutropenia with granulocyte colony-stimulating factor. N. Engl. J. Med. *320*:1306, 1989.
97. Hanahan, D. J.: Platelet activating factor: A biologically active phosphoglyceride. Annu. Rev. Biochem. *55*:483, 1986.
98. Hart, P. H., Vitti, G. F., Burgess, D. R., et al.: Potential antiinflammatory effects of interleukin-4: Suppression of human monocyte tumor necrosis factor alpha, interleukin-1 and prostaglandin E_2. Proc. Natl. Acad. Sci. U. S. A. *86*:3803, 1984.
99. Harwig, S. S. L., Ganz, T., and Lehrer, R. I.: Neutrophil defensins: Purification, characterization and antimicrobial testing. Methods Enzymol. *236*:160–172, 1994.
100. Havens, P. L., Garland, J. S., Brook, M. M., et al.: Trends in mortality in children hospitalized with meningococcal infections, 1957 to 1987. Pediatr. Infect. Dis. J. *8*:8–11, 1989.
101. Hill, H. R.: Intravenous immunoglobulin use in the neonate: Role in prophylaxis and therapy of infection. Pediatr. Infect. Dis. J. *12*:549, 1993.
102. Hill, H. R.: Additional confirmation of the lack of effect of intravenous immunoglobulin in the prevention of neonatal infection. J. Pediatr. *137*:595–597, 2000.

103. Hill, H. R., Augustine, N. H., and Jaffe, H. S.: Human recombinant interferon enhances neonatal polymorphonuclear leukocyte activation and movement, and increases free intracellular calcium. J. Exp. Med. *173*:767, 1991.
104. Hill, H. R., Estensen, R. D., Hogan, N. A., et al.: Severe staphylococcal disease associated with allergic manifestations, hyperimmunoglobulin E, and defective neutrophil chemotaxis. J. Lab. Clin. Med. *88*:796, 1976.
105. Hill, H. R., Gonzalez, L. A., and Kelsey, D. K.: The potential use of monoclonal antibodies as therapeutic modalities in neonatal infection. *In* Ballow, M. (ed.): IVIG Therapy Today. Totowa, NJ, Humana Press, 1992, pp. 29–38.
106. Hill, H. R., Gonzales, L. A., Knappe, W. A., et al.: Comparative protective activity of human monoclonal and hyperimmune polyclonal antibody against group B streptococci. J. Infect. Dis. *163*:792–798, 1991.
107. Hill, H. R., Joyner, J. L., La Pine, T. R., et al.: Defection production of IL-18 by cord blood cells in response to group B streptococci. Abstract. J. Invest. Med. *49*:72, 2001.
108. Hill, H. R., Kelsey, D. K., Gonzales, L. A., et al.: Monoclonal antibodies in the therapy of experimental neonatal group B streptococcal disease. Clin. Immunol. Immunopathol. *62*(Suppl.):87–91, 1992.
109. Hill, H. R., La Pine, T. R., Kwak, S. D., et al.: Defective production of IL-18 and IL-12 by cord blood mononuclear cells influences the TH-1 interferon-gamma response to group B streptococci. Abstract. J. Invest. Med. *50*:50, 2002.
110. Hill, H. R., Quie, P. G., Ochs, H. D., et al.: Defect in neutrophil granulocyte chemotaxis in Job's syndrome of recurrent "cold" staphylococcal abscesses. Lancet *2*:617, 1974.
111. Hill, H. R., Shigeoka, A. O., Pincus, S., et al.: Intravenous IgG in combination with other modalities in the treatment of neonatal infection. Pediatr. Infect. Dis. *5*(Suppl.):180–184, 1986.
112. Hoffmann, J. A., Kafatos, F. C., Janeway, C. A., Jr., et al.: Phylogenetic perspectives in innate immunity. Science *284*:1313–1318, 1999.
113. Hollenberg, S. M., Cunnion, R. E., and Zimmerberg, J.: Nitric oxide synthase inhibition reverses arteriolar hyporesponsiveness to catecholamines in septic rats. Am. J. Physiol. *264*:660, 1993.
114. Hoofnagle, H.: Chronic hepatitis B. N. Engl. J. Med. *323*:337, 1990.
115. Horwood, N. J., Elliott, J. , Martin, T. J., et al.: IL-12 alone and in synergy and IL-18 inhibits osteoclast formation in vitro. J. Immunol. *166*:4915, 2001.
116. Hosford, D., Koltai, M., and Braquet, P.: Platelet activating factor in shock, sepsis, and organ failure. *In* Schlag, G., and Redl, H. (eds.): Pathophysiology of Shock, Sepsis and Organ Failure. Heidelberg, Germany, Springer-Verlag, 1993, pp. 502–517.
117. Hsueh, W., Gonzalez-Crussi, F., and Arroyave, J. L.: Platelet activating factor: An endogenous mediator for bowel necrosis in endotoxemia. FASEB J. *1*:403, 1987.
118. Hsueh, W., Gonzalez-Crussi, F., and Arroyave, J. L.: Sequential release of leukotrienes and norepinephrine in rat bowel after platelet-activating factor. Gastroenterology *94*:1412, 1988.
119. Israel, E. J., Schiffrin, E., Carter, E. A., et al.: Prevention of necrotizing enterocolitis in the rat with prenatal cortisone. Gastroenterology *99*:1333–1338, 1990.
120. Itri, L. M.: The interferons. Cancer *70*:940, 1992.
121. Jacobs, L. D., Cookfair, D. L., Rudick, R. A., et al.: Intramuscular interferon beta-1a for disease progression in relapsing multiple sclerosis. The Multiple Sclerosis Collaborative Research Group (MSCRG). Ann. Neurol. *39*:285, 1996.
122. Jeppson, J. D., Jaffe, H. S., and Hill, H. R.: Use of recombinant human interferon gamma to enhance neutrophil chemotactic responses in Job's syndrome of hyperimmunoglobulinemia E and recurrent infections. J. Pediatr. *118*:383, 1991.
123. Jones, C. A., Cayabyab, R. G., Kwong, Y. C., et al.: Undetectable interleukin IL-10 and persistent IL-8 expression early in hyaline membrane disease: A possible developmental basis for the predisposition to chronic lung inflammation in preterm newborns. Pediatr. Res. *39*:966, 1996.
124. Joyner, J. L., Augustine, N. H., Taylor, K. A., et al.: Effects of group B streptococci on cord and adult mononuclear cell interleukin-12 and interferon-g mRNA accumulation and protein secretion. J. Infect. Dis. *182*:74, 2000.
125. Kawakami, K., Koguchi, Y., and Qureshi, M. H.: IL-18 contributes to host resistance against infection with *Cryptococcus neoformans* in mice with defective IL-12 synthesis through induction of IFN-g production by NK cells. J. Immunol. *165*:941, 2000.
126. Kennedy, W. A., Hoyt, M. J., and McCracken, G. H., Jr.: The role of corticosteroid therapy in children with pneumococcal meningitis. Am. J. Dis. Child. *145*:1374, 1991.
127. Kilbourn, R. G., and Griffith, O. W.: Overproduction of nitric oxide in cytokine-mediated septic shock. J. Natl. Cancer Inst. *84*:827, 1992.
128. Kilbourn, R. G., Gross, S. S., Jubran, A., et al.: NG-methyl-L-arginine inhibits tumor necrosis factor induced hypotension: Implications for the involvement of nitric oxide. Proc. Natl. Acad. Sci. U. S. A. *87*:3629, 1990.
129. Klabunde, R. E., and Helgren, M. C.: Cardiovascular actions of NG-methyl-L-arginine are abolished in a canine shock model using high dose endotoxin. Res. Commun. Chem. Pathol. Pharmacol. *78*:57, 1992.
130. Knowles, R. G., and Moncada, S.: Nitric oxide synthases in mammals. Biochem. J. *298*:249–257, 1994.
131. Kohler, G., and Milstein, C.: Continuous cultures of fused cells secreting antibody of predefined specificity. Nature *256*:495–497, 1975
132. Korenman, J., Baker, B., Waggoner, J., et al.: Long term remission of chronic hepatitis B after alpha-interferon therapy. Ann. Intern. Med. *114*:629, 1991.
133. Kotecha, S., Wilson, K., Wangoo, A., et al.: Increased interleukin IL-13 and IL-6 in bronchoalveolar lavage fluid obtained from infants with chronic lung disease of prematurity. Pediatr. Res. *40*:250, 1996.
134. Krown, S. E.: Approaches to interferon combination therapy in the treatment of AIDS. Semin. Oncol. *17*:11, 1990.
135. Krown, S. E., Gold, J. W. M., and Niedzwiecki, D.: Interferon-alpha with zidovudine: Safety, tolerance, and clinical and virological effect in patients with Kaposi sarcoma associated with the acquired immunodeficiency syndrome (AIDS). Ann. Intern. Med. *112*:812, 1990.
136. Krown, S. E., Real, F. X., Cunningham-Rundles, S., et al.: Preliminary observations on the effect of recombinant leukocyte A interferon in homosexual men with Kaposi's sarcoma. N. Engl. J. Med. *308*:1071, 1983.
137. Kubes, P., Arfovs, K. E., and Granger, D. N.: Platelet-activating factor induced mucosal dysfunction—role of oxidants and granulocytes. Am. J. Physiol. *260*:G965, 1991.
138. Kubes, P., Suzuki, M., and Granger, D. N.: Nitric oxide: An endogenous modulator of leukocyte adhesion. Proc. Natl. Acad. Sci. U. S. A. *88*:4651, 1991.
139. Lancefield, R. C.: A serologic differentiation of specific types of bovine hemolytic streptococci (group B). J. Exp. Med. *59*:441–449, 1934.
140. Lancefield, R. C.: Two serological types of group B hemolytic streptococci with related, but not identical, type-specific substances. J. Exp. Med. *67*:25–31, 1938.
141. Lancefield, R. C., McCarty, M., and Everly, W. N.: Multiple mouse-protective antibodies directed against group B streptococci. Special references to antibodies effective against protein antigens. J. Exp. Med. *142*:165–174, 1975.
142. Lane, H. C., Davey, V., Kovacs, J. A., et al.: Interferon-alpha in patients with asymptomatic human immunodeficiency virus (HIV) infection. A randomized, placebo-controlled trial. Ann. Intern. Med. *112*:805, 1990.
143. La Pine, T. R., and Hill, H. R.: Immunomodifiers applicable to the prevention and management of infectious diseases in children. Adv. Pediatr. Infect. Dis. *9*:37–58, 1994.
144. La Pine, T. R., and Hill, H. R.: Monoclonal antibodies. Semin. Pediatr. Infect. Dis. *12*:64–70, 2001.
145. Lassiter, H. A., Robinson, T. W., Brown, M. S., et al.: Effect of intravenous immunoglobulin G on the deposition of immunoglobulin G and C3 onto type III group B *Streptococcus* and *Escherichia coli* K1. J. Perinatol. *16*:346–351, 1996.
146. Lau, A. S.: Cytokines in the pathogenesis and treatment of infectious diseases. Adv. Pediatr. Infect. Dis. *9*:211–236, 1994.
147. Lau, A. S., Lehman, D., Geertsma, F. R., et al.: Biology and therapeutic uses of myeloid hematopoietic growth factors and interferons. Pediatr. Infect. Dis. J. *15*:563, 1996.
148. Lauterbach, R., Pawlik, D., Kowalczyk, D., et al.: Effect of the immunomodulating agent, pentoxifylline, in the treatment of sepsis in prematurely delivered infants: A placebo-controlled, double-blind trial. Crit. Care Med. *27*:807–814, 1999.
149. Leung, D. Y.: The immunoregulatory effects of IVIG in Kawasaki disease and other autoimmune diseases. Clin. Rev. Allergy *10*:93–104, 1992.
150. Leung, D. Y., Cotran, R. S., Kurt-Jones, E., et al.: Endothelial cell activation and high interleukin-1 secretion in the pathogenesis of acute Kawasaki disease. Lancet *1*:1298, 1989.
151. Levin, M., Quint, P. A., Goldstein, B., et al.: Recombinant bactericidal/permeability-increasing protein ($rBPI_{21}$) as adjunctive treatment for children with severe meningococcal sepsis: A randomized trial. RBPI21 Meningococcal Sepsis Study Group. Lancet *356*:961–967, 2000.
152. Levy, O., Martin, S., Eichenwald, E., et al.: Impaired innate immunity in the newborn: Newborn neutrophils are deficient in bactericidal/permeability-increasing protein. Pediatrics *104*:1327–1333, 1999.
153. Lewis, D. B., Weaver, M., Prickett, K., et al.: Restricted production of IL-4 compared to IFN-gamma by human T cells during post natal development. J. Cell. Biochem. *13*:233, 1989.
154. Lieschke, G. J., and Burgess, A. W.: Granulocyte colony-stimulating factor and granulocyte-macrophage colony-stimulating factor. N. Engl. J. Med. *327*:28, 1992.
155. Liles, W. C., and Voorhis, W. C.: Nomenclature and biological significance of cytokines involved in inflammation and host immune response. J. Infect. Dis. *172*:1573, 1995.
156. Lipsky, P., St. Clair, E. W., Furst, D., et al.: 54-wk clinical and radiographic results from the ATTRACT trial: A phase III study of infliximab in patients with active RA despite methotrexate. Arthritis Rheum. *42*(Suppl.):401, 1999.
157. Lorant, D. E., Topham, M. K., Whatley, R. E., et al.: Inflammatory roles of P-selectin. J. Clin. Invest. *92*:559, 1993.
158. Lorente, J. A., Landin, L., De Pablo, R., et al.: L-Arginine pathway in the sepsis syndrome. Crit. Care Med. *21*:1287, 1993.
159. Luce, J. M.: Introduction of new technology into critical care practice: A history of HA-1A human monoclonal antibody against endotoxin. Crit. Care Med. *21*:1233, 1993.

160. Lusk, R. P., McCabe, B. F., and Mixon, J. H.: Three-year experience of treating recurrent respiratory papilloma with interferon. Ann. Otol. Rhinol. Laryngol. *19*:158, 1987.
161. Macatonia, S. E, Hsieh, C. S., Murphy, K. M., et al.: Dendritic cells and macrophages are required for Th-1 development of $CD4^+$ T cells from ab TCR transgenic mice: IL-12 substitution for macrophages to stimulate IFN-g production is IFN-g–dependent. Int. Immunol. *5*:1119, 1993.
162. MacKendrick, W., Hill, N., Hsueh, W., et al.: Increase in plasma platelet-activating factor levels in enterally fed premature infants. Biol. Neonate *64*:89, 1993.
163. Magram, J., Connaughton, S. E., Warrier, R. R., et al.: IL-12–deficient mice are defective in IFN-g production and type 1 cytokine responses. Immunity *4*:471, 1996.
164. Mandelli, F., Avvisati, G., Amadori, S., et al.: Maintenance treatment with recombinant interferon alfa-2b in patients with multiple myeloma responding to conventional induction chemotherapy. N. Engl. J. Med. *322*:1430, 1990.
165. Mastroeni, P., Clare, S., Khan, S., et al.: Interleukin 18 contributes to host resistance and g (gamma) interferon production in mice infected with virulent *Salmonella typhimurium*. Infect. Immun. *67*:478, 1999.
166. Mathison, J. C., Wolfson, E., and Ulevitch, R. J.: Participation of tumor necrosis factor in the mediation of gram negative bacteria lipopolysaccharide-induced injury in rabbits. J. Clin. Invest. *81*:1925, 1988.
167. May, G. R., Crook, P., Moore, P. K., et al.: The role of nitric oxide as an endogenous regulator of platelet neutrophil activation within the pulmonary circulation of the rabbit. Br. J. Pharmacol. *102*:759, 1991.
168. McElvaney, N. G., Nakamura, H., Birrer, P., et al.: Modulation of airway inflammation in cystic fibrosis. In vivo suppression of interleukin-8 levels on the respiratory epithelial surface by aerosolization of recombinant secretory leukoprotease inhibitor. J. Clin. Invest. *90*:1296, 1992.
169. McEver, R. P.: Selectins. Curr. Opin. Immunol. *6*:75, 1994.
170. McInnes, I. B., Gracie, J. A., Leung, B. P., et al.: Interleukin-18: A pleiotropic participant in chronic inflammation. Immunol. Today *21*:312, 2000.
171. McIntyre, T. M., Zimmerman, G. A., and Prescott, S. M.: Leukotrienes C_4 and D_4 stimulate human endothelial cells to synthesize platelet activating factor and bind neutrophils. Proc. Natl. Acad. Sci. U. S. A. *83*:2204, 1986.
172. McIntyre, T. M., Zimmerman, G. A., Satoh, K., et al.: Cultured endothelial cells synthesize both platelet-activating factor and prostacyclin in response to histamine, bradykinin, and adenosine triphosphate. J. Clin. Invest. *76*:271, 1985.
173. Metcalf, D.: Control of granulocytes and macrophages: Molecular cellular and clinical aspects. Science *254*:529, 1991.
174. Michie, H. R., Manoque, K. R., Spriggs, D. R., et al.: Detecting circulating tumor necrosis factor after endotoxin administration. N. Engl. J. Med. *318*:1481, 1988.
175. Minami, Y., Kono, T., Miyazaki, T., et al.: The IL-2 receptor complex: Its structure, function, and target genes. Annu. Rev. Immunol. *11*:245, 1993.
176. Minty, A., Chalon, P., Derocq, J. M., et al.: Interleukin-13 is a new human lymphokine regulating inflammation and immune responses. Nature *362*:248, 1993.
177. Mitsuyasu, R. T.: Use of recombinant interferons and hematopoietic growth factors in patients infected with human immunodeficiency virus. Rev. Infect. Dis. *13*:979–984, 1991.
178. Moncada, S., Palmer, R. M., and Higgs, E. A.: Nitric oxide: Physiology, pathophysiology, and pharmacology. Pharmacol. Rev. *43*:109–142, 1991.
179. Moser, R., Fehr, J., and Bruijnzeel, P. L.: IL-4 controls the selective endothelium-driven transmigration of eosinophils from allergic individuals. J. Imunol. *149*:1432, 1992.
180. Mulligan, M. S., Polley, M. J., Bayer, R. J., et al.: Neutrophil-dependent acute lung injury. Requirement for P-selectin (GMP-140). J. Clin. Invest. *90*:1600, 1992.
181. Murray, H. W.: Interferon-gamma therapy in AIDS for mononuclear phagocyte activation. Biotherapy *2*:149, 1990.
182. Mustafa, M. M., Lebel, M. H., Ramilo, O., et al.: Correlation of interleukin-1 beta and cachectin concentration in cerebrospinal fluid and outcome from bacterial meningitis. J. Pediatr. *115*:208, 1989.
183. Natanson, C., Eichenholz, P. W., Danner, R., et al.: Endotoxin and tumor necrosis factor challenges in dogs stimulate the cardiovascular profile of human septic shock. J. Exp. Med. *169*:823, 1989.
184. Natanson, C., Hoffman, W. D., and Suffredini, A. F.: Selected treatment strategies for septic shock based on proposed mechanisms of pathogenesis. Ann. Intern. Med. *120*:771, 1994.
185. Nathan, C. F., and Hibbs, J. B., Jr.: Role of nitric oxide synthesis in macrophage antimicrobial activity. Curr. Opin. Immunol. *3*:65, 1991.
186. Nelson, S.: Role of granulocyte colony-stimulating factor in the immune response to acute bacterial infection in the nonneutropenic host: An overview. Clin. Infect. Dis. *18*(Suppl.):197, 1994.
187. Newton, J. A., Ashwood, E. R., Yang, K. D., et al.: Effect of pentoxifylline on developmental changes in neutrophil cell surface mobility and membrane fluidity. J. Cell. Physiol. *140*:427, 1989.
188. O'Garra, A.: Cytokines induce the development of functionally heterogenous T helper cell subsets. Immunity *8*:275, 1998.
189. Ohkusu, K., Yoshimoto, T., and Takeda, K.: Potentiality of interleukin-18 as a useful reagent for treatment and prevention of *Leishmania major* infection. Infect. Immun. *68*:2449, 2000.
190. Ohlsson, K., Bjork, P., Bergenfeldt, M., et al.: Interleukin-1 receptor antagonist reduces mortality from endotoxin shock. Nature *346*:550, 1990.
191. Oismüller, C., Mayer, N., Micksche, M., et al.: In-vivo modulation of human neutrophil function by pentoxifylline in patients with septic syndrome. Shock *4*:161, 1995.
192. Orlicek, S. L.: Cytokine inhibitors for sepsis and septic shock. Semin. Pediatr. Infect. Dis. *12*:24–29, 2001.
193. Peat, E. B., Augustine, N. H., Drummond, W. K., et al.: Effects of fibronectin and group B streptococci on tumor necrosis factor-a production by human culture-derived macrophages. Immunology *84*:440, 1995.
194. Perrillo, R. P.: Treatment of chronic hepatitis B with interferon: Experience in western countries. Semin. Liver Dis. *9*:240, 1989.
195. Phillips, M. L., Schwartz, B. R., Etzioni, A., et al.: Neutrophil adhesion in leukocyte adhesion deficiency syndrome type 2. J. Clin. Invest. *96*:2898, 1995.
196. Prescott, S. M., Zimmerman, G. A., and McIntyre, T. M.: Human endothelial cells in culture produce platelet-activating factor (1-alkyl-22-acetyl-sn-glycero-3-phosphocholine) when stimulated with thrombin. Proc. Natl. Acad. Sci. U. S. A. *81*:3534, 1984.
197. Present, D. H., Rutgeerts, P., Targan, S., et al.: Infliximab for the treatment of fistulas in patients with Crohn's disease. N. Engl. J. Med. *340*:1398–1405, 1999.
198. Quesada, J. R., Reuben, J., Manning, J. T., et al.: Alpha interferon for induction of remission in hairy cell leukemia. N. Engl. J. Med. *310*:15, 1984.
199. Raff, H. V., Devereux, D., Shuford, W., et al.: Human monoclonal antibody with protective activity for *Escherichia coli* K1 and *Neisseria meningitidis* group B infections. J. Infect. Dis. *157*:118–126, 1988.
200. Raff, H. V., Siscoe, P. J., Wolff, E. A., et al.: Human monoclonal antibodies to group B streptococcus. Reactivity and in vivo protection against multiple serotypes. J. Exp. Med. *168*:905–917, 1988.
201. Rambaldi, A., Torcia, M., Bettoni, S., et al.: Modulation of cell proliferation and cytokine production in acute myeloblastic leukemia by interleukin-1 receptor antagonists and lack of its expression by leukemic cells. Abstract. Blood *76*:114, 1990.
202. Richman-Eisenstat, J. B., Jorens, P. G., Hebert, C. A., et al.: Interleukin-8: An important chemoattractant in the sputum of patients with chronic inflammatory airway diseases. Am. J. Physiol. *264*:L413–L418, 1993.
203. Risso, A.: Leukocyte antimicrobial peptides: Multifunctional effector molecules of innate immunity. J. Leukoc. Biol. *68*:785–792, 2000.
204. Robbins, J. B., McCracken, G. H. Jr., Gotschlich, E. C., et al.: *Escherichia coli* K1 capsular polysaccharide associated with neonatal meningitis. N. Engl. J. Med. *290*:1216–1220, 1974.
205. Rola-Pleszczynski, M., and Stankova, J.: Differentiation-dependent modulation of TNF production by PAF in human HL-60 myeloid leukemia cells. J. Leukoc. Biol. *51*:609, 1992.
206. Rosenberg, S. A., Lotze, M. T., Muul, L. M., et al.: A progress report on the treatment of 157 patients with advanced cancer using lymphokine-activated killer cells and interleukin-2 or high doses of interleukin-2 alone. N. Engl. J. Med. *316*:884, 1987.
207. Russell, D. A., Tucken, K. K., Chinookoswoung, N., et al.: Combined inhibition of interleukin-1 and tumor necrosis factor in rodent endotoxemia: Improved survival and organ function. J. Infect. Dis. *171*:1528, 1995.
208. Sadoff, J. C.: Soluble TNF receptors. Paper presented at the Third International Congress of the Immune Consequences of Trauma, Shock and Sepsis: Mechanisms of Therapeutic Approaches, 1994, Munich.
209. Salyer, J. L., Bohnsack, J. F., Knape, W. A., et al.: Mechanisms of tumor necrosis factor alpha alteration of PMN adhesion and migration. Am. J. Pathol. *136*:831, 1990.
210. Schade, U. F., Burmeister, I., and Engel, R.: Increased 13-hydroxyoctadienoic acid content in lipopolysaccharide stimulated macrophages. Biochem. Biophys. Res. Commun. *147*:695, 1987.
211. Schedel, I., Dreikhausen, U., Nentwig, B., et al.: Treatment of gram-negative septic shock with an immunoglobulin preparation: A prospective, randomized clinical trial. Crit. Care Med. *19*:1104, 1991.
212. Schindler, R., Clark, B. D., and Dinarello, C. A.: Dissociation between interleukin-1 beta mRNA and protein synthesis in peripheral blood mononuclear cells. J. Biol. Chem. *265*:10232, 1990.
213. Schindler, R., Mancilla, J., Endres, S., et al.: Correlations and interactions in the production of interleukin-6 (IL-6), and tumor necrosis factor (TNF) in human blood mononuclear cells: IL-6 suppresses IL-1 and TNF. Blood *75*:40, 1990.
214. Sechler, J. M. G., Malech, H. L., White, C. J., et al.: Recombinant human interferon-gamma reconstitutes defective phagocyte function in patients with chronic granulomatous disease of childhood. Proc. Natl. Acad. Sci. U. S. A. *85*:4874, 1988.
215. Seki, H., Taga, K., Matsoda, N., et al.: Phenotypic and functional characteristics of active suppressor cells against IFN-gamma production in PHA-stimulated cord blood lymphocytes. J. Immunol. *137*:3158, 1986.

216. Selsted, M. E., and Ouellette, A. J.: Defensins in granules and non-phagocytic cells. Trends Cell. Biol. *5*:114–119, 1995.
217. Serogroup B meningococcal disease: Oregon, 1994. M. M. W. R. Morb. Mortal. Wkly. Rep. *44*:121–124, 1995.
218. Shigeoka, A. O., Hall, R. T., and Hill, H. R.: Blood-transfusion in group-B streptococcal sepsis. Lancet *1*:636–638, 1978.
219. Shigeoka, A. O., Jensen, C. L., Pincus, S. H., et al.: Absolute requirement for complement in monoclonal IgM antibody–mediated protection against experimental infection with type III group B streptococci. J. Infect. Dis. *150*:63–70, 1984.
220. Shigeoka, A. O., Pincus, S. H., Rote, N. S., et al.: Protective efficacy of hybridoma type-specific antibody against experimental infection with group-B *Streptococcus*. J. Infect. Dis. *149*:363–372, 1984.
221. Shigeoka, A. O., Pincus, S. H., Rote, N. S., et al.: Monoclonal antibody preparations for immunotherapy of experimental GBS infection. Antibiot. Chemother. *35*:254–266, 1985.
222. Shyur, S. D., Raff, H. V., Bohnsack, J. F., et al.: Comparison of the opsonic and complement triggering activity of human monoclonal IgG1 and IgM antibody against group B streptococci. J. Immunol. *148*:1879–1884, 1992.
223. Sirko, S., Weisman, S., and Dinarello, C. A.: Transcription, translation and secretion of IL-1 and TNF: Effect of dual cyclooxygenase/5-lipooxygenase inhibitor. Eur. J. Immunol. *21*:243, 1991.
224. Song, C.-H., Kim, H.-J., Park, J.-K., et al.: Depressed interleukin-12 (IL-12), but not IL-18, production in response to a 30- or 32-kilodalton mycobacterial antigen in patients with active pulmonary tuberculosis. Infect. Immun. *68*:4477, 2000.
225. Springer, T. A.: Traffic signals for lymphocyte recirculation and leukocyte migration: The multistep paradigm. Cell *76*:301–314, 1994.
226. Staubach, K. H., Schroder, J., Stuber, F., et al.: Effect of pentoxifylline in severe sepsis: Results of a randomized, double-blind, placebo-controlled study. Arch. Surg. *133*:94–100, 1998.
227. Stevens, P., Young, L. S., Adamu, S.: Opsonization of various (K) *E. coli* by the alternative complement pathway. Immunology *50*:497–502, 1983.
228. Stoll, S., Jonuleit, H., Schmitt, E., et al.: Production of functional IL-18 by different subtypes of murine and human dendritic cells (DC): DC-derived IL-18 enhances IL-12 dependent Th-1 development. Eur. J. Immunol. *28*:3231, 1998.
229. Talpaz, M. N., Kantarjian, H., Kurzrock, R., et al.: Interferon alpha produces sustained cytogenic responses in chronic myelogenous leukemia. Philadelphia chromosome positive patients. Ann. Intern. Med. *114*:532, 1991.
230. Talpaz, M., Kantarjian, H., McCredie, K., et al.: Hematologic remission and cytogenic improvement induced by recombinant human interferon alpha in chronic myelogenous leukemia. N. Engl. J. Med. *314*:1065, 1986.
231. Talpaz, M., Kantarjian, H. M., McCredie, K. B., et al.: Clinical investigation of human alpha interferon in chronic myelogenous leukemia. Blood *69*:1280, 1987.
232. Tracey, K. J., Fong, Y., Hesse, D. G., et al.: Anti-cachectin/TNF monoclonal antibodies prevent septic shock during lethal bacteremia. Nature *330*:662, 1987.
233. Vadhan-Raj, S., Buescher, S., Broxmeyer, H. E., et al.: Stimulation of myelopoiesis in patients with aplastic anemia by recombinant human granulocyte-macrophage colony-stimulating factor. N. Engl. J. Med. *319*:1628, 1988.
234. Valone, F. H., and Ruis, N. M.: Stimulation of tumor necrosis factor release by cytotoxic analogues of platelet-activating factor. Immunology *76*:24, 1992.
235. Van Deventer, S. J. H., Buller, H. R., Sturk, A., et al.: Endotoxin induced chain reactions. Circ. Shock *31*:246, 1995.
236. Vankayalapati, R., Wizel, B., Lakey, D. L., et al.: T cells enhance production of IL-18 by monocytes in response to an intracellular pathogen. J. Immunol. *166*:6749, 2001.
237. Wald, E. R., Kaplan, S. L., Mason, E. O., et al.: Dexamethasone therapy for children with bacterial meningitis. Pediatrics *95*:21, 1995.
238. Watson, J., and Mochizuki, D.: Interleukin 2: A class of T cell growth factors. Immunol. Rev. *51*:257, 1980.
239. Wearden, M. E.: Nitric oxide synthase inhibitors for septic shock. Semin. Pediatr. Infect. Dis. *12*:42–45, 2001.
240. Weatherstone, K. B., and Rich, E. A.: Tumor necrosis factor/cachectin and interleukin-1 secretion by cord blood monocytes from premature infants. Pediatr. Res. *25*:342, 1989.
241. Wei, X. Q., Leung, B. P., Niedbala, W., et al.: Altered immune responses and susceptibility to *Leishmania major* and *Staphylococcus aureus* infection in IL-18–deficient mice. J. Immunol. *163*:2821, 1999.
242. Weisman, L. E., Wilson, S. R., and Fischer, G. W.: Intravenous immunoglobulin (IVIG) lots used in clinical trials to prevent late-onset infection in the high risk neonate contained variable *Staphylococcus epidermidis* antibody activity. Abstract. Pediatr. Res. *139*:304, 1996.
243. Welty, S. E.: Inhibition of neutrophil adhesion and neutrophil function in sepsis. Semin. Pediatr. Infect. Dis. *12*:46–53, 2001.
244. Weyrich, A. S., Ma, X. Y., Lefer, D. J., et al.: In vivo neutralization of P-selectin protects feline heart and endothelium in myocardial ischemia and reperfusion injury. J. Clin. Invest. *91*:2620, 1993.
245. Whalen, C. M., Hockin, J. C., Ryan, A., et al.: The changing epidemiology of invasive meningococcal disease in Canada, 1985 through 1992: Emergence of a virulent clone of *Neisseria meningitidis*. J. A. M. A. *273*:390–394, 1995.
246. Whatley, R. E., Zimmerman, G. A., McIntyre, T. M., et al.: Production of platelet-activating factor by endothelial cells. Semin. Thromb. Hemost. *13*:445, 1987.
247. Williams, P. A., Bohnsack, J. F., Augustine, N. H., et al.: Production of tumor necrosis factor by human cells in vitro and in vivo induced by group B streptococci. J. Pediatr. *123*:292, 1993.
248. Wilson, C. B., Westall, J., Johnston, L., et al.: Decreased production of interferon-gamma by human neonatal cells: Intrinsic and regulatory deficiencies. J. Clin. Invest. *77*:860, 1986.
249. Winn, R. K., Vedder, N. B., Paulson, J. C., et al.: Monoclonal antibodies to P-selectin are effective in preventing reperfusion injury to rabbit ears. Circulation *86*:316, 1992.
250. Wirthmueller, U., De Weck, A. L., and Dahinden, C. A.: Platelet-activating factor production in human neutrophils by sequential stimulation with granulocyte-macrophage colony-stimulating factor and chemotactic factors C5A or formyl-methionyl-leucyl-phenylalanine. J. Immunol. *142*:3213, 1989.
251. Wong, V. K., Hitchcock, W., and Mason, W. H.: Meningococcal infections in children: A review of 100 cases. Pediatr. Infect. Dis. *8*:224–227, 1989.
252. Wright, A., Shin, S. U., and Morrison, S. L.: Genetically engineered antibodies: Progress and prospects. Crit. Rev. Immunol. *12*:125–168, 1972.
253. Yoshimoto, T., Okamura, H. Y., and Tagawa, I.: Interleukin 18 together with interleukin 12 inhibits IgE production by induction of interferon-g production from activated B cells. Proc. Natl. Acad. Sci. U. S. A. *94*:3948, 1997.
254. Zhang, P., Summer, W. R., Bagby, G. J., et al.: Innate immunity and pulmonary host defense. Immunol. Rev. *173*:39–51, 2000.
255. Zhong, Z., Burns, T., Chang, Q., et al.: Molecular and functional characteristics of a protective human monoclonal antibody to serotype 8 *Streptococcus pneumoniae* capsular polysaccharide. Infect. Immun. *67*:4119–4127, 1999.
256. Ziegler, E. J., Fischer, C. J., Jr., Sprung, C. L., et al.: Treatment of gram-negative bacteremia in septic shock with HA-1A human monoclonal antibody against endotoxin. A randomized, double-blind, placebo-controlled trial. The HA-1A Sepsis Study Group. N. Engl. J. Med. *324*:429, 1991.
257. Zimmerman, G. A., McIntyre, T. M., and Prescott, S. M.: Production of platelet-activating factor by human vascular endothelial cells: Evidence for a requirement for specific agonists and modulation by prostacyclin. Circulation *72*:718, 1985.
258. Zimmerman, G. A., Prescott, S. M., and McIntyre, T. M.: Endothelial cell interactions with granulocytes: Tethering and signaling molecules. Immunol. Today *13*:93, 1992.

PART VI

Prevention of Infectious Diseases

CHAPTER 242 Active Immunizing Agents

PENELOPE H. DENNEHY ■ GEORGES PETER

Prevention of infectious diseases in children by immunization is one of the outstanding accomplishments of medical science. Children enjoy better health today because of effective immunization programs, which in many countries have diminished the morbidity and mortality of once common contagious diseases markedly. The striking decline in the United States in vaccine-preventable childhood diseases is demonstrated in Table 242–1. The success of immunizations is further illustrated by the 1977 eradication of smallpox achieved after a 10-year effort directed by the World Health Organization (WHO) and the extraordinary progress in global elimination of poliomyelitis in the 1990s.[109, 385] To achieve this progress in child health, scientific technology and medical practice have combined efforts to (1) understand the biology of causal infectious agents; (2) purify these agents and, in some cases, their components; (3) develop and test safe and effective vaccines; (4) manufacture and administer these vaccines to appropriate segments of the population; (5) develop appropriate indications and implement schedules for immunizations; and (6) identify necessary contraindications.

Infectious diseases can be prevented through immunization by (1) stimulating an active immunologic defense (such as from humoral antibody) through the administration of antigens, usually before natural exposure to an infectious agent (i.e., active immunization), or (2) temporarily supplying preformed human or animal antibody to persons before or soon after exposure to certain infectious agents (i.e., passive immunization). Active immunizations, including the currently available vaccines, are discussed in this chapter. Major vaccines (i.e., those discussed in this chapter) and their composition and routes of administration are listed in Table 242–2.

TABLE 242–1 ■ REDUCTION IN MORBIDITY OF SOME VACCINE-PREVENTABLE DISEASES IN THE UNITED STATES*

	Maximal No. of Cases (yr)	2001	Percent Decrease
Diphtheria	206,939 (1921)	2	100.0
Pertussis	265,296 (1934)	5,396	96.3
Tetanus	1,314 (1922–1926)	27	97.2
Poliomyelitis, paralytic	21,269 (1952)	0	100.0
Measles	894,134 (1941)	108	100.0
Mumps	152,209 (1968)	231	99.8
Rubella	57,686 (1969)	19	100.0
Congenital rubella syndrome	20,000 (1964–1965)	2	99.8
Haemophilus influenzae type b	20,000 (before 1987)	183	99.1
Invasive pneumococcal disease (<5 yr)	15,933 (2000)	14,382	9.7
Hepatitis B	21,102 (1990)	8,036	61.9
Varicella†	158,364 (1992)	27,382	82.7

*Provisional data from the Centers for Disease Control and Prevention.
†Data from seven states.

Active Immunoprophylaxis—Considerations and Recommendations

VACCINES

An ideal immunizing agent should include the following characteristics: (1) the agent should be easy to produce in well-standardized preparations that are readily quantifiable and stable in immunobiologic potency, (2) it should be easy to administer, (3) it should not produce disease in the recipient or susceptible contacts, (4) it should induce long-lasting (ideally permanent) immunity that is measurable by available and inexpensive techniques, (5) it should be free of contaminating and potentially toxic substances, and (6) adverse reactions should be minimal and minor in consequences. All these objectives rarely, if ever, are met with the currently available vaccines because they are neither completely safe nor completely effective. Partial immunity or undesirable side effects or reactions, or both, including rare severe reactions, can occur. Nonetheless, vaccines in current use are highly effective and very safe.

All active immunizing agents (vaccines) contain one or more antigens that stimulate a protective immunologic response. Some are live attenuated viruses or bacteria; other vaccines consist of killed microorganisms or contain inactivated components such as exotoxins (i.e., toxoids). In some, the antigen is a highly defined, single constituent, such as meningococcal polysaccharide, whereas in other vaccines, the antigen component is less well defined (e.g., live viruses or whole-cell pertussis vaccines composed of killed *Bordetella pertussis* organisms). Immunizing agents are administered in suspending fluids such as sterile water, saline, or complex tissue culture fluid that can contain proteins or other constituents derived from the medium from which the vaccine was produced (e.g., serum proteins, egg antigens, or other tissue culture–derived antigens). With some vaccines, certain preservatives, stabilizers, or antibiotics are added, which in some cases can result in hypersensitivity reactions. To enhance immunogenicity, particularly for vaccines containing inactivated microorganisms or their extracted components, adjuvants such as specific aluminum compounds may be added.

Immunization Schedules

The age and timing of immunization are critical for the success of vaccination. The schedule by which a vaccine is provided is based on multiple factors, including the epidemiology of naturally occurring disease, the age-specific risk of complications caused by the natural disease, the anticipated immunologic response of the host to the antigens, the duration of immunity that can be induced, and often, the recommended ages for routine health care visits. In general, vaccines are recommended at the youngest age at which significant risk for the natural disease and its complications exist and at which a protective immunologic response to the vaccine will occur. An example is measles vaccine, which in the United States is recommended routinely at

TABLE 242–2 ■ AVAILABLE VACCINES IN THE UNITED STATES FOR USE IN CHILDREN AND THEIR ROUTES OF ADMINISTRATION*

Vaccine	Type	Recommended Route
BCG	Live bacteria	ID (preferred) or SC
DTaP	Toxoids and inactivated bacterial components	IM
Hepatitis A	Inactivated virus	IM
Hepatitis B	Inactivated viral antigen, yeast-derived recombinant	IM
Hepatitis B and Hib (combination)	See hepatitis B and Hib	IM
Hib	Polysaccharide-protein conjugate	IM
Hib conjugate and DTaP (combination)	See Hib and DTaP	IM
Influenza	Inactivated virus (whole virus); viral components (split virus or purified antigens)	IM
Japanese encephalitis	Inactivated virus	SC
Measles	Live virus	SC
Measles-rubella	Live viruses	SC
Meningococcal	Polysaccharide	SC
MMR	Live viruses	SC
Mumps	Live virus	SC
Pneumococcal	Polysaccharide	IM or SC
Pneumococcal conjugate	Polysaccharide-protein conjugate	IM
Poliovirus (trivalent)—IPV	Inactivated viruses	SC
Rabies	Inactivated virus	IM
Rubella	Live virus	SC
Td and DT (adsorbed)	Toxoids	IM
Typhoid		
Parenteral	Capsular polysaccharide	IM
Oral	Live bacteria	Oral
Varicella	Live virus	SC
Yellow fever	Live virus	SC

*Only major childhood vaccines and selected others are included.
BCG, bacillus Calmette-Guérin (tuberculosis); DT, diphtheria and tetanus toxoids (for children <7 yr); DTaP, diphtheria and tetanus toxoids and acellular pertussis vaccine; Hib, *Haemophilus influenzae* type b conjugate vaccine; ID, intradermal; IM, intramuscular; IPV, inactivated poliovirus vaccine; MMR, live measles, mumps, and rubella virus vaccine; SC, subcutaneous; Td, tetanus and diphtheria toxoid (for children ≥7 yr and adults).

12 to 15 months of age because many children will have residual, transplacentally acquired maternal measles serum antibody in the first year of life that will interfere with the antibody response. However, during measles outbreaks in preschool children, measles vaccination is recommended for infants as young as 6 months because the risk of complications with measles is high in children younger than 1 year.[11, 106] These infants should be vaccinated again at 12 to 15 months of age. Similarly, in countries where measles causes significant morbidity and mortality in infants younger than 9 months, the Global Advisory Group of the WHO's Expanded Programme on Immunization (EPI) has recommended giving measles vaccine to infants as young as 6 months.[214]

The recommended doses of vaccine are determined by the number necessary to achieve a uniform and predictable immunologic response and to sustain protection. Some immunizing agents require the administration of more than one dose for development of an adequate antibody response and require a booster dose to maintain protection; examples are pertussis, diphtheria, and tetanus vaccines. Intervals between doses are based on the kinetics of primary and secondary antibody responses.

Route of Administration

An example of the effect of the route of administration on immunologic response is provided by poliomyelitis vaccines. Inactivated poliovirus vaccines given intramuscularly induce systemic immunity through serum antibody production; however, they do not consistently evoke local secretory IgA antibodies in the intestinal tract and thereby effectively prevent subsequent transmission of wild-type virus. Because live-attenuated oral polio vaccine (OPV) induces optimal intestinal as well as systemic antibody, it was the preferred vaccine for routine immunization of children in the United States against poliomyelitis for 3 decades and remains the recommended vaccine by the WHO for global eradication.[385]

Vaccines containing adjuvants must be injected deep into the muscle mass because if they are administered subcutaneously or intradermally, they can cause local irritation, inflammation, granuloma formation, or necrosis.[3, 134]

Injectable vaccines should be administered in areas unlikely to cause local neural, vascular, or tissue injury.[3, 134] Although the upper, outer quadrant of the buttocks has been used as a frequent site of immunization, this area ordinarily should not be used because the gluteal region consists mostly of fat in young children and because of potential injury to the sciatic nerve. Ideally, intramuscular injections should be given in the anterolateral aspect of the upper part of the thigh or the deltoid muscle of the upper part of the arm. The anterolateral aspect of the thigh is preferred for infants because of its muscle mass relative to other sites. For older children, the deltoid muscle is usually sufficiently large for intramuscular injection. The incidence of significant pain in 18-month-old children injected intramuscularly in the thigh is greater than after deltoid injections and can result in transient limping.[238] The deltoid is generally the preferred site for intramuscular administration of vaccines in children 18 months and older, although some physicians prefer the anterolateral aspect of the thigh for toddlers.[3, 134] Subcutaneous inoculations also usually should be given in the thigh of infants and the deltoid area of older children. Intradermal vaccines generally should be administered on the volar aspect of the forearm.

Recommended routes for administration of vaccines are provided in their package inserts and are summarized in recommendations for immunizations by the Committee on Infectious Diseases of the American Academy of Pediatrics (AAP)[3] and the Advisory Committee on Immunization Practices (ACIP) of the Centers for Disease Control and Prevention (CDC).[134]

Vaccine Dose

The recommended dose of each immunizing agent is derived from theoretic considerations and vaccine trials. Because inactivated immunizing agents cannot replicate in the host, these vaccines must contain an adequate antigenic mass to stimulate the desired immunologic response. Long-lasting immunity with such vaccines requires repeated doses.

Exceeding the recommended dose can be hazardous because of excessive local or systemic concentrations of immunizing agents, whereas administration of doses smaller than those recommended may result in inadequate response and protection.[3, 134]

Lapsed Immunizations

In general, intervals between multiple doses of an antigen that are longer than those recommended do not affect the antibody responses achieved, provided that the immunization series is completed. Thus, restarting the series after interruption of the vaccine schedule or giving additional doses is not necessary.

Simultaneous Administration of Multiple Vaccines

Because most vaccines can be given simultaneously without impairment of effectiveness or safety, multiple vaccines are given to children concurrently.[253] Simultaneous administration of vaccines is particularly important for inadequately immunized children whose return for further immunization is doubtful or for patients with imminent travel plans. An inactivated vaccine and a live virus vaccine can be administered simultaneously at different sites without interference with the immune response. Exceptions are yellow fever and cholera vaccines because if administered simultaneously, antibody responses are diminished. If possible, administration of these vaccines should be separated by at least an interval of 3 weeks.[134]

In the case of live virus vaccines, the immune response to one live virus vaccine can be impaired if given within 4 weeks of another.[125, 134, 311] Thus, parenteral live virus vaccines not administered on the same day should be given at least 4 weeks apart. This consideration is the basis of the recommended minimal interval of 1 month (defined as 4 weeks) between doses of measles vaccine, such as would be the case for a previously unimmunized person entering college.

Guidelines for spacing live and killed antigen vaccines are given in Table 242–3.

TABLE 242–3 ■ GUIDELINES FOR SPACING THE ADMINISTRATION OF LIVE AND INACTIVATED ANTIGENS

Antigen Combination	Recommended Minimal Interval between Doses
2 inactivated	None. May be administered simultaneously or at any interval between doses
Inactivated and live	None. May be administered simultaneously or at any interval between doses
2 live parenteral*	4-wk minimal interval if not administered simultaneously

*Live oral vaccines, e.g., Ty21a typhoid vaccine and oral polio vaccine, can be administered simultaneously or at any interval before or after inactivated or live parenteral vaccines.

Record Keeping, Patient Information, Informed Consent, and Reporting

Accurate record keeping by physicians is required, and parents (or patients) should keep up-to-date immunization records for their children. The 1986 National Childhood Vaccine Injury Act requires that for routinely recommended childhood vaccines, health care providers record in the child's permanent medical record the date of administration of the vaccine, manufacturer, lot number, and the name of the health care provider administering the vaccines.[3]

As a general principle, all children and their parents or caregivers should be informed about the benefits and risks of any vaccines to be administered. For vaccines currently specified in the Vaccine Injury Act, Vaccine Information Statements (VISs) have been prepared by the CDC and must be used by vaccine administrators.

Informed consent should be obtained before the administration of vaccines. Some physicians and other health care providers may choose to obtain the parent's signature, but current law does not require written consent. An appropriate alternative to written consent is to note in the patient's record that the VISs have been provided and discussed with the parent, patient, or legal guardian.[3]

To increase knowledge about adverse reactions, all temporally associated events severe enough to require the patient to seek medical attention should be reported to the Vaccine Adverse Events Reporting System (VAERS). Health care providers who administer vaccines are required in the United States to report to VAERS specific adverse events in recipients of the vaccines covered by the act (Table 242–4). This system for reporting adverse events associated with vaccination was established by the Department of Health and Human Services to foster recognition of vaccine-related reactions and further study, as indicated, to establish possible causation. VAERS forms can be obtained by calling 800-822-7967 or logging onto their website, *http://www.vaers.org*.

The decrease in the occurrence of vaccine-preventable infectious diseases has resulted in a greater number of adverse events temporally related to immunization than cases of disease. Although in some cases, such as vaccine-associated paralytic poliomyelitis, vaccine has been established to be the cause, in other circumstances, such as brain damage alleged to be attributed to whole-cell pertussis vaccine, causation by vaccine has not been proved.[24]

Increased public visibility of vaccine reactions contributed to a marked increase in vaccine litigation in the 1980s as compensation was sought through the judicial system by those alleged to have suffered serious vaccine-related sequelae. A marked increase in manufacturers' actual and anticipated liability costs and subsequent escalating increases in the price of vaccines occurred concomitantly. These and other developments, such as threats to the vaccine supply, concerns by parents about vaccine safety, and recognition of the benefits derived from improved coordination and planning of vaccine programs, led to passage of the 1986 Vaccine Injury Act and the National Vaccine Injury Compensation Program, a no-fault system to compensate victims of certain presumed vaccine-related events.

The Department of Health and Human Services administers the compensation program. Decisions on compensation

TABLE 242–4 ■ REPORTABLE EVENTS AFTER IMMUNIZATION, AS REQUIRED BY THE NATIONAL CHILDHOOD VACCINE INJURY ACT*

Vaccine/Toxoid	Adverse Event	For Reporting
Tetanus in any combination: DTaP, DTP, DT, Td, or TT	Anaphylaxis or anaphylactic shock	4 hr
	Brachial neuritis	2–28 days
	Any acute complication or sequela (including death) of an illness, disability, injury, or condition referred to above for which the illness, disability, injury, or condition arose within the time period prescribed	Not applicable
Pertussis in any combination: DTaP, DTP, DTP-Hib, or P	Anaphylaxis or anaphylactic shock	4 hr
	Encephalopathy (or encephalitis)	72 hr
	Any acute complication or sequela (including death) of an illness, disability, injury, or condition referred to above for which the illness, disability, injury, or condition arose within the time period prescribed	Not applicable
Measles, mumps, and rubella in any combination: MMR, MR, M, or R	Anaphylaxis or anaphylactic shock	4 hr
	Encephalopathy (or encephalitis)	5–15 days. No limit
	Any acute complication or sequela (including death) of an illness, disability, injury, or condition referred to above for which the illness, disability, injury, or condition arose within the time period prescribed	Not applicable
Measles in any combination: MMR, MR, M	Thrombocytopenic purpura	7–30 days
	Vaccine-strain measles viral infection in an immunodeficient recipient	6 mo
	Any acute complication or sequela (including death) of an illness, disability, injury, or condition referred to above for which the illness, disability, injury, or condition arose within the time period prescribed	Not applicable
Rubella in any combination: MMR, MR, R	Chronic arthritis	7–42 days
	Any acute complication or sequela (including death) of an illness, disability, injury, or condition referred to above for which the illness, disability, injury, or condition arose within the time period prescribed	Not applicable
Oral polio (OPV)	Paralytic polio	
	In a non-immunodeficient recipient	30 days
	In an immunodeficient recipient	6 mo
	In a vaccine-associated community case	Not applicable
	Any acute complication or sequela (including death) of an illness, disability, injury, or condition referred to above for which the illness, disability, injury, or condition arose within the time period prescribed	Not applicable
Inactivated polio (IPV)	Anaphylaxis or anaphylactic shock	4 hr
	Any acute complication or sequela (including death) of an illness, disability, injury, or condition referred to above for which the illness, disability, injury, or condition arose within the time period prescribed	Not applicable
Hepatitis B	Anaphylaxis or anaphylactic shock	7 days
	Any acute complication or sequela (including death) of an illness, disability, injury, or condition referred to above for which the illness, disability, injury, or condition arose within the time period prescribed	Not applicable
Haemophilus influenzae type b (Hib) polysaccharide vaccines (unconjugated, PRP vaccines)	Early-onset Hib disease	7 days
	Any acute complication or sequela (including death) of an illness, disability, injury, or condition referred to above for which the illness, disability, injury, or condition arose within the time period prescribed	Not applicable
Haemophilus influenzae type b (Hib) polysaccharide conjugate vaccines	No condition specified	Not applicable
Varicella	No condition specified	Not applicable
Any new vaccine recommended by the CDC for routine administration to children, after publication by the secretary of a notice of coverage	No condition specified	Not applicable

*Effective April 1999. The Reportable Events Table (RET) reflects what is reportable by law (42 USC 300aa-25) to the Vaccine Adverse Event Reporting System (VAERS). In addition, individuals are encouraged to report any clinically significant or unexpected events (even if it is not certain that the vaccine caused the event) for any vaccine, regardless of whether it is listed on the RET. Manufacturers also are required by regulation (21 CFR 600.80) to report to the VAERS program all adverse events made known to them for any vaccine.

are made by the U.S. Court of Federal Claims and are based on the Vaccine Injury Table, which has been revised since passage of the original legislation in response to new findings and analysis by the several Institute of Medicine (IOM) committees. Compensation for injuries occurring after the program's effective date of October 1, 1988, is provided by excise taxes on each vaccine. The program has been successful in reducing vaccine-related litigation, stabilizing vaccine prices, and creating a favorable environment for the introduction of new vaccines.[184]

Vaccine Recommendations and Schedules

In developing recommendations for immunization, multiple factors are considered, including the vaccine's characteristics, scientific knowledge about the principles of immunization, assessment of the benefits of the vaccine, the risk of development of the disease and its complications, vaccine costs, and the risk of having adverse reactions. Changes in relative benefits and risks necessitate continued review of recommendations. In the United States, recommendations for immunization of infants and children are made by two different committees, the ACIP of the CDC and the AAP Committee on Infectious Diseases. These committees work closely together, and in most circumstances their recommendations are similar. These two committees and the American Academy of Family Practice (AAFP) issue a single vaccine schedule each year. The 2003 schedule for routine administration of childhood vaccines is given in Figure 242–1.

A major change in 1996 was the establishment of a routine pre-adolescent immunization visit at 11 to 12 years of age.[94] The first booster dose of adult tetanus-diphtheria (Td) vaccine should be given at that time rather than at 14 to 16 years of age, as previously was the case. In addition, at this pre-adolescent visit, children not previously vaccinated with hepatitis B, varicella, or the second dose of measles-containing vaccine (or any combination of these vaccines) should be given the necessary immunizations and scheduled for future visits to receive any vaccines not administered during this visit.

Other countries have similar national mechanisms for formulating immunization schedules and recommendations that are based on the local epidemiology of diseases and available vaccines. In developing countries, practices are guided by the EPI of the WHO. Current recommendations are listed in Table 242–5.

As new vaccines and scientific knowledge become available, vaccine recommendations and schedules are modified and changed. Examples of changes in the 1990s include the use of *Haemophilus influenzae* type b (Hib) conjugate vaccine beginning at 2 months of age, universal infant and adolescent hepatitis B immunization, recommendations for administration of varicella vaccine, and replacement of whole-cell with acellular pertussis vaccines.

Implementation of Vaccine Programs

In addition to the availability of safe and effective vaccines and appropriate schedules for their use, effective means of implementation and delivery are necessary for the success of vaccine programs. In the United States, high rates of immunization in school-age children have been achieved, in part because of public health programs for vaccine administration, government support for vaccine purchase, and state laws requiring immunization for school entry. In contrast to rates of approximately 95 percent or higher in school-age children, however, immunization rates in infants and young children in the 1980s were significantly lower.[388] In a survey of 21 primarily urban areas throughout the United States, 11 to 58 percent (median, 44%) of children who entered school in 1991 and 1992 were fully vaccinated by their second birthday. Failure to immunize young children was a major factor in the outbreaks of measles in major urban areas in the United States in 1989 to 1991.[355]

This epidemic and the recognition of low immunization rates prompted a national campaign to achieve the U.S. Public Health Service's goal of a 90 percent vaccine coverage rate in children by the time that they were 2 years of age. Initiatives have included improved access to vaccines, education of health care providers in the community, and the development of standards for pediatric immunization practice.[360] These standards have been endorsed by the AAP, AAFP, and other major professional organizations and serve as guidelines to be followed for improving the delivery of vaccines. They include evaluation of the immunization status of patients at all medical visits, the use of valid contraindications, simultaneous administration of all indicated vaccines, and routine audit of the immunization status of patients by providers. The standards have been updated recently[360] (Table 242–6). These and other initiatives have resulted in increasing immunization rates of young children in recent years. According to the National Immunization Survey, coverage rates in children 19 to 35 months of age in 2000 were 78 percent for completion of the four doses of DTP/DTaP/DT, three of poliovirus vaccine, and one dose of measles-mumps-rubella (MMR) vaccine.[123] Vaccination coverage rates in the United States for preschool-age children consistently have been greater than 75 percent since 1995.

Vaccine Contraindications, Precautions, and Use in Special Circumstances

Recommendations for the use of specific vaccines include contraindications and use in special circumstances, such as immunocompromised patients (from underlying disease or therapy, such as high-dose steroids) and pregnancy.[11, 106] Established, generic contraindications are moderate or severe illness, a previous anaphylactic reaction to the specific vaccine, and a severe hypersensitivity reaction to a vaccine constituent, such as anaphylaxis.

The decision to defer immunization in a febrile child should be based on the physician's assessment of the severity of the illness rather than the degree of fever. Children with minor illness and low-grade fever generally should be vaccinated, especially if a child is unlikely to return promptly for the deferred immunization.

Administration of live virus vaccines such as varicella and MMR vaccines generally is contraindicated in patients with altered immunity. However, the morbidity and mortality rates of measles and the lack of complications from vaccination of children infected with human immunodeficiency virus (HIV) have led to recommendations that these children, unless significantly immunocompromised, receive the MMR vaccine.[11, 34, 90, 106]

Because of a theoretic risk to the developing fetus, administration of live virus vaccines in most cases is not recommended for pregnant women.[4, 134] However, inadvertent administration of vaccine is not necessarily a reason for termination of the pregnancy, and some live virus vaccines, such as those for yellow fever and poliomyelitis, can be given safely to pregnant women. Inactivated bacterial and viral vaccines such as tetanus toxoids, hepatitis B, and influenza vaccine, which are composed of antigenic components or killed organisms, can and should be given during pregnancy if indicated.

Vaccines can cause severe reactions in some recipients, which may be a contraindication or precaution to subsequent administration of the specific vaccine. An example is a child in whom a fever of 40.5°C or higher develops after receiving diphtheria-tetanus-pertussis (DTP) (or diphtheria and tetanus toxoids and acellular pertussis [DTaP]) vaccine, for whom administration of further doses of pertussis-containing vaccine is not indicated in most cases. This recommendation is based on the unproven but reasonable presumption that children who experience adverse reactions after receiving pertussis immunization are at risk of having similar reactions of equal or greater magnitude on subsequent immunization.[142]

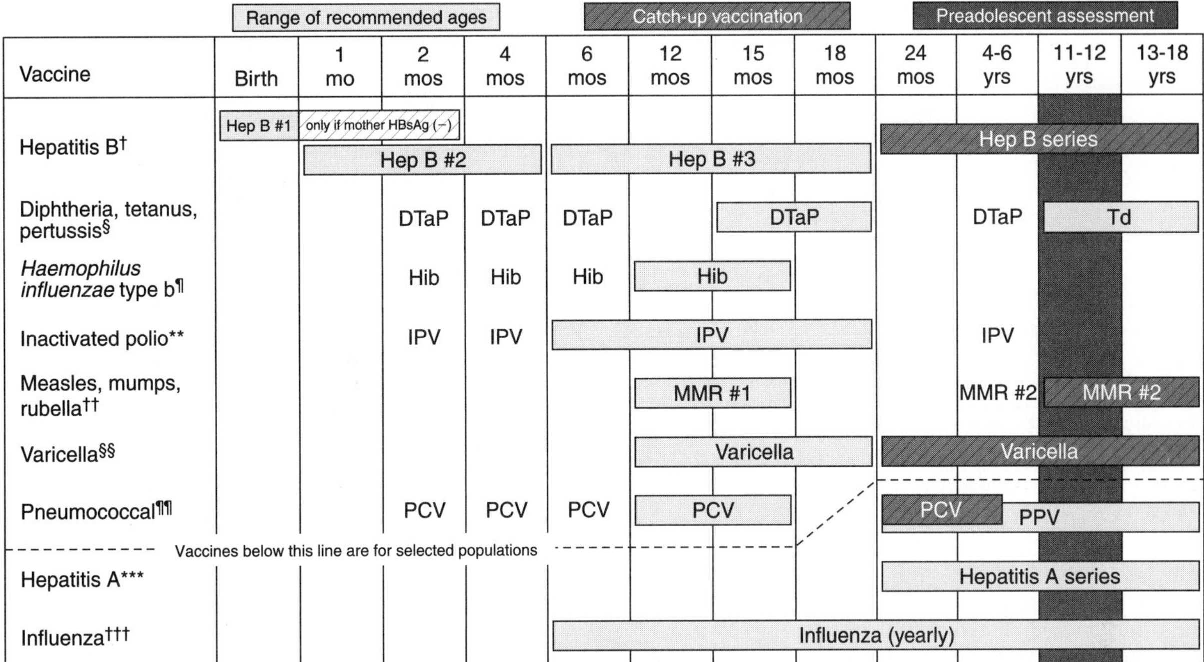

Range of recommended ages
Catch-up vaccination
Preadolescent assessment
Vaccine
Birth
1 mo
2 mos
4 mos
6 mos
12 mos
15 mos
18 mos
24 mos
4-6 yrs
11-12 yrs
13-18 yrs
Hepatitis B†
Hep B #1
only if mother HBsAg (−)
Hep B #2
Hep B #3
Hep B series
Diphtheria, tetanus, pertussis§
DTaP
DTaP
DTaP
DTaP
DTaP
Td
Haemophilus influenzae type b¶
Hib
Hib
Hib
Hib
Inactivated polio**
IPV
IPV
IPV
IPV
Measles, mumps, rubella††
MMR #1
MMR #2
MMR #2
Varicella§§
Varicella
Varicella
Pneumococcal¶¶
PCV
PCV
PCV
PCV
PCV
PPV
Vaccines below this line are for selected populations
Hepatitis A***
Hepatitis A series
Influenza†††
Influenza (yearly)

* Indicates the recommended ages for routine administration of currently licensed childhood vaccines, as of December 1, 2002, for children through age 18 years. Any dose not given at the recommended age should be given at any subsequent visit when indicated and feasible. ▨ Indicates age groups that warrant special effort to administer those vaccines not given previously. Additional vaccines may be licensed and recommended during the year. Licensed combination vaccines may be used whenever any components of the combination are indicated and the vaccine's other components are not contraindicated. Providers should consult the manufacturers' package inserts for detailed recommendations.

† **Hepatitis B vaccine (Hep B).** All infants should receive the first dose of hepatitis B vaccine soon after birth and before hospital discharge; the first dose also may be given by age 2 months if the infant's mother is HBsAg-negative. Only monovalent hepatitis B vaccine can be used for the birth dose. Monovalent or combination vaccine containing Hep B may be used to complete the series. Four doses of vaccine may be administered when a birth dose is given. The second dose should be given at least 4 weeks after the first dose except for combination vaccines, which cannot be administered before age 6 weeks. The third dose should be given at least 16 weeks after the first dose and at least 8 weeks after the second dose. The last dose in the vaccination series (third or fourth dose) should not be administered before age 6 months. Infants born to HBsAg-positive mothers should receive hepatitis B vaccine and 0.5 mL hepatitis B immune globulin (HBIG) within 12 hours of birth at separate sites. The second dose is recommended at age 1-2 months. The last dose in the vacination series should not be administered before age 6 months. These infants should be tested for HBsAg and anti-HBs at 9–15 months of age. Infants born to mothers whose HBsAg status is unknown should receive the first dose of the hepatitis B vaccine series within 12 hours of birth. Maternal blood should be drawn as soon as possible to determine the mother's HBsAg status; if the HBsAg test is positive, the infant should receive HBIG as soon as possible (no later than age 1 week).

§ **Diphtheria and tetanus toxoids and acellular pertussis vaccine (DTaP).** The fourth dose of DTaP may be administered as early as age 12 months, provided 6 months have elapsed since the third dose and the child is unlikely to return at age 15-18 months. **Tetanus and diphtheria toxoids (Td)** is recommended at age 11-12 years if at least 5 years have elapsed since the last dose of tetanus and diphtheria toxoid–containing vaccine. Subsequent routine Td boosters are recommended every 10 years.

¶ ***Haemophilus influenzae* type b (Hib) conjugate vaccine.** Three Hib conjugate vaccines are licensed for infant use. If PRP-OMP (PedvaxHIB® or ComVax® [Merck]) is administered at ages 2 and 4 months, a dose at age 6 months is not required. DTaP/Hib combination products should not be used for primary immunization in infants at age 2, 4, or 6 months, but can be used as boosters following any Hib vaccine.

** **Inactivated poliovirus vaccine (IPV).** An all-IPV schedule is recommended for routine childhood poliovirus vaccination in the United States. All children should receive 4 doses of IPV at age 2, 4, and 6-18 months, and 4-6 years.

†† **Measles, mumps, and rubella vaccine (MMR).** The second dose of MMR is recommended routinely at age 4-6 years but may be administered during any visit provided at least 4 weeks have elapsed since the first dose and that both doses are administered beginning at or after age 12 months. Those who have not previously received the second dose should complete the schedule by the visit at age 11-12 years.

§§ **Varicella vaccine.** Varicella vaccine is recommended at any visit, at or after age 12 months for susceptible children (i.e., those who lack a reliable history of chickenpox). Susceptible persons aged ≥13 years should receive 2 doses given at least 4 weeks apart.

¶¶ **Pneumococcal vaccine.** The heptavalent **pneumococcal conjugate vaccine (PCV)** is recommended for all children aged 2-23 months and for certain children aged 24-59 months. **Pneumococcal polysaccharide vaccine (PPV)** is recommended in addition to PCV for certain high-risk groups. See *MMWR* 2000;49(No. RR-9):1–38.

*** **Hepatitis A vaccine.** Hepatitis A vaccine is recommended for children and adolescents in selected states and regions, and for certain high-risk groups; consult your local public health authority. Children and adolescents in these states, regions, and high risk groups who have not been immunized against hepatitis A can begin the hepatitis A vaccination series during any visit. The two doses in the series should be administered at least 6 months apart. See *MMWR* 1999;48(RR-12);1–37.

††† **Influenza vaccine.** Influenza vaccine is recommended annually for children age ≥6 months with certain risk factors (including but not limited to asthma, cardiac disease, sickle cell disease, HIV, diabetes, and household members of persons in groups at high risk; see *MMWR* 2002;51(RR-3);1–31), and can be administered to all others wishing to obtain immunity. In addition, healthy children age 6–23 months are encouraged to receive influenza vaccine if feasible because children in these age groups are at substantially increased risk for influenza-related hospitalizations. Children aged ≤12 years should receive vaccine in a dosage appropriate for their age (0.25 mL if age 6-35 months or 0.5 mL if aged ≥3 years). Children aged ≤8 years who are receiving influenza vaccine for the first time should receive two doses separated by at least 4 weeks.

Additional information about vaccines, vaccine supply, and contraindications for immunization is available at http://www.cdc.gov/nip or at the National Immunization hotline, 800-232-2522 (English), or 800-232-0233 (Spanish). Copies of the schedule can be obtained at http://www.cdc.gov/nip/recs/child-schedule.htm. Approved by the **Advisory Committee on Immunization Practices** (http://www.cdc.gov/nip/acip), the **American Academy of Pediatrics** (http://www.aap.org), and the **American Academy of Family Physicians** (http://www.aafp.org).

FIGURE 242–1 ■ Recommended childhood immunization schedule—United States, 2003.

TABLE 242–5 ■ SCHEDULE OF THE EXPANDED PROGRAMME ON IMMUNIZATION, WORLD HEALTH ORGANIZATION

Age	Vaccines	Hepatitis B (HB)* A	or	Hepatitis B (HB)* B
Birth	BCG, OPV	HB-1		
6 wk	DTP, OPV	HB-2		HB-1
10 wk	DTP, OPV			HB-2
14 wk	DTP, OPV	HB-3		HB-3
9 mo	Measles, yellow fever†			

*Schedule A is recommended in regions where perinatal transmission of hepatitis B virus is important (e.g., Southeast Asia) and B in countries where perinatal transmission is less important (e.g., sub-regions Saharan Africa).
†In countries where yellow fever poses a risk.
BCG, bacillus Calmette-Guérin; DTP, diphtheria-tetanus-pertussis; HB, hepatitis B; OPV, oral poliovirus vaccine.

Anaphylactic reactions caused by allergenic components of a vaccine, such as gelatin or egg protein (in vaccine prepared in embryonated chicken eggs), have occurred in rare cases. Vaccines posing a potential risk for egg-sensitive persons include those against measles, mumps, inactivated influenza, and yellow fever. Before administering vaccines to persons with possible hypersensitivity to vaccine constituents, physicians should review current recommendations for these vaccines.

In other circumstances, specific immunizations may be contraindicated because of previous reactions and the child's past history, such as with DTP (e.g., evolving neurologic disorders) and MMR (e.g., immune thrombocytopenia occurring in temporal association with vaccination).[93]

TABLE 242–6 ■ STANDARDS FOR CHILD AND ADOLESCENT IMMUNIZATION PRACTICES

Vaccination services are readily available.
Vaccinations are coordinated with other health care services and provided in a medical home when possible.
Barriers to vaccination are identified and minimized.
Patient costs are minimized.
Health care professionals review the vaccination and health status of patients at every encounter to determine which vaccines are indicated.
Health care professionals assess for and follow only medically accepted contraindications.
Parents/guardians and patients be educated about the risks and benefits of vaccination in a culturally appropriate manner and in easy-to-understand language.
Health care professionals follow appropriate procedures for vaccine storage and handling.
Up-to-date, written vaccination protocols be accessible at all locations where vaccines are administered.
Persons who administer vaccines and staff who manage or support vaccine administration be knowledgeable and receive ongoing education.
Health care professionals simultaneously administer as many indicated doses as possible.
Vaccination records for patients are accurate, complete, and easily accessible.
Health care professionals report adverse events after vaccination promptly and accurately to the Vaccine Adverse Events Reporting System (VAERS) and are aware of a distinct program, the National Vaccine Injury Compensation Program (VICP).
All personnel who have contact with patients are appropriately vaccinated.
Systems are used to remind parents/guardians, patients, and health care professionals when vaccines are due and to recall those who are overdue.
Office- or clinic-based patient record reviews and vaccination coverage assessments are performed annually.
Health care professionals practice community-based approaches.

From National Vaccine Advisory Committee: Standards for Child and Adolescent Immunization Practices. Pediatrics 2003. In press.

Misconceptions

Appropriate and safe use of vaccines requires knowledge of the patient's relevant medical history, adverse reactions associated with previous receipt of vaccines, and specific indications and contraindications. Without this information, vaccines may be administered inadvertently or not given in circumstances in which immunization is indicated, thereby resulting in missed opportunities for receiving the recommended immunization and susceptibility of the child to a preventable disease. Examples of common misconceptions concerning contraindication to vaccines are given in Table 242–7.

TABLE 242–7 ■ MISCONCEPTIONS CONCERNING VACCINE CONTRAINDICATIONS

- *Mild acute illness with low-grade fever or mild diarrheal illness in an otherwise well child*
- *Current antimicrobial therapy or the convalescent phase of illness*
- *Reaction to previous DTP dose that involved only soreness, redness, or swelling in the immediate vicinity of the vaccination site or a temperature of less than 105° F (40.5° C)*
- *Prematurity*
  The appropriate age for initiating most immunizations in a prematurely born infant is the usual recommended chronologic age. Vaccine doses should not be reduced for preterm infants
- *Pregnancy of the mother or other household contact*
  Vaccine viruses in MMR vaccine are not transmitted by vaccine recipients. Although varicella virus has been transmitted by a healthy vaccine recipient to contacts, the frequency is very low, only mild or asymptomatic infection has been reported, and the use of vaccine is not contraindicated by pregnancy of either the child's mother or other household contacts
- *Recent exposure to an infectious disease*
- *Breast-feeding*
  The only vaccine virus that has been isolated from breast milk is rubella vaccine virus. No evidence indicates that breast milk from women immunized against rubella is harmful to infants
- *A history of nonspecific allergies or relatives with allergies*
- *Allergies to penicillin or any other antibiotic, except anaphylactic reactions to neomycin or streptomycin*
  These reactions occur rarely, if ever. None of the vaccines licensed in the United States contain penicillin
- *Allergies to duck meat or duck feathers*
  No vaccine available in the United States is produced in substrates containing duck antigens
- *Family history of convulsions in persons considered for pertussis or measles vaccination*
- *Family history of sudden infant death syndrome in children considered for DTaP vaccination*
- *Family history of an adverse event, unrelated to immunosuppression after vaccination*
- *Malnutrition*

DTaP, diphtheria and tetanus toxoids and acellular pertussis vaccine; DTP, diphtheria-tetanus-pertussis; MMR, measles-mumps-rubella.
Adapted from Pickering, L. K. (ed.): 2003 Red Book: Report of the Committee on Infectious Diseases. 26th ed. Elk Grove Village, IL, American Academy of Pediatrics, 2003.

International Travel

Foreign travel is often an indication for giving vaccines not routinely administered to children.[4] The risk of exposure to certain vaccine-preventable diseases may be increased relative to that in the United States, and travelers may be exposed to infections that are uncommon or do not occur in the United States. Examples include vaccines against hepatitis A, influenza, typhoid fever, yellow fever, and Japanese encephalitis (Table 242–8), depending on the location and circumstances of the person's visit. Some countries may require yellow fever vaccination for entry. The second dose of measles vaccine should be given to children and adolescents who have received only one dose (provided that 4 weeks or more has elapsed since administration of the first dose), irrespective of age, because the risk of exposure to cases of measles may be substantial in some foreign countries. In addition, children and adolescents should have received all vaccines routinely recommended for their age. Information on vaccine requirements for international travel to different countries is provided in a publication by the CDC titled *Health Information for International Travel*. It is revised annually and can be obtained from the Superintendent of Documents, U.S. Government Printing Office, Washington, D.C., 20402-9235. Information is also available from the CDC "International Travelers Hotline" by calling 404-332-4559 or on the Internet at the CDC website.

Vaccine Safety

Immunizations are among the most cost-effective and widely used public health interventions. Public health recommendations for vaccine programs and practices represent a dynamic balancing of risks and benefits. Vaccine safety or monitoring of risk is necessary to accurately weigh this balance and adjust vaccination policies.

No vaccine is perfectly safe or effective. As the incidence of vaccine-preventable diseases is reduced, public concern refocuses from the risk of contracting disease to the health risks associated with vaccines. A higher standard of safety generally is expected of vaccines than of other medical interventions because in contrast to most pharmaceutical products that are administered to ill persons for curative purposes, vaccines generally are given to healthy persons to prevent the acquisition of disease. Public tolerance of adverse reactions related to products given to healthy persons, especially healthy infants, is substantially lower than that to products administered to persons who are already ill. This lower tolerance of risk for vaccines necessitates investigating possible causes of rare adverse events after administration of vaccinations than would be acceptable for other pharmaceutical products. Because vaccination is such a common event, any health problem that occurs after immunization may be attributed to the vaccine. Health effects reported as being associated with vaccines may be true adverse reactions or may be associated with vaccination only by coincidence. Because a temporal relationship alone does not necessarily indicate causation, cause-and-effect relationships are often impossible to establish. Epidemiologic and related studies must be performed to ascertain the incidence and nature of adverse reactions to vaccines, and such studies are important in ensuring a scientific rationale for recommendations for vaccine use and optimal public and professional acceptance of vaccines.

The topic of vaccine safety became prominent during the mid-1970s with increases in lawsuits filed on behalf of patients presumably injured by the DTP vaccine.[189] Legal decisions were made and damages awarded despite the lack of scientific evidence to support claims of vaccine injury.[189] As a result of the liability, prices soared and several manufacturers halted production. A shortage of vaccines resulted, and public health officials became concerned about the return of epidemic diseases. To reduce liability and respond to public health concerns, Congress passed the National Childhood Vaccine Injury Act (NCVIA) in 1986.

The NCVIA mandated that all health care providers report certain adverse events that occur after the administration of vaccination with routinely recommended childhood vaccines. As a result, VAERS was established by the Food and Drug Administration (FDA) and the CDC in 1990. VAERS provides a mechanism for the collection and analysis of adverse events associated with vaccines currently licensed in the United States. Adverse events are defined as health effects occurring after immunization that may or may not be related to the vaccine. VAERS data are monitored continually to detect previously unknown adverse events or increases in known adverse events.[141]

The gaps that exist in the scientific knowledge of rare vaccine adverse events prompted the CDC to develop the Vaccine Safety Datalink (VSD) project.[139] This project involved forming partnerships with four large health maintenance organizations to continually monitor vaccine safety. VSD is an example of a large linked database and includes information on more than 6 million people. The VSD project allows for planned vaccine safety studies, as well as timely investigations of hypotheses.

In the late 1990s, reports in the lay press questioned the safety of routine immunizations and alarmed parents with unsupported accounts of the dangers of vaccines. One major national television network broadcast a feature piece that linked diabetes to childhood immunizations. In the United Kingdom, a report linked receipt of measles vaccine to the development of autism, and in France, hepatitis vaccine was reported to cause multiple sclerosis.

TABLE 242–8 ■ IMMUNIZATIONS FOR FOREIGN TRAVEL

In addition to the routine recommended childhood vaccines, (e.g., those against diphtheria, measles, and poliomyelitis), vaccines against the following diseases should be considered, depending on the geographic area and circumstances of the visit:
Hepatitis A
Influenza
Japanese encephalitis
Meningococcal disease
Rabies
Typhoid fever
Yellow fever

VACCINATION AND DIABETES

Classen and Classen[146] suggested that certain vaccines, if given at birth, may decrease the occurrence of type 1 diabetes, whereas if initial vaccination is performed after children are 2 months of age, the occurrence of diabetes increases. Other researchers have not found an increased risk for diabetes associated with vaccination.[243] The Classen theory is based on results from experiments in laboratory animals, as well as comparisons of rates of diabetes among countries with different immunization schedules.[146] Applying findings from laboratory animals to humans is fraught with uncertainties. Comparison of diabetes rates among countries with different vaccination policies also provides weak evidence because many factors, including vaccination schedules, may differ by country. In addition, other factors, including genetic predisposition and numerous possible environmental exposures unrelated to the administration of vaccines, may influence the development of diabetes.

The most rigorous epidemiologic study of infant vaccinations and type 1 diabetes to date found that measles vaccine was associated with a decreased risk and no association was found with bacille Calmette-Guérin (BCG), smallpox, tetanus, pertussis, rubella, or mumps vaccine.[56] In a large clinical trial of Hib vaccine conducted in Finland, no statistically significant association was found between the receipt of Hib vaccine and the development of type 1 diabetes during 10 years of follow-up.[247] The IOM Immunization Safety Committee recently reviewed the clinical and epidemiologic literature and concluded that multiple immunizations do not lead to a risk for type 1 diabetes.[237]

MEASLES VACCINE AND AUTISM

The causes of autism are unknown. Most experts agree, however, that autism is a condition that begins before birth.[325] Genetics seems to play a major role in the development of autism. Autism usually is diagnosed in children when they are 18 to 30 months old, shortly after they have received many of the recommended vaccinations. Because of this coincidence in timing, some parents of children with autism believe that an immunization may have caused their child's condition.

A 1998 report published in *The Lancet* of 12 patients who had inflammatory bowel disease and autism raised the hypothesis that a link might exist between the MMR vaccine and autism.[369] The authors speculated that MMR vaccine was the possible cause of bowel problems, with the resultant malabsorption of essential vitamins and nutrients leading to autism.

Epidemiologic studies in both the United States and Great Britain do not support a causal association between MMR and inflammatory bowel disease,[166, 291] nor do epidemiologic studies support a causal association between MMR (and other measles-containing vaccines) and autism.[58, 169, 170, 197, 287, 309, 354] A large retrospective study of California children born from 1980 to 1994 was conducted to further examine any possible association between autism and receipt of the MMR vaccine. No correlation was observed between MMR immunization coverage and the number of children with autism.[163] Expert panels convened by both the IOM and the AAP have examined the available data on autism and MMR vaccine. Both panels concluded that the available evidence does not support the hypothesis that MMR vaccine causes autism or associated disorders or inflammatory bowel disease.[217, 235]

HEPATITIS B VACCINE AND MULTIPLE SCLEROSIS

Reports of multiple sclerosis (MS) developing after receipt of hepatitis B vaccine led to the concern that immunization with hepatitis B vaccine may precipitate the onset of MS or lead to relapses. Since licensure, the safety of the hepatitis B vaccine has continued to be monitored. The several studies conducted have not found a scientific association between hepatitis B vaccination and the development of severe neurologic adverse events such as optic neuritis and Guillain-Barré syndrome (GBS). Two recently published, large epidemiologic studies examined the risk of an association between vaccines and MS. The first, a case-control study in a large cohort of nurses, demonstrated no significant association between hepatitis B vaccination and development of MS.[43] A French study of patients with MS found that vaccination did not appear to increase the short-term risk of relapse.[158]

THIMEROSAL-CONTAINING VACCINES AND NEURODEVELOPMENTAL DISORDERS

Thimerosal is a mercury-containing preservative that has been used as an additive to biologics and vaccines since the 1930s because it is effective in preventing bacterial and fungal contamination, particularly in multidose containers. The FDA Modernization Act of 1997 required a review and assessment of the risk of all mercury-containing pharmaceuticals. Assessment of vaccines led to the recognition that during the first 6 months of life some children could be exposed to a cumulative quantity of mercury that exceeds one of the federal guidelines on methylmercury. However, a significant safety margin is incorporated into all the acceptable mercury exposure limits, and no data or evidence has found that any harm was caused by the level of exposure with the existing immunization schedules. In addition, the risk posed by exposure to thimerosal, which contains ethylmercury not methylmercury, on which the federal guidelines were based, is unknown. However, to avoid any potential risk, the Public Health Service, the AAP, and vaccine manufacturers agreed in July 1999 that thimerosal-containing vaccines should be removed as soon as possible. As of March 2001, thimerosal no longer is used as a preservative in any of the pediatric vaccines given to children 6 years or younger in the United States.[119]

Mercury is a known neurotoxin. Little is known about ethylmercury in comparison to methylmercury. Preliminary studies on the effects of exposure to thimerosal in infancy from West Coast health maintenance organizations revealed dose-related evidence of an increased risk for learning disabilities, delayed speech, and other abnormalities, but no such relationship was found in an East Coast population.[364] These studies raised concern regarding the possible connection of exposure to thimerosal-containing vaccines and the development of disorders such as autism, attention-deficit/hyperactivity disorder (ADHD), and speech and language delay. At the request of the CDC and the National Institutes of Health, the Immunization Safety Review Committee of the IOM reviewed all available data and issued a report in October 2001 stating that the evidence is inadequate to accept or reject a causal relationship between exposure to thimerosal-containing vaccines and the neurodevelopmental disorders of autism, ADHD, and speech and language delay. In addition, they concluded that the hypothesis that exposure to thimerosal could be associated with the development of neurodevelopmental disorders, though not established, is biologically plausible.[236] The IOM committee recommended that thimerosal-free DTaP, hepatitis B, and Hib vaccines be used for infants, children, and pregnant women, provided that an adequate supply is available.[236]

Reference Sources

Several comprehensive sources of information about pediatric vaccines are available. The AAP publishes *The Red Book: Report of the Committee on Infectious Diseases* every 3 years. The next edition was published in 2003. In the interval between editions, the AAP publishes recommendations in its newsletter *AAP News* and subsequently in *Pediatrics*. The ACIP issues vaccine recommendations and relevant information in *Morbidity and Mortality Weekly Report*. Manufacturers provide product information for each vaccine in the FDA-approved package inserts.

Vaccines Recommended for Routine Administration

DIPHTHERIA TOXOID

The introduction of diphtheria toxoid in the 1940s led to a dramatic reduction in the incidence of diphtheria in the United States. However, diphtheria is still a potentially significant public health problem because of two factors. First, serologic surveys in the United States and England have suggested that many adults are not immune.[76, 159, 272] However, a recent study suggests that most adults in the United States do have protective concentrations of serum antitoxin.[209] Second, adequate immunization has not eliminated the potential for transmission of *Corynebacterium diphtheriae* completely because immunization does not prevent carriage of *C. diphtheriae* in the nasopharynx or on the skin.[76, 285] As a result of inadequate immunity in adults as well as in infants and children, an epidemic of diphtheria in the 1990s occurred in Russia and other countries of the former Soviet Union such as Ukraine and the central Asian republics.[191, 219] Case-fatality rates have ranged from 2.8 to 23 percent in the different states and countries. In addition, diphtheria continues to be a significant cause of morbidity and mortality in developing countries.[190]

Preparations

Diphtheria toxoid is prepared by formaldehyde treatment of *C. diphtheriae* toxin. It is available in combination with tetanus toxoid and acellular pertussis vaccine (DTaP) for routine immunization of infants and children. It also is produced in combination with tetanus toxoid (DT and Td). For children younger than 7 years, DT is given if pertussis vaccine is contraindicated, whereas Td, which contains only 15 to 20 percent (2 flocculation units [Lf] maximum) of the diphtheria toxoid in DT (6.7 to 12.5 Lf), is recommended for older children and adults because of adverse reactions related to dose and age.[6, 76] Diphtheria vaccines are adsorbed to an aluminum salt adjuvant.

Adverse Events

Other than local reactions of pain and swelling at the site of vaccine injection, immunization does not cause significant adverse events. These local reactions have been attributed to hypersensitivity reactions but do not contraindicate the administration of further vaccination if otherwise indicated.

Indications

For primary immunization, doses of diphtheria toxoid are given when children are 2, 4, and 6 months of age. A fourth dose is administered 6 to 12 months after the third dose (i.e., at 12 to 18 months of age) to maintain adequate antibody concentrations for the ensuing preschool years. For those not immunized in infancy, the first dose is followed by doses given 2 and 8 to 14 months later. A single booster dose given when the child is 4 to 6 years of age, before school entry, is indicated unless the preceding dose was given after the fourth birthday. Interruption of the recommended schedule or delay in administering subsequent doses during primary immunization does not necessitate restarting the series.

After the dose is given to the child at 4 to 6 years of age, booster doses of diphtheria toxoid (as Td) should be administered beginning at the pre-adolescent immunization visit at 11 to 12 years of age and every 10 years thereafter to maintain immunity.[94] To ensure adequate immunity, children and adults receiving tetanus toxoid for wound management should be given age-appropriate preparations of vaccines containing diphtheria as well as tetanus toxoid.[6]

Patients recovering from diphtheria infection should be immunized because infection does not confer immunity.

Precautions and Contraindications

The only contraindication to diphtheria toxoid is a history of severe hypersensitivity developing after receipt of the previous dose. Vaccination with either this or tetanus toxoid is not known to be associated with an increased risk of convulsions. Local reactions alone do not preclude continued use.

HAEMOPHILUS INFLUENZAE TYPE B VACCINE

Before the introduction of routine infant and childhood vaccination against *H. influenzae,* Hib was a major cause of invasive bacterial infections in young children in the United States. It was the most common cause of bacterial meningitis and epiglottitis and a significant cause of septic arthritis, occult febrile bacteremia, and pneumonia in children younger than 5 years, in whom it caused an estimated 12,000 cases of meningitis and 8000 additional cases of invasive Hib disease annually.[151] The cumulative risk of Hib disease was approximately 1 in every 200 American children in the first 5 years of life, with the peak incidence of Hib meningitis occurring in infants between 6 and 12 months of age. In high-risk populations, such as Native Americans, rates of disease in the absence of immunizations were higher, and a greater proportion of cases of meningitis occurred in the first year of life than in non–high-risk populations.[151, 226, 378]

Because most cases of Hib disease occur in infancy, vaccines that induce protection by the time that the child is 6 months of age are necessary for effective control of Hib disease. Realization of this goal was made possible by the development of conjugate vaccines in which the capsular polysaccharide of Hib, its major virulence factor and the antigen against which protective antibodies are directed, is chemically linked to a protein carrier. Whereas the purified capsular polysaccharide polyribosylribitol phosphate (PRP) is a poor immunogen in children younger than 18 months, PRP conjugated to a protein carrier has the antigenic properties of the protein carrier and, as a result, induces protective antibody in infants and young children and significantly greater concentrations of circulating anti-PRP at all ages than does the unconjugated polysaccharide.[323, 378] This age-dependent immunogenic characteristic of purified PRP (and other polysaccharide antigens) is that of a T-cell–independent antigen to which humoral responses are mediated by B-cell lymphocytes alone without helper T lymphocytes. In contrast, the polysaccharide-protein conjugate vaccines are T-cell–dependent antigens in which helper T-lymphocyte activation and B-cell mediation of the humoral antibody response occur. T-cell–dependent antigens also elicit booster responses, which are important to the effectiveness of polysaccharide vaccines.

The introduction of Hib conjugate vaccines in the United States, first in children 18 months and older in 1987 and for routine infant immunization in 1991, has decreased the incidence of disease dramatically. By 1995, Hib disease levels had declined by more than 95 percent below pre-immunization levels.[103, 377] The remarkably rapid reduction in incidence of disease was partly due to the ability of the vaccine to reduce nasopharyngeal carriage of the organism, thereby leading to reduced rates of exposure and infection even in those not immunized.[44]

Preparations

All Hib vaccines contain PRP, the organism's polysaccharide capsular antigen. The first vaccine licensed was purified PRP, which was recommended in 1985 for administration to children 18 to 24 months or older. Conjugate polysaccharide-protein vaccines for use in infants have replaced these products. Four conjugate vaccines have been licensed in the United States (Table 242–9). Each conjugate vaccine is composed of PRP antigen conjugated to a protein carrier and differs in the protein carrier, size of the saccharide component, and chemical linkage. Three of these vaccines, HbOC, PRP-OMP, and PRP-T, are licensed for use in early infancy; PRP-D is approved by the FDA for children 15 months and older. Of these products, only PRP-T can be mixed with DTaP for the fourth dose (see Table 242–9).

Immunogenicity and Efficacy

Placebo-controlled field trials of Hib conjugate vaccines in infants in the United States demonstrated nearly 100 percent protection and provided the basis for the initial approval of these vaccines for use in this country. In a study of HbOC in northern California, vaccine efficacy was 100 percent for infants receiving the three-dose schedule at 2, 4, and 6 months of age.[53] In a Navajo population of infants at high risk of acquiring Hib disease who were vaccinated at 2 and 4 months of age with either PRP-OMP or placebo, vaccine efficacy was 100 percent at 1 year of age and 93 percent in total.[334] Licensure of PRP-T was based on comparable immunogenicity in a three-dose schedule to that of the other two products. In addition, an efficacy trial in Great Britain and the lack of cases in trials indicate an efficacy of PRP-T comparable to that of HbOC and PRP-OMP.[57, 361]

Adverse Events

Hib vaccines are well tolerated. Local reactions occur in approximately 25 percent of recipients but typically are mild and last less than 24 hours.[168, 378] Systemic reactions, such as fever and irritability, are infrequent occurrences. When conjugate vaccines are administered concurrently with DTaP vaccine, the incidence of systemic reactions is similar to that observed when only DTaP is given.[168]

Indications[7, 74, 80]

Routine vaccination against Hib disease is recommended for all children beginning at approximately 2 months of age. Three vaccines, HbOC, PRP-T, and PRP-OMP, are licensed in the United States for use in infants. One of these products, PRP-T, can be given with DTaP, mixed in the same syringe for the fourth dose only. HbOC, PRP-T, and PRP-OMP are considered interchangeable for primary as well as booster vaccinations.

Two or three doses, depending on the product, given at 2-month intervals are indicated by the time that the child is 6 months of age. Excellent immune responses have been achieved when vaccines from different manufacturers have been interchanged in the primary series.[36, 52, 203] If PRP-OMP is administered in a series with one of the other two products licensed for infants, the recommended number of doses to complete the series is determined by the other product (and not by PRP-OMP). For example, if PRP-OMP is administered for the first dose when the child is 2 months old and another vaccine is administered at 4 months of age, a third dose of any of the three licensed Hib vaccines is recommended at 6 months of age to complete the primary series. A final dose of any product, irrespective of the previous vaccines received, is acceptable when the child is 12 to 15 months of age for completion of the Hib immunization schedule.

When feasible, the conjugate vaccine product used for the first dose should be used for subsequent doses in children younger than 12 months. When sequential doses of different products are given in the child's first year of life, three doses of any conjugate product is sufficient. A final dose of any product, irrespective of the previous vaccines received, is acceptable when the child is 12 to 15 months of age for completion of the Hib immunization schedule.

For children in whom Hib immunization has not been initiated by the time that they reach 7 months of age, the recommended schedules differ according to the child's age and the choice of conjugate vaccine.[22, 74] Previously unimmunized children who are 15 months and older should be immunized with a single dose of any licensed conjugate *Haemophilus* vaccine. For previously unimmunized children 5 years or older, immunization is indicated only if they have an underlying condition predisposing to Hib disease, such as asplenia or HIV infection.

HEPATITIS B VACCINE

Hepatitis B virus (HBV) infection is a leading cause of acute hepatitis and a major public health problem of global importance. Its incidence is especially high in many Asian and African countries. Individuals with chronic infection are at

TABLE 242–9 ■ *HAEMOPHILUS INFLUENZAE* TYPE b CONJUGATE VACCINES

Vaccine Manufacturer	Abbreviation for Vaccine (Trade Name)	Carrier Protein	Polysaccharide and Spacer	Date of Licensure in the United States
Wyeth Vaccines	HbOC (HibTITER)	CRM_{197} (a nontoxic mutant diphtheria toxin)	Small (oligo) polysaccharide and no spacer	1988
Merck & Company	PRP-OMP (PedvaxHIB)	An outer-membrane protein (OMP) complex of *Neisseria meningitidis*	Large polysaccharide and a complex spacer	1989
Aventis Pasteur	PRP-T (ActHIB,* OmniHIB†)	Tetanus toxoid	Large polysaccharide and a small 6-carbon spacer	1993

*Distributed in the United States by Aventis Pasteur.
†Distributed in the United States by Glaxo SmithKline.

risk for the development of chronic hepatitis, cirrhosis, and primary hepatocellular carcinoma. In the United States, approximately 300,000 persons are infected each year and 2 million are estimated to be chronically infected.[212] These persons not only are at increased risk for chronic and malignant liver disease but also, as chronic carriers, serve as the reservoir for transmission of HBV.

The initial strategies for prevention of hepatitis B through vaccination reflect the varying epidemiology of HBV infection in different areas of the world.[77] In the United States, for example, infection is of comparatively low endemicity and occurs primarily in adolescents and adults. The risk of acquiring infection, however, is much greater in certain populations. Examples include those born and living in areas or among groups in which HBV is highly endemic and those with lifestyles predisposing to the acquisition of HBV, such as male homosexual activity, intravenous drug abuse, and promiscuous heterosexual activity.[1] In contrast, in geographic areas in which HBV infection is highly endemic, infection usually is acquired at birth or during childhood, which has resulted in the recommendation for universal vaccination of infants.

In 1991, the CDC initiated a comprehensive hepatitis B vaccination strategy to eliminate transmission of HBV in the United States.[77] Critical elements of this strategy included preventing perinatal transmission of HBV by identifying and providing immunoprophylaxis to infants of hepatitis B surface antigen (HBsAg)-positive mothers and universal hepatitis B vaccination of infants to interrupt transmission and prevent future infection. The advantages of this approach included the existence of effective programs of routine childhood immunization, protection without any need to identify specific risk factors, and protection before significant exposure occurred. In addition, the positive effects of universal infant immunization had been observed in Taiwan, where the strategy of universal infant immunization was already being used. In Taiwan, the overall prevalence rate of HBV for children aged 1 to 10 years decreased from 9.8 percent in 1984 to 1.3 percent in 1994.[137] As a result of the implementation of this strategy in the United States, a substantial increase was seen in the percentage of children aged 19 to 35 months who had received three doses of hepatitis B vaccine, from less than 10 percent in 1991 to 84 percent in 1997.[96]

In 1994, the ACIP expanded the recommendations to include previously unvaccinated children 11 to 12 years old.[87] No nationwide vaccine coverage data are available to assess vaccine coverage in children 11 to 12 years old; however, vaccine coverage in this group is expected to increase as states implement middle-school entry requirements for hepatitis B vaccination.[102]

In October 1997, the ACIP expanded its hepatitis B vaccination recommendations still further to include all unvaccinated children 0 to 18 years old and made hepatitis B vaccine available through the Vaccines for Children (VFC) program for persons 0 to 18 years of age who are eligible for this program.[108] The other ACIP priorities for giving hepatitis B vaccination to children remained unchanged and included all infants; children in populations at high risk for acquiring HBV infection, such as Alaska Natives, Pacific Islanders, and children who reside in households of first-generation immigrants from countries where HBV infection is moderately or highly endemic; previously unvaccinated children 11 to 12 years old; and older adolescents and adults in defined at-risk groups.[77, 87] The goal of the 1997 recommendations was to increase access to hepatitis B vaccine by encouraging the vaccination of previously unvaccinated children and adolescents 0 to 18 years old whenever they are seen for routine medical visits.[95] This expansion of the recommended age group for receiving vaccination and for VFC eligibility simplifies previous recommendations and the eligibility criteria for receiving VFC vaccine.

Universal vaccination of infants and children 11 to 12 years old will result in a highly immune population and is expected to eliminate transmission of HBV in the United States. In addition, because most HBV infections in the United States occur in adults, vaccinating infants and adolescents 11 to 12 years of age alone will not lower the incidence of disease substantially for several years. Most HBV infections in adults occur in those who have defined risk factors for HBV infection, including persons with multiple sex partners (more than one partner during the preceding 6 months), men who have sex with men, and injecting drug users.[87] The primary means of preventing these infections is to identify settings where adolescents and adults with high-risk drug and sexual practices can be routinely accessed and vaccinated.

Preparations

Hepatitis B vaccines consisting of inactivated purified HBsAg derived from chronic hepatitis B plasma were introduced first in the early 1980s. In the late 1980s, two recombinant vaccines (Recombivax HB, Merck & Co. and Engerix-B, SmithKline Beecham Biologicals) were licensed in the United States. Only the recombinant vaccines are available in the United States, but plasma-derived vaccines are widely used in other areas of the world.

Immunogenicity and Efficacy[9, 108]

The recommended series of three doses of vaccine induces a protective antibody response in more than 95 percent of infants, children, adolescents, and adults younger than 40 years. In field trials, efficacy has been 80 to 95 percent and generally correlates with immunogenicity. Protection against disease is virtually 100 percent for persons who develop adequate serum antibody concentrations (anti-HBs ≥10 mIU/mL) after vaccination. Active immunization in combination with passive immunoprophylaxis with hepatitis B immune globulin (HBIG) administered shortly after birth to infants born to HBsAg-positive mothers is more than 90 percent effective in preventing transmission of HBV and infection of the infant.

Vaccine-induced protection against symptomatic infection in a normal host is prolonged and correlates with immunologic memory, which has been demonstrated in immunized children and adults for at least 12 years after vaccination. Children immunized at birth are protected for at least 10 years. Thus, a need for routine booster doses has not been demonstrated.

Adverse Events

Other than soreness at the injection site, reactions to hepatitis B vaccine rarely occur. Post-vaccination surveillance performed after licensure of the plasma-derived vaccine indicated a possible association between GBS and receipt of the first vaccine dose, but no evidence indicates an association of GBS with recombinant vaccine.[108] Anaphylaxis has been estimated to occur in 1 in 600,000 doses distributed.[108] Several nonfatal cases have been reported in children.

Indications[9, 87, 108]

HBV vaccine is recommended for all infants in the United States in a three-dose schedule administered by 18 months of age or earlier. However, in populations in which childhood infection with HBV has been highly endemic, such as Alaskan Natives, Pacific Islanders, and infants in immigrant or refugee families from countries in which HBV is of intermediate or high endemicity, the schedule should be completed by 12 months of age.

Routine screening of pregnant women for HBsAg still is recommended because of the necessity for a birth dose of vaccine and HBIG.[9, 21, 23, 77, 87, 108] Infants born to HBsAg-positive mothers should be given HBIG (0.5 mL) within 12 hours of birth at a separate injection site, as well as the birth dose of HBV vaccine.[108]

Although the recommended time for giving the first dose is shortly after birth, it may be given at any time in the first 2 months of life for infants born to HBsAg-negative mothers. For infants weighing less than 2 kg who are born to HBsAg-negative mothers, initiation of vaccine should be delayed until just before hospital discharge if the infant weighs 2 kg or more or until approximately 2 months of age when other routine immunizations are given. The 2003 *Recommended Childhood Immunization Schedule* gives a preference for administering the first dose of hepatitis B vaccine to all newborns soon after birth and before hospital discharge.[131] Administering the first dose of hepatitis B vaccine soon after birth should minimize the risk for infection because of errors in maternal HBsAg testing or reporting or from exposure to persons with chronic HBV infection in the household and can increase the likelihood of completing the vaccine series. Only monovalent hepatitis B vaccine can be used for the birth dose. Either monovalent or combination vaccine can be used to complete the series. Four doses of hepatitis B vaccine, including the birth dose, may be administered if a combination vaccine is used to complete the series. In addition to receiving HBIG and the hepatitis B vaccine series, infants of HBsAg-positive mothers should be tested for HBsAg and antibody to HBsAg (anti-HBs) at 9 to 15 months of age to identify those with chronic HBV infection or those who may require revaccination.[77] Administration of the second dose of vaccine is recommended 1 to 2 months after administration of the first dose, followed by a third dose at 6 to 18 months of age.

Universal immunization against HBV is recommended in the United States for all 11- to 12-year-old children who have not been immunized previously. In addition, vaccination is indicated for all unvaccinated children younger than 11 years who are Pacific Islanders or who reside in households of first-generation immigrants from countries where HBV is of high or intermediate endemicity. Vaccination also is recommended for those with one or more of the following risk factors for acquiring HBV infection:

- Sexually active heterosexual adolescents and adults who have a recently acquired sexually transmitted disease, are identified as prostitutes, or have had one or more sex partners in the previous 6 months.
- Sexually active men who have sex with men.
- Household contacts or sexual partners of HBsAg-positive persons.
- Injecting drug users.
- Persons at occupational risk of acquiring infection through exposure to blood or blood-contaminated body fluids, such as health care workers and public safety workers.
- Residents and staff of institutions for the developmentally disabled.
- Hemodialysis patients. Vaccination of those with early renal failure is encouraged before they require hemodialysis.
- Patients who receive clotting factor concentrates.
- Members of households with international adoptees who are HBsAg-positive.
- Travelers, especially children, to areas with high and intermediate rates of infection with HBV who have close contact with the local population or are likely to have contact with blood, such as in a medical setting, or sexual contact with residents.
- Inmates in long-term correctional facilities.

In addition to active and passive immunoprophylaxis of infants born to HBsAg-positive mothers, postexposure prophylaxis is recommended in the following circumstances:

- Sexual partner of an HBsAg-positive person. A single dose of HBIG within 14 days of the last sexual contact and initiation of the three-dose hepatitis B vaccination is recommended for susceptible persons.
- Household exposure of an unvaccinated infant younger than 12 months to a primary caregiver who has acute hepatitis B. Infants in this circumstance should receive HBIG, in addition to being vaccinated.
- Accidental percutaneous or permucosal exposure of a susceptible person to HBsAg-positive blood. This indication is most exemplified by a needle-stick or other accident involving blood in a hospital. Another example is an injury to a susceptible person caused by the bite of an HBsAg-positive child. For this indication, HBIG as well as vaccine is given. Recommendations in these circumstances are complex and based on the availability of the blood source for HBsAg testing and the hepatitis B vaccination status of the exposed person.

Booster doses are not recommended except in the case of patients undergoing hemodialysis and possibly other immunocompromised patients, in whom the need should be assessed by annual antibody testing. An additional dose is indicated for those whose serum anti-HBsAg concentration is less than 10 mIU/mL.

The current recommended doses and schedule for the use of hepatitis B vaccines licensed in the United States in infants and other age groups are shown in Table 242–10 (see elsewhere[9, 21, 23, 77, 87, 108] for more information). For completing the hepatitis B vaccine series and achieving complete vaccination for hepatitis B, the two licensed hepatitis B vaccines are interchangeable when administered in doses recommended by the manufacturers.[108]

In September 1999, the FDA approved an optional two-dose schedule of Recombivax HB for vaccination of adolescents 11 to 15 years of age. The ACIP recommended that this schedule be included in the VFC program in February 2000.[117] With the two-dose schedule, the adult dose of Recombivax HB is administered to adolescents 11 to 15 years old, with the second dose given 4 to 6 months after the first dose. In immunogenicity studies in adolescents 11 to 15 years of age, antibody concentrations and seroprotection rates were similar with the two-dose schedule and the currently licensed three-dose schedule. Follow-up data collected during the course of 2 years indicate that the rate of decline in concentration of antibody for the two-dose schedule was similar to that for the three-dose schedule. No data are available to assess long-term protection or immune memory after vaccination with the two-dose schedule, and whether booster doses of vaccine will be required is not known. Children and adolescents who have begun vaccination with a dose of the pediatric formulation should complete the three-dose series with this dose. Similarly, if the formulation administered to an adolescent at the start of a series is not known, the series should be completed with the three-dose schedule.

TABLE 242–10 ■ RECOMMENDED DOSES AND SCHEDULES OF HEPATITIS B VIRUS VACCINES IN THE UNITED STATES

	Dose of Recombivax HB (Merck & Co.)		Dose of Engerix-B (SmithKline Beecham)	
Group	μg	mL	μg	mL
Infants of HBsAg-negative mothers[1,2]	5	0.5	10	0.5
Infants of HBsAg-positive mothers[3]	5	0.5	10	0.5[4]
Children and adolescents 1–19 years[5]	5	0.5	10	0.5[6]
Adolescents 11–15 years old[7]	10	0.5	N/A	N/A
Adults ≥20 years old[5]	10	1.0	20	1.0[6]
Dialysis patients and other immunocompromised adults	40	1.0[8]	40	2.0[9,10]

1. Usual schedule: 0, 1 to 2, and 6 to 18 months of age.
2. Alternative schedule: 1 to 2, 4, and 6 to 18 months of age.
3. Usual schedule: three doses at 0, 1, and 6 months of age.
4. Alternative schedule: four doses at 0, 1, 2, and 12 to 18 months of age.
5. Usual schedule: 0, 1, and 6 months after the first dose.
6. Alternative schedule: four doses at 0, 1, 2, and 12 months after the first dose.
7. Usual schedule: 0 and 4 to 6 months after the first dose.
8. Special formulation of dialysis patients.
9. Two 1.0-mL doses given at different sites.
10. Four-dose schedule recommended at 0, 1, 2, and 12 months after the first dose.

HBsAg, hepatitis B surface antigen.

Modified from Centers for Disease Control and Prevention: A comprehensive strategy for the elimination of hepatitis B transmission in the United States through universal childhood immunization: Recommendations of the Immunization Practices Advisory Committee (ACIP). M. M. W. R. Recomm. Rep. *40* (RR-13):1–25, 1991.

Contraindications

The only contraindication is a history of anaphylaxis to a previous dose of vaccine. Although data on the safety of HBV vaccines are not available for pregnant women, these vaccines contain only HBsAg and not live virus and should not be deleterious to the developing fetus. Because HBV infection during pregnancy can result in transmission to the newborn, susceptible women at increased risk of acquiring infection should be vaccinated during pregnancy.

Inadvertent vaccination of HBsAg-positive persons has no deleterious effects.

MEASLES VACCINE

Since the introduction of both an inactivated and a live virus, attenuated measles vaccine (Edmonston B strain) in the United States in 1963, the reported incidence of measles has decreased by more than 99 percent. Although the incidence of measles has declined in all age groups, the decline has been greatest in children 5 to 14 years of age.

Measles was targeted for elimination in the United States by 1982. Efforts to eliminate measles were not successful as a result of two factors. The first was vaccine failure. In the late 1980s, outbreaks occurred in older children in schools in which immunization rates were usually greater than 95 percent.[210, 276, 294] Attack rates were 1 to 5 percent because of the accumulation of measles-susceptible individuals from vaccine failure. The recurrent measles outbreaks among vaccinated school-age children in the mid-1980s prompted both the ACIP and the AAP in 1989 to recommend that all children receive two doses of measles-containing vaccine, preferably as MMR.[20, 69] Although administration of the second dose originally was recommended either at entry to primary school (ACIP) or middle/secondary school (AAP), the ACIP, the AAP, and the AAFP now recommend that a child receive the second dose at age 4 to 6 years of age rather than delaying it until the child is 11 to 12 years old.[106] The major benefit of administering the second dose is a reduction in the proportion of persons who remain susceptible because of primary vaccine failure. Waning immunity is not a major cause of vaccine failure and has little influence on transmission of measles, and revaccination of children who have low concentrations of measles antibody produces only a transient rise in antibody concentration.[175, 273, 275, 278, 303, 370]

The second factor leading to outbreaks of measles was the failure to implement current immunization strategies, especially in the inner cities, where a high proportion of preschool children had not been vaccinated. From 1989 through 1991, the proportion of unvaccinated persons with measles increased, as reflected by outbreaks among unvaccinated inner-city preschool-age children. Multiple barriers to timely immunization of these children were identified during investigation of the measles resurgence that occurred between 1989 and 1991.

The use of a two-dose schedule combined with a major effort to increase vaccine coverage in preschool children reduced the number of cases in 1996 to 508.[96] In 2000, measles reached a record low number of 86 confirmed cases, with no measles-associated deaths.[133] The epidemiology of measles during the year 2000 suggests that measles is no longer an endemic disease in the United States, but the risk of internationally imported measles cases may give rise to indigenous transmission.

The recommended age for receiving routine vaccination with measles vaccine has been lowered in the past decade from 15 months to 12 to 15 months of age.[134] The decision to lower the age for receiving routine primary vaccination was based on the observation that most children are susceptible to measles by the time that they reach 12 months of age because of waning transplacental immunity.[271, 274] Most mothers now have vaccine-induced immunity rather than immunity conferred by infection with wild virus. Antibody concentrations induced by measles vaccination are generally lower than those induced by natural measles. Therefore, measles-specific antibodies acquired transplacentally are lower in infants of vaccinated mothers, thus resulting in these infants being susceptible at an earlier age.

Preparations

The live measles virus vaccine (Moraten strain) available in the United States is prepared in chick fibroblast cell culture. Each dose of vaccine contains neomycin, sorbitol, and hydrolyzed gelatin as a stabilizer. Preparations include a monovalent (measles only) vaccine and two combinations, measles-rubella and MMR. MMR is the vaccine of choice for use in routine vaccination programs for children and adults. In all situations in which measles vaccine is to be used, MMR should be given if the recipient is likely to be susceptible to contracting rubella or mumps.[11, 106]

Inadequate protection against measles can result from the administration of improperly stored vaccine. Before reconstitution, measles vaccine must be stored at a temperature between 2 and 8°C (35.6 to 46.4°F) or colder and must be protected from light, which may inactivate the virus. Reconstituted vaccine should be stored in a refrigerator and discarded if not used within 8 hours.

Immunogenicity and Efficacy

Immunization produces a mild or inapparent, noncommunicable infection. Measles antibodies develop in approximately 95 percent of children vaccinated at 12 months of age and in 98 percent of children vaccinated at 15 months of age.[274] Studies indicate that serologic evidence of measles immunity develops in more than 99 percent of persons who receive two doses of measles vaccine, separated by at least 1 month, on or after their first birthday.[143, 154] Although vaccine-induced antibody titers are lower than those after natural disease, persistence of protective titers for as long as 16 years after administration of vaccine has been demonstrated.[258, 275] Most vaccinated persons who appear to lose antibody have an anamnestic response after revaccination, thus indicating that they most likely are still immune.[300] A small percentage of vaccinated individuals may lose protection after several years as a result of secondary vaccine failure.[278, 390]

Adverse Events

Vaccine-associated symptoms consisting of fever higher than 39.4°C (102.9°F) occurring 5 to 10 days after immunization or transient rash develop in 5 to 15 percent of recipients.[307] Serious complications related to vaccine use occur far less frequently than after natural measles.[305]

Thrombocytopenia occurs at a rate of 1 case for every 30,000 to 40,000 doses distributed. Based on data from Sweden and Finland, the IOM concluded that a causal association exists between MMR and thrombocytopenia.[234] The decrease in platelet count presumably is caused by the measles component and is not usually clinically apparent. However, thrombocytopenic purpura occurring after vaccination has been reported.

Central nervous system disease, specifically encephalitis or encephalopathy, is reported at a rate of less than 1 case per 1 million doses of vaccine administered. Because the incidence of encephalitis or encephalopathy after the administration of measles vaccination to healthy children is lower than the observed incidence of encephalitis of unknown etiology, some or most of the reported severe neurologic disorders may be only temporally, rather than causally related to measles immunization. The risk of subacute sclerosing panencephalitis (SSPE) developing in vaccinated children is extremely low and estimated to be approximately one twelfth the risk of SSPE developing after a case of natural measles (0.7 SSPE cases per million vaccine doses versus 8.5 cases per million natural measles infections).[55, 66] Whether measles vaccine causes SSPE is unclear. Some cases of SSPE occur in children with no history of having measles or measles vaccination.[11]

Reactions to measles vaccine are not age related and occur only in susceptible vaccinees. After revaccination, reactions should be expected only in those who failed to respond to the first immunization.

Indications[11, 106]

Measles vaccine is indicated for persons susceptible to measles, unless otherwise contraindicated. The recommended age for receiving the first dose of measles vaccine is 12 to 15 months. In high-risk areas, such as those with recurrent measles transmission, the initial dose should be administered when the children reach 12 months of age. The second dose is given routinely at 4 to 6 years and no later than 11 to 12 years of age. Both doses of measles vaccine preferably should be given as MMR. The minimal interval between the two doses is 4 weeks.

Adults born before 1957 generally may be considered immune to measles because of previous natural infection. Those born after 1956 and in whom immunoprophylaxis is indicated should receive two doses of vaccine.

During outbreaks, when the likelihood of exposure to measles is high, measles vaccine should be given to infants as young as 6 months. Seroconversion rates to vaccine are significantly less in children vaccinated before reaching 1 year of age than those in older children. Children immunized before their first birthday then should be revaccinated with MMR at 12 to 15 months of age, with a third dose given according to local policy.

Measles remains endemic in many areas of the world. Although vaccination against measles is not a requirement for entry into any country, susceptible children, adolescents, and adults born after 1956 should be offered measles vaccination (usually as MMR) before embarking on international travel. Infants 6 months or older traveling to areas where measles is endemic or epidemic should be vaccinated before departure and revaccinated at 12 to 15 months. Vaccination of infants younger than 6 months is not necessary because most will be protected by maternally derived antibodies.

Exposure of susceptible individuals to measles is not a contraindication to administering vaccination; vaccine given within 72 hours of exposure may provide protection. If exposure does not result in infection, immunization will protect against future infection.

Precautions and Contraindications[11, 106]

Immunocompromised patients with conditions such as lymphoreticular or other generalized malignancy and primary or secondary immunodeficiency states should not be given live virus, attenuated measles vaccine. After cessation of their chemotherapy, these individuals generally should not receive measles vaccine for at least 3 months. However, because the intensity and type of immunosuppressive therapy, radiation therapy, underlying disease, and other factors determine when immunologic responsiveness will be restored, arriving at a definitive recommendation for an interval after cessation of immunosuppressive therapy when measles vaccine can be safely and effectively administered often is not possible.

An exception to the contraindication of administering measles vaccine to immunocompromised patients is asymptomatic HIV-infected patients, for whom measles vaccination, given as MMR at 12 to 15 months of age, is recommended. The need to protect HIV-infected persons who are at increased risk for severe complications if infected with measles has been balanced against the risk of having adverse reactions. Measles vaccine is not recommended for HIV-infected persons with evidence of severe immunosuppression. A case of progressive measles pneumonitis occurred in a person with acquired immunodeficiency syndrome (AIDS) and severe immunosuppression to whom MMR vaccine was administered,[90] and morbidity related to measles vaccination has been reported in persons with severe immunosuppression unrelated to HIV infection.[48, 279, 286, 288] In addition, the antibody response to measles vaccine in severely immunocompromised HIV-infected persons is diminished.[40] In the United States, the incidence of measles is currently very low. Among HIV-infected persons who did not have evidence of severe immunosuppression, no serious or unusual adverse events have been reported after receiving measles vaccination.[281, 298, 304, 347] Therefore, MMR vaccination is recommended for all asymptomatic HIV-infected persons who do not have evidence of severe immunosuppression and for whom measles vaccination would otherwise be indicated. MMR vaccination also should be considered for all symptomatic HIV-infected persons who do not have evidence of severe immunosuppression. Testing asymptomatic persons for HIV is not necessary before administering MMR.[34]

Systemically absorbed corticosteroids can suppress the immune system of an otherwise healthy person. However, neither the minimal dose nor the duration of therapy sufficient to cause immune suppression is well defined. Although the immunosuppressive effects of steroid treatment vary, many clinicians believe that a steroid dose equivalent to or greater than a prednisone dose of 2 mg/kg of body weight per day or a total of 20 mg/day is sufficiently immunosuppressive to raise concern about the safety of administration of live virus vaccines. Persons who have received systemic corticosteroids in doses of 2 mg/kg of body weight or 20 mg daily or on alternate days for an interval of 14 days or longer should avoid receiving vaccination with MMR and its component vaccines for at least 1 month after cessation of steroid therapy.[106] Persons who have received prolonged or extensive topical, aerosolized, or other local corticosteroid therapy that causes clinical or laboratory evidence of systemic immunosuppression also should avoid receiving vaccination with MMR for at least 1 month after cessation of therapy.[106]

The live attenuated measles virus vaccine used for immunization is not communicable. Therefore, contacts of immunocompromised patients should be vaccinated to prevent the spread of natural measles to such patients.

Although no direct evidence has demonstrated that measles vaccine is harmful to a pregnant female or her fetus, it should not be administered to women known to be pregnant or who are considering becoming pregnant because of the theoretic risk of fetal infection associated with a live virus vaccine. Women vaccinated with MMR should avoid conception for 28 days after vaccination.[126]

Because measles vaccination may diminish cutaneous manifestations of cell-mediated immunity temporarily, a tuberculin test performed several days to 6 weeks after immunization can yield a false-negative result. Although natural measles infection can exacerbate tuberculosis, no evidence indicates that measles vaccination is associated with such an effect. Therefore, tuberculin skin testing is not a prerequisite for administering measles immunization. If a tuberculin test is indicated, it should be performed on the day of immunization or postponed for 4 to 6 weeks because measles vaccination may suppress tuberculin reactivity temporarily.

In persons allergic to eggs, the risk of having serious allergic reactions such as anaphylaxis after receiving MMR vaccine is extremely low, and skin testing with vaccine is not predictive of allergic reaction to vaccination.[11, 242, 250] Therefore, a skin test is not required before administering MMR to persons who are allergic to eggs. Similarly, the administration of gradually increasing doses of vaccine is not required.[106] Data indicate that most anaphylactic reactions to measles- and mumps-containing vaccines are not associated with hypersensitivity to egg antigens but to other components of the vaccines such as the gelatin stabilizer.[204, 224, 249, 263]

Children with a previous history of thrombocytopenic purpura or thrombocytopenia may be at risk for clinically significant thrombocytopenia after immunization with MMR.[46, 234] The decision to vaccinate should be based on the benefits of immunity to measles, mumps, and rubella and the risk of reoccurrence or exacerbation of the thrombocytopenia after receiving vaccination or from natural infection with measles or rubella. For children in whom thrombocytopenia develops in the month after administration of a dose of measles-containing vaccine, withholding the second dose of measles vaccine is prudent if the incidence of measles remains low.

Receipt of antibody-containing blood products (whole blood, plasma, or parenteral immunoglobulin) may interfere with seroconversion to measles vaccine. High doses of immunoglobulin preparations can inhibit the immune response to measles vaccine for 3 or more months, depending on the dosage.[344] The length of time that such passively acquired antibody persists depends on the concentration and quantity of the blood product received[11, 134] (Table 242–11).

As in any condition that induces fever during the second year of life, children predisposed to having febrile seizures may experience seizures after receiving measles vaccination. Most convulsions that develop after measles immunization are simple febrile seizures and occur in children without known risk factors. Febrile seizures that occur after the administration of vaccinations do not increase the risk for the subsequent development of epilepsy or other neurologic disorders.[45] An increased risk of having seizures after receiving measles vaccination may occur in children with a previous history of convulsions or those with a history of convulsions in first-degree family members. Although the exact risk cannot be determined, it appears to be low. The recommendation to immunize children with a personal history of seizures or those with a history of seizures in first-degree family members is based on factors indicating that the benefits greatly outweigh the risks. Prophylactic use of anticonvulsants is not usually feasible because therapeutic concentrations of many currently prescribed anticonvulsants are not achieved for some time after the initiation of therapy.

MUMPS VACCINE

Live virus mumps vaccine became available in the United States in 1967 and was recommended for routine use in 1977. After vaccine licensure, reported mumps cases decreased rapidly. A relative resurgence of mumps occurred in 1986 and 1987. In 1989, the ACIP and AAP implemented a two-dose combined MMR schedule given at 4 to 6 or at 11 to 12 years of age. After introduction of the two-dose schedule, mumps cases declined and reached a record low of 323 cases in the year 2000.[128]

No evidence indicates waning immunity in vaccinees. The risk of mumps occurring was highest in states without comprehensive school vaccination requirements, thus providing further evidence that failure to vaccinate rather than vaccine

TABLE 242–11 ■ SUGGESTED INTERVALS BETWEEN IMMUNE GLOBULIN ADMINISTRATION AND MEASLES OR VARICELLA VACCINATION

Product/Indication	Route	Dose		Interval (mo)*
		U or mL	mg/kg	
RSV monoclonal antibody (Synagis)	IM		15	None
Tetanus (as TIG)	IM	250 U	10	3
Hepatitis A prophylaxis (as IG)				
Contact prophylaxis	IM	0.02 mL/kg	3.3	3
International travel	IM	0.06 mL/kg	10	3
Hepatitis B prophylaxis (as HBIG)	IM	0.06 mL/kg	10	3
Rabies prophylaxis (as RIG)	IM	20 IU/kg	22	4
Varicella prophylaxis (as VZIG)	IM	125 U/10 kg (maximum 625 U)	20–40	5
Measles prophylaxis (as IG)				
Standard	IM	0.25 mL/kg	40	5
Immunocompromised contact	IM	0.25 mL/kg	80	6
Blood transfusion				
Washed RBCs	IV	10 mL/kg	Negligible	None
RBCs, adenine-saline added	IV	10 mL/kg	10	3
Packed RBCs	IV	10 mL/kg	60	6
Whole blood	IV	10 mL/kg	80–100	6
Plasma/platelet products	IV	10 mL/kg	160	7
CMV-IVIG	IV		150	6
RSV-IG	IV		750 mg/kg	9
IVIG				
Replacement therapy for immune deficiencies	IV		300–400	8
ITP	IV		400	8
ITP	IV		1000	10
Kawasaki disease	IV		2000	11

*These intervals should provide sufficient time for decreases in passive antibodies in all children to allow for an adequate response to measles or varicella vaccine. Physicians should not assume that children are fully protected against measles during these intervals. Additional doses of IG or measles vaccine may be indicated after exposure to measles.

CMV, cytomegalovirus; HBIG, hepatitis B IG; IG, immune globulin; IVIG, intravenous IG; ITP, immune thrombocytopenic purpura; RBCs, red blood cells; RIG, rabies IG; RSV, respiratory syncytial virus; TIG, tetanus IG; VZIG, varicella-zoster IG.

failure primarily was responsible for the continued occurrence of mumps.[136, 152] Primary vaccine failures do occur as evidenced by outbreaks in highly vaccinated populations.[60, 138, 225]

Preparations

The live attenuated mumps virus vaccine (Jeryl Lynn strain) in current use in the United States is prepared in chick embryo cell culture and is available individually (monovalent, mumps only) and in combination as mumps-rubella vaccine and MMR. Each dose of vaccine contains neomycin, sorbitol, and hydrolyzed gelatin as stabilizers. Before reconstitution, mumps vaccine must be stored at 2 to 8° C (35.6° to 46.4° F) or colder and protected from light to avoid inactivation. After reconstitution, the vaccine should be used within 8 hours or discarded.

Immunogenicity and Efficacy

The vaccine induces an asymptomatic, noncommunicable infection. More than 97 percent of susceptible recipients develop protective antibody titers, albeit lower than those after natural infection.[376] Reported clinical vaccine efficacy has ranged from 75 to 95 percent.[136, 251] The duration of vaccine immunity is unknown, but serologic data indicate the persistence of antibody for more than 30 years.[89, 374]

Adverse Events

The use of mumps vaccine is associated with very few side effects. Parotitis and fever have been reported rarely. Hypersensitivity reactions, including rash, pruritus, and purpura, have been associated temporally with vaccination, but they are transient and generally mild. Administration of MMR is not harmful if given to an individual already immune to one or more of the viruses.[12, 106]

The frequency of reported central nervous system dysfunction after vaccination is not greater than the observed background rate in unimmunized persons.[106] The IOM concluded that evidence is inadequate to establish a causal relationship between the Jeryl Lynn strain of mumps vaccine used in the United States and aseptic meningitis, encephalitis, or sensorineural deafness.[234]

Indications[12, 106]

Routine active immunization as MMR in children 12 to 15 months of age is recommended. Most children will receive a second dose of mumps vaccine in childhood as a result of the recommendation for routine measles revaccination with MMR. Mumps revaccination is justified by the occurrence of mumps in highly vaccinated populations because substantial numbers of cases have occurred in persons with a history of mumps vaccination.[60, 138, 225]

Susceptible older children, adolescents, and adults also should be vaccinated against mumps. Adults born before 1957 generally may be considered immune to mumps as a result of previous natural infection.

Mumps remains endemic throughout most of the world. Although vaccination against mumps is not a requirement for entry into any country, susceptible children, adolescents, and adults born after 1956 should be offered mumps vaccination, usually as MMR, before engaging in international travel.

Mumps vaccine is of no proven value in the prevention of disease in susceptible individuals after exposure to mumps, probably because the time required to develop protective antibody titers after immunization exceeds the incubation period of clinical mumps. However, if the exposure did not result in infection, the vaccine confers subsequent immunity.

Precautions and Contraindications[12, 106]

Among persons who are allergic to eggs, the risk of having serious allergic reactions such as anaphylaxis after receiving MMR is extremely low, and skin testing with vaccine is not predictive of allergic reaction to vaccination.[11, 242, 250] Therefore, performing skin testing is not required before administering MMR to persons who are allergic to eggs. Similarly, the administration of gradually increasing doses of vaccine is not required.[106] Data indicate that most anaphylactic reactions to measles- and mumps-containing vaccines are not associated with hypersensitivity to egg antigens but to other components of the vaccines, such as the gelatin stabilizer.[204, 224, 249, 263]

Because of the theoretic risk of fetal damage, mumps vaccine should not be administered to women known to be pregnant or who are considering becoming pregnant. Women vaccinated with MMR should avoid conception for 28 days after vaccination.[126]

Lymphoreticular or other generalized malignancy and primary or secondary immunodeficiency states represent contraindications to the use of mumps vaccine. Exceptions are children with HIV infection who are immunized against measles with MMR (see Measles Vaccine). Because infection after vaccination is noncommunicable, susceptible close contacts of immunosuppressed patients should be vaccinated to avoid mumps exposure in such patients.

After cessation of immunosuppressive therapy, live virus mumps vaccine generally is withheld for at least 3 months. Because the intensity and type of immunosuppressive therapy, radiation therapy, underlying disease, and other factors determine when immunologic responsiveness will be restored, making a definitive recommendation for an interval after cessation of immunosuppressive therapy when mumps vaccine can be safely and effectively administered often is not possible.

The effect of immune globulin preparations on the response to mumps vaccine is unknown. High doses of immune globulin preparations can inhibit the immune response to measles vaccine for 3 or more months, depending on the dosage.[344] If mumps vaccine is given as the MMR vaccine, the recommendations for measles vaccine should be followed (see Table 242–11).

Administration of mumps vaccine should be avoided if the individual is receiving immunosuppressive dosages of systemic corticosteroids. The effects of corticosteroids vary, but many clinicians believe that a dose equivalent to either 2 mg/kg of body weight or 20 mg/day of prednisone is sufficiently immunosuppressive to raise concern about the safety of vaccination with live virus vaccines.

PERTUSSIS VACCINE

Pertussis (whooping cough) continues to cause significant morbidity and mortality worldwide among young children.[293] In the absence of vaccination, the WHO has estimated that approximately 1 million deaths would have occurred from the disease and its complications. In the United States, the number of cases has been reduced by approximately 95 percent during the vaccine era. Despite an effective vaccine, pertussis continues to occur in the United States in all age groups. Since the 1980s, its incidence has increased in cycles, with peaks every 3 to 4 years. Surveillance data from 1997 to 2000 and data from 1994 to 1996 demonstrated that the reported incidence increased 60 percent in adolescents and adults and 11 percent in infants younger than 6 months.[132] The increase in cases among young infants suggests that a true increase in pertussis circulation has occurred. The number of cases in children old enough to receive vaccine has remained stable.

The experiences of countries where rates of pertussis vaccination have markedly declined provide strong support for continuing routine immunization of infants and young children.[142] For example, in the United Kingdom as a result of adverse publicity about pertussis vaccination, a decrease in immunization rates in 2-year-old children from 77 percent in 1974 to 30 percent in 1978 was followed by an epidemic of 102,500 cases of pertussis. A similar experience occurred in Japan when 13,105 cases and 41 deaths occurred in 1979 after routine immunization had been temporarily suspended in 1975.

In the United States, publicity about alleged serious reactions to pertussis vaccine led in the 1980s to public controversy about the risk of receiving pertussis vaccine, costly litigation, escalating vaccine costs, and potential jeopardization of vaccine supply and development.[292, 310] The experience in countries such as England and Japan, the severity of pertussis in young infants, and the usually benign or self-limited sequelae of pertussis vaccination clearly justify continuation of routine childhood immunization. Several risk-benefit analyses have provided additional evidence in support of the benefits of vaccination versus the risks.[142, 227]

Effective primary preventive programs necessitate immunization of young infants, usually beginning at 2 months of age, because the morbidity and mortality of pertussis is greatest in infants, especially those younger than 6 months.[86, 142] Approximately 26 percent of reported cases in the United States occur in infants younger than 6 months. In this age group, the case-fatality rate for 1997 to 2000 was 0.8 percent; 63.1 percent were hospitalized; and complications such as pneumonia (11.8%), seizures (1.4%), and encephalopathy (0.2%) are frequent occurrences.[132] High rates of immunization in children beyond infancy may reduce the risk of infection occurring in infants further by decreasing the incidence of infection in older family members and the resultant transmission of *B. pertussis* within the household.

Preparations

Whole-cell pertussis vaccine that has been in use for many years in the United States is a suspension of inactivated *B. pertussis* and is combined with diphtheria and tetanus toxoids (DTP). To reduce the incidence of local and systemic reactions caused by whole-cell vaccines, acellular vaccines composed of one or more purified components of *B. pertussis* have been developed and combined with diphtheria and tetanus toxoids (DTaP). Multiple acellular vaccines have been formulated from the different components and methods of production and have been tested in children. All vaccines contain detoxified pertussis toxin (i.e., pertussis toxoid).[167] In addition, most vaccines have one or more of the following *B. pertussis* antigens: filamentous hemagglutinin, pertactin (a 69-kd outer-membrane protein), and fimbrial proteins that are agglutinogens.

Five acellular vaccines have been approved for the primary vaccination series during infancy (Table 242–12).

TABLE 242–12 ■ ACELLULAR PERTUSSIS VACCINES

Vaccine Manufacturer	Trade Name	No. of Pertussis Antigens	Antigenic Content	Date of Licensure	Dose Series Approved	Currently Marketed in the U.S.
Aventis Pasteur	Tripedia	2	PT, FHA	1996	5	Yes
Lederle Laboratories	Acel-Imune	3	PE, FHA, FIM	1996	5	No
Glaxo SmithKline	Infanrix	3	PT, FHA, PE	1997	4	Yes
Baxter Hyland Immuno Vaccine	Certiva	1	PT	1998	4	No
Aventis Pasteur	Daptacel	5	PT, FHA, PE, 2 FIM	2002	4	Yes

FHA, filamentous hemagglutinin; FIM, fimbriae; PE, pertactin; PT, pertussis toxin.

Two of these vaccines, Acel-Imune and Certiva, were withdrawn from the market in 2001. Of the available acellular pertussis vaccines, Tripedia is licensed for the five-dose DTaP vaccination series, whereas Infanrix and Daptacel are licensed for the first four doses of the vaccination series. The ACIP recommends that whenever feasible, the same DTaP vaccine product be used for all doses of the vaccination series. If the vaccine provider does not know or does not have available the type of DTaP previously administered, any of the available licensed DTaP vaccines may be used to complete the vaccination series.[122]

Efficacy

For both whole-cell and acellular vaccines, serologic correlates of immunogenicity have not been established for assessing efficacy. As a result, field and other epidemiologic studies must be performed to demonstrate efficacy. Studies in the United States of household contacts exposed to pertussis indicate that the efficacy of whole-cell vaccine is 80 percent or greater.[86, 142, 299] Studies reporting lower rates of vaccine efficacy often reflect different criteria for the diagnosis of pertussis and lesser effectiveness of the vaccine in protecting against mild infection than against severe disease.[186] Vaccine-induced immunity persists for at least 3 years and subsequently diminishes with time. Pertussis in those previously vaccinated is less severe than in unvaccinated persons.

In studies of the efficacy of eight acellular pertussis vaccines in infants, rates of prevention of pertussis have ranged from 58 to 93 percent.[314] Comparing efficacy between the different products, however, is often not possible because of differences in study design, vaccine schedule (specifically, the number of doses and age of administration), case definitions of pertussis, and other confounding variables. In general, these acellular vaccines appear to be similar in efficacy to most whole-cell vaccines. Whereas in two large trials in Sweden and Italy several acellular vaccines demonstrated substantially greater efficacy than noted in the one approved U.S. whole-cell vaccine, other whole-cell vaccines appeared to be slightly more effective than acellular vaccines in other trials.[177] In addition, the vaccines in these Swedish and Italian trials were given in a three-dose schedule in contrast to the four-dose primary schedule for vaccination of young children in the United States.

Adverse Events

Local and febrile reactions to whole-cell vaccines occur commonly in more than half of DTP recipients.[153] These manifestations usually develop within the first 24 hours and are brief in duration. The incidence of these febrile reactions after the administration of acellular vaccines is significantly less.[167, 314] Comparison of rates with different acellular vaccines has demonstrated similar safety profiles for each of these vaccines.[145, 337] Rates of local reactions increase with each subsequent dose of DTaP vaccine.[313, 356] Booster doses of acellular pertussis vaccine may be associated with extensive local swelling, especially with vaccines having a high diphtheria content.[321] Severe reactions to acellular vaccines are rare events.[145, 167, 314, 337]

More serious reactions to whole-cell vaccines are uncommon. Such reactions include prolonged crying of 3 hours or more (occurring in 3% of DTP recipients in a large study); unusual, distinctive, and high-pitched crying (0.1%); fever of 40.5° C or higher (0.3%); hypotonic-hyporesponsive episodes (HHEs); and seizures.[153] The incidence of convulsions and HHEs is estimated to be 1 per 1750 immunizations.[153] Most post-DTP seizures are brief, self-limited, and generalized; occur in association with fever; and usually reflect an underlying febrile convulsive disorder.[93] These seizures have not been demonstrated to result in the subsequent development of epilepsy or other neurologic sequelae. Predisposing factors include an underlying convulsive disorder, a personal history of previous convulsion, and a family history of convulsions.

Severe reactions to acellular vaccines such as prolonged crying of 3 hours or longer, unusual, distinctive, and high-pitched crying, fever of 40.5° C or higher, HHEs, and seizures are rare.[167, 202, 211, 357, 358] As with local and febrile reactions, their occurrence with acellular pertussis vaccination is significantly less than that after whole-cell vaccination.

Serious Neurologic Illness

In a large case-control study in Great Britain, the National Childhood Encephalopathy Study (NCES), the estimated occurrence of acute neurologic illness resulting in hospitalization was 1 in 140,000 DTP vaccinations.[283] Neurologic sequelae have been reported to be common occurrences in a 10-year follow-up study, but no more so than in children with unrelated, acute neurologic illness in infancy,[282] and reviews of the data have disputed the conclusion that pertussis vaccine can cause neurologic sequelae.[24, 93, 350] The role of whole-cell pertussis vaccine, if any, in causing brain damage remains unproven.[76]

Indications

Vaccination against pertussis is recommended routinely for children at 2, 4, and 6 months of age, followed by a fourth dose at 12 to 18 months of age and a fifth dose at 4 to 6 years of age.[13, 27, 88, 99] Immunization can be started when the child is as young as 6 weeks if pertussis is prevalent in the community. The interval between doses of the initial series of three doses can be as short as 4 weeks. The AAP and ACIP recommend exclusive use of acellular pertussis vaccines for all doses of the pertussis vaccine series.[115, 122] DTP is not an acceptable alternative because of its higher rates of local reactions, fever, and other common systemic reactions. However, in many countries, including several in Europe as well as in developing countries, whole-cell vaccine remains the recommended product.

Pertussis immunization is not indicated for children after they reach 6 years of age because of the diminished risk of acquiring pertussis and development of complications. Future possible strategies for enhanced control of pertussis, however, include periodic revaccination of adolescents and adults with an acellular vaccine to reduce the reservoir of infections in these age groups.

Contraindications and Precautions

The contraindications and precautions for administering pertussis vaccine are based on adverse reactions associated with whole-cell vaccine. Although reactions occurring after the administration of DTaP are much less common than those associated with DTP, at present, the contraindications and precautions for DTaP are the same.[13, 27, 88, 99]

Adverse events temporally related to pertussis immunization that contraindicate further administration of DTaP are as follows:

- An immediate anaphylactic reaction.
- Encephalopathy, defined as a severe, acute, central nervous system disorder unexplained by another cause that occurs within 7 days; it may be manifested by major alterations in consciousness or by generalized or focal seizures that persist for more than a few hours without recovery within 24 hours.

Post-vaccination reactions constituting precautions are as follows:

- A convulsion, with or without fever, occurring within 3 days of receiving DTP or DTaP vaccination.
- Persistent, severe, inconsolable screaming or crying for 3 or more hours within 48 hours.
- HHE within 48 hours.
- Temperature of 40.5°C (104.9°F) or higher, unexplained by another cause, within 48 hours.

With these adverse events occurring in temporal association with DTaP vaccination, the decision to administer additional doses of pertussis vaccine should be considered carefully. In circumstances such as a pertussis outbreak in which the potential benefits of pertussis immunization outweigh the possible risks, vaccination is indicated, particularly because these events have not been proved to cause permanent sequelae. In addition, the risk of these reactions occurring from DTaP is substantially less than after administration of DTP.

In children with an evolving neurologic disorder, pertussis immunization should be deferred until the nature and cause of the disorder have been established. A personal history of having a previous convulsion unrelated to DTaP vaccination or a family history of convulsions (in the absence of a possible evolving neurologic disorder) is not a contraindication.

PNEUMOCOCCAL VACCINE

Streptococcus pneumoniae is a leading bacterial pathogen, especially among young children, the elderly, and persons with predisposing conditions. In children, it is the most common cause of otitis media, occult bacteremia, and bacterial pneumonia requiring hospitalization. Since the widespread introduction of conjugate Hib vaccination and subsequent marked decline in occurrence of Hib meningitis, *S. pneumoniae* has become a leading cause of bacterial meningitis in children in the United States. In some populations, such as Native Alaskans, the incidence of bacteremia is markedly higher than that reported in other geographic areas of the United States.[165] High-risk groups include children with sickle-cell disease, asplenia, Hodgkin disease, congenital humoral immunodeficiency, HIV infection, and nephrotic syndrome and recipients of organ transplants. Other chronic diseases associated with an increased risk for severe pneumococcal disease include chronic cardiovascular and pulmonary diseases, diabetes mellitus, and renal failure. The role of these chronic diseases in predisposing individuals to the development of pneumococcal infection, however, has been demonstrated primarily in adults. Mortality rates are highest in those who have bacteremia or meningitis, the elderly, and patients with impaired humoral immunity or certain chronic diseases.

The purified polysaccharide vaccine has been effective in reducing severe disease in the adult population,[64] but it has had little impact in young children because the vaccine is not immunogenic in children younger than 2 years.[14] In addition, the polysaccharide vaccine has not been effective in preventing otitis media caused by *S. pneumoniae.*[14]

Several factors have made the development of new preventive strategies for pneumococcal disease a high priority.[157] Morbidity and mortality rates of pneumococcal infection appear to be particularly high in developing countries. The increasing incidence of antimicrobial-resistant pneumococci further underscores the need for developing effective pneumococcal vaccines for young children.[59] Resistance of *S. pneumoniae* to multiple antibiotics has increased rapidly in the United States and even more rapidly in other parts of the world.[246] Children younger than 2 years have the highest rate of invasive pneumococcal infection but do not develop an effective antibody response to polysaccharide vaccine. In addition, children 2 to 5 years of age may have relatively poor responses to serotypes 6B, 14, 19F, and 23F, common causes of pediatric infections and the most prevalent penicillin-resistant serotypes.

These factors have prompted the development of conjugated polysaccharide-protein vaccines. These new vaccines are similar in design to the licensed Hib conjugate vaccines. Because of the large number of serotypes of *S. pneumoniae* that cause disease, development of these conjugate pneumococcal vaccines has been more difficult than has the development of similar vaccines for Hib. Each pneumococcal antigen must be coupled to a protein carrier, and the vaccine must be prepared to ensure that enough antigen is present to induce an immune response but not enough to elicit an adverse reaction.

One potential problem with conjugate pneumococcal vaccines is the need to immunize against many different serotypes of pneumococci. Because of local reactions to the protein component, conjugate vaccines that contain more than 12 serotypes may be difficult to produce. As a result, different formulations of conjugate pneumococcal vaccine may be developed that would contain different serotypes targeted for a specific group of patients. Vaccine containing types 4, 6B, 9V, 14, 18C, 19F, and 23F would be necessary for prevention of otitis media in the United States, whereas types 1, 2, and 5 would need to be added to prevent pneumonia in developing countries. In addition, the use of conjugate vaccines against limited serotypes may lead to the emergence of pneumococcal serotypes that are currently less common and require adjustment of a vaccine's composition.[346]

Routine infant immunization using these newly developed conjugate vaccines could lead to significant reductions in the instances of *S. pneumoniae* disease. Use of conjugate vaccines has been demonstrated to reduce nasopharyngeal carriage of vaccine serotypes,[161, 162] suggesting that person-to-person transmission will be interrupted, with resulting further decreases in the incidence of disease. Colonization with other serotypes has occurred, the significance of which is unclear.

Preparations

Two vaccines are currently available. The first is a heptavalent vaccine (PCV7) containing the capsular polysaccharides from serotypes 4, 6B, 9V, 14, 18C, 19F, and 23F conjugated to mutant diphtheria toxin (CRM_{197}). This vaccine (Prevnar, Wyeth Vaccines) was licensed in the United States in 2000. Serotypes included in PCV7 and potentially cross-reactive serotypes (i.e., 6A, 9A, 9L, 18B, and 18F) accounted for 86 percent of cases of bacteremia, 83 percent of cases of meningitis, and 65 percent of acute otitis media (AOM) cases occurring in children younger than 6 years in the United States during the period 1978 to 1994.[121] The second vaccine is composed of purified, capsular polysaccharide antigens of 23 pneumococcal serotypes. Although 90 different serotypes have been identified, vaccine serotypes in the 23-valent vaccine are responsible for 85 to 90 percent of adult infections and nearly 100 percent of invasive disease and 85 percent of otitis media cases in children.[70, 195]

Immunogenicity and Efficacy

The immunogenicity of the conjugate polysaccharide vaccine appears to determined by the pneumococcal polysaccharide serotype rather than the carrier protein. Some serotypes (14, 18C, and 19F) are excellent immunogens in that they elicit antibody protection after a single dose, whereas others (6B and 23F) require three doses of vaccine.[182] Conjugate vaccine elicits immunologic memory.[185] The antibody concentrations achieved after the initial series of three doses usually are sustained for only a few months and then decline to nearly pre-immunization levels. A dose of pneumococcal vaccine, either polysaccharide or conjugate, given in the second year of life elicits an amnestic-type response.

The licensed heptavalent polysaccharide conjugate vaccine was studied in a large prospective placebo-controlled efficacy trial in northern California involving 38,000 children. The vaccine was 89 percent effective in preventing invasive disease caused by any pneumococcal serotype and 97 percent effective against disease caused by the seven vaccine serotypes.[54] For noninvasive disease, a decrease of 7 percent in cases of otitis media and 23 percent in doctor visits for recurrent otitis (six or more visits per year) occurred in vaccinated children. The study also demonstrated an 11 percent decrease in clinical cases of pneumonia in vaccinees.[343]

The ability of the heptavalent vaccine to protect children against AOM also was evaluated in an efficacy trial conducted in Finland.[183] For prevention of AOM caused by pneumococci of any serotype, efficacy was estimated to be 34 percent, whereas efficacy against AOM irrespective of etiology was 6 percent. Efficacy against AOM caused by vaccine-related serotypes was 57 percent, but an increase of 33 percent in the rate of AOM episodes caused by nonvaccine serotypes occurred in the group receiving the heptavalent vaccine in comparison to controls. However, in spite of the increase in disease caused by nonvaccine serotypes, the net effect on pneumococcal AOM was a reduction of 34 percent.

Vaccination with purified polysaccharide vaccine results in serologic type-specific antibody in most healthy adults and older children. Immunocompromised patients may respond less well. In children younger than 2 years, antibody response is poor to most serotypes, including those most likely to cause infection, such as types 6A and 14.[70, 195] Patients with AIDS have impaired antibody responses to vaccination, but asymptomatic HIV-infected adults do respond.[70]

Vaccine efficacy in preventing serious pneumococcal infection has been demonstrated for the purified polysaccharide vaccine primarily in immunocompetent adults, including the elderly and those with chronic diseases such as chronic pulmonary and cardiac disorders and diabetes mellitus, which predispose to pneumococcal infections. Efficacy against vaccine serotypes ranges from 61 to 75 percent in adults.[64, 340] Investigations in adults in whom vaccine protection against pneumococcal infection has been substantially less have been criticized for methodologic problems.[70] Efficacy in the limited studies of children has been consistent with that in adults. In children with sickle-cell disease or anatomic asplenia, an octavalent vaccine was highly effective in preventing bacteremic infection.[35]

Adverse Events

Pneumococcal conjugate vaccines appear to be safe. The reactions most commonly reported have been local reactions at the injection site, but they occur at a lower frequency than do local reactions with other childhood vaccines such as DTP.[54]

Local reactions at the injection site, such as erythema and pain, are reported in approximately 50 percent of recipients of the purified polysaccharide vaccine.[14] However, more severe local and systemic reactions, such as fever and myalgia, are rare events that occur in less than 1 percent of vaccine recipients. Severe systemic reactions such as anaphylaxis rarely have been reported. In adults who were revaccinated within 1 to 2 years in early studies, local reactions occurred more commonly than did those after initial immunization.[70] However, subsequent investigations, including studies in children, indicate no increase in the incidence or severity of local or systemic reactions upon revaccination after longer intervals.[255, 322]

Indications

Recommendations by the AAP and the ACIP for the use of PCV7 have been issued.[32, 121] The AAP and ACIP recommend universal use of PCV7 in children 23 months and younger. For children in whom pneumococcal immunization is initiated before they reach 7 months of age, four doses of PCV7 are recommended at 2, 4, 6, and 12 to 15 months of age. For children beginning PCV7 immunization between 7 months and 23 months of age, the recommended schedule differs according to the child's age (see elsewhere[32, 121] for further information). In addition, two doses of PCV7 are recommended for children 24 to 59 months of age who are at high risk of acquiring invasive pneumococcal infection and have not been immunized previously with PCV7. These children also should receive the 23-valent polysaccharide vaccine (PPV23) to expand serotype coverage. Routine immunization of children 24 months or older who are at low and moderate risk is not recommended by the AAP at this time.[32] The ACIP recommends that PCV7 be considered for all children 24 to 59 months of age, with priority given to those aged 24 to 35 months; persons of Alaskan Native, American Indian, or African American descent; and those who attend group daycare centers.[121] Children 24 to 59 months old at high risk who have not previously received PCV7 but who have already received PPV23 should be vaccinated with two doses of PCV7 given 2 or more months apart.[121] Current data do not support a recommendation to replace the PPV23 with PCV7 vaccine for older children and adults.[121]

The purified polysaccharide vaccine is recommended by the AAP[32] for children 5 years or older who have one or more of the following risk factors:

- Sickle-cell disease
- Functional or anatomic asplenia
- Nephrotic syndrome or chronic renal failure
- Immunosuppression, such as from chemotherapy, organ transplantation, or malignancy
- Cerebrospinal fluid leak
- HIV infection, symptomatic or asymptomatic

Revaccination

For previously vaccinated children 10 years or younger who are at high risk of acquiring severe pneumococcal infection, revaccination with purified polysaccharide vaccine after 3 to 5 years is recommended.[32, 121] Such children include those who have functional (e.g., sickle-cell disease) or anatomic asplenia and those who have a rapid antibody decline (e.g., nephrotic syndrome, renal failure, or organ transplantation).[196] Revaccination should be considered for high-risk older children and adults who were vaccinated 6 years or more previously.

Contraindications[32, 121]

No contraindications to initial vaccination exist. The safety of pneumococcal vaccine in pregnant women has not been evaluated, but adverse consequences to the fetus have not been observed in newborns whose mothers were vaccinated inadvertently during pregnancy. Ideally, women at high risk of acquiring pneumococcal disease should be vaccinated before pregnancy. In persons who have had a severe reaction, such as anaphylaxis or a localized, severe hypersensitivity response, revaccination should be avoided.

POLIOMYELITIS VACCINE

The widespread implementation of poliovirus vaccine programs has resulted in a dramatic reduction in the incidence of paralytic poliomyelitis throughout the world. In contrast to the pre-vaccine era, when more than 18,000 cases of paralytic disease occurred in the United States annually, the last known case in this country caused by indigenous wild-type virus occurred in 1979.[351] Other than rare imported cases, the only cases of paralytic poliomyelitis in the United States since then have been vaccine related.

The effectiveness of polio vaccination has led to major and successful initiatives by the WHO for global eradication of poliovirus infection. This effort has been successful and resulted in an 80 percent reduction in the number of reported cases worldwide since the mid-1980s. Two WHO regions have eliminated poliovirus: the region of the Americas has been polio-free since 1991, and the Western Pacific region has certified poliovirus-free since 2000. The European region is expected to be the next area to achieve eradication. Reaching the global polio eradication goal will require accelerating activities in the remaining major foci of poliovirus transmission in southern Asia and Africa.[109]

These accomplishments in the elimination of poliovirus infection have been achieved primarily through the use of OPV. This product had been the vaccine of choice for children in the United States since the early 1960s because it induced optimal intestinal immunity, was painless to administer, and secondarily immunized some contacts by fecal-oral spread of the vaccine virus and thus contributed to the immunity of the population.[65] For these same reasons, global eradication necessitates the continued use of OPV in many parts of the world.[385] However, because inactivated poliovirus vaccine (IPV) is also highly effective and does not cause vaccine-associated paralytic poliomyelitis (VAPP), it has been used for routine immunization in several European countries that have controlled or eliminated poliomyelitis, including Finland, France, and the Netherlands. In Canada, IPV replaced OPV as the vaccine of choice in the early 1990s.[315] Denmark, Israel, and the province of Prince Edward Island in Canada have used sequential schedules of IPV followed by OPV to reduce the risk of VAPP and to maintain the benefits of OPV. Because 8 to 10 cases of VAPP occur annually and the risk of exposure to wild-type poliovirus has been markedly reduced or eliminated in the United States, expanded use of IPV was recommended by the CDC and the AAP beginning in 1997.[97] In 1999, as a result of progress in the global eradication of poliomyelitis, the need for further reduction in the risk for acquiring VAPP, and the acceptance of IPV by parents and physicians,[104] IPV was recommended for the first two doses of poliovirus vaccine for routine childhood vaccination.[28, 110] To completely eliminate the risk for VAPP, in January 2000 an all-IPV schedule was recommended for routine childhood vaccination in the United States.[30, 110, 115]

Assuming that global eradication is achieved, eventual discontinuation of poliomyelitis vaccination can be anticipated. However, for the foreseeable future, immunity to poliomyelitis needs to be maintained by widespread implementation of vaccination programs.

Preparations[110]

Two types of poliovirus vaccine are licensed in the United States, OPV and IPV. Both vaccines are trivalent and consist of serotypes 1, 2, and 3. The attenuated strains of poliovirus in OPV are propagated in monkey kidney tissue. For IPV, the vaccine virus is propagated in either monkey kidney cells or human diploid (MRC-5) cell cultures before purification and formaldehyde inactivation.

Immunogenicity and Efficacy

Both OPV and IPV given in the recommended three-dose series result in immunity to all three polioviruses in nearly 100 percent of recipients.[97] No evidence suggests waning immunity with either vaccine. Most children seroconvert after two doses and often after only one. Vaccination with either vaccine results in diminished circulation of wild-type poliovirus in the community as a result of induction of mucosal immunity.[297, 315] In contrast to IPV, OPV results in not only pharyngeal immunity but also a high degree of intestinal immunity and provides a substantial degree of resistance to reinfection, which limits circulation of poliovirus from fecal-oral transmission. Intestinal immunity from IPV is incomplete.

Adverse Events[15, 110]

No serious adverse events have been associated with use of the currently available IPV vaccine. Because IPV vaccine contains trace amounts of streptomycin, neomycin, and polymyxin B, allergic reactions are possible in recipients with hypersensitivity to one or more of these antibiotics.

The OPV vaccine can cause VAPP, the overall risk of which is approximately 1 case per 2.4 million doses distributed. The rate after the first dose was approximately 1 case per 750,000 doses, including vaccine recipient and contact cases.

Indications[15, 30, 110]

All children should receive four doses of IPV at the ages of 2 months, 4 months, 6 to 18 months, and 4 to 6 years. A supplemental dose of IPV vaccine should be given before the child enters school (i.e., at 4 to 6 years of age). Administration of a fourth dose is not necessary if the third dose was given on or after the child's fourth birthday.

OPV, if available, may be used in the United States in only special circumstances, the most important of which would be vaccination campaigns if outbreaks of paralytic polio should occur. OPV also is preferred for unvaccinated children who will be traveling within 4 weeks to areas where polio is endemic or epidemic. In this situation, health care providers should administer OPV only after discussing the risk for development of VAPP with parents or caregivers.

The ACIP and AAP continue to support the global eradication initiative and use of OPV as the vaccine of choice to eradicate wild-type polio in endemic areas and during epidemics. In the immunization schedule of the EPI of the WHO, doses of OPV are recommended at birth and when the child is 6 weeks, 10 weeks, and 14 weeks of age.[3] In geographic areas with endemic polio, a dose may be given when the newborn is discharged from the hospital. Supplementary doses often are given during mass community programs in these areas. Breast-feeding does not interfere with successful immunization with OPV.

Routine immunization for adults (18 years or older) residing in the United States is not recommended because transmission of wild poliovirus no longer is occurring in this country. However, previously unimmunized persons traveling to countries where poliomyelitis is epidemic or endemic, members of communities of specific population groups experiencing wild-type poliovirus disease, health care workers in close contact with patients who may be excreting wild-type poliovirus, and laboratory workers in contact with specimens that may contain wild-type poliovirus should be vaccinated with IPV. Those who are incompletely immunized should complete the primary series with IPV, irrespective of which vaccine was given before. Previously immunized adults who are at increased risk of exposure to poliomyelitis, such as those traveling to countries where poliomyelitis is still endemic, should receive a single dose of IPV.

Precautions and Contraindications[15, 110]

IPV is contraindicated in persons who have experienced an anaphylactic reaction after receiving a previous dose of IPV or an anaphylactic reaction to one of the antibiotics in the vaccine preparation (i.e., streptomycin, polymyxin B, or neomycin).

Poliomyelitis vaccination generally is contraindicated in pregnant woman because of the theoretic risk of harm to the fetus. However, no deleterious effects from IPV administered during pregnancy have been demonstrated, and if immediate protection against poliomyelitis is needed, IPV may be given.

RUBELLA VACCINE

Rubella is a viral disease that usually is manifested as a mild febrile rash illness in adults and children; however, 20 to 50 percent of infected persons are asymptomatic. Rubella can have severe adverse effects on the fetuses of pregnant women who contract the disease during the first trimester of pregnancy; it causes a wide range of congenital defects known as congenital rubella syndrome (CRS). The primary objective of the rubella vaccination program is to prevent intrauterine rubella infection. The primary strategies for rubella control in the United States are universal childhood vaccination, prenatal screening of pregnant women for rubella immunity, and vaccination of rubella-susceptible women post partum.

In the pre-vaccine era, epidemics of rubella occurred every 6 to 9 years, with the last major epidemic in the United States taking place in 1964 to 1965. After the licensure of rubella vaccine in 1969, the incidence of rubella decreased 99 percent, from 57,686 cases in 1969 to fewer than 200 cases in 2000. As of February 2002, only 19 cases were reported in the United States in 2001. The incidence of congenital rubella in the United States has paralleled the rise and decline of rubella. Only 14 cases of congenital rubella were reported to the CDC for 1999 to 2001.

Despite high coverage rates with MMR vaccine, outbreaks still occur among groups of susceptible people with close contact.[116, 164] Because the incidence of rubella is low, even one case of rubella should be considered a potential outbreak. Most recent outbreaks were identified first in the workplace. The majority of these outbreaks have been a result of the absence of routine, recommended prevention and control efforts and the emergence of Hispanic, foreign-born persons as the main reservoirs of rubella virus in the United States.[127] Based on supplementary data reported through the national notifiable diseases surveillance system in the United States, rubella affects primarily foreign-born Hispanic adults.[319] Among rubella patients with known ethnicity in the United States, the proportion of Hispanics increased from 19 percent in 1992 to 79 percent in 1998. In Latin America, many countries only recently have introduced rubella into their routine childhood vaccination programs. For immigrants entering the United States, vaccination efforts focus on preschool-age children and students; adults are not screened or vaccinated routinely.

Prenatal screening followed by postpartum administration of vaccine against rubella is essential for the control and elimination of CRS. Though recommended by the American College of Obstetricians and Gynecologists and the ACIP,[106] prenatal screening for rubella has been discontinued in some public health clinics because of fiscal constraints. In the absence of routine prenatal serologic screening for rubella antibodies, the immune status of pregnant women potentially exposed to rubella virus is unknown. In the United States, prenatal screening and postpartum vaccination might prevent an estimated 50 percent of all CRS cases.[336] To eliminate rubella and CRS in the United States, further control efforts are needed to identify and vaccinate clusters of rubella-susceptible adults and to ensure nationwide prenatal rubella screening and postpartum vaccination of rubella-susceptible women.

Preparations

Since 1979, RA 27/3 (rubella abortus, 27th specimen/third extract) vaccine, prepared in human diploid tissue culture, has been the only vaccine available in the United States; it replaced the earlier HPV-77 and Cendehill vaccines. RA 27/3 induces higher antibody titers, more closely paralleling the immune response after natural infection than previous vaccines did.[264, 301] In addition to MMR vaccine, monovalent rubella and measles-rubella (MR) vaccines are available.

MMR vaccine generally is used for routine infant immunization programs. Rubella vaccine should be kept at 2 to 8°C (35.6 to 46.4°F) or colder during storage and should be protected from light to avoid virus inactivation. Once reconstituted, the vaccine should be used within 8 hours.

Immunogenicity and Efficacy

At least 98 percent of susceptible vaccinees 12 months or older develop antibody titers that are protective.[284] Vaccine-induced rubella antibodies have persisted in more than 90 percent of vaccinees 16 years after receiving the RA 27/3 vaccine.[144] Lifelong protection against clinical reinfection, asymptomatic viremia, or both usually results from a single dose of vaccine early in childhood.

In some cases, vaccinees exposed to natural rubella developed a rise in antibody titer unassociated with clinical symptoms. Reinfection is associated only rarely with viremia. Significant pharyngeal shedding also is observed infrequently. Person-to-person transmission, however, has not been reported. Reinfection caused by wild-type rubella virus also may be observed in individuals with previous natural rubella. The risk of CRS developing from rubella reinfection during pregnancy is extremely low.[324]

Adverse Events

Rubella vaccines are generally well tolerated. The most frequent complaints after vaccination are fever, lymphadenopathy, or rash, which occur in 5 to 15 percent of children 5 to 12 days after receiving vaccination.[16] Transient peripheral neuritis (paresthesia and pain in the arms and legs) has been observed uncommonly, primarily in older age groups.[335]

Approximately 3 percent of children have transient joint manifestations, including arthralgia and, less commonly, arthritis 1 to 3 weeks after immunization. Whereas 25 percent of adult women report having joint pain after being vaccinated, arthritis with objective clinical findings lasting less than 10 days occurs in 13 to 15 percent. Cases of persistent or recurrent joint symptoms have been reported but are rare events. In 1992, the IOM reviewed the existing data on rubella and adverse joint events and concluded that the evidence available was consistent with a causal relationship between rubella vaccination and chronic arthritis in adult women, although data on current vaccine strains are limited.[229] The incidence of joint manifestations after immunization is lower than that after natural infection at the corresponding age.

Rubella revaccination is well tolerated, even among college-age and older vaccinees, and is associated with a much lower incidence of adverse reactions than after primary rubella immunization of young adult populations. Reported rates of joint-related complaints of 4 to 18 percent after revaccination are lower than those reported after primary vaccination.[140, 338]

Indications[16, 106, 130]

Live virus rubella vaccine generally is recommended for all children 12 months or older; it is given as MMR at 12 to 15 months of age. A second dose of rubella vaccine administered as MMR is given at the recommended age for measles revaccination. The vaccine should be provided to previously unimmunized preschool-age children or older schoolchildren despite a history of having clinical rubella, unless serologic tests confirm immunity.

Emphasis should be placed on the immunization of postpubertal males and females, especially college students and those in the military. Rubella vaccine also should be administered to adolescent and adult females of child-bearing age who lack a history of previous vaccination. Other opportunities for immunization include premarital screening, routine gynecologic examinations, visits for newborn infants and well-child care, or other medical visits. The immediate postpartum period is also an excellent time for giving immunizations. Rubella vaccine may be given after administration of anti-Rho(D) immune globulin, but serologic testing to determine whether seroconversion has occurred should be performed at least 8 weeks after vaccination. When practical, potential vaccinees may be screened for susceptibility. However, vaccination of females of child-bearing age is justifiable, and may be preferable, without previous serologic testing in women not known to be pregnant.

Adults in the United States who were born in countries where rubella vaccination was not offered are at higher risk for contracting rubella and having infants with CRS. Health care practitioners who treat foreign-born adults should document their rubella immunity with a written record of rubella-containing vaccine or by serologic testing. Susceptible adults, especially women of child-bearing age, should be vaccinated. During rubella outbreaks, all susceptible persons who have no contraindications to rubella vaccine should be identified and vaccinated.

Precautions and Contraindications[16, 106, 130]

Specific contraindications to administration of live rubella vaccine include the following: (1) pregnancy; (2) severe febrile illness; (3) known history of anaphylactic reaction to rubella vaccine, gelatin, or neomycin, which are contained in the vaccine; and (4) immunodeficiency conditions (i.e., malignancy, primary immunodeficiency disease, immunosuppressive or corticosteroid therapy, and radiation therapy). Persons with mild immunosuppression, such as those with asymptomatic HIV infection or those taking short-term or low-dose corticosteroids, may be vaccinated.

Postpubertal women of child-bearing age known to be pregnant or attempting to become pregnant should not be vaccinated. Vaccinated women should be counseled about the need to avoid pregnancy for 28 days after receiving vaccination.[126] Although pregnancy is a contraindication to administering rubella vaccination, the maximal theoretic risk to the fetus is estimated to be 1.6 percent. From 1979 until 1989 the CDC registered 321 susceptible women who inadvertently had received RA 27/3 rubella vaccine within 3 months before or after conception and carried their pregnancies to term. None of their infants had defects compatible with CRS, although 2 percent had serologic evidence of intrauterine infection.[71] Because rubella virus has been isolated from the products of conception of women vaccinated during pregnancy, continued caution with respect to vaccination during pregnancy is advised. However, the evidence available indicates that inadvertent rubella vaccination during pregnancy ordinarily does not represent a reason to consider interruption of pregnancy.

Although vaccine virus may be isolated from the pharynx, vaccinees do not transmit rubella to others, except in the case of a vaccinated breast-feeding mother. In this situation, the infant may be infected through breast milk and a mild rash illness may develop, but serious adverse effects have not been noted. Infants infected through breast-feeding respond normally to rubella vaccination at 15 months of age. Breast-feeding is not a contraindication to rubella vaccination.

Concern about potential transmission of disease from immunized children to susceptible contacts, including pregnant women, has not been supported by studies of susceptible household contacts. Therefore, susceptible children whose household contacts are pregnant may be vaccinated.

Persons with a history of thrombocytopenia may experience thrombocytopenia after receipt of MMR vaccine. The decision to vaccinate should depend on the benefits of immunity versus the risk for recurrence or exacerbation of thrombocytopenia, either after vaccination or during natural infection with measles or rubella.

Rubella vaccine should not be given during an interval beginning 2 weeks before and extending 3 months after the administration of immune globulin or blood transfusion. Because rubella vaccine usually is given as MMR and recent evidence suggests that high doses of immune globulin preparations can inhibit the immune response to measles vaccine for 3 or more months, depending on the dosage, rubella vaccination with MMR necessitates deferral for longer periods (see "Measles Vaccine").[16, 106, 344]

TETANUS TOXOID

The efficacy of active immunization against tetanus was demonstrated most dramatically in military personnel during World War II, when tetanus toxoid virtually eliminated tetanus in injured servicemen.[268] Since the 1940s, routine immunization of civilians in this country with tetanus toxoid has been similarly successful in preventing tetanus. In nearly all cases, disease has been reported only in unimmunized or inadequately immunized individuals.[72] The potential for occurrence of tetanus, however, is indicated by the significant number of adults in the United States who lack protective concentrations of serum antibody.[192] Although neonatal tetanus has been nearly eliminated in the United States, it is a leading cause of morbidity in newborns in developing countries. As a result, global elimination of neonatal tetanus is a goal of the WHO.[81]

Preparations[76]

Tetanus toxoid is prepared by formaldehyde treatment of *Clostridium tetani* toxin. It has been prepared in both fluid and aluminum salt–adsorbed preparations, but in the United States, only the latter is available. Fluid toxoid preparations result in a significantly shorter duration of immunity than that induced by aluminum-adsorbed antigens; therefore, adsorbed antigens are recommended.

Tetanus toxoid is available in combination with diphtheria toxoid and acellular pertussis vaccine for routine administration to infants and children. For children in whom pertussis vaccine is contraindicated, for children 7 years and older who have not been immunized, and for booster doses, it is combined with diphtheria toxoid as either DT or Td (see "Diphtheria Toxoid"). These preparations are identical in the amounts of tetanus toxoid, but differ in the quantity of diphtheria toxoid.

Immunogenicity and Efficacy

Adequate primary immunization provides sufficient protective titers of antitoxin for at least 10 years and ensures prompt, anamnestic responses to subsequent booster injections.

Adverse Events

Local reactions of pain, swelling, and induration can occur, but in children these reactions are usually attributable to the whole-cell pertussis vaccine that is combined with tetanus toxoid. Hypersensitivity reactions can occur in adolescents and adults but very rarely are severe.

Neurologic reactions occurring after the administration of tetanus toxoid are rare events. Such reactions include brachial neuritis and GBS.

Indications

PRE-EXPOSURE.[18] For primary immunization, doses of tetanus toxoid should be given when the child is 2, 4, and 6 months of age. A fourth dose is given 6 to 12 months after the third dose (i.e., at 12 to 18 months of age) to maintain adequate serum antibody concentrations for the ensuing preschool years. For those not immunized in infancy, DTaP is given at 0 (initial dose), 2, 4, and 10 to 16 months later, followed by a single booster dose at age 4 to 6 years just before school entry. If pertussis vaccine is contraindicated, DT should be used. For persons 7 years or older, a primary series of Td given at 0, 2, and 8 to 14 months later is recommended. Interruption of the recommended schedule or delay in administering subsequent doses during primary immunization does not reduce immunity. After completion of early childhood immunization, including a dose of tetanus toxoid at 4 to 6 years of age, booster doses of Td are recommended every 10 years beginning at the 11- to 12-year-old pre-adolescent immunization visit.

ANTEPARTUM.[200] In areas of the world where the risk of acquiring neonatal tetanus is significant, previously unimmunized, pregnant women should receive two antepartum doses, properly spaced, and should complete the three-dose series subsequently. Women immunized more than 10 years previously should receive a booster dose.

POSTEXPOSURE—WOUND MANAGEMENT. The possible need for immunoprophylaxis is an integral aspect of wound management at the time of trauma or injury. The recommended use of tetanus toxoid, administered as Td, in addition to tetanus immune globulin at the time of injury is given in Table 242–13. Specific recommendations depend on the individual's immunization status, the nature of the wound, and the duration of time after the injury and before evaluation and treatment. After prophylaxis is provided, primary immunization should be completed subsequently in those lacking the recommended number of doses. This conservative approach to the frequent administration of booster

TABLE 242–13 ■ RECOMMENDED TETANUS PROPHYLAXIS IN WOUND MANAGEMENT

History of Tetanus Toxoid (Number of Doses)	Clean, Minor Wounds		All Other Wounds (Tetanus-Prone Wounds)*	
	Td†	*TIG*	*Td*†	*TIG*
Unknown or <3	Yes	No	Yes	Yes
≥3	No‡	No	No§	No

*Such as, but not limited to wounds contaminated with dirt, feces, soil, and saliva; puncture wounds; avulsions; and wounds resulting from missiles, crushing, burns, and frostbite.

†For children younger than 7 years; DTaP or DT (depending on the vaccine status of the patient) is preferred to tetanus toxoid alone.

‡Yes, if more than 10 years since the last dose.

§Yes, if more than 5 years since the last dose. More frequent boosters are not needed and can accentuate side effects.

Used with permission of the American Academy of Pediatrics: Tetanus. *In* Peter, G. (ed.): 1997 Red Book: Report of the Committee on Infectious Diseases. 24th ed. Elk Grove Village, IL, American Academy of Pediatrics, 1997.

doses of tetanus toxoid in wound management for previously immunized persons is supported by the prolonged immunity from tetanus vaccination and the increased incidence of hypersensitivity reactions associated with receipt of frequent booster injections.[17, 96, 306]

Patients convalescing from tetanus infection should complete active immunization because infection often does not confer immunity.

Precautions and Contraindications

A history of having an immediate, severe hypersensitivity reaction to tetanus toxoid–containing preparations that is severe or anaphylactic in type is a contraindication to further vaccination.[76] Persons who experience Arthus-type hypersensitivity reactions after tetanus toxoid administration usually have high serum tetanus antitoxin concentrations and should not be given doses of Td more frequently than every 10 years, even if they have a tetanus-prone wound. If an anaphylactic reaction to a previous dose of tetanus toxoid is suspected, intradermal skin testing may be helpful in determining whether to discontinue tetanus toxoid vaccination.[241] Because tetanus toxoid administration has been associated with recurrence of GBS in rare cases,[233] the decision to give additional doses in persons with a previous history of this syndrome within 6 weeks after receipt of tetanus toxoid should be based on consideration of the benefit of revaccination and the comparative risk of recurrence of GBS.[93]

VARICELLA VACCINE

Varicella is the most common childhood infectious disease in the United States. Before the availability of varicella vaccine, varicella infection was responsible for an estimated 4 million cases, 11,000 hospitalizations, and 100 deaths each year in the United States.[113] Approximately 90 percent of cases occurred in children, with the highest incidence in children 1 to 6 years of age. In recent years, severe infections with group A beta-hemolytic streptococci have complicated varicella and led to considerable morbidity and mortality in otherwise healthy individuals.[101]

Varicella is potentially severe in children with malignancies and may be fatal in as many as 4 percent of cases despite the use of prophylactic immunoglobulin and antiviral therapy.[185] Other high-risk groups of children include those with HIV and other immunocompromising conditions and those receiving high doses of systemic corticosteroids.

Varicella also may cause more severe disease in adults. Though a rare event, congenital varicella syndrome occurs in approximately 2 percent of infants born to women who contract varicella in the first or second trimester of pregnancy.[180]

Preparations

Varicella vaccine was licensed in the United States in 1995. It is a preparation of the Oka strain of varicella virus obtained from the vesicle fluid of a healthy child with varicella that has been attenuated by serial propagation in human embryo lung fibroblasts, guinea pig embryonic cells, and human diploid cell cultures. The vaccine contains trace amounts of neomycin, fetal bovine serum, sucrose, residual components of human diploid (MRC-5) cells, and gelatin. The vaccine does not contain preservatives.

Varicella vaccine is lyophilized and stored frozen at −15°C or colder until reconstituted. Any freezer that reliably maintains an average temperature of −15°C and has a separate sealed freezer door is acceptable for storing vaccine. The vaccine also may be stored at refrigerator temperature (2 to 8°C) for as long as 72 hours before reconstitution. Vaccine stored at 2 to 8°C that is not used within 72 hours should be discarded. Reconstituted vaccine should be stored at room temperature and discarded if not used within 30 minutes.

Immunogenicity and Efficacy

Varicella vaccine is highly immunogenic in susceptible children. Seroconversion has occurred in more than 96 percent of children 12 months to 12 years of age after one dose of vaccine.[380] Preexisting antibody, if present at 12 months of age, does not appear to interfere with antibody response. As with other viral vaccines, the antibody response after immunization is lower than that from natural disease. Adolescents and adults have age-related decreases in the ability to develop a primary response to varicella virus.[194] Seroconversion rates of 78 to 82 percent after one dose and 99 percent after two doses have been reported in those older than 12 years.[194, 380]

In ongoing studies in the United States and Japan, serum antibodies to varicella have been detected for as long as 10 to 20 years after immunization in more than 95 percent of immunized children.[41, 244] Antibody concentrations have persisted for at least 1 year in 97 percent of adults and adolescents who were administered two doses of vaccine 4 to 8 weeks apart.[194] Cell-mediated immunity to varicella-zoster virus (VZV) has been detected in 87 percent of children and 94 percent of adults 5 years after vaccination.[389]

Varicella vaccine has been demonstrated to be highly effective in preventing varicella in children and reducing the severity of infection if they do become infected. In pre-licensure clinical trials, vaccine was 70 to 90 percent effective in preventing varicella and more than 95 percent effective in preventing severe disease.[259, 375] Several post-licensure studies have shown similar results, with vaccine effectiveness ranging from 83 to 100 percent in preventing varicella and 87 to 100 percent in preventing severe disease.[149, 239, 363] In follow-up studies, chickenpox has developed in approximately 0.2 to 2.3 percent of vaccinated children per year after exposure to wild-type varicella virus, a rate that does not seem to increase with length of time after immunization.[365] These vaccine failure cases are mild, with fewer skin lesions, lower rates of fever, and more rapid recovery.[51, 365, 372]

In adults and adolescents who have seroconverted, varicella vaccine provides protective efficacy rates of approximately 70 percent after household exposure. In the remaining 30 percent, attenuated disease with fewer skin lesions and little or no systemic toxicity develops, as in children.[194]

The use of varicella vaccine has an impact on the epidemiology of disease. Active surveillance for varicella has been conducted at sites in Pennsylvania, Texas, and California since 1995 in a CDC-sponsored study.[339] From 1995 to 2000, vaccine coverage in 1- to 2-year-old children rose to approximately 80 percent, whereas overall cases of varicella declined 70 to 80 percent. The greatest decline was in children 1 to 4 years of age, but cases also declined in all other age groups, including infants younger than 1 year and adults, thus suggesting herd immunity. Decreasing rates of varicella also have been associated with increasing use of varicella vaccine in a daycare center population.[148]

Current estimates of vaccine efficacy and antibody persistence in vaccinees are based on observations when natural varicella infection has been highly prevalent. The extent to which boosting from exposure to natural varicella has had an impact on the efficacy of vaccine or the duration of immunity is not known. In pre-licensure clinical studies, mean serum anti-VZV levels among vaccinees continued to increase with time after vaccination, a finding attributed to immunologic boosting caused by exposure to wild-type VZV in the community. A recent study analyzed serum antibody concentrations and infection rates during 4 years of follow-up in 4631 vaccine recipients.[256] Anti-VZV titers decreased over time in high-responder subjects, but they rose in vaccinees with low titers. Among subjects with low anti-VZV titers, the frequency of clinical infection and immunologic boosting substantially exceeded the 13 percent-per-year rate of exposure to wild-type varicella. These findings suggest that vaccine strain VZV persisted in vivo and reactivated as serum antibody titers decreased after vaccination.

Adverse Events

Varicella vaccine produces relatively few adverse reactions.[341, 381] Local reactions, rash, and low grade fever occur in as many as 10 percent of vaccine recipients,[38] but rates of rash and fever have been similar in placebo groups in several studies.[181, 375] In post-licensure studies, the adverse event most frequently reported is a mild vesicular rash that occurs in approximately 5 percent of vaccinees.[113, 193] Vesicular rashes that occurred within 2 weeks of vaccination were more likely to be caused by wild-type varicella, whereas rashes that occurred more than 2 weeks after vaccination were more likely to be caused by the Oka vaccine strain.[341] One case of rash and pneumonia as a result of vaccination of a 15-month-old child infected with HIV has been reported. The child's HIV status was not known at the time of vaccination.[381]

A major concern has been whether vaccination would increase the risk for development of zoster. Based on reports to VAERS, the rate of herpes zoster after varicella vaccination is 2.6 per 100,000 vaccine doses distributed.[113] The incidence of herpes zoster after natural varicella infection in healthy persons younger than 20 years is 68 per 100,000 person-years[208] and, for all ages, 215 per 100,000 person-years.[172] However, these rates should be compared cautiously because the latter rates are based on populations monitored for longer periods than the vaccinees were. Cases of herpes zoster have been confirmed by polymerase chain reaction (PCR) to be caused by both vaccine virus and wild-type virus, thus suggesting that some herpes zoster cases in vaccinees might result from antecedent natural varicella infection.[113, 218]

Transmission of the vaccine virus occurs rarely and most often from immunocompromised vaccinees. Of the 15 million doses of varicella vaccine distributed, on only 3 occasions has transmission from immunocompetent persons been documented by PCR analysis.[261, 333] All three cases resulted in mild disease without complications. In one case, a child 12 months old transmitted the vaccine virus to his pregnant mother.[269, 333] The mother elected to terminate the pregnancy, but fetal tissue tested by PCR was negative for varicella vaccine virus. The other two documented cases involved transmission from healthy children aged 1 year to a healthy sibling aged 4½ months and to a healthy father.[113] Transmission also has occurred from a person with zoster caused by vaccine strain virus.[62] Transmission has not been documented in the absence of a vesicular rash after vaccination. No evidence indicates reversion to virulence of the vaccine strain during transmission; siblings of leukemic vaccine recipients who acquired vaccine virus had mild rash in 75 percent of cases and symptomless seroconversion in 25 percent.[38]

Indications[31, 113]

Varicella vaccine is licensed for use in individuals 12 months or older who have not had varicella. One dose of varicella vaccine is recommended for immunization of susceptible healthy children 12 to 18 months of age.[31, 113] The vaccine may be given either simultaneously with or separated from MMR by 30 days or longer.[125] In addition, one dose of vaccine is recommended for immunization of all children from the age of 19 months to the 13th birthday who lack a reliable history of having had varicella infection and who have not been vaccinated previously. Susceptible healthy adolescents who have reached their 13th birthday and adults should be immunized with two doses of varicella vaccine 4 to 8 weeks apart. If longer than 8 weeks elapses after administration of the first dose, the second dose can be administered without restarting the schedule. If an adolescent or young adult does not have a reliable history of having had varicella, serologic testing for immunity before vaccination is likely to be cost-effective because 71 to 93 percent of such individuals actually are immune.[267]

The ACIP recommendations for varicella vaccine have been expanded to promote wider use of the vaccine for susceptible children and adults.[113] Recommendations include establishing childcare and school entry requirements, use of the vaccine after exposure and for outbreak control, use of the vaccine for some children infected with HIV, and vaccination of adults and adolescents at high risk for exposure.

The ACIP recommends that all states require that children entering childcare facilities and elementary schools either have received varicella vaccine or have other evidence of immunity to varicella. Other evidence of immunity should consist of a physician's diagnosis of varicella, a reliable history of having had the disease, or serologic evidence of immunity. To prevent susceptible older children from entering adulthood without immunity to varicella, states also should consider implementing a policy that requires evidence of varicella vaccination or other evidence of immunity for children entering middle school or junior high school.

Data from both the United States and Japan indicate that varicella vaccine is effective in preventing illness or modifying the severity of varicella if used within 3 days and possibly up to as long as 5 days of exposure.[38, 42, 332, 371] The ACIP and the AAP now recommend the vaccine for use in susceptible persons after exposure to varicella.[31, 113] If the exposure results in infection, no evidence indicates that administration of varicella vaccine during the presymptomatic or prodromal stage of illness increases the risk for vaccine-associated adverse events.

Varicella outbreaks in childcare facilities, schools, and institutions can last 3 to 6 months. Varicella vaccine has been used successfully by state and local health departments and by the military for prevention and control of outbreaks. Therefore, the ACIP recommends that state and local health departments consider using the vaccine for control of outbreaks either by advising exposed susceptible persons to contact their health care providers for vaccination or by offering vaccination through the health department.[113]

The ACIP has strengthened its recommendations for susceptible persons 13 years or older who are at high risk for exposure or transmission, including designating adolescents and adults living in households with children as a new high-risk group.[113] Varicella vaccine is recommended for susceptible persons in the following high-risk groups: (1) persons who live or work in environments where transmission of VZV is likely to occur, (2) persons who live and work in environments where transmission can occur, (3) nonpregnant women of child-bearing age, (4) adolescents and adults living in households with children, and (5) international travelers. Vaccination also is recommended routinely for all susceptible health care workers.[95]

Varicella vaccine is not licensed for use in persons who have blood dyscrasias, leukemia, lymphomata of any type, or other malignant neoplasms affecting the bone marrow or lymphatic systems. The manufacturer makes free vaccine available to any physician through a research protocol for use in patients who have acute lymphoblastic leukemia (ALL) and who meet certain eligibility criteria.[92] According to current ACIP and AAP recommendations, varicella vaccine should not be administered to persons who have cellular immunodeficiencies, but persons with impaired humoral immunity may be vaccinated.[113] In addition, some HIV-infected children may be considered for vaccination. Limited data from a clinical trial in which two doses of varicella vaccine were administered to 41 asymptomatic or mildly symptomatic HIV-infected children (CDC class N1 or A1, age-specific $CD4^+$ T-lymphocyte percentage of 25% or greater)[82] indicated that the vaccine was immunogenic and effective.[113, 265] Because children infected with HIV are at increased risk for morbidity from varicella and herpes zoster than healthy children are, the ACIP recommends that after weighing potential risks and benefits, varicella vaccine be considered for asymptomatic or mildly symptomatic HIV-infected children in CDC class N1 or A1 with age-specific $CD4^+$ T-lymphocyte percentages of 25 percent or higher.[113] Eligible children should receive two doses of varicella vaccine with a 3-month interval between doses. Because persons with impaired cellular immunity are potentially at greater risk for the development of complications after vaccination with a live virus vaccine, these vaccinees should be encouraged to return for evaluation if they experience a post-vaccination varicella-like rash. The use of varicella vaccine in other HIV-infected children is being investigated.

Precautions and Contraindications[31, 113]

Varicella vaccine is contraindicated in the following situations: (1) pregnancy, (2) severe febrile illness, (3) known history of anaphylactic reaction to vaccine components, and (4) immunodeficiency states (malignancy, primary immunodeficiency disease, immunosuppressive or corticosteroid therapy, and radiation therapy).[31, 113]

Immunocompromised patients with conditions such as lymphoreticular or other generalized malignancy and primary or secondary immunodeficiency conditions should not be given live attenuated varicella vaccine. Exceptions as previously noted include (1) patients with ALL in remission, for whom a research protocol is available for immunization[78]; (2) persons with impaired humoral immunity; and (3) asymptomatic or mildly symptomatic HIV-infected children.

Administration of varicella vaccine should be avoided if the individual is receiving immunosuppressive doses of systemic corticosteroids. The effects of corticosteroids vary, but many clinicians consider a dose equivalent to either 2 mg/kg body weight or 20 mg/day of prednisone to be sufficiently immunosuppressive to raise concern about the safety of vaccination with live virus vaccines.

After cessation of immunosuppressive therapy, varicella vaccine generally is withheld for at least 1 month. Because the intensity and type of immunosuppressive therapy, radiation therapy, underlying disease, and other factors determine when immunologic responsiveness will be restored, it is often not possible to make a definitive recommendation for an interval after cessation of immunosuppressive therapy when varicella vaccine can be safely and effectively administered.

Transmission of the live attenuated varicella vaccine virus used for immunization has been documented rarely. Therefore, contacts of immunocompromised patients should be vaccinated to prevent the spread of natural varicella to such patients. Vaccinees in whom a rash develops in the month after immunization should avoid direct contact with immunocompromised, susceptible individuals for the duration of the rash.

Receipt of antibody-containing blood products (whole blood, plasma, or parenteral immunoglobulin) may interfere with seroconversion to varicella vaccine. The length of time that such passively acquired antibody persists depends on the concentration and quantity of the blood product received[134] (see Table 242–11).

Although no direct evidence demonstrates that varicella vaccine is harmful to a pregnant female or her fetus, it should not be administered to women known to be pregnant or considering becoming pregnant within the month because of the theoretic risk of fetal infection associated with a live virus vaccine. Vaccinated women should avoid conception for 1 month after receiving vaccination.

Varicella vaccine may be considered for a nursing mother. Although most live virus vaccines are not secreted in breast milk, whether varicella vaccine virus is excreted in human milk, and if so, whether the infant can be infected are unknown.

Reye syndrome has occurred in children infected with varicella who receive salicylates. Whether varicella vaccine might induce Reye syndrome is not known, but the vaccine manufacturer recommends that salicylates not be given within at least 6 weeks after administration of varicella vaccine.

Diseases for Which Combination Vaccines Are Available

An increasing number of new and improved vaccines are being introduced. Incorporation of these vaccines into already complex childhood immunization schedules poses a challenge. In the 2002 Recommended Immunization Schedule in the United States, a minimum of 19 separate injections are needed to immunize a child from birth to 6 years of age.[131] At some visits, the administration of three or four separate injections can be indicated.

Combination vaccines represent one solution to the problem of increased numbers of injections. These vaccines incorporate into a single product antigens that prevent several diseases. Combination vaccines that have been available for many years include DTP and MMR. Combinations licensed in recent years in the United States are shown in Table 242–14. In the future, combination vaccines may

TABLE 242–14 ■ COMBINATION VACCINES LICENSED IN THE UNITED STATES SINCE 1990

Vaccine	Trade Name	Manufacturer	Date of First Licensure
Hepatitis A and hepatitis B	Twinrix	Glaxo SmithKline	2001
Hib conjugate (PRP-T) and DTaP	TriHIBit	Aventis Pasteur	1996
Hib conjugate (PRP-OMP) and hepatitis B	Comvax	Merck	1996
Hib conjugate (HbOC) and DTP	Tetramune	Wyeth-Lederle	1993
IPV, DTaP, and hepatitis B	Pediarix	Aventis Pasteur	2003

include hepatitis A, *Neisseria meningitidis, S. pneumoniae,* IPV, and varicella.

The ACIP, AAP, and AAFP have indicated a preference for the use of licensed combination vaccines over separate injections of the equivalent component vaccines.[29, 112] Separate vaccines should not be combined into the same syringe for administration together unless such mixing is indicated on the package insert approved by the FDA. The safety, immunogenicity, and efficacy of unlicensed combinations are unknown.

Mixing antigens in the same syringe can result in an increase or, more commonly, a decrease in the immunogenicity of one or more components of the combination vaccine. An antigen may have chemical incompatibility with other antigens or may cause interference with the immune response to those antigens when incorporated into a single vaccine. The unpredictability of the effect of combining different products in the same syringe can be the result of interference, antigenic competition, or carrier protein interference. Interference can result from chemical incompatibility between the vaccine antigens and the stabilizers, adjuvants, or preservatives. For example, thimerosal, a preservative in DTP vaccine used in the United States, decreases the potency of poliovirus antigens in IPV. Formulations of DTP/IPV in Europe and Canada avoid interference by using a different preservative.

Antigenic competition occurs when one or more vaccine strains in a combination vaccine replicate more rapidly than the other strains do. For example, the concentration of the three vaccine strains in OPV had to be adjusted because type 2 vaccine virus replicates more rapidly than types 1 and 3 do. Administration of several doses of the vaccine also helps ensure an adequate response to all three vaccine strains.

Carrier protein interference was identified when multiple polysaccharide-protein conjugate vaccines using the same carrier protein were administered simultaneously with large doses of the carrier protein antigen. An example would be the simultaneous administration of a tetravalent pneumococcal vaccine conjugated with tetanus toxoid and a DTP-IPV-Hib-T vaccine.[160] This problem should be preventable by using different carrier proteins in new combination conjugate vaccines.

Clinical studies in infants have demonstrated that using some combination vaccine products containing Hib vaccine may induce a suboptimal immune response to the Hib vaccine component. Because of the potential for a suboptimal immune response to the Hib component,[178] the currently licensed DTaP/Hib combination product should not be used for primary vaccination in infants aged 2, 4, or 6 months.[105]

In general, vaccines from different manufacturers that protect against the same disease are interchangeable. Data are not available on the interchangeability of DTaP vaccines. Vaccines from the same manufacturer should be used throughout a series whenever feasible. Licensure of combination vaccines usually is based on studies indicating that the product's immunogenicity (or efficacy) and safety are similar to those of monovalent products licensed previously. A combination vaccine may be used interchangeably with monovalent formulations and other combination products with similar component antigens produced by the same manufacturer.

Because of the reduced frequency of adverse reactions and high efficacy, the ACIP now recommends that DTaP be used routinely for all doses of the pertussis vaccination series.[107] All major vaccine manufacturers are working, either alone or through strategic alliances, toward developing more polyvalent vaccines by adding antigens such as conjugated Hib polysaccharide, HBsAg, or IPV (or any combination) to DTaP.

Vaccines with Selective Indications for Children and Adolescents

BACILLE CALMETTE-GUÉRIN VACCINE

Effective control of tuberculosis in the United States has been achieved by the early identification and treatment of cases, followed by surveillance of household and other close contacts and institution of appropriate preventive measures for those at high risk for development of disease. In the United States, the mainstay of preventive therapy is isoniazid chemoprophylaxis, which is used in asymptomatically infected persons to prevent the progression of infection to disease. In selected instances, however, the potential for acquiring disease, poor compliance in contacts instructed to take chemoprophylaxis, or failure of chemoprophylaxis may justify the use of immunoprophylaxis.[91] Elsewhere in the world, BCG vaccine is used in more than 100 countries and is recommended routinely at birth by the WHO (see Table 242–5). Of primary concern to pediatricians is the risk to an infant born to a tuberculous mother or living within a household with other identified tuberculous individuals.[19]

Preparations

BCG is a live attenuated strain derived from *Mycobacterium bovis.* All presently available BCG vaccines are derived from the original strain at the Pasteur Institute but have been propagated by different methods in many laboratories and, therefore, vary in their immunogenic and reactogenic properties. BCG vaccines manufactured by Organon Teknika Corporation, Durham, NC, and Connaught Laboratories, Willowdale, Ontario, are licensed in the United States. Comparative evaluations of these and other BCG vaccines have not been performed. BCG is administered either percutaneously or intradermally. BCG preparations instilled in treatment of bladder cancer are not intended to be used as vaccines.[91]

Immunogenicity and Efficacy

BCG is used primarily in young infants in an attempt to prevent disseminated and other life-threatening manifestations of *Mycobacterium tuberculosis* disease. However, BCG does not prevent infection with *M. tuberculosis.* The efficacy of different BCG vaccines seems to be highly variable. Two meta-analyses of published clinical trials and case-control studies concerning the efficacy of BCG vaccines concluded that BCG has relatively high protective efficacy (approximately 80%) against meningeal and miliary tuberculosis in children.[155, 326] The protective efficacy against pulmonary tuberculosis, however, differed significantly among the studies, thus precluding a specific conclusion. Protection afforded by BCG in one meta-analysis was estimated to be 50 percent.

Adverse Events

BCG vaccination usually results in scarring at the site of injection. BCG preparations have been associated uncommonly (1 to 2% of vaccinations) with local adverse reactions such as subcutaneous abscess and lymphadenopathy, which are not generally serious. Osteitis affecting the epiphyses of long bones is a rare complication that develops in 1 per million vaccinees and may occur as long as several years after receiving BCG immunization. The rate may be higher in newborns. Disseminated fatal disease occurs rarely (0.1 to 1 case per million vaccinees), primarily in persons with severely impaired immune systems.[91, 257, 270, 349] Antituberculosis therapy, except for pyrazinamide, is recommended to treat osteitis and disseminated disease caused by BCG. Some experts also recommend treatment of chronic suppurative lymphadenitis caused by BCG. Persons with complications caused by BCG should be referred, if possible, to a tuberculosis expert for management.

Indications

In the United States, administration of BCG should be considered only in limited and select circumstances, such as unavoidable risk of exposure to *M. tuberculosis* and failure or unfeasibility of other methods of control of tuberculosis. The ACIP and the AAP have published recommendations for the use of BCG to control tuberculosis in children.[19, 91]

Healthy infants from birth to 2 months of age may be given BCG without tuberculin skin testing; thereafter, BCG is given only to children with a negative tuberculin skin test. In infants and children, BCG immunization should be considered for those who are not infected with HIV in the following circumstances:

- The child is exposed continually to a person or persons with contagious pulmonary tuberculosis resistant to isoniazid and rifampin and the child cannot be removed from this exposure.
- The child is exposed continually to a person or persons with untreated or ineffectively treated contagious pulmonary tuberculosis and the child cannot be removed from such exposure or given antituberculosis therapy.

Careful assessment of the potential risks and benefits of BCG vaccine and consultation with personnel in local area control programs for tuberculosis are strongly recommended before the use of BCG. When BCG vaccine is given, care should be taken to observe the precautions and directions for administration on the product label.

Skin Test Reactivity

Recipients of BCG should have repeat tuberculin skin tests 2 to 3 months after immunization to establish that tuberculin cellular reactivity has developed. Failure to react dictates the need for repeat BCG vaccination followed by repeat tuberculin testing.[91] The tuberculin reaction to the BCG vaccine available in the United States generally results in 7 to 15 mm of induration after vaccination and diminishes gradually during subsequent years; without revaccination or repeated exposure to *M. tuberculosis,* reactivity usually disappears within 10 years.[91] The size of the area of induration may be correlated with the number of doses of BCG.[231] However, tuberculin skin test sensitivity does not correlate with BCG efficacy.[222] In BCG recipients, differentiating between a tuberculin reaction representing acquired tuberculous infection and persisting post-vaccination reactivity is difficult. Because the degree and duration of protection against tuberculous disease afforded by BCG are uncertain, a positive tuberculin reaction always must be suspected to be indicative of disease.

Precautions and Contraindications

BCG vaccine should not be administered to individuals with burns, skin infections, and primary or secondary immunodeficiencies, including HIV infection. The use of BCG also is contraindicated in persons receiving immunosuppressive medications, including high-dose corticosteroids.

In the United States, where the risk of acquiring tuberculosis is low, BCG vaccine should not be administered to children with known or suspected asymptomatic HIV infection.[91, 296] However, in populations where the risk of contracting tuberculosis is high, the WHO has recommended that asymptomatic HIV-infected children receive BCG vaccine at birth or shortly thereafter.[383]

Although no harmful effects of BCG vaccine on the fetus have been documented, women should avoid receiving vaccination during pregnancy.

CHOLERA VACCINE

Fewer than 300 cases of cholera have been recognized in the United States in the past decade.[85] Most cases have occurred in travelers to cholera-affected areas or persons who have eaten contaminated food brought or imported from these areas.[85] Although cholera remains a significant public health concern in African, South American, and Asian countries, even in these countries the risk to U.S. travelers is low. Persons following the usual tourist itinerary who use standard accommodations in countries reporting cholera are at virtually no risk of acquiring infection.[84]

Preparations

The only vaccine currently available in the United States is prepared from a combination of phenol-inactivated whole-cell suspensions of the classic Inaba and Ogawa strains of *Vibrio cholerae* O-group 1 and is administered parenterally.[68]

Immunogenicity and Efficacy

In field trials conducted in cholera-endemic regions, the cholera vaccines currently available have been only approximately 50 percent effective in reducing the incidence of clinical illness from *V. cholerae* O1 during the 6-month period after vaccination.[68] Illness caused by the recently discovered *V. cholerae* O139 probably is unaffected by the currently available vaccines.[84]

Adverse Events

Common vaccine side effects include localized pain, erythema, and induration for 1 to 2 days at the site of injection. Fever, malaise, and headache may accompany the local reaction.[68]

Indications

Cholera vaccination is indicated only for travelers to countries that require a valid international certificate of vaccination for entry. However, the WHO no longer recommends cholera vaccination for any travelers, and vaccination is not required for entry or return into the United States.[84, 384]

Precautions and Contraindications

Extremely rare serious reactions, including neurologic reactions, have been observed and represent contraindications to revaccination.[68] The safety of immunization with cholera vaccine during pregnancy has not been established, and therefore it should not be used except in the case of substantial risk of acquiring infection.[68]

HEPATITIS A VACCINE

The occurrence of hepatitis A is highest in developing countries and reflects the primary route of transmission of fecal-oral, person-to-person spread. Hepatitis A also remains the most common cause of acute viral hepatitis in the United States and continues to cause substantial morbidity and associated costs.[114, 254]

The incidence of disease varies considerably among different populations in the United States.[114, 254, 348] Community-wide outbreaks recurring every 3 to 10 years in high-risk communities account for much of the occurrence of disease and are a primary target for control by vaccination. Rates of infection are highest among Alaskan Natives and American Indians. Other groups at increased risk include travelers to developing countries, homosexual and bisexual men, and users of illicit drugs. However, the finding that 45 percent of reported cases have no identifiable risk factor indicates that selective immunization is unlikely to have a major impact on the control of hepatitis A.

Outbreaks among children attending daycare and their staff are common and have been associated with community outbreaks.[213] However, the prevalence of hepatitis A infection in daycare center staff and in children and adolescents who previously attended daycare is not increased and suggests that infections within daycare settings most commonly reflect transmission within the community extending to these settings.[114, 241] Transmission of hepatitis A virus (HAV) also can occur in institutions for the developmentally disabled. In addition to these examples of direct person-to-person transmission, infection can be acquired by the ingestion of contaminated food or water.

Disease in the United States occurs most commonly in children 5 to 14 years of age.[114] Children and infants shed HAV for longer periods than adults do—as long as several months after the onset of clinical illness. Because children frequently have asymptomatic infections and may shed for prolonged periods, they have an important role in transmission of HAV. In one study involving adults without an identified source of infection, 52 percent of their households included a child younger than 6 years.[114] Thus, control of hepatitis A by active immunization probably will necessitate universal childhood immunization.

Preparations

Both inactivated and attenuated HAV vaccines have been developed.[171] However, only inactivated vaccines are licensed in the United States. Inactivated HAV vaccine is prepared by methods similar to those used for inactivated poliomyelitis vaccine. Virus is propagated in human diploid fibroblast cell cultures, formalin inactivated, and adsorbed to aluminum hydroxide adjuvant.[26, 114] Two such products are licensed in the United States, Havrix (SmithKline Beecham Biologicals) and Vaqta (Merck & Co.). Each vaccine has two formulations, an adult and a pediatric product with different antigen content. The pediatric formulation is indicated for persons 2 to 18 years of age. The vaccines can be used interchangeably.[63] As of June 2003, no vaccine has been approved by the FDA for children younger than 2 years.

Immunogenicity and Efficacy

Inactivated viral vaccine is highly immunogenic. After receiving a single dose, 95 percent of children and nearly all adults seroconvert within 1 month.[26, 114] After receipt of a second dose in children, seroconversion approximates 100 percent.

Concurrent administration of immune globulin and vaccine inhibits the peak serum antibody concentration achieved but not the rate of seroconversion.[367] Because antibody levels are well above the protective concentration, this inhibition is not considered to be clinically significant and supports passive-active immunoprophylaxis when indicated.

In two large clinical trials of inactivated HAV vaccine in children older than 2 years, protective efficacy has been greater than 90 percent.[232, 379] In a double-blind, placebo-controlled, randomized study in Thailand involving approximately 34,000 vaccinees, the protective efficacy against clinical hepatitis A was 94 percent after administration of two doses given 1 month apart; it was 100 percent after subsequent administration of a 12-month booster dose.[232]

Limited data indicate that most infants seroconvert after receiving a three-dose schedule.[114] However, antibody concentrations in infants with passively acquired maternal anti-HAV are relatively low.[47] The clinical significance of these diminished antibody responses is unknown, and the results of studies have been conflicting.[245, 312] Until this issue is resolved, the use of HAV vaccine in children younger than 2 years is not recommended.

Vaccination also has been demonstrated to be effective in controlling outbreaks in communities with high rates of disease.[114] For example, in a New York State community in which hepatitis A is highly endemic in children, a single dose of vaccine was 100 percent effective beginning 3 weeks after immunization in preventing symptomatic disease.[379]

The duration of protection after vaccination is likely to be prolonged. Although data on the persistence of serum antibody and protection against infection are limited to approximately 5 years of experience, adults have been demonstrated to maintain protective antibody concentrations for at least 4 years, and kinetic models of antibody decline indicate possible antibody persistence for 20 years.[362] Data in children are not available to determine whether and when booster doses are indicated.

Adverse Events

Except for rare reports of anaphylaxis and anaphylactoid reaction in adults in Europe and Asia, serious reactions to inactivated HAV vaccine have not been reported.[114] Pain, tenderness, and infection at the injection site can occur.[232]

Indications[8, 26, 114]

HAV vaccine is recommended only for persons 2 years or older who have an increased risk for infection. The indications are as follows: travel to or work in a country with a high or intermediate incidence of HAV infection, persons with clotting factor disorders, sexually active homosexual and bisexual males, illicit drug users, and persons working with infected primates or with HAV in a laboratory. Routine vaccination of persons with chronic liver disease is recommended because they may be at increased risk for fulminant hepatitis if they become infected with HAV. Children living in areas where rates of hepatitis A are at least twice the national average should be vaccinated routinely. In addition, children living in areas where rates of hepatitis A are at least greater than the national average but lower than twice the national average should be considered for routine vaccination.[114] Although the ACIP guidelines do not recommend routine vaccination of food handlers, consideration may be given to vaccination of these workers in areas where state and local health authorities or private employers determine that vaccination is cost-effective.

Vaccination also should be considered for the control of hepatitis A outbreaks in communities in which the rate of infection is increased. Production of a highly immune population reduces the incidence of hepatitis A and decreases transmission by preventing fecal shedding of HAV.[114] However, because effectiveness of vaccination has not been demonstrated in localized outbreaks occurring in institutions for the developmentally disabled, daycare centers, schools, and prisons, administration of intramuscular immune globulin currently is recommended for close contacts of infected persons in these circumstances. At present, HAV vaccine is not indicated routinely for daycare attendees and staff or for food handlers.

To control the significant public health burden of hepatitis A in the future, licensure of HAV vaccine for infants and development of combination products containing HAV and other vaccine antigens may lead to inclusion of HAV vaccine in the routine childhood immunization program.

Precautions and Contraindications[8]

HAV should not be administered to persons with a hypersensitivity reaction to any of the vaccine components, such as alum or, in the case of Havrix, phenoxyethanol. Safety data in pregnant women are not available, but the risk is considered to be low or nonexistent because the vaccine contains inactivated, purified viral proteins.

INFLUENZA VACCINE

Influenza virus infection continues to cause significant morbidity and mortality despite the availability of effective vaccines and antiviral therapy for prevention and treatment of influenza. Influenza viruses cause annual epidemics of acute respiratory diseases that affect all ages.

A major difficulty in the development and provision of satisfactory immunizing agents for the prevention of influenzal disease is the antigenic variation in these viruses. Periodic minor antigenic changes in influenza A or B virus are the major factors in the continuing occurrence of yearly influenzal disease. Although outbreaks generally are limited in magnitude, the resulting morbidity and mortality remain discouragingly high. Major antigenic changes in influenza A virus, as occurred in 1957 to 1958 (Asian strain) and again in 1968 to 1969 (Hong Kong strain), account for the pandemic spread of disease associated with greater overall morbidity and mortality, especially in high-risk populations.

Influenza outbreaks occur each year in the United States. The impact of influenza on both normal children and those with underlying high-risk conditions is appreciable. Attack rates in normal children have been estimated at 10 to 40 percent each year, and approximately 1 percent of these influenza infections result in hospitalization.[198]

Preparations

Trivalent inactivated vaccines are the only available vaccines against influenza viruses in the United States.[10, 129] These multivalent vaccines contain three virus strains (usually two type A and one type B), with the composition changed periodically in anticipation of the prevalent influenza strains expected to circulate in the United States in the following winter. Vaccines are prepared from virus grown in the allantoic sac of the chick embryo. The virus is purified by ultracentrifugation before inactivation with formalin. Vaccines available in the United States include the subvirion vaccine, which is prepared by the additional step of disrupting the lipid-containing membrane of the purified virus particle, and purified surface antigen vaccine. Whole-virus vaccine is no longer available. Febrile reactions in children younger than 13 years are minimized by the use of subvirion or purified surface antigen preparations. Influenza vaccine distributed in the United States also may contain thimerosal, a mercury-containing compound, as the preservative. Manufacturing processes differ by manufacturer. Certain manufacturers might use additional compounds to inactivate the influenza viruses, and they might use an antibiotic to prevent bacterial contamination. Package inserts should be consulted for additional information.

Of the three influenza vaccines currently licensed in the United States, two influenza vaccines (FluShield from Wyeth Laboratories, Inc., and Fluzone split from Aventis Pasteur, Inc.) are approved for use beginning at 6 months of age. One other influenza vaccine, Fluvirin (Evans Vaccines Ltd.), is approved in the United States only for persons 4 years or older because its efficacy in younger persons has not been demonstrated.

To improve the immunogenicity of inactivated influenza vaccine, several new approaches are being investigated. Cold-adapted virus vaccines have been demonstrated to be safe, immunogenic, and protective in pediatric patients.[49, 50, 150, 317] A cold-adapted, live attenuated influenza vaccine that is administered intranasally is being considered for licensure by the U.S. FDA.

Immunogenicity and Efficacy

After parenteral administration, nearly all vaccinated children and young adults develop hemagglutinin-inhibition antibody titers that are likely to be protective against infection by strains antigenically similar to those present in the preparation. However, the seroresponse of high-risk children younger than 5 years, even with two properly spaced doses of split-virus vaccine, may be erratic.[205, 206]

If provided under optimal conditions (i.e., at an appropriate time and against the appropriate prevailing influenzal strain), influenza vaccines can reduce the incidence of disease by 70 percent in healthy children and younger adults.[129] However, efficacy is dependent on the degree to which the vaccine strains share the antigens of the circulating strains of influenza virus. The protection afforded by inactivated vaccine is transient, and yearly immunization is necessary irrespective of whether significant antigenic changes have occurred in a prevailing influenza strain. Studies suggest that the use of trivalent inactivated influenza vaccine decreases the incidence of influenza-associated otitis media and the use of antibiotics in young children.[147, 223]

As determined in clinical trials with swine influenza vaccines in 1976, adequate protection generally is achieved in immunologically primed, healthy individuals given a single dose of whole-virus or split-product vaccine. In previously unimmunized populations, such as children younger than 9 years, a single dose of split-product vaccine may be significantly less immunogenic than a single dose of whole-virus preparation, and two doses may be required for a satisfactory serum antibody response.[129]

Variable immunogenicity of influenza vaccine has been reported in immunocompromised individuals, including those with malignancy. Successful immunologic responses in these populations are most likely to occur when immunized individuals have been primed previously by exposure to antigenically similar influenza strains.[207, 260] The optimal time to immunize children with malignancies who still must undergo chemotherapy is 3 to 4 weeks after chemotherapy has been discontinued and the peripheral granulocyte and lymphocyte counts are greater than 1000/mm^3.[10]

Corticosteroids administered for brief periods or every other day have only a minimal effect on the antibody response to influenza vaccine. Prolonged administration of high doses of corticosteroids (i.e., a dose equivalent to either 2 mg/kg or greater or a total of 20 mg/day of prednisone) may impair the antibody response. Influenza immunization can be deferred temporarily during the time of receipt of high-dose corticosteroids, provided that deferral does not compromise the likelihood of administering immunization before the start of the influenza season.[10]

In a study examining the reactogenicity and immunogenicity of two doses of the split-product vaccine in high-risk children 3 to 5 months of age, reactogenicity was low but seroresponse rates were variable, with a poor response to most immunizing antigens.[206] No information is available on the efficacy of influenza vaccines in infants younger than 6 months. In addition, the effect of the influenza antigens in an inactivated virus vaccine on the infant's future immune response to influenza is not known.[10]

Adverse Events

Current influenza vaccines contain only noninfectious viruses and cannot cause influenza. Respiratory disease occurring after vaccination represents coincidental illness unrelated to influenza vaccination. Influenza vaccines are generally well tolerated. Local redness or induration for 1 to 2 days at the site of injection has been reported to develop in less than one third of vaccinees. In addition, two types of systemic reactions have occurred. Fever, chills, headache, and malaise, though infrequent events, most often affect children who have had no previous exposure to the influenza virus antigens contained in the vaccine. These reactions, which are attributed to influenza antigens, generally begin 6 to 12 hours after vaccination and persist for only 1 to 2 days.[129] The second type of reaction is immediate, presumably allergic, and may involve hives, angioedema, allergic asthma, or systemic anaphylaxis. These reactions occur rarely and are probably the result of hypersensitivity to a vaccine component, most likely residual egg protein.

Influenza vaccines have been associated with a slightly increased frequency of GBS in adults. A study conducted during 1992 to 1994 showed an excess of approximately 1 GBS case per million persons immunized.[262] No cases were observed in persons younger than 45 years. GBS has not been associated with influenza immunization of children.[10]

Indications

Influenza vaccine is recommended annually for patients 6 months or older who are at high risk for acquiring disease, for medical care personnel, and for those who wish to decrease their risk of acquiring illness caused by influenza. Vaccine is most effective when it precedes exposure by no more than 2 to 4 months.

High-risk children are those at increased risk for the development of lower respiratory tract complications or death after having influenza infection and include the following[10, 129]:

- Children with chronic disorders of the pulmonary system, including children with asthma.
- Children with hemodynamically significant cardiac disease.
- Residents of institutions with patients of any age who have chronic medical conditions.
- Children who have required regular medical follow-up or hospitalization during the preceding year because of chronic metabolic diseases (including diabetes mellitus), renal dysfunction, sickle-cell anemia and other hemoglobinopathies, or immunosuppression (including HIV disease and immunosuppression caused by medications).
- Children and adolescents (6 months to 18 years of age) who are receiving long-term aspirin therapy and, therefore, might be at risk for Reye syndrome after having influenza.

Medical personnel can transmit influenza to their high-risk patients while they are incubating an infection, experiencing mild or unrecognized infection, or working despite the existence of symptoms, and they can cause nosocomial outbreaks of influenza.[199, 216] In view of the potential for introducing influenza to high-risk groups, such as patients with compromised cardiopulmonary or immune systems or infants in neonatal intensive care units, annual influenza vaccination of physicians, nurses, and other personnel who have extensive contact with these high-risk patient groups is recommended. Vaccination also is indicated for employees of nursing homes and chronic care facilities who have contact with high-risk children and for providers of home care and household members of high-risk patients, including infants with bronchopulmonary dysplasia or congenital heart disease.[129]

Infants younger than 6 months with high-risk conditions, especially those with cardiopulmonary compromise, may have the same or a greater risk than older children. Neither influenza vaccine nor prophylaxis with rimantadine, amantadine, oseltamivir, or zanamivir is recommended for this age group. Immunization and chemoprophylaxis of adults who are in close contact with high-risk infants are important means of protecting infants. In addition, household contacts and out-of-home caregivers of children 0 to 23 months of age also are encouraged to receive influenza vaccine to decrease the risk of transmitting influenza virus to these children. Vaccinating contacts of infants younger than 6 months in particular is encouraged because children of this age cannot be vaccinated and are the pediatric age group at greatest risk of requiring influenza-related hospitalization.

Other indications for vaccination include the following[129]:

- Vaccine is recommended for women who will be in the third trimester of pregnancy or early puerperium during the influenza season. Pregnant women who have medical conditions that increase their risk for complications from influenza should be vaccinated before the influenza season, regardless of the stage of pregnancy.
- Foreign travelers, especially those at risk for influenza complications, should consider receiving vaccine before they depart, depending on the season and travel destination.
- Immunization should be considered for groups of persons whose close contact facilitates rapid transmission and spread of infection that may result in disruption of routine activities. Such groups include students in colleges, schools, and other educational institutions, particularly persons who reside in dormitories or who are members of athletic teams, and persons living in residential institutions.
- The ACIP encourages, when feasible, influenza vaccination of healthy children 6 to 23 months of age because children in this age group are at substantially increased risk for influenza-related hospitalization.

Influenza vaccine may be administered to any healthy child or adolescent who wishes to reduce the chance of becoming infected with influenza. The morbidity from influenza can be appreciable in healthy children. Influenza vaccine does not adversely affect the safety of breast-feeding for mothers or infants; therefore, breast-feeding is not a contraindication to immunization.

The optimal time to vaccinate high-risk individuals is usually during October-November. However, to avoid missed opportunities for vaccination, influenza vaccine should be offered to persons at high risk when they are seen by health care providers for routine care or are hospitalized in September, provided that vaccine is available. In addition, health care providers also should continue to offer vaccine to unvaccinated persons after November and throughout the influenza season, even after influenza activity has been documented in the community.[129]

Precautions and Contraindications

Current influenza vaccines contain egg proteins and on rare occasion may induce immediate allergic reactions, including anaphylaxis. Skin testing has been used for children with severe anaphylactic reactions to eggs who are to receive influenza vaccine, but these children generally should not receive influenza vaccine because of the risk of reaction, the probable need for yearly immunization, and the availability of chemoprophylaxis against influenza infection. Less severe or local manifestations of allergy to egg or to feathers are not contraindications to influenza vaccine administration and do not warrant vaccine skin testing.[10]

Pregnancy is not a contraindication to influenza vaccine administration, and vaccination is advised for pregnant women who have an underlying high-risk condition. To avoid concern about the theoretic possibility of teratogenicity, vaccinating after the first trimester may be prudent.[129]

Persons with acute febrile illness usually should not be vaccinated until their symptoms have abated. However, minor illnesses with or without fever do not contraindicate the use of influenza vaccine, particularly in children with mild upper respiratory tract infection or allergic rhinitis.[129]

JAPANESE ENCEPHALITIS VIRUS VACCINE

Japanese encephalitis (JE) virus, the most important cause of epidemic arboviral encephalitis in Asia, has a wide clinical spectrum ranging from asymptomatic infection to permanent neurologic sequelae with a high case-fatality rate of 30 to 70 percent.[290, 359] A mouse brain vaccine has controlled JE virus infection successfully among human populations in Japan, Korea, and Taiwan since 1968.[302] A JE virus vaccine is licensed in the United States for use in persons living in or traveling to Asia.

Preparations

The JE vaccine licensed in the United States is a formalin-inactivated virus derived from purified infected mouse brain.[79] The vaccine contains gelatin as a stabilizer and thimerosal as a preservative.

Immunogenicity and Efficacy

Immunogenicity studies in the United States indicate that three doses are needed to provide protective concentrations of serum neutralizing antibody in greater than 80 percent of vaccinees.[316] Protective concentrations have been defined by animal challenge experiments.[302] The longevity of neutralizing antibody after the primary vaccination series is not known. In one Japanese study, protective antibody titers persisted for 3 years after the administration of a booster dose.[252]

A field trial of the currently licensed JE vaccine conducted in Thai children demonstrated an efficacy of 91 percent when compared with placebo.[228] The efficacy for a single year of a prototype of the currently licensed vaccine, field-tested in Taiwanese children, was 80 percent.[230]

Adverse Reactions

JE vaccination is associated with a moderate frequency of local and mild systemic side effects. Local reactions occur in approximately 20 percent of vaccines, and about 10 percent have reported systemic side effects such as fever, headache, malaise, or rash.[79]

Neurologic adverse reactions, including acute disseminated encephalomyelitis (ADE), also have been reported. In Denmark, ADE has been estimated to occur in 1 in 50,000 to 75,000 vaccinees. However, a recent review of post-marketing data in the United States from 1993 to 1999 found no serious neurologic events after JE immunization.[352]

Hypersensitivity reactions have been reported. Urticaria or angioedema of the extremities, face, and oropharynx, especially the lips, characterizes these reactions. They occur a median of 12 hours after administration of the first dose of vaccine. The interval between administration of a second dose and onset of symptoms is generally longer, with a median of 3 days and possibly as long as 2 weeks. Reactions have occurred after the administration of a second or third dose when the preceding doses did not cause symptoms. Reaction rates are similar after the administration of both first and second doses—a rate of approximately 15 to 62 per 10,000 immunizations in U.S. citizens. The vaccine component responsible for these adverse events has not been identified.[79]

Indications[79]

JE vaccine is recommended for persons, except infants, who will be residing in areas where JE is endemic or epidemic.[79] The risk for acquiring JE varies highly within endemic regions. Therefore, the incidence of JE in the area of residence, conditions of housing, the nature of activities, and the possibility of unexpected travel to high-risk areas are factors that should be considered in the decision to vaccinate.

JE vaccine is *not* recommended for all travelers to Asia. The vaccine should be offered to persons spending a month or longer in endemic areas during the transmission season, especially if travel will include rural areas. *Health Information for International Travel*, updated regularly by the CDC, provides a useful table that lists affected areas by country and notes the transmission season.

The decision to use JE vaccine should balance the risks for exposure to the virus and the development of illness, the availability and acceptability of mosquito repellents and other alternative protective measures, and the side effects of vaccination.

The recommended primary immunization series is three doses administered on days 0, 7, and 30. An abbreviated schedule of days 0, 7, and 14 can be used when a longer schedule is impractical because of time constraints. Two doses administered 1 week apart will confer short-term immunity in 80 percent of vaccinees. However, this schedule should be used only under unusual circumstances. The last dose should be administered at least 10 days before travel commences to ensure an adequate immune response and access to care if a delayed, adverse reaction occurs.[79] No data are available regarding vaccine safety and efficacy in infants.[5]

The duration of protection is unknown, and definitive recommendations cannot be given on the timing of booster doses. Booster doses may be administered after 2 years.

Precautions and Contraindications

Because generalized urticaria and angioedema can occur within minutes to as long as 2 weeks after vaccination, epinephrine, other medications, and equipment to treat anaphylaxis should be available. Vaccinees should be observed for 30 minutes after receiving vaccination and should be warned about the possibility of delayed development of urticaria and angioedema, which can occur as long as 2 weeks after vaccination. Vaccinees should be advised to remain in areas with ready access to medical care for 10 days after receiving a dose of JE vaccine.

Hypersensitivity to proteins of rodent or neural origin, to thimerosal, or to a previous dose of JE vaccine is a contraindication to receiving vaccination.

A study in U.S. military personnel found an association between reactions to JE vaccine and a past history of having urticaria. A history of urticaria should be considered when weighing the risks and benefits of vaccination.

No specific information is available on the safety of JE vaccine in pregnancy. Limited data suggest that the vaccine can be given to patients with altered immune status. Little information is available on the effect of concurrent administration of other vaccines on the safety and immunogenicity of JE vaccine.

MENINGOCOCCAL VACCINE

N. meningitidis is a leading cause of bacterial meningitis and continues to be a major public health problem, not only in the United States but also worldwide. Although the disease has a more severe impact on children and young adults, all age groups are susceptible to acquiring infection. The disease is transmitted from person to person by close contact. In the United States, an estimated 3000 cases involving meningococcal serogroups B, C, and recently Y occur each year. In other parts of the world, the number of cases is much higher. For example, in sub-Saharan Africa during the 1996 epidemics caused by serogroup A, more than 200,000 cases were reported, with 20,000 deaths. A significant proportion of children who survive infections caused by *N. meningitidis* have permanent sequelae such as deafness.

Routine immunization against meningococcal disease has not been recommended in the United States because of the limitations of the currently available vaccine and the epidemiology of the disease. Group C vaccine is poorly immunogenic in children 2 years or younger, a group accounting for 35 percent of the cases in recent surveillance data, and no vaccine is available for serogroup B, which accounts for approximately one third of cases in the United States.[327]

An increased incidence of meningococcal disease in adolescents and young adults was noted in the United States in the mid-1990s.[220, 328] A prospective surveillance study of meningococcal disease among college students by the CDC and the American College Health Association suggests that the incidence is similar to that of the general population of 18- to 22-year-olds but that dormitory residents, especially freshmen, are at increased risk.[61] In a Maryland study, the incidence of disease was significantly higher in on-campus residents than off-campus residents.[221]

Preparations

A quadrivalent vaccine containing serogroup A, C, Y, and W135 is licensed for use in the United States. Each vaccine dose contains 50 mg of each of the four purified bacterial capsular polysaccharides.[98] No vaccine is available for prevention of group B disease because unconjugated group B polysaccharide is poorly immunogenic in humans. Investigational protein-conjugated meningococcal polysaccharide vaccines that may be protective in children younger than 2 years and vaccines against group B disease are under study. In late 1999, conjugate group C meningococcal vaccine was licensed in the United Kingdom, where rates of meningococcal disease are twofold higher than those in the United States. A comprehensive public health program to vaccinate children 2 months to 17 years of age and entering college students was initiated, and within 1 year the incidence of meningitis was reduced by 92 percent in young children and by 95 percent in teenagers.[318]

Immunogenicity and Efficacy

The recommended dose is a single 0.5-mL subcutaneous injection. The vaccine may be administered concurrently with other vaccines, but at a different anatomic site. Protective antibody concentrations are achieved within 10 to 14 days after vaccination.

The antibody responses to each of the four polysaccharides in the vaccine are serogroup-specific and independent. Group A polysaccharide induces antibody in some children as young as 3 months, although a response comparable to that in adults is not achieved until the child is 4 to 5 years of age.[308] The serum antibody response to serogroup C is age-dependent, with a poor response in children younger than 2 years.[201] Serum concentrations of antibodies against group A and C polysaccharides decrease markedly during the first 3 years after receipt of a single dose of vaccine. The decrease in antibody occurs more rapidly in infants and young children than in adults.[248, 387]

Field trials of A and C meningococcal vaccines in Europe and Africa have demonstrated efficacy rates against serogroup A of 85 to 95 percent 1 year after vaccination.[308, 368] After 3 years, efficacy rates were 67 percent in older children but only 10 percent in children younger than 4 years at the time of immunization with serogroup A vaccine.[320] In an epidemic, serogroup C vaccine demonstrated clinical efficacy rates similar to those of the serogroup A vaccine.[353]

Serogroup Y and W135 antigens are immunogenic and safe in children older than 2 years. However, clinical efficacy has not been demonstrated as yet for these preparations.[2, 39, 366]

Persons with deficiencies of the terminal components of serum complement and those with anatomic or functional asplenia have antibody responses to quadrivalent meningococcal vaccines consistent with protection.[330, 331] However, the clinical efficacy of vaccination has not been evaluated in these persons.

Adverse Events

Untoward reactions have been reported infrequently and consist primarily of localized erythema and tenderness. Fever develops transiently in as many as 2 percent of young children after immunization.[25, 98]

Indications[25, 33, 120]

Immunization is recommended for certain high-risk groups, including adults and children older than 2 years with deficiencies of the terminal components of serum complement (C5 to C8) or properdin and those with anatomic or functional asplenia. Immunization also should be considered for travelers to countries in which epidemic or hyperendemic meningococcal disease is present and for Americans living in these areas.

When epidemiologic evidence indicates that an outbreak or cluster of meningococcal cases caused by a serogroup represented in the vaccine is occurring in a defined population, immunization of persons at risk may be recommended by local or state public health authorities. For close contacts such as household members, chemoprophylaxis also must be given because immunization does not prevent the development of early-onset disease.

In 2000, the ACIP and the AAP, in response to the finding of an increased risk for acquiring meningococcal disease in freshmen college students living in dormitories, recommended that college freshman dormitory residents be provided information about meningococcal infection and the benefits of vaccination and that vaccine be made available to students who wish to receive it.[33, 120]

Reimmunization should be considered after 3 to 5 years for persons at high risk for acquiring infection, such as travelers to areas where disease is epidemic. Because of the relatively poor response to vaccine in children immunized when younger than 4 years and the rapid decline in antibody concentration, revaccination should be considered after 3 years. In older children and adults, consideration of revaccination is not warranted until after 5 years. However, little information is available to accurately determine the need or timing for revaccination for persons at continued risk. A recent study in adult military personnel demonstrated the persistence of antibodies for as long as 10 years after receiving immunization.[387]

Precautions and Contraindications

Because of theoretic considerations, meningococcal polysaccharide vaccines should not be administered to pregnant women unless the risk of acquiring disease is substantial. However, evaluation of pregnant women immunized during an epidemic in Brazil demonstrated no adverse effects.[280]

RABIES VACCINE

Rabies is a viral infection transmitted in the saliva of infected mammals. The virus enters the central nervous system of the host and causes an encephalomyelitis that is almost always fatal. Postexposure prophylaxis is possible because of the long incubation period of this infection.

Rabies occurs commonly in animals, and rabies postexposure prophylaxis is frequently given. Carnivorous wild animals, especially skunks, foxes, coyotes, raccoons, and bats, are a continuing potential source of rabies; they account for most cases of animal rabies and the few cases of human rabies in the United States. Wildlife rabies occurs throughout the continental United States; only Hawaii remains consistently rabies-free. Domestic dogs and cats represent only a small proportion of proven rabid animals, but as the primary interface between the sylvan reservoir and humans, they account for most postexposure immunoprophylaxis against rabies.

Although the likelihood of human exposure to a rabid domestic animal in the United States is small, international travelers to areas where canine rabies is still endemic have an increased risk of exposure to rabies. In most of Asia, Africa, and Latin America, dogs are the most common source of rabies among humans. Twelve of the 36 human rabies deaths reported to the CDC from 1980 through 1997 appear to have been related to rabid animals outside the United States.[100, 295]

Preparations

Three inactivated rabies vaccines are licensed for pre-exposure and postexposure prophylaxis in the United States. Human diploid cell vaccine (HDCV) derived from the Pitman-Moore strain has been licensed in the United States since 1980. It is supplied now only in a formulation for intramuscular administration; the product for intradermal use is no longer available. Rabies vaccine, adsorbed (RVA), derived from the Kissling strain of rabies virus cultured in fetal rhesus lung diploid cells, was licensed in the United States in 1988. It is formulated for intramuscular administration only. A third rabies vaccine, purified chick embryo cell (PCEC) vaccine, became available in the United States in 1997.[173] It is prepared from the Flury LEP rabies virus strain grown in primary culture of chicken fibroblasts. Duck embryo rabies vaccine has not been available in the United States since 1981. Allergic reactions occurred frequently with this vaccine.

Immunogenicity and Efficacy

Essentially all HDCV recipients develop protective antibody titers that persist for at least 2 years. The immunogenicity of RVA is only slightly less than that of HDCV.

The paucity of human cases attests to the efficacy of postexposure prophylaxis with the presently recommended vaccine and immunoglobulin preparations. To date, rabies has not been reported in the United States in any patient who received the currently recommended postexposure measures. However, cases of human rabies occurring after postexposure administration of prophylaxis have resulted from failure to adhere to established guidelines, such as those of the CDC or the WHO, and may have been associated with injection of HDCV into the gluteal muscle with resulting decreased immunogenicity.[75, 174, 187, 342, 373]

Adverse Events

Reactions occurring after administration of HDCV, RVA, or PCEC vaccine are less serious and less common than those associated with the previously available vaccines.[111] Local reactions at the injection site occur in 30 to 74 percent of injections, and systemic reactions such as headache, nausea, abdominal pain, muscle aches, and dizziness occur in 5 to 40 percent of vaccine recipients. Approximately 6 percent of persons who received booster doses of HDCV had an immune complex–like reaction 2 to 21 days after administration of the booster dose.[67] This reaction occurred less frequently in persons receiving primary vaccination. The reactions have been associated with the presence of beta-propiolactone–altered human albumin in HDCV and the development of IgE antibodies to this allergen.[188]

Indications and Precautions

When used as indicated, all three types of rabies vaccine are considered equally safe and effective for both pre-exposure and postexposure prophylaxis (see the ACIP recommendations[111]). Usually, an immunization series is initiated and completed with one vaccine product. No clinical studies have been conducted that documented a change in efficacy or the frequency of adverse reactions when the series is completed with a second vaccine product.

For adults, rabies vaccination always should be administered in the deltoid area. For children, the anterolateral aspect of the thigh also is acceptable. The gluteal area never should be used for HDCV, RVA, or PCEC injections because administration of HDCV in this area results in lower neutralizing antibody titers.[187]

POSTEXPOSURE PROPHYLAXIS (Table 242–15). The essential components of rabies postexposure prophylaxis are

TABLE 242–15 ■ RABIES POSTEXPOSURE PROPHYLAXIS FOR INDIVIDUALS NOT PREVIOUSLY IMMUNIZED

Animal Type	Evaluation and Disposition of the Animal	Postexposure Prophylaxis Recommendations
Wild		
Skunk Fox Raccon Most other carnivores Bat	Regard as rabid unless animal proven negative by laboratory tests*	Consider immediate vaccination
Domestic		
Dog Cat Ferret	Healthy and available for 10 days' observation	Persons should not begin prophylaxis unless clinical signs of rabies develop in the animal†
	Rabid or suspected rabid	Immediately vaccinate
	Escaped (unknown)	Consult public health officials
Other		
Livestock Small rodents Large rodents (woodchucks and beavers) Lagomorphs (rabbit and hare) Other mammals	Consider individually	Consult public health officials. Bites of squirrels, hamsters, guinea pigs, gerbils, chipmunks, rats, mice, other small rodents, rabbits, and hares almost never require antirabies prophylaxis

*The animal should be euthanized and tested as soon as possible. Holding for observation is not recommended. Discontinue vaccine if immunofluorescence test results of the animal are negative.
†During the 10-day observation period, begin postexposure prophylaxis at the first sign of rabies in a dog, cat, or ferret that has bitten someone. If the animal exhibits clinical signs of rabies, it should be euthanized immediately and tested.
Adapted from Centers for Disease Control and Prevention: Human rabies prevention—United States, 1999. Recommendations of the Advisory Committee on Immunization Practices (ACIP). M. M. W. R. Recomm. Rep. *48*(RR-1):1–21, 1999.

wound treatment and, for previously unvaccinated persons, administration of both rabies immune globulin (RIG) and vaccine.[111] Recommendations for the management of persons with possible exposure to rabies include meticulous attention to thorough cleansing of the wound with soap and water. The decision to give rabies immunoprophylaxis depends on the circumstances precipitating the exposure, the species and condition of the animal inflicting the wound, and the prevalence of rabies in local animal populations. Bites or nonbite exposure, including scratches, abrasions, open wounds, or mucous membranes contaminated with saliva, are considered significant. Because the need for preventive measures is based on these specific circumstances, including the risk of rabies in the area, the local department of health should be consulted promptly concerning the necessity for initiating postexposure prophylaxis.

A combination of active and passive immunization is indicated for the treatment of all bites and all nonbite exposures inflicted by animals suspected or proven to be rabid. When possible, the brains of wild animals (skunks, foxes, coyotes, raccoons, and bats), stray dogs or cats, or symptomatic animals implicated in an exposure should be examined in certified laboratories for evidence of rabies. Immunization always should be initiated promptly and discontinued only if laboratory results are negative. Individuals exposed to healthy dogs or cats that are available for observation do not require immediate prophylactic treatment. Implicated healthy domestic dogs or cats should be quarantined and observed for at least 10 days. If symptoms develop that suggest rabies, the exposed individual should begin postexposure prophylaxis, and the brain of the animal should be examined. An unknown (i.e., escaped) animal must be regarded as potentially rabid.

Studies conducted in the United States by the CDC have documented that a regimen of one dose of RIG and five doses of rabies vaccine during a 28-day period was safe and induced an excellent antibody response in all recipients.[37] RIG provides rapid, passive immunity that persists for only a short time (half-life of approximately 21 days). The recommended dose of human RIG is 20 IU/kg body weight. If anatomically feasible, the full dose of RIG should be infiltrated thoroughly in the area around and into the wounds. Any remaining volume should be injected intramuscularly at a site distant from that of vaccine administration. RIG is unnecessary and should not be administered to previously vaccinated persons because an amnestic response will occur after the administration of a booster regardless of the antibody titer.[111]

Once initiated, rabies prophylaxis should not be interrupted or discontinued because of local or mild systemic adverse reactions to rabies vaccine. Usually, such reactions can be successfully managed with anti-inflammatory and antipyretic agents such as ibuprofen or acetaminophen. When a person with a history of having had serious hypersensitivity to rabies vaccine must be revaccinated, antihistamines can be administered. Epinephrine should be readily available to counteract any anaphylactic reactions, and the person should be observed carefully immediately after receiving vaccination.

PRE-EXPOSURE PROPHYLAXIS. Active immunization should be considered for high-risk groups (i.e., veterinarians, animal handlers and control officers, selected laboratory workers, persons visiting countries where rabies is hyperendemic, and persons whose pursuits may involve frequent contact with rabid animals, such as spelunkers). Persons whose risk of exposure is less but whose access to immediate competent medical care is restricted also should be considered for pre-exposure prophylaxis. The primary series consists of 3 doses at 0, 7, and 28 days given intramuscularly in the deltoid area. The primary series also may be given intradermally and consists of three doses at 0, 7, and 28 days administered in the area over the deltoid (lateral aspect of the upper part of the arm). RVA and PCEC vaccines should not be given by the intradermal route. Routine post-vaccination serologic testing for antirabies antibody after the administration of pre-exposure prophylaxis is necessary only for those suspected to be immunosuppressed. In circumstances of continued exposure, however, booster doses of rabies vaccine or serologic testing should be performed.[111]

In patients who have received adequate pre-exposure prophylaxis, postexposure prophylaxis consists of two doses of HDCV given 3 days apart. RIG is not recommended in these circumstances. Serum for antibody testing should be obtained from persons whose prophylaxis history or immune status is uncertain, and the course of postexposure active and passive immunoprophylaxis as described for nonimmune individuals should be initiated immediately. If serologic testing demonstrates adequate antirabies antibody, postexposure prophylaxis may be discontinued.

TYPHOID VACCINE

Typhoid fever remains a serious public health problem throughout the world, with an estimated incidence of 33 million cases and 500,000 deaths annually. In contrast, the incidence of the disease in the United States is low. Most reported cases occur in travelers to developing countries.[83] Hence, the primary indication for typhoid vaccination in this country is foreign travel. However, in developing countries without safe water and sanitation for the control of diarrheal diseases, mass immunization is potentially effective in the control of typhoid fever.

Preparations

Two vaccines are available in the United States.[83, 215] A parenteral heat-phenol–inactivated vaccine that had been used widely for many years is no longer available. Two new typhoid vaccines that provide significant protection without causing adverse reactions have been licensed in many countries.[266] Ty21a, an oral live attenuated vaccine consisting of a stable mutant, Ty21a, developed by chemical mutagenesis of a pathogenic *Salmonella typhi* strain, was licensed in the United States in 1991. A parenteral vaccine containing the purified Vi (virulence) polysaccharide capsular antigen of *S. typhi* was licensed in 1994.

Efficacy

Although field trials have demonstrated the efficacy of each vaccine, no comparative studies have been performed, and their efficacy in children younger than 5 years or for travelers to countries with endemic disease has not been determined.[83] Furthermore, no vaccine approaches 100 percent efficacy, and vaccine immunity can be overcome by a large inoculum of *S. typhi*. For the heat-phenol–inactivated vaccine, efficacy has been 51 to 77 percent. In trials of the Ty21a vaccine, efficacy has ranged from 42 to 96 percent after administration of the initial series of three doses, with the lower efficacies seen in trials from areas with highly endemic disease.[266, 345] The efficacy of the capsular polysaccharide vaccine (ViCPS) in clinical trials was 72 percent at 17 months and 64 percent at 21 months after administration of a single dose.[266] Additional doses of ViCPS fail to boost antibody titers. The duration of protection ranges from 2 years for ViCPS to 5 years for the oral Ty21a vaccine. Recommendations for booster doses for those whose primary immunization was with oral vaccines have not been determined. Booster doses are recommended for recipients of the parenteral vaccines.

Adverse Events

Reactions to the oral Ty21a vaccine are mild, consist of only fever or headache, and occur in less than 5 percent of recipients. Reactions to the ViCPS vaccine are also infrequent occurrences; erythema and induration at the injection site have been reported in approximately 7 percent of recipients.[83] In contrast, reactions to the inactivated, whole-cell vaccine occur more commonly and are more severe and include fever in as many as 24 percent of recipients, headache, and severe local pain or swelling in 3 to 35 percent of vaccinees. Thirteen to 24 percent of vaccinees subsequently have missed school or work.[266]

Indications[83, 215]

Typhoid vaccination in the United States is recommended only for the following groups:

- Travelers to areas where typhoid fever is endemic and in whom a risk of exposure is likely
- Persons with intimate exposure to a documented *S. typhi* carrier, such as occurs with continuing household contact
- Laboratory workers who have frequent contact with *S. typhi*

Vaccination is not recommended for persons attending summer camp or for those in areas of natural disaster or for control of common-source outbreaks.

In most circumstances, either oral Ty21a or parenteral ViCPS is the preferred vaccine because of the substantially higher rate of adverse reactions with the parenteral inactivated vaccine and similar effectiveness of the three vaccines. Because data on safety and efficacy in young children are not available, the manufacturer currently recommends that Ty21a vaccine not be given to children younger than 6 years. The parenteral heat-phenol–inactivated vaccine is the only vaccine available for children between 6 months and 2 years of age. Doses and schedules for the different typhoid vaccines are given in recommendations of the CDC.[17, 83]

Contraindications

Because the oral vaccine is a live attenuated vaccine, it should not be given to immunocompromised patients, including those with HIV infection.[83] The vaccine manufacturer also advises that Ty21a vaccine should not be administered to persons receiving antimicrobial agents within 24 hours. The only contraindication to receiving vaccination with either ViCPS or parenteral inactivated vaccine is a history of having severe local or systemic reactions after receiving a previous dose.

YELLOW FEVER VACCINE

An estimated 200,000 cases of yellow fever occur each year in South America and Africa.[289] As a result, yellow fever is an important vaccine-preventable disease among travelers to areas where yellow fever occurs on these continents. In 1996 and 1999, two U.S. and two European unvaccinated travelers to areas where yellow fever is endemic died of yellow fever viral infection.[118, 277] The risk of unvaccinated travelers acquiring yellow fever probably is increasing because potential zones of transmission of yellow fever are expanding to include urban areas with large populations of susceptible humans and abundant competent mosquito vectors. Vaccination is the most effective preventive measure against yellow fever, a disease that has no specific treatment and may cause death in 20 percent of patients.[289]

Preparations

Derived from the original 17D yellow fever vaccine strain, the live attenuated 17D-204 and 17DD yellow fever strains are the yellow fever vaccines most commonly used.[289] The 17D-204 yellow fever vaccine, which is prepared in chick embryos, is licensed in the United States.[135] Primary immunization consists of a single, subcutaneous injection of reconstituted, freeze-dried vaccine for both adults and children.

Immunogenicity and Efficacy

Seroconversion rates of 93 percent have been documented in young children receiving yellow fever vaccine.[386] Immunity acquired from immunization with the 17D strain virus has been demonstrated to persist for more than 10 years.[73, 329, 382] Revaccination is required no more frequently than every 10 years.[329]

Adverse Events

The 17D-204 and 17DD yellow fever vaccines are among the safest and most effective viral vaccines.[289] Since 1965, approximately 8 million doses of 17D-derived yellow fever vaccine have been administered to U.S. travelers, and approximately 300 million doses have been administered to persons in areas where yellow fever is endemic. Although 2 to 5 percent of persons who receive vaccine report headaches, myalgia, and low-grade fever 5 to 10 days after vaccination, less than 1 percent report curtailing their usual activities. Serious adverse events associated with yellow fever vaccine rarely occur. Historically, the most common has been post-vaccination encephalitis, which occurs primarily in young infants. Since 1965, post–yellow fever vaccination encephalitis has been reported in only one U.S. resident older than 9 months.[289] Anaphylaxis also has been reported to occur after vaccination.

From 1996 to 2001, seven cases of febrile multiple–organ system failure associated with 17D-derived yellow fever vaccination were reported.[124] All seven persons became ill within 2 to 5 days of vaccination and required intensive care; six died. None had documented immunodeficiency, and all were in their usual state of health before receiving the vaccination. Illness was characterized by fever, lymphocytopenia, thrombocytopenia, mild to moderate elevation of hepatocellular enzymes, hypotension with poor tissue perfusion, and respiratory failure. Most patients also had headache, vomiting, myalgias, hyperbilirubinemia, and renal failure requiring hemodialysis. Additional cases associated with 17DD yellow fever vaccine have occurred, including two individuals 5 and 22 years of age.

In assessing the risk for development of serious adverse events after yellow fever vaccination, the ACIP concluded that a causal association between multiple–organ system failure and 17DD yellow fever vaccination was supported by histopathologic studies of cases in which evidence of yellow fever virus was found in tissue specimens and the onset of symptoms was associated temporally with recent receipt of yellow fever vaccine. As a result, the CDC has instituted enhanced surveillance for adverse effects potentially related to yellow fever vaccine.

Indications

Yellow fever vaccine is recommended for persons 9 months or older traveling to or residing in areas where yellow fever is endemic. Because of the increased risk for neurologic complications, infants 4 to 8 months of age should be considered for vaccination only when travel to high-risk areas is required and high-level protection against mosquito exposure is not feasible. Vaccination for international travel is required. To obtain an international certificate of vaccination, a yellow fever vaccine approved by the WHO and administered at a designated yellow fever vaccine center is required. Yellow fever vaccine centers in the United States can be identified by contacting state or local health departments. The International Health Regulations require revaccination at intervals of 10 years. Revaccination may boost antibody titers; however, evidence from several studies suggests that yellow fever immunity persists for at least 30 to 35 years and probably for life.[135]

Precautions and Contraindications

Infants younger than 4 months should not receive yellow fever vaccine because of the increased risk of encephalitis developing in this age group.[5] Those between 4 and 9 months of age also should not be vaccinated unless considered necessary because of an immediate risk of disease.[135]

No adverse effects of yellow fever vaccine on the developing fetus have been demonstrated. Vaccine administration to pregnant women, however, generally is not indicated because the vaccine is a live virus. Pregnant women should be considered for vaccination only when travel to high-risk areas is required and protection against mosquito exposure is not feasible.

Yellow fever vaccine poses a theoretic risk to patients with altered immunity as a result of underlying disease or immunosuppressive therapy. These patients should not be vaccinated. If travel to an epidemic or endemic area is necessary, the patient should be instructed in ways to avoid mosquitoes and given a vaccine waiver letter.

Persons with a history of systemic anaphylaxis to eggs should not be vaccinated because the vaccines contain egg proteins and on rare occasion may induce immediate allergic reactions. Less severe or local manifestations of allergy to eggs or to feathers are not contraindications to yellow fever vaccine administration and do not warrant vaccine skin testing.[3] If international quarantine regulations are the only reason to immunize a patient known to be hypersensitive to eggs, attempts should be made to obtain a waiver. If immunization of an individual with a questionable history of egg hypersensitivity is considered essential because of a high risk of exposure, an intradermal skin test may be given as directed in the vaccine package insert.[73]

Vaccines Related to Bioterrorism

Two vaccines exist that are potentially available to protect children against bioterrorist microbiologic agents, specifically, *Bacillus anthracis* and variola. Both anthrax and smallpox vaccines are not available commercially at this time and do not have indications for children and adolescents in the absence of a bioterrorist attack. The vaccines are reviewed in the relevant disease-specific chapters.

Investigational Vaccines

Routine immunizations for children have virtually eliminated many infectious diseases from the United States.

These successes have encouraged research to develop vaccines to prevent other serious viral and bacterial diseases affecting children. A 1985 report by the IOM of the National Academy of Sciences reviewed the benefits that would be associated with the development and use of new and improved vaccines in the United States.[156] The report listed 14 diseases for which vaccines were possible. A 1999 study by the IOM notes that considerable progress has been made since the 1985 study.[157] Seven of 14 vaccines listed in the 1985 study as domestic priorities for development are now licensed. They include an acellular pertussis vaccine and vaccines against hepatitis A and B, Hib, varicella zoster, rotavirus, and pneumococcus.

The 1999 IOM report uses a new quantitative model to compare the cost and health benefits of developing candidate vaccines.[157] This model can be used to evaluate the potential impact of a new vaccine on public health. In the 1999 report, the model was used to evaluate diseases for which candidate vaccines were being developed. The report divided 26 candidate vaccines into four groups, from most to least favorable for development. The four vaccines in the top tier include a cytomegalovirus vaccine given to adolescents, a universal influenza vaccine, a group B streptococcus vaccine for high-risk adults and pregnant women, and a *S. pneumoniae* vaccine for infants and seniors. Other diseases for which vaccines would be desirable include *Chlamydia trachomatis,* enterotoxigenic *Escherichia coli,* Epstein-Barr virus, *Helicobacter pylori,* hepatitis C virus, herpes simplex virus, human papillomavirus, *M. tuberculosis, Neisseria gonorrhoeae,* respiratory syncytial virus, parainfluenza virus, *Shigella*, and groups A and B streptococcus.

Advances in biotechnology, increased understanding of the virulence factors of infectious agents, and knowledge of the host immune response have led to an explosion in the number of new approaches being used to develop vaccines.[179] The three general categories of approaches include live vaccines; killed, inactivated, or subunit vaccines; and most recently, DNA-based vaccines. In addition, new enabling technologies such as adjuvants or delivery systems and vectors can be applied to these approaches. Vaccines are being developed by the application of these vaccine technologies to a number of infectious agents for which vaccines are not currently available. Candidate vaccines are in human trials for many of the pathogens listed in the 1999 IOM report.

REFERENCES

1. Alter, M. J., Hadler, S. C., Margolis, H. S., et al.: The changing epidemiology of hepatitis B in the United States. J. A. M. A. *263*:1218–1222, 1990.
2. Ambrosch, F., Wiedermann, G., Crooy, P., et al.: Immunogenicity and side-effects of a new tetravalent meningococcal polysaccharide vaccine. Bull. World Health Organ. *61*:317–323, 1983.
3. American Academy of Pediatrics: Active immunization. *In* Pickering, L. K. (ed.): 2000 Red Book: Report of the Committee on Infectious Diseases. 25th ed. Elk Grove Village, IL, American Academy of Pediatrics, 2000, pp. 6–41.
4. American Academy of Pediatrics: Immunizations in special clinical circumstances. *In* Pickering, L. K. (ed.): 2000 Red Book: Report of the Committee on Infectious Diseases. 25th ed. Elk Grove Village, IL, American Academy of Pediatrics, 2000, pp. 54–81.
5. American Academy of Pediatrics: Arboviruses. *In* Pickering, L. K. (ed.): 2000 Red Book: Report of the Committee on Infectious Diseases. 25th ed. Elk Grove Village, IL, American Academy of Pediatrics, 2000, pp. 170–175.
6. American Academy of Pediatrics: Diphtheria. *In* Pickering, L. K. (ed.): 2000 Red Book: Report of the Committee on Infectious Diseases. 25th ed. Elk Grove Village, IL, American Academy of Pediatrics, 2000, pp. 230–232.
7. American Academy of Pediatrics: *Haemophilus influenzae* infections. *In* Pickering, L. K. (ed.): 2000 Red Book: Report of the Committee on Infectious Diseases. 25th ed. Elk Grove Village, IL, American Academy of Pediatrics, 2000, pp. 262–272.
8. American Academy of Pediatrics: Hepatitis A. *In* Pickering, L. K. (ed.): 2000 Red Book: Report of the Committee on Infectious Diseases. 25th ed. Elk Grove Village, IL, American Academy of Pediatrics, 2000, pp. 280–289.
9. American Academy of Pediatrics: Hepatitis B. *In* Pickering, L. K. (ed.): 2000 Red Book: Report of the Committee on Infectious Diseases. 25th ed. Elk Grove Village, IL, American Academy of Pediatrics, 2000, pp. 289–302.
10. American Academy of Pediatrics: Influenza. *In* Pickering, L. K. (ed.): 2000 Red Book: Report of the Committee on Infectious Diseases. 25th ed. Elk Grove Village, IL, American Academy of Pediatrics, 2000, pp. 351–359.
11. American Academy of Pediatrics: Measles. *In* Pickering, L. K. (ed.): 2000 Redbook: Report of the Committee on Infectious Diseases. 25th ed. Elk Grove Village, IL, American Academy of Pediatrics, 2000, pp. 385–396.
12. American Academy of Pediatrics: Mumps. *In* Pickering, L. K. (ed.): 2000 Redbook: Report of the Committee on Infectious Diseases. 25th ed. Elk Grove Village, IL, American Academy of Pediatrics, 2000, pp. 405–408.
13. American Academy of Pediatrics: Pertussis. *In* Pickering, L. K. (ed.): 2000 Red Book: Report of the Committee on Infectious Diseases. 25th ed. Elk Grove Village, IL, American Academy of Pediatrics, 2000, pp. 435–448.
14. American Academy of Pediatrics: Pneumococcal infections. *In* Pickering, L. K. (ed.): 2000 Red Book: Report of the Committee on Infectious Diseases. 25th ed. Elk Grove Village, IL, American Academy of Pediatrics, 2000, pp. 452–460.
15. American Academy of Pediatrics: Poliovirus infections. *In* Pickering, L. K. (ed.): 2000 Red Book: Report of the Committee on Infectious Diseases. 25th ed. Elk Grove Village, IL, American Academy of Pediatrics, 2000, pp. 465–470.
16. American Academy of Pediatrics: Rubella. *In* Pickering, L. K. (ed.): 2000 Redbook: Report of the Committee on Infectious Diseases. 25th ed. Elk Grove Village, IL, American Academy of Pediatrics, 2000, pp. 495–500.
17. American Academy of Pediatrics: *Salmonella* infections. *In* Pickering, L. K. (ed.): 2000 Red Book: Report of the Committee on Infectious Diseases. 25th ed. Elk Grove Village, IL, American Academy of Pediatrics, 2000, pp. 501–506.
18. American Academy of Pediatrics: Tetanus. *In* Pickering, L. K. (ed.): 2000 Red Book: Report of the Committee on Infectious Diseases. 25th ed. Elk Grove Village, IL, American Academy of Pediatrics, 2000, pp. 563–568.
19. American Academy of Pediatrics: Tuberculosis. *In* Pickering, L. K. (ed.): 2000 Red Book: Report of the Committee on Infectious Diseases. 25th ed. Elk Grove Village, IL, American Academy of Pediatrics, 2000, pp. 593–613.
20. American Academy of Pediatrics Committee on Infectious Diseases: Measles: Reassessment of the current immunization policy. Pediatrics *84*:1110–1113, 1989.
21. American Academy of Pediatrics Committee on Infectious Diseases: Universal hepatitis B immunization. Pediatrics *89*:795–800, 1992.
22. American Academy of Pediatrics Committee on Infectious Diseases: *Haemophilus influenzae* type B conjugate vaccines: Recommendations for immunization with recently and previously licensed vaccines. Pediatrics *92*:480–488, 1993.
23. American Academy of Pediatrics Committee on Infectious Diseases: Update on timing of hepatitis B vaccination for premature infants and for children with lapsed immunization. American Academy of Pediatrics Committee on Infectious Diseases. Pediatrics *94*:403–404, 1994.
24. American Academy of Pediatrics Committee on Infectious Diseases: The relationship between pertussis vaccine and central nervous system sequelae: Continuing assessment. Pediatrics *97*:279–281, 1996.
25. American Academy of Pediatrics Committee on Infectious Diseases: Meningococcal disease prevention and control strategies for practice-based physicians. Pediatrics *97*:404–411, 1996.
26. American Academy of Pediatrics Committee on Infectious Diseases: Prevention of hepatitis A infections: Guidelines for use of hepatitis A vaccine and immune globulin. American Academy of Pediatrics Committee on Infectious Diseases. Pediatrics *98*:1207–1215, 1996.
27. American Academy of Pediatrics Committee on Infectious Diseases: Acellular pertussis vaccine: Recommendations for use as the initial series in infants and children. American Academy of Pediatrics Committee on Infectious Diseases. Pediatrics *99*:282–288, 1997.
28. American Academy of Pediatrics Committee on Infectious Diseases: Poliomyelitis prevention: Revised recommendations for use of inactivated and live oral poliovirus vaccines. American Academy of Pediatrics Committee on Infectious Diseases. Pediatrics *103*:171–172, 1999.
29. American Academy of Pediatrics Committee on Infectious Diseases: Combination vaccines for childhood immunization: Recommendations of the Advisory Committee on Immunization Practices (ACIP), the American Academy of Pediatrics (AAP), and the American Academy of Family Physicians (AAFP). Pediatrics *103*:1064–1077, 1999.
30. American Academy of Pediatrics Committee on Infectious Diseases: Prevention of poliomyelitis: Recommendations for use of only inactivated poliovirus vaccine for routine immunization. Pediatrics *104*:1404–1406, 1999.
31. American Academy of Pediatrics Committee on Infectious Diseases: Varicella vaccine update. Pediatrics *105*:136–141, 2000.

32. American Academy of Pediatrics Committee on Infectious Diseases: Recommendations for the prevention of pneumococcal infections, including the use of pneumococcal conjugate vaccine (Prevnar), pneumococcal polysaccharide vaccine, and antimicrobial prophylaxis. Pediatrics *106*:362–366, 2000.
33. American Academy of Pediatrics Committee on Infectious Diseases: Meningococcal disease prevention and control strategies for practice-based physicians (Addendum: Recommendations for college students). Pediatrics *106*:1500–1504, 2000.
34. American Academy of Pediatrics Committee on Infectious Diseases and Committee on Pediatric AIDS: Measles immunization in HIV-infected children. American Academy of Pediatrics. Committee on Infectious Diseases and Committee on Pediatric AIDS. Pediatrics *103*:1057–1060, 1999.
35. Ammann, A. J., Addiego, J., Wara, D. W., et al.: Polyvalent pneumococcal-polysaccharide immunization of patients with sickle-cell anemia and patients with splenectomy. N. Engl. J. Med. *297*:897–900, 1977.
36. Anderson, E. L., Decker, M. D., Englund, J. A., et al.: Interchangeability of conjugated *Haemophilus influenzae* type b vaccines in infants. J. A. M. A. *273*:849–853, 1995.
37. Anderson, L. J., Sikes, R. K., Langkop, C. W., et al.: Postexposure trial of a human diploid cell strain rabies vaccine. J. Infect. Dis. *142*:133–138, 1980.
38. Arbeter, A. M., Starr, S. E., and Plotkin, S. A.: Varicella vaccine studies in healthy children and adults. Pediatrics *78*(Suppl):748–756, 1986.
39. Armand, J., Arminjon, F., Mynard, M. C., et al.: Tetravalent meningococcal polysaccharide vaccine groups A,C,Y,W135: Clinical and serological evaluation. J. Biol. Stand. *10*:335–339, 1982.
40. Arpadi, S. M., Markowitz, L. E., Baughman, A. L., et al.: Measles antibody in vaccinated human immunodeficiency virus type 1–infected children. Pediatrics *97*:653–657, 1996.
41. Asano, Y., Nagai, T., Miyata, T., et al.: Long-term protective immunity of recipients of the OKA strain of live varicella vaccine. Pediatrics *75*:667–671, 1985.
42. Asano, Y., Nakayama, H., Yazaki, T., et al.: Protection against varicella in family contacts by immediate inoculation with varicella vaccine. Pediatrics *59*:3–7, 1977.
43. Ascherio, A., Zhang, S., Hernan, M., et al.: Hepatitis B vaccination and the risk of multiple sclerosis. N. Engl. J. Med. *344*:327–332, 2001.
44. Barbour, M. L.: Conjugate vaccines and the carriage of *Haemophilus influenzae* type b. Emerg. Infect. Dis. *2*:176–182, 1996.
45. Barlow, W., Davis, R., Glasser, J., et al.: The risk of seizures after receipt of whole-cell pertussis or measles, mumps, and rubella vaccine. N. Engl. J. Med. *345*:656–661, 2001.
46. Beeler, J., Varricchio, F., and Wise, R.: Thrombocytopenia after immunization with measles vaccines: Review of the vaccine adverse events reporting system (1990 to 1994). Pediatr. Infect. Dis. J. *15*:88–90, 1996.
47. Bell, B.: Hepatitis A vaccine. Semin. Pediatr. Infect. Dis. *13*:165–173, 2002.
48. Bellini, W., Rota, J., Greer, P., et al.: Measles vaccination death in a child with severe combined immunodeficiency: Report of a case. Abstract. Lab. Invest. *66*:91, 1992.
49. Belshe, R. B., Gruber, W. C., Mendelman, P. M., et al.: Efficacy of vaccination with live attenuated, cold-adapted, trivalent, intranasal influenza virus vaccine against a variant (A/Sydney) not contained in the vaccine. J. Pediatr. *136*:168–175, 2000.
50. Belshe, R. B., Mendelman, P. M., Treanor, J., et al.: The efficacy of live attenuated, cold-adapted, trivalent, intranasal influenzavirus vaccine in children. N. Engl. J. Med. *338*:1405–1412, 1998.
51. Bernstein, H. H., Rothstein, E. P., Watson, B. M., et al.: Clinical survey of natural varicella compared with breakthrough varicella after immunization with live attenuated Oka/Merck varicella vaccine. Pediatrics *92*:833–837, 1993.
52. Bewley, K., Schwab, J., Ballanco, G., et al.: Interchangeability of *Haemophilus influenzae* type b vaccines in the primary series: Evaluation of a two-dose mixed regimen. Pediatrics *98*:898–904, 1996.
53. Black, S. B., Shinefield, H. R., Fireman, B., et al.: Efficacy in infancy of oligosaccharide conjugate *Haemophilus influenzae* type b (HbOC) vaccine in a U.S. population of 61,080 children. Pediatr. Infect. Dis. J. *10*:97–104, 1991.
54. Black, S., Shinefield, H., Fireman, B., et al.: Efficacy, safety and immunogenicity of heptavalent pneumococcal conjugate vaccine in children. Pediatr. Infect. Dis. J. *19*:187–195, 2000.
55. Bloch, A. B., Orenstein, W. A., Stetler, H. C., et al.: Health impact of measles vaccination in the United States. Pediatrics *76*:524–532, 1985.
56. Blom, L., Nystrom, L., and Dahlquist, G.: The Swedish childhood diabetes study. Vaccinations and infections as risk determinants for diabetes in childhood. Diabetologia *34*:176–181, 1991.
57. Booy, R., Moxon, E. R., Macfarlane, J. A., et al.: Efficacy of *Haemophilus influenzae* type b conjugate vaccine in Oxford region. Lancet *340*:847, 1992.
58. Bower, H.: New research demolishes link between MMR vaccine and autism. B. M. J. *318*:1643, 1999.
59. Breiman, R. F., Butler, J. C., Tenover, F. C., et al.: Emergence of drug-resistant pneumococcal infections in the United States. J. A. M. A. *271*:1831–1835, 1994.
60. Briss, P. A., Fehrs, L. J., Parker, R. A., et al.: Sustained transmission of mumps in a highly vaccinated population: Assessment of primary vaccine failure and waning vaccine-induced immunity. J. Infect. Dis. *169*:77–82, 1994.
61. Bruce, M., Rosenstein, N., Capparella, J., et al.: Risk factors for meningococcal disease in college students. J. A. M. A. *286*:688–693, 2001.
62. Brunell, P., and Argaw, T.: Chickenpox attributable to a vaccine virus contracted from a vaccinee with zoster. Pediatrics *106*:E28, 2000.
63. Bryan, J., Henry, C., Hoffman, A., et al.: Randomized, cross-over, controlled comparison of two inactivated hepatitis A vaccines. Vaccine *19*:743–750, 2000.
64. Butler, J. C., Breiman, R. F., Campbell, J. F., et al.: Pneumococcal polysaccharide vaccine efficacy. An evaluation of current recommendations. J. A. M. A. *270*:1826–1831, 1993.
65. Centers for Disease Control and Prevention: Poliomyelitis prevention: Recommendations of the Immunization Practices Advisory Committee (ACIP). M. M. W. R. Morb. Mortal. Wkly. Rep. *31*:22–26, 31–34, 1982.
66. Centers for Disease Control and Prevention: Subacute sclerosing panencephalitis surveillance—United States. M. M. W. R. Morb. Mortal. Wkly. Rep. *31*(43):585–588, 1982.
67. Centers for Disease Control and Prevention: Systemic allergic reactions following immunization with human diploid cell rabies vaccine. M. M. W. R. Morb. Mortal. Wkly. Rep. *33*(14):185–187, 1984.
68. Centers for Disease Control and Prevention: Cholera vaccine. M. M. W. R. Morb. Mortal. Wkly. Rep. *37*(40):617–624, 1988.
69. Centers for Disease Control and Prevention: Measles prevention. M.M.W.R. *38*(Suppl. 9):1–18, 1989.
70. Centers for Disease Control and Prevention: Pneumococcal polysaccharide vaccine. M. M. W. R. Morb. Mortal. Wkly. Rep. *38*(5):64–68, 73–76, 1989.
71. Centers for Disease Control and Prevention: Rubella vaccination during pregnancy—United States, 1971–1988. M. M. W. R. Morb. Mortal. Wkly. Rep. *38*(17):289–293, 1989.
72. Centers for Disease Control and Prevention: Tetanus—United States, 1987 and 1988. M. M. W. R. Morb. Mortal. Wkly. Rep. *39*(3):37–41, 1990.
73. Centers for Disease Control and Prevention: Yellow fever vaccine: Recommendations of the Immunization Practices Advisory Committee (ACIP). M. M. W. R. Recomm. Rep. *39*(RR-6):1–6, 1990
74. Centers for Disease Control and Prevention: *Haemophilus* b conjugate vaccines for prevention of *Haemophilus influenzae* type b disease among infants and children two months of age and older: Recommendations of the Immunization Practices Advisory Committee (ACIP). M. M. W. R. Recomm. Rep. *40*(RR-1):1–7, 1991.
75. Centers for Disease Control and Prevention: Rabies prevention—United States, 1991. Recommendations of the Immunization Practices Advisory Committee (ACIP). M. M. W. R. Recomm. Rep. *40*(RR-3):1–19, 1991.
76. Centers for Disease Control and Prevention: Diphtheria, tetanus, and pertussis: Recommendations for vaccine use and other preventive measures: Recommendations of the Immunization Practices Advisory Committee (ACIP). M. M. W. R. Recomm. Rep. *40*(RR-10):1–28, 1991.
77. Centers for Disease Control and Prevention: Hepatitis B virus: A comprehensive strategy for eliminating transmission in the U.S. through universal childhood vaccination: Recommendations of the Immunization Practices Advisory Committee (ACIP). M. M. W. R. Recomm. Rep. *40*(RR-13):1–25, 1991.
78. Centers for Disease Control and Prevention: Change in source of information: Availability of varicella vaccine for children with acute lymphocytic leukemia. M. M. W. R. Morb. Mortal. Wkly. Rep. *42*(25):499, 1993.
79. Centers for Disease Control and Prevention: Inactivated Japanese encephalitis virus vaccine. Recommendations of the Advisory Committee on Immunization Practices (ACIP). M. M. W. R. Recomm. Rep. *42*(RR-1):1–15, 1993.
80. Centers for Disease Control and Prevention: Recommendations for use of *Haemophilus influenzae* b conjugate vaccines and a combined diphtheria, tetanus, pertussis, and *Haemophilus* b vaccine. Recommendations of the Advisory Committee on Immunization Practices (ACIP). M. M. W. R. Recomm. Rep. *42*(RR-13):1–15, 1993.
81. Centers for Disease Control and Prevention: Progress toward the global elimination of neonatal tetanus, 1989–1993. M. M. W. R. Morb. Mortal. Wkly. Rep. *43*(48):885–887, 893–894, 1994.
82. Centers for Disease Control and Prevention: 1994 Revised classification system for human immunodeficiency virus infection in children less than 13 years of age. M. M. W. R. Recomm. Rep. *43*(RR-12):1–10, 1994.
83. Centers for Disease Control and Prevention: Typhoid immunization: Recommendations of the Advisory Committee on Immunization Practices (ACIP). M. M. W. R. Recomm. Rep. *43*(RR-14):1–7, 1994.
84. Centers for Disease Control and Prevention: Health Information for International Travel. Washington, D.C., U.S. Government Printing Office, 1995.
85. Centers for Disease Control and Prevention: Cholera associated with food transported from El Salvador—Indiana, 1994. M. M. W. R. Morb. Mortal. Wkly. Rep. *44*(20):385–386, 1995.
86. Centers for Disease Control and Prevention: Pertussis—United States, January 1992–June 1995. M. M. W. R. Morb. Mortal. Wkly. Rep. *44*(28):525–529, 1995.

87. Centers for Disease Control and Prevention: Update: Recommendations to prevent hepatitis B virus transmission—United States. M. M. W. R. Morb. Mortal. Wkly. Rep. *44*(30):574–575, 1995.
88. Centers for Disease Control and Prevention: Pertussis vaccination: Acellular pertussis vaccine for reinforcing and booster use—supplementary ACIP statement. Recommendations of the Immunization Practices Advisory Committee (ACIP). M. M. W. R. Recomm. Rep. *41*(RR-1):1–10, 1995.
89. Centers for Disease Control and Prevention: Recommended childhood immunization schedule—United States, 1995. M. M. W. R. Recomm. Rep. *44*(RR-5):1–9, 1995.
90. Centers for Disease Control and Prevention: Measles pneumonitis following measles-mumps-rubella vaccination of a patient with HIV infection, 1993. M. M. W. R. Morb. Mortal. Wkly. Rep. *45*(28):603–606, 1996.
91. Centers for Disease Control and Prevention: The role of BCG vaccine in the prevention and control of tuberculosis in the United States: A joint statement by the Advisory Council for the Elimination of Tuberculosis and the Advisory Committee on Immunization Practices. M. M. W. R. Recomm. Rep. *45*(RR-4):1–18, 1996.
92. Centers for Disease Control and Prevention: Prevention of varicella: Recommendations of the Advisory Committee on Immunization Practices (ACIP). M. M. W. R. Recomm. Rep. *45*(RR-11):1–36, 1996.
93. Centers for Disease Control and Prevention: Update: Vaccine side effects, adverse reactions, contraindications, and precautions. Recommendations of the Advisory Committee on Immunization Practices (ACIP). M. M. W. R. Recomm. Rep. *45*(RR-12):1–35, 1996.
94. Centers for Disease Control and Prevention: Immunization of adolescents: Recommendations of the Advisory Committee on Immunization Practices, the American Academy of Pediatrics, the American Academy of Family Physicians and the American Medical Association. M. M. W. R. Recomm. Rep. *45*(RR-13):1–16, 1996.
95. Centers for Disease Control and Prevention: Immunization of adolescents: Recommendations of the Advisory Committee on Immunization Practices, the American Academy of Pediatrics, the American Academy of Family Physicians, and the American Medical Association. American Academy of Pediatrics Committee on Infectious Diseases. Pediatrics *99*(3):479–488, 1997.
96. Centers for Disease Control and Prevention: Status report on the Childhood Immunization Initiative: Reported cases of selected vaccine-preventable diseases—United States, 1996. M. M. W. R. Morb. Mortal. Wkly. Rep. *46*(29):665–671, 1997.
97. Centers for Disease Control and Prevention: Poliomyelitis prevention in the United States: Introduction of a sequential vaccination schedule of inactivated poliovirus vaccine followed by oral poliovirus vaccine. Recommendations of the Advisory Committee on Immunization Practices (ACIP). M. M. W. R. Recomm. Rep. *46*(RR-3):1–25, 1997.
98. Centers for Disease Control and Prevention: Control and prevention of meningococcal disease: Recommendations of the Advisory Committee on Immunization Practices (ACIP). M. M. W. R. Recomm. Rep. *46*(RR-5): 1–10, 1997.
99. Centers for Disease Control and Prevention: Pertussis vaccination: Use of acellular pertussis vaccines among infants and young children: Recommendations of the Advisory Committee on Immunization Practices (ACIP). M. M. W. R. Recomm. Rep. *46*(RR-7):1–25, 1997.
100. Centers for Disease Control and Prevention: Human rabies—Texas and New Jersey, 1997. M. M. W. R. Morb. Mortal. Wkly. Rep. *47*(1):1–5, 1998.
101. Centers for Disease Control and Prevention: Varicella-related deaths among children—United States, 1997. M. M. W. R. Morb. Mortal. Wkly. Rep. *47*(18):365–368, 1998.
102. Centers for Disease Control and Prevention: Effectiveness of a seventh grade school entry vaccination requirement–statewide and Orange County, Florida, 1997–1998. M. M. W. R. Morb. Mortal. Wkly. Rep. *47*(34):711–715, 1998.
103. Centers for Disease Control and Prevention: Progress toward eliminating *Haemophilus influenzae* type b disease among infants and children—United States, 1987–1997. M. M. W. R. Morb. Mortal. Wkly. Rep. *47*(46):993–998, 1998.
104. Centers for Disease Control and Prevention: Impact of the sequential IPV/OPV schedule on vaccination coverage levels—United States, 1997. M. M. W. R. Morb. Mortal. Wkly. Rep. *47*(47):1017–1019, 1998.
105. Centers for Disease Control and Prevention: Unlicensed use of combination of *Haemophilus influenzae* type b conjugate vaccine and diphtheria and tetanus toxoid and acellular pertussis vaccine for infants. M. M. W. R. Morb. Mortal. Wkly. Rep. *47*:787, 1998.
106. Centers for Disease Control and Prevention: Measles, mumps, and rubella—vaccine use and strategies for elimination of measles, rubella, and congenital rubella syndrome and control of mumps: Recommendations of the Immunization Practices Advisory Committee (ACIP). M. M. W. R. Recomm. Rep. *47*(RR-8):1–57, 1998.
107. Centers for Disease Control and Prevention: Recommended childhood immunization schedule—United States, 1999. M. M. W. R. Morb. Mortal. Wkly. Rep. *48*(1):12–16, 1999.
108. Centers for Disease Control and Prevention: Update: Recommendations to prevent hepatitis B virus transmission—United States. M. M. W. R. Morb. Mortal. Wkly. Rep. *48*(2):33–34, 1999.
109. Centers for Disease Control and Prevention: Progress Toward Global Poliomyelitis Eradication—1997–1998. M. M. W. R. Morb. Mortal. Wkly. Rep. *48*(20):416–421, 1999.
110. Centers for Disease Control and Prevention: Recommendations of the Advisory Committee on Immunization Practices: Revised recommendations for routine poliomyelitis vaccination. M. M. W. R. Morb. Mortal. Wkly. Rep. *48*(27):590, 1999.
111. Centers for Disease Control and Prevention: Human rabies prevention—United States, 1999. Recommendations of the Advisory Committee on Immunization Practices (ACIP). M. M. W. R. Recomm. Rep. *48*(RR-1):1–21, 1999.
112. Centers for Disease Control and Prevention: Combination vaccines for childhood immunization. M. M. W. R. Recomm. Rep. *48*(RR-5):1–14, 1999.
113. Centers for Disease Control and Prevention: Prevention of varicella: Updated recommendations of the Advisory Committee on Immunization Practices (ACIP). M. M. W. R. Recomm. Rep. *48*(RR-6):1–5, 1999.
114. Centers for Disease Control and Prevention: Prevention of hepatitis A through active or passive immunization: Recommendations of the Immunization Practices Advisory Committee (ACIP). M. M. W. R. Recomm. Rep. *48*(RR-12):1–37, 1999.
115. Centers for Disease Control and Prevention: Notice to readers: Recommended childhood immunization schedule—United States, 2000. M. M. W. R. Morb. Mortal. Wkly. Rep. *49*(2):35–38, 47, 2000.
116. Centers for Disease Control and Prevention: Rubella among Hispanic adults—Kansas 1998, and Nebraska 1999. M. M. W. R. Morb. Mortal. Wkly. Rep. *49*(11):225–228, 2000.
117. Centers for Disease Control and Prevention: Notice to readers: Alternate two-dose hepatitis b vaccination schedule for adolescents aged 11–15 years. M. M. W. R. Morb. Mortal. Wkly. Rep. *49*(12):261, 2000.
118. Centers for Disease Control and Prevention: Fatal yellow fever in a traveler returning from Venezuela, 1999. M. M. W. R. Morb. Mortal. Wkly. Rep. *49*(14):303–305, 2000.
119. Centers for Disease Control and Prevention: Update: Expanded availability of thimerosal preservative-free hepatitis B vaccine. M. M. W. R. Morb. Mortal. Wkly. Rep. *49*(28):642, 651, 2000.
120. Centers for Disease Control and Prevention: Prevention and control of meningococcal disease and meningococcal disease and college students: Recommendations of the Advisory Committee on Immunization Practices (ACIP). M. M. W. R. Recomm. Rep. *49*(RR-7):1–20, 2000.
121. Centers for Disease Control and Prevention: Preventing pneumococcal disease among infants and young children: Recommendations of the Advisory Committee on Immunization Practices (ACIP). M. M. W. R. Recomm. Rep. *49*(RR-9):1–35, 2000.
122. Centers for Disease Control and Prevention: Use of diphtheria toxoid–tetanus toxoid–acellular pertussis vaccine as a five-dose series: Supplemental recommendations of the Advisory Committee on Immunization Practices (ACIP). M. M. W. R. Recomm. Rep. *49*(RR-13):1–8, 2000.
123. Centers for Disease Control and Prevention: National, state and urban vaccination coverage levels among children aged 19–35 months—U.S., 2000. M. M. W. R. Morb. Mortal. Wkly. Rep. *50*(30):637–641, 2001.
124. Centers for Disease Control and Prevention: Notice to readers: Fever, jaundice, and multiple organ system failure associated with 17D-derived yellow fever vaccination, 1996–2001. M. M. W. R. Morb. Mortal. Wkly. Rep. *50*(30):643–645, 2001.
125. Centers for Disease Control and Prevention: Simultaneous administration of varicella vaccine and other recommended childhood vaccines—United States, 1995–1999. M. M. W. R. Morb. Mortal. Wkly. Rep. *50*(47):1058–1061, 2001.
126. Centers for Disease Control and Prevention: Notice to readers: Revised ACIP recommendation for avoiding pregnancy after receiving a rubella-containing vaccine. M. M. W. R. Morb. Mortal. Wkly. Rep. *50*(49):1117, 2001.
127. Centers for Disease Control and Prevention: Rubella Outbreak–Arkansas, 1999. M. M. W. R. Morb. Mortal. Wkly. Rep. *50*(50):1137–1139, 2001.
128. Centers for Disease Control and Prevention: Summary of notifiable diseases, United States. M. M. W. R. Morb. Mortal. Wkly. Rep. *48*(53):1–104, 2001.
129. Centers for Disease Control and Prevention: Prevention and control of influenza: Recommendations of the Advisory Committee on Immunization Practices (ACIP). M. M. W. R. Recomm. Rep. *50*(RR-4):1–44, 2001.
130. Centers for Disease Control and Prevention: Control and prevention of rubella: Evaluation and management of suspected outbreaks, rubella in pregnant women, and surveillance for congenital rubella syndrome. M. M. W. R. Recomm. Rep. *50*(RR-12):1–23, 2001.
131. Centers for Disease Control and Prevention: Notice to readers: Recommended childhood immunization schedule—United States, 2002. M. M. W. R. Morb. Mortal. Wkly. Rep. *51*(2):31–33, 2002.
132. Centers for Disease Control and Prevention: Pertussis—United States, 1997–2000. M. M. W. R. Morb. Mortal. Wkly. Rep. *51*(4):73–76, 2002.
133. Centers for Disease Control and Prevention: Measles—United States, 2000. M. M. W. R. Morb. Mortal. Wkly. Rep. *51*(6):120–123, 2002.

134. Centers for Disease Control and Prevention: General recommendations on immunization. Recommendations of the Advisory Committee on Immunization Practices (ACIP) and the American Academy of Family Physicians (AAFP). M. M. W. R. Recomm. Rep. *51*(RR-2):1–35, 2002.
135. Centers for Disease Control and Prevention: Yellow fever vaccine: Recommendations of the Immunization Practices Advisory Committee (ACIP). M. M. W. R. Recomm. Rep. *51*(RR-17):1–11, 2002.
136. Chaiken, B. P., Williams, N. M., Preblud, S. R., et al.: The effect of a school entry law on mumps activity in a school district. J. A. M. A. *257*:2455–2458, 1987.
137. Chang, M. H., Chen, C. J., Lai, M. S., et al.: Universal hepatitis B vaccination in Taiwan and the incidence of hepatocellular carcinoma in children. Taiwan Childhood Hepatoma Study Group. N. Engl. J. Med. *336*:1855–1859, 1997.
138. Cheek, J. E., Baron, R., Atlas, H., et al.: Mumps outbreak in a highly vaccinated school population: Evidence for large-scale vaccine failure. Arch. Pediatr. Adolesc. Med. *149*:774–778, 1995.
139. Chen, R. T., Glasser, J. W., Rhodes, P. H., et al.: Vaccine Safety Datalink project: A new tool for improving vaccine safety monitoring in the United States. The Vaccine Safety Datalink Team. Pediatrics *99*:765–773, 1997.
140. Chen, R. T., Moses, J. M., Markowitz, L. E., et al.: Adverse events following measles-mumps-rubella and measles vaccinations in college students. Vaccine *9*:297–299, 1991.
141. Chen, R. T., Rastogi, S. C., Mullen, J. R., et al.: The Vaccine Adverse Event Reporting System (VAERS). Vaccine *12*:542–550, 1994.
142. Cherry, J. D., Brunell, P. A., Golden, G. S., et al.: Report of the task force on pertussis and pertussis immunization—1988. Pediatrics *81*:939–977, 1988.
143. Christenson, B., and Bottiger, M.: Measles antibody: Comparison of long-term vaccination titres, early vaccination titres and naturally acquired immunity to and booster effects on the measles virus. Vaccine *12*:129–133, 1994.
144. Chu, S. Y., Bernier, R. H., Stewart, J. A., et al.: Rubella antibody persistence after immunization. J. A. M. A. *259*:3133–3136, 1988.
145. Ciofi degli Atti, M. L., and Olin, P.: Severe adverse events in the Italian and Stockholm I pertussis vaccine clinical trials. Dev. Biol. Stand. *89*:77–81, 1997.
146. Classen, D., and Classen, J.: The timing of pediatric immunization and the risk of insulin-dependent diabetes mellitus. Infect. Dis. Clin. Pract. *6*:449–454, 1997.
147. Clements, D., Langdon, L., Bland, C., et al.: Influenza A vaccine decreases the incidence of otitis media in 6- to 30-month-old children in day care. Arch. Pediatr. Adolesc. Med. *149*:1113–1117, 1995.
148. Clements, D., Zaref, J., Bland, C., et al.: Partial uptake of varicella vaccine and the epidemiological effect on varicella disease in 11 day-care centers in North Carolina. Arch. Pediatr. Adolesc. Med. *155*:455–461, 2001.
149. Clements, D. A., Moreira, S. P., Coplan, P. M., et al.: Postlicensure study of varicella vaccine effectiveness in a day-care setting. Pediatr. Infect. Dis. J. *18*:1047–1050, 1999.
150. Clements, M., and Stephens, I.: New and improved vaccines against influenza. *In* Levine, M., Woodrow, G., Kaper, J., and Cobon, G., (ed.): New Generation Vaccines. 2nd ed. New York, Marcel Dekker, 1997, pp. 545–570.
151. Cochi, S. L., Broome, C. V., and Hightower, M. S.: Immunization of US children with *Haemophilus influenzae* type b polysaccharide vaccine. J. A. M. A. *253*:521–529, 1985.
152. Cochi, S. L., Preblud, S. R., and Orenstein, W. A.: Perspectives on the relative resurgence of mumps in the United States. Am. J. Dis. Child. *142*:499–507, 1988.
153. Cody, C. L., Baraff, L. J., Cherry, J. D., et al.: Nature and rates of adverse reactions associated with DTP and DT immunizations in infants and children. Pediatrics *68*:650–660, 1981.
154. Cohn, M. L., Robinson, E. D., Faerber, M., et al.: Measles vaccine failures: Lack of sustained measles-specific immunoglobulin G responses in revaccinated adolescents and young adults. Pediatr. Infect. Dis. J. *13*:34–38, 1994.
155. Colditz, G., Berkey, C., Mosteller, F., et al.: The efficacy of bacillus Calmette-Guérin vaccination of newborns and infants in the prevention of tuberculosis: Meta-analyses of the published literature. Pediatrics *96*:29–35, 1995.
156. Committee on Issues and Priorities for New Vaccine Development: New Vaccine Development: Establishing Priorities. Washington, D.C., National Academy Press, 1985.
157. Committee on Issues and Priorities for New Vaccine Development: Vaccines for the 21st Century: A Tool for Decisionmaking. Washington, D.C., National Academy Press, 1999.
158. Confavreux, C., Suissa, S., Saddier, P., et al.: Vaccinations and the risk of relapse in multiple sclerosis. N. Engl. J. Med. *344*:319–326, 2001.
159. Crossley, K., Irving, P., Warren, J. B., et al.: Tetanus and diphtheria immunization in urban Minnesota adults. J. A. M. A. *242*:2298–2300, 1979.
160. Dagan, R., Eskola, J., Leclerc, C., et al.: Reduced response to multiple vaccines sharing common protein epitopes that are administered simultaneously to infants. Infect. Immun. *66*:2093–2098, 1998.
161. Dagan, R., Melamed, R., Muallem, M., et al.: Reduction of nasopharyngeal carriage of pneumococci during the second year of life by a heptavalent conjugate pneumococcal vaccine. J. Infect. Dis. *174*:1271–1278, 1996.
162. Dagan, R., Muallem, M., Melamed, R., et al.: Reduction of pneumococcal nasopharyngeal carriage in early infancy after immunization with tetravalent pneumococcal vaccines conjugated to either tetanus toxoid or diphtheria toxoid. Pediatr. Infect. Dis. J. *16*:1060–1064, 1997.
163. Dales, L., Hammer, S., and Smith, N.: Time trends in autism and in MMR immunization coverage in California. J. A. M. A. *285*:1183–1185, 2001.
164. Danovaro-Holliday, M., LeBaron, C., Allensworth, C., et al.: A large rubella outbreak with spread from the workplace to the community. J. A. M. A. *284*:2733–2739, 2000.
165. Davidson, M., Schraer, C. D., Parkinson, A. J., et al.: Invasive pneumococcal disease in an Alaska native population, 1980 through 1986. J. A. M. A. *261*:715–718, 1989.
166. Davis, R., Kramarz, P., Bohlke, K., et al.: Measles-mumps-rubella and other measles-containing vaccines do not increase the risk for inflammatory bowel disease: A case-control study from the Vaccine Safety Datalink project. Arch. Pediatr. Adolesc. Med. *155*:354–359, 2001.
167. Decker, M. D., and Edwards, K. M.: Report of the nationwide multicenter acellular pertussis trial. Pediatrics *96*:547–603, 1995.
168. Decker, M. D., Edwards, K. M., Bradley, R., and Palmer, P.: Comparative trial in infants of four conjugate *Haemophilus influenzae* type b vaccines. J. Pediatr. *120*:184–189, 1992.
169. DeStefano, F., and Chen, R. T.: Negative association between MMR and autism. Lancet *353*:1987–1988, 1999.
170. DeStefano, F., and Chen, R. T.: Autism and measles, mumps, and rubella vaccine: No epidemiological evidence for a causal association. J. Pediatr. *136*:125–126, 2000.
171. D'Hondt, E.: Possible approaches to develop vaccines against hepatitis A. Vaccine *10*(Suppl.):48–52, 1992.
172. Donahue, J., Choo, P., Manson, J., et al.: The incidence of herpes zoster. Arch. Intern. Med. *155*:1605–1609, 1995.
173. Dreesen, D., Fishbein, D., Kemp, D., et al.: Two-year comparative trial on the immunogenicity and adverse effects of purified chick embryo cell rabies vaccine for pre-exposure immunization. Vaccine *7*:397–400, 1989.
174. Duvriendt, J., Staroukine, M. M., Costy, F., et al.: Fatal encephalitis apparently due to rabies: Occurrence after treatment with human diploid cell vaccine but not rabies immune globulin. J. A. M. A. *248*:2304–2306, 1982.
175. Edmonson, M., Davis, J., Hopfensperger, D., et al.: Measles vaccination during the respiratory virus season and risk of vaccine failure. Pediatrics *98*:905–910, 1996.
176. Edsall, G., Elliott, M. W., Peebles, T. C., et al.: Excessive use of tetanus toxoid boosters. J. A. M. A. *202*:17–19, 1967.
177. Edwards, K. M., and Decker, M. D.: Acellular pertussis vaccines for infants. N. Engl. J. Med. *334*:391–392, 1996.
178. Edwards, K., and Decker, M.: Combination vaccines consisting of acellular pertussis vaccines. Pediatr. Infect. Dis. J. *16*(Suppl.):97–102, 1997.
179. Ellis, R.: New technologies for making vaccines. *In* Plotkin, S., and Orenstein, W., (eds.): Vaccines. 3rd ed. Philadelphia, W. B. Saunders, 1999.
180. Enders, G., Miller, E., Cradock-Watson, J., et al.: Consequences of varicella and herpes zoster in pregnancy: Prospective study of 1739 cases. Lancet *343*:1547–1550, 1994.
181. Englund, J. A., Suarez, C. S., Kelly, J., et al.: Placebo-controlled trial of varicella vaccine given with or after measles-mumps-rubella vaccine. J. Pediatr. *114*:37–44, 1989.
182. Eskola, J., and Anttila, M.: Pneumococcal conjugate vaccines. Pediatr. Infect. Dis. J. *18*:543–551, 1999.
183. Eskola, J., Kilpi, T., Palmli, A., et al.: Efficacy of a pneumococcal conjugate vaccine against otitis media. N. Engl. J. Med. *344*:430–439, 2001.
184. Evans, G., and Marcuse, E. K.: Vaccine Injury Compensation Program update. Rep. Pediatr. Infect. Dis. *4*:22–23, 1994.
185. Feldman, S., and Lott, L.: Varicella in children with cancer: Impact of antiviral therapy and prophylaxis. Pediatrics *80*:465–472, 1987.
186. Fine, P. E. M., and Clarkson, J. A.: Reflections on the efficacy of pertussis vaccine. Rev. Infect. Dis. *9*:866–883, 1987.
187. Fishbein, D. B., Sawyer, L. A., Reid-Sanden, F. L., et al.: Administration of human diploid-cell rabies vaccine in the gluteal area. Letter. N. Engl. J. Med. *318*:124–125, 1988.
188. Fishbein, D. B., Yenne, K. M., Dreesen, D. W., et al.: Risk factors for systemic hypersensitivity reactions after booster vaccinations with human diploid cell rabies vaccine: A nationwide prospective study. Vaccine *11*:1390–1394, 1993.
189. Freed, G. L., Katz, S. L., and Clark, S. J.: Safety of vaccinations. Miss America, the media, and public health. J. A. M. A. *276*:1869–1872, 1996.
190. Galazka, A. M., and Robertson, S. E.: Diphtheria: Changing patterns in the developing world and the industrial world. Eur. J. Epidemiol. *11*:107–117, 1995.
191. Galazka, A. M., Robertson, S. E., and Oblapenko, G. P.: Resurgence of diphtheria. Eur. J. Epidemiol. *11*:95–105, 1995.

192. Gergen, P. J., McQuillan, G. M., Kiely, M., et al.: A population-based serologic survey of immunity to tetanus in the United States. N. Engl. J. Med. *332*:761–766, 1995.
193. Gershon, A. A., and LaRussa, P. S.: Varicella vaccine. Pediatr. Infect. Dis. J. *17*:248–249, 1998.
194. Gershon, A. A., Steinberg, S. P., LaRussa, P., et al.: Immunization of healthy adults with live attenuated varicella vaccine. J. Infect. Dis. *158*:132–137, 1988.
195. Giebink, G. S.: Preventing pneumococcal disease in children: Recommendations for using pneumococcal vaccine. Pediatr. Infect. Dis. *4*:343–348, 1985.
196. Giebink, G. S., Le, C. T., and Schiffman, G.: Decline of serum antibody in splenectomized children after vaccination with pneumococcal capsular polysaccharides. J. Pediatr. *105*:576–582, 1984.
197. Gillberg, C., and Heijbel, H.: MMR and autism. Autism *2*:423–424, 1998.
198. Glezen, W., Six, H., Frank, A., et al.: Impact of epidemics upon communities and families. *In* Kendal, A., and Patriaca, P., (eds.): Options for the Control of Influenza. New York, Alan R. Liss, 1986, pp. 63–73.
199. Glezen, W. P.: Consideration of the risk of influenza in children and indications for prophylaxis. Rev. Infect. Dis. *2*:408–420, 1980.
200. Global Advisory Group Expanded Program on Immunization World Health Organization: Achieving the major disease control goals. Wkly. Epidemiol. Rec. *69*:29–31, 34–35, 1994.
201. Gold, R., Lepow, M. L., Goldschneider, I., et al.: Kinetics of antibody production to group A and group C meningococcal polysaccharide vaccines administered during the first six years of life: Prospects for routine immunization of infants and children. J. Infect. Dis. *140*: 690–697, 1979.
202. Greco, D., Salmaso, S., Mastrantonio, P., et al.: A controlled trial of two acellular vaccines and one whole-cell vaccine against pertussis. N. Engl. J. Med. *334*:341–348, 1996.
203. Greenberg, D., Lieberman, J., Marcy, S., et al.: Enhanced antibody responses in infants given different sequences of heterogenous *Haemophilus influenzae* type b conjugate vaccines. J. Pediatr. *126*:206–211, 1995.
204. Greenberg, M. A., and Birx, D. L.: Safe administration of mumps-measles-rubella vaccine in egg-allergic children. J. Pediatr. *113*:504–506, 1988.
205. Groothuis, J. R., Levin, M. J., Lehr, M. V., et al.: Immune response to split-product influenza vaccine in preterm and full-term young children. Vaccine *10*:221–225, 1992.
206. Groothuis, J. R., Levin, M. J., Rabalais, G. P., et al.: Immunization of high-risk infants younger than 18 months of age with split-product influenza vaccine. Pediatrics *87*:823–828, 1991.
207. Gross, P. A., Lee, H., Wolff, J. A., et al.: Influenza immunization in immunosuppressed children. J. Pediatr. *92*:30–35, 1978.
208. Guess, H. A., Broughton, D. D., Melton, L. J., 3rd, and Kurland, L. T.: Population-based studies of varicella complications. Pediatrics *78*(Suppl.):723–727, 1986
209. Gupta, R. K., Griffin, P. J., Xu, J., et al.: Diphtheria antitoxin levels in US blood and plasma donors. J. Infect. Dis. *173*:1493–1497, 1996.
210. Gustafson, T. L., Lievens, A. W., Brunnell, P. A., et al.: Measles outbreak in a "fully immunized" secondary school population. N. Engl. J. Med. *316*:771–774, 1987.
211. Gustafsson, L., Hallander, H. O., Olin, P., et al.: A controlled trial of a two-component acellular, a five-component acellular, and a whole-cell pertussis vaccine. N. Engl. J. Med. *334*:349–355, 1996.
212. Hadler, S. C., and Margolis, H. S.: Hepatitis B immunization: Vaccine types, efficacy, and indications. Curr. Clin. Top. Infect. Dis. *12*:282–308, 1992.
213. Hadler, S. C., and McFarland, L.: Hepatitis in day care centers: Epidemiology and prevention. Rev. Infect. Dis. *8*:548–557, 1986.
214. Hall, A. J., and Greenwood, B. M.: Modern vaccines: Practice in developing countries. Lancet *335*:774–777, 1990.
215. Hall, C. B.: A single shot at *Salmonella typhi*: A new typhoid vaccine with pediatric advantages. Pediatrics *96*:348–350, 1995.
216. Hall, C. B., and Douglas, R. G., Jr.: Nosocomial influenza infection as a cause of intercurrent fevers in infants. Pediatrics *55*:673–677, 1975.
217. Halsey, N., Hyman, S., Conference Writing Panel: Measles-mumps-rubella vaccine and autistic spectrum disorder: Report from the New Challenges in Childhood Immunizations Conference Convened in Oak Brook, Illinois, June 12–13, 2000. Pediatrics *107*:e84, 2001.
218. Hammerschlag, M., Gershon, A., Steinberg, S., et al.: Herpes zoster in an adult recipient of live attenuated varicella vaccine. J. Infect. Dis. *160*:535–537, 1989.
219. Hardy, I. R. B., Dittmann, S., and Sutter, R. W.: Current situation and control strategies for resurgence of diphtheria in newly independent states of the former Soviet Union. Lancet *347*:1739–1744, 1996.
220. Harrison, L., Pass, M., Mendelsohn, A., et al.: Invasive meningococcal disease in adolescents and young adults. J. A. M. A. *286*:694–699, 2001.
221. Harrison, L. H., Dwyer, D. M., Maples, C. T., et al.: Risk of meningococcal infection in college students. J. A. M. A. *281*:1906–1910, 1999.
222. Hart, P. D. A., Sutherland, I., and Thomas, J.: The immunity conferred by effective BCG and vole bacillus vaccines, in relation to individual variations in induced tuberculin sensitivity and to technical variations in the vaccines. Tubercle *48*:201–210, 1967.
223. Heikkinen, T., Ruuskanen, O., Waris, M., et al.: Influenza vaccination in the prevention of acute otitis media in children. Am. J. Dis. Child. *145*:445–448, 1991.
224. Herman, J. J., Radin, R., and Schneiderman, R.: Allergic reactions to measles (rubeola) vaccine in patients hypersensitive to egg protein. J. Pediatr. *102*:196–199, 1983.
225. Hersh, B. S., Fine, P. E. M., Kent, W. K., et al.: Mumps outbreak in a highly vaccinated population. J. Pediatr. *119*:187–193, 1991.
226. Hetherington, S., and Lepow, M. L.: Epidemiology and immunology of *Hemophilus influenzae* type b infections in childhood: Implications for chemoprophylaxis and immunization. Adv. Pediatr. Infect. Dis. *2*:1–18, 1987.
227. Hinman, A. R., and Koplan, J. P.: Pertussis and pertussis vaccine: Reanalysis of benefits, risks and costs. J. A. M. A. *251*:3109–3113, 1984.
228. Hoke, C., Nisalak, A., Sangawhipa, N., et al.: Protection against Japanese encephalitis by inactivated vaccines. N. Engl. J. Med. *319*:608–614, 1988.
229. Howson, C. P., Katz, M., Johnston, R. B., Jr., et al.: Chronic arthritis after rubella vaccination. Clin. Infect. Dis. *15*:307–312, 1992.
230. Hsu, T. C., Chow, L. P., Wei, H. Y., et al.: A completed field trial for an evaluation of the effectiveness of mouse-brain Japanese vaccine. *In* McDHammon, W., Kitaoka, M., and Downs, W. G., (eds.): Immunization for Japanese encephalitis. Amsterdam, Excerpta Medica, 1972, pp. 285–291.
231. Ildirim, I., Hacimustafaoglu, M., and Ediz, B.: Correlation of tuberculin induration with the number of Bacillus Calmette-Guérin vaccines. Pediatr. Infect. Dis. J. *14*:1060–1063, 1995.
232. Innis, B. L., Snitbhan, R., Kunasol, P., et al.: Protection against hepatitis A by an inactivated vaccine. J. A. M. A. *271*:1328–1334, 1994.
233. Institute of Medicine: Diphtheria and tetanus toxoids. *In* Stratton, K. R., Howe, C. J., Johnston, R. B., Jr., (eds.): Adverse Events Associated with Childhood Vaccines. Washington, D.C., National Academy Press, 1994, pp. 67–117.
234. Institute of Medicine: Measles and Mumps Vaccine. *In* Stratton, K. R., Howe, C. J., Johnston, R. B., Jr., (eds.): Adverse Events Associated with Childhood Vaccines. Washington, D.C., National Academy Press, 1994, pp. 118–186.
235. Institute of Medicine, Immunization Safety Review Committee: Immunization Safety Review: Measles-Mumps-Rubella Vaccine and Autism. Washington, D.C., National Academy Press, 2001.
236. Institute of Medicine, Immunization Safety Review Committee: Immunization Safety Review: Thimerosal-Containing Vaccines and Neurodevelopmental Disorders. Washington, D.C., National Academy Press, 2001.
237. Institute of Medicine, Immunization Safety Review Committee: Immunization Safety Review: Multiple Immunizations and Immune Dysfunction. Washington, D.C., National Academy Press, 2002.
238. Ipp, M. M., Gold, R., Goldbach, M., et al.: Adverse reactions to diphtheria, tetanus, pertussis-polio vaccination at 18 months of age: Effect of injection site and needle length. Pediatrics *83*:679–682, 1989.
239. Izurieta, H. S., Strebel, P. M., Blake, P. A.: Postlicensure effectiveness of varicella vaccine during an outbreak in a childcare center. J. A. M. A. *278*:1495–1499, 1997,
240. Jackson, L. A., Stewart, L. K., Solomon, S. L., et al.: Risk of infection with hepatitis A, B or C, cytomegalovirus, varicella or measles among child care providers. Pediatr. Infect. Dis. J. *15*:584–589, 1996,
241. Jacobs, R. L., Lowe, R. S., and Lanier, B. Q.: Adverse reactions to tetanus toxoid. J. A. M. A. *247*:40–42, 1982.
242. James, J. M., Burks, A. W., Roberson, P. K., et al.: Safe administration of the measles vaccine to children allergic to eggs. N. Engl. J. Med. *332*:1262–1266, 1995.
243. Jefferson, T., and Demicheli, V.: No evidence that vaccines cause insulin dependent diabetes mellitus. J. Epidemiol. Community Health *52*:674–675, 1998.
244. Johnson, C. E., Stancin, T., Fattlar, D., et al.: A long-term prospective study of varicella vaccine in healthy children. Pediatrics *100*:761–766, 1997.
245. Kanra, G., Yalcin, S., Ceyhan, M., et al.: Clinical trial to evaluate immunogenicity and safety of inactivated hepatitis A vaccination starting a 2-month-old children. Turk. J. Pediatr. *42*:105–108, 2000.
246. Kaplan, S. L.: *Streptococcus pneumoniae:* Impact of antibiotic resistance in pediatrics. Curr. Probl. Pediatr. *27*:187–195, 1997.
247. Karvonen, M., Cepaitis, Z., and Tuomilehto, J.: Association between type 1 diabetes and *Haemophilus influenzae* type b vaccination: Birth cohort study. B. M. J. *318*:1169–1172, 1999.
248. Käyhty, H., Karanko, V., Peltolta, H., et al.: Serum antibodies to capsular polysaccharide vaccine of group A *Neisseria meningitidis* followed for three years in infants and children. J. Infect. Dis. *142*:861–868, 1980.
249. Kelso, J. M., Jones, R. T., and Yunginger, J. W.: Anaphylaxis to measles, mumps, and rubella vaccine mediated by IgE to gelatin. J. Allergy Clin. Immunol. *91*:867–872, 1993.
250. Kemp, A., Van Asperen, P., and Mukhi, A.: Measles immunization in children with clinical reactions to egg protein. Am. J. Dis. Child. *144*:33–35, 1990.

251. Kim-Farley, R., Bart, S., Stetler, H., et al.: Clinical mumps vaccine efficacy. Am. J. Epidemiol. *121*:593–597, 1985.
252. Kinamitsu, M.: A field trial with an improved Japanese encephalitis vaccine in a nonendemic area of disease. Biken J. *13*:313–328, 1970.
253. King, G. E., and Hadler, S. C.: Simultaneous administration of childhood vaccines: An important public health policy that is safe and efficacious. Pediatr. Infect. Dis. J. *13*:394–407, 1994.
254. Koff, R. S.: Seroepidemiology of hepatitis A in the United States. J. Infect. Dis. *171*(Suppl.):19–23, 1995.
255. Konradsen, H. B., Pedersen, F. K., and Henrichsen, J.: Pneumococcal revaccination of splenectomized children. Pediatr. Infect. Dis. J. *9*:258–263, 1990.
256. Krause, P. R., and Klinman, D. M.: Varicella vaccination: Evidence for frequent reactivation of the vaccine strain in healthy children. Nat. Med. *6*:451–454, 2000.
257. Kröger, L., Korppi, M., Brander, E., et al.: Osteitis caused by bacille Calmette-Guérin vaccination: A retrospective analysis of 222 cases. J. Infect. Dis. *172*:574–576, 1995.
258. Krugman, S.: Further attenuated measles vaccine: Characteristics and use. Rev. Infect. Dis. *5*:477–481, 1983.
259. Kuter, B. J., Weibel, R. E., Guess, H. A., et al.: Oka/Merck varicella vaccine in healthy children: Final report of a 2-year efficacy study and 7-year follow-up studies. Vaccine *9*:643–647, 1991.
260. Lange, B., Shapiro, S. A., Waldman, M. T. G., et al.: Antibody responses to influenza immunization of children with acute lymphoblastic leukemia. J. Infect. Dis. *140*:402–406, 1979.
261. LaRussa, P., Steinberg, S., Meurice, F., et al.: Transmission of vaccine strain varicella-zoster virus from a healthy adult with vaccine-associated rash to susceptible household contacts. J. Infect. Dis. *176*:1072–1075, 1997.
262. Lasky, T., Terracciano, G., Magder, L., et al.: Guillain-Barré syndrome and the 1992–1993 and 1993–1994 influenza vaccines. N. Engl. J. Med. *339*:1797–1802, 1998.
263. Lavi, S., Zimmerman, B., Koren, G., et al.: Administration of measles, mumps and rubella virus vaccine (live) to egg-allergic children. J. A. M. A. *263*:269–271, 1990.
264. Lerman, S. J., Bollinger, M., Brunken, J. M.: Clinical and serological evaluation of measles, mumps, and rubella (HPV-77:DE-5 and RA27/3) virus vaccines, singly and in combination. Pediatrics *68*:18–22, 1981.
265. Levin, M., Gershon, A., Weinberg, A., et al.: Immunization of HIV-infected children with varicella vaccine. J. Pediatr. *139*:305–310, 2001.
266. Levine, M. M.: Modern vaccines: Enteric vaccines. Lancet *335*:958–961, 1990.
267. Lieu, T. A., Finkler, L. J., Sorel, M. E., et al.: Cost-effectiveness of varicella serotesting versus presumptive vaccination of school-age children and adolescents. Pediatrics *95*:632–638, 1995.
268. Long, A. P., and Sartwell, P. E.: Tetanus in the U.S. Army in World War II. Bull. U.S. Army Med. Dept. *7*:371–385, 1947.
269. Long, S. S.: Toddler-to-mother transmission of varicella-vaccine virus: How bad is that? J. Pediatrics *131*:10–12, 1997.
270. Lotte, A., Wasz-Hockert, O., Poisson, N., et al.: BCG complications: Estimates of the risks among vaccinated subjects and statistical analysis of their main characteristics. Adv. Tuberc. Res. *21*:107–193, 1984.
271. Maldonado, Y. A., Lawrence, E. C., DeHovitz, R., et al.: Early loss of passive measles antibody in infants of mothers with vaccine-induced immunity. Pediatrics *96*:447–450, 1995.
272. Maple, P. A., Efstratiou, A., George, R. C., et al.: Diphtheria immunity in UK blood donors. Lancet *345*:963–965, 1995.
273. Markowitz, L., Albrecht, P., Orenstein, W., et al.: Persistence of measles antibody after revaccination. J. Infect. Dis. *166*:205–208, 1992.
274. Markowitz, L. E., Albrecht, P., Rhodes, P., et al.: Changing levels of measles antibody titers in women and children in the United States: Impact on response to vaccination. Pediatrics *97*:53–58, 1996.
275. Markowitz, L. E., Preblud, S. R., Fine, P. E., et al.: Duration of live measles vaccine–induced immunity. Pediatr. Infect. Dis. J. *9*:101–110, 1990.
276. Markowitz, L. E., Preblud, S. R., Orenstein, W. A., et al.: Patterns of transmission in measles outbreaks in the United States, 1985–1986. N. Engl. J. Med. *320*:75–81, 1989.
277. Martin, M., Tsai, T., Cropp, B., et al.: Fever and multi-system organ failure associated with 17D-204 yellow fever vaccination: A report of four cases. Lancet *358*:98–104, 2001.
278. Mathias, R. G., Meekison, W. G., Arcand, T. A., et al.: The role of secondary vaccine failures in measles outbreaks. Am. J. Public Health *79*:475–478, 1989.
279. Mawhinney, H., Allen, I., Beare, J., et al.: Dysgammaglobulinaemia complicated by disseminated measles. B. M. J. *2*:380–381, 1971.
280. McCormick, J. B., Gusmao, H. H., Nakamura, S., et al.: Antibody response to serogroup A and C meningococcal polysaccharide vaccines in infants born of mothers vaccinated during pregnancy. J. Clin. Invest. *65*:1141–1144, 1980.
281. McLaughlin, M., Thomas, P., Onorato, I., et al.: Live virus vaccines in human immunodeficiency virus–infected children: A retrospective survey. Pediatrics *82*:229–233, 1988.
282. Miller, D., Madge, N., Diamond J., et al.: Pertussis immunisation and serious acute neurological illnesses in children. B. M. J. *307*:1171–1176, 1993.
283. Miller, D., Wadsworth, J., Diamond, J., et al.: Pertussis vaccine and whooping cough and risk factors in acute neurological illness and death in young children. Dev. Biol. Stand. *61*:389–394, 1985.
284. Miller E., Hill A., Morgan-Capner P., et al.: Antibodies to measles, mumps and rubella in UK children 4 years after vaccination with different MMR vaccines. Vaccine *13*:799–802, 1995.
285. Miller, L. W., Older, J. J., Drake, J., et al.: Diphtheria immunization. Effect upon carriers and the control of outbreaks. Am. J. Dis. Child. *123*:197–199, 1972.
286. Mitus, A., Holloway, A., Evans, A., et al.: Attenuated measles vaccine in children with acute leukemia. Am. J. Dis. Child. *103*:413–418, 1962.
287. MMR vaccine is not linked to Crohn's disease or autism. Commun. Dis. Rep. C. D. R. Wkly. *8*(13):113, 1998.
288. Monafo, W., Haslam, D., Roberts, R., et al.: Disseminated measles infection following vaccination in a child with a congenital immune deficiency. J. Pediatr. *124*:273–276, 1994.
289. Monath, T.: Yellow fever. *In* Plotkin, S., Orenstein, W., (eds.): Vaccines. 3rd ed. Philadelphia, W. B. Saunders, 1999.
290. Monath, T. P.: Flaviviruses. *In* Fields, B. N., and Knipe, D. M. (eds.): Virology. New York, Raven Press, 1990, pp. 763–814.
291. Morris, D., Montgomery, S., Thompson, N., et al.: Measles vaccine and inflammatory bowel disease: A national British cohort study. Am. J. Gastroenterol. *95*:3507–3512, 2000.
292. Mortimer, E. A., Jr.: Pertussis and pertussis vaccine: 1990. Adv. Pediatr. Infect. Dis. *5*:1–33, 1990.
293. Moxon, E. R., Rappuoli, R.: Modern vaccines: *Haemophilus influenzae* infections and whooping cough. Lancet *335*:1324–1329, 1990.
294. Nkowane, B. M., Bart, K. J., Orenstein, W. A., et al.: Measles outbreak in a vaccinated school population. Epidemiology, strains of transmission and the role of vaccine failures. Am. J. Public Health *77*:434–438, 1987.
295. Noah, D., Drenzek, C., Smith, J., et al.: Epidemiology of human rabies in the United States, 1980 to 1996. Ann. Intern. Med. *128*:922–930, 1998.
296. O'Brien, K., Ruff, A., Louis, M., et al.: Bacillus Calmette-Guérin complications in children born to HIV-1–infected women with a review of the literature. Pediatrics *95*:414–418, 1995.
297. Onorato, I. M., Modlin, J. F., McBean, A. M., et al.: Mucosal immunity induced by enhanced-potency inactivated and oral polio vaccines. J. Infect. Dis. *163*:1–6, 1991.
298. Onorato, I. M., Orenstein, W. A., Hinman, A. R., et al.: Immunization of asymptomatic HIV-infected children with measles vaccine: Assessment of risks and benefits. Med. Decis. Making *9*:76–83, 1989.
299. Onorato, I. M., Wassilak, S. G., and Meade, B.: Efficacy of whole-cell pertussis vaccine in preschool children in the United States. J. A. M. A. *267*:2745–2749, 1992.
300. Orenstein, W. A., Albrecht, P., Herrmann, K. L., et al.: The plaque-neutralization test as a measure of prior exposure to measles virus. J. Infect. Dis. *155*:146–149, 1987.
301. Orenstein, W. A., Bart, K. J., Hinman, H. R., et al.: The opportunity and obligation to eliminate rubella from the United States. J. A. M. A. *251*:1988–1994, 1984.
302. Oya, A.: Japanese encephalitis vaccine. Acta Pediatr. Jpn. *30*:175–184, 1988.
303. Ozanne, G., and d'Halewyn, M.: Secondary immune response in a vaccinated population during a large measles epidemic. Clin. Microbiol. *30*:1778–1782, 1992.
304. Palumbo, P., Hoyt, L., Demasio, K., et al.: Population-based study of measles and measles immunization in human immunodeficiency virus–infected children. Pediatr. Infect. Dis. J. *11*:1008–1014, 1992.
305. Patja, A., Davidkin, I., Kurki, T., et al.: Serious adverse events after measles-mumps-rubella vaccination during a fourteen-year prospective follow-up. Pediatr. Infect. Dis. J. *19*:1127–1134, 2000.
306. Peebles, T. C., Levine, L., Eldred, M. C., et al.: Tetanus toxoid emergency boosters. A reappraisal. N. Engl. J. Med. *280*:575–580, 1969.
307. Peltola, H., and Heinonen, O.: Frequency of true adverse reactions to measles-mumps-rubella vaccine. Lancet *1*:939–942, 1986.
308. Peltola, H., Mäkelä, P. H., Käyhty, H., et al.: Clinical efficacy of meningococcus group A capsular polysaccharide vaccine in children three months to five years of age. N. Engl. J. Med. *297*:686–691, 1977.
309. Peltola, H., Patja, A., Leinikki, P., et al.: No evidence for measles, mumps, and rubella vaccine–associated inflammatory bowel disease or autism in a 14-year prospective study. Letter. Lancet *351*:1327–1328, 1998.
310. Peter, G.: Vaccine crisis: An emerging societal problem. J. Infect. Dis. *151*:981–983, 1985.
311. Petralli, J. K., Merigan, T. C., and Wilbur, J. R.: Action of endogenous interferon against vaccinia infection in children. Lancet *2*:401–405, 1965.
312. Piazza, M., Safary, A., Vegnente, A., et al.: Safety and immunogenicity of hepatitis A vaccine in infants: A candidate for inclusion in the childhood vaccine programme. Vaccine *17*:585–588, 1999.
313. Pichichero, M. E., Edwards, K. M., Anderson, E. L., et al.: Safety and immunogenicity of six acellular pertussis vaccines and one whole-cell

vaccine given as a fifth dose in four- to six-year-old children. Pediatrics *105*:e11, 2000.
314. Plotkin, S., and Cadoz, M.: The acellular pertussis vaccine trials: An interpretation. Pediatr. Infect. Dis. J. *16*:508–517, 1997.
315. Plotkin, S. A.: Inactivated polio vaccine for the United States: A missed vaccination opportunity. Pediatr. Infect. Dis. J. *14*:835–839, 1995.
316. Poland, J. D., Cropp, C. B., Craven, R. B., et al.: Evaluation of the potency and safety of inactivated Japanese encephalitis vaccine in US inhabitants. J. Infect. Dis. *161*:878–882, 1990.
317. Potter, C.: Attenuated influenza virus vaccines. Med. Virol. *4*:279–292, 1994.
318. Ramsey, M., Andrews, N., Kaczmarski, E., et al.: Efficacy of meningococcal serogroup C conjugate vaccine in teenagers and toddlers in England. Lancet *357*:195–196, 2001.
319. Reef, S., Frey, T., Theall, K., et al.: The changing epidemiology of rubella in the 1990s: On the verge of elimination and new challenges for control and prevention. J. A. M. A. *287*:464–472, 2002.
320. Reingold, A. L., Hightower, A. W., Bolan, G. A., et al.: Age-specific differences in duration of clinical protection after vaccination with meningococcal polysaccharide A vaccine. Lancet *2*:114–118, 1985.
321. Rennels, M. B., Deloria, M. A., Pichichero, M. E., et al.: Extensive swelling after booster doses of acellular pertussis-tetanus-diphtheria vaccines. Pediatrics *105*:e12, 2000.
322. Rigau-Perez, J. G., Overturf, G. D., Chan, L. S., et al.: Reactions to booster pneumococcal vaccination in patients with sickle cell disease. J. Pediatr. Infect. Dis. *2*:199–202, 1983.
323. Robbins, J. B., and Schnerson, R.: Polysaccharide-protein conjugates: A new generation of vaccines. J. Infect. Dis. *161*:821–832, 1990.
324. Robinson, J., Lemay, M., and Vaudry, W.: Congenital rubella after anticipated maternal immunity: Two cases and a review of the literature. Pediatr. Infect. Dis. J. *13*:812–815, 1994.
325. Rodier, P. M.: The early origins of autism. Sci. Am. *282*:56–63, 2000.
326. Rodrigues, L., Diwan, V., and Wheeler, J.: Protective effect of BCG against tuberculous meningitis and miliary tuberculosis: A meta-analysis. Int. J. Epidemiol. *22*:1154–1158, 1993.
327. Rosenstein, N. E., Perkins, B. A., Stephens, D. S., et al.: The changing epidemiology of meningococcal disease in the United States, 1992–1996. J. Infect. Dis. *180*:1894–1901, 1999.
328. Rosenstein, N. E., Perkins, B. A., Stephens, D. S., et al.: Meningococcal disease. N. Engl. J. Med. *344*:1378–1388, 2001.
329. Rosenzweig, E. C., Babione, R. W., and Wisseman, C. L., Jr.: Immunological studies with group B arthropod-borne viruses. IV. Persistence of yellow fever antibodies following vaccination with 17D strain yellow fever vaccine. Am. J. Trop. Med. Hyg. *12*:230–235, 1963.
330. Ross, S. C., and Densen, P.: Complement deficiency states and infection: Epidemiology, pathogenesis and consequences of neisserial and other infections in an immune deficiency. Medicine (Baltimore) *63*:243–273, 1984.
331. Ruben, F. L., Hankins, W. A., Zeigler, Z., et al.: Antibody responses to meningococcal polysaccharide vaccine in adults without a spleen. Am. J. Med. *76*:115–121, 1984.
332. Salzman, M., and Garcia, C.: Postexposure varicella vaccination in siblings of children with active varicella. Pediatr. Infect. Dis. J. *17*:256–257, 1998.
333. Salzman, M. B., Sharrar, R. G., Steinberg, S., et al.: Transmission of varicella-vaccine virus from a healthy 12-month-old child to his pregnant mother. J. Pediatr. *131*:151–154, 1997.
334. Santosham, M., Wolff, M., Reid, R., et al.: The efficacy in Navajo infants of a conjugate vaccine consisting of *Haemophilus influenzae* type b polysaccharide and *Neisseria meningitidis* outer-membrane protein complex. N. Engl. J. Med. *324*:1767–1772, 1991.
335. Schaffner, W., Fleet, W. F., Kilroy, A. W., et al.: Polyneuropathy following rubella immunization: A follow-up and review of the problem. Am. J. Dis. Child. *127*:684–688, 1974.
336. Schluter, W., Reef, S., Redd, S., et al.: Changing epidemiology of congenital rubella syndrome in the United States. J. Infect. Dis. *178*:636–641, 1998.
337. Schmitt-Grohe, S., Stehr, K., Cherry, J. D., et al.: Minor adverse events in a comparative efficacy trial in Germany in infants receiving either the Lederle/Takeda acellular pertussis component DTP (DTaP) vaccine, the Lederle whole-cell component DTP (DTP) or DT vaccine. The Pertussis Vaccine Study Group. Dev. Biol. Stand. *89*:113–118, 1997.
338. Seager, C., Moriarity, J., Ngai, A., et al.: Low incidence of adverse experiences after measles or measles-rubella mass revaccination at a college campus. Vaccine *12*:1018–1020, 1994.
339. Seward, J., Watson, B., Peterson, C., et al.: Varicella disease after introduction of varicella vaccine in the United States, 1995–2000. J. A. M. A. *287*:606–611, 2002.
340. Shapiro, E. D., Berg, A. T., Austrian, R., et al.: The protective efficacy of polyvalent pneumococcal polysaccharide vaccine. N. Engl. J. Med. *325*:1453–1460, 1991.
341. Sharrar, R., LaRussa, P., Galea, S., et al.: The postmarketing safety profile of varicella vaccine. Vaccine *19*:916–923, 2000.
342. Shill, M., Baynes, R. D., and Miller, S. D.: Fatal rabies encephalitis despite appropriate post-exposure prophylaxis: A case report. N. Engl. J. Med. *316*:1257–1258, 1987.
343. Shinefield, H., and Black, S.: Efficacy of pneumococcal conjugate vaccines in large scale field trials. Pediatr. Infect. Dis. J. *19*:394–397, 2000.
344. Siber, G. R., Werner, B. G., Halsey, N. A., et al.: Interference of immune globulin with measles and rubella immunization. J. Pediatr. *122*:204–211, 1993.
345. Simanjuntak, C. H., Paleologo, F. P., Punjabi, N. H., et al.: Oral immunisation against typhoid fever in Indonesia with Ty21a vaccine. Lancet *338*:1055–1059, 1991.
346. Spratt, B., and Greenwood, B.: Prevention of pneumococcal disease by vaccination: Does serotype replacement matter? Lancet *356*:1210–1211, 2000.
347. Sprauer, M. A., Markowitz, L. E., Nicholson, J. K., et al.: Response of human immunodeficiency virus–infected adults to measles-rubella vaccination. J. Acquir. Immune Defic. Syndr. *6*:1013–1016, 1993.
348. Steffen, R., Kane, M. A., Shapiro, C. N., et al.: Epidemiology and prevention of hepatitis A in travelers. J. A. M. A. *272*:885–889, 1994.
349. Stone, M., Vannier, A., Storch, S., et al.: Brief report: Meningitis due to iatrogenic BCG infection in two immunocompromised children. N. Engl. J. Med. *333*:561–563, 1995.
350. Stratton, K. R., Howe, C. J., Johnston, R. B., Jr. (eds.): DPT Vaccine and Chronic Nervous System Dysfunction. A New Analysis. Washington, D.C., National Academy Press, 1994
351. Strebel, P. M., Sutter, R. W., Cochi, S. L., et al.: Epidemiology of poliomyelitis in the United States one decade after the last reported case of indigenous wild virus–associated disease. Clin. Infect. Dis. *14*:568–579, 1992.
352. Takahashi, H., Pool, V., Tsail, T., et al.: Adverse events after Japanese encephalitis vaccination: Review of post-marketing surveillance data from Japan and the United States. The VAERS Working Group. Vaccine *18*:2963–2969, 2000.
353. Taunay, A. d. E., Galvao, P. A., deMorais, J. S., et al.: Disease prevention by meningococcal serogroup C polysaccharide vaccine in preschool children: Results after eleven months in Sao Paulo, Brazil. Abstract. Pediatr. Res. *8*:429, 1974.
354. Taylor, B., Miller, E., Farrington, C. P., et al.: Autism and measles, mumps, and rubella vaccine: No epidemiological evidence for a causal association. Lancet *353*:2026–2029, 1999.
355. The National Vaccine Advisory Committee: The measles epidemic. The problems, barriers, and recommendations. J. A. M. A. *266*:1547–1552, 1991.
356. Tozzi, A., Anemona, A., Stefanelli, P., et al.: Reactogenicity and immunogenicity at preschool age of a booster dose of two three-component diphtheria-tetanus-acellular pertussis vaccines in children primed in infancy with acellular vaccines. Pediatrics *107*:e25, 2001.
357. Trial synopses. International Symposium on Pertussis Vaccine Trials, Rome, October 30–November 1, 1995. Rome, Istituto Superiore di Sanità, 1995.
358. Trollfors, B., Taranger, J., Lagergard, T., et al.: A placebo-controlled trial of a pertussis-toxoid vaccine. N. Engl. J. Med. *333*:1045–1050, 1995.
359. Umenai, T., Krzysko, R., Bektimirov, T. A., et al.: Japanese encephalitis: Current worldwide status. Bull. World Health Organ. *63*:625–631, 1985.
360. National Vaccine Advisory Committee: Standards for child and Adolescent Immunization Practices. Pediatrics 2003. In press.
361. Vadheim, C. M., Greenberg, D. P., Partridge, S., et al.: Effectiveness and safety of an *Haemophilus influenzae* type b conjugate vaccine (PRP-T) in young infants. Pediatrics *92*:272–279, 1993.
362. Van Herck, K., and Van Damme, P.: Inactivated hepatitis A vaccine–induced antibodies: Follow-up and estimates of long-term persistence. J. Med. Virol. *63*:1–7, 2001.
363. Vasquez, M., LaRussa, P., Gershon, A., et al.: The effectiveness of varicella vaccine in clinical practice. N. Engl. J. Med. *344*:1007–1009, 2001.
364. Verstraeten, T.: Data presented at the Advisory Committee on Immunization Practices, Centers for Disease Control and Prevention, Atlanta, October 2000.
365. Vessey, S., Chan, C., Kuter, B., et al.: Childhood vaccination against varicella: Persistence of antibody, duration of protection, and vaccine efficacy. J. Pediatr. *139*:297–304, 2001.
366. Vodopija, I., Baklaic, Z., Hauser, P., et al.: Reactivity and immunogenicity of bivalent (AC) and tetravalent (ACW135Y) meningococcal vaccines containing o-acetyl-negative or o-acetyl-positive group C polysaccharide. Infect. Immun. *42*:599–604, 1983.
367. Wagner, G., Lavanchy, D., Darioli, R., et al.: Simultaneous active and passive immunization against hepatitis A studied in a population of travelers. Vaccine *11*:1027–1032, 1993.
368. Wahdan, M. H., Rizk, F., El-Akkad, A. M., et al.: A controlled field trial of a serogroup A meningococcal polysaccharide vaccine. Bull. World Health Organ. *48*:667–673, 1973.
369. Wakefield, A. J., Murch, S. H., Anthony, A., et al.: Ileal-lymphoid-nodular hyperplasia, non-specific colitis, and pervasive developmental disorder in children. Lancet *351*:637–641, 1998.
370. Ward, B., Boulinanne, N., Ratnam, S., et al.: Cellular immunity in measles vaccine failure: Demonstration of measles antigen-specific lymphoproliferative responses despite limited serum antibody production after revaccination. J. Infect. Dis. *172*:1591–1595, 1995.

371. Watson, B., Seward, J., Yang, A., et al.: Postexposure effectiveness of varicella vaccine. Pediatrics *105*:84–88, 2000.
372. Watson, B. M., Piercy, S. A., Plotkin, S. A., et al.: Modified chickenpox in children immunized with the Oka/Merck varicella vaccine. Pediatrics *91*:17–22, 1993.
373. Wattanasri, S., Boonthai, P., and Prasert, T.: Human rabies after late administration of human diploid cell vaccine without hyperimmune serum. Lancet *2*:870, 1982.
374. Weibel, R. E., Buynak, E. B., McLean, A. A., et al.: Persistence of antibody in human subjects for 7 to 10 years following the administration of combined live attenuated measles, mumps and rubella virus vaccines. Proc. Soc. Exp. Biol. Med. *165*:260–263, 1980.
375. Weibel, R. E., Neff, B. J., Kuter, B. J., et al.: Live attenuated varicella vaccine: Efficacy trial in healthy children. N. Engl. J. Med. *310*:1409–1415, 1984.
376. Weibel, R. E., Stokes, J., Jr., Buynak, E. B., et al.: Live attenuated mumps vaccine III. Clinical and serologic aspects in a field evaluation. N. Engl. J. Med. *276*:245–251, 1967.
377. Wenger, J.: Epidemiology of *Haemophilus influenzae* type b disease and impact of *Haemophilus influenzae* type b conjugate vaccines in the United States and Canada. Pediatr. Infect. Dis. J. *17*(Suppl. 9):132–136, 1998.
378. Wenger, J. D., Ward, J. I., and Broome, D. V.: Prevention of *Haemophilus influenzae* type b disease: Vaccines and passive prophylaxis. Curr. Clin. Top. Infect. Dis. *10*:306–339, 1989.
379. Werzberger, A., Mensch, B., Kuter, B., et al.: A controlled trial of a formalin-inactivated hepatitis A vaccine in healthy children. N. Engl. J. Med. *327*:453–457, 1992.
380. White, C. J., Kuter, B. J., Hildebrand, C. S., et al.: Varicella vaccine (VARIVAX) in healthy children and adolescents: Results from 1987–1989 clinical trials. Pediatrics *87*:604–610, 1991.
381. Wise, R., Salive, M., Braun, M., et al.: Postlicensure safety surveillance for varicella vaccine. J. A. M. A. *284*:1271–1279, 2000.
382. Wisseman, C. L., Jr., and Sweet B. H.: Immunological studies with group B arthropod-borne viruses. III. Response of human subjects to revaccination with 17D strain yellow fever vaccine. Am. J. Trop. Med. Hyg. *11*:570–575, 1962.
383. World Health Organization: Special Programme on AIDS and Expanded Programme on Immunization—joint statement: consultation on human immunodeficiency virus (HIV) and routine childhood immunization. Wkly. Epidemiol. Rec. *62*:297–299, 1987.
384. World Health Organization: Guidelines for Cholera Control. Programme for Control of Diarrheal Disease. Geneva, World Health Organization, 1991.
385. World Health Organization: Expanded Programme on Immunization: Statement on poliomyelitis eradication. Wkly. Epidemiol. Rec. *70*:345–347, 1995.
386. Yvonnet, B., Coursaget, P., Deubel, V., et al.: Simultaneous administration of hepatitis B and yellow fever vaccines. J. Med. Virol. *19*:307–311, 1986.
387. Zangwill, K. M., Stout, R. W., Carlone, G. M., et al.: Duration of antibody response after meningococcal polysaccharide vaccination in U.S. Air Force personnel. J. Infect. Dis. *169*:847–852, 1994.
388. Zell, E. R., Dieta, V., Stevenson, J., et al.: Low vaccination levels of US preschool and school-age children. Retrospective assessments of vaccination coverage, 1991–1992. J. A. M. A. *271*:833–834, 1994.
389. Zerboni, L., Nader, S., Aoki, K., et al.: Analysis of the persistence of humoral and cellular immunity in children and adults immunized with varicella vaccine. J. Infect. Dis. *177*:1701–1704, 1998.
390. Zhuji Measles Vaccine Study Group: Epidemiologic examination of immunity period of measles vaccine. Chin. Med. J. *67*:19–22, 1987.

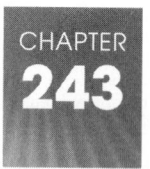

CHAPTER 243 Passive Immunization

E. RICHARD STIEHM ■ MARGARET A. KELLER

General Principles of Passive Immunity

DEFINITION

Passive immunization is the administration of antibodies from an immune subject to provide immediate protection against a microbial agent, toxic substance, or cell. Generally, passive immunization is used to provide temporary immunity in an unimmunized subject exposed to an infectious disease when active immunization is unavailable (e.g., respiratory syncytial virus [RSV] infection), is contraindicated (e.g., varicella in an immunocompromised child), or has not been given before exposure (e.g., tetanus, rabies).

Passive immunization also is used in the management of certain disorders associated with toxins (e.g., diphtheria), in certain bites (e.g., snake and spider), in drug overdose (e.g., digoxin), as a specific (e.g., Rh_0[D] immune globulin) or nonspecific (e.g., antithymocyte globulin) immunosuppressant, and in the treatment of certain infectious diseases.

Several types of preparations are used in passive immunization: (1) standard human immune serum globulin (HISG) for general use, which is available in two forms, intramuscular immune globulin (IG) and intravenous immune globulin (IVIG); (2) special IGs with a known antibody content for specific illnesses; (3) animal serums and antitoxins; and (4) monoclonal antibodies. These preparations are listed in Table 243–1. Most of the licensed special IGs are for intramuscular use only. Whole blood, plasma, and serum also can be used in passive immunization.

Passive immunization is not always effective; the duration is short and variable (1 to 6 weeks), and undesirable reactions may occur, especially if the antibody is of nonhuman origin. Hyperimmune IGs and IVIGs are identical to regular IGs and IVIGs, except that the former are derived from patients hyperimmunized or convalescing from a specific infection or the antibody content to a specific antigen is present in high titer, or both; they are useful in several disorders in which regular IG and IVIG are of little or no value.

ANIMAL SERUMS AND ANTITOXINS

Animal serums and antitoxins are derived from the serum of immunized animals, usually horses (equine). Because these serums are foreign proteins, they carry a significant risk of sensitization. Thus, they should be administered only when specifically indicated, after sensitivity tests, and by a physician prepared to deal with a hypersensitivity reaction.

A careful history must be taken before an animal serum is injected. Inquiry must be made about asthma, hay fever, urticaria, and previous injections of animal serum. Patients with a history of asthma, allergic rhinitis, or other allergic symptoms on exposure to horses may be dangerously sensitive to the corresponding serum and should be given it only with the utmost caution.

TABLE 243–1 ■ ANTIBODY PREPARATIONS AVAILABLE FOR PASSIVE IMMUNITY IN THE UNITED STATES

Product	Abbreviation(s)/Brand Name(s)	Principal Use
Standard Human Immune Serum Globulins (HISG, Gamma-Globulin)		
Immune globulin, intravenous	IVIG, IGIV	Treatment of antibody deficiency, immune thrombocytopenic purpura, Kawasaki disease, other immunoregulatory and inflammatory diseases
Immune globulin, intramuscular	IG, ISG	Treatment of antibody deficiency; prevention of measles, hepatitis A
Special Human Immune Serum Globulins for Intramuscular or Subcutaneous Use		
Hepatitis B immune globulin	HBIG	Prevention of hepatitis B
Varicella-zoster immune globulin	VZIG	Prevention or modification of chickenpox
Rabies immune globulin	RIG	Prevention of rabies
Tetanus immune globulin	TIG	Prevention or treatment of tetanus
Vaccinia immune globulin*	VIG	Prevention or treatment of vaccinia, prevention of smallpox
Rho(D) immune globulin	RhoGAM	Prevention of Rh hemolytic disease
Botulinum immune globulin	BIG	Treatment of newborn botulism
Special Human Intravenous Immune Globulins		
Cytomegalovirus immune globulin	CMV-IVIG, CMVIG, CytoGam	Prevention or treatment of cytomegalovirus infection
Respiratory syncytial virus immune globulin	RSV-IVIG, RSVIG, RespiGam	Prevention of RSV infection
Rho(D) immune globulin, intravenous	WinRho SD	Treatment of immune thrombocytopenic purpura
Animal Serums and Globulins		
Tetanus antitoxin (equine)	TAT	Prevention or treatment of tetanus (when TIG unavailable)
Diphtheria antitoxin (equine)*	DAT	Treatment of diphtheria
Botulinum antitoxin (equine)*		Treatment of botulism
Latrodectus mactans antivenin (equine)		Treatment of black widow spider bites
Crotalidae polyvalent antivenin (equine)		Treatment of most snake bites
Crotalidae polyvalent immune Fab (ovine)		Treatment of most snake bites
Micrurus fulvius antivenin (equine)		Treatment of coral snake bites
Digoxin immune Fab fragments (ovine)	Digibind, DigiFab	Treatment of digoxin or digitoxin overdose
Lymphocyte/thymocyte immune globulin (equine)	Equine ATG, Atgam	Immunosuppression
Lymphocyte/thymocyte immune globulin (rabbit)	Rabbit ATG, Thymoglobulin	Immunosuppression
Monoclonal Antibodies†		
Muromonab (anti-CD3)	OKT3	Immunosuppression
Daclizamab (anti-IL-2Rγ)	Zenapax	Immunosuppression
Basiliximab (anti-IL-2Rα)	Simulect	Immunosuppression
Infliximab (anti-TNF-α)	Ramicade	Treatment of inflammatory bowel disease, rheumatoid arthritis
Trastuzumab (anti-p185)	Herceptin	Treatment of breast cancer
Rituximab (anti-CD20)	Rituxan	Treatment of B-cell lymphoma
Gemtuzumab (anti-CD33)	Mylotarg	Treatment of acute myelocytic leukemia
Alemtuzumab (anti-CD52)	Campath	Treatment of chronic lymphocytic leukemia
Abciximab (anti-GPIIb/IIIa)	ReoPro	Prevention of thrombosis
Palivizumab (anti-RSV-F)	Synagis	Prevention of respiratory syncytial virus infection

*Available from the U.S. Centers for Disease Control and Prevention (4041635–3670).
†All are humanized mouse monoclonal antibodies except for muromonab, which is a mouse monoclonal antibody.
GP, glycoprotein; IL-2R, interleukin-2 receptor; TNF, tumor necrosis factor.

Sensitivity Tests for Animal Serum

A scratch, prick, or puncture skin test, followed by an intradermal skin test, always should be performed before any injection of animal serum, regardless of whether the patient has had the serum previously. A scratch, prick, or puncture test is performed by applying a drop of a 1:100 dilution of the serum in saline to the site of a superficial scratch, prick, or puncture on the volar aspect of the forearm and observing it for 20 minutes. A positive control (histamine phosphate, 0.1%) and negative control (saline) also should be applied. A positive reaction consists of erythema or wheal formation 3 mm greater than the control. (*Note:* Previous use of antihistamines may render results of these tests negative.)

If the scratch, prick, or puncture test result is negative, an intradermal test is performed by injecting 0.02 mL of a 1:1000 saline dilution; again, positive (histamine phosphate, 0.1%) and negative control tests should be performed. The reaction is read after 10 to 30 minutes and is positive if a wheal appears that is 3 mm greater than the negative control. If the test is negative, it should be repeated with 0.02 mL of a 1:100 dilution. For persons with negative histories of animal allergy and no previous exposure to animal sera, the 1:100 dilution may be used initially if the scratch, pick, or puncture test is negative.

Although intradermal skin tests have resulted in fatalities, scratch, prick, or puncture tests have not. Therefore, a skin test never should be performed (nor a serum injected) unless a syringe containing 1 mL of 1:1000 epinephrine is within immediate reach.

Skin tests can indicate the probability of sensitivity. However, a negative skin test is not an absolute guarantee of the absence of sensitivity. Therefore, either a specific history of allergy or a positive skin test with horse serum is sufficient reason for special caution. A positive history of sensitivity to horse dander is an indication of the need for extreme caution.

Administration of Animal Serum

If the history and sensitivity tests are negative, the indicated dose of serum may be given intramuscularly with epinephrine at hand. The patient should be watched closely for an hour for adverse reactions.

Intravenous injection may be indicated if a high concentration of circulating antibody is required rapidly, as in severe tetanus or diphtheria. The manufacturer's instructions should be consulted. If they are unavailable, a preliminary dose of 0.5 mL of serum should be diluted in 10 mL of either physiologic saline or 5 percent glucose solution. This preparation should be given intravenously over the course of 5 minutes, and the patient should be watched for 30 minutes for reactions. If no reaction occurs, the remainder of the serum, diluted 1:20, may be given at a rate not to exceed 1 mL/min.

If the skin test is positive or a history of allergy to animal serum is present and the need for the serum is unquestioned (and epinephrine is at hand), a procedure commonly called "desensitization" can be undertaken, but any significant desensitization is unlikely to occur. This procedure merely results in establishing temporary tolerance to the serum. Desensitization should be performed by trained personnel with the necessary emergency equipment and drugs immediately available.

Desensitization consists of periodic (at 15-minute intervals) injections or infusions of progressively larger doses of the serum, starting at a very low dose, until tolerance is achieved. Schedules for intravenous and intradermal-subcutaneous-intramuscular desensitization are given in the *2000 Red Book*.[9] Administration of sera after desensitization has been achieved must be continuous; protection from desensitization is lost rapidly.

Hypersensitivity Reactions to Animal Serum

Hypersensitivity reactions to animal serum may be of four general types: (1) anaphylactic reactions consisting of urticaria, other rashes, dyspnea, cyanosis, shock, and unconsciousness occurring seconds to minutes after an injection; (2) acute febrile reactions consisting of moderate or severe hyperpyrexia within 2 hours after an injection; (3) serum sickness reactions consisting of urticaria, arthritis, adenopathy, and fever occurring hours to days after an injection, depending on the dose and the presence or degree of previous sensitization (serum sickness occurs within hours or a few days after the second injection and within 7 to 12 days after the first injection); and (4) delayed reactions of varying nature, including peripheral neuritis, nephritis, Guillain-Barré syndrome, and myocarditis.

Treatment of Hypersensitivity Reactions to Animal Serum

For anaphylactic reactions, 1:1000 epinephrine at a dose of 0.01 mL/kg (0.5 mL maximum dose) is given subcutaneously or intramuscularly immediately. If improvement is not achieved immediately, 1:10,000 epinephrine at a dose of 0.01 mL/kg is given intravenously. The 1-mL 1:1000 epinephrine vials must be diluted 1:10 in physiologic saline and injected slowly. (A 1:10,000 dilution in a 10-mL vial is also available.) Administration of epinephrine may be repeated in 5 to 15 minutes if the response is not satisfactory. Vasopressors and positive-pressure oxygen are helpful. For severe urticaria or edema, particularly edema of the larynx, intramuscular injection of antihistamines and corticosteroids is indicated. Administration of serum therapy (if necessary) should be resumed 6 to 8 hours later or after all visible signs of reaction have subsided.

Mild febrile reactions (temperatures of less than 38.9° C [102° F]) are treated with aspirin or acetaminophen. Severe febrile reactions can cause convulsions and death and should be treated rigorously with sponge baths or other cooling means to reduce the temperature promptly. Serum sickness and serum neuritis generally are treated with corticosteroids.

HUMAN IMMUNE GLOBULINS (GAMMA-GLOBULIN)

HISG, or gamma-globulin, is available in two forms for general use, IG and IVIG (or IGIV). IG is used for both treatment of antibody immunodeficiencies and prevention of certain infectious disorders, as outlined in Table 243–1, whereas IVIG is used primarily in the treatment of primary and secondary antibody deficiencies and immunoregulatory disorders (e.g., immune thrombocytopenic purpura, Kawasaki disease). Although intravenous preparations theoretically could be manufactured and substituted for the high-titer intramuscular preparations, their greater expense and their limited use have inhibited this development. However, three such products, RSV-IVIG, Rh_0(D)-IVIG, and CMV-IVIG, are available.

Intramuscular Immunoglobulins

PHARMACOLOGY

IG is prepared from pooled human serum by the Cohn alcohol fractionation procedure (thus deriving its alternative name of Cohn fraction II). This procedure and viral inactivation steps remove most other serum proteins, hepatitis viruses, and human immunodeficiency viruses (HIV-1 and HIV-2), thereby providing a safe product for intramuscular injection. It is reconstituted as a sterile 16.5 percent solution (165 mg/mL) with thimerosal as a preservative.* It contains a wide spectrum of antibodies to viral and bacterial antigens.

IG is greater than 95 percent ImmunoglobulinG (IgG), but trace quantities of IgM and IgA and other serum proteins are present. The IgM and IgA are therapeutically insignificant because of their rapid half-lives (approximately 7 days) and their low concentrations in IG. IG contains all IgG allotypes (Gm and Km types).

IG is approved only for intramuscular or subcutaneous use, and intravenous injection of IG generally is contraindicated. IG aggregates in vitro to high-molecular-weight complexes (9.5S to 40S) that are strongly anticomplementary. These aggregates probably are responsible for the occasional systemic reactions to IG. The incidence of these reactions is increased if the patient has received IG previously or if it is inadvertently given intravenously. Agammaglobulinemic boys with affected male relatives (suggesting X-linked inheritance) may have a lower incidence of reactions.[194] Small intradermal injections of IG are not of value (except as a placebo), and they are contraindicated.

IMMUNE GLOBULIN IN ANTIBODY IMMUNODEFICIENCIES

The usual dosage of IG for antibody immunodeficiency is 100 mg/kg/mo, about equivalent to 0.7 mL/kg/mo of the

*A preservative-free 16 percent IG is available in Europe.

commercially available 16.5 percent (165 mg/mL) product. Two or three such injections are given at the onset of therapy as a loading dose, often over the course of a 3- to 5-day period. The maximal maintenance dosage should not exceed 20 or 30 mL/wk. Few studies on optimal dosage are available; however, the Medical Research Council Working Party[194] found that 25 mg/kg/wk (100 mg/kg/mo) was therapeutically equivalent to 50 mg/kg/wk but that 10 mg/kg/wk was inadequate. Use of IG by this route has been supplanted largely by IVIG administration.

IG should be given at multiple sites to avoid giving more than 5 mL at any one site (10 mL in a large adult). The buttocks are the preferred site, but the anterior of the thighs also can be used. Tenderness, sterile abscesses, fibrosis, and sciatic nerve injury may result from these injections. The danger of sciatic nerve injury is especially great in a small malnourished infant with inadequate muscle and fat in the gluteal regions. Large doses of IG should not be given to patients with severe thrombocytopenia because of the risk of hematoma and infection.

The injections are given initially at monthly intervals. If the patient continues to have infection or if a characteristic symptom (such as cough, conjunctivitis, diarrhea, arthralgia, or purulent nasal discharge) recurs at the end of the injection period, the interval between doses is decreased to 3 or 2 weeks. Older patients often report that they can tell when their IgG level is low and they need another injection. During acute infections, IgG catabolism increases, so extra injections of IG often are given.

Because high serum levels of IgG cannot be maintained, performing serial immunoglobulin assays is unnecessary in assessing the effectiveness of treatment. The maximal increase in serum IgG level after a standard IG injection will vary from patient to patient and from dose to dose because of different rates of absorption, local proteolysis at the injection site, and distribution within tissues. An intramuscular injection of 100 mg/kg of IG usually raises the IgG serum level by 100 mg/dL after 2 to 4 days.[425] Thus, a recent IG injection usually does not obscure the diagnosis of hypogammaglobulinemia.

ADVERSE EFFECTS OF IMMUNE GLOBULIN

Although IG is one of the safest biologic products available, rare anaphylactic reactions to intramuscular injections have been reported, particularly in patients requiring repeat injections.[92] The Medical Research Council Working Party[194] noted such reactions in 33 of 175 patients (19%) treated during a 10-year period. In all, 85 reactions occurred after approximately 40,000 injections; in 8 patients, the injections were stopped as a result of these adverse effects, and 1 death was recorded. Such reactions occurred at any stage of treatment and were unrelated to any particular lot number of IG or its anticomplementary activity. Symptoms include anxiety, nausea, vomiting, malaise, flushing, facial swelling, cyanosis, and loss of consciousness. Immediate treatment with epinephrine and antihistamines is indicated.

Persons who experience such reactions should be evaluated before receiving a repeat injection. Skin testing should be performed with several lots of IG.[119] A skin test result that is positive for an old but not a new lot of IG may indicate a particular idiosyncratic reaction to a particular lot. Under these circumstances, incremental doses of IG from a new lot are recommended. In other patients, IgE antibodies to IgG develop and result in positive immediate skin test reactions to all IG lots. In many other patients, no cause of the reactions can be found. Some of these patients will tolerate gradually increasing doses of IG, particularly if they are premedicated with a nonsteroidal anti-inflammatory agent, diphenhydramine, or corticosteroids. Finally, in a few patients, antibodies have developed to the IgA present in minute quantities in IG; these IgA antibodies can be detected by serologic means in several laboratories.[482]

Patients with selective IgA deficiency may acquire or have antibodies to IgA as a result of exposure to IgA-containing IVIG or other blood products. These antibodies can result in severe reactions to IG or IVIG because both products contain trace quantities of IgA. IVIGs low in IgA may prevent sensitization in these patients but can cause a reaction in presensitized subjects. Plasma from an IgA-deficient subject has been used in these circumstances.

Administration of exogenous gamma-globulin may inhibit the endogenous synthesis of gamma-globulin. In immunodeficiency with hyper-IgM, IG injections result in diminution of IgM levels, thus suggesting feedback inhibition of endogenous IgM synthesis.[433] In a few patients given IG from early infancy, we have noted depressed IgG levels that return to normal when the injections are stopped. Amer and colleagues reported decreased IgG levels in premature infants given monthly IG injections since birth.[8]

Immune globulin injections or infusions may inhibit antibody responses to live virus vaccines such as measles or varicella. Siber and associates[411] recommend an interval of 3 months between IVIG or IG therapy and administration of live virus vaccines after IG doses of less than 40 mg/kg, an interval of 6 months after doses of 40 to 80 mg/kg, an interval of 8 months after doses of 80 to 400 mg/kg, and an interval of 12 months after large doses (1 to 2 g/kg).

Late side effects after IG injections are uncommon; however, fibrosis of the buttocks or localized subcutaneous atrophy may develop at the site of repeated injections in some patients. Repeated injections of IG may result in high levels of mercury from the thimerosal preservative. Although symptoms of acrodynia (mercury toxicity) developed in one patient as a result of such therapy,[287] most remain asymptomatic.

Subcutaneous Immune Globulin

An alternative to intramuscular injection of IG (or infusion of IVIG) is slow subcutaneous infusion of IG or IVIG.[2, 50, 137] This route is used extensively in Europe with a 16 percent preservative-free IG. These substances are infused into the abdominal wall or thigh with a battery-operated portable infusion pump.[137] The dose is 100 to 150 mg/kg/wk, the same monthly dose as recommended for IVIG, given at a rate of 0.05 to 0.20 mL/kg/hr. Such infusions, which can be self-administered, are well tolerated, safe, and preferred by some patients.[137, 173]

Stiehm and coworkers[431] used this route successfully in patients with poor intravenous access, aseptic meningitis, anaphylactic reactions after receiving IVIG infusions, and rapid gastrointestinal (GI) protein loss; they used 10 percent IVIG because preservative-free IG is unavailable in the United States. Subcutaneous IG has been used safely in IgA-deficient adults with frequent respiratory infections,[173] during pregnancy,[51] and in children.[2]

Rapid administration of subcutaneous infusions of IG has been achieved by using two pumps at four infusion sites and increasing the rate to 20 mL/hr per pump, thereby allowing the entire infusion to be completed in little more than an hour.[137]

Intravenous Immune Globulin

IVIG is further-treated human IG that has been rendered free of complexes and is thus safe for intravenous infusion.

These products can be given in large quantities for antibody deficiencies[77] and for several autoimmune and inflammatory disorders.[37, 114] Several methods of treating Cohn fraction II, including treatment with proteolytic enzymes, ultracentrifugation, reduction of sulfhydryl bonds followed by alkylation, and incubation at low pH, have been used to eliminate high-molecular-weight complexes. Solvent/detergent treatment or pasteurization now is used to ensure viral inactivation.

Although these additional procedures increase its production cost, IVIG has several advantages over intramuscular IG, including the following: larger quantities of IgG can be given, high levels of serum IgG can be achieved rapidly, painful intramuscular injections are avoided, tissue pooling and local proteolysis are avoided, and home administration and self-administration are easier to perform (Table 243–2).

PHARMACOLOGY OF IVIG

The first IVIG produced in the United States in 1981 was Gamimune (Cutter Laboratories), a reduced and alkylated 5 percent solution containing 10 percent maltose.[24] The second IVIG produced was prepared by acidification and treatment with pepsin; the lyophilized powder could be reconstituted as a 3, 6, or 12 percent solution (Sandoglobulin, Sandoz Pharmaceuticals). Since then, several other IVIGs have been introduced by different manufacturers. Some of them are 5 to 10 percent solutions; others are lyophilized powders that are reconstituted as 3 to 12 percent solutions.[430]

Although these products vary slightly,[430] they are generally therapeutically equivalent and usually are selected on the basis of cost and convenience. Minor IgA and IgG subclass differences exist.[27, 419] Antibody titers to specific pathogens also may vary from lot to lot, as well as among different IVIGs.[130] Products low in IgA content, such as Gammagard S/D or Polygam S/D, are used to minimize reactions in patients with hypogammaglobulinemia and concurrent IgA deficiency or when anti-IgA antibodies are present in the recipient. Very sensitive patients may not tolerate any IVIG. Premixed liquids have the advantage of convenience because the reconstitution step is not required; however, most solutions must be kept refrigerated.

TABLE 243–2 ■ ADVANTAGES AND DISADVANTAGES OF INTRAVENOUS IMMUNE GLOBULIN VERSUS INTRAMUSCULAR IMMUNE GLOBULIN

Advantages of IVIG
Less painful
No pooling with tissues
No sterile abscesses
No mercury exposure
No volume limitation
Rapid attainment of high blood levels
Less frequent injections
Half-life studies feasible
Daily treatment feasible
Disadvantages of IVIG
Expensive
Venous access necessary
Longer time of administration
More frequent side effects (5–15%)
More severe side effects
Hepatitis (a few cases)
Aseptic meningitis (a few cases)
Renal insufficiency (a few cases)

All IVIG products that are currently available have adequate serum half-lives (15 to 25 days), a wide spectrum of antibody activity, and minimal anticomplementary activity, and they are free of bacterial and viral contamination.

ADMINISTRATION OF IVIG

IVIG administration requires venous access, sometimes a problem in small children or obese subjects. It also requires close monitoring during the infusion. Adverse reactions to IVIG tend to occur more frequently and are more severe than with IG injections.

IVIG is contraindicated in patients who have had an anaphylactic reaction to IVIG or other blood products. It should be administered with great caution to patients who have IgG subclass deficiencies along with IgA deficiency or anti-IgA antibodies (or both).[99]

Typically, an IVIG infusion requires 2 to 4 hours to administer.[430] The initial rate is 0.01 mL/kg/min, and if no side effects occur, it can be doubled at 20- to 30-minute intervals to a maximal rate of 0.08 mL/kg/min. Rates above 5 mL/kg/hr (0.08 mL/kg/min) are not recommended. Adverse effects tend to be associated with rapid rates of infusion in patients with concurrent acute infections, in previously untreated patients, or when significant time has elapsed between infusions (>6-week intervals).

Immediate minor reactions can be avoided or diminished by slowing the rate of infusion. Patients experiencing minor side effects such as headaches, shaking chills, nausea and vomiting, or myalgia/arthralgia can be pretreated with acetaminophen (15 mg/kg), nonsteroidal anti-inflammatory drugs, diphenhydramine (Benadryl) (1 mg/kg), or hydrocortisone (6 mg/kg) given intravenously 1 hour before the infusion. Occasionally, switching to a different product (generally one available as a solution) may alleviate the reactions.

A few investigators have given high concentrations (9% and 12% solutions) infused rapidly over a period of 20 to 40 minutes; this rapid rate can be tolerated by some patients.[397] However, it should not be done except by experienced personnel equipped to manage adverse reactions.

In responsible, older patients receiving infusions without adverse effects, infusion by home self-administration can be accomplished at great cost savings.[29, 241, 423] However, in most cases, IVIG infusions are performed in the clinic setting or by a home infusion service.

ADVERSE EFFECTS OF IVIG

Between 5 and 15 percent of IVIG infusions are associated with adverse reactions; typically, they include headaches, nausea and vomiting, flushing, chills, myalgia, arthralgia, and abdominal pain.[429, 430] Occasionally, chest tightness, hives, and severe life-threatening reactions develop. Very rarely, reactions are mediated by anti-IgA antibodies (see earlier), but they can occur in the absence of antibodies. Certain brands of IVIG may be more reactogenic; in one study involving Kawasaki disease, the two IVIGs used were equivalent therapeutically, but one had a 12-fold (2 versus 25%) increase in side effects.[374]

Serious, late, but rare reactions[111] include aseptic meningitis,[225, 476] cerebral thrombosis,[504] renal insufficiency,[361] and hemolytic anemia.[70] Thus, IVIG infusions should be supervised by individuals with the experience as well as the skill and knowledge to manage these reactions. Nurses, parents, or others who perform home infusions must be taught to recognize and treat adverse reactions.

HEPATITIS C CONTAMINATION OF IVIG

Hepatitis C has been transmitted via experimental IVIG lots,[265, 322] some European preparations,[54, 55, 263, 496] and certain commercially available U.S. lots.[333, 396] Until the report of an outbreak of hepatitis C in 1994,[333] no U.S. cases of hepatitis associated with a commercially available IVIG had been reported.

As noted, hepatitis C was transmitted by IVIG in the early 1990s, shortly after hepatitis C–seropositive donors were excluded from the donor pools used in the manufacture of IVIG. A plausible explanation for the lack of transmission before this Food and Drug Administration policy is that the hepatitis C antibodies neutralized trace amounts of hepatitis C virus not eliminated during the fractionation. As of October 1994, 137 suspected cases were reported, 88 of which were confirmed.[333, 396] Fifty-one of the 88 patients (58%) had primary immunodeficiencies, and 63 percent eventually became symptomatic.

Bjoro and associates[55] reported that immunocompromised patients had a severe and rapidly progressive course of hepatitis C infection and that responses to interferon were poor. Razvi and colleagues have not confirmed this finding in U.S. patients.[362]

The Gammagard and Polygam involved in the outbreak have been replaced with Gammagard S/D and Polygam S/D, preparation of which includes solvent/detergent treatment to inactivate hepatitis C and other membrane-enveloped viruses. Manufacturers of other preparations also have incorporated procedures such as pasteurization to inactivate hepatitis C and most other viruses. Each of the various methods seems effective, but none can guarantee total absence of infectious virus. However, no cases of HIV transmission have been reported with IVIG administration.[184, 198, 396]

IVIG IN PRIMARY IMMUNODEFICIENCIES

Administration of IVIG is indicated for patients with profound primary antibody deficiency (quantitative and qualitative), for patients with combined immunodeficiencies, and for those with secondary immunodeficiency along with significant antibody deficiency (Table 243–3). Regular infusions of IVIG can keep patients with primary antibody immunodeficiencies free of infections for long periods or lessen the severity and frequency of chronic infections. Patients with hereditary agammaglobulinemia, common variable immunodeficiency, and immunodeficiency with hyper-IgM clearly benefit from replacement therapy. In combined antibody and cellular defects and in secondary antibody immunodeficiencies, administration of IVIG serves as an important ancillary treatment, but it does not correct the associated T-cell defect or underlying cause of the secondary immunodeficiency.

The recommended dose of IVIG is 400 to 600 mg/kg/mo, usually given every 30 days.[386, 430] It can be administered in fractional doses every 2 to 3 weeks if the single dose is not tolerated or if symptoms develop late in the month between infusions. In general, the trough IgG level should be maintained at approximately 400 mg/dL higher than the pretreatment level, which will normalize the IgG level in most patients. Patients receiving these larger doses have less frequent sinopulmonary infections, improved pulmonary function, and decreased days of illness and hospitalization when compared with patients receiving lower doses (<300/mg/kg/mo).[430] Some investigators recommend even higher doses (i.e., keeping trough levels >800 mg/dL) in an effort to prevent pulmonary complications.[118, 219]

TABLE 243–3 ■ SOME IMMUNODEFICIENCIES IN WHICH HUMAN INTRAVENOUS IMMUNE GLOBULIN MAY BE BENEFICIAL

Antibody Deficiencies
Congenital agammaglobulinemia
Common variable immunodeficiency
Immunodeficiency with hyper-IgM
Transient hypogammaglobulinemia of infancy (sometimes)
IgG subclass deficiency ± IgA deficiency (sometimes)
Antibody deficiency with normal immunoglobulins

Combined Deficiencies
Severe combined immunodeficiencies (all types)
Wiskott-Aldrich syndrome
Ataxia telangiectasia
Short-limbed dwarfism
X-linked lymphoproliferative syndrome

Secondary Immunodeficiencies
Malignancies with antibody deficiencies; multiple myeloma, chronic lymphocytic leukemia, other cancers
Protein-losing enteropathy with hypogammaglobulinemia
Nephrotic syndrome with hypogammaglobulinemia
Pediatric acquired immunodeficiency syndrome
Intensive care patients: trauma, surgery, or shock
Post-transplantation
Burns
Prematurity

Some patients with severe disease do not respond to higher doses or more frequent infusions because of permanent tissue damage or deep-seated chronic infection.

IVIG also is used in patients with recurrent infections caused by antibody deficiency but with normal or nearly normal immunoglobulin levels; often, these patients need higher or more frequent doses of IVIG because their IgG catabolism is increased. Rarely, IVIG is indicated in infants with transient hypogammaglobulinemia and persistent infection that is not responsive to antibiotics. IVIG also has been used in patients with IgG subclass deficiencies, but controlled studies demonstrating efficacy are lacking.[53, 240, 413]

A syndrome of polymyositis or chronic encephalitis, or both, caused by persistent enteroviral infection in patients with agammaglobulinemia has been treated successfully with very high doses of IVIG containing specific antibody to the virus[111, 294]; however, some patients do not respond.[98]

Very high-dose IVIG (up to 2 g/kg/day) is sometimes used in patients with primary immunodeficiency and enterovirus encephalitis, parvovirus B19 infection, autoimmune disease such as immune thrombocytopenic purpura, and persistent respiratory viral infection.[430]

IVIG IN SECONDARY IMMUNODEFICIENCIES

Some patients with secondary immunodeficiencies have low immunoglobulin levels, poor antibody responses to antigenic challenge, and low levels of natural antibodies. This condition may result from loss of immunoglobulin, loss of immune cells, or the toxic effect of therapy or infection on the immune system. Table 243–3 lists diseases and conditions in which secondary antibody immunodeficiency can occur. Laboratory criteria that support the use of IVIG include significant hypogammaglobulinemia (serum IgG <200 mg/dL or total immunoglobulin [IgG + IgM + IgA] <400 mg/dL), absent or unexpectedly low titers of natural antibodies, absent or poor response to antigenic challenge (e.g., tetanus, pneumococcal vaccines), and lack of an antibody response to the infecting organism.[429]

HEMATOLOGIC AND ONCOLOGIC DISEASES. Antibody deficiencies can occur with multiple myeloma, chronic lymphocytic leukemia, lymphomata, and advanced cancer. A double-blind multicenter study concluded that the prophylactic infusion of 400 mg/kg of IVIG every 3 weeks reduced the incidence of bacterial infections in patients with chronic lymphocytic leukemia.[201] The treatment group had fewer infections with *Streptococcus pneumoniae* and *Haemophilus influenzae*, but no difference was noted in infections caused by other gram-negative bacterial, fungal, or viral infections. This beneficial effect was confirmed in a subsequent study,[136] and although concern has been raised about its cost-effectiveness,[488] IVIG also has been shown to reduce the incidence of infections in patients with multiple myeloma[88] and in those receiving chemotherapy for lung cancer.[398]

PROTEIN-LOSING ENTEROPATHY AND NEPHROTIC SYNDROME. In some pediatric patients, antibody deficiency associated with massive proteinuria (nephrosis) or diarrhea (protein-losing enteropathy) develops because of accelerated IgG catabolism. Most of these patients have minimal trouble with recurrent infection, probably because antibody synthesis is intact and most likely accelerated; however, if the loss of IgG greatly exceeds synthetic capacity, symptomatic severe hypogammaglobulinemia may result. IVIG can be used diagnostically in such cases; a large intravenous infusion, followed by serial measurements of serum IgG levels, can document an accelerated IgG half-life (i.e., <10 days).

These patients are candidates for receiving IVIG therapy if they have recurrent infections or very low IgG levels (e.g., <200 mg/dL), or both. Administration of large and repeated doses is necessary. Occasionally, antibody infusions will help control the severe diarrhea of protein-losing enteropathy.[82] Subcutaneous IG has been used in this situation because its delayed release into serum may result in higher IgG levels than can be achieved with an equivalent IVIG dose.[431]

INTENSIVE CARE PATIENTS: TRAUMA, SURGERY, AND SEPTIC SHOCK. Patients undergoing severe stress associated with trauma or extensive surgery have profound exposure and susceptibility to infection and a spectrum of immune deficiencies, including cutaneous anergy, leukocyte dysfunction, hypogammaglobulinemia, and transiently impaired antibody synthesis.[149, 308, 498] Bowel stasis and hypotension may promote gram-negative sepsis or endotoxemia, or both, along with the development of severe and often irreversible shock. Studies by Ziegler and associates[511] and Baumgartner and colleagues[45] suggested that when antisera to a mutant J5 *Escherichia coli* endotoxin with anti–lipid A activity is used in bacteremic or surgical intensive care unit (ICU) patients, the incidence and severity of severe shock could be reduced. However, Calandra and colleagues,[80] using a human IVIG to J5 *E. coli* in 71 patients with gram-negative infections and shock, could not confirm their results. They gave a single infusion of 200 mg/kg; a control group got a similar dose of regular IVIG. No differences were found in mortality, onset of time to shock, and complications.

Just and coworkers[218] administered regular IVIG and antibiotics to 50 ICU patients suspected of having infection and compared their outcome with that of 54 control patients who received antibiotics alone. Although no difference in survival occurred, they noted a trend indicating that the IVIG-antibiotic group had a shortened ICU stay, a shorter period in which respirator therapy was required, and improved renal function, as well as a favorable effect on infection (i.e., infections were a less likely cause of death in these patients). A multicenter study of 352 post-surgical patients confirmed the observation that standard IVIG (400 mg/kg at weekly intervals) reduced the incidence of infections and shortened stay in the ICU when compared with patients treated with placebo or hyperimmune core-lipopolysaccharide IG.[355]

Werdan has reviewed the use of IVIG in sepsis and suggests that certain specific subgroups may benefit (e.g., post-operative sepsis, septic shock with endotoxinemia, and sepsis with neutropenia).[492] Studies of IVIG in trauma patients requiring surgery[104, 109, 149] and in head trauma patients[498] have shown questionable efficacy.

Monoclonal antibodies to endotoxin have been tested in clinical trials of patients in septic shock, but none were of proven efficacy.[461, 493, 510] Monoclonal antibody to tumor necrosis factor–α also has shown no efficacy in the treatment of adults with septic shock.[1, 94] Monoclonal antibodies to interleukin-6 or interleukin-1 receptor likewise have not been shown to be effective in the treatment of shock.[138]

In summary, no compelling data suggest that antibody, either polyclonal or monoclonal, is of benefit in an acutely ill patient with shock.

PREMATURITY. All premature infants have low levels of maternally derived IgG at birth, and levels approaching 100 mg/dL will develop in the first months of life in most.[38] These IgG levels may be further depressed by pulmonary disease (with transudation into the lungs), stress (with increased IgG catabolism), and multiple drawing of blood.[382] In addition, their sluggish antibody responses, their concurrent IgM and IgA deficiency, and their immature complement, phagocytic, and T-cell systems render them extraordinarily susceptible to infection.[497]

Attempts to decrease infections in premature infants by using periodic IG injections date from the 1960s. Four controlled studies enrolling a total of 363 infants used IG doses of 80 to 240 mg/kg/mo during their stay in the nursery (two studies), for 4 months, and for 1 year.[8, 95, 106, 425] In two studies, a slight decrease in the number and severity of infections was noted, but no difference in survival. These mixed results suggest that IG at the doses used was not of prophylactic value in these patients.

In the last decade, the increasing rate of survival of very tiny premature infants and the availability of IVIG has reawakened interest in the use of antibody to prevent infections in premature infants. In general, IVIG is well tolerated, with minimal adverse effects, in doses of up to 1 g/kg/day.

A meta-analysis of 12 prospective, randomized, placebo-controlled prevention studies (representing 4180 infants) was performed by Jenson and Pollock.[210, 211] These studies differed in entry criteria, dose, and brand of IVIG, but most infants were less than 2000 g, given IVIG therapy within the first week of life, and received doses of at least 400 mg/kg/mo, and culture-proven sepsis was used as an end-point. Five studies showed a significant benefit of IVIG, one showed a higher incidence in the control group, and six studies showed no difference. Overall, 345 cases of sepsis occurred in 2136 infants treated with IVIG (16%) versus 408 cases in 2044 control infants (20.0%) for a p value of .02, a modest but statistically significant difference. A Cochrane review meta-analysis of 15 studies that included 5054 infants also found a 3 to 4 percent reduction in serious infections without a difference in mortality.[328]

Shamin and coworkers[403] gave sufficient IVIG for 6 months to 15 of 30 matched premature infants with severe bronchopulmonary dysplasia to maintain their IgG levels over 400 mg/dL, whereas the untreated infants had levels less than 200 mg/dL. The number of infections, notably pneumonia, was significantly reduced in the IVIG group (5 episodes of pneumonia and 4 other infections) in comparison with the control group (15 episodes of pneumonia and 12 other infections).

Thus, the evidence to date supports the 1990 National Institutes of Health (NIH) consensus statement that IVIG should not be given routinely to infants of low birth weight,[317] but that it may be of value in selected premature infants at high risk for acquiring infection.

IVIG is sometimes of benefit in premature infants with a history of serious infections and underlying lung disease; most such infants will have hypogammaglobulinemia and should be regarded as having transient hypogammaglobulinemia of infancy. Such infants also need RSV prophylaxis.

In the future, hyperimmune IVIG or monoclonal antibodies enriched in specific antibodies against *Staphylococcus epidermidis* or group B streptococcal antigens may be of special benefit to certain high-risk newborn and premature infants.

POST-TRANSPLANTATION. Conditioning regimens to eliminate or reduce the host's hematopoietic and immune systems during transplantation (bone marrow and solid organ) render these patients extremely susceptible to infection.[466]

The use of IVIG to prevent such infections, particularly sepsis, pneumonia, and GI infections, has met with limited success,[96, 157, 445–447] with the exception of preventing complications from cytomegalovirus (CMV) infection (discussed in the next section).

One report demonstrated some benefit from the infusion of IVIG in a controlled trial involving 382 bone marrow recipients.[446] The study patients received 500 mg/kg of IVIG weekly for 90 days and then monthly for 1 year, with a resultant decrease in the number of infections, number of platelet transfusions, and incidence of graft-versus-host disease (GVHD). A review from the same group of investigators concluded that IVIG has shown benefit in reducing septicemia, interstitial pneumonia, fatal CMV disease, acute GVHD, and transplantation-related mortality in adult recipients of related marrow transplants.[447] Thus, IVIG has been recommended for allogeneic marrow transplant recipients,[229, 376] but not for recipients of autologous transplants.[169, 502]

BURNS. Bacterial sepsis, particularly *Pseudomonas* and *E. coli* sepsis, is the leading cause of death in the 300,000 patients hospitalized annually in the United States for burns.[307, 308] The protein loss in these patients induces hypogammaglobulinemia in proportion to the severity of the burn. High-dose IVIG prolongs survival in experimentally burned mice infected with *Pseudomonas,* and preliminary studies of hyperimmune IG and plasma in human burn patients were encouraging, but proof of efficacy is lacking.[228, 350, 408]

INFECTION WITH THE HUMAN IMMUNODEFICIENCY VIRUS. The rationale for using IVIG in patients with advanced HIV disease is their increased susceptibility to common bacterial and viral infections, poor primary antibody responses to vaccine antigens despite hypergammaglobulinemia, and in young children, a limited antibody spectrum to common bacterial pathogens. Although the central immune defect in acquired immunodeficiency syndrome (AIDS) is a loss of helper T-cell ($CD4^+$) number and function, the polyclonal B-cell activation and defective helper T-cell function result in a significant B-cell deficiency.[52, 321] Thus, in children with AIDS, bacterial infections are more common than opportunistic infections. Immune-mediated thrombocytopenic purpura and viral diseases (e.g., RSV, parainfluenza, and CMV amenable to IVIG therapy) also may develop in patients with AIDS.

After preliminary uncontrolled studies suggested a benefit of IVIG in children with advanced HIV infection,[81, 412] two large multicenter controlled studies undertaken by the NIH-supported Pediatric AIDS Clinical Trial Group determined the efficacy of IVIG in decreasing infections and improving survival in AIDS patients.[200, 424]

In the first study, 372 children received 400 mg/kg of IVIG every 4 weeks or an albumin control for 2 years.[200] Thirty percent of all children in the IVIG-treated group had serious infections as compared with 42 percent in the placebo group. Children who were less ill (those with $CD4^+$ lymphocyte counts >200/μL) benefited in particular from IVIG. Children in this category had fewer serious infections and were hospitalized less frequently than were those in the placebo group, and their $CD4^+$ counts dropped less rapidly than did those of the placebo group. The mortality in both groups, however, was identical. Children with $CD4^+$ counts less than 200 cells/μL (i.e., those with severely impaired immunity) who were given IVIG had no significant decrease in infections, days of hospitalization, or mortality when compared with their counterparts in the placebo group.

The authors concluded that IVIG significantly reduced the risk of serious infection developing in some children with symptomatic HIV infection, primarily those with $CD4^+$ counts between 200 and 500/mL. In a follow-up study, the placebo group was allowed to cross over to receive IVIG, with a drop in the rate of serious infections and hospitalizations.[304]

In a second trial of IVIG in which all the children received zidovudine, a significant decrease in serious bacterial infections was found again, but this benefit was limited to children who did not receive trimethoprim-sulfamethoxazole prophylaxis for *Pneumocystis carinii* pneumonia.[424] A consensus of an HIV Working Group was that HIV-infected children with significant hypogammaglobulinemia or documented poor antibody formation may be candidates for receiving IVIG therapy.[26] We also recommend administering IVIG to HIV-infected children who have recurrent infections that are not controlled by antibiotics and who have chronic nonspecific diarrhea with failure to thrive.

In addition to preventing serious bacterial infections, IVIG given to children with HIV reduced the number of nonserious bacterial infections (by 60% for ear infections, 13% for skin infections, and 10% for other upper respiratory infections) and viral infections by approximately one third in both trials.[302–304, 424]

IVIG given in large doses (0.5 to 1.0 g/kg for 3 to 5 days) has been shown to be effective in reducing infection in HIV-infected adults[234] and HIV-related thrombocytopenia.[79, 256]

Regular IVIG infusions also improved left ventricular function in HIV-infected children with dilated cardiomyopathy.[270]

IVIG in Immunoregulatory Disorders

High-dose IVIG has immunosuppressive and anti-inflammatory effects that render it a valuable agent in the treatment of several autoimmune or inflammatory disorders[114] (Table 243–4). High-dose IVIG (1 to 2 g/kg/wk) may work by one or more of the following mechanisms[37, 114, 415, 455]:

1. IVIG inhibits antibody synthesis by having a direct effect on proliferating B cells, possibly through activation of the FcRII receptor.[390] This inhibition may be the mechanism in illnesses associated with a pathologic antibody such as myasthenia gravis and coagulopathy with a factor VIII inhibitor.

2. IVIG contains anti-idiotypic antibodies that can combine with autoimmune antibodies and remove them rapidly from the circulation, which may be the mechanism by which IVIG reduces anti-HLA antibodies in transplant patients.

3. IVIG binds to Fc receptors and causes an Fc receptor blockade, thus reducing the destruction of antibody-coated cells in the spleen or liver. It is the mechanism for the rapid response to IVIG noted in patients with immune thrombocytopenic purpura.

4. IVIG combines with other surface receptors to inhibit cellular activation; for example, in toxic epidermal necrolysis, IVIG prevents Fas-mediated cell death of keratinocytes by blocking the Fas receptor.[478]

5. IVIG down-regulates immune activation by decreasing inflammatory cytokine release or action. In Kawasaki disease, an immediate damping of the cytokine "storm" occurs with this illness.

6. IVIG antibodies neutralize bacterial superantigens and prevent them from activating T cells. It is the probable mechanism for its beneficial effect in toxic shock syndrome.[455]

7. IVIG combines with complement components to prevent complement-mediated tissue injury. An example is inhibition of complement-mediated myocyte damage in dermatomyositis.

8. IVIG neutralizes virus or bacterial antigens that may trigger or cause the disease. An example may be the neutralization of *E. coli* antigens in hemolytic-uremic syndrome.

The illnesses for which IVIG may be of benefit are often of unknown cause, refractory to standard treatment, somewhat responsive to steroids, and associated with local or generalized immune activation with fever, inflammatory cells, and cytokine release.[325] Large doses of IVIG (e.g., usually 1 to 2 g/kg/day) are necessary and may need to be repeated at weekly intervals. All IVIG preparations are seemingly equivalent in action. If a favorable response does not occur immediately or within a few weeks, it probably will not occur later. Proof of efficacy requires a double-blind study (e.g., as conducted for Kawasaki disease) or dramatic reversal of progressive severe disease (e.g., as noted in some cases of toxic shock syndrome). The use of IVIG in Kawasaki disease is covered earlier.

MONOCLONAL ANTIBODIES

Monoclonal antibodies specific for a single antigenic epitope have been available for laboratory use for several decades and are being developed rapidly as therapeutic agents. The first monoclonal antibody, introduced in 1984, was a murine antilymphocyte antibody (anti-CD3 [OKT3]) used for immunosuppression in transplant patients. Since then, other monoclonal antibodies have been licensed for treatment, and many others are being studied in the United States and abroad (see Table 243–1).

Most licensed monoclonal antibodies are humanized murine monoclonal antibodies containing the antibody-combining site of a mouse antibody hybridized to a human IgG1 molecule (95% of the molecule), thus rendering it less antigenic and giving it the long half-life of a human IgG molecule. One of these antibodies, palivizumab (Synagis), directed against RSV, is used in the prevention of RSV infection in high-risk infants (see later). Monoclonal antibodies against microbial antigens and inflammatory mediators will play an important role in tomorrow's battle with infectious pathogens.

TABLE 243–4 ■ AUTOIMMUNE AND INFLAMMATORY DISEASES TREATED WITH INTRAVENOUS IMMUNOGLOBULIN

Proven Benefit*
Kawasaki disease
Immune thrombocytopenic purpura (e.g., idiopathic)
Dermatomyositis
Neurologic diseases
Guillain-Barré syndrome
Chronic inflammatory demyelinating polyneuropathy
Multifocal motor neuropathy
Lambert-Eaton myasthenia syndrome
Probable Benefit†
Post-infectious thrombocytopenic purpura
Neonatal isoimmune or autoimmune thrombocytopenic purpura
Pregnancy associated with antiplatelet antibodies
Autoimmune or isoimmune neutropenia
Autoimmune hemolytic anemia
Toxic epidermal necrolysis
Neurologic diseases
Myasthenia gravis
Polymyositis
Possible Benefit‡
Toxic shock syndrome
Anticardiolipin antibody syndrome
Coagulopathy with factor VIII inhibitor
Bullous pemphigoid
Churg-Strauss vasculitis
Vasculitis with antineutrophil cytoplasmic antibodies
Other vasculitides
Graves ophthalmopathy
Uveitis
Stevens-Johnson syndrome
Solid organ transplantation
Highly HLA-sensitized patients awaiting transplantation
Prevention of antibody-mediated rejection
Prevention of allograft rejection in high-risk patients
Treatment of delayed rejection
Neurologic diseases
Multiple sclerosis
Rasmussen syndrome
Intractable pediatric epilepsy
Demyelinating neuropathy with IgM monoclonal gammopathy or anti-GAM antibodies
Acute disseminated encephalomyelitis
Cerebral infarction with antiphospholipid antibodies
HTLV-1–associated myelopathy
Lumbosacral or brachial plexitis
Stiff-man syndrome
PANDAS syndrome
Unproven or No Benefit§
Steroid-dependent asthma
Atopic dermatitis
Epidermolysis bullosa acquisita
Recurrent abortion
Hemolytic-uremic syndrome
Thrombotic thrombocytopenic pupura
Pure red cell or white cell aplasia
Acquired von Willebrand disease
Chronic fatigue syndrome
Infantile autism
Acute myocarditis
Type 1 diabetes mellitus
Rheumatoid arthritis
Lupus erythematosus
Inflammatory bowel disease
Neurologic diseases
Inclusion body myositis
Amyotrophic lateral sclerosis
POEMS syndrome
Paraneoplastic cerebellar degeneration, sensory neuropathy, encephalitis

*Controlled studies demonstrate efficacy.
†Several case reports or uncontrolled series are convincing.
‡Preliminary studies are encouraging but incomplete.
§Preliminary studies are limited, equivocal, or negative.
HTLV, human T-cell lymphotrophic virus; PANDAS, pediatric autoimmune neuropsychiatric disorder associated with streptococcal disease; POEMS, polyneuropathy, organomegaly, endocrinopathy, M protein, skin changes.

Immune Globulin Administration by Unusual Routes (Oral, Intrathecal, Aerosol)

ORAL IMMUNOGLOBULIN

Oral IG administered to provide antimicrobial activity to the GI tract mimics the action of antibody-rich colostrum and breast milk. In humans, little or no ingested IG is absorbed intact into the systemic circulation.[25] Some oral IG traverses the entire GI tract undigested, particularly in premature infants.[59] Oral IG may neutralize microorganisms, inhibit colonization, and prevent microbial attachment to the GI mucosa.

ROTAVIRUS INFECTION. Barnes and colleagues[41] fed human IG or placebo for 7 days to premature infants in a nursery in which rotavirus was endemic. Rotavirus-associated diarrhea developed in 6 of 11 babies given placebo and in 1 of 14 given oral IG.

Losonsky and coworkers[272] administered oral human IG to two children with severe combined immunodeficiency and chronic rotavirus infection and demonstrated a decrease in the amount of free rotavirus excretion and survival of the IG through the GI tract. Kanfer and associates[222] used oral human IG to treat rotavirus infection that occurred after bone marrow transplantation.

Bovine hyperimmune colostral immunoglobulin enriched in rotavirus antibodies (from immunized cows) also has been used in the prevention of rotavirus infection. Davidson and colleagues prevented rotavirus infection in 55 children admitted to an Australian hospital by administering a 10-day course of bovine colostrum; 9 of 65 control children became infected.[101] Turner and Kelsey[465] added at least 360 mL of cow colostrum to the formula of 31 term infants aged 3 to 7 months for an average of 101 days (range, 16 to 202 days). Rotavirus infections occurred in 11 (35%) of the colostrum-fed group and 14 (42%) of the control group, an insignificant difference, but symptomatic infection occurred in 1 (3%) of the infants receiving colostrum and 6 (18%) of the controls.

This product also has been used in two studies of the treatment of rotavirus diarrhea in Bangladesh.[299, 394] In both studies, less diarrhea, fewer days of illness, less stool output, and more rapid clearance of rotavirus from the stool were noted.

Guarino and coworkers[167] used oral human IG (300 mg/kg) as a single dose and observed more rapid recovery from rotavirus diarrhea. In sum, oral IG is a promising but unproven agent for the prevention and treatment of rotavirus infection.

NECROTIZING ENTEROCOLITIS. Eibl and colleagues[117] were able to prevent necrotizing enterocolitis in all 90 infants given oral IG rich in serum IgA. Six cases occurred in 91 control infants. Rubaltelli and colleagues in Italy achieved similar results with oral monomeric IgG.[377]

***CRYPTOSPORIDIUM* INFECTION.** Bovine colostrum was used successfully to treat cryptosporidial diarrhea in HIV infection.[406] Borowitz and Saulsbury[63] used oral IG to successfully treat cryptosporidial infection in a child with acute leukemia.

DIARRHEA. Oral human IG has been used in the post–bone marrow transplantation period to prevent the development of viral gastroenteritis[96] and to treat nonspecific diarrhea in immunodeficient subjects.[295]

AEROLIZED IMMUNE GLOBULIN

Aerosolized IG has been used with encouraging results in experimental models of pneumonia caused by RSV, pneumococci, staphylococci, and parainfluenza and influenza viruses.[156, 332, 359, 370]

Rimensberger and colleagues[370] conducted a placebo-controlled trial of aerosolized human IG (not RSV-IVIG) in the treatment of RSV infection. No significant benefit was found, but the treatment was well tolerated.

Heikkinen and coworkers[182] used an IgA-enriched human IG as a nasal spray twice daily for 8 weeks to reduce respiratory infections in children between 1 and 4 years of age attending daycare. A 42 percent reduction was achieved in the 19 children receiving the IG versus the 20 children in the placebo group. The authors suggested that this treatment also may decrease the incidence of otitis media.

INTRATHECAL IMMUNE GLOBULIN

Human IG has been used intrathecally for the treatment of viral encephalomyelitis in patients with antibody deficiency.[121] The use of antitoxin intrathecally in tetanus is discussed in the section on tetanus.

OTHER ROUTES

Intra-articular IG was of no clinical benefit to patients with rheumatoid arthritis.[33] We have used IG in the conjunctiva of a child with ligneous conjunctivitis without benefit.

Passive Immunity in Bacterial Infection

Antibodies have been used for a century for the prevention and treatment of infectious diseases (Table 243–5). In bacterial disease, antibodies neutralize toxins, facilitate opsonization, and with complement, promote bacteriolysis; in viral disease, antibodies block viral entry into uninfected cells, promote antibody-directed cell-mediated cytotoxicity by natural killer cells, and neutralize virus alone or with the participation of complement.

Before the use of antibiotics, antibodies were the only specific agents for the treatment of certain infections. Although this role has been supplanted largely by antibiotics, antibody still has a crucial role in the treatment of certain infectious diseases (see Table 243–5). The remainder of this chapter discusses the roles of antibody in prevention and treatment of bacterial and viral disease. Other reviews are available.[84, 85, 262]

BOTULISM, BOTULINUM ANTITOXIN, AND BOTULISM IMMUNE GLOBULIN

Botulism, a severe paralytic poisoning, results from ingestion or absorption of the neurotoxin from *Clostridium botulinum.* Three clinical variants are recognized: *food poisoning* from ingestion of contaminated canned food; *wound botulism* from a contaminated local infection; and *infant botulism* from ingestion of *C. botulinum* spores, their multiplication in the GI tract, elaboration of toxin, and subsequent absorption.[49, 87] Seven immunologic types of *C. botulinum,* designated A through G, have been identified, each elaborating an immunologically distinct toxin. Almost all human botulism has resulted from the ingestion of toxins A, B, and E, the last usually associated with fish and marine mammal products.[243, 244, 404]

Japanese studies, reviewed by Dolman and Hda,[107] indicate that antitoxin therapy is effective for type E botulism; the mortality rate associated with type E botulism was

TABLE 243–5 ■ SUMMARY OF THE EFFICACY OF ANTIBODY IN THE PREVENTION AND TREATMENT OF INFECTIOUS DISEASES

Infection	Prophylaxis	Treatment
Bacterial Infections		
Respiratory infections (streptococcal, *Streptococcus pneumoniae*, *Neisseria meningitidis*, *Haemophilus influenzae*)	Proven (NR)*	Proven (NR)
Diphtheria	Unproven (NR)	Proven
Pertussis	Unproven (NR)	Unproven (NR)
Tetanus	Proven	Proven
Other clostridial infections		
C. botulinum	Proven	Proven
C. difficile	Unproven (NR)	Probable benefit
Staphylococcal infections		
Toxic shock syndrome	Unproven (NR)	Probable benefit
Antibiotic resistance	Unproven (NR)	Possible benefit
S. epidermidis in newborns	Possible benefit	Not studied
Invasive streptococcal disease (toxic shock syndrome)	Unproven (NR)	Probable benefit
High-risk newborns	Possible benefit (NR)	Probable benefit
Shock, intensive care, and trauma	Possible benefit (NR)	Unproven
Pseudomonas infection		
Cystic fibrosis	Unproven (NR)	No benefit
Burns	Unproven (NR)	No benefit
Viral Diseases		
Hepatitis A	Proven	No benefit
Hepatitis B	Proven	No benefit
Hepatitis C	Unproven (NR)	No benefit
HIV infection	Unproven (NR)	Unproven (NR)
RSV infection	Proven	Unproven (NR)
Herpesvirus infections		
CMV	Proven	Possible benefit
EBV	Unproven (NR)	Unproven (NR)
HSV	Unproven (NR)	Unproven (NR)
VZV	Proven	Unproven (NR)
Parvovirus infection	Unproven (NR)	Proven (NR)*
Enterovirus infection	Proven (NR)*	Proven (NR)*
In newborns	Unproven	Possible benefit
Ebola	Possible benefit	Unproven
Rabies	Proven	No benefit
Measles	Proven	No benefit
Rubella	Unproven (NR)	No benefit
Mumps	Unproven (NR)	No benefit
Tick-borne encephalitis	Possible benefit	No benefit
Vaccinia	Proven	Proven

*Except for immunodeficient patients.

CMV, cytomegalovirus; EBV, Epstein-Barr virus; HIV, human immunodeficiency virus; HSV, herpes simplex virus; NR, not recommended; RSV, respiratory syncytial virus; VZV, varicella-zoster virus.

From Keller, M. A., and Stiehm, E. R. Passive immunity in prevention and treatment of infectious diseases. Clin. Microbiol. Rev. *13*:602–614, 2000.

49 percent in 135 untreated cases and 3.5 percent in 85 antitoxin-treated cases.

Tacket and associates[452] noted that 46 patients who had type A food-borne botulism and who received trivalent antitoxin had a lower mortality rate (27%) than did 13 patients who did not receive antitoxin (46% mortality). Early antitoxin administration resulted in a shorter clinical course.

The presence of toxin in the blood long after the appearance of clinical symptoms or the ingestion of toxin gives theoretic support to the use of antitoxin to prevent further binding of toxin to tissue. Some antitoxin remains in the circulation for more than 30 days, thus indicating that a single initial dose is adequate therapy.

Equine antitoxins to types A, B, and E are the primary antitoxins available in the United States. The decision to use antitoxin is complicated by its unknown efficacy and its side effects, but approximately 80 percent of patients with ingestion-type botulism receive antitoxin.[404]

Recommendations

Food-borne and wound botulism are treated with trivalent (types A, B, and E) or bivalent (types A and B) antitoxin as soon as possible after testing for sensitivity to horse serum.[9, 10, 87, 404] They are available in the United States from the Centers for Disease Control and Prevention (CDC) in Atlanta, Georgia (404-639-3670 or 2888). One vial (7500 IU of type A, 5500 IU of type B, and 8500 IU of type E) is given intravenously; additional doses are deemed unnecessary. However, with severe wound infections, higher doses may be needed, as guided by antibody titers after administration of the initial antitoxin dose. Equine antitoxin is not indicated for the treatment of infant botulism.

Antitoxin can be given prophylactically to individuals known to have ingested contaminated food. The risk of serum reactions (≈10%) developing must be weighed against the risk of contracting the disease. An investigational equine botulism heptavalent IG fragment F(ab′) also is being studied for treatment.[186]

INFANT BOTULISM

A 5-year, placebo-controlled, double-blind trial of human botulinum immune globulin (BIG) to treat infant botulism showed a significant reduction in hospital days, mechanical ventilation, and tube feedings in BIG recipients, with considerable cost savings.[10] BIG should be started immediately after the illness is suspected. It is available from the Infant Botulism Treatment and Prevention program of the California Department of Health Services under a treatment IND (investigational new drug) protocol (telephone: 510-540-2646).

CLOSTRIDIUM DIFFICILE

Clostridium difficile is an ubiquitous spore-forming anaerobe often involved in antibiotic-associated diarrhea and pseudomembranous colitis. The severity of the disease can range from an asymptomatic carrier state to fulminant colitis with toxic megacolon. Toxic strains of *C. difficile* release two antigenically distinct toxins, both of which have potent cytotoxic and inflammatory properties.[93] Infection generally leads to an antibody response to the toxins, and most individuals older than 2 years have such antibodies; thus, *C. difficile* antibodies are present in IG preparations such as IVIG.[387]

High levels of IgG antibodies acquired after colonization are associated with the asymptomatic carrier state; individuals who have persistent diarrhea have significantly lower serum IgG but not IgA to toxin A.[258] Several patients have been identified with relapsing symptomatic disease who have low IgG antibody levels to toxin A.[179, 264] Several of these patients had low levels of IgG [264] or IgG1 subclass deficiency[179] and were successfully treated with IVIG.

Recommendations

Patients with refractory *C. difficile* infections (with or without a global antibody deficiency) may be treated with 400 mg/kg of IVIG every 3 weeks.[494] Such therapy has been shown to increase antitoxin levels, help control diarrhea, and prevent relapses during the treatment period.[264, 387]

Preliminary studies with an oral anti–*C. difficile* bovine IG for both treatment and prevention are under way.[487]

OTHER CLOSTRIDIAL INFECTIONS

Gas gangrene (*Clostridium perfringens*) equine antitoxin was of unproven efficacy and no longer is available.

DIPHTHERIA AND DIPHTHERIA ANTITOXIN

Many of the adverse consequences of diphtheria result from the *Corynebacterium diphtheriae* toxin elaborated and absorbed from the diphtheritic membrane. This toxin not only has a local effect of perpetuating membrane formation but also is distributed via the blood to the heart, nervous system, kidney, and other organs. The larger the membrane, the more toxin elaborated; in addition, more toxin is elaborated from a membrane involving the pharynx and tonsils than from one involving the larynx and trachea.

Diphtheria toxin is present in three forms: (1) circulating and unbound, (2) loosely bound to tissues, and (3) firmly bound to tissues. Antitoxin neutralizes circulating toxin and competes with and partially neutralizes loosely bound toxin but has no effect on tissue-bound toxin. Thus, optimal passive immunity must be initiated at an early stage of the disease via the intravenous route so that toxin can be intercepted before it becomes tissue-bound.

Antitoxin of animal origin remains the mainstay of treatment, as it was in the pre-antibiotic era. Diphtheria was the first illness in which antiserum was used as standard therapy. Emil von Behring was awarded the first Nobel Prize in Medicine (in 1901) for this achievement.

Fibiger[127] proved the efficacy of diphtheria antitoxin in 1898 when he showed that 5 of 204 patients given horse antitoxin died whereas 14 of 201 not given antiserum died. Paschlau[340] demonstrated the importance of early administration of antitoxin in 1949; the fatality rate of 197 cases treated within 48 hours was 1.96 percent versus 8.9 percent when treatment was delayed until the fourth or fifth day. Other authors have noted similar findings.[457, 458]

Tasman and associates[457, 458] emphasized the importance of intravenous administration of antitoxin because rapid achievement of high blood levels results in rapid neutralization of antitoxin and the appearance, within 30 minutes, of antitoxin in saliva. They showed that the mortality rate and the severity of the myocarditis and neuritis in experimental diphtheria in guinea pigs could be reduced by giving antitoxin intravenously rather than intramuscularly.

McCloskey and Smilack[289] determined the antitoxin content of standard human IG. None of the lots tested contained diphtheria antitoxin in sufficient titer to allow its use for antitoxin therapy. They suggest that an IVIG with higher-titer antitoxin be developed to eliminate the risk of giving horse serum intravenously.

Recommendations

Diphtheria antitoxin of equine origin is indicated for all suspected or proven cases of diphtheria. It is available in vials containing 20,000 U from the CDC. Before administration, skin tests must be performed to determine sensitivity. If the patient has a previous history of serum reactions or these test results are positive, a schedule of desensitization must be followed as outlined earlier.

The amount of antitoxin given depends on the location and the extensiveness of the membrane, the degree of systemic toxicity, and the duration of illness. In severe and late cases, intravenous use is indicated; in mild forms, intramuscular administration will suffice. In all cases, diphtheria antitoxin should be given promptly rather than be delayed while awaiting bacterial confirmation of the diagnosis.[11]

In cutaneous diphtheria, antitoxin is of uncertain value. When used, the dose is 20,000 to 40,000 U intramuscularly to prevent toxic sequelae. In pharyngeal or laryngeal disease, 20,000 to 40,000 U is given intramuscularly; in nasopharyngeal disease, 40,000 to 60,000 U is given intramuscularly; and in extensive disease with neck edema of more than 3 days' duration, 80,000 to 120,000 U is given intravenously.[11] Although antimicrobial therapy is a valuable aid in the treatment of diphtheria, it is not a substitute for antitoxin therapy.

Routine use of antitoxin in an asymptomatic, exposed susceptible patient is not recommended. With heavy exposure or an extremely susceptible host, antitoxin, 5000 to 10,000 U intramuscularly, can be given in addition to antibiotics and diphtheria immunization; proof of efficacy is lacking, however.

PERTUSSIS

Pertussis antiserum was used in the 1930s for the treatment of pertussis.[64] Human pertussis IG was developed in the 1960s but was shown to have no additive benefit to antibiotics in the treatment of pertussis[35, 305] and no longer is available.

Granström and coworkers[158] used an experimental human hyperimmune serum from subjects immunized with a two-component acellular vaccine to treat 33 children, and an equal number received an albumin placebo. Both groups received the same antibiotic and supportive treatment. The treated children had decreased coughing and whooping, particularly if treatment was started early.

Ichimaru and colleagues[195] successfully used a high-titer human IVIG preparation to treat a severely ill 1-year-old child.

Bruss and associates[74] studied a 4 percent high-titer human pertussis IG in 26 children with pertussis and found that the product was safe at three dose levels (250, 750, and 1500 mg/kg) and provided good serum pertussis IgG levels with a half-life of 38 days. Little antibody appeared in nasal secretions. Efficacy was not evaluated in this study, but the product was effective in the treatment of aerosolized-induced pertussis in mice.[75]

RESPIRATORY AND OTHER BACTERIAL INFECTIONS

Respiratory tract infections caused by group A streptococci, *S. pneumoniae*, *H. influenzae* type b, and to a lesser extent *Neisseria meningitidis* are well recognized as occurring more frequently in patients with primary antibody deficiencies, and these infections can be markedly reduced by the regular administration of IG.[263, 323] Furthermore, specific animal antisera to these organisms were used in the early 1930s for the treatment of severe infections (e.g., meningitis), even after the introduction of sulfonamides.[7] Efficacy varied but was clearly better than no treatment at all, and a combination of sulfonamides and antibody seemed to be synergistic.[7]

Small doses of IG (100 mg/kg/mo) did not prevent or improve the course of respiratory infections in normal children.[42, 129]

Nydahl-Persson and colleagues[320] treated 24 children with repeated bacterial respiratory infection (pneumonia or otitis) with either trimethoprim-sulfamethoxazole or IVIG, 400 mg/kg/mo; both agents were effective in reducing the number of infections in comparison with a control group.

Santoshan and associates[393] administered a human intramuscular IG prepared from the sera of donors immunized with pneumococcal, meningococcal, and *H. influenzae* type b polysaccharide vaccines (termed bacterial polysaccharide immune globulin [BPIG]) to Apache Indian infants living on reservations in Arizona. The 222 infants in the study group received 80 mg/kg of BPIG at 2, 6, and 10 months of age, and the 218 infants in the control group received saline injections at the same ages. During the study period, seven cases of invasive *H. influenzae* type b disease and four cases of invasive pneumococcal disease occurred in the control group as compared with one and two cases, respectively, in the BPIG-treated group, a significant difference ($p < .05$).

Otitis

Immunologically normal otitis-prone children seem to derive little preventive or therapeutic benefit from IG given intramuscularly (100 mg/kg/mo)[216] or intravenously (200 mg/kg/mo).[220]

In patients with primary immunodeficiency, the frequency and severity of otitis are diminished dramatically by the use of IG in large doses. In children with secondary antibody deficiency associated with HIV infection, IVIG in large doses (400 mg/kg/mo) reduced the frequency of otitis by 60 percent.[303, 304] Patients with subtle immunologic abnormalities such as IgG subclass deficiencies, partial IgA deficiency, and polysaccharide antibody deficiencies may have recurrent otitis that can be reduced with large dose of IVIG (e.g., 400 mg/kg/mo).[220, 240, 320, 409, 413]

BPIG also was shown to reduce the number of episodes of pneumococcal otitis media in high-risk Indian infants.[409] It did not, however, decrease the total number of otitis media episodes. Large doses of RSV-IVIG (750 mg/kg/mo) reduced the frequency of non-RSV otitis in young infants.[416]

Ishizaka and coworkers[204] successfully treated seven children with recurrent pneumococcal otitis with IVIG.

These studies indicate that low-dose IG is ineffective in the prevention or treatment of otitis, but high doses of IVIG (e.g., >400 mg/kg/mo) may reduce the frequency and severity of otitis in immunodeficient and otitis-prone normal children, probably by reducing both virally and bacterially mediated disease. This treatment should be reserved for otitis-prone patients who have failed a trial of prophylactic antibiotics and have received pneumococcal immunization.

Sinusitis

Sinusitis is common in immunodeficient patients and is difficult to prevent or eradicate, even with optimal treatment. Mofenson and colleagues found that neither IVIG, 400/mg/kg/mo, or weekly sulfonamide prophylaxis prevented sinusitis from developing in children with HIV infection.[301]

In patients with no or subtle immune defects, high-dose IVIG sometimes may decrease the frequency and severity of sinusitis.[65, 413]

Lower Respiratory Tract Infections

Although high-dose IVIG is of proven benefit in preventing pneumonia in immunodeficient subjects, no evidence has established that it will prevent pneumonia in normal subjects. Anecdotal cases of IVIG used as adjunctive therapy for refractory viral pneumonia have been reported.[385, 437]

Cystic Fibrosis

Winnie and associates[499] suggested that IVIG may improve pulmonary function in pulmonary exacerbations of cystic fibrosis. All subjects received antibiotics, were older than 12 years, and had no long-term benefit from the IVIG. Van Wye and coworkers[475] had similar results with the use of hyperimmune *Pseudomonas* IVIG in patients with cystic fibrosis.

A controlled trial of *Pseudomonas* hyperimmune IVIG in 116 cystic fibrosis patients was discontinued because a 6-month interim analysis showed no reduction in acute pulmonary exacerbations.[352]

Burn Infections

Kefalides and associates[228] reduced the mortality rate of severely burned children by administering plasma (1 mL/kg for each 1% of surface area burned) or IG (1 mL/kg on days 1, 3, and 5) from 40 to 20 percent. They concluded that solutions containing antibodies (plasma or IG) were more effective in reducing the complications of infections than were other colloids. However, Stone and colleagues[442] could not achieve any clinical benefit from IG therapy (0.4 mL/kg every third day until skin coverage) in 60 burned subjects versus 40 controls.

Convalescent plasma, special IG with high antibody titer to *Pseudomonas,* and *Pseudomonas* vaccines also have been used in burn patients in an attempt to reduce infections, but without proof of efficacy.[97, 108, 215, 311]

Gram-Negative Infections

The most extensive use of IG for infections in adults has involved trauma/shock/postoperative patients suspected of having gram-negative infections as reviewed earlier under secondary immunodeficiency.[45, 80, 104, 149, 218, 510, 511] Some evidence indicates that IVIG has therapeutic potential in the prevention of infection in certain patients, but its routine use is not indicated.[481]

Newborn Sepsis

As noted earlier, newborns and premature infants in particular are highly susceptible to bacterial sepsis and its sequelae. In addition to antibiotics, leukocytes, granulocyte colony-stimulating factor, and IVIG have been used as adjunctive therapy.

Jenson and Pollack[210, 211] performed a meta-analysis of three prospective controlled studies involving 94 infants who received IVIG for the treatment of neonatal sepsis. The death rate in the IVIG-treated infants was 5.8 percent (3 of 52) versus 31 percent (13 of 42) in the control group, a sixfold, highly significant difference ($p = .007$).

Thus, the use of IVIG is justified for septic premature infants not responding well to conventional therapy. It may be particularly valuable for neutropenic septic infants because it may help mobilize leukocytes from the storage pool. A dose of 500 mg/kg daily for 3 days and repeated as necessary is recommended.

STAPHYLOCOCCAL INFECTIONS

Staphylococcal infections are ubiquitous and of varying severity and include superficial skin infections, deep-seated indolent cellulitis, scalded skin syndrome, and overwhelming toxic shock. Antibiotics are usually effective in controlling the infections, but in some instances, the organism is antibiotic-resistant, or the disease is rapidly progressive. IVIG may be of adjunctive benefit in some of these situations.[90]

Patients with staphylococcal toxic shock syndrome, often associated with the use of tampons by menstruating women, have a rapid onset of fever, shock, a macular desquamating rash, and multisystem organ failure.[90, 296] The pathogenesis of the disorder results from infection with a strain that releases toxic shock syndrome toxin (TSST-1).[279] Approximately 20 percent of all staphylococcal isolates carry the gene for this toxin.[273] TSST-1 is a potent superantigen that directly activates the 5 percent of T cells that have a $V_{\beta}2$ T-cell receptor[273]; such activation results in the rapid release of multiple cytokines and a clinical picture of rapidly progressive illness.

IVIG contains neutralizing antitoxins to the staphylococcal (and streptococcal) superantigens[447] and has been used successfully both in animal models of toxic shock syndrome[90] and in several patients.[43, 325, 337] Although no controlled clinical trials have been performed for staphylococcal toxic shock syndrome, most authorities recommend large IVIG doses, at least 400 mg/kg, in addition to antibiotic treatment and circulatory support.[90] IVIG also down-regulates cytokine synthesis and action and inhibits immune activation, thereby providing additional benefits.[21, 90]

Higuchi and coauthors[187] reported a large family that had recurrent episodes of staphylococcal toxic shock syndrome associated with normal immunoglobulin levels but low serum antibody titers to staphylococcal superantigens; two boys in the family achieved successful prophylaxis with regular IVIG infusions.

A second situation in which antibody may be of value is neonatal staphylococcal infection. Coagulase-negative staphylococcal infection such as with *S. epidermidis* is the most common cause of sepsis in premature infants and is aggravated in part by the use of catheters and parenteral lipid infusions.[34, 130] One controlled study showed that IVIG was of value in decreasing, but not eliminating infections,[34] but this benefit has not been found in all trials of IVIG in newborns.

This variability may be explained by differing amounts of staphylococcal antibodies present in different IVIG brands and lots, particularly opsonic antibodies, which have been shown in animal models to be the most important correlate of clinical protection.[130] Because antibody variability exists in lots of IVIG made from pools of thousands of donors, it is not surprising that Krediet and colleagues[247] could not reliably increase the opsonic titers of premature infants by administering single-donor fresh frozen plasma.

Mandy and associates[281] found that a human hyperimmune IVIG derived from donors immunized with an experimental staphylococcal vaccine increased the opsonic activity of the serum of very-low-birth-weight infants in a dose-dependent fashion; it was well tolerated at doses of 500 to 1000 mg/kg.

A final use of IG is for the treatment of antibiotic-resistant chronic staphylococcal infection, along with intravenous antibiotics. Waisbren[483] treated 16 such patients with an antibiotic–gamma-globulin combination, with recovery noted in 13 of them. We (E.R.S.) successfully treated a woman with antibiotic-resistant dissecting cellulitis of the scalp with a combination of high-dose IVIG and antibiotics. Animal studies support such a combined approach.[131]

Recommendations

Large doses of IVIG are indicated for the treatment of toxic shock syndrome. The recommended regimen is a single dose of 1 to 2 g/kg or 400 mg/kg daily for 5 days. A repeat dose may be necessary because of rapid clearance of IVIG in this illness.[21, 90]

IVIG is not recommended routinely for the prevention of infection in premature newborn infants. As noted earlier, IVIG may be of adjunctive benefit in the treatment of neonates with sepsis, particularly those with neutropenia.[211] We recommend 500 mg/kg on 3 consecutive days if the patient has not responded to optimal antibiotic and supportive management. This regimen may be repeated every week as needed.

The value of IVIG in refractory chronic staphylococcal infections is unproven, although anecdotal reports of efficacy exist.

STREPTOCOCCAL INFECTIONS

Circulating antibody may play a role in the prevention and treatment of group A streptococcal infection.[223] Newborns rarely get invasive streptococcal illness, in part because of transplacental protective antibodies.[223] Equine antitoxin was used with some success in the treatment of erysipelas and scarlet fever in the 1920s and 1930s.[275, 449] A preventive streptococcal vaccine to the M component has been proposed but as yet is unavailable.

Invasive group A streptococcal infections, including septicemia, necrotizing fasciitis or myositis, and toxic shock syndrome, are increasing in severity and frequency.[23] Streptococcal pyrogenic exotoxins (SPEs), including types A, B, and C, and mitogenic factor elaborated by certain strains of streptococci may be responsible for these serious complications of infection. SPEs are potent superantigens that activate certain T lymphocytes directly and lead to the massive production of multiple cytokines, with resultant shock, fever, and organ failure. IVIG contains neutralizing antibodies to these antigens.[318, 455]

Many case reports have attested to the value of IVIG in streptococcal toxic shock syndrome since the report by Barry and coauthors in 1992.[43, 259, 345] Kaul and colleagues[226] reported a study of 21 consecutive patients at several Canadian medical centers in 1994 and 1995 treated with IVIG and compared them with 32 similar patients not given IVIG at the same centers for the 3 preceding years. Both groups received appropriate antibiotics and were similar with regard to demographics, severity score, and timing of intervention. The median IVIG dose was 2 g/kg. The survival rate for the IVIG-treated group was significantly greater at 7 and 30 days (90% and 67%, respectively) than that in the untreated controls (50% and 34%, respectively, $p = .02$), and the days of hospitalization were insignificantly shortened (29 versus 39). Serum from the IVIG-treated patients caused a marked inhibition of lymphocyte mitogenic activity to their own bacterial isolates after a single IVIG dose.

Swedo and coauthors[448] reported a syndrome of tics or obsessive-compulsive behavior, or both, occurring in prepubertal children soon after the onset of a streptococcal infection. They termed this disorder pediatric autoimmune neuropsychiatric disorder associated with streptococcal disease (PANDAS syndrome). They reported that either IVIG or plasma exchange was of some therapeutic benefit.[352]

Recommendations

IVIG is recommended for moderate and severe cases of streptococcal toxic shock syndrome, even if the organism has not been identified. The recommended dose is 1 to 2 g/kg given in a single dose or in divided doses of 400 mg/kg. Repeat administration of IVIG may be necessary after a few days because of rapid IVIG catabolism.

IVIG is of unproven value in treating PANDAS syndrome.

TETANUS, TETANUS ANTITOXIN, AND TETANUS IMMUNE GLOBULIN

Antitoxin for the treatment of tetanus was introduced into medicine by Behring and Kitasato[342] in 1890; large doses (50 to 100 mL) of serum from horses immunized with tetanus toxin were used. The dose was increased gradually to 300 to 500 mL, equivalent to 300 to 500 U of antitoxin. As the means to increase the production and concentration of antitoxin developed and a high mortality rate persisted, the dosage of antitoxin was increased until doses as high as 200,000 IU, repeated at weekly intervals, were recommended.[342] Despite such heroic therapy, no solid proof of efficacy was obtained.

However, in 1960, Brown and colleagues,[67] using sequential analysis, found that the mortality rate was 49 percent in 41 patients with tetanus who received 200,000 U of antitoxin, a statistically significant difference that established therapeutic efficacy. Extensive controlled studies established that mortality rates did not improve when doses of 100,000 to 500,000 U were used.[274, 471–473] Similarly, Patel and associates[342] could find no difference in the mortality rates of patients with tetanus treated with antitoxin doses of 5000 to 60,000 U. Adequate blood levels of antitoxin were noted in all cases, even in fatal cases, with a dose of 10,000 U. In mild cases, no antitoxin was necessary. They and others have reported considerable differences in mortality rates, ranging from 0 to 98 percent; the rate depends primarily on the severity of illness rather than the dose of antitoxin.

Athavale[31] established that antitoxin was of benefit in tetanus neonatorum and in tetanus in children up to 12 years of age. Antitoxin affected the mortality rate in mild and moderate cases but not in severe ones. A dose of 10,000 IU was as effective as one of 30,000 IU.

The mechanism of action of antitoxin is to neutralize toxin before its transport to the nervous system via the circulation. Antitoxin also can neutralize toxin locally and prevent its systemic absorption. Thus, antitoxin can be given locally, at the site of toxin production (e.g., at the site of a wound), intravenously (in severe cases), or intramuscularly (in less severe cases).

In 1962, an estimated 750,000 annual doses of equine tetanus antitoxin were needed in the United Kingdom, which is equivalent to more than a million doses in the United States.[381] Serum sickness occurs in 6 to 14 percent and fatal anaphylaxis in 1 of every 100,000 injections. Thus, hyperimmune human tetanus immune globulin (TIG), first available in the early 1960s, gradually has replaced equine tetanus antitoxin.

Rubbo and Suri[378] and Rubinstein[381] showed that TIG given intramuscularly (5 to 10 U/kg) provides adequate circulating antitoxin levels and is maintained in the circulation for considerably longer than equine tetanus antitoxin is.

The efficacy of TIG is equivalent to that of equine tetanus antitoxin. McCracken and associates[291] compared the results of 550 U of TIG with 10,000 U of tetanus antitoxin in the treatment of tetanus neonatorum. Among the 65 infants in each treatment group, no difference was noted in severity, length of hospitalization, need for sedation or gavage feeding, or mortality rate. Blake and colleagues[56] analyzed 545 tetanus cases reported to the CDC from 1965 to 1971 and could find no difference in the outcome of patients treated with equine tetanus antitoxin versus TIG.

Gupta and associates[172] gave TIG intrathecally to alternate patients with early tetanus. Among 49 patients given intrathecal TIG (250 U), 3 got worse and 1 died; among 48 patients given intramuscular TIG (1000 U), 15 got worse and 10 died. No side effects occurred. Herrero and coworkers[185] could not prove a benefit of administering intrathecal antitoxin for tetanus neonatorum. A meta-analysis of intrathecal therapy also has cast doubt on its efficacy.[3]

TIG can be given along with tetanus toxoid (10 Lf U) for passive-active immunization. A dose of 250 U of TIG given intramuscularly at a site different from that of the toxoid does not interfere with the active antibody response.[290]

Lee and Lederman[261] measured the tetanus antitoxin titers in 29 lots of IVIG and noted considerable variability, although all lots had titers greater than 4 U/mL (mean, 21 U/mL). All lots would provide sufficient tetanus antibody if used at doses of 100 mg/kg as an alternative to TIG or tetanus antitoxin.

Recommendations

PROPHYLAXIS

If a nonimmunized person sustains a serious injury or a bite, 250 to 500 U of TIG should be given intramuscularly as soon as possible.[20] The larger dose is used in the event of an extensive wound or delay in treatment. Alum-precipitated toxoid to initiate active immunity is given at a different site with a separate syringe. If TIG is unavailable, 3000 to 5000 U of tetanus antitoxin (equine) is administered (after screening and testing for serum sensitivity).[20] TIG is available for intramuscular administration in individual vials containing 250 U. Tetanus antitoxin is available in vials containing 1500 or 20,000 U.

TREATMENT

In addition to administration of antibiotics and management of the wound, TIG should be given in doses of 3000 to 6000 IU, part infiltrated near the wound and the remainder administered intramuscularly.[20] If the wound is extensive, TIG can be diluted with saline to infiltrate the entire area. TIG also is indicated for the treatment of tetanus neonatorum.

If TIG is unavailable, equine tetanus antitoxin should be given in a single dose of 50,000 to 100,000 U, with 20,000 U given intravenously (after appropriate testing for sensitivity) and the remainder intramuscularly. Intrathecal TIG or antitoxin is unnecessary and not recommended. On recovery, primary immunization should be undertaken.

In tetanus neonatorum, McCracken and associates[291] found that 500 IU of TIG given intramuscularly and 10,000 U of equine antitoxin were equally efficacious. Intrathecal TIG has been recommended,[172] but its efficacy is unproven.[48]

Passive Immunity in Viral Infection

ENTEROVIRUSES

Poliovirus

Before the development of poliomyelitis vaccines in the mid-1950s, IG was used extensively for the prevention of poliomyelitis. Bodian[60, 61] showed that Red Cross IG had neutralizing antibody to all three strains of poliovirus in approximately equal titer and that rhesus monkeys given intramuscular poliovirus could be protected against disease by the subcutaneous administration of IG.

Bloxsom,[58] in an uncontrolled study during a 1948 Texas epidemic, gave 841 contacts an average dose of 2 mL of IG and noted only 4 cases at 1, 2, 3, and 42 days after administration of the IG injection. He suggested that the IG was given too late to prevent the first three cases and that protection had worn off in the fourth case.

A committee on immunization of the National Foundation for Infantile Paralysis recommended in March 1951 that a controlled study be conducted on the efficacy of IG for the prevention of poliomyelitis during epidemics. Hammon and associates[178] subsequently undertook a massive field study in communities in three states during poliomyelitis epidemics. Fifty-five thousand children (!) aged 1 to 11 years received either IG (average dose, 0.14 mL/lb) or gelatin in a double-blind fashion. During the first week after injection, 12 cases occurred in the IG recipients and 16 cases in the gelatin recipients. In the second week, 3 and 23 cases and, in the third to fifth weeks, 6 and 38 cases occurred in the two groups, respectively. When protection was incomplete, decreased severity was noted. Protection waned by 6 weeks and disappeared by 8 weeks. These clinical results were confirmed by isolation of virus or a rise in antibody titer in affected patients.

IG was an inefficient method of poliomyelitis prophylaxis in that it prevented only one case for every 500 to 2000 injections, and then only for a brief time. Its chief value was in close family contacts of affected children and in aborting severe local epidemics.

RECOMMENDATIONS

The use of IG rarely is indicated for the prevention of poliomyelitis. An exposed unimmunized subject can be given 0.15 mL/kg of IG. An unimmunized patient who is traveling to an endemic or epidemic area and who cannot have vaccine can be given this dose of IG for temporary protection.

An immunodeficient patient inadvertently exposed to live attenuated polio vaccine who is now excreting poliovirus in stool may be a candidate for receiving IVIG and oral IG in an effort to rid the GI tract of the virus.

Other Enteroviruses

Enteroviruses, particularly echoviruses and coxsackieviruses, can cause severe disease in neonates[203] and immunodeficient patients, particularly those with X-linked agammaglobulinemia. IG and IVIG have been used in both groups for the prevention and treatment of these infections.

Chronic enteroviral meningoencephalitis with severe neurologic findings may develop in agammaglobulinemic patients; its occurrence has decreased since routine treatment with IVIG has been instituted for these patients. IVIG does not prevent all cases, possibly because of differing titers of antibodies to different enteroviral serotypes. McKinney and coworkers[293] summarized the results of treatment of 42 patients with chronic enterovirus meningoencephalitis: 10 received IG or plasma, but only 1 survived, a patient who received high-titer human serum; 10 received IVIG, and 7 survived; and 12 received both intraventricular IVIG and systemic IVIG, and 6 improved and 10 survived.

Misbah and colleagues[298] reviewed 15 patients with chronic enteroviral meningoencephalitis not included in the McKinney report, some of whom, however, had been reported by others.[115, 245] Of 5 patients treated with IVIG, 3 survived, and of 10 treated with IVIG and intraventricular or intrathecal IVIG (only 1 patient received intrathecal, not intraventricular IVIG), 5 survived. Quartier and associates[356] reported complete clinical and virologic remission, as determined by both culture and polymerase chain reaction (PCR) assay, in one patient treated with IVIG and a brief course of pleconaril; remission was maintained for 37 months by keeping the serum IgG trough level at 800 mg/dL. A second patient was treated with IVIG and pleconaril, but intraventricular IVIG was added when cerebrospinal fluid (CSF) pleocytosis persisted after 11 months of therapy. Complete clinical and virologic remission resulted and persisted at the 20-month follow-up. This study indicated that CSF PCR assay can be used, in addition to viral culture, as a guide to successful therapy.

Severe and sometimes fatal disseminated enterovirus infection can develop in neonates.[358] Case reports have suggested benefit with the use of IVIG.[203, 214, 474] Kimura and coworkers[235] treated coxsackievirus B3 infection in four term infants with IVIG; the three who were treated early survived, but the infant treated 6 days after the onset of infection died. Abzug and associates[4] treated nine infants with echovirus and coxsackievirus B infection with IVIG but without apparent benefit; however, three of five infants who received high-titer IVIG had a shortened period of viremia. Thus, IVIG is of uncertain value, particularly if its titer against the particular virus is not known.

Nagington and colleagues[310] used IG successfully in an echovirus 11 outbreak in a special care nursery, but Kinney and coworkers[237] could not demonstrate a benefit of using IG in a similar nursery with the same virus. Pasic and associates[341] administered IVIG at 400 mg/kg prophylactically (neutralization titer, 1:32) during a nursery echovirus 6 outbreak and thought that the severity of illness was decreased, although viral transmission continued.

RECOMMENDATIONS

IVIG may be used for critically ill neonates with disseminated enterovirus infection, although its benefit is unproven. In an outbreak situation with a known serotype and the availability of IVIG with significant titer to this serotype, IVIG should be considered. Multiple doses of 500 mg/kg, as well as single doses of 750 to 1000 mg/kg, have been used.[4, 214, 235, 474]

For chronic enteroviral meningoencephalitis, McKinney and colleagues[293] recommend that sufficient IVIG be administered to maintain an IgG serum trough level of 900 to 1000 mg/dL. Even higher doses may be needed if the IVIG titer for the infecting virus is low. Quartier and coworkers[356] used 500 mg/kg of IVIG every 24 to 48 hours for 2 weeks, followed by 500 mg/kg two to three times per week for 6 weeks and then gradual reductions, but with maintenance of the trough IgG level at greater than 800 mg/dL.

Administration of IVIG by intraventricular catheter should be considered for patients without improvement despite aggressive therapy with IVIG. IVIG for intraventricular administration should have a neutral pH, be given slowly, and be at room temperature.[293] Dwyer and Erlendsson[115] used 6 percent IVIG intraventricularly starting at doses of 120 mg/day and increasing to 600 mg/day during the first week of treatment, followed by doses of 300 mg/day for 1 to 4 weeks. Quartier and colleagues[356] administered 300 mg of IVIG daily for 15 days and then 300 mg three times a week to a patient who had failed intravenous IVIG therapy. The duration and frequency of both intraventricular and intravenous IVIG must be individualized and determined by clinical and virologic response and normalization of CSF and ventricular fluid. An IVIG with a high titer to the infecting serotype should be used for both systemic and intraventricular therapy.

HEPATITIS A

The widest use for human IG has been for the prevention of hepatitis A, but this application has been decreased by the widespread use of hepatitis A vaccine. The efficacy of IG was demonstrated in 1945 by Stokes and Neefe[441] in aborting an epidemic in a children's summer camp, by Havens and Paul[180] in controlling an institutional epidemic, and by Gellis and associates[139] in preventing hepatitis A in the Mediterranean theater of operations at the close of World War II. The combined use of IG and hepatitis A vaccine and scrupulous cleanliness can be used to interrupt the intestinal-oral circuit of transmission and abort an incipient epidemic.

IG is efficacious in preventing hepatitis A if given within 2 weeks of the last exposure.[12] Protection persists for 6 to 8 weeks. Stokes and associates[438] noted that a single small dose of IG (0.02 mL/kg) provided a degree of protection for up to 9 months in individuals residing at an institution in which hepatitis A was endemic.

The effectiveness of IG in hepatitis A varies from 80 to 95 percent, depending on how soon it is administered after exposure and the severity of the exposure.[485] IG suppresses clinical manifestations of the disease, but anicteric hepatitis is not prevented, and the ratio of anicteric to icteric hepatitis may be as high as 12:1.[253] Because the period of protection exceeds the expected duration of the IG, the concept of passive-active immunity has emerged; as a result of continuous exposure, a mild illness ensues and, in turn, confers long-lasting immunity.[253, 438, 485]

The initial studies of Stokes and Neefe[441] used an IG dose of 0.15 mL/lb. Other early workers used doses of 0.06 to 0.12 mL/lb.[139, 180] Stokes and associates[438] in 1951 showed that doses as low as 0.01 mL/lb were effective in limiting spread but not in totally preventing hepatitis. Hsia and colleagues[192] in 1954 also noted that a dose of 0.01 mL/lb was effective in preventing hepatitis among family contacts. However, Ward and associates[486] in 1958 were able to reduce the incidence of hepatitis in institutionalized patients from 19.5 to 7.4 cases per 1000 with 0.01 mL/kg and to 1.7 cases per 1000 with 0.06 mL/kg. The larger dose may be particularly important in adults because they are subject to more severe disease.

The use of serologic tests for hepatitis A provides a way to determine the immunity of a subject, the presence of inapparent infection, the titer of hepatitis A virus (HAV) in lots of IG, and the validity of the passive-active immunity concept.[438, 441] In earlier studies, Krugman[248] showed that an IG preparation with a titer of 1:3200 by an immune adherence test was effective in neutralizing the infectivity of MS-1 serum, a substance known to contain HAV. Among seronegative children who received the IG–hepatitis A mixture, six remained seronegative and two became seropositive; one became ill. By contrast, hepatitis developed in 8 of 14 children who received MS-1 serum without IG.

Most current lots of IG have anti-HAV antibodies when assayed by a competitive-inhibition radioimmunoassay (RIA). Titers greater than 1:100 are protective.[420]

Recommendations

PROPHYLAXIS

HOUSEHOLD AND SEXUAL CONTACTS. Individuals, either adults or children, with a known intimate exposure to hepatitis A such as a household or sexual contact should be given a single IG dose of 0.02 mL/kg as soon as possible after exposure.[12] Hepatitis A vaccine also can be initiated. Serologic testing for hepatitis A is unnecessary and may delay the administration of IG. The use of IG longer than 2 weeks after exposure is not indicated.[12]

SCHOOL EXPOSURE. IG is not usually necessary for children and their teachers exposed to a single case of hepatitis A in the classroom of a day school. However, if several children are infected or if transmission in the school is documented, IG (0.02 mL/kg) and immunization are indicated for the students and teachers. New students and employees should be given IG and vaccine for 6 weeks after the last case is identified.[12]

IG prophylaxis is recommended for children and staff exposed at a boarding school or in a school for retarded children, where opportunities for transmission by the fecal-oral route are increased.

INSTITUTIONAL OUTBREAKS. Hepatitis A outbreaks in institutions such as boarding schools, daycare centers, facilities for the mentally retarded, or prisons require aggressive action. Other cohorts, employees, and adult members of the households of infants who wear diapers and who attend these facilities should be treated immediately with 0.02 mL/kg of IG. If recognition of an outbreak is delayed 3 or more weeks after onset of the index case or if spread to other cohorts, staff, or household contacts appears to be occurring, all personnel (staff and children) should be given IG. If an outbreak of hepatitis A is traced to a food handler, IG should be given to close contacts and other restaurant employees.[83]

HOSPITAL AND CLINIC EXPOSURE. Administration of IG to unimmunized hospital employees caring for patients with hepatitis A or to patients usually is not recommended unless evidence of an outbreak among patients or between patients and staff exists.[12]

COMMON-SOURCE EXPOSURE. These cases generally are identified too long after the exposure for IG to be effective; if an exposed person is within 2 weeks of the last exposure, IG can be given (0.02 mL/kg).[12]

COMMUNITY OUTBREAKS. Unless a source of the infection is identified, mass use of IG is ineffective and not recommended because it will not interfere with transmission.[30] Immunization is recommended.

FOREIGN TRAVEL. Ordinary tourist travel does not require IG prophylaxis or hepatitis A vaccine. However, individuals going to developing countries should receive vaccine 1 month before departure. If the departure date is less than 1 month away, 0.02 mL/kg of IG and vaccine can be used.[12] The IG will provide immediate protection and not interfere with efficacy of the vaccine. If exposure to hepatitis A will continue beyond 3 months, the IG dose should be 0.06 mL/kg and repeated every 5 months if hepatitis A exposure continues.

PRIMATE EXPOSURE. Certain subhuman primates such as chimpanzees may carry HAV. Animal handlers should observe scrupulous hygiene and be given hepatitis A vaccine. If bitten and unimmunized, they should receive 0.02 mL/kg of IG and vaccine.

NEEDLE EXPOSURE. IG is indicated for susceptible persons accidentally inoculated with blood or serum from a patient with hepatitis A. The recommended dose is 0.02 mL/kg; pregnancy is not a contraindication to the administration of IG.

NEWBORN INFANTS OF INFECTED MOTHERS. If the mother becomes symptomatic with acute hepatitis A between 2 weeks before and 1 week after delivery, the infant can be given 0.02 mL/kg of IG; efficacy has not been established, however.

HEPATITIS B AND HEPATITIS B IMMUNE GLOBULIN

Hepatitis B virus causes a wide spectrum of illness ranging from asymptomatic seroconversion to fulminant hepatitis. Although most normal subjects recover completely, the carrier state occurs commonly in exposed immunocompromised subjects such as newborns, patients taking immunosuppressive medications, and patients with primary or secondary immunodeficiencies. Transmission occurs after exposure to blood or other body fluids, through inoculation or sex, and by close personal contact such as may occur in daycare centers. The main route of transmission used to be via blood transfusion, but with donor testing, this route is no longer common in developed countries. An important route of transmission is from the mother to her newborn infant, who is likely to remain chronically infected for a lifetime. This route usually can be prevented by active and passive immunization.

Immune Globulin in Hepatitis B

In contrast to its proven efficacy in the prophylaxis of hepatitis A, IG was not reliably able to prevent post-transfusion hepatitis or hepatitis B ("serum hepatitis"). This inconsistency derived from the fact, not initially appreciated, that most (as many as 80%) cases of post-transfusion hepatitis were not caused by hepatitis B virus.

The initial study of IG in hepatitis B was conducted in 1945 by Grossman and associates,[166] who treated alternate battle casualties given whole blood or plasma with two 10-mL injections of IG 1 month apart. The incidence of icteric hepatitis was 1.3 percent in 384 IG-treated patients and 9.9 percent in 384 control patients, a highly significant difference that suggested a beneficial effect of IG. In 1947, Duncan and associates[113] reported the results from a similar study, although they gave only one 10-mL injection; hepatitis occurred in 1.2 percent of 2406 patients in the IG-treated group and in 0.9 percent of patients in the control group, an insignificant difference. However, the mean incubation period was significantly prolonged in the IG-treated group (to 103 days) as compared with the control group (87 days). Drake and associates[110] could not demonstrate a beneficial effect of IG derived from convalescent hepatitis patients when given to volunteers deliberately inoculated with blood or serum from an infected patient. The IG was ineffective when given intramuscularly or when mixed with the infective serum before injection.

Holland and associates[190] could not alter the incidence or severity of post-transfusion hepatitis in 84 open heart surgery patients given two 10-mL doses of IG 1 month apart in comparison to 83 non–IG-treated controls. These findings were confirmed in a large cooperative study of 5189 transfused cardiovascular patients given 10 mL of IG during the first, fourth, and seventh postoperative weeks.[154] Redeker and associates[364] could not demonstrate that IG protected spouses of individuals with type B hepatitis. Similarly, Kuhns and colleagues[255] could not reduce the incidence of post-transfusion hepatitis B with 20 mL of IG. Both these latter studies used IG with low titers of antibody to hepatitis B surface antigen (anti-HBs).

Several factors are probably responsible for the variation in effectiveness of IG in hepatitis B. One is the variable degree of exposure to hepatitis B virus, which can be massive (as with a blood transfusion) or minimal (e.g., a household contact). A second factor is the variable level of anti-HBs antibody in different lots of IG. Because IG does not necessarily contain high titers of anti-HBs, it no longer is recommended for hepatitis B prophylaxis.

Hepatitis B Immune Globulin

Soon after hepatitis B surface antigen (HBsAg) and its antibody (anti-HBs) were identified, researchers realized that measurement of the antibody content of IG would permit selection of lots (or donors) with high titers of anti-HBs; such selection results in IG lots with anti-HBs titers of at least 1:100,000 by RIA. This product (HBIG) has been licensed since 1978 for prevention of hepatitis B.[351, 363]

Krugman and associates[249, 250] in 1971 evaluated high-titer HBIG in institutionalized children injected with the infective serum MS-2. Hepatitis developed in all 11 children exposed to MS-2 serum; 2 became icteric, and 5 remained HBsAg carriers after 320 days. Among five children given MS-2 serum and standard IG, hepatitis developed in three, two were icteric, but none became a carrier. Of 10 children exposed to MS-2 serum and HBIG, 6 were completely protected, 1 had a transient infection, and classic hepatitis developed in 3. They concluded that HBIG was 70 percent effective under these circumstances. Their later studies confirmed that HBIG could reduce the incidence, severity, and carrier rate of HBsAg significantly after prenatal exposure to hepatitis B virus.[248]

Szmuness and associates[451] tested the efficacy of HBIG versus IG by giving either standard IG or HBIG to retarded institutionalized children at admission and at 4-month intervals for 1.5 to 2 years and comparing the incidence of hepatitis with that of untreated subjects. Both globulin-treated groups had a lower attack rate (11% versus 25% in the untreated subjects) and a lower incidence of persistent antigenemia (none in the globulin-treated group versus 13.5% in the untreated group). Thus, both IG and HBIG were effective in preventing or modifying nonparenterally transmitted hepatitis B in an endemic setting. Of note is that anti-HBs developed in 55 percent of the patients treated with standard IG whereas antibody developed in only 23 percent of the patients treated with HBIG, thus suggesting that passive-active immunity occurred more frequently in the group that received standard IG than in the group that received HBIG.

Seeff and associates[400] gave either HBIG or standard IG to 302 individuals definitively exposed orally or parenterally to material that was infectious for hepatitis B. The incidence of both clinical and subclinical hepatitis during the first 6 months was 0.7 percent in the HBIG-treated group and 6.1 percent in the IG-treated group. At 6 months, 32 percent of the IG recipients and 6 percent of the HBIG recipients had antibody, a finding indicative of minimal passive-active immunity in the HBIG-treated group; Grady[155] reported similar results with HBIG after accidental exposure. The incidence of hepatitis at 6 months was 7 percent (of 251 patients) with standard IG, 5 percent (of 208 patients) with intermediate-titer HBIG, and 2 percent (of 253 patients) with high-titer HBIG. This protection waned after 6 months, and differences in the groups became less apparent after 9 months, possibly because of re-exposure, delayed onset of infection, or failure of passive-active immunity.

Prevention of Vertical Transmission

Beasley and associates[46, 47] studied the efficacy of HBIG in preventing perinatal transmission of the hepatitis B virus carrier state from a mother to her newborn infant. HBIG or placebo was given at birth to the infants of hepatitis B early antigen (HBeAg)-positive, HBsAg-positive carrier mothers, and the infants were monitored for at least 15 months. Of 61 placebo recipients, 92 percent became carriers; of 67 infants who received 1.0 mL of HBIG at birth, 54 percent became carriers; and of 57 infants who received 0.5 mL of HBIG at birth and at 3 and 6 months, 26 percent became carriers. Passive-active immunization, indicated by the presence of anti-HBs, occurred in 27 percent of the single-dose group and in 61 percent in the three-dose group.

Based on these and other studies[212, 368] suggesting that multiple HBIG doses were more effective in interrupting vertical transmission of the HBsAg carrier state than was a single HBIG dose, advisory committees in 1981 recommended that all infants of HBsAg-positive mothers be given HBIG (0.5 mL) immediately after birth and again at 3 and 6 months. However, many of these infants became infected sometime after their last HBIG dose (i.e., in the second or third year of life), thus indicating a need for more durable active immunity.

Wong and associates[503] studied the efficacy of hepatitis B vaccine (HBV) given in conjunction with HBIG in the prevention of vertical transmission of the carrier state from mother to infant. They gave HBV (36 infants), HBV plus one dose of HBIG (35 infants), HBV plus seven monthly HBIG doses (35 infants), or placebo (35 infants) to infants of HBsAg-positive mothers. In all vaccine groups, development of a persistent carrier state was significantly reduced in comparison to the placebo group (21% with HBV alone, 2.9% with HBV plus one dose of HBIG, and 6.8% with HBV plus seven doses of HBIG versus 73.2% for placebo groups). That anti-HBs developed in all infants of the treatment groups indicated that HBIG did not interfere with active immunization.

This and other studies[92, 221, 453] indicate that HBIG given at the same time as HBV provides optimal passive-active immunity for long-lasting prevention of the carrier state, and this dose is the current recommendation. Studies in adults also confirm that HBIG given before or simultaneously with the first dose of HBV does not interfere with the antibody response to HBV.[451, 507] This approach will not prevent every case of vertical transmission because some infants may acquire the infection in utero.

HBIG is not of value in the treatment of either acute[5] or chronic[367] hepatitis B infection.

Hepatitis B Immune Globulin in Liver Transplantation

Liver transplantation in a patient infected with hepatitis B is associated with a high rate of recurrence in the new liver (≈50% in 3 years) and subsequent mortality. HBIG given intravenously (!) or by the usual intramuscular route has been used to prevent recurrence of hepatitis B.[389] In a retrospective analysis of 359 such transplants, hepatitis B recurrence was 74 ± 6 percent in 67 patients given no HBIG, 74 ± 5 percent in 83 patients given HBIG for 2 months, and 36 ± 4 percent in the 209 patients given HBIG for 6 months or longer. Grazi and coworkers[160] significantly reduced the recurrence rate in HBsAg-positive, hepatitis B virus DNA–negative cirrhotic individuals undergoing liver transplantation with the use of HBIG for 1 year after transplantation; recurrence was noted in 8 of 10 controls (80%) and 4 of 25 (16%) HBIG-treated patients.

In addition to HBIG therapy, pretransplantation and post-transplantation antiviral drugs (e.g., lamivudine, interferon-α) can be given. When administered in the immediate pretransplant period to patients with a high viral burden, these drugs may enhance the effectiveness of HBIG because less virus must be neutralized.[460]

Recommendations

PROPHYLAXIS

HBIG is recommended after parenteral or mucous membrane (oral, sexual, ophthalmic) contact with individuals with hepatitis B infection or with HBsAg-positive materials (e.g., blood, plasma) and for neonates born to HBsAg-positive mothers[13] (Table 243–6). It is available in 0.5-mL pre-filled syringes and 1- and 5-mL vials.

Exposure to Blood That Contains (or May Contain) Hepatitis B Surface Antigen

No prospective studies have tested the efficacy of a combination of HBIG and HBV in preventing hepatitis B after accidental exposure, including exposure by the percutaneous, ocular, and mucous membrane routes, as well as by human bites that penetrate the skin. Because health care workers at risk for incurring such accidents are HBV candidates and because the combination of HBIG and HBV is more effective than HBIG alone in perinatal exposure, this combination also is recommended after accidental exposure.

If the exposed patient is unimmunized and the blood or secretions come from an individual known to be HBsAg-positive or if the infection status of the source is unknown but the source is high risk, immediate prophylaxis is indicated. A single dose of HBIG (0.06 mL/kg or 5 mL for adults) should be given intramuscularly as soon as possible,

TABLE 243–6 ■ HEPATITIS B POSTEXPOSURE RECOMMENDATIONS FOR HEPATITIS B IMMUNE GLOBULIN (HBIG) AND HEPATITIS B VACCINE

	HBIG		Hepatitis B Vaccine	
Type of Exposure	**Dose**	**Recommended Timing**	**Dose**	**Recommended Timing**
Perinatal				
Infant of HBsAg⁺ mother	0.5 mL IM	Within 12 hr of birth	0.5 mL	First dose within 12 hr, repeat 2 times
Infant of mother whose HBsAg status is unknown	0.5 mL IM	Within 7 days of birth if mother is found to be HBsAg⁺	0.5 mL	First dose within 12 hr, repeat 2 times
Premature infant (<2000 g) whose mother's HBsAg status is unknown	0.5 mL IM	Within 12 hr of birth (unless maternal HBsAg test result is negative by this time)	0.5 mL	First dose within 12 hr, repeat 3 times
Mucous Membrane or Percutaneous				
Nonvaccinated	0.06 mL/kg IM	Immediately	0.5 mL*	First dose immediately, repeat 2 times
Previously vaccinated, known responder	None	None	None	
Previously vaccinated, unknown response	0.06 mL/kg IM	Test patient for anti-HBs; if anti-HBs >10 mIU/mL, omit HBIG	0.5 mL*	Test patient for anti-HBs; if anti-HBs >10 mIU/mL, omit vaccine
Previously vaccinated, known nonresponder	0.06 mL/kg IM	Immediately, may repeat in 1 mo†	0.5 mL*	Give booster immediately, repeat 2 times if necessary
Sexual				
Nonvaccinated	0.06 mL/kg IM	Immediately, but no later than 14 days	0.5 mL*	First dose immediately, repeat 2 times
Vaccinated	None	None	None	

*Dose for individuals younger than 20 years. The adult dose is 1.0 mL. The dose for immunosuppressed patients and patients undergoing dialysis varies with the vaccine used.
†See text for discussion of persons who have not responded to two vaccine series.
HBsAG, Hepatitis B surface antigen.

preferably within 24 hours of exposure.[13] HBV should be given simultaneously at a different site and repeated after 1 and 6 months (see Table 243–6). After massive exposure (i.e., via blood transfusion), much larger doses of HBIG probably are indicated.

If the exposed patient has been immunized but the serologic response is not known, anti-HBs titers should be determined and the individual managed according to the results; if nonresponsive (anti-HBs <10 mIU/kg by RIA), HBIG and a full series of vaccine should be given. In patients with a contraindication to vaccine, two doses of HBIG (0.06 mL/kg) should be used, the second administered 1 month after the first. Two doses of HBIG also should be given to an exposed health care worker who is known to have no response to two series of HBV.[13]

Perinatal Exposure

Among mothers who are HBsAg- and HBeAg-positive, 85 percent of their untreated infants will become infected and be chronic carriers, and chronic hepatitis, cirrhosis, or hepatic cancer will develop in some of them. If the mother is HBsAg-positive only, the risk of her offspring becoming a carrier is less but is still significant. Accordingly, these infants should receive HBIG prophylaxis.

INFANTS BORN TO WOMEN WHO ARE POSITIVE FOR HEPATITIS B SURFACE ANTIGEN. For optimal passive-active immunity, HBIG (0.5 mL) is given to the newborn at birth (preferably in the delivery room but within 12 hours at the latest). HBV (at a dose half that of the adult dose) is begun simultaneously and repeated at 1 and 6 months (see Table 243–6). This combination is only approximately 90 percent effective in preventing the carrier state because intrauterine infection will not be prevented.

INFANTS BORN TO MOTHERS NOT TESTED FOR HEPATITIS B SURFACE ANTIGEN. If the HBsAg status of the mother is unknown, HBV should be given to the infant within 12 hours, and HBIG should be administered as soon as the mother is shown to be a carrier. If the mother is seronegative, vaccine is continued as recommended for other infants.

HBIG effectiveness is diminished markedly if administration is delayed beyond 48 hours after birth. Nevertheless, if the mother is found to be HBsAg-positive, HBIG and HBV should be given to her infant, even if a significant delay has occurred. In this situation, the infant can be tested for HBsAg and anti-HBs at 12 to 15 months to determine the success of the HBIG and vaccine regimen. If HBsAg is present, the infant is a carrier; if anti-HBs is present, the child was successfully immunized. Administration of HBIG at birth should not interfere with polio or diphtheria-pertussis-tetanus (DPT) vaccines given at 2 months of age.

PREMATURE INFANTS. Premature infants with birth weights less than 2000 g who are born to women not tested for HBsAg should be given 0.5 mL HBIG within 12 hours unless the mother's HBsAg test results can be available within 12 hours and are negative. Immunization should be started immediately and repeated three times (rather than twice) because of the poorer response of preterm infants to the vaccine.[13]

Sexual Exposure to Hepatitis B or a Carrier of Hepatitis B

Sexual exposure to an individual who has hepatitis B or is a carrier is an indication for HBIG (0.06 mL/kg intramuscularly, 5 mL maximum) and initiation of HBV vaccination. They should be given as soon as possible but not after

14 days past exposure. If only HBIG is given, a second dose of HBIG is recommended after 30 days.

For sexual exposure (including rape victims) in which the HBsAg status of the contact is not known, HBIG (0.06 mL/kg, 5 mL maximum) is given and HBV vaccine started. Alternatively, the vaccine can be given and the HBsAg status of the contact determined; if positive, HBIG can be given within 7 days and the vaccine schedule continued.

Possible Exposure

After possible exposure (percutaneous, ingestion, sexual) to an unidentified person or body fluid in which the HBsAg status is unknown, the decision to treat with HBIG must be made individually based on the likelihood that the source is HBsAg-positive and the seriousness of the exposure. HBV should be initiated immediately.

Ideally, the source subject should be tested for HBsAg positivity; if the results are available within 7 days, HBIG (0.06 mL/kg) can be given immediately and again at 1 month if the source is HBsAg-positive. When the source subject cannot be tested or when the source is likely to be HBsAg-positive, HBIG is administered immediately and, if vaccine cannot be given, repeated in 1 month.

If the exposed individual is a high-risk patient (e.g., immunodeficient, immunosuppressed, institutionalized, or undergoing hemodialysis) or is in an environment or health care unit for which past environmental control measures have been ineffective, HBIG should be given in addition to HBV.

HBIG is not indicated on a routine basis after blood transfusions. School or hospital exposure is not an indication for HBIG.

Hepatitis B Immune Globulin in Liver Transplantation

For patients who are HBsAg-positive at the time of liver transplantation, HBIG is recommended in the preoperative period and after transplantation to prevent recurrence in the transplanted liver.[160, 306, 388, 389, 451, 460]

The exact dose, frequency, route, and duration of HBIG in this situation have not been established. At the University of California, Los Angeles, the dose of HBIG is 22,000 U on the day of transplantation and 200 to 10,000 U at 2- to 3-week intervals to keep the anti-HBs titer greater than 500 U/L for the first 3 months post-transplantation, 250 to 499 U/L for the next 3 months, and 100 to 250 U/L after 6 months. Lamivudine also is given daily. This regimen is continued indefinitely. Others use a fixed dose of 10,000 U/mo post-transplantation.

The value of assessing the achieved titers of anti-HBs as a guide to therapy also has been suggested.[306] Regardless of what regimen is followed, the dose of HBIG is very large (e.g., up to 100,000 U in the transplantation period, 100,000 U/mo thereafter) and expensive (e.g., $500 for 10,000 U!). An intravenous form of HBIG and monoclonal antibodies to HBsAg are being developed.

HEPATITIS C

Although no antibody preparation is available for the prevention of hepatitis C, past studies have suggested that polyvalent IG or HBIG provides some protection against the acquisition of non-A, non-B hepatitis (presumably hepatitis C) after heart surgery or hemodialysis.[239, 392, 418]

Two recent studies also provide some evidence for a prophylactic effect of IG. Piazza and colleagues[348] gave polyvalent IG (from pools containing antibodies to hepatitis C virus [HCV]) or placebo monthly for 4 to 20 months to the seronegative sexual partners of 884 subjects who were seropositive for HCV. One of the 450 (representing 560 subject-years) in the IG group became infected versus 6 of the 449 (500 subject-years) in the placebo group ($p = .03$; relative risk, 10.7). The authors conclude that sexual transmission of hepatitis C occurs and that IG has a protective effect.

Féray and associates[125] reviewed the records of 218 patients with hepatitis C co-infection undergoing liver transplantation who received an HBIG product that contained antibody to HCV. The incidence of HCV viremia 1 year post-transplantation was significantly lower (25 of 46 [54%]) in patients receiving HBIG than in those not receiving it (162 of 172 [94%], $p < .001$). They also reviewed 210 transplanted HCV-seronegative patients and found that hepatitis C developed within 1 year in 18 of 68 patients (26%) who received the HBIG product containing anti-HCV antibody as compared with 40 of 86 patients (47%) who did not receive HBIG, a significant difference ($p < .001$) suggesting a preventive effect.

A great need also exists to prevent recurrence of hepatitis C in hepatitis C–seropositive patients undergoing liver transplantation. Studies are under way to determine whether an experimental IG preparation enriched in hepatitis C antibodies can be used for this purpose. As noted earlier, current lots of IVIG or IG contain no hepatitis C antibodies.

HERPESVIRUSES

The common herpesviruses that cause human infection are CMV, Epstein-Barr virus (EBV), herpes simplex virus (HSV) types 1 and 2, varicella-zoster virus (VZV), and human herpesviruses 6, 7, and 8. Although these DNA viruses produce latent infection that can reactivate, particularly in immunodeficient patients, the only clear indication for administering IG is to prevent primary VZV infection. Other possible uses of antibody are considered.

Cytomegalovirus

Human antibodies to CMV in the form of CMV-IVIG (CMVIG) or IVIG have been used for more than a decade to prevent CMV in bone marrow and solid organ transplant recipients. CMVIG is prepared from the plasma of donors with high anti-CMV titers, but regular IVIG also contains anti-CMV antibodies at lower titer. Early studies used CMVIG or IVIG alone, but later studies have combined IG with antiviral agents.

Early studies in renal and liver transplant recipients showed the efficacy of CMVIG or IVIG.[78, 123, 132, 176, 354, 422] Two meta-analyses demonstrated decreased CMV mortality with the use of CMVIG or IVIG in bone marrow and solid organ transplant patients.[150, 501] Others also have shown a similar prophylactic benefit of IVIG or CMVIG.[44, 169, 297, 410] Ruutu and coworkers[384] showed no prophylactic benefit of CMVIG in CMV-seronegative bone marrow transplant (BMT) recipients. The prophylactic efficacy of CMVIG or IVIG in comparison to ganciclovir has not been studied.

Several factors have reduced the need for administering CMVIG or IVIG to transplant recipients, including the realization of a markedly reduced risk of CMV if both the recipient and donor are CMV antibody–negative, the use of ganciclovir prophylaxis, the early detection of CMV infection by PCR assay combined with early treatment with ganciclovir, and the use of CMV-seronegative or filtered blood products.

GVHD and graft rejection are important cofactors for CMV disease,[236, 379, 410] and CMV is a risk factor for graft loss.[103, 463] The value of IG prophylaxis in bone marrow transplantation may have been related in part to its immunomodulatory effect on GVHD.[236]

Another potential use of CMVIG is in the treatment of in utero CMV infection.[314] Two infusions of CMVIG were given intraperitoneally at 28 and 29 weeks' gestation to a CMV-infected fetus. The therapeutic benefit was unclear because the infant had intracranial calcifications at 2 weeks of age but was free of neurologic symptoms at 1 year of age. Nigro and associates[315] treated a pregnant women with primary CMV and in utero infection of one twin fetus with intravenous CMVIG at 30 weeks' gestation. CMVIG also was injected into the amniotic sac. The affected twin seemed to respond with better growth, decreased placental thickening, and lessened cord edema. Though born with evidence of CMV infection and hepatosplenomegaly, the child was normal at the age of 2 years. Nigro and colleagues[316] used CMVIG successfully to treat chronic cervical CMV infection associated with either recurrent abortion or infertility in three women.

RECOMMENDATIONS

Patients undergoing allogeneic human stem-cell transplantation who are at risk for acquiring CMV disease (e.g., a CMV-seropositive recipient or a CMV-seronegative recipient and a CMV-seropositive donor) should receive either prophylactic ganciclovir or preemptive ganciclovir therapy after early detection of infection by CMV PCR. CMVIG no longer is recommended for prevention of CMV disease.[170] Frequently, IVIG is used for immune modulation to prevent GVHD.

For solid organ recipients, the highest risk is a CMV-seropositive donor and a CMV-seronegative recipient, in which case antiviral prophylaxis is used. Antiviral prophylaxis rather than CMVIG or IVIG is used currently in kidney, heart, lung, and liver transplantation.[141, 209, 380, 402] Whether CMVIG or IVIG enhances protection is not known.[344] CMVIG may be used in rare situations if a patient cannot tolerate antiviral medications.

CMVIG or IVIG in combination with antiviral agents is used to treat severe CMV disease, such as pneumonia in transplant patients.[334, 343, 366, 508] For CMVIG, 400 mg/kg on days 1, 2, and 7 and 200 mg/kg on days 14 and 21 have been used in addition to antiviral therapy,[366] although others have used a lower dose (100 mg/kg every other day for 2 weeks).[140] IVIG, 500 mg/kg every other day for 10 to 59 days, followed by 500 mg/kg once or twice weekly for an extended period, also has been reported.[334]

CMVIG for in utero CMV infection is not recommended routinely but may be of some value in selected situations.

Epstein-Barr Virus

EBV, the etiologic agent of infectious mononucleosis, causes severe infection in immunocompromised patients and males with X-linked lymphoproliferative syndrome (XLP). IVIG has been given to non–EBV-infected males with XLP in an attempt to prevent EBV infection, but EBV infection developed in some of them while taking IVIG.[128]

Transplant patients with EBV-induced lymphadenopathy, lymphoproliferative syndrome, or hepatitis have been treated successfully with a combination of IVIG or CMVIG, antiviral therapy, and interferon-α.[102, 324, 454] A similar approach was not successful in XLP.[329] CMVIG was used in one case because it contained higher titers of anti-EBV antibody than IVIG did.[102] Fulminant EBV hepatitis was treated successfully with liver transplantation, antiviral therapy, and CMVIG.[124]

IVIG has been used in infection-induced hemophagocytic syndrome, for which EBV is a significant cause in children.[134, 269, 444] IVIG is of benefit in hemophagocytic syndrome without evidence of EBV.[133, 146, 153] Nagasawa and coauthors[309] reported two patients in whom IVIG may have been harmful, as evidenced by worsening symptoms of anemia and thrombocytopenia. Current treatment of EBV-induced hemophagocytic syndrome includes corticosteroids and etoposide,[197] although supplementary IVIG and cyclosporine also have been used.[196]

RECOMMENDATIONS

IVIG may be of value as adjunctive treatment of post-transplantation EBV disease. Doses of 400 to 500 mg/kg/day of IVIG or 100 mg/kg/mo of CMVIG have been used in addition to antiviral therapy.[124, 324, 454] The value of IVIG in the treatment of EBV-induced hemophagocytic syndrome is unproven.

Herpes Simplex Viruses

Antibody may have a preventive effect in HSV infection in the newborn period. Mothers with a reactivated herpes infection during delivery are 10-fold less likely to transmit HSV to their newborn infants during vaginal delivery than are mothers with primary HSV infection at delivery, presumably because of the transplacental transfer of anti-herpes antibody.[14] IVIG containing HSV antibodies has not been used in the prevention of neonatal herpes infection, although Whitley[500] has proposed that HSV monoclonal antibody or hyperimmune IGIV be evaluated for treatment of disseminated neonatal disease.

Masci and colleagues[286] compared monthly IVIG (400 mg/kg) with intermittent acyclovir treatment (800 mg twice daily, 1 week each month) in patients with recurrent genital HSV infection for 6 months and noted fewer recurrences in the IVIG-treated group.

RECOMMENDATIONS

IVIG is not recommended for the prevention or treatment of HSV infections.

Varicella-Zoster Virus and Varicella-Zoster Immune Globulin

IMMUNE GLOBULIN IN VARICELLA

After success was achieved with IG in the prevention of measles and hepatitis, IG was evaluated for the prevention of varicella. Although Funkhauser[135] in 1948 showed some beneficial effects of standard IG in the prevention of varicella in an uncontrolled study, Greenberg[162] and Schaeffer and Toomey[395] were unable to prevent chickenpox in exposed children with IG doses of 2.5 to 20 mL.

Others have reported anecdotal evidence for the efficacy of IG in large doses during the early stages of chickenpox and herpes zoster. These claims included prompt relief of pain in zoster[490] and rapid resolution of skin lesions.[260, 371] However, even high-titer IG (zoster immune globulin [ZIG]) does not prevent dissemination of herpes zoster.[427]

Ross[375] in 1962 gave 242 children IG in doses of 0.1 to 0.6 mL/lb within 3 days of exposure to chickenpox; 209 similarly exposed, uninjected children were used as controls. The attack rate was the same (97%) in both groups, thus indicating that IG does not prevent varicella under these conditions. However, with doses of IG above 0.2 mL/lb, the severity of the disease was reduced, as indicated by a decreased number of pox and reduced temperature. Children receiving the largest dose of IG (0.6 mL/lb) had maximal temperatures of 38.9°C (102°F) versus 41.1°C (106°F) for controls and 40 pox versus 207 for controls. Other investigators also have reported similar, but uncontrolled observations that IG modifies the severity of chickenpox.[202, 464]

VARICELLA-ZOSTER IMMUNE GLOBULIN IN VARICELLA

The prophylactic value of large IG doses in decreasing the incidence and severity of varicella led to a trial of high-titer plasma or IG preparations to prevent varicella.[36] These preparations include ZIG and zoster immune plasma (ZIP) from convalescing zoster patients and varicella-zoster immune globulin (VZIG) prepared from high-titer normal adults.

Brunell and associates[73] in 1969 selected convalescing zoster patients whose complement-fixing antibody titers were 1:256 or greater and prepared ZIG from their plasma; this material had titers considerably higher than standard IG did. Exposed children from six families in which chickenpox was occurring were given ZIG or IG at doses of 2 mL. In none of six children receiving ZIG did chickenpox develop, whereas it developed in all 6 children given IG. No antibody developed in the ZIG-treated group, thus indicating that the disease was prevented.

Because this dose did not prevent varicella in leukemic children or other high-risk patients, a larger dose (5 mL) was used in a later study to successfully modify or prevent varicella in eight of nine high-risk children.[71, 72] Severe varicella developed in one child given a less potent preparation of ZIG. These observations were confirmed in two later studies. Judelsohn and associates[217] gave ZIG to 56 exposed high-risk children; mild varicella occurred in 7 patients and was prevented in the others, most of whom were susceptible as determined by absence of serum antibody. Gershon and colleagues[143] gave ZIG to 15 seronegative high-risk exposed children; varicella was severe in 1, mild in 9, and subclinical in 5. Subclinical infection was determined by the acquisition of membrane antibody, as detected by fluorescent microscopy.

Orenstein and associates[331] studied 553 exposed, high-risk patients who received ZIG of two different titers (1:1280 versus 1:2560 or greater). They found that the clinical attack rate after ZIG correlated with the type of exposure (varicella developed in 36% with household exposure, 7.7% with hospital exposure, and 0% with school exposure), the rise in antibody titer (45% of patients without a fourfold titer increase became ill as compared with 22% of patients with a fourfold or greater rise in titer), and the titer of the administrated ZIG (significantly more complications and deaths occurred in recipients of the lower-titer ZIG).

Because of the limited supply of ZIG and ZIP, VZIG from normal adults has become the commercially available product in the United States. Zaia and associates[509] compared the efficacy of ZIG and VZIG in immunocompromised children exposed to varicella. Varicella attack rates and the clinical severity in recipients of VZIG and ZIG did not differ significantly. A higher incidence of subclinical infection was indicated by the rise in antibody titer in ZIG recipients (31.3%) versus that in VZIG recipients (16%). A larger dose of VZIG (2.5 mL/10 kg versus 1.25 mL/10 kg) reduced the frequency of subclinical infection (from 20% to 4.3%). Varicella developed in several high-risk patients with demonstrable serum antibody at exposure, thus indicating that history-negative seropositive patients are at risk for clinical varicella-zoster infection and should be given ZIG regardless of antibody titer.

INTRAVENOUS IMMUNE GLOBULIN IN VARICELLA PROPHYLAXIS

Paryani and colleagues[338, 339] in 1984 observed that IVIG at doses of 200 to 300 mg/kg resulted in serum VZV antibody titers comparable to those in patients receiving VZIG at standard doses. Subsequently, Chen and Liang[89] demonstrated that varicella was prevented by a single dose of IVIG at 200 mg/kg in five children with leukemia.

Immunocompromised patients who are receiving IVIG at 400 mg/kg are thought to be protected for 3 weeks after infusion and do not require additional VZIG on exposure.[22] However, Ferdman and Church[126] reported that varicella occurred in two HIV-infected children receiving 500 mg/kg of IVIG after exposure to varicella 7 and 11 days after infusion. Both had mild disease and responded well to acyclovir. They suggest that for patients with profound immunodeficiency, VZIG can be given in addition to IVIG. Kavaliotis and associates[227] found that an IVIG dose of 1 g/kg given within 6 to 24 hours of exposure was 90 percent effective in preventing varicella in an oncology unit, with no additional advantage noted with VZIG administration.

RECOMMENDATIONS

The decision to administer VZIG to prevent chickenpox is based on the patient's susceptibility, the type of exposure, and the patient's immune competence (Table 243–7).

Determination of Susceptibility

With the exception of BMT recipients, most immunocompromised individuals with previous varicella infection are considered immune; however, their immune status should be confirmed with varicella antibody titers. Healthy adults reared in the United States are considered immune even without a history of varicella or zoster, but immunocompromised children and adults without a history of varicella are considered susceptible because of their higher risk for severe infection. BMT recipients are considered susceptible regardless of the varicella history of the donor or recipient. If varicella or herpes zoster develops after transplantation, the patient then is considered to be immune.[170, 353]

An immunocompromised child without a history of chickenpox is considered susceptible even if antibody titers are present because receipt of blood products containing immunoglobulin may result in transient seropositivity. Alternatively, such patients who received VZIG may have

TABLE 243–7 ■ CANDIDATES FOR VARICELLA-ZOSTER IMMUNE GLOBULIN AFTER SIGNIFICANT EXPOSURE

Immunocompromised children without a history of varicella
Susceptible, pregnant women
Newborn infants whose mother had an onset of varicella within 5 days before delivery or within 48 hr after delivery.
All hospitalized premature infants born at less than 28 wk gestation or less than 1000 g at birth, regardless of maternal history.
Hospitalized premature infants greater than 28 wk gestation whose mother has no history of chickenpox or who is seronegative. May consider for other premature infants. See text

had asymptomatic varicella with the subsequent development of varicella antibodies, yet they may not be protected on re-exposure.[22] The value of antibody titer to determine susceptibility in these patients is controversial. VZIG is not recommended for immunodeficient patients who have been vaccinated in the past, provided that they were previously shown to have varicella antibody, even if seronegative at the time of exposure. These individuals are expected to have mild disease.[353] However, verifying varicella immunity with antibody before foregoing VZIG administration in this situation seems to be a reasonable approach.

Type of Exposure

Individuals residing in the same household as a patient with varicella, persons who have had face-to-face contact with a patient considered infectious, and patients sharing the same hospital room are considered to have significant exposure. Because the duration of exposure that results in transmission is not known, each exposure must be evaluated individually. Contact with a varicella vaccine recipient who has a varicella rash must be considered significant exposure because the vaccinee may have wild-type virus infection; vaccine strain virus rarely has been transmitted.[170]

CANDIDATES FOR VARICELLA-ZOSTER IMMUNE GLOBULIN

Normal Adults, Children, and Adolescents

Normal children, adolescents, and adults exposed to chickenpox or zoster are not usually candidates for receiving VZIG. They may be given chickenpox vaccine if older than 12 months.

Immunocompromised Children and Adults

The principal use of VZIG is to prevent chickenpox or subsequent zoster in susceptible immunocompromised children exposed to zoster or chickenpox. Immunocompromised children include those with primary immunodeficiency and those with secondary immunodeficiency, including HIV and neoplastic disease, and those receiving immunosuppressive therapy (e.g., systemic steroids, chemotherapy).[28, 326]

Term and Premature Newborns

Newborns who acquire varicella after birth are not at high risk for severe disease and are not candidates for receiving VZIG, with the possible exception of those with severe skin disease.[22] Newborn infants born to mothers in whom varicella developed within 5 days before delivery or within 2 days after delivery are at high risk for severe varicella because they have received no transplacental protective antibodies.[353]

Exposed, hospitalized premature infants born at less than 28 weeks' gestation or less than 1000 g should receive VZIG. These infants are susceptible, regardless of the maternal history of varicella, because of incomplete transplacental transfer of maternal antibody. Hospitalized premature infants with significant exposure who were born at greater than 28 weeks' gestation and whose mothers do not have a history of varicella or are seronegative also are considered candidates for receiving VZIG because transplacental antibody would not be present.[22, 353]

Gold and colleagues[151] showed that gestational age greater than 28 weeks and birth weight greater than 1000 g do not always accurately predict the presence of maternal varicella antibody. Olgivie[326] suggests that infants born before 30 weeks' gestation be given VZIG and that some infants born after 28 weeks will lose their maternal antibody by 60 days of age; she recommends antibody testing on exposure if it can be performed quickly to assess the need for VZIG. Gold and associates[151] recommended the routine use of VZIG in the neonatal ICU if the fluorescent antibody to membrane antigen (FAMA) assay is not available to determine susceptibility. Previous administration of blood products in the neonatal ICU may render these results uninterpretable.

Pregnant Women

Susceptible pregnant women are candidates for receiving VZIG because of their increased risk for severe varicella pneumonia.[421]

DOSAGE

VZIG is supplied in vials of 125 U (approximately 1.25 mL). It is produced by the U.S. Biologics Laboratories (Massachusetts) for distribution by the American Red Cross. The dose of VZIG is 125 U/10 kg intramuscularly. The minimal dose for infants is 125 U (one vial), and the maximal dose is 625 U for adults (five vials).[22, 85]

Although VZIG should be given to susceptible candidates as soon as possible after exposure for maximal protection, it can be given up to 96 hours after exposure.[85] A second dose is not needed for subsequent exposure unless it occurs beyond 3 weeks after the VZIG dose.[22] IVIG (400 mg/kg) is an acceptable alternative if the child has a bleeding diathesis and cannot receive intramuscular injections.

VZIG is not recommended for the treatment of chickenpox, zoster, disseminated varicella, or post-herpetic neuralgia[427]; it does not prevent dissemination of zoster in immunocompromised patients. Acyclovir and other antivirals are effective.

HUMAN IMMUNODEFICIENCY VIRUS

As noted earlier in the chapter, regular infusions of IVIG have been used to prevent concomitant infection in patients with HIV, notably children, who have compromised immune systems with antibody deficiencies. Attempts to use HIV-specific antibody to prevent HIV or provide an antiviral effect have met with very limited success.

These studies have used human immune plasma or hyperimmune HIV immunoglobulin (HIVIG) from asymptomatic HIV-seropositive patients, porcine antisera, or monoclonal antibodies.[435] In two of three controlled clinical trials of immune plasma in adult patients with AIDS, a modest clinical benefit was achieved as judged by decreased opportunistic infections, a slight increase in $CD4^+$ cell counts, and improved survival; however, no striking decreases in viral burden were noted.[205, 266, 480]

In a double-blind, placebo-controlled multicenter study, HIV-seropositive pregnant women receiving zidovudine were given HIVIG monthly during the last trimester of pregnancy, and one HIVIG dose was given to their newborns at birth; no effect on the rate of maternal-fetal HIV transmission versus that in a similar group given regular IVIG was found.[434] The rate of transmission in both groups was unexpectedly low (less than 5%), so the study was discontinued after 800 patients had been enrolled because the study was not statistically powered to detect a slight reduction in transmission rates.

Another study[432] examined the antiviral effect of large doses of HIVIG in 30 children with moderately advanced HIV infection who were receiving stable antiviral treatment and showed a measurable viral burden. No striking beneficial effect was observed as indicated by HIV RNA levels in plasma, cellular viral culture titers, or immunologic assays.

Despite these failures, efforts to develop antibody preparations that will neutralize the virus continue; such preparations would be particularly valuable after needle-stick or sexual exposure.[435] Under study are monoclonal antibodies to neutralizing regions of the virus, antibodies to co-receptors that may interfere with HIV attachment, or combinations of antibodies with different specificities, including combinations of HIVIG with monoclonal antibodies.[267, 268] An effective neutralizing antibody also would provide valuable information toward an effective vaccine.

MEASLES

The first successful prophylaxis of measles with convalescent serum was reported by Cenci[86] in 1907. Convalescent serum was first used in the United States in 1916 by Park, Freeman, and Zingher, who gave either 4 or 8 mL of serum to 41 recently exposed children at New York Metropolitan Hospital.[336, 512] Measles did not develop in any of the 20 children who received the 8-mL dose and developed in only 3 of the 20 children who received the 4-mL dose. Park and Freeman[336] in 1926 found that 6 to 10 mL of convalescent serum was 92 percent efficacious in preventing measles in recently exposed individuals, a finding confirmed and extended by Stillerman and associates.[436] Placental extracts containing serum antibodies also were used in the prevention and modification of measles.[292]

Stokes and colleagues[440] and Ordman and associates[330] both confirmed in 1944 that (1) large doses (0.05 mL/kg) of IG given immediately after exposure could prevent measles, (2) smaller doses (0.01 mL/kg) given immediately after exposure could modify measles, and (3) large doses (0.05 mL/kg) given in the early stages of clinical illness could lessen the severity of measles. Greenberg and coworkers in 1955 noted a lower incidence of measles encephalitis in IG-modified measles.[163]

A major use of IG in the 1960s was to diminish the side effects of the Edmonston strain of measles vaccine. Krugman and associates[251] in 1962 noted that the simultaneous administration of 0.02 mL/lb of IG at the time of Edmonston measles vaccination reduced the incidence of high fever from 40 to 14 percent and the incidence of rash from 10 to 2 percent. The mean titer of measles antibody achieved was somewhat reduced by the IG, and a slight decrease in the rate of seroconversion was noted; nonetheless, the vaccine-IG combination was 95% effective.[439] Further attenuation of measles vaccine has eliminated the necessity for concomitant IG injections.

Recommendations

IG or IVIG can be given to susceptible contacts within 6 days of exposure to prevent or modify measles. Infants younger than 1 year, immunocompromised patients, and pregnant women are at risk for severe disease and should receive immunoprophylaxis.[15] Because patients with HIV may contract measles after exposure despite immunization, they should receive passive immunoprophylaxis.[142] IG also can be given to close family contacts, although large outbreaks may limit supplies. Measles vaccine has some efficacy if given within 72 hours of exposure and is preferred for the management of outbreaks in healthy children older than 1 year.[15]

The standard dose of IG is 0.25 mL/kg (40 mg/kg) for healthy patients and 0.5 mL/kg (80 mg/kg) for immunocompromised subjects. The maximal dose is 15 mL. IVIG at doses greater than 100 mg/kg should protect for 3 weeks after administration.[15] Administration of IG to a healthy infant precludes the use of measles vaccine for 5 months, and after the administration of large doses of IVIG, longer intervals are needed (e.g., 8 to 11 months).[15]

MUMPS

Mumps IG was ineffective, and this product no longer is manufactured in the United States.[16]

PARVOVIRUS

Human parvovirus B19, the cause of the benign childhood exanthem termed fifth disease, also may cause polyarthropathy, transient aplastic crises in patients with hemolytic anemia, chronic red cell aplasia in immunocompromised patients, and hemophagocytic syndrome.[69, 199, 506] Patients susceptible to chronic parvovirus infection include those with congenital[456] or acquired immunodeficiencies,[91, 242] those receiving immunosuppressive therapy,[506] and organ transplant recipients.[224, 282] In utero parvovirus infection can result in hydrops fetalis.[462] The use of parvovirus DNA PCR has facilitated the diagnosis in immunodeficient patients unable to make antibodies or in patients who have passively acquired parvovirus antibodies.

Parvovirus B19 has a tropism for marrow erythroid progenitor cells because these cells express the blood group P antigen, the cellular receptor for the virus. Many individuals have encountered and made antibodies to parvovirus, and thus IVIG is an excellent source of antiparvovirus antibodies.[399] IVIG has been used successfully to treat parvovirus-induced red cell aplasia.[257] Patients with AIDS are particularly susceptible to this disease. Successfully treated patients have decreased viremia, reticulocytosis, and resolution of the anemia within 2 weeks. Sometimes, relapses or persistent infection occur.

Viguier and coauthors[479] reported a 33-year-old woman with parvovirus B19–associated polyarteritis nodosa and fever, palpable purpura, intense myalgia, paresthesias, and polyarthritis of the hand joints; the patient improved after receiving 1 g/kg of IVIG for 2 days.

IVIG has been used as a supplement to transfusions in severe in utero parvovirus infection with hydrops fetalis. Selbing and coworkers[401] reported a pregnant women at 24 weeks' gestation with severe pre-eclampsia whose fetus had ascites and pericardial effusion: she was given 25 g of IVIG with resolution of the ascites, effusion, and anemia.

In 1999, Rugolotto[383] treated an infant with IVIG (1 g/kg every 3 weeks for 8 months) for congenital anemia caused by intrauterine parvovirus B19 infection. Heegaard and coauthors[181] reported similar success of IVIG given to an infant postnatally, in addition to in utero transfusions. Earlier attempts to treat older infants with persistent parvovirus-induced congenital anemia with IVIG were unsuccessful.[69]

Human neutralizing monoclonal antibodies have been generated from infected individuals[145] for possible future therapeutic use.

Recommendations

Red cell aplasia caused by parvovirus infection in immunodeficient patients, including those with HIV, should be treated with IVIG, 400 mg/kg/day for 5 days or 1 g/kg/day for 2 days.[68, 242] If relapse is likely because of severe immunocompromised status, IVIG at 400 mg/kg can be given every 4 weeks.

Neonates with persistent congenital anemia caused by parvovirus B19 should receive 400 mg/kg of IVIG for 5 days, with additional doses given if the anemia does not resolve.

Pregnant women carrying fetuses with in utero hydrops fetalis caused by parvovirus B19 infection also may be candidates for IVIG therapy.

RABIES AND RABIES IMMUNE GLOBULIN

Rabies is the ideal disease for passive immunization because the exact moment, the exact source, and the exact location of exposure usually are known. Furthermore, the long incubation period and the fact that the virus remains localized to the wound for several days enhance the effectiveness of passive immunization. Although a rabies serum was prepared initially in 1889 by Babes and Lepp,[32] experiments of Habel[174] in mice, guinea pigs, and monkeys involving the use of rabbit hyperimmune serum demonstrated that antibody worked by two mechanisms: (1) neutralizing the virus while still in tissues and (2) retarding the spread of virus within the nervous system, thereby prolonging the incubation period and permitting active immunity by vaccine to become established.

On the basis of these studies, a World Health Organization Expert Committee in 1950 recommended that a field trial of the efficacy of hyperimmune rabies serum in conjunction with vaccine be conducted.[122] It was undertaken in Iran because multiple bites by a single rabid wolf coming into isolated villages were not uncommon findings, and this severe exposure had an associated 40 to 50 percent mortality. In 1954, a single rabid wolf bit 27 individuals, 17 of whom were bitten on the head. These 17 were divided into three groups: 5 received vaccine alone, 7 received vaccine and one dose of antirabies serum, and 5 received vaccine and two doses of antirabies serum.[39] Three of five persons treated with vaccine alone died of rabies, one of seven in the one-dose antiserum group died, and none of five in the two-dose antiserum group died. Antibody studies conducted on these patients indicated that a single or a double dose of antiserum, followed by 14 to 21 daily doses of vaccine, results in significant levels of circulating antibody for as long as 50 days.[175] The antibody found early is supplied passively; after the 10th day, the antibody present is a result of the vaccine. Thus, optimal treatment requires both passive and active immunization.

Before 1971, the only available antiserum was of equine origin. It is still the only product available in some countries. Since 1971, human rabies immune globulin (RIG) has been available in the United States and many other countries and is preferred because of the lessened risk of serum reactions.[414] In addition, human antibody has a half-life in the circulation twice that of equine antibody, with the result that higher levels of passive antibody are maintained. However, the antibody response to the vaccine given concomitantly is more effectively suppressed.[271]

A case of fatal rabies was reported in a 19-year-old man bitten on the finger by a rabid mongoose despite the recommended postexposure prophylaxis (RIG and five doses of human diploid cell rabies vaccine [HDCV]).[407] Possible reasons for failure included (1) inadequacy of the recommended dose of RIG; (2) vaccine injection into the gluteal region, where more fat is found than in the recommended deltoid region; and (3) decreased antibody response to the vaccine as a result of a possible immunodeficiency state.

Prevention of rabies consists of three essential components: thorough washing of the wound with a 20 percent soap solution followed by irrigation with povidone-iodine,[57] passive immunization with rabies antibody, and active immunization. Although most cases of failure are caused by lack of adherence to the aforementioned three strategies,[349] isolated cases of rabies occurring despite appropriate management have been reported.

Wilde and associates[495] reported failure of prophylaxis in five Thai children who received multiple bites on the face and head; they suggested that failure to infiltrate all wounds with IG and surgical closure before the wound was infiltrated might have been factors. Hemochudha and coauthors[183] reported failure of prophylaxis in a child with minor scratches on the nose and in a woman with a deep wound on the cheek; they suggested that direct inoculation of virus into nerve endings may have occurred.

Recommendations

RIG antiserum is recommended in nonimmunized individuals for *all bites by animals in which rabies cannot be ruled out* and for nonbite exposure to animals proved or suspected to be rabid.[357] Such treatment should be given as early as possible after exposure and followed by vaccine administration. Two human RIG products are available in the United States, BayRab and Imogam Rabies-HT; both are prepared from the plasma of hyperimmunized donors. The recommended dose of 20 IU/kg of RIG must not be exceeded because higher doses can suppress the vaccine response. If RIG is not available, the dose of equine RIG is 40 IU/kg, and desensitization is required. Researchers now recognize[193] that the entire RIG dose should be infiltrated around the wounds. If doing so is not anatomically feasible, any remaining RIG should be given intramuscularly.[17]

Wilde and colleagues,[495] recognizing the difficulty in infiltrating multiple wounds with a small volume of immune globulin, suggested diluting the RIG. The World Health Organization[505] recommends dilution of RIG twofold to threefold in saline to ensure an adequate volume for infiltration. RIG should not be frozen and, if frozen, should not be used.

Although administration of one of the three licensed vaccines should be started at the same time as RIG, the vaccine and RIG should not be administered in the same syringe or with the same syringe or needle. Vaccine should be given in the deltoid muscle or, for an infant, in the anterolateral aspect of the thigh and at an anatomic site removed from the injury or any injection sites of RIG. If RIG is not available immediately, immunization should be started and RIG given if available within 7 days.[17] If vaccine is not immediately available, RIG should be administered and the vaccine given as soon as possible. If both RIG and vaccine are delayed, both should be given whenever available, regardless of the interval between exposure and treatment.[17]

RIG is not recommended for patients who previously have received a full postexposure vaccine course of HDCV, RVA (rabies virus adsorbed), or PCEC (purified chick embryo cell) vaccines; who have received a three-dose pre-exposure intramuscular series of these vaccines; who have received a three-dose pre-exposure intradermal HDCV vaccine; or who have been immunized with any vaccine and have a documented rabies titer.[17]

Postexposure prophylaxis of immunodeficient patients has not been studied. Jaijaroensup and coauthors[208] reported poor or nondetectable neutralizing antibody in five HIV-infected patients who received intradermal vaccine and proposed that higher doses of vaccine or additional boosters be considered. Immunodeficient patients should undergo serologic testing to document seroconversion after completion of the vaccine.

RIG is not indicated for the treatment of rabies.

RESPIRATORY SYNCYTIAL VIRUS

Acute RSV infection of the respiratory tract is the most common cause of hospitalization for infants and young children and is thus a significant public health expense. For high-risk patients such as premature infants and infants with chronic lung disease, infection can be severe and life-threatening. The observation that passively transferred maternal antibody provided some protection from RSV infection[327] led to the development of passive immunity products to prevent and modify the severity of infection. No effective vaccine exists.

The first product used was RSV-IGIV (RespiGam), a 5 percent polyclonal human intravenous IG prepared from healthy donors with high RSV-neutralizing antibodies. RSV-IGIV was licensed in 1996 after studies in high-risk infants demonstrated its efficacy. Groothuis and colleagues[164] conducted a prospective, blinded, randomized trial at five centers and showed that 58 premature infants who received RSV-IVIG at 750 mg/kg/mo during the winter months had a significantly lower incidence of RSV lower respiratory tract disease than that observed in 58 premature control infants who did not receive RSV-IGIV (6.9 versus 24.1%, $p = .01$). The RSV-IVIG–treated patients also had a lower incidence of moderate to severe RSV lower respiratory tract disease ($p = .006$), fewer days of hospitalization ($p = .020$), and fewer days in the ICU ($p = .05$).

Another large RSV-IVIG multicenter, double-blind, placebo-controlled study[365] of 510 infants with either prematurity or bronchopulmonary dysplasia also demonstrated decreased hospitalizations (13.5 versus 8.0%, $p = .047$), decreased total RSV hospital days ($p = .045$), and decreased days with oxygen use ($p = .007$). RSV-IGIV also decreased hospitalization for any respiratory illness by 38 percent and total respiratory illness hospital days by 46 percent, presumably because of antibodies to other respiratory pathogens. An added benefit of RSV-IGIV prophylaxis is a decreased incidence of otitis media (number of episodes, 0.15 per patient versus 0.78 per control; $p = .003$).[416] In 1997, the American Academy of Pediatrics recommended RSV-IGIV for high-risk children with prematurity or bronchopulmonary dysplasia,[369] but not for infants with cyanotic congenital heart disease[165, 417] because of the risk of serious side effects.

In 1996, palivizumab (Synagis), a humanized IgG1 monoclonal antibody against the F (fusion) glycoprotein of RSV,[148, 443] entered clinical trials. Palivizumab neutralizes both type A and type B RSV and is 50 to 100 times more potent than RSV-IGIV.[391] A multicenter, randomized, double-blind, placebo-controlled study of 1502 high-risk infants (premature infants and infants younger than 2 years with bronchopulmonary dysplasia) demonstrated the efficacy of 15 mg/kg of palivizumab given intramuscularly every 30 days[335]; it resulted in significantly decreased RSV hospitalizations ($p < .001$), RSV hospital days ($p < .001$), and days of oxygen therapy ($p < .001$). Palivizumab was licensed in 1998, the first monoclonal antibody approved for the prevention of an infectious disease.

The safety of administering palivizumab for more than one season is not known; indeed, a theoretic risk is that an antibody to the murine component could develop and cause side effects. However, preliminary results suggest that palivizumab is safe to use for two seasons.[319]

Neither RSV-IGIV nor palivizumab is indicated for the treatment of RSV. One dose of 1500 mg/kg of RSV-IGIV was of no benefit in the treatment of RSV infection in normal and high-risk children with RSV,[372, 373] as evidenced by days in the ICU; it did, however, decrease the titer of virus in respiratory secretions. Another RSV monoclonal antibody (Medi-493), given intravenously to patients with RSV and intubated with respiratory failure, had no clinical benefit; it decreased tracheal but not nasal RSV virus titers.[280] A single dose of aerosolized human IVIG also was of no clinical benefit in the treatment of patients with RSV.[370]

DeVincenzo and associates[105] gave a single dose of RSV-IVIG (1500 mg/kg) to children who were BMT recipients after the onset of RSV infection. All but one patient also received ribavirin. Only one patient died in this small group, which compares favorably with historical controls given ribavirin therapy alone. Ghosh and coworkers[144] gave IVIG (500 mg/kg every other day) and aerosolized ribavirin to 14 adult BMT recipients with RSV upper respiratory tract infection to prevent pneumonia and death. Ten patients resolved their infection, pneumonia developed in 4, and 2 died.

Joffe and colleagues[213] examined the cost of palivizumab prophylaxis for high-risk premature infants and concluded that the cost to prevent one RSV hospitalization is $12,000; 7.4 infants would need to be treated to prevent one hospitalization. For lower-risk groups, the cost is much higher, which has led to the suggestion[238] that determination of the need for RSV prophylaxis should consider regional differences in RSV hospitalization rates. Despite the cost, palivizumab prophylaxis for high-risk infants is now the standard of practice in the United States.

Recommendations

PREVENTION

RSV-IGIV or palivizumab should be used for the prevention of RSV during the RSV season for high-risk premature infants or infants with chronic lung disease.[18] Palivizumab is preferred because of its ease of administration (intramuscular injection versus intravenous administration), efficacy, cost, and safety (avoidance of possible pathogens associated with a human plasma product). An additional advantage of palivizumab is that RSV-IGIV requires a 9-month delay in measles and varicella vaccine administration after the last dose whereas no such interval is needed for palivizumab. The duration of prophylaxis should be individualized, depending on the duration of the local RSV season.

Candidates for Prophylaxis

1. Infants younger than 24 months with chronic lung disease requiring medical treatment in the past 6 months. Two seasons of treatment may be required for some infants.

2. Premature infants without chronic lung disease who were born before 32 weeks' gestation. Infants born at 28 weeks or earlier may benefit from 12 months of prophylaxis, whereas infants born at 29 to 32 weeks' gestation may benefit most from prophylaxis for 6 months,[18] although decisions should be individualized.

3. Premature infants 32 to 35 weeks' gestation who have other high-risk factors. Such factors may include neuromuscular disorders and exposure to passive smoke, group day-care, and crowded living conditions.[391]

4. Infants with cyanotic or complicated congenital heart disease. Neither RSV-IGIV nor palivizumab is recommended for these patients. RSV-IGIV is contraindicated because of potential side effects in patients with cyanotic congenital heart disease. However, palivizumab has been recommended by some physicians for infants with congenital heart disease who are premature (<32 weeks' gestation) or have chronic

lung disease requiring therapy.[391] A multicenter study is under way.[391] Others restrict its use in these infants to those with asymptomatic and acyanotic congenital heart disease (e.g., ventricular septal defect, patent ductus arteriosus, atrial septal defect).[18]

5. Infants who are immunocompromised, particularly those requiring IVIG. These infants can receive RSV prophylaxis by substituting RSV-IGIV for regular IVIG. IVIG has only low titers of RSV antibodies and minimal protective effect.

Possible Indications

1. Palivizumab may be of value in aborting a nosocomial outbreak of RSV in the premature nursery, in addition to strict isolation practices.[391]
2. Patients with cystic fibrosis who are younger than 2 years also may be candidates for receiving prophylaxis; a multicenter study is under way.[391]
3. BMT patients with RSV upper respiratory tract infection may be candidates for receiving RSV-IVIG to prevent pneumonia.[105, 154]

Dosage and Administration

Prophylaxis with either product is given monthly from just before the start of the local RSV infection season until the end of the season.

The dose of palivizumab is 15 mg/kg/mo given intramuscularly. It is supplied in 50- and 100-mg vials.

The dose of RSV-IGIV is 750 mg/kg/mo (15 mL/kg) intravenously. The product is supplied in units of 1000 mg (20 mL) and 2500 mg (50 mL).

TREATMENT

Neither RSV-IVIG nor palivizumab is indicated for the treatment of RSV infections.

ROTAVIRUS

Recent reviews have summarized the role of oral IG in the prevention and treatment of rotavirus infection.[62, 101, 177, 489] Its effectiveness varies, in part because of differences in antibody titer in the various products.[41, 116, 167, 168, 188, 299, 394, 465] Human IG has been used to prevent rotavirus infection; Barnes and colleagues[41] gave human gamma-globulin orally to low-birth-weight infants in a nursery in which rotavirus was endemic. Patients given human IG had milder disease than placebo recipients did.

Human IG has been infused into the duodenum[168] to treat two children with prolonged rotavirus infection. One patient responded rapidly, but the other had a prolonged course. Losonsky and coworkers[272] gave human IG to three immunodeficient patients and demonstrated that it survived passage of the GI tract in an immunologically active form.

Pooled colostrum concentrate from hyperimmunized pregnant cows with high titers to several rotavirus serotypes[76] has been used in several studies. In a controlled study, bovine immune colostrum[465] did not prevent symptomatic rotavirus infection in infants, but treated patients had a decrease in the length of diarrhea. Immune bovine colostrum also was used prophylactically for 2 weeks in 10 infants in a baby care center with evidence of a protective effect.[116]

A double-blind, placebo-controlled trial of oral lyophilized rotavirus bovine colostrum in Bangladesh showed that a 4-day course decreased diarrhea, the need for oral rehydration, and viral shedding.[394] Mitra and associates[299] also showed that cow colostrum significantly shortened the duration of diarrhea and decreased stool output. Hilpert and colleagues[188] demonstrated that rotavirus colostrum decreased virus excretion in infants with rotavirus diarrhea.

Recommendation

Because rotavirus infection is usually self-limited, no commercial product has been developed, although it would be of use in developing countries. Human IG probably does not have a high enough neutralizing titer to be consistently beneficial.

RUBELLA

Rubella prevention by IG is rarely used because of its uneven efficacy. Early studies suggested some prophylactic benefit. Korns[246] in 1952 showed that one lot of IG at a dose of 0.1 mL/lb partially protected mentally handicapped institutionalized subjects against epidemic rubella. Rubella developed in 9 of 45 IG-injected subjects versus 35 of 60 noninjected controls, a significant difference. However, another IG lot was ineffective and a third was only slightly effective, thus suggesting that the titers of rubella antibodies varied significantly.

Studies in epidemic situations have shown that 5 mL of IG can prevent clinical rubella,[159] but Brody and coworkers[66] showed that an IG dose of 0.55 mg/kg resulted in a decreased clinical attack rate but also a high incidence of subclinical infection. Military recruits were protected by a 15-mL dose of IG administered before exposure.[191]

Extensive studies on IG prophylaxis of rubella conducted by Green, Krugman, and their associates[161, 252] did not demonstrate a protective effect of 0.12 to 0.2 mL of IG/lb. Lundström and coworkers[277] gave 251 exposed pregnant Swedish women 4 mL of convalescent rubella IG and 28 exposed pregnant women 24 mL of standard IG. Rubella developed in 6 of the 251 (2.4%); 3 of these 6 women aborted, and 1 had an infant with probable congenital rubella. None of the 28 women given 24 mL of standard IG contracted rubella. Their subsequent study demonstrated that convalescent rubella IG given to pregnant women with clinically manifested rubella did not protect against congenital rubella or lessen the probability of fetal damage.[278]

Recommendations

IG prophylaxis is not indicated for children and nonpregnant adults exposed to an infected contact because of the mildness of the infection.

IG is not recommended for most exposed pregnant women because the clinical syndrome may be masked and congenital rubella not prevented. For exposed pregnant women who will not consider abortion if rubella develops, a large dose of IG may be of some value. A dose of 0.55 mg/kg IG given intramuscularly is the accepted dose.[19] However, mothers who have received such prophylaxis after exposure have delivered infants with congenital rubella.[19]

VACCINIA, VARIOLA, AND VACCINIA IMMUNE GLOBULIN

Although smallpox (variola) has been eradicated from the world since 1977, the virus nonetheless exists in a few research laboratories and is, unfortunately, a potential weapon in biologic warfare. Vaccination still is used on a limited basis for members of the military and for laboratory workers who handle cultures or animals contaminated with vaccinia virus, some recombinant vaccinia viruses, and other orthopoxviruses (e.g., monkeypox virus or cowpox virus). Passive immunization is occasionally necessary after laboratory accidents, inadvertent vaccination of high-risk individuals, and exposure of high-risk individuals to a recently vaccinated individual.

Passive immunization against vaccinia was known as early as 1895, when Hlava and Honl[189] showed that schoolchildren could be protected from vaccinia by the injection of 3 to 10 mL of immune calf serum. At the same time, protective antibodies developed after vaccination, and passive transmission of these antibodies from mothers to infants was demonstrated.[426] Thereafter, effective prevention of smallpox by well-organized mass vaccine campaigns diminished interest in passive immunization.

Janeway, quoted by Enders,[120] found neutralizing vaccinia antibody in IG in 1944, and Verlinde and Spaander[477] in 1966 found high titers of such antibodies in convalescent IG from recently vaccinated individuals. Gispen and associates[147] in 1956 developed a human vaccinia immune globulin (VIG) that was shown to not interfere with active immunity, and they proposed its use with vaccine as prophylaxis against vaccinia encephalitis.

The value of human VIG in treating smallpox or disseminated vaccinia is based on the presence of viremia, which leads to secondary dissemination; administration of neutralizing antibody will prevent or limit the spread of infection and thus modify clinical expression of the disease.

A series of studies on the efficacy of VIG in treating smallpox and vaccinia complications was initiated by Kempe and colleagues in 1955.[40, 231] They used a VIG that was prepared from recently vaccinated donors with a neutralizing titer of 1:256 to 1:512, in contrast to titers of 1:16 or 1:32 in standard IG. The households of new admissions to the Madras (India) Smallpox Hospital were visited, and alternate family contacts received VIG (1.0 g in adults, 0.5 g in children).[231] After 25 days, eight cases of smallpox developed in 75 contacts not given VIG, and two cases developed in 56 contacts given VIG, a significant difference. A similar, more extensive study disclosed 21 cases of smallpox (4 severe) among 379 contacts serving as controls and 5 cases of smallpox (none severe) among 326 contacts given VIG.[232]

Kempe[230] also reported the results of 300 cases of smallpox vaccination (vaccinia) complications treated with VIG, including 62 cases of generalized vaccinia, 132 cases of eczema vaccinatum, 23 cases of vaccinia necrosum, 12 cases of vaccinia encephalitis, and 28 cases of autoinoculation. In addition, VIG was given prophylactically to 44 eczematoid children requiring smallpox vaccine (0.6 to 1.2 mL/kg). VIG did not affect the course of vaccinia encephalitis. Twenty-seven of 28 patients with autoinoculation who received VIG did well. Nine deaths occurred in the 132 patients with eczema vaccinatum given VIG; this 7 percent mortality compares favorably with the usual mortality of 30 to 40 percent with supportive care only. All 62 patients with generalized vaccinia who were given VIG did well, although 4 children required a second course.

Seven of the 23 patients with vaccinia necrosum who received VIG died (30%); however, this disease is generally fatal and immune defects were present in most of these patients.[40] These results strongly supported the efficacy of VIG and subsequently were confirmed by studies in Sweden[276] and the United Kingdom.[405]

In 1997, Kesson and coauthors reported a severely immunocompromised patient with progressive vaccinia who had inadvertently received a vaccinia melanoma oncolysate vaccination but was successfully treated with VIG and ribavirin.[233] Nanning[312] studied the effect of VIG on postvaccinia encephalitis. He gave a placebo or 2 mL of VIG to Dutch military recruits at the time of primary vaccination; 3 cases of encephalitis occurred in 43,630 vaccinated recruits given VIG as compared with 13 cases in 53,044 recruits in the control group. This 77 percent reduction is statistically significant.

Human VIG, available from the CDC, is derived from the plasma of vaccinated donors.[468] Smallpox (variola) virus is closely related antigenically to the vaccinia (cowpox) virus used for smallpox vaccination.[313]

Recommendations

Complications of vaccination are indications for the use of VIG. Accidental or intentional vaccination of a patient with a contraindication to the vaccine, autoinoculation of the eye, eczema vaccinatum, severe generalized vaccinia, and vaccinia necrosum are indications for VIG. The initial dose is 0.6 mL/kg. In adults, the dose must be divided and administered over the course of 24 to 36 hours. Repeat doses can be given at 2- to 3-day intervals for vaccine complications until recovery begins, as evidenced by no new lesions. VIG should be given as soon as possible after the diagnosis of such a complication.[468]

For unimmunized patients exposed to smallpox, VIG can be given in combination with vaccine for prevention. A dose of 0.6 mL/kg has been recommended[288, 467] and should be given within 7 days. Shorter intervals, within 1 to 3 days, are preferred.[467] Both vaccine and VIG should be given if more than 1 week has elapsed since exposure. Patients with known contraindications to the vaccine (e.g., pregnancy, eczema) who must be vaccinated because of exposure should receive VIG (0.6 mL/kg) at the time of vaccination. Recent recommendations[469] state that the current supplies of VIG would not permit its routine use in combination with vaccine for bioterrorism exposure, but that if supplies become available, the VIG dose for prophylaxis in combination with vaccine is 0.3 mL/kg.

VIG is not indicated for established smallpox infections, postvaccinia encephalitis, or hypersensitivity and toxic rashes that occur after vaccination.

VIG is contraindicated for the treatment of vaccinial keratitis because it might increase corneal scarring.[469]

REGIONAL VIRUSES

Argentine Hemorrhagic Fever

Junin virus, the etiologic agent of Argentine hemorrhagic fever, causes a febrile illness with high mortality rates from vascular or neurologic complications.[347] Patients may either improve or have severe hemorrhagic or neurologic manifestations (or both) within the first 2 weeks of illness.[279] Maiztegui and colleagues[279] found that immune plasma given before the ninth day of illness to 91 patients reduced their mortality to 1.1 percent as compared with a mortality of 16.5 percent in the 97 patients given normal plasma ($p < .01$). Ten of the patients who received immune plasma relapsed with fever and cerebellar signs after several weeks, as did 8 others who were not part of the study. The neurologic relapse was self-limited in all but one patient, who died.

Ebola

Ebola virus, a filovirus, causes severe and often fatal hemorrhagic fever; it has no effective treatment. Kudoyarova-Zubavichene and coworkers[254] reviewed the use of hyperimmune goat or equine serum in the prevention and treatment of Ebola disease. Goat hyperimmune serum protects guinea pigs from experimental infection if given less than 24 hours before exposure and provides some benefit if given within 72 hours after exposure. This product was used for emergency prophylaxis in four patients exposed by laboratory accidents. Mild infection developed in one definitely exposed patient, but Ebola disease did not develop in the other 3 patients with questionable exposure. All four patients also received recombinant human interferon alfa-2. Equine serum has protected baboons from low-dose virus challenge, but not cynomolgus monkeys from a high-dose virus challenge.[206] Equine serum given to monkeys on the day of infection and 5 days later did not prevent death.[207]

Gupta and coauthors[171] reported that a murine polyclonal immune serum protected 100 percent of normal mice and mice with severe combined immunodeficiency after incurring a lethal challenge. Thus, antibody may be a useful agent in the prevention of Ebola disease. Human monoclonal antibodies are in development.[284, 285]

RECOMMENDATION

The role of antibody in the prevention and treatment of Ebola disease is unproved, but monoclonal antibodies are being developed. Animal studies support a role for antibody in the prevention of Ebola disease.

Tick-Borne Encephalitis

Tick-borne encephalitis is caused by a flavivirus infection, which is endemic to Russia and Eastern and Central Europe. Several neurologic syndromes are associated with this infection: febrile headache, aseptic meningitis, meningoencephalitis, meningomyeloencephalitis, and postencephalitic syndrome.[112] The meningoencephalitis is the most severe form and can result in death or permanent paresis. An effective vaccine is available.[112] Passive immunization with a hyperimmune human globulin has been used for postexposure prophylaxis in endemic countries, but it may result in antibody-dependent enhancement of infection.[484] The lack of efficacy trials has led to questioning of the use of this product.[6] However, von Hedenström and colleagues[481] have recommended its use for postexposure prophylaxis in addition to immunization.

Definitive recommendations cannot be made.

Acknowledgments

The authors wish to thank Jillian le Patourel and Coralia Gomez for editorial assistance.

REFERENCES

1. Abraham, E., Wunderink, R., Silverman, H., et al.: Efficacy and safety of monoclonal antibody to human tumor necrosis factor α in patients with sepsis syndrome. J. A. M. A. *273*:934–941, 1995.
2. Abrahamsen, T. G., Sandersen, H., and Bustnes, A.: Home therapy with subcutaneous immunoglobulin infusions in children with congenital immunodeficiencies. Pediatrics *98*:1127–1131, 1996.
3. Abrutyn, E., and Berlin, J. A.: Intrathecal therapy in tetanus: A meta-analysis. J. A. M. A. *266*:2262–2267, 1991.
4. Abzug, M. J., Keyserling, H. L., Lee, M. L., et al.: Neonatal enterovirus infection: Virology, serology, and effects of intravenous immune globulin. Clin. Infect. Dis. *20*:1201–1206, 1995.
5. Acute Hepatic Failure Study Group: Failure of specific immunotherapy in fulminant type B hepatitis. Ann. Intern. Med. *86*:272–277, 1977.
6. Aebi, C., and Schaad, U. B.: TBE—immunoglobulins—a critical assessment of efficacy. Schweiz. Med. Wochenschr. *124*:1837–1840, 1994.
7. Alexander, H. E.: Treatment of *Haemophilus influenzae* infection and of meningococcic and pneumococcic meningitis. Am. J. Dis. Child. *66*:172–187, 1943.
8. Amer, J., Ott, E., Ibbott, F. A., et al.: The effect of monthly gamma globulin administration on morbidity and mortality from infection in premature infants during the first year of life. Pediatrics *32*:4–9, 1963.
9. American Academy of Pediatrics: Passive immunization. *In* Pickering, L. K. (ed.): 2000 Red Book: Report of the Committee on Infectious Diseases. 25th ed. Elk Grove Village, IL, American Academy of Pediatrics, 2000, pp. 41–53.
10. American Academy of Pediatrics: Clostridial infections. *In* Pickering, L. K. (ed.): 2000 Red Book: Report of the Committee on Infectious Diseases. 25th ed. Elk Grove Village, IL, American Academy of Pediatrics, 2000, pp. 212–219.
11. American Academy of Pediatrics: Diphtheria. *In* Pickering, L. K. (ed.): 2000 Red Book: Report of the Committee on Infectious Diseases. 25th ed. Elk Grove Village, IL, American Academy of Pediatrics, 2000, pp. 230–234.
12. American Academy of Pediatrics: Hepatitis A. *In* Pickering, L. K. (ed.): 2000 Red Book: Report of the Committee on Infectious Diseases. 25th ed. Elk Grove Village, IL, American Academy of Pediatrics, 2000, pp. 562–568.
13. American Academy of Pediatrics: Hepatitis B. *In* Pickering, L. K. (ed.): 2000 Red Book: Report of the Committee on Infectious Diseases. 25th ed. Elk Grove Village, IL, American Academy of Pediatrics, 2000, pp. 289–302.
14. American Academy of Pediatrics: Herpes simplex. *In* Pickering, L. K. (ed.): 2000 Red Book: Report of the Committee on Infectious Diseases. 25th ed. Elk Grove Village, IL, American Academy of Pediatrics, 2000, pp. 309–318.
15. American Academy of Pediatrics: Measles. *In* Pickering, L. K. (ed.): 2000 Red Book: Report of the Committee on Infectious Diseases. 25th ed. Elk Grove Village, IL, American Academy of Pediatrics, 2000, pp. 385–396.
16. American Academy of Pediatrics: Mumps. *In* Pickering, L. K. (ed.): 2000 Red Book: Report of the Committee on Infectious Diseases. 25th ed. Elk Grove Village, IL, American Academy of Pediatrics, 2000, pp. 405–408.
17. American Academy of Pediatrics: Rabies. *In* Pickering, L. K. (ed.): 2000 Red Book: Report of the Committee on Infectious Diseases. 25th ed. Elk Grove Village, IL, American Academy of Pediatrics, 2000, pp. 475–482.
18. American Academy of Pediatrics: Respiratory syncytial virus. *In* Pickering, L. K. (ed.): 2000 Red Book: Report of the Committee on Infectious Diseases. 25th ed. Elk Grove Village, IL, American Academy of Pediatrics, 2000, pp. 483–487.
19. American Academy of Pediatrics: Rubella. *In* Pickering, L. K. (ed.): 2000 Red Book: Report of the Committee on Infectious Diseases. 25th ed. Elk Grove Village, IL, American Academy of Pediatrics, 2000, pp. 495–500.
20. American Academy of Pediatrics: Tetanus. *In* Pickering, L. K. (ed.): 2000 Red Book: Report of the Committee on Infectious Diseases. 25th ed. Elk Grove Village, IL, American Academy of Pediatrics, 2000, pp. 562–568.
21. American Academy of Pediatrics: Toxic shock syndrome. *In* Pickering, L. K. (ed.): 2000 Red Book: Report of the Committee on Infectious Diseases. 25th ed. Elk Grove Village, IL, American Academy of Pediatrics, 2000, pp. 576–581.
22. American Academy of Pediatrics: Varicella-zoster infections. *In* Pickering, L. K. (ed.): 2000 Red Book: Report of the Committee on Infectious Diseases. 25th ed. Elk Grove Village, IL, American Academy of Pediatrics, 2000, pp. 624–638.
23. American Academy of Pediatrics. Committee on Infectious Diseases: Severe invasive group A streptococcal infections: A subject review. Pediatrics *101*:136–140, 1998.
24. Ammann, A. J., Ashman, R. F., Buckley, R. H., et al.: Use of intravenous gamma globulin in antibody immunodeficiency. Results of a multicenter controlled trial. Clin. Immunol. Immunopathol. *22*:60–67, 1982.
25. Ammann, A. J., and Stiehm, E. R.: Immune globulin levels in colostrum and breast milk, and serum from formula and breast fed newborns. Proc. Soc. Exp. Biol. Med. *122*:1098–1100, 1966.
26. Antiretroviral therapy and medical management of the human immunodeficiency virus–infected child. Working Group on Antiretroviral Therapy: National Pediatric HIV Resource Center. Pediatr. Infect. Dis. J. *12*:513–522, 1993.
27. Apfelzweig, R., Piszkiewicz, D., and Hooper, J. A.: Immunoglobulin A concentrations in commercial immune globulins. J. Clin. Immunol. *7*:46–50, 1987.
28. Arvin, A. M.: Varicella-zoster virus. Clin. Microbiol. Rev. *9*:361–381, 1996.
29. Ashida, E. R., and Saxon, A.: Home intravenous immunoglobulin infusion by self-infusion. J. Clin. Immunol. *6*:306–309, 1986.
30. Askenasy, O. M.: A community outbreak of hepatitis A in a religious community in Indiana: Failure of immune serum globulin to prevent the spread of the infection. Epidemiol. Infect. *124*:309–313, 2000.
31. Athavale, V. B.: Role of tetanus antitoxin in the treatment of tetanus in children. J. Pediatr. *68*:289–293, 1966.
32. Babes, V., and Lepp, M.: Recherches sur la vaccination antirabique. Ann. Inst. Pasteur *3*:385–390, 1889.

33. Bagge, E., Geijer, M., and Tarkowski, A.: Intra-articular administration of polyclonal immunoglobulin G in rheumatoid arthritis. Scand. J. Rheumatol. *25*:174–176, 1996.
34. Baker, C. J., Melish, M. E., and Hall, R. T.: Intravenous immune globulin for the prevention of nosocomial infection in low-birth-weight neonates. N. Engl. J. Med. *327*:213–219, 1992.
35. Balagtas, R. C., Nelson, K. E., Levin, S., and Gotoff, S. P.: Treatment of pertussis with pertussis immune globulin. J. Pediatr. *79*:203–208, 1971.
36. Balfour, H. H., Jr., Groth, K. E., McCullough, J., et al.: Prevention or modification of varicella using zoster immune plasma. Am. J. Dis. Child. *131*:693–696, 1977.
37. Ballow, M.: Mechanisms of action of intravenous immune serum globulin in autoimmune and inflammatory diseases. J. Allergy Clin. Immunol. *100*:151–157, 1997.
38. Ballow, M., Cates, K. L., Rowe, J. C. et al.: Development of the immune system in very low birth weight (less than 1500 g) premature infants: Concentrations of plasma immunoglobulins and patterns of infections. Pediatr. Res. *20*:899–904, 1986.
39. Baltazard, M., and Bahmanyar, M.: Essai pratique du sérum antirabique chez les mordus par loups enragés. Bull. World Health Organ. *13*:747–772, 1955.
40. Barbero, G. J., Gray, A., Scott, T. F. M., et al.: Vaccinia gangrenosa treated with hyperimmune vaccinial gamma globulin. Pediatrics *16*:609–618, 1955.
41. Barnes, G. L., Doyle, L. W., Hewson, P. H., et al.: A randomised trial of oral gammaglobulin in low birth weight infants infected with rotavirus. Lancet *1*:1371–1373, 1982.
42. Baron, S., Barnett, E. V., Goldsmith, R. S., et al.: Prophylaxis of infections by gamma globulin. Am. J. Hyg. *79*:186–195, 1964.
43. Barry, W., Hudgins, L., Donta, S. T., and Pesanti, E. L.: Intravenous immunoglobulin therapy for toxic-shock syndrome. J. A. M. A. *267*:3315–3317, 1992.
44. Bass, E. B., Powe, N. R. Goodman, S. N., et al.: Efficacy of immune globulin in preventing complications of bone marrow transplantation: A meta-analysis. Bone Marrow Transplant. *12*:273–282, 1993.
45. Baumgartner, J. D., Glauser, M. P., McCutchan, J. A., et al.: Prevention of gram negative shock and death in surgical patients by antibody to endotoxin core glycolipid. Lancet *2*:59–63, 1985.
46. Beasley, R. P., Hwang, L. Y., Stevens, C. E., et al.: Efficacy of hepatitis B immune globulin for prevention of perinatal transmission of the hepatitis B virus carrier state: Final report of a randomized double blind, placebo controlled trial. Hepatology *3*:135–141, 1983.
47. Beasley, R. P., Lin, C. C., Wang, K. Y., et al.: Hepatitis B immune globulin (HBIG) efficacy in the interruption of perinatal transmission of hepatitis B virus carrier state. Lancet *2*:388–392, 1981.
48. Begue, R. E. and Lindo-Soriano, I.: Failure of intrathecal tetanus antitoxin in the treatment of tetanus neonatorum. J. Infect. Dis. *164*:619–620, 1991.
49. Berg, B. O.: Syndrome of infant botulism. Pediatrics *59*:321–322, 1977.
50. Berger, M., Cupps, T. R., and Fauci, A.: Immunoglobulin replacement therapy by slow subcutaneous infusion. Ann. Intern. Med. *93*:55–56, 1980.
51. Berger, M., Cupps, T. R., and Fauci, A. S.: High-dose immunoglobulin replacement therapy by slow subcutaneous infusion during pregnancy. J. A. M. A. *247*:2824–2825, 1982.
52. Bernstein, L. J., Krieger, B. Z., Novic, B., et al.: Bacterial infections in acquired immunodeficiency syndrome of children. Pediatr. Infect. Dis. *4*:472–475, 1985.
53. Björkander, J., Bengtsson, U., Oxelius, V. A., et al.: Symptoms and efficacy of intravenous immunoglobulin prophylaxis in patients with low serum levels of IgG subclasses. J. Allergy Clin. Immunol. *77*:124–127, 1986.
54. Björkander, J., Cunningham-Rundles, C., and Ludon, P.: Intravenous immunoglobulin prophylaxis causing liver damage in 16 of 77 patients with hypogammaglobulinemia or IgG subclass deficiency. Am. J. Med. *84*:107–111, 1988.
55. Bjoro, K., Froland, S. S., Yun, Z., et al.: Hepatitis C infection in patients with contaminated immune globulin. N. Engl. J. Med. *331*:1607–1611, 1994.
56. Blake, P. A., Feldman, R. A., Buchanan, T. M., et al.: Serologic therapy of tetanus in the United States, 1965–1971. J. A. M. A. *235*:42–44, 1976.
57. Bleck, T. P., and Rupprecht, C. E.: Rabies virus. *In* Mandell, G. L., Bennett, J. E., and Doling, R. (eds.): Mandell, Douglas and Bennett's Principles and Practice of Infectious Diseases. 5th ed. Philadelphia, Churchill Livingstone, 2000, pp. 1811–1820.
58. Bloxsom, A.: Use of immune serum globulin (human) as prophylaxis against poliomyelitis. Tex. Med. *74*:468–470, 1949.
59. Blum, P. M., Phelps, D. L., Ank, B. J., et al.: Survival of oral human immune serum globulin in the gastrointestinal tract of low birth weight infants. Pediatr. Res. *15*:1256–1260, 1981.
60. Bodian, D.: Neutralization of three immunological types of poliomyelitis virus by human gamma globulin. Proc. Soc. Exp. Biol. Med. *72*:259–261, 1949.
61. Bodian, D.: Experimental studies on passive immunization against poliomyelitis: I. Protection with human gamma globulin against intramuscular inoculation and combined passive and active immunization. Am. J. Hyg. *54*:132–143, 1951.
62. Bogstedt, A. K., Johansen, K., Hatta, H., et al.: Passive immunity against diarrhoea. Acta Paediatr. *85*:125–128, 1996.
63. Borowitz, S. M., and Saulsbury, F. T.: Treatment of chronic cryptosporidial infection with orally administered human serum immune globulin. J. Pediatr. *119*:593–595, 1991.
64. Bradford, W. F.: Use of convalescent blood in whooping cough. Am. J. Dis. Child. *50*:918–928, 1935.
65. Brodsky, L., Afshani, E., Pizzuto, M., et al.: Open trial of intravenous immune serum globulin for chronic sinusitis in children. Ann. Allergy Asthma Immunol. *79*:119–124, 1997.
66. Brody, J. A., Sever, J. L., and Schiff, G. M.: Prevention of rubella by gamma globulin during an epidemic in Barrow, Alaska in 1964. N. Engl. J. Med. *272*:127–129, 1965.
67. Brown, A., Mohamed, S. D., Montgomery, R. D., et al.: Value of a large dose of antitoxin in clinical tetanus. Lancet *2*:227–230, 1960.
68. Brown, K. E.: Parvovirus B19. *In* Mandell, G. L., Bennett, J. E., and Doling, R. (eds.): Mandell, Douglas and Bennett's Principles and Practice of Infectious Diseases. 5th ed. Philadelphia, Churchill Livingstone, 2000, pp. 1685–1693.
69. Brown, K. E., Green, S. W., Antunez de Mayolo, J., et al.: Congenital anaemia after transplacental B19 parvovirus infection. Lancet *343*:895–896, 1994.
70. Brox, A. G., Courmoyer, D., Sternbach, M., et al.: Hemolytic anemia following intravenous immunoglobulin administration. Am. J. Med. *83*:633–635, 1987.
71. Brunell, P. A., and Gershon, A. A.: Passive immunization against varicella zoster infections. J. Infect. Dis. *127*:415–423, 1973.
72. Brunell, P. A., Gershon, A. A., Hughes, W. T., et al.: Prevention of varicella in high risk children: A collaborative study. Pediatrics *50*:718–722, 1972.
73. Brunell, P. A., Ross, A., Miller, L. H., et al.: Prevention of varicella by zoster immune globulin. N. Engl. J. Med. *280*:1191–1194, 1969.
74. Bruss, J. B., Malley, R., Halperin, S., et al.: Treatment of severe pertussis: A study of the safety and pharmacology of intravenous pertussis immunoglobulin. Pediatr. Infect. Dis. J. *18*:505–511, 1999.
75. Bruss, J. B., and Siber, G. R.: Protective effects of pertussis immunoglobulin (P-IGIV) in the aerosol challenge model. Clin. Diagn. Lab. Immunol. *6*:464–470, 1999.
76. Brüssow, H., Hilpert, H., Walther, I., et al.: Bovine milk immunoglobulins for passive immunity to infantile rotavirus gastroenteritis. J. Clin. Microbiol. *25*:982–986, 1987.
77. Buckley, R. H., and Schiff, R. I.: The use of intravenous immune globulin in immunodeficiency diseases. N. Engl. J. Med. *325*:110–117, 1991.
78. Bulinski, P., Toledo-Pereyra, L. H., Dalal, S., and Hernandez, G.: Cytomegalovirus infection in kidney transplantation: Prophylaxis and management. Transplant. Proc. *28*:3310–3311, 1996.
79. Bussel, J. B., and Himi, J. S.: Isolated thrombocytopenia in patients infected with HIV: Treatment with intravenous gammaglobulin. Am. J. Hematol. *28*:79–84, 1988.
80. Calandra, T., Glauser, M. P., Schellekens, J., et al.: Treatment of gram negative septic shock with human IgG antibody to *Escherichia coli* J5: A prospective, double blind, randomized trial. J. Infect. Dis. *158*:312–319, 1988.
81. Calvelli, T. A., and Rubinstein, A.: Intravenous gamma globulin in infant acquired immunodeficiency syndrome. Pediatr. Infect. Dis. *5*(Suppl.): 207–210, 1986.
82. Cannon, R. A., Blum, P. M., Ament, M. E., et al.: Reversal of enterocolitis associated combined immunodeficiency by plasma therapy. J. Pediatr. *101*:711–717, 1982.
83. Carl, M., Francis, D. P., and Maynard, J. E.: Food borne hepatitis A: Recommendations for control. J. Infect. Dis. *148*:1133–1135, 1983.
84. Casadevall, A.: Passive antibody therapies: Progress and continuing challenges. Clin. Immunol. *93*:5–15, 1999.
85. Casadevall, A., and Scharff, M. D.: Return to the past: The case for antibody-based therapies in infectious diseases. Clin. Infect. Dis. *21*:150–161, 1995.
86. Cenci, F.: Alcune esperienze di sieroimmunizzazione e sieroterapia nel morbillo. Riv. Clin. Pediatr. *5*:1017–1025, 1907.
87. Centers for Disease Control: Botulism in the United States, 1899–1977. Handbook for Epidemiologists, Clinicians and Laboratory Workers. Atlanta, Centers for Disease Control, May 1979.
88. Chapel, H. M., Lee, M., Hargreaves, R., et al.: Randomized trial of intravenous immunoglobulin as prophylaxis against infection in plateau-phase multiple myeloma. Lancet *343*:1059–1063, 1994.
89. Chen, S. H., and Liang, D. C.: Intravenous immunoglobulin prophylaxis in children with acute leukemia following exposure to varicella. Pediatr. Hematol. Oncol. *9*:347–351, 1992.
90. Chesney, P. J., and Davis, J. P.: Toxic shock syndrome. *In* Feigin, R. D., and Cherry, J. D. (eds.): Textbook of Pediatric Infectious Diseases. 4th ed. Philadelphia, W. B. Saunders, 1998, pp. 830–850.
91. Chuhjo, T., Nakao, S., and Matsuda. T.: Successful treatment of persistent erythroid aplasia caused by parvovirus B19 infection in a patient with common variable immunodeficiency with low-dose immunoglobulin. Am. J. Hematol. *60*:222–224, 1999.

92. Chung, W. K., Yoo, J. Y., Sun, H. S., et al.: Prevention of perinatal transmission of hepatitis B virus: A comparison between the efficacy of passive and passive active immunization in Korea. J. Infect. Dis. *151*:280–286, 1985.
93. Cleary, R.: *Clostridium difficile*–associated diarrhea and colitis: Clinical manifestations, diagnosis, and treatment Dis. Colon Rectum *41*:1435–1449, 1998.
94. Cohen, J., and Carlet, J.: INTERSEPT: An international, multicenter, placebo-controlled trial of monoclonal antibody to human tumor necrosis factor-alpha in patients with sepsis. Crit. Care Med. *24*:1431–1440, 1996.
95. Conway, S. P., Gillies, D. R. N., and Docherty, A.: Neonatal infection in premature infants and use of human immunoglobulin. Arch. Dis. Child. *62*:1252–1256, 1987.
96. Copelon, E. A. and Tutschka, P. J.: Immunoglobulin in bone marrow transplantation. *In* Morell, A., and Nydegger, U. E. (eds.): Clinical Use of Intravenous Immunoglobulins. New York, Academic Press, 1986, pp. 117–121.
97. Craig, R. D. P.: Immunotherapy for severe burns in children. Plast. Reconstr. Surg. *35*:263–270, 1965.
98. Crennan, J. M., Van Scoy, R. E., McKenna, C. H., et al.: Echovirus polymyositis in patients with hypogammaglobulinemia: Failure of high dose intravenous gammaglobulin therapy and review of the literature. Am. J. Med. *81*:35–42, 1986.
99. Cunningham-Rundles, C., Bjorkander, J., and Hanson, L. A.: Therapeutic use of an IgA-depleted intravenous immunoglobulin patient. *In* Morell, A., and Nydegger, U. E. (eds.): Clinical Use of Intravenous Immunoglobulins. New York, Academic Press, 1986, pp. 87–96.
100. Davidson, G. P.: Passive protection against diarrheal disease. J. Pediatr. Gastroenterol. Nutr. *23*:207–212, 1996.
101. Davidson, G. P., Whyte, P. B., Daniels, E., et al.: Passive immunisation of children with bovine colostrum containing antibodies to human rotavirus. Lancet *2*:709–712, 1989.
102. Delone, P., Corkill, J., Jordan, M., et al.: Successful treatment of Epstein-Barr virus infection with ganciclovir and cytomegalovirus hyperimmune globulin following kidney transplantation. Transplant. Proc. *27*(Suppl. 1):58–59, 1995.
103. De Otero, J., Gavalda, J., Murio, E., et al.: Cytomegalovirus disease as a risk factor for graft loss and death after orthotopic liver transplantation. Clin. Infect. Dis. *26*:865–870, 1998.
104. DeSimone, C., Delogu, G., and Corbetta, G.: Intravenous immunoglobulins in association with antibiotics: A therapeutic trial in septic intensive care unit patients. Crit. Care Med. *16*:23–26, 1988.
105. DeVincenzo, J. P., Hirsch, R. L., Fuentes, R. J., and Top, F. H., Jr.: Respiratory syncytial immune globulin treatment of lower respiratory tract infection in pediatric patients undergoing bone marrow transplantation—a compassionate use experience. Bone Marrow Transplant. *25*:161–165, 2000.
106. Diamond, E. F., Purugganan, H. B., and Choi, H. J.: Effect of prophylactic administration on infection morbidity in premature infants. Illinois Med. J. *130*:668–670, 1966.
107. Dolman, C. E., and Hda, H.: Type E botulism: Its epidemiology, prevention and specific treatment. Can. J. Public Health *54*:293–308, 1963.
108. Donta, S. T. P., Peduzzi, A. S., Cross, J., et al.: Immunoprophylaxis against *Klebsiella* and *Pseudomonas aeruginosa* infections. J. Infect. Dis. *174*:537–543, 1996.
109. Douzinas, E. E., Pitaridis, M. T., Louris, G., et al.: Prevention of infection in multiple trauma patients by high-dose intravenous immunoglobulins. Crit. Care Med. *28*:8–14, 2000.
110. Drake, M. E., Barondess, J. A., Bashe, W. J., Jr., et al.: Failure of convalescent gamma globulin to protect against homologous serum hepatitis. J. A. M. A. *152*:690–693, 1953.
111. Duhem, C., Dicato, M. A., and Ries, F.: Side-effects of intravenous immune globulins. Clin. Exp. Immunol. *97*:79–83, 1994.
112. Dumpis, U., Crook, D., Oksi, J.: Tick-borne encephalitis. Clin. Infect. Dis. *28*:882–90,1999.
113. Duncan, G. G., Christian, H. A., and Stokes, J., Jr.: An evaluation of immune serum globulin as a prophylactic agent against homologous serum hepatitis. Am. J. Med. Sci. *213*:53–57, 1947.
114. Dwyer, J. M.: Manipulating the immune system with immune globulin. N. Engl. J. Med. *326*:107–116, 1992.
115. Dwyer, J. M., and Erlendsson, K.: Intraventricular gamma-globulin for the management of enterovirus encephalitis. Pediatr. Infect. Dis. J. *7*(Suppl.):30–33, 1988.
116. Ebina, T.: Prophylaxis of rotavirus gastroenteritis using immunoglobulin. Arch. Virol. Suppl. *12*:217–223, 1996.
117. Eibl, M. M., Wolf, H. M., Furnkranz, H., Rosenkranz, A.: Prevention of necrotizing enterocolitis in low-birth-weight infants by IgA-IgG feeding. N. Engl. J. Med. *319*:1–7, 1988.
118. Eijkhout, J. W., Van Der Meer, J. W. M., Cees, G. M., et al.: The effect of two different dosages of intravenous immunoglobulin on the incidence of recurrent infections in patients with primary hypogammaglobulinemia: A randomized, double-blind, multicenter crossover trial. Ann. Intern. Med. *135*:165–174, 2001.
119. Ellis, E. F., and Henney, C. S.: Adverse reactions following administration of human gamma globulin. J. Allergy *43*:45–54, 1969.
120. Enders, J. F.: Chemical, clinical, and immunological studies on the products of human plasma fractionation. X. The concentrations of certain antibodies in globulin fractions derived from human blood plasma. J. Clin. Invest. *23*:510–530, 1944.
121. Erlendsson, K., Swartz, T., and Dwyer, J. M.: Successful reversal of echovirus encephalitis in X-linked hypogammaglobulinemia by intraventricular administration of immunoglobulin. N. Engl. J. Med. *312*:351–353, 1985.
122. Expert Committee on Rabies: Hyperimmune antirabies serum. W. H. O. Tech. Rep. Ser. *28*:23–25, 1950.
123. Falagas, M. E., Snydman D. R., Ruthazer, R., et al.: Cytomegalovirus immune globulin (CMVIG) prophylaxis is associated with increased survival after orthotopic liver transplantation. Clin. Transplant. *11*:432–437, 1997.
124. Feranchak, A. P., Tyson, R. W., Narkewicz, M. R., et al.: Fulminant Epstein-Barr viral hepatitis: Orthotopic liver transplantation and review of the literature. Liver Transpl. Surg. *4*:469–476, 1998.
125. Féray, C., Gigou, M., Samuel, D., et al.: Incidence of hepatitis C in patients receiving different preparations of hepatitis B immunoglobulin after liver transplantation. Ann. Intern. Med. *128*:810–816, 1998.
126. Ferdman, R. M., and Church, J. A.: Failure of intravenous immunoglobulin to prevent varicella-zoster infection. Pediatr. Infect. Dis. J. *19*:1219–1220, 2000.
127. Fibiger, J.: Om serum behandling af difteri. Hospitalstidende *6*:337–339, 1898.
128. Filipovich, A. H., Gross, T., Jyonouchi, H., et al.: Immune-mediated hematologic and oncologic disorders, including Epstein-Barr virus infection. *In* Stiehm, E. R. (ed.): Immunologic Disorders in Infants and Children. 4th ed. Philadelphia, W. B. Saunders, 1996, pp. 855–888.
129. Finkel, K. C., and Haworth, J. C.: Clinical trial to assess the effectiveness of gamma globulin in acute infections in young children. Pediatrics *25*:798–806, 1960.
130. Fischer, G. W., Cieslak, T. J., Wilson, S. R., et al.: Opsonic antibodies to *Staphylococcus epidermidis:* In vitro and in vivo studies using human intravenous immune globulin. J. Infect. Dis. *169*:324–329, 1994.
131. Fisher, M. W.: Synergism between human gamma globulin and chloramphenicol in the treatment of experimental bacterial infections. Antibiot. Chemother. *7*:315–321, 1956.
132. Flynn, J. T., Kaiser, B. A., Long, S. S., et al.: Intravenous immunoglobulin prophylaxis of cytomegalovirus infection in pediatric renal transplant recipients. Am. J. Nephrol. *17*:146–152, 1997.
133. Fort, D. W., and Buchanan, G. R.: Treatment of infection-associated hemophagocytic syndrome with immune globulin. J. Pediatr. *124*:332, 1994.
134. Freeman, B., Rathore, M. H., Salman, E., et al.: Intravenously administered immune globulin for the treatment of infection-associated hemophagocytic syndrome. J. Pediatr. *123*:479–481, 1993.
135. Funkhouser, W. L.: The use of gamma globulin antibodies to control chickenpox in a convalescent hospital for children. J. Pediatr. *32*:257–259, 1948.
136. Gamm, H., Huber, C., Chapel, H., et al.: Intravenous immune globulin in chronic lymphocytic leukemia. Clin. Exp. Immunol. *97*(Suppl.):17–20, 1994.
137. Gardulf, A., Hammarstrom, L., and Smith, C. I. E.: Home treatment of hypogammaglobulinaemia with subcutaneous gammaglobulin by rapid infusion. Lancet *338*:162–166, 1991.
138. Gaur, S., Kesarwala, H., Gavai, M., et al.: Clinical immunology and infectious diseases. Clin. Immunol. *41*:745–782, 1994.
139. Gellis, S. S., Stokes, J., Jr., Brother, G. M., et al.: The use of human immune serum globulin (gamma globulin) in infectious (epidemic) hepatitis in the Mediterranean theater of operations. I. Studies on prophylaxis in two epidemics of infectious hepatitis. J. A. M. A. *128*:1062–1063, 1945.
140. George, M. J., Snydman, D. R., Werner, B. G., et al.: Use of ganciclovir plus cytomegalovirus immune globulin to treat CMV pneumonia in orthotopic liver transplant recipients. Transplant. Proc. *25*(Suppl. 4):22–24, 1993.
141. Gerbase, M. W., Dubois, D., Rothmeier, C., et al.: Costs and outcomes of prolonged cytomegalovirus prophylaxis to cover the enhanced immunosuppression phase following lung transplantation. Chest *116*:1265–1272, 1999.
142. Gershon, A. A.: Measles virus (rubeola). *In* Mandell, G. L., Bennett, J. E., and Doling, R. (eds.): Mandell, Douglas and Bennett's Principles and Practice of Infectious Diseases. 5th ed. Philadelphia, Churchill Livingstone, 2000, pp. 1801–1809.
143. Gershon, A. A., Steinberg, S., and Brunell, P. A.: Zoster immune globulin. A further assessment. N. Engl. J. Med *290*:243–245, 1974.
144. Ghosh, S., Champlin, R. E., Englund, J., et al.: Respiratory syncytial virus upper respiratory tract illnesses in adult blood and marrow transplant recipients: Combination therapy with aerosolized ribavirin and intravenous immunoglobulin. Bone Marrow Transplant. *25*:751–755, 2000.

145. Gigler, A., Dorsch, S., Hemauer, A., et al.: Generation of neutralizing human monoclonal antibodies against parvovirus B19 proteins. J. Virol. *73*:1974–1979, 1999.
146. Gill, D. S., Spencer, A., and Cobcroft, R. B.: High-dose gamma-globulin therapy in the reactive haemophagocytic syndrome. Br. J. Haematol. *88*:204–206, 1994.
147. Gispen, R., Lansberg, H. P., and Nanning, W.: The effect of antivaccinia gamma globulin on smallpox vaccination in view of a proposed attempt to prevent postvaccinal encephalitis. Antonie van Leeuwenhoek *22*:89–102, 1956.
148. Givner, L. B.: Monoclonal antibodies against respiratory syncytial virus. Pediatr. Infect. Dis. J. *18*:541–542, 1999.
149. Glinz, W., Grob, P. V. J., Nydegger, U. E., et al.: Polyvalent immunoglobulins for prophylaxis of bacterial infections in patients following multiple trauma. Intensive Care Med. *11*:288–294, 1985.
150. Glowacki, L. S., and Smaill, F. M.: Use of immune globulin to prevent symptomatic cytomegalovirus disease in transplant recipients—meta-analysis. Clin. Transplant. *8*:10–18, 1994.
151. Gold, W. L., Boulton, J. E., Goldman, C., et al.: Management of varicella exposure in the neonatal intensive care unit. Pediatr. Infect. Dis. J. *12*:954–955, 1993.
152. Gooding, A. M., Bastian, J. F., Peterson, B. M., and Wilson, N. W.: Safety and efficacy of intravenous immunoglobulin prophylaxis in pediatric head trauma patients: A double-blind controlled trial. J. Crit. Care *4*:212–216, 1993.
153. Goulder, P., Seward, D., and Hatton, C.: Intravenous immunoglobulin in virus-associated haemophagocytic syndrome. Arch. Dis. Child. *65*:1275–1277, 1990.
154. Grady, G. F.: Prevention of post transfusion hepatitis by gamma globulin: Preliminary report. A cooperative study. J. A. M. A. *214*:140–142, 1970.
155. Grady, G. F.: Hepatitis B immune globulin prevention of hepatitis from accidental exposure among medical personnel. N. Engl. J. Med. *293*:1067–1070, 1975.
156. Graham, B. S., Tang, Y., and Gruber, W. C.: Topical immunoprophylaxis of respiratory syncytial virus (RSV)-challenged mice with RSV-specific immune globulin. J. Infect. Dis. *171*:1468–1474, 1995.
157. Graham-Pole, J., Camitta, B., Casper, J., et al.: Intravenous immunoglobulin may lessen all forms of infection in patients receiving allogeneic bone marrow transplantation for acute lymphoblastic leukemia: A Pediatric Oncology Group study. Bone Marrow Transplant. *3*:559–566, 1988.
158. Granström, M. A., Olindor-Nielson, A. M., Holmblad, P., et al.: Specific immunoglobulin for treatment of whooping cough. Lancet *338*:1230–1233, 1991.
159. Grayston, J. T., and Watten, R. H: Epidemic rubella in Taiwan, 1957–1958. III. Gamma globulin in the prevention of rubella. N. Engl. J. Med. *261*:1145–1150, 1959.
160. Grazi, G. L., Mazziotti, A., Sama, C., et al.: Liver transplantation in HBsAg-positive HBV-DNA–negative cirrhotics: Immunoprophylaxis and long-term outcome. Liver Transpl. Surg. *2*:418–425, 1996.
161. Green, R. H., Balsamo, M. R., Giles, J. P., et al.: Studies of the natural history and prevention of rubella. Am. J. Dis. Child. *110*:348–365, 1965.
162. Greenberg, M.: Gammaglobulin in pediatrics. Med. Clin. North Am. *May*:602–608, 1947.
163. Greenberg, M., Pellitteri, O., and Eisenstein, D. T.: Measles encephalitis. I. Prophylactic effect of gamma globulin. J. Pediatr. *46*:642–647, 1955.
164. Groothuis, J. R., Simoes, E. A., Hemming, V. G.: Respiratory syncytial virus (RSV) infection in preterm infants and the protective effects of RSV immune globulin (RSVIG). Respiratory Syncytial Virus Immune Globulin Study Group. Pediatrics *95*:463–467, 1995.
165. Groothuis, J. R., Simoes, E. A., Levin, M. J., et al.: Prophylactic administration of respiratory syncytial virus immune globulin to high-risk infants and young children. N. Engl. J. Med. *329*:1524–1530, 1993.
166. Grossman, E. B., Stewart, S. G., and Stokes, J. P.: Post-transfusion hepatitis in battle casualties. J. A. M. A. *129*:991–994, 1945.
167. Guarino, A., Canani, R. B., Russo, S., et al.: Oral immunoglobulins for treatment of acute rotaviral gastroenteritis. Pediatrics *93*:12–16, 1994.
168. Guarino, A., Guandalini, S., Albano, F., et al.: Enteral immunoglobulins for treatment of protracted rotaviral diarrhea. Pediatr. Infect. Dis. J. *10*:612–614, 1991.
169. Guglielmo, B. J., Wong-Beringer, A., and Linker, C. A.: Immune globulin therapy in allogeneic bone marrow transplant: A critical review. Bone Marrow Transplant. *13*:499–510, 1994.
170. Guidelines for preventing opportunistic infections among hematopoietic stem cell transplant recipients. M. M. W. R. Recomm. Rep. *49*(RR-10):1–125, 2000.
171. Gupta, M., Mahanty, S., Bray, M., et al.: Passive transfer of antibodies protects immunocompetent and immunodeficient mice against lethal Ebola virus infection with complete inhibition of viral replication. J. Virol. *75*:4649–4654, 2001.
172. Gupta, P. S., Kapoor, R., Goyal, S., et al.: Intrathecal human tetanus immunoglobulin in early tetanus. Lancet *2*:439–440, 1980.
173. Gustafson, R., Gardulf, A., Granert, A., et al.: Prophylactic therapy for selective IgA deficiency. Lancet *350*:865, 1997.
174. Habel, K.: Seroprophylaxis in experimental rabies. Public Health Rep. *60*:545–560, 1945.
175. Habel, K., and Koprowski, H.: Laboratory data supporting the clinical trial of antirabies serum in persons bitten by a rabid wolf. Bull. World Health Organ. *13*:773–779, 1955.
176. Ham, J. M., Shelden, S. L., Godkin, R. R., et al. Cytomegalovirus prophylaxis with ganciclovir, acyclovir, and CMV hyperimmune globulin in liver transplant patients receiving OKT3 induction. Transplant. Proc. *27*(Suppl. 1):31–33, 1995.
177. Hammarström, L.: Passive immunity against rotavirus in infants. Acta Paediatr. Suppl. *430*:127–132, 1999.
178. Hammon, W. M., Coriell, L. L., Stokes, J., Jr., et al.: Evaluation of Red Cross gamma globulin as a prophylactic agent for poliomyelitis (5 parts). J. A. M. A. *150*:739–760, 1950; *151*:1272–1285, 1953; *156*: 21–27, 1954.
179. Hassett, J., Meyers, S., McFarland, L., et al.: Recurrent *Clostridium difficile* infection in a patient with selective IgG1 deficiency treated with intravenous immune globulin and *Saccharomyces boulardii*. Clin. Infect. Dis. *20*(Suppl. 2):266–268, 1995.
180. Havens, W. P., Jr., and Paul, J. R.: Prevention of infectious hepatitis with gamma globulin. J. A. M. A. *129*:270–271, 1945.
181. Heegaard, E. D., Hasle, H., Skibsted, L., et al.: Congenital anemia caused by parvovirus B19 infection. Pediatr. Infect. Dis. J. *19*:1216–1218, 2000.
182. Heikkinen, T., Ruohola, A., Ruuskanen, O., et al.: Intranasally administered immunoglobulin for the prevention of rhinitis in children. Pediatr. Infect. Dis. J. *17*:367–372, 1998.
183. Hemachudha, T., Mitrabhakdi, E., Wilde, H., et al.: Additional reports of failure to respond to treatment after rabies exposure in Thailand. Clin. Infect. Dis. *28*:143–144, 1999.
184. Henin, Y., Marechal, V., Barre, F., et al.: Inactivation and partition of HIV during Kistler and Nitschmann fractionation of human blood plasma. Vox Sang *54*:78–83, 1988.
185. Herrero, J. I. H., Beltrán, R. R., and Sánchez, A. M. M.: Failure of intrathecal tetanus antitoxin in the treatment of tetanus neonatorum. J. Infect. Dis. *164*:619–620, 1991.
186. Hibbs, R. G., Weber, J. T., Corwin, A., et al.: Experience with the use of an investigational $F(ab')_2$ heptavalent botulism immune globulin of equine origin during an outbreak of type E botulism in Egypt. Clin. Infect. Dis. *23*:337–340, 1996.
187. Higuchi, S., Awata, H., Nunoi, H., et al. A family of selective immunodeficiency with normal immunoglobulins: Possible autosomal dominant inheritance. Eur. J. Pediatr. *153*:328–332, 1994.
188. Hilpert, H., Brüssow, H., Mietens, C., et al.: Use of bovine milk concentrate containing antibody to rotavirus to treat rotavirus gastroenteritis in infants. J. Infect. Dis. *156*:158–166, 1987.
189. Hlava, J., and Honl, I.: Serum vaccinicum und seine Wirkungen. Wien. Klin. Rundschau *9*:625–627, 1895.
190. Holland, P. V., Rubenson, R. M., Morrow, A. G., et al.: Gamma globulin in the prophylaxis of post transfusion hepatitis. J. A. M. A. *196*:471–474, 1966.
191. Houser, H. B., and Schalet, N.: Prevention of rubella with gamma globulin. Clin. Res. *6*:281–282, 1958.
192. Hsia, D. Y., Lonsway, M., Jr., and Gellis, S. S.: Gamma globulin in the prevention of infectious hepatitis. Studies on the use of small doses in family outbreaks. N. Engl. J. Med. *250*:417–419, 1954.
193. Human rabies prevention—United States, 1999. Recommendations of Advisory Committee on Immunization Practices (ACIP). M. M. W. R. Recomm. Rep. *48*(RR-1):1–21. 1999.
194. Hypogammaglobulinemia in the United Kingdom. Summary report of a Medical Research Council working-party. Lancet *1*:163–169, 1969.
195. Ichimaru, T., Y. Ohara, Y., Hojo, M., et al.: Treatment of severe pertussis by administration of specific gamma globulin with high titers anti-toxin antibody. Acta Paediatr. *82*:1076–1078, 1993.
196. Imashuku, S.: Advances in the management of hemophagocytic lymphohistiocytosis. Int. J. Hematol. *72*:1–11, 2000.
197. Imashuku, S., Hibi, S., Ohara T., et al.: Effective control of Epstein-Barr virus–related hemophagocytic lymphohistiocytosis with immunochemotherapy. Blood *93*:1869–1874, 1999.
198. Imbach, P., Perret, B., Babington, R. et al.: Safety of intravenous immunoglobulin preparations. Vox Sang *61*:1–4, 1991.
199. Inoue, S., Kinra, N. K., Mukkamala, S. R., et al.: Parvovirus B19 infection: Aplastic crisis, erythema infectiosum and idiopathic thrombocytopenic purpura. Pediatr. Infect. Dis J. *10*:251–253, 1991.
200. Intravenous immune globulin for the prevention of bacterial infections in children with symptomatic human immunodeficiency virus infection. The National Institute of Child Health and Developments Intravenous Immunoglobulin Study Group. N. Engl. J. Med. *325*:73–80, 1991.
201. Intravenous immunoglobulin for the prevention of infection in chronic lymphocytic leukemia. A randomized, controlled clinical trial. Cooperative Group for the Study of Immunoglobulin in Chronic Lymphocytic Leukemia. N. Engl. J. Med. *319*:902–907, 1988.

202. Iriarte, P. V., Tangco, A., Jagasia, K. H., et al.: Effect of gamma globulin on modification of chickenpox in children with malignant disease. Cancer *18*:112–116, 1965.
203. Isacsohn, M., Eidelman, A. I., Kaplan, M., et al.: Neonatal Coxsackie virus group B infections: Experience of a single department of neonatology. Isr. J. Med. Sci. *30*:371–374, 1994.
204. Ishizaka, A., Sakiyana, Y., Otsu, M., et al.: Successful intravenous immunoglobulin therapy for recurrent pneumococcal otitis media in young children. Eur. J. Pediatr. *153*:174–178, 1994.
205. Jacobson, J. M., Colman, N., Ostrow, N. A., et al.: Passive immunotherapy in the treatment of advanced human immunodeficiency virus infection. J. Infect. Dis. *168*:298–308, 1993.
206. Jahrling, P. B., Geisbert, J., Swearengen, J. R., et al.: Passive immunization of Ebola virus–infected cynomolgus monkeys with immunoglobulin from hyperimmune horses. Arch. Virol. Suppl. *11*:135–140, 1996.
207. Jahrling, P. B., Geisbert, T. W., Geisbert, J. B., et al.: Evaluation of immune globulin and recombinant interferon-a2b for treatment of experimental Ebola virus infections. J. Infect. Dis. *179*(Suppl.):224–234, 1999.
208. Jaijaroensup, W., Tantawichien, T., Khawplod, P., et al.: Postexposure rabies vaccination in patients infected with human immunodeficiency virus. Clin. Infect. Dis. *28*:913–914, 1999.
209. Jassal, S. V., Roscoe, J. M., Zaltzman J. S., et al.: Clinical practice guidelines: Prevention of cytomegalovirus disease after renal transplantation. J. Am. Soc. Nephrol. *9*:1697–1708, 1998.
210. Jenson, H. B., and Pollock, B. H.: Meta-analyses of the effectiveness of intravenous immune globulin for prevention and treatment of neonatal sepsis. Pediatrics *99*(2):E2, 1997.
211. Jenson, H. B., and Pollock, B. H.: The role of intravenous immunoglobulin for the prevention and treatment of neonatal sepsis. Semin. Perinatol. *22*:50–63, 1998.
212. Jhaveri, R., Rosenfeld, W., Salazar, D., et al.: High titer multiple dose therapy with HBIG in newborn infants of HBsAg positive mothers. J. Pediatr. *97*:305–308, 1980.
213. Joffe, S., Ray, G. T., Escobar, G. J., et al.: Cost-effectiveness of respiratory syncytial virus prophylaxis among preterm infants. Pediatrics *104*:419–427, 1999.
214. Johnston, J. M., and Overall, J. C., Jr.: Intravenous immunoglobulin in disseminated neonatal echovirus 11 infection. Pediatr. Infect. Dis. J. *8*:254–256, 1989.
215. Jones, R. J., Roe, E. A., and Gupta, J. L.: Controlled trial of *Pseudomonas* immunoglobulin and vaccine in burn patients. Lancet *2*:1263–1265, 1980.
216. Jorgensen, F., Andersson, B., Hanson, L. A., et al.: Gamma-globulin treatment of recurrent acute otitis media in children. Pediatr. Infect. Dis. J. *9*:389–394, 1990.
217. Judelsohn, R. G., Meyers, J. D., Ellis, R. J., et al.: Efficacy of zoster immune globulin. Pediatrics *53*:476–480, 1974.
218. Just, H. M., Voge, W., Metzger, M., et al.: Treatment of intensive care unit patients with severe nosocomial infections. *In* Morell, A., and Nydegger, U. E. (eds.): Clinical Use of Intravenous Immunoglobulins. New York, Academic Press, 1986, pp. 346–352.
219. Kainulainen, L., Varpula, M., Liippo, K., et al.: Pulmonary abnormalities in patients with primary hypogammaglobulinemia. J. Allergy Clin. Immunol. *104*:1031–1036, 1999.
220. Kalm, O., Prellner, K., and Christensen, P.: The effect of intravenous immunoglobulin treatment in recurrent acute otitis media. Int. J. Pediatr. Otorhinolaryngol. *11*:237–246, 1986.
221. Kanai, K., Takehiro, A., Noto, H., et al.: Prevention of perinatal transmission of hepatitis B virus (HBV) to children of e antigen positive HBV carrier mothers by hepatitis B immune globulin and HBV vaccine. J. Infect. Dis. *151*:287–290, 1985.
222. Kanfer, E. J., Abrahamson, G., Taylor, J., et al.: Severe rotavirus-associated diarrhoea following bone marrow transplantation: Treatment with oral immunoglobulin. Bone Marrow Transplant. *14*:651–652, 1994.
223. Kaplan, E. L., and Gerber, M. A.: Group A, group C, and group G beta-hemolytic streptococcal infections. *In* Feigin, R. D., and Cherry, J. A. (eds.): Textbook of Pediatric Infectious Diseases. 4th ed. Philadelphia, W. B. Saunders, 1998, pp. 1106–1116.
224. Kariyawasam, H. H., Gyi, K. M., Hodson, M. E., and Cohen, B. J.: Anaemia in lung transplant patient caused by parvovirus B19. Thorax *55*:619–620, 2000.
225. Kato, E., Shindo, S., Eto, Y., et al.: Administration of immune globulin associated with aseptic meningitis. J. A. M. A. *259*:3267–3271, 1988.
226. Kaul, R., McGeer, A., Norrby-Teglund, A., et al.: Intravenous immunoglobulin for streptococcal toxic shock syndrome—a comparative observational study. Clin. Infect. Dis. *28*:800–807, 1999.
227. Kavaliotis, J., Loukou, I., Trachana, M., et al.: Outbreak of varicella in a pediatric oncology unit. Med. Pediatr. Oncol. *31*:166–169, 1998.
228. Kefalides, N. A., Arana, J. A., Bazan, A., et al.: Role of infection in mortality from severe burns. Evaluation of plasma, gamma globulin, albumin, and saline solution therapy in a group of Peruvian children. N. Engl. J. Med. *267*:317–323, 1962.
229. Keller, T., McGrath, K., Newland, A., et al.: Indications for use of intravenous immunoglobulin. Recommendations of the Australasian Society of Blood Transfusion consensus symposium. Med. J. Aust. *159*:204–206, 1993.
230. Kempe, C. H.: Studies on smallpox and complications of smallpox vaccination. Pediatrics *26*:176–189, 1960.
231. Kempe, C. H., Berge, T. O., and England, B.: Hyperimmune vaccinial gamma globulin: Source, evaluation, and use in prophylaxis and therapy. Pediatrics *18*:177–188, 1956.
232. Kempe, C. H., Bowles, C., Meiklejohn, G., et al.: The use of vaccinia hyperimmune gamma globulin in the prophylaxis of smallpox. Bull. World Health Organ. *25*:41–48, 1961.
233. Kesson, A. M., Ferguson, J. K., Rawlinson, W. D., and Cunningham, A. L.: Progressive vaccinia treated with ribavirin and vaccinia immune globulin. Clin. Infect. Dis. *25*:911–914, 1997.
234. Kiehl, M. G., Stoll, R., Broder, M., et al.: A controlled trial of intravenous immune globulin for the prevention of serious infections in adults with advanced human immunodeficiency virus infection. Arch. Intern. Med. *156*:2545–2550, 1996.
235. Kimura, H., Minakami, H., Harigaya, A., et al.: Treatment of neonatal infection caused by coxsackievirus B3. J. Perinatol *19*:388–390, 1999.
236. King, S. M.: Immune globulin versus antivirals versus combination for prevention of cytomegalovirus disease in transplant recipients. Antiviral Res. *40*:115–137, 1999.
237. Kinney, J. S., McCray, E., Kaplan, J. E., et al.: Risk factors associated with echovirus 11 infection in a hospital nursery. Pediatr. Infect. Dis. J. *5*:192–197, 1986.
238. Kneyber, M. C. J., Moll, H. A., and de Groot, R.: Treatment and prevention of respiratory syncytial virus infection. Eur. J. Pediatr. *159*:399–411, 2000.
239. Knodell, R. G., Ginsburg, A. L., Conrad, A. L., et al.: Efficacy of prophylactic gamma-globulin in preventing non-A non-B post transfusion hepatitis. Lancet *1*:557–561, 1976.
240. Knutsen, A. P.: Patients with IgG subclass and/or selective antibody deficiency to polysaccharide antigens: Initiation of a controlled clinical trial of intravenous immunoglobulin. J. Allergy Clin. Immunol. *84*:640–647, 1989.
241. Kobayashi, R. H., Kobayashi, A. D., Lee, N., et al.: Home self administration of intravenous immunoglobulin therapy in children. Pediatrics *85*:705–709, 1990.
242. Koduri, P. R., Kumapley, R., Valladares, J., and Teter, C.: Chronic pure red cell aplasia caused by parvovirus B19 in AIDS: Use of intravenous immunoglobulin—a report of eight patients. Am. J. Hematol. *61*:16–20, 1999.
243. Koenig, M. G., Drutz, D. J., Mushlin, A. I., et al.: Type B botulism in man. Am. J. Med. *42*:208–219, 1967.
244. Koenig, M. G., Spickard, A., Cardella, M. A., et al.: Clinical and laboratory observations on type E botulism in man. Medicine (Baltimore) *43*:517–545, 1964.
245. Kondoh, H., Kobayashi, K., Sugio, Y., and Hayashi, T.: Successful treatment of echovirus meningoencephalitis in sex-linked agammaglobulinaemia by intrathecal and intravenous injection of high titer gammaglobulin. Eur. J. Pediatr. *146*:610–612, 1987.
246. Korns, R. F.: Prophylaxis of German measles with immune serum globulin. J. Infect. Dis. *90*:183–192, 1952.
247. Krediet, T. G., Beurskens, F. J., Van Dijk, J., et al.: Antibody responses and opsonic activity in sera of preterm neonates with coagulase-negative staphylococcal septicemia and the effect of the administration of fresh frozen plasma. Pediatr. Res. *43*:645–651, 1998.
248. Krugman, S.: Effect of human immune serum globulin on infectivity of hepatitis. J. Infect. Dis. *134*:70–74, 1976.
249. Krugman, S., and Giles, J. P.: Viral hepatitis, type B (MS 2 strain): Further observations in natural history and prevention. N. Engl. J. Med. *288*:755–760, 1973.
250. Krugman, S., Giles, J. P., and Hammond, J.: Viral hepatitis, type B (MS 2 strain): Prevention with specific hepatitis B immune serum globulin. J. A. M. A. *218*:1665–1670, 1971.
251. Krugman, S., Giles, J. P., Jacobs, A. M., et al.: Studies with live attenuated measles virus vaccine. Am. J. Dis. Child. *103*:353–363, 1962.
252. Krugman, S., and Ward, R.: Demonstration of neutralizing antibody in gamma globulin and re-evaluation of the rubella problem. N. Engl. J. Med. *259*:16–19, 1958.
253. Krugman, S., Ward, R., Giles, J. P., et al.: Infectious hepatitis: Studies on the effectiveness of gamma globulin and on the incidence of inapparent infection. J. A. M. A. *174*:823–830, 1960.
254. Kudoyarova-Zubavichene, N. M., Sergeyev, N. N., Chepurnov, A. A., and Netesov, S. V.: Preparation and use of hyperimmune serum for prophylaxis and therapy of Ebola virus infections. J. Infect. Dis. *179*(Suppl. 1): 218–223, 1999.
255. Kuhns, W. J., Prince, A. M., Brotman, B., et al.: A clinical and laboratory evaluation of immune serum globulin from donors with a history of hepatitis: Attempted prevention of post transfusion hepatitis. Am. J. Med. Sci. *272*:255–261, 1976.
256. Kurtzberg, J., Friedman H. S., Kinney P. R., et al.: Management of human immunodeficiency virus–associated thrombocytopenia with

intravenous gammaglobulin. Am. J. Pediatr. Hematol. Oncol. *9*:299–301, 1987.
257. Kurtzman, G., Frickhofe, N., Kimball, J., et al.: Pure red cell aplasia of 10 years duration due to persistent parvovirus B19 infection and its cure with immunoglobulin therapy. N. Engl. J. Med. *321*:519–523, 1989.
258. Kyne, L., Warny, M., Qamar, A., et al.: Asymptomatic carriage of *Clostridium difficile* and serum levels of IgG antibody against toxin A. N. Engl. J. Med. *342*:390–397, 2000.
259. Lamothe, F., D'Amico, P., Ghosn, P., et al.: Clinical usefulness of intravenous human immunoglobulins in invasive group A streptococcal infections: Case report and review. Clin. Infect. Dis. *21*:1469–1470, 1995.
260. Lea, W. A., Jr., and Taylor, W. B.: Gamma globulin in the treatment of herpes zoster. Tex. Med. *54*:594–596, 1958.
261. Lee, D. C., and Lederman, H. M.: Anti-tetanus toxoid antibodies in intravenous gamma globulin: An alternative to tetanus immune globulin. J. Infect. Dis. *166*:642–645, 1992.
262. Lee, M. L., Gale, R. P., and Yap., P. L.: Use of intravenous immunoglobulin to prevent or treat infections in persons with immune deficiency. Annu. Rev. Med. *48*:93–102, 1997.
263. Lehner, P. J., and Webster, A. D.: Hepatitis C from immunoglobulin infusion. B. M. J. *306*:1541–1542, 1993.
264. Leung, D. Y. M., Kelly, C. P., Boguniewicz, M., et al.: Treatment with intravenously administered gamma globulin of chronic relapsing colitis induced by *Clostridium difficile* toxin. J. Pediatr. *118*:633–637, 1991.
265. Lever, A. M., Webster, A. D. B., Brown, D., et al.: Non-A, non-B hepatitis occurring in agammaglobulinaemic patients after intravenous immunoglobulin. Lancet *2*:1062–1064, 1984.
266. Levy, J., Youvan, T., Lee, M. L., et al.: Passive hyperimmune plasma therapy in the treatment of acquired immunodeficiency syndrome: Results of a 12-month multicenter double-blind controlled trial. Blood *84*:2130–2135, 1994.
267. Li, A., Baba, T. W., Sodroski, J., et al.: Synergistic neutralization of a chimeric SIV/HIV type 1 virus with combinations of human anti-HIV type 1 envelope monoclonal antibodies or hyperimmune globulins. AIDS Res. Hum. Retroviruses *13*:647–656, 1997.
268. Li, A., Katinger, H., Posner, M. R., et al.: Synergistic neutralization of simian-human immunodeficiency virus SHIV- vpu+ by triple and quadruple combinations of human monoclonal antibodies and high-titer anti–human immunodeficiency virus type 1 immunoglobulins. J. Virol. *72*:3235–3240, 1998.
269. Lim, M. E., and Kim, K. S.: Hemophagocytic lymphohistiocytosis. Pediatr. Infect. Dis. J. *18*:154–155, 1999.
270. Lipshultz, S. E., Orav, E. J., Sanders, S. P., et al.: Immunoglobulins and left ventricular structure and function in pediatric HIV infection. Circulation *92*:2220–2225, 1995.
271. Loofbourow, J. C., Cabasso, V. J., Roby, R. E., et al.: Rabies immune globulin (human). Clinical trials and dose determination. J. A. M. A. *217*:1825–1831, 1971.
272. Losonsky, G. A., Johnson, J. P., Winkelstein, J. A., et al.: Oral administration of human serum immunoglobulin in immunodeficient patients with viral gastroenteritis: A pharmacokinetic and functional analysis. J. Clin. Invest. *76*:2362–2367, 1985.
273. Lowy, F.: *Staphylococcus aureus* infections. N. Engl. J. Med. *339*:520–532, 1998.
274. Lucas, A. O., Willis, A. J., Mohamed, S. D., et al.: A comparison of the value of 500,000 I.U. tetanus antitoxin with 200,000 I.U. in the treatment of tetanus. Clin. Pharmacol. Ther. *6*:592–597, 1965.
275. Lucchesi, P. F., and Bowman, J. E.: Antitoxin versus no antitoxin in scarlet fever. J. A. M. A. *103*:1049–1051, 1930.
276. Lundström, R.: Complications of smallpox vaccination and their treatment with vaccinia immune globulin. J. Pediatr. *49*:129–140, 1956.
277. Lundström, R., Thorén, C., and Blomquist, B.: Gamma globulin against rubella in pregnancy. I. Prevention of maternal rubella by gamma globulin and convalescent gamma globulin: A follow up study. Acta Paediatr. *50*:444–452, 1961.
278. Lundström, R., Thorén, C., and Blomquist, B.: Gamma globulin against rubella in pregnancy. II. Manifest maternal rubella in early pregnancy treated with convalescent gamma globulin: A follow up study. Acta Paediatr. *50*:453–456, 1961.
279. Maiztegui, J. I., Fernandez, N. J., and De Damilano, A. J.: Efficacy of immune plasma in treatment of Argentine haemorrhagic fever and association between treatment and a late neurological syndrome. Lancet *2*:1216–1217, 1979.
280. Malley, R., DeVincenzo, J., Ramilo, O., et al.: Reduction of respiratory syncytial virus (RSV) in tracheal aspirates in intubated infants by use of humanized monoclonal antibody to RSV F protein. J. Infect. Dis. *178*:1555–1561, 1998.
281. Mandy, G. T., Weisman, L. E., Horwith, G., et al.: Safety of a *Staphylococcus aureus* (SA) intravenous immune globulin (AltaStaph) in very-low-birth-weight (VLBW) infants. Abstract. Pediatr. Res. *47*:343, 1999.
282. Marchand, S., Tchernia, G., Hiesse, C., et al.: Human parvovirus B19 infection in organ transplant recipients. Clin. Transplant. *13*:17–24, 1999.
283. Marrack, P., and Kappler, J.: The staphylococcal enterotoxins and their relatives. Science *248*:705–711, 1990.
284. Maruyama, T., Parren, P. W., Sanchez, A., et al.: Recombinant human monoclonal antibodies to Ebola virus. J. Infect. Dis. *179*(Suppl.): 235–239, 1999.
285. Maruyama, T., Rodriquez, L. L., Jahrling, P. B., et al.: Ebola virus can be effectively neutralized by antibody produced in natural human infection. J. Virol. *73*:6024–6030, 1999.
286. Masci, S., De Simone, C., Famularo, G., et al.: Intravenous immunoglobulins suppress the recurrences of genital herpes simplex virus: A clinical and immunological study. Immunopharmacol. Immunotoxicol. *17*:33–47, 1995.
287. Matheson, D. S., Clarkson, T. W., and Gelfand, E. W.: Mercury toxicity (acrodynia) induced by long term injection of gamma globulin. J. Pediatr. *97*:153–155, 1980.
288. McClain, D. J.: Smallpox. *In* Sidell, F. R., Takafuji, E. T., Franz, D. R. (eds.): Medical Aspects of Chemical and Biological Warfare. Washington, D. C., Borden Institute, Walter Reed Army Medical Center; Falls Church, VA, Office of the Surgeon General, U. S. Army; Fort Sam Houston, TX, U. S. Army Medical Department Center and School; Fort Detrick, Frederick, MD, U. S. Army Medical Research and Material Command; Bethesda, MD, Uniformed Services University of the Health Sciences, 1997, pp. 539–559.
289. McCloskey, R. V., and Smilack, J.: Diphtheria antitoxin content of human immune serum globulins. Ann. Intern. Med. *77*:757–758, 1972.
290. McComb, J. A., and Dwyer, R. C.: Passive active immunization with tetanus immune globulin (human). N. Engl. J. Med. *268*:857–862, 1963.
291. McCracken, G. H., Jr., Dowell, D. L., and Marshall, F. N.: Double blind trial of equine antitoxin and human immune globulin in tetanus neonatorum. Lancet *1*:1146–1149, 1971.
292. McKhann, C. F., Green, A. A., and Coady, H.: Factors influencing the effectiveness of placental extract in the prevention and modification of measles. J. Pediatr. *6*:603–614, 1935.
293. McKinney, R. E., Jr., Katz, S. L., and Wilfert, C. M.: Chronic enteroviral meningoencephalitis in agammaglobulinemic patients. Rev. Infect. Dis. *9*:334–356, 1987.
294. Mease, P. J., Ochs, H. D., and Wedgwood, R. J.: Successful treatment of echovirus meningoencephalitis and myositis fasciitis with intravenous immune globulin therapy in a patient with X-linked agammaglobulinemia. N. Engl. J. Med. *304*:1278–1281, 1981.
295. Melamed, I., Griffiths, A. M., and Roifman, C. M.: Benefit of oral immune globulin therapy in patients with immunodeficiency and chronic diarrhea. J. Pediatr. *3*:486–489, 1991.
296. Melish, M. E., Murata, S., Fukunaga, C., et al.: Vaginal tampon model for toxic shock syndrome. Rev. Infect. Dis. *11*(Suppl. 1):238–246, 219–228, 1989.
297. Messori, A., Rampazzo, R., Scroccaro, G., and Martini, N.: Efficacy of hyperimmune anti-cytomegalovirus immunoglobulins for the prevention of cytomegalovirus infection in recipients of allogeneic bone marrow transplantation: A meta-analysis. Bone Marrow Transplant. *13*:163–167, 1994.
298. Misbah, S. A., Spickett, G. P., Ryba, P. C. J., et al.: Chronic enteroviral meningoencephalitis in agammaglobulinemia: Case report and literature review. J. Clin. Immunol. *12*:266–270, 1992.
299. Mitra, A. K., Mahalanabis, D., Ashraf, H., et al.: Hyperimmune cow colostrum reduces diarrhoea due to rotavirus: A double-blind, controlled clinical trial. Acta Pediatr. *84*:996–1001, 1995.
300. Mofenson, L. M., Bethel, J., Moye, J., et al.: Effect of intravenous immunoglobulin (IVIG) on CD4+ lymphocyte decline in HIV-infected children in a clinical trial of IVIG infection prophylaxis. J. Acquir. Immune Defic. *6*:1103–1113, 1993.
301. Mofenson, L. M., Korelitz, J., Pelton, S., et al.: Sinusitis in children infected with human immunodeficiency virus: Clinical characteristics, risk factors, and prophylaxis. Clin. Infect. Dis. *21*:1175–1181, 1995.
302. Mofenson, L. M., and Moye, J., Jr.: Intravenous immune globulin for the prevention of infections in children with symptomatic human immunodeficiency virus infection. Pediatr. Res. *33*(Suppl.):80–89, 1992.
303. Mofenson, L. M., Moye, J., Bethel, J., et al.: Prophylactic intravenous immunoglobulin in HIV-infected children with $CD4^+$ counts of $.20 \times 10^9$/L or more: Effects on viral, opportunistic, and bacterial infections. J. A. M. A. *268*:483–488, 1992.
304. Mofenson, L. M., Moye, J., Korelitz, J., et al.: Crossover of placebo patients to intravenous immunoglobulin confirms efficacy for prophylaxis of bacterial infections and reduction of hospitalizations in human immunodeficiency virus–infected children. Pediatr. Infect. Dis. J. *13*:477–484, 1994.
305. Morris, D., and McDonald, J. C.: Failure of hyper-immune globulin to prevent whooping cough. Arch. Dis. Child. *32*:236–239, 1957.
306. Müller, R., Gubernatis, G., Farle, M., et al.: Liver transplantation in HB_S antigen (HB_SAg) carriers: Prevention of hepatitis B virus (HBV) recurrence by passive immunization. Hepatology *13*:90–96, 1991.
307. Munster, A. M.: Immunologic response of trauma and burns. Am. J. Med. *7*:142–145, 1984.
308. Munster, A. M.: Infections in burns. *In* Morell, A., and Nydegger, U. E. (eds.): Clinical Use of Intravenous Immunoglobulins. New York, Academic Press, 1986, pp. 339–344.

309. Nagasawa M., Okawa, H., and Yata, J.: Deleterious effects of high dose γ-globulin therapy on patients with hemophagocytic syndrome. Letter. Int. J. Hematol. *60*:91–93, 1994.
310. Nagington, J., Gandy, G., Walker, J., and Gray, J. J.: Use of normal immunoglobulin in an echovirus 11 outbreak in a special-care baby unit. Lancet *2*:443–446, 1983.
311. Nance, F. C., Hines, J. L., Fulton, R. E., et al.: Treatment of experimental burn wound sepsis by post burn immunization with polyvalent *Pseudomonas* antigen. Surgery *68*:248–253, 1970.
312. Nanning, W.: Prophylactic effect of anti-vaccinia gamma globulin against post vaccinial encephalitis. Bull. World Health Organ. *27*:317–324, 1962.
313. Neff, J. M.: Introduction to Poxviridae. *In* Mandell, G. L., Bennett, J. E., and Doling, R. (eds.): Mandell, Douglas and Bennett's Principles and Practice of Infectious Diseases. 5th ed. Philadelphia, Churchill Livingstone, 2000, p. 1552.
314. Negishi, H., Yamada, H., Hirayama, E., et al.: Intraperitoneal administration of cytomegalovirus hyperimmunoglobulin to the cytomegalovirus-infected fetus. J. Perinatol. *18*:466–469, 1998.
315. Nigro, G., La Torre, R., Anceschi, M. M., et al.: Hyperimmunoglobulin therapy for a twin fetus with cytomegalovirus infection and growth restriction. Am. J. Obstet. Gynecol. *180*:1222–1226, 1999.
316. Nigro, G., Mazzocco, M., Aragona, C., et al.: Hyperimmunoglobulin therapy for cytomegalovirus-associated infertility: Case reports. Fertil. Steril. *74*:830–831, 2000.
317. NIH Consensus Development Conference: Diseases, doses, recommendations for intravenous immunoglobulin. HLB Newsletter. Natl. Inst. Heart Lung Blood Dis. *6*:73–78, 1990.
318. Norrby-Teglund, A., Basma, H., Anderson, J., et al.: Varying titers of neutralizing antibodies to streptococcal superantigens in different preparations of normal polyspecific immunoglobulin G: Implications for therapeutic efficacy. Clin. Infect. Dis. *26*:631–638, 1998.
319. Null, D. M., Connor, E. M., and Palivizumab Study Group: Evaluation of immunogenicity and safety in children receiving palivizumab for a second RSV season. Abstract. Pediatr. Res. *45*:170, 1999.
320. Nydahl-Persson, K., Petterson, A., and Fasth, A.: A prospective, double-blind, placebo-controlled trial of IV immunoglobulin and trimethoprim-sulfamethoxazole in children with recurrent respiratory tract infections. Acta Paediatr. *84*:1007–1009, 1995.
321. Ochs, H. D.: Intravenous immunoglobulin in the treatment and prevention of acute infections in pediatric acquired immunodeficiency syndrome patients. Pediatr. Infect. Dis. *6*:509–511, 1987.
322. Ochs, H. D., Fischer, S. H., Virant, F. S., et al.: Non-A non-B hepatitis and intravenous immunoglobulin. Lancet *1*:404–405, 1985.
323. Ochs, H. D., and Winkelstein, J.: Disorders of the B-cell system, *In* Stiehm E. R. (ed.): Immunologic Disorders in Infants and Children. 4th ed. Philadelphia, W. B. Saunders, 1996, pp. 296–338.
324. Oettle, H., Wilborn, F., Schmidt, C. A., and Siegert, W.: Treatment with ganciclovir and Ig for acute Epstein-Barr virus infection after allogeneic bone marrow transplantation. Blood *82*:2257–2262, 1993.
325. Ogawa, M., Ueda, S., Anzai, N., et al.: Toxic shock syndrome after staphylococcal pneumonia treated with intravenous immunoglobulin. Vox Sang *68*:59–60, 1995.
326. Ogilvie, M. M.: Antiviral prophylaxis and treatment in chickenpox, a review prepared for the UK Advisory Group on chickenpox on behalf of the British Society for the Study of Infection. J. Infect. *36*(Suppl. 1): 31–38, 1998.
327. Ogilvie, M. M., Vathenen, S., Radford, M., et al.: Maternal antibody and respiratory syncytial virus infection in infancy. J. Med. Virol. *7*:263–271, 1981.
328. Ohlsson, A., and Lacy, J. B.: Intravenous immunoglobulin for preventing infection in preterm and/or low birth-weight infants (Cochrane Review). The Cochrane Library, Oxford. Issue 1, 2001.
329. Okano, M., Pirruccello, S. J., Grierson, H. L., et al.: Immunovirological studies of fatal infectious mononucleosis in a patient with X-linked lymphoproliferative syndrome treated with intravenous immunoglobulin and interferon-a. Clin. Immunol. Immunopathol. *54*:410–418, 1990.
330. Ordman, C. W., Jennings, C. G., Jr., and Janeway, C. A.: Chemical, clinical and immunological studies on the products of human plasma fractionation. XII. The use of concentrated normal human serum gamma globulin (human immune serum globulin) in the prevention and attenuation of measles. J. Clin. Invest. *23*:541–549, 1944.
331. Orenstein, W. A., Heymann, D. L., Ellis, R. J., et al.: Prophylaxis of varicella in high risk children: Dose response effect of zoster immune globulin. J. Pediatr. *98*:368–373, 1981.
332. Ottolini, M. G., Hemming, V. G., Piazza, F. M., et al.: Topical immunoglobulin is an effective therapy for parainfluenza type 3 in a cotton rat model. J. Infect. Dis. *172*:243–245, 1995.
333. Outbreak of hepatitis C associated with intravenous immunoglobulin administration—United States, October 1993–June 1994. M. M. W. R. Morb. Mortal. Wkly. Rep. *43*(28):505–508, 1994.
334. Paar, D. P., and Pollard, R. B.: Immunotherapy of CMV infections. Adv. Exp. Med. Biol. *394*:145–151, 1996.
335. Palivizumab, a humanized respiratory syncytial virus monoclonal antibody, reduces hospitalization from respiratory syncytial virus infection in high-risk infants. The IMpact-RSV Study Group. Pediatrics *102*:531–537, 1998.
336. Park, W. H., and Freeman, R. G., Jr: The prophylactic use of measles convalescent serum. J. A. M. A. *87*:556–558, 1926.
337. Parsonnet, J.: Nonmenstrual toxic shock syndrome: New insights into diagnosis, pathogenesis and treatment. Curr. Clin. Top. Infect. Dis. *16*:1–20, 1996.
338. Paryani, S. G., Arvin, A. M., Koropchak, C. M., et al.: Varicella zoster antibody titers after the administration of intravenous immune serum globulin or varicella zoster immune globulin. Am. J. Med. *76*(3A):124–127, 1984.
339. Paryani, S. G., Arvin, A. M., Koropchak, C. M., et al.: Comparison of varicella zoster antibody titers in patients given intravenous immune serum globulin or varicella zoster immune globulin. J. Pediatr. *105*:200–205, 1984.
340. Paschlau, V. A.: Zur umstrittenen Wirksamkeit des Diphtherie Heilserums. Dtsch. Med. Wchenschr. *74*:1569–1573, 1949.
341. Pasic, S., Jankovic, B., Abinun, M., and Kanjuh, B.: Intravenous immunoglobulin prophylaxis in an echovirus 6 and echovirus 4 nursery outbreak. Pediatr. Infect. Dis. J. *16*:718–720, 1997.
342. Patel, J. C., Mehta, B. C., Nanavati, B. H., et al.: Role of serum therapy in tetanus. Lancet *1*:740–743, 1963.
343. Paya, C. V.: Role of immunoglobulin and new antivirals in treatment of cytomegalovirus infection. Transplant. Proc. *27*:28–30. 1995.
344. Paya, C. V.: Prevention of cytomegalovirus disease in recipients of solid-organ transplants. Clin. Infect. Dis. *32*:596–603, 2001.
345. Perez, C. M., Kubak, B. M., Cryer, H. G., et al.: Adjunctive treatment of streptococcal toxic shock syndrome using intravenous immunoglobulin: Case report and review. Am. J. Med. *102*:111–113, 1997.
346. Perlmutter, S. J., Leitman S. F., Garvey M. A., et al.: Therapeutic plasma exchange and intravenous immunoglobulin for obsessive-compulsive disorders in childhood. Lancet *354*:1153–1158, 1999.
347. Peters, C. J.: Lymphocytic choriomeningitis virus, Lassa virus and the South American hemorrhagic fevers. *In* Mandell, G. L., Bennett, J. E., and Doling, R. (eds.): Mandell, Douglas and Bennett's Principles and Practice of Infectious Diseases. 5th ed. Philadelphia, Churchill Livingstone, 2000, pp. 1855–1862.
348. Piazza, M., Sagliocca, L., Tosone, G., et al.: Sexual transmission of the hepatitis C virus and efficacy of prophylaxis with intramuscular immune serum globulin. Arch. Intern. Med. *157*:1537–1544, 1997.
349. Plotkin, S. A.: Rabies. Clin. Infect. Dis. *30*:4–12, 2000.
350. Pollack, M.: Antibody activity against *Pseudomonas aeruginosa* in immune globulins prepared for intravenous use in humans. J. Infect. Dis. *147*:1090–1098, 1983.
351. Postexposure prophylaxis of hepatitis B. M. M. W. R. Morb. Mortal. Wkly. Rep. *33*(21):285–290, 1984.
352. Press Release NABI: Discontinuation of phase II clinical trial of Hypergam+™ CF. Boca Raton, FL, July 1996.
353. Prevention of varicella, recommendations of the Advisory Committee on Immunization Practices (ACIP). M. M. W. R. Recomm. Rep. *45* (RR-11): 1–36, 1996.
354. Prian, G. W., and Koep, L. J.: Elimination of cytomegalovirus disease in liver transplant patients treated prophylactically with combination cytomegalovirus hyperimmune globulin and ganciclovir. Transplant. Proc. *26*(Suppl. 1):54–55, 1994.
355. Prophylactic intravenous administration of standard immune globulin as compared with core-lipopolysaccharide immune globulin in patients at high risk of postsurgical infection. The Intravenous Immunoglobulin Collaborative Study Group. N. Engl. J. Med. *327*:234–240, 1991.
356. Quartier, P., Foray, S., Casanova, J.-L., et al.: Enteroviral meningoencephalitis in X-linked agammaglobulinemia: Intensive immunoglobulin therapy and sequential viral detection in cerebrospinal fluid by polymerase chain reaction. Pediatr. Infect. Dis. J. *19*:1106–1108, 2000.
357. Rabies prevention—United States, 1984. M. M. W. R. Morb. Mortal. Wkly. Rep. *33*(28):393–402, 407–408, 1984.
358. Rabkin, C. S., Telzak, E. E., Ho, M.-S., et al.: Outbreak of echovirus 11 infection in hospitalized neonates. Pediatr. Infect. Dis. J. *7*:186–190, 1988.
359. Ramisse, F., Binder, P., Szatnik, M., et al.: Passive and active immunotherapy for experimental pneumococcal pneumonia by polyvalent human immunoglobulin or $F(ab')_2$ fragments administered intranasally. J. Infect. Dis. *173*:1123–1128, 1996.
360. Ramisse, F., Szatanik, M., Bider, P., et al.: Passive local immunotherapy of experimental staphylococcal pneumonia with human intravenous immunoglobulin. J. Infect. Dis. *168*:1030–1033, 1993.
361. Rault, R., Piraino, B., Johnston, J. R., et al.: Pulmonary and renal toxicity of intravenous immunoglobulin. Clin. Nephrol. *36*:83–86, 1991.
362. Razvi, S., Schneider, L., Jonas, M. M., et al.: Outcome of intravenous immunoglobulin-transmitted hepatitis C virus infection in primary imunodeficiency. Clin. Immunol. *101*:284–288, 2001.
363. Recommendations for protection against viral hepatitis. M. M. W. R. Morb. Mortal. Wkly. Rep. *34*(22):313–324, 329–335, 1985.
364. Redeker, A. G., Mosley, J. W., Gocke, D. J., et al.: Hepatitis B immune globulin as a prophylactic measure for spouses exposed to acute type B hepatitis. N. Engl. J. Med. *293*:1055–1059, 1975.

365. Reduction of respiratory syncytial virus hospitalization among premature infants and infants with bronchopulmonary dysplasia using respiratory syncytial virus immune globulin prophylaxis. The PREVENT Study Group. Pediatrics *99*:93–99, 1997.
366. Reed, E. C., Bowden, R. A., Dandliker, P. S., et al.: Treatment of cytomegalovirus pneumonia with ganciclovir and intravenous cytomegalovirus immunoglobulin in patients with bone marrow transplants. Ann. Intern. Med. *109*:783–788. 1988.
367. Reed, W. D., Eddleston, A. L. W. F., Cullens, H., et al.: Infusion of hepatitis B antibody in antigen positive active chronic hepatitis. Lancet *2*:1347–1351, 1973.
368. Reesink, H. W., Reerink Brongers, E. E., Lafeber Schut, B. J. T., et al.: Prevention of chronic HBsAg carrier state in infants by HBsAg positive mothers by hepatitis B immunoglobulin. Lancet *2*:436–438, 1979.
369. Respiratory syncytial virus immune globulin intravenous: Indications for use. American Academy of Pediatrics Committee on Infectious Diseases, Committee on Fetus and Newborn. Pediatrics *99*:645–650, 1997.
370. Rimensberger, P. C., Burek-Kozlowska A., Morell, A., et al.: Aerosolized immunoglobulin treatment of respiratory syncytial virus infection in infants. Pediatr. Infect. Dis. J. *15*:2009–2016, 1996.
371. Rodarte, J. G., and Williams, B. H.: Treatment of herpes zoster and chickenpox with immune globulin. Arch. Dermatol. *73*:553–556, 1956.
372. Rodriguez, W. J., Gruber, W. C., and Groothuis, J. R.: Respiratory syncytial virus immune globulin treatment of RSV lower respiratory tract infection in previously healthy children. Pediatrics *100*:937–942, 1997.
373. Rodriguez, W. J., Gruber, W. C., Welliver, R. C., et al.: Respiratory syncytial virus (RSV) immune globulin intravenous therapy for RSV lower respiratory tract infection in infants and young children at high risk for severe RSV infections: Respiratory Syncytial Virus Immune Globulin Study Group. Pediatrics *99*:454–461, 1997.
374. Rosenfeld, E. A., Shulman, S. T., Corydon, K. E., et al.: Comparative safety and efficacy of two immune globulin products in Kawasaki disease. J. Pediatr. *126*:1000–1003, 1995.
375. Ross, A. H.: Modification of chickenpox in family contacts by administration of gamma globulin. N. Engl. J. Med. *267*:369–376, 1962.
376. Rowe, J. M., Ciobanu, N., Ascensao, J., et al.: Recommended guidelines for the management of autologous and allogeneic bone marrow transplantation. Ann. Intern. Med. *120*:143–158, 1994.
377. Rubaltelli, F., Benini, F., and Sala, M.: Prevention of necrotizing enterocolitis in neonates at risk by oral administration of monomeric IgG. Dev. Pharmacol. Ther. *17*:138–143, 1991.
378. Rubbo, S. D., and Suri, J. C.: Passive immunization against tetanus with human immune globulin. B. M. J. *2*:79–81, 1962.
379. Rubin, R. H.: Cytomegalovirus disease and allograft loss after organ transplantation. Clin. Infect. Dis. *26*:871–873, 1998.
380. Rubin, R. H.: Prevention and treatment of cytomegalovirus disease in heart transplant patients. J. Heart Lung Transplant. *19*:731–735, 2000.
381. Rubinstein, H. M.: Studies on human tetanus antitoxin. Am. J. Hyg. *76*:276–292, 1962.
382. Ruderman, J. W., Peter, J. B., Gall, R. C., et al.: Prevention of hypogammaglobulinemia of prematurity with intravenous immune globulin. J. Perinatol. *10*:150–155, 1988.
383. Rugolotto, S.: Intrauterine anemia due to parvovirus B19: Successful treatment with intravenous immunoglobulins. Haematologica *84*:668–669, 1999.
384. Ruutu, T., Ljungman, P., Brinch, L., et al.: No prevention of cytomegalovirus infection by anti-cytomegalovirus hyperimmune globulin in seronegative bone marrow transplant recipients. Bone Marrow Transplant. *19*:233–236, 1997.
385. Sabroe, I., McHale, J., Tait, D. R., et al.: Treatment of adenoviral pneumonitis with intravenous ribavirin and immunoglobulin. Thorax *50*:1219–1220, 1995.
386. Sacher, R. A., and Gelfand, E.: Consensus of the use and safety of IVIG. Conference summary sponsored by Georgetown University Medical Center and Interactive Information Solutions. 2000, pp. 1–20.
387. Salcedo, J., Keates, S., Pothoulakis, C., et al.: Intravenous immunoglobulin therapy for severe *Clostridium difficile* colitis. Gastroenterology *41*:366–370, 1997.
388. Samuel, D., Bismuth, A., Serres, C., et al.: HBV-infection in liver transplantation in HBsAg positive patients: Experience with long-term immunoprophylaxis. Transplant. Proc. *23*:1492–1494, 1991.
389. Samuel, D., Muller, R., Alexander, G., et al.: Liver transplantation in European patients with the hepatitis B surface antigen. N. Engl. J. Med. *329*:1842–1847, 1993.
390. Samuelsson, A. T., Towers, T. L., and Ravetch, J. V.: Anti-inflammatory activity of IVIG mediated through the inhibitory Fc receptor. Science *291*:484–486, 2001.
391. Sanchez, P. B.: Immunoprophylaxis of respiratory syncytial virus disease. Pediatr. Infect. Dis. J. *19*:791–801, 2000.
392. Sanchez-Quijano, A., Pireda, J. A., Lissen, E., et al.: Prevention of post-transfusion non-A, non-B hepatitis by non-specific immunoglobulin in heart surgery patients. Lancet *1*:1245–1249, 1988.
393. Santoshan, M., Reid, R., Ambrosino, D. N., et al.: Prevention of *Haemophilus influenzae* type b infections in high risk infants treated with bacterial polysaccharide immune globulin. N. Engl. J. Med. *317*:923–929, 1987.
394. Sarker, S. A., Casswall, T. H., Mahalanabis, D., et al.: Successful treatment of rotavirus diarrhea in children with immunoglobulin from immunized bovine colostrum. Pediatr. Infect. Dis. J. *17*:1149–1154, 1998.
395. Schaeffer, M., and Toomey, J. A.: Failure of gamma globulin to prevent varicella. J. Pediatr. *33*:749–752, 1948.
396. Schiff, R. I.: Transmission of viral infections through intravenous immune globulin. N. Engl. J. Med. *331*:1649–1650, 1994.
397. Schiff, R. I., Sedlak, D., and Buckley, R. H.: Rapid infusion of Sandoglobulin in patients with primary humoral immunodeficiency. J. Allergy Clin. Immunol. *88*:61–67, 1991.
398. Schmidt, R. E., Hartlapp, J. H., Niese, D., et al.: Reduction of infection frequency by intravenous gammaglobulins during intensive induction therapy for small cell carcinoma of the lung. Infection *12*:167–170, 1984.
399. Schwarz, T. F., Roggendorf, M., Hottenträger, B., et al.: Immunoglobulins in the prophylaxis of parvovirus B19 infection. J. Infect. Dis. *162*:1214, 1990.
400. Seeff, L. B., Zimmerman, H. J., Wright, E. C., et al.: Efficacy of hepatitis B immune serum globulin following "needlestick" exposure: A preliminary report of the Veterans Administration Cooperative Study. Lancet *2*:939–941, 1975.
401. Selbing, A., Josefsson, A., Dahle, L. O., and Lindgren, R.: Parvovirus B19 infection during pregnancy treated with high-dose intravenous gammaglobulin. Lancet *345*:660–661, 1995.
402. Seu, P., Winston, D. J., Holt, C. D., et al.: Long-term ganciclovir prophylaxis for successful prevention of primary cytomegalovirus (CMV) disease in CMV-seronegative liver transplant recipients with CMV-seropositive donors. Transplantation *64*:1614–1617, 1997.
403. Shamim, M., Giacola, G. P., and West, K.: The use of intravenous immunoglobulin (IVIG) to prevent infection in bronchopulmonary dysplasia: Report of a pilot study. J. Perinatol. *40*:239–244, 1991.
404. Shapiro, R. L., Hatheway, C., and Swerdlow, D. L.: Botulism in the United States: A clinical and epidemiologic review. Ann. Intern. Med. *129*:221–228, 1998.
405. Sharp, J. C. M., and Fletcher, W. B.: Experience of antivaccinia immunoglobulin in the United Kingdom. Lancet *1*:656–659, 1973.
406. Shield, J., Melville, C., Novelli, V., et al.: Bovine colostrum immunoglobulin concentrate for cryptosporidiosis in AIDS. Arch. Dis. Child. *69*:451–453, 1993.
407. Shill, M., Baynes, R. D., and Miller, S. D.: Fatal rabies encephalitis despite appropriate post exposure prophylaxis. N. Engl. J. Med. *316*:1257–1258, 1987.
408. Shirani, K. Z., Vaughan, G. M., McManus, A. T., et al.: Replacement therapy with modified immunoglobulin G in burn patients: Preliminary kinetic studies. Am. J. Med. *76*:175–180, 1984.
409. Shurin, P. A., Rehmus, J. M., Johnson, C. E., et al.: Bacterial polysaccharide immune globulin for prophylaxis of acute otitis media in high-risk children. J. Pediatr. *123*:801–810, 1993.
410. Siadak, M. F., Kopecky, K., and Sullivan, K. M.: Reduction in transplant-related complications in patients given intravenous immune globulin after allogeneic marrow transplantation. Clin. Exp. Immunol. *97*(Suppl. 1):53–57, 1994.
411. Siber, G. R., Werner, B. G., Halse, N. A., et al.: Interference of immune globulin with measles and rubella immunization. J. Pediatr. *122*:204–211, 1993.
412. Siegel, F. P., and Oleske, J.: Management of the acquired immune deficiency syndrome: Is there a role for immune globulins? *In* Morell, A., and Nydegger, U. E.(eds.): Clinical Use of Intravenous Immunoglobulins. New York, Academic Press, 1986, pp. 373–384.
413. Silk, H. J., Abrosino, D., and Geha, R. S.: Effect of intravenous gammaglobulin therapy in IgG2 deficient and IgG2 sufficient children with recurrent infections and poor response to immunization with *Hemophilus influenzae* type b capsular polysaccharide antigen. Ann. Allergy *64*:21–25, 1990.
414. Sikes, R. K.: Human rabies immune globulin. Public Health Rep. *84*:797–801, 1969.
415. Silvestris, F., Cafforio, P., and Dammacco, F.: Pathogenic anti-DNA idiotype-reactive IgG in intravenous immunoglobulin preparations. Clin. Exp. Immunol. *97*:19–25, 1994.
416. Simoes, E. A. F., Groothuis, J. R., Tristram, D. A., et al.: Respiratory syncytial virus–enriched globulin for the prevention of acute otitis media in high risk children. J. Pediatr. *129*:214–219, 1996.
417. Simoes, E. A. F., Sondheimer, H. M., Top, F. H., Jr., et al.: Respiratory syncytial virus immune globulin for prophylaxis against respiratory syncytial virus disease in infants and children with congenital heart disease. J. Pediatr. *133*:492–499, 1998.
418. Simon, N.: Prevention of non-A, non-B hepatitis in haemodialysis patients by hepatitis B immunoglobulin. Lancet *2*:1047, 1984.
419. Skavaril, F., and Gardi, A.: Differences among available immunoglobulin preparations for intravenous use. Pediatr. Infect. Dis. *7*(Suppl.):43–48, 1988.
420. Smallwood, L. A., Tabor, E., Finlayson, J. S., et al.: Antibodies to hepatitis A virus in immune serum globulin. J. Med. Virol. *7*:21–27, 1981.

421. Smego, R. A. Jr., and Asperilla, M. O.: Use of acyclovir for varicella pneumonia during pregnancy. Obstet. Gynecol. *78*:1112–1116, 1991.
422. Snydman, D. R., Werner, B. G., Heinze-Lacey, B., et al.: Use of cytomegalovirus immune globulin to prevent cytomegalovirus disease in renal-transplant recipients. N. Engl. J. Med. *317*:1049–1054, 1987.
423. Sorensen, R. U., Kallick, M. D., and Berger, M.: Home treatment of antibody deficiency syndromes with intravenous immunoglobulin. J. Allergy Clin. Immunol. *80*:810–815, 1987.
424. Spector, S. A., Gelber, R. D., McGrath, N., et al.: A controlled trial of intravenous immune globulin for the prevention of serious bacterial infections in children receiving zidovudine for advanced human immunodeficiency virus infection. N. Engl. J. Med. *331*:1181–1187, 1994.
425. Steen, J. A.: Gamma globulin in preventing infections in prematures. Arch. Pediatr. *77*:291–294, 1960.
426. Steinberg, G. M.: Wissenschaftliche Untersuchungen uber das spezifische Infektionsagens der Blattern und die erzeugung kunstlicher Immunitat gegen Diese. Krankheit. Zentralbl. Bakt. 1. *19*:857–868, 1896.
427. Stevens, D. A., and Merigan, T. C.: Zoster immune globulin prophylaxis of disseminated zoster in compromised hosts. Arch. Intern. Med. *140*:52–54, 1980.
428. Stiehm, E. R.: The use of human intravenous immune globulin in immunoregulatory disorders and in the newborn period. Immunol. Allergy Clin. North Am. *8*:39–50, 1988.
429. Stiehm, E. R.: Recent progress in the use of intravenous immunoglobulin. Curr. Probl. Pediatr. *22*:335–348, 1992.
430. Stiehm, E. R.: Human intravenous immunoglobulin in primary and secondary antibody deficiency diseases. Pediatr. Infect. Dis. J. *16*:696–707, 1997.
431. Stiehm, E. R., Casillas, A. M., Finkelstein, J. Z., et al.: Slow subcutaneous human intravenous immunoglobulin in the treatment of antibody immunodeficiency: Use of an old method with a new product. J. Allergy Clin. Immunol. *101*:848–849, 1998.
432. Stiehm, E. R., Fletcher, C. V., Mofenson, L. M., et al.: Use of human immunodeficiency virus–intravenous immunoglobulin (HIV-IVIG) in HIV-1 infected children (Pediatric AIDS Clinical Trials Group Protocol 273). J. Infect. Dis. *181*:548–554, 2000.
433. Stiehm, E. R., and Fudenberg, H. H.: Clinical and immunologic features of dysgammaglobulinemia type I. Report of a case diagnosed in the first year of life. Am. J. Med. *40*:805–815, 1966.
434. Stiehm, E. R., Lambert, J. S., Mofenson, L. M., et al.: Efficacy of zidovudine and human immunodeficiency virus (HIV) hyperimmune immunoglobulin for reducing perinatal HIV transmission from HIV-infected women with advanced disease: Results of Pediatric AIDS Clinical Trials Group Protocol 185. J. Infect. Dis. *179*:567–575. 1999.
435. Stiehm, E. R., Mofenson, L., Zolla-Pazner, S., et al.: Summary of the workshop on passive immunotherapy in the prevention and treatment of HIV infection. The Passive Antibody Workshop Participants. Clin. Immunol. Immunopathol. *75*:84–93, 1995.
436. Stillerman, M., Marks, H. H., and Thalhimer, W.: Prophylaxis of measles with convalescent serum. Am. J. Dis. Child. *67*:1–14, 1944.
437. Stogner, S. W., King, J. W., Black-Payne, C., et al.: Ribavirin and intravenous immune globulin therapy for measles pneumonia in HIV infection. South. Med. J. *86*:1415–1418, 1993.
438. Stokes, J., Jr., Farquhar, J. A., Drake, M. E., et al.: Infectious hepatitis: Length of protection of immune serum globulin (gamma globulin) during epidemics. J. A. M. A. *147*:714–719, 1951.
439. Stokes, J., Jr., Hilleman, M. R., Weibel, R. E., et al.: Efficacy of live, attenuated measles virus vaccine given with human immune globulin. N. Engl. J. Med. *265*:507–513, 1961.
440. Stokes, J., Jr., Maris, E. P., and Gellis, S. S.: Chemical, clinical and immunological studies on the products of human plasma fractionation. XI. The use of concentrated normal human serum in the prophylaxis and treatment of measles. J. Clin. Invest. *23*:531–540, 1944.
441. Stokes, J., Jr., and Neefe, J. R.: The prevention and attenuation of infectious hepatitis by gamma globulin. J. A. M. A. *127*:144–145, 1945.
442. Stone, H. H., Graber, C. D., Martin, J. D., Jr., et al.: Evaluation of gamma globulin for prophylaxis against burn sepsis. Surgery *58*:810–814, 1965.
443. Storch, G. A.: Humanized monoclonal antibody for prevention of respiratory syncytial virus infection. Pediatrics *102*:648–651, 1998.
444. Su, I.-J., Wang C.-H., Cheng, A.-L., and Chen R.-L.: Hemophagocytic syndrome in Epstein-Barr virus–associated T-lymphoproliferative disorders: Disease spectrum, pathogenesis, and management. Leuk. Lymphoma *19*:401–406, 1995.
445. Sullivan, K. M.: Immunoglobulin therapy in bone marrow transplantation. Am. J. Med. *83*(Suppl. 4A):34–35, 1987.
446. Sullivan, K. M.: Intravenous immune globulin prophylaxis in recipients of a marrow transplant. J. Allergy Clin. Immunol. *84*:632–639, 1989.
447. Sullivan, K. M., Kopecky, K. J., Jocom, J., et al.: Immunomodulatory and antimicrobial efficacy of intravenous immunoglobulin in bone marrow transplantation. N. Engl. J. Med. *323*:705–712, 1990.
448. Swedo, S. E., Leonard, H. L., Garvey, M., et al.: Pediatric autoimmune neuropsychiatric disorders associated with streptococcal infections: Clinical description of the first 50 cases. Am. J. Psychiatry *155*:264–271, 1998.
449. Symmers, D., and Lewis, K.: The antitoxin treatment of erysipelas. J. A. M. A. *99*:1082–1084, 1932.
450. Szmuness, W., Prince, A. M., Goodman, M., et al.: Hepatitis B immune serum globulin in prevention of non parenterally transmitte hepatitis B. N. Engl. J. Med. *290*:701–706, 1974.
451. Szmuness, W., Stevens, C. E., Oleszko, W. R., et al.: Passive active immunisation against hepatitis B: Immunogenicity studies in adult Americans. Lancet *1*:575–577, 1981.
452. Tacket, C. O., Shandera, W. X., Mann, J. M., et al.: Equine antitoxin use and other factors that predict outcome in type A foodborne botulism. Am. J. Med. *76*:794–798, 1984.
453. Tada, H., Yanagida, M., Mishina, J., et al.: Combined passive and active immunization for preventing perinatal transmission of hepatitis B virus carrier state. Pediatrics *70*:613–619, 1982.
454. Taguchi, Y., Purtilo, D. T., and Okano, M.: The effect of intravenous immunoglobulin and interferon-alpha on Epstein-Barr virus–induced lympho-proliferative disorder in a liver transplant recipient. Transplantation *57*:1813–1815, 1994.
455. Takei, S., Arora, Y. K., and Walker, S. M.: Intravenous immunoglobulin contains specific antibodies inhibitory to activation of T cells by staphylococcal toxin superantigens. J. Clin. Invest. *91*:602–607, 1993.
456. Tang, M. L., Kemp, A. S., and Moaven, L. D.: Parvovirus B19–associated red blood cell aplasia in combined immunodeficiency with normal immunoglobulins. Pediatr. Infect. Dis. J. *13*:539–541, 1994.
457. Tasman, A., and Landsberg, H. P.: Problems concerning the prophylaxis, pathogenesis and therapy of diphtheria. Bull. World Health Organ. *16*:939–973, 1957.
458. Tasman, A., Minkenhof, J. E., Vink, H. H., et al.: Importance of intravenous injection of diphtheria antiserum. Lancet *1*:1299–1304, 1958.
459. Tchervenkov, J. I., Tector, A. J., Barkun, J. S., et al.: Recurrence-free long-term survival after liver transplantation for hepatitis B using interferon-alpha pretransplant and hepatitis B immune globulin posttransplant. Ann. Surg. *226*:356–368, 1997.
460. Terrault, N. A., Zhou, S., Combs, C., et al.: Prophylaxis in liver transplant recipients using a fixed dosing schedule of hepatitis B immunoglobulin. Hepatology *24*:1327–1333, 1996.
461. The French National Registry of HA-1A (Centoxin) in septic shock. A cohort study of 600 patients. The National Committee for the Evaluation of Centoxin. Arch. Intern. Med. *154*:2484–2491, 1994.
462. Torok, T. J.: Human parvovirus B19. *In* Remington, J. S., and Klein, J. O. (eds.): Infectious Diseases of the Fetus and Newborn Infant. 4th ed. Philadelphia, W. B. Saunders, 1995, pp. 668–702.
463. Toupance, O., Bouedjoro-Camus, M.-C., Carquin, J., et al.: Cytomegalovirus-related disease and risk of acute rejection in renal transplant recipients: A cohort study with case-control analyses. Transpl. Int. *13*:413–419, 2000.
464. Trimble, G. X.: Attenuation of chickenpox with gamma globulin. Can. Med. Assoc. J. *77*:697–699, 1957.
465. Turner, R. B., and Kelsey D. K.: Passive immunization for prevention of rotavirus illness in healthy infants. Pediatr. Infect. Dis. J. *12*:718–722, 1993.
466. Tutscha, P. J.: Diminishing morbidity and mortality of bone marrow transplantation. Vox Sang *51*(Suppl. 2):87–94, 1986.
467. U.S. Army Medical Research Institute of Infectious Diseases: Smallpox. *In* Medical Management of Biological Casualties Handbook. 4th ed. http://www.nbc-med.org/SiteContent/HomePage/WhatsNew/MedManual/Feb01/ handbook.htm, 2001.
468. Vaccinia (smallpox) vaccine recommendations of the Advisory Committee on Immunization Practices (ACIP). M. M. W. R. Recomm. Rep. *40*(RR-14):1–10, 1991.
469. Vaccinia (smallpox) vaccine, recommendations of the Advisory Committee on Immunization Practices (ACIP). M. M. W. R. Recomm. Rep. *50*:1–25, 2001.
470. Vaishnava, H., Goyal, R. K., Neogy, C. N., et al.: A controlled trial of antiserum in the treatment of tetanus. Lancet *2*:1371–1374, 1966.
471. Vakil, B. J., Tulpule, T. H., Armitage, P., et al.: A comparison of the value of 200,000 I.U. tetanus antitoxin with 50,000 I.U. in the treatment of tetanus. Clin. Pharmacol. Ther. *4*:182–187, 1963.
472. Vakil, B. J., Tulpule, T. H., Armitage, P., et al.: A comparison of the value of 200,000 I.U. tetanus antitoxin (horse) with 20,000 I.U. in the treatment of tetanus. Clin. Pharmacol. Ther. *5*:695–698, 1964.
473. Vakil, B. J., Tulpule, T. H., Armitage, P., et al.: A comparison of the value of 200,000 I.U. of tetanus antitoxin (horse) with 10,000 I.U. in the treatment of tetanus. Clin. Pharmacol. Ther. *9*:465–471, 1968.
474. Valduss, D., Murray, D. L., Karna, P., et al.: Use of intravenous immunoglobulin in twin neonates with disseminated coxsackie B_1 infection. Clin. Pediatr. (Phila.) *32*:561–563, 1993.
475. Van Wye, J. E., Collins, M. S., Baylor, M., et al.: *Pseudomonas* hyperimmune globulin passive immunotherapy for pulmonary exacerbations in cystic fibrosis. Pediatr. Pulmonol. *9*:7–18, 1990.
476. Vera-Ramirez, M., Charlet, M., and Parry, G. J.: Recurrent aseptic meningitis complicating intravenous immunoglobulin therapy for chronic inflammatory demyelinating polyradiculoneuropathy. Neurology *42*:1636–1637, 1992.

477. Verlinde, J. D., and Spaander, J.: Neutralisatie van vaccine virus door gamma globuline. Ned. Tijdschr. Geneesk. *93*:2958–2962, 1949.
478. Viard, I., Wehrli, P., Bullani, R., et al.: Inhibition of toxic epidermal necrolysis by blockade of CD95 with human intravenous immunoglobulin. Science *282*:490–493, 1998.
479. Viguier, M., Guillevin, L., and Laroche, L.: Treatment of parvovirus B19–associated polyarteritis nodosa with intravenous immune globulin. Letter. N. Engl. J. Med. *344*:1481–1482, 2001.
480. Vittecoq, D., Chevret, S., Morand-Joubert, L., et al.: Passive immunotherapy in AIDS: A double-blind randomized study based on transfusions of plasma rich in anti-human immunodeficiency virus-1 antibodies vs. transfusions of seronegative plasma. Proc. Natl. Acad. Sci. U. S. A. *92*:1195–1199, 1995.
481. Von Hedenström, M., Heberle, U., and Theobald, K.: Vaccination against tick-borne encephalitis (TBE): Influence of simultaneous application of TBE immunoglobulin on seroconversion and rate of adverse events. Vaccine *13*:759–762, 1995.
482. Vyas, G. N., Perkins, H. A., and Fudenberg, H. H.: Anaphylactoid transfusion reactions associated with anti IgA. Lancet *2*:312–315, 1968.
483. Waisbren, B. A.: The treatment of bacterial infections with the combination of antibiotics and gamma globulin. Antibiot. Chemother. *7*:322–332, 1957.
484. Waldvogel, K., Bossart, W., Huisman, T., et al.: Severe tick-borne encephalitis following passive immunization. Eur. J. Pediatr. *155*:775–779, 1996.
485. Ward, R., and Krugman, S.: Etiology, epidemiology and prevention of viral hepatitis. Prog. Med. Virol. *4*:87–118, 1962.
486. Ward, R., Krugman, S., Giles, J. P., et al.: Infectious hepatitis. Studies of its natural history and prevention. N. Engl. J. Med. *258*:407–416, 1958.
487. Warny, M., Fatimi, A., Bostwick, E. F., et al.: Bovine immunoglobulin concentrate–*Clostridium difficile* retains *C. difficile* toxin neutralizing activity after passage through the human stomach and small intestine. Gut *44*:212–217, 1999.
488. Weeks, J. C., Tierney, M. R., and Weinstein, M. C.: Cost-effectiveness of prophylactic intravenous immune globulin in chronic lymphocytic leukemia. N. Engl. J. Med. *325*:81–86, 1991.
489. Weiner, C., Pan, Q., Hurtig, M., et al.: Passive immunity against human pathogens using bovine antibodies. Clin. Exp. Immunol. *116*:193–205, 1999.
490. Weintraub, I.: Treatment of herpes zoster with gamma globulin. J. A. M. A. *157*:1611, 1955.
491. Weisman, L. E., Schuman, R. E., Lukomska, E., et al.: Effectiveness and pharmacokinetics of an anti-lipoteichoic acid humanized mouse chimeric monoclonal antibody. Abstract. Pediatr. Res. *49*:301, 2001.
492. Werdan, K.: Supplemental immune globulins in sepsis. Clin. Chem. Lab. Med. *37*:341–349, 1999.
493. Wheeler, A. P., and Bernard, G. R.: Treating patients with severe sepsis. N. Engl. J. Med. *340*:207–214, 1999.
494. Wilcox, M.: Treatment of *Clostridium difficile* infection. Antimicrob. Chemother. *41*(Suppl. C):41–46, 1998.
495. Wilde, H., Sirikawin, S., Sabcharoen, A., et al.: Failure of postexposure treatment of rabies in children. Clin. Infect. Dis. *22*:228–232, 1996.
496. Williams P. E., Yap P. L., Gillon J., et al.: Transmission of non-A or non-B hepatitis by pH 4–treated intravenous immunoglobulin. Vox Sang *57*:15–18, 1989.
497. Wilson, C. B., Louis, D. B., and Penix, L. A.: The Physiologic immunodeficiency of immaturity. *In* Stiehm, E. R. (ed.): Immunologic Disorders in Infants and Children. 4th ed. Philadelphia, W. B. Saunders, 1996, pp. 253–295.
498. Wilson, N. W., Ochs, H. D., Peterson, B., et al.: Abnormal primary antibody responses in pediatric trauma patients. J. Pediatr *115*:424–427, 1989.
499. Winnie, G. B., Cowan, R. G., and Wade, N. A.: Intravenous immune globulin treatment of pulmonary exacerbations in cystic fibrosis. J. Pediatr. *114*:309–314, 1989.
500. Whitley, R. J.: Neonatal herpes simplex virus infections: Is there a role for immunoglobulin in disease prevention and therapy? Pediatr. Infect. Dis. J. *13*:432–439, 1994.
501. Wittes, J. T., Kelly, A., and Plante, K. M.: Meta-analysis of CMVIG studies for the prevention and treatment of CMV infection in transplant patients. Transplant. Proc. *28*(Suppl. 2):17–24, 1996.
502. Wolff, S. N., Fay, J. W., Herzig, R. H., et al.: High-dose weekly intravenous immunoglobulin to prevent infections in patients undergoing autologous bone marrow transplantation or severe myelosuppressive therapy. A study of the American Bone Marrow Transplant Group. Ann. Intern. Med. *118*:937–942, 1993.
503. Wong, V. C., Ip, H. M. H., Reesink, H. W., et al.: Prevention of the HBsAg carrier state in newborn infants of mothers who are chronic carriers of HBsAg and HBeAg by administration of hepatitis B vaccine and hepatitis B immunoglobulin. Lancet *1*:921–926, 1983.
504. Woodruff, R. K., Griff, A. P., Firkin, F. L., et al.: Fatal thrombotic events during treatment of autoimmune thrombocytopenia with intravenous immunoglobulins in elderly patients. Lancet *2*:217–219, 1986.
505. World Health Organization: WHO recommendations on rabies postexposure treatment and the correct technique, part 1. *In* Guide for Rabies Post-Exposure Treatment. Geneva, World Health Organization, 1997, pp. 1–10.
506. Young, N. S.: Parvovirus infection and its treatment. Clin. Exp. Immunol. *104*(Suppl. 1):26–30, 1996.
507. Zachoval, R., Jilg, W., Lorbeer, B., et al.: Passive/active immunization against hepatitis B. J. Infect. Dis. *150*:112–117, 1984.
508. Zaia, J. A.: Prevention and treatment of cytomegalovirus pneumonia in transplant recipients. Clin. Infect. Dis. *17*(Suppl. 1):392–399, 1993.
509. Zaia, J. A., Levin, M. J., Preblud, S. R., et al.: Evaluation of varicella zoster immune globulin: Protection of immunosuppressed children after household exposure to varicella. J. Infect. Dis. *147*:737–743, 1983.
510. Ziegler, E. J., Fisher, C. J., Jr., Sprung, C. L., et al.: Treatment of gram negative bacteremia and septic shock with HA 1A human monoclonal antibody against endotoxin. N. Engl. J. Med. *324*:429–436, 1991.
511. Ziegler, E. J., McCutchan, J. A., Fierer, J., et al.: Treatment of gram negative bacteremia and shock with human antiserum to a mutant *Escherichia coli*. N. Engl. J. Med. *307*:1225–1230, 1982.
512. Zingher, A.: Convalescent whole blood, plasma, and serum in prophylaxis of measles. J. A. M. A. *82*:1180–1187, 1924.

SECTION XXV

Other Preventive Considerations

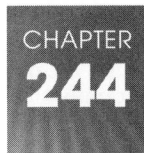

CHAPTER 244

Public Health Considerations

STEVEN L. SOLOMON ■ DAVID W. FRASER ■ SHELDON L. KAPLAN

Public health can be defined as those aspects of health and disease that are determined by the interaction of people and their environment, including but not limited to circumstances in which the condition of one person or group of persons affects that of others. These diseases may be nutritional, toxic, or infectious, but they are alike in that they all have an exogenous source. Because the source is exogenous, cases of diseases that fall under public health tend to occur in clusters, patterns of which are determined by the interplay of exposure and susceptibility. The main thrusts of disease control in public health are (1) prevention of additional cases by identification and elimination of the source of exposure or prevention of transmission from it and (2) identification of the high-risk susceptible group and reduction of its susceptibility.

Tools for control of public health problems fall into two categories: recognition/evaluation and intervention. Foremost among the tools for recognition and evaluation is surveillance, which can be defined as the systematic collection of information about the occurrence of disease in a community. When an unusual cluster of disease is recognized through surveillance or serendipity, an epidemic investigation is required and includes a description of the disease, determination of the pattern of its occurrence in the community, formulation of hypotheses of the cause of the unusual frequency, testing of the hypotheses, and framing of control methods. Of assistance in both surveillance and epidemic investigation is the recognition of common patterns of disease spread either within groups of people or from the environment to people.

Many tools are available for intervention. Two important categories are not considered in this chapter because they are addressed at length elsewhere in this book; one is immunization (active and passive) (Chapters 237 and 238), and the other is treatment of individual patients. Tools that are discussed here include isolation, chemoprophylaxis, water and food sanitation (including the special situation of international travel), and vector control.

Surveillance

The primary purpose of surveillance is to permit timely recognition of new public health problems through monitoring the pattern of occurrence of disease in the community, with the ultimate aim being to effect early control of these problems.[161] A secondary purpose is to answer defined questions about the pattern of occurrence of disease, but the ultimate goal is the same.

Surveillance involves the collection, collation, and analysis of data and feedback of information. When used properly, this information helps in directing disease control activities and evaluating their impact. In the primary collection of information, three major factors must be defined.[26] The first is the population to be surveyed, which may be circumscribed geographically (e.g., the United States) or restricted to a certain age group (e.g., infants, for the surveillance of birth defects) or to a certain institution (e.g., a school, a hospital, the U.S. Army). Second, the data to be monitored can be as crude as the number of cases of disease or deaths from a disease. Additional information that could be collected and be useful epidemiologically includes the characteristics of ill persons with regard to age, sex, place of residence, occupation, and so on, or detailed characteristics of the organisms involved, such as antibiotic sensitivity, serogroup, or site of the body from which an isolate was recovered. The third and most important element of the reporting system is the primary reporting source. Unless a report of disease is initiated—by a physician, infection control practitioner, or laboratory—no information is generated. Incentives to the primary reporting source to maintain good reporting are essential for maintaining a useful surveillance system.

In each state, reporting of specified infectious diseases is required by law. However, state laws vary with regard to the persons who are responsible for reporting, the diseases or conditions that are reportable, and the circumstances under which reporting is to occur.[52, 99] Specific information is generally available on request from state or local health agencies.

Collection of surveillance information on the occurrence of disease is pointless unless the data are used to initiate or modify control actions. The first step is collation and analysis, which may be done at the level of the local health department, the state health department, or the federal government. If this step is performed in a timely fashion, problems can be recognized early and a response made.

After this information is collated and analyzed, the results are fed back to the primary reporting source and to others interested in the data. Such feedback serves to maintain interest in the reporting system and thereby maintains the quality of data obtained and continuously updates persons at each level of the surveillance system about the changing patterns of occurrence of disease and new strategies for disease control.

One vehicle for the feedback of national surveillance information is the *Morbidity and Mortality Weekly Report*, which is published by the Centers for Disease Control and Prevention (CDC). Also published by the CDC are periodic summaries of surveillance activities relating to specific diseases. Regular summaries of surveillance activities also are published by the World Health Organization and by many state health departments.

Identification of a disease problem in the course of surveillance should prompt an attempt to control the problem. Control may involve the initiation of an epidemic investigation if surveillance data suggest an unusual frequency of occurrence of a disease or the adjustment in a public health program if, for example, surveillance data suggest that vaccine is not being given to a particular age group of susceptible people.

Epidemic Investigation

When faced with a possible outbreak, a useful approach is for the investigator to address the inquiry systematically.

1. *Verify the diagnosis.* Review of available clinical and laboratory information and examination of a few patients will permit the creation of a list of possible diagnoses and will suggest additional diagnostic specimens that may be needed to secure the diagnosis. The investigation may proceed without a microbiologic diagnosis if a clearly defined clinical syndrome can be identified. With or without microbiologic confirmation, a firm case definition is needed.
2. *Confirm the existence of an epidemic.* Through the use of an objective case definition, the baseline incidence of the illness before the apparent occurrence of an epidemic should be determined by review of appropriate microbiologic, serologic, or clinical records. Armed with these data, the investigator can decide whether recent events indicate an unusual clustering of illness (i.e., whether an epidemic exists).
3. *Describe the time, place, and person.* Graphic display of the distribution of cases in time not only confirms the existence of an epidemic but also indicates whether the outbreak is waxing or waning. It may permit judgment about whether the outbreak is spread from person to person or from a common source of exposure and an estimate of the incubation period. Comparison of the characteristics of cases with regard to age, sex, geographic location, and other relevant factors with those of persons who reasonably might have been considered to have been at risk but who did not become ill forms the basis for making epidemiologic hypotheses. Determining the attack rate (number ill/[number ill + number well]) is a useful method of describing the risk of development of illness in various groups.
4. *Frame an epidemiologic hypothesis.* By taking the diagnosis (presumed or confirmed) and the pattern of occurrence of disease into account, the investigator may hypothesize one or several possible common sources of infection and one or more modes of spread (food- or water-borne, airborne, vector-borne, or by a particular therapeutic or diagnostic procedure). Alternatively, the hypothesis may be of person-to-person spread.
5. *Identify the control group or groups.* Central to the epidemiologic process is identification of a group of persons in whom illness might have developed but did not.[66] The activities and exposures that set well persons apart from sick persons often point to the source of the outbreak. For gastroenteritis occurring after a church supper, one control group might be those who went to the supper but did not get sick, and another control group might be residents of the same community who did not attend the supper. For histoplasmosis in schoolchildren occurring after a school clean-up program, controls might be the well children.
6. *Test the hypothesis epidemiologically.* The attack rates of illness among persons exposed or not exposed to a hypothesized source then are compared by using the number of cases and controls in each group. A true common source should be associated with a higher attack rate in those exposed to it than in those not so exposed. Statistical tests are useful for assessing the significance of differences observed in attack rates of those exposed and not exposed.
7. *Explain the outliers.* Any case that occurs in a person apparently not exposed to an implicated common source needs to be explained. As an example, if vanilla ice cream is implicated as the common source in a food-borne outbreak and ill persons are found who ate only chocolate ice cream, one might hypothesize reasonably that cross-contamination of the ice cream scoop has occurred. Faulty memory of exposure to a common source and the simultaneous occurrence of endemic cases unrelated to the outbreak may complicate this stage of the investigation.
8. *Confirm the hypothesis microbiologically.* Cultures of the implicated common-source material may permit recovery of the infectious agent. When a microorganism is isolated, typing methods may be used to support the epidemiologic hypothesis by demonstrating that the same strain was responsible for disease in all affected patients and can be recovered from the common source. Traditional methods for typing microorganisms—serotyping, biotyping, antimicrobial sensitivity testing, and immunoblotting—remain very useful. In recent years, these techniques have been supplemented and, in some settings, replaced by DNA-based typing methods such as plasmid profile analysis, pulsed-field gel electrophoresis of chromosomal DNA, and polymerase chain reaction assay for identifying DNA segments.[118, 160] However, culturing the agent from a particular site without any epidemiologic implication of that site as a source of infection provides little or no information needed to direct control measures.
9. *Implement control measures.* Knowledge of the agent, source, and mode of spread permits drafting of control measures and their implementation. Without careful attention to this step, the investigation is an academic exercise only.
10. *Measure the impact of control measures.* This step doubles as the ultimate test of the epidemiologic hypothesis and as an assessment of the design and implementation of the control measures. Surveillance for the occurrence of disease in groups shown to be at high risk is the most common technique used for this measurement, and a decrease in the attack rate to zero or to the baseline incidence is the measure of success.

An example of the process is the investigation of an epidemic of postoperative group A streptococcal wound infections. In November 1970, the CDC was informed by the staff of a 140-bed hospital that a large number of streptococcal wound infections had occurred in the preceding 2 weeks and that two patients had died. In his subsequent investigation, Conrad Fulkerson determined that group A streptococci had been isolated (step 1) and that the number of patients in the hospital with group A streptococcal isolates from wounds increased from two in September to seven in October and to four in the first 10 days of November. Earlier months had averaged one case per month (step 2). He found that the 13 infected patients came from six preoperative wards in the hospital, had widely ranging ages, underwent a variety of surgical procedures, and included members of both sexes. The interval from surgery to the onset of wound infection was 0.5 to 2 days for 10 patients; 2 of the 3 patients who had intervals greater than 2 days had been given prophylactic systemic antibiotics at surgery (step 3).

Because group A streptococci almost invariably are spread from person to person, because patients came from many wards, and because most cases occurred shortly after surgery, Dr. Fulkerson hypothesized that spread had occurred from one of the operating room personnel to the patients during surgery (step 4). Dr. Fulkerson chose as the control group all persons who underwent major operations during the epidemic period (step 5). They were listed in the operating room log in chronologic order. To reduce this list to a more workable size, Table 244–1 includes only every fifth member of the actual control group, as well as the 13 cases. You may wish to execute step 6 yourself by using the data in Table 244–1. Once convinced that you have identified the source by epidemiologic methods, you may wish to speculate on step 7 and design an investigation to satisfy step 8 before turning to the Appendix at the end of this chapter for the dénouement.

Common Patterns of Disease Spread

DISEASE SPREAD FROM ANIMALS TO PEOPLE

Many infectious diseases are transmitted from other animals to humans. Physicians who routinely inquire about animal contacts as part of the clinical and epidemiologic history of an ill patient frequently find valuable clues to an obscure diagnosis.[1] Table 244–2 lists infectious disease agents for which some suggestive or definitive evidence exists that disease can be spread from animal to human, either directly or via a vector. A distinctive disease name associated with the organism also is listed, as are the various animal groups that have been suggested or shown to act as sources of transmission to humans. The frequency with which an animal group serves as a source of infection for humans and the frequency with which a vector is involved

TABLE 244–1 ■ OPERATING ROOM LOG EXCERPT FROM EPIDEMIOLOGIC INVESTIGATION

Surgical Case No.	Sex	Surgeon	Assistant	Anesthesiologist	Circulating Nurse	Scrub Nurse
1709	F	Zellner	Pane	Mutsen	Land	Roman
1719	F	Wilson	Toulson	Sutterfield	Roman	Bartt
1726*	F	Dryden	Zellner	Sutterfield	Grasser	Bartt
1733	F	Dryden	Walker	Taylor	Hodge	Roman
1744	M	Wilson	—	—	Peak	Bartt
1760	F	Polson	Riley	Mutsen	Jones	Land
1773	F	Martin	Riley	Sutterfield	Hodge	Roman
1788	F	Stein	Wilson	Mutsen	Hodge	Bartt
1795	F	Polson	Pane	Mutsen	Jones	Bartt
1807	M	Dryden	Riley	Sutterfield	Jones	Roman
1831	F	Kirk	Toulson	Taylor	Peak	Land
1847	F	Martin	Wright	Mutsen	Peak	Roman
1865	F	Wilson	Dryden	Taylor	Hodge	Roman
1874	F	Bear	Zellner	Taylor	Swift	Roman
1895	F	Berger	Sartorius	Sutterfield	Swift	Hodge
1905*	F	Zellner	Ballson	Sutterfield	Jones	Roman
1918	M	Wilson	Toulson, Martin	Sutterfield	Jones	Hodge
1938	F	Berger	Toulson	Sutterfield	Jones	Hodge
1942*	M	Berger	Caroll	Sutterfield	Jones	Hodge
1953	F	Kirk	Toulson	Taylor	Peak	Roman
1964*	F	Bear	Dryden	Sutterfield	Hodge	Roman
1968	F	Berger	—	Mutsen	Peak	Land
1982	F	Stein	Toulson	Sutterfield	Peak	Grasser
1996*	M	Ballson	Inger	Sutterfield	Hodge	Roman
1999	F	Martin	Pane	Taylor	Peak	Roman
2017*	F	Zellner	Bear	Sutterfield	Jones	Roman
2019*	F	Zellner	Bear	Sutterfield	Jones	Roman
2023	F	Martin	Able	Sutterfield	Swift	Roman
2039	M	Ballson	Dryden	Sutterfield	Swift	Peak
2050	F	Martin	Toulson	Sutterfield	Jones	Bartt
2069*	F	Dryden	Martin	Sutterfield	Jones	Peak
2074	F	Zellner	Bear	Taylor	Jones	Land
2083	F	Wilson	—	—	Land	—
2093*	F	Bear	Caroll	Mutsen	Hodge	Roman
2101	M	Martin	Toulson	Sutterfield	Peak	Roman
2119	F	Bear	Zellner	Taylor	Hodge	Peak
2134	F	Avis	—	Sutterfield	Peak	—
2148	M	Kirk	Pool	Sutterfield	Peak	Swift
2162*	F	Martin	Riley	Taylor	Swift	Bartt
2166	F	Bear	Zellner	Taylor	Land	Peak
2173	M	Martin	Ballson	Taylor	Jones	Land
2183	F	Wilson	Toulson	Taylor	Land	Roman
2194*	F	Berger	Wilson	Taylor	Peak	Roman
2200*	F	Polson	Dryden	Sutterfield	Jones	Roman
2202	F	Wilson	—	Taylor	Hodge	Bartt
2208	F	Martin	Pool	Sutterfield	Land	—
2224	F	Bear	Caroll	—	Land	Bartt

*Patients in whom postoperative streptococcal wound infection developed.

TABLE 244–2 ■ INFECTIOUS DISEASE SPREAD FROM ANIMALS TO HUMANS*

		Animal Source†																
Organism	**Disease**	*Vector-borne*‡	*Dogs*	*Cats*	*Cattle*	*Horses*	*Swine*	*Sheep, Goats*	*Domestic Fowl*	*Pigeons*	*Parrots, Parakeets*	*Mice, Rats*	*Rabbits*	*Fish*	*Shellfish*	*Turtles*	*Nonhuman Primates*	*Other*
Bacterial Diseases																		
Spirochetes and Curved Bacteria																		
Borrelia species	Relapsing fever	++			?	?						2					?	Opossums ? Squirrels 2 Small rodents 2 Armadillos ?
Borrelia burgdorferi	Lyme disease	++	?	?	?							2	?					Deer 2 Birds ? Other rodents 2 Other carnivores ?
Leptospira interrogans	Leptospirosis		2	1	2	1	2	1				2	?					Skunks 1 Squirrels 1 Raccoons 1 Many animals 2
Spirillum minus	Rat-bite fever											3						Carnivores 1 Other rodents ?
Gram-Negative Rods																		
Aeromonas species															2			
Burkholderia pseudomallei	Melioidosis	?	?			?												
Burkholderia mallei	Glanders		?			3		?										Mules 3 Wolves ? Asses 3
Brucella abortus	Brucellosis				3													
Brucella suis					2		3											
Brucella melitensis								3										
Brucella canis			3															
Bordetella bronchiseptica			2	1								?	2					Guinea pigs 2
Francisella tularensis	Tularemia	+							2			2	2					Muskrats 2 Beaver 1 Other rodents 1 Squirrels 1 Hamsters 2
Campylobacter species			1	1	2			1	3			1						
Salmonella species			1	1	1	1	1	1	3	1	1	1	1	1	1	2	2	Many 1, 2
Shigella species																	2	
Yersinia pestis	Plague	++	1	2								2	1					Ground squirrels 2 Prairie dogs 2 Wild carnivores 1 Tree squirrels 1 Other rodents 1
Yersinia pseudotuberculosis			1	1									?					Canary 1 Hamster ? Guinea pig ?
Yersinia enterocolitica			1				3											
Vibrio parahaemolyticus															?			
Vibrio vulnificus															3			
Pasteurella multocida			2	2	2	1	2		1				1					Opossum 1
Pasteurella haemolytica																		Deer 1
Pasteurella pneumotropica			2	2														
Capnocytophaga canimorsus			2															Coyotes ? Bears ? Tigers ?
Streptobacillus moniliformis	Rat-bite fever											2						
Bartonella henselae	Bacillary angiomatosis, ? cat-scratch disease			3														
Gram-Positive Cocci																		
Staphylococcus aureus							?							?				
Group A streptococci				1														

TABLE 244-2 ■ INFECTIOUS DISEASE SPREAD FROM ANIMALS TO HUMANS*—cont'd

		Animal Source[†]																
Organism	**Disease**	***Vector-borne***[‡]	***Dogs***	***Cats***	***Cattle***	***Horses***	***Swine***	***Sheep, Goats***	***Domestic Fowl***	***Pigeons***	***Parrots, Parakeets***	***Mice, Rats***	***Rabbits***	***Fish***	***Shellfish***	***Turtles***	***Nonhuman Primates***	***Other***
Group B streptococci				?														
Group C streptococci						2												
Group R streptococci							2											
Group S streptococci							2											
Gram-Positive Rods																		
Bacillus anthracis	Anthrax				2	2		2										
Clostridium tetani	Tetanus				?	?												
Listeria monocytogenes					1			1	1									Whales 1
Erysipelothrix insidiosa							3		2			?		2	2			Seals 1
Corynebacterium equi					?		?	?										
Corynebacterium pyogenes								?										
Corynebacterium pseudotuberculosis								?										
Mycobacterium tuberculosis	Tuberculosis		1	1	1												2	
Mycobacterium bovis			1	1	3													
Micobacterium avium							?											
Mycobacterium marinum														2				Dolphins 1 Poikilotherms 1
Mycobacterium leprae	Leprosy	?																Armadillo ?
Dermatophilus congolensis					?	?		?										
Rickettsiae																		
Ehrlichia chaffeensis	Human ehrlichiosis	++																?
Rickettsia prowazekii	Louse-borne typhus	++			?	?	?	?										
Rickettsia typhi	Murine typhus	++		1								3						
Rickettsia ricketsii	Rockey Mountain spotted fever	++	2	2								2	2					Other rodents 2 Birds ?
Rickettsia siberica	North Asian tick typhus	++										3						Birds ?
Rickettsia conorii	Fièvre boutonneuse	++	2									2						Birds ?
Rickettsia australis	Queensland tick typhus	++										2						Small marsupials 2
Rickettsia akari	Rickettsialpox	++										3						
Rickettsia tsutsugamushi	Scrub typhus	++										3						Birds ?
Coxiella burnetii	Q fever	+			2			3										Small mammals 2 Birds ?
Chlamydiae																		
Chlamydia psittaci	Psittacosis	?		1	?				2	2	2							Other birds 2 Muskrats ?
Fungal Diseases																		
Microsporum canis	Ringworm		2	2														
Microsporum equinum	Ringworm					2												
Microsporum nanum	Ringworm						2											
Trichophyton equinum	Ringworm					2												
Microsporum gallinae	Ringworm								2									
Trichophyton mentagrophytes var. *quinckeanum*												2						
Trichophyton mentogrophytes var. *erinacei*	Ringworm																	Hedgehogs 2
Trichophytan mentogrophytes var. *mentographytes*	Ringworm		2									2						
Trichophytan verrucosum	Ringworm				2													
Parasitic Diseases																		
Helminths																		
Angiostrongylus species												2		3	3[§]			Amphibians 3 Reptiles 3
Capillaria hepatica			1	1								2						
Capillaria philippinensis														3				
Dioctophyma renale														2				Mink and other fish-eating mammals 2

Continued

TABLE 244–2 ■ INFECTIOUS DISEASE SPREAD FROM ANIMALS TO HUMANS*—cont'd

		Animal Source†																
Organism	**Disease**	***Vector-borne‡***	***Dogs***	***Cats***	***Cattle***	***Horses***	***Swine***	***Sheep, Goats***	***Domestic Fowl***	***Pigeons***	***Parrots, Parakeets***	***Mice, Rats***	***Rabbits***	***Fish***	***Shellfish***	***Turtles***	***Nonhuman Primates***	***Other***
Trichinella spiralis				?			3											Bears 1, seals 1, walruses 1, whales 1
Filaria																		
Brugia malayi	Filariasis	++		2													2	Other carnivores 2
Dirofilaria immitis	Heartworm	++	3															
Dirofilaria tenuis		++																Raccoons 3
Dirofilaria repens		++	2	2														
Nematodes																		
Ascaris lumbricoides							1											
Ascaris suum							1											
Baylisascaris procyonis																		Raccoons 3
Ancylostoma braziliense	Cutaneous larva migrans		2	3														
Ancylostoma caninum	Cutaneous larva migrans		2															
Ancylostoma ceylonicum	Cutaneous larva migrans		2	2														
Uncinaria stenocephala	Cutaneous larva		2	2														Foxes 1
Gnathostoma spinigerum	Visceral and cutaneous larva migrans		2	2					2					2				Frogs 1 Snakes 1 Racoons 2
Toxocara canis	Visceral larva migrans		3															Other canids 2
Toxocara cati	Visceral larva migrans			3														
Anisakis species														3				Marine mammals 2
Strongyloides stercoralis			2	2												?		
Trichostrongylus species					2	2		2										Donkeys 2
Trematodes																		
Schistosoma haematobium															3		3	
Schistoma japonicum			2	2	2	2	2	2				2			3			
Schistosoma mansoni												?			3			Baboons 2
Clinostomum complanatum														2				
Clonorchis sinensis	Oriental liver fluke		2	2										3	3			
Dicrocoelium dendriticum					2			2							2			Ants 2
Dicrocoelium hospes					2			2							2			Ants 2
Echinostoma species			1	1			1		2	2		1		1	2			
Fasciola gigantica	Liver fluke				2	2		2							2			
Fasciola hepatica	Liver fluke				2			2							2			
Fasciolopsis buski	Liver fluke						2								2			
Gastrodiscoides hominis							2								2	3		
Haplorchis species			2											3	2			Numerous birds and mammals 2
Heterophyes species			2	2								2		3	3			Other birds 2 Other carnivores 2
Metagonimus species															3	2		Numerous birds and mammals 2
Opisthorchis felineus				2										3	2			Numerous other birds, reptiles, and mammals 2
Paragonimus species															3			Numerous mammals 2
Heterophids																		
Centrocestus formosanum			2	2								2		3	2			Other birds 2
Stellantchasmus species			2	2										3	2			
Cestodes																		
Taenia saginata	Taeniasis				3													
Taenia solium	Taeniasis/cysticercosis		2				3											
Echinococcus granulosus	Hydatid disease		3				3											Other carnivores 2
Echinococcus multilocularis	Hydatid disease		3	2								2						Foxes 2
Bertiella species	Tapeworm	++															1	
Diphyllobothrium latum	Fish tapeworm													3				Other carnivores 2

TABLE 244–2 ■ INFECTIOUS DISEASE SPREAD FROM ANIMALS TO HUMANS*—cont'd

		Animal Source[†]																
Organism	**Disease**	***Vector-borne***[‡]	***Dogs***	***Cats***	***Cattle***	***Horses***	***Swine***	***Sheep, Goats***	***Domestic Fowl***	***Pigeons***	***Parrots, Parakeets***	***Mice, Rats***	***Rabbits***	***Fish***	***Shellfish***	***Turtles***	***Nonhuman Primates***	***Other***
Dipylidium caninum	Tapeworm	++	3	2														
Hymenolepis diminuta	Tapeworm	++										2						
Hymenolepis nana	Tapeworm	?										2						Hamsters ?
Mesocestoides species	Tapeworm	?	2	2														Snakes 1 Birds 1 Other carnivores 2
Spirometra species	Sparganosis		1	1			1		1			1						Frogs 2 Copepods 1 Snakes 1
Protozoa																		
Trypanosoma cruzi	Chagas disease	++	2	2									2					Raccoons 2 Guinea pigs 2 Opossum ? Armadillo ? Numerous small mammals 2
Trypanosoma gambiense	Gambian sleeping sickness	++	1				1											
Trypanosoma rhodesiense	Rhodesian sleeping sickness	++			2													Bushback 2
Leishmania brasiliensis	Espundia, uta, etc.	++										2						Other rodents 2 Sloths ? Anteater ?
Leishmania mexicana	Espundia, uta, etc.	++										2						Small mammals 2
Leishmania donovani	Kala-azar	++	2	?	?	?		?				2						Jackals 2 Foxes 2
Leishmania chagasi	Kala-azar	++	2									2						Foxes Other rodents 2
Leishmania tropica	Oriental sore	++	2									2						Gerbils 2 Other rodents 2
Leishmania major	Oriental sore, etc.	++																Gerbils 2 Other rodents 2
Leishmania aethiopica	Oriental sore, etc.	++																Hyrax 2 Other rodents 2
Plasmodium knowlesi	Malaria	++															2	
Plasmodium simium	Malaria	++															?	
Babesia divergens	Babesiosis	++			2													
Babesia microti	Babesiosis	++										2						Deer 2
Pneumocystis carinii												?						
Sarcocystis species					?		?	?									1	
Toxoplasma gondii		?		2	2		2	2	?			?						
Cryptosporidium species	Cryptosporidiosis		?	?	2	?	?	?	?		?	?	?	?			?	Deer ?
Viral Diseases																		
Herpesvirus simiae	Monkey B encephalitis																3	
Cowpox					3													
Pseudocowpox	Milker's nodule				3													
Orf								3										
Bovine papular stomatitis					3													
Monkeypox																	3	
Vesicular stomatitis		?			2													
Junin fever	Argentine hemorrhagic fever											3						
Machupo	Bolivian hemorrhagic fever											3						
Hantaan	Korean hemorrhagic fever											3						Shrews 1, voles 1 Other rodents 1
Sin Nombre	Hantavirus pulmonary syndrome											3						
Lassa												3						
Lymphocytic choriomeningitis												2						Hamsters 2

Continued

TABLE 244–2 ■ INFECTIOUS DISEASE SPREAD FROM ANIMALS TO HUMANS*—cont'd

		Animal Source†															
Organism	**Disease**	*Vector-borne*‡	*Dogs*	*Cats*	*Cattle*	*Horses*	*Swine*	*Sheep, Goats*	*Domestic Fowl*	*Pigeons*	*Parrots, Parakeets*	*Mice, Rats*	*Rabbits*	*Fish*	*Shellfish*	*Turtles*	*Nonhuman Primates*	*Other*
Hepatitis A															2		2	
Influenza A/swine	Swine influenza						2											
Newcastle									3									
Foot and mouth disease					1			1										
Marburg																	2	
Ebola																	1	
Rabies			2	1	1													Wolf 2 Bat 1, fox 1 Skunk 1 Mongoose 1 Racoon 1 Jackal 1
Arboviruses																		
Chikungunya		++															2	
O'nyong-nyong		++															?	
Sindbis		++							?	?								Other birds 2
Eastern equine encephalitis		++																Other birds 2
Western equine encephalitis		++																Other birds 3
Venezuelan equine encephalitis		++				2						2						
Yellow fever		++															2	
Japanese encephalitis		++				?	2											Other birds 2
Murray Valley encephalitis		++																Other birds 2
Wesselsbron		+						3										
West Nile		++								?								Other birds 3
Zika		++															2	
St. Louis encephalitis		++							?	?								Other birds 3
Ilheus		++																Other birds ?
Kyasanur Forest disease		++										2					2	
Louping II		++							3									Other birds ?
Omsk hemorrhagic fever		++			?							?						Muskrat ?
Powassan		++										?						Birds ? squirrels ? Woodchucks ?
Tick-borne encephalitis		++			2			2				2						Other birds 2
Dengue		++															?	
Bwamba		++															?	
LaCrosse		++																Chipmunks 2 Foxes 2 Squirrels 2
California encephalitis		++											?					Squirrels 2
Oropouche		++															?	Other birds ? Sloth ?
Kemerovo		++			2	?						2						Other birds ?
Congo/CHF	Crimean hemorrhagic fever	++			2	2						2	2					Other birds 2
Colorado tick fever		++										1						Ground squirrels 3 Porcupines ?
Nairobi sheep disease		++						3										
Rift Valley fever		++			2			2				?						
Ross River		++					?	?										Kangaroos ?
Mayaro		++																Other mammals ?
Group C fevers		++										3					1	Other birds ?

*Certain rare or accidental infectious diseases omitted.

†Animal species that seem to be sources, either directly or through a vector, or microbial agents that infect humans: 3, typical source of human infection; 2, common source of human infection; 1, rare source of human infection; ?, speculative source of human infection. Many diseases and many animal species are omitted for which evidence is lacking that infection is transmitted from lower animals to humans.

‡Disease acquired through bites from, contact with, or ingestion of insects or arachnids: ++, disease typically vector-borne: +, disease occasionally vector-borne: ?, speculation that disease occasionally may be vector-borne.

§Numbers in italics indicate intermediate hosts for certain parasitic diseases.

are indicated in semiquantitative fashion. Perhaps the most recent disease recognized to be spread from animals to humans in the United States is West Nile virus. West Nile virus was introduced first in the northeastern part of the United States in the summer and fall of 1999. By 2001, West Nile virus activity detected in mosquitoes, people, dead birds, captive sentinel animals, and other sources had been reported from 359 counties in 27 states.[46] Omitted are many species that may be infected with the organism but do not appear to act as a source of human infection. Also omitted are certain rare or accidental infectious diseases. The complex life cycles of some parasites are difficult to display in tabular form; intermediate animal hosts are designated in Table 244–2 to facilitate interpretation. Details of the clinical manifestations, differential diagnosis, and treatment of the zoonoses are found in the appropriate chapters elsewhere in this book. For a complete description of the circumstances under which each agent is spread from animal to person, consult a textbook of zoonoses.[1, 16]

Excluded from Table 244–2 are several interesting groups of infectious diseases in which human beings and animals appear to interact but in which infection does not spread from animals to people. The first group includes organisms that infect both animals and humans from a common source in nature. Such organisms include *Burkholderia pseudomallei, Blastomyces dermatitidis,* and *Aspergillus* spp., which can infect a wide variety of animal species, including humans, from soil or other inanimate sources.

A few diseases typically are spread from humans to animals. Perhaps the most prominent example is *Herpesvirus hominis,* which can cause fatal encephalitis in nonhuman primates when spread from humans.[96] Tuberculosis also can spread from humans to nonhuman primates, as well as the reverse.

Cryptococcus neoformans lives in animal feces but does not infect animals. From the fecal material, these organisms may spread to infect people.

Some organisms can be transmitted by fomites of animal origin. They act as mechanical carriers, and the process does not involve infection of the animals. Examples include *Histoplasma capsulatum,* which has been observed to be spread by chicken feathers, and *Coccidioides immitis,* which can be spread in bales of wool contaminated with fungus-laden dust.

Another group of diseases are spread from person to person but through an insect vector, either typically or on occasion. Filariasis caused by *Wuchereria bancrofti* is a prime example of a disease in which vector-borne person-to-person spread is the rule. Typhoid and yaws have been shown to be spread by vectors on occasion. Evidence that *Mycobacterium leprae* can be recovered from mosquitoes that have fed on patients with lepromatous leprosy exists, as does speculation that such mosquitoes may serve as vectors of transmission.

DISEASE SPREAD FROM PERSON TO PERSON

As members of groups—including the family, school, camp, daycare center, and church—children are at risk of acquiring or spreading infectious agents that are transmitted from person to person. Knowledge of the typical patterns of spread can be useful in planning surveillance or in designing control measures. For example, recognition that diarrhea commonly results from person-to-person spread in daycare centers and that it can indicate inadequate hygienic practices may justify specific surveillance for diarrhea in that setting. Documentation of secondary cases in various categories of contacts of cases of meningococcal disease permits focusing the delivery of chemoprophylaxis on just the high-risk groups.

In this section, spread in the family and schools is discussed, but several groups of interest are omitted. The important areas of transmission of disease within daycare centers and within hospitals are discussed in separate chapters. Maternal transmission of specific infections to the fetus or neonate also is reviewed elsewhere in this book. Spread, especially of enteric diseases, within institutions for the mentally retarded is recognized widely as an important problem, but it does not impinge directly on the practice of most pediatricians.

Of course, perhaps infection caused by human immunodeficiency virus (HIV) or acquired immunodeficiency syndrome (AIDS) is one of the areas for which public health surveillance is most critical. The CDC has reported that during 1994 to 2000, HIV infection was diagnosed in more than 128,800 persons in 25 states that have been conducting surveillance for HIV infection for this time frame.[47] The number of persons in whom HIV infection without AIDS initially was diagnosed declined 21 percent from 1994 to 2000. Approximately 1 percent of the HIV (n = 1073) or AIDS (n = 224) cases between 1994 and 2000 occurred in children younger than 13 years. The numbers of new pediatric cases remained steady during this time interval. In contrast, cases occurring in persons between 25 and 44 years of age declined by approximately 33 percent. Maternal transmission and person-to-person spread of HIV infection are at the top of the list of public health concerns and are covered extensively in Chapter 192.

The Family

Spread of disease agents in the family can be considered in two stages: introduction of the agent into the family, usually by a single member ("index case" or "index carrier"), and spread to other family members. Spread to other members can be described in terms of rapidity and intensity, the latter commonly measured by the secondary infection rate (or secondary attack rate), which is defined as the proportion of the contacts of the index carrier or index case who become infected (or ill) in a given interval after exposure. The secondary infection rate varies from agent to agent and may be affected by the age and sex of the introducer; the size of the family; crowding; the age of household contacts; previous immunity; and interventions attempted, including isolation, treatment, and chemoprophylaxis. The ratio of the secondary attack rate to the incidence of disease in the community is a measure of the importance of the family as a focus of disease.[76]

Of the bacteria spread by the respiratory route, pneumococci, group A streptococci, meningococci, and *Haemophilus influenzae* have been studied most completely. In a study of English families of five persons each (mother, father, and three children, the youngest of whom was younger than 5 years), type-specific introduction of pneumococci was attributed most frequently to the middle child.[18] The oldest and middle children were the most efficient spreaders of pneumococci to other family members. Among household contacts, children were more likely than their parents to become infected. The overall secondary infection rate was 9 percent. Routine administration of pneumococcal conjugate vaccine to young infants probably will alter the epidemiology of pneumococcal colonization, as well as invasive infection, similar to what has been observed with the conjugate vaccine for *H. influenzae* type b (Hib). Children with group A streptococcal infection in members of families in Cleveland,

Ohio, were even more important than children with pneumococcal infection as introducers and recipients of intrafamilial transmission.[102] The pattern of spread of meningococcal infection has been reported to be strikingly different. The most common introducers of meningococci into families are men, followed distantly and in decreasing order of frequency by women, girls, and boys.[83] Once meningococci are introduced, all family members may become infected, although studies of carriers in household transmission of meningococcal disease in Brazil suggest that spread may proceed from an adult to older children and only thereafter to infants.[132]

Children younger than 5 years have the greatest risk of acquiring serious disease from Hib infection. Overall carriage rates are less than 5 percent, although high rates of colonization have been reported in settings such as daycare, where young children are in close contact, and in families with a child who has invasive Hib disease.[126] Among unvaccinated contacts of persons with Hib disease, children younger than 5 years have the highest carriage rates (30 to 40%), with rates dropping progressively with increasing age.[9] However, the epidemiology of Hib disease has been changed markedly by the use of vaccines; the annual incidence of disease in children younger than 5 years fell more than 99 percent (from 100/100,000 to 0.3/100,000) from 1990 to 2000 after the introduction of conjugate vaccines.[2, 43] Unlike earlier polysaccharide vaccines, conjugate vaccines appear to prevent colonization as well as disease; one study using a matched case-control analysis showed that conjugate vaccines had 81 percent efficacy in decreasing colonization.[133]

Bordetella pertussis spreads easily within families. In a study of 21 families in Finland, 83 percent of the family members of primary cases showed serologic evidence of secondary infection.[125] Secondary attack rates for symptomatic disease were lower in older children and adults. Children 2 to 15 years of age were more likely to introduce pertussis into the family than were younger children or family members older than 15 years. Adults may be of increasing importance as reservoirs of *B. pertussis* leading to infection in infants.[113, 134] A study in Germany of 122 households with an index case of pertussis showed that index cases who were adults were as likely to spread pertussis within the family as were index cases who were children. Fourteen (78%) of 18 adults and 74 (71%) of 104 children spread pertussis to at least 1 other family member.[172] Outbreaks have been reported in which an adult with persistent bronchitis acted as a source of pertussis for children.[108, 114] In the United States during 1997 to 2000, of the pertussis cases reported to the CDC for which the age of the person was known, 20 percent occurred in persons 20 years or older.[42]

Both tuberculosis and leprosy usually are acquired by children from adults who introduce the mycobacteria into the household.[69] These introducers typically shed large numbers of bacteria from the respiratory tract (especially from the nose in lepromatous leprosy) for months or years. Secondary attack rates are similar for the two diseases and are highest for tuberculosis in children younger than 5 years.[148] For leprosy, children of all ages beyond the neonatal period are at significant risk.

Introducers who are ill tend to be more efficient spreaders of bacteria in the respiratory tract. In the Cleveland study, spread of group A streptococci was 2.7 times as frequent when the introducer was symptomatic as when the introducer was asymptomatic. Spread of group A streptococci was observed in Egyptian families particularly frequently if the person who introduced the strain into the household was ill enough to seek medical care or if the strain persisted in the respiratory tract of the introducer for 3 or more months.[67] Nasal shedders have been shown to be more efficient spreaders,[119] and nasal shedding commonly is found early in illness. In 14 (56%) of the 25 episodes of transfer of pneumococci observed in Virginia families, the spreader experienced sneezing, rhinorrhea, nasal congestion, or cough during the 2-week period in which transfer occurred, whereas such symptoms were present in 159 (37%) of the other 423 2-week periods of observation.[84] Again, this finding may relate to higher rates of recovery of pneumococci from the nose during symptoms of upper respiratory tract infection.

Crowding has been observed inconsistently to affect spread of pneumococci. English families living in only two rooms had a secondary infection rate of 16.0 percent, whereas those living in four or more rooms had an 11.2 percent secondary infection rate.[18] Floor space was not shown to affect spread in families in Syracuse, New York,.[62] Severe overcrowding, inadequate ventilation, and altered host susceptibility were important factors in an outbreak of pneumococcal disease in a large urban jail.[93] Limited ventilation of houses seems to promote the spread of meningococci in the meningitis belt in Africa.[79] In a population-based case-control study, household crowding was shown to be a risk factor for *H. influenzae* disease.[53] Ill children were 2.6 times more likely to live in households containing one or more persons per room than were well children in control families. The magnitude of risk associated with crowding increased as the extent of crowding increased.

Carriage of meningococci[83] and group A streptococci[102] may persist for many months, resulting in multiple cases of disease in a family widely separated in time. Typically, however, half the secondary cases of meningococcal and Hib disease occur within 5 days of that of the index case.[74, 82, 132]

The changing epidemiology of measles and mumps demonstrates the impact of vaccines on the transmission of viral diseases spread by the respiratory route. The age at which a person is most at risk for acquiring one of these diseases is determined largely by the communicability of the virus and the completeness of immunity. Hope-Simpson[94] calculated that disease developed in 75 percent of susceptible family contacts exposed to a case of measles, whereas the corresponding figures for varicella and mumps were 61 and 31 percent, respectively. In that study, the mean ages at which infection occurred were 5.6, 6.7, and 11.5 years for measles, varicella, and mumps, respectively, typical of figures obtained in the prevaccine era. Spread of measles before the introduction of vaccine occurred primarily in younger school-age children (5 to 9 years of age) within the community, with secondary spread to siblings within the family. From 1960 to 1964, 53 percent of all measles cases occurred in children 5 to 9 years of age and 37 percent in children younger than 5 years.[72] However, transmission now is most likely to occur in older school-age children and college students, whereas preschoolers, especially those too young to receive vaccine, constitute a continuing pool of susceptible persons.[117] In 1994, only 10 percent of the measles cases were reported in children 5 to 9 years of age; 40 percent occurred in children and adolescents 10 to 19 years of age, and 26 percent were in children younger than 5 years.[33] A comparable change has been seen in the epidemiology of mumps, with a decreasing proportion of cases in younger school-age children and an increasing proportion in older children, adolescents, and young adults.[54, 164] Although varicella vaccine has been shown to be more than 85 percent effective in preventing varicella in clinical practice, it is too soon to know what effect the vaccine will have on the epidemiology of this infection.[165]

For respiratory syncytial virus, secondary attack rates of infants have been estimated at 45 percent, higher than the corresponding rate of 27 percent for all family contacts.[85] The infant's older sibling is the most frequent introducer of respiratory syncytial virus into the family. In the study of Cleveland families, common respiratory diseases (including the common cold, rhinitis, laryngitis, and bronchitis) occurred more often in young school-age children than in preschool children and, in the latter, more frequently in siblings of school-age children than in preschool children without such siblings.[60] Secondary attack rates of common respiratory diseases averaged 25 percent, were highest in children younger than 5 years (37 to 49%), and were similar in preschool children with or without siblings in school.

The epidemiology of some acute respiratory diseases also may be changing. Transmission varies both with levels of immunity and with opportunities for exposure of susceptible persons. A comparison of the Cleveland family study data with data from a more recent longitudinal study of children in daycare suggested that out-of-home childcare may be lowering the age of first exposure to and infection with acute respiratory pathogens.[59] Young children in daycare are more likely than children in home care to have more than six upper respiratory tract infections per year and more than 60 days of illness per year.[167] In a study of lower respiratory tract infections in children younger than 2 years, children hospitalized with lower respiratory tract infection were three times more likely to have received care in a daycare center attended by six or more children.[7] Crowding in the child's home also was observed to be an independent factor that increased the risk of acquiring respiratory disease.

In the Seattle Virus Watch study of family spread of influenza virus, school-age children were the most likely family members to acquire community-acquired infection and then to introduce the infection into the household; they also were most at risk for spread from other family members (57 to 63% secondary attack rate).[71] However, secondary attack rates among all household members were highest (70 to 75%) when the introducer was younger than 5 years. For infants in the first year of life, the risk of influenza developing is related to the number of siblings in the household.[80]

Parvovirus B19 infection appears to be transmitted effectively within families, with a secondary attack rate of 50 percent among close contacts[27]; the risk of transmission seems to decrease with advancing age.[105] The risk of pregnant women acquiring acute parvovirus B19 infection increases with an increasing number of children in the household. Having children 6 to 7 years old resulted in the highest risk for acquiring acute infection in these mothers.[163] Preschool-age children, especially those in daycare, may introduce cytomegalovirus into the family, infect seronegative mothers, and thereby pose a risk to the fetus if the mother is pregnant.[140] The risk of transmission from child to mother is greatest if the child is younger than 20 months.[3]

The spread of some enteric diseases within the family also has been studied. In two community outbreaks of shigellosis, Weissman and associates[169] found that in 86 percent of families the bacterium was introduced by a child younger than 10 years. The secondary attack rate averaged 31 percent and was highest in children younger than 5 years. The secondary attack rate was significantly higher in families with an initial case in a preschool-age child than in families with an initial case in an older person. Spread within the family did not correlate with family size or household crowding but appeared to be highly dependent on whether an ill preschool-age child was in the family.

After a food-borne outbreak of Norwalk gastroenteritis associated with a school cafeteria, secondary transmission occurred in 44 percent of the households with a primary case. In households with a primary case, the risk of secondary illness was twice as high among preschool-age children (70% attack rate) as among adults (31%).[90]

Poliovirus seems to spread more readily than *Shigella* in families. Gelfand and associates[77] studied household contacts of children found to have wild poliovirus infection. Among household contacts, evidence of recent infection, usually no later than 1 month after that in the index child, was found in 73 percent of adults, 96 percent of older siblings, and 84 percent of younger siblings. By studying the spread of live poliomyelitis vaccine virus strains in families, they found a secondary infection rate among susceptible persons of 53 percent in a lower economic group and 9 percent in a higher economic group.[78] Secondary infection rates were higher with type 3 (77%) than with types 1 (47%) or 2 (36%). Virus appeared to spread more readily from those with pharyngeal excretion and less readily from adults than from children.

In the study of Cleveland families, "infectious gastroenteritis" was found to be introduced most commonly by children younger than 6 years.[60] The secondary attack rate averaged 11 percent and was highest in children younger than 8 years. The secondary attack rate was related directly to the number of major gastrointestinal symptoms (vomiting, diarrhea, and abdominal pain) suffered by the index case: 10 percent for contacts of those with one symptom, 16 percent for contacts of those with two, and 32 percent for contacts of those with all three.

Helicobacter pylori infections cluster within families.[63] Families of children with *H. pylori* infection identified in the gastric antrum after endoscopy were studied for positive serology to *H. pylori* antibody. Seventy-four percent of the parents of infected children were seropositive as compared with 24 percent of the parents of uninfected children; 82 percent of the siblings of infected children also were positive. A study of 215 adults in England found an association between seropositivity for *H. pylori* antibodies and a history of crowded living conditions in childhood.[123]

In a community-wide study of rotavirus transmission, children younger than 2 years were most likely to introduce the infection into the family.[106] Persons living in households with a child younger than 2 years had a risk of becoming infected that was 2.9 (for adults) to 3.5 times (for children 10 to 17 years of age) higher than that for persons of comparable age in other families.

Young children attending daycare also are likely to introduce into their families infections associated with parasitic enteropathogens. A study in Houston, Texas, found a 17 percent secondary attack rate for *Giardia* enteritis in families with a child who became infected in daycare.[141] At least one secondary case of giardiasis was identified in 47 percent of all households with a *Giardia*-infected child during an outbreak at a Washington, D.C., daycare center.[144] During an outbreak of diarrheal disease at a daycare center in Oklahoma, stool samples were positive for *Cryptosporidium* in 23 percent of the household contacts of children with confirmed *Cryptosporidium* infection.[88] Young children may acquire an asymptomatic hepatitis A infection in daycare and transmit this infection to adult household contacts, who may become quite ill.[166]

International adoptees may introduce infectious diseases that are endemic in the child's country of origin into families that might otherwise not be at risk. In one study, parents of hepatitis B surface antigen (HBsAg)-seropositive adopted children were five times more likely to have serologic evidence of hepatitis B virus infection than were parents of HBsAg-seronegative adoptees.[75] Children from various countries also have been shown to have tuberculosis, cytomegalovirus infection, congenital syphilis, and infection with enteric pathogens when joining their adopted families.[95] Careful screening has been recommended for such children to identify and treat these infections.

Schools

In general, infectious disease agents spread much less readily from child to child in schools than in daycare centers. Jacobson and associates[101] showed during an epidemic of meningococcal disease in Brazil that young elementary school classmates of a student with meningitis seemed not to be placed at increased risk of acquiring meningitis. Low carriage and acquisition rates for classroom contacts of meningococcal carriers similarly were demonstrated during a study of primary schoolchildren in England.[24] However, small outbreaks can occur in schools. A review of serogroup C meningococcal outbreaks in the United States found four outbreaks that occurred in elementary or junior high schools in the period from 1980 to 1993.[100] The number of cases involved in each outbreak, ranging from 3 to 7, generally was less than those of community outbreaks, although attack rates (233 to 1028/100,000 students) usually were higher than those of community outbreaks. The relatively high attack rates and the short interval between cases in these outbreaks led to rapid institution of vaccination programs, which may have had a role in limiting spread. Another CDC study of meningococcal disease in schools between January 1989 and June 1994 identified 22 clusters in 15 states.[175] The estimated incidence of secondary meningococcal disease among schoolchildren aged 5 to 18 years was 2.5 per 100,000 population, a relative risk of 2.3. More than 70 percent of secondary cases occurred within 2 weeks of the index case. College students, particularly freshmen living in dormitories, have an increased risk of acquiring meningococcal disease, and the recommendation of the American Academy of Pediatrics (AAP) is that these students and their parents be informed of this increased risk and that vaccination with the quadrivalent meningococcal vaccine be offered.[4]

Attack rates of shigellosis during a group of outbreaks in elementary schools ranged from 0.4 to 1.1 percent; the higher values occurred in schools with larger numbers of children younger than 8 years.[162] Enforced handwashing and disinfection of items potentially contaminated with feces have been associated with control of a shigellosis outbreak in an elementary school.[14]

Typically, spread in schools is less than that in families. In a measles outbreak that involved children in 20 of 26 classrooms in one school, the attack rate in unimmunized pupils with no history of measles was only 16 percent.[57] Landrigan[109] observed in a community outbreak that measles spread most quickly in situations in which unvaccinated children were brought together for the first time; in urban areas, such spread occurred in daycare centers and nursery schools, whereas in rural areas, where children seldom attended daycare, it occurred in elementary schools.

Schools may serve to spread infection from family to family. In outbreaks of measles, mumps, and pertussis, children infected within classroom settings appear to have spread disease to younger siblings at home. These outbreaks have occurred in school settings in which a high proportion of students have been immunized previously.[19, 50, 57, 117, 120, 128] In outbreaks of measles and mumps, failure of the vaccine to evoke a protective immunologic response (primary vaccine failure) has been a more significant factor resulting in susceptibility to infection than has waning immunity from previous successful vaccination (secondary vaccine failure). Waning immunity has been shown to be a particular problem leading to susceptibility to pertussis in adolescents and adults.

Occasionally, person-to-person spread in a school appears to be very efficient. Miller and associates[127] described a diphtheria outbreak in an elementary school in which 34 percent of all students were found to be infected and clinical diphtheria developed in 30 percent of the unimmunized students. The reason for the intense spread was not found. In a measles outbreak in a high school, 69 secondary cases occurred in a single generation; aerosolization of virus by vigorous coughing in the index case and inadequate levels of immunity in a cohort of students were identified as probable factors leading to a high level of transmission.[42]

Multiple outbreaks of tuberculosis in children have been reported.[103] In most cases, the outbreaks occurred in schools. In one outbreak in an elementary school, a physical education teacher with cavitary pulmonary tuberculosis was identified as the source case.[92] Of 343 students in the school, 176 were found to be skin test–positive. Infection was associated with frequency of contact with the teacher. Abnormal chest radiographs were found in 32 children, and active disease was associated with having a low body mass index. Although occasional outbreaks of tuberculosis can occur in schools and in daycare homes,[103, 135] children younger than 12 years rarely spread the infection and are more likely to be sentinels of infection in the adults with whom they are in contact. Widespread tuberculin skin test screening of school-age children has been shown to not be cost-effective[129]; screening is recommended only for groups of children considered to be at high risk for infection.[55]

Settings that result in a greater level of person-to-person contact than found in typical classroom settings, such as participation in school sports[13, 131] or attendance at a boarding school (or summer camp), also can result in more efficient transmission of disease.[20, 152] In one report, an outbreak of pleurodynia probably caused by coxsackievirus B1 in high school football players was associated with drinking from the team cooler or eating ice cubes from the team ice chest.[97]

Food-Borne Illnesses

Food-related disease develops in an estimated 76 million people each year in the United States, thus rendering food safety one of the most important objectives of public health officials. The most common clinical manifestations of food-borne illness are gastrointestinal. In 2001, the incidence per 100,000 of the most common food-borne illnesses in the United States based on active surveillance by the CDC (FoodNet data) was 15.1 for *Salmonella*, 13.8 for *Campylobacter*, 6.4 for *Shigella*, 1.6 for *Escherichia coli* O157, and 1.5 for *Cryptosporidium*.[44] Outbreaks of food-borne illness are very common and often result in investigations by local, state, or federal epidemiologists (or all three). The CDC publishes annual reports on surveillance of food-borne disease and outbreaks related to food. Physicians must work in conjunction with public health officials so that food-borne outbreaks can be recognized in timely fashion and thus control and prevent these illnesses most effectively.[41]

Bioterrorism

Unfortunately, a very important responsibility of public health officials is to help in preparing the nation for the possibility of biologic or chemical terrorism. Thus, in April 2000, the CDC issued a strategic plan for preparedness and response to biologic and chemical terrorism.[37] Eighteen months later in October 2001, the first case of intentional exposure to *Bacillus anthracis* was reported in Palm Beach County, Florida. Eventually, 23 cases of anthrax were identified as a result of intentional exposure, predominantly through envelopes containing or contaminated with highly purified anthrax spores. Eleven cases were inhalational and 12 cutaneous; 1 cutaneous case was laboratory acquired. Four individuals died.[45, 104] Public health officials had to address the public's fear and hysteria after the initial cases were reported. Guidelines for the proper handling of mail and recommendations for rational use of antibiotics, including prophylaxis, were developed quickly and disseminated.[39] Special recommendations were required for children and breast-feeding mothers because ciprofloxacin was the agent of choice for adults.[40] Many more cases of anthrax probably were prevented in part as a result of the rapid response and recommendations of public health officials to this bioterrorist attack.

CDC also identified smallpox virus as a likely bioterrorism agent and developed guidelines for preparations in case of a threat related to smallpox: Centers for Disease Control and Prevention Interim Smallpox Response Plan & Guidelines (*http://www.bt.cdc.gov/DocumentsApp/Smallpox/RPG/index.asp*). On June 21, 2002, the Advisory Committee on Immunization Practices of the CDC made the following recommendations with respect to smallpox vaccination:

> Under current circumstances, with no confirmed smallpox and the risk of an attack assessed as low, vaccination of the general population is not recommended, as the potential benefits of vaccination do not outweigh the risks of vaccine complications.
>
> Smallpox vaccination is recommended for persons pre-designated by the appropriate bioterrorism and public health authorities to conduct investigation and follow-up of initial smallpox cases that would necessitate direct patient contact.
>
> Smallpox vaccination is recommended for healthcare personnel at risk for exposure to the initial smallpox cases in facilities that are pre-designated to receive these patients.
>
> http://www.cdc.gov/nip/smallpox/policy-updt-7-8-02.htm

Undoubtedly, as the situation changes and perhaps improved vaccines against smallpox virus and other biologic agents are developed, the CDC and other public health agencies will issue updated recommendations and guidelines for combating and preventing infections related to bioterrorism.

Control Methods

ISOLATION

Indications for isolation of patients with infectious diseases have changed greatly in this century with increasing knowledge of modes of spread and with antimicrobial therapy, which rapidly renders patients with many diseases noninfectious. Isolating patients with diphtheria was shown to be of value in Providence, Rhode Island, in 1904 to 1913 and probably remains so today. The attack rate among family contacts of diphtheria patients treated at home was 6.5 percent, whereas that among contacts of patients treated in the hospital was 4.3 percent; after adjusting for the ages of contacts in the two groups, hospitalization was associated with a 43 percent decrease in cases among household contacts.[61] Specific therapy has made such institutional isolation unnecessary for some diseases. Isolation of patients with bacilliferous leprosy, which once was a central part of leprosy control, no longer is necessary because dapsone and rifampin quickly kill most *M. leprae;* therapy rapidly prevents any further risk of transmission.

Indications for and techniques of isolating patients in hospitals to prevent nosocomial transmission are discussed elsewhere in this book. An extensive, practical discussion of disease control strategies, including isolation, is readily available in *Control of Communicable Diseases Manual*,[51] which can be purchased in paperback from the American Public Health Association, 800 I Street, N.W., Washington, D.C., 20001-3710 (www.apha.org). In most instances, the need for isolating children without hospitalization is occasioned by bacterial respiratory disease, diarrhea, acute viral diseases of childhood, conjunctivitis, contagious skin diseases, and arthropod-borne diseases.

For bacterial respiratory diseases for which therapy rapidly and consistently renders a patient noninfectious, isolation of infected children may be as brief as 1 or 2 days (as for group A streptococcal pharyngitis or meningococcal infections). Isolation of patients known to have whooping cough still is recommended for at least 5 days after the initiation of erythromycin therapy. For patients with infection or colonization by vancomycin-resistant enterococcus, standard and contact precautions remain in force until culture results from multiple sites (stool, wound, perineal area, etc.) are negative on three separate series of cultures obtained at least 1 week apart.[34] The Red Book from the Committee on Infectious Diseases of the AAP is also an important resource for information about isolation recommendations.

An attempt should be made to limit contamination with the feces of children with diarrhea. Careful handwashing is of great importance, both for the children and for those who take care of them. Clothing and linen contaminated with excreta should be laundered. Adults who are infected with and may be excreting *Salmonella, Shigella, Yersinia enterocolitica,* hepatitis A virus, or other enterically transmitted pathogens should be excluded from preparing food or providing direct care to young children. (See Chapter 240 for recommendations for excluding children from daycare.)

Indications for isolating patients with acute viral diseases of childhood depend on the severity of the illness and the degree of contagiousness. No value of isolation for the common acute viral respiratory diseases has been established. For rubella, isolation is recommended only from women in early pregnancy. Isolation of patients with poliomyelitis within the home is of little value because spread occurs most commonly during the prodrome. The same holds true for measles, which spreads efficiently, although the period of communicability can extend until 4 days after the onset of rash, and children with measles should be kept home from school at least that long. Attempts are made to isolate children with varicella and mumps from school for 7 and 9 days, respectively, after the onset of typical illness; these diseases spread less efficiently than measles does.[94]

Children with conjunctivitis caused by transmissible agents should be excluded from school during the acute phase of illness. This form of isolation may help limit the spread of *H. influenzae* biogroup *aegyptius,* pneumococci, picornavirus, adenovirus, and *Chlamydia trachomatis.*

Children with contagious skin diseases should avoid having skin contact with other children outside their family. Those with molluscum contagiosum, herpes simplex, or impetigo should avoid engaging in wrestling or other contact sports.[13] Those with scabies should be excluded from school until the day after treatment. Children with tinea corporis should avoid gymnasia, swimming pools, and contact sports.

Children in the early phases of arthropod-borne diseases, when the infecting organism still may be in the blood, should avoid being bitten by the vector. The wide variety of such illnesses includes arboviral diseases, bartonellosis, leishmaniasis, microfilarial infections, malaria, and African trypanosomiasis.

CHEMOPROPHYLAXIS

The word *chemoprophylaxis* is used loosely in this section to describe the use of antimicrobial drugs to prevent infection (as with falciparum malaria), to treat asymptomatic infection and thereby prevent disease (as with isoniazid treatment of tuberculin skin test–positive children), and to treat disease and thereby prevent complications of the disease (as with primary prevention of acute rheumatic fever). In each situation, however, the primary purpose is to prevent a disease by administering an antimicrobial agent that affects the causative microorganism.

The decision to initiate chemoprophylaxis and the choice and dosage of agents require careful consideration of both the child's clinical status and the epidemiologic factors that may place the child at risk for acquiring the disease. Local health departments should be notified of exposure to communicable diseases; they often can provide useful additional information on recommended treatment regimens. In addition, they may need to conduct an investigation to ensure that all exposed persons have been identified and, when necessary, treated or placed under observation.

A summary of 13 diseases for which chemoprophylaxis may be administered to children is given in Table 244–3. Some special situations, such as chemoprophylaxis for immunodeficient children and mass prophylaxis to abort epidemics, are omitted from the discussion. For more detailed discussion of antimicrobial drug use in prevention of disease, one should consult the regularly updated *Red Book: Report of the Committee on Infectious Diseases* of the AAP.[56]

Acute rheumatic fever that occurs after streptococcal pharyngitis can be prevented in 90 percent of patients despite a delay in drug administration of as much as 9 days after the onset of sore throat.[25, 58] Rates of success are related directly to eradication of streptococci and are highest with administration of repository penicillin. Provision of neighborhood health centers (and presumably delivery of primary prophylaxis) has been associated with a significant decrease in rates of acquisition of acute rheumatic fever in an urban population.[81] Secondary prophylaxis also can be up to 90 percent effective and depends largely on the faithfulness with which an effective drug is taken.

One study has suggested that antibiotics will prevent the development of acute glomerulonephritis after group A streptococcal pharyngitis,[147, 168] but the apparent reduction in incidence was not statistically significant.[168] No evidence indicates that administration of antibiotics will prevent the development of acute glomerulonephritis after streptococcal skin infection. Studies to determine the effectiveness of chemoprophylaxis and optimal drug regimens are needed.

Among untreated household contacts of endemic meningococcal cases, secondary cases develop at a rate of 0.4 percent; in epidemics, this figure may rise to 5 percent.[124] Daycare center and other intimate contacts also are at risk. Rifampin is the drug of choice for treatment of contacts. However, rifampin is associated with adverse side effects, is teratogenic, and may not eliminate carriage.[150] Ceftriaxone is an alternative agent. For individuals 18 years and older, a single oral dose of ciprofloxacin is another choice. Because of the emergence of sulfonamide-resistant strains of *Neisseria meningitidis,* the use of sulfadiazine as a prophylactic agent now is limited to outbreaks in which the causal microorganism is known to be sulfonamide-susceptible.

Gonococcal ophthalmia can be contracted by an infant from an infected mother during birth. Silver nitrate, erythromycin, or tetracycline instilled into the eyes is effective in preventing this potential cause of corneal ulceration and blindness.[48, 86] Silver nitrate, in use since the 19th century, is less costly than the antibiotics but may be associated with a higher incidence of chemical conjunctivitis. These agents do not appear to be effective in preventing neonatal conjunctivitis caused by *C. trachomatis,* although some studies have produced contradictory results. In one study, the incidence of neonatal chlamydial ophthalmia among infants born to mothers with chlamydial infection was 20 percent in those who received silver nitrate prophylaxis and 14 percent and 11 percent in those receiving erythromycin and tetracycline, respectively.[86] Despite having received appropriate prophylaxis, gonococcal ophthalmia developed in 0.06 percent of the infants born in that hospital during the study period. A study of 3117 infants in Kenya showed that the use of a 2.5 percent solution of povidone-iodine as prophylaxis against ophthalmia neonatorum resulted in fewer infections (13.1% of treated infants) than occurred with either 0.5 percent erythromycin ointment (15.2%) or 1 percent silver nitrate solution (17.5%).[98] As demonstrated in previous studies, the presence of maternal vaginal infection was correlated highly with infectious conjunctivitis. Screening for and treatment of gonococcal and chlamydial infections in pregnant women are the best ways to prevent neonatal disease.[48]

Isoniazid prophylaxis can prevent infection in uninfected tuberculin-negative contacts of tuberculosis cases.[5, 153, 155] Children usually are infected as a result of exposure to an adult with infectious tuberculosis. Children with negative skin tests who have been close contacts of infectious persons (e.g., household contacts) should receive preventive therapy for a minimum of 12 weeks after the last contact with the infectious source. If the result on repeat skin testing remains negative, preventive therapy may be discontinued unless the child has continuing exposure to the infectious source. If the result of a repeat skin test is positive, therapy should be continued for a total of 9 months.[5] Isoniazid prophylaxis also has been shown to decrease the incidence of disease in tuberculin-positive children.[68] When compared with adults or older children, young children have a greater risk of tuberculous disease developing when infected, are more likely to have disseminated disease, and are less susceptible to isoniazid hepatitis when treated with that drug. Thus, young children generally have a high priority for receipt of isoniazid prophylaxis.

The risk of development of leprosy in children who are household contacts of a lepromatous patient was shown in one double-blind trial to be halved by 3 years of dapsone prophylaxis.[136] Community-wide prophylaxis in hyperendemic areas also has been successful.

In a study of 37 households with a primary case of pertussis during a community outbreak, administration of erythromycin prophylaxis to contacts was associated with a decreased likelihood of secondary cases.[154] Delays in beginning erythromycin treatment of primary cases and prophylaxis of contacts were associated with increased secondary spread. Similarly, in a study of a pertussis outbreak in an institutionalized population, erythromycin was shown to be effective in reducing the attack rate and severity of disease among exposed persons.[156] Because the disease may be fatal in infants, this group is most in need of receiving effective prophylaxis. Azithromycin and clarithromycin are probably as effective as erythromycin for prophylaxis of household and other close contacts of patients with pertussis, but no large studies have documented the efficacy of these drugs for this indication.[8]

TABLE 244–3 ■ CHEMOPROPHYLAXIS AGAINST COMMUNICABLE DISEASE IN CHILDREN

Disease	Target Group	Value for Chemoprophylaxis	Recommended Drug*	Regimen*	Vaccine for Target Group	Ref.
Acute glomerulonephritis	Those with group A streptococcal infection in nephritis outbreak	Proposed	Benzathine penicillin G IM	≤27 kg: 600,000 U >27 kg: 1,200,000 U	No	39, 143
			Penicillin V PO	Children: 250 mg 2–3 times daily × 10 days Adolescents: 500 mg 2–3 times daily × 10 days		
			Erythromycin estolate PO	20–40 mg/kg day in 2–4 divided doses (not to exceed 1 g/day) × 10 days		
			Erythromycin ethyl succinate PO	40 mg/kg/day in 2–4 divided doses (not to exceed 1 g/day) × 10 days		
Acute rheumatic fever (ARF)	Those with group A streptococcal infection (not impetigo)	Shown	See above	See above	No	39
	Those with previous ARF	Shown	Benzathine penicillin G IM	1,200,000 U every 3–4 wk		
			Penicillin V PO	250 mg twice a day		
			Sulfadiazine PO	≤27 kg: 0.5 g daily >27 kg: 1 g daily		
			Erythromycin PO	250 mg twice a day		
Cholera	Household contacts of a case	Shown	Tetracycline PO	≥9 yr: 50 mg/kg/day in 4 divided doses × 3 days	No	14, 37, 138
			Doxycycline PO	≥9 yr: 6 mg/kg in a single dose		
			Trimethoprim-sulfamethoxazole PO	8–10 mg/kg/day trimethoprim, 40–50 mg/kg/day sulfamethoxazole in 2 divided doses × 3 days		
Diphtheria	Household, day care center, or other close contacts of a case	Proposed	Erythromycin PO	40–50 mg/kg/day in divided doses (not to exceed 2 g/day) × 7 days	Yes	37, 99
			Benzathine penicillin G IM	<30 kg: 600,000 U ≥30 kg: 1,200,000 U		
Gonorrhea	Neonates	Shown	Silver nitrate	1% aqueous solution	No	31
			Erythromycin	0.5% ophthalmic ointment		
			Tetracycline	1% ophthalmic ointment		
			All instilled into the eye			
Haemophilus influenzae disease	Household contacts of a case when ≥1 susceptible contact is <4 yr old	Shown	Rifampin PO	<1 mo: 10–20 mg/kg/day once daily × 4 days ≥1 mo: 20 mg/kg/day once daily × 4 days (maximal dose, 600 mg/day)	Yes	7, 37
	Daycare center contacts of a case	Proposed	Rifampin PO	<1 mo: 10–20 mg/kg/day once daily × 4 days ≥1 mo: 20 mg/kg/day once daily × 4 days (maximal dose, 600 mg/day)		
Leprosy	Household contacts of lepromatous and dimorphous case	Shown	Dapsone PO	1 mg/kg/day	Yes	37

Continued

TABLE 244–3 ■ CHEMOPROPHYLAXIS AGAINST COMMUNICABLE DISEASE IN CHILDREN—cont'd

Disease	Target Group	Value for Chemoprophylaxis	Recommended Drug*	Regimen*	Vaccine for Target Group	Ref.
Malaria	Travelers to malarious areas without chloroquine-resistant strains	Shown	Chloroquine phosphate PO	5 mg/kg base (8.3 mg/kg salt) once/wk (not to exceed 300 mg base/wk); start 1–2 wk before entering malarious area, continue during travel and for 4 wk after leaving such areas	No	27, 111
			Hydroxychloroquine sulfate PO	5 mg/kg base (6.5 mg/kg salt) once/wk (not to exceed 310 mg base/wk); start 1–2 wk before entering malarious area continue during travel and for 4 wk after leaving such areas		
	Travelers to malarious areas with chloroquine-resistant strains		Mefloquine PO	<15 kg: 5 mg/kg/wk 15–19 kg: 1/4 tablet/wk 20–30 kg: 1/2 tablet/wk 31–45 kg: 3/4 tablet/wk >45 kg: 1 tablet/wk; start 1–2 wk before entering malarious area, continue during travel and for 4 wk after leaving such areas		
			Doxycycline PO	>8 yr: 2 mg/kg of body weight/day (not to exceed 100 mg/day); start 1–2 days before entering malarious area, continue during travel and for 4 wk after leaving such areas		
			Chloroquine PO plus proguanil PO	See above <2 yr: 50 mg/day 2–6 yr: 100 mg/day 7–10 yr: 150 mg/day >10 yr: 200 mg/day; take daily during exposure and continue for 4 wk after last exposure		
Meningococcal disease	Household, day care center, nursery school, or other close contacts of a case	Suggested	Rifampin PO	<1 mo: 5–10 mg/kg twice a day × 2 days ≥1 mo: 10 mg/kg (not to exceed 600 mg/day) twice a day × 2 days	Yes (if group A, C, or Y or W-135)	37, 130
			Ceftriaxone IM	<12 yr: 125 mg in a single dose ≥12 yr: 250 mg in a single dose		
			Ciprofloxacin PO	Single 500-mg dose for those ≥18 yr old		
Pertussis	Close contacts irrespective of vaccine status	Proposed	Erythromycin PO	40–50 mg/kg/24 hr (not to exceed 2 g) in 4 divided doses × 14 days	Yes	37, 134
Plague	Contacts of pneumonic cases	Proposed	Tetracycline PO	≥9 yr: 15–20 mg/kg/24 hr in 4 divided doses × 7 days	No	

TABLE 244–3 ■ CHEMOPROPHYLAXIS AGAINST COMMUNICABLE DISEASE IN CHILDREN—cont'd

Disease	Target Group	Value for Chemoprophylaxis	Recommended Drug*	Regimen*	Vaccine for Target Group	Ref.
			Trimethoprim-sulfamethoxazole PO	8 mg/kg/day trimethoprim 40 mg/kg/day sulfamethoxazole in 2 divided doses × 7 days		122, 145
Tuberculosis	Exposed, skin test-negative	Shown	Isoniazid PO	10–15 mg/kg daily (maximum, 300 mg); continue for 12 wk after last contact with infectious source; may discontinue if skin test remains negative after 12 wk	BCG?	
	Skin test-positive	Shown	Isoniazid PO	10–15 mg/kg daily (maximum, 300 mg) for 9 mo		4
	Skin test-positive contacts of cases with isoniazid-resistant rifampin-susceptible organisms	Proposed	Rifampin PO	10–20 mg/kg daily (maximum, 600 mg) for 9 mo		
Yaws	Close contact of a case	Shown	Benzathine penicillin G IM	<10 yr: 600,000 U ≥10 yr: 1,200,000 U	No	19

*Some recommended drugs and dosages are subject to change.
BCG, bacille Calmette-Guérin; IM, intramuscularly; PO, orally.

Erythromycin and benzathine penicillin G have been shown to be effective in eliminating pharyngeal carriage of *Corynebacterium diphtheriae* in 92 and 84 percent, respectively, of those treated.[121] The effectiveness of these drugs as chemoprophylaxis against diphtheria has not been studied. However, the high incidence of diphtheria in nonimmune household contacts of cases,[61] the side effects of diphtheria antitoxin, and delay associated with and the possible false negativity of cultures are points in favor of giving chemoprophylaxis. Because the vaccine is directed against the toxin, immunized persons still may be carriers and become infected; thus, chemoprophylaxis should be administered to all close contacts regardless of immunization status. All close contacts should be cultured and kept under surveillance for 7 days. Patients with positive cultures should complete a full course of antimicrobial treatment. Previously immunized contacts should receive a booster dose of vaccine. Active immunization should be initiated for those who have not been immunized fully in the past.

Individuals with primary or secondary pneumonic plague are potential sources of person-to-person spread. Tetracycline, sulfonamides (including sulfadiazine and trimethoprim-sulfamethoxazole), streptomycin, and chloramphenicol all have been used for treatment and variously suggested as agents for prophylaxis.[143, 170, 171] Doxycycline is the drug of choice for contacts older than 8 years, whereas trimethoprim-sulfamethoxazole is recommended for exposed children younger than 8 years. Chemoprophylaxis in contacts generally is practiced, and recent experience in the United States has not been associated with failure; however, the efficacy of chemoprophylaxis has not been determined.[143, 171]

Cholera typically is not spread from person to person in households. However, in developing countries, if the household secondary attack rate is known to be high, family contacts may be treated prophylactically with tetracycline or doxycycline to prevent illness.[159] In the United States, prophylactic treatment is not recommended unless a high likelihood exists of secondary transmission as a result of unusually poor sanitary or hygienic conditions. After the first day of prophylaxis, tetracycline prophylaxis for 5 days is associated with a 12.6 to 0.3 percent decrease in cholera cases in contacts.[122] Some strains of cholera are tetracycline-resistant; alternative drugs include trimethoprim-sulfamethoxazole, erythromycin, and furazolidone. Tetracyclines cause staining of developing teeth and should not be used in children younger than 8 years.

Mass campaigns of treatment of patients with yaws and their community contacts have been successful in markedly decreasing the prevalence of the disease, although transmission has not been stopped completely.[21] Similar campaigns have been even more effective in the control of hyperendemic nonvenereal syphilis.

Chloroquine is effective prophylaxis against malarial parasitemia caused by *Plasmodium vivax, Plasmodium ovale, Plasmodium malariae,* and chloroquine-sensitive strains of *Plasmodium falciparum;* however, chloroquine resistance of *P. falciparum* has spread to most areas of the world with malaria.[36, 49] Mefloquine is an effective prophylactic agent against drug-resistant *P. falciparum,* but it is not approved for children weighing less than 15 kg or for pregnant women. However, for children weighing less than 15 kg, the CDC Traveler's Health website recommends a mefloquine dose of 4.6 mg/kg base (5 mg/kg salt) orally once a week (*www.cdc.gov/travel/mal_kids_hc.htm*). Alternative regimens, including doxycycline and proguanil, are contraindicated in small children and pregnant women or are incompletely effective. Thus, persons anticipating travel to areas with chloroquine-resistant *P. falciparum* must weigh carefully the risks of acquiring disease and the problems associated with prophylaxis for small children and pregnant women.[29, 36, 49] Detailed recommendations for preventing malaria are available 24 hours a day from the CDC by telephone at 877-394-8747 (toll-free voice information system) or 888-232-3299 (toll-free facsimile request line) or on the Internet at *http://www.cdc.gov/travel/diseases.htm#malaria.*

P. vivax and *P. ovale,* which have an extra-erythrocytic form, may relapse after chloroquine therapy has been stopped. Primaquine, taken as terminal prophylaxis after leaving the malarious area, decreases the risk of having relapses; however, it may cause severe hemolysis in persons with glucose-6-phosphate dehydrogenase deficiency.[49] Deciding whether to give terminal prophylaxis with primaquine depends on individual factors, including the degree of the traveler's risk of acquiring *Plasmodium* with an extra-erythrocytic form and the potential for having adverse reactions; primaquine generally is indicated for persons who have had prolonged exposure in endemic areas.

WATER PURIFICATION

The average per capita use of water in the United States is approximately 600 L/day. Provision of a safe and plentiful water supply is a major factor in preventing some communicable diseases. Purification of water occurs both naturally and through human intervention. Natural methods include evaporation and condensation, filtration through the earth, and a series of processes acting during the flow of a stream or on standing: aeration, light-accelerated plant growth, gravity, and oxidation and reduction of organic material by bacteria.[137] Municipal water treatment programs use a variety of measures, including protection of the watershed, chemical disinfection, and filtration of surface water supplies such as lakes and rivers, to ensure the safety of community water supplies.[32] Failure in one of these systems can result in widespread outbreak of water-borne disease. Although many such outbreaks involve a few dozen to a few hundred persons, more than 400,000 cases of illness may have resulted from an outbreak of cryptosporidiosis in Milwaukee, Wisconsin, in 1993.[115] The outbreak was associated with a marked increase in turbidity of the water supply and failure of coagulation and filtration at the water treatment plant to remove oocysts of *Cryptosporidium* from the treated water.

Since 1971, the CDC and the Environmental Protection Agency have maintained a voluntary surveillance system for the reporting of water-borne disease outbreaks. Figure 244–1 shows the annual number of outbreaks of disease associated with water intended for drinking that were reported from 1971 to 1998 in the United States.[89, 111, 130] After 1983, the number of reported outbreaks of water-borne disease in which an etiologic agent has been identified appears to have diminished.[38] The factors apparently resulting in these outbreaks were treatment deficiencies, untreated ground water, deficiencies in the distribution system, untreated surface water, and unknown or multiple factors. Outbreaks more commonly occurred in the summer; 25 percent of the outbreaks occurred in the month of July.

An increasingly important problem is the occurrence of outbreaks of water-borne disease associated with recreational water use, as for swimming or wading and in hot tubs or spas.[23, 28, 116, 130, 145] From 1997 to 1998, 18 states reported 32 outbreaks associated with recreational water.[38] The median outbreak size was 11 persons (range, 1 to 650). Nine of the 18 outbreaks of gastroenteritis were caused by parasites, 4 by bacteria, and 2 by viruses. Fifteen were associated with fresh water and 17 with treated water. Diseases transmitted in this manner include shigellosis, cryptosporidiosis, Norwalk virus diarrhea, viral conjunctivitis, giardiasis, legionellosis, and *Pseudomonas* dermatitis. Deaths may occur, especially with cases of primary amebic meningoencephalitis caused by *Naegleria* infection in persons who recently have been swimming.[31]

MILK SANITATION

Milk has been demonstrated as the vehicle of transmission in outbreaks of brucellosis, tuberculosis, and diphtheria, as well as outbreaks of diseases caused by group A streptococci, *Salmonella, Shigella, Campylobacter, Listeria, Y. enterocolitica,* and staphylococcal toxin.[146] Although the quality of milk has improved steadily in the United States—largely

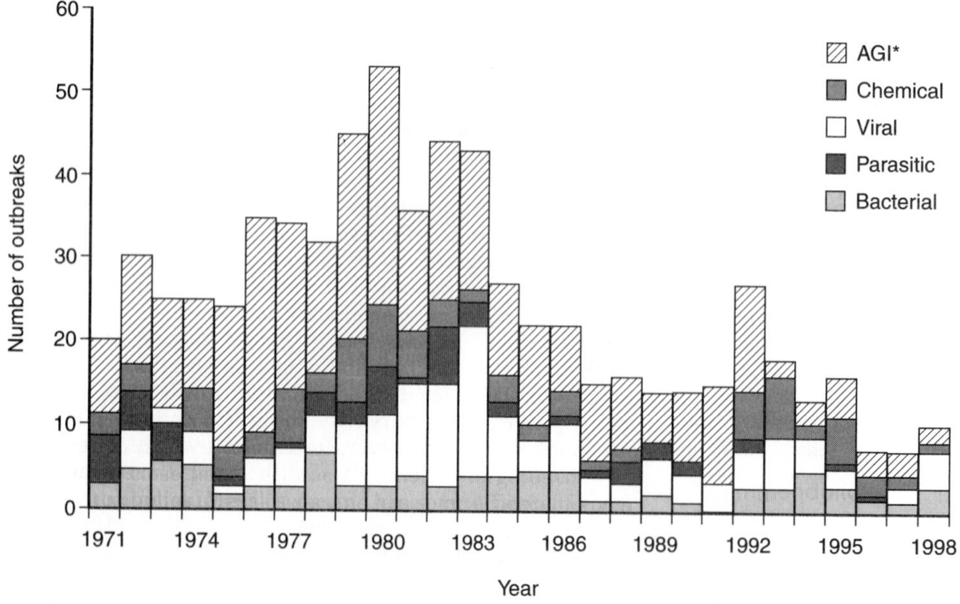

FIGURE 244–1 ■ Number of water-borne disease outbreaks associated with drinking water by year, United States, 1971–1998. (From Barwick, R. S., Levey, D. A., Craun, G. F., et al.: Surveillance for water-borne disease outbreaks—United States, 1997–1998. In CDC Surveillance Summaries, May 26, 2000. M. M. W. R. *49*[SS-4]:1–35, 2000.)

*Acute gastrointestinal illness of unknown etiology.

through mechanization and sanitation of milking operations, pasteurization, and cold storage—the use of raw milk as a "health food" continues to account for outbreaks of disease, particularly outbreaks caused by *Salmonella* and *Campylobacter*.[146] Children sometimes drink raw milk while visiting dairy farms on school field trips or other youth activities; a retrospective survey of state health departments identified 20 outbreaks involving a total of 458 cases of *Campylobacter* enteritis occurring as a result of such activities during the period 1981 to 1990.[173]

The quality of milk is monitored by a standard bacterial plate count, the phosphatase test (an assay for prior pasteurization), and measurement of the density of coliform organisms.[73] Nonetheless, pasteurized milk has been associated with outbreaks of enteric disease.[70, 149] Both post-pasteurization contamination at the dairy[149] and intrinsic contamination with survival of organisms despite adequate pasteurization[70] have been suggested as possible mechanisms of transmission.

The incidence of outbreaks of milk-borne disease has decreased greatly in the past 40 years in the United States.[11, 12, 41] From 1917 to 1941, 168 outbreaks (7 per year) were traced to raw milk in New York State alone.[64] From 1993 to 1997, fewer than three milk-borne outbreaks per year were reported for the entire country.[138] The most common etiologic agent was *Salmonella.* One outbreak, caused by antimicrobial-resistant *Salmonella typhimurium* that contaminated pasteurized 2 percent milk, was the largest outbreak of *Salmonella* infection ever identified in the United States; an estimated 200,000 people were affected.[149]

FOOD SANITATION

Foods other than milk have been shown to be the vehicle of transmission in outbreaks caused by 10 or more genera of bacteria, hepatitis A virus, Norwalk-like viruses, and a variety of parasites, in addition to a wide range of toxic chemicals. Major public health programs in the United States involving inspection of meat and poultry, shellfish sanitation, and inspection of public eating and drinking places have had a significant impact, notably in reduction of the incidence of tuberculosis and brucellosis in cattle and limitation of spread of typhoid and hepatitis A by contaminated shellfish. Significant problem areas remain, however. Contamination of meat, poultry, and eggs with *Salmonella, Yersinia, E. coli* O157:H7, *Listeria,* and other pathogens and deficiencies in food storage and preparation both in eating establishments and in the home still contribute to outbreaks and sporadic cases.[12, 15, 110, 151, 157] Several outbreaks of *E. coli* O157:H7 infection and hemolytic-uremic syndrome have been related to apple juice.[91] In addition, new problems can result from changes in the food industry and in patterns of food consumption.[87] In recent years, several large outbreaks of salmonellosis have been associated with the widespread distribution of fresh produce, a previously rare vehicle of *Salmonella* transmission. These outbreaks have occurred after notable increases during the past 2 decades in the per-capita consumption of fresh fruits and vegetables in the United States.[30, 87] Larger, centralized production and processing facilities with extensive distribution networks may increase the number of persons affected when commercial products do become contaminated.[12, 15, 112, 149] In a global economy, the importation of food from resource-poor countries is another source of contaminated food. For example, multistate outbreaks have been linked to the importation of foods, such as cyclosporiasis associated with raspberries from Guatemala.[35] Adequate cooking of foods, proper canning techniques (both commercial and home), and refrigeration are major contributors to control of outbreaks of food-borne disease. In approximately half of the outbreaks of food-borne disease, one or more food preparation practices are reported to be contributing factors; improper storage or holding temperature is reported in approximately two thirds of these outbreaks and poor personal hygiene of the food handler in approximately two fifths.[11, 12]

Although the number of outbreaks reported to public health authorities represents only a small fraction of those that occur, these reports can provide important insight into the epidemiology of food-borne disease. From 1993 to 1997, the number of outbreaks and the number of cases reported annually remained relatively constant[138] (Table 244–4). The specific cause is confirmed in approximately 30 percent of all outbreaks, and of these, bacterial pathogens, particularly *Salmonella,* account for the majority. Other infectious etiologic agents include *Clostridium botulinum, Clostridium perfringens, Campylobacter, Shigella, Vibrio cholerae,* hepatitis A virus, *Giardia,* and *Trichinella spiralis.* From 1993 to 1997, *Salmonella enteritidis* remained the most commonly isolated cause of outbreaks of food-borne disease.[138]

HEALTH INFORMATION FOR INTERNATIONAL TRAVEL

International travel, whether by child or adult, necessitates preparation beforehand to obtain the proper immunizations, contingency plans for the possibility of encountering

TABLE 244–4 ■ FOOD-BORNE DISEASE OUTBREAKS AND CASES REPORTED IN THE UNITED STATES, 1993–1997, BY ETIOLOGY

	1993	1994	1995	1996	1997
Total number of outbreaks/cases reported	484/17,477	653/16,234	628/17,800	477/22,607	504/11,940
Total number of reported outbreaks with a confirmed cause	168	197	194	151	168
Percent of all reported outbreaks with a confirmed cause	34	30	31	32	33
Number of outbreaks/cases caused by bacterial diseases	135/10,402	148/5487	155/10,017	112/14,219	105/3696
Number of outbreaks/cases caused by *Salmonella*	68/7122	70/2858	90/8449	69/12,450	60/1731
Percent of all bacterial outbreaks caused by *Salmonella*	50	47	58	62	57
Number of outbreaks/cases caused by chemical agents	21/75	37/161	29/133	26/85	35/122
Number of outbreaks/cases caused by viral diseases	10/757	10/612	9/512	10/1420	17/765
Number of outbreaks/cases caused by parasitic diseases	2/16	2/22	1/9	3/1588	11/690

Adapted from Olsen, S. J., MacKinnon, L. C., Goulding, J. S., et al.: Surveillance for foodborne-disease outbreaks: United States, 1993–1997. Morb. Mortal. Wkly. Rep. C. D. C.. Surveill. Summ. *49* (SS-1):1-62, 2000.

unsanitary food or water during the travel, and the realization that illnesses acquired abroad may not be manifested until return home, with consequent diagnostic difficulty.[10]

Needs for active and passive immunization are covered elsewhere in this book and are summarized fully in two continuously updated CDC publications to which the reader is referred: *Health Information for International Travel*[33] (which can be purchased from the Superintendent of Documents, U.S. Government Printing Office, Washington, D.C., 20402) and the *Morbidity and Mortality Weekly Report.* The CDC travel Web site also is very helpful as a source of up-to-date information for travelers (www.cdc.gov/travel).

Safe water may be found in many hotels in large cities throughout the world, but only water from adequately chlorinated sources can be considered truly safe. Where chlorinated water is not available, canned or bottled carbonated beverages and beverages made from boiled water (as well as beer or wine) may be safe. Transmission of cholera by uncarbonated bottled mineral water has been described.[17] Ice made from unchlorinated water may contaminate an otherwise safe beverage, either directly or by leaving contaminated water on the outside of the container. Although heat treatment by boiling is the most reliable method to render questionable water potable, chemical treatment also can be used.[33]

HEAT

1. Bring the water to a vigorous boil. Allow to cool at room temperature—do not add ice. At very high altitudes, for an extra margin of safety, boil for several minutes or use chemical disinfection.
2. Adding a pinch of salt to each quart or pouring the water from one clean container to another several times will improve the taste.

CHEMICALS

1. Tincture of iodine. Follow the directions in Table 244–5. Let stand for at least 30 minutes.
2. Tetraglycine hydroperiodide tablets (can be purchased at pharmacies and sporting goods stores). The manufacturer's instructions should be followed. If the water is cloudy, the number of tablets should be doubled; if the water is extremely cold, an attempt should be made to warm the water, and the recommended contact time should be increased to achieve reliable disinfection.

Cloudy water should be strained through a clean cloth into a container to remove any sediment or floating matter before treatment with heat or iodine. Although chlorine has been used for chemical disinfection, its germicidal activity varies greatly with pH, temperature, and the organic content of the water to be purified, and therefore it is less reliable than iodine.

TABLE 244–5 ■ TREATMENT OF WATER WITH TINCTURE OF IODINE

Tincture of Iodine	Drops* to Be Added per Quart or Liter of	
	Clean Water	Cold or Cloudy Water†
2%	5	10
1. Let stand for 30 minutes.		
2. Water is safe to use.		

*One drop is 0.05 mL.
†Very turbid or very cold water may require prolonged contact time; let stand up to several hours before use, if possible.
Adapted from Centers for Disease Control and Prevention: Health Information for International Travel 1995. HHS Publication No. (CDC) 95-8280, 1995.

Food should be selected carefully. In areas of the world where hygiene and sanitation are poor, the traveler should avoid intake of salads, uncooked vegetables, unpasteurized milk, and milk products such as cheese and should eat only food that can be peeled by the traveler or has been cooked and is still hot.

Children 0 to 2 years of age have a high risk of acquiring traveler's diarrhea.[36, 142] Immediate medical attention should be sought for an infant or child with blood or mucus in the stool, fever with rigors, or persistent vomiting or diarrhea with dehydration. Because infants and small children are especially at risk for becoming dehydrated, parents need to be aware of the signs of dehydration (Table 244–6) and be prepared to use oral rehydration therapy as a preventive measure while medical attention is being obtained. Replacing fluid losses may be achieved best by the use of an oral rehydration solution containing appropriate concentrations of electrolytes and glucose.[36, 65, 139] Oral rehydration solution packets are available at stores or pharmacies in almost all developing countries. The solution is prepared by adding one packet to the appropriate volume of boiled or treated water.[139]

Although prophylaxis with several different agents, including trimethoprim-sulfamethoxazole, doxycycline, fluoroquinolone antibiotics, and bismuth subsalicylate, may prevent some cases of traveler's diarrhea in adults, no drug has been shown to be both safe and effective for this purpose in children. Iodoquinol (Entero-Vioform) is especially dangerous because of its association with subacute myelo-optic neuropathy. Administration of bismuth subsalicylate may lead to salicylate toxicity.

VECTOR CONTROL

Techniques of environmental control of vectors responsible for the transmission of disease have included eradication of habitats for mosquito larvae, construction of rat-proof houses, and elimination of rodent habitats.[174] In some instances, dam construction, large-scale irrigation projects, and deforestation have led to increases in the density of vectors responsible for the transmission of schistosomiasis, onchocerciasis, and mosquito-borne diseases.

Chemical control of vectors, which seemed so attractive a few years ago, has been complicated by environmental contamination by undegraded chemicals and by the appearance of vectors resistant to the organochlorine insecticides (DDT, dieldrin), organophosphorus insecticides (malathion, fenitrothion), and carbonates (propoxur, carbaryl). The persistence of DDT and dieldrin in the environment has resulted in their being banned in some countries and their use being severely restricted in others. The use of ultra-low-volume spraying, as with malathion in the control of malaria, has permitted the use of minimal amounts of insecticide while still effecting a decrease in the incidence of disease over a considerable area.[107]

The rising incidence of tick-borne diseases, especially Lyme disease, has led to an increased interest in methods for the control of ticks and their animal hosts. Area-wide spraying of pesticides in residential areas may reduce tick populations but also may pose health or environmental risks if these chemicals are applied improperly. Personal protection includes avoiding vector-infested areas, wearing protective clothing, using insect repellents applied to skin (e.g., *N,N*-diethyl-*meta*-toluamide) or to clothing (permethrin), and frequently inspecting for and promptly removing attached

TABLE 244–6 ■ ASSESSMENT OF DEHYDRATION LEVELS IN INFANTS

	Signs of Dehydration		
	Mild	Moderate	Severe
General condition	Thirsty, restless, agitated	Thirsty, restless, irritable	Withdrawn, somnolent, or comatose
Pulse	Normal	Rapid and weak	Rapid and weak
Anterior fontanelle	Normal	Sunken	Very sunken
Eyes	Normal	Sunken	Very sunken
Tears	Present	Absent	Absent
Urine	Normal	Reduced and concentrated	None for several hours
Weight loss	4–5%	6–9%	≥10%

Adapted from Centers for Disease Control and Prevention: Health Information for International Travel 1995. HHS Publication No. (CDC) 95-8280, 1995.

ticks. These individual preventive measures can be practiced in any circumstance where exposure to infected ticks may occur.[6]

Experimental work with genetic and biologic control of vectors has had limited success, as with the use of larvivorous fish, chemosterilized male mosquitoes, and parasites that attack the vector.[6, 22]

Appendix

The attack rate was considerably higher in patients attended by any of eight people (four surgeons, an anesthesiologist, and three nurses) than in patients who were not. Only for Sutterfield, the anesthesiologist, however, was the difference so marked that the probability of the association's occurring by chance alone was less than 0.05 (Table 244–7). The attack rate in patients when Sutterfield was listed in the operating room log as the anesthesiologist was 43 percent (10/23), as opposed to an attack rate of 13 percent (3/24) when Sutterfield was not listed. (Note that these attack rates are artificially high because four fifths of the actual controls have been omitted, but the comparison is still valid.) This finding appears to implicate Sutterfield as the source of infection (step 6).

The three patients who became ill but for whom Sutterfield's name did not appear in their record must be explained. Interviews with the anesthesiology staff determined that frequently, one anesthesiologist would spell another for brief periods during a long procedure without recording the fact on the operating room log; this policy may explain the three outliers (step 7).

To confirm the hypothesis microbiologically, cultures were made from throat, nose, skin, and anus specimens from two surgeons, Sutterfield, and three nurses. Only from Sutterfield, and only from his anus, were group A streptococci recovered; the strain was M nontypable T 28, the same strain isolated from the patients (step 8). Subsequently, Sutterfield was treated with antibiotics, and his streptococcal carriage was eradicated (step 9). Prospective surveillance for group A streptococcal wound infections in the hospital showed none in the subsequent several months (step 10).

TABLE 244–7 ■ RECORDED INTRAOPERATIVE CARE BY ANESTHESIOLOGIST SUTTERFIELD AMONG CASES OF GROUP A STREPTOCOCCAL WOUND INFECTION AND CONTROLS

		Cases	Controls	Total
Recorded contact with Sutterfield	Yes	10	13	23
	No	3	21	24
	Total	13	34	47

χ^2 is 5.63, 1 d.f.; *p* is 0.18.

REFERENCES

1. Acha, P. N., and Szyfres, B.: Zoonoses and Communicable Diseases Common to Man and Animals. 2nd ed. Washington, D.C., Pan American Health Organization, 1987.
2. Adams, W. G., Deaver, K. A., Cochi, S. L., et al.: Decline of childhood *Haemophilus influenzae* type b (Hib) disease in the Hib vaccine era. J. A. M. A. *269*:221–226, 1993.
3. Adler, S. P.: Cytomegalovirus transmission and child day care. Adv. Pediatr. Infect. Dis. *7*:109–122, 1992.
4. American Academy of Pediatrics, Committee on Infectious Diseases: Meningococcal disease prevention and control strategies for practice-based physicians. (Addendum: Recommendations for college students.) Pediatrics *106*:1500–1504, 2000.
5. American Thoracic Society: Treatment of tuberculosis and tuberculosis infection in adults and children. Am. J. Respir. Crit. Care Med. *149*: 1359–1374, 1994.
6. Anderson, J. F.: Preventing Lyme disease. Rheum. Dis. Clin. North Am. *15*:757–766, 1989.
7. Anderson, L. J., Parker, R. A., Strikas, R. A., et al.: Day-care center attendance and hospitalization for lower respiratory tract illness. Pediatrics *82*:300–308, 1988.
8. Bace, A., Zrnic, T., Begovac, J., et al.: Short-term treatment of pertussis with azithromycin in infants and young children. Eur. J. Clin. Infect. Dis. *18*:296–298, 1999.
9. Band, J. D., Fraser, D. W., and Ajello, G.: *Hemophilus influenzae* disease study group: Prevention of *Hemophilus influenzae* type b disease. J. A. M. A. *251*:2381–2386, 1984.
10. Barry, M.: Medical considerations for international travel with infants and older children. Infect. Dis. Clin. North Am. *6*:389–404, 1992.
11. Bean, N. H., Goulding, J. S., Lao, C., et al.: Surveillance for foodborne-disease outbreaks—United States, 1988–1992. Morb. Mortal. Wkly. Rep. C. D. C. Surveill. Summ. *45*(SS-5):1–66, 1996.
12. Bean, N. H., Griffin, P. M., Goulding, J. S., and Ivey, C. B.: Foodborne disease outbreaks, 5-year summary, 1983–1987. Morb. Mortal. Wkly. Rep. C. D. C. Surveill. Summ. *39*(1):15–57, 1990.
13. Becker, T. M., Kodsi, R., Bailey, P., et al.: Grappling with herpes: Herpes gladiatorum. Am. J. Sports Med. *16*:665–669, 1988.
14. Beer, B., O'Donnell, G. M., and Henderson, R. J.: A school outbreak of Sonne dysentery controlled by hygienic measures. Monthly Bull. Ministry Health (Lond.) *25*:36–41, 1966.
15. Bell, B. P., Goldoft, M., Griffin, P. M., et al.: A multistate outbreak of *Escherichia coli* O157:H7-associated bloody diarrhea and hemolytic uremic syndrome from hamburgers: The Washington experience. J. A. M. A. *272*:1349–1353, 1994.
16. Beran, G. W. (ed.-in-chief): Handbook of Zoonoses. 2nd ed. Boca Raton, FL, CRC Press, 1994.
17. Blake, P. A., Rosenberg, M. L., Florencia, J., et al.: Cholera in Portugal, 1974. II. Transmission by bottled mineral water. Am. J. Epidemiol. *105*:344–348, 1977.
18. Brimblecombe, F. S. W., Cruickshank, R., Masters, P. L., et al.: Family studies of respiratory infections. B. M. J. *1*:119–128, 1958.

19. Briss, P. A., Fehrs, L. J., Parker, R. A., et al.: Sustained transmission of mumps in a highly vaccinated population: Assessment of primary vaccine failure and waning vaccine-induced immunity. J. Infect. Dis. *169*:77–82, 1994.
20. Broome, C. V., LaVenture, M., Kaye, H. S., et al.: An explosive outbreak of *Mycoplasma pneumoniae* infection in a summer camp. Pediatrics *66*:884–888, 1980.
21. Brown, S. T.: Therapy for nonvenereal treponematoses: Review of the efficacy of penicillin and consideration of alternatives. Rev. Infect. Dis. *7*(Suppl.):318–326, 1985.
22. Bruce-Chwatt, L. J.: Malaria and its control: Present situation and future prospects. Annu. Rev. Public Health *8*:75–110, 1987.
23. Caldwell, G. G., Lindsey, N. J., Wulff, H., et al.: Epidemic of adenovirus type 7 acute conjunctivitis in swimmers. Am. J. Epidemiol. *99*:230–234, 1974.
24. Cann, K. J., Rogers, T. R., Jones, D. M., et al.: *Neisseria meningitidis* in a primary school. Arch. Dis. Child. *62*:1113–1117, 1987.
25. Catanzaro, F. J., Stetson, C. A., Morris, A. J., et al.: The role of *Streptococcus* in the pathogenesis of rheumatic fever. Am. J. Med. *17*:749–756, 1954.
26. Centers for Disease Control and Prevention: Guidelines for evaluating surveillance systems. M. M. W. R. Morb. Mortal. Wkly. Rep. *37*(Suppl. 5):1–18, 1988.
27. Centers for Disease Control and Prevention: Risks associated with human parvovirus B19 infection. M. M. W. R. Morb. Mortal. Wkly. Rep. *38*(6):81–88, 93–97, 1989.
28. Centers for Disease Control and Prevention: Swimming-associated cryptosporidiosis—Los Angeles County. M. M. W. R. Morb. Mortal. Wkly. Rep. *39*(20):343–345, 1990.
29. Centers for Disease Control and Prevention: Change of dosing regimen for malaria prophylaxis with mefloquine. M. M. W. R. Morb. Mortal. Wkly. Rep. *40*(4):72–73, 1991.
30. Centers for Disease Control and Prevention: Multistate outbreak of *Salmonella poona* infections—United States and Canada, 1991. M. M. W. R. Morb. Mortal. Wkly. Rep. *40*(32):549–552, 1991.
31. Centers for Disease Control and Prevention: Primary amebic meningoencephalitis—North Carolina, 1991. M. M. W. R. Morb. Mortal. Wkly. Rep. *41*(25):437–440, 1992.
32. Centers for Disease Control and Prevention: Assessment of inadequately filtered public drinking water—Washington, D.C., December 1993. M. M. W. R. Morb. Mortal. Wkly. Rep. *43*(36):661–669, 1994.
33. Centers for Disease Control and Prevention: Health Information for International Travel 1995. HHS Publication No. (CDC) 95-8280, 1995.
34. Centers for Disease Control and Prevention: Recommendations for preventing the spread of vancomycin resistance. Recommendation of the Hospital Infection Control Practices Advisory Committee (HICPAC). M. M. W. R. Recomm. Rep. *44*(RR-12):1–13, 1995.
35. Centers for Disease Control and Prevention: Outbreak of cyclosporiasis—Ontario, Canada, May, 1998. M. M. W. R. Morb. Mortal. Wkly. Rep. *47*(38):806–809, 1998.
36. Centers for Disease Control and Prevention: Summary of Notifiable Diseases—United States, 2000. M. M. W. R. Morb. Mortal. Wkly. Rep. *49*(53):1–100, 2000.
37. Centers for Disease Control and Prevention: Biological and chemical terrorism: Strategic plan for the preparedness and response. Recommendations of the CDC Strategic Planning Workgroup. M. M. W. R. Recomm. Rep. *49*(RR-4):14, 2000.
38. Centers for Disease Control and Prevention: M. M. W. R. Surveillance summaries. Surveillance for waterborne-disease outbreaks. Morb. Mortal. Wkly. Rep. C. D. C. Surveill. Summ. *49*(SS-4):1–35, 2000.
39. Centers for Disease Control and Prevention: Update: Investigation of bioterrorism-related anthrax and interim guidelines for exposure management and antimicrobial therapy, October 2001. M. M. W. R. Morb. Mortal. Wkly. Rep. *50*(42):909–919, 2001.
40. Centers for Disease Control and Prevention: Update: Interim recommendations for antimicrobial prophylaxis for children and breastfeeding mothers and treatment of children with anthrax. M. M. W. R. Morb. Mortal. Wkly. Rep. *50*(45):1014–1016, 2001.
41. Centers for Disease Control and Prevention: Diagnosis and management of foodborne illnesses. A primer for physicians. M. M. W. R. Recomm. Rep. *50*(RR-2):1–69, 2001.
42. Centers for Disease Control and Prevention: Pertussis—United States, 1997–2000, M. M. W. R. Morb. Mortal. Wkly. Rep. *51*(4):73–76, 2002.
43. Centers for Disease Control and Prevention: Progress toward elimination of *Haemophilus influenzae* type b invasive disease among infants and children—United States, 1998–2000. M. M. W. R. Morb. Mortal. Wkly. Rep. *51*(11):234–237, 2002.
44. Centers for Disease Control and Prevention: Preliminary FoodNet data on the incidence of foodborne illnesses—selected sites, United States, 2001. M. M. W. R. Morb. Mortal. Wkly. Rep. *51*(15):325–329, 2002.
45. Centers for Disease Control and Prevention: Update: Cutaneous anthrax in a laboratory worker—Texas, 2002. M. M. W. R. Morb. Mortal. Wkly. Rep. *51*(22):482, 2002.
46. Centers for Disease Control and Prevention: West Nile virus activity—United States, 2001. M. M. W. R. Morb. Mortal. Wkly. Rep. *51*(23): 497–501, 2002.
47. Centers for Disease Control and Prevention: Diagnosis and reporting of HIV and AIDS in states with HIV/AIDS surveillance—United States, 1994–2000. M. M. W. R. Morb. Mortal. Wkly. Rep. *51*(27):595–598, 2002.
48. Centers for Disease Control and Prevention: 2002 Sexually transmitted diseases. Treatment guidelines. M. M. W. R. Recomm. Rep. *51*(RR-6): 1–78, 2002.
49. Centers for Disease Control and Prevention: Malaria Surveillance—United States, 2000. Morb. Mortal. Wkly. Rep. C. D. C. Surveill. Summ. *51*(SS-5):2–21, 2002.
50. Chen, R. T., Goldbaum, G. M., Wassilak, S. G. F., et al.: An explosive point-source measles outbreak in a highly vaccinated population. Am. J. Epidemiol. *129*:173–182, 1989.
51. Chin, J. (ed.): Control of Communicable Diseases Manual. 17th ed. Washington, D.C., American Public Health Association, 2000.
52. Chorba, T. L., Berkelman, R. L., Safford, S. K., et al.: Mandatory reporting of infectious diseases by clinicians. J. A. M. A. *262*:3018–3026, 1989.
53. Cochi, S. L., Fleming, D. W., Hightower, A. W., et al.: Primary invasive *Haemophilus influenzae* type b disease: A population-based assessment of risk factors. J. Pediatr. *108*:887–896, 1986.
54. Cochi, S. L., Preblud, S. R., and Orenstein, W. A.: Perspectives on the relative resurgence of mumps in the United States. Am. J. Dis. Child. *142*: 499–507, 1988.
55. Committee on Infectious Diseases, American Academy of Pediatrics: Screening for tuberculosis in infants and children. Pediatrics *93*:131–134, 1994.
56. Committee on Infectious Diseases, American Academy of Pediatrics: 2000 Red Book: Report of the Committee on Infectious Diseases. 25th ed. Elk Grove Village, IL, American Academy of Pediatrics, 2000.
57. Currier, R. W., Hardy, G. E., Jr., and Conrad, J. L.: Measles in previously vaccinated children: Evaluation of an outbreak. Am. J. Dis. Child. *124*:854–857, 1972.
58. Dajani, A. S., Taubert, K., Ferrieri, P., et al.: Treatment of acute streptococcal pharyngitis and prevention of rheumatic fever: A statement for health professionals. Pediatrics *96*:758–764, 1995.
59. Denny, F. W., Collier, A. M., and Henderson, F. W.: Acute respiratory infections in day care. Rev. Infect. Dis. *8*:527–532, 1986.
60. Dingle, J. H., Badger, G. F., and Jordan, W. S., Jr.: Illness in the Home: A Study of 25,000 Illnesses in a Group of Cleveland Families. Cleveland, Western Reserve University, 1964.
61. Doull, J. A.: Factors influencing selective distribution in diphtheria. Prev. Med. *4*:371–404, 1930.
62. Dowling, J. N., Sheehe, P. R., and Feldman, H. A.: Pharyngeal pneumococcal acquisition in "normal" families: A longitudinal study. J. Infect. Dis. *124*:9–17, 1971.
63. Drumm, B., Perez-Perez, G. I., Blaser, M. J., et al.: Intrafamilial clustering of *Helicobacter pylori* infection. N. Engl. J. Med. *322*:359–363, 1990.
64. Dublin, T. D., Rogers, E. F. H., Perkins, J. E., et al.: Milkborne outbreaks due to serologically typed hemolytic streptococci. Am. J. Public Health *33*:157–166, 1943.
65. Duggan, C., Santosham, M., and Glass, R. I.: The management of acute diarrhea in children: Oral rehydration, maintenance, and nutritional therapy. M. M. W. R. Recomm. Rep. *41*(RR-16):1–20, 1992.
66. Dwyer, D. M., Strickler, H., Goodman, R. A., et al.: Use of case-control studies in outbreak investigations. Epidemiol. Rev. *16*:109–123, 1994.
67. El Kholy, A., Fraser, D. W., Guirguis, N., et al.: A controlled study of penicillin therapy of group A streptococcal acquisitions in Egyptian families. J. Infect. Dis. *141*:759–771, 1980.
68. Ferebee, S. H.: Controlled chemoprophylaxis trials in tuberculosis: A general review. Adv. Tuberc. Res. *17*:38–106, 1970.
69. Filice, G. A., and Fraser, D. W.: Management of household contacts of leprosy patients. Ann. Intern. Med. *88*:538–542, 1978.
70. Fleming, D. W., Cochi, S. L., MacDonald, K. L., et al.: Pasteurized milk as a vehicle of infection in an outbreak of listeriosis. N. Engl. J. Med. *312*:404–407, 1985.
71. Fox, J. P., Cooney, M. K., Hall, C. E., et al.: Influenza virus infections in Seattle families, 1975–1979. II. Pattern of infection in invaded households and relation of age and prior antibody to occurrence of infection and related illness. Am. J. Epidemiol. *116*:228–242, 1982.
72. Frank, J. A., Jr., Orenstein, W. A., Bart, K. J., et al.: Major impediments to measles elimination: The modern epidemiology of an ancient disease. Am. J. Dis. Child. *139*:881–888, 1985.
73. Frank J. F., and Barnhart M. H.: Food and dairy sanitation. *In* Last, J. M., and Wallace R. B. (eds.): Maxcy-Rosenau-Last Public Health and Preventive Medicine. 13th ed. E. Norwalk, Appleton & Lange, 1992, pp. 589–618.
74. Fraser, D. W.: *Haemophilus influenzae* in the community and the home. *In* Sell, S. H., and Wright, P. F. (eds.): *Haemophilus influenzae:* Epidemiology, Immunology and Prevention of Disease. New York, Elsevier Biomedical, 1982.
75. Friede, A., Harris, J. R., Kobayashi, J. M., et al.: Transmission of hepatitis B virus from adopted Asian children to their American families. Am. J. Public Health *78*:26–29, 1988.
76. Frost, W. H.: The familial aggregation of infectious diseases. Am. J. Public Health *28*:7–13, 1938.

77. Gelfand, H. M., LeBlanc, D. R., Fox, J. P., et al.: Studies on the development of natural immunity to poliomyelitis in Louisiana. II. Description and analysis of episodes of infection observed in study group households. Am. J. Hyg. *65*:367–385, 1957.
78. Gelfand, H. M., Potash, L., LeBlanc, D. R., et al.: Intrafamilial and interfamilial spread of living vaccine strains of polioviruses. J. A. M. A. *170*: 2039–2048, 1959.
79. Ghipponi, P., Darrigol, J., Skalova, R., et al.: Study of bacterial air pollution in an arid region of Africa affected by cerebrospinal meningitis. Bull. World Health Organ. *45*:95–101, 1971.
80. Glezen, W. P., Taber, L. H., Frank, A. L., et al.: Influenza virus infections in infants. Pediatr. Infect. Dis. J. *16*:1065–1068, 1997.
81. Gordis, L.: Effectiveness of comprehensive-care programs in preventing rheumatic fever. N. Engl. J. Med. *289*:331–335, 1973.
82. Granoff, D. M., and Daum, R. S.: Spread of *Haemophilus influenzae* type b: Recent epidemiologic and therapeutic considerations. J. Pediatr. *97*: 854–860, 1980.
83. Greenfield, S., Sheehe, P. R., and Feldman, H. A.: Meningococcal carriage in a population of "normal" families. J. Infect. Dis. *123*:67–73, 1971.
84. Gwaltney, J. M., Jr., Sande, M. A., Austrian, R., et al.: Pneumococcal spread in families. II. Transfer colds and serum antibody. J. Infect. Dis. *132*:62–68, 1975.
85. Hall, C. B., Geiman, J. M., Biggar, R., et al.: Respiratory syncytial virus infections within families. N. Engl. J. Med. *294*:414–419, 1976.
86. Hammerschlag, M. R., Cummings, C., Roblin, P. M., et al.: Efficacy of neonatal ocular prophylaxis for the prevention of chlamydial and gonococcal conjunctivitis. N. Engl. J. Med. *320*:769–772, 1989.
87. Hedberg, C. W., MacDonald, K. L., and Osterholm, M. T.: Changing epidemiology of food-borne disease: A Minnesota perspective. Clin. Infect. Dis. *18*:671–682, 1994.
88. Heijbel, H., Slaine, K., Seigel, B., et al.: Outbreak of diarrhea in a day care center with spread to household members: The role of *Cryptosporidium*. Pediatr. Infect. Dis. J. *6*:532–535, 1987.
89. Herwaldt, B. L., Craun, G. F., Stokes, S. L., et al.: Waterborne-disease outbreaks, 1989–1990. Morb. Mortal. Wkly. Rep. C. D. C. Surveill. Summ. *40*(SS-3):1–21, 1991.
90. Heun, E. M., Vogt, R. L., Hudson, P. J., et al.: Risk factors for secondary transmission in households after a common-source outbreak of Norwalk gastroenteritis. Am. J. Epidemiol. *126*:1181–1186, 1987.
91. Hilborn, E. D., Mshar, P. A., Fiorentino, T. R., et al.: An outbreak of *Escherichia coli* O157:H7 infections and haemolytic uraemic syndrome associated with consumption of unpasteurized apple cider. Epidemiol. Infect. *124*:31–36, 2000.
92. Hoge, C. W., Fisher, L., Donnell, H. D., Jr., et al.: Risk factors for transmission of *Mycobacterium tuberculosis* in a primary school outbreak: Lack of racial difference in susceptibility to infection. Am. J. Epidemiol. *139*:520–530, 1994.
93. Hoge, C. W., Reichler, M. R., Dominguez, E. A., et al.: An epidemic of pneumococcal disease in an overcrowded, inadequately ventilated jail. N. Engl. J. Med. *331*:643–648, 1994.
94. Hope-Simpson, R. E. H.: Infectiousness of communicable diseases in the household (measles, chicken pox, and mumps). Lancet *2*:549–554, 1952.
95. Hostetter, M. K., Iverson, S., Dole, K., et al.: Unsuspected infectious diseases and other medical diagnoses in the evaluation of internationally adopted children. Pediatrics *4*:559–564, 1989.
96. Huemer, H. P., Larcher, C., Czedik-Eysenberg, T., et al.: Fatal infection of a pet monkey with human herpesvirus 1. Emerg. Infect. Dis. *8*: 639–641, 2002.
97. Ikeda, R. M., Kondracki, S. F., Drabkin, P. D., et al.: Pleurodynia among football players at a high school. An outbreak associated with coxsackievirus B1. J. A. M. A. *270*:2205–2206, 1993.
98. Isenberg, S. J., Apt, L., and Wood, M.: A controlled trial of povidone-iodine as a prophylaxis against ophthalmia neonatorum. N. Engl. J. Med. *332*:562–566, 1995.
99. Istre, G. R.: Disease surveillance at the state and local level. *In* Halperin, W., Baker, E. L., and Monson, R. R. (eds.): Public Health Surveillance. New York, Van Nostrand Reinhold, 1992, pp. 42–55.
100. Jackson, L. A., Schuchat, A., Reeves, M. W., et al.: Serogroup C meningococcal outbreaks in the United States: An emerging threat. J. A. M. A. *273*:383–389, 1995.
101. Jacobson, J. A., Camargos, P. A. M., Ferreira, J. T., et al.: The risk of meningitis among classroom contacts during an epidemic of meningococcal disease. Am. J. Epidemiol. *104*:552–555, 1976.
102. James, W. E. S., Badger, G. F., and Dingle, J. H.: A study of illness in a group of Cleveland families. XIX. The epidemiology of the acquisition of group A streptococci and of associated illnesses. N. Engl. J. Med. *262*:687–694, 1960.
103. Jereb, J. A., Kelly, G. D., and Porterfield, D. S.: The epidemiology of tuberculosis in children. Semin. Pediatr. Infect. Dis. *4*:220–231, 1993.
104. Jernigan, J. A., Stephens, D. S., Ashford, D. A., et al.: Bioterrorism-related inhalational anthrax: The first 10 cases reported within the United States. Emerg. Infect. Dis. *7*:933–944, 2001.
105. Koch, W. C., and Adler, S. P.: Human parvovirus B19 infections in women of childbearing age and within families. Pediatr. Infect. Dis. *8*:83–87, 1989.
106. Koopman, J. S., Monto, A. S., and Longini, I. M.: The Tecumseh study. XVI. Family and community sources of rotavirus infection. Am. J. Epidemiol. *130*:760–768, 1989.
107. Krogstad, D. J., Joseph, V. R., and Newton, L. H.: A prospective study of the effects of ultralow volume (ULV) aerial application of malathion on epidemic *Plasmodium falciparum* malaria. Am. J. Trop. Med. Hyg. *24*:199–205, 1975.
108. Kurt, T. L., Yeager, A. S., Guenette, S., et al.: Spread of pertussis by hospital staff. J. A. M. A. *221*:264–267, 1972.
109. Landrigan, P. J.: Epidemic measles in a divided city. J. A. M. A. *221*:567–570, 1972.
110. Lee, L. A., Gerber, A. R., Lonsway, D. R., et al.: *Yersinia enterocolitica* 0:3 infections in infants and children, associated with the household preparation of chitterlings. N. Engl. J. Med. *322*:984–987, 1990.
111. Levine, W. C., Stevenson, W. T., and Craun, G. F.: Waterborne disease outbreaks, 1986–1988. Morb. Mortal. Wkly. Rep. C. D. C. Surveill. Summ. *39*(1):1–14, 1990.
112. Linnan, M. J., Mascola, L., Lou, X. D., et al.: Epidemic listeriosis associated with Mexican-style cheese. N. Engl. J. Med. *319*:823–829, 1988.
113. Linnemann, C. C., Jr., and Nasenbeny, J.: Pertussis in the adult. Annu. Rev. Med. *28*:179–185, 1977.
114. Linnemann, C. C., Jr., Perlstein, P. H., Ramundo, N., et al.: Use of pertussis vaccine in an epidemic involving hospital staff. Lancet *2*:540–541, 1975.
115. MacKenzie, W. R., Hoxie, N. J., Proctor, M. E., et al.: A massive outbreak in Milwaukee of *Cryptosporidium* infection transmitted through the public water supply. N. Engl. J. Med. *331*:161–167, 1994.
116. Makintubee, S., Mallonee, J., and Istre, G. R.: Shigellosis outbreak associated with swimming. Am. J. Public Health *77*:166–168, 1987.
117. Markowitz, L. E., Preblud, S. R., Orenstein, W. A., et al.: Patterns of transmission in measles outbreaks in the United States, 1985–1986. N. Engl. J. Med. *320*:75–81, 1989.
118. Maslow, J. N., Mulligan, M. E., and Arbeit, R. D.: Molecular epidemiology: Application of contemporary techniques to the typing of microorganisms. Clin. Infect. Dis. *17*:153–164, 1993.
119. Master, P. L., Brumfitt, W., and Mendez, R. L.: Bacterial flora of the upper respiratory tract in Paddington families, 1952–1954. B. M. J. *1*:1200–1205, 1958.
120. Matson, D. O., Byington, C., Canfield, M., et al.: Investigation of a measles outbreak in a fully vaccinated school population including serum studies before and after revaccination. Pediatr. Infect. Dis. J. *12*:292–299, 1993.
121. McCloskey, R. V., Green, M. J., Eller, J., et al.: Treatment of diphtheria carriers: Benzathine penicillin, erythromycin, and clindamycin. Ann. Intern. Med. *81*:788–791, 1974.
122. McCormack, W. M., Chowdhury, A. M., Hahangir, N., et al.: Tetracycline prophylaxis in families of cholera patients. Bull. World Health Organ. *38*:787–792, 1968.
123. Mendall, M. A., Goggin, P. M., Molineaux, N., et al.: Childhood living conditions and *Helicobacter pylori* seropositivity in adult life. Lancet *339*:896–897, 1992.
124. Meningococcal Disease Surveillance Group: Meningococcal disease secondary attack rate and chemoprophylaxis in the United States, 1974. J. A. M. A. *235*:261–265, 1976.
125. Mertsola, J., Ruuskanen, O., Eerola, E., et al.: Intrafamilial spread of pertussis. J. Pediatr. *103*:359–363, 1983.
126. Michaels, R. H., and Norden, C. W.: Pharyngeal colonization with *Haemophilus influenzae* type b: A longitudinal study of families with a child with meningitis or epiglottitis due to *H. influenzae* type b. J. Infect. Dis. *136*:222–228, 1977.
127. Miller, L. W., Older, J. J., Drake, J., et al.: Diphtheria immunization: Effect upon carriers and the control of outbreaks. Am. J. Dis. Child. *123*:197–199, 1972.
128. Mink, C. A., Sirota, N. M., and Nugent, S.: Outbreak of pertussis in a fully immunized adolescent and adult population. Arch. Pediatr. Adolesc. Med. *148*:153–157, 1994.
129. Mohle-Boetani, J. C., Miller, B., Halpern, M., et al.: School-based screening for tuberculous infection: A cost-benefit analysis. J. A. M. A. *274*:613–619, 1995.
130. Moore, A. C., Herwaldt, B. L., Craun, G. F., et al.: Surveillance for waterborne disease outbreaks: United States, 1991–1992. Morb. Mortal. Wkly. Rep. C. D. C. Surveill. Summ. *42*(SS-5):1–22, 1993.
131. Moore, M., Baron, R. C., Filstein, M. R., et al.: Aseptic meningitis and high school football players. J. A. M. A. *249*:2039–2042, 1983.
132. Munford, R. S., Taunay, A. E., Morais, J. S., et al.: Spread of meningococcal infection within households. Lancet *1*:1275–1278, 1974.
133. Murphy, T. V., Pastor, P., Medley, F., et al.: Decreased *Haemophilus* colonization in children vaccinated with *Haemophilus influenzae* type b conjugate vaccine. J. Pediatr. *122*:517–523, 1993.
134. Nelson, J. D.: The changing epidemiology of pertussis in young infants: The role of adults as reservoirs of infection. Am. J. Dis. Child. *132*:371–373, 1978.
135. Nolan, C. M., Barr, H., Elarth, A. M., et al.: Tuberculosis in a day-care home. Pediatrics *79*:630–632, 1987.

136. Noordeen, S. K.: Chemoprophylaxis in leprosy. Lepr. India *41*:247–254, 1969.
137. Okun, D. A.: Water quality management. *In* Last J. M., and Wallace R. B. (eds.): Maxcey-Rosenau-Last Public Health and Preventive Medicine. 13th ed. E. Norwalk, CT, Appleton & Lange, 1992, pp. 619–648.
138. Olsen, S. J., MacKinnon, L. C., Goulding, J. S., et al.: Surveillance for foodborne-disease outbreaks—United States, 1993–1997. Morb. Mortal. Wkly. Rep. C. D. C. Surveill. Summ. *49*(1):1–62, 2000.
139. Oral rehydration solutions. Med. Lett. Drugs Ther. *25*:19–20, 1983.
140. Pass, R. F., Little, E. A., Stagno, S., et al.: Young children as a probable source of maternal and congenital cytomegalovirus infection. N. Engl. J. Med. *316*:1366–1370, 1987.
141. Pickering, L. K., Evans, D. G., DuPont, H. L., et al.: Diarrhea caused by *Shigella* rotavirus and *Giardia* in day-care centers: Prospective study. J. Pediatr. *99*:51–56, 1981.
142. Pitzinger, B., Steffen, R., and Tschopp, A.: Incidence and clinical features of traveler's diarrhea in infants and children. Pediatr. Infect. Dis. J. *10*:719–723, 1991.
143. Poland, J. D., Quan, T. J., and Barnes, A. M.: Plague. *In* Beran, G. W. (ed.-in-chief): Handbook of Zoonoses. 2nd ed. Boca Raton, FL, CRC Press, 1994, pp. 93–112.
144. Polis, M. A., Tuazon, C. U., Alling, D. W., et al.: Transmission of *Giardia lamblia* from a day care center to the community. Am. J. Public Health *76*:1142–1144, 1986.
145. Porter, J. D., Ragazzoni, H. P., Buchanon, J. D., et al.: *Giardia* transmission in a swimming pool. Am. J. Public Health *78*:659–662, 1988.
146. Potter, M. E., Kaufmann, A. F., Blake, P. A., et al.: Unpasteurized milk: The hazards of a health fetish. J. A. M. A. *252*:2050–2054, 1984.
147. Rammelkamp, C. H., Jr.: Epidemic nephritis. Trans. Assoc. Am. Physicians *67*:276–282, 1954.
148. Rees, R. J. W., and Meade, T. W.: Comparison of the modes of spread and the incidence of tuberculosis and leprosy. Lancet *1*:47–49, 1974.
149. Ryan, C. A., Nickels, M. K., Hargrett-Bean, N. T., et al.: Massive outbreak of antimicrobial-resistant salmonellosis traced to pasteurized milk. J. A. M. A. *258*:3269–3274, 1987.
150. Schwartz, B.: Chemoprophylaxis for bacterial infections: Principles of and application to meningococcal infections. Rev. Infect. Dis. *13*(Suppl. 2):170–173, 1991.
151. Schwartz, B., Broome, C. V., Brown, G. R., et al.: Association of sporadic listeriosis with consumption of uncooked hot dogs and undercooked chicken. Lancet *2*:779–782, 1988.
152. Schwartz, B., Harrison, L. H., Motter, J. S., et al.: Investigation of an outbreak of *Moraxella* conjunctivitis at a Navajo boarding school. Am. J. Ophthalmol. *107*:341–347, 1989.
153. Snider, D. E., Rieder, H. L., Combs, D., et al.: Tuberculosis in children. Pediatr. Infect. Dis. *7*:271–278, 1988.
154. Sprauer, M. A., Cochi, S. L., Zell, E. R., et al.: Prevention of secondary transmission of pertussis in households with early use of erythromycin. Am. J. Dis. Child. *146*:177–181, 1992.
155. Starke, J. R., Jacobs, R. F., and Jereb, J.: Resurgence of tuberculosis in children. J. Pediatr. *120*:839–855, 1992.
156. Steketee, R. W., Wassilak, S. G. F., Adkins, W. N., et al.: Evidence for a high attack rate and efficacy of erythromycin prophylaxis in a pertussis outbreak in a facility for the developmentally disabled. J. Infect. Dis. *157*:434–440, 1988.
157. St. Louis, M. E., Morse, D. L., Potter, M. E., et al.: The emergence of grade A eggs as a major source of *Salmonella enteritidis* infections: New implications for the control of salmonellosis. J. A. M. A. *259*:2103–2107, 1988.
158. Straker, E., Hill, A. B., and Lovell, R.: A study of the nasopharyngeal bacterial flora of different groups of persons observed in London and southeast England during the years 1930 to 1937. Reports on Public Health and Medical Subjects 90. London, His Majesty's Stationery Office, 1939, pp. 7–51.
159. Swerdlow, D. L., and Ries, A. A.: Cholera in the Americas: Guidelines for the clinician. J. A. M. A. *267*:1495–1499, 1992.
160. Tenover, F. C., Arbeit, R., Archer, G., et al.: Comparison of traditional and molecular methods of typing isolates of *Staphylococcus aureus*. J. Clin. Microbiol. *32*:407–415, 1994.
161. Thacker, S. B., and Berkelman, R. L.: Public health surveillance in the United States. Epidemiol. Rev. *10*:164–190, 1988.
162. Thomas, M. E. M., and Tillett, H. E.: Sonne dysentery in day schools and nurseries: An eighteen-year study in Edmonton. J. Hyg. *71*:593–602, 1973.
163. Valeur-Jensen, A. K., Pedersen, C. B., Westergaard, T., et al.: Risk factors for B19 infection in pregnancy. J. A. M. A. *281*:1099–1105, 1999.
164. Van Loon, F. P. L., Holmes, S. J., Sirotkin, B. I., et al.: Mumps surveillance—United States, 1988–1993. Morb. Mortal. Wkly. Rep. C. D. C. Surveill. Summ. *44*(SS-3):1–14, 1995.
165. Vazquez, M., LaRussa, P. S., Gershon, A. A., et al.: The effectiveness of the varicella vaccine in clinical practice. N. Engl. J. Med. *344*:955–960, 2001.
166. Venczel, L. V., Desai, M. M., Vertz, P. D., et al.: The role of child care in a community-wide outbreak of hepatitis A. Pediatrics *108*:E78, 2001.
167. Wald, E. R., Dashefsky, B., Byers, C., et al.: Frequency and severity of infections in day care. J. Pediatr. *112*:540–546, 1988.
168. Weinstein, L., and LeFrock, J.: Does antimicrobial therapy of streptococcal pharyngitis or pyoderma alter the risk of glomerulonephritis? J. Infect. Dis. *124*:229–231, 1971.
169. Weissman, J. B., Schmerler, A., Weiler, P., et al.: The role of preschool children and day-care centers in the spread of shigellosis in urban communities. J. Pediatr. *84*:797–802, 1974.
170. Werner, S. B., Weidmer, C. E., Nelson, B. C., et al.: Primary plague pneumonia contracted from a domestic cat at South Lake Tahoe, Calif. J. A. M. A. *251*:929–931, 1984.
171. White, M. E., Gordon, D., Poland, J. D., et al.: Recommendations for the control of *Yersinia pestis* infections. Infect. Control *1*:326–329, 1980.
172. Wirsing von König, C. H., Postels-Multani, S., Bock, H. L., et al.: Pertussis in adults: Frequency of transmission after household exposure. Lancet *346*:1326–1329, 1995.
173. Wood, R. C., MacDonald, K. L., and Osterholm, M. T.: *Campylobacter* enteritis outbreaks associated with drinking raw milk during youth activities: A 10-year review of outbreaks in the United States. J. A. M. A. *268*:3228–3230, 1992.
174. World Health Organization: Ecology and Control of Vectors in Public Health. Geneva, Technical Report Series No. 561, 1975.
175. Zangwill, K. M., Schuchat, A., Riedo, F. X., et al.: School-based clusters of meningococcal disease in the United States. Descriptive epidemiology and a case-control analysis. J. A. M. A. *277*:389–395, 1997.

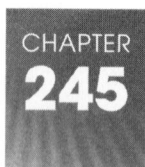

CHAPTER 245 Infections in Daycare Environments

ELLEN R. WALD

The ever-increasing number of young women in the work force has contributed to the large number of infants and toddlers receiving out-of-home care. Current estimates are that approximately 75 percent of the mothers of children younger than 5 years work outside the home and that 13 million children receive some form of child daycare. About half of these children receive care in their own homes provided by parents or relatives. Twenty percent receive care in family daycare and 28 percent in daycare centers. As children grow older, families increasingly rely on center care and decrease the use of parental care.[22]

The term *daycare* is used to describe a variety of different options for the supervision of children in the absence of their parents. Types of daycare include (1) large daycare centers housed in nonresidential settings that provide care for at least seven children in one location (included here are situations in which the parent's employer is the sponsor of the daycare, frequently at the site of employment, and also preschool and nursery schools in which childcare is provided in a structured, primarily educational setting), (2) daycare homes in which care is provided in a residential setting for six or fewer children, (3) before- and after-school care designed to bridge the gap between organized schools (such as preschool or public or private school) and parental departure for or return from work, and (4) cooperatives in which childcare is rendered by parents who alternate in caring for their own children as well as other enrolled children.

The quality of care provided to children attending various daycare facilities varies widely. Although daycare centers are licensed in most states, only 23 percent of children in out-of-home care are enrolled in these facilities.[182] State regulations vary from state to state; some are quite lenient in setting suggested ratios for staff to child, whereas others have no regulations governing group size. Even if impeccable regulations and well-trained caregivers were available, the regulations would not protect the vast majority of children who are in unlicensed facilities.

Many factors contribute to the transmission of infectious agents in the daycare setting (Table 245–1), the most important of which are host factors relating to the immunologic susceptibility of young children. Once infection is established, it is transmitted easily because of the natural tendency for intimacy in an age group that has not established acceptable toileting practices and is ignorant of basic hygienic practices. Respiratory and gastrointestinal pathogens frequently contaminate toys.

Caregivers may have received insufficient training in infection control practices. A lack of policy regarding immunization and health care screening of employees may contribute to the spread of infection. In addition, overcrowding, understaffing, and poorly designed physical environments foster transmission of infectious agents in daycare facilities. A lack of or inadequate number of handwashing facilities for both children and providers creates an almost insurmountable barrier to infection control.

Major risk factors for spread of infection are related to the age of the participants, the number of children, and the ratio of staff to children. The last is determined in part by the age of the children and the experience of the daycare provider. In overcrowded situations with inadequate staff, infection is spread easily because of inadequate washing of hands and attention to other facets of infection control.

Factors identified as particularly important in the spread of gastrointestinal organisms are large numbers of diaper-age children in centers where staff members who diaper children are also responsible for food preparation.[13, 64] Separating diaper-aged children from those who are older is important to limit spread of enteric illness. If meals are prepared in the daycare setting, separating this activity from toilet areas is essential. If food is brought from home, it should be transported properly and stored to avoid spoilage. Lack of attention to this issue may result in additional illness. Daycare centers that operate for profit are also at higher risk for having infectious disease outbreaks, probably as a result of lower staff-to-children ratios.[101] Finally, parents may not withdraw ill children from attendance at daycare voluntarily because of the expense and inconvenience of creating alternate childcare arrangements.

TABLE 245–1 ■ RISK FACTORS FOR INFECTIOUS DISEASE IN DAYCARE

Children
Immunologic susceptibility to infectious agents
Lack of toilet training
Natural tendency to intimacy
Frequent oral contact with environment
Lack of awareness and practice of good hygiene
Caregivers
Insufficient training in infection control
Lack of policy regarding immunization
Inadequate screening for infectious diseases
Environmental and Economic Problems
Inappropriate staff-child ratios
Overcrowding
Failure to separate age groups
Poorly designed physical layout
Inadequate or poorly placed sinks
Failure to separate toilet areas from areas of food preparation
Parental pressure to admit sick children to daycare

Modes of Transmission of Infectious Diseases

The most important pathogens and their modes of transmission of infection in daycare are shown in Table 245–2. Respiratory infections are by far the most common cause of illness in infants, toddlers, and preschoolers, regardless of whether they attend daycare.

RESPIRATORY

For some microbiologic species causing infection, the mode of transmission is the airborne route. The organism is aerosolized and remains in the air like cigarette smoke. Direct contact with the infected individual is not necessary for spread of the infection. Illnesses known to be transmitted by this means include measles, varicella, pertussis, and tuberculosis.

Most commonly, respiratory organisms are spread by the production of droplets laden with infective particles. These droplets may be transmitted directly from mucosa to mucosa when close physical contact occurs. More often, droplets land on nonporous surfaces (e.g., cribs, tables, chairs) or on clothes and paper (fomites) and remain infective for minutes to hours. Hand contact with contaminated surfaces and fomites can result in infection if the hands touch the nasal or conjunctival mucosa.[67] Agents that can be transmitted by droplet spread (mucosa to mucosa), from finger to mucosa, or by fomites include most respiratory viruses (respiratory syncytial, rhinovirus, influenza, parainfluenza, adenovirus, parvovirus B19, measles, mumps, rubella, and varicella), *Haemophilus influenzae* type b (Hib), *Streptococcus pneumoniae, Neisseria meningitidis,* and *Streptococcus pyogenes.*[56, 58, 63, 66, 67] Finger-to-mucosa spread of respiratory pathogens is the most important and common mechanism for transmission of viral and bacterial infections.[72] Consequently, handwashing is an essential element of preventing spread of infection.

GASTROINTESTINAL

Spread of gastrointestinal organisms is by fecal-oral transmission. The number of organisms required to produce infection will determine whether infection occurs by person-to-person spread or whether a food or fluid intermediary is required. For example, rotavirus, *Giardia lamblia,* and *Shigella* spp. are transmitted readily in very small numbers of organisms on the hands (without obvious gross contamination) after person-to-person contact or by touching infected surfaces. In contrast, *Salmonella*, rarely a cause of diarrheal outbreaks in the daycare setting, requires large numbers of organisms to produce infection. Accordingly, an intermediary step of food or beverage contamination is

TABLE 245–2 ■ PATHOGENS AND MODES OF TRANSMISSION OF INFECTION IN DAYCARE

Mode of Transmission	Bacteria	Viruses	Parasites
Respiratory	*Haemophilus influenzae* type b *Streptococcus pneumoniae* *Neisseria meningitidis* *Streptococcus pyogenes* *Bordetella pertussis* *Mycobacterium tuberculosis*	Adenovirus Influenza A & B Measles Mumps Parainfluenza Parvovirus B19 Respiratory syncytial Rhinovirus Rubella Varicella	
Fecal-oral	*Campylobacter* organisms *Clostridium difficile* *Escherichia coli* O157:H7 *Salmonella* organisms *Shigella* organisms	Enteroviruses Hepatitis A Rotavirus Calicivirus	*Cryptosporidium parvum* *Enterobius vermicularis* *Giardia lamblia*
Person to person via skin contact	*Streptococcus pyogenes* *Staphylococcus aureus*	Herpes simplex	*Pediculus capitis* *Sarcoptes scabei* *Trichophyton* species *Microsporum* species
Contact with blood, urine, or saliva		Cytomegalovirus Hepatitis B Herpes simplex Human immuno-deficiency virus	

Adapted from American Academy of Pediatrics: Children in out-of-home child care. *In* Pickering, L. (ed.): 2000 Red Book: Report of the Committee on infectious Diseases. 25th ed. Elk Grove Village, IL, American Academy of Pediatrics, 2000, p. 107.

required to allow organisms to replicate up to the necessary inocula.

Numerous studies have demonstrated fecal organisms on daycare center environmental surfaces with which infants and toddlers have had contact, as well as on the hands of care providers.[46, 91, 183, 190] Contamination of the environment is highest when the daycare children are younger than 3 years. This age predilection correlates with the number of children still wearing diapers.[184] Important pathogens, including fecal bacteria, rotavirus, hepatitis A virus (HAV), and *G. lamblia* cysts, are able to survive on environmental surfaces for periods ranging from hours to weeks.[29, 97]

SKIN

Bacterial, viral, and parasitic infections of the skin can be transmitted from person to person by direct contact. Bacterial pathogens such as *S. pyogenes* and *Staphylococcus aureus* usually are not primarily invasive unless a break in the integument occurs, such as after minor trauma (e.g., insect bites). Herpes simplex virus may be transmitted from skin or mucosa to skin by direct contact, again only if the skin is broken. Infestations such as scabies and lice are transmitted from person to person by mobile parasites. The superficial dermatophytes responsible for tinea infections (*Trichophyton, Microsporum,* and *Epidermophyton*) are transmitted from person to person or by contact with infected fomites such as combs, hairbrushes, and hats.

BLOOD, URINE, AND SALIVA

Hepatitis B virus (HBV), hepatitis C virus (HCV), human immunodeficiency virus (HIV), and cytomegalovirus (CMV) can be transmitted by blood and sexual activity (presumably resulting in microtrauma, thereby leading to blood exposure). Transmission of HCV by sexual activity is uncommon, however. Although both HBV and HIV can be demonstrated in urine and saliva, exchange of these body fluids is very unlikely to transmit infection. At daycare centers, transmission of CMV probably occurs between attendees by contamination of toys with saliva. Mothers and care providers can become infected with CMV by the finger-to-mucosa route after contamination of hands by urine or saliva.

Patterns of Infection in Daycare

Children in daycare experience several different patterns of occurrence of infection[61] (Table 245–3). Most of the increased infectious disease burden found in daycare centers is experienced by the children themselves. They have an excess of

TABLE 245–3 ■ PATTERNS OF OCCURRENCE OF INFECTIONS EXPERIENCED IN DAYCARE

Patterns of Occurrence	Examples
Clinical manifestation of infection primarily in children	Respiratory syncytial virus, rotavirus infections
Infection affects children, daycare staff, and close family members	Shigellosis, giardiasis *Neisseria meningitidis* infection
Inapparent infection in children with clinically important infection in adult contacts	Hepatitis A
Inapparent or mild infection in children and adults but may have serious consequences for fetus in pregnant contact	Cytomegalovirus infection Rubella Parvovirus B19 infection Coxsackievirus A16 infection

Modified from Goodman, R. A., Osterholm, M. T., Granoff, D. M., et al.: Infectious diseases and child day care. Pediatrics *74*:134–139, 1984.

respiratory and gastrointestinal infections when compared with children who are in home care.[187] Certain specific infections, such as those due to Hib, rotavirus, and respiratory syncytial virus (RSV), are shouldered almost exclusively by the children. However, on occasion, adult personnel working as providers will experience some of the same respiratory and gastrointestinal infections as in the children. Examples of infections for which daycare attendees and staff share an increased burden include shigellosis, giardiasis, and invasive meningococcal disease.

Several infections barely recognizable in a daycare child (because they are mild or asymptomatic) cause significant repercussions when spread to adults—either parents or daycare providers. The most notable of these diseases is hepatitis A, which in adults tends to be an illness of moderate severity and often leads to extended absences from work.

Finally, with some infections, clinical manifestations in adults are mild, but the infection may have potential effects on the fetus if the childcare provider or mother of a daycare attendee is pregnant. CMV and rubella virus are associated with severe birth defects if infection occurs in the first trimester. Infection with parvovirus B19 during pregnancy poses a risk for the development of nonimmune hydrops in the fetus.

Infectious Agents in Daycare

INFECTIONS SPREAD BY THE RESPIRATORY ROUTE

Viral Upper Respiratory Infections

Respiratory viruses (rhinovirus, RSV, parainfluenza, influenza, adenoviruses, and Epstein-Barr) are the most common cause of infection in preschool-age children.[15, 42, 56] The range of clinical manifestations includes asymptomatic infection, simple upper respiratory infection (rhinitis), acute otitis media, pharyngitis, croup, tracheitis, bronchiolitis, and pneumonitis. Disease may be mild or severe and involve single or more than one level of the respiratory tree. Children may experience multiple infections with each agent because of antigenic diversity within virus subtypes (e.g., influenza A virus), multiple subtypes (e.g., rhinoviruses), and failure of immunity to develop after a single exposure (e.g., RSV). Viruses are shed from the site of infection (conjunctiva, nose, throat), even before clinical symptoms develop, thereby rendering control of the spread of these infections in daycare difficult. Documentation that children in daycare (family or large daycare centers) experience more respiratory infections than those noted in children in home care is ample.[43, 52, 78, 103–105, 164, 166, 187] The risk of acquiring infection for children in group or family care is intermediate between that for large daycare centers and home care.[187]

The most common bacterial complication of viral upper respiratory infection is acute otitis media. The peak age incidence of otitis media is between 6 and 18 months, similar to that of viral upper respiratory tract infections. Most children have had at least one episode of acute otitis media by the time that they reach their second birthday, and approximately a third will have had at least three episodes by that time.[176] Not surprisingly, as the frequency of viral respiratory infections is increased in children attending daycare, these children experience a notable increase in the frequency of otitis media.[143, 164, 166, 168, 187] Two recent reviews strongly support the notion that attendance at daycare is a major risk factor for acquiring acute otitis media.[149, 181] Table 245–4 shows a comparison of the annualized rates of acute respiratory tract infection, otitis media, and antibiotic treatment among children in various modes of child care. Wald and colleagues[187] provided data indicating that the risk of hospitalization for performance of myringotomy with tube placement was highest for children in large daycare environments.

TABLE 245–4 ■ COMPARISONS OF ANNUALIZED RATES OF ACUTE RESPIRATORY TRACT INFECTIONS, OTITIS MEDIA, AND ANTIBIOTIC TREATMENT AMONG CHILDREN IN VARIOUS MODES OF CHILDCARE

Study	Length of Time Observed	Annual Rate of Acute Respiratory Infection (per Child-Year)	Annual Rate of Otitis Media (per Child-Year)	Annual Rate of Antibiotic Treatment (per Child-Year)
Wald et al.[187]*				
DCC (n = 33)	12–18 mo	6.3		
DCH (n = 23)	12–18 mo	5.1		
HC (n = 97)	12–18 mo	3.9		
Strangert[168]†				
DCC (n = 108)	8 mo	7.5	1.2	1.9
DHC (n = 42)	8 mo	7.5	1.3	1.6
HC (n = 57)	8 mo	3.0	0.5	0.8
Stahlberg[164]‡				
DCC (n = 23)	8 wk	13.8	2.3	4.8
DCC (n = 23)	8 wk	12.0	0.9	2.8
HC (n = 23)	8 wk	9.9	1.1	1.4
Reves and Jones[143]§				
DCC (n = 42)	8 wk	8.1	6.0	9.1
DCH (n = 72)	8 wk	2.6	1.6	2.7
HC (n = 156)	8 wk	3.0	1.6	2.5

*Telephone interview every 2 weeks.
†Active surveillance in DCC; telephone call every 4 months for children in DCH and HC.
‡Daily diary in all groups.
§Health maintenance organization abstraction covering an 8-week period for each child.
DCC, daycare center; DCH, daycare home; HC, cared for at home.
Modified from Reves, R. R., and Jones, J. A.: Antibiotic use and resistance patterns in day care centers. Semin. Pediatr. Infect. Dis. *1*:212–221, 1990.

Likewise, the risk of contracting recurrent acute otitis media and persistent middle ear effusion is also higher for children in daycare than for those who receive care at home.[35, 50, 165, 179]

Researchers do not recommend that children with mild respiratory infections be excluded from daycare or be separated from the group of well children because this strategy has not been shown to achieve an overall reduction in infections for children in daycare facilities.

Systemic Viral Infections

CYTOMEGALOVIRUS

CMV is a common cause of infection in preschool-age children. Most often, the infection is completely asymptomatic.[79] Rarely, the child may experience a febrile illness with lymphadenopathy and hepatosplenomegaly. Sources of CMV in the daycare setting are infants and children who have been infected by their mothers via vertical transmission either in utero (1–2%), perinatally (2–3%), or postpartum through breast-feeding (approximately 6%). Strangert[166] reported the isolation of CMV from 7 of 10 children between 21 and 30 months of age in one daycare center. Strom[169] found that 13 of 18 (72%) children between 24 and 36 months of age in a single nursery excreted CMV. Urine cultures frequently were persistently positive for CMV for many months. Other investigators have demonstrated that peak rates of infection occur between 1 and 3 years of age, when viral excretion may be documented in as many as 70 percent of children in daycare, as shown in Table 245–5.[1, 80, 88, 117, 128, 130]

Infection in preschool-age children leads to viral shedding documented by positive CMV cultures obtained from swabs of the throat (thereby contaminating saliva) and urine. Transmission probably occurs through fomites (toys and blankets) contaminated with saliva rather than by respiratory droplets.[162] Shedding of CMV is as chronic among infected toddlers in daycare centers as it is in children with perinatal or congenital infection.[129, 130]

CMV is a problem if acquisition of infection occurs during early pregnancy in daycare providers or mothers of children attending daycare.[1–4] Such acquisition may lead to clinically evident congenital CMV infection (microcephaly, hepatosplenomegaly, chorioretinitis, psychomotor retardation, and deafness) in approximately 5 percent of infected children. Another 10 to 15 percent of infants experience occult, but potentially damaging infection that results in milder degrees of hearing loss and learning disabilities.[163]

PARVOVIRUS B19

Parvovirus B19, the etiologic agent of erythema infectiosum, or fifth disease, is spread by the respiratory route. Viral replication, viremia, and nasopharyngeal shedding occur approximately 1 week before the development of clinical symptoms. This benign disease of childhood (in a normal host) may occur in preschool- and school-age children. The clinical illness is characterized by an erythematous rash on the face that gives a "slapped-cheek" appearance. Patients usually do not have fever or other constitutional symptoms. The rash progresses after the first day and spreads as a maculopapular eruption beginning on the proximal ends of the extremities and extending to the distal portions and trunk. After several days, these lesions develop into a lacy reticular pattern on the proximal parts of the extremities and then fade. Unrecognized in immunocompetent hosts is an infection of the erythrocyte precursor that leads to transient red blood cell aplasia.

In adults, parvovirus B19 infection frequently causes arthralgia and arthritis. Its clinical importance in the context of daycare infections is transmission from an infected preschool-age child to a pregnant mother or daycare provider.[58] In a large outbreak of erythema infectiosum in Connecticut, 19 percent of susceptible adult school personnel became infected; the highest rates of seroconversion were observed in personnel in contact with large numbers of young children. Infection of the fetus may lead to nonimmune hydrops secondary to infection of erythrocyte progenitor cells. Estimates of fetal loss when a pregnant woman of unknown antibody status is exposed to parvovirus are 2.5 percent after household exposure and 1.5 percent after occupational exposure in a school or daycare facility.[10]

TABLE 245–5 ■ EXCRETION OF CYTOMEGALOVIRUS IN URINE FROM CHILDREN IN DAYCARE

Study	No. of Daycare Centers Studied	Age of Children Studied (mo)	No. of Children Studied	No. (%) with CMV in Urine
Strangert[167, 168]	1	21-30	10	7 (70)
	13	6-36	40	9 (23)
Strom[169]	1	24-36	18	13 (72)
Pass et al.[128]	1	3-12	11	1 (9)
		13-24	18	15 (83)
		25-36	16	10 (63)
		36-60	25	10 (40)
Pass et al.[128]	1	0-60	103	59 (57)
Hutto et al.[80]	3	<12	10	0 (0)
		12-24	38	14 (37)
		25-36	35	27 (77)
		38-48+	143	36 (25)
Jones et al.[88]	11	<12	33	8 (21)
		12-24	51	15 (29)
Adler[1]	1	25-48	52	9 (17)
		0-24	31	8 (25)
		24-60	34	7 (20)
Murph et al.[117]	1	0-9	8	2 (25)
		12-24	12	8 (67)
		25-36	14	4 (29)
		37-48+	39	3 (8)

COXSACKIEVIRUS A16

Epidemics of infection with coxsackievirus A16 cause hand, foot, and mouth disease, a clinical syndrome characterized by a vesicular exanthem on the distal parts of the extremities and mild stomatitis. Two outbreaks have been reported in children attending daycare.[48, 49] The disease is mild in children but has a high attack rate. Its importance relates to the possibility of infection during pregnancy, which may lead to spontaneous abortion.[49, 121]

Local Bacterial Infections

STREPTOCOCCUS PYOGENES OR GROUP A STREPTOCOCCI

Group A streptococci (GAS) are a frequent cause of respiratory and skin infections. The most common expression of infection with GAS is the development of pharyngitis and fever in an elementary school–age child. Usually, the throat infection is accompanied by tender anterior cervical nodes. In classic infection, none of the usual signs of viral upper respiratory disease—coryza, cough, and conjunctivitis—are present. Illness peaks in the late winter and spring. In contrast, streptococcal infection of a preschool child or child in daycare takes the form of a protracted upper respiratory infection. Specifically, these patients have low-grade fever, persistent nasal discharge, anorexia, and cervical adenopathy.

Although exposure of daycare children to an index case of streptococcal pharyngitis can be assumed to result in secondary cases, relatively few epidemics of GAS infection have been reported in daycare facilities.[47, 76, 160] An outbreak occurred in a daycare center in which preschool children shared facilities with kindergarten children in an "after" school program.[160] During a 3-month period, 47 percent of the daycare population had positive cultures for GAS or positive results on a rapid antigen-detection test. Outbreaks of scarlet fever and perianal cellulitis each have been reported recently from daycare centers.[116] Children with GAS infections of the throat or skin should be excluded from daycare for 24 hours after the initiation of appropriate antibiotic treatment.

Invasive Bacterial Disease

HAEMOPHILUS INFLUENZAE TYPE b

Hib used to be the major bacterial pathogen of childhood and was responsible for meningitis, epiglottitis, pneumonia, facial cellulitis, and septic arthritis. These infections occurred in children between 2 months and 5 years of age, with a peak between 6 and 18 months of age. The organism colonizes the nasopharynx before becoming blood-borne; hematogenous dissemination results in a distant focus of infection. Infected children usually have a several-day history of mild upper respiratory symptoms followed by an abrupt onset of high fever and localized symptoms indicating the site of infection (e.g., irritability or seizures in central nervous system infection, cutaneous findings in cellulitis). Colonized individuals who lack anticapsular antibody are susceptible to the development of invasive disease.[62]

In the 1980s, considerable debate ensued regarding whether children in daycare had a higher risk than those in home care for having primary episodes of infection with Hib. The risk of primary disease developing in an individual child is defined as the risk of Hib disease in that child in the absence of known contact with another case in the previous 60 days. Many Hib infections have occurred in children attending daycare centers,[28, 53, 60, 82, 119, 141, 173] with estimates of 28 to 40 percent in several studies.[82, 141] However, the presence and magnitude of the increased risk have shown significant variation that was dependent on the age of the child, the type and size of the daycare facility, and the geographic location of the facility. In general, studies have found that the risk of contracting primary Hib infection is highest in younger children (≤23 months of age) during their first month of enrollment in daycare and in children attending a larger daycare center as opposed to a daycare home.[82, 141]

An additional concern was whether the risk of development of secondary cases of Hib infection in the daycare setting was significantly elevated. Although several studies have substantiated an increased risk for secondary cases of invasive Hib infection in daycare attendees exposed to another attendee infected with Hib,[11, 52, 106] others have not.[118, 125] Based on available data,[11, 52, 106, 118, 125] the risk of secondary disease developing in daycare classroom contacts of a child with invasive Hib was probably higher than that in children of similar age in the general population; however, the magnitude was not well defined and depended on the characteristics and geographic location of the daycare center. Management of daycare attendees younger than 2 years who were exposed to an individual with invasive Hib infection was controversial.[37]

The availability and universal use (in infancy) of effective vaccines for the prevention of Hib infection have changed the epidemiology of infections caused by this pathogen dramatically.[158] Schulte and coworkers[153] reviewed the pattern of invasive Hib infection in New York State. They demonstrated a dramatic decline in the incidence of Hib disease in children younger than 5 years, both those in daycare and those in home care. The decrease in cases of infection attributable to Hib occurred in children attending daycare centers before being observed in non-daycare attendees, perhaps because of the requirement for Hib vaccine before enrollment in daycare. The virtual disappearance of this once common and serious problem and the high immunization rates with Hib vaccine obviate a lengthy discussion regarding the need for rifampin prophylaxis after exposure to cases of invasive disease. In the rare instance of a case of invasive Hib disease occurring in a family daycare center housing other susceptible children (<4 years of age), all daycare contacts (adults and children) should receive rifampin, 20 mg/kg/day once daily for 4 days, to a maximum dose of 600 mg.

NEISSERIA MENINGITIDIS

N. meningitidis is a gram-negative, polysaccharide-encapsulated diplococcus found colonizing the nasopharynx. It is the second leading cause of meningitis in the United States. Other manifestations of infection include pericarditis, sepsis, and pneumonia. Similar to that in patients experiencing infection with Hib, the attack rate is highest in children 2 months to 5 years of age, with a peak between 6 and 12 months of age. The pathogenesis is hematogenous dissemination from the nasopharynx as a site of colonization. Household contacts exposed to patients with meningococcal disease have a significantly higher risk of acquiring that disease than that in the general population.[38, 112, 115]

Secondary spread of infection with *N. meningitidis* has been recognized as a potential risk, especially in situations of crowding such as in military barracks and college dormitories. In addition, reports suggest that the risk of acquiring secondary disease caused by *N. meningitidis* is increased in the daycare setting.[41, 85, 100, 150] In a Belgian report,[41] exposure in a daycare nursery during a prolonged meningococcal epidemic conferred a risk for infection that was 76 times greater than that in children of similar age who received care at home. Prompt institution of rifampin prophylaxis is the recommended strategy for management of all intimate child contacts of a person with invasive *N. meningitidis* disease to prevent secondary or associated illness. A single oral dose of ciprofloxacin (500 mg) or an intramuscular dose of ceftriaxone (250 mg) is an alternative for adult contacts. Physicians do not recommend that throat cultures be performed to identify those who require rifampin prophylaxis. The cultures may be insensitive, and waiting for results will delay the administration of appropriate management.

STREPTOCOCCUS PNEUMONIAE

Pneumococci are the most common cause of bacterial infections of the upper and lower respiratory tracts, including otitis media, sinusitis, and pneumonia.[154] As respiratory pathogens, they also cause other upper respiratory tract infections, such as conjunctivitis, and important systemic illnesses, including occult bacteremia, bacteremic periorbital cellulitis, and meningitis.

Multiply antibiotic-resistant *S. pneumoniae,* a problem that began in the 1960s, is now widespread in South Africa and large parts of Europe. It has been steadily increasing in the United States since 1990.

Although *S. pneumoniae* is the most common cause of otitis media and otitis media is the most common infection caused by *S. pneumoniae,* the rarity of performing tympanocentesis (despite the frequency of otitis media in children in daycare) explains the delayed appreciation of the fact that *S. pneumoniae* is spread easily in the daycare setting. The ease of transmission of penicillin-resistant *S. pneumoniae* (tracked by antibiotic resistance patterns, capsular types, and genetic patterns) in the daycare setting now has been demonstrated amply.[44, 71, 138, 139] In addition, although the increased risk of children acquiring secondary cases of pneumococcal disease in daycare versus home care is unknown, several outbreaks of invasive *S. pneumoniae* disease in daycare centers have brought increased attention to this issue.[32, 139] A study of children in an Ohio daycare center[142] showed that prophylactic doses of antibiotics and frequent use of antibiotics were risk factors for nasopharyngeal carriage of antibiotic-resistant *S. pneumoniae.* A cluster of cases of invasive pneumococcal disease occurring in young children in childcare[25] involved a 12F serotype of pneumococcus that was penicillin-sensitive; three of six children in the daycare facility experienced bacteremic infections. In the most recent outbreak of disease, three cases of meningitis caused by multidrug-resistant serotype 14 *S. pneumoniae* occurred at a daycare center over a period of 5 days.[32]

Several reports claim that rifampin is ineffective or only partially effective in eradicating carriage of *S. pneumoniae.*[139, 142] However, this finding may be explained by inadequacy of the dose of rifampin,[139] lack of compliance with drug administration, or inappropriate timing for test-of-cure cultures.

A pneumococcal conjugate vaccine containing seven common serotypes of *S. pneumoniae* was licensed in March 2000. The vaccine is administered to children at 2, 4, and 6 months of age and again between 12 and 15 months. In a large field trial conducted at the Kaiser Permanente Vaccine Study Center, the vaccine performed very well. The trial achieved a 93 percent reduction in invasive disease (meningitis and bacteremia), 73 percent reduction in consolidative pneumonia, and 7 percent reduction in episodes of otitis media.[19] Use of the vaccine in all children will reduce the most serious manifestations of infection with *S. pneumoniae* substantially.[8]

MYCOBACTERIUM TUBERCULOSIS

Reported cases of tuberculosis have been on the decline in the United States since 1992, including a decrease in the number of infected children. In general, children with tuberculosis are not generally infectious. Rather, an adult in the environment invariably has active disease. Three clusters of cases of tuberculosis in children have been traced to attendance at daycare.[90, 99, 120] Screening of all daycare personnel, both staff and volunteers, with tuberculin skin testing is essential to eliminate this problem. A recent case of tuberculosis in a 9-year-old boy resulted in positive tuberculin skin tests in 79 percent of his classroom contacts and 16 percent of his daycare contacts.[34]

INFECTIONS OF THE GASTROINTESTINAL TRACT

Giardia lamblia

G. lamblia is one of the most common causes of diarrhea in the daycare setting.[18, 140, 155] Infection can be caused by the ingestion of as few as 10 cysts. Transmission most commonly results from person-to-person spread, although water-borne outbreaks have been documented.[92] Parents of daycare attendees are at risk for acquiring infection.[135] Demonstration of *G. lamblia* cysts on environmental surfaces indicates additional potential for transmission.[29] Infection with this parasite causes infestation of the duodenum and proximal jejunum and results in asymptomatic carriage more often than clinical disease.[81] After an incubation period of approximately 2 weeks, symptomatic patients experience diarrhea, intermittent abdominal pain, anorexia, and flatulence. The most notable feature of the infection is its tendency to become protracted, thereby leading to weight loss, failure to thrive, and anemia. The diagnosis is made by recovery of the organism from stool or occasionally by examination of duodenal aspirates or intestinal biopsy specimens.[86, 177] After resolution of the symptoms, either by virtue of treatment or by spontaneous cure, patients may continue to shed cysts for a very long time.[81] Treatment is not recommended for asymptomatic individuals shedding *G. lamblia* cysts. For symptomatic individuals, treatment may be undertaken with metronidazole, furazolidone, or quinacrine. Relapses occur in approximately 15 percent of patients.

Cryptosporidium

Cryptosporidium is a cause of severe diarrhea in immunocompromised hosts but usually causes self-limited illness in immunocompetent children and adults.[31] The parasite may be spread from person to person or via food or water. The usual clinical symptoms are watery diarrhea and low-grade fever with abdominal pain and weight loss. Vomiting occurs in approximately 30 percent of patients.

Cryptosporidium, like *G. lamblia,* has a very low infectious dose for humans. Ninety percent of infant nonhuman primates will become infected with 10 to 50 oocysts.[113] Spread of infection is facilitated in daycare centers because oocysts shed in the feces of infected persons are highly resistant to common disinfectants. Many outbreaks of diarrhea caused by *Cryptosporidium* have been reported from daycare centers.[5, 6, 30, 33, 70, 175] Asymptomatic children and adults shed oocysts for weeks after infection.[31]

The diagnosis is made by examination of stool for oocysts with special stains. Treatment is supportive. Exclusion from daycare is recommended until the patient is asymptomatic.

Shigella

Infection with *Shigella* organisms causes illness of variable severity but easy transmissibility. Accordingly, *Shigella* is one of the most common causes of diarrhea outbreaks in the daycare population,[114, 132, 134, 172, 188, 189] and *Shigella* infection was among the first enteric diseases recognized to be spread in daycare centers. Infection can be caused by as few as 10 to 100 organisms. Although a low inoculum is sufficient to cause infection, the organism does not survive well outside the human host. Person-to-person transmission is considered more important than environmental contamination.[188] Although infection with *Shigella* may be caused by one of four species (*Shigella sonnei, Shigella flexneri, Shigella dysenteriae,* and *Shigella boydii*), *S. sonnei* and *S. flexneri* are the most common.

Shigellosis is primarily a disease of young children. In outbreaks, younger children have the highest attack rate and are the most effective transmitters of infection.[178] Daycare personnel and family contacts also experience high attack rates.[75, 174] After an incubation period of several days, fever and watery diarrhea followed by crampy abdominal pain, tenesmus, and mucoid bloody stools occur in patients with classic disease. In many cases, the illness is mild and indistinguishable from other causes of gastroenteritis. The presence of fecal leukocytes on examination of stool provides supportive information; stool culture is diagnostic.

Treatment of shigellosis with an appropriate antimicrobial effectively terminates the illness. Susceptibility varies, but sulfamethoxazole-trimethoprim for 5 days is most often effective in the United States. Antimicrobial treatment decreases the duration of symptoms and fecal shedding. Untreated persons continue to excrete organisms for several weeks.

Campylobacter jejuni

Campylobacter jejuni is the most common cause of bacterial diarrhea in children in the United States, but it is less likely than *Shigella* to cause outbreaks of diarrheal disease in daycare centers.[83, 98, 127] Most often, a high inoculum of *Campylobacter* is required to produce infection, thereby necessitating a food or water vehicle. Less often, transmission can occur by person-to-person spread of smaller numbers of organisms. The clinical findings are variable, but the usual onset includes fever, abdominal pain, and diarrhea. Many cases resemble classic shigellosis. Watery diarrhea and low-grade fever with only modest constitutional signs of illness also may be observed. The illness usually lasts between 3 and 7 days. The diagnosis can be made by culture of stool; examination of stool by darkfield microscopy or direct smear may be very informative if performed by an experienced observer.

Treatment with erythromycin is effective in terminating excretion of the infective organism, which may be important in controlling epidemics or outbreaks. The impact of erythromycin on the clinical course of disease is variable.

Salmonella

Salmonella is the most common cause of bacterial diarrhea in many parts of the United States, but it is an uncommon cause of gastroenteritis outbreaks in daycare centers.[102] Because the organism is widespread in nature and has 2200 different serotypes, it has been very difficult to control. Infection usually occurs after the ingestion of contaminated food or beverages. Person-to-person spread seldom occurs, except in infancy when the infective dose is low.[193]

The most common expression of infection with *Salmonella* is uncomplicated gastroenteritis. The illness begins approximately 12 to 36 hours after exposure and often is characterized initially by vomiting and subsequently by diarrhea. Abdominal pain and fever are frequent accompaniments; occasionally, stools will contain mucus and blood. Although most cases are self-limited, *Salmonella* can be distinguished from other causes of gastroenteritis by its occasionally protracted course. The diagnosis is made by culture of stool. In general, antimicrobials are not recommended unless bacteremia is documented. Management of special hosts, such as neonates and immunocompromised patients, is controversial. Although some authors recommend antimicrobial therapy for these groups, few data support this recommendation. Exclusion from daycare is recommended until the diarrhea resolves. Once stools are normal, little reason exists to restrict attendance. Obtaining stool cultures from daycare contacts or the index case in convalescence is not necessary.[178] If anyone in the household is a food handler, the appropriate procedure is to check their stool for *Salmonella* carriage.

Clostridium difficile

C. difficile is the classic cause of pseudomembranous colitis in patients who have received or are receiving antimicrobial agents, and it rarely causes disease unassociated with antimicrobial use. The organism, a gram-positive, spore-forming rod, is distributed widely in soil and in the gastrointestinal tract of humans. It frequently is found colonizing asymptomatic newborns. Disease is a consequence of the elaboration of toxin or toxins by vegetative organisms. Hospital environments and daycare facilities are reservoirs for the organism.[93, 94] During outbreaks of *C. difficile* diarrhea in daycare centers, environmental contamination is increased, as is recovery of *C. difficile* from the hands of children and staff.[94]

Clinical symptoms include fever, diarrhea, and abdominal cramps. Stools may contain blood and mucus. The illness varies in severity from mild to life-threatening. The diagnosis of *C. difficile* gastroenteritis is made by recovery of the toxin from a stool sample. Treatment includes cessation of antibiotics and supportive care. Specific antimicrobial therapy with oral vancomycin or metronidazole may be necessary to achieve clinical cure. Metronidazole is favored in an era of concern regarding the development of vancomycin-resistant enterococci after the use of oral vancomycin. Children and personnel should be excluded from daycare until they are asymptomatic.

Escherichia coli

Several outbreaks of diarrhea caused by various *E. coli* strains have been associated with significant morbidity and mortality in the childcare setting. In 1986, an outbreak of diarrhea caused by *E. coli* O157:H7 was reported from a daycare attended by 107 children.[161] Thirty-four percent of attendees became ill, with a significant increase in risk for younger children. Approximately a third of the children with diarrhea had bloody stools, and hemolytic-uremic syndrome developed in three. Although infection with *E. coli* O157:H7 usually occurs after the ingestion of contaminated beef, person-to-person spread of infection most likely occurred in this epidemic. The diarrheal illness also was documented in family members of ill children. Subsequent epidemiologic studies in Minnesota have confirmed the mode of transmission for *E. coli* O157:H7 to be person to person in the daycare setting.[16] Accordingly, symptomatic children should be excluded from daycare until stools are formed and culture-negative for *E. coli* O157:H7. Unfortunately, fecal shedding of *E. coli* 0157:H7 may be quite prolonged in young children.[171]

E. coli O157:H7 is recovered from stool samples after being plated on MacConkey-sorbitol agar. Sorbitol-negative colonies of *E. coli* are picked and screened with O157 antisera by tube agglutination. Antibiotic treatment is not recommended for persons with diarrhea caused by *E. coli* O157:H7.[194] Hemolytic-uremic syndrome develops in approximately 5 to 10 percent of children infected with *E. coli* O157:H7.

Outbreaks of diarrhea caused by enteropathogenic *E. coli* in the childcare setting have been characterized by chronic, often relapsing diarrhea in infants and toddlers.[21, 131] The diarrheal illness has had a high attack rate (56–90%) and has led to prolonged hospitalization in 8 to 30 percent of affected children.

Rotavirus

Rotavirus is the most common etiologic agent of gastroenteritis in infants and children and the leading cause of hospitalization for gastroenteritis in industrialized countries, including the United States.[20, 107] It is an important cause of diarrhea in developing countries as well and contributes substantially to the worldwide mortality figures for gastroenteritis. It is the pathogen most commonly present in daycare settings.[39]

Rotavirus frequently is recovered from asymptomatic hosts, especially neonates and infants.[24] It is shed in large numbers in the stool of symptomatic patients, thereby contributing to the high prevalence of the virus on environmental surfaces during outbreaks.[192] Viral shedding occurs both before and after symptoms have appeared[133]; only a low inoculum is needed to cause infection.

Most illnesses caused by rotavirus occur in the winter in temperate climates but year-round in tropical areas. The peak attack rate is in the 6- to 24-month-old age group. After a brief incubation period of 2 to 3 days, patients may have prodromal respiratory symptoms (coryza and cough) and then varying combinations of vomiting, diarrhea, and low-grade fever that last 3 to 5 days. The range of severity is broad, and dehydration occasionally may be profound. Spread of rotavirus infection is extremely common in hospitals[147]; not surprisingly, transmission within a daycare center is very rapid, and many outbreaks have been reported in this setting.[14, 123, 124, 133, 134, 146] In prospective studies of diarrheal illness in children attending daycare, rotavirus was implicated in 6 to 24 percent of cases of gastroenteritis[13, 74, 170] and in 20 to 40 percent of outbreaks.[14, 134] Daycare workers and family contacts are at risk for acquiring rotavirus infection.

Rotavirus cannot be cultivated easily in tissue culture in a viral diagnostic laboratory. The diagnosis is made with an antigen-detection method on a stool specimen. Treatment is supportive, and exclusion from daycare is recommended until the diarrhea resolves.

Hepatitis A Virus

HAV, an enterovirus, is the most common cause of acute hepatitis in children. As with other enteric pathogens, this organism is transmitted by the fecal-oral route. Manifestations of infection vary remarkably according to age. In young children (<6 years), infection with HAV may be entirely asymptomatic or associated with relatively mild and nonspecific symptoms such as low-grade fever, anorexia, nausea, vomiting, and diarrhea in 30 percent of patients.[7] Jaundice, a more specific marker of liver disease, occurs in less than 10 percent of children younger than 6 years.[59] In contrast, adults with hepatitis A are often icteric in conjunction with other gastrointestinal symptoms. Infection, when symptomatic, usually lasts several weeks but occasionally can become protracted.

HAV is shed in high density in the stool of infected persons from 2 weeks before until 1 week after the onset of clinical symptoms. Transmission is primarily from person to person, but fomites may play an important role because the organism can persist and remain infective in the dried state for months.[108] The diagnosis usually is made by detecting serologic evidence of marker antibodies against HAV (IgM anti-HAV). Treatment is symptomatic. Prevention of illness in contacts can be accomplished with intramuscular immune serum globulin and most recently with hepatitis A vaccine.[191] A study conducted among children residing in a Hasidic Jewish community in New York State demonstrated the efficacy of inactivated hepatitis A vaccine in preventing hepatitis A during 7 months of follow-up after vaccination.[126] Further study is under way to determine the duration of immunity and the need for boosters.

HAV can be spread easily in daycare centers with diaperage children because of the facility of person-to-person transmission.[65] Spread of infection is barely noticeable until symptomatic HAV infection develops in an adult contact (usually a parent or daycare worker). Other contacts, including siblings, extended family members, and babysitters, also are affected frequently. Clusters of cases of hepatitis A in communities have been traced to a single daycare center. The risk of a hepatitis outbreak occurring in a daycare center has been shown to be related directly to the number and age of children in attendance and the hours that the center is open. Larger centers with longer hours and diaperage children have the highest rates of infection and greatest spread to the community.[64]

INFECTIONS SPREAD BY SKIN CONTACT

Group A Streptococci

GAS have become a less common cause of impetigo and pyoderma in children during the last decade, with a concomitant rise in cases caused by *S. aureus*. Nonetheless, these organisms still can cause superficial infection of traumatized skin (insect bites, scratches), erysipelas, and cellulitis. The latter infections can result in an abrupt onset of fever and dramatic cutaneous erythema and tenderness often accompanied by regional adenopathy. An outbreak of perianal *S. pyogenes* infection in a daycare center was reported recently. Typical signs and symptoms include perianal inflammation, itching, rectal pain, and blood-streaked stool. Four documented cases in three children and two presumed cases were treated without obtaining specific cultures.[152] The diagnosis of streptococcal skin infection can be made by careful performance of wound or surface cultures (obtained after carefully cleansing the periwound area) or examination of tissue aspirates. Spread of typical impetigo occurs commonly within families and presumably also would occur within daycare centers. Children should be excluded from daycare until they have completed 24 hours of appropriate antimicrobial therapy (of a 10-day course).

Scabies

Scabies is an infection of the skin caused by infestation with the female mite *Sarcoptes scabiei*. Transmitted person to person by an infested individual, the mite buries itself beneath the stratum corneum and burrows along for its 30-day life span while laying two to three eggs per day. The larval and nymphal mites scatter after hatching to embed themselves in skin at distant sites. Some 3 to 6 weeks later, a pruritic eruption (worse at night) develops and leads to excoriation, bleeding, and crusting. The distribution of lesions varies with age. In adults and older children, the eruption, which consists of papules, vesicles, and nodules, occurs commonly in the interdigital spaces of the hands, on the extensor surface of the elbows, and around the umbilicus, waist, axillary lines, and genital area. In infants and young children, vesicular and eczematous lesions are found on the hands and feet, as well as on the face and head.

The diagnosis is made by scraping the lesions and demonstrating the mite, ova, or mite feces. Treatment of the index case should be undertaken with a scabicide, preferably 5 percent permethrin, applied to the entire body. Alternative, less desirable drugs are lindane and crotamiton. Asymptomatic contacts should be treated simultaneously because they might be infected unknowingly and may be capable of transmitting the mite during this asymptomatic period. Clothing and bed linen should be washed, dry-cleaned, or stored for a week to ensure that they are not infectious.

Although scabies is spread primarily by intimate personal contact, skin-to-skin transmission can occur after prolonged casual contact, as occurs in institutional settings, nursing homes, and daycare centers.[151] Mites can survive for 2 to 3 days on inanimate surfaces, which permits transmission via fomites such as clothes, bed linen, and furniture. An outbreak of scabies recently was reported in a hospital-affiliated daycare facility.[151] Elimination of the problem required a coordinated effort with simultaneous treatment of all potentially infected individuals. An infected child should be excluded from daycare for 24 hours after treatment is undertaken. More commonly, transmission occurs within the family setting.

Head Lice

Head lice infestation occurs commonly in daycare and school-age children as a consequence of infection with *Pediculus capitis*. The insect, a hemophagocytic ectoparasite, obtains nourishment by sucking capillary blood from the scalp. Female lice attach egg cases (nits) to the hair shafts at or very near the scalp. The eggs hatch 8 to 11 days later, with three louse nymphs released.

The diagnosis is made when the symptoms of scalp pruritus, excoriation, pyoderma, and regional lymphadenopathy cause the caregiver to inspect the scalp closely. Nits are observed readily, although live lice may be difficult to see, especially in light infestations. Transmission is by direct contact with or spread by fomites of live lice. The latter is facilitated with common storage of hats and coats.

Treatment is with permethrin shampoos to eradicate the lice. Nits can be removed mechanically with spiral combs after preparation of the hair with vinegar soaks or a commercially prepared rinse. All clothing and infested bedding can be disinfected by machine washing or drying (at temperatures of at least 128.3°F [53.5°C]), dry cleaning, or storage in plastic bags for approximately 10 days.

INFECTIONS SPREAD BY CONTACT WITH BLOOD, URINE, AND SALIVA

Hepatitis B Virus

HBV is a DNA-containing virus that causes infections with a wide range of clinical manifestations from asymptomatic seroconversion to fatal hepatitis. Infection in children is more likely to be asymptomatic than that in adults.[110] Common symptoms include fever, fatigue, anorexia, malaise, and jaundice. Other gastrointestinal symptoms, such as nausea, vomiting, and diarrhea, may be prominent. Joint symptoms (arthritis and arthralgias) and cutaneous lesions (papular acrodermatitis) may be noted early in the illness.

The most common modes of transmission of HBV in adults are contact with blood and sexual activity. Young children usually acquire infection with HBV by vertical transmission from their mother at delivery. The maternal infection may be acute or chronic. Infection acquired vertically by an infant is usually asymptomatic, but it leads to chronic carriage of hepatitis B surface antigen in most cases. With increasing immigration and adoption of infants from HBV-endemic areas, more HBV carrier children will be identified.[68]

Transmission of HBV within the daycare setting has been documented twice in the United States[40, 156] and once in Australia.[109] In one case, the probable source was a bite by a child who was a carrier of HBV.[156] In the other, a daycare worker with chapped hands was exposed to the blood of a child who was an HBV carrier.[40] The case in Australia involved an aggressive 21-month-old infant with weeping dermatitis and a history of biting other children. Three other investigations have failed to demonstrate transmission in daycare facilities despite long-term contact, including one situation with a high potential for blood exposure.[40, 156, 157] The most recent surveillance activity showed only 1 of 496 HBV-infected children in daycare to be without a family member as a potential source.[55] In Japan, where the background prevalence of hepatitis B surface antigen carriage is higher than that in the United States, data suggest that transmission of HBV most probably occurs among children in nursery schools.[69] Implementation of the current recommendation to screen all parturients for HBV and to undertake universal immunization against hepatitis B in infancy should curtail spread of this infection in the future. A study to assess progress in hepatitis B vaccination of children showed an impressive increase from 1994 through 1996 (from 41% to 84%) and a plateau of 84 to 85 percent in 1996/1997.[195] Because of the low risk of transmission within the daycare setting, the American Academy of Pediatrics (AAP), the American Public Health Association, and the Centers for Disease Control and Prevention (CDC) do not recommend exclusion of HBV-infected children from daycare or HBV screening of children as a criterion for entry.[7]

Cytomegalovirus

CMV can be transmitted by blood, urine, and saliva, as described earlier.

Human Immunodeficiency Virus

To date, HIV infection has not been reported to be transmitted in a daycare center. In light of its rare horizontal transmission to nonsexual contacts within households with an infected member, HIV would not be expected to spread in daycare.[57, 87] The risk of transmission of HIV is less than 1 in 500 exposures, even when direct inoculation with HIV-infected blood has occurred by needle-stick injury to a health care worker. The risk of exposure other than by direct inoculation is far less than 1 in 500. The risk in daycare is even lower. Potential high-risk situations might involve HIV-positive children who are persistent biters or who have extensive weeping skin lesions.

One example of possible transmission of HIV between siblings was reported from Germany.[186] In this case, a bite may have been the source, although complete information on other interactions between the brothers was not available. Other reports have indicated a lack of transmission to 35 individuals bitten or scratched by a person infected with HIV.[45, 159, 180] In addition, a study of family members of children infected with HIV reported no seroconversion to HIV in nine contacts bitten by HIV-infected children and seven uninfected children who bit children infected with HIV.[148] These studies support the lack of evidence for transmission of HIV in the daycare setting.

Vaccine-Preventable Diseases

DIPHTHERIA

Diphtheria is now a very rare disease in the United States; fewer than five cases a year have been observed recently. The infection can cause nasal symptoms, membranous pharyngitis, obstructive laryngotracheitis, or skin manifestations. The prominent symptoms are usually a severe sore throat and croup accompanied by toxemia.

Corynebacterium diphtheriae is spread by droplets from people with infection or carriers after intimate contact. Individuals are susceptible if they have not been immunized or have been immunized only partially. Treatment is with antitoxin and antibiotics (erythromycin or penicillin). Prophylaxis can be accomplished with erythromycin or penicillin if an individual is found to be a carrier. Immunization with diphtheria-tetanus-pertussis or diphtheria-tetanus vaccine is effective in preventing disease and spread of infection.

VARICELLA-ZOSTER

Varicella-zoster, or chickenpox, is a common, highly contagious infection of childhood that affects more than 80 percent of the population by the time that they reach 10 years of age. The infection is spread easily by the airborne route and by respiratory droplets. It is characterized by a pruritic, generalized vesicular rash that occurs in one to six crops, each crop separated by 24 to 36 hours. Fever is usually mild. The most common complication is secondary bacterial pyoderma. Varicella-zoster virus remains latent in the body after primary infection but can be reactivated as herpes zoster or "shingles," in which case it is manifested as a vesicular eruption involving one to three sensory dermatomes. If infection is acquired in early pregnancy, a varicella embryopathy (limb bands or amputation) has been noted in a small fraction of offspring.

Rates of varicella peak during the preschool and kindergarten years (3 to 6), with only 20 percent of children remaining susceptible to chickenpox after 8 years of age. Data on the relative risk of varicella's developing in children in daycare are minimal.[51, 89] However, outbreaks of varicella in daycare centers are known to occur commonly, and the prevalence of varicella in children who attend daycare appears to be higher than that documented for the general population.[54] Children with varicella are excluded from daycare but may return 6 days after the onset of rash or when all their lesions are crusted.

In 1995, varicella vaccine became available for universal use in children between 12 and 15 months of age. The availability of this vaccine has altered the epidemiology of varicella in the United States dramatically. The vaccine has been demonstrated to be highly effective during outbreaks of varicella in daycare[27, 84] and in clinical practice in general.[185] The effectiveness of the vaccine is 83 to 86 percent against all forms of the disease and 97 to 100 percent against moderate to severe disease.

MEASLES

Measles (rubeola) is a highly contagious respiratory infection. After many years of decline, it again reached epidemic proportions in impoverished and medically underserved inner-city areas in the United States between 1989 and 1992. Although susceptibility to measles virus infection occurs when maternal antibody wanes, the peak age group for measles in the pre-immunization era was school-age children between 5 and 9 years old. More recently, outbreaks have involved preschool children, thus setting the stage for outbreaks in daycare facilities.

Measles virus is spread by droplets, hand transmission, and the airborne route. The illness is usually moderate to severe; high fever and prominent respiratory symptoms (cough and coryza) and conjunctivitis are present for several days before onset of the rash. Diarrhea occasionally may be a prominent feature. After the rash erupts, the fever and respiratory symptoms persist for several more days. Pneumonia and encephalitis are complications of measles virus infection; each occurs at an incidence of 1 per 1000 cases.

Measles is prevented effectively by immunization. Current recommendations are to immunize twice: once between 12 and 15 months of age and again at 4 to 6 years or 10 to 14 years of age.[7, 111] In epidemic situations, primary immunization may be given before a child is 12 months of age. In such cases, another vaccination is given between 12 and 15 months of age, and the first is not counted toward the two required for full protection.

When measles is diagnosed in a child attending daycare after several days of illness, intramuscular immune serum globulin is the most effective way to prevent secondary cases in susceptible contacts. When there has been a single recent exposure to a case of measles, administration of measles-mumps-rubella (MMR) vaccine within 3 days of exposure should be effective in preventing natural infection.

RUBELLA

Rubella, another exanthematous disease of childhood, is much milder than rubeola but attacks a similar age group. As with measles, until recently rubella nearly had been eradicated by routine universal immunization with MMR vaccine.

Clinically, rubella is characterized by mild fever, lymphadenopathy (postauricular and occipital), and rash. The illness is difficult to distinguish from other viral exanthems. Infection may be completely asymptomatic. Children with documented rubella should be excluded from daycare until 5 days after the onset of illness.

If rubella is contracted during the first or early second trimester of pregnancy, a severe fetal infection resulting in microcephaly, deafness, congenital heart defects, eye disorders, and psychomotor retardation may result. Acquisition of infection during pregnancy may be a potential hazard for daycare personnel or mothers of children who attend daycare if an outbreak of rubella occurs in the daycare setting. Recently, a large outbreak of rubella occurred in Nebraska. Fourteen children (9 of whom were younger than 12 months) and 2 parents acquired their infection in a daycare center.[36]

Congenital rubella syndrome can be minimized by appropriate immunization of preschoolers and personnel. No specific recommendations exist for care after exposure of a susceptible pregnant adult.

PERTUSSIS

Pertussis, or whooping cough, is a highly communicable respiratory disease caused by *Bordetella pertussis*. The attack rate and severity of disease are highest in the first year of life. The illness classically is divided into three phases: catarrhal, paroxysmal, and convalescent. In the first stage, the child has no fever but has symptoms, primarily rhinorrhea and a cough. When the nasal symptoms resolve, however, the cough becomes and remains very prominent for many weeks. The cough is characterized by paroxysms that are followed by an inspiratory effort (whoop) or leave the child exhausted and occasionally apneic. The convalescent stage is the many weeks necessary for complete recovery. Treatment with erythromycin is effective in decreasing the shedding of organisms, but it does not alter the course of the disease.

Complete immunization with sequential use of whole killed pertussis vaccine and acellular pertussis vaccine or a five-dose series of acellular pertussis vaccine is effective in preventing most cases of pertussis, although illness does occur in partially and occasionally in fully immunized children.[26] After exposure to a case, erythromycin for 14 days provides effective prophylaxis, despite its negligible clinical effect after the paroxysmal stage begins. It is recommended for exposure in daycare.[12] If appropriate, booster doses of acellular diphtheria-tetanus-pertussis vaccine should be given to exposed children in a daycare or household setting. A child with pertussis should be excluded from daycare until 5 days of a 14-day course of erythromycin has been received.[26]

POLIOMYELITIS

Poliovirus is an enterovirus that now rarely causes disease in the United States. Although most infections with poliovirus are subclinical, in the pre-immunization era, polio was the major cause of acquired paralytic disease, especially in older children and young adults. In some developing countries, it remains a major health problem.

Poliomyelitis is prevented effectively by use of either the live oral poliovirus vaccine or the inactivated, enhanced-potency parenteral vaccine (IPV).[137] The Advisory Committee on Immunization Practices of the CDC and the AAP recommend a four-dose all-IPV vaccine schedule for routine immunization of all infants and children in the United States.

MUMPS

Mumps is a relatively benign infection of childhood that is often asymptomatic. The most prominent clinical feature is parotitis. Occasionally, a clinically significant central nervous system infection causes unilateral sensorineural deafness. This infection virtually has been eliminated by widespread use of the MMR vaccine. Children with mumps should be excluded from the daycare setting until the parotid swelling subsides or, if the swelling is prolonged, until 9 days after the onset of swelling.

HEPATITIS B

HBV is a vaccine-preventable infection that is spread by contact with blood, urine, and saliva, as described earlier.

Management of Infections

EXCLUSION POLICY

The AAP and the American Public Health Association have reached a consensus regarding exclusion policies for children attending daycare.[9] The recommendations reflect the understanding that when children have moderate to severe illnesses, they should not be allowed to participate in usual activities or may require more individualized care than available and that the spread of certain communicable diseases within the daycare center will be reduced by the exclusion of people with infections. Accordingly, children known to have highly infectious illnesses should not be allowed to attend daycare until treatment is initiated (as for head lice or GAS infections) or the symptoms have resolved (e.g., diarrhea caused by *Shigella*, rotavirus, or *Giardia*) or until transmissibility has waned, as in pertussis, varicella, measles, and mumps. In addition, children should be excluded if the contagiousness of their illness is uncertain (e.g., if a child has a high fever and a rash). A complete list of recommendations for exclusion is presented in Table 245–6.

Important conditions that do not necessarily require exclusion from daycare include (1) asymptomatic excretion of an enteropathogen, (2) nonpurulent conjunctivitis, (3) a rash without a fever or behavioral change, (4) CMV infection, (5) the carrier state of HBV infection, (6) HIV infection, and (7) parvovirus B19 infection in an immunocompetent host. Any exceptions to this statement are found in the

TABLE 245–6 ■ RECOMMENDATIONS FOR EXCLUSION FROM DAYCARE

Symptoms

Illness that prevents the child from comfortably participating in program activities
Illness that results in a greater need for care than the staff can provide without compromising the health and safety of other children
The child has any of the following conditions; fever, lethargy, irritability, persistent crying, difficulty breathing, or other manifestations of possible severe illness
Diarrhea or stools that contain blood or mucus
Escherichia coli 0157:H7 or *Shigella* infection, until the diarrhea resolves and 2 stool cultures are negative for these organisms
Vomiting 2 or more times during the previous 24 hours, unless the vomiting is determined to be due to a noncommunicable condition and the child is not in danger of dehydration
Mouth sores associated with drooling, unless the child's physician or local health department authority states that the child is noninfectious
Rash with fever or behavior change, until a physician has determined that the illness is not a communicable disease

Specific Diseases

Purulent conjunctivitis (defined as pink or red conjunctiva with white yellow eye discharge, often with matted eyelids after sleep and eye pain or redness of the eyelids or skin surrounding the eye), until examined by a physician and approved for re-admission, with treatment
Tuberculosis, until the child's physician or local health department authority states that the child is noninfectious
Impetigo, until 24 hours after treatment has been initiated
Streptococcal pharyngitis, until 24 hours after treatment has been initiated
Head lice (pediculosis), until after the first treatment
Scabies, until after treatment has been given
Varicella, until all lesions have dried and crusted (usually 6 days)
Pertussis, until 5 days of appropriate antibiotic therapy (which is to be given for a total of 14 days) has been completed
Mumps, until 9 days after the onset of parotid gland swelling
Measles, until 4 days after the onset of rash
Hepatitis A virus infection, until 1 week after the onset of illness or jaundice (if symptoms are mild)

Used with permission of the American Academy of Pediatrics: Children in out-of-home child care. *In* Pickering, L. (ed.): 2000 Red Book: Report of the Committee on Infectious Diseases. 25th ed. Elk Grove Village, IL, American Academy of Pediatrics, 2000, p. 108.

individual discussions of the infectious agents. For many infections, the highest risk of transmission of disease occurs before the appearance of recognizable symptoms. Once illness occurs, other children already have been exposed and exclusion is a less effective strategy, which explains why exclusion has not been shown to be successful in reducing the frequency of viral upper respiratory tract infections.

PROPHYLAXIS OF INFECTION

Prophylaxis is a strategy that may be helpful in the management of some infections that occur in daycare centers. For example, if a child has had invasive disease caused by *N. meningitidis,* rifampin prophylaxis for all daycare contacts may prevent secondary or associated cases. If a child has pertussis, exposed children may be protected by a booster immunization if appropriate and administration of erythromycin for prophylaxis. Intramuscular immune serum globulin may be used to protect susceptible contacts after exposure to measles or hepatitis A.

VACCINATION

Vaccination can be used as a strategy to prevent infection during epidemics in a community. For example, immunization with MMR vaccine is successful in terminating epidemics of measles in elementary or high school. Varicella vaccine also can be used community-wide and up to 3 days after exposure to curtail the spread of chickenpox. Hepatitis A vaccine is an appropriate intervention for controlling an outbreak of hepatitis A in daycare centers and other settings.[77]

HBV rarely has been reported to be transmitted in a daycare setting in the United States. Hepatitis B vaccine, now recommended for universal use in infancy, protects against transmission of infection if a carrier of HBV is identified.

Prevention of Infections

VACCINATION

Currently, the 12 vaccine-preventable diseases for a preschool child are diphtheria, tetanus, pertussis, polio, measles, mumps, rubella, varicella, Hib infection, *S. pneumoniae* infection, hepatitis A, and hepatitis B. The timely and appropriate use of immunizations will eliminate or dramatically reduce these problems from the daycare setting. Recommendations for the use of hepatitis A vaccine in children are awaited. Studies have shown that children who attend registered daycare facilities are more likely to be up-to-date in their immunizations than are children cared for at home.[73] Laws requiring age-appropriate vaccination of children attending licensed child daycare programs exist in almost all states.[23]

EDUCATION

An integral part of the control of infection within a daycare center is education of staff and families. The staff must understand the general principles of infection transmission and control. Education before job placement and frequent inservice seminars reinforce the importance of some basic techniques, especially handwashing. Supervision is essential to ensure compliance with policies.[95] Two recent studies have shown a modest benefit of increased attention to handwashing in preventing respiratory infections in children younger than 2 years and in preventing episodes of diarrhea in children older than 2 years.[144, 145]

Parents should be educated regarding recognition of illness, especially illnesses for which the child receives the best care at home. The rationale and importance of compliance with center rules should be emphasized. The childcare program should inform parents of the need to share information about communicable illnesses in the child or a family member.

WRITTEN POLICIES

Each daycare facility should have written policies for managing child and employee illness.[9] It should have written procedures for handwashing, personal hygiene policies, environmental sanitation policies and procedures, and policies for filing and updating immunization records. Employees should be screened for tuberculosis by skin testing when hired and annually if the skin test is initially negative. If the skin test result is positive, a chest radiograph should be obtained. Other recommendations regarding immunization of daycare employees are shown in Table 245–7. Screening daycare attendees or employees for HIV, HBV, or CMV is not necessary.

PHYSICAL PLANT CHARACTERISTICS

In the planning of daycare facilities, areas for infants and toddlers should be separated from those for older children. Because fecal contamination is related strongly and inversely to age, having physical premises large enough to separate children younger than 3 years from older children is important. If such separation cannot be achieved, an age restriction should be placed on admission. The kitchen and food storage areas should be separated from the toilet space. Because contamination of hands is the most critical factor in transmission of infection, handwashing facilities must be available to staff and children. Such facilities are especially important in the diaper-changing and food preparation areas. The handwashing facility preferably should be pedal-operated and in easy reach of soap and towel dispensers.

When construction materials are selected, the choice should be based on durability and ease of cleaning. Diaper-changing areas should be made of materials that can be

TABLE 245–7 ■ IMMUNIZATIONS FOR DAYCARE EMPLOYEES

Vaccine	Personnel	Schedule
Diphtheria, tetanus	All	Every 10 yr
Measles-mumps-rubella	All	If born after 1955, evidence of previous infection or 2 doses at least 1 mo apart
Varicella	Nonimmune	Two doses 1 mo apart
Polio	All	Primary immunization with inactivated poliovirus vaccine if needed. Consider booster if previously immunized
Influenza A/B	If older than 55 yr	Annually
Hepatitis B	Advised	0, 1, and 6 mo
Hepatitis A	All	Two doses 1 mo apart

cleaned easily and light-colored so that soilage can be detected. A pedal-operated, closed receptacle is ideal for disposal of soiled diapers. Only paper diapers should be used. The toddler area should be equipped with training toilets and junior-sized toilets. The use of potty chairs should be discouraged. If they are used, they should be emptied into the toilet, cleaned in a utility sink, and disinfected after each use.[9] These areas must be cleaned frequently.

HYGIENIC STANDARDS

The key factor in prevention of disease in the daycare setting is maintenance of optimal hygienic standards based on recognized mechanisms of transmission of infection. Handwashing is considered the single most important preventive measure[12, 17, 61, 95, 135] in recognition of the fact that both respiratory and enteric pathogens are spread by contaminated hands.

REFERENCES

1. Adler, S. P.: The molecular epidemiology of cytomegalovirus transmission among children attending a day care center. J. Infect. Dis. *152*:760–768, 1985.
2. Adler, S. P.: Molecular epidemiology of cytomegalovirus: Evidence for viral transmission to parents from children infected at a day care center. Pediatr. Infect. Dis. J. *5*:315–318, 1986.
3. Adler, S. P.: Cytomegalovirus transmission among children in day care, their mothers and caretakers. Pediatr. Infect. Dis. J. *7*:279–285, 1988.
4. Adler, S. P.: Molecular epidemiology of cytomegalovirus: Viral transmission among children attending a day care center, their parents, and caretakers. J. Pediatr. *112*:366–372, 1988.
5. Alpert, G., Bell, L. M., Kirkpatrick, C. E., et al.: Cryptosporidiosis in a day care center. N. Engl. J. Med. *311*:860–861, 1984.
6. Alpert, G., Bell, L. M., Kirkpatrick, C. E., et al.: Outbreak of cryptosporidiosis in a day-care center. Pediatrics *77*:152–157, 1986.
7. American Academy of Pediatrics: Children in out-of-home child care. *In* Pickering, L. (ed.): 2000 Red Book: Report of the Committee on Infectious Diseases. 25th ed. Elk Grove Village, IL, American Academy of Pediatrics, 2000, p. 113.
8. American Academy of Pediatrics. Committee on Infectious Diseases. Policy Statement: Recommendations for the prevention of pneumococcal infections, including the use of pneumococcal conjugate vaccine (Prevnar), pneumococcal polysaccharide vaccine, and antibiotic prophylaxis. Pediatrics *106*:362–366, 2000.
9. American Public Health Association and American Academy of Pediatrics: Caring for our children. *In* National Health and Safety Performance Standards: Guidelines for Out-of-Home Child Care Programs. Washington, DC, American Public Health Association, 2000.
10. Anderson, L. J.: Human parvoviruses. J. Infect. Dis. *161*:603–608, 1990.
11. Band, J. D., Fraser, D. W., and Ajello, G.: *Haemophilus influenzae* disease study group: Prevention of *Haemophilus influenzae* type b disease by rifampin prophylaxis. J. A. M. A. *251*:2381–2386, 1984.
12. Bartlett, A. V., Broome, C. V., Hadler, S. C., et al.: Public health considerations of infectious diseases in child day care centers. J. Pediatr. *105*:1683–701, 1984.
13. Bartlett, A. V., Moore, M., Gary, G. W., et al.: Diarrheal illness among infants and toddlers in child day care centers. J. Pediatr. *107*:495–502, 1985.
14. Bartlett, A. V., Reves, R. R., and Pickering, L. K.: Rotavirus in infant-toddler day care centers: Epidemiology relevant to disease control strategies. J. Pediatr. *113*:435–441, 1988.
15. Beem, M. O.: Acute respiratory illness in nursery school children: A longitudinal study of the occurrence of illness and respiratory viruses. Am. J. Epidemiol. *90*:30–44, 1969.
16. Belongia, E. A., Osterholm, M. T., Soler, J. T., et al.: Transmission of *Escherichia coli* O157:H7 infection in Minnesota child day care facilities. J. A. M. A. *269*:883–888, 1993.
17. Black, R. E., Dykes, A. C., Anderson, K. E., et al.: Handwashing to prevent diarrhea in day-care centers. Am. J. Epidemiol. *113*:445–451, 1981.
18. Black, R. E., Dykes, A. C., Sinclair, S. P., et al.: Giardiasis in day-care centers: Evidence of person-to-person transmission. Pediatrics *60*:486- 491, 1977.
19. Black, S., Shinefield, H., Fireman, B., et al.: Efficacy, safety and immunogenicity of heptavalent pneumococcal vaccine in children. Pediatr. Infect. Dis. J. *19*:187–195, 2000.
20. Blacklow, N., and Greenberg, H. B.: Medical progress: Viral gastroenteritis. N. Engl. J. Med. *325*:252–264, 1991.
21. Bower, J. R., Congeni, B. L., Cleary, T. G., et al.: *Escherichia coli* O114: Non-motile as a pathogen in an outbreak of severe diarrhea associated with a day care center. J. Infect. Dis. *160*:243–247, 1989.
22. Cain, V. S.: Child care and child health: Use of population surveys. Pediatrics *94*:1096–1098, 1994.
23. Centers for Disease Control and Prevention: State Immunization Requirements, 1991–1992. Washington, DC, U. S. Department of Health and Human Services, CDC, 1992.
24. Champsaur, H., Questiaux, E., Prevot, J., et al.: Rotavirus carriage, asymptomatic infection and disease in the first two years of life. 1. Virus shedding. J. Infect. Dis. *149*:667–673, 1984.
25. Cherian, T., Steinhoff, M. C., Harrison, L. H., et al.: A cluster of invasive pneumococcal disease in young children in child care. J. A. M. A. *271*:695–697, 1994.
26. Christie, C. D., Marx, M. L., Daniels, J. A., and Adcock, M. P.: Pertussis containment in schools and day care centers during the Cincinnati epidemic of 1993. Am. J. Public Health *87*:460–462, 1997.
27. Clements, D. A., Moreira, S. P., Coplan, P. M., et al.: Post licensure study of varicella vaccine effectiveness in a day-care setting. Pediatr. Infect. Dis. J. *18*:1047–1050, 1999.
28. Cochi, S. L., Fleming, D. W., Hightower, A. W., et al.: Primary invasive *Haemophilus influenzae* type b disease: A population-based assessment of risk factors. J. Pediatr. *108*:887–896, 1986.
29. Cody, M. M., Sottnek, H. M., and O'Leary, V. S.: Recovery of *Giardia lamblia* cysts from chairs and tables in child day care centers. Pediatrics *94*(Suppl.):1006–1008, 1994.
30. Combee, C. L., Collinge, M. L., and Britt, E. M.: Cryptosporidiosis in a hospital associated day care center. Pediatr. Infect. Dis. J. *5*:528–532, 1986.
31. Cordell, R. L., and Addiss, D. G.: Cryptosporidiosis in child care settings: A review of the literature and recommendations for prevention and control. Pediatr. Infect. Dis. J. *13*:310–317, 1994.
32. Craig, A. S., Erwin, P. C., Schaffner, W., et al.: Carriage of multi-drug resistant *Streptococcus pneumoniae* and impact of chemoprophylaxis during an outbreak of meningitis at a day care center. Clin. Infect. Dis. *29*:1257–1264, 1999.
33. Crawford, F. G., Vermund, S., Ma, J. Y., et al.: Asymptomatic cryptosporidiosis in a New York City day care center. Pediatr. Infect. Dis. J. *7*:806–807, 1988.
34. Curtis A. B., Ridzon, R., Vogel, R., et al.: Extensive transmission of *Mycobacterium tuberculosis* from a child. N. Engl. J. Med. *341*:1491–1495, 1999.
35. Daly, K., Giebink, S., Le, C. T., et al.: Determining risk for chronic otitis media with effusion. Pediatr. Infect. Dis. J. *7*:471–475, 1988.
36. Danovaro-Holliday, M. C., LeBaron, C. W., Allensworth, C., et al.: A large rubella outbreak with spread from the workplace to the community. J. A. M. A. *284*:2733–2739, 2000.
37. Dashefsky, B., Wald, E., and Li, K.: Commentary: Management of contacts of children in day care with invasive *Haemophilus influenzae* type b disease. Pediatrics *78*:939, 1986.
38. DeMaeyer-Aeempoel, S., Reginster-Hancuse, G., Dachy, A., et al.: Meningococcal disease in Belgium: Secondary attack rate among household, day-care nursery, and pre-elementary school contacts. J. Infect. *3*(Suppl. 1):63–70, 1981.
39. Dennehy, P. H.: Transmission of rotavirus and other enteric pathogens in the home. Pediatr. Infect. Dis. J. *19*(Suppl.):103–105, 2000.
40. Desoda, C. C., Shapiro, C. N., Carroll, K., et al.: Hepatitis B virus transmission between a child and staff member at a day care center. Pediatr. Infect. Dis. J. *13*:828–830, 1994.
41. DeWals, P., Hertoghe, L., Borlée-Grimée, I., et al.: Meningococcal disease in Belgium: Secondary attack rates among household, day-care nursery and pre-elementary school contacts. J. Infect. *1*(Suppl.):53–61, 1981.
42. Dingle, J. H., Badger, G. F., and Jordan, W. S., Jr.: Illness in the Home. Cleveland, Press of Western Reserve University, 1964.
43. Doyle, A. B.: Incidence of illness in early group and family day-care. Pediatrics *58*:607–613, 1976.
44. Doyle, M. G., Van, R., and Pickering, L. K.: Penicillin-resistant *Streptococcus pneumoniae* in children in home care and day care. Pediatr. Infect. Dis. J. *11*:831–835, 1992.
45. Drummond, J. A.: Seronegative 18 months after being bitten by a patient with AIDS. J. A. M. A. *256*:2342–2343, 1986.
46. Ekanem, E. E., DuPont, H. L., Pickering, L. K., et al.: Transmission dynamics of enteric bacteria in day-care centers. Am. J. Epidemiol. *118*:562–572, 1983.
47. Falck, G., and Kjellander, J.: Outbreak of group A streptococcal infection in a day care center. Pediatr. Infect. Dis. J. *11*:914–919, 1992.
48. Ferson, M. J.: Infections in day care. Curr. Opin. Pediatr. *5*:35–40, 1993.
49. Ferson, M. J., and Bell, S. M.: Outbreak of Coxsackie A16 hand, foot and mouth disease in a child day care center. Am. J. Public Health *81*:1675–1676, 1991.
50. Fiellau-Nikolajsen, M.: Tympanometry in 3-year old children. ORL J. Otorhinolaryngol. Relat. Spec. *41*:193–205, 1979.
51. Finger, R., Hughes, J. P., Meade, B. J., et al.: Age specific incidence of chickenpox. Public Health Rep. *109*:750–755, 1994.

52. Fleming, D. W., Cochi, S. L., Hightower, A. W., et al.: Childhood upper respiratory tract infections: To what degree is incidence affected by day care attendance? Pediatrics *79*:55–60, 1987.
53. Fleming, D. W., Leibenhaut, M. H., Albanea, D., et al.: Secondary *Haemophilus influenzae* type b in day care facilities: Risk factors and prevention. J. A. M. A. *254*:509–514, 1985.
54. Foscarelli, P.: Infectious conditions in day care: There is more than enteritis and rhinitis. Am. J. Dis. Child. *144*:955–956, 1990.
55. Foy, H. M., Swenson, P. D., and Freitag-Koontz, M. J., et al.: Surveillance for transmission of hepatitis B in child day care. Pediatrics *94*(Suppl.):1002–1004, 1994.
56. Frenck, R. W., and Glezen, W. P.: Respiratory tract infections in children in day care. Semin. Pediatr. Infect. Dis. *1*:234–244, 1990.
57. Friedland, G. H., Saltzman, B. R., Rogers, M. F., et al.: Lack of transmission of HTLV-III/LAV infection to household contacts of patients with AIDS or AIDS-related complex with oral candidiasis. N. Engl. J. Med. *314*:344–349, 1986.
58. Gillespie, S. M., Cartter, M. L., Asch, S., et al.: Occupational risk of human parvovirus B19 infection for school and day care personnel during an outbreak of erythema infectiosum. J. A. M. A. *263*:2061–2065, 1990.
59. Gingrich, G. A., Hadler, S. C., Elder, H. A., et al.: Serologic investigation of an outbreak of hepatitis A in a rural day care center. Am. J. Public Health *73*:1190–1193, 1983.
60. Ginsburg, C. M., McCracken, G. H., Jr., Rae, S., et al.: *Haemophilus influenzae* type b disease: Incidence in a day-care center. J. A. M. A. *238*: 604–607, 1977.
61. Goodman, R. A., Osterholm, M. T., Granoff, D. M., et al.: Infectious diseases and child day care. Pediatrics *74*:134–139, 1984.
62. Granoff, D. M., Gilsdorf, J., Gessert, C. E., et al.: *Haemophilus influenzae* type b in a day care center: Relationship of nasopharyngeal carriage to development of anticapsular antibody. Pediatrics *65*:65–68, 1980.
63. Gwaltney, J. M., Moskalski, P. B., and Hendley, J. O.: Hand-to-hand transmission of rhinovirus colds. Ann. Intern. Med. *88*:463–467, 1978.
64. Hadler, S. C., Erben, J. J., Francis, D. P., et al.: Risk factors for hepatitis A in day-care centers. J. Infect. Dis. *145*:255–261, 1982.
65. Hadler, S. C., Webster, H. M., Erbin, J. J., et al.: Hepatitis A in day-care centers: A community-wide assessment. N. Engl. J. Med. *302*:1222–1227, 1980.
66. Hall, C. B., and Douglas, R. G.: Modes of transmission of respiratory syncytial virus. J. Pediatr. *99*:100–103, 1981.
67. Hall, C. B., Douglas, R. G., and Geimann, J. M.: Possible transmission by fomites of respiratory syncytial virus. J. Infect. Dis. *141*:98–102, 1980.
68. Hayani, K. C., and Pickering, L. K.: Screening of immigrant children for infectious diseases. Adv. Pediatr. Infect. Dis. *6*:91–110, 1990.
69. Hayashi, J., Kashiwagi, S., Nomura, H., et al.: Hepatitis B transmission in nursery schools. Am. J. Epidemiol. *125*:492–498, 1987.
70. Heijbel, H., Slaine, K., Seigel, B., et al.: Outbreak of diarrhea in a day care center with spread to household members: The role of *Cryptosporidium*. Pediatr. Infect. Dis. J. *6*:744–749, 1987.
71. Henderson, F. W., Gilligan, P. H., Wait, K., et al.: Nasopharyngeal carriage of antibiotic resistant pneumococci by children in group day care. J. Infect. Dis. *157*:256–263, 1988.
72. Hendley, J. O., Wenzel, R. P., and Gwaltney, J. M.: Transmission of rhinovirus colds by self-inoculation. N. Engl. J. Med. *288*:1361–1364, 1973.
73. Hinman, A. R.: Vaccine-preventable diseases and child day care. Rev. Infect. Dis. *8*:573–583, 1986.
74. Hjelt, K., Paerregaard, A., Nielson, O. H., et al.: Acute gastroenteritis in children attending day care centers with special reference to rotavirus infections. I. Aetiology and epidemiology aspects. Acta Paediatr. *76*:754–762, 1987.
75. Hoffman, R. E., and Shillam, P. J.: The use of hygiene, cohorting, and antimicrobial therapy to control an outbreak of shigellosis. Am. J. Dis. Child. *144*:219–221, 1990.
76. Hsueh, P. R., Teng, L. J., Lee, P. I., et al.: Outbreak of scarlet fever at a hospital day care center: Analysis of strain relatedness with phenotypic and genotypic characteristics. J. Hosp. Infect. *36*:191–200, 1997.
77. Hurwitz, E. S., Desada, C. C., Shapiro, C. N., et al.: Hepatitis infections in the day care setting. Pediatrics *94*(Suppl.):1023–1024, 1994.
78. Hurwitz, E. S., Gunn, W. J., Pinsky, P. F., et al.: A nationwide study of the risk of respiratory illness associated with day care attendance. Pediatrics *87*:62–69, 1991.
79. Hutto, C., Little, E. A., Ricks, R., et al.: Isolation of cytomegalovirus from toys and hands in a day care center. J. Infect. Dis. *154*:527–530, 1986.
80. Hutto, C., Ricks, R., Garvie, M., et al.: Epidemiology of cytomegalovirus infections in young children: Day care vs. home care. Pediatr. Infect. Dis. J. *4*:149–152, 1985.
81. Ish-Horowicz, M., Korman, S. H., Shapiro, M., et al.: Asymptomatic giardiasis in children. Pediatr. Infect. Dis. J. *8*:773–779, 1989.
82. Istre, G. R., Conner, J. S., Broome, C. V., et al.: Risk factors for primary invasive *Haemophilus influenzae* disease: Increased risk from day-care attendance and school age household members. J. Pediatr. *106*:190–195, 1985.
83. Itoh, T., Saito, K., Maruyama, T., et al.: An outbreak of enteritis due to *Campylobacter fetus* subspecies *jejuni* at a nursery school in Tokyo. Microbiol. Immunol. *24*:371–379, 1980.
84. Izurieta, H. S., Strebel, P. M., and Blake, P. A.: Postlicensure effectiveness of varicella vaccine during an outbreak in a child care center. J. A. M. A. *278*:1495–1499, 1997.
85. Jacobson, J. A., Filice, G. A., and Holloway, J. T.: Meningococcal disease in day-care centers. Pediatrics *59*:299–300, 1977.
86. Janoff, E. N., Craft, J. C., Pickering, L. K., et al.: Diagnosis of *Giardia* infections by detection of parasite specific antigens. J. Clin. Microbiol. *27*:431–435, 1989.
87. Jones, D. S., and Rogers, M. F.: Human immunodeficiency virus infection in children in day care. Semin. Pediatr. Infect. Dis. *1*:280–286, 1990.
88. Jones, L. A., Duke-Duncan, P. M., and Yeager, A. S.: Cytomegalovirus infections in infant-toddler centers: Centers for the developmentally delayed versus regular day care. J. Infect. Dis. *151*:953–955, 1985.
89. Jones, S. E. E., Armstrong, C. B., Bland, C., et al.: Varicella prevalence in day care centers. Pediatr. Infect. Dis. J. *14*:404, 1995.
90. Kaupas, V.: Tuberculosis in a family day-care home: Report of an outbreak and recommendations for prevention. J. A. M. A. *228*:851–854, 1974.
91. Keswick, B. H., Pickering, L. K., DuPont, H. L., et al.: Survival and detection of rotavirus on environmental surfaces in day care centers. Appl. Environ. Microbiol. *46*:813–816, 1983.
92. Keystone, J. S., Krayden, S., and Warren, M. R.: Person-to-person transmission of *Giardia lamblia* in day care nurseries. Can. Med. Assoc. J. *119*:241–242, 247–248, 1978.
93. Kim, K., Dupont, H. L., and Pickering, L. K.: Outbreaks of diarrhea associated with *Clostridium difficile* and its toxin in day care centers: Evidence of person-to-person spread. J. Pediatr. *102*:376–382, 1983.
94. Kim, K. H., Fekety, R., Batts, D. H., et al.: Isolation of *Clostridium difficile* from the environment and contact of patients with antibiotic-associated colitis. J. Infect. Dis. *143*:42–46, 1981.
95. Kotch, J. B., Weigle, K. A., Weber, D. J., et al.: Evaluation of a hygienic intervention in child day care centers. Pediatrics *94*(Suppl.):991–994, 1994.
96. Krugman, S., Katz, S., Gershon, A. A., et al.: Infectious Diseases of Children. 5th ed. St. Louis, C. V. Mosby, 1985, pp. 71–73.
97. Laborde, D. J., Weigle, K. A., Weber, D. J., et al.: The frequency, level, and distribution of fecal contamination in day care center classrooms. Pediatrics *94*(Suppl.):1008–1011, 1994.
98. Lauwers, W., DeBoeck, S. M., and Butzler, J. P.: *Campylobacter* enteritis in Brussels. Lancet *1*:604–605, 1978.
99. Leggiadro, R. J., Baddour, L. M., Frasch, C. E., et al.: Invasive meningococcal disease: Secondary spread in a day care center. South. Med. J. *82*:511–513, 1989.
100. Leggiadro, R. J., Callery, B., Dowdy, S., et al.: An outbreak of tuberculosis in a family day care home. Pediatr. Infect. Dis. J. *8*:52–54, 1989.
101. Lemp, G. F., Woodward, W. E., Pickering, L. K., et al.: The relation of staff to the incidence of diarrhea in day care centers. Am. J. Epidemiol. *120*:750–758, 1984.
102. Lieb, S., Gunn, R. A., and Taylor, D. N.: Salmonellosis in a day care center. J. Pediatr. *100*:1004, 1982.
103. Loda, F. W., Glezen, W. P., and Clyde, W. A., Jr.: Respiratory disease in group day care. Pediatrics *49*:428–437, 1972.
104. Louhiala, P. J., Jaakkola, N., Ruotsalainen, R., and Jaakkola, J. J.: Form of day care and respiratory infections among Finnish children. Am. J. Public Health *85*:1109–1112, 1995.
105. Lundgren, K., Ingvarsson, L., and Olofsson, B.: Epidemiologic aspects in children with recurrent otitis media. *In* Lim, D. J., Bluestone, C. D., Klein, J. O., et al. (eds.): Recent Advances in Otitis Media with Effusion. Philadelphia, B. C. Decker, 1984, pp. 22–25.
106. Makintubee, S., Istre, G. R., and Ward, J. I.: Transmission of invasive *Haemophilus influenzae* type b disease in day care settings. J. Pediatr. *111*:180–186, 1987.
107. Matson, D. O., and Estes, M. K.: Impact of rotavirus infection at a large pediatric hospital. J. Infect. Dis. *162*:598–604, 1990.
108. McCaustland, K. A., Bond, W. W., Bradley, D. W., et al.: Survival of hepatitis A virus in feces after drying and storage for 1 month. J. Clin. Microbiol. *16*:957–958, 1982.
109. McIntosh, E. D. G., Bek, M. D., Burgess, M. A., et al.: Molecular evidence of transmission of hepatitis B in a day-care center. Lancet *347*:118–119, 1996.
110. McMahon, B. J., Alward, W. L. M., Hall, D. B., et al.: Acute hepatitis B virus infection: Relation of age to the clinical expression of disease and subsequent development of the carrier state. J. Infect. Dis. *151*:599–603, 1985.
111. Measles prevention. M. M. W. R. Morb. Mortal. Wkly. Rep. *38*(Suppl. 9):1–18, 1989.
112. Meningococcal disease. Secondary attack rate and chemoprophylaxis in the United States, 1974. J. A. M. A. *235*:261–265, 1976.
113. Miller, R. A., Bronsdon, M. A., and Morton, W. R.: Experimental cryptosporidiosis in a primate model. J. Infect. Dis. *161*:312–315, 1990.
114. Multiply-resistant shigellosis in a day-care center—Texas. M. M. W. R. Morb. Mortal. Wkly. Rep. *35*(48):753–755, 1986.
115. Munford, R. S., de Morais, J. S., Tauney, A. E., et al.: Spread of meningococcal infection in households. Lancet *1*:1275–1278, 1974.

116. Muotiala, A., Saxen, H., and Vuopio-Varkila, J: Group A streptococcal outbreak of perianal infection in a day-care center. Adv. Exp. Med. Biol. *418*:211–215, 1997.
117. Murph, J. R., Bale, J. F., Murray, J. C., et al.: Cytomegalovirus transmission in a Midwest day care center: Possible relationship to child care practices. J. Pediatr. *109*:35–39, 1986.
118. Murphy, T. V., Clements, J. F., Breedlove, J. S., et al.: Risk of subsequent disease among day-care contacts of patients with systemic *Haemophilus influenzae* type b disease. N. Engl. J. Med. *316*:5–10, 1987.
119. Murphy, T. V., Osterholm, M. T., and Granoff, D. M.: Risk of *H. influenzae* type b (HIB) disease (DIS) in children attending day care in Dallas County, Texas (DAL), and Minnesota (MN). Abstract. Pediatr. Res. *25*:103, 1989.
120. Nolan, C. M., Barr, H., Elarth, A. M., et al.: Tuberculosis in a day-care home. Pediatrics *79*:630–631, 1987.
121. Ogilvie, M. M., and Tearne, C. F.: Spontaneous abortion after hand-foot-and-mouth disease caused by Coxsackie virus A16. B. M. J. *281*:1627–1628, 1980.
122. O'Ryan, M., and Matson, D. O.: Viral gastroenteritis pathogens in the day care center setting. Semin. Pediatr. Infect. Dis. *1*:252–262, 1990.
123. O'Ryan, M., Matson, D. O., Estes, M. K., et al.: Molecular epidemiology of rotaviruses in children attending day care centers in Houston. J. Infect. Dis. *162*:810–816, 1990.
124. Osterholm, M. T.: Lack of efficacy of *Haemophilus* b polysaccharide vaccine in Minnesota. J. A. M. A. *260*:1423–1428, 1988.
125. Osterholm, M. T., Pierson, L. M., White, K. E., et al.: The risk of subsequent transmission of *Haemophilus influenzae* type b disease among children in day care. N. Engl. J. Med. *316*:1–5, 1987.
126. Osterholm, M. T., Reves, R. R., Murph, J. R., et al.: Infectious diseases and child day care. Pediatr. Infect. Dis. J. *11*:531–541, 1992.
127. Pai, C. H., Sorger, S., Lackman, L., et al.: *Campylobacter* enteritis in children. J. Pediatr. *94*:589–591, 1979.
128. Pass, R. F., August, A., Dworsky, M. E., et al.: Cytomegalovirus infection in a day-care center. N. Engl. J. Med. *307*:477–479, 1982.
129. Pass, R. F., and Hutto, C.: Group day care and cytomegalovirus infections of mothers and children. Rev. Infect. Dis. *8*:599–605, 1986.
130. Pass, R. F., Hutto, S. C., Reynolds, D., et al.: Increased frequency of cytomegalovirus infection in children in group day care. Pediatrics *74*:121–126, 1984.
131. Paulozi, L. J., Johnson, K. E., Komahele, L. M., et al.: Diarrhea associated with adherent enteropathogenic *Escherichia coli* in an infant and toddler center, Seattle, Washington. Pediatrics *77*:296–300, 1986.
132. Pickering, L. K.: Bacterial and parasitic enteropathogens in day care. Semin. Pediatr. Infect. Dis. *1*:263–269, 1990.
133. Pickering, L. K., Bartlett, A. V., Reves, R. R., et al.: Asymptomatic excretion of rotavirus before and after rotavirus diarrhea in children in day care centers. J. Paediatr. *112*:361–365, 1988.
134. Pickering, L. K., Evans, D. G., Dupont, H. L., et al.: Diarrhea caused by *Shigella*, rotavirus, and *Giardia* in day-care centers: Prospective study. J. Pediatr. *99*:51–56, 1981.
135. Pickering, L. K., and Woodward, W. E.: Diarrhea in day care centers. Pediatr. Infect. Dis. J. *1*:47–52, 1982.
136. Pickering, L. K., Woodward, W. E., Dupont, H. L., et al.: Occurrence of *Giardia lamblia* in children in day care centers. J. Pediatr. *104*:522–526, 1984.
137. Plotkin, S. A.: Inactivated polio vaccine for the United States: A missed vaccination opportunity. Pediatr. Infect. Dis. J. *14*:835–839, 1995.
138. Radetsky, M. S., Istre, G. R., Johansen, T. L., et al.: Multiply-resistant pneumococcus causing meningitis and its epidemiology within a day care center. Lancet *2*:771–773, 1981.
139. Rauch, A. M., O'Ryan, M., Van, R., et al.: Invasive disease due to multiple resistant *Streptococcus pneumoniae* in a Houston, Texas, day-care center. Am. J. Dis. Child. *144*:923–927, 1990.
140. Rauch, A. M., Van, R., Bartlett, A. V., et al.: Longitudinal study of *Giardia lamblia* infection in a day care center population. Pediatr. Infect. Dis. J. *9*:186–189, 1990.
141. Redmond, S. R., and Pichichero, M. E.: *Haemophilus influenzae* type b disease: An epidemiologic study with special reference to day-care centers. J. A. M. A. *252*:2581–2584, 1984.
142. Reichler, M. R., Allphin, A. A., Breiman, R. F., et al.: The spread of multiply resistant *Streptococcus pneumoniae* at a day care center in Ohio. J. Infect. Dis. *166*:1346–1353, 1992.
143. Reves, R. R., and Jones, J. A.: Antibiotic use and resistance patterns in day care centers. Semin. Pediatr. Infect. Dis. *1*:212–221, 1990.
144. Roberts, L., Jorm, L., Patel, M., Smith, W., et al.: Effect of infection control measures on the frequency of diarrheal episodes in child care: A randomized, controlled trial. Pediatrics *105*:743–746, 2000.
145. Roberts, L., Smith, W., Jorm, L., et al.: Effect of infection control measures on the frequency of upper respiratory infection in child care: A randomized, controlled trial. Pediatrics *105*:738–742, 2000.
146. Rodriguez, W. J., Kim, H. W., Brandt, C. D., et al.: Common exposure outbreak of gastroenteritis due to type 2 rotavirus with high secondary attack rate within families. J. Infect. Dis. *140*:353–357, 1979.
147. Rogers, M., Weinstock, D. M., Eagan, J., et al.: Rotavirus outbreak on a pediatric oncology floor: Possible association with toys. Am. J. Infect. Control *28*:378–380, 2000.
148. Rogers, M. F., White, C. R., Sanders, R., et al.: Lack of evidence of transmission of human immunodeficiency virus from infected children to their household contacts. Pediatrics *85*:210–214, 1990.
149. Rovers, M. M., Zielhius, G. A., Ingels, K., and VanderWitt, G. J.: Day care and otitis media in young children: A critical overview. Eur. J. Pediatr. *158*:1–6, 1999.
150. Saez-Nieto, J. A., Perucha, M., Casamayor, H., et al.: Outbreak of infection caused by *Neisseria meningitidis* group C type 2 in a nursery. J. Infect. *8*:49–55, 1984.
151. Sargent, S. J., and Martin, J. T.: Scabies outbreak in a day-care center. Pediatrics *94*(Suppl.):1012–1013, 1994.
152. Saxén, H., Muotiala, H., Rostila, T., and Vuopio-Varkila, J.: Outbreak of perianal *Streptococcus pyogenes* infection in a day-care center. Pediatr. Infect. Dis. J. *16*:247–249, 1997.
153. Schulte, E. E., Birkhead, G. S., Kondraki, S. F., et al.: Patterns of *Haemophilus influenzae* type b invasive disease in New York State, 1987 to 1991: The role of vaccination requirements for day-care attendance. Pediatrics *94*(Suppl.):1014–1015, 1994.
154. Schwartz, B., Giebink, G. S., Henderson, F. G. W., et al.: Respiratory infections in day care. Pediatrics *94*(Suppl.):1018–1020, 1994.
155. Sealy, D. P., and Schuman, S. H.: Endemic giardiasis and day care. Pediatrics *72*:154–158, 1983.
156. Shapiro, C. N., McCaig, L. F., Gensheimer, K. F., et al.: Hepatitis B virus transmission between children in day care. Pediatr. Infect. Dis. J. *8*:870–875, 1989.
157. Shapiro, E. D.: Lack of transmission of hepatitis B in a day care center. J. Pediatr. *110*:90–92, 1987.
158. Shapiro, E. D., Murphy, T. V., Wald, E. R., et al.: The protective efficacy of *Haemophilus* b polysaccharide vaccine. J. A. M. A. *269*:1419–1422, 1988.
159. Shirley, L. R., and Ross, S. A.: Risk of transmission of human immunodeficiency virus by bite of an infected toddler. J. Pediatr. *114*:425–427, 1989.
160. Smith, T. D., Wilkinson, V., and Kaplan, E. L.: Group A *Streptococcus*-associated upper respiratory tract infections in a day care center. Pediatrics *83*:380–384, 1989.
161. Spika, J. S., Parson, J. E., Nordenberg, D., et al.: Hemolytic uremic syndrome and diarrhea associated with *Escherichia coli* O157:H7 in a day care center. J. Pediatr. *109*:287–291, 1986.
162. Stagno, S., and Cloud, G. A.: Working parents: The impact of day care and breast feeding on cytomegalovirus infections in offspring. Proc. Natl. Acad. Sci. U. S. A. *91*:2384–2389, 1994.
163. Stagno, S., Pass, R. F., Cloud, G., et al.: Primary cytomegalovirus infection in pregnancy: Incidence, transmission to fetus and clinical outcome. J. A. M. A. *256*:1904–1908, 1986.
164. Stahlberg, M. R.: The influence of form of day care on occurrence of acute respiratory tract infections among young children. Acta Pediatr. Suppl. *282*:1–87, 1980.
165. Stahlberg, M. R., Ruuskanen, O., and Virolainen, E.: Risk factors for recurrent otitis media. Pediatr. Infect. Dis. J. *5*:30–32, 1986.
166. Strangert, K.: Respiratory illness in preschool children and different forms of day care. Pediatrics *57*:191–196, 1976.
167. Strangert, K., Carlstrom, G., Jeansson, S., et al.: Infections in preschool children in group day care. Acta Paediatr. *65*:455–463, 1976.
168. Strangert, K.: Otitis media in young children in different types of day care. Scand. J. Infect. Dis. *9*:119–123, 1977.
169. Strom, J.: Study of infections and illnesses in a day nursery based on inclusion-bearing cells in the urine and infectious agent in faeces, urine and nasal secretion. Scand. J. Infect. Dis. *11*:265–269, 1979.
170. Sullivan, P., Woodward, W. E., Pickering, L. K., et al.: Longitudinal study of occurrence of diarrheal disease in day care centers. Am. J. Public Health *74*:987–991, 1984.
171. Swerdlow, D. L., and Griffin, P. M.: Duration of fecal shedding of *Escherichia coli* O157:H7 among children in day-care centers. Lancet *348*:745–746, 1997.
172. Tacket, C. O., and Cohen, M. L.: Shigellosis in day care centers: Use of plasmid analysis to assess control measures. Pediatr. Infect. Dis. J. *2*:127–130, 1983.
173. Takala, A. K., Eskola, J., Palmgren, J., et al.: Risk factors of invasive *Haemophilus influenzae* type b disease among children in Finland. J. Pediatr. *115*:694–701, 1989.
174. Taute, R. V., Johnson, K. E., Boase, J. C., et al.: Control of day care shigellosis: A trial of convalescent day care in isolation. Am. J. Public Health *76*:627–630, 1986.
175. Taylor, J. P., Perdue, J. N., Dinley, D., et al.: Cryptosporidiosis outbreak in a day care center. Am. J. Dis. Child. *39*:1023–1025, 1985.
176. Teele, D. W., Klein, J. D., Rosner, B., et al.: Epidemiology of otitis media during the first seven years of life in children in greater Boston: A prospective cohort study. J. Infect. Dis. *160*:83–94, 1989.
177. Thompson, S. C.: *Giardia lamblia* in children and the child care settings: A review of the literature. J. Paediatr. Child. Health *30*:202–209, 1994.

178. Thompson, S. C.: Infectious diarrhea in children: Controlling transmission in the child care setting. J. Paediatr. Child. Health *30*:210–219, 1994.
179. Tos, M., Poulsen, G., and Borch, J.: Tympanometry in 2-year-old children. ORL J. Otorhinolaryngol. Relat. Spec. *40*:77–85, 1978.
180. Tsoukas, C., Hadjis, T., Shuster, J., et al.: Lack of transmission of HIV through human bites and scratches. J. Acquir. Immune Defic. Syndr. *1*:505–507, 1988.
181. Uhari, M., Mantysaari, K., and Niemela, M.: A meta-analytic review of the risk factors for acute otitis media. Clin. Infect. Dis. *22*:1079–1083, 1996.
182. U. S. Bureau of the Census: Who's minding the kids? Child care arrangements: Winter 1984–85. Current Population Reports. Series P-70, No. 9. Washington, DC, U. S. Government Printing Office, 1987.
183. Van, R., Morrow, A. L., Reves, R. R., et al.: Environmental contamination in child day care centers. Am. J. Epidemiol. *133*:460–470, 1991.
184. Van, R., Wun, C. C., Morrow, A. L., et al.: The effect of diaper type and overclothes on fecal contamination in day care centers. J. A. M. A. *265*:1840–1844, 1991.
185. Váquez, M., LaRussa, P. S., Gershon, A. A., et al.: The effectiveness of the varicella vaccine in clinical practice. N. Engl. J. Med. *344*:955–960, 2001.
186. Wahn, V., Kramer, H. H., Voit, T., et al.: Horizontal transmission of HIV infection between two siblings. Lancet *2*:694, 1986.
187. Wald, E. R., Dashefsky, B., Byers, C., et al.: Frequency and severity of infections in day care. J. Pediatr. *112*:540–546, 1988.
188. Weissman, J. B., Gangarosa, E. J., Schmerler, A., et al.: Shigellosis in day care centers. Lancet *1*:88–90, 1975.
189. Weissman, J. B., Schmerler, A., Weiler, P., et al.: The role of preschool children and day care centers in the spread of shigellosis in urban communities. J. Pediatr. *84*:797–802, 1974.
190. Weniger, B. G., Ruttenber, J., Goodman, R. A., et al.: Fecal coliforms on environmental surfaces in two day care centers. Appl. Environ. Microbiol. *45*:733–735, 1983.
191. Werzberger, A., Meusch, B., Kuter, B., et al.: A controlled trial of formalin inactivated hepatitis A vaccine in healthy children. N. Engl. J. Med. *327*:453–457, 1992.
192. Wilde, J., Van, R., Pickering, L., et al.: Detection of rotaviruses in the day care environment by reverse transcriptase polymerase chain reaction. J. Infect. Dis. *166*:507–511, 1992.
193. Wilson, R., Feldman, R. A., Davis, J., et al.: Salmonellosis in infants: The importance of intrafamilial transmission. Pediatrics *69*:436–438, 1982.
194. Wong, C. S., Jelacic, S., Habeeb, R. L., et al.: The risk of the hemolytic-uremic syndrome after antibiotic treatment of *Escherichia coli* O157:H7. N. Engl. J. Med. *342*:1930–1936, 2000.
195. Yusuf, H. R., Coronado, V. G., Averhoff, F. A., et al.: Progress in coverage with hepatitis B vaccine among US children, 1994–1997. Am. J. Public Health *89*:1684–1689, 1999.

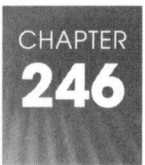

CHAPTER 246 Human and Animal Bites

CHAPTER 246A

Human Bites

ELLIE J. C. GOLDSTEIN

Human bites have been recorded since the biblical era and currently are a common cause of serious medical and surgical disease. They are the third most frequent type of bite after dog and cat bites. Reports of secondary infection occurring after a human bite in children have been noted in the United States since at least 1910.[41] Approximately 30 percent of human bites are accidental and result from injuries that are self-inflicted (such as bitten lips and nail biting) or from injuries suffered while playing sports or games, during falls, during dental therapy, and during treatment of seizures. They also may be intentional, with 70 percent resulting from aggressive behavior. Fighting is the primary cause of human bites, but aggressive bites also may occur during play (especially in the childcare setting). In addition, bite wounds may be incurred in the course of restraining impaired patients, as a consequence of criminal or police activities, or from child abuse and child battering.[22] Sexual bites or "love nips" account for 5 to 20 percent of human bite wounds and may be either intentional or accidental and occur in children of all ages.[1, 61, 72, 73]

Incidence and Epidemiology

In 1977, the New York City Department of Health altered its reporting system to include human bites. From that year's data of 892 reports, Marr and colleagues[49] noted an incidence of 10.7 human bites per 100,000 population per year, with a range of 0.9 to 60.9 per 100,000 population for different geographic areas. Although a bias was suggested that median income, population density, and younger age might have been factors in this geographic variance, it could not be substantiated. Human bites have their peak incidence in the spring and early summer for both children[3] and adults[49] and on Saturdays, especially for the 15- to 30-year-old age group. Alcohol and drug abuse may play a role in some of these instances. For children[12] and adults,[49] bites occur more commonly in males than in females (1.35 to 1.5:1), except for the 15- to 20-year-old and the 55- to 60-year-old age groups, in which females are bitten more frequently; human bites occur most often in men 20 to 25 years of age. Most bites in teenagers are associated with aggressive behavior. This pattern was documented in 1936 by Welch,[71] who reported that teenagers accounted for 5 of 13 human bite cases, some of which resulted in amputations. Farmer and Mann[17] noted that 12 percent of their patients with bites at a large urban hospital were younger than 20 years. Bites to the lip occurred most often in women (78% in women versus 22% in men) and to the lower lip (65%) more often than the upper lip (35%).[68] Baker and Moore[3] reported that of 322 children who suffered human bites, 21 percent were younger than 5 years, 21 percent were 5 to 10 years of age, and 58 percent were older than 10 years. When corrected for gender, 64 percent of the girls and 39 percent of the boys were 12 years of age or older.

Biting is common in the childcare center setting, in which it is the third most frequently reported injury. The incidence peaks in mid-morning and during the early school year in

September. Toddlers from 13 to 30 months of age are bitten more often than infants and other preschoolers,[65] and males are bitten more frequently than females.[21] Bites account for 3 and 6 percent of reported injuries in boys and girls, respectively,[19] and may be self-inflicted in many cases.[12] Other researchers have noted that approximately 50 percent of all children enrolled in daycare suffer bite wounds, with a rate of 3.9 bites per child per year in general, but 9.4 bites per male child per year for full-time enrollees.[21, 64] Garrard and colleagues[21] reported that 104 of 224 children (46%) experienced 347 bites in a single year, and Solomons and Elardo[64] noted that 66 of 133 children (50%) experienced 224 bites in a 42-month period. Fortunately, most of these bites are minor and do not break the skin. A higher proportion of bites in younger children (such as preschoolers) are to the face, whereas most bites in adolescents are on the upper extremities and hands.

Paronychial infections are not actual bites, but when infection occurs, it is related to contamination by oral flora when children bite or suck their fingers. Brook[9] noted children from 2 to 9 years of age (mean age, 5 years, 8 months) who were treated at a children's hospital for paronychial infection and reported the bacteriologic and clinical findings of these infections.

Bites as harbingers or signs of child abuse are noted more commonly in the 0- to 4-year-old age group[66]; the age of the abusing parents was younger than 20 years for mothers and younger than 22 years for fathers. An attempt should be made to identify the biter and measure distances between circular bite marks to ascertain the spread. In addition, biting children may have learned this behavior from abusive adults and may themselves be victims of human bites.

Bacteriology

The bacteriology of these wounds, including occlusional bites, clenched-fist injuries, and paronychia, reflects the human oral flora of the biter and has been the focus of various studies.[5, 10, 24, 32, 34, 36] Human saliva and dental plaque can contain more than 42 different species of bacteria in concentrations of 10^8 colony-forming units per milliliter. Table 246–1 lists common human bite wound isolates and their relative frequency of isolation. Alpha-hemolytic streptococci are the most frequent isolates. Other common bacterial isolates include *Streptococcus pyogenes, Staphylococcus aureus, Haemophilus* spp., *Eikenella corrodens,* and oral anaerobes, especially *Prevotella* and *Porphyromonas* spp. Cultures of virtually all infected bite wounds grow bacterial pathogens; wound cultures of patients who are initially seen less than 8 hours after injury, before the development of clinical infection, yield potential bacterial pathogens in 85 percent of cases.[23, 32] The bacteriology of early-treated, colonized wounds is remarkably similar to the bacteria isolated from wounds evaluated later with established infection. The average bite wound yields between 3.4 and 5.4 bacterial isolates per wound, including 1.7 to 2.4 aerobes and 1.7 to 3.0 anaerobes.[10, 32] Anaerobes were recognized as important pathogens and markers for serious bite infections, especially bite infections involving the hand, as early as 1936.[4, 8, 28, 54, 55, 71] Anaerobes are isolated from more than 50 percent of human bite wounds, almost always in mixed culture with aerobes, and they are associated more often with more serious infections, amputation, and the presence of abscesses.[28, 32] Many of the anaerobes isolated from human bite wounds, especially *Prevotella* and *Porphyromonas* spp., are β-lactamase producers.[10, 36]

E. corrodens, a capnophilic, gram-negative rod that is part of the normal human oral flora, has been recognized as an important pathogen in approximately 20 percent of clenched-fist injuries.[24, 34] It has an unusual antimicrobial susceptibility pattern in that it is susceptible to penicillin but resistant to first-generation cephalosporins, β-lactamase–stable penicillins (such as oxacillin), and erythromycin.[25, 33] When unrecognized or treated with the incorrect antibiotic, *E. corrodens* has been associated with therapeutic failure.[24] Usually isolated in mixed culture, it may be missed by microbiologists because of its slow growth characteristics and overgrowth of other bacterial colonies. *E. corrodens* produces a small colony that "pits" or "corrodes" the agar surface and has a light yellow pigment and an odor like that of hypochlorite bleach.

The bacteriology of paronychial infections is similar to that of other human bite infections, except that aerobes and anaerobes each have been isolated in pure culture in 27 percent of cases.[9] Brook[9] found a total of 3.6 isolates per specimen: 1.4 aerobes, 2.0 anaerobes, and 0.2 *Candida albicans;* β-lactamase-producing organisms, including isolates of *Prevotella melaninogenica* and *Prevotella oralis,* were found in 45 percent of the wounds.

In addition to oral bacterial infection, human bites have been associated with viral infections such as those due to herpes simplex virus,[20, 50] cytomegalovirus,[50] hepatitis B virus,[11, 14] hepatitis C virus,[16] and possibly human immunodeficiency virus (HIV),[1, 42, 50, 60, 63] as well as syphilis,[18] tuberculosis,[23] actinomycosis,[7] and tetanus.[52, 59]

Clinical Manifestations

Human bites may be categorized into three groups: (1) bites resulting in paronychial infection, (2) occlusional bites, and (3) clenched-fist injuries. Patients in the latter two categories may be seen early (<8 hours after injury) for wound care or tetanus boosters or late (>8 hours after injury), usually because of established infection or infectious complications. All share the predominance of oral aerobic and anaerobic bacteria as primary etiologic pathogens. Noninfectious complications may include injury to tendons and nerves or fractures. Potential complications of human bites are noted in Table 246–2. Table 246–3 lists some of the diseases acquired as a result of human bites. The incidence of infection developing after human bites is estimated to be 10 to 30 percent. Because of the typically superficial nature of human bite wound injuries in children, the infection rate in children is estimated to be approximately 10 percent.

BITES RESULTING IN PARONYCHIAL INFECTION

Paronychia is an infection (inflammation) of the structures of the distal phalanx, either those surrounding the nail or the bone itself. Most are caused by finger sucking in younger children but may be caused by accidental biting. The area is red, tender, and swollen and may have some underlying purulence.

OCCLUSIONAL BITES

Occlusional bites occur when the teeth actually contact any part of the human anatomy. Human bite wounds occur most often on the upper extremity (18–71%), the head and neck (4–33%), the thorax and abdomen (6–25%), the breasts or genitals (3–25%), and the lower extremity (3–11%).[3, 21, 32, 49, 69] Vale and Noguchi[69] reported the anatomic distribution of

TABLE 246–1 ■ APPROXIMATE PREVALENCE AND BACTERIOLOGY OF ISOLATES FROM HUMAN BITE WOUND INFECTIONS

Isolate	Prevalence (%)	Present in OB	Present in CFI
Aerobes			
Streptococci			
Alpha-hemolytic	28–90	+	+
Beta-hemolytic			
Group A	17–26	+	+
Other	12	+	+
Gamma-hemolytic	3–33	+	–
Enterococci	11	–	+
Staphylococcus aureus	13–50	+	+
Coagulase-negative staphylococci	11–53	+	+
Haemophilus influenzae	6	+	+
Haemophilus species (other)	11–20	+	+
Eikenella corrodens	10–29	+	+
Micrococcus species	3–5	–	+
Moraxella species	3	+	–
Neisseria species	11–15	+	+
Corynebacterium species	28–41	+	+
Acinetobacter calcoaceticus	4–6	–	+
Escherichia coli	6	+	–
Klebsiella pneumoniae	3–6	+	+
Enterobacter species	3–4	+	–
Nocardia species	3	–	+
Anaerobes			
Acidaminococcus species	2	+	+
Actinomyces species	4	+	+
Bacteroides ovatus	6	–	+
Bacteroides ureolyticus	3–11	+	–
Bacteroides species (unspeciated)	12–33	+	+
Bifidobacterium species	11	–	+
Clostridium perfringens	4	+	–
Prevotella (Bacteroides) melaninogenica	15–22	+	+
Prevotella (Bacteroides) intermedia	11–26	+	+
Prevotella (Bacteroides) oralis	6–17	+	+
Prevotella buccae	15	+	+
Prevotella disiens	3	–	+
Prevotella loeschii	3	+	+
Eubacterium species	3–11	+	+
Fusobacterium nucleatum	12–33	+	+
Fusobacterium necrophorum	6	–	+
Fusobacterium species (other)	17	–	+
Peptostreptococcus anaerobius	3	+	–
Peptostreptococcus asaccharolyticus	22	+	+
Peptostreptococcus intermedius	3	+	–
Peptostreptococcus magnus	3–17	+	+
Peptostreptococcus micros	12	+	+
Gamella (Peptostreptococcus) morbillorum	3	+	–
Peptostreptococcus prevotii	3	+	–
Peptostreptococcus species (other)	3–22	+	+
Veillonella parvula	9–11	+	+
Veillonella species (other)	6–18	+	+
Spirochetes	5–30	+	+

OB, occlusional bite wounds; CFI, clenched-first injuries.
+, present; –, absent.
Based on a compilation of data from references 5, 10, 27, 35, and 53.

bite marks in 67 forensically evaluated cases, including 13 (19%) cases in children younger than 15 years. They noted more than one bite mark in 40 percent of victims and that female victims were bitten most frequently on the breasts, arms, and legs whereas bites to males more often were on the upper extremities and shoulders. Marr and colleagues[49] did not differentiate the location of bites by sex of the victim but noted that 15 percent were to the head and neck, 12 percent were to the thorax and abdomen, 61 percent were to the upper extremities, 4 percent were to the lower extremities, and 9 percent were to unknown locations. Our experience with teenagers and adults is similar to that of Marr and colleagues,[49] perhaps because of a selection bias involving patients who seek medical care or come to the attention of infectious disease consultants. When the hand is involved, wounds tend to occur most frequently on the terminal phalanx of the middle (long) finger of the dominant hand.[6, 15, 27, 67] Bites to the upper extremities occur most frequently in toddlers (66%), infants (71%), and preschoolers (46%)[21] and in children overall (42%).[3]

Most wounds are minor and require routine care with cleansing and bandaging. The infection rate after occlusional

TABLE 246–2 ■ POTENTIAL COMPLICATIONS OF HUMAN BITE WOUNDS

Abscess
Cellulitis
Compartment syndrome
Fracture
Necrotizing fasciitis
Nerve severance/injury
Osteomyelitis
Scarlet fever
Sepsis
Septic arthritis
Tendon severance/injury
Tenosynovitis
Toxic shock syndrome

bite wounds has been estimated to be 10 to 30 percent, 87 percent of which may require hospitalization.[3, 44] Wounds to the hand and with any edema or crush injury and those that involve a bone or a joint have a greater potential to become infected. Infections, when they occur, usually are manifested as cellulitis. If the child is treated early,[15, 44] these injuries rarely result in serious complications. Patients in whom treatment is delayed (>12 hours after injury) probably have a preselection bias because they usually seek attention for an already established infection. These infections generally spread proximally and not distally and in less than 5 percent of cases have associated fever, lymphangitis, or lymphadenopathy. A malodorous discharge or abscess may be present if anaerobes are involved.

Complications may be limited to skin defects (when skin avulsion has occurred), but septic arthritis and osteomyelitis may develop if the joint or bone is involved.[37] In immunocompromised hosts, such as those with hematologic malignancy or neutropenia, sepsis may occur. Amputation may be necessary as a result of the initial bite in approximately 2 to 5 percent of cases or as a result of serious chronic infection in 0 to 18 percent of cases.[4, 15, 44, 46, 51, 53, 71] Tendon injury, primary nerve injury and tenosynovitis, compartment syndrome, and resultant secondary nerve damage may occur.[56]

CLENCHED-FIST INJURIES

Clenched-fist injuries, or "fight bites," are the most serious of human bite wounds and occur when the closed fist of one person strikes another in the teeth and a break in the skin occurs.[38] The most common cause is a fight, although cases can occur during contact sports or boxing if gloves are not worn. The metacarpophalangeal joint (knuckle) of the middle (long) finger of the dominant hand is involved most frequently.[24, 34, 62] The break in the skin may be only 2 to 5 mm in length but often results in penetration into the joint or even the bone. Patients and physicians may underestimate the potentially serious nature of these wounds. During the initial contact, bacteria penetrate the knuckle area and, on relaxation of the hand, are carried by the tendons further back into the potential spaces of the hand. Infection may spread laterally, between the collateral and accessory ligaments, or dorsally into the thin-walled bursa overlying the metacarpal head or into the palmar deep spaces of the hand. The typical patient avoids seeking attention because of the circumstances surrounding the injury and often wakes up 6 to 8 hours later with a painful, throbbing, swollen, infected hand and then seeks medical attention. Often, the patient has a purulent exudate emanating from the injury, which may be foul-smelling if *P. melaninogenica* or other anaerobes are present, and the patient comes to the physician with the hand elevated to diminish the pain. The swelling usually spreads proximally and not distally from the site of injury. The physician should take samples for both aerobic and anaerobic cultures and secure the assistance of a surgeon experienced in hand cases. Chuinard and D'Ambrosia[13] and others[47, 48, 57] have outlined the surgical management of these wounds; such management includes a determination, under a bloodless field, of whether penetration of the joint capsule has occurred or whether only localized cellulitis is present. Complications occur frequently, and in our experience, these patients have a 50 percent chance of development of septic arthritis, osteomyelitis, or both. The range of motion of the hand usually is limited by swelling and edema but also may be limited as a result of tendon or nerve injury or severance. Permanent limitation of range of motion and joint stiffness are frequent results of osteomyelitis in the affected joints. Osteomyelitis, which usually involves the small bones of the hand, often is manifested as continued pain, swelling, and erythema with or without drainage at 10 days to 3 weeks after the injury has occurred.[17] Osteomyelitis and septic arthritis caused by *E. corrodens,* often in association with alpha-hemolytic streptococci, are frequently insidious and persistent and may lead to amputation, especially if treated with the wrong antibiotics.[24] Other complications include fracture, collar-button abscess, and muscle atrophy.

TABLE 246–3 ■ DISEASES TRANSMITTED BY HUMAN BITE WOUNDS

Actinomycosis
Cytomegalovirus infection
Hepatitis B virus infection
Hepatitis C virus infection
Herpesvirus infection
HIV infection
Invasive group A streptococcal infection
Syphilis
Tetanus
Toxic shock syndrome
Tuberculosis
Whitlow

Potential for Transmission of the Human Immunodeficiency Virus

Reports[42, 63, 67] have noted the transmission of HIV from biter to victim. HIV is isolated uncommonly from the saliva of infected persons, and when recovered, it has been in low number. Consequently, the possibility of HIV transmission is considered unlikely, though negligible.[58, 60] Rickman and Richman[60] reviewed instances of reported HIV transmission via human bites and concluded that "no well documented case of HIV transmission through bites exists"; the risk of HIV transmission is possible biologically but appears to be negligible. A review and commentary of professional sports-related injuries also noted the unlikely possibility of HIV transmission via sporting events and outlined similar commonsense control measures.[50] Most schools allow preschool-age children with HIV to attend childcare centers unless a significant, real risk exists in an individual's behavior or hygienic habits.

TABLE 246–4 ■ MANAGEMENT PROCEDURES FOR HUMAN BITE WOUNDS

Obtain history from patient
- Situation leading to injury
- Place of occurrence
- Patient allergies
- Other medications (potential interactions)

Perform evaluation of patient
- Nerve function
- Tendon function
- Vascular integrity
- Range of motion
- Potential bone and joint involvement

Diagram or photograph wound
Mark leading edge of cellulitis
Culture wound (if infected)
Irrigate wound
Débride wound cautiously
Drain abscess
Administer antimicrobial agents
- Prophylactic therapy, 3 to 5 days
- Longer duration for established infection

Elevate injured area
Immobilize wound area (3 days for hands)
Have the patient exercise the injured area (if previously immobilized)
Close the wound
- Primary for face and head
- Delayed for early wounds
- Secondary intent for infected wounds

Administer tetanus toxoid
Obtain radiograph (if indicated)
Submit health department report (if required)

Treatment

The basic elements of management are outlined in Table 246–4. They include a complete history of the circumstances of the injury, with an attempt to identify the biter. If the biter is identified, some questions about the presence of herpes and other potentially orally transmitted viral diseases should be asked. Awareness of the potential for child abuse or battering must be considered, and a search should be performed for other associated injuries. The examination must include an evaluation of range of motion if a hand or joint is involved; determination of the integrity of tendons, nerves, and the vascular supply; and a diagram of the location of the bite marks. Because most victims have multiple wounds, a thorough search of the entire body should be made, and the wounds should be measured. Special attention must be paid to any wound close to bones or joints, especially when it involves the hands, and the possibility of bone or joint penetration should be considered. Radiographic studies of the hand should be obtained for all clenched-fist injuries or in any situation in which suspicion of fracture or the potential for osteomyelitis exists. Magnification radiography may be helpful in identifying bone penetration. If tetanus immunization is not current, a toxoid booster should be given. If the patient has no record of immunization, tetanus immunoglobulin and tetanus toxoid should be administered.

The wound should be cleansed with normal saline, and any foreign body or debris and necrotic tissue should be removed. Cautious débridement is indicated for some wounds, with care taken to not create a potential skin defect. The wound then is irrigated, with a syringe and needle/catheter tip used as a high-pressure jet to diminish the bacterial inoculum. Aerobic and anaerobic cultures should be obtained and Gram stain performed if infection is present. In cases of clenched-fist injury, a hand surgeon should examine the patient to determine whether the joint capsule or bone has been compromised.[13] With many hand infections, especially after exploration of clenched-fist injuries, immobilization in a plaster splint is recommended. Elevation of a swollen or inflamed part is crucial to healing. The elevation should be maintained above the level of the heart. Promises made by patients or family to "keep the hand up" should not be accepted unless a properly fitting sling is issued or made from a scarf; in addition, a tubular stockinette and an intravenous pole may be used. Legs and hands also can be elevated with pillows. The use and value of topical agents have not been studied, although most patients have applied them before seeking medical attention.[32]

Antimicrobial agents should be selected empirically according to the most likely pathogens and their usual susceptibility patterns to antimicrobial agents.[26, 27, 35, 39, 40] If cultures are performed, therapy should be adjusted according to the organisms isolated and their specific susceptibility to antimicrobial agents. The activity of antibiotics commonly used against the usual human bite wound pathogens is outlined in Table 246–5. Common pathogens that need to be considered in the selection of antimicrobial therapy include streptococci, *S. aureus*, *Haemophilus* spp., *E. corrodens*, and β-lactamase–producing oral anaerobes. The oral

TABLE 246–5 ■ COMPARATIVE IN VITRO ANTIMICROBIAL ACTIVITY OF SELECTED ORAL ANTIMICROBIAL AGENTS AGAINST COMMON HUMAN BITE WOUND PATHOGENS

Agent	*Staphylococcus aureus*	Streptococci	*Haemophilus*	*Eikenella corrodens*	Anaerobes
Amoxicillin	–	+	v	+	v
Amoxicillin-clavulanic acid	+	+	+	+	+
Cephalexin	+	+	–	–	–
Cefaclor	+	+	+	–	–
Cefuroxime	+	+	+	+	–
Cefprozil	+	+	+	–	–
Loracarbef	+	+	+	–	–
Dicloxacillin	+	+	–	–	–
Erythromycin	v	+	v	–	–
Azithromycin	+	+	+	+	v
Clarithromycin	+	+	+	–	–
Trimethoprim-sulfamethoxazole	+	v	+	+	–
Chloramphenicol	v	v	v	+	+

Note: Because of contraindications in pediatric patients, tetracyclines and fluoroquinolones are not included.
+, active; –, poorly active or inactive; v, variable.

agent of choice is amoxicillin–clavulanic acid; for penicillin-allergic children, a combination such as trimethoprim-sulfamethoxazole plus clindamycin can be substituted. Many other combination regimens may be used, including cefuroxime plus clindamycin or metronidazole. The intravenous agents of choice are ampicillin-sulbactam and ticarcillin-clavulanate.[2] For penicillin-allergic children, combination therapy with an extended-spectrum cephalosporin or trimethoprim-sulfamethoxazole plus clindamycin should be administered.[2] Additional potentially useful intravenous agents include cefoxitin, cefotetan, imipenem, and combinations of such agents as cefuroxime or cefotaxime plus metronidazole. First-generation cephalosporins are of limited utility because of poor activity against *E. corrodens* and some anaerobes[25, 33] and should not be used as empirical monotherapy. Erythromycin also has poor activity against *E. corrodens* and *Fusobacterium nucleatum,*[31] and its use as monotherapy can lead to therapeutic failure. Newer macrolides, including azithromycin, show improved activity when compared with erythromycin against the spectrum of bite wound pathogens, but *F. nucleatum* remains relatively resistant.[27, 35]

The quinolones, particularly gatifloxacin, exhibit broad activity against the pathogens implicated in bite wounds, except that fusobacteria are sometimes resistant.[30] The risk-to-benefit ratio should be considered before administration because the quinolones are not approved for use in children younger than 18 years. Linezolid, a new oxazolidinone, appears to be more active than the macrolides against the gram-positive organisms and fusobacteria isolated from human bite wounds, but some aerobic gram-negative organisms are at the susceptibility breakpoint.[29] Once patient-specific cultures return, antimicrobial therapy should be adjusted in accordance with the patient's individual isolates and susceptibility pattern. The duration of antimicrobial therapy is determined by the type and severity of infection. Prophylactic antimicrobial agents typically are given for 3 to 5 days, whereas the course for established infection is usually longer, such as 10 to 14 days for cellulitis and 4 to 6 weeks for septic arthritis and osteomyelitis. If any question exists about the prompt filling of a prescription because of financial or other concerns, a dose of intramuscular or intravenous antibiotics should be administered and hospitalization considered.

Patients' wounds should be re-examined within 24 to 48 hours. If outpatient therapy is initiated and the cellulitis advances, hospitalization is indicated. Table 246–6 lists the reasons for hospitalization of patients with human bite wounds. Such indications include patient noncompliance and virtually all clenched-fist injuries.

Infected wounds should not be closed. However, the value and risks associated with primary closure in patients who are initially seen less than 8 hours after injury and without any symptoms or signs of established infection have not been studied in a prospective or randomized manner. Exceptions are wounds to the face and neck and losses of the lip, for which early primary closure has been successful.[68, 70] However, the information about those wounds is probably not applicable to bite wounds to the hands or other parts of the body for several reasons: (1) head and face wounds are débrided and copiously irrigated with as much as a liter of normal saline, which diminishes the bacterial inoculum; (2) most surgeons give a course of 5 or more days of antibiotics; (3) the blood supply to the head and face area is superior to that of most other anatomic areas; and (4) these areas are rarely dependent, and therefore edema and swelling resolve more rapidly or do not develop. The use of primary wound closure in early-treated, uninfected wounds remains at the physician's discretion. Wounds to the hands should be observed and left open for either delayed primary or secondary closure.

TABLE 246–6 ■ INDICATIONS FOR HOSPITALIZATION OF A VICTIM OF A HUMAN BITE INJURY

Clenched-fist injury
Immunocompromised host
Asplenia (diagnostic or traumatic)
Cirrhosis
Leukemia
Lupus/steroids
Mastectomy (radical or modified radical)
Crush injury
Edema
Preexisting in the injured area or developed during therapy
Cirrhosis
Mastectomy
Malnutrition
Congestive heart failure
Fever (>100.5° F)
Lymphadenopathy
Patient noncompliance
Failure to take medication
Failure to elevate the injured area
Osteomyelitis
Septic arthritis
Progression of infection despite outpatient therapy

In general, hyperbaric oxygen therapy for human bite wounds remains of unproven benefit. Lehman and colleagues[43] prospectively studied the use of a portable hyperbaric oxygen chamber in 16 of 43 patients admitted to the hospital for human bite infections of the hand, almost all caused by clenched-fist injuries. They found that no benefit was obtained for mild or moderate infections, but the duration of the hospital stay was shortened (4.7 versus 11.2 days) in patients with severe infections. Although the authors thought that return of function was more rapid in the hyperbaric group, limitations in follow-up precluded evaluation, and the institution of an early, aggressive exercise program may have been an important factor.

Prevention

Mast and colleagues[50] reviewed both risk and prevention strategies for the transmission of blood-borne pathogens during sports. Prevention strategies include appropriate infection control measures in the sports setting and education of young athletes, as well as their coaches and trainers. Bites may occur in the daycare setting, even "when caregivers are vigilant." The use of "disciplinary techniques," including a developmentally appropriate curriculum ("busy, happy children are less likely to get into serious mischief"), avoidance of too much open space in classrooms, and discipline that pays attention to redirected positive behavior, has been advocated.[64, 65] More attention should be given to the victim than to the aggressor; teachers should work with the biter on behavior modification with reinforcement, extinction, and punishment strategies, which should be limited to "time-out" procedures.

REFERENCES

1. Al Fallouji, M.: Traumatic love bites. Br. J. Surg. 77:100–101, 1990.
2. American Academy of Pediatrics: Bite wounds. *In* Pickering, L. K. (ed.): 2000 Red Book: Report of the Committee on Infectious Diseases. 25th ed. Elk Grove Village, IL, American Academy of Pediatrics, 2000, pp. 155–159.

3. Baker, M. D., and Moore, S. E.: Human bites in children. Am. J. Dis. Child. *41*:1285–1290, 1987.
4. Barnes, M. N., and Bibby, B. G.: A summary of reports and a bacteriologic study of infections caused by human tooth wounds. J. Am. Dent. Assoc. *26*:1163–1170, 1939.
5. Barnham, I.: Once bitten, twice shy: Microbiology of bites. Rev. Med. Microbiol. *2*:31–36, 1991.
6. Bassadre, J. O., and Parry, S. W.: Indications for surgical débridement in 125 human bites to the hands. Arch. Surg. *126*:65–67, 1991.
7. Blinkhorn, R. J., Strimbu, V., Effron, D., et al.: "Punch" actinomycosis causing osteomyelitis of the hand. Arch. Intern. Med. *148*:2668–2670, 1988.
8. Boland, F. K.: Morsus humanus: Sixty cases of human bites in Negroes. J. A. M. A. *116*:127–131, 1941.
9. Brook, I.: Bacteriologic study of paronychia in children. Am. J. Surg. *141*:703–705, 1981.
10. Brook, I.: Microbiology of human and animal bite wounds in children. Pediatr. Infect. Dis. J. *6*:29–32, 1987.
11. Cancio-Bello, T. P., deMedina, M., Shorey, P., et al.: An institutional outbreak of hepatitis B related to a human biting carrier. J. Infect. Dis. *146*:652–656, 1982.
12. Chang, A., Lugg, M. M., and Nebedum, A.: Injuries among preschool children enrolled in day-care centers. Pediatrics *83*:272–277, 1989.
13. Chuinard, R. G., and D'Ambrosia, R. D.: Human bite infections of the hand. J. Bone Joint Surg. Am. *59*:416–418, 1977.
14. Davis, L. G., Weber, D. J., and Kemon, S. M.: Horizontal transmission of hepatitis B virus. Lancet *1*:889–893, 1989.
15. Dreyfuss, U. Y., and Singer, M.: Human bites of the hand: A study of one hundred and six patients. J. Hand Surg. [Am.] *10*:884–889, 1985.
16. Dusheiko, G. M., Smith, M., and Schever, P. F.: Hepatitis C virus transmitted by human bite. Lancet *336*:503–504, 1990.
17. Farmer, C. B., and Mann, R. J.: Human bite infections of the hand. South. Med. J. *59*:515–518, 1966.
18. Fiumara, N. J., and Exnor, J. H.: Primary syphilis following a human bite. Sex. Transm. Dis. *8*:21–82, 1981.
19. Fuller, E. M.: Injury-prone children. Am. J. Orthopsychiatry *18*:708–723, 1948.
20. Fuortes, L., and Melson, E.: Brief report: Primary and recurrent herpes simplex infection in a pediatric nurse resulting from a human bite. Infect. Control Hosp. Epidemiol. *10*:120, 1989.
21. Garrard, J., Leland, N., and Smith, D. K.: Epidemiology of human bites to children in a day-care center. Am. J. Dis. Child. *142*:643–650, 1988.
22. Gold, M. H., Roenigk, H. H., Jr., Smith, E. S., et al.: Evaluation and treatment of patients with human bite marks. Am. J. Forensic Med. Pathol. *10*:140–143, 1989.
23. Goldstein, E. J. C.: Bite wounds and infection. Clin. Infect. Dis. *14*:633–640, 1991.
24. Goldstein, E. J. C., Barones, M. F., and Miller, T. A.: *Eikenella corrodens* in hand infections. J. Hand Surg. *8*:563–566, 1983.
25. Goldstein, E. J. C., and Citron, D. M.: Susceptibility of *Eikenella corrodens* to penicillin, apalcillin, and twelve cephalosporins. Antimicrob. Agents Chemother. *26*:947–948, 1984.
26. Goldstein, E. J. C., and Citron, D. M.: Comparative activities of cefuroxime, amoxicillin–clavulanic acid, ciprofloxacin, enoxacin, and ofloxacin against aerobic and anaerobic bacteria isolated from bite wounds. Antimicrob. Agents Chemother. *32*:1143–1148, 1988.
27. Goldstein, E. J. C., and Citron, D. M.: Comparative susceptibilities of 173 aerobic and anaerobic bite wound isolates to sparfloxacin, temafloxacin, clarithromycin and older agents. Antimicrob. Agents Chemother. *37*:1150–1153, 1993.
28. Goldstein, E. J. C., Citron, D. M., and Finegold, S. M.: Role of anaerobic bacteria in bite wound infections. Rev. Infect. Dis. *6*(Suppl):177–783, 1984.
29. Goldstein, E. J. C., Citron, D. M., and Merriam, C. V.: Linezolid activity compared to those of selected macrolides and other agents against aerobic and anaerobic pathogens isolated from soft tissue bite infections in humans. Antimicrob. Agents Chemother. *43*:1469–1474, 1999.
30. Goldstein, E. J. C., Citron, D. M., Merriam, C. V., et al.: Activity of gatifloxacin compared to those of five other quinolones versus aerobic and anaerobic isolates from skin and soft tissue samples of human and animal bite wound infections. Antimicrob. Agents Chemother. *43*:1475–1479, 1999.
31. Goldstein, E. J. C., Citron, D. M., Vagvolgyi, A. E., et al.: Susceptibility of bite wound bacteria to seven oral antimicrobial agents, including RU-985, a new erythromycin: Considerations in choosing empiric therapy. Antimicrob. Agents Chemother. *29*:556–559, 1986.
32. Goldstein, E. J. C., Citron, D. M., Wield, B., et al.: Bacteriology of human and animal bite wounds. J. Clin. Microbiol. *8*:667–672, 1978.
33. Goldstein, E. J. C., Gombert, M. E., and Agyare, E. O.: Susceptibility of *Eikenella corrodens* to newer beta-lactam antibiotics. Antimicrob. Agents Chemother. *18*:832–833, 1980.
34. Goldstein, E. J. C., Miller, T. A., Citron, D. M., et al.: Infections following clenched-fist injury: A new perspective. J. Hand Surg. *3*:455–457, 1978.
35. Goldstein, E. J. C., Nesbit, C. A., and Citron, D. M.: Comparative in vitro activities of azithromycin, Bay y 3118, levofloxacin, sparfloxacin, and 11 other oral antimicrobial agents against 194 aerobic and anaerobic bite wound isolates. Antimicrob. Agents Chemother. *39*:1097–1100, 1995.
36. Goldstein, E. J. C., Reinhardt, J. F., Murray, P. M., et al.: Animal and human bite wounds: A comparative study of augmentin vs. penicillin +/− dicloxacillin. Postgrad. Med. J. Special Suppl. 105–110, 1984.
37. Gonzalez, M. N., Papierski, P., and Hal, R., Jr.: Osteomyelitis of the hand after a human bite. J. Hand Surg. [Am.] *18*:520–522, 1993.
38. Griego, R. D., Rosen, T., Orengo, I. F., et al.: Dog, cat and human bites: A review. J. Am. Acad. Dermatol. *33*:1019–1029, 1995.
39. Guba, A. M., Mulliken, J. B., and Hoopes, J. E.: The selection of antibiotics for human bites of the hand. Plast. Reconstr. Surg. *56*:538–541, 1975.
40. Haughey, R. E., Lammers, R. L., and Wagner, D. K.: Use of antibiotics in the initial management of soft-tissue hand wounds. Ann. Emerg. Med. *10*:187–192, 1981.
41. Hultgen, J. D.: Partial gangrene of the left index finger caused by symbiosis of the fusiform *Bacillus* and the *Spirochaeta denticola*. J. A. M. A. *10*:887–890, 1910.
42. Khajotia, R. R., and Lee, E.: Transmission of human immunodeficiency virus through saliva after a lip bite. Arch. Intern. Med. *157*:1901, 1997.
43. Lehman, W. L., Jr., Jones, W. W., Allo, M. D., et al.: Human bite infections of the hand: Adjunct treatment with hyperbaric oxygen. Infect. Surg. *14*:460–465, 1985.
44. Lindsey, D., Christopher, M., Hollenbach, J., et al.: Natural course of human bite wound: Incidence of infection and complications in 434 bites and 803 lacerations in the same group of patients. J. Trauma *27*:45–48, 1987.
45. Long, W. T., Filler, B., Cox, E., et al.: Toxic shock syndrome after a human bite to the hand. J. Hand Surg. [Am.] *13*:957–959, 1988.
46. Loro, A., and Franceschi, F.: Human bites and finger infections: A survey at Dodoma Regional Hospital, Tanzania. Trop. Doctor *22*:24–26, 1992.
47. Malinowski, R. W., Strate, R. G., Perry, J. F., Jr., et al.: The management of human bite injuries of the hand. J. Trauma *19*:655–659, 1979.
48. Mann, R. J., Hoffeld, T. A., and Farmer, C. B.: Human bites of the hand: Twenty years of experience. J. Hand Surg. *2*:97–104, 1977.
49. Marr, J. S., Beck, A. M., and Lugo, J. A., Jr.: An epidemiologic study of the human bite. Public Health Rep. *94*:514–521, 1979.
50. Mast, E. E., Goodman, R. A., Bond, W. W., et al.: Transmission of bloodborne pathogens during sports: Risk and prevention. Ann. Intern. Med. *122*:283–285, 1995.
51. Mennen, U., and Howells, C. J.: Human fight-bite injuries of the hand: A study of 100 cases within 18 months. J. Hand Surg. [Br.] *16*:431–435, 1991.
52. Muguti, G. I., and Dixon, M. S.: Tetanus following human bite. Br. J. Plast. Surg. *45*:614–615, 1992.
53. Muguti, G. I., Zvomuya-Ncube, M., and Bvuma, E. T.: Experiences with human bites in Zimbabwe. Cent. Afr. J. Med. *37*:294–298, 1991.
54. Murphy, R., Katz, S., and Massaro, D.: *Fusobacterium* septicemia following a human bite. Arch. Intern. Med. *111*:97–99, 1963.
55. Narsete, T. A., Omer, G. E., and Moneim, M. S.: Hand infections from human saliva. Orthop. Rev. *12*:81–84, 1983.
56. Nunley, D. L., Sasaki, T., Atkins, A., et al.: Hand infections in hospitalized patients. Am. J. Surg. *140*:374–376, 1980.
57. Peeples, E., Boswick, J. A., Jr., and Scott, F. A.: Wounds of the hand contaminated by human and animal saliva. J. Trauma *20*:383–389, 1980.
58. Pretty, I. A., Anderson, G. S., and Sweet, D. J.: Human bites and the risk of human immunodeficiency virus transmission. Am. J. Forensic Med. Pathol. *20*:232–239, 1999.
59. Prevots, R., Sutter, R. W., Strebel, P. M., et al.: Tetanus surveillance—United States, 1989–1990. M. M. W. R. CDC Surveill. Summ. *41*(SS-8): 1–9, 1992.
60. Rickman, K. M., and Richman, L. S.: The potential for transmission of human immunodeficiency virus through human bites. J. Acquir. Immun. Defic. Syndr. *6*:402–406, 1993.
61. Schweich, P., and Fleisher, G.: Human bites in children. Pediatr. Emerg. Care *1*:51–53, 1985.
62. Shields, C., Patzakis, M. J., Meyers, M. H., et al.: Hand infections secondary to human bites. J. Trauma *15*:235–236, 1975.
63. Shirley, L. R., and Ross, S. A.: Risk of transmission of human immunodeficiency virus by bite of an infected toddler. J. Pediatr. *114*:425–427, 1989.
64. Solomons, H. C., and Elardo, R.: Bite injuries at a day care center. Early Child Res. Q. *4*:89–96, 1989.
65. Solomons, H. C., and Elardo, R.: Biting in day care centers: Incidence, prevention and intervention. J. Pediatr. Health Care *5*:191–196, 1991.
66. Sperber, N. D.: Bite marks, oral and facial injuries: Harbingers of severe child abuse. Pediatrician *16*:207–211, 1989.
67. Transmission of HIV by human bite. Lancet *2*:522, 1987.
68. Uchendu, B. O.: Primary lip closure of human bite losses of the lip. Plast. Reconstr. Surg. *90*:841–845, 1992.
69. Vale, G. L., and Noguchi, T. T.: Anatomical distribution of human bite marks in a series of 67 cases. J. Forensic Sci. *28*:61–69, 1983.
70. Weinstein, R. A., Stephen, R. J., Morof, A., et al.: Human bites: Review of the literature and report of a case. J. Oral Surg. *31*:792–794, 1973.
71. Welch, C. E.: Human bite infections of the hand. N. Engl. J. Med. *215*:901–908, 1936.
72. Wolf, J. S., Gomez, R., and McAninch, J. W.: Human bites to the penis. J. Urol. *147*:1265–2067, 1992.
73. Wolf, J. S., Turzan, C., Cattolica, E. V., et al.: Dog bites to the male genitalia: Characteristics, management and comparison with human bites. J. Urol. *149*:286–289, 1993.

CHAPTER **246B**

Animal Bites

MORVEN S. EDWARDS

Many children delight in teasing dogs, and without caution go too near them, by which they get miserably torn and mangled. . . . What these boys had been doing to enrage the dog we cannot tell, but suspect they had been tormenting him in some way, thinking that as he was chained he could not injure them. But they were mistaken in this, and one of them is likely to be bitten very severely.[6]

Author unknown, 1830

Historical Aspects

Although the agents causing infection were undefined, the consequences to children of bites resulting from provoking dogs, as noted in the opening quotation, were of concern in the 19th century just as they are today.[33] In early reports concerning bite wound infections, the wounds were found to contain fusiform bacilli and spirochetal organisms.[68, 74, 117] More recently, researchers have become aware that a vast array of aerobic and anaerobic organisms making up the normal flora of the biting animal must be considered potential pathogens in an infected bite wound.

The importance of surgical débridement and drainage in the treatment of infected bite wounds was well recognized in the era before the advent of antibiotics. However, in spite of this mode of treatment, wound infections were associated with high morbidity.[115] In a report from 1936, amputation was required in one third of cases in which treatment was delayed for 24 hours or longer.[139] Adjuncts to cleansing, such as electrocauterization[93] and even radiation therapy, were used in an effort to prevent or treat infection, but not until the introduction of penicillin was the outcome of bite wound infections improved over that achieved by symptomatic therapy alone.[115]

Epidemiology

Approximately 108 million cats and dogs are kept as pets in the United States.[58] The estimated annual incidence of animal bites is 1 to 2 million dog bites, 400,000 cat bites, and 45,000 snake bites.[48, 57, 67, 86, 137] Researchers have estimated that the direct medical charges annually for dog bites alone are $165 million.[118] Species of animals that cause at least 1 percent of bite injuries are rabbits, skunks, squirrels, horses, rats, hogs, and monkeys.[32, 40, 133, 134] Numerous severe facial injuries have been inflicted because of unprovoked pet ferret attacks.[110] Considered together, however, bites from nondomestic animals, generally thought to pose a higher risk for transmission of rabies, constitute less than 1 percent of reported bites.[129] The right arm is the site most frequently bitten, presumably because of attempts by victims to use their dominant arm for defense. At least three quarters of all bites are located on the extremities.[70, 92, 134] Facial bites account for only 10 percent of bites, but most of them (58 to 64%) are sustained by children younger than 10 years.[70, 86]

Children are the most common victims of animal bites. From half to three fourths of dog bites are reported in persons younger than 20 years.[70, 129] The peak incidence occurs in children 5 to 14 years of age.[15, 129] An estimated nearly 2 percent of children 5 to 9 years of age are bitten annually. In one survey, 15 percent of 531 children had been bitten by a mammal by the time that they had reached 1 year of age.[32] Many of these bites did not require a visit to the physician and were not reported. Among cases that are reported, the number of children bitten exceeds the rate of all reportable childhood diseases.[20] Thus, one is not surprised that as many as 1 percent of all pediatric emergency room visits during the summer months are for treatment of animal bites.[38, 81, 86] Most bites occur during the late afternoon and early evening hours. Boys sustain dog bites twice as often as girls do, but girls are bitten more frequently by cats.[70, 86, 99]

Large dogs with an average weight of 50 lb or more account for most animal bites[70] and are implicated most frequently in bites with a fatal outcome. Ten to 20 fatal human attacks occur yearly in the United States. At least 25 breeds of dogs were implicated in 238 fatalities from dog bites during the past 20 years, but pit bull–type dogs and rottweilers were involved in more than half the deaths.[123] These animals can exert a biting force (1500 psi) several times that of a German shepherd. The severity of wounds inflicted by pit bull breeds also is due to their tendency to inflict multiple bites and to bite and grind their molars into tissue. Ninety-four percent of pit bull injuries in one study were the consequence of unprovoked attacks.[10] In most instances (75%), the dog's owner is known by the victim, although only a small percentage of bites are caused by a family-owned dog.[70] Stray dogs account for only 10 percent of bites inflicted.[70, 86] When the circumstances are known, most mammalian bites are provoked, although the victim may not have agitated the animal intentionally.[30, 86, 126]

Infection is a common complication of animal bites. Between 3 and 20 percent of dog bites and 20 and 50 percent of cat bites for which medical care is sought become infected.[1, 27, 58, 86, 137] With the exception of monkey bites, which have a high (25%) infection rate, infection developing after other mammalian bites is uncommon.[1, 40] Factors influencing the risk for infection include patient age, wound type, wound location, and length of time between the bite and initiation of treatment.[19, 26] Children younger than 4 years are reported to have an increased incidence of wound infection by some, but not all investigators, and infection occurs more commonly in patients older than 50 years.[26] Wounds of the hand are more likely to become infected (30–36%) than those of the arm (17–27%), leg (15–17%), or face (4–11%).[26, 27] Puncture wounds are more likely to become infected than lacerations, superficial wounds, or wounds with skin and soft tissue defects.[1, 26, 27, 133] Infection is likely to develop when wounds are repaired surgically or when care is delayed more than 24 hours after injury.[26, 133]

Microbiology

Researchers have suggested that the mammalian mouth can be viewed as a microbial incubator supporting the growth of some 200 species of facultative organisms and obligate anaerobes.[46] The normal oral flora of the animal, rather than the skin flora of the victim, is the source of most bacteria isolated from bite wound cultures,[65, 99] but each may be viewed as a potential source of infection. Infections are usually polymicrobial and contain mixed aerobic-anaerobic isolates. Table 246–7 enumerates bacterial isolates from the wounds of 50 patients with dog bites and 57 with cat bites that were infected at the time of arrival at

TABLE 246–7 ■ BACTERIA ISOLATED FROM 50 DOG AND 57 INFECTED CAT BITES

Bacteria	Number of Patients (%)	
	Dog Bite	Cat Bite
Aerobes		
Pasteurella	25 (50)	43 (75)
Streptococci	23 (46)	26 (46)
Staphylococcus aureus	10 (20)	2 (4)
Other staphylococci	13 (23)	18 (31)
Neisseria	8 (16)	11 (19)
Corynebacterium	6 (12)	16 (28)
EF-4b	5 (10)	9 (16)
Moraxella	5 (10)	20 (35)
Enterococcus	5 (10)	7 (12)
Bacillus	4 (8)	6 (11)
Pseudomonas	3 (6)	3 (5)
Actinomyces	3 (6)	2 (4)
Brevibacterium	3 (6)	2 (4)
Weeksella	2 (4)	4 (7)
Eikenella corrodens	1 (2)	1 (2)
Capnocytophaga	1 (2)	4 (7)
Acinetobacter	0	4 (7)
Other	19 (38)	19 (33)
Anaerobes		
Fusobacterium	16 (32)	19 (33)
Bacteroides	15 (30)	16 (28)
Porphyromonas	14 (28)	17 (30)
Prevotella	14 (28)	11 (19)
Propionibacterium	10 (20)	10 (18)
Peptostreptococcus	8 (16)	3 (5)
Eubacterium	2 (4)	1 (2)
Others	1 (2)	5 (9)

Adapted from Talan, D. A., Citron, D. M., Abrahamian, F. M., et al.: Bacteriologic analysis of infected dog and cat bites. N. Engl. J. Med. *340*:85–92, 1999.

an emergency department for care.[131] A median of five bacterial isolates were found per culture. Slightly more than half the wounds yielded both aerobes and anaerobes, and anaerobes alone were isolated from slightly more than a third. *Pasteurella* spp. were the isolates most frequently found in dog and cat bites (50% and 75%, respectively), with *Pasteurella canis* being isolated most commonly from dog bites and *Pasteurella multocida* subspecies *multocida* and *septica* the most common isolates from cat bites. *Pasteurella* carrier rates range as high as 66 percent for dogs and 90 percent for cats, so one is not surprised that this organism is associated so commonly with bite wound infections.[9] Infection is not restricted to the bite of house cats; it also has been reported after lion,[25, 130] cougar,[87] and tiger bites.[25] The type of wound commonly inflicted (i.e., puncture by cats versus laceration by dogs) might explain the species-specific disparity in infection rates.

Other aerobic agents commonly isolated from infected dog or cat bites include streptococci, staphylococci, *Moraxella, Neisseria,* and corynebacteria. Although streptococci are often beta-hemolytic, *Streptococcus pyogenes* was isolated from only 12 percent of dog bites and none of the infected cat bites in one large series.[131] Similarly, *Staphylococcus aureus* was isolated frequently from infected dog bites but infrequently from cat bite wounds. Species such as *Weeksella zoohelcum, Capnocytophaga canimorsus,* and *Neisseria weaveri,* which previously were classified under the Centers for Disease Control and Prevention alphanumeric system, are notable because numerous infections reported in association with these species have occurred in

TABLE 246–8 ■ SYSTEMIC INFECTIONS TRANSMISSIBLE BY ANIMAL BITES

Infection	Type of Bite	Representative References
Viral		
Arbovirus (Rio Bravo infection)*	Bat	80
Cytomegalovirus	Chimpanzee	107
Hemorrhagic fever with renal syndrome†	Rodent	41
Monkeypox	Chimpanzee	108
Rabies	C, D, O	32, 42, 132
B virus (*Herpesvirus simiae*) encephalitis	Monkey	80
Venezuelan equine encephalitis‡	Bat	132
Bacterial		
Brucellosis	D	119
Cat-scratch disease	C, D, monkey	29
Leptospirosis	D, mouse, rat	80, 95, 113
Plague	C	54
Rat-bite fever§	D, rat, mouse, squirrel, weasel, gerbil	55, 142
Tetanus	D	129
Tularemia	C, D, O	7, 31, 47, 80, 97
Mycobacterial		
M. marinum	Dolphin	53
M. fortuitum	D	8
Fungal		
Blastomycosis	D	56, 75, 83
Parasitic		
Trypanosomiasis‡	Bat	132

*Caused by a California bat salivary gland virus.
†Murine virus nephropathy.
‡Possible or questionable transmission.
§Both Haverhill fever caused by *Streptobacillus moniliformis* and sodoku caused by *Spirillum minus.*
C, cat; D, dog; O, other mammals.

splenectomized persons or those with immunocompromising conditions.[5, 23, 77]

Animal bites have been implicated as the vehicle for transmission of an extensive array of systemic infectious diseases caused by viruses, fungi, and mycobacteria, in addition to bacteria[46] (Table 246–8). For some of these infections, the list of "other animals" that may transmit the infection via biting is extensive. For example, tularemia may be transmitted by the bite of a wild boar, coyote, hog, lamb, muskrat, opossum, raccoon, rat, skunk, squirrel, snapping turtle, or weasel.[80]

Clinical Manifestations

Signs of bacterial infection after animal bites develop within hours to several days after injury. As noted by Goldstein and associates,[60] infection is the usual reason that patients seek medical attention more than 12 hours after injury, whereas those seen earlier are more concerned with prophylaxis or surgical repair. Symptoms suggestive of wound infection include localized swelling, erythema, and pain with or without serosanguineous or purulent drainage (Fig. 246–1). The clinical findings vary with the infecting organism, site of injury, and type of bite.

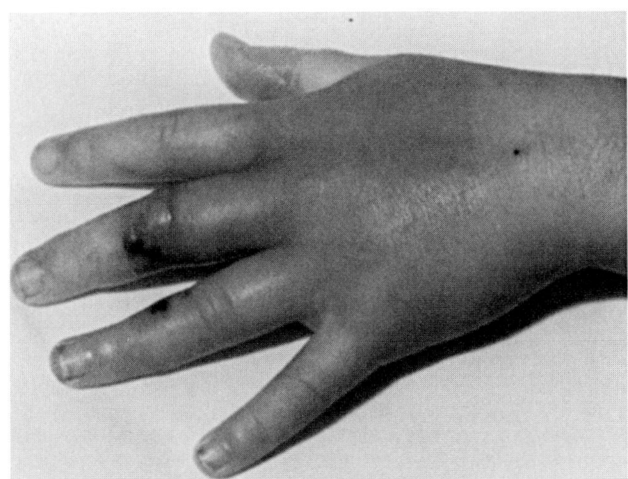

FIGURE 246–1 ■ Dog bite wound–associated tenosynovitis in a 4-year-old girl. Group D *Streptococci* were isolated from the wound culture.

In patients with *P. multocida* infection, the characteristic clinical syndrome of intense pain, swelling, and erythema develops rapidly, often within hours after injury.[94] Intense cellulitis is usually evident within 24 to 36 hours after the bite,[9, 36, 76, 94] but occasionally it may be delayed for 3 to 5 days.[36, 76] Despite these intense local symptoms, patients are generally afebrile, and less than 20 percent have lymphangitis and regional adenitis. In contrast, patients with wound infection caused by staphylococci or streptococci usually experience less intense pain, have a delay between injury and the onset of symptoms of days rather than hours, and may have a more diffuse, less fiery cellulitis. Extensive gas in the tissues of the forearm clinically suggestive of clostridial gas gangrene has been described in infections caused by *Streptococcus anginosus* and *Streptococcus mutans* after horse bite lacerations.[101] Wound infection clinically resembling that caused by *P. multocida* from which the related but more unusual gram-negative rod *Actinobacillus lignieresii* was isolated has been reported in a child who sustained a facial bite by a horse.[37]

"Seal finger" deserves mention because failure to initiate appropriate therapy may result in permanent sequelae. The etiologic agent is unknown, but a possible role has been suggested for *Mycoplasma.*[11] Infection may result from contact through a skin laceration with the skin of a seal or from a seal tooth- or claw-associated puncture wound.[100, 104] The incubation period averages 4 to 8 days, and infection is characterized by severe pain and often massive swelling, moderate erythema, and in some cases, regional adenopathy and ascending lymphangitis. It has a predilection for involvement of the joint closest to the inoculation site.[100] Once the diagnosis is made, treatment should be initiated with tetracycline, which is the drug of choice.[100, 104] The use of other antibiotics, including ampicillin, erythromycin, and cephalosporins, produces no effect and has been associated with progression of infection and joint destruction.[104]

In patients with systemic infections transmitted by an animal bite, the incubation period and clinical manifestations vary with the causative agent. For example, streptobacillary rat-bite fever occurs after an incubation period of less than 1 week, whereas spirillary rat-bite fever, or sodoku, has a 2-week asymptomatic interval after the bite. However, rat-bite fever caused by *Spirillum minor* and *Streptobacillus moniliformis* can occur together. The term squirrel-bite fever has been suggested for a syndrome clinically similar to streptobacillary rat-bite fever that has been described after the bite of the ground squirrel *Xerus erythropus.*[105] For most of the infections listed in Table 246–8, the bite wound serves as the site of inoculation and has healed completely during the incubation period. For example, fatal encephalitis has resulted from the bite or scratch of a monkey that is actively shedding B virus (*Herpesvirus simiae*). Institution of acyclovir treatment intravenously at the time of injury may abort progression of the disease.[13, 91] The systemic symptoms heralding the onset of systemic infections caused by animal bites do not depend on the mode of transmission and are discussed in their respective chapters. A high index of suspicion may be required to trace the infection to the animal source. For example, most cases of human plague in the United States result from bites by infected fleas, but contact with a *Yersinia pestis*–infected domestic cat can be the source of infection.[54] With tularemia, an ulcerative[118] or pustular[49] lesion develops at the bite site 4 to 7 days after injury in association with fever, chills, and painful regional adenopathy. In a case of *Mycobacterium marinum* infection after a dolphin bite, one of several discrete fluctuant masses containing the isolate developed in an area just proximal to the original wound.[53] With cat-scratch disease caused by *Bartonella henselae,* a papule or pustule may be present at the original bite site when systemic signs develop.

The jaws and teeth of dogs are likely to produce multiple puncture wounds, as well as jagged lacerations with devitalized tissue. These lesions may be associated with depressed skull fractures, sometimes in more than one cranial region.[141] Puncture wounds, particularly those inflicted by cat bites, are often deceptively innocuous. Inoculation of organisms deep into poorly vascularized areas, such as tendon sheaths, fascia, joints, and bones, is likely to result in an infected wound.[22]

Some of the complications that have resulted from direct extension or generalized spread of infection caused by animal bites are summarized in Table 246–9. Tenosynovitis caused by *P. multocida* may be apparent within hours after injury,[22] or the diagnosis may be delayed for days to weeks after the bite until the persistence of swelling, tenderness or pain with motion, and a mass overlying the involved tendon sheath suggest the diagnosis.[94] The development of *Pasteurella* osteomyelitis after cat bites was reported first in 1942.[2] Both acute[82, 94] and chronic[9, 17, 36, 82, 94] disease subsequently has been described, and each is characterized by pain, swelling, and tenderness over the involved bone. In patients with chronic infection, draining sinuses or a persistently draining wound is a frequent initial sign. When the periosteum has been entered, osteomyelitis may develop despite early local care and antibiotic treatment. Although combined osteomyelitis and septic arthritis have been reported, septic arthritis alone shows a predilection for previously damaged joints.[47] Feline incisors are more likely to penetrate the periosteum than canine incisors are, but osteomyelitis may occur as a complication of dog bites as well.[82, 96]

Bites to the cranium occur with relative frequency in small children because their heads are at the level of the mouth of medium to large dogs. Complications of perforating cranial bites that have been described in children include compound depressed skull fractures, dural lacerations, and extensive intracerebral injuries, which may prove fatal.[25, 141] Brain abscess and meningitis may occur as complications of these injuries (see Table 246–9).

Generalized or systemic complications from animal bites occur usually, but not exclusively in hosts with altered immune status. For example, the three most common underlying findings in infections associated with *Capnocytophaga canimorsus* are splenectomy, alcoholism, and

TABLE 246–9 ■ SOME INFECTIOUS COMPLICATIONS OF ANIMAL BITES

Complications	Isolates	Type of Bite	Representative References
Direct Extension			
Arthritis	*Pasteurella multocida*	D, C, lion	25, 48
Brain abscess	*Peptococcus*	D	3
	P. multocida	D	88
	Streptococcus bovis	Rooster	14
	Clostridium tertium		
	Aspergillus niger		
	*Capnocytophaga canimorsus**	D	79
Endophthalmitis	*P. multocida*	C	145
Orbital cellulitis	Not specified	Rat	39
Osteomyelitis	*Haemophilus hemoglobinophilus*	D	90
	P. multocida	D, C, lion	2, 9, 17, 25, 36, 48, 82, 94, 96
	VE-2, EF-4,† *P. multocida*	D	82
	Acinetobacter calcoaceticus	D	49
	Acinetobacter anitratus	Hamster	102
	Enterococcus	Monkey	49
Synovitis	*Mycobacterium fortuitum*	D	8
Tendonitis, tenosynovitis	*Pseudomonas aeruginosa*	D	49
	P. multocida	C, D	22, 72
Generalized			
Endocarditis	*P. multocida*	D	124
	Pasteurella spp.	C	69
	Erysipelothrix rhusiopathiae	D	16
	P. multocida	C	140
	Unclassified, GNR	D	84, 125
Generalized Shwartzman reaction	*P. multocida*†	D	106
Meningitis ± sepsis‡	Unclassified, GNR	D	18, 21
	P. multocida	D, tiger	12, 25
	Streptobacillus moniliformis	D	55
Mycotic aneurysm	*P. multocida*	C	66
Pneumonia	*P. multocida*	C	73
Sepsis ± coagulopathy	*Bacteroides* spp.	D	50
	P. multocida	D, C	85, 143
	C. canimorsus	D	84
Sepsis, infected knee joint prostheses	*P. multocida, P. aeruginosa*	C	109
Sepsis, post-splenectomy	Unclassified GNR, including *C. canimorsus*	D	51, 103

*Formerly dysgonic fermenter type 2, DF-2.
†Isolates possibly associated with infection.
‡Includes some probable direct extension cases.
C, cat; D, dog; GNR, gram-negative rods.

chronic lung diseases.[51, 84, 103, 116] Disseminated intravascular coagulation, hypotension, cutaneous gangrene, and renal failure also have been described in patients with leukemia or lymphoma and in association with steroid therapy.[84, 146] Symptoms ensue 1 day to 2 weeks after dog or, occasionally, cat bites; the overall mortality rate from *C. canimorsus* septicemia exceeds 20 percent.[35] However, bacteremia and fatal endocarditis caused by this organism have occurred in immunocompetent patients. Although removal of bilaterally affected knee joint prostheses was required to achieve cure of infection caused by *P. multocida* and *Pseudomonas aeruginosa* in one report,[109] cure also has been achieved with antibiotics and drainage with the prosthesis remaining in situ.[48]

Diagnosis and Treatment

The most important aid in the diagnosis of infection after animal bite wounds is the proper use of wound cultures. A culture need not be obtained from children initially seen in the immediate postinjury period (the first 8 hours) unless the bite is located on the face or hand or signs of infection are present. The isolates from an uninfected, but contaminated wound reflect the normal flora of the biting animal and do not predict the future development of infection.[19, 26] Routine determination of the microorganisms colonizing bites on the face or hands is a useful precaution because of the potentially devastating consequences of infection at these locations. After the wound has been cleansed, culture should be performed routinely when patients are initially seen at an interval exceeding 8 hours from the time of injury, except for wounds evaluated more than 24 hours after injury in which no signs of infection are present.

When material is obtained for wound culture, the microbiology laboratory should be informed that the source of the specimen is an animal bite wound. This information should optimize accuracy because *P. multocida* may be mistaken morphologically for *Neisseria* or *Haemophilus influenzae*,[94, 134] appropriate media must be used for the isolation of anaerobes, and gram-negative rods should be considered pathogens. A blood culture should be performed when the elevation in temperature is substantial (greater than 38.9° C [102° F] rectally) or if systemic toxicity is evident, although associated bacteremia is a rare occurrence.[49] Radiographic evaluation of the bite-injured area is indicated when possible or if the periosteum definitely has been penetrated. A computed tomographic study may be an aid to detecting periosteal defects, particularly in children with cranial bite wounds. For patients in whom a wound infection has extended locally, sutures, if present, should be removed and material from the involved tissue compartment harvested for study. Material should be aspirated from areas of cellulitis or drained from areas of frank abscess formation. If osteomyelitis is suspected, a diagnostic bone biopsy specimen should be submitted for Gram stain, culture, and histopathologic evaluation. If the course of the wound infection is indolent, acid-fast stains and mycobacterial cultures should be performed. Serum for serologic testing should be obtained from patients with symptoms suggesting cat-scratch disease, tularemia, syphilis, or blastomycosis. The details of the indicated diagnostic evaluation for systemic infections transmissible by animal bite (see Table 246–8) are specified in the appropriate chapters.

The first step in care of the wound is to cleanse it and the surrounding area.[71] Visible dirt should be sponged away gently to avoid further damage to traumatized tissue. The wound should be irrigated copiously with normal saline. Cleansing by high-pressure syringe irrigation with a 25-mL syringe and 19-gauge needle is effective.[28, 128, 136] This method of irrigation decreased the incidence of infection associated with wounds from dog bites by fivefold, from 69 to 12 percent.[26] Puncture wounds should be cleansed but not irrigated because irrigation may damage tissues further.

Devitalized tissues should be débrided. Callaham[26] found that further careful trimming of the wound edge in nonpuncture wounds was associated with a significant decrease in the rate of infection. Others investigators contend that wound excision should not be considered standard treatment.[43] The issue of bite wound closure has been controversial because of concern that sutured wounds have an increased rate of infection. Callaham,[28] in a retrospective study, found that infection rates were significantly lower in sutured than in nonsutured wounds. However, the same investigator found no difference in the infection rate in 57 patients assessed prospectively, with the exception of those suffering hand bites, which were more likely to become infected when sutured.[27] After appropriate cleansing and débridement, most nonpuncture animal bite wounds except those involving the hand apparently can be treated by primary closure without increasing the incidence of infection.[26, 28, 86, 98, 133]

Data with which to assess the use of prophylactic antibiotics after animal bites are sparse. One investigator found that oxacillin did not reduce the incidence of infection after dog bite wounds[44] but did after cat bites.[45] In another study, a trend toward a reduced rate of infection, particularly for hand wounds, was shown for patients receiving penicillin prophylactically after incurring dog bites.[27] In a well-designed, prospective study limited to children with nonfacial dog bites that did not require closure, prophylactic penicillin at a dose of 250 mg four times daily for 5 days did not affect the rate of infection significantly.[19] Prophylactic dicloxacillin, cephalexin, or erythromycin was not beneficial therapy for low-risk dog bite wounds in another prospective study. The infection rates for wounds in the antibiotic and control groups were 1.1 and 5.1 percent, respectively.[38]

A meta-analysis of eight randomized trials totaling 783 patients with dog bite wounds found that prophylactic antibiotics did reduce the incidence of infection.[34] The estimated cumulative incidence of infection was 16 percent in controls, and the relative risk was 0.56 (95% confidence interval, range 0.38 to 0.82) in patients given antibiotics. Treatment of approximately 14 patients was required to prevent one infection. Thus, one view is that prophylaxis has a role, but it should be used selectively.[30] Alternatively, some researchers consider antibiotic use therapeutic rather than prophylactic in this setting and suggest that antibiotic therapy be given in all cases of dog bites except those initially evaluated more than 24 hours after injury with no clinical signs of infection.[140]

Until additional data are available, a reasonable approach appears to be administration of prophylactic antibiotics in the following circumstances: (1) dog bites more than 8 hours old; (2) moderate to severe dog bites less than 8 hours old, especially if edema or crush injury is present; (3) puncture wounds, particularly if bone or joint penetration may have occurred; (4) facial wounds; (5) all hand bites; (6) wounds in the genital area; and (7) wounds in immunocompromised persons.[58, 99, 136, 138]

Empiric treatment should be directed toward the most common infecting organisms: *P. multocida,* staphylococci, streptococci, and anaerobes.[99] Amoxicillin-clavulanate is active against almost all species of bacteria found in bite wounds and is the drug of choice for empiric oral treatment.[4, 24, 59] The recommended dosage is 40 mg/kg/day administered at 8-hour intervals. Erythromycin is only moderately active against *P. multocida.*[99, 127] A recommended oral regimen for penicillin-allergic children is trimethoprim-sulfamethoxazole (10 and 50 mg/kg/day) plus clindamycin (30 mg/kg/day).[4] Numerous other combination regimens such as cefuroxime axetil (30 mg/kg/day) plus clindamycin or metronidazole (30 mg/kg/day) may be used. For hospitalized patients requiring prophylaxis, ampicillin-sulbactam (200 mg/kg/day) and ticarcillin-clavulanate (200 mg/kg/day) are the drugs of choice.[4] Imipenem (80 mg/kg/day) is an alternative choice. For penicillin-allergic children, combination therapy with an extended-spectrum cephalosporin or trimethoprim-sulfamethoxazole plus clindamycin should be administered.[4]

Newer macrolides, including azithromycin, show improved activity (versus erythromycin) against the organisms causing animal bite wound infections, but some strains of staphylococci and fusobacteria are resistant.[63] Azithromycin is more active than clarithromycin against all *Pasteurella* spp.[61] To date, clinical trials documenting its efficacy are not available, and the use of regimens for which clinical experience exists is advisable. Similarly, the quinolones and, in particular, gatifloxacin exhibit broad activity against the spectrum of pathogens isolated from bite wounds, with the exception of fusobacteria.[64] However, the risk-to-benefit ratio should be considered before its administration in children because it is approved for use only for those 18 years or older.

Penicillin is the drug of choice for *P. multocida* infection. This organism has a median minimal inhibitory concentration to penicillin G of 0.1 to 0.8 μg/mL.[48, 49] Other active antibiotics in vitro are ampicillin, tetracycline, chloramphenicol, cephalothin,[127] trimethoprim-sulfamethoxazole, and third-generation cephalosporins.[49] Cefuroxime is potentially useful and more active than cephalexin.[59] Antibiotics with poor activity against *P. multocida* include the penicillinase-resistant penicillins, clindamycin, and aminoglycosides.[127]

As a general guideline, a suggested duration of therapy, assuming that proper drainage has been established, is 10 days for cellulitis or localized abscess, 2 to 3 weeks for tenosynovitis, and 3 to 4 weeks for osteomyelitis. When improvement is evident, treatment can be completed orally. At least 4 weeks of intravenous therapy should be administered to patients with endocarditis. Although the number of patients is too small to establish the required dosage with certainty, ampicillin (400 mg/kg/day) has been used successfully for the treatment of *P. multocida* meningitis.[12]

The antimicrobial therapy for wound infections should be adjusted according to the susceptibility of organisms isolated from the wound cultures.

In every child sustaining a bite wound, immunization status should be determined to assess the need for tetanus prophylaxis and whether rabies prophylaxis should be undertaken (see the appropriate chapters).

Reptile Bites

Approximately 8000 people in the United States are bitten yearly by poisonous snakes.[135] Approximately half of these bites occur in people younger than 20 years. The curiosity of children may contribute to this exposure because many are bitten while handling poisonous snakes.[111] Between 9 and 15 persons die of snake bites each year.[89]

Venomous snakes are divided into four families, two of which, the Crotalidae (rattlesnakes, copperheads, and water moccasins) and the Elapidae (coral snakes), are found in the United States. Snake venoms are among the most complex of proteins. The local effects of the venom of pit vipers (Crotalidae), which is rich in proteolytic activity, include swelling, pain, edema, ecchymosis, and tissue necrosis with the formation of bullae.[121] The venom of the eastern coral snake causes minimal local tissue destruction. The systemic effects of crotalid envenomation result from increased blood vessel permeability and hemolysis and may include hematuria, hematemesis, and disseminated intravascular coagulopathy.[121] The venom of the eastern coral snake is a neurotoxin that produces paresthesia of the involved extremity, followed by involvement of the cranial nerves and bulbar paralysis.

Since the pre-antibiotic era, researchers have recognized that the oral flora of snakes' mouths frequently consists of multiple organisms, particularly gram-negative bacilli, staphylococci, and anaerobes.[112, 144] Goldstein and associates[62] isolated 58 aerobic and 28 anaerobic organisms after culturing the venom from 15 rattlesnakes. The aerobes most commonly isolated were *P. aeruginosa, Proteus* spp., and *Staphylococcus epidermidis*. Among the anaerobes, *Clostridium* spp. were the isolates found most frequently; *Bacteroides fragilis* also was recovered. The defecation of prey during ingestion has been suggested to be responsible for this preponderance of gastrointestinal flora. By cleansing the fangs carefully before collection, these investigators demonstrated that the venom itself is sterile, thus indicating that bacterial isolates potentially contaminating snake bite wounds are a reflection of the oral flora.

In persons sustaining alligator bite wounds, infection is caused most commonly by *Aeromonas hydrophila*. A report of mixed infection with *A. hydrophila, Enterobacter agglomerans,* and *Citrobacter diversus* and the frequency with which *Proteus vulgaris* and *Pseudomonas* spp. are isolated from alligator mouths suggest that treatment of alligator bites should be directed at gram-negative species.[52] *Vibrio* infection should be suspected in victims of shark bites, as well as all wounds exposed to salt water.[114] *Aeromonas* spp. and other gram-negative bacilli, as well as *S. aureus* and anaerobes, all can infect shark bites.[120]

The exotic pet industry is growing in the United States, and the common green iguana is a popular pet. Few cases of infections from iguana bites have been reported because these creatures are generally nonaggressive, but *Serratia marcescens* cellulitis has been observed.[78]

The role of empiric antibiotics after reptile wounds is undefined, as is the incidence of infection and subsequent complications. The problem in defining the incidence of infection after snake bites stems from the fact that the inflammatory changes of envenomation may be difficult to differentiate from those of infection.[92] At least one instance of osteomyelitis as a complication of an infected snake bite has been documented.[122] Russell[122] suggests that a broad-spectrum antibiotic be used for injuries with severe tissue involvement but not for bites with minor or minimal envenomation. Other experts suggest that antibiotics be withheld unless evidence of bacterial infection develops.[135] Amoxicillin-clavulanate is an appropriate oral antimicrobial and ampicillin-sulbactam plus gentamicin an appropriate parenteral regimen for empiric treatment of reptile bite wounds.[4] The oral alternatives for penicillin-allergic children are the same as those given for other animal bite wounds; one parenteral regimen for a penicillin-allergic child is clindamycin plus gentamicin. Treatment should be guided by the results of Gram stain and susceptibility testing.

REFERENCES

1. Aghababian, R. V., and Conte, J. E.: Mammalian bite wounds. Ann. Emerg. Med. *9*:79–83, 1980.
2. Allin, A. E.: Cat-bite wound infection. Can. Med. Assoc. J. *46*:48–50, 1942.
3. Alpert, G., and Sutton, L. N.: Brain abscess following cranial dog bite. Clin. Pediatr. (Phila.) *23*:580, 1984.
4. American Academy of Pediatrics: Bite wounds. *In* Pickering, L. K. (ed.): 2000 Red Book: Report of the Committee on Infectious Diseases. 25th ed. Elk Grove Village, IL, American Academy of Pediatrics, 2000, pp. 155–159.
5. Andersen, B. M., Steigerwalt, A. G., O'Conner, S. P., et al.: *Neisseria weaveri* sp. nov., formerly CDC group M-5, a gram-negative bacterium associated with dog bite wounds. J. Clin. Microbiol. *31*:2456–2466, 1993.
6. Anonymous: The Book of Accidents: Designed for Young Children. New Haven, CT, Sidney's Press, 1830.
7. Arav-Boger, R.: Cat-bite tularemia in a seventeen-year-old girl treated with ciprofloxacin. Pediatr. Infect. Dis. J. *19*:583–584, 2000.
8. Ariel, H., Haas, H., Weinberg, H., et al.: *Mycobacterium fortuitum* granulomatous synovitis caused by a dog bite. J. Hand Surg. *8*:342–343, 1983.
9. Arons, M. S., Fernando, L., and Polayes, I. M.: *Pasteurella multocida:* The major cause of hand infections following domestic animal bites. J. Hand Surg. *7*:47–52, 1982.
10. Avner, J. R., and Baker, M. D.: Dog bites in urban children. Pediatrics *88*:55–57, 1991.
11. Baker, A. S., Ruoff, K. L., and Madoff, S.: Isolation of *Mycoplasma* species from a patient with seal finger. Clin. Infect. Dis. *27*:1168–1170, 1998.
12. Belardi, F. G., Pascoe, J. M., and Beegle, E. D.: *Pasteurella multocida* meningitis in an infant following occipital dog bite. J. Fam. Pract. *14*:778–782, 1982.
13. Benson, P. M., Malane, S. L., Banks, R., et al.: B virus (*Herpesvirus simiae*) and human infection. Arch. Dermatol. *125*:1247–1248, 1989.
14. Berkowitz, F. E., and Jacobs, D. W. C.: Fatal case of brain abscess caused by rooster pecking. Pediatr. Infect. Dis. *6*:941–942, 1987.
15. Berzon, D. R., and DeHoff, J. D.: Medical cost and other aspects of dog bites in Baltimore. Public Health Rep. *89*:377–381, 1974.
16. Bibler, M. R.: *Erysipelothrix rhusiopathiae* endocarditis. Rev. Infect. Dis. *10*:1062–1063, 1988.
17. Bjorkhölm, B., and Tönnes, E.: *Pasteurella multocida* osteomyelitis caused by cat bite. J. Infect. *6*:175–177, 1983.
18. Bobo, R. A., and Newton, E. J.: A previously undescribed gram-negative bacillus causing septicemia and meningitis. Am. J. Clin. Pathol. *65*:546–569, 1976.
19. Boenning, D. A., Fleisher, G. R., and Campos, J. M.: Dog bites in children: Epidemiology, microbiology, and penicillin prophylactic therapy. Am. J. Emerg. Med. *1*:17–21, 1983.
20. Borchelt, P. L., Lockwood, R., Beck, A. M., et al.: Attacks by packs of dogs involving predation of human beings. Public Health Rep. *98*:57–66, 1983.
21. Bracis, R., Seibers, K., and Julien, R. M.: Meningitis caused by group II J following a dog bite. West. J. Med. *131*:438–440, 1979.
22. Branson, D., and Bunkfeldt, F., Jr.: *Pasteurella multocida* in animal bites of humans. Am. J. Clin. Pathol. *48*:552–555, 1967.
23. Brenner, D. J., Hollis, D. G., Fanning, G. R., et al.: *Capnocytophaga canimorsus* sp. nov. (formerly CDC group DF-2), a cause of septicemia following dog bite, and *C. cynodegmi* sp. nov., a cause of localized wound infection following dog bite. J. Clin. Microbiol. *27*:231–235, 1989.
24. Brook, I.: Human and animal bites. J. Fam. Pract. *28*:713–718, 1989.
25. Burdge, D. R., Scheifele, D., and Speert, D. P.: Serious *Pasteurella multocida* infections from lion and tiger bites. J. A. M. A. *253*:3296–3297, 1985.
26. Callaham, M.: Treatment of common dog bites: Infection risk factors. J. Am. Coll. Emerg. Physicians *7*:83–87, 1978.
27. Callaham, M.: Prophylactic antibiotics in common dog bite wounds: A controlled study. Ann. Emerg. Med. *9*:410–414, 1980.

28. Callaham, M.: Dog bite wounds. J. A. M. A. *244*:2327–2328, 1980.
29. Callaham, M.: Human and animal bites. Top. Emerg. Med. *4*:1–15, 1982.
30. Callaham, M.: Prophylactic antibiotics in dog bite wounds: Nipping at the heels of progress. Ann. Emerg. Med. *23*:577–579, 1994.
31. Capellan, J., and Fong, I. W.: Tularemia from a cat bite: Case report and review of feline-associated tularemia. Clin. Infect. Dis. *16*:472–475, 1993.
32. Carithers, H. A.: Mammalian bites of children. Am. J. Dis. Child. *95*:150–156, 1958.
33. Cone, T. E., Jr.: Book of accidents. Excerpt VIII. Worrying dogs. Pediatrics *47*:460, 1971.
34. Cummings, P.: Antibiotics to prevent infection in patients with dog bite wounds: A meta-analysis of randomized trials. Ann. Emerg. Med. *23*:535–540, 1994.
35. Dankner, W. M., Davis, C. E., and Thompson, M. A.: DF-2 bacteremia following a dog bite in a 4-month-old child. Pediatr. Infect. Dis. *6*:695–696, 1987.
36. DeBoer, R. G., and Dumler, M.: *Pasteurella multocida* infections: A report of six cases. Am. J. Clin. Pathol. *40*:339–344, 1963.
37. Dibb, W. L., Digranes, A., and Tønjum, S.: *Actinobacillus lignieresii* infection after a horse bite. B. M. J. *283*:583–584, 1981.
38. Dire, D. J., Hogan, D. E., and Walker, J. S.: Prophylactic oral antibiotics for low-risk dog bite wounds. Pediatr. Emerg. Care *8*:194–199, 1992.
39. Diwan, R., Sen, D. K., and Sood, G. C.: Rat bite orbital cellulitis. Br. J. Ophthalmol. *54*:211, 1970.
40. Douglas, L. G.: Bite wounds. Am. Fam. Physician *11*:93–99, 1975.
41. Dournon, E., Moriniere, B., Matheron, S., et al.: HFRS after a wild rodent bite in the Haute-Savoie: And risk of exposure to Hantaan-like virus in a Paris laboratory. Lancet *1*:676–677, 1984.
42. Edlich, R. F., Spengler, M. D., and Rodeheaver, G. T.: Mammalian bites. Compr. Ther. *9*:41–47, 1983.
43. Elenbaas, R. M., McNabney, W. K., and Robinson, W. A.: Prophylactic antibiotics and dog bite wounds. J. A. M. A. *246*:833–834, 1981.
44. Elenbaas, R. M., McNabney, W. K., and Robinson, W. A.: Prophylactic oxacillin in dog bite wounds. Ann. Emerg. Med. *11*:248–251, 1982.
45. Elenbaas, R. M., McNabney, W. K., and Robinson, W. A.: Evaluation of prophylactic oxacillin in cat bite wounds. Ann. Emerg. Med. *13*:155–157, 1984.
46. Elliot, D. L., Tolle, S. W., Goldberg, L., et al.: Pet-associated illness. N. Engl. J. Med. *313*:985–995, 1985.
47. Evans, M. E., McGee, Z. A., Hunter, P. T., et al.: Tularemia and the tomcat. J. A. M. A. *246*:1343, 1981.
48. Ewing, R., Fainstein, V., Musher, D. M., et al.: Articular and skeletal infections caused by *Pasteurella multocida*. South. Med. J. *73*:1349–1352, 1980.
49. Feder, H. M., Shanley, J. D., and Barbera, J. A.: Review of 59 patients hospitalized with animal bites. Pediatr. Infect. Dis. *6*:24–28, 1987.
50. Fiala, M., Bauer, H., Khaleeli, M., et al.: Dog bite, *Bacteroides* infection, coagulopathy, renal microangiopathy. Ann. Intern. Med. *87*:248–249, 1977.
51. Findling, J. W., Pohlmann, G. P., and Rose, H. D.: Fulminant gram-negative bacillemia (DF-2) following a dog bite in an asplenic woman. Am. J. Med. *68*:154–156, 1980.
52. Flandry, F., Lisecki, E. J., Domingue, G. J., et al.: Initial antibiotic therapy for alligator bites: Characterization of the oral flora of *Alligator mississippiensis*. South. Med. J. *82*:262–266, 1989.
53. Flowers, D. J.: Human infection due to *Mycobacterium marinum* after a dolphin bite. J. Clin. Pathol. *23*:475–477, 1970.
54. Gage, K. L., Dennis, D. T., Orloski, K. A., et al.: Cases of cat-associated human plague in the western US, 1977–1998. Clin. Infect. Dis. *30*:893–900, 2000.
55. Gilbert, G. L., Cassidy, J. F., and Bennett, N. M.: Rat-bite fever. Med. J. Aust. *2*:1131–1134, 1971.
56. Gnann, J. W., Jr., Bressler, G. S., Bodet, C. A., III, et al.: Human blastomycosis after a dog bite. Ann. Intern. Med. *98*:48–49, 1983.
57. Goldstein, E. J. C.: Management of human and animal bite wounds. J. Am. Acad. Dermatol. *21*:1275–1279, 1989.
58. Goldstein, E. J. C.: Bite wounds and infection. Clin. Infect. Dis. *14*:663- 640, 1992.
59. Goldstein, E. J. C., and Citron, D. M.: Comparative activities of cefuroxime, amoxicillin–clavulanic acid, ciprofloxacin, enoxacin, and ofloxacin against aerobic and anaerobic bacteria isolated from bite wounds. Antimicrob. Agents Chemother. *32*:1143–1148, 1988.
60. Goldstein, E. J. C., Citron, D. M., and Finegold, S. M.: Dog bite wounds and infection: A prospective clinical study. Ann. Emerg. Med. *9*:508–512, 1980.
61. Goldstein, E. J. C., Citron, D. M., Gerardo, S. H., et al.: Activities of HMR 3004 (RU 64004) and HMR 3647 (RU 66647) compared to those of erythromycin, azithromycin, clarithromycin, roxithromycin, and eight other antimicrobial agents against unusual aerobic and anaerobic human and animal bite pathogens isolated from skin and soft tissue infections in humans. Antimicrob. Agents Chemother. *42*:1127–1132, 1998.
62. Goldstein, E. J. C., Citron, D. M., Gonzalez, H., et al.: Bacteriology of rattlesnake venom and implications for therapy. J. Infect. Dis. *140*:818–821, 1979.
63. Goldstein, E. J. C., Citron, D. M., Hudspeth, M., et al.: In vitro activity of Bay 12-8039, a new 8-methoxyquinolone, compared to the activities of 11 other oral antimicrobial agents against 390 aerobic and anaerobic bacteria isolated from human and animal bite wound skin and soft tissue infections in humans. Antimicrob. Agents Chemother. *41*:1552–1557, 1997.
64. Goldstein, E. J. C., Citron, D. M., Merriam, C. V., et al.: Activity of gatifloxacin compared to those of five other quinolones versus aerobic and anaerobic isolates from skin and soft tissue samples of human and animal bite wound infections. Antimicrob. Agents Chemother. *43*:1475–1479, 1999.
65. Goldstein, E. J. C., Citron, D. M., Wield, B., et al.: Bacteriology of human and animal bite wounds. J. Clin. Microbiol. *8*:667–672, 1978.
66. Goldstein, R. W., Goodhart, G. L., and Moore, J. E.: *Pasteurella multocida* infection after animal bites. N. Engl. J. Med. *315*:460, 1986.
67. Goldstein, E. J. C., and Richwald, G. A.: Human and animal bite wounds. Am. Fam. Physician *36*:101–109, 1987.
68. Guba, A. M., Jr., Mulliken, J. B., and Hoopes, J. E.: The selection of antibiotics for human bites of the hand. Plast. Reconstr. Surg. *56*:538–541, 1975.
69. Gump, D. W., and Holden, R. A.: Endocarditis caused by a new species of *Pasteurella*. Ann. Intern. Med. *76*:275–278, 1972.
70. Harris, D., Imperato, P. J., and Oken, B.: Dog bites: An unrecognized epidemic. Bull. N. Y. Acad. Med. *50*:981–1000, 1974.
71. Hawkins, J., Paris, P. M., and Stewart, R. D.: Mammalian bites: Rational approach to management. Postgrad. Med. *73*:52–64, 1983.
72. Hawkins, L. G.: Local *Pasteurella multocida* infections. J. Bone Joint Surg. Am. *51*:363–365, 1969.
73. Henderson, J. A. M., and Rowsell, H. C.: Fatal *Pasteurella multocida* pneumonia in an IgA-deficient cat fancier. West. J. Med. *150*:208–210, 1989.
74. Hennessy, P. H., and Fletcher, W.: Infection with the organisms of Vincent's angina following man-bite. Lancet *2*:127–128, 1920.
75. Hiemenz, J. W., Coccari, P. J., and Macher, A. M.: Human blastomycosis from dog bites. Ann. Intern. Med. *98*:1030, 1983.
76. Holloway, W. J., Scott, E. G., and Adams, Y. B.: *Pasteurella multocida* infection in man: Report of 21 cases. Am. J. Clin. Pathol. *51*:705–708, 1969.
77. Holmes, B., Steigerwalt, A. G., Weaver, R. E., et al.: *Weeksella zoohelcum* sp. nov. (formerly group II-J) from human clinical specimens. Syst. Appl. Microbiol. *8*:191–196, 1986.
78. Hsieh, S., and Babl, F. E.: *Serratia marcescens* cellulitis following an iguana bite. Clin. Infect. Dis. *28*:1181–1182, 1999.
79. Hsu, H.-W., and Finberg, R. W.: Infections associated with animal exposure in two infants. Rev. Infect. Dis. *11*:108–115, 1989.
80. Hubbert, W. T., McCulloch, W. F., and Schnurrenberger, P. R. (eds.): Diseases Transmitted from Animals to Man. 6th ed. Springfield, IL, Charles C Thomas, 1975, pp. 1117–1128.
81. Jaffe, A. C.: Animal bites. Pediatr. Clin. North Am. *30*:405–413, 1983.
82. Jarvis, W. R., Banko, S., Snyder, E., et al.: *Pasteurella multocida* osteomyelitis following dog bites. Am. J. Dis. Child. *135*:625–627, 1981.
83. Jaspers, R. H.: Transmission of blastomyces from animals to man. J. Am. Vet. Med. Soc. *164*:8, 1974.
84. Job, L., Horman, J. T., Grigor, J. K., et al.: Dysgonic fermenter-2: A clinico-epidemiologic review. J. Emerg. Med. *7*:185–192, 1989.
85. Jones, A. G. H., and Lockton, J. A.: Fatal *Pasteurella multocida* septicaemia following a cat bite in a man without liver disease. J. Infect. *15*:229–235, 1987.
86. Kizer, K. W.: Epidemiologic and clinical aspects of animal bite injuries. J. Am. Coll. Emerg. Physicians *8*:134–141, 1979.
87. Kizer, K. W.: *Pasteurella multocida* infection from a cougar bite: A review of cougar attacks. West. J. Med. *150*:87–90, 1989.
88. Klein, D. M., and Cohen, M. E.: *Pasteurella multocida* brain abscess following perforating cranial dog bite. J. Pediatr. *92*:588–589, 1978.
89. Kurecki, B. A., III, and Brownlee, H. J., Jr.: Venomous snake bites in the United States. J. Fam. Pract. *25*:386–392, 1987.
90. Lavine, L. S., Isenberg, H. D., Rubins, W., et al.: Unusual osteomyelitis following superficial dog bite. Clin. Orthop. *98*:251–253, 1974.
91. Leads from the MMWR. B-virus infection in humans—Pensacola, Florida. J. A. M. A. *257*:3192–3193, 3198, 1987.
92. Ledbetter, E. O., and Kutscher, A. E.: The aerobic and anaerobic flora of rattlesnake fangs and venom: Therapeutic implications. Arch. Environ. Health *19*:770–778, 1969.
93. Lowry, T. M.: The surgical treatment of human bites. Ann. Surg. *104*:1103–1111, 1936.
94. Lucas, G. L., and Bartlett, D. H.: *Pasteurella multocida* infection in the hand. Plast. Reconstr. Surg. *67*:49–53, 1981.
95. Luzzi, G. A., Milne, L. M., and Waitkins, S. A.: Rat-bite acquired leptospirosis. J. Infect. *15*:57–60, 1987.
96. Maccabe, A. F., and Conn, N.: The isolation of *Pasteurella septica* following dog and cat bites: A report of 5 cases. Scott. Med. J. *13*:242–244, 1968.
97. Magee, J. S., Steele, R. W., Kelly, N. R., et al.: Tularemia transmitted by a squirrel bite. Pediatr. Infect. Dis. *8*:123–125, 1989.
98. Maimaris, C., and Quinton, D. N.: Dog-bite lacerations: A controlled trial of primary wound closure. Arch. Emerg. Med. *5*:156–161, 1988.

99. Marcy, S. M.: Special series: Management of pediatric infectious diseases in office practice. Infections due to dog and cat bites. Pediatr. Infect. Dis. *1*:351–356, 1982.
100. Markham, R. B., and Polk, B. F.: Seal finger. Rev. Infect. Dis. *1*:567–579, 1979.
101. Marrie, T. J., Bent, J. M., West, A. B., et al.: Extensive gas in tissues of the forearm after horsebite. South. Med. J. *72*:1473–1474, 1979.
102. Martin, R. W., Martin, D. L., and Levy, C. S.: *Acinetobacter* osteomyelitis from a hamster bite. Pediatr. Infect. Dis. J. *7*:364–365, 1988.
103. Martone, W. J., Zuehl, R. W., Minson, G. E., et al.: Postsplenectomy sepsis with DF-2: Report of a case with isolation of the organism from the patient's dog. Ann. Intern. Med. *93*:457–458, 1980.
104. Mass, D. P., Newmeyer, W. L., and Kilgore, E. S., Jr.: Seal finger. J. Hand Surg. *6*:610–612, 1981.
105. McMillan, B., and Boulger, L. R.: Squirrel-bite fever. Trans. R. Soc. Trop. Med. Hyg. *62*:567, 1968.
106. Meyers, B. R., Hirschman, S. Z., and Sloan, W.: Generalized Shwartzman reaction in man after a dog bite: Consumption coagulopathy, symmetrical peripheral gangrene, and renal cortical necrosis. Ann. Intern. Med. *73*:433–438, 1970.
107. Muchmore, E.: Possible cytomegalovirus infection in man following chimpanzee bite. Lab. Anim. Sci. *21*:1080–1081, 1971.
108. Mutombo, M. W., Arita, I., and JeZek, Z.: Human monkey pox transmitted by a chimpanzee in a tropical rain forest area of Zaire. Lancet *1*:735–737, 1983.
109. Orton, D. W., and Fulcher, W. H.: *Pasteurella multocida*: Bilateral septic knee joint prostheses from a distant cat bite. Ann. Emerg. Med. *13*: 1065–1067, 1984.
110. Paisley, J. W., and Lauer, B. A.: Severe facial injuries to infants due to unprovoked attacks by pet ferrets. J. A. M. A. *259*:2005–2006, 1988.
111. Parrish, H. M.: Analysis of 460 fatalities from venomous animals in the United States. Am. J. Med. Sci. *245*:129–141, 1963.
112. Parrish, H. M., MacLaurin, A. W., and Tuttle, R. L.: North American pit vipers: Bacterial flora of the mouths and venom glands. Va. Med. *83*: 383–385, 1956.
113. Parry, W. H., and Seymour, M. W.: An unusual case of leptospirosis. Practitioner *210*:791–793, 1973.
114. Pavia, A. T., Bryan, J. A., and Maher, K. L.: *Vibrio carchariae* infection after a shark bite. Ann. Intern. Med. *111*:85–86, 1989.
115. Peeples, C., Boswick, J. A., Jr., and Scott, F. A.: Wounds of the hand contaminated by human or animal saliva. J. Trauma *20*:383–389, 1980.
116. Pers, C., Gahrn-Hansen, B., and Frederiksen, W.: *Capnocytophaga canimorsus* septicemia in Denmark, 1982–1995: Review of 39 cases. Clin. Infect. Dis. *23*:71–75, 1996.
117. Peters, W. H.: Hand infection apparently due to *Bacillus fusiformis*. J. Infect. Dis. *8*:455–462, 1911.
118. Quinlan, K. P., and Sacks, J. J.: Hospitalizations for dog bite injuries. J. A. M. A. *281*:232–233, 1999.
119. Robertson, M. G.: *Brucella* infection transmitted by dog bite. J. A. M. A. *225*:750–751, 1973.
120. Royle, J. A., Isaacs, D., Eagles, G., et al.: Infections after shark attacks in Australia. Pediatr. Infect. Dis. J. *16*:531–532, 1997.
121. Russell, F. E.: Venomous animal injuries. Curr. Probl. Pediatr. *3*:1–47, 1973.
122. Russell, F. E.: Snake venom poisoning in the United States. Annu. Rev. Med. *31*:247–259, 1980.
123. Sacks, J. J., Sinclair, L., Gilchrist, J., et al.: Breeds of dogs involved in fatal human attacks in the United States between 1979 and 1998. Am. J. Vet. Med. Assoc. *217*:836–840, 2000.
124. Sannella, N. A., Tavano, P., McGoldrick, D. A., et al.: Aortic graft sepsis caused by *Pasteurella multocida*. J. Vasc. Surg. *5*:887–888, 1987.
125. Shankar, P. S., Scott, J. H., and Anderson, C. L.: Atypical endocarditis due to gram-negative bacillus transmitted by dog bite. South. Med. J. *73*:1640–1641, 1980.
126. Spence, G.: A review of animal bites in Delaware, 1989 to 1990. Del. Med. J. *62*:1425–1429, 1990.
127. Stevens, D. L., Higbee, J. W., Oberhofer, T. R., et al.: Antibiotic susceptibilities of human isolates of *Pasteurella multocida*. Antimicrob. Agents Chemother. *16*:322–324, 1979.
128. Stevenson, T. R., Thacker, J. G., Rodeheaver, G. T., et al.: Cleansing the traumatic wound by high pressure syringe irrigation. J. Am. Coll. Emerg. Physicians *5*:17–21, 1976.
129. Strassburg, M. A., Greenland, S., Marron, J. A., et al.: Animal bites: Patterns of treatment. Ann. Emerg. Med. *10*:193–197, 1981.
130. Swartz, M. N., and Kunz, L. J.: *Pasteurella multocida* infections in man. Report of two cases: Meningitis and infected cat bite. N. Engl. J. Med. *261*:889–893, 1959.
131. Talan, D. A., Citron, D. M., Abrahamian, F. M., et al.: Bacteriologic analysis of infected dog and cat bites. N. Engl. J. Med. *340*:85–92, 1999.
132. Thomas, J. G., Jr., and Harlan, H. J.: Vampire bat bites seen in humans in Panama: Their characterization, recognition, and management. Mil. Med. *146*:410–412, 1981.
133. Thomson, H. G., and Svitek, V.: Small animal bites: The role of primary closure. J. Trauma *13*:20–23, 1973.
134. Tindall, J. P., and Harrison, C. M.: *Pasteurella multocida* infections following animal injuries, especially cat bites. Arch. Dermatol. *105*: 412–416, 1972.
135. Treatment of snakebite in the USA. Med. Lett. Drugs Ther. *24*:87–89, 1982.
136. Trott, A.: Care of mammalian bites. Pediatr. Infect. Dis. *6*:8–10, 1987.
137. Underman, A. E.: Bite wounds inflicted by dogs and cats. Vet. Clin. North Am. *17*:195–207, 1987.
138. Weber, D. J., and Hansen, A. R.: Infections resulting from animal bites. Infect. Dis. Clin. North Am. *5*:663–680, 1991.
139. Welch, C. E.: Human bite infections of the hand. N. Engl. J. Med. *215*:901–908, 1936.
140. Wiggins, M. E., Akelman, E., and Weiss, A.-P. C.: The management of dog bites and dog bite infections to the hand. Orthopedics *17*:617–623, 1994.
141. Wilberger, J. E., Jr., and Pang, D.: Craniocerebral injuries from dog bites. J. A. M. A. *249*:2685–2688, 1983.
142. Wilkins, E. G. L., Millar, J. G. B., Cockcroft, P. M., et al.: Rat-bite fever in a gerbil breeder. J. Infect. *16*:177–180, 1988.
143. Williams, E.: Septicaemia caused by an organism resembling *Pasteurella septica* after a dog-bite. B. M. J. *2*:169–171, 1960.
144. Williams, F. E., Freeman, M., and Kennedy, E.: The bacterial flora of the mouths of Australian venomous snakes in captivity. Med. J. Aust. *2*:190–193, 1934.
145. Yokoyama, T., Hara, S., Funakubo, H., et al.: *Pasteurella multocida* endophthalmitis after a cat bite. Ophthalmic Surg. *18*:520–522, 1987.
146. Zumla, A., Lipscomb, G., Corbett, M., et al.: Dysgonic fermenter-type 2: An emerging zoonosis: Report of two cases and review. Q. J. Med. *257*(New Series 68):741–752, 1988.

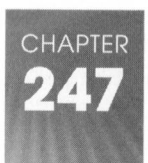

CHAPTER 247 Bioterrorism

ROBERT J. LEGGIADRO

The intentional delivery of *Bacillus anthracis* spores through mailed letters or packages established the clinical reality of bioterrorism in the United States in autumn 2001.[5, 27] An understanding of the epidemiology, clinical manifestations, and management of the more credible biologic agents is critical to limiting morbidity and mortality from a bioterrorism attack.[11, 20, 25, 33]

Implementation of an effective response to deliberate release of biologic agents by terrorists requires detection and reporting of cases as soon as possible.[4, 7] Prompt recognition of unusual clinical syndromes and increases above seasonal levels in the incidence of common syndromes or deaths from infectious agents is critical to an effective response.[4, 18, 25, 31]

History

The concept of biologic warfare or terrorism is not a new one. In 1346, the Tatar force attacking Kaffa (now Feodossia, Ukraine) was struck by a plague epidemic.[8] To take advantage of this development, the Tatars catapulted the corpses of their plague victims into Kaffa. Although an outbreak of plague did occur in the city, whether the disease was a result of the Tatars' action is unclear.

Smallpox first was used as a biologic weapon during the French and Indian War of 1754 to 1767.[8] Apparently, British troops deliberately infected Native Americans with smallpox by giving them blankets from infected patients.

A secret branch of the Japanese army, Unit 731, reportedly caused outbreaks of plague by dropping plague-infected fleas over populated areas of China in World War II.[23] Bomb experiments of weaponized anthrax spores were conducted by the Allies on uninhabited Gruinard Island near the coast of Scotland and resulted in heavy contamination in 1942.[38] Viable anthrax spores persisted until the island was decontaminated with formaldehyde and seawater in 1986.

In response to a perceived German biologic warfare threat, the United States began research into the offensive use of biologic agents in 1943 at Camp Detrick (renamed Fort Detrick in 1956) in Frederick, Maryland.[16] President Nixon stopped all offensive biologic and toxin weapon research and production by executive order in 1969. Included among the agents destroyed as a result of this action were *B. anthracis,* botulinum toxin, *Francisella tularensis, Coxiella burnetii,* Venezuelan equine encephalitis virus, *Brucella suis,* and staphylococcal enterotoxin B. Begun in 1953, the U.S. defensive program at Fort Detrick continues today as the U.S. Army Medical Research Institute of Infectious Diseases (USAMRIID).

The Biological and Toxin Weapons Convention was ratified in 1972 and went into effect in 1975.[44] It prohibits the development, production, stockpiling, or transfer of biologic weapons agents (microbial pathogens and toxins) for other than peaceful purposes and any devices used to deliver these agents. One hundred forty-three states are parties to the convention, with an additional 18 signatories. Unfortunately, the treaty was not accompanied by effective provisions for verification.

Although the Soviet Union signed the convention at its inception in 1972, it formed and funded an organization known most recently as Biopreparat (Chief Directorate for Biological Preparations) 2 years later.[13] This organization was designed to carry out offensive biologic weapons research, development, and production concealed behind legal and civil biotechnology research. Its capacity for production of biologic weapons included plague, tularemia, glanders, brucellosis, anthrax, smallpox, and Venezuelan equine encephalomyelitis.[1]

An incident at a military microbiology facility in Sverdlovsk (now Yekaterinburg) in the former Soviet Union in 1979 proved to be a grim warning of the dangers of biologic weapons science.[34] An accidental aerosolized release of anthrax spores resulted in at least 79 cases of anthrax, including 68 deaths. This largest reported outbreak of inhalational anthrax occurred in people living or working within a 4-km zone downwind of the facility.

Iraq's biologic warfare program commenced in earnest in 1985 after initial explorations in the late 1970s.[46] By the end of the Persian Gulf War in 1991, Iraqi scientists had investigated the biologic warfare potential of five bacterial strains, one fungal strain, five viruses, and four toxins. The United Nations Special Commission suspects that from 1991 to 1995, Iraq actively preserved biologic weapons capability, including botulinum toxin, anthrax, and *Clostridium perfringens* spores.[13]

The Japanese cult Aum Shinrikyo made several unsuccessful attempts at disseminating anthrax from rooftops and trucks in central Tokyo in the early 1990s before successfully releasing sarin nerve gas into Tokyo's subways and killing a dozen people in 1995.[45] A large community outbreak of salmonellosis was caused by the intentional contamination of restaurant salad bars for political reasons by members of a religious commune in The Dalles, Oregon, in 1984.[42]

Epidemiology

Potential biologic weapons share several characteristics. Ease of acquisition and production is a primary consideration. Other ideal properties include the potential to be aerosolized (particle size, 1 to 10 μm) and dispersed over a wide geographic area, as well as resistance to sunlight, desiccation, and heat. The potential to cause lethal or debilitating disease and person-to-person transmission are important features, as is lack of effective therapy or prophylaxis.[19, 20, 33]

Any small or large outbreak of disease merits evaluation as a potential biologic event.[35] Unusually high rates of disease, as well as unusual clinical syndromes, should signal a warning (e.g., a cluster of life-threatening pneumonia cases in previously healthy adults). Once definition of the cause and rate of attack has been determined, an epidemic curve based on the number of cases during a specific time can be calculated. The epidemic curve in a biologic event triggered by a point-source exposure most likely would be compressed, with a peak in a matter of hours or days. A second curve peak would be possible with contagious agents as a result of person-to-person transmission. The steep epidemic curve expected in a bioterrorism attack is similar to what would be seen with other point-source exposures such as food-borne outbreaks.

Several epidemiologic clues may be helpful in determining whether further investigation into an outbreak as a potential biologic attack is warranted. A large epidemic, especially in a discrete population, more severe disease than expected for a given pathogen, and a disease unusual for a given geographic area (e.g., pulmonic tularemia in an urban setting) are major indicators. Multiple simultaneous epidemics of different diseases, outbreaks with both human and zoonotic consequences, and unusual strains or susceptibility profiles are additional helpful parameters. Variable attack rates as a function of agent release relative to the interior or exterior of a building also would be useful.[35] Although most bioterrorism attacks will be covert,[4, 7] intelligence revealing plans for an attack, terrorist claims of deliberate release, or direct physical evidence of an attack obviously would point to a biologic event.

The emergence of mosquito-borne West Nile virus encephalitis in New York City in the summer of 1999 is an example of a naturally occurring outbreak that had elements of a potential bioterrorist attack.[4, 18, 40] This outbreak represented a disease occurring in an unusual (previously nonendemic) area, as well as one with zoonotic (birds) in addition to human consequences. It marked the first documented appearance of West Nile virus in the Western Hemisphere and the first arboviral outbreak in New York City since the yellow fever epidemics of the 19th century.[18] A large avian die-off, affecting primarily crows, preceded the outbreak in humans by at least several weeks.

Critical Biologic Agents

In addition to anthrax, critical biologic agents include brucellosis, plague, Q fever, and tularemia; smallpox, viral encephalitis, and viral hemorrhagic fever; and illnesses

TABLE 247–1 ■ CRITICAL BIOLOGIC AGENTS

Bacteria
Anthrax
Plague
Q fever
Tularemia
Brucellosis
Viruses
Smallpox
Viral encephalitis
Viral hemorrhagic fevers
Toxins
Botulinum toxin
Staphylococcal enterotoxin B

related to botulinum and staphylococcal enterotoxin B toxins[4, 28, 31] (Table 247–1). The five more credible biologic agents are discussed further.

ANTHRAX

B. anthracis is a large sporulatory, gram-positive rod with three distinct life cycles featuring multiplication of spores in soil, animal (herbivore) infection, and human infection.[29] Anthrax continues to occur in developing countries where the organism is highly endemic and the use of animal anthrax vaccine is not comprehensive (e.g., Iran, Iraq, Turkey, Pakistan, and sub-Saharan Africa). Human cases may be classified as either agricultural or industrial. Herders, butchers, and slaughterhouse workers in direct contact with infected animals are susceptible to agricultural infection, and workers in mills that process animal hair and those handling bone meal may acquire industrial infection.[36]

The three forms of human anthrax are cutaneous, inhalational, and gastrointestinal. The most common form is cutaneous, which is acquired through contact with an infected animal or animal products. The much less common inhalational form results from the deposition of spores in the lungs, and gastrointestinal anthrax occurs after the ingestion of infected meat. Because human-to-human transmission of anthrax has not been reported, standard precautions are recommended for hospitalized patients with all forms of anthrax infection.[24, 41]

In the United States, 224 cases of cutaneous anthrax were reported between 1944 and 1994.[24] Most cases in recent decades were a result of exposure to wool or animal hair.[36]

The clinical features and course of the first 10 confirmed cases of inhalational anthrax associated with bioterrorism in the United States in fall 2001 have been reported.[27] Epidemiologic investigation indicated that the outbreak was a result of intentional delivery of *B. anthracis* spores through mailed letters or packages. The median incubation period was 4 days and ranged from 4 to 6 days. Several clinical features of these patients were not emphasized in earlier reports of inhalational anthrax, a previously rare disease. Drenching sweating, nausea, and vomiting were common manifestations of the initial phase of illness in this outbreak. Pleural effusions were a remarkably consistent clinical feature. No predominant underlying diseases or conditions were noted.

None of the 10 patients had an initially normal chest radiograph. In addition to characteristic mediastinal widening (Fig. 247–1), paratracheal or hilar fullness, pleural effusions, and parenchymal infiltrates were noted. Computed tomography of the chest was more sensitive than chest radiography in revealing mediastinal lymphadenopathy, and

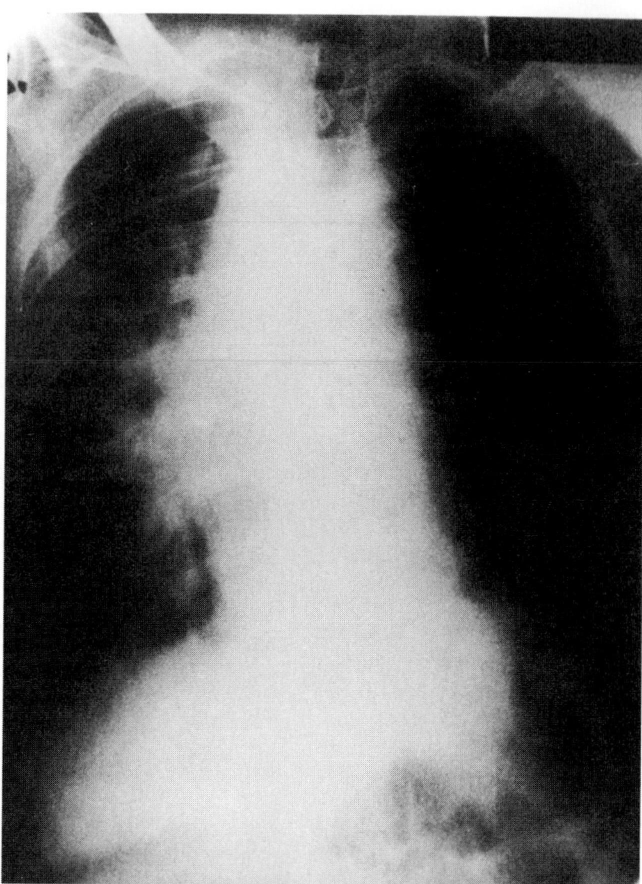

FIGURE 247–1 ■ Chest radiograph showing a widened mediastinum secondary to hemorrhagic mediastinitis in a patient with a fatal case of inhalation anthrax. (From LaForce, F. M., Bumford, F. H., Feeley, J. C., et al.: Epidemiologic study of a fatal case of inhalation anthrax. Arch. Environ. Health *18*:798–805, 1969. Reprinted with permission of Helen Dwight Reid Educational Foundation. Published by Heldref Publications, 1319 Eighteenth St., NW, Washington, DC 20036-1802. Copyright 2000.)

an elevation in the proportion of neutrophils or band forms represented an early diagnostic clue.

Inhalational anthrax previously was reported to be a biphasic illness with influenza-like symptoms such as fever, cough, malaise, fatigue, and chest discomfort in the first phase, followed briefly by 1 to 2 days of improvement before development of the acute phase 2 to 5 days later.[10] However, this brief period of improvement between the initial and fulminant phases of illness was not observed in the first intentional outbreak associated with mail.[27]

The 60 percent survival rate in this series was higher than previously reported (<15%). Limited data on treatment of survivors suggest that early treatment with a fluoroquinolone and at least one other active drug (e.g., rifampin, clindamycin, or vancomycin) may improve survival.[5, 27, 41]

Nasal congestion, rhinorrhea, and sore throat, infrequently seen in this series, might help distinguish influenza-like illness from inhalational anthrax.[12] Newer diagnostic methods for *B. anthracis* infection include polymerase chain reaction (PCR), immunohistochemistry, and sensitive serologic tests. Optimal management, including combination antimicrobial regimens, as well as adjunctive therapy such as immunoglobulin antitoxin and corticosteroids, remain to be defined.[5, 27, 41]

Cutaneous anthrax is characterized by a skin lesion evolving from a papule, through a vesicular stage, to a depressed black eschar, often surrounded by significant edema and erythema.[15, 39, 41] The lesion, which may mimic a spider bite, is usually painless and located on exposed parts of the body (i.e., face, neck, and arms). The incubation period ranges from 1 to 12 days but is commonly less than 7 days. Fatalities are rare (<1%) with effective antimicrobial therapy.

The organism grows readily on sheep blood agar and forms rough, gray-white colonies 4 to 5 mm in size with characteristic comma-shaped or "comet tail" protrusions.[29] *B. anthracis* is differentiated from other *Bacillus* spp. by an absence of the following: hemolysis, motility, growth on phenylethyl alcohol blood agar, gelatin hydrolysis, and salicin fermentation. Biosafety level 2 conditions for safe specimen processing in the microbiology laboratory and prompt confirmation of suspected isolates at the Centers for Disease Control and Prevention (CDC) or the USAMRIID in Fort Detrick are warranted.[24, 36]

Postexposure vaccination with an inactivated, cell-free anthrax vaccine may be indicated along with ciprofloxacin, doxycycline, or amoxicillin chemoprophylaxis after a proven biologic event.[41, 43] Pre-exposure vaccination may be indicated for the military and other select populations or for groups for which a calculable risk can be assessed.

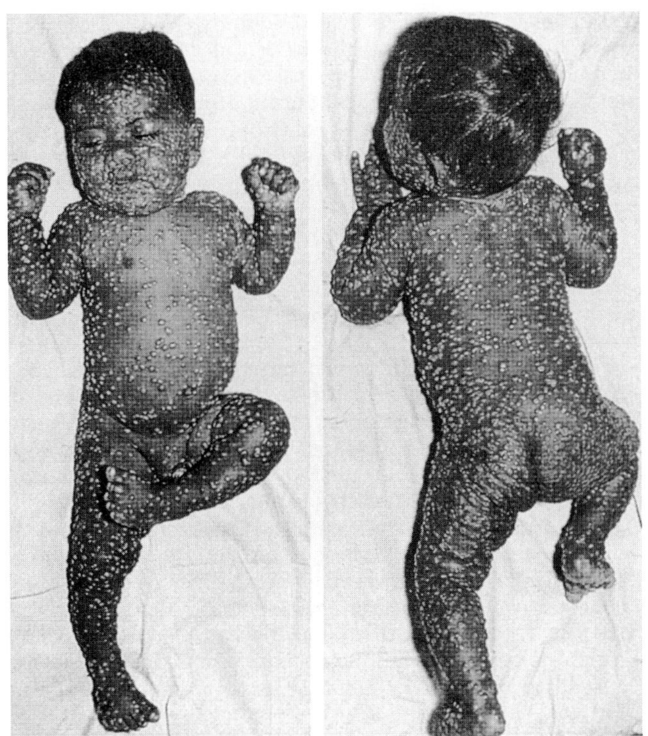

FIGURE 247–2 ■ The lesions of smallpox are at the same stage of development on each area of the body, are deeply embedded in the skin, and are more densely concentrated on the face and extremities. (From Henderson, D. A.: Smallpox: Clinical and epidemiologic features. Emerg. Infect. Dis. *5*:537–539, 1999.)

SMALLPOX

After a worldwide eradication program, the last known endemic case of smallpox occurred in Somalia in 1977, and the World Health Organization declared smallpox eradicated in 1980.[22] No animal reservoir exists. Current recognized stocks of variola virus are authorized only at the CDC in Atlanta and a Russian state laboratory in Koltsovo. However, it is speculated that additional variola isolates, either long held unreported or acquired through security breaches, also may exist. Because vaccination against smallpox ceased in the United States in 1972, virtually the entire population now would be considered susceptible because immunity wanes over time. Release of an aerosol would be the most likely route of transmission during an act of bioterrorism.

Smallpox is transmitted by respiratory secretions and requires close person-to-person contact. The incubation period is generally 12 to 14 days, with a range of 7 to 17 days. The prodromal illness of classic variola major features an acute onset of malaise, fever, rigors, vomiting, headache, and backache. Two to 3 days later, a discrete rash appears on the face, hands, forearms, and mucous membranes; it spreads to the legs and then centrally to the trunk during the second week of illness. Lesions progress from macules to papules to pustular vesicles during the course of 1 to 2 days. Umbilicate scabs form 8 to 14 days after onset and leave depressions and depigmented scars.[21]

In contrast to varicella (chickenpox), the rash of smallpox is centrifugal, with a concentration of lesions on the face and extremities, including the palms and soles, versus the trunk in varicella (Fig. 247–2). Smallpox lesions are also synchronous in stage of development, whereas the lesions of chickenpox appear in crops every few days, which results in lesions at very different stages of maturation in different areas of the skin. Any confirmed case of smallpox represents an international emergency and must be reported to national authorities through local and state health departments.[22]

Historically, the mortality associated with smallpox was 30 percent for unvaccinated contacts, and currently no antiviral therapy of proven efficacy has been developed. Supplies of vaccinia vaccine and vaccinia immune globulin are available only through the CDC.[22] Postexposure vaccination and strict quarantine are indicated for all household and other face-to-face contacts of suspected smallpox cases.[22]

In a limited outbreak with few cases, hospitalized patients should receive care in negative-pressure rooms with high-efficiency particulate air filtration. In addition, precautions using gloves, gowns, and masks are indicated. Home isolation and care are appropriate for most patients in larger outbreaks.[22]

PLAGUE

Plague, a zoonotic illness caused by the gram-negative bacillus *Yersinia pestis,* is primarily a disease of rodents, with transmission occurring through infected fleas. Human disease is acquired through rodent flea vectors, as well as respiratory droplets from animals to humans and humans to humans. Transmission of plague to humans in the United States primarily is via the bites of fleas from infected rodents. From 1970 to 1995, 341 cases of human plague were reported in the United States, most commonly from Arizona, California, Colorado, and New Mexico.[37] Indications of a deliberate release of plague bacilli would include the occurrence of cases in locations not known to have enzootic infection, in persons without known risk factors, and in the absence of previous rodent deaths.[23]

The three clinical forms of human plague are bubonic, primary septicemic, and pneumonic. Bubonic plague, characterized by the development of an acute regional lymphadenopathy, is the most frequent clinical form and accounts for 80 to 90 percent of U.S. cases.[37] However, the pneumonic form would be the most likely manifestation as a result of release of an aerosol during a biologic attack.[19, 23] This clinical form is the least common, but it has the highest mortality; it is almost always fatal if antibiotics are not begun within 24 hours of the onset of symptoms. Septicemic plague without obvious lymphadenopathy may be more difficult to diagnose than bubonic plague because of nonspecific manifestations (i.e., fever, chills, abdominal pain, nausea, vomiting, diarrhea, tachycardia, tachypnea, and hypotension).[23] Delay in diagnosis and appropriate therapy may lead to death.[23, 32]

The incubation period for primary pneumonic plague is 1 to 3 days. Fever, chills, headache, and rapidly progressive weakness are characteristic of all clinical forms of plague. Cough, dyspnea, and hemoptysis are distinctive of primary pneumonic plague. The sudden appearance of a large number of previously healthy patients with fever, cough, shortness of breath, chest pain, and a fulminant course leading to death should suggest the possibility of pneumonic plague or inhalational anthrax immediately. The presence of hemoptysis would strongly suggest plague.[3, 23]

Y. pestis may be identified in clinical specimens by Gram, Wright-Giemsa, Wayson, and immunofluorescence staining methods, in addition to standard bacterial culture. Appropriate clinical specimens include lymph node aspirates and blood, as well as tracheal washes or sputum smears if pneumonic plague is suspected. Tests that would be used to confirm a suspected diagnosis, including antigen detection, IgM enzyme immunoassay, and PCR assay, are available only through state health departments, the CDC, and military laboratories.[23]

Effective therapy is available in the form of streptomycin, gentamicin, chloramphenicol, doxycycline, and ciprofloxacin.[23] Parenteral aminoglycoside therapy is recommended in a contained casualty setting (modest number of patients requiring treatment); oral therapy is recommended in a mass casualty scenario.[23] The potential benefits of doxycycline and ciprofloxacin in the treatment of pneumonic plague infection in children substantially outweigh the risks.[7, 23] An inactivated, whole-cell *Y. pestis* vaccine was discontinued by its manufacturers in 1999 and is no longer available.[23]

In addition to standard precautions, droplet precautions are indicated for all patients with suspected plague until pneumonia is excluded and appropriate therapy has been initiated. Droplet precautions should be continued in patients with confirmed pneumonic plague for 48 hours after the initiation of appropriate therapy.[23] Only standard precautions are recommended for bubonic plague.

TULAREMIA

The etiologic agent of this zoonotic illness is *F. tularensis*, a gram-negative coccobacillus. The disease may be acquired from ticks and deer flies, contact with animals such as rabbits and rodents, ingestion of contaminated water, or inhalation of aerosols. In a bioterrorist event, inhalation of an aerosol would be the most likely route of infection.[3, 14] Human-to-human transmission of tularemia has never been reported. The annual incidence of tularemia in the United States is less than 200 cases; all suspected or confirmed cases must be reported to health authorities.

Clinical forms of the disease include ulceroglandular, glandular, oculoglandular, oropharyngeal, pneumonic, and typhoidal, the type reflecting the organism's portal of entry.[17, 26] Either pneumonic alone or typhoidal, with or without a pneumonic component, would be the most likely clinical manifestation of tularemia as a result of aerosol release during a biologic attack.[3, 14] The incubation period for tularemia is 3 to 6 days, with a range 1 to 21 days. Typhoidal tularemia may manifest as fever of unknown origin. Standard precautions are indicated for hospitalized patients with all forms of tularemia.[14]

The diagnosis is established most often by serologic testing, and isolation of *F. tularensis* from clinical specimens requires cysteine-enriched media or inoculation of laboratory mice. In addition to a need for special media, the laboratory should always be informed when tularemia is suspected because of the potential hazard to laboratory personnel. Suspected isolates should be confirmed by the CDC or USAMRIID through local or state health departments.[14]

Effective therapeutic agents include streptomycin, gentamicin, tetracycline, ciprofloxacin, and chloramphenicol; postexposure prophylaxis with doxycycline or ciprofloxacin may be considered.[14] The benefits of tetracycline or ciprofloxacin therapy may outweigh the risks for children younger than 8 years in select clinical situations, including tularemia.[14, 30] A live attenuated vaccine for pre-exposure use is available through the USAMRIID.[9]

BOTULISM

Seven distinct but related neurotoxins, A through G, are produced by different strains of *Clostridium botulinum*, an anaerobic gram-positive rod. The most common types in U.S. food-borne outbreaks are A, B, and E; outbreaks with unusual botulinum toxin types (i.e., C, D, F, and G, or E not acquired from an aquatic food) would suggest deliberate release.[2] Classic neuroparalytic disease is acquired through the ingestion of preformed neurotoxin. Other forms include localized infection (wound botulism) and *C. botulinum* intestinal colonization in infants with in vivo toxin production (infant botulism). Botulism in the United States is seen most often in small clusters or single cases associated with home-canned foods. Although airborne transmission of botulinum neurotoxin does not occur naturally, aerosolization of preformed toxin would be the most likely route of transmission in a bioterrorism event.[2, 19] Sabotage of food supplies is also possible. Botulism is not transmitted from human to human; standard precautions are recommended for hospitalized patients.

The incubation period for food-borne botulism is generally 12 to 36 hours (range, 6 hours to 8 days). The clinical manifestations of disease acquired by inhalation would be the same as those for food-borne botulism. Early manifestations include blurred vision, diplopia, and dry mouth.

Later clinical features indicative of more severe disease include dysphonia, dysarthria, dysphagia, ptosis, and symmetric, descending, progressive muscular weakness with respiratory failure.[2] Clinical suspicion is critical because a recognized source of exposure may be absent in a biologic attack. Botulism is a reportable disease.

A toxin neutralization bioassay in mice is used to identify botulinum toxin in serum, stool, or food. *C. botulinum* also may be cultured from stool and food. Electromyography can be helpful diagnostically. Botulinum antitoxin of equine origin, available from the CDC and state or municipal health departments, should be administered as soon as possible to patients symptomatic with botulism after testing for hypersensitivity to equine sera.[2, 16] A pentavalent toxoid of *C. botulinum* toxin types A, B, C, D, and E is available as a vaccine under investigational drug status through the CDC or Department of Defense.[2, 9]

Preparedness and Response

Being prepared for a bioterrorist attack or any other large-scale infectious disease outbreak relies on similar critical elements.[18, 25, 40] Clinician awareness and education are paramount. Because practicing physicians most likely will be the first group to encounter diseases caused by biologic weapons, they must be familiar with the signs and symptoms of the more credible biologic agents (e.g., smallpox and anthrax).[25] Recognition of an unusual case or cluster of illnesses should prompt a report to the local public health authorities.[6, 18] Improved communication between human and animal health authorities is warranted because many potential bioterrorist agents, such as anthrax, brucellosis, Q fever, plague, and tularemia, are zoonotic diseases.[18] Knowledge of the processes by which either the hospital laboratory, the local or state health department, or the CDC performs diagnostic studies to implicate or exclude biologic agents is also important.[4, 18, 25] Local, state, and federal public health agencies must coordinate plans for dealing with a large-scale outbreak caused by a biologic event.[4, 6, 18, 40] They should address rapid investigation of the outbreak, public education, mass distribution of antibiotics and vaccines, the capacity to care for mass casualties, and proper, expeditious treatment of the dead.[4, 18, 25, 40]

REFERENCES

1. Alibek, K.: Biohazard. New York, Random House, 1998, pp. 298–300.
2. Arnon, S. S., Schechter, R., Inglesby, T. V., et al.: Botulinum toxin as a biological weapon. Medical and public health management. J. A. M. A. *285*:1059–1070, 2001.
3. Bartlett, J. G., Dowell, S. F., Mandell, L. A., et al.: Practice guidelines for the management of community-acquired pneumonia in adults. Clin. Infect. Dis. *31*:347–382, 2000.
4. Biological and chemical terrorism: Strategic plan for preparedness and response. Recommendations of the CDC Strategic Planning Workshop. M. M. W. R. Recomm. Rep. *49*(RR-4):1–14, 2000.
5. Bush, L. M., Abrams, B. H., Beall, A., and Johnson, C. C.: Index case of fatal inhalational anthrax due to bioterrorism in the United States. N. Engl. J. Med. *345*:1607–1610, 2001.
6. Campbell, G. L., and Hughes, J. M.: Plague in India: A new warning from an old nemesis. Ann. Intern. Med. *122*:151–153, 1995.
7. Chemical-biological terrorism and its impact on children: A subject review. American Academy of Pediatrics. Committee on Environmental Health and Committee on Infectious Diseases. Pediatrics *105*:662–670, 2000.
8. Christopher, G. W., Cieslak, T. J., Pavlin, J. A., and Eitzen, E. M.: Biological warfare. A historical perspective. J. A. M. A. *278*:412–417, 1997.
9. Cieslak, T. J., Christopher, G. W., Kortepeter, M. G., et al.: Immunization against potential biological warfare agents. Clin. Infect. Dis. *30*:843–850, 2000.
10. Cieslak, T. J., and Eitzen, E. M.: Clinical and epidemiologic principles of anthrax. Emerg. Infect. Dis. *5*:552–555, 1999.
11. Cole, L. A.: The specter of biological weapons. Sci. Am. *275*:60–65, 1996.
12. Considerations for distinguishing influenza-like illness from inhalational anthrax. M. M. W. R. Morb. Mortal. Wkly. Rep. *50*(44):984–986, 2001.
13. Davis, C. J.: Nuclear blindness: An overview of the biological weapons programs of the former Soviet Union and Iraq. Emerg. Infect. Dis. *5*:509–512, 1999.
14. Dennis, D. T., Inglesby, T. V., Henderson, D. A., et al.: Tularemia as a biological weapon. Medical and public health management. J. A. M. A. *285*:2763–2773, 2001.
15. Dixon, T. C., Meselson, M., Guilliemin, J., and Hanna, P. C.: Anthrax. N. Engl. J. Med. *341*:815–826, 1999.
16. Eitzen, E., Pavlin, J., Cieslak, T., et al. (eds.): Medical Management of Biological Casualties. 3rd ed. Fort Detrick, MD, U.S. Army Medical Research Institute of Infectious Diseases, 1998.
17. Evans, M. E., Gregory, D. W., Schaffner, W., and McGee, Z. A.: Tularemia: A 30-year experience with 88 cases. Medicine (Baltimore) *64*:251–269, 1985.
18. Fine, A., and Layton, M.: Lessons from the West Nile viral encephalitis outbreak in New York City, 1999: Implications for bioterrorism preparedness. Clin. Infect. Dis. *32*:277–282, 2001.
19. Franz, D. R., Jahrling, P. B., Friedlander, A. M., et al.: Clinical recognition and management of patients exposed to biological warfare agents. J. A. M. A. *278*:399–411, 1997.
20. Henderson, D. A.: Bioterriorism as a public health threat. Emerg. Infect. Dis. *4*:488–492, 1998.
21. Henderson, D. A.: Smallpox: Clinical and epidemiologic features. Emerg. Infect. Dis. *5*:537–539, 1999.
22. Henderson, D. A., Inglesby, T. V., Bartlett, J. G., et al.: Smallpox as a biological weapon. Medical and public health management. J. A. M. A. *281*:2127–2137, 1999.
23. Inglesby, T. V., Dennis, D. T., Henderson, D. A., et al.: Plague as a biological weapon. Medical and public health management. J. A. M. A. *283*:2281–2290, 2000.
24. Inglesby, T. V., Henderson, D. A., Bartlett, J. G., et al.: Anthrax as a biological weapon. Medical and public health management. J. A. M. A. *281*:1735–1745, 1999.
25. Inglesby, T. V., O'Toole, T., and Henderson, D. A.: Preventing the use of biological weapons: Improving response should prevention fail. Clin. Infect. Dis. *30*:926–929, 2000.
26. Jacobs, R. F., and Narain, J. P.: Tularemia in children. Pediatr. Infect. Dis. *2*:487–491, 1983.
27. Jernigan, J. A., Stephens, D. S., Ashford, D. A., et al.: Bioterrorism-related inhalational anthrax: The first 10 cases reported in the United States. Emerg. Infect. Dis. *7*:933–944, 2001.
28. Kortepeter, M. G., and Parker, G. W.: Potential biological weapons threats. Emerg. Infect. Dis. *5*:523–527, 1999.
29. LaForce, F. M.: Anthrax. Clin. Infect. Dis. *19*:1009–1014, 1994.
30. Leggiadro, R. J.: Tetracycline for Rocky Mountain spotted fever. Pediatrics *87*:124–125, 1991.
31. Leggiadro, R. J.: The threat of biological terrorism: A public health and infection control reality. Infect. Control Hosp. Epidemiol. *21*:53–56, 2000.
32. Mann, J. M., Shandler, L., and Cushing, A. H.: Pediatric plague. Pediatrics *69*:762–767, 1982.
33. McDade, J. E., and Franz, D.: Bioterrorism as a public health threat. Emerg. Infect. Dis. *4*:493–494, 1998.
34. Meselson, M., Guillemin, J., Hugh-Jones, M., et al.: The Sverdlovsk anthrax outbreak of 1979. Science *266*:1202–1208, 1994.
35. Pavlin, J. A.: Epidemiology of bioterrorism. Emerg. Infect. Dis. *5*:528–530, 1999.
36. Pile, J. C., Malone, J. D., Eitzen, E. M., and Friedlander, A. M.: Anthrax as a potential biological warfare agent. Arch. Intern. Med. *158*:429–434, 1998.
37. Prevention of plague: Recommendations of the Advisory Committee on Immunization Practices (ACIP). M. M. W. R. Recomm. Rep. *45*(RR-14): 1–15, 1996.
38. Regis, E.: The Biology of Doom. The History of America's Secret Germ Warfare Project. New York, Henry Holt, 1999, pp. 27–31.
39. Roche, K. R., Chang, M. W., and Lazarus, H.: Cutaneous anthrax infection. N. Engl. J. Med. *345*:1611, 2001.
40. Schoch-Spana, M.: Implications of pandemic influenza for bioterrorism response. Clin. Infect. Dis. *31*:409–413, 2000.
41. Swartz, M. N.: Recognition and management of anthrax—an update. N. Engl. J. Med. *345*:1621–1626, 2001.
42. Torok, T. J., Tauxe, R. V., Wise, R. P., et al.: A large community outbreak of salmonellosis caused by intentional contamination of restaurant salad bars. J. A. M. A. *278*:389–395, 1997.
43. Use of anthrax vaccine in the United States. M. M. W. R. Recomm. Rep. *49*(RR-15):1–20, 2000.
44. Wheelis, M.: Investigating disease outbreaks under a protocol to the biological and toxin weapons convention. Emerg. Infect. Dis. *6*:595–600, 2000.
45. WuDunn, S., Miller, J., and Broad, W. J.: How Japan germ terror alerted world. New York Times, May 26, 1998, pp. 1 and 6.
46. Zilinskas, R. A.: Iraq's biological weapons. J. A. M. A. *278*:418–424, 1997.

PART VII

Guides to the Diagnosis of Infection

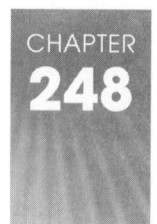

Use of the Bacteriology, Mycology, and Parasitology Laboratories

SHELDON L. KAPLAN ■ EDWARD O. MASON, JR.

An efficient and proficient bacteriology laboratory is of preeminent importance in the care of patients with infection. Well-trained personnel and a laboratory supervisor or director with expertise in microbiology, mycology, and serology are more important than expensive equipment and a large armamentarium of tests and services. The laboratory should strive continually to meet the needs of patients and physicians by producing prompt and accurate data. This goal requires cooperation and communication between the physician and laboratory personnel.

Specimen Collection

The physician, after evaluating the clinical and epidemiologic circumstances of a given infection, usually suspects various etiologic possibilities. Appropriate samples for culture should be obtained and submitted promptly to the laboratory along with relevant clinical and epidemiologic data.

Whenever possible, specimens should be obtained before the initiation of antibiotic therapy and directly from the site of infection, even if an invasive procedure, needle aspiration, or surgical drainage is required. Surface specimens obtained from the general area of a deep infection seldom are helpful. For example, isolates from the sinus tract may not reflect the primary etiologic agent of osteomyelitis or deep-seated abscesses.

When transport of specimens to the laboratory could be delayed, carrier media should be used. If unusual or fastidious microorganisms are suspected, the laboratory should be notified in advance so that appropriate materials or media can be made available for specimen collection (e.g., Thayer-Martin medium for gonococci or prereduced media for anaerobes).

The attending physician as well as the laboratory director must insist that specimens submitted to the laboratory be of sufficient quality and quantity for adequate evaluation. Sputum specimens that do not contain purulent material should not be processed. The time of collection of clean voided urine specimens should be recorded so that if their arrival at the laboratory is delayed unduly, repeat specimens can be requested. In most instances, stool specimens are preferable to rectal swabs for isolation of enteric pathogens. If purulent material is drained or aspirated, a volume of the material, rather than swab specimens, should be submitted. Surgical specimens should be submitted in sterile bottles without fixative. In some instances, the preferred procedure is for the attending physicians to obtain samples personally and transport them to the laboratory. If an unusual microorganism is suspected, the laboratory should be notified so that the specimen can be placed on appropriate media (e.g., cysteine nutrient agar for *Francisella tularensis*).

Specimen Inspection and Staining

Laboratory personnel should inspect specimens carefully before proceeding with culturing and staining. Sputum specimens must contain purulent material. Stool specimens should be inspected for gross evidence of blood, mucus, and pus. Body fluids should be examined for turbidity. Purulent material and exudates should be inspected for color, consistency, odor, and evidence of granules (e.g., sulfur granules).

GRAM STAIN: PROCEDURE AND INTERPRETATION

A Gram-stained smear is probably the single most important laboratory procedure in the diagnosis of infectious diseases. Virtually all clinical specimens should be Gram-stained as a routine part of the laboratory evaluation. This procedure serves three functions: it further documents the quality of the specimen, it alerts laboratory personnel to the presence of microorganisms that might require special media for isolation, and it provides the physician with clues about the etiologic agent so that initial antibiotic therapy can be selected intelligently.

The specimen is applied to a clean, glass microscope slide with a loop or swab and allowed to air-dry. It is then heat-fixed by passage once or twice through a burner flame. Overheating must be avoided because it causes morphologic distortion of bacteria and cellular elements and may induce crystallization of the dye, thereby obscuring interpretation. One or two extra slides should be prepared and saved to be available for staining if the initial procedure is inadequate technically.

A variety of Gram-staining methods have been described. An adequate procedure is as follows:

1. Air-dry and *lightly* heat-fix.
2. Flood the slide with crystal violet. Allow to stand 30 seconds.
3. Wash with tap water.
4. Flood the slide with iodine. Allow to stand 30 seconds.
5. Wash with tap water.
6. Destain with an acetone-alcohol mixture until dye ceases to run from the edge of a thin part of the specimen.
7. Wash with tap water.
8. Counterstain with safranin for 30 seconds.
9. Wash with tap water and blot dry.

Interpretation of a Gram-stained smear requires some skill and practice. When the procedure is performed properly, background material and cellular elements stain red or pink. If they stain blue or purple, the smear has not been decolorized adequately. If microorganisms that morphologically resemble staphylococci or streptococci stain red rather than dark blue, the smear probably has been overdecolorized. Bizarre morphologic forms may result from too much heat fixation, as well as from previous antibiotic therapy.

Interpretation of a Gram-stained smear includes noting the quantity and characteristics of cellular elements, estimating the overall number of microorganisms, and judging the predominant microorganism. Gram-positive bacteria are seen easily, and one must take care to search the background for gram-negative organisms, especially intracellular organisms. However, a Gram stain can be misinterpreted by inexperienced observers; a common error is to think that deposits of crystal violet are gram-positive cocci. False-positive results also may be obtained because of contaminating viable or nonviable microorganisms in the materials used for the procedure or in specimen tubes. Morphologic terms should be used to describe what is seen on the smear instead of attempting to arrive at species designations. Distinguishing among *Streptococcus* spp., between *Staphylococcus aureus* and *Staphylococcus epidermidis,* among *Neisseria* spp., and among various gram-negative enteric bacteria on a Gram-stained smear is impossible. If the initial smear reveals no bacteria, centrifuging the specimen and staining a thick smear of the sediment is helpful.

The Gram stain remains one of the most important techniques by which to rapidly identify a bacterial pathogen in a patient's specimen. Although the Gram stain does not provide definite proof that a particular microorganism is present, when the technique is performed and interpreted properly, the probable causative agent is demonstrated in many cases, particularly staining of cerebrospinal fluid (CSF) in children with bacterial meningitis. For instance, in *Streptococcus pneumoniae* meningitis, a Gram stain of CSF is reported as positive in as many as 90 percent of patients in most studies.[5, 83]

The greater the density of microorganisms in CSF ($>10^5$ colony-forming units [CFU]/mL), the more likely that the Gram stain is positive. Previous antimicrobial therapy may decrease the density of *Haemophilus influenzae* type b or *Neisseria meningitidis* in CSF and thus render the Gram stain negative.[45] In addition, gram-positive organisms have a tendency to appear gram-negative in selected cases in which antibiotics have been administered before lumbar puncture is performed.

Gram stain of urine can detect significant bacteriuria rapidly, with approximately 90 percent accuracy. Two or more gram-negative rods per high-power field of unspun urine are associated with quantitative urine cultures exceeding 10^5 CFU/mL.[48]

Typical morphologic features of *Campylobacter* (slender curved rods, "seagull" or "equivalent sign" appearance) may be observed in stool specimens by Gram or carbolfuchsin stain.[162] Gram stain of undiluted blood drawn back through a central catheter may permit a presumptive diagnosis of catheter-related sepsis.[113] These are just a few examples of how the Gram stain can provide valuable information inexpensively and rapidly.

ACRIDINE ORANGE STAIN

Acridine orange is a fluorochrome that stains the nucleic acids of bacteria, other microorganisms, and background material in clinical specimens, and this stain can be an important aid for rapidly discerning the presence of bacteria in specimens in low numbers. The stain is simple and rapid but requires the use of a fluorescent microscope. In practice, the specimen is scanned at low power, and the presence of brightly fluorescing bacteria is seen easily against the yellow to pale green appearance of human cells under a fluorescent microscope. The shape but not the Gram stain reaction then is confirmed at higher magnification. The procedure is especially useful when the specimen background is high, as often encountered with gram-negative bacteria in low numbers in thick exudates or in blood culture bottles. Furthermore, intracellular bacteria are detected more readily by acridine orange than by Gram stain. Kleiman and associates[91] noted that the acridine orange stain was superior to Gram stain in detecting bacteria in CSF, including specimens collected from children who had been receiving antibiotics. Acridine orange stain is especially valuable for examining clinical specimens that are negative by Gram stain, and it also has proved valuable in detecting bacteria in buffy coats in neonates with septicemia.[90] As with the Gram stain technique, experience in interpretation of the acridine orange stain is required for an accurate result.

ACID-FAST STAIN: PROCEDURE AND INTERPRETATION

Acid-fast stains of sputum or CSF should be performed if pulmonary tuberculosis or tuberculous meningitis is suspected. Because the gastric contents and urine often are contaminated by saprophytic mycobacteria, acid-fast smears of these specimens are of little value. The procedure for the Ziehl-Neelsen acid-fast stain is as follows:

1. Cover the smear with filter paper and flood the slide with carbolfuchsin.
2. Steam (do not boil) the slide for 5 minutes, with more carbolfuchsin added as necessary.
3. Rinse the slide with a gentle stream of tap water.
4. Decolorize with acid alcohol until no more color appears in the washings; rinse with tap water.
5. Counterstain with aqueous methylene blue for 30 seconds, rinse with tap water, and air-dry.

Mycobacterium and *Nocardia* spp. stain red, whereas other organisms and background material stain blue. *Mycobacterium* spp. sometimes have a beaded appearance, and *Nocardia* spp. often stain unevenly.[11] For *Nocardia,* destaining with acid alcohol should *not* exceed 5 to 10 seconds; as an alternative, 2 percent sulfuric acid can be used in place of acid alcohol and allowed to stand on the smear for 1 minute. The laboratory always should be informed of any suspicion of *Nocardia* infection when stains are requested, and the physician should be assured that the proper destaining procedure was used if the acid-fast stain is reported as negative and the clinical picture indicates *Nocardia* infection.

Many laboratories use fluorescence microscopy with auramine-rhodamine stain for the detection of *Mycobacterium* spp. in clinical specimens because of the ease and speed of performing the technique.

MICROSCOPIC EXAMINATION FOR FUNGI

Unfixed specimens of pus, sputum, or tissue scrapings may be examined as a wet mount in a drop of 10 percent potassium hydroxide. This procedure cleans the specimen, with the more resistant fungal structures left intact. Caution is necessary to avoid confusing artifacts with fungi; however, the procedure may give the physician rapid presumptive information.

Specimens from suspected fungal infections also should be fixed and stained with procedures that distinguish fungi specifically. The hematoxylin and eosin stain is not suitable as a fungal stain, although careful examination may demonstrate hyphal elements in tissues. More suitable fungal stains are the periodic acid–Schiff stain and the Gomori methenamine silver stain. The former stains fungal elements purple-red; the latter stains them black. One or both should be requested when fungal disease is suspected.

Calcofluor white specifically binds to chitin or cellulose and is brightly fluorescent when viewed by ultraviolet light, which renders the stain useful for detecting fungi in tissues and wet-mount specimens.[65] It can be used with 10 percent potassium hydroxide to view yeasts and hyphal elements in skin scrapings or on specimens previously stained by the periodic acid–Schiff or methenamine silver techniques if those stains require confirmation.

Countercurrent Immunoelectrophoresis

Countercurrent immunoelectrophoresis demonstrates bacterial antigens most successfully in the rapid detection of capsular polysaccharides of *H. influenzae* type b, *S. pneumoniae, N. meningitidis,* and group B *Streptococcus.* Countercurrent immunoelectrophoresis is predicated on the principle that when placed in agar of correct pH and ionic strength, polysaccharide antigens are charged negatively and antibodies are charged less negatively. When an electric current is passed through the agar, the antigen migrates toward the anode and the antibody diffuses to the cathode by endosmosis (carried along by buffer ions). If an antibody is directed against an antigen, a line of precipitation forms between the antibody- and antigen-containing wells. This technique has been replaced by latex agglutination in most laboratories.

Latex Agglutination

Latex agglutination is easier and faster to perform and is a more sensitive technique for detecting antigens from many microorganisms than countercurrent immunoelectrophoresis is. Numerous latex agglutination kits are available commercially, either in a combination form or for individual antigens. Antiserum to specific antigen is adsorbed onto latex particles of uniform diameter, usually 0.8 μm. After washing, the coated latex particles are resuspended to a proper dilution. Control latex particles are prepared similarly but with control sera. When the antigen to which the antiserum is directed is added to the latex particles, visible agglutination of latex particles occurs. Control latex particles should not agglutinate. Both positive and negative control specimens should be included with each patient specimen. Sera containing rheumatoid factor are associated with false-positive latex agglutination test results. The optimal fluid for latex agglutination testing is CSF because nonspecific agglutination of latex particles rarely occurs with CSF. However, urine and sera have been associated with nonspecific agglutination, as noted by agglutination of the control latex particles, which prevents interpretation of the test. In addition, agglutination of more than one type of antiserum may occur and also results in an uninterpretable test. Heating and diluting sera and urine avoid some of these nonspecific reactions, and manufacturers of commercial latex agglutination kits recommend various means by which to avoid having nonspecific reactions with their products.

Latex agglutination has been found to be a sensitive method by which to detect *H. influenzae* type b, *S. pneumoniae, N. meningitidis,* group B *Streptococcus,* and *Cryptococcus neoformans* in CSF.[8] Latex particles coated with either murine monoclonal antibody or rabbit antisera to *N. meningitidis* group B are available commercially, but results obtained with the group B serotype are not satisfactory. In almost all comparative studies, latex agglutination is superior to countercurrent immunoelectrophoresis for detecting the capsular polysaccharide antigen of the three major meningeal pathogens in CSF. The sensitivity of latex agglutination for purified group B streptococcal polysaccharide is 63 ng/mL, as compared with 500 ng/mL for countercurrent immunoelectrophoresis.[7]

Latex agglutination tests for *Clostridium difficile,* which actually detect glutamate dehydrogenase produced by toxigenic and nontoxigenic *C. difficile,* are not sufficiently sensitive to be used alone.[136]

Coagglutination of *Staphylococcus aureus*

The Cowan strain of *S. aureus* contains protein A in its outer membrane, which binds the Fc portion of IgG, thus leaving the Fab fragment free to bind with antigen. In the presence of homologous antigen, antibody-coated *S. aureus* visibly agglutinates. *S. aureus* protein A coagglutination requires the same controls as latex agglutination does, namely, *S. aureus* coated with normal sera from the same animal used to develop specific antisera to serve as a control suspension, as well as positive and negative control specimens. As with latex agglutination, coagglutination has been evaluated mainly for detecting antigen in CSF for the major pathogens causing bacterial meningitis in children.[192] Nonspecific agglutination with uninterpretable test results also occurs with the coagglutination test.

Diagnosis of Meningitis

In general, latex agglutination is more sensitive than countercurrent immunoelectrophoresis for detection of the three major meningeal pathogens in CSF. Detection of the capsular polysaccharide of *H. influenzae* type b in CSF is more reliable than for *N. meningitidis* or *S. pneumoniae.*[27, 34, 78, 83, 126, 183] Urine may remain positive for several days after the initiation of large-dose antibiotics, thus allowing identification of a causative agent, even when all cultures are negative. Urine is the best antigen source for bacteremic non-meningitis infections such as pneumonia or for cellulitis caused by *H. influenzae* type b.[28] However, *H. influenzae* type b capsular polysaccharide can be detected in urine by latex agglutination for several days after immunization with certain *H. influenzae* type b protein-conjugate vaccines.[106, 169] Thus, a history of recent *H. influenzae* type b immunization should be sought to exclude this possibility. Because high densities of bacteremia may develop in children with anatomic or functional asplenia during overwhelming sepsis, these immunologic techniques may detect antigen in sera from such patients.

The routine use of rapid antigen-detection techniques for examining the CSF of children with suspected bacterial meningitis is not warranted, although in selected circumstances such tests can be useful.[110] With the decline in bacterial meningitis caused by *H. influenzae* type b in developed countries, false-positive results may outnumber true-positive results and lead to unnecessary hospitalization and treatment.[135] If a child with bacterial meningitis has been treated with an oral or parenteral agent before undergoing lumbar puncture, Gram stain and culture of CSF may be negative for the causative pathogen in some patients. In children who are severely ill and too unstable for lumbar puncture, several days of parenteral antibiotics is likely to render the CSF sterile on culture. In such cases, antigen detection can be helpful. However, in the vast majority of children with suspected bacterial meningitis, the initial antibiotic therapy is not influenced or changed as a result of an antigen-detection test. The presence or quantity of antigen in the sera or CSF of patients with bacterial meningitis correlates with the severity of illness and the prognosis.[7, 63, 83, 84, 196]

In patients with cryptococcal meningitis, the titer of cryptococcal antigen by latex agglutination in CSF or serum may provide prognostic information. Diamond and Bennett[33] found that patients who died with active disease during therapy had significantly higher titers ($p < .001$) of cryptococcal antigen in CSF and serum than did patients who were cured. Furthermore, a high antigen titer in CSF at the beginning of therapy, as well as failure of a positive antigen titer to decrease or turn negative, was correlated with treatment failure. Similarly, Bennett and associates,[13] in a large, collaborative study, noted that the geometric mean cryptococcal antigen titer in CSF was higher in unsuccessfully treated patients than in improved or cured patients at the beginning of therapy (1:676 versus 1:95; $p < .01$) and at the completion of treatment (1:137 versus 1:12; $p < .02$).

Enzyme Immunoassays

Enzyme immunoassays have been developed for the detection of a wide variety of microbial antigens in clinical material. Advantages of enzyme immunoassay include a sensitivity with in vitro standards that is superior to that of other immunologic techniques (however, it may not translate into superior performance with clinical specimens), the use of diluted reagents that are relatively cheap (expensive equipment and radioactive material are unnecessary), and the ability to be automated.

Most types of enzyme-linked immunosorbent assays (ELISAs) are the direct or indirect variety and are based on the fact that when an antibody and enzyme are linked covalently, their respective immunologic and enzymatic activities are retained. ELISA takes advantage of the ability of a single enzyme molecule to catalyze the alteration of many molecules of substrate, which can intensify an antibody-antigen reaction.[202] Antibody to a specific antigen is bound to a solid phase, such as a polyvinyl microtitration plate or plastic bead, usually by absorption. Unbound antibody is removed, and the solid phase either can be used immediately or can be stored until needed. The clinical specimen containing the microbial antigen is placed in the well and incubated for a variable period, during which antigen is bound to the solid-phase antibody. The wells are washed, and in the direct ELISA, an enzyme-labeled antibody to the same antigen is applied. With the indirect method, unlabeled antibody from an animal species different from the solid-phase antibody is used. Then, enzyme-linked antibody directed against the globulin of the second antibody is applied. The plates are washed, and the substrate for the enzyme is added. The substrate is catalyzed by the linked enzymes, and the rate of reaction, usually monitored by a color change, depends on the amount of enzyme-labeled antibody, which is related directly to the quantity of antigen in the clinical specimen. The change in color can be read visually or quantitated with a spectrophotometer. The indirect technique avoids the need for having a separate enzyme-linked antibody for each antigen and is somewhat more sensitive than the direct method, but it adds another step to the procedure. Alkaline phosphatase and horseradish peroxidase are just two of the enzymes that are suitable for ELISA. Membrane-bound antigen capture simplifies these techniques and can be performed in minutes in a self-contained disposable device.

Selected antigens for which ELISA has been described are outlined in Table 248–1. Perhaps the ELISA technique has its greatest application for the rapid detection of viral infections. Enzyme immunoassays for bacterial detection are available commercially for *Neisseria gonorrhoeae, Chlamydia trachomatis,* group A *Streptococcus, Cryptosporidium,* and *Aspergillus* (galactomannan assay).

TABLE 248–1 ■ SELECTED MICROBIAL ANTIGENS DETECTABLE BY ENZYME IMMUNOASSAY

Bacteria
Haemophilus influenzae type b[29]
Streptococcus pneumoniae[63, 69, 165]
Neisseria meningitidis type A[165]
Neisseria gonorrhoeae[131,137,170]
Group A *Streptococcus*[35,36]
Group B *Streptococcus*[114,142,166]
Helicobacter pylori[112,168]
Legionella pneumophila[86]
Leptospira interrogans[155]
Mycobacterium tuberculosis[154,190]
Staphylococcus aureus[97]
Chlamydia trachomatis[105]
Vibrio cholerae 01[70]
Clostridium difficile[58]
Mycoplasma pneumoniae[108]
Escherichia coli O157[37]
Fungi
Candida albicans[4, 98,128,163]
Aspergillus fumigatus[104,153]
Coccidioides immitis[187]
Histoplasma capsulatum[203]
Parasites
Giardia lamblia[150,159]
Taenia solium[44]
Cryptosporidium parvum[149]
Entamoeba histolytica[199]

Immunofluorescence

Immunofluorescent techniques have been used for several years for the rapid detection of viral and bacterial infections. This procedure requires high-quality antisera, fluorescein conjugates, a fluorescent microscope, and most important, an experienced microscopist for reliable and reproducible results to be achieved. The immunofluorescence procedure is not well suited for large volumes of specimens but has been used successfully in both clinical and research laboratories for the rapid diagnosis of selected bacterial pathogens.

Bordetella pertussis infection can be diagnosed tentatively by immunofluorescence procedures rapidly on nasopharyngeal swabs.[107] However, as with any immunofluorescence technique, the source of antibody and the experience of the observer greatly influence the reliability of the results. In many instances, the immunofluorescence test result is positive but cultures are negative for *B. pertussis* in children with suspected whooping cough. Unfortunately, *B. pertussis* may be difficult to isolate, even when a nasopharyngeal swab is streaked immediately on appropriate media at the patient's bedside.

Fluorescent antibody stains of sputum, pleural fluid, or lung tissue for *Legionella pneumophila* or skin biopsy material for *Rickettsia rickettsii* have been applied successfully to the diagnosis of these infections in children.[21, 47] Immunofluorescent stains have been developed for the rapid identification of *Pneumocystis carinii,*[181] *Escherichia coli* O157:H7,[132] *Shigella dysenteriae,*[2] and *Giardia lamblia.*

DNA Hybridization

DNA technology has been applied to the rapid identification of numerous different microorganisms and involves the detection of specific segments of microbial DNA in clinical specimens.[133, 152] This technique is based on homologous DNA-DNA binding, in which a single-stranded, cloned DNA probe generally is labeled with a labeled nucleotide. Biotin-labeled DNA probes or other non-radioactive labels avoid the use of radioactive material. Clinical specimens are treated to free nucleic acids and then placed on nitrocellulose paper and allowed to dry (dot blot). The nitrocellulose paper is incubated with the labeled probe DNA for hybridization. The paper is subjected to autoradiography to expose radiographic film for radiolabeled probes or other detector systems, depending on the label used. DNA probes are available for *N. gonorrhoeae,*[26] *C. trachomatis,*[31] *L. pneumophila,*[133] *Mycoplasma pneumoniae,*[71] and *Mycobacterium tuberculosis.*[40] *Listeria monocytogenes* also has been detected with DNA probes.[30]

Polymerase Chain Reaction

Amplifying sequences of target DNA for detecting the presence of specific microorganisms is an incredibly powerful and sensitive tool.[41, 141, 160] The techniques are well established, and the reagents and instrumentation are widely available. The one major requirement for polymerase chain reaction (PCR) is specific oligonucleotides to act as primers for amplification of the DNA. Synthesis of these oligonucleotides requires detection of a well-characterized region of the genetic sequence of the microorganism. Oligonucleotides from a wide variety of microorganisms have been synthesized, and new applications are being introduced with extraordinary speed (Table 248–2). Virtually any organism can be detected by PCR techniques. Because the technique is so sensitive, any slight contamination may lead to false-positive results. Thus, great care must be taken during the procedure so that foreign DNA is not introduced into the assay. PCR is being applied routinely in many clinical microbiology laboratories. It is becoming the gold standard by which infections with *B. pertussis* or *N. meningitidis* are documented.[182]

TABLE 248–2 ■ DETECTION OF PATHOGENS BY POLYMERASE CHAIN REACTION

Bartonella henselae[61]
Bordetella pertussis[99]
Borrelia burgdorferi[148]
Chlamydia trachomatis[122]
Enteroinvasive *Escherichia coli*[50]
Helicobacter pylori[168]
Legionella pneumophila[171]
Leptospira species[10]
Mycobacterium leprae[197]
Mycobacterium tuberculosis[39]
Mycoplasma pneumoniae[16]
Neisseria meningitidis[123]
Pneumocystis carinii[25]
Rickettsia rickettsii[185]
Shigella[50]
Streptococcus pneumoniae[152]
Toxoplasma gondii[24]
Treponema pallidum[64]
Trypanosoma cruzi[115]

Identification-Speciation

Most diagnostic bacteriology laboratories now use one of the multitest systems for microbial identification, which by a variety of methods, correctly and consistently allow rapid identification to the genus and species level. Smaller laboratories that do not or cannot provide this information routinely should have arrangements with a qualified reference laboratory capable of identification to this level. More specific identification, such as serotyping, chromosomal restriction enzyme analysis, or other molecular techniques, is seldom necessary for treatment of an individual patient but may be important for hospital epidemiology.[179] Thus, a system whereby isolates from significant infections, or isolates with unexpected susceptibility patterns, are retained for a reasonable amount of time in the event that further identification is required would seem to be a prudent practice.

Individual laboratories define significant isolates that they routinely report from nonsterile sites differently, depending on agreements reached between the laboratory director and the medical staff. In general, only group A streptococci are reported from throat cultures. If infection caused by *Corynebacterium diphtheriae* or *B. pertussis* is suspected, the physician must notify the laboratory so that appropriate culture media and identification techniques can be used. Other similar potential sources of confusion exist and can be averted consistently through communication with the laboratory.

Bacterial taxonomy is changing continually to reflect advances in technology that allow more precise definition of the relationships between genera and species of bacteria.[175] The reader should be familiar with sources that constantly update bacterial names, such as the website List of Bacterial Names with Standing in Nomenclature, *http://www.bacterio.cict.fr/.*

Selected Organisms or Infections

BACTERIA

Neisseria gonorrhoeae

Gram stain of a urethral discharge in a male with urethritis is highly specific (>90%) and sensitive (96–98%) for the diagnosis of *N. gonorrhoeae* infection. In females and asymptomatic males, the usefulness of Gram stain is not as great. A commercially produced enzyme immunoassay for detecting *N. gonorrhoeae* antigen (Gonozyme, Abbott Laboratories, Abbott Park, IL) can be performed in 2 hours, and urethral or endocervical specimens can be stored for as long as 30 days without affecting the results.[131, 170] Antigen can be detected in the face of negative culture results because of previous or concurrent administration of antibiotics. Stamm and associates[170] found the Gonozyme test to be 94 percent sensitive and 98 percent specific in comparison to culture results in men, but it was no better than Gram stain in diagnosing gonorrhea. On the other hand, in women, the enzyme immunoassay was 78 percent sensitive and 98 percent specific in comparison to cervical culture, but it had significantly better sensitivity than cervical Gram stain did (78% versus 40%, $p < .001$).

Detection of *N. gonorrhoeae* by DNA probe has been reported by several groups.[26] A probe assay that is commercially available has a sensitivity exceeding 90 percent, which culture does not. Positive predictive values also approach 90 percent. Nucleic amplification tests are available to detect *N. gonorrhoeae* and *C. trachomatis* simultaneously in endocervical, urine, and vaginal specimens.[23] DNA applications may be particularly valuable in detecting pharyngeal infection by *N. gonorrhoeae.*[129]

Group A Beta-Hemolytic *Streptococcus*

Throat culture is the time-honored manner by which to confirm group A streptococcal pharyngitis, despite the variables that may affect culture results.[87] Cultures require 36 to 48 hours for final identification, and the clinician frequently feels obligated to administer antibiotics before knowing the culture results. Techniques for the rapid identification of group A *Streptococcus* in the throat involve nitrous acid extraction of throat swabs followed by incubation of the extracted fluid with the test reagents. Tests that use latex agglutination and enzyme immunoassay technology are available. A commercially produced chemiluminescent DNA probe for group A *Streptococcus* is also available.[72] Many different rapid streptococcal antigen tests that have been compared with blood agar culture of throat swabs are available.[35, 53–55] In general, the sensitivity of the rapid tests varies between 70 and 90 percent in comparison to blood agar cultures. The specificity of the tests is excellent. Thus, for any of the tests, a positive result is a reliable indicator of group A streptococcal pharyngitis. However, which test to use in the office or laboratory setting is an individual decision based on personal experience, cost, and the need for other equipment, as well as the sensitivity and specificity of the technique. The accuracy of the test results when the test is performed by properly trained nurses is equivalent to that of a laboratory technologist in a pediatric satellite laboratory setting.[36] In one study, an optical immunoassay for group A beta-hemolytic streptococcal pharyngitis was more sensitive than blood agar plate cultures when performed in pediatricians' offices.[56] Other studies have not confirmed these findings.[140] At the present time, a routine throat culture should be performed when the rapid test result is negative, no matter which rapid antigen test is used.

Group B *Streptococcus*

Latex agglutination tests for group B *Streptococcus* are most useful on the CSF of babies with suspected meningitis, but in most instances they do not influence selection of the initial empiric antibiotics.[38, 191] If the CSF culture is negative because the patient previously received parenteral therapy, antigen detection may be the only method by which an etiologic diagnosis can be established. The use of rapid antigen tests for detecting group B streptococci in urine is not recommended because of the high rate of false-positive results.[157] The use of group B streptococcal rapid antigen tests as a strategy for preventing early-onset group B streptococcal infection in neonates is not recommended by the American Academy of Pediatrics.[3] At some point, DNA-based PCR approaches for rapid real-time detection of group B streptococci in pregnant women may be useful for targeting chemoprophylaxis.[14]

Mycobacterium tuberculosis

The diagnosis of tuberculous meningitis in children frequently is based on typical CSF (pleocytosis, mononuclear predominance, depressed glucose concentrations) and clinical findings. In many instances, an acid-fast stain and culture of CSF are negative, or the culture does not become positive until many weeks after therapy has been initiated. A rapid method for detecting mycobacterial antigens in CSF could be extremely beneficial when one encounters a child in whom tuberculous meningitis is suspected. ELISA and other techniques used to detect mycobacterial antigen in CSF have not proved satisfactory. Adenosine deaminase activity may be increased in the CSF of patients with tuberculous meningitis, but it is not a specific test.

Numerous laboratories have described PCR assays for the diagnosis of tuberculosis from sputum specimens.[49, 124, 158] The sensitivity, specificity, and false-positive and false-negative rates are not known, and these tests are not approved yet for commercial diagnostic evaluation.[32] In pediatrics, the value of using PCR for detecting *M. tuberculosis* from gastric aspirates is unclear. Several laboratories using different PCR strategies and DNA sequences for probes have reported detection of *M. tuberculosis* products in CSF from patients with tuberculous meningitis.[95, 101] In one study, an in-house PCR was compared with Amplicor and conventional culture in 251 specimens (235 gastric aspirates, 16 bronchoalveolar lavage samples) from 88 children. When assessed with the final clinical diagnosis, the in-house PCR had a sensitivity of 60 percent and a specificity of 97 percent versus 44 percent and 94 percent for the Amplicor, respectively.[60] Some false-positive results were noted for both PCR tests. Commercial amplification tests have demonstrated sensitivities of 33 to 60 percent.[17, 94] This application would be a valuable addition to routine diagnostic studies for rapid diagnosis because only a minority of children with tuberculous meningitis have positive acid-fast bacterial stains of CSF. Currently, nucleic acid–based amplification tests are adjunctive measures for establishing the diagnosis of tuberculosis in children.

Urinary Tract Infections

Since the 1980s, automated methods have been available to detect bacteriuria more quickly and perhaps more cheaply than with the conventional agar plate culture technique.[138, 139] In several studies, urine specimens with 10^5 CFU/mL of a single pathogen could be identified within 5 hours. The negative predictive value for the automated urine screening methods is close to 100 percent for greater than 10^5 CFU/mL; however, the positive predictive value is only between 20 and 40 percent. Thus, a negative automated urine screen virtually eliminates the possibility of bacteriuria exceeding 10^5 CFU/mL. These automated techniques generally require expensive equipment and are practical only for screening large numbers of urine specimens.

Strips for indicating nitrites (product of bacterial metabolism) or leukocyte esterase are available for screening urine for infection.[184] Urine is screened best for nitrate on the first morning void. Leukocyte esterase strips may not be as sensitive in febrile children as in adult women. The presence of bacteria on Gram stain of uncentrifuged urine (any bacteria per oil immersion field) plus 10 or more white blood cells/mm^3 in urine obtained by catheter in febrile children younger than 2 years was found to be an excellent predictor of urine cultures containing 50,000 CFU/mL or greater.[75] In a meta-analysis of screening tests for urinary tract infections in children, Gorelick and Shaw[62] concluded that Gram stain and dipstick analysis for nitrite and leukocyte esterase are equivalent and superior to routine microscopic analysis for pyuria.

FUNGI

One of the most difficult and perplexing problems for the clinician is the decision of when to initiate therapy for fungal infections such as candidiasis or aspergillosis in an immunocompromised host.[172] Frequently, no clinical signs or laboratory evidence of disseminated fungal infection is present, and yet fungi are demonstrated throughout the body at necropsy. Even when cultures are positive for some of these ubiquitous fungi, their meaning is unclear. Positive cultures simply may represent surface colonization. Because making the diagnosis of fungal infection is so difficult, antifungal treatment is delayed commonly and, therefore, is frequently ineffective. Serologic techniques that demonstrate serum antibodies or precipitins to *Candida* or *Aspergillus* are not reliable and are difficult to interpret. Furthermore, the very patients in whom these tests would be most valuable may be unable to mount an antibody response because of immunosuppression.

Candida

As a result of problems with the rapid serodiagnosis of fungal infections, several investigators have developed methods to detect fungal antigens, such as *Candida* mannan.[79] *Candida* mannan has been detected by countercurrent immunoelectrophoresis,[88] enzyme immunoassay,[163] and latex agglutination[52] in the sera of patients with invasive candidiasis. Antibody to *Candida* antigens was produced in rabbits by the individual laboratories in each case. In general, these procedures are specific when positive but lack sensitivity (mannan was detected in the sera of 50 to 60% of patients with proven disseminated *Candida* infection). A commercially produced latex agglutination kit is available for detecting *Candida* antigens of unknown composition (Cand-Tec, Ramco Laboratories, Houston). Initial studies of this test appeared promising; however, subsequent evaluations have reported unacceptably low sensitivity and specificity for the diagnosis of invasive candidiasis.[6, 43, 51, 96, 120] No information exists on the value of the Cand-Tec test in children, and this test cannot be recommended for the rapid or early diagnosis of invasive candidiasis in immunocompromised children.[161]

Walsh and associates[189] described a double-sandwich liposomal immunoassay to detect circulating *Candida* enolase, a 48-kd cytoplasmic antigen. They used multiple serum samples and detected enolase in 11 of 13 cases of deep-tissue infection and in 7 of 11 cases of fungemia, all occurring in neutropenic cancer patients. The specificity of the test was 96 percent, but this test has never been pursued commercially. PCR technology for detecting *Candida* spp. has been applied by several groups, and the preliminary results are encouraging.[82] As expected, some *Candida* DNA may be detected in the serum of patients at risk for systemic candidiasis but with negative blood cultures. Whether they represent true-positive or false-positive results is yet to be determined.[188] PCR may be helpful in diagnosing *Candida* endophthalmitis.[74]

Cryptococcus neoformans

The latex agglutination test has been a valuable method for detecting and quantitating cryptococcal polysaccharide in CSF and sera. In comparative evaluations, certain commercial *Cryptococcus* latex agglutination kits were more reliable than others.[177, 201] When proper controls are included, latex agglutination for cryptococcal antigen is highly specific and sensitive (100%), although as with latex agglutination tests in general, rheumatoid factor and other interfering proteins may cause false-positive results. Pretreatment of specimens with pronase reduces false-negative rates and increases the cryptococcal antigen titer by eliminating proteins that interfere with the reaction.[66] Some experts warn that cryptococcal antigen titers of 1:8 or less in CSF should be interpreted cautiously.[76] Furthermore, false-negative results appear to occur more commonly in normal than in immunocompromised hosts with cryptococcal meningitis.[15] False-positive latex agglutination tests are rare (<0.3%) but have been reported as a result of contamination of CSF with surface condensation from agar (syneresis fluid).[18] India ink mount can detect *C. neoformans* in CSF rapidly and conveniently and is positive in approximately 60 percent of patients with cryptococcal meningitis. However, this technique requires experienced laboratory personnel to distinguish the cryptococcal organism from mononuclear white blood cells. Both the India ink preparation and the latex agglutination test may remain positive after the CSF is culture-negative and even subsequent to apparent cure of cryptococcal meningitis. A commercial enzyme immunoassay (EIA) is also available for detecting cryptococcal polysaccharide antigen.

Aspergillosis

Invasive aspergillosis is a fungal infection, predominantly of immunocompromised hosts, that has approximately an 80 percent mortality rate. As in systemic candidiasis, early diagnosis and treatment are mandatory if the outcome is to be favorable. Antibody determination for invasive aspergillosis is also unreliable in immunocompromised patients, and antigen-detection techniques hold the greatest promise for making a rapid early diagnosis. Initially, investigators used radioimmunoassay techniques to detect *Aspergillus fumigatus* antigen.[193] ELISA techniques have been the most sensitive to detect galactomannan antigen in the serum and urine of patients with invasive or disseminated aspergillosis.[164] In one study, this procedure was 95 percent specific and 95 percent sensitive for *Aspergillus* infections, although multiple specimens may be required and antisera directed against *A. fumigatus* may cross-react with *Aspergillus flavus*. Several groups have developed PCR techniques to detect *Aspergillus* spp. Specimens such as blood and bronchoalveolar lavage fluid that are PCR-positive have high specificity for invasive aspergillosis.[144, 145] In other studies, positive results were reported in patients whose respiratory tracts only probably were colonized.[104] Further studies are necessary to define the value of detecting *Aspergillus* by PCR.

Histoplasma capsulatum

Wheat and associates[195, 203] have developed radioimmunoassay and ELISA techniques for detecting the polysaccharide antigen of *H. capsulatum*. Antibody to *H. capsulatum* was produced by immunizing rabbits with formalinized live yeast cells. Antigen was detected in serum and urine (90% of patients tested) obtained from persons with disseminated histoplasmosis. When the test was evaluated in patients with acquired immunodeficiency syndrome (AIDS) and disseminated histoplasmosis, high levels of antigen were detected in the urine of 97 percent of patients and in the sera of 79 percent of patients.[194] Antigen levels decreased during and after antifungal therapy. Widespread availability of this test should lead to earlier diagnosis and perhaps superior monitoring of disseminated histoplasmosis, especially for patients with AIDS.

PARASITES

Pneumocystis carinii

The most reliable method by which to diagnose *P. carinii* pneumonitis is lung biopsy. Obviously, this invasive procedure should be considered cautiously in terms of its risk-to-benefit ratio when the physician is faced with an immunocompromised patient with interstitial pneumonitis.

A rapid method for the reliable detection of circulating antigen from *P. carinii* possibly could avoid the necessity for lung biopsy, but to date, such a method is not available.

Stains of induced sputum or fluid obtained by bronchoalveolar lavage may demonstrate *P. carinii* cysts in patients with AIDS and *P. carinii* pneumonia.[125] Immunofluorescent staining of these specimens with monoclonal antibodies enhances the detection of cysts when compared with Giemsa-like (Diff-Quick) or toluidine blue D stains.[93] Calcofluor white staining of respiratory specimens is quick but not as sensitive as the immunofluorescent stain.[174, 181] However, with the immunofluorescent stain, *P. carinii* cysts may be detected in asymptomatic patients with AIDS; thus, the laboratory and clinical findings must be considered together carefully.[122]

PCR can detect *P. carinii* in bronchoalveolar lavage fluid, induced sputum, and even blood.[100, 151] In one study, PCR was more sensitive than conventional staining techniques for induced sputum but was not superior to conventional stain for bronchoalveolar lavage fluid.[151] As with immunofluorescent staining, some asymptomatic carriage of *P. carinii* may be identified by PCR. *P. carinii* was detected by nested PCR in blood specimens, which might suggest disseminated infection. PCR of blood is especially of interest in a young infant with suspected *P. carinii* infection, in whom an induced sputum sample is difficult to obtain. However, *P. carinii* DNA was detected in necropsy lung samples from 13 of 75 (17%) children with non–*P. carinii* pneumonitis.[85] Thus, current PCR for *P. carinii* is less specific for true infection than conventional techniques are for diagnosis.

Chlamydia trachomatis

Bell and associates[12] found a direct fluorescent monoclonal antibody stain to be specific and sensitive for establishing the diagnosis of *C. trachomatis* conjunctivitis. Fluorescing elementary bodies were seen within epithelial cells, and the procedure required approximately an hour to complete. Positive immunofluorescent smears were found in specimens from all 21 infants who were culture-positive when inflamed eyes were examined. Other investigators have documented the excellent sensitivity and specificity of commercially available fluorescent monoclonal antibody stains for detecting *C. trachomatis* in conjunctival specimens obtained from infants with conjunctivitis.[146, 147] Paisley and associates[130] reported that this technique correlated well with culture results of nasopharyngeal secretions obtained from infants younger than 6 months with pneumonitis.

Enzyme immunoassays are also available for the rapid identification of *C. trachomatis* in conjunctival and nasopharyngeal specimens.[67, 68] For both enzyme immunoassay and fluorescent antibody tests, specimens that are rapid test–positive but culture-negative have been reported. However, these results do not seem to be false-positive findings but, rather, instances in which the rapid tests are more sensitive than the culture techniques. Care must be taken in the proper use of these commercially available laboratory tests. The tests appear to be good for respiratory specimens but lack specificity for chlamydial infection of the vagina in prepubertal girls and, thus, should not be used for the evaluation of sexual abuse.[143]

DNA amplification for detecting *C. trachomatis* in vaginal or urine specimens is well studied in adults, but few studies have been performed in children, particularly in the setting of suspected sexual assault. Urine testing by ligase chain reaction is attractive for young females because of the ease of collection, along with greater sensitivity than with conventional vaginal cultures by swab for *C. trachomatis*.[57]

Antibiotic Susceptibility Testing

Antibiotic susceptibility testing is an important function of the microbiology laboratory and should be performed on all bacteria isolated from serious infections. Instances in which the susceptibility of an isolate can be predicted accurately without susceptibility testing are, unfortunately, diminishing to the point that *Streptococcus pyogenes* and *Streptococcus agalactiae* remain predictably susceptible to penicillins and other β-lactam antibiotics.[178] This worldwide emergence of antibiotic resistance in previously susceptible bacteria is creating problems for physicians and the laboratory alike. Before 1979, reports of antibiotic-resistant *S. pneumoniae* were sporadic.[92] Subsequently, pneumococci resistant to penicillin, the third-generation cephalosporins, erythromycin, trimethoprim-sulfamethoxazole, and chloramphenicol have been reported increasingly and are associated with treatment failure with these agents.[20, 92, 109, 167] Delayed responses to penicillin therapy in patients with meningitis caused by *N. meningitidis* have been reported from Spain and the United States and linked to strains with modified penicillin-binding proteins.[22, 186, 200] Multiply antibiotic-resistant enterococci may be resistant to vancomycin, thus seriously diminishing the ability to treat nosocomial infections caused by these organisms.[116, 180] Methicillin resistance among community-acquired isolates of *S. aureus* is a major problem in many areas of the United States.[73] Thus, increasing antibiotic resistance renders the selection of empiric antibiotics more difficult, raises the cost of therapy, and forces the microbiology laboratory to test more bacteria with an increasing number of antibiotics in an effort to determine effective antibiotic therapy accurately.

Selection of one of the several methods available for susceptibility testing varies with such factors as the size of the hospital, the patient population, and the laboratory budget.[80, 156] The agar diffusion test, or the Kirby-Bauer test, is one of the oldest and most standardized methods of susceptibility testing and probably will remain a reliable primary as well as backup system for several reasons.[46, 156] It is cost-efficient; it is easy to perform, control, and interpret; and it allows customized selection of the antimicrobials tested to reflect physician preferences, the hospital formulary, and changing resistance patterns. The results of disk diffusion reported as susceptible, intermediate, and resistant are qualitative, but the interpretation of susceptibility and resistance is defined clearly by published guidelines and well understood by all physicians. The disk diffusion test allows the laboratory to optimally characterize macrolide and clindamycin susceptibility for *S. aureus*, especially methicillin-resistant isolates that are community acquired.[1] Isolates with complete zones of inhibition around the clindamycin disk that are resistant to erythromycin probably have an efflux mechanism of resistance for macrolides but remain susceptible to clindamycin. However, isolates demonstrating a flattening of the clindamycin zone in the area adjacent to the erythromycin disk have an inducible MLS_B mechanism of resistance and should be considered resistant to macrolides and clindamycin (Fig. 248–1).

Quantitative methods or broth dilution procedures (macro and micro) give more precise results in the form of a minimal inhibitory concentration (MIC), but they generally are needed only for difficult infections, such as meningitis, osteomyelitis, or endocarditis, and the results are interpreted best by physicians with infectious disease training (Fig. 248–2). Automated versions of the microbroth procedure are restricted further by an inability to specify antibiotics included in the commercial panels and a lack of clinically useful end-points applicable to all pathogens and

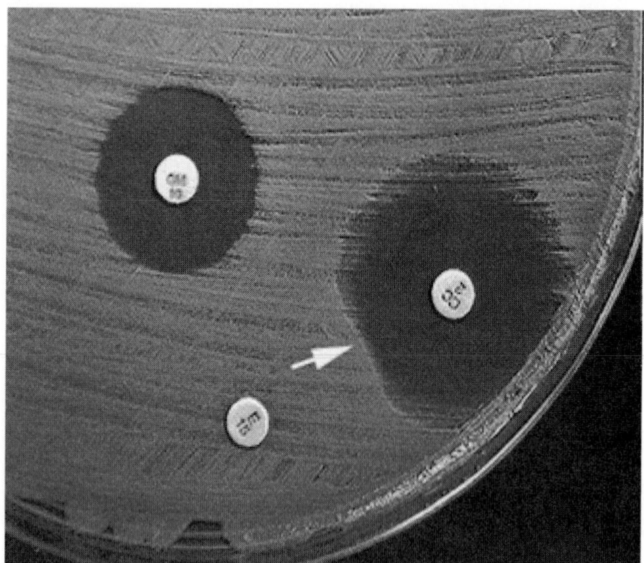

FIGURE 248–1 ■ "D-zone." A methicillin-resistant *Staphylococcus aureus* isolate demonstrating flattening of the clindamycin zone of inhibition around the clindamycin disk *(arrow)* in the area adjacent to the erythromycin disk. The isolate has inducible MLS_B phenotype resistance to clindamycin.

antibiotic–bacterial species combinations for which results can be unreliable.[46] All antibiotic susceptibility test results are influenced by a number of factors, including the growth media, cation content, inoculum concentration, antibiotic concentration, incubation time, and incubation temperature. Standardization of these factors is addressed for the disk diffusion and microbroth dilution procedures in methods recommended by the Subcommittee on Antimicrobial Susceptibility Testing of the National Committee for Clinical Laboratory Standards (NCCLS).[119] Proper performance of the procedure with an appropriate control strain of known susceptibility should be adhered to strictly for accurate reproducible results and is required by all laboratory-accrediting agencies.

Automated quantitative antibiotic susceptibility systems are widely available and affordable. Frequently, the cost-effectiveness of these systems is increased by combining identification and antibiotic susceptibility on the same test plate and by freeze-drying the contents of the plates, thus significantly increasing their shelf life. Instrument failure can occur, and thus backup systems are required for both identification and antibiotic susceptibility. In addition to the benefits of automation, these systems often provide same-day susceptibility results, which is claimed by some physicians to lead to more effective antibiotic management, although this matter remains controversial.[46] Major deficiencies of automated systems are a limitation of the numbers of antibiotics and concentration ranges of the antibiotics tested. Custom-prepared panels with specified concentrations of antibiotics are available but are more expensive. Additionally, automated systems often deliver erroneous results for nutritionally fastidious bacteria or those with difficult-to-detect resistance mechanisms, such as methicillin-resistant *S. aureus* and the newly emerging vancomycin-resistant strains of enterococci. Media supplements provided by the manufacturers to correct these deficiencies are often inadequate, and *S. aureus, S. pneumoniae, Enterococcus* spp., and *Haemophilus* spp. require manual systems for accurate testing.

E-TEST

The E-test (AB Biodisk, Solna, Sweden) is performed just as a disk diffusion test is, but by placing an antibiotic concentration gradient on a plastic strip, the resulting elliptical zone of inhibition is interpreted as a quantitative MIC (Fig. 248–3). The advantage is a quantitative result with a diffusion test that allows any antibiotic to be tested on media containing nutritional supplements, thereby permitting testing of fastidious as well as nonfastidious bacteria and anaerobes.[127] Studies have verified the accuracy of the procedure with most bacteria,[9] including *S. pneumoniae,*[102] *H. influenzae,*[81] and *N. meningitidis.*[59, 77] Although the E-test is relatively expensive, judicious selection of relevant antibiotics by the physician should allow this procedure to become a useful tool in antibiotic susceptibility testing.

Dilution Susceptibility—MIC and MBC

Minimal Inhibitory Concentration (MIC) = the smallest concentration of an antibiotic that inhibits visible growth of the patient's infecting bacteria after overnight incubation

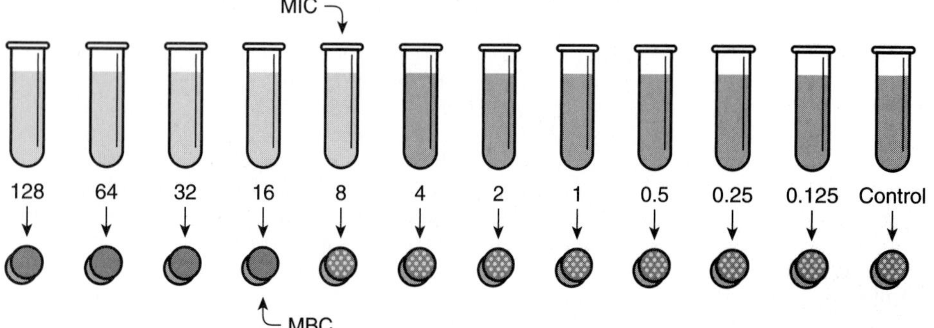

Minimum Bactericidal Concentration (MBC) = the smallest concentration of an antibiotic that kills 99.9% of the patient's infecting bacteria as seen by lack of growth following subculture to non-antibiotic–containing solid media

FIGURE 248–2 ■ Quantitative dilution susceptibility. The initial antibiotic concentration is obtained by quantitative preparation of antibiotic from standard powder obtained from the manufacturer. Twofold dilutions are made to obtain antibiotic concentrations, and a standard inoculum is added to each tube, including the antibiotic-free control tube. The minimal inhibitory concentration volume is read after 24 hours of incubation. Tubes with no visible turbidity are subcultured to antibiotic-free solid media, and the minimal bactericidal concentration volume is read after an additional 24 hours of incubation.

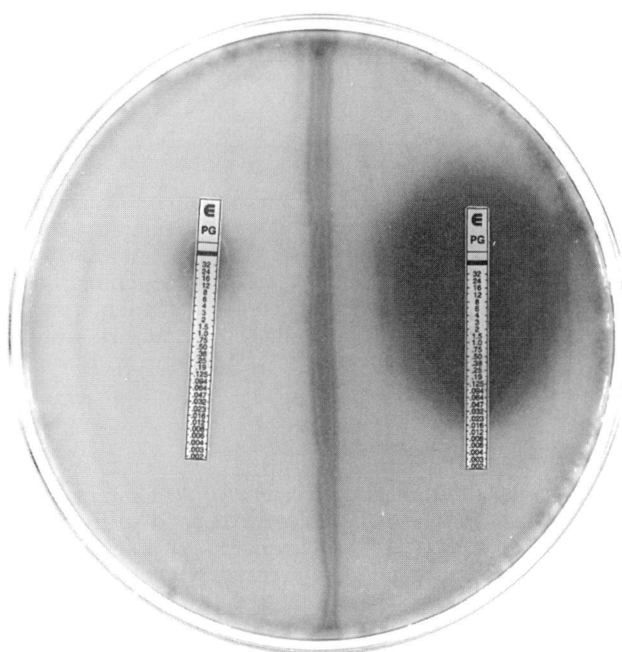

FIGURE 248–3 ■ E-test. Plastic strips containing an antibiotic gradient are placed on a lawn of bacterial inoculum, and the plate is incubated for 24 hours. In this figure, two pneumococcal strains are being tested for susceptibility to penicillin. The strain on the *right* is susceptible with a minimal inhibitory concentration value of 0.032 μg/mL. The strain on the *left* is resistant with a minimal inhibitory concentration value of 16 μg/mL.

β-LACTAMASE TEST

Detection of the β-lactamase enzyme responsible for the inactivation of ampicillin, penicillin, and other β-lactam antibiotics affords a rapid method for assessing the susceptibility of several bacteria to these compounds. In the microbiology laboratory, detection of β-lactamase enzymes has clinical value in the prediction of resistance by *H. influenzae, N. gonorrhoeae, Moraxella catarrhalis, S. aureus, Enterococcus* spp., and *Bacteroides* spp. These rapid tests (1 to 60 minutes) can be accomplished by acidometric, iodometric, or chromogenic cephalosporin methods (nitrocefin). The last is available commercially and is useful for all the species listed (it is the only reliable method for testing *M. catarrhalis).* When testing this group of bacteria, a positive test signifies resistance to penicillin, ampicillin, and other aminopenicillins. It does not imply resistance of *S. aureus* to the β-lactamase–stable penicillins (oxacillin, nafcillin, methicillin) or resistance of *H. influenzae* and *N. gonorrhoeae* to the extended-spectrum cephalosporins. In addition, although β-lactamase is the primary mechanism of resistance for most *H. influenzae* and *N. gonorrhoeae* organisms, cases have been reported of resistance to these compounds by mechanisms involving modification of penicillin-binding proteins that this test does not detect. β-Lactamase results do not always predict susceptibility or resistance to the penicillin class antibiotics in the Enterobacteriaceae and *Pseudomonas* spp.[176]

Extended-spectrum β-lactamases (ESBLs) are enzymes with expanded spectra of activity, including activity against oxyimino-cephalosporins such as cefotaxime and ceftazidime.[19] ESBLs are noted especially in isolates of *Klebsiella* and *E. coli*, but they can occur in many different genera of Enterobacteriaceae and *Pseudomonas aeruginosa.* These organisms may produce ESBLs but be susceptible to extended-spectrum cephalosporins by standard testing using NCCLS breakpoints. However, in some studies, treatment failures with these cephalosporins have been documented in association with such isolates. Strains of *Klebsiella* and *E. coli* should be screened for the potential production of ESBLs and confirmed with additional tests (cefotaxime and ceftazidime alone and in the presence of clavulanic acid) (Fig. 248–4). ESBL-producing isolates are best treated with a carbapenem and should be considered resistant to all penicillins, cephalosporins, and aztreonam.[134]

Special Studies

A variety of specialized antibiotic-related studies may be offered by the microbiology or infectious disease laboratory or may be available through a reference laboratory. Most of them are expensive to perform and labor-intensive, and some may be influenced by concurrent antibiotic therapy. Request for and interpretation of these tests should be limited in most cases to physicians with special training in infectious diseases.

ANTIBIOTIC ASSAY

Assay procedures for determining blood levels of potentially toxic antibiotics should be available in or accessible to all hospital bacteriology laboratories. This information is vital in the management of infections in patients with compromised renal function. Standardized immunologic and radiometric assays are available for determining levels of aminoglycosides and vancomycin. Bioassay procedures

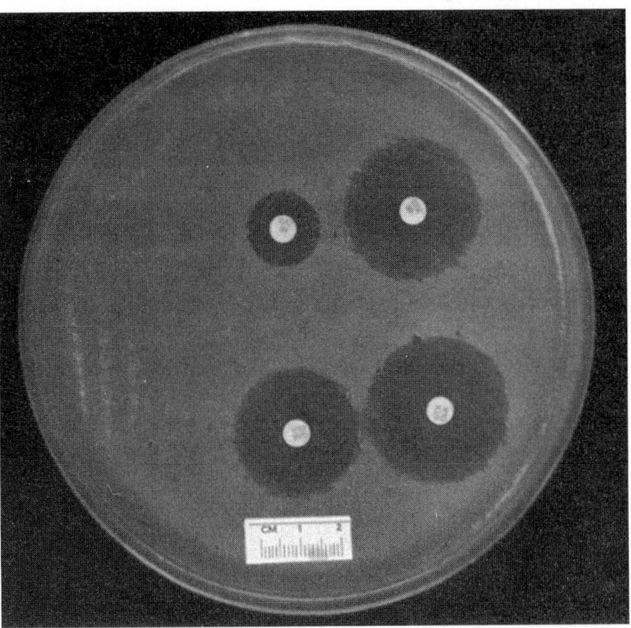

FIGURE 248–4 ■ Extended-spectrum β-lactamase (ESBL) confirmatory test. An *Escherichia coli* isolate is plated on Mueller-Hinton agar that contains ceftazidime *(upper left)* and ceftazidime plus clavulanic acid disks *(lower left),* as well as cefotaxime *(upper right)* and cefotaxime plus clavulanic acid disks *(lower right).* A greater than 5-mm increase in zone diameter for either antibiotic tested in combination with clavulanic acid in comparison to its zone when tested alone indicates ESBL production.

based on diffusion of the antibiotic in agar seeded with an indicator organism or high-pressure liquid chromatography assays are available in reference or research laboratories for unique instances when antibiotic levels are needed and no commercial assay kit is available. Often, the bioassays are restricted by being valid only if the patient is receiving no other antibiotic concurrently.

SERUM BACTERICIDAL TEST

The serum bactericidal test is performed by diluting the patient's serum and determining the minimal dilution that has inhibitory and bactericidal activity against the bacteria isolated from the infection (Fig. 248–5). In practice, it is much like performing quantitative susceptibility studies on that patient's infecting bacteria, except that in addition to measuring total metabolized antibiotics, it also measures the effects of serum factors in the blood. The test is easy to perform in that only a sample of serum, usually obtained at the nadir (trough) and the peak of the anticipated dose cycle, and the infecting bacteria from the patient are all that are required.[117, 137] However, substantial controversy exists regarding the performance, interpretation, and relevance of the bactericidal titer.[103, 173] Until recently, no standard procedures similar to the standards developed for quantitative susceptibility existed for the performance of bactericidal titers, and interlaboratory as well as intralaboratory variations were significant. The NCCLS has published guidelines for performance, which include the use of 50 percent serum in the broth media to simulate in vivo conditions more closely.[117, 119] Although these efforts are necessary to minimize variation, some question remains regarding how the addition of a serum source different from the patient's truly reflects individual patient serum. In addition, this requirement adds to the logistics and expense of performing the test. Alternative guidelines for the procedure omit the use of a serum diluent. Interpretation of the test results is also controversial.[103] Disagreement exists about how much the peak or trough level must exceed the MIC/minimal bactericidal concentration of the bacteria to be optimally therapeutic and whether maintaining the peak or the trough above a given level is more advantageous.[198] As one would suspect, clinical data to support all these variables are difficult to obtain. Finally, an important note is to realize that the bactericidal titer reflects conditions in the serum, and data to guide interpretation of the results when the site of infection is other than blood are incomplete.

SYNERGY

In special instances, combinations of antibiotics may be tested in vitro to confirm synergy or to detect antagonistic activity between two antibiotics. All these tests are labor-intensive and require special expertise in design and interpretation; furthermore, their therapeutic value remains questionable. Thus, they should be performed only in carefully selected circumstances.[42, 89] Several methods are available.

Fixed Combinations

Several compounds are tested regularly in combination (sulfamethoxazole-trimethoprim, erythromycin-sulfisoxazole, amoxicillin– and ticarcillin–clavulanic acid, piperacillin-tazobactam, and ampicillin-sulbactam). Standard disks are available for testing these compounds by disk diffusion methods. Quantitative susceptibility testing is performed best by a reference laboratory regularly engaged in testing these compounds.

Checkerboard

One method of obtaining a quantitative assessment of antibiotic activity in the presence of another antibiotic is the broth dilution method, most often with the use of microdilution plates. The tests are labor-intensive and require experienced personnel and proper controls. The results of these tests are expressed as fractional inhibitory concentrations of one drug in the presence of the other. In general, a combination is considered synergistic if the fractional inhibitory concentration is 0.5 or less, and it is antagonistic if the fractional inhibitory concentration is 4.0 or greater.[89]

Growth Curve

The growth curve is also a labor-intensive method of assessing the effects of antibiotic combinations in vitro. The bacteria are grown in broth containing appropriate dilutions of

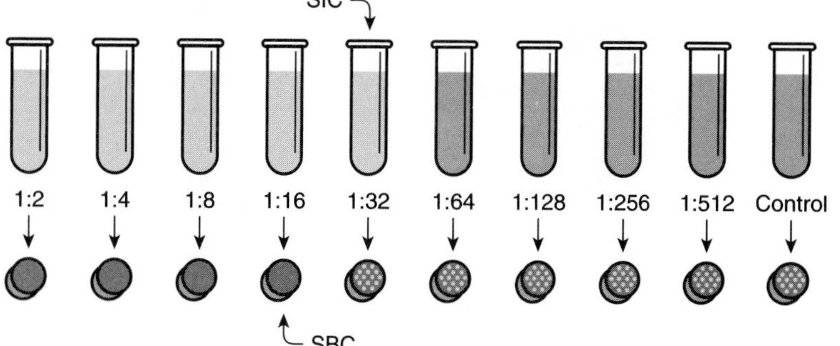
Serum Bactericidal Concentration
Dilutions of serum which inhibit growth are subcultured to solid media without antibiotics to determine the bactericidal dilution
SIC
1:2
1:4
1:8
1:16
1:32
1:64
1:128
1:256
1:512
Control
SBC
The highest dilution of the patient's serum that kills 99.9% of the patient's infecting bacteria

FIGURE 248–5 ■ Serum bactericidal concentration (SBC). Serum obtained from a patient while receiving antibiotic therapy is diluted twofold to obtain concentration ranges. A carefully controlled bacterial inoculum is added to all tubes and incubated for 24 hours. The serum inhibitory concentration (SIC) is the greatest dilution that inhibits growth, as judged by the lack of visible turbidity. Tubes with no visible growth are subcultured to antibiotic-free solid media, and the SBC is read after an additional 24 hours of incubation.

the antibiotics, alone and in combination. Viable cells are counted at the beginning and at several points during the experiment. Increased killing in the presence of the combination is considered synergistic, and decreased killing is considered antagonistic. Again, several controversial issues exist with regard to this method of testing: the concentration of the antibiotics to be tested, the length of time for the test, and the similarity of test conditions and in vivo conditions. Tolerance to antibiotics also can be documented by growth curves, which by definition show a less than 2-log drop in colony-forming units per milliliter after 5 hours of incubation with the antibiotic of interest. Isolates of *S. pneumoniae* tolerant to vancomycin may be responsible for treatment failures or relapse in patients receiving vancomycin.[111] Growth curve studies may be the only readily available means to document tolerance to vancomycin.[121]

Screening *(Enterococcus)*

Synergy between β-lactam antibiotics and the aminoglycosides may be of significant therapeutic benefit in treating infections caused by enterococci. This synergy with β-lactam antibiotics is not universal among strains of enterococci but is predictable by demonstrating the absence of high-level aminoglycoside resistance.[119] Such demonstration can be made by using a single tube containing 500 μg/mL of gentamicin and 1000 μg/mL of streptomycin and observing the presence or absence of growth. Although synergy with a β-lactam is ruled out by the determination of high-level aminoglycoside resistance (growth in the screen tube), synergy with that aminoglycoside cannot be assumed universally.

REFERENCES

1. Acar, J. F., and Goldstein, F. W.: Disk susceptibility test. *In* Lorian, L. (ed): Antibiotics in Laboratory Medicine. 3rd ed. Baltimore, Williams & Wilkins, 1991, pp. 42–44.
2. Albert, M. J., Ansaruzzaman, M., Abu, R. M. A., et al.: Fluorescent antibody staining test for rapid diagnosis of *Shigella dysenteriae* 1 infection. Diagn. Microbiol. Infect. Dis. *15*:359–361, 1992.
3. American Academy of Pediatrics: Group B streptococcal infections. *In* Pickering, L. D. (ed.): 2000 Red Book: Report of the Committee on Infectious Diseases. 25th ed. Elk Grove Village, IL, American Academy of Pediatrics, 2000, p. 537.
4. Araj, G. F., Hopfer, R. L., Chestnut, S., et al.: Diagnostic value of the enzyme-linked immunosorbent assay for detection of *Candida albicans* cytoplasmic antigen in sera of cancer patients. J. Clin. Microbiol. *16*:46–52, 1982.
5. Arditi, M., Mason, E. O., Jr., Bradley, J. S., et al.: Three-year surveillance of pneumococcal meningitis in children: Clinical characteristics and outcome related to penicillin susceptibility and dexamethasone use. Pediatrics *102*:1087–1097, 1998.
6. Bailey, J. W., Sada, E., Brass, C., et al.: Diagnosis of systemic candidiasis by latex agglutination for serum antigen. J. Clin. Microbiol. *21*:749–752, 1985.
7. Baker, C. J., and Rench, M. A.: Commercial latex agglutination for detection of group B streptococcal antigen in body fluids. J. Pediatr. *102*:393–395, 1983.
8. Baker, C. J., Webb, B. J., Jackson, C. V., et al.: Countercurrent immunoelectrophoresis in the evaluation of infants with group B streptococcal disease. Pediatrics *65*:1110–1114, 1980.
9. Baker, C. N., Stocker, S. A., Culver, D. H., et al.: Comparison of the E test to agar dilution, broth microdilution, and agar diffusion susceptibility testing techniques by using a special challenge set of bacteria. J. Clin. Microbiol. *29*:533–538, 1991.
10. Bal, A. E., Gravekamp, C., Hartskeerl, R. A., et al.: Detection of leptospires in urine by PCR for early diagnosis of leptospirosis. J. Clin. Microbiol. *32*:1894–1898, 1994.
11. Beaman, B. L., Saubolle, M. A., and Wallace, R. J.: *Nocardia, Rhodococcus, Streptomyces, Oerskovia,* and other aerobic actinomycetes of medical importance. *In* Murray, P. R., Baron, E. J., Pfaller, M. A., et al. (eds.): Manual of Clinical Microbiology. 6th ed. Washington, D.C., American Society for Microbiology, 1995, pp. 379–399.
12. Bell, T. A., Kuo, C.-C., Stamm, W. E., et al.: Direct fluorescent monoclonal antibody stain for rapid detection of infant *Chlamydia trachomatis* infections. Pediatrics *74*:224–228, 1984.
13. Bennett, J. E., Dismukes, W. E., Duma, R. J., et al.: A comparison of amphotericin B alone and combined with flucytosine in the treatment of cryptococcal meningitis. N. Engl. J. Med. *301*:126–131, 1979.
14. Bergeon, M. G., Danbing, K., Ménard, C., et al.: Rapid detection of group B streptococci in pregnant women at delivery. N. Engl. J. Med. *343*:175–179, 2000.
15. Berlin, L., and Pincus, J. H.: Cryptococcal meningitis: False-negative antigen test results and cultures in nonimmunosuppressed patients. Arch. Neurol. *46*:1312–1316, 1989.
16. Bernet, C., Garret, M., Barbeyrac, B. D., et al.: Detection of *Mycoplasma pneumoniae* by using the polymerase chain reaction. J. Clin. Microbiol. *27*:2492–2496, 1989.
17. Bonington, A., Strang, J. I., Klapper, P. E., et al.: Use of Roche Amplicor *Mycobacterium tuberculosis* PCR in early diagnosis of tuberculous meningitis. J. Clin. Microbiol. *36*:1251–1254, 1998.
18. Boom, W. H., Piper, D. J., Ruoff, K. L., et al.: New cause for false-positive results with the cryptococcal antigen test by latex agglutination. J. Clin. Microbiol. *22*:856–857, 1985.
19. Bradford, P. A.: Extended-spectrum β-lactamases in the 21st century: Characterization, epidemiology, and detection of this important resistant threat. Clin. Microbiol. Rev. *14*:933–951, 2001.
20. Bradley, J. S., and Connor, J. D.: Ceftriaxone failure in meningitis caused by *Streptococcus pneumoniae* with reduced susceptibility to beta-lactam antibiotics. Pediatr. Infect. Dis. J. *11*:871–873, 1991.
21. Brady, M. T.: Nosocomial legionnaires' disease in a children's hospital. J. Pediatr. *115*:46–50, 1989.
22. Buck, G. E., and Adams, M.: Meningococcus with reduced susceptibility to penicillin isolated in the United States. Pediatr. Infect. Dis. J. *13*:156–157, 1994.
23. Buimer, M., Doornum, G. J. J., Ching, S., et al.: Detection of *Chlamydia trachomatis* and *Neisseria gonorrhoeae* by ligase chain reaction–based assays with clinical specimens from various sites: Implications for diagnostic testing and screening. J. Clin. Microbiol. *34*:2395–2400, 1996.
24. Burg, J. L., Grover, C. M., Pouletty, P., et al.: Direct and sensitive detection of a pathogenic protozoan, *Toxoplasma gondii,* by polymerase chain reaction. J. Clin. Microbiol. *27*:1787–1792, 1989.
25. Cartwright, C. P., Nelson, N. A., and Gill, V. J.: Development and evaluation of a rapid and simple procedure for detection of *Pneumocystis carinii* by PCR. J. Clin. Microbiol. *32*:1634–1638, 1994.
26. Chapin-Robertson, K., Reece, E. A., and Edberg, S. C.: Evaluation of the Gen-Probe PACE II assay for the direct detection of *Neisseria gonorrhoeae* in endocervical specimens. Diagn. Microbiol. Infect. Dis. *15*:645–649, 1992.
27. Colding, H., and Lind, I.: Counterimmunoelectrophoresis in the diagnosis of bacterial meningitis. J. Clin. Microbiol. *5*:405–409, 1977.
28. Coonrod, J. D.: Urine as an antigen reservoir for diagnosis of infectious diseases: Infectious Diseases Symposium. Am. J. Med. *75*(Suppl. 1B): 85–92, 1983.
29. Crosson, F. J., Winkelstein, J. A., and Moxon, E. R.: Enzyme-linked immunosorbent assay for detection and quantitation of capsular antigen of *Haemophilus influenzae* type b. Infect. Immun. *22*:617–619, 1978.
30. Datta, A. R., Wentz, B. A., and Hill, W. E.: Detection of hemolytic *Listeria monocytogenes* by using DNA colony hybridization. Appl. Environ. Microbiol. *53*:2256–2259, 1987.
31. Dean, D., Palmer, L., Pant, C. R., et al.: Use of a *Chlamydia trachomatis* DNA probe for detection of ocular chlamydia. J. Clin. Microbiol. *27*:1062–1067, 1989.
32. Diagnosis of tuberculosis by nucleic acid amplification methods applied to clinical specimens. M. M. W. R. Morb. Mortal. Wkly. Rep. *42*(35):686, 1993.
33. Diamond, R. D., and Bennett, J. E.: Prognostic factors in cryptococcal meningitis. Ann. Intern. Med. *80*:176–181, 1974.
34. Dirks-Go, S. I. S., and Zanen, H. C.: Latex agglutination, counterimmunoelectrophoresis, and protein A co-agglutination in diagnosis of bacterial meningitis. J. Clin. Pathol. *31*:1167–1171, 1978.
35. Dobkin, D., and Shulman, S. T.: Evaluation of an ELISA for group A streptococcal antigen for diagnosis of pharyngitis. J. Pediatr. *110*:566–569, 1987.
36. Donatelli, J., Macone, A., Goldmann, D. A., et al.: Rapid detection of group A streptococci: Comparative performance by nurses and laboratory technologists in pediatric satellite laboratories using three test kits. J. Clin. Microbiol. *30*:138–142, 1992.
37. Dylla, B. L., Vetter, E. A., Hughes, J. G., et al.: Evaluation of an immunoassay for direct detection of *Escherichia coli* O157 in stool specimens. J. Clin. Microbiol. *33*:222–224, 1995.
38. Edwards, M. S., Kasper, D. L., and Baker, C. J.: Rapid diagnosis of type III group B streptococcal meningitis by latex particle agglutination. J. Pediatr. *95*:202–205, 1979.
39. Eisenach, K. D., Cave, M. D., Bates, J. H., et al.: Polymerase chain reaction amplification of a repetitive DNA sequence for *Mycobacterium tuberculosis*. J. Infect. Dis. *161*:977–981, 1990.
40. Eisenach, K. D., Crawford, J. T., and Bates, J. H.: Repetitive DNA sequences as probes for *Mycobacterium tuberculosis*. J. Clin. Microbiol. *26*:2240–2245, 1988.

41. Eisenstein, B. I.: New molecular techniques for microbial epidemiology and the diagnosis of infectious diseases. J. Infect. Dis. *161*:592–602, 1990.
42. Eliopoulos, G. M., and Eliopoulos, C. T.: Antibiotic combinations: Should they be tested? Clin. Microbiol. Rev. *1*:139–156, 1988.
43. Escuro, R. S., Jacobs, M., Gerson, S. L., et al.: Prospective evaluation of a candida antigen detection test for invasive candidiasis in immunocompromised adult patients with cancer. Am. J. Med. *87*:621–627, 1989.
44. Estrada, J. J., and Kuhn, R. E.: Immunochemical detection of antigens of larval *Taenia solium* and anti-larval antibodies in the CSF of patients with neurocysticercosis. J. Neurol. Sci. *71*:39–48, 1985.
45. Feldman, W. E.: Effect of prior antibiotic therapy on concentrations of bacteria in CSF. Am. J. Dis. Child. *132*:672–674, 1978.
46. Ferraro, M. J.: Automated antimicrobial susceptibility testing: What the infectious diseases subspecialist needs to know. Curr. Clin. Top. Infect. Dis. *14*:103–119, 1994.
47. Fleisher, G., Lennette, E. T., and Honig, P.: Diagnosis of Rocky Mountain spotted fever by immunofluorescent identification of *Rickettsia rickettsii* in skin biopsy tissue. J. Pediatr. *95*:63–65, 1979.
48. Forbes, B. A., and Granato, P. A.: Processing specimens for bacteria. *In* Murray, P. R., Baron, E. J., Pfaller, M. A., et al. (eds.): Manual of Clinical Microbiology. 6th ed. Washington, D.C., American Society for Microbiology, 1995, pp. 265–281.
49. Forbes, B. A., and Hicks, K. E. S.: Direct detection of *Mycobacterium tuberculosis* in respiratory specimens in a clinical laboratory by polymerase chain reaction. J. Clin. Microbiol. *31*:1688–1694, 1993.
50. Frankel, G., Riley, L., Giron, J. A., et al.: Detection of *Shigella* in feces using DNA application. J. Infect. Dis. *161*:1252–1256, 1990.
51. Fung, J. C., Donta, S. T., and Tilton, R. C.: *Candida* detection system (CAND-TEC) to differentiate between *Candida albicans* colonization and disease. J. Clin. Microbiol. *24*:542–547, 1986.
52. Gentry, L. O., Wilkinson, I. D., Lea, A. S., et al.: Latex agglutination test for detection of *Candida* antigen in patients with disseminated disease. Eur. J. Clin. Microbiol. *2*:122–128, 1983.
53. Gerber, M. A.: Comparison of throat cultures and rapid strep tests for diagnosis of streptococcal pharyngitis. Pediatr. Infect. Dis. J. *8*:820–824, 1989.
54. Gerber, M. A., Randolph, M. F., Chantry, J., et al.: Antigen detection test for streptococcal pharyngitis: Evaluation of sensitivity with respect to true infection. J. Pediatr. *108*:654–658, 1986.
55. Gerber, M. A., Spadaccini, L. J., Wright, L. L., et al.: Latex agglutination tests for rapid identification of group A streptococci directly from throat swabs. J. Pediatr. *105*:702–705, 1984.
56. Gerber, M. A., Tanz, R. R., Kabat, W., et al.: Optical immunoassay test for group A beta-hemolytic streptococcal pharyngitis. An office based, multicenter investigation. J. A. M. A. *277*:899–903, 1997.
57. Girardet, R. G., McClain, N., Lahoti, S., et al.: Comparison of the urine-based ligase chain reaction test to culture for the detection of *Chlamydia trachomatis* and *Neisseria gonorrhoeae* in pediatric sexual abuse victims. Pediatr. Infect. Dis. J. *20*:144–147, 2001.
58. Girolami, P. C. D., Hanff, P. A., Eichelberger, K., et al.: Multicenter evaluation of a new enzyme immunoassay for detection of *Clostridium difficile* enterotoxin A. J. Clin. Microbiol. *30*:1085–1088, 1992.
59. Gomez-Herruz, P., Gonzalez-Palacios, R., Romanyk, J., et al.: Evaluation of the E-test for penicillin susceptibility testing of *Neisseria meningitidis*. Diagn. Microbiol. Infect. Dis. *21*:115–117, 1995.
60. Gomez-Pastrana, D., Torronteras, R., Caro, P., et al.: Comparison of Amplicor, in-house polymerase chain reaction, and conventional culture for the diagnosis of tuberculosis in children. Clin. Infect. Dis. *32*:17–22, 2001.
61. Goral, S., Anderson, B., Hager, C., Edwards, K. M.: Detection of *Rochalimaea henselae* DNA by polymerase chain reaction from suppurative nodes of children with cat-scratch disease. Pediatr. Infect. Dis. J. *13*:994–997, 1994.
62. Gorelick, M. H., and Shaw, K. N.: Screening tests for urinary tract infection in children: A meta-analysis. Pediatrics *104*(5):e54, 1999. http://www.pediatrics.org/cgi/content/full/104/5/e54.
63. Greenwood, B. M., Whittle, H. C., and Dominic-Rajkovic, O.: Countercurrent immunoelectrophoresis in the diagnosis of meningococcal infections. Lancet *2*:519–521, 1971.
64. Grimprel, E., Sanchez, P. J., Wendel, G. D., et al.: Use of polymerase chain reaction and rabbit infectivity testing to detect *Treponema pallidum* in amniotic fluid, fetal and neonatal sera, and CSF. J. Clin. Microbiol. *29*:1711–1718, 1991.
65. Hageage, G. J., and Harrington, B. J.: Use of calcofluor white in clinical mycology. Lab. Med. *15*:109–112, 1984.
66. Hamilton, J. R., Noble, A., Denning, D. W., and Stevens, D. A.: Performance of cryptococcus antigen latex agglutination kits on serum and CSF specimens of AIDS patients before and after pronase treatment. J. Clin. Microbiol. *29*:333–339, 1991.
67. Hammerschlag, M. R., Gelling, M., Roblin, P. M., et al.: Comparison of Kodak Surecell *Chlamydia* Test Kit with culture for the diagnosis of chlamydial conjunctivitis in infants. J. Clin. Microbiol. *28*:1441–1442, 1990.
68. Hammerschlag, M. R., Roblin, P. M., Cummings, C., et al.: Comparison of enzyme immunoassay and culture for diagnosis of chlamydial conjunctivitis and respiratory infections in infants. J. Clin. Microbiol. *25*:2306–2308, 1987.
69. Harding, S. A., Scheld, W. M., McGowan, M. D., et al.: Enzyme-linked immunosorbent assay for detection of *Streptococcus pneumoniae* antigen. J. Clin. Microbiol. *10*:339–342, 1979.
70. Hasan, J. A. K., Huq, A., Tamplin, M. L., et al.: A novel kit for rapid detection of *Vibrio cholerae* 01. J. Clin. Microbiol. *32*:249–252, 1994.
71. Hata, D., Kuze, F., Mochizuki, Y., et al.: Evaluation of DNA probe test for rapid diagnosis of *Mycoplasma pneumoniae* infections. J. Pediatr. *116*:273–276, 1990.
72. Heiter, B. J., and Borubeau, P. P.: Comparison of the Gen-Probe group A streptococcus direct test with culture and a rapid streptococcal antigen detection assay for diagnosis of streptococcal pharyngitis. J. Clin. Microbiol. *31*:2070–2073, 1993.
73. Herold, B. C., Immergluck, L. C., Maranan, M. C., et al.: Community-acquired methicillin-resistant *Staphylococcus aureus* in children with no identified predisposing risk. J. A. M. A. *279*:593–598, 1998.
74. Hidalgo, J. A., Alangaden, G. J., Eliott, D., et al.: Fungal endophthalmitis diagnosis by detection of *Candida albicans* DNA in intraocular fluid by use of a species-specific polymerase chain reaction assay. J. Infect. Dis. *181*:1198–1201, 2000.
75. Hoberman, A., Wald, E. R., Reynolds, E. A., et al.: Pyuria and bacteriuria in urine specimens obtained by catheter from young children with fever. J. Pediatr. *124*:513–519, 1994.
76. Hopfer, R. L., Perry, E. V., and Fainstein, V.: Diagnostic value of cryptococcal antigen in the CSF of patients with malignant disease. J. Infect. Dis. *145*:915, 1982.
77. Hughes, J. H., Biedenbach, D. J., Erwin, M. E., et al.: E test as susceptibility test and epidemiologic tool for evaluation of *Neisseria meningitidis* isolates. J. Clin. Microbiol. *31*:3255–3259, 1993.
78. Ingram, D. L., Pearson, A. W., and Occhiuti, A. R.: Detection of bacterial antigens in body fluids with the Wellcogen *Haemophilus influenzae* b, *Streptococcus pneumoniae,* and *Neisseria meningitidis* (ACYW135) latex agglutination tests. J. Clin. Microbiol. *18*:1119–1121, 1983.
79. Jones, J. M.: Laboratory diagnosis of invasive candidiasis. Clin. Microbiol. Rev. *3*:32–45, 1990.
80. Jorgensen, J. H.: Antimicrobial susceptibility testing of bacteria that grow aerobically. Infect. Dis. Clin. North Am. *7*:393–409, 1993.
81. Jorgensen, J. H., Howell, A. W., and Maher, L. A.: Quantitative antimicrobial susceptibility testing of *Haemophilus influenzae* and *Streptococcus pneumoniae* by using the E-test. J. Clin. Microbiol. *29*:109–114, 1991.
82. Kan, V. L.: Polymerase chain reaction for the diagnosis of candidemia. J. Infect. Dis. *168*:779–783, 1993.
83. Kaplan, S. L.: Antigen detection in CSF: Pros and cons: Infectious Diseases Symposium. Am. J. Med. *75*(Suppl. 1B):109–118, 1983.
84. Kaplan, S. L., Mason, E. O., Mason, S. K., et al.: Prospective comparative trial of moxalactam versus ampicillin or chloramphenicol for treatment of *Haemophilus influenzae* type b meningitis in children. J. Pediatr. *104*:447–453, 1984.
85. Kasolo, F., Lishimpi, K., Chintu, C., et al.: Identification of *Pneumocystis carinii* DNA by polymerase chain reaction in necropsy lung samples from children dying of respiratory tract illnesses. J. Pediatr. *140*:367–369, 2002.
86. Kazandjian, D. R., Chiew, L., and Gilbert, G. L.: Rapid diagnosis of *Legionella pneumophila* serogroup 1 infection with the Binax enzyme immunoassay urinary antigen test. J. Clin. Microbiol. *35*:954–956, 1997.
87. Kellogg, J. A.: Suitability of throat culture procedures for detection of group A streptococci and as reference standards for evaluation of streptococcal antigen detection kits. J. Clin. Microbiol. *28*:165–169, 1990.
88. Kerkering, T. M., Espinel-Ingroff, A., and Shadomy, S.: Detection of candida antigenemia by counterimmunoelectrophoresis in patients with invasive candidiasis. J. Infect. Dis. *140*:659–664, 1979.
89. King, T. C., Schlessinger, D., and Krogstad, D. J.: The assessment of drug combinations. Rev. Infect. Dis. *3*:627–633, 1981.
90. Kleiman, M. B., Reynolds, J. K., Schreiner, R. L., et al.: Rapid diagnosis of neonatal bacteremia with acridine orange–stained buffy coat smears. J. Pediatr. *105*:419–421, 1984.
91. Kleiman, M. B., Reynolds, J. K., Watts, N. H., et al.: Superiority of acridine orange stain versus Gram stain in partially treated bacterial meningitis. J. Pediatr. *104*:401–404, 1984.
92. Klugman, K. P.: Pneumococcal resistance to antibiotics. Clin. Microbiol. Rev. *3*:171–196, 1990.
93. Kovacs, J. A., Ng, V. L., Masur, H., et al.: Diagnosis of *Pneumocystis carinii* pneumonia: Improved detection in sputum with use of monoclonal antibodies. N. Engl. J. Med. *318*:589–593, 1988.
94. Lang, A., Feris-Iglesias, J., Pena, C., et al.: Clinical evaluation of the Gen-Probe Amplified Direct Test for detection of *Mycobacterium tuberculosis* complex organisms in CSF. J. Clin. Microbiol. *36*:2191–2194, 1998.
95. Lee, B. W., Tan, J. A., Wong, S. C., et al.: DNA amplification by the polymerase chain reaction for the rapid diagnosis of tuberculous meningitis: Comparison of protocols involving three mycobacterial DNA sequences, IS6110, 65kDa antigen, and MPB64. J. Neurol. Sci. *123*:173–179, 1994.

96. Lemieux, C., St.-Germain, G., Vincelette, J., et al.: Collaborative evaluation of antigen detection by a commercial latex agglutination test and enzyme immunoassay in the diagnosis of invasive candidiasis. J. Clin. Microbiol. *28*:249–253, 1990.
97. Lentino, J. R., and Rytel, M. W.: Detection of circulating free and complexed staphylococcal antigens by enzyme-linked immunosorbent assay. J. Clin. Microbiol. *16*:1019–1024, 1982.
98. Lew, M. A., Siber, G. R., Donahue, D. M., et al.: Enhanced detection with an enzyme-linked immunosorbent assay of *Candida* mannan in antibody-containing serum after heat-extraction. J. Infect. Dis. *145*:45–56, 1982.
99. Li, Z., Jansen, D. L., Finn, T. M., et al.: Identification of *Bordetella pertussis* infection by shared-primer PCR. J. Clin. Microbiol. *32*:783–789, 1994.
100. Lipschick, G. Y., Gill, V. J., Lundgren, J. D., et al.: Improved diagnosis of *Pneumocystis carinii* infection by polymerase chain reaction on induced sputum and blood. Lancet *340*:203–206, 1992.
101. Liu, P. Y.-F., Shi, Z.-Y., Lau, Y.-J., et al.: Rapid diagnosis of tuberculous meningitis by a simplified nested amplification protocol. Neurology *44*:1161–1164, 1994.
102. Macias, E. A., Mason, E. O., Jr., Ocera, H. Y., et al.: Comparison of E test with standard broth microdilution for determining antibiotic susceptibilities of penicillin-resistant strains of *Streptococcus pneumoniae*. J. Clin. Microbiol. *32*:430–432, 1994.
103. MacLowry, J. D.: Perspective: The serum dilution test. J. Infect. Dis. *160*:624–626, 1989.
104. Maertens, J., Verhaegen, J., Demuynck, H., et al.: Autopsy-controlled prospective evaluation of serial screening for circulating galactomannan by a sandwich enzyme-linked immunosorbent assay for hematological patients at risk for invasive aspergillosis. J. Clin. Microbiol. *37*:3223–3238, 1999.
105. Magder, L. S., Klotz, K. C., Bush, L. H., et al.: Effect of patient characteristics on performance of an enzyme immunoassay for detecting cervical *Chlamydia trachomatis* infection. J. Clin. Microbiol. *28*:781–784, 1990.
106. Marchant, C. D., Band, E., Froeschle, J. E., et al.: Depression of anticapsular antibody after immunization with *Haemophilus influenzae* type b polysaccharide–diphtheria conjugate vaccine. Pediatr. Infect. Dis. J. *8*:508–511, 1989.
107. Marcon, M. J.: *Bordetella. In* Murray, P. R., Baron, E. J., Pfaller, M. A., et al. (eds.): Manual of Clinical Microbiology. 6th ed. Washington, D.C., American Society for Microbiology, 1995, pp. 566–573.
108. Marmion, B. P., Williamson, J., Worswick, D. A., et al.: Experience with newer techniques for the laboratory detection of *Mycoplasma pneumoniae* infection: Adelaide, 1978–1992. Clin. Infect. Dis. *17*(Suppl. 1):90–99, 1993.
109. Mason, E. O., Jr., Kaplan, S. L., Lamberth, L. B., et al.: Increased rate of isolation of penicillin-resistant *Streptococcus pneumoniae* in a children's hospital and in vitro susceptibilities to antibiotics of potential therapeutic use. Antimicrob. Agents Chemother. *36*:1703–1707, 1992.
110. Maxson, S., Lewno, M. J., and Schutze, G. E.: Clinical usefulness of CSF bacterial antigen studies. J. Pediatr. *125*:235–238, 1994.
111. McCullers, J. A., English, B. K., and Novak, R.: Isolation and characterization of vancomycin-tolerant *Streptococcus pneumoniae* from the CSF of a patient who developed recrudescent meningitis. J. Infect. Dis. *181*:369–373, 2000.
112. Monteiro, L., Gras, N., and Megraud, F.: Magnetic immuno-PCR assay with inhibitor removal for direct detection of *Helicobacter pylori* in human feces. J. Clin. Microbiol. *39*:3778–3780, 2001.
113. Moonens, F., El Alami, S., Gossum, A. V., et al.: Usefulness of Gram staining of blood collected from total parenteral nutrition catheter for rapid diagnosis of catheter-related sepsis. J. Clin. Microbiol. *32*:1578–1579, 1994.
114. Morrow, D. L., Kline, J. B., Douglas, S. D., et al.: Rapid detection of group B streptococcal antigen by monoclonal antibody sandwich enzyme assay. J. Clin. Microbiol. *19*:457–459, 1984.
115. Moser, D. R., Kirchhoff, L. V., and Donelson, J. E.: Detection of *Trypanosoma cruzi* by DNA amplification using the polymerase chain reaction. J. Clin. Microbiol. *27*:1477–1482, 1989.
116. Murray, B. E.: The life and times of the *Enterococcus*. Clin. Microbiol. Rev. *3*:46–65, 1990.
117. National Committee for Clinical Laboratory Standards: Methodology for the Serum Bactericidal Test: Approved Guideline. NCCLS Document M21-A. Villanova, PA, NCCLS, 1999.
118. National Committee for Clinical Laboratory Standards: Methods for Determining Bactericidal Activity of Antimicrobial Agents: Approved Guideline. NCCLS Document M26-A. Villanova, PA, NCCLS, 1999.
119. National Committee for Clinical Laboratory Standards: Methods for Dilution Antimicrobial Susceptibility Tests for Bacteria That Grow Aerobically. 5th ed. Approved Standard. NCCLS Document M7-A5. Villanova, PA, NCCLS, 2000.
120. Ness, M. J., Vaughan, W. P., and Woods, G. L.: *Candida* antigen latex test for detection of invasive candidiasis in immunocompromised patients. J. Infect. Dis. *159*:495–502, 1989.
121. Normark, B. H., Novak, R, Örtqvist, Å., et al.: Clinical isolates of *Streptococcus pneumoniae* that exhibit tolerance of vancomycin. Clin. Infect. Dis. *32*:552–558, 2001.
122. Ng, V. L., Yajko, D. M., McPhaul, L. W., et al.: Evaluation of an indirect fluorescent-antibody stain for detection of *Pneumocystis carinii* in respiratory specimens. J. Clin. Microbiol. *28*:975–979, 1990.
123. Ni, H., Knight, A. I., Cartwright, K., et al.: Polymerase chain reaction for diagnosis of meningococcal meningitis. Lancet *340*:1432–1434, 1992.
124. Nolte, F. S., Metchock, B., McGowan, J. E., Jr., et al.: Direct detection of *Mycobacterium tuberculosis* in sputum by polymerase chain reaction and DNA hybridization. J. Clin. Microbiol. *31*:1777–1782, 1993.
125. Ognibene, F. P., Gill, V. J., Pizzo, P. A., et al.: Induced sputum to diagnose *Pneumocystis carinii* pneumonia in immunosuppressed pediatric patients. J. Pediatr. *115*:430–433, 1989.
126. Olcen, P.: Serological methods for rapid diagnosis of *Haemophilus influenzae, Neisseria meningitidis,* and *Streptococcus pneumoniae* in CSF: A comparison of co-agglutination, immunofluorescence, and immunoelectroosmophoresis. Scand. J. Infect. Dis. *10*:283–289, 1978.
127. Olsson-Liljequist, B., and Nord, C. E.: Methods for susceptibility testing of anaerobic bacteria. Clin. Infect. Dis. *18*(Suppl. 4):293–296, 1994.
128. Ostergaard, L., Birkelund, S., and Christiansen, G.: Use of polymerase chain reaction for detection of *Chlamydia trachomatis*. J. Clin. Microbiol. *28*:1254–1260, 1990.
129. Page-Shafer, K., Graves, A., Kent, C., et al.: Increased sensitivity of DNA amplification testing for the detection of pharyngeal gonorrhea in men who have sex with men. Clin. Infect. Dis. *34*:173–176, 2002.
130. Paisley, J. W., Lauer, B. A., Melinkovich, P., et al.: Rapid diagnosis of *Chlamydia trachomatis* pneumonia in infants by direct immunofluorescence microscopy of nasopharyngeal secretions. J. Pediatr. *109*:653–655, 1986.
131. Papasian, C. J., Bartholomew, W. R., and Amsterdam, D.: Validity of an enzyme immunoassay for detection of *Neisseria gonorrhoeae* antigens. J. Clin. Microbiol. *19*:347–350, 1984.
132. Park, C. H., Hixon, D. L., Morrison, W. L., et al.: Rapid diagnosis of enterohemorrhagic *Escherichia coli* O157:H7 directly from fecal specimens using immunofluorescence stain. Am. J. Clin. Pathol. *101*:91–94, 1994.
133. Pasculle, A. W., Veto, G. E., Krystofiak, S., et al.: Laboratory and clinical evaluation of a commercial DNA probe for the detection of *Legionella* spp. J. Clin. Microbiol. *27*:2350–2358, 1989.
134. Patterson, D. L., Ko, W. C., Gottberg, A. V., et al.: Outcome of cephalosporin treatment for serious infections due to apparently susceptible organisms producing extended-spectrum β-lactamases: Implications for the clinical microbiology laboratory. J. Clin. Microbiol. *39*:2206–2212, 2001.
135. Perkins, M. D., Mirrett, S., and Reller, L. B.: Rapid bacterial antigen detection is not clinically useful. J. Clin. Microbiol. *33*:1486–1491, 1995.
136. Peterson, L. R., and Kelly, P. J.: The role of the clinical microbiology laboratory in the management of *Clostridium difficile*–associated diarrhea. Infect. Dis. Clin. North Am. *7*:277–293, 1993.
137. Peterson, L. R., and Shanholtzer, C. J.: Tests for bactericidal effects of antimicrobial agents: Technical performance and clinical relevance. Clin. Microbiol. Rev. *5*:420–432, 1992.
138. Pezzlo, M. T.: Automated methods for detection of bacteriuria. Am. J. Med. *75*:71–78, 1983.
139. Pezzlo, M. T., Wetkowski, M. A., Peterson, E. M., et al.: Evaluation of a two-minute test for urine screening. J. Clin. Microbiol. *18*:697–701, 1983.
140. Pitetti, R. D., Drenning, S. D., and Wald, E. R.: Evaluation of a new rapid antigen detection kit for group A beta-hemolytic streptococci. Pediatr. Emerg. Care *14*:396–398, 1998.
141. Podzorski, R. P., and Persing, D. H.: Molecular detection and identification of microorganisms. *In* Murray, P. R., Baron, E. J., Pfaller, M. A., et al. (eds.): Manual of Clinical Microbiology. 6th ed. Washington, D.C., ASM Press, 1995, pp. 130–134.
142. Polin, R. A., and Kenneth, R.: Use of monoclonal antibodies in an enzyme-linked inhibition assay for rapid detection of streptococcal antigen. J. Pediatr. *97*:540–544, 1980.
143. Porder, K., Sanchez, N., Roblin, P. M., et al.: Lack of specificity of Chlamydiazyme for detection of vaginal chlamydial infection in prepubertal girls. Pediatr. Infect. Dis. J. *8*:358–360, 1989.
144. Raad, I., Hanna, H., Huaringa, A., et al.: Diagnosis of invasive pulmonary aspergillosis using polymerase chain reaction–based detection of aspergillus in BAL. Chest *121*:1171–1176, 2002.
145. Raad, I., Hanna, H., Sumoza, D., and Albitar, M.: Polymerase chain reaction on blood for the diagnosis of invasive pulmonary aspergillosis in cancer patients. Cancer *94*:1032–1036, 2002.
146. Rapoza, P. A., Quinn, T. C., Kiessling, L. A., et al.: Assessment of neonatal conjunctivitis with a direct immunofluorescent monoclonal antibody stain for chlamydia. J. A. M. A. *255*:3369–3373, 1986.
147. Roblin, P. M., Hammerschlag, M. R., Cummings, C., et al.: Comparison of two rapid microscopic methods and culture for detection of *Chlamydia trachomatis* in ocular and nasopharyngeal specimens from infants. J. Clin. Microbiol. *27*:968–970, 1989.
148. Rosa, P. A., and Schwan, T. G.: A specific and sensitive assay for the Lyme disease spirochete *Borrelia burgdorferi* using the polymerase chain reaction. J. Infect. Dis. *160*:1018–1029, 1989.
149. Rosenblatt, J. E., and Sloan L. M.: Evaluation of an enzyme-linked immunosorbent assay for detection of *Cryptosporidium* spp. in stool specimens. J. Clin. Microbiol. *31*:1468–1471, 1993.

150. Rosenblatt, J. E., Sloan, L. M., and Schneider, S. K.: Evaluation of an enzyme-linked immunosorbent assay for the detection of *Giardia lamblia* in stool specimens. Diagn. Microbiol. Infect. Dis. *16*:337–341, 1993.
151. Rowx, P., Laxrard, I., Poirot, J. L., et al.: Usefulness of PCR for detection of *Pneumocystis carinii* DNA. J. Clin. Microbiol. *32*:2324–2326, 1994.
152. Rudolph, K. M., Parkinson, A. J., Black, C. M., et al.: Evaluation of polymerase chain reaction for diagnosis of pneumococcal pneumonia. J. Clin. Microbiol. *31*:2661–2666, 1993.
153. Sabetta, J. R., Miniter, P., and Andriole, V. T.: The diagnosis of invasive aspergillosis by an enzyme-linked immunosorbent assay for circulating antigen. J. Infect. Dis. *152*:946–953, 1985.
154. Sada, E., Lopez-Vidal, Y., Ruiz-Palacios, G. M., et al.: Detection of mycobacterial antigens in CSF of patients with tuberculous meningitis by enzyme-linked immunosorbent assay. Lancet *11*:651–652, 1983.
155. Saengjaruk, P., Chaicumpa, W., Wyatt, G., et al.: Diagnosis of human leptospirosis by monoclonal antibody–based antigen detection in urine. J. Clin. Microbiol. *40*:480–489, 2002.
156. Sahm, D. F., Neuman, M. A., Thornsberry, C., et al.: Cumitech 25: Current concepts and approaches to antimicrobial agent susceptibility testing. *In* McGowan, J. E., Jr. (ed.): Washington, D.C., American Society for Microbiology, 1988.
157. Sanchez, P. J., Siegel, J. D., Cushion, N. B., et al.: Significance of a positive urine group B streptococcal latex agglutination test in neonates. J. Pediatr. *116*:601–606, 1990.
158. Savic, B., Sjöbring, V., Alugupalli, S., et al.: Evaluation of polymerase chain reaction, tuberculostearic acid analysis, and direct microscopy for the detection of *Mycobacterium tuberculosis* in sputum. J. Infect. Dis. *166*:1177–1180, 1992.
159. Scheffer, E. H., and Van Etta, L. L.: Evaluation of rapid commercial enzyme immunoassay for detection of *Giardia lamblia* in formalin-preserved stool specimens. J. Clin. Microbiol. *32*:1807–1808, 1994.
160. Schochetman, G., Ou, C.-Y., and Jones, W. K.: Polymerase chain reaction. J. Infect. Dis. *158*:1154–1157, 1988.
161. Schreiber, J. R., Maynard, E., and Lew, M. A.: *Candida* antigen detection in two premature neonates with disseminated candidiasis. Pediatrics *74*:838–841, 1984.
162. Schwartz, R. H., Bryan, C., Rodriguez, W. J., et al.: Experience with the microbiologic diagnosis of *Campylobacter* enteritis in an office laboratory. Pediatr. Infect. Dis. J. *2*:298–301, 1983.
163. Segal, E., Berg, R. A., Pizzo, P. A., et al.: Detection of *Candida* antigen in sera of patients with candidiasis by an enzyme-linked immunosorbent assay: Inhibition technique. J. Clin. Microbiol. *10*:116–118, 1979.
164. Shaffer, P. J., Kobayashi, G. S., and Medoff, G.: Demonstration of antigenemia in patients with invasive aspergillosis by solid phase (protein A–rich *Staphylococcus aureus*) radioimmunoassay. Am. J. Med. *67*:627–630, 1979.
165. Sippel, J. E., Prato, C. M., Girgis, N. I., et al.: Detection of *Neisseria meningitidis* group A, *Haemophilus influenzae* type b, and *Streptococcus pneumoniae* antigens in CSF specimens by antigen capture enzyme-linked immunosorbent assays. J. Clin. Microbiol. *20*:259–265, 1984.
166. Skoll, M. A., Mercer, B. M., Baselski, V., et al.: Evaluation of two rapid group B streptococcal antigen tests in labor and delivery patients. Obstet. Gynecol. *77*:322–326, 1991.
167. Sloas, M. M., Barrett, F. F., Chesney, P. J., et al.: Cephalosporin treatment failure in penicillin- and cephalosporin-resistant *Streptococcus pneumoniae* meningitis. Pediatr. Infect. Dis. J. *11*:662–666, 1992.
168. Snyder J. D., and Zanten, V.: Novel diagnostic tests to detect *Helicobacter pylori* infection. A pediatric perspective. Can. J. Gastroenterol. *13*:585–589, 1999.
169. Sood, S. K., Ballanco, G. A., Mather, F. J., et al.: Distribution and excretion of capsular antigen after immunization with *Haemophilus influenzae* type b polysaccharide–*Neisseria meningitidis* outer membrane protein conjugate vaccine. J. Infect. Dis. *161*:574–577, 1990.
170. Stamm, W. E., Cole, B., Fennell, C., et al.: Antigen detection for the diagnosis of gonorrhea. J. Clin. Microbiol. *19*:399–403, 1984.
171. Starnbach, M. N., Falkow, S., and Tompkins, L. S.: Species-specific detection of *Legionella pneumophila* in water by DNA amplification and hybridization. J. Clin. Microbiol. *27*:1257–1261, 1989.
172. Stevens, D. A.: Diagnosis of fungal infections: Current status. J. Antimicrob. Chemother. *49*(Suppl. 1):11–19, 2002.
173. Stratton, C. W.: Serum bactericidal test. Clin. Microbiol. Rev. *1*:19–26, 1988.
174. Stratton, N., Hryniewicki, J., Aarnoes, S. L., et al.: Comparison of monoclonal antibody and calcofluor white stains for the detection of *Pneumocystis carinii* from respiratory specimens. J. Clin. Microbiol. *29*:645–647, 1991.
175. Summanen, P.: Microbiology terminology update: Clinically significant anaerobic gram-positive and gram-negative bacteria (excluding spirochetes). Clin. Infect. Dis. *21*:273–276, 1995.
176. Swenson, J. M., Hindler, J. A., and Peterson, L. R.: Special tests for detecting antibacterial resistance. *In* Murray, P. R., Baron, E. J., Pfaller, M. A., et al. (eds.): Manual of Clinical Microbiology. 6th ed. Washington, D.C., American Society for Microbiology, 1995, pp. 1356–1367.
177. Tanner, D. C., Weinstein, M. P., Fedozciw, B., et al.: Comparison of commercial kits for detection of cryptococcal antigen. J. Clin. Microbiol. *32*:1680–1684, 1994.
178. Tenover, F. C.: Novel and emerging mechanisms of antimicrobial resistance in nosocomial pathogens. Am. J. Med. *91*(Suppl. 3B):76–81, 1991.
179. Tenover, F. C., Arbiet, R. D., Goering, R. V., et al.: Interpreting chromosomal DNA restriction patterns by pulse-field gel electrophoresis: Criteria for bacterial strain typing. J. Clin. Microbiol. *33*:2233–2239, 1995.
180. Tenover, F. C., Tokars, J., Swenson, J., et al.: Ability of clinical laboratories to detect antimicrobial agent–resistant enterococci. J. Clin. Microbiol. *31*:1695–1699, 1993.
181. Tiley, S. M., Marriott, D. J. E., and Harkness, J. L.: An evaluation of four methods for the detection of *Pneumocystis carinii* in clinical specimens. Pathology *26*:325–328, 1994.
182. Tilley, P. A., Kanchana, M. V., Knight, I., et al.: Detection of *Bordetella pertussis* in a clinical laboratory by culture, polymerase chain reaction, and direct fluorescent antibody staining; accuracy and cost. Diagn. Microbiol. Infect. Dis. *37*:17–23, 2000.
183. Tilton, R. C., Dias, F., and Ryan, R. W.: Comparative evaluation of three commercial products and counterimmunoelectrophoresis for the detection of antigens in CSF. J. Clin. Microbiol. *20*:231–234, 1984.
184. Todd, J. K.: Management of urinary tract infections: Children are different. Pediatr. Rev. *16*:190–196, 1995.
185. Tzianabos, T., Anderson, B. E., and McDade, J. E.: Detection of *Rickettsia rickettsii* DNA in clinical specimens by using polymerase chain reaction technology. J. Clin. Microbiol. *27*:2866–2868, 1989.
186. van Esso, D., Fontanls, D., Uriz, S, et al.: *Neisseria meningitidis* strains with decreased susceptibility to penicillin. Pediatr. Infect. Dis. J. *6*:438–439, 1987.
187. Wack, E. E., Dugger, K. O., and Galgiani, J. N.: Enzyme-linked immunosorbent assay for antigens of *Coccidioides immitis:* Human sera interference corrected by acidification-heat extraction. J. Lab. Clin. Med. *111*:560–565, 1988.
188. Wahyuningsih, R., Freisleben, H.-J., Sonntag, H.-G., and Schnitzler, P.: Simple and rapid detection of *Candida albicans* DNA in serum by PCR for diagnosis of invasive candidiasis. J. Clin. Microbiol. *38*:3016–3021, 2000.
189. Walsh, T. J., Hathorn, J. W., Sober, J. D., et al.: Detection of circulating candida enolase by immunoassay in patients with cancer and invasive candidiasis. N. Engl. J. Med. *324*:1026–1031, 1991.
190. Watt, G., Zaraspe, G., Bautista, S., et al.: Rapid diagnosis of tuberculous meningitis by using an enzyme-linked immunosorbent assay to detect mycobacterial antigen and antibody in CSF. J. Infect. Dis. *158*:681–686, 1988.
191. Webb, B. J., and Baker, C. J.: Commercial latex agglutination test for rapid diagnosis of group B streptococcal infection in infants. J. Clin. Microbiol. *12*:442–444, 1980.
192. Webb, B. J., Edwards, M. S., and Baker, C. J.: Comparison of slide coagglutination test and countercurrent immunoelectrophoresis for detection of group B streptococcal antigen in CSF from infants with meningitis. J. Clin. Microbiol. *11*:263–265, 1980.
193. Weiner, M. H., Talbot, G. H., Gerson, S. L., et al.: Antigen detection in the diagnosis of invasive aspergillosis: Utility in controlled, blinded trials. Ann. Intern. Med. *99*:777–782, 1983.
194. Wheat, L. J., Connolly-Stringfield, P., Kohler, R. B., et al.: *Histoplasma capsulatum* polysaccharide antigen detection in diagnosis and management of disseminated histoplasmosis in patients with acquired immunodeficiency syndrome. Am. J. Med. *87*:396–400, 1989.
195. Wheat, L. J., Kohler, R. B., and Tervari, R. P.: Diagnosis of disseminated histoplasmosis by detection of *Histoplasma capsulatum* antigen in serum and urine specimens. N. Engl. J. Med. *314*:83–88, 1986.
196. Whittle, H. C., Greenwood, B. M., Davidson, N. M., et al.: Meningococcal antigen in diagnosis and treatment of group A meningococcal infections. Am. J. Med. *58*:823–828, 1975.
197. Williams, D. L., Gillis, T. P., Booth, R. J., et al.: The use of a specific DNA probe and polymerase chain reaction for the detection of *Mycobacterium leprae*. J. Infect. Dis. *162*:193–200, 1990.
198. Wolfson, J. S., and Swartz, M. N.: Serum bactericidal activity as a monitor of antibiotic therapy. N. Engl. J. Med. *312*:968–975, 1985.
199. Wonsit, R. N., Thammapalerd, N., Tharavanij, S., et al.: Enzyme-linked immunosorbent assay based on monoclonal and polyclonal antibodies for the detection of *Entamoeba histolytica* antigen in faecal specimens. Trans. R. Soc. Trop. Med. Hyg. *86*:166–169, 1992.
200. Woods, C. R., Smith, A. L., Wasilauskas, B. L., et al.: Invasive disease caused by *Neisseria meningitidis* relatively resistant to penicillin in North Carolina. J. Infect. Dis. *170*:453–456, 1994.
201. Wu, T. C., and Koo, S. Y.: Comparison of three commercial cryptococcal latex kits for detection of cryptococcal antigen. J. Clin. Microbiol. *18*:1127–1130, 1983.
202. Yolken, R. H.: Enzyme immunoassays for the detection of infectious antigens in body fluids: Current limitations and future prospects. Rev. Infect. Dis. *4*:35–68, 1982.
203. Zimmerman, S. E., Stringfield, P. C., Wheat, R. B., et al.: Comparison of sandwich solid-phase radioimmunoassay and two enzyme-linked immunosorbent assays for detection of *Histoplasma capsulatum* polysaccharide antigen. J. Infect. Dis. *160*:678–685, 1989.

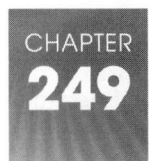

Use of the Diagnostic Virology Laboratory

MARJORIE J. MILLER ■ JAMES D. CHERRY

In the present era of readily available, sophisticated, and complex equipment to aid in medical diagnosis, as well as the availability of exciting new therapeutic programs, a sad note is that practical, clinical, and diagnostic virologic services are available in only a modest number of hospitals and, where available, frequently are not used appropriately by physicians. Because of the present renewed interest in useful viral diagnosis, several innovative methods for the rapid identification of viral infections have been developed. However, laboratories have been supplying useful clinical and viral diagnostic services for more than 30 years. The major problem during the last 3 decades has been the lack of a positive attitude and indoctrination, not the lack of adequate methods.

Clinical bacteriology and mycology evolved slowly over a span of more than a century, whereas virology made a comparable advance in a 10-year period with the advent of tissue culture techniques. Initially, virology developed as a tool of the researcher; during the decade 1950 to 1960, many of the major virus-disease associations that we know today were first recognized, and both polioviruses and measles virus were attenuated for vaccine development. During this period of rapid development, research funds were readily available, so young persons with an interest in virology gravitated to investigative endeavors. Also, hospital clinical microbiology laboratories were operated primarily by persons trained as bacteriologists and pathologists, who in general thought that because the new virologic techniques were so different, introducing them into the setting of a hospital laboratory would be impractical. This idea also was fostered by epidemiologists and researchers. Because of the lack of diagnostic services locally, state and federal facilities instituted viral diagnostic services. In addition, many research programs offered limited diagnostic services for special cases.

Although the services of state laboratories and the research units contributed to our understanding of the spectrum of viral illness, their methods of operation did much to hinder the ultimate development of useful clinical viral diagnostic laboratory services. Because these units were directed by epidemiologists and others interested in the dynamics of disease rather than in individual patients, services were not geared to the welfare of the patient. Specimens were collected routinely from patients, but viral diagnostic procedures were performed only if the physician provided acute- and convalescent-phase sera. This procedure always led to such a delay that most physicians lost interest; they directed their concerns to more pressing problems.

Progress in virology continued at a remarkable rate. However, by the mid-1960s, the major share of research in virology shifted from epidemiologic considerations and clinical disease associations to more basic laboratory virology. With this change in research emphasis, the attitude that we have learned all there is to know about clinical diseases associated with viral infections prevailed. More alarming is the fact that few medical school departments of microbiology presently staff persons qualified to teach the clinical aspects of virology. The result is that few students today receive any practical training in this sphere.

Another aspect that greatly contributes to the lack of and failure to use viral diagnostic services relates to medical economics and the delivery of health care. At present, major research efforts are directed toward health care systems. Although these programs are necessary, all seem flawed. No research program takes into consideration the fact that even the simplest aspect of clinical medicine (such as respiratory infection) is dynamic and not static; most health care evaluation systems seem to assume that nothing more can be learned about routine medical problems. This attitude is deplorable because, of course, we still have much to learn about "simple" problems such as upper respiratory infections. Even more important, care suffers when physicians are denied the chance to be inquisitive about the problems they confront.

Because diagnosis is the foundation of all medical care, justifying an accurate diagnosis of specific viral diseases should be unnecessary. However, as is apparent from the preceding discussion, the values of viral diagnosis need emphasis. Specific reasons why clinical virologic laboratory services should be routinely available are listed in Table 249–1. Routine viral diagnostic laboratories should be similar to bacteriology laboratories and specialize in the identification of specific etiologic agents as rapidly as possible. Serologic study in cases of possible viral disease often can be relegated to reference laboratories, as is done when serologic studies are performed for possible bacterial and fungal infections. At present, some laboratories routinely provide effective viral diagnostic services; laboratory reports of viral isolates reach physicians almost as rapidly as bacterial

TABLE 249–1 ■ WHY CLINICAL VIROLOGIC LABORATORY SERVICES SHOULD BE AVAILABLE ON A ROUTINE BASIS

Knowledge of etiology in the clinical setting tunes the physician's interest and leads to better care.
Knowledge of viral infection reduces inappropriate antibiotic administration.
Knowledge of viral etiology reduces the cost and discomfort of unnecessary diagnostic procedures and lengthy hospital stays.
Virologic diagnosis is critical for the use of presently available antiviral drugs. As new drugs are developed, such diagnosis becomes even more important.
Wider use of viral diagnostic services leads to a better understanding of disease processes: viral-bacterial interactions and the relationship of viruses to "noninfectious diseases" such as myocardial infarction and pancreatitis.
Success and failure of viral vaccines are monitored more accurately.
Better patient awareness results from specific viral study. Patients like to know their illness, and such knowledge can be useful historically when future medical illnesses occur.
More accurate prognosis of disease outcome is possible when the specific etiologic agent is known.
The routine availability and use of viral diagnostic services make the physician more aware of priorities in medical research. The morbidity and mortality associated with specific viral agents, such as respiratory syncytial virus, should lead to interest in the development of new vaccines.

reports do, and charges are similar to those for conventional bacteriologic procedures.[112, 113, 184, 220]

This chapter presents general aspects of viral diagnosis, including specimen selection, collection, and transport; conventional and modified culture for virus isolation and identification; and rapid detection of viral antigens and nucleic acids directly in specimens. Specific aspects of viral diagnosis are presented in the respective chapters covering the particular agents.

Specimen Collection and Transport

Currently, many well-equipped state public health laboratories use traditional as well as more recently developed technologies that should ensure successful recovery of viruses from a high percentage of submitted specimens. However, the isolation rates in these facilities are frequently poor because of suboptimal collection and transport of specimens. In contrast, some small hospital-based laboratories offering a limited variety of procedures often have high isolation rates because of efficient, rapid collection and transport of specimens.

SPECIMEN COLLECTION SITES

The selection of appropriate sites for specimen collection as early in the acute phase of the illness as possible is critical to the recovery of viruses. A guide to recommended collection sites for specific viral syndromes is presented in Table 249–2. In general, the extent of the diagnostic investigation should be dictated by the characteristics of the illness being studied. For example, in common respiratory illnesses such as

TABLE 249–2 ■ SPECIMEN COLLECTION GUIDE FOR THE DIAGNOSIS OF VIRAL INFECTIONS BASED ON THE VIRAL SYNDROME AND ETIOLOGIC AGENT SUSPECTED

		Specimen Collection Source			
Main Location or Category of Illness	**Clinical Diagnosis**	*Most Practical*	*Most Definitive*	**Other Sources**	**Etiologic Agent Suspected***
Upper respiratory tract	Common cold, nasopharyngitis	Nasopharynx/nose	Nasopharynx/nose	Nasal wash, stool, blood	Rhinoviruses, coronaviruses, parainfluenza viruses, respiratory syncytial virus, enteroviruses, adenoviruses
	Pharyngitis	Throat	Throat	Stool, blood	Adenoviruses, enteroviruses, Epstein-Barr virus, influenza viruses, parainfluenza viruses
	Herpangina, other enanthems	Throat	Lesions	Stool, blood	Enteroviruses, herpes simplex virus
	Laryngitis, laryngotracheitis	Throat	Larynx or trachea	Nasal wash	Parainfluenza viruses, influenza viruses
	Parotitis, other salivary gland enlargement	Throat	Stensen duct	Urine, blood, cerebrospinal fluid	Mumps virus, enteroviruses
Lower respiratory tract	Bronchitis, bronchiolitis, pneumonia	Throat	Bronchoalveolar lavage, bronchial washing, biopsy	Stool, blood	Respiratory syncytial virus, parainfluenza viruses, adenoviruses, influenza viruses
	Pleurodynia	Throat	Throat	Stool	Enteroviruses
	Pleural effusion	Pleural fluid	Pleural fluid	Throat, stool, blood	Enteroviruses, adenoviruses
Heart	Myocarditis, pericarditis, conduction defects	Throat	Pericardial fluid, biopsy	Stool, blood, urine	Enteroviruses influenza viruses, adenoviruses
Central nervous system	Meningitis	Throat	Cerebrospinal fluid	Stool, blood, urine	Enteroviruses, mumps virus, arboviruses, herpes simplex virus type 2, lymphocytic choriomeningitis virus
	Encephalitis	Throat	Brain biopsy	Cerebrospinal fluid, stool, blood, urine	Arboviruses, mumps virus, enteroviruses, herpes simplex virus type 1, influenza viruses
	Guillain-Barré syndrome, cerebellar ataxia, transverse myelitis, poliomyelitis	Throat	Throat	Stool, blood, cerebrospinal fluid	Influenza viruses, arboviruses, enteroviruses, Epstein-Barr virus
Genital tract	Orchitis, epididymitis	Throat	Testicular biopsy	Stool, blood, urine	Mumps, enteroviruses, lymphocytic choriomeningitis virus
	Herpes genitalis	Lesions	Lesions	Vagina, cervix, urethra	Herpes simplex virus
Urinary tract	Cytomegalovirus infection	Urine	Urine	Throat, blood	Cytomegalovirus
	Hematuria and/or pyuria	Throat, urine	Urine	Blood, stool	Arboviruses, enteroviruses, mumps virus, adenoviruses

Continued

TABLE 249–2 ■ SPECIMEN COLLECTION GUIDE FOR THE DIAGNOSIS OF VIRAL INFECTIONS BASED ON THE VIRAL SYNDROME AND ETIOLOGIC AGENT SUSPECTED—cont'd

		Specimen Collection Source			
Main Location or Category of Illness	**Clinical Diagnosis**	*Most Practical*	*Most Definitive*	**Other Sources**	**Etiologic Agent Suspected***
Gastrointestinal tract	Nausea and/or vomiting	Throat	Throat	Stool, blood	Enteroviruses, influenza viruses, Norwalk-like agents
	Diarrhea	Stool	Stool	Throat	Rotaviruses, Norwalk-like agents, enteroviruses, adenoviruses
	Abdominal pain	Throat	Throat	Stool, blood	Enteroviruses, adenoviruses
	Acute abdomen, mesenteric adenitis	Throat	Mesenteric lymph node biopsy, peritoneal fluid	Stool, blood	Enteroviruses, adenoviruses
	Hepatitis	Throat	Liver biopsy	Stool, blood	Hepatitis A, B, C, E, and G viruses, Epstein-Barr virus, adenoviruses, enteroviruses, cytomegalovirus
	Pancreatitis	Throat	Duodenal fluid	Stool, blood	Enteroviruses
	Reye syndrome	Throat	Liver biopsy	Blood	Influenza viruses, varicella virus
Reticuloendothelial system	Hepatosplenomegaly	Throat	Blood, liver biopsy	Stool, urine	Adenoviruses, enteroviruses, Epstein-Barr virus, cytomegalovirus
	Generalized lymphadenopathy	Throat	Blood, lymph node biopsy	Stool, urine	Adenoviruses, enteroviruses, Epstein-Barr virus, cytomegalovirus
	Immune deficiency	Blood	Blood	Lymph nodes	HIV
Bone or joints	Osteomyelitis	Bone	Bone	Throat, blood, urine, skin lesion	Rubella virus, vaccinia virus
	Arthritis	Joint fluid	Joint fluid	Throat, blood, urine	Rubella virus, arboviruses
Muscle	Myositis	Throat	Muscle biopsy	Stool, blood	Influenza viruses, enteroviruses
Skin	Exanthematous disease	Throat	Vesicular fluid, skin biopsy	Stool, blood, urine, eye	Measles virus, rubella virus, varicella virus, enteroviruses
Eye	Conjunctivitis, including pharyngoconjunctival fever	Eye	Eye	Throat, stool	Adenoviruses, enteroviruses
Fever	Nonspecific febrile illness (human-to-human transmission)	Throat	Blood	Stool, urine, cerebrospinal fluid	Enteroviruses, influenza viruses, adenoviruses, cytomegalovirus
	Nonspecific febrile illness (arthropod vector)	Blood	Blood	Throat, urine, cerebrospinal fluid	Arboviruses
	Fever of unknown origin	Blood	Blood	Urine, stool, throat	Hepatitis A, B, C, E, and G viruses, cytomegalovirus, herpes simplex virus, Epstein-Barr virus, adenoviruses
Congenital infection	Rubella virus, cytomegalovirus infections	Throat	Blood	Urine, nasopharynx, biopsy material, cerebrospinal fluid	Rubella virus, cytomegalovirus
	HIV infection	Blood	Blood	Lymph node	HIV
Perinatal and neonatal infections	Herpes simplex virus, cytomegalovirus, enterovirus infections	Throat	Blood	Urine, nasopharynx, stool, skin lesions, cerebrospinal fluid	Enteroviruses, respiratory syncytial virus, influenza viruses, herpes simplex virus, cytomegalovirus

*This listing includes only the more commonly associated agents; it is likely that with more general use of viral diagnostic services, new virus-disease associations will be made.

pharyngitis or croup, collection of a single specimen from the throat is all that is usually necessary. In other situations in which an illness is severe or unique, collection of specimens from multiple sites is important. In addition, in unusual cases, serum should be obtained for frozen storage in case subsequent serologic studies are required.

In unusual and severe illnesses, invasive procedures (e.g., brain, cardiac, liver, lung biopsies; needle aspiration of body fluids) are frequently necessary to obtain material for laboratory study. Many medical specialists argue against using these invasive procedures because little can be done to treat viral illnesses. However, in our experience, the knowledge gained from a positive viral identification justifies some risk incurred in collecting specimens. At present, antiviral drugs are similar to antibacterial and antifungal agents in that they generally can be used effectively only after definitive identification of the etiologic agent. Demonstration of a viral etiologic agent in diseases such as encephalitis, pneumonia, or cardiac disease can prevent the unnecessary administration of antibiotics and steroids. In many cases, overutilization of services, patient trauma, and overall cost can be reduced when a viral etiologic agent is confirmed. Finally, the prognosis of a particular illness is more accurate when the specific etiologic agent is known.

COLLECTION OF SPECIMENS

Specimens for virus culture or direct examination generally are obtained as for other microbiologic studies. The primary purpose of a transport medium is to provide a protective protein, neutral pH, and antibiotics for control of microbial contamination and, most importantly, for prevention of desiccation. Many viral transport and storage media are available commercially or are prepared readily in the laboratory; their utility has been reviewed.[13, 41, 134] Convenient and practical collection devices, such as the Culturette (Becton Dickinson, Cockeysville, MD) or the Virocult (Medical Wire and Equipment Co., Victory Gardens, NY), consist of a swab, usually Dacron or rayon, on a plastic or aluminum shaft accompanied by a self-contained transport medium (Stuart or Amies), and they are routinely available in most hospitals for bacteriologic culture. Calcium alginate swabs, which are toxic to herpes simplex virus (HSV), and wooden shafts, which may be toxic to viruses as well as the cell culture system itself, should not be used. Saline or holding media that contain serum also should be avoided. Useful liquid transport media (2-mL aliquots in screw-capped vials) consist of tryptose phosphate broth with 0.5 percent bovine albumin; Hanks balanced salt solution with 5 percent gelatin or 10 percent bovine albumin; or buffered sucrose phosphate (0.2 mol/L, 2-SP),[118, 134] which has been used as a combined transport medium for viral, chlamydial, and mycoplasmal culture requests[269] and is appropriate for long-term frozen storage of specimens and isolates.[118]

Some of these transport media also have been evaluated and found acceptable for use in rapid methods (e.g., enzyme-linked immunosorbent assay [ELISA][209, 305] and polymerase chain reaction [PCR]).[190]

Throat

Specimens from the throat should be obtained with a swab in a manner similar to that used for bacterial culture. The posterior pharyngeal wall and tonsillar surfaces, any inflamed or erythematous areas, and any visible lesions are swabbed firmly without contact with the tongue and anterior oral cavity.

Nose and Nasopharynx

Specimens should be collected with nasopharyngeal swabs that have thin, flexible wire shafts by inserting the swab into the nasopharynx and rotating it to obtain the maximal number of ciliated, columnar epithelial cells and then placing the swab in transport medium. Alternatively, a flexible nasal probe with a cupped tip may be used (Rhinoprobe, Rhinotechnics, San Diego, CA).[131, 309] Nasopharyngeal cultures can be obtained from infants by the wash technique described by Hall and Douglas.[106] In this method, a small amount of sterile phosphate-buffered saline (3 to 7 mL) is squeezed into the nose with a nasal bulb aspirator (1 oz, tapered) and then immediately withdrawn and placed in a sterile, screw-capped container. Alternatively, nasopharyngeal aspirates may be obtained with a mucus collection device. An appropriately sized catheter is inserted nasally into the posterior of the nasopharynx; intermittent suction is applied as the catheter is withdrawn. Aspirate is washed through the tubing with 5 to 8 mL of transport medium or sterile phosphate-buffered saline. Washes and aspirates (versus swabs) are preferred for direct antigen detection because more epithelial cells are obtained with this method.[3]

Other Respiratory Specimens (Sputum, Tracheal Aspirates, Bronchial Washings, Bronchoalveolar Lavage)

Collection depends on the volume obtained. Volumes of 0.5 mL or larger should be placed in a sterile container and sealed tightly. If the volume is less than 0.5 mL, the specimen is placed in 2 mL of transport medium.

Eye

Exudate or pus should be removed first with a sterile swab. Conjunctival specimens may be obtained by pressing a swab premoistened with sterile saline firmly against the inflamed areas. The swab is returned to the self-contained transport device, or the tip is broken off into 2 mL of transport medium. Corneal scrapings should be obtained by an ophthalmologist or other trained person and placed in transport medium immediately.

Body Fluids Other Than Blood

Body fluids such as urine (clean voided, 10 to 20 mL), cerebrospinal fluid (CSF) (2 to 5 mL), pleural effusion, and peritoneal, pericardial, or joint fluid should be collected under sterile conditions and placed in securely sealed, sterile containers. For small volumes (<0.5 mL), the specimen may be placed in transport medium.

Lesions

For lesions, fresh vesicles should be selected because recovery of virus from older lesions decreases significantly. Gently swab the area with sterile saline. Rupture the vesicle and collect both fluid and cells from the base of the lesion. Material obtained from several lesions may be pooled. Desiccation must not be allowed to occur; swabs should be submitted moistened with their self-contained transport medium or, if that is unavailable, placed in 2 mL of transport medium. Specimens may be collected with a swab or aspirated with a 26-gauge needle attached to a tuberculin syringe. Aspirated fluid should be rinsed into 1 to 2 mL of transport medium.

For direct antigen detection by immunofluorescence (IF) (direct fluorescent antibody [DFA]), the vesicle is ruptured as previously described and epithelial cells are collected by firmly swabbing the base of the lesion. Cells are transferred to a clean glass slide by firmly rolling the swab back and forth over a 5- to 10-mm area (dime size); for differentiation of HSV types 1 and 2 (HSV-1 and HSV-2) and varicella-zoster virus (VZV), three areas should be prepared.

Stool and Rectal Specimens

Because of initial studies with polioviruses and other enteroviruses, culture of fecal material has been overemphasized in virology. Both enteroviruses and adenoviruses can be recovered readily from stool, but because these agents are carried in the lower gastrointestinal tract for considerable periods after acute infection, use of this source for the diagnosis of specific illnesses is limited. A specimen of fecal material is practical only when the specific primary diagnosis is diarrhea or when concomitant serologic study with paired sera can be performed.

For recovery of enteroviruses, fresh stool specimens are better than rectal swabs; transfer 2 to 5 g (2 to 3 tsp) of formed or liquid specimen to a sterile, leak-proof container. However, from a practical point of view, a rectal swab is the simplest method of specimen collection. A rectal swab can be obtained immediately, whereas collection of a stool specimen usually entails considerable delay. Of importance is that the swab contain visible stool; insert the swab 3 to 5 cm into the rectum, roll the swab against the mucosa, and then transport in a Culturette or similar device.

Blood

Some viruses can be recovered from serum or red blood cells (RBCs), but in general, leukocytes are a better source of virus. Fresh blood (optimally 5 mL) is collected in a suitable anticoagulant (heparin, ethylenediaminetetraacetic acid [EDTA], acid citrate dextrose) and transported to the laboratory for processing by density gradient centrifugation[119] or other methods to enrich for leukocytes. EDTA is the anticoagulant of choice because it is an acceptable transport for culture as well as molecular methods such as hybridization and PCR.

Bone Marrow

Aspirate about 2 mL into a tube or syringe containing heparin anticoagulant, mix thoroughly to prevent clotting, and transport without further additives or diluents.

Biopsy Specimens

For biopsy specimens, fresh tissue obtained from the affected site should be placed in 2 mL of transport medium to prevent desiccation.

Autopsy Specimens

Most postmortem specimens are almost useless for viral cultivation because of the manner in which autopsies usually are performed. If labile agents are to be recovered, the autopsy should be performed within 4 hours of death. All tissues (1- to 2.5-cm cubes) for study should be obtained aseptically, and individual tissue should be collected with sterile instruments and placed in separate sterile containers. Because the usual autopsy routine entails fixation of specimens, of vital importance is that specimens for viral isolation not be placed in containers with fixatives such as formalin or other preservatives.

TRANSPORT TO THE LABORATORY

The method of handling specimens from the time of collection to laboratory processing is critical for preservation of virus infectivity and subsequent recovery in culture. In general, the less time that transpires between collection and inoculation into cell culture, the greater the chance of virus recovery. Specimens should not be frozen or exposed to temperatures higher than 22° C. For short-term storage (<5 days) of most viruses, the specimen should be held at 4° C until it can be processed in the laboratory. For transport to the laboratory, this temperature can be achieved with the use of cold packs or simply by placing one ice cube next to the specimen container within an aluminum foil wrapping.

Although the degree of sensitivity varies, all viruses are inactivated by ultraviolet light. Therefore, shielding specimens from sunlight is important and can be accomplished by using opaque transport boxes or wrapping individual specimens in aluminum foil or opaque paper.

When considerable delay between collection and culture will elapse (transport to other laboratories, holiday schedules, and so on), special preparation is necessary. Such preparation needs to be individualized and based on the most likely viral cause of a particular illness. For example, when an enteroviral etiologic agent is suspected, freezing the specimen (−70° C) and shipping with dry ice are satisfactory. In contrast, a urine specimen from a patient with possible cytomegalovirus (CMV) infection should not be frozen. It should be shipped under wet ice at 4° C because CMV in urine is stable for several days at this temperature. In addition, media that protect viruses against the deleterious effects of temperature fluctuations, particularly freeze-thawing, are available for transport as well as long-term storage.[118, 134] For specific characteristics of individual viruses, see Chapters 157 to 193 and the general references at the end of this chapter.[165, 198, 258, 271]

Laboratory Diagnosis of Viral Infections

Previously, the perception that isolation of virus was difficult, nonproductive, and too slow to be of clinical utility, combined with the lack of consistently available reliable reagents, discouraged the use of diagnostic virology services. Since the mid-1980s, a dramatic increase has occurred in the quality and availability of diagnostic reagents, primarily monoclonal antibodies, which has significantly improved the turnaround time of reporting virology results. Direct detection of viral antigens in clinical specimens—for example, the herpes group viruses (HSV, VZV, CMV), respiratory syncytial virus (RSV), influenza viruses, adenoviruses, and rotaviruses, usually by IF, an immunoperoxidase (IP) test, or ELISA—has become routine and has made obtaining same-day results a reality. In addition, detection of viral antigens in cell culture by the application of IF/IP staining or ELISA, before the appearance of cytopathic effect (CPE), has greatly reduced the time needed to report a positive result. More recently, molecular techniques for the direct detection and quantitation of viral nucleic acids in specimens[60, 129, 217] have begun the transition from research tool to routine use in the clinical laboratory as commercial reagents become readily available, methods are simplified and standardized, and some assays are manufactured in kit format. Methods for the laboratory diagnosis of specific viral infections are presented in Chapters 157 to 193, and detailed methods are provided in the general references at the end of this chapter.[129, 165, 198, 237, 258, 271] Table 249–3 summarizes specific methods for the laboratory identification of viruses, in addition to indications for serologic study of selected viruses.

VIRUS ISOLATION

Despite technologic advances and innovations, culture remains the cornerstone of the diagnostic virology laboratory. Culture still is among the most sensitive of diagnostic methods because theoretically, a single infectious virus can be detected. Unlike rapid methods, which are limited to the detection of a specific viral antigen or nucleic acid, culture is open ended and permits the detection of unexpected viruses, new viruses, or multiple viruses within the same specimen. In addition, a broad range of specimens can be evaluated, whereas rapid methods usually are approved or licensed for use with specimens collected from specific sites. Viruses that can be isolated and identified readily include adenoviruses,

TABLE 249–3 ■ COMMON LABORATORY METHODS FOR VIRUS ISOLATION, IDENTIFICATION, AND DIRECT DETECTION AND MOST USEFUL METHOD FOR DIAGNOSIS OF SPECIFIC VIRAL ILLNESSES

	Culture/Direct Detection	Identification of Isolates	Serology	Most Useful Method for Diagnosis of Specific Viral Illness
Adenoviruses	Primary HEK, A549, WI-38, HEp-2, HeLa, KB cell culture/FA, ELISA	Group identified by characteristic CPE and/or FA; type identified by neutralization with specific antiserum	CF on paired sera, ELISA, HAI	Virus isolation
Arboviruses of North America	Suckling mouse intracerebral inoculation, Vero, BHK-21, LLC-MK2 cell culture	Neutralization with specific antiserum	CF on paired sera, HAI, indirect FA, IgM antibody capture ELISA	CF on paired sera
Coronaviruses	Human embryo tracheal organ culture, HEK	Neutralization with specific antiserum	Neutralization, CF, HAI on paired sera	No practical method presently available
Rhinoviruses	WI-38, MRC-5 cell culture	Characteristic CPE; stability on exposure to lipid solvents and inactivation at pH 3	Neutralization on paired sera	Virus isolation
Enteroviruses	MK, WI-38 cell culture, suckling mouse inoculation (intracerebral and intraperitoneal)/ PCR	Group identified by characteristic CPE in cell culture or illness or pathology in mice; type identified by neutralization with specific antiserum; FA for some serotypes	Neutralization, CF, HAI on paired sera	Virus isolation
Cytomegalovirus	WI-38, MRC-5, foreskin cell culture/FA, IP, PCR, hybrid capture	Characteristic CPE; FA/IP for definitive identification	CF on paired sera, ELISA, LA, indirect FA	Virus isolation
Epstein-Barr virus (EBV)	Practical method not available/PCR	Practical method not available	Indirect FA against viral capsid antigen on paired sera; indirect FA against early antigen in single serum	Infectious mononucleosis rapid slide tests; rarely, EBV-specific FA test
Herpes simplex viruses	WI-38, MRC-5, primary RK cell culture/FA, IP, ELISA, PCR	Characteristic CPE; FA, IP, ELISA for definitive identification	CF on paired sera, ELISA, indirect FA	Virus isolation; antigen detection by FA, ELISA
HIV	ELISA, PCR, bDNA	ELISA, Western blot	ELISA, Western blot, indirect FA	ELISA
Influenza viruses	MK, LLC-MK2, MDCK cell culture and chicken embryo (amniotic sac and allantoic cavity) inoculation/FA, ELISA	HA or hemadsorption of guinea pig or chicken erythrocytes and inhibition with specific antiserum for type/strain identification; FA for identification of type	CF, HAI; ELISA on paired sera	Virus isolation; antigen detection by FA, ELISA
Measles virus	Primary MK, HEK cell culture/FA	Hemadsorption and HA of monkey erythrocytes and inhibition with specific antiserum or identification by FA	CF, HAI on paired sera; identification of measles-specific IgM antibody by ELISA, indirect FA	Identification of measles-specific IgM antibody by ELISA, indirect FA or CF/HAI antibody titer rise
Parainfluenza viruses, mumps virus	Primary MK, LLC-MK2, HEK cell culture/FA	Hemadsorption and HA of guinea pig erythrocytes; specific identification by FA	CF, HAI on paired sera, ELISA, indirect FA	Virus isolation; antigen detection by FA
Respiratory syncytial virus	HEp-2, WI-38 cell culture/FA, ELISA	Characteristic CPE in absence of hemadsorption; specific identification by FA	CF on paired sera, ELISA, indirect FA	Detection of viral antigen by FA/ELISA; virus isolation

Continued

TABLE 249–3 ■ COMMON LABORATORY METHODS FOR VIRUS ISOLATION, IDENTIFICATION, AND DIRECT DETECTION AND MOST USEFUL METHOD FOR DIAGNOSIS OF SPECIFIC VIRAL ILLNESSES—cont'd

	Culture/Direct Detection	Identification of Isolates	Serology	Most Useful Method for Diagnosis of Specific Viral Illness
Rabies virus (animal infections)	Demonstration of Negri bodies by microscopic examination of brain or demonstration of viral antigen by FA, mouse inoculation	Demonstration of Negri bodies or antigen by FA	Neutralization, ELISA	Antigen detection by FA
Reoviruses	Primary MK, HEK, HeLa cell culture/EM	CPE; neutralization with specific antiserum; HAI, FA	Neutralization, HAI on paired sera	Virus isolation
Rubella virus	African green monkey kidney cell culture	Interference of enteroviral CPE, neutralization with specific antiserum	HAI on paired sera; identification of rubella-specific IgM antibody by ELISA, indirect FA	Identification of rubella-specific IgM antibody by ELISA, indirect FA or HAI antibody titer rise
Poxviruses	MK, WI-38 cell culture/FA, EM	Characteristic CPE; FA or appearance on EM	Not useful for diagnosis	Antigen detection by FA, EM
Varicella-zoster virus	WI-38, MRC-5 cell culture/FA, PCR	Characteristic CPE; FA for definitive identification	CF on paired sera, EIA, LA, IHA, IAHA, ACIF, FAMA	Detection of viral antigen by FA; virus isolation
Hepatitis A virus	Demonstration of antigen by ELISA, IEM, RIA	ELISA, IEM, RIA	ELISA, RIA, HAI	Identification of HAV-specific IgM by ELISA, RIA
Hepatitis B virus	Demonstration of antigen by ELISA, RIA, HA; demonstration of DNA by hybridization, PCR	ELISA, RIA, HA	ELISA, RIA, HA	Demonstration of antigen, nucleic acid
Hepatitis C virus	Demonstration of RNA by PCR or bDNA	Practical method not available	ELISA, RIBA	ELISA, RIBA, demonstration of viral RNA
Norwalk-like agents	Demonstration of antigen by IEM, RIA	IEM, RIA	ELISA, RIA-BL; serology not used routinely	Demonstration of antigen
Rotavirus	Demonstration of antigen by ELISA, LA, EM	EM, ELISA	ELISA; serology not used routinely	Demonstration of antigen
Adenovirus 40/41	Demonstration of antigens by ELISA	ELISA	CF, ELISA on paired sera; serology not used routinely	Demonstration of antigen

For details, see Chapters 173 to 193.

ACIF, anticomplement immunofluorescence; A549, human lung carcinoma; bDNA, branched-chain DNA; BHK-21, continuous baby hamster kidney cell line; CF, complement fixation; CPE, cytopathic effect; ELISA, enzyme-linked immunosorbent assay; EM, electron microscopy; FA, immunofluorescent antibody; FAMA, fluorescent antibody to membrane antigen; HA, hemagglutination; HAI, hemagglutination inhibition; HAV, hepatitis A virus; HEK, human embryonic kidney; HEp-2, human laryngeal carcinoma cells; IAHA, immune adherence hemagglutination assay; IEM, immune electron microscopy; IHA, indirect hemagglutination; IP, immunoperoxidase test; KB, oral cavity carcinoma; LA, latex agglutination; LLC-MK2, continuous line of rhesus MK; MDCK, Madin-Darby canine kidney; MK, monkey kidney; PCR, polymerase chain reaction; RIA, radioimmunoassay; RIA-BL, radioimmunoassay blocking test; RIBA, recombinant immunoblot assay; RK, rabbit kidney; Vero, continuous line of African green MK; WI-38, MRC-5, human fetal diploid lung fibroblasts.

HSV, VZV, CMV, enteroviruses, rhinoviruses, influenza and parainfluenza viruses, RSV, rubella virus, mumps virus, and measles virus. The number and type of isolates encountered depend on the patient population, season, and type of specimens submitted. For optimal laboratory diagnosis, indicating the virus suspected on the requisition is important because some viruses require specific cell lines, procedures for identification, or both. Cultures are maintained for different time frames before finalizing a report of negative results, depending on the virus being sought; for example, HSV cultures usually are observed for 5 to 7 days, CMV for 1 month, and all others for 2 to 4 weeks. Improvements and modifications in culture methods have resulted in more rapid identification of isolates, with greater than 70 percent being reported within 5 days.[58, 124]

Traditional Culture

Although animals such as suckling mice and chicken embryos originally were the only means of isolating viruses, most laboratories now use cell culture exclusively. A variety of cell lines capable of supporting the growth of a broad spectrum of viruses can be obtained fresh weekly from commercial sources. After inoculation of the specimen, cultures are observed at regular intervals for evidence of viral infection characterized by the appearance of CPE or the ability to hemadsorb or hemagglutinate RBCs. Adenoviruses, CMV, HSV, VZV, rhinoviruses, and enteroviruses can be identified and reported by their characteristic CPE. The mean time between inoculation of a specimen and the appearance of CPE is usually 1 week or less for most of this group except CMV and some adenoviruses, which may require longer incubation. Cultures containing HSV and enteroviruses are often positive within 1 to 2 and 3 to 5 days, respectively. In the event of atypical or questionable CPE, IF with monoclonal antibodies can be used to identify CMV, VZV, HSV-1, HSV-2, adenoviruses, enteroviruses, and some select coxsackieviruses and echoviruses in infected cell cultures. Though rarely performed, the neutralization test is used to definitively identify adenoviruses and enteroviruses if serotyping is requested for epidemiologic or other reasons.[129, 258]

Respiratory viruses, including parainfluenza and influenza viruses, which may or may not produce CPE, generally can be detected within 5 to 7 days of specimen inoculation with the traditional hemadsorption method, in which a suspension of guinea pig RBCs is added to the cell culture. The RBCs are observed to adhere to tissue culture cells infected with these viruses, usually 3 to 5 days after the inoculation of specimens for most isolates.[196] An adaptation of this method uses cell culture medium and guinea pig RBCs in a microtiter plate format to detect viral hemagglutinins in suspension. The results are similar to those observed with hemadsorption, but the adapted method is more rapid and simple to perform when screening numerous specimens.[138] RSV is identified presumptively, usually within 3 to 5 days of specimen inoculation, by its typical CPE (syncytium formation) and inability to hemadsorb/hemagglutinate guinea pig RBCs. This group of viruses is identified definitively by IF with monoclonal antibodies.[129, 258]

Finally, the traditional method for isolation and identification of rubella virus uses primary African green monkey kidney cells in conjunction with the interference assay. After specified intervals following inoculation, cultures are challenged with a second virus, usually echovirus 11, incubated for an additional 3 to 4 days, and examined for CPE. The presence of rubella virus interferes with growth of the challenge virus, and no CPE is observed; on the other hand, if the challenge virus grows and produces CPE, the specimen is considered negative for rubella virus. Final identification of the isolate requires neutralization of the interference with specific rubella antibody.[198, 258]

Serologic diagnosis is recommended for viruses that are difficult or impossible to isolate in commonly available cell cultures or that require special techniques for detection of their presence. For instance, in most cases of arbovirus infection, the study of paired sera for antibody development is the most rewarding for diagnosis. Human immunodeficiency virus (HIV) infection generally is identified best by the demonstration of serum antibody or antigen with the use of ELISA. Measles virus is relatively difficult to grow, and identification can take considerable time; when measles is suspected, the diagnosis is confirmed most easily by serologic study. Paired sera collected 1 week apart usually reveal a fourfold antibody titer rise. Alternatively, demonstration of specific IgM antibody allows diagnosis with the use of a single serum sample. Similarly, serology is useful for the diagnosis of mumps virus. Although mumps virus can be isolated in the same cell lines used for other paramyxoviruses and detected by hemadsorption/hemagglutination as previously described, such requests are rare. Rubella virus requires 2 or more weeks for isolation and specific identification. Because of this delay, rubella virus infection, other than that acquired congenitally, is confirmed best by serologic study. In all instances of suspected congenital rubella, virus isolation should be attempted.

Modified Culture

A variety of physical and chemical methods have been evaluated for their ability to enhance the rapid detection of virus in culture.[124] These methods include the effect of low- and high-speed rolling of cultures, centrifugation, chemicals such as dimethyl sulfoxide, hormones such as dexamethasone, and enzymes such as trypsin on the isolation of viruses. Early detection of viral antigens in culture by IF and IP, before the appearance of CPE, also has been evaluated.[79, 191, 221, 243] A technique that entails the physical method of centrifugation with early antigen detection in cell culture and is called variously the shell vial assay (SVA), the spin-amplified technique, or culture-amplified antigen detection is used routinely in most laboratories to decrease the time to detection of a positive culture. Cell lines are propagated on 12-mm round coverslips in 1-dram shell vials. An aliquot of specimen is inoculated into the vial, centrifuged at 700×*g* for 1 hour, and incubated 1 to 3 days, depending on the virus being sought. Antigen typically is detected by IF or occasionally by IP staining with monoclonal antibodies directed against a specific virus.

SVA was described initially and evaluated extensively for HSV[78, 98, 173, 219, 224, 247] and CMV,[80, 92, 96, 97, 164, 214, 215, 229] and its use since has been extended to the rapid identification of VZV,[93, 255] adenovirus,[8, 69, 174, 291] RSV,[20, 268] influenza virus,[75, 193, 262, 277] parainfluenza virus,[254] and measles virus[194] antigens in culture. Pooled antibodies directed against seven commonly isolated respiratory viruses (adenovirus, influenza viruses A and B, parainfluenza virus types 1, 2, and 3, and RSV) also have been evaluated.[180, 210, 228] In addition, SVA has been applied to the detection of enteroviruses[146, 168] and human herpesvirus type 6.[188] Recently, the application of mixed cell lines in tube and shell vial culture has resulted in several improvements in isolation of virus. Combination cell lines in a single tube or shell vial broaden the range of culturable viruses, reduce the requirement for multiple single cell lines, and decrease the time to detection of a positive result, with sensitivity similar to that of conventional culture. Mixed cell lines are useful for rapid isolation of respiratory viruses,[11, 82, 122, 324] enteroviruses,[10, 85, 123] and herpes group viruses.[121] The sensitivity of mixed cell versus conventional single cell lines for virus detection ranges from 92 to 100 percent for respiratory viruses[11, 82, 122, 324] to 85 to 97 percent for enteroviruses,[85, 123] with time to detection of a positive result reduced from an average of 5 to 10 days to 1 to 2 days for respiratory viruses and 1 to 3 days for enteroviruses.

Though rapid, sensitive, and specific, SVA is an adjunct to and not a substitute for traditional culture. When compared with traditional culture, the sensitivity of SVA averages approximately 85 percent (range, 70–100%) and depends on numerous variables, including the cell line,[333] the age of cells,[80] the concentration of virus,[333] the type of specimen,[164, 214] the number of vials inoculated,[214] and the type of reagents used.[73, 98, 191, 219, 247] Table 249–4 summarizes the typical time to detection of a positive result in traditional culture and SVA, the sensitivity of SVA versus culture, and the turnaround time for each.

Other culture modifications include hybridization[73, 84] and ELISA[8, 55, 187, 306, 313] for rapid detection of viruses. A modification of cell culture for the rapid detection of HSV is the enzyme-linked virus-inducible system (ELVIS).[273, 274] This system consists of a mixture of modified baby hamster kidney cells and MRC-5 cells. The modified baby hamster kidney cells contain an HSV-inducible promoter and an *Escherichia coli LacZ* reporter gene that produces β-galactosidase only when cells are infected with HSV. After the addition of a substrate for the β-galactosidase, infected cells stain blue whereas uninfected cells remain colorless. ELVIS appears to be comparable to culture for the detection of HSV-positive specimens (95–100% sensitivity) in a similar time frame, 1.4 to 1.7 days.[34, 177] This system may have future application in antiviral susceptibility testing.[260]

TABLE 249–4 ■ DETECTION OF VIRUS IN TRADITIONAL CULTURE AND SHELL VIAL ASSAY

	Traditional Culture		Shell Vial Assay	
Virus	*Usual Day Positive, Range*	*Negative Turnaround Time*	*Day Stained (Range)*	*% Sensitivity vs. Culture*
Adenovirus	4–10	2–3 wk	2 (1–3)	92–100
CMV	7–14	1 mo	2 (1–3)	75–100
Enterovirus	1–7	2–3 wk	3	85–100
HSV	1–3	5–7 days	1	70–100
HHV-6	NA	2–3 wk	3 (2–3)	86
Influenza	3–7	2–3 wk	2 (1–3)	92–100
Parainfluenza	3–7	2–3 wk	2 (1–3)	92–100
RSV	3–7	2–3 wk	2 (1–3)	92–100
VZV	5–10	2–3 wk	3 (2–5)	80–100

CMV, cytomegalovirus; HHV-6, human herpesvirus type 6; HSV, herpes simplex virus; RSV, respiratory syncytial virus; VZV, varicella-zoster virus.

DIRECT DETECTION

Cytology

Historically, rapid detection of viral infection relied on light microscopy and evaluation of tissues and exfoliated cells for viral inclusions or other CPEs. Cytologic identification of virus is most useful in illnesses with vesicular exanthems, such as HSV or VZV infection. A scraping of the base of an HSV or VZV lesion (Tzanck smear) reveals multinucleated giant and balloon cells when stained with hematoxylin and eosin, Wright, or Giemsa stain. In contrast, vesicular lesions caused by enteroviral infections do not contain giant or balloon cells, and allergy-related lesions contain eosinophils. Cytologic study of urine in congenital CMV infection reveals cells with the characteristic "owl's eye" intranuclear inclusions in 25 to 50 percent of cases, and nasal or pharyngeal smears in measles may reveal typical giant cells (see Fig. 183–5). These types of stains no longer are performed routinely in most diagnostic virology laboratories because they have been replaced by IF, which is more sensitive and specific.[37, 38] Whereas the Tzanck smear cannot differentiate HSV from VZV and the presence of multinucleated giant cells is necessary to make the diagnosis, IF can identify the causative agent specifically, and the presence of viral antigen in balloon or giant cells is diagnostic.

Antigen Detection

Antigen-detection methods are available for most commonly isolated viruses. Advantages of these methods include speed; the use of standardized reagents and kits; the ability to detect nonviable, nonculturable, or difficult-to-grow viruses; and the ability to detect antigen when culture may be negative late in the course of infection. Generally, for viruses that can be cultured, these methods are not as sensitive as optimized culture; thus, culture backup is recommended. These tests also are approved for specific specimen types. DFA, indirect immunofluorescent assay (IFA), and ELISA are used most commonly for antigen detection in the clinical laboratory.

Immunofluorescence

Antigen detection by IF requires collection of the appropriate cell types (i.e., those in which the virus propagates) in adequate numbers for evaluation. In some cases, the specimen is placed on the slide directly (e.g., HSV or VZV detection), but usually the sample is transported to the laboratory for processing and slide preparation (e.g., for respiratory virus detection).

DFA methods use a virus-specific monoclonal antibody labeled with fluorescein dye to detect antigen and usually require approximately 30 to 45 minutes to complete. If processing of the specimen is required and slides are prepared in the laboratory, additional time is necessary. For IFA, unlabeled monoclonal antibody is added to the sample and incubated for 30 minutes, followed by a wash and the addition of fluorescein-labeled antimouse immunoglobulin. After an additional 30 minutes' incubation and a wash step, the slide can be examined for typical fluorescence (for excellent photographic examples, see Rossier and colleagues[237]). IFA can be completed in 2 to 3 hours, depending on specimen-processing requirements and the number of viral antigens being sought. The advantage of using DFA or IFA is the ability to determine specimen adequacy and perform small-batch and demand testing. A high-quality microscope and skilled, experienced personnel are required for optimal preparation and evaluation of the specimen.

The first DFA reagent available for use in the diagnostic laboratory was for the detection of HSV[99] in genital, dermal, oral, and anal lesions. The test has not been validated for the detection of HSV in CSF, asymptomatic genital specimens, tracheal aspirates, or bronchoalveolar lavage (BAL) specimens from immunocompromised patients. The sensitivity of DFA versus culture for HSV detection ranges from 72 to 92 percent[153, 223] and, like culture, depends on the stage of the lesion.[37, 38] The ability to detect HSV by DFA or culture decreases with the stage and age of the lesion. DFA or culture detected HSV in 96.7 percent of vesicles, 79.2 percent of pustules, 44.7 percent of ulcers, and 16.7 percent of crusts; HSV was detected in 82 percent of lesions less than 24 hours old, 77 percent of lesions 25 to 72 hours old, 50 percent of lesions 73 to 121 hours old, and 15 percent of lesions older than 122 hours.[37]

DFA is an excellent method for detecting VZV in lesion material, and because the virus is labile, the sensitivity of DFA is superior to that of culture.[33, 59, 93, 255, 259] In a comparison of DFA and culture for the detection of VZV in skin lesions, the sensitivity and negative predictive values were 97.5 and 96.8 percent for DFA and 49.4 and 60.4 percent for culture, respectively. Because of the sensitivity of DFA, culture backup is not necessary.

Rapid detection of CMV antigen in lung tissue or BAL specimens[64, 105, 175, 308, 315] and in liver tissue[213] for the diagnosis of CMV pneumonia or hepatitis also has been evaluated. The sensitivity is less than that of culture or SVA and ranges from 56 to 100 percent; results were best when a mixture of antibodies directed against early and late viral antigens was used.[308] Sensitivity may be reduced further because BAL specimens virtually have replaced lung biopsy for the diagnosis of CMV pneumonia. A comparison of the cellular portion, supernate, and whole BAL for isolation of CMV in culture suggested that in most BAL specimens, CMV is associated with the cell-free rather than the cellular component.[32]

The antigenemia assay[302, 303] is a sensitive, specific, and rapid method for detecting CMV viremia. Antigenemia has been used for the early diagnosis of CMV infection[67, 68, 158]; to monitor patients at high risk for acquiring CMV disease, including bone marrow,[16] heart transplant,[91] renal transplant,[301] and liver transplant patients,[299] as well as those with acquired immunodeficiency syndrome (AIDS)[181]; and to monitor the treatment of severe disease after organ transplantation.[91, 300] Clinically, it has been useful in detecting infection before the onset of symptoms, and through quantitation

TABLE 249–5 ■ SUMMARY OF RAPID INFLUENZA A AND B ASSAYS

	Directigen Flu A	Directigen Flu A + B	FLU OIA	ZstatFlu	QuickVue
Manufacturer	Becton Dickinson	Becton Dickinson	Biostar, Inc	ZymeTx, Inc	Quidel Corp
Detects influenza	A	A and B	A/B*	A/B	A/B
Acceptable specimens	NP wash/aspirate; NP, throat swab	Same as Flu A plus lower nasal swab, BAL	Nasal aspirate, NP swab, throat swab, sputum	Throat swab	Nasal wash, aspirate, or swab
Specimen storage	2–8° C	2–8° C	2–8° C, 24 hr	0–40° C, 24 hr	2–8° C, 1 hr
Assay time	15–20 min	15–20 min	15–20 min	20–30 min	10–15 min
Sensitivity	64–90%	47–86%	54–88%	41–87%	73–94%
Specificity	80–100%	90–100%	52–97%	90–100%	90–98%
References	139, 155, 208, 245, 311	244, 281	19, 39, 115	108, 208	9, 244

*A/B, does not differentiate A from B.
BAL, bronchoalveolar lavage.

of viral load it has enabled differentiation of disease from asymptomatic infection.[89, 156, 288] The assay consists of separation of leukocytes from whole blood, spotting or cytocentrifuging of cells onto microscope slides, fixation and permeabilization, staining with monoclonal antibodies, and detection by fluorescein- or peroxidase-labeled secondary antibodies. Antigen-positive leukocytes are quantitated. Once the assay was optimized,[17, 89, 90] standardized IFA[158] and IP[67, 68] kits became available commercially. Antigenemia is more sensitive than traditional culture or SVA for detecting CMV viremia. Antigenemia results were positive in 91 percent (90 of 99) of confirmed active CMV infections as compared with 34 percent (34 of 99) for culture[158]; another study yielded similar antigenemia results: 91 percent sensitivity versus 66 and 57 percent sensitivity for culture and SVA, respectively.[68] Disadvantages of the assay are that it is labor-intensive, time-consuming, and subjective; the leukocyte suspension must be adjusted to 10^6/mL, and the specimen must be processed quickly because storage for longer than 6 hours results in inaccurate quantitation of positive cells.[17, 156]

Finally, DFA and IFA are useful for the rapid detection of common respiratory virus antigens[183, 185, 231, 270, 279, 310, 312, 321] in nasopharyngeal washes, aspirates, and suctions. DFA for RSV has been evaluated extensively,[27, 140, 183, 195, 231, 279, 289] and its sensitivity in comparison to that of optimized culture ranges from 80 to 97 percent. As is the case for VZV, RSV is relatively labile, and antigen detection actually may be more sensitive than culture; thus, culture backup usually is not required. However, culture still may be advisable because 5 to 25 percent of specimens submitted for the diagnosis of RSV contain other viruses.[15] The sensitivity of DFA and IFA for detection of influenza virus A and B, parainfluenza virus 1, 2, and 3, and adenovirus antigens varies when compared with that of culture (ranging from 29 to 100%[8, 126, 157, 180, 183, 270, 279]), so culture must be performed for optimal diagnosis.

Enzyme-Linked Immunosorbent Assay

Standardized, well-characterized commercial kits for the detection of viral antigen by ELISA are available for HSV, RSV, influenza virus A, rotavirus, adenovirus, and hepatitis B virus (HBV). Intracellular as well as extracellular antigen can be detected, the method is simple technically, and sub-optimal specimen handling still may yield positive results. ELISAs come in two basic formats, either a classic microtiter/tube system or the more recently developed self-contained membrane assays. The microtiter/tube format uses antibodies lining the surface of the solid phase to capture viral antigen, which in turn is reacted with an enzyme-labeled secondary antibody followed by detection with the addition of substrate and color development. Results are read spectrophotometrically and thus are objective, thereby eliminating some of the difficulties inherent in microscopic techniques, which require technical skill and expertise for evaluation of specimens. These tests are relatively inexpensive, can be automated, are suitable for processing large numbers of specimens, and generally can be completed within 2 to 4 hours. Specimens normally are batched and cannot be tested on demand as previously described for IF. In addition, the adequacy of the specimen cannot be ascertained. In contrast, membrane assays use the membrane as the solid support to retain viral antigen. Enzyme-labeled antibodies are added to react with trapped antigen, and antigen-antibody complexes are detected via a chromogenic substrate. The results are read visually. Though rapid (15 to 20 minutes) and simple to perform, these tests are more expensive, require more hands-on time, and do not result in objective end-points. False-positive results and interpretation can be a problem.

Numerous studies have evaluated the performance of ELISA for detection of HSV in genital, dermal, oral, and ocular specimens.[36, 45, 95, 100, 136, 209, 263, 305, 307] Herpchek (DuPont Pharmaceuticals, Wilmington, DE) has been investigated most frequently and, when compared with culture, yields sensitivities and specificities ranging from 72 to 99 percent and 92 to 100 percent, respectively (the average sensitivity is approximately 90%). An automated system, VIDAS (bioMerieux, Hazelwood, MO), also has shown promise, with a sensitivity, specificity, positive predictive value (PPV), and negative predictive value (NPV) of 92, 89, 83, and 95 percent, respectively.[136] Results obtained with another assay (Ortho ELISA) yielded an unacceptably low sensitivity of 35 percent, but the specificity, PPV, and NPV were 100, 100, and 85 percent, respectively,[100] thus illustrating the substantial differences among assays and the need for evaluation and validation by the laboratory. Membrane assays are less sensitive than microwell ELISA, with a reported sensitivity, specificity, PPV, and NPV of 73, 99, 97, and 84 percent, respectively, and therefore they are used infrequently.[57, 334]

Detection of RSV antigen in nasopharyngeal aspirates, washes, suctions, and swabs, like HSV, also has been evaluated extensively in standard[81, 107, 137, 160, 289, 298, 309] and membrane* ELISA formats. The reported sensitivity, specificity,

*See references 56, 107, 148, 178, 189, 241, 282, 289, 298, 323.

PPV, and NPV for standard ELISA ranged from 71 to 91, 87 to 100, 95, and 94 percent, respectively, and for membrane enzyme immunoassay (EIA), from 57 to 94, 73 to 100, 38 to 100, and 75 to 97 percent, respectively. When the results of TestPack RSV (Abbott Laboratories, Abbott Park, IL) and Directigen RSV (Becton Dickinson) membrane EIAs are compared, TestPack appears to be more sensitive and specific for the detection of RSV antigen; the mean sensitivity, specificity, PPV, and NPV for TestPack and Directigen were 87, 93, 89, and 92 percent and 76, 81, 63, and 89 percent, respectively. In many of these studies, antibody-blocking assays confirmed the specificity of ELISA. The recent introduction of antiviral therapy for influenza A and B has increased the demand for rapid diagnosis, thus prompting the development of several new assays. Table 249–5 summarizes the features of these five assays. The assays are rapid and require 15 to 40 minutes to perform. Directigen Flu A (Becton Dickinson) detects influenza A only, whereas Directigen Flu A + B is the only assay that differentiates influenza A from B; the other assays detect both viruses but do not differentiate them. In general, these rapid assays are expensive, are best suited to small-batch testing, require subjective interpretation, and are less sensitive than culture or rapid IF detection. Sensitivity is variable and highly dependent on the type and quality of the specimen.[19, 39, 135, 155, 245, 281, 311] Directigen Flu A and culture were compared for the detection of influenza A in nasopharyngeal washes, throat gargles, nasopharyngeal swabs, and throat swabs obtained from experimentally infected volunteers. Culture yielded 3.6, 1.2, 1.8, and 0.6 log of virus from these sources, respectively. The sensitivity of Directigen Flu A versus culture was 75, 22, and 64 percent for nasopharyngeal washes, throat gargles, and combined throat and nasopharyngeal swabs, respectively.[139] For optimal diagnosis, these devices should not be used when disease prevalence is low (at a 1–2% prevalence, the predictive value of a positive result is <15%) or in the off-season, adequate specimen collection must be emphasized, and negative results should be backed up by culture or IF testing.

For the diagnosis of rotavirus and adenovirus 40/41 infection, ELISA is the only rapid test available in the clinical laboratory. Rotavirus antigen detection by standard ELISA has been studied thoroughly.[42, 47, 149, 290] Many of the assays have excellent sensitivity (93–100%) and specificity (98–100%) when compared with that of electron microscopy (EM), although the best results were obtained with monoclonal (versus polyclonal) antibody–based kits (see elsewhere[48, 179] for a review of available tests). Some assays can be read either visually or spectrophotometrically, so instrumentation is not always necessary. Several membrane EIAs are also available for rotavirus antigen detection (TestPack, Abbott Laboratories; ImmunoCard, Meridian Diagnostics, Cincinnati, OH) and, as is typical of this format, are somewhat less sensitive than standard ELISA, with approximately 2 to 4 × 10^7 virions/mL required for detection of a positive specimen. The reported sensitivity and specificity versus EM are 94 to 100 percent and 90 to 100 percent, respectively.[21, 29, 48] An excellent ELISA for detection of adenovirus 40/41 in stool specimens is available and yields a reported sensitivity, specificity, PPV, and NPV of 96, 96, 95, and 96 percent, respectively.[114, 133, 322]

Latex Agglutination

Latex agglutination (LA) has been used primarily to diagnose rotavirus infection,[47, 179, 211, 248, 249] although assays are also available for detection of adenovirus[103] and HSV[278] antigens. LA is the least technically demanding of the tests described thus far, is rapid (2 to 5 minutes for rotavirus, 25 minutes for HSV), and is adequate for testing specimens collected early in the course of infection, but it is not as sensitive as standard ELISA, with 10^7 virions/mL required for detection of a positive specimen. The sensitivity, specificity, PPV, and NPV for detection of rotavirus antigen by LA range from 70 to 93, 80 to 100, 76 to 100, and 85 to 95 percent, respectively (see elsewhere[47, 179] for review); those for HSV were 73, 89, 89, and 72 percent, respectively.[278] The sensitivity and specificity of LA versus EM for detection of adenovirus were 95 and 100 percent, respectively.[103]

Nucleic Acid Detection

Molecular methods for the detection, identification, and characterization of microorganisms are being adapted increasingly for use in the clinical laboratory.[147, 216–218, 222, 286, 287, 316, 318, 319] The two broad categories for detecting nucleic acids are direct detection via labeled DNA or RNA probes and hybridization or amplification of selected nucleic acid targets followed by detection of the amplified product. Direct hybridization formats include solid-phase (slot/spot/dot blot, microwell/bead capture, Southern/Northern blot), solution-phase, and in situ hybridization.[65, 147, 217, 287, 319] Nucleic acid amplification techniques are characterized as target (PCR), probe (ligase chain reaction), or signal (branched-chain DNA [bDNA]) amplification types.[65, 217, 286, 319] Some of this methodology is moving from the research to the clinical laboratory for the following reasons: (1) replacement of radiolabels with enzyme, chemiluminescent, or affinity labels (e.g., biotin); (2) replacement of more cumbersome, labor-intensive detection methods with simplified, objective, ELISA-like formats; (3) simplified specimen preparation methods for releasing and exposing target nucleic acid; (4) the availability of standardized, optimized, and quality-controlled reagents and kits; and (5) the publication of guidelines and recommendations for the use of molecular testing in infectious disease diagnosis.[65] A few of these techniques are described in the following section with respect to their application for the diagnosis and monitoring of certain viral infections. Table 249–6 lists various methods and their relative analytic sensitivity for the detection of viruses, viral antigen, or viral nucleic acid.

IN SITU HYBRIDIZATION

In situ hybridization is a type of solid-phase hybridization assay in which whole cells or tissue sections fixed to

TABLE 249–6 ■ COMPARISON OF ANALYTIC SENSITIVITIES

Detection Method	Approximate Detection Limit of Assay (Virions or Copies/mL)
Culture	1–10
Antigen	
IF-, IP-stained cells	1–10
Microwell ELISA	10^3 to 10^6
Membrane ELISA	10^7
Latex agglutination	10^7
Electron microscopy	10^6 to 10^7
Nucleic acid	
Radiolabeled oligonucleotide probes	10^6
Radiolabeled full-length probes	10^4
Enzyme-labeled probes	10^4
Chemiluminescent probes	10^4
Compound or branched probes	50 to 10^3
Nucleic acid amplification	≤10 to 10^3

ELISA, enzyme-linked immunosorbent assay; IF, immunofluorescence; IP, immunoperoxidase.

microscope slides are taken through the hybridization process within the morphologic context of infected tissue. Cell suspensions and fresh-frozen and formalin-fixed, paraffin-embedded tissue sections have been used as the starting material for hybridization. The target nucleic acid is made accessible for hybridization via proteases and heat to increase availability of the target while preserving cellular architecture and morphology through the use of fixatives such as formalin, paraformaldehyde, or glutaraldehyde.[217] Detection systems include radiolabeled as well as enzyme-, biotin-, and digoxigenin-labeled probes. Some commercial kits are available, but methods are often optimized individually, thereby leading to variations in sensitivity among laboratories. In situ hybridization has been applied to the study and diagnosis of numerous infections,[217, 293, 295] particularly CMV viremia,[44, 276] pneumonia,[94, 199, 315] hepatitis,[70, 213] and HSV infection.[83, 159, 232, 280] In some cases, culture,[94] immunocytochemistry,[280] and histopathology[70] had equivalent or superior sensitivity in comparison to hybridization. Although in situ hybridization is probably one of the first molecular techniques applied to the diagnosis of viral infections, lack of sensitivity, cost, and complexity have precluded its widespread use in diagnostic virology laboratories. In addition, the technique is related more closely to routine histologic staining and immunocytochemistry and, thus, is suited better to other areas of the pathology laboratory.[294, 295]

SIGNAL AMPLIFICATION

In signal amplification, target nucleic acid is hybridized with complementary DNA or RNA probes, captured onto a solid surface such as a microtiter well or test tube, and in an assay similar to ELISA, detected after the addition of enzyme-labeled probes and substrate. The attachment of multiple enzyme-labeled probes to each captured target molecule allows for amplification of the signal rather than the target nucleic acid itself. Thus, the signal generated is approximately proportional to the quantity of target nucleic acid in the sample, which is determined from a standard curve. Two signal amplification systems that have become commercially available are bDNA assays (Quantiplex, Bayer Corp., Norwood, MA [formerly Chiron Corp., Emeryville, CA]) and Hybrid Capture System (HCS) (Digene Corp., Gaithersburg, MD).

bDNA

Quantiplex assays have been developed for the detection of HBV,[28, 111, 331] hepatitis C virus (HCV),[49, 171, 207] and HIV[51, 233] viremia. Virus is concentrated from plasma or serum; the target nucleic acid is released by disruption, hybridized with target and capture probes, and incubated overnight. The captured complex is hybridized with bDNA, incubated and washed, hybridized with alkaline phosphatase–labeled probes, and detected via a chemiluminescent substrate.[47] As many as 3000 alkaline phosphatase–labeled probe molecules can be incorporated onto each target molecule, thereby amplifying the signal and increasing the sensitivity of detection.[217] Because the signal is proportional to the quantity of nucleic acid in the specimen, the assay can be used to quantitate viral burden. Although the analytic sensitivity of bDNA is less than that obtained with PCR (10^1 to 10^5 copies/mL versus 10^1 to 10^2 copies/mL, respectively), bDNA's ability to quantitate viral burden by using a relatively simple and reproducible method has made it useful for the diagnosis and prognosis of HBV,[26, 28, 111, 120, 331] HCV,[49, 120, 207] and HIV[12, 125, 161, 162, 253, 267] infections, as well as for monitoring the response to antiviral therapy.

Hybrid Capture System

HCS assays have been developed for the detection and monitoring of human papilloma virus, HBV,[7, 26, 117] HSV,[170, 176] and CMV[12, 125, 127, 161, 172, 182, 191, 253, 267] infections. Briefly, specimens are treated to release viral DNA, target DNA combines with specific RNA probes to create RNA/DNA hybrids, hybrids are captured onto a test tube or microwell coated with capture antibody specific for the RNA/DNA hybrids, and captured hybrids are detected with multiple antihybrid antibodies conjugated to alkaline phosphatase. The bound alkaline phosphatase is detected with a chemiluminescent substrate. Similar to the case with bDNA, as many as 3000 alkaline phosphatase molecules can bind to each captured hybrid, and the signal generated is proportional to the quantity of nucleic acid in the original sample.

HCS has been evaluated for the detection and quantitation of CMV viremia; correlation to symptomatic infection; and response to therapy in renal,[12, 125, 161, 162, 253, 267] liver,[161, 162, 172] heart,[161, 162] and bone marrow transplant[161] and HIV-positive patients.[127, 182, 192] HCS was more sensitive than traditional tube culture, SVA, or both, and it was useful for the early detection of CMV infections. Higher DNA concentrations correlated with clinically significant disease or progression, and quantitative DNA was useful in monitoring antiviral therapy. As with all quantitative methods, the threshold levels that predict disease must be determined in various patient populations. The lower limit of detection is 600 copies/mL, levels similar to those detected by PCR.

TARGET AMPLIFICATION BY POLYMERASE CHAIN REACTION

Of the molecular techniques developed recently, probably none has had a greater impact on basic and clinical research than has PCR. PCR has been applied to the detection and study of numerous, if not most bacteria, fungi, parasites, and viruses. PCR is a target amplification technique in which a specific nucleic acid sequence is replicated by repeated cycles of denaturation, annealing, and extension directed by an oligonucleotide primer pair that defines the region of interest.[217, 319] Target nucleic acid is produced in sufficient quantities to render it detectable by a variety of methods. The most practical and adaptable detection methods use an ELISA-like format with 96-well microtiter plates. These methods entail the use of biotinylated primers in the amplification step, which are incorporated into the PCR product and subsequently detected via avidin-biotin interaction. In one scheme (Roche Diagnostic Systems, Indianapolis, IN), the biotinylated PCR product is captured through hybridization with a specific probe attached to the microwell and detected with avidin–horseradish peroxidase conjugate. This system also features enzymatic prevention of carryover contamination.[142, 151, 171, 207, 233, 240, 261, 314, 328] Another system (Digene Corp.) uses solution hybridization with specific RNA probes to form RNA/DNA hybrids that are captured onto streptavidin-coated microwells. Bound PCR product then is detected by the addition of alkaline phosphatase–conjugated antibodies directed against RNA/DNA hybrids. This universal product detection system has been used to detect amplified CMV,[74, 152] HBV,[297] and HIV[167] and can be adapted for the detection of numerous targets with the use of specific primer/probe sets. Issues that surround the implementation of PCR diagnostics include the production of diagnostic kits, the availability of standardized kits approved by the Food and Drug Administration (FDA), guidelines for use and interpretation, standardization and quality control of test procedures and specimen preparation, qualitative versus quantitative PCR, validation of test protocols, participation in proficiency

TABLE 249–7 ■ CLINICAL USE OF POLYMERASE CHAIN REACTION FOR THE DIAGNOSIS OF SELECTED VIRAL INFECTIONS

Virus	Clinical Utility
CMV	Diagnosis of CNS infection, diagnosis of neonatal/congenital infection, diagnosis of ocular infections, diagnosis and monitoring of active infection/viral load in immunocompromised hosts
EBV	Diagnosis of active EBV infection, diagnosis of CNS infection, diagnosis and monitoring of EBV-related lymphoproliferative disorders in liver and bone marrow transplants undergoing suppression
Enteroviruses	Rapid diagnosis of CNS infection
HBV	Early detection of infection, confirmation of infectivity, monitoring of viral load and therapeutic efficacy in chronic hepatitis
HCV	Detection before seroconversion, resolution of indeterminate or ambiguous serology, monitoring of viral load and therapeutic efficacy in chronic infection
HHV-6	Confirmation of infection
HIV	Detection before seroconversion, resolution of indeterminate immunoblot results, evaluation of suspected prenatal and intrapartum HIV infection, monitoring of viral load to evaluate therapeutic efficacy and disease progression
HSV	Diagnosis of HSV encephalitis, confirmation of neonatal HSV infection, detection of virus in late lesions, diagnosis of ocular infections
HTLV-I/II	Detection of HTLV-I in adult T-cell leukemia and lymphoma and tropical spastic paraparesis/HTLV-I-associated myelopathy
Parvovirus B19	Detection of infection, early detection before seroconversion
VZV	Diagnosis of CNS infection, detection of virus in late or atypical lesions, diagnosis of ocular infections

CMV, cytomegalovirus; CNS, central nervous system; EBV, Epstein-Barr virus; HBV, hepatitis B virus; HCV, hepatitis C virus, HHV-6, human herpesvirus type 6; HIV, human immunodeficiency virus; HSV, herpes simplex virus; HTLV-I/II, human T-cell lymphotropic virus types I and II; VZV, varicella-zoster virus.

surveys such as the College of American Pathologists survey, and re-evaluation of the gold standard. Although PCR is a powerful and sensitive technique, as with all other diagnostic tests, interpretation of results must integrate the clinical features, patient history, supporting laboratory data, and treatment records. PCR is a rapid, sensitive, and specific tool that is clinically useful for the diagnosis of particular viral infections in select situations. PCR is useful (1) when culture is too insensitive, lengthy, expensive, difficult, impractical, or unavailable; (2) for confirmation of infection; (3) for early detection of infection; (4) for detection late in disease; (5) for resolution of indeterminate serology results; (6) to monitor the status of disease; and (7) to monitor response to therapy (Table 249–7). Use of PCR for the diagnosis of certain viral infections is addressed in the following section.

PCR has been used to detect HSV DNA in a variety of clinical specimens, including CSF and brain biopsy material,* skin lesions,[200, 201] genital lesions,[35, 52, 110] and ocular samples.[130, 326] The application of PCR to CSF specimens for the diagnosis of HSV encephalitis (HSE) has received a great deal of emphasis. Brain biopsy remains the gold standard for diagnosis. However, it rarely is performed, and patients are treated empirically. Traditional laboratory methods, including culture, antigen detection, intrathecal antibody production, CSF and serum antibodies, and the serum/CSF antibody ratio, lack sensitivity or specificity or are too slow and most useful for retrospective diagnosis. Numerous reports have documented the utility of CSF PCR for diagnosing HSE in a timely manner, with sensitivity and specificity greater than 95 and 100 percent, respectively.* Most of these studies have used some combination of traditional methods along with clinical observation and radiodiagnostic studies for case definition. Lakeman and Whitley[154] compared CSF PCR and brain biopsy in 101 patients, 54 with biopsy-proven HSE and 47 who were biopsy culture–negative. The sensitivity and specificity of CSF PCR were 98 percent (53 of 54) and 94 percent (44 of 47), respectively. The PCR-positive, biopsy-negative specimens remained PCR-positive in repeat assays with two different primer pairs and were considered true-positive; culture failures were perhaps due to sampling problems. The PCR-negative, biopsy-positive sample remained PCR-negative after DNA extraction and was not inhibitory to PCR. Patients also were monitored after acyclovir treatment; 100, 98, 47, and 21 percent of CSF specimens were PCR-positive at times 0, 0 to 7, 8 to 14, and greater than 15 days, respectively, after brain biopsy and initiation of therapy. The authors concluded that PCR should be the standard for diagnosis of HSE because its sensitivity and specificity were adequate for the diagnosis of focal biopsy-proven HSE; its usefulness for defining the spectrum of HSV infection of the central nervous system (CNS) continues to be investigated. Detection of HSV DNA in skin and genital lesions has shown that PCR is more sensitive than culture, is able to identify asymptomatic HSV, detects the presence of HSV for a longer period (in older lesions and even fixed tissue), and has greater diagnostic value than culture and clinical observations do for assessing genital HSV and treatment efficacy in patients with recurrent genital HSV.[35, 52, 110, 200, 201] PCR is also useful for the diagnosis of ocular infections caused by specific viruses or as supporting information in the clinical diagnosis of specific ocular disease syndromes.[130, 326]

PCR has been used to diagnose cutaneous,[53, 143, 150, 200, 201] ocular,[204, 326] CNS,[227, 265] and congenital VZV infection[128] and as a tool for studying the natural history of primary and reactivated disease.[53, 143, 150] The principal clinical use of PCR in VZV disease is for the diagnosis of VZV CNS infection because isolation of virus is rarely successful and intrathecal antibodies cannot be used as an early diagnostic tool.[227, 265]

Significant morbidity and mortality are associated with CMV infection, primarily in organ transplant recipients and patients with AIDS, and surveillance and monitoring for infection or disease by culture or antigenemia are required. Increasingly, PCR is being used to detect CMV DNA in blood,* CSF,[2, 6, 31, 102, 320] urine,[46, 190] and the same spectrum of specimens submitted for culture.[190] Whole blood, peripheral blood leukocytes, serum, and plasma have been evaluated extensively for detection of infection, association with

*See references 4, 50, 104, 144, 154, 225, 226, 242, 256, 292, 296, 317.

*See references 22, 61, 62, 87, 91, 101, 132, 190, 202, 264, 272, 314, 335.

clinical disease, and therapeutic monitoring. Although PCR was positive earlier, remained positive longer, and was more sensitive than culture or antigenemia for the detection of CMV infection in whole blood or peripheral blood leukocytes, in the absence of a positive culture or antigenemia, PCR was not always associated with clinical symptoms and did not necessarily predict or correlate with the appearance of clinical disease, although it did predict a risk of relapse.[62, 91, 132, 335] Detection of CMV DNA in serum or plasma, however, correlated with viremia, clinical disease, or both in patients with CMV infection,[22, 272, 314] including congenital CMV infection.[202] Detection of mRNA in peripheral blood leukocytes by reverse transcriptase PCR also has been used to assess active productive CMV infection and to identify patients at risk for symptomatic infection.[14, 101] Detection of CMV viremia by PCR is likewise useful for monitoring antiviral therapy, both for the early initiation of treatment and as a predictor of treatment efficacy.[61, 91, 314, 335] In addition, commercial kits (Roche Diagnostic Systems) are being evaluated for the qualitative and quantitative detection of CMV DNA from plasma.[18, 23, 266, 314] PCR is also useful for the diagnosis of CMV CNS infection, primarily in AIDS patients,[6, 31, 102, 320] with reported sensitivity ranging from 79 to 100 percent.[6]

Conventional diagnostic methods are not generally useful in the evaluation of Epstein-Barr virus (EBV)-related disorders in immunosuppressed patients. Culture is not practical or useful, and serology is difficult to interpret in the setting of immunosuppression. PCR offers the possibility of rapid detection of EBV in a variety of clinical specimens and allows a semiquantitative or quantitative estimate of viral load. PCR has been used for the diagnosis of AIDS-related CNS lymphoma,[5] EBV-related lymphoproliferative disorders,[40, 145, 176, 203, 275, 285] and other EBV-associated diseases (e.g., infectious mononucleosis, fatal infectious mononucleosis, chronic active EBV infection, and EBV-associated hemophagocytic syndromes) in which increased DNA concentrations are associated with more severe clinical categories.[325] PCR is particularly useful for the early identification and diagnosis of lymphoproliferative disorders in pediatric patients after liver transplantation, for monitoring EBV levels so that immunosuppression can be adjusted, and as a prognostic marker.[40, 145, 176, 203, 275, 285]

PCR is useful for the early detection of HIV infection, resolution of indeterminate Western blot results, evaluation of suspected prenatal and intrapartum infection, and monitoring of the viral load for prognosis and evaluation of therapeutic efficacy.[116, 142, 151, 186, 233, 234] Qualitative[142, 151] (for detection of proviral DNA in peripheral blood leukocytes) and quantitative[63, 66, 197, 233, 246] (for detection of viral RNA in plasma) kits are available commercially (Roche Diagnostic Systems), and the quantitative assay has FDA approval. Quantitative PCR is useful for correlating RNA levels to disease stage, predicting clinical outcome, and monitoring response to therapy.[116, 186] However, guidelines for the optimal use of PCR and other quantitative assays (bDNA, nucleic acid sequence–based amplification [NASBA]) still are evolving.[246] In a comparison of PCR, NASBA, and bDNA,[188] no significant differences in sensitivity were found for baseline measurement of HIV-1 RNA levels in the three assays. In addition, changes in RNA levels in response to therapy were comparable. The lower limit of detection for PCR, NASBA, and bDNA was 200, 4000, and 10,000 copies/mL, respectively; the turnaround time was 6 hours, 5 hours, and 1.5 days, respectively. Improvements in PCR and bDNA assays have lowered the limits of detection to 50 copies/mL.[63, 66, 197] Commercial kits (Roche Diagnostic Systems) are also available for the detection of HCV RNA in plasma.[171, 207, 240, 261, 332] Detection of HCV RNA is useful for the diagnosis of acute hepatitis before seroconversion, for detection of chronic HCV in seronegative patients, for resolution of indeterminate serologic test results, and to monitor patients receiving therapy. PCR was more sensitive than bDNA,[171, 207] with approximately 11 percent of true-positives undetected by bDNA.[207] The analytic sensitivity of PCR and bDNA was 400 and 3.5×10^5 copies/mL, respectively.[207] Modifications to the Quantiplex HCV version 3.0 bDNA assay have lowered the detection limit to 2500 copies/mL with a linear detection range of 2500 to 50,000,000 copies/mL. The unit of measure for HCV PCR assays has been converted from copies per milliliter to international units per milliliter, with lower limits of detection of 600 and 50 IU/mL for the quantitative and qualitative assays, respectively.[163] The qualitative assay is the first HCV assay to receive FDA approval.

With regard to enteroviruses, PCR has been used to diagnose enteroviral CNS[25, 235, 236, 238, 239, 250, 257, 328] and neonatal infections[1, 43, 236] and to identify vaccine[327] and wild-type[30] poliovirus infections. Major emphasis, however, has been placed on developing a rapid, sensitive method for diagnosing aseptic meningitis because as many as 25 to 35 percent of specimens from patients with characteristic enterovirus infection are negative and, when positive, require an average of 4 to 8 days for detection in culture.[238, 250, 328] CSF evaluation for pleocytosis is not always reliable because specimens with no pleocytosis also may be culture- or PCR-positive.[235, 250] PCR for the diagnosis of enteroviral CNS infections has a sensitivity, specificity, PPV, and NPV of 95 to 100, 97 to 100, approximately 98, and 98 percent, respectively.[235, 236, 238, 239, 250, 257] Commercial kits also have become available and yield rapid (<6 hours), sensitive, and specific results.[24, 239, 250, 283, 328, 329] In addition, rapid diagnosis by PCR will have an effect on patient management with regard to days of hospitalization, antibiotic treatment, and therefore, overall cost.[109, 230, 235, 257]

Increased use of PCR for the diagnosis of disease has stimulated several recent developments, including automation of nucleic acid extraction, amplification, detection, and reporting and interpretation of results. Automation of specimen processing significantly improves the PCR process by rapidly and efficiently providing standardized, reproducible nucleic acids for amplification, comparable to those obtained with more labor-intensive manual methods.[72, 197] Roche has developed numerous qualitative and quantitative PCR assays for the COBAS, an instrument that automates PCR amplification and detection and yields results similar to those of manual methods. Assays that have been developed for the COBAS include HCV,[54, 88, 330] HBV,[141, 206] CMV,[18, 23, 266] and HIV.[197] In addition to increased automation is a trend to obtain more rapid, clinically relevant results through the use of real-time PCR. Amplification and detection are integrated in real-time PCR and occur simultaneously, in contrast to conventional PCR, in which these processes are separate. Turnaround time for conventional PCR ranges from 4 to 48 hours, depending on the detection system, whereas real-time PCR can be completed in 20 minutes to 2 hours, depending on the system and instrumentation used. In addition, concern regarding contamination is reduced in real-time PCR because amplification and detection occur in a closed system. For quantitative assays, real-time PCR also offers linearity over a broader dynamic range (5 to 6 logs) than possible with conventional PCR (2 to 3 logs). Real-time PCR has been used for the qualitative and quantitative detection of CMV,[86, 205, 251, 252, 284] HSV,[71, 77] VZV,[76] EBV,[145, 203, 275] HBV,[169, 212] and influenza A and B[304] from a variety of specimens.

Summary

Methods for the laboratory diagnosis of viral infections, including culture, SVA, antigen detection, and molecular diagnostic methods, have been reviewed. The use of these tests in some combination is most practical because a single test may not yield a diagnosis. For many viruses, culture has been the gold standard or reference method for evaluation of the new, rapid tests. However, culture is not 100 percent sensitive nor always diagnostic of symptomatic infection. With the newer methods, particularly molecular diagnostic methods, the gold standard is changing, and evaluation of new techniques must be compared against a spectrum of laboratory and clinical data. Standards for performance and guidelines for the use and interpretation of molecular techniques are becoming available. Quantitative (versus qualitative) viral results may be useful for interpreting tests, particularly with regard to viruses causing latent infection, or for monitoring therapy or disease progression. Finally, interpretation of any result requires integration of the clinical history and findings, a variety of laboratory data, treatment records, and observation of trends over time.

REFERENCES

1. Abzug, M. J., Loeffelholz, M., and Rotbart, H. A.: Diagnosis of neonatal enterovirus infection by polymerase chain reaction. J. Pediatr. *126*:447–450, 1995.
2. Achim, C. L., Nagra, R. M., Wang, R., et al.: Detection of cytomegalovirus in cerebrospinal fluid autopsy specimens from AIDS patients. J. Infect. Dis. *169*:623–627, 1994.
3. Ahluwalia, G., Embree, J., McNicol, P., et al.: Comparison of nasopharyngeal aspirate and nasopharyngeal swab specimens for respiratory syncytial virus diagnosis by cell culture, indirect immunofluorescence assay, and enzyme-linked immunosorbent assay. J. Clin. Microbiol. *25*:763–767, 1987.
4. Ando, Y., Kimura, H., Miwata, H., et al.: Quantitative analysis of herpes simplex virus DNA in cerebrospinal fluid of children with herpes simplex encephalitis. J. Med. Virol. *41*:170–173, 1993.
5. Arribas, J. R., Clifford, D. B., Fichtenbaum, C. J., et al.: Detection of Epstein-Barr virus DNA in cerebrospinal fluid for diagnosis of AIDS-related central nervous system lymphoma. J. Clin. Microbiol. *33*:1580–1583, 1995.
6. Arribas, J. R., Storch, G. A., Clifford, D. B., et al.: Cytomegalovirus encephalitis. Ann. Intern. Med. *125*:577–587, 1996.
7. Aspinall, S., Steele, A. D., Peenze, I., et al.: Detection and quantitation of hepatitis B virus DNA: Comparison of two commercial hybridization assays with polymerase chain reaction. J. Viral Hepatol. *2*:107–111, 1995.
8. August, M. J., and Warford, A. L.: Evaluation of a commercial monoclonal antibody for detection of adenovirus antigen. J. Clin. Microbiol. *25*:2233–2235, 1987.
9. Bankowski, M. J., Varica, S., and Moore, B.: Evaluation of the Quidel QuickVue influenza test for the direct detection of influenza virus type A and B. Abstract S22. Paper presented at the 17th Annual Clinical Virology Symposium, 2000, Clearwater Beach, FL.
10. Barenfanger, J., Drake, C., Mueller, T., et al.: Combination of mixed cell lines E-Mix A and E-Mix B supports growth of all clinical enterovirus isolates tested. Abstract M21. Paper presented at the 15th Annual Clinical Virology Symposium, 2000, Clearwater, FL.
11. Barenfanger, J., Drake, C., Mueller, T., et al.: R-Mix cells are faster, at least as sensitive and marginally more costly than conventional cell lines for the detection of respiratory viruses. J. Clin. Virol. *22*:101–110, 2001.
12. Barrett-Muir, W., Breuer, J., Millar, C., et al.: CMV viral load measurements in whole blood and plasma—which is best following renal transplantation? Transplantation *70*:116–119, 2000.
13. Bettoli, E. J., Brewer, P. M., Oxtoby, M. J., et al.: The role of temperature and swab materials in the recovery of herpes simplex virus from lesions. J. Infect. Dis. *145*:399, 1982.
14. Bitsch, A., Kirchner, H., Dupke, R., et al.: Cytomegalovirus transcripts in peripheral blood leukocytes of actively infected transplant patients detected by reverse transcription–polymerase chain reaction. J. Infect. Dis. *167*:740–743, 1992.
15. Blanding, J. G., Hoshiko, M. G., and Stutman, H. R.: Routine viral culture for pediatric respiratory syncytial specimens submitted for direct immunofluorescence testing. J. Clin. Microbiol. *27*:1438–1440, 1989.
16. Boeckh, M., Bowden, R. A., Goodrich, J. M., et al.: Cytomegalovirus antigen detection in peripheral blood leukocytes after allogeneic marrow transplantation. Blood *80*:1358–1364, 1992.
17. Boeckh, M., Woogerd, P. M., Stevens-Ayers, T., et al.: Factors influencing detection of quantitative cytomegalovirus antigenemia. J. Clin. Microbiol. *32*:832–834, 1994.
18. Boivin, G., Belanger, R., Delage, R., et al.: Quantitative analysis of cytomegalovirus (CMV) viremia using the pp65 antigenemia assay and the COBAS AMPLICOR CMV MONITOR PCR test after blood and marrow allogeneic transplantation. J. Clin. Microbiol. *38*:4356–4360, 2000.
19. Boivin, G., Hardy, I., and Kress, A.: Evaluation of a rapid optical immunoassay for influenza viruses (Flu OIA Test) in comparison with cell culture and reverse transcription–PCR. J. Clin. Microbiol. *39*:730–732, 2001.
20. Bromberg, K., Tannis, G., and Daldone, B.: Early use of indirect immunofluorescence for the detection of respiratory syncytial virus in HEp-2 cell culture. Am. J. Clin. Pathol. *96*:127–129, 1991.
21. Brooks, R. G., Brown, L., and Franklin, R. B.: Comparison of a new rapid test (TestPack Rotavirus) with standard enzyme immunoassay and electron microscopy for the detection of rotavirus in symptomatic hospitalized children. J. Clin. Microbiol. *27*:775–777, 1989.
22. Brytting, M., Xu, W., Wahren, B., et al.: Cytomegalovirus DNA detection in sera from patients with active cytomegalovirus infections. J. Clin. Microbiol. *30*:1937–1941, 1992.
23. Caliendo, A. M., Schuurman, R., Yen-Lieberman, B., et al.: Comparison of quantitative and qualitative PCR assays for cytomegalovirus DNA in plasma. J. Clin. Microbiol. *39*:1334–1338, 2001.
24. Carroll, K. C., Taggart, B., Robison, J., et al.: Evaluation of Roche AMPLICOR enterovirus PCR assay in the diagnosis of enteroviral central nervous system infections. J. Clin. Virol. *19*:149–156, 2000.
25. Casas, I., Klapper, P. E., Cleator, G. M., et al.: Two different PCR assays to detect enteroviral RNA in CSF samples from patients with acute aseptic meningitis. J. Med. Virol. *47*:378–385, 1995.
26. Chan, H. Y., Leung, N. W. Y., Lau, T. C. M., et al.: Comparison of three sensitive assays for hepatitis B virus DNA in monitoring of responses to antiviral therapy. J. Clin. Microbiol. *38*:3205–3208, 2000.
27. Cheeseman, S. H., Pierik, L. T., Leombruno, D., et al.: Evaluation of a commercially available direct immunofluorescence staining reagent for the detection of respiratory syncytial virus in respiratory secretions. J. Clin. Microbiol. *24*:155–156, 1986.
28. Chen, C. H., Wang, J. T., Lee, C. Z., et al.: Quantitative detection of hepatitis B virus DNA in human sera by branched-DNA signal amplification. J. Virol. Methods *53*:131–137, 1995.
29. Chernesky, M., Castriciano, S., Mahony, J., et al.: Ability of TESTPACK ROTAVIRUS enzyme immunoassay to diagnose rotavirus gastroenteritis. J. Clin. Microbiol. *26*:2459–2461, 1988.
30. Chezzi, C.: Rapid diagnosis of poliovirus infection by PCR amplification. J. Clin. Microbiol. *34*:1722–1725, 1996.
31. Cinque, P., Vago, L., Brytting, M., et al.: Cytomegalovirus infection of the central nervous system in patients with AIDS: Diagnosis by DNA amplification from cerebrospinal fluid. J. Infect. Dis. *166*:1408–1411, 1992.
32. Clarke, L. M., Daidone, B. J., Inghida, R., et al.: Differential recovery of cytomegalovirus from cellular and supernatant components of bronchoalveolar lavage specimens. Am. J. Clin. Pathol. *97*:313–317, 1992.
33. Coffin, S. E., and Hodinka, R. L.: Utility of direct immunofluorescence and virus culture for detection of varicella-zoster virus in skin lesions. J. Clin. Microbiol. *33*:2792–2795, 1995.
34. Cole, L. J., Campbell, M. B., and Gleaves, C. A.: Detection of HSV from clinical specimens using the ELVIS™ tube culture test as compared to standard cell culture. Abstract M20. Paper presented at the 12th Annual Clinical Virology Symposium, 1996, Clearwater, FL.
35. Cone, R. W., Hobson, A. C., Palmer, J., et al.: Extended duration of herpes simplex virus DNA in genital lesions detected by the polymerase chain reaction. J. Infect. Dis. *164*:757–760, 1991.
36. Cone, R. W., Swenson, P. D., Hobson, A. C., et al.: Herpes simplex virus detection from genital lesions: A comparative study using antigen detection (HerpChek) and culture. J. Clin. Microbiol. *31*:1774–1776, 1993.
37. Corey, L.: Laboratory diagnosis of herpes simplex virus infections: Principles guiding the development of rapid diagnostic tests. Diagn. Microbiol. Infect. Dis. *4*(Suppl):111–119, 1986.
38. Corey, L., and Spear, P. G.: Infections with herpes simplex viruses. N. Engl. J. Med. *314*:686–691, 749–757, 1986.
39. Covalciuc K. A., Webb, K. H., and Catlson, C. A.: Comparison of four clinical specimen types for detection of influenza A and B viruses by optical immunoassay (Flu OIA Test) and cell culture methods. J. Clin. Microbiol. *37*:3971–3974, 1999.
40. Cox, K. L., Lawrence-Miyasaki, L. S., Garcia-Kennedy, R., et al.: An increased incidence of Epstein-Barr virus infection and lymphoproliferative disorder in young children on FK506 after liver transplantation. Transplantation *59*:524–529, 1995.
41. Crane, L. R., Gutterman, P. A., Chapel, T., et al.: Incubation of swab materials with herpes simplex virus. J. Infect. Dis. *141*:531, 1980.
42. Cromien, J. L., Himmelreich, C. A., Glass, R. I., et al.: Evaluation of new commercial enzyme immunoassay for rotavirus detection. J. Clin. Microbiol. *25*:2359–2362, 1987.
43. Dagan, R.: Nonpolio enteroviruses and the febrile young infant: Epidemiologic, clinical and diagnostic aspects. Pediatr. Infect. Dis. J. *15*:67–71, 1996.

44. Dankner, W. M., McCutchan, J. A., Richman, D. D., et al.: Localization of human cytomegalovirus in peripheral blood leukocytes by in situ hybridization. J. Infect. Dis. *161*:31–36, 1990.
45. Dascal, A. J., Chan-Thim, J., Morahan, M., et al.: Diagnosis of herpes simplex virus infection in a clinical setting by a direct antigen detection enzyme immunoassay. J. Clin. Microbiol. *27*:700–704, 1989.
46. Demmler, G. J., Buffone, G. J., Schimbor, C. M., et al.: Detection of cytomegalovirus in urine from newborns by using polymerase chain reaction DNA amplification. J. Infect. Dis. *158*:1177–1184, 1988.
47. Dennehy, P. H., Gauntlett, D. R., and Tenle, W. E.: Comparison of nine commercial immunoassays for the detection of rotavirus in fecal specimens. J. Clin. Microbiol. *26*:1630, 1988.
48. Dennehy, P. H., Hartin, M., Nelson, S. M., et al.: Evaluation of the ImmunoCardSTAT! Rotavirus assay for detection of group A rotavirus in fecal specimens. J. Clin. Microbiol. *37*:1977–1979, 1999.
49. Detmer, J., Lagier, R., Flynn, J., et al.: Accurate quantification of hepatitis C virus (HCV) RNA from all HCV genotypes by using branched-DNA technology. J. Clin. Microbiol. *34*:901–907, 1996.
50. DeVincenzo, J. P., and Thorne, G.: Mild herpes simplex encephalitis diagnosed by polymerase chain reaction: A case report and review. Pediatr. Infect. Dis. J. *13*:662–664, 1994.
51. Dewar, R. L., Highbarger, H. C., Sarmiento, M. D., et al.: Application of branched DNA signal amplification to monitor human immunodeficiency virus type 1 burden in human plasma. J. Infect. Dis. *170*:1172–1179, 1994.
52. Diaz-Mitoma, F., Ruben, M., Sacks, S., et al.: Detection of viral DNA to evaluate outcome of antiviral treatment of patients with recurrent genital herpes. J. Clin. Microbiol. *34*:657–663, 1996.
53. Dlugosch, D., Eis-Hubinger, A. M., Kleim, J. P., et al.: Diagnosis of acute and latent varicella-zoster virus infections using the polymerase chain reaction. J. Med. Virol. *35*:136–141, 1992.
54. Doglio, A., Laffont, C., Caroli-Bosc, F. X., et al.: Second generation of the automated Cobas Amplicor HCV assay improves sensitivity of hepatitis C virus RNA detection and yields results that are more clinically relevant. J. Clin. Microbiol. *37*:1567–1569, 1999.
55. Doller, G., Schuy, W., Tjhen, K. Y., et al.: Direct detection of influenza virus antigen in nasopharyngeal specimens by direct enzyme immunoassay in comparison with quantitating virus shedding. J. Clin. Microbiol. *30*:866–869, 1992.
56. Dominguez, E. A., Taber, L. H., and Couch, R. B.: Comparison of rapid diagnostic techniques for respiratory syncytial and influenza A virus respiratory infections in young children. J. Clin. Microbiol. *31*:2286–2290, 1993.
57. Dorian, K. J., Beatty, E., and Atterbury, K. E.: Detection of herpes simplex virus by Kodak SureCell herpes test. J. Clin. Microbiol. *28*:2117–2119, 1990.
58. Drew, W. L.: Controversies in viral diagnosis. Rev. Infect. Dis. *8*:814–824, 1986.
59. Drew, W. L., and Mintz, L.: Rapid diagnosis of varicella-zoster virus infection by direct immunofluorescence. Am. J. Clin. Pathol. *73*:699–701, 1980.
60. Ehrlich, G. D., and Greenberg, S. J.: PCR-Based Diagnostics in Infectious Disease. Boston, Blackwell, 1994.
61. Einsele, H., Ehninger, G., Steidle, M., et al.: Polymerase chain reaction to evaluate antiviral therapy for cytomegalovirus disease. Lancet *338*:1170–1172, 1991.
62. Einsele, H., Steidle, M., Vallbracht, A., et al.: Early occurrence of human cytomegalovirus infection after bone marrow transplantation as demonstrated by the polymerase chain reaction technique. Blood *77*:1104–1110, 1991.
63. Elbeik, T., Charlebois, E., Nassos, P., et al.: Quantitative and cost comparison of ultrasensitive human immunodeficiency virus type 1 RNA viral load assays: Bayer bDNA Quantiplex versions 3.0 and 2.0 and Roche Amplicor Monitor version 1.5. J. Clin. Microbiol. *38*:1113–1120, 2000.
64. Emmanuel, D., Peppard, J., Gold, J., et al.: Rapid immunodiagnosis of cytomegalovirus pneumonia by bronchoalveolar lavage using human and murine monoclonal antibodies. Ann. Intern. Med. *104*:476–481, 1986.
65. Enns, R. K., Bromley, S. E., Day, S. P., et al.: Molecular Diagnostic Methods for Infectious Diseases: Approved Guideline. NCCLS Document MM3-A. Villanova, PA, National Committee for Clinical Laboratory Standards, 1995.
66. Erice, A., Brambilla, D., Bremer, J., et al.: Performance characteristics of the QUANTIPLEX HIV-1 RNA 3.0 assay for detection and quantitation of human immunodeficiency virus type 1 RNA in plasma. J. Clin. Microbiol. *38*:2837–2845, 2000.
67. Erice, A., Holm, M. A., Gill, P. C., et al.: Cytomegalovirus (CMV) antigenemia assay is more sensitive than shell vial cultures for rapid detection of CMV in polymorphonuclear blood leukocytes. J. Clin. Microbiol. *30*:2822–2825, 1992.
68. Erice, A., Holm, M. A., Sanjuan, M. V., et al.: Evaluation of CMV-vue antigenemia assay for rapid detection of cytomegalovirus in mixed-leukocyte blood fractions. J. Clin. Microbiol. *33*:1014–1015, 1995.
69. Espy, M. J., Hierholzer, J. C., and Smith, T. F.: The effect of centrifugation on the rapid detection of adenovirus in shell vials. Am. J. Clin. Pathol. *88*:358–360, 1987.
70. Espy, M. J., Paya, C. V., Holley, K. E., et al.: Diagnosis of cytomegalovirus hepatitis by histopathology and in situ hybridization in liver transplantation. Diagn. Microbiol. Infect. Dis. *14*:293–296, 1991.
71. Espy, M. J., Ross, T. K., Teo, R., et al.: Evaluation of LightCycler PCR for implementation of laboratory diagnosis of herpes simplex virus infections. J. Clin. Microbiol. *38*:3116–3118, 2000.
72. Espy, M. J., Rys, P. N., Wold, A. D., et al.: Detection of herpes simplex virus DNA in genital and dermal specimens by LightCycler PCR after extraction using the IsoQuick, MagNA Pure, and BioRobot 9604 methods. J. Clin. Microbiol. *39*:2233–2236, 2001.
73. Espy, M. J., and Smith, T. F.: Detection of herpes simplex virus in conventional tube cell cultures and in shell vials with a DNA probe kit and monoclonal antibodies. J. Clin. Microbiol. *26*:22–24, 1988.
74. Espy, M. J., and Smith, T. F.: Comparison of SHARP signal system and Southern blot hybridization analysis for detection of cytomegalovirus in clinical specimens by PCR. J. Clin. Microbiol. *33*:3028–3030, 1995.
75. Espy, M. J., Smith, T. F., Harmon, M. W., et al.: Rapid detection of influenza virus by shell vial assay with monoclonal antibodies. J. Clin. Microbiol. *24*:677–679, 1986.
76. Espy, M. J., Teo, R., Ross, T. K., et al.: Diagnosis of varicella-zoster virus infections in the clinical laboratory by LightCycler PCR. J. Clin. Microbiol. *38*:3187–3189, 2000.
77. Espy, M. J., Uhl, J. R., Mitchell, P. S., et al.: Diagnosis of herpes simplex virus infections in the clinical laboratory by LightCycler PCR. J. Clin. Microbiol. *38*:795–799, 2000.
78. Espy, M. J., Wold, A. D., Jesperson, D. J., et al.: Comparison of shell vials and conventional tubes seeded with rhabdomyosarcoma and MRC-5 cells for the rapid detection of herpes simplex virus. J. Clin. Microbiol. *29*:2701–2703, 1991.
79. Fayram, S. L., Aarnaes, S., and de la Maza, L. M.: Comparison of CultureSet to a conventional tissue culture fluorescent antibody technique for isolation and identification of herpes simplex virus. J. Clin. Microbiol. *18*:215–216, 1983.
80. Fedorko, D. P., Ilstrup, D. M., and Smith, T. F.: Effect of age of shell vial monolayers on detection of cytomegalovirus from urine specimens. J. Clin. Microbiol. *27*:2107–2109, 1989.
81. Flander, R. T., Lindsay, P. D., Chairez, R., et al.: The evaluation of clinical specimens for the presence of respiratory syncytial virus antigen using an enzyme immunoassay. J. Med. Virol. *19*:1–9, 1986.
82. Fong, K. Y., Lee, M. K., and Griffith, B. P.: Fresh cells in shell vials for detection of respiratory viruses. J. Clin. Microbiol. *38*:4660–4662, 2000.
83. Forghani, B., Dupuis, K. W., and Schmidt, N. J.: Rapid detection of herpes simplex virus DNA in human brain tissue by in situ hybridization. J. Clin. Microbiol. *22*:656–658, 1985.
84. Forman, M. C., Merz, C. S., and Charache, P.: Detection of herpes simplex virus by a nonradiometric spin-amplified in situ hybridization assay. J. Clin. Microbiol. *30*:581–584, 1992.
85. Garber, M., Vestal, D. and Body, B. A.: Comparison of E-Mix A and E-Mix B fresh cells and conventional tissue tube culture for the detection of enteroviruses. Abstract S32. Presented at the 17th Annual Clinical Virology Symposium, 2001, Clearwater, FL.
86. Gault, E., Michel, Y., Dehee, A., et al.: Quantification of human cytomegalovirus DNA by real-time PCR. J. Clin. Microbiol. *39*:772–775, 2001.
87. Gerdes, J. C., Spees, E. K., Fitting, K., et al.: Prospective study utilizing a quantitative polymerase chain reaction for detection of cytomegalovirus DNA in the blood of renal transplant patients. Transplant. Proc. *25*:1411–1413, 1993.
88. Gerken, G., Rothaar, T., Rumi, M. G., et al.: Performance of the COBAS AMPLICOR HCV MONITOR test, version 2.0, an automated reverse transcription–PCR quantitative system for hepatitis C virus load determination. J. Clin. Microbiol. *38*:2210–2214, 2000.
89. Gerna, G., Revello, M. G., Percivalle, E., et al.: Quantification of human cytomegalovirus viremia by using monoclonal antibodies to different viral proteins. J. Clin. Microbiol. *28*:2681–2688, 1990.
90. Gerna, G., Revello, M. G., Percivalle, E., et al.: Comparison of different immunostaining techniques and monoclonal antibodies to the lower matrix phosphoprotein (pp65) for optimal quantitation of human cytomegalovirus antigenemia. J. Clin. Microbiol. *30*:1232–1237, 1992.
91. Gerna, G., Zipeto, D., Parea, M., et al.: Monitoring of human cytomegalovirus infections and ganciclovir treatment in heart transplant recipients by determination of viremia, antigenemia and DNAemia. J. Infect. Dis. *164*:488–498, 1991.
92. Gleaves, C. A., Hursh, D. A., and Meyers, J. D.: Detection of human cytomegalovirus in clinical specimens by centrifugation culture with a nonhuman cell line. J. Clin. Microbiol. *30*:1045–1048, 1992.
93. Gleaves, C. A., Lee, C. F., Bustamante, C. I., et al.: Use of murine monoclonal antibodies for laboratory diagnosis of varicella-zoster virus infection. J. Clin. Microbiol. *26*:1623–1625, 1988.
94. Gleaves, C. A., Myerson, D., Bowden, R. A., et al.: Direct detection of cytomegalovirus from bronchoalveolar lavage samples by using a rapid in situ DNA hybridization assay. J. Clin. Microbiol. *27*:2429–2432, 1990.
95. Gleaves, C. A., Rice, D. H., and Lee, C. F.: Evaluation of an enzyme-immunoassay for the detection of herpes simplex virus (HSV) antigen

from clinical specimens in viral transport media. J. Virol. Methods *28*:133–139, 1990.

96. Gleaves, C. A., Smith, T. F., Shuster, E. A., et al.: Rapid detection of cytomegalovirus in MRC-5 cells inoculated with urine specimens by using low speed centrifugation and monoclonal antibody to an early antigen. J. Clin. Microbiol. *19*:917–919, 1984.
97. Gleaves, C. A., Smith, T. F., Shuster, E. A., et al.: Comparison of standard tube and shell vial cell culture techniques for detection of cytomegalovirus in clinical specimens. J. Clin. Microbiol. *21*:217–222, 1985.
98. Gleaves, C. A., Wilson, D. J., Wold, A. D., et al.: Detection and serotyping of herpes simplex virus in MRC-5 cells by use of centrifugation and monoclonal antibodies 16 h postinoculation. J. Clin. Microbiol. *21*:29–32, 1985.
99. Goldstein, L. C., Corey, L., McDougall, J. K., et al.: Monoclonal antibodies to herpes simplex viruses: Use in antigenic typing and rapid diagnosis. J. Infect. Dis. *147*:829–837, 1983.
100. Gonik, B., Seibel, M., Berkowitz, A., et al.: Comparison of two enzyme-linked immunosorbent assays for detection of herpes simplex virus antigen. J. Clin. Microbiol. *29*:436–438, 1991.
101. Gozlan, J., Salord, J. M., Chouaid, C., et al.: Human cytomegalovirus (HCMV) late mRNA detection in peripheral blood of AIDS patients: Diagnostic value for HCMV disease compared with those of viral culture and HCMV DNA detection. J. Clin. Microbiol. *31*:1943–1945, 1993.
102. Gozlan, J., Salord, J. M., Roullet, E., et al.: Rapid detection of cytomegalovirus DNA in cerebrospinal fluid of AIDS patients with neurologic disorders. J. Infect. Dis. *166*:1416–1421, 1992.
103. Grandien, M., Pettersson, C. A., Svensson, L., et al.: Latex agglutination test for adenovirus diagnosis in diarrheal disease. J. Med. Virol. *23*:311, 1987.
104. Guffond, T., Dewilde, A., Lobert, P. E., et al.: Significance and clinical relevance of the detection of herpes simplex virus DNA by the polymerase chain reaction in cerebrospinal fluid from patients with presumed encephalitis. Clin. Infect. Dis. *18*:744–749, 1994.
105. Hackman, R. C., Myerson, D., Meyers, J. D., et al.: Rapid diagnosis of cytomegalovirus pneumonia by tissue immunofluorescence with a murine monoclonal antibody. J. Infect. Dis. *151*:325, 1985.
106. Hall, C. B., and Douglas, R. G., Jr.: Clinically useful method for the isolation of respiratory syncytial virus. J. Infect. Dis. *131*:1–10, 1975.
107. Halstead, D. C., Todd, S., and Fritch, G.: Evaluation of five methods for respiratory syncytial virus detection. J. Clin. Microbiol. *28*:1021–1025, 1990.
108. Hamilton, M. S., Abel, D., Ballam, Y., et al.: Zstat FLU-LITE assay compared to Directigen FLU A+B and tissue culture of nasal aspirates in a children's hospital, 2000/2001. Abstract T18. Paper presented at the 17th Annual Clinical Virology Symposium, 2001, Clearwater, FL.
109. Hamilton, M. S., Jackson, M. A., and Abel, D.: Clinical utility of polymerase chain reaction testing for enteroviral meningitis. Pediatr. Infect. Dis. J. *18*:533–537, 1999.
110. Hardy, D. A., Arvin, A. M., Yasukawa, L. L., et al.: The successful identification of asymptomatic genital herpes simplex infection at delivery using the polymerase chain reaction. J. Infect. Dis. *162*:1031–1035, 1990.
111. Hendricks, D. A., Stowe, B. J., Hoo, B. S., et al.: Quantitation of HBV DNA in human serum using a branched DNA (bDNA) signal amplification assay. Am. J. Clin. Pathol. *104*:537–546, 1995.
112. Hermann, E. C., Jr.: Experience in providing a viral diagnostic laboratory compatible with medical practice. Mayo Clin. Proc. *42*:112–123, 1967.
113. Hermann, E. C., Jr.: The tragedy of viral diagnosis. Postgrad. Med. J. *46*:545–550, 1970.
114. Herrmann, J. E., Perron-Henry, D. M., and Blacklow, N. R.: Antigen detection with monoclonal antibodies for the diagnosis of adenovirus gastroenteritis. J. Infect. Dis. *155*:1167–1171, 1987.
115. Hindiyeh, M., Goulding, C., Morgan, H., et al.: Evaluation of BioStar FLU OIA assay for rapid detection of influenza A and B viruses in respiratory specimens. J. Clin. Virol. *17*:119–126, 2000.
116. Ho, D. D.: Viral counts count in HIV infection. Science *272*:1124–1125, 1996.
117. Ho, S. K., Chan, T. M., Cheng, I. K., et al.: Comparison of the second-generation Digene hybrid capture assay with the branched-DNA assay for measurement of hepatitis B virus DNA in serum. J. Clin. Microbiol. *37*:2461–2465, 1999.
118. Howell, C. L., and Miller, M. J.: Effect of sucrose phosphate and sorbitol on infectivity of enveloped viruses during storage. J. Clin. Microbiol. *18*:658–662, 1983.
119. Howell, C. L., Miller, M. J., and Martin, W. J.: Comparison of rates of virus isolation from leukocyte populations separated from blood by conventional and Ficoll-Paque/Macrodex methods. J. Clin. Microbiol. *10*:533–537, 1979.
120. Hu, K.-Q., and Vierling, J. M.: Molecular diagnostic techniques for viral hepatitis. Gastroenterol. Clin. North Am. *23*:479–537, 1994.
121. Huang, Y. T., Hite, S., Duane, V., et al.: Application of mixed cell lines for the detection of viruses from clinical specimens. Clin. Microbiol. Newsl. *22*:89–92, 2000.
122. Huang, Y. T., and Turchek. B. M.: Mink lung cells and mixed mink lung and A549 cells for rapid detection of influenza virus and other respiratory viruses. J. Clin. Microbiol. *38*:422–423, 2000.
123. Huang, Y. T., Yam, P., and Jollick, J. A.: $CaCO_2$ and engineered BGMK mixed cells for the detection of enteroviruses. Abstract S31. Paper presented at the 17th Annual Clinical Virology Symposium, 2001, Clearwater, FL.
124. Hughes, J. H.: Physical and chemical methods for enhancing rapid detection of viruses and other agents. Clin. Microbiol. Rev. *6*:150–175, 1993.
125. Imbert-Marcille, B.-M., Cantarovich, D., Boedec, S., et al.: Evaluation of a new quantification method for cytomegalovirus DNA in leucocytes: Clinical value in renal transplant recipients. Scand. J. Infect. Dis. *99*(Suppl.):15–16, 1995.
126. Irmen, K. E., and Kelleher, J. J.: Use of monoclonal antibodies for rapid diagnosis of respiratory viruses in a community hospital. Clin. Diagn. Lab. Immunol. *7*:396–403, 2000.
127. Isada, C., Kohn, D., Lazar, J. G., et al.: Rapid diagnosis of cytomegalovirus (CMV) using the Digene Hybrid Capture System: A comparison with tissue culture and polymerase chain reaction (PCR). Abstract S19. Paper presented at the 12th Annual Clinical Virology Symposium, 1996, Clearwater, FL.
128. Isada, N. B., Paar, D. P., Johnson, M., et al.: In utero diagnosis of congenital varicella zoster infection by chorionic villus sampling and polymerase chain reaction. Am. J. Obstet. Gynecol. *165*:1727–1730, 1991.
129. Isenberg, H. D. (ed.): Clinical Microbiology Procedure Handbook. Washington, D. C., American Society for Microbiology, 1992, Supplement No. 1, 1994.
130. Jackson, R., Morris, D. J., Cooper, R. J., et al.: Multiplex polymerase chain reaction for adenovirus and herpes simplex virus in eye swabs. J. Virol. Methods *56*:41–48, 1996.
131. Jalowayski, A. A., Walpita, P., Puryear, B. A., et al.: Rapid detection of respiratory syncytial virus in nasopharyngeal specimens obtained with the rhinoprobe scraper. J. Clin. Microbiol. *28*:738–741, 1990.
132. Jiwa, N. M., van Gemert, G. W., Raap, A. K., et al.: Rapid detection of human cytomegalovirus DNA in peripheral blood leukocytes of viremic transplant recipients by the polymerase chain reaction. Transplantation *48*:72–76, 1989.
133. Johansson, M. E., Uhnoo, I., Svensson, L., et al.: Enzyme-linked immunosorbent assay for detection of enteric adenovirus 41. J. Med. Virol. *17*:19–27, 1985.
134. Johnson, F. B.: Transport of viral specimens. Clin. Microbiol. Rev. *3*:120–131, 1990.
135. Johnston, S. L. G., and Bloy, H.: Evaluation of a rapid enzyme immunoassay for detection of influenza A virus. J. Clin. Microbiol. *31*:142–143, 1993.
136. Johnston, S. L. G., Hamilton, S., Bindra, P., et al.: Evaluation of an automated immunodiagnostic assay system for direct detection of herpes simplex virus antigen in clinical specimens. J. Clin. Microbiol. *30*:1042–1044, 1992.
137. Johnston, S. L. G., and Siegel, C. S.: Evaluation of direct immunofluorescence, enzyme immunoassay, centrifugation culture, and conventional culture for the detection of respiratory syncytial virus. J. Clin. Microbiol. *28*:2394–2397, 1990.
138. Johnston, S. L. G., Wellens, K., and Siegel, C.: Comparison of hemagglutination and hemadsorption tests for influenza detection. Diagn. Microbiol. Infect. Dis. *15*:363–365, 1992.
139. Kaiser, L., Briones, M. S., and Hayden, F. G.: Performance of virus isolation and Directigen Flu A to detect influenza A virus in experimental human infection. J. Clin. Virol. *14*:191–197, 1999.
140. Kellog, J. A.: Culture vs. direct antigen assays for detection of microbial pathogens from lower respiratory tract specimens suspected of containing the respiratory syncytial virus. Arch. Pathol. Lab. Med. *115*:451–458, 1991.
141. Kessler, H. H., Stetzl, E., Daghofer, E., et al.: Semiautomated quantification of hepatitis B virus DNA in a routine diagnostic laboratory. Clin. Diagn. Lab. Immunol. *7*:853–855, 2000.
142. Khadir, A., Coutlee, F., Saint-Antoine, P., et al.: Clinical evaluation of Amplicor HIV-1 test for detection of human immunodeficiency virus type 1 proviral DNA in peripheral blood mononuclear cells. J. Acquir. Immune Defic. Syndr. Hum. Retrovirol. *9*:257–263, 1995.
143. Kido, S., Ozaki, T., Asada, H., et al.: Detection of varicella-zoster virus DNA in clinical samples from patients with VZV by the polymerase chain reaction. J. Clin. Microbiol. *29*:76–79, 1991.
144. Kimura, H., Futamura, M., Kito, H., et al.: Detection of viral DNA in neonatal herpes simplex virus infections: Frequent and prolonged presence in serum and cerebrospinal fluid. J. Infect. Dis. *164*:289–293, 1991.
145. Kimura, H., Morita, M., Yabuta, Y., et al.: Quantitative analysis of Epstein-Barr virus load by using real-time PCR assay. J. Clin. Microbiol. *37*:132–136, 1999.
146. Klespies, S. L., Cebula, D. E., Kelley, C. L., et al.: Detection of enteroviruses from clinical specimens by spin amplification shell vial culture and monoclonal antibody assay. J. Clin. Microbiol. *34*:1465–1467, 1996.

147. Kohne, D. E.: The use of DNA probes to detect and identify microorganisms. Adv. Exp. Med. Biol. *263*:11–35, 1990.
148. Kok, T. W., Barancek, K., and Burrell, C. J.: Evaluation of the Becton Dickinson Directigen Test for respiratory syncytial virus in nasopharyngeal aspirates. J. Clin. Microbiol. *28*:1458–1459, 1990.
149. Kok, T. W., and Burrell, C. J.: Comparison of five enzyme immunoassays, electron microscopy and latex agglutination for detection of rotavirus in fecal specimens. J. Clin. Microbiol. *27*:364, 1989.
150. Koropchak, C. M.: Investigation of varicella-zoster virus by polymerase chain reaction in the immunocompromised host with acute varicella. J. Infect. Dis. *163*:1016–1022, 1990.
151. Kovacs, A., Xu, J., Rasheed, S., et al.: Comparison of a rapid nonisotopic polymerase chain reaction assay with four commonly used methods for the early diagnosis of human immunodeficiency virus type 1 infection in neonates and children. Pediatr. Infect. Dis. J. *14*:948–954, 1995.
152. Krajden, M., Shankaran, P., Bourke, C., et al.: Detection of cytomegalovirus in blood donors by PCR using the Digene SHARP signal system assay: Effects of sample preparation and detection methodology. J. Clin. Microbiol. *34*:29–33, 1996.
153. Lafferty, W. E., Kroftt, S., Remington, M., et al.: Diagnosis of herpes simplex virus by direct immunofluorescence and viral isolation from samples of external genital lesions in a high prevalence population. J. Clin. Microbiol. *25*:323, 1987.
154. Lakeman, F. D., and Whitley, R. J.: Diagnosis of herpes simplex encephalitis: Application of polymerase chain reaction to cerebrospinal fluid from brain-biopsied patients and correlation with disease. J. Infect. Dis. *171*:856–863, 1995.
155. Landry, M. L., Cohen, S., and Ferguson, D.: Impact of sample type on rapid detection of influenza virus A by cytospin-enhanced immunofluorescence and membrane enzyme-linked immunosorbent assay. J. Clin. Microbiol. *38*:429–430, 2000.
156. Landry, M. L., and Ferguson, D.: Comparison of quantitative cytomegalovirus antigenemia assay with culture methods and correlation with clinical disease. J. Clin. Microbiol. *31*:2851–2856, 1993.
157. Landry, M. L., and Ferguson, D.: SimulFluor respiratory screen for rapid detection of multiple respiratory viruses in clinical specimens by immunofluorescence staining. J. Clin. Microbiol. *38*:708–711, 2000.
158. Landry, M. L., Ferguson, D., Stevens-Ayers, T., et al.: Evaluation of CMV Brite kit for detection of cytomegalovirus pp65 antigenemia in peripheral blood leukocytes by immunofluorescence. J. Clin. Microbiol. *34*:1337–1339, 1996.
159. Langenberg, A., Zbanysek, R., Dragavon, J., et al.: Detection of herpes simplex virus DNA from genital lesions by in situ hybridization. J. Clin. Microbiol. *26*:933–937, 1988.
160. Lauer, B. A., Masters, H. A., Wren, C. G., et al.: Rapid detection of respiratory syncytial virus in nasopharyngeal secretions by an enzyme-linked immunosorbent assay. J. Clin. Microbiol. *22*:782, 1985.
161. Lazar, J., Salim, H., Scearce, L., et al.: Improved detection of CMV viremia: A multicenter trial of the Hybrid Capture™ CMV DNA assay. Paper presented at the San Diego Nucleic Acids Conference, American Association of Clinical Chemistry, 1995.
162. Lazzarotto, T., Campisi, B., Galli, S., et al.: A quantitative test (HCMV Hybrid Capture) to detect human cytomegalovirus DNA in the blood of immunocompromised patients compared with antigenemia and polymerase chain reaction. Paper presented at the Fifth International Cytomegalovirus Conference, 1995, Stockholm.
163. Lee, S. C., Antony, A., Lee, N., et al.: Improved version 2.0 qualitative and quantitative AMPLICOR reverse transcription–PCR tests for hepatitis C virus RNA: Calibration to international units, enhanced genotype reactivity, and performance characteristics. J. Clin. Microbiol. *38*:4171–4179, 2000.
164. Leland, D. S., Hansing, R. L., and French, M. L. V.: Clinical experience with cytomegalovirus isolation using both conventional cell cultures and rapid shell vial techniques. J. Clin. Microbiol. *27*:1159–1162, 1989.
165. Lennette, E. H., and Smith, T. F. (eds.): Laboratory Diagnosis of Viral Infections. 3rd ed. New York, Marcel Dekker, 1999.
166. Leonardi, G. P., Leib, H., Birkhead, G. S., et al.: Comparison of rapid detection methods for influenza A virus and their value in health care management of institutionalized geriatric patients. J. Clin. Microbiol. *32*:70–74, 1994.
167. Lin, H. J., Haywood, M., and Hollinger, F. B.: Application of a commercial kit for detection of PCR products to quantification of human immunodeficiency virus type 1 RNA and proviral DNA. J. Clin. Microbiol. *34*:329–333, 1996.
168. Lipson, S. M., David, K., Shaikh, F., et al.: Detection of precytopathic effect of enteroviruses in clinical specimens by centrifugation-enhanced antigen detection. J. Clin. Microbiol. *39*:2755–2759, 2001.
169. Loeb, K., Jerome, K., Goddard, J., et al.: High-throughput quantitative analysis of hepatitis B virus DNA in serum using the TaqMan fluorogenic detection system. Hepatology *32*:626–629, 2000.
170. Long, C., Cullen, A., Cox, T., et al.: Rapid detection and typing of herpes simplex virus using the Hybrid Capture system. Abstract M25. Paper presented at the 12th Annual Clinical Virology Symposium, 1996, Clearwater, FL.
171. Lunel, F., Mariotti, M., Cresta, P., et al.: Comparative study of conventional and novel strategies for the detection of hepatitis C virus RNA in serum: Amplicor, branched-DNA, NASBA and in-house PCR. J. Virol. Methods *54*:159–171, 1995.
172. Macartney, M., Gane, E., and Williams, R.: Comparison of Hybrid Capture CMV DNA assay with PCR, IgM detection, cell culture and DEAFF test in liver transplant patients. Paper presented at the Fifth International Cytomegalovirus Conference, 1995, Stockholm.
173. MacDonald, R. L., Hughes, B. L., Aarnaes, S. L., et al.: Evaluation of a shell vial centrifugation method for the detection of herpes simplex virus. Diagn. Microbiol. Infect. Dis. *9*:51, 1988.
174. Mahafzah, A. M., and Landry, M. L.: Evaluation of immunofluorescent reagents, centrifugation, and conventional cultures for the diagnosis of adenovirus infection. Diagn. Microbiol. Infect. Dis. *12*:407–411, 1989.
175. Martin, W. J., II, and Smith, T. F.: Rapid detection of cytomegalovirus in bronchoalveolar lavage specimens by a monoclonal antibody method. J. Clin. Microbiol. *23*:1006–1008, 1986.
176. Martinez, O. M., Villanueva, J. C., Lawrence-Miyasaki, L., et al.: Viral and immunologic aspects of Epstein-Barr virus infection in pediatric liver transplant recipients. Transplantation *59*:519–524, 1995.
177. Mason, T., Bloom, G., and Leland, D.: Evaluation of ELVIS HSV Gold, a commercially available tube culture system featuring a genetically engineered cell line and a histochemical assay for detection of herpes simplex virus (HSV). Abstract M24. Paper presented at the 12th Annual Clinical Virology Symposium, 1996, Clearwater, FL.
178. Masters, H. B., Bate, B. J., Wren, C., et al.: Detection of respiratory syncytial virus antigen in nasopharyngeal secretions by Abbott Diagnostics enzyme immunoassay. J. Clin. Microbiol. *26*:1103–1105, 1988.
179. Mathewson, J. J., Winsor, D. K., DuPont, H. L., et al.: Evaluation of assay systems for the detection of rotavirus in stool specimens. Diagn. Microbiol. Infect. Dis. *12*:139–141, 1989.
180. Matthey, S., Nicholson, D., Ruhs, S., et al.: Rapid detection of respiratory viruses by shell vial culture and direct staining by using pooled and individual monoclonal antibodies. J. Clin. Microbiol. *30*:540–544, 1992.
181. Mazzulli, T., Rubin, R. H., Ferraro, M. J., et al.: Cytomegalovirus antigenemia: Clinical correlations in transplant recipients and in persons with AIDS. J. Clin. Microbiol. *31*:2824–2827, 1993.
182. Mazzulli, T., Wood, S., Chua, R., et al.: Evaluation of the Digene Hybrid Capture system for the detection and quantitation of human cytomegalovirus viremia in human immunodeficiency virus–infected patients. J. Clin. Microbiol. *34*:2959–2962, 1996.
183. McDonald, J. C., and Quennec, P.: Utility of a respiratory virus panel containing a monoclonal antibody pool for screening of respiratory specimens in nonpeak respiratory syncytial virus season. J. Clin. Microbiol. *31*:2809–2811, 1993.
184. McIntosh, K.: Recent advances in viral diagnosis. Arch. Pathol. Lab. Med. *104*:3–6, 1980.
185. McQuillin, J., Madeley, C. R., and Kendal, A. P.: Monoclonal antibodies for the rapid diagnosis of influenza A and B virus infections by immunofluorescence. Lancet *2*:911, 1985.
186. Mellors, J. W., Rinaldo, C. R., Jr., Gupta, P., et al.: Prognosis in HIV-1 infection predicted by the quantity of virus in plasma. Science *272*:1167–1176, 1996.
187. Michalski, F. J., Shaikh, M., Sahraie, F., et al.: Enzyme-linked immunosorbent assay spin amplification technique for herpes simplex virus antigen detection. J. Clin. Microbiol. *24*:310–311, 1986.
188. Milburn, G. L., Carrigan, D., Dienglewicz, R., et al.: Diagnosis of active human herpesvirus six (HHV-6) infection in immunocompromised patients with a rapid shell vial assay. Abstract C136. Paper presented at the 96th General Meeting of the American Society of Microbiology, 1996, New Orleans.
189. Miller, H., Milk, R., and Diaz-Mitoma, F.: Comparison of the VIDAS RSV assay and the Abbott Testpack RSV with direct immunofluorescence for detection of respiratory syncytial virus in nasopharyngeal aspirates. J. Clin. Microbiol. *31*:1336–1338, 1993.
190. Miller, M. J., Bovey, S., Pado, K., et al.: Application of PCR to multiple specimen types for diagnosis of cytomegalovirus infection: Comparison with cell culture and shell vial assay. J. Clin. Microbiol. *32*:5–10, 1994.
191. Miller, M. J., and Howell, C. L.: Rapid detection and identification of herpes simplex virus in cell culture by a direct immunoperoxidase staining procedure. J. Clin. Microbiol. *18*:550–553, 1983.
192. Miller, M. J., Wagar, E. A., Moe, A. A., et al.: Comparison of nucleic acid hybridization, culture, and shell vial assay for detection of CMV in blood. Abstract C89. Paper presented at the 96th General Meeting of the American Society of Microbiology, 1996, New Orleans.
193. Mills, R. D., Cain, K. J., and Woods, G. L.: Detection of influenza virus by centrifugal inoculation of MDCK cells and staining with monoclonal antibodies. J. Clin. Microbiol. *27*:2505–2508, 1989.
194. Minnich, L. L., Goodenough, F., and Ray, C. G.: Use of immunofluorescence to identify measles virus infection. J. Clin. Microbiol. *29*:1148–1150, 1991.
195. Minnich, L. L., and Ray, C. G.: Comparison of direct and indirect immunofluorescence staining of clinical specimens for detection of respiratory syncytial virus antigen. J. Clin. Microbiol. *15*:969, 1982.

196. Minnich, L. L., and Ray, C. G.: Early testing of cell culture for detection of hemadsorbing viruses. J. Clin. Microbiol. *25*:421–422, 1987.
197. Murphy, D. G., Cote, L., Fauvel, M., et al.: Multicenter comparison of Roche COBAS AMPLICOR MONITOR version 1.5, Organon Teknika Nuclisens QT with extractor, and Bayer Quantiplex version 3.0 for quantification of human immunodeficiency virus type 1 RNA in plasma. J. Clin. Microbiol. *38*:4034–4041, 2000.
198. Murray, P. R., Baron, E. J., Pfaller, M. A., et al. (eds.): Manual of Clinical Microbiology. 7th ed. Washington, D.C., American Society for Microbiology, 1999.
199. Myerson, D., Hackman, R. C., and Meyers, J. D.: Diagnosis of cytomegalovirus pneumonia by in situ hybridization. J. Infect. Dis. *150*: 272–277, 1984.
200. Nahass, G. T., Goldstein, B. A., Zhu, W., et al.: Comparison of Tzanck, viral culture, and DNA diagnostic methods in detection of herpes simplex and varicella zoster infection (PCR). J. A. M. A. *268*:2541–2544, 1992.
201. Nahass, G. T., Mandel, M. J., Cook, S., et al.: Detection of herpes simplex and varicella zoster infection from cutaneous lesions in different clinical stages with the polymerase chain reaction. J. Am. Acad. Dermatol. *32*:730–733, 1995.
202. Nelson, C. T., Istas, A. S., Wilkerson, M. K., et al.: PCR detection of cytomegalovirus DNA in serum as a diagnostic test for congenital cytomegalovirus infection. J. Clin. Microbiol. *33*:3317–3318, 1995.
203. Niesters, H. G., van Esser, J., Fries, E., et al.: Development of a real-time quantitative assay for detection of Epstein-Barr virus. J. Clin. Microbiol. *38*:712–715, 2000.
204. Nishi, M., Hanashiro, R., Mori, S., et al.: Polymerase chain reaction for the detection of the varicella zoster genome in ocular samples from patients with acute retinal necrosis. Am. J. Ophthalmol. *114*:603–609, 1992.
205. Nitsche, A., Steuer, N., Schmidt, C. A., et al.: Different real-time PCR formats compared for the quantitative detection of human cytomegalovirus DNA. Clin. Chem. *45*:1932–1937, 1999.
206. Noborg, U., Gusdal, A., Pisa, E. K., et al.: Automated quantitative analysis of hepatitis B virus DNA by using the Cobas Amplicor HBV monitor test. J. Clin. Microbiol. *37*:2793–2797, 1999.
207. Nolte, F. S., Thurmond, C., and Fried, M. W.: Preclinical evaluation of AMPLICOR hepatitis C virus test for detection of hepatitis C virus RNA. J. Clin. Microbiol. *33*:1775–1778, 1995.
208. Noyola, D. E., Clark, B., O'Donnell, F. T., et al.: Comparison of a new neuraminidase detection assay with an enzyme immunoassay, immunofluorescence, and culture for rapid detection of influenza A and B viruses in nasal wash specimens. J. Clin. Microbiol. *38*:1161–1165, 2000.
209. Ogburn, J. R., Hoffpauir, J. T., Cole, E., et al.: Evaluation of new transport medium for detection of herpes simplex virus by culture and direct enzyme-linked immunosorbent assay. J. Clin. Microbiol. *32*:3082–3084, 1994.
210. Olsen, M. A., Shuch, K. M., Sambol, A. R., et al.: Isolation of seven respiratory viruses in shell vials: A practical and highly sensitive method. J. Clin. Microbiol. *31*:422–425, 1993.
211. Pai, C. H., Shahrabad, M. S., and Ince, B.: Rapid diagnosis of rotavirus gastroenteritis by a commercial latex agglutination test. J. Clin. Microbiol. *22*:846–850, 1985.
212. Pas, S. D., Fries, E., De Man, R. A., et al.: Development of a quantitative real-time detection assay for hepatitis B virus DNA and comparison with two commercial assays. J. Clin. Microbiol. *38*:2897–2901, 2000.
213. Paya, C. V., Holley, K. E., and Wiesner, R. H.: Early diagnosis of cytomegalovirus hepatitis in liver transplant recipients: Role of immunostaining, DNA hybridization, and culture of hepatic tissue. Hepatology *12*:119, 1990.
214. Paya, C. V., Wold, A. D., Ilstrup, D. M., et al.: Evaluation of number of shell vial cell cultures per clinical specimen for rapid diagnosis of cytomegalovirus infection. J. Clin. Microbiol. *26*:198–200, 1988.
215. Paya, C. V., Wold, A. D., and Smith, T. F.: Detection of cytomegalovirus infections in specimens other than urine by the shell vial assay and conventional tube cell cultures. J. Clin. Microbiol. *25*:755–757, 1987.
216. Persing, D. H.: Polymerase chain reaction: Trenches to benches. J. Clin. Microbiol. *29*:1281–1285, 1991.
217. Persing, D. H., Smith, T. F., Tenover, F. C., et al. (eds.): Diagnostic Molecular Microbiology, Principles and Applications. Washington, D.C., American Society for Microbiology, 1993.
218. Peter, J. B.: The polymerase chain reaction: Amplifying our options. Rev. Infect. Dis. *13*:166–171, 1991.
219. Peterson, E. M., Hughes, B. L., Aarnaes, S. L., et al.: Comparison of primary rabbit kidney and MRC-5 cells and two stain procedures for herpes simplex virus detection by a shell vial centrifugation method. J. Clin. Microbiol. *26*:222–224, 1988.
220. Peterson, L. R., Moore, B. M., Edelman, C. K., et al.: Primary virus isolation by a satellite laboratory. Arch. Pathol. Lab. Med. *104*:9–10, 1980.
221. Phillips, L. E., Magliola, R. A., Stehlik, M. L., et al.: Retrospective evaluation of the isolation and identification of herpes simplex virus with CultureSet and human fibroblasts. J. Clin. Microbiol. *22*:255–258, 1985.
222. Podzorski, R. P., and Persing, D. H.: PCR: The next decade. Clin. Microbiol. Newsl. *15*:137–143, 1993.
223. Pouletty, P., Chomel, J. J., Thourvenot, D., et al.: Detection of herpes simplex virus in direct specimens by immunofluorescence assay using a monoclonal antibody. J. Clin. Microbiol. *25*:958–959, 1987.
224. Pruneda, R. C., and Almanza, I.: Centrifugation–shell vial technique for rapid detection of herpes simplex virus cytopathic effect in Vero cells. J. Clin. Microbiol. *25*:423–424, 1987.
225. Puchhammer-Stockl, E., Heinz, F. X., Kundi, M., et al.: Evaluation of the polymerase chain reaction for diagnosis of herpes simplex virus encephalitis. J. Clin. Microbiol. *31*:146–148, 1993.
226. Puchhammer-Stockl, E., Heinz, F. X., and Kunz, C.: Evaluation of three nonradioactive DNA detection systems for identification of herpes simplex DNA amplified from cerebrospinal fluid. J. Virol. Methods *43*:257–266, 1993.
227. Puchhammer-Stockl, E., Popow-Kraupp, T., Heinz, F., et al.: Detection of varicella-zoster virus DNA by polymerase chain reaction in the cerebrospinal fluid of patients suffering from neurological complications associated with chicken pox or herpes zoster. J. Clin. Microbiol. *29*:1513–1516, 1991.
228. Rabalais, G. P., Stout, G. G., Ladd, K. L., et al.: Rapid diagnosis of respiratory viral infections by using a shell vial assay and monoclonal antibody pool. J. Clin. Microbiol. *30*:1505–1508, 1992.
229. Rabella, N., and Drew, W. L.: Comparison of conventional and shell vial cultures for detecting cytomegalovirus infection. J. Clin. Microbiol. *4*:806–807, 1990.
230. Ramers, C., Billman, G., Hartin, M., et al.: Impact of a diagnostic cerebrospinal fluid enterovirus polymerase chain reaction test on patient management. J. A. M. A. *283*:2680–2685, 2000.
231. Ray, C. G., and Minnich, L. L.: Efficiency of immunofluorescence for rapid detection of common respiratory viruses. J. Clin. Microbiol. *25*:355, 1987.
232. Redfield, D. C., Richman, D. D., Albanil, S., et al.: Detection of herpes simplex virus in clinical specimens by DNA hybridization. Diagn. Microbiol. Infect. Dis. *1*:117–128, 1983.
233. Revets, H., Marissens, D., DeWit, S., et al.: Comparative evaluation of NASBA HIV-1 RNA QT, AMPLICOR-HIV Monitor, and QUANTIPLEX HIV RNA assay, three methods for quantification of human immunodeficiency virus type 1 RNA in plasma. J. Clin. Microbiol. *34*:1058–1064, 1996.
234. Rogers, M. F., Ou, C. Y., Rayfield, M., et al.: Use of the polymerase chain reaction for early detection of the proviral sequences of human immunodeficiency virus in infants born to seropositive mothers. N. Engl. J. Med. *320*:1649, 1989.
235. Romero, J. R., Hinrichs, S. H., Cavalieri, S. J., et al.: Potential health care cost saving from PCR-based rapid diagnosis of enteroviral meningitis. Abstract. Paper presented at the Society of Pediatric Research Annual Meeting, May 6–10, 1996, Washington, D.C.
236. Romero, J. R., and Rotbart, H. A.: PCR based strategies for the detection of human enteroviruses. *In* Ehrlich, G. D., and Greenberg, S. J. (eds.): PCR-Based Diagnostics in Infectious Disease. Boston, Blackwell, 1994, pp. 341–374.
237. Rossier, E., Miller, H. R., and Phipps, P. H.: Rapid Viral Diagnosis by Immunofluorescence: An Atlas and Practical Guide. Ottawa, Canada, University of Ottawa Press, 1989.
238. Rotbart, H. A.: Enteroviral infections of the central nervous system. Clin. Infect. Dis. *20*:971–981, 1995.
239. Rotbart, H. A., Sawyer, M. H., Fast, S., et al.: Diagnosis of enteroviral meningitis by using PCR with a colorimetric microwell detection assay. J. Clin. Microbiol. *32*:2590–2592, 1994.
240. Roth, W. K., Lee, J. H., Ruster, B., et al.: Comparison of two quantitative hepatitis C virus reverse transcriptase PCR assays. J. Clin. Microbiol. *34*:261–264, 1996.
241. Rothbarth, P. H., Hermus, M. C., and Schrijnemakers, P.: Reliability of two new test kits for rapid diagnosis of respiratory syncytial virus infection. J. Clin. Microbiol. *29*:824–826, 1991.
242. Rowley, A. H., Whitley, R. J., Lakeman, F. D., et al.: Rapid detection of herpes simplex virus DNA in cerebrospinal fluid of patients with herpes simplex encephalitis. Lancet *335*:440–441, 1990.
243. Rubin, S. J., and Rogers, S.: Comparison of Culture Set and primary rabbit kidney cell culture for the detection of herpes simplex virus. J. Clin. Microbiol. *19*:920–922, 1984.
244. Ruest, A., Michaud, S., Deslandes, S., et al.: Comparison of Directigen Flu A+B with QuickVue and with culture for influenza diagnosis. Abstract T15. Paper presented at the 17th Annual Clinical Virology Symposium, 2001, Clearwater, FL.
245. Ryan-Poirier, K. A., Katz, J. M., Webster, R. G., et al.: Application of Directigen Flu-A for the detection of influenza A virus in human and nonhuman specimens. J. Clin. Microbiol. *30*:1072–1075, 1992.
246. Saag, M. S., Holodniy, M., Kuritzkes, D. R., et al.: HIV viral load markers in clinical practice. Nat. Med. *2*:625–629, 1996.
247. Salmon, V. C., Turner, R. B., Speranza, M. J., et al.: Rapid detection of herpes simplex virus in clinical specimens by centrifugation and immunoperoxidase staining. J. Clin. Microbiol. *23*:683–686, 1986.
248. Sambourg, M. A., Goudeau, A., Courant, C., et al.: Direct appraisal of latex agglutination testing, a convenient alternative to enzyme immunoassay for the detection of rotavirus in childhood gastroenteritis,

by comparison of two enzyme immunoassays and two latex tests. J. Clin. Microbiol. *21*:622–625, 1985.
249. Sanders, R. C., Campbell, A. D., and Jenkins, M. F.: Routine detection of human rotavirus by latex agglutination: Comparison with enzyme-linked immunosorbent assay, electron microscopy, and polyacrylamide gel electrophoresis. J. Virol. Methods *13*:285, 1986.
250. Sawyer, M. H., Holland, D., Aintablian, N., et al.: Diagnosis of enteroviral central nervous system infection by polymerase chain reaction during a large community outbreak. Pediatr. Infect. Dis. J. *13*:177–182, 1994.
251. Schaade, L., Kockelkorn, P., Ritter, K., et al.: Detection of cytomegalovirus DNA in human specimens by LightCycler PCR. J. Clin. Microbiol. *38*:4006–4009, 2000.
252. Schalasta, G., Eggers, M., Schmid, M., et al.: Analysis of human cytomegalovirus DNA in urines of newborns and infants by means of a new ultrarapid real-time PCR-system. J. Clin. Virol. *19*:175–185, 2000.
253. Schirm, J., Kooistra, A., van Son, W. J., et al.: Comparison of the Murex Hybrid Capture CMV DNA (v2.0) assay and the pp65 CMV antigenemia test for the detection and quantitation of CMV in blood samples from immunocompromised patients. J. Clin. Virol. *14*:153–165, 1999.
254. Schirm, J., Luijt, D. S., Pastoor, G. W., et al.: Rapid detection of respiratory viruses using mixtures of monoclonal antibodies on shell vial cultures. J. Med. Virol. *38*:147–151, 1992.
255. Schirm, J., Meulenberg, J., Pastoor, G., et al.: Rapid detection of varicella zoster virus in clinical specimens using monoclonal antibodies on shell vials and smears. J. Med. Virol. *28*:1–6, 1989.
256. Schlesinger, Y., Buller, R. S., Brunstrom, J. E., et al.: Expanded spectrum of herpes simplex encephalitis in childhood. J. Pediatr. *126*:234–241, 1995.
257. Schlesinger, Y., Sawyer, M. H., and Storch, G. A.: Enteroviral meningitis in infancy: Potential role for polymerase chain reaction in patient management. Pediatrics *94*:157–162, 1994.
258. Schmidt, N. J., and Emmons, R. W. (eds.): Diagnostic Procedures for Viral, Rickettsial, and Chlamydial Infections. 6th ed. Washington, D.C., American Public Health Association, 1989.
259. Schmidt, N. J., Gallo, D., Devlin, V., et al.: Direct immunofluorescence staining for detection of herpes simplex and varicella zoster virus antigens in vesicular lesions and certain tissue specimens. J. Clin. Microbiol. *12*:651–655, 1980.
260. Scholl, D. R., Dul, J. C., McHard, K. D., et al.: ELVIRA (TM) HSV promoter cell clone for rapid antiviral resistance testing. Abstract M29. Paper presented at the 12th Annual Clinical Virology Symposium, 1996, Clearwater, FL.
261. Seme, K., and Poljak, M.: Use of a commercial PCR kit for detection of hepatitis C virus. Eur. J. Clin. Microbiol. Infect. Dis. *14*:549–552, 1995.
262. Seno, M., Kanamoto, Y., Takao, S., et al.: Enhancing effect of centrifugation on isolation of influenza virus from clinical specimens. J. Clin. Microbiol. *28*:1669–1670, 1990.
263. Sewell, D. L., and Horn, S. A.: Evaluation of a commercial enzyme linked immunosorbent assay for the detection of herpes simplex virus. J. Clin. Microbiol. *21*:457–458, 1985.
264. Shibata, D., Martin, W. J., Appleman, M. D., et al.: Detection of cytomegalovirus DNA in peripheral blood of patients infected with human immunodeficiency virus. J. Infect. Dis. *158*:1185–1192, 1988.
265. Shoji, H., Honda, Y., Murai, I., et al.: Detection of varicella zoster virus DNA by polymerase chain reaction in cerebrospinal fluid of patients with herpes simplex meningitis. J. Neurol. *239*:69–70, 1992.
266. Sia, I. G., Wilson, J. A., Espy, M. J., et al.: Evaluation of the COBAS AMPLICOR CMV MONITOR test for detection of viral DNA in specimens taken from patients after liver transplantation. J. Clin. Microbiol. *38*:600–606, 2000.
267. Siennicka, J., Durlik, M., Litwinska, B., et al.: Usefulness of hybridization and PCR methods in monitoring of CMV infection in renal transplant recipients. Ann. Transplant. *5*:21–24, 2000.
268. Smith, M. C., Creutz, C., and Huang, Y. T.: Detection of respiratory syncytial virus in nasopharyngeal secretions by shell vial technique. J. Clin. Microbiol. *29*:463–465, 1991.
269. Smith, T. F., Weed, L. A., Pettersen, G. R., et al.: Recovery of *Chlamydia* and genital *Mycoplasma* transported in sucrose phosphate buffer and urease colortest medium. Health Lab. Sci. *14*:30–34, 1977.
270. Spada, B., Biehler, K., Chegas, P., et al.: Comparison of rapid immunofluorescence assay to cell culture isolation for the detection of influenza A and B viruses in nasopharyngeal secretions from infants and children. J. Virol. Methods *33*:305–310, 1991.
271. Specter, S., Hodinka, R. L., and Young, S. A. (eds.): Clinical Virology Manual. 3rd ed. Washington, D.C., ASM Press, 2000.
272. Spector, S. A., Merrill, R., Wolf, D., et al.: Detection of human cytomegalovirus in plasma of AIDS patients during acute visceral disease by DNA amplification. J. Clin. Microbiol. *30*:2359–2365, 1992.
273. Stabell, E. C., and Olivo, P. D.: Isolation of a cell line for rapid and sensitive histochemical assay for the detection of herpes simplex virus. J. Virol. Methods *38*:195–204, 1992.
274. Stabell, E. C., O'Rourke, S. R., Storch, G. A., et al.: Evaluation of a genetically engineered cell line and a histochemical β-galactosidase assay to detect herpes simplex virus in clinical specimens. J. Clin. Microbiol. *31*:2796–2798, 1993.
275. Stevens, S. J., Pronk, I., and Middeldorp, J. M.: Toward standardization of Epstein-Barr virus DNA load monitoring: Unfractionated whole blood as preferred clinical specimen. J. Clin. Microbiol. *39*:1211–1216, 2001.
276. Stockl, E., Popow-Kraupp, T., Heinz, F. X., et al.: Potential of in situ hybridization for early diagnosis of productive cytomegalovirus infection. J. Clin. Microbiol. *26*:2536–2540, 1988.
277. Stokes, C. E., Bernstein, J. M., Kyger, S. A., et al.: Rapid diagnosis of influenza A and B by 24-h fluorescent focus assays. J. Clin. Microbiol. *26*:1263–1266, 1988.
278. Storch, G. A., Reed, C. A., and Dula, Z. A.: Evaluation of a latex agglutination test for herpes simplex virus. J. Clin. Microbiol. *26*:787, 1988.
279. Stout, C., Murphy, M. D., Lawrence, S., et al.: Evaluation of a monoclonal antibody pool for rapid diagnosis of respiratory viral infections. J. Clin. Microbiol. *27*:448–452, 1989.
280. Strickler, J. G., Manivel, J. C., Copenhaver, C. M., et al.: Comparison of in situ hybridization and immunohistochemistry for detection of cytomegalovirus and herpes simplex virus. Hum. Pathol. *21*:443, 1990.
281. Swierkosz, E. M., Brown, P., Berger, J., et al.: Directigen RSV and Directigen Flu A+B are insensitive for detection of RSV and influenza virus in nasopharyngeal swab specimens. Abstract T22. Paper presented at the 17th Annual Clinical Virology Symposium, 2001, Clearwater, FL.
282. Swierkosz, E. M., Flander, R., Melvin, L., et al.: Evaluation of the Abbott TEST PACK RSV enzyme immunoassay for detection of respiratory syncytial virus in nasopharyngeal swab specimens. J. Clin. Microbiol. *27*:1151–1154, 1989.
283. Taggart, B., Crist, G., Carroll, K., et al.: Enterovirus (EV) detection by reverse transcription–polymerase chain reaction (RT-PCR) using commercially available reagents on cerebrospinal fluid (CSF). Abstract S37. Paper presented at the 17th Annual Clinical Virology Symposium, 2001, Clearwater, FL.
284. Tanaka, N., Kimura, H., Iida, K., et al.: Quantitative analysis of cytomegalovirus load using real-time PCR assay. J. Med. Virol. *60*:455–462, 2000.
285. Telenti, A., Marshall, W. F., and Smith, T. F.: Detection of Epstein-Barr virus by polymerase chain reaction. J. Clin. Microbiol. *28*:2187–2190, 1990.
286. Templeton, N. S.: The polymerase chain reaction: History, methods, and applications. Diagn. Mol. Pathol. *1*:58–72, 1992.
287. Tenover, F. C.: Diagnostic deoxyribonucleic probes for infectious diseases. Clin. Microbiol. Rev. *1*:82–101, 1988.
288. The, T. H., van der Ploeg, M., van der Berg, A. P., et al.: Direct detection of cytomegalovirus in peripheral blood leukocytes: A review of the antigenemia assay and the polymerase chain reaction. Transplantation *54*:193–198, 1992.
289. Thomas, E. E., and Book, L. E.: Comparison of two rapid methods for detection of respiratory syncytial virus (TestPack RSV and Ortho ELISA) with direct immunofluorescence and virus isolation for the diagnosis of pediatric RSV infection. J. Clin. Microbiol. *29*:632–635, 1991.
290. Thomas, E. E., Puterman, M. L., Kawano, E., et al.: Evaluation of several immunoassays for detection of rotavirus in pediatric stool samples. J. Clin. Microbiol. *26*:1189–1193, 1988.
291. Trabelsi, A., Pozzetto, B., Mbida, A. D., et al.: Evaluation of four methods for rapid detection of adenovirus. Eur. J. Clin. Microbiol. Infect. Dis. *11*:535–539, 1992.
292. Troendle-Atkins, J., Demmler, G. J., and Buffone, G. J.: Rapid diagnosis of herpes simplex virus encephalitis by using the polymerase chain reaction. J. Pediatr. *123*:376–380, 1993.
293. Unger, E. R.: In situ and northern hybridizations: Technical considerations guiding clinical application. Cancer *69*:1532–1535, 1992.
294. Unger, E. R., and Brigati, D. J.: Colorimetric in situ hybridization in clinical virology: Development of automated technology. Curr. Top. Microbiol. Immunol. *143*:21–31, 1989.
295. Unger, E. R., Budgeon, L. R., Myerson, D., et al.: Viral diagnosis by in situ hybridization: Description of a rapid simplified colorimetric method. Am. J. Surg. Pathol. *10*:1–8, 1986.
296. Uren, E. C., Johnson, P. D. R., Montanaro, J., et al.: Herpes simplex virus encephalitis in pediatrics: Diagnosis by detection of antibodies and DNA in cerebrospinal fluid. Pediatr. Infect. Dis. J. *12*:1001–1006, 1993.
297. Valentine-Thon, E.: Evaluation of SHARP signal system for enzymatic detection of amplified hepatitis B virus DNA. J. Clin. Microbiol. *33*:477–480, 1995.
298. Van Beers, D., DeFoor, M., DiCesare, L., et al.: Evaluation of a commercial enzyme and immunomembrane filter assay for detection of respiratory syncytial virus in clinical specimens. Eur. J. Clin. Microbiol. Infect. Dis. *10*:1073–1076, 1991.
299. Van den Berg, A. P., Klompmaker, I. J., Haagsma, E. B., et al.: Antigenemia in the diagnosis and monitoring of active cytomegalovirus infection after liver transplantation. J. Infect. Dis. *164*:265–270, 1991.
300. Van den Berg, A. P., Tegzass, A. M., Scholten-Sampson, A., et al.: Monitoring antigenemia is useful in guiding treatment of severe cytomegalovirus disease after organ transplantation. Transplant. Infect. *5*: 101–107, 1992.
301. Van den Berg, A. P., van der Bij, W., van Son, W. J., et al.: Cytomegalovirus antigenemia as a useful marker of symptomatic cytomegalovirus infection after renal transplantation: A report of 130 consecutive patients. Transplantation *48*:991–995, 1989.

302. Van der Bij, W., Schirm, J., Torensma, R., et al.: Comparison between viremia and antigenemia for detection of cytomegalovirus in blood. J. Clin. Microbiol. *26*:2531–2535, 1988.
303. Van der Bij, W., Torensma, R., van Son, W. J., et al.: Rapid immunodiagnosis of active cytomegalovirus infection by monoclonal antibody staining of blood leukocytes. J. Med. Virol. *25*:179–188, 1988.
304. Van Elden, L. J., Nijhuis, M., Schipper, P., et al.: Simultaneous detection of influenza viruses A and B using real-time quantitative PCR. J. Clin. Microbiol. *39*:196–200, 2001.
305. Verano, L., and Michalski, F. J.: Herpes simplex virus antigen direct detection in standard virus transport medium by DuPont HerpChek enzyme-linked immunosorbent assay. J. Clin. Microbiol. *28*:2555–2558, 1990.
306. Verano, L., and Michalski, F. J.: Spin-amplified culture followed by enzyme immunoassay for detection of herpes simplex virus in patient specimens: A comparative study. Clin. Diagn. Virol. *1*:23–28, 1993.
307. Verano, L., and Michalski, F. J.: Comparison of direct antigen enzyme immunoassay, HerpChek, with cell culture for detection of herpes simplex virus from clinical specimens. J. Clin. Microbiol. *33*:1378–1379, 1995.
308. Volpi, A., Whitley, R. J., Ceballos, R., et al.: Rapid diagnosis of pneumonia due to cytomegalovirus with specific monoclonal antibodies. J. Infect. Dis. *147*:1119–1120, 1983.
309. Waecker, N. J., Jr., Shope, T. R., Weber, P. A., et al.: The Rhino-Probe nasal culturette for detecting respiratory syncytial virus in children. Pediatr. Infect. Dis. J. *12*:326–329, 1993.
310. Walls, H. H., Harmon, M. W., Slagle, J. J., et al.: Characterization and evaluation of monoclonal antibodies developed for typing influenza A and influenza B viruses. J. Clin. Microbiol. *23*:240–245, 1986.
311. Waner, J. L., Todd, S. J., Shalaby, P., et al.: Comparison of Directigen Flu-A with viral isolation and direct immunofluorescence for the rapid detection and identification of influenza A virus. J. Clin. Microbiol. *29*:479–482, 1991.
312. Waner, J. L., Whitehurst, N. J., Downs, T., et al.: Production of monoclonal antibodies against parainfluenza 3 virus and their use in diagnosis by immunofluorescence. J. Clin. Microbiol. *22*:535, 1985.
313. Warford, A. L., Chung, J. W., Drill, A. E., et al.: Amplification techniques for detection of herpes simplex virus in neonatal and maternal genital specimens obtained at delivery. J. Clin. Microbiol. *27*:1324–1328, 1989.
314. Warford, A. L., Kao, S. Y., Valantine, H., et al.: Evaluation of CMV plasma PCR for monitoring of heart transplant recipients receiving both ganciclovir and Cytogam prophylaxis. Abstract S18. Paper presented at the 12th Annual Clinical Virology Symposium, 1996, Clearwater, FL.
315. Weiss, R. L., Snow, G. W., Schumann, G. B., et al.: Diagnosis of cytomegalovirus pneumonitis on bronchoalveolar lavage fluid: Comparison of cytology, immunofluorescence, and in situ hybridization with viral isolation. Diagn. Cytopathol. *7*:243–247, 1990.
316. White, T. J., Madej, R., and Persing, D. H.: The polymerase chain reaction: Clinical applications. Adv. Clin. Chem. *29*:161–196, 1992.
317. Whitley, R. J., and Lakeman, F.: Herpes simplex virus infections of the central nervous system: Therapeutic and diagnostic considerations. Clin. Infect. Dis. *20*:414–420, 1995.
318. Williams, S. D., and Kwok, S.: Polymerase chain reaction: Applications for viral detection. *In* Lennette, E. H. (ed.): Laboratory Diagnosis of Viral Infections. 2nd ed. New York, Marcel Dekker, 1992, pp. 147–173.
319. Wolcott, M. J.: Advances in nucleic acid based detection methods. Clin. Microbiol. Rev. *5*:370–386, 1992.
320. Wolf, D. G., and Spector, S. A.: Diagnosis of human cytomegalovirus central nervous system disease in AIDS patients by DNA amplification from cerebrospinal fluid. J. Infect. Dis. *166*:1412–1415, 1992.
321. Wong, D. T., Welliver, R. C., Riddlesberger, K. R., et al.: Rapid diagnosis of parainfluenza virus infection in children. J. Clin. Microbiol. *16*:164–167, 1982.
322. Wood, D. J., Bijlsma, K., de Jong, J. C., et al.: Evaluation of a commercial monoclonal antibody–based enzyme immunoassay for detection of adenovirus types 40 and 41 in stool specimens. J. Clin. Microbiol. *27*:1155–1158, 1989.
323. Wren, C. G., Bate, B. J., Masters, H. B., et al.: Detection of respiratory syncytial virus antigen in nasal washings by Abbott TestPack enzyme immunoassay. J. Clin. Microbiol. *28*:1395–1397, 1990.
324. Yam, P., Cornish, N., and Kruger, R.: The use of mixed shell vials for respiratory virus detection from clinical specimens. Abstract S17. Paper presented at the 15th Annual Clinical Virology Symposium, 1999, Clearwater, FL.
325. Yamamoto, M., Kimura, H., Hironaka, T., et al.: Detection and quantification of virus DNA in plasma of patients with Epstein-Barr virus–associated diseases. J. Clin. Microbiol. *33*:1765–1768, 1995.
326. Yamamoto, S., Pavan-Langston, D., Kinoshita, S., et al.: Detecting herpes virus DNA in uveitis using the polymerase chain reaction. Br. J. Ophthalmol. *80*:465–468, 1996.
327. Yang, C. F., De, L., Holloway, B. P., et al.: Detection and identification of vaccine-related polioviruses by the polymerase chain reaction. Virus Res. *20*:159–179, 1991.
328. Yerly, S., Gervaix, A., Simonet, V., et al.: Rapid and sensitive detection of enteroviruses in specimens from patients with aseptic meningitis. J. Clin. Microbiol. *34*:199–201, 1996.
329. Young, P. P., Buller, R. S., and Storch, G. A.: Evaluation of a commercial DNA enzyme immunoassay for detection of enterovirus reverse transcription–PCR products amplified from cerebrospinal fluid specimens. J. Clin. Microbiol. *38*:4260–4261, 2000.
330. Yu, M. L., Chuang, W. L., Dai, C. Y., et al.: Clinical evaluation of the automated COBAS AMPLICOR HCV MONITOR test version 2.0 for quantifying serum hepatitis C virus RNA and comparison to the Quantiplex HCV version 2.0 test. J. Clin. Microbiol. *38*:2933–2939, 2000.
331. Zaaijer, H. L., ter Borg, F., Cuypers, H. T. M., et al.: Comparison of methods for detection of hepatitis B virus DNA. J. Clin. Microbiol. *32*:2088–2091, 1994.
332. Zeuzem, S., Ruster, B., and Roth, W. K.: Clinical evaluation of a new polymerase chain reaction assay (Amplicor HCV) for detection of hepatitis C virus. Z. Gastroenterol. *32*:342–347, 1994.
333. Zhao, L., Landry, M. L., Balkovic, E. S., et al.: Impact of cell culture sensitivity and virus concentration on rapid detection of herpes simplex virus by cytopathic effects and immunoperoxidase staining. J. Clin. Microbiol. *25*:1401–1405, 1987.
334. Zimmerman, S. J., Moses, E., and Sofat, N.: Evaluation of a visual, rapid, membrane enzyme immunoassay for the detection of herpes simplex virus antigen. J. Clin. Microbiol. *29*:842–845, 1991.
335. Zipeto, D., Revello, M. G., Silini, E., et al.: Development and clinical significance of a diagnostic assay based on the polymerase chain reaction for detection of human cytomegalovirus DNA in blood samples from immunocompromised patients. J. Clin. Microbiol. *30*:527–530, 1992.

CHAPTER

250 Use of the Serology Laboratory

EDWARD O. MASON, JR.

Serologic diagnosis of infectious diseases may be accomplished either by demonstration of a specific antibody response in the patient's serum or by detection of antigens of the infecting agent in tissue or body fluids with the use of hyperimmune sera of known specificity. These two diagnostic approaches often are used simultaneously and may be performed in the same laboratory. This chapter, however, is concerned primarily with interpretation of the serologic response of the patient in order to diagnose infectious diseases. Appropriate use and interpretation of antigen-detection tests are presented in Chapters 248 and 249.

Selection of optimal serologic procedures for the diagnosis of an infectious agent involves considerations of sensitivity, specificity, antigen availability, time, and cost. A variety of techniques have been developed and applied to the serologic diagnosis of infectious diseases. Before any one procedure is adopted, the advantages, disadvantages, and performance of each of the many tests (Table 250–1) should be considered carefully. Evaluation of new procedures begins with comparison of the sensitivity and specificity of the proposed assay with results obtained by testing the same samples by established serologic techniques.[3] Once the reliability and reproducibility of the new assay have been determined, the value of the new procedure in predicting the presence or absence of disease must be determined by validation studies.

Serologic diagnoses are made either by demonstrating a fourfold rise in antibody titer between acute and convalescent serum samples or by detecting specific immunoglobulin (Ig) antibodies (indicating a recent infection) elicited by the infecting agent. The laboratory must be prepared to document the time of collection of serum samples accurately and preserve them adequately until companion samples can be obtained and tested together. Interfering substances caused by improper handling and storage of samples can be minimized by prompt removal of serum from the clot and storage at −20° C or below. Even when circumstances do not permit immediate freezing, separation of serum often allows future analysis. Likewise, the samples must be protected adequately from further deterioration in antibody content when they are referred to outside laboratories.

The purity of any serologic reagent is a limiting factor in the usefulness of any assay. The availability of specific monoclonal antiglobulin for use in indirect fluorescent antibody (IFA) tests, enzyme-linked immunosorbent assays (ELISAs), and radioimmunoassays (RIAs) has permitted standardization of many procedures that quantitate the primary IgM antibody response, which allows rapid diagnosis of infection with only a single determination. The availability and interpretation of serologic tests for the diagnosis of bacterial, fungal, parasitic, and viral infections are discussed in the paragraphs that follow.

TABLE 250–1 ■ SEROLOGIC PROCEDURES

Agglutination reactions
Bacterial
Latex
Hemagglutination
Hemagglutination inhibition
Precipitin reactions
Tube precipitation
Gel immunodiffusion
Countercurrent immunoelectrophoresis
Immunofluorescence
Indirect immunofluorescence
Indirect complement fixation
Enzyme-linked immunosorbent assay
Radioimmunoassay
Complement fixation
Neutralization
Viral
Toxin
Western blot (immunoblot)

Serodiagnosis of Bacterial Infections

BORRELIA SEROLOGY

Infection caused by *Borrelia burgdorferi* (e.g., Lyme borreliosis, Lyme disease, erythema chronicum migrans) is a clinical diagnosis. After identification and isolation of the spirochetal etiologic agent in 1982, an IFA method for serologic diagnosis was developed and reported to be both specific and sensitive.[14, 144] Experience with the test, however, has revealed that cross-reactions occur in the sera of patients with other spirochetal and tick-borne diseases.[95] The results of the test are often negative in early primary Lyme disease, and the antibody response to different antigens varies with the stage of infection.[94, 95] Subsequently, ELISA was reported to be more specific, sensitive, and less dependent on subjective variables inherent in the IFA test.[24, 96] ELISA has become the test of choice in many laboratories, yet this test is also subject to poor interlaboratory reproducibility.[93] Immunoblotting of extracts of *B. burgdorferi* allows analysis of the immunologic response to the individual components of the spirochete and has been shown to be the most sensitive method for detecting antibody responses during the early stages of infection.[39, 54, 93] Children with well-documented, resolved Lyme arthritis remain seropositive for at least 6 months after therapy, thus rendering borreliosis a tempting diagnosis for many unexplained symptoms.[129]

At least 45 first-step assays (ELISAs, IFAs, or immunodot procedures) and 8 supplemental second-step assays (Western blot) are currently licensed by the Food and Drug Administration (FDA) for testing blood, serum, or plasma only. Although the FDA recommends that manufacturers evaluate and report the performance of the assay on a 40-item serum panel reflecting a variety of manifestations and collection times relative to the disease state, many manufacturers decline to participate.[176] Hence, the laboratory's selection of methodology and manufacturer is of great importance. Accuracy and clinical usefulness are further compounded by the timing of collection in the natural course of the disease, the presence or lack of symptoms, the prevalence of the disease in the geographic area, and the patient's vaccine status now that a licensed vaccine is available.[11] The only role of serology in borreliosis is in support of the clinical diagnosis of Lyme disease, and commercially available kits are not reliable as a primary diagnostic criterion.[11]

BRUCELLA SEROLOGY

Serodiagnosis of brucellosis is useful because members of the genus *Brucella* often cause insidious infections and are difficult to culture in the laboratory. The first antibody response to infection with *Brucella* is by IgM, followed by an IgG response.[42] The standardized tube agglutination test can demonstrate both these antibodies separately or together reliably when it is performed according to a strictly standardized protocol. *Brucella* antigen obtained from the U.S. Department of Agriculture National Animal Disease Center in Ames, Iowa, is prepared with a single strain of *Brucella abortus* but reacts with antibodies to *Brucella suis* and *Brucella melitensis,* as well as *B. abortus.*[141] A tube agglutination titer of 1:160 or greater or a fourfold rise in agglutination titer is diagnostic of brucellosis.[180] Vaccination or natural disease caused by *Vibrio cholerae, Francisella tularensis,* or *Yersinia enterocolitica* evokes cross-reacting antibodies; however, the titers are not usually as high as those encountered in brucellosis. The agglutination procedure outlined by the National Research Council Committee on the Public Aspects of Brucellosis requires the dilution scheme to be performed at least to a titer of 1:320 to avoid false-negative reactions caused by a "prozone" effect related to the presence of heat-labile blocking substances.[180]

In contrast to serologic responses in other diseases, the IgM antibody induced by infection with *Brucella* may persist indefinitely.[177] IgG antibody, which appears later in the course of the disease, declines rapidly with appropriate antibiotic therapy. The presence of IgG antibody in serum therefore signifies present or recent infection.[177] The persistence of or an increase in IgG antibody is correlated with inadequate treatment and is highly prognostic.[126] The standard tube agglutination test measures both IgG and IgM responses. Treatment of serum with 2-mercaptoethanol dissociates IgM and permits measurement of the IgG response alone[12] but lowers the sensitivity of the test. The use of 2-mercaptoethanol to measure IgG antibody should be considered as a secondary procedure after a positive titer is obtained by the standard agglutination test.[12]

Efforts to establish the utility of ELISA for the diagnosis of human brucellosis have found that although the results are encouraging, the technique requires further study in prospective trials to establish the confidence retained by the older tube agglutination techniques.[26] Differentiation of relapsing and chronic disease, however, which is difficult with standard agglutination tests, seems to be accomplished more readily by ELISA measurement of rises in IgA and IgG antibody.[113, 178]

Infection of humans by a fourth species of *Brucella, Brucella canis,* is a rare occurrence; nonetheless, at least 30 cases (2 in children) have been reported since 1967.[155, 177] Standard *Brucella* antibody tests do not detect infection with *B. canis.* When such infection is suspected, serum should be referred to a state reference laboratory. Infection with *B. canis* in humans usually results in antibody titers greater than 1:100.[19]

LEPTOSPIRA SEROLOGY

The definitive serologic test for leptospirosis is the microagglutination test performed with live leptospire antigens representing 12 to 16 individual serotypes.[41, 148] Maintaining viable stock cultures of these organisms is difficult, which renders the test impractical for all but large reference or research facilities. Antibodies elicited in response to acute leptospiral infection do not appear until day 6 to 12 after infection and reach their peak by week 3 to 4 of infection.[174] The following points should be considered when interpreting serologic results:

1. A fourfold rise in titer may not be present if the serum sample is obtained late in the course of disease and the titer has reached a peak.
2. Negative titers do not rule out leptospirosis because the infecting strain may not be represented in the antigen panel used to screen for antibody.
3. Prompt initiation of antibiotic therapy can suppress the serologic response.

Many laboratories perform leptospiral serologic testing by the macroagglutination technique, which entails the use of four pools containing three serotypes each of killed antigen preparation. This slide agglutination test is easy to perform and rapid but, unfortunately, is of very low specificity.[147] The slide agglutination test is hampered further by the inconsistent quality of the killed antigens available and cross-reactions among these antigens.

An indirect hemagglutination assay (IHA) for detection of leptospiral antibodies that uses an alcohol extract of a single leptospiral strain as a sensitizing antigen has been reported.[147] The sensitivity of IHA was 92 percent versus 69 percent for the macroagglutination test. The specificity of IHA was 95 percent, whereas the specificity of the macroagglutination test was 83 percent. Although IHA seems to offer improved serologic testing for leptospirosis, it does not reliably detect antibodies late in the course of disease.[147]

Two procedures, IgM-specific dot-ELISA, modified from the original procedure described by Pappas and colleagues,[111] and the genus-specific microscopic agglutination test, have been found comparable in sensitivity and specificity to the classic macroagglutination procedure for the diagnosis of leptospirosis. A modification of this procedure by Ribeiro and associates[127] found that use of the dot-ELISA with a proteinase K–resistant antigen detected antibody activity in 43 percent of acute-phase sera that were missed by the microscopic agglutination test. Both tests use a single, broadly reactive antigen derived from the nonpathogenic strain of *Leptospira biflexa* serovar Patoc 1 to replace the battery of serotype antigens used in the macroagglutination procedure.[163]

MYCOPLASMA SEROLOGY

Detection of infection with *Mycoplasma pneumoniae* often is based on clinical symptoms rather than isolation of the pathogen.[17, 18] The presence of serum cold agglutinins is a nonspecific indication of *Mycoplasma* infection.[51, 151] Because *Mycoplasma* has a long incubation period, serum cold agglutinins appear earlier than the more specific complement-fixation (CF) titers and often are elevated by the first week after the development of symptoms. Cold agglutinins also may be elicited in several viral diseases, as well as in noninfectious illnesses.[43] Thus, a serum cold agglutinin titer greater than 1:64 is only suggestive of *Mycoplasma* infection. The severity of the infection also is reflected in the magnitude of the serum cold agglutination response, and mild infections may not elicit an increase in cold agglutinin titer.

Screening serum for cold agglutinins before titration for quantification eliminates the need to evaluate negative samples.[51] A rapid method of qualitative screening for cold agglutinins can be performed away from the laboratory by using a few drops of capillary blood (finger-stick) and a small citrated collection tube. Positive results, seen by clumping of red blood cells when the tube is placed on ice and dissolution of the clumps when the tube is warmed, should be confirmed by quantitative determination of the titer in the laboratory.[51]

Although several specific serologic tests are available for *M. pneumoniae* (growth inhibition test, immunofluorescence, IHA, and RIA), the only test available in non-research laboratories is the CF test using a glycolipid antigen. A single titer greater than 1:256 is only suggestive evidence of a recent infection, and a fourfold rise in titer is required for definitive diagnosis of *Mycoplasma* infection.[18] Because CF antibody titers rise slowly and peak 1 month after infection, repeating titers on paired specimens at weekly intervals may be necessary.

Studies in 92 children comparing polymerase chain reaction (PCR), IgM IFA, culture, and CF prospectively identified nine patients with *M. pneumoniae* infection and found that only the combination of PCR and CF testing allowed the diagnosis of all cases.[30] Evidence provided by retrospective analysis of a small group of patients with both clinical and CF titer evidence of *Mycoplasma* disease demonstrated IgM antibodies in 70 percent of acute and 100 percent of convalescent sera with use of urease-conjugated ELISA.[21] Two rapid qualitative assays that detect IgM antibodies are available commercially. One, an enzyme-linked immunobinding assay using a protein antigen, was as sensitive as the CF test but currently is recommended only as a rapid screening procedure.[153]

RICKETTSIA SEROLOGY

The Weil-Felix test is a nonspecific serologic test that uses *Proteus vulgaris* strains OX-19, OX-2, and OX-K to detect agglutinins in the serum of patients who may have one of several rickettsial diseases.[57] *Proteus* agglutination is easy to perform, and the reagents are readily available commercially. Although clinical suspicion together with high (>1:160) OX-19 or OX-2 titers is highly suggestive of the diagnosis of Rocky Mountain spotted fever, the results of the Weil-Felix test should be confirmed by other specific rickettsial serologic procedures.[59] Conversely, negative Weil-Felix test results do not rule out rickettsial infection, especially in cases in which antibiotic therapy is instituted promptly, because antibody titers may not appear for 2 to 3 weeks. Low Weil-Felix titers can be evoked in response to infections with *Proteus, Leptospira,* and other rickettsiae or in severe hepatitis.[59]

The CF test uses group-specific rickettsial antigens to distinguish between the typhus group and the spotted fever group of diseases. The CF test lacks sensitivity, and detection of antibody also can be delayed by antibiotic therapy.[84] In addition, because the Centers for Disease Control and Prevention (CDC) have stopped distribution of the CF antigen, performance and standardization of the CF test are in jeopardy.[159] The micro-indirect IFA test is reported to be as specific and more sensitive than the CF test.[56, 118] By spotting four different antigens on the same circle of an immunofluorescence slide, the test can measure the specific antibody titer to four rickettsial antigens simultaneously with the same drop of diluted serum.[58] Latex-agglutination (LA) tests using *Rickettsia rickettsii* antigens are as specific and sensitive as the micro-indirect IFA test.[57] LA test materials are available commercially, and a rapid ELISA kit for detection of IgG and IgM antibodies to *Rickettsia typhi* is being evaluated.[82] IFA testing for rickettsial disease is limited to public health, research, or reference laboratories.[159]

SALMONELLA SEROLOGY

Improvements in the ability to isolate *Salmonella* have reduced the importance of detecting *Salmonella* agglutinins (Widal test). The many variables that affect this test (stage of disease, effects of antibiotics, normal agglutinins, and previous vaccinations) render interpreting and defining a diagnostic Widal titer difficult. No single titer can be considered diagnostic, and a fourfold rise between acute and convalescent sera should be interpreted as diagnostic only if the sera are tested together.[46]

The original Widal test is a tube agglutinin test that uses commercially available O (somatic) and H (flagellar) *Salmonella* antigens.[173] The slide agglutination test cannot replace the tube agglutination procedure, although some manufacturers of antigen preparations describe this rapid modification as an alternative procedure.[46] Testing for antibodies to both the O and H antigens is necessary for proper interpretation. Tests using antigens other than *Salmonella typhi* or *Salmonella enteritidis* bioserotypes A, B, or C should not be performed because (1) salmonellae other than these rarely are associated with enteric fever illness and (2) gastrointestinal infections alone rarely evoke antibody responses.[46]

Demonstration of antibody to the capsular polysaccharide Vi antigen has been associated with carrier states after infection with *S. typhi.*[173] Agglutination tests for Vi antibodies, however, are of low specificity and sensitivity.[9] The use of purified Vi antigen[106] in ELISA[5] may improve the serologic identification of typhoid carriers.

STAPHYLOCOCCUS SEROLOGY

The diagnosis of endocarditis, osteomyelitis, and other systemic infections caused by *Staphylococcus aureus* that cannot be confirmed by culture may be aided by serologic procedures to detect antibodies to teichoic acid. Detection of teichoic acid antibodies by agar gel diffusion in the serum of patients has been reported to be specific for systemic *S. aureus* infection.[171] Unfortunately, the sensitivity of the procedure is only 36 percent.[103] The use of counterimmunoelectrophoresis (CIE) to detect teichoic acid antibodies improves the sensitivity but lowers the specificity of the assay.[103] ELISA is reported to be a specific and sensitive method for detection of antibodies to teichoic acid in *S. aureus* systemic infections. Thisyakorn and associates[154] reported that a serum ELISA titer greater than 1:3200 has a sensitivity of 93 percent and a specificity of 89 percent in children with culture-proven *S. aureus* infection.

The teichoic acid antigen is either a sonicate or an extract of the Lafferty strain of *S. aureus,* and variations in preparations have hampered comparisons of results among laboratories.[170] This single antigen preparation detects all strains of *S. aureus.*[135] One preparation available commercially (Endo-Staph, Meridian Diagnostics, Cincinnati, OH) with a standardized teichoic acid antigen is reported to be reliable.[170] Regardless of the test used, an antibody response is detected only 10 to 14 days after infection and may not be detected at all in immunocompromised patients. Studies have demonstrated that immunodiffusion (ID) tests and ELISA show a higher immune response to teichoic acid in patients with endocarditis and bacteremia caused by *S. aureus* than do control sera from patients without staphylococcal disease.[7] The serologic response does not, however, distinguish between endocarditis and bacteremia caused by *S. aureus*. Likewise, attempts to use antibody responses to another *S. aureus* surface antigen, protein A, were not sufficiently sensitive or specific for diagnosis.[49]

STREPTOCOCCUS SEROLOGY

Infection by *Streptococcus pyogenes* (group A *Streptococcus*) may elicit antibodies to different bacterial extracellular enzymes, depending on the *Streptococcus* strain, the age of the host, the site of the infection, and the duration of the antigenic stimulus.[116] The measure of antibody response to *S. pyogenes* infection used most frequently is the antistreptolysin O (ASO) reaction. Antibody to streptolysin O, an oxygen-labile extracellular hemolysin, can be detected within 2 to 4 weeks in 85 percent of patients after pharyngeal streptococcal infection.[76] However, ASO antibodies are elevated only slightly or undetected after pyodermal streptococcal infection.[161] Thus, serologic responses to other streptococcal antigens (DNase B, hyaluronidase, NADase, and streptokinase) are necessary to document antecedent streptococcal disease and nonsuppurative complications. Because assessment of antibodies to these individual antigens is costly and laborious, a screening procedure (Streptozyme, Wampole Laboratories, Stamford, CT) often is used to detect an elevation in antibodies to any one of these several antigens. The Streptozyme test is an IHA that uses erythrocytes that have been sensitized to several extracellular enzymes of a strain of *S. pyogenes*. The test is not quantitative, and positive results should be confirmed by determining antibodies to the individual antigens. Mild elevations in individual antibody titers may not be detected by the Streptozyme test.[60] The Streptozyme test is the only test available commercially that is sufficiently sensitive (100% in this case) to detect elevations in ASO antibodies but is less sensitive (22%) in detecting anti-DNase B antibodies.[72] Different lots of erythrocyte antigens used in the Streptozyme procedure may vary in strength, and other streptococci may produce identical enzymes. Thus, when strong clinical suspicion of streptococcal disease is not supported by Streptozyme screening tests, individual antibody determinations must be performed.[78] The significance of single titers should be established by each laboratory after analysis of baseline values for noninfected children of different age groups in that area. In any test, however, a rise of two (0.3 log) or more dilutions between acute and convalescent sera is significant.

SYPHILIS SEROLOGY

Nontreponemal serologic tests for syphilis are the CF tests described by Wasserman and Kolmer and the newer Venereal Disease Research Laboratory (VDRL) and rapid plasma reagin (RPR) flocculation tests. The nontreponemal tests are suited for mass screening procedures but are limited by lack of sensitivity in early and late disease.[138] In addition, a high percentage of false-positive results are associated with aging, autoimmune disorders, pregnancy, drug addiction, and malignancy. For this reason, positive results by one of the nontreponemal tests should be confirmed by a treponemal test such as the *Treponema pallidum* immobilization test, the fluorescent treponemal antibody test, the fluorescent treponemal antibody absorption (FTA-ABS) test, or the microhemagglutination *T. pallidum* (MHA-TP) antibody test.

Nontreponemal Tests

Most laboratories perform either a VDRL or an RPR test because of the ease and ready commercial availability of the test reagents. The results of both tests are comparable, and both can be quantified, but only the VDRL test is suitable for detecting antibody in cerebrospinal fluid (CSF) for the diagnosis of neurologic syphilis. The antibody titers measured by the VDRL and RPR tests decrease with the institution of proper antibiotic therapy and revert to negative when the patient has completed successful therapy. The antigen used in these tests is a cardiolipin-lecithin-cholesterol complex that detects antibody elicited by infections caused by other bacterial or viral pathogens, by collagen vascular disease, by hepatitis, or by drug addiction.[115] These biologic false-positive titers are usually 1:8 or less and generally disappear in 6 months. In contrast, false-positive titers in sera may persist longer than 6 months in patients with certain chronic diseases such as autoimmune disorders and connective tissue disease.[172] Specific treponemal antibody test results are usually negative in these cases.

Treponemal Tests

The FTA-ABS and MHA-TP tests are specific tests with technical difficulties and costs that render them unsuitable for routine screening.[85] The primary function of the FTA-ABS test is to confirm the specificity of a nontreponemal test; quantification of the FTA-ABS test has not proved prognostic in that the antibody titer does not decrease with treatment. In addition, the value of the FTA-ABS test for detecting antibody in CSF has not been established. Lack of sensitivity has hampered development of the FTA-ABS IgM test that exclusively detects IgM antibody to *T. pallidum*. The diagnosis of congenital syphilis is complicated further by maternal IgG crossing the placental barrier and reacting with the VDRL and RPR tests, which detect primarily IgG antibodies. The low sensitivity of the FTA-ABS IgM test renders confirmation of congenital syphilis especially difficult in asymptomatic neonates.[138] Fractionation of *T. pallidum* antigens plus the use of polyacrylamide gel electrophoresis with Western blotting to nitrocellulose has shown that neonatal IgM directed against a 47-kd antigen of *T. pallidum* may be a better diagnostic predictor of congenital syphilis.[90, 131] IgM capture EIA has been found to be more sensitive than the FTA-ABS test for the diagnosis of congenital syphilis when interpreted along with the mother's clinical history.[85, 89] This same commercially available system using IgG capture also has been found to be as sensitive and specific as the RPR test for syphilis screening.[137]

The MHA-TP test is a treponemal test with a specificity similar to that of the FTA-ABS test. The MHA-TP test is easier to perform technically, and interpretation of the end-point is less subjective. Although the MHA-TP test is slightly less sensitive in detecting antibodies in early primary syphilis, it appears to be a reasonable alternative to the FTA-ABS test, which is technically more demanding.[35] None of the treponemal tests distinguishes between syphilis and other treponematoses (yaws, pinta, and bejel).

Serodiagnosis of Fungal Infections

ASPERGILLUS SEROLOGY

Invasive aspergillosis is almost exclusively a disease of immunocompromised patients. The diagnosis is difficult to make, and tissue for culture frequently requires biopsy.

Because these patients are often the least able to tolerate such invasive procedures, numerous serologic methods have been developed in an attempt to lessen the risk associated with biopsy. Antibodies to *Aspergillus* antigens rarely are found in the serum of healthy persons, even though species of *Aspergillus* are abundant in the environment.[92] ID tests and the more sensitive ELISAs can demonstrate antibodies to *Aspergillus* reliably with 70 to 90 percent sensitivity in non-immunocompromised patients with either aspergilloma or allergic aspergillosis.[92, 114] However, the value of serodiagnosis of invasive aspergillosis remains controversial.[27, 67] Young and Bennett[179] reported a complete lack of serologic response to *Aspergillus* antigens in 16 immunocompromised patients with histologically confirmed aspergillosis. Detection of antibody is more prognostic than diagnostic in that an increase in antibody after immunosuppression is associated with recovery and low or declining antibody suggests a poor prognosis.[86] Unfortunately, the purified antigens required for these tests must be prepared in research laboratories and thus have restricted availability.

BLASTOMYCES SEROLOGY

The CF test with yeast-phase antigen was the first test used in the serodiagnosis of infection by *Blastomyces dermatitidis*. Although this test is still widely available in clinical laboratories, it is of little diagnostic or prognostic value in this disease.[132, 133] CF test results are positive (>1:8) in only 50 percent of patients with histologically proven blastomycosis, and significant cross-reactions occur in serum from patients with confirmed histoplasmosis and coccidioidomycosis.[15] Although few reports of blastomycosis in pediatric patients exist, one study found that similar to the findings in infected adults, only 5 of 12 children infected with *B. dermatitidis* had a positive CF response.[120]

Kaufman and associates[81] described an ID test for blastomycosis that relies on the presence of specific precipitin bands (A and B) as a more sensitive and specific indication of active infection by this fungus. The A band alone or together with the B band was present in 79 percent of sera from persons with proven blastomycosis. No instances of false-positive results have been reported, and disappearance of the bands may correlate with successful therapy. Detection of this A band depends on carefully prepared antigens and the use of control sera containing the A and B precipitins, which are not often available, and at least one kit available commercially has been found unreliable.[132, 133]

CANDIDA SEROLOGY

Methods other than culture would be useful to distinguish invasive candidiasis from colonization with *Candida albicans* in that 15 to 40 percent of cases of disseminated candidiasis diagnosed at necropsy cannot be confirmed by culture before the death of the patient.[38] Tests for invasive candidiasis must detect antibody responses to antigens that distinguish between colonized and infected persons.[121] Measurement of antibody to a variety of *Candida* antigens can be achieved by whole-cell agglutination, gel diffusion, IHA, LA, CIE, and more recently, RIA and ELISA.[28] Comparing the efficacy and usefulness of these procedures is difficult because (1) investigators are not consistent in their definition of invasive candidiasis, (2) most patients are immunosuppressed, thus rendering antibody detection unreliable, (3) many antigen preparations are undefined, and (4) experimental methods and study designs are different.

The CIE, ID, and LA tests for antibody to *C. albicans* were compared in a collaborative, nonclinical study of immunocompetent patients with systemic candidiasis and were shown to have sensitivities of 80 percent or greater.[100, 157] These tests can be of value in the diagnosis of invasive candidal disease but rely heavily on the use of standardized reagents that are not yet commercially available. Furthermore, studies using more sensitive RIA and ELISA techniques have shown that cell wall mannan antibodies are a consistent component of human serum in immunocompetent persons.[50] Immunoblot analysis of cell wall mannan-free protein extracts of *C. albicans* in sera from neutropenic patients detected these proteins in 25 to 70 of the sera tested.[99] A study in Sweden found elevated IgG, IgM, and IgA to three different antigens in 10 of 10 children actively infected with *C. albicans* and little response in 280 healthy control children. In addition to the small number of infected children studied, the report did not include any clinical information on which the value of the findings could be judged.[90] Although sensitivity and specificity were similar to other tests, statistical significance was shown for low antibody levels and mortality in a recent study using IHA procedures.[75] Regardless, because of technical inadequacies in antigen purity, availability, and specificity, as well as the absence of an antibody response in the patient population most at risk for acquiring invasive candidiasis, the use of antibody tests for the diagnosis of systemic candidiasis is of little clinical value.[77]

COCCIDIOIDES SEROLOGY

Unlike their use in many of the other mycoses, serologic procedures in the diagnosis and prognosis of disease caused by *Coccidioides immitis* have established value. Two antigens, coccidioidin (a mycelial-phase antigen) and spherulin (an endospore antigen), are detected in response to infection by this fungus. The most useful tests are tube precipitin (TP) tests, LA tests, CF tests, and gel ID using coccidioidin antigen.[110] Both the TP and LA tests measure IgM, but the LA test is more sensitive in that it detects 71 versus 13 percent[73, 74] of positive specimens. The LA test, however, does have a 6 to 10 percent false-positive rate.[22] Many patients with asymptomatic pulmonary disease may never have a positive TP test result, which may explain the added sensitivity of these LA test results. Also possible is that testing of sera from patients in the later stages of disease can result in false-negative reactions in both these tests because of the disappearance of IgM antibodies. Neither test is quantitative. The LA test is available commercially, is easy to perform, and is faster than the TP test (4 minutes versus 3 days). Because the low protein content of CSF destabilizes the latex/coccidioidin particles and causes nonspecific agglutination,[108] the LA test is not suitable for detecting antibody in spinal fluid. Neither the LA nor the TP test should ever be used for the diagnosis of coccidioidal meningitis.[33]

If the coccidioidin antigen is heated and used in the ID test, it is known as the IDTP test. It detects IgM antibody, as in the LA and TP tests, and is of intermediate sensitivity between these two tests. The LA test and the IDTP test are considered screening tests, and positive results should be confirmed with a standard TP test or followed with a CF test.

Both the CF and the ID tests (using unheated, ultrafiltered coccidioidin—IDCF) detect IgG responses to infection by *C. immitis*. The CF test is both diagnostic and prognostic and, despite its difficulty in performance, is invaluable in the management of symptomatic coccidioidomycosis. In as many as 60 percent of patients with asymptomatic pulmonary coccidioidomycosis, CF antibodies may fail to develop.[33] In patients in whom antibodies do develop, a low and stable titer may indicate mild morbidity, and a declining titer usually is associated with clinical improvement or a favorable response to therapy.[139, 140] A rising CF titer is associated with dissemination and has a poor prognosis.[110] For cases in which rising or declining titers may be of clinical importance, researchers have suggested that aliquots of serum from each serologic determination be frozen and all specimens be retested together to avoid the variations inherent in CF test procedures.[33, 109]

Detection of antibody to *C. immitis* by the CF, IDTP, or IDCF tests in CSF is specific for coccidioidal meningitis. Previous studies showed that the CF test detected antibodies in the CSF of 76 percent of 92 patients with coccidioidal meningitis.[109] Overnight incubation of the antigen-antibody complex at 4° C (39.2° F) improved the sensitivity of the CF test. This modification allowed detection of *C. immitis* antibodies in the CSF of 96 percent of 265 patients with culture-proven meningitis.[107]

EIA using both TP and CF antigens is approved by the FDA and is available commercially. It has been shown to be reliable and rapid and overcomes problems encountered with serum that is anticomplementary. The test can be used to detect antibody in both serum and CSF. Because it uses specific anti-IgG and anti-IgM, the results are more specific than those of the ID and CF tests. At present, it is approved only for qualitative results from serum, but the optical density units correlate well with CF titer antibody levels.[98]

CRYPTOCOCCUS SEROLOGY

Cryptococcosis is diagnosed rapidly and accurately by the detection of cryptococcal capsule polysaccharide in CSF or serum by the LA test.[79] Although several methods are available for detection of the serologic response of patients to *Cryptococcus neoformans,* they are of primary utility for the seroepidemiology of cryptococcosis and of little value in the clinical diagnosis or prognosis of the disease.[48]

HISTOPLASMA SEROLOGY

In cases of primary acute pulmonary *Histoplasma capsulatum* infection, serologic evidence of infection is often all that is available to the clinician. Unfortunately, serodiagnosis is not sufficiently specific or sensitive to be of unrestricted usefulness. The CF test can be performed with two antigens: a yeast-phase extract and a filtrate of the mycelial phase (histoplasmin).[81] Antibodies to the yeast antigen are usually positive (≥1:32) in patients with uncomplicated histoplasmosis within 4 weeks of exposure to the agent.[81] The CF test using the yeast-phase antigen has been reported to have a specificity and sensitivity of 90 to 94 percent.[6, 80] Use of the mycelial antigen in CF tests, on the other hand, has a specificity of 99 percent but a greatly reduced sensitivity of 68 to 80 percent.[6, 80] Titers of 1:8 and 1:16 are difficult to interpret and often are found in patients with other pulmonary mycoses.[81]

The ID test, first described by Heiner,[61] has advantages over the CF test in that anticomplementary sera can be tested and the technical difficulties of the CF test are avoided. The ID test is less sensitive than the CF test and is not quantitative, but it is specific. The original studies found six precipitin bands in serum from patients with histoplasmosis by using the histoplasmin (mycelial) antigen. Two of these bands, designated M and H, were found to be of diagnostic significance. The H band is specific for active histoplasmosis and is unaffected by skin testing. Unfortunately, it may not be present in the serum of many patients with active histoplasmosis.[61] The M band appears before the H band in patients with histoplasmosis, persists after recovery, and also may appear as a result of previous use of the skin test antigen. The presence of M and H bands together is highly suggestive of active histoplasmosis (sensitivity, 90%; specificity, 94%) and is comparable with a CF yeast antigen titer of 1:32 or greater.[168] Current recommendations are that the CF test using the yeast-phase antigen and the ID test using histoplasmin be performed together for the serodiagnosis of histoplasmosis.[6] Contrary to serologic titers in coccidioidomycosis, persistence of elevated titers to *Histoplasma* antigens does not correlate with disseminated disease.[168] However, one incident involving a common exposure of multiple persons in a bat cave demonstrated that the serologic response correlates with the severity of acute infection.[166]

Lack of specificity caused by cross-reactions with antibodies present in other fungal and bacterial diseases has been a major problem in the reliable serodiagnosis of histoplasmosis. Studies have demonstrated a wider range of cross-reactions than was recognized previously, which renders proper interpretation more difficult.[167] CF test results were positive for histoplasmosis in 18 percent of patients with other fungal infections and in 34 percent of patients with tuberculosis. The percentage of false-positive reactions was even greater with the use of an RIA procedure that previously was shown to be more sensitive than the CF or ID reaction in detecting early histoplasmosis.[169] As with serologic tests for most mycoses, especially in immunocompromised patients, lack of an immune response does not rule out histoplasmosis.[114]

Evidence has shown that both the CF test and the ID test are useful in detecting antibody in the CSF of patients with disseminated histoplasmosis and meningitis.[119] This antibody appears to be produced locally in the central nervous system. Three patients with disseminated histoplasmosis but without meningitis did not have detectable antibody to *H. capsulatum* in CSF by any test. Performing CF and ID tests for histoplasmosis on the CSF of patients with suspected histoplasmosis and clinical signs of meningitis would seem a reasonable approach.

Serodiagnosis of Parasitic Infections

Serodiagnosis of parasitic infections is of less value than similar diagnostic procedures for viral, bacterial, and fungal pathogens, primarily because of the complex nature and multiplicity of parasite antigens. Because of these features, sensitive and specific serologic tests have been difficult to develop. Interpreting tests is complicated because most parasitic diseases are chronic, thus rendering the precise stages of illness difficult to identify. The development of newer serologic methods, as well as the availability of chemically defined antigens, has enhanced the reliability of serodiagnosis in several parasitic diseases. Most of these serologic tests are available only through research/reference laboratories or the CDC laboratory.

TOXOPLASMA SEROLOGY

The Sabin-Feldman dye test remains the standard technique for demonstrating antibodies elicited by infection with *Toxoplasma gondii.*[130] Unfortunately, it is technically difficult and time consuming, and it requires live trophozoites, which must be propagated biweekly in mice. Introduction of the IFA test for toxoplasmosis led to ease of performance and good correlation with dye test titers. Killed whole *Toxoplasma* trophozoites fixed on microscope slides (commercially available) are exposed to dilutions of the test serum. After incubation, unreacted serum is removed by washing, and fluorescein-tagged antihuman globulin is allowed to incubate on the cells. After removal of any unreacted antiglobulin, the slides are examined with an ultraviolet light microscope. The presence of antibody to *Toxoplasma* is demonstrated by observing a smooth ring of fluorescence surrounding the crescent-shaped *Toxoplasma* trophozoite. A minor difficulty in the interpretation of some reactions by the IFA technique is the occasional instance of "polar" fluorescence caused by the nonspecific binding of immunoglobulin to the Fc receptors found on the surface of the parasite.[13]

The dye test is reliable, specific, and extremely sensitive; however, the titer peaks in 6 to 8 weeks and can remain high for life. Rising titers seldom can be demonstrated, and the test is suitable only for the detection of previous infection.[165] The IFA test using anti-IgG or antiglobulins is also of use in detecting previous infection, and a titer of 1:256 or greater is highly suggestive of recent or current infection.

The IFA IgM test is useful and reliable in predicting recent or ongoing infection with *T. gondii*.[105] IgM titers may rise with the onset of symptoms and begin to disappear in 4 to 6 months.[104] Thus, demonstration of an IgM response of 1:64 or greater is evidence of recent infection. ELISA also has been shown to be useful in the diagnosis of recent *Toxoplasma* infection and, in addition, is more sensitive and specific than the IFA procedure. An ELISA IgM titer of 1:256 or greater is equivalent to an IFA IgM titer of 1:64 and is highly indicative of recent infection.[29] The use of a "double-sandwich" technique in IgM ELISA further improves sensitivity and avoids problems of interference by other globulins in serum.[136] Demonstration of anti-*Toxoplasma* IgM in umbilical cord serum or the serum of neonates by either procedure is diagnostic of congenital toxoplasmosis. However, failure to demonstrate IgM titers does not rule out congenital infection.

Demonstration of anti-*Toxoplasma* IgA and IgE by ELISA is a reliable indication of acute infection or congenital infection in the fetus or infant. It does not identify patients with chronic infection or patients with acquired immunodeficiency syndrome (AIDS) and toxoplasmic encephalitis.[145, 175]

Serodiagnosis of Viral Infections

Because of the acute nature of most viral infections, serologic testing is generally helpful in the diagnostic setting in confirming the specific agent responsible after resolution of the disease. Rapid and reliable methods of determining serologic evidence of past infection by a variety of agents are essential in blood transfusion and organ transplantation. As vaccines against such viruses become available, the immune status of potential vaccine recipients will be important in developing a cost-effective strategy for immunization programs involving hepatitis A and B virus and varicella virus vaccines. Adequate quantities of acute and convalescent sera always should be obtained and held for future viral serologic study. Of importance is that those responsible for saving this sera understand that it must be separated promptly from the clot, carefully labeled, and stored at −20° C or below. Failure to care for the samples properly may render performance of subsequent serologic examinations impossible.

Because of the multiple serotypes found in many viral groups, neutralization titers against the patient's isolate are often the only means of confirming that the virus isolated was responsible for the illness. For neutralization tests, the viral isolate and acute and convalescent sera must be forwarded to a laboratory capable of performing such procedures. Viral diseases that require confirmation by neutralization are infections with rhinovirus, echovirus, and coxsackievirus. Other viral diseases can be diagnosed either by neutralization tests or by serologic tests using antigens that are commercially available or prepared in the laboratory (Table 250–2).

CYTOMEGALOVIRUS SEROLOGY

Techniques for the detection of antibodies to cytomegalovirus (CMV) include neutralization tests, CF tests, IHAs, ELISAs, RIAs, immunoprecipitation tests, immunofluorescence tests, and anticomplement immunofluorescence tests.[69, 70] The use of nine serologic techniques and 14 different antigen preparations renders interpreting serologic data in the diagnosis of CMV infection difficult. Interpretation is hampered further by the difficulty in correlating the time that the serum sample was obtained with the precise stage of the disease process. Although CF tests are the basis for much of the earlier data, ELISAs are more sensitive and are now standard laboratory procedures.[10, 101, 124]

A conclusive diagnosis of congenital CMV infection is made by culture of the virus from urine or other body fluids during the newborn period. Although this procedure is reliable, results may not be known for 1 to 3 weeks. Rapid serodiagnosis of infection in these patients is difficult to accomplish. CF antibody titers (with CMV strain AD 169 antigen) for detecting IgG are often the only tests

TABLE 250–2 ■ COMMONLY AVAILABLE VIRAL SEROLOGIC TESTS

	CF	HAI	NEUT	IFA	RIA	ELISA	Immunoblot
Adenovirus	X		X				
Arbovirus	X	X	X	X			
Coxsackievirus			X				
Cytomegalovirus	X	X	X	X			
Echovirus			X				
Epstein-Barr virus				X			
Hepatitis A virus					X	X	
Hepatitis B virus					X	X	
Hepatitis C virus						X	X
Herpes simplex virus	X		X				
Influenza virus	X	X	X				
Measles virus	X	X					
Mumps virus	X	X					
Poliovirus	X		X				
Rabies virus			X				
Respiratory syncytial virus	X	X	X	X		X	
Rhinovirus			X				
Rubella virus	X	X	X				
Smallpox virus	X	X					
Varicella-zoster virus	X						
Yellow fever virus	X	X	X		X		

CF, complement-fixation test; ELISA, enzyme-linked immunosorbent assay; HAI, hemagglutination-inhibition test; IFA, indirect fluorescent antibody assay; NEUT, neutralization test; RIA, radioimmunoassay.

performed. IgG antibodies to CMV in the newborn are unreliable in predicting congenital infection because these titers may represent transplacentally acquired maternal IgG elicited by previous exposure. Thus, serodiagnosis of congenital infection requires demonstration of the persistence of CF antibody after the loss of maternal IgG at 3 to 6 months of age. Alternatively, demonstration of specific IgM antibody in a single serum specimen is diagnostic of congenital CMV infection.[62] The effectiveness of IFA techniques, however, is hampered by the inconsistent quality of commercial anti-IgM sera, the lower sensitivity of the IFA procedure (attributed partly to the subjectiveness of reading the results), and the high prevalence of false-positive results caused by the interference of antinuclear antibody.[87, 142, 143] Infection of test cells with CMV in the preparation of antigen slides for use in the IFA test causes the induction of Fc receptors on the surface of the cells, which then can bind IgG nonspecifically. This nonspecific interference can be avoided in IFA tests by using an anticomplement immunofluorescence procedure[31] or ELISA.[36] The use of antigens derived by recombinant technology may be helpful in the standardization of antigens and may lead to more useful serologic assays.[158] The use of RIA for detecting CMV IgM antibody increases the sensitivity of IgM detection to 89 percent, and detection of IgM in umbilical cord serum by RIA is diagnostic of congenital CMV infection.[52] Evidence is also available that elevated RIA IgM titers are correlated with more severe symptoms. Unfortunately, the rheumatoid factor present in serum often interferes with the detection of CMV-specific antibodies in the RIA IgM test. Removal of this rheumatoid factor by adsorption or fractionation of serum is time consuming, thus restricting this test to research laboratories.

Primary CMV infection is accompanied by the transient production of CMV-specific IgM antibody, which persists for as long as 4 months. Detection of this IgM is diagnostic of a primary infection.[53] Although the IgM response is specific for primary infection, IgM may result from reactivation of CMV, continual exposure to different strains of the virus, or both.[32] Seroconversion (as demonstrated by tests that measure IgG) is also evidence of a primary infection with CMV, and measurement of low-avidity IgG antibodies likewise may indicate primary infection.[8] The IgM response is specific for primary infection and has not been demonstrated in patients who are known to have been infected with CMV previously. No serologic procedure was found that could differentiate active from chronic infection as measured by viral culture or antigen detection in patients with AIDS.[88] Thus, the presence of an antibody titer to CMV of the IgG class with the absence of an IgM response indicates past exposure to CMV.

EPSTEIN-BARR VIRUS (INFECTIOUS MONONUCLEOSIS) SEROLOGY

Infectious mononucleosis can be serodiagnosed by demonstration of specific antibodies to Epstein-Barr virus (EBV) or by demonstration of nonspecific heterophile antibodies. Heterophile antibodies may appear in the course of mononucleosis or serum sickness or can occur idiopathically, and they can be demonstrated by the agglutination of sheep erythrocytes.[112] Such agglutination is nonspecific and without diagnostic significance unless the serum is adsorbed first with beef erythrocyte antigen and guinea pig kidney antigen. After adsorption with guinea pig kidney antigen, serum from patients with infectious mononucleosis continues to agglutinate the sheep cells, whereas adsorption of the same serum with beef cell antigen abolishes the agglutination reaction. The Monospot test, a commercial modification of the heterophile test, improves the sensitivity of heterophile antibody testing by using horse erythrocytes. Nonetheless, the serum used in Monospot tests also must be adsorbed to be specific for mononucleosis. Newer tests available commercially based on immunochromatographic assay and LA are rapid and simple to perform and have sensitivities between 91 and 96 percent, respectively, and specificities of 99 percent.[40] Heterophile antibodies, however, do not appear in the serum of 10 to 15 percent of patients with typical mononucleosis syndromes, and further testing is indicated.

EBV can infect cells in tissue culture, and growth of the cells can be stopped at different stages of the infective process. By manipulating expression of the antigens present in the cell cultures, one can use IFA testing to demonstrate antibodies to at least three important antigens that are helpful in determining the stage of illness.[47] IgG antibodies to the viral capsid (EBV VCA) appear with the onset of symptoms and persist for life.[63] The presence of IgG anti-VCA represents past exposure to EBV and is of little diagnostic significance. IgM anti-VCA, in the absence of rheumatoid factor, usually suffices for the diagnosis of acute EBV infection.[149] This diagnosis is reinforced by the absence of an antibody titer to nuclear antigen and the presence of antibodies to the D component of the EBV early antigen, although these antibodies cannot be detected in 10 to 20 percent of children with acute EBV infection.[149] Primary infection also is indicated by finding a titer against IgG antinuclear antigen because antibodies to this antigen do not appear until late in the course of mononucleosis[4, 45, 64] (Table 250–3).

HEPATITIS VIRUS SEROLOGY

Hepatitis A Virus

Antibody to hepatitis A virus (HAV) can be detected accurately by RIA, a hemagglutination-inhibition (HAI) test, or EIA. These tests are available commercially and can detect either total immunoglobulin or IgM antibody alone. Infection with HAV produces lifelong immunity, as evidenced by a persistent IgG antibody titer.[20] Detection of IgG alone is useful to determine individual immunity to HAV in cases in which immunoglobulin prophylaxis is to be administered to susceptible persons after exposure or to vaccine candidates. Acute HAV infection can be diagnosed by detecting anti-HAV IgM in a single serum sample.[34, 44] IgM antibody appears 12 to 15 days after infection and often is elevated at the time of the onset of symptoms. IgG rises later in the course of illness and peaks while IgM is declining. A newly developed solid-phase antibody capture hemadsorption assay for IgM antibody is reported to be equally or more sensitive and specific than RIA, can produce results in 6 hours, and can be read visually as agglutination of goose red blood cells.[150]

TABLE 250–3 ■ INTERPRETATION OF EPSTEIN-BARR VIRUS SEROLOGY

	IgM-VCA	IgG-VCA	Anti-NA	Anti-EA
Current infection	+	+	–	–/+
Recent infection	–/+	+	–/+	+
Past infection	–	+	+	–

+, Antibody present; –, antibody absent; –/+, no antibody or seroconversion.

EA, early antigen; NA, nuclear antigen; VCA, viral capsid antibody.

Hepatitis B Virus

Tests for hepatitis B virus (HBV) antigen and antibody are used to monitor the course and prognosis of HBV infection and to determine postexposure immune status; in addition, they are used as cost-effective guides to immunization[20] (Table 250–4). Three antigens may be detected during the course of illness in patients infected with HBV:

1. The surface antigen (HBsAg), formerly known as the Australia antigen, is the outer envelope protein of the virus particle. It can be detected in blood during the incubation period before symptoms appear and during acute infection.[160] HBsAg disappears during recovery, but it does so at variable rates in individual cases.[68]
2. The core antigen (HBcAg) is the nucleocapsid of the virion. This antigen can be detected in the hepatocytes of patients with HBV infection by using immunofluorescent techniques. HBcAg is not detected in serum and, thus, is of little diagnostic importance.[128]
3. The e antigen (HBeAg) is a soluble protein component of the nucleocapsid. Its presence in blood is correlated with large quantities of circulating virus, greater infectivity, and more active liver disease. Persistence of circulating HBeAg is prognostic of chronic hepatitis.[68]

Antibody to these antigens can be detected by RIA and ELISA systems and is also useful in the diagnosis and prognosis of HBV infection.

1. Anti-HBs (antibody to the surface antigen) is present during all acute and chronic hepatic disease as well as in most patients who have recovered from HBV infection. Chronic HBV carriers may have both HBsAg and anti-HBs circulating simultaneously. Vaccination with HBsAg gives rise to anti-HBs alone and indicates immunity to HBV.[152]
2. Anti-HBc (antibody to the core antigen) IgM is present in high titer in acute disease and in lower titer in chronic disease and thus enables distinction between these two manifestations of disease.[23]
3. Anti-HBe (antibody to the e antigen) may be prognostic in that its early appearance (before 6 weeks) is correlated with uncomplicated recovery. Delay in the appearance of anti-HBe may be prognostic of the development of chronic hepatitis.[2]

Hepatitis C Virus

Detection of infection with hepatitis C virus (HCV) is important in screening blood donors and managing patients with HCV. Serologic procedures are performed with cloned antigens and are referred to as first-, second-, and third-generation ELISAs or immunoblot tests.[25] First-generation ELISAs detected antibody in most non-A, non-B post-transfusion patients with hepatitis but lacked sensitivity in the early stages of disease and gave false-positive reactions when used in blood donor screening programs. The development of second-generation ELISAs permitted earlier detection of infection and resulted in greater specificity.[97] The third-generation ELISAs incorporate additional recombinant antigens but with only minor improvements in sensitivity and specificity.[97] Immunoblot assays are useful in the analysis of cross-reactions seen with other infections and results that are interpreted as indeterminate by ELISA.[37] Detection of IgM antibodies in patients with HCV does not differentiate acute from chronic infection.[181] In many cases, serologic tests must be performed sequentially over time for accurate assessment of disease.[134]

TABLE 250–4 ■ MARKERS OF HEPATITIS TYPE B VIRUS INFECTION

		Chronic			
Marker	**Acute HBV**	**Active**	**Persistent**	**Carrier**	**Vaccinated**
HBsAg	+	+	+	+	–
HBeAg	+	+/–	+/–	+/–	–
Anti-HBs	+/–	–	–	–	+
Anti-HBc	+	+	+	+	–
Anti-HBe	+	+/–	+/–	+/–	–
Symptoms	+	+	–	–	–

+, Detectable in serum; –, not detectable in serum; +/–, detection depends on the stage of illness.
HBc, hepatitis B core antigen; HBeAg, hepatitis B e antigen; HBsAg, hepatitis B surface antigen; HBV, hepatitis B virus.

HIV-1 SEROLOGY

ELISAs for antibody to human immunodeficiency virus type 1 (HIV-1), originally developed in 1985 for blood donor screening,[122] now have been modified to screen for both HIV-1 and HIV-2 alone or together for the clinical diagnosis of AIDS.[65, 91] The significance of the detection of antibody without clinical symptoms and in patients without obvious risk factors requires careful clinical correlation and additional confirmatory testing. The ability to culture the virus and to find viral products via PCR technology is also of value in the interpretation and prognosis of the infection.

Originally, an ELISA using inactivated, disrupted whole virus was licensed to several commercial sources. The sensitivity of this test was determined to be between 93 and 95 percent, and it has a demonstrated specificity greater than 99 percent.[117, 164] Newer ELISA reagents containing specific viral protein antigens derived from recombinant gene technology were reported to be more specific (second-generation tests). Western blot analysis is used to confirm repeatedly positive ELISA results.[125, 146] Because of the ability of early antiretroviral treatment to decrease the risk of perinatal HIV transmission, rapid HIV testing during labor is used with good results.[102] The rapid test has a sensitivity and specificity similar to those of the standard ELISA, and the negative predictive value is such that a negative test does not require confirmation. A positive test, however, should be confirmed.[156] Patients with negative ELISA results who are symptomatic or who have one or more risk factors, regardless of symptoms, should undergo serum testing by Western blot analysis and procedures to isolate the virus or its products. In Western blotting, proteins of the disrupted virus are separated by molecular weight electrophoretically and transferred from polyacrylamide gel to nitrocellulose paper. These discrete protein bands are reacted first with the patient's serum and then reacted with enzymatically labeled anti-immunoglobulins and visualized by the addition of an enzyme substrate to produce colored bands on the nitrocellulose.[66] Interpretation of the results has been the subject of some confusion in that the opinions of at least four agencies or committees and the one licensed manufacturer differ on the significance of reactive proteins in a positive test result. The World Health Organization has made recommendations on the interpretation of Western blot analysis for HIV-1.[1] Among these recommendations are that (1) laboratories should report test results as positive, indeterminate, or negative; (2) negative results are those that detect *no* bands; (3) positive results detect any two of the proteins labeled p24, gp41, and gp120/gp160; and (4) patients with results interpreted as indeterminate must undergo repeat testing at intervals determined by the physician, who must evaluate the indeterminate results as part of the entire clinical history of the patient. Probably a prudent measure is for the laboratory report to list the individual bands detected so that the physician is aware of the criteria used in interpretation of the test.

MEASLES VIRUS SEROLOGY

Indirect ELISAs and IgM capture assays now are used to routinely diagnose acute measles and to assess immunity in individuals. Testing can be performed with materials available commercially or most often though state and regional public health laboratories.[162] A significant rise in titer of fourfold or greater between acute and convalescent sera is indicative of infection, but acute infection is preferably assessed by the demonstration of a single IgM titer. IgM seropositivity is best demonstrated, regardless of the test used, when the specimen is collected 6 to 14 days after the onset of symptoms.[16]

Subacute sclerosing panencephalitis, a severe manifestation of persistent measles virus infection, can be diagnosed accurately by detecting measles antibody in CSF. In this disease, measles antibody titers in CSF often exceed 1:1280.[71]

RUBELLA VIRUS SEROLOGY

IHA has been supplanted by other tests to determine immune status and infection by rubella virus.[162] Newer tests available commercially include ELISA, which is used most commonly, but IFA and LA are also available. All are suitable for determining immunity status, and a significant titer rise must be observed between acute and convalescent sera to diagnose infection. Rubella virus titers are variable, and testing paired sera with the same assay is imperative. Congenital infection can be diagnosed by testing serum for IgM-specific antibody.[55, 123]

REFERENCES

1. AIDS: Proposed WHO criteria for interpreting Western blot assays for HIV-1, HIV-2, and HTLV-I/HTLV-II. Bull. World Health Organ. *69*:127–133, 1991.
2. Aldershvile, J., Frosner, G. G., Nielsen, J. O., et al.: Hepatitis B e antigen and antibody measured by radioimmunoassay in acute hepatitis B surface antigen–positive hepatitis. J. Infect. Dis. *141*:293–298, 1980.
3. Alonzo, T. A., and Pepe, M. S.: Using a combination of reference tests to assess the accuracy of a new diagnostic test. Stat. Med. *18*:2987–3003, 1999.
4. Andiman, W. A.: Epstein-Barr virus–associated syndromes: A critical reexamination. Pediatr. Infect. Dis. J. *3*:198–203, 1984.
5. Barrett, T. J., Snyder, J. D., Blake, P. A., et al.: Enzyme-linked immunosorbent assay for detection of *Salmonella typhi* Vi antigen in urine from typhoid patients. J. Clin. Microbiol. *15*:235–237, 1982.
6. Bauman, D. S., and Smith, C. D.: Comparison of immunodiffusion and complement fixation tests in the diagnosis of histoplasmosis. J. Clin. Microbiol. *2*:77–80, 1975.
7. Bayer, A. S., Lam, K., Ginzton, L., et al.: *Staphylococcus aureus* bacteremia: Clinical, serologic, and echocardiographic findings in patients with and without endocarditis. Arch. Intern. Med. *147*:457–462, 1987.
8. Blackburn, N. K., Besselaar, T. G., Schoub, B. D., et al.: Differentiation of primary cytomegalovirus infection from reactivation using the urea denaturation test for measuring antibody avidity. J. Med. Virol. *33*:6–9, 1991.
9. Bokkenheuser, V., Smity, P., and Richardson, N.: A challenge to the validity of the Vi test for the detection of chronic typhoid carriers. Am. J. Public Health *54*:1501–1503, 1964.
10. Booth, J. C., Hannington, G., Bakir, T. M. F., et al.: Comparison of enzyme-linked immunosorbent assay, radioimmunoassay, complement fixation, anticomplement immunofluorescence and passive haemagglutination techniques for detecting cytomegalovirus IgG antibody. J. Clin. Pathol. *35*:1345–1348, 1982.
11. Brown, S. L., Hansen, S. L., and Langone, J. J.: Role of serology in the diagnosis of Lyme disease. J. A. M. A. *282*:62–66, 1999.
12. Buchanan, T. M., and Faber, L. C.: 2-Mercaptoethanol *Brucella* agglutination test: Usefulness for predicting recovery from brucellosis. J. Clin. Microbiol. *11*:691–693, 1980.
13. Budzko, D. B., Tyler, L., and Armstrong, D.: Fc receptors on the surface of *Toxoplasma gondii* trophozoites: A confounding factor in testing for anti-*Toxoplasma* antibodies by indirect immunofluorescence. J. Clin. Microbiol. *27*:959–961, 1989.
14. Burgdorfer, W., Barbour, A. G., Hayes, S. F., et al.: Lyme disease: A tick-borne spirochetosis? Science *216*:1317–1319, 1982.
15. Busey, J. F.: North American blastomycosis. Gen. Pract. *30*:88–95, 1964.
16. Canadian Communicable Disease Report. Measles surveillance: Guidelines for laboratory support. Can. Commun. Dis. Rep. *25*:201–216, 1999.
17. Cassell, G. H.: Severe *Mycoplasma* disease—rare or underdiagnosed? West. J. Med. *162*:172–175, 1995.
18. Cassell, G. H., and Cole, B. C.: Mycoplasmas as agents of human disease. N. Engl. J. Med. *304*:80–89, 1981.
19. Centers for Disease Control: Brucellosis Surveillance: 1975. Surveillance Annual Summary. Atlanta, U.S. Department of Health, Education, and Welfare, July 1976, p. 14.
20. Chernesky, M. A., Escobar, M. R., Swenson, P. D., et al.: Laboratory diagnosis of hepatitis viruses. *In* Specter, S. (ed.): Cumitech 18. Washington, D.C., American Society for Microbiology, 1984, pp. 1–12.
21. Chia, W. K., Spence, L., Dunkley, L., et al.: Development of urease conjugated enzyme-linked immunosorbent assays (EIA) for the detection of IgM and IgG antibodies against *Mycoplasma pneumoniae* in human sera. Diagn. Microbiol. Infect. Dis. *11*:101–107, 1988.
22. Chick, E. W., Baum, G. L., Furcolow, M. L., et al.: Scientific assembly statement: The use of skin tests and serologic tests in histoplasmosis, coccidioidomycosis, and blastomycosis. Am. Rev. Respir. Dis. *108*:156–159, 1973.
23. Cohen, B. J.: The IgM antibody response to the core antigen of hepatitis B virus. J. Med. Virol. *3*:141–150, 1978.
24. Craft, J. E., Grodzicki, R. L., and Steere, A. C.: The antibody response in Lyme disease: Evaluation of diagnostic tests. J. Infect. Dis. *149*:789–795, 1984.
25. Cuthbert, J. A.: Hepatitis C: Progress and problems. Clin. Microbiol. Rev. *7*:505–532, 1994.
26. De Klerk, E., and Anderson, R.: Comparative evaluation of the enzyme-linked immunosorbent assay in the laboratory diagnosis of brucellosis. J. Clin. Microbiol. *21*:381–386, 1985.
27. de Repentigny, L.: Serodiagnosis of candidiasis, aspergillosis, and cryptococcosis. Clin. Infect. Dis. *14*(Suppl.):11–22, 1992.
28. de Repentigny, L., and Reiss, E.: Current trends in immunodiagnosis of candidiasis and aspergillosis. Rev. Infect. Dis. *6*:301–312, 1984.
29. Desmonts, G., Naot, Y., and Remington, J. S.: Immunoglobulin M-immunosorbent agglutination assay for diagnosis of infectious diseases: Diagnosis of acute congenital and acquired *Toxoplasma* infections. J. Clin. Microbiol. *14*:486–491, 1981.
30. Dorigo-Zetsma, J. W., Zaat, S. A., Wertheim-van Dillen, P. M., et al.: Comparison of PCR, culture, and serological tests for diagnosis of *Mycoplasma pneumoniae* respiratory tract infection in children. J. Clin. Microbiol. *37*:14–17, 1999.
31. Drew, W. L.: Diagnosis of cytomegalovirus infection. Rev. Infect. Dis. *10*(Suppl.):468–476, 1988.
32. Drew, W. L., Sweet, E., Miner, R. C., et al.: Multiple infections with cytomegalovirus in patients with acquired immunodeficiency syndrome: Documentation by Southern blot hybridization. J. Infect. Dis. *150*:952, 1984.
33. Drutz, D. J., and Catanzaro, A.: Coccidioidomycosis: Part 1. Am. Rev. Respir. Dis. *117*:559–585, 1978.
34. Duermeyer, W., Wielaard, F., and van der Veen, J.: A new principle for the detection of specific IgM antibodies applied in an EIA for hepatitis. Am. J. Med. Virol. *4*:25–32, 1979.
35. Dyckman, J. D., Storms, S., and Huber, T. W.: Reactivity of microhemagglutination, fluorescent treponemal antibody absorption, and Venereal Disease Research Laboratory tests in primary syphilis. J. Clin. Microbiol. *12*:629–630, 1980.
36. Dylewski, J. S., Rasmussen, L., Mills, J., et al.: Large-scale serological screening for cytomegalovirus in homosexual males by enzyme-linked immunosorbent assay. J. Clin. Microbiol. *19*:200–203, 1984.
37. Ebeling, F., Naukkarianen, R., and Leikola, J.: Recombinant immunoblot assay for hepatitis C virus antibody as predictor of infectivity. Lancet *335*:982–983, 1990.
38. Edwards, J. E., Lehrer, R. I., Stiehm, E. R., et al.: Severe candidal infections: Clinical perspective, immune defense mechanisms, and current concepts of therapy. Ann. Intern. Med. *89*:91–106, 1978.
39. Engstrom, S. M., Shoop, E., and Johnson, R. C.: Immunoblot interpretation criteria for serodiagnosis of early Lyme disease. J. Clin. Microbiol. *33*:419–427, 1995.
40. Farhat, S. E., Finn, S., Chua, R., et al.: Rapid detection of infectious mononucleosis–associated heterophile antibodies by a novel immunochromatographic assay and a latex agglutination test. J. Clin. Microbiol. *31*:1597–1600, 1993.
41. Farr, R. W.: Leptospirosis. Clin. Infect. Dis. *21*:1–6, 1995.

42. Farrell, I. D., Robertson, L., and Hinchliffe, P. M.: Serum antibody response in acute brucellosis. J. Hyg. *74*:23–28, 1975.
43. Finland, M., Peterson, O. L., Allen, E., II, et al.: Cold agglutinins. I. Occurrence of cold isohemagglutinins in various conditions. J. Clin. Invest. *24*:451, 1945.
44. Flehmig, G., Ranke, M., Berthold, H., et al.: A solid-phase radioimmunoassay for detection of IgM antibodies to hepatitis A virus. J. Infect. Dis. *140*:169–175, 1979.
45. Fleisher, G., Henle, W., Henle, G., et al.: Primary infection with Epstein-Barr virus in infants in the United States: Clinical and serologic observations. J. Infect. Dis. *139*:553–558, 1979.
46. Freter, R.: Agglutinin titration (Widal) for the diagnosis of enteric fever and other enterobacterial infections. *In* Rose, N. R., and Friedman, H. (eds.): Manual of Clinical Immunology. Washington, D.C., American Society for Microbiology, 1976, pp. 285–288.
47. Ginsburg, C. M., Henle, W., Henle, G., et al.: Infectious mononucleosis in children: Evaluation of Epstein-Barr virus–specific serological data. J. A. M. A. *237*:781–785, 1977.
48. Goldman, D. L., Khine, H., Abadi, J., et al.: Serologic evidence for *Cryptococcus neoformans* infection in early childhood. Pediatrics *107*:E66, 2001.
49. Greenberg, D. P., Bayer, A. S., Turner, D., et al.: Antibody responses to protein A in patients with *Staphylococcus aureus* bacteremia and endocarditis. J. Clin. Microbiol. *28*:458–462, 1990.
50. Greenfield, R. A., Bussey, M. J., Stephens, J. L., et al.: Serial enzyme-linked immunosorbent assays for antibody to *Candida* antigens during induction chemotherapy for acute leukemia. J. Infect. Dis. *148*:275–283, 1983.
51. Griffin, J. P.: Rapid screening for cold agglutinins in pneumonia. Ann. Intern. Med. *70*:701–705, 1969.
52. Griffiths, P. D., Stagno, S., Pass, R. F., et al.: Congenital cytomegalovirus infection: Diagnostic and prognostic significance of the detection of specific immunoglobulin M antibodies in cord serum. Pediatrics *69*:544–549, 1982.
53. Griffiths, P. D., Stagno, S., Pass, R. F., et al.: Infection with cytomegalovirus during pregnancy: Specific IgM antibodies as a marker of recent primary infection. J. Infect. Dis. *145*:647–652, 1982.
54. Grodzicki, R. L., and Steere, A. C.: Diagnosing early Lyme disease by immunoblotting: Comparison with indirect ELISA using different antigen preparations. J. Infect. Dis. *157*:790–797, 1988.
55. Gupta, J. D., Peterson, V., Stout, M., et al.: Single-sample diagnosis of recent rubella by fractionation of antibody on Sephadex G-200 column. J. Clin. Pathol. *24*:547–550, 1971.
56. Hechemy, K. E.: Laboratory diagnosis of Rocky Mountain spotted fever. N. Engl. J. Med. *300*:859–860, 1979.
57. Hechemy, K. E., Anacker, R. L., Philip, R. N., et al.: Detection of Rocky Mountain spotted fever antibodies by a latex agglutination test. J. Clin. Microbiol. *12*:144–150, 1980.
58. Hechemy, K. E., and Michaelson, E. E.: Rocky Mountain spotted fever: A resurgent problem. Lab. Management *Oct.*:29–40, 1981.
59. Hechemy, K. E., Stevens, R. W., Sasowski, S., et al.: Discrepancies in Weil-Felix and microimmunofluoresence test for Rocky Mountain spotted fever. J. Clin. Microbiol. *9*:292–293, 1979.
60. Hederstedt, B., Holm, S. E., and Wadstrom, T.: Discrepancy between results of the Streptozyme test and those of the antideoxyribonuclease B and antihyaluronidase tests. J. Clin. Microbiol. *8*:50–53, 1978.
61. Heiner, D. C.: Diagnosis of histoplasmosis using precipitin reactions in agar gel. Pediatrics *22*:616–627, 1958.
62. Hekker, A. C., Brand-Saathof, B., Vis, J., et al.: Indirect immunofluorescence test for detection of IgM antibodies to cytomegalovirus. J. Infect. Dis. *140*:596–600, 1979.
63. Henle, G., Henle, W., and Horwitz, C. A.: Antibodies to Epstein-Barr virus–associated nuclear antigen in infectious mononucleosis. J. Infect. Dis. *130*:231–239, 1974.
64. Henle, W., Henle, G., and Horwitz, C. A.: Epstein-Barr virus–specific diagnostic tests in infectious mononucleosis. Hum. Pathol. *5*:551–565, 1974.
65. Hess, G., Avillez, F., Lourenco, M. H., et al.: Diagnosis of human immunodeficiency virus (HIV) infection: Multicenter evaluation of a newly developed anti-HIV 1 and 2 enzyme immunoassay. J. Clin. Microbiol. *32*:403–406, 1994.
66. Hirsch, M. S., Wormser, G. P., Schooley, R. T., et al.: Risk of nosocomial infection with human T-cell lymphotropic virus III (HTLV-III). N. Engl. J. Med. *312*:1–4, 1985.
67. Holmberg, K., Berdischewsky, M., and Young L. S.: Serologic immunodiagnosis of invasive aspergillosis. J. Infect. Dis. *141*:656–664, 1980.
68. Hoofnagle, J. H.: Serological markers of hepatitis B virus infection. Annu. Rev. Med. *32*:1–11, 1981.
69. Hopson, D. K., Niles, A. C., and Murray, P. R.: Comparison of the Vitek Immunodiagnostic Assay System with three immunoassay systems for detection of cytomegalovirus-specific immunoglobulin G. J. Clin. Microbiol. *30*:2893–2895, 1993.
70. Horodniceanu, F., and Michelson, S.: Assessment of human cytomegalovirus antibody detection techniques. Arch. Virol. *64*:287–301, 1980.
71. Horta-Barbosa, L., Krebs, H., Ley, A., et al.: Progressive increase in cerebrospinal fluid measles antibody levels in subacute sclerosing panencephalitis. Pediatrics *47*:782–783, 1971.
72. Hostetler, C. L., Sawyer, K. P., and Nachamkin, I.: Comparison of three rapid methods for detection of antibodies to streptolysin O and DNase B. J. Clin. Microbiol. *26*:1406–1408, 1988.
73. Huppert, M.: Serology of coccidioidomycosis. Mycopathol. Mycol. Appl. *41*:107–113, 1970.
74. Huppert, M., Pererson, E. T., Sun, S. H., et al.: Evaluation of a latex particle agglutination test for coccidioidomycosis. Am. J. Clin. Pathol. *49*:96–102, 1968.
75. Ibanez-Nolla, J., Torres-Rodriguez, J. M., Nolla, M., et al.: The utility of serology in diagnosing candidosis in non-neutropenic critically ill patients. Mycoses *44*:47–53, 2001.
76. Janeff, J., Janeff, D., Taranta, A., et al.: A screening test for streptococcal antibodies. Lab. Med. *2*:38–40, 1971.
77. Jones, J. M.: Laboratory diagnosis of invasive candidiasis. Clin. Microbiol. Rev. *3*:32–45, 1990.
78. Kaplan, E. L., and Huwe, B. B.: The sensitivity and specificity of an agglutination test for antibodies to streptococcal extracellular antigens: A quantitative analysis and comparison of the Streptozyme test with the anti-streptolysin O and anti-deoxyribonuclease B tests. J. Pediatr. *96*:367–372, 1980.
79. Kaufman, L.: Serodiagnosis of fungal disease. *In* Rose, N. R., and Friedman, H. (eds.): Manual of Clinical Immunology. Washington, D.C., American Society for Microbiology, 1976, pp. 363–381.
80. Kaufman, L.: Laboratory methods for the diagnosis and confirmation of systemic mycoses. Clin. Infect. Dis. *14*(Suppl.):14–29, 1992.
81. Kaufman, L., McLaughlin, D. W., Clark, M. J., et al.: Specific immunodiffusion test for blastomycosis. Appl. Microbiol. *26*:244–247, 1973.
82. Kelly, D. J., Chan, C. T., Paxton, H., et al.: Comparative evaluation of a commercial enzyme immunoassay for the detection of human antibody to *Rickettsia typhi*. Clin. Diagn. Immunol. *2*:355–360, 1995.
83. Klingspor, L., Eberhared, T. H., Stintzing, G., et al.: Antibody response to *Candida* and its use in clinical practice. Mycoses *37*:199–204, 1994.
84. Lackman, D. B., and Gerloff, R. K.: The effect of antibiotic therapy upon diagnostic and serologic tests for Rocky Mountain spotted fever. Public Health Lab. *11*:97–99, 1953.
85. Larsen, S. A., Steiner, B. M., and Rudolph, A. H.: Laboratory diagnosis and interpretation of tests for syphilis. Clin. Microbiol. Rev. *8*:1–21, 1995.
86. Latge, J. P.: *Aspergillus fumigatus* and aspergillosis. Clin. Microbiol. Rev. *12*:310–350, 1999.
87. Lazzarotto, T., Casa, B. D., Campisis, B., et al.: Enzyme-linked immunosorbent assay for detection of cytomegalovirus-IgM: Comparison between eight commercial kits, immunofluorescence, and immunoblotting. J. Clin. Lab. Anal. *6*:216–218, 1992.
88. Lazzarotto, T., Dal Monte, P., Boccuni, M. C., et al.: Lack of correlation between virus detection and serologic tests for diagnosis of active cytomegalovirus infection in patients with AIDS. J. Clin. Microbiol. *30*:1027–1029, 1992.
89. Lefebre, J., Bertrand, M., and Bauriaud, R.: Evaluation of the Captia enzyme immunoassays for detection of immunoglobulins G and M to *Treponema pallidum* in syphilis. J. Clin. Microbiol. *28*:1704–1707, 1990.
90. Lewis, L. L., Taber, L. H., and Baughn, R. E.: Evaluation of immunoglobulin M Western blot analysis in the diagnosis of congenital syphilis. J. Clin. Microbiol. *28*:296–302, 1990.
91. Lin, H. J.: Laboratory tests for human immunodeficiency viruses. J. Int. Fed. Clin. Chem. *7*:61–66, 1995.
92. Longbottom, J. L.: Immunologic aspects of infection and allergy due to *Aspergillus* species. Mykosen *116*:207–217, 1978.
93. Luger, S. W., and Krauss, E.: Serologic tests for Lyme disease: Interlaboratory variability. Arch. Intern. Med. *150*:761–763, 1990.
94. Magnarelli, L. A., Anderson, J. F., and Johnson, R. C.: Cross-reactivity in serological tests for Lyme disease and other spirochetal infections. J. Infect. Dis. *156*:183–188, 1987.
95. Magnarelli, L. A., Dumler, J. S., Anderson, J. F., et al.: Coexistence of antibodies to tick-borne pathogens of babesiosis, ehrlichiosis, and Lyme borreliosis in human sera. J. Clin. Microbiol. *33*:3054–3057, 1995.
96. Magnarelli, L. A., Meegan, J. M., Anderson J. F., et al.: Comparison of an indirect fluorescent-antibody test with an enzyme-linked assay for serological studies of Lyme disease. J. Clin. Microbiol. *20*:181–184, 1984.
97. Marcellin, P., Martino-Peignoux, M., Gabriel, F., et al.: Chronic non-B, non-C hepatitis among blood donors assessed with HCV third generation tests and polymerase chain reaction. J. Hepatol. *19*:167–170, 1993.
98. Martins, T. B., Jaskowski, T. D., Mouritsen, C. L., et al.: Comparison of commercially available enzyme immunoassay with traditional serological tests for detection of antibodies to *Coccidioides immitis*. J. Clin. Microbiol. *33*:940–943, 1995.
99. Matthews, R. C., Burnie, J. P., and Tabaqchali, S.: Immunoblot analysis of the serological response in systemic candidosis. Lancet *2*:1415–1418, 1984.

100. Merz, W. G., Evans, G. L., Shadomy, S., et al.: Laboratory evaluation of serological tests for systemic candidiasis: A cooperative study. J. Clin. Microbiol. *5*:596–603, 1977.
101. Middeldorp, J. M., Johgsma, J., ter Haar, A., et al.: Detection of immunoglobulin M and G antibodies against cytomegalovirus early and late antigens by enzyme-linked immunosorbent assay. J. Clin. Microbiol. *20*:763–771, 1984.
102. Mofenson, L. M.: Technical report: Perinatal human immunodeficiency virus testing and prevention of transmission. Committee on Pediatric AIDS. Pediatrics *106*:E88, 2000.
103. Nagel, J. G., Tuazon, C. U., Cardella, T. A., et al.: Teichoic acid serologic diagnosis of staphylococcal endocarditis. Ann. Intern. Med. *82*:13–17, 1975.
104. Naot, Y., Guptill, D. R., and Remington, J. S.: Duration of IgM antibodies to *Toxoplasma gondii* after acute acquired toxoplasmosis. J. Infect. Dis. *145*:770, 1982.
105. Naot, Y., and Remington, J. S.: An enzyme-linked immunosorbent assay for detection of IgM antibodies to *Toxoplasma gondii:* Use for diagnosis of acute acquired toxoplasmosis. J. Infect. Dis. *142*:757–766, 1980.
106. Nolan, C. M., Feeley, J. C., White, P. C., Jr., et al.: Evaluation of a new assay for Vi antibody in chronic carriers of *Salmonella typhi*. J. Clin. Microbiol. *12*:22–26, 1980.
107. Pappagianis, D.: Coccidioidomycosis. *In* Samter, M. (ed.): Immunological Diseases. Boston, Little, Brown, 1978, p. 652.
108. Pappagianis, D., and Crane, R.: Survival in coccidioidal meningitis since introduction of amphotericin B. *In* Ajello, L. (ed.): Coccidioidomycosis: Current Clinical and Diagnostic Status. Miami, Symposia Specialists Medical Books, 1977, pp. 223–237.
109. Pappagianis, D., Krasnow, R. I., and Beall, S.: False-positive reactions of cerebrospinal fluid and diluted sera with the coccidioidal latex-agglutination test. Am. J. Clin. Pathol. *66*:916–921, 1976.
110. Pappagianis, D., and Zimmer, B. L.: Serology of coccidioidomycosis. Clin. Microbiol. Rev. *3*:247–268, 1990.
111. Pappas, M. G., Ballou, W. R., Gray, M. R., et al.: Rapid serodiagnosis of leptospirosis using the IgM-specific dot-ELISA: Comparison with the microscopic agglutination test. Am. J. Trop. Med. Hyg. *34*:346–354, 1985.
112. Paul, J. R., and Bunnell, W. W.: The presence of heterophile antibodies in infectious mononucleosis. Am. J. Med. Sci. *183*:90–104, 1932.
113. Pellicer, T., Ariza, J., Foz, A., et al.: Specific antibodies detected during relapse of human brucellosis. J. Infect. Dis. *157*:918–924, 1988.
114. Penn, R. L., Lambert, R. S., and George, R. B.: Invasive fungal infections: The use of serologic tests in diagnosis and management. Arch. Intern. Med. *143*:1215–1220, 1983.
115. Peter, C. R., Thompson, M. A., and Wilson, D. L.: False-positive reactions in the rapid plasma reagin-card, fluorescent treponemal antibody-absorbed, and hemagglutination treponemal syphilis serology tests. J. Clin. Microbiol. *9*:369–372, 1979.
116. Peter, G., and Smith, A. L.: Group A streptococcal infections of the skin and pharynx. N. Engl. J. Med. *297*:311–317, 1977.
117. Petricciani, J. C.: Licensed tests for antibody to human T-lymphotropic virus type III: Sensitivity and specificity. Ann. Intern. Med. *103*:726–729, 1985.
118. Philip, R. N., Casper, E. A., Ormsbee, R. A., et al.: Microimmunofluorescence test for the serological study of Rocky Mountain spotted fever and typhus. J. Clin. Microbiol. *3*:51–61, 1976.
119. Plouffe, J. F., and Fass, R. J.: *Histoplasma* meningitis: Diagnostic value of cerebrospinal fluid serology. Ann. Intern. Med. *92*:189–191, 1980.
120. Powell, D. A., and Schuit, K. E.: Acute pulmonary blastomycosis in children: Clinical course and follow-up. Pediatrics *63*:736–740, 1979.
121. Preisler, H. D., Hasenclever, H. F., Levitan, A. A., et al.: Serologic diagnosis of disseminated candidiasis in patients with acute leukemia. Ann. Intern. Med. *70*:19–30, 1969.
122. Provisional Public Health Service inter-agency recommendations for screening donated blood and plasma for antibody to the virus causing acquired immunodeficiency syndrome. M. M. W. R. Morb. Mortal. Wkly. Rep. *34*:1–5, 1985.
123. Punnarugsa, V., and Mungmee, V.: Detection of rubella virus immunoglobulin G (IgG) and IgM antibodies in whole blood on Whatman paper: Comparison with detection in sera. J. Clin. Microbiol. *29*:2209–2212, 1991.
124. Rawlinson, W. D.: Broadsheet. Number 50: Diagnosis of human cytomegalovirus infection and disease. Pathology *31*:109–115, 1999.
125. Recommendations for assisting in the prevention of perinatal transmission of human T-lymphotropic virus type III/lymphadenopathy-associated virus and acquired immunodeficiency syndrome. M. M. W. R. Morb. Mortal. Wkly. Rep. *34*(48):721–726, 731–732, 1985.
126. Reddin, J. L., Anderson, R. K., Jenness, R., et al.: Significance of 7S and macroglobulin *Brucella* agglutinins in human brucellosis. N. Engl. J. Med. *272*:1263–1267, 1965.
127. Ribeiro, M. A., Souza, C. C., and Almeida, S. H. P.: Dot-ELISA for human leptospirosis employing immunodominant antigen. J. Trop. Med. Hyg. *98*:452–456, 1995.
128. Rizzetto, M., Shih, J. W. K., Verme, G., et al.: A radioimmunoassay for HBcAg in the sera of HBsAg carriers: Serum HBcAg, serum DNA polymerase activity, and liver HBcAg immunofluorescence as markers of chronic liver disease. Gastroenterology *80*:1420–1427, 1981.
129. Rose, C. D., Fawcett, P. T., Gibney, K. M., et al.: Residual serologic reactivity in children with resolved Lyme arthritis. J. Rheumatol. *23*:367–369, 1996.
130. Sabin, A. E., and Feldman, H. A.: Dyes as microchemical indicators of a new immunity phenomenon affecting protozoan parasite *(Toxoplasma)*. Science *108*:660–663, 1948.
131. Sanchez, P. J., McCracken, G. H., Jr., Wendel, G. D., et al.: Molecular analysis of the fetal IgM response to *Treponema pallidum* antigens: Implications for improved serodiagnosis of congenital syphilis. J. Infect. Dis. *159*:508–517, 1989.
132. Sarosi, G. A., and Davies, S. F.: Blastomycosis. Am. Rev. Respir. Dis. *120*:911–938, 1979.
133. Sarosi, G. A., Davies, S. F., Klein, B., et al.: Recent developments in blastomycosis. Am. Rev. Respir. Dis. *134*:817–818, 1986.
134. Schneider, L., and Geha, R.: Outbreak of hepatitis C associated with intravenous immunoglobulin administration: United States, October 1993–June 1994. M. M. W. R. Morb. Mortal. Wkly. Rep. *43*:505–509, 1994.
135. Sheagren, J. N., Menes, B. I., Han, D. P., et al.: Technical aspects of the *Staphylococcus aureus* teichoic acid antibody assay: Gel diffusion and counterimmunoelectrophoretic assays, antigen preparation, antigen selection, concentration effects, and cross-reactions with other organisms. J. Clin. Microbiol. *13*:293–300, 1981.
136. Siegel, J. P., and Remington, J. S.: Comparison of methods for quantitating antigen-specific immunoglobulin M antibody with a reverse enzyme-linked immunosorbent assay. J. Clin. Microbiol. *18*:63–70, 1983.
137. Silletti, R. P.: Comparison of Captia syphilis G enzyme immunoassay with rapid plasma reagin test for detection of syphilis. J. Clin. Microbiol. *33*:1829–1831, 1995.
138. Singh, A. E., and Romanowski, B.: Syphilis: Review with emphasis on clinical, epidemiologic, and some biologic features. Clin. Microbiol. Rev. *12*:187–209, 1999.
139. Smith, C. E.: Coccidioidomycosis. Pediatr. Clin. North Am. *2*:109–125, 1955.
140. Smith, C. E., Saito, M. N. T., and Simons, S. A.: Pattern of 39,500 serologic tests in coccidioidomycosis. J. A. M. A. *160*:546–552, 1956.
141. Spink, W. W., McCullough, N. B., Hutchings, L. M., et al.: A standardized antigen and agglutination technique for human brucellosis: Report No. 3 of the National Research Council Committee on Public Aspects of Brucellosis. Am. J. Clin. Pathol. *24*:496–498, 1954.
142. Stagno, S., Pass, R. F., Reynolds, D. W., et al.: Comparative study of diagnostic procedures for congenital cytomegalovirus infection. Pediatrics *65*:251–257, 1980.
143. Stagno, S., Reynolds, D. W., Tsiantos, A., et al.: Comparative serial virologic and serologic studies of symptomatic and subclinical congenitally and natally acquired cytomegalovirus infections. J. Infect. Dis. *132*:568–577, 1975.
144. Steere, A. C., Grodzicki, R. L., Kornblatt, A. N., et al.: The spirochetal etiology of Lyme disease. N. Engl. J. Med. *308*:733–740, 1983.
145. Stepick-Bick, P., Thulliez, P., Araujo, F. G., et al.: IgA antibodies for diagnosis of acute congenital and acquired toxoplasmosis. J. Infect. Dis. *162*:270–273, 1990.
146. Sullivan, M. T., Jucke, H., Kadey, S. D., et al.: Evaluation of an indirect immunofluorescence assay for confirmation of human immunodeficiency virus type 1 antibody in U.S. blood donor sera. J. Clin. Microbiol. *30*:2509–2510, 1992.
147. Sulzer, C. R., Glosser, J. W., Rogers, F., et al.: Evaluation of an indirect hemagglutination test for the diagnosis of human leptospirosis. J. Clin. Microbiol. *2*:218–221, 1975.
148. Sulzer, C. R., and Jones, W. L.: Leptospirosis: Methods in Laboratory Diagnosis. Publication No. (CDC) 74-8275. Atlanta, Centers for Disease Control, U.S. Department of Health, Education, and Welfare, 1974.
149. Sumaya, C. V.: Epstein-Barr virus serologic testing: Diagnostic indications and interpretations. Pediatr. Infect. Dis. J. *5*:337–342, 1986.
150. Summers, P. L., Dubois, D. R., Cohen, W. H., et al.: Solid-phase antibody capture hemadsorption assay of detection of hepatitis A virus immunoglobulin M antibodies. J. Clin. Microbiol. *31*:1299–1302, 1993.
151. Sussman, S. J., Magoffin, R. L., Lennette, E. H., et al.: Cold agglutinins, Eaton agent, and respiratory infections of children. Pediatrics *38*:571–577, 1966.
152. Szmuness, W., Stevens, C. E., Harley, E. J., et al.: Hepatitis B vaccine: Demonstration of efficacy in a controlled clinical trial in a high-risk population in the United States. N. Engl. J. Med. *303*:833–841, 1980.
153. Thacker, W. L., and Talkington, D. F.: Comparison of two rapid commercial tests with complement fixation for serologic diagnosis of *Mycoplasma pneumoniae* infections. J. Clin. Microbiol. *33*:1212–1214, 1995.
154. Thisyakorn, U., Shelton, S., Lin, T., et al.: Detection of teichoic acid antibodies in children with staphylococcal infections. Pediatr. Infect. Dis. J. *3*:222–225, 1984.
155. Tosi, M. F., and Nelson, T. J.: *Brucella canis* infection in a 17-month-old child successfully treated with moxalactam. J. Pediatr. *101*:725–727, 1982.

156. Update: HIV counseling and testing using rapid tests—United States, 1995. M. M. W. R. Morb. Mortal. Wkly. Rep. *47*(11):211–215, 1998.
157. van Deventer, A. J., van Vliet, H. J., Voogd, L., et al.: Increased specificity of antibody detection in surgical patients with invasive candidiasis with cytoplasmic antigens depleted of mannan residues. J. Clin. Microbiol. *31*:994–997, 1993.
158. Vornhage, R., Plachter, B., Hinderer, W., et al.: Early serodiagnosis of acute human cytomegalovirus infection by enzyme-linked immunosorbent assay using recombinant antigens. J. Clin. Microbiol. *32*:981–986, 1994.
159. Walker, D. H.: Diagnosis of rickettsial diseases. Pathol. Annu. *23*:69–96, 1988.
160. Wands, J. R., Bruns, R. R., Carlson, R. I., et al.: Monoclonal IgM radioimmunoassay for hepatitis B surface antigen: High binding activity in serum that is unreactive with conventional antibodies. Proc. Natl. Acad. Sci. U. S. A. *79*:1277–1281, 1982.
161. Wannamaker, L.: Differences between streptococcal infections of the throat and of the skin. N. Engl. J. Med. *282*:23–31, 1970.
162. Watson, J. C., Haddler, S. C., Dykewicz, C. A., et al.: Measles, mumps, and rubella—vaccine use and strategies for elimination of measles, rubella, and congenital rubella syndrome and control of mumps: Recommendation of the Advisory Committee on Immunization Practices (ACIP). M. M. W. R. Recomm. Rep. *47*(RR-8):1–57, 1998.
163. Watt, G., Alquiza, L. M., Padre, L. P., et al.: The rapid diagnosis of leptospirosis: A prospective comparison of the dot enzyme-linked immunosorbent assay and the genus-specific microscopic agglutination test at different stages of illness. J. Infect. Dis. *157*:840–842, 1988.
164. Weiss, S. H., Goedert, J. J., Sarngadharan, M. G., et al.: Screening test for HTLV-III (AIDS agent) antibodies. J. A. M. A. *253*:221–225, 1985.
165. Welch, P. C., Masur, H., Jones, T. C., et al.: Serologic diagnosis of acute lymphadenopathic toxoplasmosis. J. Infect. Dis. *142*:256–264, 1980.
166. Wheat, L. J.: Laboratory diagnosis of histoplasmosis: Update 2000. Semin. Respir. Infect. *16*:131–140, 2001.
167. Wheat, J., French, M. L. V., Kamel, S., et al.: Evaluation of cross-reactions in *Histoplasma capsulatum* serologic tests. J. Clin. Microbiol. *23*:493–499, 1986.
168. Wheat, J., French, M. L. V., Kohler, R. B., et al.: The diagnostic laboratory tests for histoplasmosis: Analysis of experience in a large urban outbreak. Ann. Intern. Med. *97*:680–685, 1982.
169. Wheat, J. J., Kohler, R. B., French, M. L. V., et al.: IgM and IgG histoplasmal antibody response in histoplasmosis. Am. Rev. Respir. Dis. *128*:65–70, 1983.
170. Wheat, J., Kohler, R. B., Garten, M., et al.: Commercially available (Endo-Staph) assay for teichoic acid antibodies: Evaluation in patients with serious *Staphylococcus aureus* infections and in controls. Arch. Intern. Med. *144*:261–264, 1984.
171. Wheat, L. J., and White, A. C.: Rapid diagnosis of staphylococcal infections. *In* Rytel, M. W. (ed.): Rapid Diagnosis in Infectious Diseases. Boca Raton, FL, CRC Press, 1979, pp. 115–124.
172. Wilfert, C., and Gutman, L.: Genitourinary tract infections: Syphilis. *In* Feigin, R. D., and Cherry, J. D. (eds.): Textbook of Pediatric Infectious Diseases. Philadelphia, W. B. Saunders, 1981, pp. 388–400.
173. Wilson, G. S., and Miles, A. A. (eds.): Enteric infections. *In* Topley and Wilson's Principles of Bacteriology and Immunity. Baltimore, Williams & Wilkins, 1975, pp. 2005–2039.
174. Wong, M. L., Kaplan, S., Dunkle, L. M., et al.: Leptospirosis: A childhood disease. J. Pediatr. *90*:532–537, 1977.
175. Wong, S. Y., Hajdu, M. P., Ramirez, R., et al.: Role of specific immunoglobulin E in diagnosis of acute *Toxoplasma* infection and toxoplasmosis. J. Clin. Microbiol. *31*:2952–2959, 1993.
176. Wormser, G. P., Aguero-Rosenfeld, M. E., and Nadelman, R. B.: Lyme disease serology: Problems and opportunities. J. A. M. A. *282*:79–80, 1999.
177. Young, E. J.: Human brucellosis. Rev. Infect. Dis. *5*:821–842, 1983.
178. Young, E. J.: An overview of human brucellosis. Clin. Infect. Dis. *21*:283–290, 1995.
179. Young, R. C., and Bennett, J. E.: Invasive aspergillosis: Absence of detectable antibody response. Am. Rev. Respir. Dis. *104*:710–716, 1971.
180. Yow, M. D.: Brucellosis. *In* Feigin, R. D., and Cherry, J. D. (eds.): Textbook of Pediatric Infectious Diseases. Philadelphia, W. B. Saunders, 1981, pp. 828–833.
181. Zaaijer, H. L., Mimms, L. T., Cuyers, H. T., et al.: Variability of IgM response in hepatitis C virus infection. J. Med. Virol. *40*:184–187, 1993.

PART VIII

Biostatistics Applicable to the Subspecialty of Infectious Diseases

CHAPTER

251 Epidemiology and Biostatistics

EUGENE D. SHAPIRO

Clinicians care for individual patients, each of whom has certain unique problems. Clinicians base their decisions on a panoply of factors that include features of the acute and chronic medical problems of the patients, as well as features of both their personalities (e.g., How likely are they to comply with a certain therapeutic regimen?) and their private lives (e.g., Can they afford a certain medication? Are they planning to travel out of the country in the next few days?).

In contrast, epidemiologists study groups of people. They draw conclusions from studies of large numbers of patients and usually base conclusions on probabilities and biostatistical analyses of average (mean) outcomes.

Fortunately, these two approaches—the individualistic approach of the clinician and the probabilistic approach of the classic epidemiologist—are not incompatible. Indeed, each can illuminate the other. So it is that a chapter on epidemiology and biostatistics is included in a clinical textbook of pediatric infectious diseases. The goal of this chapter is not to make the reader an expert in these fields—courses and textbooks are designed for that purpose.[5, 8–11, 18–20] Instead, the goal is to summarize how selected key aspects of epidemiology and biostatistics can be applied to understand studies that will improve our ability to evaluate and treat children with infectious diseases.

Epidemiology

DESIGN OF STUDIES

Overview

Epidemiologic studies generally are designed to be either descriptive or analytic. In *descriptive* studies, the goal is to describe a population (e.g., the clinical manifestations and prognosis of children with tuberculosis). In *analytic* studies, the goal is to assess associations between two or more variables (e.g., In children who receive an experimental vaccine, is the infection that the vaccine is intended to prevent less likely to develop than in controls?). Indeed, analytic studies usually are designed to assess whether a causal association exists between the variables (e.g., Is a vaccine efficacious? Do children who attend daycare centers have a higher risk for infections caused by certain bacteria or viruses?). Of course, categorizing a study so easily may not be possible. In a primarily descriptive study, causal associations within subgroups may be assessed (e.g., in a study of the clinical epidemiology of tuberculosis in children, the investigators may compare the mortality rates of younger children with those of older children or the mortality rates of children with tuberculous meningitis with those of children who have infection at other sites).

Most studies, whether descriptive or analytic, seek to reach conclusions about the particular group that is being assessed (e.g., children with tuberculosis). However, because studying all persons with the condition of interest is not possible, investigators inevitably study a *sample* of persons and hope that the conclusions drawn from studying the sample apply to the entire population of interest (the *target population*). The *validity* of a study refers to the extent to which the results are true (accurate). The extent to which the conclusions drawn from the study sample (e.g., children with tuberculosis at Bellevue Hospital in New York City) are valid for the target population (e.g., all children with tuberculosis in New York City) is a measure of the study's *internal validity*. The extent to which the conclusions drawn from the study sample are valid for a less restrictively defined, larger population (e.g., all children with tuberculosis in the United States) is a measure of the study's *external validity,* which also is called its *generalizability.* To ensure that a study is both valid and generalizable, investigators must take steps to protect against a variety of potential biases (discussed later) that may distort the results of a study.

Elements of an Analytic Study

Epidemiologists refer to the major elements of an analytic study as the *exposure* and the *outcome.* The *exposure* is the factor that the investigator hypothesizes is related causally to the outcome of interest. In this context, the term *exposure* is not used in the classic sense of potential contact with an infectious agent; rather, it is any factor (e.g., living at a certain altitude, race, receipt of either a vaccine or a medication, smoking cigarettes) that may be associated causally with the outcome. The *outcome* is the effect (e.g., disease caused by a particular bacterium) that putatively is related causally to the exposure. The putative association may be one in which the exposure either causes or prevents the outcome of interest.

Before the specific type of study is defined, several additional elements of a study must be considered. One is how the *sample* for the study is selected. In general, investigators select a sample of the population based either on exposure (e.g., patients who either received or did not receive a vaccine or who either attend or do not attend group daycare) or on outcome (e.g., patients who either had or did not have pneumococcal bacteremia or patients who either died or survived). Another key element is the *timing* of the study in relation to the timing of exposure and outcome. In studies in which the timing is *historical,* both the exposure and the outcome occurred before the study was initiated (e.g., a case-control study of a vaccine's efficacy in which cases with disease are identified from historical logbooks and antecedent receipt of the vaccine is determined from medical records). Timing may be *concurrent*—that is, both the exposure and the outcome occur after the study is initiated (e.g., a randomized clinical trial of the efficacy of a new antibiotic). Timing also may be *mixed,* a mixture of historical and concurrent (e.g., a study of the current IQ of children who previously had aseptic meningitis).

A final important element of a study is its *direction.* Direction is used to describe the order in which outcome and exposure are assessed. It may be done in a *forward* direction, from exposure to outcome (e.g., in a clinical trial of a vaccine's efficacy, the exposure [receipt or nonreceipt of the experimental vaccine] occurs first, and the occurrence of the outcome [the infection that the vaccine is designed to prevent] is determined subsequently). Alternatively, a study's direction may be *backward,* from outcome to exposure (e.g., in a case-control study, the outcome [e.g., pneumococcal bacteremia] is determined first, and exposure [e.g., previous receipt of pneumococcal vaccine] is determined subsequently). Alternatively, exposure and outcome may be determined simultaneously (e.g., a survey in which determination of whether subjects have sickle-cell disease and whether they are taking penicillin occurs at the same time). A study's direction can have important implications for inferences about causal associations; for example, even though a strong statistical association may exist between sickle-cell disease and the use of penicillin, concluding that the penicillin caused the sickle-cell disease would be erroneous. Although such an inference is obviously not plausible in this instance, the dangers of making erroneous inferences about causality are very real when exposures and outcomes that are less well understood are studied.

Although the terms *prospective* and *retrospective* are used widely, substantial variability exists in how they are applied. The term *prospective* is used to describe studies in which selection of the sample is based on the exposure, in which the timing is concurrent, or in which the direction of the study is forward (from exposure to outcome). The term *retrospective* is used to describe studies in which selection of the sample is based on the outcome, in which the timing is historical, or in which the direction of the study is backward (from outcome to exposure). Referring to the specific elements of the study is preferable to using the terms *prospective* and *retrospective,* which are applied so imprecisely.

Types of Studies

Epidemiologic studies may be classified as either experimental or observational. In *experimental studies,* the exposure is assigned by the investigators (e.g., in a clinical trial of an experimental vaccine, the investigator assigns subjects to receive either the experimental vaccine or a placebo). In *observational studies,* the exposure occurs naturally (e.g., rainfall in a study that assesses the effect of the amount of rainfall on rates of mosquito-borne infections), is selected by the subjects or their parents (e.g., attendance at group daycare in a study that assesses the frequency of infectious illnesses in children who attend and others who do not attend group daycare), or is assigned in the course of regular medical care (e.g., receipt of an approved vaccine in a case-control study of the protective efficacy of the vaccine). Observational studies also are called *surveys.*

EXPERIMENTAL STUDIES

The paradigm for an experimental study is the *randomized clinical trial,* which is a special type of a *longitudinal cohort study* in which the exposure is assigned randomly to the subjects by the investigators. In randomized trials, the direction of the study always is forward, selection (or categorization) of subjects always is based on exposure (i.e., exposure is determined at the time of randomization), and timing always is concurrent (both exposure and outcome are determined during the real period of the study). Randomized trials are the sine qua non for evaluating the effect of new agents designed either to prevent (e.g., vaccines, prophylactic drugs) or to treat (e.g., antimicrobials) diseases. By randomly allocating subjects to receive or not receive the agent that is being tested, potential bias is minimized. Theoretically, if the size of the sample is adequate, the only difference between the groups is whether they received the experimental agent. Consequently, if the study is conducted properly, inferring that statistically significant differences in outcomes between the groups were related causally to the experimental agent is reasonable. For this reason, in most instances, the efficacy of new therapeutic agents or new vaccines must be demonstrated in clinical trials before the Food and Drug Administration will approve them (although in some instances new products are approved if criteria for safety and for some surrogate end-point are met, such as a serologic correlate of immunity).

The advantages and disadvantages of randomized trials are summarized in Table 251–1. Although clinical trials are the gold standard for investigators who wish to design a scientifically valid study, they do have numerous limitations. A major problem is that clinical trials are usually expensive. Subjects need to be selected, enrolled, and monitored longitudinally to detect the outcomes. When the outcome is a disease that is relatively rare (e.g., pneumococcal bacteremia), large samples are needed to provide adequate statistical power. Because sponsors of clinical trials usually want to test a new drug or an experimental vaccine under conditions that will maximize the chance that it will be found to be efficacious, patients with comorbid conditions (e.g., sickle-cell disease, asplenia, metastatic cancer) that might affect their response to the new agent often are excluded from the study. If the subjects who are excluded are an important part of the target population for the new agent (e.g., the patients with comorbid conditions are likely to be at high risk for serious complications of the disease and thus potentially could benefit greatly from an effective new intervention), the generalizability of the results of the clinical trial may be impaired.

Most randomized clinical trials are conducted in a double-blind manner; that is, neither the investigators nor the subjects know whether they received the experimental intervention (e.g., a new drug) or the comparison agent (e.g., either a placebo or an agent used in the standard manner). Double blinding helps ensure lack of bias in ascertainment of the outcome because neither the subject nor the investigator can be influenced to (or not to) either seek medical care or undergo diagnostic tests based on which of the interventions was received.

Randomized clinical trials may pose difficult ethical problems because the new (and potentially efficacious) agent is not given to the controls. By the time that clinical trials are begun, usually some evidence suggests that the agent is efficacious (e.g., preliminary studies showing that a new vaccine

TABLE 251–1 ■ RANDOMIZED CLINICAL TRIALS

Advantages
Gold standard for scientific validity
Randomization ensures unbiased allocation of the exposure (e.g., a new drug or an experimental vaccine)
Blinding ensures unbiased assessment of outcomes
Disadvantages
Poor statistical power for rare diseases
Requires large samples
Requires longitudinal follow-up
Logistically complex and expensive
Impaired generalizability when the study population differs from the ultimate target population
Ethical issues
Requires informed consent
Difficult to use to evaluate approved (presumably efficacious) products

induces antibodies). Accordingly, some patients and patient advocates might suggest that withholding a potentially efficacious therapeutic agent or a vaccine from persons at risk is not ethical; consequently, it may be difficult to have persons agree to be potential controls in studies of a promising new therapy.

Problems also may arise when approval of a product for the target population is based on studies that are conducted in a different population. For example, polyvalent pneumococcal polysaccharide vaccine was approved in the United States for the elderly and for adults with chronic conditions, such as chronic obstructive pulmonary disease and congestive heart failure, that put them at increased risk of acquiring serious pneumococcal infections. However, the data on which approval was based were derived from clinical trials conducted among young gold miners in South Africa who were at risk not because of their age or underlying illnesses but because of the conditions in which they lived and worked. Reports of vaccine failure and poor antibody response to the vaccine in the target population in the United States led to questions about the vaccine's efficacy.[4] However, once the vaccine was approved, conducting a randomized clinical trial in the target population was difficult ethically because it would mean withholding, on a random basis, an approved (and presumably efficacious) vaccine from patients at risk. Consequently, all but one of the postlicensure studies of this vaccine's efficacy were observational studies.

Conducting an experimental study in which the exposure is not assigned randomly is possible. For example, one might conduct an experimental cohort study in which volunteers receive a certain intervention (e.g., a new drug) while controls receive no intervention. Both groups would be monitored forward in time while undergoing surveillance for the outcome event. Although such a study incorporates some of the features of a randomized clinical trial, because the intervention is not assigned randomly, such studies are subject to significant biases.

OBSERVATIONAL STUDIES

Observational Cohort Studies

The direction of cohort studies always is forward, and the selection (or categorization) of subjects always is based on exposure; however, the timing may be concurrent, historical, or mixed. Thus, a cohort study may identify a cohort of subjects at a point (or at several points) in time in the recent or remote past, categorize them regarding their status with respect to the exposure (e.g., receipt of either a vaccine or a drug), and then monitor them forward in time for the occurrence of the outcome event (e.g., an infection) until a certain point in time, which could be in the past, present, or future. As in a clinical trial, subjects must not have the outcome at the onset of the study.

Cohort studies share many of the disadvantages of randomized clinical trials (see Table 251–1) but have the additional disadvantage that because they are not experimental, they are subject to many potential biases. On the other hand, cohort studies have many practical advantages (e.g., the timing can be historical, so conducting a 30-year follow-up study in just months is possible), and because they are observational studies, they usually have fewer potential ethical problems than a randomized trial does. In addition, for rare exposures, a critical factor is to be able to base selection of subjects on exposure.

Case-Control Studies

In both clinical trials and observational cohort studies, the selection of subjects is based on their exposure, and they are monitored in a forward direction until the outcome is determined. In *case-control studies,* the process is reversed. Subjects are selected on the basis of an outcome. The cases have the outcome, usually a disease; the controls do not have the outcome. The direction of the study is backward—the previous exposure is ascertained after the subjects are selected. The timing of case-control studies usually is historical, but it may be mixed; the timing of the exposure always is historical, but the timing of the outcome may be either historical or concurrent. For example, an investigator may conduct a case-control study of a vaccine's efficacy in which persons who are infected (cases) are identified concurrently through active surveillance of a microbiology laboratory. Because case-control studies are nonexperimental and the exposure (and, sometimes, the outcome) occurred in the past, the potential for bias is great, both in selection of the sample and in ascertainment of both the exposure and the outcome. The advantages and disadvantages of case-control studies are shown in Table 251–2.

Cross-Sectional Studies

Unlike cohort studies (both experimental and observational), in which subjects are monitored forward from exposure to outcome, and case-control studies, in which subjects are monitored backward from outcome to exposure, in cross-sectional studies, outcome and exposure are determined at the same point in time. In cohort studies, causal inference is made from cause to effect, whereas in case-control studies, causal inference is made from effect to cause. In cross-sectional studies, determining whether the exposure preceded the outcome may not be possible. Consequently, making valid causal inferences from a cross-sectional study also may not be possible.

Selection of subjects for a cross-sectional study may be based on outcome, exposure, or neither. However, because cross-sectional studies include only persons with prevalent outcomes, they are particularly problematic for studies of infectious diseases because patients whose illnesses (outcomes) either resolved or resulted in death before the point in time at which the study is conducted are not counted as having the outcome. Consequently, cross-sectional studies are more suitable to the study of chronic conditions and rarely are used in studies of infectious diseases.

ANALYSIS OF EPIDEMIOLOGIC STUDIES

The results of epidemiologic studies with dichotomous exposures and outcomes often are displayed in a 2×2 *contingency table.* However, the way that the results are analyzed statistically depends on the type of study.

Cohort Studies

Analysis of longitudinal cohort studies (both experimental trials and observational studies) is shown in Table 251–3.

TABLE 251–2 ■ CASE-CONTROL STUDIES

Advantages
Statistically powerful method to assess outcomes that are rare or delayed
Logistically easier and more efficient than large experimental or observational cohort studies
No longitudinal follow-up, so it can be completed relatively quickly and inexpensively
Ethically acceptable because it is an observational study
Disadvantage
Subject to many potential biases

TABLE 251–3 ■ ANALYSIS OF EXPERIMENTAL OR OBSERVATIONAL COHORT STUDIES

	Outcome Present	Outcome Absent	Total
Exposed	a	b	a + b
Unexposed	c	d	c + d
Total	a + c	b + d	

Risk in exposed subjects: a/(a + b)
Risk in unexposed subjects: c/(c + d)
Relative risk: (a/a + b) ÷ (c/c + d)
Attributable risk: (a/a + b) − (c/c + d)

The measure of association between the exposure and the outcome is the *relative risk* (sometimes called the *risk ratio),* which is an expression of the *magnitude* of this association in the study sample and represents an *estimate* of the association in the population from which the study sample was drawn. A relative risk of 1 indicates that no association exists between the exposure and the outcome, a relative risk greater than 1 indicates that the exposure is associated with an increased risk of the outcome, and a relative risk less than 1 indicates that the exposure is associated with a decreased risk of the outcome. The *attributable risk* (the risk of the outcome that is attributable to the exposure) is calculated as the risk in exposed subjects minus the risk in unexposed subjects. Of course, testing the statistical significance of any association is necessary because the relative risk could be greater than 1 or less than 1 by chance (see later sections on stochastic statistics and confidence intervals).

These analyses assume that no attrition exists among the subjects in the study. However, because of death, migration out of the study area, and loss to follow-up, as well as variation in the time of enrollment (enrollment in either a clinical trial or an observational cohort study may occur over a prolonged period or, indeed, throughout a study), variation virtually always exists among subjects in the duration of time that they are at risk for the outcome. If the average time at risk among the exposed and the unexposed subjects is equal, the analysis shown in Table 251–3 is likely to be valid. However, if a great deal of irregular attrition or new enrollment occurs during the study, the denominator is expressed better as person-time at risk (e.g., person-months, person-years) rather than as the number of persons in the group. When this method is used, the rate then is called the *incidence density rate* and the index of comparison is called the *incidence density ratio.*

In studies of infectious diseases, the outcome event is often the occurrence of an infection. Frequently, persons who become infected recover and may remain at risk for the outcome event again. Nevertheless, a subject usually should be censored (i.e., removed from the study) once the outcome event occurs. The fact that the outcome occurred may indicate that the subject has an increased risk for the outcome, independent of the exposure that is being assessed. For example, consider a study of the protective efficacy of a conjugate pneumococcal vaccine in which one of the subjects (whether the subject is a vaccinee or a control does not matter) experiences three or four episodes of invasive infection caused by pneumococci (perhaps because the subject has a previously unrecognized underlying condition, such as acquired immunodeficiency syndrome [AIDS] or an immunoglobulin deficiency). The estimate of the vaccine's efficacy would be distorted substantially if each of the outcome events were counted. Certainly, in a primary analysis, only the initial event should be counted. Another reason to censor the subject is that in some instances, the outcome event may be fatal. If some subjects die of the outcome (and therefore must be censored), not censoring subjects with the outcome who survive is, in effect, incorporating an assessment of the exposure's effect on prognosis and not just on the risk of the outcome event.

Using a different method to adjust for unequal durations of follow-up in a study may be necessary, particularly when a long latent period exists between exposure and outcome (a condition that often is met when the study involves the effect of a potential carcinogen, for example). In such instances, simply to sum the total person-times of exposure may be misleading because the outcome is more likely to occur many years after exposure. For example, although the total person-time at risk would be the same, the risk of an outcome developing clearly may be substantially different for 500 persons, each of whom is monitored for 2 years after exposure, than it may be for 40 persons, each of whom is monitored for 25 years. In such situations, the analyses must be adjusted for variation in the length of follow-up, which can be done with the use of *survival analysis* (also known as *life-table analysis*). The two basic methods of survival analysis, the *actuarial* method and the *Kaplan-Meier (product-limit)* method, are described in detail elsewhere.[12]

Case-Control and Cross-Sectional Studies

Analysis of a case-control study (with dichotomous outcomes and exposures) is shown in Table 251–4. Because selection of subjects is based on their outcomes, one cannot calculate the risk of development of the outcome, as one would in a longitudinal study (such as a clinical trial). Instead, one calculates the proportion of each group (cases and controls) that is exposed. The measure of association in a case-control study is the *odds ratio.* The *odds* of some occurrence is the probability that it will occur divided by the probability that it will not occur. In a case-control study, we are interested in the odds of exposure. The odds ratio is the ratio of the odds of exposure among cases (a/c) divided by the odds of exposure among controls (b/d). For rare events, the odds ratio closely approximates the relative risk of exposure that would be found in a longitudinal study of the same association. Cross-sectional studies are analyzed either like a case-control study (if the selection of subjects was based on their outcomes) or like a cohort study (if the selection of subjects was based on their exposures).

Bias

Bias occurs when the estimate of the association between the exposure and the outcome in the sample differs systematically from the true value in the population. Bias in the estimate of the association is different from bias in the measurement of individual variables. The latter bias (which may

TABLE 251–4 ■ ANALYSIS OF CASE-CONTROL STUDIES

	Cases (Outcome Present)	Controls (Outcome Absent)
Exposed	a	b
Unexposed	c	d

Proportion of exposed cases: a/(a + c)
Proportion of exposed controls: b/(b + d)
Odds of exposure among cases: a/c
Odds of exposure among controls: b/d
Odds ratio: (a/c) ÷ (b/d) or (ad) ÷ (bc)

occur, for example, if an instrument such as a thermometer is calibrated incorrectly) may or may not affect the estimate of association in an epidemiologic study. Biased measurements usually affect the exposed and the unexposed groups equally. By contrast, *analytic bias* is the effect of *differential error (nonrandom error)* on the assessment of the relationship between exposure and outcome. Analytic bias can occur because of *information bias* (as a result of differential error in ascertainment of either the exposure or the outcome), *sample distortion bias* (because the joint distribution of the exposure and the outcome in the sample chosen for the study is not representative of the distribution of these factors in the target population), and *confounding bias* (because the joint distribution of one or more variables that independently are related both to the exposure and to the outcome is unequal in the groups that are being compared). Ensuring that bias does not affect a study is critical to its validity. Furthermore, although using statistical methods to adjust for certain sources of bias (particularly for confounding bias) in analysis of the results of a study sometimes is possible, adjustment for bias after the fact may be impossible.

An example of information bias is *detection bias,* which occurs when differential detection of the outcome exists in the exposed and the unexposed groups. For example, numerous studies in which clinical scales to assess whether children with fever have a serious illness have been developed.[13] Often, however, the "serious illness" may include certain abnormal laboratory test results (such as an abnormal radiograph of the chest or a low concentration of sodium in serum). Because children with high scores on these scales were more likely to undergo diagnostic tests, detection bias may have occurred because similar abnormalities (such as a "silent" pneumonia or a mildly depressed concentration of sodium in serum) might go undetected in the "unexposed" group (children with lower scores on the clinical scale), a much smaller proportion of whom underwent a diagnostic test to detect a possible outcome. The best way to avoid having information bias is to use standardized, consistent methods to ascertain both the exposure and the outcome and to blind subjects and investigators to ensure that no differential ascertainment of either the outcome (in longitudinal studies) or the exposure (in case-control studies) occurs.

Sample distortion bias occurs when the sample in a study is not representative of the target population. However, a nonrepresentative sample does not lead to bias necessarily; bias in an assessment of the association between exposure and outcome occurs only if differential distribution of the exposure (or differential risk of the outcome) occurs in the subjects who are selected for the study versus the overall target population. This distribution can be the result of *selection bias.* For example, consider a case-control study of the protective efficacy of an approved vaccine in which the control subjects (the uninfected patients) were chosen from private practices in affluent suburbs whereas the case subjects (the infected patients) were any patients in whom a serious infection developed and who were hospitalized. The association between antecedent vaccination and infection probably is biased because the controls are not a representative sample of the population from which the cases emerged, and the proportion of them likely to have been vaccinated is higher than in the group of all uninfected persons in the population. Another possible source of sample distortion bias is differential loss to follow-up in a longitudinal study. The potential for sample distortion bias can be minimized by maximizing the probability that a representative sample will be selected, ideally by random sampling (or some other kind of unbiased sampling), and by minimizing loss to follow-up in longitudinal studies.

Confounding bias occurs when the association between exposure and outcome is distorted by a variable (a *confounder*) that is distributed unequally between the groups, is associated independently with both the exposure and the outcome, and is not in the causal pathway from exposure to outcome. One example of confounding bias is *susceptibility bias,* which occurs when the risk of the subjects (to development of the outcome) differs in the exposed and the unexposed groups, independent of the exposure. For example, imagine a longitudinal study of the protective efficacy of a vaccine against *Haemophilus influenzae* type b in infants. Ensuring that an equal proportion of subjects in the vaccinated and the unvaccinated groups attended group daycare is important because attendance at group daycare is associated with an increased risk for infection with *H. influenzae* type b. If a substantially higher proportion of vaccinees than of controls attended group daycare, their attendance might confound assessment of the vaccine's efficacy and result in a biased (lower) estimate of the effect of the vaccine. By contrast, if a disproportionate number of controls attended group daycare, the estimate of the vaccine's efficacy might be biased in the opposite direction (it would be erroneously high because controls would have a disproportionately higher risk of infection with *H. influenzae* type b than vaccinees would).

In the previous example, adjusting for the effect of the confounder might be possible by either stratification or multivariable analysis (see later). However, identifying confounders may not always be possible. Random allocation of subjects probably is the best strategy to protect against confounding, especially potential confounders that cannot be identified.

Statistics

SUMMARY STATISTICS

Perhaps the most basic use of statistical analysis is to summarize data. This type of statistical analysis often is called either *summary* or *descriptive* statistics. The specific summary measures that are used depend, in part, on whether the variables being summarized are *continuous* (variables with equal distance between intervals) or *categorical* (variables with two or more discrete categories). Age, weight, height, temperature, concentration of creatinine in serum, and the number of hours spent in group daycare are all examples of continuous variables (sometimes called *dimensional* or *quantitative* variables). Race, sex, country of residence, and whether a patient is being ventilated artificially are examples of categorical variables (sometimes called *discrete* variables). Of course, continuous variables can be analyzed categorically (e.g., age can be divided into either a *dichotomous* variable [<45 years or ≥45 years] or a *polychotomous* variable [20 to 44 years, 45 to 59 years, or ≥60 years]).

Continuous Variables

A *frequency distribution* is classification of the values of a sample of continuous variables into successive categories (e.g., for a sample of different ages, one might place each value into different 5-year [0 to 4 years, 5 to 9 years, etc.], 3-year [0 to 2 years, 3 to 5 years, etc.], or 1-year [0 years, 1 year, 2 years, 3 years, etc.] categories) and expression of the frequency of values within each category.

A sample of values of a continuous variable also can be summarized mathematically by describing its central tendency, shape, and spread. The *central tendency* can be expressed as a *mean* (or *average*), a *median* (the middle value of the sample), or a *mode* (the most frequent value in the sample). The mean value is calculated by summing all the individual values in the sample and dividing by the number of individual values. Thus, for a sample that is composed of subjects aged 1, 1, 2, 2, 2, 3, 3, 4, 10, and 12 years, the mean age is 4 years (40/10), the median age (the age for which half the subjects are older than and half are younger than its value—if the number of subjects is even, the median is the mean of the two middle values) is 2.5 years [(2 + 3)/2], and the mode is 2 years. These summary measures provide only a limited view of the data. For example, the mean of a distribution can be shifted in the direction of extreme outlying values; in the example, the mean is 4 years even though 70 percent of the subjects are younger than 4 years. Likewise, from the median value alone, one would not know whether outlying values existed. Consequently, describing the spread of a distribution is important.

The *spread* of a sample may be expressed by its *range* and by its *standard deviation*. The range of a sample is the interval between the highest and the lowest value in its distribution. In the example, the range is from 1 to 12 years. Another useful way of mathematically summarizing the spread of a distribution is to express the interval between each individual value and the mean value of the sample. To summarize these values, one cannot simply sum all the differences because the sum always equals zero (the sum of the positive differences equals the sum of the negative differences). To avoid this problem, the standard deviation of a sample is used. This parameter is calculated by taking the square root of the *variance* of the sample. The variance is the sum of the squares of the differences from the mean of each individual value, divided by the number of *degrees of freedom* of the sample (which is equal to the number of values in the sample minus one, or $N - 1$). The sum of the squares is divided by the number of degrees of freedom of the sample ($N - 1$), rather than by N (the actual number in the sample), because this calculation is thought to more accurately represent the true variance of the population from which a sample is taken.

To calculate the standard deviation of the sample in the example, one must determine the variance, which is the sum of the squares of the difference of each individual value from the mean of the sample:

$$(2[4-1]^2 + 3[4-2]^2 + 2[4-3]^2 + [4-4]^2 + [4-10]^2 + [4-12]^2) \div (10-1)$$

which equals 132/9, or 14.6667 years. The standard deviation simply is the square root of the variance, which is 3.8297 years.

In the medical literature, investigators often use the *standard error of the mean* (which is the square root of the variance divided by the square root of the number in the sample) to express the spread of the frequency distribution of a sample. However, the standard error actually is designed to be a measure of the standard deviation of the means of repeated samples from a single source population. Because the standard error always is smaller than the standard deviation of a single sample, it gives the erroneous impression that the spread of a sample is smaller than it actually is. A large sample with a large spread (and a large standard deviation) may have a small standard error. The standard error should not be used to describe the spread of a single sample.

The general shape of the frequency distribution can be inferred from the parameters given earlier. The characteristics of the most important distribution in statistics, the familiar bell-shaped curve of the normal distribution, are shown in Figure 251–1 and are discussed in a later section about diagnostic tests. The peak value of any distribution is the mode. A distribution may be bimodal, trimodal, and so on if it has two or more modes. A frequency distribution may be asymmetric, or *skewed*. If the mean is greater than the median (as in the example), the distribution is skewed to the right; conversely, if the mean is less than the median, the distribution is skewed to the left.

An investigator may want to summarize the relationship between two different continuous variables, which can be done with the use of linear regression, in which a straight line is constructed to represent the relationship between a continuous *dependent variable* (y) and a continuous *independent variable* (x). An equation ($y = a + bx$) can be created that represents the best "fit" to describe the relationship between the actual values of y and x, in which a (the *intercept*) is the value of y when x equals zero and b (the *regression coefficient*) is the slope of the line. Such an equation allows us to summarize the relationship between these variables and to extrapolate the value of each variable for conditions that may not have been observed in the sample. For example, one can calculate the incremental value of y for each interval change in the value of x.

Categorical Variables

The measure generally used to summarize categorical data is called a *rate* or a *proportion*. Rates consist of a numerator and a denominator. The numerator represents the actual number of persons in the sample who have the characteristic of interest (e.g., those with fever, those with tuberculosis, those who received a vaccine), and the denominator is the total number of persons in the sample. The persons in the

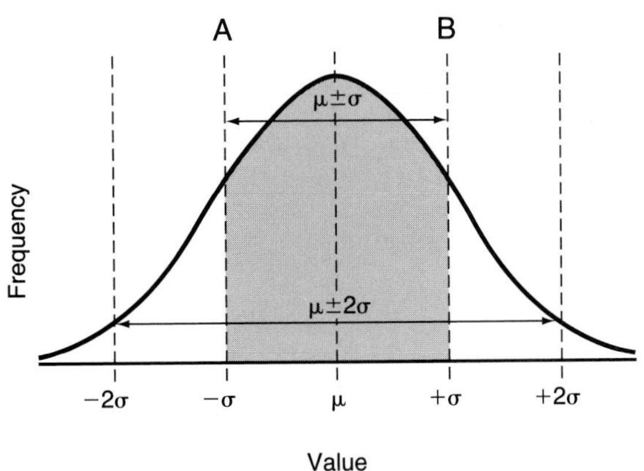

FIGURE 251–1 ■ Theoretic normal (gaussian) distribution showing where 1 and 2 SD above and below the mean would fall. The Greek letter mu (μ) stands for the mean in the theoretic distribution, and the Greek letter sigma (σ) stands for the standard deviation in the theoretic population. In this figure, the area under the curve represents all the observations in the distribution. One standard deviation above and below the mean, shown in dark gray and represented by the distance from point A to point B, is equivalent to 68 percent of the area under the curve, and therefore 68 percent of the observations in a normal distribution fall within this range. Two standard deviations above and below the mean, represented by the areas shown in dark and light gray, are equivalent to 95.4 percent of the area of the curve or 95.4 percent of the observations in a normal distribution. (From Jekel, J. F., Elmore, J. G., and Katz, D. L.: Epidemiology, Biostatistics, and Preventive Medicine. Philadelphia, W. B. Saunders, 1996, p. 118.)

numerator must be included in the group that the denominator represents, and the persons in the denominator must be able to have the characteristic that the numerator represents. For example, if one were interested in the rate of testicular cancer in the population, women should not be included in the denominator because they cannot have testicular cancer. Some experts believe that rates, by definition, should include a time factor (e.g., incident cases per person-months or per year). However, the term is used widely to refer to a proportion of a sample, as described earlier.

One of the most important rates that is calculated in epidemiologic studies is the *incidence rate,* which is the number of persons in whom a certain outcome develops divided by the number of persons in whom the outcome could have developed during a specified period. For example, a comparison may be made of the incidence rates of an infection over time in two groups in which the interventions given to prevent an infection differed (e.g., a vaccine and a placebo).

Another important rate, the *prevalence rate,* is the number of persons in whom a certain outcome develops divided by the total number of persons in the group at a specific point in time. In calculating the incidence rate, persons who at *zero time* (before the study begins) already have the outcome (e.g., prevalent cases) are excluded from both the numerator and the denominator. At time zero, the numerator of the incidence rate is zero. Thus, if one were interested in the incidence rate of lung cancer, persons who had lung cancer at the beginning of the study period would be excluded. The prevalence rate, by contrast, is measured at one point in time, and the numerator includes all persons with the outcome at that time.

Certain features of many infectious diseases affect both the prevalence rate and the incidence rate as measures of the occurrence of disease. The prevalence rate of any condition is related to its chronicity and the mortality rate associated with it; conditions that are common and chronic but are not associated necessarily with immediate mortality (e.g., atherosclerotic heart disease) have a relatively high prevalence rate. On the other hand, the prevalence rates are relatively low of conditions that either have a low mortality rate and resolve completely (such as many infectious illnesses) or have a high short-term mortality rate. To get a reliable estimate of the importance of such conditions, one must determine their incidence rates.

STOCHASTIC STATISTICS

Statistical Significance

Stochastic statistics deals with probability. Most readers are familiar with the use of "*p* values" to assess the *statistical significance* of a finding from a study. Usually, the threshold used to separate "significant" from "nonsignificant" results is a probability (*p* value) of less than 0.05, which means that (arbitrarily, by convention) if a result is likely to be observed by chance less than 1 in 20 times, the finding is considered to be "statistically significant." It must be emphasized, however, that statistical significance and clinical significance are very different. A statistically significant result means that the result is considered unlikely to be attributable to chance alone. As we shall see, the *p* value is related not only to the magnitude of the difference between the things that are being compared (e.g., a characteristic of either the exposed and the unexposed groups in a longitudinal study or the cases and the controls in a case-control study) but also to the size of the sample. Consequently, differences that are clinically unimportant (e.g., a difference in mean weight of 0.2 kg between two groups, a difference of 4% in the distribution of whites between two groups) can be statistically significant if the size of the sample is large. Of importance is to remember that a statistically significant finding may be of no clinical significance.

By the same token, the "magic" *p* value of 0.05 itself may be misleading because it is an arbitrary threshold; in fact, usually little difference exists in the results associated with a *p* value of 0.04 and one associated with a *p* value of 0.06. If the size of a sample is small, a large, clinically important difference may not be statistically significant. One should not automatically dismiss the importance of a finding for which the *p* value is 0.05 or higher.

Hypothesis Testing

In most epidemiologic studies, stochastic tests are used to check the validity of a hypothesis. By convention, one tests the validity of the *null hypothesis* that no difference exists in either the mean value of the characteristic (for continuous variables) or the frequency distribution of the characteristic (for categorical values) between the groups being compared. In essence, one is testing the probability that the two samples being compared (exposed subjects versus unexposed subjects or cases versus controls) emerged from the same population—that is, whether a difference between the groups could have been the result of chance if the two samples were selected randomly from the same population or whether the difference is so great that it probably (less than 1 chance in 20, or a *p* value of <0.05) did not occur by chance; that is, the samples probably actually represent a true difference in the populations of either exposed subjects versus unexposed subjects or cases versus controls.

Hypotheses can be either *bidirectional (nondirectional)* or *unidirectional (directional).* A nondirectional hypothesis asks whether an association exists between exposed and unexposed subjects, but it does not assume in which direction the association will occur. For example, one might ask whether an association exists between the height of fever and the outcomes of children with typhoid fever without specifying whether the association would be in the direction of better or worse outcomes (perhaps high fever indicates a more severe infection, or perhaps it indicates a more vigorous immune response). In such instances, the associated *p* value should be interpreted in a bidirectional, or *two-tailed,* manner because the distribution of the test statistic contains two "tails," one at either end of the curve; the *p* value represents the sum of the area under the two tails of the curve. In effect, one is specifying that for a result to be statistically significant, the probability of the result being in a positive direction is less than 2.5 percent and the probability of the result being in a negative direction is less than 2.5 percent. Most tables of *p* values provide results that are to be interpreted in a two-tailed manner (because this is the most conservative approach to testing a hypothesis), so the *p* value for a given test statistic can be read directly from the table.

In some instances, however, one might have good reason to suspect that an exposure is associated with an outcome in a unidirectional manner (e.g., that possession of a handgun is associated with an increased risk of sustaining a gunshot wound). If, in advance, the investigator decides to test this hypothesis in a unidirectional manner (the null hypothesis for which would be that ownership of a gun is not associated with an increased risk of incurring a gunshot wound), interpreting the results of a test statistic in a unidirectional, or *one-tailed,* manner might be appropriate. To derive a one-tailed *p* value, the two-tailed value is divided by 2. Thus, if the two-tailed *p* value is 0.06, the one-tailed value for the same result is 0.03. Clearly, obtaining statistically significant results by testing hypotheses in a unidirectional manner is easier. However, of importance is to specify before the study is conducted the *a priori* plan for how the results of statistical tests will be interpreted. Furthermore, although many hypotheses might seem to lend themselves to unidirectional analyses (e.g., one might think that an experimental vaccine that has been shown to be immunogenic could only be beneficial), in fact, unidirectional analyses are used only rarely. First, the possibility that an exposure may have an effect opposite that expected usually cannot be ruled out in advance. For example, researchers found that persons who were immunized with a vaccine composed of inactivated respiratory syncytial virus had an increased risk for symptomatic infection with the virus. In addition, because two-tailed interpretation of data is more conservative, many authorities (such as editors of journals and such licensing agencies as the Food and Drug Administration) demand two-tailed analyses.

Type I Error, Type II Error, and Statistical Power

Two types of errors can be made when testing the validity of a null hypothesis. The first occurs when the null hypothesis is true but is rejected erroneously, which leads to an erroneous conclusion that a difference exists between the exposed and unexposed subjects; this kind of mistake is termed a *type I error,* or *alpha error.* If a test statistic with a *p* value of less than 0.05 is accepted as statistically significant (and the null hypothesis is rejected on that basis), approximately 5 percent of the time a type I error is made because if no difference actually exists between the groups, that result will occur by chance 1 in 20 times. By contrast, if the *p* value is less than 0.001, a type I error will occur less than 1 in 1000 times if the null hypothesis is rejected.

The other kind of error, *type II error,* or *beta error,* occurs when the null hypothesis erroneously is not rejected even though a difference between the two groups truly exists. If the *p* value associated with the result is 0.05 or greater, the probability that the null hypothesis is false is not sufficiently low to reject it (even though the probability that the observed result could have occurred by chance may be only 6%).

Type I and type II errors are mutually exclusive. If one rejects the null hypothesis, one risks committing a type I error, the probability of which is equal to the *p* value. In such instances, a type II error cannot occur. If one accepts (i.e., fails to reject) the null hypothesis, one may commit a type II error (in which case a type I error cannot occur). The probability of committing a type II error is not related directly to the observed *p* value. Instead, one can estimate the probability of committing a type II error (beta error) before the study begins based on an assumed (clinically important) degree of association between the exposure and the outcome. Certain assumptions also must be made about the magnitude of the effect among the exposed subjects and the frequency of the outcome in the unexposed subjects. One is calculating a unidirectional probability that, by chance, the study will fail to detect an association equal to or greater than the magnitude that is specified for what is, in effect, an *alternative hypothesis* (i.e., that an association truly exists between the exposure and the outcome). The *statistical power* of a study (the unidirectional probability that the null hypothesis will be rejected given a specified degree of type I error—usually $<5\%$) is equal to 1 minus beta.

In designing a study, adequate statistical power is critical to ensure that a true association between the exposure and the outcome is not missed erroneously. The probability of a type II error depends on the size of the sample, the degree of variance within the sample, and the magnitude of the association that one wants to be able to detect: the smaller the sample, the larger the variance, and the smaller the magnitude of the association that one wants to detect, the larger the beta error (type II error) and the lower the statistical power of the study to detect an association. Of these factors, the investigator usually has control over only the size of the sample (because in the population the variance is generally a relatively fixed attribute of the characteristic being measured and the magnitude of association that is chosen is usually the minimal association that is clinically meaningful; for example, to design a study of an experimental vaccine so that it could detect as little as 30 percent efficacy would not make sense because in most instances, such a product would not be approved unless the magnitude of its effect was much greater).

Exactly what constitutes adequate power is debatable. Because enrolling a large number of subjects in a study is often expensive and time consuming, frequently the power that a study is designed to have depends on both the financial resources and the time available to conduct the study. A statistical power of 80 percent often is chosen as a reasonable compromise between ensuring that the study has a sufficient number of subjects to answer the research hypothesis and the realities of logistic and financial exigencies. On the other hand, if a pharmaceutical company has invested many years and millions of dollars to develop a new drug or a new vaccine, it may demand that a pivotal clinical trial of the product have at least 90 percent power to detect a clinically meaningful effect in an attempt to ensure that the product will be approved if it is efficacious.

Multiple Comparisons

Another more subtle problem in interpreting results arises when more than one hypothesis is assessed in a single study. If multiple tests of statistical significance are performed in a study, the probability that by chance alone the *p* value associated with any one variable will be less than 0.05 is substantially greater than 5 percent. In fact, the probability that by chance at least one test will be associated with a *p* value less than 0.05 is equal to $1 - (0.95)^k$, with k equal to the number of independent tests of statistical significance that are performed. Thus, if 10 different hypotheses are tested, a 40 percent probability exists that at least 1 of them will be statistically significant (i.e., that at least 1 of the tests will have a *p* value of <0.05). Of course, this matter violates the arbitrary rule that we only consider a finding to be statistically significant if it is likely to have occurred by chance less than 5 percent of the time. If multiple different associations in a study have *p* values less than 0.05, determining which occurred by chance and which truly are statistically significant is difficult.

On the other hand, studies are often expensive, time consuming, and logistically difficult to conduct. Therefore, sometimes a reasonable approach is to try to increase efficiency by assessing more than one hypothesis in a single study. To address this problem, one can specify in advance the *primary hypothesis* and the *secondary* and *tertiary hypotheses.* One then might give most credence to the statistical test of the primary hypothesis. Another approach is to lower the threshold used to define statistical significance by dividing 0.05 by the number of different tests that are performed. Thus, if five independent hypotheses are tested, any one would have to be associated with a p value of less than 0.01 before the null hypothesis would be rejected. However, this approach might be too stringent because the different hypotheses that are being tested often are not truly independent, and the probability that two or more associations will be statistically significant may be greater than the product of their individual probabilities. For example, one might assess whether infection is associated both with diarrhea and with vomiting; if it is associated with one of these symptoms, usually a higher than chance probability exists that it also is associated with the other. At the least, an investigator should acknowledge this potential problem and its consequences before drawing conclusions from the study.

Tests of Statistical Significance

Going into detail about the many different stochastic tests that are available is beyond the scope of this chapter. However, several general comments as well as descriptions of a few commonly used tests are in order.

Tests of statistical significance are either parametric or nonparametric. The test statistic of a *parametric* test is based on the assumption that the frequency distribution of the characteristic being assessed in the source population follows certain parameters. For example, for certain tests, one assumes that the characteristic in the population has a normal distribution. If the assumption is violated (e.g., the characteristic is not distributed normally), the statistical test will not be valid. In such instances, an appropriate approach might be to use a test based on a different, skewed distribution, such as the *Poisson distribution* for rare events, that might reflect more accurately the distribution of the characteristic in the population.

Alternative approaches to assess the statistical significance of differences between groups, if the distribution of the characteristic in the population is known to be highly skewed, include transforming the data so that they are normalized, usually by converting the values to their logarithmic equivalent, or using a *nonparametric* test.[21] Nonparametric tests, such as the *Mann-Whitney U-test* and the *Wilcoxon ranked sum test,* do not depend directly on the numerical values of the data; instead, the individual values are ranked in order of their values, and the statistical analyses are based on the relative ranks of the values in the different groups rather than on an assumed distribution in the population or in the sample.

For large samples, parametric tests are usually valid and are often easier to calculate than nonparametric tests. For smaller samples and for samples with highly skewed distributions, nonparametric tests or tests that use log-transformed data may be preferable.

Continuous Variables

To test the statistical significance of differences between groups in continuous variables (such as degree of fever, IQ, age, or a score on a standardized questionnaire), the mean values of the different groups can be compared.[22] The tests of statistical significance use the magnitude of the difference of the means and the variance in the sample to assess the probability that the difference could occur by chance. If more than two groups are being compared for a single variable, the procedure is called *one-way analysis of variance.* The null hypothesis is that the mean values from each group are the same (i.e., that the different groups are random samples from the same population). The total variance in all the subjects is separated into the amount that is attributable to differences between the groups of subjects (the *intergroup variance*) and the amount that is attributable to differences among the subjects within each group (the *intragroup variance*). The greater the quotient of the intergroup variance divided by the intragroup variance (the *F-ratio*), the more likely that differences between the groups are statistically significant (i.e., that they are not due to chance variation). The statistical significance of the F-ratio can be determined from the *F-test* table of p values. When this type of test is performed to assess the statistical significance of the simultaneous effects of two factors (by stratifying into additional groups), the test is called *two-way analysis of variance.*

The familiar *t-test* is just a special form of one-way analysis of variance in which the means of just two groups are compared. A *one-sample t-test* assesses whether the mean value of the study sample is statistically significantly different from the mean value in the source population. It assumes that the mean value in the source population is known and is calculated by dividing the difference of the mean of the sample minus the mean of the population by the quotient of the variance of the sample divided by the square root of the number in the sample.

A more common use of the t-test is to assess the statistical significance of the difference between the mean values of either a characteristic or an outcome of subjects in two different samples (e.g., of the exposed and the unexposed groups in a study). The null hypothesis of this *two-sample t-test* is that the mean values of the two samples are not statistically significantly different (i.e., that they could be random samples from the same population). The t-test statistic is equal to the difference in the mean values of the two samples divided by the square root of the pooled variance of the samples (the standard error of the difference of the means of the two groups). The p value of the result (t) is read from the table of the t distribution, with the degrees of freedom equal to the sum of the number of subjects in each sample minus 2.

Categorical Values

The chi-square statistic (χ^2) commonly is used to assess the statistical significance of differences in categorical values between groups.[6] Most often, proportions of two different groups (e.g., the proportions of the exposed and of the unexposed groups in which the outcome developed) are compared. Typically, the data are displayed in a *2 × 2 contingency table* (Table 251–5). The null hypothesis is that no association exists between the exposure and the outcome (or whatever the rows and columns represent)—that is, that the two groups could be random samples from the same population. This hypothesis is tested statistically by comparing the number of subjects who would be expected to be in a given cell by chance with the actual frequency (the observed frequency). The expected frequency can be calculated from the total number of subjects in the rows and the columns (the marginal totals) and is equal to the product of the number of subjects in the row times the number of subjects in the column divided by the total number of subjects in the sample.

TABLE 251–5 ■ 2 × 2 CONTINGENCY TABLE

	Outcome Present	Outcome Absent	Total
Exposed	a	b	a + b
Unexposed	c	d	c + d
Total	a + c	b + d	N

$\chi^2 = [(ad - bc)^2 N] \div [(a + b)(a + c)(b + d)(c + d)]$

The value of χ^2 (with N equal to the total number of subjects) is shown in Table 251–5. The statistical significance of χ^2 can be determined by reading the p values from a table of the χ^2 distribution. The larger the value of χ^2, the less likely that the observed proportions could have occurred by chance. Unfortunately, the assumption that the probability that the observed proportions of a random sample of subjects will follow the χ^2 distribution is not necessarily accurate if the expected frequency of any cell is small. Consequently, many experts use a *continuity correction* (sometimes called the *Yates correction*) to adjust for the deviation from the smooth, continuous theoretic distribution of χ^2 when the discrete values of small numbers of expected subjects disrupt the validity of the assumed distribution. The equation for χ^2 with the continuity correction is

$$\chi_c^2 = [(ad - bc - (N/2))^2 N] \div [(a + b)\,(a + c)(c + d)\,(b + d)]$$

If the expected frequency in any cell is very small (often defined as <5), the χ^2 test, even with the continuity correction, is not a valid estimate of the probability that the observed values could have occurred by chance. In such instances, the *Fisher exact test,* which is based on a hypergeometric distribution, should be used to assess the statistical significance of differences in categorical values.

Confidence Intervals

Although the validity of a null hypothesis typically is tested by stochastic tests and the use of p values, construction of a *confidence interval* (usually a *95% confidence interval*) has the advantage of providing information about both the *precision* of the estimate of the association (the narrower the confidence interval, the more precise the estimate) and its statistical significance.[3] Confidence intervals have become a standard component of reports of the results of epidemiologic studies.

Analyses of studies are concerned with both estimation (of the "true" value of the association between the exposure and the outcome in the population) and hypothesis testing (i.e., What is the probability that any association that is observed could have occurred by chance alone?). A sample of the population is enrolled in any study. The association observed in the study is hoped to be an accurate estimate of the true value of the association in the entire population. However, if an unbiased study were repeated many times, by chance alone the results will vary (because of random *sampling error*). A confidence interval is a range of values, based on the estimate and the spread of the data from a single study, within which the true value of the association in the population is likely to lie with a specified probability (i.e., 95% of the time for a 95% confidence interval, 99% of the time for a 99% confidence interval). Confidence intervals provide information about both the magnitude of associations (so that the clinical significance of the estimate can be assessed) and their statistical significance. If the confidence interval is calculated for a single outcome and if the 95 percent confidence interval for the difference between two groups does not include zero, the outcome is statistically significant (i.e., <5% probability that the null hypothesis of no difference between the groups is true). If the confidence interval is for a risk ratio or an odds ratio, the association will be statistically significant if the 95 percent confidence interval for the association does not include 1 (i.e., <5% probability that the null hypothesis of no association is true). Confidence intervals can be calculated with both continuous and categorical data, as well as for estimates of a single proportion and for differences (or associations) between two groups.

Adjustment for Potential Confounding Variables

The effect of confounding variables on the associations between exposure and outcome may be controlled in either the design or the analysis of a study. Random allocation of subjects to the exposed and the unexposed groups is a common strategy to avoid the effect of confounding in longitudinal studies. Although randomization actually ensures only lack of bias if a confounding variable is distributed unevenly between the groups (because an uneven distribution is as likely to favor the exposed group as the unexposed group), randomization is likely to be effective in preventing confounding if the size of the sample is large (which renders substantial inequalities between groups in the distribution of an independent variable unlikely to occur). Nevertheless, an investigator must check to ensure that confounding does not occur, even in a randomized clinical trial.

Another way to ensure that a potential confounding variable does not affect the results of a study is to *match* on that variable. Subjects in the exposed and the unexposed groups (or, in a case-control study, the cases and the controls) can be matched on certain variables that are known to be associated independently with both the exposure and the outcome. Such matching can be achieved either by matching subjects individually or by *frequency matching* (i.e., ensuring that the overall frequency distribution of the potential confounder is the same among the cases and the controls). Matching can ensure that the matched variable (e.g., race, age) does not affect the observed association between exposure and outcome.

One disadvantage of matching is that the effect of the matched variable on the association between exposure and outcome cannot be assessed as it might be if either stratification or multivariable analysis were used to control for confounding. If matching is used in the design of the study, analyzing the data with special tests for matched designs is necessary. For example, in a matched-pairs case-control study, only discordant pairs (matched pairs in which the cases and controls differ in their exposure status) provide information. Calculation of the matched odds ratio and the associated test of statistical significance (*McNemar* χ^2) is shown in Table 251–6.

Adjusting for the effect of potential confounders in the analyses is also possible. One way to accomplish this adjustment is with *stratification,* which is performed by dividing the data into different groups, or *strata,* according to the potential confounder. For example, a study may indicate that children whose parents both work were three times more likely to become febrile during the course of a study than were children whose parents both do not work. We may suspect, however, that it is not having both parents at work,

TABLE 251–6 ■ ANALYSIS OF A MATCHED CASE-CONTROL STUDY

	Cases	
Controls	Exposed	Unexposed
Exposed	a	b
Unexposed	c	d

Matched odds ratio: b/c
McNemar χ^2:$(b - c)^2/(b + c)$
McNemar χ^2 (with continuity correction: $(b - c - 1)^2/(b + c)$

per se, that results in this increased risk for fever; rather, another factor probably is related independently to the risk for fever and to the probability that both parents work. Attendance at group daycare is such a factor. If we stratified the results of the study by whether the children attended group daycare, we most likely would find that a disproportionate number of children whose parents both work also attended group daycare. When the risk ratios in the two different strata are combined (by using the *Mantel-Haenszel technique*), we probably would find that the apparent association between having both parents work and the risk of fever disappears when the effect of attendance at group daycare is controlled by stratification.

Advantages of stratification are that it can be understood easily and it can be performed without changing the design of the study after it is completed. One disadvantage is that it requires being able to identify and accurately to measure potential confounders (which is not necessary if one allocates subjects to different groups randomly). In addition, if several different potential confounders exist, performing the calculations may be difficult and time consuming, and the sizes of the individual strata may be so small that the ability to make statistical inferences is poor.

Finally, one can adjust for confounding with the use of one of many *multivariable statistical techniques,* such as *multiple linear regression* (if both the dependent and the independent variables are continuous) or *logistic regression* (if the dependent variable is dichotomous and the independent variables are either categorical or continuous). Providing a detailed description of multivariable techniques is beyond the scope of this chapter. However, in general, these techniques involve creating a mathematic model that fits the data and then using that model to analyze various associations.[1, 2, 5, 20] Although multivariable techniques are a powerful tool for both assessing the effects of and controlling for potential confounding variables, they depend on mathematic assumptions that may not always be valid and use techniques that are not intuitively obvious.

META-ANALYSIS

The term *meta-analysis* refers to a number of different types of analysis. The common feature of all meta-analyses is that they summarize the results of two or more different studies. The term often is used to refer to a quantitative technique in which the results of different studies are combined after they are weighted in the calculations according to the sizes of their samples and the variances of their results. The term also sometimes refers to a qualitative analysis of a group of studies, including critical analyses that rate the methodologic soundness of different studies but do not combine their results quantitatively. For example, one might review a group of studies that reached different conclusions about a topic. If the methodologically rigorous studies had similar results that differed from those of the weaker studies, one might conclude that the results of the more rigorous studies were more likely to be valid.

The concept of producing a single, statistically valid result by combining the results of different, often contradictory studies has great appeal. However, quantitative meta-analysis has many shortcomings. Perhaps chief among them is that no distinction is made between studies that are sound methodologically and those that are not. Thus, the results of a meta-analysis may be dominated by a large, but methodologically questionable study, whereas a superbly performed, but smaller study may fail to override the impact of the larger study in the meta-analysis. Another major problem is the selection of studies to include in a meta-analysis. Should only published, peer-reviewed studies be included (although clearly a bias exists that studies with positive results are more likely to be published than studies with negative results)? Should the analysis be limited only to studies that meet certain basic criteria for methodologic rigor (and who should decide on the criteria and whether they are met), or should only randomized clinical trials be included? What formula should be used to weight the different studies? Is combining the results of methodologically different studies valid? Results of meta-analyses should be interpreted with great circumspection.[23]

Diagnostic Tests

Although clinicians typically order diagnostic tests many times each day, misinterpretation and misuse of diagnostic tests are extremely common.[17] The widespread practice of interpreting continuous values (e.g., the total white blood cell count) in a dichotomous manner (so that the result is either "normal" or "abnormal") and failure to appreciate fully the difference between the accuracy of a diagnostic test (i.e., its sensitivity and specificity) and its predictive value are major factors in the misuse of diagnostic tests.

WHAT IS NORMAL?

In most instances, the "cutoff" for an abnormal test of a continuous variable, such as the total white blood cell count or the concentration of antibodies against an infectious agent, is based on the distribution of the results of the test in the population. One usually assumes that the distribution of most such results in the population will follow a gaussian (or "normal") distribution, which is illustrated by the bell-shaped curve in Figure 251–1. Gauss and other statisticians used the term *normal* to refer to the shape of this curve. However, in medicine, the term *normal* long has been used to mean something very different—the dichotomy between a state of health *(normal)* and one of disease *(abnormal).* Unfortunately, the different meanings of these terms often have been used interchangeably, which has added to confusion in the interpretation of diagnostic tests.

In a normal distribution, the mode (the most frequent value) is the mean value, and 68.3 percent, 95.4 percent, and 99.7 percent of the values lie within (plus or minus) 1, 2, and 3 SD from the mean value, respectively. The cutoff for an abnormal test result often is defined arbitrarily as any value that is more than 2 SD from the mean of a normally distributed population; thus, 5 percent (actually 4.6%) of the population would be categorized as abnormal. Half the people with abnormal results will be 2 SD below the mean, and half will be 2 SD above the mean. Thus, 2.5 percent (actually 2.3%) of the population will have abnormally high values. In some instances, 3 SD (or some other arbitrary parameter) is used to determine the cutoff. However, of importance is to realize that these definitions of normal and abnormal are merely statistical models that should not necessarily be translated to mean that 2.5 percent of the population is "diseased." As noted earlier, with this kind of statistical logic, the diagnosis of disease may be related to the number of tests performed because if multiple tests are conducted, the likelihood that the result of any one will be abnormal is increased. If 15 independent tests are performed on a patient, the probability that any one of the test results will be abnormal by chance is 54 percent.

Other statistical models might be more appropriate for assessing a diagnostic test. For example, interpreting diagnostic tests would be relatively easy if two separate, non-overlapping normal distributions of diseased and disease-free patients existed. Unfortunately, although this model may apply for some rare conditions (such as genetic disorders in which affected persons are missing an enzyme that metabolizes certain substances, which leads to uniquely high concentrations of the substance in persons with the disorder), the model rarely is applicable. A model that is more appropriate for most infectious illnesses is shown in Figure 251–2. In this model (the example of which uses levels of serum calcium), the diseased and nondiseased populations have separate, partially overlapping distributions. The specificity of a diagnostic test is related directly to the degree to which the two distributions overlap.

ACCURACY OF A DIAGNOSTIC TEST

Two important characteristics of a diagnostic test—its *reproducibility* and its *validity*—are the key components of its accuracy. The reproducibility (sometimes called *reliability* or *precision)* of a test simply is the degree to which retesting yields the same result. A test that provides results that are not reproducible is of little diagnostic value. The validity of the results of a diagnostic test may be divided into two components: *sensitivity* and *specificity* (Table 251–7). The *sensitivity* of a test is the proportion of persons with disease who are identified accurately by the test as having disease (true positives/[true positives + false negatives]). The *specificity* of a test is the proportion of persons without disease who are identified accurately by the test as not having disease (true negatives/[true negatives + false positives]). The ideal test has both a specificity and a sensitivity of 1. Of course, no diagnostic tests are that accurate. Indeed, a trade-off exists between sensitivity and specificity—usually, the more sensitive a test is, the less specific it is, and vice versa.

Although the sensitivity and specificity of a given test often are considered to be absolute characteristics of a test, in fact, these characteristics do depend on the types of patients included in the studies in which the indices of the test were developed. Indeed, tests that appear to be both highly sensitive and highly specific in preliminary studies commonly prove to be much less so when used in actual clinical practice because the preliminary studies that establish a test's sensitivity and specificity frequently are affected by problems of spectrum and bias.[16] If the patients enrolled in studies used to assess the test (both those with disease and those without disease) have a relatively narrow spectrum of clinical manifestations, both the sensitivity and the specificity of a diagnostic test may appear to be better than they actually are. For example, if one were to assess the sensitivity of a differential heterophile test to diagnose infection with Epstein-Barr virus (EBV), its sensitivity would appear to be far better if all the subjects infected with EBV were teenagers with severe pharyngitis (a high proportion of whom will have a positive heterophile test result) than if it included subjects with a broader spectrum of manifestations of EBV infection (such as toddlers with symptoms of an infection of the upper respiratory tract, who are much less likely to have a positive heterophile test result when infected with EBV). Likewise, the specificity of a diagnostic test may appear to be better when only asymptomatic, healthy persons are used as nondiseased subjects instead of including patients with other illnesses that produce symptoms similar to those of the target illness.

In addition, of importance is to realize that the cutoffs for classifying results as either normal or abnormal are usually somewhat arbitrary and may depend on how the test is used, as well as the nature of the disease that one is trying to detect. If a diagnostic test is being used to screen a population for a relatively mild disorder with a low prevalence, one would want to use a cutoff that results in high specificity to avoid having a large number of false-positive results, even at the expense of lower sensitivity. On the other hand, if the diagnostic test is for a serious disorder or is used not for screening but for diagnosis in a targeted population with at least a moderate prevalence of the disorder (e.g., a white blood cell count in cerebrospinal fluid to detect possible bacterial meningitis in febrile children), one might want to err on the side of overdiagnosis and therefore use a cutoff with a high sensitivity at the expense of lower specificity.

PREDICTIVE VALUE OF A DIAGNOSTIC TEST

Sensitivity and specificity are important characteristics of a diagnostic test, but to calculate them, one must know whether the patients do or do not have the disease; clearly,

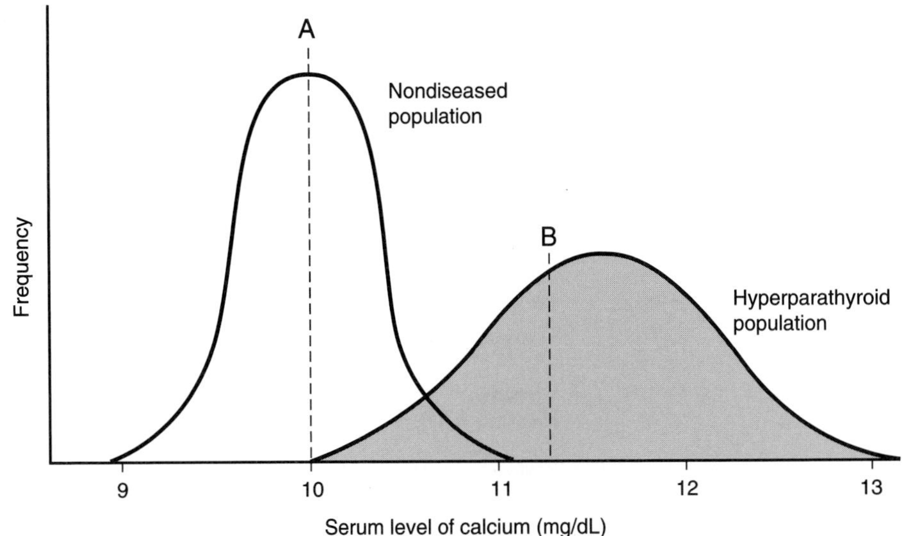

FIGURE 251–2 ■ Overlap in values of randomly performed tests in a population in which most of the people are healthy (curve on the *left*) but some of the people are diseased (curve on the *right*). A person with a level of calcium below point A would be unlikely to have hyperparathyroidism. A person with a level of calcium above point B would be likely to have an abnormality in calcium metabolism, possibly hyperparathyroidism. A person with a level of calcium between point A and point B may or may not have an abnormality in calcium metabolism. (*Note:* The normal range of calcium depends on the method used in a specific laboratory. In some laboratories, the range is from 8.5 to 10.5 mg/dL. In others, as in this illustration, it is from 9 to 11 mg/dL.) (From Jekel, J. F., Elmore, J. G., and Katz, D. L.: Epidemiology, Biostatistics, and Preventive Medicine. Philadelphia, W. B. Saunders, 1996, p. 88.)

TABLE 251–7 ■ STATISTICAL INDICES OF A DIAGNOSTIC TEST

Result of Test	Disease	No Disease
Positive	a	b
Negative	c	d
True positives: a	Sensitivity = a/(a + c)	
False positives: b	Specificity = d/(b + d)	
True negatives: d	Positive predictive value = a/(a + b)	
False negatives: c	Negative predictive value = d/(c + d)	

if a physician already has this knowledge, the test does not need to be performed in the first place. From the perspective of a clinician who is caring for an individual patient, the key characteristic of a diagnostic test is its *predictive value* (Table 251–7). That is, if a test result is positive, what is the probability that the patient has the disease (*positive predictive value*)? Conversely, if a test result is negative, what is the probability that a patient does not have the disease (*negative predictive value*)? However, unlike sensitivity and specificity, the predictive value of a test depends critically on the prevalence of the disease among the subjects who are tested.

This concern is illustrated by the example in Table 251–8. In example *a,* the prevalence of the disease in the sample is 1 percent and the positive predictive value of a positive test result is only 8.8 percent. By contrast, as shown in examples *b* and *c,* when the prevalence of disease in the sample rises to 10 percent and to 50 percent, respectively, the positive predictive value of a positive test result rises to 51.4 percent and to 90.5 percent, respectively, even though the sensitivity and the specificity of the test are constant. By the same token, as the prevalence of disease in the sample that is tested rises, the predictive value of a negative test result falls, although the negative predictive value remains reasonably good until the prevalence of disease becomes high.

Of importance for clinicians is to be aware of these epidemiologic truths when ordering diagnostic tests for patients. Sometimes a physician orders tests to "rule out" the possibility that a patient's symptoms are caused by a disease that, based on the patient's history, physical examination, and previous laboratory tests, is unlikely to be the cause of the problem (i.e., the "prior probability" that the patient has the disease is low). Unless the specificity of such tests approaches 100 percent (which is unlikely for most serologic tests), in such situations the great majority of positive test results will be falsely positive; the physician then will be in the unfortunate position of ignoring the result, ordering additional diagnostic tests, or treating the patient for a disease that probably is not the cause of the symptoms. Consequently, clinicians should be selective in ordering diagnostic tests.

Assessment of the Protective Efficacy of a Vaccine

The protective efficacy (PE) of a vaccine may be assessed with either experimental or observational studies. The classic way to assess a vaccine's efficacy is in an experimental, randomized, double-blind clinical trial. The major observational designs available are cohort studies and case-control studies, although a large variety of hybrid designs such as household exposure studies and indirect cohort studies are available, but complete descriptions of them are beyond the scope of this chapter.[14, 15] Table 251–9 illustrates calculation of the PE of a pneumococcal vaccine with data from clinical trials, cohort studies, and case-control studies.

CLINICAL TRIALS

In a randomized clinical trial, subjects at risk of acquiring the infection in question would be assigned randomly either to receive the vaccine (vaccinees) or not to receive the vaccine (controls). Subsequently, all subjects would be observed for occurrence of the infection during an appropriate period of follow-up. At the conclusion of the study, the *protective efficacy* of the vaccine, an index devised by Greenwood and Yule[7] to indicate the proportionate reduction in the frequency of disease attributable to the vaccine, would be calculated. PE is defined as follows:

$$\text{PE} = (\text{Risk of infection in controls} - \text{Risk of infection in vaccinees}) \div \text{Risk of infection in controls}$$

TABLE 251–8 ■ PREDICTIVE VALUE OF A DIAGNOSTIC TEST WITH 95% SENSITIVITY AND 90% SPECIFICITY WITH DIFFERENT PREVALENCE OF DISEASE IN THE SAMPLE

	Test	Disease	No Disease	Total
a*	Positive	95	990	1085
	Negative	5	8910	8915
	Total	100	9900	10,000
	Positive predictive value = 8.8%		Negative predictive value = 99.9%	
b†	Positive	950	900	1850
	Negative	50	8100	8150
	Total	1000	9000	10,000
	Positive predictive value = 51.4%		Negative predictive value = 99.4%	
c‡	Positive	4750	500	5250
	Negative	250	4500	4750
	Total	5000	5000	10,000
	Positive predictive value = 90.5%		Negative predictive value = 94.7%	

*Prevalence of disease: 1%.
†Prevalence of disease: 10%.
‡Prevalence of disease: 50%.

TABLE 251–9 ■ CALCULATION OF PROTECTIVE EFFICACY (PE) OF PNEUMOCOCCAL VACCINE

Clinical Trial or Cohort Study	Pneumococcal Infection	No Pneumococcal Infection	Total
Vaccinated	a	b	a + b
Not vaccinated	c	d	c + d
PE = [(c/c + d) − (a/(a + b)] ÷ (c/c + d) = 1 − [(a/(a + b) ÷ (c/c + d)]*			

Case-Control Study	Pneumococcal Infection (Cases)	No Pneumococcal Infection (Controls)
Vaccinated	a	b
Not vaccinated	c	d
PE = 1 − [(ad) ÷ (bc)]†		

*The expression [(a/(a+b) ÷ (c/c+d)] also is known as the relative risk of infection in vaccinated versus unvaccinated persons.
†The expression [(ad) ÷ (bc)] is the odds ratio relating vaccination to infection. In a case-control study, the odds ratio approximates the relative risk if the outcome is rare.

A PE of 100 percent indicates complete protection against infection, a PE of 0 percent indicates no protection, and negative values indicate that a greater risk of acquiring infection existed among vaccinees than among controls. By rearranging terms, PE equals 1 minus the risk of infection in vaccinees divided by the risk of infection in controls. Because the ratio in this equation is the relative risk of infection developing in vaccinees versus controls, PE is, by definition, equal to 1 minus the relative risk.

OBSERVATIONAL COHORT STUDIES

In a cohort study, subjects at risk would be selected on the basis of whether they had been vaccinated or had been left unvaccinated during routine clinical care. The vaccinated and unvaccinated groups then would be monitored longitudinally to assess frequencies of infection. The analysis of a vaccine's PE for cohort studies is similar to that for clinical trials, but because the study is nonexperimental, the results are more subject to bias than those of a well-conducted, randomized clinical trial.

CASE-CONTROL STUDIES

In a case-control study, patients with antecedent conditions that place them at high risk for pneumococcal infection would be eligible to be subjects. Patients with serious pneumococcal infection would become subjects in the case group. The control group would consist of subjects with similar high-risk conditions but without pneumococcal infection. The two groups then would be compared for the frequency of antecedent vaccination with pneumococcal vaccine.

In a case-control study, the strength of the relationship between vaccination and subsequent infection is measured by an odds ratio (the ratio of the odds of vaccination in the case subjects to the odds of vaccination in the controls). Because the odds ratio in a case-control study closely approximates the relative risk of pneumococcal infection in a longitudinal study and because PE is defined as 1 minus the relative risk, the value (1 − odds ratio) closely approximates the PE that would be calculated from a longitudinal study.

REFERENCES

1. Breslow, N. E., Day, N. E., and Davis, W. (eds.): Statistical Methods in Cancer Research. Vol. I. The Analysis of Case-Control Studies. Lyon, International Agency for Research on Cancer, 1980.
2. Breslow, N. E., Day, N. E., and Heseltine, E. (eds.): Statistical Methods in Cancer Research. Vol. II. The Design and Analysis of Cohort Studies. Lyon, International Agency for Research on Cancer, 1987.
3. Bulpitt, C. J.: Confidence intervals. Lancet *1*:494–497, 1987.
4. Clemens, J. D., and Shapiro, E. D.: The pneumococcal vaccine controversy: Are there alternatives to randomized clinical trials? Rev. Infect. Dis. *6*:589–600, 1984.
5. Feinstein, A. R.: Clinical Epidemiology: The Architecture of Clinical Research. Philadelphia, W. B. Saunders, 1985.
6. Fleiss, J.: Statistical Methods for Rates and Proportions. 2nd ed. New York, John Wiley & Sons, 1981.
7. Greenwood, M., and Yule, U. G.: The statistics of anti-typhoid and anti-cholera inoculations, and the interpretation of such statistics in general. Proc. R. Soc. Med. *8*:113–194, 1915.
8. Jekel, J. F., Elmore, J. G., and Katz, D. L.: Epidemiology, Biostatistics, and Preventive Medicine. Philadelphia, W. B. Saunders, 1996.
9. Kahn, H. A., and Sempos, C. T.: Statistical Methods in Epidemiology. Vol. 12. Monographs in Epidemiology and Biostatistics. New York, Oxford University Press, 1989.
10. Kelsey, J. L., Thompson, W. D., and Evans, A. S.: Methods in Observational Epidemiology. Vol. 10. Monographs in Epidemiology and Biostatistics. New York, Oxford University Press, 1986.
11. Kleinbaum, D. G., Kupper, L. L., and Morgenstern, H.: Epidemiologic Research: Principles and Quantitative Methods. Belmont, CA, Lifetime Learning Publications Division, Wadsworth, 1982.
12. Lee, E. T.: Statistical Methods for Survival Data Analysis. Belmont, Lifetime Learning Publications Division, Wadsworth, 1980.
13. McCarthy, P. L., Sharpe, M. R., Spiesel, S. Z., et al.: Observation scales to identify serious illness in febrile children. Pediatrics *70*:802–809, 1982.
14. Orenstein, W. A., Bernier, R. H., Dondero, T. J., et al.: Field evaluation of vaccine efficacy. Bull. World Health Organ. *63*:1055–1068, 1985.
15. Orenstein, W. A., Bernier, R. H., and Hinman, A. R.: Assessing vaccine efficacy in the field: Further observations. Epidemiol. Rev. *10*:212–241, 1988.
16. Ransahoff, D. F., and Feinstein, A. R.: Problems of spectrum and bias in evaluating the efficacy of diagnostic tests. N. Engl. J. Med. *299*:926–930, 1978.
17. Riegelman, R. K., and Hirsch, R. P.: Studying a Study and Testing a Test: How to Read the Medical Literature. 2nd ed. Boston, Little, Brown, 1989.
18. Sackett, D. L., Haynes, R. B., Guyatt, G. H., et al.: Clinical Epidemiology: A Basic Science for Clinical Medicine. 2nd ed. Boston, Little, Brown, 1991.
19. Schlesselman, J. J.: Case-Control Studies: Design, Conduct, Analysis. Monographs in Epidemiology. New York, Oxford University Press, 1982.
20. Selvin, S.: Statistical analysis of epidemiologic data. *In* Kelsey, J. L., Marmot, M. G., Stolley, P. D., et al. (eds.): Monographs in Epidemiology and Biostatistics. Vol. 17. New York, Oxford University Press, 1991.
21. Siegel, S.: Nonparametric Statistics for the Behavioral Sciences. McGraw-Hill Series in Psychology. New York, McGraw-Hill, 1956.
22. Snedecor, G. W., and Cochran, W. G.: Statistical Methods. 7th ed. Ames, Iowa State University Press, 1980.
23. Thompson, S. G., and Pocock, S. J.: Can meta-analyses be trusted? Lancet *338*:1127–1130, 1991.

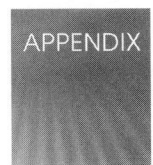

APPENDIX

Molluscum Contagiosum*

Molluscum contagiosum is a common viral skin disease in children. The disease now is being seen with increasing frequency in sexually active and immunodeficient individuals.[1, 3] The infection may occur at any age, with the highest incidence reported to be in patients younger than 5 years of age[2, 8] in some studies and at school age in others.[4, 7] The infection is two to three times more common in school age and sexually active males than in females.[2, 3, 8] Transmission is via close contact, including routine play, sports, sexual activity, and breast feeding.[3, 4, 7, 8] Spread by fomites also is possible.[1, 2, 7] The incidence of disease is highest in warm climates and in areas of overcrowding.[2, 3, 7, 8]

Clinical Manifestations

The incubation period for molluscum is between 2 and 7 weeks; however, there has been a report of an infant presenting with molluscum contagiosum at 1 week of age.[3, 8] The typical lesions of molluscum contagiosum are 1 to 5 mm, dome-shaped, white, skin-colored, or pink papules with a distinctive central umbilication. Giant molluscum up to 1 to 2 cm can be seen.[2, 6, 7] Usually, 2 to 30 lesions are present.[3, 8] In children, molluscum most commonly is seen on the face, neck, trunk, and extremities but may be seen on any part of the body, including the mucous membranes.[3] Periocular molluscum may lead to a secondary keratoconjunctivitis or trachoma.[3, 10] Molluscum least commonly is seen on the palms and soles.[3, 4] In some cases, molluscum contagiosum is a sexually transmitted disease, raising the issue of sexual abuse when infection is seen in the genital area. The most common etiology of genital molluscum is autoinoculation; however, if the lesions occur solely in the genital area or there is a question about the patient's social situation, the possibility of abuse should be explored.[7, 8]

Atypical molluscum lesions are being seen more commonly, especially with the improved survival of patients with acquired immunodeficiency syndrome (AIDS) and other immunocompromised patients. The incidence of molluscum contagiosum in patients infected by the human immunodeficiency virus (HIV) is 5 to 18 percent,[3, 6, 11] with the highest incidence in individuals with CD4 counts lower than 100 cells/mm^3.[3]

Molluscum lesions in immunocompromised patients often are large, are situated more deeply in the epidermis, and may number in the hundreds.[6, 11] The results of one study that evaluated molluscum contagiosum in immunocompromised children indicated that it was not more common or more severe in this population.[5] However, this study included only six patients (five with various cancers and one with AIDS), and two of the patients were described as being disease-free and immunocompetent at the time of onset of molluscum contagiosum. The results of this and other studies suggest that the presence and degree of cellular immunodeficiency may be important in the presentation of molluscum contagiosum.[5, 11]

*This material is taken from a chapter by Stacey E. Gallas and Moise L. Levy that appeared in the fourth edition.

Patients with atopic dermatitis also may be predisposed to more severe molluscum contagiosum virus (MCV) infection.[4, 5] There is not enough available information to know whether this is related to the eczema itself, which may alter the skin barrier, or to the use of corticosteroids. The term *molluscum dermatitis*, more commonly seen in patients with atopic dermatitis, is used to describe an eczematous reaction that may occur around molluscum contagiosum lesions and is felt to represent a delayed type hypersensitivity reaction to viral antigens in the dermis.[2, 12]

Diagnosis

The diagnosis of molluscum contagiosum almost always is clinical. However, there are situations in which the virus manifests atypically, and microscopic diagnosis is useful. Structurally, the molluscum lesion is formed by one or more epidermal lobules extending into the dermis with an opening onto the surface.[3] The basement membrane is intact, and dermal inflammation is rare.[2, 3] The central umbilication is filled with molluscum bodies and keratin fragments.[3] The characteristic microscopic finding is a lobular collection of large, round keratinocytes with characteristic intracytoplasmic inclusion bodies, termed *molluscum bodies*.[7, 8, 12] The contents of a papule can be expressed and smeared on a slide and then stained with Wright, Giemsa, Gram, or Papanicolaou stains to illustrate these structures.[2, 8, 12] The molluscum bodies (also called *Henderson-Patterson bodies*) are spherical, eosinophilic hyaline masses, which become more basophilic in the upper epidermis and contain viral colonies.[2, 7, 12]

Antibodies to molluscum are produced in most immunocompetent patients with MCV infection.[3] These antibodies have been identified in various studies by immunofluorescence, gel filtration, and other techniques. Antibody detection currently is not a clinically relevant method of diagnosis.

Differential Diagnosis

Molluscum contagiosum, especially atypical forms, can be difficult to differentiate from many other disorders. Molluscum may be confused with verrucae, furuncles, juvenile xanthogranulomas, syringomas, and hidrocystomas.[2, 7, 8] Large lesions may mimic basal cell carcinoma or keratoacanthomas.[7, 8, 12] Lesions around the eye may be mistaken for chalazion, granulomata, adnexal tumors, and lid abscesses.[7, 8] Cryptococcosis and other deep fungal infections are important clinical considerations, especially in the immunocompromised patient.[7, 9]

Treatment

Many different modalities, including benign neglect, ultimately result in the resolution of molluscum contagiosum in the immunocompetent patient. Treatment may be undertaken to avoid autoinoculation and spread to others and for cosmetic reasons. Superficial curettage or expression of the plug after a superficial incision is made is an effective but often frightening method of treatment in young children. In some cases, application of a topical local anesthetic, such as EMLA (eutectic mixture of lidocaine-prilocaine), may be necessary before treatment takes place. Cryotherapy using liquid nitrogen also is effective.[1, 2, 7, 8] Application of local irritants, such as cantharidin 0.7 to 0.9 percent in flexible collodion, podophyllin in tincture of benzoin, 0.05 to 0.1 percent tretinoin, trichloracetic acid, or 10 percent benzoyl peroxide, also can be used either alone or after superficial incision.[2, 3, 7, 8, 12] These treatments can be dangerous around the eye, and, in many cases, lesions in this location should be allowed to resolve spontaneously. Systemic treatment of molluscum contagiosum has been tried with griseofulvin and methisazone (a compound with activity against variola and vaccinia), but neither has shown definitive or consistent effectiveness.[3] In the vast majority of cases, molluscum contagiosum resolves without treatment in 4 weeks to several months.

Treatment of molluscum in the immunocompromised patient can be problematic. No one treatment has been shown to be effective or has prevented recurrences universally. Trichloracetic acid peels were shown to be helpful in reducing lesion counts in one study of HIV-positive patients.[3] Combination therapy using cantharidin, tretinoin, and curettage controlled MCV infection in about 50 percent of HIV-positive patients with CD4 counts lower than 200 cells/mm^3.[3, 11] However, zidovudine has not been helpful in controlling molluscum contagiosum in other HIV-positive patients.

Prevention

Because of the generally benign nature of infection, no specific isolation is needed for individuals with molluscum contagiosum. Spread of infection can be decreased by treatment and by avoidance of close contact with infected individuals.

REFERENCES

1. Epstein, W. L.: Molluscum contagiosum. Semin. Dermatol. *11*:184–189, 1992.
2. Frieden, I. J., and Penneys, N. S.: Viral infections. *In* Schachner, L. A., and Hansen, R. C. (eds.): Pediatric Dermatology. New York, Churchill Livingstone, 1988, pp. 1371–1413.
3. Gottlieb, B. L., and Myskowski, P. L.: Molluscum contagiosum. Int. J. Dermatol. *33*:453–461, 1994.
4. Highet, A. S.: Molluscum contagiosum. Arch. Dis. Child. *67*:1248—1249, 1992.
5. Hughes, W. P., and Parham, D. M.: Molluscum contagiosum in children with cancer or acquired immunodeficiency syndrome. Pediatr. Infect. Dis. J. *10*:152–156, 1991.
6. Izu, R., Manzano, D., Gardezabal, J., et al.: Giant molluscum contagiosum presenting as a tumor in an HIV-infected patient. Int. J. Dermatol. *33*:266–267, 1994.
7. Janniger, C. K., and Schwartz, R. A.: Molluscum contagiosum in children. Cutis *52*:194–196, 1993.
8. Landau, J. W., and Gurevitch, A. W.: Molluscum contagiosum. *In* Feigin, R. D., and Cherry, J. D. (eds.): Textbook of Pediatric Infectious Diseases. 3rd ed. Philadelphia, W. B. Saunders, 1992, pp. 818–820.
9. Prose, N. S., and Resnick, S. D.: Cutaneous manifestations of systemic infection in children. Curr. Probl. Pediatr. *21*:92–113, 1991.
10. Robinson, M. R., Lidell, I. J., Garber, P. P., et al.: Molluscum contagiosum of the eyelid in patients with acquired immune deficiency syndrome. Ophthalmology *99*:1745–1747, 1992.
11. Schwartz, J. J., and Myskowski, P. L.: Molluscum contagiosum in patients with human immunodeficiency virus infection. J. Am. Acad. Dermatol. *27*:583–588, 1992.
12. Williams, L. R., and Webster, G.: Warts and molluscum contagiosum. Clin. Dermatol. *9*:87–93, 1991.

INDEX

Note: Page numbers followed by the letter f refer to figures; those followed by the letter t refer to tables.

F

J

N

O

P

T

W